# MEDICAL-SURGICAL NURSING

## *Concepts and Clinical Practice*

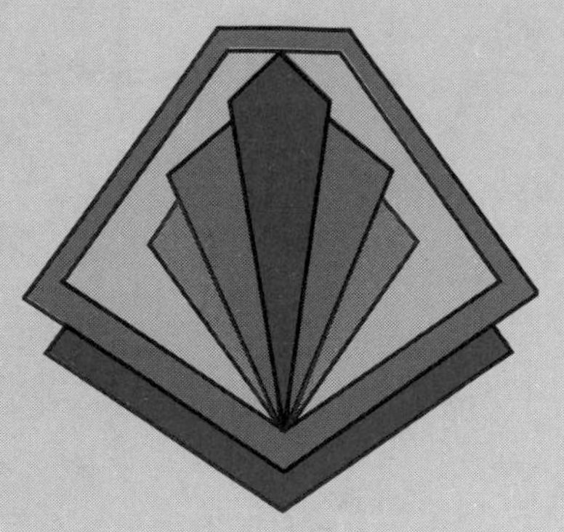

# MEDICAL-SURGICAL NURSING

## CONCEPTS AND CLINICAL PRACTICE


EDITED BY

**WILMA J. PHIPPS, PhD, RN, FAAN**
Professor Emeritus of Medical-Surgical Nursing
Frances Payne Bolton School of Nursing
Case Western Reserve University
Cleveland, Ohio

**VIRGINIA L. CASSMEYER, PhD, RN, CS**
Associate Professor and Academic Coordinator
School of Nursing, University of Kansas Medical Center
Kansas City, Kansas

**JUDITH K. SANDS, EdD, RN**
Associate Professor and Director of Undergraduate Studies
University of Virginia School of Nursing
Charlottesville, Virginia

**†MARY KAY LEHMAN, MSN, RN**
Doctoral Candidate, Director Student Services
Frances Payne Bolton School of Nursing
Case Western Reserve University
Cleveland, Ohio

†Deceased.


**FIFTH EDITION**
***with* 1250 *illustrations***


Mosby

St. Louis Baltimore Berlin Boston Carlsbad Chicago London Madrid
Naples New York Philadelphia Sydney Tokyo Toronto

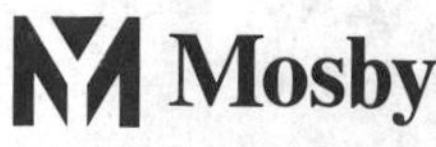

Dedicated to Publishing Excellence

Publisher: Nancy L. Coon
Editor: Michael S. Ledbetter
Senior Developmental Editor: Teri Merchant
Developmental Editor: Kathy Sartori
Project Manager: Patricia Tannian
Senior Production Editor: Betty Hazelwood
Senior Book Designers: Jeanne Wolfgeher and Gail Morey Hudson
Manufacturing Supervisor: Betty Richmond



**FIFTH EDITION**



A NOTE TO THE READER:

The author and publisher have made every attempt to check dosages and nursing content for accuracy. Because the science of pharmacology is continually advancing, our knowledge base continues to expand. Therefore we recommend that the reader always check product information for changes in dosage or administration before administering any medication. This is particularly important with new or rarely used drugs.



Printed in the United States of America

Composition by Graphic World, Inc.
Printing/binding by Rand McNally

Mosby–Year Book, Inc.
11830 Westline Industrial Drive
St. Louis, Missouri 63146



**Library of Congress Cataloging in Publication Data**

Medical-surgical nursing : concepts and clinical practice / edited by Wilma J. Phipps . . . [et al.].—5th ed.
p. cm.
Includes bibliographical references and index.
ISBN 0-8016-7888-9
1. Nursing. 2. Surgical nursing. I. Phipps, Wilma J.
[DNLM: 1. Nursing Care. 2. Nursing Process. 3. Surgical Nursing.
WY 150 M4894 1994]
RT41.M49 1994
610.73—dc20
DNLM/DLC
for Library of Congress 94-36432
CIP

94 95 96 97 98 / 9 8 7 6 5 4 3 2

*This fifth edition of*

**Medical-Surgical Nursing: Concepts and Clinical Practice**

*is dedicated to the memory of*

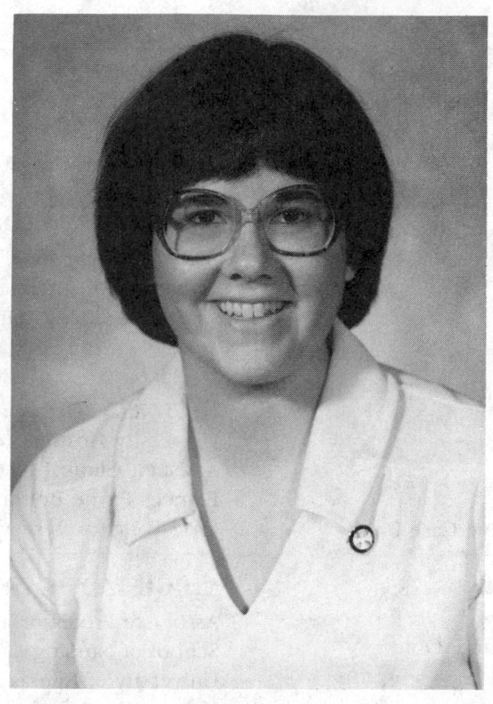

**Mary Kay Lehman,** MSN, RN
Doctoral Candidate
Case Western Reserve University
Cleveland, Ohio

whose untimely death on January 28, 1994, saddened us all. Mary Kay died at the age of 36 from a ruptured splenic aneurysm in the eighth month of her pregnancy.

Mary Kay had joined us as an editor of this edition after being an author or coauthor of chapters in the third and fourth editions. She was involved in the planning for this edition, which included selecting contributors and consulting with them as they developed their chapters. She also completed three of her own chapters.

Mary Kay contributed much to her chosen profession. She was a skillful practitioner, an able administrator, an excellent teacher and role model for students, an author, and a researcher. She had an impact on the lives of all who knew her. We will remember always her sunny disposition, ready smile, kindness to others, willingness to seek out new challenges, and devotion to her parents, husband, and 6-year-old son.

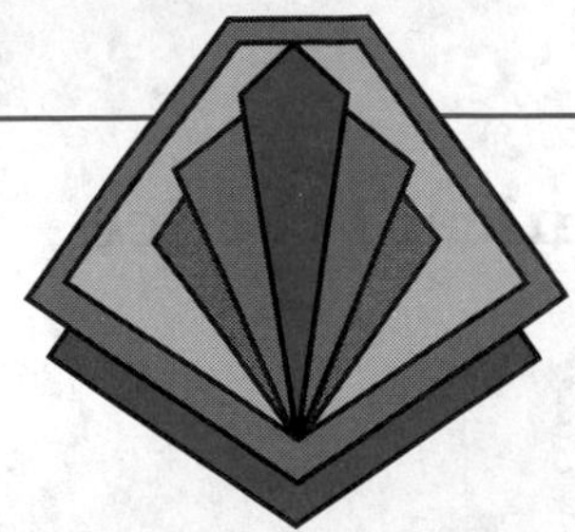

# Contributors


**TERRI ABRAHAM,** MSN, RN, CCRN
Nurse Manager, Intensive Care Unit
Mercy Hospital, Miami, Florida

**MARION ALLEN,** PhD, RN
Professor of Nursing
University of Alberta, Edmonton,
Edmonton, Alberta, Canada

**MARTHA L. ALLEN,** MSN, RN
Head Nurse, Cardiac and Medical Intensive Care Units
University Hospitals of Cleveland;
Clinical Instructor
Frances Payne Bolton School of Nursing
Case Western Reserve University, Cleveland, Ohio

**BARBARA ASTLE,** MSN, RN
Nurse Educator, Orbis International
New York, New York

**NANCY K. BARR,** BSN, RN, MSN (cand)
Clinical Nurse II, Emergency Department
St. Joseph Health Center, Kansas City, Missouri

**MARILYN ROSSMAN BARTUCCI,** MSN, RN, CS, CCTC
Head Nurse Manager, Transplant Center
University Hospitals of Cleveland;
Clinical Instructor
Frances Payne Bolton School of Nursing
Case Western Reserve University, Cleveland, Ohio

**PATRICIA A. BETRUS,** PhD, RN
Assistant Professor, Department of Psychosocial Nursing
University of Washington School of Nursing
Seattle, Washington

**DOROTHY R. BLEVINS,** MSN, RN
Associate Professor of Nursing
Kent State University School of Nursing
Kent, Ohio

**CYNTHIA F. BROGDON,** MSN, RN, OCN
Clinical Nurse Specialist, AMGEN
Kansas City, Missouri

**JOSEPHINE JACOBS BRUCIA,** PhD, RN
Assistant Professor
University of Virginia School of Nursing
Charlottesville, Virginia

**PATRICIA S. BUERGIN,** BSN, RN
Head Nurse, Orthopaedics
University Hospitals of Cleveland;
Assistant Clinical Instructor
Frances Payne Bolton School of Nursing
Case Western Reserve University, Cleveland, Ohio

**VIRGINIA L. CASSMEYER,** PhD, RN, CS
Associate Professor and Academic Coordinator
School of Nursing
University of Kansas Medical Center
Kansas City, Kansas

**BARBARA J. DALY,** PhD, RN, FAAN
Assistant Professor
Frances Payne Bolton School of Nursing
Case Western Reserve University;
Co-Director, Clinical Ethics Service
University Hospitals of Cleveland, Cleveland, Ohio

**GLADYS E. DETERS,** MSN, RN
Assistant Professor of Nursing
University of Virginia School of Nursing
Charlottesville, Virginia

**Sr. KARIN DUFAULT,** SP, PhD, RN
Administrator, St. Elizabeth Medical Center
Yakima, Washington

**GEORGE ANN EAKS,** MN, RN, ARNP, CDE
Clinical Nurse Specialist, Assistant Director,
Cray Diabetes Management Center
University of Kansas Medical Center
Kansas City, Kansas

**ELIZABETH CAMERON ECKSTEIN,** MSN, RN, CIC
Infection Control Nurse
Cleveland Veterans Administration Hospital
Cleveland, Ohio

**CAROLYN W. EDDINS, MSN, RN, ET**
Assistant Professor of Nursing
University of Virginia School of Nursing
Charlottesville, Virginia

**KATHERINE A. FLETCHER, PhD (cand), RN, CS**
Clinical Instructor, School of Nursing
University of Kansas Medical Center
Kansas City, Kansas

**DIANE BROADBENT FRIEDMAN, MSN, RN, CS**
Research Coordinator, Department of Vascular Surgery
Milton S. Hershey Medical Center
Pennsylvania State University
Hershey, Pennsylvania

**DIANE E. FRITSCH, MSN, RN, CCRN, CS**
Clinical Nurse Specialist, Trauma Critical Care Nursing
MetroHealth Medical Center
Cleveland, Ohio

**GREER GLAZER, PhD, RN**
Associate Professor
Kent State University School of Nursing
Kent, Ohio

**MARGARET HEITKEMPER, PhD, RN, FAAN**
Professor, Department of Physiological Nursing
School of Nursing, University of Washington
Seattle, Washington

**MAURA A. HOPKINS, MSN, RN**
Assistant Director of Nursing for Specialty Services
Kaiser Permanente Medical Center
Santa Rosa, California

**ARLENE W. KEELING, PhD, RN**
Assistant Professor
University of Virginia School of Nursing
Charlottesville, Virginia

**Maj. DEBORAH J. KENNY, MSN, EdM, RN, CCRN**
Head Nurse, Hematology Oncology
US Army Nurse Corps, Aurora, Colorado

**DENISE M. KRESEVIC, MSN, RN, CS**
Clinical Nurse Specialist
University Hospitals of Cleveland;
Clinical Instructor, Doctoral Candidate
Frances Payne Bolton School of Nursing
Case Western Reserve University, Cleveland, Ohio

**†MARY KAY LEHMAN, MSN, RN**
Doctoral Candidate, Director Student Services
Frances Payne Bolton School of Nursing
Case Western Reserve University, Cleveland, Ohio

**JO ANN LIERMAN, MN, EdS, RN, CS, ARNP**
Clinical Nurse Specialist
University of Kansas Medical Center;
Assistant Clinical Professor, School of Nursing
University of Kansas Medical Center, Kansas City, Kansas

**RUTH A. LINCOLN, MSN, RN, RNC**
Formerly Advanced Clinical Nurse
University Hospitals of Cleveland;
Clinical Instructor
Frances Payne Bolton School of Nursing
Case Western Reserve University, Cleveland, Ohio

**MOLLY LONEY, MSN, RN, OCN**
Oncology Clinical Nurse Specialist
Saint Luke's Medical Center;
Clinical Instructor
Frances Payne Bolton School of Nursing
Case Western Reserve University, Cleveland, Ohio

**BARBARA C. LONG, MSN, RN**
Associate Professor Emeritus of Medical-Surgical Nursing
Frances Payne Bolton School of Nursing
Case Western Reserve University, Cleveland, Ohio

**MARILYN S. LOTTMAN, MSN, RN, OCN**
Instructor in Nursing
Frances Payne Bolton School of Nursing
Case Western Reserve University, Cleveland, Ohio

**JANE F. MAREK, MSN, RN**
Research Nurse, Motion Study Laboratory
Cleveland Veterans Administration Medical Center;
Clinical Instructor, Meridia Huron School of Nursing
Cleveland, Ohio

**PAMELA HOLSCLAW MITCHELL, MS, ARNP, CNRN, FAAN**
Professor, Department of Physiological Nursing
School of Nursing
University of Washington
Seattle, Washington

**DIANA LYNN MORRIS, PhD, RN**
Assistant Professor
Frances Payne Bolton School of Nursing
Case Western Reserve University, Cleveland, Ohio

**GRACE A. MURO, MSN, RN**
Clinician IV, Operating Room
University of Virginia Health Sciences Center
Charlottesville, Virginia

**MARY KAY NACCAROTO, MSN, RN, CCRN**
Associate Director of Research
Metropolitan Health System, Cleveland, Ohio

†Deceased.

**JANICE NEVILLE, DSC, RD**
Professor of Nutrition
Case Western Reserve University, Cleveland, Ohio

**KYLE M. PASKERT, MSN, RN**
Formerly Clinical Nurse Specialist
University Hospitals of Cleveland;
Clinical Instructor
Frances Payne Bolton School of Nursing
Case Western Reserve University, Cleveland, Ohio

**WILMA J. PHIPPS, PhD, RN, FAAN**
Professor Emeritus of Medical-Surgical Nursing
Frances Payne Bolton School of Nursing
Case Western Reserve University, Cleveland, Ohio

**SANDRA JEAN FULTON PICOT, PhD, RN**
Assistant Professor
Frances Payne Bolton School of Nursing
Case Western Reserve University, Cleveland, Ohio

**DEBORAH POWER, MN, RN**
Formerly Lecturer, Department of Physiological Nursing
School of Nursing
University of Washington
Seattle, Washington

**JANET PRIMOMO, PhD, RN**
Senior Research Fellow
School of Nursing
University of Washington
Seattle, Washington

**DORA RICE, MSN, RN**
Infection Control Nurse
Cleveland Veterans Administration Hospital
Cleveland, Ohio

**REBECCA ANNE ROBERTS, MSN, RN, ET**
Clinical Nurse Specialist, University Hospitals of Cleveland;
Clinical Instructor
Frances Payne Bolton School of Nursing
Case Western Reserve University, Cleveland, Ohio

**JUDITH K. SANDS, EdD, RN**
Associate Professor and Director of Undergraduate Studies
University of Virginia School of Nursing
Charlottesville, Virginia

**HELEN A. SCHAAG, MSN, MA, RN**
Health Care Consultant
Human and System Development
Kansas City, Missouri

**ELIZABETH ANNE SCHENK, MSN, RNC, CRRN**
Formerly Vice President of Nursing
Heather Hill, Inc., Munson, Ohio

**LINDA T. SCHURING, MSN, RN**
Nurse Director, Balance Disorder Clinic
Warren Otologic Group, Warren, Ohio

**CAROL E. SMITH, PhD, RN**
Professor and Research Coordinator, School of Nursing
University of Kansas Medical Center
Kansas City, Kansas

**DEBERA JANE THOMAS, DNS, RN**
Assistant Professor
Frances Payne Bolton School of Nursing
Case Western Reserve University, Cleveland, Ohio

**KATHRYN SABO THOMPSON, MSN, RN**
Project Leader, Special Care Unit
University Hospitals of Cleveland, Cleveland, Ohio

**LYNN VALENTINE, DNSc, RN**
Associate Professor of Nursing
Piedmont Virginia Community College
Charlottesville, Virginia

**M. EILEEN WALSH, MSN, RN**
Vascular Clinical Nurse Specialist, Jobst Vascular Center
The Toledo Hospital, Toledo, Ohio

**JUDITH H. WATT-WATSON, BScN, MScN**
Clinical Associate Professor, Faculty of Nursing
University of Toronto, Toronto, Canada

**VICKIE WEAVER, MN (cand), BSN, RN, CETN**
Enterostomal Therapist, Nurse Clinician
University of Kansas Medical Center, Kansas City, Kansas

**ANITA L. WINGATE, PhD, RN**
Associate Professor, Academic Coordinator
School of Nursing, University of Kansas Medical Center
Kansas City, Kansas

**E. RONALD WRIGHT, PhD**
Associate Professor of Nursing and Biology
Frances Payne Bolton School of Nursing
Case Western Reserve University, Cleveland, Ohio

**LYNNE C. YURKO, BSN, RN**
Unit Manager, Burn Intensive Care Unit
MetroHealth Medical Center, Cleveland, Ohio

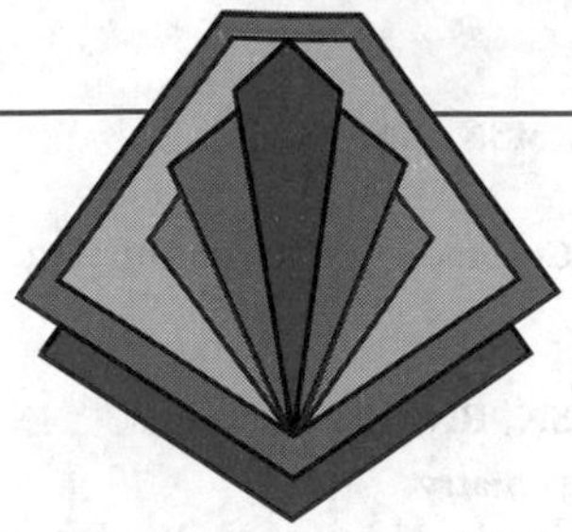

# Reviewers

**SARAH E. ANGERMULLER, MEd, MSN, RN**
Associate Professor of Nursing, Columbus College
Columbus, Georgia

**ARDELINA A. BALDANADO, PhD, RN**
Associate Professor and Chairperson
Department of Medical-Surgical Nursing
Niehoff School of Nursing
Loyola University, Chicago
Chicago, Illinois

**BETTY L. BELL, MSN, RN**
Associate Professor, Nursing
Community College of Allegheny County
Pittsburgh, Pennsylvania

**SANDRA HAGEN BENSON, MS, RN**
Assistant Professor, Adult Health Nursing
College of Nursing, University of North Dakota
Grand Forks, North Dakota

**SUSAN BROWN, MS, RN**
Instructor and Chairperson, Medical-Surgical Nursing II
Harbor Hospital School of Nursing
Baltimore, Maryland

**TERRI CRANFORD, MBA, BSN, RN**
Nursing Instructor, Tarleton State University
Stephenville, Texas

**ANGELISE DAVIS, DSN, RN, AHNP**
Associate Professor of Nursing
University of South Carolina, Spartanburg
Spartanburg, South Carolina

**JANET DELGADO, MN, RN**
Assistant Professor, Neuroscience Specialist
Rush-Presbyterian-St. Luke's Medical Center
Chicago, Illinois

**PAT DOLAN, MS, RN**
Associate Professor of Nursing
University of Massachusetts School of Nursing
North Dartmouth, Massachusetts

**MARY LYNN DROUGHTON, MSN, RN**
Clinical Nurse Specialist, Head and Neck Oncology
Cleveland Clinic Foundation, Cancer Foundation
Cleveland, Ohio

**SHEILA A. DUNN, MSN, RN**
Adjunct Instructor
St. Louis University School of Nursing
St. Louis, Missouri

**SIOBHAN DUNNAVANT, BSN, RN**
Intensive Care Unit and Home Health Nurse
University of Virginia
Charlottesville, Virginia

**LORI GEISMAN, MSN(R), RN**
Staff Nurse, Medical Intensive Care Unit
Barnes-Jewish Health System
Washington University Medical Center
St. Louis, Missouri

**SUSAN K. GIULIANETTI, MSN, RN**
Clinical Director, Bolton Scholar BSN Program
Frances Payne Bolton School of Nursing
Case Western Reserve University, Cleveland, Ohio

**SHIRLEY HEMMINGER, MSN, RN**
Instructor, Kent State University School of Nursing
Kent, Ohio

**MARY REUTHER HERRING, MSN, RN**
Occupational Health Nurse; Instructor
University of Phoenix, Phoenix, Arizona

**FRANK HICKS, MS, RN, CCRN**
Assistant Professor, Medical-Surgical Nursing
Niehoff School of Nursing
Loyola University, Chicago, Chicago, Illinois

**BARBARA E. HIRSCH, JD, BSN**
Nurse-Attorney, Freeman and Jenner, P.C.
Bethesda, Maryland

**Sr. ESTHER D. HOLZBAUER, MSN, RN**
Assistant Professor of Nursing
Mount Marty College, Yankton, South Dakota

**PAM IDZIOREK, MS, MA, BA**
Assistant Professor of Nursing
College of St. Scholastica, Duluth, Minnesota

**PATRICIA A. JABLONSKI, MS, RN**
Instructor of Nursing
Hudson Valley Community College, Troy, New York;
Clinical Nurse Specialist, Trauma and Surgery
Albany Medical Center, Albany, New York

**NOURA KASSIS, EdD, RN**
Instructor of Nursing
Mt. San Antonio Community College
Walnut, California

**PATRICIA J. KELLY, MS, RN, CEN**
Chairman, Medical-Surgical I
School of Nursing, Harbor Hospital Center
Baltimore, Maryland

**LINDA LEA KERBY, MA, RNC**
Educational Consultant
Leawood, Kansas

**JANE KOECKERITZ, PhD, RN**
Assistant Professor of Nursing, Health and Human Services
University of Northern Colorado, Greeley, Colorado

**ANTOINETTE K. LEDBETTER, MS, RN**
Trauma Coordinator
St. John's Mercy Medical Center
St. Louis, Missouri

**JUDITH R. LENTZ, PhD, RN**
Adjunct Instructor of Nursing
St. Louis University, St. Louis, Missouri

**JoANN LOWDON, MA, RN**
Professor of Nursing
Blue Ridge Community College, Weyers Cave, Virginia

**JACKIE MANGNALL, MS**
Assistant Professor of Nursing
Jamestown College, Jamestown, North Dakota

**DORIS MARSHALEK, MSN, RN**
Professor of Nursing
Community College of Allegheny County;
Staff Nurse, Intensive Care Unit, Divine Providence Hospital
Pittsburgh, Pennsylvania

**ESTHER MATASSARIN-JACOBS, PhD, RN, OCN**
Associate Professor
Medical-Surgical Nursing Department
Loyola University, Chicago, Chicago, Illinois

**MARJORIE MATZEN, MS, RN**
Director, School of Nursing
Jennie Edmundson Memorial Hospital
Council Bluffs, Iowa

**DIANE C. MEADOR, MSN, RN**
Instructor of Nursing
University of Northern Colorado School of Nursing
Greeley, Colorado

**JEFFREY MILLER, MSN, RN**
Project Coordinator, Psychiatry
Medical College of Wisconsin, Milwaukee, Wisconsin

**DONNA J. MULLEN, MS, RNCS**
Nursing Instructor
Southwest Wisconsin Technical College
Fennimore, Wisconsin

**ELIZABETH NAUGLE, MS, RN**
Instructor, Applied Sciences
Mission College, Santa Clara, California

**ANN W. OBERLE, MN, RN**
Assistant Professor of Nursing
Northwestern State University
Natchitoches, Louisiana

**KRISTINE A. PILOSKI, MSN, RN**
Staff Nurse, Surgical Intensive Care Unit
Barnes-Jewish Health System
Washington University Medical Center
St. Louis, Missouri

**LENORA RICHARDSON, DSN, RN**
Assistant Professor of Nursing
University of North Carolina at Greensboro
Greensboro, North Carolina

**FRANCINE ROBERTS, MSN, RN**
Assistant Professor of Nursing
George Mason University, Fairfax, Virginia

**LOIS ROBINSON, MSN, RN**
Associate Professor and Chairman, Medical-Surgical Nursing
School of Nursing, Kansas Newman College
Wichita, Kansas

**BOBI ROSE, BSN, RN**
Baptist Memorial Hospital School of Nursing
Memphis, Tennessee

**CAROL RUSCIN, MSN, RN**
Clinical Nurse Specialist
Nursing Administration Department
University of Central Arkansas, Conway, Arkansas

**TERRY S. SAVAN, MA, RN**
Nurse Specialist, Emergency Department
California Pacific Medical Center and
University of California, San Francisco;
Research Assistant, School of Pharmacy
University of California, San Francisco
San Francisco, California

**BRUCE SCOTT, MSN, RN**
Lecturer, School of Nursing
Los Angeles County Medical Center
Los Angeles, California

**E. MARIAN SIMON, MS, RN**
Assistant Professor of Nursing
College of St. Scholastica, Duluth, Minnesota

**CESARINA THOMPSON, PhD, RN**
Associate Professor of Nursing
Southern Connecticut State University
New Haven, Connecticut

**ROBYN THOMPSON, MSN, RN**
Nursing Department, Umpqua Community College
Roseburg, Oregon

**PATRICIA K. TRINOSKY-LIND, MS, RN**
Assistant Professor of Nursing
Beth-El College of Nursing
Colorado Springs, Colorado

**MARY CATHERINE TUCKER, MSN, RN**
Formerly Clinical Educator
Missouri Baptist Medical Center
St. Louis, Missouri

**BARBARA VAN DROOF, MN, RNC**
Professor of Nursing, Shoreline Community College
Seattle, Washington

**GAYLE P. VARNELL, PhD, RN, CPNP**
Nursing Instructor, El Centro College
Dallas, Texas

**GERALDINE VARRASSI, EdD, RN**
Medical-Surgical Nursing Instructor
Department of Nursing Education
North Shore University Hospital
Manhasset, New York

**DOROTHY A. WATSON, MSN, RN**
Assistant Professor of Nursing
Roane State Community College
Harriman, Tennessee

**JUANITA WATSON, PhD, RN**
Assistant Professor of Nursing, Rutgers University
Camden College of Arts and Sciences
Camden, New Jersey

**PAMELA BECKER WEILITZ, MSN(R), RN**
Manager, Care Paths, Barnes-Jewish Health System
Washington University Medical Center
St. Louis, Missouri

**NANCY E. WHITE, PhD, RN**
Professor of Nursing
University of Northern Colorado
Greeley, Colorado

**LAUREL WIERSEMA, MSN, RN, CS**
Surgery Clinical Nurse Specialist
Barnes-Jewish Health System
Washington University Medical Center
St. Louis, Missouri

**ROSEMARY WITTSTADT, EdD, RN**
Professor of Nursing, Towson State University
Towson, Maryland

**JEAN M. WORTOCK, MSN, ARNP**
Professor of Nursing
St. Petersburg Junior College
St. Petersburg, Florida

**LINDA M. WRAY, MSN, RN**
Assistant Professor, Baccalaureate Nursing
Eastern Kentucky University, Richmond, Kentucky

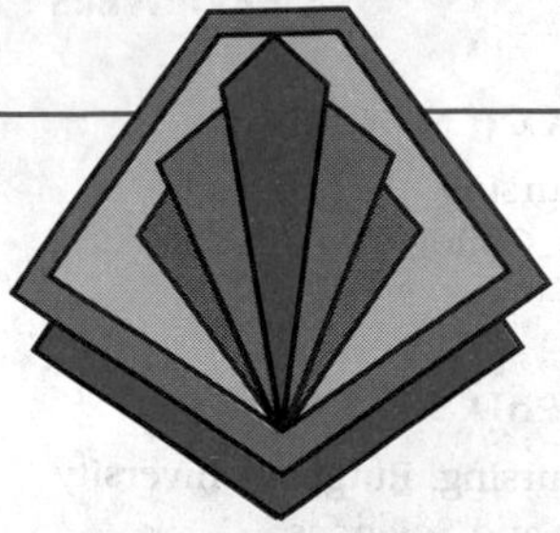

# Preface

There seems to be no better word to describe what is going on today in nursing and in health care than *change.* As we move toward the twenty-first century, the changes in health care delivery are many, with many more yet to come when Congress passes a health care reform bill. The changes in nursing necessary to meet the changes in society and in the delivery of health care in the United States are reflected in this fifth edition. Some new chapters have been added, some chapters have been deleted, and some chapters have been combined so that the information provided is relevant to today's medical-surgical nursing practice. We continue to believe, as we did when the first edition was published, that nurses need an up-to-date textbook that incorporates information from nursing and a variety of other disciplines. To accomplish this, we have sought out clinical experts to write each of the chapters. Some of the authors are first-time contributors to this book, and others have been contributors to several editions. We also have new editors from different regions of the country (Kansas and Virginia), which expands the nursing viewpoints presented in the fifth edition.

As in the fourth edition, we refer to recipients of the services of nurses as *patients* rather than *clients.* Although *client* is widely used in the nursing community, we have been interested in the distinction between the two terms. The article, "Complexities and clarity in nurse-client and nurse-patient relationships," by L. Nowakowski, published in the July-August 1985 issue of the *Journal of Professional Nursing,* addresses this subject well. Using her framework, we think the use of *patient* in this book seems appropriate. We found her article to be useful and thought-provoking, and we recommend the article to the reader.

## ORGANIZATION

The 72 chapters in this edition are divided into two parts: Part One, Perspectives for Nursing Practice with Ill Adults; and Part Two, Alterations in Human Functioning. Part One, divided into five units, provides the foundations for nursing practice associated with the care of ill adults.

Unit I, Perspectives for Health and Illness, contains seven chapters. Chapter 1 addresses changes in the population of the United States in terms of multiculturalism and the aging of the population. Managed care and what it means to the role of nurses are also discussed in Chapter 1, along with the changes in nursing education designed to prepare nurses to function in an everchanging health care system. Chapter 2, Ethical Decision Making in Nursing, a new chapter written by a nurse-ethicist, focuses on understanding the process for analyzing and addressing ethical dilemmas. The content about ill adults has been divided into two chapters, Nursing Practice with Young and Middle-Aged Adults and Nursing Practice with Elders. Another new chapter in this unit is Healthy Life-Styles: Nutrition, Exercise, Rest, and Sleep, which emphasizes the importance of health promotion. Chapter 7, Stress, Stressors, and Stress Management, describes the body's responses to stress that impact on health or illness.

Unit II, Common Concepts for Care of Ill Adults, has been revised extensively to reflect today's nursing practice. For example, Chapter 8, Chronic Illness and Rehabilitation, has increased content on rehabilitation. The same is true for Chapter 9, Body Image and Self-Esteem, where concepts about self-esteem have been added. Chapter 10 added concepts on grief, reflected in the title change to Loss, Grief, and Dying. Chapter 11, Human Sexuality, incorporates content that in previous editions was covered in the unit on Alterations in Sexuality and Reproduction. Because this content is relevant for care to *all* patients, it was moved to Unit II. Chapter 12, Alterations in Consciousness in the Hospitalized Adult, is a new chapter designed to help students understand the changes in mental status seen in medical-surgical patients. Chapter 13, Inflammatory and Immune Responses, incorporates content found in previous editions in the chapter entitled Biologic Defense Mechanisms.

Unit III, Common Problems Encountered in the Care of Ill Adults, consists of nine chapters. Chapter 14, Fatigue, is a new chapter focusing on the management of this major health concern, common among ill adults. The chapters on infection, cancer, and pain are thoroughly revised to reflect the latest information. Chapter 18, Sleep Disorders, was moved from the unit on Alterations in Cognition, Sensation, and Motion in previous editions to Unit III of the fifth edition. Chapter 19, Substance Abuse, now incorporates key content about eating disorders. Chapters on fluid and electrolyte imbalance, acid-base imbalance, and shock complete this unit.

Unit IV, Surgery: Perioperative Nursing, has three chapters: Preoperative Nursing, Intraoperative Nursing, and Postoperative Nursing. These chapters are organized as in previous editions and provide the most up-to-date content reflecting current practice.

Unit V, Special Environments of Care, is the last unit of Part One and contains three chapters. These chapters, Critical Care Environment, Home Care Environment, and Emergency Care Environment, were moved forward from the end of the book in the fourth edition. All have been revised to reflect the latest concepts and clinical practice. Chapter 27, Home Care Environment, addresses the needs of patients who require the use of complex technology in the home. Current health care trends are moving more toward patients spending fewer days in the hospital. In response, persons with complex medical-surgical problems are being cared for in their homes. This presents a challenge both to nurses in the hospital, who have only a short time to prepare the patient and family for discharge to the home, and to the nurse providing care in the home. This chapter should help the student understand the transition from hospital care to home care.

Part Two, Alterations in Human Functioning, contains six units focusing on detailed discussions of the care of patients with alterations within body systems. Each system is discussed within a consistent format, beginning with a separate assessment chapter, followed by one or more chapters on the management of persons with disorders associated with the system.

Unit VI, Alterations in Fluid and Gas Transport, contains nine chapters dealing with the *cardiovascular system, hematologic system,* and *respiratory system.* As in previous editions, the cardiovascular content is presented in three chapters in addition to the assessment chapter. New to this edition, the *hematologic system* includes a separate assessment chapter. Also new to the fifth edition, coverage of the *respiratory system* has been incorporated into three chapters. The content on common interventions for respiratory problems previously in a separate chapter has been integrated into Chapter 36, Management of Persons with Problems of the Upper Airway, and Chapter 37, Management of Persons with Problems of the Lower Airway. Both chapters have been extensively revised to reflect changes in therapy and current approaches to care.

Unit VII, Alterations in Metabolism, has retained the organization of three chapters on the *endocrine system* and two chapters on the *hepatic system.* These chapters have been revised to reflect changes in the care of patients with these problems.

Unit VIII, Alterations in Digestion and Elimination, has been condensed to 8 chapters from 11 chapters in the previous edition. Content in the previous edition on nutritional assessment and dietary counseling has been incorporated into Chapter 6. Section One covers the *gastrointestinal, biliary,* and *exocrine pancreatic systems.* Content about the *renal system* is presented in Section Two.

Unit IX, Alterations in Reproduction and Sexuality, has five chapters. With the exception of the material on human sexuality, which is now in Chapter 11, this unit is organized as it was in the previous edition. All chapters have been extensively revised to reflect advances in these areas.

Unit X, Alterations in Cognition, Sensation, and Motion, has been condensed to 10 chapters from 12 in the fourth edition. Content changes are most evident in Section One on the *nervous system.* In addition to the assessment chapter, the nervous system contains two distinct chapters: Chapter 57, Management of Persons with Problems of the Brain; and Chapter 58, Management of Persons with Problems of the Spinal Cord and Peripheral Nerves. The content related to altered levels of consciousness, which was a separate chapter in earlier editions, is incorporated into Chapter 57 and Chapter 12. The chapter, Sleep Disorders, previously covered with the nervous system, has been moved to Unit III. Unit X continues with detailed coverage of the *visual system, auditory system,* and *musculoskeletal system.* Revisions in the musculoskeletal system section have been extensive and include the latest orthopedic surgical techniques and the resulting changes associated with the preoperative and postoperative care of these patients.

Unit XI, Alterations in Defense and Protection, covers two body systems: the *integumentary system* and the *immune system.* In Section One on the integumentary system, content on common interventions for skin problems, in a separate chapter in previous editions, has been integrated into Chapter 67, Management of Persons with Problems of the Skin. Section Two on the immune system includes a new chapter, Chapter 72, Management of Persons with Organ/Tissue Transplants. In previous editions, transplantation was discussed with each of the organ problems for which transplantation is a possible treatment. That content was deleted from those chapters and incorporated into this new chapter. Because the principles related to transplantation are common to all organ transplants, we believe the reader will benefit by having all this content in one chapter.

## FEATURES

Each chapter begins with detailed **Learning Objectives,** followed by a list of **Key Terms.** The key terms are in bold-face and defined within the chapter. The chapter concludes with a **Chapter Summary, Questions to Consider,** and **Critical Thinking Activities.** The Chapter Summary is categorized by appropriate internal chapter headings for accessibility to content.

Questions to Consider, as in the fourth edition, test the students' ability to apply knowledge of the material covered in the chapter. New to the fifth edition are Critical Thinking Activities designed to help the students reflect on the material learned in the chapter.

To help readers keep abreast of the changes in health care and the delivery of nursing care, several new or updated features are incorporated throughout the fifth edition, including the following:

- The goals for health promotion and disease prevention as set in *Healthy People 2000,* the 1991 US Department of Health and Human Services, Public Health Service publication are incorporated throughout the text.
- Updating and expansion to more than 30 *nursing care plans.*
- Eighteen *critical pathways* are included for the common problems found in hospitalized ill adults. These pathways provide the student with examples of collaborative clinical tools based on DRGs with defined time lines for achieving patient outcomes. Most critical pathways have an associated nursing care plan for the same patient problem.
- **Nursing diagnoses** and their **possible etiologic factors** are included in the management chapters. The nursing diagnoses used in this edition are from the Eleventh NANDA Conference, 1994. The authors of the chapters have listed the diagnoses in the priority they would be used in implementing nursing care.
- Management of symptoms, a major function of nursing, is discussed in several chapters, and the guidelines recently published by the Agency for Health Care Policy and Research (AHCPR) are introduced as a valuable source of information about the management of symptoms, such as pain and incontinence. A complete list of guidelines and how to obtain the publications are found inside the back cover.

## FORMAT

The management of the most common diseases or disorders are discussed in the body systems chapters. The more common disorders are discussed in more detail using a long format that includes, in most instances, the following: **Etiology, Epidemiology, Pathophysiology, Prevention, Medical Management,** and, if appropriate, **Surgical Management. Nursing Management** is the heart of discussion for each disorder and in the long format follows the five-step nursing process framework: assessment, nursing diagnosis, expected patient outcomes, interventions, and evaluation. Integrated in the nursing interventions section you will find a new feature, wherever appropriate: **Managing Critical Care.**

Following Nursing Management are **Gerontologic Patient Considerations—**a section that delineates special assessments or interventions for elderly patients with a specific disorder. **Home Care Considerations** are included here when home care is an option for a specific disorder. **Complications** are listed when appropriate to help students learn to anticipate possible problems and to prevent them whenever possible.

## TEACHING/LEARNING PACKAGE

For this edition an extensive array of ancillary products for instructors and students to use in class and clinical settings is offered.

### INSTRUCTOR'S RESOURCE MANUAL

This valuable resource manual, prepared by Carol J. Green and Penny L. Marshall, follows the textbook chapter by chapter and includes chapter outlines, chapter overviews, and teaching suggestions to help in lecture preparation. The two new key components to this edition are classroom applications and practice applications. These focus on teaching strategies to help students apply what they have learned in the classroom and clinical settings. Also included is a thoroughly revised *Test Bank,* containing more than 1500 questions in NCLEX format accompanied by an answer key with page references.

### STUDY GUIDE

New to the fifth edition, this comprehensive and challenging study guide was prepared by Carol J. Green and Penny L. Marshall. This valuable study tool helps students assess their knowledge by testing their clinical skills and emphasizing critical thinking.

### OVERHEAD TRANSPARENCIES

One hundred two-color transparency acetates provide visual reinforcement of key illustrations and concepts from the text. Many of the transparencies are new to this edition and feature new computer artwork.

### QUICK REFERENCE FOR IV THERAPY

New to this edition is *Quick Reference for IV Therapy* by Cynthia Hermey, a handy, pocket-sized resource that accompanies every copy of the text. This accessible clinical tool features information on IV solutions, equipment, techniques, and an IV compatibility chart.

### COMPUTEST

Available in both IBM and Macintosh formats, *Computest* is the computerized version of the *Test Bank* from the *Instructor's Resource Manual.* Complete with a user's guide, *Computest* allows instructors to edit, add, delete, or select questions on the computer.

## CLINICAL MANUAL OF MEDICAL-SURGICAL NURSING

The third edition of *Clinical Manual of Medical-Surgical Nursing,* prepared by Judith K. Sands and Pamela Dennison, is a practical and concise clinical reference presented in an accessible format. It covers over 300 common medical-surgical conditions within a nursing process framework. Each chapter begins with patient history, physical assessment, and diagnostic tests for each major disorder. New to the third edition are two chapters: Substance Abuse and Immune System. Also new are gerontologic considerations and home care integrated in the text or in boxes, where appropriate.

## ACKNOWLEDGMENTS

With this edition we welcome Judith K. Sands as a new editor. Dr. Sands has not been involved in this textbook before, but she is the author of the *Clinical Manual of Medical-Surgical Nursing,* which is a companion reference for this textbook, and thus she is very familiar with the content and goals of this book.

Mary Kay Lehman was also a new editor until her untimely death in January 1994 (see Dedication, p. v).

Many experts have contributed to this fifth edition. For some, this is their first appearance as an author or coauthor of a chapter in this text. Several other contributors have been involved in one or more editions, and some have been contributors since the first edition. All of them have helped us make the fifth edition as up-to-date as possible. We are indebted to each of them for sharing their knowledge and expertise with our readers.

We are also indebted to all the readers and reviewers who made comments and suggestions during the development of the fifth edition. We found their comments to be helpful, and we trust that they will be pleased with the changes made in this edition.

The new illustrations for the fifth edition are the work of Nancy Burgard of Cleveland and Jack Reuter of St. Louis. Nadine Sokol of St. Louis created the computer-generated art. We are pleased with their contribution to the visual appeal and educational value of this text.

We are grateful to Michael Ledbetter, Kathy Sartori, Teri Merchant, and Betty Hazelwood of Mosby for their support and assistance during the preparation of this fifth edition.

**Wilma J. Phipps**
**Virginia L. Cassmeyer**
**Judith K. Sands**

Special and personal thanks to the following:
Sondra Patrizi, Dorothy Kontos, Jennifer Mann, and Sandy Wyper for helpful preparation of parts of this manuscript.

WJP

Helen Schaag for support and assistance in preparing this edition.

VLC

My colleagues at the University of Virginia School of Nursing for their support for this project, and Eric and David for their pride and pleasure in Mom's work.

JKS

## SPECIAL ACKNOWLEDGMENT

This is the first edition of this textbook that does not carry the names of Barbara C. Long and Nancy Fugate Woods as editors. Both have withdrawn to give more time to other pursuits. Since the publication of the first edition in 1979, Nancy Woods moved from Duke University to the University of Washington. There she pioneered research in women's health, which culminated in her being designated outstanding young nurse researcher in 1994.

Barbara Long has remained in Cleveland, and she and I have been involved in many projects together. Now she wants more time to travel with her husband and to pursue other interests, especially genealogy research. Barbara had not planned to be involved in this fifth edition, but volunteered her assistance after the sudden death of Mary Kay Lehman. I can never thank her enough for all her help.

I wish to thank both of them for all they contributed to the first four editions of this textbook, and I wish them well in their future endeavors.

**Wilma J. Phipps**

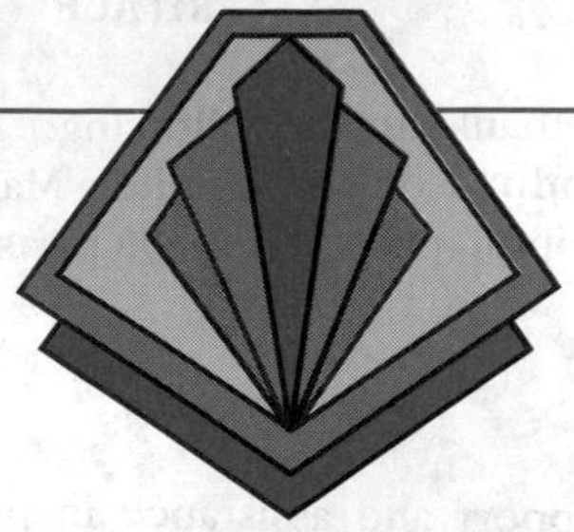

# To the Student

Because medical-surgical nursing is the heart of your nursing education, we have developed a student-friendly format for this text that emphasizes nursing responsibilities and helps you learn the material easily and assess your learning.

Guidelines boxes 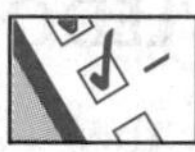 focus on nursing responsibilities, including preparing patients for diagnostic tests, nursing care after specific surgeries, patient teaching, and discharge planning.

Because elderly patients are the fastest growing segment of the population, an entire chapter focuses on care of elders, and specific considerations for care of gerontologic patients have been integrated throughout the body systems chapters. This logo 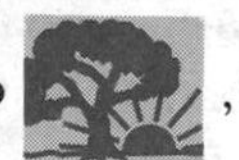, which appears both in boxes and in text, alerts you to specific assessments and interventions to remember when your patient is elderly.

Many medical-surgical problems are associated with pathologic states that require critical care; therefore the critical care environment, including hemodynamic monitoring and ventilator support, is introduced in Chapter 26. In addition, information related to managing critical care is emphasized in appropriate discussions in the text, such as fat embolism syndrome, with this logo.

Home health care is becoming a part of the nursing care of many patients because of shortened hospital stays. Thus home health care is featured in a separate chapter, as well as being incorporated in appropriate discussion in the book, such as persons with laryngectomy, with this logo.

The references for this book include both classic and current sources. All references cited in a particular chapter are listed in alphabetical order at the end of the chapter. At the end of the book on pages B1 to B65, literature sources are organized by topics for each chapter. This type of organization should allow for rapid identification of resources for specific topics within one area of nursing care of adults with specific pathologic conditions. Again both classical and current references are included in the bibliography.

We have provided you with many self-assessment aids for testing your knowledge of medical-surgical nursing. Because we want you to develop skill in making clinical decisions, **Critical Thinking Questions** at the end of each chapter ask for your judgment concerning a short patient care situation. No answers are given, but you can discuss the situations with your classmates. The **Questions to Consider** at the end of the chapters are another way to test your learning. The **Study Guide** that accompanies this text includes primarily critical thinking questions, but also adds true-false, short answer, and matching questions and answers.

**Wilma J. Phipps**
**Virginia L. Cassmeyer**
**Judith K. Sands**

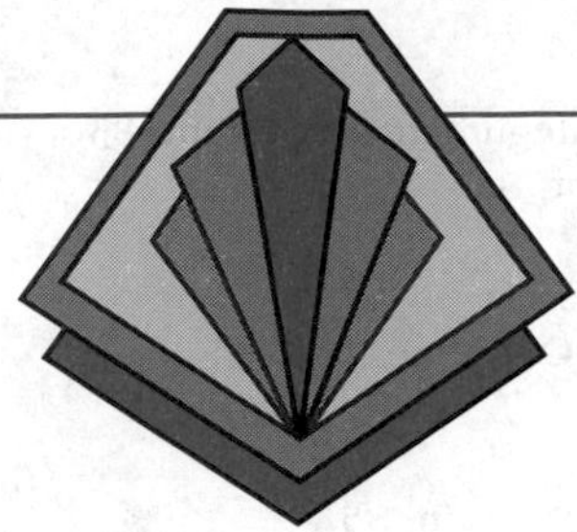

# Contents

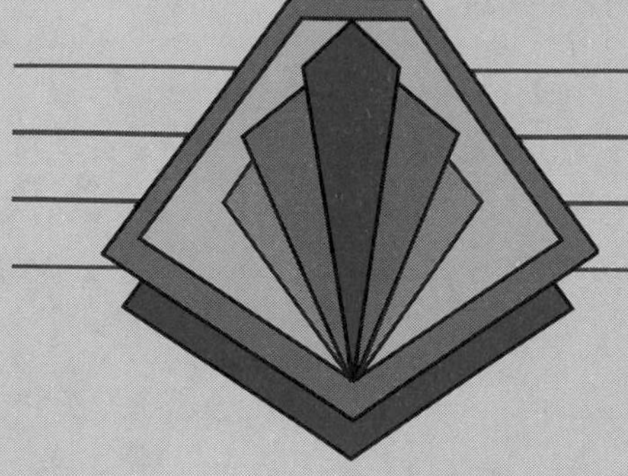

P A R T   O N E

# *Perspectives for Nursing Practice With Ill Adults*

U N I T   I

*Perspectives for Health and Illness*

U N I T   I I

*Common Concepts for Care of Ill Adults*

U N I T   I I I

*Common Problems Encountered in Care of Ill Adults*

U N I T   I V

*Surgery: Perioperative Nursing*

U N I T   V

*Special Environments of Care*

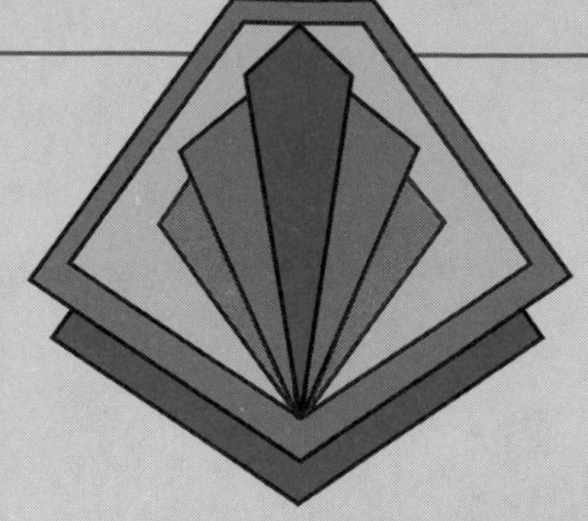

UNIT I

# Perspectives for Health and Illness

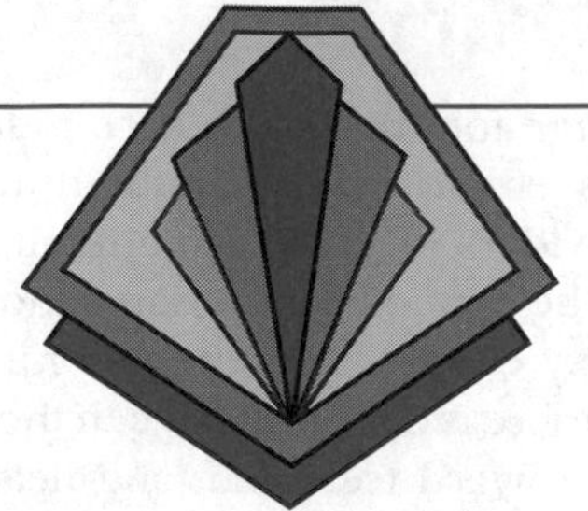

CHAPTER 1

# Nursing Practice With Ill Adults: Context, Structure, Process, and Outcomes

***Helen A. Schaag***
***Wilma J. Phipps***

## CHAPTER OBJECTIVES

***After studying this chapter, the learner should be able to do the following:***

1 Identify changing characteristics of American society and implications for nursing.
2 Recognize the impact of growth of the elderly population, growth of multiculturalism, new health care problems, and technologic advances on health care delivery systems, nursing practice, nursing roles, and nursing education.
3 Identify factors that have affected the evolution of the health care system in the United States.
4 Define health care from a systems approach.
5 Discuss the evolution of health care insurances, including prepaid types, preferred provider organizations (PPOs), health maintenance organizations (HMOs), and governmental plans, and their effect on health care facilities, physician practice, and nursing practice.
6 Discuss the reasons for the proliferation of ambulatory care centers, home health care services, and long-term care facilities.
7 Discuss the differences between total patient care, team or functional nursing, primary nursing, and case management nursing care.
8 Differentiate between managed care and case management.
9 Identify characteristics of potential nursing students and factors that will influence their choice of nursing as a profession.
10 Describe characteristics of nursing schools and nursing practitioners in the twenty-first century.
11 Identify three reasons why TQM and CQI are important aspects of the practice of nursing.
12 Describe six standards of clinical nursing practice developed by the American Nurses Association (ANA).
13 Describe how patient outcome variances are used to improve quality of care.

## KEY TERMS

case management care
clinical nurse specialist (CNS)
collaboration
community health agency
cost-benefit analysis
cost effective
critical pathway
DRGs
HMOs
home health agency
horizontal integration
Independent Practice Association (IPA)
indicator monitoring system
JCAHO
Medicaid
medical practice acts
Medicare
medigap
nurse practice acts
nurse practitioner (NP)
nursing case management
outcome-oriented care
peer review
point of service (POS)
PPOs
precertification approval
primary health care
primary nursing
Professional Review Organization (PRO)
prospective payment system (PPS)
quality assurance (QA)
total quality management/continuous quality improvement (TQM/CQI)
variances
vertical integration

Rapid changes in society during the past decade have had profound effects on the health care industry in the United States. Access to care, quality of care, and cost of health care are the most complex and debated issues in the country. These issues have significant implications for the role of nurses and how nursing is practiced in the future. This chapter focuses on several major factors that affect these issues and discusses anticipated trends and changes.

## CHANGES IN AMERICAN SOCIETY

### GROWTH OF THE ELDERLY POPULATION AND ITS CARE

Elderly persons, those individuals 65 years of age and older, are the fastest growing segment of our population, and persons 85 years of age and older are the fastest growing portion of the elderly population.[83] By the year 2000, the "old-old" population—those 85 years of age and older—will increase by 30% to a total of 4.6 million. At that time, 35 million people, or 13% of population, will be 65 years of age or older. By the year 2020, it is expected this number could increase to 51 million. From 1946 to 1964, the most recent baby-boom period, there were 76 million births. This baby-boom generation will be entering the elderly age range beginning in the year 2011. By the year 2030, there will be only three active workers for each retired person as compared with five workers for every retired person today.

The increase in longevity and a simultaneous decline in the birth rate are being experienced by all Western societies. Because of these changes in society, it has been suggested by some lawmakers that the eligibility age for retirement under Social Security and access to Medicare coverage be raised from 65 to 67 years of age. If this suggestion should become law, it would have profound effects on our culture, health care needs, the make-up of the work force, and the work environment itself.

For the aging who remain in their own homes or elsewhere in the community, it is evident that additional facilities for their care and well-being, including health care, must be provided. In addition to home health care services, a comparatively new development—the day-care center for the chronically ill and the elderly adult—shows evidence of becoming an important part of the health care scene. Such centers would be welcomed by adult working children who care for elderly parents and find it difficult to provide a supervised and structured environment for them. At present, there is minimal third-party reimbursement for this type of service. Medicare does not usually provide reimbursement even though it could be more cost effective to pay for this type of care than to pay for care in the person's home or in a nursing home.

### GROWTH OF MULTICULTURALISM

The rapid growth of multiculturalism in the United States is another change dramatically affecting the health care industry. The challenge for the health care industry is twofold: hospitals as employers of multicultural staff members and as providers of care to multicultural patients. In addition to the expected communication problems, cultural diversity creates the potential for significant problems when there is conflict between the values, beliefs, and attitudes toward treatment and health-promotion practices.[29] Currently, 71% of the United States population is white, 12% is African-American, 9% is Hispanic, 7% is of Asian–Pacific Islands origin, and less than 1% is Native American and Inuit.[77] By the year 2000 there will be a decrease to 62% for the white population, with increases to 10% for the Hispanic and 9% for the Asian–Pacific Islands groups.[78] Not only will the work force be older; it will be more racially and ethnically diverse.[12,68]

### NEW HEALTH CARE PROBLEMS

Besides the pressure for health care reform, several patient care challenges will have a profound effect on nursing and the health care industry in the United States. The four most significant challenges are care of HIV-positive and AIDS patients, ethical dilemmas in health care, violence and abuse, and the poor and homeless. Discussion of each of these follows.

#### HIV Infection and AIDS

Although acquired immunodeficiency syndrome (AIDS) emerged in 1981 as an unidentified killer of young men, there is still neither a cure for the disease nor a preventive vaccine. The human immunodeficiency virus (HIV) was identified in 1986 as the virus that caused AIDS. The diseases associated with HIV-positive status and AIDS are pandemic (worldwide). At this time 14 million persons worldwide are HIV positive and, of these, more than 3 million are women of childbearing years. Worldwide, 2.5 million people have AIDS.[65]

At present, the largest proportionate increase in reported cases of AIDS is among women, and it is the fourth leading cause of death among women 25 to 44 years of age in the United States. Heterosexual contacts account for the largest proportionate increase in reported cases of AIDS, whereas the incidence of AIDS among homosexual and bisexual persons has decreased. Although homosexual/bisexual men and injecting-drug users still constitute the largest populations in the United States who are HIV positive or have AIDS, the heterosexual population is the most rapidly growing group to become infected.[87,88]

In light of the already existing crisis in health care in the United States, the cost associated with providing the necessary care for persons with HIV infection or AIDS is significant. (See Chapter 71 for a detailed discussion of HIV infection and AIDS.)

#### Health Care Ethical Dilemmas

The administrators and board of directors of each health care facility must identify the basic culture and operating values of the institution to provide the basis for the overall direction and values of the organization. This includes beliefs about how personnel will be managed and valued and how the organization and its personnel will value and treat patients. Patient care outcomes that are unmet or ethical issues that occur can be identified through continuous quality improvement (CQI) activity, which is discussed in more detail later in this chapter.

There are several reasons to focus ethical decision making on CQI activity. First, the rapidly increasing opportunities in patient care will provide more options for patients and providers. Heart transplantation for one patient, for example, may mean that a family must agree that the heart of a comatose patient who is on a ventilator can be sacrificed. Balancing individual rights with social good will become more frequent and more difficult in the future. Second, as resources continue to diminish, problems of distributive justice will arise. It is quite possible that in the future some type of health care rationing will exist. For example, who should receive what services? How much? Who should pay? As public policymakers attempt to reduce all care choices to **cost-benefit analysis,** the nurse must be able to see beyond these calculations and the inability of them to account for human pain and suffering.

Third, nurses, as well as other health care professionals, must participate in ethical decision making or risk losing their unique influence. For example, in cases of the comatose, terminally ill patient, **peer review** would focus not only on the clinical aspects of death but also on the human dimension. Did the health care provider keep the patient or family members, or both, totally informed? Were the providers guided by the wishes of the patient and family? Did the provider seek competent, objective, and relevant third-party opinions? None of these decisions can be made irrespective of federal or state laws, but questions of quality lie within the realm of CQI activity.

*The Patient Self-Determination Act of 1990* provides persons 18 years of age and older the right to make decisions about their care, including the right to accept or refuse treatments and the right to formulate advance directives.[61,66] This law strengthens the patient's legal right to make treatment decisions. Advance directives are documents completed in advance of serious illness that indicate an individual's treatment choices during illness or that name someone to make these choices if one becomes incapacitated. *Advance directives,* such as *living wills* and *durable powers of attorney for health care decisions, provide legal directives for the kind of life-prolonging medical care* when one becomes terminally ill and unable to make decisions. Most states have their own living-will laws and forms, and these laws vary somewhat from state to state. Although the Patient Self-Determination Act, a federal law, became effective December 1991, most individuals have not completed the formal paperwork that is now asked upon admission to a health care facility.[95] The law requires hospital staff members to ask all persons admitted to a hospital with the capacity to understand the question if they have completed an advance directive; if they have not, they are asked if they would like to do so. If patients have their advance directive form, they are asked if the directives are still current and a copy of the form is placed in their medical record. If a person wants to complete advance directives after a hospital admission, representatives will assist the patient to do so. A patient may change his or her mind about specific requests in the directives at any time the person has the capacity to make changes.

Ethical decision making is discussed more fully in Chapter 2.

## Violence and Abuse

The United States is rapidly becoming a more violent society. Public health officials describe a virtual epidemic of youth violence in the past 5 years, spreading from the inner cities to the suburbs. For example, in 1993, on average, more than six young people were murdered every day in the United States, which resulted in more than 2200 violent deaths for the year.[33] Handgun violence is the second leading cause of death in the teen population in the United States. Death from handgun violence is the leading cause of death in men ages 18 to 45 years. Each year for the past several years approximately 50,000 people were murdered in the United States, and a woman is physically abused every 18 seconds. The incidence of rape also is increasing at an alarming rate. Almost all these victims of violence go to emergency centers for treatment and, typically, many of the victims of violence do not have any health insurance coverage.

## The Poor and The Homeless

A population at risk that has always been of concern to nurses is the poor. A new population that is of equal concern and that overlaps the poor population is the homeless. Most of the poor and homeless are women and children. There is a greater distance now than in the past between the "haves" and the "have nots" of our society. The number of persons able to pay for increasingly expensive health care insurance is decreasing. Among the 37 million Americans who do not have health care insurance are those who have lost their jobs, those who work at low-paying jobs or who can find only part-time work (without health care insurance), and those who may be unemployed for variable periods.

Many poor people are homeless, often as a result of job loss or discharge from a mental institution or from another custodial living arrangement without proper follow-up care. Nurses have been and continue to be concerned with these problems.[1] One result of such concern is a clinic established in Atlanta by three nurses, two of them nurse practitioners, for care of the homeless of that city.[76]

Nurses cannot escape being involved in any of the

issues just mentioned. However, many nurses need support in clarifying their own values, especially when they may differ from those of the persons for whom they are caring. Inservice education programs for nurses related to these topics are helpful. Knowledge about the details of pertinent laws is essential. Ability to use an ethical decision-making model and apply ethical principles in practice is also necessary. As mentioned earlier, a detailed discussion on ethical decision making can be found in Chapter 2.

### TECHNOLOGIC ADVANCES

Technologic advances have changed medical care in the United States in many significant ways. Technology has saved the lives of patients with conditions that only a few years ago would have proved fatal. Diagnostic advancements (1) in the laboratory with new diagnostic screens, (2) in medical imaging with expanded CT scans, MRIs, and ultrasonic equipment, and (3) in pharmaceuticals agents have contributed to the rapid growth in the health care industry. Perhaps the technology that has had the most dramatic impact on health care in the past few years is in the field of fiberoptic scoping, especially laparoscopic procedures for exploratory surgeries, cholecystectomies, and hysterectomies and orthoscopic procedures. This technology has significantly reduced the number of inpatient days and decreased the number of days lost from work. The expense of all these technologic advances has "driven up" health care costs dramatically. Increasingly, questions are being raised about how health care monies should be allocated.

Many of the questions have ethical implications and will require hard decisions. For example, will money be allocated to treat chronic illnesses such as end-stage renal disease? Will money be used to treat illnesses associated with life-styles such as tobacco and alcohol abuse? Will the United States decide on allocation of resources as has been done in Great Britain or Canada, where age is an important variable that determines eligibility for certain procedures?

Another issue related to technology includes the ability to prolong life. At present, billions of dollars are spent annually on neonatal intensive care units that keep extremely small, underdeveloped babies alive. If these babies survive, many have lifetime physical problems that require long-term medical care. At the other end of the life span, prolongation of life—especially for those persons who have not communicated their preference about continuing life by artificial means—continues to be a problem. Approximately 28% of Medicare dollars is spent on persons in their last year of life.

Other technologic advances such as joint replacements and organ transplantation are widely discussed issues related to health care. Both of these advances are costly. In addition, organ transplantation raises questions about who will receive an organ when the demand for organs always exceeds the supply. Although a law became effective in the late 1980s requiring hospital staff members to ask family members before a patient's death for appropriate organs and tissues for transplantation, the supply of organs remains significantly below the demand.

Will better informed consumers of health care continue to demand the latest in health care technology, despite cost? Evidence indicates that the demand for new technology will continue to increase. This demand, in turn, will continue to drive up medical costs. For this reason and others the federal government and other third-party payers have begun to exert controls to prevent further escalation of health care costs.

## COST OF HEALTH CARE

In 1992 the cost to the U.S. government of health care exceeded $830 billion, or about 14% of the gross national product (GNP).[50] By the year 2000, at the projected rate with no changes in the health care system, annual health care costs would be $1.6 trillion, or about 16.5% of the GNP.[79] If this projection becomes a reality, nearly one sixth of the total GNP will be spent on health care, as compared with one sixteenth of the total GNP in 1965. The growing concern about cost is coupled with a growing uneasiness that the United States has the most expensive health care system in the world but its population is not more healthy than people in other developed countries.

At present, those 65 years of age and older account for a third of the health care consumption in the United States. It is estimated that people older than 65 years of age comprise almost half of all hospital admissions. The average length of stay (LOS) for this age-group is 8.3 days, approximately 3 days more than for persons younger than 65 years of age.[27] As just mentioned, about one fourth of Medicare dollars is spent in the person's last year of life.[39] "Old-old" persons use more than 10 times the health care resources used by persons under 85 years of age, and more than 22% of these persons require institutionalization of some kind.

The nursing home population rose by 24% in the 1980s with most of the growth being from those in the old-old group.[56] In 1990 most of the 1.8 million people in nursing homes were women, outnumbering men by a ratio of almost 3 to 1. Also, the old-old population occupied 42% of all nursing home beds, an increase of 34% from 1980. Of persons 95 years of age and older, 47% are in nursing homes. About half the population in nursing homes suffer from dementia. It is estimated that by 2001, between 14 and 27 million older adults in the United States will need some type of nursing home care.

Long-term care costs are projected to triple from $42 billion to $120 billion between 1988 and 2018. Data indicate that millions of elderly persons are living at home, usually alone rather than with family members. As a result, they often require some type of assisted-living arrangements. The amount and type of assistance required range from Meals-on-Wheels for persons in their own homes, to apartments with special services for elders, to group living homes, to skilled caregivers or home aide assistance in the patient's home.

Many elderly persons could not survive without Social Security. The Social Security system (including Medicare and Medicaid) continues to be viewed by some legislators as consuming too much of the GNP, and these legislators are looking for ways to reduce benefits or to freeze increases. The Social Security Act of 1935 was amended in 1965 to include **Medicare** health care insurance for those 65 years of age and older and for the permanently disabled. The expanded legislation also established **Medicaid,** a state and federal cost-sharing program to provide medical services for those meeting certain eligibility criteria linked to income as determined by the individual states. Medicare reimbursement has been frozen or reduced several times, and the deductible cost (amount not reimbursed by Medicare) has increased almost yearly since the Medicare program began in 1965. Medicare has two parts: Part A and Part B.

For Part A of Medicare (which covers inpatient care and skilled nursing care) the individual currently is required to pay an annual deductible amount of $696 for each episode of illness. From days 61 to 90 of hospitalization, the patient pays $174 per day as coinsurance. Skilled nursing care coverage (for persons who medically qualify for it) extends for 20 days. If additional care is needed, the individual must pay $88 per day as coinsurance for days 21 to 100. Beyond 100 days of skilled nursing care the patient pays all costs.[43] Most persons carry coinsurance such as a medigap policy, which usually pays for all of the amount not paid by Medicare.

Part B of Medicare (which covers outpatient expenses, physician office fees, home health care, and other defined services) provides reimbursement of 80% of Medicare's schedule for cost after the individual pays an annual deductible amount of $100.[43] Coinsurance usually pays for the 20% not paid by Medicare.

The rates for Part A and Part B usually increase every year. Persons 65 years and older are urged to carry private health insurance, referred to as **medigap** insurance. Those who cannot afford to purchase medigap insurance may be able to receive Medicaid assistance. The financial implications of a growing society of elders, advances in health care technology, and a declining work force to finance the cost raise questions about how health care for elders will be financed in the future.

Another significant factor that has increased the cost of health care is the practice of "defensive medicine," in which providers order many expensive diagnostic tests and perhaps unnecessary medications to protect themselves from malpractice law suits. A recent American Medical Association (AMA) report shows that 8 of 10 physicians (80%) routinely practice defensive medicine.

## HEALTH CARE IN THE UNITED STATES

The tremendous diversity in this country is reflected in the beliefs, expectations, and sociocultural traditions related to health and health care. The words *health, wellness,* and *illness* mean different things to different people. On a health-illness continuum, a person's own concept often defines his or her state of wellness. The term *health,* as used in health care and health insurance, in reality usually means *illness* in our society.

### HISTORICAL PERSPECTIVE

Because social systems exist for the protection and well-being of their members, it would seem that planning for and providing health care would be of great importance. However, the Constitution of the United States makes no provision for the health care of its citizens. In the eighteenth century, health and illness were considered to be individual concerns and were taken care of within the family or community. For many years thereafter, waves of immigrants brought with them their own ways of maintaining health and coping with illness, much of which was outside of organized medical care.

Over time, government at several levels became involved in health care. In the early years the federal government established a hospital for merchant seamen, which became the nucleus of the United States Public Health Service. Individual states have been semiautonomous from the beginning of the nation, and they soon found it essential to establish rules and regulations to protect public health in such areas as safe drinking water and food and the threat of communicable diseases. Some cities, especially those on the eastern seaboard, established hospitals to care for homeless immigrants and others who became public charges because of communicable diseases or mental or other illnesses. For example, New York City developed a complex hospital system that was publically supported from its beginnings.

Today the Social Security Administration, which has overall responsibility for Medicare and Medicaid, is within the Department of Health and Human Services. The Department of Veterans Affairs, which operates one of the largest hospital and ambulatory care services in the world, became a cabinet-level agency in 1991. The legal responsibility for all of these services lies within the domain of the United States Congress.

Another factor in the evolution of health care in the United States is the philosophy of individual initiative and private enterprise. Except for those conditions that threaten the health of large segments of the population and thus come under the aegis of public health, the delivery of health care traditionally has been on a fee-for-service basis.

Every industrialized country in the world today, except the United States, has some kind of national health system that guarantees a basic level of care to all its citizens. In developing countries, the provision of basic health care is usually one of their early goals. National health systems begin with the premises that (1) there should be a minimum of health care services for all citizens, (2) whatever health care is available should be equally available to all, and (3) resources above the minimum should be distributed according to need—with any deviation permitted only if those worse off would be made better off.

## SYSTEMS APPROACH TO HEALTH CARE

In the United States a large aggregate of illness care systems, often poorly articulated with each other, continue to exist. There have been many attempts to establish some kind of an organized system, at least to the extent that everyone would be entitled to basic care. In 1965 Medicare, a form of health insurance for persons 65 years of age and older was established under Title XVIII of the Social Security Act. Medicaid, a health insurance plan for welfare recipients that is administered by individual states, was established under Title XIX of the same act. These entitlements still left large segments of the population without any assurance that they would receive essential care when ill or in need.

During the 1970s some form of national health insurance for U.S. citizens seemed inevitable, even though it was not determined how soon or how broad such a plan would be.[4,34] However, countervailing forces—most of them economic concerns of physicians, hospitals, and other providers—prevailed and no national plan was agreed on. During the 1970s and 1980s health care cost increased dramatically for a variety of reasons, including inflation, cost shifting of hospital expenses to private payers, and the introduction of more sophisticated technology. In 1971 comprehensive health insurance cost $9 per month for an individual and $25 per month for a family. In 1993 this same kind of coverage cost at least $150 per month for an individual and $425 per month for a family.[26] In response to these increased health care costs, some employers reduced health care benefits, others increased copayments for employees, and some canceled all health care benefits. At the same time, as new technology became available, everyone expected to benefit from it no matter what the cost.

By the early 1990s legislators and taxpayers acknowledged that not only are the health care systems in the United States out of control relative to cost, but approximately 37 million Americans have no health insurance and another 35 million are believed to be underinsured. The reality of these data can be seen in the number of persons who use emergency departments (the most expensive place to receive health care) as their only access to health care. A recent survey in four metropolitan areas in the United States indicates that one third to one half of all emergency room patients were seeking help for primary care needs.[59] Health-wellness data in the United States reveal that infant mortality is almost as bad as that of third-world countries, and many illnesses that previously were not problematic are now becoming public health crises.

Health care costs have escalated to the point that in 1993 health care accounted for about 14% of the GNP. The effects of inflation escalating the cost of health care have become a national concern as the annual inflation rate for the health care industry has been two to four times more than that of the national inflation rate.

## ILLNESS CARE

Most health care in the United States is really illness care provided by physicians in solo or group practices, operating on a fee-for-service basis. However, more and more physicians are being employed by hospitals, health maintenance organizations **(HMOs)**, private insurance companies, public health services (federal, state, and local), the Veterans Administration, and the military services. All physicians must be licensed by the state in which they practice, and they continue to be the "gatekeepers" for illness care in the existing health care systems.

Most hospitals in the United States were built during the first decades of the twentieth century when scientific medicine was developing rapidly and physicians and surgeons needed a workplace for their activities. Even the smallest communities believed they needed a hospital, and they worked hard to obtain one. Fund drives, private philanthropy, and taxes were used to build, maintain, and add to hospitals to meet community needs. The Hill-Burton Act of 1946 provided more than $3 billion of federal tax money to communities over a 25-year span to build or to improve hospitals throughout the country. As a result of this Act, great medical complexes were developed—sometimes more than one in a large city. Medical care became more and more concentrated in large cities while rural areas were underserved. Within these large medical complexes (often associated with schools of medicine), research and technology were producing the miracles of modern medical science.

In the 1960s and 1970s health care insurance began to assume more and more importance as health care costs, both in and out of hospitals, rose sharply. Initially, health insurance was purchased by employers for their employees or by individuals for themselves and their families. Then it was purchased by groups to share cost and spread liability.

Recently there has been a dramatic shift of more patient care activity to outpatient areas. Although hospital admission traditionally has been through the patient's personal physician, the number of hospital admissions from hospital emergency departments has increased dramatically. During the 1970s the appearance of alternative, nontraditional access to health care occurred, such as storefront clinics, shopping mall clinics, and mobile screening vans.[45,58]

## HEALTH CARE INSURANCE

During the past decade major changes have occurred in the health care insurance options for subscribers and employers. As the cost of health care benefits for employees began to escalate, employers sought ways to reduce these expenditures. Some asked their employees to share some of the costs and introduced the "80-20" plans, which required employees to pay 20% of the cost of their health insurance. Other employers contracted with health maintenance organizations (HMOs) or preferred provider organizations (PPOs) to provide health care services to their employees. By 1992 only 4% of workers in public or private settings with more than 200 employees selected a "traditional" type of health care insurance that used no form of precertification or managed care.[22] On the other hand, 43% of subscribers belonged to a traditional type of health care insurance that used precertification or other utilization controls. Of the remaining subscribers 23% belonged to HMOs, 21% belonged to PPOs, and 3% belonged to a point of service (POS) plan. In 1976 only 6 million people belonged to an HMO, whereas in 1992 more than 39 million people belonged to an HMO.[22]

## Prepaid Health Care Insurance

The traditional type of health care insurance, such as that offered by Blue Cross and other insurance companies, played a large role in the interplay of health and illness care in the United States. At one time prepaid health insurance represented a small segment of the insurance industry. Blue Cross first offered the prepaid health care insurance plan in 1929. Rapid growth in health insurance coverage, however, did not occur until after World War II. Originally, Blue Cross paid the hospital for all service charges, and Blue Shield paid physicians an agreed amount. With this type of coverage, the subscriber usually had to pay no additional cost and no questions were asked about the necessity for treatment or surgery. Although this type of coverage is still available, fewer people use it because of its higher premiums.

Health care insurance plans paid for all health care expenses submitted by hospitals with no questions asked. Health care insurance companies continued to raise their premiums to cover their expenses. Employers began to offset their health care expenses by increasing the share of the premium paid by employees. Eventually, some businesses could no longer afford health care coverage as a benefit for employees and dropped the benefit; thus employees were left with no coverage unless they paid for their own health insurance. Although traditional health insurance is still available, the number of subscribers has been declining as other options became more cost-efficient for the employer and employee.

## Prospective Payment System and Diagnosis-Related Groups

From 1965 to 1983 hospitals were paid for the full costs they incurred in caring for Medicare patients. Whatever the cost, Medicare paid the full hospital bill without question. In 1983 Medicare changed the reimbursement system for hospitals from a retrospective payment system to a **prospective payment system (PPS).** As part of the PPS, hospitals were notified how much they would be reimbursed for Medicare patients based on patient diagnoses. The diagnoses were grouped into diagnosis-related groups **(DRGs),** and a specific payment and length of stay (LOS) were predetermined for each DRG. If hospitals were able to provide treatment and care for patients for the specified reimbursement, they would break even financially. If hospitals were able to treat and discharge patients earlier than the predetermined LOS, they were paid the specified amount for the DRG and were able to make money that they could keep. However, if hospitals could not discharge patients within the specified LOS, they lost money because they were not reimbursed for the additional days of care. Originally there were 467 DRGs. Because some of the DRGs did not reflect the care needs of all patients in that group, additional DRGs were added. Currently there are 496 DRGs with specific reimbursement rates identified by Medicare.

The DRG and PPS arrangement has been in existence for about 10 years. In examining how successful hospitals have been in reducing costs, it becomes clear that some of them are becoming more and more competitive as they seek to attract the patient on whom they can make money (such as patients undergoing cardiac catheterization) and avoid admitting those patients on whom they will lose money. As hospitals learned how to operate within the DRG system, some hospitals would transfer patients on whom they would lose money to other hospitals under the pretext that the patient required more sophisticated care than they could provide. This practice is known as "dumping." Many such patients were transferred from community hospitals to teaching hospitals in large medical centers. Dumping became such a large problem that Congress enacted Public Law 99-272 to prevent this practice. This law, referred to as the "anti-dumping" law, is part of the Consolidated Omnibus Budget Reconciliation Act (COBRA) of 1986. This law mandates that heavy fines will be levied against an agency that violates the law.

Despite the changes made to control health care costs, it is evident that there is a health care crisis. As mentioned earlier, it is estimated that at least 37 million Americans have no health care insurance. Some are uninsured because of major layoffs, which terminated their health care coverage. Others have been dropped by their insurer because they have conditions that require large amounts of expensive care, such as that required by patients with malignancies, HIV and AIDS, or chronic conditions such as diabetes. These persons are then unable to obtain insurance from another carrier because of their preexisting conditions.

The need for health care reform has been identified by many Americans, and it was a major factor in determining the outcome of the 1992 presidential election. President Clinton has proposed a national plan that would provide health care insurance for all Americans. There are two major provisions of the plan. The first is that the insurance is to be portable and no one who is laid off or changes employment can lose this coverage. The second provision of the plan is that no one can be denied insurance because of a preexisting condition. To make insurance of patients who require large amounts of expensive care more equitable, all insurance carriers would be required to insure some of these patients so that the risk is spread among insurers.

As this chapter is being written, the health care plan has not been finalized, but several ideas are being considered as means by which health care cost can be contained. One of the options under discussion is *managed care,* which is discussed below.

## Managed Care Options

The managed care concept evolved out of need to control ever-escalating health care costs. Managed care, which has been evolving for many years, refers to a system of insured health care delivery that offers health care coverage but limits the enrollees' choice of providers and self-referrals. In return, employers and enrollees save money on premiums and copayments. In 1980, only 5% of employees enrolled in a managed care option, whereas by 1991, 55% of employees enrolled in a managed care option.[81]

Most health care insurance companies now offer managed care options along with traditional health care insurance plans. The focus of managed care is to provide **cost-effective, outcome-oriented care.** Through the use of existing patient outcome data, managed care promotes the identification of expected outcomes, time frames for accomplishing these outcomes, processes, and resources required to achieve the expected outcomes before the patient enters the health care system. Thus the provider and the enrollee know in advance the expected and reasonable outcomes. As with all types of managed care and with Medicare and Medicaid, criteria for patient admission, intensity of service, and severity of illness must be stated before approval for admission is granted. This process is referred to as **precertification approval.** An insurance company can negotiate with selected physicians and hospitals to provide health care to a large number of enrollees at reduced charges. This approach guarantees physicians and hospitals a volume of potential patients.

Today there are two major types of managed care plans: HMOs and PPOs.[60]

### Health maintenance organizations

The HMO philosophy is to promote wellness and prevent illness in the enrollees and to provide incentives to the health care provider to minimize the use of expensive inpatient care. Enrollees have access to all services but have a limited choice of physicians, self-referrals, and hospitals. Providers usually are paid on a per capita basis. Enrollees pay a set fee for regular preventive and screening services, as well as for illness care. Fees are prepaid, usually on a monthly or yearly basis similar to other insurance plans. Although HMOs have been in existence for more than 50 years, their rapid growth began only about 20 years ago. The HMO model has been adopted by many third-party insurers and by some private medical practice groups, many of which use nurse practitioners as providers.[25] HMOs fare best financially when enrollees are helped to stay well and kept out of the hospital. There are more than 500 HMOs across the country with approximately 39 million enrollees, which is about 15% of the total U.S. population.[22] The success and profitability associated with HMOs have led to the development of many more of these organizations. At present, Kaiser-Permanente's HMO (which is one of the oldest HMOs) has the largest number of enrollees in the United States. Continuous quality improvement (CQI) becomes an important issue in HMOs, because there may be a perceived or actual decrease in quality in favor of cost savings and profits.

### Preferred provider organizations

The rapid growth of **PPOs** is directly attributable to several factors. These include (1) the response of fee-for-service physicians to the competition from HMOs and (2) actions by third-party health insurance providers to offer PPO services at a reduced rate to their subscribers. In return, the contracted physicians and hospitals are guaranteed that a large number of patients will use their health care services. PPOs provide members with a greater range of choice in selecting "preferred" physicians, hospitals, and providers than do HMOs. Also, enrollees can use a provider or facility not on the preferred list by paying additional money for the services. This variation of a PPO is referred to as the **point-of-service (POS)** option. In this variation, members have the option of seeking care outside the plan at an additional fee.[22]

### Variations of HMOs and PPOs

Many hybrids and mixed models are emerging from HMOs and PPOs. Thus the names and initials are constantly evolving to reflect a new incentive or plan.

A variation of the HMO is the **independent practice association (IPA)** option. Within an IPA, physicians provide care out of their own offices instead of a central site.[22] Concerns with the IPA are that it may not be as efficient as an HMO and patient records may become decentralized rather than kept in one location.

## Managed Competition

*Managed competition* is a phrase commonly used today to describe what the probable national health care reform package will look like. Soon after President Clinton's inauguration in 1993, he began a process to revamp the health care system in the United States so that it addresses the problems identified with the current system, including bringing the national debt under control. Although the regional version of managed competition is not completely defined at this time, the organizing principles are directed at improving quality, managing costs, promoting competition among health care plans, and increasing cost-consciousness on the part of consumers. The underlying goals are to make health care cost effective and accessible to all.[17] In a limited way many large cities currently are practicing many of the principles of managed competition. The health care reform package probably will use price controls, cost sharing, more family and nurse practitioners, and so on to achieve the goals. The so-called universal coverage may resemble the health care reform systems developed in Canada, Minnesota, Hawaii, and Florida or may result in some combination of these.[85] It is well-known that health care costs can be reduced by focusing on promotion of health and prevention of illness.[23]

## HEALTH CARE DELIVERY SYSTEMS

All hospitals or health care delivery systems can be classified into one of two types of ownerships: private and government. On the private side, ownership can be grouped into not-for-profit and for-profit organizations. On the government side, ownership can be grouped into federal, state, or local.

### Not-For-Profit and For-Profit Hospitals

The two categories of private hospitals are *not-for-profit* and *for-profit.* All hospitals or health care delivery systems seek to make a profit, that is, an excess of income over expenses. It is how the profits are used that differentiates the two types. Not-for-profit hospitals use profits to enhance the content or quality of health services or to control costs. In the United States, more hospitals are not-for-profit than are for-profit.

The goal of for-profit hospitals is to make a profit that is paid to owners/investors. Most often these are large corporations that own several hospitals in a region or across the country. Recently, Galen Health Care, Inc., previously known as Humana Hospital Corporation, was purchased by Columbia Hospital Corporation to become Columbia Health Care, Inc., the largest for-profit chain of hospitals in this country. Although some for-profit hospitals have existed for a long time, they have proliferated in recent years and have become an important segment of the competitive scene in the health care industry. Typically they have concentrated on providing medical and surgical services to those patients who are able to finance their own care, either because they are well insured or because they are financially able to pay for their care. Generally these corporations provide minimal or no care to the medically indigent. They have attracted well-qualified physicians by providing them with the latest technology and equipment, office space attached to their hospitals, an office support system at a reasonable cost, joint ventures, and so on. They also have the resources to build modern, up-to-date hospitals with amenities that are aimed at attracting the paying consumer. Because of their ability to buy supplies and equipment in volume and because of their centralized accounting and billing services, these corporations have been able to control costs and provide a profit for their investors. It appears that they will continue to proliferate and prosper, often at the expense of those hospitals that provide care to all segments of society, regardless of the patients' ability to pay for their care.

### Vertical and Horizontal Integration

Hospitals continue to grow larger and more complex each year. To remain competitive they have had to review their methods of offering services. During the past 10 to 15 years two major changes have occurred in how hospitals organize their delivery of services: vertical and horizontal integration.

**Vertical integration** of the delivery of care within one hospital involves providing "full-service" delivery of care, including all inpatient care services, skilled nursing care, outpatient care, long-term care, and home health care services. **Horizontal integration** involves the consolidation of several hospitals into multihospital complexes, which allows for sharing of technology, facilities, and expertise, resulting in economies of scale and increased influence in the health care market.

### Ambulatory Care and Home Health Care Services/Long-Term Care

The areas of health care delivery that have experienced the most rapid growth (as a result of DRGs, managed care plans, and other cost control measures) are ambulatory care and home health care services.[27] (See Chapter 27 for a detailed discussion of home health care of the ill adult.)

Until the early decades of this century and before the great boom in hospital construction and use, nearly all illness care was managed in the physician's office or in the patient's home. People were born and died at home. Several agencies for the care of ill people at home developed from the early days of this nation. Many visiting nurse associations (VNAs) were founded to offer help to persons who were ill at home. Many tax-supported public health agencies also provided some care for the ill in their homes, although their first mission was controlling and preventing communicable disease and protecting the health of the public. The term **community health agency** is an overall designation, with the added **home health agency** used to indicate that many expanded services—such as physical therapy and homemaker care—also are available. Many of these agencies began or expanded their services because Medicare paid for the delivery of certain kinds of home health care to the homebound.

The original focus of most public health agencies was the care of infants and children and their mothers. In the early years of our nation most people did not live to be as old as persons do today and those who did usually were cared for by their own families. However, as mentioned earlier, people are living longer and the care of the elderly population has become a national concern as more and more people are living into the eighth and ninth decades of life. Although fewer than 5% of those persons older than 65 years are now institutionalized, it is clear that health problems increase as one ages and that elders need a larger share of the health care resources. As mentioned, the number of "old-old," those 85 years and older, is now the fastest growing age-group in the United States; in other words, the elderly group is itself aging. Initiation of DRGs provided Medicare recipients with increased home health care coverage, and thus, almost immediately, home health care emerged as a giant industry. The growing Medicare population, the number of Medicare recipients with chronic health problems, and advances in technology that permit the home use of ventilators, dialysis, and intravenous therapy are the major reasons for this boom.[74] In 1979 Medicare spent about $592 million for home health care services, and by 1991 the cost had increased to $1.6 billion.[13] There are now about 10,000 home health agencies in the United States.

Hospice care is a rapidly growing segment of home health care. From its beginnings in a small, homelike institutional setting, it has developed, especially in the United States, almost entirely into a home care service. Most communities in the United States have some services that make it possible for persons with a terminal illness who have fewer than 6 months to live to remain in their own homes. Much planning is necessary for this to occur, and nursing is the logical professional group to coordinate and provide hospice care. Enormous patient and family satisfaction is reported by those who have been through the hospice experience.[29] In addition, hospice care has helped to control costs by reducing occupancy of expensive hospital beds.

Ambulatory care or outpatient care is the fastest growing method of providing health care, whereas inpatient utilization in community hospitals continues to decrease. Total outpatient visits to community hospitals increased by 6.1% in 1992 while total admissions to community hospitals decreased by 1.1%.[27] The increase in outpatient growth represents all areas, including surgery, diagnostic procedures, and nonsurgical treatments. These trends are anticipated to continue, especially as more tests and procedures are available in the outpatient department and more health insurance plans will reimburse for tests and procedures performed only on an outpatient basis.

# NURSING IN THE UNITED STATES

## HISTORICAL PERSPECTIVE

Professional nursing in the United States is about 100 years old, and it has assumed an indispensable role in every aspect of health care delivery. It is the largest professional group involved in health care. Nurses are employed in acute and chronic care hospitals, long-term care facilities, home health care services, HMOs, and health care insurance companies. The greatest number of professional nurses continue to work in acute care facilities.

## NURSING CARE DELIVERY SYSTEMS

After World War II the hospital and health care industry began its tremendous growth as more and more patients entered hospitals for care. As nursing services in hospitals matured, different types of nursing care delivery systems were developed.

The objectives of nursing care delivery systems include assessing the patient, identifying patient needs, providing the necessary nursing care, and evaluating the effectiveness of the nursing care. The patient care goals are short, usually extending only through hospitalization, and are based on nursing diagnosis. From the 1940s to the 1990s some remarkable trends, evolutions, and repackaging of nursing care delivery systems have occurred. There have been many attempts to find the ideal way of providing nursing care to groups of persons designated as ill or in need of care. It is likely that all of these models of nursing care delivery systems are used in one form or another, even coexisting within the same organization.

### Total Patient Care

Before World War II *total patient care* was the usual type of nursing care delivery system. Registered nurses worked almost exclusively in hospitals, and RNs and nursing students gave complete care to patients. At present, total patient care is the typical nursing care delivery system used in intensive care units (ICUs). This seems appropriate because intensive care patients are critically ill, have an unstable health status, and thus require the expertise and knowledge provided by RNs.

### Team or Functional Nursing

During World War II many women volunteered to work in hospitals under the sponsorship of the Red Cross. These women were known as "gray ladies" because of their gray uniforms. Many of these volunteers were socially prominent women who had the time to volunteer as their part of the war effort. Because of the nursing shortage, they were taught basic tasks, such as bathing patients, making beds, and transferring and repositioning patients. After the war, when these women left hospitals, aides were trained on the job to do these tasks, inasmuch as the gray ladies had demonstrated that lay persons could be taught to do these tasks. At this point there was no secretarial help on the nursing unit and RNs were responsible for transcribing orders and charting on all patients.

As the nursing shortage continued, team nursing was introduced as a method to deliver patient care and to make the best use of the limited number of RNs. In team nursing, RNs served as team leaders. They were responsible for assessing all the patients on their team and deciding which ones needed their professional expertise and which ones could be assigned to nursing aides, nursing students, or in some hospitals, practical nurses. The team leader was responsible for developing a nursing care plan for each patient assigned to his or her team.

The nursing care plan was written to provide guidance to non-RN caregivers. The RN administered all medications and treatments for these patients. She or he also gave direct patient care to patients who were judged to have the most complex needs—not always in terms of physical care but often those with the greatest emotional, teaching, and rehabilitation needs. The team held daily nursing conferences to discuss the needs of individual patients. All persons involved with a particular patient attended the conference, reviewed the nursing care plan, and evaluated the care given. New data supplied by direct caregivers were used by the RN team leader to revise the patient's plan of care. A characteristic of functional nursing that differentiates this model from team nursing is the practice of having specific patient care tasks completed on some or all patients by different direct caregivers.

In reality, team nursing usually did not work as conceptualized. The main problems were fragmented care for patients, the lack of time needed by the team leader for effective team planning, and the difficulty of team leaders finding time to supervise and coordinate the care provided by their team members. Although team or functional nursing continued for many years and even to the present, both models generally are considered by health care providers and by patients to be unsatisfactory because of the fragmentary nature of care.

## Primary Nursing

In the late 1970s and in the 1980s primary nursing evolved as the method to best care for the increased number of acutely ill patients in hospitals. Primary nursing must be distinguished from primary care, which is discussed later. In the **primary nursing** model, a professional nurse is completely responsible for assessing, planning, implementing, and evaluating the nursing care given to a relatively small number of patients during their total hospitalization. The essence of primary nursing is to establish a therapeutic relationship between the nurse and the patient to help the patient achieve his or her goals. The primary nurse assumes 24-hour responsibility for all aspects of the patient's care, from admission to discharge on that unit. The designated primary care nurse cares for the same patient throughout the stay on the unit and is accountable for the outcomes of care that result from nursing interventions.

To those who were active in nursing before World War II this does not appear to be a new method but a coming to full circle. The model was demonstrated early at the Loeb Center for Nursing and Rehabilitation in New York City, where for many years nurses had been providing care through the primary nursing model.[11] Many agencies have since moved to primary nursing because studies indicate that it is more satisfying both to patients and to nurses and it is more cost effective than team nursing. It also makes the RNs accountable for the care the patient receives, and this is most important with the emphasis on quality assurance. In the nursing care delivery systems previously mentioned, accountability is hard to determine and sometimes it appears as if "everyone who cares for the patient is equally accountable; thus no one is really accountable." Manthey et al. define primary nursing as a way of organizing work and staff members in a common-sense system based on professional principles.[41] Studies have clearly demonstrated that in addition to the satisfaction of patients and nurses, physicians and other health care providers also are more satisfied with primary nursing, because it is clear with whom they should communicate their questions and suggestions about the patient.

Primary nursing has markedly changed the role of the head nurse, who in the past in some institutions was the only person who gave and received all communications regarding patients. With the complexity of patient care today, especially in larger hospitals and medical centers, it is clearly impossible for one person, the head nurse, to know all that is necessary to know about 30 or more patients.

Although many positive aspects about primary nursing make it a desirable model as a nursing care delivery system, several problems emerge. Ideally, only RNs should be primary nurses and associate nurses. The fiscal restraints on nursing services today make it almost impossible to employ a sufficient number of RNs to be primary and associate nurses. In addition, the supply of RNs in some areas of the country is not adequate to meet the demand. Thus many hospitals have substituted LPNs for RNs as primary nurses or associate nurses. In some facilities, primary nursing is delivered during the day shift when RNs function as the primary nurse, and another type of nursing care delivery system is employed on the other shifts. With these alterations, the objectives of primary nursing are soon lost.

The second problem encountered with the primary nursing model is the impact of 12-hour shifts and the increasing number of RNs who work part-time. Twelve-hour shifts are popular because they allow nurses the flexibility of full-time status by working 3 days a week, with 4 days off to meet personal and family needs. The reality of a primary nurse working 3 days a week means, at best, that the RN will care for a patient only 3 of the 5 days of an average length of stay. The same problem exists when RNs work part-time because these nurses are available only during a part of the average hospital stay. Thus it is impossible for a nurse who works only 1 to 3 days per week to be responsible for patients 24 hours a day, from admission to discharge.

## Case Management Care

**Case management care** is the process of identifying, coordinating, and monitoring the implementation of services needed to achieve desired patient care outcomes within a specified period.[93,96] Managed care health insurance plans are effective in controlling the cost of health care because of their ability to regulate the amount and type of health care provided and to control its cost. Contracted physicians agree on the reimbursement rate for such services as office visits, hospital visits, and surgeries. Contracted hospitals agree on cost-per-day rates for hospital stays, for cost of inpatient and outpatient tests, and so on. Multiple mandatory preapproval processes are involved for many medical interventions, such as for most diagnostic procedures, for second opinions before surgeries, for admission to hospitals, and for many therapeutic interventions. Most of these controlling activities occur before a patient is admitted to a hospital. After the patient is admitted, managed care plans expect physicians and hospital services to provide quality care that is effective and efficient. If physicians and hospitals maintain this expectation, their contracts most likely will be renewed. If physicians and hospital services do not provide quality care that is effective and efficient, it is more than likely that their contracts will not be renewed. Many hospitals have established case management programs to ensure that effective, efficient, and high-quality care is given throughout the patient's hospitalization. The essence of achieving case management goals lies within the nursing case management delivery system. Managed care and case management have the capacity to improve patient care by using nurses throughout the health care delivery system.[18]

### Nursing case management

Nursing case management is the latest nursing care delivery system, and it is rapidly gaining in popularity. This system complements the expectations of managed care programs: cost efficiency, effective interventions, and assured quality.[37,92,93,95,96] On a unit level, nursing case management is a patient care delivery system that combines some of the best qualities from the previously mentioned delivery systems. Nursing case management acknowledges fiscal limitations with staffing dollars and utilizes all levels of nursing positions. Nurse case managers who are RNs are the key team members. They coordinate, communicate, collaborate, and facilitate all the care given to their case load of patients.

**Nursing case management** organizes patient care by case type or major diagnosis and focuses on achievement of predetermined outcomes within specific time frames and resources. The major components of nursing case management are (1) collaboration of care with *all* health care team members, (2) integration of anticipated patient outcomes with time frames to evaluate clinical practice (use of *critical pathways*), (3) utilization of principles of continuous quality improvement (CQI) and variance analysis, and (4) promotion of professional practice.[46] Many nurses, physicians, patients, and hospital administrators have been highly satisfied with this new delivery system.

Nursing case management is based on predetermined practice patterns for specified types of patients. The results of care tend to reduce the length of stay for patients, reduce unnecessary diagnostic procedures, and ensure continuous quality of care to patients. These predetermined practice patterns are put into written form in a tool generically referred to as a **critical pathway** (several chapters in Part II of this book give examples of critical pathways). Critical pathways are developed by the appropriate members of the health care team, including physicians, in a collaborative manner for groups of patients with a specified medical condition. Priority for the development of critical pathways is given to patients with medical diagnoses that represent a high volume of admissions, patients with medical conditions that frequently result in complications and increased lengths of stay, and patients with conditions that cause the hospital to lose money.[94]

Nurse case managers (NCMs) are the key to the success of this nursing care delivery system.[15,20,51,80,84] It is highly recommended that NCMs be clinical nurse specialists or master's-prepared nurses who can function as collaborators, problem solvers, communicators, facilitators, and enhancers of patient care.[67,80,84] The NCM is usually responsible for a case load of 10 to 15 patients from admission to discharge as they move from unit to unit throughout the hospital. NCMs work 8-hour shifts and collaborate with all health team members, including physicians, to ensure that practice patterns reflect the predetermined interventions agreed on in the critical pathways. The activities of NCMs, the implementation of the system, and the follow-up of any variances from the critical pathways are coordinated by a case management coordinator (CMC). The NCM has a team that includes RNs, LPNs, and NAs to provide direct care to patients. The NCM reviews the critical pathway and the patient's response to interventions, with the nurse providing care to ensure that all desired outcomes are achieved on time and, if not, to determine what is preventing them from being achieved. The NCM also solves any system, provider, or patient problems that are hindering the achievement of the desired patient outcomes stated in the critical pathway. If the problem is a patient problem—for example, development of a complication such as a cerebrovascular accident (CVA)—the NCM documents the problem and in a collaborative manner modifies the critical pathway to match the patient status. Any problems affecting the achievement of the goals of the critical pathway (system, provider, or patient) are handled as **variances,** and these variances are followed up with total quality management/continuous quality improvement (TQM/CQI) activities through the case management committee, which is led by the case management coordinator. Although NCMs are the key to the success of the nursing case management program, the visible support and the involvement of the chief executive officer (CEO), the chief nurse executive (CNE), the chief financial officer (CFO), and the chief of staff (COS) are paramount to the overall success of the case management program (Figure 1-1).

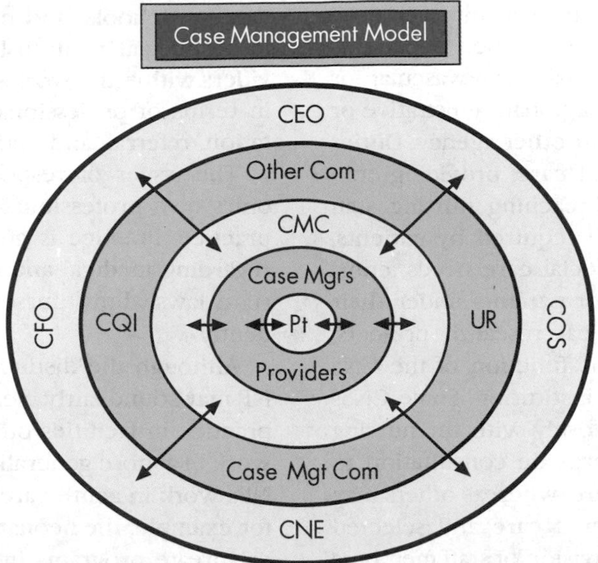


**FIGURE 1-1** Case management model demonstrating the central role of patient *(Pt).* The key role of nurse case managers *(Case Mgrs)* and care providers *(Providers)* is emphasized by the central placement of these persons and the arrows showing the continuous interaction. Nurse case managers assist, when necessary, with the coordination, facilitation, and problem solving of the day-to-day interventions. The need for support by committees and other persons/offices is demonstrated by the outside rings. The arrows demonstrate that the case management coordinator *(CMC)* is the person responsible for integrating all activities, analyzing patient outcome variances, and identifying system, provider, and patient problems. The chief executive officer *(CEO),* chief of staff *(COS),* chief nurse executive *(CNE),* and chief financial officer *(CFO)* provide the essential visible and ongoing support. The CMC interacts with various committees: continuous quality improvement *(CQI)* committee; case management committee *(Case Mgt Com),* which is chaired by the CMC; utilization review *(UR)* committee; and other committees *(Other Com)* as needed. Providers include physicians, nurses, pharmacists, dietitians, respiratory therapists, social service workers, and others. (Case management model developed by Helen A. Schaag.)

## ADVANCED PRACTICE NURSES

The four categories of advanced practice nurses (APNs) are the clinical nurse specialist (CNS), the nurse practitioner (NP), the certified nurse midwife (CNM), and the certified registered nurse anesthetist (CRNA).[46] Advanced practice nurses involved in the nursing care of medical-surgical patients are the NP and CNS. A discussion of these two roles follows.

In the late 1980s and 1990s changes in the federal laws governing reimbursement of health care providers in federally operated programs enabled advanced practice nurses to be directly reimbursed for their services.[46] Direct reimbursement for APNs is still limited to these federally operated programs. Significant barriers to their practice remain, however, in the areas of legal scope of practice, reimbursement, and prescriptive authority.[46,53] Direct reimbursement gives APNs, as primary care providers, recognition, credibility, and visibility. It is estimated that somewhere between $6.4 billion and $8.75 billion could be saved in the United States annually if APNs were used to their fullest potential as primary health care providers.[63] It is believed to be only a question of time before third-party payment for health care services provided by APNs becomes widely accepted, because research data indicate positive public acceptance, quality care, and cost effectiveness of their practice.[25,36,60]

**Primary health care** is a term used to describe the kind of care needed by most of the people most of the time. It generally denotes the patient's first contact with the health care system. It may be preventive, including identification of health problems at an early stage, or it may be the care of minor, noncritical, and chronic illnesses. Results of a recent study revealed that within their areas of competence, certified nurse midwives provide a quality of care that is equivalent to the quality of care provided by physicians. Patients were more satisfied with the care provided by NPs than the care provided by physicians relative to the amount of information conveyed, the reduction of professional mystique, and the cost of care.

### Clinical Nurse Specialists

The **clinical nurse specialist (CNS)** is a registered nurse who has completed a master's degree program in a clinical specialty—usually with a specified population of patients, such as medical-surgical, maternity, geriatric, or psychiatric patients, or with a population of patients with specific problems, such as renal, cardiovascular, or diabetic. Typically, the CNS is in a nonadministrative or a staff position within a hospital or other agency. Duties may include giving direct patient care, providing consultation to nursing personnel, teaching nursing staff members about the special care required by patients, teaching patients about their special care needs, coordinating nursing care services for patients under their jurisdiction, implementing clinical research projects, and acting as change agents. The function of the CNS varies and is determined by the institution. Some CNSs are unit-based and work most closely with the nursing staff on a specific unit; others provide consultation to several units. Some give direct care, whereas others may provide a combination of selected care and selected consultation, teaching, and supervision of staff members who are giving direct care. Some CNSs assume administrative or line positions and are in charge of a unit such as intensive care. When this transition occurs, the CNS usually assumes a title that reflects the administrative position.

Although some hospitals and other agencies employ nurses who are called clinical nurse specialist regardless of their educational background, the American Nurses Association (ANA) standards for CNS state that the title of *clinical nurse specialist* is limited to nurses with a Master of Science degree in nursing.[5] Further, a nurse must hold this degree to be eligible to sit for the CNS certification examination.

### Nurse Practitioners

The title of **nurse practitioner (NP)** was first used in 1965 when pediatric nurse practitioners were prepared to work in rural areas of Colorado to provide primary health care to children in areas seriously underserved by physicians. Although in the past NPs have been educated in a variety of ways—from very short certificate-awarding programs to master's degree programs—the trend now is toward the latter, because of the broad background of knowledge needed by the practitioner. There are different clinical specialty areas for NPs. The most common ones are pediatric NP, women's health NP, family NP, adult NP, and gerontology NP.[47] Nurse practitioners typically work in primary care settings, providing direct care to prevent illnesses and to treat noncritical, nonacute, minor, or stable chronic illnesses. NPs often manage the medical treatment of patients, using protocols established with physician colleagues.

Until recently, mainly because of the fee-for-service problem, it was more common to find the nurse practitioner in a group practice with physicians and other professional health care providers. This is changing, and many NPs are practicing alone or in groups with other NPs.[25,46,63,69] Many are employed by HMOs, mental health centers, schools, and nursing homes. Their practice is in a collegial relationship with other health care providers within the work setting: the NP is a team member in terms of professional expertise in practice, consultation, referral, and planning.

The issues of responsibility and accountability for one's own professional actions are vital in this type of practice. Practice is governed by individual state laws regarding medical and nursing practice, although most state laws allow nurses to practice *nursing* independently.

Although the distinctions between the CNS and the NP may sound fairly clear, it is not always so. Many CNSs practice in facilities other than acute care settings and work in a more generalist role. On the other hand, many NPs work in acute care settings with a specialty group, for example, the neonatal NP. Because graduates of baccalaureate programs in nursing are prepared to obtain health histories and to perform routine physical assessment and many of them are obtaining master's degrees, combining the NP and CNS roles may become easier. Some authorities believe that there will be a merging of the two titles (NP and CNS) over time.[14,28,82]

## NATIONAL CERTIFICATION

Many nursing specialty organizations offer certification examinations for nurses practicing in their specialty. Each of these organizations sets its own criteria; many require a certain level of education to sit for the certification examination in a particular area. In many instances the educational requirement is becoming stricter. This is particularly true for nurse practitioner certification and for all certification examinations administered by the ANA. At present the ANA has 23 areas in which a nurse can receive national certification, including certification examinations for clinical nurse specialists.[8] Some certifying organizations such as the American Association of Critical-Care Nurses (AACN) do not require a master's degree but candidates must meet other criteria. It is predicted that in the future the increasing sophistication of nursing and health care will demand higher educational preparation of nurses sitting for any certification examination.

# CHALLENGES TO NURSES AND NURSING

Factors to be considered by nurses and the nursing profession in this changing health care environment are the ways in which nurses can have the greatest impact on the health care delivery system. Nurses will have to be risk takers in identifying areas where nursing input can affect the health care delivery system. This includes entrepreneurship and incorporation by groups of nurses to provide a variety of services in a wide variety of settings.

## COLLABORATION BETWEEN NURSES AND PHYSICIANS

The relationship between nurses and physicians has a significant impact on patient care outcomes.[2,21,58,72] This relationship is receiving more and more attention as health care organizations look at systems and models to deliver effective and efficient quality care. Health care organizations are realizing that the relationship between nurses and physicians significantly affects the provision of effective and efficient care.

The most desirable relationship between nurses and physicians is a collaborative relationship. **Collaboration** is defined as a relationship of interdependence; the ability to work together collaboratively involves trust and respect not only of each other but of the work and perspectives each contributes to the care of patients.[21,64] Collaborative relationships between nurses and physicians improve patient outcomes and, in many situations, reduce patient costs.[44,75] Collaboration is essential to effectively evaluate patient care outcomes, analyze variances in outcomes, and modify necessary practice patterns. This results in improved quality of patient care.

## COLLABORATION BETWEEN NURSING PRACTICE AND NURSING EDUCATION

The many changes in the health care delivery system and pressures on educational institutions are forcing the issue of increased collaboration between education and practice.[57] There has been some movement toward such collaboration for at least 25 years, but today's pressures are causing both nursing service directors and nurse educators to examine the issue even more seriously.

There are several good reasons for this, some of which are that (1) both groups of nurses have the patient as their focus, (2) nursing education requires a practice laboratory for students, and (3) health care agencies must rely on nursing schools to produce practitioners to work in their agencies. Also, nurses engaged in practice may not have the preparation or time to carry out their own nursing research, but they can work closely with nursing faculty engaged in research to identify phenomena encountered in practice that should be systematically studied.

An increasing number of nurses are receiving PhD degrees in nursing. This is accelerating the amount of research in areas germane to nursing practice. In this regard the National League for Nursing (NLN) recommended in 1993 that the emphasis for nursing research shift to an increase in the number of studies concerned with health promotion and disease prevention at the group and community levels.[55] The findings of nursing research will form a knowledge base for the science of nursing. Nursing scholars are examining the results of this research, identifying theories, and organizing the knowledge derived from research. These results will be incorporated into nursing education and practice as nursing moves toward the future. At present, nurses are examining the use of conceptual frameworks for nursing practice and will be expected to use a conceptual framework to guide their practice. Classification systems and nursing diagnoses will be used to help describe the nursing care delivered to patients. This will be essential if the impact of nursing care on a patient's recovery is to be delineated and documented.

As Naisbitt[49] pointed out, the increase in "high tech" demands a concomitant increase in "high touch." There is no setting in which this is more evident than in intensive care units, where some nurses have asked whether they are nursing patients or machines.

## ISSUES IN NURSING EDUCATION

### Nursing Schools in the Twenty-First Century

All the changes discussed will affect nursing education now and in the future. In 1993 the National League for Nursing (NLN)[54] and the American Association of Colleges of Nursing (AACN)[3] issued proposals for preparing nurses for the twenty-first century. Both proposals reflect recommendations made in *Nursing Agenda for Health Care Reform,*[6] published by the ANA, and in the surgeon general's report, *Healthy People 2000.*[89]

With increasing emphasis on health promotion and prevention of illness, the focus of nursing education needs to change from the hospital to the community. This does not mean that students will have no experience in acute care but that they will have increased experience in community-based, community-focused health care settings. Several schools of nursing have developed community nursing centers, and others are moving to do so. These "nurse-managed care agencies" provide cost-effective, easily accessible, quality primary care with focus on disease prevention and "wellness" care. By the end of 1993, more than 66 nursing schools had established community nursing centers[52] (Figure 1-2). These centers serve as practice sites where students learn from advanced practice preceptors how to function in a community-based, community-focused health care system. It is estimated that 250 centers are needed to meet the diverse requirements of individual organizations and communities.[52] Other possible community practice sites are patients' homes, schools, workplaces, ambulatory settings, long-term care facilities, shelters for the homeless, and other places in the community where persons gather. The sites used will reflect the community in which they are based and ideally will offer experiences with culturally diverse populations. Because many university faculties are not prepared to function in the community, the preceptors for students often will be advanced practice nurses (APNs) holding master's degrees in nursing.

Other skills that students will need to develop are critical thinking, collaboration, shared decision making, a socioepidemiologic viewpoint, and ability to analyze

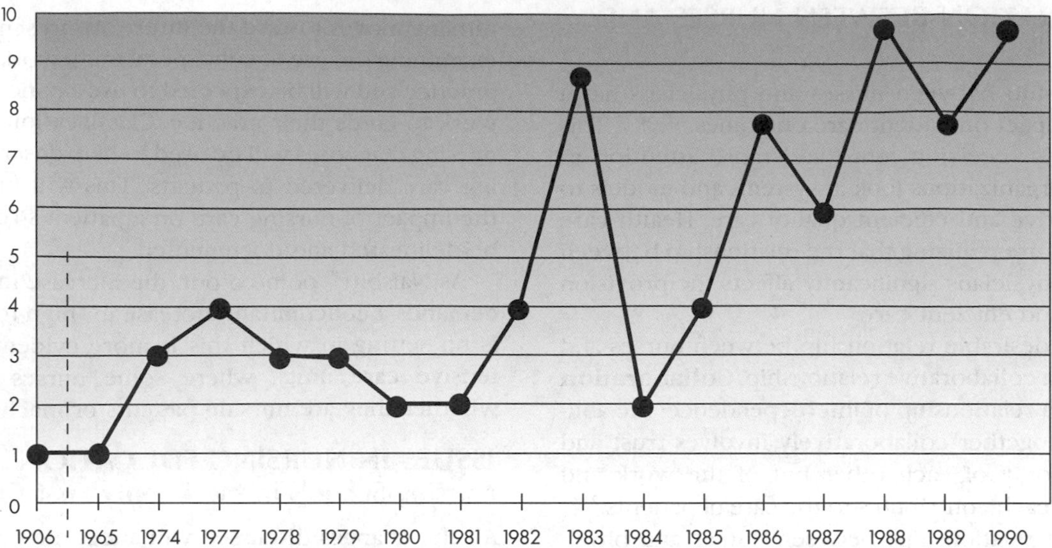


**FIGURE 1-2** The recent increase in the number of nursing centers founded per year, based on the NLN/Metropolitan Life sample. (From National League for Nursing: *PRISM—the NLN Research and Policy Quarterly* 1(1):1, 1993.)

the effectiveness of interventions in terms of outcomes for individuals, groups, and the community.

To be prepared to function in a new health care delivery system, nurses with baccalaureate degrees desiring to serve as APNs will require advanced degrees.[78]

Because of changes in how information is processed, it can be expected that all nursing students will be computer literate. Much of the basic information that nurses need to know will be transmitted by computer-assisted instruction (CAI) and less by textbooks, lectures, and so on. Currently, many nursing programs use CAI materials and new materials continue to be developed. In addition, several researchers are studying how nurses make clinical decisions.[10,62] This knowledge will help nursing students to acquire the vast amount of knowledge they must master to use in their practice. There is no doubt that all nursing programs will need to address the question of how nurses can assist those they serve to *attain, maintain,* or *regain* the highest level of health possible. Although nursing students will gain experience working with patients of all ages in a variety of settings, emphasis needs to be placed on the health care of the rapidly increasing number of elderly persons and on what nurses can do to assist them.

In addition, there is a movement within the profession to move preparation of nursing to the postbaccalaureate level.[70] Case Western Reserve University established the first doctorate of nursing (ND) program in 1979,[40] the second program was instituted at Rush University in 1989, and a third program was founded at the University of Colorado in 1990. In addition, several other schools are now considering instituting ND degrees. Continued interest in promoting ND programs was evidenced by a conference on ND education sponsored by the University of Colorado in the spring of 1994. At present many universities (Yale, Pace) offer a generic master's degree.

## The ND Degree

The basis for the ND degree is the belief that preservice preparation for nursing should be built on a strong undergraduate base as is true in other professions such as medicine, dentistry, pharmacy, or law.[73] In this respect, the establishment of the ND degree is an evolutionary process similar to that which has occurred in comparable professions.

For example, a remarkable increase in the last 20 years has occurred in the number of programs leading to the PharmD degree. Although some universities continue to offer both the bachelor's degree and the doctorate in pharmacy, others have phased out their undergraduate program.

The following reasons support the prediction that the number of ND programs will increase by the end of this century:

1. The recognition that current nursing education is too vocational and narrow as it tries to encompass both liberal and professional education in one program[70]
2. The move to have nursing recognized as an autonomous health profession
3. The need to prepare nurses who will be able to function at a higher level and compete for positions in a much more competitive health care system
4. The need to provide nurses with more parity with other health professionals, especially physicians; symbols such as degrees and titles of address (Dr.) are becoming even more important in today's society

**BOX 1-1 Factors Influencing Choice of Nursing as a Profession**

1. Status and image of nursing
2. Remuneration when compared with other professions
3. Autonomy
4. Opportunities for practice
5. The recognition that persons making a midlife career change to nursing who already hold a baccalaureate or a postbaccalaureate degree in other fields need a degree different from the BSN, which would give them a second baccalaureate degree

## Characteristics of Nursing Students

The population of nursing students is more heterogeneous today than it was 25 years ago and this will continue. Thus the need to recruit more culturally diverse students and faculty is ongoing. It can be hoped that an increasing number of men will be attracted to nursing, as well as women and men who are selecting nursing as a midlife career change. Future students will be more concerned with what the nursing profession has to offer them. Some of the factors that will determine whether potential students will be interested in nursing as a profession are listed in Box 1-1.

## Nursing Supply and Demand

### Staff nurses

Although some experts believe that a nursing shortage persists, (ranging from 8% to 12%), in some areas of the country new graduates are having difficulty finding jobs in acute care hospitals. The decrease in hospital nursing positions is the result of several factors. First, the decreased length of stay (LOS) of hospitalized patients has reduced the demand for acute care beds. Second, the number of acute care hospitals throughout the country continues to decrease. Third, the number of acute care beds in hospitals continues to be reduced as hospitals "downsize" their operations. Most troubling to nursing, however, is the substitution of less well–prepared workers for RNs.[9] In some institutions whose nursing staff comprised almost 100% RNs, the new goal is a 60% RN and 40% LPN/NA mix.

The rationale for this change is the need to reduce hospital costs, which is achieved primarily by reducing salary costs. Among the troubling issues related to this trend is the threat to quality of care. If RNs are to monitor and supervise staff members who are not registered nurses, they will spend more time in nonpatient care activities and less time providing direct care to patients. In addition, shorter LOSs and more intensely ill patients in hospitals will make it more difficult for fewer RNs to effectively assess, analyze, coordinate, and collaborate in care for more patients during shorter LOSs and yet maintain quality of care. To maintain quality of care the entire organization must be committed to total quality management (TQM) and support an effective continuous quality improvement (CQI) program. As organizations consider changing the RN staffing mix, an objective means to measure quality of patient care is imperative.

With the shift of health care from hospitals to the community, some experts predict that acute care hospitals will soon consist only of intensive care beds. At present, experienced critical care nurses are in demand, and this demand can be expected to continue because less well–prepared workers are not able to function effectively in these units.

### Nurses with additional preparation

By the year 2005 the shortage of nurses is estimated to be 600,000: 400,000 at the baccalaureate level and 200,000 at the master's and doctorate levels.[78] The need for more nurse gerontologists is obvious in view of the growing number of elders. At present, at least 50% of all adult patients in acute care facilities are 65 years of age or older. Further, the intensity of nursing care required in acute care facilities continues to increase as length of stay decreases. Nurses must be able to think critically and solve a diversity of problems. Nurses in long-term facilities must provide not only "high touch" care but also "high-tech" care and have the appropriate knowledge base to direct and manage the complex health care needs of their patients.

There also is a need for additional *advanced practice nurses* (APNs). This need is based on the fact that the United States does not have enough primary care providers. It is estimated that about 250,000 primary care providers will be needed to manage the goals of the health care reform plan. At this time there are only 55,000 to 60,000 primary care physicians in the United States, and the medical profession can add only an additional 2400 primary care physicians a year. At this rate it would take about 100 years to reach the goal for primary care physicians. At present more than 100,000 APNs are already providing primary care as NPs, CNMs, CRNAs, and CNSs. An additional 400,000 RNs either are delivering primary care or could be trained to do so in 18 months or less.[47] Thus the nursing profession is at a pivotal point in assuming a major role as primary health care providers throughout the total health care reform plan.[48]

It is crucial that nursing education be equipped to prepare more nurses to function as nurse practitioners. Failure to do so will open the door to other groups such as physician assistants, who will be happy to assume the role of primary care providers if nurses do not meet this need.

In the fall of 1993, several nursing programs began offering special courses in primary nursing care for nurses already holding the MSN degree. These programs are two to four semesters in length depending on the background of the individual student. In addition, most nursing programs are reorienting their master's programs to include more emphasis on primary care and preparation of the graduates to function as nurse practitioners.

The nursing profession needs to continue supporting the evolution of differentiated nursing practice.[35] Differentiated practice legitimizes and rewards the expert who is practicing nursing at an advanced level of competency and responsibility. The nurse with an Associate Degree in Nursing (ADN) should function in roles that provide patients with physiologic care and comfort. The nurse with a Bachelor of Science in Nursing (BSN) degree should plan the care, provide patient education, and evaluate the effectiveness of interventions in terms of patient outcomes. Advanced education at the Master of Science in Nursing (MSN) and doctoral levels is highly specialized and prepares nurses for a variety of increasingly complex roles, responsibilities, and broadened career choices. Education at the advanced level incorporates the primary components of theory, special clinical practice, consultation experiences, education principles and research expertise. The expectation is that nurses with the master's degree and those with doctorates have the ability not only to apply these theories and principles in their practice but to refine and generate new theories and principles.[24]

## EVALUATION OF THE OUTCOMES OF PATIENT CARE

### HEALTH CARE REGULATORS

The individual states, as part of their powers (the power to protect the health, safety, and welfare of the public), have enacted legislation to license certain types of health care facilities such as hospitals, nursing homes, and ambulatory care centers. It is essential for health care facilities to be licensed by federal, state, and/or local authorities. However, states cannot regulate the activities of federal health facilities within their state because of a stipulation in the Constitution that separates these two levels of government. On the federal level the Health Care Financing Administration (HCFA), a component of the Department of Health and Human Services (HHS), is responsible for administering Medicare and Medicaid programs. The need for safe quality care resulted in the development of review organizations and accreditation agencies.

### PROFESSIONAL REVIEW ORGANIZATION

Since the Medicare program began in 1965, the federal government has made several efforts to ensure appropriate use of Medicare funds and to contain costs while maintaining quality. In 1972 Congress created the Professional Standards Review Organization (PSRO), a program designed to review the medical necessity of services provided to Medicare patients. This program proved to be unsuccessful. Subsequently, a state-level agency, the **Professional Review Organization (PRO),** was created by the Social Security Act Amendments of 1983. It is responsible for monitoring quality assurance and cost containment. The purpose of the PRO, like its predecessors, is to determine whether hospitals will receive payment for care given to Medicare patients. PRO staff members randomly select medical records of patients receiving Medicare to determine whether they meet certain criteria (Box 1-2). If the PRO review panel finds that the criteria were not met, the hospital is informed in writing of the discrepancies. If the hospital is unable to provide an acceptable explanation for the discrepancies or cannot supply data acceptable to the panel, the PRO will either deny payment for all or part of the hospital days and/or levy penalty points against the hospital. If a hospital accumulates a specified number of points in a defined period of time, the percentage of Medicare records reviewed at random is increased. If similar discrepancies are found at the next review, additional punitive measures are levied against the hospital.

**BOX 1-2 Questions Addressed in a PRO Review**

1. Did the patient meet predetermined parameters for hospital admission?
2. Was the patient medically ready for discharge?
3. Was the care delivered to the patient appropriate?
4. Did the care delivered meet professionally accepted standards of quality?

In 1990 the Institute of Medicine completed a congressionally mandated study that recommended a new approach for ensuring quality of care, referred to as the *health care quality improvement initiative* (HCQII). Under this plan, Medicare's PRO is *committed to quality improvement* with a focus on *improving patient care outcomes* and *creating a cooperative,* rather than confrontational, *exchange among the HCQII reviewer, hospitals, and physicians.* The new format devotes fewer resources to case-level review, using instead statistical analyses of the overall patterns of outcomes. If standards of care are not met the PRO will continue to deny payment for care.

#### Accreditation

Without a doubt, no other voluntary organization has had as much impact on the health care industry as has the Joint Commission on Accreditation of Healthcare Organizations **(JCAHO),** formerly known as the Joint Commission on Accreditation of Hospitals (JCAH). In 1918 the American College of Surgeons (ACS) established a standardization program to improve the hospital-based practice of medicine. In 1952 JCAH was formed.

The American Osteopathic Hospital Association has

a similar national accrediting process for osteopathic hospitals. Its review organization is the American Osteopathic Association (AOA).

The importance of JCAH or AOA accreditation took on special significance with the passage of the Medicare Act in 1965. Congress mandated that hospitals would have to be accredited by either JCAH or AOA to receive Medicare reimbursement. Although seeking JCAH or AOA accreditation was voluntary and not the same as licensure or certification by the state or local authorities, the congressional action made it appear that it was mandatory. In the late 1980s, the Joint Commission's name change reflected the total spectrum of health care organizations accredited by them. Accreditation has come to be recognized as a benchmark of quality and is used by some regulatory agencies as one criterion for licensure or certification and by some insurance agencies as a condition for honoring reimbursement claims. Acknowledging the importance of accreditation by the Joint Commission, many AOA-accredited hospitals also are accredited by the Joint Commission.

In 1987 the Joint Commission initiated its *Agenda for Change,* which refocused its standards for accreditation toward patient outcomes instead of how care is given to patients. Since 1987 the Joint Commission has been collecting patient care data from several hundred of its accredited hospitals around the country. The data will be used to establish baseline parameters for outcomes of care for a variety of patient care areas, such as infection control, obstetrics, anesthesia, cardiovascular care, home infusion therapy, medication use, and so on. Some consider the development of the Joint Commission's **indicator monitoring system** the most significant quality assessment tool within the Agenda for Change era.

By 1994 any hospital accredited by the Joint Commission could voluntarily submit its outcomes of patient care within specified care areas to the commission. By 1996 participation in the indicator monitoring system will be mandatory for accreditation. The expectation is that the requested data will be submitted on a quarterly basis. A hospital will then receive information on how its outcomes of patient care compare with those of other hospitals in its region and to all hospitals in the nation. Thus hospitals will receive continuous feedback on their performance. When a hospital has negative outcome indicators, a dialogue between the Joint Commission and the hospital will address the problems, clarifying them and, if necessary, outlining the process to correct the problems. Another change in the commission's standards is the transition from a quality assurance (QA) system to a continuous quality improvement (CQI) system. The change of focus from reviewing the process of care to reviewing the outcomes of care complements the Agenda for Change model.

In 1993, for the first time in the Joint Commission's history, a registered nurse was appointed to the board of directors for a 3-year term.[86]

**BOX 1-3 ANA's Standards of Clinical Nursing Practice**

| | |
|---|---|
| **Standard I.** | ***Assessment:*** The nurse collects client health data. |
| **Standard II.** | ***Diagnosis:*** The nurse analyzes the assessment data in determining diagnosis. |
| **Standard III.** | ***Outcome identification:*** The nurse identifies expected outcomes individualized to the client. |
| **Standard IV.** | ***Planning:*** The nurse develops a plan of care that prescribes interventions to attain expected outcomes. |
| **Standard V.** | ***Implementation:*** The nurse implements the interventions identified in the plan of care. |
| **Standard VI.** | ***Evaluation:*** The nurse evaluates the client's progress toward attainment of outcomes. |

From American Nurses Association: *Standards of clinical nursing practice,* Washington, DC, 1991, The Association.

Accreditation by either organization—the Joint Commission or AOA—is required today by all health care facilities that seek certification in care for Medicare and Medicaid patients.

## Professional Standards

In 1991 the ANA released a revised *Standards of Clinical Nursing Practice* for the purpose of ensuring the public of quality nursing care (Box 1-3).[7] The primary responsibility for implementing these standards, however, rests with the individual nurse, who bears the responsibility for ensuring that these criteria are met in his or her own practice setting. To fulfill this responsibility, professional nurses must be familiar with both the generic (general) and the specific standards pertinent to the care of the patient population for which the nurse is responsible. These standards identify the elements of nursing care that must be met to ensure quality care. They also provide a baseline for measuring that quality.

Three other sets of professional standards also must be considered: nurse practice acts, medical practice acts, and the standards set by the JCAHO. At present, all states have nurse practice and medical practice acts; both constitute sources on which to base standards for nursing practice. Taken together they define and delineate the content and scope of practice of medicine and nursing from a legal standpoint.

**Nurse practice acts** define nursing practice and identify those activities that fall within the province of nursing. **Medical practice acts** further delineate nursing practice by outlining those areas that constitute the exclusive province of the physician. Such exclusions restrict the activities in which nurses may engage. Neither act sets actual standards for practice; rather the acts designate general areas of activity for both professions, and they establish the legal relationship of the nurse to society and to other health care professions.

The Joint Commission is a highly influential external

**BOX 1-4 The Joint Commission's Standards for Quality Assessment and Improvement**

1. The organization's leaders set expectations, develop plans, and implement procedures to assess and improve the quality of the organization's governance, management, clinical, and support processes.
2. The organization has a written plan for assessing and improving quality that describes the objectives, organization, scope, and mechanisms for overseeing the effectiveness of monitoring, evaluation, and improvement activities.
3. There is a planned, systematic, and ongoing process for monitoring, evaluating, and improving the quality of care and of key governance, managerial, and support activities.
4. The administration and coordination of the hospital's approach to assessing and improving quality are designed to assure that activities described are undertaken.

From Joint Commission on Accreditation of Healthcare Organizations. In *Accreditation manual for hospitals,* Chicago, 1993, The Commission.

source of nursing standards. In 1976 the Joint Commission added a section on quality of professional services to its *Accreditation Manual for Hospitals,* which is revised yearly. The standard delineates the characteristics of patient care evaluation programs. It includes an effective review and evaluation of the quality and appropriateness of patient care. In 1993 the Commission added a section to the manual designated "Quality Assessment and Improvement" (Box 1-4), which prescribes standards based on the following principles[30]:

1. Leadership's role
2. Focus on processes to improve patient outcomes
3. Customer focus
4. Continuous improvement
5. Hospital-wide involvement
6. Statistical measurements of processes and outcomes
7. Emphasis on prevention

Consequently, the hospital's major goal should be to help each employee improve the processes in which he or she is involved—at the same time fulfilling its responsibility to address serious problems involving deficits in knowledge or skill of staff members.

## TRANSITION FROM QUALITY ASSURANCE TO TOTAL QUALITY MANAGEMENT/ CONTINUOUS QUALITY IMPROVEMENT

**Quality assurance (QA)** is defined as a *process that involves evaluating the degree of excellence of the observable and measurable characteristics of delivered nursing care.* Quality assurance can be described on two levels. In its strictest sense it is described as a set of techniques for assuring the maintenance and improvement of standards and the efficiency and effectiveness of nursing care. More broadly, it is an effort to control nursing practice. As such, it involves relationships between nurses and consumers and between nurses and governmental bodies.

**TABLE 1-1 Comparisons Between Quality Assurance and Total Quality Management/Continuous Quality Improvement**

| QA | TQM/CQI |
|---|---|
| **FOCUS** | |
| Problem | Patient |
| Provider/employee | System |
| Single issue | Multiple issues |
| Solve problem | Improve process/outcome |
| Management control | Provider/employee control |
| Inspection driven | Process driven |
| **TIMING** | |
| Retrospective | Prospective |
| Reactive | Proactive |
| Episodic based on problems | Continuous goal to maintain quality |
| **INVOLVEMENT** | |
| Limited staff involved | Many staff involved |
| Top-down directed | Bottom-up directed |
| External-to-problem | Internal-to-problem |
| **QUALITY** | |
| Not assured when problem solved | Integrated in process |

Developed by Helen A. Schaag.

For many reasons the transition in health care motivated hospital administrators, providers, and insurance companies to focus on outcomes of patient care as the way to measure quality. The Joint Commission, too, changed its focus for measuring quality. The primary focus had been on reviewing the process of care, such as staff members' consistency in using appropriate policies and procedures for providing care. Thus the QA program of many hospitals focused on how will certain standards for care were met. The Joint Commission's Agenda for Change requires a continuous quality improvement program that focuses on patient outcomes, that is, why patient outcomes were not achieved. Thus **total quality management/continuous quality improvement (TQM/CQI)** is a commitment by the organization to provide quality care to achieve expected and predetermined patient outcomes (see Table 1-1 for a comparison of QA and TQM/CQI).

An example that will help differentiate the two systems is a review of patient falls. The QA approach would examine "why" the patient fell, and the manager would focus on altering the causes for these patient falls. The cause might be inadequate supervision of patients by staff, poor lighting (especially at night), beds not lowered to their lowest position, or patients' mobility problems. The TQM/CQI focus is on "why" the patient fell and allowing the staff members, multidisciplinary when necessary, caring for patients to determine how they will reduce patient falls. TQM/CQI focuses on the system and all issues involved with falls, such as staff-patient ratio, environment, types of patients, situations preceding the fall, and the ways to avoid or reduce the frequency of these falls. TQM/CQI looks at falls and other problems in general and not at one situation. TQM/CQI is carried out by all staff members and is not management-directed. TQM/CQI builds in checks to assess whether problems are solved. QA activity, on the other hand, usually focused only on the employee or employees involved with the problem and the manager would work to change the deficient behavior or procedures; other staff members were not involved in analyzing and resolving the probem. Naturally, the interaction between the manager and the staff member causing the problem occurred some time after the incident. Although the responsible person might not cause this problem again, there was no assurance that falls would not recur. As it evolves, TQM/CQI seems to be a less threatening and more effective problem-solving approach than QA.

QA activity was used during the 1970s and 1980s and achieved the goals it was designed to meet. It served a valuable function in that it was the first organized system to review and document patient care problems.

Three major concerns prompted the health care industry to make the transition from QA to TQM/CQI: (1) the Joint Commission's new requirements to adopt some form of CQI activity (see preceding details), (2) the demand by health insurance programs and employers paying high premiums to ensure quality coverage for the money being spent, and (3) consumer demand for improved quality of health care. Consumerism was the spark that began the patients' rights movement in hospitals, acknowledging the right of patients to participate in their care and to make their own health care decisions. This movement has resulted in an increased knowledge base that has made consumers better informed about the business of health care and about treatment and diagnostic options. More knowledgeable consumers have become more confident in asking physicians about the care they are receiving or would like to have. In addition, data banks that contain information on the performance of physicians and hospitals are beginning to be released to the public—for example, data comparing hospitals in geographic areas as to the number of deaths from open heart surgery, providing the name of the cardiac surgeon, the number of patient deaths in general by hospital, the costs for specific diagnostic tests, the number of cesarean sections performed, and so on. These data are used by some businesses to determine which hospitals and physicians will be covered in their health insurance plans.

An important reason to adopt the TQM/CQI system is that it is estimated that 94% of all errors made in the hospital are because of "system" problems versus provider or employee problems.[19] The main focus of TQM/CQI is on patient outcomes and the systems that support attaining these outcomes.

## Definition of TQM/CQI

After World War II, a then unknown engineer named W. Edwards Deming was unsuccessful in his attempts to introduce to the leaders of this country's largest industries a new method for ensuring quality control. Businesses and industries were booming and no one in the United States was interested. At the same time Japan was struggling with its postwar problems, including the worldwide perception that Japanese products were of inferior quality. The Japanese believed they could not compete with American-made products. Deming accepted an invitation to help Japanese business leaders improve the quality of their products. Today "everyone" in the United States is studying and adopting Deming's management model,[19,42,90] and it has been recognized as the single most important factor responsible for transforming large American companies into global competitors. It is estimated that at least 80% of all manufacturing companies in the United States incorporate some form of quality improvement in their businesses.[71]

*Total quality management (TQM)* is the philosophy of an organization, it is customer driven, and the focus is on every aspect of an organization.[31,32] TQM, which uses the scientific method, continuously strives to exceed customer expectations.

Continuous quality improvement (CQI) complements the philosophy of TQM. The focus of CQI is on the need for an organization such as a hospital to continually seek opportunities to enhance the quality of its services by use of statistical analyses of these services. The overall expectations are that both quality and efficiency of care will be enhanced with the adoption of TQM and CQI because they force the organization to systematically examine its practices.

To be successful in using TQM and CQI, organizations must undergo a shift in the way they think about quality improvement. The mind set of "If it ain't broken, don't fix it" must be changed to "If it ain't broken, that's the best time to make it better."[38] TQM provides a mechanism for organizations to be proactive; that is, its ongoing review of all systems prevents crises from developing. With CQI, quality meets or exceeds the patient's or customer's needs. Figure 1-3 is a CQI flow chart that focuses on the prevention of patient falls.

### Total quality management

Many TQM models have been described in the literature. Deming's management model[19] consists of 14 points that guide the process (Box 1-5).

### Continuous quality improvement

The goal of CQI is to identify variations in patient care outcome and to reduce or eliminate as many specific variations as possible. The case management process

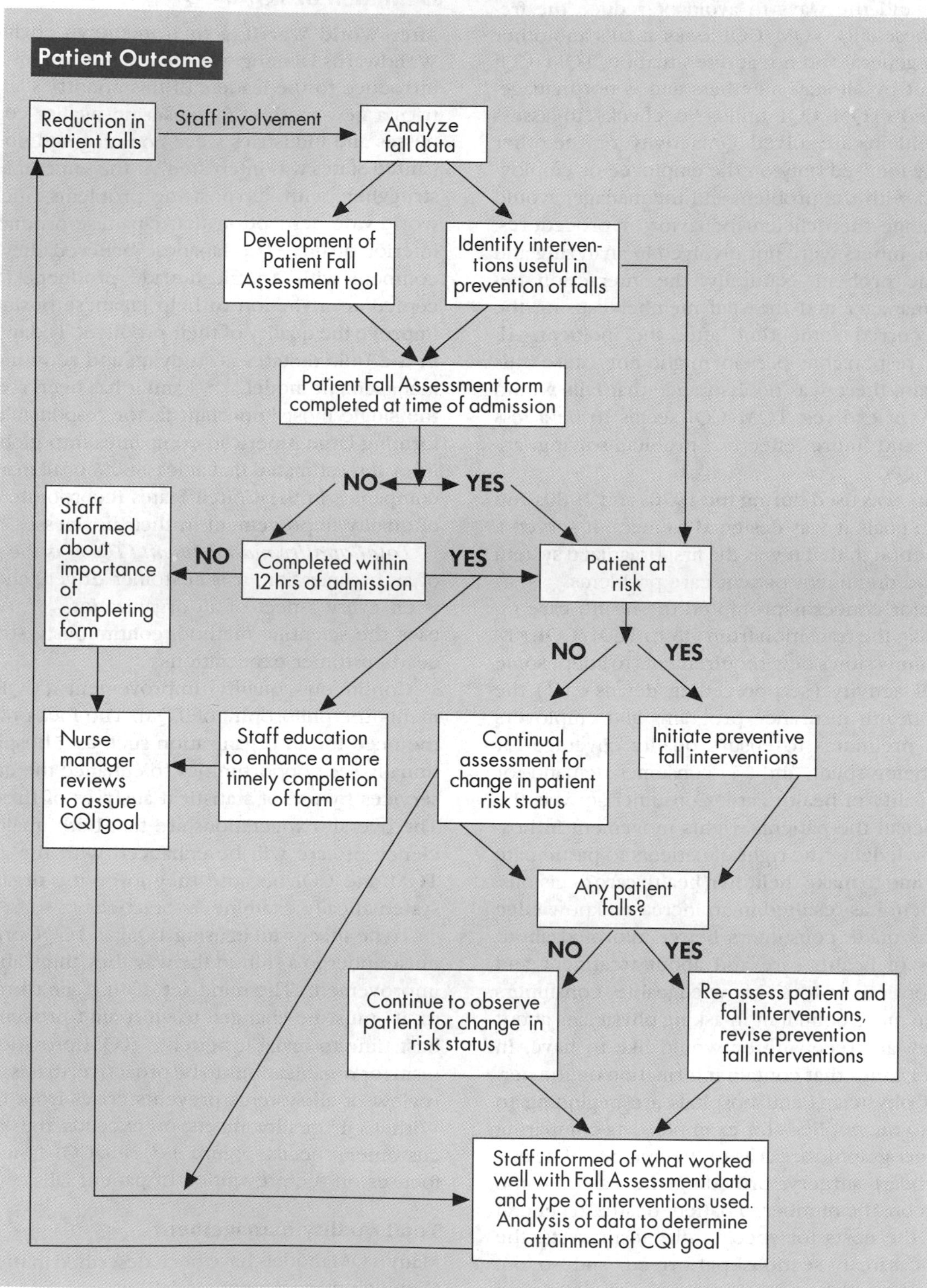


**FIGURE 1-3** Flow chart for continuous quality improvement (CQI) focused on reduction of patient falls. Note that CQI starts with a goal. Also note the continual reassessment and "grass roots" level of nursing staff involvement. (Developed by Helen A. Schaag.)

**BOX 1-5 Deming's 14 Points to Improved Quality of Care (Revised 10 January 1990)**

1. Create and publish to all employees a statement of the aims and purposes of the company or other organization. The management must demonstrate constantly their commitment to this statement.
2. Learn the new philosophy, top management and everybody.
3. Understand the purpose of inspection, for improvement of processes and reduction of cost.
4. End the practice of awarding business on the basis of price tag alone.
5. Improve constantly and forever the system of production and service.
6. Institute training.
7. Teach and institute leadership.
8. Drive out fear. Create trust. Create a climate for innovation.
9. Optimize toward the aims and purposes of the company the efforts of teams, groups, staff areas.
10. Eliminate exhortations for the work force.

11a. Eliminate numerical quotas for production. Instead, learn and institute methods for improvement.

11b. Eliminate Management by Objective. Instead, learn the capabilities of processes, and how to improve them.

12. Remove barriers that rob people of pride of workmanship.
13. Encourage education and self-improvement for everyone.
14. Take action to accomplish the transformation.



uses critical pathways to identify **variances** in patient care outcomes. The health care professionals on the case management committee differentiate between random, nonspecific variations and nonrandom, specific variations. There needs to be ongoing documentation of the continuous improvement activities used to correct the nonrandom, specific variations.

The Shewhart cycle is a TQM technique used to test innovations.[19] The process is referred to as the *P-D-C-A cycle,* an ongoing interaction using four steps: *P,* plan what to do; *D,* do it; *C,* check effect of action; and *A,* act. It is a helpful tool to keep the focus on outcomes and on the process. That is, it initiates actions that had positive results or revises actions that had unwanted results, and then the P-D-C-A cycle activity is resumed.

## UTILIZATION REVIEW

The utilization review (UR) program for hospitals was first mandated by JCAH in 1978. It has as its primary goal the appropriate allocation of a hospital's resources and patient length of stay (LOS). In most acute care facilities the activities of UR have merged with the case management program's activities.

## INFECTION CONTROL

All employees who have direct contact with patients are involved in programs to monitor and control infection rates. An infection control report provides monthly data on the number and types of nosocomial infections on a given hospital unit. Questions can then be raised about procedures or practices used not only by nursing personnel but also by physicians, respiratory therapists, phlebotomists, and so on. Variances from patient care outcomes (identified through critical pathways) that deal with nosocomial infections are analyzed and appropriate CQI activity initiated. (See Chapter 15 for more information about infection control.)

## RISK MANAGEMENT

The focus of risk management (RM) is on decreasing the probability of incurring an adverse outcome and thus reducing the organization's exposure to risk in the form of litigation. The goals of RM, which closely parallel the goals of CQI, focus on increasing the probability of achieving desired (patient care) outcomes. Although exposure to litigation will never be totally eliminated, everyone in the organization has a role in identifying and reporting risk incidence and in designing CQI activities to reduce or eliminate risks that could result in the hospital or physicians being sued.

## CONFIDENTIALITY

Confidentiality of all data is an issue usually associated with risk management. The availability and use of evaluative data about a patient or groups of patients have always been of concern to health professionals. The increasing use of computerized data has generated enormous concern for the potential threats to the privacy of sensitive information. Most quality review activities and case management analysis can be conducted without recording patients' names and are reported in terms of aggregate data. Review of care provided to a particular patient requires constant vigilance to ensure the protection of the patient's identity, as well as protection of the identity of the health care team members. Confidentiality of employee data is another sensitive issue that needs to be protected. Maintaining confidentiality should be a constant goal of everyone in health care.

# FUTURE CONCERNS

Changes in the delivery of health care and how monies are allocated undoubtedly will receive the attention of most persons in the United States over the next few years. Increasingly the public is expressing concern that the quality of health care may take second place to the cost of that care. Properly designed and executed TQM programs and CQI activities are vital feedback mechanisms that can help assure the "customers" of health care—patients, health care insurance plans, physicians, nurses, and others—that an acceptable quality of health care is maintained.

## QUESTIONS TO CONSIDER

- What are the reasons for the increased utilization of alternative health care facilities?
- What are the responsibilities associated with attaining the status of advanced nurse practitioner?
- Why is differentiated practice necessary?
- What are the major differences between the goals of quality assurance (QA) and the goals of continuous quality improvement (CQI)?
- How could the variances identified by the continuous quality improvement process be used in research?

## CRITICAL THINKING ACTIVITIES

- What are the major values and dilemmas that have led to the current health care crisis?
- How do you believe money should be allocated for health in the United States?

## CHAPTER SUMMARY

### CHANGES IN AMERICAN SOCIETY

- American society is aging, and the greatest increase is in persons older than 85 years of age, called the "old-old."
- Questions are being raised about the ability of a proportionately smaller working population to support Social Security for elders.
- Technologic advances have dramatically changed medical care and driven up costs.
- Ethical problems arise in the use of technological advances such as organ transplantation and life-sustaining interventions.

### COST OF HEALTH CARE

- There has been no decision in the United States concerning how health care reform is to be financed.

### HEALTH CARE IN THE UNITED STATES

- The United States is the only industrial society that does not have some form of national health insurance.
- The many changes in health care insurance coverage include the health maintenance organization (HMO) and the preferred provider organization (PPO). Clinical nurse specialist and nurse practitioner are types of advanced practice positions in nursing.
- Patients are being discharged sooner from the hospital as the result of DRGs and other cost-containment measures, resulting in an increased need for ambulatory care, home care services, and skilled nursing units.

### NURSING IN THE UNITED STATES

- Several methods have been used to deliver nursing care in the hospital, including team, total, and primary nursing, and case management.
- Primary nursing, which clearly defines accountability for the care of each primary patient to the assigned primary nurse, requires a greater proportion of RNs.
- Alternate health care settings such as hospice care are rapidly growing in the United States.
- Health promotion is becoming a major focus of nursing care, with individuals expected to assume more responsibility for their own health.
- A major concern to nurses is that the United States is rapidly moving toward a two-tier health care system—one for the "haves" and another for the "have nots."

### CHALLENGES TO NURSES AND NURSING

- Collaboration, viewed as a positive move, is increasing between nursing practice and nursing education.
- The increase in "high tech" in hospitals demands an increase in "high touch." Nurses are being challenged to provide high touch to patients who are attached to highly complex equipment.
- The demand for nurses continues to increase even though more nurses are employed now than ever before.
- Nursing schools are changing to reflect the changes in society, for example, the need for all students to be computer literate.
- Some nursing schools are advancing the preparation of nurses to the postbaccalaureate level, which is what other professions (such as pharmacy) are choosing to do.
- More attention should be paid to factors that influence the choice of nursing as a profession.
- Nursing's commitment to professional excellence includes monitoring the quality of care given.
- Four factors that have influenced quality of practice in nursing are (1) health care legislation, (2) changes in third-party reimbursement, (3) economic factors, and (4) professional standards.
- The ANA's *Standards of Clinical Nursing Practice* includes six standards to be followed by all nurses who provide nursing care.

### EVALUATION OF THE OUTCOMES OF PATIENT CARE

- The Joint Commission on the Accreditation of Healthcare Organizations is a voluntary organization that accredits hospitals and other health care organizations. It publishes an annual accreditation manual that includes a standard for quality of professional services. This standard provides the basis for evaluating patient care.

- The Joint Commission has replaced quality assessment (QA) with continuous quality improvement (CQI) as the system to ensure that quality of care is continuously improved by focusing on patient care outcomes.
- The main goals of CQI are to improve patient care by focusing on patient care outcome variances and by reducing or eliminating specific, nonrandom variances.
- Case management is a patient care delivery system that organizes patient care by specific case types and that focuses on achievement of outcomes within specific time frames and resources.
- The main goals of case management are to increase quality of care, nurse/patient/family satisfaction, and collaborative care and to decrease length of stay and use of resources.
- Critical pathways are patient outcome–focused tools that require a collaborative approach of a multidisciplinary team to identify usual interventions for high-volume or high-risk patient diagnostic groups. The tool is designed to provide specific interventions on specific time frames throughout the hospital stay.

## REFERENCES


1. Aiken L: *Am Nurse* 17(4):18, 1985 (editorial).
2. Alpert HB et al: 7 Gryzmish: toward an understanding of collaboration, *Nurs Clin North Am* 27(1):47-59, 1992.
3. American Association of Colleges of Nursing: *Position statement: nursing education's agenda for the 21st century,* Washington, DC, 1993, The Association.
4. American Nurses Association: *A national policy for health care: principles and positions,* Washington, DC, 1977, The Association.
5. American Nurses Association: *The role of the clinical nurse specialist,* Washington, DC, 1986, The Association.
6. American Nurses Association: *Nursing's agenda for health care reform,* Washington, DC, 1991, The Association.
7. American Nurses Association: *Standards of clinical nursing practice,* Washington, DC, 1991, The Association.
8. American Nurses Credentialing Center: *Am Nurse,* p 29, July-Aug 1993.
9. Anderson CA: From the editor: making the invisible visible, *Nurs Outlook* 41(6):246-247, 1993.
10. Benner P: *From novice to expert,* Menlo Park, Calif, 1984, Addison-Wesley.
11. Bower-Ferres S: Loeb center and its philosophy of nursing, *Am J Nurs* 75:810-815, 1975.
12. Cejka S: The changing healthcare workforce: a call for managing diversity, *Healthc Exec,* pp 20-23, Mar-Apr 1993.
13. Champlin L: Home healthcare: word to the wise for the 21st century providers, *Kansas City Health Care Times* 2(2):9, 1993.
14. Cook S: Breaking with tradition, *Academic Nurs,* pp 19-21, summer 1993.
15. Cronin CJ, Maklebust J: Case-management care: capitalizing on the CNS, *Nurs Manage* 40(3):38-47, 1989.
16. Crosby PB: *Quality is free: the art of making quality certain,* New York, 1979, McGraw-Hill.
17. Curtin L: Health reform: the shape of things to come, *Nurs Manage* 24(4):28-32, 1993.
18. delBueno DL: Paradigm shifts—what's good and not so good for health care, *Nurs Health Car* 14:100-101, 1993.
19. Deming WE: *Out of crisis,* Cambridge, Mass, 1986, Center for Advanced Engineering Study, Massachusetts Institute of Technology.
20. Dunstron J: How managed care can work for you, *Nursing 90* 20(10):56-59, 1990.
21. Fagin CM: Collaboration between nurses and physicians: no longer a choice, *Nurs Health Care* 13:354-363, 1992.
22. Friedman E: Managed care: where will your hospital fit in? *Hospitals* 67(7):18-23, 1993.
23. Fries JF et al: Reducing health care costs by reducing the need and demand for medical services, *N Engl J Med* 329:321-325, 1993.
24. Frik SM, Pollock SE: Preparation for advanced nursing practice, *Nurs Health Care* 14:190-195, 1993.
25. Griffith H: Who will become the preferred providers? *Am J Nurs* 85:539-542, 1985.
26. Handley T: Need for reform is in the numbers, *Kansas City Health Care Times* 2(7):5, 1993.
27. Hull K: Outpatient acceleration: 1992 survey traces continued ambulatory care growth, *Hospitals* 67(9):40-41, 1993.
28. Jackson LE: Looking toward an NP/CNS merger by the year 2000, *Nurs Pract* 18(4):15-19, 1993.
29. Jackson LE: Understanding, eliciting and negotiating clients' multicultural health beliefs, *Nurs Pract* 18(4):30-43, 1993.
30. Joint Commission on Accreditation of Healthcare Organizations: Quality assessment and improvement. In *Accreditation manual for hospitals,* Chicago, 1993, The Commission.
31. Juran JM: *Juran on quality leadership: how to go from here to there,* Wilton, Conn, 1987, Juran Institute.
32. Juran JM: *Juran on planning for quality,* New York, 1988, Free Press.
33. Kantrowitz B: Wild in the streets, *Newsweek,* pp 40-46, Aug 2, 1993.
34. Kennedy EM: Congress and the national health policy (Rosenhause lecture), *Am J Public Health* 68:241-244, 1978.
35. Koerner J: Differentiated practice: the evolution of professional nursing, *J Prof Nurs* 8:335-341, 1992.
36. Kotthoff E: Current trends and issues in nursing in the U.S.: the primary health care nurse practitioner, *Int Nurs Rev* 28:24-28, 1981.
37. Ling K: Initiation and evolution of managed care at the Johns Hopkins Hospital, *Nurs Adm Q* 17(3):54-58, 1993.
38. Lopresti J, Whetstone WR: Total quality management: doing things right, *Nurs Manage* 24:34-36, 1993.
39. Lubitz LD, Riley GF: Trends in medicare payments in the last year of life, *N Engl J Med* 328:1092-1096, 1993.
40. Lutz EM, Scholtfeldt RM: Pioneering a new approach to professional education, *Nurs Outlook* 33:139-143, 1985.
41. Manthey M et al: Primary nursing—a return to the concept "my nurse" and my "patient," *Nurs Forum* 9:65-83, 1970.
42. McCabe WJ: Total quality management in a hospital, *QRB* 18:134-140, 1992.
43. *Medicare: 1994 highlights,* Baltimore, 1994, US Department of Health and Human Services.
44. Michelson EL: The challenge of nurse-physician collaborative practices: improved patient care provision and outcomes, *Heart Lung* 17:390-391, 1988 (editorial).
45. Milio N: *The store front that didn't burn,* Ann Arbor, 1970, University of Michigan Press.
46. Mittelstadt PC: Federal reimbursement of advanced practice nurses' services empowers the profession, *Nurs Pract* 18(1):43-49, 1993.
47. Morgan WA: Using state board of nursing data to estimate the number of nurse practitioners in the United States, *Nurs Pract* 18(2):65-74, 1993.
48. Mundinger MO: Health care reform: nursing's vision of change, *Hospitals* 67(8):20-24, 1993.
49. Naisbitt J: *Megatrends,* New York, 1982, Warner Books.
50. National Center for Health Statistics: Health United States 1991, Hyattsville, Md, 1992, US Public Health Service.
51. National League for Nursing: Legislative initiatives: removing barriers to nursing practice, *PRISM—the NLN Research and Policy Quarterly* 1(1):6-10, 1993.

52. National League for Nursing: Nursing centers enter policy arena, *PRISM—the NLN Research and Policy Quarterly* 1(1):1-2, 1993.
53. National League for Nursing: A promising trend in the American care system, *PRISM—the NLN Research and Policy Quarterly* 1(1):3-5, 1993.
54. National League for Nursing: *A vision for nursing education,* New York, 1993, The League.
55. Newman M, Lamb GS, Michaels C: Nurse case management: the coming together of theory and practice, *Nurs Health Care* 12(8):404-408, 1991.
56. Nursing homes' population up, *Kansas City Star,* p 6A, June 28, 1993.
57. O'Koren ML: Reflections on facilitating collaboration between nursing services and nursing education, *J Prof Nurs* 2:72-74, 1986 (editorial).
58. Olendski MC: *Cautionary tales,* Wakefield, Mass, 1973, Contemporary Publications.
59. One in 3 ED patients is seeking primary care, *Am J Nurs* 93(8):9, 1993 (headlines).
60. Packard NJ: The price of choice: managed care in America, *Nurs Adm Q* 17(3):8-15, 1993.
61. Patient self-determination act, *Omnibus Reconciliation Act of 1990,* Washington, DC.
62. Paulen A: A time for reassessment, *Cancer Nurs* 9:2, 1986 (editorial).
63. Pearson LJ: 1992-93 update: how each state stands on legislative issues affecting advanced nursing practice, *Nurs Pract* 18(1):23-26, 1993.
64. Pike AW et al: A new architecture for quality assurance: nurse-physician collaboration, *J Nurs Care Qual* 7(3):1-8, 1993.
65. Projections of the number of persons diagnosed with AIDS and the number of immunosuppressed HIV-infected persons—United States, 1992-1994, *MMWR* 41(RR-18):1-29, 1992.
66. Put it in writing: *Questions and answers on advance directives,* Chicago, March 1991, American Hospital Association.
67. Robinson JA, Robinson KJ, Lewis DJ: Balancing quality of care and cost-effectiveness through case management, *Am Nephrol Nurs Assoc J* 19(2):182-188, 1992.
68. Sabatino F: Culture shock: are U.S. hospitals ready? *Hospitals* 67(10):23-28, 1993.
69. Safriet BJ: Health care dollars and regulatory sense: the role of advanced practice nursing, *Yale J of Regulation* 9(2):419-487, 1992.
70. Sakalys JA, Watson J: Professional education: post-baccalaureate education for professional nursing, *J Prof Nurs* 2:91-97, 1986.
71. Saldon R, Tanner FW: Quality management program boosts financial performance, *Provider* 18(10):56-57, 1992.
72. Sandrick K: Collaboration: a prerequisite to effective reform, *Health Care Exec* 8:17-19, 1993.
73. Scholotfeldt RM: The professional doctorate: rationale and characteristics, *Nurs Outlook* 26:302-311, 1978.
74. Schondelmeyer B: Home health care is a growing business, *Kansas City Health Care Times* 2(2):4, 1993.
75. Schull DE, Tosch P, Wood M: Clinical nurse specialists as collaborative care managers, *Nurs Manage* 23(3):30-33, 1992.
76. Selby T: Nurses establish clinic for the homeless, *Am Nurse* 17:1,20, 1985.
77. Sherer JL: Crossing cultures: hospitals begin breaking down the barriers to care, *Hospitals* 67(10):29-31, 1993.
78. Sherer JL: Nursing education: addressing post-reform needs, *Hospitals* 67(10):25, 1993.
79. Should health care cost concern you? *AIDE Magazine,* pp 6-9, Apr 1993.
80. Simmons FM: Developing the trauma nurse case manager role, *Dimen Crit Care Nurs* 11(3):164-170, 1992.
81. Solomon J et al: Why wait for Hillary? *Newsweek* pp 38-40, June 28, 1993.
82. Spross J, Hamrick AB: A model for future clinical specialist practitioner. In Hamrick AB, Spross J, editors: *The clinical nurse specialist in theory and practice,* New York, 1983, Grune & Stratton.
83. Suzman R, Riley NW: Introducing the oldest old: health and society, *Milbank Q* 63:177-186, 1985.
84. Trinidad EA: Case management: a model of CNS practice, *Clin Nurse Spec* 7(4):221-223, 1993.
85. Turque B: Experimental states, *Newsweek,* pp 38-39, May 17, 1993.
86. Update: nurse chosen to fill Joint Commission Board seat, *J Nurs Adm* 22(12):9, 1992.
87. Update: acquired immunodeficiency syndrome—United States, 1992, *MMWR* 42(28), 1993.
88. Update: mortality attributable to HIV infection/AIDS among persons aged 25-44 years—United States, 1990 and 1991, *MMWR* 42(25):481-486, 1993.
89. US Department of Health and Human Services, Public Health Service: Healthy people 2000: *National health promotion and disease prevention objectives,* Washington, DC, 1990, US Government Printing Office.
90. Wakefield DS, Wakefield BJ: Overcoming the barriers to implementation of TQM/CQI in hospitals: myths and realities, *QRB* 19:83-88, 1993.
91. Ward-Evans S, Hodges LC, Smith J: A new role for neuroscience nurses: the case manager, *J Neurosci Nurs* 23(4):256-260, 1991.
92. Weber G: Tips on implementing the patient self-determination act, *Nurs Health Care* 14:86-91, 1993.
93. Zander K: Managed care within acute care settings: design and implementation via nursing case management, *Health C Supervisor* 6(2):27-43, 1988.
94. Zander K: Nursing case management, *Nurs Clin North Am* 23(3):503-520, 1988.
95. Zander K: Nursing case management: strategic management of cost and quality outcomes, *J Nurs Adm* 18(5):23-30, 1988.
96. Zander K: Critical pathways. In Melum MM, Simioris MK, editors: *Total quality management,* Chicago, 1992, American Hospital Association.

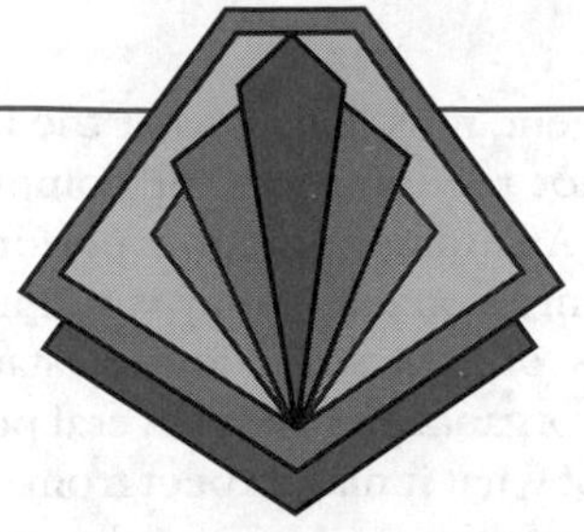

C H A P T E R 2

# Ethical Decision Making in Nursing

*Barbara J. Daly*

## CHAPTER OBJECTIVES

***After studying this chapter, the learner should be able to do the following:***

1 Explain how laws, policies, professional codes, and personal values may contribute to moral judgments in specific circumstances.
2 Apply the concepts of autonomy, beneficence, and justice in examining specific ethical dilemmas.
3 Use a five-step process in analyzing ethical dilemmas.
4 Compare and contrast the living will with the durable power of attorney for health care.
5 Describe nursing responsibilities in caring for a patient with treatment-limitation orders.
6 Identify potential resources to assist the nurse in addressing ethical issues in the workplace.

## KEY TERMS

advance directive
advocate
autonomy
beneficence
coherence
competency
consequentialist
deontological
durable power of attorney for health care
ethical
ethical dilemmas
ethics
informed consent
justice
laws
living will
moral
moral agent
morally relevant differences
nonconsequentialist
paternalism
Patient Self-Determination Act
reasonable person standard
utilitarianism
values

**Ethics** is the study of the reasoned process of making moral decisions. When we ask ethical questions, we are asking about the morally correct action in a specific situation or about how we ought to behave to live a good or worthy life. Although some make a distinction between the terms **ethical** and **moral,** these words are used interchangeably in this chapter to refer to actions and beliefs that express normative judgments about right and wrong, goodness and evil.

**Ethical dilemmas** are situations in which there seems to be no right answer. Typically these cases involve conflicts between two mutually exclusive rules or principles, such as might occur when a nurse tries to protect a patient's ability to make his or her own choices about care and yet feels an obligation to prevent the harm that might occur from an unwise choice.

We encounter ethical questions in our everyday lives. Debates regarding the morality of capital punishment or abortion, justification for civil disobedience, and instances of racial discrimination are examples of ethical issues that affect us all. In addition to our involvement in these issues, health care professionals are likely to face further situations that call for reasoned ethical analysis. Technologic advances have made it possible to intervene in health and illness in ways that raise new questions about right courses of action. For example, our ability to prolong life through the use of sophisticated technology sometimes raises doubts about the quality of the life prolonged; discoveries in the field of genetic mapping have created new questions about how to properly use information concerning an individual's genetic predispositions; and improvement in organ transplantation techniques has led to questions about the acceptability of methods to encourage donation.

The current interest in addressing ethical questions also reflects the public's growing awareness of and interest in becoming active participants in these debates. The consumer movement of the 1960s and 1970s, in addition to creating a gradual disillusionment with medicine and science in general, contributed to changing societal norms regarding health care. The recognition and acceptance of patients' rights have fostered new beliefs about the importance of involving patients in decisions about their care, informing them of all options in treatment approaches, and joining with them in mutual attempts to meet their health care needs.

Anyone who attempts to *understand an ethical issue* and reach a thoughtful decision about the *morally correct course of action* is acting as a **moral agent.** The purpose of this chapter is to review some of the common principles used by moral agents in ethical reasoning and to consider practical features of health care environments that influence the nurse's ability to make ethical decisions. Situations commonly encountered are discussed.

## MORAL AGENCY

Although moral decisions ultimately must stem from the individual's own decision making, two external sources of direction are relevant to any consideration of how we should resolve an ethical dilemma. These are the law and the professional code. Although these formal rules should never take the place of individual decision making, they must be considered as part of the process.

Many ethical dilemmas involve questions that have legal aspects. For example, when a nurse considers a patient's request that life support be discontinued, it is appropriate and even necesssary to take into account the current laws regarding treatment discontinuation. **Laws** *represent formalized societal norms regarding specific actions,* and nurses, like all citizens, are obligated to respect the laws of our country. Knowledge of the law, however, does not always answer moral questions. In many instances laws are too general to be of assistance. In other instances the law is merely silent on the question of what should be done in a specific situation. For example, we generally believe that the nurse has an obligation to be truthful when speaking to the patient; yet there is no actual law forbidding deception.

In many ways the nurse should use an understanding of the law in the same way that he or she uses knowledge of hospital policy in decision making. These external rules tell the nurse what society (in the case of laws) or the hospital (in the case of policies) expects in terms of standards of behavior. These laws and policies describe obligations of the nurse as citizen and employee and in some instances may constrain the options available to the nurse. It is essential, however, that the nurse recognize from the outset that laws and policies, like any kind of general rule, may be unwise, outdated, or just not applicable in a given situation. For this reason the nurse, as moral agent, must know what the laws and policies are but cannot rely on them for complete justification for action. An immoral action performed in accordance with an unreasonable policy is still immoral.

Professional codes of ethics are formal statements made by professional organizations for several purposes. They inform society of what it may expect from a profession, provide guidance to the members of the profession in decision making, and provide standards that the profession can use in judging and regulating members.[28] The *code for nurses,* developed by the Committee on Ethics of the American Nurses Association[2]—rather than providing an explicit set of rules— expresses the values, goals, and moral commitments of the profession.[3] The broad statements and principles contained in the code are intended to serve as a framework within which individual decision making can take place. For example, the code states in the preamble that the most fundamental principle to be used in making clinical judgments is respect for persons. Eleven specific responsibilities are then described, including such factors as confidentiality, public safety, competence, accountability, and collaboration. The nurse must be aware of the profession's code and should use it for guidance in solving ethical problems (Box 2-1).

In addition to appreciating the role of laws, policies, and professional codes in ethical decision making, it is essential that the nurse understand the difference between value judgments and moral decisions. **Values** are *expressions of individual preferences and beliefs* about things that are important or worthwhile. One's values may include material goods, such as a nice home, or more abstract goods, such as meaningful personal relationships. Values are important determinants of behavior because we tend to act in a way that will help us achieve or obtain the things we think are important in life.

Students are routinely assisted in clarifying their own values and cautioned to avoid imposing their values on others. *Values clarification* is important in helping us to understand our own behavior, and it is necessary before we can begin to resolve both intrapersonal conflicts among our own values and interpersonal conflicts between our values and the values of others. By avoiding the imposition of our values on others we avoid interfering in others' pursuit of what they believe a good or worthwhile life to be. This is required because most of us do not ordinarily examine every value we hold; rather, we simply accept that everyone has ideas that are important to them without asking if some of these values are based on false beliefs or are imprudent or more justifiable than others.

In moral issues, however, we must move beyond the level of simply recognizing personal preferences. The entire history of morality is founded on the conviction that there is meaning to the basic concepts of "right" and "wrong," "good" and "evil." This belief entails the recognition that some actions, although they stem from sincerely held values, are morally wrong and should not

**BOX 2-1 ANA Code for Nurses**

1. The nurse provides services with respect for human dignity and the uniqueness of the client, unrestricted by considerations of social or economic status, personal attributes, or the nature of health problems.
2. The nurse safeguards the client's right to privacy by judiciously protecting information of a confidential nature.
3. The nurse acts to safeguard the client and the public when health care and safety are affected by the incompetent, unethical, or illegal practice of any person.
4. The nurse assumes responsibility and accountability for individual nursing judgments and actions.
5. The nurse maintains competence in nursing.
6. The nurse exercises informed judgment and uses individual competence and qualifications as criteria in seeking consultation, accepting responsibilities, and delegating nursing activities to others.
7. The nurse participates in activities that contribute to the ongoing development of the profession's body of knowledge.
8. The nurse participates in the profession's efforts to implement and improve standards of nursing.
9. The nurse participates in the profession's efforts to establish and maintain conditions of employment conducive to high quality nursing care.
10. The nurse participates in the profession's effort to protect the public from misinformation and misrepresentation and to maintain the integrity of nursing.
11. The nurse collaborates with members of the health professions and other citizens in promoting community and national efforts to meet the health needs of the public.

Courtesy Committee on Ethics, American Nurses Association, Washington, DC, 1985.

be performed and that other actions, even if not ordinarily preferred, are morally obligatory.

Bandman and Bandman[5] discuss the need to move beyond values clarification and begin to seek justification for values as one attempts to resolve moral problems. Recognizing that a nurse, physician, or patient holds a certain value does not mean that the value or preference should be acted upon. It may be the case that the value in question is not justified. For example, many people in our country still value segregation between races. They believe that there are differences among people of different races, and they value institutions and practices that promote discrimination. If we examine this value and find, after careful reflection, that it is not justified, that it is based on mistaken beliefs, and that acting on it involves violating important moral principles, then we should not respect or even allow those actions to be taken. This does not mean that we cease to respect the person nor that we judge the person to be evil; it does mean that we make a judgment that certain actions are morally wrong regardless of the values of the person performing the action.

The caution regarding imposing our own values on others is most important when we interact with others who hold values very different from our own. For example, it could be the case that the nurse may value a life-style quite different from that valued by the gay patient with AIDS (acquired immunodeficiency syndrome). The nurse may believe strongly that traditional heterosexual relationships are more valuable and may have difficulty understanding why someone might adopt other patterns of behavior. In this case the nurse must be cautious to avoid interacting with the patient in such a way as to convey condemnation of the patient's chosen life-style or the message that this patient is less deserving of care than other patients because of his or her values. Although the nurse sincerely disagrees with the patient's values, this difference is a matter of personal belief and should have no impact on the caring relationship. However, to be alert to inappropriate ways in which our values may affect our behavior, we must first understand what values we hold.

As can be seen, the process of examining values for justification and making decisions about what actions are morally correct is quite complicated. To make these judgments the individual must use both an understanding of basic moral theories and principles and insight into personally held values and beliefs. Because nurses also must fulfill obligations to their patients and sometimes to the other professionals with whom they work, nurses must be knowledgeable about practical steps that can be effective in obtaining the desired outcome of ethical dilemmas. Each of these issues is discussed further in the remainder of this chapter.

## ETHICAL THEORIES AND PRINCIPLES

Ethical theories, like all theories, provide a framework for understanding the phenomena existing within a certain domain. Theories provide us with definitions of the relevant concepts and explain the relationship between concepts. In the study of ethics we are seeking answers to questions like "What types of acts are right?" "Which traits are praiseworthy?" "What makes certain values justified?" "Which rules should I use to guide my behavior?"[24] Ethical theories offer us a way to answer these general questions by directing the method or approach to use in addressing any ethical issue.

Although many specific theories exist, most can be classified under two headings. One group of theories is termed **consequentialist** because these ideas instruct us to evaluate the consequences of actions to judge the rightness or wrongness of the action. The other group of theories is referred to as **nonconsequentialist** because the beliefs are based on concepts of fundamental rights and duties, rather than consequences, in choosing the right course of action.

Of all of the consequentialist theories, *utilitarianism* is the most prominent today. Contemporary versions of utilitarianism define right action as any action that promotes human well-being or welfare. When we are confronted with a choice between two actions, we are to assess the expected utility of each action (hence the name **utilitarianism**) and choose that action which is most likely to produce the largest benefit, or least harm, for the greatest number of people. Everyone's welfare, including the person choosing, counts equally.

Nonconsequentialist theories, also referred to as **deontological,** argue that consequences are not the standard by which we should judge actions. Rather, there are fundamental duties and rights that stem from our nature as rational beings or, in some theories, as beings subject to the rules of God or a divine power. The morality of any action can be judged according to the dictates of these rights and duties.

All moral theories make use of principles and rules. Although the justification for the principles is quite different among theories and the strength or rigidity with which we are to follow the rules varies, there is considerable agreement about the importance of several broad principles as guides to action. These principles are general statements about ideals that should be valued, such as honesty and kindness, and they serve as the basis for more specific rules, such as "Always tell the truth." In actual practice it is these principles and rules to which we turn in addressing ethical problems rather than to the more abstract theories that underlie them. Although many different principles are components of each theory, the *three* that are *most common* and *relevant to nursing practice* are *autonomy, beneficence,* and *justice.*

## AUTONOMY

Autonomy is a term that is derived from the Greek words *autos*, meaning self, and *nomos*, meaning rule or law. The central notion of **autonomy** is that of self-rule or liberty to follow one's own will.[32] The principle of autonomy is crucial to the study of ethics for three reasons. *First*, without some sense of persons as autonomous or free, rational decision makers, we have no basis for assigning responsibility for actions. Without this sense that we are responsible for our choices, behaviors, and consequences of actions there is no point to ethical inquiry. Our understanding of human beings as entities at least potentially capable of autonomous decisions and actions underlies all of ethics.

*Second,* recognition of the principle of autonomy imposes some very important duties on us. If it is the case that people have a right to make autonomous choices, then we have a duty not to interfere with these choices. We can interfere with free choice by simply not permitting someone to make a choice, but we also can limit the ability to choose by such acts as withholding necessary information. All of these forms of interference violate the principle of autonomy and will be discussed in more detail.

The *third* reason autonomy is a significant concept in ethics is that it provides a way of classifying actions that has important implications for other duties. Even if we accept the general rule that we should respect a person's free, rational decisions, what are we to do when someone makes a decision that is clearly not rational? For example, if we believe that someone is acting under the influence of drugs, we generally do not perceive an obligation to facilitate or respect these choices. In fact, in many cases we believe we should actually protect the person from acting on these unwise decisions. Thus we need to be able to differentiate autonomous choices from nonautonomous choices as part of our determination of our own responsibilities toward others.

When we think about autonomy, a tendency exists to confuse the notion of an autonomous person with autonomous choices and autonomous actions. Although it makes sense to ask if someone is ordinarily capable of autonomy, we know that even normally rational adults may at times lose their capacity for autonomy because of an injury, period of emotional disturbance, or ingestion of mind-altering substances. It makes no difference if someone ordinarily is capable of autonomous choices if the particular decision at hand is made while the person is impaired in some way. Consequently it is more helpful to concentrate our discussion on autonomous decisions and autonomous actions rather than autonomous persons.

An autonomous decision is one that (1) is based on the decision maker's values, (2) utilizes adequate information and understanding, (3) is free from coercion or restraint, and (4) is based on reason and deliberation.[34] *Autonomous actions* are those that stem from autonomous decisions, rather than from the person being forced to act or restrained from acting in a certain way. When we think about why anyone, even ourselves, makes certain choices or behaves in a certain way, we realize that we are all under varying amounts of influence from many sources. At any one time we may have other people asking us to do something or telling us we must behave in a certain way. In addition, practical limits always affect the choices available because of factors such as time, access to opportunities, or sometimes the monetary costs associated with certain choices. If we thought that one had to be completely free to make absolutely any choice one wished, then we would have to say that none of us has ever made completely autonomous decisions. This would make the concept of autonomy meaningless. Therefore, what we are interested in is determining whether the individual in a given situation was making a decision or taking an action that was "substantially autonomous."[6] That is, we want to ensure that the individual was aware of the right to make a choice, was physically, emotionally, and mentally able to make some evaluation of the options, and had the information necessary to do so.

Both consequentialist and nonconsequentialist thinkers place great importance on autonomy. Consequentialists argue that, in general, each individual is the best judge of what will make his or her life go well, of what choices will contribute most to well-being. As a rule of thumb, then, we should refrain from interfering in the choices of others, even if these choices seem unwise or imprudent to us, up to the point where actions begin to harm or threaten the well-being of others. Nonconsequentialists believe that the respect we owe to each person entails respecting their choices of life-styles and life projects. By interfering in the decisions others make or forcing them to act in ways not freely chosen, we are expressing disrespect for the person himself or herself.

The broad principle of autonomy yields many specific rules for health care providers. The best known of these is the rule of **informed consent,** which specifies that we must obtain permission from the patient before we do anything to him or her. Although we generally are most conscious of obtaining explicit consent in the form of a written document before invasive or risky procedures, the principle of autonomy actually means that we cannot do anything, even very ordinary treatments and procedures, without the patient's agreement. For example, when patients refuse medication or diagnostic tests, we are morally obligated to respect that decision and to refrain from coercing or in any way forcing the patient to take the medicine or accept the test.

Autonomy also can serve as the basis for duties of truth telling. One way in which we can interfere with a person's right to make free choices is by withholding important information or by deceiving the person in some way. To make decisions that will promote our well-being, as conceived by each of us, we have to have accurate information. In making treatment decisions in particular we need to know something about the disease or health problem itself, the range of options for intervention, and the likely benefits and risks associated with each option. If we withhold some of this information, we are interfering in the patient's ability to make a rational decision that is in line with his or her values and preferences, and we are thus violating the principle of autonomy.

As the phrase implies, informed consent has two parts, an informational component and a volitional or consensual component.[15] If we are to feel confident that a patient has given truly informed consent, we must be confident that the requirements of both components have been met. An individual, to be "informed," not only must have been provided with all the relevant information about a proposed action or decision but also must have a certain level of understanding or comprehension. For example, if we were to provide a patient with information about a proposed drug regimen by reading the package insert regarding actions and side effects, we would certainly have given some factual information. However, by providing it in a form that is incomprehensible to most lay persons, we would have no reason to think that the patient had any level of comprehension. Thus, even if the patient consented to take the drug, we could not say that this consent was informed.

The volitional component of informed consent is met by ensuring that the patient's agreement is free of coercion or duress. This means that the individual must be able to agree or disagree without fear of reprisal or punishment. Someone could be literally forced to sign a consent form by holding a gun to the person's head or threatening harm if he or she did not consent; clearly the person's signature on a consent form in these cases would not mean that consent had been given freely. For patients, coercion or duress may take the form of fear that health care providers will abandon them or give up on them for not agreeing to the treatment the physicians and nurses think is best. Another common violation of this part of informed consent occurs when patients feel threatened to make decisions quickly, without the opportunity to think things over. When the patient inadvertently is led to believe that a decision has to be made immediately or the opportunity to receive that treatment will be lost or the health problem will become much worse, a subtle form of coercion may be perceived.

As can be seen, it is the process of obtaining consent to treatment that is morally important, not the simple act of obtaining a signature on a form. Rules about informed consent, based on the principle of autonomy, are so important in our society that they have been formalized in law. Because the concept of informed consent is not a simple one, however, disputes and even lawsuits have arisen regarding the question of whether informed consent was properly obtained before treatment was begun. Although these cases have usually involved physicians and consent for surgical interventions, the nurse is subject to the same requirement to obtain informed consent before initiating nursing actions. Consequently nurses also need to be certain that patients agree to receive the care offered and that this agreement is based on accurate and meaningful information.

This requirement, of course, raises the question of how we are to determine how much information is necessary and how complete the patient's understanding must be before we can feel confident that informed consent has been given. This question has been much debated, and no very specific answer will be correct for all circumstances.[6,15,24] It is certainly unreasonable to expect that absolutely every fact that is known about a proposed intervention be provided to the patient. This is not only a practical impossibility but, as mentioned in the earlier example, probably would be ineffective in that it is likely to confuse most people who do not have the background necessary to understand complex pharmacology or pathophysiology. The ideal might be to try to provide exactly as much information as the individual patient needs in a particular instance to understand the proposed treatment and make a reasoned decision. Although this approach seems right, we have no way of determining in advance exactly how much information and which pieces of information would represent the ideal for every individual. Instead, we need a general guideline that will be appropriate for most cases, recognizing that we will need to tailor this general rule for situations that fall outside the norm.

The guideline that is currently used to judge whether informed consent has been given is termed the **reasonable person standard.**[6] According to this standard, our obligation in obtaining informed consent is to provide the information that a hypothetic "reasonable person" would wish to have to make a decision about a proposed treatment. Most people, for example, probably would want to know about the expected benefits and the more common risks and complications of a given surgical treatment, as well as all other options with their attendant benefits and risks. In approaching patients to seek permission for interventions, then, we are to provide them with the amount and kind of information that we would expect the average person in this situation to need to know.

Two common issues that arise related to informed consent are the suggestion that, because patients have come to us seeking care, they have already given their consent to treatment, and the worry that we should refrain from giving advice or our opinion about which treatment is best for fear of unduly influencing patients' choices. Regarding the first concern, it seems valid to assume that patients come to the hospital or health care facility because they wish to have some kind of treatment or assistance. However, that tells us nothing about their wishes regarding specific interventions. Patients may come to the hospital just for nursing care, for pain relief, or for aggressive, invasive therapies aimed at cure. Until we talk with them, we have no basis for presuming consent. This does not mean that we have to ask explicitly for consent before we do anything, even common interventions such as turning a patient in bed or bathing. It does mean that the *nurse must be cognizant of two particular rules. First,* as *interventions become more invasive, risky, or burdensome,* we must begin to *explicitly ask patients* if they consent to the intervention to be certain that we have given them the opportunity to refuse. *Second, whenever the competent patient does refuse an intervention, we must heed his or her refusal and stop what we are doing.*

The *second concern*—that we may inadvertently pressure patients into making the decisions we want if we tell them what we think they should do—can be addressed by again thinking about what a reasonable person would want to know. Given the fact that the health care provider is more knowledgeable about health, illness, and possible treatments, most people would want to know what the provider thinks about each option, how they evaluate each, and what courses of action they believe to be best, all things considered. This can be done in such a way as to avoid coercing the patient by being careful to be open about our reasons for recommending a particular intervention and by offering clear reassurance that we will continue to care for the patient regardless of which option is chosen.

All the discussion of autonomy and the rules of informed consent hinge on the belief that the patient is competent to make an informed, autonomous decision. **Competency** *is a legal term* and refers to a court's judgment that an individual is capable of exercising the right of self-determination.[11] The most important component of this judgment is the assessment of decision-making capacity and the absence of seriously impaired mental status. This determination is often made by psychiatrists, although each of us informally makes this assessment when we decide to accept or reject a patient's decision.

The question of an individual's capacity to make autonomous decisions is a crucial one because it determines whether we have a strict obligation to refrain from interfering in the patient's choices. Although patients often make choices that we wish they would not—choices that we believe are not in their best interests—we may not act contrary to these choices as long as the person understands his or her condition, knows the consequences of the decision, and has reasons that make some sense to us.[11]

## BENEFICENCE

In situations in which we believe an individual cannot make an autonomous decision, we rely on the principle of beneficence to direct our actions. **Beneficence** *is the duty to do good, to prevent harm, or to reduce harm where it is present.* Some include within beneficence the principle of nonmaleficence, or the duty to refrain from doing harm, whereas others treat nonmaleficence as a separate and even more important principle. Although beneficence and nonmaleficence are duties of some importance for everyone, they are especially significant for health care professionals. Part of the core meaning of "professional" is the commitment to act for the good of society in general and individual clients or patients in particular.[30] Nurses feel a particular responsibility to protect patients and to act in their best interests.

For nurses, the notion of *advocacy* is prominent today as an avenue for both supporting patient autonomy and fulfilling duties of beneficence. An **advocate** is one who speaks for the patient as part of a broader effort to protect the patient's rights. As a description of a particular role or activity, "advocacy" is a somewhat vague term, lacking precise definition.[33] It does capture an important function of nurses—that of acting as an interface between the patient and the complex health care bureaucracy. There is no question that nurses are particularly suited, as Winslow notes, to serve as patient confidante, to assist patients in making their wishes known, and to ensure, through education, that patients are properly informed.[33] However, the current emphasis on advocacy does not provide much direction to the nurse who perceives a conflict between the duty to foster patient autonomy and yet to prevent harm and produce benefit.

When patients make choices that clearly will lead to physical dangers to their health, all care providers face a dilemma. For example, patients often object to being restrained or having their side rails up, even after the nurse has carefully explained the danger of falling out of bed. To ignore the patient's wishes seems to be a clear violation of the patient's autonomy. Yet to follow the patient's wishes seems to fail to protect the patient from harm. Dilemmas such as this involve the possibility of paternalistic action.

**Paternalism** consists of actions that, to benefit or protect a person, override that person's wishes, usually with the justification that one "knows better" what is in the patient's interest.[6] Benjamin and Curtis use the term *parentalism* to reflect the origins of this kind of action in the parent-child model of relationships.[7] The question of when, if ever, we are justified in overriding a patient's wishes regarding treatment is a major issue in health care.

This is one reason why determination of decision-making capacity is so important. If the patient lacks the capacity to make informed decisions, regardless of whether this is a permanent or temporary impairment, the principle of autonomy is an inadequate guide for us in determining what to do. It is fortunate if friends or family members can speak on the patient's behalf. If not, then we are obligated to act according to the principle of beneficence. This moral guideline, as can be seen, does not tell us exactly what to do or how to judge what would be in the best interest of the patient, but it does serve as the basis for our duty to help those who cannot speak for themselves.

When the dictates of autonomy and beneficence appear to conflict, rights of autonomy generally take precedence. The right of patients to accept or reject care has been repeatedly reaffirmed by the courts, and all care providers are both morally and legally obligated to respect the wishes of competent patients regarding their treatment. It may be helpful to the nurse who experiences the conflict to recall that the principle of beneficence directs us to promote good, but it does not specify what that good is. There are many ways in which something might be judged to be "good." For example, a treatment that contributed to physiologic stability is a certain kind of good, and production of happiness or relief of suffering is another type of good. Each of these is a rather limited or narrow conception of "good." Most of us, if asked, could identify a higher or more important good. For some this might be ensuring that our family is well cared for, whereas for others it might be retaining a sense of dignity, living in accordance with God's laws, or simply being in control of what happens. In situations in which the nurse finds it impossible to follow the patient's wishes without seeming to act in a way that does not contribute to physiologic good, it can be helpful to remember that there are many kinds of goods. Autonomy simply directs us to let the patient's conception of the highest good be most important in our decision making. Thus, when we act to support the patient's choice, thereby helping the individual achieve his or her personal conception of "good," we are acting in accord with both autonomy and beneficence.

## JUSTICE

The third principle that is relevant to health care is justice. Justice is a very broad principle that has many implications. In the most basic sense, justice merely means treating equals equally and unequals unequally.[26] That is, **justice** demands that we have equal respect and concern for the rights of others and that differences in how we treat people be in proportion to morally relevant differences. This requirement has important implications for how we treat people generally and particularly for how we distribute scarce resources.

Anytime we are faced with a shortage of valuable resources, we are dealing with a justice problem. For example, the nurse who must decide how to divide a limited amount of time among several patients must decide the fair or just way to apportion this time. The nurse could simply divide the 8-hour shift equally, with each of four patients having 2 hours. This makes no sense, however, because we believe that the degree of need is a morally relevant difference. Instead, it seems fair to divide the time according to how much care is needed, with the patients who have the greater needs receiving more time and the patients who need less receiving less time. Although the nurse is treating people differently, the difference is in proportion to a morally relevant property—need for care. On the other hand, if the nurse divided his or her time according to something we think is morally irrelevant, such as the race or age of the patient, we would say that this is unfair or unjust. **Morally relevant differences** are those factors or characteristics of individuals that have some logical relation to the resources that are to be distributed or to the treatment in question. In the example just given, a person's race has nothing to do with why he became ill, the reason he came to the hospital, the burdens of illness, or the benefits of treatment. Race is thus a *morally irrelevant factor* to consider in distributing health care resources.

Although justice problems thus can occur even at the bedside, *the most serious issue for justice today is the national health care distribution system.* Health care in our country is currently distributed in a very uneven fashion. Although some care is provided through social welfare programs (Medicaid and Medicare), many Americans do not qualify for these programs. For those who do not, health care is distributed as a market good. This means that access to care is determined by ability to pay, just as access to cars, houses, clothing is determined by one's ability to purchase the goods in a free market. The current estimate is that about 37 million Americans do not qualify for either Medicare or Medicaid but also cannot afford to purchase private health insurance.[12]

The question of how our health care system should

be reformed to make it more just is a complex one that involves moral issues such as the establishment of a right to care, economic questions about the best way to pay for this care, and practical concerns about how to structure a universal access program. Consideration of these issues would take us beyond the scope of this chapter, but several points are important for the student.

First, as shown by the earlier example, the principle of justice has implications for the individual. Whenever we are faced with deciding how to apportion a scarce resource, such as our time, the last bed in the intensive care unit, or the last open time on the operating room schedule, we must be aware of the patient characteristics we are using in our decision. We should ask ourselves if the criteria for our decisions are fair and if we would be willing to say that resources always should be distributed according to these criteria. Regarding the larger issue of health reform, the nurse must be informed about proposed legislation and be prepared to contribute to these changes at least through knowledgeable use of voting power.

## RESOLVING ETHICAL DILEMMAS

As the reader has probably noted in the earlier section, understanding the moral principles does not in itself provide answers to dilemmas. Rather, the theories, principles, and rules provide us with tools to use in the process of reaching a decision about what to do. There are many suggested approaches to ethical decision making, usually involving a series of steps much like the nursing process.[14,16,17,23,24] An organized process to guide one's thinking is particularly helpful when the nurse is unfamiliar with ethical analysis. Although there is some variation among models of decision making, most utilize the five steps discussed in Box 2-2.

**BOX 2-2 Steps in Ethical Decision Making**

1. Review the facts.
2. Define the problem.
3. List the choices.
4. Decide on the action.
5. Evaluate the choice.

### REVIEWING THE FACTS

As with any reasoned problem-solving process, the first step is to collect data and be certain of the facts. Applying ethical theories correctly requires that we know all the relevant facts about a situation, including such factors as data about the patient's condition, patient and family preferences, patient competence, and relevant hospital policies and laws. *Formally reviewing the facts with everyone involved in the ethical dilemma is essential for two reasons.*

*First,* we want to be sure that we are proceeding on a full and correct data base. In particular, we need to know something about why the individuals involved hold the views they do. Simply knowing that a patient wants to leave the hospital against medical advice (AMA), for example, is not enough. Does the patient want to leave because he or she believes that care is not being effective, because there is some problem at home that needs to be addressed, because there is concern over the cost of care, because there has been a disagreement with the nurse or physician, or because the patient has consciously and competently decided that the benefits of treatment are not worth the burdens? The answer to this question would have important implications for action.

*Second,* it often happens that different individuals in the situation have different pieces of information at their disposal. What initially may be thought to be an ethical disagreement may turn out to be different beliefs about the facts or unjustified assumptions. For example, one nurse may believe that chemotherapy should be stopped because it is not working and is causing the patient unnecessary suffering. Another nurse may have had a discussion with the oncologist about the latest bone marrow biopsy results that showed a reduction in leukemic cells, suggesting that the therapy was in fact beginning to work. If these two nurses did not review the facts together, each might come to a different conclusion about what was in the patient's best interest. This would be a disagreement stemming from different data bases, not a disagreement over moral principles.

### DEFINING THE PROBLEM

Defining the problem consists of making a concise statement specifying the central issues or questions. This might take the form of statements such as, "This competent patient wishes to stop life-supporting treatment. Are we obligated to respect this wish and remove the ventilator?" or "The family members of this incompetent patient disagree about what is in the patient's best interest. How should we resolve this question, and what are the implications of this for treatment of the patient?"

Explicit statement of the problem serves several purposes. It focuses discussion on the exact situation, which may help care givers concentrate on the case at hand rather than becoming distracted by a debate of the more abstract general issues, such as whether autonomy, overall, is more important than beneficence. The theoretic issues are, of course, important, but it is neither possible nor necessary to reach complete agreement on these to resolve individual patient problems.

Defining the issue also clarifies that the problem is a moral one and starts to narrow the field of inquiry to the relevant moral questions. For example, the aforementioned problems suggest situations that involve questions about patients' rights to refuse life-supporting treatment in the one case and questions about who should speak for incompetent patients in the second case. Other moral principles, such as duties related to justice, truth telling, and confidentiality, are not involved. Thus describing the problem in one or two sentences helps everyone to focus on the central issue of the particular situation at hand.

### LISTING THE CHOICES

When we confront difficult decision-making situations, particularly those in which disagreement among the participants is obvious from the outset, views often become polarized. For example, in the situation in which a patient is requesting the removal of the life-supporting ventilator, members of the health care team might find themselves initially divided into two camps—those who think the patient's wishes should be followed and those who think not. If we are not careful first to consider what all of the options might be, we may miss consideration of some actions that actually are better solutions. In our example the complete range of options might include removing the ventilator today, removing it for a short trial period and then allowing the patient to reconsider his or her decision, asking the patient to allow the care givers a defined period of time to continue selected interventions before making the decision to stop ventilation, or offering the option of going home on the ventilator.

Listing the choices also reminds us that ethical dilemmas always involve choices among several actions. We cannot solve actual problems by choosing values or principles alone. Each of the possible resolutions to a dilemma involves a decision about which course of *action* is morally justified.

### DECIDING ON THE ACTION

In reaching a decision the nurse uses the tools of ethical theories and principles discussed earlier. To decide which of all the available options is the morally justified one, the nurse must be able to refer to fundamental principles and rules that direct action, usually specifying duties and rights. To make a choice between supporting a patient's decision to cease treatment or overriding that decision, the nurse must have access to an articulated moral system that specifies the principle, such as autonomy, that takes priority in situations of conflict.

In making a choice, the nurse also will be making use of the facts identified in the first step of the process. We began with outlining all of the relevant data because we need to have these data readily available as part of our justification for action. Even the strongest-held principles and the most important rules have reasonable exceptions. To examine whether an exception is justified in a specific case, we usually appeal to facts about the situation. We might, for example, believe that patients have a right to full information about their condition, and yet choose to put off telling a particular male patient the results of his diagnostic tests if we know that in a few days his closest relative will be arriving in town and will be able to support him as he hears disappointing news.

### EVALUATING THE CHOICE

As with any decision-making process, the last step is to evaluate the choice made. In ethical decision making, the nurse examines the choice for its consistency and coherence with other moral decisions. *Decisions* that are *consistent* are said to be *universalizable* in that the *same decision* should be made *in any situation* that was *similar in morally relevant ways.* Thus the nurse who chooses to respect a patient's wishes in one situation, believing that autonomy is the most important principle, should expect to make the same decision in all situations involving similar conflicts.

**Coherence** refers to the degree to which the specific decision fits within a fully developed moral system. For example, the moral system of the nurse who chooses to respect the patient's wish to have life-supporting treatment discontinued could not logically support a view in which life itself is thought to be the ultimate value.

These evaluative steps are helpful in two ways. Moral dilemmas take place in complicated real-life situations in which the nurse is subject to many influences, including external constraints of law and policy, the opinion of peers and supervisors, and the nurse's own personal preferences and needs. These influences can make it difficult at times to be sure that the decisions reached are truly the result of thoughtful deliberation rather than the pressure to conform or to choose the option that creates the least controversy.

Taking the step of conscious evaluation also assists the nurse in learning more about his or her own moral values and encourages the process of seeking justification for these values. By asking ourselves if we are being consistent in how we choose to solve problems, if we are willing to commit ourselves to this same answer in all situations like this one, and if this answer "fits" with our other values, we can begin to develop a comprehensive moral system that can direct action in a variety of situations.

## COMMON ETHICAL ISSUES IN ACUTE CARE

Although the preceding steps are intended to be used in any situation, two issues are so common in acute care that review of their current status will be helpful to the student. These are the issues of advance directives and treatment withdrawal.

### ADVANCE DIRECTIVES

**Advance directive** refers to any document that is enacted by an individual before becoming ill, specifying one's wishes regarding treatment should one be unable to express them later on.[4,19] Although one could make an advance directive simply by writing down one's treatment preferences, the two forms of advance directives formally recognized by law in most states are the living will and the durable power of attorney for health care.[13,27]

**Living wills** generally take effect only when the patient is terminally ill and is unable to voice his or her wishes. Under these two conditions, the living will directs that no life-sustaining treatment is to be administered. In addition, some living will forms include more specific directions regarding the individual's wishes for withholding food and fluid or other specific treatment modalities. The presence of a living will can be quite helpful to care givers who are faced with treatment decisions for patients who can no longer speak for themselves, but they do not take the place of timely communication. One of the shortcomings of living wills is that, unless we have the opportunity to discuss the document with the patient while the patient is still able to communicate, we cannot be certain of precisely what the patient's wishes were in conditions other than terminal illness. For example, some persons who have experienced a significant neurologic insult, such as a massive cardiovascular accident (CVA), might wish that life-sustaining treatment not be carried out. However, because a CVA does not generally produce a "terminal" condition, the living will is not applicable.

A second type of advance directive, the **durable power of attorney for health care** (DPAHC), is more broad and flexible than a living will, and many people choose to have both instruments. The DPAHC transfers all rights that the individual normally has regarding health care decisions—such as accepting and refusing treatment, inspecting the medical record, accepting or changing physicians—to another person called the "agent" or "attorney in fact."[1] Like a living will, the DPAHC goes into effect only when the individual has lost decision-making capacity. This, however, is the only criterion for activation. Thus, even if the individual is unconscious only for a short time, the DPAHC is in effect during that period; it is not limited to conditions of terminal illness. In addition, because the agent has all decision-making powers, the DPAHC is helpful in seeking any decision about care, including not only life-supporting treatments but also questions related to blood transfusions, antibiotic therapy, and surgical procedures.

Although the DPAHC is applicable in many more situations than is a living will, it does have the disadvantage of leaving all decision making in the hands of the agent. For this reason many people prefer to have both forms of advance directives. A living will is completed to indicate the patient's own wishes and relieve others of the burden of decision making in cases of terminal illness, and the DPAHC is completed to designate someone to make all other decisions.

The **Patient Self-Determination Act** (PSDA), part of the Omnibus Budget Reconciliation Act of 1991, is a federal law that makes it essential for all nurses to be familiar with the living will and DPAHC laws in their states. The PSDA requires all hospitals, nursing homes, hospices, and home health care agencies to inform all patients on admission to the facility of their rights under state law to utilize advance directives and of hospital policy regarding these directives and to ask if the patient has any advance directives in effect.[18,22,27] The response must be documented in the medical record. Hospitals have chosen several ways to comply with this law. In some facilities admissions clerks or social workers ask patients about advance directives, whereas in others the nurse who admits the patient to the hospital has this responsibility. Regardless of who raises this subject with the patient initially, the nurse caring for the patient must be prepared to discuss the topic with the patient, answer questions, or obtain other resources to assist patients. Both living wills and DPAHC forms should be available for patients to complete while hospitalized, if they so desire.

## TREATMENT LIMITATION

Decisions to limit treatment in some way are always associated with potential ethical concerns. There are legal, moral, and practical aspects to these decisions, which often become intertwined. The fundamental principles involved in situations of limitation of treatment are quite clear. Patients have an almost absolute legal and moral right to make decisions to limit treatment in any way, regardless of whether that treatment is a life-sustaining one.[20,31] The only exception to this position occurs with pregnant women; in these cases courts have sometimes ruled that the concern for the welfare of the fetus justifies overriding the wishes of the mother regarding treatment.

It is important for the student to be aware of attempts that have been made in the past to differentiate acceptable forms of treatment limitation from unacceptable. At various times some have suggested that extraordinary treatments were not obligatory, whereas it was mandatory to administer "ordinary" treatments, that treatments could be withheld but not withdrawn, and that complex technologic interventions could be withheld but that hydration and nutrition must always be provided.[25] The arguments involving each of these distinctions are complex, and the reader is referred to texts on bioethics for further discussion.[9] It is important, however, to understand that all these distinctions currently are viewed as unimportant and that any intervention to which a competent patient does not consent must be withheld or withdrawn if already being administered.

Although there is relatively complete consensus regarding the moral acceptability of limiting treatments that the patient wishes to stop or that are futile, no such agreement exists regarding acts of active euthanasia. Intervening with the primary intention to cause death, with patient consent, motivated by the wish to end suffering, is considered to be a form of active euthanasia. Similarly, acts of physicians that provide the patient with the means to end his or her own life are termed *aid-in-dying* or *physician-assisted suicide.* Opponents of such acts argue that in these cases, unlike situations in which medical treatment is withheld or withdrawn, the cause of death is not the illness itself but the person who intervenes. Deliberately causing death in this way is prohibited by law in some states and by all professional codes. Opponents argue that there is no morally relevant difference between withdrawing a treatment such as a mechanical ventilator, with the certain knowledge that death will occur, and administering a drug that will lead to a painless death.[10,25] Sufficient public concern about people who are made to suffer prolonged, painful deaths has resulted in proposed legislation that would legalize aid-in-dying in two states (Washington and California). Although neither state has yet secured passage of the legislation, this trend is certain to continue.

The nurse must become knowlegeable about the moral issues involved and decide on a personal position on the question. Although it is more common for patients to request assistance with ending their life from physicians, nurses often are involved in these discussions with patients and families as they confront terminal illness. Consequently the nurse should be prepared to answer patients' questions about aid-in-dying and discuss the patient's concerns and fears about it.

When a situation occurs in which treatment limitation is an issue, one practical factor that often causes confusion is communication. Any decision to limit treatment in any way must be documented in the physician's orders. The most common form of such treatment limitation orders is the "do not resuscitate" (DNR) order. This order reflects a decision to withhold cardiopulmonary resuscitation in the event of an arrest. Unless additional treatment restriction orders are written, a DNR order does not limit other forms of aggressive treatment, and patients with a DNR order should continue to receive close monitoring and any therapy necessary to prevent an arrest. One of the most important responsibilities of the professional nurse in caring for the patient with a DNR order is to be certain that the exact intention of the DNR order is understood. Vague phrases such as "no heroics" should not be used because it is unclear to what specific interventions the word *heroics* refers.

The role of the nurse also includes being an active participant in discussions with patients and families regarding their wishes for treatment. It is essential that these discussions be documented and communicated to all persons involved in the patient's care.[21] It is not uncommon for the patient or the patient's family to first mention their thoughts about limiting or withdrawing treatment to the nurse, and the nurse can be instrumental in assisting the patient and family members in raising this issue with the patient's physician. Because issues such as patient requests for treatment termination often are complicated by differing views and uncertainty about the moral principles involved, it is helpful for the nurse to be aware of resources available.

## RESOURCES

Today many hospitals have ethics committees. These committees are multidisciplinary, and their purpose is to provide consultation to clinicians regarding specific ethical problems. They usually include physicians, nurses, hospital lawyers and administrators, social workers, and clergy. The conclusions of the committee generally are expressed as recommendations, and clinicans are not obligated to follow their advice.[8] Typically, anyone can request that the ethics committee consider a case. These committees are quite helpful in providing an objective review of the situation by personnel who are familiar with ethics and are knowledgeable about ethical analysis.

In addition to formal committees, some hospitals have ethics consultation services. These services consist of several persons who have expertise in addressing ethical dilemmas and in helping others to resolve them. Consultation services are somewhat more flexible than committees in that the consultant usually can go to the patient care area on rather short notice to meet with the patient and family, perform an independent assessment of the situation, and meet immediately with the care givers to offer advice.[29]

Even in hospitals in which the nurse does not have access to these formal resources, several general guidelines are available to the nurse who recognizes an ethical dilemma. It is almost always helpful for the nurse to discuss the ethical issue with at least one other person. This action helps ensure that all the data have been considered and that all options have been reviewed. Because ethical dilemmas frequently involve disagreements and controversy, it is beneficial for the nurse to have the support of peers.

In addition to colleagues, nurses must feel free to express ethical concerns to supervisors and others in the administrative hierarchy. Although most cases can be resolved through thoughtful reflection and clear, planned communication, some issues require administrative action. Policies such as those related to DNR orders, treatment withdrawal, refusal to care for certain patient groups, and concerns about appropriate staffing levels are examples of issues that cannot be resolved by individuals acting alone.

Most important, nurses must continue to develop their understanding of ethical principles and to become comfortable with analyzing ethical dilemmas. This process involves gaining knowledge of specific theories, gaining insight into their own moral beliefs, and being willing to examine these beliefs for justification.

## QUESTIONS TO CONSIDER

- What is the difference between making value judgments and making a moral judgment?
- What is the major difference between consequentialist and deontological theories?
- In what ways is the process recommended for addressing ethical dilemmas similar to the process of problem solving?
- Why are we obligated to respect patients' wishes regarding treatment?
- What resources are available in confronting ethical dilemmas?

## CRITICAL THINKING ACTIVITIES

- Why is knowledge and application of hospital policy alone inadequate for analyzing moral dilemmas?
- How can you, as a nurse, assist patients in making decisions about their future health care?

## CHAPTER SUMMARY

- Ethics is the study of the reasoned process of making moral decisions.
- Ethical dilemmas are situations in which there is a conflict between mutually exclusive rules or principles that appears to lack a correct or "right" answer.

### MORAL AGENCY

- Acting as a moral agent involves thoughtful consideration of principled reasons for actions, understanding of relevant laws and policies, and knowledge of the professional code of ethics.
- Unlike value judgments, moral judgments reflect evaluation of values and a search for justification. Judgments that involve the concepts of right and wrong, good and evil, go beyond personal preference and are impersonal.

### ETHICAL THEORIES AND PRINCIPLES

- Ethical theories provide a method for answering questions about right courses of action. The two major categories of ethical theories are consequentialist and nonconsequentialist.
- Virtually all theories emphasize the importance of three principles—autonomy, beneficence, and justice—although the justification for these principles differs.
- Autonomy refers to the right of self-determination. It depends on the possession of decision-making capacity and underlies specific rules of informed consent.
- Beneficence is a duty to benefit or do good. The obligation to help others is particularly important for professionals and directs us to promote the welfare of others when they cannot make autonomous choices. Acting in such a way as to benefit others while overriding or violating their right to make their own decisions constitutes paternalistic action.
- Justice is generally understood as the obligation to treat equals equally through equal concern and respect for their rights. The most important application of principles of justice today is the need for reform of the health care distribution system.

### RESOLVING ETHICAL DILEMMAS

- A five-step process for resolving ethical dilemmas is recommended. These steps include (1) reviewing the facts, (2) defining the problem, (3) listing the choices, (4) deciding on the action, and (5) evaluating the choice.

### COMMON ETHICAL ISSUES IN ACUTE CARE

- *Advance directives* is a term that refers to written instructions from the patient regarding his or her future health care. It includes both the living will and durable power of attorney for health care.
- "Do not resuscitate" orders reflect the decision to withhold resuscitation should a cardiopulmonary arrest occur. They do not have implications for withholding or withdrawing other treatments, although additional interventions also may be limited by specific orders.
- There is currently much controversy regarding the moral status of patient requests for aid-in-dying, also called active euthanasia or assisted suicide. Professional codes and some state laws currently do not support involvement of nurses or physicians in active euthanasia.
- In caring for any patient for whom treatment limitation is being considered, the nurse should be an active participant in discussions and can play an important role in assisting patients and families in decision making.
- Ethics committees and ethics consultation services can be helpful resources to nurses and others in dealing with ethical problems.
- Documentation, communication, and gaining the support of peers and supervisory personnel are important steps in the process of seeking resolution.

## REFERENCES

1. Abrams FR: Advance directives: When the patient cannot communicate. In Monagle JF, Thomasma DC, editors: *Medical ethics,* Rockville, Md, 1988, Aspen.
2. American Nurses Association: *Code for nurses,* Washington, DC, 1985, The Association.
3. American Nurses Association: *Ethics in nursing,* Washington, DC, 1988, The Association.
4. Badzek LA: What you need to know about advance directives, *Nurs 92*(6):58-59, 1992.
5. Bandman EL, Bandman B: *Nursing ethics through the life span,* ed 2, Norwalk, Conn, 1992, Appleton & Lange.

6. Beauchamp TL, Childress JF: *Principles of biomedical ethics,* ed 3, New York, 1989, Oxford University Press.
7. Benjamin M, Curtis, J: *Ethics in nursing,* ed 3, New York, 1992, Oxford University Press.
8. Blake DC: The hospital ethics committee, *Hastings Cent Rep* 22(1):6-11, 1992.
9. Brock D: Death and dying. In Veatch RM: *Medical ethics,* Boston, 1989, Jones & Bartlett.
10. Brock D: Voluntary active euthanasia, *Hastings Cent Rep* 22(2):10-22, 1992.
11. Chell B: Competency: what it is and what it isn't. In Monagle JF, Thomasma DC: *Medical ethics,* Rockville, Md, 1988, Aspen.
12. Committee on Ways and Means, U.S. House of Representatives: *Health care resources book,* Washington, DC, 1991, US Government Printing Office.
13. Emanuel L: Advance directives: what have we learned so far? *J Clin Ethics* 4:(1):8-16, 1993.
14. Fowler MD: Piecing together the ethical puzzle: operationalizing nursing ethics in critical care. In Fowler MD, Levine-Ariff J, editors: *Ethics at the bedside,* Philadelphia, 1987, JB Lippincott.
15. Gorovitz S: Informed consent and patient autonomy. In Callahan JC: *Ethical issues in professional life,* New York, 1988, Oxford University Press.
16. Haggarty MC: Ethics: nurse patron or nurse advocate? *Nurs Manage* 16(5) (critical care edition):34O-34U, 1985.
17. Halloran MC: Rational ethical judgments utilizing a decision-making tool, *Heart Lung* 11(6):566-570, 1982.
18. Idemoto B et al: Implementing the Patient Self-Determination Act, *Am J Nurs* 93(1):21-25, 1993.
19. Lo B: The clinical use of advance directives. In Monagle JF, Thomasma DC: *Medical ethics,* Rockville, Md, 1988, Aspen.
20. Meisel A: The legal consensus about foregoing life-sustaining treatment: its status and prospects, *Kennedy Inst Ethics J* 2(4):309-346, 1992.
21. Meyer C: End-of-life care: patients' choices, nurses' challenges, *Am J Nurs* 93(2):40-47, 1993.
22. Mezey M, Latimer B: The Patient Self-Determination Act, *Hastings Cent Rep* 23(1):16-20, 1993.
23. Novak J: An ethical decision-making model for the neonatal intensive care unit, *J Perinat Nurs* 1(3):57-67, 1988.
24. Purtillo R: *Ethical dimensions in the health professions,* ed 2, Philadelphia, 1993, WB Saunders.
25. Rachels J: Euthanasia. In Regan T: *Matters of life and death,* New York, 1986, Random House.
26. Rakowski E: *Equal justice,* Oxford, 1991, Clarendon Press.
27. Schwarz JK: Living wills and health care proxies, *Nurs Health Care* 13(2):92-96.
28. Silva MC: The American Nurses Association's code for nurses: purposes, content, and enforceability, *Health Matrix* 11(2):55-63, 1989.
29. Simpson KH: The development of a clinical ethics consultation service in a community hospital, *J Clin Ethics* 3(2):124-130, 1992.
30. Veatch RM: Models for ethical medicine in a revolutionary age, *Hastings Cent Rep* 2(3):5-7, 1972.
31. Veatch RM: Foregoing life-sustaining treatment: limits to the consensus, *Kennedy Inst Ethics J* 3(1):1-20, 1993.
32. Wiens AG: Patient autonomy in care: a theoretical framework for nursing, *J Prof Nurs* 9(2):95-103, 1993.
33. Winslow GR: From loyalty to advocacy: a new metaphor for nursing, *Hastings Cent Rep* 14(3):32-39, 1984.
34. Wright RA: *Human values in health care,* New York, 1987, McGraw-Hill.

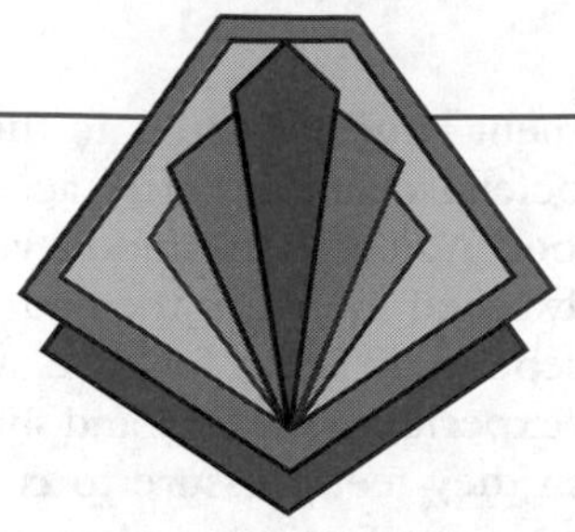

CHAPTER 3

# Nursing Practice With Young and Middle-Aged Adults

***Diana Lynn Morris***
***Janet Primomo***

## CHAPTER OBJECTIVES

***After studying this chapter, the learner should be able to do the following:***

1 Analyze physical, psychosocial, spiritual, sexual, and cognitive aspects of development in early and middle adulthood.
2 Describe potential effects of injury and illness on adult development.
3 Propose health promotion and health risk prevention plans appropriate to adult developmental requirements for selected patients.

## KEY TERMS

adulthood
blended family
core middle years
early adulthood
early adult transition
empty nest syndrome
human growth and development
maturity
middle adulthood
partner
sandwich generation

## OVERVIEW OF ADULT DEVELOPMENT

**Adulthood** is not a static period of life. The subtle intrinsic and adaptive sequence of changes that evolves over the adult years must be understood to provide optimum nursing care. Indeed, there is a great deal of variation in the ways people cope and adapt to illness. Physical changes and neurologic status are important in helping nurses evaluate the patient's self-care potential. The sphere of psychosocial development includes family, social, and occupational tasks that normally accompany a specific period in the life span. Sexuality differs across the life span and may be threatened by certain illnesses. Cognitive changes in adulthood such as problem-solving ability and intellectual capacity have implications for how nurses teach patients about health care. Spiritual changes over the years include the ability to find meaning in life and accept the inevitable end of life.

Development in each of the spheres does not happen independently, but rather the changes are linked together and can influence each other. A developmental perspective gives nurses a road map to help them understand the many physical and psychosocial changes that occur during the adult years. In this chapter, development during the adult years is reviewed, and implications for nursing care are identified. A developmental perspective helps highlight the salient issues that people face at specific points in the life span. A person's development may influence how that individual copes with a situation brought on by illness. For example, a woman in her mid-thirties who has young children and an elderly ill parent to care for may find it very difficult to find the time to take care of her own health needs. Rather than identify the woman as "noncompliant," nurses—to plan and provide sensitive and appropriate nursing care—must consider the developmental processes and needs of adults as they experience health and illness.

## THE PROCESS OF HUMAN GROWTH AND DEVELOPMENT

The process of **human growth and development** continues throughout the life span. The human being's growth and development comprise an integration of physical, psychosocial, cognitive, sexual, and spiritual aspects. Physical growth, caused by the development and integration of differentiated cells, is a continuous process from the moment of conception until maturity. *Growth* results in a change in body structure or size.

*Development* denotes increases in functional capacity evolving from physical and mental maturation and learning. Development also implies expansion in detail and growth into an advanced state.

Adulthood often is characterized as a period of stability, developmental potential, and ultimately decline in later years. Dramatic physical changes are few, but changes do occur. Psychologic changes also occur during the adult years, but there is relative *stability* in *values, attitudes,* and *feelings about self and others.* The stability of such personal features does not necessarily indicate a lack of development. Rather, stable personal features may represent the foundation of prior developmental achievements upon which present and future maturation is built. Thus, as people grow older, their personality remains basically the same, but they may become increasingly mature. *Maturity* in adulthood is marked by the capacity for *acceptance of self, intimacy with others,* and a *sense of meaning in one's life experience.*

One cautionary note relative to understanding the human growth and developmental process in practice should be mentioned. Although discussions of growth and development often provide chronologic age markers for achieving certain developmental stages and tasks, it is important to remember that such markers are merely guidelines. Chronologic age is not necessarily a predictor of a developmental stage, particularly during early and middle adulthood—a period of some 47 to 52 years. The growth and development process ebbs and flows for each individual. The process does not occur in isolation but is influenced by interpersonal and social factors, life events, life-style choices, and ethnicity, as well as political and economic events.

In the past the adult years have been divided into three general stages: young adulthood, middle adulthood, and older adulthood. More recently, one can find discussions of *four stages of adult development* as a result of *increased longevity: early adulthood* (ages 18 to 40), *middle adulthood* (ages 40 to 65), *older adulthood* (ages 65 to 85), and *old-old adulthood* (age 85 and older). The focus of this chapter is on early and middle adulthood, and Chapter 4 addresses the older and old-old adulthood stages of development. For each general stage, normative growth and development, health promotion needs, and health concerns will be discussed. Health promotion and health concerns address health goals and issues identified with each developmental stage described in the U.S. Public Health Service report, *Healthy People 2000,*[40] and related to nursing practice.

## DEMOGRAPHIC TRENDS

Although most of society's attention to growth and development has been on children and more recently on older adults, increasing attention is being given to the growth and development issues of adults in their early and middle years. Societal changes partly account for the interest in adulthood. Adults in the middle years may find themselves "sandwiched" between their parents and their children who depend on them for care. Adults in the middle years may experience chronic and short-term illness at a time when they feel pressure to contribute to society by functioning as a family member, caring for both the younger and the older generations, and maintaining occupational productivity. The more we understand about adults in their middle years, the better we can help them cope with the challenges they face during a period of illness.

Demographic changes that have occurred over the past few decades also account for the interest in adulthood (Table 3-1). A major trend is the increasing growth rate of the population over age 65.[38] In fact, the number of persons 75 years of age or older is increasing proportionately faster than the total group over age 65. In 1986, 12% of the U.S. population, or 29.1 million people, were older than 65 years of age. By the year 2000, it is estimated that 13% of the population—34.8 million people—will be 65 years of age or older.[38] There will be more older adults to be cared for by the young and middle-aged adults in society. The increasing number of elderly persons has resulted primarily from the dramatic increase in the life expectancy of Americans. At the turn of the century, life expectancy for women was about 48 years, and for men it was about 46 years. By 1986 it had increased to 78.3 years for women and 71.3 years for men. The decrease in infant mortality, the prevention and control of communicable disease during childhood, the improved treatment of acute and chronic disease, and improvements in medical care in general contributed to the increased life expectancy in this country. At the same time the birth rate in the United States is declining.

The 1990 census report indicated that the median age of the U.S. population was 32.9 years.[39] There were 154 million Americans in early and middle adulthood, representing 61.8% of the total population. Persons

**TABLE 3-1 Adult Population by Age (in millions)**

| | ACTUAL | | PROJECTED |
|---|---|---|---|
| AGE (YR) | 1986 | 1990 | 2000 |
| 18-24 | 27.7 | 26.3 | 25.2 |
| 25-44 | 75.9 | 80.7 | 81.0 |
| 45-54 | 22.8 | 25.2 | 37.2 |
| 55-64 | 22.2 | 21.1 | 24.2 |
| 65-74 | 17.3 | 18.1 | 18.2 |
| ≥75 | 11.8 | 13.1 | 16.6 |

From US Bureau of the Census: *1990 census of population and housing,* Washington, DC, 1991, US Government Printing Office.

younger than 18 years of age comprised 25.6% of the population whereas persons 65 years of age and older comprised 12.6% of the population.

Other dramatic demographic trends include the lower rates of life expectancy for nonwhite persons compared with white persons and the higher number of elderly women than men. In 1991 life expectancy was 72.5 years for African-American women and 79.3 years for white women. In 1986 African-American men had a life expectancy of 66 years compared with 72.6 years for white men. Although the proportions of both men and women in the over-65 age-groups will increase over the next decade, the population of women older than age 65 outnumbers that of men by about 6.1 million. It is projected that in the year 2000, 59% of those over 65 years of age will be women.[38]

## HEALTH GOALS FOR YOUNG AND MIDDLE-AGED ADULTS

### *Healthy People 2000*

Health goals and health risks for Americans of all ages were addressed by the Public Health Service in the 1990 report *Healthy People 2000: National Health Promotion and Disease Prevention.*[40] The goals and risks for *early* and *middle adulthood* identified in the report are discussed in the appropriate sections of this chapter. The following is a brief discussion of the publication and its significance for nursing.

*Healthy People 2000* provides a vision of quality of life and well-being for all citizens as we approach the twenty-first century. The report takes into consideration anticipated changes in the population of the United States. The population is expected to increase by 7% to 270 million people with only about one half of the households having traditional husband-wife partnerships. The median age will be 36 years, with the age of older adults continuing to increase, particularly among those 85 years of age and older. The racial and ethnic composition of the United States will continue to change, with an increase in the number of Hispanic and African-American persons, as well as increases in other minority groups. In the next century, those entering the work force are more likely to be women from all racial and ethnic groups and persons from what we currently identify as minority groups.

The authors considered the following factors in the development of *Healthy People 2000:* projected population characteristics, the current state of health care, health technology, health care access, changes in longevity, health-risk patterns, and social, economic, and political factors that have contributed to the current health status of the people of the United States. It is important to note that the prevailing goal for all persons—no matter their age, ethnicity, or economic status—is to increase the period of healthy functioning life.

### SIGNIFICANCE FOR NURSING

The U.S. Public Health Service report *Healthy People 2000* is a guide for health professionals and the citizen-consumer. The document provides guidelines for nurses in their daily practice as they provide care to patients. Nurses can anticipate that this report will be used to provide direction for national health policies and future health care priorities and reimbursement. The publication provides a common ground for collaboration with other health care professionals and health service agencies.

The strength of *Healthy People 2000* is that it focuses on health promotion and disease prevention, which traditionally have been emphasized in nursing. All nurses can use this document to support the care and education of patients in all types of settings, no matter the disease process being treated. The report also provides information about the health promotion and disease prevention needs of specific groups according to characteristics such as age, race and ethnicity, and economic status.

## EARLY ADULTHOOD

**Early adulthood** extends from the ages of 18 to 40 years. These age boundaries are arbitary and are used as guidelines rather than absolute markers of developmental processes. Early adulthood focuses on the definition of "self" as an adult in society, achievement of personal goals, and development of the capacity for intimacy with oneself and others.[38] Early adulthood is a time of personal and social expansion, including career development and establishment of a family system.[4,37] In the following section, early adult development is reviewed and health promotion and health risk concerns are discussed.

### PHYSICAL DEVELOPMENT

Full growth and development is completed by the mid-twenties, and most body systems are functioning at maximum levels.[17,27] Of the physical changes that occur in adulthood, some begin early and others begin in middle age; some are abrupt, and some are gradual. Cardiac output and stroke volume begin to decrease. Vital capacity of the respiratory system decreases. As a person grows older, the gastrointestinal system slows down so that digestion, absorption, and elimination of food takes longer. Changes in weight and muscle mass occur primarily because of alterations in diet and exercise. Thinning and graying of hair and wrinkling of skin occur as the young adult years progress. After age 25, visual acuity begins to decline. Finally, fertility in women declines with the passing years.[17]

### PSYCHOSOCIAL DEVELOPMENT

Adulthood often is equated with **maturity;** it is characterized by a sense of responsibility, the maintenance of appropriate impulse control, the ability to plan and

**TABLE 3-2 Summary of Selected Theories of Psychosocial Development in Adulthood**

| AGE | ERIKSON[16] | STEVENSON[39] | LEVINSON[23] | LOEVINGER[24] |
|---|---|---|---|---|
| Young adulthood | Intimacy versus isolation<br>Significant objects—persons, causes<br>Virtue: love | Young adulthood (18-30)<br>Achieving independence | Early adult transition (17-22)<br>Entering adult world (22-28) | Conformist<br>Identification with group<br>Conscientious<br>Increased sense of personal responsibility |
| Adulthood | Generativity versus stagnation<br>Significant persons—spouse, family, friends<br>Virtue: care | Core middle years (30-50)<br>Assist older and younger generations | Age 30 transition (28-33)<br>Settling down (33-40)<br>Midlife transition (40-45)<br>Entering middle adulthood (45-50) | Autonomous<br>Mutual interdependence, coping with conflict<br>Integrated<br>Cherishing individual difference |
| | | New middle years (50-70)<br>Assume primary responsibility for cultural and social survival | Age 50 transition (50-55)<br>Culmination of middle adulthood (55-60) | |
| Maturity | Integrity versus disgust, despair<br>Significant persons—spouse, family<br>Virtue: wisdom | | Late adult transition (60-65)<br>Late adulthood (65+) | |

implement realistic goals, the development of a career, and the capacity to enter into intimate relationships. Everyone does not arrive at early adulthood with the same level of maturity; therefore age-related norms may be misleading. Psychosocial development, emotional maturity, intellectual ability, and physical characteristics may vary from person to person, men to women, and culture to culture.

Developmental markers and outcomes may be expected to change with increased life expectancy and with changing social, economic, and health patterns. Thus developmental expectations for specific age-groups may differ, and it is necessary to review developmental theories and be aware of the need to support systematic study to determine their adequacy. In addition, psychosocial development in "young" adults who experience illness, especially chronic illness, may be altered. Conversely, the experience of illness may be shaped by the person's development. Theories of psychosocial development and their implications for nursing are reviewed in the following section.

Table 3-2 shows selected theories of psychosocial development especially relevant to nursing practice. Most of the theories include sequential stages and developmental tasks, but they vary in the number of stages and types of processes involved. Erikson emphasized the conflicts or turning points that the individual must cope with at different stages of the life span. Failure to successfully resolve the tasks at one stage affects development in the next stage. Erikson identified an alternative to each stage that would occur if the person did not successfully complete the tasks relevant to that stage.[16] The two outcomes indicated for each of Erikson's stages, however, should not be interpreted as dichotomous or polar opposites. For example, the earliest stage of development focuses on trust versus mistrust, with trust being the most desired outcome. Nevertheless, it is desirable and even healthy for one not to trust, or to mistrust, in certain situations. In fact, it may be necessary to one's survival.

In Erikson's *eight ages of man,* the first adult stage is characterized by *intimacy versus isolation*[16] (see Table 3-2). Intimacy implies sharing the self to form a commitment to an intense, lasting relationship with another person, a cause, or a creative effort without fearing the loss of identity. Intimacy requires responsibility, impulse control, the ability to plan, and also the ability to trust. Erikson suggests that the virtue of love is acquired as a result of developing the capacity to be intimate with another, whereas inability to develop some form of intimacy draws the person into increasing feelings of isolation, alienation, and self-absorption.

Stevenson, a nurse theorist, identified early adulthood as the time for achieving independence from parents, assuming adult responsibility, and beginning a family.[39] The tasks of new parenthood add another dimension to the adult's life. Stevenson's delineation of tasks for this stage of adulthood represents traditional patterns in our culture. It should be noted that social, cultural, and economic factors may alter what we have assumed to be "normal" developmental tasks. No longer can we expect everyone to assume parenting roles or become independent of his or her parents during early adulthood.

Levinson emphasized the life structures or tasks and the transitions that occur in the adult years.[23] **The early adult transition** is the bridge between preadulthood and early adulthood when a person leaves home and establishes independence. In early adulthood the person explores adult roles, makes interpersonal commitments, and builds and maintains an adult life-style. The early adult years are a time of great energy when people try to find their niche in society. There are many rewards during this period of life, including satisfaction with love, family, work, and life-style. However, the competing demands for a person's time, creativity, and energy may have a cost. Levinson's work, which focused on adult men, may have particular value for a professional working with men. Again, as with most developmental models, the theory may need to be modified for persons in nontraditional roles and for those with alternative life-styles.

Loevinger presented a somewhat different view of psychosocial development. Rather than identifying developmental stages according to social tasks, her theory emphasizes how a person's overall perception of the world varies across the life span and influences behavior and attitudes. Loevinger, who focused on the development of the "ego" or self,[24] described milestones of ego development that can be considered stages. The stages are marked by sources of conflict, and each successive stage is more complex. At each stage the person's frame of reference and attitudes about life vary. In other words, a person's behavior and perception of the world reflect the developmental stage of the individual. Loevinger's theory differs from other theories in that age norms are not specified, and all individuals may not reach the highest stage.

## Developmental Tasks

Psychologic and social aspects of the young adult's development can be gleaned from the developmental tasks common to this period (Box 3-1). The developmental tasks of early adulthood are most concretely seen in the choice of a vocation and a partner, which clearly involve a certain choice of life-style. Although fairly clear boundaries have been established between self and parents by this time, parental attitudes and value systems have been internalized in young adults and become a salient part of their identity, thus affecting future life choices.

### Occupational choice

An occupation represents much more than a set of skills and functions or a way to earn a living. It is a way of life that determines much of the environment, both physical and social, in which a person lives. Occupational choice plays a significant part in further shaping the person by providing a social system, status, roles, and a life-style. The choice of an occupation often requires consideration of appropriate educational preparation, and thus educational goals and achievements become a very important part of this choice.

**BOX 3-1 Tasks of Early Adulthood**

- Achieving self-identity separate from parents
- Developing a sense of responsibility for one's own life
- Developing a sense of social, civic, and economic responsibility
- Choosing a life-style
- Choosing and starting an occupation or a vocation
- Choosing a partner
- Choosing to become a parent
- Managing a home

During the early adult years (ages 18 to 40) when involvement in an occupation is of prime importance, unemployment may cause the individual to feel unneeded or unwanted, thus fostering feelings of inadequacy and failure. Furthermore, unemployment has dire consequences for the person involved and the family, including poverty, homelessness, and limited access to health care. The nurse must be sensitive to concerns and anxieties regarding unemployment or changes in employment because of illness, accidents, and altered ability to conduct former work. Vocational counseling or rehabilitation may be recommended for persons with disabilities who need to restructure their vocation after illness or injury.[15] Those who are temporarily or permanently unable to work should be referred to social service agencies that can help them obtain public assistance, housing, and access to health care.

During the past few decades, social and economic forces have changed the composition of the work force in this country. In fact, well over 50% of women are in the labor force today.[38] The feminist movement exerted a significant influence on women's occupational choices. In addition, it is an economic reality that many women, especially single parents, must work outside the home and provide for the economic needs of their families. Among young adults there is a growing tendency to delay having children until career goals are solidified. Overall, employment outside the home has been seen as having a positive influence on women's lives.[32] Employed women who are responsible for dependent children or aging parents may be burdened with additional demands such as child care or adult day-care. Therefore when a woman is ill, she may have concerns about the welfare of her family as well as employment-related concerns. This is true also for fathers who are single parents and men who are care givers of adult family members.

### Choice of partner

A major decision in early adulthood is that of choosing a **partner.** This decision is based on sexual orientation and social and cultural norms. The choice of a partner often includes or is followed by decisions about marriage and whether to raise children. It is important that nurses respect the life-style choices of the young adults they care for. Specifically, it is critical that nurses recognize the important role a patient's partner plays in the patient's life, well-being, and recovery from illness.

The dominant society continues to strongly support marriage between young, heterosexual adults. From this perspective marriage has a legal definition and in many jurisdictions includes only heterosexual partnerships. Some people also choose not to marry, preferring to remain single or to engage in a partnership that is not legally recognized. In such circumstances, partners may make a personal commitment to one another that for some includes a religious or public ceremony. No matter what the composition of or legal standing of the partnership, it is a close and loving relationship between two people. The *partnership* is a place where intimacy and affection exist in a free and equal relationship.

### Choice to parent

Today both single young adults and those in a marital or partner relationship make decisions about whether to become parents through childbirth or adoption. The arrival of the first child transforms the partners into parents, and they take on the roles and parenting behavior learned from other parents.[25] Parenthood is experienced as a joy as well as a crisis. The arrival of a child necessitates adjustments in daily routine and life-style, which often are seen as a burden. Courses designed to prepare persons for parenthood have not been widely available in our society. It is therefore difficult for couples to anticipate many of the stresses of being parents and the changes required of them and their relationship. If the nurse assesses that an individual is experiencing undue stress and an inability to cope, referrals to private professionals or agencies providing such assistance can be made.

### Life choices and family

Although the institutions of marriage and the family are the most socially acceptable, there is an increasing tolerance for diversity in living patterns. Alternatives to traditional family life that are increasingly common include cohabitation with members of the same or opposite sex, living alone, becoming a single parent, remaining a childless couple, and communal living. Other alternative family structures include homosexual couples who make a lifelong commitment and choose to raise a family. Divorce, a common occurrence today, is a highly stressful event that often creates a crisis. Today almost half of all marriages end in divorce. The young adult may perceive divorce as a failure to achieve intimacy, one of the normal developmental tasks. Most adults who are divorced, however, go on to marry again. In fact, in more than 45% of all marriages, one or both partners were married previously, with either or both spouses having children from previous marriages, resulting in what is called a **blended family.**[10] These couples may also have children of their own. Role adjustment for all family members will be necessary.

Although personality characteristics and interpersonal problems are primary sources of difficulties in adjustment to marriage and parenthood, cultural and societal variables often make these adjustments difficult. For instance, the mobility of our society results in a dispersal of family members and close relatives, with less available help from these significant others in times of need and stress. Nurses should be in touch with their attitudes about varying life-styles and choices and remain nonjudgmental in caring for patients.

Developmental theory is useful in exploring the possible effects that chronic or life-threatening health conditions may have at different points in the life span. During the intimacy versus isolation stage of young adulthood, a chronic condition may be viewed as a limiting factor in finding a mate.[15,22,32] In one study, Primomo found that some young women with diabetes mellitus were concerned about disclosing their illness to prospective partners for fear that they would "frighten them away."[32] When faced with a chronic illness, people may question their ability to provide for and raise children.[1] Having a health condition that can be passed on to children can influence a person's decision to have a family. An altered body image may be perceived as affecting relationships with peers. Young adults with physical disabilities and chronic conditions that are stigmatized by society may have limited opportunities to achieve intimacy and sexual and vocational fulfillment.[12] A young adult who experiences an illness may need parental assistance at a time when freedom and independence are desired. Family roles may have to be adjusted and redefined.[15] Theories of psychosocial development that focus on developmental tasks are useful in helping nurses to recognize the "normal" activities that young adults engage in. When an individual is faced with a long-term threat to health that requires emotional, physical, vocational, and social adaptation on the part of the person and family, the nurse can listen carefully to the concerns expressed and acknowledge that distress is a normal reaction. Information can be provided, and referrals for counseling can be made.

Loevinger's theory provides an alternative developmental framework for considering how people adapt to illness and the intervention strategies used. Rigid treatment approaches may be less effective than strategies that take into account the unique characteristics of the individual. For example, at higher stages of development the needs of others, as well as the individual's own needs, are considered even when the needs are conflicting. Therefore nurses must find out how patients think an illness situation affects those around them so that treatment strategies can include concern for others. Since the early 1980s researchers have studied how development in women is different from that in men.[5,19] Interdependence with others and interpersonal relationships are especially significant for women in their early adult years.[18,19] Again, the importance of taking women's concerns into account and including family members in planning treatment strategies may increase the nurse's effectiveness in caring for patients with chronic conditions.

The successful resolution of the early adult phase of the life cycle depends on a positive self-concept. How people feel about themselves affects relationships as well as the choices made during this period. A person who feels adequate and competent in setting and achieving goals tends to experience more positive outcomes than one whose self-concept is that of inadequacy and incompetency. These negative feelings tend to foster withdrawal and inability to mobilize resources for positive gains.[36] In caring for the young adult it is therefore important to assess the individual's self-perception. These data not only provide information about motivation potential but also are a basis for nursing interventions that help to increase the individual's self-esteem.

Sexuality is an integral part of self-concept. Competence in the area of sexuality is of prime importance during the adult years. Sexuality may be defined as a "deep pervasive aspect of the total person, the sum total of one's feelings and behavior as a male or female, the expression of which goes beyond genital response."[27] Early adulthood is normally the time when the body's sexual response is powerful, and there is a need to find adequate and satisfactory ways to express it. It is known that a man reaches his peak sexual capacity at about 18 years of age, whereas a woman reaches her peak of sexual capacity in her early thirties.

If the expression of sexual feelings is restricted, perhaps because of illness or injury, causing a felt or imagined change in body image, sexual concerns may become paramount. Nurses frequently are asked by young adults for assistance with marital or sexual concerns. Unless the nurse is secure in his or her own sexual identity and has had adequate preparation to deal with such matters, the person should be referred to appropriate personnel who can deal with these concerns.

Body image, an important aspect of self-concept, is a mental picture of the body's appearance as well as the attitudes, emotions, and personality of the individual. At a period of life when acceptance by others is most important, and with society's emphasis on youth, beauty, and physical fitness, any alteration in body function or structure poses a threat to a positive body image. Adaptation to these alterations depends on the nature and meaning of the threat to the person and his or her coping mechanisms and available support systems.

In summary, nursing interventions to help someone deal with a threat to or change of body image involve (1) careful assessment of the individual's perception of the condition, (2) assistance in helping the individual maintain a realistic perception of the threat in relation to the person's total self-image, (3) assistance in identifying useful coping mechanisms, and (4) identification of support systems.

## COGNITIVE DEVELOPMENT

Cross-sectional studies have shown that the highest overall intelligence test performance occurs at some time between the late teens and late twenties. People in their thirties, forties, and fifties tend to score somewhat lower. Longitudinal evidence has shown, however, that general intelligence either remains the same or increases slightly during the adult years.[35] Certain factors, such as education and other sociocultural advantages, may influence intellectual development and performance.

It should be noted that the measure of one's intelligence is more than a score on a standardized examination. Intelligence can include a person's capacity for creativity and understanding of how systems work. Traditionally, young adults are described as having achieved the highest level of cognitive development in the use of formal operations.[31] More recently, authors have suggested developmental stages beyond those of Piaget's formal operations[21] and have proposed that the cognitive development of women may be different. Nurses should consider styles of cognitive development when they assess an individual and develop health education materials.

## SPIRITUAL DEVELOPMENT

Spiritual development focuses on the meanings one attaches to life, particularly one's own life experience. For some individuals, spirituality includes a connection with and commitment to a particular religious orientation and religious institution. However, belonging to a church or belief in specific religious dogma may not be part of a person's spirituality. Bianchi[6] describes aging as a "spiritual journey" that synthesizes a person's inner contemplative experience and external human concerns. Although the search for the meaning of one's life often is described as a focus in *middle adulthood,* nurses should consider their patient's spiritual development during early adulthood. Spiritual development during middle and older adulthood is built on experiences of childhood, adolescence, and early adulthood. Spirituality is represented by the meaning one attaches to life experiences at any age and represents a holistic integration of physical, social, psychologic, cultural, sexual, and theologic experiences. Spiritual development during early adulthood is of particular concern for persons who experience illness. The experience of physical illness and life crises can precipitate a transforming spiritual change or cause a patient to become more introspective and contemplative. The nurse can help a patient to explore the meaning of a particular physical or life crisis, thus supporting the patient's spiritual development. For many young adults this process means helping patients

**RESEARCH**

Ragsdale D, Kortarba JA, Morrow JR: Quality of life of hospitalized persons with AIDS, *Image* 24(4):259, 1992.

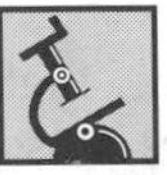

The purpose of this study was to examine the quality of everyday life from the perspective of hospitalized adults with AIDS. Thirteen men and one woman on a specialized AIDS unit in a community hospital participated in the study. The participants ranged in age from 26 to 61 years and were evenly divided between blue-collar workers and professionals. Participants were asked about how they felt, what a typical hospital day was like, and the quality of their interactions with nurses, physicians, and other personnel. Five management or coping styles were used by the participants to create and maintain a sense of control. The participants' need for control focused on efforts to understand and interpret events during their hospitalization and to be able to provide input into their assessment and care. *Management styles* included *the loner, the activist, the victim, the time keeper,* and *the mystic,* which reflect the meanings different patients attach to an illness experience. The findings suggest that nurses should include assessment of the meanings clients attach to being hospitalized with AIDS. Further, care plans should be developed with that particular person's coping style incorporated into the plan.

to find meaning in their lives through definitions of self and personhood that go beyond physical abilities, attributes, and work roles (see Research box above).

## HEALTH PROMOTION

Early adulthood covers a number of years when adults are establishing health patterns—and sometimes risk behaviors—that can determine life expectancy and functional health.[40] These years, during which physical growth ceases, may involve experimentation with life-styles and life-style changes. Chronic or life-threatening illnesses may occur, and high-risk behaviors, particularly in those between the ages of 18 and 24 years, may result in death.[11,26,40] Patterns and attitudes are established that influence health and productivity, as well as social and personal relationships. It is a time when nurses can have a major influence on a patient's health behaviors and health outcomes that will affect the person's middle and late life. The following topics address selected health promotion needs and health risks for young adults.

### Nutrition

Nutrition needs of early adulthood are somewhat different from those of the growing adolescent because of the cessation of physical growth.[17,27] Men should increase their consumption of foods high in vitamins C, E, $B_6$, and riboflavin. Men need only 10 mg of iron in their daily diets, whereas women require 18 mg. In young women the need for protein and vitamins A, E, $B_6$, $B_{12}$, and riboflavin remains about the same as in earlier years, but the need for vitamin C and calcium increases. For example, women need 1000 mg of calcium daily along with vitamin D to prevent osteoporosis. Furthermore, women who are pregnant or breast-feeding have additional nutritional requirements.

Dietary modification may be indicated, depending on whether the young adult has a chronic illness. For example, diabetes mellitus is partially controlled by diet. Modifications in diet are recommended for those at risk for illnesses that are considered to be diet-related, such as cancer, heart disease, atherosclerosis, hypertension, and type II diabetes. In fact, the surgeon general recommends that all Americans eat a balanced diet of the minimum number of calories needed to maintain desirable weight; lower their intake of saturated fat, cholesterol, sugar, and salt; and increase consumption of complex carbohydrates (whole grains, fruits, and vegetables), fish, poultry, and legumes.

Nutritional problems of young adults may result from their life-styles; for example, busy schedules, limited income, and increased family, job, or educational demands may contribute to poor nutritional choices and habits. Eating disorders such as anorexia (extreme self-imposed food restriction and exercise) and bulimia (recurrent episodes of binge eating followed by self-induced vomiting or laxative abuse) that primarily affect adolescent girls may be identified in young women and men as well. Nurses can be alert to signs and symptoms of nutritional deficits and help the young adult understand the importance of adequate nutrition for maintaining well-being, preventing illness, and recovering from illness. Nurses and dietitians can assist young adults in developing nutritionally balanced meal plans that are tailored to their health status, income, life-styles, and preferences.

### Exercise

Exercise serves several functions during early adulthood. It helps to regulate appetite, burn calories, control fat accumulation, improve or maintain muscle tone, enhance cardiac function, release tension, aid sleep, and improve overall well-being. To be most beneficial, exercise should be regularly scheduled three or four times weekly for at least 30 minutes. The type of exercise should be appropriate to the individual's overall health status. For example, a woman with diabetic neuropathy may find swimming to be a safer form of exercise than running.

Many activities such as walking, jogging, bicycling, swimming, tennis, rowing, aerobic water exercise, and jumping rope provide exertion that benefits the cardiopulmonary system. However, intermittent exercise is not as effective as a regular, planned exercise program, because sporadic exertion produces sudden demands on the cardiopulmonary systems without allowing the body to adequately adjust. When an individual begins an exercise program, a gradual increase in the intensity of exertion is recommended to allow the body to adapt to the physical demands. Continued and regular exercise contributes to the sustained maintenance and optimal functioning of body systems.

### Rest and Sleep

Sleep is a basic requirement for all human beings. Sufficient sleep is needed to maintain energy levels, physical appearance, and well-being. For adults, approximately 6 to 8 hours of uninterrupted sleep per day is considered adequate.[17] Although an individual can adjust to a lack of sleep for a short time, prolonged periods of decreased sleep and rest can contribute to anxiety, fatigue, irritability, lack of concentration, reduced alertness, and slowed recovery from illness.[34] The sleep patterns of young adults may be altered because of family responsibilities such as caring for growing children, work roles that include jobs requiring night and rotating shifts, social activities, and career development such as further education.

## HEALTH RISKS

The health of adults depends on a complex set of social and environmental circumstances, including life-style and health practices. There is increasing recognition that social and economic conditions can influence health status. Research has shown that the death rates from cancer, diabetes, tuberculosis, heart disease, and multiple sclerosis in urban populations are higher for those of lower income than for the more economically advantaged, suggesting that environmental conditions such as poverty may be important determinants in these diseases. Injuries and illnesses that restrict normal activity may create social and economic problems for the young adult. As mentioned earlier, dependence on others, especially parents, during injury or illness may create conflict for the young adult's quest for independence.

The *Healthy People 2000* report indicates that the death rate during early adulthood as a result of heart disease and cancer needs to be decreased. The three leading causes of death and injury, however, are accidental trauma, homicide, and suicide.[40] There has been a recent upward trend in unintentional injuries and death. Unintentional injuries most often involve automobiles, and at least 50% of these injuries are related to alcohol use. Homicide is the second leading cause of death in early adulthood and the number one cause of death in African-American males. In fact their risk of homicide in early adulthood is seven times that of white males.[40] Socioeconomic status is a major predictor of violent death. Alcohol use (50%)—and less often other drugs—may be a factor. Most homicides are committed by a relative or acquaintances of the victim and involve the use of firearms.[11] Reports indicate that the suicide rate in early adulthood is rising among those between the ages of 20 and 24 years.[26] As with homicide, firearms are the predominant means (60%) used in suicide.

During early adulthood other threats to health include tobacco use, drug and alcohol abuse, stress-related disorders, and preexisting chronic conditions such as heart disease, epilepsy, and diabetes. Sexual concerns include sexually transmitted diseases (including *Chlamydia trachomatis* and HIV), contraception, unwanted pregnancy, sexual identity conflicts, and guilt related to parental and societal values about sexual practices.

Major health-risk behaviors in early adulthood are connected with sexual activity and substance use. Sexually transmitted diseases are on the rise in young adults, and of particular concern is the incidence of HIV on college campuses and in young minority populations. Sexually transmitted diseases are discussed in Chapter 52, and HIV infection and AIDS are discussed in Chapter 71.

The use of tobacco, alcohol, and drugs not only is related to immediate health risks but can increase the risk of acute and chronic illnesses in later life. Although the use of alcohol is slowly decreasing, it remains a major health and social problem.[28] The use of illicit drugs continues to be a problem in early adulthood, including the "social" use of cocaine and crack (see Chapter 19).

According to the National Center for Health Statistics, the most common chronic conditions in early adulthood are chronic sinusitis, hay fever or allergic rhinitis, and deformities or orthopedic impairments.[29] The most effective nursing interventions might be to assist young adults in managing these chronic conditions through self-care. Upper respiratory tract infections are common among young adults; environmental pollutants, occupational exposure to agents, smoking, and child rearing may contribute to the problem because of the frequency of upper respiratory infections in children. The nurse's primary responsibility lies in teaching preventive measures. Prevention is directed at supporting the body's own defenses through basic health practices (adequate rest and sleep, exercise, and a balanced diet). Reducing the susceptibility to and risk of illness can be accomplished by encouraging health-promoting behaviors, maintaining weight, limiting alcohol intake, stopping smoking, practicing safe sex to reduce sexually transmitted diseases, managing stress, maintaining safety measures at work and while engaging in sports and other leisure activities, using seat belts, and practicing self-care such as breast self-examination.

Physiologic and psychologic changes resulting in unusual or disturbed adaptive behavior patterns may occur when the young adult has difficulty coping with newly acquired tasks and responsibilities. Mate selection, marriage, childbearing, college, job demands, social expectations, financial worries, and independent decision making are all stressors, carrying the threats of insecurity and some degree of failure. Some stress reactions take the form of physical illness. Related to the stresses of achievement in the young adult years is the occurrence of gastric and duodenal ulcers. Prevention here is directed at reinforcement of appropriate diet, exercise, and rest. When stressors are perceived as overwhelming, the result may be self-destructive behavior such as drug abuse and addiction, alcoholism, excessive smoking, and suicide (ranked as one of the leading causes of death in this age-group).

Sensitivity to the many pressures and responsibilities facing the young adult is vital to good nursing care. The patient's major concern often is not self-directed. The person may be the breadwinner of a family. How is the family being supported during the illness? How are the medical bills to be paid? The patient may be a parent of small children. Who will care for them? When hospitalized, the patient often is concerned about how the family is getting along at home. The patient may have no family nearby. Who will look in on the patient if he or she is ill at home? Who will provide care during convalescence? These are only a few of the problems frequently facing the young adult patient. Some problems of hospitalized patients may be alleviated by providing the use of a telephone or by arranging a visit with a family member, friend, or business associate. Help needed by the patient may be available through other support systems such as social services in the hospital or through family service or community health agencies. The nurse in a physician's office or clinic also should be alert for persons who need this kind of assistance.

## MIDDLE ADULTHOOD

***Middle adulthood*** extends from the ages of 40 to 65 years. The arbitrary definition of middle adulthood by an age criterion has changed over the years. For example, at one time the end of the middle years was 45 years of age. With increased life expectancy, however, the criterion has changed, and a few authors have begun to suggest that middle adulthood could extend to 70 years of age.

Middle adulthood is characterized as a time of few physical changes unless an illness, which may create profound changes in every aspect of the person's life, is experienced. Middle adulthood is a time rich in psychosocial alterations. The middle years are approached with a sharpened sense of awareness as adults begin to evaluate their lives. Ideally, there is a sense of self-acceptance and a willingness to revise aspirations on the basis of the realities of one's current life situation. In the following sections middle adult development is reviewed, and health promotion and health risks are discussed.

### PHYSICAL DEVELOPMENT

Physically the adult usually enters this phase of life functioning at near-peak efficiency.[23] As the middle years progress, physiologic changes occur gradually. If a chronic condition or illness is experienced, the resulting physical changes must be taken into account because they may influence how a person adapts during this period of life.

Some of the physical changes during the middle adult years are a continuation of changes that began during the end of the young adult period.[33] The loss of elasticity and the changes in arterial structure may contribute to cardiovascular problems. As activity and metabolism slow down, the weight gain that often results may have detrimental effects on other body systems. These factors put adults at risk for cardiovascular disease, hypertension, atherosclerosis, diabetes, kidney disease, cancer, and gallstones. The decreased elasticity of the lungs contributes to certain chronic respiratory diseases. A redistribution of fatty tissue occurs, regardless of any change in diet or exercise patterns. A loss of muscle strength, especially in the back and legs, is noted, and muscle and joint stiffness can occur. The individual may become aware of the appearance of gray hairs, little creases or lines in the face, and dry skin that begins to show signs of decreasing elasticity.[17]

The sense organs undergo change in the middle years. One of the most noticeable conditions affects the eyes. ***Presbyopia***, a reduction in elasticity of the lens of the eye, results in decreased accommodation for near points of vision and acuity in darkness.[17] Many adults need to wear bifocals, trifocals, or reading glasses to correct this problem. During the middle years a gradual deterioration and hardening of the auditory cells and nerves result in some loss of hearing.

In women, menopausal changes that affect hormonal levels take place between 40 and 55 years of age. Some women may experience mood swings, nervousness, headaches, heart palpitations, insomnia, fatigue, and mild depression.[42] As ovarian function gradually diminishes, decreased amounts of estrogen and progesterone are produced by the ovaries. Small amounts of estrogen continue to be produced by other tissues for several years after ovarian function ceases. Some of the symptoms associated with "the change of life" are hot flashes, night sweats, and atrophic vaginitis in which the vaginal mucosa becomes thin and dry, contributing to itching, burning, and possible discharge.[42] Osteoporosis is not necessarily a result of menopause, but it often accompanies or follows menopause as bone demineralization accelerates in the absence of estrogen.

The psychologic changes that sometimes accompany menopause may not be precipitated by the hormonal deficiency but may be more appropriately related to the personal and life-style adjustments that occur in the middle years. For example, the loss of fertility or the experience of a chronic or life-threatening illness may be a significant cause for grief. Life-style changes also may be the result of positive events such as the decision to have children. This decision, however, requires special supervision of the mother's physical status after age 40. Thus changes in the family system such as children leaving home, divorce, illness or death of a spouse, and the illness or death of parents may contribute to the emotional difficulties women experience during this phase of life.

Physical changes in the male reproductive organs are minimal. Hypertrophy of the prostate gland can cause urinary frequency, dribbling, and urinary retention. Controversy exists over whether a male climacteric occurs. Although there are some emotional changes in men during the middle adult years, they are not believed to be the result of hormonal changes because androgen levels decline very slowly.[42] In fact, reproductive capabilities continue into the later years. Any loss of sexual desire or potency may be the result of psychologic changes, stress, illness (particularly diabetes), disability, or medications (especially antihypertensive drugs), rather than physiologic changes of aging.

## PSYCHOSOCIAL DEVELOPMENT

Numerous theories of adulthood have furthered the notion that middle adulthood is a distinct phase of life with specific inner growth and developmental tasks. Many of the changes during middle adulthood involve role transitions that may alter self-image, life-style, values, and attitudes. The ability to give up roles and adapt to new roles may contribute to a creative and productive life during the middle years and beyond (Box 3-2).

**BOX 3-2 Tasks of Middle Adulthood**

- Choosing to be a parent
- Assisting children to become responsible adults
- Coping with role transition
- Renewing and redeveloping earlier relationships
- Maintaining involvement in occupational, social, and civic spheres
- Assisting in the care of aging parents
- Reevaluating life's goals
- Developing adult leisure-time activities

Erikson, one of the first theorists to study the universal dilemmas faced during adulthood, described this stage in terms of resolving the generativity versus stagnation crisis (Table 3-2). Generativity involves the creation and guidance of children, products, or ideas; it includes productivity, creativity, and concern for others in the broadest sense.[16]

The virtue acquired during this developmental stage is care—for family, friends, and society at large. Similarly, Stevenson described this as a stage of social productivity in which the individual focuses on bringing up a family and contributing to society to ensure its survival.[37] For some this is a time of beginning a family or taking on the role of the sandwich generation—that is, caring for both the younger and the older generations.[2,8,9,20] According to Erikson, when this enrichment and fulfillment is not experienced, stagnation and personal impoverishment occur, causing isolation and preoccupation with the self. If a person fails to be a productive adult who tries to improve society or influence future generations, life may be tedious and devoid of further development. The mobilization of inner resources, however, generates the creativity and productivity that encourage continued growth throughout the remaining years.

In Levinson's description of the "seasons of life" or the life course, the midlife transition is the period when adults become more compassionate, more evaluative, more tolerant and loving of themselves and others, and less driven by external demands and conflicts than in previous stages.[23] This external orientation to the world contrasts with the internal orientation of young adults who are preoccupied with achieving goals, obtaining independence, and gaining approval from the outside world. Midlife is a time when renewal and full development of relationships can occur. Once children are grown, child-centered patterns are altered and the intimate relationship between a couple can be nurtured. However, mutual support, open communication, and an awareness of each other's needs are necessary ingredients for an enriching relationship. Although the person may be enjoying the enrichment of a new and renewed relationship, there is the inevitable experience of loss of significant others. Death may take friends, parents, family, or spouse, necessitating alterations in relationships and life-styles.

*Middle adulthood* is thought to be a time of continued social influence, prosperity, economic success, and stability. Because work is an important part of the middle adult years, job loss or change may threaten one's self-concept and can result in altered health status. Unless illness or injury causes a setback, most persons become the "senior member" in their particular world niche. This means that middle adults must be responsible for their own work, the work of others, and the mentorship of younger adults. For many adults the middle years are approached with a sense of frustration and failure if goals and expectations set in earlier years have not been reached and are not realistically attainable. The realization that the time has passed for achieving status and success is often a crisis-producing situation. Reevaluation tends to result in ambivalence and uncertainty regarding everyday tasks, reflecting a change in values and attitudes. The adult who once considered daily responsibilities to be fulfilling and enjoyable may begin to complain about being trapped. It is likely that the job or situation has not changed, but that the person has.

Stevenson described the **core middle years** (ages 30 to 50) as years concerned with assisting both the younger and older generations.[37] The term **sandwich generation** is used to refer to adults who are caught between the needs of their growing children and aging parents. For adults who delayed childbearing, parenting roles must be learned. Families with children experience predictable stages such as the preschool years, school-age years, teen years, and the launching period, each with its own unique challenges.[14] With the maturation of children comes the need to let go of parenting roles so that children can achieve independence and establish adult relationships. In situations in which life revolved solely around the children, parents may experience a profound sense of loss when the children depart.

The loss of the parenting role, often called the "empty nest syndrome," can affect both parents and may even result in symptoms of depression. Given the current economic and employment difficulties, parents may face a different type of life-style change and stress because children and grandchildren return to the nest or do not leave the parental home. *Middle adulthood* also is a time when some couples or individuals may decide to become parents through birth or adoption. New parents face the same psychosocial adjustments and stresses as younger adults—but in the context of social expectations and developmental issues of middle-aged adults.

This may also be a time when the health status of the adult's parents is changing. Illness and perhaps impending death often necessitate assuming the role of parent to one's own parent(s). Middle-aged adults are faced with difficult decisions regarding their parent's care. If the parent is no longer able to continue living independently, the family must consider options such as intermittent or live-in care at the parent's home, having the parents live with a family member, or institutionalization. These decisions may have profound emotional, life-style, and economic effects on the entire family.[15]

Although Loevinger's theory of psychosocial development does not provide age norms, the stages are consistent with those of some other theories. Younger adults and persons in Loevinger's *conscientious stage* tend to strive for independence, mastery, and achievement of goals.[24] As human beings get older, however, characteristics of higher stages of development, such as interdependence with others and the ability to cope with conflicting demands in relationships, are present.

The developmental milestones or achievements described are generalizations and do not occur for every adult according to the age-related guidelines. For example, the timing of developmental tasks may be altered depending on when the childbearing years begin. If a chronic or life-threatening illness strikes a person in the middle adult years, limitations posed by the illness or its treatment may alter the developmental schedule and require the person and family to adapt.[15] Although an illness could make it difficult for the person to achieve the "expected" tasks, knowledge of developmental theory helps nurses to assist patients. For example, a man who develops cardiac disease may decide to make a vocational change because of the stress in his job situation. His marital partner may adjust, too, by increasing her employment from part-time to full-time to supplement the family income. She might join him in an exercise routine that will help reduce stress, and they may seek joint counseling to help them work through the changes they experience. By recognizing norms, the nurse can assist family members experiencing an illness as they strive to maintain a fulfilling family life and community involvements.

Patients and their families often adjust to the challenges of illness by reformulating goals and roles so that generativity can be achieved. The grown family of a woman in her middle years who develops metastatic breast cancer may find that the traditional roles played by the father in the family have changed. Over the course of the mother's illness, the father learns to run a household, grocery shop, and do laundry, in addition to being a caregiver. Together, family members may struggle with the mother's limited life span and may plan special family events and celebrations that take into account the mother's limited physical functioning so that she has the opportunity to pass along family history and the wisdom she has acquired with age.

Sexuality in the middle years is affected by several factors, including the physical aspects of aging, general health status, preexisting illness, family and work pressures common to this phase of the life span, and attitudes about sexuality and sexual functioning. It is a myth, however, that with middle age comes the end of physical attractiveness and a decline in sexual interest and capacity for competent sexual functioning.[42] Youth-oriented sociocultural influences have perpetuated the notion that aging brings sexual decline. The adult who approaches the middle years with self-acceptance, an understanding about normal changes in sexuality, and alternatives to traditional ways of expressing sexuality is apt to have a satisfying and fulfilling sexual life in later years.

Some of the physical changes that accompany menopause may affect the pleasure of sexual intercourse. For example, delay in the production of vaginal lubrication caused by the decrease in steroids may result in some discomfort during intercourse, and on occasion the irritation may cause cystitis. There may be a tendency to refrain from sexual activity because of discomfort. If such problems exist, the nurse can explain their causes, suggest use of a water-soluble lubricant during intercourse, and advise the woman to consult her health care practitioner.

As men age, certain social and psychologic factors influence their sexual responsiveness. Masters and Johnson noted several recurrent themes in interviews concerned with waning of sexual responsiveness: monotony in the sexual relationship or a feeling of being taken for granted, concerns with economic or career pursuits, mental and physical fatigue, personal or spousal physical or mental illness, overindulgence in food or drink, and fear of failure. They suggest that practice of sexual activity contributes to the quality of the sexual relationship, as well as to the continuation of sexual activity into the later years.[7,42] In another study of individuals from 45 to 69 years of age, previous satisfaction with sexual experience was the most significant contributing factor to current sexual functioning, including interest in, frequency of, and enjoyment of sexual relations.[13]

Because of prevailing cultural attitudes about waning sexual interest in the middle years, sexual concerns often are ignored in the care and rehabilitation of the middle-aged adult. It is important that health care providers become knowledgeable about and sensitive to the sexual needs of patients, particularly those who experience injury or illness that restricts physical activity. The nurse also should be aware of the sexual and psychosocial needs of gay and lesbian patients and their partners as they age together.[7] It is important to remember that their relationships—like those of heterosexual couples—are similarly affected by injury and illness.

The nurse must recognize that certain illnesses and medications can interfere with sexual functioning.[42] Patients can be monitored for side effects, and alterations in treatment regimens can be made so that patients do not experience undesirable side effects. Nurses can help the patient cope with anxieties regarding sexual functioning by providing the opportunity to discuss these concerns with a urologist, gynecologist, or nurse trained in sexual counseling.

Finally, with the recognition that sexual functioning continues throughout the adult years, all women and men who are sexually active and not in a long-term monogamous relationship should be instructed to practice safer sex to help prevent HIV and other sexually transmitted diseases.

## COGNITIVE DEVELOPMENT

Creativity, productivity, and cognitive capacity remain stable in the middle years, contrary to some popular beliefs.[37] Researchers who have studied intellectual functioning in this group suggest that there is little or no decline in learning capability and memory function.[3,35] Active use of mental capacity throughout life contributes to mental productivity in the later years. Encouraging adults to maintain activities that are intellectually stimulating is an important aspect of health promotion for middle adulthood.

## SPIRITUAL DEVELOPMENT

Spiritual development in middle adulthood is described as a major task for those experiencing midlife transition.[6] The spiritual growth and meaning achieved during middle adulthood can result in spiritual change that manifests by changes in a person's attitudes and priorities. Bianchi[6] describes the midlife search for meaning as a blend of Jung's description of the inward dialogue that leads to confronting one's own mortality and Erikson's theory of the psychosocial stage of generativity. Rather than a blend, such spiritual development may be more properly characterized as a synthesis and integration of various aspects of development in the context of life experiences. It is suggested that the spiritual journey of aging is grounded in childhood and family experiences.[6] During the middle years, persons become more introspective and contemplative as they deal with issues of self-identity, the world of work and social responsibility, and intimacy and relationships. Such personal reflection takes place in the context of real or anticipated changes in the physical body and physical attributes. The *inward focus* of *middle adulthood* is not as egocentric as in early adulthood; the meaning of life is understood in connection with other human beings and the broader society as one moves toward old age and death. As with younger adults, life crises such as acute, chronic, and life-threatening illnesses can be catalysts for spiritual development and can even force patients to face their own mortality and the meaning of their lives. The nurse can be instrumental in helping patients express themselves and find meaning in the illness experience. The nurse can provide nonjudgmental support and advocacy for patients and their families as they seek meaning within the illness experience. For some patients the nurse may need to accommodate the visits of a minister, priest, or rabbi, whereas other patients may need the nurse to assist them with life-review activities. Most important, the nurse needs to be aware of his or her own spiritual development, which includes an ability to be open to and facilitate the spiritual development of patients whose stage of development and whose meanings differ from the nurse's. This ability is particularly significant because the nurse is most likely to be interacting with patients at a time of spiritual crisis and transformation (see Research box, p. 52).

## HEALTH PROMOTION

Because many of the causes of death during the adult years are at least partially preventable, *middle adulthood* is a time to focus on life-style patterns that promote health and reduce health risks.[40] For example, changes in health behaviors and life-styles have led to decreased mortality as a result of motor vehicle accidents[30] and fewer deaths from heart disease.[28] Life-style changes to promote and maintain health at this stage of development can affect both longevity and the number of years of healthy functioning in old age.

During middle adulthood, adults may experience increased disability because of illness, chronic conditions, occupational factors, stress, and life-style. However, health promotion and maintenance in the middle adult years can be very important in promoting optimal functioning and recovery from illness. The following sections address health-promotion needs and health risks in middle adulthood.

### Nutrition

Adults in the middle years require fewer calories because of reduced energy requirements. Excessive caloric intake relative to physical demands contributes to obesity and atherosclerosis, which are risk factors for coronary artery disease, hypertension, renal failure, and diabetes.[17,27] Adults in their middle years need to be aware that biologic changes necessitate a reduction in calories, saturated fats, and cholesterol. The diet should contain the four basic food groups, and the caloric intake should be based on age, body build, size, and activity patterns. Diet counseling should include specific examples of polyunsaturated oils, dairy products, and chicken or fish that can be substituted for red meats high in saturated fats and cholesterol. Adequate fluid intake will help prevent constipation, and a balanced diet will maintain weight control.

The calcium needs of middle adults, especially women, increase because of bone reabsorption. To prevent osteoporosis, daily calcium requirements for premenopausal women are 1000 to 1200 mg/dl, and 1500 to 2000 mg/dl for postmenopausal women. Because chronic disease is more prevalent in the middle years than among younger adults, diets may need to be tailored to the individual's specific health conditions.

### Exercise

Consistent exercise may minimize some of the physical changes associated with growing older. Throughout the adult years, exercise helps to maintain and improve muscle tone, strength, coordination, and weight. It improves work performance, reduces chronic fatigue, increases the efficiency of the cardiopulmonary system, and promotes relaxation. The regularity of exercise is important; sporadic exercise is not as effective. Exercise activities that are performed incorrectly and cause overexertion can be detrimental to a person's health. Adults in the middle years should increase exercise gradually, exercise consistently, and avoid overexertion.[27] Heart and respiratory rates should return to their normal status within 10 minutes after the exercise is stopped.

Before any exercise program is begun, a thorough health assessment, including preexisting health conditions, should be conducted. An assessment of daily activity patterns and a discussion about exercise preferences are useful in planning the specific kind and amount of exercise program desired. Consultation with specialists is recommended if the person is overweight, has a personal or family history of cardiovascular or respiratory illness, or has lead a physically inactive life.

Exercise programs are an important part of treatment in many chronic diseases. For some persons with type II diabetes, the illness is managed with diet and exercise. After cardiac illness, monitored exercise is prescribed as part of the treatment regimen. Nurses can play an important role as part of the health care team involved in the management of chronic conditions by assisting patients with exercise regimens.

### Rest and Sleep

Rest and sleep must be balanced with physical activity to keep the body functioning at its best. Sleep requirements remain the same during the middle and young adult years—between 6 and 8 hours daily.[17] After 40 years of age, adults experience some differences in sleep cycles and patterns, such as less deep sleep and frequent awakening during the night.[38] Subsequently, they may feel less rested.

It is important that such a change in pattern is not considered abnormal but viewed as a developmental change that adults in the middle years can incorporate into their daily schedules. Sleep and rest also may be affected by work schedules, stress, and illness. If a person experiences sleep difficulties, nurses can recommend decreased caffeine intake, reduction of stress, warm baths, and relaxation exercises to promote sleep.

## HEALTH RISKS

The leading cause of death in middle adulthood is malignant neoplasm.[28] The lung, rectum, breast, cervix, and oropharynx are the most common sites of malignant neoplasms in this age group. Lung cancer is the most common cause of death for both men and women, with breast cancer as the second leading cause of cancer deaths in women. The incidence of colorectal cancer has increased in African-American men, and African-American women have three times the cervical cancer death rate of white women.

Heart disease is the second leading cause of death in middle adulthood, followed by injuries, stroke, and suicide. Smoking is a major risk factor in the development of lung cancer, heart disease, chronic obstructive pulmonary disease, stroke, bladder cancer, and peptic ulcer. Certain dietary patterns are thought to contribute to the incidence of heart disease, some types of cancer, diabetes, and hypertension. Work-related hazards, including dust and chemicals, radiation, and environmental pollutants, are believed to contribute to the risk of cancer development.

The most common chronic conditions that affect persons in middle adulthood are arthritis, hypertension, and chronic sinusitis.[29] Obesity, alcoholism, substance abuse, anxiety, and depression also may create serious problems for this group and their families. Gum disease or periodonitis, which is caused by bacterial plaque, is the leading cause of tooth loss for persons older than 35 years. Loss of teeth can lead to altered self-image and nutritional deficits. Accidents and injuries are common acute health problems of this period of life. Fractures and dislocations (often occupation-related) are leading causes of injury to both sexes.

Prevention of illness and injury is the most effective means of dealing with these problems. Education tailored to the person's level of understanding, unique psychosocial circumstances, and cultural background should include information on diet, exercise, the need for routine health examinations and screening, and

## BOX 3-3 University Hospitals Nursing Assessment Tool*

Date: ______ Patient: ______ ID: ______
Informant: ______ Relationship: ______
Presenting problem: ______

### MENTAL STATUS

Appearance: ______

Mood, affect (including check for depression, orientation): ______

Cognitive function (examples): ______

Communication: ______

### SLEEPING

Does patient sleep well? ______ Feel well rested? ______
If not, explain: ______
Ease of falling asleep: ______ Nap pattern: ______
Hours per night/times up during the night: ______
Concerns of patient/family: ______

### SENSES

Sight: ______
Hearing: ______
Taste: ______ Smell: ______
Touch: ______

### ACTIVITIES OF DAILY LIVING

| | Independent | Dependent | Circle dependent activities |
|---|---|---|---|
| Bathing | | | Initiation of bath<br>Type of bathing (tub, shower, sponge)<br>Bath preparation<br>Get in/out of tub<br>Ability to wash self<br>Hair washing |
| Dressing | | | Clothing selection<br>Putting on garments<br>Doing up buttons, etc.<br>Appropriateness of attire<br>Undressing<br>Laundry |
| Transfer | | | From bed to chair<br>From chair to standing |
| Toileting | | | Able to find bathroom<br>Able to use toilet appropriately<br>Hygiene |
| Bowel continence | | | Frequency and control<br>Constipation |
| Feeding | | | |

*Courtesy University Hospitals of Cleveland, Cleveland, Ohio.

*Continued.*

**BOX 3-3 University Hospitals Nursing Assessment Tool—cont'd**

## INSTRUMENTAL ACTIVITIES OF DAILY LIVING

| | Alone | Assist | Never (N/A) | No longer | |
|---|---|---|---|---|---|
| Telephone | | | | | Look up number<br>Dial |
| Medication | | | | | Preparation<br>Taking |
| Outside of home | | | | | Organization<br>Getting lost |
| Driving | | | | | |
| Housework | | | | | Organization<br>Doing (List what able to do.) |
| Food preparation | | | | | Planning<br>Shopping<br>Preparing |
| Finances | | | | | Banking<br>Paying bills<br>Balancing checkbook |

## URINARY CONTINENCE

Does patient have "accidents"? (If "yes," when?) ______
Patient's knowledge of accidents: ______ Frequency: ______
Urgency: ______ Can patient get to bathroom in time? ______
Does patient wet when coughing or sneezing or at other times? ______
Where is center of concern about wetting (patient, family, both)? ______
Other concerns: ______

## MOBILITY

Walking ability (use of assistive devices): ______
Distance able to walk (and frequency): ______
Gait, posture: ______
Stiffness (morning, after inactivity, evening, where?): ______

What does patient do to maximize mobility? ______
Hand dexterity and function: ______
Problems with feet and shoes: ______
Other concerns of patient/family: ______

## NUTRITION

No. of meals per day: ______ No. of glasses of fluid: ______
Indigestion, nausea/vomiting, change in bowels: ______
Dentition: ______
Appetite: ______ Weight stability: ______
Concerns of family (need for referral to nutritionist): ______

**BOX 3-3 University Hospitals Nursing Assessment Tool—cont'd**

**MEDICATIONS**

List medications as prescribed and how they are taken in ( ) (Note how long patient has been on medication.)

Patient's knowledge of medications (reason for, side effects, precatuions)

Nonprescription medications:

Allergies (medications): (other):

Person responsible for medication administration:

Alcohol intake (past/present): Smoking history:

**SAFETY**

Is patient alone at any time? Gets lost?

Kitchen safety:

Household safety (rugs, cords, railings, stairs):

Other concerns:

**CARE GIVER**

Name of formal care giver: Relationship:

Informal care-giving system:

Care giver's role/function:

Impact of care giving on care giver/family:

Assessment of stability/security provided in present care environment:

**SUMMARY**

Completed by:

proper dental care. Moderate use of alcohol, not smoking, and safety-related practices such as using seat belts are effective means of preventing illness and injury in adults. Health problems of older adulthood are discussed in Chapter 4.

## HEALTH ASSESSMENT

A critical component of health promotion and risk prevention for adults in the middle years is regular health assessment. Periodic assessments also provide the opportunity to identify chronic illnesses that are associated with old age and may result in early disability. This is of particular concern in later midlife for African-Americans, Hispanics, or Native Americans (see Chapters 4 and 8). Adults in midlife should have a thorough yearly health examination that includes a detailed medical history, occupational history, physical assessment of body systems, blood and urine tests, electrocardiogram, chest x-ray examination, and rectal or proctoscopic examination. Men should have testicular exams, and women should have Pap smear tests, breast examinations, and mammography as indicated. Routine dental, vision, and hearing examinations should be done because periodontal disease, glaucoma, and hearing loss may be prevented or treated if detected early.[41]

## NURSING ASSESSMENT

As people develop and change through the life span, so do their health needs. A developmental perspective is helpful for understanding the physical and psychosocial factors that influence health at various points in the life span. When working with an adult who is experiencing physical or emotional stress, the nurse must assess the medical problems at hand, as well as the physical, psychosocial, and situational factors relative to the person's developmental status.

The assessment also should include a mental health assessment, with emphasis on screening for the presence of alcohol and drug abuse, symptoms of depression, and suicidal thoughts. Such mental health concerns may be exacerbated by or secondary to chronic and acute illnesses. It is often the nurse in the acute care setting who has the opportunity to identify mental health problems, provide immediate intervention, and request follow-up referrals. Box 3-3 provides an example of a comprehensive assessment tool, including an adapted Katz's activities of daily living scale, Barthel's instrumental activities scale, and a mental health assessment scale.

Data from the nursing assessment provide guidance in understanding those factors that may be affecting the person's response to stress, feelings and attitudes about recovery, and potential to adapt. When a person's goals and expectations are thwarted by illness or disability, a crisis may result. This crisis affects members of the family, as well as the individual, and may require adaptation on their part also. The nurse should demonstrate acceptance of the person's behaviors and attitudes, realizing that this may be the individual's unique manner of coping with stress. When stress is intense, problem-solving abilities may be diminished. The nurse can help the individual and family make decisions by offering options and referral to resources. In this way, their needs can be met while the nurse fosters and maintains their independence by facilitating participation in care planning and decision making.

## QUESTIONS TO CONSIDER

- Using the theories and stages identified in Table 3-2, choose the developmental stage that best describes you at this point in your life. What are the typical developmental tasks associated with your present stage?
- Think about a middle-aged adult patient with whom you have recently worked. How did the patient's illness situation affect the achievement of developmental tasks (or how might the illness have affected developmental tasks)?
- Think about a young adult you know. Describe the person's behavior on the basis of Erikson's theories.

## CRITICAL THINKING ACTIVITIES

- Connie, age 30, was diagnosed in her teens with diabetes mellitus and is regulated on daily insulin and diet. She is single and lives with her parents. Renee, age 45, was recently diagnosed with cancer of the breast. She has 3 children ages 10, 13, and 17. Compare and discuss the effect that a chronic illness has on the young versus middle-aged adult.
- Discuss why it may be misleading to rigidly adhere to specific developmental expectations for specific age groups when planning nursing care.

## CHAPTER SUMMARY

### THE PROCESS OF HUMAN GROWTH AND DEVELOPMENT

- Each human being grows and develops physically and psychosocially in a unique way during the adult years.

### EARLY ADULTHOOD

- Psychosocial stages in young adults can be characterized by an emphasis on gaining and maintaining individual goals and independence.

### MIDDLE ADULTHOOD

- In middle adulthood the focus of development is on concern for others, productivity, and creativity rather than external demands and expectations.

### HEALTH ASSESSMENT

- Human behavior is extremely complex, and it is difficult to predict how patients might respond to illness situations. Theories of life-span development combine physical, psychosocial, sexual, cognitive, and spiritual aspects of the growth process; they provide nurses with general guidelines about specific periods of the life span that are useful in planning nursing care for adults of all ages.

### NURSING ASSESSMENT

- Although implications for nursing care of young adults and those in midlife can be suggested, it is critical to include the patient in the decision-making process to individualize the plan of care to each person's unique personal, family, and social situation.
- Physiologically, young adults are functioning at peak efficiency. As the adult years progress, normal changes occur very gradually.

## REFERENCES


1. Ahlfield J, Soler N, Marcus S: The young adult with diabetes: impact of the disease on marriage and having children, *Diabetes Care* 8(1):52-56, 1985.
2. Austin JK: Family adaptation to a child's chronic illness. In Fitzpatrick JF, Taunton RL, Jacox AK, editors: *Annual review of nursing research,* vol 10, New York, 1991, Springer.
3. Baltes P: Theoretical propositions of life-span developmental psychology: on the dynamics between growth and decline, *Dev Psychol* 23(5):611-626, 1987.
4. Bee H, Mitchell S: *The developing person: a life-span approach,* ed 2, New York, 1984, Harper & Row.
5. Belenky M et al: *Women's ways of knowing,* New York, 1986, Basic Books.
6. Bianchi EC: *Aging as a spiritual journey,* New York, 1990, Crossroad.
7. Boston Women's Health Book Collective: *The new revised our bodies, ourselves,* New York, 1992, Simon & Schuster.
8. Bowers B: Intergenerational caregiving: adult caregivers and their aging parents, *Adv Nurs Sci* 9(2):20-31, 1987.
9. Brody E: Parent care as a normative stress, *Gerontologist* 25(1):19, 1985.
10. Carter B, McGoldrick M, editors: *The changing family life cycle,* Boston, 1989, Allyn & Bacon.
11. Centers for Disease Control: *Homicide surveillance: high risk racial and ethnic groups, blacks and Hispanics, 1970 to 1983,* Atlanta, 1985, Center for Health Promotion and Education.
12. Dimond M, Jones S: *Chronic illness across the life span,* Norwalk, Conn, 1983, Appleton-Century-Crofts.
13. Dresen SE: The middle years: the sexually active middle adult, *Am J Nurs* 75:1001-1005, 1975.
14. Duvall EM: *Marriage and family development,* ed 5, Philadelphia, 1977, JB Lippincott.
15. Eisenberg M, Sutkin L, Jansen M, editors: *Chronic illness and disability through the life span,* New York, 1984, Springer.
16. Erikson EH: *Childhood and society,* ed 2, New York, 1963, WW Norton.
17. Gallagher L, Kreidler MC: *Nursing and health: maximizing human potential throughout the life cycle,* Norwalk, Conn, 1987, Appleton & Lange.
18. Giele JZ: *Women in the middle years,* New York, 1982, John Wiley & Sons.
19. Gilligan C: *In a different voice: psychological theory and women's development,* Cambridge, 1982, Harvard University Press.
20. Given BA, Given CW: Family caregiving for the elderly. In Fitzpatrick JF, Taunton RL, Jacox AK, editors: *Annual review of nursing research,* vol 10, New York, 1991, Springer.
21. Koplowitz H: A projection beyond Piaget's formal-operations stage: a general system stage and unitary stage. In Commons ML, Richards FA, Armon C, editors: *Beyond formal operations: late adolescent and adult cognitive development,* New York, 1984, Praeger.
22. Lancaster L: Impact of chronic illness over the life span, *ANNA J* 15(3):164-198, 193, 1988.
23. Levinson D: *The seasons of a man's life,* New York, 1978, Ballantine/Del Rey/Fawcett Books.
24. Loevinger J: *Ego development: conceptions and theories,* San Francisco, 1976, Jossey-Bass.
25. McBride A: The experience of being a parent. In Werley H, Fitzpatrick J, Taunton R, editors: *Annual review of nursing research,* vol 2, New York, 1984, Springer.
26. Mecham PJ et al: *Suicide attempts among young adults.* Paper presented at the thirty-ninth annual Epidemic Intelligence Service conference, Atlanta, 1990.
27. Murray R, Zentner J: *Nursing assessment and health promotion through the life span,* ed 5, Englewood Cliffs, NJ, 1993, Prentice-Hall.
28. National Center for Health Statistics: *Health, United States, 1989 and prevention profile,* Department of Health and Human Services Pub No (PHS) 90-1232, Hyattsville, Md, 1990, US Department of Health and Human Services.
29. National Center for Health Statistics, Collins J: *Prevalence of selected chronic conditions, United States, 1983-1985: advance data from vital and health statistics,* No 155, Department of Health and Human Services Pub No (PHS) 88-1250, Hyattsville, Md, 1988, US Public Health Service.
30. National Center for Statistics and Analysis: *Occupant protection facts,* Washington, DC, 1989, US Department of Transportation.
31. Piaget J: The stages of intellectual development of the child, *Bull Menninger Clin* 26(4103):120, 1962.
32. Primomo J: *Patterns of chronic illness management, psychosocial development, family and social environment, and adaptation among diabetic women,* doctoral dissertation, Seattle, 1989, University of Washington.
33. Rossman I: *Clinical geriatrics,* ed 3, Philadelphia, 1986, JB Lippincott.
34. Shaver JLF, Giblen EC: Sleep. In Fitzpatrick JF, Taunton RL, Benoliel JQ, editors: *Annual review of nursing research,* vol 7, New York, 1989, Springer.
35. Sorensen A, Weinert F, Sherrod L, editors: *Human development and the life course: multidisciplinary perspectives,* Hillsdale, NJ, 1987, Lawrence Erlbaum Associates.
36. Stanwyck D: Self-esteem through the life span, *Fam Community Health* 6(2):11-28, 1983.
37. Stevenson J: Adulthood: a promising direction for future research. In Werley H, Fitzpatrick J, Taunton R, editors: *Annual review of nursing research,* vol 1, New York, 1983, Springer.
38. US Bureau of the Census: *Statistical abstracts of the United States, 1988,* annual ed 108, Washington, DC, 1988, US Government Printing Office.
39. US Bureau of the Census: *1990 Population of census and housing,* Washington, DC, 1991, US Government Printing Office.
40. US Department of Health and Human Services, Public Health Services: *Healthy people 2000: national health promotion and disease prevention objectives,* Washington, DC, 1990, US Government Printing Office.
41. Wolanin MD, Philips LRF: *Confusion, prevention, and care,* St Louis, 1981, Mosby.
42. Woods NF: *Human sexuality in health and illness,* ed 3, St Louis, 1984, Mosby.

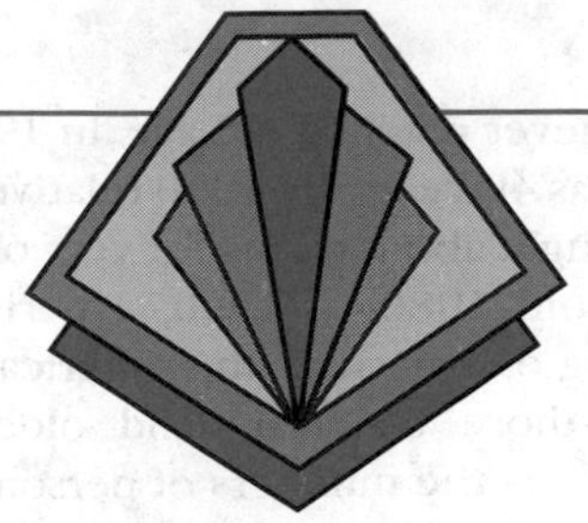

CHAPTER 4

# Nursing Practice With Elders

***Denise M. Kresevic***
***Ruth A. Lincoln***

## CHAPTER OBJECTIVES

***After studying this chapter, the learner should be able to do the following:***

1. Distinguish between primary and secondary changes of aging.
2. Describe psychosocial aspects of aging.
3. Compare health concerns of elderly adults with those of younger adults.
4. Describe health-promotion strategies for the older adult.
5. Describe special precautions for hospitalized elders.

## KEY TERMS

| | | |
|---|---|---|
| activities of daily living (ADLs) | dysfunctional syndrome | orthostatic hypotension |
| Alzheimer's disease | gerontology | pressure sore |
| delirium | incontinence | primary aging |
| dementia | instrumental activities of daily living | secondary aging |
| durable power of attorney | living will | shearing lesion |

## HISTORICAL PERSPECTIVES

Human beings have the longest life span of any animal species. Yet for centuries mystery and myth have surrounded the phenomenon of aging. Hippocrates believed that the vital life force was heat. The ancient Greeks believed that this innate heat was gradually used up in the normal process of aging. They observed then, as has been confirmed today, that old people are subject to a host of health problems, including dyspnea, joint pains, dizzy spells, insomnia, and visual and hearing losses. The teachings of Sir Francis Bacon (1561-1626) marked the beginning of the scientific approach to aging. Bacon believed that the effects of aging accounted for the physical decline of joints and vision. According to Bacon, factors slowing or accelerating the effects of aging included physical stature, temperament, environment, diet, and heredity. These factors remain important correlates that affect health even today. Metchnikoff (1845-1916) regarded aging as a natural physiologic process beginning at the moment of conception, and Nasher (1863-1944) argued that age-related diseases were distinct from aging as a normal process. In 1909 Nasher used the word *geriatrics* to refer to diseases of old age. In 1927 Rybrikov, a Russian psychologist, referred to the aging process as the study of **gerontology.** Over time, the following *five basic characteristic patterns of aging* have been identified:

1. Increased mortality with age
2. Changes in the chemical composition of the body, including a decrease in lean body mass, an increase in fats and lipofuscins, and cross-linking of collagen tissues
3. Progressive deteriorative changes demonstrated in cross-sectional longitudinal studies
4. Reduced ability to adapt to environmental changes
5. Increased vulnerability to multiple diseases

Nurses have cared for elders and their family members throughout history. In 1904 the *American Journal of Nursing* published an article on old age and disease. The American Nurses Association (ANA), guided by an understanding of normal aging, the unique needs of elders, and a commitment to scientific care, established a division of geriatric nursing in 1966 to develop standards of nursing care for elders. These standards are used to

**BOX 4-1 Standards of Geriatric Nursing Practice**

1. All gerontological nursing services are planned, organized, and directed by a nurse executive. The nurse executive has a baccalaureate or master's preparation and has experience in gerontological nursing and administration.
2. The nurse participates in the generation and testing of theory as a basis for clinical decisions. The nurse uses theoretical concepts to guide the effective practice of gerontological nursing.
3. The health status of the older person is regularly assessed in a comprehensive, accurate and systematic manner. Information obtained in the health assessment is shared with appropriate members of the interdisciplinary health care team including the older person and family.
4. The nurse uses health assessment data to determine nursing diagnosis.
5. The nurse develops the plan of care in conjunction with the older person, mutually setting goals to address preventive, restorative, and rehabilitative needs of the older person. The plan of care helps the older person attain and maintain the highest level of health, well-being and quality of life achievable, as well as a peaceful death. The plan of care facilitates continuity of care over time as the client moves to various settings.
6. The nurse intervenes to provide care to restore the older person's functional capabilities and to prevent complications and excessive disability.
7. The nurse continually evaluates the client's and family's response to interventions, to determine attainment of goals and needed revisions.
8. The nurse collaborates regularly with the health care team.
9. The nurse participates in research to generate knowledge development, and dissemination of findings into practice settings.
10. The nurse is guided by the ANA code of ethics.
11. The nurse assumes responsibility for professional development, including peer review.

From American Nurses Association.

guide clinical care, knowledge development, and research endeavors. In 1981 the ANA published standards of care to guide generalist and advanced practice nurses caring for elders. These standards, which serve as a model for practice, apply to all settings and can be used to evaluate care (Box 4-1).

This chapter discusses the characteristics of elders from a health perspective. Major health needs of elderly persons and the role of the nurse in assisting them with health promotion and health problems are addressed. The chapter focuses on assisting elderly persons to improve their quality of life.

Two groups constitute those who are collectively referred to as elders. These are persons in late adulthood (ages 65 to 85 years) and the old-old group (persons 85 years of age and older).

## DEMOGRAPHIC TRENDS

America is a nation of aging people. In colonial times, half the population was younger than 16 years of age and most Americans never reached old age. In 1900 life expectancy at birth was 49 years. By 1950 relatively few American families thought about caring for very old, frail persons. However, from 1980 to 1990, a period described as "the graying of America," the American population of *old-old*—those 85 years and older—increased by 38%, whereas the numbers of persons aged 65 to 84 years increased only 20% and those younger than 65 years of age increased by only 8%. By 1990 the so-called baby boomers (persons born between 1946 and 1964) constituted one third of the population of the United States and the number of elders reached 30 million. It is predicted that by 2010 the number of elders will reach 39 million and by 2030, 66 million. This age-group, which comprised 4% of the population in 1900, will increase 23% by the year 2030, with the largest growth occurring among those older than 85 years. Americans indeed reflect an aging population, with four-generational families becoming common as more and more Americans live into their 100s (Figure 4-1).

These demographic trends have had a significant impact not only on families and the labor force but also on the health care system. More and more elders are living longer with chronic illnesses and functional disability and are surviving catastrophic acute illnesses. The health care needs of these persons will continue to increase. Those caring for this aging population will need increased knowledge and skills to help this group to maintain health and function and to avoid complications—all of which will affect the quality and cost of care for elders.

Improving the quality of life, rather than searching for means to increase longevity, becomes of utmost importance. According to *Healthy People 2000* the major goal for the 1990s is to increase the span of *healthy life* for all Americans.

## BIOLOGIC THEORIES OF AGING

Several biologic theories of aging have been proposed. Although none of these theories adequately explains the complex phenomenon of aging, they do add significantly to our understanding of the process. Biologic theories of aging attempt to explain cellular function and mutation throughout the life cycle. Five of these theories are discussed here.

The *error theory* focuses on the phenomenon of decreased bonding of protein cells that occurs spontaneously or in response to stressors such as radiation. This stressor results in errors in the synthesis of RNA and DNA and produces cells with impaired function.

The *somatic mutation theory,* similar to the error theory, suggests that cells exposed to chemicals or radiation result in alterations within the DNA molecule. Mutations result from these alterations, accumulate over time, and become more evident with age and increasing cellular impairment. Some studies support this theory. Aging cells of the immune system have been noted to

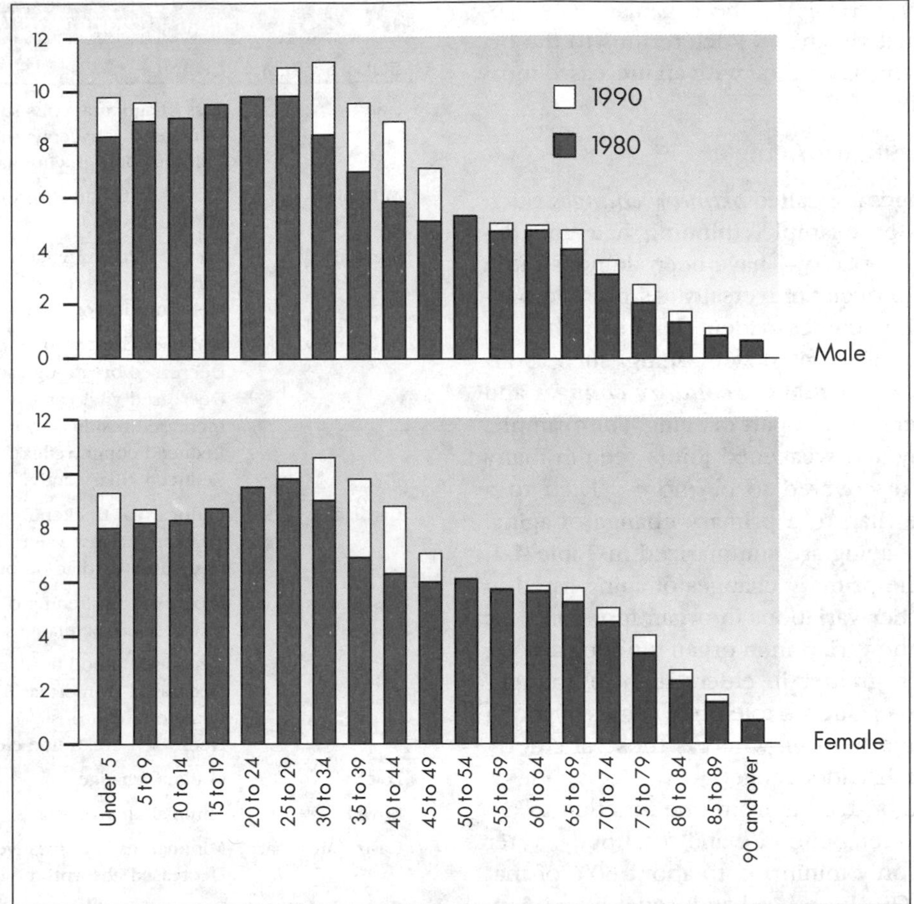


**FIGURE 4-1** Graphs showing that 1 in 8 Americans are elderly. *Top,* Male population by age in 1980 and in 1990. *Bottom,* Female population by age in 1980 and in 1990. (From U.S. Bureau of the Census, U.S. Department of Commerce, 1991.)

become increasingly diversified, and they progressively lose normal self-regulatory functions, including antibody function. Therefore the mutation theory provides a greater understanding of such well-known aging changes as those manifested in the autoimmune abnormalities common in elders.

The *cross-link theory* postulates that chemical reactions create bonds between molecular structures that normally are separate. Cross-linking occurs in aging collagen tissue. Collagen maintains tissue structure form, support, and strength. Cross-linking also occurs in connective tissues, resulting in a loss of elasticity. This cross-link theory provides an explanation for the aging changes that occur in the skin and muscles, including the heart, in which elasticity is replaced with more rigid and fragile tissues.

The *free radical theory* postulates that the oxidation of proteins, fats, and carbohydrates results in unpaired ions or free radicals. These free radicals attach to other cells and jeopardize normal cellular functions. Scientists have postulated that vitamins A and C, as well as niacin, usually low in elders, can function as scavengers for the free radicals.

The *wear and tear theory* of aging, first described by Sir Francis Bacon, is relevant even today. Bacon noted that cells subjected to repeated injury or overuse responded with injurious metabolic by-products, cellular dysfunction, and ultimately cellular death. It is of interest that this theory offers a basic explanation for the aging changes seen in striated, skeletal, cardiac, and nerve cells that may be destroyed by mechanical or chemical wear and tear.

## GENERAL RESPONSES TO AGING

Many of the physical changes that begin gradually during adulthood continue through the later adult years. **Biologic aging** leads to some general responses in the older person. First, there is a gradual decline in functional ability, particularly where multisystem coordination is required. These age decrements are greater in performances that require more complex functioning than in those involving individual system functions.

The research on biologic aging has generated a body of knowledge regarding the normal and abnormal changes associated with the aging process. Normal aging changes are those that are (1) universal to all members of the species, (2) intrinsic to the organism, (3) progressive and cumulative, and (4) deleterious to the organism as a whole and associated with an increased mortality.

## Primary and Secondary Aging

Normal aging changes are called *primary changes.* Such effects of aging—for example, thinning hair and decreased pulmonary capacity—have been demonstrated through research to occur universally. As more knowledge is generated, it becomes evident that many changes once thought to be associated with aging, such as arthritis and senility, are actually *secondary changes* and do not occur universally as a part of aging. For example, the muscle atrophy and weakened joints seen in many elders have been discovered to be more related to a sedentary life-style than to a primary change of aging. Primary changes of aging are summarized in Table 4-1.

In addition to the primary changes of aging listed in Table 4-1, some other variations in organ function bear mentioning. First, the variation in organ function among individuals is much greater in elders than in younger persons. For example, glucose tolerance values of young adults cluster around a norm, whereas those of elderly persons have a much wider range.

Second, the rate of decline from one function to another varies. Basal metabolic rate and total body water of elders decrease only minimally to about 80% of that of young adults.[38] On the other hand, renal blood flow and maximum breathing capacity show a significant decline in most elderly persons.

A third major change related to the aging process occurs in response to stress. Although an aged person may have adequate cardiac output at rest, stress in the form of an infection, exertion, or emotional shock will decrease cardiac output, and it will take much longer for it to return to the person's baseline level. In addition, there is a loss of reserve capacity related to a decline in coordination of brain interactions. This decline causes a slowing of reaction time and a greater susceptibility to infection and accidents.

**TABLE 4-1 Primary Changes of Aging**

| BODY SYSTEM | CHANGE |
|---|---|
| Skin | Loss of subcutaneous supportive tissue<br>Decreased sebaceous secretions<br>Thinning and graying hair |
| Muscular | Increased fat substitution for muscle<br>Muscle atrophy |
| Skeletal | Loss of calcium from bones<br>Shrinkage of vertebral disks<br>Deterioration of cartilage |
| Pulmonary | Reduced chest wall compliance<br>Decreased breathing capacity<br>Decreased vital capacity<br>Increased residual volume<br>Reduced cough reflex<br>Reduced ciliary activity |
| Cardiac | Endocardial thickening<br>Thickened heart valves<br>Decreased cardiac output (under stress) |
| Vascular | Progressive stiffening of arteries<br>Atherosclerotic plaques |
| Renal | Decreased blood flow<br>Decreased glomerular filtration rate<br>Reduced nephrons<br>Decreased creatinine clearance |
| Liver | Minimal change |
| Bowel | Minimal change |
| Gastrointestinal | Minimal loss of digestive enzymes<br>Decreased absorption |
| Endocrine | Decreased utilization of insulin<br>Cessation of progesterone<br>Decline, then plateau of estrogen<br>Gradual decline in testosterone |
| Vision | Deterioration in ability of lens to focus<br>Loss of color sensitivity<br>Decreased dark adaptation<br>Decreased peripheral vision<br>Decreased sensitivity to glare |
| Hearing | Increased threshold for high frequencies<br>Difficulty in speech discrimination<br>Degeneration of cochlea and auditory pathways |
| Sexual | Minimal change in amount of sexual response<br>Increase in time for full sexual response<br>Decreased vaginal lubrication<br>Increased refractory period for males |

From Rossman I: *Clinical geriatrics,* ed 3, Philadelphia, 1986, JB Lippincott.

## PSYCHOSOCIAL DEVELOPMENT IN OLDER ADULTS

Loevinger's description of the higher stages of development gives us a better understanding of how people might adjust to the later years of life. As people age and increasingly depend on others for assistance, they also may provide assistance to those who help them. There are many examples of this mutual interdependence. When grandparents provide child care assistance to the childrearing family, all three generations benefit mutually. The grandparents have an opportunity to share their wisdom, the parents have tangible assistance while they pursue their vocational roles, and the children receive love and nurturance. Some older adults who want to maintain their independence as long as possible choose to live in retirement complexes where assistance is available if needed. The decision to enter a residential facility may result in inner conflict concerning giving up and moving out of one home, establishing a new home, and accepting the possibility of future dependence.

Emotional and psychologic responses to aging have been explored by numerous researchers. In one survey elderly persons were asked what they considered essential for happiness. They mentioned good health, a place to live, enough money to live comfortably, recognition by others, and the opportunity for a variety of experiences.[15,16] Reed, a nurse scientist, identified four dimensions of development in older adults: (1) transcendence, the orientation toward purposes greater than the self, (2) temporal awareness, the awareness of time and that a person's time is limited, (3) plasticity, the ability to make changes, and (4) the maintenance of physical integrity.[26] Cummings and Henry described the elderly person's response to the reality of death as one of release, characterized by "a mutual withdrawal or disengagement."[8] Either the individual or the social system might initiate the withdrawal. The outcome of this response might be a movement away from involvement, achievement, and productivity on the part of the older adult.

Many younger people falsely assume that older persons have no interest in sex and lack the ability to perform sexually. Men and women of all ages are capable of sexual arousal and orgasm. Masters and Johnson emphasize that one of the primary factors in maintaining sexual activity in old age is the frequency of sexual performance.[23] Studies conducted at the Duke University Center for the Study of Aging revealed sexual activity in the eighth and ninth decades. Often the aged person becomes sexually inactive because of lack of an acceptable partner or the presence of symptoms associated with chronic disease (pain, dyspnea, chronic fatigue) that are common in the old old.

The primary nursing focus of meeting the psychosocial needs of elderly persons is to help them make the adjustments necessary to achieve the desired goals. A first step is to understand the needs of the person. The desires of elders and the difficulties that must be overcome to obtain them should both be considered in planning their nursing care. Success in meeting this objective depends on the nurse developing a plan that reflects the following concepts of normal aging and individual variations: (1) emotional development continues in the older adult years and is associated with new tasks of living, (2) each elderly individual has different expectations of a life that is worth living, (3) each will react differently to the limitations and frustrations that are imposed on achieving and maintaining this worthwhile existence, and (4) elderly persons often will react (cope) essentially as they have reacted to other stresses throughout their lives. (See Chapter 3 for other theories that underlie the psychosocial development of adults, especially Table 3-2, which presents a summary.)

As mentioned in Chapter 3, human beings have a tremendous potential to grow and change during every phase of life. Psychosocial development is a lifelong process that is reflected in how human beings perceive the nature of the world.[2,26] The tasks of later adulthood are listed in Box 4-2. Knowledge of developmental changes and events that occur in the later adult years is useful in understanding how people adapt to health and illness. Knowledge of developmental processes is vital to understanding behavioral changes throughout the life span, interpreting behaviors of older adults, and assisting them with their health and developmental needs.

**BOX 4-2 Tasks of Later Adulthood**

- Assuming responsibility for sharing the wisdom of age
- Reminiscing and participating in life review
- Putting affairs in order
- Accepting life with serenity
- Adjusting to new limitations of declining physical strength and declining health
- Adjusting to reorganized family patterns
- Adjusting to a new pattern of social and civic responsibilities
- Adjusting to death of spouse and other loved ones
- Establishing affiliation with one's age-group
- Maintaining satisfactory living arrangements
- Accepting death with serenity and assisting others to accept death

## ASSESSMENT OF ELDERS

Assessment is a critical step in effective nursing care for elders. The global aspects of health in elders can be separated into *three major concepts: absence of disease, performance of basic self-care activities,* termed **activities of daily living (ADLs),** and *performance of more complex activities,* called **instrumental activities of daily living.**

Beginning as early as the late 1800s, information on functional health as an estimate of morbidity was obtained in Europe and the United States. During the 1940s, classifications of disability included self-care activities of dressing, toileting, and ambulation. Since that time, three self-maintenance components have consistently been identified: *basic activities of daily living* (bathing, eating, toileting), *more complex social activities of living* (shopping, managing finances, cooking, housekeeping, transportation, managing medications), and the ability to use a telephone and cope with other aspects of one's environment—that is, *instrumental activities of daily living.*

Functional disability has been demonstrated to correlate with physical illness, self-care ability, complications during hospitalization, rehabilitation potential, and even mortality. Therefore the concept of *functional ability in elders has become a valuable health indicator.* Measures of functional status that examine the ability to function independently despite disease are the most useful clinical and research indicators of elders with multiple chronic and acute illnesses.

In addition to assessing the respiratory, cardiovascular, digestive, neurologic, and other body systems of the elderly patient, the nurse must carefully assess the elder's *functional self-care ability.* Subtle changes in appetite or ambulation or even the onset of urinary incontinence may be the initial and only clinical indicator of infections such as pneumonia, urinary tract infections, or even myocardial infarctions. Several functional assessment tools and scales have been widely used in a variety of clinical settings, including the Katz ADL scale and the Bathel index. (See Chapter 3, Box 3-3, for an example of an assessment tool developed by clinical gerontologic nurse specialists in one institution.) See Research box below.

## UNIQUE PATTERNS OF ILLNESS AMONG ELDERS

A hallmark of gerontology is that disease may have atypical presentations in elders (Table 4-2). Often acute illnesses are superimposed on several chronic illnesses complicated by the effects of primary aging. A careful history, as well as knowledge about the unique clinical presentation in elders, aids the clinician in assessment, in establishing nursing diagnoses, and in effective interventions. In assessing the health and illness patterns of elders, some general factors must be recognized. *First,* age-related decline in immune function results in a less rapid and less effective response to infections and in an increased incidence of autoimmune and malignant disease.[17] *Second,* stress situations (either physiologic or psychosocial) produce more pronounced reactions in elderly persons and require a longer time for readjustment. *Third,* complex functions that require multisystem coordination show the most obvious decline and require the greatest compensation and support. *Fourth,* elders frequently have atypical manifestations of an illness. Pain may be less pronounced, and some typical symptoms may be either missing or the opposite of what is expected (when compared with what is seen in younger age-groups). Confusion, restlessness, or other altered mentation is a common occurrence in the presence of illness. Obscure or unexplained deterioration of health or function should not be accepted as normal aging and must be evaluated carefully.

Multiplicity and chronicity of diseases are common among elders, and many patients have several chronic ailments. Most have developed slowly. Heart disease, cancer, renal disease, vascular disease such as cerebrovascular accident, chronic obstructive pulmonary disease such as emphysema, and accidents are the most common problems that bring elderly persons to the hospital. Other common chronic ailments such as arthritis, skin disorders, mild neuromuscular conditions, and hearing impairments usually are cared for while the person is ambulatory. The most common diseases are ar-

### RESEARCH

Sholes D et al: Tracking progress toward national health objectives in the elderly: what do restricted activity days signify? *Am J Public Health* 81(4):485-588, 1991.

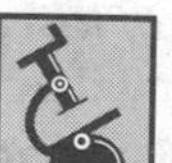

This study evaluated restricted activity days (RAD) as an outcome measure in a random study of 2300 health maintenance organization enrollees. RAD is the measure by which the health objectives for 1990 for prevention of functional disability in older adults were evaluated. RAD was correlated more with physical disability measures than with mental, social, and global self-perceived health.

**TABLE 4-2 How Illness Changes With Age**

| PROBLEM | CLASSIC PRESENTATION IN YOUNG PATIENT | PRESENTATION IN ELDERLY |
|---|---|---|
| Urinary tract infection | Dysuria, frequency, urgency, nocturia | Dysuria often *absent;* frequency, urgency, nocturia sometimes present. Incontinence, confusion, anorexia are other signs. |
| Myocardial infarction | Severe substernal chest pain, diaphoresis, nausea, shortness of breath | Sometimes no chest pain, or atypical pain location such as in jaw, neck, shoulder. Shortness of breath may be present. Other signs are tachypnea, arrhythmia, hypotension, restlessness, syncope. |
| Pneumonia (bacterial) | Cough productive of purulent sputum, chills and fever, pleuritic chest pain, elevated white blood cell count | Cough may be productive, dry or absent; chills and fever and/or elevated white count also may be absent. Tachypnea, slight cyanosis, confusion, anorexia, nausea and vomiting, tachycardia may be present. |
| Congestive heart failure | Increased dyspnea (orthopnea, paroxysmal nocturnal dyspnea), fatigue, weight gain, pedal edema, night cough and nocturia, bibasilar rales | All of the manifestations of young adult and/or anorexia, restlessness, confusion, cyanosis, falls. |
| Hyperthyroidism | Heat intolerance, fast pace, exophthalmos, increased pulse, hyperreflexia, tremor | Slowing down (apathetic hyperthyroidism), lethargy, weakness, depression, atrial fibrillation and congestive heart failure. |
| Depression | Sad mood and thoughts, withdrawal, crying, weight loss, constipation, insomnia | Any of classic signs, plus memory and concentration problems, weight gain, increased sleep. |

Modified from Henderson ML: *Am J Nurs* 85(10):110, 1985.

thritis, heart disease, hypertension, and diabetes.[7] The *three most common causes of death in older adults are heart disease, malignant neoplasms, and cerebrovascular accidents.*[17,24] Changes in two of the body systems are discussed next.

## CARDIOVASCULAR SYSTEM

The Framingham heart study, which has followed up more than 5000 persons for over 40 years, suggests that *acute myocardial infarction* in elders often *is not accompanied by pain.* More common symptoms include weakness and confusion. Pulmonary edema, congestive heart failure, and conduction defects such as heart block or atrial fibrillation that often occur with a myocardial infarction are not common in elders, whose only symptom may be confusion.

Asymptomatic drops in blood pressure are common in elders after position changes or ingestion of meals. These episodes of hypotension place elders at significant risk because as one ages, counterregulatory mechanisms to protect from such blood pressure drops are less effective than in younger persons.

## IMMUNE SYSTEM

In aging, changes in immune function alter the presentation of infections such as pneumonia, urinary tract infections, and even acute appendicitis. Elders often have a subnormal temperature so that temperature elevations are not recognized as a fever. The aging immune system may not be able to produce the high levels of white blood cells needed to fight an infection. Fever and elevated WBC counts frequently accompany infections in young and middle-aged adults. In elders, however, fever and elevated WBC counts are less common. Pathologic conditions such as pneumonia may manifest clinically as congestive heart failure, confusion, weakness, or falls. In some elders incontinence and poor appetite may be the first and only clinical indicators of urinary tract infections. *Tuberculosis,* a common geriatric infection, especially among nursing home patients, *may be present without a positive skin test reaction because of the decreased ability of the elderly immune system to produce an antigen-antibody reaction.* Because a high percentage of elders have a positive tuberculin test result, they are at risk for reactivation of tuberculosis secondary to debility, poor nutrition, and diseases such as diabetes mellitus or to treatment with certain medications, especially the steroids. (For more information on tuberculosis see Chapter 37.)

In summary, hallmarks of acute illness in elders include weakness, confusion, falls, poor appetite, and incontinence. Laboratory values also vary, as can be seen in Table 4-3.

# MAJOR HEALTH PROBLEMS OF ELDERS

Although many elderly persons maintain independent life-styles, they usually are affected by one or more health problems. The number of problems increases proportionately as the person ages. This section addresses the systems most likely to show effects of primary and secondary aging. The nursing process is the framework used for each system.

# COGNITIVE-PERCEPTUAL PROBLEMS

Elders differ from their younger counterparts in several aspects of cognitive and perceptual function. *The most dramatic changes occur in the central nervous system; the peripheral motor neurons and the autonomic nervous system remain relatively constant throughout the life span.*

**TABLE 4-3 Reference Ranges of Laboratory Values That Are Appreciably Different in Old Age***

| VALUE | RANGE FOR ADULTS | RANGE FOR ELDERLY |
|---|---|---|
| Albumin | 37-51 g/L | 33-49 g/L |
| Globulin | 19-33 g/L | 20-41 g/L |
| Potassium | 3.6-4.7 mmol/L | 3.6-5.2 mmol/L |
| Urea | 3.2-7.2 mmol/L | 3.9-9.9 mmol/L |
| Creatinine | 62-123 μmol/L (0.7-1.4 mg/dl) | 52-159 μmol/L (0.6-1.8 mg/dl) |
| Uric acid (men) | 4.0-7.6 mg/dl | 3.1-7.8 mg/dl |
| Uric acid (women) | 2.6-6.2 mg/dl | 2.1-7.7 mg/dl |
| Calcium (men) | 2.25-2.60 mmol/L | 2.19-2.59 mmol/L |
| Calcium (women) | 2.18-2.55 mmol/L | 2.18-2.68 mmol/L |
| Alkaline phosphatase (men) | 19-75 IU/L | 22-81 IU/L |
| Alkaline phosphatase (women) | 14-67 IU/L | 22-83 IU/L |
| Erythrocyte sedimentation rate (women) | 0-7 mm/hr | 6-69 mm/hr |
| Leukocyte count | 4000-11,000/mm³ | 3100-8900/mm³ |

Modified from Hazzard W et al: *Principles of geriatric medicine,* New York, 1990, McGraw-Hill.

*Ranges given are likely to vary slightly from those of many American laboratories, which often do not adjust ranges for gender or age.

**BOX 4-3 Aging Changes Affecting Cognition and Perception**

- Decreased brain weight
- Diminished enzyme activity
- Slowed reflexes
- Decreased sensory receptors for temperature, pain, and tactile discrimination
- Weakening of interneuron connections
- Increased response time
- Chronic hypoxia

The changes listed in Box 4-3 affect complex processes such as learning, memory, language, and mentation. Although loss of memory is not considered a primary aging change, many older persons have progressively increasing problems with short-term memory. Pain and temperature, taste, and touch are all dulled to some extent as one ages. Hearing and vision become less acute as the elder experiences *presbyopia* and *presbycusis* (see Chapter 60). Long-distance vision is less acute, as well as in night vision, and tolerance for glare decreases. The older person has more difficulty hearing high tones and discriminating speech in noisy situations.

## NURSING MANAGEMENT

### ♦ ASSESSMENT

#### Subjective Data

Data to be collected to determine the patient's orientation include information about long- and short-term memory, judgment, abstract thinking, insight, loss of vision and hearing, changes in ability to recognize hot and cold, and pain.

#### Objective Data

Data to be collected to assess the patient's cognitive-perceptual status establish the person's ability to discriminate between hot and cold objects, as well as hearing and visual losses. See Box 4-4 for the many variables that can be associated with confusion in elders.

Although delirium (temporary) is the more common form of confusion, the nurse should be aware that *chronic dementia* may be present. The most common dementia is Alzheimer's disease, which afflicts 50% to 60% of those who have organic brain disease (see Chapter 57). This devastating condition progressively affects the memory until the patient no longer remembers how to eat, dress, or toilet and is unable to recognize loved ones' faces. ***The patient and family need great support and encouragement when the patient with Alzheimer's disease is hospitalized for an acute illness.***

Using a modified mental status examination (Box 4-5), the nurse can efficiently determine the amount of orientation and judgment the elder retains.

**BOX 4-4 Variables Associated With Confusion in Elders**

**PHYSIOLOGIC**
- Pulmonary disease
- Cardiovascular disease
- Anemia
- Infections
- Trauma
- Dehydration
- Electrolyte imbalance
- Hypoglycemia/hyperglycemia

**MEDICATIONS**
- Sedatives/hypnotics
- Narcotic analgesics
- Antihypertensives
- Antidysrhythmics
- Anticonvulsants
- Diuretics
- Digitalis
- Tagamet

**ENVIRONMENTAL**
- Strange equipment
- Unfamiliar surroundings
- Restraints
- Tubings (IV, Foley)
- Strange people

**SENSORY LIMITATION**
- Decreased vision
- Decreased hearing
- Sensory overload
- Sensory deprivation

**EMOTIONAL STRESSORS**
- Loss of health
- Loss of loved ones
- Loss of home
- Loss of cherished possessions
- Loss of pets
- Expectations of sick role

Modified from Roberts B, Lincoln R: *Nurs Res* 35(2):126-127, 1986 (abstract).

### ♦ NURSING DIAGNOSES

Nursing diagnoses are determined from analysis of patient data. Nursing diagnoses for the patient with cognitive-perceptual problems may include but are not limited to the following:

| Diagnostic Title | Possible Etiologic Factors |
|---|---|
| Thought processes, impaired | Acute confusional states, chronic dementia (Alzheimer's disease), stress |
| Sensory/perceptual alteration | CVA, dementia, diabetes, neuromuscular diseases |

### ♦ EXPECTED PATIENT OUTCOMES

Expected patient outcomes for the person with a cognitive-perceptual problem may include but are not limited to the following:

1. Maintains orientation.
2. States that he or she understands procedures and routines.
3. Remains free from harm during hospitalization.
4. Communicates with persons in immediate environment.

### ♦ INTERVENTIONS

#### Promoting Orientation

Imagine a relatively independent 72-year-old woman who comes to the hospital with pneumonia. She is stripped of her belongings, taken to a strange room, jabbed with needles, and barraged by questions from strangers. A needle is placed in a vein for antibiotics;

**BOX 4-5 Mental Status Examination**

**ORIENTATION**

What day is it?
What season is it?
What is the holiday closest to today? (past or future)

**LONG-TERM MEMORY**

How old are you?
What is your birth date?
What happened at Pearl Harbor? *or* What happened to President Kennedy?

**SHORT-TERM MEMORY**

What was the last meal you ate?

**ABSTRACT THINKING**

What is 2 plus 2? 5 minus 3?

**INSIGHT**

What do you think is wrong with you?

**JUDGMENT**

What would you do if you spilled your tray on the floor? *or* What would you do if you had to go to the bathroom?

From Lincoln R: University Hospitals of Cleveland, 1986.

her hands are restrained to keep her from pulling it out. Her glasses and hearing aid are in the drawer. She compensates adequately until nightfall. Then she cannot distinguish shapes or outlines. She becomes quite agitated, thrashing about. A sedative does not help her. Suddenly she cries out, loosens her wrists, gets out of bed, and falls. The many stressors have overtaxed her hypoxic brain, and she has become confused and delirious.

The nurse can prevent or at least minimize these common effects by following a few simple measures. Give patients detailed, repeated explanations of where they are and what is being done to them. Place glasses and hearing aid on the patient while he or she is awake. Maintaining adequate hydration and pain control is often sufficient to clear a confused state. ***A friend or relative staying through the night could eliminate the need for restraints, and an antihistamine that causes drowsiness is preferable to a sedative for sleep.***[36]

When caring for confused patients, the nurse should endeavor to maintain as structured an environment as possible. Fitting the patient's usual routine to that of the hospital may be difficult, but any adaptations that can be made help to maintain the elder's orientation. Competing stimuli should be kept to a minimum. The following general guidelines may prove helpful in caring for a confused or demented patient:

1. Use the first name of the patient, and ask the patient to call you by your first name.
2. Give simple one-step directions; repeat as necessary.
3. Encourage any remaining social skills.
4. Promote reminiscence and life review.
5. Use distraction for negative behavior (never scold or argue).
6. Decrease physical stressors such as pain or full bladder.
7. Allow rest or "time-out" periods that alternate with physically active periods.
8. Speak slowly and distinctly in one- or two-syllable words.
9. Avoid tranquilizers and sedatives as much as possible.
10. Reduce extraneous stimuli such as TV, radio, or large groups of people.

## Promoting Communication

The ability to communicate is often impaired in patients with cognitive deficits. ***Those who know what the nurse is asking but have trouble following directions need physical guidance, such as laying out the articles for the bath. Persons who have difficulty understanding what is being said need verbal prompts and someone to show them the desired behavior. When attention disorders are present, the nurse may need to prompt the patient frequently.***[18]

## Reducing Agitation

Agitation in an elderly demented patient can be one of the most difficult behaviors for the nurse to manage. Agitated patients may pull out intravenous lines, disrupt dressings, remove catheters, fall out of bed, wander about, and generally create problems. Strategies to prevent and treat agitation are similar to those used in promoting orientation, promoting communication, and preventing fatigue.

Looking for the possible meaning of the behavior gives clues to interventions. Removal of clothing may indicate a need for toileting. Respond to kicking and biting by removing as many stimuli as possible, including other persons in the environment. If the person is agitated at bath time, the nurse should leave and return when the patient is less agitated. The same advice is true for giving medications. A minimum of physical and chemical restraints should be used.[27]

## Using Touch

***Touch is of great value in caring for confused patients.***[18] Even the most demented person, who has lost the ability to understand verbal communication, can recognize the tender healing touch of a compassionate nurse. Elderly persons who have been alone or institutionalized may suffer most from lack of physical contact. The nurse who uses touch for comfort, protection, and affection finds this an important part of the care of all elderly persons.

### Maintaining Sensory Function

#### Vision

Changes occur in the eyes with aging, such as a decrease in the conjunctival secretions, and sometimes the lower lid droops (ectropion), causing the moistening fluid of the eye to be lost.[4,7] Therefore irritation of the conjunctivae and tearing are common complaints of elders. Smoke also may be more irritating to their eyes than to those of younger persons. Isotonic solution eyedrops frequently are ordered as a comfort measure.

An accumulation of secretions at the inner canthus of the eye may be present, particularly on awakening, and may be a prodromal sign of infection. A sterile cotton sponge moistened with a physiologic solution of sodium chloride can be used to cleanse the eyes. Care must be taken not to press on the eyeballs or to irritate any exposed conjunctiva. Cataracts, failing vision, and actual blindness are common in elders. The lens of the eye loses its ability to accommodate effectively as aging progresses. Most persons older than 50 years need glasses, at least for reading. In the hospital or nursing home setting, care of glasses is important. Glasses should be labeled with the patient's name, and they should be kept clean and accessible to the elderly person. If glasses are worn by the hospital patient, but were lost, broken, or left at home at the time of hospital admission, arrangements should be made to have new glasses made or the existing ones brought to the hospital. No patient education, rehabilitation (such as ambulation activities), or increased self-care measures can be initiated in the treatment plan until the person is using his or her maximum visual skill with the aid of the glasses.

The eyes of older persons adjust more slowly to changes in light. Bright lights or sunlight may be almost unbearable; therefore blinds may need to be partially drawn. Many elderly persons see poorly in the dark; night lights are used to reduce confusion and to prevent accidents among those who get up during the night. Many older persons require glasses or contact lenses. These visual aids must be protected from damage or loss and need to be kept clean for best use.

#### Hearing

The major changes that affect the hearing of elderly adults are difficulties with speech discrimination, loss of ability to hear high-pitched tones, and problems with background noises. Nurses should make certain that any hearing aids are functioning correctly and are used when the patient is awake.

Pocket talkers are available for the hearing impaired. When speaking, talk slowly and face the patient with good lighting so the patient can see your face as you talk.

## ♦ EVALUATION

To evaluate the effectiveness of nursing interventions, compare patient behaviors with those stated in the expected patient outcomes. Successful achievement of patient outcomes to improve a cognitive-perceptual problem is indicated by the following:

1. Regains or maintains orientation to the surroundings.
2. Can state understanding of the treatment regimen.
3. Remains free from injury during hospitalizations.
4. Is able to hear and see well enough to communicate with others.

# ALTERATIONS IN THE GASTROINTESTINAL SYSTEM

The aging changes in the gastrointestinal system can affect the mouth, teeth, and gums; the esophagus and stomach; and the large and small intestines (Box 4-6).

## NUTRITIONAL NEEDS

Nutritional requirements of elders are essentially the same as for other adults, except that calorie needs diminish because of a decrease in lean body mass relative to fat (which burns fewer calories).[6] Fiber (i.e., fruits, vegetables, whole-grain bread, cereals), although undigestible, is an important constituent in the diet. Fiber holds water in the fecal mass, which softens the stools and enhances regular evacuation. The incidence of diverticulitis, colon cancer, or gallstones is thought to be influenced by diets chronically low in fiber. Although one might argue that low dietary fiber as a risk factor for these diseases is more relevant to those in their middle and earlier years, persons at or near age 65 may still have a life expectancy of 15 or more years during which dietary fiber deficiencies might play a role in development of colon cancer, diverticulitis, or gallstones. Because the latter disorders and constipation are common problems in elders, it is important that moderate amounts of fiber be regularly included in the diet.[6,38]

Water is vital for function and temperature regulation. A number of situations may predispose elders to a deficiency in body water. Approximately 50% of the body's water supply is obtained from solid foods; therefore a reduction in calorie intake may mean that water intake from food sources is not adequate. Some elders, especially those who are chronically ill, may have a defective thirst sensation mechanism, resulting in a diminished awareness of the body's signal to increase fluid intake. Finally, the elderly person may lose water from com-

**BOX 4-6 Aging Changes of Gastrointestinal System**

| | |
|---|---|
| Decreased motility | Decreased salivation |
| Decreased enzyme activity | Decreased taste |
| Atrophied musculature | Decreased sphincter tone |
| Decreased absorption | Decreased metabolism |

monly occurring conditions such as diarrhea, excessive perspiration, or polyuria or from the use of diuretics. In the event of a water deficit, elderly people should be encouraged to consume more fluids, particularly water (minimum of 1500 to 2000 ml/day unless contraindicated by conditions such as congestive heart failure).

Many elders, especially those who are ill, frequently are malnourished and have inadequate levels of energy expenditure through regular activity or exercise. Diets often are deficient in calcium, vitamins A and C, iron, and zinc. A vitamin-mineral supplement may be indicated.[37] Other than acute and chronic illnesses, possible causes of malnutrition are changes in taste, vision, smell, or dentition; limited financial resources; psychologic factors such as boredom and lack of companionship when eating; edentia; lifelong faulty eating patterns; fads and misconceptions regarding certain foods; lack of energy to prepare food; inability to feed oneself; and lack of sufficient knowledge of the essentials of a well-balanced diet. Living arrangements may affect dietary patterns; elderly men who live alone were found to have less adequate diets than older women living alone.[9]

Because malnutrition may be related to a number of coexisting factors, promotion of optimal nutrition depends heavily on accurate identification of the involved factors. Improved nutritional states more likely will occur if (1) the elderly individual has participated in the development of a plan to resolve the problems and (2) there are regularly scheduled intervals for evaluation and modification of these plans. Nursing interventions should be focused on resolving the specific problem. Interventions may include (1) experimentation with varying types of foods and seasonings to improve the range of food group options that are palatable and suitable to the individual's food preparation and serving capabilities, (2) referral to a dentist for dental problems (in many communities low income or mobile dental units are available for poor and homebound elders, which may be identified by contacting the state dental association or a local senior information center), (3) use of educational sessions and literature to improve the individual's understanding of the relationship between nutrition and health (involvement of family, friends, or others who live with the person or help in food preparation will increase the likelihood of a sustained change in nutritional intake), (4) referral to Meals on Wheels or another similar program in the community, (5) referral to hot lunch programs at senior centers for those who are not homebound and desire the opportunity for companionship and social interaction at meals, or (6) referral to or consultation with an occupational therapist specializing in elders who can provide suggestions or specific adaptive devices for persons who have difficulty with food handling or feeding caused by functional deficits (i.e., decreased vision, impaired joint mobility associated with arthritis, hemiparesis associated with cerebrovascular accidents).

Some elderly persons are obese even though they may be undernourished. Excess weight burdens the heart, liver, kidneys, and musculoskeletal system and should be avoided. Weight reduction for the elderly person, however, should be gradual. The weight loss program should be coordinated by the nurse through the physician and the nutritionist (if one is available). Sudden loss of weight is poorly tolerated by many elderly persons whose vascular system has become adjusted to the excess weight. Sudden weight reduction may lead to serious consequences, including confusion associated with lowered blood pressure, exhaustion, and vasomotor collapse.

Elderly persons often enter the hospital in a poorly nourished state because of chronic illness or other factors previously described. Trauma, surgery, or sepsis may increase nutritional demands and cause further nutritional deficiencies, particularly in protein and calories, to develop rapidly. Often, a poor state of nutrition upon admission, increased nutritional needs, and decreased appetite coexist in hospitalized elders. A nutritional assessment, including a record of food intake over several days and weight on admission with regular weight checks thereafter, should be a priority in nursing to detect deficiencies early.

General nursing care should include planning diagnostic tests between meals when possible; helping with tray setup and feeding when needed; encouraging the consumption of variety and quantity in the various food groups, and providing between-meal, high-protein, high-calorie snacks, especially if the person becomes easily satiated and consumes only small quantities at meals. Family members can be consulted about the patient's favorite foods and encouraged to bring special foods from home unless contraindicated by medical treatment.

"Liquid meals" are available (the type may vary depending on changes in market products and hospital and nutrition department preference) that are usually very palatable. These liquid drinks are often successful forms of supplemental nourishment for the person who has difficulty chewing or has a poor appetite.

The nurse should consult the physician if there is a sustained poor intake of food over several days and/or greatly increased nutritional demands on the body. On the basis of a full evaluation, the physician may consider intervention in the form of parenteral or enteral nutritional supplementation. The placement of a nasogastric feeding tube is an invasive procedure that may cause the patient discomfort at the time of insertion and while in place. Despite these concerns, other measures often fail, and the elderly person simply cannot eat enough to keep up with bodily demands, in many cases because of extreme fatigue. Therefore the risks and benefits of nasogastric feeding must be carefully considered in the early phases of nutritional deficits in the elderly patient if prompt resolution of nutritional problems is to occur.

## FLUID INTAKE

Unless high fluid intake is definitely contraindicated, the elderly patient should be urged to take sufficient fluids to dilute urine and decrease its irritating properties. Fluids may be limited in the evening if nocturia is interfering with sleep. If the patient is weak or has mobility problems, a urinal or bedpan should be offered during the night.

Elderly women have relaxation of perineal structures, which may interfere with complete emptying of the bladder and predispose to bladder infection. Some elderly patients have decreased sensation and do not realize when the bladder must be emptied.[7] Periodic dribbling of urine suggests that the bladder is not being emptied completely. The nurse should observe the very elderly patient for distention of the bladder and consult the physician.

**Incontinence** is common in the elders, especially among elderly women. This problem is embarrassing to the woman and should be brought to the health care provider's attention. Incontinence is never normal. It may be a sign of an infection or another easily reversible condition. The nurse can assist the patient by assessing voiding patterns, instituting regular toileting regimens, and suggesting that women perform Kegel's exercise to strengthen the muscles in the pelvic floor.[36] Involutional changes in the lining of the vagina lead to lessened resistance to invasion by organisms. Mild infections with troublesome symptoms and discharge are not unusual in elderly women. This condition should be reported to the physician, who may order specific therapy for it. Frequent bathing of the perineum may be helpful in allaying itching. Embarrassment may prevent the elderly patient from reporting symptoms. The nurse should be aware of the symptoms of this condition and watch for them.

Almost all elderly men have hypertrophy of the prostate gland, which makes urination difficult. The nurse must report or must urge the patient to report such complaints to his physician, because specific treatment often is necessary and can be administered safely even when the patient is far advanced in years.

## CARE OF MOUTH AND TEETH

Oral health in elders is important for several reasons. First, the mouth is the portal for nutritional intake, and any problems here could affect overall ability to meet the nutritional needs of cells and tissues throughout the body. Second, lesions or disorders of the mucous membranes, gums, or teeth may lead to severe discomfort, affecting both the person's emotional and social status (e.g., inability to partake in usual activities, including dining with others). Third, debilitated persons who are unable to perform mouth care regularly and have a poor cough reflex are at increased risk for pneumonia caused by aspiration of bacteria-laden oral secretions.

With increasing age there is a recession of the gums (gingivitis) and exposure of the root surface, which results in an increase in the prevalence of root (cervical) caries. The occurrence of caries can be a source of discomfort and expensive to repair; if it affects the anterior teeth, it poses an aesthetic problem. Because more than 65% of elders have an edentulous jaw, dental caries is not a concern of most older persons.[38] However, future generations are more likely to retain their teeth throughout late adulthood because of the current emphasis on preventive dental care and the advances in disease prevention and dental technology. Teaching preventive care to minimize caries in the elders must be considered a priority in dental care.

Lesions of the oral mucosa may result from a number of causes (e.g., infections, drug reactions, cancer). Especially noteworthy are oral neoplasms and lesions caused by dentures. Because cancerous and benign lesions look similar, any lesion of the oral mucosa that is not directly attributable to irritation from dentures or another identifiable source should be referred to a specialist for diagnosis.[38] Care of dentures, prevention of denture-associated problems, and prevention of denture loss is part of the general care of elders. Poorly fitting dentures may cause chronic irritation to areas on the gums or oral mucosa and cause ulcerations or hyperkeratosis. Denture use and fit should be a part of the general nursing assessment. Persons with recent significant weight loss that may alter the oro-facial tissue contour or who have a disease (e.g., anemia) or are on a drug regimen (e.g., chemotherapy) that may affect oral tissue integrity are at risk for denture-associated lesions.[4]

Persons with loose-fitting dentures also are at risk for airway obstruction during sleep and should be instructed to wear dentures only when awake. General care and teaching should include (1) cleaning dentures after each meal, (2) soaking dental plates in tap water or a denture solution when not in use, and (3) strategies to avoid loss or mix-ups, including placing dental plates in a safe, convenient place and putting the name or other identification marking on the dentures.

There is some recent evidence that older persons, particularly those without teeth, may normally experience changes in the muscles used to masticate food.[7] These changes may prevent the elderly person from chewing food adequately before swallowing. In addition, the older person is more willing to swallow larger-size particles than is the younger person and may be less aware of this functional change. Complaints such as "slow chewing" or "hard to chew" or avoiding certain foods may suggest oral muscular weakness or difficulties. Oral motor dysfunction may occur because of pathologic conditions such as paresis associated with a cerebrovascular accident or tardive dyskinesia associated with phenothiazine use. The consequences of such motor dysfunction can include choking, apnea, or regurgitation.[7] The nursing assessment should include an evaluation of oral muscle function and development of a plan of care if a problem exists. This individualized plan might include patient education regarding selection and preparation of foods that require less chewing without sacrificing essential nutrients or a pleasing taste and appearance. The person should maintain a sitting position when eating, avoid talking while eating, and avoid eating in stressful situations. Finally, when possible, the elderly person should be encouraged to eat when others are present to assist if choking does occur.

## BOWEL AND BLADDER ELIMINATION

A common concern for many elders is bowel function. Many factors contribute to constipation. The absence of routines, a different environment, decreased physical activity, reduced dietary roughage, decreased fluid intake, and the routine use of enemas may result in reduced bowel function and contribute to constipation. Any marked change in bowel habits, however, and any unusual reactions to normal doses of laxatives should be reported because malignant disease of the large bowel and diverticulitis are fairly common in this age-group.

Nursing intervention to manage constipation in elders includes increasing dietary fiber, fluids, and activity. Antacids that can cause constipation and laxatives should be avoided. Frequency in elimination is important because it provides regular stimulus to evacuate the bowel. Therefore attempts should be made to establish regular toileting patterns. The very elderly and somewhat confused patient should be reminded to go to the bathroom after meals. The addition of bran to a person's daily food intake has been found to be helpful in preventing constipation and resultant impaction. If the patient is constipated, it may be necessary occasionally to carefully insert a gloved finger into the rectum to be certain impaction has not occurred.

Frequency of voiding is common with aging (caused in part by a smaller bladder capacity) and becomes a problem during illness. It may be necessary to catheterize the patient to check for residual urine. One of the first signs of diminishing or failing kidney function is frequency of micturition during the night. Frequency, urgency, and burning on urination are symptoms of bladder infection.

## GASTROINTESTINAL PROBLEMS

## NURSING MANAGEMENT

### ♦ ASSESSMENT

#### Subjective Data

Data to be collected to assess the patient with gastrointestinal problems include inquiries about appetite, dysphagia, choking, condition of teeth and gums, types of foods and liquids taken, symptoms after meals, problems with constipation, indigestion, and bowel habits.

#### Objective Data

Objective data are collected by assessing the condition of the patient's mouth and mucous membranes, the presence of gag reflex, and chewing and swallowing ability and by performing an abdominal assessment.

### ♦ NURSING DIAGNOSES

Nursing diagnoses are determined from analysis of patient data. Nursing diagnoses for the patient with gastrointestinal problems may include but are not limited to the following:

| Diagnostic Title | Possible Etiologic Factors |
|---|---|
| Nutrition, altered: less than body requirements | Poorly fitting dentures, tooth loss, lack of sensation, hiatal hernia, loss of taste or smell, anorexia |
| Constipation | Lack of muscle tone, reliance on use of laxatives/enemas, lack of bulk in diet, low fluid intake |

### ♦ EXPECTED PATIENT OUTCOMES

Expected patient outcomes for the patient with gastrointestinal problems may include but are not limited to the following:

1. Maintains/regains weight.
2. States satisfaction with diet.
3. Has normal bowel movements and patterns.

### ♦ INTERVENTIONS

#### Maintaining/Regaining Weight

*For the person who tends to choke, check the fit of dentures and suggest slower eating with smaller bites and alternating liquids with solids.*

If the patient has a poor appetite, determine high-protein, high-calorie foods that appeal to him or her; offer small frequent meals. Persons with a hiatal hernia and/or esophageal reflux can be helped by avoiding cold liquids, sitting up for 1 to 2 hours after meals, and taking small doses of antacids and $H_2$ antagonists such as cimetidine or ranitidine. Teach the patient to keep the head raised during sleep by elevating the head of the bed on 3-inch blocks.

#### Preventing Aspiration

To prevent aspiration in a patient with decreased sensation in the mouth and throat, try giving soft foods such as custard, gelatin, and applesauce rather than liquids. Give small bites and wait between mouthfuls. Ask the patient to keep the head bent forward. Put the utensil in the patient's hand, giving verbal directions, to promote independence. If a patient needs help, sit beside him or her and tell him/her each food that will be fed.

### Promoting Alternative Feeding Methods

For patients who are unable to chew or swallow, two main feeding alternatives are available. The easiest and least complicated is the percutaneous enterostomal gastrostomy (PEG) (see Chapter 45). Under local anesthesia, a small tube is placed directly into the stomach through the abdominal wall and stitched in place. After 24 hours, the tube is used to give enriched formula feedings either continuously or in several bolus feedings. Another alternative is a Dobhoff tube placed through the nose into the stomach through which feedings can be given. Patients must be observed closely for the possibility of aspiration, the head is kept elevated during feeding, and small amounts are given at first to test tolerance. One complication of tube feedings is diarrhea. This can be managed by slowing down the feeding and giving high-fiber formulas. The dietitian or nutritionist can be consulted about the type of tube feeding.

All patients receiving tube feedings should be given 200 to 600 ml of water daily per tube. This is in addition to water used to flush the tube.

### Relieving Constipation

More than 700 constipation remedies exist, and some studies report that over 50% of elderly persons use laxatives regularly. In many cases, the use of laxatives may cause rather than cure constipation. They hinder the absorption of vitamins and may upset the patient's electrolyte balance.

Teaching should focus on developing or maintaining normal habits. Because of decreased sphincter control, removing laxatives from the patient's routine may be difficult, but normal patterns can be resumed with use of stool softeners and bulk-forming agents such as Metamucil. Patients should be advised to use natural substances to help aid elimination, such as prunes and prune juice. Adding bran to cereal or other foods is sometimes helpful. Elders often neglect to drink enough fluids for fear of incontinence or because limited mobility creates problems getting to the toilet. Sometimes by merely increasing the intake of water, the person can relieve constipation.

When trying to regain normal bowel habits, the patient should go to the bathroom after breakfast and other meals to take advantage of the gastrocolic reflex. Sometimes the use of a mild glycerine suppository may stimulate the bowels. The elderly person should be encouraged to keep trying to regain normal habits; after years of laxative abuse, sometimes the process takes several weeks. Use enemas only as a last resort. If the stool is very hard and impacted, use an oil-retention enema before the cleansing enema to soften the stool. Use greater caution when giving cleansing enemas to the elderly than to younger adults. The rectal mucosa may be very friable and easily traumatized. Elderly persons are much more prone to electrolyte imbalances and can become very weak and hypokalemic after administration of multiple enemas.

### ♦ EVALUATION

To evaluate the effectiveness of nursing interventions, compare patient behaviors with those stated in the expected patient outcomes. Successful achievement of patient outcomes to improve gastrointestinal function is indicated by the following:

1. Maintains or increases weight.
2. States satisfaction with diet.
3. Has more normal bowel patterns and states satisfaction with amount and frequency of bowel movements.

## DEHYDRATION

Dehydration is a common problem among elders and is a frequent cause of admission to the hospital.

## NURSING MANAGEMENT

### ♦ ASSESSMENT

#### Subjective Data

Data to be collected to assess the patient with dehydration include information about usual fluid intake, types of fluids preferred, thirst, ability to handle fluid containers, swallowing ability, usual pattern of consumption, changes in intake related to illness, and any indications that affect intake and output (diuretics, laxatives).

#### Objective Data

Objective data are collected by assessing the patient for skin turgor, texture, fragility, temperature; condition of mucous membranes; weakness; and orientation.

### ♦ NURSING DIAGNOSES

Nursing diagnoses are determined from analysis of patient data. Nursing diagnoses for the patient with dehydration may include but are not limited to the following:

| Diagnostic Title | Possible Etiologic Factors |
|---|---|
| Fluid volume deficit or Fluid volume deficit, high risk for | Dysphagia, congestive heart failure, medications, dementia, depression, stroke, hypertension, use of diuretics, inability to obtain fluids, fear of incontinence, fever, diarrhea, renal failure |

### ♦ EXPECTED PATIENT OUTCOMES

Expected patient outcomes to promote good hydration may include but are not limited to the following:

1. Takes 2000 ml of fluid in 24 hours.
2. Achieves greater intake than output for 48 hours.
3. Manifests skin and mucous membranes that are intact and moist.
4. Produces urine that is light amber in color and is clear.

## ♦ INTERVENTIONS

### Promoting Hydration

The nurse can take several steps to promote hydration: encourage fluid intake of 7 to 8 glasses a day; offer a variety of fluids, especially juices; weigh the patient daily; keep accurate intake and output records; and provide cups and pitchers that the person can handle.

### Facilitating Learning

Instruct the patient in the importance of maintaining adequate fluid intake. Teach which fluids are best: soup and fruit juices may have high sodium content; milk increases phlegm; alcohol depresses the CNS; coffee, tea, and colas contain caffeine, which is a stimulant; soft drinks and gelatins are high in sugar.

## ♦ EVALUATION

To evaluate the effectiveness of nursing interventions, compare patient behaviors with those stated in the expected patient outcomes. Successful achievement of patient outcomes to promote good hydration is indicated by the following:

1. Drinks adequate volume of fluids.
2. Has greater intake than output.
3. Manifests skin and mucous membranes that are moist, pink, and intact.
4. Produces normal color and consistency of urine.

# ALTERATIONS IN THE URINARY SYSTEM

Although aging leads to decreased kidney function, most elders can maintain normal voiding. *Incontinence* is always a result of pathologic process and not of primary aging (Box 4-7).

## NURSING MANAGEMENT

## ♦ ASSESSMENT

### Subjective Data

Data to be collected to assess the patient with an alteration in the urinary system include information about usual urinary patterns, any changes in habits, pain, hesitancy, burning, urgency, and loss of control. If incontinence exists, assess amount, frequency, type of management, and loss of control with sneezing, coughing, or movement.

**BOX 4-7 Aging Changes of the Urinary System**

Reduced renal blood flow
Decreased glomerular filtration rate
Decreased bladder muscle tone

### Objective Data

Objective data are collected by observing the patient's urine for color, consistency, amount, and presence of blood. If cloudy, or if sediment is present, send urine for culture and sensitivity.

## ♦ NURSING DIAGNOSES

Nursing diagnoses are determined from analysis of patient data. Nursing diagnoses for the patient with urinary problems may include but are not limited to the following:

| Diagnostic Title | Possible Etiologic Factors |
| --- | --- |
| Incontinence, functional | Altered environment, sensory, cognitive, or mobility deficits |

## ♦ EXPECTED PATIENT OUTCOMES

Expected patient outcomes to improve urinary elimination may include but are not limited to the following:

1. Increases time between voidings.
2. Achieves ability to toilet independently.
3. Decreases number of incontinent episodes.

## ♦ INTERVENTIONS

### Minimizing Functional Incontinence

Elderly persons are especially susceptible to functional incontinence. Factors affecting this condition are urinary infections, inability to get to the bathroom, and altered fluid intake caused by illness and hospitalization. Use of restraints and attachment of multiple tubes often hinder the ability of the person to accomplish independent toileting. The presence of cognitive impairment and limited mobility complicates the situation.

The nurse can assist the patient getting to the bathroom independently through modification of the environment. This may involve moving furniture and equipment to clear a path to the bathroom or arranging for a bedside commode to be placed near enough to the patient's bed for easy use. Sometimes providing a cane or walker is all that is necessary, as well as giving the patient some privacy. If special equipment presents a hindrance, the nurse can teach the patient how to manipulate intravenous tubing or machinery and urge the patient to call for assistance.

It is important for the nurse to remember that incontinence is embarrassing and shameful for the patient. The patient should be treated in a matter-of-fact manner, never scolded, and helped to avoid future incidents. The nurse may tell the patient that urinary control in the hospital is much more difficult where the surroundings are unfamiliar and assure the patient that when he or she returns home, continence may be regained or improved.

Continuous intravenous fluids, having nothing orally because of diagnostic studies, and altered eating schedules may interfere with voiding patterns. Whenever possible, fluids should be encouraged, up to 2 L/day, with the bulk of the liquids given between 8 AM and 7 PM. Limiting the fluids at night helps prevent incontinent episodes during sleeping hours. If the patient is restrained or hindered by intravenous or other tubings, he or she should be offered opportunities to void before and after meals and at bedtime. Urinary tract infections are common and should be treated with the appropriate antibiotics.

Some elderly men can void only when standing. Others may have urinary frequency and hesitancy because of an enlarged prostate, which is common in older men. Assistance should be provided as necessary to handle these difficult problems. Maintaining as much independence as possible is important in keeping the elderly person from losing functional capacity.

### Promoting Urinary Elimination

Foley catheters may be placed in some patients to monitor and accurately record urinary output. After the catheter is removed, the elderly patient may have trouble regaining bladder control, especially if mild incontinence was present previously.

The best approach for urinary retention after catheter removal is to do a straight catheterization every 6 to 8 hours until the person is able to void voluntarily. This is preferable to reinserting the indwelling catheter. For the person who is *incontinent, teaching Kegel strengthening exercises may help tone the pelvic floor muscles.* The patient should be reassured that most incontinence ceases after a routine of fluids and voiding has been reestablished. To assist in a more complete emptying of the bladder, women can be taught to lean forward as far as possible at the end of voiding. This motion usually results in additional urine being voided.

For any elderly person who has problems with incontinence, it is important for the nurse to determine what type of incontinence is present. In many cases, stress and urge incontinence is exaggerated by functional incontinence. *Urinary incontinence is never a normal part of aging.* The nurse may be the first person to discover the patient's problem, and referrals for incontinence studies can be a vital part of the nursing care.

A critical need is to teach patients about the management and treatment of incontinence. The Agency for Health Care Policy and Research (AHCPR) has issued a clinical practice guideline, *Urinary Incontinence in Adults.* They also published a patient guide, *Urinary Incontinence in Adults.* Information about procuring these materials can be found on the inside back cover of this text.

### ♦ EVALUATION

To evaluate the effectiveness of nursing interventions, compare patient behaviors with those stated in the expected patient outcomes. Successful achievement of patient outcomes to promote satisfactory urinary elimination is indicated by the following:

1. Indicates a decrease in the number of incontinent episodes.
2. Is able to toilet independently.
3. States satisfaction with control of incontinent episodes.

## ALTERATIONS IN THE MUSCULOSKELETAL SYSTEM

One of the most common problems of secondary aging is joint and muscle disease (Box 4-8). *Osteoarthritis, rheumatism,* and *osteoporosis are prevalent among elders.* As joints stiffen and muscle tone decreases, the person may develop an awkward, halting gait. The ability to rise from a chair or to get in and out of cars or buses decreases. Impaired gait, cardiovascular changes, sensory deficits, and osteoporosis make elders susceptible to falls. The factors contributing to falls are listed in Box 4-9. Falls account for 23% of deaths and injuries in persons older than 65 years of age.

## NURSING MANAGEMENT

### ♦ ASSESSMENT

### Subjective Data

Data to be collected to assess the patient with musculoskeletal problems include information about limitations of joint and muscle movement, ability to walk, turn, and go up stairs. Learn about problems the patient has with bathing, dressing, toileting, grooming, eating, and carrying out household tasks.

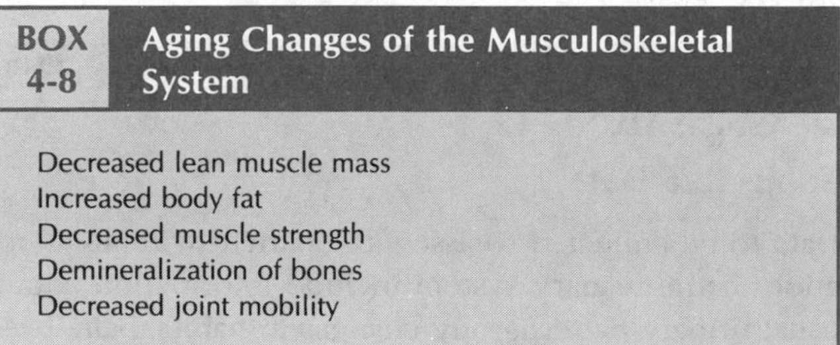
**BOX 4-8 Aging Changes of the Musculoskeletal System**

- Decreased lean muscle mass
- Increased body fat
- Decreased muscle strength
- Demineralization of bones
- Decreased joint mobility

**BOX 4-9 Factors Associated With Falls**

| INTRINSIC | EXTRINSIC |
|---|---|
| Limited mobility | Poor lighting |
| Decreased vision | Unfamiliar environment |
| Confused mental state | Loose slippers |
| Orthostatic hypotension | Room cluttered with equipment and furniture |
| Decreased ability to maintain equilibrium | |

### Objective Data

Objective data are collected by checking muscle tone and strength, joint flexibility, range-of-motion, and gait, and whether the patient uses assistive aids such as a cane, walker, or crutches.

## ♦ NURSING DIAGNOSES

Nursing diagnoses are determined from analysis of patient data. Nursing diagnoses for the patient with musculoskeletal problems may include but are not limited to the following:

| Diagnostic Title | Possible Etiologic Factors |
|---|---|
| Mobility, impaired physical | Arthritis, osteoporosis, neuromuscular diseases, stroke |
| Self-care deficit | Same as above |

## ♦ EXPECTED PATIENT OUTCOMES

Expected patient outcomes to improve musculoskeletal problems may include but are not limited to the following:

1. Transfers from the bed to the chair independently.
2. Walks in the hall at least three times daily, gradually increasing the distance.
3. Washes own face, hands, and trunk, and feeds self after tray is set up.
4. Maintains joint mobility by performing range-of-motion exercises daily.
5. Uses assistive device (cane) correctly, seeking help with ambulation as necessary.
6. Is safe from harm and injury.

## ♦ INTERVENTIONS

### Promoting Mobility

Physical therapists and occupational therapists are involved early in the hospitalization to arrange a program of care that maintains as much independence for the patient as possible. Sometimes providing a cane or walker and raising a toilet seat is all that is necessary to maintain functional independence. In other cases, assistive devices, such as long-handled spoons and reachers, facilitate a person's dressing and self-feeding.

*Elders often have fragile bones and joints from osteoarthritis and osteoporosis.* Use caution when working with them. Do not lift an elderly person under the armpits when assisting to move, stand, walk, or transfer from one surface to another. Support the person's trunk and joints as the person is moved. Transfer and lifting sheets are helpful and may allow one caregiver to move or transfer the patient without additional help.

*Active and passive range-of-motion exercises* are as important for the elderly person as for the younger adult. Because elders may have more limitations of joint motion, great care must be taken not to move the joint past the point of resistance or pain.

Progressive activity, such as getting the patient out of bed soon after admission, and progressive ambulation are essential aspects of nursing care that help maintain independence and function. The term **dysfunctional syndrome** as applied to elders *refers to a loss of function through imposed bedrest and altered nutrition patterns during hospitalization.*[22] This decline occurs despite improved medical health and is attributable to a lack of aggressive measures designed to maintain the person's baseline function.

Prevention of dysfunctional syndrome includes early ambulation, arrangements for independence in toileting, dining in a central location in a social situation, and encouraging independence in bathing, grooming, and dressing. Fulfilling the goal of functional independence necessitates ingenuity and patience on the part of the nurse. It involves spending more time allowing elders to do for themselves instead of doing it for them. This may require increased staffing.

### Preventing Injury

Nurses have often used restraints on the elderly person with the mistaken idea that injurious falls can be prevented with these devices. *The restraints themselves are often more dangerous than any falls that may be prevented. When patients are held down with waist belts and extremity restraints, decreased functional capacity, loss of independence, incontinence, and decreased musculoskeletal and cardiovascular tone can result.* Far worse, however, is the psychologic impact resulting from the use of restraints. *Anger, fear, humiliation, embarrassment, discomfort, and demoralization are some of the undesirable effects documented when restraints are used.*[3]

*Removing restraints from patients in long-term care facilities is part of the requirements of the Omnibus Budget Reconciliation Act of 1987.* In facilities where this has been achieved, *falls* have been *reduced by* 30%, and less danger of strangulation and injury from restraints has occurred.[3]

Nursing strategies to maintain patient safety are complex and must be individually determined. *Nurses should assess the needs of each patient and determine the relative risks of "tying down" over risk of falling.* Family members can play a significant role in understanding the patient's needs as well as participating in the care of the elder.

*Changes* can be made *in the environment* to protect patients. Some of these changes are *low beds, half side rails, carpeted or cushioned floors, bed alarms,* and *chairs adapted to accommodate patients of various heights and weights.*[5]

If all attempts fail to maintain safety of the elder and restraints become necessary as a last resort, the following measures should be taken:

1. Use the least amount of restraint possible; for example, wrist versus chest restraints.

2. Reevaluate the need for the restraint every 4 to 8 hours.
3. Monitor the patient closely for chafing, redness, tenderness, and circulation under the restraint.
4. Follow manufacturer's directions carefully when applying restraints.
5. Remember that the patient needs increased nursing care while restrained; for example, offering bedpan/urinal, feeding, and turning.
6. *Remove the restraint every 2 hours to exercise the part restrained.*
7. Always explain the need for the restraint to the patient, no matter how much cognitive impairment may be present—for example, for his or her protection and not for punishment.
8. Continue to seek alternatives and remove the restraint as soon as possible.

## Preventing Orthostatic Hypotension

**Orthostatic hypotension** is a special problem of some elders that increases the risk of falling. This condition is caused by an inadequate baroreceptor response to sudden changes of position or changes during the digestive process. When the person gets out of bed, rises from a hot bath, or eats a large meal, blood pressure may drop precipitously, causing the patient to become faint and fall.

The nurse should *teach the following measures to prevent orthostatic hypotension*[1]:

1. Sleep with the head of bed elevated 8 to 12 inches.
2. Get up slowly from lying position in three stages: sit up, dangle feet over side of bed, then stand up.
3. Do not bend all the way to the floor or stand up quickly.
4. Postpone grooming activities, such as shaving and bathing, to 1 hour after arising.
5. Wear support hose at night.
6. Get out of a hot bath slowly.
7. Wait for an hour or so after a meal to engage in strenuous activity.
8. Be cautious with position changes 1 hour after taking antihypertensive medications.
9. Use a rocking chair to increase circulation.
10. Avoid the Valsalva maneuver.

## ♦ EVALUATION

To evaluate the effectiveness of nursing interventions, compare patient behaviors with those stated in the expected patient outcomes. Successful achievement of patient outcomes to improve musculoskeletal function is indicated by the following:

1. Is able to transfer independently.
2. Can walk farther each day.
3. Is able to feed self, dress self, bathe self, and toilet self.
4. Is maintaining joint mobility by regular exercise.
5. Is maintaining safety in use of assistive devise.

**BOX 4-10 Aging Changes of the Respiratory and Cardiovascular Systems**

**RESPIRATORY SYSTEM**

Decreased elasticity of lungs and chest wall
Decreased recoil of lungs
Increased residual lung volume
Decreased forced expiratory volume
Decreased oxygen pressure ($Po_2$) ($Po_2$ decreases about 4 mm Hg/decade)

**CARDIOVASCULAR SYSTEM**

Decreased elasticity of blood vessels
Decreased cardiac output
Possible blocking of blood vessels by fatty deposits (atherosclerosis)
Increased peripheral vascular resistance leading to increased blood pressure
Slowed circulation
Decreased efficiency of valves in veins of lower extremities

# ALTERATIONS IN THE CARDIOPULMONARY SYSTEM

One of the most pronounced changes that occurs as a person ages is the decline in pulmonary function. Although the changes in the cardiovascular system are not as dramatic, some differences exist between the older and the younger adult (Box 4-10).

## NURSING MANAGEMENT

## ♦ ASSESSMENT

### Subjective Data

Data to be collected to assess the patient with cardiopulmonary problems include information about fatigue, especially with normal routines, breathlessness, palpitations, swollen ankles, need to sleep with several pillows, persistent cough, falls with dizziness, chest pain, confusion, and medication history.

### Objective Data

Objective data are collected by checking the patient's vital signs, orthostatic blood pressure, edema, use of accessory breathing muscles, condition of legs and feet, capillary refill, temperature of hands and feet, and peripheral pulses.

## ♦ NURSING DIAGNOSES

Nursing diagnoses are determined from analysis of patient data. Nursing diagnoses for the patient with cardiopulmonary problems may include but are not limited to the following:

| Diagnostic Title | Possible Etiologic Factors |
|---|---|
| Breathing pattern, ineffective | Chronic obstructive pulmonary disease (COPD), sedentary life-style, bronchitis, pneumonia |
| Cardiac output, decreased | Congestive heart failure (CHF), stress |
| Activity intolerance | Sedentary life-style, immobility |

## ♦ EXPECTED PATIENT OUTCOMES

Expected patient outcomes for the person with cardiopulmonary changes may include but are not limited to the following:

1. Uses an effective breathing pattern, taking twice as long to exhale as to inhale.
2. Walks the length of the room without dyspnea using portable oxygen.
3. Maintains normal respiratory rate.
4. Accomplishes own ADLs with a minimum of fatigue.

## ♦ INTERVENTIONS

### Decreasing Fatigue

The primary focus of the nurse in caring for the patient with an ineffective breathing pattern, decreased cardiac output, or activity intolerance is coping with the residual effects of fatigue. Energy-saving techniques are valuable for the patient who becomes breathless with exertion or who has chronic fatigue.

1. Sit rather than stand for grooming or household chores.
2. Take frequent rest periods between activities.
3. Avoid extremes of temperature.
4. Wear loose clothing and use long-handled reachers.
5. Have friends or family help with household chores.
6. Plan meals in advance and organize cooking activities.
7. Sit down while preparing meals.
8. Practice relaxation exercises.
9. Remove self from stressful situations.
10. Use portable oxygen as necessary when walking longer distances.

### Facilitating Learning

Smoking and exposure to secondary passive smoke are the biggest risk factors in the development of pulmonary disease at any age. The nurse can promote a smoke-free environment by encouraging smokers to stop smoking and referring them to programs such as SmokeEnders. Even the elderly patient can enjoy improved health with the cessation of smoking.[21]

The nurse should teach the patient to report any unusual signs or symptoms. Cardiopulmonary disease often has an atypical presentation in elders. Therefore symptoms that seem insignificant may indicate a serious problem. Some *symptoms to watch for are chronic indigestion, heartburn, confusion, tingling or numbness in the extremities, shortness of breath, and edema not alleviated by elevating the feet.* Frequent blood pressure checks are important. Other tips are to avoid tight garters and crossing legs and to engage in a suitable exercise (conditioning) program (see primary prevention, p. 94).

Medications should be reviewed frequently because elders are more prone to side effects and drug interactions, especially when taking heart medications.

## ♦ EVALUATION

To evaluate the effectiveness of nursing interventions, compare patient behaviors with those stated in the expected patient outcomes. Successful achievement of patient outcomes to improve cardiopulmonary function is indicated by the following:

1. Walks a prescribed distance without dyspnea using portable oxygen when necessary.
2. Maintains normal respiratory rate.
3. Can accomplish ADLs successfully with a minimum of fatigue.

# ALTERATIONS IN THE INTEGUMENTARY SYSTEM

The primary aging changes that occur in the integumentary system are the ones most noticeable to the lay person and are commonly associated with "growing old" (Box 4-11).

The skin changes occur as the basal membrane flattens and epidermal turnover rate diminishes. These changes cause a decrease in the barrier function of the skin, making it more susceptible to irritants and allergens. As the hair follicles decrease in number and melanocytes become less active, the hair becomes gray and thin. Decreased sweat production and decreased subcutaneous fat lead to altered thermoregulation, making elders more prone to hypothermia in the winter and heat exhaustion in the summer. Wrinkling is due to loss of elasticity and decreased subcutaneous fat. Fingernails and toenails become brittle and thick, with many deformities resulting from trauma and circulatory impairment.[21]

**BOX 4-11 Aging Changes of the Integumentary System**

- Graying hair
- Loss of connective tissue
- Decreased vascularity
- Liver spots
- Senile purpura
- Decreased seborrheic secretions
- Seborrheic keratoses
- Decreased venous circulation
- Decreased elasticity of skin
- Loss of subcutaneous fat
- Decreased skin turgor
- Tooth loss
- Malodorous breath
- Receding gums
- Hardened nails
- Corns, calluses

## NURSING MANAGEMENT

### ♦ ASSESSMENT

#### Subjective Data

Data to be collected to assess the patient with integumentary system problems include information about dry skin, pruritus, skin and nail infections, tooth loss and decay, gum disease, bathing patterns, use of emollients, skin-care habits, mouth-care habits, and foot problems.

#### Objective Data

Objective data are collected by assessing the patient for dryness of skin, skin turgor (test over sternum, not on forearm), rashes and skin lesions, condition of hair, nails, gums, and mouth, and capillary refill.

### ♦ NURSING DIAGNOSES

Nursing diagnoses are determined from analysis of patient data. Nursing diagnoses for the patient with integumentary system problems may include but are not limited to the following:

| Diagnostic Title | Possible Etiologic Factors |
|---|---|
| Skin integrity, impaired | Dehydration, immobility, shearing, poor venous circulation, incontinence |
| Mucous membrane, altered oral | Gingivitis, stomatitis, tooth loss |

### ♦ EXPECTED PATIENT OUTCOMES

Expected patient outcomes for the person with integumentary system problems may include but are not limited to the following:

1. Skin remains intact and free of lesions.
2. No signs of infection are present.
3. Feet remain in good condition (intact skin and clipped toenails).
4. Mucous membranes are pink, moist, and intact.

### ♦ INTERVENTIONS

#### Maintaining Skin Integrity

##### Dryness and itching

Elders are especially prone to very dry, itching skin, called **senile pruritus.** The best treatment is frequent use of creams and emolients. Elderly persons do not need daily baths, but they should include more sponge baths in their routine and decrease the use of soap. Liquid cleansers made for sensitive skin are often recommended in place of soap. Hot showers or baths should be avoided, and skin should be patted instead of rubbed dry. Perfumed creams and perfumes that contain alcohol can be drying and irritating to already compromised skin texture.

##### Skin tumors

Both benign and malignant skin tumors are common in elders, especially those persons who have prolonged exposure to the sun. Elderly persons should be advised to see a physician if they have any changes in their skin, especially changes in moles or pigmented areas. The major concern is that a skin lesion might be a *malignant melanoma.* If found early, these tumors can be removed with no further complications. Teaching should include daily inspection of skin, wearing protective clothing for work or leisure activities out-of-doors, and avoiding exposure to the ultraviolet rays of the sun. When out in the sun, elders should wear a sunscreen lotion with a skin protection factor of at least 15.

#### Preventing Pressure Sores and Shearing Lesions

Elderly patients who are bed bound for all or part of the day are especially susceptible to **pressure sores** and **shearing lesions.** Pressure sores are ischemic areas of breakdown that occur when fragile tissue is compressed between a bony prominence (sacrum, heels, scapulae) and a firm surface such as a mattress or a chair. Shearing lesions arise from loss of outer layers of skin, resulting from friction when a person is moved or turned in bed. Treatment of deep pressure sores can cost thousands of dollars. Nurses can help prevent this serious complication.

Prevention requires meticulous attention to relief of pressure through regular turning schedules (as often as every 2 hours) and pressure-reducing devices. Maintaining clean, dry skin that is free of abrasions, adequate hydration (up to 2400 ml/day), and supplemental nutrition for those who are malnourished is encouraged. These measures are critical to the prevention of pressure sores.

#### Promoting Proper Foot Care

Elderly persons have more corns, calluses, bunions, hammer toes, and horny toenails than do younger persons. They are taught to wear protective footwear, clean and inspect feet daily, and guard against frostbite and burns. For difficult toenails or other foot problems, a podiatrist should be consulted. Diabetic patients should never cut their own toenails but should have a professional attend to foot care.

#### Preventing Intravenous Therapy Injury

Elderly persons create special challenges for the phlebotomist and intravenous therapist. Their veins are fragile and inelastic, making it difficult to enlarge them with a tourniquet. Hematomas form quickly. Sometimes anatomic markings are not in the usual places. When choosing a vein, use the network on the back of the forearm, the cephalic vein on the thumb side of the hand, and the basilar vein on the posterior arm.[14]

Select as small a cannula as possible, protect the skin with proper skin preparation, and use the indirect method of entering the vein. Maintain traction on the skin during insertion. Always remove the needle gently so as not to damage the vein.[14]

### Maintaining Mucous Membranes and Dental Health

Tooth decay is not a serious problem among elders; they are much more afflicted by periodontal disease. Periodontal disease is responsible for most tooth loss after age 35. Gingivitis (gum disease) and periodontitis (bone disease) occur when plaque develops in gum crevices; then the bacterial growth causes receding gums and invasion of the bone.

For sore receding gums, broken teeth, ill-fitting dentures, or malodorous breath, the nurse should refer the patient to a dentist or oral health clinic. Other helpful measures include the following:

1. Frequent mouth care for patients who are using oxygen, are taking nothing by mouth, or are immunosuppressed
2. Use of emolients on lips and nares for patients who are using oxygen or nasogastric and Dobhoff tubes
3. Frequent suctioning of secretions for those who cannot handle secretions themselves
4. Treatment of yeast (thrush) infections

## ♦ EVALUATION

To evaluate the effectiveness of nursing interventions, compare patient behaviors with those stated in the expected patient outcomes. Successful achievement of patient outcomes to improve problems of the integumentary system is indicated by the following:

1. Maintains skin integrity.
2. Shows no signs of infection or pressure sores.
3. Has intact skin on feet and toenails are clipped.
4. Has intact mucous membranes.

# ALTERATIONS IN COMFORT: PAIN

## NURSING MANAGEMENT

## ♦ ASSESSMENT

Assessment of pain in the elderly person is more complex than in the younger adult. Pain may appear in atypical forms. Conditions that normally cause pain in young persons may not do so in elders.

The nurse assesses for location, quality, intensity, onset, duration, and physical manifestations of pain in the same manner as for any patient. In addition, the nurse must attend to the impact of pain on activities of daily living, gait, and behavior.

Factors that affect pain in elders differ from those affecting younger persons. Impaired vision and hearing, problems expressing oneself, inability to concentrate, and cognitive changes may interfere with assessment. More attention must be paid to nonverbal expressions, as well as soliciting comments from family members.

The belief system of the elderly person affects his or her expression of pain. Some believe that pain is a normal part of the aging process and must be endured stoically. If the person fears loss of autonomy, she or he may deny having pain. A fear of serious illness may lead to denial of pain. Some ethnic groups believe showing pain is not acceptable, whereas others may be more vocal when they experience pain.

An atypical presentation of pain is much more common in elders. For example, one half of patients with myocardial infarctions have no pain. Diseases usually associated with severe pain, such as peptic ulcer, appendicitis, and pneumonia, may provoke only mild pain in older persons. Some abdominal emergencies manifest as chest pain at first. Depression masks pain, and pain may be difficult to assess, especially if the patient is also cognitively impaired.

Taking all these factors into consideration, the nurse must establish rapport with the elderly person by taking plenty of time and phrasing questions in several different ways. For the asphasic patient, a pain chart with a drawing of a body to which the patient may point may be helpful. Patients may be asked to rate their pain using a pain scale numbered 1 to 10, with 10 being the most severe pain ever felt and 1 for the least severe pain (see Chapter 17 for more information). Showing concern for the patient and his or her suffering rather than dismissing the pain as "part of growing old" assists immeasurably in gathering accurate data.

## ♦ NURSING DIAGNOSES

Nursing diagnoses are determined from analysis of patient data. Nursing diagnoses for the patient with pain may include but are not limited to the following:

| Diagnostic Title | Possible Etiologic Factors |
|---|---|
| Pain | Pathophysiologic changes, trauma/diagnostic tests, immobility, improper positioning, disability |

## ♦ EXPECTED PATIENT OUTCOMES

Expected patient outcomes for the person with pain may include but are not limited to the following:

1. States pain is decreased.
2. Exhibits fewer nonverbal signs of pain.
3. Is more independent in ADLs.

## ♦ INTERVENTIONS

### Alleviating/Minimizing Pain

In the care of the elders, the nurse should consider a variety of modifications in managing pain that differ from those used with the younger adult. Elderly persons are more prone to mild arthritis and fibrositis. The incidence of osteoporosis, especially involving the spine and femur, is very high in elderly women. Great care must be taken to protect the joints, back, and shoulders when transferring, moving, and turning. Whereas one nurse could handle a younger adult, two persons may be needed to move the older patient in bed or to help him or her walk.

Protective adipose tissue under the skin disappears with age, and the volume of circulating blood, particularly to the small outer arteries, may be diminished. This affects the ability to withstand cold without discomfort. Several layers of light-weight clothing are warmer than fewer heavy layers when the person is cold. Many elderly persons wish to wear socks and additional clothing in bed. Provision must be made to prevent drafts in the room while maintaining good air circulation.

Elderly patients may tolerate smaller doses of pain medications than do younger adults (see secondary prevention, p. 96). *Bizarre reactions to pain medications may occur, such as hallucinations, delirium, aggravated pain, and agitation.* Great caution should be used in starting and/or changing dosages of narcotics to prevent reactions and interactions. The nonsteroidal antiinflammatory medications are gaining in popularity for treating pain from arthritis and neuralgias. These drugs create fewer side effects, and elderly patients tolerate them better (see Chapter 65 for more information about these medications).

### ♦ EVALUATION

To evaluate the effectiveness of nursing interventions, compare patient behaviors with those stated in the expected patient outcomes. Successful achievement of patient outcomes to reduce pain is indicated by the following:

1. Shows less evidence of pain.
2. Rates pain between 2 and 3.
3. Is able to do ADLs more independently.

## ALTERATIONS IN SLEEP PATTERNS

Certain changes in sleep and sleep patterns seem to occur as part of normal aging. These include a prolonged sleep latency (time it takes to fall asleep), an increase in the number of awakenings during the sleep period, a decrease in slow-wave sleep (thought to be associated with physical restoration), and a decrease in rapid eye movement (REM) sleep that occurs in advanced old age (thought to be associated with mental restoration).[7] These changes often result in more fragmented sleep than that experienced in earlier years. Although many elders adapt to these normal sleep changes, others experience acute or chronic insomnia. Physical problems that cause pain, shortness of breath, frequency of urination, incontinence, impairment of mobility, or confusion may disrupt sleep. Other contributing factors include certain drugs (e.g., some antihypertensives) and environmental factors such as temperature, light, noise, and type of bed and its location.

Because quality of sleep can have far-reaching effects on the individual's general well-being, an essential component of the nurse's health assessment of elders must include an evaluation of sleep. If a sleep problem is identified, it should be analyzed as to its onset, subjective complaint (how the problem is described by the patient), previous treatments and effectiveness, and sleep patterns prior to the onset of the problem.

### PROMOTING SLEEP

Promotion of sleep in the elders includes identification and treatment of the specific sleep problem when one exists. Health care settings (hospital, nursing home, retirement home) should be planned so that individual sleep needs can be preserved. Flexibility such as providing areas for night persons to enjoy activities is a prerequisite to planning.

Nursing interventions that teach manipulation of the environment may be part of the treatment plan for acute insomnia or chronic insomnia. The goal of this strategy is to promote restoration of the sleep-wake cycle by identifying the specific factors that are disrupting sleep, and minimizing or eliminating them. If the person has pain, the pain must be controlled; if there is nocturia, the cause should be found and treated; if there is a disruptive partner, beds or rooms should be changed. Warm milk or a snack at bedtime will aid in inducing sleep naturally. The elderly person should be allowed nap times during the day. In addition, mind-stimulating activities and exercise should not be engaged in before bedtime.

Usual nighttime routines help prepare the patient for sleep. Keep a low night light on, lower the bed, and provide adequate supervision at night to prevent accidents. If the person is likely to get up for toileting, place a bedside commode next to the bed and teach the person how to use it safely. Sedatives are prescribed with caution in elders because they interfere with REM sleep and may cause increased confusion, coordination impairment, and decreased mental alertness. An antihistamine that causes drowsiness is the sleeping medication of choice.

## SPECIAL NEEDS

### PSYCHOSOCIAL NEEDS

Psychosocial development in older adults is centered around integrating life experiences, sense of identity, and realistic perspectives of future opportunities and events.[10,15,26] Ideally, the goal of aging for each person is the congruence of life experiences and self-identification with the environment.[26] To meet patient needs, the combination of environmental resources and inner strengths that has helped the patient become a "survivor" should be considered.

Resources include the wisdom that comes from a lifetime of effective coping, a realistic perspective of time, religion (spirituality), and the process of reminiscence.[26] Effective movement through developmental crises and challenges during the first half of life as well as during middle age provides a variety of effective approaches to new challenges and experiences. In essence, elderly men and women are survivors; they have proved their stamina for adaptation by virtue of having attained old age.

To develop nursing interventions that promote psychologic health, nurses must understand what is needed from the patient's perspective. Meeting the needs of older adults is enhanced by an understanding of the general developmental processes and changes of aging. What losses has the person experienced? What is the person's health status? Who does the person consider to be available for emotional support and assistance with day-to-day living? When planning care for elders, the available personal, family, and social resources that can be mobilized to assist the patient should be considered. By providing the patient with a range of choices, it is often possible to negotiate care plans in such a way that minimal or acceptable life pattern change is required. Nursing interventions should focus on facilitating the use of previous coping styles; promoting the preferred, established life-style; and supporting maximum independence, particularly when this is threatened by hospitalization or the probability of nursing home placement.[32] Emotional stress and maladaptation may result in problems related to stimulation, self-image, socialization, life review, self-control, losses, dying, and death.

Nursing intervention should be aimed at avoiding overstimulation or understimulation, both of which can lead to confusion, depression, or anxiety. The basic level of stimulation must include *regular* daily activation of each of the senses (sight, hearing, touch, smell, taste). The nurse should identify interventions that will both stimulate the senses and provide variety. Understimulation is most likely to occur when the person's ability to move independently in the environment is restricted and sensory input becomes limited or nonvaried, or both. Fractured hips, strokes, widespread arthritis, and generalized weakness associated with severe malnutrition or chronic illness are but a few of the health problems that may result in a loss of independent movement.

Overstimulation often occurs when the elder is hospitalized or institutionalized and is being cared for by many new people in a strange environment with high levels of activities and noises. The nurse can explore possible ways to more evenly distribute activities to avoid or minimize days of tightly scheduled tests and therapies.

Self-image is a basic element for emotional health. Threats to self-image occur as a result of perceived losses in physical powers, emotional or financial security, and roles. Nursing care should be designed to maintain or enhance the elderly person's perceived needs for a healthy self-image. Perceived needs for physical appearance may include aspects such as makeup, jewelry, hair style, or clothing styles; body integrity and shape (threatened by invasive procedures such as mastectomy, amputation, fluctuations in weight); and physical agility. Perceived needs for emotional comfort may include physical contact, privacy, communication with loved ones (including pets), productivity, opportunities to help others, and participation in pleasurable activities.

Because socialization needs are individualized, they vary in older persons just as they do in those who are younger. Some persons have always been extroverts whereas others are more introverted. Unfortunately, what happens in many health care settings is that the extroverted person's life-style is usually considered the normal, healthy pattern, whereas the person who prefers less socialization is suddenly and obtrusively encouraged or required to adopt a pattern of socialization that is emotionally uncomfortable. This practice (of encouraging increased socialization) may occur because of the myth that all older people are lonely because they have lost family or friends and/or the ability to "connect" with others because of illness or immobility. This is often true for the extroverted person who is at greater risk for loss of social opportunities, but it is not true for those who prefer to be alone. The nurse must be aware of previous social patterns of the person and should foster surroundings (socialization) that approximate preferred patterns.

Life review is a healthy activity in achieving emotional integrity in the later years.[6,26,32] Nursing interventions can include providing the opportunity to verbalize past achievements and experience. Volunteers and clergy can assist the person in a life review. The opportunity for life review may occur naturally in the nurse's process of gathering assessment data and in the provision of day-to-day nursing care. Tasks that do not require focused attention can be done while engaging in conversation that allows the person to talk about his or her past. Life review may trigger unexpected feelings of loss (e.g., of career, family, or social contacts). If this occurs, it is important to allow the person to discuss the loss and express emotion if desired.

Death and the process of dying are life events that elicit a multitude of emotional responses. Elderly patients are usually aware of death as an imminent possibility, and some see this as a welcome natural event. Others who may not have achieved a sense of wholeness and closure to their lives in later years may anticipate their death with concern and fear. Nursing interventions should include the opportunity to discuss death and dying with appropriate persons—the nurse, a member of the clergy, family members, or physician. Often the opportunity to talk about death and putting life in order (estates, etc.) is more important to elders than their medical treatment.

## SEXUALITY

Both men and women maintain interest in sexual activity into the late adulthood years. More women cease having sexual activity after age 65 than do men. The primary reasons for the cessation are lack of an acceptable sexual partner for widows or an ailing husband for married women (rather than lack of interest).[23]

Cultural attitudes toward the elderly influence both genders. Older men and women frequently are thought of as sexually unattractive and lacking in ability to engage in sex. However, Masters and Johnson[23] have found that although sexual responses are slower, elders still have the same phases of excitement, plateau, orgasm, and resolution as younger persons. Men, in particular, can expect adequate sexual performance up to and beyond the eighth decade (see Chapter 51).

Sexual problems occur more frequently for the elders. Women may have dyspareunia as a result of vaginal thinning and decreased lubrication. These factors are caused by postmenopausal steroid starvation. Men tend to be affected by secondary impotence related to performance anxiety and low self-esteem. Diabetes, alcohol, and medications for hypertension are other prominent causes of impotence.

Masters and Johnson report a condition known as "widower's syndrome."[23] After an extended period of sexual inactivity, a man cannot achieve or maintain an erection. An equivalent condition occurs in women: the vagina constricts and undergoes atrophic changes. The conclusion is that those who do not engage in sexual activity lose the ability to do so.

Sexuality is more than the physical act of intercourse. Elderly persons continue to need human companionship and the sharing of love and affection. Nurses need to be aware of the components of sexuality and how elders may be affected by chronic illness, loss of a partner, and need for touch. Being sensitive to family dynamics is just as important for a newly married couple in their seventies as for a young couple.[33] Through counseling the nurse can explain aging changes, suggesting vaginal lubrication for women, and extra physical stimulation for men. Changes in sexual position and styles of lovemaking are appropriate for those with disabling diseases. Nurses have a vital role in enabling elderly persons to express their needs for love and affection.

Unfortunately, elders are susceptible to sexually transmitted disease, although not in the same numbers as younger adults. Acquired immunodeficiency syndrome (AIDS) is becoming increasingly prevalent in elders as the epidemic spreads among all age-groups. The "at risk" categories differ for elders (e.g., not as many are intravenous drug abusers).[30] However, other risk factors are present: the decline in the ability of the immune system to ward off infections makes elders more susceptible to organisms of sexually transmitted diseases. Women in particular are more vulnerable because of the friable vaginal lining that occurs with aging. "Safe sex" education and counseling for those at risk should not be overlooked just because the person is older than 65 years of age.[30]

# ACUTE ILLNESS IN ELDERS

## HOSPITALIZED ELDERS

Elders enter acute care hospitals more frequently, stay longer, and experience more adverse consequences than do younger adults. Frequently hospitalization of elders occurs in response to a crisis situation such as a fall that results in a fracture or a decline in cognitive status. These acutely ill elders require attention to the following areas of nursing care: prevention of iatrogenesis, discharge planning, mobility, nutrition, skin care, and prevention of confusion. The prevention of *iatrogenic* illness is a key to maintaining functioning. Iatrogenic illness can result from many common hospital-related factors, such as restricted mobility and nutrition, as well as the use of multiple medications.

### TEAM APPROACH

A multidisciplinary team approach to care affords the opportunity to review all aspects of the patient's care, including progress toward goals and prevention of complications. Physician members of the team should communicate about the patient's medical problems, the usefulness of medications planned, diagnostic procedures, and estimated length of stay (LOS) in the hospital. The nurse should assess and communicate about the person's functional status, nutritional intake, cognitive status, patient and family educational needs, and responses to or side effects of medications and other treatments. The social worker may provide an assessment of the patient's support system, including financial resources and community services. Other team members may include physical and occupational therapists, dietitians, and home care nurses who provide additional assessments, as well as interventions planned to achieve the goals of care.

Ongoing and open communication between the team and the patient and family is critical. Within the framework of the team approach, difficult decisions about interventions or the withholding of interventions can be carefully made. Tentative plans for discharge from the hospital should be made at the time of admission (if not before hospitalization), if at all possible. In many instances the discharge of an elderly family member may require family members to take time off from work to provide assistance until the older person is able to regain strength and independence in activities of daily living. Discharge planning should include an estimation of the length of stay, anticipated outcomes, and posthospitalization needs. A family conference often is helpful in gathering sufficient information to assist with discharge planning. A family conference also fosters communication, promotes trust, and provides support for the family.

### MOBILITY

Bedrest and immobility should be avoided whenever possible because they contribute to weakness and decreased functional ability. Patients should be encouraged to ambulate at least twice a day while wearing firm walking shoes. Patients and family members should be taught range-of-motion exercises, pumping the feet to prevent postural hypotension, and coughing and deep-breathing exercises. Independent mobility should be promoted through the avoidance of physical restraints or medications that make the patient drowsy or dizzy. Whenever patients are identified as having activity limitations, con-

## RESEARCH

Hirsch CH et al: The natural history of functional morbidity in hospitalized older patients, *J Am Geriatr Soc* 38:1296-1303, 1990.

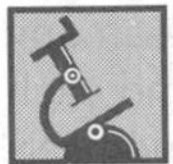

This study revealed that changes in functional health status of older patients was associated with acute hospitalizations. Assessments of functional status included mobility, transfer, toileting, incontinence, feeding, grooming, and mental status. Between baseline (or 2 weeks before hospitalization) and day 2, statistically significant deteriorations occurred for the overall functional score and for the individual scores for mobility, transfer, toileting, feeding, and grooming. None of these scores improved significantly by discharge. The authors conclude that greater efforts to prevent functional decline in hospitalized elders is warranted. In addition, an awareness of this decline is important in planning for discharge and postdischarge care needs.

sultation with physical and occupational therapists early in the admission can serve to reverse decline and restore function. Hospital environments should be assessed carefully for safety. Hand rails, elevated toilet seats, sturdy chairs with arms, adequate lighting, and accessible nurse call bells are critical environmental adaptations that promote independence and safety. Elderly patients should be assessed on admission and daily for safe mobility. Those patients assessed as being at risk for falls should have planned interventions to reverse or ameliorate the factors that place them at risk. Patients with weakness should be taught a paced exercise program that may include ambulatory aids such as a cane or a walker. Patients with postural hypotension should be taught leg exercises and instructed about adequate fluid and sodium intake. See the Research box above for a study of functional morbidity in hospitalized elders.

Physical (mechanical) restraints are devices used to inhibit free motion. These devices include vests, belts, mittens, jackets, and wrist and ankle restraints. Restraints can be dangerous. In addition to limiting movement, their use has been associated with increased agitation, pressure sores, incontinence, muscle deconditioning, and strangulation. The decision to use restraints should be evaluated carefully by the interdisciplinary team. Factors to consider before using restraints are alternatives to restraints, goals of therapy, and monitoring for safety. Patients and families need clear explanations about the risks and benefits of restraint use. The need to continue the use of restraints should be reevaluated at least every shift, with the goal being to remove the restraints as soon as it is safe to do so. (See p. 81.)

## NUTRITION

Many elders enter the hospital in a malnourished state. Nutritional goals during hospitalization should include adequate caloric and fluid intake and the maintenance or restoration of ideal weight. Interventions to prevent imbalances and complications such as aspiration of food or fluids include oral care before meals, getting out of bed for meals, and sitting up for 30 minutes after completion of meals. Elders often have poor appetites even when not acutely ill. High-calorie snacks should be available around the clock. Family members may be persuaded to supply preferred foods and socialization during meal times. Nurses should assess elderly patients daily to detect weight loss and assess food and fluid intake. Early consultation with dietitians may prevent severe malnutrition and dehydration and their complications. Often patients may need dietary restrictions for diagnostic tests, surgery, or treatment of illness. During such times diligent monitoring by the nurse and the dietitian, with communication among the team members, can prevent unnecessary restrictions and complications.

## CONTINENCE

To promote independent urinary function and prevent infections, indwelling catheters should be avoided whenever possible. Adequate hydration of at least 1200 ml of fluid should be ensured to stimulate normal stretch receptors in the bladder. Patients should be taught the value of a planned toileting schedule based on fluid intake, bladder capacity, and treatment regimens. Incontinence is not a normal aging change and may reflect illness, such as infections or an enlarged prostate gland. Incontinence has been associated with infections, pressure sores, depression, and increased nursing home placement.

## SKIN CARE

Elders have fragile skin caused by primary aging changes. Pressure sores may begin with falls or immobility that occurs before hospitalization. Poor nutrition, the use of intravenous catheters, and diuretics may all contribute to the development of new pressure sores, infections, or further deterioration of skin integrity. Careful daily assessment of skin integrity is important for all elderly hospitalized patients. Patients and families should be taught how to care for dry, aging skin to prevent breakdown. These interventions include the use of lotions, pressure-release mattresses, and a turning schedule. Extensive pressure sores may require the consultation of a clinical nurse specialist or physician.

## PSYCHOSOCIAL CHANGES

### General Care

In dealing with psychosocial changes the nurse assesses the physiologic changes, the diseases present, and the person's emotional make-up and apparent adjustment to the particular situation. Older persons frequently talk at length about their families and the past; their conversations may give clues to interests that should be encouraged and to problems confronting them. Plans

**BOX 4-12 Community Support Services for Older Persons**

**SENIOR CITIZEN CENTERS**
Social, nutritional, educational, and counseling services

**GERIATRIC DAY-CARE CENTERS**
Assistive daytime nursing care and social, nutritional, and rehabilitative services may be available

**ADULT FOSTER HOME CARE**
Care in private home for the older person who is unable to live alone

**MEALS ON WHEELS**
Meals delivered to the person's home

**HOMEMAKING SERVICE**
Household chores, shopping, and so on

**TRANSPORTATION SERVICE**
Arranged pickup by public transportation system

**HOME HEALTH SERVICE**
Skilled home nursing care

**LEGAL SERVICES**
Will, settlement of estate

**RESPITE CARE**
Short-term care to support primary caregiver, provided by hospitals, extended care facilities, or Visiting Nurses' Association

**COUNSELING SERVICES**
Private, governmental, public services for patient and caregivers

**SUPPORT GROUPS**
Private, nonprofit groups related to specific diagnosis

**REHABILITATION SERVICES**
Physical and occupational therapy in home or hospital

should be made to help them maintain as much independence as possible despite their limitations. Community resources are available to assist older persons to maintain independence and meet their social needs (Box 4-12).

Elderly patients are often lonely and appreciate just talking with others. Volunteers may provide a service by visiting with elders. Many patients appreciate visits with a member of the clergy. When visiting with elderly persons, it should be remembered that, although they commonly talk about events and activities in their own past, they usually are interested in the activities of younger persons and of the world around them.

The need to be useful is important to all persons. There are many tasks in which even the elderly person who is ill may be able to participate. At home elders may be able to help with the dishes or with meal preparation. They may be interested in crafts or making useful items. The older person may be quite slow, and great care must be taken not to show impatience, which may discourage further participation.

**RESEARCH**

Frierson R: Suicide attempts by the old and very old, *Arch Intern Med* 151(1):141-144, 1991.

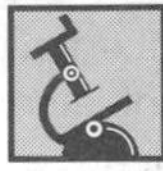

A study of suicide attempts was made among 95 elderly patients (ages 60 to 90), and each person was evaluated by a consultation service after a suicide attempt. The subjects differed significantly when compared with those in younger age-groups who attempted suicide, but persons in the younger age-groups were similar to the elders who successfully committed suicide. Recommendations are increased detection and treatment of depression and alcoholism, early psychiatric referral, limited access to firearms, and strategies to decrease social isolation.

Depression is not uncommon, and elders may be suicidal. Nurses need to be alert to signs of depression and thoughts of suicide, especially in older persons who are lonely and may not have a social support system. The Research box above presents a study of suicide attempts by elders.

Elderly persons usually are aware of death as an imminent possibility and sometimes see it as a welcome event. The issue should not be avoided. If the patient shows genuine concern about impending death, the nurse can encourage discussion of feelings (see Chapter 10). Family members also may need opportunities to discuss their feelings about death.

## Psychosocial Interventions

Healthy social and psychologic function can be promoted through environmental engineering, reality orientation, maintenance of normal sleep-wake cycles, and interactive activities. Socialization is important in maintaining cognitive status and preventing boredom and depression. Visits from family members and friends should be encouraged. Whenever possible, socialization with other elderly patients should be promoted. Because drugs are metabolized more slowly in elders, they are at high risk for adverse drug effects, especially with the use of multiple medications. In general, psychoactive or anticholinergic drugs often used for anxiety, agitation, and sleep are most commonly associated with adverse effects. The administration of any drugs, but most important, benzodiazipines, neuroleptics, tricyclic antidepressants, and anticholinergics, demand special attention to doses, side effects, and interactions with other drugs they are taking. (See Table 4-6, p. 98.)

**Delirium** or *an acute confusional state,* which is one of the most commonly encountered types of confusion in the acutely ill, occurs in 20% to 35% of all hospitalized elders. Delirium manifests by global cognitive impairments, disturbances of attention, reduced level of consciousness, increased or decreased psychomotor activity, and disturbances in sleep-wake cycles. Elderly patients should be assessed daily for orientation, the ability to recall words or recent events, and disturbances in language, attention, vision, or hearing. *Agitation,* which frequently accompanies delirium, often is more pronounced at night. Causes of delirium often are multiple and include cerebral diseases such as strokes and dementia and systemic diseases such as infections, neoplasms, electrolyte and metabolic disturbances, cardiovascular diseases, the effects of medications (especially in the hospital), and alcohol or drug withdrawal. Some medications given to relieve agitation may have a reverse effect in the compromised elder. Patients with cognitive impairments such as **dementia** may suffer further cognitive decline along with the delirium.

The management of delirium includes treating the underlying causes and providing supportive care. All medications should be carefully reviewed. Decreased doses of short-acting medications may offer temporary help in accomplishing diagnostic testing and other procedures. It is important to remember that the *delirious patient is a frightened patient.* Nursing care should focus on reality orientation. Environmental cues such as clocks, calendars, and daily newspapers, along with pictures and familiar objects from home, can be helpful in reducing agitation and allaying fears. In addition, special attention should be given to activity, socialization, and nutrition. The presence of family members through the evening and night hours may be helpful. Those who communicate with the patient should use simple, repetitive words and gestures. In many cases the use of restraints increases agitation. Thus restraints, because they are a potentially hazardous intervention, should be used with extreme caution with agitated patients. Delirious patients who are restrained should be monitored closely. (See Research box above for a study of deaths caused by restraints.)

**RESEARCH**

Miles ST, Irvine P: Deaths caused by physical restraints, *Gerontologist* 32(6):762-766, 1992.

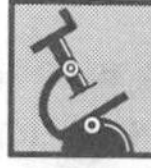

A retrospective analysis of 122 deaths caused by vest and strap restraints was undertaken. Victims were found suspended from chairs (42%) or beds (58%). Detailed analysis of 19 cases revealed that all victims were demented, the median age was 81 years, and 14 of the 19 had recently tried to escape from a restraint or had been found in a dangerous position while restrained. The authors conclude that restraint-related deaths are underrecognized, underreported, and avoidable.

## SPECIAL PROBLEMS

### Diagnostic Tests

Diagnostic testing can create a stressful situation for the elderly patient and the family who may experience a number of fears regarding the tests. Thus the actual procedures for testing should be explained and ample opportunities allowed for asking questions. Both the patient and family members may experience distress caused by the uncertainty of the test results and the patient's future. If the patient desires, family members should be allowed to be with the patient for as much of the testing as possible.

Elderly patients who are undergoing diagnostic tests that require withholding of meals or the use of enemas or cathartics should be attended unless they are in their beds, because they often become quite weak and dizzy. No elderly patient should ever be left unattended on a treatment table, and such patients should be helped on and off the table. Because the person may be dizzy, it is advisable for him or her to rise slowly and sit on the edge of the table for a few moments before standing. The dizziness may be caused by the slow compensation of inelastic blood vessels. Older patients with cardiovascular disease also may be orthopneic and cannot tolerate lying flat for examinations.

Because of the rapidity with which they develop pressure ulcers, elderly patients who must lie on x-ray, treatment, or operating room tables for lengthy periods need pads placed under the normal curves of their backs and a pad of material such as sponge rubber placed under bony prominences. On return to the unit, the patient's skin should be checked for pressure areas, and, if any signs of pressure are evident, these areas should be massaged gently until the tissue appears normal in color.

If the patient is placed in lithotomy position, care must be taken to place both legs in the stirrups at the same time to prevent undue pull on unresilient muscles. The same approach applies to removing the legs from the stirrups. Care also must be taken to prevent hyperextension and hyperflexion of the joints, because many elderly patients have arthritis and reduced flexibility.

### Anesthesia and Surgery

For the patient who is undergoing surgery, age in itself is not a risk factor. The risk factors for elders are the presence and severity of any underlying disease, such as congestive heart failure, renal disease, ischemic heart problems, or chronic obstructive lung disease.[17] The surgeon and anesthesiologist study the patient carefully to determine how much risk is involved. Their recommendations are made according to the type of surgery and concerns about cardiopulmonary function.

During the preoperative period, the nurse assists the patient in restoring fluids that have been lost through dehydration, bowel disease, or blood loss. In addition, the nurse provides basic preoperative teaching. Teaching is particularly important for an elderly person with cognitive deficits who may need extra time and patience to understand the procedures that have been planned. Family members may be concerned that the person's age makes him or her a poor risk. They need careful detailed explanations of the surgery and the intraoperative procedures.

When choosing anesthesia for elders, the anesthesiologist is most likely to use a regional anesthetic. If general anesthesia is necessary, then shorter-acting anesthetic agents are best. With underlying cardiopulmonary disease, the risks are greater for aspiration, shock, pulmonary edema, and myocardial infarction.[17]

After surgery elders are more prone to confusion and sleepiness. Other common problems are *hypothermia, respiratory depression, fluctuations in blood pressure, and renal failure.*

Postoperative nursing care focuses careful attention on vital signs, especially early signs of shock or hypertension. Warm blankets are even more important for elderly persons than for the younger adult. Urinary output, BUN, and creatinine levels require careful monitoring. The person who is confused may require frequent reorientation and repetition of instructions. Having a familiar family member at the bedside helps the elderly patient who is frightened and confused. Although they should be used as little as possible, restraints may be necessary in the early postoperative period to keep the person from tugging at intravenous lines, nasogastric tubes, and oxygen tubes. Attendance by a significant other may eliminate the need for restraints.

The postoperative course may be longer for the elderly patient. Because the functional reserve capacity is decreased, the patient may be more susceptible to urinary and pulmonary infections. Return to baseline function requires more effort on the part of both the nurse and the patient. If the patient is discharged while still below his or her normal-function level, relatives or home nursing services will be needed to meet the patient's needs until full recuperation is accomplished (see Chapter 27 for more information on home care).

## Diabetes

Elderly persons are more susceptible to abnormalities in glucoregulation than are younger persons. In elders, the presenting sign is not an elevated blood sugar level but microvascular changes that go undetected until signs and symptoms of complications, such as neuropathy, nephropathy, or retinopathy, occur. The fasting blood sugar level may be normal, and a glucose-tolerance test is needed for a definite diagnosis. Factors that lead to a decline in glucose tolerance in elders are obesity, deconditioning, decreased muscle mass, poor diet, coexisting diseases, and medications.[17]

The diagnosis is often made when the patient is under care for some other condition such as an infection, workup for surgery, or other complicating illness. Non–insulin-dependent diabetes is seen most often in obese patients older than 50 years of age who have had significant glucose intolerance for several years before it is detected.

The goal of medicine is not vigorous treatment of the hyperglycemia but rather adequate control in the hope of minimizing organ complications. About half of elderly diabetics need sulfonylurea drugs, and fewer than half require insulin.[4] The nurse teaches the patient the significance of weight loss (80% of elderly diabetics are overweight), aerobic exercise, and good foot and skin care. (See Chapter 40 for more information about diabetes.)

# ❦ HOME CARE CONSIDERATIONS

## Discharge Planning

After hospitalization the younger adult most frequently returns home to an independent life-style, whereas the older adult must be evaluated for ability and resources to manage at home. The following factors are considered:

1. Has the patient been functioning independently before hospitalization?
2. If the patient is independent, has function returned to baseline?
3. Are appropriate caregivers or support persons at home?
4. Are other dependent disabled persons in the home?
5. What is the health of the primary caregiver?
6. How capable are the caregivers emotionally, physically, and mentally?
7. What financial resources are available for home care, such as supplies and equipment?

The patient who has declining function and requires increasing amounts of assistance with activities of daily living usually has three choices for discharge placement:

1. Home with family caregiver
2. Home with family and/or professional nursing services or other assistance (see Chapter 27)
3. Nursing home or extended-care facility

The nurse often becomes the coordinator for the discharge planning for the elderly patient who needs assistance after discharge. For the patient returning home, the nurse must teach transfer techniques, physical care, use of special equipment, and knowledge of medications. If the patient needs home nursing services, the nurse makes the appropriate referral, listing all the patient's needs. Social work services are necessary for the patient who must be transferred to an extended-care facility or who needs financial assistance.

In the case of the patient who may need institutional care, the nurse has a key role. First, the patient's functional abilities must be evaluated thoroughly to determine if placement is really necessary. Then the nurse and social worker help family members choose the appropriate facility by giving them a list of available places and teaching them how to evaluate each one. This is frequently a difficult task for family members, who may feel guilty about removing the patient from the home. The nurse gives emotional support during the decision-making process to both the family and the patient, who may view the decision negatively because he or she is losing autonomy.

The nurse may be caught in a controversy between the patient's wishes to return home and the wishes of the family and physician to institutionalize the patient. It is not unusual for the patient to deny the amount of care needed. In such a situation, ethical principles must be carefully considered.

Patient autonomy may need to be weighed against the greatest good for the greatest number (the family). The process involves listing alternatives, predicting consequences, and selecting the solution based on those consequences. For example, a positive consequence results if a patient with declining physical function is returned home. However, harm could occur from a fall, and continued physical decline might result (negative consequence). Therefore the protected environment of the nursing home would be a positive consequence, and the family would be relieved of the burden of care.[19]

Each case must be decided individually with as much input from all parties as possible. The nurse is obligated to support the process and the chosen solution, no matter what her or his personal values. In many cases the options are limited, and the solution brings sadness to all involved.

### TERMINATING TREATMENT

The nurse frequently is involved in decisions about initiating or withholding treatments for the elderly person who is terminally ill. No simple legislated answers exist to the questions, "Who should have treatment?" or "Is withholding fluids and food a form of passive euthanasia?" Some states have legal provision for a **living will,** but even this document does not guarantee that the patient's wishes will be followed in the event he or she is incompetent or unable to make known his or her desires.

Some experts recommend that a **durable power of attorney** for health care be obtained while the person is mentally competent. Then when the patient becomes ill or incapacitated, the person with the durable power of attorney can act on the patient's behalf and ensure that the patient's wishes are carried out.

When a patient has no living will or durable power of attorney, the health care team must consider the following factors when making decisions regarding withholding of treatments[17]:

1. Did the patient express any wishes when competent?
2. What are the wishes of the family?
3. Does the giving of treatment represent a disproportionate burden to others?
4. What is the quality of life for the individual?

The nurse can act as advocate for the patient by interviewing family members, supporting the decision-making process, and encouraging the parties involved to make the decisions without haste. Wishes the patient expresses while competent should be carefully documented in the patient's record. (See Chapter 2 for further discussion of this and other ethical issues.)

## HEALTH PROMOTION: PREVENTION

Chronic diseases are a major health problem and are much more common among the elderly population (Box 4-13). Estimates show that 85% of elders have one or more chronic diseases. Heart disease and hypertension are the most prevalent, with 50% of persons older than the age of 65 years having observable signs of heart disease. Gastrointestinal disorders, rheumatism, and arthritis affect large numbers of elders. Visual problems, atherosclerosis, lung disease, and hypertension appear to be associated with lower socioeconomic status.

The figures on prevalence of health problems may be misleading. The important issues are what is normal functioning and how disabling are the chronic conditions?

Despite chronic disease, 83% of persons older than 65 years of age have little difficulty carrying out activities of daily living. Only 5% live in nursing homes, although 35% will be in a nursing home at one time or another. Another 5% are homebound.

The following factors are important considerations in evaluating the physical capacities of elders:

1. Organ systems have a great compensatory ability, despite loss of cells and tissue through aging (such as in the brain, kidney, heart, and liver).
2. Compensatory mechanisms may fail when the organism is stressed through illness and disease (e.g., renal failures can occur with urinary tract infection).
3. The body takes a longer time to return to normal after a stressful event.
4. Once a stressful event has occurred, the individual may not return to baseline function.
5. The immune system is decreasingly effective as the person ages, causing increased susceptibility to in-

**BOX 4-13 Major Health Problems of Late Adulthood**

Heart disease
Hypertension
Cancer
Renal disease
Chronic obstructive pulmonary disease
Acute pulmonary disease (pneumonia, pulmonary edema)
Vascular disease (cerebrovascular accident, peripheral vascular disease)
Arthritis
Skin disorders
Accidents
Alcoholism

**BOX 4-14 Stressful Life Changes for Elders**

Loss of driver's license
Multiple relocations
Hemiplegia
Sensory deficits
Hospitalization
Institutionalization
Mechanical speech difficulties
Loss of children and friends
Dispersal of significant belongings
Incompetency proceedings
Inheritance conflicts
Birth of grandchildren
Moving to a nursing home
Inadequate health insurance coverage

fection. Elders are much more prone to pneumonia, skin infections, urinary tract infection, and sepsis.

6. The symptoms of a particular disease often are atypical in elders (e.g., a myocardial infarction without severe crushing chest pain, an infection without a fever, a gastrointestinal hemorrhage without severe stomach pain).
7. The most typical sign that an elder has had a change in physical well-being is sudden onset of confusion.

Stress situations (Box 4-14) may produce more pronounced reactions in elders and require a longer period of readjustment.

## PRIMARY PREVENTION

The goal of health care for elders is to keep them functioning at the optimal level for their age. Health promotion is just as important for the elderly person as for the young person. Nurses in any health care setting have an ideal opportunity to assist elderly persons with health promotion.

Even in the acute care setting where the focus is on illness, the nurse should identify priority needs and introduce an educational program designed to enhance the person's life-style after hospitalization.

The four main areas the nurse should address are ***health habits*** (smoking and drinking), ***exercise, nutrition,*** and ***immunizations.*** This section also addresses general principles in teaching elders.

### Health Habits

Nursing assessment in any setting should include questions regarding smoking and alcohol use. Smoking cessation can have positive health benefits for a person at any age—for example, reduced incidence of respiratory infections and improved ventilatory capacity. A smoking history should reveal not only the number of packs smoked per day but also the meaning of smoking to the person, habits connected with smoking (e.g., eating and drinking, reading, answering the telephone), and attempts made to stop in the past. The nurse can help the elder to analyze his or her smoking behavior to find ways to cut down or quit, as well as encourage the use of special programs, such as SmokeEnders or Smokestoppers.

Alcohol abuse is a largely unrecognized problem among elders. The signs and symptoms are similar to other secondary aging processes: tremors, sleep difficulties, gait abnormalities, depression, and malnutrition. The elderly person and his or her family may deny the seriousness of the problem, and health professionals may neglect to assess the individual for alcohol abuse.

Elderly persons have a decreased tolerance for alcohol because of a declining ability of the liver to detoxify and metabolize it. Loneliness and depression may intensify the feelings that lead to drinking. Heavy drinking contributes to confusion, injuries from falls, self-neglect, and malnutrition.[13]

The nurse should always be alert to symptoms that suggest alcohol abuse and should ask questions regarding drinking habits. Patients should be taught about aging changes that aggravate the effect of alcohol and informed about community agencies that are available to assist with alcohol problems. Many of these agencies have chapters of Alcoholic Anonymous. (For more information on alcohol abuse see Chapter 19.)

### Exercise

An exercise program has many benefits for older persons, whether or not they have engaged in exercise in the past. Exercise increases endurance, strengthens the muscles, enhances the cardiovascular system, reduces stress, and promotes relaxation. Table 4-4 shows the benefits to the body systems.

For elders who are experiencing normal aging changes and chronic health problems that contribute to diminished physical capacity, fitness will be more critical to maintenance of their independent function and ability to pursue enriching leisure activities. In one study, elders reported a problem with physical ability three times more often than other problems (i.e, lack of transportation, no money) as the main factor deterring their pursuit of leisure activities (walking, gardening, fishing, or driving).[31]

As with other age-groups—and perhaps even more—elders vary considerably in their physical abilities and overall physical fitness. One may distinguish between (1) "active" elders (those persons who seem little affected by their age and continue with lifelong activity habits), (2) "inactive" elders (those persons who are hindered by a variety of age-related problems that mentally or physically limit their physical ability), and (3) "very active" elders (those persons who have maintained a high degree of fitness and still participate in competitive sports events).[31]

Because fitness levels vary among elders, the focus of nursing care is either (1) to promote continued activity in those already engaged in moderate to high levels of

**TABLE 4-4 Benefits of Exercise**

| SYSTEM | BENEFIT |
|---|---|
| Cardiovascular | Increased maximum oxygen consumption<br>Increased cardiac output<br>Reduced mean blood pressure |
| Pulmonary | Reduced loss of $Vo_2$ maximum |
| Musculoskeletal | Increased bone mineral content<br>Decreased loss of calcium<br>Preservation of lean muscle mass |
| Regulatory system | Increased basal metabolic rate<br>Increased hemoregulation |
| Nervous system | Decreased sleeplessness<br>Decreased anxiety |

From Schilke J: *J Gerontol Nurs* 17(5):5-9, 1991.

activity or (2) to motivate and assist less active elders to engage in physical activities that are appropriate for their abilities and needs and are of interest to them. For the group of moderately to highly active persons, the nurse's responsibility is to promote and support their preferred activities.

In local communities groups or organizations such as YMCAs or senior centers often provide opportunities for elders to exercise in the form of protected and appropriately challenging hiking trails, swimming facilities, or other group exercise programs. By becoming familiar with the local exercise resources, the nurse is readily able to direct elders to appropriate resources. Whatever the type of program, the following guidelines are important[31]:

1. Seek the advice of a physician before starting a strenuous exercise program.
2. Do not exercise to the point of dyspnea or pain.
3. Stop if signs of activity intolerance appear: dizziness, nausea, palpitations, or fatigue.[26]

When advising elderly persons about an exercise program, the nurse should instruct them in taking their pulse rate and teach them to aim for 75% to 85% of the maximum heart rate.[23] Aerobic exercise, which increases oxygen uptake and strengthens the cardiovascular system, should be performed three or more times weekly for maximum benefit.

If the active individual becomes hospitalized or admitted to an extended-care facility for rehabilitation, all members of the interdisciplinary team (e.g., occupational and physical therapists, physiatrists) will involve the elder in assessing a prescribed plan of activity that will help restore the person's physical abilities and overall health. This prescribed plan will most likely consist of formal physical or occupational therapy sessions with the specialists in these areas, as well as a more informal plan that outlines the elder's participation in self-care activities and mobilization. The latter area requires considerable input from the nurse, who is in the best position to assess, implement, and evaluate individual activity patterns on a sustained basis.

For the less active elder who may be in a nursing home or at home and using home care resources (e.g., skilled nursing service, homemaker), prescribed rehabilitation activities often will be needed. However, there are additional general nursing measures to be considered in planning activity for persons who are partially or fully immobilized. When the individual is confined to bed, proper body alignment, frequent repositioning, and range-of-motion exercises will aid in maintaining comfort and maximum range of motion of the joints. Unless there is some particular contraindication, exercises for the arms and legs, exercises to keep abdominal and gluteal muscles in good tone, and exercises to strengthen the extensor muscles of the spine should be performed several times each day by every bed-restricted patient. The patient is taught to flex, abduct, adduct, and extend each leg separately and both legs simultaneously. The heel of one foot can be placed on the knee of the opposite leg and then the heel passed slowly down the leg to the ankle. This can then be repeated, alternating the legs. Arms, hand, neck, and shoulder movements can be encouraged by having the patient first raise and lower the head, neck, and shoulders from a flat supine position without a pillow and then by having the patient extend the arms in front of the chest, followed by raising them above the head. The person should be encouraged to do as many of the exercises as possible and to take deep breaths and exhale fully in coordination with the exercises. Daily exercises should be supervised by the nurse or caregiver. The regular performance of exercises helps to prevent the loss of muscle tone that occurs in all bed-restricted patients, regardless of age. If the person is unable to do active range-of-motion exercises independently, the nurse should help with them or do passive range-of-motion exercises.

Because immobile elders are at high risk for orthostatic hypotension, osteoporosis, venous stasis and thrombus formation, pneumonia and other respiratory infections, and sensory deprivation, the nursing care plan should include regular daily intervals out of bed spent walking with assistance or sitting in a chair.

## Nutrition

Nutritional requirements of elderly persons differ from those of younger adults. The physical changes associated with aging and changes in the gastrointestinal tract, the digestive enzymes, and metabolism all affect nutritional status. Social factors may have as much impact on the person's nutrition as physical changes. Some of these are loneliness, difficulty obtaining food, difficulty in preparing food, and social isolation. Malnutrition is common (Box 4-15). The following are the nutritional needs of elderly persons[20]:

- Calories should be reduced by 5% per decade between ages 55 and 75; 7% after 75 years of age.
- Carbohydrate levels should be maintained but should be obtained from fruits, vegetables, cereals, and

**BOX 4-15 Causes of Malnutrition in Elders**

Acute and chronic illness
Limited financial resources
Psychologic factors such as boredom and lack of companionship while eating
Loss of teeth
Faulty eating patterns
Fads and notions regarding certain foods
Lack of energy to prepare foods
Lack of knowledge of appropriate nutrition
Decreased digestive enzymes

From Reed P: *ANS* 6:18-25, 1983.

breads. Only moderate amounts of foods with refined sugars (e.g., candy, cake, cookies) should be consumed.

- Protein consumption should be reduced, especially red meats and high-fat dairy products. Fish, poultry, and combinations of plant foods should be increased.
- Fat levels should be maintained, but fats should make up no more than 25% to 30% of daily caloric intake.
- Vitamin supplements are not necessary unless dietary intake is poor. Absorption and storage capacity of vitamins decline. Vitamin D deficiency occurs occasionally.
- Mineral supplements are not needed unless a physician diagnoses deficiencies. Those older than 85 years are often deficient in calcium and zinc.
- Water consumption should not change, but dehydration is common among elders. Six to seven glasses of fluid should be taken per day.

### Immunizations

Persons older than 65 years should be advised to have yearly immunizations against influenza and a one-time immunization against pneumonia as part of the annual physical examination (Box 4-16). As the immunologic system ages, the elderly person becomes more susceptible to acute communicable diseases. The reserve capacity to recover from stress declines as well. Persons at high risk are those with chronic disorders of the pulmonary and cardiovascular systems. Immunizations for influenza change annually as different strains of the influenza virus are identified. The best advice is to have patients check with their physician. Some communities offer influenza immunizations through the local health department.

### Health Education

The elderly adult learner presents an interesting challenge to the nurse in any setting. The same teaching-learning principles apply to the older person as to a younger adult, with some additional guidelines. As with any adult learner, the environment must be comfortable and familiar, so as not to distract from the learning process. For the elderly person this means the nurse must take particular care to ensure that the patient is warm, relaxed, and free from pain and other discomforts. The older adult may have a hearing or vision impairment that inhibits the learning process, and the nurse must take this into consideration when planning teaching methods.

**BOX 4-16 Immunizations for Elders**

Pneumococcal 23-valent vaccine; given one time
Influenza vaccine; given annually in the fall
Tetanus vaccine, for penetrating injuries, or booster dose given every 10 years.

From Reed P: *ANS* 6:18-25, 1983.

The nurse should present the content of any teaching plan in several short sessions, focusing on single elements of the topic and reinforcing previous learning. This is especially important if the person has a short attention span or is distracted by the treatments and equipment in the environment.

One problem the nurse may overlook in the elderly patient is low literacy.[20] When a patient has cognitive and sensory impairments, the lack of good reading and vocabulary skills may hamper well-intentioned educational efforts. Low literacy provokes several reactions. The person may say she or he understands the teaching when in fact he or she does not, resulting in withdrawal from the situation or disregarding complicated instructions. The following are hints for teaching patients with low literacy:

1. Use simple one- or two-syllable words.
2. Use large-print materials.
3. Use pictures with colors and symbols.
4. Divide teaching sessions into segments.
5. Reinforce previous learning.
6. Give positive rewards for mastering content (e.g., praise, attention, touch).
7. Involve other family members in the teaching process.[20]

## SECONDARY PREVENTION

### Health Screening

Health screening is as important for the elderly as for the younger adult. The elderly person should have an annual physical examination. Box 4-17 lists the recommended screening procedures for both sexes.

### Medications

The most common treatment modality for illness, especially chronic illness, is the use of prescribed medications.[25] The use of both prescribed and nonprescribed medications increases with age. Elders consume disproportionately more of all kinds of drugs than do middle

**BOX 4-17 Recommended Health Screening**

| | |
|---|---|
| **COMPLETE PHYSICAL EXAMINATION** | |
| Women (breast examination) | |
| Self | Monthly |
| Professional | Annually |
| Mammogram | Annually until age 70, then discretionary |
| Pap and pelvic | Annually |
| Men (penis, scrotum, testicles) | |
| Self | Monthly |
| Professional | Annually |
| **RECTAL EXAMINATION** | |
| Both men and women | Annually |
| Proctosigmoidoscopy | Every 3-5 yr after two consecutive negative annual test results |
| Stool for occult blood | Annually |
| **DENTAL EXAMINATION** | Every 6-12 mo |
| Oral screen for cancer | Every 6-12 mo |

Modified from Pastorino C, Dickey T: *Orthop Nurs* 9(6):36, 1990.

adults, partly because older adults experience more chronic illness. Medications provide tremendous benefits to older adults, but they also can create problems for the patient, family, and health care provider. The medication regimen may be complex and troublesome for the patient or family to administer. Some medications may be difficult to tolerate and can cause unpleasant side effects; others may produce adverse reactions and interactions or unpredictable responses in the elders.[25]

### Drug absorption

Numerous age-related physical changes in older adults affect the response to medications. The *absorption* of drugs may be influenced by the presence or absence of nutrients or by the decrease of hydrochloric acid that normally occurs with aging; drugs that depend on an acid medium may be absorbed less effectively. Absorption also may be altered because the rate of transit through the gastrointestinal system tends to slow with age.

### Drug distribution

The *distribution* of drugs within the body is affected by the loss of lean body mass and the increased proportion of body fat. Fat-soluble drugs tend to be stored in fat, thereby decreasing the intensity of the reaction while increasing the duration. Within the bloodstream the distribution of drugs is affected by the amount of serum protein, specifically the albumin, available as binding sites for drugs. In aging persons, the serum albumin levels tend to be lower, resulting in altered concentrations of bound (inactive) and unbound (active) drugs. Unbound drugs in the circulation are active in producing the effects of the drug. The unbound drug can be excreted by the kidneys or metabolized by the liver. A principal mechanism of drug interaction seems to be the displacement of one drug by another from these protein-binding sites. For example, warfarin may be displaced by aspirin, indomethacin, and other drugs, causing increased anticoagulation activity.

### Drug metabolism

The *metabolism* of drugs in elders may be altered by lower levels of enzyme activity in the liver. The result of prolonged or incomplete metabolism is an increase in the half-life of some drugs, which allows the drug to exert its effect over a longer period of time.

### Drug excretion

The kidney is the primary route of excretion of drugs. *Aging* changes such as decreased renal plasma flow to the kidney, the decreased glomerular filtration rate, and the decreased number of functional tubules combine to result in inefficient excretion of active drug. This increases the risk of accumulation of drugs to potentially toxic levels because of decreased renal clearance. The decreased rate of excretion and the changes in binding sites in the blood unite to prolong the elevated blood level and activity of many drugs. Digoxin has a narrow margin of safety and is an example of a drug that is critically affected by the change in renal excretion.

Medications have a definite place in the therapeutic regimen for the older adult, but they must be handled carefully. One general principle in medication therapy is that the drug level should be built up gradually, and the lowest dose and fewest possible number of drugs should be used. In prescribing medications for elders, it is wise to "start low and go slow" because standard doses typically have been developed for younger groups.[11] Nurses should check for untoward reactions to medications and report them to the health care provider. If a patient is emaciated or elderly, medication should be prescribed with caution and the use of a full adult dose of any drug should be questioned. Most elders take three or more therapeutic agents, and drug reactions and interactions are far more prevalent. Table 4-5 shows the pharmacokinetic changes that occur in the elderly person.

As part of the health care team, nurses can assist patients and families in developing strategies to improve medication-taking behaviors. In one study of home care clients, nurses identified medication-taking behavior as the number one problem with clients.[25] Some common problems elders have with medication administration include forgetfulness, regulation of dosages, poor storage, sharing medications, outdated prescriptions, diffi-

**TABLE 4-5 Pharmacokinetic Changes in Elders**

| PROCESS | CHANGE | POSSIBLE RESULT |
|---|---|---|
| Absorption | Decrease in HCL in stomach | Inadequate absorption of weak acid drugs |
| | Delay in gastric emptying | Prolonged exposure of drug to mucosa leads to possible overdosage and toxicity |
| Distribution | Decrease in cardiac output | Slower circulation of drug to desired sites of action and elimination |
| | Decrease in body muscle mass | Onset and duration of action of many drugs change |
| | Increase in body fat | Fat-soluble drugs have delayed onset of action |
| | Decrease in body water | More sensitive to water-soluble drugs |
| | Decrease in serum albumin | Increase in amount of free-active (usually protein bound) drugs<br>Increased potential for drug interactions |
| | Slowing of active transport systems | Delayed drug action |
| | Increased sensitivity to CNS drugs | Possible seizures, excitation, certain drugs (barbiturates) cause confusion |
| Biotransformation | Impaired liver function | Elevated plasma levels of drugs because of a decrease in first pass effect and in biotransformation<br>Elevated levels of active metabolites of drugs |
| Excretion | Impaired kidney function | Elevated plasma levels of drugs |

From Gray M: *Orthop Nurs* 9(6):49, 1990.

**TABLE 4-6 Drug Interactions and Their Potential Results**

| DRUG A | DRUG B | POTENTIAL RESULTS |
|---|---|---|
| Digoxin | Furosemide | Reduced potassium produced by B could increase risk of arrhythmia produced by A |
| Warfarin | Aspirin | Protein displacement of A by B could increase risk of bleeding |
| Tetracycline | Antacid | Absorption impairment of A by B could reduce the antibiotic efficacy of A |

From Hershey L, Whitney C. In Kart C, Metress E, Metress S, editors: *Aging, health, and society,* Boston, 1988, Jones & Bartlett.

culty in reading and understanding labels, and inability to open child-proof containers. Nursing assessment to determine the patient's ability to independently administer medications involves observation and interviews with the patient and family.

■ ■ ■

*Four problems affect elders* as they take medications: ***drug interactions, adverse reactions, drug and food interactions,*** and ***medication errors.*** Each category is detailed in the following discussion.

### Drug interactions

Some medications interact with others, causing harmful effects. Table 4-6 shows some of the possible combinations that are problems for elders.

### Adverse reactions

Medications that cause no problems for middle-aged adults may be harmful for elders because of the physiologic changes mentioned previously. Table 4-7 shows typical medications taken by elders and the most common adverse reactions.

**TABLE 4-7 Typical Medications and Their Effects**

| MEDICATION | EFFECT ON ELDERS |
|---|---|
| Tranquilizers | CNS effects (sleepiness) |
| Aminoglycoside antibiotics | Ototoxicity, nephrotoxicity |
| Anticoagulants | Risk of bleeding |
| Phenothiazines | Risk of tardive dyskinesia |
| Beta blockers | Lightheadedness, slowed heart rate |
| Digoxin | Confusion |

Modified from Hershey L, Whitney C. In Kart C, Metress E, Metress S, editors: *Aging, health, and society,* Boston, 1988, Jones & Bartlett.

Beta blockers can be particularly problematic for elders because these commonly prescribed agents depress cardiac contractility, leading to lethargy and dyspnea. Elderly persons are more prone to orthostatic hypotension, hypoglycemia, thyroid dysfunction, arthritic changes, and depression, all of which are possible side effects of beta blockers.

### Drug and food interactions

Some foods may inhibit or change the effect of a particular medication more dramatically in elderly than middle-aged persons. Levodopa taken by patients with Parkinson's disease has a reduced effect if taken with a high-protein meal. The antidepressants in the monoamine oxidase (MAO) inhibitor group are affected by red wine, blue cheese, and herring, causing malignant hypertension.[25]

### Medication errors

**Medication errors** are common among elders and include omitting prescribed drugs, taking drugs at the wrong times, and taking medications without fully knowing why they are prescribed. ***In studies of medication errors, the persons most likely to err were those who took the most medications, those who lived alone, and those who were relatively less well-educated.***[21]

**BOX 4-18 Patient Medication History**

**GENERAL QUESTIONS**

What medications do you take every day?
What are they used for?
Have you taken any other medications during the past month? Past year?
What do you take for pain? How often?
What do you take to help you sleep? How often?
What do you take for constipation? How often?
Do you take any vitamins and health food preparations?
What medications do you share with your family? Friends?
What alcoholic beverages do you consume? How often? How much?
Do you smoke? How often?
Have you used any home remedies to treat this problem? Any other problem?

**ADVERSE/ALLERGIC RESPONSES**

Have you ever had an allergic response to medication?
Can you describe how it affected you?
Did you have this reaction in a hospital? At home?
What was done when you had this reaction?

**QUESTIONS ABOUT TAKING MEDICATIONS**

When do you take your medications? (time of day and number of times)
What happens if you miss a medication?
Are there any medications you take differently than the prescription says?
Do you have trouble reading the regular labels?
Do you have trouble removing the cap on the medication?
Do you have trouble in pouring or drawing up medication?
Do you have trouble swallowing any of your medications?

**CARE OF MEDICATIONS**

Where do you store your medications?
What happens with leftover medications?
Do you purchase medications in large quantities?

**OBTAINING PRESCRIPTION MEDICATIONS**

Have your medications been prescribed by more than one doctor?
Where do you get your prescriptions filled?

**PSYCHOSOCIAL ASPECTS**

With whom do you live?
Have you ever omitted medications because they were too expensive?
How do you pay for your medications?

Modified from Gray M: *Orthop Nurs* 9(6):49, 1990.

### Facilitating learning about medications

First, the nurse should make a detailed and thorough assessment in all contacts with elders. Questions included in medication history are presented in Box 4-18.

Education is based on the strengths and deficits revealed in the medication history. If the patient does not know the name of the drug but remembers the pink "heart" pill, the nurse emphasizes the pink digoxin (Lanoxin) pill for the heart when discussing the medication. When administering medications in the acute care setting, the nurse is obligated to repeat the name, dose,

**BOX 4-19 Resources Concerning Older Adults**

American Association of Retired Persons (AARP)
Program Resources Department
1909 K Street, N.W.
Washington, DC 20049
(202) 872-4700
Provides information, including a list of reading materials, educational programs, and numerous booklets for patient teaching on many topics. (AARP is the nation's largest and oldest organization of Americans 50 years and older, retired or not.)

Children of Aging Parents
2761 Trenton Road
Levittown, PA 19056
Offers lists of support groups for some states, information about case-management workers, and caregiving booklets.

Department of Health and Human Services
Public Health Service
Agency for Health Care Policy and Research
Publications Clearinghouse
P.O. Box 8547
Silver Spring, MD 20907
1-800-358-9295
(301) 495-3453
Publishes clinical practice guidelines and a patient's guide for several patient problems of concern to medical-surgical nurses.

National Council on Aging
NCOA Publications
P.O. Box 7227
Ben Franklin Station
Washington, DC 20044
(202) 479-1200
Write for listing of books and pamphlets.

National Institute on Aging (NIA)
NIA Information Center
2209 Distribution Circle
Silver Spring, MD 20910
(301) 495-3455
Publication list and information on health topics of interest to older people are available. (NIA is part of U.S. Department of Health and Human Services, Public Health Services, National Institutes of Health)

**AUDIOVISUAL RESOURCES**

*Aging:* 54-minute color VHS videocassette, 1988.
PBS Video
1320 Braddock Place
Alexandria, VA 22314-1698
PBS Video
475 L'Enfant Plaza, S.W.
Washington, DC 20024
1-800-344-3337 or
1-800-424-7963

*Aging:* 16-mm color film
CRM educational films
1104 Camino Del Mar
Del Mar, CA 92014
PBS Video
475 L'Enfant Plaza, S.W.
Washington, DC 20024
1-800-344-3337 or
1-800-424-7963

*Continued.*

**BOX 4-19 Resources Concerning Older Adults—cont'd**

*Be well: health in the later years,* 24-minute 16-mm color film, 1983.
Churchill Films
662 North Robertson Blvd.
Los Angeles, CA 90069
1-800-334-7830 or
(213) 657-5110

*Feeding techniques for adult dysphagic patients,* Chicago, Rehabilitation Institute of Chicago. (Videotape)

*Into aging,* ed 2, Thorofare, NJ, 1991, Slack Publishers. (Boxed simulation game)

*Peege,* Princeton, NJ, Phoenix Films. (Film)

*Presentation of illness in the elderly,* Philadelphia, 1988. JB Lippincott. (Videotape)

and desired effect of the drugs. Through repetition, even persons with cognitive and learning impairments start to gain name recognition for their medications.

Whenever possible, patients should be allowed to take their own medications in the hospital setting. Self-medication allows the nurse to assess the patient's understanding of the drugs and their timing. It also provides an opportunity to observe side effects, such as lethargy or hypotension.

When teaching the patient how to take medications at home, the nurse must allow sufficient time for adequate learning. The following hints assist the nurse:

1. Teach in several short sessions spread over 1 to 2 days rather than one crammed session as the patient is being discharged.
2. Simplify medication schedules; for example, use colored stickers for different bottles.
3. Use large-print instructions.
4. Coordinate times for medications with the person's daily schedule, for example with meals, when reading paper, before or after brushing teeth.
5. Use pictures for a person who cannot read well, for example, use a drawing of a clock with hands showing the medication time.
6. Use special containers as reminders for a forgetful person. For example, egg cartons labelled with days/times or a medication box with compartments (found in drugstores and pharmacies).
7. Emphasize important reminders: take with food, take all the medication; keep out of reach of children.
8. Remind elders to carry a list of medications with them and show it to any physician, at any clinic, or when coming to the hospital.

## RESOURCES

Some helpful resources for nurses and others working with elders are listed in Box 4-19.

## QUESTIONS TO CONSIDER

- Talk with and observe persons older than 65 years of age. How do you and they differ in terms of physical development and major concerns in your lives?
- Review the eating patterns of an elderly person of your acquaintance; compare his or her food intake with your understanding of an adequate diet. If there are inadequacies, what are some possible reasons?
- From what you have read in newspapers and heard discussed, what would you select as major problems of elderly people in your community?
- What services are available for elders in your community?
- Compare your grandparents or other elderly relatives with elderly acquaintances for differentiation in primary and secondary aging.
- Describe some measures you can take to improve memory in an older adult who has a decline in cognition.

## CRITICAL THINKING ACTIVITIES

- You are caring for two patients in the same room. One is an elderly lady with rheumatoid arthritis. The other is a young lady with acute appendicitis. Both are experiencing pain. How will the care of these patients differ?
- A committee to write standardized nursing care plans addresses the topic of elderly patients. Several nurses express their ideas on how the plan of care should be written. Why would a standardized plan of care for all elderly, regardless of circumstances, not be ideal?
- The daughter of an elderly patient confides in you that she is disturbed about her mother. You learn that the patient has been told that she has a terminal illness. The daughter feels her mother is not disturbed about this news and almost seems relieved. Based on developmental tasks of older adulthood, what explanation could be given to the daughter about her mother's reaction to such news?

## CHAPTER SUMMARY

### HISTORICAL PERSPECTIVES

- Persons in late adulthood focus on life accomplishments and look toward life's end while maintaining autonomy and dignity.
- Elderly adults often have more than one chronic illness, with the incidence increasing with age.
- Nursing care must be tailored according to the specific physical, psychologic, sexual, and social effects of any disease or illness on the individual.

### ASSESSMENT OF ELDERS

- Nurses need to be cognizant of the differences between primary and secondary aging changes in elders.

- Nursing care should be predicated on the belief that late adulthood is a time of diversity, richness, and increasing complexity.
- Health promotion is as important for older age-groups as for younger persons in maintaining a high quality of life.
- The strengths of the older person should be given the same consideration as their disabilities when devising health care strategies.

### MAJOR HEALTH PROBLEMS OF ELDERS

- Many conditions in elders have the initial symptom of confusion.
- Elders are more susceptible to falls, but restraints are not an adequate intervention.
- Elders often are malnourished because of physiologic and social aging changes.
- Constipation is a secondary aging change and can be controlled with diet and habit training.
- Urinary incontinence is a secondary aging change. The most common form is functional incontinence.
- Hearing and vision defects affect the ability of elders to communicate adequately.
- Elders experience many minor discomforts, but some do not have pain as a typical symptom of disease.
- Dehydration is common in many elders admitted to the acute-care setting.
- Helping elders and their families with discharge planning is an important priority.
- Supporting decision making in an ethical context is a challenge for the nurse who works with elderly persons.
- Geriatric nursing standards provide a context of care for the nurse.

## REFERENCES


1. Aronson L, Carlson-Wolfe N, Schoener S: Pressures that fall on rising, *Geriatr Nurs* 12(2):58-60, 1991.
2. Bee H, Mitchell S: *The developing person: a life-span approach,* ed 2, New York, 1984, Harper & Row.
3. Blakeslee J et al: Making the transition to restraint-free care, *J Gerontol Nurs* 17(2):4-8, 1991.
4. Brokiehurst JC: *Textbook of geriatric medicine and gerontology,* New York, 1985, Churchill Livingstone.
5. Brower T: Alternatives to restraints, *J Gerontol Nurs* 17(2):18-20, 1991.
6. Burnside I: *Nursing and the aged: a self-care approach,* ed 3, New York, 1988, McGraw-Hill.
7. Cassel CK, Walsh JR, editors: *Geriatric medicine,* vols 1 and 2, New York, 1984, Springer.
8. Cummings E, Henry WE: *Growing old,* New York, 1955, Basic Books.
9. Davis MA et al: Living arrangements and dietary patterns of older adults, *J Gerontol* 40(4):434-442, 1985.
10. Erikson EH: *Childhood and society,* ed 2, New York, 1963, WW Norton.
11. Gallagher L, Kreidler MC: *Nursing and health: maximizing human potential throughout the life cycle,* Norwalk, Conn, 1987, Appleton & Lange.
12. Gibaldi M: Drug dosage and the elderly, *Perspect Clin Pharmacol* 5(2):9-16, 1987.
13. Gray M: Polypharmacy in the elderly, *Orthop Nurs* 9(6):49, 1990.
14. Hadaway L: Intravenous tips, *Geriatr Nur* 12(2):78, 1991.
15. Havinghurst RJ et al: Psychology of aging, Bethesda conference, *Public Health Rep* 70:837-856, 1955.
16. Havinghurst RJ: Perspectives on health care for the elderly, *J Gerontol Nurs* 3(2):21-24, 1977.
17. Hazzard W et al: *Principles of geriatric medicine,* New York, 1990, McGraw-Hill.
18. Heacock P et al: Caring for the cognitively impaired, *J Gerontol Nurs* 17(3):22-26, 1991.
19. Hogstel M: Safety or autonomy, *J Gerontol Nurs* 17(3):5-10, 1991.
20. Hussey L: Overcoming the clinical barrier of low literacy and medication noncompliance among elderly, *J Gerontol Nurs* 17(3):27-29, 1991.
21. Kart C, Metress E, Metress S: *Aging, health, and society,* Boston, 1988, Jones & Bartlett.
22. Landefeld S, Palmer R, Kresevic D: Dysfunctional syndrome, *GAS Abstracts,* 1990.
23. Masters W, Johnson V: *Human sexual response,* Boston, 1966, Little, Brown & Co.
24. Pastorino C, Dickey T: Health promotion for the elderly, *Orthop Nurs* 9(60):36, 1990.
25. Patsdaugher C, Pesznecker B: Medication regimens and the elderly home care client, *J Gerontol Nurs* 14(10): 30-34, 1988.
26. Reed P: Implications for life-span developmental framework for well-being in adulthood and aging, *ANS* 6:18-25, 1983.
27. Reed P: Mental health of older adults, *West J Nurs Res* 11(2):143-163, 1989.
28. Roper J, Shapiro J, Chang B: Agitation in the demented patient, *J Gerontol Nurs* 17(3):17, 1991.
29. Rossman I: *Clinical geriatrics,* ed 3, Philadelphia, 1986, JB Lippincott.
30. Scura K, Whipple B: Older adult as an HIV positive risk group, *J Gerontol Nurs* 16(1):6-10, 1990.
31. Smith E, Sergass RC: *Exercise and aging: the scientific basis,* Hillside, NJ, 1981, Enslow Publishers.
32. Stevenson J: Adulthood: a promising direction for future research. In Werley H, Fitzpatrick J, Traunton R, editors: *Annual review of nursing research,* vol 1, New York, 1983, Springer Publishing.
33. Thorson JA, Thorson JR: How accurate are stress scales? *J Gerontol Nurs* 12(1):21-24, 1986.
34. Travis S: Older adults' sexuality and remarriage, *J Gerontol Nurs* 13(16):8-14, 1987.
35. US Bureau of the Census: *Statistical abstracts of the United States, 1990,* Washington, DC, 1990, US Government Printing Office.
36. Wolanin MD, Philips LRF: *Confusion, prevention, and care,* St Louis, 1981, Mosby.
37. Woods NF: *Human sexuality in health and illness,* ed 3, St Louis, 1984, Mosby.
38. Young E: Nutrition, aging and the aged, *Med Clin North Am* 67(2):295-313, 1983.

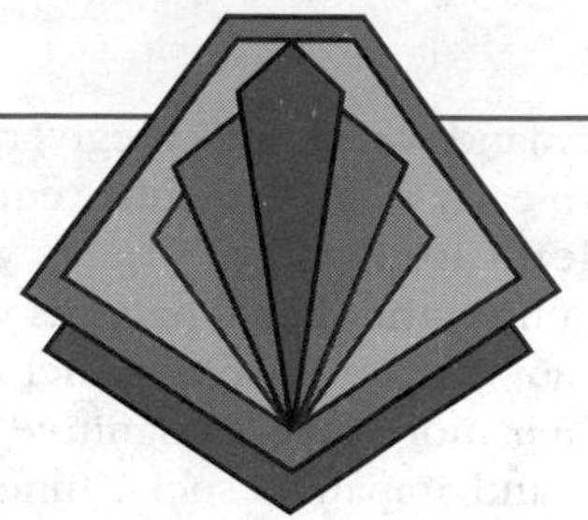

C H A P T E R 5

# Family and Cultural Influences on Illness

*Sandra Jean Fulton Picot*

## CHAPTER OBJECTIVES

***After studying this chapter, the learner should be able to do the following:***

1 Judge the appropriateness of selected theoretic frameworks to explain how families from various cultures function when a stressor such as illness is present.
2 Compare the impact on family members caring for an ill family member during the early diagnostic, acute, chronic, and terminal stages of illness.
3 Identify ways that nurses can support families caring for an ill family member.
4 Analyze the experiences of nurses and persons from different social and cultural perspectives.
5 Apply the strategies of cultural awareness, cultural knowledge, cultural skills, and cultural encounter to provide culturally competent nursing care.

## KEY TERMS

caregivers
cultural awareness
cultural encounter
cultural knowledge
cultural skill
culture
ecologic environment
ecology framework
emic
ethnic groups
etic
exosystem
family
family stress theory
family systems theory
illness trajectory
macrosystem
mesosystem
microsystem
minority
race

With advances in medical technology, people are living longer. As a consequence, the number of persons 65 years of age and older is growing rapidly. Demographers predict that the number of persons 65 and older will more than double from 32 million in 1990 to 69 million in the year 2030.[5,142,149] Notable is the growth of racial and ethnic groups, resulting in increasing racial and ethnic diversity among our elders. The proportion of the total elderly population who are African-American will increase from 8% to 14%, the proportion of races other than white or African-American will increase from 2% to 7%, and Hispanics will increase from fewer than 4% to nearly 12%. Ethnic groups are distinctive from the majority population (white) not only in racial and/or national background but also in shared history and cultural values,[7,161] beliefs, and practices. These ethnocultural differences may result in different perceptions of and responses to similar health and illness situations.

Nursing has been defined as the diagnosis and treatment of individual and group responses to actual or potential health problems.[1] Thus it behooves nurses to become knowledgeable about how culture filters and colors individual and family responses to health and illness. Application of this knowledge helps to avoid misunderstandings that result from the use of culturally ineffective strategies by nurses—no matter how well intended.

Living longer increases the probability that chronic illness will develop. Chronic illnesses include arthritic conditions, Parkinson's disease, emphysema, multiple sclerosis, heart disease, stroke, diabetes, and cancer. More than 75% of elderly persons die of heart disease, cancer, or stroke—with heart disease as the number one cause of death for this population.[5] African-American men have the highest rates of death as a result of heart disease and cancer, followed by white men. For cerebrovascular diseases, African-Americans have significantly higher death rates than do white persons of both sexes until the oldest ages. Often persons with chronic diseases experience periods of acute exacerbations that require hospitalization. However, with the continued focus on curbing rising health care costs, especially among elders, whose Medicare costs make up a large portion of the nation's health care budget, patients are being discharged sooner and sicker. These earlier discharges of patients with more complex home care regimens are putting new levels of demands on families.

Among the 85-year-olds living in a household, one in five is unable to carry on a major activity and two in five have a condition that limits their activities. Despite the common belief that our current societal norms foster less reliance on family members for assistance in crises than in the past, it has been well documented that families play a vital role in providing physical, emotional, social, and economic support to ill relatives. Research shows that from 1982 to 1989, two thirds of elders received all required help from family and friends, with only a modest increase in the use of formal services over that period.[142] Persons who live alone, do not have children nearby, are unmarried and less disabled and who have higher incomes, as well as white women generally, are most likely to use formal care exclusively.[72] Formal care is care paid for by the family or the patient. Informal care is not paid for by the family or the patient and usually is provided by the family, neighbors, and friends.

It is clear from the changing trends in the American population that nurses must become culturally competent to care for and work with more elderly and ethnically diverse patients and families in the future. Thus this chapter examines the effects of culture and family on the nursing management of a patient's experience of health and illness.

## BACKGROUND

The illness of a family member poses one of the most challenging situations facing families. Each member of the family may be affected as routines are altered, family members' responsibilities change, and heightened concern and anxiety occur. The impact that illness has on families may depend on the illness itself and family characteristics.

Illnesses affect the physical and mental status of patients in different ways and in turn affect their family caregivers differently. **Caregivers** often are family members but not always. The differences in the effects on both the family caregivers and care recipients result from differences in these disease/illness characteristics: (1) time demands of care, (2) prognosis for care, and (3) patient response to care.[91] The impact that illness has on families also may depend on whether the illness is short-lived (acute) or long-term (chronic). Although acute illness may demand rapid, intense mobilization of family resources, chronic illness allows families to adjust more slowly but may require a long-term commitment of family resources.

Physical, social, psychologic, and cognitive disabilities place different demands on family caregivers.[131] For example, patients with early-stage dementia require less assistance with physical care than do patients with hip fracture or stroke. On the other hand, patients with dementia require more supervision than do other types of patients because of their more severe cognitive deficits, disruptive behaviors, and impaired social functioning. Furthermore, the supervision required by patients with dementia is less amenable to planning than that for other patients. Barring the possibility of severe aphasia, patients with stroke and hip fracture can express gratitude for provided care. In contrast, patients with dementia have increasingly limited abilities to make such expressions of gratitude. The patient's inability to express gratitude contributes to a lack of perceived rewards by the caregiver[14] and to negative health consequences. The overall course of dementia is one of continual decline in the patient's functioning. Most patients with stroke and hip fracture improve or at least stabilize in their functional capacities. Therefore dementia caregivers (e.g., Alzheimer's caregivers) experience a unique set of stressors.[14,61]

The negative consequences of caregiving have been extensively studied over recent years. Factors such as the caregiver's lack of perceived rewards, awareness of the continued decline in patient functioning,[131] disruptive behaviors, agitation, hallucinations, dangerous or embarrassing behaviors, and impaired social functioning[35] contribute to caregiver depression.[61] In contrast, limitations on the elder's activities of daily living (ADLs) have the strongest effect on the caregiver's activity restrictions and physical health. See Research box, p. 105.

Although the patient's mental and physical impairments or diagnosis may contribute to negative consequences for the caregiver, so can the type of caregiving activities that the caregiver performs. (Box 5-1 depicts common caregiving activities.) Often caregivers attempt to protect their relative from an awareness of cognitive decline by maintaining the person's positive self-image, and thus they have found protective caregiving to be the most stressful caregiving activity.[12] Nevertheless, as the intensity and frequency of instrumental caregiving activities increase, the caregiver also becomes more stressed.[134]

In summary, the mental impairment of patients with dementia, especially disruptive behavior and social-functioning deficits, appears more stressful to family caregivers than the physical impairment of patients with illnesses and/or self-care deficits. Self-care deficits, however, also appear to contribute to family caregiver stress by restricting social activities. The degree to which these care-recipient behaviors, self-care deficits, and caregiving activities add to caregiver stress is influenced by the caregiver's ethnocultural background. To understand the influence culture has on the patient and family coping with illness, culture and related terms need to be defined.

**RESEARCH**

Haley, W et al: Stress, appraisal, coping, and social support as predictors of adaptational outcome among dementia caregivers, *Psychol Aging* 2(4):323-330, 1987.

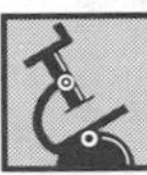

In a sample of 44 primary caregivers (i.e., daughters, wives, sons, husbands, and other relatives) of senile dementia patients and 44 matched control subjects), Haley and associates assessed the specific effects of stress on caregiver psychologic, social, and health functioning. Also, an attempt was made to compare caregivers in terms of race, age, gender, marital status, education, and income. The authors reported that caregivers had significantly higher levels of depression and negative affect toward their relatives and lower life satisfaction than control subjects. Furthermore, caregivers experienced significant restriction of their social activities and reported poorer health, more prescription medication use, and higher use of health care than did noncaregivers. The caregivers did not differ significantly on major demographic variables.

**BOX 5-1 Common Caregiving Activities**

**ANTICIPATORY CAREGIVING**
Making decisions, doing activities based on anticipated needs of a care recipient; often occurs at a distance

**PREVENTIVE CAREGIVING**
Performing activities for the purpose of preventing illness, injury, complications, and physical and mental deterioration of the care recipient

**SUPERVISORY CAREGIVING**
Arranging for, checking up, making sure, setting up, and checking out the care recipient

**INSTRUMENTAL CAREGIVING**
Doing for, assisting, providing, and giving—the "hands-on" caregiving. Its purpose is to maintain the care recipient's physical integrity and health status

**PROTECTIVE CAREGIVING**
Protecting the care recipient from the consequences of that which was not or could not be prevented

From Bowers B: *Adv Nurs Sci* 9(2):20-31, 1987.

## CULTURAL DIMENSIONS

**Culture** has been defined as a learned, shared, and symbolically transmitted design for living. Culture also has been described as shared and learned assumptions, beliefs, symbols, and ways of behaving that characterize a human society, as explicit and implicit rules for living, and as a shared way of life.[2] Chrisman[29] describes culture as a set of perspectives that influences how we view the world: ourselves, those close to and distant from us, and the nature of life around us. Health preservation, sickness prevention, causes of sickness, treatment, coping, caring, dying, and death are part of the health component of every culture.[51] Primarily, culture helps us make sense out of life. Culture is shared, both stable and dynamic, pervasive, and mostly unconscious. Culture also provides the range of possibility of action, meaning, and interpretation. In other words, culture addresses beliefs, values, and practices of human beings.

Culture helps the family and patient to interpret symptoms as signs of illness or signs of health. Although culture is universal to human beings and some aspects of particular cultures may be shared, no two cultures are identical. Culture sometimes is misunderstood as belonging only to someone different from oneself or being an attribute of foreign persons or those of racial or ethnic minorities. Having culture is part of being human, and thus culture influences all human activities, including nursing the sick and participating in scientific and other types of scholarly research.

Societies, particularly heterogeneous societies like the United States, contain many subcultural groups. A subculture may be defined as a recognized social group that maintains a distinctive set of beliefs and behaviors but shares some cultural traits with the mainstream society. An example of a type of American subculture is the ethnic group. **Ethnic groups** are collectives of persons sharing a common (often foreign) ancestry. Specific beliefs of particular ethnic groups vary both within and among groups. Having "Irish blood" or having facial features that appear Swedish or Chinese does not necessarily determine one's membership in or affiliation with an ethnic group; social relations and personal identification with such a group determine ethnic group membership. Other types of subcultures may be regional (New Englanders), religious (the Amish or Evangelical Christians), based on location (urban, suburban, rural), age-related, or based on sexual preference (the gay or lesbian community).[46]

**Race** is another important social subgroup among North Americans. Races often are described as biologic rather than social categories, although little evidence supports the notion of racial groups. Genetic differences between two individuals of the same racial group may range in the tens of thousands, whereas genetic differences among different races are relatively small, fewer than two dozen. Distinguishing pure racial types also is problematic. People considered "white" in one sociocultural setting may be considered "African-American" in another. This is true also for racially mixed persons.

The notion of what is a biologic race may differ from century to century as well. In the early part of this century, Irish-Americans were considered racially (biologically) distinct from white Americans of English descent and were thought to be genetically more susceptible to

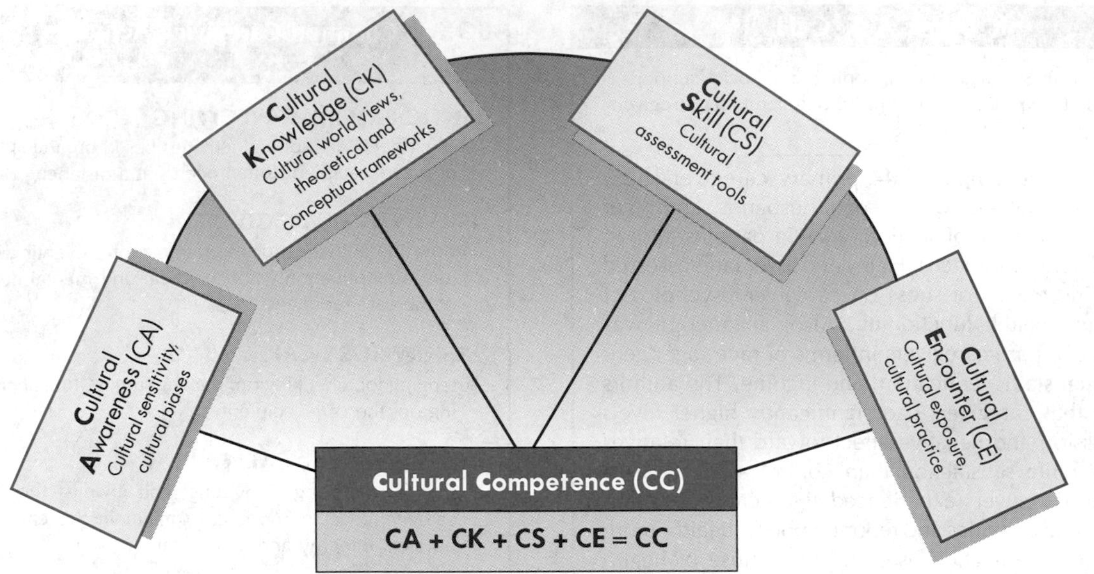


**FIGURE 5-1** A culturally competent model of care. (Redrawn from Campinha-Bacote J: *The process of cultural competence: a culturally competent model of care,* Wyoming, Ohio, 1991, Transcultural C.A.R.E.)

rheumatic fever. As work and living conditions for Irish-Americans improved, this susceptibility was reduced. Poor and working class African-Americans inherited not only the substandard working and living conditions of the Irish-American but also the genetic susceptibility to rheumatic fever. This example illustrates the danger of confusing social groups and social phenomena with nature.[65]

The names by which various ethnic and racial groups identify themselves also change with the sociohistoric context. Most North Americans who were formerly known as Oriental now prefer the terms Asian or Asian-American or prefer a more specific term, for example, Japanese-American. Similarly, persons formerly described as Negro now prefer black American or African-American,[6] and white persons may prefer European American. Patients' rights to choose and name themselves should be respected, regardless of whether the patient's appearance or race/ethnicity coincides with the nurse's preconceptions.

The term **minority** is used to describe any group that constitutes less than a numerical majority of the population.[52] Often racial, religious, or occupational groups compose a minority group. Usually associated with this minority designation is a lack of power (subordinate position in society), assumed inferior traits, and/or supposedly undesirable characteristics. The nurse needs to be aware that the minority designation of a family and patient can sometimes affect access to health care resources or their assertiveness in pursuing health care services. Being aware that the cultural identity of the family and patient influences the illness response can help the nurse effectively work within the cultural context of individuals, families, or communities from diverse cultural/ethnic backgrounds.[22]

Numerous service-delivery models have been proposed for the integration of culture awareness into practice,[56] including ethnic-competence,[37,56] cross-cultural awareness practice,[56] ethnic minority practice,[96] and cultural-specific care.[90] Campinha-Bacote[22] has proposed another model, the ***culturally competent model of care.*** She describes this culturally competent model of care as practice-oriented; cultural awareness, cultural knowledge, cultural skill, and cultural encounter are dimensions of cultural competence (Figure 5-1). Campinha-Bacote has recently suggested that a dimension she terms *cultural desire,* that is the desire to become knowledgeable about other cultures, precedes the process of acquiring cultural knowledge (Campinha-Bacote, personal communication, Jan. 29, 1994).

## CULTURALLY COMPETENT MODEL OF CARE

**Cultural awareness** is the process by which nurses become sensitive to other cultures by examining their own biases and prejudices toward other cultures. **Cultural knowledge** is the process through which the nurse obtains a sound educational foundation concerning the world views of other cultures by learning their specific theoretic and conceptual frameworks. Ideally the nurse should enroll in a formal transcultural nursing program. **Cultural skill** involves the process of learning how to assess the patient and family's cultural values, beliefs, and practices to provide culturally relevant services. This process requires the nurse to acquire the skill of conducting a "culturologic" assessment. Last, **cultural encounter** encourages the nurse to *directly* engage in cross-cultural interactions with patients from diverse cultural backgrounds. As a result, the nurse validates, negates, or modifies existing cultural knowledge and gains a culturally relevant knowledge base. From this culturally relevant base, the nurse can develop culturally specific interventions for the patient and family. Application of the model is discussed throughout the remainder of this chapter.[22] However, before continuing the discussion of family and cultural influences on illness, it is important to discuss the definition of family and appropriate theoretic frameworks to guide the nursing process.

# FAMILY INFLUENCES ON ILLNESS

## DEFINITION OF FAMILY

The definition of **family** has changed over time. In the past the concept of family as extended family was considered the societal norm. With the advent of urbanization, the norm became the nuclear family (mother, father, and children). Today the concept of family includes the single-parent family, the reconstituted family, and the gay or lesbian couple, among others. Family may be defined according to geographic proximity, as in shared households or residential retirement homes. Family also may be defined by shared emotional bonds between individuals or by one's support network. For this reason, throughout this chapter family is regarded as those people whom the ill individual or spokesperson identifies as family. A flexible definition of the family is especially important among ethnic families such as African-Americans and Mexican-Americans. African-American elders often consider blood, marriage, or friendship relationships as equivalent, and caregivers treat personal care aides of the same cultural background as kin.[77] These nonblood relationships are referred to as *fictive kin.*[27] In addition, Mexican-Americans use a "compadre" system or coparent who assumes the parenting role should anything happen to the natural parents.[52]

## THEORETIC MODELS OF FAMILY FUNCTIONING

Theoretic models of family functioning provide ways of thinking about the family that allow one to understand and predict behavior. Models are useful because they suggest ways that families may be helped. The three models described here are useful to nurses when they think about how families cope with illness. When selecting a theoretic framework of family functioning to address an ethnically diverse population, the nurse needs to determine if the definition of the family addresses changes in today's family compositions.[152] For example, family systems theory assumes that family members must be together to have relationships. However, family members who live at a distance may be just as intimate as those who live together. Anthropologic and developmental perspectives suggest that family must be legally sanctioned or that all families go through the same stages at the same time. Because these two perspectives fail to address nonblood relationships or the earlier ages at which many minority families go through some of the developmental stages, they provide less guidance to the nurse for planning interventions. Despite the limitations of family systems theory, it is still one of the most frequently used family theories because of its focus on the interaction of the family members with the external environment.[87] Therefore family systems theory, along with family stress theory and the ecologic framework, are discussed next.

### Family Systems Theory

The family systems perspective is derived from general systems theory (GST), as described in the work of Ludwig von Bertalanffy.[151] **Family systems theory** conceptualizes the family as an open system that functions within the broader context of the environment. The more open the family system, the greater is the exchange of information with the environment. Within the boundary of the family, dynamic interactions between the members or subsystems (such as the subsystem of parents or children) are governed by the family's organization. The organization of the family system is characterized by roles, relationships, expectations, and rules.

The terms *roles, relationships, expectations,* and *rules* are used to define organization in the family systems literature. Family members occupy and function in roles in relationship to one another. They seem to function in these roles according to the expectations of the whole family. Thus one family member may take on the role of breadwinner, whereas another may take on the role of homemaker. One family member may be the decision maker, and another may be the primary caregiver for the small children.

The term *rules* applies to the family expectations about how each person in his or her role relates to other family members; this becomes a standard for behavior over time. Whether spoken or implicit, these rules result in patterns of relating that characterize the family's interpersonal relationships and attempt to maintain equilibrium.

The dynamic interactions that take place within the family are governed by the family's organization. According to family systems theory, the interactions are directed toward achieving and maintaining equilibrium within the system. Homeostasis reflects the family's striving to maintain equilibrium in the face of internal or external changes. More recently, family theorists have refined the thinking on homeostasis with development of the concepts of morphogenesis and morphostasis.[73,136] Morphostasis describes maintenance of the status quo within the family system, and morphogenesis reflects the ability of the family to change its basic structure and organization to survive and remain viable. Morphogenesis and morphostasis describe the family system as existing in a dynamic balance between change and stability in response to the environment.[98]

Certain principles describe the characteristics of a system. The principle of circular causality describes family as a group of individuals who are interrelated such that changes in one member evoke changes in another, which in turn affect the first individual. That is to say, individuals living in a family do not exist in a vacuum. They are constantly affected by the behavior of others in the family, which in turn affects their own behavior.

The principle of nonsummativity holds that the family as a whole is more than the sum of the individuals who make up that family. A family cannot be described by the characteristics of its individuals alone because this does not allow for the interaction among them. Thus one cannot look at each member of a family individually and have an appreciation of the characteristics of the family as a whole.

Understood within the framework of family systems theory is the idea that the organism of the family is constantly moving toward goals. The principle of equifinality states that different outcomes may have the same beginnings and that the same beginnings may lead to different outcomes. Because families are open systems, they are constantly exchanging information with the larger environment. Thus the outcome of the system is affected by more than just its initial conditions.

The family systems framework suggests several key assessment areas for the nurse:

1. What are the family rules related to the patient, caregiver, and all other identified family member roles?
2. How flexible is each family member in creating and adapting roles to accommodate changes in the patient's health?
3. What are the patient and family goals related to the illness?
4. What environmental sources of information and support are known and unknown to the family?

## Family Stress Theory

**Family stress theory** stems from the work of Hill,[69,70] who described families' responses to dealing with the loss of the father-husband after he was drafted into the armed services. Hill's ABC = X conceptualization of the family's response to stress serves as the foundation for investigation and theory building in the area of family stress research. Although researchers have made some modifications over the years to provide clarity and empiric support to the framework, it has remained essentially unchanged. This family crisis framework can be stated as follows:

A (the event) + Interacting with B
(the family's crisis-meeting resources) +
Interacting with C (how the family defines the event) =
X (the crisis)

The A factor represents the stressor event, which can be either external or internal to the family. It can result from normative changes or catastrophic events. In the case of an illness, the illness itself is the stressor event to the family.

The B factor represents family resources, which may be of two types. Resources may be (1) those already available to the family or (2) coping resources strengthened or developed in response to the crisis event. Resources already available to the family might include a family member who is a health care professional or who has had previous experience in caring for an ill person.

The C factor represents the family's perception of the crisis. This is related to the family's view of the event's seriousness as well as what the event means to the family. If a family has experienced the death of a member from a stroke, the family might view a stroke in a second family member more seriously than would another family.

The X factor represents the crisis as experienced by the family. It is the outcome of the stressor event for the family after it is interacted on by family resources and perceptions.

The family's resources, the B factor, represent the area of the family stress framework that has received the most attention by researchers. Family resources may include the family member's personal resources and the family system's internal resources, social support, and coping skills. Two of the most important internal resources are the adaptability and cohesion of the family unit.

### Adaptability and cohesion

Family adaptability is the family's ability to reorganize and change roles, rules, and patterns of interaction in response to either situational or developmental stress. Adaptability refers to how flexible family members are in changing roles to accommodate changes in the family. Is the wife-mother able to compensate for her husband's roles of co-breadwinner and co-disciplinarian if he is no longer able to fulfill his role? Can the children accept the mother as the new family disciplinarian? To the extent that family members can be flexible in their roles, rules, and patterns of interaction, the family can successfully manage changes brought about by having a chronically ill member. Families who cannot make the necessary changes in their role structure and who have difficulty changing family rules are described as being rigid. Families at the opposite end of the adaptability continuum are described as being chaotic; they experience such dramatic role shifts and dramatic changes in rules that family members often do not know what rules apply.[110,111]

Family cohesion describes the extent to which family members feel bonded to each other and concerned and committed to the family. As with adaptability, cohesion is conceptualized as being on a continuum. Extreme cases of cohesion are (1) enmeshment, an over-involvement of family members in each other's lives and, at the other end, (2) disengagement, in which family members are detached from the family and have little commitment to it. Healthy families lie somewhere between these two extremes. A sense of commitment in family members is vital if the ill member is to be cared for and the family is to continue.

### Characteristics of families

Particular qualities either increase the family's resources or add to the "pileup," a term used to describe the family experience of having additional stressors at the time of a stressor event. The nurse's awareness of a family's characteristics can give insight into the amount of burden families experience and the resources families have in caring for an ill member. These characteristics include but are not limited to the ones discussed in the following paragraphs.

**Familial relation to the patient.** Spouses and adult children experience caregiving in different ways. Spouses are more concerned about their health and see their physicians more often, rate their health poorer, report more stress symptoms, and use more psychotropic medications than do adult children. The negative effects on the spouse caregiver's health may be related to the spouse's hesitancy to make use of respite services. Respite services are designed to give a few hours to several days of relief from caregiving activities. Thus the nurse must assess the caregiver's awareness of services and the cultural acceptability of these services and encourage the use or creation of respite by the caregiver. To minimize potential guilt feelings, the nurse should stress the importance of respite for the caregiver's health and continued quality of patient care.

In contrast, adult children are more concerned about family, time, and emotional conflicts. Consequently, adult children often express more burden[78] and place their parents in nursing homes more readily than do spouse caregivers. The fact that adult children perceive more burden may be related to the infrequent visits of family and friends and time spent relaxing.[49] Nevertheless, adult children use respite services more readily and report more benefits than do spouses. Finally, wives are more bothered by their cognitively impaired husband's frequent dangerous behaviors and embarrassing acts, and adult children are more stressed by a parent's inability to bathe himself or herself or stay alone.

**Gender.** Just as differences exist between spouses and adult children, so do differences exist between the genders.[44,71,75,124,165] Wives tend to be more distressed/burdened during the initial stages of their caregiving role than are husbands,[44,165] and some women throughout the experience describe the situation as more confining and oppressive than do men.[124] Nevertheless, with the passage of time, some wives perceive less burden and reflect attitudes comparable with those of husband caregivers.[165]

Sons perform and experience the caregiving role differently and do not sense any major caregiving problems.[71] This low perception of problems probably is related to the fact that sons often delegate the physically intimate caregiving activities to their wives (i.e., the daughter-in-law) and focus on managing their parents' financial concerns. Daughters usually do not have the opportunity to delegate these activities. Therefore daughters may sense more caregiving problems.

The family-life cycle also affects family responses. The family may have the additional burden of caring for both young children and elderly parents, although sometimes older children or young adults can share in the caregiving. Middle-aged daughters are more likely than older wives to have parental, employment, and marital obligations competing with caregiving. As the patient's level of impairment increases and need for the daughter's assistance increases, so does the daughter's sense of burden[49] and rewards.[83,162] Older husbands are more likely than sons to experience burden as caregivers because older men are likely to be full-time caregivers and sons are more likely to be part-time caregivers.[4] Noting where the family is in its life cycle can assist the nurse in identifying potential areas of needed support.

**Ethnicity.** When focusing on diseases such as Alzheimer's disease, the nurse needs to consider the patient and family's ethnic heritage.[150] The patient's ethnic heritage may produce different human responses to the same phenomenon. Individual responses to catastrophic illness are filtered through differing belief systems and practices.[112] Consequently nurses need to consider the influence of family culture on the selection of coping strategies. White caregivers are more burdened when the patient has dementia and is unable to perform instrumental daily living tasks.[103] Instrumental daily living tasks include preparing meals, laundering clothes, shopping, and paying one's bills. In contrast, African-American caregivers are less burdened by the amount of supervision needed by Alzheimer's patient than are white caregivers.[119] Instead, African-American caregivers are more burdened by a variety of physical disabilities that require more physical labor. The higher level of burden from physical disabilities among African-American caregivers may reflect their overall poorer health status compared with that of white caregivers. Nevertheless, white caregivers are more likely to institutionalize persons with a dementia than are African-American caregivers.

Family composition also affects the family response. It may be a large family, with several persons who can share in the caregiving, or it may be a single-parent household already pressed to care for its members. The nurse must assess not only the actual participation of household members in caregiving activities but also the caregiver's perceived helpfulness of these acts of caregiver support. A large household does not always mean shared caregiving, and a small household does not always mean more limited support.

**Socioeconomic status.** This determines whether a family can afford to hire extra help to compensate for the loss of the ill member's job and whether the cost of the illness places an added financial strain on the family.

**Employment status.** The employment situation of the caregiver is also important. The female caregiver may have been forced to quit her job or decrease her productivity/income because of caregiving demands. Women who continue to work experience absences, work interruptions, loss of pay, decreased energy to do their jobs well, limited job choices, and a desire to not work.[15] Often women who are forced to quit their jobs score the lowest on mental health measures, which suggests that work may provide some respite for caregivers. Obviously, as the caregiving family's income decreases, the ability to purchase services to support the caregiver will decrease. A nurse referral of the family to a social worker may be helpful to the family at this point.

**Problem solving.** This is another important aspect to consider. Family members may or may not have the knowledge and ability to do the necessary problem solving required to care for an ill member and meet the family's demands. The perceived caregiver costs, rewards, and the helpfulness of available social support are majors factors in the ability to cope.[74,115]

**Family health.** Family health is also important. The caregiver may have a chronic illness as well, which often occurs in a family of elderly persons. African-American caregivers often have as many as four chronic illnesses.[81]

**Support network.** A support network composed of persons external to the family who can help the members carry out their tasks and give them emotional support is important for coping. African-American elders living in the South have larger, more diverse support networks composed of family, relatives, friends, and fictive kin than African-American elders living in the North.[27,34] Fictive kin or "para-kin are unrelated individuals with whom interpersonal relationships are so close that they [the fictive kin] are viewed as family members."[48] In addition, fictive kin have the same familial obligations as "blood" relatives.[27] Living in the South tends to increase the actual frequency of support. Not only does region of the country affect the family's caregiver activity, it also affects the type of services used. African-American urban elders use more health services than do rural African-American elders.[23,159] Rural elders turn first to their families in the case of illness, but urban elders turn to the hospital. The generally higher incomes of urban elders make services more affordable for them than for rural elders. Furthermore, African-Americans, Native Americans, poor white persons, and others living in small towns and rural areas are far more dependent on unpaid family members and friends than on public and private service-delivery agencies for meeting their everyday needs in life. Also, there are fewer of these services in their area.[153]

**Social support.** It is important to determine whether the family is receiving help with the care needs of the patient, the family's emotional needs, and activities outside of the household. Can the family identify persons who visit them, call them, provide respite to them, and/or assist them with decision making? The caregiver's perception of social support decreases the feelings of burden and social isolation.*

**Religion.** The nurse should never overlook the role of the patient and family's religion during a hospitalization. Religion can affect the patient's practices, acceptable treatments, and attire.[47] Prayer is especially important in the lives of African-Americans and Muslims. For many African-Americans, frequent prayer demonstrates their belief in the power of God to cure any disease in a faithful person. If the person is not cured, then the person failed to demonstrate sufficient faith. Similarly, devout Muslims must pray to Allah, their supreme being, five times a day. The Muslim patient may be found kneeling on a prayer rug facing Mecca, the Holy Land, during these times. It is important for nursing staff members to assess and arrange for the times the patient will need privacy for prayer. Failure to integrate prayer times into the patient's treatment plan may result in tension between the family and health care professionals. Sometimes the patient's faith that God will provide a cure may interfere with the patient's ability to realize that God sends cure through the hands of health care professionals. Health care professionals may need to employ the assistance of a local religious leader to stress this point.

At other times a patient's religion may forbid the acceptance of a treatment. For example, Jehovah's Witnesses refuse blood transfusions and Orthodox Jews refuse the use of anything electrical on the Sabbath. For Jehovah's Witnesses, to accept a blood transfusion means choosing to give up eternity with Jehovah. Although the health care professional may disagree with the Jehovah's Witness patient's beliefs, he or she must still respect and support the patient. For the Orthodox Jew, the Sabbath begins at sundown Friday and ends at sundown Saturday. During the Sabbath, work of any kind is prohibited, including driving, using the telephone, handling money, and even pushing an elevator button. While caring for one Orthodox Jewish woman with renal failure, the nurses on her medical floor rearranged the time of her hemodialysis on Friday afternoon to the morning hours. Consequently, when the Sabbath began, this patient al-

*References 27, 28, 118, 143, 144, 164.

ready had returned to her room and was not in need of the electric elevator for transportation. Furthermore, the patient used battery-powered candles so that she did not have to operate the electric lights. Finally, when the patient needed the head of her bed raised, although she was capable of operating the bedside switches, the nurse brought the patient a bedside bell so that she could use the bell rather than the push-button call bell.

Observance of the Sabbath has ramifications for discharge planning also. Because of the prohibition against operation of a vehicle on the Sabbath, it is important to plan discharge of the Orthodox Jewish patient before or after the Sabbath. Otherwise the patient's family has to find a non-Orthodox Jew to pick up the patient from the hospital. The only exception to strict adherence to these practices is in a situation of life or death. For example, a young Jewish boy was severely injured one Saturday afternoon while playing football. He needed to go to the hospital immediately. The only person available to take him was his Orthodox Jewish grandfather, who drove him the 25 miles to the hospital. Once the boy was safely admitted, his grandfather walked home.[47]

Sometimes patients wear religious symbols, which the nurse must treat respectfully. These religious symbols include rosaries for Catholics, sacred threads around necks or arms of Hindus, medicine bundles for Native Americans, red ribbon for Mexican children, and mustard seed, which is worn by some Mediterranean people to ward off the evil eye.[128] When a medical procedure needs to be performed, removal of these religious symbols may be a problem. After explaining the rationale for removing the symbol in a calm, soothing tone, the nurse should gently place the symbol in close contact with the patient or at least within eyesight of the patient.

These are just a few cultural characteristics of families that can affect the family's experience as caregivers for a chronically ill member. As positive attributes, they can be indicators of family resources. As negative attributes, they may be predictors of deficits in family coping.

The family stress theory suggests several key assessment areas for the nurse:

1. What does the illness mean to the family? Are there different meanings among family members?
2. What family characteristics serve as indicators of possible coping resources?
3. What family characteristics suggest possible deficits in family coping?
4. Has the illness increased or decreased the family's cohesion?
5. Which religious beliefs and practices must be integrated into the plan of care?

## The Ecology Framework

The ecology framework comes from biologic ecology in which plants were studied in the context of their environment. The **ecology framework** defines the family as a bonded unit of interrelated and interdependent persons who have common goals, shared resources, and at one point a shared living space. This definition allows recognition of families whose members may not all share the same household.

The **ecologic environment** is conceived as a set of nested structures (concentric circles), each inside the next like a set of Russian dolls. The microsystem, mesosystem, exosystem, and macrosystem are the nested structures that make up the ecologic environment. The **microsystem** is a pattern of activities, roles, and interpersonal relations *experienced* by the developing person (e.g., the patient) in a given setting with particular physical and material characteristics.[17] Activities are the tasks or operations in which the person sees himself, herself, or others as engaging. Interpersonal relations are the perceived interconnections among the individuals in the setting as members of a group engage in common, complementary, or relatively independent undertakings. Role consists of a set of behaviors and expectations associated with a position in society, such as patient, wife, husband, or child.

The **mesosystem** consists of the interrelations among two or more settings in which the developing person actively participates. For the patient, interrelations exist among family, work, and visiting nurses. A mesosystem is formed every time a person moves into a new setting.

The **exosystem** is composed of one or more settings that do not involve the developing person as an active participant but in which events occur that affect or are affected by what happens in the setting that contains the developing person. One of the best examples of an exosystem is this: the family of an alcohol-dependent man with esophageal varices has joined Al-Anon. The events that occur in Al-Anon can affect him even though he is not an active participant in Al-Anon. Thus Al-Anon is part of his exosystem. Any organization that the family of a patient participates in can become part of the patient's exosystem, and often these organizations undertake legislative activities that can affect the patient and the family.

The **macrosystem** is composed of the consistencies that exist at cultural and subcultural levels, including beliefs and values. In addition, there is a focus on the impact of socioeconomic changes on the persons. For example, the impact of any health care reform changes made by the administration or United States Congress is likely to affect the patient, the family, and the mesosystem. Therefore the ecologic framework views the individual, the family, the community, and the larger society as concentric circles, with the individual as the inner circle followed by the family, the community, and the larger society.[106]

The ecology framework suggests that every human being has a physical, social, psychologic, and cultural environment. All of these environments interact to determine personality development within the family. As a member of this ecosystem, the family (microsystem) must interact with systems outside the family (exosystems) to carry out its roles. These exosystems affect how well the family can carry out its roles. Social policies can determine whether the family experiences difficulty in coping. Health-related economic policies can affect the ability of the family to function (e.g., Medicare and Medicaid policies).[18] Recognition of the constant transactions between the family and its environment and vice versa is one of the major strengths of the ecology framework.

Additional concepts that are pertinent to the effects of family on illness include reciprocity between the person and systems at all levels, the importance of social support at all levels, the impact of culture on family functioning, and the importance of the person's perception and interpretation of his or her environment. Examination of roles and positions is important in evaluating the effect of the illness on the family and vice versa. The framework suggests that individuals influence their own role, as well as other family members' implementation of their roles. Thus the nurse needs to focus on the previous role of the patient and new or changed roles for the family members. Environments furnish the resources necessary for family life, and the nurse should assess which resources are available and unavailable to the patient and family.

*Energy* is another very useful concept; this refers to an information exchange in the form of symbols, messages, and signs exchanged among systems. Different amounts of energy are needed for family interactions and for coping with stress. Families exhibit different degrees of selectivity and patterns in their intake of energy and information. In other words, families can be described on a continuum of energy/information intake from very open to very closed. For example, some African-American family members who care for cognitively impaired relatives desire to participate in support groups to obtain additional information, but other caregivers do not. The former caregiver group could be described as open whereas the latter group is more closed. Further, the energy exchange can range from very little to overload and can affect the family and patient as well. Identifying the patient's and the family's comfort levels with energy exchange is a key component of the nursing assessment.

Finally, the ecology framework focuses on the stages of development of the individual and the family and the influence of these stages on functioning. Development is defined as what is perceived, what is thought about, and what is acquired as knowledge and how these factors change with environmental exposure and interaction. Families and patients construct their own realities based on their own perceptions. The nurse's understanding of the transactions of the family and patient with their environment is key to analyzing, describing, and predicting family/patient behavior and understanding the interrelatedness of the family with its community and society. The ecology framework suggests several key assessment areas for the nurse:

1. How does the social, economic, and physical environment affect family members and the patient and their interpersonal interactions? For example, whether a patient is insured or uninsured can affect family/patient interpersonal interactions.
2. How does the environment (e.g., hospital, home) shape family and patient behavior?
3. How does the context of the setting influence family relationships?
4. How do relationships change over time? For example, when an illness becomes a chronic illness, how do relationships change?
5. What are the critical aspects of the environment that mediate functional or dysfunctional transactions in various situations?

Now let us turn our attention to the course of illness and its interaction with the culture of the family.

## SOCIAL AND BIOCULTURAL DIMENSIONS OF HEALTH AND ILLNESS

### SOCIAL DIMENSIONS

The nurse must understand not only the impact of culture on definitions of health, disease, illness, and disorder but also the unique diseases, illnesses, and physical characteristics of various ethnic/racial groups. Such a focus involves *cultural knowledge,* the first component of the culturally competent model.

#### Illness, Disease, and Disorder

The experience of sickness has been described as both a personal and a collective experience.[51] Determination of the presence and manifestations of sickness is influenced by culture and is itself a part of culture. Hahn has introduced the concept of suffering as a universal human experience, usually considered unfortunate. Suffering includes three dimensions[14]:

1. *Illness*—the experience and perspective of the patient
2. *Disease*—the perspective of professional biomedical practitioners (such as nurses, physicians, physiologists)
3. *Disorder*—the perspectives of folk or other than biomedical health practitioners (such as *curanderas* and practitioners of Chinese medicine)

Sickness, disease, and illness often are used interchangeably, but the focus in the biomedical model (i.e., Western medicine) is on the pathway of the disease or injured part or diseased mind. Often the professional interpretation of the patient's symptoms is that of a disease. In contrast, the patient may interpret sickness as an illness, that is, the experiencing of a disease or injury or psychologic disorder in its personal, interpersonal, and cultural dimensions. Similarly, the folk healer may label the symptoms as a disorder. Consequently, the sick person could have a disease and be either ill or not ill or have a disorder and not have a disease.[51] Thus it becomes essential for the nurse to assess how the patient and family's culture influences the interpretation of the symptoms. Although there are certain cultural interpretations of symptoms, the nurse should note that education, occupation, income, residential location, and religion can lead to differences in the symptom interpretation within the same group.[51]

Hahn uses the three dimensions of suffering to describe and explain sickness. He questions the validity and appropriateness of one best explanatory system. Considerable variation occurs even within the various systems. Professional-sector biomedical beliefs and practices are influenced by cultural factors, varying considerably among the United States, England, Germany, and France, for example.[14]

Further, not all sickness can be classified under the biomedical system. *Susto,* roughly defined as soul loss and present as part of the folk belief systems of many Latin cultures, may have physical, biomedically recognized symptoms. Yet it is incompletely described and treated outside the cultural belief system in which it occurs. Illnesses identified in some cultures, such as hot/cold imbalances, do not have an equivalent in Western medicine.[51] Ignoring, devaluing, or ridiculing the patient's beliefs are all examples of poor nursing care in which patients are given labels (hypochondriac, malingerer, or hysterical) instead of appropriate treatment. The respectful consideration of the patient's perspective of the illness leads the health care team, instead, to consult family members, community resources, and a folk healer. Thus the health care team learns that suffering from *susto* is a shared cultural belief, not an idiosyncratically held one. The biomedical health care team provides necessary care in the area of its expertise and, additionally, provides emotional support and validation for the patient and family. The folk healer may then be called in as a "specialist" to take care of the *susto.*

## Cross-Cultural Comparative Approaches

Planning health care for various subcultural groups in American society requires identification of traditional beliefs and practices and determination of the extent of practice of these traditions within a group. Information may then be used to deliver culturally competent health care. One way to facilitate identification of the universal features of human responses to illness, as well as responses unique to a group or subculture, is by means of a cross-cultural comparative approach.

A comparative approach is developing within nursing. One nurse-anthropologist advocates a transcultural nursing approach, which offers a frame of reference that "can offer insight, new relationships, new foci, and new dimensions of caring about one's own culture in relation to another."[25] Transcultural health care is defined as an evolving body of knowledge and practices regarding health-illness caring patterns from a comparative perspective of two or more cultures to determine major care features and the health services of cultures.

The comparison of illness-referral systems discussed in the preceding section offers one approach for the comparison and contrast of the social processes by which people make initial diagnosis and seek therapy. Cultural categories and criteria for defining illness also may be studied and compared by use of ethnographic or ethnoscientific strategies or techniques. Culture is uniquely human. All human groups have a culture, but it is in the analysis of detailed differences and similarities within and among groups that subtle relationships and understanding emerge.[120]

The ethnographic approach is a naturalistic comparative method aimed at studying human behavior, beliefs, and attitudes through observation and interviews in the natural setting.[120] Ethnoscience or ethnoscientific analysis comprises one aspect of the ethnographic approach. The suffix *science,* which refers to classification or taxonomy, is not used in the usual sense. Ethnoscience refers to a system of cognition or classification typical of a given culture. The terms *emic* and *etic* are used for arriving at a cultural group's classification system. **Emic** categories are culturally specific; *etic* categories are universal, that is, common to more than one culture. Emic analysis seeks to discover significant distinctions made by members of a particular culture and avoids the use of a priori definitions or categories.[145b] The **etic** perspective concerns observations and definitions of the situation by the observer and not the member of a cultural group. Etic analysis, composed of externally derived criteria, permits the observer to compare and theorize across several cultures. Etic features are considered culture-free because they can be applied across cultures; emic features are culturally unique. Categories derived from Western biomedicine use etic classification or explanatory systems.

Ethnographies or ethnographic descriptions take into account the perspective of members of a social or cultural group and include the beliefs, behaviors, and values that underlie and organize the activities related to health maintenance and restoration. They rely on observations and formal and informal interviews to elicit peoples' interpretations and responses to health-threatening or health-enhancing situations. There are an increasing number of ethnographic studies initiated by nurses[35,50,59,146,148] that would facilitate a comparative study of lay persons' responses (emic) with those of the health professional (etic) for a number of illness entities or phenomena.

In addition to differentiation of lay persons and professional perspectives by an emic-etic analysis, there are a number of constructs that are similar in analytic

**TABLE 5-1 Puerto Rican Hot/Cold Classifications**

| *FRIO* (COLD) | *FRESCO* (COOL) | *CALIENTE* (HOT) |
|---|---|---|
| **ILLNESSES AND BODILY CONDITIONS** | | |
| Arthritis<br>Colds and upper respiratory symptoms (including asthma)<br>*Empacho**<br>Menstrual period<br>Muscular spasm *(pasmo)*<br>Pain in the joints<br>Upset stomach (*frialdad del estomago* or *frio en el estomago*) | None | Constipation<br>Diarrhea<br>Rashes<br>Tenesmus *(pujo)*<br>Ulcers |
| **MEDICINES AND HERBS** | | |
| None | Bicarbonate of soda<br>Linden flowers *(flor de tilo)*<br>Mannitol *(mand de manito)*<br>Mastic bark *(almacigo)*<br>$MgCO_3$ *(magnesia boba)*<br>Milk of magnesia<br>Nightshade *(yerba mora)*<br>Orange-flower water *(agua de azahar)*<br>Sage | Anise<br>Aspirin<br>Castor oil<br>Cinnamon<br>Cod-liver oil<br>Iron tablets<br>Penicillin<br>Rue *(ruda)*<br>Vitamins |
| **FOODS** | | |
| Avocado<br>Bananas<br>Coconut<br>Lima beans<br>Sugar cane<br>White beans | Barley water<br>Bottled milk<br>Chicken<br>Fruits<br>Honey<br>Raisins<br>Salt cod *(bacalao)*<br>Watercress | Alcoholic beverages<br>Chili peppers<br>Chocolate<br>Coffee<br>Corn meal<br>Evaporated milk<br>Garlic<br>Kidney beans<br>Onions<br>Peas<br>Tobacco |

Modified from Harwood A: *Ethnicity and medical care,* Cambridge, Mass, 1981, Harvard University Press.
*Characterized by nausea, vomiting, and/or diarrhea, mainly in children, *empacho* is attributed to an obstruction in the stomach or intestines caused by either a bolus of undigested food or saliva swallowed by a teething baby.

and interpretive power. Examples include folk-modern, little tradition–great tradition, common sense models–biomedical, and lay explanatory models–biomedical. The constructs enable nurses to make distinctions between the perspective of the popular or lay person and that of the orthodox or professional person. Comparison and contrasts are facilitated, and nursing interventions can be planned to decrease the gap or culture lag between lay persons and professionals. Nurses can then frame questions about the consequences of beliefs and behaviors that differ from the modern, biomedical, or professional criteria.

Tables 5-1 and 5-2 depict the hot/cold classification system used by urban Puerto Ricans and interventions appropriate for professionals working within the hot/cold framework.[19]

## BIOCULTURAL DIMENSIONS

The existence of ethnicity and race as social rather than biologic groupings does not rule out differences in morbidity, mortality, and some physical traits among (as well as within) different ethnic and racial groups. Biologic variations among various racial groups can occur along several dimensions, including body structure, skin color and other physical characteristics, enzymatic and genetic variations, electrocardiographic patterns, susceptibility to disease, nutritional preferences and deficiencies, and psychologic characteristics.[52] Of these possible variations, however, skin color is perhaps the most relevant dimension for providing nursing care. Becoming knowledgeable about the specific biologic variations of the racial groups frequently seen in the nurse's clinical setting is essential for delivering culturally competent care. As the illness trajectory is discussed, additional examples will be provided.

The construct *adaptation* relates to a particular environment or the possession of traits or attributes that make it possible for persons to function effectively and to reproduce in this environment.[9] Adaptation, however, may be bought at a high price, and certain peculiarities that are assets in some geographic areas may be handicaps in others. The sickle cell hemoglobin condition, which may have evolved as a protection against malaria, is an example of such a change. Cancer, heart disease,

**TABLE 5-2 Management Issues with Puerto Rican Patients Who Follow Hot/Cold Theory**

| GENERAL PROBLEM | EXAMPLE | RECOMMENDED SOLUTION WITHIN HOT/COLD FRAMEWORK |
|---|---|---|
| Patient fails to take prescribed medication or eat recommended foods because they directly contradict notions of good therapy within hot/cold framework. | Pregnant women avoid "hot" foods and medications to prevent their babies from being born with a rash or red skin. As a result, they do not take prescribed iron or vitamin supplements. | When patient rejects "hot" substances, use neutralization principle.<br>When patient rejects "cool" medication, use an alternative drug not classified in the hot/cold system. |
| Patient on maintenance dose of a "hot" medication stops therapy when he experiences a "hot" symptom<br>Patient on maintenance dose of a "cool" medication stops therapy when a "cold" symptom develops. | Patient on prophylactic program of penicillin stops therapy when he experiences diarrhea or constipation and may discontinue therapy entirely to prevent a recurrence. | With "hot" medications, follow neutralization principle and advise patients to take them with a "cool" substance.<br>With "cool" medications, use a drug not classified in the hot/cold system or prescribe an equivalent "hot" drug until the "cold" symptom subsides. |
| Patient discontinues "hot" or "cold" foods in a dietary regimen if symptoms within the same category develop. | Patients on diuretics who are told to eat dried fruits, oranges, and bananas (all "cold" or "cool" foods) as sources of potassium will stop these foods should "cold" symptoms develop. Since these symptoms include menstruation, women are most at risk. | For any dietary recommendation, provide options from all three categories of the hot/cold system. (For example, "hot" cocoa or peas might also be suggested as sources of potassium.) |
| Substances traditionally used to "refresh" the stomach (that is, to neutralize "hot" foods) may be harmful in themselves. | To protect babies from developing rashes or other "hot" symptoms from formula made with evaporated milk, some mothers add "cool" $MgCO_3$ or mannitol to the bottle, often in quantities sufficient to cause diarrhea. | Stress use of harmless "cool" additives (barley water, fruit juice) in place of potentially harmful ones. |

From Harwood A: *Ethnicity and medical care,* Cambridge, Mass, 1981, Harvard University Press.

and diabetes have all been referred to as diseases of civilization. Many types of *neoplastic disease* have been traced to environmental factors. The incidence of cancer has been shown to vary according to culture and social class.[9,32] Lung cancer is a common cause of death in the United States, England, Wales, and several other Western countries where cigarette smoking is common. Stomach cancers account for 50% of cancer among men in Iceland and Japan but only 10% in the United States. Liver cancer accounts for half of all causes of death among the Bantu in Africa and less than 4% in Europe. Breast cancer is eight times more common in Israel than in Japan.[9] Regional variations have been found in the incidence of skin and lip cancer in the United States and Russia. In both countries more cases occur in the south than in the north.

The etiologic factors in *diabetes, a chronic disease,* are still poorly understood. Some epidemiologic and genetic evidence suggests that a virus may be involved in causing at least one type of diabetes.[26] Both genetic and environmental factors are believed to play an important role in the high incidence of diabetes in some cultural groups, for example, some Native American tribes and Hispanics.[52,123] The high incidence of obesity among some populations is also correlated with the prevalence of diabetes. Changes in the specific components of a cultural group's diet and activity patterns have been identified as leading to an increased expression of diabetes.[29,38,106] The incidence of the three types of diabetes varies with race, gender, and age. Insulin-dependent diabetes mellitus peaks between the ages of 10 to 14 years, affecting boys and white persons at a somewhat higher rate than girls and nonwhites. In contrast, the occurrence of non-insulin dependent diabetes mellitus increases with age and occurs more frequently among nonwhites. It accounts for 80% to 90% of the cases. Gestational-onset diabetes mellitus, however, has been linked to increasing maternal age but not to race.[52] The accumulating data about geographic and cultural differentials in the incidence of diabetes and pathologic complications raise questions relative to the nature of human adaptation to culture change and cultural domination. The increased incidence of diabetes reported for rural migrants to urban centers in Israel,[31,106] South Africa,[85,123] and Canada[47,129] has led some to label diabetes a disease of civilization.

The relationship between increasing urbanization and diabetes morbidity reinforces Neel's hypothesis[106] of diabetes as a "thrifty" genotype. The theory holds that in prehistoric times the prediabetic person was better equipped to adapt to the environment. The gene or genes responsible for diabetes mellitus predisposed a person to gaining extra weight during times of relative plenty and thus enhanced survival during times of famine. Once these factors no longer existed, the diabetes gene once considered functional for survival became a liability.

Hypertension is another chronic illness for which there is a higher incidence among African-Americans than in white persons. Not only is there an increased incidence, but also an increased severity of the symptoms and complications. Data indicate that primary hypertension occurs in African-Americans almost 15 times more often than in non–African-Americans.[52] Therefore to assist with early detection it is essential that the nurse be cognizant of the risk factors for hypertension.

Studies of the differences in population frequencies of *lactose intolerance* suggest a genetic, as well as an acquired, basis.[16,17,66] Adults of cultures as diverse as the Thai, Japanese, Andean Indians, and Chinese have reduced levels of lactase. In the United States the rate for lactose intolerance among adults of predominantly European ancestry is between 10% and 20%. This contrasts with 70% lactose intolerance among adults of African descent.[16] The geographic distribution of the trait supports the hypothesis that primary adult lactose intolerance occurred after the cultural practice of domesticating milk-producing animals and initiating large-scale milk production was established.

Given the high nutritional value placed on milk in the United States and its inclusion in special diets, a reassessment of milk consumption is indicated. Persons with the enzyme deficiency suffer discomforts such as flatulence, bloating, severe abdominal cramping, and diarrhea after ingesting milk; thus, contrary to the popular slogan, some persons, especially those of African and Asian origin, do outgrow their need for milk. There is evidence that many lactose-intolerant adults in the milk-drinking culture of the United States simply restrict the amount of milk they drink at any one time to an amount that does not provoke symptoms. In this way they derive some benefits without suffering adverse effects.[17] In addition, cheese, yogurt, sour milk, and other milk products with a lower lactose content may be substituted.

Another significant enzymatic deficiency disorder is glucose-6-phosphate dehydrogenase (G6PD) deficiency, which is more prevalent among African-Americans, Chinese, Southeast Asians, Greeks, Sardinians, and Sephardic Jews. Under conditions of metabolic stress and ingestion of certain medications, severe hemolytic anemia may result because of G6PD deficiency. Situations that can precipitate hemolytic anemia include ingestion of medicines such as quinine, aspirin, phenacetin, chloramphenicol, probenecid, sulfonamides, and thiazide diuretics; eating fava beans; and the presence of infection.[52] Again, it is essential that the nurse be knowledgeable about situations likely to precipitate hemolytic anemia secondary to G6PD deficiency.

Differences in mortality and morbidity among white persons, African-Americans, and other population groups continue to the present decade. Much attention has been paid to sickle cell anemia, a genetically transmitted condition found primarily in African-Americans. Deaths from sickle cell anemia account for about 17% of the excess mortality of African-American over white persons.[149] A study by the Task Force on Black and Minority Health, reported by the Department of Health and Human Services in 1985, revealed that African-Americans have the highest incidence of cancer and mortality rates of any population group. Cancer incidence is 25% higher among African-American males than white males; African-American females have a 4% higher incidence rate for cancer than do white females. The prevalence of diabetes is significantly greater among African-Americans, Hispanics, Native Americans, and Asian and Pacific Islanders than among white persons, and the coronary heart disease rate among African-American women is twice that for white women, whereas stroke deaths among African-American men are nearly double those of white men. Although minorities generally have poorer health rates than do white persons, in some areas they actually do better. The overall cancer rate for Asian-Americans—Chinese, Japanese, and Filipinos—is lower than that for the white population. Native Americans have the lowest mortality from all cancers combined. Although it is essential that nurses be knowledgeable about ethnic and racial differences in the morbidity and mortality of various diseases, it is equally important that they focus on the impact of culture on the trajectory of illnesses.

## ILLNESS TRAJECTORY

The course an illness takes has been termed the **illness trajectory.**[9] The trajectory involves not only the physical manifestations and interpretation of the illness, but also the work involved in managing it, its impact, and the changes it demands in the lives of the ill individual and family members. Thinking of it as a line on paper, an illness trajectory takes on different shapes depending on the phases the illness passes through or the overall trend of the illness (Figure 5-2). These phases include the original health status followed by a preillness phase, acute (prediagnosis and diagnosis) phase, comeback (treatment) phase, alternating stable and unstable phases, and downward (terminal) phase.

### PHASES

Before a patient and family enter the institutional health care setting, there is a *preillness phase.* Unless an acute emergency exists, patients will use their "hierarchy of resort" before seeking professional medical care.[51] Kleinman et al.[85] estimate that 70% to 90% of self-recognized episodes of sickness are treated outside the formal health care system. Thus, during this preillness phase, the patient and family evaluate the meaning of the symptoms on the basis of their culture, religion, past experiences, support network, and the availability of folk healers. Symptoms may be interpreted as a death sentence, an unlucky deal of the cards of life, an outrage that thwarts

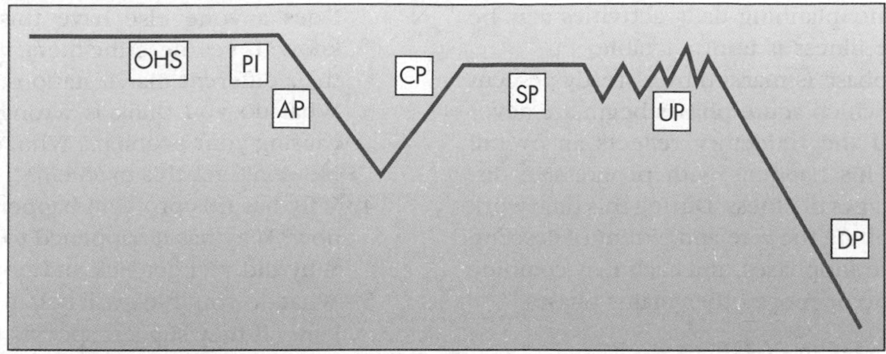


**FIGURE 5-2** Illness trajectories. *OHS,* Original health status; *PI, preillness phase; AP,* acute (prediagnosis and diagnosis) phase; *CP,* comeback (treatment) phase; *SP,* stable (chronic) phase; *UP,* unstable phase; *DP,* downward (terminal) phase.

life goals, failure of the government to control a polluted environment, the will of God, punishment for sin, personal failure to stop health-risk behavior (e.g., smoking, unprotected sexual intercourse), a challenge to accomplish certain goals, a curse from a long-time enemy, or spirit possession.[21,51] The patient and family's interpretation of the symptoms affects at which time in the progression of symptoms they will enter the professional health care system— if at all. However, the professional health care system is just one part of the health care system available to the patient.

Kleinman et al. have developed a three-part model of the health care system: professional, folk, and popular sectors. The *professional sector* includes formally educated, state-licensed practitioners of Western-style scientific medicine, also referred to as *biomedicine.* Professional-sector practitioners include physicians, nurses, and physical therapists. The *folk sector* of the health care system includes healers, whose education is often obtained through apprenticeship and whose practice is based on a traditional medical system. These healers often display inborn or spirit-given talent. The third sector, the *popular sector,* includes the sharing of health and illness information among family members, friends, and other knowledgeable, informal helpers.[85] Lock[95] makes a further distinction between *folk medical systems,* which are derived from a nonbiomedical, scholarly medical tradition and require formal education of practitioners (such as traditional Chinese medicine or the East Indian Ayurvedic medicine), and *local folk medical systems,* which are less sophisticated and organized (such as the local Japanese folk practitioners who practice moxibustion, which is the burning of an herb on specific, strategic sites on the body).

Knowledge and practice of medicine from each of the sectors mutually influence each other, and many health beliefs and practices are not limited to one sector. Knowledge of scientific medicine is readily available to many lay persons through health teaching, television, and print media. The 12-step recovery program of Alcoholic Anonymous, which may be considered "folk" practice, is used within hospitals, which are biomedical institutions. Physicians and nurses who believe in and practice scientific medicine may also use home remedies learned from parents and grandparents.

Popular and folk remedies may be tried, including extra rest, dietary changes such as special soups, over-the-counter medication or use of one's own or another's previously prescribed medications; self-help groups; herbs; poultices, amulets, religious practices and rituals, or use of folk healers such as medicine men or shamans.[51] The preillness phase follows the straight line representing the original health status before the sharp downward turn of the acute phase.

The *acute phase* is characterized by a line turning sharply downward and then upward. Depending on the extent of recovery, the upward line may be the same length (if health returns to preillness status), shorter (if a health deficit exists when compared with the preillness status), or longer (if health status exceeds the preillness level). During this phase, work is directed at obtaining and receiving immediate medical attention, stabilizing the illness, and promoting recovery. It may coincide with the diagnosis of a chronic illness characterized by an acute episode, such as a heart attack.

The *comeback phase* is marked by a line angling upward. This phase represents the recovery that may occur after an acute phase. Work is directed at regaining functional ability and reconciling any residual disability. This occurs in—although it is not limited to—the treatment stage, as when a person is treated immediately after a heart attack.

The *stable* phase is depicted by a straight line, which describes a period when changes occur gradually over years. Work by family members is directed at maintaining stability. This is the chronic stage of an illness.

The *unstable* phase can occur at any time during the course of an illness. During this time the illness is continuously out of control, and work is directed at finding the source of instability. An unstable phase of an illness occurs, for example, when cancer recurs or when an infection exacerbates an already existing health problem. During this time, planning daily activities may be difficult because the illness is unpredictable.

The *downward* phase is marked by a steady descent on a line; points at which acute phases begin are never really regained, and the trajectory reflects an overall downward trend. This happens with progressive disability or terminal stages of illness. During this time work is directed at controlling the rate and extent of descent. Each phase may have subphases, and each may combine or alternate with one or more other major phases.[10]

## EARLY DIAGNOSTIC STAGE

The early diagnostic period of an illness or injury may be triggered by a sudden event—for example, a heart attack or accident that results in the victim being rushed to the emergency room. Another scenario might involve someone visiting a physician's office to confirm or discount the meaning of a symptom. A third situation might result from a routine physical examination that points to serious illness. Although we are aware that the ill person is experiencing and reacting to the events, we are often less aware that the family members also are experiencing their own set of reactions. All patients and families have cultural backgrounds that must be considered if culturally competent care is to be delivered. Thus it is essential for the nurse to assess the patient and family's perceptions of the meaning of an injury or illness.

### Nursing Interventions for the Prediagnosis Phase

#### Culturologic assessment

The nurse needs to employ the third component of the culturally competent model of care, *cultural skill.* The use of cultural skill assumes that the nurse has already begun and continues the processes of *cultural awareness* and *cultural knowledge* through a personal examination of biases and prejudices toward other cultures and continues to become more educated about the perspectives of the different cultural groups represented in the practice setting. Cultural skill is reflected by the nurse's use of culturologic assessment to evaluate the patient and family members' beliefs, values, practices, and accepted interventions. Numerous culturologic assessment tools are designed to capture the patient's culture so that relevant data can be considered in planning culturally competent services.* For example, Pfifferling[114] developed the cultural status examination, which consists of the following questions (p. 207):

1. How would you describe the problem that has brought you to me, hospital, or agency? Is there anyone else with you that I can talk to about your problem? (If yes, to significant other: Can you describe X's problem?) Has anyone else in your family/friend network helped you with this problem?
2. How long have you had this (these) problem(s)? Does anyone else have this problem that you know? Is yes, describe them, how old are they, and their different manifestations.
3. What do you think is wrong, out of balance, or causing your problem? Who, or what kind of people don't get this problem?
4. Why has this problem happened to you, and why now? Why has it happened to (the involved part)? Why did you get sick and not someone else?
5. What do you think will help to clear up your problem? (If they suggest specific tests, procedures, or drugs, ask them to further define what they are and how they will help.)
6. Apart from me, who else do you think can help you get better? Are there things that make you feel better or give you relief, that doctors don't know about?

This next-to-last question assumes that the patient/family perceives the health care professional as being the one to help them. Campinha-Bacote,[22] however, suggests the following more open-ended approach, "As a *(fill in the blank),* what can I do to assist you with your problem?" The health care provider fills in the appropriate discipline. Nurses should incorporate the aforementioned questions into their admission assessment on *all* patients, regardless of the patient and family's ethnic/racial background.

Corbin and Strauss[33] have described the early diagnostic period as a "diagnostic quest" involving a prediagnostic phase, announcement phase, and postdiagnostic phase. Each phase may be long or short; each requires an expenditure of physical and emotional energy from family members. The whole process may need to be repeated many times as new symptoms appear throughout the course of the illness.

The onset of chronic illness is often insidious. Small discomforts are explained away or adapted to over time without the person being fully aware of making life changes. As symptoms become harder to ignore, they may become visible to family members or a greater concern to the ill person. The initial response of family members may be to read about the symptoms and compare them to symptoms friends have experienced. Depending on the severity of the symptoms, reactions may range from feeling that nothing is wrong to fear of death. At some point, when the symptoms can no longer be ignored, a visit is made to the physician and the diagnostic work begins.[117]

Frustrations are inherent in the diagnostic process. Having tests scheduled in a timely manner, undergoing multiple diagnostic tests, and receiving inconclusive findings and false-positive results can all add to emotional strain for family members as well as for the patient. Research has consistently shown that families rate supportive resources, environmental conveniences, information, frequent visitation, and empathic interactions as very important needs during critical illness of a family

*References 9, 11, 22, 76, 85, 90, 113, 114, 147.

## RESEARCH

Reeder J: Family perception: a key to intervention, *AACN Clin Issues* 2(2):188-194, 1991.

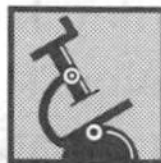

Using family stress theory in her study of 112 families of persons who had received severe injuries, Reeder reported that families used these words to describe how they felt about their family member being injured: "hurt, sad, afraid, worried, devastated," and "shocked." The family's perception of a critical illness or injury was key to the family coping and nursing intervention. When families were asked the most important thing for them to know *right now* about their injured family member, they replied, "information and hope." Informational needs were as follows: (1) to have questions answered honestly, (2) to know the prognosis, (3) to know specific facts concerning the patient's progress, (4) to have explanations given in understandable terms, (5) to receive information about the patient once a day, (6) to be called at home about changes in the patient's condition, and (7) to know why things were done for the patient.

member.[92] Of these needs, information is reported as the most important.[24,122] Although these needs are relevant during the early diagnostic phase, they also are relevant during any unstable period in the patient's illness. (See Research box, above.)

### Physical assessment

In addition to conducting a culturologic assessment, the nurse performs a physical assessment during the early diagnostic phase, which includes assessment of skin color. Because patients have varying amounts of the pigment melanin in their skin, the nurse must know the proper techniques to evaluate cyanosis, pallor, and jaundice in patients with very dark skin color. Suggested techniques for proper assessment of skin color in dark-skinned persons are noted in Box 5-2.

## BOX 5-2 Physical Assessment of Skin Color in Dark-Skinned Persons

**PALLOR**

Establish the patient's baseline skin color using daylight or a 60-watt bulb as the light source. Patients with dark skin tones should be assigned the bed near the window, when possible. Observe those skin surfaces having the least amount of pigmentation, which include the volar surfaces of the forearms, the palms of the hands, the soles of the feet, the abdomen, and the buttocks. Note the underlying red tone that is typical of all skin, regardless of how dark its color. Absence of this red tone may be indicative of pallor. Also, assess the mouth, conjunctiva, and nailbeds for pallor.

**JAUNDICE**

Observe the hard palate, sclera, or lips, which will be yellow in the presence of jaundice.

**PETECHIAE**

Observe the conjunctiva for the presence of petechiae.

**CYANOSIS**

The lips can be used to assess for cyanosis. However, the lip color of some persons with very dark skin may have a naturally bluish cast. As in persons with a lighter skin tone, the nailbed can be used to assess for cyanosis by noting how quickly the color returns to the nailbeds after pressure is released from the free edge of the nail.

**RASHES/INFLAMMATION**

Gently palpate the skin for rashes; note signs of inflammation such as swelling, increased warmth, and ecchymosis; and observe for facial reactions such as grimacing.

**HYPERPIGMENTATION**

It is normal to find hyperpigmentation of the oral mucosa and tongue, as well as scleral brown freckles and yellow fatty deposits.

### Family responses during prediagnostic phase

Family members' involvement in this prediagnostic phase may require them to rearrange their lives. For instance, they may need to take time off from work, schedule child care, or juggle other tasks. A financial burden may result from loss of work, the cost of child care, and the expense of testing, all of which may have a significant impact on family resources. All these stressors place additional emotional and physical strains on family members.

Many factors influence how the diagnosis is relayed and received. There may be barriers to communicating these informational needs to patients and families whose cultural group differs from that of the health care professionals. One's culture influences how feelings are assessed and what verbal and nonverbal expressions are appropriate.[52] The nurse must know the styles and types of feedback unique to certain cultural groups. For example, a Vietnamese may say "yes," which does not necessarily mean understanding but may simply be an attempt to avoid a confrontation and to appease. Similar behavior can be observed in elderly African-Americans. Culture also influences to whom communications should be directed. For example, in some Hispanic families, the male head of the household must give his permission for the performance of procedures. Under such circumstances, female members will attempt to delay decision making until the male member is present. Similarly, some Navajos believe it is not proper to answer questions about another person.[52] Consequently, they may attempt to avoid answering some assessment questions. Other communication dimensions that the nurse must consider are appropriateness of touch, proximity when speaking to a person, use of silence, and literal interpretation of some English words by some patients/families, as well as eye contact, voice quality, and body posture. Depending on diagnostic test results and the physician's style, the information may be given compassionately or bluntly. The diagnosis may be certain or tentative, and a prognosis may or may not be given. Some physicians may be selective about what information is given to the patient and what information is given to the family. This can sometimes be difficult for family members because it makes communication with the patient more problematic.[68] Hoping to protect the patient, some family members may ask the physician to withhold information. Sometimes the same information may be given but heard differently by various members of the family.[33]

The diagnosis often brings shock and disbelief.[54,127] One person said, "I threw my arms around Connie, crying bitterly. I had always found it difficult to cry. That night I could not seem to stop. 'CJ, it isn't true; the doctor's wrong. It isn't happening.' "[126] Other family members may feel relief because the ambiguity of the diagnostic period has ended.[89]

Family members may have numerous questions. Is surgery necessary before a diagnosis can be confirmed? Should a second opinion be sought to either validate or disprove it? (This may result in additional diagnostic procedures, and the process starts again.) What are the treatment options? What will be the extent of disability? What changes in day-to-day living will have to be made? What will life be like for the family in 6 months, 1 year, 5 years? All these unanswered questions and concerns create a tremendous amount of uncertainty for the patient and family members. Nurses need to employ numerous strategies to facilitate communication during all phases of the patient's illness. These strategies include the following[52,154]:

1. Assess personal beliefs surrounding persons from different cultures.
2. Assess communication variables from a cultural perspective.
3. Plan care based on the communicated needs and cultural background.
4. Modify communication approaches to meet cultural needs.
5. Understand that respect for the patient and communicated needs are central to the therapeutic relationship.
6. Communicate in a nonthreatening manner.
7. Use validating techniques in communication.
8. Be considerate of the reluctance to talk when the subject involves sexual matters.
9. Adopt special approaches when the patient speaks a different language.
10. Use interpreters to improve communication.

Unfortunately, sometimes the use of an interpreter can compound the communication problems. If the interpreter misunderstands the communication from the nurse and consequently changes the initial meaning, the response from the patient and family may be inappropriate.

In an effort to preserve family life as it was before the illness and to close off uncertainty, some family members may deny that the patient has a serious illness.[155] They may persist in the notion that the illness has been misdiagnosed or that the situation is not as serious as portrayed. They may choose not to hear what they have been told. Some argue that denial of the problem's seriousness can be a valuable first response to a situation and can provide the person with time to pull resources together before dealing with the problem.[88]

Hearing the diagnosis may be accompanied by feelings of guilt, fear, and remorse. Family members may wonder if they could have detected the illness earlier or what they might have done to contribute to its onset.[40,58,116,138] One man stated, "The uncertainty of Martha's future filled me with stone-cold fear. Mingled with it was an aching remorse: I should have insisted that she have the biopsy when the lump was first discovered. Failing that, I should have insisted on a biopsy when the tumor couldn't be aspirated just a few weeks before."[104] Often a diagnosis of cancer may trigger terror from memories of others who suffered from cancer.[54,55]

In addition to trying to gain an understanding of the illness and how it will affect family life, family members often attempt to find meaning in the illness and understand why this has happened to them. They may spend energy researching the illness in an effort to understand how the illness developed and what behaviors or characteristics of the patient led to it. Family members not only attempt to find meaning for the illness event but also wish to assure themselves that the same condition will not strike another member of the family.[53]

Family members may employ various strategies in coping with the diagnosis. They may cope by taking some form of action, such as providing support and assistance or obtaining information. They may also seek out an empathic listener,[99] seek direction from an authority such as the physician, or try to find something favorable about the situation.[89]

### Family participation in treatment selection

In addition to coping with the diagnosis, family members are faced with how to share the information with others. They must decide how much to tell, when, and with whom to share information about the diagnosis.[53]

The role family members play in making a decision about treatment may vary. As discussed earlier, the family's culture dictates which and to what extent family members will be involved in the decision making. Lack of involvement should not necessarily be construed as disinterest. To ensure the involvement of the patient and family members in the decisions related to the treatment plan—to the extent that is culturally prescribed and/or desired—the nurse must use a collaborative framework.

**Collaborative framework.** The *collaborative framework* means determining whether each self-care remedy is detrimental and whether it will antagonize a patient's therapeutic regimen.[21] If the remedy is not harmful, instead of negating a culturally relevant folk treatment and implementing a culturally incompatible regimen, the practice should be incorporated. These practices may involve drinking herb tea; eating certain foods; using natural products, special vitamins, or over-the-counter drugs; or engaging in other practices. Treatments that are culturally incompatible will be promptly discontinued on the patient's discharge, resulting in the label of noncompliant patient/family. Charonko[26] argues that there is no such patient as the "noncompliant" patient—only a patient for whom this collaborative approach was not used. Nevertheless, sometimes patients and families want to use remedies or practices that, after an analysis of the benefits and risks, are determined to be detrimental. Then health care professionals must make an effort to validate their understanding of the family's rationale for wanting to use the practice and explain in lay persons' terms the risks involved in employing that practice. The key is to demonstrate respect for cultural beliefs and practices even if they cannot be used in the treatment plan. The following story provides an example of the use of the collaborative approach by health care professionals. A 35-year-old white man of the Pentecostal faith who was dependent on a ventilator requested that his wife be allowed to put special herbs through his nasogastric tube and play gospel tapes in his room. After the herbs were determined to be harmless and because the patient was in a private room, both requests were successfully negotiated by the patient, wife, and the health care team.

Some family members may be highly involved in helping the patient negotiate a treatment plan. Family members may become active participants, researching options and alternatives for treatment and accompanying the patient for second opinions. Some family members choose to be passive, assuming that they have no right to voice an opinion inasmuch as it is not their body nor their illness. Passive approaches may also be taken by those who believe "the doctor knows best what to do."

In disengaged families, reactions may include unconcern or disinterest. Wellisch, Jamison, and Pasnau[157] reported that men who had been highly involved in the decision-making process regarding their partners' mastectomies thought that their relationships were sound and rewarding, whereas those who were relatively uninvolved identified the decision-making time as the point at which emotional disruption began in the relationship. In addition, most of these men wished in retrospect that they had been more involved in the decision-making process.

A major challenge for the family is to decide how to continue with their lives while accommodating the illness. The response to this ongoing uncertainty often is to continue researching, reading, and talking with others.

## TREATMENT STAGE

Depending on the illness and the regimen negotiated, treatment may take place in a hospital, outpatient clinic, rehabilitation center, or at home. Technical advances in treatment protocols and the economic impact of diagnosis-related groups (DRGs) are resulting in shorter hospital stays, necessitating that family members become increasingly involved in providing care during the treatment phase.[25,109]

When illnesses require the person to be hospitalized for treatment, this period can be a particularly distressing time for family members. The time during and immediately after surgery has been reported by partners of mastectomy patients as very stressful.[140,156] Stolar[140] speculated that these men confronted the possibility of their spouse's death during this time. In addition to spending time visiting and offering support to the patient, family members may need to manage home and child care, as well as work responsibilities.[107,108,163]

Family members' participation in the delivery of treatment may extend from being a supportive presence to actually providing care. Treatment regimens may be simple or complex, may be quickly accomplished, or may take hours to complete, as in dialysis. Family members may have to spend considerable time learning specialized procedures. Although family caregivers experience rewards through the provision of care to their relatives,[83,115] the nurse must be observant of signs of caregiver burden, stress, and strain. These signs include anxiety, depression, fatigue, unkempt physical appearance, irregular meals, little absence from the patient's bedside or waiting room, presence of children too young to visit in the hospital waiting room on a consistent basis, irritability, arrival in an inebriated state or with the smell of alcohol on the breath, little evidence of the social support network providing the caregiver a break, and a lack of funds to pay for toiletries, food, or transportation.

Concern about the caregiver is especially important in cases in which the caregiver will be taking the patient home and will continue to provide care. In such cases it is important for the nurse to communicate to the caregiver permission not to visit and provide care every day and to make a referral to the social service department to gain additional support for the family.[45] However, the caregiver's culture and the perceived quality of the care being delivered by the health care professionals to the patient will dictate the person's acceptable visitation and care restrictions. For example, some Native American tribes believe that if a patient is critically ill, he or she should not be left alone.[52] Further, if the family notices that health care professionals prioritize the delivery of care on the basis of which patients have family members present, the perception may be that their presence is necessary to ensure that the relative receives care promptly.

In the critical care setting, family participation is limited and families often may feel excluded from the focus of care.[135] In reaction to restricted visiting hours, one family member stated, "Don't they know how important visiting is to us? It infuriates me that they are unwilling to bend a little. Why can't we just sit quietly in a corner?"[122] Because the issues of visitation and participation in care of family members in critical care settings continue to be a source of stress for both nursing staff and families,[92,122] it is important for nurses to carefully evaluate the reasons for these restrictions. Reeder[122] suggests that nurses should consider whether their lack of comfort with more frequent visitation and participation may relate to one of the following factors: (1) a nurse's lack of skills in family support and intervention, (2) a nurse's anxiety about personal well-being when families with a history of street violence are present, (3) the availability of support from hospital security personnel for visitor control, and (4) the availability of psychosocial services to support families with complex needs. The unit's design, with little extra space, also can serve as a deterrent to family visitation.[92]

In situations in which patients do not experience many side effects and are otherwise feeling well enough to carry on with regular activities, the impact of treatment may be minimal. For other caregivers, however, providing transportation to treatment,[109] following through on protocols at home, and managing side effects of treatment can be an emotionally and physically demanding time. Attempting to provide this care to the ill person while continuing with already existing responsibilities may be difficult at best. Often families need to redefine their roles, rules, and responsibilities to accommodate the illness. Also, while all this is taking place, uncertainty regarding treatment outcomes remains a major concern for all.

## CHRONIC STAGE

The chronic stage of illness is characterized by a relatively stable trajectory. The ill family member may experience a gradual decline in health, which may be interrupted occasionally with acute episodes. Family members adapt to this period by making changes in their day-to-day living arrangements to accommodate caring for the ill member and taking over role responsibilities as needed. As the chronic period continues, sometimes for years, the physical and emotional demands of caregiving may take their toll on the family.

### Caregiver Strain

#### Physical strain

The caregiving role frequently is assumed by the spouse of the ill person. If the couple is elderly, the caregiving spouse is not only aged, but may have chronic health problems as well.[130] When an ill person is divorced or widowed, the caregiving role often falls to an adult daughter. Many women work full-time in addition to raising young children. Assuming a caregiving role for a chronically ill relative while contending with personal health problems or while working and raising children can create significant stress and strain.

The family caregiver may experience a constant drain on physical energies. The patient may be incapable of self-care and may require total physical care. Often the patient's dependency needs allow the caregiver little personal time.[58,67] In addition, caregiving responsibilities may continue throughout the night, leaving the caregiver constantly deprived of much-needed sleep.

Imagine this scenario. You and the man or woman you chose out of all the world because you loved and trusted and admired this person are walking in the woods. The one you love steps in a bear trap and lies there bleeding and in pain. You both work on the trap, but this is long, long ago and far off in the woods and neither rocks nor fingernails are strong enough to open the trap. Your loved one is cold and hungry. You build a shelter and look for berries. That's one day. The leg rots. The pain increases. It snows. That's one year. It snows again. You plant a few pumpkin seeds and slap a little mud on the shelter. At what point, exactly, do you say "So long, Charlie"?[141]

#### Financial strain

Depending on the family's financial situation, considerable stress may be generated by loss of income.[10,40,58] Because of a family member's illness, the caregiver may no longer be able to work. In addition, home responsibilities and fatigue may make outside employment impractical for the family caregiver. Even when the household does not lose income, financial hardship may result from medical expenses.[20] In a study of 83 African-American female caregivers of persons with a dementia, 66.2% (n = 55) reported the available caregiver household income to be under $10,000 annually.[115]

#### Role strain

Family members may experience a range of stresses resulting from increased or changed responsibilities. The roles of family members may be radically altered. They may need to learn new skills. They may find that an increase in caregiving responsibilities leaves less time for other role responsibilities.[10,40,41,84] Sometimes the caregiver is unable to cope psychologically with the caregiving demands. One elderly African-American woman whose husband had a severe impaction, with abdominal distention and projectile vomiting, could not psychologically ready herself to administer the prescribed enema to her husband despite his obvious discomfort. The visiting nurse had to administer the enema.

Perceived caregiver costs, rewards, and helpfulness of social support were the best predictors of the caregiver's coping in a recent study of African-American female caregivers.[115] Although these caregivers turned most frequently to God and family for social support, health care professionals were more important than family to the patient's physical care. These findings have implications for discharge planning. Referring to the information gathered during the cultural assessment, the nurse and patient/family can negotiate mutually acceptable discharge regimens. The nurse will need to help the family identify the specific care demands of the regimen, the cultural and individual acceptance of the care demands, and the availability and helpfulness of social support to the caregiver. Sometimes caregivers may have large social networks, but the persons and agencies that compose the social network may not be perceived by the caregiver as helpful. Some caregivers report that some persons who attempt to provide help are more of a nuisance than a help.[115] If the caregiver is an older daughter, caregiving responsibilities may leave her less time for her own family and her role as a mother. A caregiver may be required to undergo a reversal in roles with the ill family member or a role change, perhaps becoming head of the household for the first time in a long-term marriage.[58,64] The role changes are likely to require additional decision making on the part of the caregiver, often without the benefit of input from the ill family member. Thus, in addition to the increased role responsibilities inherent in caregiving, family members may be required to take on additional responsibilities once belonging to the patient.[40,41,84]

### Interfamilial relationship strain

Additional stresses within the family context may be caused by conflicts stemming from care issues. Family members may differ in their goals for the patient and the best way to meet these goals. Interfamilial conflict may arise around such issues as need for institutionalization versus home care.[58] Interfamilial conflict also may surface when a family member looks to other relatives for assistance or respite. When help is not forthcoming, the caregiver may perceive this as a lack of support for dealing with the increased responsibilities of caregiving.[10]

### Emotional strain

The losses experienced by family members may impose a tremendous emotional strain. These losses are dictated largely by the nature of the patient's illness. For some families the loss may include the mental as well as the physical capabilities of the patient[39,40] and with those, the loss of a best friend and confidant.[58] Some family members report that their interactions with the ill person are no longer satisfying and supportive because of the patient's increased dependence on them for emotional and physical care and they have to depend less on the patient in these areas.[10,116] One family member stated, "All that stuff that we shared before is now my responsibility. Being emotionally strong and not falling apart is also my responsibility. If I'm home and I cry, Joel asks me not to because it gets him upset. So I either have to go out to the sidewalk and cry, wait until he is out, or not cry at all."[125] Another potential loss experienced by partners of chronically ill persons is that of a sexual partner.[82,94,137]

### Social relationship strain

As a result of increased responsibilities, family members may find they have less time for relationships outside of the home.[41,58,132] Many family members experience a loss of time for self. In cultural groups in which religion plays a major role, the inability to attend and participate in church activities can be stressful for the family.[161] Therefore the nurse should determine if family members would like their religious leader to be contacted. Many families may lose their financial security and may need to put aside plans made for the future.[40] Living without the ill family member may be yet another loss the caregiver anticipates if the illness is life-threatening.[10] The uncertainty of treatment outcomes can cause ongoing stress in dealing with many chronic illnesses, especially life-threatening ones.[93] For the family the losses may affect every aspect of life.

For some family members these losses lead to increased feelings of resentfulness, anger, anxiety, impatience, frustration, guilt, and ambivalence. Resentfulness may arise as an outgrowth of increased worries and responsibilities. Some may express anger at the illness and the situation in which the family now finds itself. This anger comes from crushed expectations and the loss of quality time that could have been spent together.[40] Guilt may arise as family members continue to blame themselves for the patient's illness or for their inability to prevent the illness.[40,62,116] Many family members express concern that they are not doing enough for the patient.[10,40,67] Ambivalence may surface as family members feel anger at the situation created by the illness and their desire for it to end, and yet they do not want the ill member to die. This ambivalence may be a source of tension and guilt.[93]

Long-term caregiving can result in health risks for family members. Because of the time involved in the caregiving role, they may experience social isolation. An intact support system has been demonstrated to be of prime importance in helping persons cope with stress.[62,79,80] A lack of supportive relationships, particularly in times of crisis and transition, places family members at risk for developing physical and emotional illness and even premature death.[8,30,80] In addition to the health risk created by lack of support, caregivers are also at risk from the stress and strains inherent in caregiving.[3,40,84,132]

Family members of chronically ill persons have a tremendous need for information regarding the course, duration, outcome, and potential impact of the illness.[42] Studies of caregiving demands during advanced disease often show that problems arise in information exchanges with health care professionals.[139,160] As previously described, many factors influence the course of chronic illnesses, and concrete answers may not be possible.

However, needs such as being informed of the patient's condition or any changes in condition and being assured that the patient is comfortable have been identified as important information needs by family members of persons with advanced disease.[122,160]

For adolescent members of the family, adjusting to the changes in responsibility imposed by the illness may be difficult. Developmentally, adolescence is a time for moving away emotionally and physically from the home and family. These activities run counter to the demands placed on the adolescent as a result of the illness, which may include helping with chores, being increasingly involved with family, and providing emotional support.[93,156] When a parent is ill, the inherent role modeling that usually occurs for children may be compromised.[116] A parent who is tired, is always in bed, or is depressed may be sending unintended messages. Last, children of all ages may be sensitive and fearful about their parent's health, harboring worries and concerns about death and its implications.

## TERMINAL STAGE

One of the greatest challenges families face is caring for a dying family member. For many family members this may be their first intimate experience with death. Members are forced to face issues that they may have long avoided, even in the face of a long-term illness. Suddenly their relationship with the health care system may seem more problematic as the focus of care moves from prolonging life to controlling symptoms and enhancing the quality of life that remains.

When a family member is dying, other family members need information so that they can make decisions and plan and provide care. However, in a complex health care setting that involves numerous physicians, family members may not even be able to identify the primary physician.[86]

As family members confront the reality of losing a loved one, they are asked to make major decisions about care and perhaps to take on more of that care. They may be asked to decide where their family member will die. Can the patient's symptoms be managed at home by family members with the help of home health nurses, or is home care not a feasible option? Sometimes a nursing home is the appropriate choice, particularly if the terminal period is prolonged. Admission to an inpatient hospice for symptom control or terminal care may be desirable. Each choice has its advantages and costs to family members. Some evidence suggests that if communication between the patient and family is poor, the family is more apt to choose for the patient to die in the hospital rather than at home.[86] If the family member is to remain at home, who will do the caregiving, and what assistance will that person need? All this is further complicated because often these decisions are not clear-cut, and family members continue to wrestle with the question of ongoing treatment or exactly how much will be done to prolong the patient's life.

At a time when family members need most to share their feelings and concerns, communication among them may become most troublesome. They may find themselves responding differently to the situation, and tension may arise as they find their feelings and concerns at odds with others in the family and with the ill member. One family member may still want to explore treatment as a possibility, whereas another may be trying to accept the finality of the illness. Another family member may feel angry with the physicians or nurses for their handling of the care, and another family member may be working hard to keep peace within the family. The dying person may have strong feelings about remaining at home to die, but family members may not be able to provide the care. Family members may not have previously talked with each other about their feelings. Many do not talk about death, even with the patient.[86] The final stages of an illness may come after a long period of family members' giving physical care and expending much emotional energy. Somehow family members must find the reserves to carry on with even greater intensity.

When an ill person is in the terminal stage of illness, family members often begin to anticipate what lies ahead. The term *anticipatory grief* has been used to describe this experience. This allows family members to absorb the reality of the loss over time, attend to unfinished business with the dying person (express feelings, resolve past conflicts), begin to change assumptions about life and identity, and make plans for the future so that they will not feel they betrayed their loved one once he or she has died.[121] Multiple losses, including what the person's death will mean to each person as well as to the family, may surface as these aspects of the terminal period are addressed. One way the nurse can support the family during the terminal stages of a patient's illness is to assist with the implementation of cultural rituals related to death and dying. (Ideally, the nursing staff should have identified these rituals during the early diagnostic phase of the patient's illness.) Practices related to the terminal stage of a patient's life vary both among cultural and religious groups and between individual members. Thus it is critical that the nurse document family and patient preferences. Generally, during the dying process Mexican Americans prefer family and clergy to be present, but most Japanese Americans do not want the presence of family, and only one half of Japanese Americans, African-Americans, and white Americans want a clergyman present.[13] White persons are less in contact with the dying process than are African-Americans, Japanese Americans, and Mexican Americans. Table 5-3 provides some general religious guidelines related to death and dying. However, the nurse must assess for individual and family differences.

Throughout the early diagnostic, treatment, chronic, and terminal stages of the patient's illness, the nurse is involved in **cultural encounter,** the final component of the culturally competent model of care. Cultural encounter requires the nurse to interact directly with pa-

**TABLE 5-3 Religious Guides Related to Death and Dying**

| RELIGION/ISSUE | BELIEFS AND PRACTICES |
|---|---|
| **BAHA'I FAITH** | |
| *Prolongation of life* | Premature ending of life is rarely permissible |
| *Autopsy* | Acceptable, if medically necessary or legally required |
| *Donation of body* | Acceptable for medical research and restorative purposes |
| **BUDDHISM** | |
| *Prolongation of life* | If there is hope for recovery and continued pursuit of enlightenment by the patient, all means of support are encouraged |
| *Autopsy* | It is a matter of individual preference |
| *Donation of body* | If donation of the entire body or a part will help another, donation is encouraged |
| **CATHOLICISM (ROMAN RITE)** | |
| *Prolongation of life* | During illness, the basic rite of the Sacrament of the Sick is practiced. Members must take ordinary means to prolong life (e.g., intravenous medication) but are not obligated to take extraordinary means (e.g. cardiopulmonary resuscitation) |
| *Autopsy* | Permissible as long as body is shown proper respect and there is sufficient reason for performing the autopsy |
| *Donation of body* | Permissible |
| **CHRISTIAN SCIENCE** | |
| *Prolongation of life* | Medical means to prolong life indefinitely are not usually pursued |
| *Autopsy* | Unlikely (deduced from donation of body approach) |
| *Donation of body* | Most Christian Scientists prefer to contribute to medical science through an alternative way |
| **CHURCH OF JESUS CHRIST OF LATTER-DAY SAINTS (MORMONS)** | |
| *Prolongation of life* | The sick are blessed in a ritual for the sick by a first and second elder; whenever possible, medical and faith healing are used to reverse illnesses that threaten life. If death is inevitable, a peaceful and dignified death is promoted |
| *Autopsy* | Permitted with the consent of next of kin and within local laws |
| *Donation of body* | Organ donation is permitted |
| **HINDUISM** | |
| *Prolongation of life* | No religious custom or restriction |
| *Autopsy* | Permissible |
| *Donation of body* | Acceptable |
| **ISLAM** | |
| *Prolongation of life* | Any attempt to shorten one's life or terminate it is prohibited; dead body is washed and rinsed by same-sex persons and placed in three pieces of clean white cloth |
| *Autopsy* | Permitted only for medical and legal purposes |
| *Donation of body* | Acceptable |
| **JEHOVAH'S WITNESS** | |
| *Prolongation of life* | The use of extraordinary means is a matter of individual conscience, but transfusions are prohibited |
| *Autopsy* | Acceptable only if required by law |
| *Donation of body* | Forbidden |
| **JUDAISM** | |
| *Prolongation of life* | Current measures should not be discontinued, but no new therapeutic measures need to be initiated |
| *Autopsy* | Permitted only in special circumstances, and decision makers must include family, rabbi, and physician |
| *Donation of body* | If it seems necessary, then consultation with the rabbi is required |
| **MENNONITE CHURCH** | |
| *Prolongation of life* | When hope of a meaningful recovery no longer exists, most Mennonites believe the health care team should consult the family to determine if life-sustaining measures should be withheld |
| *Autopsy* | Acceptable |
| *Donation of body* | Acceptable |
| **SEVENTH-DAY ADVENTISTS** | |
| *Prolongation of life* | The pastor and church elders pray for and anoint the sick person with oil; no official position on prolonging life, but generally prolongation of life is promoted |
| *Autopsy* | Acceptable |
| *Donation of body* | Acceptable |
| **UNITARIAN/UNIVERSALIST CHURCH** | |
| *Prolongation of life* | Favor the right to die with dignity |
| *Autopsy* | Recommended |
| *Donation of body* | Acceptable |

Modified from Andrews M, Hanson P. In Boyle J, Andrews M: *Transcultural concepts in nursing care,* Glenview, Ill, 1989, Scott, Foresman.

tients from diverse cultural groups to refine or remodify existing knowledge about those cultural groups.

## NURSING MANAGEMENT

### ♦ ASSESSMENT

Assessment of the family is discussed in the sections on family systems, family stress, ecologic frameworks, and culturologic assessment. The key areas to assess include ethnicity and degree of adherence to cultural values, beliefs, and practices, religious beliefs and practices, family composition, social network, social support, adaptability, cohesion, family-life cycle, socioeconomic status, and identified environmental resources.

### ♦ NURSING DIAGNOSES

Nursing diagnoses are determined from analysis of family data. Nursing diagnoses related to family and cultural concerns during an illness may include but are not limited to the following.

| Diagnostic Title | Possible Etiologic Factors |
|---|---|
| Coping, family: compromised | Inadequate or incorrect information or understanding, preoccupation by significant other with personal reactions, temporary family disorganization, role changes and crises; prolonged disability of significant other |
| Coping, family: disabling | Maladaptive coping styles, highly ambivalent family relationships, maladaptive behaviors |
| Home maintenance management, impaired | Individual/family member disease/injury, insufficient family resources, impaired cognitive functioning, lack of knowledge, role modeling, inadequate support systems |
| Role strain, high risk for caregiver | Situational crises, inadequate support services, caregiver fatigue or physical limitations |
| Noncompliance | Patient value system (health beliefs, cultural influences, values), patient-provider relationships, treatment side effects, cognitive/perceptual alterations |

### ♦ EXPECTED FAMILY OUTCOMES

Expected family outcomes for the social support of families managing the illness of a family member may include but are not limited to the following:

1a. Discusses the meaning of the patient's illness (e.g., symptoms) with family members and the nurse.
 b. Compares the family's perception of the illness with the health care professional's diagnosis.
 c. Discusses health and care concerns with the nurse.
 d. Accurately describes how cultural or religious beliefs and practices will affect selected treatment.
2. Identifies family characteristics that enhance and disable family coping.
3a. Identifies knowledge and skills needed to manage the home care of the patient.
 b. Negotiates with health care team acceptable ways to meet and evaluate the treatment needs of the patient.
4a. Discusses patient and primary caregiver needs with support network and the nurse.
 b. Identifies available support network and community resources for treatment or assistance.
5. Demonstrates competence with the negotiated treatment regimen.

### ♦ INTERVENTIONS

More than ever before, families are being asked to care for family members at home with the use of sophisticated technology. Nurses are often in a position to bridge the gap for families between the home and hospital settings. An important role of the nurse working with the chronically ill patient is to see how the family manages the illness on a day-to-day basis. This knowledge, along with an understanding of the illness, creates the foundation for nursing intervention. If the nurse attributes meaning to the symptoms only from the professional's world view, interventions may be inappropriate and the family/patient may be inappropriately labeled as noncompliant.

#### Translation Process Model

Wenger[158] has developed a translation process model that focuses on the search for cultural meaning in understanding patient symptoms. There are four components of the translation process, including (1) analyzing the reported symptoms within the family/patient's cultural context, (2) transferring the analyzed data into the biomedical (i.e., nurse's) perspective, (3) restructuring the clinical picture of the symptoms, integrating the cultural meaning of the patient's symptoms with the nurse's knowledge, identifying a fit or misfit, and finally, (4) negotiating the clinical care and cure actions among the patient, family members, and nurse.

*Analysis of the reported symptoms* within the family/patient's cultural context requires the nurse to solicit their world view. The nurse gathers cultural information about what the patient and family members believe is causing the symptoms, when the symptoms started and why they began at that time, how the symptoms work in the body, the expected course of the symptoms, and what should be done to treat the symptoms. In addition, other family/patient health and care concerns are shared with the nurse. It is vital that the nurse suspend any judgment while collecting, validating, and analyzing this shared information.

After the analysis of the information, ***the nurse shares with the family/patient the biomedical perspective on the symptoms.*** The nurse allows the family/patient time to reflect on the nurse's prescription of the cultural meaning of the symptoms. Next the nurse restructures the clinical picture of the symptoms, incorporating the cultural meaning of the patient's symptoms with professional knowledge that identifies fit or misfit. From this translation process, the patient, family, and nurse will together identify the problematic symptoms and knowledge deficits and select culturally appropriate care and cure actions.

### Promoting effective family coping

The nurse reviews with the family and patient the data related to family composition, social support network, social support, adaptability, cohesion, family-life cycle, socioeconomic status, known community resources, and the treatment regimen to help them identify areas of needed support from family, friends, church, and community organizations. One of the major needs identified by family members across all illness periods is the need for information. In the critical care setting, family members want their questions answered honestly and want facts regarding the patient's progress, treatment changes, and prognosis. Families also want explanations that are understandable.[91,99,101,122] When a family member is being treated for cancer, the family members need to know what symptoms the disease or treatment can cause and when to expect symptoms to occur.[145] Hospitalization during the course of a chronic illness can be a difficult time for family members. They are used to providing care and making day-to-day decisions about that care. When the patient is hospitalized, this role is taken over by the health care system. Providing family members with maximal opportunities to be involved in treatment and care helps foster a sense of control.[97] Nurses should encourage family members to maintain physical closeness to the patient, despite the presence of equipment and machines, and to give as much physical care as they wish. The need to ensure that the ill family member is comfortable and receiving the best possible care is an important aspect of the hospital experience for family members.[63,91,99,101,133] Family members feel reassured when they are certain that the patient is comfortable. Nurses must be open with family members about the care being provided and how the patient's needs are being met.

During interactions with the family and patient, the nurse pays attention to the family's communication. Family members may be distressed about the tension among members during their communications. The nurse should ensure that family members know that this tension is normal and that it is important that they communicate openly, honestly, and with respect for differing viewpoints. However, the nurse's specific intervention in the facilitation of effective communication must be culturally sensitive. Effective communication among family members is an important family strength and builds family cohesion.[43] Family cohesion can act as a buffer for families during the illness by building the family's sense of competence and self-worth. A strong sense of family cohesion can help family members find meaning in the illness experience and some positive outcomes. Open discussions allow family members to share concerns and feelings, which assists with problem solving and decision making. The nurse can facilitate this type of communication by helping to clarify issues, by encouraging discussion, and by being an empathic listener. Family members need to talk about what is happening with someone whom they feel understands their plight. Even when the family has an open pattern of communication among members, the nurse can listen to thoughts and feelings too sensitive to share with the patient. This type of intervention is essential when treatment goals are being determined. During the terminal period of an illness—when the decision to prolong or terminate treatment must be made—the nurse can play a key role in helping family members understand each other's wishes.

### Supporting effective home management

If family members are to care for the patient at home, they will need the help of nurses in learning new skills related to caregiving. Family members report that they need assistance in learning to help the patient walk, manage the patient's bowels and dietary needs, manage pain, and increase the patient's comfort level.[57] In addition, they may have to learn how to care for wounds, to suction, or to manage parenteral narcotics. They may need referral to other sources of information to assist them in decision making or in managing the illness and resulting strains. For instance, nurses can make a referral to a social worker to assist with handling the financial burden of the illness or to a home health agency to acquire the services of a home care nurse or home health aide. Specific community services that can be helpful to families are listed in Box 5-3. Most of these services can be located through the local area agencies on aging or departments of aging, Visiting Nurses' Association, Department of Social Services, or information and referral services.

### Promoting compliance

In complex health care settings, such as teaching hospitals, family members may not know who the primary health care professionals are or how to access them. Helping family members to understand the roles of different health care professionals and how to access them is necessary if families are to function comfortably and effectively in the health care setting. One of the most useful interventions nurses can provide is to act as interpreter in helping family members understand information given by other health care professionals. The nurse can then help families identify what information they still need to make appropriate decisions. Families

**BOX 5-3 Community Services to Support Families**

**ADULT DAY-CARE SERVICES**

Agencies provide structured supervision of adults during the day outside the family's home. Often these agencies specialize in the supervision of elderly patients.

**COMMUNITY MENTAL HEALTH SERVICES**

Agencies provide support for families or individual family members dealing with communication issues, depression, anxiety, and other mental health concerns.

**COMPANION SERVICES**

Agencies provide a person who routinely visits an elderly person and provides companionship, letter writing, and other mutually agreed upon services. Often area agencies on aging provide these services.

**FINANCIAL SERVICES**

Social service departments should be consulted for help with applying for financial assistance to caregivers and with applications for Medicaid, Medicare, Social Security Disability Income, and other grants.

**HOME CHORE SERVICES**

Assistance with light housekeeping and meal preparation is provided by agency chore workers.

**HOME HEALTH AIDES**

These aides can provide assistance with basic physical activities of daily living, including bathing, grooming, dressing, toileting, and ambulating the patient.

**HOME MEAL SERVICES**

Meals are delivered to the home of an elderly person (i.e., over age 60) by the local area agency on aging or other organizations.

**HOME NURSING SERVICES**

Agencies such as the Visiting Nurses' Association can provide nurses to assist with skilled care procedures and teach new knowledge and skills.

**HOSPICE SERVICES**

These services help provide either in-the-home or out-of-the-home services to facilitate the family's management of a terminally ill patient.

**INFORMATION AND REFERRAL SERVICES**

Information and referral service organizations provide a wealth of information regarding community resources and services.

**LEGAL SERVICES**

Often legal services can be found through free legal clinics, legal aid societies, universities with law schools, and the area agencies on aging.

**PHYSICAL THERAPY/OCCUPATIONAL THERAPY**

Therapy provides assistance with rehabilitation of the patient in the areas of mobility or self-care skills.

**RESPITE SERVICES**

These services provide the family a couple of hours to several days of either in-home or out-of-home relief from caregiving responsibilities.

**SUPPORT GROUPS**

Consultation with the local Alzheimer's Disease and Related Disorders Association, for example, can be helpful for families managing the care of a person with a dementia (e.g., impairment in cognition, judgment, language). Other support groups exist for persons who have had cancer, strokes, etc.

**TRANSPORTATION SERVICES**

In urban areas, tickets for public transportation or specially equipped vehicles for wheelchairs often can be purchased at a reduced rate for disabled and elderly persons.

may have to make many decisions about care and treatment in the course of a chronic illness, and they must have an accurate understanding of the information they receive. Sometimes the family perceives an unwillingness of the physician team to take into consideration their cultural beliefs and practices. Although it is not nursing's role to serve as mediator of the physician-patient relationship, the nurse can be an advocate for the integration of beneficial folk practices and explanations into the treatment regimen. This may mean coaching both family members and physician in the respective cultural views. Most important, discharge planning that integrates the explanatory models of both the family and biomedical cultures can result in reduced recidivism and better adherence to the treatment goals.[158]

The need for a sense of hope is an important aspect of coping with illness.[105,122] Hope allows one to envision the idea of a future. Fostering hope within a family is another aspect of the nurse's role. Hope, at different stages of the illness, takes on different meanings for the family. The nurse who can be with family members and help them cultivate a sense of hope also helps them deal with feelings of despair.[53,97]

### Preventing caregiver role strain

The stresses and strains of caregiving over time are extensive for family members. Often they may feel uncomfortable about leaving the ill member in the care of others or may feel guilty about wanting time for themselves. Nurses can teach family members to pace themselves and share the caregiving burden with others. Also important is the nurse's acknowledgment that "time away" is an important and legitimate activity for caregivers.[40,121] Nurses can inform families about such important resources as caregiver support groups and respite care.

## ♦ EVALUATION

To evaluate the effectiveness of nursing interventions, compare the family's behaviors with those in the expected family outcomes. Successful achievement of family outcomes for the social support of the family managing the illness of a family member is indicated by the following:

1a. Discusses the meaning of the patient's illness with other family members and the nurse.
b. Identifies areas of commonality and difference in the family's perception of the illness and the medical diagnosis.
2. Accurately identifies family characteristics that enhance and disable family coping.
3a. Identifies areas of needed knowledge and skills to implement the treatment regimen.
b. Identifies strategies to address the caregiver's health, knowledge, and skill needs.
c. Demonstrates psychomotor skills and knowledge needed to implement negotiated treatment.
4. Initiates discussion of social support resources with social support network and the community organizations.
5. Identifies at least one acceptable treatment alternative for unacceptable treatment requirements.
   a. When identification of an acceptable alternative is not possible, expresses the implications of not implementing the treatment.

Nurses are in a key position to help families manage illness. Assessing family strengths and weaknesses, identifying knowledge deficits, providing information, and teaching caregiving skills are important activities for nurses. Nurses can refer families to available resources to help meet their needs. In addition, nurses can help families deal with their concerns by being available to listen and by facilitating family communication and problem solving.

## QUESTIONS TO CONSIDER

- How does the stress of illness affect other family members? What resources do families have to help them cope with illness?
- What effects can a family's past have on how they respond to illness in a member?
- What effects can the family's culture have on how they respond to illness in a member?
- What characteristics of families are most relevant to consider when a member has an illness?
- What is the difference in family members' experiences in caring for an ill member during the diagnostic, treatment, chronic, and terminal states?
- How does the illness trajectory affect the family's abilities to cope with the illness?
- Have you experienced an illness in a family member? What did people do for you that was helpful? Not helpful? Based on your experiences, would you agree or disagree with the family functioning and cultural service-delivery models presented in this chapter? Justify your position.

## CRITICAL THINKING ACTIVITIES

- Why is it important for the nurse to understand the importance of how race, ethnicity, and social factors can contribute to the morbidity and mortality of some diseases?
- In what ways do caregivers differ from individuals who are not providing care for an ill family member, in regard to health and employment status?
- Sarah has had a nagging cough for the past several months. She attributed the cough to allergies and took antihistamines, which have been of little value. Certain that she needs stronger medication, she seeks medical attention to confirm her allergic condition. Make a judgment about the stage of the patient within the illness trajectory, and explain how the nurse can be of assistance.

## CHAPTER SUMMARY

### BACKGROUND

- As persons live longer and the American society becomes more culturally diversified, nurses must be prepared to deliver culturally competent care to families.
- Because nurses have not always known what factors to consider in planning and delivering care to different cultures, theoretic models of family functioning and service-delivery models for the integration of culture into practice have been proposed.

### FAMILY INFLUENCES ON ILLNESS

- Family systems theory, family stress theory, and the ecology framework provide a basis for understanding the effect of a family member's illness on family functioning.
- Selection of the appropriate model of family functioning depends on the model's definition of family that most closely matches the culture of the family.
- Theoretic models of family fuctioning provide ways of thinking about the family that allow the nurse to understand and predict behavior and subsequently plan interventions.
- The family systems theory describes the family as an open system that exchanges information with the larger environment.
- Interactions among the family members are governed by roles, relationships, expectations, and rules.
- The key assessment areas for nurses include a determination of the family rules, roles, expectations, and relationships that have been affected by the patient's illness. As a result, the nurse can determine what environmental sources of information and support are needed by the family.

- The family stress theory proposes that family reactions to an illness are based on characteristics of the illness, the family's resources for meeting the crisis created by the illness, and the meaning of the illness to the family.
- Two important family resources include adaptability, which is the family's ability to reorganize and change roles, rules, and patterns of interaction in response to a stress, and cohesion, which is the extent the family members feel bonded to each other and concerned and committed to family.
- Various family characteristics can affect the family's degree of adaptability and cohesion and include familial relation to the patient, gender, family-life cycle, ethnicity, family composition, socioeconomic status, employment status of the family members, problem-solving ability, family health, support network, social support, and religion.
- The family stress theory emphasizes the importance of the nurse's assessment of the cultural meaning of the illness to the family, the family's adaptability and cohesion on the basis of family characteristics, and important religious beliefs and practices.
- The ecology framework focuses on the interdependence of four systems, the microsystem, mesosystem, exosystem, and macrosystem.
- The microsystem is a pattern of activities, roles, and interpersonal relations experienced by the patient in a given setting.
- The mesosystem consists of the interrelations among two or more settings in which the patient and family participate.
- The exosystem includes one or more settings that do not involve the patient but that do involve the family. Events within that exosystem still affect the patient.
- The macrosystem focuses on the cultural, political, and socioeconomic characteristics of the larger society and their influence on the family unit.
- The ecology framework suggests that nurses need to focus on identifying the various environments (systems) that affect the family and how these may change over time.
- Campinha-Bacote has proposed the culturally competent model of care as one service-delivery model for the integration of culture into practice.
- Culture is a learned, shared, and symbolically transmitted design for living, including beliefs about the meaning, existence, and appropriate treatment of illness.
- The culturally competent model of care is a dynamic model that represents the process of striving for cultural competence.
- In addition to the culturally competent care constructs of cultural awareness, cultural knowledge, cultural skill, and cultural encounter, Campinha-Bacote has suggested that a nurse must have a cultural desire to gain more knowledge about other cultures. All of these constructs are interactive and cyclic in nature.
- Cultural awareness focuses on the nurse becoming more sensitive to other cultures by increased awareness of personal biases and prejudices toward other cultures.
- Cultural knowledge is the process of acquiring a sound foundation in the world views of other cultures.
- Cultural skill describes the assessment approaches to identify the family's cultural values, beliefs, and practices for integration into practice.
- Cultural encounter encourages direct engagement of the nurse in cross-cultural interactions to facilitate validation, negation, or modification of the nurse's existing cultural knowledge.

#### SOCIAL AND BIOCULTURAL DIMENSIONS OF HEALTH AND ILLNESS

- Health and illness have both social and biocultural dimensions. The social dimension addresses how symptoms may be interpreted from various perspectives: the patient/family's as an illness, the health professional's as disease, and the folk healer's as a disorder.
- An attempt must be made to understand illness, disease, and disorder to facilitate negotiation of a culturally competent response.
- The biocultural dimension of health and illness highlights the importance of the nurse's recognition of the biologic variations among different ethnic and racial groups.
- Variations can occur along several dimensions, encompassing body structure, skin color, enzymatic and genetic variations, electrocardiographic patterns, susceptibility to disease, nutritional preferences and deficiencies, and psychologic characteristics.
- The nurse must strive to accurately assess the family's definition of the symptoms and to identify pertinent biologic variations.

#### ILLNESS TRAJECTORY

- The way families respond to illness is a function of the family's characteristics and the illness trajectory.
- The illness trajectory consists of four major stages—early diagnostic, treatment, chronic, and terminal. Each stage presents the family with different emotional and physical challenges.
- During the early diagnostic phase the nurse assesses the meaning of the symptoms, using the techniques of culturologic and physical assessment.
- Negotiation of appropriate care and cure actions can be facilitated by the nurse's use of the collaborative framework.
- Using the collaborative framework, family members and the nurse determine whether or not each proposed self-care remedy will conflict with the proposed therapeutic regimen or vice versa. Only those approaches that are mutually agreed on are incorporated into the treatment plan. Such an approach decreases

the incidence of noncompliance with the treatment regimen.

- Although family members report the importance of supportive resources, environmental conveniences, frequent visitation, empathic interactions, and information during the diagnostic stage, they consider accurate and timely information as critical to their effective coping.
- Facilitation of the family's obtaining culturally relevant information communicated in a culturally responsive manner is a key role of the nurse.
- The treatment stage requires the family and the nurse to have negotiated a culturally relevant treatment plan. During this stage, families often are confronted by complex treatment regimens and hospital regulations regarding visitation. Family involvement in care, to the extent that is culturally desired, is incorporated into the treatment plan.
- Recognition of the multiple demands on the family members' time is essential to the nurse's recognition of the potential for caregiver strain and impaired home maintenance as nursing diagnoses during this time.
- Strategies that help the family to identify needed knowledge, skills, and internal family resources, as well as external community services, are important now and in the chronic stage.
- The chronic stage of the illness is a relatively stable period in the illness trajectory but may include a gradual decline in health with occasionally interspersed acute episodes.
- The family members may experience physical, financial, role, interfamilial relationship, emotional, and social relationship strains.
- The strategies employed during the treatment stage are still appropriate throughout the chronic stage.
- An important role of the nurse is to bring to the attention of the family the variety of community resources and support services available. Next the nurse and family can discuss their cultural acceptability.
- Sometimes the patient's illness trajectory continues downward to the terminal stage.
- Two nursing functions during the terminal stage are the facilitation of family communication and the incorporation of cultural rituals related to death and dying.

### NURSING MANAGEMENT

- As family members move through the illness experience, the nurse plays an important role in supporting them by assessing their culture and resources, providing information and facilitating family coping.
- Major nursing diagnoses during the illness trajectory stages include but are not limited to ineffective family coping, impaired home maintenance, caregiver strain, and noncompliance.
- Consideration of the effect that the family and its culture has on illness and its management is an important aspect of a nurse's role and can result only in improving the effectiveness of nursing care and in increasing family and patient satisfaction.

## REFERENCES


1. American Nurses Association: *Nursing: a social policy statement,* Kansas City, Mo, 1980, The Association.
2. Andrews M: Cultural perspectives on nursing in the 21st century, *J Prof Nurs* 8(1):7-15, 1992.
3. Archbold P: Impact of parent caring on middle aged offspring, *J Gerontol Nurs* 6(2):79-85, 1980.
4. Barresi C, Smerglia V: *Older male primary caregivers and the homemaker role.* Paper presented at the thirty-fourth annual meeting of the American Society on Aging, San Diego, Calif, March 1988.
5. Bass S, Kutza E, Torres-Gil F: *Diversity in aging* (professional books on aging), Glenview, Ill, 1990, Scott, Foresman.
6. Bell P, Evans J: *Counseling the black client,* Center City, Minn, 1981, Hazelden Educational Materials.
7. Bengtson V: Ethnicity and aging: problems and issues in current social inquiry. In Gelfand D, Kutzik A, editors: *Ethnicity and aging: theory, research, and policy,* New York, 1979, Springer.
8. Berkman L, Syme S: Social networks, host resistance, and mortality: a nine-year follow-up study of Alameda county residents, *Am J Epidemiol* 109(2):80-85, 1977.
9. Berlin E, Fowkes W: A teaching framework for cross-cultural health care, *West J Med* 139(6):934-938, 1982.
10. Blank J et al: Perceived home care needs of cancer patients and their caregivers, *Cancer Nurs* 12(2):78-84, 1989.
11. Bloch B: Bloch's assessment guide for ethnic/cultural variations. In Orque M, Bloch B, Monroy L, editors: *Ethnic nursing care,* St Louis, 1983, Mosby.
12. Bowers B: Intergenerational caregiving: adult caregivers and their aging parents, *Adv Nurs Sci* 9(2):20-31, 1987.
13. Boyle J, Andrews M: *Transcultural concepts in nursing care,* Glenview, Ill, 1989, Scott, Foresman.
14. Brody E: The family at risk. In Light E, Lebowitz B, editors: *Alzheimer's disease treatment and family stress: directions for research,* Rockville, Md, 1989, National Institute of Mental Health.
15. Brody E et al: Work status and parent care: a comparison of four groups of women, *Gerontologist* 27(2):201-208, 1987.
16. Brody S, Poulshock S, Masciocchi C: The family caring unit: a major consideration in the long-term support system, *Gerontologist* 18(6):556-561, 1978.
17. Bronfenbrenner U: *The ecology of human development,* Cambridge, Mass, 1979, Harvard University Press.
18. Buckley W: Society as a complex adaptive system. In Buckley W, editor: *Modern systems research for the behavioral scientist,* Chicago, Ill, 1968, Aldine.
19. Burr W: Families under stress. In McCubbin H, Cauble A, Patterson J, editors: *Family stress, coping, and social support,* Springfield, Ill, 1973, Charles C Thomas.
20. Burton L, Dilworth-Anderson P: The intergenerational family roles of aged black Americans, *Marriage Fam Rev* 16(3/4):311-330, 1991.
21. Bushy A: Cultural considerations for primary health care: where do self-care and folk medicine fit? *Holistic Nurs Pract* 6(3):10-18, 1992.
22. Campinha-Bacote J: *The process of cultural competence: a culturally competent model of care,* Wyoming, Ohio, 1991, Transcultural C.A.R.E.
23. Capitman JA: *Long-term care use by minority elders: an eldercare information packet,* Waltham, Mass, 1992, Brandeis University.
24. Cassileth B, Hamilton J: The family with cancer. In Cassileth B, editor: *The cancer patient,* Philadelphia, 1979, Lea & Febiger.

25. Cawley M, Gerdts E: Establishing a cancer caregivers program, *Cancer Nurs* 11(5):267-273, 1988.
26. Charonko C: Cultural influences in "noncompliant" behavior and decision making, *Holistic Nurs Pract* 6(3):73-78, 1992.
27. Chatters L, Taylor R, Jackson J: Size and composition of the informal helper networks of elderly blacks, *J Gerontol* 40(5):605-614, 1985.
28. Chatters L, Taylor R, Jackson J: Aged blacks: choices for an informal helper network, *J Gerontol* 41(1):94-100, 1986.
29. Chrisman NJ: Culture-sensitive nursing care. In Patrick M et al, editors: *Medical surgical nursing*, Philadelphia, 1991, JB Lippincott.
30. Cobb S: Social support as a moderator of life stress, *Psychosom Med* 38(5):300-314, 1976.
31. Cohen AM: Prevalence of diabetes among different ethnic Jewish groups in Israel, *Metabolism* 10:50, 1961.
32. Cooper R: The biological concept of race and its applications to public health and epidemiology, *J Health Polit Policy Law* 11(6):97-116, 1986.
33. Corbin J, Strauss A: *Unending work and care: managing chronic illness at home*, San Francisco, 1988, Jossey-Bass.
34. Croog S, Lipson A, Levine S: Help patterns in severe illness: the roles of kin network, nonfamily resources, and institutions, *J Marriage Fam* 34(1):32-41, 1972.
35. Deimling G, Bass D: Symptoms of mental impairment among elderly adults and their effects on family caregivers, *J Gerontol* 41(6):778-784, 1986.
36. Dellasege C: Health in the sandwich generation, *Geriatr Nurs* 10(5):242-243, 1989.
37. Devore W, Schlesinger EG: *Ethnic-sensitive social work practice*, St Louis, 1981, Mosby.
38. Dubos R: *Man, medicine and environment*, New York, 1968, Mentor Books.
39. Elipoulos C: Chronic care and the elderly: impact on the client, the family, and the nurse, *Top Clin Nurs* 3(1):71-83, 1981.
40. Farkas S: Impact of chronic illness on the patient's spouse, *Health Soc Work* 5(4):39-46, 1980.
41. Fengler A, Goodrich N: Wives of elderly disabled men: the hidden patients, *Gerontologist* 19(2):175-183, 1979.
42. Finlayson A, McEwen J: *Coronary heart disease and patterns of living*, New York, 1977, Prodist.
43. Fisher B, Sprenkle D: Therapists' perceptions of healthy family functioning, *Int J Fam Counseling* 6(2):9-18, 1978.
44. Fitting M et al: Caregivers for dementia patients: a comparison of husbands and wives, *Gerontologist* 26(3):248-252, 1986.
45. Foxall F, Eckberg J, Griffith N: Spousal adjustment to chronic illness, *Rehabil Nurs* 11(2):13-16, 1986.
46. Frankenberg R: Growing up white: feminism, racism and the social geography of childhood. In Alarcon N et al, editors: *The third wave: feminist perspectives on racism*, New York, 1989, Kitchen Table Women of Color Press.
47. Galanti G-A: *Caring for patients from different cultures*, Philadelphia, 1991, University of Pennsylvania Press.
48. George L: Social participation in later life: black-white differences. In Jackson JS, editor: *The black American elderly: research on physical and psychosocial health*, New York, 1988, Springer.
49. George L, Gwyther L: Caregiver well-being: a multidimensional examination of family caregivers of demented adults, *Gerontologist* 26(3):253-259, 1986.
50. German C: *The cancer unit: an ethnographic study*, Wakefield, Mass, 1979, Nursing Resources.
51. Germain C: Cultural care: a bridge between sickness, illness, and disease, *Holistic Nurs Pract* 6(3):1-9, 1992.
52. Giger J, Davidhizar R: *Transcultural nursing: assessment and intervention*, St Louis, 1991, Mosby.
53. Glacquinta B: Helping families face the crises of cancer, *Am J Nurs*, 77(10):1585-1588, 1977.
54. Gotay C: The experience of cancer during early and advanced stages: the views of patients and their mates, *Soc Sci Med* 19(7):605-613, 1984.
55. Gould A, Toghill P: How should we talk about acute leukaemia to adult patients and their families? *Br Med J* 282(6259):210-212, 1981.
56. Green JW: *Cultural awareness in the human services*, Englewood Cliffs, NJ, 1982, Prentice-Hall.
57. Grobe M, Ilstrup D, Ahmann D: Skills needed by family members to maintain the care of an advanced cancer patient, *Cancer Nurs* 4(5):371-375, 1981.
58. Gwyther L, Matteson M: Care for the caregivers, *J Gerontol Nurs* 9(2):72-95, 110, 116, 1983.
59. Hagey R: Drumming and dancing, *Can Nurs* 79(4):28-31, 1983.
60. Haley W et al: Psychological, social, and health consequences of caring for a relative with senile dementia, *J Am Geriatr Soc* 35(5):405-411, 1987.
61. Haley W et al: Stress, appraisal, coping, and social support as predictors of adaptational outcome among dementia caregivers, *Psychol Aging* 2(4):323-330, 1987.
62. Hamburg D, Killilea M: Relation of social support, stress, illness, and the use of health services. In US Department of Health, Education and Welfare: *Healthy people: the surgeon general's report on health promotion and disease prevention*, Washington DC, 1979, US Government Printing Office.
63. Hampe S: Needs of the grieving spouse in a hospital setting, *Nurs Res* 24(2):113-119, 1975.
64. Hansen D, Hill R: Families under stress. In Christensen H, editor: *Handbook of marriage and the family*, Chicago, 1964, Rand McNally.
65. Harris M: One man's food is another man's whitewash, *Nat Hist* 81(3):12-13, 1972.
66. Harrison GG: Primary adult lactase deficiency: a problem in anthropologic genetics, *Am Anthropol* 77(5):812-835, 1975.
67. Hartford M, Parson R: Groups with relatives of dependent older adults, *Gerontologist* 22(3):394-398, 1982.
68. Herskovits MJ: *Cultural anthropology*, 1955, New York, Alfred A. Knopf.
69. Hill R: *Families under stress*, New York, 1949, Harper & Brothers.
70. Hill R: Generic features of families under stress, *Soc Casework* pp 139-150, 1958.
71. Horowitz A: Sons and daughters as caregivers to older parents: differences in role performance and consequences, *Gerontologist* 25(6):612-617, 1985.
72. Jackson B: *Family caregiving: still going strong?* Paper presented at the Changing Face of Informal Caregiving, US Department of Health and Human Services Office of the Assistant Secretary for Planning and Evaluation, Berkeley Springs, W Va, Oct 1992.
73. Jackson D: The question of homeostasis, *Psychiatr Q Suppl* 31:79-90, 1954.
74. Jackson D: The study of the family, *Fam Process* 4:1-20, 1965.
75. Jackson J: Sex and social class variations in black aged parent-adult-child relationships, *Aging Hum Dev* 1(6):96-107, 1971.
76. Jacobsen F: Ethnocultural assessment. In Comas-Diaz L, Griffith E, editors: *Clinical guidelines in cross cultural mental health*, New York, 1988, John Wiley & Sons.
77. Johnson C, Barer B: Families and networks among older inner-city blacks, *Gerontologist* 30(6):726-733, 1990.
78. Johnson C, Catalano D: A longitudinal study of family supports to impaired elderly, *Gerontologist* 23(6):612-618, 1983.
79. Kahn R, Antonucci T: Convoys over the life course: attachment, roles, and social support, *Life Span Dev Behav* 3(2):253-286, 1980.

80. Kaplan B, Cassel J, Gore S: Social support and health, *Med Care 15*(suppl):47-58, 1977.
81. Kauffman C et al: ***Characteristics and needs of black caregivers and their elderly clients in personal care homes*** (preliminary report), Washington, DC, 1987, American Red Cross.
82. Kavanagh T, Shephard R: Sexual activity after myocardial infarction, *Can Med Assoc J* 116(11):1250-1253, 1977.
83. Kinney J, Stephens M: Hassles and uplifts of giving care to a family member with dementia, *Psychol Aging* 4(4):402-408, 1989.
84. Klein R, Dean A, Bogdonoff M: The impact of illness upon the spouse, *J Chronic Dis* 20:241-248, 1967.
85. Kleinman A, Eisenburg L, Good B: Culture, illness and care: clinical lessons from anthropologic and cross-cultural research, *Ann Intern Med* 88(2):251-258, 1978.
86. Krant M, Johnston L: Family perceptions of communications in late stage cancer, *Int J Psychiatry Med* 8(2):203-217, 1977-1978.
87. L'Abate L, Ganahl G, Hansen J: ***Methods of family therapy,*** Englewood Cliffs, NJ, 1986, Prentice-Hall.
88. Lazarus R: The costs and benefits of denial. In Monat A, Lazarus R, editors: ***Stress and coping: an anthology,*** New York, 1985, Columbia University Press.
89. Leahy M, Wright L: ***Families and life-threatening illness,*** Springhouse, Penn, 1987, Springhouse.
90. Leininger M: ***Transcultural nursing: concepts, theories and practices,*** New York, 1978, John Wiley & Sons.
91. Leske J: Needs of relatives of critically ill patients: a follow-up, *Heart Lung* 15(2):189-193, 1986.
92. Leske J: Comparison ratings of need importance after critical illness from family members with varied demographic characteristics, *Crit Care Nurs Clin North Am* 4(4):607-613, 1992.
93. Lewis F, Ellison E, Woods N: The impact of breast cancer on the family, *Semin Oncol Nurs* 1(3):206-213, 1985.
94. Lilius H, Valtonen E, Wikstrom J: Sexual problems in patients suffering from multiple sclerosis, *J Chronic Dis* 29(10):643-647, 1976.
95. Lock M: ***East Asian medicine in urban Japan: varieties of medical experience,*** Berkeley, Calif, 1980, University of California Press.
96. Lum D: ***Social work practice and people of color: a process-stage approach,*** Monterey, Calif, 1986, Brooks/Cole.
97. Martocchio B: Family coping: helping families help themselves, *Semin Oncol Nurs* 1(4):292-297, 1985.
98. McCubbin H, Patterson J: Family adaptation to crisis. In McCubbin H, Cauble A, Patterson J, editors: ***Family stress, coping, and social support,*** Springfield, Ill, 1982, Charles C Thomas.
99. Millar B: Critical support in critical care, *Nurs Times* 85(16):31-33, 1989.
100. Miller FJW: The epidemiological approach to the family as a unit in health statistics and the measurement of community health, *Soc Sci Med* 8(9):479-482, 1974.
101. Molter N: Needs of relatives of critically ill patients: a descriptive study, *Heart Lung* 8(2):332-339, 1979.
102. Moos R, Moos B: A typology of family social environments, *Fam Process* 15(4):357-371, 1976.
103. Morycz R et al: Racial differences in family burden: clinical implications for social work, *J Gerontol Social Work* 10 (1-2):133-154, 1987.
104. Murcia A, Stewart B: ***Man to man: when the woman you love has breast cancer,*** New York, 1989, St Martin's Press.
105. Murdaugh C: Coping responses of spouses of M.I. patients and of hemodialysis patients as measured by the Jalowiec coping scale, *J Cardiovasc Nurs* 2(1):67-74, 1987.
106. Neel JV: Diabetes mellitus: a "thrifty" genotype rendered detrimental by progress, *Am J Hum Genet* 14:353-362, 1962.
107. Northouse L, Swain M: Adjustment of patients and husbands to the initial impact of breast cancer, *Nurs Res* 36(4):221-225, 1987.
108. Oberst M, James R: Going home: patient and spouse adjustment following cancer surgery, *Top Clin Nurs* 7(1):46-57, 1985.
109. Oberst M et al: Caregiving demands and appraisal of stress among family caregivers, *Cancer Nurs* 12(4):209-215, 1989.
110. Olsen D, McCubbin H: Circumplex model of marital and family systems. V. Application to family stress and crisis intervention. In McCubbin H, Cauble A, Patterson J, editors: ***Family stress, coping, and social support,*** Springfield, Ill, 1982, Charles C Thomas.
111. Olsen D, Sprenkle D, Russell C: Circumplex model of marital and family systems. I. Cohesion and adaptability dimensions, family types and clinical applications, *Fam Process* 18(7):3-28, 1979.
112. Olsen E: The impact of serious illness on the family system, *Postgrad Med* 47(2):169-174, 1970.
113. Pedersen P: ***A handbook for multicultural awareness,*** Arlington, VA, 1988, American Association for Counseling and Development.
114. Pfifferling JH: A cultural prescription for mediocentrism. In Eisenburg L, Kleinman A, editors: ***The relevance of social science for medicine,*** Boston, 1981, D. Rudel.
115. Picot S: The relationship between the rewards, costs, and coping strategies of black family caregivers, *Diss Abstr Int* 52(11):5760-B, 1992.
116. Piening S: Family stress in diabetic renal failure, *Health Soc Work* 9(2):134-141, 1984.
117. Pitzele S: ***We are not alone: learning to live with chronic illness,*** Minneapolis, Minn, 1985, Thompson & Co.
118. Pratt C et al: Burden and coping strategies of caregivers to Alzheimer's patients, *Fam Relations* 34(5):27-33, 1985.
119. Pratt C, Wright S, Schmall V: Burden, coping and health status: a comparison of family caregivers to community dwelling and institutionalized Alzheimer's patients, *Gerontol Social Work* 10(1/2):99-112, 1987.
120. Ragucci AT: Ethnographic approach and nursing research, *Nurs Res* 21(6):485-490, 1972.
121. Rando T: ***Grief, dying, and death: clinical interventions for caregivers,*** Champaign, Ill, 1984, Research Press.
122. Reeder J: Family perception: a key to intervention, *AACN Clin Issues* 2(2):188-194, 1991.
123. Remoin DL: Ethnic variability in glucose tolerance and insulin secretion, *Arch Intern Med* 124:695-700, 1969.
124. Robinson B, Thurnher M: Taking care of aged parents: a family life cycle transition, *Gerontologist* 19(6):586-593, 1979.
125. Rosenberg M: ***Patients: the experience of illness,*** Philadelphia, 1980, WB Saunders.
126. Ryan C, Ryan K: ***A private battle,*** New York, 1979, Fawcett.
127. Sabo D, Brown J, Smith C: The male role and mastectomy: support groups and men's adjustment, *J Psychosoc Oncol* 4(1/2):19-31, 1986.
128. Schaefer O: When the Eskimo came to town, *Nutr Today* 6(2):8-16, 1971.
129. Schaefer O: The changing health picture in the Canadian North, *Can J Ophthalmol* 8(10):196-204, 1973.
130. Sexton D, Munro B: Impact of a husband's chronic illness (COPD) on the spouse's life, *Res Nurs Health* 8(1):83-90, 1985.
131. Silliman R, Sternberg J: Family caregiving: impact of patient functioning and underlying causes of dependency, *Gerontologist* 28(3):377-382, 1988.
132. Skippe J, Fink S, Hallenbeck P: Physical disability among married women: problems in the husband-wife relationship, *J Rehabil,* pp 16-19, Sept-Oct 1968.
133. Skorupka P, Bohnet N: Primary caregivers' perceptions of

nursing behaviors that best meet their needs in a home care hospice setting, *Cancer Nurs* 5(5):371-374, 1982.
134. Smallegan M: There was nothing else to do: needs for care before nursing home admission, *Gerontologist* 25(4):364-369, 1985.
135. Speedling E: Social structure and social behavior in an intensive care unit: patient-family perspectives, *Soc Work Health Care* 6(2):1-15, 1980.
136. Speer D: Family systems: morphostasis and morphogenesis, or "Is homeostasis enough?" *Fam Process* 9(3):259-278, 1970.
137. Steele T, Finkelstein S, Finkelstein F: Hemodialysis patients and spouses, *J Nerv Ment Dis* 162(4):225-237, 1976.
138. Stern J, Pascale L: Psychosocial adaptation postmyocardial infarction: the spouse's dilemma, *J Psychosom Res* 23(1):83-87, 1979.
139. Stetz K: Caregiving demands during advanced cancer: the spouse's needs, *Cancer Nurs* 10(5):260-268, 1987.
140. Stolar E: Coping with mastectomy: issues for social work, *Health Soc Work* 7(1):26-34, 1982.
141. Strong M: *Mainstay: for the well spouse of the chronically ill,* Boston, 1988, Little, Brown & Co.
142. Taeuber C: Sixty-five plus in the U.S.A., Washington, DC, 1990 US Bureau of the Census.
143. Taylor R: The extended family as a source of support to elderly blacks, *Gerontologist* 25(5):488-495, 1985.
144. Taylor R: Receipt of support from family among black Americans: demographic and familial differences, *J Marriage Fam* 48(1):67-77, 1986.
145. Tringali C: The needs of family members of cancer patients, *Oncol Nurs Forum* 13(4):65-70, 1986.
145b. Tripp RT: Reconceptualizing the construct of health: integration of *emic* and *etic* perspectives, *Res Nurs and Health* 6(5):101-109, 1984.
146. Tripp-Reimer T: Retention of folk healing practice *(Matiasma)* among four generations of urban Greek immigrants, *Nurs Res* 32(2):97-101, 1983.
147. Tripp-Reimer T, Brink P, Saunders J: Cultural assessment: content and process, *Nurs Outlook* 32(2):78-82, 1984.
148. Tripp-Reimer T, Doughtery M: Cross-cultural nursing research, *Ann Rev Nurs Res* 3:77-104, 1985.
149. US Bureau of the Census: *Statistical abstract of the United States, 1981,* ed 102, Washington, DC, 1982, US Government Printing Office.
150. Valle R: Cultural and ethnic issues in Alzheimer's disease family research. In Light E, Lebowitz B, editors: *Alzheimer's disease treatment and family stress: directions for research,* Rockville, Md, 1989, National Institute of Mental Health.
151. von Bertalanffy L: General systems theory and psychiatry. In Arieti S, editor: *American handbook of psychiatry,* ed 2, New York, 1974, Basic Books.
152. Walsh F: Conceptualizations of normal family functioning. In Walsh F, editor: *Normal family processes,* New York, 1982, Guilford.
153. Watson W: *Strengthening family caregivers and the delivery of social services to older blacks in the south: final report* (Award No 90AT0131/01), Washington, DC, 1987, Administration on Aging, Office of Human Development Services.
154. Watzlawick P, Bavelas J, Jackson D: *Pragmatics of human communication* New York, 1967, WW Norton.
155. Weisman A: *The coping capacity,* New York, 1984, Human Services Press.
156. Wellisch D: Family relationships of the mastectomy patient: interactions with the spouse and children, *Isr J Med Sci* 17(9-10):993-996, 1981.
157. Wellisch D, Jamison K, Pasnau R: Psychosocial aspects of mastectomy. II. The man's perspective, *Am J Psychiatry* 135(5):543-546, 1978.
158. Wenger A: Cultural meaning of symptoms, *Holistic Nurs Pract* 7(2):22-35, 1993.
159. Wood J: *Coping with the absence of perceived control: ethnic and cultural issues in family caregiving for patients with Alzheimer's disease,* doctoral dissertation, Richmond, Va, 1987, Virginia Commonwealth University.
160. Wright K, Dyck S: Expressed concerns of adult cancer patients' family members, *Cancer Nurs* 7(5):371-374, 1984.
161. Yee D, Kamikawa O: *Diversity among elders: implications for research on aging.* Paper presented at the Summer Institute in Research on Minority Aging, sponsored by the National Institute on Aging, Warrenton, Va, 1992.
162. Young R, Kahana E: Specifying caregiver burden outcomes: gender and relationship aspects of caregiver strain, *Gerontologist* 29(5):660-666, 1989.
163. Zahlis E, Shands ME: Breast cancer: illness demands experienced by the partner. Unpublished manuscript, 1989.
164. Zarit S, Reever K, Bach-Peterson J: Relatives of the impaired elderly: correlates of feelings of burden, *Gerontologist* 20(6):649-655, 1980.
165. Zarit S, Todd P, Zarit J: Subjective burden of husbands and wives as caregivers: a longitudinal study, *Gerontologist* 26(3):260-266, 1986.

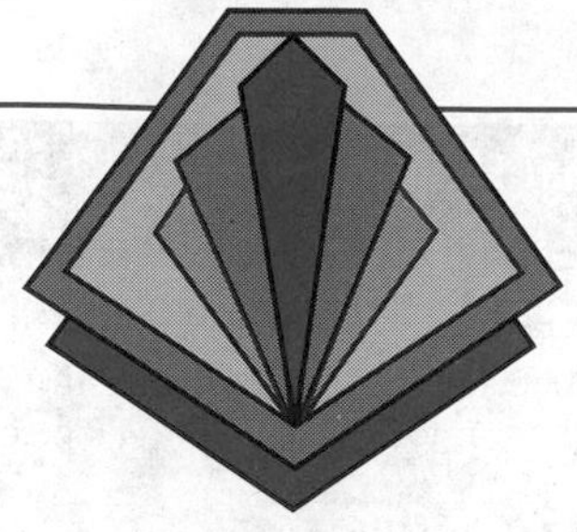

C H A P T E R 6

# Healthy Life-Styles: Nutrition, Exercise, Rest, and Sleep

*Barbara C. Long*

## CHAPTER OBJECTIVES

***After studying this chapter, the learner should be able to do the following:***

1 Describe factors and approaches that affect and facilitate health-promoting behaviors.
2 Differentiate among nutrient standards, food guides, and dietary guidelines in terms of purpose and content.
3 Explain the contribution of the seven dietary guidelines recommended by the Department of Health and Human Services.
4 Differentiate among cholesterol and saturated, monounsaturated, and polyunsaturated fats in terms of definition and recommendations for health.
5 Use the daily food guide to evaluate adequacy of nutrient intake.
6 Describe physiologic and psychosocial factors that influence obesity.
7 Explain approaches to facilitate weight loss, weight gain, and control of dietary fats and cholesterol.
8 Describe the benefits and components of a healthy exercise program.
9 Explain normal sleep patterns and interventions to improve sleep.

## KEY TERMS

aerobic exercise
anaerobic exercise
behavior modification
body mass index (BMI)
carbohydrates
cholesterol
dietary fiber
fat
health promotion
health protection
ideal body weight
isometric exercise
isotonic exercise
minerals
non–rapid eye movement (non-REM) sleep
nutrition
obesity
protein
rapid eye movement (REM) sleep
recommended dietary allowances
self-confrontation
sleep
starch
underweight
vitamins

The healthiest people usually are those who have chosen a healthy life-style; they carry out activities that promote and protect health and prevent illness. This chapter discusses health-promoting activities related to nutrition, exercise, and sleep. Disease prevention is discussed in chapters on specific body systems (Units VI through XI of this text).

Health promotion and disease prevention have become major focuses of health care in the United States. In 1979 the surgeon general presented a document that described a national public health agenda for the first time. This was followed in 1980 by the *1990 Health Objectives* that established measurable objectives in areas of health status, risk reduction, public and professional awareness, health services and protective measures, and surveillance and evaluation. Although progress was noted, many of the objectives were not being met by the late 1980s.[35] Therefore the Department of Health and Human Services has developed a new set of objectives in its report *Healthy People 2000,*[31] which contains four major sections: health promotion, health protection, preventive services, and surveillance and

**BOX 6-1 Year 2000 National Health Objectives: Priority Areas**

**HEALTH PROMOTION**

Physical activity and fitness
Nutrition
Tobacco
Alcohol and other drugs
Family planning
Mental health and mental disorders
Violent and abusive behavior
Educational and community-based programs

**HEALTH PROTECTION**

Unintentional injuries
Occupational safety and health
Environmental health
Food and drug safety
Oral health

**PREVENTIVE SERVICES**

Maternal and infant health
Heart disease and stroke
Cancer
Diabetes and chronic disabling conditions
HIV infection
Sexually transmitted diseases
Immunization and infectious diseases
Clinical preventive services

**SURVEILLANCE AND DATA SYSTEMS**

From US Department of Health and Human Services, Public Health Service: *Healthy people 2000: national health promotion and disease prevention objectives,* Washington, DC, 1990, US Government Printing Office.

data systems (Box 6-1). Note that the first two categories of health promotion are *physical activity* and *fitness* and *nutrition.* (For additional information on national health objectives for the year 2000 see Chapter 8.)

## HEALTH PROTECTION

**Health protection** (see Box 6-1) as part of a healthy life-style bears mention here although activities that promote health protection are not detailed in this chapter. Health protection can be defined as activities that shield the individual from danger. It is a defense against injury. *Unintentional injuries* can be prevented by monitoring home safety. Accidents in and about the home cause almost one fourth of all accidental deaths, with *falls* accounting for about half this number and *fires* and *poisonings* the remainder. Elderly persons are especially susceptible to falls, and their environment should be monitored for risk factors leading to falls (see Chapter 4). Homes should be equipped with functioning smoke alarms in strategic places, such as kitchen, bedrooms, halls, and basement. The largest number of accidental injuries and deaths, however, result from motor vehicle accidents. Many lives can be saved by the wearing of seat belts, an important life-style change everyone can make. Statistics show that between 1990 and 1993, motor vehicle deaths have decreased from 2.5 to 1.8 deaths per 100,000 miles driven.[8] Part of this decreased mortality rate is the result of the increased use of seat belts and the "designated driver" plan for those drinking alcohol.

**BOX 6-2 Occupational Health Risks**

Work-related injury or death
Lung diseases: pneumonoconiosis, asbestos-related lung disease, occupational asthma, toxic lung injury, lung cancer
Toxic liver disease
Gas/smoke irritation of oral passageways
Dermatitis
Leukemia
Eye injuries from foreign bodies
Hearing loss (noise-induced)

Protective actions pertaining to *occupational safety and health* include evaluation of and measures to decrease exposure to harmful substances that may cause diseases of the lung, liver, oral passageways, skin, or blood (Box 6-2). Prevention of occupational lung diseases is discussed in Chapter 37. Protection of the eyes and ears from injury is also important (Chapters 60 and 62). Activities that promote *environmental health* are described frequently in the literature. A healthy life-style includes activities that promote a clean environment—one that provides air that is free of toxic agents. Nurses can be leaders in their communities in this effort. Progress can be seen in the many communities that have mandated smoke-free environments. Smoke can affect the heart, lungs, gastrointestinal tract, bladder, and blood vessels (see appropriate text chapters). An encouraging sign has been a decrease in the prevalence of smoking from 1990 to 1993 among Americans, from 29% to 22.7% of the population.[8]

*Food and drug safety* includes decreasing the incidence of alcoholism, drug abuse, and eating disorders (see Chapter 19). *Oral health* is important in preventing diseases of the teeth and gums, which influences food intake and thus nutrition. Preventive actions include dental hygiene, dental care, and water fluoridation.

## HEALTH PROMOTION

Because the goal of nursing is to assist people to achieve optimal health, nurses are among the leaders of health professionals working toward meeting the national health objectives. The American Nurses Association (ANA) has placed new emphasis on health promotion, health teaching, and self-care.[21] Nurses are well prepared as health teachers and health advocates. Therefore health promotion is one aspect of medical-surgical nursing.

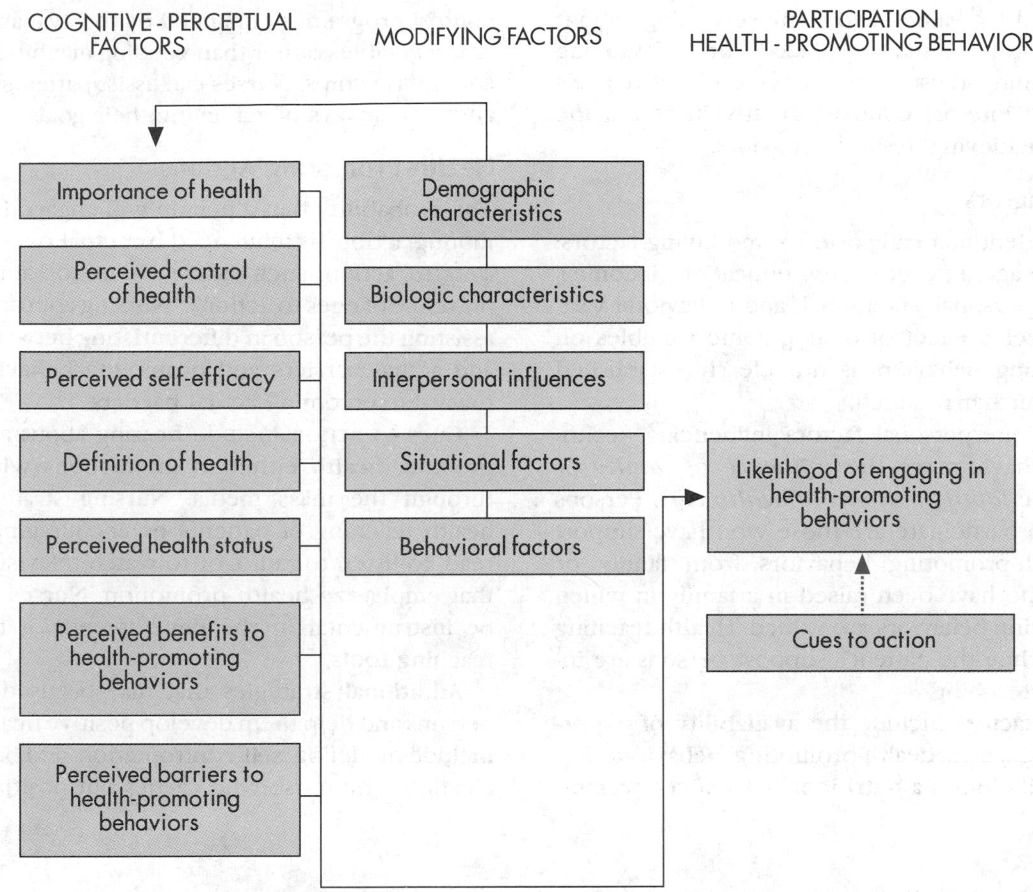


**FIGURE 6-1** Pender's health promotion model. (Redrawn from Pender NJ: *Health promotion in nursing practice,* ed 2, East Norwalk, Conn, 1987, Appleton & Lange.)

**Health promotion** can be defined as activities directed toward helping persons maintain or achieve a high level of functioning and well-being. Health promotion is an integral part of nursing care for all types of patients and clients in all types of environments of care. In ambulatory care centers and in home health care, health promotion assumes a major focus. In acute care centers the major focus is assisting patients to regain their health (illness care). However, health care also must be considered; that which is healthy must be promoted or maintained.

Health promotion strengthens the person's capacity to withstand physical and emotional stress. Thus the person who is in an excellent nutritional state, has good physical endurance, has adequate sleep patterns, and copes well with stress is at less risk of developing a pathophysiologic disorder and has resources to use in regaining optimal functioning more quickly if illness or disease does occur.

## FACTORS AFFECTING HEALTH-PROMOTING BEHAVIORS

Why do some persons take actions that promote a high level of functioning, whereas others do not? Pender[22] has identified factors that (1) affect the individual's perceptions, (2) modify behaviors, and (3) influence the likelihood of health-promoting actions (Figure 6-1).

### Individual Perceptions

Motivation to participate in health-promoting behaviors is influenced by the person's perceptions about health and perceptions about self:

1. Perceptions about health
   a. Value placed on health by the person
   b. Desire for the highest achievable health level versus that for maintaining status quo
   c. Evaluation of present health status
   d. Perceived benefits of the health-promoting behaviors
2. Perceptions about self
   a. Perceived control over own behavior (internal versus external control)
   b. Desire for mastery of the environment
   c. Self-concept
   d. Self-esteem

Thus persons who do not value health nor see a need to improve their health status, who are not self-motivated, or who have a poor self-concept are less likely to engage in health-promoting behaviors. Nursing approaches in these situations include helping these persons identify their values and explore feelings about themselves with emphasis placed on identifying strengths. Helping these persons set their own goals (thus exerting internal control) greatly increases the likelihood of achieving desired behaviors.

## Modifying Factors

Pender[22] has identified categories of modifying factors: demographic (age, sex, ethnicity, education, income), biologic, interpersonal, situational, and behavioral variables. The specific effect of demographic variables on health-promoting behaviors is not clearly established and requires further research.

The major interpersonal factors influencing health-promoting behaviors are the *influence of family or friends* and the *family patterns of health care.* Persons more likely to participate are those who have support for the health-promoting behaviors from family or friends and who have been raised in a family in which health-promoting behaviors are valued. Health teaching is enhanced when the patient's support persons are included in the teaching.

Situational factors include the availability of opportunities to engage in health-promoting behaviors. For example, facilitation of a nutritionally balanced weight-control program is enhanced by the availability of fruits and vegetables rather than vending machines with candy and potato chips. Nurses can assist patients in exploring alternative ways of achieving their goals.

## Health-Promoting Actions

The probability that a person will engage in health-promoting actions is influenced by actual or perceived barriers to action, such as cost, time, or ability, and the presence of cues to action.[22] Nursing approaches include assisting the person in differentiating between perceived and actual barriers and promoting behaviors directed toward overcoming actual barriers.

Cues to action include hearing about activities that promote health either in interactions with others or through the mass media. Nursing strategies include health teaching of patients or encouraging patients to read, to listen to radio, or to watch television programs that emphasize health promotion. Nurses also need to be instrumental in the development of these health-teaching tools.

Additional strategies that may be used to motivate persons and help them develop positive health behaviors include modeling, self-confrontation, and behavior modification. The nurse who carries out positive health be-

**TABLE 6-1 Recommended Dietary Allowances[a]**

| | | | | | | | FAT-SOLUBLE VITAMINS | | | |
|---|---|---|---|---|---|---|---|---|---|---|
| | | WEIGHT[b] | | HEIGHT[b] | | | | | | |
| CATEGORY | AGE (yr) OR CONDITION | (kg) | (lb) | (cm) | (in) | PROTEIN (g) | VITAMIN A (µg RE)[c] | VITAMIN D (µg)[d] | VITAMIN E (mg α-TE)[e] | VITAMIN K (µg) |
| Infants | 0.0–0.5 | 6 | 13 | 60 | 24 | 13 | 375 | 7.5 | 3 | 5 |
| | 0.5–1.0 | 9 | 20 | 71 | 28 | 14 | 375 | 10 | 4 | 10 |
| Children | 1–3 | 13 | 29 | 90 | 35 | 16 | 400 | 10 | 6 | 15 |
| | 4–6 | 20 | 44 | 112 | 44 | 24 | 500 | 10 | 7 | 20 |
| | 7–10 | 28 | 62 | 132 | 52 | 28 | 700 | 10 | 7 | 30 |
| Males | 11–14 | 45 | 99 | 157 | 62 | 45 | 1,000 | 10 | 10 | 45 |
| | 15–18 | 66 | 145 | 176 | 69 | 59 | 1,000 | 10 | 10 | 65 |
| | 19–24 | 72 | 160 | 177 | 70 | 58 | 1,000 | 10 | 10 | 70 |
| | 25–50 | 79 | 174 | 177 | 70 | 63 | 1,000 | 5 | 10 | 80 |
| | 51+ | 77 | 170 | 173 | 68 | 63 | 1,000 | 5 | 10 | 80 |
| Females | 11–14 | 46 | 101 | 157 | 62 | 46 | 800 | 10 | 8 | 45 |
| | 15–18 | 55 | 120 | 163 | 64 | 44 | 800 | 10 | 8 | 55 |
| | 19–24 | 58 | 128 | 164 | 65 | 46 | 800 | 10 | 8 | 60 |
| | 25–50 | 63 | 138 | 163 | 64 | 50 | 800 | 5 | 8 | 65 |
| | 51+ | 65 | 143 | 160 | 63 | 50 | 800 | 5 | 8 | 65 |
| Pregnant | | | | | | 60 | 800 | 10 | 10 | 65 |
| Lactating | 1st 6 months | | | | | 65 | 1,300 | 10 | 12 | 65 |
| | 2nd 6 months | | | | | 62 | 1,200 | 10 | 11 | 65 |

From the Food and Nutrition Board, National Academy of Sciences—National Research Council, revised 1989.

[a]Designed for the maintenance of good nutrition of practically all healthy people in the United States. The allowances, expressed as average daily intakes over time, are intended to provide for individual variations among most normal persons as they live in the United States under usual environmental stresses. Diets should be based on a variety of common foods in order to provide other nutrients for which human requirements have been less well defined. See text for discussion of other nutrients not tabulated.

[b]Weights and heights of reference adults are actual medians for the U.S. population of the designated age, as reported by the National Health and Nutrition Examination Survey (1976-1980) (NHANES II). The median weights and heights of those under 19 years of age were taken from Hamill et al. (1979) (see pp 16-17). The use of these figures does not imply that the height-to-weight ratios are ideal.

haviors, such as exercising regularly, serves as a *model* that others may emulate. Modeling positive health behaviors is an important nursing role function that, unfortunately, is not carried out to the degree that it should if health promotion is truly valued. **Self-confrontation** includes helping persons identify inconsistencies in health beliefs, values, or behaviors; dissatisfaction with these inconsistencies that follow the awareness may lead to behavioral changes.[22]

**Behavior modification,** or operant conditioning, consists of changing the behavior by means of a cognitive plan that is made by the person with the health care professional and that rewards positive behaviors. Positive reinforcement of desired behaviors increases the likelihood of desirable behavior repetitions. The person is involved throughout the process. Behavior modification is accomplished over a period of time by the following self-actions:

1. Setting own goals
2. Self-monitoring
3. Developing a personal reward system
4. Obtaining positive feedback
5. Developing a new self-concept
6. Developing and implementing an activity program

Behavior modification has been useful in weight-reduction programs (p. 153). (See references 22 and 33 for in-depth discussion of these and other methods that facilitate health promotion.)

Health promotion includes eating a well-balanced diet, with emphasis on weight control, regular exercise, sufficient sleep and rest, and reduction of stress. Stress management is discussed in Chapter 7. Health promotion also includes practices that decrease the risk of disease, such as not smoking and eating a low-fat, low-salt, high-fiber diet. Specific aspects of health promotion are also discussed in various chapters, such as those for cancer and for respiratory and cardiovascular disorders. The following discussion focuses on nutrition, exercise, sleep and rest.

## NUTRITION*

**Nutrition** refers to all the processes involved with the intake into the system of proper foods. Excesses and imbalances of certain food components are of as much concern in the United States as are nutrient deficiencies.

*The author thanks Janice Neville, DSc, Professor of Nutrition, Case Western Reserve University, Cleveland, Ohio, for her contributions to this portion of the chapter.

| WATER-SOLUBLE VITAMINS | | | | | | | MINERALS | | | | | | |
|---|---|---|---|---|---|---|---|---|---|---|---|---|---|
| VITAMIN C (mg) | THIAMIN (mg) | RIBOFLAVIN (mg) | NIACIN (mg NE)[f] | VITAMIN $B_6$ (mg) | FOLATE (μg) | VITAMIN $B_{12}$ (μg) | CALCIUM (mg) | PHOSPHORUS (mg) | MAGNESIUM (mg) | IRON (mg) | ZINC (mg) | IODINE (μg) | SELENIUM (μg) |
| 30 | 0.3 | 0.4 | 5 | 0.3 | 25 | 0.3 | 400 | 300 | 40 | 6 | 5 | 40 | 10 |
| 35 | 0.4 | 0.5 | 6 | 0.6 | 35 | 0.5 | 600 | 500 | 60 | 10 | 5 | 50 | 15 |
| 40 | 0.7 | 0.8 | 9 | 1.0 | 50 | 0.7 | 800 | 800 | 80 | 10 | 10 | 70 | 20 |
| 45 | 0.9 | 1.1 | 12 | 1.1 | 75 | 1.0 | 800 | 800 | 120 | 10 | 10 | 90 | 20 |
| 45 | 1.0 | 1.2 | 13 | 1.4 | 100 | 1.4 | 800 | 800 | 170 | 10 | 10 | 120 | 30 |
| 50 | 1.3 | 1.5 | 17 | 1.7 | 150 | 2.0 | 1,200 | 1,200 | 270 | 12 | 15 | 150 | 40 |
| 60 | 1.5 | 1.8 | 20 | 2.0 | 200 | 2.0 | 1,200 | 1,200 | 400 | 12 | 15 | 150 | 50 |
| 60 | 1.5 | 1.7 | 19 | 2.0 | 200 | 2.0 | 1,200 | 1,200 | 350 | 10 | 15 | 150 | 70 |
| 60 | 1.5 | 1.7 | 19 | 2.0 | 200 | 2.0 | 800 | 800 | 350 | 10 | 15 | 150 | 70 |
| 60 | 1.2 | 1.4 | 15 | 2.0 | 200 | 2.0 | 800 | 800 | 350 | 10 | 15 | 150 | 70 |
| 50 | 1.1 | 1.3 | 15 | 1.4 | 150 | 2.0 | 1,200 | 1,200 | 280 | 15 | 12 | 150 | 45 |
| 60 | 1.1 | 1.3 | 15 | 1.5 | 180 | 2.0 | 1,200 | 1,200 | 300 | 15 | 12 | 150 | 50 |
| 60 | 1.1 | 1.3 | 15 | 1.6 | 180 | 2.0 | 1,200 | 1,200 | 280 | 15 | 12 | 150 | 55 |
| 60 | 1.1 | 1.3 | 15 | 1.6 | 180 | 2.0 | 800 | 800 | 280 | 15 | 12 | 150 | 55 |
| 60 | 1.0 | 1.2 | 13 | 1.6 | 180 | 2.0 | 800 | 800 | 280 | 10 | 12 | 150 | 55 |
| 70 | 1.5 | 1.6 | 17 | 2.2 | 400 | 2.2 | 1,200 | 1,200 | 320 | 30 | 15 | 175 | 65 |
| 95 | 1.6 | 1.8 | 20 | 2.1 | 280 | 2.6 | 1,200 | 1,200 | 355 | 15 | 19 | 200 | 75 |
| 90 | 1.6 | 1.7 | 20 | 2.1 | 260 | 2.6 | 1,200 | 1,200 | 340 | 15 | 16 | 200 | 75 |

[c]Retinol equivalents. 1 retinol equivalent = 1 μg retinol or 6 μg β-carotene.
[d]As cholecalciferol. 10 μg cholecalciferol = 400 IU of vitamin D.
[e]α-Tocopherol equivalents. 1 mg d-α tocopherol = 1 α-TE.
[f]1 NE (niacin equivalent) is equal to 1 mg of niacin or 60 mg of dietary tryptophan.

Dietary factors are associated with four of the ten leading causes of death in American adults: heart disease, cancer, stroke, and diabetes. (The remaining six leading causes of adult deaths are chronic obstructive pulmonary disease, accidents, pneumonia, suicide, HIV infection, and homicide.) Specific dietary objectives in *Healthy People 2000* include the following[31]:

1. Reduce the number of overweight adults (age 20 and older) to no more than 20% of the adult population.
2. Reduce dietary fat intake to less than 30% of calories and saturated fat intake to less than 10% of calories.
3. Increase daily intake of complex carbohydrates and fiber-containing foods to five or more servings for fruits and vegetables (including legumes) and six or more servings for grain products.
4. Decrease salt and sodium intake so that
   - More than 65% of home meals are prepared without adding salt
   - More than 80% of persons avoid using salt at the table
   - More than 40% of adults regularly purchase foods modified or lower in sodium

## NUTRITION REQUIREMENTS

Good nutritional status exists when protein, fat, carbohydrate, vitamins, and minerals are consumed in sufficient amounts and are used appropriately by the body to meet needs regardless of age, sex, life-style, or state of health. All persons need the same basic nutrients throughout life. The amounts required vary in predictable patterns. Growth, basal metabolic needs, and physical activity are the major factors responsible for changing nutrient needs. Changes in amounts of nutrients recommended from infancy throughout life are illustrated in Table 6-1. Disease, trauma, variations in metabolism (normal and abnormal), medications, and treatments also can affect needs.

All nutrients are of equal importance, although they are not required in equal amounts. The nutrients that provide energy (protein, fats, carbohydrates) and water are required in much larger quantities than are vitamins that regulate body processes. The differences in the quantities of the various required nutrients are much greater than the changes in amounts of any one nutrient over the life cycle. If a person consumed vitamin A in the quantities recommended for calcium or phosphorus, toxicity would result.

When food is used as the source for nutrients, such imbalances are unlikely to occur; however, nutrients are available in concentrated forms as dietary supplements, over-the-counter preparations, and prescription drugs. There is an *unsupported* intuitive feeling, enhanced by advertising, that nutritional supplements are essential. Persons respond to these supplements when the persons have been relatively nutrition-deficient, eating foods marginal in nutrient value, and when the supplement provides the specific nutrients that are deficient. There is a point beyond which supplementation does not help the person and *may actually cause harm.* Continued intake of vitamins and minerals at levels from 10 to 100 times the recommended dietary allowance (RDA) (less than 10 times for vitamin A) is associated with chronic toxicity.

### Energy Needs

The body has a constant need for energy to maintain circulation, respiration, muscle tone, and body temperature. Depending on mass and physical activity, great differences can exist in the amount of energy needed to maintain appropriate body weight (Table 6-2). Persons of similar gender and body composition have similar *basal* energy requirements. The requirement is related to the amount of muscle tissue and can be predicted from body weight (excluding excess body fat because adipose tissue is relatively inert).

The total energy requirement may vary widely depending on physical activity (Table 6-3). The best method for determining the adequacy of energy intake for the person is to evaluate weight for height (and rate of growth for children) in relation to energy intake, which is assessed from dietary information.

A person's daily energy requirements are large and are measured in thousands of calories. Adequate but not excessive energy must be supplied to meet individual needs; also of importance is the source of the energy.

### Energy Sources

Most foods are mixtures of carbohydrates, protein, and fat. The relative contributions of these nutrients to the fuel value of the diet (Table 6-4) can vary within wide limits without harm. There is a basic requirement for some **carbohydrate** in the diet as starch and sugar (to prevent ketosis) and as fiber. As much as 80% of dietary calories may be supplied by carbohydrate in persons whose major food staple is grain. This pattern is seen in some persons, although it is not typical. The usual American food patterns include generous use of animal foods, fats, oils, and sugars. Current emphasis on dietary guidelines has resulted in positive change, however, such as decreased fat intake.

The provision of 10% to 15% of required calories by **protein** intake from a variety of foods (animal and plant) generally is sufficient to meet needs for protein of good quality—that is, containing the essential amino acids and sufficient nitrogen for body needs when caloric intake is sufficient to meet needs. This is not true of low-calorie diets. As much as 25% of total calories may come from protein in self-selected diets, but this is a maximum. Levels above this are rare because the diet becomes unpalatable and expensive.

Some **fat** in the diet is needed to provide the essential fatty acids and to ensure adequate supplies and efficient absorption of fat-soluble vitamins. Dietary fats are concentrated sources of energy (providing 9 kcal/g, as com-

**TABLE 6-2 Median Heights and Weights and Recommended Energy Intake**

| CATEGORY | AGE (yr) OR CONDITION | WEIGHT (kg) | WEIGHT (lb) | HEIGHT (cm) | HEIGHT (in) | REE† (kcal/day) | AVERAGE ENERGY ALLOWANCE (kcal)* MULTIPLES of REE | AVERAGE ENERGY ALLOWANCE (kcal)* PER kg | AVERAGE ENERGY ALLOWANCE (kcal)* PER day‡ |
|---|---|---|---|---|---|---|---|---|---|
| Infants | 0.0-0.5 | 6 | 13 | 60 | 24 | 320 | | 108 | 650 |
| | 0.5-1.0 | 9 | 20 | 71 | 28 | 500 | | 98 | 850 |
| Children | 1-3 | 13 | 29 | 90 | 35 | 740 | | 102 | 1300 |
| | 4-6 | 20 | 44 | 112 | 44 | 950 | | 90 | 1800 |
| | 7-10 | 28 | 62 | 132 | 52 | 1130 | | 70 | 2000 |
| Males | 11-14 | 45 | 99 | 157 | 62 | 1440 | 1.70 | 55 | 2500 |
| | 15-18 | 66 | 145 | 176 | 69 | 1760 | 1.67 | 45 | 3000 |
| | 19-24 | 72 | 160 | 177 | 70 | 1780 | 1.67 | 40 | 2900 |
| | 25-50 | 79 | 174 | 177 | 70 | 1800 | 1.60 | 37 | 2900 |
| | 51+ | 77 | 170 | 173 | 68 | 1530 | 1.50 | 30 | 2300 |
| Females | 11-14 | 46 | 101 | 157 | 62 | 1310 | 1.67 | 47 | 2200 |
| | 15-18 | 55 | 120 | 163 | 64 | 1370 | 1.60 | 40 | 2200 |
| | 19-24 | 58 | 128 | 164 | 65 | 1350 | 1.60 | 38 | 2200 |
| | 25-50 | 63 | 138 | 163 | 64 | 1380 | 1.55 | 36 | 2200 |
| | 51+ | 65 | 143 | 160 | 63 | 1280 | 1.50 | 30 | 1900 |
| Pregnant | | | | | | | | | |
| First trimester | | | | | | | | | +0 |
| Second trimester | | | | | | | | | +300 |
| Third trimester | | | | | | | | | +300 |
| Lactating | | | | | | | | | |
| First 6 mo | | | | | | | | | +500 |
| Second 6 mo | | | | | | | | | +500 |

From Food and Nutrition Board, National Academy of Sciences—National Research Council, 1989.
*In the range of light to moderate activity, the coefficient of variation is ±20%.
†Resting energy expenditure.
‡Figure is rounded.

pared with 4 kcal/g provided by carbohydrates and protein); they are useful in providing calories for persons unable to consume large volumes of food. Too much dietary fat, especially saturated fats, is undesirable (see p. 146).

## Vitamins and Minerals

**Vitamins** are not equally distributed in foods. Certain fruits or vegetables must be selected to ensure adequate intake of vitamins C and A. Animal products contribute vitamins $B_{12}$ and D, although some ready-to-eat cereals and some soy products may be fortified with these vitamins. Fortified milk is one food source for many vitamins, as well as high-quality protein. Green leafy vegetables are superior sources of vitamins A and C and of iron and other minerals. Sunshine provides additional vitamin D, and our symbiotic relationship with intestinal flora appears to provide biotin and vitamin K. In contrast to vitamin C, thiamin is found in most foods, but no one food is superior in content. When persons substitute sugars and sweets (including honey) or alcohol for other foods, they obtain concentrated sources of energy that yield small levels of vitamins or minerals.

Major **minerals** include calcium, phosphorus, sodium, potassium, magnesium (see Chapter 20), iron (see Chapter 33) and zinc. Major food sources include milk and milk products, eggs, meats, grains, legumes, and green leafy vegetables.

**TABLE 6-3 Comparison of Calories Used in 1 Hour for Different Types of Physical Activity (exclusive of basal energy needs)**

| ACTIVITY | CALORIES EXPENDED PER HOUR: WOMAN (121 lb) | CALORIES EXPENDED PER HOUR: MAN (143 lb) |
|---|---|---|
| Lying quietly | 6 | 7 |
| Sitting | 22 | 26 |
| Standing | 28 | 32 |
| Ironing, dishwashing, driving car | 55 | 65 |
| Working in office, painting furniture | 82 | 98 |
| Walking, slow dancing, bicycling | 138 | 162 |
| More active walking, skating, fast dancing | 220 | 260 |
| Running, climbing stairs, sawing wood | 358 | 422 |
| High-speed walking, swimming | 468 | 552 |

A warning is needed. This discussion of the importance of careful choice in kinds of foods might tempt one to conclude that it is simpler to rely on vitamin and mineral supplements. Data from the second U.S. Health and Nutrition Examination Survey (NHANES II) show that vitamin and mineral supplements are among the most common nonprescription drugs consumed in this country. Almost 35% of the adult population take supplements regularly, and persons with the highest nutrient intakes from food tend to be the ones who take supplements.[17] The ready availability of vitamin and mineral supplements, as well as their popularity as placebos or miracle workers, increases the possibility that *toxic effects may occur.* Many of the over-the-counter vitamin preparations provide excess amounts of vitamins that are relatively inexpensive to produce and minimal quantities of others. It is not an uncommon occurrence for a person to be carefully taking a diet supplement that does not provide the nutrient really needed.

***Calcium*** is an important supplement to prevent *osteoporosis* (see Chapter 65), a major public health problem among older women. Men also are at risk from osteoporosis because they are now living longer. Calcium intake of 1500 mg is safe.[16] Adolescents need at least 1200 mg/day of calcium to maintain peak bone mass. Premenopausal women should have at least 800 mg/day and estrogen-deficient women 1200 mg/day. The best dietary sources of calcium are dairy products, dark-green leafy vegetables, sardines, clams, and oysters. Excluding dairy products, the average adult American diet provides about 300 mg calcium per day.[25] Each milk product exchange (see food guide pyramid, Figure 6-2) provides another 300 mg. Supplements can be used to complete the total requirement. It is important to note that increasing calcium intake without increasing vitamin D is not the answer. Vitamin D promotes absorption of calcium; sources include sunshine and fortified milk. Some calcium supplements include vitamin D. Osteoporosis cannot be prevented by calcium intake alone, however. *Weight-bearing exercise* is required to maintain peak bone mass. Rapid bone loss in postmenopausal women during the early years after menopause can be diminished by estrogen replacement (see Chapter 65).

**TABLE 6-4 Summary of Major Food Nutrients**

| NUTRIENT | SOURCES | FUNCTIONS | RECOMMENDED DIETARY ALLOWANCES | MALNUTRITION SIGNS |
|---|---|---|---|---|
| Protein | Meat, fish, poultry, legumes, nuts, milk, cheeses | Provides amino acids for tissue growth and repair, helps maintain osmotic pressure, facilitates serum transport, provides immunoglobulin renewal, provides source of energy (4 kcal/g) | 0.75g/kg body weight/day (adults) | Stunted growth, negative nitrogen balance, weakness, nutritional edema, decreased resistance |
| Carbohydrate | Grains, fruits and vegetables, milk and milk products, sugar, honey | Major energy source (4 kcal/g), protein-sparing action; facilitates fat metabolism, provides fiber to promote elimination | Grains and legumes: 6+ servings<br>Fruits: 2-3 servings<br>Vegetables: 3-5 servings | Underweight, overweight, fatigue |
| Fat | Visible fat on meats/poultry, processed meats, bacon, whole milk/cheese, egg yolks, butter, margarine, oils, salad dressings, baked goods | Concentrated form of energy (9 kcal/g), storage form of energy; insulates and protects body organs, facilitates transport of fat-soluble vitamins | 30% or less of total daily calories | Overweight, underweight; risk factor for coronary heart disease, cancer of breast, colon, rectum, prostate |
| Vitamins | Fruits and vegetables, milk and milk products, fish and sunlight (vitamin D), cereal, grains, meat, fish, poultry, nuts, seeds | Regulates metabolism, helps convert carbohydrate and fat to energy, promotes tissue and bone formation | Variable (see Table 6-1) | Rarely seen with general food intake; signs specific to type of vitamin deficiency |
| Minerals | Milk and milk products, eggs, meats, grains, legumes, green leafy vegetables | Maintains acid-base balance and osmotic pressure, regulates metabolism of many enzymes, maintains nerve and muscle irritability, oxygen transport (iron) | Variable (see Table 6-1) | Altered acid-base balance, edema, neuromuscular dysfunction; other signs specific to type of mineral deficiency |

### Nutritional Needs of Elderly Persons

Elderly persons may have a high risk for malnutrition. Contributing factors include decreased physical activity, changes in the gastrointestinal tract, chronic illness, poor dentition, and limited access to health care. At increased risk for malnutrition are elderly persons who are physically disabled, isolated, depressed, and who live alone or in nursing homes. Many older adults drink less than recommended amounts of water and may have a decreased intake of calcium, iron, zinc, copper, thiamin, riboflavin, folate, and vitamins $B_{12}$ and D.[1] (See Chapter 4 for further discussion on nutritional needs of elderly persons and activities to promote good nutrition.)

## NUTRITIONAL GUIDELINES

It is helpful to have some guidelines to follow in deciding on types and amounts of food to eat for maintaining health. Three types of nutritional guidelines for health promotion are nutrient standards, food guides, and dietary guidelines.

### Nutrient Standards

Nutrient standards are designed for the maintenance of good nutrition of practically all healthy people in the United States.[34] **Recommended dietary allowances** (RDAs) are accepted nutrient standards for proteins, vitamins, and minerals. The RDAs differ for age-groups of children, men, and women on the basis of weight and height (see Table 6-1).

#### Food labeling

Food labels are useful as a basis for food choices. Labels on some packaged foods have provided a variety of information in the recent past. In 1990 the U.S. Congress passed the Nutrition Labeling and Education Act requiring the U.S. Food and Drug Administration (FDA) to develop a new system to be applied to nearly all food packages in supermarkets. The date for meeting the requirements was postponed from May 1993 to May 1994. The purposes of the new regulations are to (1) standardize serving portions, (2) mandate a standard chart of nutrients for all packages, (3) provide enforceable definitions for commonly used terms, and (4) strictly limit health claims linking foods to specific diseases.[13] A discussion of these four purposes follows.

**Standardized serving portions.** Serving sizes on the new labels are required to be consistent with similar foods. For example, all similar dry cereals should have the same serving size for easy comparison. The FDA has proposed standard portions for 131 categories of foods.[5]

**Standardized chart of nutrients.** The new standard food labels contain information on calories and selected nutrients. *Calories* are listed as *total calories* and *calories from fat.* This detail will help persons who are trying to limit their calories from fat to the recommended level of less than 30% of their total calories, as well as those who are trying to control their total intake. The label section noted as % *daily values* shows the percentages provided by the nutrient based on a 2000-calorie diet by one serving of the food product. The following nutrients are included in this section, with information provided in both grams (gm) or milligrams (mg) and % daily value: *fat* (total and saturated), *cholesterol, sodium, total carbohydrate, dietary fiber, sugars, and protein.* Information on vitamins and minerals has been limited to those most likely to be low in the usual American diet: *vitamins A and C, calcium, and iron.* The values are based on percent of RDAs. Niacin, riboflavin, and thiamin information is optional because these B complex vitamins are in good supply in the American diet.

**Standardized terms.** Many terms that have been used on food labels to describe and promote food products are ambiguous. The FDA has defined terms that are acceptable and has provided the standards to be met for correct usage. The new definitions of food terms are listed in Box 6-3.

**BOX 6-3 Definitions of FDA Food Labeling Terms**

*High* (rich in, excellent source): contains ≥20% of recommended daily intake for the nutrient
*Good source:* contains 10%-19% of the daily value/serving for a desirable nutrient
*More* (fortified, enriched, added): contains ≥10% of daily value for protein, vitamins, minerals, dietary fiber, or dietary potassium than the reference food; may not be used as a claim on meat or poultry items
*Low* (little, few, low source): foods that can be eaten in reasonable amount without exceeding dietary guidelines
- Low calorie: ≤40 kcal/serving
- Low fat: ≤3 g/serving; low saturated fat: ≤1 g/serving and <15% of calories from saturated fat
- Low cholesterol: ≤20 mg/serving
- Low sodium: ≤140 mg/serving; very low sodium: ≤35 mg/serving

*Free* (without, no, zero): contains very small or insignificant amounts of one or more of the following—fat, saturated fat, cholesterol, sodium, sodium/salt, sugars, or calories
*Light/lite:* one-third fewer calories or 50% less fat; also may be used to describe texture or color (must be specified on label)
*Reduced, less, fewer:* food has been changed to contain at least 25% less of a nutrient or calories than the reference food
*Lean:* <10 g fat, <4 g saturated fat, <95 mg cholesterol/serving per 100 g of meats, poultry, seafood, or game meats
- Extra lean: <5 g fat, <2 g saturated fat, <95 mg cholesterol per 100 g of meats, poultry, seafood, or game meats

*Fresh:* raw or unprocessed food never frozen, heated, or preserved (milk and bread excepted)
- Fresh frozen: allowed on foods that have been quickly frozen while fresh

Modified from American Dietetic Association: *Understanding food labels* [pamphlet], Chicago, 1993, The Association.

**Limited health claims.** Numerous health claims have been made on food products, most of which have not been proved. The FDA has tried to consider all claims and identify those with scientific bases. The following health claims have been accepted for use on food labels, provided the following requirements are met:

1. Calcium and osteoporosis—product must contain ≥20% of daily value for calcium (200 mg/serving)
2. Fat and cancer—must meet definition for extra lean
3. Saturated fat/cholesterol and coronary heart disease—must meet definition for low saturated fat, low cholesterol, and low fat
4. Fiber-rich products and cancer—must contain fruit, vegetable, or grain products and meet definition for low fat and good source of fiber
5. Fiber-rich products and risk of heart disease—must contain fruit, vegetable, or grain products and meet definition for low fat, low saturated fat, and low cholesterol and contain (without fortification) at least 0.6 g soluble fiber per serving
6. Sodium and high blood pressure—≤140 mg/serving
7. Fruits and vegetables and cancer—must meet definitions of low fat and a good source (without fortification) of at least one of the following: fiber, vitamin A, or vitamin C

## Food Guides

Food guides provide a *practical* approach for organizing food intake to ensure the needed variety and balance of required nutrients. Two examples of food guides are the food guide pyramid (Figure 6-2) and *food exchange lists* commonly used with dietary control of diabetes mellitus (see Chapter 40).

## Dietary Guidelines

Dietary guidelines are general statements to help persons plan a healthy diet. The guidelines are directed not only toward promoting general health but also reducing risk of disease. Therefore they reflect the current emphasis on prevention of the major diseases, such as heart disease and cancer. The dietary guidelines for the American public developed by the Department of Health and Human Services (DHHS) and the nutrition section of the U.S. Department of Agriculture are a good example:

1. Eat a variety of foods
2. Maintain ideal weight
3. Avoid too much fat, saturated fat, and cholesterol
4. Eat foods with adequate starch and fiber
5. Avoid too much sugar
6. Avoid too much sodium
7. If you drink alcohol, do so in moderation

These seven guidelines are detailed in the following discussion.

### Eating a variety of foods

The only food that comes close to providing a wide variety of essential nutrients is milk. The greater the variety of foods consumed, the more likely that the individual will receive the required nutrients. One method to ensure a good variety of food is to follow the food guide pyramid.

### Maintaining ideal weight

Weight control is a major concern of many Americans; at least one of every four Americans follows a weight-reducing diet at any given time.[34] **Ideal body weight** (IBW) is difficult to identify because of individual vari-

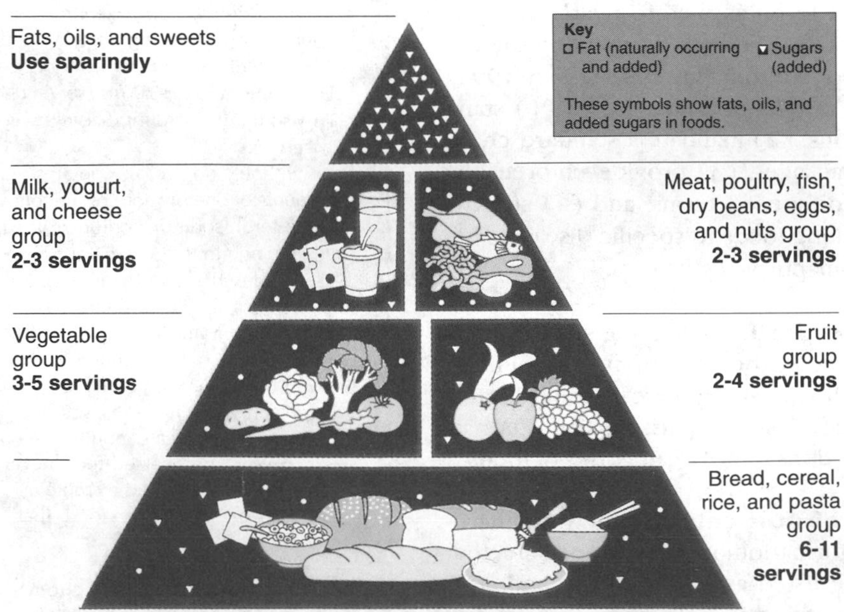


**FIGURE 6-2** Food Guide Pyramid. (US Department of Agriculture, Washington, DC.)

ations, such as sex, age, genetic framework, and metabolic needs. Two men of the same age may weigh the same, but one may be an athlete and have large amounts of muscle with little fat, whereas the other may have considerable fat. However, height and weight tables are practical guides for determining a *general* weight range (Table 6-5). The height and weight table must be used with caution because it is based on "averages" and the "average person" does not exist.

**Overweight/Obesity.** The body mass index (BMI) is used to determine fatness; it is determined by dividing measured body weight in kilograms by the height in meters squared (see p. 149). Normal BMI is 20 to 25 kg/m$^2$. **Obesity** refers to BMI above 27.5 kg/m$^2$. The National Institutes for Health has divided obesity into three levels: mild (BMI 27.5 to 30 kg/m$^2$), moderate (BMI 30 to 40 kg/m$^2$), and severe or morbid obesity (BMI >40 kg/m$^2$).[30] *Morbid* obesity places the person at a high risk for numerous disorders. Individuals with moderate or morbid obesity have higher mortality and morbidity rates than their peers of normal weight.[30] It has not yet been proved that overweight or mild obesity places persons at risk for disease.[34] Many persons, however, do not feel at their optimal level of fitness and self-esteem when they are overweight.

Obesity usually does not result from a single cause but rather from a complex interrelationship of numerous physiologic, psychologic, and social factors. Old age is not a factor; most elderly persons are not severely obese. Mild overweight is considered to be beneficial for elderly persons because it provides an available source of nutrients during periods of stress or illness.

***Physiologic factors.*** Obesity results from the intake of foods in amounts exceeding body needs; the excess is stored as fat. There may be a genetic influence in the predisposition to obesity. In persons of normal weight who gain weight, fat is deposited by hypertrophy of existing fat cells in adipose tissue. This group responds well to weight-reduction regimens. Fat cells also can increase in number (hyperplasia); this process usually is irreversible, and being overweight tends to be a life-long condition.[15] Weight reduction in persons with hyperplastic obesity is difficult to achieve and to maintain. Some persons can eat large quantities of caloric foods and not gain significant weight. Other persons gain weight with only slight increases in caloric intake. The difference apparently is the result of the ability to use the calories more or less efficiently.

***Metabolic*** abnormalities have been noted in persons with severe or massive obesity (Table 6-6). Triglycerides are stored in fat deposits in adipose tissue. When fatty acids are needed for energy, triglycerides are released and circulated in the bloodstream. The obese person has increased serum triglyceride levels that may predispose the person to atheromatous plaques. Obese persons have a high risk of diabetes. Increased serum glucose places a stress on the pancreas to produce more insulin, and hyperinsulinism occurs. The pancreatic islet cells may first exhibit hyperplasia but then fail. An increased *resistance-to-insulin* effect also results from the large number of fat cells with a diminished number of insulin receptors.[15]

Selected *hormones* can influence the use of ingested calories. Thyroid hormones stimulate basal metabolism,

**TABLE 6-5 Metropolitan Life Insurance Company Height and Weight Table**

| MEN* | | | | | WOMEN† | | | | |
|---|---|---|---|---|---|---|---|---|---|
| HEIGHT | | | | | HEIGHT | | | | |
| FEET | INCHES | SMALL FRAME | MEDIUM FRAME | LARGE FRAME | FEET | INCHES | SMALL FRAME | MEDIUM FRAME | LARGE FRAME |
| 5 | 2 | 128-134 | 131-141 | 138-150 | 4 | 10 | 102-111 | 109-121 | 118-131 |
| 5 | 3 | 130-136 | 133-143 | 140-153 | 4 | 11 | 103-113 | 111-123 | 120-134 |
| 5 | 4 | 132-138 | 135-145 | 142-156 | 5 | 0 | 104-115 | 113-126 | 122-137 |
| 5 | 5 | 134-140 | 137-148 | 144-160 | 5 | 1 | 106-118 | 115-129 | 125-140 |
| 5 | 6 | 136-142 | 139-151 | 146-164 | 5 | 2 | 108-121 | 118-132 | 128-143 |
| 5 | 7 | 138-145 | 142-154 | 149-168 | 5 | 3 | 111-124 | 121-135 | 131-147 |
| 5 | 8 | 140-148 | 145-157 | 152-172 | 5 | 4 | 114-127 | 124-138 | 134-151 |
| 5 | 9 | 142-151 | 148-160 | 155-176 | 5 | 5 | 117-130 | 127-141 | 137-155 |
| 5 | 10 | 144-154 | 151-163 | 158-180 | 5 | 6 | 120-133 | 130-144 | 140-159 |
| 5 | 11 | 146-157 | 154-166 | 161-184 | 5 | 7 | 123-136 | 133-147 | 143-163 |
| 6 | 0 | 149-160 | 157-170 | 164-188 | 5 | 8 | 126-139 | 136-150 | 146-157 |
| 6 | 1 | 152-164 | 160-174 | 168-192 | 5 | 9 | 129-142 | 139-153 | 149-170 |
| 6 | 2 | 155-168 | 164-178 | 172-197 | 5 | 10 | 132-145 | 142-156 | 152-173 |
| 6 | 3 | 158-172 | 167-182 | 176-202 | 5 | 11 | 135-148 | 145-159 | 155-176 |
| 6 | 4 | 162-176 | 171-187 | 181-207 | 6 | 0 | 138-151 | 148-162 | 158-179 |

From Stein JH: *Internal medicine*, ed 4, St. Louis, 1994, Mosby.

*Weights at ages 25 to 59 based on lowest mortality. Weight in pounds according to frame (in indoor clothing weighing 5 lb, shoes with 1 in heels).

†Weights at ages 25 to 59 based on lowest mortality. Weight in pounds according to frame (in indoor clothing weighing 3 lb, shoes with 1 in heels).

**TABLE 6-6 Physiologic Effects of Obesity**

| PARAMETER | METABOLIC EFFECT | ASSOCIATED DISORDER |
|---|---|---|
| Increased fatty acid | Hypertriglyceridemia | Atherosclerosis, hypertension, emboli |
| | Increased cholesterol synthesis | Gallstones, atherosclerosis |
| Increased glucose | Hyperinsulinism leading to pancreatic β-cell failure | Diabetes mellitus |
| Increased body mass | Cumulative trauma to weight-bearing joints | Osteoarthritis |
| | Increased workload for heart | Angina, sudden death |
| | Decreased thorax expansion with decreased tidal volume | Respiratory insufficiency |

requiring energy and calorie expenditure; thus the person who has a thyroid deficiency may experience weight gain. Decreased insulin in diabetes mellitus and increased cortisone production with Cushing's syndrome also lead to overweight.

***Psychosocial factors.*** Eating is a social custom. Some ethnic groups perceive that "fat is beautiful" and encourage the eating of large amounts of food. Parents who are socialized to eat large quantities of food pass on this practice to their children. Western societies often feed their infants high-caloric milk and cereals at a time when there is a greater chance for an increased number of fat cells to be produced.

Social gatherings usually involve eating or drinking high-calorie foods. In recent years there has been greater emphasis on serving low-calorie foods such as sliced raw vegetables at social functions. Diet drinks also have increased in popularity.

A person may attach symbolic meanings to foods as a result of experiences. During times of stress, some people eat more food or more highly caloric foods and thus gain weight. Compulsive eating may occur, leading to severe obesity.

Obese persons who have tried many times unsuccessfully to lose weight may become sensitive to suggestions to eat low-caloric foods. Some have reported deliberately choosing high-caloric foods as a means of establishing control of their own identity. Body image is an important factor in obesity and may help to prevent weight gain by motivating a person to lose weight.

**Underweight. Underweight** is described as 20% below the accepted weight and height standards (BMI <20kg/m$^2$). Unplanned weight loss may be an early sign of a medical disorder, and medical evaluation should be sought. Some weight loss may be due to inadequate calorie intake or failure to increase calorie intake when physical activity is increased. Weight loss associated with eating disorders (anorexia nervosa, bulimia nervosa) are discussed in Chapter 19. Undernutrition leads to nutritional deficits that affect growth and development, metabolism, and the body's protective mechanisms. *Hospitalized patients are at risk for malnutrition* for several reasons. First, stress and increased metabolic rates from certain disorders deplete nutrient stores. Second, the patient is less active and may be relatively immobile. Third, the patient may not be ingesting the required nutrients because of anorexia, nausea/vomiting, missed meals because of tests or surgery, or prescribed restrictive diets. Ongoing assessment of the patient's nutrient status is important.

### Avoiding too much fat, saturated fats, and cholesterol

Excess calories lead to fat deposition, adding to body weight. Research strongly supports a relationship between dietary fat and coronary heart disease and with the incidence of cancer, especially cancer of the breast, colon, rectum, and prostate.[6]

The phrase "avoid too much fat, saturated fat, and cholesterol" is vague; therefore more direction is needed. The 1991 nutritional guidelines developed by the National Cholesterol Education Program (NCEP) of the National Heart, Lung, and Blood Institute (and consistent with national objectives for the year 2000 and with guidelines set by other health agencies) are as follows:

| Total Fat | To Average ≤30% of Calories |
|---|---|
| Saturated | <10% |
| Monounsaturated | 10% to 15% |
| Polyunsaturated | Up to 10% |
| Cholesterol | <300 mg/day |

The different types of fats are defined in Box 6-4. Note that the more hydrogen found in the fatty acid, the more it is saturated. Although saturated fats are of animal origin, unsaturated oils can be hardened commercially by injection of hydrogen gas to saturate them, producing margarines. About 40% of fats are visible in foods; the remainder is hidden, especially in red meats. **Cholesterol** is essential as a precursor to body steroids, for the development of bile acids, and as a component of cell membranes. Excess serum cholesterol that is not excreted contributes to the formation of atheromatous plaques in linings of blood vessels, especially the coronary arteries, leading to blocking of the blood vessels. Recommended foods with lower cholesterol are listed on p. 154.

The American public is becoming better informed about the effects of high levels of serum cholesterol as a risk factor for coronary heart disease. From the time of the National Health and Nutrition Examination Survey

**BOX 6-4 Definitions of Terms Pertaining to Fats and Cholesterol**

**Lipids** A group of fatty substances that are insoluble in water

**Triglycerides** Simple lipids that are composed of one molecule of glycerol linked to three molecules of fatty acids

**Saturated fats** Triglycerides whose fatty acids have no double bonds in the carbon chains; the fatty acid is filled (saturated) with hydrogen atoms

**Monounsaturated fats (MUFA)** Fatty acids that have one double bond (one less hydrogen atom); of plant origin (e.g., olive oil)

**Polyunsaturated fats (PUFA)** Fatty acids that have two or more double bonds (fewer hydrogen atoms); of plant origin (e.g., corn or sunflower oils)

**Lipoproteins** The form in which fats are carried in the bloodstream; the unsoluble fat is wrapped in a water-soluble protein; may be very-low-density lipoprotein (VLDL), low-density lipoprotein (LDL), or high-density lipoprotein (HDL)

**Cholesterol** A steroid that is found in animal fats and body tissue; most cholesterol is synthesized in the body; carried in bloodstream primarily attached to low-density lipoproteins; produced by the liver in human beings

(NHANES II) (1976-1980) to the NHANES III (1988-1991) the proportion of adults with high blood cholesterol levels (≥240 mg/dl) fell from 26% to 20% while the proportion with desirable levels (<200 mg/dl) rose from 44% to 49%.[28] A 1990 survey found that 65% of adults reported having had their cholesterol levels tested; however, only 24% stated that they were trying to lower their cholesterol levels through dietary means.[26] The NCEP lists the following guidelines for adults:

1. Have cholesterol level measured every 5 years.
2. Know your cholesterol level.
3. Take steps to lower the cholesterol, if elevated.

The NCEP has established the following criteria for evaluating total serum cholesterol levels[11]:

<200 mg/dl—desirable
200-239 mg/dl—borderline
≥240 md/dl—high

Two lipoproteins (see Box 6-4), high-density lipoprotein (HDL) and low-density lipoprotein (LDL), are significant factors in evaluating persons with high cholesterol levels. The lower the level of LDL (<130 mg/dl is desirable; 130-159 mg/dl is borderline) the less the risk of coronary heart disease. Levels of HDL above 35 mg/dl are desirable.[11] (For further discussion of these lipoproteins, see Chapter 30).

### Eating foods with adequate starch and fiber

**Starch** is a polysaccharide (complex carbohydrate) found primarily in cereal grains, legumes, and vegetables (especially potatoes). Carbohydrates are an important energy source for the body. The suggested national objectives for the year 2000 include increasing the daily intake for grain products and legumes to 6 or more daily servings, which is consistent with the food guide pyramid recommendations.

**Dietary fiber** contains cellulose and some noncellulose polysaccharides. Cellulose is not digestible; therefore it remains in the gastrointestinal tract, providing bulk to help stimulate peristalsis in the intestines. The noncellulose polysaccharides absorb water to add to the bulk. Noncellulose substances also bind dietary cholesterol, preventing its absorption. Dietary fiber therefore is important to promote normal bowel elimination and to decrease dietary cholesterol absorption. In addition, dietary fiber has been shown to have an inverse association with colon cancer; that is, a high intake of dietary fiber decreases the risk for colon cancer.[6] Sources of dietary fiber include whole grains (wheat, rye, oats) used in cereals and breads, and bran and fiber found in fruits and vegetables.

The current intake of dietary fiber in the United States is approximately 10 to 15 g daily. The National Cancer Institute recommends *increasing daily fiber intake to 20 to 30 g,* with an upper limit of 35 g to avoid adverse effects.[6] The suggested national objectives for the year 2000 are to increase daily servings of *fruits and vegetables to 5 or more and grain/legumes products to 6 or more.* These suggested servings will provide 20 to 30 g of dietary fiber.[31]

### Avoiding too much sugar

Excess amounts of sugar add to caloric intake without supplying nutrients; sugars also contribute to formation of dental caries. In general, sugars in American diets average about 20% of daily calories.[34] Persons who diet by cutting out sugar but continue to consume fats deceive themselves because fats provide almost double the amount of calories. Use of artificial sweeteners does not necessarily reduce caloric intake because the artificial sweeteners do not relieve the desire for "something sweet," and the person then may turn to fats to achieve the feeling of satiety.[34] Substituting complex carbohydrates for some of the sugars provides for greater intake of essential nutrients and feelings of satiety.

### Avoiding too much sodium

Sodium, a major body electrolyte (see Chapter 20), can affect blood pressure levels. Although the cause of hypertension is unknown, a decreased sodium intake can help decrease blood pressure in persons with hypertension. Sodium in the form of salt-cured or salt-pickled foods has been associated with the increased incidence of gastric cancer.[6] Foods that are high in sodium are listed in Box 6-5. Most American diets are high in sodium, and dietary recommendations suggest that sodium intake be decreased to promote health. The suggested national health objectives for the year 2000 include the following:

- Increase to at least 50% the proportion of households that purchase foods low in sodium, prepare

**BOX 6-5 Foods High in Sodium**

Salt-preserved foods: ham, bacon, sausage, hot dogs, cold cuts
Salted or smoked fish
Salted snacks: crackers, popcorn, pretzels, potato chips, nuts
Spices/condiments: meat tenderizer, bouillon cubes, celery salt, garlic salt, MSG, pickles, olives, Worcestershire sauce, soy sauce
Cheese

**BOX 6-7 Medications to Be Taken with Food**

| | |
|---|---|
| Aminophylline | Phenylbutazone (Butazolidin) |
| Chlorothiazide (Diuril) | Phenytoin (Dilantin) |
| Indomethacin (Indocin) | Prednisolone |
| Metronidazole (Flagyl) | Reserpine (Serpasil) |
| Nitrofurantoin (Macrodantin) | Triamterene (Dyrenium) |

foods without adding salt, and do not add salt at the table.

**Limiting alcohol**

Alcohol is high in calories but low in nutrients. Excess alcohol intake leads to medical disorders and possible alcohol abuse (see Chapter 19). Persons who drink excessively often do not eat balanced meals and therefore experience malnutrition. A large percentage of automobile accidents (a major public health problem) are caused by drivers who have been drinking alcohol. All health guidelines suggest that those who drink alcohol should do so in moderation.

## Food-Drug Interactions

Some medications may affect nutritional status if taken over a period of time (Box 6-6). Conversely, food can interfere with absorption of oral medications.

Drugs are absorbed more readily if the gastrointestinal tract is free of food. Drugs taken with water when the stomach is empty move rapidly into the small intestine, where much drug absorption takes place. Fatty foods delay gastric emptying for as long as 2 hours; therefore drugs that are absorbed in the small intestine have delayed absorption if taken with a meal high in fat. Food particularly delays the absorption of antimicrobial drugs, specifically the tetracyclines, the penicillins, and the sulfonamides. However, medications that have a gastric irritant effect may be enhanced if taken with food (Box 6-7).

Drugs that are normally slightly acidic, such as aspirin or barbiturates, usually ionize and are absorbed in the stomach. If the stomach pH increases, such as by milk or antacids, the rate and extent of absorption of these drugs decrease. Alteration in stomach acidity also may break down the protective coating of spansules or enteric-coated tablets, resulting in premature release of contents. Acidic liquids, such as lemon, pineapple, or cranberry juices or dry ginger ale, may inactivate acid-unstable drugs such as ampicillin, potassium, penicillin G, cloxacillin, and erythromycin.

Food components can interact with oral medication by the chemical or physical binding of one substance on another, thus interfering with absorption of either the food component or the drug. Tetracycline becomes bound with calcium, aluminum, or magnesium ions when it is taken with milk or antacids. This decreases absorption of tetracycline. The effects can be controlled by timing intake of food and drug. Foods that contain tyramine (cheeses, wines) may interact with monoamine oxidase (MAO) inhibitors, such as the antidepressants phenelzine (Nardil) or tranylcypromine (Parnate), and cause hypertensive reactions.

**BOX 6-6 Effect of Some Drugs on Nutritional Status**

| | |
|---|---|
| **Antacids** | Malabsorption of iron, phosphorus |
| **Aspirin** | Malabsorption of folate<br>Excretion of vitamin C |
| **Barbiturates** | Malabsorption of thiamin, vitamin $B_{12}$<br>Excretion of vitamin C |
| **Corticosteroids** | Malabsorption of calcium, zinc, phosphorus; increased cholesterol and glucose |
| **Hydralazine** | Excretion of pyridoxine |
| **Methotrexate** | Malabsorption of vitamin $B_{12}$, folate, fat |
| **Mineral oil** | Malabsorption of fat-soluble vitamins, calcium, phosphorus |
| **Neomycin** | Malabsorption of major nutrients |
| **Oral contraceptives** | Possible decreased absorption of vitamin C, B-complex vitamins, magnesium, zinc |
| **Penicillin** | Loss of potassium |
| **Tetracycline** | Malabsorption of calcium, iron, magnesium, pyridoxine<br>Excretion of vitamin C, riboflavin, niacin, folic acid |
| **Thiazides** | Excretion of potassium, magnesium, zinc, riboflavin |

# NURSING MANAGEMENT

## ♦ ASSESSMENT

To assess nutritional status it is necessary to determine the supply of available nutrients, the sources available for metabolic processes, body size, and physical signs. To assess possible changes in dietary patterns, information on the person's perceptions and desires also are collected.

### Subjective Data

Data to be collected to determine nutritional status include the following[9]:

Food intake
 Typical day food/fluid pattern (type, amount)
 Recent changes in amount and type of intake
 Recent changes in appetite
Eating ability
 Dentures (fit, comfort)
 Problems with chewing or swallowing
Weight
 Usual and current weight
 Patient's perception of weight level
  If overweight/underweight: lifetime patterns, feelings about weight, reasons for recent change
Food supplements, medications, drugs (types, duration)

### Food intake

In collecting data about nutrition, it is especially important to phrase the questions so that patients describe what they typically eat rather than what they think they should. For example, the question, "Do you usually drink orange juice for breakfast?" implies (1) that breakfast is a desirable or expected behavior and (2) that orange juice is essential. Thus the patient may answer "yes," believing that is the expected answer, when in fact neither orange juice nor breakfast usually is taken. A better approach is to say, "Tell me what you typically eat and drink in a day. What do you usually eat or drink first?" Questioning should elicit a picture of total food consumption for a day, including all snacks. Designation by meals or snacks is not really necessary and may bias answers by implying value judgments.

Identification of amount consumed is as important as the type of food. Often people find this difficult to estimate. Persons familiar with cooking may be able to estimate in terms of tablespoons or cups. For the hospitalized patient the equipment or portions on the tray can be used as a basis for comparison.

Changes in appetite or in the amount or type of food or fluids ingested may be the result of illness (e.g., anorexia, nausea, vomiting, or pain), self-imposed dietary regimens, or emotional or physical stress.

### Additional data for persons with obesity

1. Person's perception of his or her weight. Many persons who are slightly overweight perceive that they are moderately or severely overweight; severely overweight persons who do not perceive their status may not be motivated to lose weight.
2. Duration of weight gain. A person with a recent weight gain will respond more positively to a weight-reduction program than will one with a lifelong pattern of obesity.
3. Perception of the cause of weight gain.
4. Family history of obesity.
5. Person's reasons for losing weight and the weight goal. The goals may or may not be realistic and may indicate a lack of knowledge about obesity.
6. Weight-reduction approaches used in the past, effectiveness of the approaches, and ideas about present approaches to be used.
7. Eating patterns (meals and snacks).
8. Exercise patterns.
9. Stressors that may be present (home, job, community, or personal).
10. Medications currently taken. Some medications cause weight gain (glucocorticoids, oral contraceptives, tricyclic antidepressants, antithyroid preparations, and phenothiazines).
11. Perceptions of self-worth; example: "What do you think about yourself as a person?"

### Additional data for inadequate intake

1. Food and fluid likes and dislikes.
2. Financial resources.
3. Facilities and ability for purchasing, storing, and preparing food.
4. Problems with prescribed diets.

## Objective Data

Data to be collected to determine nutritional status include the following.

### Height and weight

Height and weight are easily measured and are important data to obtain and use. The most reliable weight measurement is in the morning after voiding and before eating or drinking fluids. The patient's weight or height is compared with a table of recommended values (see Table 6-5). Interpretation of the table requires knowing frame size.

### Body mass index

A relative index of body fatness can be determined by calculating the **body mass index (BMI)** using the following formula:

$$\text{BMI} = \frac{\text{Weight (kg)}}{\text{Height (m)}^2}$$

Divide the number of pounds by 2.2 to determine weight in kg. Divide the number of inches by 39.37 to determine height in meters; then multiply this number by itself to square it. For example, the BMI calculation of a person who weighs 125 pounds and is 5 feet 3 inches tall is as follows:

$$125 \div 2.2 = 56.8 \text{ kg}$$
$$5 \text{ ft } 3 \text{ in} = 63 \text{ in}; 63 \div 39.37 = 1.6; 1.6 \times 1.6 = 2.56$$
$$\text{Therefore the BMI} = 56.8 \div 2.56 = 22.18 \text{ kg/m}^2$$

For health maintenance, the BMI range suggested for adults is 20 to 25 kg/m$^2$.[30] The person in the sample calculation is not overweight and has a normal body fat level.

**Skinfold measurement**

Body fat can be estimated by skinfold measurements. Calipers are used to measure skinfolds by compressing the skin and subcutaneous fat, not muscle, into a fold at specific body sites (e.g., biceps, subscapsular, suprailiac, thigh, and periumbilical areas).

## Analysis of Food Intake

Food guides developed to help people choose the kinds and amounts of food to eat for health can be used for rapid evaluation of adequacy of the diet eaten at home or food intake in the hospital. Many different food guides are available, because to be effective they must be devised for a specific country or culture and feature the foods readily available and acceptable to the persons being evaluated.

Servings and nutrients supplied by the food guide pyramid used in the United States are shown in Table 6-7. The guide groups staple food items rich in protein, vitamins, and minerals into five major classes according to their major nutrient contributions. Recommendations are made for the number and size of servings to be selected from each food group. To evaluate a diet quickly, one checks to see if the recommended types of food and servings are included in the usual dietary pattern.

Because foods are mixtures of nutrients, the protein, vitamin, and mineral requirements are substantially met when the daily intake includes the recommended servings from each group.

The absence of any one food group from the diet or particular types of food should alert the nurse that the person has a potential nutrition problem. Box 6-8 is an assessment and an example of an analysis of food intake using the daily food guide.

The food guide pyramid also can be used for evaluating vegetarian diets. Many people are vegetarians, and their reasons vary (e.g., religion, food cost, philosophy). The diets vary as well. Generally the lactoovovegetarian (includes milk products and eggs) diet is nutritionally sound when a variety of foods is included. Persons on more restricted vegetarian (vegan) diets should be considered at nutritional risk and candidates for more detailed study (refer to dietitian). One potential problem with the vegan diet is vitamin $B_{12}$ insufficiency unless fortified cereal or a dietary supplement is taken. The young adult who has changed to a vegan diet may use body stores of $B_{12}$ for a time (a 5-year store is possible) but is at potential risk, especially if intake of folacin in vegetables is high, masking the signs of megaloblastic anemia.

**TABLE 6-7 Serving Sizes and Nutrients Supplied by Food Groups**

| FOOD GROUP (servings/day) | SERVING SIZES | NUTRIENTS SUPPLIED |
|---|---|---|
| **Bread, cereals, pasta, rice** (6-11) | Bread, 1 slice<br>Dry cereal, 30 g<br>Cooked rice/pasta, ½ cup | Complex carbohydrates, protein, iron, thiamin, riboflavin, niacin |
| **Vegetables** (3-5) | ½ cup or usual portion, e.g., medium potato | Fiber; vitamins, especially A (dark-green and deep-yellow vegetables) and C (tomato, cabbage, pepper); minerals |
| **Fruits** (2-4) | Usual portion, e.g., medium apple, ¼ cantaloupe, ½-1 banana | Fiber; vitamins, especially C (citrus fruits, cantaloupe, strawberries); minerals |
| **Milk, yogurt, cheese** (2-3) | Milk, 1 cup (8 oz)<br>Yogurt 1 cup<br>Cheese, 40 g (1½ oz)<br>Ice cream, 1¾ cup | Calcium, phosphorus; protein (high quality); vitamins and minerals, especially riboflavin; carbohydrates and fat |
| **Meat, poultry, fish, dry beans, eggs, nuts** (2-3) | Lean meat, poultry, fish, 60-75 g (2-3 oz)<br>Eggs, 2<br>Cooked beans, lentils, peas, 1 cup<br>Peanut butter, 4 Tbsp | High-quality protein; fat; B-complex vitamins (plant products lack vitamin $B_{12}$) |
| **Fats** (natural, added) and **sugar** (added) | Use sparingly | Fats; simple sugar |

## ♦ NURSING DIAGNOSES

Nursing diagnoses are determined from analysis of patient data. Nursing diagnoses for the patient with or at risk for nutritional imbalance may include but are not limited to the following:

| Diagnostic Title | Possible Etiologic Factors |
|---|---|
| Knowledge deficit | Lack of information |
| Nutrition, altered: high risk for more than body requirements | Dysfunctional eating behaviors |
| Nutrition, altered: more than body requirements | Dysfunctional eating behaviors, lack of exercise |
| Nutrition, altered: less than body requirements | Dysfunctional eating behaviors, anorexia, decreased intake because of tests or surgery |

## ♦ EXPECTED PATIENT OUTCOMES

Expected patient outcomes to promote good nutritional status may include but are not limited to the following:

1. Describes desired servings for each food group to meet basic nutritive needs.
2. Maintains weight within desired weight range.
3. Describes modifications in dietary intake to cor-

**BOX 6-8 Assessment of a Diet History**

45-year-old woman with obesity and hypertension; meals eaten at home

**7 AM**
1 c cooked oatmeal
2 tsp sugar
1 c skim milk (fortified)
3 c coffee, plain

**10:15 AM**
2 c coffee, plain

**1 PM**
Sandwich
- 2 slices white bread, enriched
- ½ tsp margarine
- ½ tsp mayonnaise
- 60 g (2 oz) meatloaf or luncheon meat

4 cookies (fig bars, gingersnaps)
3 c coffee, plain

**4 PM**
7 cookies
½ c unsweetened fruit (canned, frozen, or fresh)
2 c tea, plain

**10 PM**
8 soda crackers
60 g (2 oz) American cheese
360 ml (12 oz) cola (sweet)
½ c homemade bread-and-butter pickles

**Midnight**
2 aspirin
1 c tea, plain

**Assessment**

| *Food group* | *Servings* |
|---|---|
| Milk | |
| Skim milk | 1 |
| Cheese | 1 |
| Meat (protein) | |
| Meatloaf | 1 |
| Fruits, vegetables | |
| Fruit | 1 |
| Vegetable | 1 |
| Bread, cereal | |
| Oatmeal | 2 |
| Bread, enriched | 2 |
| Crackers | 2 |
| Sweets | |
| Cookies | 11 |
| Cola (360 ml [12 oz]) | |
| Pickles, cucumber | |
| Fats | |
| Margarine | |
| Mayonnaise | |

***Evaluation***

Choice from milk group adequate. Meat intake low. Fruit and vegetable intake very low. Bread intake is minimal. Intake of sweets, particularly cookies, high. Use of pickles and soda crackers questionable, inasmuch as patient reports that low-sodium diet was prescribed for her several years ago.

Dietitian was asked to check caloric value. Intake is 1500 to 1600 calories/day, which includes 800 calories from basic food items; remainder from sweets and fat. Protein levels adequate, although source of protein could be improved.

**To the reader:** Identify nutritional risks for this person; identify appropriate interventions and behavioral goals for her.

rect existing or potential nutritional deficits or excesses.

The person must be involved in the planning if expected outcomes are to be accomplished. The person is guided to set realistic outcomes. Therapy for the obese person should have three objectives: (1) reduction of the body fat component, (2) reduction of total body weight when indicated, and (3) maintenance of desirable body size and composition. Far too often, both patient and therapist look only at the pounds of weight lost or the rate of loss. No differentiation is made as to whether the pounds represent water, muscle, or fat. Very rapid weight loss is satisfying to both patient and therapist, whether the loss is in body fat or water and whether the loss is permanent or not. Rapid weight loss usually results from loss of water rather than fat.

## ♦ INTERVENTIONS

### Facilitating Learning

Teaching patients with specific knowledge deficits includes identification of the patient's motivation to learn. Patients with extensive lack of knowledge about food preparation, particularly with ways of preparing nutritionally balanced meals at low cost, may profit from the services of a dietitian.

The food guide pyramid is a useful tool for teaching persons a method of evaluating their own food intake. The dietitian may be helpful in developing a specific food guide for persons whose cultural patterns or personal preferences (e.g., vegetarians) do not fit the standard food guides.

Persons who have been prescribed a dietary modification may need interpretation of the rationale for the diet and assistance in planning acceptable meals using the prescribed dietary plan. The dietitian usually initiates the discussion of a new home-going diet, but the nurse serves as interpreter to the patient by providing explanations about the diet and feedback on how to make changes in current dietary patterns to meet the dietary prescription. Because the patients are the ones who must implement the dietary changes, they need to internalize the need for a behavior change. This takes active participation in all phases of the learning process. The person who does the cooking (if not the patient) also needs to be involved in the learning process. Dietary changes are more likely to be implemented if the changes can be easily adjusted to the family's usual meal plans.

## Facilitating Weight Control

Weight reduction is not achieved simply by lowering the fuel value of the person's diet. A deficit must be produced between energy expenditure and fuel intake so that body stores of fuel will be mobilized. The deficit may be achieved by increasing energy expenditures or decreasing caloric intake, as shown in Figure 6-3.

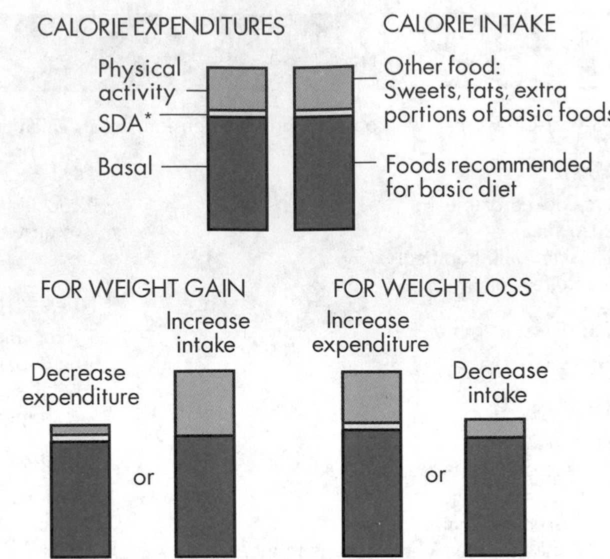


**FIGURE 6-3** Calorie balance in an average adult.

The purpose of therapy for obese persons is *weight control throughout the life span;* therefore most obese persons have to learn new patterns of eating and exercise. Physicians may prescribe medication as part of a weight-reduction program. Surgery also may be performed for the massively obese person when all other methods fail, although long-term weight control may not be effective (see Chapter 45).

### Diet

Diet is the most important method of weight reduction. Dieting has been widely reported, even among those who are not overweight. Diet plans vary, however, from balanced, low-calorie diets to nutritionally poor fad diets. Books are written favoring various plans, not all of which are either appropriate or nutritionally sound. Many persons have tried different approaches but do not keep to one diet for any period of time. Weight usually is regained within 1 to 2 years unless eating patterns have changed.[30]

Persons consuming high levels of calories before weight-reduction therapy are likely to be successful in achieving rapid weight loss, because the calorie deficit between weight-maintenance requirements and the recommended diet is large. Men have a reputation for being more cooperative than women because they lose weight more rapidly. If both a man and a woman are instructed to adhere to a 1000 calorie intake, however, the man would be expected to lose at a faster rate because his calorie deficit is larger.

Weight loss for some persons may be achieved by eating three average, balanced meals a day, including groups from the food guide pyramid, and avoiding fried foods, sweets, and between-meal snacks. Some persons achieve better results with planned, frequent small meals. Some obese persons omit breakfast but then snack frequently and thus ingest more calories and fewer required nutrients. *Changes in eating patterns* therefore are usually required for permanent weight loss.

One pound of adipose tissue has an energy potential of 3500 calories. To lose 1 pound of adipose tissue per week, a calorie deficit of 500 calories per day must be induced. If a person requires only 1500 calories to maintain current weight, that person should not be expected to lose more than 1 pound of body fat per week when adhering to a 1000 calorie diet. Weight loss is more rapid when lean body tissue is catabolized, because lean tissue has an energy potential of about 1850 calories. If a deficit of 500 calories per day were met by catabolizing lean tissue, the rate of loss would be about 2 pounds per week. Dehydration produces very rapid weight loss from loss of water. Water has no calorie value per se, but 1 L of water weighs approximately 1 kg.

When caloric intake is severely reduced, there is often a large initial weight loss as a result of loss of water. A plateau in observable weight loss is then reached when fat (which weighs less than water) is being lost. This plateau usually lasts 7 to 10 days and may discourage the dieter. Observable weight loss will then be noted after this period but will not be as rapid because of the body's adaptation by decreased metabolic rate and fuel utilization.

Adhering to a diet plan is often difficult. The dieter tends to become preoccupied with food. There may be social pressure to eat, and it is difficult to resist available calorie-rich foods. Support from others is important and is the basis for more positive results when a person joins a weight-control group such as Weight Watchers.

**BOX 6-9 Risks of Fasting Diets**

| | |
|---|---|
| Ketosis | Hepatic impairment |
| Metabolic acidosis | Polyneuritis |
| Hypokalemia | Wernicke's syndrome |
| Hyperuricemia | Ulcerative colitis |
| Hypotension | Renal insufficiency and death in some instances |
| Nephrolithiasis | |

Diets are planned on an individual basis, with the caloric intake planned at a level below the person's caloric need for maintaining weight. The calorie intake should come from complex carbohydrates and proteins. A protein intake of about 1 g/kg of ideal body weight should be maintained. Fats must be decreased. Salt-free diets are of no permanent value because the weight loss relates to water loss, and the weight will return when salt is added to the diet.

*Fasting* diets are controversial. Rapid weight loss may be necessary in some instances; however, weight gain after the fasting period is a common occurrence. Most fasting programs use a high-protein liquid; some commercial products use hydrolyzed collagen that is low in nutritional value. Close medical supervision is imperative for fasting diets because risks are high (Box 6-9). To prevent false advertising the FDA has placed constraints on fasting programs.

### Exercise

Exercise is the second part of every weight-reduction program. Although the actual number of calories used varies, the combination of diet and exercise promotes loss of fat rather than lean tissue. Exercise has added benefits, which include influencing plasma insulin and lipid levels, promoting muscle tone, increasing coronary perfusion, and creating psychologic well-being. *Brisk* walking is encouraged and is more easily tolerated if done with another person. The distance walked is progressively increased. Group exercise and swimming programs designed for obese persons also are effective.

### Medication

The use of appetite suppressants is controversial because of long-term inefficiency and in some cases, such as with amphetamines, possible drug abuse.

Most over-the-counter dietary aids contain phenylpropanolamine and bulk-producing agents.[7] Phenylpropanolamine is a sympathomimetic with anorectic action similar to amphetamine but with no untoward CNS effects. Its usefulness as a weight control drug in humans has been questioned, however. The drug should not be used for more than 3 months and should not be taken concurrently with antihypertensive drugs or with monoamine oxidase (MAO) inhibitors. Nervousness, restlessness, insomnia, headache, nausea, and hypertension may be side effects of phenylpropanolamine.

Bulk-producing agents, such as methylcellulose, expand the stomach and provide a sense of fullness. The same effect can be produced by drinking 2 to 3 glasses of water before each meal.[7] Bulk-producing agents have a laxative effect.

### Behavior modification for weight control

The purpose of behavior modification is to help the person achieve the change in eating and exercise patterns that is necessary if weight reduction is to be maintained. Behavior-modification programs may be offered by health clinics, self-help groups, or by commercial programs. Group sessions are more effective.

The technique of behavior modification for weight control is based on four approaches[33]:

1. Self-monitoring of eating behavior
   a. Purpose is to increase dieter's awareness of calories consumed and associated eating behaviors
   b. Recording of all food/fluids consumed and the time and circumstances related to eating (daily log)
2. Control of environmental stimuli for eating
   a. Elimination of enticements to eating; for example:
      1. Eliminating snacks around the house
      2. Avoiding reading or watching TV while eating
   b. Replacement by positive stimuli; for example:
      1. Eating only at the table
      2. Using special dishes for eating
3. Teaching to enhance behavior change in eating to decrease intake
   a. Putting fork down between bites
   b. Taking smaller bites
   c. Eating chewy rather than soft foods to prolong the eating period but not increase the intake
   d. Drinking water with meals
4. Rewards for progress
   a. Short-term rewards: points or coins directed toward long-term goals or a small treat
   b. Long-term rewards: special big treat, such as new wardrobe or travel

The therapist's emphasis should be on what the individual has chosen as the outcome of the weight-reduction plan.

## Facilitating Weight Gain

Persons who are underweight or have inadequate nutritional stores need encouragement to eat the right nutrients and calories. Motivating a person with anorexia to eat can be a challenge. Interventions that can correct the cause lead to improved appetite. Determining the person's likes and dislikes, providing an environment conducive to eating, and providing several small meals

**TABLE 6-8 Guidelines for Decreasing Dietary Fats and Cholesterol**

| FOOD GROUPS | USE | DECREASE |
|---|---|---|
| Meat | Fish, skinned poultry, lean cuts of meat | Fatty meats, sausages, hot dogs, cold cuts |
| Milk products | Skimmed or 1% milk, low-fat cheeses, and low-fat yogurt | Whole milk, whole-milk yogurt, natural cheeses, sour cream, frozen dairy desserts, whole-milk ice cream |
| | Egg whites | Egg yolks |
| Fruits | All fruits | Fruits cooked in pies, desserts |
| Vegetables | All vegetables | Butter or sauces added to vegetables |
| Bread/cereal | Low-fat crackers and cookies, angel food cake, homemade baked goods with limited saturated fats | High-fat crackers and cookies, commercially baked goods, foods made with saturated fats |
| | | Refined breads/cereals; egg noodles |
| | Whole grain breads/cereals; rice, pasta | High-fat sauces on pasta |
| Fats/oils | Canola, corn, safflower, sesame, soybean, and sunflower oils | Coconut and palm kernel oil; butter, saturated fat, bacon fat |
| | Seeds and nuts (limited) | Coconut |

From Expert Panel: *Arch Intern Med* 148:36-69, 1988.

rather than three large meals a day may facilitate an adequate nutritional intake.

If the patient can eat, a high-calorie, high-protein diet is indicated to provide energy and amino acids for tissue building. The diet is essentially a normal one with added protein and supplementary high-calorie feedings. New types of liquid feedings are available. High-protein diets may be contraindicated if a patient has liver disease, because protein catabolism takes place in the liver. For persons with protein-calorie malnutrition, enteral and parenteral feedings are frequently necessary.

## Facilitating Control of Dietary Fats and Cholesterol

As cited previously (see p. 147), adults should know their cholesterol levels and should take measures to decrease the level if it is greater than 200 mg/dl. The usual American diet is 10% to 15% of kcal ***higher*** in total fats (10% higher in saturated fats, 5% higher in monounsaturated fats, and slightly higher in polyunsaturated fats) than the recommended levels. The cholesterol level of the average American diet is ***two to two and one-half times*** that of the recommended level of less than 300 mg/day.[10] Therefore it is necessary for everyone to modify these intakes to the recommended levels (see p. 146). Guidelines for decreasing fats and cholesterol are listed in Table 6-8.

Maintaining a low–saturated fat, low-cholesterol diet is not always easy because it involves deleting some well-liked foods, such as high-fat cheeses and cold cuts. Learning to eat a diet that is lower in saturated fats and cholesterol, as with other types of permanent diet changes, requires a ***change in eating behavior*** patterns (behavior modification). People need to know the differences among the types of fats, cholesterol and fat content of foods, and how to read food labels (p. 143).[20] For example, many producers of plant-based products advertise that their product has zero cholesterol; this is in fact true, but one must remember that cholesterol comes only from animal products.

Suggestions for decreasing or modifying fat intake include the following[14]:

1. Eat fish or shellfish at least twice a week; clams, scallops, and oysters contain less cholesterol than crab, shrimp, or lobster.
2. Eat chicken without skin. Light meat contains less cholesterol than dark meat. Trim away loose fat.
3. Eat only lean, well-trimmed meat; avoid marbled cuts of beef such as ribeye; use leaner cuts of meat such as round or tenderloin. Look for "lean" labels on meat packages. Pour off melted fat during cooking.
4. Broil, roast, or bake foods rather than frying.
5. Use low-fat dairy products.
6. Use tub margarines, which are lower in saturated fats than stick margarines.
7. Consider using substitutes, such as frozen egg substitute, cream-flavored powders, or cooking sprays.
8. Use non-fat or low-fat salad dressings in place of regular dressings (read labels carefully).
9. Use oils low in saturated fat, such as canola or safflower.

## ♦ EVALUATION

To evaluate the effectiveness of nursing interventions, compare patient behaviors with those stated in the expected patient outcomes. Successful achievement of patient outcomes to promote good nutritional status and weight control is indicated by the following:

1. Correctly describes foods within each food group and serving sizes of the recommended daily food guide.
2. Weighs no more than 20% above or below desirable weight (see Table 6-5).

**BOX 6-10 Benefits of Aerobic Exercise**

Sense of well-being
Enhanced coping with stress
Decreased anxiety or depression
More restful sleep
Maintenance of physiologic functioning at optimal level
Enhanced weight control
Decreased risk of osteoporosis
Decreased risk factors for coronary artery disease
Better control of hypertension and diabetes mellitus
Decreased risk of colon cancer
Assistance with reduction of addictive behavior (e.g., smoking, overeating, or drinking)

3. Gradually loses weight if planned (average of 0.5 kg [1 lb] per week).
4. Correctly describes ways to decrease dietary fats and cholesterol, especially if cholesterol is greater than 200 mg/dl.

## EXERCISE

Regular physical activity can help a person feel well, cope with stress, enhance normal body functioning, and decrease risk factors for some diseases. Physical activity and fitness is the first listed category of health promotion in *Healthy People 2000*.[31] When the 1990 objectives for physical activity and fitness were evaluated, it was found that the actual number of adults who participated in moderate daily activity or in vigorous exercise at least three times a week was far below the desired level.[24] Much health teaching and active promotion of exercise and fitness are necessary, therefore, if the following objectives for the year 2000 are to be met:

Increase to more than 30% the proportion of persons older than 6 years of age who engage regularly, preferably daily, in light to moderate activity for at least 30 minutes per day.

Increase to more than 20% the proportion of persons older than age 18 who engage in vigorous physical activity for more than 20 minutes, 3 or more days a week.

Although a positive trend has developed toward increased exercise in recent years, most adults live a sedentary life-style. People are aware that activity or mobility is necessary for health, but many still do not make the effort to increase their activity level. Persons who do not value exercise as a means of maintaining optimal health often find excuses for not participating in a planned exercise program on an ongoing basis. Exercise does imply effort; if exercise is not valued, the effort is not made.

### BENEFITS OF EXERCISE

A program of regular exercise can have both psychologic and physiologic benefits (Box 6-10). A physically fit person also tends to have greater endurance and faster recovery time (return to resting rate), which can contribute to more rapid recovery from illness.

**BOX 6-11 Physiologic Effects of Exercise**

**MUSCULOSKELETAL SYSTEM**

Maintains muscle strength
Maintains joint flexibility
Maintains endurance (tolerance to continue an activity)
Increases mineral content of bones

**NEUROSENSORY SYSTEM**

Maintains coordination
Maintains orientation to environment

**CIRCULATORY SYSTEM**

Maintains a more constant average workload on heart
Maintains normal blood pressure regulatory adjustment to transient position changes
Promotes venous return through contraction of muscles
Contributes to improved cardiovascular health: lower total cholesterol levels, with increased high-density lipoprotein and decreased low-density lipoprotein values

**RESPIRATORY SYSTEM**

Contributes to ease of breathing
Provides stimulus to deep breathing and aeration of alveoli
Provides movement of secretions

**GASTROINTESTINAL SYSTEM**

Maintains elimination through muscle activity and visceral reflex patterns
Encourages the person to heed defecation reflex

**URINARY SYSTEM**

Promotes urine formation
Promotes complete emptying of bladder

Exercise is important *regardless of age.* Some elderly persons believe they are too old to begin an active fitness program, but these programs are possible even for those with chronic illness. The fitness program is individually planned and based on the person's interests, capabilities, and limitations.

Physically, exercise enhances cardiovascular fitness, endurance, muscle strength, flexibility, and weight control. It has positive effects on the musculoskeletal, neurosensory, circulatory, respiratory, gastrointestinal, and urinary systems (Box 6-11).

### CLASSIFICATION OF EXERCISE: AEROBIC/ANAEROBIC

**Aerobic exercises** are those activities that are supported by aerobic metabolism (the breakdown of carbohydrates and fats to carbon dioxide and water in the presence of oxygen, i.e., the Krebs cycle). Aerobic exercise is characterized by activities that involve large muscle groups and that are performed in a rhythmic and continuous nature for more than 15 minutes. Examples of aerobic exercise include brisk walking, jogging, running, bicycling, swimming, skating, cross-country skiing, and aerobic dancing.

**Anaerobic exercises** involve anaerobic metabolism (the breakdown of glucose to lactic acid in the absence of oxygen). This occurs at the beginning of any exercise period and with high-intensity activities in which the available oxygen is used up and the anaerobic pathways are then used to provide the necessary additional energy. Anaerobic exercise is characterized by bursts of energy of short duration. Types of exercises include weight lifting and competitive sports, such as football, soccer, basketball, baseball, volleyball, and hockey. Greater benefits to overall physical fitness and well-being are achieved with aerobic rather than with anaerobic exercises.

## RECOMMENDATIONS FOR PHYSICAL FITNESS

### Preliminary Testing

There is a difference of opinion concerning who needs a physical examination before beginning an exercise program. The American Heart Association recommends that all persons should have a physical examination within 2 years of starting an exercise program. The American College of Sports Medicine suggests those not needing to do so are the apparently healthy persons younger than the age of 45 years without significant cardiac risk factors (history of hypertension, hypercholesterolemia, diabetes mellitus, cigarette smoking, or abnormal resting electrocardiogram, or family history of coronary heart disease).[18] Any person with a history or signs of medical illness or who is 45 years of age or older should have a preliminary physical examination with exercise testing.

Exercise testing can determine the maximum amount of oxygen that can be used by the body—that is, maximum oxygen consumption ($MVO_2$). The maximum aerobic capacity to provide the most cardiovascular benefits is 60% to 80% of $MVO_2$. This correlates with 70% to 85% of the maximal heart rate.[2] *Maximal heart rate* is the rate measured at the highest exercise intensity attained by exercise testing. *Target heart rate* is the desirable rate for achieving the most aerobic benefits, or 70% to 85% of maximal heart rate. Other methods of measuring exercise-intensity capacity include the percentage of maximum MET levels (metabolic equivalent of the task, a measure of oxygen consumption) or subjective measurement of perceived exertion using rate of perceived exertion (RPE) charts.[19]

If the maximal heart rate has not been calculated from exercise testing, it can be *estimated* by subtracting age from 220. For example, the target heart rate for a 20 year old would be 70% to 85% of 200 (220 − 20), that is, within a range of 140 to 170 beats/min. This method underestimates the target heart rate by about 15%.[3]

### Types of Exercises

**Isometric exercise**

With **isometric exercises,** opposing muscles are contracted, thus increasing the tone of the muscle fibers but not changing muscle length or moving the joints. The purpose of these exercises is to *maintain muscle strength and tone.* There is very little effect on cardiovascular or respiratory conditioning, and isometric exercises may not be easily tolerated by persons with coronary artery disease. Examples of isometric exercises for hospitalized patients are quadriceps-setting exercises and gluteal sets to maintain muscle strength in the thighs and buttocks for walking.

Persons doing isometric exercises should be taught to *exhale while exerting effort.* Many persons tend to hold their breath while bearing down (Valsalva's maneuver). This increases intrathoracic pressure, causing a decrease in venous return to the heart. When the breath is then released, the intrathoracic pressure decreases, causing a large surge of blood return to the heart and increasing the cardiac workload. Exhaling while exerting effort can prevent the Valsalva effect.

**Isotonic exercises**

With **isotonic exercises,** muscle length changes and joint movements occur. There is less muscle tension than with isometric exercises. Isotonic exercises *maintain and increase muscle strength.* Aerobic exercises are one form of isotonic exercises. Some types of isotonic exercises for the hospitalized patient include moving and turning in bed, ambulating, and moving arms and legs against light resistance.

### Exercise Prescriptions: Frequency, Intensity, Duration

Exercising should be done on a regular basis; one of the year 2000 national objectives is "at least 20 minutes of exercise three times a week by all persons."[31] The American College of Sports Medicine (ACSM) recommends the following[3]:

| | |
|---|---|
| Frequency | 3 to 5 days per week |
| Intensity | 60% to 90% of maximal heart rate |
| Duration | 20 to 60 minutes of *continuous* aerobic exercise |

There should be no more than 2 days between each exercise period. Persons at low fitness levels and those in weight-reduction programs should exercise at least 5 days a week.[3]

An *intensity* of 60% to 90% of maximal heart rate is a wide range suitable for most persons. In most healthy persons, less than 60% of maximal heart rate will not provide sufficient aerobic benefits. The suggested target heart rate to achieve the most benefits for the average healthy person is 70% to 85%. The pulse should be counted after about 3 to 5 minutes of continuous exercise, using either a radial or carotid pulse.[19] The heart rate must be counted quickly during a pause in the

**BOX 6-12 Signs of Overexertion**

Angina, chest pain, or discomfort
Irregular heart rate
Persistent shortness of breath after exercise
Dizziness
Excessive fatigue
Nausea or vomiting
Muscle or joint swelling
Abnormal muscle soreness

exercise regimen because it rapidly begins to slow down when exercise is reduced. A 10-second pulse count (multiplied by 6) is recommended.[3]

*Duration* is related to intensity; the greater the intensity, the less is the duration required to achieve cardiovascular conditioning. For example, high-intensity aerobic dancing achieves about the same effect in 30 minutes that brisk walking may achieve in about 60 minutes.

The better conditioned the person, the longer is the duration that can be tolerated. Therefore persons in *low physical conditioning* should begin exercising at a lower intensity for the duration that can be tolerated. If the target heart rate is exceeded or the recovery period extended, the exercise is too strenuous. As conditioning improves, intensity and duration are increased until the desired target heart rate is achieved. With inactivity there is a loss of 20% conditioning within 2 to 3 weeks and up to 50% loss by 1 month.[3] Return to physical activity after inactivity means starting at a lower level and working up gradually. A person who has symptoms should stop exercising and seek health advice (Box 6-12).

### Phases of Exercising

Any exercise program should consist of the following three phases:

1. Warm-up phase (5 to 10 minutes): range of motion (ROM) and stretch exercises to increase flexibility, decrease muscle injury, and ready the cardiovascular system. Examples of activities: ROM of shoulder, knee bends, twisting side to side, stretch to touch toes, raise arms over head and bend side to side, put one foot forward and bend that knee while stretching other leg.
2. Aerobic exercise phase (20 to 60 minutes): performed continuously at target heart rate.
3. Cool-down phase (5 to 10 minutes): a slowing down of activity using large muscles, such as walking slowly or pedaling without resistance. Heart rate should slow down gradually to usual level.

## EXERCISES FOR ELDERLY PERSONS

It is important that elderly persons, even frail persons, perform some exercises to prevent loss of strength and flexibility. Increased activity in this group results in decreased risk of coronary heart disease, fewer osteoporotic fractures, fewer depressive signs and symptoms, and decreased mortality.[32] Young elders may be able to continue previous patterns of exercising by lowering their heart rate target to 60% to 75%. If they can participate in special group exercises planned for their abilities, they may gain added benefits of increased social interactions and expanded interests. Exercises can be performed in standing, sitting, or lying-down positions. Persons in wheelchairs can do upper-body exercises. Aged or frail persons can do exercises that use slow easy movements for full joint range of motion, as well as light muscle strengthening such as leg lifts or walking. (Suggestions for exercise programs for elderly persons can be found in reference 12.)

## EXERCISES FOR CHRONICALLY ILL PERSONS

Exercises often are prescribed for *rehabilitation* of persons with chronic illness, such as for coronary heart disease, chronic obstructive pulmonary disease (COPD), diabetes mellitus, obesity, hypertension, peripheral vascular disease, and osteoarthritis. Exercising has been shown to increase the person's social activity, increase toleration to activities of daily living (ADLs), increase appetite, decrease fear of exercise, decrease anxiety, and promote adjustment to disability in persons with chronic illness.[3]

The exercise programs are especially tailored to each person's needs and abilities. Duration, intensity, and frequency of exercises are modified. Exercises are begun slowly at a low intensity, but at greater frequency. As tolerance to activity increases, duration and intensity are increased. Brisk walking, cycling, and swimming often are fairly well tolerated.

*Obese* persons have special problems and are susceptible to lightheadedness and fainting during exercise sessions. Bicycle and other weight-supported activities (such as swimming or water aerobics) are recommended to minimize orthopedic problems and to encourage patient participation.

Isometric and high-intensity exercise are *not* recommended for persons with *hypertension* because of blood pressure increases during these activities. Antihypertensive medications also may affect the person's response to exercise (Box 6-13). For persons with *peripheral vascular disease,* the intensity of exercises must be balanced between moderate discomfort and the prescribed target heart rate. A recommended prescription for these patients is to exercise twice a day for a minimum of 5 days a week.[3]

Persons with *osteoarthritis* should avoid excessive stress on arthritic joints but should exercise to a slight pain level to maintain maximum range of motion. Water-based exercises are good for persons with arthritis because the joints are supported. Special exercise prescriptions for persons with *coronary heart disease,*

**BOX 6-13 Effects of Antihypertensive Medications With Exercise**

**Diuretics** Hypokalemia with dysrhythmias
**Beta blockers** Hyperkalemia, hyperuricemia
**Vasodilators** Reflex tachycardia, angina
**ACE* inhibitors** No effects
**Calcium channel blockers** Alter heart rate and hemodynamic variables (differs among drugs)
**Centrally acting** Hypotension, dizziness, syncope
**Peripheral alpha blockers** No effects

Modified from American College of Sports Medicine: *Guidelines for exercise testing and prescription,* ed 3, Philadelphia, 1986, Lea & Febiger.
**ACE,* Angiotensin-converting enzyme.

*COPD,* and *diabetes mellitus* are discussed in appropriate text chapters.

## ENHANCEMENT OF SUCCESS IN EXERCISING

Getting started is probably the biggest hurdle in developing a regular exercise program. The following are some suggestions:

1. Identify types of physical activity that are most preferable. If you like what you are doing, then you are more apt to continue doing it. Exercise should be pleasurable.
2. Develop a weekly plan that sets *specific time periods* for the activity, which is based on desires and daily schedule. For example, it may be easier to exercise before or immediately after work or during a lunch period. Once you are at home and relaxed, it is often more difficult to get up and get going. Scheduled exercises are more likely to be carried out than just planning three times a week.
3. Begin the activity for short periods at a low level; then increase time and effort toward the desired goal. If you do too much initially and ache or become overtired, you are more apt to give up the activity.
4. Share the activity with others; you are more likely to continue the activity if other persons are involved. Doing exercises at home alone on a regular basis requires considerable willpower to continue for any period of time. Get a friend to walk with you; the time goes faster and is more enjoyable if socialization occurs concurrently. Some community agencies have scheduled aerobic classes such as low-impact aerobics or water exercises that are fun. If you pay for the class, you are more likely to attend to get your money's worth.
5. Set small goals toward meeting the long-term goal. Achievement of small goals increases feelings of self-esteem. Reward yourself when you achieve each goal, such as each time you add an additional mile to your walk.
6. If for some reason, such as illness, you have had to stop your exercise program, start back with the activity at a lower level than when you ended. Muscle strength and tone are lost with only a short absence of activity. Then work toward achieving your desired level.

# SLEEP AND REST

A healthy life-style requires more than eating the correct type and amount of food and exercising regularly. Activity must be balanced with rest to provide energy for physical and mental activities. Sleep is the most important form of rest; quantity and quality of sleep are good indicators of the general state of wellness.

## SLEEP

### Physiologic Patterns of Sleep

**Sleep** consists of two different physiologic states: (1) **non–rapid eye movement (non-REM) sleep,** which consists of four stages and is characterized by *light sleep* (stages I and II) and *slow-wave* or *deep sleep* (stages III and IV); and (2) **rapid eye movement (REM) sleep** during which most dreaming occurs. There are cycles of non-REM and REM throughout the night, with most of the slow-wave sleep occurring in the first third of the night and most REM sleep in the last third. During *non-Rem sleep,* respirations are deep and slow, heart rate is regular and slow, eyes show occasional slow movement, and muscle movements are decreased from wakefulness. During *REM sleep,* respirations and heart rate are variable, eyes show rapid movement, and muscle movements are almost absent although twitches may occur; brain blood flow and oxygen consumption increase.

### Theories of Sleep

Why do we need sleep? Despite all the research on sleep, its precise function is not known. There are, however, two major theories concerning the function of sleep, conservation of energy and recuperation/restoration.

The *conservation of energy* theory suggests that the energy spent during the day is balanced by low-energy demands during slow-wave sleep. Research has shown that sleep deprivation is followed by increased amounts of slow-wave sleep.[29]

The more popular theory suggests that sleep is a period of *recuperation* or *restoration.* Physiologic signs supporting this theory are that (1) catabolism is decreased and anabolism is increased during slow-wave sleep, (2) growth hormones are released at night during slow-wave sleep and people sleep more during periods of increased growth, and (3) protein synthesis and adenosine triphosphate (ATP) concentrations increase during sleep. Slow-wave sleep therefore appears to be important for macromolecular synthesis and REM sleep for maintaining synaptic connections and cognitive functions.[29]

Other theories regarding the function of sleep include its role in consolidation of memory, binocular vision, thermoregulatory evolution, and routine cell maintenance. A newer theory suggests that instead of one sleep center, different parts of the brain sleep at different times and that the purpose of sleep is for maintenance of vital groups of nerve cells.[23]

### Sleep Requirements

The *amount* of sleep individuals require varies with age. At the beginning of life the newborn sleeps about 22 hours a day; this amount decreases rapidly during the first year to about 14 hours a day, including naps. Most young children require about 11 to 12 hours a day, the amount decreasing to about 8 or 9 hours a day in older children. Adults generally sleep about 7 to 9 hours a day, although some can get along well with only about 5 hours a day, whereas others may require more than 9 hours a day. Elderly persons tend to sleep less at night but nap more frequently during the day. This information provides only *averages;* there is considerable variation within age-groups. Most persons know how many hours of sleep they require to feel rested and restored of energy.

*Type* of sleep also varies with age. Infants have the highest percentage of REM sleep; the ratio of REM to non-REM changes from 50:50 in young children to 20:80 in adults. Elderly persons spend more time in light sleep and have less slow-wave and REM sleep. Because they sleep more lightly, elderly persons have a pattern of frequent awakenings during the night and may nap more during the day.

Not all persons have the same sleep patterns. Some persons fall asleep quickly, awaken early, and feel at their highest energy peak early in the day. Other persons take longer to fall asleep and their peak energy period occurs later in the day. Both patterns are "normal." Having difficulty going to sleep or waking up frequently (other than in elderly persons) is termed *insomnia;* this is discussed in Chapter 18.

Sleep patterns can be affected by *drugs,* including hypnotic drugs, antianxiety drugs, ethyl alcohol, and anorectic agents. *Hypnotic drugs,* which are taken for insomnia, suppress REM sleep; when the drug is withdrawn, there is a rebound in REM sleep, with vivid dreams and frequent awakenings. Anxiety from REM rebound may lead the individual to take increasingly larger drug doses, with the potential for drug abuse.[7] *Antianxiety drugs* and *alcohol* can have the same effects if taken in large enough doses. Some *anorectics* (drugs used to control obesity) have the same effects as amphetamines, but with fewer side effects; one side effect includes insomnia from increased wakefulness. Lack of sleep leads to changes in non-REM/REM sleep patterns. *Over-the-counter sleep aids* contain antihistamines, which tend to cause drowsiness. Some persons find these drugs helpful but many do not.

### Measures to Enhance Sleep

Measures other than taking drugs are recommended to enhance sleep and include the following suggestions:

1. Follow a consistent schedule for retiring and arising to promote regulation of circadian rhythms.
2. Exercise daily but avoid strenuous exercise near bedtime. Exercise contributes to physical fatigue and promotes readiness and quality of sleep; overfatigue, however, may produce insomnia.
3. Read or watch a relaxing television show before going to sleep, but avoid stimulating or anxiety-producing activities. Relaxation promotes falling asleep, but strong mental stimulation or worry leads to insomnia.
4. Avoid heavy meals shortly before bedtime; gastric discomfort may interfere with sleep.
5. Bedtime snacks may help some persons because feelings of hunger may interfere with going to sleep. Some persons find drinking milk helpful; milk contains L-tryptophan, which is a sleep-inducer.[27]
6. Caffeine-containing drinks should be avoided late in the day by most persons; caffeine is a stimulant, promoting wakefulness.
7. Provide an environment conducive to sleep: relative darkness, room at comfortable temperature, and noise kept to a minimum. Eye shades and ear plugs may be helpful for eliminating excessive light or noise that cannot be controlled.
8. Morning napping does not usually interfere with night sleep, but late-day naps can disturb sleep.
9. Avoid thinking about the previous day's activities or planning for the next day when trying to go to sleep. Imaging, light fantasizing, or relaxation exercises (see Chapter 7) may provide sufficient relaxation to induce sleep.

## REST

Rest is essential to provide energy for physical and mental activities. When we are "rested," we are ready to take on life's activities. In a sense, the opposite of being rested is being tired, either physically or mentally, or both. (Fatigue is discussed in Chapter 14.) The problem with the concept of rest is that it means different things to different people. There is very little research concerning rest, other than the aspect of sleep.

*Physical rest* is fairly easy to understand. ATP is the fuel used for all types of activities; because it is not stored in large amounts in the body, it must be produced continuously. During physical activity there is an increased demand for ATP; if supply does not keep up with demand, the person must rest to replenish the supply. If we are tired from physical activity, we can get off our feet, relax the large muscles, and give the body time to replenish ATP levels.

Rest also includes *mental rest,* the readiness to pursue activities and enjoyment of life. People report many different activities they find relaxing, such as forms of entertainment and participating in sports, gardening, taking walks, and reading. A healthy life-style therefore includes participating in activities (other than job-related) that the person enjoys and finds refreshing.

## CONCLUSION

Promoting a healthy life-style is an important part of medical-surgical nursing in all settings. The nurse also needs to consider serving as a role model for a healthy life-style: eating a well-balanced, low-fat, low-salt, high-fiber diet, controlling weight, avoiding smoking, supporting a healthy environment, participating in a planned exercise program, obtaining sufficient sleep and rest, and reducing stress.

### QUESTIONS TO CONSIDER

- Select a health behavior that you do not follow. How does this behavior relate to your definition of health? What factors can you identify that may be barriers to the desired behaviors?
- In what ways do your eating behaviors differ from the seven recommended dietary guidelines? What measures could you take to meet or maintain each of the guidelines?
- Why would it be ineffective to tell an overweight person to lose weight?
- How often do you engage in 15 minutes or more of aerobic activities each week? What changes, if any, could you make to meet recommendations for health promotion?

### CRITICAL THINKING ACTIVITIES

- Nancy is 35 years old and mother of four children. She works full-time and finds it very difficult to meet financial obligations on a monthly basis. She often buys TV dinners and fast-food items as a matter of convenience, since she works more than 40 hours/week. The children get home from school at different hours and are hungry at different times. Nancy doesn't particularly like to cook, since she is often tired after work. Differentiate between actual and possible perceived barriers to changing the family eating habits.
- Rebecca is 65 years old and complains of insomnia. She states she has difficulty falling asleep and wakes up frequently through the night. Make 3 or 4 suggestions that may facilitate sleep for Rebecca. Develop several questions that would help assess possible causes of Rebecca's insomnia.

## CHAPTER SUMMARY

### HEALTH PROTECTION

- Factors that influence health-promoting behaviors include perceptions about health and self, demographic factors, influence of family or friends, family patterns of health care, availability of opportunities to engage in health-promoting behaviors, and actual or perceived barriers to health-promoting actions.

### HEALTH PROMOTION

- Health-promoting strategies include health teaching, modeling, self-confrontation, and behavior modification.

### NUTRITION

- All persons need the same nutrients throughout life; the amounts required vary in predictable patterns.
- Excess dietary supplementation of vitamins and minerals may cause harm; continued intake at levels from 10 to 100 times the RDA is associated with chronic toxicity.
- Good nutrition requires a balanced complement of protein and calories. Protein not needed for synthesis is used for fuel.
- Persons of similar body composition and sex have similar basal energy requirements; the total energy requirement varies depending on physical activity.
- Three types of nutritional guidelines are nutrient standards (recommended dietary allowances—RDAs), food guides (the food guide pyramid and food exchange lists), and dietary guidelines.
- A recommended dietary guideline includes (1) eating a variety of foods, (2) maintaining ideal weight, (3) avoiding too much fat, saturated fat, and cholesterol, (4) eating foods with adequate starch and fiber, (5) avoiding too much sugar, (6) avoiding too much sodium, and (7) consuming alcohol in moderation.
- New food labels provide standard serving portions, standardized information on total calories, calories from fat, cholesterol, sodium, total carbohydrate, dietary fiber, sugars, protein, vitamins A and C, calcium, and iron.
- Normal body mass index (BMI) is 20 to 25 kg/m$^2$; obesity refers to BMI >27.5 kg/m$^2$ and underweight <20 kg/m$^2$.
- Guidelines for fat intake include total fat less than 30% of calories, saturated fat less than 10%, monounsaturated 10% to 15%, and polyunsaturated up to 10%.
- Guidelines for cholesterol awareness and actions include having cholesterol measured every 5 years, knowing one's cholesterol level, and taking steps to lower an elevated cholesterol level.
- Dietary fiber provides bulk to help stimulate intestinal peristalsis, binds dietary cholesterol to prevent absorption, and is a factor in reducing risk for cancer of the colon. A daily intake of 20 to 30 g of dietary fiber is recommended.
- Recommendations for decreasing sodium intake include eating foods low in sodium, preparing foods without adding salt, and not adding salt at the table.
- Medications may affect nutritional status; food can, in turn, affect absorption of oral medications.
- The dietary food guide is useful for a quick dietary assessment and for use in health teaching.

**EXERCISE**

- Methods of weight reduction include diet, exercise, and behavior modification.
- Exercise enhances cardiovascular fitness, endurance, muscle strength, flexibility, weight control, sense of well-being, sleep, and ability to cope with stress. Exercise also has a positive effect on the body systems, decreases risk factors of coronary artery disease, provides better control of hypertension, and assists in reducing addictive behaviors.
- Aerobic exercises are those that involve large muscle movements in a continuous and rhythmic manner for more than 15 minutes. Anaerobic exercises are high-intensity activities that use up available oxygen and are supported by anaerobic pathways.
- A recommended exercise program consists of 20 to 60 minutes of continuous aerobic exercise at 60% to 90% of maximal heart rate, three to five times a week. The exercises should have a 5- to 10-minute warm-up and cool-down periods.
- Activity tolerance of healthy active adults can be assessed by a pulse rate of 70% to 85% of maximal heart rate during exercise that returns to normal within 5 minutes.

**SLEEP AND REST**

- Sleep is the most important form of rest; the amount required varies with age. Sleep patterns can be affected by disturbances in circadian rhythms, overfatigue, worry, hunger or gastric discomfort, caffeine, uncomfortable sleeping environment, and evening naps.
- Drugs that can affect sleep patterns include hypnotics, antianxiety drugs, anorectics, and alcohol.

## REFERENCES

1. Ahmed FE: Effect of nutrition on the health of the elderly, *J Am Diet Assoc* 92:1102-1108, 1992.
2. Allan JD: Exercise program. In Bulichek GM, McCloskey JC, editors: *Nursing interventions,* ed 2, Philadelphia, 1992, WB Saunders.
3. American College of Sports Medicine: *Guidelines for exercise testing and prescription,* ed 3, Philadelphia, 1986, Lea & Febiger.
4. American Dietetic Association: *Understanding food labels* [pamphlet], Chicago, 1993, The Association.
5. An end to label hype? *Consumer Rep* 57:32-33, 1992.
6. Butrum RR, Clifford CK, Lanza E: NCI dietary guidelines: rationale, *Am J Clin Nutr* 48:888-895, 1988.
7. Clark JB, Queener SF, Karb VB: *Pharmacologic basis of nursing practice,* ed 4, St Louis, 1993, Mosby.
8. Collier J: Good and bad news on health, *Plain Dealer* (Cleveland), p. E-6, Sept 14, 1993.
9. Curtas S, Chapman G, Meguid MM: Evaluation of nutritional status, *Nurs Clin North Am* 24(2):301-312, 1989.
10. Expert Panel: Report of the National Cholesterol Education Program Expert Panel on detection, evaluation, and treatment of high blood cholesterol in adults, *Arch Intern Med* 148:36-69, 1988.
11. Expert Panel: Summary of the second report of the National Cholesterol Education Program (NCEP) Expert Panel on detection, evaluation, and treatment of high blood cholesterol in adults, *JAMA* 269(23):3015-3023, 1993.
12. Flatter K, Wilhite B, Reyes-Watson E: *Exercise activities for the elderly,* New York, 1988, Springer.
13. Food labels: new and improved? *Consumer Rep* 57:654-655, 1992.
14. Greene JM, Feldman EB: Physician's office guide to a lipid-lowering diet, *J Am Coll Nutr* 10:443-452, 1991.
15. Groer MW, Shekleton ME: *Basic pathophysiology,* ed 3, St Louis, 1989, Mosby.
16. Heaney RP: Effect of calcium on skeletal development, bone loss, and risk of fractures, *Am J Med* 91 (suppl 5B):23S-28S, 1991.
17. Koplan JR et al: Nutrient intake and supplementation in the United States (NHANES II), *Am J Public Health* 76:287-289, 1986.
18. Levine GN, Balady GJ: The benefits and risks of exercise training, *Adv Intern Med* 38:57-79, 1993.
19. Maynard T: Exercise. II. Translating the exercise prescription, *Diabetes Educ* 17(5):384-393, 1991.
20. McCann BS: Promoting adherence to low-fat, low-cholesterol diets: review and recommendations, *J Am Diet Assoc* 90: 1408-1414, 1990.
21. Molloy D: Now is the time to advocate wellness, *Am Nurse* 23(4):4, 1991.
22. Pender NJ: *Health promotion in nursing practice,* ed 2, East Norwalk, Conn, 1987, Appleton & Lange.
23 Powers M: A new theory on why we sleep, *Plain Dealer* (Cleveland), p. E-1, Sept 13, 1993.
24. Progress toward achieving the 1990 national objectives for physical fitness and exercise, *MMWR* 38(26):449-453, 1989.
25. Riggs L, Melton LJ III: The prevention and treatment of osteoporosis, *N Engl J Med* 327:620-627, 1992.
26. Schectman G et al: Dietary intake of Americans reporting adherence to low-cholesterol diet (NHANES II), *Am J Public Health* 80:698-703, 1990.
27. Schirmer MS: When sleep won't come, *J Gerontol Nurs* 9:16-20, 1983.
28. Sempos CT et al: Prevalence of high blood cholesterol among U.S. adults, *JAMA* 269(23):3009-3014, 1993.
29. Shapiro CM, Flanigan MJ: Function of sleep, *Br Med J* 306 (6974):383-385, 1993.
30. Tierney LM et al: *Current medical diagnosis and treatment,* ed 32, East Norwalk, Conn, 1993, Appleton & Lange.
31. US Department of Health and Human Services, Public Health Service: *Healthy people 2000: national health promotion and disease prevention objectives,* Washington, DC, 1990, US Government Printing Office.
32. Wagner EH et al: Effects of physical activity on health status of older adults. I. Observational studies, *Annu Rev Public Health* 13:451-468, 1992.
33. White JH: Behavioral intervention for the obese client, *Nurs Pract* 11:27-34, 1984.
34. Williams SR: *Essentials of nutrition and diet therapy,* ed 6, St Louis, 1994, Mosby.
35. Year 2000 national health objectives, *MMWR* 38(37):629-623, 1989.

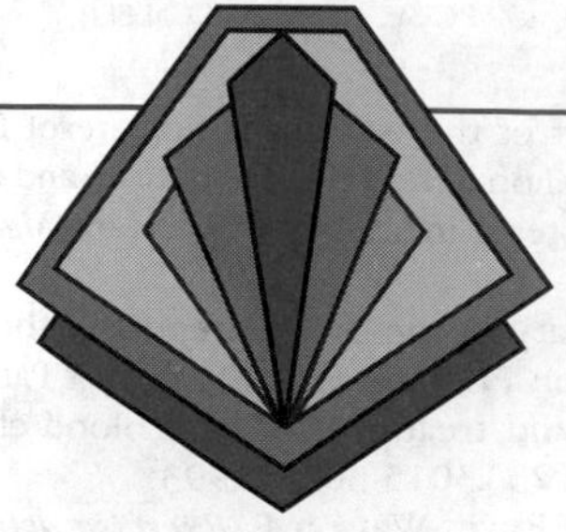

C H A P T E R 7

# Stress, Stressors, and Stress Management

*Virginia L. Cassmeyer*
*Pamela Holsclaw Mitchell*
*Patricia A. Betrus*

## CHAPTER OBJECTIVES

***After studying this chapter, the learner should be able to do the following:***

1. Define adaptation, stress, and coping.
2. Differentiate between stressors and stress response.
3. Explain the relationship of dealing with stressors to optimal functioning and growth.
4. Describe the neuroendocrine response to stressors.
5. Describe behavioral responses to stressors.
6. Describe types of coping strategies.
7. Identify assessment parameters of anxiety.
8. Describe interventions for persons with anxiety.
9. Describe approaches to crisis intervention.
10. Describe methods of stress management.

## KEY TERMS

adaptation
aggression
anxiety
autogenic training
Benson's relaxation response
biofeedback
coping
crisis
defense mechanisms
denial
depression
general adaptation syndrome (GAS)
local adaptation syndrome (LAS)
maladaptation
meditation
neuroendocrine response
progressive relaxation
rational-emotive therapy
regression
stress
stress management
stressor
stress response
systematic desensitization
withdrawal

*Stress, adaptation,* and *coping* are words commonly used in both lay and professional literature to refer to problematic biophysical-chemical or psychosocial-cultural situations. These words also are used to describe the body's response to or the ways of dealing with problematic situations. These terms are entrenched in nursing literature to the extent that it is now axiomatic that a major function of nursing is to help people cope with stressors and adapt to stressful situations.

Yet, when attempting to define these terms to study and understand them better, we find that there is no scientific consensus as to their meanings. Thus how can these terms be used professionally to understand the nature of human problem-solving behavior? Why have they come to such prominence in the helping professions? Is there a set of related phenomena that these terms describe, or should they be abandoned as jargon?

The position taken here is that these terms are in the literature to stay and that they describe phenomena regarding the ways human beings deal with life's changing events. Each term provides a general reference point to approach common experiences of persons interacting with their environments even though precise definitions acceptable to most investigators have been elusive. At best, one may recognize common themes that emerge from the multiple perspectives of those who have tried to define these terms precisely.

**Stress** is a general term describing patterns of psychologic and physiologic responses to a variety of emotional and physical stimuli. Stress responses occur when the ordinary capacity to adapt to life's demands is taxed. Stress can thus be seen *as a subset of the concept adaptation*—or the processes of maintaining psychobiologic equilibrium during interaction with the environment. **Coping** comprises those strategies by which adaptation to ordinary or extraordinary environmental demands is accomplished. In this chapter the common themes that have emerged from the scientific study of stressors, stress, adaptation, and coping are presented. These themes are then applied as a framework for management.

## ADAPTATION

Human beings can be conceptualized as open systems that respond to stimuli from the internal and external environments.[49] This process of interaction can be termed **adaptation.** In this context, adaptation has neither positive nor negative values. However, many prefer to use the term in a positive sense to mean the process of interaction with the environment that promotes homeostasis or dynamic equilibrium and growth. The process that leads to inadequate functioning is then termed **maladaptation** or *ineffective adaptation.* Within the nursing field, the concept of adaptation is most closely associated with Roy.[40]

Human beings adapt biologically, psychologically, emotionally, and socially. The goal of biologic adaptation is survival or stability of internal processes. When the ability to maintain this equilibrium is lost, pathophysiologic disorders result. Psychologic and emotional adaptation is directed toward preservation of self-identity and self-esteem. The person adapting in these modes is mentally healthy, whereas maladaptation leads to mental illness. Social adaptation depends on the sociocultural expectations of the society of which the person is a member. A maladaptive or socially deviant behavior in one society may be acceptable in another.

Although any changing environmental stimuli can initiate the need for adaptation, stressors create major adaptive demands for humans. As shown in Figure 7-1, the neuroendocrine responses, coping behaviors, defense mechanisms, and behavioral responses are major strategies available for meeting adaptive demands associated with stressors. Nurses help patients adapt at many levels:

1. To identify and remove stressors that require adaptive demands
2. To support healthy strategies that meet the adaptive demands of stressors
3. To use higher-level defense mechanisms
4. To deal with the psychologic responses to stressors
5. To develop alternative coping behaviors or behavioral responses to stressors
6. To deal with the illnesses that result if adaptation is not effective

## STRESS

### HISTORICAL PERSPECTIVE

The term **stress** has been used colloquially for centuries to refer to mental and emotional strain or pressure. In physics, stress has a precise mechanical meaning—the force put on an object. The resulting deformation or response is designated as *strain.* Selye[44] was the first to use the term *stress* in a biologic context—the nonspecific response of the body to a variety of noxious stimuli. He termed the stimulus the **stressor.** Initially, Selye[42] avoided the term *stress* because of its common use in connoting emotional turmoil. However, as he came to see that many strong stimuli were capable of provoking the general adaptation syndrome, he postulated that emotional stimuli were equivalent to physical stressors (e.g., heat, cold, trauma) in evoking the response, and he began to use stress as synonymous with the general adaptation syndrome.[44]

The notion of a general integrated and mutually interacting biologic and psychologic response to a variety of environmental stimuli was not unique to Selye. In fact, his work was preceded by the philosophic writings of James,[21] who proposed that the perception of visceral responses to emotional events *was* the emotion; by the experiments of Cannon,[6] who observed the similarity of

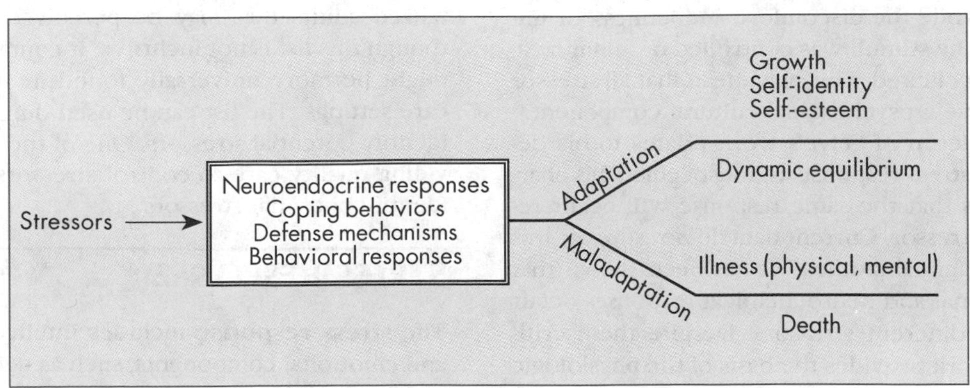


**FIGURE 7-1** Responses to stressors may lead to adaptation or maladaptation.

physiologic responses of the sympathetic nervous system during a variety of emotional states; and by Jacobsen,[20] who documented responses of the sympathetic nervous system and skeletal muscles to emotional states.

## GENERAL ADAPTATION SYNDROME

Selye's work led him to label the nonspecific response to various agents as the **general adaptation syndrome (GAS).**[44-46] GAS became known as the stress syndrome and was viewed by Selye as having three stages:

1. *The alarm reaction,* during which protective resources are mobilized
2. *The stage of resistance* that occurs when the full syndrome is in place and the stressor is being controlled
3. *The stage of exhaustion* that occurs when the body is not able to control the stressor

Selye[43,46] also proposed that the hormones produced during the GAS were responsible for the "diseases of adaptation." The stress response or GAS involves the sympathetic branch of the autonomic nervous system and the pituitary and adrenal glands. Selye also described the **local adaptation syndrome (LAS),** which is the response to a locally applied stimulus. The inflammatory process is an example of the LAS.

Some major criticisms of Selye's work should be noted. First, in his early work Selye did not acknowledge that psychologic events could serve as stressors, although his later writings included this acknowledgment.[45] The work of various persons as early as the 1950s[18] revealed that the GAS could be elicited in response to psychologic stimuli.

Another criticism of Selye's work was the idea that stimuli that serve as stressors were stressors for everyone. The work of Lazarus[26] and Cox[9] pointed out that a stimulus must be perceived as a stressor before the GAS response is elicited. Important in this perception process is the analysis of the stimulus in terms of the person's resources and the perception of the stimulus as controllable or uncontrollable.

Another important factor in relation to psychologic and emotional influences on physiologic stressors is that in some experiments[30-33] in which physical stressors were induced while the discomfort, suddenness, or unpleasantness of the stimuli was controlled or minimized, the GAS was not elicited. This may mean that all stressor stimuli must have a psychosocial-cultural component.

One last criticism of Selye's work relates to his description of the stress response as nonspecific. This characteristic means that the same response will occur regardless of the stressor. Current data do not support this assumption. In animal studies[28] it has been shown that different hormonal and neurochemical responses occur in response to different stressors. Despite these criticisms, Selye's work provides the basis of the physiologic response that can be elicited by stressors and an appreciation of the various stimuli that may serve as stressors in many persons.

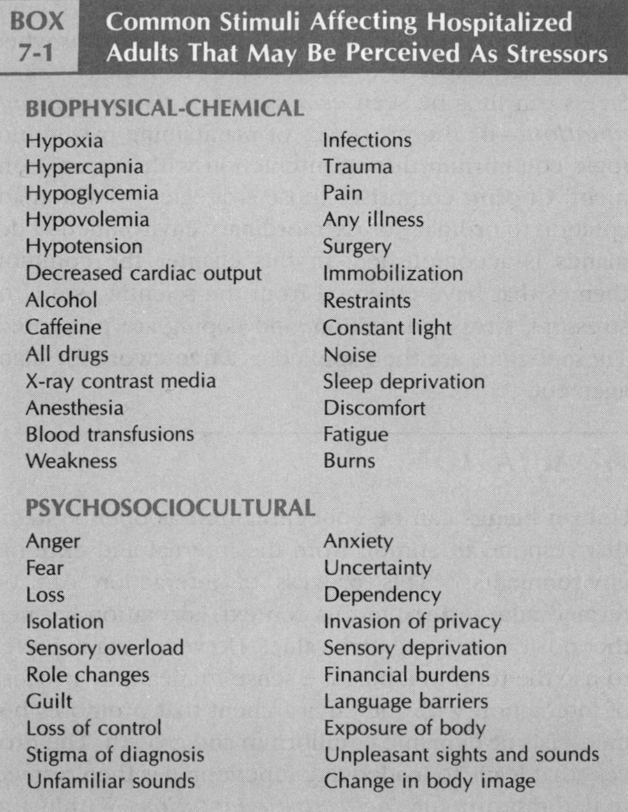

**BOX 7-1 Common Stimuli Affecting Hospitalized Adults That May Be Perceived As Stressors**

**BIOPHYSICAL-CHEMICAL**

| | |
|---|---|
| Hypoxia | Infections |
| Hypercapnia | Trauma |
| Hypoglycemia | Pain |
| Hypovolemia | Any illness |
| Hypotension | Surgery |
| Decreased cardiac output | Immobilization |
| Alcohol | Restraints |
| Caffeine | Constant light |
| All drugs | Noise |
| X-ray contrast media | Sleep deprivation |
| Anesthesia | Discomfort |
| Blood transfusions | Fatigue |
| Weakness | Burns |

**PSYCHOSOCIOCULTURAL**

| | |
|---|---|
| Anger | Anxiety |
| Fear | Uncertainty |
| Loss | Dependency |
| Isolation | Invasion of privacy |
| Sensory overload | Sensory deprivation |
| Role changes | Financial burdens |
| Guilt | Language barriers |
| Loss of control | Exposure of body |
| Stigma of diagnosis | Unpleasant sights and sounds |
| Unfamiliar sounds | Change in body image |

### STRESSORS

Many different studies have shown that stressors can be biologic, physical, chemical, social, developmental, cultural, or psychologic stimuli.[3,13,19,52] Stressors can vary from an alarm clock that does not go off on time, to an approaching deadline, to the onset of the common cold in a relatively healthy person, to major burns over 50% of the body. The stressors that nurses deal with vary depending on the patient population. Nurses in outpatient settings, in home health care, or in discharge planning may focus more on daily irritations and primary health care problems. Nurses working with patients during the acute or critical stages of illness may deal with more severe physiologic stressors.

Box 7-1 lists some common stimuli affecting hospitalized adults that may be perceived as stressors. Although this list is not inclusive, it contains stressors that might be more universally found in acute and critical care settings. The list can be used during assessment to identify potential stressors. One of the first steps in providing quality care to control stressors is to be able to identify potential stressors.

# STRESS RESPONSE

The **stress response** includes intellectual, behavioral, and emotional components, such as decision-making activities, withdrawal, and anger, as well as physiologic components. The physiologic components involved in the stress response include the central nervous system,

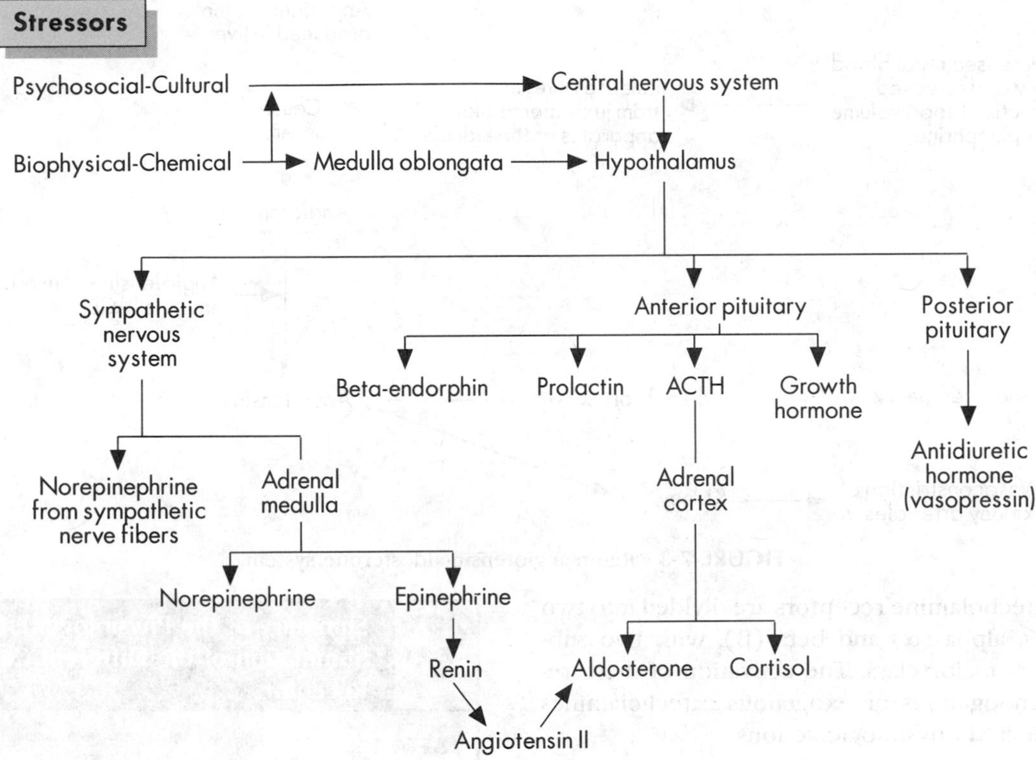


**FIGURE 7-2** Physiologic components involved in the neuroendocrine response to stressors.

the hypothalamus, the sympathetic nervous system, the anterior and posterior pituitary glands, the adrenal medulla, and the adrenal cortex. The physiologic components and their secretions (hormones and catecholamines) are responsible for the **neuroendocrine response** to stressors. As discussed earlier in this chapter, not all of these components will necessarily be involved in the response to every stressor; however, to provide holistic nursing care, the nurse must know the effects of stimulation of each of these components of the neuroendocrine response to stressors. Understanding the response is critical to (1) identify persons at high risk for impaired ability to deal with stressors, (2) understand how prolonged or repeated stressors can result in disease, and (3) understand how the neuroendocrine component of the stress response eventually can become a threat to health.

The physiologic components of the neuroendocrine stress response are diagramed in Figure 7-2. Stressors—either perceived at the level of the central nervous system or on an unconscious level by baroreceptors, chemoreceptors, or glucoreceptors, which transfer information to the medulla oblongata—serve as the afferent input. This information eventually is forwarded to the hypothalamus, which coordinates the response. The hypothalamus activates the sympathetic nervous system and the anterior and posterior pituitary glands. The adrenal medulla is an extension of the sympathetic nervous system and thus is activated when the sympathetic nervous system is stimulated.

The hypothalamus stimulates the anterior pituitary gland by releasing hormones such as corticotropin-releasing hormone (CRH), growth hormone–releasing hormone (GHRH), and prolactin-releasing hormone (PRH). Some anterior pituitary hormones will be released when the hypothalamus diminishes its secretion of inhibiting hormones. For example, dopamine acts as a prolactin-inhibiting hormone (PIH), and thus prolactin secretion is increased when dopamine secretion is decreased.

Adrenocorticotropic hormone (ACTH), which is released from the anterior pituitary gland, stimulates the release of cortisol from the adrenal cortex. The adrenal cortex also releases the hormone aldosterone in response to ACTH secretion. However, the major control of aldosterone secretion is the renin-angiotensin system, which is shown in Figure 7-3.

The last endocrine gland activated by the hypothalamus is the posterior pituitary gland. The posterior pituitary gland, when stimulated, releases antidiuretic hormone (ADH) or vasopressin. The effects of stimulation of the sympathetic nervous system, anterior and posterior pituitary glands, adrenal medulla, and adrenal cortex are mediated by the catecholamines and hormones released by the nervous system or the glands.

## CATECHOLAMINES

The catecholamines, epinephrine and norepinephrine, act by stimulating receptors unique to them. The receptors are located on various cells throughout the

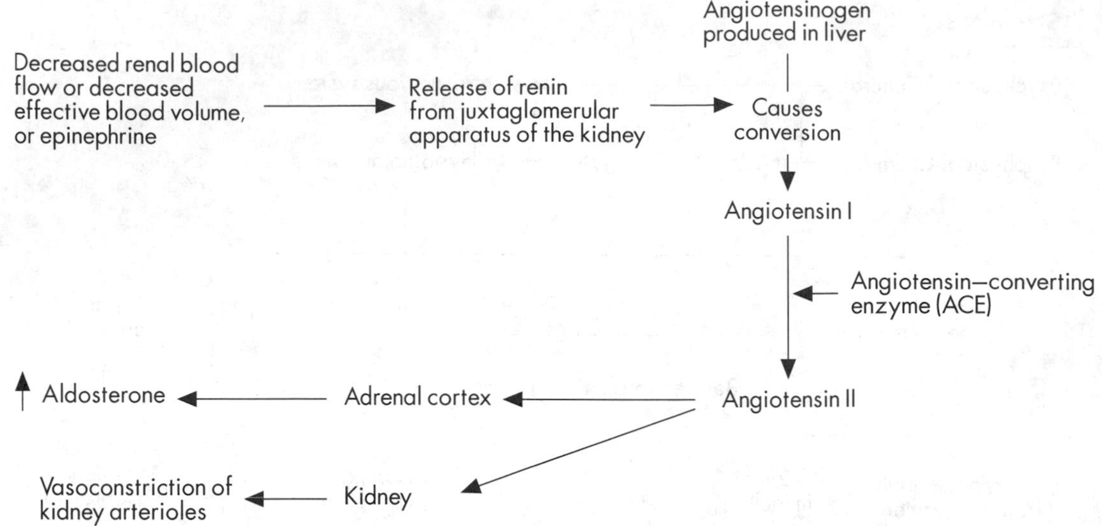


**FIGURE 7-3** Renin-angiotensin-aldosterone system.

body. The catecholamine receptors are divided into two major classes, alpha (α) and beta (β), with two subclasses of each major class. The activation of these receptors by endogenous or exogenous catecholamines results in selected physiologic actions

Stimulation of $\alpha_1$-adrenergic receptors is associated primarily with excitation or stimulation, and stimulation of $\alpha_2$-adrenergic receptors is primarily associated with relaxation or inhibition. Stimulation of $\beta_1$-adrenergic receptors primarily is associated with stimulation of cardiac activity, and stimulation of $\beta_2$-adrenergic receptors is associated with all other effects related to beta receptors, such as bronchial dilation. (See Box 7-2 for a more detailed description of functions associated with stimulation of specific receptor types.)

During the neuroendocrine response to stressors, both norepinephrine and epinephrine are released. Norepinephrine binds primarily to α-adrenergic receptors, whereas epinephrine activates both α-adrenergic and β-adrenergic receptors. The effects of catecholamines during the stress response then are due to a combination of the actions of both catecholamines and activation of several different receptors. The effects seen with the release of catecholamines during the stress response are summarized in Table 7-1.

**BOX 7-2 Summary of the Physiologic Effects of Stimulation of the Different Catecholamine Receptors**

**BETA 1**

Increased heart rate (chronotropic), increased contractility of atria and ventricles (inotropic), increase in automaticity and conduction of ventricular electrical system; lipolysis

**BETA 2**

Dilation of the smooth muscles of the coronary, skin, skeletal muscle, and pulmonary arterioles and systemic veins; relaxation of bronchial smooth muscle; decreased motility of stomach and intestines; relaxation of bladder muscle; secretion of renin; increased gluconeogenesis and hepatic and muscle glycogenolysis; increased secretion of insulin and glucagon

**ALPHA 1**

Contraction of smooth muscles of coronary, skin, mucosa, skeletal muscle, cerebral, pulmonary, mesenteric, renal, and salivary glands; and arterioles and systemic veins; Contraction of radial muscle of eye (mydriasis); contraction of sphincters of gastrointestinal tract; contraction of sphincter of bladder and urethra; ejaculation; contraction of pilomotor muscles; increased secretion of localized sweat glands

**ALPHA 2**

Decreased motility of gastrointestinal tract; decreased insulin secretion; platelet aggregation; possibly decreased secretion of intestinal tract

Data from Granner D. In Murray RK et al, editors: *Harper's biochemistry,* ed 21, New York, 1988, Lange; McCance KL, Huether SE, *Pathophysiology: the biologic basis for disease in adults and children,* ed 2, St Louis, 1994, Mosby; Shoemaker W et al, editors: *Textbook of critical care,* ed 2, Philadelphia, 1989, WB Saunders.

## CORTISOL

Cortisol is released from the adrenal cortex under the control of ACTH and CRH. Cortisol has major effects on glucose, protein, and fat metabolism and on fluid and electrolyte balance; it also has antiinflammatory and immunosuppressant effects. It enhances the activity of other hormones and works with epinephrine, glucagon, and growth hormone in elevating the blood glucose level. Cortisol also augments the effects of other hormones and catecholamines in maintaining cardiac output and blood pressure. Detailed information of the effects of cortisol on the body is presented in Box 7-3.

Cortisol's effect on metabolism, body fluids, and electrolytes, as well as its permissive effect on other hormones, seems logical in response to the body's needs in the presence of stressors; however, the antiinflammatory and immunosuppressant effects seem illogical in that they appear to be more detrimental than helpful. Munck, Guyre, and Holbrook[35] have suggested that the major

**TABLE 7-1 Systemic Effects of Epinephrine and Norepinephrine Released During the Neuroendocrine Response to Stressors**

| ORGAN | PHYSIOLOGIC EFFECTS | ASSESSMENT FINDINGS |
|---|---|---|
| Brain | Blood vessels dilated; blood flow increased; metabolism increased | Patient more alert or restless |
| Eyes | Dilation of pupils | Pupils dilated; patient appears startled |
| Heart | Coronary blood vessels dilated; increased heart rate; increased contractility; cardiac output and stroke volume increased | Tachycardia, increased cardiac output |
| Vascular system | Constriction of arterioles to skin, mucosa, kidneys, and abdominal viscera; increased constriction of veins; ischemia with result of tissue death may occur | Skin pale, cool; urine output decreased; toe temperature decreased. With ischemia of kidneys, fluid retention, increased blood urea nitrogen, and increased serum creatinine level are seen. With ischemia of GI tract decreased bowel sounds |
| Lungs | Dilation of pulmonary vascular bed; bronchodilation; increased rate and depth of respiration; increased $O_2$ uptake and increased $CO_2$ excretion | Tachypnea; hyperventilation; respiratory alkalosis (decreased $PCO_2$ and increased pH) |
| Gastrointestinal tract | Decreased motility and secretion; decreased production of mucus; decreased blood flow to GI tract | Blood in GI secretions (NG or stool) |
| Exocrine pancreas | Decreased enzyme, fluid, and electrolyte secretions | |
| Endocrine pancreas | Decreased insulin secretion | Elevated blood glucose |
| Liver | Increased gluconeogenesis and glycogenolysis; decreased glycogen synthesis; decreased glucose uptake | Elevated blood glucose |
| Adipose tissue | Increased lipolysis and fatty acid production | Increased serum triglycerides and lipoproteins |
| Skeletal muscle | Increased muscle glycogenolysis; decreased glucose uptake; increased contractility | Generalized muscle tension |
| Skin, sweat glands | Decreased blood flow; increased localized secretion of sweat; piloerection | Skin cool, pale, moist; goosebumps present |

**BOX 7-3 Systemic Effects of Cortisol Release During the Neuroendocrine Response to Stressors**

**METABOLIC EFFECTS**

1. Maintains blood glucose by increasing gluconeogenesis and decreasing glucose uptake by many body cells, particularly muscle
2. Increases protein catabolism, which provides substrate for glucose formation
3. Promotes lipolysis to provide alternative nutrient sources

**FLUID AND ELECTROLYTE EFFECTS**

1. Promotes sodium and water retention
2. Promotes potassium excretion

**ANTIINFLAMMATORY/IMMUNOSUPPRESSIVE EFFECTS**

1. Decreases eosinophils, basophils, monocytes, and lymphocytes in the circulation
2. Increases neutrophils (polymorphonuclear leukocytes) by movement from bone marrow and circulatory pools
3. Decreases leukocyte accumulation at inflammatory sites
4. Inhibits release of inflammatory substances (kinins, prostaglandins, leukotrienes)
5. Degrades collagen
6. Decreases scar tissue formation
7. Decreases lymphoid tissue mass, participation of T lymphocytes in cellular-mediated immunity, and production of interleukins

**BOX 7-3 Systemic Effects of Cortisol Release During the Neuroendocrine Response to Stressors—cont'd**

**MISCELLANEOUS EFFECTS**

1. Maintains emotional stability
2. Increases red blood cell formation
3. Possibly increases platelet formation
4. Increases gastric acid and pepsin production
5. Is permissive for other hormones and catecholamines (i.e., cortisol is necessary for the full functioning of some hormones and catecholamines), particularly in relation to effects of epinephrine and norepinephrine on blood pressure control, cardiac output, and metabolism

beneficial effect of cortisol release during the neuroendocrine response to stressors is to inhibit, or turn off, the body's protective response to stressors when it is no longer needed so that the response does not damage the body.

## ALDOSTERONE

Aldosterone primarily is released from the adrenal cortex in response to activation of the renin-angiotensin system as diagramed in Figure 7-3. Some aldosterone also is released in response to ACTH from the anterior pituitary gland. Aldosterone acts on the distal kidney tubule cells and causes reabsorption of sodium and water and excretion of potassium and hydrogen ions. Aldosterone helps to maintain vascular volume and blood pressure.

## ANTIDIURETIC HORMONE

Antidiuretic hormone (ADH) or vasopressin is released from the ends of axons of hypothalamic neurons that terminate in the posterior pituitary gland. ADH acts on the distal tubules and collecting ducts of the kidneys and causes an increase in the size of pores within the cell membrane so that water can be reabsorbed. Water is reabsorbed in response to the osmotic gradient established by the difference in osmolality of the tubular fluid and the medullary interstitial fluid. ADH controls the osmolality of body fluid. ADH in high concentration can result in arteriole vasoconstriction and can help to increase blood pressure. Vasopressin also stimulates the release of ACTH and thus influences the pituitary-adrenocortical response to stressors.[14]

## OTHER PITUITARY HORMONES

*Endogenous opiates* (β-endorphins) are released as part of the neuroendocrine response to stressors. These endogenous opiates may be involved in the pituitary-adrenocortical response to stressors,[14] and they are known to increase tolerance to painful stimuli. Release of endogenous opiates in stressful situations may account for the analgesic effect present in persons who experience major traumas.

*Growth hormone* is released from the anterior pituitary during the neuroendocrine response to stressors. Hypoglycemia and strenuous exercise are two stressors associated with an increase in growth hormone. Growth hormone helps to provide nutrients for the energy needs of various cells and tissues during the stress response. Growth hormone decreases glucose use and is an insulin antagonist; thus it helps to maintain the blood glucose level, which provides glucose for the nervous tissue. Growth hormone increases lipolysis, free fatty acid levels, and ketone formation, which furnish nutrients for various tissues, such as skeletal and cardiac muscles.

*Prolactin*[33] also is released in the presence of certain stressors. The function of prolactin in relation to dealing with stressors is unknown.

## EFFECTS OF STRESS RESPONSE

The catecholamines, ACTH, cortisol, ADH, endogenous opiates, and growth hormone released during the neuroendocrine response to stressors provide through their various actions a total body response that allows the individual to cope with stressors or to withdraw from the stressors *(fight or flight response).* The total body response includes the following:

1. Increase in blood levels of substrates necessary for energy—glucose for nervous tissue and fatty acid substrates for other tissues
2. Increase in oxygen uptake to provide oxygen for metabolic processes
3. Maintenance of vascular volume and increase in cardiac function for transport of nutrients and oxygen to tissues and for removal of waste products
4. Increase in respiratory activity for the elimination of excessive carbon dioxide that will be produced while the person is coping with the stressor and for the delivery of more oxygen
5. Increase in muscle activity and alertness that might allow for flight from the stressor
6. Increase in blood flow to brain that might allow for critical decision making, activation of psychologic defense mechanisms, or problem solving

The intensity of the stress response depends on a combination of (1) intensity of stimulus, (2) duration of stimulus, and (3) perception of control over the stimulus.

### Intensity of Stimulus

Intense physical and psychologic stimuli such as trauma, forceful immobilization, and strong fear lead to stress responses in most human beings. Animal research has revealed a graduated multisystem response to graduated increases in intensity of the trauma.[41] A similar graded response is at least partially evident in human response to various traumas and surgical procedures. For example, the metabolic response to a burn over 40% of the body area is considerably greater than that to a hernia repair. The psychologic component (threat, fear, inescapability, lack of control) also is greater for the patient with a burn than for the person experiencing elective surgery.

### Duration of Stimulus

Some investigators have suggested that although most organisms may have similar emergency responses to acute and intense stimuli, ongoing stimuli may elicit different individual responses. The adaptive response of one organism to ongoing stimuli may either resemble or differ from the response of another organism. The works with colonies of mice by Henry and Ely is the most extensive long-term investigation of the physiologic responses of animals to their ordinary social interactions.[17] As these animals established their social dominance hierarchy, those who became the dominant animals exhibited primarily sympathetic–adrenal medullary activation, characterized biochemically by elevated catecholamine levels, behaviorally by muscular activity, and symptomatically by hypertension. In contrast, the animals at the bottom of the social hierarchy showed primarily a pituitary-adrenocortical response: elevated corticosteroid levels, withdrawn behavior, and ultimately enlarged adrenal glands and stomach ulcers.

The animals who challenged the dominant animals had profiles midway between the two groups. Although this study is not intended to suggest that socially dominant persons will become hypertensive, it does support the notion that in ordinary daily living, organisms, including human beings, tend to respond in a characteristic mode. This mode depends partially on genetic factors, social position, and learned modes of coping with or responding to everyday events.

### Perception of Control

Perception of control over a situation and relevant feedback regarding the effect of one's behavior on the stimulus appear to be potent factors regulating the multihormonal stress response. When a dominant animal from Henry's mouse colony was put into a colony in which dominance had already been established, the previously dominant mouse became submissive and its behavior and physiologic response became that of the submissive mice. One could argue that the mouse perceived itself as no longer being in control. Parachutists in training in Norway exhibited all the characteristic neuroendocrine stress responses before their first jump but rapidly returned to baseline values in subsequent jumps. Their subjective fear decreased as their sense of mastery and control over the task increased.[29] Weiss[54] presents an excellent summary of animal research demonstrating that control over aversive stimuli (shock) and relevant feedback regarding one's efforts reduced and even prevented pathologic physiologic stress responses in a variety of situations.

The concepts of hardiness and resilience in human beings have been shown to be important factors in maintaining health in stressful situations.[22,29] Perception of control over life situations is a key component of these concepts. Stress has been linked both in the popular press and in scientific literature with disease, presumably caused by prolonged or excessive physiologic responses to a variety of situations. It should be evident from the foregoing, however, that it is not the situations by themselves that create the stress response but rather the combination of psychologic appraisal and sense of control.[11,24] These concepts lead logically to the notion of coping with change: the perception and appraisal of some relevant but challenging situation and the psychobiologic responses emanating from that perception.[27,39]

## COPING

The definitions of *coping* are as many and varied as those for adaptation and stress. White[55] considers **coping** the *strategies* of adaptation—the means by which adaptation takes place. It often is defined as involving problem-solving efforts in situations that are perceived as being highly relevant to the individual and that tax adaptive resources.[27] Although many persons explicitly or implicitly consider coping to be primarily a cognitive process, some authors recognize the interrelationship between physiologic and cognitive responses to adverse circumstances. Levine, Weinberg, and Ursin[29] define the ultimate goal of coping processes to be reduction of physiologic activation, whereas Murphy[37] divides coping processes into coping I, the capacity to deal with the changing environment (action and cognition), and coping II, the capacity to maintain the internal environment.

In general, then, coping refers to *processes or skills that individuals use to deal with events, circumstances, or situations that are out of the ordinary.* It is an integrated psychobiologic process. The stimuli that elicit coping may arise in the external environment in the form of physical stimuli, interpersonal relationships, or community and international events. Similarly, stimuli may arise in the internal environment in terms of thoughts, feelings, and physical illness.

### GENERAL THEMES IN COPING

Coping processes enable us to learn from new situations some strategies that may be useful in the future, and they emerge from what has been learned in the past. Coping processes may thus be considered the major means for growth in the continual process of adaptation. When various perspectives in coping are evaluated, recurrent themes are evident: (1) coping stems from appraisal of relevant situations; (2) there is motivation to change; (3) information must be sought and used; (4) either action is practiced and tried or attitudes are changed; (5) there must be relevant feedback regarding coping efforts; and (6) coping takes place in a social context that defines appropriate and inappropriate coping and that transmits coping strategies from one generation to the next. People tend, over time, to develop coping styles, using strategies that have served them well in the past to reduce physiologic arousal and to meet the developmental challenges of maturation.

Coping strategies have been categorized as those involving direct action on oneself or on the environment or involving intrapsychic processes.[27] With direct action one may change the environment or oneself or in some way directly confront, avoid, or sidestep the situation out of which the need to cope arises. Intrapsychic processes are largely cognitive ways of changing the meaning of the situation or of dealing with the emotions that arise from the situation. Many investigators have found that those who are judged as coping most successfully with a variety of situations are flexible in using strategies from both categories rather than rigidly repeating the same strategies in each new situation.[53]

### COPING IN ILLNESS AND DISABILITY

Illness often represents a crisis that challenges comfortable coping styles. Chronic illness and physical disability demand the development of new coping skills. As with all coping, the individual's appraisal of the meaning of the illness and disability determines the extent to which these situations represent a crisis. However, the characteristics of a given illness or disability together with societal expectations of related behaviors add a new dimension to previously learned coping skills.

Adams and Lindemann[1] define four mechanisms fundamental to successful coping with the environment: movement, sensing, energy production, and cerebral integration. Impairment of any of these leaves an individual with a diminished capacity to cope with the environment and thus with a disability. All acute and chronic illnesses affect one or more of these fundamental functions and thus by their nature diminish the available capacity for coping. When experiencing acute or chronic illness, people have two sets of adaptive tasks, as defined by Moos[34]: general tasks, as in any life crisis, and illness-related tasks. The *general tasks* defined by many authors include maintaining a sense of personal worth or self-esteem, maintaining a reasonable emotional balance, maintaining or restoring relationships with significant persons, and preparing for an uncertain future. *Illness-related tasks* include dealing with pain and incapacitation, enhancing the recovery of body functions, dealing with the hospital environment, and developing adequate relationships with hospital personnel.

*Chronic illness* or *disability* imposes additional adaptive tasks.[51] These tasks include the prevention of medical crises, control of ongoing systems, carrying out treatment regimens, adjustment to changes in the disease course, maintaining self-esteem, obtaining funding for survival and ongoing treatment, adapting to or preventing social isolation, normalizing relationships with others, and confronting psychologic, marital, and familial problems (see Chapter 8).

A number of coping skills are as relevant to dealing with illness and disability as they are to general crisis situations. They relate to both action (problem-focused) or intrapsychic (emotion-focused) strategies.

*Action-focused strategies* include seeking relevant information about the illness or disability, learning procedures or tasks specifically related to it, setting concrete and realistic goals, and rehearsing alternative outcomes.[34] For example, a person faced with long-term hemodialysis for renal failure may cope with this major change in life-style and threat to life by learning everything possible about home dialysis, how others have managed, and the procedures that must be mastered to safely accomplish it. Information regarding expected energy levels, time required for dialysis, and duration between treatments may help the person set realistic goals for employment or education. Although the intended goal of home dialysis is to allow continued life and reasonable functioning, it is possible that the condition will worsen and less and less time off dialysis will be possible. Rehearsal of alternative outcomes is a strategy by which such possible outcomes are thought about, discussed, and possible options considered (e.g., kidney transplantation or death). Rehearsal is one strategy by which all of us "practice" behaviors for anticipated circumstances.

Other *intrapsychic strategies* include reframing the problem or finding some meaning or general purpose in it. If the event is explicable in the context of some larger purpose or understanding of life, distressing emotions may become more manageable and energy can be freed to focus on the problem itself. Simultaneously, one may be requesting reassurance and emotional support from others in the environment. Such support helps reaffirm a sense of personal worth in the face of major change.

There is no one specific or best way to cope with any given situation. What is useful to one individual may be inappropriate for another. The nature of the particular illness, the person's state of development, the social and cultural environment, and the physical and interpersonal resources available influence the style and effectiveness of coping strategies. In nursing, as in other helping relationships, it is most useful to assist a person to cope in ways that are congruent with previously established styles. Weisman[53] suggests seven simple questions that can provide a great deal of information about coping strategies:

1. What problems, if any, do you see this illness creating?
2. How do you plan to deal with them?
3. When faced with a problem you must do something about, what do you do?
4. How does it usually work out?
5. To whom do you turn when you need help?
6. What has happened in the past when you have asked for help?
7. What kinds of problems usually tend to get you upset or down?

These questions establish perception of the current problem, usual style of dealing with problems, sources of help and response to help, and recurrent trouble areas.

## DEFENSE MECHANISMS

Coping strategies are not entirely rational. Emotional responses to crises are dominant and interact with action responses at all points. *Emotional strategies* that serve to protect us, consciously or unconsciously, from severe distress or anxiety are often called **defense mechanisms.** Defense mechanisms are processes that evolve during personality development and serve to protect the personality, satisfy emotional needs, maintain harmony between conflicting tendencies, and reduce tension or anxiety by modifying reality to make it more acceptable. Defense mechanisms are compromise solutions.

There are two levels of defense mechanisms: those that are considered more primitive and those that are of a higher level (Box 7-4). Defense mechanisms are used by both mentally healthy and mentally unhealthy persons. In the mentally healthy, defense mechanisms are used less frequently, and those mechanisms of a more primitive kind are avoided. Defense mechanisms be-

**BOX 7-4 Defense Mechanisms**

**HIGHER LEVEL: LESS PRIMITIVE MECHANISMS**

**Repression**
Ideas painful to consciousness are forced into the unconscious.

**Suppression**
Thoughts or desires are consciously inhibited.

**Sublimation**
Energy of repressed tendencies is transformed and directed to socially acceptable goals.

**Identification**
Person assumes the personal qualities or elements of the personality of another.

**Compensation**
Person makes up, covers up, or disguises real or fancied inadequacies in another area.

**Displacement**
An emotion is transferred or displaced from its original object to a more acceptable substitute that is less threatening.

**Rationalization**
Plausible explanations are given to account for a belief or behavior motivated from unconscious sources.

**LOWER LEVEL: MORE PRIMITIVE MECHANISMS**

**Denial**
Intolerable thoughts, feelings, or wishes are disavowed; person refutes external elements of reality that are unpleasant or painful.

**Regression**
Person reverts to a pattern of behavior belonging to an earlier stage of development.

**Conversion**
Painful emotional experience is repressed and later is expressed in the form of a physical symptom.

**Projection**
That which is emotionally unacceptable within the self is rejected and attributed to others.

**Introjection**
Person absorbs the emotional attitudes, wishes, ideals, or personality of others into self; the aspirations and self-restraints of others are incorporated into the personality.

**Reaction Formation**
Person adopts attitudes and behavior that are opposites of the impulses to which he or she is reacting.

come pathologic when they are overused.

A defense mechanism is effective when it succeeds in easing intrapsychic tensions. When lower level defense mechanisms fail, a more pathologic process evolves, and the person exhibits psychiatric symptoms. All defense mechanisms are unconscious with the exception of suppression. The hospitalized patient frequently manifests two defense mechanisms, denial and repression, which are discussed in more detail in the following sections.

## DENIAL

One of the defense mechanisms used frequently in dealing with illness is **denial.** This mechanism occurs during the early stages of crisis after the initial stressful impact. Denial of the illness helps the person deal with increased tension by protecting the self from reality. The pattern used by the person is similar to games played by children when they close their eyes and believe no one can see them. "It's not there because I don't see it." That which cannot be perceived is therefore not painful.

During denial intolerable thoughts are disowned. The ego gets rid of unwelcome facts (such as an illness) while still retaining its faculty for reality testing. The person manifests denial by disowning any body changes. For example, patients with coronary disease may deny they have had heart attacks and blame their discomfort on indigestion. Patients may even deny the severity of the pain and act as though the pain were not present.

Denial works well for the person who has been independent and has a self-image of a strong, self-made individual or who views sickness as a sign of weakness. Denial can be complete or partial and includes a "splitting" of thoughts, feelings, and actions; for example, the patient may own the thoughts but deny the feelings.

Approaches that may be useful in working with the person exhibiting denial include the following:

1. Explore fears and anxieties underlying the denial.
2. Avoid direct confrontation of denial.
3. Assist person in controlling selected aspects of care.
4. Provide reassurance of the person's worth as a human being despite being in a dependent state.
5. Reinforce behaviors indicating reality acceptance.
6. Set limits kindly but firmly when denial behavior interferes with treatment.

## REGRESSION

**Regression** is a defense mechanism often seen in persons who are ill, because regression facilitates acceptance of the patient role. Regression makes a dependency relationship possible because of the individual's reversion to behavior patterns of an earlier level of development. Illness necessitates patients' placing themselves in the hands of competent others. They often become self-centered and concerned only with their own needs and interests. These interests focus on what is happening to the person and on their acceptance or rejection by caregivers. Often regression helps patients promote conservation of energy.

Approaches that may be useful in working with the person exhibiting regression include the following:

1. Explore the observable behavior with the patient.
2. Discuss the patient's goals.
3. Discuss the patient's unreadiness to attain goals, and revise as appropriate.

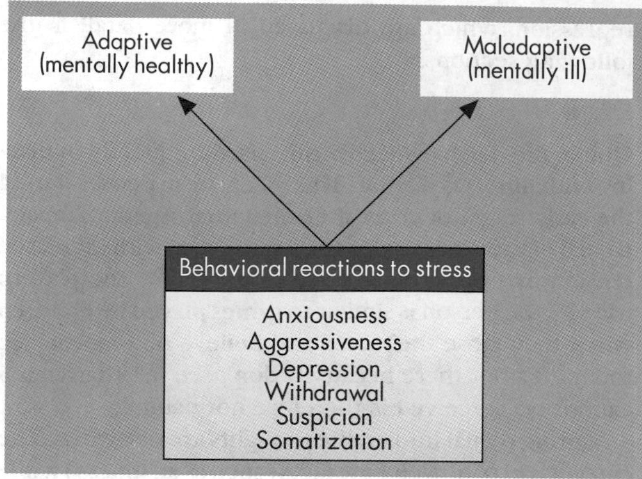


**FIGURE 7-4** Behavioral responses of persons experiencing anxiety from stress, such as illness, range from adaptive to maladaptive behavior.

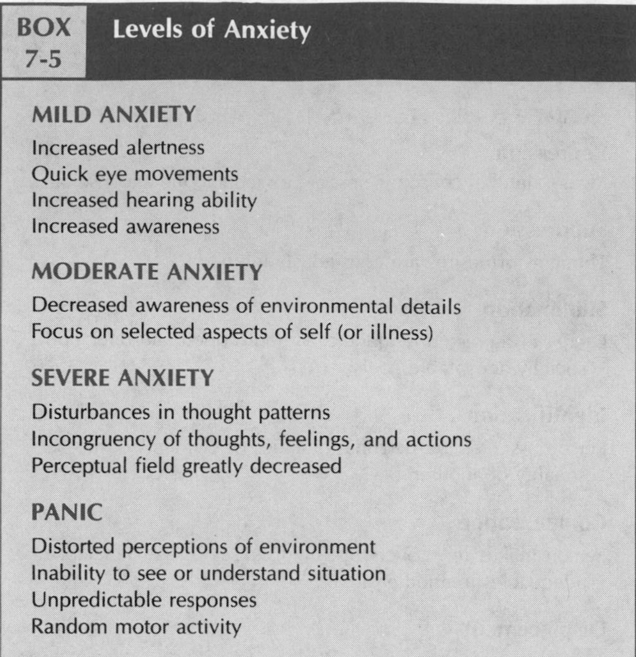

**BOX 7-5 Levels of Anxiety**

**MILD ANXIETY**

Increased alertness
Quick eye movements
Increased hearing ability
Increased awareness

**MODERATE ANXIETY**

Decreased awareness of environmental details
Focus on selected aspects of self (or illness)

**SEVERE ANXIETY**

Disturbances in thought patterns
Incongruency of thoughts, feelings, and actions
Perceptual field greatly decreased

**PANIC**

Distorted perceptions of environment
Inability to see or understand situation
Unpredictable responses
Random motor activity

## SPECIFIC BEHAVIORAL RESPONSES

Stressors and the stress response lead to behaviors that are either adaptive or maladaptive. Persons who display adaptive behavior are those who make appropriate use of their coping mechanisms and do not exhibit symptoms of psychologic disturbance. Those with maladaptive behavior are at the end of the spectrum (Figure 7-4); their psychiatric symptoms are a way of dealing with the increased stress. (For further information on maladaptive behavior consult a psychiatric–mental health text.) Anxiety and other common behaviors resulting from the stress of illness are discussed in the following section.

### ANXIETY

**Anxiety** is a psychologic response to stressors that has both physiologic and psychologic components. Anxiety is a feeling of dread or uneasiness from an unrecognized source. It differs from fear, which is a feeling of dread focused on a recognized source. Anxiety results when a person perceives a threat to the self either physically or psychologically (such as to self-esteem, body image, or identity). Anxiety manifests in different levels, ranging from mild to severe.[38] Box 7-5 presents the behavioral changes that are commonly associated with the different levels of anxiety. Awareness, which is heightened with mild anxiety, begins to decrease until the panic stage, in which perceptions of the environment become distorted. Persons can vacillate among the several kinds of anxiety. The level of anxiety engendered and its manifestations depend on the individual's maturity, understanding of need, level of self-esteem, and coping mechanisms.

Anxiety is a psychologic response that cannot be seen; it is only implied by actions. The state of *anxiousness* manifested by behavioral changes is communicated interpersonally. Highly anxious persons can transmit the sense of anxiousness to others; for example, very anxious patients can heighten family members' anxieties and vice versa.

Although the ego attempts to deal with anxiety through the use of defense mechanisms, certain degrees of anxiety are reflected in behaviors resulting from a discharge of energy necessary to restore equilibrium. These responses range from behavior that is adaptive to behavior that is considered, by our social standards, maladaptive (Figure 7-5). The types of behavioral reactions that occur are influenced by psychosocial-cultural factors, basic personality development, past experiences, values, and economic status. The conclusion that a person is demonstrating anxious behavior can be made when several signs of anxiety are present. With mild anxiety the signs are fewer and less prominent. Signs of anxiety are more overt in persons who are experiencing severe anxiety or panic.

Subjective data to be collected to determine the patient's anxiety level include the following:

1. Statements of feeling apprehensive, uncertain, fearful, out of control, helpless, or anxious
2. Statements of fears of unspecific consequences
3. Statements of feeling overexcited, rattled, distressed, or jittery
4. Statements of feeling tired and having difficulty sleeping

Data from the inital nursing history and the situation (such as proposed surgery, diagnostic tests) may provide clues to possible causes of anxiety.

Objective data related to anxiety are listed in Box 7-6; observations are made about the behavior in addition to the physiologic signs. The physiologic signs result

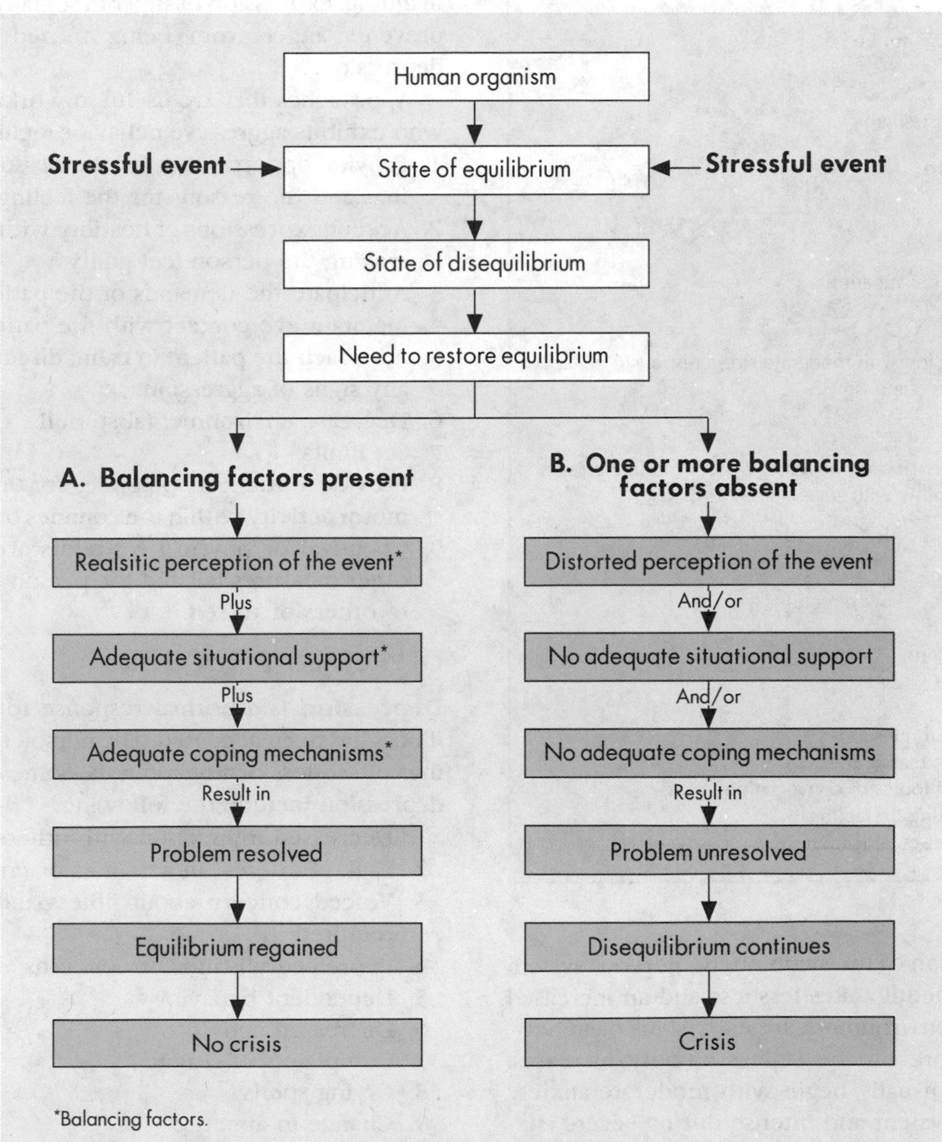


**FIGURE 7-5** Paradigm: effect of balancing factors in a stressful event. (From Aguilera DC: *Crisis intervention: theory and methodology,* ed 7, St Louis, 1994, Mosby.)

**BOX 7-6 Signs of Anxiety**

**PHYSIOLOGIC RESPONSE**

**Skin**
Pale or ashen, moist

**Pupils**
Dilated

**Respirations**
Deeper; may or may not be faster

**Pulse**
Increased rate and strength

**Body temperature**
Slightly increased

**GI tract**
Anorexia, nausea, constipation

**Urinary Tract**
Frequency of urination with moderate stress response, oliguria with severe stress response

**Motor System**
Restlessness, frequent hand movements with moderate stress response; immobility with severe stress response

**BEHAVIOR**

Decreased attention span
Decreased ability to follow directions
Increased acting out
Increased somatization

**INTERACTION**

Increased number of questions
Constant seeking of reassurance
Frequent shifting of topics of conversation
Avoidance of focusing on feelings
Focus on equipment or procedures

from the stimulation of the sympathetic nervous system and the adrenal medulla. Restlessness and an increased awareness of the environment are early signs of anxiety. Persons focus more on the self as anxiety increases. Physiologic signs usually begin with moderate anxiety and are more prevalent and intense during severe anxiety and panic.

Approaches that prove to be useful in working with persons exhibiting anxious behaviors include the following:

1. Decrease stimuli.
2. Maintain a calm approach.
3. Provide structure.
4. Explain situation.
5. Help patients use coping mechanisms to bring the anxiety level down to a controllable level.
6. Promote exploration of feelings.
7. Avoid asking patients to make choices.

## AGGRESSIVE BEHAVIOR

The person whose self-concept is threatened may respond with aggression, which is a way to feel less helpless and more powerful. **Aggression** involves acting in a hostile manner or launching an attack. Aggression is one way of handling anxiety. People are often angry at the loss of health status and question what is happening to them. They become irritable and uncooperative and may project their anger on others and become demanding. Expression of anger in socially acceptable ways prevents anger from being turned inward, causing depression.

Approaches that are useful in working with a person who exhibits aggressive behavior include the following:

1. Provide opportunities for the person to express feelings and the reasons for the feelings.
2. Accept expressions of hostility without retaliation or making the person feel guilty.
3. Anticipate the demands of the patient.
4. Maintain eye contact with the patient.
5. Approach the patient in calm, direct manner without any signs of aggression.
6. Decrease environmental stimuli.
7. Set limits.
8. Provide outlets, if possible, for increased psychomotor activity within the confines of the hospital unit.
9. Chemical or physical restraints are used only if all other measures fail and the person becomes harmful to others or to self.

## DEPRESSED BEHAVIOR

**Depression** is a normal response to illness, once the illness has been accepted. The person may describe feelings of sadness or unhappiness. Some common signs of depression include the following:

1. Decreased interaction with others
2. Lack of interest in activities or environment
3. Voiced concern about illness and amount of care required
4. Expressed wish for or concerns about dying
5. Dependent behavior
6. Decreased activity
7. Complaints of fatigue
8. Crying spells
9. Change in appetite
10. Change in sleep pattern

Any expressions about suicide should be taken seriously and the person referred for immediate counseling.

Approaches useful when working with a person exhibiting depressed behavior include the following:

1. Approach the patient in a serious mood.
2. Convey by action and communication an understanding of what the person must be feeling.
3. Help the person express feelings.
4. Convey acceptance of the right to feel sad.
5. Listen to the person so that the anger can be turned outward.

## WITHDRAWN BEHAVIOR

**Withdrawal** is commonly noted during illness. Withdrawal permits the person to conserve mental and physical energy needed to deal with stressors and to promote repair and restoration. Withdrawn patients usually do not pose many problems and are apt to be labeled "good" patients. They demand little from others and thus may be overlooked. Withdrawn patients regress more easily to earlier levels of behavior at which they can accept the patient role. They may have feelings of low self-worth.

Approaches that may be useful in working with the withdrawn person include the following:

1. Spend time with the patient to increase the person's self-worth—even if you are both silent.
2. Provide gentle encouragement to talk, express feelings, and relate to others.
3. Express acceptance of the withdrawn person.

## SUSPICIOUS BEHAVIOR

A sense of powerlessness or lack of control as a result of stressors and the stress response and anxiety may lead to behavior that reflects the patient's **suspiciousness**. Suspicious patients have difficulty with trust and may have had experiences in which they learned to distrust others. They often are suspicious of health care staff members, health care routines, medicines, and procedures. Overheard conversations may reinforce the person's suspicion that others are talking about him or her.

Approaches that may be useful in working with a patient exhibiting suspiciousness may include the following:

1. Let the person talk about concerns, but do not insist.
2. To promote trust, keep promises made to the person.
3. Avoid an overzealous approach, which may make the person more suspicious.
4. Provide explanations of procedures and routines so that the person knows what to expect.
5. Avoid whispering or talking softly within the person's hearing.

## SOMATIC BEHAVIOR

A familiar reaction to illness is one that can be called *flight into illness.* Patients somatize their concerns; that is, they have learned to express anxiety through complaints about a variety of physical symptoms. They may be preoccupied with body functions and feelings of pain. Vague complaints of backache, headache, or fatigue are expressed to legitimize the *attention needed.* Staff members often become angry at patients who use somatic behavior because of the frequent vague complaints. Staff members feel "caught" if they minimize the symptoms, because there is always the possibility that the complaints are truly connected with an illness. Staff guilt persists for some time if a complaining patient who was ignored is diagnosed as having a physical illness.

Approaches that may be useful for the person exhibiting somatic behavior may include the following:

1. Accept all symptoms and report them.
2. Spend time with the person and listen to physical complaints with some limit setting.

# STRESS MANAGEMENT THERAPEUTICS

Many strategies have been developed for stress management. These strategies utilize physiologic, cognitive, or behavioral techniques to diminish the effects of stress. Stress management as a therapeutic process has proliferated in the past two decades. Many of its techniques have been scrutinized carefully, and research documents the efficacy of these procedures in the management of stress.

The traditional mode of care in nursing has focused on providing direct care to patients. The direct care mode focuses on the nurse's knowledge and ability to identify and intervene to promote patient health. Patient health in this mode reflects the action and ability of the nurse to monitor, direct, and control the change process.

Effective stress reduction is a function of everyday living. It is under the control of the individual patient. Intervention by direct care is inadequate for stress reduction except for brief time-limited problems, such as control of anticipatory vomiting in cancer patients. For stress management to be effective in health maintenance and promotion, another mode of care must be implemented.

**Stress management** embraces a self-management orientation, emphasizing individual responsibility and participation in treatment.[23] The nurse's treatment goal is to provide the behavioral, cognitive, and psychophysiologic skills necessary for individuals to manage their own stress responses. In contrast to the traditional relationship between the patient and the nurse, which focuses on "compliance," patients who learn stress management strategies are active change agents. The nurse is cognizant of the limitations of his or her own therapeutic role. Ideally, the nurse is a proficient therapist who acts as an instigator, facilitator, and model to assist the patient to acquire relaxation and related stress management skills. The nurse assumes the responsibility for designing a structured, realistic program of change, but it is the patient's responsibility to implement and maintain the program.[25] Table 7-2 compares the use of direct care and self-management.

## GENERAL INTERVENTION STRATEGIES

General interventions for persons experiencing stressors include various activities, which are described here.

### Supporting Protective Mechanisms

Rest is essential to maintain energy supply for metabolic functions when a person experiences stressors and stress responses. The patient is kept comfortably warm but never overly warm, because overheating causes vaso-

**TABLE 7-2 Contrast of Direct Care and Self-Management According to Care Characteristics**

| | DIRECT CARE | SELF-MANAGEMENT |
|---|---|---|
| Locus of control | Professional dominance | Predominantly patient, but nurse takes responsibility for imparting knowledge, skills, and feedback |
| Problem awareness and assessment | Usually depends on clinical observations and judgment of nurse | Self-awareness and self-assessment, with guidance from nurse |
| Goal setting | Most care based on end goal determined by nurse | Negotiation of goals of both patient and nurse |
| Change agent | Action by nurse is medium by which changes are generated | Predominantly patient action or skills to achieve changes |
| Knowledge | Predominantly nurse; knowledge is premise for care | Knowledge is transmitted to patient to use for developing skills to generate care |
| Feedback | Not central for effectiveness of care | Crucial for effectiveness of care and promoting change |

From Kogan H, Betrus P: *Adv Nurs Sci* 6(4):55-73, 1984.

dilation and counteracts the arteriolar constriction necessary to ensure an adequate blood supply to vital organs.

Even minor stress responses can cause annoying discomforts such as backaches, generalized muscle tension, and headaches. These discomforts can act as additional stressors, and comfort measures such as back rubs, position changes, and back supports to relax muscles are indicated. Pain should be alleviated as much as possible, and noise and disturbance should be kept to a minimum. During severe stress responses, oral food and fluids may need to be withheld until nausea subsides and gastrointestinal tract activity returns to normal.

## Providing Structure

Structure decreases anxiety and is helpful for persons experiencing mild or moderate anxiety. Explanations are one method of providing structure. New experiences should be explained and, if possible, related to other familiar experiences. The higher the level of anxiety, the more simple the explanations need to be.

If patients are to have treatments or tests, they need to be given some ideas of what will be done, the preparations involved, and the reasons procedures are necessary. To remove water pitchers and inform patients that they cannot have any more water until after x-ray examinations can generate many anxious thoughts: "What x-ray examination?" "I wonder when it is" "What will it be like?" "It must be something special if I can't have any water." Anxiety caused by lack of knowledge reflects lack of consideration for patients' rights.

Explanations should be given in terms understood by patients, at appropriate times, and repeated as necessary. If patients are very anxious, repeated explanations are necessary because extreme anxiety reduces intellectual function, including memory. Until the problem is resolved, it is useful to give explanations to patients who are severely anxious or sedated or to those who have high temperatures or severe pain. Repetition often is required for older persons and children because of shorter attention spans or poor recent memory.

Time spent in giving explanations to relatives is not wasted. Not only does it relieve anxieties, which may be transmitted to patients, but it also saves having to untangle misinformation. Often family members are helpful in interpreting necessary instructions to patients in a manner that patients understand and accept.

## Promoting Exploration of Feelings

In most instances a large part of the nurse's work is to encourage patients to express anxieties, to help them identify the fears in their situations, to help them seek outlets for their fears and tensions, and to allay negative feelings whenever possible. Nurses provide opportunities for patients to talk, but they should not probe. There is a difference between prying into patients' thoughts and beliefs and eliciting information that aids in the understanding of behavior and in planning for care. Without seeming unduly curious, one usually can find topics of interest to patients that provide openings. A picture on the bedside table may be such an example. Nurses who listen with sincere interest and without making judgments may begin to gain insight into patients as persons. More important, patients may begin to speak about personal fears.

As soon as a patient begins to talk about feelings, nurses should encourage conversations, taking cues from what the patient offers. Nurses who feel inadequate or anxious may cut off conversations. For instance, if a patient says, "You know, I don't think I'll ever get to see my little boy again," a common response is, "Oh, don't say that, certainly you will; you're going to be all right"—when the patient very well may not be all right. A better response is, "What makes you feel this way?" Such a response allows exploration of subjects and leaves opportunities for the patient to examine concerns. Nurses willing to listen to patients, to be guided by their reactions, and to work with them rather than to make decisions for them will provide needed emotional support. Solving patients' problems, even if it were possible, is not the aim of nursing. Indeed, it would make patients less healthy psychologically.

The art of meaningful communication involves more than just listening; it includes moving conversations so that the patient's attempt to communicate is assisted. Observing patients for facial changes and general body movements provides opportunities for the nurse to discover the full meanings of a situation. For example, consider the patient who sucks in air while talking. The mouth becomes drier and drier, and the tongue seems to stick in the mouth. This patient is not at ease, and even innocuous words may belie anxiety. A simple statement and question such as, "Your mouth seems very dry. Would a glass of water help?" allow the nurse to clarify observations. Such an approach provides an opportunity to tell what the patient is feeling and to gain understanding by talking about it.

The nurse helps patients examine those problems that they are able to bring into awareness. Underlying problems should be handled by professionals trained in psychotherapy. A nurse needs to recognize normal anxiety reactions and to report exaggerated reactions that may indicate the need for psychiatric referral.

When anxiety increases to a high level, the nurse may need to sit with the patient. The nurse's presence is often reassuring. If possible, the patient is helped to recognize the anxiety by the nurse's asking, "Are you uncomfortable?" or "What are you feeling?" In severe anxiety and panic, being there is most important, and touch may be used as a means of reassurance. Some severely anxious persons, however, view touching as an intrusion of their personal boundary, and the nurse needs to keep this in mind. When the pateint is able to talk, the nurse helps the patient describe what is happening, what has happened, and what is expected to happen.

## RESEARCH

Munro BH et al: Effect of relaxation therapy on post-myocardial infarction patient's rehabilitation, *Nurs Res* 37:231-235, 1988.

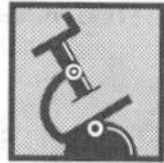

This experimental study involved 57 subjects (27 experimental, 30 control) who were participants in a cardiac rehabilitation program. The study was designed to measure whether practicing Benson's relaxation techniques resulted in improvement in psychosocial functioning as measured by Sickness Impact Profile, aerobic conditioning level (MET level), systolic and diastolic blood pressure, or heart rate. The study also explored the influence of behavioral style on the outcome measures.

The major finding was that diastolic blood pressure was reduced and maintained over a 3-month period. Systolic blood pressure also was reduced, but the reduction was not statistically significant. Subjects in this study showed improvement in psychosocial functioning, aerobic conditioning, and heart rates, but the practice of the relaxation techniques did not enhance these improvements. Behavioral style was not related to outcome measures.

The lack of significant findings for some of the outcome measures may have been related to the nonspecificity of the measures. For example, the measure of behavior style did not contain many items regarding hostility and anger, which may be the most important factors of personality type related to coronary risk. The measure used to evaluate psychosocial functioning focused on illness rather than overall psychosocial functioning.

### Facilitating Problem Solving

Some persons solve problems in a haphazard manner, whereas others are highly structured in their approach to problem solving. Problem solving can be a means for coping with stressors and the stress response and is more effective if the problem-solving steps are consciously followed. The steps include the following:

1. Gathering data
2. Identifying the problem (or effect of stressor)
3. Identifying the factors affecting the problem or stressor
4. Determining goals
5. Exploring alternative ways and consequences to achieve the goals
6. Implementing actions
7. Evaluating effectiveness of actions

If the stressor has been identified, the nurse first assists the patient in exploring feelings and reactions associated with the stressor. Often persons are not consciously aware of what they are feeling and therefore may select inappropriate actions. Persons vary in their ability to identify problems and in their desire to discuss personal feelings, although it is widely accepted that talking does help. If the patient is urged indiscriminately to talk about problems, the relationship becomes superficial and mechanical. The identification of the consequences of actions often is omitted, but it is an important component if problem solving is to be effective.

Problem solving reduces ambiguity and feelings of loss of control. Persons who do not generally employ conscious problem solving as a means of coping with stressors may benefit from learning about problem solving as a strategy for coping with stress.

### Teaching Relaxation Techniques

Relaxation exercises are developed from the concept that the stress response of anxiety does not and cannot exist when the muscles of the body are relaxed. Relaxation exercises do not "cure" the stressors or the stress response but do help to minimize effects of the stress response and give the person a sense of control. A daily program of relaxation exercises has an effect on physiologic responses to stressors (e.g., lowering of elevated blood pressure or elevated blood sugars), as well as psychologic responses to stressors (e.g., decreased level of anxiety) (see Research box above). These exercises also are helpful on a short-term basis when anxiety occurs.

There are four basic components of relaxation techniques:

1. *Quiet environment:* eliminating all possible noise and distractions
2. *Comfortable position:* sitting with no undue muscle tension
3. *Passive attitude:* emptying all thoughts from the conscious mind
4. *Mental device:* focusing on a sound, word, phrase, mental image, object, or breathing pattern to shift the mind from logical, externally oriented thoughts

The important factor is that the person empties his or her mind of all thoughts and concentrates on the mental device. It is natural for the mind to wander. When this occurs, a person simply redirects thoughts back to the mental device. Each relaxation session should take approximately 20 minutes.

There are several approaches to performing relaxation exercises. Two approaches that can be carried out by nursing instructions to patients, without use of special equipment and without physician's orders, are **progressive relaxation** and **Benson's relaxation response.**

**Progressive relaxation** consists of tensing and relaxing muscle groups and focusing on the feelings of relaxation (Box 7-7). The systematic application of progressive relaxation has three major effects, as follows[8]:

### Progressive relaxation

1. Muscle groups are relaxed more and more with each practice.
2. Each of the major muscle groups is relaxed one after the other. As a new muscle group is added, the previously relaxed portions also relax.
3. More total body relaxation is experienced as the person moves into the relaxation phase. The relaxed state is maintained beyond the relaxation period.

**Benson's relaxation response** omits the muscle tensing. It is particularly helpful for muscle relaxation in patients who are experiencing pain or discomfort. It is important to remain with the patient to coach and encourage relaxation,[4] as follows:

### Benson's relaxation response

1. Assume a comfortable sitting position in a quiet room.
2. Close eyes.
3. Relax body muscles (i.e., "let go").
4. Concentrate on breathing; repeat a word or sound such as "one" or "um-m" after each exhalation.
5. Continue for about 20 minutes.
6. Open eyes.
7. Take time to adjust to surroundings before moving.

For some acute stressors, such as those experienced by hospitalized adults, the nurse may use abridged forms of relaxation techniques that can be implemented more rapidly. Effective abridged relaxation techniques include deep breathing or squeezing and relaxing the hands.

## Implementing Music Therapy

Music therapy is an intervention that can help patients achieve relaxation and promote coping with stressors and the stress response. Music therapy has been used successfully in various environments, including intensive care units, dentists' offices, and surgery units.[16,50] Music therapy has been used with patients who have acute and chronic health problems.

When music therapy is used, the patient's preference must be considered, because the type of music that is relaxing and pleasant for one person may be irritating and unpleasant for another. Instrumental music is better than vocal music because words often evoke various emotional responses. In addition, the use of headphones is advocated to help decrease other stimuli. The patient should be able to control the volume.

Music therapy is easily accessible. Only a source of music (tapes, CDs) and a machine are required. Cassette tapes and players are used most frequently because they are least expensive, most portable, and easily available in a variety of clinical settings. Because of the large selection in tapes, individual preferences are easy to accommodate. Unlike other relaxation interventions, neither nurses nor patients need special skills to use music therapy. All that is needed is an enjoyment of music.

## Providing Antianxiety Medications

In some instances, the patient may be prescribed an antianxiety medication to reduce anxiety symptoms. Antianxiety agents may be divided into two groups, the

### BOX 7-7 Progressive Relaxation

1. Assume a comfortable position in a quiet room.
2. Begin by focusing on easy breathing.
3. Tense specific muscle groups (see step 5) for 5 to 7 seconds, then relax quickly.
4. Concentrate for 10 seconds on the sensations of the relaxed muscles.
5. Follow a sequence, repeating each muscle group, tensing two or three times
   a. Hand and arm: clench fist, pull elbow tightly, pull arms tightly into body
   b. Face: wrinkle forehead, close eyes tightly, wrinkle nose, purse lips, smile with teeth tightly clenched
   c. Neck; pull chin to chest
   d. Trunk: pull shoulder blades together, tighten stomach and buttocks
   e. Leg and foot: push down with leg, point toes upward (dorsiflexion) dominant leg first
6. Repeat process in any areas in which increased tension has been identified.

benzodiazepines and the nonbenzodiazepines (Table 7-3). Note that the dosage of benzodiazepines is less for elderly persons, who metabolize the drugs slowly, which can result in a prolonged depressant effect. Dosage also should be reduced for persons with impaired liver or kidney function.

The benzodiazepines are the most frequently prescribed antianxiety agents. These drugs act by inhibiting transmission of stimuli from the limbic system of the brain (septum, amygdala, and hippocampus). Side effects include drowsiness, dizziness, and weakness.

Antianxiety agents produce muscle relaxation and a sense of well-being. The drugs are prescribed for short-term relief of anxiety but not for anxiety from daily stressors. Long-term therapy leads to increased tolerance and dependence; larger doses are then needed to produce the desired effects and drug abuse may ensue.

Persons taking antianxiety agents are cautioned not to drink alcohol or take other CNS depressants during therapy because of serious complications, even death, as a result of synergistic effects. They also need to be cautious when driving or working around heavy machinery because of possible dizziness.

## CRISIS INTERVENTION

Awareness of what occurs during a crisis helps the nurse understand the accompanying behavior. When the ego is met with overwhelming anxiety created by biologic, psychologic, or social threats to the self, a **crisis** ensues. The ego is not able to cope successfully with the sudden disequilibrium, and the person needs assistance to use the situation as a growth experience.

A crisis occurs when a person faces for a time what seems to be an insurmountable obstacle to an important life goal and is unable to use customary methods of coping. A period of disorganization ensues—a period of upset during which many abortive attempts at solutions are made.

Shontz[48] describes several phases or stages that occur during crisis. These stages are similar to the stages of death and dying described by Kübler-Ross.

1. *Initial impact.* During this phase the person experiences shock and depersonalization as reality is clearly perceived. Functioning is organized and automatic, with individual centering and docility.
2. *Realization.* In the second phase the existing self-structure collapses. Reality seems overwhelming, and the person experiences high anxiety, panic, and helplessness. There is inability to plan, reason, or understand the situation.
3. *Defensive retreat.* The third phase is one of regression in which an attempt is made to establish previous identity—to return to better times. Reality is avoided, and denial and wishful thinking may help to relieve the anxiety. When challenged, the ego reacts with anger and the person may experience rage and disorientation. Thinking is situation-bound, and change is resisted.
4. *Acknowledgment.* This is the "yes" stage: "It has happened to me." The individual experiences depression and self-depreciation. Reality imposes itself again and looms large in relating the event to one's life. Without intervention the person may become more disorganized, depressed, and suicidal.
5. *Adaptation.* This is the stage in which change occurs if help is adequate. New identity appears along with hope and renewed sense of personal worth. Anxiety is subsequently decreased and satisfaction is increased as a result of the stabilization and reorganization. Functional improvement is noted without actual change in disability status.

The model just offered is a useful approach for explaining what a person experiences during an illness

**TABLE 7-3 Antianxiety Agents**

| GENERIC NAME | TRADE NAME | USUAL ADULT DOSAGE | DOSAGE FOR ELDERS |
|---|---|---|---|
| **BENZODIAZEPINES** | | | |
| Alprazolam | Xanax | 0.25-0.5 mg tid | 0.25 mg bid/tid |
| Chlordiazepoxide | Librium, Libritabs | 5-25 mg tid/qid | 5 mg bid/qid |
| Clorazepate | Tranxene | 7.5-15 mg bid/qid | 7.5-15 mg qd |
| Diazepam | Valium | 2-10 mg bid/qid | 2-2.5 mg qd or bid |
| Halazepam | Paxipam | 20-40 mg tid/qid | 20 mg qd or bid |
| Lorazepam | Ativan | 1-3 mg bid/tid | 0.5-1 mg bid |
| Oxazepam | Serax | 10-30 mg tid/qid | 10-15 mg tid |
| Prazepam | Centrax | 10 mg tid or 20-40 mg at bedtime | 5 mg bid/tid or 15 mg at bedtime |
| **NONBENZODIAZEPINES** | | | |
| Hydroxyzine HCl | Atarax | 25-100 mg tid/qid | Same as adult dosage |
| Meprobamate | Equanil, Meprospan, Miltown | 400 mg bid/tid or 600 mg bid | Same as adult dosage |

crisis, even though reactions to crisis are individual. People are not equally vulnerable to all categories of stressors, but there is thought to be some commonality in the reactions. Knowledge about the commonalities can facilitate plans for nursing intervention.

The essential element of crisis intervention is the intensive nature of support required to help the ego maintain its integrity and its ability to use coping mechanisms. Crisis, according to Caplan,[7] is self-limiting. Early intervention can prevent maladaptive behavior, and the individual can emerge a stronger person. Acute or catastrophic illness often precipitates a crisis reaction. The outcome of a crisis is governed by the kind of interaction that takes place between the individual and key figures in the environment during the time of crisis.

Often because of changes in society, previous guidelines for behavior in stressful situations render the individual helpless. In crisis the individual is helped to find ways to facilitate efforts to learn from the experience. A state of disequilibrium produces a felt need to reduce anxiety. The following balancing factors[2] have been identified as being necessary to resolve the problem and avert a crisis:

1. A realistic perception of the event
2. Adequate situational support (staff and family)
3. Adequate coping mechanisms

When one or more of these balancing factors are absent, the result is an increase in anxiety, with immobilization and an inability to avert the crisis (see Figure 7-5).

In crisis, help should be immediate. Staying with the person, talking through the situation, and encouraging catharsis facilitate recognition and expression of feelings and subsequent relief of guilt. Strengthening coping mechanisms is crucial in preventing the development of symptoms. Personal growth is facilitated by using problem-solving skills.

## SPECIFIC SUPPORT APPROACHES

Persons who are having difficulty coping because of severe or multiple stressors may be referred for individual or group counseling. Some may need assistance and support from the nurse in seeking out and initiating counseling.

*Therapeutic groups* consist of persons who are experiencing common stressors. Peer support is given because the participants share the common experience. Persons often are able to express their feelings more easily when they know that the group members understand what they are experiencing. Approaches found helpful in solving the common problems also are shared. Therapeutic groups may be self-help groups or be directed by health professionals. Examples of therapeutic groups are Al-Anon (for family member of alcohol-dependent persons), Parents Without Partners, Reach to Recovery (postmastectomy), "ostomy" groups, bereavement groups, and the American Cancer Society's "I Can Cope" program.

## ADDITIONAL STRESS MANAGEMENT THERAPIES

In dealing with some stressors, particularly chronic stressors or diseases associated with stressors and the stress response, the nurse may use some stress management therapies that require special training or equipment. These are implemented over a long-term basis and usually in outpatient settings. Stress management therapists help patients design and implement structured programs of change to enable them to control and deal more effectively with stressors and the stress response. Some of the therapies include biofeedback, meditation, attitudinal restructuring, autogenic training, behavioral change programs, and systematic desensitization.

### Biofeedback

**Biofeedback**[10] is a system of learning voluntary control over autonomically regulated body functions so that an individual is able to monitor the physiologic stress response and to replace it with a nonstressful response. For example, if after a stressful day you notice soreness and muscle tension in your shoulders, you can sit quietly and concentrate on relaxing the shoulder muscles to feel the tension slip away.

With biofeedback, machinery is used to "train" the person to monitor certain parameters. For example, muscle activity can be monitored with an electromyograph (EMG) and the stimuli converted into a visual or auditory signal. Using this biofeedback, the person can learn how to replace muscle tension with muscle relaxation. Machines also can be used to measure skin temperature or sweat activity, and a similar feedback approach is used. The person is then weaned from the machine to produce the desired effects without machinery. A comprehensive biofeedback program includes feedback from multiple systems and sites.

### Meditation

For centuries the art of **meditation** has been practiced in the East. Proponents of meditation techniques claim that meditators can control physiologic processes, some as dramatic as voluntarily stopping heartbeats.[4] There are many different types of meditation, with differing goals and focuses, including Zen Buddhism, yoga, and transcendental meditation (TM). Research has focused on TM because it is one of the most practiced forms of meditation in the West.

TM is not a complicated process. One is given a word, a mantra—which is to be repeated silently while one sits in a comfortable position and focuses attention on breathing and repeating the mantra. The purpose of the mantra is to enhance a passive attitude and prevent distracting thoughts. Meditators are instructed to practice twice daily for at least 20 minutes. The physiologic relaxation that is produced during meditation is carried over into everyday life as a protection against the effects of the stress response.

## Attitudinal Restructuring

The basic premise of **rational-emotive therapy**, developed by Ellis,[12] is that much if not all emotional suffering (stress response) is due to the irrational ways people perceive the world. The assumptions that people make lead to self-defeating internal dialogues or negative self-talk. The goal of therapy is to replace negative self-statements with positive self-statements. Changing self-talk involves three steps: identifying self-talk, evaluating it, and replacing it with more appropriate self-talk.

Detection of self-talk may be difficult at first because it is "inaudible." Detection of self-talk usually involves keeping a daily log to identify specific thoughts and feelings.

Self-talk often causes a person to distort reality or arrive at false conclusions. The following five questions are useful in examining self-talk and the situations that are antecedent to it:

1. Have I disregarded an important aspect of the situation?
2. Have I exaggerated the meaning of an event?
3. Are my perceptions of the situation overly simplified or rigid?
4. Have I drawn conclusions where evidence is lacking or where evidence supports a contrary conclusion?
5. Have I overgeneralized or generated a false conclusion?

The answers to the five questions should reveal when self-talk is inappropriate and how to restructure it. Negative internal dialogues probably are a major source of stress to many persons.[5]

## Autogenic Training

**Autogenic training** teaches cognitive behavioral change together with physiologic behavioral change through passive concentration to decrease sympathetic nervous system activity. The person repeats a statement verbally with the physiologic state that is being practiced. The physiologic states are heaviness and warmth of extremities, calm and regular heartbeat and breathing, abdominal warmth, and cooling of forehead. The methods are similar to that of TM.

## Behavioral Change Programs

Some specific stress-related behaviors, such as smoking or overeating, may be eliminated by behavioral conditioning. The programs consist of the following:

1. Self-monitoring to identify characteristics and situations associated with the behaviors
2. Identifying outcome criteria in precise behavioral terms
3. Developing a formal contract with the therapist stating short-term goals with rewards and frequency of evaluation

The overall goal is a change in behavior. Behavioral change programs are most effective with highly motivated persons who sincerely *want* to change behavior.

## Systematic Desensitization

**Systematic desensitization** provides specific stressors (such as those related to phobias) in increasing doses while the individual practices relaxation skills. The person is first taught effective relaxation skills. Stimuli eliciting anxieties are then presented in increasing intensity, starting at a minimal level while relaxation techniques are used. Then the person is instructed to relax while imagining the situation in more threatening circumstances. The principle of systematic desensitization is to train the person to behave (relax) in a manner opposite to anxiety behavior (tension). A low initial stimulus that increases in intensity gives the person a sense of control in coping with the undesirable stimulus, thus decreasing the anxiety.

## QUESTIONS TO CONSIDER

- Should you try to lead a life that is free from stressors? Explain.
- Think back over several situations in which your patients experienced the stress response. What type of physical symptoms did they experience? What is the physiologic reason for each symptom experienced? Were the symptoms always the same? If not, why?
- In what way(s) do you cope with stressors? What other coping strategies might be useful for you?
- Identify from your experience patient situations in which you think relaxation exercises might have been useful nursing interventions. Were relaxation exercises used? If not, why?

## CRITICAL THINKING ACTIVITIES

- Pam, 32 years old with 3 children, is trying to work part-time and care for her children without using child care. Her husband works overtime to make ends meet. She often finds herself easily distracted, and she has difficulty concentrating and sleeping. Paul, 40 years old, travels every week and spends only short periods each weekend with his 8-month-old son and 2-year-old daughter. His wife frequently confronts him about his travel and leaving her to care for the children. Paul's boss confronted him last week about some recent paperwork mistakes. He wakes up early every morning, unable to sleep. Based on these two situations, can any generalizations be made about individuals experiencing stress?
- Jim, 22 years old, was recently diagnosed with testicular cancer. On admission assessment the nurse notes that Jim is quite defensive. When asked to explain why he was being hospitalized, Jim angrily responds, "I just want to go back to college with my friends and get on with my life." After her interview, the nurse concludes that Jim is experiencing an illness crisis. Analyze this situation, and offer suggestions on how best to handle it.

## CHAPTER SUMMARY

### ADAPTATION

- Adaptation is a process of interaction with the environment that promotes homeostasis and growth. Maladaptation leads to inadequate functioning.

### STRESS

- Responses to stressors include neuroendocrine response, coping behaviors, defense mechanisms, and specific behavioral responses.
- Response to stressors is influenced by the type of stimuli, the intensity and duration of stressors, the meaning of the stressor, perception of stressor, sense of control, coping resources, and health status.
- The general adaptation syndrome consists of three stages: alarm reaction, resistance, and exhaustion. The first two stages occur frequently throughout life; death may ensue from exhaustion.

### STRESS RESPONSE

- The physiologic stress response consists of stimulation of the sympathetic nervous system, adrenal medulla, anterior and posterior pituitary glands, and the adrenal cortex.
- The neuroendocrine stress response is integrated by the hypothalamus.
- During the stress response, norepinephrine is released and causes vasoconstriction of blood vessels to skin, mucous membranes, and the organs of the abdomen and pelvis.
- The blood shifted from the vasoconstricted vessels flows to the dilated blood vessels of the heart, lung, and brain.
- In addition to dilating selected blood vessels, epinephrine increases cardiac function, dilates bronchial smooth muscles, and alters metabolism to provide substrates for energy needs.
- Cortisol, acting in concert with catecholamines, growth hormone, and glucagon, helps to mobilize substrates for energy.
- Cortisol may serve a major function by its antiinflammatory and immunosuppressive actions, thus dampening the stress response to prevent overactivity.
- Water and sodium balance, osmolality, and blood volume are protected by the action of aldosterone and ADH, which are released during the neuroendocrine response to stressors.

### COPING

- Types of coping strategies include action, cognitive, intrapsychic, interpersonal, and emotional strategies.

### DEFENSE MECHANISMS

- Defense mechanisms are unconscious mechanisms human beings use to adjust to life stressors. Mentally healthy persons occasionally use defense mechanisms, avoiding more primitive mechanisms.

### SPECIFIC BEHAVIORAL RESPONSES

- Some specific behavioral responses to stressors include anxiety, aggressive behavior, depressed behavior, withdrawn behavior, suspicious behavior, and somatic behavior.
- Anxiety results when a person perceives a threat to the self, either physically or psychologically.
- Anxiety may be mild, moderate, severe, or a state of panic. When anxiety increases, awareness of the environment decreases and physiologic signs increase.

### STRESS MANAGEMENT THERAPEUTICS

- Rest and relief of discomfort conserve energy for coping with stressors and the stress response; providing explanations provides structure, which helps to decrease anxiety. Exploration of feelings helps to relieve tension associated with the stress response, and problem solving reduces feelings of loss of control associated with the stress response.
- Relaxation is the opposite of the tension associated with the stress response; it also gives the person a sense of control. Basic components of relaxation techniques are quiet environment, comfortable position, passive attitude, and a mental device to remove externally oriented thoughts.
- Music therapy is an easy-to-apply intervention to decrease stress.
- The most frequently prescribed antianxiety agents are the benzodiazepines. Alcohol or other CNS depressants should be avoided when one takes antianxiety agents.
- Crisis occurs when anxiety overwhelms the self and the person is unable to use coping mechanisms. Crisis is self-limiting. Balancing factors necessary to resolve crises include a realistic perception of the event, adequate situational support, and adequate coping mechanisms.
- Other stress management therapies requiring special expertise include meditation, attitudinal restructuring, biofeedback, autogenic training, behavioral change programs, and systematic desensitization.

## REFERENCES

1. Adams J, Lindemann E: Coping with long-term disability. In Coehlo GV, Hamburg DA, Adams JE, editors: *Coping and adaptation,* New York, 1974, Basic Books.
2. Aguilera DC: *Crisis intervention: theory and methodology,* ed 7, St Louis, 1994, Mosby.
3. Ballard KS: *Identification of environmental stress for patients in the surgical intensive care unit,* master's thesis, Kansas City, 1979, University of Kansas School of Nursing.
4. Benson H: *The relaxation response,* New York, 1975, William Morrow.
5. Betrus P, Kogan H: Stressors in nursing: causes, results and

interventions. In *Stressors in nursing: responses and resolutions,* Seattle, 1981, University of Washington Press.

6. Cannon WB: *The wisdom of the body,* New York, 1939, WW Norton.
7. Caplan G: *Principles of preventative psychiatry,* New York, 1964, Basic Books.
8. Carlson CE, editor: *Behavioral concepts and nursing interventions,* ed 2, Philadelphia, 1978, WB Saunders.
9. Cox T: *Stress,* New York, 1978, Macmillan.
10. Danskin D, Crow M: *Biofeedback: an introduction and guide,* Palo Alto, Calif, 1981, Mayfield Publishing.
11. Dixon JP, Dixon JK, Spinner J: Perceptions of life-pattern disintegrity as a link in the relationship between stress and illness, *Adv Nurs Sci* 11(2):1-11, 1989.
12. Ellis A: *Reason and emotion in psychotherapy,* New York, 1962, Lyle Stuart.
13. Frain M, Valiga T: The multiple dimensions of stress, *Top Clin Nurs* 1(1):43-57, 1979.
14. Gaillard RC, Al-Damleiji S: Stress and the pituitary-adrenal axis, *Baillieres Clin Endocrinol Metab* 1:319-354, 1987.
15. Granner D: Hormones of the adrenal medulla. In Murray RK et al, editors: *Harper's biochemistry,* ed 23, New York, 1993, Lange Medical Books.
16. Guzzetta C: Effect of relaxation and music therapy on patients in a coronary care unit with presumptive acute myocardial infarction, *Heart Lung* 18:609-616, 1989.
17. Henry JP, Ely DL: Physiology of emotional stress: specific responses, *J SC Med Assoc* 75:501-508, 1979.
18. Hetzel BS et al: Changes in urinary 17-hydroxy-corticosteroid excretion during stressful life situations in man, *J Clin Endocrinol* 15:1057-1068, 1955.
19. Hornberger CA: *Perceived stressors, perceived stress response, and level of cardiac reactivity in wellness sample,* master's thesis, Kansas City, 1989, University of Kansas School of Nursing.
20. Jacobsen E: *Progressive relaxation,* Chicago, 1938, University of Chicago Press.
21. James W: What is emotion? *Mind* 9:188-205, 1884.
22. Kadner KD: Resilience: responding to adversity, *J Psychosoc Nurs* 27(7):20-25, 1989.
23. Kanfer F, Goldstein A: *Helping people change,* New York, 1975, Pergamon Press.
24. Kemp VH, Hatmaker DD: Stress and social support in high-risk pregnancy, *Res Nurs Health* 12:331-336, 1989.
25. Kogan H et al: *Therapeutic manual for the management of stress response,* Seattle, 1980, University of Washington.
26. Lazarus RS: *Psychological stress and the coping process,* New York, 1966, McGraw Hill.
27. Lazarus RS, Folkman S: *Stress, appraisal and coping,* New York, 1984, Springer.
28. Lenox RH et al: Specific hormonal and neurochemical responses to different stressors, *Neuroendocrinology* 30:300-308, 1980.
29. Levine S, Weinberg J, Ursin H: Definition of the coping process and statement of the problem. In Ursin H, Baade E, Levine S, editors: *Psychobiology of stress: a study of coping men,* New York, 1978, Academic Press.
30. Mason JW: A re-evaluation of the concept of nonspecificity in stress theory, *J Psychiatr Res* 8:323-333, 1971.
31. Mason JW: Specificity in the organization of neuroendocrine response profiles. In Seeman P, Brown GM, editors: *Frontiers in neurology and neuroscience research* (First International Symposium of the Neuroscience Institute) Toronto, 1974, University of Toronto.
32. Mason JW: A historical view of the stress field, *J Human Stress* 1(1):6-12; 1(2):22-36, 1975.
33. McCance KL, Huether SE: *Pathophysiology: the biologic basis for disease in adults and children,* ed 2, St Louis, 1994, Mosby.
34. Moos R: *Coping with physical illness,* ed 2, New York, 1985, Plenum.
35. Munck A, Guyre PM, Holbrook NJ: Physiological functions of glucocorticoids in stress and their relation to pharmacological actions, *Endocr Rev* 5:25-44, 1984.
36. Munro BH et al: Effect of relaxation therapy on post-myocardial infarction patient's rehabilitation, *Nurs Res* 37:231-235, 1988.
37. Murphy LP: Coping, vulnerability and resilience in childhood. In Coehlo GV, Hamburg DA, Adams JE, editors: *Coping and adaptation,* New York, 1974, Basic Books.
38. Peplau H: A working definition of anxiety. In Burd S, Marshall M, editors: *Some clinical approaches to psychiatric nursing,* New York, 1963, Macmillan.
39. Pollock SE: The hardiness characteristic: a motivating factor in adaptation, *Adv Nurs Sci* 11(2):53-62, 1989.
40. Roy C, Roberts SL: *Theory construction in nursing: an adaptation model,* Englewood Cliffs, NJ, 1981, Prentice-Hall.
41. Salo M: Endocrine response to anaesthesia and surgery. In Watkins J, Salo M, editors: *Trauma, stress and immunity inanaesthesia and surgery,* Boston, 1982, Butterworth.
42. Selye H: A syndrome produced by diverse nocuous agents, *Nature* 138:32-35, 1936.
43. Selye H: The general adaptation syndrome and the diseases of adaptation, *J Clin Endocrinol* 6:117-230, 1946.
44. Selye H: *The stress of life,* New York, 1956, McGraw-Hill.
45. Selye H: The stress syndrome, *Am J Nurs* 65:97-99, 1965.
46. Selye H: *Stress in health and disease,* Boston, 1976, Butterworth.
47. Shoemaker W et al, editors: *Textbook of critical care,* ed 2, Philadelphia, 1989, WB Saunders.
48. Shontz F: *The psychological aspects of physical illness and disability.* New York, 1975, Macmillan.
49. Simpson GG: Behavior and evolution. In Roe AR, Simpson GG, editors: *Behavior and evolution,* New Haven, Conn, 1958, Yale University Press.
50. Stevens K: Patients' perception of music during surgery, *J Adv Nurs* 15:1045-1051, 1990.
51. Strauss A et al. *Chronic illness and the quality of life,* ed 2, St Louis, 1984, Mosby.
52. Sutterley DC: Stress and health: a survey of self-regulation modalities, *Top Clin Nurs* 1(1):1-29, 1979.
53. Weisman A: *Coping with cancer,* New York, 1979, McGraw-Hill.
54. Weiss JM: Psychological factors in stress and disease, *Sci Am* 226(6):104-113, 1972.
55. White RD: Strategies of adaptation: an attempt at systematic description. In Coehlo GV, Hamburg DA, Adams JE, editors: *Coping and adaptation,* New York, 1974, Basic Books.

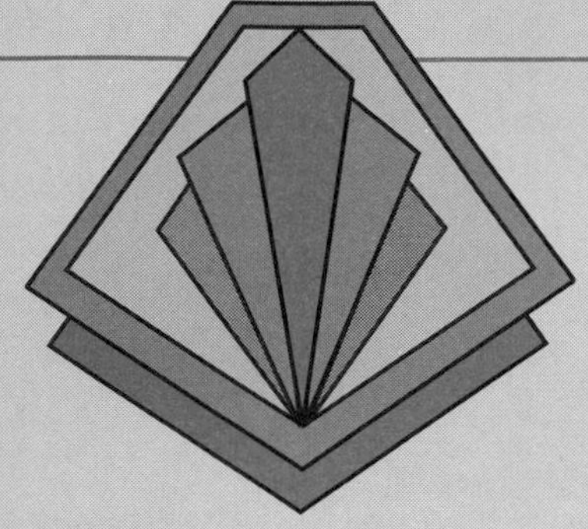

UNIT II

# Common Concepts for Care of Ill Adults

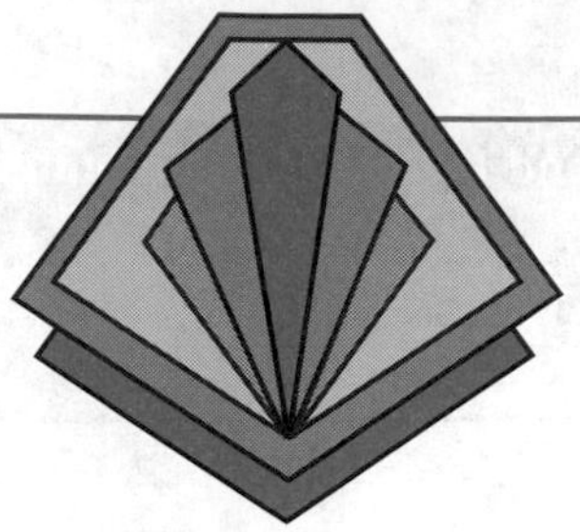

C H A P T E R 8

# Chronic Illness and Rehabilitation

***Wilma J. Phipps***

## CHAPTER OBJECTIVES

***After studying this chapter, the learner should be able to do the following:***

1. Differentiate between acute and chronic illness.
2. Describe factors that influence chronic illness.
3. Identify areas of assessment for the chronically ill person.
4. Describe physical and psychosocial interventions for the person with a chronic illness.
5. Define rehabilitation and the roles of the patient and team members (especially the nurse).
6. Describe different patterns and facilities for continuing care.
7. Describe provisions of the Americans With Disabilities Act.
8. Identify major health goals related to chronic health problems to be achieved by the year 2000.

## KEY TERMS

acute illness
ambulatory care
chronic grief
chronic illness
disability
exacerbation
home care
home health aide
incidence
limitation of activity
prevalence
primary prevention
rehabilitation
remission
respite care
restriction of activity
secondary prevention
tertiary prevention

## IMPACT OF CHRONIC ILLNESS ON SOCIETY

Prevention and control of chronic disease constitute a major aspect of the health problems in the United States today. In the past the impact of chronic diseases on individuals, families, and communities has been overlooked. Currently, there is increasing awareness in the United States of great pockets of unmet needs among persons with long-term health problems. These individuals have needs that extend beyond the strictly medical. Their problems demand the use of multiple sources of help and care. In many cases the coping capacities of chronically ill persons are reduced because of advancing age, serious functional impairment and disability, and limited personal, social, and financial resources.

*Chronic disease is not an entity in itself but an umbrella term that encompasses long-lasting diseases, which often are associated with some degree of disability.* Each chronic illness is unique and has a different impact on the individual, family, and community. Nevertheless, common problems and complications that accompany the various chronic health problems can be studied in general to help the nurse understand and care for persons with specific long-term illnesses.

The incidence and prevalence of chronic diseases have increased since the beginning of the twentieth century. **Incidence** refers to the number of cases of illness that had their onset during a specified period of time. Health statistics commonly report the number of new cases for a calendar year. **Prevalence** refers to the total number of cases at a given point in time. Thus prevalence rates are higher than incidence rates because they include all persons (cases) with a specified condition (old cases) and those who acquired the condition during a specified period of time (new cases).

The reason that both the incidence and prevalence are increased for chronic diseases is because fewer per-

**TABLE 8-1 Persons With Activity Limitation, by Selected Chronic Conditions and Income, United States, 1980 and 1985 (Figures in Millions of Persons Affected)**

| | | | FAMILY INCOME FOR 1985 ONLY | | |
|---|---|---|---|---|---|
| | 1980 | 1985 | UNDER $20,000 | $20,000-$34,999 | $35,000 AND OVER |
| **AGE (YEARS)** | | | | | |
| All ages | 31.4 | 32.7 | | | |
| Under 45 | 10.2 | 11.6 | 16.6 | 7.1 | 4.7 |
| 45-64 | 10.4 | 10.4 | | | |
| 65 years and over | 10.8 | 10.7 | | | |
| **SEX** | | | | | |
| Male | 15.5 | 15.3 | | | |
| Female | 15.9 | 17.4 | | | |

Latest available figures. From US Department of Commerce, Bureau of the Census: *Statistical abstract of the United States 1990*, Washington DC, 1990.

sons are dying from acute diseases. There is decreased mortality from infectious diseases such as whooping cough and chickenpox in children and tuberculosis and pneumonia in persons of all ages. Improved sanitation, the introduction of effective vaccines and mass immunizations, and the discovery of antibiotics have all contributed to this decrease in deaths from infectious diseases. Unfortunately measles immunization rates for children have declined recently, and in 1991 several young children died from the consequences of measles. Most of these deaths were in children living under the poverty level with limited access to medical care. Also, several states stopped providing free immunization services because of budget restrictions at the federal and state levels.

The latest available figures from the U.S. Bureau of the Census show that the number of persons with some limitation in activity has been increasing each year. Another finding of interest is that the number of persons with limited activity decreased as family income increased (Table 8-1). This last finding seems to indicate that persons from higher income levels may be better educated about preventive health measures and that they are able to afford better diet, better housing, and better medical care.

**Disability** refers to any long- or short-term *reduction of activity* as the result of an acute or a chronic condition. **Limitation of activity** is used to describe a *long-term reduction* in a person's ability to perform the kind or amount of activity associated with a particular age-group. **Restriction of activity** is generally used to refer to a relatively short-term reduction in a person's activity below his or her normal capacity.

Death rates from heart disease decreased so dramatically in persons 45 to 64 years of age from 1970 until the present that heart disease is no longer the leading cause of death in persons in that age-group. Cancer has replaced it as the leading cause of death in persons between 25 and 65 years of age.[2]

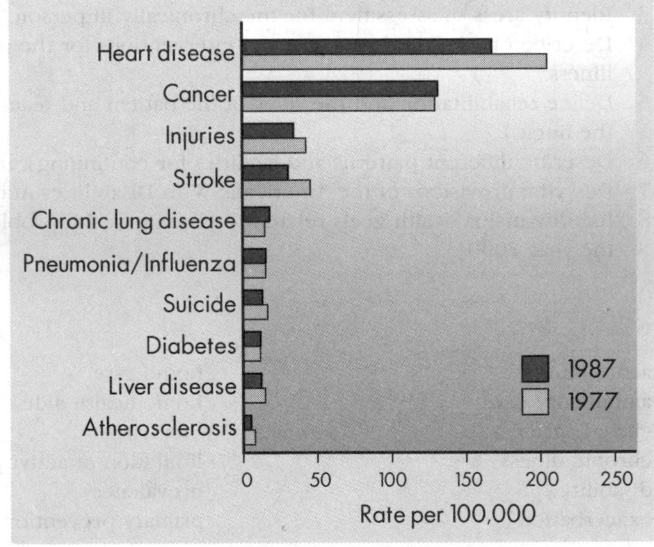


**FIGURE 8-1** Comparison of leading causes of death 1977 and 1987. (From US Department of Health and Human Services, Public Health Service: *Healthy people 2000: national health promotion and disease prevention objectives,* Washington, DC, 1990, US Government Printing Office.)

While death rates from heart disease were decreasing dramatically, death rates from other conditions were increasing. The death rate from AIDS increased 12.7% from 1989 to 1990.[5] In 1991 it moved up from tenth to ninth place. AIDS was the leading cause of death in black men from 25 to 44 years of age and the third leading cause of death in black women in the same age-group. Seven times as many deaths from AIDS occurred among men of all races than among women. The other leading causes of death in 1991 were *stroke, chronic obstructive pulmonary disease, accidents, pneumonia and influenza, diabetes, suicide,* and *homicide* (Figure 8-1). All the leading causes of death have risk factors associated with life-style, and many of these diseases could be prevented by effective control of smoking, blood pressure, diet, and alcohol consumption.

Several factors may have contributed to the increase in suicide and homicide: *increases in substance abuse, access to handguns, poverty, urbanization* and *crowding*, and *family disruption* and *disorganization.*[5] Deaths from homicides increased by 23% from 1987 to 1990. Most of this increase occurred among young black men from 15 to 24 years of age and has been attributed to the preceding factors.

Death rates also increased for diabetes, with an increase of 23% from 1984 to 1990; 15% of this increase occurred between 1988 and 1990 alone, among persons from 55 to 85 years of age.

For the first time the National Health Survey of 1982 identified major disparities in the health of African-Americans and other minorities in the United States compared with the white population. As a result of these findings, the secretary of the U.S. Department of Health and Human Services (DHHS) established a task force on black and minority health.[23] The findings of the task force are discussed on p. 190.

According to the surgeon general's report, 80% of the over-65 population have one or more chronic diseases.

## DEFINITION OF ACUTE AND CHRONIC ILLNESS

An **acute illness** is one caused by a disease that produces symptoms and signs soon after exposure to the cause, that runs a short course, and from which there is usually a full recovery or an abrupt termination in death. An acute ilness may become chronic. For example, a common cold may develop into chronic sinusitis. A **chronic illness** is one caused by disease that produces symptoms and signs within a variable period of time, that runs a long course, and from which there is only partial recovery. The National Health Survey defines chronic conditions as follows: (1) the conditions were first noticed 3 months or more before the date of the interview or (2) they belong to a group of conditions (including heart disease, diabetes, and others) that are considered chronic regardless of when they began.[25] This follows the pattern of the *Commission on Chronic Illness,* which in 1949 *defined chronic illness as any impairment or deviation from normal that has one or more of the following characteristics.*

1. The illness or impairment is permanent.
2. The illness or impairment leaves residual disability.
3. The illness or impairment is caused by nonreversible pathologic alteration.
4. The illness or impairment requires a long period of supervision, observation, or care.

This definition is still in use more than 40 years later.

The symptoms and general reactions caused by chronic disease may subside with proper treatment and care. The period during which the disease is controlled and symptoms are not obvious is known as **remission.** However, at a future time the disease may become active again with recurrence of pronounced symptoms. This is known as an **exacerbation** of the disease.

**BOX 8-1 Problems Faced by Persons With Chronic Illness**

1. Preventing and managing medical crises
2. Controlling symptoms
3. Following prescribed regimen
4. Maintaining normal interactions with others
5. Adjusting to recurrent patterns in the course of the disease
6. Arranging payment for treatment

From Strauss AL: *Chronic illness and the quality of life,* ed 2, St Louis, 1984, Mosby.

Exacerbations of chronic disease often cause the patient to seek medical attention and may lead to hospitalization. The needs of a patient who has an acute illness may be very different from those of the patient with an acute exacerbation of a chronic disease. For example, a young person may enter the hospital with complaints of fever, chest pain, shortness of breath, fatigue, and a productive cough. If the diagnosis is pneumonia, the patient usually can be assured of recovery after a period of rest and a course of antibiotic treatment. If, however, the diagnosis is rheumatic heart disease and the patient is being admitted to the hospital for the third, fourth, or fifth time, the desired reassurance will not be so definite, clear-cut, or easy to give. In such a case it is necessary to begin planning care that will extend beyond the period of hospitalization, taking into consideration many aspects of the patient's total life situation. The concerns of the patient who has repeated attacks of illness will be very different from the concerns of the one who has a short-term illness.

Further, the needs of patients who are admitted to the hospital with an acute illness but who also have an underlying chronic condition must not be overlooked. For example, elderly patients who enter the hospital with pneumonia may receive treatment for the pneumonia and recover from their illness. However, they may still be hampered by the arteriosclerotic heart disease and arthritis that they have had for years. Also, these two chronic conditions may have been aggravated by the acute infection, or the return to former activity may be hindered by joint stiffness resulting from bedrest and inactivity. Consideration of a patient's several diagnoses can help in preventing new problems associated with the chronic illness.

Strauss,[21] a well-known medical sociologist, has described some problems experienced by persons with chronic illness (Box 8-1).

According to the National Health Survey of 1990, 80 million people have one or more chronic conditions.[25] *The survey classified chronic conditions in the following categories:* (1) *selected skin and musculoskeletal conditions,* (2) *impairments (visual, hearing, speech, paralysis, deformity, or orthopedic impairment),* (3) *selected digestive conditions,* (4) *selected conditions of the genitourinary, nervous, endocrine, metabolic, and blood and blood-forming systems,* (5) *selected circulatory conditions,* and (6) *selected respiratory conditions.*[25]

Many of these conditions cause a limitation of activity, which affects the life-style of those who are chronically ill. One of the trends that has been documented is that the impact of acute illness has diminished, whereas the burden of chronic health problems and related disability has increased. *Limitation of activity is a measure of long-term disability resulting from chronic health problems or impairment and is defined as the inability to carry on the major activity for one's age-group, such as cooking, keeping house, going to school, or going to work.*

Approximately 14% of the population experiences some activity limitations, whereas almost half of the persons over 65 years of age are limited in their activities by one or more chronic conditions. Some activity limitations are associated with mental disabilities, but most are the result of physical handicaps caused by heart conditions and arthritis. *Because chronic disability increases in direct proportion to age, persons older than 65 years of age are most prone to severe chronic disability.*

As the population of the United States ages, the number of persons with chronic illness will continue to increase. The inability to work or to move about greatly influences the kind of medical treatment and health supervision needed by persons who have a chronic illness. Some persons need only periodic medical examination and perhaps continuing treatment with medications; others may require complete physical care. Some have a disease that progresses very slowly without remissions, whereas others may have episodes of acute illness and then seem comparatively well for a time. Each person requires a thorough assessment to determine the stage of the illness, the course the illness is likely to take, the type of care needed, and the method by which that care will be delivered if the individual is to be helped appropriately.

## FACTORS THAT INFLUENCE CHRONIC ILLNESS

### Age

Different age-groups have different kinds of experience with acute and chronic diseases. The young are more likely to experience short, intense, acute conditions that are quickly over. Elderly persons are more likely to have long, drawn-out chronic diseases; nevertheless, it is true that anyone can have either an acute or a chronic disease at any age. Chronic illness and disability may date from birth (e.g., spina bifida with neurologic damage), or it may originate in childhood, adolescence, or early adult life (e.g., multiple sclerosis, rheumatoid arthritis). *The major chronic illnesses among those 65 years and older identified in the National Health Survey were arthritis, diabetes, heart disease,* and *hypertension.*[25]

Because of strides made in pediatric medicine, children who 30 years ago would have died of diseases such as cystic fibrosis are living longer. The reduction in death rates among the younger age-groups has allowed a higher percentage of the population to reach the age of greatest risk from chronic diseases. Cancer develops far more frequently in older persons. Because the average age of our population continues to rise, about 30% of persons now alive will eventually contract cancer.[2]

*Much remains to be learned about interactions of the normal, pathologic, and physiologic changes of aging with various diseases.* A common question that is asked is "When does aging end and illness begin?" Differences found in age-groups or changes found in individuals as they age represent normal aging—that is, a universal, intrinsic process of growth and development that is inevitable, irreversible, unpreventable, but ultimately detrimental. Even though aging, a normal process, is distinct from chronic disease, a pathologic process, *chronic illness often accompanies aging.* The problems of aging and chronic disease are influenced in major ways by each other; for example, the social problems confronting elders are strongly influenced by the presence and severity of chronic disabilites. Remissions and exacerbations are possibilities with chronic illness; they are not with aging.

*Healthy People 2000*[22] makes the following observations about age and chronicity. Persons in the United States who reach the age of 65 years can now expect to live into their 80s. However, it is not likely that all those years will be active and independent ones. Thus, *improving the functional independence* and *not just the length of later life* is an important element in promoting the health of this age-group.

One measure of health that considers quality as well as the length of life is the years of healthy life. Whereas people aged 65 years and older have 16.4 years of life remaining on average, it is estimated that they have about 12 years of healthy life remaining. *Thus quality of life is determined by the individual's ability to perform activities of daily living so that he or she can be independent.*

### Race and Ethnicity

Race or ethnic group membership is a factor that influences chronic health problems. Race-specific rates measure the association between disease occurrence and race. Data on specific conditions indicate not only that some problems are more prevalent among nonwhites (African-Americans, Native Americans, and Asians) but also that many nonwhites fail to receive necessary care.[5] *For example, nonwhites are more than three times more likely to die of hypertension than whites of the same age-group. The findings of the Task Force on*

***Black and Minority Health, which were released late in 1985, found that 60,000 excess deaths occur each year in minority populations.***[23]

The excess number of preventable deaths is derived by calculating the difference between the number of deaths in the African-American population and the number that would have been expected to occur by applying the average annual age-specific rates of the U.S. white population to the U.S. midperiod black population (as of 1983).[8] ***This means that there would be no excess black deaths if the mortality rates of black and white persons were the same.***

Seven causes of death were identified that together account for more than 80% of the excess mortality. The following health problems related to excess deaths are listed in alphabetic order[8]:

- Cancer—16% of excess mortality among African-American men younger than 70 years of age.
- Cardiovascular disease and stroke—24% of excess mortality among African-American men and 41% among African-American women. Most of these deaths were due to hypertensive heart disease.
- Chemical dependency (measured by deaths resulting from cirrhosis of the liver, associated with excessive use of alcohol—13% of excess mortality among Native American men and 22% among Native American women younger than 70 years of age.
- Diabetes—38% of excess deaths among Mexican-born Hispanic women.
- Homicides and accidents (unintentioned injuries)—60% of excess mortality among Hispanics younger than 65 years of age.
- Infant mortality—of excess deaths among African-American females up to age 45 years, death in the first year of life account for 35%.
- Unintentional injuries cause 44% of excess deaths among male and 30% among female Native Americans. Homicides and unintentional injuries account for 19% of excess mortality among African-American men younger than 70 years of age and 38% among those younger than age 45. The figures for African-American women are 6% and 14%, respectively. A substantial portion of excess deaths in this category may be associated with excessive use of alcohol and other drugs.

Table 8-2 compares the rates of four major chronic illnesses for white and black Americans.

The life expectancy for both black and white populations in the United States increased from 1980 to 1990 for all age categories except for black males between 15 and 24 years of age (Table 8-3).

## Cultural Values

***Western culture tends to be cure-oriented; therefore, health care for acute conditions is often more valued than is health care for the chronically ill.*** In contrast to the exciting aspects of sophisticated and mechanical technology, caring for chronically ill persons is often considered boring. The continued struggle to cope with day-to-day living soon becomes tedious for ill persons, their families, and health professionals. ***The rewards of treating chronic illness cannot be measured by a cure but by the prevention of complications and by helping persons function at their optimal level.***

The cultural context has many symbolic meanings, beliefs, and values that health professionals need to understand to meet individual health needs. Some persons may view their chronic disease as a form of punishment from God (see Chapter 5). Thus they may experience a sense of guilt. Those who view their chronic disease as a "leper phenomenon" may experience a sense of social rejection. Others may see their chronic illness as a destructive force without meaning or simply as a physical response of the body. Appreciation of the person's beliefs and behavior in the context of his or her cultural heritage rather than denial of the cultural influence increases understanding between the health professional and the chronically ill person. Differences need not imply deviance. It is possible to introduce health practices in a manner congruent with the individual's cultural values (see Chapter 5).

**TABLE 8-2 Number of Selected Reported Chronic Conditions per 1000 Persons by Race and Age: United States, 1989**

| | WHITE | | BLACK | |
|---|---|---|---|---|
| CHRONIC CONDITIONS | 65-74 | 75 YEARS AND OVER | 65-74 | 75 YEARS AND OVER |
| Arthritis | 431.7 | 562.8 | 520.4 | 525.3 |
| Diabetes | 80.2 | 82.0 | 148.2 | 196.0 |
| Heart disease | 234.7 | 366.7 | 207.8 | 243.3 |
| Hypertension | 367.8 | 366.9 | 534.0 | 490.1 |

From National Center for Health Statistics, Division of Interview Health Statistics. Data from National Health Interview Survey, 1989.

**TABLE 8-3 Comparison of Life Expectancy for the Black and White Populations From 1980 to 1991**

| | LIFE EXPECTANCY IN YEARS | |
|---|---|---|
| POPULATION | 1980 | 1991 |
| Black males* | 63.8 | 64.6 |
| White males | 70.7 | 72.9 |
| Black females | 72.5 | 73.8 |
| White females | 78.1 | 79.6 |

From National Center for Health Statistics, Division of Interview Health Statistics. Data from National Health Interview Survey, 1991.
*Increase in life expectancy for all except those 15-24 years of age, in whom the death rate increased each year since 1980.

### Cost of Disability

Chronically ill persons and their families are subjected to great personal and emotional losses that must be dealt with—loss of self-esteem, loss of status within the family, loss of independence, feeling of rejection, and feelings of helplessness are only a few. These can be more devastating than economic deprivation, which is a constant problem.

The economic cost to the patient and family is considerable. The cost of hospitalization rises yearly. Frequent or extended hospitalization and medical expenses can be ruinous if patients are inadequately insured or if they cannot afford medical insurance or have been dropped by an insurance company because of the chronicity of their condition. In 1993 it was estimated that 37 million Americans had no medical insurance.

Many are forced to seek public assistance merely to survive. Placement in quality nursing homes, which commonly costs $3000 or more a month, is financially impossible for most patients or their families to manage. The cost of medications to control or maintain a patient's health status may require a major portion of the family budget. Additional expenses may include special diets and equipment, home modifications (e.g., ramps or widening of doors for wheelchairs), transportation, and support services provided by homemakers, day or live-in attendants, or nurses.

The ability of the individual family to pay its own way is determined in part by which member of the family becomes disabled. Older studies showed that the family suffered less economic deprivation if the wife was disabled. In those studies, three fourths of the chronically ill persons unable to carry out their jobs were men. Today, however, more and more households are headed by women who are single parents and are the only wage earners for the family. Women who head households will need additional help and support, and nurses should be sensitive to their needs.

Some financial assistance is provided by Medicare. This federally administered program provides hospital and medical insurance protection for persons 65 years of age and older, as well as for those younger than 65 years who are disabled and eligible for Social Security benefits. Persons under age 65 who are medically indigent because of health problems may be eligible for assistance through the Medicaid program.

Recent changes in federal funding have altered Medicare and Medicaid programs. Persons aged 65 years and older receiving Social Security benefits have a higher fee deducted from their monthly payments to pay for their Medicare premiums. Medicare Part A pays for hospitalization; Medicare Part B covers medical expenses and physician care. Since Jan. 1, 1994, Medicare Part A pays all but $676 for the first 60 days of hospitalization and Medicare Part B covers physician bills, physical therapy treatments, rental of wheelchairs, and so on. Part B does not cover the cost of medicines, eyeglasses, hearing aids, or dentures. Medicare reimbursement is commonly 80% of the amount billed. Most persons covered by Medicare purchase supplemental health insurance (coinsurance) to cover the expenses not reimbursed by Medicare.

There have been severe cutbacks in Medicaid, which is administered by state governments. For example, persons seeking Medicaid assistance in Ohio are not eligible if they have assets of more than $1500. Until recently a person was allowed to keep his or her home if a spouse was living in it. However, some persons who were financially well-off were advised by lawyers to "spend down their assets" to become eligible for Medicaid. That is, they were advised to transfer their assets to children or other relatives so that it appeared they were unable to pay for nursing home care. Because Medicaid was intended to be a program for the indigent, several governors have proposed more stringent eligibility standards and some states have passed laws that make it impossible for well-to-do persons to receive Medicaid after they have "spent down their assets." In Ohio a person is allowed to keep his or her home if a spouse is still living in it; however, the house will be sold by the state after the death of the spouse to recover the amount of Medicaid assistance received by one or both spouses. Because of large state budget deficits beginning in the 1990s, several governors proposed even more stringent eligibility standards for Medicaid.

Thus persons with chronic illnesses may have considerable difficulty in paying for prescribed therapy. For example, antiinflammatory agents used to treat arthritis are very expensive. Many of these medications cost between $0.75 and $1.25 each, and the usual dose is three times daily. Persons with other chronic conditions such as Parkinson's disease may be taking even more expensive drugs (costing as much as $1200/month). It is not uncommon for persons with limited resources to have to decide whether to purchase medications or food because there is not enough money for both.

At this writing, President Clinton's proposal for health care reform in the United States is being debated by Congress. His proposal would provide health insurance for all Americans, would be portable (i.e., would go with the person from one job to another), and would provide assistance with the cost of prescription medications for those receiving Medicare.

## EPIDEMIOLOGY

Epidemiology examines the distribution of chronic disease, as well as the measurement of health status in the general population. It is both a body of knowledge and a method for obtaining knowledge. As a methodology, epidemiology can be used to assist in explaining the multifactorial causal patterns of chronic diseases.

## PROBLEMS IN DETERMINING CAUSALITY OF CHRONIC DISEASES

Some of the factors that contribute to the difficulty of studying the cause of chronic disease are the following:

1. *Multifactorial nature of etiologic factors.* The operation of multiple factors is particularly important in chronic diseases. The interaction of factors may be purely additive or synergistic; that is, the combined potential for harm of many risk factors is more than the sum of the individual potentials. They interact, reinforce, and even multiply each other. Asbestos workers, for example, have increased lung cancer risk. Asbestos workers who smoke have 30 times more risk than co-workers who do not smoke and 90 times more risk than persons who neither smoke nor work with asbestos.

2. *Absence of a known agent.* Because no specific diagnostic test exists for many chronic diseases, the distinction between persons with a disease and those free of disease may be more difficult to establish than in most infectious diseases.

3. *Long latent period.* Many chronic diseases have a long latent period, which is the equivalent of the incubation period in infectious disease except that it is generally longer. Because of the extended latency, it is often difficult to link antecedent events with outcomes. However, increasing evidence shows that onset of ill health is strongly linked to influences of physical, social, economic, and family environments. It is easy to identify the common exposure to chickenpox in a school setting, but it is much more difficult to identify the impact of drastic alterations in family circumstances and resulting mental disorders or slow-onset physical illnesses.

4. *Indefinite onset.* The problem of pinpointing the initial occurrence of the disease exists with many chronic conditions, such as degenerative diseases and mental illnesses. Because of the vague onset of chronic illnesses, it is difficult to collect statistics on the number of new cases in any given year.

5. *Differential effect of factors on incidence and course of disease.* Factors in the socioeconomic environment that affect health include income level, housing, employment status, culture, and life-style. For example, Mormons who abstain from smoking and alcohol have lower cancer rates than the general population as a whole.

6. *Disease-specific mortality rates.* These rates are difficult to determine with chronic illness because the cause of death may result from factors other than the chronic disease itself.

One approach for studying chronic illness from an epidemiologic viewpoint is to emphasize that interrelated factors determine illness; that is, disease is a process that results from the breakdown of a multiplicity of factors: biologic, cultural, economic, emotional, and social. The multiple interactions involving the *host,* the *environment,* and the *agent* sometimes are described as the "web of causation." With this approach an attempt is made to identify the multiple related factors that lead to the disease process. *Until a disease can be understood as a web of causation, it is difficult to make rational decisions regarding therapeutic interventions, and it is even more difficult to identify early preventive actions.* To develop a chain of causation, one must identify first the natural history of disease by systematic studies of groups of people.

## NATURAL HISTORY OF DISEASE

All diseases have a natural history. For example, chronic diseases extend over time and develop through a sequence of stages. When people speak of the epidemiology of a disease, they are referring to its natural history. That is, the outcomes of a particular disease are observed over time, and the numbers of the affected persons developing each outcome are measured. This information is used to predict an individual's possible future health. Knowledge of the natural history of disease allows us to intervene to prevent or limit the effects of diseases. The stages involved in the natural history include the following:

1. *Stage of susceptibility.* The disease has not yet developed, but the groundwork has been laid by the presence of factors that favor its occurrence. These may be referred to as *risk factors.* The need to identify such factors is becoming more apparent as awareness grows that chronic diseases present our major health challenge. Some major risk factors are environmental and behavioral and therefore are amenable to change; for example, smokers can be persuaded to give up smoking.

2. *Stage of presymptomatic disease.* No manifestation of disease is present, but pathologic changes have begun. An example of presymptomatic disease is atherosclerotic changes in coronary vessels before any overt signs or symptoms of illness appear.

3. *Stage of clinical disease.* By this stage sufficient anatomic or functional changes have occurred so that recognizable signs of disease exist. At present the natural history of many diseases is incompletely understood. For example, it is not known why some individuals with several risk factors do not progress to clinical disease, whereas others with fewer risk factors develop disease.

4. *Stage of disability.* Disability, which can result from an acute or a chronic condition, reduces a person's activity. The extent of protracted disability resulting from chronic disease is very significant to the person and society because of the person's reduced income, the impact on psychosocial rules, and the burden on community resources.

The subtlety of the natural history of chronic diseases often leaves the person unaware of a disease process for an extended period. Recently, *predisposing characteristics or habits that help identify the person at risk to develop a particular chronic disease have been studied*

***extensively. By altering habits of eating, rest, activity, or smoking, the course of certain chronic illnesses*** such as emphysema, hypertension, or heart disease ***may be changed.*** Unfortunately, many chronic conditions begin without the individual's awareness of significant physiologic changes. An important step in prevention is early detection of these changes.

## PREVENTION

Because chronic disease evolves over time and pathologic changes may become irreversible, the goal is to detect risk factors as early as possible. Although the degenerative diseases differ from their infectious disease predecessors in having more complex causes, it is now clear that many are preventable.

Generally, prevention means inhibiting the development of a disease before it occurs. More specifically, the term includes several levels of prevention to interrupt or slow the progression of disease: (1) primary prevention, (2) secondary prevention, and (3) tertiary prevention.

**Primary prevention,** appropriate in the stage of susceptibility, is concerned with health promotion and specific protection against diseases. **Secondary prevention,** applied in presymptomatic and clinical disease, includes early detection and prompt intervention to halt the progression of the disease. **Tertiary prevention,** appropriate in the stage of disability, uses rehabilitation activities to prevent further complications and to restore optimal functioning as much as possible.

Another way of looking at prevention has been identified by Albee.[1] He has developed a "prevention equation" for preventing dysfunction:

$$\text{Incidence of dysfunction} = \frac{\text{Stress} + \text{Constitutional vulnerabilities}}{\text{Social supports} + \text{Coping skills} + \text{Competence}}$$

The two major strategies for preventing dysfunction are decreasing the values in the numerator (i.e., decreasing stress or constitutional vulnerabilities) and increasing the values in the denominator (i.e., increasing social supports, coping skills, and competence). It is more difficult to have an impact on the numerator of the prevention equation because stress in our lives cannot always be controlled; however, creative ways to decrease individual and societal stress must continually be sought. It is easier to affect the denominator by strengthening social supports, coping skills, and competence.[1] (For more information on stress see Chapter 7.)

One valuable tool that has been developed to assist persons to identify their own risk factors and change their life-styles is the health hazard appraisal (HHA).[17] The HHA is a screening process that includes a comprehensive questionnaire and the taking of certain physical measurements. On the basis of probability tables, a risk assessment is then calculated from each person's profile along with goals that would result in risk reduction. Counseling and follow-up are provided to reinforce the data.

## CHRONICALLY ILL PERSONS AND THEIR FAMILIES

***The effects of chronic illness on the affected person and family members are numerous and varied. The first impact of the disability may nearly immobilize them.*** Time must be provided for them to talk through their concerns and fears before they can be expected to begin coping with their new situation.

Marked changes are often required in family living as a result of chronic illness. Some families may find themselves drawn closer together. Other families may drift apart, the individual members being incapable of helping one another. At times, chronic illness may threaten a person's basic emotional stability, and the whole situation may be unbearable to others. Sometimes the person's emotional needs may not have been apparent to family members early in the illness, but when such needs grow obvious, relatives feel inadequate to cope with the situation. ***The length of illness, periodic hospitalizations, and increased financial, emotional, and social burdens are stressors that threaten the family's integrity.***

Many persons struggle on their own to assume the full financial burden of the illness and consequently expose other members of the family to lower standards of nutrition, housing, and care. Many times relatives move in with one another, arguments develop, and family ties are strained or broken. Public assistance may be acceptable to some families, whereas others find it impossible to accept.

Chronic illness imposes additional problems of learning how to cope with restrictions on activities of daily living, how to prevent or identify medical crises that occur, and how to carry out treatment regimens as delineated by the health care provider. Family members also need to learn about the restrictions, not only to be of assistance to the chronically ill person but also to adjust to resultant disruptions in their own activity patterns.

***Because chronic illness may have periods of exacerbation when symptoms become more acute and medical crises may occur, patients and family members need to know which symptoms must be reported to the health care provider as well as the time interval for reporting these symptoms.*** They also need to know how to contact the provider and what measures to take if a medical crisis occurs. For example, if a person has a history of myocardial infarction, family members must know what to do if the person experiences severe chest pain. Should the person be taken immediately to a hospital emergency room or should the physician be contacted first? Patient and family members should plan in

## RESEARCH

Burckardt CS et al: Quality of life of adults with chronic illness: a psychometric study, *Res Nurs Health* 12(6):347-354, 1989.

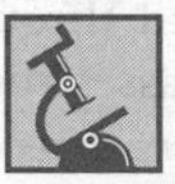

This study was designed to look at the quality of life of middle-aged to older adults with one of four chronic conditions: diabetes mellitus, ostomy secondary to colon cancer or colitis, osteoarthritis (OA), or rheumatoid arthritis (RA). Four instruments, including the quality of life scale (QOLS), and open-ended questions were used to collect data. All four groups of subjects identified the areas that were important to their quality of life. The major areas identified were independence, being physically active, being able to care for self, being healthy, having a sense of security, and maintaining positive interactions and relationships with others. Persons with OA also emphasized freedom from pain whereas those with diabetes emphasized being in control. These findings suggest that nurses need to be aware of the importance the persons they are caring for attach to the factors identified in this study.

advance the sequence of actions to take during a medical crisis, depending on the nature and extent of the presenting symptoms.

## COMPLIANCE AND NONCOMPLIANCE

Persons with chronic illness often are labeled as "compliant" or "noncompliant" in carrying out regimens prescribed for them. There are many factors that influence the person's ability or motivation to carry out the prescribed regimen. If the person does not carry out the regimen (noncompliant), it does not necessarily mean that the individual is refusing to do so deliberately, although this may sometimes occur.

Before the nursing diagnosis of noncompliance is made, the nurse needs to assess the situation to determine the reasons that the patient is not complying with therapeutic recommendations. The etiology of noncompliance includes the patient's value system (health beliefs, cultural influence, spiritual values).[12] The following are some possible reasons for nonadherence to a prescribed therapy[15]:

1. Failure to understand or internalize the reason for the recommendations
2. Procedures that are difficult to learn and carry out
3. Time required to carry out therapy
4. Inability to pay for prescribed therapy
5. Side effects of therapy (e.g., medications, exercises)
6. Embarrassment about carrying out regimen in front of others
7. Social isolation and lack of support and positive reinforcement

Conflicts occur within the family structure when one family member recognizes the importance of carrying out the prescribed regimen but another does not. For example, a wife may see the need for continuing checkups and medication for her husband's hypertension, whereas he may perceive this as a needless expense because he feels well and has no symptoms. Persons vary from time to time in the extent of compliance. Those who are not hospitalized are their own health care agents and they (or their significant others) determine the actions that are taken.

*Coping mechanisms that have been developed should not be tampered with unless, based on a thorough understanding of the situation, viable and more appropriate alternatives can be proposed.* If the goal of maintaining the chronically ill person in the optimal state of health is being interfered with by the individual's or the family's attitudes or capacities, a change in those attitudes or capacities is necessary, but it must be a change that is mutually acceptable. In preparation for giving the highest level of care to persons with a chronic illness, the nurse may find it helpful to review research in this area.[14,18-20,27] See Research box on left.

# ASSESSMENT OF THE PERSON WITH A CHRONIC ILLNESS

Before a plan of care can be devised for the chronically ill person, a thorough assessment of needs and capabilities must be carried out. Included in such an assessment are the individual's *physical, psychologic, social,* and *financial status.*

## PHYSICAL STATUS

Because medical diagnoses do not accurately reflect the physical status and functioning of the chronically ill person, the use of a profile system or assessment tool may be instituted as a guide for those working with the patient. One such tool[17] provides a guide for grading the patient in six different categories: (1) physical condition, including cardiovascular, pulmonary, gastrointestinal, genitourinary, endocrine, or cerebrovascular disorders, (2) upper extremities—structure and function—including the shoulder girdle and cervical and upper dorsal spine, (3) lower extremities—structure and function—including the pelvis and lower dorsal and lumbar sacral spine, (4) sensory components relating to speech, vision, and hearing, (5) excretory function, including the bowels and bladder, and (6) mental and emotional status. The ability of the person to carry out activities of daily living (e.g., dressing, feeding, bathing, brushing teeth, combing hair, toileting, and moving from place to place) specifically needs to be assessed. The completed assessment should indicate in what areas the patient has difficulty and the extent of that difficulty. Such a guide can be used in planning goals for care, both immediate and long term, and will be useful in assisting the individual and the family to make realistic plans for care.

Because a chronic condition is not static, reassessment should be carried out at regular intervals to establish whether there is improvement or regression. The assessment tool on p. 206 covers the areas just mentioned.

The impact of chronic illness on the person's desire for or ability to participate in sexual activities should be assessed. Changes in body appearance, shortness of breath, and musculoskeletal or neurologic impairments cause some persons to think that they can no longer be sexually active. In addition, the side effects of certain medications tend to decrease sexual desire or cause impotence. The nurse should determine if concern about sexual ability is a problem for the person, and if it is, appropriate action including referral can be taken. (See Chapter 51 for more information about sexuality in health and illness.)

## PSYCHOLOGIC STATUS

***Assessment of the person's psychologic needs and capabilities includes determining attitudes and stage of adaptation to the illness, feelings concerning how illness affects the family or significant others, and the person's own goals in regard to living with an illness.*** For example, those who are almost totally helpless as a result of an accidental spinal cord injury may seem to have no interest in learning ways to help themselves. Family members may react in the same manner and be of little help to them. Both the affected person and family need interest and support from nurses and other professionals as they learn to cope with the change in their life situations.

***Feelings of anxiety, frustration, irritability, bitterness, and guilt may be expressed by some chronically ill persons who face unending pain and loss of economic and social security.*** Some persons become obsessed with their health problems and spend much of each day thinking about what will happen and what to do. Guilt may result from being unable to work and support oneself or from the belief, as a result of a search for some purpose or reason for the affliction, that one must deserve the suffering. *Depression is common among chronically ill persons, especially those who feel powerless. Powerlessness can be the result of feeling unable to control or overcome what has happened to one.*[13] Patients who are depressed may be suicidal, and the nurse should be alert to cues that the patient may be contemplating suicide.

## SOCIAL AND FINANCIAL STATUS

Social and financial status must be considered because both relate specifically to the kind of support and resources available to meet the person's goals. It would be unrealistic, for example, to plan for a hydraulic bathtub chair if the patient could not afford it, if family members were unavailable to help operate it, or if the patient's apartment manager would not permit it to be installed. Alternative methods of helping the patient to take a tub bath would have to be explored.

The social assessment includes living arrangements, family roles, support of significant others, cultural and social group memberships, education, and vocational and avocational activities. The data collected through the performance of this kind of thorough assessment should make it possible to devise a ***plan of care directed toward the accomplishment of attainable goals that are mutually acceptable to the patient, the family, and the caregivers.***

## ♦ NURSING DIAGNOSES

Nursing diagnoses are determined from analysis of patient data. Nursing diagnoses for the patient with a chronic illness may include but are not limited to the following (these diagnoses are listed in alphabetical order and not in order of priority):

| Diagnostic Title | Possible Etiologic Factors |
|---|---|
| Activity intolerance | Bedrest, immobility, generalized weakness, sedentary life-style |
| Adjustment, impaired | Disability requiring change in life-style; inadequate support systems; impaired cognition, sensory overload; altered locus of control; incomplete grieving |
| Anxiety | Threat to self-concept; threat of change in health status, socioeconomic status, and role functioning |
| Breathing pattern, ineffective | Neuromuscular impairment, pain, musculoskeletal impairment |
| Communication, impaired verbal | Aphasia, physical impairment |
| Constipation | Change in life-style, immobility, inadequate nutrition, inadequate fluid intake |
| Coping, ineffective family: compromised | Inadequate or incorrect information, temporary family disorganization and role changes, prolonged disability of significant person |
| Diversional activity deficit | Long-term hospitalization |
| Fear | Loss of body part, long-term illness, pain, life-style changes |
| Health maintenance, altered | Altered communication skills, decreased motor skills |
| Home maintenance management, impaired | Insufficient family resources, lack of knowledge/role modeling, inadequate support systems |
| Hopelessness | Prolonged activity restriction, failing physical condition, long-term stress |
| Incontinence, functional | Altered environment; sensory, cognitive, or mobility deficits |
| Incontinence, reflex | Neurologic impairment |
| Injury, high risk for | Sensory/motor deficits, lack of awareness of environmental hazards |
| Knowledge deficit | Lack of exposure/recall, cognitive limitation |

| Diagnostic Title | Possible Etiologic Factors |
|---|---|
| Mobility, impaired physical | Intolerance to activity; decreased strength/endurance; pain/discomfort; cognitive, neuromuscular, or musculoskeletal impairment; depression; severe anxiety |
| Nutrition, altered: less than body requirements | Chewing or swallowing difficulties, inability to obtain food |
| Pain | Immobility, improper positioning, pressure points |
| Powerlessness | Health care environment, illness-related regimen, lifestyle of helplessness |
| Self-care deficit, bathing/hygiene, dressing/grooming, feeding/toileting | Intolerance to activity/fatigue, pain/discomfort, perceptional/cognitive impairment, musculoskeletal impairment, depression |
| Self-esteem disturbance | Severe trauma, change in body appearance, change in social involvement |
| Sexual dysfunction | Altered body structure, physiologic limitations |
| Skin integrity, impaired | Mechanical forces (pressure, shearing), immobility |
| Social interaction, impaired | Poor communication skills, self-concept disturbance, absence of supportive others, altered thought processes |

## ♦ EXPECTED PATIENT OUTCOMES

Because outcomes for specific chronic diseases are discussed in the chapters dealing with those diseases, not all possible outcomes will be discussed here. However, in general it may be stated that on discharge from the hospital or other care facility, patients with chronic disease or their family members should be able to do the following:

1. Demonstrate or explain those measures that must be taken to avoid further preventable disability.
2. Demonstrate or explain those self-care activities of which they are capable.
3. Identify those activities for which help is needed.
4. Explain who will be available to help with those activities and on what basis that help will be available.
5. Recognize the effect that change in body appearance and social involvement have on self-esteem.
6. Recognize the need to work on coping skills of patient and family.
7. Explain what community resources are available and how to obtain them.
8. Discuss in reasonable detail their plans for follow-up care and reevaluation.

## ♦ INTERVENTIONS

### Limiting Disability

The first focus in intervention for the chronically ill person is on preventing and reducing disability and enabling the person to remain a socially functioning individual in every respect. Some disabilities among chronically ill persons might have been prevented if prompt, aggressive, suitable medical and nursing care had been available at the onset of the illness. *Many of the difficulties that limit these persons may not have been caused by the disease itself but may have developed because of immobility during the acute phase of the illness.*

Keeping the person's body in good alignment, maintaining joint range and strength, and preventing decubitus ulcers are physical measures that constantly must be borne in mind. (For further information, see Chapter 67.) A careful plan of rest and activity helps preserve physical resources and makes the day purposeful. If assistance is needed, it should be given until the person can manage the activity by himself or herself or until an alternative method of management can be taught.

### Promoting Self-Care

Asking the person to identify what is meaningful is a primary step toward helping develop self-care. Physical needs are of paramount importance for chronically ill persons. Meeting these physical needs provides a way to convey to such individuals an interest in their progress and welfare. For chronically ill persons who must be hospitalized, it is important that they be allowed to perform as much of their own care as possible. Persons who have been independent in self-care before hospitalization should not be allowed to regress in these abilities if at all possible. Helping them to take their own baths, attend to toilet needs, and groom themselves can give some sense of accomplishment and help them maintain their self-respect. Helping them to be dressed appropriately promotes a sense of wellness. Success in performing portions of their own self-care may be stimulating enough to strengthen ill persons' motivation; they and their families then may make amazing strides in thinking through and working out future problems themselves. For their planning to be realistic and ultimately functional, all health care personnel must teach chronically ill persons the total physiologic ramifications of their disability, as well as methods of coping with those ramifications.

Persons who are in their homes or in substitute homes should be encouraged to dress in regular, comfortable street clothing rather than pajamas or gowns. Visitors to the home and family members who constantly see such individuals dressed in bedclothes think of them as sick and are reminded of their illness. Seeing them dressed as usual helps to maintain normal attitudes, relationships, and expectations.

### Promoting Self-Esteem

The care of chronically ill persons requires alertness in feeling, seeing, and hearing. Continued warmth and interest are necessary to the self-esteem of any chronically ill person. Very often a relationship based on an understanding of these requirements promotes self-esteem and helps the individual to become highly motivated. It may be taxing to listen to the same questions and say the same things day after day, but the nature of chronic illness may require this attention, and the manner in which responses are given will convey warmth and interest. The world of chronically ill persons, whether they are in the hospital or elsewhere, becomes narrowed and circumscribed. They treasure and are interested in those things and those people who are close to them. Their conversations may be largely about themselves, their immediate environment, a few close objects, and the persons who are close to them. Although they may be confined to bed and to their room, others can keep them up-to-date on outside news. Depending on their level of adaptation to their illness, they may welcome hearing about outside events, or they may not be able to think beyond themselves. When they reach the stage of being able to look beyond themselves, newspapers, magazines, radio, television, or creating something with their own hands may help to keep up their interest in others and in outside events.

## Supporting Coping Skills

Coping skills may be challenged by persistent, ongoing problems such as chronic pain, recurring medical expenses, or continuing difficulties in carrying out activities of daily living. Usual coping methods may become impossible; for example, a person who usually copes by *expending energy in physical activity* may become unable to do so. The person who *usually copes by discussing problems with family members* will need to find an alternative method if family communication patterns break down. The person can be helped to identify usual coping methods and to explore alternative approaches when necessary.

It is important to recognize that chronically ill persons or their families may suffer from unresolved sadness known as **chronic grief.** Chronic grief may be defined as accumulated or prolonged grief. It extends over long periods, with permanent characteristics developing in many persons, and carries with it a potential for decreased functioning. The causes are varied, and new waves of grief are constantly triggered. One example is grief caused by the losses associated with aging: youth, dreams, jobs, hair, friends, family, health, visual acuity, social role, money, body parts, and mobility. Each loss is accompanied by grief, which builds on previous grief, just as individual bricks create a wall. In chronic grief the person may be faced with repeated acute episodes. These episodes may coincide with exacerbation of the condition, facing a new limitation, or meeting new indignities. Each new episode requires a renewed struggle back and forth through the various stages of grief.[18]

The nurse can assist by listening and helping the person explore feelings and the content related to these feelings. Because the grief is ongoing, family members also can be helped to identify their feelings and strengthen the communication patterns within the family structure for normal support of its members.

## Clarifying Nurse-Patient Values

Before nurses can work effectively with chronically ill persons they need to be able to distinguish between their own values, standards, and goals and those of the patient. In day-to-day contact with individuals who are making little or no progress, it is tempting to make plans for their future because of a sincere interest in helping them. This is particularly true when the patient's age is similar to one's own. There may be a feeling that something must be done to speed progress. One may become frustrated by the feeling of wanting to do something or wanting to see some marked change. However, the nurse must recognize that *management of chronically ill persons requires a slow-moving, persistent pace* with *possibly little or no change for a long time.* The person's physical and mental condition must be maintained at its present level or improved, and efforts must be made to progress and encourage the family's adaptation to the patient's condition. Eagerness and readiness to progress will be determining factors for the future. The *"doing" in the care of the chronically ill person is not always a physical action with the hands. Often the maintenance of a positive approach and attitude and a demonstration of real interest are the greatest help to the patient.* Teaching patients to perform activities related to their own care independently rather than performing those activities for them also may lead to progress.

## Supporting the Person With a Progressive Disability

Health care personnel must be prepared to provide care for patients whose disease will follow a course of progressive disability, as in multiple sclerosis or rheumatoid arthritis. In these instances, goals of care must be modified to retard the downhill progression of disability rather than to achieve maintenance or improvement of physical status. Helping the patient and family cope with progressive deterioration and in some cases eventual death is a demanding task. Those who wish additional information relating to this aspect of care are referred to the literature on this subject.[21]

Persons with a disability, whether obvious to others or unrecognizable, should be viewed not from the standpoint of the disability alone but for their abilities as well. Usually the greatest need is for comprehensive health services and continuing care. Comprehensive care is provided to patients according to their needs in an appropriate, continuous, and dynamic pattern. Accommodating the plan of care to the needs and goals of individual patients rather than to those of the providers is the essence of comprehensive care.

### Providing Community Resources

There has been increasing interest in providing programs for chronically ill persons and in assisting them and disabled persons to assume a more active role in their communities. Volunteer workers may act as readers both in hospitals and in homes or may assist with other diversional activities (Figure 8-2). Institutions receiving federal funds are required to make aids such as ramps available to persons who are unable to climb stairs or who are in wheelchairs. (See p. 214 for discussion of Americans With Disabilities Act.) With the development of structural changes that facilitate mobility, some persons with physical limitations are more involved in local activities and associations. Nurses can assist by supporting the further development of these structural changes in all community buildings and by encouraging the participation of chronically ill persons in community activities of interest. Various information sources may be obtained from national organizations involved with chronic illness and disability. Many of these agencies have services available in the community (Box 8-2). Programs, facilities, and legislation of this nature reflect the public's increasing awareness of the difficulties faced by chronically ill and disabled persons.

## ♦ EVALUATION

To evaluate the effectiveness of nursing interventions, compare patient behaviors with those stated in the expected patient outcomes. Successful achievement of patient outcomes for patients with chronic disease or their family members is indicated by the following:

1. Can demonstrate or explain the measures necessary to avoid further preventable disability.
2. Can demonstrate or explain the self-care activities of which the patient is capable.
3. Can identify the activities for which help is needed.
4. Can explain who will be available to help with the aforementioned activities and on what basis they will be available.
5. Can verbalize the effect that change in body appearance and social involvement has had on self-esteem.
6. Give evidence that they have been working to improve their coping skills.
7. Can explain what community resources they are using and how they obtained them.
8. Can discuss plans for follow-up care and reevaluation.

## REHABILITATION

Rehabilitation is the process of assisting the individual with a handicap to realize his or her particular goals, physically, mentally, socially, and economically. As such, **rehabilitation** is *an active concept* and *must be clearly differentiated from the concept of maintenance care.* After a thorough assessment of patients' disabilities and capabilities, assumptions can be made regarding the potential for improving their conditions. If improvement can be made, patients are candidates for rehabilitation. If improvement cannot be made, care is directed toward maintaining the current condition, that is, preventing further disability. The process of rehabilitation can be viewed more appropriately as *patient education* rather than *patient care.* One must remember, however, that the rehabilitation of every patient will reach an end point, that is, a point at which no further progress is possible. At that time the focus of care reverts to that of maintenance.

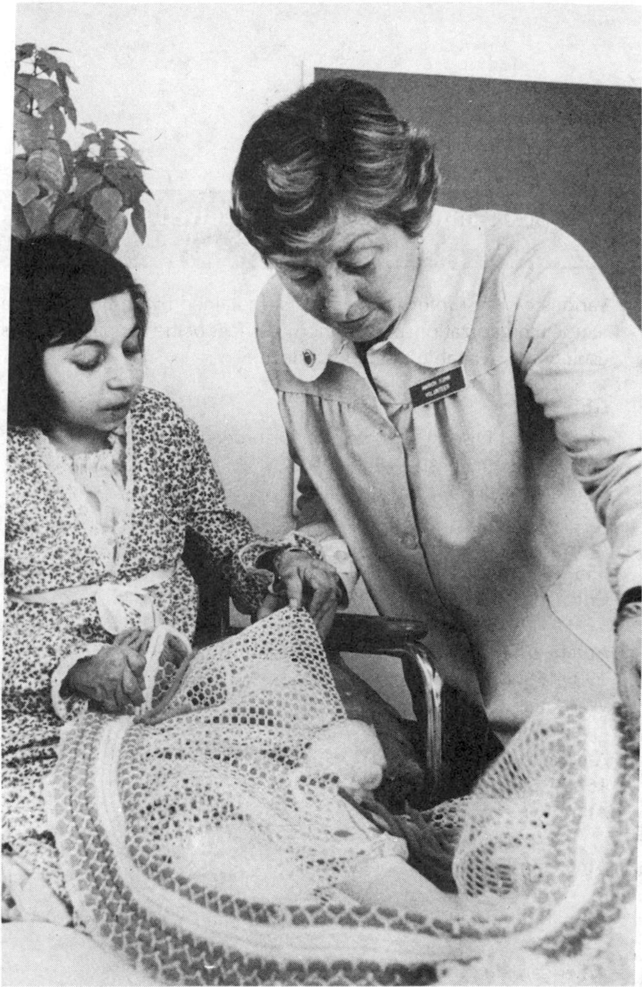

**FIGURE 8-2** Volunteer helping patient who has a chronic illness with some handwork.

The purpose or extent of rehabilitation ranges from employment or reemployment for the handicapped person to the more limited achievement of developing self-care abilities. This latter accomplishment can be just as important to the individual as earning money and may represent that person's greatest life achievement. This might be true, for example, for a person who was born with a severe physical handicap such as cerebral palsy.

**BOX 8-2** **Community Resources Involved in Chronic Health Problems**

Various types of information may be obtained by writing to these national organizations. In addition, services of the various agencies usually are available at the local level.

### GENERAL

Alzheimer's Disease and Related Disorders Association
360 N. Michigan Ave., Suite 601
Chicago, IL 60641

American Association of Diabetes Education
3553 W. Peterson Ave.
Chicago, IL 60659

American Association of Retired Persons
1909 K St., N.W.
Washington, DC 20006

American Cancer Society
1599 Clifton Rd., N.E.
Atlanta, GA 30329

American Diabetes Association
1 W. 48th St.
New York, NY 10020

American Heart Association
44 E. 23rd St.
New York, NY 10010

American Lung Association
1740 Broadway
New York, NY 10019

American Parkinson Disease Association
147 E. 50th St.
New York, NY 10022

Arthritis Foundation
221 Park Ave. S.
New York, NY 10003

Easter Seal Society for Crippled Children and Adults
2023 W. Ogden Ave.
Chicago, IL 60612

Juvenile Diabetes Foundation
23 E. 26th St.
New York, NY 10010

Leukemia Society of America, Inc.
211 E. 43rd St.
New York, NY 10017

Mental Health Materials Center
419 Park Ave. S.
New York, NY 10016

Muscular Dystrophy Association, Inc.
810 7th Ave.
New York, NY 10019

National Aid to Retarded Citizens
(formerly N.A.R. Children)
2709 E. St.
Arlington, TX 76011

National Association for Down's Syndrome
628 Ashland Ave.
River Forest, IL 60305

National Association for Mental Health, Inc.
1800 N. Kent St.
Rosslyn Station
Arlington, VA 22209

National Association for Sickle Cell Disease, Inc.
945 S. Western Ave., Suite 206
Los Angeles, CA 90006

National Association for Visually Handicapped
305 E. 24th St.
New York, NY 10010

National Asthma Center
875 Avenue of the Americas
New York, NY 10001

National Council on Aging
1828 L. St. NW
Washington, DC 20036

National Cystic Fibrosis Research Foundation
3379 Peachtree Rd., N.E.
Atlanta, GA 30326

National Epilepsy League
6 N. Michigan Ave.
Chicago, IL 60602

**BOX 8-2 Community Resources Involved in Chronic Health Problems—cont'd**

National Foundation—March of Dimes
1275 Mamaroneck Ave.
White Plains, NY 10605

National Genetics Foundation
250 W. 57th St.
New York, NY 10019

National Head Injury Foundation
333 Turnpike Rd.
Southborough, MA 01772

National Hemophilia Foundation
25 W. 39th St., Rm. 903
New York, NY 10018

National Kidney Foundation
116 E. 27th St.
New York, NY 10016

National Multiple Sclerosis Society
205 E. 42nd St.
New York, NY 10017

Nutrition Foundation, Inc.
489 5th Ave.
New York, NY 10017

Parents of Down's Syndrome Children
11507 Yates St.
Silver Spring, MD 20902

Shriners Hospital for Crippled Children
323 N. Michigan Ave.
Chicago, IL 60601

Stroke Clubs of America
805 12th St.
Galveston, TX 77550

United Cerebral Palsy Association, Inc.
66 E. 34th St.
New York, NY 10066

United Ostomy Association
1111 Wilshire Blvd.
Los Angeles, CA 90017

**REHABILITATION**

American Coalition of Citizens with Disabilities
1346 Connecticut Ave. N.W., Rm. 817
Washington, DC 20036

Architectural and Transportation Barriers Compliance Board
330 C St. W.W., Rm. 1010
Washington, DC 20201

Closer Look, National Information Center for the Handicapped
Box 1492
Washington, DC 20013

Mainstream, Inc.
1200 15th St., N.W., Rm. 403
Washington, DC 20005

National Center for a Barrier-Free Environment
8401 Connecticut Ave.
Washington, DC 20015

National Center for Law and the Handicapped
1235 N. Eddy St.
South Bend, IN 46617

National Congress of Organizations of the Physically Handicapped
7611 Oakland Ave.
Minneapolis, MN 55432

National Paraplegia Foundation
333 N. Michigan Ave.
Chicago, IL 60601

Paralyzed Veterans of America
7315 Wisconsin Ave. N.W.
Washington, DC 20014

President's Commission on Employment of the Handicapped
111 20th St. N.W., Rm. 636
Washington, DC 20210

Success in learning to adjust to living with a disability depends on the *person's premorbid personality, total life experience,* and *premorbid family relationships,* as well as the *person's current behavior and motivation.* Certainly, some rehabilitation can occur in any health agency; nevertheless, the greater the number of rehabilitation disciplines made available as needed to individuals, the greater is their chance of achieving their highest potential. The rehabilitation process, as with any form of education, is involved as deeply in the motives and purposes of the teacher as in those of the learner.

Persons with disabilities, whether obvious to others or unrecognizable, should not be viewed from the standpoint of their disability alone. Usually the greatest need is for comprehensive health services and continuing care. *Comprehensive care is that which is provided to patients according to their needs in an appropriate, continuous, and dynamic pattern.* Accommodating the plan of care to the needs and goals of individual patients rather than to those of the providers of care is the essence of comprehensive care.

## INTERDISCIPLINARY APPROACH

The number of professional persons required to assist the patient and family with rehabilitation will vary. *Most often the patient, the family, the physician, and the nurse can work out a practical plan.* If a patient's problems are complex, other members may be added to the team. Typically, such a team consists of a physician, nurse, discharge coordinator, medical social worker, vocational counselor, psychologist, speech pathologist, occupational and physical therapists, and a caseworker from the patient's social agency. Figure 8-3 shows members of an interdisciplinary team planning care for a patient. Teamwork requires that members of the team be able to use their special knowledge and skill and understand the value of their contribution to the patient's care. In addition, team members need some understanding of each other's professional functions and contributions. *One of the cooperative efforts of the involved team members is to meet regularly to evaluate patients and their abilities thoroughly. On the basis of this assessment, each patient and the team devise a plan to foster readjustment, compensation, and the learning of new ways to manage self-care and living.*

## REHABILITATION CENTERS

Persons with very complex problems of rehabilitation may need to receive care at specialized centers for rehabilitation, or they may receive care at home combined with visits to day rehabilitation centers. The variety of specialized centers includes teaching and research centers (centers located in and operated by hospitals and medical schools), community centers with facilities for inpatients, community outpatient centers, insurance centers, skilled nursing homes with an active rehabilitation service and staff including physical and occupational therapists, and vocational rehabilitation centers. In addition to centers that provide multiple services for the physically disabled, specialized centers provide rehabilitation for blind, deaf, mentally ill, and mentally retarded persons. Most centers offer a wide range of services that usually fall into the following three areas:

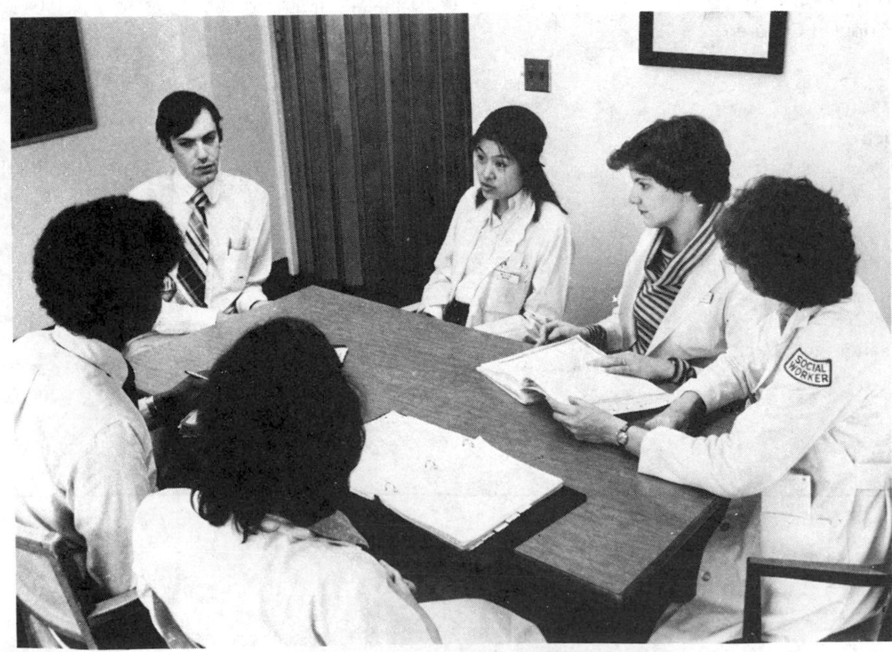


**FIGURE 8-3** The team approach to rehabilitation is essential. Here, physicians, nurse, physical therapist, and social worker review a patient's program and progress.

**Physical area**
- Physical, nursing, and medical evaluation
- Physical therapy
- Occupational therapy
- Speech therapy
- Medical and nursing supervision of appropriate activities

**Psychosocial area**
- Evaluation
- Personal counseling
- Social service
- Psychometrics
- Psychiatric service
- Recreational therapy

**Vocational area**
- Work evaluation
- Vocational counseling
- Prevocational experience
- Industrial fitness of programs
- Trial employment in sheltered workshops
- Vocational training
- Terminal employment in sheltered workshops
- Job placement

Several advantages exist for patients participating in organized programs for rehabilitation. They have an opportunity to see and be with others who have similar or more extensive disabilities. Often they progress more rapidly when they realize that others have similar difficulties and are overcoming them. Group therapy often arouses a competitive spirit, and a formerly reluctant person may become willing and diligent. On the other hand, all personnel need to be alert to those patients who have the opposite reaction. Patients who see others advance in activity while they either do not improve or progress very slowly may become so discouraged that they give up trying. In some cases the person becomes very depressed and may be suicidal. The nurse should be aware of changes in the person's behavior and be sensitive to any expression of suicidal ideas.

*On a rehabilitation unit activities are scaled so that individuals can see their own progress in comparison with their beginning abilities. Patients may take an active interest in keeping their own scores.* After a program of therapy has been planned and is scheduled as to time of day, patients can help to keep themselves on the schedule by having a copy of it at the bedside. Patients can then be assisted to gradually assume more responsibility for readying themselves for scheduled activities. In addition, a master plan of activities for all patients on the unit can be a useful device for nurses, physicians, and therapists. The plan can be kept in a central place on the unit and should list name, activity, and time of activity for each patient. This type of plan is also helpful when a patient's progress is to be reevaluated.

A public program for vocational rehabilitation has been serving the United States since 1920. The program involves a partnership between the state and the federal governments. Services for disabled persons are provided by state divisions of vocational rehabilitation. The federal government, through the Social and Rehabilitation Service (SRS), administers grants-in-aid and provides technical assistance and national leadership for the program. Opportunities and services are available in all 50 states, the District of Columbia, and Puerto Rico. All persons of working age with a substantial job handicap resulting from either physical or mental impairment are eligible for help or assistance. The purpose of this service is to *preserve, develop,* or *restore* the ability of disabled persons to earn their own livings. The individual services offered are medical care, counseling and guidance, training, and job finding. All 50 states have separate rehabilitation programs for blind persons. Application for such services can be made to the SRS or to the agency in the state for serving the blind.

## ROLE OF THE PATIENT

*The most important contributions to patients' rehabilitation are made by the patients themselves. The patient, his or her family, the nurse, the physician, the social worker, the occupational therapist, and sometimes others planning together can arrive at the best plans for the future,* but the *patient's attitudes, acceptance,* and *motivation are the most important considerations.* If the patient cannot adjust to the disability, whatever it is and however extensive, attempts at rehabilitation usually are hindered. Patients must make the decisions and they change at their own pace. If they are agreeable to suggestions but make little or no effort to try them, one should question if they really have accepted them.

The importance of motivation in rehabilitation was demonstrated recently by Dennis Byrd, a professional football player for the New York Jets, who was injured in a collision with another player during a game in November 1992. The seriousness of his injury was impressed on those watching the game on television by the extreme caution with which he was positioned on a backboard while his head was held in midline.

His prognosis was grave, and there was doubt that he would walk again. Yet, less than a year later he was able to walk unaided into the stadium on opening day of the 1993 football season, where he greeted his teammates and fans. From the beginning he believed that he would walk again and he worked hard to achieve this goal. In his book about his rehabilitation, *Rise and Walk,* he discusses the superb support he received from his wife, young daughter, and others and the role that his religious faith played in his recovery. His first-hand report gives the reader an insight into the role his motivation played in his recovery.

Self-care is encouraged within existing limitations. The patient's behavior from day to day can be the first indication of the direction of positive motivation. For example, if the patient makes every effort to resume normal daily activities such as feeding, bathing, and dressing, one can be certain that the person has a sincere desire to be independent. As patients become ready for more advanced activities, such as ambulation and work in the occupational therapy shop, they need continuing genuine interest and support (Figures 8-4 and 8-5). As obstacles arise, patients may be able to accept and eventually overcome them. Patients who are truly motivated toward helping themselves never seem to give up, finding ways of accomplishing activities that professional personnel might believe impossible. Each person working with the chronically ill patient has seen that many times life has meaning for the individual even though it may not be readily apparent to others. Some patients, however, when faced with an added burden, cannot accept it and give up trying. Guidance and support for the families of such patients become tremendously important. Health care personnel who understand these attitudes and behaviors can help make life satisfying for the chronically ill person and can positively influence the behaviors of the family, professional co-workers, and the public.

## ROLE OF THE NURSE

The concepts of comprehensive nursing care and rehabilitation can be considered synonymous. Helping the patient and family members to help themselves is an integral part of nursing care. Nurses who work with patients who have disabilities have two major responsibilities: (1) *to ensure that disability from disease or disuse is limited* as much as possible and (2) to *see that*

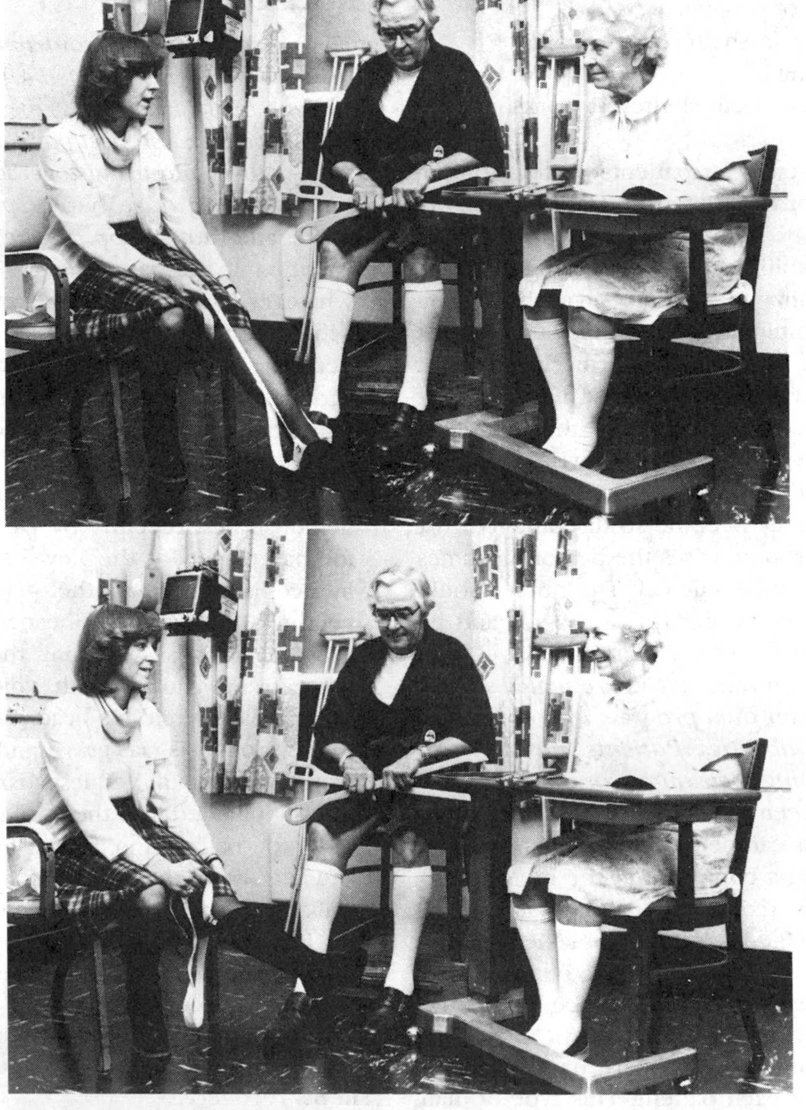

**FIGURE 8-4** The occupational therapist is concerned with helping patients make necessary adaptations in activities of daily living to permit independent functioning. Here the occupational therapist demonstrates the use of a stocking aid that, to the delight of patients, really works.

*a rehabilitation program is planned* and implemented. Details of the nurse's role and responsibilities are listed in Box 8-3.

## Limiting Disability

*Limitation of disability* is the *nurse's first responsibility* and *requires attention to the prevention of complications, to the early recognition of symptoms of exacerbations or complications, and to the prevention of deformity.* For patients with chronic illnesses, the onset of exacerbations or complications is frequently subtle, marked by minute changes in functional ability or general performance or attitude. Nurses, working closely with such patients and understanding the pathophysiology of their diseases, are frequently the first to recognize initial signs of difficulty and make provision for appropriate intervention.

## Planning and Implementing a Rehabilitation Program

The second responsibility, planning and implementing a program of rehabilitation in *accordance with the patient's goals,* is a process with which nurses are immediately involved. The first step in planning is to take a careful health history in four categories: physical/functional, psychosocial, economic/vocational, and spiritual. A tool for gathering these data can be found in Figure 8-6. Nursing personnel are likely to be in contact with a patient and the family for a longer period each day than are members of any other discipline on the reha-

*Text continued on p. 211.*

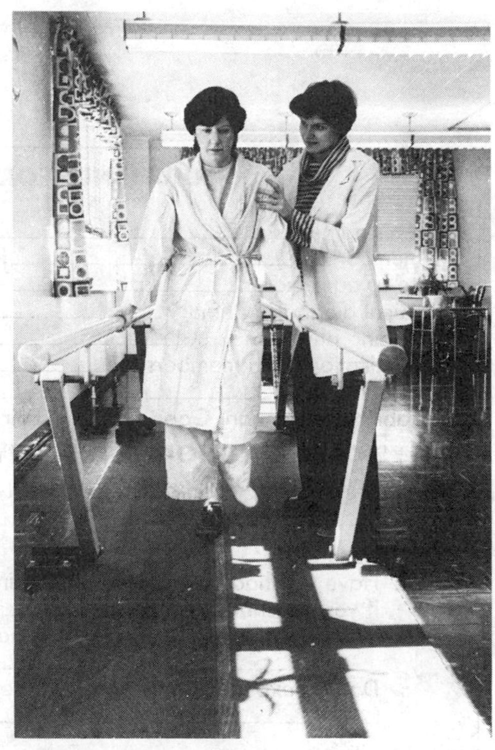

**FIGURE 8-5** A physical therapist begins a patient's ambulation training by teaching her to walk with the support of parallel bars. The patient wears no shoe on her left foot to remind her not to bear weight on it.

**BOX 8-3 The Nurse's Role and Responsibilities in Rehabilitation**

- I. Limit disability from disease as much as possible.
  - A. Prevent complications.
    - 1. Ensure early recognition of symptoms including patient's condition worsening.
      - a. Review signs and symptoms and pathology of the chronic illness to recognize changes.
      - b. Review signs and symptoms of complications frequently associated with the chronic illness, such as infection.
    - 2. Prevent deformities.
      - a. Maintain proper body alignment.
      - b. Position limbs to prevent contractures.
      - c. Turn frequently; keep skin clean and dry to prevent skin breakdown.
      - d. Provide adequate nutrition.
      - e. Provide adequate fluid intake to maintain bladder and bowel program.
      - f. Take precautions to prevent infection.
- II. Plan and implement rehabilitation program appropriate to patient.
  - A. Determine patient's own goals for rehabilitation.
  - B. Plan appropriate nursing interventions based on mutually agreed-on goals.

    Early in rehabilitation nurse may have to assume total responsibility for assisting with activities of daily living (ADLs): bathing, dressing, intake of food and fluids, bowel and bladder programs, maintaining skin integrity, turning patient, and so on.
  - C. Plan nursing interventions that encourage patient to assume responsibility for own ADLs as soon as possible.
    - 1. Set short-term goals with patient.
    - 2. Goals should be realistic and attainable.
    - 3. Reinforce patient's progress (no matter how small) with positive feedback.
    - 4. Work with other members of the rehabilitation team in providing a consistent, coordinated rehabilitation plan.
    - 5. Keep patient's significant others informed of patient's progress so they can give positive feedback to patient.
    - 6. Reassess goals periodically and set new goals as appropriate.
    - 7. Teach patient, family, and, if necessary, employer about patient's limitations and rehabilitative expectations.

## GUIDELINES FOR RECORDING HEALTH HISTORY

Client's name ________ Date of birth ________ Age ________
ID number ________ Race/ethnic origin ________
Date of admission ________ Date of initial assessment ________
Medical diagnosis: Primary ________ Secondary ________
Attending physician ________ Primary nurse ________
Rehabilitation team members ________
Informant: Client ________ Family member ________
Reliability of historian: Good ________ Fair ________ Poor ________

### PHYSICAL/FUNCTIONAL HISTORY

1. How would you describe your general health? Excellent ________ Very good ________ Good ________ Fair ________ Poor ________
2. Breathing
   a. Have you had any difficulty breathing before or with this admission? No ________ Yes ________
   If yes, describe the difficulty ________
   b. What can be done during your rehabilitation to make breathing easier for you? ________
   c. Do you expect any difficulties in breathing when you return home? ________
3. Nutrition
   a. How would you describe your nutrition? Excellent ________ Very good ________ Good ________ Fair ________ Poor ________
   b. Describe a typical day's food intake ________
   c. What is your weight? ________
   d. What foods do you like the best? ________
   e. What foods do you like the least? ________
   f. Are you now or have you ever been on a special diet? No ________ Yes ________
   If yes, what was the diet? ________
   g. At what times do you usually eat?
   h. Have you needed any assistance to eat? No ________ Yes ________
   If yes, what types of assistance? ________
   i. What is the condition of your mouth? Good ________ Cavities ________ Gum disease ________ Other ________ Specify other ________
   j. Do you wear dentures? No ________ Yes ________ Upper ________ Lower ________ Partial ________
4. Elimination
   a. Bladder
      (1) Have you had any difficulty passing urine? No ________ Yes ________
      If yes, what was the problem? ________
      what did you do about it? ________
      what treatment, if any, did you receive? ________
      (2) Do you frequently experience any of the following symptoms?

| | | | |
|---|---|---|---|
| Incontinence | ________ | Foul-smelling urine | ________ |
| Urgency | ________ | Cloudy urine | ________ |
| Frequency | ________ | Burning on urination | ________ |
| Pain on urination | ________ | Bloody urine | ________ |

If yes, to any of the above problems, what was done about it? ________

**FIGURE 8-6** Guidelines for recording health history. (From Dittmar SS: *Rehabilitation nursing: process and application,* St Louis, 1989, Mosby.)

**PHYSICAL/FUNCTIONAL HISTORY—cont'd**

(3) Do you need any assistance with bladder elimination? No _______ Yes _______
If yes, what type of assistance do you need? _______

b. Bowel

(1) How would you describe your bowel habits? Regular _______ Irregular _______

(2) How often do you usually have a bowel movement? Every day _______ Every other day _______
Twice a week _______ Once a week _______ Other _______

(3) What time of day do you usually have a bowel movement? Morning _______ Afternoon _______
Evening _______

(4) Tell me if you do any of the following things to assist you in having a bowel movement:
Eat certain foods _______ Specify _______
Drink certain fluids _______ Specify _______
Take medications _______ Specify _______
Insert suppositories _______ Specify _______
Perform digital stimulation _______ Perform Valsalva maneuver _______
Specify other _______

(5) Do you frequently experience any of the following problems?
Diarrhea _______ Impaction _______
Constipation _______ Incontinence _______
Specify other _______
If yes to any of the above, what did you do about the problem? _______
_______
What treatment, if any, did you receive? _______
_______

(6) Do you need any assistance in getting to the bathroom? No _______ Yes _______
If yes, what type of assistance? _______

5. Skin integrity

a. How would you describe the condition of your skin? Excellent _______ Very Good _______
Good _______ Fair _______ Poor _______

b. Do you bruise easily? No _______ Yes _______

c. Have you ever had open sores or ulcers that are slow to heal? No _______ Yes _______

d. Have you ever had rashes? No _______ Yes _______

e. Have you ever had moles that have grown? No _______ Yes _______

f. Do you sweat easily? No _______ Yes _______

g. Have you ever had itchy skin? No _______ Yes _______

h. If yes to any of the above problems, describe the circumstances and what you did about the problem?
_______
_______

6. Rest/comfort

a. Rest

(1) How would you describe the amount of rest you get? Always enough _______ Enough _______
Sometimes enough _______ Never enough _______

(2) What time do you usually go to bed? _______ Get up in the morning? _______

(3) Do you have any difficulty going to sleep at night? Always _______ Usually _______
Sometimes _______ Never _______

(4) Do you awaken during the night? Always _______ Usually _______ Sometimes _______
Never _______

(5) Do you take naps? No _______ Yes _______ If Yes, when? _______

(6) What aids, if any, do you use to go to sleep at night?
Drink warm liquids _______ Read _______
Take an alcoholic beverage _______ Turn night light on in room _______
Watch television _______ Take sleeping pills _______

**FIGURE 8-6, cont'd** Guidelines for recording health history.

*Continued.*

**PHYSICAL/FUNCTIONAL HISTORY—cont'd**

b. Comfort
(1) How would you describe your physical comfort? Always very comfortable ______
Usually comfortable ______ Sometimes comfortable ______ Never comfortable ______
(2) Have you experienced discomfort in the past? No ______ Yes ______
If yes, describe ______
______
What did you do about it? ______
Did it help? No ______ Yes ______ Partially ______
(3) If you have discomfort during your rehabilitation program, what would you like the nurse or therapists to do about it? ______
______

7. Personal hygiene/grooming
a. Have you needed the help of another person with:

| | | | |
|---|---|---|---|
| Bathing | ______ | Shaving | ______ |
| Brushing/combing your hair | ______ | Applying makeup | ______ |
| Brushing your teeth | ______ | Feminine hygiene | ______ |
| Applying deodorant | ______ | Dressing: Uppers ______ Lowers ______ Both | ______ |

b. Have you used any adaptive aids to assist with any personal hygiene or grooming activities?
No ______ Yes ______
If yes, specify ______

8. Communication
a. Vision
(1) How would you describe your vision? Excellent ______ Very good ______ Good ______
Fair ______ Poor ______
(2) Do you wear glasses? All the time ______ For reading ______ Never ______
(3) Do you wear contact lenses? All the time ______ While awake ______ Sometimes ______
Never ______
b. Hearing
(1) How would you describe your hearing?
Right ear: Excellent ______ Very good ______ Good ______ Fair ______ Poor ______
Left ear: Excellent ______ Very good ______ Good ______ Fair ______ Poor ______
(2) Have you ever had pain in either ear? No ______ Yes ______
(3) Have you ever had ringing in your ears? No ______ Yes ______
(4) Have you ever had a discharge from either ear? No ______ Yes ______
(5) If yes to any of these problems, describe ______
______
What did you do about it? ______
What treatment, if any, did you receive? ______
______
c. Sensation/perception
(1) Do you have any difficulties with feeling pain? No ______ Yes ______
With feeling temperature? No ______ Yes ______
(2) Do you have any intolerance to temperature? No ______ Yes ______
(3) If yes to 1 or 2, describe ______
______
What do you do about the problem? ______
d. Speech/language
(1) How would you describe your ability to express yourself? Excellent ______ Very good ______
Good ______ Fair ______ Poor ______
(2) How would you describe your ability to understand others? Excellent ______ Very good ______
Good ______ Fair ______ Poor ______

**FIGURE 8-6, cont'd** Guidelines for recording health history.

**PHYSICAL/FUNCTIONAL HISTORY—cont'd**

(3) Have you ever had difficulty expressing yourself? No ______ Yes ______
If yes, describe the circumstances ______
(4) Have you ever had difficulty understanding others? No ______ Yes ______
If yes, describe the circumstances ______

9. Mobility (ask questions appropriate to client's mobility status)
   a. How would you describe your ability to get out of or into a bed or chair? Excellent ______ Very good ______ Good ______ Fair ______ Poor ______
   b. How would you describe your ability to get into the bathtub? Excellent ______ Very good ______ Good ______ Fair ______ Poor ______
   c. How would you describe your ability to walk/navigate a wheelchair? Excellent ______ Very good ______ Good ______ Fair ______ Poor ______
   d. Have you ever had difficulty moving about? No ______ Yes ______
      If yes, describe the difficulty ______
      How did you manage? ______
   e. Do you expect to have any difficulty getting around when you leave the rehabilitation unit? No ______ Yes ______
      If yes, what do you expect to do about it? ______

10. Sexuality (ask questions according to client's martial status)
   a. How would you describe your sex life? Very satisfactory ______ Satisfactory ______ Not very satisfactory ______
   b. Has there been or do you expect differences in your ability to be a:
      Husband No ______ Yes ______
      Father No ______ Yes ______
      Wife No ______ Yes ______
      Mother No ______ Yes ______
      Significant other No ______ Yes ______
      If yes, describe what you expect the differences to be ______
      ______
   c. Do you expect your sexual functioning to be changed in any way after your rehabilitation? No ______ Yes ______
      If yes, describe expected changes ______
      ______
   d. Do you want the nurse to obtain more information about sexual function for you? No ______ Yes ______
      If yes, specify interests ______
      Refer you to a sex counselor? No ______ Yes ______

**PSYCHOSOCIAL HISTORY**

1. What is your marital status? Married ______ Divorced ______ Separated ______ Widowed ______ Never married ______
2. Do you have any children? No ______ Yes ______
   If yes, how many? ______ What are their ages? ______
3. What type of housing do you live in? Upper apartment ______ Lower apartment ______ Ranch ______ Two or more story dwelling ______
4. How many people live in your home? ______
5. Where do you sleep? ______
6. Where is the bathroom located? ______
7. How would you describe your relationships with others living in your home? Excellent ______ Very good ______ Good ______ Fair ______ Poor ______
   If fair or poor, would you like to tell me anything about these relationships? ______
   ______

**FIGURE 8-6, cont'd** Guidelines for recording health history. *Continued.*

**PSYCHOSOCIAL HISTORY—cont'd**

8. Do you have any interests or hobbies? No ______ Yes ______
   If yes, describe ______
9. How far did you go in school?
   Grammar school ______ College graduate ______
   Some high school ______ Some graduate school ______
   High school graduate ______ Graduate school degree ______
   Some college ______
10. What are your habits?
    Smoking ______ How long? ______ How many packs/day? ______
    Drinking ______ How long? ______ How much? ______
    Drugs ______ How long? ______ How much? ______
    Coffee ______ How many cups/day? ______
    Exercise ______ Type ______ How often? ______ How long? ______
11. Coping
    a. How would you describe your coping abilities? Excellent ______ Very good ______ Good ______
       Fair ______ Poor ______
    b. What do you do when you are upset? ______
    c. Does it help? No ______ Yes ______
12. Relationships
    a. Who is the most important person to you? ______
    b. How many close friends do you have? ______
    c. What effect has your disability had on your family and friends? ______
    d. Do you expect your family and friends to visit during your rehabilitation program? ______
    e. Who of your friends or family would you most like to assist with your rehabilitation program? ______
    f. Who should be notified in case of an emergency? ______
       Telephone number ______
       Address ______

**ECONOMIC/VOCATIONAL HISTORY**

1. What is your occupation? Present ______ Past ______
   Unemployed ______ If unemployed, are you retired? No ______ Yes ______
2. How would you describe your financial resources? Excellent ______ Very good ______ Good ______
   Fair ______ Poor ______
3. How will you pay for your rehabilitation program?
   Self, family ______ Vocational rehabilitation agency ______
   Insurance plan ______ Medicaid ______
   Worker's compensation ______ Medicare ______
   Specify other ______

**SPIRITUAL HISTORY**

1. Do you practice a religion? No ______ Yes ______
   If yes, what denomination? Catholic ______ Protestant ______ Jewish ______
   Specify other ______
   a. Do you attend a place of worship regularly? No ______ Yes ______
   b. Do you have any dietary restrictions as part of your religious practices? No ______ Yes ______
   c. Would you like to see a chaplain while you are here? No ______ Yes ______
2. Do you feel your spiritual needs are met? Yes ______ No ______
   If no, is there anything the nurse can do to assist you in meeting your spiritual needs? ______

**FIGURE 8-6, cont'd** Guidelines for recording health history.

**OTHER**

1. What do you know about your current health concerns? ______________________________

2. Do you have any questions right now about your current health concerns? ______________________________

Thank you for answering all my questions. I will be back later to see if we agree on your major health concerns and sit down to establish goals with you for your rehabilitation program.

**FIGURE 8-6, cont'd** Guidelines for recording health history.

bilitation team. Both in the hospital and in the home, nurses are in an excellent position to assist the patient in planning a reasonable care program, as well as to teach the patient, the family, and, if necessary, the employer, about the patient's limitations and rehabilitative expectations.

Much of the nursing activity in the rehabilitation process is no different from the nursing care given to all patients. Measures such as appropriate bowel and bladder programs, providing proper diet and fluid requirements, implementing new methods of bathing, and maintaining skin integrity fall within the domain of nursing concern and knowledge. Initially, nursing personnel may assume almost total responsibility for performing these activities for the patient. After assessing patient abilities in these areas, nurses formulate, implement, and evaluate a teaching plan in much the same way as do therapists from other disciplines. The assistance nurses can give the patient and family depends on nurses' ability to understand themselves, personal feelings, and personal behavior as well as the behavior of the patient, family, and other professional team members.

One of the most important aspects of giving continuing care to a patient with a disability is the nurse's own attitude, perseverance, and expectations. Improvement may be slow, and patients may reach a plateau in their progress. Such a time can be critical for patients because they may become discouraged and not wish to continue with their program of care. *Realistic encouragement can often sustain patients so that they will not regress before some improvement is noted.*

Patients in a rehabilitation program must often learn and practice special physical techniques to strengthen muscles and to improve mobility. Such measures as physical exercise to improve walking, activities to improve self-care abilities, and the use of prostheses require the special knowledge and skills of physical and occupational therapists. *To be effective in the rehabilitation process, nurses must have an understanding of the techniques used by the various therapists so that they can plan and work cooperatively with them in caring for the patient. This knowledge is also used to help the patient employ appropriate techniques in carrying out activities of daily living.*

## CONTINUING CARE

Traditionally, health care professionals have assumed responsibility for the patient's well-being within the hospital and little to no responsibility for the patient and family in the home setting. This dichotomy between health care in the home and hospital facility made little sense. With chronically ill persons the dichotomy interferes with a smooth transition from hospital to home. *The major portion of health care for persons with chronic illnesses occurs in the home; thus ongoing communications must exist between the patient and health professionals.* Strauss et al.[21] advocate that sick persons participate more in their care within health facilities and that health care professionals play a greater role in aiding chronically sick persons *and* their families to cope with their problems at home. Social forces such as shorter hospital stays have made it necessary for nurses to be more aware of home health care needs.

### SELF-HELP GROUPS

Self-help groups are associated with self-care. These groups may or may not include the guidance of health care providers. They provide social support to their members through the creation of a caring community, and they increase members' coping skills through the sharing of information, experiences, and problem solutions. Examples of self-help groups include those for women who have had mastectomies and those for persons who have colostomies, diabetes, or obesity. There are now self-help groups or clubs for patients with a variety of conditions. Nurses should learn what groups are available to patients in their community. A telephone call to a health agency such as the American Cancer Society, American Heart Association, or American Lung Association can elicit information about clubs available to patients who have the specific condition served by the agency.

In some hospitals and nursing homes nurses have been instrumental in setting up support groups for families of patients with chronic health problems such as Alzheimer's disease.

It can be expected that more support groups, both those for patients and those for families, will be developing in the future. Some of the impetus for these groups can be traced to changes in health care reimbursement. With prospective reimbursement and the use of diagnosis-related groups (DRGs) as a basis for reimbursement for patients whose care is being paid for with federal dollars (Medicare and Medicaid), the need for such groups has increased. Prospective reimbursement has resulted in shorter hospital stays for both patients with acute illnesses and patients with chronic illnesses. As a result, patients and their families need to be better prepared to care for the patient in the home because patients are sent home sooner than in the past and their needs for continuing care are greater.

## FACILITIES FOR CONTINUING CARE

It is impossible to include here all the facilities that provide continuing care. Each of the programs mentioned has its own criteria for acceptance of patients for the services it renders. *Before application for service is made and before the program is discussed with the patient and family, the individual patient's eligibility for that service should be determined.*

### Ambulatory Care

The term **ambulatory care** is used interchangeably with *outpatient care* and *refers to first-contact health care services as well as to continuing contact services in settings that do not require overnight stays.* The use of ambulatory care facilities has expanded because of the increase in chronic illness and the increase in cost of inpatient services. A good ambulatory care service constitutes one of the most important elements of the hospital's contribution to community health. There is a trend toward development of ambulatory care facilities in neighborhood health centers to assist disabled, aged, or disadvantaged persons to obtain needed health care. An ambulatory care center usually provides long-term follow-up care needed by the person with a chronic illness, in addition to preventive health care, diagnostic work-ups, and treatment of acute illnesses for which hospitalization is unnecessary.

### Home Care

Before World War II the home was the place where medical treatment was given. Well-to-do persons rarely went to a hospital; instead, they received the services of a private physician in their own home, and the family or nurses employed by the family were responsible for the day-to-day care. Poor families were among the first persons to use hospitals. The philosophy of home care can be traced as far back as 1796, when the Boston Dispensary provided medical care to the sick poor in their homes.

One of the most obvious reasons for the development of home care programs was to provide care to patients with long-term illnesses who did not need the around-the-clock services of an institution and yet who were too ill to go to an outpatient center. Caring for patients at home is often desired by the individual and family, and it also releases hospital beds for use by acutely ill patients. (See Chapter 27 for more information about home care of the adult.)

Today **home care** is being provided for acutely ill patients discharged from the hospital earlier than in the past. Prospective reimbursement for hospitals on the basis of DRGs has meant that many patients are being discharged while they still need skilled nursing care. As a result, many hospitals have set up *home care programs* to supply nursing care and other services to their patients after discharge. Hospitals that have not set up their own programs are contracting with the Visiting Nurse Association and other nursing agencies to supply nursing care for their patients after discharge.

Frequently the issue arises as to who should pay for home health services and who should be reimbursed for health care provided. The American Nurses Association's position is that reimbursement systems should foster care of individuals in their homes on the basis of the following premises[3]:

1. Home health care is humane and respectful of the individual's dignity and integrity.
2. Home care or care within the community can be less costly than institutional care.
3. Nursing care is the primary element in home care.
4. Payment systems for home care should recognize nurses as the major providers of home care, and nurses should be reimbursed on their own authority.

Home care may not be possible for all patients. For those living in smaller dwellings, adequate space for the patient, necessary equipment (oxygen, intravenous fluids, and so on), and for other members of the family may be at a premium. The choice of home care, independent living center, or institutional care depends not only on the desires of the patient and the family but also on the ability to finance the care.

Some states are testing pilot programs to keep selected elders in their own homes instead of sending them to a nursing home. Carefully selected patients whose needs can be met at home—as long as nursing and other services are available to them—are enrolled in these programs, which are financed by Medicaid funds. The premise for these projects is that keeping patients in their own homes would make it possible to contain

Medicaid costs and reduce the number of expensive nursing home beds.

Despite many inconveniences, some families wish to have the patient with them. The family members' understanding of the patient and their ability to assist one another will make a great difference in choosing between home care and other living arrangements. Not only may space be inadequate, but many times it is impossible to have a family member at home with the patient during the day. Family members who work cannot afford to sacrifice jobs to stay with the patient. However, many families find it easier financially to have the patient at home and are able to make satisfactory arrangements even though their facilities are limited.

Many communities now provide portable meals (Meals on Wheels) for homebound persons. Most programs provide one hot meal daily and food that does not need to be heated for at least one other meal. The cost differs widely and depends on the services offered, such as special diets, and on the sponsorship of the plan. Volunteer groups frequently deliver the meals. This service alone often makes it possible for a chronically ill or aged person to remain at home.

#### Home health aide services

Home health aide services were increased when Medicare came into existence. The greater number of persons eligible for such services under Medicare spurred their growth. The early discharge of patients from hospitals has increased the need for these services even more. **Home health aides** provide physical care to the patient after a registered nurse evaluates the home situation and the patient's need for physical personal care. They are also responsible for keeping the patient's environment clean and for preparing the patient's meals. Ongoing supervision of the home health aide is the responsibility of the registered nurse assigned by the agency providing the home care.

#### Homemaker services

Homemaker services also have developed with the increased use of home care. These services are increasingly in demand in many communities and may be sponsored by a public or voluntary health or welfare agency or by a private agency that bills the family. Homemakers provide service to families with children and to the person who is convalescing, aged, or acutely or chronically ill. Homemakers are trained to assist in homes where the responsible family manager is temporarily unable to perform his or her usual responsibilities because of illness or absence.

#### Day-care centers

In many communities some senior centers and nursing homes are expanding their facilities and services to include day-care centers. Many chronically ill persons are able to live with their families but require 24-hour attendance. Often the caretaker in the family has to work. Homemaker or home health care aides services are generally not available for the time the caretaker is at work. Day-care centers provide a place where the chronically ill person can be looked after on a daily basis. Nursing services, physical and occupational therapy, recreational therapy, meals, and, in some instances, transportation to and from the center are provided. This form of service may allow a person to remain at home with the family rather than having to resort to institutional care.

#### Respite care services

Some nursing homes and some community hospitals maintain a specified number of beds for **respite care.** As the name implies, these beds are available on a short-term basis to provide respite for families who have a chronically ill person at home. The day-to-day care of the patient, often 24 hours a day, is a very trying experience for any family. To provide the family or primary caretaker with a period free of this responsibility, respite care may be the answer. Usually the cost of respite care is not reimbursable; however, it may be the only alternative if the primary caregiver cannot continue to care for the family member without a break.

Community health agencies, such as the Visiting Nurse Association, are providing respite services in some cities. They supply respite care in the patient's own home for part of a day, for 24 hours, or for extended periods depending on need. As mentioned, the cost of this service is usually not covered by health insurance.

### Independent Living Centers

Some persons with chronic illnesses may be unable to cope with the demands of maintaining a home but wish to live as independently as possible. Various options are available in some communities; these range from living units, where persons cook their meals but have the unit maintained, to assisted living units, where persons can have their own physical living area but where one or more meals a day and other services are available. Living units are designed with such features as handrails for support in ambulation, wide doors to facilitate passage of wheelchairs, and emergency call systems.

### Foster Homes

Care in foster homes is a service that is now being widely used in many communities. Carefully selected families volunteer to take chronically ill persons into their own homes and provide the nonprofessional care needed. The family is paid either by the patient or the patient's family, from public funds, or by some social agency. The plan is primarily for those patients who have no family and cannot live alone but who neither desire nor need institutional care.

### Institutional Care

Institutional care may be necessary when alternatives are not available, or the type of care needed by the patient requires close professional supervision. This includes chronic disease hospitals, skilled care facilities, convalescent homes, rest homes, homes for the aged, and nursing homes. Veterans Administration hospitals provide services for men and women who have served in one of the U.S. armed forces. The patient's potential for rehabilitation, the need for maintenance care, or the level of physical disability are factors that determine eligibility for placement in any of these facilities. A large or limited selection of outside facilities may be available, depending on the community.

## ROLE OF THE NURSE IN CONTINUING HEALTH CARE

A nurse may be involved in continuing health care in several ways: (1) as an independent nurse practitioner or clinical nurse specialist assisting the person with chronic illness to cope with problems incurred by the illness, (2) as a public health nurse or visiting nurse involved in a primary rehabilitative program in the home, (3) as a supervisor of home health aides, or (4) as a nurse in a hospital concerned about the care patients will be receiving after they leave the hospital, particularly when the patient's rehabilitation program is not completed before discharge or when rehabilitation is not possible. Any of these nurses also may be involved in research pertaining to chronic illness. Some concepts that need further study in the area of chronic disease include social stigmatization, effects of isolation, and effects of chronic illness on the family, marriage, and domestic and occupational roles. Research can make a major contribution to clarification of these general concepts by identifying their relationship to chronic health problems.

Nurses must know the community resources available to patients to inform them and their families about what resources they might obtain, the types of service from which they may benefit, and what referrals they need for obtaining those services (see Box 8-2 for a list of community resources). The hospital nurse should clearly communicate to the continuing care agency the data pertinent to the patient's care so that continuity is ensured. Teamwork and continuity are the keys to successful rehabilitation and management services for patients, and they must be practiced at all stages of care if patients are to realize their fullest potential.

## FOCUS ON THE FUTURE

### AMERICANS WITH DISABILITIES ACT

In 1990 Congress passed the Americans With Disabilities Act (ADA), which some call the Civil Rights Act for the disabled. This law provides protection to the estimated 48 million Americans with disabilities. It has *four main components,* which *address employment, public services, public accommodations* and *services operated by private entities,* and *telecommunication services.* The provisions under each of the components are listed in Box 8-4.

**BOX 8-4 Provisions of Americans With Disabilities Act**

1. Employers may not discriminate against a qualified person with a disability in hiring or promotion.
2. Employers can ask about the person's ability to perform a job but may not ask if someone has a disability or use tests that tend to screen out persons with disabilities.
3. Employers need to provide "reasonable accommodation" to individuals with disabilities, including job restructuring and modification of equipment.
4. Employers do not need to provide accommodations that impose an "undue hardship" on business operations.
5. Employers with 25 or more employees were to comply by July 26, 1992.
6. Employers with 15 to 24 employees were to comply by July 26, 1994.

**TRANSPORTATION**

1. New public transit buses ordered after Aug. 26, 1990, must be accessible to persons with disabilities.
2. Transit authorities must provide comparable paratransit or other special transportation services to persons with disabilities who cannot use fixed route bus service, unless an undue burden would result.
3. Existing rail systems must have an accessible car per train by July 26, 1995.
4. New rail cars ordered after Aug. 26, 1990, must be accessible.
5. New bus and train stations must be accessible.
6. Key stations in rapid, light, and commuter rail systems were to be made accessible by July 26, 1993, with extensions up to 20 years for commuter rail (30 years for rapid and light rail).
7. All existing Amtrak stations must be accessible by July 26, 2010.

**PUBLIC ACCOMMODATIONS**

1. Restaurants, hotels, and retail stores may not discriminate against persons with disabilities, effective Jan. 26, 1992.
2. Auxiliary aids and services must be provided to persons with hearing or vision impairments or other persons with disabilities, unless an undue burden would result.
3. Physical barriers in existing facilities must be removed, if removal is readily achievable. If not, alternative methods of providing the service must be offered, if they are readily achievable.
4. All new construction and alterations of facilities must be accessible.

**TELECOMMUNICATIONS**

Companies offering telephone service must offer telephone relay services to persons who use telecommunication devices from the deaf (TTDs) or similar devices, effective July 26, 1993.

**STATE AND LOCAL GOVERNMENTS**

State and local governments may not discriminate against qualified persons with disabilities.

### Implications for Nursing

It is important for nurses to know about the provisions of the Disability Act so that they can inform the disabled about their rights under the law.

Nurses working in the rehabilitation settings will be able to employ nursing interventions that will assist the disabled person to function at his or her highest possible level. The role of the nurse in rehabilitation is discussed earlier in this chapter (see p. 205).

All nurses as citizens can be advocates for the disabled and help articulate their needs to the general public. Nurses can be active in their own communities to ensure that the public accommodations and public service provisions are carried out.[26]

A copy of the Americans With Disabilities Act, Public Law 101-239, may be obtained free from the U.S. Government Documents Office in Washington, D.C., or from one's congressional representative.

## CENTER FOR MEDICAL REHABILITATION RESEARCH

Another event that should have a favorable impact on persons with disabilities was the signing into law a bill that created the Center for Medical Rehabilitation Research. The Center, which is within the National Institute of Child Health and Development, will be involved in basic, clinical, and applied rehabilitation research. It is expected to have a significant impact on the development of medical rehabilitation therapies and services.[7]

## HEALTH CARE GOALS FOR THE YEARS 1990 AND 2000

In 1979 the surgeon general's report established five goals concerned with reducing death rates in the United States by 1990.[22] Tables 8-4 and 8-5 show the progress made in meeting the 1990 goals. As can be seen from the percentage figures in Table 8-5, there was progress in all health-promotion areas. Because these areas are crucial to promoting personal responsibility for one's health, they are included in the goals for the year 2000.[24]

As follow-up to the 1990 goals, work was begun in 1987 on developing health care goals for the year 2000, which are published in *Healthy People 2000: National Health Promotion and Disease Prevention Objectives.*[24]

The development of the year 2000 goals was a national effort that involved health professionals, citizens, private organizations, and public agencies from every part of the United States. Almost 300 national membership organizations and health departments from the 50 states were involved, with nurses represented by the American Nurses Association, the National League for Nursing, and several specialty organizations.

Before discussing the goals for the year 2000, it is important to describe the changes in the U.S. population that are expected to occur between now and 2000.

### Profile of Americans in the Year 2000

*Healthy People 2000* describes the demographic changes that will occur between 1990 and 2000.

1. By the year 2000 the population of the United States will have grown about 7% to approximately 270 million people. The slowest growth rate in the history of the country is projected to occur between 1995 and 2000. Average household size is expected to decline from 2.69 in 1985 to 2.48 in 2000, with husband-wife households decreasing from 58% to 53% of all households.
2. By the year 2000 the American population will be older, with a median age of more than 36 years, compared with 29 years in 1975. The number of children younger than 5 years of age will decline from more than 18 million to fewer than 17 million between 1990 and 2000.
3. By the year 2000, 35 million persons older than 65 years of age will represent 13% of the population as compared with 8% in 1950. The "oldest old"—those over age 85—will increase to 30% to a total of 4.6 million by 2000.
4. By the year 2000, the racial and ethnic composition

**TABLE 8-4 Progress in Meeting 1990 Health Goals by Age-Group**

| LIFE STAGE | 1990 GOALS | 1990 STATUS |
|---|---|---|
| Infants | 35% lower death rate | Achieved—35% lower |
| Children | 20% lower death rate | Exceeded—29% lower |
| Adolescents/young adults | 20% lower death rate | Not met—9% lower |
| Adults | 25% lower death rate | Achieved—25% lower |
| Older adults | 20% fewer days of restricted activity | Not met—14% lower |

From McGinnis JM et al: *JAMA* 268(18):2545-2552, 1992.

**TABLE 8-5 Progress in Meeting 1990 Health-Promotion Objectives**

| PRIORITY HEALTH-PROMOTION AREA | NO PROGRESS (%) | PARTIALLY ACHIEVED (%) | ACHIEVED (%) |
|---|---|---|---|
| Smoking and health | 22 | 39 | 39 |
| Misuse of alcohol and drugs | 15 | 20 | 65 |
| Nutrition | 6 | 88 | 6 |
| Physical fitness and exercise | 9 | 45 | 45 |
| Control of stress and violent behavior | 44 | — | 56 |

Modified from McGinnis JM et al: *JAMA* 268(18):2545-2552, 1992.

**BOX 8-5 Three Broad Goals for the Year 2000**

1. Increase the span of healthy life for all Americans.
2. Reduce health disparities among Americans.
3. Achieve access to preventive services for all Americans.

From US Department of Health and Human Services, Public Health Service: *Healthy people 2000: national health promotion and disease prevention objectives,* Washington, DC, 1990, US Government Printing Office.

**TABLE 8-6 Target Populations—Years of Healthy Life by Year 2000**

| POPULATIONS | 1980 BASELINE | 2000 TARGET |
|---|---|---|
| African-Americans | 56 | 60 |
| Hispanics | 62 | 65 |
| People 65 and older—years of healthy life remaining | 12 | 14 |

From US Department of Health and Human Services, Public Health Service: *Healthy people 2000: national health promotion and disease prevention objectives,* Washington, DC, 1990, US Government Printing Office.

of the American population will change. The number of white persons will decline from 76% to 72% of the population. The forecast is that the number of Hispanic persons will increase from 8% to 11.3%, that is, to more than 31 million by the year 2000. The number of African-Americans will increase from 12.4% to 13.1%. Other racial groups, including Native Americans, Native Alaskans, and persons of Asian and Pacific Islands extraction will increase from 3.5% to 4.3% of the total population.

5. By the year 2000, the working population will reflect changes in racial and ethnic populations and more nonwhite than white groups will enter the work force. Women of all racial and ethnic groups will be the major source of new entrants into the labor force. The women in the work force will comprise 47% of the total working population as compared with 45% in 1988. White men will make up only 25% of the net growth of the labor force.

6. Occupations most likely to grow include service, professional, technical, sales, and executive and management positions.

7. By the year 2000 the American population may increase through immigration by as much as 6 million people. This immigration will be to certain states and cities, with the greatest number settling on the east and west coasts.

The purpose of the *Healthy People 2000* report was to commit the nation to the attainment of three broad goals that will bring us as a nation to our full potential (Box 8-5).

The goals to be achieved by the year 2000 are divided into 22 priority areas. The first 21 of these goals are grouped into three broad categories: *health promotion, health protection,* and *preventive services.* It seems clear that the achievement of the three broad goals would reduce the number of people in the United States with chronic health problems. These goals and the three approaches to them *require that individuals take more responsibility for their own health and for preventing chronic illnesses.* At the same time, health professionals are called on not only to treat disease but to prevent disease and conditions that result in premature death and chronic disability.

The challenge spelled out in *Healthy People 2000* is for communities to translate these national objectives into state and local action.

Not all the goals for 2000 can be discussed in this chapter. Only those objectives related to chronic conditions are presented. Other goals related to persons with specific health problems are discussed in the appropriate chapters of this text.

## Health Status Objectives Related to Chronic Disabling Conditions

Health status objectives related to chronic disabling conditions include the following:

1. Increase years of healthy life to at least 65 years from an estimated baseline of 62 years in 1980. Special target populations are listed in Table 8-6.

2. Reduce to no more than 8% (from a baseline of 9.4% in 1988) the proportion of persons who experience a limitation in major activity because of a chronic condition. Special target populations for this objective are presented in Table 8-7.

3. Reduce to no more than 90 per 1000 people the proportion of persons aged 65 and older who have difficulty in performing two or more personal care activities (bathing, dressing, using the toilet, getting in and out of bed) thereby preserving independence. The baseline was 111 per 1000 population in 1984-1985. The special target population for this objective is people aged 85 years and older.

4. Reduce to no more than 10% the proportion of persons with asthma who experience activity limitation as compared with a baseline of 19.4% in 1986 to 1988.

5. Reduce activity limitation resulting from chronic back conditions to a prevalence of no more than 19 per 1000 by the year 2000 as compared with a baseline of 21.9 per 1000 in 1986-1988.

6. Reduce significant hearing impairment to a prevalence of no more than 82 per 1000 persons by the year 2000, from a baseline of 88.9 per 1000 persons during 1986-1988. Special target population is persons 45 years and older in whom a prevalence of hearing impairment would be no more than 180 per 1000 as compared with a baseline of 203 per 1000 in 1986-1988.

7. Reduce significant visual impairment to a preva-

**TABLE 8-7 Prevalence of Disability in Special Population Targets**

| PREVALENCE OF DISABILITY | 1989 BASELINE (%) | 2000 TARGET (%) |
|---|---|---|
| Low-income persons (annual family income: $10,000 in 1988) | 18.9 | 15 |
| Native-Americans/Alaskan natives | 13.4 | 11 |
| African-Americans | 11.2 | 9 |

From US Department of Health and Human Services, Public Health Service: *Healthy people 2000: national health promotion and disease prevention objectives,* Washington, DC, 1990, US Government Printing Office.

lence of no more than 30 per 1000 persons by the year 2000, from a baseline average of 34.5 per 1000 during 1986-1988. Special target population is people aged 65 and older in whom a prevalence of visual impairment would be 70 per 1000 as compared to 87.7 in 1986-1988.

8. There are several objectives related to diabetes. These are presented in Chapter 40.

### Services and Protection Objectives

Services and protection objectives related to the health status objectives[24] include the following:

1. Increase to at least 60% the proportion of providers of primary care for older adults who routinely evaluate people aged 65 and older for urinary incontinence; impairments of vision, hearing, and cognition; and functional status. Baseline data were not available.

2. Increase to at least 90% the proportion of premenopausal women who have been counseled about the benefits and risks of estrogen replacement therapy (combined with progestin, when appropriate) for prevention of osteoporosis. Baseline data were not available.

3. Increase to at least 75% the proportion of work sites with 50 or more employees that have a voluntarily established policy or program for hiring persons with disabilities. The baseline was 37% of medium and large companies in 1986. This objective reflects the intentions of the Americans With Disabilities Act (see p. 214).

4. Increase to 50 the number of states that have service systems for children at risk of chronic conditions, as required by Public Law 101-239 (Americans With Disabilities Act (p. 214).

All nurses need to be aware of the goals spelled out in *Healthy People 2000* and the plans developed in the state in which they are residing for bringing these goals to fruition. The goals, if met, should assist all persons in the United States to have as healthy a life as possible.

## MANAGEMENT SYSTEM FOR PERSONS WITH CHRONIC CONDITIONS

In reviewing health care for the chronically ill in the United States, it seems obvious that some changes need to be made. One consultant to hospitals has suggested that hospitals need to look at their focus on acute care and give higher priority to care of the chronically ill.[11] He recommends that hospitals develop chronic disease centers just as they have developed ambulatory service centers. He points out that the present health care delivery system is oriented to intervening in the disease process and "fixing" the condition whereas persons with a chronic condition are trying to minimize their chronic condition and live as normal lives as possible.

The consultant also suggests that chronic disease centers could become the primary care provider for persons with chronic conditions. His suggestion will not be acceptable to all care providers, including many nurses who believe that clinical nurse specialists and nurse practitioners are the ideal health care providers for these patients because much of their care involves teaching and counseling, which are central to the nursing role.

## QUESTIONS TO CONSIDER

- What types of patients do you think are most in need of rehabilitation? Outline the rehabilitation needs of a patient you are now caring for or have cared for in the past.
- What proportion of the patients on the hospital unit to which you are assigned has a chronic illness as either a primary or secondary diagnosis? What proportion has more than one chronic health problem? What age-group is affected most by more than one chronic health problem?
- What resources are available in your community for the care of the chronically ill? Are the facilities adequate for the number of persons needing care? How are these facilities supported financially?
- From what you have learned in anatomy, outline in detail the physical movements necessary to rise from a sitting position in a chair to a standing position. Describe how you would assist a patient to stand while allowing him or her to be as independent as possible.

## CRITICAL THINKING ACTIVITIES

- You are caring for two patients both of whom have advanced, progressive multiple sclerosis. One family adapts well to the debilitated state of their family member while the other family members drift and are unable to offer their support to the patient. Offer an explanation for this difference in family reaction.
- How may the care of one person with a chronic illness be generalized to the care of other persons with chronic illnesses?
- On admission to the hospital of a patient with a chronic illness, the nurse performs a thorough physical assessment but makes no mention of psychological assessment of the patient. Should this oversight be called to her attention or is the physiological assessment more important?

## CHAPTER SUMMARY

### IMPACT OF CHRONIC ILLNESS ON SOCIETY

- Chronic health problems constitute a major area of health problems in the United States.
- The incidence and prevalence of chronic diseases have increased in this century and can be expected to increase even more as the population ages.
- The Bureau of the Census estimates that approximately 110 million persons in the United States have one or more chronic illnesses.
- There are major disparities in the health of African-Americans and other minorities in the United States when compared with the white population.
- The characteristics of chronic illnesses include one or more of the following: (1) illness or impairment that is permanent, (2) residual disability, and (3) nonreversible pathologic alteration, which requires a long period of care.
- Chronic illnesses may be present from birth or can develop during childhood, adolescence, early adult life, or old age.
- Today some children with chronic illnesses such as cystic fibrosis live into early adulthood because of more effective treatment.
- Major chronic illnesses of adults include arthritis, diabetes, heart disease, and hypertension. The rates for arthritis and hypertension are higher in black than in white persons.
- Cultural values determine how both nurses and patients view chronic illness.
- The economic costs of chronic illness are considerable, and many persons will require some type of financial assistance.

### PREVENTION

- It is important that nurses be involved in prevention of chronic illness.
- There are three levels of prevention: primary, secondary, and tertiary, and the nurse has an important role to play at each level.
- Primary prevention involves health promotion and specific protection against disease (such as immunization against childhood diseases).
- Secondary prevention includes early detection of disease and prompt intervention to halt progression of disease.
- Tertiary prevention includes rehabilitation appropriate to the stage of disability, prevention of further disability, and restoration of functioning to the highest possible level.

### CHRONICALLY ILL PERSONS AND THEIR FAMILIES

- Failure to understand or internalize the reason for therapeutic recommendations, procedures that are difficult to learn and carry out, time necessary to carry out therapy, side effects of therapy, inability to pay for prescribed therapy, and social isolation and lack of support and positive reinforcement are possible reasons why a person may be noncompliant with therapeutic recommendations.

### ASSESSMENT OF THE PERSON WITH A CHRONIC ILLNESS

- Depression is common among chronically ill persons, especially those who feel powerless about controlling or overcoming what has happened to them.

### REHABILITATION

- Rehabilitation is best carried out in a setting in which an interdisciplinary team of nurses, physicians, physical and occupational therapists, social workers and, if necessary, speech therapists are available to work together in planning the therapeutic regimen for the patient and in assisting and supporting the patient with the prescribed therapy.
- The two major roles of the nurse working with persons with disabilities are (1) to limit disability from disease as much as possible and (2) to see that the rehabilitation program is planned and implemented.
- The nurse should be familiar with community facilities for continuing care and the eligibility requirements for each facility.

### FOCUS ON THE FUTURE

- The Americans With Disabilities Act passed by Congress in 1990 provides protection for the disabled in terms of employment, public services, public accommodations, services operated by private entities, and telecommunication services.
- *Healthy People 2000* is a publication prepared for the surgeon general of the United States. It presents more than 300 objectives to improve the health of U.S. citizens by the year 2000.
- Nurses need to be aware of the plans of the state in which they reside for meeting the goals for the year 2000.

## REFERENCES

1. Albee G: In Curtis N, editor: *Self Help Reporter* 3(4), 1977.
2. American Cancer Society: 1993 cancer facts and figures, Atlanta, 1993, The Society.
3. American Nurses Association: *A national policy for health care: principle and positions,* Kansas City, Mo, 1977, The Association.
4. Burckardt CS et al: Quality of life of adults with chronic illness: a psychometric study, *Res Nurs Health* 12:347-354, 1989.
5. Centers for Disease Control: Years of potential life lost before age 65: United States, 1990 and 1991, *MMWR* 42(13):252-253, 1993.
6. Council on Ethical and Judicial Affairs: Black-white disparities in health care, *JAMA* 263(17):2344-2346, 1990.
7. DeLisa JA, Jain SS: Physical medicine and rehabilitation, *JAMA* 265(23):358-359, 1991.

8. Desencios JC, Hahn RA: Years of potential life lost before age 65, by race, Hispanic origin, and sex—United States, 1986-1988, *MMWR* 41(SS-6):13-23, 1992.
9. Dittmar S: *Rehabilitation nursing process and application,* St Louis, 1989, Mosby.
10. Foxall MJ, Ekberg JY: Loneliness of chronically ill adults and their spouses, *Issues Ment Health Nurs* 10(2):149-167, 1989.
11. Henry WF: Chronic care needs to be a higher priority, *Hospitals* 20, p 68, Feb 20, 1991.
12. Kim MJ, McFarland GK, McLane AM: *Pocket guide to nursing diagnoses,* ed 5, St Louis, 1993, Mosby.
13. Lambert VA, Lambert CE, editors: Psychosocial impacts created by chronic illness, *Nurs Clin North Am* 22:527-533, 1987.
14. Leidy NK: A structural model of stress, psychosocial resources, and symptomatic experiences in chronic physical illness, *Nurs Outlook* 34(4):230-236, 1990.
15. Leslie PM: Nursing diagnosis: use in long-term care, *Am J Nurs* 81:1012-1014, 1981.
16. McGinnis JM et al: Health progress in the United States: results of the 1990 objectives for the nation, *JAMA* 268(18):2545-2552, 1992.
17. Moskowitz E, McCann CB: Classification of disability in the chronically ill and aging, *J Chronic Dis* 5:342-346, 1957.
18. Pollock SE: Human response to chronic illness: physiologic and psychosocial adaptation, *Nurs Res* 35:90-95, 1986.
19. Primomo J, Yates BC, Woods NF: Social support for women during chronic illness: the relationship among sources and types to adjustment, *Res Nurs Health* 13:153-161, 1990.
20. Raleigh EDH: Sources of hope in chronic illness, *Oncol Nurs Forum* 19(3):443-448, 1992.
21. Strauss AL et al: *Chronic illness and the quality of life,* ed 2, St Louis, 1984, Mosby.
21a. US Department of Commerce, Bureau of the Census: *Statistical abstract of the United States 1990,* Washington, DC, 1990.
22. US Department of Health, Education and Welfare: *Healthy people: surgeon general's report on health promotion and disease prevention,* Washington, DC, 1979, US Government Printing Office.
23. US Department of Health and Human Services: *Secretary's task force on black and minority health,* Washington, DC, 1985, US Government Printing Office.
24. US Department of Health and Human Services, Public Health Service: *Healthy people 2000: national health promotion and disease prevention objectives,* Washington, DC, 1990, US Government Printing Office.
25. US Department of Health and Human Services: *Vital and health statistics: current estimates from the national health interview survey, 1990,* Washington, DC, 1991, US Government Printing Office.
26. Watson PG: The Americans With Disabilities Act: more rights for people with disabilities, *Rehab Nurs* 15(6):325-328, 1990.
27. Woog P, editor: *The chronic illness trajectory framework—the Corbin and Strauss nursing model,* New York, 1992, Springer.

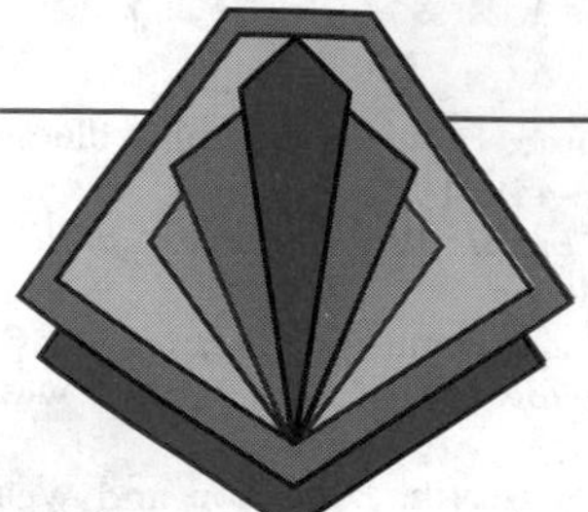

C H A P T E R 9

# Body Image and Self-Esteem

***Lynn Valentine***

## CHAPTER OBJECTIVES

***After studying this chapter, the learner should be able to do the following:***

1 Analyze the concepts of self-esteem and body image.
2 Identify conditions that may cause disturbances in self-esteem or body image.
3 Implement nursing actions to care for patients with disturbances in self-esteem or body image.

## KEY TERMS

adaptive responses
body image
body image disturbances
body monitoring
self-esteem
self-image

Burnard and Morrison[7] suggest that the terms **self-esteem, self-image,** and **self-concept** are all closely related and that if people are happy with their physical selves (body image or physical appearance), they are more likely to experience positive feelings of self-esteem.

This chapter focuses on (1) self-esteem and body image, (2) causes of disturbance in self-esteem and body image, (3) the individual's response to disturbances, and (4) nursing management when disturbances occur.

Threats to body image may disrupt usual life activities of work and play and may affect relationships with others.[49,50,74] Preventing body image alterations and thus self-esteem disturbances is an important nursing activity. The content of this chapter is limited to acquired body image disturbances (see pediatric texts for information about congenital problems).

## SELF-ESTEEM

Rogers defines self-concept as an organized configuration of perceptions of the self that are admissible to awareness.[58] Self-esteem is the evaluative component of self-concept. It is defined as the extent to which a person feels positive, negative, or neutral regarding judgments about one's self-concept.[51] It is a self-evaluation of the extent to which one believes oneself to be capable, significant, and worthy.[41] Although self-concept is a descriptive term and self-esteem is an evaluative term, the two terms often are used interchangeably.[30] Self-esteem is closely related to personal satisfaction and worth.[53] It is a vital component of effective human functioning[11] and has been identified as one factor important to adaptation in general.[26] Contemporary self-concept theories emphasize the multidimensional nature of the self.[30] In the normal adult, self-concept remains relatively stable in the absence of major personal or environmental changes.

Self-esteem, like body image, is derived from social, emotional, and physical components. It is determined by relationships with peers and significant others; physical ability and physical appearance are key components. Self-esteem develops early and is influenced by opportunities to accomplish age-appropriate tasks.[56] If developmental tasks cannot be achieved, an assault on self-esteem occurs. For example, a chronic illness may lead to regression, dependence, and feelings of being different. Positive self-esteem is a major objective because of its lasting impact on behavior.[56] For decades research has suggested that persons with high self-esteem are happier and better able to meet environmental demands.[11] Recent research in the area has explored self-esteem in patients with spinal cord injuies,[53] in halo braces,[51] and in pulmonary rehabilitation programs.[30]

## BODY IMAGE

**Body image** is the mental idea a person has of his or her body at any moment based on past as well as present perceptions. This mental picture of one's body develops over time and is derived from internal sensations, postural changes, contact with outside objects and people, emotional experiences, and fantasies.[62] Body image is formed by the interaction between the perceptual pool and the experiential pool.[21,49] The perceptual pool consists of all present and past sensory experiences, whereas the experiential pool consists of all experiences, affects, and memories.

Although the literature contains a great deal of research regarding body image, there is not one uniformly accepted theory or model to explain or predict body image. Nurses have drawn from psychosocial sciences to understand the nature of body image changes and to develop appropriate interventions.

It is helpful to remember that internal factors may affect external appearances. Neurologic, metabolic, and hormonal influences affect body image. Examples include hirsutism as a consequence of Cushing's syndrome or skin texture changes because of hypothyroidism. Other experiences that affect body image are motor, cognitive, perceptual, and personality variables. Physical characteristics and how the body actually "feels" contribute to the development of body image. Factors in the environment that may influence body image include peer-group attitudes, cultural variables, and attitudes of parents, significant others, and society.[4] Modification of one's body image occurs with new percepts and new experiences.[47] Throughout all stages of growth and development and with changes in health stage, body image is continually being altered.

Body image makes up one aspect of the individual's self-concept. The importance of body image within the self-concept will vary mainly according to the nature and intensity of values and emotions invested in it.[61] Self is what a person is, whereas self-image is what a person thinks of self. An essential factor in the development of self-image is body image. Body image is an intrapersonal experience of the body, including one's attitudes and feelings. One's body image becomes a standard that influences performance and self-concept.

Many societal and cultural standards influence the development of body image.[50] The attitudes of society, parents, and peers will be reflected in the way persons view their bodies. There has been much discussion of the emphasis on youth, wholeness, and beauty in the American culture. Body image includes both reality and ideality[16]; thus body image does not always coincide with objective body[3]. Components of a person's ideal body image may be youth, slenderness, or beauty. Individuals may incorporate so much ideal into their body image that when confronted by the reality of a videotape or a mirror, they are genuinely shocked. They do not feel older, and the face in the mirror does not seem to belong.[16]

Because body image is a dynamic, constantly changing perception, change in the structure, function, or appearance of the body requires modification of the image an individual has. The idea of **body image disturbances** arises from observations that persons with altered structure, function, or appearance may fail to perceive the changes and to adapt to the body as it exists.

Problems with body image related to illness and disability have been widely studied. Current clinical literature related to persons with altered structure, function, or appearance includes studies of patients with alopecia,[1,67,74] amputation,[23,44] breast and gynecologic cancer,[12,36,67] depression,[46] facial disfiguration,[14,25] heart attack,[71] obesity,[17,20] bulimia,[10,22,32] anorexia nervosa,[5,70] stomas,[63] lactation,[28] and pregnancy.[18] Such studies frequently have direct application to patient assessment and intervention by a variety of the health professions involved in rehabilitation of the physically disabled. Body image alterations are a concern in critical as well as chronic illness.[6,54,55,57] A major assumption underlying this chapter is that physical disability or a change in body structure that results in altered function or appearance, or both, is accompanied by an alteration in the person's body image and may cause a disturbance in self-esteem. Interventions by the health care team to help the patient manage the results of the physical change must include help in the psychosocial areas of life also affected. Much of the effort made in this latter area is focused on helping the patient recognize, accept, and live with the change in self-concept, which includes both body image and self-esteem. These conditions occur not only in the young but also in the older person.

Alteration in body function or appearance usually is not an isolated problem. People often are faced with high hospital costs and long-term use of medications and prosthetic devices. The chronicity of the problem may affect the entire family. Change in body image often creates anxiety, distortion of self, self-deprecation, and mourning for a loss.[34]

## LIFE-SPAN CONSIDERATIONS

Health problems have different meanings at different stages in the life cycle; however, the same problem may be perceived quite differently by persons of the same age. By 4 years of age body image is becoming stabilized and can be affected by body changes. Special care must be taken to assess a child's perception of body image, because it influences personality organization and ego strength. The level of psychosocial development, the quality of the child's relationship with the parents, and previous adjustment are important.

In adolescence the body image undergoes a massive upheaval. Physical changes in the body as a result of accident or illness place an enormous strain on the coping abilities of the young person, who already may be overwhelmed by the "normal" changes occurring within his or her body.

The young adult needs independence. The nurse who "does for" the young adult rather than permitting self-care may precipitate conflicts. Young war veterans with disabling injuries that occur at a time of peak physical abilities find adjustment very difficult, and aggressive behavior is common. Concern for sexual identity is prominent.

Middlescence causes another period of body image and self-esteem evaluation. Graying or thinning hair, sagging breasts, and appearance of crow's-feet are visible signs of aging. Internal changes also are occurring. For example, the onset of menopause may cause decreased vaginal lubrication; thus women in this age-group who adjust to the body image change incorporate supplemental lubrication into their self-care regimen.

Older persons face the changes of aging: physical deterioration, social losses, and death. Esberger[16] describes a phenomenon known as **body monitoring** found most often in older persons, because the body at this time requires more care to maintain adequate performance. Because older persons have more health problems, they often require daily medications, more frequent contacts with health care agencies, special diets, and prosthetic aids. It often becomes more difficult for the older person to maintain activities and hobbies that contribute to positive self-concept.

One existing stereotype—that aging leads to a diminished body image—was investigated.[8] Researchers noted a steady decline of interest in appearance as age increased, with the exception that women older than 60 years of age became more interested in their appearance. Respondents did not report a poorer body image as they got older; rather young women were the most dissatisfied with their bodies. The authors suggested that as people get older, they shift their standards appropriately. Elders also report less emphasis and satisfaction with their fitness and more emphasis and satisfaction with their health.

## Disturbances in Self-Esteem and Body Image

Nurses most commonly deal with challenges to body image that, if not processed, can lead to self-esteem disturbances. Changes that may cause a disturbance in self-esteem or body image include (1) altered structure or appearance, (2) altered function, (3) changes in mobility, and (4) pain or disease. These changes rarely occur independently. For example, a colostomy changes both the appearance and the function of the body. A disturbance in self-esteem might occur if a male patient experienced a loss of sexual functioning, thereby feeling less of a man. Generally these changes occur as a result of trauma, disease, and weight gain or loss (Box 9-1). See Research box at right.

### Altered Appearance

Body image changes can occur from alterations in appearance that may or may not alter function. Traumatic injury to the external ear that leaves hearing unimpaired but requires repair of facial lacerations is an example.

**BOX 9-1 Selected Causes of Disturbances in Body Image**

**Injuries from trauma**
Amputation
Burns
Lacerations
Fractures

**Manifestations of disease**
Cancer
Neurologic impairments
Sensory deficits
Endocrine disorders

**Change in body weight**
Obesity
Anorexia
Cushing's syndrome
Pregnancy

**RESEARCH**

Salter MJ: What are the differences in body image between patients with a conventional stoma compared with those who have had a conventional stoma followed by a continent pouch? *J Adv Nurs* 17:841-848, 1992.

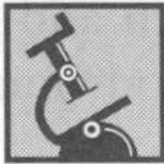

A qualitative study of seven patients explored the perceptions of body image in patients with a conventional stoma compared with those who had a conventional stoma followed by a continent pouch. The outcome of this study, which used a phenomenologic approach, indicated that patients with stomas expressed difficulties in coming to terms with an ostomy and had a negative body image. Patients with the continent pouch were of the opinion that such a procedure enhanced their lives over an ileostomy. Most patients, however, still considered the experience traumatic, and the changes caused by stoma surgery affected their perception of body image negatively.

Alopecia (loss of hair) also affects appearance, yet does not affect function as do scars without contractures from burns, some surgeries, aging, pregnancy, and increase or decrease of body weight.

### Altered Function

Physical disability often is associated with a change in body image and can cause loss of function while not necessarily altering the individual's appearance. Loss of function occurs in paraplegia, hemiplegia, and chronic renal failure. Partial loss of function occurs in chronic respiratory insufficiency and chronic cardiac disease. Renal, respiratory, and cardiac problems show relatively few visible signs of their presence until the problems are far advanced. Function and eventually appearance are modified in paraplegia as the muscles of the legs atrophy and contractures occur. Facial muscles may droop, and the hands may appear flaccid or spastic on the affected side of a patient with hemiplegia. Enucleation of the eye and amputation of an extremity cause marked changes in both function and appearance.

### CHANGES IN MOBILITY

Loss of mobility may alter body image and decrease self-esteem. Persons with spinal cord injuries may become socially isolated as a result of limited mobility.[53] Feelings of isolation and hopelessness, depression, and loss of independence may occur.[45] The patient who cannot get to the toilet quickly enough to meet the need, thereby soiling the bed, may suffer an insult to self-esteem. A contracture from a burn, an improperly healed fracture, or any other condition that limits mobility also can alter body image or decrease self-esteem.

### PAIN OR DISEASE

Alterations in body image may occur as a result of pain or disease.[50] Disease alters one's perceptions of the body by producing new sensations and different motor actions.[65] The cause for these alterations may not be always visible—for example, impaired cardiac function after myocardial infarction, chronic renal failure, diabetes, or some types of cancer for which the only treatment is palliative care. Rheumatoid arthritis is an example of a condition that combines loss of function, altered appearance, decreased mobility, and pain. All aspects of daily living are affected. Inability to sew or complete housework may alter a housewife's self-esteem; a painter who can no longer hold a brush needs help in seeking a new role. Deformity occurs as a result of progressive joint destruction. Loss of joint motion limits mobility. Joints are hot, swollen, painful, and not easily moved. Eating, sleeping, working, and even dressing activities such as zipping and buttoning can cause pain. This chronic illness can cause a loss of independence and may affect employment or relationships at home.

Studies conducted in the 1960s and 1970s indicated that women were more vulnerable than men to body image distortions in that society forces the female to be more concerned with physical appearance. Therefore women were often concerned about cosmetic effects.[33,42,66,68] However, the multiple changes that have occurred in female roles make it unclear how valid these conclusions are for the 1990s. In addition, a study by Cash, Winstead, and Janda[8] compares data from body image surveys done in 1972 and 1985. Respondents in 1985 were considerably more dissatisfied with their bodies, and particularly for men, the pressure to look good seems to have intensified. The authors believe that men do not feel as free as women to talk about their looks. Further research is needed.

The self-concept is closely linked to sexuality and perception of body image. The response to mastectomy is in part a response to the culture's preoccupation with the breast as a symbol of femininity. This represents the integration of the ideal into the body image. Thus the loss of a breast often is followed by lowered self-esteem, postoperative depression, and concerns of the woman's psychosexual role and sexual functioning. The ability of a woman to accept the trauma of loss of her breast depends on her reactions (real, perceived, or anticipated) and the acceptance of her partner.[36,67] Her response reflects the value she assigns to the loss, to rehabilitation and reinforcement from health professionals, and to positive role models.

Women as well as men often are concerned about their ability to work and their earning capacity. The loss of earning power and the resultant loss of self-esteem are important determinants of family relationships. Dyk and Sutherland[15] reported that after ostomy surgery, the reduction in housework seemed to be more acceptable to wives than the reduction in gainful employment was to husbands. Most men expressed fears of dependence on spouse or children. The thought of getting old and being ill can be disabling; however, when fears of ostomy spillage and other problems are added, the older person with a stoma may view the burden as insurmountable. Work is important to a sense of achievement, and many persons express who they are in terms of their work.

Social interactions also are affected. Dropkin[14] reported that social interactions decreased after head and neck surgery as the deformity became more pronounced. To varying degrees everyone has a need to feel that the presentation of one's body is acceptable to others. The person who has sustained facial alterations may feel isolated, excluded, stigmatized, helpless, or ashamed. Physical unattractiveness often is associated with social devaluation, denied opportunities, inaccurate judgments of worth, and low self-esteem. The individual with a low need for social approval does not rely as heavily on others to maintain body image, but a low need for social approval does not preclude fear of social rejection. This person, however, may show earlier signs of integration through early efforts toward self-care.[14]

## IMPORTANT DETERMINANTS OF RESPONSES TO CHANGES IN BODY IMAGE

Regardless of the body image alteration, the response of the person will depend on (1) the personal meaning and the significance of the change, (2) the responses of significant others, (3) the availability of help for the person and the family, (4) previous coping behaviors, (5) the availability of positive role models, (6) the time period in which the change occurred, and (7) temporary or permanent status of the alteration. The outcome of the alteration in body image also is influenced by the physiologic status of the person, that is, the amount of pain present, the extent of the change or disability, and the realistic expectations of therapy. The physiologic status is relatively fixed for the specific disability; therefore this section explores the broader psychosocial factors that are amenable to intervention by health care professionals.

## MEANING OF THE CHANGE TO THE INDIVIDUAL

The value the individual assigns to what was lost, the visibility and meaning the part or the function has, and the intensity of the person's feelings about the loss all influence how the individual will respond. A person may attribute successes in life to specific body features. When there is an overvaluation and reliance on security through physical beauty or activity, alteration in the body image is likely to cause severe emotional disturbances. Human beings are disturbed when serious threats to or actual deficits in the structure, function, mobility, or appearance of the body occur. They must revise long-accepted assumptions about their bodies, and life patterns may need to be changed. They face problems regarding work, social activities, and family; for example, sexual activities may require modification. They may believe that goodness is lost, the ability to accomplish is lost, and that valued skills and talents are impaired. They may feel they are receiving "deserved punishment." One reaction that may interfere with recovery is expectation of rejection and separation. The person also may feel vulnerable, resigned, rebellious, defiant, rejected, dependent, avoided, resentful, timid, self-conscious, unhappy, humiliated, stigmatized, inferior, and hypersensitive. Indecision, decreased self-respect, bitterness, and cynicism also occur. The hostility of a disabled person toward the healthy may interfere with communication. The attitudes of disabled persons toward themselves are more important than the nature of their disabilities.

## RESPONSES OF SIGNIFICANT OTHERS

Satisfactory social adaptation to a body change depends to a great extent on family relationships and cultural attitudes toward the body structure involved. The sociocultural milieu plays an important role in the acceptance of the change.

What are the attitudes of others, including parents, siblings, and peers, toward physical disability? What are the specific body values of the subculture of the patient? What prejudices are there that are related to wholeness, independence, and attractiveness?

The source of the change, its type, and the opinions of others are important. Hirschfield and Behan[27] describe acceptable and unacceptable disability after accidents. Changes resulting from heroic sacrifice are viewed differently from changes resulting from socially unacceptable activities. The loss of a leg saving a comrade in battle is viewed quite differently from loss of a leg in a motorcycle accident during a high-speed chase from the scene of a crime. Sterility as a result of a sexually transmitted disease may be viewed as deserved punishment, whereas sterility caused by exposure to prescribed radiation therapy carries no stigma. The cause of the disability (active combat injury vs. the sequelae of veneral disease), the type of disability (paralysis vs. weakness or anxiety), and the opinion of others (sympathy vs. scorn) make a difference in the meaning of the disability.

Does stigma accompany the change? A stigma is an attribute that is deeply discrediting. Goffman[24] discusses the idea of being discredited (having a disability fairly readily noted) and being discreditable (having a disability that may be discovered).

Myths and misconceptions abound regarding the person whose body is scarred or mishapen by disease or is distorted during movement. An overabundance of largely unfounded opinion and folklore surrounds physical disability. A strange belief exists that suffering and misfortune somehow make one "a better person." It also is believed that the disabled person mysteriously develops untapped assets and achieves a new depth of understanding and sensitivity.

## HELP AVAILABLE TO PATIENT AND FAMILY

How the patient deals with the loss may well depend on the kind of help available. The help available from the health care team and specifically the nurse's role in helping clients with altered body image is discussed later in this chapter. Much of the outcome will depend on whether the client can and does make use of the help offered.

The rehabilitation program generally has as its goal the recovery of physical function. Psychosocial diagnoses and psychosocial therapy are often secondary. The person needing rehabilitation should be viewed as a complete person with a partial disability. Attempts should be made to strengthen the individual's inner resources and the relationship between the individual and the immediate family. A family assessment should be made and family therapy instituted, if necessary.

The family needs help from health care providers to be supportive during this time of change. The reactions of patients discussed earlier also apply to the family. Their reaction will depend on the meaning of the threat, their coping patterns, available resources, and positive role models. They also are frightened by the altered appearance of the patient or the loss of function. They wonder and speculate about the significance of the change in their lives. Because their response plays a significant role for the patient in the integration of the body image alteration and rehabilitation, the family cannot be ignored.

Patient care conferences that involve physicians, nurses, social workers, and the family are extremely beneficial in delineating the reality of the situation and the available resources. Rehabilitation centers often use these conferences appropriately when the patient is admitted. More acute care centers are also holding patient care conferences throughout the patient's hospitalization. Involvement of the patient and family is encouraged.

## COMMUNITY RESPONSES

Society values youth and beauty, attractive facial features, physical wholeness, and activeness. Social discrimination against those who are different is common. Physical disability provokes stereotyped responses in the public. The type of deformity rather than its severity evokes the stereotypic response. Subtle and overt negative reactions occur. Repulsion, revulsion, rejection, contempt, ridicule, taunts, discrimination, patronizing aversion, tactless curiosity, staring, questioning, and devaluing pity are frequent.

Reactions to one who is physically disabled may range from overly sympathetic to unsympathetic. Because one takes on the attitude of others toward one's body, negative feelings already present about one's body may be reinforced by society.

Visible handicaps alter social and psychologic functioning in important ways. Confronting a damaged face disrupts one's sense of inner security. The thought of disfigurement or scarring causes fear of public reaction in most people, and not without cause. Social ostracism is a real possibility. Physical disability is accompanied by a fear of being unable to perform one's regular routines and the fear of loss of control. If the disability is not visible, it may not be considered important by others.

The part of the body that is lost or nonfunctioning also influences the reactions of others. People are usually very uncomfortable discussing ostomies or the wearing of a pouch. Nor is loss of sexual function easily accepted. Others will often respond with comments such as "He should be thankful he's alive," showing a lack of concern for the values of the individual.

Some body image alterations are more acceptable than others. Breast cancer and mastectomies have received national television coverage. Several movies have been made about recoveries after spinal cord injuries. Yet many other body image alterations are poorly understood by the public (e.g., Kaposi's sarcoma and the butterfly rash of systemic lupus erythematosus).

## HEALTH CARE TEAM RESPONSES

Each member of the health care team must work through personal feelings regarding loss, disability, and disfigurement and examine behavior used in coping with such threats. If this conscious self-examination is omitted, feelings and behaviors may interfere with the patient's rehabilitation and may result in the professional's leaving this field of service. Responses of staff members to persons with disability should be honest, patient, consistent, realistic, and firm but not hostile. Often they must be acceptant of a patient who is hostile and rejecting. Every effort must be made to avoid reinforcing the person's low self-esteem. Special preparation is needed for open, honest discussion of the patient's probems with sexuality. Consistent support promotes the trust vital to learning to cope with altered structure, function, and appearance and provides the patient with a sense of hope.

Members of the health care team are not immune to negative attitudes toward the disabled. They may subscribe to certain stereotypes, especially with regard to sexual functioning in persons with disabilities. Condescension, resentment, insensitivity, and aloofness can be found in those "dedicated to help." Members of the health care team may expect a passive, compliant, dependent patient. They may feel protective, or they may react with superiority. Examples of negative attitudes are reflected in the use of such labels as "unmotivated" as justification for closing a case. The disabilities that people have should not be used to describe them. The use of stereotypic labels—"CPs," "CVAs," "quads"—reflects obvious disregard for the individuality of the patient. The reactions of health care professionals may include embarrassment, undefined anxiety, relief if the patient is cheerful, abandonment by disregarding stress signals, and maintenance of a superficial atmosphere of being thoughtful, understanding, and helpful. Anger at being unable to help is a recurring phenomenon.

Health care professionals can contribute to a patient's lowered self-esteem when they express openly or covertly negative reactions to a patient's change in structure, function, or appearance. A patient's loss of control threatens the professional's control. Sarcasm covered with saccharine sweetness and testing may be signs of displaced anger. People reject what they cannot cope with, and they may withdraw from the situation. Health care professionals should honestly explore their feelings toward the patient with body changes.

Little investigation of health care team attitudes has been undertaken. This is unfortunate, because the health care team probably is more important in shaping the patient's response than is any other group.[38] Tucker[73] noted that the rehabilitation teams' negative feelings, attitudes, and behaviors had a powerful negative impact on the patient's adjustment to disability. Persons who

### RESEARCH

Brillhart B, Hazel J, Wyers ME: Attitudes toward people with disabilities, *Rehabil Nurs* 15(2):80-85, 1990.

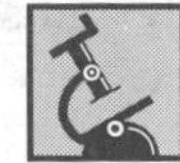

Attitudes toward people with disabilities are learned, emotionally toned predispositions. This study compares such attitudes held by nursing faculty, beginning nursing students, graduating nursing students, registered nurses, and persons with disabilities. Results indicate that persons with disabilities were significantly more positive in their attitudes. Faculty members held the least positive attitude, closely followed by graduating nursing students.

work with the disabled should try to be as sensitive and perceptive as possible about their own responses to disability and the disabled and about the patient's emotional reactions to problems. Recently, group experiences have been made possible so that health care providers can explore their feelings and be better able to facilitate rehabilitation. Specialization in certain areas has occurred within nursing as professionals identify those patients with whom they are best capable of working. Values clarification is one method of helping nurses identify their values and the effect of personal values on the care provided. See Research box, p. 225.

### PREVIOUS COPING BEHAVIORS

As a result of their life history, all persons have a well-developed and predictable pattern of coping with threats, real or perceived. Some people immediately begin to problem solve, looking for alternatives; others are immobilized and require help to return to a balance.[72]

### AVAILABILITY OF POSITIVE ROLE MODELS

The use of positive role models in the rehabilitation plan after body image alteration has increased significantly. Trained visitation programs sponsored by the American Cancer Society have resulted in Reach to Recovery, Ostomy Visitors, and Laryngectomy Visitors. The value of visitors and self-help groups is readily apparent in the growth of these services around the country.

Patients gain from talking with someone who has been through a similar situation and has coped and adapted well. One important aspect is the timing of the visit. The nurse needs to assess each person carefully and offer the choice of a preoperative or postoperative visit. If possible, it would be best if the visitor were close to the patient's age and had a similar diagnosis and surgery. Most important, the visitor should have reached a successful level of rehabilitation, know how to talk with others, and be prepared for a mixed reaction from the patient.

### TIME FRAME

The time period in which the change occurred is an important determinant of response. A sudden posttrauma amputation elicits different feelings from those a diabetic patient might experience with a planned amputation. Samonds and Cammermeyer[64] measured body image of persons with multiple sclerosis (MS) and found that those who reported satisfaction with body and self tended to be older and to have had MS longer.

### PERMANENCE OF CHANGE

The meaning of the disability is influenced by the expected duration of the change and its permanence. A colostomy may be more acceptable if the patient expects colostomy closure within 3 months. A body image alteration resulting from a diagnosis of cancer involves the fear of recurrence or death. The alteration in the body function or structure may be of lesser significance if the person equates the change with an extension or saving of life.

## ADAPTIVE RESPONSES TO CHANGES IN BODY IMAGE

Those responses in which the patient works through and accepts the loss are considered **adaptive**. Any situation perceived by a person as resulting in a major body change and profoundly affecting body image may precipitate a crisis. Most commonly the period of crisis is followed by unrealistic defenses, gradual acceptance, and then reduction of the problem to manageable proportions. Responses depend on the number and intensity of the stresses in terms of the degree of emotional support and the strength of personal attributes. Patients are helped to meet the challenge of disability if they are mature and secure from the start. An acute sense of proportion helps them recognize reality. A sense of humor helps them live with reality. The urge to fight back and pick up the pieces of an interrupted life may even motivate the patient.

Several authors note that the loss of a valued body part or function is followed by a period of reaction and adjustment that can be compared with the grief and mourning process that follows the death of a loved one (see Chapter 10). Grief is the subjective state of one who has sustained the loss of a valued object—in this instance, physical function or body appearance, or both. Mourning is the psychologic process by which one works through to acceptance (ideally) of the loss. The subjective reactions to grief include helplessness, loneliness, hopelessness, sadness, guilt, and anger. Mourning usually leads to relinquishing that which was lost. Eventually the person looks at the past realistically and comfortably.

Rubin[60] describes the losses associated with body image change as the loss of the *capacity for functioning* and the loss of the capacity for *control of functioning* in time and place. A sense of shame accompanies such losses. This reaction reflects a private judgment of failure. The intensity of the emotional response seems to be related to the intensity of the struggle to maintain control.

An individual facing a real or threatened change or loss may experience several stages of adaptation, including (1) impact, (2) defensive retreat, (3) acknowledgment, and (4) reconstruction.[57] During the first stage the person may be unable to understand or comprehend the event, its meanings, and its implications. During defensive retreat the person acknowledges the event but is unable to cope with the meaning and implications. The retreat provides time and distance and may appear as denial. Acknowledgment is the recognition of the reality of the situation, its meaning, and its significance. Reconstruction is the integration of the change or loss in a way that is supportive of functional living. The person is realistic about the event, its meaning, and its significance.

The reactions of individuals are different throughout the adaptation process. Some persons may lack initiative at first but will demonstrate goal-directed behavior later. Others may feel helpless, angry, guilty, or lost.

## Maladaptive Responses to Changes in Body Image

When a person is unable to accept the reality of a situation, the response is maladaptive. Patients may deny the change in appearance or the loss of function. They may completely deny the change, may appear withdrawn and aloof, may joke and laugh, or may present a pseudo–self-confidence. They may use a variety of defense mechanisms such as denial, projection, repression, or regression.

The loss may be acknowledged but its significance denied and the situation intellectualized. The person may project concern onto others: "My wife is very upset about my having to change jobs." Tasks may be avoided. Overcompensation for the loss may occur. Patients may project hostile feelings that interfere with acceptance. The resumption of a social, sexual, and emotional life may be impossible. Some may reject others out of a fear of being rejected themselves.[29]

Some persons may try to hide the body image change in an attempt to forget it, and they often pay a high price for such a futile endeavor. Exaggerated independence, overdependence, and pseudocooperation are responses that interfere with the necessary acceptance of help from the family and health care team.

Occasionally, the body image alteration may be used as a crutch, and if the defect is corrected, problems may occur. For example, a person may attribute failures in life to an external facial feature; when this feature is changed by plastic surgery, the person may be forced to examine the realities. A similar situation may exist after changes resulting from illness and injury, and in both cases extreme emotional upsets are possible.

Another strategy is to focus attention on a healthy part to deny or shut out the damaged part. Idealizing normal standards commits the disabled person to repeated feelings of inferiority. On the other hand, overidentification with the disabled may limit efforts toward achievable levels of rehabilitation. The patient may use the body image alteration as the excuse for early retirement. A return to work can thus be avoided. Another defensive response is the illusion of restoration of the part (phantom). A complete rejection of reality is a psychotic response and may require intense therapy.

The effects of the body image alteration may spread beyond the specific structure, function, or change in appearance to other areas of life and activity and increase the patient's limitations. Perceptions of being incompetent, unlovable, insecure, and unworthy reflect low self-esteem. The person's perception of the situation, the responses received from others, and previous experience with losses determine the level of self-esteem and affect coping mechanisms.

The initial response of the family to the loss depends on many factors already discussed. The *rapidity of onset,* the *specific loss,* and *its meaning* are especially important. The patient is the center of attention, and the family is unified by dread, numbness, a sense of unreality, and the shared threat of loss. During the time the patient is denying the situation, the family also may be denying it. Fear and anger may be directed at staff members. The family may lose interest and patience. They may urge the patient to make a more rapid recovery.

The *degree and quality of support* are important. Sometimes families deal well with the immediate threat, but they have difficulty with the kinds of long-term help needed. Family members must acknowledge the change in the patient, their way of life, and the patient's reactions. Family conflicts over the prescribed regimen occur. Families may use the patient's changed state to keep the patient dependent. Rejection by the family complicates the life of a disabled person. Family members may attempt to conceal the defect by avoiding and isolating the patient. They may be angry, blaming, and rejecting or indifferent. Ambivalence is not uncommon.

Family members must acknowledge the change in the patient and deal with changes in the interpersonal reactions within the family. Constructive, supportive attitudes in the family increase the possibilities for successful adaptation and for compensatory development without personality disorder. As patients move to reorganize their lives, their families should reexamine interactions, modify living arrangements, encourage social activities, and try to improve family relationships.

## Nursing Management

### ♦ Assessment

Self-esteem remains relatively stable in the absence of major personal or environmental changes.[30] However, illness, hospitalization, and changes in physical ability and appearance may affect self-esteem. Any patient who has undergone a change in body structure, function, appearance, and degree of mobility or who has been diagnosed with a disease or condition, painful or nonpainful, is at risk for body image disturbance. Assessment focuses on the patient's ability to adjust in a positive manner to the change from the "old" body to the "new" body.

#### Subjective Data

The nurse is alert for questions or comments from the patient that may indicate a desire to discuss his or her feelings. While a colostomy appliance is being changed, a patient's comment such as "It smells so bad, doesn't it?" warrants more than a yes or no answer. One helpful response might be "Yes, there is an odor, but remember that it's normal for stool to have an odor." Continued exploration might reveal the patient's embarrassment at what is considered a private experience, or the patient may be using the nurse as a test for society's reaction. Honest answers to questions generally build trust.

The same comment from a burn patient during a dressing change might relay different concerns. Fear of infection or further surgery resulting in even more scarring may be the patient's real concern. Through exploration of the patient's feelings and perceptions, an accurate assessment can be obtained.[2]

In general, any verbalizations by the patient that indicate a negative perception about the self or self-capabilities can be used to support a diagnosis of self-esteem disturbances.[31,40,48]

### Objective Data

Observation and associated exploration of feelings and perceptions are excellent assessment techniques.[64] For example, the nurse might say, "Mrs. A., I notice you turn your head away when I change your colostomy appliance. Is it hard for you to look at your colostomy?"

During dressing changes or during procedures, observe the patient's facial expression and body position. Describe the expression you see to the patient, for example, "Mrs. A., you seem to be frowning." After validating your observation, explore the patient's feelings further. Also observe the patient's use of a mirror. Some patients avoid using a mirror because they are not ready to see the suture line, dressing, or appliance. Because self-esteem influences behavior, the nurse must validate with the patient the meaning of any given behavior.

The assessment includes the patient, family members, and significant others, including direct observation of their interactions if possible. Identify the patient's support system. Consider culture, religious restraints, and the general environment.

In addition to observation, verbalization, clarification, and validation, various instruments to measure self-esteem and body image may prove useful. The Likert scale is popular. In this method of measurement, respondents are presented with statements and asked how much they agree or disagree. Two popular tools based on the Likert scale are the Rosenberg self-esteem scale[59] and the Tennessee self-concept scale.[19] Rosenberg's scale has 10 items and is intended as an unidimensional measure of self-esteem. The Tennessee self-concept scale uses 100 descriptive statements in which subjects rate themselves on a Likert type of scale. The score is a composite of nine subscales that include identity, self-satisfaction, behavior, physical self, moral and ethical self, personal and family self, social self, and self-criticism. A high score indicates increased self-concept. The test-retest reliability coefficient is 0.80 to 0.90.[19] The Perlow self-esteem scale[52] has recently been developed and tested for reliability and validity. Further use in clinical settings is being investigated.

A wide variety of instruments have been used to measure the concept of body image.[13] Questionnaires, interview guides, drawings, and video techniques have proved useful.[37] The body cathexis scale, a widely used tool, allows subjects to rate 46 different areas of the body.[68] It is reliable and easily administered and interpreted in the clinical setting (Box 9-2). If an instrument to measure body image or self-esteem is used, make sure it is the best tool available for the specific clinical situation. Consider time constraints, ease in administration, and the patient's ability to complete the tool. See Research box above.

**BOX 9-2 Body-Cathexis, Self-Cathexis Scale: Sample Content***

| BODY CATHEXIS ITEMS | SELF-CATHEXIS ITEMS |
|---|---|
| Hair | General knowledge |
| Skin texture | Self-confidence |
| Weight | Emotional control |
| Body build | Happiness |
| Elimination | Capacity for work |

Modified from Secord PF, Jourard SH: *Consulting Psychology* 17:343-347, 1953.

*Subjects rate their level of satisfaction with physical traits and personal characteristics on a scale of 1-5, with a high score indicating strong, secure body image.

**RESEARCH**

Piazza D et al: Hope, social support and self-esteem of patients with spinal cord injuries, *J Neurosci Nurs* 23(4):224-230, 1991.

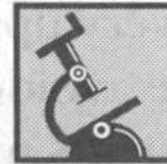

A descriptive study was conducted to determine if a relationship existed among the variables of hope, social support, and self-esteem in persons with spinal cord injuries. Three instruments were used, including the Rosenberg self-esteem scale; 77 subjects participated. There was a statistically significant relationship between hope and social support, hope and self-esteem, and social support and self-esteem. By multiple regression analysis, the best predictors of hope in the subjects were self-esteem, social support, and education.

## ♦ NURSING DIAGNOSES

Nursing diagnoses are determined from analysis of patient data. Nursing diagnoses for the patient with body image disturbance or altered self-esteem may include but are not limited to the following:

| Diagnostic Title | Possible Etiologic Factors |
|---|---|
| Body image disturbances | Changes or losses in body structure, function, appearance, mobility, disease, and pain |
| Self-esteem disturbance | Overevaluation or underevaluation |
| Self-esteem, situational low | Temporary condition, significant loss |
| Self-esteem, chronic low | Negative reinforcers from childhood |

## ♦ EXPECTED PATIENT OUTCOMES

Expected outcomes for the patient with body image disturbance or altered self-esteem may include but are not limited to the following[39]:

1. Shows awareness of loss or change; expresses grief; resolves fear and anxiety; acknowledges changes; expresses constructive integration of body image.
2. Perceives self positively.
3. Perceives the situation realistically and acknowledges factors that decrease self-esteem; engages in corrective activities to restore/improve self-esteem.
4. Increases the frequency of positive statements pertaining to self.

## ♦ INTERVENTIONS

The patient's perception of the situation and usual pattern of adapting must be considered in planning nursing intervention. How does the patient deal with stress? What threats are seen as dangerous? What are the patient's goals? Consider the patient's personality, values, needs, and readiness for learning.

### Providing Anticipatory Guidance

If possible, work to prevent body image disturbances. Anticipatory guidance, counseling, and education are nursing actions that may be effective. Proper preparation before surgery may alter the degree of body image disturbance a patient experiences after surgery.

Transitional points of entry and termination are critical points of emotional adjustment—they reflect periods of change. The move from rehabilitation center to home for a patient with paraplegia or the first hemodialysis treatment at home for a patient with chronic renal failure are examples of such points.

Nurses can assist the patient and family to adjust to these changes by preparing them in advance. The use of books, audio material, and videotapes or other educational materials may be helpful. Help the patient find the facts; speculation can be worse than the truth.

### Facilitating Expression of Grief

The person with a change in body image needs understanding. Assume that such patients are coping with an overwhelming experience, support the self-esteem necessary for them to reorganize the body image, and permit crying in such a manner that patients still have a sense of self-respect and worthiness. Give patients time, and help them confront the problem in manageable steps. Acknowledge appropriate feelings, recognize assets and strengths, and provide support to the extent needed, that is, the degree mutually agreed upon.

Be accepting within appropriate limits. Assure the patient that grief is normal. The patient also must accept the fact that some goals will remain unattainable. Privacy and a safe environment are necessary for the patient to achieve control of a lost or altered body function. Avoid overprotection and unnecessary restrictions. Work on exploring realistic alternatives rather than being overly optimistic or pessimistic.

### Restoring Self-Esteem

Let the patient ventilate, helping clarify misconceptions. Promote a sense of trust, respect, security, and comfort. It is essential for the patient to come to terms with the change. Reassurance that "you'll be as good as new" delays adjustment and raises false hopes. Do not encourage the patient to blame others; rather, assist the patient to accept help with everyday tasks. Counteract the effects of deprivation and immobilization by helping the patient understand what is occurring and by maintaining the remaining body integrity.

General interventions include being nonjudgmental at all times, being consistent and genuine, and demonstrating concern, interest, and understanding.[39] Nurses can provide a positive outlook and attitude.[53] The focus of care is on the patient's ability not the disability. Although it may interfere with nursing care, encourage patients to wear their own clothes, shave, use make-up or toiletries, nail polish, hair curlers—anything that is part of their normal grooming patterns.

### Referral

When basic nursing actions are not effective, more specific strategies may be used by advanced practitioners. Clinical nurse specialists, psychologists, psychiatrists, and other clinical experts are available to meet both short-term and long-term patient needs. Strategies include letter writing from the patient to his or her body, group feedback to help patients begin to accept distortions about their bodies, and self-disclosure exercises with a group of peers.[43]

Nursing interventions for patients experiencing disturbances in body image and self-esteem are summarized in the Guidelines box, p. 230.

## ♦ EVALUATION

Positive attitudes of the patient toward rehabilitation, staff members, and program of help are desirable. Acceptance and use of prosthetic devices are expected. Desired patient outcomes include self-assurance, confident behavior, self-reliance, stable motivation, self-ac-

### Guidelines for Management of Disturbances in Body Image and Self-Esteem

Refer to body part with proper name.
Accept initial need for concealment of change.
Provide gentle persuasion to explore altered body part.
Help significant others to support and assist the patient.
Offer opportunities for social contacts with persons who have had similar experiences.
Introduce patient to support groups.
Assist the patient to express anger, frustration, and disappointment.
Actively listen.
Assist the patient to engage in problem-solving activities.
Identify behaviors that will help to restore self-esteem.
Assist the patient to develop strategies to help cope with loss, stress, or environmental factors that can cause low self-esteem.

Modified from McFarland GK, McFarlane EA: *Nursing diagnosis and intervention,* ed 2, 1993, St Louis, Mosby.

ceptance, and adequate social interactions. It is generally accepted that a person is happier if involved in productive activities.

Siller[69] suggests that one outcome measure of the acceptance of the loss is the degree to which the reconstituted self is oriented toward self-approval and is responsive to reality.

Some dependency may be legitimate, and some physical help may be needed. Retirement from gainful employment may be required, or reduced household responsibilities and a sharp curtailment of social activities may be unavoidable.

Litman's study[35] of family disruption because of disability shows no significant relationship between the degree of family solidarity and rehabilitation response. Family support during rehabilitation, however, has a significant effect on the patient's response to the program. Family members consequently reexamine and probably reorient interpersonal relationships and readjust living arrangements.

Employment, school attendance, or home responsibilities are insufficient measures of outcomes for many patients. Areas to be considered include cognition, activities of daily living, home activities, activities outside the home, and social interaction.

Champion, Austin, and Tzeng[9] examined the interrelationships between concept and body image to provide a base for developing nursing interventions. Because patients are not regularly tested, behavioral responses usually are used to evaluate the effectiveness of the integration of a change in body image. A therapeutic relationship established early in the rehabilitative phase is often beneficial in evaluating change.

If a specific measure to enhance body image or self-esteem was used before implementation of nursing interventions, repeat the measure and evaluate the changes in the score. Of course, patient verbalizations and expressions of positive thoughts and feelings about themselves are useful during the evaluation phase. If possible, observe interactions with significant others for desired changes.

The change in body image does not occur quickly. Adaptation to a change may take a year or longer, but that does not signify maladaptation. The integration of a new mental image takes time and a reorganization of thoughts and images.

## QUESTIONS TO CONSIDER

- How might a patient's response differ if a below-the-knee amputation was caused by a motor vehicle accident as compared with a similar amputation for diabetic gangrene in one foot?
- How might the family response differ if the cause of a patient's altered function was related to alcoholism versus long-term employment in a textile mill?
- What interventions might be particularly useful for a patient scheduled for an ileostomy?
- What types of activities might increase a patient's self-esteem?

## CRITICAL THINKING ACTIVITIES

- Charlotte is a 21 year old hospitalized for anorexia nervosa. She is severely underweight, malnourished, and depressed. She states, "My mother is very upset about my weight. She thinks I'm mentally ill." Analyze this situation and differentiate between the adaptive and maladaptive responses.
- Carla, 57, is recovering from colorectal surgery. She was diagnosed with adenocarcinoma and required a permanent colostomy. In her discharge discussion with her nurse, Carla states, "I'm sure glad the ostomy nurse will be visiting me at my home. My husband and I want to learn how to care for this thing and get on with our lives." Analyze this situation and differentiate between the adaptive and maladaptive responses.

## CHAPTER SUMMARY

### SELF-ESTEEM

- Self-esteem is an evaluative term.

### BODY IMAGE

- Body image is a dynamic, changing perception.
- Changes in structure, function, appearance, mobility, disease and pain require modification in body image.
- Changes in body image may influence self-esteem.
- The patient's perception of the situation and pattern of coping affect his or her responses.

### IMPORTANT DETERMINANTS OF RESPONSES TO CHANGE IN BODY IMAGE

- The family's response and ability to support the patient are important to outcomes.
- The patient and family responses determine the nature of assistance needed.

### ADAPTIVE RESPONSES TO CHANGES IN BODY IMAGE

- Adaptation to changes in body image takes time.

## REFERENCES


1. Baxley KO et al: Alopecia: effect on patient's body image, *Cancer Nurs* 7(6):499-503, 1984.
2. Bernado LM, Conway A, Bove M: The ABC method of emotional assessment and intervention: a new approach in pediatric emergency care, *J Emerg Nurs* 16(2):70-76, 1990.
3. Bernstein NR, Cope O: *Emotional care of the facially burned and disfigured,* Boston, 1976, Little, Brown & Co.
4. Brown MS: Normal development of body image. In Bower F, editor: *Wiley nursing concept modules,* New York, 1977, John Wiley & Sons.
5. Brown T, Cash T, Lewis R: Body image disturbances in adolescent female binge-purgers: results of a national survey, *J Child Psychol Psychiatry* 30:605-613, 1989.
6. Brundage DJ: Self-concept alterations: theory and assessment. In Thelan LA, Urden LD, Davie JK, editors: *Nursing diagnosis in critical care,* St Louis, ed 2, 1993, Mosby.
7. Burnard J, Morrison L: Body image and physical appearance, *Surg Nurse* 3(4):4-8, 1990.
8. Cash TF, Winstead BA, Landa LH: The great American shape-up, *Psychol Today,* pp 30-37, April, 1986.
9. Champion VS, Austin JK, Tzeng O: Assessment of relationship between self-concept and body image using multivariate techniques, *Issues Ment Health Nurs* 4(4):299-315, 1982.
10. Cooper P, Taylor M: Body image disturbance in bulimia nervosa, *Br J Psychiatry* 153(suppl 2):32-36, 1988.
11. Coopersmith S: *The antecedents of self-esteem,* New York, 1967, WH Freeman.
12. Derogatis LR: The unique impact of breast and gynecologic cancers on body image and sexual identity in women: a reassessment. In Vaeth JM, editor: *Body image, self-esteem, and sexuality in cancer patients,* ed 2, Basel, 1986, Karger.
13. Diekmann JM: Measuring body image. In Frank-Stromberg M, editor: *Instruments for clinical nursing research,* Norwalk, Conn, 1988, Appleton & Lange.
14. Dropkin MJ: Rehabilitation after disfigurative facial surgery, *Plast Surg Nurs* 5(4):130-134, 1985.
15. Dyk RB, Sutherland A: Adaptation of the spouse and other family members to the colostomy patient, *CA* 9:123-125, 1956.
16. Esberger K: Body image, *J Gerontol Nurs* 4(4):35-38, 1978.
17. Faubel M: Body image and depression in women with early and late onset obesity, *J Psychol* 123(4):385-395, 1989.
18. Fawcett J et al: Spouses' body image changes during and after pregnancy: a replication and extension, *Nurse Res* 35(4):220-223, 1986.
19. Fitts W: *Tennessee self-concept scale manual,* third rev, Los Angeles, 1983, Western Psychological Services.
20. Fowler B: The relationship of body image perception and weight status to recent changes in weight status of the adolescent female, *Adolescence* 24:557-568, 1989.
21. Fujita MT: The impact of illness or surgery on the body image of the child, *Nurs Clin North Am* 7:641-649, 1972.
22. Gardner B, Moncriefe C: Body image distortion in anorexics as a non-sensory phenomenon: a signal detection approach, *J Clin Psychol* 44(2):101-107, 1988.
23. Garrett JF, Levine ES: *Rehabilitation practices with the physically disabled,* New York, 1973, Columbia University Press.
24. Goffman E: *Stigma: notes on the management of spoiled identity,* Englewood Cliffs, NJ, 1963, Prentice-Hall.
25. Goin JM, Goin MK: *Changing the body: psychological effects of plastic surgery,* Baltimore, 1981, Williams & Wilkins.
26. Hamburg DA, Coelho GV, Adams FE: *Coping and adaptation: steps toward a synthesis of biological and social perspectives,* New York, 1974, Basic Books.
27. Hirschfield AH, Behan RC: The accident process: disability, acceptable and unacceptable, *JAMA* 197:85-89, 1966.
28. Hughes R: Satisfaction with one's body image and success in breastfeeding, *Issues Compr Nurs* 7:141-153, 1984.
29. Kaplan SP: Some psychological and social factors present in the condition of obesity, *J Rehabil* 45(3):52-54, 1979.
30. Kersten L: Changes in self-concept during pulmonary rehabilitation. I. *Heart Lung* 19(5):456-461, 1990.
31. Kim MJ, McFarland GK, McLane AM: *Pocket guide to nursing diagnoses,* ed 5, St Louis, 1993, Mosby.
32. Laessle R et al: The specific psychopathology of bulimia nervosa: a comparison with restrained and unrestrained (normal) eaters, *Consult Clin Psychol* 57(6):772-775, 1989.
33. Lerner RH, Brackney BE: The importance of inner and outer body parts attitudes in the self-concept of late adolescents, *Sex Roles* 4:225-238, 1978.
34. Liss JL: Psychiatric issues in ostomy management. In Broadwell DC, Jackson BS: *Principles of ostomy care,* St Louis, 1982, Mosby.
35. Litman TJ: The family and physical rehabilitation, *J Chronic Dis* 19:211-217, 1966.
36. May HJ: Psychosexual sequelae to mastectomy: implications for therapeutic and rehabilitative intervention, *J Rehabil* 46(1):29-31, 1970.
37. McCrea CW, Summerfield AB, Rosen B: Body image: a selective review of existing measurement techniques, *J Med Psychol* 55:225-233, 1982.
38. McDaniel JW: *Physical disability and human behavior,* New York, 1969, Pergamon Press.
39. McFarland GK, McFarlane EA: *Nursing diagnosis and intervention: planning for patient care,* ed 2, St Louis, 1993, Mosby.
40. McFarland GK et al: Self-esteem disturbance. In Thompson JM et al: *Mosby's clinical nursing,* ed 3, St Louis, 1993, Mosby.
41. McGlashan R: Strategies for rebuilding self-esteem for the cardiac patient, *Dimen Crit Care Nurs* 7(1):28-38, 1988.
42. Meisner A, Thoreson R, Butler A: The impact of obvious physical handicap on male and female self-concept, *Percept Mot Skills* 24:1099-1105, 1967.
43. Miller KD: Body-image therapy, *Nurs Clin North Am* 26(3):727-736, 1991.
44. Mital MA, Peirce DS: *Amputees and their prostheses,* Boston, 1971, Little, Brown & Co.
45. Nelson AL: Normalization: the key to integrating the spinal cord-injured patient into the community, *SCI Nurs* 4:3-6, 1987.
46. Noles SW, Cash TF, Winstead BA: Body image, physical attractiveness and depression, *J Consult Clin Psychol* 53(1):88-94, 1985.
47. Norris CM: The professional nurse and body image. In Carlson CE, Blackwell B, editors: *Behavioral concepts and nursing intervention,* ed 2, Philadelphia, 1978, JB Lippincott.
48. Norris J, Kunes-Connell M: Self-esteem disturbance: a clinical validation study. In McLane AM: *Classification of nursing diagnoses, proceedings of the seventh conference,* St Louis, 1987, Mosby.
49. Nortridge J: Teaching the concept of body image: use of affective and cognitive domains, *J Enterstom Ther* 14:255-258, 1987.

50. O'Brien J: Mirror, mirror, why me? *Nurs Mirror* 150(17):36-37, 1980.
51. Olson B, Ustanko L, Warner S: The patient in a halo-brace: striving for normalcy in body image and self-concept, *Orthop Nurs* 10(1):44-50, 1991.
52. Perlow M: Validity and reliability of the PSES, *West J Nurs Res* 14(2):201-210, 1992.
53. Piazza D et al: Hope, social support and self-esteem of patients with spinal cord injuries, *J Neurosci Nurs* 23(4):224-230, 1991.
54. Platzner H: Body image. I. A problem for intensive care patients, *Intensive Care Nurs* 3:61-66, 1987.
55. Platzner H: Body image. II. Helping patients to cope with changes—a problem for nurses, *Intensive Care Nurs* 3:125-132, 1987.
56. Reasoner RW: Enhancement of self-esteem in children and adolescents, *Fam Community Health* 6:51-64, 1983.
57. Roberts SL: *Behavioral concepts and the critically ill patient,* ed 2, East Norwalk, Conn, 1986, Appleton & Lange.
58. Rogers C: *Client-centered therapy,* Boston, 1951, Houghton Mifflin.
59. Rosenberg M: *Conceiving the self,* New York, 1979, Basic Books.
60. Rubin R: Body image and self esteem, *Nurs Outlook* 16:20-23, 1968.
61. Safilios-Rothschild C: *The sociology and social psychology of disability and rehabilitation,* New York, 1981, University Press of America.
62. Salkin J: *Body ego technique,* Springfield, Ill, 1973, Charles C Thomas.
63. Salter MJ: What are the differences in body image between patients with a conventional stoma compared with those who have had a conventional stoma followed by a continent pouch? *J Adv Nurs* 17:841-848, 1992.
64. Samonds RJ, Cammermeyer M: Perceptions of body image in subjects with multiple sclerosis: pilot study, *J Neurosci Nurs* 21(3):190-194, 1989.
65. Shilder P: The body image. In Bender L, editor: *Contributions to developmental neuropsychiatry,* New York, 1964, International Universities Press.
66. Schoenburg B et al, editors: *Loss and grief: psychological management in medical practice,* New York, 1970, Columbia University Press.
67. Scott DW: Quality of life following the diagnosis of breast cancer, *Top Clin Nurs* 4(4):20-37, 1983.
68. Secord PF, Jourard SH: The appraisal of body cathexis: body cathexis and the self, *J Consult Psychol* 17:343-347, 1953.
69. Siller J: Psychosocial aspects of physical disability. In Mesilin J: *Rehabilitation medicine and psychiatry,* Springfield, Ill, 1976, Charles C Thomas.
70. Slade P: Body image in anorexia nervosa, *Br J Psychiatry* 153(suppl 2):20-22, 1988.
71. Smith C: Body image changes after myocardial infarction, *Nurs Clin North Am* 7:663-688, 1972.
72. Sultenfuss S: Psychosocial issues and therapeutic intervention. In Broadwell DC, Jackson BS: *Principles of ostomy care,* St Louis, 1982, Mosby.
73. Tucker SJ: The psychology of spinal cord injury: patient-staff interaction, *Rehabil Lit* 41:114-121, 1980.
74. Williamson ML: The nursing diagnosis of body image disturbance in adolescents dissatisfied with their physical characteristics, *Holistic Nurs Pract* 1(4):52-59, 1987.

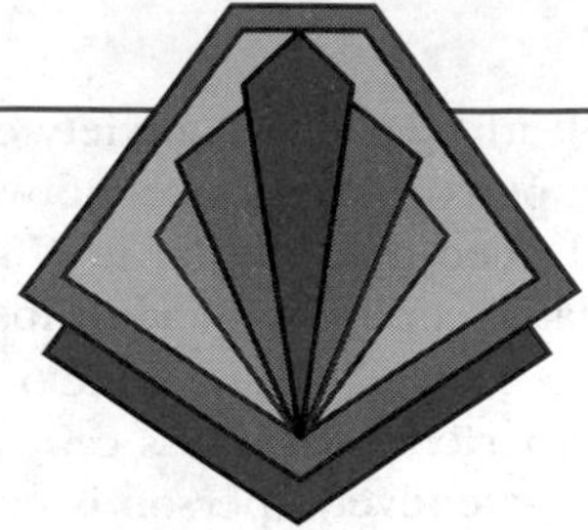

C H A P T E R 10

# Loss, Grief, and Dying

***Molly Loney***
***Sr. Karin Dufault***

## CHAPTER OBJECTIVES

***After studying this chapter, the learner should be able to do the following:***

1 Recognize how loss affects the individual, family, and nurse during life changes and the dying process.
2 Identify death as a significant loss and transition in human development.
3 Describe the process of normal grieving and the behavioral manifestations of each phase.
4 Compare bereavement theories in terms of key tasks for the individual and the family working toward grief recovery.
5 Identify behaviors that place the dying person and family at risk for poor bereavement outcomes.
6 Identify prevailing societal attitudes that influence how nurses, patients, and families respond to situations in which someone is dying or has died.
7 Describe nursing strategies useful in assessing and intervening with individuals and families who are grieving.
8 Discuss factors that affect quality of life for the individual and family during the dying process.
9 Describe self-care strategies for nurses to use in surviving the stress of caring for the dying.

## KEY TERMS

advance directives
bereavement
death
durable power of attorney
dying
euthanasia
grief
informed consent
living will
loss
mental capacity
mourning
reconciliation
recovery

Throughout time people have been concerned with questions regarding life and death and mortality and immortality. Philosophers, poets, and scientists have attempted to understand and even to control death. Death, however, remains a part of life. The fact that humans are finite beings creates anxiety but also gives meaning to life.

The thoughts people have about death affect living in many ways. Some are beneficial and inspiring, whereas others are anxiety provoking and threatening. Koestenbaum[49] reiterates the many ways that death beneficially affects perceptions of life:

Death helps one savor life.
It provides an opposing standard against which to judge being alive.
It gives a sense of individual existence.
It helps give meaning to life.
It allows one to evaluate personal achievements.
It allows retrospective analysis of one's life.
It gives one strength to express convictions.
It reveals the importance of intimacy.

On the other hand, thoughts of death, especially one's own death or the deaths of close friends or relatives, can be anxiety provoking. Conceiving of a time with no future arouses anxiety. In our culture, death threatens all that we know and value.

Our personal thoughts about death and how we adapt to these thoughts significantly influence our lives, feelings, and behavior. Some people refuse to talk about death or acknowledge its existence. Consequently they may avoid attending funerals or other death-related events, as well as having annual physical examinations or participating in other health-promoting activities and making a will.

People recognize mortality in different ways. Some perceive life on earth to be a transient state, a prelude to a better and more joyful life; thus they downplay the importance of worldly goods and emphasize the tenets of a particular religious group that include a life after death.

Other people seek to control death. They may place themselves in dangerous situations occupationally or socially. They may ignore signs of illness or instructions about how to care for a serious illness.

Still others accept the finite nature of their lives but search for immortality in other ways. They may leave a legacy of artistic works or a long line of heirs, or they may search for a means to preserve their bodies after death so that they can be revived at a future time.

One thing is certain: all persons react to the knowledge that life is finite, and how they react to this knowledge influences how they live *and* die.[51] Reactions of health care professionals to dying, death, loss, and grief also affect the care given dying persons and their families.

Even though dying and grief are personal and vary from one individual to another, it is the purpose of this chapter to share understandings and to offer general guidelines that assist in caring for persons who are dying and in helping family members who are sharing the experience. Loss is the underlying theme. Perhaps the most beneficial way to learn to effectively care for dying persons and their families is to understand our own perspectives and those of others on loss, dying, and death.

## THE LOSS EXPERIENCE

Loss is a natural part of human existence. It is a universal experience that is interwoven into daily life, and its pattern is repeated as one faces change or development challenge.[11] As a child learns to become progressively more independent in terms of feeding, going to school, making friends, surviving puberty, driving, and wage-earning, loss occurs.

Loss is an important force in a person's life because it implies the removal of someone or something that had meaning to an individual.[7] It has been defined as any change that reduces the probability of reaching some desired goal or that deprives a person suddenly of a valued possession or relationship.[8] Although it can be caused by a negative change or a positive developmental event, loss always represents some form of deprivation.[71] According to Viorst,[87] persons grow by having to give up some deep attachment or cherished part of themselves to gain a new level of autonomy and mastery.

Bowlby[8] views loss within a framework of early childhood attachment. During periods of high vulnerability and uncertainty, as in childhood, persons develop strong bonds of affection with significant others who meet their basic needs. These significant others offer safety and security beyond simply meeting physical needs for food and shelter. If attachment bonds are threatened or broken, as with maternal death, separation anxiety ensues.[7] The ways in which the person learns to cope with this loss of attachment and need gratification in childhood can be a predictor of later coping with adult loss.[90]

Whether a person faces separation or some other significant life changes, experience with loss can result in a crisis. A crisis occurs whenever a person is unable to manage stress and meet basic needs in the usual way. If past coping skills become ineffective or the stress overwhelming, the individual perceives a threat to self-integrity and a loss of control. Feelings of vulnerability and anxiety trigger an adaptive response, and the person tries to resolve the stress by avoidance, finding support, or becoming immobilized.[4] The tension and uncertainty that accompany crisis and loss can motivate regression or growth, depending on the presence of key balancing factors.[59] Mastery involves balancing the stressors with realistic perceptions, using available supports, and regaining some control by tapping constructive coping skills.[4] Growth results when a person develops more resilience in managing life changes in the face of the loss.[37]

### TYPES OF LOSS

As a component of crisis, **loss** can be categorized as developmental or situational (Box 10-1). Developmental loss involves any predictable change in status, role, relationships, or bodily function that normally occurs in life. Although developmental losses require adaptation, we are socially and culturally prepared for making social and biologic transitions in reaching a new level of growth and maturity.[4] Situational loss involves an unanticipated change in roles, relationships, or function. The person lacks preparation or role modeling in terms of effective adaptation, except through experience with previous situational losses.[37] Natural disasters, accidents, unemployment, and illnesses are situations that challenge the person's usual adaptive response and may precipitate life crises. Any illness represents several losses occurring simultaneously in all areas of one's life. Situational losses can overwhelm the individual, with each component involving a "small death" and bringing the inevitable reality of one's own mortality into closer focus.[17]

Loss also can be conceptualized as *simple, symbolic,* or *compound.* A simple loss involves the loss of a familiar object, such as misplacing a favorite pair of earrings. The

**BOX 10-1 Types of Losses**

| DEVELOPMENTAL LOSS | SITUATIONAL LOSS |
|---|---|
| Predictable change | Unanticipated change |
| Part of life process | Part of life events |
| Social and cultural preparation | Trial-and-error preparation |
| Potential for crisis | Potential for crisis |
| Observable or anticipated | Observable |

loss carries little attachment value and can easily be replaced. If, however, the earrings were a gift from a grandmother, the loss becomes symbolic and carries with it special meaning. Symbolic losses are secondary losses of simple loss and signify cherished roles, relationships, or identities. Compound loss involves several symbolic losses occurring together. If the earrings were the gift of a deceased grandmother with whom the person had a special relationship, then the loss becomes a compound loss.[26] Examples of compound loss in this situation include loss of history, support, friend, maternal figure, self-image, and childhood innocence. Although initially difficult to identify, symbolic losses are important to recognize because they account for the meaning behind the loss.[77]

Loss can be felt whether it is observable or perceived. Depending on the degree of threat to self or others, anticipation of loss can trigger an adaptive response similar to an actual loss.[52] Anticipatory loss experienced during a progressive and terminal illness can be as challenging and painful as the death of a loved one as the person confronts uncertainty over an inevitably tragic future.[76] Although uncertainty can serve as a motivating force, it also can overwhelm and deplete a person's adaptive reservoir for coping with loss.[80]

## FACTORS INFLUENCING LOSS

Individuals differ in their ability to adapt to loss in growth-producing ways, especially when the loss is perceived as a major life change. The meaning and extent of loss are interpreted by each person on the basis of personality, background, and coping resources. The extent to which a loss is intensified depends on factors such as the importance of the attachment, the possibility of replacing the object or relationship, the point in time of the person's development, the amount of personal and social disruption caused by the loss, and the availability of a supportive environment[7,17,71,90] (Box 10-2). The more cumulative and meaningful a loss is, the greater its threat to integrity of self and the greater its intensity. Aging, terminal illness, and death represent multiple and often overwhelming losses for any person, regardless of his or her adaptive resources.[26]

In addition to intensity and meaning, timing is an important factor in determining how loss is perceived. If a person is preoccupied with mastering a developmental task, such as accepting retirement, his or her ability to deal with other life changes will be reduced (Table 10-1). If the same person is also confronted with the sudden death of his wife, he may experience greater difficulty in adaptation. Each loss requires time and effective coping skills for successful integration. Loss cannot be managed in global terms because one type of loss can be symbolic or representative of other losses.[90] The loss experience can be viewed as analogous to an onion, with multiple, interfacing layers. To understand the experience, each layer needs to be peeled away and examined, even if it is painful.

Each loss in life is experienced uniquely in terms of the person's developmental stage, as well as the experience's meaning, relationship to other losses, intensity, and timing.[71] Individuals also vary in the length of time needed to adapt to or recover from the loss experience. Although a year has been used as a time frame for measuring recovery from a significant loss, current research suggests that true recovery may take years, depending on influencing factors.[91]

## LOSS AND THE FAMILY

Loss challenges the family to find ways to adapt to life changes while maintaining the integrity of the family unit. An individual's perception of loss can become magnified as each family member and the family as a whole search for meaning in the experience.[20] The meaning changes over time with the family as it does with individuals, because loss makes demands in managing uncertainty over roles, relationships, and responsibilities.[76] How successful a family is in adapting to loss depends on the factors influencing individual members, as well as family patterns, such as the family's stage of development, rules, belief system and cultural ties, communication patterns, perceived threat to the family's integrity, role flexibility, coping skills, and use of community supports.[7] If loss confronts a family during reorganization or high stress, adaptation becomes difficult and the family is at risk for an ongoing crisis.[4]

## FACING DEATH: THE FINAL LOSS

Although death can be defined as a normal life crisis and a fact of life,[84] it is the most significant loss experienced by an individual or family in today's society.[7] It represents not only separation from an important relationship, but also an inevitability that we all face. Despite awareness of our own mortality, death in our culture usually is perceived as untimely and incongruent with laws of nature, especially when caused by an illness or an accident.[48] Death challenges individuals and families to

**BOX 10-2 Factors Influencing Loss**

| INDIVIDUAL | FAMILY |
|---|---|
| Personality | Individual factors *plus* |
| Developmental level | Family's stage of development |
| Past experience | Family rules and roles |
| Role modeling | Belief system |
| Perception of intensity of loss | Patterns of communication |
| Meaning of attachment | Perception of threat to family integrity |
| Types of loss | Flexibility in roles |
| Replaceability | Repertoire of coping skills |
| Timing of experience | Relationship to community |
| Disruption from loss | Use of community supports |
| Threat to self and significant other(s) | |
| Coping skills | |
| Availability of supports | |

**TABLE 10-1 Developmental Impact of Loss and Death**

| AGE | DEVELOPMENTAL STAGE* | CONCEPT OF DEATH | IMPACT OF LOSS |
|---|---|---|---|
| 0-1½ yr | Trust vs. mistrust | Self-centered and center of world | Separation |
| 1½-3 yr | Autonomy vs. shame and doubt | Unable to think concretely about abstract concepts | Disappearance |
| 3-5 yr | Initiative vs. guilt | Very temporary | Fear of not being loved |
| 5-12 yr | Industry vs. inferiority | Other-oriented<br>Concrete and logical (sees possible causes and as final)<br>Thinks can outwit its inevitability | Punishment for not measuring up to expectations<br>Threat of bodily harm |
| 9-18 yr | Identity vs. role diffusion | Peer-oriented<br>Abstract thinking (sees as inevitable and irreversible part of life)<br>Problem-solves and predicts | Threat to independence<br>Sign of being different from peers |
| Young adulthood (18-25 yr) | Intimacy vs. isolation | Abstract | Disruption of life-style<br>Separation |
| Adulthood (21-45 yr) | Generativity vs. stagnation | Abstract | Disruption of family unit<br>Threat to history or future |
| Maturity (45 to death) | Integrity vs. despair | Abstract<br>Philosophic | Separation<br>Part of life cycle<br>Reward |

Modified from Brice C: *Am J Psychoanal* 42(4):315-325, 1982; DeSpelder L, Strickland A, *The last dance: encountering death and dying,* ed 3, Mountain View, Calif, 1992, Mayfield.
*According to Erikson E: *Identity, youth, and crisis,* New York, 1968, Norton.

search for meaning in terms of their belief systems and life-styles. Because of such searching, death always implies several interfacing losses that serve only to remind the survivor(s) of the loved one's death.[51] Concomitant losses of role relationships, normalcy, shared future, identity as a unit (as with a couple or family), sense of control over life events, intimacy, social support, role model, and social approval can all be symbolic of a loved one's death.[71] As a point of transition and potential for growth, death's intensity and complexity challenge the individual's and the family's coping skills. Supportive nursing interventions often are needed to promote the transition from crisis to growth.

### LOSS AND THE NURSE

Occupational stress involving loss is part of the daily experience of nurses, especially those who work with patients facing terminal illnesses and death.[25] To remain caring and empathic, nurses become vulnerable to identifying with their patients' and families' losses.[5] The observable loss of a patient's independence after learning that cancer has caused irreversible spinal cord compression can symbolize both personal losses in the nurse's own family history, as well as professional helplessness.[20] With today's medical emphasis on using technology for cure, nurses are at risk for loss of control, fear of failure, and loss of professional satisfaction when their patients are beyond cure.[7]

Because loss is a universal phenomenon that is experienced by patients, their families, and the nurses who support them, it becomes important to understand the process of adaptation.

## BEREAVEMENT: AN ADAPTIVE RESPONSE TO LOSS

Grief and bereavement are frequent companions of adulthood experience as loss is faced with increasing frequency in the life cycle. Each loss affects the individual and the family by prompting an adaptive response.[4] (Figure 10-1 is an illustrative diagram of adaptation to the loss experience.) Separation from something or someone of value triggers certain instinctive behaviors through which the person tries to hold onto the loss object. Such behaviors are the basis for the bereavement response.[8]

### DEFINITIONS

**Bereavement** is the subjective state of having suffered the loss of a person or object with whom a significant relationship existed. Although used interchangeably with bereavement, grief is the normal, expected process of adapting to any loss. It is the total response to the separation or emotional suffering caused by the loss. As a total response, its manifestations include psychologic, cognitive, social, and somatic dimensions.[71,77,90]

What makes grief difficult to conceptualize is its universal but individual nature. Grief is based on each person's unique perception of loss. Not only can grief manifest differently from one individual to another, but also

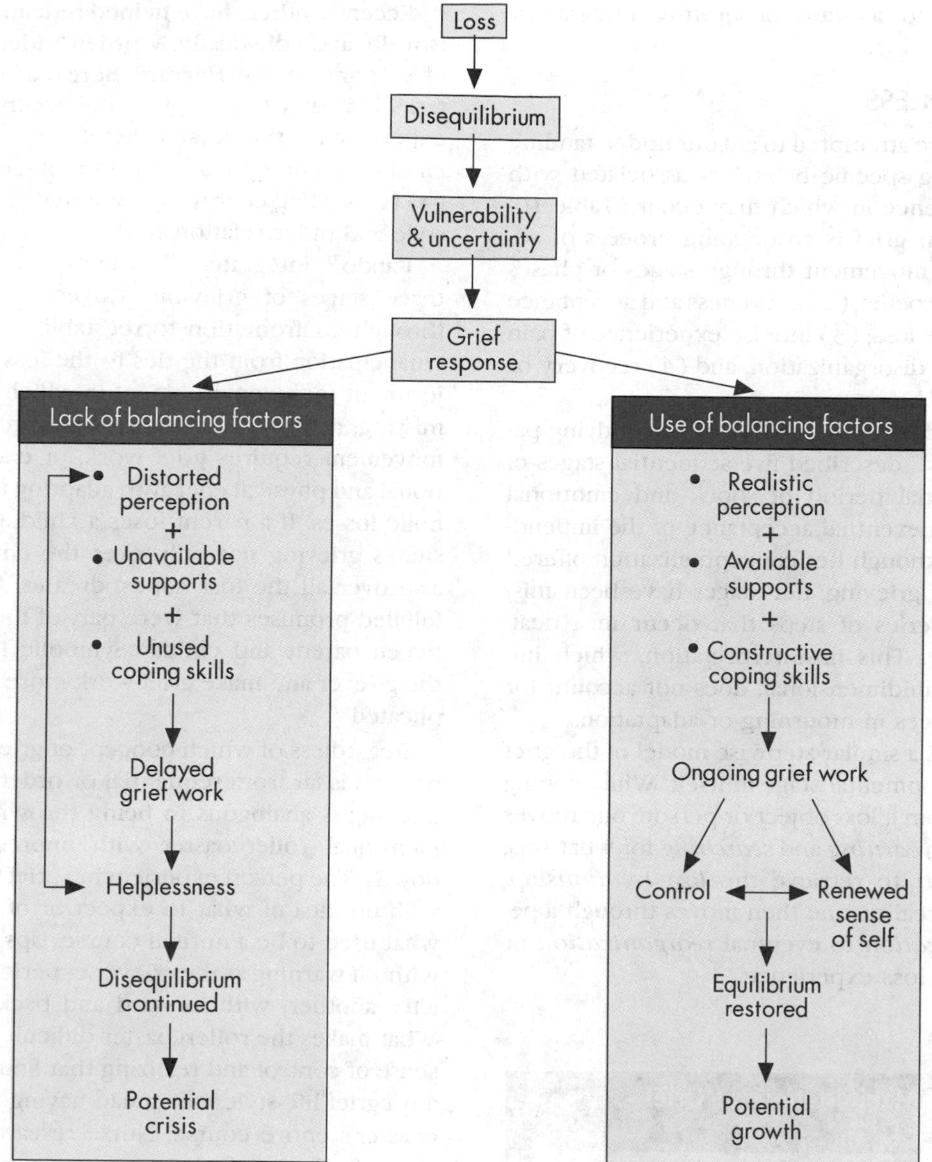


**FIGURE 10-1** Adaptation to the loss experience. (Modified from Aguilera D, Messick J: *Crisis intervention: theory and methodology,* ed 6, St Louis, 1990, Mosby.)

an individual's manifestations of grief can change over time. Because loss is a component of human development, grieving can help a person to adapt to a loss, as well as to grow from the experience.[17,37,51]

**Mourning** is the cultural and social response to loss, which includes any manifestation of grief. It is learned through role modeling and socialization during childhood. *Mourning* is an important term because it often implies how grief is expressed by the individual and family within their cultural norms.[71,77]

## HISTORICAL PERSPECTIVE

In 1915 Freud[32] described grief as a process of gradual withdrawal of the energy that ties the bereaved person to the lost object or person who died. Eliot[27,28] studied grief reactions in the 1930s and 1940s. Observations of victims of fire and war led Lindemann[53] to define **grief** as an *adaptive syndrome* with both *psychologic* and *somatic symptoms* that could be resolved with psychotherapy. Engel[29] further legitimized grief as an important field of study by classifying it as a discrete syndrome with common etiologic factors and universal manifestations. Grief, as a disease, temporarily reduces a person's ability to function and requires time for healing.

Later authors[47,55,72,77] have described general patterns of the grief process, suggesting an uncomplicated and naturally occurring syndrome that has a more or less predictable course of behavior. Such behavior can include a period of shock and somatic distress, feelings of hostility, guilt, and abandonment, interruption of life's usual activities, preoccupation with thoughts of the deceased, and finally, a recovery period of working through loss to a state of healthy integration (Box 10-3).

## THE GRIEF PROCESS

Several authors have attempted to aid our understanding of grief by defining specific behaviors associated with grief and the sequence in which they occur (Table 10-2). Most agree that grief is an ongoing process of adaptation involving movement through stages or phases of (1) shock and disbelief, (2) awareness and acceptance of the reality of the loss, (3) intense experience of pain over the loss, with disorganization, and (4) recovery or reestablishment of homeostasis.

In working to identify the unique needs of dying patients, Kübler-Ross[50] described five sequential stages of grief, from an initial period of shock and emotional numbness through eventual acceptance of the impending or past loss. Although her conceptualization offered a tangible view of grieving, her stages have been misinterpreted as a series of steps that occur in a neat, chronologic order. This misinterpretation, which implies that grief is unidimensional, does not account for individual differences in mourning or adaptation.

Bowlby[8] offered a similar stepwise model of the grief process as a developmental stage in itself. While coping with separation from a loss object or person, one moves from *numbing* to *yearning* and *searching* for what was, almost in an effort to retrieve the *lost relationship.* When faced with reality, one then moves through a period of *disorganization* to eventual *reorganization* or *recovery* from the loss experience.

**BOX 10-3 Common Manifestations of Grief**

| PHYSIOLOGIC | PSYCHOLOGIC |
|---|---|
| Anorexia | Numbing and dulling of senses |
| Tightness in throat | Foglike feeling |
| Sighing | Anger |
| Insomnia | Sadness |
| Crying | Yearning |
| Exhaustion | Loneliness |
| Feeling of emptiness or heaviness | Guilt |
| Shortness of breath | Visual hallucinations |
| Lack of sexual desire or hypersexuality | Lack of concentration |
| Restlessness | Disorganization |

Recently others have helped redefine grief more realistically and holistically. Worden[90] identified basic tasks of grieving in the Harvard Bereavement Study. These tasks include (1) accepting the reality of the loss, (2) experiencing the total pain of loss, (3) withdrawing emotional energy from the loss object or person, and (4) reinvesting energy in resuming an independent life-style and other relationships.

Rando[71] integrated Worden's concepts of tasks in three stages of grieving. Movement from avoidance through confrontation to reestablishment involves (1) emancipation from the ties to the loss object, (2) readjustment to the environment in which the loss object is missing, and (3) formation of new relationships. Such movement requires grief work, or exerting both emotional and physical energy in adapting to actual and symbolic losses. If a parent loses a child, grief work necessitates grieving not only over the child's absence but also over all the lost hopes, dreams, fantasies, and unfulfilled promises that were part of the relationship between parent and child.[71] Symbolic losses are real to the griever and make grief work more intense and complicated.

Regardless of which concept of grief one follows, the process is far from sequential or orderly. In many ways, grieving is analogous to being thrown onto a three-dimensional rollercoaster with unpredictable ups and downs. The person experiencing grief feels "off balance" with no idea of what to expect or of how to return to what used to be a normal course. Ups and downs occur without warning as the griever experiences one emotion after another, with forward and backward movement. What makes the rollercoaster difficult is regaining some sense of control and realizing that finding a way back to a pregrief life-style may mean having to ride the rollercoaster's entire course. Nurse researchers have begun to study the grief phenomenon in terms of a nursing theory framework. See Research box, p. 239, left-hand column.

## DEATH AND GRIEF

Not all losses are attributable to death, but because of the many life changes imposed on the survivors, the most disruptive losses are associated with the death of loved ones. The most profound loss is the death of a spouse or a child because of the closeness and intertwining of the relationship.[17,77]

**TABLE 10-2 Comparison of Grief Theories**

| STAGE | LINDEMANN | KÜBLER-ROSS | BOWLBY | WORDEN | RANDO |
|---|---|---|---|---|---|
| Initial | Shock and disbelief | Shock and denial | Numbing | Accepting reality | Avoidance |
| Acute grief | Acute mourning | Anger<br>Bargaining<br>Depression | Yearning and searching<br>Disorganization | Experiencing the pain<br>Withdrawing | Confrontation |
| Recovery | Resolution | Acceptance | Reorganization | Reinvesting | Reestablishment |

## RESPONSES BY SURVIVORS

Understanding the process of grieving and recognizing the behavioral manifestations that usually occur can assist the nurse to prepare survivors for what they can expect or to help them make sense of their feelings or somatic symptoms. Timing of the sharing of information, as well as the type and amount of information given at any one session, is important. Understanding the various processes and behaviors, both anticipated and unexpected, of bereaved persons may help to avert misunderstandings, strengthen the survivors, and help them to grow during the period of grieving. Grieving persons are helped by sharing their experiences. Recognizing the "normal" nature of the experiences, even those that seem somewhat bizarre, opens the way for sharing. Nurse researchers are beginning to develop sensitive assessment tools that are consistent with nursing theory. See Research box below, right-hand column.

### Shock and Disbelief

The initial response begins at the time of death and usually lasts for several weeks beyond the funeral.[33,77,90] Regardless of whether the death was anticipated or not, the immediate response is shock, numbness, and disbelief. The survivors may feel a sense of unreality, and as a consequence, they may appear to be "taking the death well." After the funeral this feeling of unreality or numbness changes to feelings of pain and separation. Survivors may experience some somatic symptoms, including muscular weakness, tremors, and tightness of the throat. They may experience diaphoresis, sigh deeply, have cold or clammy sensations, become anorexic, or feel exhausted. Bereaved persons exhibit extremes of behavior. They may become sedentary and do little or nothing except nap. On the other hand, they may be so hyperactive that they are unable to sit quietly or to sleep. They may experience extremes of mood such as profound sadness, anger, depression, or guilt or find themselves laughing without an explanation. They may have difficulty in concentrating. Coupled with these extremes in mood and behavior may be a continuance of disbelief, although the death is comprehended intellectually. "Searching behaviors" are common. These include dreams in which the deceased is alive and experiences of "seeing" the deceased or "feeling" the deceased's touch. During this phase, offers of comfort are often rejected because the bereaved is focusing on the deceased.[55,90]

### Yearning and Protest

For several weeks the bereaved have feelings of yearning and protest. They may feel anger toward the deceased for leaving them, toward God for allowing the death to occur, toward the caregivers for not returning the deceased to health. They may be jealous of others who still have their loved ones. They may wish they had been the one to die. During this period they may find it difficult to share their feelings or thoughts with others because they question their own sanity. Knowing that others have had similar thoughts and feelings sometimes is helpful.[71,77]

### Anguish, Disorganization, and Despair

As the bereaved begin to focus more on themselves and as the numbness and rage begin to fade, the reality and permanence of the loss begin to be recognized. New feelings and accompanying behaviors emerge. The bereaved may experience a sense of confusion, aimlessness, an inability to make decisions, a loss of motivation or interest, and a loss of confidence. During this period they feel lonely and depressed and experience a general loss of meaning to their lives.

All the experiences that they formerly shared with the deceased now seem irrelevant. They experience extremes of mood. The intensity of their feelings often is frightening to them. Memory lapses and difficulty in concentrating, although common and temporary, increase their feelings of anguish. They fear they will lose emotional control and as a defense become centered on themselves. Family members and friends may interpret this behavior as selfish and either reprimand them or withdraw. Neither behavior is helpful to the bereaved.

The experience of anguish leads to a new awareness of the preciousness of life. Life appears fragile. The be-

**RESEARCH**

Pilkington F: The lived experience of grieving the loss of an important other, *Nurs Sci Q* 6(3):130-138, 1993.

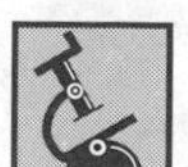

Using Parse's theory of nursing, the lived experience of grieving the loss of an important other was examined. Five participants described their grief in detail. Their narratives were analyzed to identify common themes. Results indicated consistency with Parse's theory as a means to further define the complex, highly unique grief experience.

**RESEARCH**

Lev E, Munro B, McCorkle R: A shortened version of an instrument measuring bereavement, *Int J Nurs Stud* 30(3):213-226, 1993.

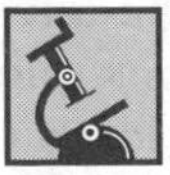

The authors developed a tool useful for measuring the grief experience by revising a more complex questionnaire, the Grief Experience Inventory. Parkes' bereavement research was used as a theoretic framework; 418 subjects who had been primary caregivers for significant others before their death completed the revised grief experience questionnaire. Results demonstrated the tool's sensitivity as a concise, valid, and reliable measurement of the highly individual experience of grief.

reaved may display intense fears of their being hurt or worry over the welfare of family members. At the same time they may smoke or excessively use chemicals such as drugs or alcohol. Other health-risking behaviors, such as lack of rest, may occur.

The wish and need to cry fulfill an important function in acknowledging the loss and in receiving support from others. Memories and mental images of the deceased are void of negative characteristics. Feelings of guilt, remorse, fear, and regret may surface. Opportunities to reminisce and to share feelings with others are helpful.[56,77,90]

### Identification

The bereaved may adopt the behavior, admired qualities, and mannerisms of their lost beloved ones. Some may take on the symptoms of the last illness of the lost loved one. Care must be taken to distinguish symptoms associated with physical illness from those associated with loss. Symptoms associated with loss will abate as the loss is resolved.[35,55,71]

### Reorganization and Restitution

The feelings and symptoms of grieving gradually subside; they do not suddenly disappear. Bereaved persons tell us they have periods of depression, as well as periods of well-being as life begins to make sense once again. Reorganization and restitution generally begin approximately 6 months after the loss and last for a few years. The process may be considerably longer or shorter and still be within normal range. Contrary to old popular beliefs, although life stabilizes, the pain of loss may remain for a lifetime. Reactions to loss recur around circumstances that are poignant reminders of the deceased—birthdays, anniversaries, and holidays.[55,90]

## FACTORS AFFECTING GRIEF RESPONSE

Many factors combine to affect the degree of stress and the particular response of survivors to a death. The major factors include (1) the type of relationship lost, (2) the nature of the death, (3) the characteristics of the survivor, (4) the social and cultural milieu, and (5) the nature of the support network.

### Type of Relationship

The loss of someone—spouse, parent—upon whom one has been dependent leaves an expected void and feelings of helplessness. Not as expected is the intense void that accompanies the loss of the survivor's role as a caring wife, husband, or daughter when the loved one dies.

The greater the reliance on the lost person for validation of self, identity, role, meaningful activities, and links to social and friendships networks, the greater the impact on life-style and the more profound the feelings of loss. Generally, therefore, the loss of a spouse is the most emotionally devastating.[18,31,39,88]

### The Bereaved and Deceased

Identities and roles are related. A survivor—widow, widower, daughter, son—is left with incomplete skills because the usual divison of labor in everyday life is lost. Loss of children creates its own special problems. The normal course of life events is disrupted when the young die before the old. Feelings of guilt and self-blame may be more pronounced.[90]

### Nature of the Death

The nature of the death and the circumstances after a death affect the grieving process. The closer the circumstances are to what the survivors perceive as a "good" death, the more comforting it will be. Anticipatory grieving or grieving that began before loss may ease the transition once a loss is complete. However, too much anticipation and repeated cycles of anticipatory grief may deplete a survivor's energy to complete the grieving process when the death finally occurs.[76,83]

### Personal Characteristics and Risk Factors

Individual characteristics of survivors such as age, personality attributes, physical and mental health, and the number and nature of grief and crises experienced have impact on grief responses. Various factors associated with high risk in widowers and widows have been identified from the literature[56]:

1. Loss of socioeconomic status
2. Poor health before the loss

**BOX 10-4 Signs of Poor Bereavement Outcomes**

Overactivity without a sense of loss
Taking on symptoms belonging to the deceased
Development of psychosomatic illness
Withdrawal from relationships with close friends and family members
Hostility and rage against persons associated with the death or loss
Wooden and formal conduct that masks rage and hostility
Lasting loss of social interaction skills
Destructive behavior (e.g., giving away one's belongings, substance abuse)
Prolonged and agitated depression, with risk of suicide
Feelings of worthlessness, self-blame, and need for punishment
Intense feeling that death or loss occurred yesterday
Inability to talk about the deceased without emotional distress a year after the loss
A relatively minor event triggers intense grief
False euphoria after the loss
Overidentification with the deceased
Phobias about illness or death
History of prolonged grieving
Inability to carry out usual activities of daily living

From Houseman C, Pheifer W: *Arch Psychiatr Nurs* 2:296-301, 1988; Kübler-Ross E: *On death and dying*, New York, 1969, Macmillan; Worden W: *Grief counseling and grief therapy*, ed 2, New York, 1991, Springer.

3. Sudden death or short illness
4. Perceived lack of social support
5. Perceived lack of supportive family
6. Family who discourage expression of grief
7. Extreme clinging to the deceased before death
8. Preoccupation with the image of the deceased
9. Strong reactions of anger, distress, or self-reproach
10. History of psychiatric illness or suicidal ideation

A person's success in grieving at a given point in time will affect future experiences of loss and adaptation. With any loss comes the reliving or resurfacing of old issues involving separation and helplessness. If these issues are not acknowledged in some way and their associated feelings worked through, the griever may carry the pain of the experience into the future.[71,77] Cumulative, unresolved loss has been identified as a significant risk factor for morbidity after bereavement.[67,90] It not only can change perception, but also can confront the person with overwhelming feelings of grief at some future time. When needs for grief work are ignored or denied, even a minor change in the person's routine can serve as a catalyst to resurrect the intensity and burden of past losses.[90] Unresolved loss or grief that is ignored becomes a crisis for the affected individual and family and causes impairment of the usual activities of daily living (Box 10-4).

## GRIEF RESOLUTION

Although theorists have described ending stages or tasks in the grief process, debate exists over whether one can ever recover from the experience of loss.[91] Lindemann[53] suggests that grief resolution can occur within a few weeks of the loss. Recent research findings, however, recognize that grief is more appropriately measured in years.

Because grieving is such an individual process, with a wide range of possible manifestations, how can it be determined if and when an individual has successfully completed grief work? Engel[30] defined successful mourning as the ability to remember comfortably and realistically both the pleasures and disappointments of the lost relationship. Graininger[36] identified a change in perspective as the key to grief recovery. This change in perspective occurs when the person can rise above the emotions of the loss and view the situation more objectively, while finding some meaning in the loss experience.

Silverman and Worden[81] further clarified what is meant by grief recovery. **Recovery** is not simply letting go of the loss object or person. Instead, it is the negotiating and renegotiating of the meaning of the loss over time. Their view reinforces that loss may be permanent and unchanging, but, like development, the grief process is ongoing.

Wolfelt[89] offered **reconciliation** as the term that best describes how acute grief is processed or worked through. Reconciliation means moving on with life even without the presence of the loss object. In reconciliation, there is a renewed energy and a sense of confidence, an ability to fully acknowledge the loss, and a capacity to become reinvolved in normal activities of daily living. Reconciliation involves acknowledging that loss is a difficult yet necessary or growth-facilitating part of life. Wolfelt's view focuses on *reconciliation as a process, not as an event or outcome.* As human beings, we never get over grief; rather we become reconciled to it.

## NURSING MANAGEMENT

Jackson[42] states that the role of the caregiver is to assist the griever in releasing emotional ties to the deceased despite the discomfort and sorrow it causes and in subsequently replacing the type of interaction lost. The griever must be persuaded to participate in grief work that entails *accepting the pain of looking realistically and actively at the loss.* A number of strategies are available to assist grievers. Rando[71] groups these in broad phases that roughly correspond to the process of grief—from shock to reintegration. These activities are useful to health professionals *in helping others* to help the bereaved. Some are neither feasible nor appropriate for health professionals to perform themselves.

### ♦ ASSESSMENT

Planning interventions for helping grieving persons help themselves must be preceded by accurate assessment of where persons are in their grief, as well as what factors are influencing their grief.[55] The preceding sections—responses by survivors and factors affecting the survivors' responses—provide a framework for gathering subjective and objective data associated with grief. Intervening without understanding the grieving situation and the factors influencing it can introduce more harm than good. Raphael[72] suggests the following assessments of the bereaved that yield information but also facilitate the expression of emotion and promote the grieving process:

1. Tell me a little about the death. What happened?
   These questions give the griever permission to talk about the death while providing information about the nature and circumstances of the death. At the same time the griever's feelings, ability to talk about the death, stresses related to it, and whether the griever had the opportunity to say good-bye can be evaluated.
2. Tell me about (name the deceased) and about your lives together or relationship together from the beginning.
   This opening allows the caregiver to evaluate the relationship, its quality, and the interactions associated with it. It also provides the opportunity to evaluate a griever's degree of denial of the loss and the degree to which he or she speaks of the

loss in realistic terms. In addition, risk factors can be assessed.

3. What has been happening since the death? How have things been with your family and friends?
This question provides the opportunity to explore patterns of family and social support that the bereaved perceive to be available. It also provides the opportunity to assess other crises that may affect the grieving process.
4. Have you been through any other bad times recently or when you were younger?
This offers the opportunity to explore past experiences and concurrent crisis. It also opens the way to help the bereaved identify past successful ways of coping and new ways of coping.

Any assessment needs to be continually updated and revised. Fluctuations in the experiences of the bereaved are to be expected. Interventions that are appropriate for one person are not useful or may even be harmful to another person. Reassessment may address such major topics as:

1. Acceptance of the reality of the loss
2. Evaluation for need for medical attention and treatment
3. Identification of unresolved grief
4. Detection of illogical thoughts

People, especially under stress, attempt to impute cause. They may believe their actions in some way contributed to the death; for example, they did not get to the hospital soon enough, or they did not prepare a diet properly. Such beliefs can lead to unresolved feelings of guilt.[56]

Instruments have been developed to identify persons at risk for difficulty in the grieving process or to identify the problems of persons who experienced prolonged bereavement-related distress in widowhood. The grief resolution index, a screening instrument developed by Remondet and Hansson,[73] includes four measures of short-term adjustment (survival expectation, fear, preparation, and desperation indexes) and four measures of long-term adjustment (depression inventory, anxiety, adjustment to widowhood, and health indexes). Assessment tools that are consistent with nursing theory are being developed.

## ♦ NURSING DIAGNOSES

Human responses to the loss of a loved one are varied. Although other nursing diagnoses may be applicable, the most commonly recognized one among persons who experience loss is *grieving*. Grieving is an appropriate diagnostic category for those seeking to promote wellness and to facilitate healing associated with significant loss. At the same time, normal grieving may be associated with dysfunctional or distorted behaviors[1] that can be recognized in a variety of secondary diagnoses. Nursing diagnoses are determined from analysis of patient data. Nursing diagnoses for the person experiencing the loss of a loved one may include but are not limited to the following:

| Primary Diagnostic Title | Possible Etiologic Factors |
|---|---|
| Grieving | Loss of loved one |
| **Secondary Diagnostic Title** | **Possible Etiologic Factors** |
| Anxiety | Loneliness, social isolation; self-reproach; fear of the unknown; financial insecurity; fear of own death |
| Self-care deficit | Depression; anxiety; fatigue; social isolation |
| Nutrition, altered | Anxiety; grief; loss of mealtime companion; inertia because of fatigue; feeling of tightness in throat |
| Coping, ineffective (individual) | Depression in response to loss |
| Social isolation | Withdrawal; uncontrolled anger; knowledge deficit regarding support resources; housebound state (unemployed, young children); rejection by significant others |
| Spiritual distress | Inability to understand meaning of loss; anger at God; anxiety; depression |
| Hopelessness | Separation from significant other; inability to achieve goals in life associated with loss; loss of belief in God's care |
| Thought processes, impaired | Grief, anxiety, insomnia; guilt; loneliness; substance abuse; hallucinations |
| Self-esteem disturbance | Hallucinations centered on the deceased; anger; anxiety; preoccupation with the deceased; social isolation; substance abuse; fear of loss of control |
| Sleep-pattern disturbance | Anxiety; hyperactivity; agitation; fear of nightmares; substance abuse |

Grieving is the ultimate price of loving, of attachment, of a meaningful relationship.[55,80] In some instances the person is unable to mourn in a manner that allows for resolution of the grief and reinvestment in life, and this may result in dysfunctional grief.

NANDA has approved two independent nursing diagnostic categories in relationship to grieving: (1) anticipatory grieving and (2) dysfunctional grieving.[21] *Anticipatory grieving* is defined as "a condition in which the individual grieves before an actual loss,"[21] and *dysfunctional grieving* is defined as "a condition in which the individual experiences delayed or exaggerated response to a perceived, actual, or potential loss."[21]

| Diagnostic Title | Possible Etiologic Factors |
|---|---|
| Grieving, anticipatory | Perceived loss of a significant other, physiopsychosocial well-being, personal possessions |

| Diagnostic Title | Possible Etiologic Factors |
|---|---|
| Grieving, dysfunctional | Actual or perceived object loss; thwarted grieving response to loss; absence of anticipatory grieving; chronic fatal illness; loss of others; loss of physio/psychosocial well-being; prolonged denial; intense pining and yearning; ambivalent relationship with the deceased; severe self-reproach; multiple crises; lack of support from family |

For some, the grieving process is extended or excessively intense, making reorganization and restitution improbable or impossible.[67] The bereaved in this situation has been described as "dying of a broken heart." The anger, guilt, depression, and self-blame are more intense, and time offers no relief. Carpentino[12] defined the nursing diagnosis of unresolved grief as a "pathological response of prolonged denial of the loss or a profound psychotic response." Inasmuch as the range of normality differs in each case of grief, it is difficult to describe dysfunctional grief. Much research remains to be done to clarify the expected duration of uncomplicated grief, the phenomenology of unresolved grief, and valid and reliable methods of assessing grief.

## ♦ EXPECTED PATIENT OUTCOMES

The expected outcomes associated with grief and the work that is entailed in the grieving process include remembering the loved one without emotional pain and reinvesting emotional energy in life so that the capacity to love is not lost. Cantor[11] speaks of the same outcome as "enriched remembrance," which may not preclude sadness. To achieve these outcomes, the grieving person must accomplish the six "tasks" of grief work:[43]

1. Face the pain.
2. Permit the emotional expression of the full range of feeling.
3. Achieve emancipation from bondage to the deceased.
4. Adjust to an altered environment.
5. Renew or form new relationships.
6. Be able to live with memories.

## ♦ INTERVENTIONS

Understanding the grieving process as a normal part of loving provides the basis for nursing assessments and interventions. Nursing actions in response to the bereaved call for a delicate blending of being present, listening, expressing honest feelings, and inviting the bereaved to share their experiences and emotions.[56]

Some interventions are appropriately directed at supporting the caregivers and alleviating their stress while caring for the needs of dying relatives, which in turn enhances or promotes the caregiver's health after the death.[64] Bereavement interview data collected in the National Hospice study revealed that health problems in the bereaved before the loved one's death was the key determinant of health care use and morbidity after the death.[62] In addition to assessing health of the caregiver before the death, nurses can learn about other existing resources available to the caregiver and reinforce them before and after the death. These resources include interpersonal support (provision of information, material goods and services, emotional support), religious-spiritual beliefs, and intrapersonal coping (cognitive and behavioral strategies).[75]

After the death, the following nursing interventions may be appropriate:

1. Make contact and assess.
   a. Establish a relationship; simply be present.
   b. Assess the bereaved in her or his grief to plan appropriate future interventions.
2. Reach out.
   a. Take the initiative; reach out in a concrete way. Don't say "call me if you need me." Do be specific in how you can assist or get others to assist. For example: "How about if I call your sister to accompany you to select the casket?" "Suppose I arrange for you to attend a widow-to-widow meeting?"
   b. Do not take refusals personally or give up.
   c. Repeat offers of assistance. Grievers initially may be unable to respond to and appreciate offers of help but will benefit over time.
3. Be physically and emotionally present to offer security and support.
   a. Do use physical contact, hugging, touching, handholding, as appropriate. These actions are important early in the process to convey that the griever is not alone. There may be exceptions. Some people do not like to be touched. You can sit nearby if you perceive that that will be more comforting.
   b. Social supports generally are decreased weeks or months after a death, when the bereaved is forced to resume life without the loved one. Encourage family members to be present after all the intensity of the funeral has subsided.
   c. Encourage regular expression of feelings to help minimize the tendency to become overwhelmed and unable to function.
   d. Encourage others to take charge of routine functions and responsibilities of the bereaved, for example, run errands, prepare meals.
   e. Provide for security through direction concerning meals, rest, priorities of activities for the day or week.
   f. Help family members focus on one problem at a time.
   g. Address problems to which practical solutions can be found before addressing more complicated problems.

4. Give people "permission" to grieve.
   a. Display nonjudgmental attitudes and behaviors. Be neutral.
   b. Communicate compassionate support through verbal and nonverbal behavior; for example, when the griever's voice cracks, facial muscles quiver, eyes water, and the bereaved turns to the caregiver, lean forward, relax, do not turn away or offer them a tissue, allow the griever to cry. Display your comfort and approval through your body language; your actions will speak louder than your words.
5. Do not allow grievers to remain isolated.
   a. Be present and have others present.
   b. Suggest self-help groups and assist grievers to attend.
6. Maintain a family perspective.
   a. Remember that the family is changed.
   b. Help the bereaved reassess.

## ♦ EVALUATION

Progress in grieving is difficult to measure because of its ongoing nature and wide range of manifestations.[13] Any assessment needs to be continually updated and revised. Fluctuations in the experiences of the bereaved are to be expected. Interventions that are appropriate for one person may not be useful or may even be harmful to another person.

The grief experience can present an overwhelming challenge to the grieving person, family, and nurse. To face the challenge, measurable outcomes need to be preestablished for *each* person on the basis of the individual's sociocultural situation. The outcomes serve as a yardstick of progress. They offer hope that the intensity of grieving does not last forever.

Examples of progressive bereavement outcomes for the grieving person and family include the following:

1. Acknowledging the loss and its impact in changing roles and/or relationships.
2. Talking about the *reality* of the loss (e.g., son's deceased father will not be taking him to the park to play ball anymore).
3. Beginning to incorporate the reality of the loss (e.g., wife no longer sets place at table for deceased husband).
4. Displaying *some* sign(s) of grieving, (e.g., cognitive, social, physical, and/or psychologic).
5. Indicating an absence of
   a. Destructive behavior (e.g., suicidal thoughts, alcohol or drug abuse).
   b. Signs of poor bereavement outcomes.
6. Using some constructive means to express feelings with a significant other or health care professional about the loss.
7. Establishing and maintaining an ADL routine in meeting own needs (i.e., rest, nutrition, fluids, elimination).
8. Identifying at least one grief support in significant other or health care professional.
9. Beginning to set some goals for own future and decreasing preoccupation with the loss.

Evaluation methods that can be useful in measuring grief recovery include the following:

1. Perceptions of the grieving person and family about the experience
2. Observations of responses to nursing interventions
3. Comparisons of current grief behavior with baseline behavior
4. Functional status of the grieving person and family in maintaining life-style
5. Mutual discussion of goals and ways to work toward goal achievement
6. Perceptions of the nurse about own grief history

When unresolved grief is evident, psychiatric intervention may be required. Parkes[66] identified the following behaviors that require psychiatric care:

1. An extreme depressive reaction manifested by persistent sadness with no shifts to a normal state; an unresponsiveness to warmth; extreme expressions of guilt and identification symptoms
2. Psychotic break with reality (neurotic anxiety; obsessions; phobic, hysteric, or schizophrenic reactions; acting and speaking as though the deceased were still present)
3. Suicidal tendencies (self-punitive acts, often to expiate guilt)
4. Excessive drinking, drug abuse, or promiscuity (as substitutes for the deceased)

Although the discussion in this section focuses primarily on the survivors, all involved are experiencing loss. The dying person, perhaps, is facing the greatest loss of all. Everyone involved is grieving. The principles apply to all from different perspectives. Nursing care of dying persons includes several patients and multiple processes.

Dying persons and their families and friends may or may not experience the grieving process in the same way. Dying persons may grieve over the loss of physical function, the loss of past abilities, the ultimate loss of life, and separation from all they know and love. At the same time, significant others may grieve over the potential loss of the loved one, the hurt they feel, and the emptiness they anticipate.[51,57,71]

# FACING DEATH: THE FINAL LOSS

## DYING: A PART OF LIVING

Despite the amazing advances of science, technology, nursing, and medical knowledge, dying is and will continue to be a part of living. The fact is that at some future time we will cease "to be." In a sense we are dying even as we are living. To conceptualize living and dying as the opposite ends of a continuum creates a false dichotomy. Living and dying are not opposite ends of a continuum; they *are* the continuum. When we interact with persons who are known to have a life-threatening illness, we are more directly confronted with their dying and our own finiteness. This confrontation evokes anxiety, and thus we become more aware of the dying component of living. Although we may identify with the suffering and sorrow of persons as they live their dying, we interact with living persons. To appreciate our own and others' responses to loss, dying, and death, we need an understanding of the context in which they occur and of our own views and reactions within varying contexts.

## SOCIETAL, CULTURAL, AND SOCIAL PERSPECTIVES

### Dying and Death: The Differences

Dying is different from death. **Dying,** a part of living, is a process—the process of coming to an end. **Death,** the permanent cessation of all vital functions—the end of human life—is an event and a state. The event is the moment of death; the state is that of being dead.

Both dying and death have unique aspects that evoke fears, anxieties, and uncertainties. Some aspects of dying such as physical and emotional pain, the loss of others, and the inability to function in familiar ways may also occur under other circumstances (e.g., illness, retirement, or relocation) and therefore are not unique to dying. The unique aspect of dying is that it ends in death. People have no prior experiences to help them understand what it means to be dead. Questions surface: Can dead persons think? Do they have feelings? What is it like to be dead? Is there another life? Where will they go?

At the same time that death is a unique event, it is universal. Because it is universal, each society has had to develop its own beliefs, norms, mores, restrictions, and standards related to loss, dying, and after-death practices. Appropriate ways to respond in one societal or cultural group may be inappropriate in another. Each society dictates the standards and practices that it will support. Thus members of a society have a prescribed set of behaviors from which to choose.[60]

In general, the dominant view of dying, death, and loss of members of any one society is a function of how death fits into the teleologic view of life. Individual responses reflect the dominant societal view. However, the repertoire of responses of dying persons or the survivors also is determined by personal beliefs and subcultural group (e.g., social, cultural, religious) affiliations. For instance, Americans may view dying similarly, but their responses may be influenced by their religious beliefs, their views of life after death, their social class, and their occupations.

### Prevailing Societal Attitudes

*Death denial, death defiance, death acceptance, and desire for death* are four prevailing societal attitudes toward death. As these general attitudes are discussed, it is important to remember that they may vary in different situations, depending on whose death is involved.

Recognition of the prevailing attitudes and their differences helps health care professionals to understand the process of dying, guides them when interacting with others, helps them to avoid conflicts among themselves, and, most important, enhances their communication abilities and thus their patient care. Quality care for dying persons and family members must remain the constant goal of health care professionals.

No attitude is good or bad; attitudes are merely different. Our behavior reflects our attitudes. If we recognize our own attitudes toward dying and death in a particular situation, as well as those of other persons involved, we may better understand why all of us feel the way we do and why we are acting the way we are. This recognition and understanding may not always lead to agreement, but it can contribute to modifications of behavior and to decreased conflict in decision making. These attitudes are explored briefly in the following sections.

#### Death denial

Western society has been described as a *death-denying* society.[6] Many people avoid the subject of dying and death. Health care professionals, particularly physicians, have been described as being unwilling to talk to patients about their dying.[31] Both health care professionals and family members often justify their stance by expressing the belief that they are "protecting" the dying person.

The question is, whom are they really protecting? In most situations they are protecting themselves; that is, consciously or unconsciously, they weigh the impact on themselves and decide—or choose—not to act because of fear of the reaction or response. The following questions often arise: What will happen to me? Will I lose emotional control? Will the other person shout, cry, or become angry? Will family members become angry? Will the physician become angry? Will I know what to do or say? What if they do not react at all?

In nursing, a death-denying attitude has taken on a negative connotation. But *no attitude in and of itself is good or bad—it just is.* The actions and consequences of an attitude can be evaluated as good or bad. For example, a death-denying attitude may contribute to a lack of open communication about dying, but it also may contribute to continuing to give care in bleak situations. On the other hand, a behavior or action such as continuation of care may reflect more than one attitude; for example, it may reflect both death denial and death defiance.

#### Death defiance

*Death defiance* is a part of the Judeo-Christian heritage. Throughout the ages people have fought for causes or ideologies, even though they knew that they might die in the attempt. This attitude is reflected in hospitals, especially in critical care units or during emergency situations. The cause is saving a life; the battle is with death.

Although it is not the staff members who die in the battle, they are open to loss. If the patient dies, staff members live with the sense of a battle lost. Moreover, they face once again the finiteness of their own lives and the inevitability of death, despite modern technology.

Death defiance is helpful as we fight for life. It is not helpful when we do not also attend to the realities of the situation.

### Death acceptance

*Death acceptance* is viewing death as a normal, natural, and integral part of living. Becker,[6] a prominent philosopher, defined the resignation to and acceptance of our limited existence as the central task for achieving maturity. With this acceptance, death becomes the conclusion of life's plan. It sounds so simple. Intellectually it calms the fears and pains of dying and of facing our own mortality. Like other attitudes toward death, however, this attitude is not a panacea. In fact, Schneidman[79] helps us to regain our perspective when he points out how romantic this attitude can be.

For some, death acceptance is the ultimate achievement of maturation, a form of self-actualization. The dying person must achieve this attitude himself or herself; it cannot be forced on him or her by others.

The value of the death-acceptance attitude can be judged by actions and behaviors of the dying person.

### Desire for death

The fourth attitude, the *desire for death,* is more common in our society than people generally know or like to admit. People may desire their own deaths or the death of others.

Many circumstances give rise to the desire to die or for someone else to die. One major reason is the search for relief from misery. Misery takes many forms; pain, loneliness, disability, fear, uncertainty, and economic and emotional crises are but a few.

Other reasons that contribute to the desire to die may be associated with a relief from misery but are expressed in a different way. Some persons search for reunion with loved ones. Still others look forward to death as a last phase in the fulfillment of life.

Recognition of how people express their desire to die is important. In many instances the expression of the desire to die is the dying person's or family member's way of confirming his or her recognition that death is inevitable within a predictable period of time in the near future.

## Meaning of Death

The knowledge that death is imminent or probable within a predicted period of time adds reality to feelings of fear, anxiety, and uncertainty.[45,54] As a result, persons facing imminent death experience these emotions differently than do healthy persons who are speculating about what it is like to be dying. Healthy persons speak of death in the abstract; they talk about the death of another or project it into the distant future. Casual comments such as, "We all have to die someday," "We are all dying from the time we are born," or "Everyone has to die of something," reflect what Freud[32] called "unconscious immortality." The fact that people can continue to think about others who have died causes them to unconsciously believe in their own immortality. Hearing of someone else's dying or death, however, forces them to face their own finiteness.

Neither the casual comments nor the unconscious belief in our own immortality are good or bad in and of themselves. However, they offer little in the way of understanding or support when made to a dying person or to his or her family. The statements usually are in response to the discomfort we feel when someone tells us that death is imminent. A more understanding response might be "I'm sorry to hear that."

Views toward dying and death vary considerably, depending on whether the discussion is about "my death" or "your death" or whether the discussion is about a member of "my family" or "your family" or someone dear to me or to you. Even when we are discussing hypothetical situations, our closeness to dying or to a dying person can influence our views and our responses.[66] The same data are seen differently from different perspectives. We can use age as a common factor and consider how our responses may change. For example, my father is 75 years old, and your father is 75 years old. When death appears imminent, our thoughts may vary, depending on the referent of my father or your father. For example, my father is still young; your father has lived a long and a good life.

It is important to identify the referent under discussion whether we are talking in theoretic terms or about practical situations. In other words, from whose perspective are we evaluating the situation: my perspective, your perspective, the patient's perspective, or a family member's perspective? Lack of recognition of different perspectives leads to poor communication, faulty nursing judgments, and inappropriate nursing interventions.

### Quality of life

What constitutes *quality of life?* Who can predict what quality of life is or will be during the dying process? Can one person judge the quality of life of another, especially if the other is dying?

Much has been written on what constitutes quality of life from the research perspective, but there is little on what constitutes quality of life for the dying person. In fact, it has been suggested that, if the known instruments were used to measure quality of life, most dying persons would receive low scores, because most instruments focus on objective physical, behavioral, psychologic, and economic results of disease and treatment and less on measures of a general sense of well-being, happiness, or satisfaction.[57] Dying persons may perceive quality of life differently than those who are living with an acute or chronic illness or who are well. What constitutes quality of life differs from person to person and for any one person during the various stages of life. What contributes to the *meaningfulness of life* may be a more cogent question than what constitutes quality of life in considering the dying person.[71] For example, depression can be expected but how much and for how long? A person can live with pain, anxiety, and fear but how much and for how long? How much control does the person have over the situation? Can we increase the control he or she can have in the situation, although the person has lost control over dying? Do the symptoms detract from the meaning of life from the perspective of the dying person? Sometimes trials and tribulations contribute to a person's growth.

Dying persons must have freedom to choose a style of dying and then be assisted in that choice. Patients preferences are important because they make explicit the values of personal autonomy and self-determination.[57]

**Informed consent,** then, becomes an important factor in supporting meaningfulness of life. It includes giving dying people sufficient information about their diagnoses, prognoses, and possible therapies so that they make informed choices about how they will live or die and about who will help them and in what ways. Informed consent is a person's agreement to allow something to happen on the basis of a full disclosure of facts needed to make an intelligent decision.[86] Informed consent reinforces the value of personal autonomy. It assumes that the person has the emotional and mental ability to understand, to process data, to assess benefits and burdens, and to make decisions. This ability is sometimes referred to as competence or **mental capacity.**

*Competence* and *incompetence* are used in many ways in everyday life to infer that a person is capable in some way, that is, clinically competent. Actually, the terms *competence* and *incompetence* are best reserved as legal terms. As such they infer reasoning ability and emotional stability sufficient to appreciate the nature and consequences of making decisions regarding such things as wills, contracts, or being a parent. A judge or other proper legal authority makes the judgment of whether or not a person is competent. If a person is judged incompetent, he or she is assigned a guardian. The guardian may be responsible for all decisions for another person, or his or her power may be restricted to *one area* of the dying person's affairs. For example, a person may be deemed incompetent in matters of business but may retain the mental capacity that allows autonomy in decisions about medical treatment.

In the health care setting, use of the term *mental capacity* rather than *competence* or *incompetence* offers some clarity. *Mental capacity* refers to the ability to understand the situation and voluntarily make decisions about it. The mentally capable dying person has the right to refuse or to request treatment. When the request is based on an informed choice, it should be respected, thus reinforcing the value of autonomy. As in other situations, it is not a simple matter. What makes a person mentally capable or incapable? Box 10-5 suggests some of the components of a systematic assessment of mental capacity or mental incapacity and factors that could influence judgments. Nurses can enhance the mental capacity of dying patients by educating them about their illnesses and treatments and assisting them to formulate questions for the health care team. They also can provide a safe environment for patients as they deal with uncertainty.

**BOX 10-5 Assessment of Mental Capacity and Factors Influencing Judgment**

Orientation to time, place, person, and situation
Ability to recall recent and past events, to logically sequence events, to understand abstract ideas, to make reasoned judgments
Psychologic state, mood, and affect that may affect the ability to make choices, e.g., anxiety, fear, depression, suicidal ideation, hallucinations, delusions, illusions
Prior history of psychiatric disorders that could affect present judgments

## QUALITY OF DEATH

### Rights of Dying Persons

Some health care consumers are demanding that dying and death no longer be hidden behind closed doors. As a consequence, there is a movement to recognize that dying persons have rights. One right of dying persons is the right to know that they are seriously ill and that they may die. The assumption is that such information ensures that they will have more control over what happens to them. As a result, they can participate more fully in decisions about their care and will have the opportunity to complete unfinished business.

Another right is the right to die in an atmosphere of hopefulness. Persons have a right to die in peace and dignity, surrounded by loved ones and unencumbered by tubes and machines. They have a right to privacy. Dying persons are entitled to be cared for by sensitive, caring, knowledgeable people who attempt to understand them and their loved ones. They are entitled to die as free from pain or other discomforts as is possible.[82] Comfort contributes to dying with a sense of self-esteem and gives meaning to life.[55]

#### Advance directives

Concern that patients be allowed to die in a dignified manner has led to the development of the living will, or **advance directive,** in state statutes, in which it is referred to as the *Natural Death Act.* **Living wills** direct decisions for withholding or withdrawing of life-sustaining treatment when the patient is in a terminal condition and death is imminent. Traditionally, life-sustaining treatment has included cardiopulmonary resuscitation and mechanical treatment such as a ventilator. However, with the growing number of court cases, questions have arisen about inclusion of nutrition and hydration.[24,44]

Living wills are written documents that instruct anyone who may become responsible for the person's health, welfare, or affairs, such as family members, lawyers, physicians, clergy, or representatives of any medical facility in which the person may be. These documents advise them on health care preferences. Living wills include directives to physicians and a durable power of attorney for health care.

Living wills generally request that under conditions in which (1) an individual can no longer take part in decisions about his or her own future and (2) there is no reasonable expectation for recovery, the person be allowed to die and not be kept alive through the use of artificial or extraordinary means. Most living wills also request that the person be kept free of suffering and pain, even though the medications administered for pain relief may hasten the moment of death.

Several states have enacted legislation that permits designation of a **durable power of attorney** for health care, a form of advance directive that enables one to choose an agent to act as decision maker if one becomes too incapacitated to responsibly participate in one's own health care decisions. Included are special directions for life-sustaining treatments and hydration/nutrition issues.

At the present time, living wills are not legally enforceable in all states. In addition, there are many questions related to the conditions under which a living will can or should be honored. What is important for purposes of this chapter is that a living will can help caregivers and family members know what the dying person's wishes were, at least at the time of the writing.

Copies of living wills usually are given to family members, physicians, the person's attorney, and the person's religious advisor. People are advised to sign and date them at least yearly. The wills are likely to be honored if they are written or signed immediately before a person becomes unable to express his or her own wishes about dying care.

In those states where advance directives are included in state law, mandated forms may be required. The state statute should be consulted before one advises patients or acts on the directive. Ordinarily, other documents or statements of one's choosing can be added to the mandated form.[19]

A sharing with loved ones and primary health care providers of one's philosophy of life and desires related to the process of dying is perhaps the most effective way of ensuring a meaningful death—or what has been referred to as a "good" death.[23]

## Good Death/Bad Death

Many nurses, in fact people in general, express concern over dying with dignity or dying a "good" death. Is there such a thing as a good death? There is no one good death; rather there are many. There is no one right way to die, just as there is no one right way to live. Dying with dignity, or a good death, is really an ideal. The terms offer little in the way of guiding care.

There are many views about what constitutes a good death: to die as one lived, to die without pain, to die in the company of loved ones are all answers.

There are many ways to die well. A good death involves individual perceptions of the living-dying process, as well as shared observations of the death event. *A death is more likely to be labeled as good when dying is viewed as a part of living* and not as a separate phenomenon. A good death also is associated with the way all persons involved interact with each other preceding and during the event—that is, if there is harmony rather than conflict.

Sometimes nurses refer to deaths as normal or abnormal. Deaths are perceived as normal or good when most or all persons involved perceive that all was done that could be done and that the wishes of the patient were respected and accepted by most persons involved. In these instances there is a sense of loss, but the loss is accompanied by a sense of fulfillment and closure. Nurses label deaths as *bad* or *abnormal* when there is conflict over the type or length of treatment and when the wishes of the patient are ignored and there are bad feelings about a lack of honesty, especially with family members.

Whether a death is seen as good or bad does not always have to do entirely with the way the person died. Sometimes it has to do with who is present and how they interpret what is happening in the situation. People's attitudes toward dying and when people should die, as well as the characteristics of the dying person, influence how they interpret the situation and how they act and interact with others.

## Age and Premature Death

There was a time when people did not make a connection between aging, loss of body function, and general progressive debilitation and dying. For example, primitive people believed that if there were no accidents or magically induced illnesses, no one would die.

The expectations of living have changed as life expectancies have changed. During the Roman period, life expectancy was 20 years; it increased to about 35 years during the Middle Ages. By the late 1800s Americans could anticipate living 50 years; few persons lived past the age of 60 or 70. In contemporary American life, people not only anticipate living more than 70 years; they expect to do so as active, functioning individuals.

Many people believe that any age is too young to die. In contemporary society death is perceived as premature and clinically unnecessary. The concept of clinical death is well entrenched. Some perceive that people do not die of natural causes or of old age; people die as a result of accidents, homicides, and suicides. They die while receiving treatment for a recognized, diagnosed clinical problem such as heart disease, stroke, disseminated intravascular coagulation (DIC), or total body failure. As a consequence, most deaths can be interpreted as avoidable, unnecessary, and premature. If death always is interpreted as avoidable, unnecessary, or premature, it follows that someone must be blamed. Who can be blamed—the physician, the hospital, society? Perhaps it is the fault of the person who died for not seeking help sooner. It is this interpretation of death as always being avoidable that contributes to conflict and guilt. People die; death is a part of living. People can receive the best care possible and still die. In fact, sometimes the very treatments that save lives create dilemmas by prolonging life or perhaps even by prolonging dying.

### Prolonged Dying

Just as there is concern over premature death, there is concern over prolonged dying. Through modern technology and therapy we have become adept at maintaining life in the desperately ill person. Unfortunately, at times the same techniques used to maintain life during temporary crises create dilemmas related to what constitutes life. When are we prolonging dying rather than life? Our ability to prolong dying leads to many moral and ethical issues related to life and death.

### Dying: An Achievement or a Failure

Although most dying people express resentment, fear, or sorrow over the major changes that are forced on their lives by their progressive debilitation, some view dying as an achievement.

Some persons, especially those with a prolonged course of living with dying, focus on living their dying so as to die well. They speak about their dying to selected persons and at selected times. People who believe that dying well is an achievement sometimes are described by health professionals as denying or defying death. These people recognize their dying but choose therapy or choose to go home and participate in their customary activities. If you listen carefully to what they tell you, you will see that they intend to live their dying the way they wish, and thus from their own perspective they die well. These persons seem to do more than adjust or accommodate. They rise to an unseen challenge and in so doing expand their living rather than extend their dying.

A small number of persons may perceive dying as a personal failure or may attribute it to external forces. Some dwell on all they could have accomplished were it not for their illness. They usually exude a sense of powerlessness and futility and express overt anger. Others appear depressed, helpless, and resigned to their situation.

Remember that how people perceive their dying may change throughout the course of their dying. Attitudes, like physical capabilities, do not remain static. Dying encompasses the whole person; it is an emotional, behavioral, and physical process.[66,75]

## FUNERALS AND AFTER-DEATH RITUALS

All societies have funeral practices associated with care and disposal of the body and with the expected behavior of the bereaved. Although there have been scathing attacks on the funeral industry,[61] funerals and after-death rituals serve many positive functions for the bereaved. They include the following:

1. Focus on the bereaved by a gathering of friends and family offers sympathy, a recognition of the loss, communication of caring—in short, social support. Wakes, viewings, and visitations are forms of gatherings for family and friends. Nurses and other health care professionals accomplish similar tasks by reviewing together what occurred and sharing past experiences about the person who died or others who have died.
2. Use of ritual, which is often religious in nature, offers some reason or lends some meaning to death.
3. Visual display of the dead body assists survivors with reaching closure or accepting the finality of death.
4. There is opportunity to display grief publicly in a procession that ends at the place of final disposition.
5. Burial, entombment, cremation, or some kind of sanitary disposition of the body reinforces the idea of preservation of life on earth and for some provides a place to return for prayer or reminiscence.
6. Material expenditure for funerals is one way to communicate "the loss of the bereaved to society."

All major changes in life have rituals to help individuals and society adapt to the changed state and cope with the disequilibrium that occurs during the transition from one state to another (e.g., birth, marriage, and death). Funerals serve as a rite of passage[85] from life to death. They function to validate the life of the deceased[71] and act as a testimony that a life has been lived.

During the funeral the bereaved begins the process of emancipation from the bondage of the deceased, readjustment to an environment in which the deceased is missing, and incorporation to a new state. The bereaved publicly appears without the living loved one, to be reincorporated into their previous social group in a changed state. The deceased is removed from the social group and admitted to the land of the dead by internment, entombment, or cremation. The relationships are publicly declared changed.

During the funeral, society bestows rank on the deceased for the last time. The specifics of the ritual (e.g., 21-gun salute), the number of mourners, and the impact of the death on society all reflect the value of the deceased individual.

Funerals meet the needs of mourners and society.

They are for the living, not the dead. They offer spiritual, psychologic, and social benefits to the survivors and therefore are important.

## THE DYING PROCESS

Thus far we have discussed dying and death in somewhat general terms. Now let us turn more directly to a discussion of dying persons and their characteristics, which will form a basis for nursing assessment.

### Chronicity of Dying

The nature of dying has changed. Because of modern therapies and technology, patterns of illness have shifted from acute infectious diseases to chronic conditions; as a result, dying has become a chronic process. With the exception of some acute problems such as myocardial infarction, severe infections, fatal accidents, homicides, and suicides, most dying persons experience chronic problems with multiple pathophysiologic alterations. These alterations usually are permanent and result in disability, with a need to adjust to loss and to accommodate to change. Multiple series of losses can affect a person's behavioral responses and ability to cope.[41,55]

Dying takes on many characteristics of chronic illness. Dying persons, just as do other chronically ill persons, express feelings of being socially displaced or isolated. They grieve over the loss of former activities and abilities. They express sorrow over the continued loss of friends, business associates, and acquaintances. They talk of being alive and yet not able to live. They are expected to be present-oriented rather than future-oriented.[68,75]

Whenever the anticipated life span is *perceived* as *shortened,* persons, even though they are healthy, may be viewed as chronically ill or dying and treated accordingly. For example, some elderly persons are perceived and perceive themselves as not having enough time left to make future-oriented plans or decisions. The same perception is associated with some persons with diagnoses of such illnesses as cancer, stroke, and multiple sclerosis. Some people with shortened life spans may perceive themselves or be perceived by others as not deserving of services or not being worthy of the efforts of others, because they will not live long; thus they may become displaced, isolated individuals, not allowed to live their living. Furthermore, the chronicity of their dying may force them into experiencing a *social death* while they are functionally and biologically very much alive. Many factors contribute to promoting social dying long before the event of death; these factors are discussed in the next section.

### The Living-Dying Interval

The theoretic stages and phases of dying are sensitizing schemes to help us remain open to assessing what is "going on" in a situation so that we may understand it better. Our ultimate goal is quality care for dying persons and their families. Understanding, observation, and assessment assist in determining appropriate intervention to better achieve that goal. Another tool to help understand the nature of grief and dying is the patterns of living-dying.[22,56,58]

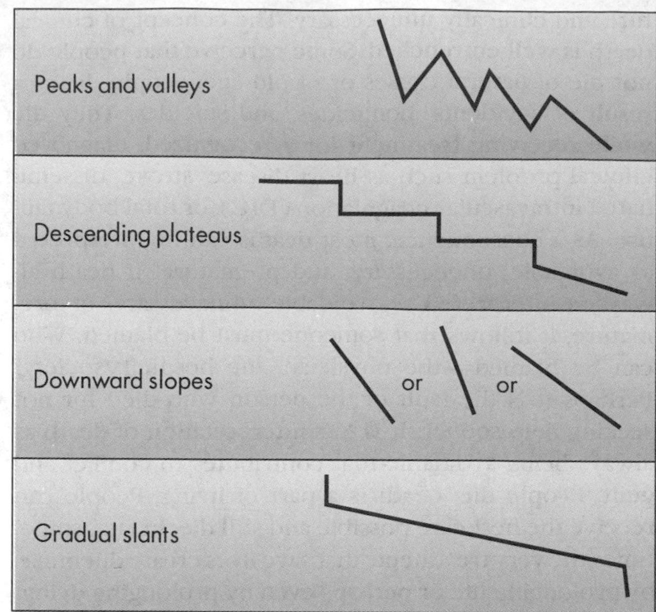


**FIGURE 10-2** Martocchio's patterns of living-dying.

The four major patterns and their various combinations are based on the clinical courses of dying patients (Figure 10-2). They describe what has occurred, not what will occur. In other words, they are descriptive, not predictive. They are useful for understanding the variations of behavior among dying persons. They also demonstrate the futility of expecting persons to pass through a series of stages of behavior in any fixed sequence.

#### Peaks and valleys pattern

The *pattern of peaks and valleys* is characterized by periods of greater health (peaks) and periods of crises (valleys). Dying persons refer to the peaks as *"hopeful highs"* and the valleys as *"terrible or depressing lows."* Although there are times of greater health, the overall course is downward to the event of death. Many hospitalizations and many moments of increased expectation and dashed hopes are associated with the experience of dying in this pattern. The uncertainties are great; fluctuations in behavior and difficulties in planning and adjustment are to be expected as goals and plans change.

#### Descending plateaus pattern

The pattern of *descending plateaus* is characterized by an unpredictable number of progressive degenerative steps, with *plateaus* (periods of stable health) lasting an indeterminate period of time. Again, the overall general course is downward. People do not return to their former level of health or functioning after each crisis. Like the peaks and valleys pattern, the course is fraught with uncertainty and anxiety about whether another crisis will occur and cause more debilitation.

This pattern is associated with expressions of futility and anger. Dying persons and their families grieve over the fact that functional ability is lost in spite of concerted rehabilitative efforts to maintain or regain it.

**Downward slopes pattern**

The *downward slopes pattern* is characterized by a consistent, persistent, easily discernible downward course. Unlike the other patterns, death is expected within a predictable period of time measured in hours or days. In most instances the dying person loses consciousness, and there is little time to prepare family members for the death of their loved one. These deaths usually occur in critical care units.

**Gradual slants pattern**

The fourth pattern of living-dying, *gradual slants,* is characterized by a low ebb of life, gradually and almost imperceptibly culminating in death. Generally these persons experience a debilitating bodily insult from which there is little recovery. In many instances the person is no longer conscious, and life is maintained by life-support systems such as ventilators. This pattern is associated with many of the following questions:

When should life-support system be discontinued?
Where should these persons be cared for?
Who should be responsible for their care?

In reality, many combinations of the four patterns may occur in one person's experience of living-dying. For example, a person's pattern may change from peaks and valleys to a downward slope or from a downward slope to a gradual slant.

## Choice: A Need and a Right

All dying persons eventually learn of their fate. They should be free to choose what role, if any, they will play in the circumstances and manner in which they learn.[23]

Dying persons describe a system of filtering out or listening only to what they want to know or to realize. They tell us of how they listen to or look at the facts initially but do not hear or see them until later. They allow the facts to permeate their minds at their own pace. Dying persons, or any person facing an extreme crisis, can describe reaching an emotional readiness when they suddenly hear or see the facts and wonder how long they have been there. Sometimes facts have to be introduced more than once by various persons and in various ways. Sometimes patients look for confirmation of what they heard or what they saw—that is, of what they think they know.

The person who recognizes that death is imminent but is not allowed to talk about it is locked behind an impermeable wall of silence with no way to escape to the comfort of loving arms or to the closeness of a relationship with a loved one. No one should be condemned to such total isolation. No rationalization or self-protection exists to support such punishment of dying persons or their loved ones.[56]

How does this happen? Fear is probably the greatest cause. Families and health care providers blunder into subterfuge and thus tragedy. No one anticipates all the additional lies that will be needed to support the first lie. No one anticipates the energy that will be spent futilely guarding the secret that all, including the patient, know.

There is tremendous hurt and anger when the truth is recognized. Would the person have chosen to live differently during the time that can never be returned? What happens to the confidence the person may have had in the nurses, physicians, and health system—the confidence that has been betrayed?

On the other hand, there are patients who sincerely choose not to see or to hear—who choose not to know. If that is their *informed* choice, then it is inappropriate to push them to know that which they do not want to see or hear. To force them to see or hear what they wish to deny is as cruel and inhumane as the conspiracy of silence. The refusal of the patient to know or to discuss the facts creates its own set of problems. The foremost problems, both with lying to patients and with refusal by patients to acknowledge or discuss the facts of dying, are the creation of barriers to comforting and supporting care and communication among interactors and the inability to share feelings and concerns on the basis of the reality of the situation.[56]

## Role of Confidant

Nurses can introduce the element of choice by fulfilling the patient's need for a *confidant* who will initiate and allow honest talk. The role of confidant is a necessary but difficult role. Talking of dying is not easy, and periods of awkwardness and expressions of fear are inevitable.

Dying persons look to the confidant for honesty and acceptance as they search for understanding of their state. They are not searching for pity, consolation, or sympathy. They are uncomfortable with the helplessness that they see in the eyes of others. The length of time that relationships exist with patients who have long-term chronic illnesses provides both the opportunity and the obligation for nurses to establish *authentic relationships* with dying patients, relationships in which nurses can be viewed as confidants.[57]

The confidant is one to whom patients can voice their deepest fears. They do not voice such fears to business associates; they cannot expect casual friends to understand. They do not reveal their most terrible anxieties to those they love; they protect loved ones from their panic. There are great risks in seeking information about that which they most dread because what they most dread might be confirmed. There is also the superstition that lurks in their minds that what is said aloud might happen or come true; therefore, if they do not talk about it, it will not happen. The result may be fear and silence.

The *role of the confidant* is primarily *to listen* and *to reassure* as the dying person grapples with the experience of dying. The confidant can help to make the period of shifting from living to dying a time for a deepening feeling of closeness, a time for reinforcing family relationships, and a time to do and say what needs to be done and said.

Acting as a confidant does not mean that the relationship with the patient is a friendship. A true friendship is characterized by mutuality, with each party having equal rights and equal obligations to be sensitive and concerned for the needs and desires of the other. In contrast, in the nurse/patient relationship, the needs and desires of the patient are the primary concern and provide direction for interaction. Although not a friendship, an atmosphere of emotional closeness is a significant part of the relationship. Within this context, patients can develop and share their agendas for the future, for quality of life, and for what they truly want, without the need to protect the nurse from difficult truths.[57]

Dying persons do not confide in every nurse, nor will the person they select as confidant necessarily be a nurse. Dying persons, just as any other persons, will be selective. Nurses are obligated to offer opportunities to be selected; to demand to serve in the role of confidant is not only inappropriate, but impossible. Nurses who may not be a confidant can support the chosen confidant and learn information that can be useful in guiding care.

## Impact on the Family

Thus far we have focused on the dying person, but the impact of the knowledge that death is imminent extends beyond the dying person to his or her family, social groups, and the society in which he or she lives.

### Cohesive or disruptive force

The experience of dying may serve as a cohesive force in some families and a disruptive force in others. In general, families who have responded to stressors or crises as a unified force in the past will offer each other strength and support. For families who have strained relationships, the dying experience may promote further strain.

Family members generally express remorse over the fact that a family member had to come face-to-face with death before they realized how much they needed each other or cared for each other. But unless this recognition is coupled with assistance in learning how to make the relationship grow, it will not necessarily lead to greater social and emotional solidarity.[58]

### Family control

Dying persons at times use their dying to control the behaviors of family members. When dying persons use dying as a means of control for self-gain or as a weapon, the result is anger, resentment, and perhaps retaliation by family members. Retaliation usually takes the form of not visiting, not phoning, or visiting for only short periods. It is an attempt to protect themselves from the tyranny of the dying person even while they wish to be close and loving.

The problem becomes more serious for the family members and the dying person alike if the dying person is being cared for at home. The dying person usually recognizes the antagonism of family members but may interpret it as inappropriate, because, after all, he or she is dying. More frequently, the dying person may feel rejected and unloved and may not understand that the family loves him or her but not the behavior.

Family members may recognize their own behavior as a response to the dying person's manipulation, but at the same time they feel guilty about their responses because the other person is dying and because they do care. The problem is best addressed openly and honestly, but it is usually difficult to resolve. It is difficult to deal with expressions of anger, resentment, and long-term depression under the best of circumstances. They are almost impossible to deal with when one person is dying. In either case, the focus must be on love for the dying person but displeasure with the offending behavior.[57]

### An unreasonable situation

Although biomedical technologic advances continue to shift the locus of dying to the hospital, the hospice movement is attempting to deinstitutionalize dying. The American Nurses Association's *Standards and Scope of Hospice Nursing Practice*[3] provides an overview of hospice care in the United States and describes nursing as the cornerstone of hospice care. The standards provide a useful guide to those interested in understanding the special responsibilities of hospice nurses and the criteria for evaluating hospice care.

With the increased emphasis on hospice care and the pressures by Medicare and other insurers to discharge patients as soon as aggressive treatment is discontinued, more and more persons are encouraged to die in the privacy of their own homes surrounded by family.

To have those we love die at home, cared for by family, may fulfill the romantic ideas we have surrounding dying; however, it takes proper, careful, and advanced planning. Two major factors usually are considered: the economic situation and the dying person's wishes. Other important factors to be considered that pertain to environment and available caretakers are addressed in Box 10-6. Unless all factors are discussed in advance, family members may be ill-prepared to deal with the most simple tasks. They may not know how to change an occupied bed. They may be concerned about how, what, or even whether to feed the dying person. Nurses choose to become nurses and have been educated to nurse. Family members are expected suddenly to assume nursing responsibilities that they may not

**BOX 10-6 Factors to Consider in Home Care of the Dying Person**

Who will be the caretakers?
Who will relieve the caretakers?
How is the home arranged?
Are the doors large enough to accommodate a wheelchair?
Can rooms be arranged to accommodate a commode or other necessary equipment?
Would a hospital bed or other hospital equipment be helpful?
Are the people in the home prepared for the changes they must make in their own life-styles?
Was the decision made a family decision?

desire or feel prepared to do, such as change dressings, irrigate wounds, and administer medications.

When families are asked to do more than they believe they can accomplish, especially when they do not have readily available assistance, they may feel trapped in an unreasonable situation. Feelings of entrapment lead to anger, frustration, depression, fear, and despair.

Family members who are prepared to care for dying persons in the home need planned times for their own social activities, as well as for grocery shopping and other necessities. Visitors and other family members, as well as the dying person, need help in actively supporting the caretaker.

Nurses can help caregivers by providing time off and giving them acknowledgment for what they are doing.

## NURSING CARE OF THE DYING PATIENT AND FAMILY

Although each person's experience of dying and grieving is unique and personal, there are similarities. Knowledge of the uniqueness of the perceived experience coupled with knowledge of some expected common responses assist nurses in assessing each situation, planning care, intervening, and evaluating both the plan of care and the interventions for dying people and their families and friends. Nurses who do not consider family members, as well as the dying person, as the focus of their care will not achieve the best possible quality of care for the dying person.

### A Realistic Perspective

To be of most assistance to dying persons and their families, nurses must be realistic about how much they can relieve suffering. Nurses cannot stop the dying process or bring back the dead loved one. Nor can they take away the pain of loss. A realistic perspective helps make the experience better and facilitates appropriate grief. Nurses can *reach out* if they objectively accept the fact that pain and the often volatile responses to it are a natural part of the interaction.

**BOX 10-7 Nursing Assessment**

**INPUT FROM DYING PERSON AND SIGNIFICANT OTHERS**

**General Perception of Each Individual**

Awareness of clinical diagnosis and prognosis
Philosophy of living while dying and views regarding dying
Perceptions of self and effect on self of the dying process
Expected physiologic and behavioral changes
Past experiences with major illnesses or crises
Shared experiences with major illnesses or crises

**Perceived Strengths, Desires, and Hopes**

Personal abilities and coping techniques
Personal support systems
Availability of resources
Beliefs; religious convictions; cultural views of dying, death, and bereavement
Past experiences with death
Expectations about care and dying, use of life supports (present and future)

**INPUT FROM NURSE**

Beliefs, values, attitudes, responses
Support systems: personal and professional
Expertise, including incorporating others in care

### Assessment: Your Perspectives

The role of the nurse is to help the dying person and family members to cope.[16] Philosophic or religious tenets (e.g., "It's God's will," and "Everything happens for a reason") may assuage the nurse's feelings but are not helpful to others who need to ventilate their feelings and thoughts. A difficult situation is made less difficult by being honest and forthright, that is, by acknowledging that the situation is painful and does not make sense. It is not improved by rationalizing or trying to paint a rosy picture. It is good to plant seeds of hope regarding the meaning of life at a future time while acknowledging the despair of the present. Sometimes it helps to show emotion, to allow others to cry, or to ask the dying person or family members privately and as a group to talk about what is happening or will happen. By listening, the nurse can then help them separate fact from fiction. It may be a helpful way to begin an assessment.

## NURSING MANAGEMENT

### ♦ ASSESSMENT

Nursing assessment is an ongoing process throughout the term of the dying person–family-nurse relationship. It will continue and become the family-nurse relationship at the death of the patient. A thorough initial assessment with direct input from the dying person and significant others provides the basis for relationships. Assessment criteria are listed in Box 10-7.

## ♦ NURSING DIAGNOSES

As one reviews the various nursing assessment criteria in caring for dying persons and their significant others, it becomes clear that analyses of the data may lead to identification of nearly all the NANDA nursing diagnoses over the course of the dying process. The complex physiologic, psychologic, social, and spiritual dynamics that accompany dying help explain the presence of the multiple primary and secondary nursing diagnoses. Perhaps the greatest challenge to nurses is prioritizing—which nursing diagnoses should be addressed and in which order?

Among the most important diagnoses to address are those related to symptom management and anticipatory grief. The physical symptoms that accompany the dying process depend on the particular pathophysiology of the disease responsible for the life-threatening state and the interface with other preexisting emotional and physical health problems. Assessing and understanding the cause of the symptoms is central to determining appropriate interventions. Following is a brief outline of some of the most common nursing diagnoses associated with care of dying persons as they relate to major symptoms/problems. A more complete discussion of the topic can be found in Amenta and Bohnet.[1]

| Diagnostic Title | Possible Etiologic Factors |
|---|---|
| *Anorexia problems* | |
| Nutrition; altered; less than body requirement | Nausea and vomiting secondary to chemotherapy, medication interactions, obstructions in the gastrointestinal tract, anxiety; altered taste secondary to dysphagia, weakness, depression |
| *Body movement problems* | |
| Activity intolerance, high risk for | Depression, shortness of breath |
| Injury (trauma), high risk for | Secondary to metastases to bone, confusion, seizures |
| Mobility, impaired physical | Weakness, contractures, pain, infection, semicomatose/comatose state |
| *Bowel elimination problems* | |
| Constipation | Medication reaction, poor fluid-dietary intake, immobility |
| Diarrhea | Impaction, disease process |
| Incontinence, bowel | Secondary to weakened state; semicomatose/comatose state |
| *Fluid balance problems* | |
| Fluid volume deficit | Low fluid intake secondary to weakness, fever, reduced extracellular fluid volume, dysphagia, gastrointestinal fluid losses, oliguria, polyuria |
| Fluid volume excess | Altered cardiac output; effects of medication |
| *Mouth symptoms* | |
| Mucous membrane, altered, oral | Disease secondary to impaired immune system, decreased protein intake; effects of treatment such as chemotherapy, radiation, and continuous oxygen |
| Pain | Stomatitis secondary to dehydration, continuous mouth breathing and local trauma; dysphagia |
| *Respiratory/ventilation symptoms* | |
| Airway clearance, ineffective | Inability to eliminate secretions |
| Breathing pattern, ineffective | Dyspnea, pain, rales/rhonchi, obstruction, semicomatose/comatose state |
| Gas exchange, impaired | Shortness of breath |
| Tissue perfusion, altered (respiratory) | Respiratory distress syndrome |
| *Skin problems* | |
| Skin integrity, impaired | Edema, immobility, urinary incontinence, sweating, cachexia, fungating tumors<br>Complications of treatment, reaction to medications<br>Poor tissue perfusion secondary to infrequent turning/repositioning; circulatory impairment |
| *Sleep and rest problems* | |
| Sleep-pattern disturbance | Fear of dying, uncertainty about the future, pain, shortness of breath, metabolic effects of disease, drug interactions/untoward drug reactions, night sweats, restlessness, depression |
| *Temperature problems* | |
| Temperature, high risk for altered body | Medication reaction, decreased fluid intake, altered metabolic rate, sedation; neurologic and/or circulatory alterations |
| *Urinary problems* | |
| Urinary elimination, pattern, altered | Reaction to medications, obstruction of the urinary tract, reduced fluid intake, nausea, urinary tract infection |

In addition to the nursing diagnoses associated with physical symptoms, other nursing diagnoses associated with dying persons relate to psychosocial and spiritual dimensions. The following are examples that may be evident:

| Diagnostic Title | Possible Etiologic Factors |
|---|---|
| Coping, compromised (family) | Conflicting perceptions among members, maladaptive coping styles |
| Coping, ineffective (individual) | Pain, effects of medication, lack of family or social support |
| Diversional activity deficit | Total focus on pain, effects of medication |
| Family processes, altered | Patient's or other family members' inability to fulfill accustomed roles secondary to pain and disability |
| Grieving, anticipatory | Association of existence of pain and dysfunction with imminent death |

| Diagnostic Title | Possible Etiologic Factors |
|---|---|
| Knowledge deficit | Patient's and family's lack of awareness of availability of modern methods of palliation |
| Powerlessness | Dependence on others for care secondary to pain and effects of medication |
| Social isolation | Inability of patient to focus away from symptoms, discomfort of others when confronted with patient's symptoms and dying |
| Spiritual distress | Association of symptoms with punishment, imminence of death, and sense of abandonment by God |

## ♦ PLANNING

As with assessment, planning is a joint venture. Successful planning incorporates the goals of the family and the dying person, as well as goals of nurses and other health care providers.

The expertise of the nurse is of special importance in anticipating the dying person's various needs as his or her physical state declines. This expertise is needed to identify the neighbors, church groups, and family members who may serve as support persons and to help them to know when and how they may be of assistance to the dying person and to each other. These persons can participate with the nurses in planning the timing of nursing interventions (Box 10-8) and identifying alternative interventions.

Nurses need to plan for their own health maintenance (Box 10-9). This planning is achieved in relation to each individual situation involving a dying person or the significant others of dying persons.

The care of dying persons and their families is best accomplished by a team of caregivers. Planning care—if comprehensive care is to be achieved—therefore must include obtaining input from and relying on and listening to others in the situation.

**BOX 10-8 Planning Times for Nursing Interventions**

- Times for physical care
- Social interaction times
- Times for privacy for family members and patient
- Quiet times alone for reflection, grieving, or rest
- Times for reassessment
- Times for group planning and evaluation

**BOX 10-9 Plans for Nurse's Health Maintenance**

- Time commitments
- Support from other professionals or own significant others
- Considerations of actual or potential value conflicts and means of dealing with conflicts

## ♦ INTERVENTIONS

The nursing needs of dying persons are the nursing needs of living persons. The range of activities are as broad as for any diverse population of patients, family, and significant others. Nursing intervention may occur in a variety of settings, either at home or in various institutional settings.

Direct physical care is a major part of caring for dying persons. Maintenance of comfort, both physical and emotional, is of the essence. Teaching others involved in direct care how to maintain the patient's comfort allows their participation and promotes their feelings of competence and well-being.

Health teaching may include teaching such measures as breathing exercises, relaxation techniques, and coping strategies to the dying person and to significant others for use throughout their grieving process. Teaching how dying persons may use medication for comfort and at the same time dispelling expressed fears of patient addiction may help the dying person and family alike. One should recognize and respect cultural differences and fears about addiction. Addiction in dying persons is improbable and in the last days of living, inconsequential.

Another nursing responsibility is to be well-informed about organized support systems, agencies, and independent resources within the community and to be prepared to assist patients and their families in contacting and using these resources. Inquiries related to the many alternative modes of care for dying persons, such as hospice and other forms of home care, nursing home care, and other forms of institutional care, should be answered openly and honestly. If the nurse cannot answer the patient's or family's questions, they should be referred to those who can supply the answers.

Nursing intervention may include participation in resuscitative efforts and the maintenance of dying patients on life-support systems. Along with direct patient care in these circumstances, nurses are responsible for communicating with and supporting family members or for ensuring that someone is providing this service.

In essence, nurses assist patients and families in maintaining control over their individual lives as much as is possible to ensure dignity and self-esteem. This control is accomplished through the aforementioned actions.[33,56]

If nurses are to care effectively for patients and families, they need to maintain their own well-being. Planned confidential sessions to discuss thoughts and feelings about a particular situation may be helpful. Recognition that others (other health professionals, volunteers, and family members) have much to contribute and are as committed and concerned about the patient's welfare is of importance. There is a tendency for each person to believe he or she is alone in the situation.

Withdrawal from a situation may be necessary in some rare situations, but it should occur only when other nursing personnel are available to maintain the care of the patient and significant others.

### ♦ EVALUATION

Each nurse is responsible for evaluating his or her own practice as it relates to each situation. Comfort and satisfaction of the patient may be used as criteria. Nursing interventions may be evaluated through a preestablished evaluation system. Use of these systems contributes to the nurse's development and well-being by affording support in the decision process.

1. Evaluation methods in the care of dying persons
   a. Care of patient and significant others
   b. Observation of responses to interventions
   c. Discussion of goals and how they have been achieved
   d. Discussion of alternative methods to achieve goals more effectively or with more comfort for patient
   e. Mutual evaluation of continued appropriateness of goals
   f. Mutual identification of new or revised goals and means to achieve these goals
2. Preestablished nursing evaluation systems
   a. Formal and informal peer review of goals and interventions
   b. Open discussion of problems
   c. Venting of feelings
   d. Sharing of positive responses
   e. Special criteria developed by groups of nurses involved in caring for dying persons

A nurse will experience loss when a nurse-patient relationship concludes with the death of the patient. Evaluation of his or her contribution to the relationship gains importance, especially for each nurse's well-being. Recognition of specific successful interventions and contributions leads to feelings of achievement and success. Lack of this recognition may lead to perceiving consecutive losses as a sign of failure.[13,56]

Peer support is most beneficial to nurses caring for dying persons. Peer support may be accomplished through formal and informal groups. In addition to groups, one-to-one interactions with a trusted peer or personal significant other may alleviate some of the stress related to working with dying persons.[25] More important, such relationships serve as an appropriate avenue for recognizing and reinforcing the inherent rewards of providing nursing care for persons who are living their dying and for those who are sharing the experience.

## SPECIAL ISSUES IN BEREAVEMENT

### ETHICAL PERSPECTIVES

To help a person die well is to support that person's sense of self-respect, dignity, and choice until the last moment of life. Achievement of this goal entails skilled and compassionate nursing care to maximize comfort and minimize suffering. The goal is to provide calm, sensitive, individualized nursing care to each person so that dying, the final human experience, is as free from pain and anxiety as possible.[2]

Historically the profession and activities of nursing have been concerned with life and based on two fundamental principles. These principles are that all people should (1) live as whole persons and (2) should live long and healthful lives. The expectation has been that nurses and physicians would help to fulfill these principles.

In the past, nurses and physicians fulfilled their obligations by striving to save lives. There were no miracle drugs, life-sustaining machines, transplantation surgeries, or radiation therapies. Intensive and continuous nursing care was the main hope of saving lives. Modalities such as heat, cold, food, fluid, rest, exercise, and maintenance of a sanitary environment were used. Physicians and nurses relied on the natural healing powers of the body. If a body failed to heal despite the efforts of nurses and physicians, the patient died. The power of medicine and nursing simply was no match for the diseases that people experienced. Death often was caused by infection and communicable disease. Many people died at young ages.

With the advent of miracle drugs and advances in anesthesia, surgical techniques, and life-sustaining technologies, persons who would have succumbed to life-threatening illnesses now seek treatment to restore health and function. The capacity to prolong life and to ease the pain and suffering of seriously ill persons has improved to a great extent. The improvement has been accompanied by some difficult consequences. Increasingly, deaths occur in institutions. In many instances, deaths occur in critical care units to the sound of monitors. More and more often death is caused by someone's decision rather than the failure of the heart to pump blood or the lungs to breathe.

Death become impersonal when the body and the tubes and machines become one and when there is only a deteriorating organ system present. The situation becomes so confusing that those involved have conferences to determine whether life or death is being prolonged.

When a dying person has been termed a nonperson and seems neither dead nor alive, all involved persons search for resolution of a situation in which neither grief nor hope is appropriate. Family members long to return to normal living. They search for help in making life and death decisions for loved ones who are no longer able to contribute to decision making. Staff members search for relief from a situation fraught with dilemmas.

The dying person does not have to be completely incoherent or comatose for ethical issues to arise. Many ethical issues are inherent in the situation. For example, modern technology has made possible successful treatment of diseases that formerly resulted in fairly immediate death. Now cures from diseases such as cancer are possible. In many instances there are no cures, but there are temporary reprieves; for example, the mechanical ventilator can prolong life. In some situations the result of therapy is ambiguous—for example, therapy that is associated with great discomfort to the patient or the family, such as with bone marrow transplantation, or that involves great expense and limited supply, such as in the case of organ transplantation.

Discussions of such issues as "quality of life," "right to die," "death with dignity," "living wills," and "informed consent" in lay as well as professional literature demonstrate the extent and awareness of the conflicts associated with modern therapies that extend life but at great cost. Concern over decisions regarding life and death issues has led to the development of organizations that represent differing views. The Hemlock Society,[39] the Society for the Right to Die,[70] and the Americans United for Life are examples of a few of these organizations.

The question of who should decide under what circumstances is important. There are other important questions. What is death? What constitutes informed consent? When are therapies ordinary and when are they extraordinary? Should all life be preserved, regardless of quality? Should pain be treated, even though the medication may decrease the life span? What constitutes euthanasia? Is there a distinction between active and passive euthanasia? Is suicide a person's right? All these questions create ethical issues that are discussed in Chapter 2.

## MORAL JUDGMENT AND NURSING ASSESSMENT

In general, good clinical nursing is ethical nursing. Ethics are inextricably linked to a nurse's primary task—that of deciding on and carrying out the best nursing care for a particular person in a particular environment under a particular set of circumstances. Just as systematic assessments are completed to decide on appropriate nursing diagnoses and related actions, organized systematic assessment can assist in making moral judgments or ethical decisions. (See Chapter 2 for information on ethical decision making.)

## ETHICAL ISSUES

Many ethical issues evolve around indications for medical and nursing interventions. These issues arise from such questions as the following: When should medical therapies be started or stopped? When should life supports be discontinued? What constitutes death? Who should decide?

### Withholding or Withdrawing Treatment

Appropriate consideration of withholding or withdrawing specific therapy occurs when (1) the therapy offers no reasonable expectation of the patient's attaining any human awareness, (2) the therapy is proving medically ineffective and useless after sufficient trial, or (3) therapy is perceived from the expressed point of view of the patient (or the decision-making representative) to be cumulatively a greater burden than a benefit.[63]

When decisions are made to withhold or withdraw life-sustaining treatment, the goal of medical and nursing care focuses on keeping the patient comfortable, avoiding suffering and pain, and providing support, comfort, and care on a physical, emotional, and spiritual level. To distinguish which procedures are not directed to supportive care and may be omitted becomes more difficult once medical procedures designed to prolong life are withheld or withdrawn. Perhaps the most controversial area is that of determining the proportionate benefit and burden of medical (artificial) nutrition and hydration.[38,44,65] The issue of withdrawing treatment, once it is started, is also present.

The American Nurses Association Committee on Ethics has prepared guidelines to assist nurses in sorting through the concerns related to withdrawing or withholding food and fluids.[5] The document reflects principles of the Nursing Code of Ethics, as well as other ethical, medical, and legal considerations. Examining questions of if and when to discontinue treatment presents issues surrounding euthanasia.

### Euthanasia

**Euthanasia** comes from the Greek words meaning good or pleasant death. It implies that under some circumstances a person may prefer death to life. Euthanasia, or "mercy killing," is a topic surrounded by controversy. At the present time, there is no agreement on whether death is ever preferable to life or on what constitutes euthanasia. In fact, Curtin and Flaherty[14] provide 16 different definitions of the term.

The more common distinctions made when discussing euthanasia are those of ***active and passive*** and ***voluntary and involuntary*** (Box 10-10). Active euthanasia refers to an act that directly and intentionally shortens a person's life. It is an act of commission. Passive euthanasia, an act of omission, usually refers to letting death occur either by withholding or by withdrawing a treatment that might prolong a person's life.

In looking at questions related to euthanasia, there is a continuum ranging from a strict belief in the sanctity of life (antieuthanasia, treating at all costs) to passive euthanasia (letting die) to active euthanasia (ending life, killing) (see Box 10-10).

**BOX 10-10 Euthanasia**

| DISTINCTIONS | CONTINUUM |
|---|---|
| Active/passive | Antieuthanasia: treating at all costs |
| Commission/omission | Passive euthanasia: letting die |
| Killing/letting die | Active euthanasia: ending life |
| Voluntary/involuntary | |

A persistent moral issue is the question of whether letting death occur is morally equivalent to killing, or omission equivalent to commission. Remember, no action is an action. Both active and passive euthanasia are intentional choices. The distinction seems to be that of the intent of the action. The 1986 statement by the AMA Council on Ethical and Judicial Affairs holds that the patient and/or immediate family can decide to "discontinue all means of life-prolonging medical treatment" even "if death is not imminent but a patient's coma is beyond doubt irreversible."[2] The New Jersey Supreme Court implicitly invoked this distinction when it held that judgments about therapy should be made in terms of the degree of invasiveness of the treatment and its chance of success.[9] Ethicists have distinguished ordinary treatment from extraordinary treatment by stating that ordinary treatments offer a reasonable prospect of benefit for the patient without excessive pain, expense, or inconvenience.[14]

In more direct terms, killing is wrong, but letting die in the sense of not instituting extraordinary efforts or by discontinuing extraordinary treatments is morally permissible. In fact, most physicians accept that killing a patient is morally wrong and thus not permissible, but in some circumstances it may become morally required to let a patient die.[9] Nurses generally accept the same view.

## Suicide

Quality of living and quality of dying may be closely associated. A person with terminal illness may assess the situation and decide that living with pain, disability, or despair is not living. He or she may ask the question: Is it better to take measures to bring about a peaceful death than to continue in such a state?

Suicide or voluntary euthanasia carried out by the individual on his or her own behalf has been seen as an affirmation of life, a denial of life, and a questioning of life. The traditional religious teaching of the Western world since St. Augustine has condemned all forms of self-destruction. Suicide was and still is considered by some to be a sin and an interference with God's will.[15] According to Kant,[46] human beings do not have the power of disposal of their bodies. They can only treat their bodies as they choose in relation to self-preservation. These views are being challenged in society today as they have been in the past. According to Engel, suicide is no longer considered a crime.[30] Heifetz and Magel[38] suggest that under some circumstances, when death is imminent, persons who are severely ill should be helped by their physicians to commit suicide. They distinguish this element of the population from the lonely, elderly, and physically handicapped, for whom they do not advocate assisted euthanasia. They point out that, although laws do not exist in the United States covering physician participation, they do exist in Uruguay, Switzerland, Peru, Japan, and Germany. Some cultures such as the Japanese and, regardless of culture, some individuals favor suicide over other negative values such as dishonor. Brutus preferred suicide to the disgrace of being marched through Rome as a vanquished hero.

Individual and societal views and practices regarding suicide run the gamut from opposition to suicide under all conditions and at all costs, to suicide as justifiable under some conditions, to suicide as a person's right. The question of an individual's right to autonomy or self-determination is a basic consideration in discussing suicide. Those who oppose suicide under all conditions usually use some form of the argument that "life is a gift, and no one has the right to take a life." Those at the opposite end of the continuum argue that a person has the right to determine his or her own fate, even if it means destroying his or her own life. Other considerations in arguments opposing suicide include viewing suicide as cowardly, a crime against society, an insult against humanity, and an act that brings great pain to the survivors.

Suicide is of particular concern to health care professionals who may be in a position to offer other alternatives and thus prevent it. It is difficult to evaluate what constitutes suicide. Is refusal to eat or to continue with prescribed therapies a form of suicide, or must there be an overt act such as an overdose of medications? Is suicide always a voluntary act, or is a person driven to suicide by rejection of others or by pain that might have been controlled? When is suicide justifiable in the person known to be dying? What do you do when a patient who is dying all too slowly and painfully asks for your assistance in ending it all? Of interest is Rollin's[76] account of what she did when her mother, who was slowly dying of cancer and in unrelenting pain, expressed her desire to commit suicide and asked her to assist. Rollin did assist—to her own peace of mind and satisfaction—as well as her mother's.

Nurses and physicians, however, are committed to another imperative—that is, to *never abandon care.*[65] Never to abandon care includes ensuring that a dying person is not alone, that others are aware of his or her dying, and that he or she is free from pain and anxiety. It is not an obligation to assist in ending life. In fact, the ethical basis for suicide prevention is the psychologic thesis that a suicide attempt is often a cry for help rather than an unambivalent decision to end one's life. Thus nurses and physicians have a legal and ethical obligation to assess and recognize suicidal risk and depression in patients and to make efforts to assist them in receiving counseling.[78] Often suicide is not an act of autonomy but rather is caused by impaired capacity that, in turn, is caused by an underlying emotional conflict or extreme physical discomfort. But what about instances of prolonged dying when it is medically impossible to control pain in spite of the positive impact of the hospice movement? Life for some dying people does become more of a burden than a gift.

The impact of pain is really a quality of life question

that can best be evaluated by the dying individual bearing the pain. If quality of life is determined by the person living the life, is suicide a purely personal decision? It seems that the quality of life of survivors also should be considered. When the survivors have had no prior warning or a part in the decision, and when the suicide is not perceived as an action to achieve comfort, the anguish to the survivors is great. For some the anguish never ends. Their grief is compounded by guilt, shame, and even anger. In some instances the survivors become victims of a society that condemns the act as a crime.

Even in such a limited discussion of suicide, and even when addressing persons known to be dying, it becomes evident that suicide is an issue about which health professionals and others disagree. It is an issue to be discussed with understanding and openness to better determine appropriate interventions.

Suicide may be a form of control by the dying person, or it may be a form of escape. Some dying people seek an escape from loss of control over the event of dying; others seek an end to suffering. Nurses can be influential in providing dying persons and their families a sense of control by assisting with such problems as pain control, bowel and bladder control, and depression. They can decrease the uncertainty of the situation by explaining what the dying person and family can anticipate over the coming days. In other words, they can assist in promoting quality of life.[56]

### Definitions of Death

Much controversy surrounds the question, "What is death?" Is death the irreversible cessation of respiration and circulation, or is death the irreversible cessation of all functions of the entire brain, including the brainstem?

The term *brain dead,* in use for some time, still causes much confusion. Originally it referred to a person whose heart and lungs were activated by a ventilator but whose centers in the brainstem were destroyed. Removal from the support system would end in death as a result of the inability of the person to resume spontaneous breathing. In addition, brain dead means that the person is dead in the sense that a functioning brain is the seat of identity. What decision can be made about persons in a "persistent vegetative state"? They show no evidence of cortical functioning but continue to have sustained capacity for spontaneous breathing and heartbeat.

Advocates use definitions that reflect their values and provide them with a rationale to act. Each appeal or action has its own consequences. For example, the use of some definitions of brain dead provides more latitude for organ transplantation and experimentation. The rationale for this latitude is that the removal of organs from the person who is brain dead aids the living. A worthy endeavor, but does retrieving organs lead to violation of the dead? What are the constraints? Are the bodies being used with the consent of the donor, or is consent necessary once a person is brain dead?

There are no clear rules that dictate decisions in these matters. Decisions depend on discretion and are reflections of basic values. They are accompanied by conflict, insecurity, and discomfort. The conflict and emotions that accompany decisions about the life or death of another are entirely appropriate because they are irreversible.

The important factor in any ethical issue, regardless of whether it is dealing with euthanasia, suicide, or treatment decisions, is to be aware of the values or forces that lead us to make the decisions we do. An understanding of our own values and perspectives, as well as of formal ethical systems, does not give explicit answers to dilemmas. It does, however, help us to be consistent and to communicate with others in a way that is understandable.[13] This does not ensure agreement, but it does facilitate discussion and attention to multiple perspectives and to the consequences of actions.

## QUESTIONS TO CONSIDER

**SITUATION**

- Ron is a 29-year-old, unemployed man with a 5-year history of AIDS and recent development of lymphoma. Since his diagnosis he has withdrawn from any social activities with friends and has refused to return to working as a bus driver. He is currently hospitalized with anorexia and meningitis, which have caused urinary incontinence, weakness, and inability to bear weight. Over the past year he has lost 60 pounds and says he is "wasting away."
- Ron learned yesterday that his mother, with whom he has lived since his diagnosis, cannot continue to care for him. She has been diagnosed with advanced lung cancer. Most of his former friends have died of AIDS, including his partner.
- When you enter Ron's room to check his vital signs, he cries out "Can't you help me? I want to die. . . . I can't go on living like this. I'm not worth nothing to nobody. I asked my Mom to bring me some sleeping pills so I can pass on—but she won't even come to see me. Please give me a shot or something and put me out of my misery."

**QUESTIONS**

- Identify three losses that Ron and his mother are facing.
- What influencing or balancing factors are affecting Ron's perception of loss and grieving?
- Where is Ron in the grief process? Identify the stage, which theory you are using, and your rationale.
- Identify at least three ethical issues or conflicts in Ron's current situation.
- Describe briefly four supportive nursing interventions for helping Ron and his mother in their grieving.
- Define the meaning of death versus the dying process in reflecting on Ron's situation.

## CRITICAL THINKING ACTIVITIES

- At this stage in your own life, do you think it is possible to define "quality of life" for yourself as a dying person? Why or why not?
- Assisting individuals to cope with the death of a loved one is challenging and difficult. Discuss nursing strategies that are most effective in facilitating the grieving process.
- Discuss how aspects of the dying process are similar to such events as retirement or relocation.

## CHAPTER SUMMARY

### THE LOSS EXPERIENCE

- Coping with loss and dying is an integral part of living.
- Prevailing societal attitudes toward death include death denial, death defiance, death desire, and death acceptance.
- Living wills and advance directives are vehicles used to communicate one's desires related to the process of dying.
- With advances in modern therapies, dying has taken on many characteristics of chronic illness with its resultant challenges.
- Understanding the stages and phases of grief and dying can aid in assessing the diversity of responses among dying persons and their families.
- Discussions with family members and patients are critical in determining the likelihood of families being able to offer care in the home during the final phases of dying.
- The complex physiologic, psychologic, social, and spiritual dynamics accompanying dying help explain the presence of the multiple primary and secondary nursing diagnoses and challenge nurses to prioritize them for interventions.

### BEREAVEMENT: AN ADAPTIVE RESPONSE TO LOSS

- Bereavement is the subjective state that occurs as a result of having suffered the loss of a significant person, whereas grief is the total response (thoughts, feelings, and behaviors) to the emotional suffering caused by a loss.

### DEATH AND GRIEF

- Normal grieving includes behavioral manifestations—of shock and disbelief, yearning and protest, anguish, disorganization and despair, identification, reorganization and restitution—that are often frightening and misunderstood by the grieving person.
- Some individual characteristics of survivors are associated with a high risk for problems with the grieving process.

### SPECIAL ISSUES IN BEREAVEMENT

- Many ethical issues and dilemmas surround the care and treatment of dying persons and their families and call for an exploration of the values, perspective, and ethical systems involved in the making of decisions.

## REFERENCES


1. Amenta MO, Bohnet NL: *Nursing care of the terminally ill,* Boston, 1986, Little, Brown & Co.
2. American Nurses Association: *Nursing practice in the care of the dying,* Kansas City, Mo, 1982, The Association.
3. American Nurses Association: *Standards and scope of hospice nursing practice,* Kansas City, Mo, 1987, The Association.
4. Aquilera D, Messick J: *Crisis intervention: theory and methodology,* ed 6, St Louis, 1990, Mosby.
5. Assimacopoulos L: Realizing empathy in loss, *J Psychosoc Nurs* 25(11):26-29, 1992.
6. Becker E: *The denial of death,* Riverside, NJ, 1973, The Free Press.
7. Benoliel J: Loss and terminal illness, *Nurs Clin North Am* 20(2):438-447, 1985.
8. Bowlby J: Attachment and loss: retrospect and prospect, *Am J Orthopsychiatry* 52(4):644-677, 1972.
9. Branson J, Casebeer K: The Quinlan decison: observing the role of the physician, *Hastings Cent Rep* 6(1):8-11, 1976.
10. Brice C: Mourning throughout the life cycle, *Am J Psychoanal* 42(4):315-325, 1982.
11. Cantor RC: *And a time to live: toward emotional well being during the crisis of cancer,* New York, 1978, Harper & Row.
12. Carpenito LJ: *Nursing diagnosis: application to clinical practice,* ed 3, Philadelphia, 1989, JB Lippincott Co.
13. Cooley M: Bereavement care: a role for nurses, *Cancer Nurs* 15(2):125-129, 1992.
14. Curtin L, Flaherty MJ: *Nursing ethics: theories and pragmatics,* Bowie, Md, 1982, Robert J Brady.
15. Davis AJ, Aroskar MA: *Ethical dilemmas and nursing practice,* ed 2, New York, 1983, Appleton-Century-Crofts.
16. Davis B, Oberle K: Dimensions of the supportive role of the nurse in palliative care, *Oncol Nurs Forum* 17(1):87-94, 1990.
17. DeSpelder L, Strickland A: *The last dance: encountering death and dying,* ed 3, Mountain View, Calif, 1992, Mayfield.
18. Diamond M: Bereavement and the elderly: a critical review with implications for nursing practice and research, *J Adv Nurs* 6:461-470, 1981.
19. Dimond E: The oncology nurse's role in patient advanced directives, *Oncol Nurs Forum* 19(6):891-896, 1992.
20. Donovan ML, Girton SE: *Cancer care nursing,* ed 2, New York, 1984, Appleton-Century-Crofts.
21. Duespohl TA: *Nursing diagnosis manual for the well and ill client,* Philadelphia, 1986, WB Saunders.
22. Dufault K: *Hope and elderly persons with cancer,* doctoral dissertation, Cleveland, 1981, Case Western Reserve University.
23. Dufault K: Helping patients and families make life-sustaining treatment decisions, *AORN J* 39(7):1132-1133, 1984.
24. Dufault K: What is nurse's role when adults forego treatment? *Am Nurse* 16(2):5, 23, 1984.
25. Eakes G: Grief resolution in hospice nurses, *Nurs Health Care* 11(5):243-248, 1988.
26. Ebersole P, Hess P: *Toward healthy aging: human needs and nursing response,* ed 3, St Louis, 1990, Mosby.
27. Eliot T: The adjustive behavior of bereaved families: a new field of research, *Soc Forces* 8:543-549, 1930.
28. Eliot T: The bereaved family, *Ann Am Acad Polit Soc Sci* 160:184-190, 1932.
29. Engel G: Is grief a disease? *Psychosom Med* 3(1):18-22, 1961.

30. Engel G: A life setting conducive to illness: the giving-up given-up complex, *Ann Intern Med* 69:355-365, 1968.
31. Feifel H: *The functions and attitudes toward death and dying: attitudes of patient and doctor,* New York, 1965, Group for Advancement of Psychiatry.
32. Freud S: *Instincts and their vicissitudes: collected papers,* New York, 1915, Basic Books.
33. Gifford B, Cleary B: Supporting the bereaved, *Am J Nurs* 90(2):49-54, 1990.
34. Glass B: The role of the nurse in advanced practice in bereavement care, *Clin Nurs Spec* 7(2):62-66, 1993.
35. Glick I, Weiss RS, Parkes CM: *The first year of bereavement,* New York, 1974, John Wiley & Sons.
36. Graininger R: Successful grieving, *Am J Nurs* 90(9):12-15, Sept 1990.
37. Haber J et al: *Comprehensive psychiatric nursing,* ed 4, St Louis, 1992, Mosby.
38. Heifetz MS, Magel C: *The right to die,* New York, 1975, GC Putnam & Sons.
39. Hemlock Society: *Supporting the option of active voluntary euthanasia for the terminally ill,* Los Angeles, 1985, The Society.
40. Houseman C, Pheifer W: Potential for unresolved grief in survivors of persons with AIDS, *Arch Psychiatr Nurs* 2:296-301, 1988.
41. Hull M: Coping strategies of family caregivers in hospice homecare, *Oncol Nurs Forum* 19(8):1179-1187, 1992.
42. Jackson EN: *Understanding grief: its roots, dynamics and treatment,* Nashville, Tenn, 1957, Abingdon Press.
43. Jackson EN: Grief. In Grollman E: *Concerning death: a practical guide for living,* Boston, 1974, Beacon Press.
44. Johnson SH: The Cruzan case: who has the right to decide, *Health Prog* 89(11):22-25, 1989.
45. Kalish RA: Death and dying in a social context. In Binstock RH, Shanes E: *Handbook of aging,* New York, 1976, Van Nostrand Reinhold.
46. Kant I: Duties towards the body in regard to life. In Gorovitz S et al: *Moral problems in medicine,* Englewood Cliffs, NJ, 1976, Prentice-Hall.
47. Kaprio J et al: Mortality after bereavement: a prospective study of 95,647 widowed persons, *Am J Pub Health* 77:283-287, 1987.
48. Kastenbaum R: *The psychology of death,* ed 2, New York, 1992, Springer.
49. Koestenbaum P: *Is there any answer to death?* Englewood Cliffs, NJ, 1976, Prentice-Hall.
50. Kübler-Ross E: *On death and dying,* New York, 1969, Macmillan.
51. Kübler-Ross E: *Death: the final stage of growth,* Englewood Cliffs, NJ, 1975, Prentice-Hall.
52. Lev E, Munroe B, McCorkle R: A shortened version of an instrument measuring bereavement, *Int J Nurs Stud* 30(3):213-226, 1993.
53. Lindemann E: Symptomatology and management of acute grief, *Am J Psychiatry* 101:141-148, 1944.
54. Martocchio BC: *Living while dying,* Bowie, Md, 1982, Robert J Brady.
55. Martocchio BC: Family coping: helping families help themselves, *Semin Oncol Nurs* 1(4):11-16, 1985.
56. Martocchio BC: Grief and bereavement: healing through hurt, *Nurs Clin North Am* 20(2):327-341, 1985.
57. Martocchio BC: Agendas for quality of life, *Hospice J* 2(1):11-21, 1986.
58. Martocchio BC, Dufault K: Dying, a part of living. In Diamond M, editor: *Advances in geriatrics: long-term care nursing,* vol 1, New York, 1983, Pro Scientia.
59. Maslow A: *Motivation and personality,* New York, 1954, Harper & Brothers.
60. McGoldrick M, et al: *Ethnicity and family therapy,* New York, 1982, The Guilford Press.
61. Mitford J: *The American way of death,* New York, 1963, Simon & Schuster.
62. Mor V, McHorney C, Sherwood S: Secondary morbidity among the recently bereaved, *Am J Psychiatry* 143(2):158-163, 1986.
63. Mumma CM: Withholding nutrition: a nursing perspective, *Nurs Adm Q* 10(3):31-38, 1986.
64. Norris FH, Murrell SA: Older adult family stress and adaptation before and after bereavement, *J Gerontol* 42(6):606-612, 1987.
65. Otte DM, Allen KS: Ethical principles in the nursing care of the terminally ill adult, *Oncol Nurs Forum* 14(5):87-91, 1987.
66. Parkes CM: The first year of bereavement: a longitudinal study of the reaction of London widows to the death of their husbands, *Psychiatry* 33:444-457, 1970.
67. Parkes CM, Weiss RS: *Recovery from bereavement,* New York, 1983, Basic Books.
68. Pattison EM: *The experience of dying,* Englewood Cliffs, NJ, 1977, Prentice-Hall.
69. Pilkington F: The lived experience of grieving the loss of an important other, *Nurs Sci Q* 6(3):130-138, 1993.
70. Rachels J: Active and passive euthanasia, In Levine C, editor: *Taking sides: clashing views on controversial bioethical issues,* Guilford, Conn, 1984, Dashkin.
71. Rando TA: *Grief, dying and death,* Champaign, Ill, 1983, Research Press.
72. Raphael B: *The anatomy of bereavement,* New York, 1983, Basic Books.
73. Remondet JH, Hansson RO: Assessing a widow's grief—a short index, *J Gerontol Nurs* 13(4):30-34, 1987.
74. Richter JM: Support: a resource during crisis of mate loss, *J Gerontol Nurs* 13(11):18-22, 1987.
75. Rolland J: Anticipatory loss: a family systems developmental framework, *Fam Process* 29(3):229-243, 1990.
76. Rollin B: *Last wish,* New York, 1985, Simon & Schuster.
77. Sanders C: *Grief: the mourning after,* New York, 1989, John Wiley & Sons.
78. Saunders JM, Valente SM: Cancer and suicide, *Oncol Nurs Forum* 15:575-581, 1988.
79. Schneidman ES: On the deromantization of death, *Am J Psychoanal* 25:4-17, 1971.
80. Selder F: Life transition theory: the resolution of uncertainty, *Nurs Health Care* 10(8):437-451, 1992.
81. Silverman P, Worden W: Detachment revisited: the child's reconstruction of a dead parent, *Am J Orthopsychiatry* 62(4):494-503, 1992.
82. Society for the Right to Die: *Support of dying with dignity,* New York, 1985, The Society.
83. Steele L: The death surround: factors influencing the grief experience of survivors, *Oncol Nurs Forum* 15(5):575-581, 1990.
84. Temes R: *Living with an empty chair,* New York, 1992, New Horizons.
85. Van Jennap A: *The rites of passage,* Chicago, 1960, University of Chicago Press.
86. Varricchio CG, Jassak P: Informed consent: an overview, *Semin Oncol Nurs* 5(2):95-98, 1989.
87. Viorst J: *Necessary losses,* New York, 1986, Simon & Schuster.
88. Waltman R: When a spouse dies, *Nursing '92* 92(7):40-51, 1992.
89. Wolfelt A: Resolution versus reconciliation: the importance of semantics, *Thanatos,* pp 22-25, Winter 1987.
90. Worden W: *Grief counseling and grief therapy,* ed 2, New York, 1991, Springer.
91. Wortman C, Silver R: The myths of coping with loss, *J Consult Clin Psychol* 57(3):349-357, 1989.

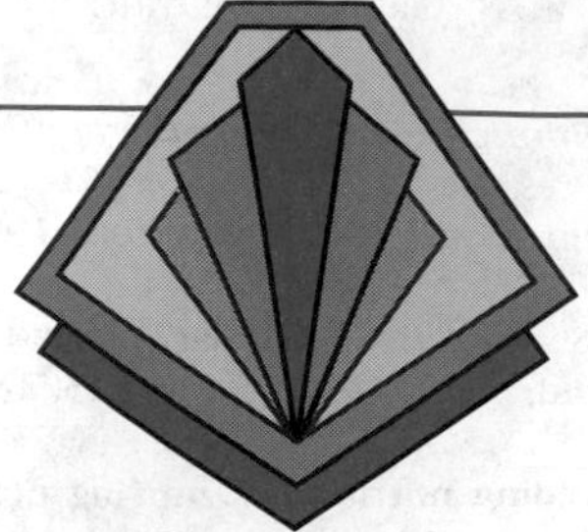

C H A P T E R 11

# Human Sexuality

***Judith K. Sands***

## CHAPTER OBJECTIVES

***After studying this chapter, the learner should be able to do the following:***

1. Describe the physiologic and psychosocial components of human sexual response.
2. Compare the myths and facts of sexual response in later life.
3. Discuss the major symptoms of menopause and their management.
4. Describe the imbalances in bone metabolism that result in osteoporosis and options for management.
5. Identify common illness- and treatment-related factors that have an impact on sexuality.
6. Describe four strategies to facilitate sexual assessment.
7. Offer specific examples of each level of the PLISSIT model for sexuality intervention.

## KEY TERMS

biologic sex
dyspareunia
ejaculation
estrogen replacement therapy (ERT)
gender identity
gender role
homosexuality
human sexuality
menopause
orgasm
osteoporosis
plateau phase
resolution phase
sexual function
sexual health
sexual relationship

## SEXUALITY AND HEALTH

Humans are sexual beings from the moment they are conceived. **Biologic sex** is well established by the twelfth week of fetal life. An infant is born with an established biologic sex, but both gender role and identity are established after birth. **Gender identity** is the feeling that one is male or female. This identity is gradually established by parental behaviors and then steadily reinforced by all elements of the larger society. Gender identity is typically solidified in the child by the age of 3. **Gender role** is the outward expression of one's gender and is also learned early in life. The distinctions between male and female behavior are established socially and culturally, and they vary substantially among various cultures. Gender role includes such diverse elements as dress and manner, appearance and style, and occupational and recreational activities. Gender roles used to be rigidly defined, but the distinctions are becoming less clear in Western society, which increasingly recognizes that androgynous behavior is compatible with mentally healthy gender role behavior. When developmental processes proceed normally, the person's biologic sex is congruent with both gender identity and gender role. This complex set of biologic and psychosocial variables, which is set in motion by conception, has a pervasive influence on our entire lives.

**Human sexuality** encompasses the total person and involves the complex interplay of biologic, psychologic, and sociocultural variables. However, the concept of sexual health is an elusive one that defies easy definition. The classic World Health Organization definition states that "sexual health is the integration of the somatic, emotional, intellectual, and social aspects of sexual being, in ways that are positively enriching and that enhance personality, communication and love."[18]

The concept of **sexual health** is not restricted to a discrete state but involves consideration of sexual function, gender role and identity, and sexual relationships over time. **Sexual function** refers to the person's capacity to engage in and experience pleasure from sexual activity. It encompasses not only the ability to experience orgasm, but also a wide range and variety of other sexual behaviors. Gender role and identity encompass social roles and behavior and also our sense of physical body image related to sexuality. **Sexual relationships** incorporate those interpersonal relationships with others that include shared sexual activity. Sexual health is obviously multifaceted, and maintaining a balance is not easy for many individuals. A wide variety of physical, emotional, social, and cultural factors may upset this delicate balance and cause sexual health to become an elusive goal.

## HUMAN SEXUAL RESPONSE

The various components of sexual functioning develop and change in subtle and significant ways throughout life. Many of the basic sexual functions are clearly evident in infants and children, such as the ability to have erections and orgasms, and persist into the last days of life.

Masters and Johnson, pioneers in the scientific study of the physiologic aspects of sexual behavior, demonstrated that sexual response is a cyclic phenomenon consisting of four phases. The **excitement phase** develops from sexually arousing stimuli, such as touch, and is characterized by an increase in sexual tension. The **plateau phase,** a consolidation period, occurs next and involves an intensification of the sexual tension. The involuntary climax of sexual tension, **orgasm,** follows and involves only a small portion of the sexual response cycle. During this period, changes attributable to muscular tension and congestion of blood vessels reach a peak and begin to dissipate. During the **resolution phase**—an involuntary period—the changes involving the blood vessels, sexual organs, and muscular tension are reversed. Women may at this time begin another sexual response cycle immediately; men cannot be restimulated to higher levels of sexual tension immediately.

The physiologic changes seen during human sexual response depend on two main principles: myotonia and vasocongestion. The congestion of pelvic blood vessels and the involuntary muscular contractions in the pelvic organs and other parts of the body are responsible for arousal and orgasmic experience. Sexual response is a total body response, involving nearly every body system. Phase-specific descriptions of the sexual response cycle follow.

### Excitement

The hallmark of sexual arousal in females is vaginal lubrication. It is believed to result from the movement of a mucuslike substance across the vaginal mucosa and begins to appear within seconds of sexual stimulation. The vagina becomes longer and wider as the uterus begins to elevate in the pelvis. Vasocongestive changes are also seen in the external genitalia: the clitoris becomes longer and wider, and the labia minora flatten and separate from the vaginal opening. As the labia minora become vasocongested, they actually extend outward, lengthening the vagina. Extragenital changes are also seen with sexual excitement. The woman's nipples become erect, the areolae become engorged, venous patterns in the breast become more evident, and breast size actually increases. The sex flush—which looks like a red, maculopapular rash—appears over the chest in some persons.

The hallmark of sexual arousal in the male is the rapid engorgement and erection of the penis. The scrotal sac tenses, and the testes begin to rise toward the perineum. Men's nipples may also become erect. An increase in both heart rate and blood pressure occurs in both genders, which parallels the level of sexual excitement.

### Plateau

During the plateau phase, the clitoris retracts upward beneath the clitoral hood. Clitoral stimulation may still occur indirectly with traction on the labia. The orgasmic platform, the extremely vascular tissue at the outer portion of the vagina and the labia minora, becomes increasingly congested. The uterus continues to elevate in the pelvis, which creates a tenting effect in the innermost portion of the vagina. Externally, the labia majora become more congested, and the labia minora deepen in color as a result of vasocongestion. A few drops of mucoidlike material are secreted from Bartholin's glands, probably to assist with the lubrication of the outermost portion of the vagina. The woman's areolae may become so engorged that it is difficult to see the erect nipple. The sex flush continues to spread, sometimes involving the neck, face, and arms.

The diameter of the penis continues to increase, especially at the coronal ridge, and the testes increase in size to 50% over their unstimulated state as they elevate closer to the perineum. A few drops of mucoid material are secreted from Cowper's glands.

Hyperventilation occurs in both males and females, along with heart rates of 100 to 175 beats per minute, and significant elevations of both systolic and diastolic blood pressure.[12]

### Orgasm

Orgasm involves the climactic release of sexual tension and is evident in contractions throughout the body. The woman's orgasmic platform contracts rapidly, and expulsive contractions along the entire male urethra propel semen from the vas out through the penis **(ejaculation).** During orgasm, the internal bladder sphincter in men contracts, thus preventing semen from being propelled backward into the bladder. Uterine contractions are also noted in women with orgasm, much like those characteristic of labor. The rectal sphincter also contracts rapidly in both men and women during orgasm.

The female orgasmic response is highly variable from individual to individual, as well as from orgasm to orgasm in the same individual. Multiple orgasms may occur when sexual tension does not fall and stimulation is continued.

Recent research indicates that some women appear to ejaculate a glandular secretion during orgasm. The process seems to be triggered by stimulation of the Grafenberg spot, an area in the anterior vaginal wall. One study reported a rate of female ejaculation as high as 54% in the study population.[2]

Vital sign changes reach their peak during orgasm in both sexes. Hyperventilation to 40 breaths per minute, heart rates of from 110 to 180 beats per minute, and blood pressure increases of 30 to 100 mm Hg systolically and 20 to 50 mm Hg diastolically are frequently recorded.

### Resolution

During this phase, vasocongestion is lost gradually from the clitoris and breasts but rapidly from the orgasmic platform. The clitoris quickly returns to its usual position under the clitoral hood. Vasocongestion of the labia dissipates, nipple erection recedes, and the uterus descends to its usual position in the pelvis. Cardiovascular and respiratory rates quickly return to normal. In men, there is initially a rapid loss of erection to 1 to 1.5 times the size of the penis in its unstimulated state. Later there is a slower resolution of vasocongestion until the penis returns to prestimulation size. The scrotum and testes lose their vasocongestive changes, and the testes rapidly descend into the scrotum. Occasionally, a thin film of perspiration may appear over the entire body.

## NEUROPHYSIOLOGIC COMPONENTS OF SEXUAL RESPONSE

Although the Masters and Johnson description of human sexual response is the most widely used, it is clearly possible to look at this complex process from other perspectives. Different neurophysiologic systems are involved in the various aspects of sexual response, and an understanding of them can be useful in explaining and treating the various etiologic factors that may impair sexual function.

Sexual desire is perhaps the most elusive component. The stimuli that cause individuals to seek sexual contact are activated by neural systems of the brain, possibly involving the limbic system and nuclei of the hypothalamus. These centers are theorized to be connected chemically or neurally with the brain's pleasure and pain centers, which serve to either reinforce or inhibit the activity. Testosterone, luteinizing hormone (LH), and the neurotransmitters serotonin and dopamine are all mediators of sexual desire. Serotonin acts as an inhibitor, whereas dopamine acts as a facilitator of desire. A wide variety of stimuli—including sights, smells, and other sensory cues—are capable of stimulating sexual desire. Many of these stimuli are learned behaviors and conditioned by the culture or society. Fear and pain are classic inhibitors of sexual desire unless alternately conditioned.

Reflex vasodilation underlies the excitement and plateau phases of sexual desire. Two centers in the spinal cord at $S_2$ to $S_4$ and $T_{11}$ to $L_2$ cause the arterioles to dilate, which engorges the genitalia for sexual activity. The reflex vasodilation is primarily a parasympathetic response. Intense sympathetic activity can lead to an instant loss of erection. Although the exact function of the thoracic/lumbar center is not understood, it appears that it responds primarily to psychic stimulation, whereas the sacral center responds to tactile stimulation of the genitals.

Orgasm involves genital reflexes controlled by spinal centers that trigger reflex contractions of the genital muscles. Sensory stimuli enter the spinal cord via the pudendal nerve in the sacral cord. Efferent fibers exit from $T_{11}$ to $L_2$. Various vascular and neurologic disorders may produce inadequate ejaculatory control, or orgasmic dysfunction.

### Subjective Component of Sexual Response

Despite an ever-increasing knowledge base concerning the neurophysiology of sexual response, it is clear that there is enormous subjectivity in sexual experience. Masters and Johnson have demonstrated that the experience of orgasm in women may be primarily vaginal, primarily uterine, or a blend of the two. Subjective descriptions of orgasm are as varied as the individuals describing the experience. The experience of orgasm has slightly more consistency in description for men but remains a sensory experience that eludes word descriptions.

## VARIATIONS IN SEXUAL EXPRESSION

People experience sexual pleasure in a wide variety of ways. An individual's culture strongly influences the nature and type of sexual behaviors that are considered to be acceptable. What is considered "normal" varies significantly, but most cultures do clearly establish parameters for both sexual modesty and acceptable behavior. Incest taboos are virtually universal, although the definition of incest may vary. Cultural variations in sexual behavior encompass approaches to sexual stimulation, which partner acts as the initiator, the duration and frequency of sexual acts, and positions commonly used for intercourse. Heterosexuality and monogamy are the most pervasive patterns worldwide, but they are clearly not the only ones. Homosexuality, bisexuality, and multiple partners are other common variations. Transvestism, fetishism, voyeurism, exhibitionism, sadism, and masochism are other less common and more dramatic variants of sexual expression. Health professionals must be prepared to encounter a wide range of sexual behaviors in their practice. Some of these behaviors are likely to be distasteful or even repugnant to the individual's own code of morality or sexual conduct. The health professional is not in the position to judge or reject individuals in their care because of their sexual values or behaviors. However, it is appropriate for the health professional to explore the meaning of specific behaviors for individuals and whether these behaviors impoverish or enrich their lives and overall health.

### Homosexuality

Homosexuality is the most common sexual variation. Although many children and young adults engage in some type of homosexual behavior, only 10% of the adult population actually identify themselves as being homosexual in their sexual orientation. **Homosexuality,** by definition, involves erotic attraction to individuals of the same gender. Although male and female homosexuals compose a significant proportion of the general population, homosexuality remains poorly understood by health professionals and vocally rejected by much of the majority culture. Homosexuality has been regarded at various times in Western society as a criminal offense, mental illness, and life-style choice. Despite the blatant rejection, the various Kinsey sexual behavior studies have consistently demonstrated that about 40% of men and 15% of women have had at least one homosexual experience that led to orgasm.[9] A continuum is frequently proposed for sexual behavior with exclusive heterosexuality at one end, exclusive homosexuality at the other end, and a vast middle ground representing various combinations of the two.

Many explanations have been proposed to explain the origins of homosexuality, none of which have proved satisfactory. Neither sociologic nor psychologic origins are explanatory. Current research is focusing on chromosomal variants that may find expression in subtle but powerful differences in brain structure or hormone balance. The dilemma is compounded by the fact that homosexuality in American society frequently composes a life-style, rather than just a choice of sexual partner. Within homosexuality there is as much variation in sexual practices as in the population at large. Homosexuals cannot be typified as sexually hyperactive or hypoactive, and they do not consistently behave in any way that conforms to widely held stereotypes. The psychologic adjustment of homosexuals in stable relationships is equivalent to that of heterosexuals in similar relationships.

Homosexual life-styles vary significantly for men and women. Gay men tend to have more partners than do lesbian women, but both groups express a preference for stable, loving relationships. Masters and Johnson compared the physiology of sexual response in homosexuals and heterosexuals and found no demonstrable differences in the sexual response cycles.[12]

Although homosexuals have many of the same health care needs as do heterosexual patients, health care professionals should recognize certain unique factors. Many gay and lesbian patients approach the entire health care system with distrust, fearing rejection by another segment of society. They may be reluctant to acknowledge their sexual orientation or discuss problems that may be related to it. Gay men may experience concerns over genitourinary problems, anal disorders, and bowel dysfunction that can be adequately addressed only within the context of their sexual practices. The incidence and spread of STDs among this population is of particular concern.

The AIDS epidemic, which began in the 1980s, has had an immeasurable effect on the homosexual community in the United States and will continue to do so until a cure or effective treatment is developed. Homosexuals have watched their life-style and sexual practices become front-page news; have stood by helplessly and watched countless numbers of their friends, lovers, and colleagues die of the disease; have borne the brunt of a tidal wave of blame and rejection from the heterosexual community; and live with the spectre of premature, horrible death. The toll of AIDS on this community and our society at large is difficult to overestimate. The unrelenting spread of AIDS is forcing health care professionals to become knowledgeable about the unique problems and challenges of homosexuality, as they attempt to provide holistic and effective health care to this formerly invisible segment of the population. AIDS is discussed in detail in Chapter 71.

## AGING AND SEXUALITY

Aging has not been positively regarded in the United States, and this general negativity has clearly included attitudes toward sexuality in older adults. Society has frequently not genuinely acknowledged or validated the role of sexual activity in the elderly population. It has been assumed that sexuality is not a concern for older people. Research on sexuality and aging, however, emphatically contradicts these stereotypes. Although functional declines clearly occur, there is no single point in the life cycle at which sexual activity or interest automatically ceases. Instead, sexual activity is an important dimension of being alive and may persist well into the eighth and ninth decades of life. It is increasingly recognized that balanced well-being and health in later life should include active sexual activity for as long as possible.

Myths and stigmas concerning the sexuality of elderly persons do exist and have varied explanations. Before this century, it was relatively unusual for individuals to live significantly beyond their childbearing years. Sexuality in later life was rarely an issue or possibility. An emphasis on sex as a purely procreative function also excluded the older adult from inclusion or consideration. Current preoccupations with sex as an activity reserved exclusively for the young and beautiful have also impaired our ability to acknowledge the sexuality needs of elders. The life-style of many older adults makes active sexuality even more difficult. Many older women lack partners and may either live alone or be forced to move in with their children, who are typically very reluctant to view their parents as sexual beings. The physical arrangements of nursing homes and assisted living situations frequently condemn an elderly person to a life of celibacy by their absolute lack of privacy. Masturbation may become an increasingly important aspect of sexual expression for the older adult, but it may not be acceptable within the value system of the individual. Tact and sensitivity must be used to explore this and any other sexual option with elderly persons. See Research box below.

## CHANGES IN SEXUAL RESPONSE

The capacity for sexual pleasure persists throughout life, but there are age-related changes in both the sexual organs and sexual response. A comparison of middle-aged and older adults, however, shows many more similarities than differences. Sexual activity is clearly decreased, and some of that change is attributable to the biologic changes of aging. However, most of the decrease in sexual activity can be attributed to changes related to chronic illnesses and medications, social situations enforcing loneliness and isolation, and behavioral responses to diminished physical capacities and altered life circumstances. The physiologic processes essential for sexual response generally occur more slowly with advancing age, and some of the phase-specific changes may be less intense. Common changes in sexual response in elderly persons are summarized in Box 11-1.

As women age, there is a gradual change in their genitalia and breasts, paralleling the changes in estrogen levels associated with menopause (see p. 267). There is a decrease in clitoral erection, engorgement of the labia and breasts, and vaginal ballooning with sexual stimulation. The vagina both shortens and decreases in diameter. There is often a delay in the production of vaginal lubrication, although this appears to be much less of a problem for women who have been consistently sexually active throughout their lives.

Elevation and tenting of the uterus during sexual excitement are less marked, and vasocongestive changes in the labia and breasts are less evident. Vasocongestion of the orgasmic platform is less apparent, and during orgasm, the frequency of contraction of the orgasmic platform is less than that for younger women. Orgasms therefore tend to be slightly shorter and less intense.[13] Management of these changes is fairly straightforward. Water-soluble lubricants can readily compensate for the decrease in vaginal secretions, and frequent sexual stimulation appears to help sustain the body's natural lubricating ability. Additional time for foreplay before intercourse is another effective method of compensation.

Age-related changes in sexual response in men parallel those changes in women. The time necessary to experience an erection increases, and the erection is likely to be less full than earlier in life. There is usually less profound evidence of vasocongestion in the scrotum and testes. Because the plateau phase of the sexual response cycle is prolonged, the aging man attains better control of ejaculation. Orgasm encompasses a shorter time span. The intensity of the ejaculation decreases, and a man may feel satisfied, ejaculating every second or third time he has intercourse.

Physical assessment in the male tells little about sexual performance. Aging causes few changes, except for a slight decrease in the size of the testicles and thinning of the pubic hair. Erectile dysfunction is not a normal consequence of aging and should always be investigated for a treatable cause. Satisfactory sexual relations can frequently be resumed when co-morbid conditions and medications are appropriately managed or adjusted.

### RESEARCH

Dickey RM: Nursing staff low in sexual knowledge, *Nurs Homes* 39(6):31-32, 1990.

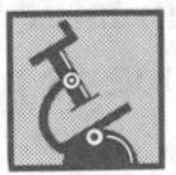

This study was designed to assess the sexual knowledge level of nursing home nursing staff. The Sexual Knowledge and Attitude Test (SKAT) was administered to 62 nursing home personnel, including 49 nursing assistants and 12 LPNs. The mean scores of the study participants were found to be significantly lower than reported scores for medical students, professional nursing students, and other population groups.

### BOX 11-1 Changes in Sexual Response With Aging

**FEMALE**

Decrease in the following:
- Clitoral erection
- Breast engorgement
- Labial engorgement
- Vaginal ballooning with stimulation
- Vaginal secretions
- Frequency and intensity of orgasmic contractions

**MALE**

- Longer interval to achieve erection and ejaculation
- Less firm erections
- Decreased vasocongestion in scrotum and testes
- Decreased semen volume
- Shorter and less intense ejaculation
- Increased duration of refractory period

## MENOPAUSE

The medical term **menopause** refers to a single, specific physical event in a woman's life—the occurrence of the last menstrual period. As such, it is an event that can be diagnosed only retrospectively, usually after 1 year has passed without spontaneous bleeding. In reality, the term is used much more broadly to refer to the 12- to 18-month climacteric or transitional phase between the end of reproductive ability and the beginning of the nonreproductive phase. Increasingly, menopause research has expanded its view to include the entire perimenopausal period, which may extend from age 35 to as much as 60 years of age. This is the period in which physical changes can be clearly linked to altered levels of hormones.

The personal and cultural meanings that are attached to menopause clearly influence how women will respond to the changes in their bodies, how others respond to them, and the kind of health care that is provided. Both sexism and ageism have tainted our understanding and management of the physical challenges of menopause, which have been viewed very negatively in our society. Feminist literature encourages women to accept menopause as a natural process that does not require medical intervention. The opposite interventionist view approaches menopause as a straightforward estrogen deficiency that should be managed with replacement in the same way that diabetes is managed with insulin. These polar opposites in approach each have their vocal champions, and the obvious controversy makes it difficult for many women to make informed choices about such issues as estrogen replacement therapy.

The importance of understanding and managing menopause appropriately is underscored by current population statistics. Of the female population in the United States, 50% are 50 years of age or older, and this figure continues to grow.[5] This translates into nearly 50 million individuals. Four million women each year turn 40, and with current life expectancies, a woman can expect to live nearly one third of her life *after* menopause. By virtue of numbers alone, problems of menopausal and postmenopausal women must be regarded as major public health concerns.

### Physical Changes of Menopause

Natural menopause may occur in women between the ages of 35 and 60 years of age. The average age is 49 to 51 years in Western societies. This average has remained quite stable over time, despite fairly significant changes in the average age of onset for menstruation.[16] According to statistics, 25% of all women experience menopause before age 45, 50% between 45 and 50 years of age, and 25% after age 50.[16] Chronic, heavy cigarette smoking is one of the only variables clearly associated with the early onset of menopause.[11] Age at menarche, childbearing status, height, weight, and use of oral contraceptives do not appear to influence the onset of menopause. The term *premature ovarian failure* is used to describe the onset of menopause in women younger than age 40. It occurs in 0.9% to 5% of women and has no identifiable cause.[11] Menopause may be artificially induced by surgical removal or irradiation of the ovaries, severe infections, and the effects of certain chemotherapeutic agents. The removal of the uterus, hysterectomy, results in a cessation of menses but does not itself result in menopause, as long as the ovaries are left intact.

The changes of menopause are primarily related to a gradual decline in ovarian production of estrogen. Although menopause is defined by a cessation of menses, the process is rarely abrupt. Over a period of years, the menses become more scanty and may become irregular or spaced further apart until they eventually stop. The ovaries produce three different forms of estrogen. Estriol is produced during pregnancy. Estradiol is produced in the ovulatory follicle and is the primary estrogen of premenopausal women. Ovulation begins to decline between 38 and 42 years of age. The third form, estrone, is a by-product of the metabolism of estradiol and is also produced and held in adipose tissue. It is the primary postmenopausal estrogen and has a potency of only one-tenth that of estradiol. Cellular estrogen receptors are found in organs throughout the body, so a decline in estrogen triggers a wide variety of potential symptoms. The severity of symptoms is thought to be basically related to the rapidity of changes in estrogen level. Symptom severity may be mediated somewhat by the fat content of the body and the meaning attached to the specific symptoms by the woman. Women with higher fat stores in their bodies will retain a storage pool of estrogen to buffer them through the early transition period. Commonly reported symptoms of menopause are summarized in Box 11-2.

#### Vasomotor responses

Hot flashes or flushes are by far the most commonly reported symptom of menopause. Approximately 10% of women experience severe vasomotor symptoms, and 25% to 30% report symptoms serious enough to require medical attention. A woman's overall attitude toward

**BOX 11-2 Common Menopausal Symptoms**

**VASOMOTOR**
- Hot flashes
- Hot flushes
- Perspiration
- Palpitations

**VAGINAL**
- Dryness
- Vulvar itching or burning
- Dyspareunia

**URINARY**
- Frequency or urgency
- Stress incontinence

**PSYCHOLOGIC**
- Sleep disorders/insomnia
- Irritability
- Mood swings
- Depression

## RESEARCH

Wilbur JE et al: The relationship among menopausal status, menopausal symptoms and physical activity in midlife women, *Fam Community Health* 13(3):67-78, 1990.

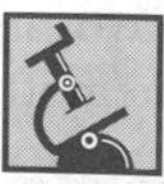

The study sample included 386 women, ranging in age from 34 to 62, who were screened for participation in a Bone Density Research Program. The subjects completed four questionnaires on demographics, health, calcium intake, and physical activity. Bone density was measured, hormonal assays were obtained, and aerobic fitness was assessed by bicycle ergometer.

Data were collected about common perimenopausal symptoms, such as vasomotor responses; nervous symptoms; and general health symptoms, such as joint pain and backache. Menopausal status was clearly related to the incidence of vasomotor symptoms, whereas nervous symptoms were not. The incidence of general health symptoms increased with menopause. Physical activity was negatively correlated with the incidence of nervous and general health symptoms. A significant positive relationship was found between occupational activity (energy expenditure, not mere hours) and nervous and general health symptoms. Physical activity had no relationship to the incidence or severity of vasomotor symptoms.

menopause is clearly linked to her willingness to report distressing menopausal symptoms.[5] See Research box above.

A hot flash is experienced as a sudden sensation of extreme warmth, primarily involving the head and torso, and may vary significantly in intensity. Hot flashes are typically followed by a hot flush, an actual and observable change in skin temperature that is accompanied by perspiration. Their cause remains unclear, but they are theorized to result from an instability between the hypothalamus and catecholamine levels in the autonomic nervous system triggered by the decrease in estrogen. Hot flashes may be so mild that they are barely noticed, or they may be severe and distressing. Their duration ranges from seconds to minutes or even an hour. Their frequency varies from one or two per hour to one or two per week. Hot flashes that occur at night result in night sweats, which can seriously impair normal sleep patterns. At least 85% of women experience hot flashes—usually for about 1 year. However, in severe cases they may persist for as long as 5 years or more.

Hot flashes may be triggered by a wide variety of stimuli, including alcohol use, spicy food, stress and excitement, exercise, and excess clothing. Despite their disrupting effects, hot flashes do not pose a health hazard to women. A variety of methods have been used in the attempt to control hot flashes. The most common method involves supplementing the diet with vitamins E and B complex. Although anecdotal reports of improvement are widespread, scientific research is not available to support this claim. Estrogen replacement therapy has proved effective in relieving severe vasomotor symptoms.

### Urogenital changes

The decline in estrogen causes classic changes in the genitalia. The linings of the vagina and urethra are rich in estrogen receptors, and they are very sensitive to declining estradiol levels. The vagina becomes thin and pale, and the production and volume of natural secretions decrease significantly, resulting from a decline in function of the Bartholin's glands. Slow atrophy and a loss of elasticity may result in pain during intercourse **(dyspareunia),** vaginal dryness, burning, itching, and occasional slight bleeding. Vaginal secretions gradually become more alkaline, which may result in an increase in vaginal infections. Atrophic changes in the urethra and the pH changes in the vagina also increase the frequency of urinary tract infections, and they may trigger urinary frequency, urgency, and stress incontinence. The changes in fat and glandular tissue also affect the breasts, which become less full and hang more loosely.

### Osteoporosis

The effects of estrogen depletion on the development and severity of osteoporosis in postmenopausal women is being carefully studied. The problem is complex and is discussed in more detail on pp. 270-274. The role of estrogen replacement in preventing the development of postmenopausal osteoporosis provides the most compelling argument for the widespread use of estrogen supplementation in older women.

## Nursing Interventions During Menopause

Menopause marks the end of a woman's reproductive capacity, but it in no way signals an end to a woman's productivity, attractiveness, or sexuality. Sexual pleasure does not depend on the continued release of ova. But to large numbers of women, this single, predictable, physiologic change in their lives has been allowed to be coupled with an end to their youth and attractiveness. The complex interaction of physiologic changes, anatomic factors, and psychosocial/cultural variables that characterize menopause provides multiple opportunities for the nurse to intervene and support healthful adjustments and transitions.

Virtually all women have heard of the "change of life." Women learn to respond to menopause from the framework of their culture. In the United States, this traditionally has not been a positive framework. Instead, the negative image of menopause is reinforced by media, books, advertising, and health professionals. Although the negative culture of menopause has been readily absorbed, it cannot be assumed that the average woman possesses factual knowledge about either the process or outcomes of menopause. Most older women began their

**BOX 11-3 Health Teaching for Menopause**

1. Knowledge about menopause
   a. Cessation of ovarian function, with cessation of menstruation over 12 to 18 months
   b. Average age is 49-51 years
   c. Changes in reproductive ability
      (1) Conception still possible during the period of change
         (a) Contraception should be used for 1 year after last menstrual period
         (b) Rhythm method is an unreliable contraceptive method during this period
      (2) Ability to conceive ceases when menopause is completed
   d. Sexual ability still present
   e. Physical symptoms vary from mild to severe; estrogen therapy may be given to relieve severe symptoms
2. Promotion of health and physical appearance
   a. Moderate exercise to maintain muscle tone and help prevent osteoporosis
   b. Calcium supplement to prevent osteoporosis
   c. Dietary control to prevent weight gain
   d. Activities that encourage self-esteem and interest outside of self
   e. Peer support groups during menopause, if necessary
3. Prevention of discomfort
   a. Relief of vasomotor reactions (hot flashes)
      (1) Moderation of factors identified by patient as exacerbating hot flashes (excitement, alcoholic beverages, heavy eating, excessive clothing, impairment of heat loss in hot weather)
      (2) Vitamin E or B-complex vitamins
      (3) Estrogen, Bellergal
   b. Prevention of dyspareunia: local application of lubricant or vaginal cream
   c. Relief of vaginal itching: vitamin E or estrogen therapy

reproductive years without adequate education about their bodies and end those years with the same deficiencies. Nurses must identify women who can profit from education about menopause and provide anticipatory guidance to women in their 40s before the onset of climacteric. Women need to understand what menopause is, why and when it occurs, the effects it has on reproductive and sexual functioning, how to control common symptoms, and what symptoms require medical attention. Health teaching concerning menopause is summarized in Box 11-3.

### Managing symptoms

The nurse begins by carefully assessing the patient's life-style and the effects of menopausal symptoms. Life-style factors and attitudes are clearly related to a woman's willingness to report symptoms and the frequency and severity of some symptoms. Women with multiple satisfying life roles, positive marital relationships, and active physical life-styles are most likely to report mild and infrequent menopausal symptoms. The exception appears to be the frequency and severity of hot flashes, which cannot be predicted based on other factors.

The management of hot flashes is discussed on p. 268. The nurse encourages the woman to assess her own symptom pattern and explore the effectiveness of simple, unproved methods of controlling symptoms, such as avoiding overeating, alcohol use, and excess stress or exercise. Vaginal problems are the second most common symptom of menopause. The nurse encourages the woman to use a water-soluble lubricant as needed for adequate comfort during intercourse. Vitamin E appears to have some effectiveness in alleviating dryness of vaginal tissue over time. Estrogen creams will restore elasticity and moisture, but they are absorbed systemically and must be used with caution. The nurse encourages the woman to be scrupulous concerning perianal hygiene, to avoid douching, and to seek prompt treatment if symptoms of urinary tract infection (UTI) or vaginal infection develop.

Some women may feel that they are less attractive after menopause. Research has refuted the presumed link between menopause and depression,[17] but the nurse can help to support a woman's self-concept and body image by encouraging moderate exercise for bone building, improved general health, and physical appearance. Improved fitness has been shown to decrease all menopausal symptoms except vasomotor ones and is particularly effective in improving sleep pattern and overall mental outlook.[17] Peer support during menopause may be helpful.

The nurse who works with perimenopausal women needs to be alert to issues of contraception. Although most women are clearly aware of the risks of unplanned pregnancy during middle age, a recent study found that more than 20% of women between 40 and 44 years of age used no means of contraception.[16] This is a higher percentage than for any other age-group. During this period, menstrual cycles and ovulation may become irregular and a highly reliable means of contraception is necessary. The rhythm method is unreliable with irregular cycles. Contraception should be continued for 1 year after a woman's last menstrual period.

**Estrogen replacement therapy. Estrogen replacement therapy (ERT)** after menopause has been one of the most hotly debated interventions in medicine. Advantages and disadvantages have been discussed constantly in the media. The role of ERT in the prevention and management of osteoporosis has not received as much attention as has been paid to the increased incidence of uterine and breast cancer that is associated with the use of pure estrogen products. As a result, both women and health care providers are ambivalent about the general use of ERT. The decision needs to be an informed choice. The nurse can help the woman evaluate personal risk factors, examine the data, and choose an option. Once the decision is made, the focus shifts to supporting the woman and teaching her about mon-

**RESEARCH**

Harris RB et al: Are women using postmenopausal estrogens? A community survey, *Am Public Health* 80(10):1266-1268, 1990.

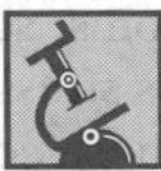

In a California community, a telephone survey was conducted of 954 women, ages 50 to 65 years, concerning current use of estrogen replacement therapy. Of the women interviewed, 32% were using postmenopausal estrogens, with 18% also taking a progestin. Premarin was the most frequently named drug. Women who were taking ERT were younger and thinner than other sample members. They were also more likely to be married and were usually caring for fewer persons in their households than were nonusers. Widowed women were the least likely to be using ERT.

The study findings showed a discrepancy between the enthusiasm for ERT found in the current medical literature and a low reported use by women.

itoring for side effects and complications of either choice. The use of ERT in osteoporosis is discussed on p. 272. ERT is also an extremely effective intervention for managing other menopausal symptoms, such as hot flashes and vaginal atrophy. See Research box above.

The occurrence of menopause is confirmed before ERT is initiated. Serum estradiol levels of below 40 pg/ml, with FSH and LH levels of above 100 mIU/ml, indicate menopause. If estrogens are prescribed, they are usually taken for extended periods but may be tapered and discontinued at any time if a woman so desires. The use of combination estrogen and progestin products is standardly recommended. These combination products appear to lower significantly the risk of associated endometrial cancer and lower the risk of breast cancer slightly. However, they do alter the lipoprotein ratios and slightly decrease the protective effects estrogen has on heart disease. Because the incidence of uterine cancer is universally higher in this age-group, postmenopausal women should have uterine screening examinations for cancer at least once a year, whether or not they are receiving ERT. The nurse advises all women that bleeding after menopause is an important warning sign that must be evaluated by a physician.

Guidelines for ERT are general, because the risks and benefits need to be evaluated on an individual basis. Because some of the risks of menopause are present whether or not ERT is used, women need to receive enough information to make informed decisions. Estrogen can be administered in an oral form, in vaginal creams, and by transdermal patches. The general policy is to use the lowest possible dose that relieves symptoms. Absolute contraindications to ERT include venous thromboembolic disease, a history of endometrial or breast cancer, recent MI or CVA, and estrogen-related gallbladder or pancreatic disease. Relative contraindications include heavy smoking, morbid obesity, and cystic breast disease or a family history of breast cancer, diabetes, hypertension, gallbladder, or liver disease.

## OSTEOPOROSIS

### Etiology/Epidemiology

**Osteoporosis** can be defined as a disorder in which bone mass is lost to the point where the skeleton is no longer able to withstand unexpected or normal mechanical forces.[6] It is the most common skeletal disorder and is second only to arthritis as a cause of musculoskeletal morbidity in elderly persons.[14] Osteoporosis has its origins in young adulthood but typically does not manifest itself until much later in life. It affects an estimated 25 million Americans and causes 1.5 million fracture episodes each year, at an annual cost of $7 to $10 billion.[10] More than half of individuals older than age 45 have evidence of osteoporosis, and the disease is present in more than 90% of individuals over 75 years of age. It is estimated that one in four females will experience an osteoporosis-related fracture by age 65.

The continuing aging of the American population makes osteoporosis statistics and projections even more compelling. The current annual incidence of 200,000 to 250,000 hip fractures is projected to increase to more than 350,000 annually by the end of the first decade of the twenty-first century. These hip fractures carry a projected price tag of $30 to $60 billion annually.[3] The average 50-year-old woman is projected to have a 16% risk of hip fracture, a 15% risk of forearm fracture, and a 32% risk of vertebral fracture in her lifetime, whereas her male counterpart's risk is approximately 5% for all forms of fracture.[6] Hip fracture and its sequelae cause the most concern. An estimated 15% of individuals experiencing hip fracture die within a short period, 30% die of secondary complications, and a full 50% experience a significant loss of independence and self-care ability, often necessitating admission to a long-term care facility.[10] It is difficult to overemphasize the importance of osteoporosis as a threat to independence and quality of life in an aging population.

The bones of the body undergo a constant cyclic pattern of remodeling. The remodeling process is a complex and highly integrated activity that strategically balances the forces of resorption or breakdown with the process of bone building. The osteoblastic or building forces predominate throughout childhood and young adulthood, until peak bone mass is reached at about age 35. After a variable period of relative balance, the resorptive breakdown forces begin to predominate and they continue to dominate throughout the remainder of a person's life. In osteoporosis, the bone itself is essentially normal but there is not enough of it to withstand mechanical stresses. Simple bone mass is the major determinant of bone strength and accounts for about 75% to 85% of its variance.

**Risk factors**

Any factor that influences the complex process of bone remodeling can increase the rate and severity of osteoporosis development. Bony loss occurs universally with aging, which makes aging the primary risk factor. At the point of peak bone mass, men have—on the average—30% more bone mass than women, making gender the second major risk factor. Racial differences are reflected in the fact that African-Americans typically have about 10% greater bone mass than do whites. Light-skinned whites of northern European or Scandinavian descent are at greatest risk, followed by Asians and Orientals. A strong hereditary link also seems clear.

Additional identified risk factors are more directly related to hormonal balance. The loss of natural estrogen at menopause appears to increase dramatically the process of bony resorption, although the mechanisms of this change are not well understood. Chronic calcium deficiency is a common problem in the aging population, and adequate calcium is essential to bone production. The mechanism of intestinal absorption of calcium becomes less efficient with advancing age, increasing the demand for calcium. Diets high in fat appear to decrease calcum absorption, and excess protein ingestion—particularly animal protein—increases the excretion of calcium by the kidney. Alcohol and possibly caffeine also increase calcium excretion, and chronic smoking appears to both lower body estrogen levels and block calcium absorption.

Lack of exercise is the final essential risk factor. The body responds to vigorous muscle pulls and stresses by producing a bony skeleton that is capable of bearing functional loads. Chronic immobility is accompanied by well-documented and ongoing increases in the resorptive activities in the bone. In normal daily life-styles, this translates into an increased risk of osteoporosis for individuals with small frames, low body weight, and a sedentary activity pattern.

Osteoporosis can also be a secondary effect of a variety of other disorders, particularly those involving hormonal imbalance or treatment. Identified risk factors are summarized in Box 11-4.

**BOX 11-4 Risk Factors for Osteoporosis**

**MAJOR RISK FACTORS**

- Aging
- Female
- White race
- Family history
- Postmenopause—surgical or natural
- Chronic calcium deficiency
- Sedentary life-style
- Small frame, low body weight

**RELATED RISK FACTORS**

- Chronic smoking
- Diet high in protein and fat
- Chronic alcohol use
- Excessive caffeine intake (possible)

**SECONDARY CONTRIBUTING FACTORS**

- Endocrine disorders, e.g., diabetes mellitus, Cushing's syndrome, hyperthyroidism, parathyroidism
- GI disorders, e.g., malabsorption syndromes, alcoholism
- Rheumatoid arthritis
- COPD
- Drug therapy, e.g., with glucocorticoids, heparin, anticonvulsants, loop diuretics (e.g., furosemide), barbiturates

## Pathophysiology

Osteoporosis may exist as a primary disorder or occur as a secondary response to another disease process or treatment modality. Primary osteoporosis is typically classified as type I or type II. The pathology overlaps extensively, but the initiating factors and target areas of the bony skeleton show striking differences.

**Type I** osteoporosis, also called *rapid bone loss,* is primarily osteoclast mediated and is triggered by the losses of estrogen resulting from menopause. **Type II** osteoporosis, termed *slow bone loss,* is primarily osteoblast mediated and is associated with advanced age—after age 70. The process of type II osteoporosis affects both males and females fairly equally.

Although there are a wide variety of types of bones in the body, they all share a similar basic structure. Approximately 80% of the bone is cortical (compact bone—dense and hard), composed of groups of bony layers packed tightly together on the outer surfaces and shafts of the bone. The remaining 20% is trabecular (cancellous or medullary), which is found inside the bone and has a spongy appearance. As a unit it forms a strong supporting network, and it also contains the marrow-filled spaces.

After the fourth decade of life, bone resorption predominates in the ongoing bone remodeling process. Resorption continues at a rate of about 0.3% to 0.5% annually in both men and women for the duration of life. Therefore the most powerful overall predictor of bone density is chronologic age. At menopause the loss of estrogen triggers a dramatic increase in the rate of bone resorption. The rate of bone resorption averages 2% to 3% annually and continues for a minimum of 5 to 8 years and perhaps as long as 10 to 15 years after menopause before it tapers to the more normal aging pattern.[7]

Type I osteoporosis affects primarily trabecular bone and particularly targets the vertebrae and radius. Type II osteoporosis affects both the cortical and trabecular bone, particularly targeting the femur and humerus. Both the rate and depth of resorptive cratering are dramatically increased. Simultaneously, the action of the osteoblasts in filling and remodeling the pits and holes in the bone is inadequate. Bones gradually become thinner and more porous.

Calcium absorption and utilization are important components of osteoporosis. Calcium salts are laid down in a protein framework to form the osteoid matrix. It is thought that a deficiency of 1,25-dihydroxyvitamin $D_3$, a hormone that controls calcium absorption, may be a crucial component of osteoblastic deficiency in elderly persons.[8] The net result is that women in advanced age may have lost 50% of their trabecular bone and 35% of their cortical bone, whereas elderly men lose up to 25% of each.[6] The differences in outcome are self-evident from the fracture incidence statistics.

The final major pathophysiologic component of osteoporosis is hormonal. When bone resorption increases, the serum calcium level rises slightly, because the bones and teeth are the reservoirs for 99% of total body calcium. Even a minor elevation in the serum calcium level causes PTH secretion by the parathyroids to decrease. Renal calcium excretion increases in response to the decline in PTH, and intestinal absorption of calcium decreases.

Osteoporosis begins in early to middle adulthood, but its clinical manifestations take many years to develop. Fractures that occur in response to normal activity or minimal trauma are the classic feature. Although any bones can be affected by osteoporosis, the classic fracture sites include the vertebrae and ribs, proximal femur, proximal humerus, and distal radius (Colles' fracture). Vertebral fractures that occur in younger postmenopausal woman are typically accompanied by acute pain, whereas those that occur in elderly persons may cause mild discomfort or be completely asymptomatic. This is particularly true when fractures occur in the midthoracic region. Back pain is by far the most common clinical manifestation. Unless the fracture is acute, the pain is usually described as a chronic, dull aching that may be difficult to distinguish from osteoarthritis. A loss of standing height of greater than 2 inches and the development of the typical kyphosis (dowager's hump) are other classic signs. Clinical manifestations of osteoporosis are summarized in Box 11-5.

**BOX 11-5 Clinical Manifestations of Osteoporosis**

Back pain (compression fracture of vertebrae)
- Chronic dull aching
- Sudden onset of acute pain greatly intensified by coughing, sneezing, or movement

Fracture
- Proximal femur (minimal or no trauma)
- Distal radius (outstretched arm to break a fall)
- Proximal humerus
- Ribs

Thoracic kyphosis (dowager's hump)

Loss of more than 2 inches standing height

## Medical Management

Osteoporosis is a pathophysiologic process that cannot be reversed or cured. The most effective management strategies are preventive, focusing on building peak skeletal mass in young adults and minimizing age-associated losses. Osteoporosis is a community-based health problem, because patients are hospitalized only to deal with the fracture complications of the disease.

### Diagnostic tests

Definitive diagnosis of osteoporosis usually is not made until complicating fractures develop. General laboratory studies usually are of minimal value, because they are typically within normal limits, but urine calcium and serum calcium, phosphate, alkaline phosphatase, and PTH levels may be evaluated. Conventional x-ray examinations cannot show the effects of osteoporosis until 30% to 50% of the bone is lost. If it is considered essential to measure bone density, single or dual photon absorptiometry may be used. CT scans of the lumbar vertebrae provide excellent data about bone density, but they are extremely expensive.

### Medication

Drug therapy is the primary medical treatment for osteoporosis. The various drugs that are prescribed attack this complex problem from several different perspectives.

**Estrogen replacement therapy.** The use of estrogen for postmenopausal women has been extensively researched and hotly debated over the past decade. The use of estrogen is an important clinical decision that should be made in collaboration with the woman. The use of estrogen definitely slows rapid bone losses when it is started in the early postmenopausal period, and it has been shown to reduce the incidence of fractures by 50%.[6] It must be used long term, however, because the accelerated losses begin again immediately when it is discontinued. It does not influence the slower type II losses that are purely age related. The exact mode of action of estrogen in the prevention of osteoporosis is not understood, and the relatively small but real associated cancer risks must be considered. The increased incidence of breast and uterine cancers are very real concerns. Combination progestin products are therefore recommended, which lessen the risk of uterine cancer, but the use of progestin products does not appear to significantly lower the risk of breast cancer. The mortality from breast cancer is not affected by ERT, but the incidence *is* increased with the use of all estrogen preparations. The continuation of menstrual bleeding makes these drugs unacceptable to some women. It is generally agreed that ERT is indicated in all patients with high-risk profiles and in most women who experience menopause before age 50.[19] The importance of estrogen replacement in osteoporosis prevention is so widely rec-

**TABLE 11-1 Estrogen Replacement Therapy**

| DRUG | MINIMUM EFFECTIVE DOSE | SIDE EFFECTS | GENERAL CONSIDERATIONS FOR ERT |
|---|---|---|---|
| Conjugated estrogen (Premarin) | 0.625 mg/day PO given cyclically for 25 days of each cycle, followed by 5-10 mg of progestin for 10-14 days; combination preparations are available | Anorexia, bloating, breast tenderness | Proven effectiveness in controlling menopause-related symptoms and slowing type I osteoporosis.<br>Estrogen cuts the risk of cardiovascular disease in half.<br>Progestin use reverses this protective balance to some degree. |
| Estropipate (Ogen) | 0.625 mg/day PO given cyclically as above | Same as for conjugated estrogen | Link between estrogen use and breast cancer remains controversial. |
| Estradiol (Estrace) | 2.0 mg/day PO given cyclically as above; combination preparations are available | Same as for conjugated estrogen | The risk is clear but small, except when undiagnosed tumors are estrogen dependent. |
| Estradiol (Estraderm) | 0.05-0.100 mg/day as a slow-release transdermal patch—used for 3 weeks of cycle and replaced twice a week | Less GI distress as bypasses intestinal absorption; skin redness and irritation possible | Estrogen multiplies the risk of endometrial cancer by 4 times.<br>Adding progestin reduces this risk dramatically by promoting shedding of uterine lining.<br>Regular PAP smears, uterine biopsy if indicated, and mammograms are encouraged. |

ognized now that it is included in the *Healthy People 2000* goals as the following:

Increase to at least 90 percent the proportion of perimenopausal women who have been counseled about the benefits and risks of estrogen replacement therapy (combined with progestin when appropriate) for prevention of osteoporosis.[4]

The cardiovascular protective effects of estrogen are another definite plus to its use. Table 11-1 summarizes the major options for estrogen replacement.

**Calcium supplementation.** The exact role of calcium in osteoporosis treatment is unclear. Calcium does not increase bone density or prevent fracture, but it is essential to osteoblastic activity to rebuild bone in the remodeling cycle. The average American diet is clearly deficient in calcium. Daily calcium requirements are estimated at 1000 mg in early adulthood and 1500 mg after menopause. The average adult diet contains 400 to 800 mg.[3]

The major obstacles to calcium supplementation are absorption and the percentage of elemental calcium contained in the preparation. Absorption depends on interaction with hydrochloric acid (HCl), so the supplement should be taken with or after meals. Calcium carbonate is composed of 40% elemental calcium and is the standard preferred form. Calcium phosphate contains 31% elemental calcium; lactate, 13%; and gluconate, 9%. A full glass of water is recommended with each dose, although the risk of stones and hypercalcemia is very small. Because vitamin D is essential for calcium absorption in the intestine, a standard multivitamin is usually also recommended. Calcium is also known to interfere with the action of a variety of medications. The individual woman is counseled to consult a pharmacist or physician about potential drug interactions with prescription medications before initiating calcium supplementation.

**Calcitonin.** Calcitonin is a hormone secreted by the thyroid gland that has been found to decrease osteoclast activity significantly. It may be prescribed for women at high risk for osteoporosis who cannot take estrogen. Salmon calcitonin may be used, which is more potent and longer acting. The dosage is 50 to 100 IU daily or every other day. The major drawback is that the drug loses its effectiveness after 18 to 24 months of treatment. It also is extremely expensive and must be administered by subcutaneous injection, although clinical trials with intranasal sprays are ongoing.

**Sodium fluoride.** Sodium fluoride has a proven effect on osteoblast activity and has been extensively researched. It clearly is able to stimulate the development of new bone, but the quality and tensile strength of that bone appear to be inadequate. No positive effect on the incidence of fractures has been demonstrated by its use.[8]

**Etidronate disodium (Didronel).** This drug has been shown to decrease osteoclast activity. Current research trials are focused on using it in cycles to attempt to mimic the normal remodeling cycle of the bone, thereby suppressing the resorptive phase.[7]

**Thiazide diuretics.** Electrolyte changes typically occur with the use of thiazide diuretics. These include a definite decrease in the urinary excretion of calcium. Targeted clinical trials in osteoporosis show an early indication of a decreased incidence of hip fracture.[15]

## NURSING MANAGEMENT

The goal of all nursing interventions for patients with osteoporosis is to prevent or delay the destructive bone changes that are characteristic of the disease. Successful prevention of osteoporosis begins in childhood and continues throughout life. The individual needs to incorporate preventive strategies into the full course of the life span to promote a healthy and active old age.

### Promoting calcium intake

Although the exact role of calcium in osteoporosis therapy is uncertain, there is little doubt about its importance in building peak bone mass. There is also little doubt that Americans, particularly American women, are chronically deficient in their daily intake. Supplements are one route, but most nutritionists recommend obtaining the element from foods in the diet. Calcium is liberally present in a wide variety of dairy foods, but these foods typically fall out of favor once adulthood is reached. They tend to be avoided as high calorie and cholesterol sources.

The nurse explores the individual's usual dietary plan and evaluates its adequacy for calcium. The nurse teaches the woman about the role of calcium in bone building and the importance of osteoporosis prevention in early adulthood, decades before the symptoms of osteoporosis may appear. Table 11-2 identifies the calcium content of common foods that can be used to plan an adequate intake. The absorption of calcium is impaired by the presence of a high amount of fat or fiber, and its renal excretion is heightened in the presence of a high amount of protein. The nurse assists the individual to adjust his or her meal pattern as needed to compensate for these factors. The essential component of the teaching is the understanding that milk and milk products are needed for more than just childhood growth, and their use does not need to result in a high calorie or high fat intake.

**TABLE 11-2 Major Dietary Sources of Calcium**

| FOOD | QUANTITY | CALCIUM (mg) |
|---|---|---|
| **MILK** | 1 cup (240 ml) | |
| Skim | | 302 |
| 1% | | 300 |
| 2% | | 297 |
| **ICE CREAM** | 1 cup | |
| Hard | | 176 |
| Soft | | 236 |
| **ICE MILK** | 1 cup | |
| Hard | | 176 |
| Soft | | 274 |
| **CHEESE** | | |
| Cheddar | 1 oz | 204 |
| Swiss | 1 oz | 272 |
| American | 1 oz | 150 |
| Cottage | 1 cup | 155 |
| **BEANS** | | |
| Pinto (cooked) | 1 cup | 86 |
| Soy (cooked) | 1 cup | 131 |
| Navy (cooked) | 1 cup | 95 |
| Green (cooked) | 1 cup | 80 |
| **VEGETABLES** | | |
| Turnip greens (cooked) | 1 cup | 249 |
| Broccoli (cooked) | 1 cup | 90 |

### Promoting exercise

Active weight-bearing exercise is the second major emphasis of osteoporosis prevention. As with diet adjustment, the role of exercise is primarily preventive and must be incorporated into the individual's life-style throughout the life span. Active exercise puts mechanical stresses on the skeleton, thereby stimulating bony growth. Immobility or continued sedentary activity at any time of life increases the rate of bone resorption slightly but significantly. For peak effect, exercise needs to be initiated before peak bone mass is reached in the mid-30s. Active exercise is particularly important for slight, thin women whose body mass in itself is insufficient to stimulate bone growth. Particular concern rests with highly trained female athletes of small body mass, such as gymnasts and marathon runners. Periods of amenorrhea are common in these women, and concern exists over the long-term effect on bone mass and

**RESEARCH**

Zhang J, Feldblum PJ, Fortney JA: Moderate physical activity and bone density among perimenopausal women, *Am J Public Health* 82(5):736-738, 1992.

This study involved 352 white women, ages 40 to 54, in North Carolina. They completed a questionnaire covering health history, reproductive history, past and current exercise patterns, and past and current diet. A personal activity computer was used to determine exercise and energy expenditures over several days. Bone mineral density (BMD) was measured at the second to fourth lumbar vertebrae and at the mid and distal radius.

Spinal BMD decreased slightly with age and was substantially lower in postmenopausal women. Lumbar BMD was found to be significantly higher in women who had breast-fed infants. Women with higher physical activity as measured by the computer were found to also have significantly higher BMDs at the spine and distal radius. This effect remained significant, even when other determinants of BMD were taken into account.

strength from periods of estrogen depletion. See Research box, p. 274.

The duration and extent of exercise needed for bone health is basically unknown. The general recommendation is 30 to 40 minutes of active exercise three times a week, which matches heart healthy guidelines. Brisk walking or hiking, aerobics, tennis, and ballroom dancing are all possibilities. The essential component is that the exercise be resistive and gravitational and involve vigorous muscle pulls. Swimming, although excellent aerobic exercise and recommended for persons with arthritis, is essentially weightless and does not meet the criteria for resistance needed for prevention of osteoporosis.

Another focus of exercise is promoting strength and balance in elderly persons. Most osteoporosis-related fractures involve minimal trauma. The nurse encourages the individual to wear low-heeled, soft-soled shoes and to carefully evaluate the home for hazard risks, such as polished floors, throw rugs, and loose wires. The Osteoporosis Foundation has prepared an exercise guide that specifically targets the vulnerable vertebrae. Sample exercises are shown in Figure 11-1. Individuals at high risk for osteoporosis should avoid spine flexion exercises, such as sit-ups, and focus on maintaining full extension capability. The Osteoporosis Foundation is an excellent source of high-quality literature for patients about the disease and strategies for prevention.

## Persons at Risk for Sexual Concerns or Problems

The experience of illness and its treatment can influence an individual's sexuality in a wide variety of ways. Potential threats to sexual health include direct anatomic or physiologic changes that may affect the person's ability to engage in sexual activity, body image changes that alter the person's self-concept as a sexual being, and environmental and behavioral problems that may trigger changes in sexual arousal, desire, or relationships. Sexual response is vulnerable to interference from life changes and challenges, even in the presence of optimal health. The addition of health-related problems causes most persons encountered in clinical practice to be at least "at risk" for sexual concerns or problems.

People with acute or chronic illness can develop a wide variety of sexual problems, ranging from mild anxiety to sexual dysfunction. The range of true sexual dysfunction includes loss of desire or arousal, impotence, orgasmic dysfunction, and gender identity disorders. These problems are complex and multifaceted and are beyond the scope of practice of most nurses. Patients with true sexual dysfunction are best referred to highly trained specialists for assessment and treatment. The treatment is beyond the scope of this discussion. Treatment alternatives for physiologic impotence are presented in Chapter 53.

Sexual concerns that accompany illness and its treatment typically begin with worry, discomfort, or dissatisfaction. These concerns will not in themselves cause significant problems in either sexual relationships or performance. Over time, however, misinformation, guilt, and difficulty communicating about sexual issues can significantly alter sexual patterns and satisfaction. Although some individuals can readily identify and discuss their sexual concerns and problems, most persons cannot. It is important for the nurse to be aware of the nature and scope of common sexual concerns associated with illness and its treatment and to be committed to their inclusion in the normal range of patient care.

### PROBLEM SITUATIONS

#### Pharmacologic Effects

The potential effect of pharmacologic agents on sexuality has only recently been openly acknowledged. The effects of alcohol are perhaps the most widely recognized. In small doses, alcohol promotes initial relaxation and release of inhibition. In larger doses, however, this positive effect is lost, and alcohol causes central nervous system depression and interference with motor activity, which have negative effects on sexual function.

Several other categories of commonly used drugs are known to have negative effects on sexual function. These include antihypertensives, antidepressants, antihistamines, sedatives and tranquilizers, antispasmodics, sex hormone preparations, and some narcotic and psychoactive drugs. Potential effects on sexuality include a decrease in sex drive or libido, the inability to attain or sustain an erection, and impaired orgasm or ejaculation. Noncompliance with the prescribed pharmacologic treatment regimen is a common problem with hypertension therapy, and it is frequently attributed to drug-induced sexual dysfunction. Antihypertensive agents that cause direct vasodilation or block the actions of the sympathetic nervous system cause the most significant problems. It is critical that all health care providers inform patients about possible sexual side effects of prescribed medications and assess openly for problems. Drug or dosage changes frequently can alleviate the problems, but only if the reality of sexual side effects of drugs is openly acknowledged. Table 11-3 summarizes the major drugs affecting sexual behavior.

#### Physiologic Changes

Many illnesses can alter the physiologic processes necessary for sexual response, including nerve transmission, vasocongestion, hormonal metabolism, and the perception of pleasurable sensation. In general, it appears that both the severity of the disorder and its duration or chronicity primarily determine the frequency and severity of associated sexual problems. Although the range of potential physiologic interference with sexual function is very wide, as shown in Table 11-4, diabetes mellitus is the most widely acknowledged disease process.

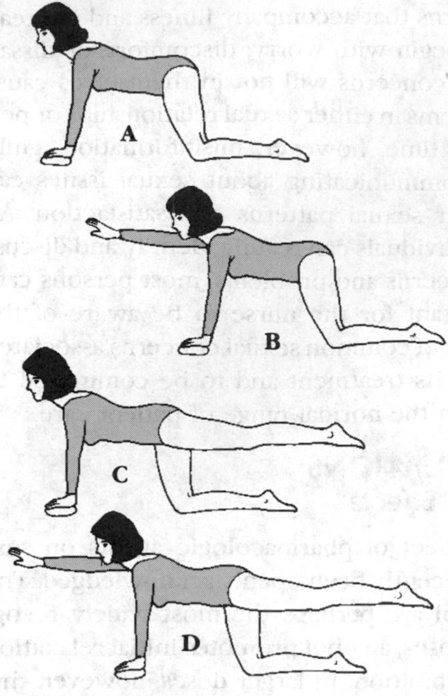


**All fours arm/leg lifts**
Position yourself on your hands and knees, with your hands directly under your shoulders and your knees directly under your hips (A). Your back should be flat or slightly arched. Lift one arm and hold for 3 seconds (B). Repeat with the other arm. Then lift one leg and hold for 3 seconds (C). Repeat with the other leg. If you can do these exercises comfortably, try lifting your right arm and left leg simultaneously (D), and then your left arm and right leg.

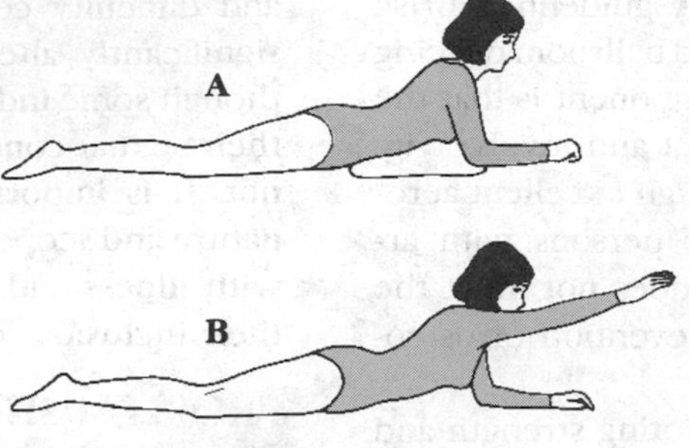


**The elbow prop**
Lie on your stomach, with your elbows holding the weight of your upper body (A). Stay in this position for 5 minutes the first day; gradually increase the time to half an hour. You may be more comfortable if you put a pillow under your stomach. The elbow prop position helps reverse the effects of bad posture by passively decompressing the vertebrae and disks. To exercise the back as well, reach the right arm forward (B), then the left, and repeat.

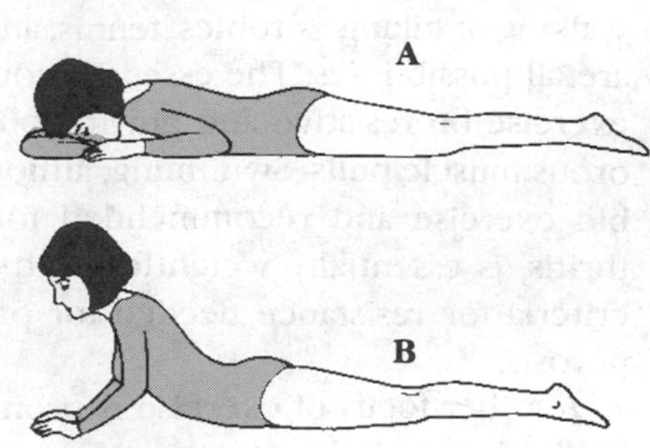


**Prone press-ups with deep breathing**
Start out in a conventional "push-up" position (A). Arch your back, pinching your shoulder blades together (B). As you push up, inhale; as you lie down, exhale. Keep elbows partially bent to protect the back. Make sure you don't lift your pelvis.

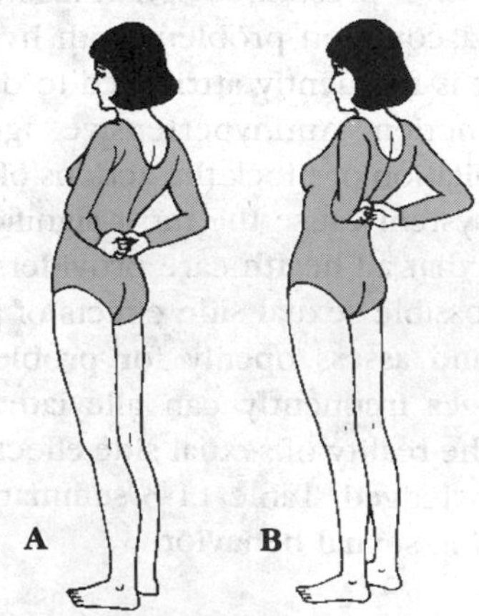


**Standing back bend**
Put your firsts on your lower back. Arch backwards slowly while taking a deep breath (A). Relax and put your arms down, then repeat, this time with the fists on the middle back (B).

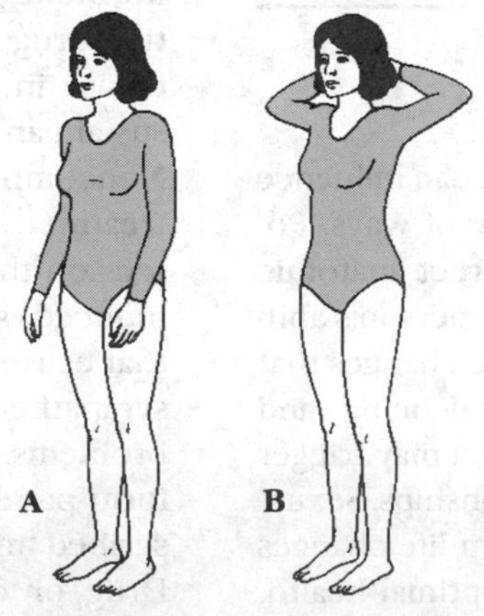


**Isometric posture correction**
Stand as tall as you can, with your chin in, not up (A). Place your palms against the back of your head. Simultaneously push your hands against your head while pinching your shoulder blades together (B). Hold for 3 seconds, then relax for 3 seconds. Maintain an erect posture throughout the exercise.

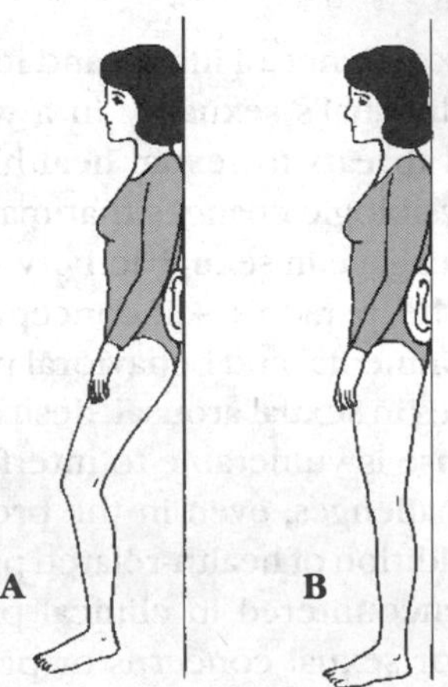


**Standing and pelvic tilt**
Stand with your feet about a foot from the wall, with your knees slightly bent and your back straight (A). Use a towel to support your lower back. Slide up and down, keeping the back straight and the stomach muscles contracted. You should be able to plant your feet closer to the wall as you improve.

**FIGURE 11-1** Exercises for osteoporosis prevention. (From *Boning up on osteoporosis: a guide to prevention and treatment,* Washington, DC, 1990, National Osteoporosis Foundation.)

**TABLE 11-3 Drug Effects on Human Sexual Behavior**

| DRUG OR DRUG CATEGORY | EFFECT | PROBABLE MECHANISM OF ACTION |
|---|---|---|
| **ANTIHYPERTENSIVES** | | |
| Clonidine (Catapres)<br>Guanethidine (Ismelin)<br>Methyldopa (Aldomet)<br>Propranolol (Inderal)<br>Reserpine (Serpasil) | May cause impotence and erectile and orgasmic dysfunction | Central and peripheral blockage of nervous innervation |
| **ANTIDEPRESSANTS** | | |
| Amitriptyline (Elavil)<br>Desipramine (Norpramin, Pertofrane)<br>Imipramine (Tofranil)<br>Nortriptyline (Aventyl)<br>Pargyline (Eutonyl)<br>Phenelzine sulfate (Nardil)<br>Protriptyline (Vivactil)<br>Tranylcypromine sulfate (Parnate) | Possible decreased libido and transient impotence | Central depression; peripheral blockade of nervous innervation |
| **ANTIHISTAMINES** | | |
| Chlorpheniramine (Chlor-Trimeton)<br>Diphenhydramine (Benadryl)<br>Promethazine (Phenergan) | Decreased libido; decreased vaginal lubrication | Blockade of parasympathetic nervous innervation |
| **ANTISPASMODICS** | | |
| Glycopyrrolate methobromide (Robinul)<br>Hexocyclium (Tral)<br>Methantheline (Banthine)<br>Poldine (Nacton) | Erectile and vaginal lubrication problems | Ganglionic blockade of nervous innervation |
| **SEDATIVES AND TRANQUILIZERS** | | |
| Benperidol<br>Chlordiazepoxide (Librium)<br>Chlorpromazine (Thorazine, Megaphen)<br>Chlorprothixene (Taractan)<br>Diazepam (Valium)<br>Mesoridazine (Serentil)<br>Methaqualone (Quaalude)<br>Phenoxybenzamine (Dibenzyline)<br>Prochlorperazine (Compazine)<br>Thioridazine (Mellaril) | Decreased libido | Central sedation; blockade of autonomic innervation; suppression of hypothalamic and pituitary function<br>Tranquilization and relaxation |
| **NARCOTICS AND PSYCHOACTIVE DRUGS** | | |
| Methadone<br>Morphine | Decreased libido; impaired potency | Central depression |
| Amphetamines<br>Cocaine | Transiently positive | Release of inhibitions |
| **SEX HORMONE PREPARATIONS** | | |
| Cyproterone acetate<br>Methandrostenolone (Dianabol)<br>Nandrolone phenpropionate (Durabolin)<br>Norethandrolone (Nilevar) | Loss of libido; decreased potency | Antiandrogenic effects on sexual function |

**TABLE 11-4 Physiologic Interferences with Sexual Health**

| PHYSIOLOGIC INTERFERENCES | HYPOTHESIZED MECHANISM OF ACTION |
|---|---|
| **SYSTEMIC DISEASES** | |
| Pulmonary disease<br>Renal disease<br>Malignancies<br>Infections<br>Arthritis<br>Some cardiovascular diseases<br>Degenerative neurologic diseases (MS, ALS) | Debility, pain, and depression probably interfere with sexual libido, as well as expression. |
| **METABOLIC DISRUPTIONS** | |
| Cirrhosis<br>Hepatitis<br>Diabetes mellitus<br>Hypothyroidism<br>Addison's disease<br>Hypopituitarism<br>Acromegaly<br>Cushing's disease | Hepatic problems in men result in estrogen buildup from inability of liver to conjugate estrogens; similar processes occur in women along with general debility.<br>By depression of CNS function, general debilitation, and depression, libido may be decreased, and impaired erectile abilities in men may result. |

Sexual dysfunction is extremely common among those with diabetes and reflects its widespread hormonal, vascular, and neuropathic effects. The microvascular and neuropathic changes of diabetes combine to produce impotence in as many as 50% of men with diabetes. Comparable changes occur in women, but their effects have not been documented as thoroughly through research. Chronic vaginitis is a common complaint. The incidence of sexual problems is related directly to the duration of the disease. It is hoped that early detection and treatment of complications and improved glucose control will gradually decrease the incidence of sexual dysfunction. Surgical interventions for male impotence are discussed in Chapter 53.

Painful conditions may also make it difficult for an individual to engage satisfactorily in sexual activity. Degenerative and rheumatoid arthritis are by far the most common examples. Joint mobility is commonly impaired, and positioning for sex is difficult. Chronic pain by its relentless presence may seriously impair both desire and satisfaction. Body image may also be adversely affected by the joint swelling and distortions. Pain-free sexual activity requires careful planning, creativity, and open communication by both partners. The chronicity of the disease and the lack of a cure frequently are demoralizing to the patient and partner. Partners will face frustration and frequently guilt over the existence of their own sexual desires in the face of the patient's obvious pain. The sexual relationship is a common victim of this chronic disease. Transient depression frequently accompanies chronic illness and also may cause decreased interest in sexual function or even the inability to function sexually.

Although some conditions do not interfere directly with sexual function, their perceived seriousness or accompanying symptoms may discourage persons from engaging in their usual sexual practices. One very common example is associated with cardiac disease, particularly myocardial infarction. Although marital coitus does not demand a great energy expenditure, many persons are fearful of attempting sexual intercourse after a heart attack. In general, a person who has had a myocardial infarction may gradually return to regular sexual activity, as long as care is taken to avoid concurrent conditions that increase cardiac workload. Heavy food or alcohol consumption, temperature extremes, and extreme anxiety are common examples. Specific guidelines concerning sexual rehabilitation for cardiac patients are discussed in Chapter 30.

Often a change in health is accompanied by malaise or fatigue. As a consequence, the person experiences a decrease in sexual desire or difficulty becoming aroused. This effect may not be a direct function of the disease itself, but rather the consequence of an incompatibility between "feeling bad" and the stimulating thoughts and feelings an individual associates with sexual response. This is particularly true for patients undergoing treatment for cancer. Patients experience severe fatigue and treatment side effects, such as nausea, bruising, stomatitis, and alopecia. Yet research clearly indicates the need of these patients for physical closeness, comfort, and caring from their partners. The desire for sexual intercourse may be lacking, but the desire for nondemanding physical love and comfort is ongoing.

Similar outcomes affect individuals with end-stage liver or renal disease. Every body system is affected. In addition to the overwhelming physical changes, the patient also faces enormous challenges to role functioning and self-esteem. Impotence, sterility and a decline in libido are all common outcomes and usually are not very responsive to treatment. Both patient and partner will need a great deal of support to maintain communication and a functional relationship.

## Structural Changes

A variety of injuries and surgeries may result in structural changes that interfere with sexuality. Although spinal cord injury is probably the best known and most widely studied, it is by no means the only or most common problem. Cancers involving the prostate, bladder, colon, and rectum are standardly treated with wide surgical excision in the pelvic region. This treatment inevitably damages nerves in the pelvis, which then interferes with the sensory and motor aspects of the sexual response. Male impotence is a common result. New treatments that attempt to spare the pelvic nerves are discussed in Chapters 47 and 53. Structural changes resulting from

## RESEARCH

Girts C: Nursing attitudes about sexuality needs of spinal cord injury patients, *Rehab Nurs* 15(4):205-206, 1990.

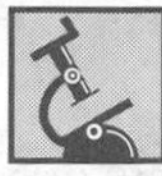

This study assessed the differences in attitudes toward the sexuality needs of spinal cord patients among nurses in acute care and rehabilitation practice settings. A convenience sample was obtained from among 72 nurses in four different settings. Forty questionnaires were analyzed—20 each from acute care and rehabilitation settings.

Sixty percent of nurses in both settings accepted the responsibility for sexual reeducation of their patients. Sixty seven percent of acute care nurses and 90% of rehabilitation nurses believed that sexual reeducation should take place in the rehabilitation setting. Ninety five percent of the nurses in both groups acknowledged a need to improve their own knowledge base concerning sexuality in SCI. Neither group of nurses believed that their own sexuality beliefs were reflected in their counseling, but only 50% of each group reported feeling comfortable with topics such as oral sex or masturbation. All of the study participants agreed that spouses and partners should be included in the education effort.

obstetric trauma and reproductive tract surgery are other examples of problems that may impair sexual function.

The challenges and dilemmas of the patient with a spinal cord injury have helped to underscore the importance of including sexuality in a total rehabilitation care plan. Men and women alike express great concern about the future of their sexuality, but most of the research concerning sexual functioning after spinal cord injury has focused on men. Little information is available to date about women's experiences. It is important to recognize that fertility usually is retained in women with a spinal cord injury, whereas sperm may not be viable in men with such an injury. Contraception measures must be included in the plan of care, and normal pregnancy is possible if desired. See Research box above.

The presence of a caring partner is without a doubt the essential key to satisfactory sexual activity for a person with a spinal cord injury. Genital sexual functioning and cognitive eroticism become separated. Sexual function specifically depends on the number of nerve fibers that were damaged and the level of the injury. These factors determine the ability of the patient to achieve reflexive or psychogenic erection and reach orgasm or ejaculation. Reflex erections are common with upper cord injury and rare with lumbar and sacral injury. Ejaculation is rare with complete cord injuries, but an orgasmlike experience may occur in other parts of the body, such as the breasts in women. Work with imagery and fantasy has enabled some individuals to channel their thoughts and feelings to produce a psychic experience similar to orgasm. Specific suggestions for sexual activity reflect the individual patient's unique strengths and weaknesses, including upper extremity strength, hip flexibility, and the presence of urinary drainage appliances, as well as the sexual value system of both partners. Spinal cord rehabilitation is discussed in more detail in Chapter 58.

**BOX 11-6 Health Problems Associated With Body Image Changes That Frequently Affect Sexuality**

| SURGICAL | OTHER |
|---|---|
| Mastectomy | Dermatologic disorders |
| Ostomy | Scarring—burn, trauma |
| Hysterectomy | Obesity |
| Amputation | Spinal cord injury |
| Prostatectomy | Rheumatoid arthritis |
| Laryngectomy/neck dissection | |

## Body Image Changes

The extent to which body image changes influence an individual's sexuality depends on both the perceptions of the person and those of others, particularly significant others. The meaning and significance that are attached to the changed body part is particularly important and can be understood only from the individual's perspective. This individual perspective has been particularly important in understanding body image changes related to mastectomy and hysterectomy. The organs involved are closely intertwined in our society with notions of femininity and sexual attractiveness. The visibility of a change also plays an important role. Aversion and rejection from friends and strangers alike can have profound effects on all aspects of a person's social interactions, including sexual functioning. The health care professional must first understand the meaning of the body change for the individual before attempting to plan any type of intervention. Common situations causing body image problems are listed in Box 11-6. See Chapter 9 for a more complete discussion of body image and self-esteem.

## Environmental Factors

Some persons cannot reintegrate their sexuality with the role changes that often accompany illness and hospitalization. Lack of privacy is a significant obstacle, particularly in the institutional setting. Partners also find themselves in confusing situations. Normal sexual interest may need to be suppressed or ignored, or it may trigger feelings of guilt or selfishness. The necessity to assume the role of caretaker frequently impairs the ability to sustain the parallel role of lover. The fact of chronic illness makes these challenges long term, and a pattern of silence or poor communication between partners may seriously interfere with sustaining a successful sexual relationship.

## NURSING MANAGEMENT

### ♦ ASSESSMENT

Many nurses are not experienced in taking a sexual history and may be uneasy about doing so. Social changes over the past 20 years, however, have made sexuality and sexual concerns increasingly public. As a result, professional nurses are increasingly expected to be informed, willing to discuss sexual concerns, and able to educate and counsel patients on basic issues related to sexuality.

No single approach to taking a sexual history is appropriate for every situation, but strategies for increasing the comfort of both the patient and the nurse will increase the likelihood of success. The nurse ensures privacy through such measures as closing the door to the patient's room and establishes an atmosphere of trust and confidentiality. If possible, the sexual history is begun during the initial nursing assessment. This communicates to the patient that sexuality is a legitimate concern in health care. The process of obtaining data about sexuality also provides permission for the individual to discuss sexual concerns with the nurse and validates their normalcy and acceptability. The nurse's own level of comfort with sexual issues is important also. It is appropriate for nurses to explore and define their own value systems and attitudes concerning sexual matters so that the influence of these personal values can be recognized. Sexual assessment demands an attitude of openness on the part of the nurse. It is not essential that the nurse be completely knowledgeable about all aspects of sexuality or capable of directly intervening to problem solve. Expecting to feel completely at ease is also not reasonable, especially in early attempts to assess for sexual concerns. But it is essential that the nurse be able to initiate the process, convey an attitude of openness and concern to the patient, and listen carefully. Skill in sexuality assessment is developed through practice and critique, just as it is for any other form of assessment.

It is important to use language that the individual understands, and it may be necesssary to spend time validating and defining terms. "Street language" may be unfamiliar to the nurse, and "medical language" may be confusing to the patient. It usually is preferable to move from less sensitive to more sensitive areas, such as exploring sexual role before discussing the ability to achieve orgasm or taking a menstrual history before a history of actual sexual experiences. Other specific strategies for approaching a sexual history are summarized in the Guidelines box above.

A brief sexual assessment can be easily incorporated into the standard nursing history with three basic questions. The questions can be modified to specifically deal with illness, hospitalization, life events, and any other element that may influence or interfere with sexual health.

- Has your (illness, surgery, hospitalization . . . ) affected your being a (husband, wife, mother . . . )?
- Has your (heart attack, mastectomy, ostomy . . . ) affected the way you see yourself as a (woman, man . . . )?
- Has your (diabetes, medication, chemotherapy . . . ) affected your ability to function sexually (or your sex life)?

These questions are nonthreatening and place sexuality within its proper context of self-concept, self-esteem, and role performance. They deemphasize sexual activity and emphasize the effect of problems on the whole person. These questions can also be used to elicit fears and concerns about changes that may result from impending procedures and surgeries. They invite patients to share their concerns in a very low-key and nonthreatening way.

When sexual problems are found to exist, it is important to elicit a description of the problem in the individual's own words, including onset, nature, and duration. It is important to explore the person's understanding of the nature and cause of the problem and any attempts at treatment or evaluation that have already been explored. Finally, it is appropriate to explore the individual's desires and expectations related to treatment, because common ground must be established before any interventions are attempted.

Any sexual assessment today must also explore the individual's current practices in regard to preventing the transmission of AIDS and other sexually transmitted diseases. This includes both knowledge of the principles of safe sex and incorporation of them into sexual habits and routines. Box 11-7 summarizes some sexual practices by their degree of safety or risk. Individuals are safest when they restrict their sexual acts to one healthy partner.

Physical assessment of the male and female reproductive systems is discussed in Chapter 51.

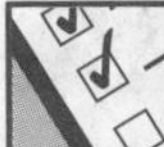

**Guidelines for Facilitating a Sexual History**

Ensure privacy for history taking.
Use language the individual understands—clarify "street" or "medical" terms.
Move from less sensitive to more sensitive topics.
Unload the question: "Some women have intercourse daily, others weekly, etc. On the average how often do you . . . "
Make questions all inclusive—use "how" and "when" rather than "did you ever."
Indicate that practices are not unusual—"Many people experience . . . "
Encourage questions and comments from the individual.
Respect the individual's right to not participate in the sexual history.

**BOX 11-7 Safety of Sexual Practices**

**PROBABLY SAFE**
Dry kissing, hugging
Mutual masturbation on healthy skin
Unshared sex toys
Massage, touching, fantasy
Sex between healthy, monogamous partners

**POSSIBLY SAFE**
Deep kissing
Intercourse (vaginal or anal) with a condom
Oral sex with a condom
Urine-to-skin contact

**UNSAFE**
Intercourse without a condom (vaginal or anal)
Oral sex without a condom
Oral-anal contact or anal intercourse
Fingers or hand in rectum
Shared sex toys
Urinating into mouth, vagina, or rectum

## ♦ NURSING DIAGNOSES

Nursing diagnoses are determined from analysis of patient data. Nursing diagnoses related to sexual concerns may include but are not limited to the following:

| Diagnostic Title | Possible Etiologic Factors |
|---|---|
| Sexuality patterns, altered | Decreased libido |
| | Body image changes |
| | Pain or fatigue |
| | Effects of medical or surgical conditions |
| | Poor communication with partner |
| | Lack of privacy |
| | Loss of mobility |
| Sexual dysfunction | Erectile dysfunction |
| | Effects of medical or surgical conditions |
| | Effects of prescription drugs |

## ♦ EXPECTED PATIENT OUTCOMES

Expected patient outcomes for patients with sexual concerns may include but are not limited to the following:

1a. Identifies factors that compromise sexual functioning.
b. Accurately describes how illness or treatment will affect sexual functioning.
c. Discusses feelings and concerns with partner.
d. Identifies strategies and techniques to enhance sexual expression.

2a. States alternative sexual practices in the presence of physiologic impotence.
b. Discusses limitations and problems with partner.
c. Identifies available community resources for treatment or assistance.
d. Expresses sexual feelings in a manner consistent with personal values and beliefs.

## ♦ INTERVENTIONS

Sexual problems or concerns can be approached from a variety of perspectives. Annon[1] has presented a model that organizes the various types of potential interventions for persons with sexual concerns or problems by levels. The model has been widely accepted for use in clinical practice. The levels of intervention are permission, limited information, specific suggestions, and intensive therapy (PLISSIT). Nurses in general practice generally will employ strategies from the first three levels. Intensive therapy requires specific educational preparation in sex therapy theory and techniques.

### Offering Permission

Individuals often want merely to know that their sexual feelings, concerns, and practices are normal, acceptable, and not perverted. They may use health professionals for this validation. The intervention level of permission takes a variety of forms and may be used preventively, as well as therapeutically. Permission applies to thoughts and feelings, as well as actual behaviors. Examples of the use of permission include the following:

- Permission to discuss alternative approaches to sexual pleasure when physiologic or structural changes interfere with normal practices—for example, alternatives to standard intercourse for the patient with a spinal cord injury or variations on common positions for intercourse for persons with arthritis
- Permission to be concerned about sexual issues—for example, after a heart attack, childbirth, or hysterectomy
- Permission *not* to engage in certain behaviors or activities—for example, adolescents who do not wish to be sexually active or engage in unsafe sex
- Permission to grieve over losses—for example, after mastectomy or ostomy surgery

The act of initiating the brief sexual history is perhaps the most powerful form of permission used by the nurse. By initiating this process, the nurse directly acknowledges sexuality as a valid and important topic of concern and indicates a willingness to work with the patient in this sensitive and potentially difficult area.

The assessment process is the first permission intervention. But patients may not always feel ready or able to discuss their concerns related to sexuality so early in the nurse-patient relationship. It is important for the nurse to leave the door open for discussion at a later date. All inclusive statements, such as "Many women undergoing (mastectomy) have concerns about the effects of the surgery . . ." reinforce the appropriateness of the concern. Following up with statements that clearly indicate that the issue will not be forgotten can be helpful. The nurse might add, "If questions or concerns do arise, I'll be happy to discuss them with you." This simple statement keeps the issue of sexuality concerns open. The nurse might also provide the patient with written materials or pamphlets that address sexuality, such as "The Sensuous Heart" from the American Heart Association or "Living and Loving" from the Arthritis Foundation. These booklets are a powerful reinforcer of the permission to be concerned about sexuality.

## Providing Limited Information

This level of intervention involves providing information to patients that is directly relevant to their particular concern or problem. It may be used to provide new information or to counter or refute myths related to the body and sexuality. The strategy may be used therapeutically, but it can also be used preventively as individuals move through predictable life-style and developmental changes. Examples of the use of limited information include the following:

- Basic sex education about masturbation, pregnancy, contraception, and the relationship of breast or penis size to sexual pleasure
- Information about sexuality during and after pregnancy or during menopause
- Information about sexuality after hysterectomy, ostomy, or prostatectomy

The nature and seriousness of the current AIDS epidemic mandates that all nurses include limited information about safe sex practices and reducing risks of transmission of STDs in virtually every patient contact, regardless of the underlying basic problem.

Providing limited information can free the individual from anxieties connected with sexual performance or assumptions about the negative effects of health-related conditions on sexual activity. Combating popular myths about sexuality can be an important health-promoting intervention for nurses in any practice setting.

## Making Specific Suggestions

Interventions associated with offering permission and providing limited information are straightforward and should be part of any nurse's fund of general knowledge for nursing practice. The level of specific suggestions presupposes that a problem related to sexual functioning has already been identified and recognized. Interventions are targeted directly at managing or alleviating the problem and therefore demand a specialty knowledge base from the nurse. No nurse can be prepared to make specific suggestions for all of the potential problems related to sexual functioning that may occur in medical-surgical nursing practice. However, competent and expert practice in a specialty area must include the knowledge of strategies for dealing with common associated sexual concerns. Specific suggestions related to sexuality are included in this text in the various problem chapters. Common examples of specific suggestions include the following:

**RESEARCH**

Hahn K: Sexuality and COPD, *Rehab Nurs* 14(4):191-195, 1989.

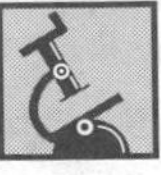

A support group program designed to help persons with chronic obstructive pulmonary disease (COPD) become more knowledgeable and confident discussing sexual matters was evaluated by participants. Group members wanted health professionals to ask matter-of-factly about their sexual concerns. They agreed unanimously that a simple, direct question would help them talk about their sexual needs. Dyspnea, coughing, energy management, sexual self-concept, and problems communicating about sex were addressed in the group. Participants were asked what had changed about their sex life since their breathing problems began. They indicated decreased mouth kissing, increased resting after position changes, and changed positions. They described apprehension about sexual activity and fear of provoking dyspnea by both the patient and partner. The most frequently mentioned consequences of role changes were decreased sexual activity, frequency of intercourse, and threat to sexual self-concept.

- Suggestions for altering positions for intercourse to accommodate hip, knee, or back involvement in arthritis
- Suggestions for incorporating sexual rehabilitation into the overall cardiac rehabilitation plan
- Suggestions for modifications to accommodate urinary drainage catheters during intercourse for patients with a spinal cord injury

See Research box above.

Partner communication is one specific suggestion that cuts across practice areas. The responsibility for successfully adapting a sexual relationship to altered health circumstances remains with the individual and sexual partner. The largest stumbling block frequently is the inability of the two individuals to honestly discuss their needs and concerns. The nurse plays a major role in giving permission to the couple to be concerned about sexual matters and then facilitating and encouraging improved partner communication to constructively problem solve toward the goal of restoring or maintaining sexual pleasure for both parties.

A number of organizations have developed specific teaching materials related to sexuality, including arthritis, heart disease, cancer care, ostomies, and spinal cord injury. Nurses working with these specialty populations should maintain files of these excellent materials, which can serve as an excellent springboard for patient teaching. They also serve as yet another reinforcement of permission that it is both okay and appropriate to be concerned about sexual functioning in the midst of serious illness.

### Referring for Intensive Therapy

Intensive sexual therapy combines techniques and concepts of psychotherapy with special approaches to intervention for individuals or couples having sexual problems. The problems involved are usually one or more of the sexual dysfunctions. These forms of therapy usually require intensive preparation beyond that provided in most schools of nursing. However, an awareness of the common sexual dysfunctions will enable nurses to refer persons with complex problems to trained therapists.

## ♦ EVALUATION

To evaluate the effectiveness of nursing interventions, compare the patient's behavior with those stated in the expected patient outcomes. Successful achievement of patient outcomes for the patient with sexual concerns is indicated by the following:

1a. Identifies factors that impair sexual functioning.
 b. Accurately describes effects of illness or treatment plan on sexuality.
 c. Initiates discussion with partner related to sexual concerns.
 d. Selects two or three new techniques to incorporate into sexual activity.

2a. Identifies two alternative strategies for sexual pleasure, despite physiologic impotence.
 b. Expresses comfort with nature and use of alternative sexual approaches.
 c. Initiates discussion of sexual dysfunction with partner.
 d. Has contact address and phone number for community resource or treatment center.

## QUESTIONS TO CONSIDER

- What behaviors by a nurse would enhance your comfort in discussing your sexual history? What behaviors would cause you to feel uncomfortable?
- How would you counsel a menopausal woman who asks you, "Should I take estrogen replacement therapy for my hot flashes?"
- Design a brief program to provide limited information to clients with cancer, diabetes, or heart disease. What information would you include? How will you present it? What adaptations will you make relating to individual clients?
- Review the records of five patients you have cared for. Did any receive medications that might interfere with their sexual functioning? How might their medical diagnoses affect their sexual self-concept? sexual relationships? sexual functioning?

## CRITICAL THINKING ACTIVITIES

- While hospitalized for an unrelated condition, Mrs. Planter, 54, complains of going through the "change" and experiencing hot flashes. What can the nurse suggest to her that may decrease her discomfort and does not require a physician order?
- Mrs. Planter also complains that she has frequent vaginal yeast infections and occasionally experiences pain with intercourse. She asks if this is normal. What explanation may be given to Mrs. Planter about her symptoms?
- Differentiate between gender identity and gender role, citing factors that help contribute to each.

## CHAPTER SUMMARY

### SEXUALITY AND HEALTH

- Sexual health is multidimensional, including sexual function, sexual self-concept, and sexual relationships.
- Human sexuality is the result of complex physiologic, psychosocial, and cultural influences.
- Human sexual response is a total body response based on myotonia and vasocongestion. Desire, arousal, and orgasm result from different neurophysiologic systems in response to physical, interpersonal, and contextual stimuli.
- Variations in sexual experience and sexual expression reflect human development and individual differences. Homosexuality and heterosexuality represent common variations of sexual expression and experience and exist on a continuum.

### AGING AND SEXUALITY

- Although sexual interest and sexual activity may decline as people age, many continue an active sexual life well into their later years. Activity levels appear to be related to sexual activity during younger years.
- Societal prejudices, lack of privacy, and lack of partners are common barriers to active sexuality among elderly persons.
- Age-related sexual changes include decreased lubrication and slower and less intense sexual response and orgasm.
- Approximately 10% of women have pronounced symptoms during menopause. Although many symptoms have been associated with menopause, the three major symptoms are osteoporosis, hot flashes, and vaginal dryness.
- Controversy surrounds the use of estrogen replacement therapy (ERT) with many experts encouraging all women to take ERT to prevent or retard osteoporosis. It is of proven benefit in slowing rapid bone loss.

- Nonpharmacologic methods of menopause symptom relief include exercise, vitamins E and B-complex, ginseng, adequate nutrition, and local application of a vaginal cream.
- Osteoporosis is the most common musculoskeletal disorder in older adults.
- Type I osteoporosis involves rapid bone loss and is caused primarily by estrogen depletion, resulting in increased osteoclast activity.
- Type II osteoporosis is related to general aging and is primarily associated with decreased osteoblast activity. It affects men and women about equally.
- ERT with progestins minimizes the associated risks of breast and uterine cancer.
- Most adult American diets are seriously deficient in calcium. RDAs are 1000 to 1500 mg daily. Dietary replacement is preferred, but supplements may be necessary.
- Calcium carbonate has the highest percentage of elemental calcium. It is taken with meals and requires adequate vitamin D levels for absorption.
- Active weight-bearing exercise is essential throughout life to minimize bone loss from osteoporosis.

### PERSONS AT RISK FOR SEXUAL CONCERNS OR PROBLEMS

- Illness may affect sexuality and sexual function through changes in body structure and function, effects of pharmacologic agents, body image changes, or environmental restrictions (privacy, competing stimuli, partner segregation).
- Sexual concerns and difficulties generally do not produce profound problems in sexual response, although they may interfere temporarily with sexual functioning.

### NURSING MANAGEMENT

- Levels of intervention for persons with sexual problems include giving permission for engaging or not engaging in sexual behaviors, providing limited information directly related to the particular problems or concerns, giving specific suggestions, or providing intensive sexual therapy. The type of intervention depends on the nature of the problem and the level of expertise of the provider.

## REFERENCES


1. Annon J: *The behavioral treatment of sexual problems,* Honolulu, 1974, Enabling Systems.
2. Bullough B: Subjective reports of female orgasmic expulsion of fluid, *Nurse Pract* 9:55-59, 1984.
3. Erickson GP, Jones JA: Osteoporosis risk assessment of mature working women, *AAOHN* 40(9):423-428, 1992.
4. DHHS/PHS: *Heathy people 2000: summary report,* Boston, 1992, Jones & Bartlett.
5. Fishbein EG: Women at midlife—the transition to menopause, *Nurs Clin North Am* 27(4):951-957, 1992.
6. Fleming LA: Osteoporosis: clinical features, prevention and treatment, *J Gen Inter Med* 7:554-558, 1992.
7. Hay EK: That old hip—the osteoporosis process, *Nurs Clin North Am* 26(1):43-51, 1991.
8. Kaplan FS: Prevention and treatment of osteoporosis, *Hosp Med* 27(3):65-77, 1991.
9. Kinsey AC: *Sexual behavior in the human male,* Philadelphia, 1948, WB Saunders.
10. Liscum B: Osteoporosis: the silent disease, *Orthop Nurs* 11(4):21-25, 1992.
11. Maddox MA: Women at midlife—hormone replacement therapy, *Nurs Clin North Am* 27(4):959-969, 1992.
12. Masters W, Johnson V: *Human sexual response,* Boston, 1966, Little, Brown & Co.
13. McCraw RK: Psychosexual changes associated with the perimenopausal period, *J Nurse Midwife* 36(1):17-23, 1991.
14. National Osteoporosis Foundation: *Boning up on osteoporosis,* Washington DC, 1990, The Foundation.
15. Scharbo-DeHaan M, Brucker MC: The perimenopausal period, *J Nurse Midwife* 36(1):9-15, 1991.
16. Tolstoi LG, Levin RM: Osteoporosis—the treatment controversy, *Nutr Today* 27(4):6-12, 1992.
17. Wilbur J et al: The relationship among menopausal status, menopausal symptoms and physical activity in midlife women, *Fam Community Health* 13(3):67-78, 1990.
18. World Health Organization: *Education and treatment in human sexuality,* Geneva, Switzerland, 1975, The Organization.
19. Youngkin EQ: Estrogen replacement therapy and the estraderm transdermal system, *Nurse Pract* 15(5):19-31, 1990.

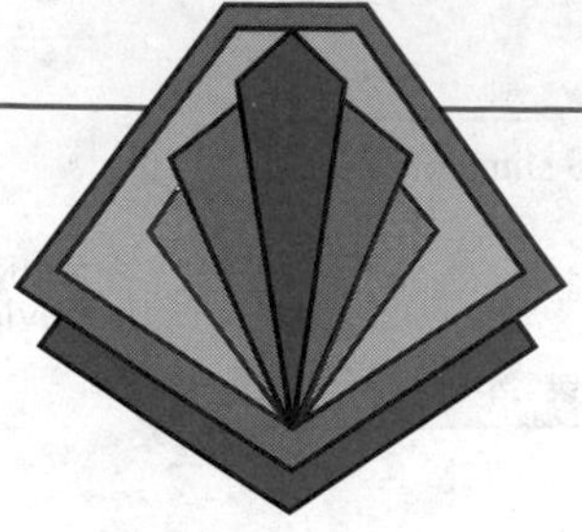

CHAPTER 12

# Alterations in Consciousness in the Hospitalized Adult

**Helen A. Schaag**

## CHAPTER OBJECTIVES

***After studying this chapter, the learner should be able to do the following:***

1. Describe the sensory process, particularly explaining the role of the reticular formation.
2. Differentiate between level of consciousness or arousal and content of consciousness or awareness.
3. Identify the four states and six stages of consciousness.
4. Differentiate the two types of confusion.
5. Identify how depression can mask the behaviors associated with acute or chronic confusion.
6. Describe the behaviors usually associated with acute confusion and delirium.
7. Explain the association between acute confusion and alterations in consciousness.
8. Describe the behaviors associated with chronic confusion and dementia.
9. Explain the association between chronic confusion and alterations in consciousness.
10. Identify four broad causes of alterations in consciousness and one or two specific pathologies for each cause.
11. Identify the most common etiologies of alterations in level of consciousness, acute confusion or delirium, and chronic confusion or dementia.
12. Assess the consequences of sensory overload and sensory deprivation for the elderly patient.
13. Discuss the management for patients experiencing an alteration in level or content of consciousness.
14. List the major laboratory tests for patients with alterations in level of consciousness or acute confusion.
15. Discuss the nursing assessment and immediate management of a person at high risk for changes in level of consciousness.
16. Discuss the nursing assessment and management for patients experiencing an alteration in content of consciousness.
17. Identify five key interventions to protect from injury the patient with alterations in level or content of consciousness.

## KEY TERMS

acute confusion
alertness
arousal
awareness
chronic confusion
confusion
consciousness
content of consciousness
delirium
dementia
depression
disorientation
level of consciousness (LOC)
perception
perceptual deprivation
reticular activating system (RAS)
reticular formation (RF)
sensory deprivation
sensory overload
unconsciousness

Managing persons with actual or potential changes in consciousness is a frequent role of nurses working with ill adults. Changes in consciousness may result from factors in the health care setting, from underlying illnesses, or from a combination of both. The purpose of this chapter is to explore acute and chronic changes in consciousness, identify causes common to hospitalized adults, and discuss selected aspects of medical and nursing management.

## SENSORY PROCESS

Persons continuously interact with their internal and external environments. Their boundaries, as unique systems, have been developmentally defined through their sensory apparatuses. It is through their senses that persons learn to distinguish themselves as separate entities.

Because sensation is such an integral part of the ability to perceive and interact with the external environment, it follows that any alterations of sensation will result in the potential for system disequilibrium. As open systems, persons constantly receive input or cues from the external environment. If this input were suddenly diminished or increased radically in some way, the normal method of receiving environmental cues would be affected and adaptation would be necessary. If an individual is unable to adapt, disequilibrium results.

The reception and organization of stimuli are collectively known as *sensory perception.* The process of sensory perception depends on several factors: a stimulus, adequate sensory receptors, intact neural pathways, and adequate processing by the brain to interpret the stimulus input.

Stimuli are received by sensory receptors, which then synapse with cranial or peripheral nerves. These nerves then synapse either with sensory nerve tracts in the spinal cord or with neuronal structures of the brain. The exact mechanism by which the brain interprets sensory input is not known. However, it is known that rather than experiencing sensory stimuli individually and discretely, multiple stimuli are integrated into a single perception; for example, one can identify perfusion to skin just by touch. It is also known that the **reticular formation (RF)** has an integral role in processing sensory input.

The organization of the RF is vague; however, it does contain some distinct nuclei with long, overlapping fibers and dendrites. The RF network of neurons extends from the medulla of the lower brainstem up to the thalamus in the diencephalon. Within the RF is the **reticular activating system (RAS).** This is a special core of gray matter that begins in the midpons and extends into the hypothalamus and thalamus. Impulses from the RAS are necessary for arousal. General central nervous system (CNS) activity and selectivity of arousal, awareness, and attention are controlled by the RF. In addition, conscious behavior depends on an intact, functioning cerebrum.

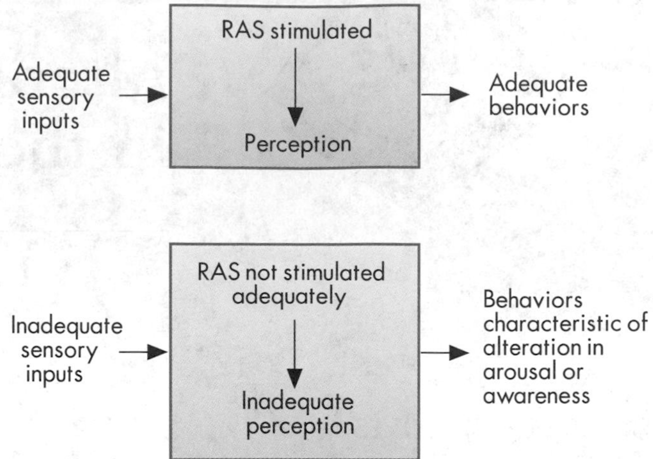


**FIGURE 12-1** Relationship between sensory inputs and outcome. *RAS,* Reticular activating system.

The RF can be stimulated by two major sources of stimuli, external and internal. External stimuli include cortical impulses and input from tactile, visual, auditory, and olfactory sources; internal stimuli include input from somatic and visceral sources (muscles, joints).

The RF serves a monitoring function for both input and output to the human system. It is believed that the RF, in conjunction with other structures, collects and combines sensory input. **Perception** takes place when the sensory input is received, decoded (synthesized), and interpreted by the cortex. When interpretation occurs, a conscious awareness of sensation begins. Perception provides the individual with an awareness of the external environment, which then serves as a basis for determining what response is required to maintain equilibrium.

It is important to note that without the function of the RF, perception and thus interpretation do not occur. For example, in a person under barbiturate anesthesia, the sensory pathways can conduct messages to the primary receiving areas but discrimination and perception do not occur. Thus it is seen that the RF not only has an important role in providing a mechanism for general arousal and alertness of the individual, but also must be stimulated for perception and awareness to take place.

If sensory input is adequate and the RF is functioning and is stimulated, an alert, aroused state is created in the individual. If the RF is inadequately stimulated or not functioning, restlessness, listlessness, drowsiness, disorientation, confusion, and so on occur (Figure 12-1). From a systems perspective, the stimulus serves as an input; the sensory receptors, neural pathways, and cerebral decoding necessary for processing are "throughput," and the resulting adaptive response or behavior of the individual is "output" (Figure 12-2).

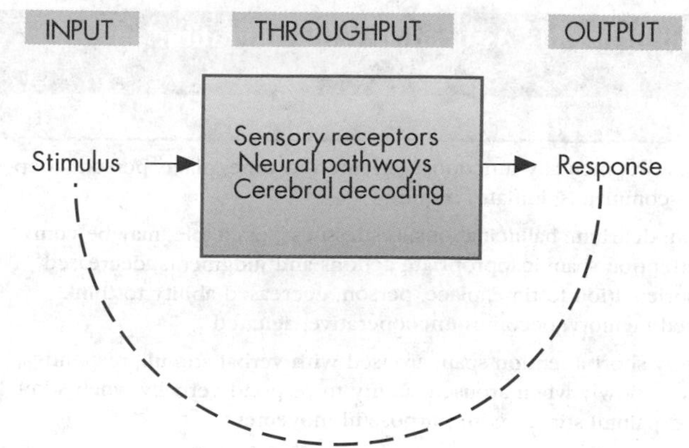


**FIGURE 12-2** Sensory process from a systems perspective.

## CONSCIOUSNESS AND ALTERATIONS IN CONSCIOUSNESS

The conscious state refers to a state of being in which the patient is able to respond to sensory stimuli, has subjective experiences, exercises will, and is capable of thought and reasoning. **Consciousness** may be defined as self-awareness, awareness of the external environment, the ability to function mentally and physically in a manner appropriate to the level of one's normal ability, and the ability to experience life to the fullest degree. The cerebrum has the central role in these higher functions.

**Unconsciousness** implies that there is an impairment in response to sensory stimuli; no thinking, feelings, or emotions are apparent. The unconscious person is not aware of what is going on in the environment and may not be arousable with any stimuli. Between these two extremes are various other states and stages of consciousness.

The two aspects of consciousness that must be considered are **arousal/alertness** or level and awareness or content.[10] **Arousal** or **level of consciousness (LOC)** is a physiologic function associated with wakefulness. It involves a primitive set of responses located entirely within the brainstem and synchronized by a network of fibers of the RAS. **Awareness** or **content of consciousness** is the sum of all cognitive and affective functions. Awareness involves a higher level integration of multiple sensory input that allows meaningful understanding of self and environment.

When an insult or its effect impinges on the RF, consciousness is altered. As the severity of the insult increases, there is increasing impairment of responsiveness to events in the internal and external environments. The nurse caring for the ill adult must be able to identify persons at high risk for alterations in level or content of consciousness, identify subtle changes in behavior indicating impairment in consciousness, and intervene as appropriate. The conscious state cannot be measured directly, but only through behavior. Any impairment, reduction, or absence of consciousness indicates a serious dysfunction of the brain in terms of level or content of consciousness.

### ALTERATIONS IN LEVEL OF CONSCIOUSNESS

The nurse will work with patients who have temporary or permanent decreases in LOC or arousal, as well as with persons who are at risk for changes in LOC because of injury, illness, or exogenous agents. Every patient with head trauma or other intracranial problems is at risk for impairment in LOC. In addition, temperature alterations, metabolic disturbances, hypoxic conditions, and multiple drugs may alter LOC.

Although it is better to avoid labels, the nurse must have an understanding of the gradations of LOC, that is, the degrees of behavior between consciousness or arousal/alertness and unconsciousness or deep coma. LOC frequently is divided into four states: conscious-aware, clouded consciousness, semiconscious-semicomatose, and unconscious-comatose. These four states are further divided into six stages:

1. Alertness
2. Confusion
3. Drowsiness
4. Stupor
5. Light coma
6. Deep coma

Particular behaviors have been identified for each stage (Table 12-1). The behaviors listed are those identified in the clinical setting. The use of the different labels for states and stages allows for succinct, clearer communication among caregivers.

### ALTERATIONS IN CONTENT OF CONSCIOUSNESS

Normal awareness or content of consciousness allows for meaningful interaction with the external environment. Alteration in awareness may occur in the presence of a clear or clouded LOC. Alterations in awareness or content of consciousness may precede alterations in LOC and may or may not progress to alterations in LOC.

Alterations in content of consciousness or awareness may be acute or chronic in nature. Box 12-1 presents some of the more common labels used to describe alterations in content of consciousness or awareness. The next section presents more detailed information on the concepts of confusion, acute confusion, delirium, chronic confusion, and dementia.

#### Confusion

**Confusion** is an ambiguous term that in its broadest sense defines a state of alteration in LOC or arousal *and*

**TABLE 12-1 Common Labels To Describe States, Stages, and Behaviors Associated With Alterations in Consciousness**

| STATE | STAGE | BEHAVIORS |
|---|---|---|
| Conscious-aware | Alert | Normal activity; aware, mentally functional; oriented to time, place, person; cooperative; follows commands; initiates requests |
| Clouded consciousness | Confused | Poor coordination; delirium; hallucinations; restlessness; excitable; may be combative; short attention span; inappropriate actions and judgments; decreased awareness; disorientation to time, place, person; decreased ability to think clearly; impaired memory; becomes uncooperative; agitated |
| Semiconscious/semicomatose | Obtunded, drowsy | Sleepy/listless; very short attention span; aroused with verbal stimuli; responds appropriately but slowly when aroused; ability to respond verbally when stimulated; fends off painful stimuli with purposeful movement |
| | Stupor | Apathetic; slow-moving; blank expression; drooping head; staring; arousal only to vigorous stimuli; incomplete arousal to painful stimuli; no verbal response or moaning; response to verbal communication inconsistent and vague |
| Unconscious/comatose | Light coma | Response only by grimace or withdrawing limb from pain; primitive and disorganized response to painful stimuli |
| | Deep coma | Absence of response to even most painful stimuli; no reflex response |

**BOX 12-1 Labels Applied to Acute or Chronic Alterations in Awareness or Content of Consciousness**

**ACUTE ALTERATIONS**

Acute confusion
Delirium
Encephalopathy
Organic mental disorder
Psychosis (intensive care unit [ICU] or postcardiotomy)
Toxic brain syndrome
Toxic confusional state

**CHRONIC ALTERATIONS**

Chronic confusion
Dementia
Organic mental disorder
Sundowner syndrome

a state of alteration in content of consciousness or awareness. In a more narrow sense, it is used to describe behaviors characteristic of selected pathologic states. Although any person who is acutely ill can experience confusion, the exact incidence of confusion is unknown. The following data provide an appreciation of the potential magnitude of the problem of confusion.

Confusion occurs more often in persons older than 65 years. Approximately 50% of adults in acute care hospitals are older than 65. Thus the incidence of confusion in these older adults can be a significant problem for any hospital because an estimated 20% to 80% of persons of this age-group in critical care units experience acute confusion during hospitalization.[4,6,8] In addition, data indicate that those patients who experience acute confusion are five times more likely to die than those patients who do not.[13] It is estimated that chronic confusion or dementia affects as many as 10% of Americans over age 65.[12]

One of the reasons the incidence of confusion may be underestimated is that depression can occur as a comorbid problem with confusion. Symptoms associated with depression such as changes in sleep patterns, psychomotor alterations, and decreased attention span may mask confusion (Box 12-2). This overlapping of symp-

**BOX 12-2 Diagnostic Criteria for a Major Depressive Episode**

A. Presence of at least *five* of the following symptoms during the same 2-week period, representing a change from previous functioning; must include at least *one of the first two* symptoms:
 1. Depressed mood
 2. Greatly diminished interest or pleasure
 3. Significant weight loss or weight gain
 4. Insomnia or hypersomnia
 5. Psychomotor agitation or retardation
 6. Fatigue
 7. Feelings of worthlessness or excessive guilt
 8. Decreased concentration
 9. Recurrent thoughts of death or suicide
B. Symptoms do not meet criteria for a mixed episode
C. Symptoms cause clinically significant distress in functioning
D. Symptoms are not the result of the physiologic effect of substance or general medical condition or of bereavement

Modified from American Psychiatric Association: *Diagnostic and statistical manual of mental disorders,* ed 4 rev, Washington, DC, 1994, The Association.

**BOX 12-3 Manifestations of Acute Confusion**

- Decreased attention span
- Memory loss
- Disorientation
- Disorganized thinking
- Distorted perception
- Disturbed sleep-wake cycles
- Fluctuating levels of alertness ranging from clouded consciousness to stupor
- Altered psychomotor behavior, including agitation and restlessness or lethargy
- Inappropriate actions or judgment

**RESEARCH**

Yeaw EMJ, Abbate JH: Identification of confusion among the elderly in an acute care setting, *Clin Nurs Specialist* 7:192-197, 1993.

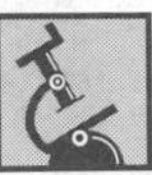

This descriptive study was conducted with a group of 25 staff nurses on medical-surgical units at a large acute care hospital to determine (1) what descriptors were used by staff nurses to arrive at a diagnosis of confusion and (2) which descriptors were perceived as most significant for diagnosis. These nurses used cognitive descriptors more frequently than behavioral descriptors to describe confusion in elderly persons, although most nurses used a combination. The most frequent descriptors used were disorientation (to time, place, person, date, objects) and inappropriate verbal expression. For more effective assessment and management, a need exists to standardize assessment parameters.

toms decreases the ability of health care professionals to identify confusion correctly. Major depression affects almost 10 million Americans, but more than 70% of those affected never receive treatment.[11] These data reflect the large numbers of patients who potentially may experience confusion during hospitalization and make managing confused patients a real challenge for every health care professional and facility providing care for adults.

### Acute confusion

**Acute confusion** is associated with variable manifestations and varies over time.[3] The major fact about acute confusion is that it is a transient condition lasting from hours to less than a month.[5] When confused, a patient can be alert with some clouding of consciousness and yet perceives phenomena incorrectly; thinking and reasoning are inappropriate, and remembering is difficult. The patient with acute confusion may experience or demonstrate a variety of behaviors. Box 12-3 presents common manifestations of acute confusion. Although the terms *confusion* and *disorientation* are sometimes used interchangeably, acute confusion is defined as a state in which there is transient impairment in content of consciousness with a clouded LOC, whereas **disorientation** is a behavior that indicates confusion. The patient who is unable to identify the season of the year or his or her location is assessed as being disoriented to time and place and labeled as being confused.

Acute confusion has a sudden onset. Behaviors associated with confusion vary and reflect the severity of confusion—from mild confusion to severe confusion. Behaviors associated with mild confusion include poor coordination, short attention span, and disorientation to time, place, and person. These behaviors may be difficult to assess when they first occur because they may be subtle or appear only periodically (see Research box above, right).

Mild acute confusion does not always progress to more severe acute confusion. The most important issue with confusion, regardless of severity, is early detection so the appropriate interventions can be implemented in a timely manner to reserve or minimize the serious effects of acute confusion.

**Delirium** is a term frequently used interchangeably with acute confusion. Behaviors associated with delirium include perceptual disturbances, either ***illusions*** (misinterpretation of sensory impressions) or ***hallucinations*** (false perception with no relation to reality) and significant memory impairment. These behaviors usually develop over a few hours to 1 to 2 days and tend to fluctuate throughout the day, diurnally. Various types of tremors typically are present. Autonomic signs such as flushed face, sweating, increased blood pressure and pulse, and dilated pupils are common with delirium.[1] (See Box 12-4 for criteria used to diagnose delirium.) Etiologic factors for acute confusion, whether mild or severe, are the same.

Unfortunately, it is often difficult for health care professionals to identify the exact onset of acute confusion. The reasons for this delay in diagnosis may result from the following:

1. Although the onset of acute confusion may be abrupt, some behaviors exhibited by the patient may be subtle (depending on the cause).
2. Some health care professionals may have a misconception that being elderly implies a decreased capacity to think clearly, and thus some behaviors may be overlooked.[9]
3. Manifestations of depression or chronic confusion may mimic acute confusion or overshadow behaviors of acute confusion and may result in incorrect labeling and thus incorrect interventions for the patient.[8]

### Chronic confusion

**Chronic confusion** is usually an irreversible change in content of consciousness or awareness without a change

**BOX 12-4 Diagnostic Criteria for Delirium (with multiple etiologic factors)**

A. Disturbance of consciousness with reduced ability to focus, sustain, or shift attention
B. Change in cognition (e.g., memory deficit, disorientation) or development of a perceptual disturbance that is not the result of dementia
C. Disturbance that develops over a short period and tends to fluctuate during the course of the day
D. Evidence (from history, physical examination, or diagnostic results) that the delirium has more than one etiologic factor, such as several medical conditions or a medical condition and withdrawal from or intoxication with a drug*

Modified from American Psychiatric Association: *Diagnostic and statistical manual of mental disorders,* ed 4, Washington, DC, 1994, The Association.

*If evidence supports only substance intoxication, the delirium is labeled as *substance intoxication delirium.* If the underlying medical condition is known and is the single etiologic factor, the delirium is labeled as *delirium caused by a specific medical condition.*

**BOX 12-5 Diagnostic Criteria for Dementia (Alzheimer's type)**

A. Development of multiple cognitive deficits, which include the following:
   1. Memory impairment
   2. At least one of the following cognitive disturbances
      a. Aphasia (language disturbance)
      b. Apraxia (inability to carry out motor activities)
      c. Agnosia (failure to recognize objects)
      d. Disturbance in executive function (e.g., planning, abstracting)
B. Cognitive deficits as described above cause significant disruption and represent a significant decline in functioning
C. Course characterized by gradual onset and continued cognitive decline
D. Cognitive deficits in criteria A-1 and A-2 are *not* caused by the following:
   1. Other CNS conditions that cause progressive deficits in memory and cognition
   2. Systemic conditions that are known to cause dementia
E. Deficits do not occur exclusively during the course of a delirium
F. Disturbance is *not* the result of major psychiatric disorder such as depression or schizophrenia

Modified from American Psychiatric Association: *Diagnostic and statistical manual of mental disorders,* ed 4, Washington, DC, 1994, The Association.

in LOC. This term is most frequently used interchangeably with dementia. **Dementia** is a syndrome characterized by various manifestations.[1] A major characteristic of dementia and chronic confusion is deterioration in intellectual functioning in the presence of a normal LOC. Dementia or chronic confusion progresses over time and causes changes in cognitive function, personality characteristics, and psychomotor behavior. Dementia, although progressing over time, is not always irreversible.[2] Box 12-5 presents the diagnostic criteria for dementia.

A major difficulty facing the nurses working with the patient who is chronically confused or demented is that acute confusion or delirium may occur in the presence of chronic confusion. The manifestations of acute confusion may be subtle and thus may be missed.

## ETIOLOGY

Multiple causes exist for alterations in level or content of consciousness. For this reason, nurses working in many different environments must be able to initiate appropriate assessment to detect alterations in level or content of consciousness and to provide appropriate care for patients with these alterations, regardless of the cause. Box 12-6 presents a summary of the etiologic factors causing alterations in consciousness in general.

Generally, causes of alterations in consciousness can be divided into four broad categories: (1) primary brain injury or disease, (2) systemic conditions, (3) psychologic conditions, or (4) environmental causes. However, the most common etiologies vary depending on the type of alteration in consciousness. The most common causes for changes in LOC or general arousal/alertness are head trauma, hypoxia, anesthetic agents, and acute drug or alcohol intoxication.

The most common causes of acute confusion or delirium are drugs with anticholinergic or CNS effects, systemic infections, sodium and potassium imbalances, and metabolic disturbances.[7] The most common causes of chronic confusion or dementia are Alzheimer's disease, multi-infarct dementia, drug and alcohol toxicity, and endocrine abnormalities.[2] The most common etiologic factors vary with the patient population.[7] In surgical patients, decreased temperature and blood loss are significant etiologic factors; in patients with diabetes mellitus treated with insulin, hypoglycemia is a significant factor; and in patients with human immunodeficiency virus (HIV) infections, acquired immunodeficiency syndrome (AIDS) dementia is a significant factor.

Predisposing factors are important in the occurrence of alterations in consciousness (see first Research box, p. 291). A major predisposing factor for both acute and chronic confusion is age. The number of co-morbid conditions and the severity and length of the illness also are important predisposing factors. Most incidents of acute confusion or delirium have multiple causes. Other predictors of acute confusion are pain, use of narcotics, decreased mobility, and increased number of errors on the mental status test (see second Research box, p. 291).

## PATHOPHYSIOLOGY

The various causes of alterations in consciousness are discussed in detail in the relevant chapters of this book. Next, the four broad categories listed in Box 12-6 are discussed.

**BOX 12-6 Possible Causes of Alterations in Consciousness**

1. Resulting from primary brain injury or disease
   a. Trauma (concussion, contusion, laceration, or traumatic intercerebral hemorrhage, subdural hematoma, epidural hematoma)
   b. Vascular disease (intracerebral hemorrhage, subarachnoid hemorrhage, infarction)
   c. Infections (meningitis, encephalitis, abscess, human immunodeficiency virus [HIV])
   d. Neoplasms (primarily intracranial, metastatic, or nonmetastatic complication of malignancy)
   e. Seizures
   f. Degeneration (Alzheimer's disease)
2. Resulting from systemic conditions that secondarily affect the brain
   a. Metabolic encephalopathies (hypoglycemia, diabetic ketoacidosis, hyperglycemic nonketotic hyperosmolar states, uremia, hepatic encephalopathy, hyponatremia, hypokalemia, myxedema, acid-base imbalances, hypercalcemia)
   b. Urinary or respiratory infections
   c. Hypoxic encephalopathies (severe congestive heart failure with decompensation, severe anemia, hypertensive encephalopathies, hemorrhage)
   d. Toxicity (drugs, especially alcohol, anticholinergics, those with CNS effects)
   e. Physical causes (heatstroke, hypothermia)
   f. Nutritional causes (Wernicke's encephalopathy)
3. Resulting from psychologic causes that affect the brain
   a. Stress
   b. Depression
   c. Anxiety
4. Resulting from environmental conditions that affect the brain
   a. Sensory deprivation
   b. Sensory overload

## PRIMARY BRAIN INJURY OR DISEASE

Alterations in either level or content of consciousness may be the first sign of brain injury or disease. Depending on the rapidity with which structural and functional changes in brain tissue occur with injury or disease, persons may primarily demonstrate changes in awareness (content) or the manifestations may progress rapidly to more severe depression in LOC (arousal). Neurologic injuries or diseases associated with increased intracranial pressure frequently cause the state of consciousness to move from alertness to confusion to obtunded to coma rapidly. If brain injury or disease is severe enough, permanent irreversible loss of cognitive ability may result. Degenerative disease, vascular disease, and HIV infection result in slow but progressive loss of intellectual function.

## SYSTEMIC CONDITIONS

Decreased levels of oxygen or glucose have very rapid, dramatic affects on cerebral function. The brain is extremely sensitive to hypoxia. Only a few seconds of anoxia can lead to altered awareness and decreased LOC.

**RESEARCH**

Williams-Russo P et al: Post-operative delirium: predictors and prognosis in elderly orthopedic patients, *J Am Geriatr Soc* 40:759-767, 1992.

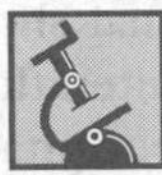

Fifty-one patients underwent bilateral knee replacement under epidural anesthesia. The mean age of 28 women and 23 men was 68 years, with the range from 48 to 84. No patient manifested preoperative dementia. The incidence of acute postoperative delirium was 41%, with a difference that resulted from the type of postoperative analgesic prescribed. Predictors of delirium were age (mean age was 6 years older for delirious group), gender (more men than women), and history of alcohol use (more than three drinks a week). All cases of delirium resolved within 1 week. Length of hospitalization was similar for those who had delirium and those who did not.

**RESEARCH**

Williams M et al: Predictors of acute confusional states in hospitalized elderly patients, *Res Nurs Health* 8:31-40, 1985.

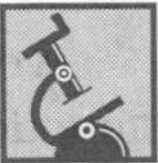

In this study, 170 elderly (mean age, 78.8 years) patients from four hospitals with no prior history of mental impairment were evaluated during the first 5 postoperative days to determine the incidence of acute confusional state. More than half (51.5%) demonstrated some postoperative confusion. On the basis of admission data, older persons, those who made more errors on the mental status test given on admission, and those with lower levels of activity before injury were most likely to experience confusion. In addition, data obtained during the hospitalization also were used to predict confusion. Based on treatment and clinical progress data, the best set of predictors included age and performance on the mental status test, the previous day's confusion score, pain, narcotics, and mobility.

The amount of oxygen available to cells of the cerebral cortex depends on adequacy of blood flow, blood oxygen tension ($PO_2$), hemoglobin concentration, oxygen saturation, and arterial pH. Coma usually results when the $PO_2$ level falls below 25 mm Hg.

*Infections* typically cause depression in LOC and impairment in content of consciousness, particularly in elderly persons. Urinary tract infections and lower respiratory tract infections, the most common sites of nosocomial infections, can produce very subtle behavioral manifestations of acute confusion. The subtle behavioral manifestations include difficulty concentrating, restlessness, and disorientation.

Several metabolic events can precipitate an episode of alteration in level or content of consciousness. *Metabolic encephalopathies,* such as those associated with diabetic ketoacidosis, precipitate many changes in behavior, including inappropriate judgment, decreased awareness, and mental lethargy, which can progress to coma if untreated. Cerebral function is very sensitive to decreased glucose. The CNS has no reserve of glucose and depends on the blood level. Even minimal short-term decreases in serum glucose can result in alterations in awareness or arousal. Hypoglycemia precipitates changes in patient consciousness that may occur rapidly, moving quickly to coma, or that may be subtle and include poor judgment. These changes can prevent the initiation of self-care measures to correct the blood glucose level.

*Alterations in thyroid function* may cause lethargy or depression. *Fluid and electrolyte imbalances* can occur in those patients who are on a regimen of diuretics, who experience acute periods of diarrhea, who become dehydrated from the effects of heat, who depend on others for providing fluids, or who retain abnormal amounts of fluid and electrolytes. All these situations can cause sodium or osmolar imbalance. These changes in sodium or osmolarity can lead to acute or chronic confusion, weakness, and depressed arousal. Potassium changes also can lead to changes in arousal, as well as weakness.

*Hypoxic encephalopathies* result from adverse changes in the cardiopulmonary systems. Malfunctions of the heart and respiratory systems, such as dysrhythmias, congestive heart failure, or chronic obstructive pulmonary disease, affect cardiac output or effective circulatory volume, which leads to diminished cerebral blood flow and acute or chronic confusion or decreased arousal.

*Drug* and *other toxicities* can cause confusion in multiple ways.[17] Drugs can reduce cardiac output or decrease blood glucose levels. Drug toxicity can alter the metabolic activity of brain cells, suppress the respiratory center, or alter the oxygen supply to the brain. The activity of neurotransmitters in the brain and the amino acids needed by the brain can be changed. Importantly, in elderly patients the half-life of many drugs increases, which leads to a higher incidence of drug toxicity. Drugs typically associated with acute or chronic confusion include anticholinergic agents and drugs with CNS effects, such as psychoactive drugs, antihypertensive agents, and CNS depressants, including alcohol.

## PSYCHOLOGIC CAUSES

A common psychologic cause precipitating or mimicking alterations in content or level of consciousness is **depression.** It is important to differentiate depression from confusion as quickly as possible. Typically, the onset of depression is linked to a major change or loss, whereas the onset of acute or chronic confusion may be subtle and uncertain or unrelated to any significant event. The administration of antidepressants frequently can differentiate depression from acute or chronic confusion because the drugs will alter and alleviate the behaviors associated with depression.

*Anxiety* or *stress* also can cause a person to become disoriented, have decreased ability to concentrate, and have altered ability to perceive correctly; thus these two states must be identified as possible causes of acute confusion.

## ENVIRONMENTAL CAUSES

Sensory input affects every hospitalized adult. Any patient in a health care facility is at risk for becoming acutely confused from either sensory overload or sensory deprivation. Information about the environment is gathered through all senses, including vision, hearing, touch, and smell. The term *sensory deprivation* has been used synonymously in the literature with many different terms, ranging from social deprivation to restricted stimulation and solitude. The patient who does not have enough stimuli, either because of poor vision or hearing or because of minimal contact, may sleep all the time or at nonscheduled times. For the purposes of this discussion, **sensory deprivation** is defined as a state of being in which the amount or intensity of sensory input is below the individual's range of tolerance. Tolerance is the unique range each person has for coping with a type of sensation, which promotes healthy functioning.

Deprivation refers to the general concept of decreased sensory input. In the specific case of a reduction in the pattern of meaningfulness of stimuli, the term **perceptual deprivation** is used. It should be emphasized that sensory deprivation and perceptual deprivation refer to a reduction of stimulation from a previous level and not the total absence of stimulation. An example of sensory deprivation is isolation in a room without outside windows. With isolation, the amount

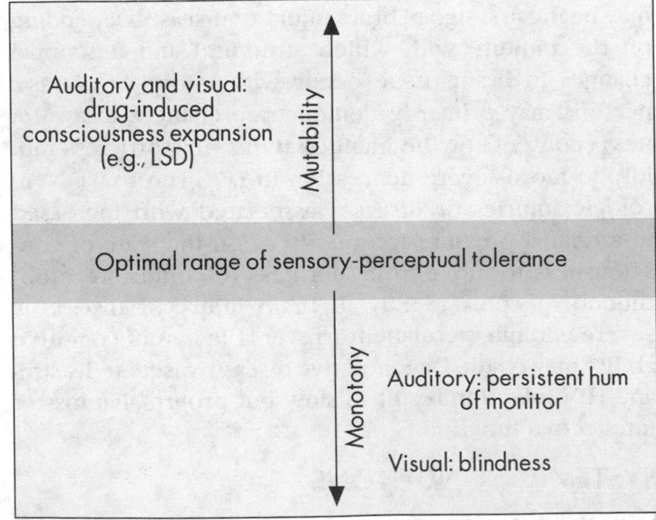


**FIGURE 12-3** Sensory/perceptual deprivation. Change in pattern of sensory input may create mutability or monotony.

of sensory input could be decreased from normal. An example of perceptual deprivation is the consistent hum of a monitor in the intensive care unit (ICU). With a consistent hum, the pattern of the sensory stimuli does not change. Sensory stimuli below the individual's optimal range of tolerance is defined as *monotony* (Figure 12-3).

When sensory input exceeds the optimal range of tolerance, **sensory overload** can occur. The state of being in which the patterning of sensory input is above the optimal range is termed *mutability* (Figure 12-3). When too many stimuli exist—as in ICUs, with overhead pages, loud talking day and night, and lights on 24 hours of day—or when the pattern of sensory input is above the optimal range of tolerance, the patient will not be able to rest and sleep adequately. These situations usually result in patients becoming disoriented, experiencing hallucinations, and becoming combative. Either mild or severe acute confusion can occur with either sensory overload or sensory deprivation.

## MEDICAL MANAGEMENT

Regardless of the underlying etiology and pathophysiology of confusion, some common management techniques must be applied to every patient. Medical management of the patient with actual or potential alteration in LOC or content of consciousness has three primary focuses: (1) that focused on identifying the cause of alterations in consciousness, (2) that directed toward the specific causative factor, and (3) that focused on support of the patient. The first focus of care is implementation of the appropriate diagnostic tests to assist in correctly diagnosing the etiology for the alteration in level or content of consciousness. Diagnostic testing is very important for the patient with a decreased LOC or potential for decreased LOC or for the patient with acute confusion, since these are emergency conditions and, if not identified and treated, can lead to irreversible damage or death. Routine laboratory tests are performed, including those noted in Box 12-7. Diagnostic testing for chronic confusion is important but does not have the same level of emergency.

For patients with alterations of LOC and acute confusion, a toxicology screen is obtained in blood, urine, and gastric aspirate for drugs and alcohol. Other studies that are helpful to determine the cause and nature of primary brain injury or disease include the following:

1. Skull roentgenograms
2. Computed tomographic (CT) scan of the head
3. Magnetic resonance imaging (MRI) of head
4. Lumbar puncture (if there is suspicion of intracranial infection)
5. Electroencephalogram (EEG)
6. Cerebral angiography
7. Evoked potentials

For alterations in LOC or content of consciousness caused by systemic conditions, the patient's history often provides necessary clues to etiologic factors. However, if the cause of alteration in LOC or acute confusion is not apparent, extensive studies of cardiac, respiratory, hepatic, and metabolic functioning may be necessary. For chronic confusion, a thorough history and physical examination constitute the first assessment, followed by general blood hematology and chemistry studies. Specialized tests, particularly of the neurologic system, often are necessary.

The management directed toward the specific etiologic factor is discussed in relevant chapters throughout this text. Supportive care for the patients with altered consciousness involves support of the patient to maintain total body function. This care includes meeting the fluid, electrolyte, metabolic, protective, oxygenation, elimination, skin integrity, comfort, and interaction needs. (See Chapter 57 for a detailed description of diagnostic tests and medical management of neurologic problems and other relevant chapters for management of other diseases.)

**BOX 12-7 Important Laboratory Tests for Patients With Alterations in Consciousness**

**PRIMARY TESTS**

Arterial blood gases
Blood cultures
Blood glucose
Blood urea nitrogen (BUN)
Calcium
Complete blood count (CBC)
Serum creatinine
Serum electrolytes (sodium, potassium, chloride, bicarbonate)
Urinalysis

**SECONDARY TESTS**

Cerebrospinal fluid studies
Liver function tests
Serum enzymes
Serum osmolarity

## NURSING MANAGEMENT

*Assessment* is the major focus of nursing care for persons with actual or at high risk for alterations in LOC or content of consciousness. This assessment must be initiated at the time of admission to provide baseline data for future comparison. Early baseline data can be gathered while other admission data are collected. However, it may be difficult to obtain accurate information from the patient who has alterations in level or content of consciousness. In addition, whatever information is obtained from the patient, essential history should always be obtained from the family or significant other.

Although time is of essence in gathering data, one cannot overlook the importance of establishing rapport and communication with the patient. Pausing a few moments to do this will probably not only reduce the anxiety the patient or family is experiencing, but also produce a more open, nonthreatening data-collecting process. A good way to attract the patient's attention and to provide comfort is through use of touch. Once the contact is made, speak in a calm, quiet, unhurried manner. To help maintain normal awareness or arousal or to minimize anxiety, eliminate other stimuli such as the radio and television, which tend to clutter the sensory field and prevent clear communication between the nurse and patient.

The following data need to be gathered:

1. What may have precipitated the alterations in consciousness
2. Time of onset of changes in consciousness
3. Exact behaviors related to level or content of consciousness present
4. Patient's awareness of condition
5. Presence of manifestations of primary brain injury or disease, such as pain, discomfort, stiff neck, headache, visual changes, focal neurologic deficits, and decreased motor strength
6. Presence of manifestations of any systemic diseases, such as fever, history of infection, alterations in fluid intake and output, nutritional changes, and cardiac, respiratory, hepatic, or endocrine complaints
7. History of head trauma
8. Listing of all patient's medications, prescribed and over the counter, and times of last doses
9. Amount of daily/weekly alcohol intake
10. Exposure to extreme temperatures

In addition to this information, the nurse needs to obtain the following physical examination data for baseline reference:

1. Vital signs
2. Pupillary signs: size, equality, and reactivity
3. Focal motor or sensory signs: presence, symmetry, and character of movements, sensation, eye movements, and reflexes
4. Presence of vomiting or hiccoughing
5. Retinal changes, including papilledema
6. Speech pattern
7. Mental status, including appearance, behavior, language, memory and recall, attention and calculation, and registration
8. Odor of breath (a clue to diabetic ketoacidosis, recent alcohol intake, etc.)

A pattern of reassessment of these eight areas is established. Reassessment at 15- to 60-minute intervals may be necessary. Any changes in these areas are reported immediately. Changes in any of these areas of assessment from baseline help to identify current therapeutic needs, and changes over time help to identify additional therapeutic need.

Frequent observation and examination of the patient must be possible to allow for early detections of changes in alterations in consciousness. Any actual change in sensory/perceptual ability or in thought processes increases the patient's dependency on the nurse to meet basic needs such as safety, nutrition, fluids, elimination, and prevention of infection.

In addition to incorporating the necessary interventions as identified from the previous data, nursing management of the patient with actual or at high risk for alterations in level or content of consciousness also focuses on the following ***nursing diagnoses:***

Injury, high risk for
Sensory/perceptual alterations: input deficit
Sensory/perceptual alterations: input excess
Thought processes, impaired
Knowledge deficit
Anxiety (degree)

A major focus of care is patient safety and prevention of injuries. Patients with acute confusion or delirium may put themselves at danger by pulling at tubes, lines, or catheters or climbing out of bed. Some patients may become very agitated. For patients with chronic confusion, climbing out bed and wandering are two behaviors that put them at risk for injury. For the acutely confused patient, explaining about tubes, moving devices out of the ranges of vision, covering intravenous lines as much as possible, and using touch are some of the ways to decrease anxiety and agitation and increase awareness. For patients who wander, exercise and stimulation can help decrease the wandering behavior.

The overall philosophy to achieve safety is to prevent injury using the least restrictive device to protect the patient. If the presence of side rails disturbs the patient, as they sometimes do, a judgment must be made whether to use them and risk increased agitation or not use them and risk a fall. It may be necessary to use a bed-check alarm device or place the patient on continuous observation. Importantly, most patients with alterations in LOC, acute confusion, or chronic confusion can be protected without the use of physical or chemical restraints.

When alterations in sensory/perceptual or thought processes, as well as anxiety, are present, frequent nurse-patient contact and frequent reorientation to the environment are necessary. A quiet, calm environment will decrease worsening of changes in consciousness and anxiety. To maintain orientation, explain in advance what you will do. Include the patient as much as possible in planning and discussions; however, it is advisable to keep decision making at a minimum for the patient with alterations in consciousness. See that the room is well lighted. Keep a large calendar and clock in view. Talk slowly and distinctly and use short statements. Face the patient and stay within a conversational distance of 4 feet. When talking with the patient, apply the principles as described earlier. When possible, provide consistency by having the same staff members care for the patient every day.

The nurse can decrease the onset of acute confusion by recognizing environmental stimuli likely to precipi-

## RESEARCH

Williams M et al: Reducing acute confusional states in elderly patients with hip fractures, *Res Nurs Health* 8:329-337, 1985.

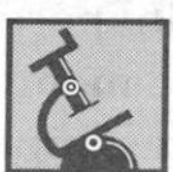

Interpersonal and environmental nursing interventions were carried out with 57 elderly (older than 60 years) patients on orthopedic units in three hospitals to reduce the incidence of acute confusional state. Preventive approaches were related to strange environment, altered sensory input, loss of control and independence, disruption in elimination patterns. Ameliorative approaches were related to mild behaviors suggestive of confusion, sundowning, unsafe behavior, hallucinations or illusions, and fright. The overall incidence of confusion was 51.5% for the nonintervention sample and 43.9% for the intervention sample. The difference was especially apparent for moderate to severe confusion, for which the incidence rates for the nonintervention and intervention groups were 16% and 8.8%, respectively.

tate acute confusion and teaching the patient and staff how to eliminate or reduce these stimuli. Emphasize to the patient and family that physical and environmental factors are contributing to the acute confusion, fears, and memory loss; reassure the patient that the confusional state will eventually pass. Preventing both sensory and perceptual deprivation or overload is critical. Keeping the environment simplified and well organized, placing noisy machines as far from the patient's head as possible, dimming lights to facilitate sleep, organizing care to provide the longest possible sleep periods, placing familiar personal objects within view, and using touch judiciously are some measures that will decrease environmental stimuli that predispose to acute confusion (see Research box, above).

Knowledge deficit may be a major problem. Because most alterations in consciousness in hospitalized adults are acute situations with many interventions being initiated rapidly, the patient needs clear, concise explanations of what is happening, what is to be done, why, when, and so on. If the patient has a high anxiety level, a decreased LOC, or altered content of consciousness, teaching must be repetitive. Information must be given in clear, simple terms and in small amounts. In general, some teaching can be accomplished with a patient who has alterations in consciousness. Family members also need much help and understanding, as well as teaching about the disease process and care involved. Help family members or significant others to understand what is happening and what such behavior might imply. Let them know that their presence provides a familiar stabilizing force. Let them make plans for the patient's care in the hospital and at home. Support their decisions as much as possible.

(See Guidelines box above, right, for a summary of care for the patient with altered level or content of consciousness.)

### Guidelines for Nursing Care of Persons With Alteration in Consciousness

1. Promote communication.
   a. Touch may be useful to establish communication.
   b. Use calm, quiet, and unhurried voice to talk to patient.
   c. Talk slowly and distinctly and use short sentences.
   d. Face patient when talking and stay within conversational range.
2. Promote orientation.
   a. Explain procedures in advance.
   b. Environment should be well lighted.
   c. Keep large calendar and clock in view.
   d. Introduce self when caring for patient.
   e. Keep sensory stimulation to a minimum.
   f. Provide consistency in staff members caring for patient.
   g. Keep decision making to a minimum.
3. Support family.

## FUTURE CONCERNS

Several reasons explain the increased incidence of alteration in consciousness in hospitalized patients. First, the largest growing group of persons consists of those older than 65 years, and the fastest growing segment is composed of those 85 years and older. At least 50% of all adult patients in hospitals are older than 65. Thus the largest number of hospitalized patients are elderly persons. Second, many of these older patients have multiple diagnoses and are undernourished or malnourished. Their general conditions easily become compromised. All these factors predispose to the occurrence of acute confusion. The incidence of chronic confusion or dementia is age related; the older the person, the greater the possibility for dementia to occur. Thus, there will be more patients in hospitals who experience acute confusion and more patients who have dementia.

Nurses need to be knowledgeable about the care needs and problems common to the elderly patient. The focus of this knowledge must be on the special needs of the elderly patient and how to assess and implement nursing interventions to make the hospitalization safe and uncomplicated.

## QUESTIONS TO CONSIDER

- How would you assess a patient's level of cognition?
- How would you design the care for an adult who is admitted with a current history of excessive alcohol consumption?
- How would you design the care for an adult who has a diagnosis of dementia? What would you consider the most difficult aspect of this patient's care?
- What are some sources of sensory overload or sensory deprivation in your clinical environment?

## CRITICAL THINKING ACTIVITIES

- While working on a medical-surgical unit, you are assigned to care for four patients: Mr. Wayne, 69, is being treated for respiratory failure secondary to COPD; Mrs. Janes, 53, is being treated for diverticulitis; Mr. Russell, 37, is recovering from a colon resection; and Mrs. Cordera, 79, was admitted for control of her diabetes. Which, if any of your patients should be observed for behaviors that may indicate the development of confusion or a change in level of consciousness? Support your choice(s).
- Ms. Lynn was admitted to the hospital for pneumonia. While obtaining Ms. Lynn's history from her daughter, you learn that Ms. Lynn has suffered dementia for several years and is unable to care for herself or be left alone. During the course of her hospitalization, Ms. Lynn frequently is incontinent of urine and stool and cries when she soils herself. You observe that she often babbles nonsensical words for a while just before being incontinent. What is your assessment of this situation, and what could you do to assist Ms. Lynn?

## CHAPTER SUMMARY

### CONSCIOUSNESS AND ALTERATIONS IN CONSCIOUSNESS

- Consciousness is the process of awareness of the self and the environment.
- Impaired consciousness may result from conditions that depress or destroy the brainstem or the cerebrum.
- Arousal or level of consciousness is a physiologic function associated with wakefulness.
- Awareness is the sum of all cognitive and affective functions of the body.
- The presence of consciousness depends on a normally functioning interplay among certain neurons, the brain, and the reticular activating system (RAS).
- Stages of LOC are alertness, confusion, drowsiness, stupor, light coma, and deep coma.
- Alterations in content of the consciousness or awareness result in acute or chronic confusion.
- Depression may mask confusion because of overlapping behaviors.
- Alterations in content of consciousness may be associated with alterations in LOC or may occur alone.
- Acute confusion or delirium has a sudden onset, is transient, and is associated with changes in attention, memory loss, disorientation, impairment in thinking and judgment, sleep-cycle alterations, and altered psychomotor activity.
- Manifestations of acute confusion vary within the same person, throughout the day, among patients, and with different etiologic factors.
- Delirium is a term used interchangeably with acute confusion, particularly severe acute confusion.
- Delirium is diagnosed based on the presence of a complex set of manifestations, including decreased attention, disorganized thinking, disturbance in perceptions, disturbance in sleep patterns, impaired memory, sudden onset, and presence of actual or presumptive etiologic factors.
- Chronic confusion or dementia is a progressive loss of cognitive ability.
- Dementia is a symptom complex manifested by loss of memory, impairment in thinking and judgment, disturbance in higher cortical function, changes in personality, interference with social and work activities, occurrence in the absence of delirium, and evidence of actual or presumptive causative factors.
- The subsequent course of dementia depends on the etiologic factor.

### ETIOLOGY

- The causes of alterations in level or content of consciousness can be categorized into primary brain injury or disease, systemic conditions that secondarily affect the brain, psychologic causes, and environmental conditions.
- The primary causes of alterations in LOC are head injury, hypoxia, anesthetic agents, and acute drug or alcohol intoxication.
- The major cause of acute confusion is drug toxicity, respiratory and urinary tract infections, and electrolyte imbalances.
- Chronic confusion or dementia most frequently results from Alzheimer's disease or cerebrovascular changes.
- Aging is a major predisposing factor for acute or chronic confusion.

### MEDICAL MANAGEMENT

- Medical management of the patient with alteration in consciousness focuses on identifying the causes, treating the etiologic factors, and supporting the patient.

### NURSING MANAGEMENT

- Nursing focuses first on assessment, particularly emphasizing behaviors, presence of neurologic or systemic diseases, drug and alcohol intake, neurologic physical examination, and mental status examination.
- Baseline assessment data is essential to compare with changes in any future data; this includes objective data and subjective data from patient and family members.
- Important nursing measures for the patient with altered level or content of consciousness include maintaining stimulation, nutrition, elimination, circulation, safety, activity, skin integrity, normal body temperature, and good hygiene.

- Although the unconscious or confused patient may not be aware of the severity of the situation, family members or significant others are aware and need support and education.
- With depressed levels of consciousness or acute or chronic confusion, it is essential for the nurse to provide a safe environment for the patient and protect from self-injury.
- Maintain a calm environment with appropriate stimuli to reduce the possibility of precipitating confusion states.

### FUTURE CONCERNS

- The growing elderly population and the high percentage of patients over age 65 in hospitals demand attention from health care providers to care appropriately for these patients, who are at high risk for becoming confused during their hospitalization.

## REFERENCES


1. American Psychiatric Association: *Diagnostic and statistical manual of mental disorders,* ed 4, Washington, DC, 1994, The Association.
2. Davies HD: Dementia and delirium. In Chenitz WC, Stone JT, Salisbury SA, editors: *Clinical gerontological nursing,* Philadelphia, 1991, WB Saunders.
3. Foreman MD: Acute confusional states in the hospitalized elderly: a research dilemma, *Nurs Res* 35:34-38, 1986.
4. Foreman MD: Confusion: incidence, onset and associated factors, *Res Nurs Health* 12:21-29, 1989.
5. Foreman MD: The cognitive and behavioral nature of acute confusional states, *Scholarly Inquiry Nurs Pract* 5(1):3-16, 1991.
6. Foreman MD: Adverse psychologic responses of the elderly to critical illness, *AACN J* 3(1):64-72, 1992.
7. Foreman MD: Acute confusion in the elderly. In Fitzpatrick J, Stevenson JS, editors: *Annual review of nursing research,* New York, 1993, Springer.
8. Foreman MD, Gillies DA, Wagner D: Impaired cognition in the critically ill elderly patient: clinical implications, *Crit Care Nurs Q* 12(1):61-73, 1989.
9. Lipowski ZJ: *Delirium: acute confusional states,* New York, 1990, Oxford University.
10. Plum F, Posner JB: *Diagnosis of stupor and coma,* Philadelphia, 1980, FA Davis.
11. Simpson SG, DePaulo JR Jr: Are you recognizing depression in your patients? *Postgrad Med* 94(3):85-93, 1993.
12. Stewart JT: Managing the care of patients with dementia, *Postgrad Med* 90(4):45-49, 1991.
13. Weddington WW Jr: The mortality of delirium: an underappreciated problem, *Psychosomatics* 23:1232-1235, 1982.
14. Williams M et al: Predictors of acute confusion states in hospitalized elderly patients, *Res Nurs Health* 8:31-40, 1985.
15. Williams M et al: Reducing acute confusional states in elderly patients with hip fractures, *Res Nurs Health* 8:329-337, 1985.
16. Williams-Russo P et al: Post-operative delirium: predictors and prognosis in elderly orthopedic patients, *J Am Geriatr Soc* 40:759-767, 1992.
17. Wolanin MD, Phillips LR: *Confusion: prevention and care,* St Louis, 1981, Mosby.
18. Yeaw EMJ, Abbate JH: Identification of confusion among the elderly in an acute care setting, *Clin Nurs Specialist* 7:192-197, 1993.

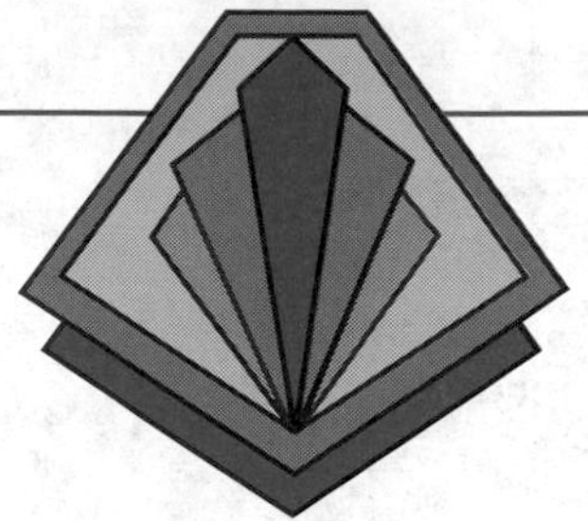

CHAPTER 13

# Inflammatory and Immune Responses

***Anita L. Wingate***
***E. Ronald Wright***

## CHAPTER OBJECTIVES

***After studying this chapter, the learner should be able to do the following:***

1 Differentiate between the concepts of self and nonself.
2 Identify the external and internal nonspecific biologic defense mechanisms.
3 Describe the mechanism and function of the complement cascade.
4 Describe the steps of the inflammatory process and biologic basis of symptoms.
5 Define immunogens and immunoglobulins, and identify the site, structure, and function of each immunoglobulin.
6 Identify the cells involved in the provision of specific immune responses and their genesis, location, and function.
7 Describe the humoral and cell-mediated immune responses, and differentiate between primary and secondary immune responses.
8 Explain the immunologic bases for passive and active immunizations, cancer, human immunodeficiency virus (HIV) infection, tissue transplantation, and monoclonal antibodies.

## KEY TERMS

active immunization
antibodies
antigen-presenting cell
antigen-processing cell
antigens
carrier
cell-mediated system
cellular exudation
complement
cytokines
external
fluid exudation
humorally mediated system
immune response
immune tolerance
immunogens
immunoglobulins
inflammation
interferons
internal
microbial antagonism
mononuclear phagocytic system
nonself
nonspecific
passive immunization
pathogenic
phagocytic
self
skin
specific
susceptibility

## CONCEPT OF BIOLOGIC DEFENSE

The human body exists in a milieu of antagonistic environmental forces that are constantly attacking and threatening its integrity. In response to these onslaughts, the body exhibits a wide array of adaptations (structures, mechanisms, responses) designed to provide a defense against these threats and to protect the body from both external and internal deleterious agents. This chapter deals with those anatomic and biologic mechanisms that provide protection against environmental factors that physically threaten the patient's body. The implications and applications of the functions of these systems also are discussed.

Knowledge of the basic structures and mechanisms that provide this protection helps in the understanding of (1) resistance to infectious disease, (2) diagnosis of disease and physiologic state, (3) rejection of tissue transplants, (4) prevention of the development of malignant growths, (5) adaptations in the aging process, (6) immunization against infectious disease, (7) expression of disease of autoimmunity or immunodeficiency, (8) development of allergic reaction, and (9) significance of the localized or systemic inflammatory re-

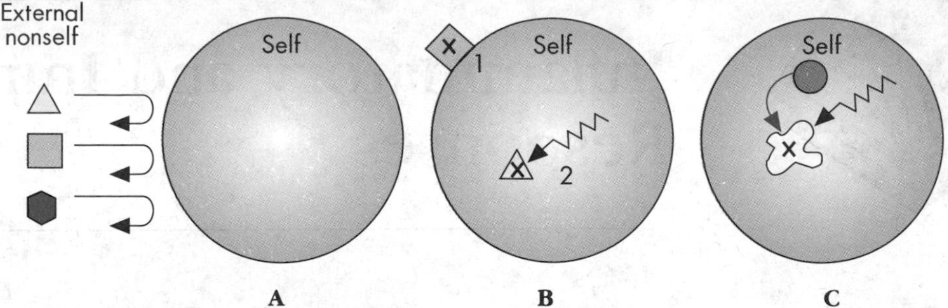


**FIGURE 13-1** Mechanisms of biologic defense in the human body. **A,** Exclusion of external nonself. **B,** Destruction of external nonself by *(1)* nonspecific external mechanisms and *(2)* nonspecific or specific internal mechanisms. **C,** Destruction of altered self. *X* indicates nonspecific mechanisms; → indicates specific mechanisms.

sponse. Much of preventive and restorative nursing practice is built on the maintenance or restoration of the cells, systems, and mechanisms that provide defenses against harmful factors in the external and internal environment.

## SELF VERSUS NONSELF

Each human being can be regarded as a genetically and immunologically unique collection of cells and molecules that make up a biologic unit of **self.** It is the function of the biologic defense mechanisms of the body to protect the integrity of self from encroachment by **nonself** (or foreign) materials. These mechanisms (Figure 13-1) serve to protect the self from both external and internal destructive agents in the following ways:

1. *Exclusion* of harmful agents from the body
2. *Recognition* of harmful agents within the body
3. *Response* designed to dispose of the harmful agents that gain access to the body

The sources of these harmful nonself materials are generally external. These external agents include nonliving materials of the environment such as potentially harmful inorganic chemicals and compounds produced by other living organisms. The most serious external threats to biologic integrity, however, come from the living organisms that constantly surround the body. Some of these organisms pose no real threat because the mechanical, biochemical, and metabolic processes of the human body will not support them or offer them shelter. There are myriad living forms, on the other hand, for which the human body is an ideal haven for growth and survival. Most of these organisms, if allowed to penetrate the body, would wreak havoc on the normal functionings of the body. The living forms that come to mind in this regard are the organisms classified as **pathogenic** (disease-causing). Although the progress of these organisms in the body can be altered by external agents such as antibiotics, the eradication of the offending organism from the body must be accomplished by the host's own adaptive mechanisms.

In addition to protection against external agents, the defense mechanisms also offer protection against the accumulation of damaged or dysfunctional self material. Without these processes to carry out the systematic, specific removal of damaged or worn-out cellular material, the body would become clogged with debris. Another general function of these systems is recognition of a self's alteration to a potentially dangerous state. When this defense function falters, the tragedy of malignancy (cancer) may result.

## RECOGNITION OF SELF FROM NONSELF

The preceding discussion shows that a critical feature of the protective mechanisms of the human body's immune response system is the ability to discriminate between self and nonself materials. This is accomplished by certain specific protein molecules embedded in the cell membrane of all human body cells, which serve as a cellular fingerprint because the proteins are unique to that individual (Figure 13-2). The recognition process then occurs at the cell membrane surface. Immunoresponsive cells (lymphocytes) have specific protein molecules embedded in their membranes that recognize foreign (nonself) proteins. A person's own immunoresponsive cells recognize nonself proteins on cells that are genetically different, and this triggers a sequence of cellular reactions within the immune response system. This sequence of cellular reactions leads to the elaboration of materials and cells that attack the nonself materials. Contact with self proteins (markers) does not produce an immune attack; that is, there is self-tolerance. This explains why cells from different species or genetically dissimilar members of the same species cannot be transplanted from one host to another without triggering an immunologic attack and rejection of the tissue.

In summary, immune system cells have a unique ability to examine the cell surface proteins on any cell or organism with which they come in contact. They interpret these cell surface proteins as either self or nonself and react accordingly.

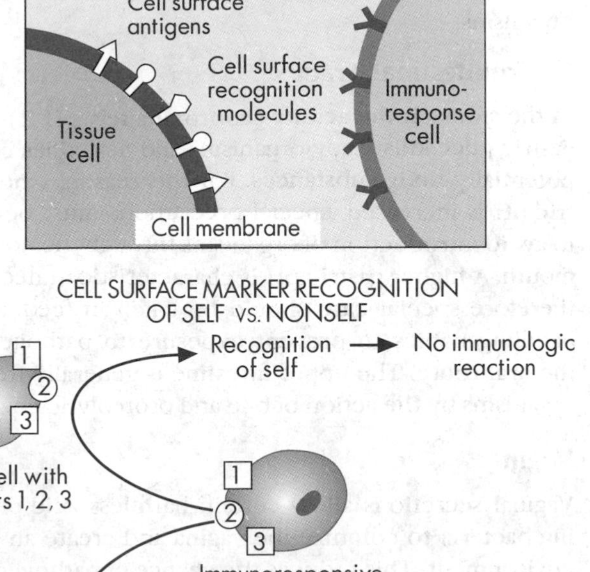


**FIGURE 13-2** Cell surface markers for recognition of self versus nonself.

**TABLE 13-1 Biologic Defense Mechanisms**

| NONSPECIFIC MECHANISMS | SPECIFIC MECHANISMS |
|---|---|
| **EXTERNAL** | |
| Mechanical exclusion | Immunoglobulin A |
| Physical structures | In mucosal secretions |
| Skin | In mucosal cells |
| Mucous membranes | |
| Specialized structures | |
| Physical actions | |
| Biochemical factors | |
| Body secretions | |
| pH | |
| Lysozyme | |
| Microbial antagonism | |
| **INTERNAL** | |
| Mononuclear phagocytic system | Antigen processing by macrophage |
| | Primary immune response |
| Blood | Humoral immune response |
| Cellular components | Synthesis of circulating immunoglobulins by B cells |
| Fluid components | Interaction of immunoglobulins with antigen |
| Complement | |
| Acute-phase proteins | |
| Phagocytosis | Cell-mediated immune response |
| Inflammatory response | Activation of T cell response |
| Interferons | Lymphokines |
| | Combined immune response |
| | Secondary immune response |

## SCOPE OF DEFENSE MECHANISMS

The array of defense mechanisms that have been adapted to protect the normal human body is formidable and complex. For the sake of orderly presentation, they may be divided into **nonspecific** and **specific** mechanisms (Table 13-1). The specific and nonspecific mechanisms can be further divided on the basis of where the lines of defense are formed—that is, **external** for the mechanisms of mechanical exclusion, biochemical destruction, and microbial competition and **internal** for the physiologic reactions. The nonspecific mechanisms are nonselectively directed against *any* foreign substance. The specific mechanisms are specifically elicited by *unique* substances to which the body has *acquired* the ability to respond.

# EXTERNAL NONSPECIFIC DEFENSE MECHANISMS

## ANATOMIC STRUCTURES AND MECHANICAL ACTIONS

### Skin and Mucous Membranes

The first line of defense against penetration by foreign materials, including pathogenic microorganisms, is the **skin.** When the skin is intact, it serves as an extremely efficient physical barrier to harmful agents and environmental forces such as heat, cold, and trauma. This protection is afforded by the keratinized surface cells, which provide a tough, dense, waterproof covering. Beneath this outermost layer is a dense layer of highly vascularized connective tissue (see Figure 66-1).

Even though some of the fatty acids derived from sebaceous gland secretions have antimicrobial activity, the environment provided by the skin allows the growth of microorganisms on its upper layers and within hair follicles and sweat glands. These resident microorganisms are mainly nonpathogenic; however, when these organisms gain entrance to the tissues of a host exhibiting reduced resistance, they may cause significant problems. Because thorough scrubbing with soap and water removes only the surface organisms, the skin can never be considered sterile.

Any time the physical integrity of the skin is broken—such as occurs during surgery, indwelling venous catheterization, or physical irritation or trauma—there is significant risk of microorganisms gaining entrance to the body. The skin must be kept relatively dry inasmuch as the continued presence of moisture tends to cause maceration of the skin. Further, when essential oils are lost from the skin surfaces, they should be supplemented by lotions to maintain the resilience and unbroken texture of the surface cells. Adequate care of the skin of the hospitalized patient is not just a luxury but a necessity for the provision of an extremely important aspect of biologic defense.

Mucous membranes protect the eye and line all body tracts that have external openings. When intact, the mucous membranes, as with the skin, are basically impervious to foreign materials and microorganisms. The surfaces are covered by a viscous secretion that tends to trap and inactivate microorganisms. The mucous membrane of the respiratory tract is further protected by the surface activity of the ciliated epithelial cells, which sweep foreign material out of the tract. The mucous membranes are highly vascularized so that the internal defense mechanisms are readily available to attack any microorganisms that do gain access to the surface of these cells.

Also found in the mucosal secretions and in high concentration within the secretory mucosal cells of the respiratory and intestinal tracts is a specific class of immunoglobulins (antibodies) known as immunoglobulin A (IgA) (see p. 314 and Table 13-5). These specific antibodies are secreted from the mucosal cells and have antibacterial, antiviral, and antitoxic properties. These antibodies serve to prevent microbial adherence and colonization of these tracts by pathogens. As seen in Table 13-1, these could be considered a specific immune mechanism in the external line of defense.

### Specialized Structures and Mechanical Functions

Other structures and functions of the human body that generally are taken for granted actually serve extremely important roles in defense. The filtration action of the nasal hairs serves to trap particles and microorganisms. The flushing action of saliva and urine prevents the build-up of organisms. The eyes are protected from dirt particles and organisms by the lids and lashes. Foreign material that does gain entrance to the eye tends to be washed out by tears. The constant movement of foods through the stomach and intestines prevents the build-up of organisms and toxic waste products. Even the action of vomiting and the watery stools of diarrhea are active mechanisms of removal of harmful products from the gastrointestinal (GI) tract. Dysfunction or blockage of any of these processes means that special measures must be taken to protect against the establishment of pathogenic organisms and the build-up of toxic materials.

## BIOCHEMICAL FACTORS

Many areas of the body are protected not only by mechanical barriers but also by specific antimicrobial chemicals that provide added protection.

### Skin

The acetic acid and salt concentration of perspiration is toxic to many pathogenic microorganisms. Some of the fatty acids released to the skin surface by the sebaceous glands also serve to inhibit the growth of some microorganisms.

### Gastrointestinal Tract

In the stomach the acidity (approximately pH 2) of the gastric juice kills many organisms and detoxifies certain potentially toxic substances. For this reason, when gastric pH is increased, special precautions must be taken to avoid introduction of organisms through the nose and mouth. A higher gastric pH is characteristic in neonates; therefore special care should be taken in feeding and handling babies to prevent exposure to pathogens by the oral route. The upper intestine is generally freed of organisms by the action of bile and proteolytic enzymes.

### Vagina

Vaginal secretions allow certain harmless acid-producing bacteria to colonize the vagina and create an acidic environment. This reduces the chance of pathogens colonizing the vagina. When either the amount or the acidity of the vaginal secretions is reduced, a much greater chance exists that a vaginal infection will develop. Because vaginal secretions are not present before puberty and are greatly reduced after menopause, both young girls and older women are more prone to vaginitis. The use of certain types of oral contraceptives may cause a shift in the composition and pH of the vaginal secretions, which increases the possibility of colonization of the vagina, especially by the causative agent of gonorrhea, *Neisseria gonorrhoeae*.

### Lysozyme

The most ubiquitous antimicrobial factor in the body is the bactericidal enzyme lysozyme. It is capable of lysing (splitting) the bacterial cell wall of many gram-positive organisms and causing their destruction. The enzyme is present in mucus, tears, saliva, and skin secretions and is also found in many of the internal fluids and cells of the body. Within the body lysozyme tends to work in combination with complement and other blood factors to destroy bacteria directly.

## MICROBIAL ANTAGONISM

The skin and mucosal surfaces offer varying nutritional and environmental conditions for the growth and multiplication of certain microbial cells. Although the surfaces of the body are constantly exposed to temporary contamination by organisms from the environment, most of these organisms, known as *transient flora*, do not find conditions suitable for colonization in the body; however, many microorganisms do colonize the skin and mucosal surfaces. These organisms make up what is known as the *normal microbial flora*. Although this normal flora varies from site to site within the body and may vary in response to environmental, hygienic, and physiologic changes, it is capable of reestablishment and

**TABLE 13-2 Distribution of Normal Microbial Flora**

| REGION OF BODY | STERILE AREAS | NONSTERILE AREAS | MICROORGANISMS |
|---|---|---|---|
| Skin | None | All skin | *Staphylococcus, Bacillus, Corynebacterium, Mycobacterium, Streptococcus,* transient environmental organisms |
| Respiratory tract | Larynx, trachea, bronchi, bronchioles, alveoli, sinuses | Nose, throat, mouth | *Staphylococcus, Candida, Streptococcus, Neisseria, Pneumococcus,* oral organisms |
| GI tract | Esophagus, stomach, upper small intestine | Esophagus and stomach (transiently), large intestine | Gram-negative rods, *Streptococcus, Bacteroides, Proteus, Clostridium, Lactobacillus* |
| Genitourinary tract | Cervix, uterus, fallopian tubes, ovaries, prostate gland, epididymides, testes, bladder, kidneys | External genitalia, anterior urethra, vagina | Skin organisms, *Lactobacillus, Bacteroides* |
| Body fluids and cavities | Blood, pleural fluid, synovial fluid, spinal fluid, lymph, etc. | None | |

reflects a fairly predictable pattern. Table 13-2 provides an overview of the body areas normally colonized and shows which organisms most often make up the normal flora of the various areas.

The maintenance of this balanced microbial flora makes it difficult for pathogenic organisms to establish themselves on the body surfaces. Because the normal flora have a selective advantage in their environmental niche, they compete for nutrients and space. Some release antimicrobial substances to retard the growth of transient organisms seeking to occupy the same site. These microbial interferences are known as **microbial antagonism.**

Most of the normal microbial flora are basically nonpathogenic; however, some overtly pathogenic organisms such as *Staphylococcus aureus* and *Streptococcus pyogenes* can be part of the normal flora. The individual who harbors such organisms without demonstrating any symptoms of disease is known as a **carrier.** This carrier state is significant because the carrier may unknowingly be shedding organisms into the environment and infecting others.

The protective effects of the normal microbial flora become most apparent when something upsets the microbial balance within the body. The extended use of broad-spectrum antibiotics sometimes creates such an effect. The imbalance may allow a segment of the normal flora to gain ascendency, causing adverse reactions. An example of this phenomenon occurs when certain oral antibiotics induce marked shifts in the normal intestinal flora, allowing organisms generally suppressed by the growth of competitors to thrive to an unusual degree. This imbalance may induce uncomfortable GI tract problems or even allow gastroenteritis to develop.

## INTERNAL NONSPECIFIC DEFENSE MECHANISMS

Once a foreign agent (living or nonliving) penetrates the external resistance barriers, it is met by an even more complex array of defense mechanisms, which provides for the recognition, capture, and disposal of the foreign material. The key to this process is the specific recognition and vigorous action taken against the foreign material and at the same time the protection of the host tissues from extensive damage. The physiologic reactions that serve to contain and inactivate the foreign agent are carried out through interactions of cells and molecules of the mononuclear phagocyte system, blood, vascular system, and body tissues.

### MONONUCLEAR PHAGOCYTE SYSTEM

The **mononuclear phagocyte system (MPS)** was formerly known as the reticuloendothelial system. It is a widespread system of **phagocytic cells** (devouring cells) scattered throughout various body tissues (Fig. 13-3). The role of these cells is to ingest foreign particulate matter and damaged host tissues. Some of the phagocytic cells are *fixed* in a variety of tissues such as lymphoid tissue, liver, spleen, bone marrow, lungs, and blood vessels. Within the different tissues these anchored cells have been given unique names (Table 13-3). The function of the fixed cells is to capture and destroy foreign materials found in the fluids of their environment.

Other cells making up the phagocytic network are not stationary and are called *wandering macrophages.* Depending on where they are found, they may be known as *monocytes* (in the bloodstream) or *histiocytes* (in loose connective tissues). The wandering macrophages carry out the important role of final cleanup of a damaged site in preparation for repair. The cells have the capacity to engulf and destroy virtually any type of foreign material or debris within the body. The macrophages also play an important role in the specific response mechanisms discussed later in this chapter.

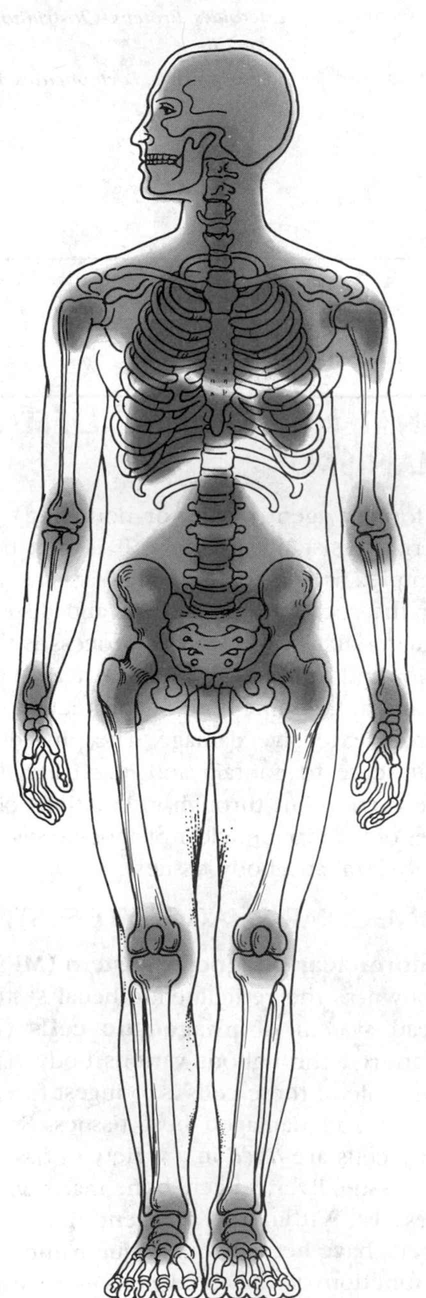

**FIGURE 13-3** Mononuclear phagocyte system (MPS). Note anatomic distribution of maximal activity in system, as indicated by shaded areas over body. To produce such an image, certain radioactive colloidal particles are given to the patient, and radiation detection techniques delineate tissue uptake. Note definition of liver, spleen, and active bone marrow in axial skeleton and proximal parts of long bones.

## BLOOD

Blood is one of the primary sources of elements designed to provide protection against injurious agents. The blood transports these active factors to the site of an injury or intrusion and through specific vascular changes concentrates these materials at the site. Both the fluid and the cellular constituents of blood contain these factors.

### Cellular Components

The important cellular components of blood in this nonspecific response include granulocytes, lymphocytes, monocytes, and thrombocytes (platelets) (see Figure 13-11). The granulocytes, also referred to as *polymorphonuclear leukocytes* (PMNs), and the monocytes are the most important because of their phagocytic activity.

One of the key methods of nonspecific defense is the ingestion of microorganisms and other particulate matter by the phagocytic white blood cells (WBCs). The phagocytes carry out the process of *phagocytosis* in several discrete steps (Figure 13-4). Most infecting microbes are quickly and efficiently destroyed by phagocytosis; however, some pathogens can escape this destruction. Some bacteria, such as strains of streptococci and staphylococci and *Bacillus anthracis* (anthrax), actually produce factors that will kill the phagocyte. Other organisms resist ingestion or digestion. Some organisms may survive within the phagocytes and multiply there. This may lead to the transport of the organism to other sites in the body or may serve as a chronic focus of continued infection.

The granulocytes can be divided on the basis of their structure and function into neutrophils, eosinophils, and basophils. The "granules" found within these cells represent discrete packets of degradative enzymes used to digest the ingested materials. The neutrophils are the most numerous in circulation and are the most efficient and responsive phagocytic cells involved in the inflammatory process. Where there is adequate blood supply to a region, the phagocytes are constantly available to move from the blood vessels to the site of injury or infection. The neutrophils and monocytes are actually attracted to the scene by chemicals released during infection or injury. This cellular response to chemical at-

**TABLE 13-3 Distribution and Names of Macrophages in Various Tissue Sites**

| TISSUE | NAME |
|---|---|
| Peripheral blood | Monocyte |
| Loose connective tissue | Histiocyte |
| Liver | Kupffer's cells |
| Spleen, MPS | Wandering or fixed macrophage |
| Lung | Alveolar macrophage or dust cell |
| Granulomatous tissue | Epithelioid and giant cells |
| Peritoneal cavity, pleural cavity, bone | Macrophages |

tractants is known as *chemotaxis,* and the substances released are called *chemotactic substances.*

## Fluid Factors

The fluid portion of uncoagulated blood is called *plasma.* Some of the components of plasma provide important constituents for the internal defense mechanisms. Plasma transports the *circulating immunoglobulins* produced in specific response to antigen stimulation. These immunoglobulins bind to the specific antigens against which they are formed. The antigens become coated with these immunoglobulins. The phagocytic cells can recognize the immunoglobulin bound to the antigen through receptors on the surface of the phagocyte, thereby greatly enhancing the ability of the cell to engulf the antigen. This process of enhanced phagocytosis is known as *opsonization.* Through this process the specific immune response mechanism contributes to the nonspecific mechanism and makes it significantly more efficient.

Another plasma constituent, *fibrin,* may create a meshwork around the injured area, sealing it off. Microorganisms may also become trapped within this meshwork, where they are more easily captured by the phagocytic cells.

## COMPLEMENT

One of the most important constituents of plasma is a complex series of proteins known by the singular name of **complement.** There are as many as 20 different protein components, with 11 designated as major components in the complement cascade. The liver is the primary site of synthesis of the components of complement. The primary role of complement is to provide specific lysis (rupturing) of cell membranes. The initiation of the *complement cascade* most often is triggered by the binding of the first complement protein to complement-binding immunoglobulins that have already bound to their antigens. Thus complement serves to accentuate or complete the action of an immunoglobulin. The immunoglobulin by itself cannot produce cell lysis, but with the recruitment of complement in the reaction, the cell may be ruptured. However, other nonimmune substances also can activate complement. Complement is considered a nonspecific component of the plasma because it is not increased by immunization. In addition to its cy-

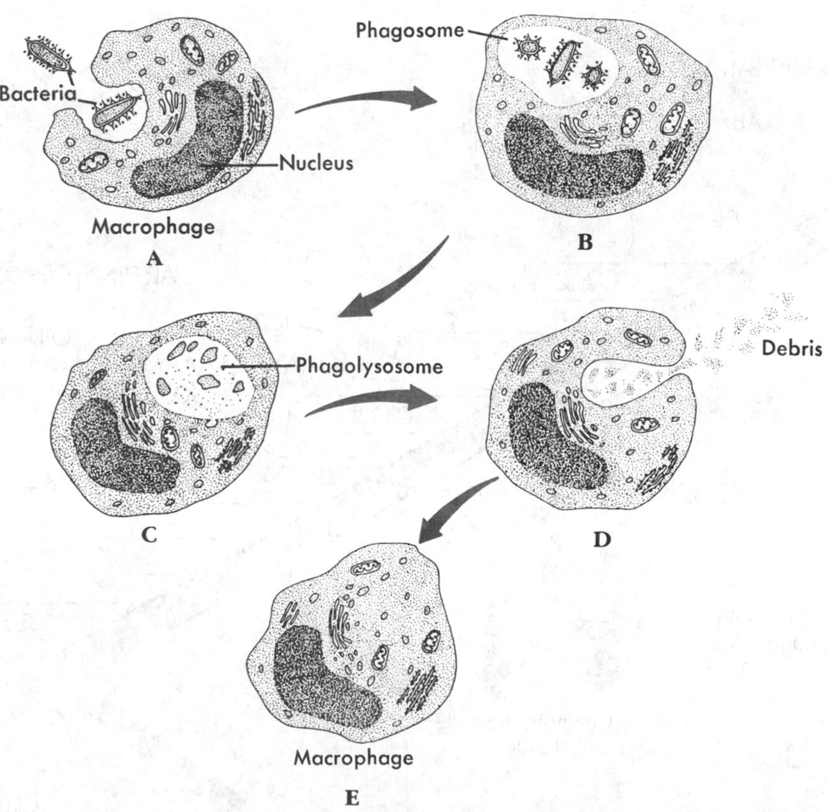


**FIGURE 13-4** Phagocytosis sketched in macrophage. **A,** Opsonized bacteria engulfed by phagocyte (macrophage). **B,** Phagosome formed. **C,** Phagosome becomes phagolysosome; bacteria digested. (To this point the process of phagocytosis is comparable to either macrophage or neutrophil, not shown.) **D,** Debris is egested. (Neutrophil would succumb here.) **E,** Macrophage returns to resting state. (From Smith AL: *Microbiology and pathology,* ed 12, St Louis, 1980, Mosby.)

tolytic effects, complement is involved in leukocyte chemotaxis, release of histamines, enhancement of phagocytosis by PMNs, viral neutralization, and bactericidal activity.

The classic activities ascribed to complement depend on the sequential interaction of nine protein subunits (C1 to C9), the first component of which consists of three subfractions termed C1q, C1r, and C1s (thereby accounting for the 11 separate proteins). The C1q, C1r, and C1s components constitute the recognition unit, inasmuch as this unit is capable of recognizing the antibody and fixing to the Fc (for fragment, crystallizable) (see Figure 13-9) portion of the antibody. When the first component, C1, is bound by an antigen-immunoglobulin complex on the surface of a cell, it acquires the enzymatic ability to activate many molecules of the next components in the sequence, C4 and C2, to form an active C42 complex (Figure 13-5). (Unfortunately, the numbering system of the complement components reflects their order of discovery and not their sequential additive pattern.) Each of the activated C42 complexes (the activation units) is then able to act on multiple molecules of the next components and so on, producing a cascade effect (a chain reaction) and greatly amplifying the reaction. As each component is added, new enzymatic activity is created to initiate the next step. This cascade effect is similar to that of blood coagulation. The final component, C5b6789, has the ability to create a lesion in the cell membrane, and if enough lesions are created on the membrane, cell death results. This complex is sometimes called the ***membrane attack unit.*** The intermediate stages in the complement sequence also give rise to complexes and fragments with other significant biologic activities. Figure 13-5 depicts the generation of some of these activities, which include the following:

1. ***Histamine release.*** Histamines cause an extreme increase in vascular permeability and contraction of smooth muscle. A fragment (C3a) split off during the activation of C3 and another fragment (C5a) created by the activation of C5 are released into the surrounding tissues, where they cause the release of histamine from mast cells. The histamines in turn exert their physiologic effects on the smooth muscle tissues and vascular system. Because these histamine-mediated reactions are the same as those created during anaphylactic shock (see Chapter 70), these fragments are called ***anaphylatoxins.***
2. ***Enhanced phagocytosis.*** Neutrophils and macrophages have receptors for C3b on their cell surfaces, which adds to the opsonization effect. Complement activation at the site of infection labels foreign ma-

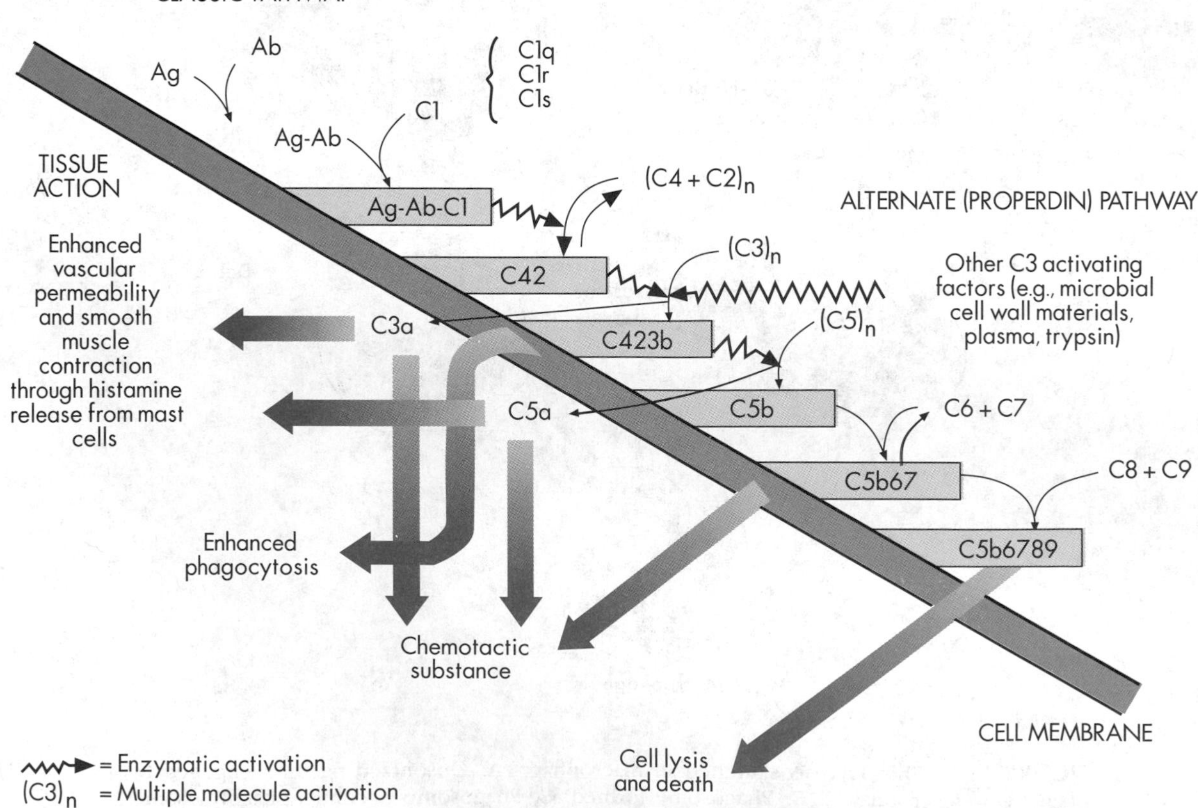


**FIGURE 13-5** Classic and alternate complement cascade. Sequence of complement activation generates multiple biologically active intermediate molecules, which are active in the inflammatory response.

terials with the C3b fragments and makes them more subject to phagocytosis. The contribution of the process to protection is most apparent in persons with a genetic deficiency in the synthesis of the C3 protein. Such individuals suffer from recurrent bacterial infections and septicemia.

3. *Chemotactic substance formation.* Several of the fragments and intermediate factors serve as chemotactic substances to attract phagocytes to the site of the reaction.

All these activities are central to the inflammatory response.

The plasma fraction contains several proteins that inhibit the action of the activated components of complement in the fluid phase. Such inhibitors serve to focus the attack on the microorganism's membrane surface and thereby prevent damage to host cells.

In addition to the activated C42 complement complex, several other enzymes exhibit C3 *convertase* activity. These include trypsin, plasmin, and thrombin, as well as bacterial endotoxins and a factor derived from cobra venom. Each leads to alterations in C3 that are similar, if not identical, to those produced by the complement cascade–derived C3 convertase. These activations are mediated through a plasma component known as *properdin* and are referred to as the *alternative,* or *properdin, pathway.*

The effects of age on the function of the complement system are not clear. There appears to be an increase in the number of complement components or the amount of complement activity from birth to old age, with synthesis beginning as early as the first month of gestation. An increased incidence of conditions whose activities are mediated by complement is seen in elderly persons.[2]

## ACUTE-PHASE PROTEINS

**Acute-phase proteins** are serum proteins with concentrations that increase dramatically in the serum of persons suffering from any type of severe inflammatory response. Both infectious and noninfectious inflammations trigger an increase of these proteins in plasma. Interleukin-1, a cytokine secreted by macrophages, stimulates the liver secretion of acute-phase proteins. These proteins include liver-synthesized haptoglobin, fibrinogen, complement proteins, ceruloplasmin, and C-reactive protein. Because C-reactive protein is more prevalent and is easily measured, it is often used interchangeably with acute-phase proteins. C-reactive protein derives its name from its ability to bind to the C protein of the cell walls of *Streptococcus pneumoniae.* C-reactive protein binds to a variety of bacteria and fungi and has the property of activating the complement C3 protein to initiate the subsequent steps in the complement cascade on the surface of the foreign cells, leading to their destruction. C-reactive proteins, by binding to lymphocytes, may modulate their function.

The amount of acute-phase proteins found in the serum is roughly proportional to the severity of the inflammation; therefore a test for these proteins is useful in the diagnosis and management of diseases that are difficult to differentiate and have a hidden inflammatory aspect, such as bacterial endocarditis, cryptic abscesses, rheumatic fever, and certain types of cancer.

## INTERFERONS

**Interferons** comprise a group of proteins produced by various human cells, usually in response to the viral infection of the cell. When a cell is infected by a virus, the infected cell begins to make interferon almost immediately (Figure 13-6). The interferon is released into its surrounding environment, where it induces uninfected cells to produce alterations that protect those cells from viral multiplication. This antiviral action is exerted before the synthesis of immunoglobulins specific for the virus reach protective levels. The elaboration of interferons from virally infected cells continues for a few hours (up to about 24 hours) after infection, thereby playing a significant role in isolating the infective foci in many, but not all, viral infections.

Although viruses seem to be the most potent agents for the induction of interferon, production is not restricted to viral infection of cells. Other intracellular parasites such as rickettsia, bacteria, and parasites may also trigger the formation of interferon. Even bacterial and fungal extracts, as well as such other materials as double-stranded ribonucleic acid (RNA), synthetic polymers, and plant extracts, may serve as signals.

Three distinct types of interferons are produced by different cell types in the human body, and each type seems to exert different protective effects. *Alpha-interferon* is produced by lymphocytes and seems to have antiviral activity. *Beta-interferon* is formed by fibroblasts, epithelial cells, and macrophages; it is definitely antiviral. *Gamma-interferon* is produced by T lymphocytes of the specific immune response system and has an immunoregulatory effect.[3] In addition to their antiviral activities, the interferons are capable of inhibiting cell growth; therefore they are being used widely in clinical trials as an *antitumor agent.*

In general the production of interferon occurs regardless of the viral agent that initiated its formation; thus interferon is said to be *virus-nonspecific.* It does not inhibit all viruses equally. Among the viruses that seem to be especially sensitive are the arboviruses, influenza virus, and smallpox virus. Most vertebrate species seemingly are capable of producing interferons; however, each animal species' interferon is protective against viral infection only in that species. This means the bovine (cow) interferon has only limited protective value in the human, and vice versa. The term *species specificity* is used to describe this quality. This characteristic limited early research into the effects of interferon, because it was difficult to obtain enough human interferon to conduct clinical trials. Through the use of

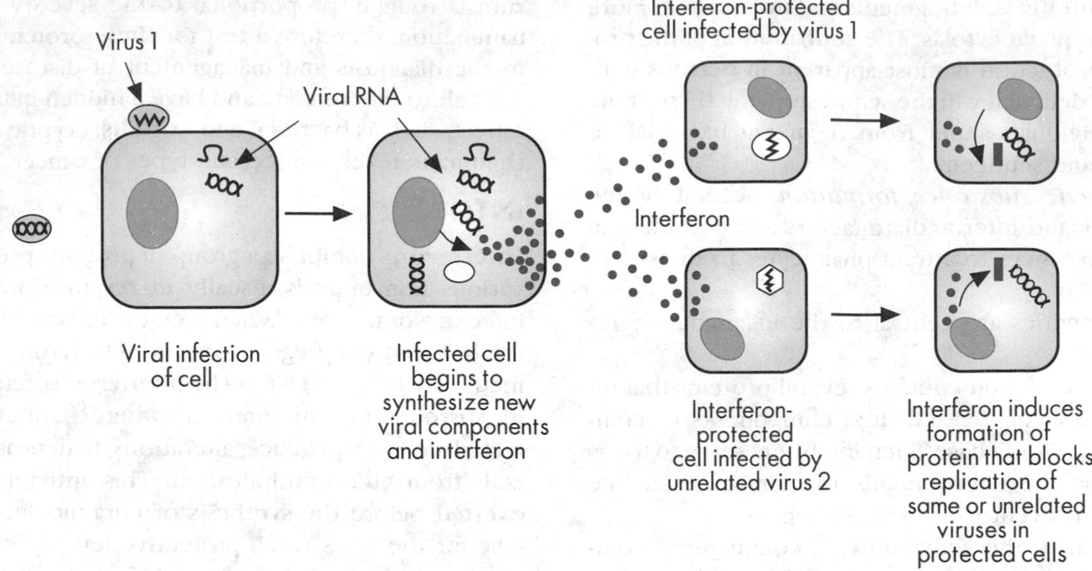


**FIGURE 13-6** Mechanism of interferon action.

recombinant deoxyribonucleic acid (DNA) technology, the human interferon gene has been introduced into bacterial cells. By growing such bacteria in culture, large amounts of specific types (alpha [α], beta [β], and gamma [γ]) of interferon can be harvested, purified, and used in clincal studies. The other benefit of this application of genetic engineering is to greatly reduce the cost of the purified interferon.

Interferons provide cancer therapy by slowing down cell replication and by enhancing natural killer cell activity. Alpha-interferon was approved for the treatment of hairy cell leukemia in 1986 and Kaposi's sarcoma and hepatitis C in 1988.[4]

## INFLAMMATORY RESPONSE

When injury occurs in the body, all the nonspecific and to some degree the specific defense mechanisms are directed toward localizing the effects of the injury, protecting against microbial invasion at the site, and preparing the site for repair. This process is called **inflammation.**

The inflammatory response can be initiated by any type of injury: heat, cold, irradiation, chemicals, trauma, infection, immunologic injury, or neoplasia. Whatever the stimulus, the response of the body is the same, but the extent of the involvement of the nonspecific response system's various facets depends on the degree and severity of the injury.

### Steps in the Response

Three major physiologic responses occur during the inflammatory process: vascular response, fluid exudation, and cellular exudation (Table 13-4). The *vascular response* consists of a transitory vasoconstriction (stress response) followed immediately by vasodilation. This occurs as a result of chemical substances such as histamine or kinins released at the site of injury or invasion. The amount of blood flow to the area is thus increased *(hyperemia),* causing redness and heat. Blood flow slows as the capillaries dilate. Increased permeability of the capillary walls facilitates fluid and cellular exudation. The extra fluid in the tissues may act to dilute toxins and microorganisms that are in the area.[5]

**Fluid exudation** from the capillaries into the interstitial spaces begins immediately and is most active during the first 24 hours after injury or invasion. Initially the fluid exudate is primarily serous fluid, but as the capillary wall becomes more permeable, protein (albumin) is lost into the interstitial spaces. This increases the colloid osmotic pressure in these spaces, which encourages more fluid exudation. The swelling of the tissue from the fluid in the interstitial spaces is called *edema.*

**Cellular exudation** refers to the migration of WBCs (leukocytes) through the capillary walls into the affected tissue. An increased number of WBCs are attracted to the vessels in the affected area as a result of chemotactic substances being released from the tissues by cell injury and complement activation. The WBCs adhere to the capillary wall and then pass in ameboid fashion through the widened endothelial junctions of the capillary wall. Neutrophils (PMNs), which make up about 60% of the circulating WBCs, are the first leukocytes to respond, usually within the first few hours. The neutrophils ingest the bacteria and dead tissue cells (phagocytosis); then they die, releasing proteolytic enzymes that liquefy the dead neutrophils, dead bacteria, and other dead cells (pus). Monocytes and lymphocytes appear later. The macrophages continue the phagocytosis, and the lymphocytes play a role in the antigen-antibody response at the site.

**TABLE 13-4 Summary of the Steps in the Inflammatory Response**

| STEPS | MEDIATORS | OUTCOME |
|---|---|---|
| 1. Injury | Physical, chemical, biologic, immunologic stimulus | Cell and tissue injury |
| 2. Vascular response | | |
| a. Vascular dilation | Histamine, plasmin, serotonin, kinins, prostaglandins released or activated by injury | Dilation of vessels, causing stasis of blood and margination of leukocytes |
| b. Fibrin clot formation | Activation of clotting mechanism | Containment of irritants |
| 3. Fluid exudation | Histamine, kinins, prostaglandins cause opening of venule–endothelial cell junction | Fluid exudation into tissues |
| 4. Cellular exudation | | |
| a. Leukocyte exudation | Chemotactic substances released by complement activation, clot formation, injured cells | Passage of leukocytes from blood to site of injury and accumulation there |
| b. Attack and engulfment of foreign materials | Neutrophils, macrophages | Removal and digestion of bacteria, foreign particles, damaged tissues |
| 5. Healing | Fibroblasts produce collagen fibers, tissue regeneration | Resolution of inflammation, formation of scar tissue |

## Local Manifestations of Inflammation

The five cardinal symptoms of inflammation were identified many centuries ago. These are redness *(rubor)* and heat *(calor)* caused by the hyperemia, swelling *(tumor)* caused by the fluid exudate, pain *(dolor)* caused by the pressure of the fluid exudate and by chemical (bradykinin, prostaglandins) irritation of the nerve endings, and *loss of function* of the affected part caused by the swelling and pain.

The inflammatory response prepares the tissue for healing and contains the spread of bacterial invasion. To prevent the spread of bacteria, fibroblasts are attracted to the area and secrete fibrin, a threadlike substance that encircles the affected area to wall it off from healthy tissue. If interference occurs with this walling-off process, bacteria can spread into the surrounding tissue. This explains why an abscess should not be incised and drained until it has "come to a head" or until the walling-off process is completed.

## Regional Lymph Node Manifestations

Bacteria may fail to be contained locally and may spread to other parts of the body by means of the lymph system or bloodstream. If picked up by the lymph stream, the bacteria will be carried to the nearest lymph node. These nodes are located along the course of all lymph channels, and bacteria can be ingested and destroyed here as well. If the bacteria are virulent enough to resist the action of the lymph nodes, leukocytes are brought in by the bloodstream to attack and engulf the bacteria in the node. The node then becomes swollen and tender because of the accumulation of phagocytes, bacteria, and destroyed lymphoid tissue. This is known as *lymphadenitis.* Swollen lymph nodes can be palpated primarily in the neck, axilla, and groin.

## Systemic Manifestations

Moderate to severe inflammatory responses can produce generalized systemic manifestations. The three major manifestations are (1) increase in body temperature *(fever),* (2) increase in WBCs in peripheral circulation *(leukocytosis),* and (3) increased *erythrocyte sedimentation rate* (ESR).

Fever is produced by the release of substances known as *endogenous pyrogens* at the inflammatory site. These pyrogens come from injured cells, materials released by WBCs that accumulate at the site, and components of the bacterial cell wall. The pyrogens include prostaglandins, leukotrienes, bacterial endotoxins, and interleukin-1. The substances are carried to the temperature-regulating center in the hypothalamic region of the brain, where they signal a resetting of the body temperature set-point. The body responds by increasing heat production and decreasing heat loss. As long as the pyrogens remain in circulation, the set-point will be elevated. The fever response is designed as part of the defense mechanism and helps increase production of antimicrobial agents such as interferon. It also tends to support increased phagocytic activity of some cells, including fixed and wandering macrophages.

Leukocytosis develops when agents released from damaged cells and WBCs accumulating at the inflammatory site are carried by the circulation to the bone marrow, where WBCs are produced. These agents are known as *leukopoietins.* When these agents reach the bone marrow, they signal the release of mature neutrophils held in reserve there. This leads to an immediate rise in the WBC count in the peripheral circulation to greater than 10,000/$mm^3$. The chemotactic agents draw these cells to the inflammatory site. Leukopoietins also increase the production of WBCs in the bone marrow.

With prolonged inflammation the bone marrow stores of WBCs are depleted, and the synthesis of mature WBCs may not be able to keep pace with the needs of the inflammatory site; thus the marrow releases more immature neutrophils as the inflammation continues. These less mature cells, known as *bands,* become more prevalent in the peripheral circulation and indicate a significant ongoing inflammation. The condition sometimes is referred to as a "shift to the left." This clinical phrase was derived from the past clinical laboratory method of counting the less mature cells and tabulating them in the left-hand columns of differential count forms.

With inflammation an increased blood sedimentation rate also occurs; that is, when an anticoagulant is added to the blood in the laboratory, the red blood cells (RBCs) settle to the bottom of a test tube more rapidly than normal. This increase in the ESR is believed to be caused by an increase in fibrinogen, a blood protein essential to the healing process. The ESR is elevated during the acute inflammatory stage of infection, which indicates that the body's defense mechanisms for the repair of damaged tissue are operating.

Inflammations can be classified as acute or chronic. *Acute* inflammations are characterized by a sudden onset and an increase in the fluid exudative response. *Chronic* inflammations have a slower, more insidious onset and are characterized by increased cellular exudation.

Knowledge of the physiologic changes that occur during the inflammatory process helps the nurse to understand the changes that occur in a variety of diseases. For example, whenever cells die as a result of injury or disease *(necrosis),* such as during a myocardial infarction, the inflammatory process occurs. Fat deposits *(atheromas)* on blood vessel walls cause injury to the lining of the vessel wall and initiate an inflammatory response. Irritation of the peritoneum by trauma or bacterial invasion can cause inflammation of the peritoneum *(peritonitis).*

## Repair and Healing

No healing will occur until inflammation has subsided and pus and dead tissue have been removed. Pus is a local accumulation of dead phagocytes, dead bacteria, and dead tissue. The bacteria most frequently causing this reaction are staphylococci, streptococci, *Neisseria* organisms, and *Pseudomonas aeruginosa (P. pyocyanea).* A collection of pus that is localized by a zone of inflamed tissue is called an *abscess* (Figure 13-7). An inflammation that involves cellular or connective tissue is called *cellulitis,* whereas an inflammation in which pus collects in a preexisting cavity such as the pleura or gallbladder is called *empyema.* When infection forms an abscess within the body, develops a suppurating channel, and ruptures onto the surface or into a body cavity, it is called a *sinus.* If the infection forms a tubelike passage from an epithelium-lined organ or normal body cavity to the surface or to another organ or cavity, it is called a *fistula.*

After the infected area is clean, new cells are produced to fill in the space left by the injury. They may be the normal structural cells, or they may be fibrotic tissue cells known as *scar tissue.* If they are fibrotic cells, they will not function as the cells functioned formerly but only serve to fill in the injured area. Some body cells readily regenerate; for instance, after the bowel has healed, it is almost impossible to find the injured area. The respiratory tract also regenerates its tissues readily. Liver tissue has the capacity to regenerate, but over a longer period. Nerve cells are always replaced with fibrous tissue. If a large amount of tissue is destroyed, structural cells may not be replaced, regardless of the type of tissue. (See Chapter 25 for discussion of wound healing.)

Some persons, especially those with brown or black skin, are prone to excessive scar formation. Such tissue formation, known as a *keloid,* is hard and shiny in appearance and may enlarge to a surprising degree. It may

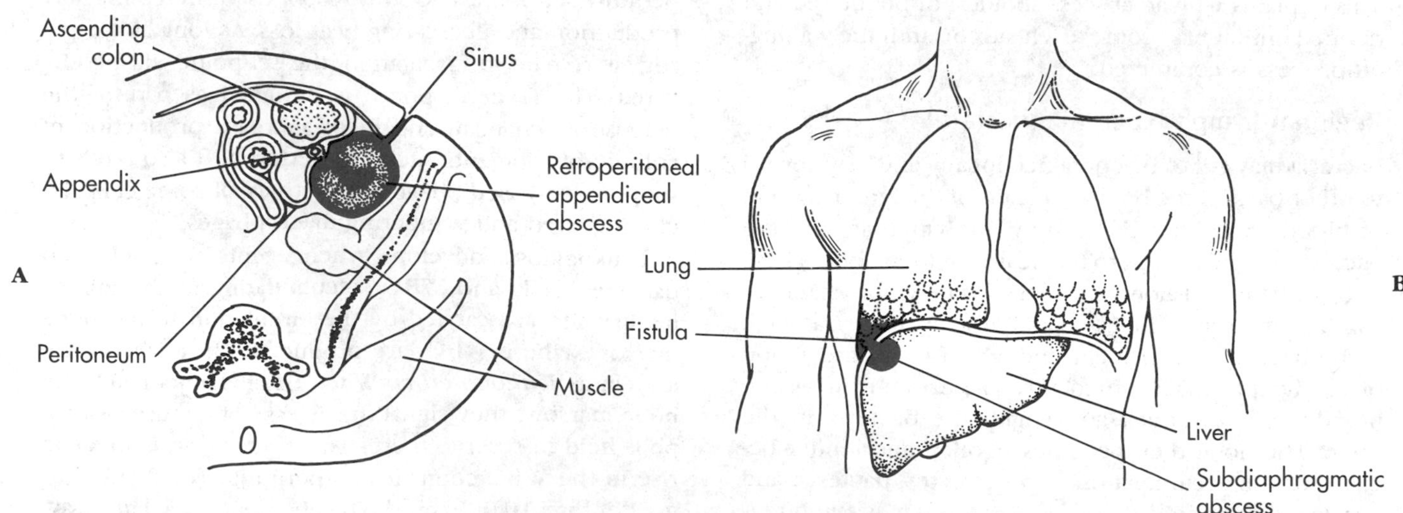


**FIGURE 13-7** **A,** Cross section of torso showing appendiceal abscess with sinus that has developed through abdominal wall. **B,** Subdiaphragmatic abscess that has developed fistula opening into pleural cavity.

cause disfigurement or undergo malignant degeneration and thus is usually excised surgically. Serous membranes sometimes become adherent during inflammatory and healing processes, and as the inflammation subsides, fibrous tissue forms, holding the membranes together. This fibrous tissue is called an *adhesion*. Adhesions may occur in the pleura, in the pericardium, about the pelvic organs, and in many other parts of the body. They often occur in and around the intestinal tract, where they may cause an obstruction.

Instead of healing, necrosis (death of the tissue) may occur. Bacteria, both pathogens and nonpathogens, often invade the necrotic tissue and cause decomposition, which is called *gangrene*. The body defenses are useless in preventing or curing gangrene because no blood can get to the area. Gangrenous tissue must be completely removed before healing can occur.

## SPECIFIC DEFENSE MECHANISMS

### CONCEPTS OF AN ADAPTIVE SPECIFIC IMMUNE SYSTEM

Specific defense mechanisms within the body provide specific protection against a particular microorganism or molecular entity. This mechanism of protection leads to what is termed *specific immunity*. Depending on the relative levels of protection, the body may be able to defend itself totally or only partially from damage by the agent. The *immune system* is composed of many of the same organs, cells, and molecular entities operating to provide nonspecific defense. It works with the nonspecific mechanisms to focus and amplify the general mechanisms of defense against specifically recognized foreign materials.

The fundamental nature of the specific **immune response** is characterized by diversity, specificity, recognition, memory, and action. Among the most intriguing aspects of immune response is its *diversity of ability to respond* while at the same time responding with *specificity of action*. Almost any conceivable organic molecular array on the surface of a molecule has been shown to be able to induce a series of cellular events culminating in the production of **antibodies (immunoglobulins).*** These antibodies combine with the inducing **antigen (immunogen)** by virtue of combining sites on the immunoglobulin molecule that exhibit an extremely narrow specificity. The remainder of the immunoglobulin molecule is chemically and structurally similar to all other antibody molecules with distinctly different combining-site specificities.

*Recognition* and *memory* are two other aspects of this system that make it unique. The normal organism recognizes its own antigenic make-up and will not produce antibodies against its own antigens. This is known as *recognition of self* or **self-tolerance.** At the same time this intricate system of self-recognition must be able to detect extremely subtle changes in its own cells when incipient tumors that differ only slightly in antigenic constitution are forming. Further, once the immune system has responded to an antigen, subsequent encounters with that antigen produce an even more vigorous and rapid response. This response includes a wide variety of mechanisms designed to take *action* against the offending agent. Many of these actions are among the most potent biochemical and cellular reactions that the body can produce; yet they are focused so discretely that the foreign agent is rapidly destroyed with a minimum of damage to the host.

### BASIC DESIGN OF THE SYSTEM

The basic design of the specific immune response system is such that the body provides itself with cells and molecules that can respond to and thwart encroachment of nonself materials rapidly and efficiently. The system has two major interactive divisions: (1) a humorally mediated system of specifically designed proteins known as *antibodies* or *immunoglobulins* and (2) a cell-mediated system of specifically reactive WBCs known as *activated lymphocytes* or *T cells*. Both arms of the system usually are triggered to respond to encroachment; however, only one of the systems may provide the most protection against certain types of encroachment.

The **humorally mediated system** provides major immunity against (1) bacteria that produce acute infection (such as *Staphylococcus, Streptococcus, Haemophilus* organisms), (2) bacterial exotoxins (diphtheria, botulinus, and tetanus toxins), (3) viruses that must enter the bloodstream to reach their target tissues (e.g., poliomyelitis, hepatitis virus), and (4) organisms that enter the body from the mucosal tissues (e.g., cold viruses, enteroviruses, influenza viruses). Even though circulating antibodies may be produced against other organisms (such as tuberculosis, HIV, fungi), these antibodies do not protect the body from infection.

The **cell-mediated system,** on the other hand, offers protection from (1) chronic bacterial infections (e.g., syphillis, tuberculosis, leprosy), (2) many viral infections (e.g., measles, herpesvirus infections, chickenpox), (3) fungal infections (e.g., candidiasis, histoplasmosis, cryptococcis), (4) parasitic infections (e.g., leishmaniasis, toxoplasmosis, *Pneumocystis carinii*), and (5) transplanted or transformed cells (e.g., tissue transplants, some transformed cells of cancer).

One or both of these systems can be immunodeficient

*The terms *antibody* and *immunoglobulin* can be used more or less interchangeably and are used that way throughout this chapter. Specifically, *antibody* is the original, more general term describing serum agents that inactivate foreign substances in the body. It was coined in the early part of this century before the specific proteins of the serum had been identified as the globulin proteins of the $\gamma$-globulin fraction. The term *immunoglobulin* more specifically identifies the molecules of the serum that have antibody activity. In the same way, *antigen* is the original, more general term for foreign materials that elicit the immune response reaction; the newer, more accurate and interchangeable term for such materials is *immunogen*.

(see Chapter 70). When one system is not functioning properly, the person becomes susceptible to infection or encroachment by the agents against which that system provided primary protection. For example, infection with the HIV reduces the protection afforded by the cell-mediated system, making the individual susceptible to fungal infections (candidiasis), protozoan infections (*Pneumocystis carinii* pneumonia), viral infections (herpesvirus infection), and cancers (Kaposi's sarcoma, lymphoma). Alternatively, the loss of the humorally mediated system that occurs in Bruton's agammaglobulinemia is accompanied by increased incidence of acute bacterial infections, respiratory tract infections, and GI tract problems. If both systems are lost or compromised, the individual is fully susceptible to infectious agents and cannot survive in an unprotected, nonsterile environment.

## IMMUNE RESPONSE SYSTEM

### Immunogens and Immunoglobulins

#### Immunogens (antigens)

An **immunogen** is defined as a substance that, when introduced into an animal, elicits the formation of antibodies, or specifically sensitized cells. The antigen must be recognized as nonself or foreign material within the body. Although most antigens are naturally occurring proteins of at least 10,000 molecular weight, other substances, such as polysaccharides, nucleoproteins, lipoproteins, and glycoproteins, also may serve as antigens. The bulk of the antigen consists of subsurface molecular structures that do not elicit an immune response but do serve as carriers for the multiple *antigenic determinants* on the surface. Most antigens have many antigenic determinants and are termed *multivalent antigens;* however, some molecules may be monovalent.

Because of their small size, certain molecules cannot induce the synthesis of antibodies; however, when coupled with a high-molecular-weight carrier, they can serve as antigenic determinants. These molecules are *incomplete antigens,* or *haptens.* They take on specific significance in the consideration of hypersensitivities, which are allergies to low-molecular-weight compounds such as certain drugs and antibiotics (see Chapter 70).

#### Immunoglobulins (antibodies)

The body's response to the introduction of an immunogenic substance is the production of a specific, soluble immunoglobulin or a sensitized (antigen-reactive) lymphocyte population. The type of antigen introduced determines the immune response: antibody synthesis or antigen-reactive lymphocyte, or a combination of both.

The circulating antibodies represent modified (e.g., antigen-specific) globulin proteins found in blood serum. The serum contains several distinct protein fractions, which are separable on the basis of their net electrical charge, molecular size, and molecular conformation into several fractions: albumin, α-globulins, β-globulins, and γ-globulins (Figure 13-8). The antibody activity of the serum is characteristically associated with the γ-globulin and β-globulin fractions. Those γ-globulins with the ability to bind antigens are called *immunoglobulins.* The immunoglobulins can be further subdivided into different *classes* on the basis of structure and function of the molecules. The generic symbol for immunoglobulins is Ig, and each of the classes is designated by a letter of the alphabet: IgA, IgD, IgE, IgG, and IgM (Table 13-5).

The basic pattern of structure for all immunoglobulins is based on a four-peptide chain monomeric unit (Figure 13-9). Two of the chains are of higher molecular weight

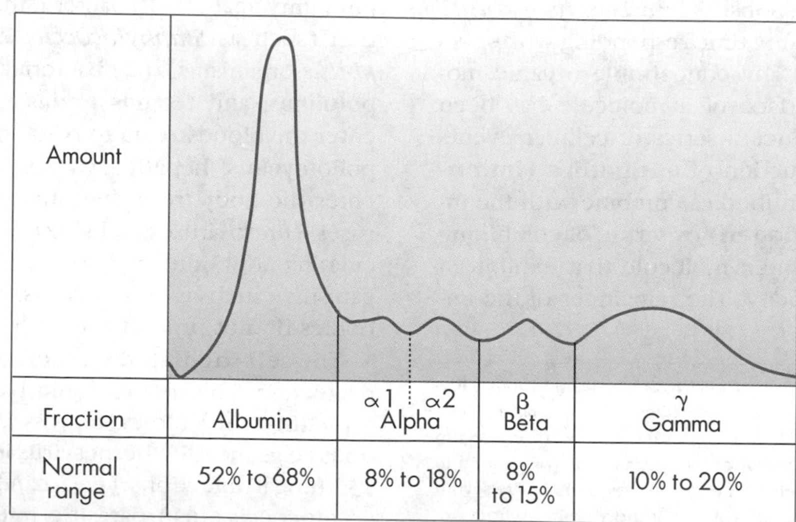


**FIGURE 13-8** Electrophoretic separation of major serum proteins. Most antibody activity lies within the gamma-globulin fraction. This fraction rises with active synthesis of antibodies in response to antigenic stimulation.

and are termed *heavy* (H) *chains;* two are of lower molecular weight and are called *light* (L) *chains.* Each L chain is linked by disulfide (—ss—) bonds to an H chain, and in turn the H chains are linked to each other by disulfide bonds. When immunoglobulin monomers are visualized by means of electron microscopy, they are seen to have a Y-shaped structure. At the ends of the two arms of the Y are the sites where antigen is bound. Both the H and L chains participate in the formation of these *antigen-binding sites.* Thus most monomers of immunoglobulin have two antigen-binding sites and are termed *bivalent.* The two arms of the Y are designated the *Fab* (for fragment, antigen-binding) *regions.* The base of the Y is called the *Fc region* (for fragment, crys-

**TABLE 13-5 Properties of Immunoglobulin Classes**

| | IMMUNOGLOBULIN CLASS | | | | |
|---|---|---|---|---|---|
| PROPERTY | IgG | IgM | IgA | IgE | IgD |
| Physiochemical | | | | | |
| Percentage of Ig | 75-85 | 7 | 10 | 0.002 | 1 |
| Configuration | Monomer | Pentamer | Monomer, dimer | Monomer | Monomer |
| Half-life in serum (days) | 23 | 5 | 6 | 2 | 3 |
| Functional antigen-binding sites | 2 | 5 | 2 | 2 | 2 |
| Biologic | | | | | |
| Principal site found | Internal body fluids | Serum | Serum and exocrine secretions | Tissue bound | Bound to lymphocyte surface |
| Fixed complement | Yes | Yes | No | No | No |
| Crosses placenta | Yes | No | No | No | No |
| Principal functions | Agglutination, detoxification, virus neutralization; enhancement of phagocytosis | Agglutination, cytolysis; enhancement of phagocytosis | Protection of mucosal surfaces | Mediation of immediate type of hypersensitivity | Control of lymphocytic activation and suppression |

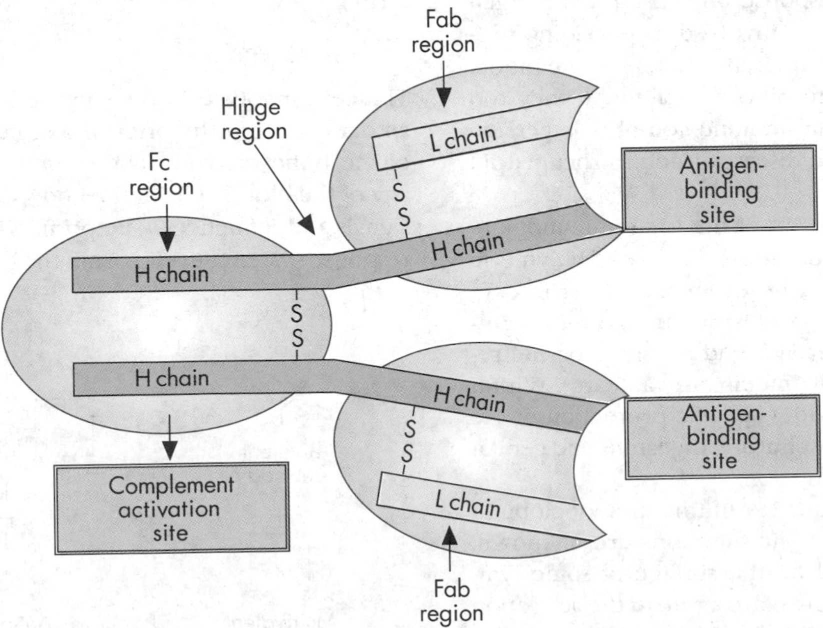


**FIGURE 13-9** Basic structure of IgG monomer. All immunoglobulin classes are composed of variations of this basic structure with combinations to form dimers (IgA) or pentamers (IgM).

tallizable). The Fc fragment binds to complement and to white blood cells, including macrophages. In the region of the disulfide bond joining the H chains, the molecule seems to be flexible, and this region is known as the "hinge" region.

The predominant class of immunoglobulins in normal adult serum is *IgG.* It makes up about 75% to 85% of the immunoglobulin fraction. Because of its structure and biologic activity, it is also found in the extravascular fluids of the body (see Table 13-5). IgG is capable of crossing the placenta to provide the newborn with temporary natural passive immunity to those diseases against which the mother has circulating antibodies. It functions primarily in the processes of toxin neutralization and viral and bacterial inactivation and in the formation of antigen-antibody-complement immune complexes associated with certain types of hypersensitivity (see Chapter 70). IgG is the immunoglobulin class primarily responsible for the rise in serum antibodies during a secondary (anamnestic, booster) response (see p. 321).

*IgM* structurally is composed of five monomeric units attached to each other at the Fc region. Thus the star-shaped molecule with the antigen-binding sites pointed outward that results from this macromolecular arrangement is termed a *pentamer.* Sometimes this immunoglobulin class, which constitutes about 7% of the immunoglobulin in serum, is called the *macroglobulin* because of its molecular size. As a result of its size, it is confined primarily to the intravascular fluids. IgM, as with IgG, is capable of binding the C1 component of complement and initiating the complement cascade. In each antigenic stimulation, IgM antibodies are the first to appear, but they neither reach the levels of IgG nor exhibit an anamnestic response on subsequent antigen contact. They are primarily involved in providing protection against viral and bacterial invaders in the blood. Because of their ability to bind complement, they too are responsible for certain immune complex hypersensitivities and autoimmune diseases, such as rheumatoid arthritis.

*IgA* constitutes about 10% of the total immunoglobulin in serum. It can be found in a variety of polymeric forms (primarily monomer in serum and dimer in exocrine secretions). IgA is also termed the *secretory immunoglobulin* because it is found in the exocrine secretions of the body (milk, mucin, saliva, tears). Within these secretions IgA provides specific protection of the mucosal surfaces of the respiratory, digestive, and genital tracts from pathogenic invasion.

*IgD* makes up only about 1% of the immunoglobulin fraction of serum. Its biologic functions are unknown. Most of the IgD is found on the surface of some lymphocytes, where it probably plays a role in the activation and suppression of lymphocyte function. It may also modify the activity of IgM.

*IgE* is present in the serum in extremely small amounts (0.002%), a sparsity that results from this immunoglobulin's predilection for attachment to the surface of mast cells and basophils. When bound by the Fc region of the monomer to the surface of these cells, which are rich in the potent, physiologically active substances histamine, kinins, and serotonin, IgE serves to mediate the severe and occasionally fatal anaphylactic type of hypersensitivities. These include anaphylactic shock, allergic asthma, and hay fever (see Chapter 70). The protective role of this immunoglobulin is not clear, but it may be effective in providing protection against certain parasitic worms.

**Immunogen-immunoglobulin interactions**

When an immunoglobulin comes in contact with its specific antigen, a physical interaction occurs between the two, causing a reversible binding of the antibody to the antigen. The antibody's affinity for the antigen and the avidity, or tightness, of the binding depend on the location and spatial arrangement of the antigenic determinants on the antigen's surface and how well the antigen-combining site on the antibody molecule "fits" the antigenic determinant. Inasmuch as the antigen usually is multivalent and the antibody generally is at least bivalent, the antigen molecules may be cross-bound and clumped (agglutinated, precipitated) by antibody molecules (Figure 13-10).

Within the body the binding of antibody to the antigen can have direct beneficial effects, such as detoxification of toxins, inactivation of viruses, or, coupled with complement, the direct lysis of cells. In most cases, however, the antigen-antibody combination initiates and facilitates the nonspecific defense mechanisms (phagocytosis, complement, inflammatory response, and so forth).

## Cells Involved

The cells involved in the specific immune response are all derived from the original undifferentiated stem cells of the bone marrow. The stem cell may develop into any of the blood cells of the body, depending on various signals and influences. The primary cells of the immune response system develop from the lymphocytic cell pop-

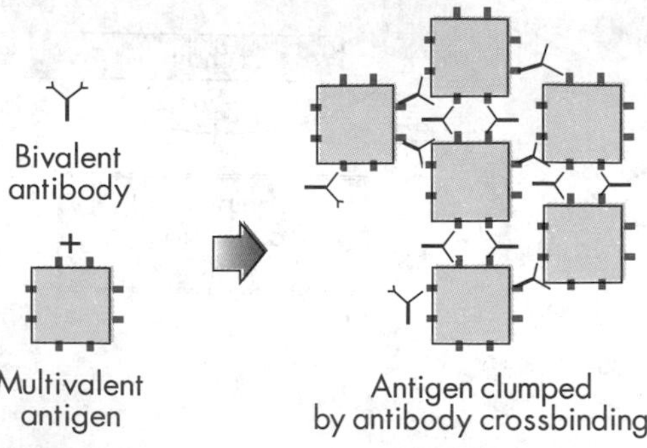


**FIGURE 13-10** Clumping of multivalent antigen by its specific antibody.

ulation (Figure 13-11). One population of lymphocytic cells undergoes differentiation under the influence of the thymus gland and becomes *thymus-dependent lymphocytes,* or *T cells.* These cells become responsible for facilitating the *cell-mediated immunity* (CMI) *response.* Another population of lymphocytes matures in a site other than the thymus and is known as *thymus-independent lymphocytes,* or *B cells.* The designation B cell comes from the fact that in the chicken, where this process was first detected, a single site exists where this differentiation occurs, that is, the *bursa of Fabricius.* No such singular lymphoid organ is found in human beings, but it is believed that the process occurs in the bone marrow or possibly the gut-associated lymphoid tissues (tonsils, Peyer's patches of the intestines, appendix). Because the exact site in humans has not been unequivocably identified, it often is referred to as the *bursa equivalent.* The B cells are responsible for production of the immunoglobulins and provision of the *humoral immune response.*

The role of the lymphocytes (B or T cells) is to recognize the presence of an antigen and to initiate specific mechanisms of disposal. Just as important, the lymphocyte must recognize a component of host tissues as *self* and protect that tissue from immunologic response reactions.

B and T lymphocytes can be differentiated from each other on the basis of specific *markers* (membrane-bound proteins) on the surface of the cells. For instance, T cells have a marker that causes the binding of sheep RBCs, whereas B cells are lacking such protein. B cells, on the other hand, usually have immunoglobulins displayed on their cell surface. By the identification of the specific markers on the cell surface, cells can be divided into B or T cell types and even further subdivided into subtypes (see later discussion on helper and suppressor T cells).

A third type of cell is directly involved in the immune response, the **antigen-presenting cell** (APC) (also called **antigen-processing cell**). The macrophage of the bloodstream and lymphoid tissues is the cell type

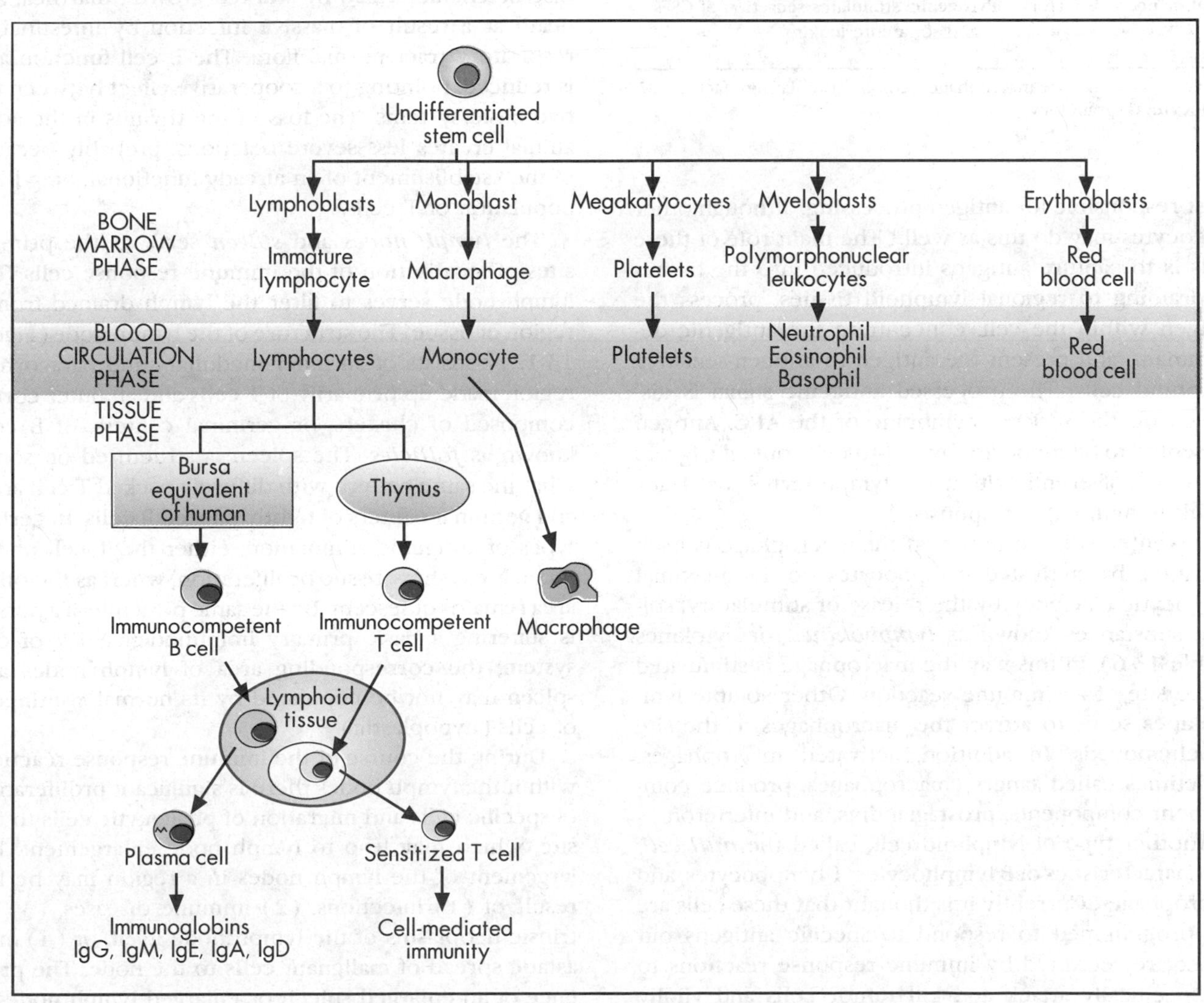


**FIGURE 13-11** Development of B and T lymphocytes.

**TABLE 13-6 Cytokines Liberated in the Immune Response**

| CYTOKINE | FUNCTION |
|---|---|
| Interferon | Inhibits viral replication<br>Activates macrophages and neutrophils<br>Activates natural killer cells |
| GM-CSF | Stimulates growth and differentiation of myeloid stem cells |
| M-CSF | Stimulates production of monocytes and macrophages |
| G-CSF | Stimulates production of neutrophils |
| Interleukin-1 | Pyrogenic; stimulates helper T cells and B lymphocytes |
| Interleukin-2 | Stimulates production of T lymphocytes |
| Interleukin-3 | Stimulates production of bone marrow stem cells |
| Interleukin-4 | Stimulates growth of B lymphocytes |
| Interleukin-5 | Stimulates growth of eosinophils and function of plasma cells |
| Interleukin-6 | Stimulates growth of B lymphocytes and stem cell production |
| Tumor necrosis factor | Pyrogenic; stimulates secretion of CSFs and some interleukins |

*GM-CSF,* Granulocyte-macrophage colony-stimulating factor; *M,* monocyte; *G,* granulocyte.

most responsible for antigen processing, although other leukocytes may do this as well.[1] The main role of these cells is to capture antigens introduced into the tissues or draining to regional lymphoid tissues, process the antigen within the cell, concentrate the antigenic determinant, and present the antigen to antigen-sensitive lymphoid cells. The processed antigenic signal is displayed on the surface membrane of the APC. Antigen presented to lymphocytes by cell-to-cell contact triggers the series of events within the lymphocytes that leads to full immunologic response.

It is interesting to note that the macrophage is itself activated by activated lymphocytes to its maximal phagocytic efficiency by the release of stimulatory, soluble substances known as *lymphokines,* or cytokines (Table 13-6). In this way the macrophage is stimulated at the site of an immune reaction. Other soluble lymphokines serve to attract the macrophages to the site by chemotaxis. In addition, activated macrophages, sometimes called "angry" macrophages, produce complement components, prostaglandins, and interferon.

Another type of lymphoid cell, called the *null cell,* has characteristics of B lymphocytes, T lymphocytes, and macrophages. Currently it is thought that these cells are not programmed to respond to specific antigens but rather are recruited by immune response reactions to nonspecifically attack and kill tumor cells and virally infected cells. When activated and directed against foreign cells, these are referred to as *natural killer* (NK) *cells.* After destroying target cells, the NK cell is able to survive unharmed and attack other target cells.

## Organs and Tissues Involved

The organs and tissues of the specific immune response system include the central organs (bone marrow, thymus) and the peripheral organs (lymph nodes, spleen, lymphatic vessels). Within the central organs the immune response cells are synthesized and matured, whereas within the peripheral organs the mature cells are concentrated.

The *thymus* serves as the control organ of the immune system. It is the differentiation site of the T cell lymphocytic populations and, through certain soluble thymic hormones, serves to regulate the overall immune system. The activity of the thymus reaches its peak in childhood, and the organ begins to shrink in size after puberty. If the thymus is removed (thymectomy) very early in an animal's life, a severe state of immunodeficiency is induced and T cell–mediated immunity never develops. The thymectomized animal develops a wasting disease characterized by stunted growth, diarrhea, and death as a result of massive infection by intestinal or respiratory tract normal flora. The B cell function also is reduced, pointing to a cooperative effect between the two basic systems. The loss of the thymus in the adult animal creates less severe reactions, probably because of the establishment of an already functional, long-lived population of T cells.

The *lymph nodes* and *spleen* serve as the primary sites of localization of the immune response cells. The lymph node serves to filter the lymph drained from a region of tissue. The structure of the lymph node (Figure 13-12) consists of an inner medullary and paracortical region made up primarily of T cells and an outer cortex composed of clusters, or germinal centers, of B cells known as *follicles.* The spleen is structured on somewhat the same pattern with diffusely packed T cell areas and germinal centers of tightly packed B cells. In certain types of antigenic stimulation, either the T cell or the B cell areas show tissue proliferation, whereas the other area remains quiescent. By the same principle, if a person is suffering a basic primary immunodeficiency of one system, the corresponding area of lymph nodes and spleen may not be populated by its normal contingent of cells (hypoplastic).

During the course of the immune response reaction, within the lymph nodes there is significant proliferation of specific cells and migration of phagocytic cells to the site, which may lead to lymph node enlargement. Enlargement of the lymph nodes in a region may be the result of (1) infections, (2) immune diseases, (3) intrinsic neoplasms of the lymph node itself, or (4) metastatic spread of malignant cells to the node. The presence of an enlarged spleen or enlarged lymph nodes is almost always an important clinical finding.

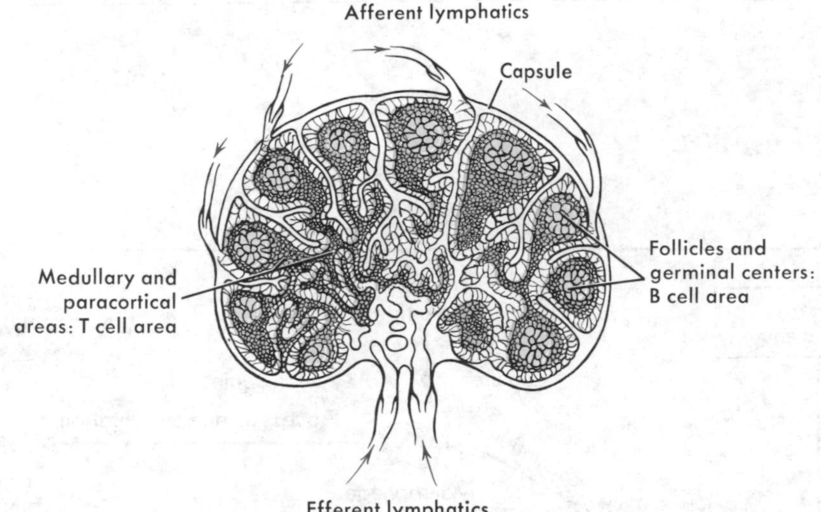


**FIGURE 13-12** B and T cell areas of lymph node.

The presence of other nonencapsulated lymphoid tissues is associated with the mucosal surfaces of the body, such as the gastrointestinal, respiratory, and urogenital tracts. These immune response tissues are referred to as the *mucosal-associated lymphoid tissues.* The function of these tissues is similar to that of the encapsulated regional lymph nodes, but they may be especially involved in the synthesis of the secretory immunoglobulin, IgA, which is important in providing total immune protection of mucosal surfaces.

## Primary Immune Response

### Antigenic challenge

When an antigen is introduced into the body, it can trigger a wide or narrow spectrum of response mechanisms. The specific pattern of response depends on (1) the amount of antigen introduced, (2) the site of introduction, and (3) the type of antigen introduced.

Small amounts of a noninvasive, large, particulate antigen introduced at a single body site are quickly and efficiently handled at a local site with little or no systemic involvement beyond the local lymph node. Because the inflammatory response and local lymph node can localize the spread of the antigen, the immune response may go completely unnoticed by the host organism. Larger, particulate antigens are readily cleared, but small, soluble antigens are more difficult to clear from the circulation.

Large amounts of an antigen may allow the antigen to escape from the local site simply by overwhelming the local defense mechanisms. Even though the lymph nodes and MPS can clear 80% to 90% of an antigen on a single pass, if the amount of the antigen is extremely large, some antigen may escape the local site. An excessively large, sustained antigen dose can exhaust not only the local site but the entire MPS as well. This greatly reduces the body's ability to respond to even minor invasive challenges and renders the host vulnerable to secondary infections.

Highly invasive antigens (e.g., bacteria such as *S. aureus* or *S. pyogenes*) or those introduced directly into the bloodstream by blood transfusion, intravenous catheterization, or injection can immediately establish a systemic type of immune response. This is why extreme care must be exercised in the use of any type of medical procedure that would allow the introduction of antigens into the general circulation. The localization action of the immune response is critical to efficient functioning of the response.

### Antigenic processing and presentation

When an antigenic substance is introduced into the body, either it is carried directly by lymphocytic circulation to a regional lymphoid tissue, where it is engulfed by an APC, or an APC engulfs the antigen at the site of introduction and carries the antigen to the lymphoid tissues. In the APC the complex antigen is degraded, and the antigenic determinants are attached to one of the cell membrane proteins on the APC known as a *major histocompatability complex* (MHC) antigen on its surface. These same MHC antigens are the markers on the surface of the cell that allow recognition of self versus nonself cells (see Figure 13-2). The APC, with the concentrated antigenic determinants, then *presents* this antigenic signal to specifically reactive B or T cells in the regional lymph node. This is accomplished by a cell-to-cell contact. With this interaction the specific B or T cell is stimulated to undergo proliferation (cell division) and differentiation (change in structure and function). A soluble material known as ***interleukin 1*** (IL-1) released from the APC signals the lymphocyte to divide and differentiate.

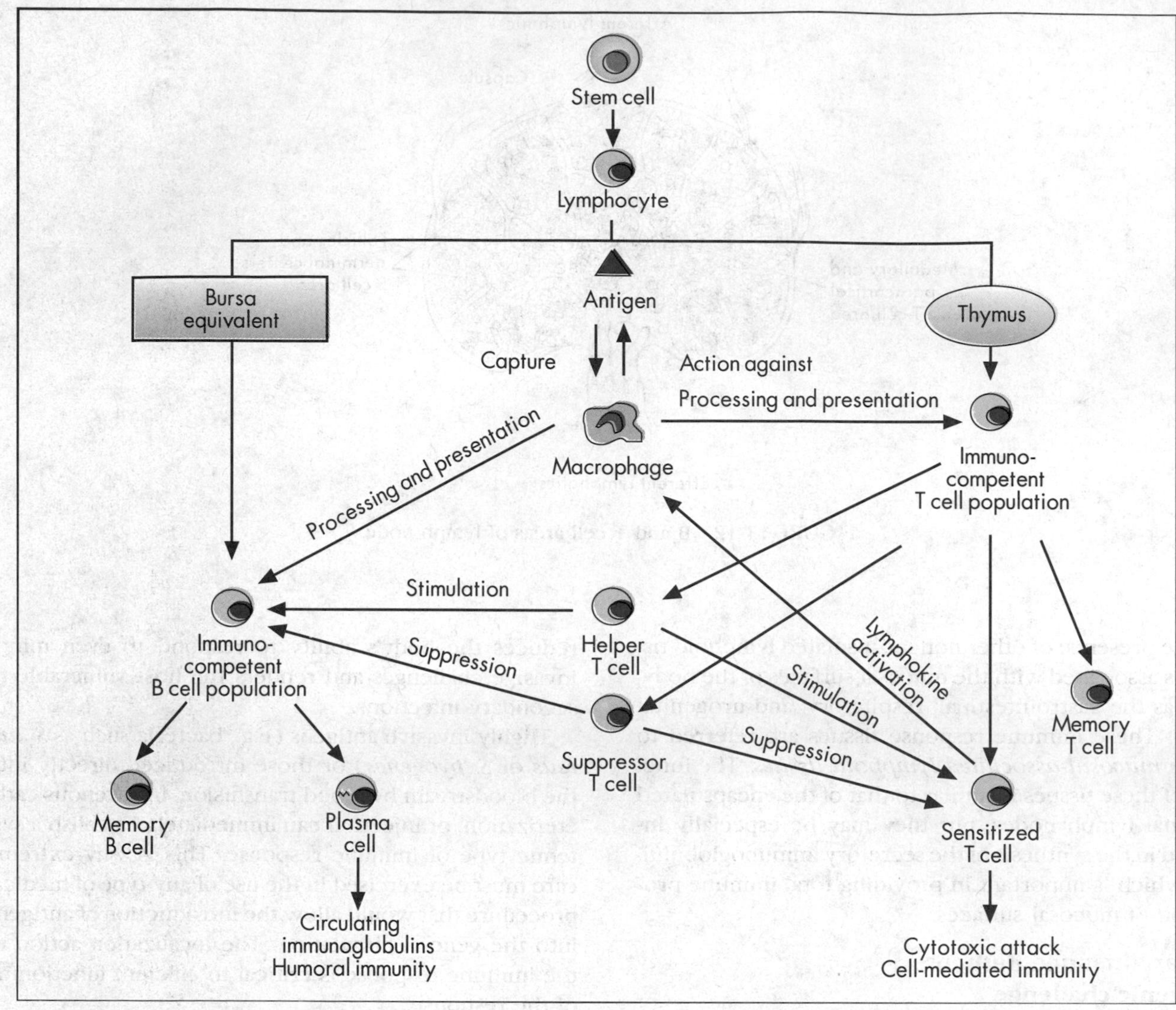


**FIGURE 13-13** Combined response of B and T cell systems.

## Humoral response

When the antigen is introduced for the first time, one of three basic mechanisms of response is elicited: (1) a response mediated primarily by B cells, the humoral response, (2) a response in which the T cells are primarily involved, the CMI, or (3) a combined type of response.

If the antigen is the type that triggers a humoral response, the first time the body is exposed to the antigen, the B cell system responds with the synthesis of circulating immunoglobulins (Figure 13-13).

Antigen-specific B cells bear receptors to their surface, which allow them to recognize their antigenic stimulant. These receptors are the antigen-specific immunoglobulin molecules that the cell is programmed to produce. They are embedded in the membrane by the Fc region of the monomer with their antigen-binding sites extended out. Seemingly only a few lymphocytes within a lymph node have the ability to respond to the antigen. The stimulated B cell then begins a process of proliferation and differentiation. The progeny of the stimulated cell increases in number within the lymph node, forming *clones* of specifically adapted lymphocytes. With each generation of new cells within the clone, the lymphocytes become more differentiated toward a cell population ideally suited for the synthesis and release of immunoglobulin. These cells are known as *plasma cells.*

With the development of the plasma-cell population in the lymph node (several days after the introduction of the antigen), antibodies can be detected in the lymph node. It is not until about 7 days after the antigenic challenge, however, that detectable levels of specific antibodies appear in the serum. The plasma cell population of the lymph node and the levels of antibody in the blood continue to increase for another 2 to 3 weeks,

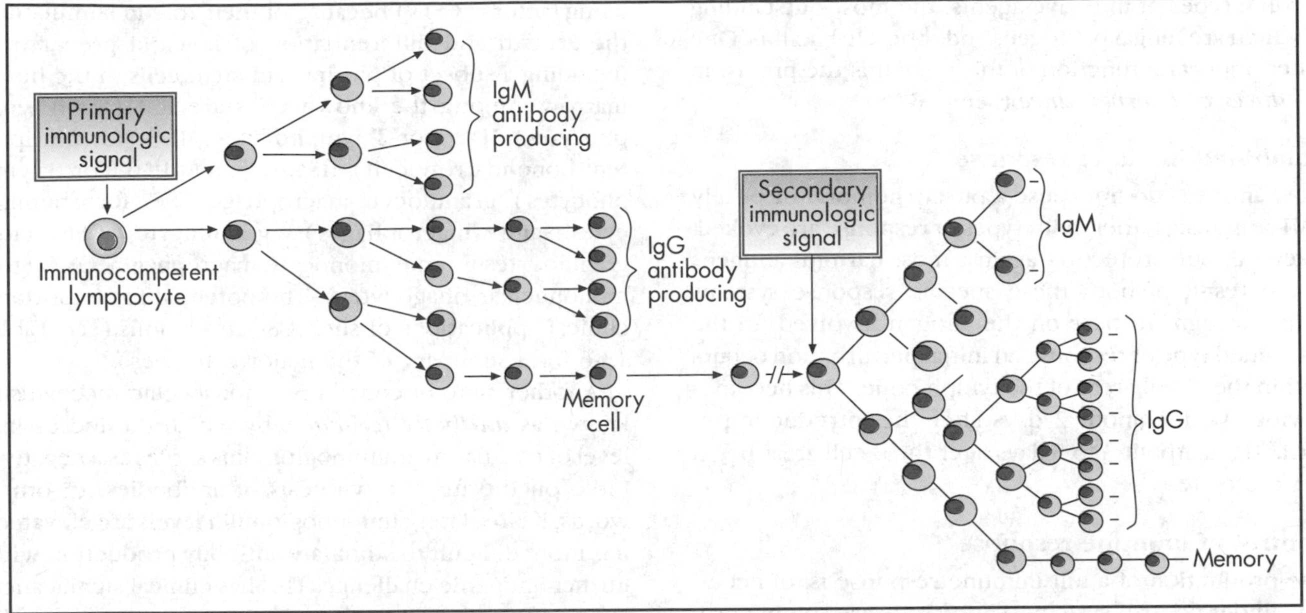


**FIGURE 13-14** Response of memory cells to antigen signal.

and then both begin to retreat. Some of the lymphocytes of the activated clone become "memory cells," which are much more responsive, both in time of reaction and efficiency of antibody synthesis, to subsequent contact with the antigen (Figure 13-14).

The humoral response serves to protect the body from such agents as microbial toxins, bacteria within the extravascular spaces in the blood and on mucosal surfaces, and viruses that must pass through the circulatory system to reach their site of infection (e.g., poliomyelitis virus).

### Cell-mediated immune response

Certain antigens trigger a response mediated by T cell proliferation and reaction. A T cell that has received its antigenic stimulus is referred to as a *sensitized T cell lymphocyte* (see Figure 13-13).

The initial steps of the CMI response—those involving the antigen processing by the macrophage, or APC—seem to be the same as in the humoral response. After the presentation of the antigenic stimulus to lymph node T cells, proliferation in the T cell domain occurs. Circulating antibodies are not released; rather, sensitized lymphocytes are released into the circulation. These cells migrate to the site of the antigen's entrance into the body, where the invading agent or residual antigen is found. These activated lymphocytes, along with macrophages, infiltrate the regions of the tissue and begin a direct attack on the antigen or tissue cells labeled with the antigen. The T cells participating in this direct attack are known as *cytotoxic T cells.*

To amplify the site reaction further, the sensitized lymphocytes activate the nonspecific phagocytotic cells (macrophages, PMNs, null cells) in the region of the antigen. This is accomplished through the release of the soluble cytokines (see Table 13-6), which marshall this additional cellular involvement to attack the antigenic materials.

The observable results of this attack of antigen-labeled tissues are classically illustrated by a positive tuberculin test reaction. In this case the inflammation (erythema, induration) observed at the site of the intradermal injection of a small amount of cell wall extract of *Mycobacterium tuberculosis* represents a T cell attack on the antigen-labeled cells. The positive test result is actually mediated by a secondary immune response (see following discussion) produced by prior exposure to *M. tuberculosis.* With the introduction of the antigen, it is engulfed, processed, and presented by the APC to responsive clones of T cells in the regional lymph node. That clone of cells is stimulated to undergo proliferation, and activated T cells are released into circulation. The activated T cells seek out the antigen (at the site of injection) and begin to accumulate at the site, where they release cytokines (lymphokines) that stimulate null cells and macrophages to attack the tissues at the focal site. The lag time (24 to 48 hours) required for the development of the inflammation at the site is consistent with the time needed to trigger the release of the responsive cells from the regional lymph node and their accumulation at the site of the antigen-labeled tissues.

The CMI response is especially effective in protection against diseases that grow and do their damage intracellularly, where the circulating immunoglobulins cannot reach them. Diseases of this type include viral and rickettsial diseases and those produced by certain chronic types of infective agents, the most outstanding of which are fungal pathogens and tubercle bacillus. One other important function of this system is the provision of *cancer cell surveillance* (see p. 326).

### Combined immune response

Most antigens do not cause a purely humoral or purely CMI response; rather, both types of response are evoked. Likewise, our protection against most harmful antigens is the result of both these specific response systems being brought to bear on the antigen involved. In the combined type of response an initial perturbation occurs within the T cell areas of the lymph node. This becomes obvious within about 2 days after the introduction of the antigen. About 3 to 5 days later the B cell areas begin to proliferate.

### Control of immune response

The production of a full immune response is, of necessity, under control systems. **Cytokines** are soluble protein mediators that induce and regulate various aspects of immunity. They act as hormones and are synthesized by a variety of cells: macrophages, neutrophils, eosinophils, monocytes, and T lymphocytes. These protein mediators have been called by various names as information about them was uncovered. Initially they were termed *lymphokines* when it was recognized that many of them were produced by activated T lymphocytes. When it was generally acknowledged that other cells secreted them as well, they were termed *cytokines.* An even more specific name, *interleukins,* recognizes that the major function of many of the cytokines is communication among various leukocytes. As many as 14 interleukins have been recognized, with specific functions and structures.

Interleukin-1 is produced by macrophages when they come into contact with bacterial products, the helper T cell, or tumor necrosis factor. Interleukin-1 is an endogenous pyrogen; it increases the proliferation of helper T cells, stimulates growth and differentiation of B lymphocytes, and induces the secretion of other interleukins. Interleukin-2 (IL-2) is produced by helper T cells; it increases the growth and differentiation of T lymphocytes and also stimulates increased production of more IL-2 from activated lymphocytes. In addition, it increases nonspecific cytotoxic functions in natural killer cells (lymphokine-activated killer [LAK] cells). Interleukin-3 (IL-3), produced by helper T cells, stimulates production of immature bone marrow stem cells in the presence of infection. Interleukin-4 and interleukin-5 (IL-4 and IL-5) also are produced by helper T cells; IL-4 stimulates growth and proliferation of B lymphocytes, whereas IL-5 stimulates their differentiation into actively producing antibody cells. Interleukin-6 (IL-6), made by both macrophages and T cells, is thought to have antiviral and possibly antitumor effects. IL-6 stimulates the growth of activated B lymphocytes.

Some of these interleukins are called colony-stimulating factors (CSFs) because of their role in stimulating the growth and differentiation of myeloid precursors, including a subset of pluripotent stem cells in the bone marrow. Among the known CSFs are IL-1 (for B lymphocytes), IL-2 (for T lymphocytes), IL-3 (for pluripotent bone marrow cell), IL-4, IL-5, and IL-6 (for B lymphocytes), granulocyte-macrophage CSF (for granulocytes and macrophages), granulocyte CSF (for granulocytes), and monocyte-macrophage CSF (for mononuclear phagocytes). The potential for important clinical applications of such CSFs is obvious (see Table 13-6 for a summary of the major cytokines).

Another type of control is a nonspecific mechanism known as *antibody feedback,* by which the increasing level of circulating immunoglobulins serves as a negative force on the further synthesis of antibodies. In other words, if circulating immunoglobulin levels are elevated, it is more difficult to stimulate antibody production with further antigenic challenge. This has clinical significance in the case of abnormal antibody production by individuals suffering from gammopathies, such as multiple myeloma or macroglobulinemia (see Chapter 70). These diseases are marked by significant elevation of the $\gamma$-globulin fraction of the blood and a seemingly paradoxic increased susceptibility to infection. The high levels of nonspecific $\gamma$-globulin exert an immunosuppressive effect on further specific antibody synthesis when the host is challenged by a pathogen.

The immune response system also is controlled by the presence of specific regulator T cells. A subset of the T cell population of the body is known as *helper T cells* (designated $T_H$ or $T_4$ cells). The function of these cells is to cooperate with the B cells and T cells to allow the full expression of a B cell or T cell response. If a B cell clone required the aid of a helper T cell clone and the $T_H$ cell clone is missing, the B cell clone will not undergo proliferation and differentiation to form plasma cells that produce the specific immunoglobulin. On the other hand, the presence of *suppressor T cell* clones (designated $T_S$ or $T_8$ cells) prevents or suppresses the full development of the immunoresponsive clones (see Figure 13-13).

If for some reason the normal balance between immunoresponsive T or B cells and $T_S$ and $T_H$ cells is disrupted, control over proper immune response reactions may be lost. The classic example of this problem can be observed in AIDS, in which a disproportionate ratio occurs in the number of $T_S$ ($T_8$) cells compared with $T_H$ ($T_4$) cells in peripheral circulation; this results from destruction of the $T_H$ cells caused by HIV infection. In other conditions, such as some autoimmune diseases, the loss of certain $T_S$ clones may allow the production of antibodies against self antigens.

## Secondary Immune Response

As emphasized at the outset of this section, one of the touchstone characteristics of the specific response system is its ability to remember prior contact with an

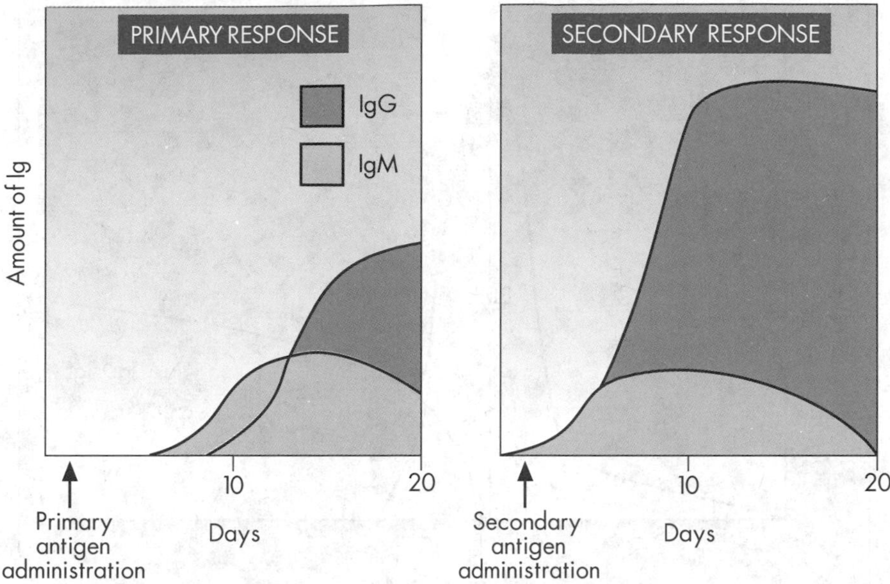


**FIGURE 13-15** Primary and secondary humoral responses.

antigen and to provide a more rapid and efficient protective reaction on subsequent contact. The first contact between the immune response system and an antigen leads to the primary response, as just described. When antibody synthesis is measured in a primary response, there is significant lag time to the appearance of antibodies in the circulation (Figure 13-15). Immunoglobulins of the IgM class are the first to appear, but they maintain protective levels for only a short period. Specific IgG antibodies follow and reach protective levels within 12 to 14 days, but they also fall off fairly quickly with only this initial exposure. When the "primed" immune response system encounters the antigen again, a secondary response ensues, which is more rapid, of greater intensity, and longer lasting than the primary response. This secondary response is termed an *anamnestic response.* This "remembered" response is a characteristic of both the B and T cell systems. The prior contact with the antigen is stored in special memory cells of both cell lines. As illustrated in Figure 13-14, the memory cells respond immediately to the antigenic signal, so that the lag time between exposure to the antigen and production of protective antibody levels is greatly reduced. This phenomenon provides the basis for active immunization and "booster" doses to maintain the protective levels of immunity. In an immunized person the memory cells elicit the rapid response in time for the immune system to overwhelm the pathogen or toxin before it can produce its damage. These memory cells are long-living lymphocytes, surviving and able to respond for years after their development.

## IMMUNE TOLERANCE

**Immune tolerance** is defined as the state of immunologic nonresponsiveness. By some mechanisms the body becomes tolerant to self while maintaining responsiveness to foreign materials. Evidence establishes that self-tolerance is acquired primarily during embryonic development; however, the exact mechanisms by which it develops remain an issue. During fetal development the immune system is presented with antigens from the developing tissues. These become identified as self antigens; thus, when exposed to these antigens postnatally, the individual is tolerant of them.

One proposed mechanism by which this state could be induced is known as the *clonal selection theory.* This theory states that when potentially responsive clones of B or T cells come into contact with an antigen prenatally, the responsive cell line is killed or controlled, thus eliminating the responsiveness to that antigen from the body. This produces a state of *natural tolerance.* This theory is supported by experimental data that show that, by exposing experimental animals to foreign antigens in utero, a tolerance to that antigen is developed; however, some antigens introduced in this manner are found to be more *tolerogenic* (capable of inducing tolerance) than others. Further, the clonal selection theory does not explain how it is possible to break tolerance in adults, as indicated in certain experimental studies or with certain autoimmune diseases (see Chapter 70). In some cases at least, tolerance is not caused by the total elimination of specifically reactive cells but by the blocking of expression or temporary inactivation of the responsive cells. The action of suppressor T cells or the failure of mobilization by helper T cells has been shown to play a significant role in maintaining the state of self-tolerance.

## DEVELOPMENTAL ASPECTS OF IMMUNE RESPONSE

Lymphoid cells first appear in the fetus as stem cells in the fetal liver at about the end of the first trimester. The

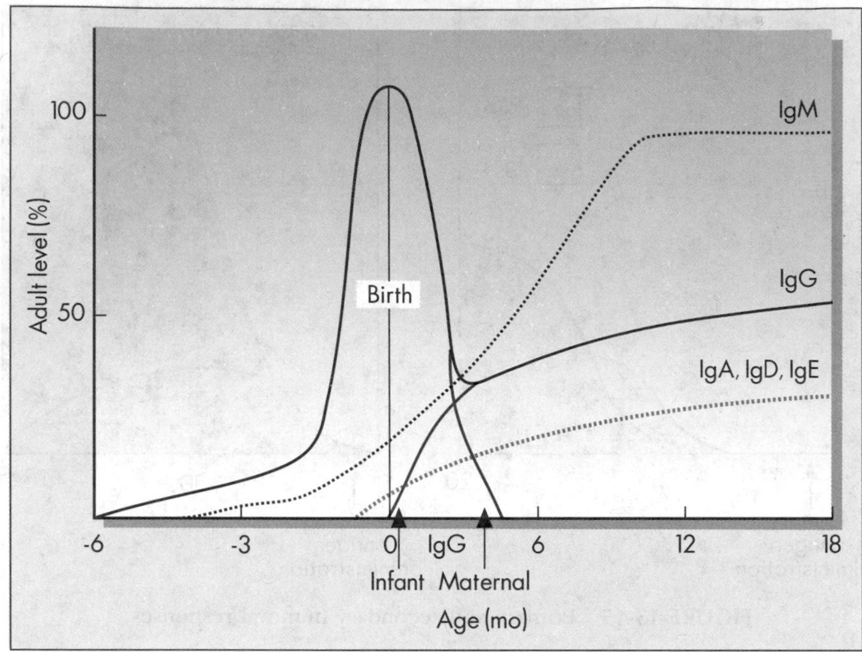


**FIGURE 13-16** Immunoglobulin levels in fetus and neonate.

lymphoid tissues of the thymus also develop fairly early in the fetus. At birth, however, the lymph nodes and spleen are still underdeveloped, but T and B cell responsiveness is fully functional. The fetus is capable of some immune response if challenged by an in utero (within the uterus) infection, such as congenital syphilis or rubella. Unless the fetus has been exposed to a congenital infection, at birth the synthesized immunoglobulin levels of the neonate are low (Figure 13-16). The newborn has high levels of transplacentally acquired maternal IgG antibodies. These maternal antibodies have a half-life of about 30 days in the child; this, coupled with the increase in blood volume in the growing infant, leads to a drop in the IgG levels of the blood over the first 3 months. Thereafter the rate of the child's own synthesis of IgG provides for a steady increase in the immunoglobulin concentration within the serum. IgM levels reach adult concentrations by about age 9 months.

Numerous studies in both animals and humans have shown that during the aging process a progressive loss of immunologic vigor occurs. The prime immunologic age probably is achieved during the late adolescent years, when virtually the full complement of immunities has been developed and the responsiveness of the system peaks. The middle years are characterized by a plateau and slowly falling curve until the later years of life, when a sharp decline becomes evident. This decline is seen in both CMI and humoral response systems. This decrease in immunologic sensitivity is associated with an increasingly less effective and more misdirected immune response. There is an increasing frequency of autoimmune disease, susceptibility to pathogenic and opportunistic microorganisms, and incidence of cancer.

## NEUROENDOCRINE FACTORS INFLUENCING IMMUNE RESPONSE

The cells of the immune response system are influenced by and in turn influence the other regulatory communication systems in the body, that is, the endocrine and neural systems. The immune response cells have receptors on their surface to receive modifying input from the full array of hormones: insulin, growth hormone, glucocorticoids, estrogen, testosterone, and so on. Some of these hormone signals (glucocorticosteroids, testosterone, estrogen, progesterone) have been shown to depress immune function. Other hormones (growth hormone, thyroxine, insulin) tend to improve immune function. Other neurotransmitters and hormones found in lower doses in the body also influence immune response cell function. The negative effects of the corticosteroids are so great that they are widely used as pharmacologic agents to suppress immune function (see Chapters 70 and 72).

The thymus gland functions as an endocrine organ, releasing hormones that influence not only immunoresponsive cells and lymphoid tissues but other body cells that have receptors for these hormones. Interleukin 1 and other cytokines have been shown to stimulate glucocorticosteroid synthesis by influencing the pituitary gland to release adrenocorticotropic hormone (ACTH). The thymus and lymphoid tissues receive direct innervation from autonomic and sensory neurons that control blood circulation to these organs and also seem to exercise more direct control over the immune response cells themselves.

The physiologic control of the neuroendocrine function has long been recognized in the immunosuppressive effects produced by the stress response. Growing evidence suggests that this immunosuppression also is produced indirectly through neural signals to the immunoresponsive tissues.

These interconnections among the three major communication systems of the body has led to the development of the following concept: although many aspects of each system can be considered to stand alone, a broader, more holistic perspective views them as functioning as an interrelated complex. The term *psychoimmunoendocrine system* has been developed to reflect this more inclusive conceptualization. With this perspective in mind, psychotherapeutic methods and cognitive visualization have been increasingly used as adjunctive therapy in immune-related diseases and cancer. However, because most of the connections between these systems are fairly indirect and because our understanding of the control functions of each is still tenuous, these therapies should never be relied on as a primary approach. Also, some potential danger exists in leading patients to believe that they can exercise direct cognitive control over their pathologic conditions. When they are not successful, patients may become disillusioned and lose hope, which then removes whatever positive aspects might be derived from the indirect betterment of their overall improved immune state. The emphasis should be on the general and broad improvement of their general immune state.

# APPLICATIONS AND IMPLICATIONS OF IMMUNE RESPONSE

## CONCEPT OF SUSCEPTIBILITY AND IMMUNITY

The objective of the biologic defense mechanisms is to provide the host with protection. The ultimate protection would be total resistance to encroachment or damage by an organism or agent; this usually is termed *absolute immunity.* Absence of such protective barriers is called **susceptibility.** Although these terms generally are applied to immunity from infectious organisms, they can be used to describe the relative susceptibility to encroachment by an external agent. As described earlier, nonspecific immunity, or innate immunity, is provided when the external and internal nonspecific defense mechanisms serve as the barrier excluding or destroying the invading agent. Specific immunity protects against a single, unique agent through the development of specific antibodies or responsive cells in the body. It is acquired from prior contact with the agent (antigen) or through the introduction of specifically protective antibodies or cells into the body.

The acquisition of specific immunity may result from a natural encounter or artificial introduction. Immunity acquired *naturally* results from such natural conditions as recovery from a disease. Immunity acquired *artificially* means that the antigen or protective antibodies were purposely introduced into the body by vaccination. The immunity may be active or passive. When an individual is producing the antibodies within the body, the immunity is termed *active.* When an individual receives the protective antibodies from some other source, the immunity is termed *passive.* Thus, when antibodies are transferred from the mother across the placenta, the child is said to have a natural passive immunity. When a vaccine is given so that antibodies are produced within the body, the immunized person is characterized as having an artificial active immunity. Table 13-7 summarizes the different types of acquired specific immunities.

Specific or nonspecific immunity to harmful agents is a relative state. The effects of different dosages of an infectious organism or the toxic products of such organisms in experimental studies clearly demonstrate that administration of sufficiently large numbers of an organism or high dosages of a toxin can overwhelm even the most highly immunized animal. Further, when the normal mechanisms of defense are breached, even in the highly resistant host, disease can result. Thus acquired immunity to infection is not always an absolute condition but depends on many complex variables. These include not only the defense mechanisms of the host but also the dosage, route of contact, and virulence of the harmful agent.

## IMMUNIZATION

Long before the mechanisms of immune response were worked out, it was recognized that recovery from certain diseases conferred protection against subsequent exposure to that disease. Dating from the days of Jenner's vaccination with cowpox exudate to protect against smallpox (1798) through the success of Pasteur with anthrax and rabies (1880s), and up to the present, the specific protective mechanisms of the immune system have been used to protect against serious infectious diseases.

### Passive Immunization

Temporary protection, usually measured in days or at most weeks, is afforded by the acquisition of preformed antibody from another host. This process is referred to as **passive immunization**. As the acquired antibodies are used up through binding with antigen or by being catabolized, the protection is lost.

*Natural passive immunization* occurs transplacentally through the transfer of IgG antibodies from the maternal circulation across the placenta to the fetal blood. Some acquisition of immunoglobulins also occurs through the colostrum of the mother's milk. A common misconception is that infants acquire large amounts of circulating antibodies from breast milk that are added to their own. Most of the protective immunoglobulins passed in maternal milk are of the IgA class and offer some protection to the infant's GI tract. Antimicrobial factors other than immunoglobulins also are present in the milk and probably account for most of the decreased

**TABLE 13-7 Types of Acquired Specific Immunity**

| TYPE OF IMMUNITY | ACQUISITION OF IMMUNITY | PROTECTION | EXAMPLES |
|---|---|---|---|
| **ACTIVE** | | | |
| Antibodies synthesized by body in response to antigenic stimulation | *Natural:* natural contact with antigen through clinical or subclinical case | *Development:* develops slowly; protective levels reached in a few weeks<br>*Duration:* long-term; often lifetime<br>*Spectrum:* specific to antigen contacted | Recovery from childhood diseases (e.g., chickenpox, measles, mumps) |
| | *Artificial:* immunization with antigen | *Development:* develops slowly; protective levels reached in a few weeks<br>*Duration:* several years; extended protection with "booster" doses<br>*Spectrum:* specific to antigen immunized against | Immunization with live or killed vaccines; toxoid immunization |
| **PASSIVE** | | | |
| Antibodies produced in one individual transferred to another | *Natural:* transplacental and colostrum transfer from mother to child | *Development:* immediate<br>*Duration:* temporary; several months<br>*Spectrum:* all antigens that mother has immunity to | Maternal immunoglobulins in neonate |
| | *Artificial:* injection of serum from immune human or animal | *Development:* immediate<br>*Duration:* temporary; several weeks<br>*Spectrum:* all antigens that source has immunity to | Injection of pooled human γ-globulin; injection of animal hyperimmune sera |

incidence of infections observed in breast-fed versus bottle-fed infants.

*Artificial passive immunization* may be necessary if the individual to be immunized has suffered exposure to a serious infectious agent to which he or she has no immunity or if the individual's own immune system is impaired or deficient. The sources of these preformed antibodies are pooled human adult γ-globulin or heterologous (from another species) globulin fractions. Pooled human γ-globulin has been used to modify the effects of measles, particularly in premature infants, in children with primary immunodeficiencies, and in patients undergoing immunosuppressive therapies. Individuals who have contact with persons with hepatitis and smallpox also may be protected by this method. It should be noted, however, that isolated γ-globulin preparations tend to form small protein aggregates; if injected intravenously, these could lead to severe anaphylactic reactions (see Chapter 70). For this reason the material is always administered *intramuscularly.*

The most frequently used heterologous antibody fractions are antitetanus and antidiphtheria antisera derived from horse globulins. Because these are foreign proteins, they can lead to the development of serum sickness (see Chapter 70). Serum sickness is more likely to occur in subjects already primed by previous contact with horse globulin; thus multiple use of heterologous sera is to be avoided.

## Active Immunization

The objective of **active immunization** is to provide effective long-term immunity by establishing within the individual's own body the capacity (1) to produce effective levels of immune response and (2) to establish a population of sensitive cells that can respond to a subsequent antigenic contact.

*Immunizing agents* ideally should be noninjurious to the individual being immunized. To accomplish this, the pathogenic effects must be modified, and at the same time the antigenicity of the agent must be maintained. Bacteria exotoxins such as those produced by diphtheria and tetanus bacteria can be successfully detoxified by formaldehyde treatment without destroying the major antigenic determinants on the protein molecule. Such detoxified antigenic materials are called *toxoids.* The use of *killed vaccines* of viruses and bacteria also can provide a safe antigen for immunization. Killed vaccines include those for pertussis (whooping cough), typhoid and cholera, and the Salk poliomyelitis vaccine. The protection conferred by these vaccines generally is inferior to that produced by live vaccines. Some of the most successful vaccines consist of living organisms that have been modified so that they are nonvirulent. The *attenuated live vaccines* provide excellent protection, but some risk exists in their use because of the possibility of reversion to the virulent form of the organism. Live vaccines of importance are those for measles, mumps, and tuberculosis (bacille Calmette-Guérin [BCG]) and the Sabin poliomyelitis vaccine.

The provision of protective levels of residual immunity depends on the inducement of (1) the right type of response (i.e., cell mediated or humoral), (2) in sufficient amounts, (3) at the right place (i.e., where the immune response can contact the antigen), and (4) against the right antigenic determinants (i.e., the antibodies formed produce an inactivating effect). Simply inducing an immune response is not sufficient to provide protection. For example, the early killed virus measles vaccines elicited a splendid production of circulating antibodies against the measles virus, but protection against measles is most effectively mediated by cellular immune responses. The humoral production did not prevent infection.

Another problem of immunization for which provision must be made is the *interference* that one antigen may have with another if the two are given simultaneously. The live virus vaccines occasionally interfere with each other; when measles and smallpox vaccines are administered at the same time, they each interfere with the development of immunity by the other. This is probably the result of interferon production. Some live virus vaccines contain more than one strain of the virus, and these can cross-inhibit. In the case of the Sabin oral polio vaccine, three separate doses are required because three strains exist within the same vaccine. With the initial dose, immunity to only one strain may develop if the strain interferes with the other two.

## Complications of Immunization

Although immunization is the most successful approach to control many infectious diseases, minimal but potentially serious risks are involved. The development of postvaccination encephalitis or other neural autoimmune complications is a serious risk with such vaccines as those for smallpox or rabies. Children with immunodeficiencies may be overwhelmed by vaccination with live vaccine. With viral vaccines, which are produced in the monkey kidney of human cell culture, a slight risk exists of introducing oncogenic (cancer-causing) viruses. A fetus may be significantly at risk if the mother receives a live virus vaccine during pregnancy. Such live vaccines should never be administered to a pregnant woman.

In addition to these rather serious risks, general discomfort is to be expected from some forms of immunization. The typhoid vaccine, for instance, is composed of large numbers of killed *Salmonella* bacteria; because the endotoxic cell wall materials of these cells is a pyrogenic (fever-producing) substance, fever and malaise

**TABLE 13-8 Effect of Selected Drugs on the Immune System**

| DRUG | IMMUNE SYSTEM IMPAIRMENT | INDICATIONS FOR IMMUNOSUPPRESSIVE THERAPY |
|---|---|---|
| Corticosteroids | Impairment of T cell function<br>Catabolism of immunoglobulins (decreased IgG)<br>Lymphocytopenia<br>Type 1 hypersensitivity: vasoconstriction, eosinopenia<br>Type 3 hypersensitivity: decreased vascular permeability<br>Type 4 hypersensitivity: decreased macrophage function | Diseases for which immune disorder is unknown<br>Tissue and organ transplantation<br>Autoimmune diseases |
| Antimetabolites (azathioprine) | Interference with RNA, DNA, and protein synthesis<br>Depression of bone marrow and antibody reproduction<br>Decreased primary immune response | Autoimmune diseases<br>Tissue transplantation<br>Dermatologic disease (pemphigus, psoriasis)<br>Neoplasia |
| Alkylating agents (cyclophosphamide) | Interference with DNA, RNA, and protein synthesis<br>Lymphocytolytic effect<br>Suppression of primary immune response | Autoimmune disease<br>Tissue transplantation<br>Inflammatory disease of unknown cause |
| Antilymphocyte serum (ALS), antilymphocyte globulin (ALG) | Inhibition of lymphocyte stimulation by specific antigens<br>Inhibition of lymphocyte mobility<br>Agglutination and lysis of lymphocytes in the presence of complement | Renal transplantation<br>Bone marrow transplantation<br>Autoimmune diseases |
| Antibiotics (actinomycin D, chloramphenicol, tetracycline, cyclosporine) | Interference with DNA-directed RNA synthesis<br>Suppression of primary immune response<br>Inhibition of protein synthesis | Cyclosporine for tissue transplantation |

are possible sequelae. The influenza vaccines often produce febrile reactions in children.

## TISSUE TRANSPLANTATION

The transfer of healthy tissues and organs from one individual to replace damaged or diseased tissues in another has been surgically possible for many years. Early attempts failed because the body rejected the foreign cells and tissues. With the growing knowledge of the immune response, the mechanisms of this rejection process became more apparent. It is now possible to make judgments and predictions concerning the likelihood of transplantation success. The course of the graft transfer process now can be controlled to favor the acceptance of the transplanted tissue.

The antigenic determinants of the tissues that lead to graft rejection are primarily found on the surface of the cells within the transplanted tissues. These antigens are known as *histocompatibility antigens* and are controlled by independently segregating genes on chromosome 6 within the chromosomal structure of the human being. They also are called *human leukocyte antigen* (HLA). Some of the histocompatibility antigens are more antigenic than others; thus some antigens are referred to as major and others as minor. The major transplantation antigens are those of the ABO and Rh blood groups and the HLA (see Chapter 72).

Graft rejection can be minimized by use of chemical (drug) or physical (radiation) agents that nonspecifically or specifically interfere with the development of an immune response reaction against the foreign tissue. Clinically, four types of chemical immunosuppressive agents are effective in providing the transitional protection needed to promote establishment of the graft (Table 13-8).

*Glucocorticoids,* especially prednisone, are significantly antiinflammatory and impair lymphocyte (B and T cell) activation and function. Prednisone exerts a wide spectrum of activity against all immune response and inflammatory response mechanisms. Although it suppresses the cell-mediated system more than the humoral system, the continued high dosage needed to maintain cell-mediated suppression creates significant risks in reducing the responsiveness of the humoral system. Often lower dosages of prednisone and azathioprine are used together because they seem to act synergistically.

*Antimetabolites and alkylating agents,* such as azathioprine and cyclophosphamide, act nonspecifically against rapidly dividing cells within the body, and thus they are used for cancer chemotherapy. They interfere with DNA synthesis and with the B and T cell systems.

A more specific immunosuppression of the T cell system is achieved with *antilymphocyte serum* (ALS). ALS blocks the action of the synthesized cells in circulation while leaving the lymph node B cell system only slightly suppressed. This preserves the host's protection against the humorally safeguarded infectious agents while suppressing the most active rejection system, the cell-mediated immune response.

*Cyclosporine* (cyclosporin A), is an antibiotic derived from fungi that exerts its action on the T lymphocytes. Success with this drug has greatly improved the prognosis after transplantation.

## CANCER IMMUNOLOGY

One of the primary functions of the CMI system seems to be the recognition and destruction of cancer cells within the body. By the same mechanisms operative in allograft rejection, it is postulated that the immune system continually protects against the establishment of tumor growths, providing immune surveillance. The recognition of tumor cells as nonself is based on the appearance of "new" surface antigens that allow identification. A growing body of evidence supports the view that this is a vital function of the immune system. Patients in whom the cellular immune system is impaired (immunosuppressed) or defective (immunodeficient) for significant periods are at especially high risk for the development of certain neoplastic diseases. To these data is coupled the observation that cancers are most prone to appear early in life, before the immune system is fully functional, or in later life as the system becomes less effective.

Cancers may become established in the body by escaping the surveillance mechanisms or by growing so rapidly that they outdistance the immune system's ability to respond. Experiments have demonstrated that if a few thousand tumor cells are transferred from a cancerous animal to a noncancerous animal, the latter is capable of responding and destroying the tumor; however, if the tumor cell load is increased to several billion cells, the tumor may become established. The humoral immune system may actually serve to protect the developing cancer by producing noncytotoxic antibodies *(enhancing antibodies)* that coat the tumor cell surfaces and mask the surface from recognition by sensitized lymphocytes. As a tumor grows, it is capable of both specific and nonspecific suppression of the immune system. This further reduces the effectiveness of a response.

Some of the new surface antigens, known as *tumor-specific transplantation antigen* (TSTA), appearing on the cancerous cell are shed into the circulation and can be immunologically detected there. Some of these antigens, such as carcinoembryonic antigen (CEA) and alpha-fetoprotein (AFP), are present during fetal development but are not expressed in the adult. Their reappearance lends support to the theory that cancer represents a dedifferentiation to a more primitive cell. These antigens, termed *oncofetal antigens* (OFA), are of some significance in early detection, diagnostic confirmation, and determination of malignant disease progress.

Some very early progress has been made in stimulat-

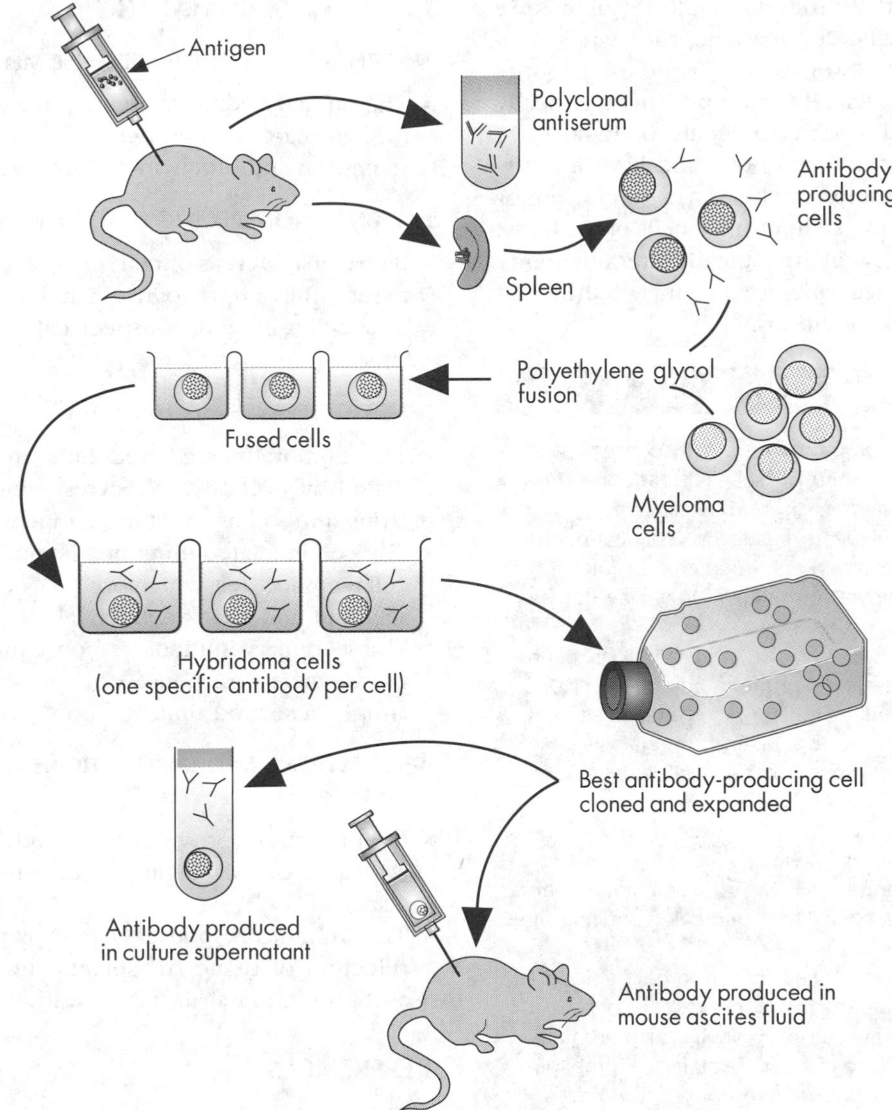


**FIGURE 13-17** Production of a monoclonal antibody. (From Baron EJ, Finegold SM: *Bailey and Scott's diagnostic microbiology,* ed 8, St Louis, 1990, Mosby.)

ing, both specifically and nonspecifically, the body's immunologic response to cancers in the hope of preventing further growth of the tumors. The use of biologic response modifiers (BRMs) has created a complex use for cytokines that normally regulate the immune system. Some of the cytokines used in cancer therapy are the interferons, interleukins, colony-stimulating factors (CSFs), and tumor necrosis factor (TNF). With further knowledge of both the cancer process and the immune response mechanisms, the possibility of using immunotherapy, immunoprophylaxis, and immunodiagnosis as specific tools against malignancies seems realistic.

## MONOCLONAL ANTIBODIES

With use of a tissue culture technique, it is possible to develop and isolate antibodies of great specificity for single antigenic determinants. Normally, immunoglobulins that are produced in the body in response to antigenic challenge bind to various antigenic determinants introduced on the multivalent antigen. The antibodies themselves are produced by a variety of B cells responding to the antigen signal; thus 90% of the antibodies produced have little or no avidity for specific antigenic determinants. By a technique for the production of immortal clones of *hybridoma* cells (made by the fusion of normal antibody-producing B cells with an appropriate B cell tumor line) and selection of single clones of cells producing only a single, highly specific antibody, large quantities of highly antigen-specific antibodies can be isolated (Figure 13-17). These immunoglobulins are known as *monoclonal antibodies.*

The clinical and diagnostic implications for the use of monoclonal antibodies are enormous. It is now possible to identify individual cell types (such as $T_H$ versus

$T_S$ lymphocytes, partially differentiated versus mature cells) with very specific cell markers, to diagnose malignant transformed cells, or to type tissue using monoclonal antibodies for each HLA subtype. Therapeutically it is possible to bind a toxic molecule or radioactive isotope to the monoclonal antibody and have it delivered specifically to a tumor cell bearing a specific tumor cell marker, thus sparing all nontumor cells of the body. Monoclonal antibodies will dramatically alter our ability to identify, characterize, and treat many of the most significant pathologic conditions.

## QUESTIONS TO CONSIDER

- What would happen if the immune response system did not properly distinguish "self" cells and inappropriately labeled them as "nonself"?
- We have come to regard fever and leukocytosis as negative pathologic responses that call for intervention, such as antipyretic therapy. Why may this be an inappropriate perspective?
- Several years ago, David, the child who had been raised throughout his entire life in a germ-free, controlled environment in Houston, died after an attempt to transplant bone marrow taken from his sister. He represented a most severe case of altered immune response.
  a. What is the usual fate of children born with the same alteration as David?
  b. Why was bone marrow transplantation attempted? What was the medical team hoping would happen?
  c. Why was David's sister chosen to be the donor?
  d. After David's death, an autopsy revealed a cancer caused by the Epstein-Barr virus, which normally does not produce cancer. Explain the probable reason for the cancerous response in David.

## CRITICAL THINKING ACTIVITIES

- Analyze the following patient situations: Mr. Jackson has third-degree burns over one fourth of his body; Baby Miles is one month premature and is being fed diluted formula via a nasogastric tube; Ms. Tyler has smoked two packs of cigarettes/day for 40 years and is being treated for COPD. What conclusions can be drawn about these patients as a whole, and individually?
- David was born without the ability to produce adequate numbers of antibodies. Diane has a disease in which her T helper cells are being destroyed. What assumption(s) can be made about these individuals and why?

## CHAPTER SUMMARY

### EXTERNAL NONSPECIFIC DEFENSE MECHANISMS

- The human body is protected from encroachment by foreign materials and cells by a system of protective structural and biochemical barriers.

### INTERNAL NONSPECIFIC DEFENSE MECHANISMS

- If foreign materials or cells gain access to internal body tissues, they are recognized and attacked by a system of specifically and nonspecifically responding mechanisms.

### SPECIFIC DEFENSE MECHANISMS

- The humorally mediated immune response is mediated by B cell lymphocytes, which produce circulating antibodies that bind antigens.
- The cell-mediated immune response is mediated by T cell lymphocytes, which produce activated T cells that seek out and attack antigen-labeled cells.
- The secondary immune response provides a faster and more efficient response on contact with the specific antigen a second time.

### APPLICATIONS AND IMPLICATIONS OF IMMUNE RESPONSE

- Immunization provides the body with protection against tissue-damaging infections and toxic substances.
- The immune response system plays a direct role in rejection of tissue transplants and in recognition of and protection against neoplastic transformation.

## REFERENCES

1. Abbas A, Lichtman A, Pober J: *Cellular and molecular immunology,* Philadelphia, 1991, WB Saunders.
2. Nelson DS, editor: *Natural immunity,* Sydney, 1989, Academic Press.
3. Reynolds CW, Wiltrout RH, editors: *Functions of the natural immune system,* New York, 1989, Plenum Press.
4. Rumsey KA, Reiger PT, editors: *Biological response modifiers: a self-instruction manual for health professionals,* Chicago, 1992, Precept Press.
5. Workman ML, Ellerhorst-Ryan J, Hargrave-Koertge V: *Nursing care of the immunocompromised patient,* Philadelphia, 1993, WB Saunders.
6. Wujcik D: An odyssey into biologic therapy, *Oncol Nurs Forum* 20(6):879-887, 1993.

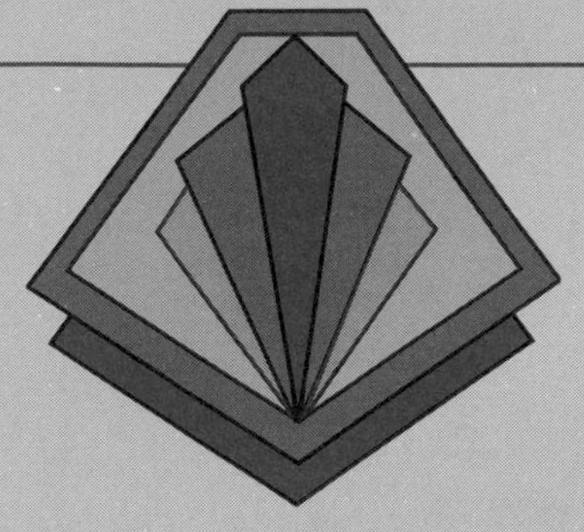

UNIT III

# Common Problems Encountered in Care of Ill Adults

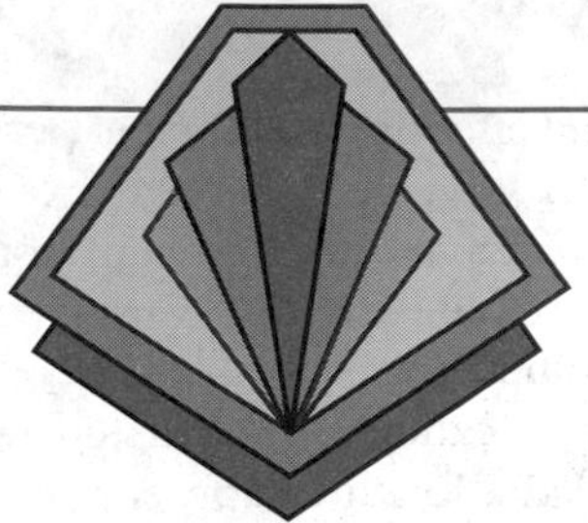

# CHAPTER 14

# Fatigue

*Virginia L. Cassmeyer*

## CHAPTER OBJECTIVES

***After studying this chapter, the learner should be able to do the following:***

1. Describe the phenomenon of fatigue, emphasizing the commonalities as presented by various authors.
2. Describe the central and peripheral mechanisms postulated to underlie muscle fatigue.
3. Describe the biobehavioral framework of fatigue, incorporating examples of situations where resources and activities are not in balance.
4. Describe the medical management, including diagnostic tests, for persons with fatigue.
5. Develop a nursing care plan for a patient with fatigue that incorporates assessment, patient counseling, and promotion of healthy life-style, including adequate sleep, nutrition, exercise, and stress management.

## KEY TERMS

central fatigue
chronic fatigue syndrome (CFS)
fatigue
peripheral fatigue
postinfectious fatigue syndrome (PIFS)

Fatigue is a major health concern that nurses will manage in a variety of clinical situations. Fatigue is one of the most common complaints of persons seeking primary care.[32] Of importance, many persons seeking help for fatigue report no improvement with care.[27] Fatigue is an accepted nursing diagnosis available to describe nursing diagnostic judgments.[16]

## DEFINITION

### FATIGUE IN GENERAL

Although **fatigue** is a common complaint, the phenomenon is poorly defined. Carpenito[7] defines fatigue as a subjective feeling of being drained that is pervasive and cannot be eliminated. According to Carpenito, fatigue is different from tiredness, which is transient and temporary. Gordon[16] defines fatigue as an "overwhelming, sustained sense of exhaustion and decreased capacity for physical and mental work." Other clinicians and researchers defined fatigue from various perspectives, including mechanisms of fatigue, related pathophysiologic states, and ability to work. A review of relevant literature reveals the following common assumptions about fatigue across disciplines, clinicians, and researchers. Fatigue:

1. Is a subjective perception
2. Varies over a continuum
3. Consists of "normal" and "abnormal" components
4. May be acute or chronic
5. Has psychologic, social, and physiologic aspects, both in terms of antecedents and consequences
6. May be protective

### CHRONIC FATIGUE SYNDROME

A distinct form of fatigue, **chronic fatigue syndrome (CFS),** has been strictly defined by the Centers for Disease Control and Prevention (CDC).[21] The definition is restrictive and was designed for the purpose of providing guidance for future epidemiologic and clinical studies.[21] (See Box 14-1 for a summary of the criteria for diagnosis of CFS.) Major complaints with this restrictive definition include the exclusion of patients with minor psychiatric problems.[31] The term *chronic fatigue syndrome* replaces such other names as chronic Epstein-Barr virus syndrome, chronic mononucleosis syndrome, chronic mononucleosis-like syndrome, and chronic fatigue immune dysfunction syndrome.[6,21]

Because of dissatisfaction with the CDC's definition, specialists from various fields developed and published guidelines from a consensus meeting that defines CFS slightly differently. These experts defined CFS as char-

**BOX 14-1 Diagnostic Criteria for Chronic Fatigue**

**MAJOR CRITERIA**

Both major criteria must be present.

1. New, debilitating, persistent, or relapsing fatigue that does not improve with rest and that has impaired daily activities by 50% over 6 months or longer.
2. Absence of other conditions that produce similar symptoms. These include autoimmune diseases, cardiac disease, cancer, human immunodeficiency virus (HIV) or other infections, gastrointestinal dysfunction, hepatic problems, endocrine dysfunction, neuromuscular complaints, psychiatric problems, and so forth.

**MINOR CRITERIA**

Six or more of the 11 symptoms with two or more of the three signs or eight or more of the 11 symptoms must be present.

**Symptoms**

Symptoms must have started after fatigue onset and persisted or recurred for 6 months or longer.

1. Mild fever (37.5° to 38.6° C)
2. Sore throat
3. Cervical or axillary adenopathy
4. Generalized muscular weakness
5. Myalgia
6. Prolonged fatigue (≥24 hours) after exercise that was previously tolerated
7. New onset of generalized headache
8. Noninflammatory arthralgia
9. Complaints of one or more of the following: photophobia, transient visual scotomata, forgetfulness, excessive irritability, confusion, difficulty thinking, inability to concentrate, or depression
10. Insomnia or hypersomnia
11. Onset of symptoms over a few hours to a few days

**Signs**

Signs must be documented by a physician on two occasions at least 1 month apart.

1. Low-grade fever
2. Nonexudative pharyngitis
3. Palpable/tender cervical or axillary lymph nodes of 2 cm or less

Modified from Holmes GP et al: *Ann Intern Med* 108:387-389, 1988.

acterized by a primary symptom of fatigue that is severe, is disabling, causes physical and mental dysfunction, and has been present 50% of the time for 6 months or more. Other symptoms, such as mood disturbances, muscle aches, and sleep disturbances, may be present. These same experts defined a separate entity, **postinfectious fatigue syndrome (PIFS).** This syndrome is characterized by the criteria for CFS previously listed that are present a minimum of 6 months after an infection. The infection must be corroborated by laboratory evidence and be present before the fatigue.[40,44]

## EPIDEMIOLOGY

The exact incidence and prevalence of fatigue are unknown. Fatigue is an expensive problem costing millions of dollars each year and affecting millions of persons.[26,35] One longitudinal study revealed that 24% of patients seeking primary care had a major complaint of fatigue.[27] Fatigue is found or associated with a variety of pathophysiologic states, including:

1. Breast and other cancers,[4,24] particularly with chemotherapy, radiation therapy, or biotherapy treatment[23,25,36]
2. Human immunodeficiency virus (HIV) infections and acquired immunodeficiency syndrome (AIDS)
3. Postoperative states[9]
4. Renal failure[42]
5. Congestive heart failure[11]
6. Various neuromuscular problems, particularly multiple sclerosis[28]
7. Various autoimmune or rheumatoid conditions, such as rheumatoid arthritis or fibromyalgia[33,43]
8. Metabolic problems such as hypothyroidism, Addison's disease, and Cushing's syndrome
9. Diabetes mellitus[8]
10. Mineral and electrolyte imbalances, such as calcium,[38] sodium, and potassium[13]
11. Ventilator dependency resulting from unsuccessful weaning[34]
12. Low back pain[12]
13. Deconditioned states, such as those associated with sedentary life-style, obesity, or chronic illnesses
14. Depression or other mood disorders
15. Multiple prescribed drugs

Besides being present concurrently with the multiple disease states just listed, fatigue and exhaustion have been shown to be predictive of future myocardial infarctions independent of the risk factors of age, blood cholesterol level, glucose tolerance, blood pressure, or smoking.[2] Last, fatigue is of major concern to nurses working with caregivers of acutely, chronically, or terminally ill persons, since caregiver fatigue may affect the patient as well as the caregiver.[15,45]

## MECHANISMS

Although fatigue is associated with many disease states; with environmental factors such as alterations in rest, sleep, work, or other activities; with nutrition; and with psychobiologic factors such as depression, anxiety, and stress, the mechanisms responsible for fatigue are unknown. This section discusses some possible mechanisms.

### CENTRAL-PERIPHERAL MECHANISM

Researchers in the area of muscle physiology have described central and peripheral mechanisms that may contribute to fatigue. Central components responsible for fatigue include alterations in recruitment of motor units, impulse transmission, or the spinal reflexes. In addition, changes in neurotransmitters, alterations in substances such as ammonia, and acid-base changes may contribute to **central fatigue.** Motivation can influence the occurrence of central fatigue.[30]

**Peripheral fatigue** can result from possible changes at three sites: (1) the level of the neuromuscular junction and muscle cell membrane, (2) the level of the transverse tubular system and sarcoplasmic reticulum with release of calcium, and (3) the level of actin-myosin cross-bridge formation and muscle contraction. At this last level, two hypotheses[41] have been proposed for muscle fatigue: the *accumulation hypothesis* and the *exhaustion hypothesis.*

The accumulation within the muscle of hydrogen ions, ammonia, and inorganic phosphates can result in changes in energy metabolism, force, and contractility and result in peripheral fatigue.[30] The exhaustion of metabolites such as adenosine triphosphate (ATP), phosphocreatine, and glycogen or an imbalance in supply and demand because of enzyme changes may result in fatigue.[22,30]

Because of the complexity of muscle activity, peripheral fatigue most likely involves the interaction of accumulation and depletion processes along with either alterations at the neuromuscular junction or transverse tubular and sarcoplasmic reticulum.[30] Last, central and peripheral mechanisms that allow the release of cytokines and lymphokines (substances from white blood cells that alter the immune, neuroendocrine, and other systems) may have a role in fatigue, at least in some situations.[36]

Although detailed, the central-peripheral model of fatigue does not integrate the roles of psychologic, social, and personality factors, as well as biologic factors.

## BIOBEHAVIORAL FRAMEWORK

The Center for Biobehavioral Management of Fatigue at the University of Kansas School of Nursing conceptualizes fatigue as an imbalance between resources and activity[1,5] (Figure 14-1). Resources include biopsychosocial resources such as cellular glycogen levels, blood glucose and oxygen levels, coping mechanisms, economic support, and family support. Activities include any task, whether physical, mental, or emotional, that needs to be accomplished. Resource deficit can occur if production or utilization is impaired or if demand exceeds availability. An imbalance between resources and activity can occur in multiple ways. Persons with diabetes mellitus have impairment in utilization and restoration. Persons with multiple sclerosis, although producing adequate resources, utilize them ineffectively. Persons with severe infections may lack sufficient resources to meet the needs of the immune and inflammatory processes and other activities. Persons who are deconditioned also may utilize resources ineffectively so that demand exceeds supply. Caregivers may lack the family support needed to cope with their own needs and those of the care recipient. Regardless of how it occurs, when an imbalance between resources and activity is present, fatigue occurs.

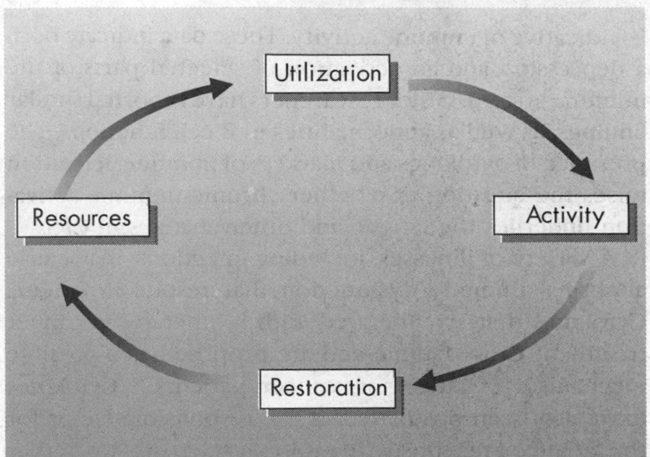


**FIGURE 14-1** Biobehavioral framework of fatigue. (From the Center for Biobehavioral Management of Fatigue, School of Nursing, University of Kansas, Kansas City, Kan.)

The Center's framework[1,5] also proposes that self-monitoring and self-regulation are ongoing. When fatigue is perceived on a conscious or nonconscious level, compensatory mechanisms are initiated to resolve or at least control the fatigue. These compensatory mechanisms also may occur at the conscious and nonconscious levels. If the compensatory mechanisms do not work, fatigue will continue and may actually worsen.

The biobehavioral framework allows different perspectives and definitions of fatigue to be explored. As experienced by persons with various pathophysiologic or psychologic problems, fatigue can be examined. Intervention studies for fatigue in general and yet unique to individual populations also can be explored.

## INFECTIVE AND IMMUNOLOGIC MECHANISMS

The role of infections and immune changes have been explored by multiple researchers in relation to CFS. Infections with various organisms, mostly viral, have been associated with chronic fatigue and explored as possible factors in CFS.[6,39,44] Organisms associated with some cases of CFS include Epstein-Barr virus, coxsackie B virus, herpes simplex virus, cytomegalovirus, measles virus, and retrovirus.[39] However, no consistent relationship exists between viral infections and CFS.

The role of the immune system in CFS also has been explored by several researchers.[29,36,39] Although conflicting data exist, some of the conflicts may result from CFS having been defined differently in different studies. Of importance, laboratory data of immune dysfunction are present in most persons with CFS. Gupta and Vayuvegula,[18] who used the CDC's definition of CFS, found that persons with CFS had decreased numbers of natural killer (NK) cells and a decreased response of T cells and antibodies to antigens. They also found increased expression of specific antigens (markers) on lymphocytes and monocytes. The expression of these markers is indicative of immune activity. These data indicate both a depression and an activation of selected parts of the immune system. Other researchers have reported similar findings, as well as abnormalities in B cell function.[3] The presence of cytokines and markers of immune activation raises the question of whether chronic immune activation underlies the fatigue and other changes in CFS.

A variety of illnesses, including infections, may cause abnormal immune dysfunction that results in fatigue. Cytokines that are liberated with biotherapy in cancer treatment cause fatigue and are proposed as a possible mechanism of fatigue in cancer patients.[36] Cytokines have also been postulated as the responsible factor for the fatigue of persons with multiple sclerosis.[35] Whether chronic activation of immune mechanisms has a role in fatigue associated with other pathophysiologic, social, or psychologic states remains unknown.

### MOOD CHANGES AND NEUROENDOCRINE MECHANISMS

Depression is a major condition associated with the fatigue state in CFS and other pathophysiologic states.* What is not clear is the time sequence of fatigue and depression. Hickie et al.[20] have reported that the presence of major depression before the diagnosis of CFS was no greater than for any other patients. Of particular relevance to the role of depression in fatigue is that Demitrack et al.[10] have found alterations in the hypothalamic-pituitary-adrenal axis in persons with CFS. Both Cushing's syndrome and Addison's disease are associated with depression. Alterations in the hypothalamic-pituitary-adrenal axis may be the link between fatigue and depression or other affective symptoms.[37]

## MANIFESTATIONS

Besides the major manifestation, persistent fatigue, other indications include expressions of tiredness that is overwhelming, no energy, worn out, and so forth. Complaints of emotional lability and disinterest are common. The person may complain of inability to do normal activities and at times the inability to "get out of bed." Persons frequently report increased sleeping, as well as changes in mental alertness and sharpness.

Physical examination may reveal evidence of fatigue, including lethargic appearance, slowing of responses or activity, drowsiness, and a lack of vitality.[19] The face may be dull and expressionless. The body may slump.

Other manifestations, both subjective and objective, may be present because of the presence of underlying pathophysiology. No common laboratory indications of fatigue exist, although abnormalities from the underlying pathophysiology may be present.

*References 3, 17, 24, 27, 32, 43.

**BOX 14-2 Recommended Diagnostic Tests for Persons with Chronic Fatigue Syndrome**

- Body weight over time
- Body temperature over time
- Complete blood count with differential
- Serum electrolytes (sodium, potassium, chloride, bicarbonate)
- Serum calcium and phosphorus
- Serum glucose
- Serum creatinine and blood urea nitrogen
- Serum enzymes (aspartate aminotransferase, alanine aminotransferase, alkaline phosphatase, creatine kinase)
- Total serum bilirubin
- Endocrine studies (thyroid-stimulating hormone, $T_4$, $T_3$)
- Immune studies (erythrocyte sedimentation rate, antinuclear antibodies, HIV antibodies, mononucleosis tests, skin tests)
- Urinalysis
- Stool hemoccult
- Chest roentgenogram and electrocardiogram

Modified from Holmes GP et al: *Ann Intern Med* 108:387-389, 1988.

## MEDICAL MANAGEMENT

Because no known mechanism for fatigue exists, medical management focuses on diagnoses. The diagnostic process focuses on identification of any related pathophysiologic states. Besides a thorough history and physical examination, persons with suspected CFS should have the tests listed in Box 14-2.

If the diagnosis reveals an underlying pathophysiologic state, medical management focuses on improvement of that condition. Treatment for CFS has included use of a variety of pharmacologic agents,[14] such as acyclovir, immune globulin, antibacterials, antifungals, and immune modifiers to treat potentially infective agents; glucocorticoids and nonsteroidal antiinflammatory drugs to treat myalgia and other symptoms of inflammation; and antidepressants and anxiolytics for associated mood changes. Vitamins and minerals have been used. Most of this pharmacologic therapy is considered experimental. Additional medical treatment in any person with fatigue focuses on improvement of nutrition and conditioning, promotion of adequate sleep, and symptom management.

## NURSING MANAGEMENT

### ASSESSMENT

Assessment of the person with fatigue consists of a thorough history and physical examination. The intensity, severity, and duration of fatigue need to be assessed. In addition, the fatigued person should be assessed for related sensory and affective changes and the effects of the fatigue on performance of daily activities. The temporal aspects of fatigue should be elicited. These subjective aspects of fatigue can be quantified by use of various scales that measure fatigue. The mood state, the presence of other symptoms, and sleep pattern effectiveness must also be assessed. Again, tools to quantify these subjective phenomena are available. The nursing assessment should focus on potential contributing factors, such as nutritional patterns, sleep patterns, activity and exercise patterns, stressors, coping skills, and social support. Last, a history of any previous or current illnesses, along with treatment, should be elicited.

## INTERVENTIONS

Interventions focus on any related pathophysiologic or psychosocial state, patient counseling and education, and promotion of a healthy life-style. A major focus is to help patients gain an awareness of the fatigue in their lives.[19] Patients need to identify potential triggers of fatigue for themselves and manifestations common to themselves. Each patient must be able to identify the unique way in which fatigue starts and progresses. Some type of diary that incorporates checklists to rate the fatigue phenomenon and its characteristics and space for written comments may be very helpful. The patient would keep these diaries for 1 or 2 weeks. The diaries would be repeated to evaluate the effectiveness of any interventions.

After the patient gains an awareness of the personal pattern of fatigue, the principles related to adequate rest, sleep, nutrition, and exercise need to be taught (see Chapter 6). Again, before changing behavior, the individual needs to gain insight into current patterns of rest, sleep, nutrition, and exercise. One area where persons with fatigue may need much encouragement is the development of a healthy pattern of activity and exercise. Exercise may seem to be contradictory in the presence of fatigue. Exercise improves conditioning and resource utilization and can improve resource restoration. Exercise enhances the performance of every body system. The patient must have an individualized program that incorporates a gradual increase in intensity and duration of exercise. The nurse must continually help patients incorporate exercise in a manner that does not exacerbate fatigue and that promotes regular participation.

The last area of care focuses on stress reduction techniques, including use of relaxation, meditation, massage, imagery, touch, music, biofeedback, and positive affirmation.[19] (See Chapter 7 for these and other measures to help reduce stress.)

In summary, because fatigue affects the total body by some as yet undefined mechanism, a holistic approach to the patient with fatigue is necessary. This holistic approach needs to be incorporated into both the assessment and the interventions.

## QUESTIONS TO CONSIDER

- What questions about the fatigue experience would you include in a fatigue diary?
- Although no laboratory evidence of fatigue is known, multiple laboratory tests are done. Why are many tests done? Relate each test to pathophysiologic states.
- What are some ways to quantify the fatigue experience?
- How and what type of activity modulation would decrease fatigue in persons with type II diabetes mellitus, AIDS, rheumatoid arthritis, and ventilator dependency?

## CRITICAL THINKING ACTIVITIES

- Your neighbor recently underwent coronary artery bypass surgery and is now recovering at home. While you are visiting him, he tells you that he doesn't have as much energy as he thought he would have after surgery. His wife asks you why. How would you answer her?
- While caring for Joe, a patient with severe multiple sclerosis, you note that Martha, his wife, is very fatigued. What is the relationship between Joe's disability and Martha's fatigue? What interventions may be necessary to reduce Martha's fatigue?

## CHAPTER SUMMARY

- Fatigue occurs in a variety of persons and currently is not well treated.

### DEFINITION

- Fatigue is a subjective symptom of pervasive and overwhelming exhaustion with a decrease in work (physical or mental).
- Fatigue occurs along a continuum; has psychologic, social and physiologic aspects; and at times may be protective.
- Chronic fatigue syndrome (CFS) has been defined very strictly and includes the presence of fatigue for at least 6 months, the exclusion of any other pathophysiologic states that could cause fatigue, and a constellation of signs and symptoms.
- No laboratory tests exist for fatigue.

### EPIDEMIOLOGY

- Fatigue is associated with cancers and their treatment, HIV infections and AIDS, postoperative status, renal failure, congestive heart failure, neuromuscular problems, autoimmune problems, metabolic problems, electrolyte imbalance, ventilator dependence, low back pain, mood disorders, deconditioned states, drug therapy, and caregiver burden.

- Fatigue may be predictive of future myocardial infarctions.

## MECHANISMS

- Central and peripheral changes in muscle control and function constitute one model of fatigue.
- An imbalance between resources and activity caused by impaired utilization or restoration or demand exceeding availability are the bases of a biobehavioral framework of fatigue.
- Immune abnormalities are found in most persons with CFS.
- Chronic immune activation may be a common underlying mechanism for fatigue regardless of the associated pathophysiologic or psychosocial state.
- Depression is a common mood disorder in persons with fatigue.
- Alterations in the hypothalamic-pituitary-adrenal axis may be the link between fatigue and affective symptoms.

## MANIFESTATIONS

- Manifestations of fatigue include verbal complaints of exhaustion or no energy, along with changes in appearance.

## MEDICAL MANAGEMENT

- Medical management of fatigue includes diagnosis, management of related pathophysiologic states, experimental pharmacologic therapy, improvement of nutrition and conditioning, promotion of adequate sleep, and symptom management.

## NURSING MANAGEMENT

- Nursing assessment includes a thorough history and physical examination, quantification of the fatigue experience, and exploration of potential contributing factors.
- Nursing interventions focus on those directed toward related pathophysiologic states, patient counseling and education to promote self-awareness of the fatigue experience, and promotion of a healthy life-style with adequate nutrition, sleep, exercise, and reduction of stress.

## REFERENCES


1. Aaronson L: Exploratory Center for Biobehavioral Studies of Fatigue Management, University of Kansas School of Nursing, grant from NINR, NIH (P20NR03270), 1992-1995.
2. Appels A, Mulder P: Excess fatigue as a precursor of myocardial infarction, *Eur Heart J* 9:758-764, 1988.
3. Bell DS: Chronic fatigue syndrome, *Postgrad Med* 91(6):245-252, 1992.
4. Blesch KS et al: Correlates of fatigue in people with breast or lung cancer, *Oncol Nurs Forum* 18(1):81-87, 1991.
5. Cahill C et al: Conceptual framework for biobehavioral management of fatigue (in preparation).
6. Calabrese L et al: Chronic fatigue syndrome, *Am Fam Phys* 45(3):1205-1213, 1992.
7. Carpenito LJ: *Nursing diagnosis: application to clinical practice,* Philadelphia, 1992, JB Lippincott.
8. Cassmeyer VL: Fatigue, physical activity and metabolic control in non-insulin dependent diabetes mellitus, Presentation to Kansas Regional Research Exchange, Wichita, 1993.
9. Christensen T et al: Fatigue and cardiac and endocrine metabolic response to exercise after abdominal surgery, *Surgery* 105(1):46-50, 1989.
10. Demitrack M et al: Evidence of impaired activation of the hypothalamic-pituitary-adrenal axis in patients with chronic fatigue syndrome, *J Clin Endocrinol* 73:1224-1234, 1991.
11. Feinstein AR, Fisher MB, Pigeon JG: Changes in dyspnea-fatigue ratings as indicators of quality of life in the treatment of congestive heart failure, *Am J Cardiol* 64(7):50-55, 1989.
12. Feuerstein M, Carter RL, Papciak AS: A prospective analysis of stress and fatigue in recurrent low back pain, *Pain* 31:333-344, 1987.
13. Friedland J, Paterson, D: Potassium and fatigue, *Lancet* 2:961-962, 1988 (letter to editor).
14. Gantz NM, Holmes GP: Treatment of patients with chronic fatigue syndrome, *Drugs* 38(6):855-862, 1989.
15. Goldstein V, Regnery G, Wellin E: Caretaker role fatigue, *Nurs Outlook* 29(1):24-30, 1981.
16. Gordon M: *Manual of nursing diagnosis: 1991-1992,* St Louis, 1991, Mosby.
17. Gorensek MJ: Chronic fatigue and depression in the ambulatory patient, *Prim Care* 18(2):397-419, 1991.
18. Gupta S, Vayuvegula B: A comprehensive immunological analysis in chronic fatigue syndrome, *Scand J Immunol* 33:319-327, 1991.
19. Hart LK, Freel MI, Milde FK: Fatigue, *Nurs Clin North Am* 25(4):967-976, 1990.
20. Hickie I et al: The psychiatric status of patients with the chronic fatigue syndrome, *Br J Psychiatry* 156:534-540, 1990.
21. Holmes GP et al: Chronic fatigue syndrome: a working case definition, *Ann Intern Med* 108:387-389, 1988.
22. Hultman E, Bergstrom J: Local energy-supplying substrates as limiting factors in different types of leg muscle work in normal man. In Keul J, editor: *Limiting factors of physical performance,* Stuttgart, 1971, Thieme.
23. Irvine DM et al: A critical appraisal of the research literature investigating fatigue in the individual with cancer, *Cancer Nurs* 14(4):188-199, 1991.
24. Jamar SC: Fatigue in women receiving chemotherapy for ovarian cancer. In Funk S et al: *Key aspects of comfort,* New York, 1989, Springer.
25. King KB et al: Patient's descriptions of the experience of receiving radiation therapy, *Oncol Nurs Forum* 12(4):55-61, 1985.
26. Kirk J et al: Chief complaint of fatigue: a prospective study, *J Fam Pract* 30(1):33-41, 1990.
27. Kroenke K et al: Chronic fatigue in primary care, *JAMA* 260(7):929-934, 1988.
28. Krupp LB et al: Fatigue in multiple sclerosis, *Arch Neurol* 45:435-437, 1988.
29. Landay AL et al: Chronic fatigue syndrome: clinical conditions associated with immune activation, *Lancet* 338:707-712, 1991.
30. Maclaren DP et al: A review of metabolic and physiological factors in fatigue, *Exerc Sport Sci Rev* 17:29-66, 1989.
31. Manu P, Mathews D, Lane T: The mental health of patients with a chief complaint of chronic fatigue: a prospective evaluation follow-up, *Arch Intern Med* 84:118-121, 1991.
32. Nelson E et al: Chief complaint fatigue: a longitudinal study from the patient's perspective, *Fam Pract Res J* 6(4):175-188, 1987.

33. Neuberger G et al: Correlates of fatigue in rheumatoid arthritis clients, *Arthritis Care and Research* 6(4): 517 (abstract 45), 1994.
34. Pierce J, Claney R, Trank J: *Biochemical and contractile properties of diaphragm fatigue*. Presentation to Midwest Nursing Research Society, Milwaukee, Wis, 1994.
35. Piper BF: Fatigue. In Carrieri-Kohlman V, Lindsey AM, West CM, editors: *Pathophysiological phenomena in nursing: human responses to illness,* Philadelphia, 1993, WB Saunders.
36. Piper BF et al: Recent advances in the management of biotherapy-related side effects: fatigue, *Oncol Nurs Forum* 16(suppl 6):27-34, 1989.
37. Potempa KM: Chronic fatigue, *Annu Rev Nurs Res* 11:57-76, 1993.
38. Richardson JH, Palmerton T, Chenan M: The effect of calcium on muscle fatigue, *J Sports Med* 20:149-151, 1980.
39. Shafran SD: The chronic fatigue syndrome, *Am J Med* 90(6):730-739, 1991.
40. Sharpe MC et al: A report—chronic fatigue syndrome: guidelines for research, *J R Soc Med* 84:118-121, 1991.
41. Simonson E: *Physiology of work capacity and fatigue,* Springfield, Ill, 1971, Charles C Thomas.
42. Srivastava RH: Fatigue in end-stage renal disease patients. In Funk S et al: *Key aspects of comfort,* New York, 1989, Springer.
43. Tack BB: Fatigue in rheumatoid arthritis: conditions, strategies, and consequences, *Arthritis Care Res* 3(2):65-70, 1990.
44. Wallace PG: Epidemiology: a critical review, *Br Med Bull* 47(4):942-951, 1991.
45. Williams P: *Caregiver fatigue and at-risk infants at home: preliminary findings*. Presentation to Kansas Regional Research Exchange, Hays, Kan, 1994.

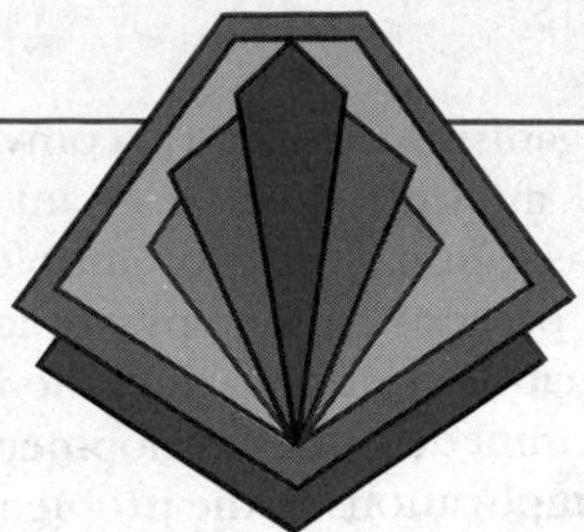

C H A P T E R 15

# Infection

***Dora Rice***
***Elizabeth Cameron Eckstein***

## CHAPTER OBJECTIVES

***After studying this chapter, the learner should be able to do the following:***

1 Describe the chain of infection.
2 Identify high-risk factors for infection.
3 Describe white blood cell response to infection.
4 Identify community approaches to infection control, including immunization programs.
5 Identify measures to prevent and control nosocomial infections (e.g., bacteremia; urinary, wound, and respiratory infections).
6 Compare category-specific isolation precautions and body substance isolation, including major components of each.

## KEY TERMS

active immunity
airborne transmission
antibodies
bacteremia
booster dose
carrier
causative agent
colonization
common vehicle transmission
community acquired infection
convalescent
differential count
direct contact transmission
droplet transmission
endemic
fomite
herd immunity
incubation period
infection
isolation
normal flora
nosocomial
passive immunity
pathogen
pyrexia
reservoir
subclinical
superinfection
vector-borne transmission

## HISTORICAL PERSPECTIVE

Infection control has become a recognized discipline only in the past 25 years, although the principles governing it have been in existence for some time. In the middle of the nineteenth century Semmelweiss, an obstetrician in Vienna, demonstrated the significance of handwashing in combating the transmission of infection. He observed that the incidence of puerperal fever, a major cause of postpartum mortality, was much higher on the ward where the medical students trained than on the ward attended by the midwives. Although the role of microorganisms in causing infection was not yet realized, Semmelweiss believed that somehow the medical students could be transmitting disease from the autopsy suite to maternity patients. He showed that when the students and physicians were required to wash their hands and rinse them in a chlorinated lime solution before a delivery, the incidence of puerperal fever decreased greatly. The idea that handwashing alone could prevent the spread of disease met with much opposition by his colleagues. Better acceptance came after Pasteur, Lister, and Koch developed the germ theory of disease and related asepsis to the prevention of the spread of disease. At about the same time, Nightingale made significant contributions to sanitation and isolation practices. From this evolved an era in which medical asepsis was practiced more by ritual than with true understanding of the specific principles on which it was based.

A turning point came during World War II, when the sulfonamides and penicillin were first used successfully to treat infections. As new antibiotics were developed, a false sense of security developed about infection control. It soon became apparent, however, that antibiotics were not the sole answer to infection control. Organisms once well controlled by antibiotics demonstrated the ability to develop resistant strains. In the late 1950s and the 1960s, outbreaks of penicillin-resistant *Staphylo-*

*coccus aureus* infections were common, and gram-negative organisms such as *Pseudomonas,* which were previously considered nonpathogenic (incapable of producing disease), were suddenly implicated as the cause of infections acquired in the hospital. Along with drug resistance and the emergence of newly recognized pathogens, the number of persons at risk of secondary infections increased. A longer life expectancy, the use of immunosuppressive agents, and an increase in the use of invasive procedures to diagnose and treat disease increased the risk of infection in certain persons.

The rise in hospital infections made it necessary to examine preventive and control measures, including a reemphasis on aseptic techniques. In 1970 an international conference to address the problem of hospital-acquired *(nosocomial)* infections was held in Atlanta. As a result, the Centers for Disease Control (CDC) in Atlanta set forth guidelines for prevention and control of infections in hospitals. The CDC is constantly updating and revising its recommendations based on epidemiologic studies and research findings. The American Hospital Association (AHA) and the Joint Commission on Accreditation of Hospitals (JCAH—renamed the Joint Commission on Accreditation of Healthcare Organizations [Joint Commission]), a major private accrediting agency, looked at the ethical and economic issues concerning nosocomial infections and established standards for programs in infection control. The purpose of these programs is to decrease morbidity and mortality from infections, as well as reduce the cost of infections that could have been prevented. Consumer awareness of the problem also contributed to the attention given the issue of infection control. In the early 1970s only 10% of hospitals in the United States had infection surveillance and control programs; by the end of the decade nearly all had them.

The field of infection control is challenging, with the identification of new pathogens and advances in research uncovering new information that may change current thinking and practices. Discovery of the human immunodeficiency virus (HIV) as the pathogen responsible for the current epidemic of acquired immunodeficiency syndrome (AIDS) has provided the incentive to develop safer practices to protect health caregivers from all blood-borne pathogens. Determining the modes of transmission of HIV has helped the CDC and infection control practitioners (ICPs) to develop new systems (universal precautions and body substance isolation) for personnel to use when caring for all patients. It is well documented that HIV is not transmitted by casual contact and that it is easily killed by household disinfectants. Hospital personnel are most at risk for infection with HIV from needlestick injuries. Programs to prevent needlestick injuries and to present factual information are essential. (See Chapter 71 for detailed information about HIV infection and AIDS.)

In the late 1980s and early 1990s, antimicrobial-resistant organisms became more prevalent in both the developing world and in hospitals in the United States.[6] Examples of such organisms include vancomycin-resistant enterococci and multiple drug–resistant tuberculosis (MDR-TB). Indiscriminate use of antibiotics and noncompliance with prescribed therapy are largely responsible for this situation. Unfortunately the high cost of drug research has impeded the development of new antibiotics. Nursing implications of the problem include adherence to infection control practices to prevent the spread of resistant organisms from patient to patient.

ICPs serve as a valuable resource as they interact with hospital departments, surveying for infections and teaching prevention and control. When a question or problem about infection control arises, the ICP should be contacted without hesitation. Questions may deal with clinical procedures, products for cleaning and disinfection, waste disposal, isolation systems, or personnel health issues.

All health care facilities should have infection control policies that address the issues of employee health and safety and patient care practices. Incorporated in these policies are Occupational Safety and Health Administration (OSHA) guidelines to protect health caregivers from exposure to blood-borne pathogens such as hepatitis B and HIV.[1]

This chapter presents an overview of the role of the nurse in the prevention and control of infection. For further information regarding a specific infectious disease, the reader should consult the chapter in which the site of the disease is discussed, for example, Chapter 42 for hepatitis, Chapter 37 for tuberculosis, and so on.

## INFECTIOUS DISEASE PROCESS

### DEFINITIONS

A **pathogen** is a microorganism or substance that is capable of producing disease. This discussion is concerned with microorganisms as pathogens. Factors that affect the microorganism's *pathogenicity,* or capacity to infect and produce disease, are listed in Box 15-1.

**Infection** is the presence in the body of a pathogen that multiplies and produces effects that are injurious to the host. This injury may result from the presence and spread of the microorganism through the body tissues, known as the pathogen's *invasiveness,* or from the effects on the body of toxins produced by the microorganism, known as its *toxigenicity.* Some organisms, such as pneumococci, are highly invasive and virtually nontoxigenic, whereas others, such as *Clostridium tetani,* present the other extreme of high toxicity but low in-

**BOX 15-1 Factors Affecting Pathogenicity of a Microorganism**

- Ability to live and multiply outside its host
- Its virulence
- Its host specificity
- Resistance of the host

vasiveness. An infection may be *apparent,* thus causing clinical signs and symptoms, or *inapparent,* in which no perceivable signs or symptoms are present (asymptomatic).

Pathogenic organisms that are present in the body but do not produce injury or incite an injurious body response are said to be **colonizing** the body. **Colonization** with microorganisms often occurs in patients who have an endotracheal or tracheostomy tube in place. Another example is the person whose nasal passages or skin surfaces are colonized with *Staphylococcus aureus.* The question of whether a person has an infection or colonization can be difficult to answer. What is important to realize is that persons in whom either colonization or infection occurs can easily serve as a source of infection to themselves and others at risk.

## CHAIN OF INFECTION

Essential to appropriate intervention in the prevention and control of infection is an understanding of the infectious disease process. With all infectious diseases, a common sequence of events occurs (Figure 15-1).

First, a **causative agent,** or pathogen, must exist. This can be a bacterium, virus, fungus, rickettsial organism, protozoa, or helminth (worm). Second, there must be a **reservoir** where the agent can be found. The reservoir can be animate (human, animal) or inanimate (soil, water, intravenous solutions, equipment, and so on). Human reservoirs can be persons with an acute clinical infection or with colonization or who are symptomless carriers. Carriers can (1) be *incubating* the agent before the onset of signs and symptoms, (2) have an inapparent **(subclinical)** infection, (3) be in the **convalescent stage** of an infection, or (4) be **chronic carriers** of the agent. Viral hepatitis B is an example of an infectious disease that can be transmitted by human carriers in all these stages. Often the reservoir of an agent responsible for an outbreak of an infection is not readily apparent and may never be identified. If the process of infection is well understood, however, appropriate and effective control measures can be instituted, even though the original source of the causative agent is not known.

The agent must have a *means of exit* from the reservoir. If the reservoir is human, the exit can be (1) the respiratory tract, (2) the gastrointestinal (GI) tract, (3) the genitourinary tract, (4) open lesions on the skin, or (5) across the placenta.

Once the agent has left the reservoir, it needs a *mode of transmission* to a host. Transmission can be by direct contact, by airborne vehicle, or by vectors. *Contact transmission* includes direct, indirect, or droplet contact. **Direct contact transmission** occurs when there is spread of infection from the source to the host without the presence of an intermediate object. This happens

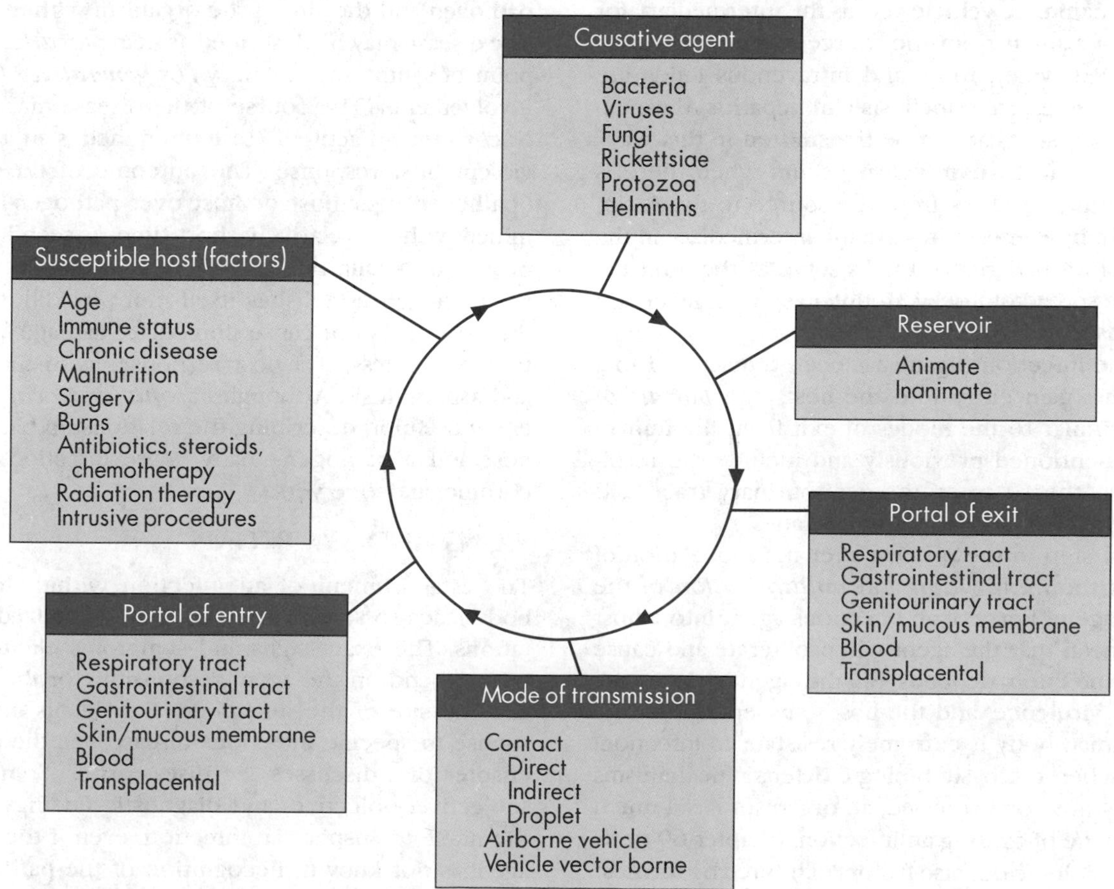


**FIGURE 15-1** The infectious disease process.

when there is physical contact with or skin shedding onto the host. Gonorrhea is an example of a disease transmitted by direct contact.

*Indirect contact transmission* has an intermediate object between the source and the host. This intermediary can be the contaminated hands of a person who has had contact with an infected source and then touches a susceptible host without washing the hands. An inanimate object that has been contaminated by an infectious source is known as a **fomite.** Bed linen, respiratory therapy equipment, tissues, and silverware are examples of fomites that can be responsible for the indirect transmission of an infectious agent.

**Droplet transmission** occurs when the infectious agent is expelled from the reservoir in the form of droplets, as happens with a sneeze or cough in the direction of a nearby recipient. These droplets do not become airborne but settle on surfaces about 3 to 4 feet from their source. Meningococcal meningitis and influenza are examples of diseases transmitted in this manner.

**Airborne transmission** occurs when the infectious agent expelled from the source remains suspended in the form of *droplet nuclei* or dust in the air. The agent is then inhaled by a host. These droplet nuclei are 1 to 5 μm in size and are smaller than the droplets discussed in droplet transmission, and they can thus be carried by air currents. Chickenpox (varicella zoster) and tuberculosis are diseases that can be spread by this route.

**Common vehicle transmission** occurs when a contaminated inanimate vehicle acts as the intermediary for the infectious agent from the source to multiple hosts. Contaminated water, food, and intravenous fluids are common vehicles. Salmonellosis and hepatitis A are examples of diseases that can be transmitted in this way.

**Vector-borne transmission** occurs when there is an animate intermediary from the source to the recipient. For example, mosquitos are the intermediary in the transmission of malaria, and ticks serve as the intermediary in the spread of Rocky Mountain spotted fever and Lyme disease.

Once the infectious agent has been transmitted to a host, it must gain entry into the host. The *portals of entry* are similar to the modes of exit from the human reservoir mentioned previously and include the respiratory tract, the GI tract, the genitourinary tract, and breaks in the skin or mucous membranes.

The final step in the process after the inoculation of the host is the *maturation* and *multiplication* of the infectious agent. Entry of an infectious agent into a host does not mean that the agent will proliferate and cause infection. Infection depends on the agent's dose, the organism's virulence, and the host's susceptibility. The healthy human body is extremely resistant to infection; however, when the basic biologic defense mechanisms of the body are compromised, an organism has a much greater chance of causing an infection. Chapter 69 deals with many biologic defense factors exhibited by the host to prevent infection and injury. Some of the factors that affect host susceptibility to infection are (1) age (very young and very old persons being more susceptible), (2) immune status (certain disease states such as HIV infection, diabetes, cancer, or other chronic diseases can impair the immune status), (3) therapeutic treatments such as radiation and certain drugs, especially antibiotics, steroids, and chemotherapeutic agents, (4) surgery, (5) burns, (6) poor nutritional status, and (7) invasive procedures (intravenous catheters, chest tubes, urinary catheters) that break through the normal external defense barriers.

From this discussion of the infectious disease process, it becomes evident that no one factor is responsible for an infection. Rather, such variables as the *agent,* the *environment,* and the *host* determine the outcome. To be able to intervene effectively in the disease process, it is important that all these concepts be understood.

## CLINICAL MANIFESTATIONS

Once a pathogen gains access to a susceptible host, a time known as the **incubation period** passes before the clinical symptoms of the disease appear. During this period the organism is establishing itself, spreading to target organs or tissues, and proliferating within various body sites. This incubation period varies depending on the condition of the host but is often predictable and diagnostically significant. The appearance of symptoms depends on the type of injury elicited by the virulent pathogen and the site of the organism within the body. The disease may be described as being *localized* (a focal point of symptoms or injury) or *generalized* (systemic involvement). The course of the disease may be *acute* or *chronic.* An acute disease often incites an immediate violent host response. The outcome of the infection (pathogen over host or host over pathogen) is determined within a relatively short time, as seen in mumps, plague, or smallpox. Conversely, in a chronic infection the pathogen establishes itself more insidiously within the host, does not cause immediate damage, and tends to provoke less of a host response, as in tuberculosis and aspergillosis. Although *chronic and acute* are generally useful in describing the relationship between the host and a pathogen, many acute infections become chronic, and vice versa.

## SIGNS AND SYMPTOMS

The establishment of an infection within the human body leads to several specific and generalized manifestations. The exact signs and symptoms elicited in the host depend on the agent responsible for the infection and the site of the infection. (For details on host response to specific infectious disease, see the particular chapter that discusses the disease site.) Some general subjective, objective, and diagnostic findings can alert the nurse to suspect an infection, even if the causative agent is not known. Recognition of the patient with a suspected infection is a crucial step in initiating early prevention and control measures.

Examples of data that would make the nurse suspect the patient may be developing an infection are listed in Box 15-2.

For generalized infections the symptoms may be even more vague. The earliest clinical manifestations of an infection generally are sensed within the host as nondescript, nonspecific reactions such as weakness, headache, lightheadedness, congestion, muscle aches, pain in the joints, decreased appetite, or malaise. These sensations are broadly referred to as *prodromal symptoms* (preceding the infection). As the infection progresses, other manifestations develop. These include fever, increased pulse rate, hypotension, altered mental status, or even jaundice, shock, confusion, and convulsions.

Of all the clinical symptoms mentioned, fever **(pyrexia)** is one of the most valuable diagnostic indicators of infection, although not all fevers are the result of an infectious process. Most persons with an infectious disease develop fever as a generalized response to the infectious agent.

Another systemic response to infection is the variation in leukocytes (white blood cells [WBCs]) in peripheral circulation. The normal WBC count in blood is 5000 to 10,000 WBCs/$mm^3$. With the presence of a serious infection the number of WBCs rises above 10,000/$mm^3$ in response to the infectious inflammation. Leukocyte values between 10,000 and 20,000 are considered slightly elevated; 20,000 to 40,000 moderately elevated; and more than 40,000 greatly elevated. In a few infectious diseases the number of WBCs in circulation actually drops, which is also significant diagnostic data.

Five types of mature WBCs are found in circulation: ***neutrophils, eosinophils, basophils, lymphocytes,*** and ***monocytes.*** Each type plays a more or less specific role in body defense (see Chapter 69); therefore different diseases produce different reactions among the WBC populations in the blood. These changes in patterns of distribution are detected not only by counting the total number of WBCs in a stained blood smear, but also by classifying them according to morphology and calculating the relative percentage of each cell type present. This type of count is known as a **differential count.** For example, an increase in the number of immature neutrophils is commonly referred to as a ***shift to the left*** and may indicate an acute infection. The differential count may provide information that can be correlated with other clinical data to help diagnose an infection. Table 15-1 provides some general correlations between leukocyte response and infectious diseases.

None of the signs and symptoms present in localized or generalized infections is diagnostic by itself. Many can be demonstrated by other disease processes. They can, however, serve as helpful clues in the diagnosis of a suspected infectious process.

**BOX 15-2 Subjective and Objective Data Suggesting Infection**

**LOCALIZED INFECTION**

| **Subjective** | **Objective** |
|---|---|
| Pain | Inflammation |
| Tenderness | Edema |
| Warmth | Redness |
| Swelling | Warmth |
| Itching | Exudate or drainage |
| | Amount |
| | Color |
| | Consistency |

**RESPIRATORY TRACT INFECTION**

| **Subjective** | **Objective** |
|---|---|
| Sore throat | Redness of throat |
| Congestion | Rales |
| Cough | Rhonchi |
| Sputum production | Cough |
| Chest pain | Type |
| Stuffy nose | Frequency |
| Runny nose | Sputum |
| | Amount |
| | Color |
| | Consistency |

**GI TRACT INFECTION**

| **Subjective** | **Objective** |
|---|---|
| Anorexia | Vomitus |
| Nausea | Frequency |
| Vomiting | Amount |
| Diarrhea | Color |
| | Consistency |
| | Diarrhea |
| | Frequency |
| | Amount |
| | Color |
| | Consistency |

**GENITOURINARY TRACT INFECTION**

| **Subjective** | **Objective** |
|---|---|
| Urgency | Frequency |
| Frequency | Amount |
| Burning or painful urination | Color |
| | Odor |
| Change in color or smell of urine | Purulent, foul discharge |
| | Presence of WBCs and bacteria |
| Flank or pelvic pain | Urinalysis |
| Discharge | Culture |
| Itching | |

**GENERALIZED INFECTION**

| **Subjective** | **Objective** |
|---|---|
| Malaise | Fever |
| Muscle aches | Elevated WBC count |
| Headache | Hypotension |
| Weakness | Altered mental status |
| Joint pain | Confusion |
| Anorexia | Convulsions |
| | Shock |
| | Tachycardia |

**TABLE 15-1 White Blood Cell Response to Infections**

| LEUKOCYTE RESPONSE | ASSOCIATED INFECTIOUS PROCESS |
|---|---|
| Increase in neutrophils (neutrophilia) | Typical in many acute local and systemic infections caused by bacteria (especially pyogenic bacteria), rickettsia, some viruses, and a few protozoa |
| Decrease in neutrophils (neutropenia) | Frequent in salmonellosis, brucellosis, whooping cough, overwhelming bacterial infections, influenza, infectious mononucleosis, hepatitis A infection, mumps, rubella, rubeola, and some rickettsial and protozoan diseases |
| Increase in eosinophils (eosinophilia) | Frequent in allergic reactions, chronic skin disease, helminthic infections, and scarlet fever |
| Increase in lymphocytes (lymphocytosis) | Frequent in chickenpox, mumps, measles, infectious mononucleosis, influenza, whooping cough, syphilis, tuberculosis, salmonellosis, viral hepatitis, and viral pneumonia; sometimes in convalescent phase of acute bacterial infection |
| Increase in monocytes (monocytosis) | Common in tuberculosis, chickenpox, brucellosis, mumps, syphilis, and certain rickettsial diseases; may occur in certain viral and protozoan diseases and in convalescent phase of acute bacterial infections |
| Decrease in lymphocytes (lymphocytopenia) | HIV |

## DIAGNOSTIC TESTS

Diagnostic tests are an important adjunct in the diagnosis of an infection. Some of the diagnostic tests used to obtain data include skin tests, radiologic tests, gallium scans, ultrasound, computed tomography (CT scan), magnetic resonance imaging (MRI), microbiologic cultures, serologic antibody titers, and complete blood cell (CBC) count. Examples of data obtainable from such tests include leukocytosis; anemia; increase in erythrocyte sedimentation rate (ESR); appearance of C-reactive protein; proteinemia; positive bacterial, viral, and fungal cultures; and positive radiologic findings, all of which may indicate the presence of an infection.

Proper collection and handling of laboratory specimens are essential to ensure accurate laboratory results. Inappropriate collection or handling of specimens may lead to unnecessary delays in test results or inaccurate results, thus affecting the patient's therapy. When an infection is suspected, culture specimens are obtained from the suspected site. In the patient who has a fever and in whom the site of infection is unknown, culture specimens typically are obtained from the blood, urine, sputum, and any other possible sites of infection. This may include spinal fluid cultures, aspirates of body fluid, or intravenous catheter tips. *It is imperative that these cultures be obtained before the initiation of antibiotic therapy because antibiotics can suppress any bacteria present and give inaccurate or false-negative culture results.* Cultures should be obtained in a manner that avoids contamination. Aseptic preparation of the culture site, observance of aseptic technique, and placement of specimens in an appropriate container are crucial factors to be observed in ensuring the best sample. Once obtained, the specimen must be properly stored and transported promptly to the laboratory. Each institution should have guidelines for the proper method for collecting and handling specimens for the laboratory. All specimens must be accompanied by the correct requisition and include the following information: (1) patient's name, (2) date and time of collection, (3) test requested, (4) type of specimen, (5) how specimen was obtained (clean void or catheter urine, expectorated sputum, tracheal aspirate), and (6) where the results are to be sent. A record of all tests is kept to avoid unnecessary duplication of tests.

Interpretation of laboratory results is sometimes difficult. Certain body sites have bacteria known as **normal flora,** which reside there in a commensal (intimate) relationship with the host. The skin, upper respiratory tract, vagina, urethra, and bowel are examples of body sites in which normal bacterial flora can be found. The bacteria found vary from site to site, and knowledge of the normal flora is helpful in discerning the significance of laboratory culture results. *A Clinician's Dictionary of Bacteria and Fungi*[5] is an excellent publication that lists in detail the normal flora of various sites. It must be emphasized that laboratory results alone cannot be used to make diagnostic and therapeutic decisions. Rather, they are used in conjunction with the patient's clinical status to make appropriate diagnostic and therapeutic decisions.

Knowledge about the infectious disease process and how to recognize or suspect an infectious process is vital to the prevention and control of infectious diseases in both community and hospital settings. Prevention and control of disease are addressed in the remainder of this chapter.

## INFECTION CONTROL IN THE COMMUNITY

An infectious disease is termed a *communicable disease* when it is highly transmissible to other persons. Smallpox is an example of a communicable disease that, through cooperative efforts worldwide, has been successfully eradicated.[3] The methods used to eradicate smallpox throughout the world can serve as a model of how to eliminate other communicable diseases. The eradication of smallpox also demonstrates the importance of accurate reporting of communicable diseases to the proper authorities so that appropriate prevention and control measures can be instituted.

Efforts are now under way to eliminate rubella and measles (rubeola) in the United States. Rubella vaccine was licensed in 1969, and since then widespread epidemics of rubella and congenital rubella syndrome (CRS) have been successfully prevented. The continued occurrence of rubella in women of childbearing age has led to recommendations for immunization of both men and women in institutional settings such as hospitals and colleges to prevent outbreaks.

The original vaccine against rubeola licensed in 1963 was successful in reducing the incidence of measles by 99% until 1986. Since 1986 the outbreaks have increased, especially among unvaccinated preschool children and among vaccinated school-age children and college students. Outbreaks in students vaccinated before 1978 to 1980 are thought to result from instability of the vaccine manufactured before 1980. Current recommendations are for a two-step vaccination for infants in inner-city areas (at 9 and 15 months) and for revaccination of students in outbreaks (if vaccinated before 15 months of age or before 1980). Many schools and colleges now require proof of immunization before enrollment.

On the international level the World Health Organization (WHO), a special agency of the United Nations, has as its primary purpose the improvement and standardization of measures to prevent and control disease throughout the world. Its Epidemiological Intelligence Service in Geneva receives immediate notification of large-scale outbreaks of infectious diseases throughout the world and advises the world community of impending epidemics. *The Weekly Epidemiological Record* is an official publication of the agency.

On the national level, the Centers for Disease Control and Prevention (CDC) is responsible for programs for the prevention and control of communicable and other preventable disease in the United States. The CDC provides epidemiologic and laboratory services to state health facilities on request. It enforces quarantine regulations and conducts foreign quarantine activities; administers international activities for the control of malaria, smallpox, and measles; and provides consultation to other nations in the control of preventable diseases. It also collects, tabulates, and assesses data on reportable diseases from state health departments and publishes the findings in the *Morbidity and Mortality Weekly Report (MMWR)*. Through its continuous surveillance, the CDC is able to detect new cases of diseases and intervene to control disease outbreaks. In addition, the CDC is instrumental in providing guidelines and recommendations for infection control.

In the United States the control of infectious diseases is the responsibility of each state. State health officers usually delegate this responsibility to a division of communicable diseases. A staff of physicians, nurses, veterinarians, and sanitary engineers works closely with a state epidemiologist in detection, assessment, and control of specific reportable diseases.

Local public health departments work in conjunction with their state health departments in this effort. The community health nurse plays a vital role in the collection of data, surveillance activities, immunization programs, education, and other control measures. Physicians and health care facilities have a responsibility to report communicable diseases promptly to the health department. Health agencies in the community can use the reported data to determine potential or real problems, identify the causative agent and hopefully its source, and identify the population at risk. A method to control the problem, care for those exposed, and protect the population at risk can then be devised and implemented.

## PREVENTION AND CONTROL MEASURES

One method of prevention and control of disease in the community involves environmental control measures such as sanitation techniques that ensure a pure water supply and proper disposal of sewage and other potentially infectious materials. These measures have been legislated into building codes, state laws, and federal regulations. Similarly, regulations address health practices in institutions that handle, package, and prepare foods. Another environmental control measure is spraying a designated area to kill mosquitos, which are implicated in the spread of viral encephalitis. Spraying usually is done only after an outbreak has been identified.

Depending on the communicable disease, care of exposed persons and protection of the population at risk for contracting the disease may entail prophylaxis, immunization, or only careful monitoring of new cases. Often, simple adherence to basic principles of hygiene is sufficient. Determination of additional required measures should be made by the local or state health department. Attempts are made to reach those at risk and inform them of the preventive measures. Education of the public is a key component of these efforts.

In the United States a marked reduction has occurred in the incidence of infectious diseases that can be prevented by immunization. Because of accessibility and cost, however, there has been a decline in the number of children being immunized. In addition, many persons are concerned that federal monies used to support local immunization efforts have been reduced to such a level that free immunizations are no longer equally available in all 50 states. In 1993 President Clinton requested additional funds for the immunization program. Infections formerly seen only in children are now occurring more frequently in adults because of the failure of the population to develop acquired immunity during early childhood. This reduction in childhood infections is believed to be directly related to improved sanitary conditions.

Because of air travel, a more recent concern is the elimination of the barriers of time and distance. Thus a person with an infectious disease may be brought from a remote area of the world to a major population center where the disease can be readily spread to a susceptible public.

Several infectious diseases have been dramatically controlled by the development and use of various *inactivated vaccines* and *live attenuated antigens.* The potential for eradication of common infectious diseases brings with it major responsibilities for public health agencies, physicians, and nurses. Ways must be found not only to carry out planned programs of immunization but also to educate the public about the hazards of apathy and failure to maintain proper levels of immunization. Continued progress in control and eradication requires continued commitment to increase knowledge about immunization patterns, to evaluate effectiveness and risks of antigens used, and to monitor levels of protection in a population.

## IMMUNIZATION PROGRAMS

Immunization programs have played and continue to play a primary role in the control of infectious disease throughout the world. The body can be stimulated to produce antibodies against some specific diseases without actually having the disease *(active artificial immunity).* Temporary protection sometimes can be provided by injecting antibodies produced by other persons or animals into the bloodstream of a human being *(passive artificial immunity).*

Recommendations concerning current immunization schedules are found in *Morbidity and Mortality Weekly Reports,* which presents recommendations of the U.S. Public Health Service's Advisory Committee on Immunization Practices (ACIP). The reader should refer to this resource when questions arise about proper immunization practices, prophylaxis, interruption in immunization schedules, or adverse reactions and side effects.

### Active Immunization

**Active immunity** can be acquired by artificially injecting small numbers of attenuated (weakened) or dead organisms of specific types or modified toxins from the organisms (toxoids) into the body. This procedure is known as *inoculation.* If 90% of the population is protected against organisms that require continued passage through humans to reproduce and live, the disease caused by the organism can be virtually eliminated because there are too few susceptible hosts for organism spread. Smallpox has been eliminated from the world in this way. This type of group protection is called **herd immunity.** It is ineffectual, however, against organisms such as tetanus bacilli that can exist indefinitely (in the soil), and in this instance each person must be immunized to be protected. If the disease is not prevalent in the environment, such as diphtheria in the United States, or is not spread from person to person by direct contact, such as tetanus, the inoculation must be repeated at regular intervals to maintain protection. This inoculation is called a **booster dose,** and usually one tenth of the original inoculating dose is sufficient.

An inoculation often causes a local tissue response. Symptoms of *inflammation* (redness, tenderness, swelling, sometimes ulcerations) appear at the site of the injection, and symptoms of *widespread tissue involvement* (slight febrile reactions, general malaise, muscle aching) for 1 or 2 days are common. The initial inoculation produces delayed symptoms because the immune response system must become sensitized to the antigen. Usually an accelerated, less severe systemic reaction to subsequent inoculations occurs because the immune response is stimulated at once. The local reaction also is less severe than that after the initial inoculation because the organisms have less opportunity to produce inflammation.

*Active artificial immunization* against many bacilli and viruses is now available. All persons should be encouraged to avail themselves of the protection advised by local health officials. They also should be advised to keep a permanent record of the date of each immunization.

In the United States the ACIP recommends that all children be immunized against diphtheria, pertussis (whooping cough), tetanus, mumps, rubella, poliomyelitis, measles, *Haemophilus influenzae,* and hepatits B.

## PRIMARY IMMUNIZATION SCHEDULES

The immunization schedule for diphtheria, pertussis, tetanus (DPT) begins with one dose of combined toxoid and vaccine when an infant is 6 weeks to 2 months old (Table 15-2). The next two doses are given at 4- to 8-week intervals thereafter. The fourth dose is administered about 1 year after the third dose. This schedule maintains adequate antibody levels until the child enters kindergarten, when a booster immunization is given. Thereafter, booster doses of tetanus and diphtheria are given only every 10 years (see Table 15-2).

Oral poliovirus vaccine (OPV), trivalent, is a live vaccine containing all three strains of poliomyelitis virus. OPV is the vaccine recommended for infants and children. Inactivated poliovirus vaccine (IPV) is preferred after age 18 years. IPV is also preferred for immunocompromised persons and their household contacts because it eliminates the theoretic risk to the *vaccinee* and prevents the spread of vaccine virus to immunocom-

**TABLE 15-2 Recommended Schedule for Active Immunization of Normal Infants and Children***

| RECOMMENDED AGE | VACCINE | COMMENTS |
|---|---|---|
| Birth | HB vaccine | |
| 2 mo | DTP No. 1, OPV No. 1<br>HbCV No. 1, HB vaccine | Can be given earlier in endemic areas |
| 4 mo | DTP No. 2, OPV No. 2<br>HbCV No. 2 | 6-wk to 2-mo interval desired between OPV doses |
| 6 mo | DTP No. 3, HbCV No. 3<br>HB vaccine No. 3 | An additional dose of OPV at this time is optional in areas with a high risk of polio exposure |
| 15 mo | MMR, DTP No. 4<br>OPV No. 3,<br>HbCV booster | Completion of primary series |
| 4-6 yr | DTP No. 5, OPV No. 4 | At or before school entry |
| 14-16 yr | Td† | Repeat every 10 yr throughout life |

Data from *MMWR* 38(13):210, 1989; *MMWR* 40(RR-1), 1991; *MMWR* 40(RR-13), 1991.
*HB,* Hepatitis B vaccine; *DTP,* diphtheria, tetanus, pertussis; *OPV,* oral polio vaccine; *HbCV,* vaccine composed of *Haemophilus* b polysaccharide antigen conjugated to a protein carrier; *MMR,* measles, mumps, rubella.
*See individual ACIP recommendations for details.
†Tetanus and diphtheria toxoids, adsorbed (for use in persons aged 7 years and older); contains same amount of tetanus toxoid as DTP or DT but a reduced dose of diphtheria toxoid.

promised persons. The primary series of OPV consists of three doses. The first usually is given at the same time the DPT series is begun (6 to 12 weeks of age). The next dose is administered 6 to 8 weeks later, and the third dose at least 6 weeks and preferably 8 to 12 months after that. A fourth dose is given just before entry into school.

A single dose of measles, mumps, rubella (MMR) virus vaccine, live, is given when the child is 15 months old. As mentioned previously, in urban outbreaks the first dose of monovalent measles vaccine, a live attenuated vaccine, may be given at age 9 months, followed by a dose of MMR at 15 months. Children who have not been vaccinated as infants can be vaccinated at any age.

Mumps vaccine, also live attenuated, should not be administered before 12 months of age because of the persistence of maternal antibodies, which may interfere with seroconversion. Mumps vaccine usually is given in a combined vaccine with measles and rubella (MMR) at 15 months of age. All susceptible children, adolescents, and adults should be vaccinated.

A single dose of rubella vaccine as part of MMR is recommended for children after 12 months of age for maximal seroconversion. As previously discussed, most cases of measles are now seen in young adults, whereas before the vaccine became available in 1969, most cases occurred in school-age children. Women in childbearing years should be tested for rubella antibodies if they cannot document immunization, because rubella infection in the first trimester of pregnancy is associated with neonatal morbidity and mortality (congenital rubella syndrome). If antibodies are not present, vaccination is recommended. Because of the theoretic risk to the fetus, women of childbearing age are vaccinated only if they are not pregnant, and they are counseled not to become pregnant for 3 months after vaccination.

*Haemophilus influenzae* b vaccine with polysaccharide conjugated to protein (HbCV) is recommended at 2, 4, and 6 months of age with a booster dose at 15 months.

Routine vaccination against *smallpox* is no longer recommended by the Public Health Service because the side effects and complications of the vaccine are greater than the danger of acquiring the disease. The vaccine is indicated only for laboratory workers who are directly involved with smallpox or closely related orthopox viruses.

At present, immunization against *typhoid fever* is recommended only when exposure to a typhoid carrier occurs in the household, when an outbreak of typhoid occurs in a community, or when a person travels to countries where typhoid is **endemic** (always present).

Immunization to protect against other diseases is given on a selective basis; that is, groups at a high risk are immunized.

Because of the prevalence of *influenza* and its potential for causing death, the ACIP recommends immunization against influenza for all persons at increased risk of adverse consequences from infection of the lower respiratory tract. This includes persons older than 60 years of age and those more than 2 years of age who have chronic cardiac, respiratory, metabolic, or renal disease or diseases that impair the immune system. Protection is obtained by giving an injection of influenza vaccine beginning in October or November. Infants and children up to 9 years old who are at risk are given a subvirion (split-virus) vaccine in two doses 4 weeks apart. A yearly booster dose is needed to maintain and update immunity. Persons who are allergic to eggs or egg products should not be immunized because of the danger of hypersensitivity reactions.

The newest pneumococcal vaccine is a 23-valent polysaccharide vaccine licensed in 1983. It is recommended for adults and children 2 years of age and older with chronic illness who are at increased risk for pneumococcal disease or its complications. It also is rec-

**TABLE 15-3 Description of Selected Vaccines**

| VACCINE | DESCRIPTION | COMMENTS |
|---|---|---|
| DPT | | |
| Diphtheria | Toxoid<br>Inactivated<br>Diphtheria toxin | Booster dose every 10 years |
| Tetanus | Inactivated<br>Tetanus toxoid | Booster dose every 10 years<br>For contaminated wound management, additional booster given if more than 5 years since last booster dose |
| Pertussis | Killed whole *Bordetella pertussis* | Not recommended for persons older than 7 years of age because risk of pertussis low and reaction possibly severe |
| Measles | Live attenuated virus vaccine | Contraindications: pregnancy, immunocompromised state, history of anaphylactic reaction to eggs |
| Mumps | Live attenuated virus vaccine | Contraindications: pregnancy, immunocompromised state, history of anaphylactic reaction to eggs |
| Rubella | Live attenuated rubella virus grown in human diploid cells | Contraindications: pregnancy, immunocompromised state |
| Polio | | |
| OPV | Live attenuated oral poliovirus vaccine | Contraindications: pregnancy, immunocompromised state |
| IPV | Inactivated poliovirus vaccine | Administered by subcutaneous injection, contraindicated in pregnancy |
| Influenza | Inactivated whole or disrupted (split) influenza viruses | Antigenic content annually changed to reflect influenza A and B virus strains in circulation; administered annually; contraindication: history of anaphylactic hypersensitivity to eggs |
| Pneumococcal | Purified preparation of 23 different types of pneumococcal capsular polysaccharide | Should be given only once to adults because of possible adverse reactions; data are not currently available regarding revaccination of children; should be given only to children 2 years and older who have chronic illnesses specifically associated with increased risk for pneumococcal disease |
| Hepatitis B | | |
| Recombinant deoxyribonucleic acid (DNA) | Purified surface antigen of virus produced by recombinant yeast cells | Given in series of three injections; first followed by other two 1 and 6 months later; indicated for persons who have routine or frequent contact with blood and body fluids; contraindicated for persons allergic to yeast |
| Human serum | Purified, inactivated surface antigen of virus from plasma of human carriers | Administration schedule same as for recombinant DNA form; recommended for hemodialysis patients |
| *Haemophilus influenzae* b (HbCV) | Bacterial polysaccharide conjugated to protein | Administration schedule may vary depending on brand of vaccine used |

ommended for adults older than 65 years of age who are otherwise healthy and for persons of any age with asymptomatic or symptomatic HIV infection. In general, revaccination of persons who received the previous 14-valent vaccine is not recommended because of the reported increase in adverse reactions.

Table 15-3 summarizes various vaccines.

## Passive Immunization

**Antibodies** produced by other persons or by animals such as the horse, cow, and rabbit can be introduced into a person's bloodstream for protection against attack by a pathogen. This protection is *temporary,* usually lasting only a few weeks, and stimulates no production of antibodies by the recipient. It is called *artificial* **passive immunity.** Artificial passive immunization is given to a person who has been exposed to a disease and has no natural or artificial active immunity. It usually is administered before the disease develops but may be given to modify disease symptoms. However, for effectiveness after the disease has developed, it must be administered early, before extensive damage to body tissue.

Passive immunization usually is reserved for persons to whom the disease would be detrimental. For example, it rarely is given to prevent a disease such as chickenpox or mumps in children because they are at an optimal age for the body to respond immunologically with minimal inflammatory response. On the other hand, an adult exposed to the same diseases often would be given antibodies because adults may have a severe pathologic response. Immunization is given to all age-groups exposed to pathogens that cause serious diseases such as hepatitis, poliomyelitis, diphtheria, tetanus, or rabies. *Antivenins,* which are given to persons bitten by poisonous snakes or black widow spiders, are other examples of passive immunologic products.

Products used for passive immunization may be specific to the disease. *Antitoxins* and *immune animal* and *human sera* are examples. These materials contain elevated levels of immune globulins, which can specifically detoxify the toxin, neutralize the virus, or inactivate the bacterium. The whole blood of a patient who has recently recovered from a disease against which antibodies are produced also may be used. Antitoxins are available for diphtheria, tetanus, botulism, gas gangrene, and the venom of snakes. Human immune serum is available for mumps, measles, pertussis, poliomyelitis, tetanus, and rabies.

*Immune serum globulin* (ISG), or gamma globulin ($\gamma$-globulin), is an antibody-rich fraction of pooled plasma from normal donors. The rationale for pooling plasma is that someone among the donors will have had the diseases and will have developed antibodies against them. The *globulin fraction* of the plasma carries the antibodies, and because it is known not to transmit the virus of hepatitis, it is considered safe to use. Because of occasional side effects, it is now recommended that the use of ISG be limited to those disorders in which its efficacy has been definitely established. These are measles prophylaxis or modification, viral hepatitis type A prophylaxis or modification, and immunodeficiency diseases. ISG is considered to be of questionable value in the following situations: (1) prevention of rubella in the first trimester of pregnancy, (2) prevention or modification of varicella in certain high-risk patients, (3) prevention or modification of viral hepatitis type B (serum hepatitis) after accidental inoculation, and (4) life-threatening bacterial infections.

*Special human ISGs* are derived from the sera of persons previously immunized or convalescing from specific diseases. Tetanus immune globulin (human) is of value in prophylaxis and treatment of tetanus in persons who have not received prior immunization. Pertussis immune globulin (human) and mumps immune globulin (human) are of uncertain or unproved value in the prevention and treatment of pertussis and mumps, respectively. Hepatitis B immune globulin (human) is available for prophylaxis after exposure to hepatitis B. Zoster immune globulin (human) is available for restricted use for prophylaxis against chickenpox.

## Nursing Responsibilities in Immunization

Probably the greatest responsibility of the nurse in immunization programs is to teach the public the advantages of immunization and encourage widespread participation in programs recommended by the local public health officer.

### Teaching

In teaching it is advisable to provide the public with the following information: against what disease protection is being given, why immunization is desirable, and when booster doses should be obtained. The relative safety of the immunization and the advantages of immunization early in life also should be stressed.

The nurse is responsible for assessing persons before immunization because some contraindications exist to receiving certain immunizing substances. Those that are prepared in chicken or duck embryos may cause an allergic reaction in persons allergic to eggs. Many people are allergic to horse serum, and substances containing horse serum, such as tetanus antitoxin, should never be given unless a small amount of the substance has been injected intradermally (a *sensitivity test*) and no "hive" reaction about the injection site has been produced after 20 minutes. *Active immunologic products* should not be given while a person has a cold or other infection because the inflammatory reaction from the immunization will be greater than usual.

Children with histories of allergy often are *not* given routine immunization against diseases for which there is herd immunity because the danger of severe allergic response to the immunization is greater than the danger of contracting the disease. These children should be immunized against diseases such as tetanus, however, and immunization is achieved by giving the vaccine or toxoid in small doses over several weeks or months. The package inserts accompanying the immunologic product should always be read carefully to determine the indications, precautions, and side effects.

Live attenuated virus vaccines should not be given to persons with alterations in the immune status, because virus replication after administration may be unchecked in these individuals. As noted earlier, OPV viruses are excreted by the recipient of the vaccine and are communicable to other persons. Thus individuals who live with an immunocompromised person should receive IPV instead of OPV. Other factors to be considered in the administration of vaccines are listed in Box 15-3.

Before leaving the clinic, the person or family members should be instructed as to the expected effects of an inoculation and told to contact the physician or to report to a hospital emergency room if any other symptoms develop. The person is cautioned not to scratch any lesion produced by an inoculation. If a severe local reaction with redness, swelling, and tenderness occurs, the physician may order the application of hot, wet dressings. If the lesion is open, these dressings should be sterile.

**BOX 15-3 Additional Considerations for Vaccine Administration**

In general, inactivated vaccines and live vaccines (except cholera and yellow fever) can be administered simultaneously in separate sites.

Whenever possible, live vaccines should be administered on the same day or at least 30 days apart.

Purified protein derivative (PPD) testing for tuberculosis can be done on the same day as live virus vaccines are given or 4 to 6 weeks later.

Live attenuated vaccines should not be given at the same time as passive immunization because passively acquired antibodies can interfere with the response to live attenuated virus vaccines.

Pregnant women should not receive live attenuated vaccines because of the theoretic risk to the fetus.

If a person has a febrile illness, it is usually best to wait until recovery before vaccination.

***When antitoxins, antisera, or antivenins are given, the patient is kept under observation for 20 to 30 minutes. Symptoms of severe allergic response usually will appear within that time. Epinephrine 1:1000 should be available for immediate administration if an allergic response occurs.***

Persons employed in health care facilities should be evaluated for immunity against chickenpox, rubella, measles, polio, diphtheria, tetanus, and hepatitis B. Persons at risk for occupational hepatitis B infection should be offered vaccine at the time of employment. Persons with negative tuberculin skin tests should be retested every 6 to 12 months, depending on the prevalence of tuberculosis in the area. Yearly chest roentgenograms are no longer recommended for the routine management of persons with positive tuberculin test reactions. After the initial roentgenogram following a skin test conversion, annual films have not been shown to be of significant clinical value and are not cost effective in monitoring persons for early disease.

### HOME CARE

Persons with infections frequently are cared for at home. The community health nurse often is asked to teach family members how to care for the patient and how to protect family members, friends, and neighbors. Many of the same principles of infection control apply in the home as in the hospital. Some general principles for home care of persons with an infection are discussed here.

Handwashing is considered the most effective measure in preventing the spread of infection in the home. Hands should be washed before care and after contact with body substances (blood, urine, feces, sputum, vomitus, wound drainage, and so on). Caregivers should wear a smock or coverall to protect their clothes. Gloves should be worn when handling body substances. Soiled dressings, used disposable gloves, and other disposable items that contain body substances should be put in plastic bags before being discarded in the trash. All liquid waste can be flushed down the toilet. Used needles and syringes should be put in a puncture-resistant plastic container or can, which is tightly closed before discarding in the trash. Disposable dishes are not required. Dishes and linen should be washed in hot soapy water. A cup of bleach should be added to the detergent to disinfect laundry soiled with blood. Blood and body substance spills should be cleaned up using an effective household disinfectant. If gloves are not available, plastic bags can be worn to protect the caregiver's hands. All persons should be taught to cover the nose and mouth when coughing. In general, it is not considered necessary for the caregiver to wear a mask in the home. The special problems the nurse encounters in controlling hospital-acquired infections are the focus of the remainder of this chapter.

## INFECTION CONTROL IN THE HOSPITAL

### SCOPE OF THE PROBLEM

A **nosocomial** infection is not present or incubating when a person is admitted to the hospital but develops after admission. A **community-acquired infection** is present or incubating at the time of admission to the hospital. The nurse should be aware of the problem of nosocomial infections; their effects on patient morbidity, mortality, and increased hospital costs; and the related legal aspects. The nurse also should be knowledgeable about the types of infections seen most often, the common pathogens and how they are transmitted, factors that predispose a patient to a nosocomial infection, how to recognize persons at risk of infection, and the prevention and control measures necessary to decrease the incidence of nosocomial infections.

At least 2 million persons, or about 5% of all patients admitted to hospitals in the United States each year, develop nosocomial infections. In addition to the considerable morbidity and mortality caused by these infections, their diagnoses and treatment, including additional days of hospitalization, cost more than $4.5 billion per year (Table 15-4).[4] The Joint Commission develops and publishes standards for infection control in the *Accreditation Manual for Hospitals.* These standards are designed to help an institution improve its quality of patient care. The Joint Commission requires that those institutions seeking accreditation have an effective, hospital-wide program for surveillance, prevention, and control of infection. In addition, infection control indicators (performance measures) are being studied. These indicators would allow the Joint Commission to standardize the survey and accreditation process.[15] The AHA and the CDC have developed guidelines for the prevention and control of infectious diseases for use

TABLE 15-4 Estimated Average Number of Extra Days, Average Amount of Extra Charges per Infection, and Deaths Caused by and Contributed to by Nosocomial Infections—United States 1992

| | | | DEATHS DIRECTLY CAUSED BY INFECTIONS | | DEATHS TO WHICH INFECTIONS CONTRIBUTED | |
|---|---|---|---|---|---|---|
| TYPE | EXTRA DAYS | EXTRA CHARGES* | TOTAL | (%) | TOTAL | (%) |
| Surgical wound infection | 7.3 | $3,152 | 3,251 | (0.6) | 9,726 | (1.9) |
| Lower respiratory tract infection | 5.9 | $5,683 | 7,087 | (3.1) | 22,983 | (10.1) |
| Bloodstream infection | 7.4 | $3,517 | 4,496 | (4.4) | 8,844 | (8.6) |
| Urinary tract infection | 1.0 | $ 680 | 947 | (0.1) | 6,503 | (0.7) |
| Other types | 4.8 | $1,617 | 3,246 | (0.8) | 10,036 | (2.5) |
| **All types†** | **4.0** | **$2,100** | **19,027** | **(0.9)** | **58,092** | **(2.7)** |

From *MMWR* 41(42):783, 1992.
* 1992 dollars.
†Some infections were weighted differently in computing these averages *(3)*.

in patient care centers. Because of these external forces, as well as to provide the best possible care for their patients, hospitals are recognizing the need to increase infection surveillance and upgrade programs to prevent nosocomial infections.

The incidence of *nosocomial* infections varies with the type of hospital. This can be attributed to differences in the size of hospitals, the severity of illness in the patient population, susceptibility of the patient population, and the number of staff members who have hands-on contact with the patients. The patient with the greatest risk of developing a nosocomial infection has a chronic illness, a prolonged hospital stay, and the most direct contact with various hospital personnel (physicians, students, nurses, therapists, and so on). These factors hold true for variations in infection rates not only from institution to institution but also within an institution. Certain patient care areas are considered to be ***high-risk areas*** for the development of nosocomial infections. These areas are where patients who have decreased host defenses or who receive invasive procedures and devices are given care. Areas generally considered to be high risk are (1) intensive care units (including neonatal units), (2) burn units, (3) dialysis units, and (4) oncology units. The infection rate in these areas may be well over 20%.

## Persons at Risk

The nurse must recognize patients at the greatest risk of a nosocomial infection. Some of the factors that predispose a person to infection were mentioned previously. Briefly, these include (1) the age of the patient, the very young and the very old being the most susceptible; (2) impairment of normal immune defenses because of an underlying disease process, such as cancer, chronic renal disease, chronic lung disease, diabetes, or AIDS; (3) impairment of the normal immune defenses because of the therapy being given, such as radiation, steroids, or chemotherapy; (4) use of antibiotics, which can eliminate the patient's normal flora, providing opportunity for colonization with pathogenic and drug-resistant organisms that may then progress to cause infection; (5) use of invasive diagnostic and therapeutic procedures and devices, which bypass the patient's normal defense barriers and thus provide a portal of entry into the body (e.g., indwelling urinary catheters, monitoring devices, intravenous catheters, respiratory assistive devices); (6) surgery; (7) burns; and (8) length of hospitalization. Probably the most important factor that predisposes a patient to acquiring a nosocomial infection is the severity of the patient's underlying disease.

A patient admitted to the hospital with an infection may develop a **superinfection** with another organism during the hospitalization. Often this superinfection is with a more virulent or drug-resistant organism. For example, a patient admitted with a leg ulcer infected with *Staphylococcus aureus* may develop further infection (not colonization) with *Pseudomonas aeruginosa.* Furthermore, if this infection progresses to involve the bloodstream, a ***secondary bacteremia*** has occurred. Infection can occur secondary to (1) an existing infection, (2) an underlying disease process, or (3) an anatomic defect that may be causing obstruction. An example of this is the man with benign prostatic hypertrophy (BPH) who develops a urinary tract infection secondary to the obstruction caused by the BPH. These concepts are the most helpful ones when seeking to determine the cause of a particular infection.

Hospitals participating in the National Nosocomial Infection Study (NNIS) provide the only source of recurring nationwide data on nosocomial infections. In 1986, NNIS revised its surveillance protocols. These now include nosocomial surveillance by service, site of infection, pathogen, device, patient risk factors, and type of hospital.[16]

The most common site for a nosocomial infection is the urinary tract; 75% of these infections are related to instrumentation, including indwelling urinary catheters, catheterizations, and urologic procedures. Infected surgical wounds, followed by lower respiratory tract infections, cutaneous infections, and bloodstream infections (some associated with the use of intravascular lines), are the next most frequently encountered types of nosocomial infections. Together these sites account for about 35% of all nosocomial infections.

## Pathogens Causing Nosocomial Infections

The types of pathogens typically responsible for nosocomial infections and their usual reservoirs are listed in Table 15-5. NNIS data from 1986-1990 show that the most frequently reported nosocomial pathogens are *Escherichia coli, Staphylococcus aureus, Enterococcus faecalis, Pseudomonas aeruginosa,* and coagulase-negative staphylococci.

*E. coli* continues to account for most reported nosocomial urinary tract infections on medical services, and *S. aureus* is the main organism causing nosocomial surgical wound infections. *P. aeruginosa* is the most common pathogen causing nosocomial pneumonia. Coagulase-negative staphylococci and *S. aureus* are the pathogens most frequently causing nosocomial primary bacteremia.

**TABLE 15-5 Modes of Transmission of Some Common Pathogens**

| PATHOGEN | COMMON RESERVOIR |
|---|---|
| Gram-positive cocci | |
| *Staphylococcus aureus* | Contaminated objects, hands, and nasal tracts of health care workers, air, self |
| Group A streptococci | Direct contact, air, hands, rarely objects |
| Enterococcus group | Self, hands of health care workers, environmental surfaces |
| Gram-negative rods | |
| *Escherichia, Klebsiella, Enterobacter* | Self, hands of health care workers, contaminated solutions |
| *Proteus, Salmonella, Providencia, Serratia, Citrobacter* | Contaminated food and water, hands of health care workers, self |
| *Pseudomonas* | Contaminated environment, hands, self |
| Anaerobic bacteria | |
| *Clostridium, Bacteroides* | Self, contaminated environment, hands |
| Fungal organisms | |
| Yeasts | Self, hands of health care workers |
| Fungi | Air, contaminated environment |
| Viruses | |
| Varicella | Air, direct contact |
| Herpes | Self, direct contact, air |
| Rubella | Direct contact, air |
| Hepatitis B | Contaminated instruments or injectables, direct contact |

The reservoirs for *S. aureus* are the respiratory tract and skin. From 10% to 15% of the general population can be persistent carriers of this organism, which is harbored in the anterior nares. Among persons working in hospitals, the carrier rate may be as high as 25% to 30%. Nasal carriers, especially those with respiratory tract infections, are potential sources of environmental and human contact contamination. Methicillin-resistant *S. aureus* (MRSA) especially causes concern among caregivers. Methicillin is one of the penicillins specifically developed to treat *S. aureus* infections. *S. aureus* is a common surgical wound and cutaneous pathogen. Although MRSA is no more virulent than methicillin-sensitive *S. aureus* (MSSA), it is more difficult and expensive to treat. The antibiotic of choice for treating MRSA infection is vancomycin. This antibiotic is available only for intravenous administration, which contributes to overall treatment cost. Because of fear of cross-transmission, long-term care institutions have refused admission to patients with MRSA colonization. Institutions have used various strategies in an attempt to eradicate MRSA colonization in their patient populations. These strategies include new admission cultures, periodic surveillance cultures, isolation, and various antibiotic protocols. All have proved to be largely ineffective.

Group A streptococci *(Streptococcus pyogenes)* are gram-positive organisms seen in nosocomial infections. Strains of these organisms cause streptococcal sore throat, scarlet fever, and streptococcal skin infections. Streptococci are found in animate reservoirs, particularly the pharynx and nares of personnel and patients.

Other organisms involved in nosocomial infections include gram-negative coliforms, *Escherichia, Klebsiella,* and *Enterobacter,* which live in the human intestinal tract. Although these organisms usually are susceptible to antibiotics, they have the capacity to develop antibiotic resistance. The large reservoir of coliform organisms within the general population can be a source for self-infection or for cross-infection from the hands of hospital personnel through the ingestion of foods or through the contamination of other materials. Some strains of these organisms are more likely than others to produce infection. The more pathogenic strains seem to gain ascendency in patients who are receiving antibiotic therapy; immunodeficient patients are particularly susceptible to infection by the coliforms.

Although *Salmonella* organisms usually are acquired outside the hospital, the organism is readily transmissible and can be the cause of nosocomial infection. It is transmitted by direct or indirect contact with an infected person or through food (especially raw eggs), dairy products, or water contaminated with the organism. The CDC recommends that no one eat raw eggs. Patients with sickle cell disease, HIV, or malignancies are more vulnerable to infection from these organisms.

*P. aeruginosa,* a gram-negative organism, is present throughout the hospital environment, especially where water is always present (in sinks, irrigating solutions, nebulizers). It is more frequently found in patients with *leukopenia* secondary to burns, leukemia, cystic fibrosis, and various immunodeficiency syndromes. It also is known to be a significant cause of infection in patients receiving prolonged courses of antibiotics, immunosuppressive drugs, and inhalation therapy. *P. aeruginosa* can be a threat to patients undergoing instrumentation (tracheostomy, urinary tract catheterization) and receiving renal transplants. Neonates, particularly premature infants, as well as elderly and debilitated persons, are the most vulnerable.

*Serratia marcescens* and *S. liquefaciens* are gram-negative organisms seen in nosocomial infections. The reservoirs for these organisms are soil and water, and they are found in the hospital in similar reservoirs as *Pseudomonas.* Previously thought to be nonpathogenic, *S. marcescens* was used because of its red pigmentation to mark air flow and settling patterns of bacteria. It is now recognized as a pathogen that can cause severe infection in a susceptible host. One problem with *Serratia* organisms has been their ability to develop resistance to antibiotics rapidly. This can have devastating consequences in an intensive care or burn unit when an outbreak occurs. Because its mode of transmission is through direct or indirect contact on the hands of personnel or on contaminated articles, good handwashing and aseptic techniques are the most effective measures to prevent outbreaks of infection.

*Candida albicans* is a yeastlike fungus that can cause infection, especially in immunocompromised patients or those receiving antibiotics. These patients have a decrease in the normal flora, which provides a niche for the *Candida* organisms to settle in and proliferate. Antibiotics suppress bacterial growth but do not affect fungal growth; special antifungal agents are necessary to control these infections unless the normal flora return after discontinuance of the antibiotics.

## PREVENTION AND CONTROL MEASURES

In the hospital many potential sources of infection exist, including patients, personnel, visitors, equipment, linen, and so on. Patients may become infected with organisms either from the external environment *(exogenous)* or, as is often seen in the severely immunocompromised host, from their own internal organisms *(endogenous).* Virtually any microorganism can be a potential pathogen to the immunocompromised patient. Most of the causative organisms are present in the patient's external environment and are introduced into the body through direct contact or contaminated materials. In many instances nosocomial infections could be prevented by strict aseptic technique when giving care and by greater restraint in the use of invasive procedures and antibiotics. Some specific infection control measures follow.

### Control of External Environment

Health care providers should be in good health and keep their immunization status up to date. They should report to the employee health service when they feel ill. Visitors also should be in good health and their number should be limited to prevent overcrowding in the patient's room. Staff members should wear clean clothing and observe good personal hygiene practices, especially *thorough handwashing,* which decreases transient and resident flora on the hands and thus acts as a deterrent to cross-infection by the hands. Friction and rinsing are the two most important components of good handwashing. Ample handwashing facilities are necessary throughout the hospital and should be used by all personnel before and after patient contact; after contact with excretions, secretions, wound drainage, or any contaminated articles; and before any clean or sterile procedure or contact with clean or sterile equipment. *Handwashing is the most effective method for preventing nosocomial infection.*[2] Dermatologic conditions of the hands should be corrected, because dry, cracked skin can more readily become colonized with pathogens and broken skin is more difficult to rid of transient and resident flora. The person with a skin problem on the hands also tends to avoid proper handwashing, because it can further increase dryness and irritation. The person with active herpes simplex infection of the hand *(herpetic whitlow)* should not give direct patient care until the lesion has healed.

Housekeeping and sanitation practices should be strictly observed to reduce dust and environmental reservoirs of organisms, especially in high-risk areas such as nurseries, operating rooms, and intensive care units. Spills of blood or other body fluids should be cleaned up promptly with an approved hospital disinfectant or a 1:10 dilution of 5.25% sodium hypochlorite (household bleach and water). Linens should be changed with as little contact with the nurse's uniform as possible; linen should not be thrown on the floor or shaken in the air, because this not only will further contaminate the linen but also will stir up dust particles and create air currents that can transmit pathogens. Waste products should be disposed of in the appropriate receptacle. State and federal laws regulate the disposal of infectious waste from health care institutions. Items such as needles and syringes, laboratory cultures and tissue specimens, and other disposable items that are saturated with blood or body substances are considered regulated infectious waste. *Regulated infectious waste must be incinerated or treated (to render it noninfectious) before disposal.* Other waste materials from patient rooms may be disposed of as regular trash. Proper cleaning and sterilization of contaminated reusable articles and equipment are essential. A program should exist to monitor the effectiveness of these practices; however, routine culturing of the environment is not advocated.

Air is generally not considered an important factor in nosocomial cross-infection. However, in the case of *Aspergillus* spores and *Mycobacterium tuberculosis,* adequate air exchanges are necessary to reduce the number of organisms. Minimal standards for air exchanges in patient care areas are published by the Department of Health and Human Services. Minimal air changes of outdoor air per hour range from 2 in patient rooms to 15 in operating rooms.

## Control of Internal Environment

Reducing the *endogenous* sources of infection is more difficult than control of the external environment. Often the source is the patient's own normal flora, and these infections are not directly preventable by the nurse. Preventive measures are aimed at increasing the patient's defense mechanisms and thus decreasing the risk of the infection. Teaching the patient about good nutrition and personal hygiene is a practical measure that is part of nursing care. Maintaining the patient's normal flora and preventing colonization with pathogens that can serve as a source of infection are other effective measures. These, however, are not always possible when patients are receiving antibiotics or undergoing chemotherapy, because these measures may disrupt the normal flora and promote colonization. Appropriate use of antibiotics for prophylaxis and treatment helps prevent colonization with pathogens and decreases the incidence of infection with drug-resistant organisms. Good handwashing by all who have contact with the patient decreases the possibility of the patient's inoculation with pathogenic organisms. Staff members should develop the habit of working from clean procedures to dirty procedures when delivering patient care. For example, the nurse should adjust the intravenous infusion rate and check the intravenous site *before* changing the bed of an incontinent patient. A summary of some prevention and control measures is provided in the Guidelines box at right.

### Guidelines for Preventing and Controlling Nosocomial Infections

**CONTROL OF EXTERNAL ENVIRONMENT (EXOGENOUS SOURCES OF INFECTION)**

**Health Care Providers**

1. In good health—do not care for patients when ill
2. Keep immunizations current
3. Practice effective handwashing between each patient
   - If skin dry, rough, or broken, seek appropriate attention
   - If active herpes simplex infection of hand (herpetic whitlow), do not give direct patient care until lesion healed
4. Wear gloves when contact with any body substance is anticipated

**Housekeeping and Sanitation**

1. Bed linens not shaken in air or thrown on floor
2. Proper disposal of wastes—solid and liquid
3. Proper cleaning and sterilization of contaminated articles
4. Proper ventilation for adequate air exchanges
   - Modern hospitals—patients' room air is under negative pressure
   - Negative pressure keeps air from patients' rooms from moving into hallways
5. Proper mopping and damp dusting to remove dust and other environmental reservoirs of infection

**CONTROL OF INTERNAL ENVIRONMENT (ENDOGENOUS SOURCES OF INFECTION)**

1. Preventive measures aimed at increasing patient's defense mechanisms and thus reducing risk of infection
   - Teach patient about good nutrition
   - Teach patient about personal hygiene, especially handwashing
2. Be aware that normal flora of patient can be disrupted when patient is receiving antibiotics or chemotherapy and colonization may occur
   - Give antibiotics on time as scheduled
   - Teach patient about appropriate use of antibiotics and dangers of taking them when not prescribed by physician

## Prevention of Urinary Tract Infections

As mentioned previously, urinary tract infections (UTIs) are the most common nosocomial infections seen in the hospital. Most of these infections are associated with catheterization and instrumentation of the urinary tract. Urinary catheters should be used only when absolutely necessary. If a catheter must be used, it should be discontinued as soon as medically feasible, because the longer the catheter is in place, the greater the risk of developing an infection. To prevent transmission of bacteria into the bladder, strict aseptic technique is necessary during insertion of the catheter. Bacteria that are present around the catheter-meatal junction also can be transmitted on the tip of the catheter into the bladder along the thin layer of mucus that surrounds the catheter in the urethra. For this reason the catheter should be securely anchored to prevent it from moving in and out of the urethra. Movement of the catheter can track bacteria into the urethra and up into the bladder along the mucous sheath. Furthermore, the catheter-meatal junction should be kept clean; the patient incontinent of stool can pose a problem in this regard. In some institutions, antiseptic agents are used to cleanse the meatus, and antimicrobial agents are applied around the catheter-meatal junction. *Both these practices are considered controversial.* Good handwashing techniques by personnel, cleansing of the patient's meatal area with soap and water, and proper anchoring of the catheter are considered effective ways to reduce the incidence of UTIs in patients with indwelling catheters.

Another portal of entry for bacteria is through the

distal catheter–proximal drainage tube junction. Every time the system is disconnected, the risk of introducing bacteria into the system increases; thus a closed drainage system should be maintained. Bladder irrigations should not be a routine practice. If irrigation is necessary, a sterile disposable syringe and sterile solution should be used. If frequent irrigations are necessary, such as in patients who have had a transurethral prostatectomy (TURP), in which blood clots are common, a three-way catheter drainage system with continuous bladder irrigation is recommended. In this way a closed system is maintained. Urine specimens should be obtained from the rubber portal on the drainage tubing. The portal should be cleansed with an antiseptic before insertion of the needle into the portal.

Another portal of entry of bacteria into the system is through the collection bag. The bag should be kept below the bladder level at all times to prevent reflux of urine into the bladder. It also should be kept off the floor, and the emptying spout should be cleansed with an antiseptic after the urine is emptied from the bag. The container used to collect the urine from the bag must be used for only one patient; it should not be shared among patients.

A final control measure in preventing nosocomial UTIs is to place patients with urinary catheters in separate rooms. This is helpful in preventing cross-infection among patients.

## Prevention of Surgical Wound Infections

Surgical wound infection is primarily related to (1) the degree of contamination, endogenous or exogenous, during the surgical procedure and (2) specific host factors (underlying illnesses and the presence of a remote untreated infection at the time of surgery). The degree of contamination is related to the anatomic wound site, the wound classification, and the duration of surgery. Procedures involving the abdominal cavity, as well as wounds classified as contaminated or dirty, increase the patient's risk of surgical wound infection. Surgical procedures lasting longer than 2 hours have been shown to be the second best predictors of postoperative infection after controlling for the anatomic location of the surgery.[9] The duration of the procedure often is considered a function of the surgeon's skill and experience. The surgical wound infection rate rarely is affected by the postoperative nursing care because the closed wound serves as a barrier to further contamination from exogenous organisms. However, handwashing and aseptic technique during dressing changes are important for all staff members having contact with the surgical wound.

Studies have shown that the most effective approach to reducing surgical wound infection in both high- and low-risk patients involves two components. The first consists of (1) an ongoing surgical wound infection surveillance and control program and (2) the routine reporting of surgical wound infection rates back to the surgeons. The second component is the use of a hospital epidemiologist with specific training in hospital infection control who is an active member of the hospital infection control committee. Findings from the Project Study on the Efficacy of Nosocomial Infection Control demonstrated that hospitals with programs featuring both components had a 35% reduction in high-risk and 41% reduction in low-risk surgical wound infection rates.[10] Keeping the surgeons and operating room nurses informed about specific infection rates heightens awareness of the importance of aseptic technique and efficiency during surgery. Other measures that minimize the risk of infection include the appropriate use of prophylactic antibiotics, limiting the preoperative hospital stay, preoperative bathing with antiseptics, hair removal (preferably by depilatory or clipping) immediately before surgery, and traffic control in the operating room. A summary of surgical wound classification appears in Table 15-6.

**TABLE 15-6 Surgical Wound Classification**

| WOUND CLASSIFICATION | DESCRIPTION AND EXAMPLE |
|---|---|
| Clean | Wounds in which the GI or respiratory tract is not entered; no inflammation or break in aseptic technique<br>Cholecystectomy, hysterectomy |
| Clean contaminated | Clean operation in which the GI or respiratory tract is entered<br>Colon resection |
| Contaminated | Nonpurulent inflammation, gross spillage from GI tract, fresh traumatic wounds, or major breaks in sterile technique<br>Gunshot wound |
| Dirty or infected | Old traumatic with dead tissue, pus encountered, or perforated viscus found<br>Ruptured abscess |

## Prevention of Respiratory Tract Infections

*Nosocomial pneumonia* occurs in approximately 0.6% of hospitalized medical patients (6 cases per 1000 hospital discharges) and is associated with the highest mortality rate of all nosocomial infections.[16] A major risk factor is respiratory intubation inasmuch as endotracheal, nasotracheal, and tracheostomy tubes bypass the patient's defense mechanisms of the upper respiratory tract. The importance of proper maintenance and decontamination of respiratory therapy equipment in preventing nosocomial pneumonias is well established. Handwashing is essential before and after contact with patients and respiratory assist devices, which contain moisture and are ideal reservoirs for organisms, especially gram-negative species such as *Pseudomonas* and *Serratia*. Suctioning is a sterile procedure necessitating the use of sterile equipment and irrigants (see Chapter 37). Surgical procedures that lead to impaired coughing also are a risk factor. Preoperative patient teaching that stresses the importance and proper technique of coughing and deep breathing is essential to the success of postoperative pulmonary toilet. Inappropriate use of antibiotics should be avoided to minimize oropharyngeal colonization with gram-negative bacteria; if aspirated, these may lead to a more serious pneumonia. Debilitated patients should be protected from the hazards of aspiration, especially while eating.

### Prevention of Bacteremias

Many blood infections **(bacteremias)** occur secondary to infections at another site; thus prevention may depend greatly on control of the underlying infection. Some bacteremias result from the use of intravascular devices and systems. The sources of infection in these instances are the hands of staff members, the patient's skin, or infusions contaminated either from mishandling by hospital personnel or, less often, at the time of manufacture. Intravenous and intraarterial catheters should be inserted under aseptic conditions, and catheter insertion sites should be cared for aseptically. The insertion site is treated as an open wound and is inspected frequently for any sign of infection, such as redness, swelling, exudate, purulence, or warmth. The patient also may complain of pain at the site.

Central lines should have a sterile dressing to prevent contamination of the insertion site. A controversy exists over the use of transparent dressings rather than gauze dressings. Some studies have shown an increase in site colonization and catheter-related infection with the use of transparent dressings.[7] However, other studies show no increase in the incidence of site infections with the use of transparent dressings.[17]

Peripheral catheters should be changed every 72 hours or more often if a complication such as infiltration or phlebitis occurs. The catheter is secured to prevent in-and-out movement and tracking of bacteria into the cannula site. Aseptic technique should be followed during the mixing and adding of drugs, changing the infusion, or manipulating connections or stopcocks. It is recommended that the tubing also be changed every 72 hours.[14]

Before hanging a solution, the nurse should check it for turbidity, particulate matter, and leaks in the system. Solutions should be discarded after 24 hours. Hyperalimentation solutions require special adherence to these practices because they are composed of nutrients that provide an excellent culture medium for organisms. *Candida* infections occur frequently in patients receiving hyperalimentation, particularly those who are immunocompromised.

## PROTECTION BY ISOLATION

The purpose of **isolation** is to protect both the caregiver from exposure to infectious agents and the patient from cross-infection. In 1983 the CDC published revised guidelines for isolation precautions in hospitals. Two systems were offered for use. One was based on categories of isolation, and the other listed disease-specific isolation precautions. Hospitals were advised to choose the system most appropriate for their needs. Hospitals also were given the option of devising their own system of isolation using the information and recommendations in these guidelines. The system listed seven major categories of isolation: *strict, contact, respiratory, tuberculosis (AFB), enteric, drainage/secretion,* and *blood/body fluids.* Protective isolation was eliminated as a category because it has not been shown to reduce the risk of infection in the immunocompromised patient.

The current AIDS epidemic has emphasized *the need for caregivers to consider the blood and body fluids of all patients as potentially infectious.* Although it has been shown that the risk of HIV transmission to caregivers is low, other pathogens (hepatitis A virus, hepatitis B virus, non-A, non-B hepatitis virus, cytomegalovirus, herpes simplex virus, Epstein-Barr virus, *S. aureus*) are more easily transmitted in health care settings. Infections with these agents frequently are undiagnosed at the initial contact with the patient. Therefore, taking precautions with the body fluids of all patients will protect the caregiver and reduce nosocomial transmission of pathogens. In August 1987 the CDC published new recommendations for the prevention of HIV transmission in health care settings. These guidelines recommended the elimination of a separate blood/body fluid category because these precautions are to be taken with all patients. Many hospitals have eliminated all the isolation categories and implemented a system called *body substance isolation* (BSI). Following BSI principles will protect both the caregiver and the patient because it does not depend on diagnosis to initiate precautions. The following sections explain (1) category-specific isolation with universal blood/body fluid precautions and (2) BSI.

Table 15-7 lists information about isolation for patients with specific diseases.[5]

### Category-Specific Isolation with Universal Blood/Body Fluid Precautions

#### Strict isolation

Strict isolation is recommended only for highly transmissible diseases that are spread by direct contact and airborne routes of transmission. Some examples of disease requiring strict isolation are burn or skin wounds infected with *S. aureus* or group A streptococcus organisms in which the wound drainage cannot be adequately contained by a dressing; diphtheria; disseminated herpes zoster; and staphylococcal pneumonia. Strict isolation requires that (1) the patient be in a private room with the door kept closed; (2) gowns, masks, and gloves are worn by all persons entering the room; (3) hands are washed on entering and leaving the room; and (4) all articles in the room must be placed in durable

**TABLE 15-7 Disease/Category-Specific Isolation with Universal Blood/Body Fluid Precautions**

| DISEASE | CATEGORY | INFECTIVE MATERIAL | DURATION OF PRECAUTIONS |
|---|---|---|---|
| Abscess, minor or limited | Drainage/secretion | Pus | Duration of illness (DOI) |
| AIDS | * | Blood/body fluids | DOI |
| Amebic dysentery | Enteric | Feces | DOI |
| Babesiosis | * | Blood | DOI |
| Burn infection, minor or limited | Drainage/secretion | Drainage | DOI |
| Cholera | Enteric | Feces | DOI |
| Colorado tick fever | * | Blood | Duration of hospitalization |
| Conjunctivitis | | | |
| Pink eye | Drainage/secretion | Purulent exudate | DOI |
| Gonococcal | Drainage/secretion | Purulent exudate | For 24 hours after start of effective therapy |
| Coxsackievirus disease | Enteric | Feces, respiratory secretions | For 7 days after onset |
| Creutzfeldt-Jakob disease | * | Blood, brain tissue, cerebrospinal fluid | DOI |
| Decubitus ulcer, infected, minor or limited | Drainage/secretion | Pus | DOI |
| Dengue | * | Blood | Duration of hospitalization |
| Diarrhea, acute, infectious cause suspected | Enteric | Feces | DOI |
| Diphtheria | | | |
| Cutaneous | Contact | Lesion secretion | Until two lesion cultures (taken 24 hours apart after antibiotics discontinued) are negative for *Corynebacterium diphtheriae* |
| Pharyngeal | Strict | Respiratory secretions | Same as cutaneous, except cultures obtained from nose and throat |
| Echovirus disease | Enteric | Feces, respiratory secretions | For 7 days after onset |
| Encephalitis, infectious cause suspected | Enteric | Feces | DOI or for 7 days after onset |
| Endometritis, group A *Streptococcus* | Contact | Vaginal discharge | For 24 hours after start of effective therapy |
| Enterocolitis: *Clostridium difficile* or *Staphylococcus* | Enteric | Feces | DOI |
| Enteroviral infection | Enteric | Feces | For 7 days after onset |
| Epiglotitis caused by *Haemophilus influenzae* | Respiratory | Respiratory secretions | For 24 hours after start of effective therapy |
| Erythema infectiosum | Respiratory | Respiratory secretions | For 7 days after onset |
| Gastroenteritis | Enteric | Feces | |
| *Campylobacter* | | | DOI |
| *Clostridium difficile* | | | DOI |
| *Cryptosporidium* species | | | DOI |
| *Dientamoeba fragilis* | | | DOI |
| *Escherichia coli* (enteropathogenic, enterotoxic, or enteroinvasive) | | | DOI |
| *Giardia lamblia* | | | DOI |
| Rotavirus | | | DOI |
| *Salmonella* species | | | DOI |
| *Shigella* species | | | Until three consecutive stool cultures (taken after antimicrobials discontinued) are negative |
| *Vibrio parahaemolyticus* | | | DOI |
| Viral | | | DOI |
| *Yersinia enterocolitica* | | | DOI |
| Hand-foot-and-mouth disease | Enteric | Feces | DOI |
| Hepatitis, viral | | | |
| Type A (infectious) | Enteric | Feces | For 7 days after onset of jaundice |
| Type B (serum, including hepatitis B surface antigen [$HB_sAG$] carrier) | * | Blood/body fluids | Until $HB_sAG$ negative |
| Non-A, non-B | * | Blood/body fluids | DOI |
| Herpangina | Enteric | Feces | For 7 days after onset |

From Garner JS, Simmons BT: *Infect Control* 4:261-283, 1983.

*Previously listed as blood/body fluid precaution category. Implementation of universal blood/body fluid precautions for all patients eliminates the need for this category.

*Continued.*

| TABLE 15-7 Disease/Category-Specific Isolation with Universal Blood/Body Fluid Precautions—cont'd | | | |
|---|---|---|---|
| **DISEASE** | **CATEGORY** | **INFECTIVE MATERIAL** | **DURATION OF PRECAUTIONS** |
| Herpes simplex | | | |
| Disseminated, primary, or severe | Contact | Lesion secretion | DOI<br>Until all lesions are crusted |
| Mucocutaneous, recurrent (skin, oral, genital) | Drainage/secretion | Lesion secretion | Until all lesions are crusted |
| Herpes zoster (varicella zoster): disseminated or localized in immunocompromised patient | Strict | Lesion secretion and possibly respiratory secretions | DOI<br>Until all lesions are crusted |
| Impetigo | Contact | Lesions | For 24 hours after start of effective therapy |
| Lassa fever | Strict | Blood/body fluids, respiratory secretions | DOI |
| Leptospirosis | * | Blood, urine | Duration of hospitalization |
| Malaria | * | Blood | DOI |
| Measles (rubeola) | Respiratory | Respiratory secretions | For 4 days after start of rash; DOI in immunocompromised patients |
| Meningitis | | | |
| Aseptic | Enteric | Feces | For 7 days after onset |
| *H. influenzae* | Respiratory | Respiratory secretions | For 24 hours after start of effective therapy |
| *Neisseria meningitidis* (meningococcal) | Respiratory | Respiratory secretions | For 24 hours after start of effective therapy |
| Meningococcal pneumonia | Respiratory | Respiratory secretions | For 24 hours after start of effective therapy |
| Meningococcemia | Respiratory | Respiratory secretions | For 24 hours after start of effective therapy |
| Multiply resistant bacteria, infection or colonization at any site with any of the following:<br>1. Gram-negative bacilli resistant to all aminoglycosides tested<br>2. *Staphylococcus aureus* resistant to methicillin<br>3. Pneumococcus resistant to penicillin<br>4. *H. influenzae* resistant to ampicillin | Contact | Site of positive culture | Until antimicrobials discontinued and culture negative |
| Mumps | Respiratory | Respiratory secretions | For 9 days after onset of swelling |
| Pediculosis | Contact | Infested area | For 24 hours after start of effective therapy |
| Plague, pneumonic | Strict | Respiratory secretions | For 3 days after start of effective therapy |
| Pleurodynia | Enteric | Feces | For 7 days after onset |
| Pneumonia | | | |
| *S. aureus* | Strict | Respiratory secretions | For 48 hours after start of effective therapy |
| *Streptococcus,* group A | Strict | Respiratory secretions | For 24 hours after start of effective therapy |
| Poliomyelitis | Enteric | Feces | For 7 days after onset |
| Rabies | Contact | Respiratory secretions | DOI |
| Rat-bite fever | * | Blood | For 24 hours after start of effective therapy |
| Relapsing fever | * | Blood | DOI |
| Ritter's disease (staphylococcal scalded skin syndrome) | Contact | Lesions | DOI |
| Rubella | Contact | Respiratory secretions | For 7 days after onset of rash |
| Scabies | Contact | Infested area | For 24 hours after starting effective therapy |
| Skin, wound, or burn infection | | | |
| Minor or limited | Drainage/secretion | Pus | DOI |
| Major | Contact | Pus | DOI |
| Smallpox | Strict | Lesions, respiratory secretions | DOI<br>Room with special ventilation required |
| Syphilis, primary and secondary with skin and mucous membrane lesions | * | Lesions, blood | For 24 hours after start of effective therapy |
| Tuberculosis, pulmonary | Tuberculosis (AFB) | Airborne droplet nuclei | Usually within 2-3 weeks after chemotherapy begun and guided by clinical response and reduction of AFB on sputum smear; private room with special ventilation required |
| Typhoid fever *(Salmonella typhi)* | Enteric | Feces | DOI |
| Varicella (chickenpox) | Strict | Lesions, respiratory secretions | Until all lesions are crusted |
| Viral pericarditis | Enteric | Feces, possibly respiratory secretions | For 7 days after onset |

plastic or paper bags and double bagged for disinfection or sterilization.

### Respiratory isolation

Respiratory isolation is recommended to prevent transmission of infectious diseases that primarily are carried for only short distances through the air (droplet transmission). Direct and indirect contact transmission occurs with some infections in this category but infrequently. The precautions to be practiced in respiratory isolation include placing a patient in a private room; however, patients infected with the same organism generally may share the same room. Masks are to be worn by staff members who come close to the patient, usually estimated to be within an arm's length. Gown and gloves are not indicated. Contaminated articles should be discarded or placed in a labeled plastic bag before being sent for decontamination. Staff members must wash their hands after touching the patient or potentially contaminated articles and before taking care of another patient.

### Tuberculosis isolation (AFB isolation)

Tuberculosis isolation is indicated for patients with suspected or confirmed pulmonary tuberculosis who show positive results on a sputum smear for AFB or whose chest roentgenogram strongly suggests active tuberculosis. Laryngeal tuberculosis also is included in this isolation category. (See Chapter 37 for discussion and care of the patient with pulmonary tuberculosis.) In general, infants and young children with active pulmonary tuberculosis do not require isolation because they rarely cough and their bronchial secretions do not contain many AFBs.[8]

The precautions to be practiced in tuberculosis isolation include placing the patient in a private room with the door closed. The room should be equipped with negative pressure ventilation so that the room air is exhausted to the outside and not recirculated through the hospital. Ultraviolet (UV) lights may be used to disinfect the air. Particulate respirators are special masks recommended for use by staff members who provide patient care. Patients should be instructed to cover their nose and mouth when they cough or sneeze and wear a mask if they must be out of the isolation room for procedures. Access to the isolation room should be restricted. Gowns and gloves are not routinely indicated. Proper handwashing is required before touching articles. Procedures such as bronchoscopy and dental examinations generally are postponed until the patient has received approximately 2 weeks of appropriate antituberculosis therapy and is no longer considered infectious.

### Contact isolation

Contact isolation is designed to prevent transmission of infectious diseases or multiple resistant microorganisms that are spread by close or direct contact. Staff members are advised to wear a mask, gown, and gloves when in close or direct contact with a patient who has an infection or colonization that requires contact isolation. A private room is required; however, patients with the same infections may share the same room. Patients colonized with epidemiologically important, multiply resistant microorganisms (e.g., vancomycin-resistant enterococcus, methicillin-resistant *S. aureus*) generally require contact isolation for the duration of the hospital stay. The infection control practitioner can help ascertain which patients have the same strains, as determined by an identically matching antibiotic-sensitivity pattern, plasmid analysis, or restriction-endonuclease analysis.

### Enteric precautions

Enteric precautions are designed to prevent transmission of disease through direct or indirect contact with infected feces or heavily contaminated articles. Pathogens are spread from contaminated hands to mouth, where they are ingested. Precautions to be practiced primarily consist of thorough handwashing after any patient contact. Gloves should be worn when handling infective excreta or objects contaminated with feces. Masks are not required. Gowns are indicated only if clothing may be soiled with feces. A private room is required when the patient does not practice good hygiene measures, such as handwashing after using the bathroom.

### Drainage and secretion precautions

Drainage and secretion precautions are designed to prevent the transmission of microorganisms from direct contact with a patient's wound drainage. The infectious diseases included in this category result in the production of purulent drainage from any body site that does not require more extensive precautions. Infected wounds are generally minor or limited, in which the drainage is contained within the dressing. Staff members are advised to wear gloves when in direct contact with the infective material. Contaminated articles should be discarded or placed in a plastic bag (which is labeled) before sending for decontamination. Gowns are indicated if clothing is likely to become contaminated with the infective material. Masks are not required. The patient does not require a private room for this category of isolation.

### Universal blood and body fluid precautions

*Universal precautions are intended to protect health caregivers from exposure to blood-borne pathogens.* The body fluids to which universal precautions apply are blood, semen, vaginal secretions, cerebrospinal fluid, synovial fluid, pleural fluid, peritoneal fluid, pericardial fluid, amniotic fluid, tissues, and other body fluids that contain visible blood. These precautions are to be used in the care of all patients. This practice consists of wearing protective barriers and depends on the anticipated

**TABLE 15-8 Body Substance Isolation (BSI) Techniques**

| ITEM | PRECAUTIONS |
|---|---|
| Gloves | Worn for contact with mucous membranes, nonintact skin, and moist body substances; changed after each patient contact |
| Gown or plastic apron | Worn if soiling of clothing is likely |
| Mask and eye protection | Worn if mucous membranes may be splashed with body substances |
| Private room* | Indicated if personal hygiene is poor or if body substances contaminate the environment |
| Needles | Disposed of uncapped and unbent at point of use in puncture-resistant container |
| Soiled linen | Placed in leak-proof bags: gown and gloves worn by laundry workers sorting all soiled linen |
| Reusable equipment | Bagged for transport to decontamination area; gowns, gloves, masks, and eye protection worn by decontamination workers |
| Trash | Bagged to prevent leakage; sharp items, laboratory waste, and disposable items saturated with body substances discarded in regulated infectious waste containers |

Modified from Lynch P, Jackson M: *Infect Control Forum* 8(4):2-5, 1986.

*Airborne-transmitted diseases still necessitate private patient room with sign to alert persons entering. Special ventilation such as negative pressure indicated. A particulate respirator is required to enter room of patient with pulmonary tuberculosis. A mask is required before entering room of patient with meningococcal disease. Only immune persons should enter room of patient with chickenpox.

contact with blood and the body fluids mentioned. Gloves are worn for touching blood and body fluids and are changed after each patient contact. Masks and protective eyewear or face shields should be worn during procedures likely to generate droplets of blood or body fluids to prevent exposure of mucous membranes of the mouth, nose, and eyes. Gowns or aprons are worn during procedures likely to cause splashes of blood or body fluids. Hands and other body surfaces should be washed if contaminated with these fluids. Care should be taken to prevent injuries from needles or other contaminated sharp instruments. Contaminated needles should not be recapped, bent, or broken; removed from disposable syringes; or otherwise manipulated by hand. A one-hand or device-assisted recapping may be employed when use of remaining medication is anticipated or when disposal is delayed. Used needles and other sharp items (scalpel blades, lancets) should be placed in puncture-resistant containers, which should be located as close to the point of use as possible.

## Body Substance Isolation

Jackson et al. and Lynch et al.[11-13] described a system of isolation that emphasizes precautions with the body substances (blood, sputum, urine, feces, pus, drainage, and so on) of *all* patients. They recognized that the colonized patient, not only the diagnosed patient, is a potential source of cross-infection. Therefore the practice of BSI provides better protection for patients and caregivers against the transmission of unrecognized communicable disease. (See Table 15-8 for BSI techniques.)

Precautions should be determined by the anticipated interactions with a patient's body substances. Under this system, designation of patients with diagnosed infections would be a hindrance and support a double standard of practice. For example, a double standard exists when caregivers wear gloves when handling the urine of a patient with diagnosed *Serratia* UTI but not when handling the urine of other patients. Colonization with this or other resistant pathogens, which is never diagnosed unless a urine culture is obtained, can occur in any patient.

## General Principles of Isolation

Some general principles apply regardless of the type of isolation. Barriers such as gowns, gloves, and masks should be used only once and then discarded in an appropriate receptacle before leaving the patient's room. These barriers should be conveniently available for each patient room. *Hands must be washed before and after each patient contact even when gloves are worn.*

One can see the similarities between the CDC's universal blood and body fluid precautions and BSI. The difference is that BSI does not require the other categories except for airborne-transmitted diseases because BSI technique will prevent the transmission of diseases in the other categories. Redundancy exists in the CDC's category-specific and universal blood and body fluid precaution system. Nurses will need to determine which system is being used in their health care setting.

## QUESTIONS TO CONSIDER

- Define the following terms: (1) active immunity, (2) passive immunity, and (3) herd immunity.
- What is the danger in giving live virus vaccines to immunocompromised persons?
- List six factors that place a hospitalized patient at risk for the development of a nosocomial infection.
- What is the most common nosocomial infection? What measures could nurses take to reduce the incidence of this nosocomial infection?
- What measures can nurses take to prevent occupationally acquired infectious diseases?
- Analyze one ethical issue that can arise when caring for a patient with AIDS.

## CRITICAL THINKING ACTIVITIES

- Mary's husband has cancer and is being treated with chemotherapy. Both Mary and her husband want to have a child because they fear he will not survive his diseases. Before getting pregnant, Mary has a measles antibody titer drawn, which is low. Should Mary be given a measles vaccination? Provide rationale for your decision.
- As a nurse working in a local acute care facility, how can you be effective in preventing the spread of disease in your community?
- Your neighbor tells you that she is happy that her 3-year-old daughter has had all of her immunizations because she cannot stand to see the baby cry. You know that further immunizations are necessary. How would you best approach this neighbor without appearing judgmental?

## CHAPTER SUMMARY

### HISTORICAL PERSPECTIVE

- Infection control programs exist to decrease morbidity, mortality, and cost of nosocomial infections.

### THE INFECTIOUS DISEASE PROCESS

- The sequence of events in the chain of infection involves (1) a causative agent, (2) a reservoir, (3) a portal of exit, (4) a mode of transmission, (5) a portal of entry, and (6) a susceptible host.
- Modes of transmission are (1) contact (direct, indirect, droplet), (2) airborne, (3) vehicle, and (4) vector.
- Fever and a WBC count greater than 10,000/mm$^3$ may indicate a generalized infection.
- When possible, appropriate cultures should be obtained before initiating antibiotic therapy.

### INFECTION CONTROL IN THE COMMUNITY

- In the United States the ACIP recommends that children be immunized against diphtheria, tetanus, pertussis (DTP); measles, mumps, rubella (MMR); poliomyelitis (OPV); *Haemophilus influenzae* (HbCV); and hepatitis B.
- Health caregivers who have frequent contact with blood and body fluids should be immunized against hepatitis B virus.
- Passive immunity is temporary, lasting a few weeks without stimulating antibody production in the recipient.
- In general, live attenuated virus vaccines should not be given to persons with alterations in immune status.

### INFECTION CONTROL IN THE HOSPITAL

- A nosocomial infection is one that is not present or incubating when a person is admitted to the hospital but develops after admission.
- Handwashing is the most important measure in preventing cross-infection.
- Urinary catheterization is associated with increased risk for nosocomial urinary tract infection.
- Nosocomial pneumonia occurs in approximately 0.6% of hospitalized medical patients and is associated with the highest mortality rate of all nosocomial infections.
- Aseptic technique is an important factor in preventing nosocomial infection.
- Two systems of isolation are (1) category-specific isolation with universal blood/body fluid precautions and (2) body substance isolation (BSI).
- Adherence to universal blood/body fluid precautions or BSI is the best protection caregivers have from occupationally acquired blood-borne infections.
- Caregivers should direct problems concerning any aspect of infection control to the infection control nurse, the hospital epidemiologist, or the infection control committee in their institution.

## REFERENCES

1. American Hospital Association: *OSHA's final bloodborne pathogens standard: a special briefing*, Chicago, Feb 1992, The Association.
2. Bennett JV, Brachmann PS, editors: *Hospital infections,* Boston, 1992, Little, Brown & Co.
3. Centers for Disease Control: Recommendations of the ACIP: smallpox vaccine, *MMWR* 34(23):341-342, 1985.
4. Centers for Disease Control and Prevention: Public health focus: surveillance, prevention, and control of nosocomial infections, *MMWR* 41(42):783-787, 1992.
5. *Clinician's dictionary of bacteria and fungi,* Indianapolis, Ind, 1986, Eli Lilly Co.
6. Cohen ML: Epidemiology of drug resistance: implications for a post-antimicrobial era, *Science* 257:1050-1055, 1992.
7. Conly JM, Grieves K, Peters B: A prospective, randomized study comparing transparent and dry gauze dressings for central venous catheters, *J Infect Dis* 159(2):310-319, 1989.
8. Garner JS, Simmons BP: Guideline for isolation precautions in hospitals, *Infect Control* 4(4):245-325, 1983.
9. Haley RW: Nosocomial infections in surgical patients: developing valid measures of intrinsic patient risk, *Am J Med* 91(suppl 3B):145S-151S, 1991.
10. Haley RW et al: The efficacy of infection surveillance and control programs in preventing nosocomial infections in U.S. hospitals, *Am J Epidemiol* 121(2):182-205, 1985.
11. Jackson MM, Lynch P: Infection control: too much or too little? *Am J Nurs* 84:208-210, 1984.
12. Jackson MM et al: Why not treat all body substances as infectious? *Am J Nurs* 87(3):1137-1139, 1987.
13. Lynch P et al: Implementing and evaluating a system of generic infection precautions: body substance isolation, *Am J Infect Control* 18:1-12, 1990.
14. Maki DG et al: Prospective study of replacing administration sets for intravenous therapy at 48 vs 72 hour intervals, *JAMA* 258:1777, 1987.
15. Nadzam DM: Infection control indicators in critical care settings, *Heart Lung* 21(5):477-481, 1992.
16. Nosocomial infection rates for interhospital comparison: limitations and possible solutions, *Infect Control Hosp Epidemiol* 12:609-621, 1991.
17. Petrosino BP, Becker H, Christian B: Infection rates in central venous catheter dressings, *Oncol Nurs Forum* 15(6):709-717, 1988.

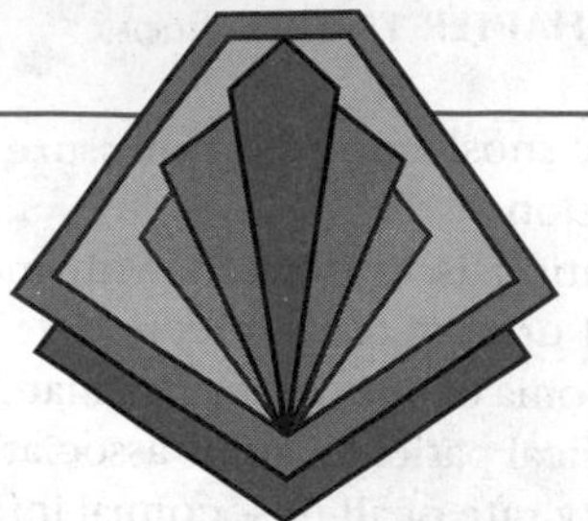

# CHAPTER 16

# Cancer

***Gladys E. Deters***

## CHAPTER OBJECTIVES

***After studying this chapter, the learner should be able to do the following:***

1. Describe epidemiologic factors related to cancer.
2. Identify the nurse's role in prevention of cancer and in health education.
3. Describe the pathophysiology of cancer, including the characteristics of malignant cells, growth of neoplasms, and nature of metastases.
4. Identify the factors related to carcinogenesis.
5. Relate the pathophysiologic changes that cause clinical manifestations of cancer.
6. Apply the nursing process to identify care of the patient in the diagnostic and treatment phases of cancer.
7. Explain the rationale for the four major types of cancer therapy and discuss nursing care of patients receiving these therapies.

## KEY TERMS

afterloading
anaplasia
antibody
biologic response modifier therapy
biotherapy
brachytherapy
cachexia
cancer
carcinogens
carcinoma
cellular differentiation
doubling time
dysplasia
hyperplasia
immunotherapy
interferons
metaplasia
metastasis
mutation
oncogenes
palliative treatment
paraneoplastic syndrome
radiosensitivity
radiotherapy
sarcoma
staging
stem cells
teratoma

## NATURE OF THE PROBLEM

Cancer was recognized in ancient times by skilled observers who gave it the name "cancer" (L., *cancri,* crab) because it stretched out in many directions like the legs of a crab. **Cancer** is an "umbrella" word used to describe a group of more than 270 diseases in which cells multiply without restraint, destroy healthy tissue, and endanger life.

Few diseases cause greater feelings of anxiety and apprehension than cancer. Its physiologic and psychologic impact on patients and their families results in profound changes in their life-styles. Cancer may spell death to some and mutilation to others. The legends surrounding malignant disease, often focusing on incurability, help foster feelings of hopelessness and dread. Yet much progress has been made in prevention, early detection, and treatment of cancer, and research continues in these areas.

Nurses too may have the same negative attitudes that exist in society. For this reason it is extremely important that all nurses examine their own feelings about cancer and try to work through them, both by increasing their knowledge of the disease and its treatment and by discussing feelings openly with members of the health care team. Nurses who have resolved their own feelings are more able to help patients and their familes than are nurses who have not done so.

Cancer nursing has been recognized as a subspecialty in the nursing profession since 1975. Oncology nurses must have a broad base of knowledge in both pathophysiology and the psychosocial arena. They care for patients of all ages, both sexes, and in a variety of settings that range from the acute care hospital to health-promotion centers, ambulatory care clinics, home care agencies, and hospice care. The oncology nurse fills the role of care provider, manager, researcher, teacher, and consultant. To provide comprehensive care the nurse must have correct knowledge of the prevention, control, and treatment of cancer. Teaching about cancer is not limited to the practice setting but may take place in industry, at PTA meetings, and at other public forums. In addition to teaching about prevention, the nurse has an active role in treatment and control programs in all settings in which patients are found. Patients and their families look to the nurse for assistance and guidance in all phases of this illness, from detection to terminal care.

To be effective as a helping person the nurse must be aware of the emotional impact that the diagnosis of cancer has on the patient and family because this emotional response affects every aspect of nursing care. Cancer nursing is a challenge to the creativity, skill, and commitment of the nurse.

# ETIOLOGY

## MULTISTEP PROCESS OF CARCINOGENESIS

Comprehension of cellular kinetics is necessary to understanding the multistep process of cancer development: *initiation, promotion,* and *progression.* Initiation begins with exposure of normal cells to **carcinogens**—substances that can cause cancer. Carcinogens such as radiation, chemicals, drugs, and viruses cause irreversible genetic damage that is referred to as **mutation.** Promotion, the second step, may last for many years. Promoting factors can include cigarette smoking, alcohol abuse, or dietary components that act repeatedly over time on the already transformed cell. Promoters enhance the structural changes within the cell and are thought to facilitate the rate of these spontaneous mutations that are passed on through mitosis, producing ever-increasing numbers of abnormal cells.[16] Progression, the final step, is the uncontrolled growth of a malignant tumor capable of metastatic activity. Research into the carcinogenesis of colorectal cancer reveals that a sequence of events directed at five genes is required as the tumor progresses to invasion and metastasis.[49]

Carcinogenesis is a dynamic process that is influenced by many independent and poorly defined variables. The initial molecular changes are irreversible. Etiologic agents may be co-carcinogens. A genetic predisposition for a "weak" immune system along with a viral infection may lead to cancer, or oncogenic viruses may act as suppressants of the immune system. Chemical carcinogens may activate latent viral genes or inhibit the immune system's effectiveness in destroying cancer cells. Figure 16-1 illustrates the multistep process of cancer development.

## FACTORS INHIBITING TUMOR GROWTH

Some tumor growth may be checked by lack of vascularization. Tumor cells compete with normal cells and tissue for blood supply. As tumor cells grow, they stimulate vascularization (angiogenesis) with the establishment of new capillary sprouts. Until the capillaries penetrate the tumor, growth is slow and the tumor is termed *avascular.* After capillary penetration occurs, the tumor begins to grow rapidly, is capable of distant metastasis, and is said to be in a *vascular* stage. Carcinoma in situ

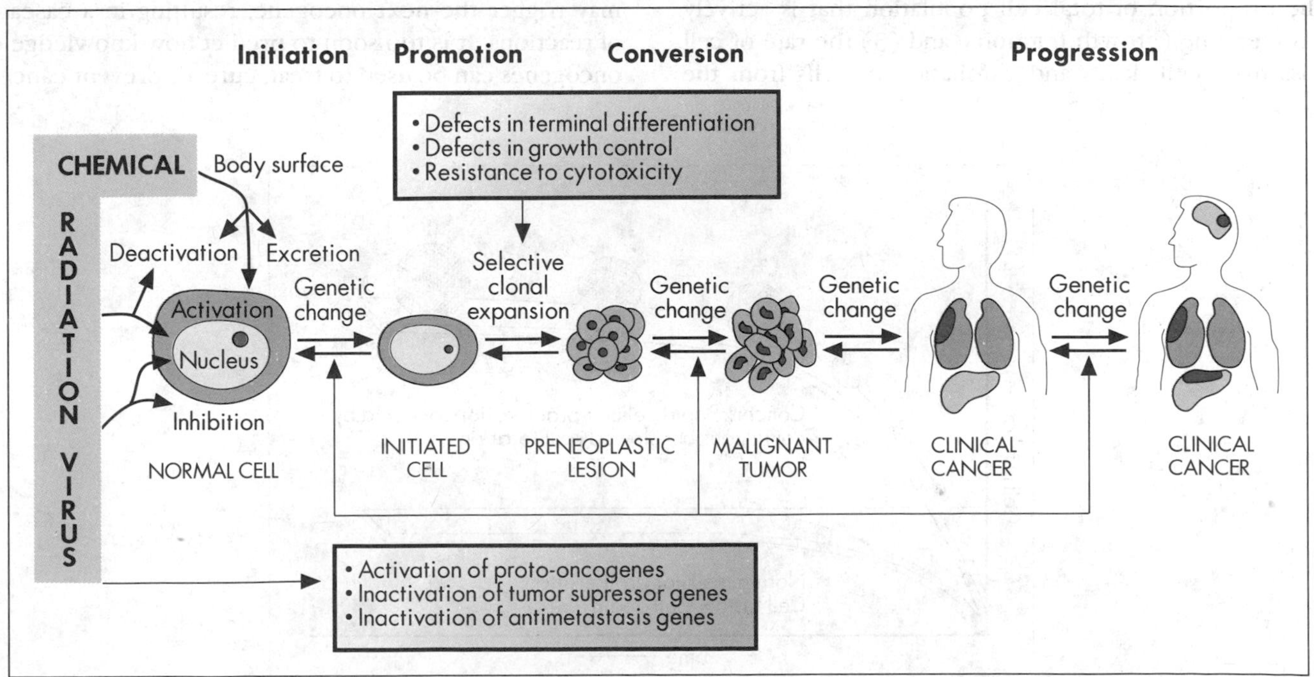


**FIGURE 16-1** Multistage process of carcinogenesis evolving from a single transformed cell to a malignant cell. (Modified from Harris CC: *Cancer Res* 51:5023-5044, 1991.)

lesions are in the avascular phase of development, which accounts for their slow and localized growth.

Growth of tumors that arise in tissues regulated by sex hormones may be affected in positive or negative ways. For example, breast cancers that occur during pregnancy often grow rapidly but tend to grow less rapidly after delivery.

Although it is rare, tumors have regressed spontaneously, in some cases as a result of maturation and differentiation of tumor cells. This happens most frequently in neuroblastoma, a tumor of embryonic neuroblasts. The cause and physiologic action of spontaneous maturation are not known.

## FACTORS AFFECTING RATE OF TUMOR GROWTH

The rate of growth of a tumor is expressed in terms of **volume-doubling time.** Human tumors generally have a long doubling time, from 1 week to more than 1 year, with median time of about 60 days. Because tumors contain many different types of cells, the length of the cell cycle (median generation time) varies from 2 to 3 days among the various cells.

In normal adult tissue, cell birth is equal to cell death. In contrast, cancer cell division continues indefinitely. When the tumor is small and growing rapidly, a relatively high proportion of cells are undergoing division and tumor doubling time is rapid. As the tumor increases in size with a larger cell population, a larger doubling time is needed. This growth pattern is known as *gompertzian function* (Figure 16-2).

Three factors affect *rate* of tumor growth: (1) the rate of replication of proliferating cells (cell cycle time), (2) the proportion of total cell population that is actively proliferating (growth fraction), and (3) the rate of cell loss from cell death and exfoliation of cells from the tumor surface. Cell cycle time is relatively constant in tumors with similar histology, but there is considerable difference between normal and tumorous tissue. For a given cycle time, a tumor with a high growth fraction will double faster than a tumor with a low growth fraction.

Knowledge of cell kinetics is important because the sensitivity of the cell to chemotherapy and radiotherapy depends heavily on the proliferative state of the cell at a specific time. In addition, study of cell cycle kinetics helps increase understanding of tumor growth and regulation, laying the foundation for better methods of controlling cancer cells.

## ROLE OF ONCOGENES

In the early 1970s **oncogenes** (specific genes that can trigger cancer cell growth) were discovered. Thirty of these cancer genes have now been identified. These oncogenes are similar, if not identical, to genes normally present in the cell, called *proto-oncogenes*. It appears now that these normal genes—when activated by radiation, chemicals, or viruses—are transformed to a malignant state. It is unclear yet if oncogenes are involved in all or just some cancers or how they fit into the overall pattern of carcinogenesis.

The cancer-causing genes and normal genes appear to be virtually the same, but their functions are drastically different. Although the activation of an oncogene may be part of the process of carcinogenesis, it is not in itself enough to cause cancerous growth. It is possible that tumors grow from the concerted effort of a number of oncogenes, each representing one of the multiple steps of carcinogenesis. The activation of one oncogene may trigger the next oncogene, resulting in a cascade of reactions. It is too soon to predict how knowledge of oncogenes can be used to treat, cure, or prevent cancer.

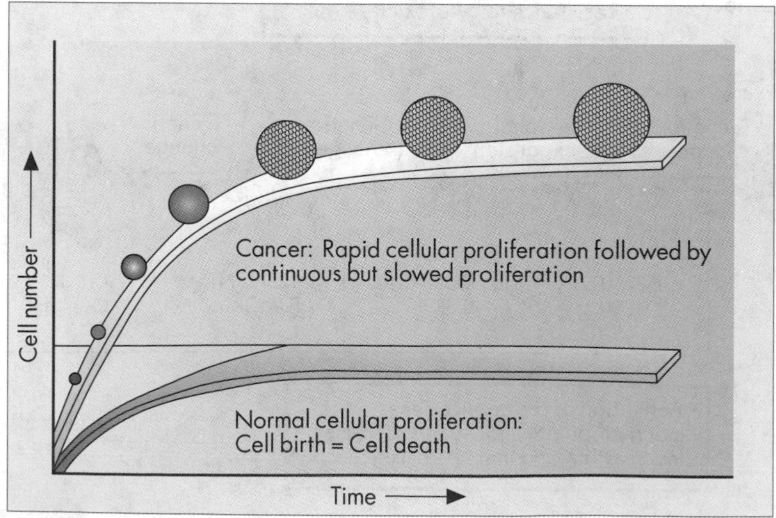


**FIGURE 16-2** Gompertzian function. (Modified from *Cancer: chemotherapy and care,* Part I, Syracuse, NY, Bristol Laboratories.)

## HOST SUSCEPTIBILITY

### Genetic Factors

Certain conditions and predispositions of the individual person seem to contribute to the development of cancer. Studies of genetic factors have focused on specific cancer sites and the disease in general. Research seems to indicate that in inherited disorders the deranged gene, chromosomal defect, translocation (genetic material moved from one chromosome to another), or altered DNA may result in changes that render the cell vulnerable to malignant transformation.[35] As a direct consequence of this single genetic change, all future descendants of the transformed cell will be malignant and the trait will be inherited by all future generations.

Hereditary cancer has certain general characteristics: (1) an early age of onset, occurring 20 or more years earlier than in the general population, (2) a marked incidence of bilateral cancer in paired organs—for example, breasts, kidneys, thyroid glands, (3) multiple primary or multicentered cancers with greater frequency than expected, and (4) well-established autosomal recessive sex-linked and cytogenic cancer and precancerous disorders. In addition, in many cases there is evidence of vertical transmission in consecutive generations with autosomal dominant inheritance.

Leukemia is an example of a malignant condition associated with chromosomal alterations. Chronic myelogenous leukemia is associated with Philadelphia chromosome 22 translocation, whereas trisomy 21 found in Down syndrome has been shown to be a risk factor for leukemia development. It is also possible to inherit a condition that increases a person's risk for the eventual development of a certain type of cancer. Ulcerative colitis, if left untreated, can result in cancer of the colon. In familial polyposis, an inherited disease, colon cancer is expected in 100% of all untreated cases.

True "cancer families" are rare and differ from normal families in whom many cancers seem to develop. Cancer families tend to inherit the same kind of cancer and develop the disease at an early age (Table 16-1). Studies have shown that the pattern of inheritance is not usually that of a single mendelian gene, and it is still not known whether the incidences of many specific cancers are a result of a combination of genetic or environmental factors.

**TABLE 16-1 Cancers Associated with Genetic Factors**

| TYPE OF CANCER | CHARACTERISTICS |
|---|---|
| Wilms' tumor | Purely hereditary |
| Familial polyposis of colon | Precursor of cancer |
| Breast cancer | High incidence in vertical line of descent (mother to daughter) |
| Bronchogenic cancer | Seems to develop from synergistic effect of heredity and cigarette smoking |
| Cancer family syndrome (CFS): adenocarcinoma of colon and endometrium; sometimes of stomach, breast, and ovaries | Autosomal dominant inheritance; transmitted vertically |
| Familial atypical multiple mole–melanoma (FAMMM) syndrome | Familial disease; genetic factors predispose individuals |
| Xeroderma pigmentosum and disseminated superficial actinic porokeratosis | Autosomal recessive disorders; skin cancer precursors |

### Hormonal Factors

Some evidence suggests that hormones may in some way be connected with the development of certain cancers. In addition, some metabolites of cancers may also act as antihormones or have new physiologic effects. Hormones do not appear to be primary carcinogens but rather seem to influence carcinogenesis in three ways: (1) by a preparative action on the target tissues, making them susceptible to the carcinogenic agent, (2) by a "permissive" influence on carcinogenesis, allowing the process to progress, and (3) by a conditioning effect on the tumor. Hormones are capable of restraining or enhancing growth of tumors that have developed. Hormone therapy and some surgical therapies (hypophysectomy and oophorectomy) are based on this fact.

There is evidence that tissues that are endocrine-responsive (e.g., breasts, endometrium, and prostate) do not develop cancer unless they are stimulated by their growth-promoting hormones. Estrogens have been associated with such cancers as adenocarcinoma of the vagina, hepatic tumors, breast tumors, and uterine cancer.

In addition to tissue stimulation by the hormone, carcinogenesis may be determined by the length of time of the hormonal effect. The longer the preparative influence of the hormone, the greater is the chance of cancer development.

### Precancerous Lesions

Certain benign lesions and tumors have a tendency toward malignant change. These cancers are preventable if minor precursor conditions are located and treated early. These precancerous conditions include polyps of the colon and rectum, certain pigmented moles, dysplasias of the cervical epithelium, Paget's disease of the bone, and radiodermatitis and senile keratosis.

Senile (solar) keratoses are thickened patches on the skin of the face and hands of those who are exposed to sunlight. Xeroderma pigmentosum, a rare congenital hypersensitivity to light, results in warty precancerous elevations of the skin in childhood. Epidermal carcinoma or malignant melanoma frequently develops. Leukoplakia, precancerous white thickened patches, may occur on the mucous membranes of the lips, mouth, tongue, vulva, and cervix.

Precancerous lesions belong to a large and heterogeneous group; in some, cancer is inevitable, whereas in others the risk is so low that medical management disregards the cancer risk. For example, the risk of cancer is high in xeroderma pigmentosum but low in leukoplakia of mucous membranes, especially of the oral cavity, larynx, and vulva.

## Chronic Irritation

The role of trauma, chronic irritation, or inflammation has been considered as a causative factor in cancer. Scientific proof has been difficult to demonstrate. Nevertheless it is prudent to be alert to the possible consequences of trauma or chronic irritation to any part of the body. Effort is being made in industry to protect workers from coal-tar products known to contain carcinogens. Masks and gloves are recommended in some instances, and workers are urged to wash their hands and arms thoroughly to remove all irritating substances at the end of the day's work.

Any kind of chronic irritation to the skin should be avoided, and moles that are in locations where they may be irritated by clothing should be removed. Shoelaces, shoetops, belts, girdles, brassieres, and shirt collars are examples of clothing that may be a source of chronic irritation. Glasses, earrings, dental plates, and pipes that are in repeated contact with skin and mucous membrane may contribute to cancer. Chewing food thoroughly is recommended to lessen irritation in the throat and stomach. Cancer of the mouth sometimes is associated with constant irritation of the oral mucous membrane by rough, jagged teeth. The habit of drinking scalding hot or freezing cold liquids is also thought to be irritating to the mouth and to the esophagus. Indiscriminate use of laxatives is believed to have possible carcinogenic effects on the large bowel.

## Immunologic Factors

Immunologists have been increasingly aware of the role of the immune system in the natural history of malignant disease. It may be possible that failure of the normal immune mechanism may predispose one to certain cancers. The change from normal to malignant cells is relatively common. These new cells are antigenically different and are recognized as such by the body's immune system. If the immune response is initiated, the malignant cell will be destroyed. That a kind of immune surveillance system may exist is suggested by the following evidence. (1) The two peaks of high incidence of tumors in humans are in early childhood and old age—periods when the immune system is weak. (2) Increased evidence of tumor development exists in persons with rare immunodeficiency diseases in which there is a defect in cellular immunity. (3) Persons who are receiving cyclosporine, the major immunosuppressive drug used to prevent organ transplant rejection, have an increased evidence of neoplasia such as lymphoma, Kaposi's sarcoma, and carcinoma of the kidney.[34]

The question arises: if a surveillance system exists, why do initial tumor cells progress to clinical cancer? There are no clear-cut answers, but some are suggested. Some tumors arise in areas that are poorly served by the immune system—areas such as the central nervous system or the retrobulbar aspect of the eye. Some tumors do not stimulate antibody formation because they are so similar to normal cells. The normally occurring system, composed of suppressor lymphocytes, which checks the immune response, may become overly active and overwhelm the immune system. The problem may reside in persons who do not have the same genetic ability for immune response that others have—just as not all have the same physical strength.

The normal immune system is capable of detecting and destroying as many as 10 million cancer cells at a time. However, when a tumor mass grows at a rate faster than the normal immunologic response can effectively handle it, the tumor will continue to grow undetected. Typically, a tumor mass is at least 1 cm in size before it can be detected by present conventional diagnostic methods. Unfortunately a tumor 1 cm in diameter already contains more than 1 billion malignant cells. It is anticipated that as research on the immune system progresses, more definitive answers will be revealed as to the interplay of immune function and surveillance and cancer development. (The role of immune system and cancer therapy is discussed later in this chapter and in detail in Chapter 13.)

## Drug Effects

The International Agency for Research on Cancer has identified a number of drugs that are known to have carcinogenic potential in human beings. The list includes some over-the-counter (OTC) drugs easily purchased by consumers, such as mixtures containing phenacetin, as well as a variety of commonly prescribed medications (Box 16-1).

Oral contraceptives, classified as having carcinogenic potential for breast cancer, are now recognized as having a protective effect against ovarian and endometrial cancers.[10] In 1971 a rare form of vaginal cancer in women

**BOX 16-1 Drugs That May be Oncogenic to Human Beings**

1. Cytotoxic agents
2. Immunosuppressive agents
3. Estrogens
4. Oral contraceptives
5. Androgenic anabolic steroids
6. Methoxsalen
7. Phenacetin-containing analgesics

was linked to the ingestion by their mothers of diethylstilbestrol (DES), which was prescribed to prevent spontaneous abortion.

Cancer therapy itself may increase the risk for other cancers. Intensive alkylating agent therapy is accompanied by significant subsequent risk of acute leukemia. Consequently its use is limited to those cases for which no comparable alternative therapy exists. Further research on disease response to drugs is needed to prevent long-term risks of cancer treatment.

## Environmental Factors

As long ago as 1775 the incidence of prostate cancer was recognized in men employed as chimney sweeps in English homes where coal was burned as fuel. Coal tar, an end product of coal combustion, is now acknowledged as the first occupational chemical carcinogen. The importance of the link between environment and cancer development increases when patterns of incidence and mortality are studied. As people move from place to place throughout the world, the baseline incidence rates and mortality for each type of cancer change. It is thought that environmental factors play a causative role in 90% of cancers seen today.[27]

The Occupational Safety and Health Act of 1970 authorized the Occupational Safety and Health Administration to enforce maximal allowable concentrations of exposure to carcinogens (threshold limit values [TLVs]). The National Institute for Occupational Health and Safety at present believes that it is not possible to show precise tolerance levels of chemical carcinogens and consequently stresses that exposure to any known or suggested carcinogens must be reduced to the least possible level by any means available.

Numerous environmental factors are implicated directly or indirectly in cancer development. Two major factors are diet and tobacco use. Also included are ionizing and ultraviolet radiation, occupational hazards (chemicals, air pollution), alcohol, drugs, sexual behavior, and possibly individual personality traits (Table 16-2).

### Ionizing radiation

Radiography and radium may cure cancer, but in other cases they cause it. Ionizing radiation consists of electromagnetic waves or material particles that have sufficient energy to ionize atoms or molecules (i.e., remove electrons from them) and thereby alter their chemical behavior. In adequate amounts it destroys the cells.

Every living thing from the beginning of time has been exposed to small amounts of radiation from the sun and from certain natural elements in the earth, such as uranium, that emit gamma rays ($\gamma$-rays) in the process of their decay. This is known as natural background radiation. No problem regarding radiation existed until after 1895, when the roentgen-ray (x-ray) machine was developed and became widely used in diagnosis of disease. The development of this machine was followed by the discovery of radium and the use of both radium and radiography for treatment of diseases such as cancer.

Radiologists working with early radiographic equipment showed a higher than normal incidence of skin cancer. Workers employed in painting radium on watch dials had high rates of oral and sinus carcinomas and osteosarcomas. It is well known that survivors of the atomic bombs dropped on the Japanese cities of Hiroshima and Nagasaki during World War II were exposed to high doses of radiation. Within a 10-year period after

**TABLE 16-2 Summary of Cancer-Associated Environmental Factors**

| FACTOR | SITES CONSIDERED IN DRAWING THE ESTIMATES | RANGE OF ESTIMATES ASSOCIATED WITH FACTOR* |
|---|---|---|
| Tobacco | Upper respiratory tract, bladder, esophagus, kidney, pancreas | 22%-30% (30%) |
| Alcohol | Upper digestive tract, larynx, liver | 3%-5% (3%) |
| Natural radiation | Skin, breast, thyroid, lung, bone, blood (leukemia) | 1%-3% (1%) |
| Medical drugs and radiation | Breast, endometrium, ovary, thyroid, bone, lung, blood (leukemia) | 1%-4% (1%) |
| Occupation, all exposures | Upper respiratory tract, others | 4%-38% (4%-10%) |
| Diet | Digestive tract, breast, endometrium, ovary | 35%-50% (35%) |
| Sexual development, reproductive patterns, and sexual practices | Breast, endometrium, ovary, cervix | 1%-13% (7%) |
| Pollution | Lung, bladder, rectum | 1%-5% (2%) |
| Consumer products (e.g., cosmetics, clothing) | Possibly all sites | <1% |
| Infection | Uterine cervix, prostate, and other sites | 1%-15% (10%) |
| Unknown associations | All sites | 1%-10% |

From Kupchella CE: *Semin Oncol Nurs* (3):162, 1986.

*Values in parentheses refer to the most commonly cited "best" estimate.

exposure, a variety of cancers higher than the normal incidence rates developed in this population.[30]

Radiation in the environment as a result of nuclear testing and the well-publicized nuclear power plant "leaks" in the United States and Russia caused widespread fear and debate over the use of nuclear energy. No one really knows how much exposure to radiation is safe for persons working with patients and for patients having repeated radiographs taken for various purposes. Relatively small amounts of exposure have produced serious damage in experimental animals, but human beings have not lived through enough generations of relatively high exposure for conclusive evidence of safe levels to be established. It is reasonable to assume that the less exposure one has the better.

The ionizing effect of radiation on the body cells remains, so that exposure is cumulative throughout life. Exposure of the entire body enormously increases the amount of radiation received. For this reason all of the body except the part being treated is protected from exposure when relatively high doses are given for therapeutic purposes.

There is now conclusive evidence of a link between prenatal radiation exposure and tumor development, not only early in life but throughout adulthood. The radiation causes breaks in the DNA strands in the exposed cells during the prenatal period so that when these same cells are later exposed to promoting agents such as more radiation or drugs, cancer will occur.[43] The amount of exposure the patient receives from a series of radiographs taken for diagnostic purposes depends on the machine used and the technical skill involved. Usually, the fluoroscopic examination entails more exposure than the use of radiography. The exposure of the average nurse working in a hospital and occasionally assisting a patient while a radiograph is taken is almost negligible.

Systemic reactions to excessive radiation exposure are leukopenia, leukemia, bone cancer, and sterility or damage to the reproductive cells. Because of the increased risk, badges are worn by persons whose daily work exposes them to radiation. The badge, which contains photographic film capable of absorbing radiation, is developed each month. A darkening or blackening of the film indicates excessive exposure. Personnel who are becoming overexposed are removed, at least temporarily, from direct contact with radiation.

Because of the danger to the fetus, particularly between the second and sixth weeks of life, radiographs are seldom taken of pregnant women. If radiographs must be taken, the lower portion of the abdomen is carefully protected. Also, pregnant women usually are not employed in radiology departments or in caring for patients receiving radioactive materials internally.

### Effects of the sun

Our society at times seems sun-addicted, and a tanned skin is eagerly sought by many. The carcinogenic effect of sunlight, although not completely understood, appears to be related to ultraviolet B (UVB) radiation. There is speculation that depletion of the ozone may be a factor in the rising rates of skin cancer.[30] The answer will come from research efforts now under way.

Skin cancer occurs mostly in persons who work in the open air, such as sailors, construction workers, and farmers, and on areas of the body most exposed to sunlight. Light-complexioned individuals are the most cancer-susceptible.

### Radon and electromagnetic field effects

Radon exposure in the environment is an increasing concern as a cause of cancer. Radon is an inert gas that emanates from the ground and stone building materials. It results from the decay of uranium, taking the form of radon gas and alpha particles. When the particles are inhaled into the respiratory tract, the resultant alpha irradiation to the bronchial epithelium can result in lung cancer. The radon gas is not as much of a factor in cancer development as the alpha particles. The first known association of radon exposure and lung cancer was found among uranium miners. Coal miners, not exposed to the same high levels of radon radioactivity, do not have increased rates of lung cancer.[41]

Whether the same potential risks apply to the general population through indoor exposure remains unknown, but the possibility is a concern. The leakage of radon is irregular and depends on the condition of both the building structure and the ground beneath. It is believed that the use of central heating and improvements made in building insulation now allow high concentrations of radon to remain indoors instead of escaping into the environment. Studies conducted in many parts of the world indicate that lung cancer risk is increased with exposure to elevated indoor radon levels.[41] A well-ventilated indoor environment is a necessary first step in the elimination of radon risk. Radon detection kits are available to test home levels. It is recommended that detectors be used in several areas of a building, such as in the basement and on each floor level. Studies have shown that radon concentrations are about two to five times less on the first floor than those found in the basement. Measuring several areas will provide a more reliable *average level* to which occupants are exposed. However, because radon levels vary from season to season and room to room, screening indicates only the potential for radon problems. Users of these detection kits should seek professional assistance in interpreting results.[22]

The effects of exposure to persons living or working near electromagnetic fields (EMFs) is another recent environmental concern that requires more study. Exposure to EMFs can come from household appliances, from electrical wiring found in the home, and even from living near electrical power lines and electricity-generating facilities. Electrical transmission lines generate both electric and magnetic fields. The intensity of the EMF is in proportion to the electrical energy running through the lines. The nearer one is to the source (within 20 meters), the greater will be the exposure. Whether EMFs are carcinogenic remains unclear, but a weak association in leukemia incidence has been shown in children who live near high-voltage electric transmission lines. Electronic engineers and power line workers also may have a greater leukemia risk as a result of their occupation.[41] In addition, the use of cellular telephones is being studied as a source (and thus a risk) of EMF exposure. At present no one can predict what the long-term effects of EMF exposure will be or what rate of exposure is detrimental. Until a definitive answer is found, the public should be made aware of the potential risks related to occupation and location of residence.

#### Air pollution

The long-range consequences of air pollution and cancer causation are not now completely understood. Two areas of greatest concern are the depletion of the ozone layer as a result of increasing levels of pollutants from heavy industry and the presence of gases such as carbon dioxide, nitrous oxide, methane, and chlorofluorocarbons that are known to produce "acid rain." The carcinogenic effects are most clearly associated with an increased risk of lung or skin cancers inasmuch as they are inhaled or have direct contact with exposed skin. At this time, however, the multitude of pollutants present in the air we breathe and the complexity of possible interactions make it difficult to identify other organ systems that might be at risk for cancer after exposure.

#### Chemical pollutants

Exposure to chemicals has been blamed for the rising incidence of cancer in the twentieth century. Polycyclic hydrocarbons, for example, have been recognized as carcinogenic (Box 16-2).

Many nitrosamines cause a variety of cancers in different species. Nitrates are commonly used as food additives, whereas nicotine may be a source of amines. A liver carcinogen, aflatoxin 13, has been isolated from a common mold that grows on peanuts, soybeans, fruit, some meats, and mild and cheddar cheese.

Cyclamates previously used as a sugar substitute have been banned because they may be potentially carcinogenic. Saccharin also has been identified as being carcinogenic in a study of rats, and the Food and Drug Administration (FDA) has recommended that it not be used as an artificial sweetener. Some hair dyes have been implicated in certain cases of cancer.

It is argued that some degree of carcinogenic risk is acceptable; others say that no level is acceptable and that all risks must be eliminated from the environment—no matter what the cost. Most agree that some level of regulation is necessary, but the mechanisms and standards for these regulations have not been delineated. Agencies such as the Environmental Protection Agency, Occupational Safety and Health Association (OSHA), and trade unions are aware of the health risks and together have begun formulating guidelines for prevention and protection of workers and the general public.

### Life-Style Practices

#### Smoking and tobacco use

Cigarette smoking is linked to the increased incidence of lung cancer. More reports are appearing that incriminate moderate and heavy cigarette smoking as a predisposing factor in the development of lung cancer. In 1993 lung cancer killed approximately 170,000 persons in the United States. In addition, 2.6 million persons will die each year worldwide as a result of smoking.[1] Although the rate of lung cancer in men has been alarming, studies have noted a proportionately greater rise in the rate of lung cancer in women. The rise appears to parallel an increase in recent years of women smokers, particularly young girls.

It also has been demonstrated that a correlation exists between cancer mortality and the number of cigarettes smoked daily, the number of years a person has smoked, and the age at which he or she began to smoke cigarettes. Smokers of two or more packs a day have a lung cancer mortality rate 15 to 25 times greater than that of a nonsmoker. Smoking also has been connected with esophageal cancer and possibly bladder cancer.[1] If smoking is discontinued even after a habit of 30 years, the incidence of lung cancer decreases.

Many smokers have changed to filtered cigarettes, pipe smoking, or the use of smokeless tobacco (plug, leaf, snuff) in the misguided belief that their cancer risk will be lessened or eliminated. Evidence is abundant that there is no "safe" cigarette and that smokeless tobacco is equally unsafe because it places the user at a high risk for head and neck cancers.

The carcinogenic effects of tobacco smoke released into the environment—environmental tobacco smoke (ETS)—have been thoroughly investigated. Results show that ETS contains most of the same carcinogenic compounds that have been identified in mainstream

**BOX 16-2 Chemical Carcinogenic Agents**

Polycyclic aromatic hydrocarbons (tar, pitch): skin cancer
Arsenic: skin cancer
Aromatic amines: bladder cancer
Chromium compounds: skin cancer
Asbestos: respiratory and lung cancer
Benzene inhalation: leukemia
Nitrosamines (food additives, nicotine)
Chloromethyl methyl ether and vinyl chloride (polyvinyl plastics)
Some hair dyes

smoke.[2] Consequently nonsmokers inhaling the ambient air near a cigarette smoker are exposed to the same carcinogens as the smoker and increase their risk for lung cancer, cardiovascular disease, and other respiratory conditions. The American Academy of Pediatrics estimates that 9 million children younger than the age of 5 years are exposed to the effects of ETS. As a result, these children have an increased frequency of respiratory infections and other respiratory ailments.[1]

Since January 2, 1971, no cigarette advertising has been permitted on either television or radio. On the same date the warning on packages was changed from "Caution: cigarette smoking may be hazardous to your health" to either "Warning: the surgeon general has determined that cigarette smoking is dangerous to your health" or a more definitive statement asserting that smoking may cause cancer, heart disease, and emphysema. Although the campaign to convince people to stop smoking has been slow and arduous, changes have been noted in smoking patterns. Two thirds of the population are nonsmokers, and many have been active and in some instances successful in getting legislation passed to prevent smoking in public places such as on domestic flights and in public buildings. Now with the existence of solid scientific evidence of the effects of ETS on nonsmokers, the regulation and restriction of public smoking and the sale of tobacco products in places of public assembly can advance on both the local and national levels. Box 16-3 lists various strategies concerned persons can use to eradicate or at least limit smoking.

### Nutrition

Second to the elimination of hazards from tobacco use, the most significant life-style change to reduce cancer risk relates to dietary habits. Nutrition research has increased steadily over the past decade, and a variety of studies indicate a relationship between dietary components and the development of cancer. Some estimate that dietary modification might reduce stomach and colon cancer death rates by 90% and endometrial, gallbladder, pancreas, and breast cancer by 50%.[25]

Obesity, the usual outcome of overnutrition, has been suggested as a risk factor in several cancers. The relationship between diets high in fat and calories and the development of breast, colon, and prostate cancer has been widely studied. These cancers are more prevalent in developed countries such as the United States and European nations. These cancer risks may be related more to affluence and overnutrition than specifically to high fat consumption.[25] However, increasing evidence points to a relationship between ingestion of animal fat and an increase in colon cancer risk.[48] Studies suggest that a fatty diet enhances the body's ability to synthesize cholesterol and bile acid in the liver, thus increasing their metabolic levels in the colon. These metabolites then may act as promoters in the development of colon cancer. Data gathered by the National Health and Nutrition Examination Survey (NHANES) have not as yet demonstrated a definite link between high fat ingestion and breast cancer.[25] Postmenopausal women, however, are recognized as being at a greater risk of breast and endometrial cancers. Their vulnerability is the result of prolonged tissue exposure to high levels of estrogen, which is stored in body fat. Large-scale long-term studies of the effect of dietary fat on women are needed to determine the role fat plays in causing cancer.

Diets high in fiber content appear to offer protection against colon cancer. Fiber is believed to reduce cancer risk by diluting colon contents, thus limiting contact with any carcinogens present; by reducing the amount of carcinogens and promoters present, such as bacteria or bile salts; and by lowering fecal pH and mutagens.[25] Fruits, vegetables, and whole grain foods, which are sources of vitamins C and D, beta carotene, and selenium, appear to have a cancer-deterrent effect. These vitamins and minerals, known as *antioxidants,* assist in cellular repair of damage caused by *free radicals.* Free radicals damage the genetic make-up of the cell and thus its natural ability to resist cancer development.

Research continues to provide definitive information

**BOX 16-3 Methods to Control Smoking**

- Encourage young people not to start.
- Educate the public on the hazards of smoking, with the aim of getting the smoker to quit.
- Provide self-help materials.
- Work with the media.
- Recruit ex-smoker volunteers to provide one-to-one help for smokers trying to quit.
- Encourage industries, hospitals, and organizations to conduct their own stop-smoking programs.
- Make available Fresh Start, the American Cancer Society quit-smoking program.
- Support legislation to restrict smoking and the sale of tobacco products in public places.

**BOX 16-4 Nutritional Practices to Prevent Cancer**

- Maintain a desirable weight and adequate energy balance by eating moderately and avoiding obesity.
- Reduce fat consumption to less than 30% of total calories.
- Increase consumption of fruits, cruciferous vegetables (cabbage, broccoli, Brussels sprouts, cauliflower), whole grain cereals, breads, and pasta.
- Limit or eliminate the consumption of alcohol.

Modified from American Cancer Society: *1993 Cancer facts and figures,* New York, 1993, The Society; Benito E, Giacosa A: *Public education on diet and cancer,* Dordrecht, Netherlands, 1991, Kluwer.

about the role of diet in cancer risk and cancer prevention. It is important to recognize that nutrition research studies are difficult to plan, implement, and interpret. Results rely heavily on self-report from questionnaires or complex diet diaries and are fraught with problems of participant noncompliance. Adhering to a prescribed diet involves many changes not often anticipated, such as the need for new patterns of meal planning, food purchasing, and preparation, as well as lengthy commitments of time. Substitutions of one dietary component for one that is not under study can compromise results. The substitution may even present an increase in another dietary risk factor.[31] As a result of nutrition research, dietary recommendations have been established that may reduce or prevent cancer[1] (Box 16-4).

A significant association exists between high alcohol intake and cancer of the mouth, pharynx, larynx, and esophagus. Heavy beer consumption has been linked to an increase in colon and bladder cancers.[26] However, alcoholism often is associated with smoking and with vitamin and dietary deficiencies, whose etiologic roles in cancer development are not fully known. It is speculated that alcohol consumption and nutritional deficiencies enhance carcinogenesis by increasing the metabolic activities of specific tobacco carcinogens. Tumors of the involved sites occur with greater frequency in men, blacks, lower socioeconomic groups, increasingly urbanized societies, and elderly persons.

**Sexual practices**

Carcinoma of the uterine cervix is less common in virgins than in married women. The incidence is higher in those who have first coitus at an early age, who have an early first marriage, and who have had multiple sex partners. Teen-age women are said to be at greater risk for cervical dysplasia, a precursor stage in the development of cancer of the squamocolumnar junction. The use of barrier contraceptives and more frequent Papanicolaou (Pap) testing should be advocated to reduce the risk.

Carcinoma of the penis is virtually unknown among circumcised men. The means by which circumcision provides protection is not clear, but it is probably related to better hygiene. It is no longer believed that coitus with an uncircumcised partner places a woman at risk for cervical cancer.

The correlation between sexual activity and breast cancer is the reverse of that for the uterine cervix. Women in whom breast cancer develops tend to marry and become pregnant later in life. However, a woman's age at the birth of a first child is a relevant factor in the later development of breast cancer. Women who give birth to their first child before age 20 have only one-third the risk of women older than age 35 who deliver a first child. This fact should be used not to advise against pregnancy at an early age but to make an informed decision on when to begin a family.[42] (Box 16-5 summarizes cancer-related factors.)

**BOX 16-5 Summary of Factors Related to Cancer Causation**

- Genetic predisposition
- Hormonal effects
- Precancerous lesions
- Chronic irritation, trauma, or inflammation
- Immune system function
- Drug therapy
- Environmental factors:
  - Ionizing radiation
  - Sun exposure
  - Radon and electromagnetic field effects
  - Chemical pollutants
  - Air pollution
- Life-style practices:
  - Smoking and tobacco use
  - Nutrition
  - Alcohol consumption
  - Sexual practices
- Viruses
- Psychosocial factors:
  - Personality traits and attitudes
  - Social support system

## Viruses

Studies in animals have established a viral role in carcinogenesis, but proof that human beings are affected has not been definitely ascertained. Viruses have been isolated and identified as the cause of cancer in mice, rabbits, and frogs.

Cervical cancer may result from a virus introduced into the cervix during sexual intercourse. This virus may be a member of the herpes group, Herpesvirus hominis (HV-II), and is more frequently found in women with dyplasia of the uterine cervix.

Herpes-like viruses have been visualized by use of electron microscopy in Burkitt's tumor and Hodgkin's disease cells. Investigators, however, have been unable to demonstrate human oncogenic viruses from human tumors. This may be a technical problem inasmuch as the ideal laboratory conditions for the isolation of tumor viruses have not been found. In addition, the long latency period in humans makes study of viruses difficult.

## Psychosocial Factors

Stressors such as life changes, loss of a significant other, and personality variables have been suggested as etiologic factors in the development of cancer. A "cancer-prone" personality also has been suggested, but considerable research is needed to determine if there is such a personality. Some researchers believe that even if such a personality is identified, there is little possibility of practical application of the information because it is extremely difficult to change behavior.

The role of "psychologic" treatments in "curing" cancer has as yet had little investigation. Information about the relationship of a positive attitude to the outcome of cancer is sparse, one study finding no relationship between the two factors. Little is known, also, about the effect of states of mind on the immune or hormonal systems that may affect the disease. Some evidence suggests that psychosocial variables can affect the immune response. For example, the activity of natural killer (NK) cells may be altered and in some manner influence cancer development. Further studies in psychoneuroimmunology may yet reveal the mechanism for these complex interactions.[6]

Social support in the form of institutions, family, and friends also may be an important variable. The person with minimal social support and maximal need may be at a higher risk for developing cancer. In addition, lack of social support may adversely affect coping responses to therapy and to the illness. At present, however, how one defines the nature of social support and the degree to which it is present or lacking are unclear.

## EPIDEMIOLOGY

The study of epidemiology is essential to identify patterns of cancer occurrence that help determine research, treatment, and financial priorities in cancer care. Cancer affects human beings wherever they live and whatever their race, color, cultural background, or economic status.

Cancer ranks second to heart disease as the cause of death in the United States, but significant progress has been made in prevention and treatment. Success can be attibuted to (1) the diagnosis of more cancers in the early localized stage, (2) the treatment of more patients within 4 months of diagnosis, and (3) the development of new diagnostic and treatment modalities, especially chemotherapy.

Despite these advances, 526,000 persons died of cancer in 1993. According to 1993 population figures it was estimated that approximately 85 million Americans, or one in three persons now alive, will have cancer in their lifetime. These statistics, however, reflect the growing number of persons who have survived other diseases and who are "available" or at risk for the development of cancer. More than 8 million Americans are alive today who have a diagnosis of cancer, and, of those, 5 million are considered cured of their disease. "Cure" refers to those persons who have no evidence of active disease and have a life expectancy comparable to that of a person who has never had cancer. Although in general cancer reflects no distinctions on the basis of economic or social status, there are some variables with regard to gender, site, age, race, and geographic location.

### GENDER AND SITE

The chance for developing cancer is greater in males than in females. White males now show the highest probability at birth of eventually developing cancer. By site, the highest probabilities are for the development of lung, skin, and prostate cancers in males. Women, on the other hand, are at risk for breast, colorectal, and lung cancer. In both groups the largest increases are seen for lung cancer and cancer of the colon-rectum (Table 16-3).

Overall survival rates for some cancers have increased, such as those for cervical cancer, whereas rates for most other cancers have leveled off in the past 30 years. Increases in survival have occurred for cancers of the prostate gland, uterine corpus, thyroid gland, kidney, bladder, and larynx and for melanoma of the skin, Hodgkin's disease, and chronic leukemia. The survival rates for lung cancer have improved only slightly over a 10-year period; only 13% of these patients live 5 or more years after diagnosis.[1]

The average cancer mortality in developed countries is higher for men than for women. During the past 40 years a decrease in mortality from cancer among American women is a result of a sharp reduction in the number of deaths caused by uterine cancer. It is revealing to note that while the incidence of lung cancer has decreased in men, there has been a corresponding increased incidence in women. In 1987 lung cancer surpassed breast cancer as the number one killer of women. This appears to be related in part to increased cigarette smoking by American women.[1]

The death rate from cancer involving the female genital tract has dropped from between one-third to one-half the rate of 25 years ago. There is ample evidence that the increased use of the Pap test to detect lesions of the cervix before symptoms develop has resulted in early treatment and a higher rate of cure. Figure 16-3 compares cancer incidence and deaths in 1993 by site and gender.

### AGE

Cancer has been called a disease of aging. Some researchers believe that if people live long enough, they will eventually develop cancer. Although cancer is the leading cause of death in women 35 to 74 years of age, the three most prevalent malignancies (lung, breast, colorectal) peak between ages 55 and 74 years. In men, this same age span, 55 to 74 years, reflects the years in which the most deaths occur from lung, colorectal, and prostate cancer.

Today the average life expectancy for women is 78.9 years and for men it is 72 years. The elderly population has been growing and now comprises about 12% of the population in the United States. In fact, those aged 80 and older constitute the fastest-growing age-group in our society at present. If predictions hold true, the greatest rise will occur among Hispanics and Asian-Americans.

**TABLE 16-3 Reference Chart: Leading Cancer Sites, 1993***

| SITE | ESTIMATED NEW CASES 1993 | ESTIMATED DEATHS 1993 | WARNING SIGNALS (IF YOU HAVE ONE, SEE YOUR DOCTOR) | SAFEGUARDS | COMMENT |
|---|---|---|---|---|---|
| Breast | 184,000 | 46,300 | Lump or thickening in breast or unusual discharge from nipple | Regular checkup, monthly breast self-examination, mammograms | Second leading cause of cancer death in women |
| Colon and rectum | 152,000 | 57,000 | Change in bowel habits, bleeding | Regular checkup including digital examination, stool blood test, proctoscopy, especially for those over 50 | Considered a highly curable disease when digital and proctoscopic examinations are included in routine checkups |
| Lung | 170,000 | 149,000 | Persistent cough or lingering respiratory ailment | 80% of lung cancers would be prevented if no one smoked cigarettes | Leading cause of cancer death among men and women |
| Oral (including pharynx) | 29,800 | 7700 | Sore that does not heal, difficulty in swallowing, lump or thickening | Regular checkup | Many more lives should be saved because the mouth is easily accessible to visual examination by physicians and dentists |
| Skin | 32,000† | 6800 | Sore that does not heal or change in wart or mole | Regular checkup, avoidance of overexposure to sun | Skin cancer readily detected by observation and diagnosed by simple biopsy |
| Uterus | 44,500‡ | 10,000 | Bleeding outside normal menstrual period or after menopause, unusual vaginal discharge | Regular checkup including pelvic examination with Papanicolaou test | Uterine cancer mortality has declined 70% during the last 40 years with wider application of Papanicolaou test; postmenopausal women with abnormal bleeding should be checked |
| Kidney and bladder | 79,500 | 20,800 | Urinary difficulty, bleeding, in which case consult physician at once | Regular checkup with urinalysis | Protective measures for workers in high-risk industries are helping to eliminate one of the important causes of these cancers |
| Larynx | 12,600 | 3800 | Hoarseness, difficulty in swallowing | Regular checkup including laryngoscopy | Readily curable if caught early |
| Prostate gland | 165,000 | 35,000 | Urinary difficulty | Regular checkup including palpation | Occurs mainly in men over 60; disease can be detected by palpation at regular checkup |
| Stomach | 24,000 | 13,600 | Indigestion | Regular checkup | 63% decline in mortality in 25 years for reasons yet unknown |
| Leukemia | 29,300 | 18,600 | Leukemia is a cancer of blood-forming tissues and is characterized by the abnormal production of immature white blood cells. Acute lymphocytic leukemia strikes mainly children and is treated by drugs that can cure or extend life from a few months to many years. Chronic leukemia usually strikes after age 25 and progresses less rapidly. | | |
| Other blood and lymph tissue | 63,700 | 31,400 | These cancers arise in the lymph system and include Hodgkin's disease, non-Hodgkin's lymphoma, and multiple myeloma. Some patients with lymphatic cancers can lead normal lives for many years. Five-year survival rate for Hodgkin's disease is 77%. Prognosis for non-Hodgkin's lymphoma has improved over past 30 years from 31% to 51%. | | |

Modified from American Cancer Society: *1993 cancer facts and figures,* New York, 1993, The Society.

*All figures rounded to nearest 1000. Incidence estimates based on rates from NCI SEER Program (National Cancer Institute Surveillance, Epidemiology, and End Results), 1987-1989.

†Melanoma only.

‡Invasive cancer only.

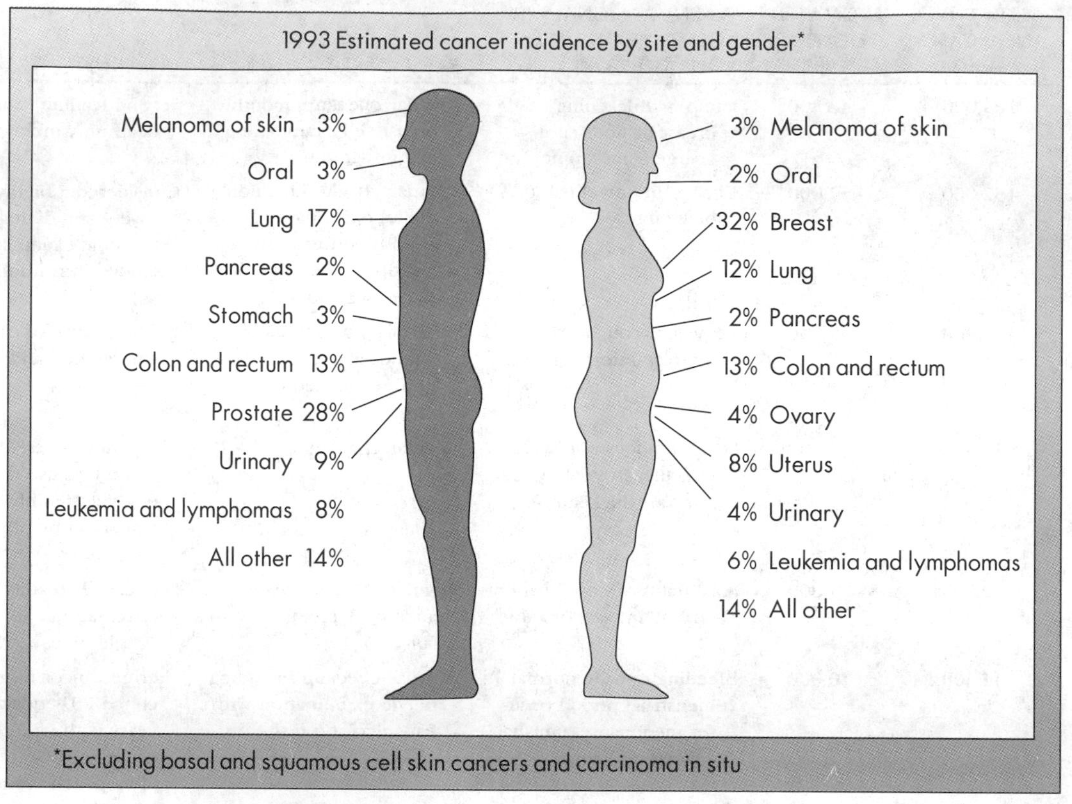


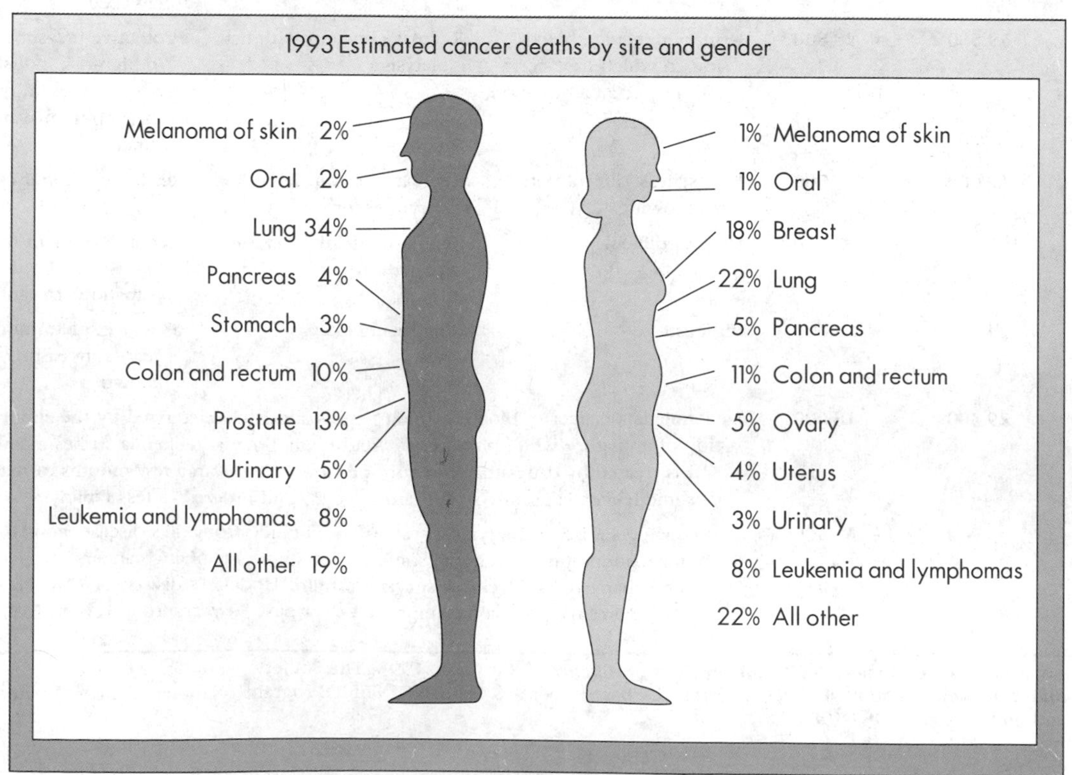


**FIGURE 16-3** Comparison of cancer incidence and deaths by site and gender (1993 estimates). (Modified from *CA* Jan/Feb, 1993.)

Thus the "graying of America" will have immense impact on our present health care system and health care policies. The elderly population now uses a disproportionate amount of health care resources, especially physician time, medications, and hospital admissions when compared with other age-groups. In addition, other problems confront this ever-growing segment of our population. Access to health care for many elders is influenced by several factors: financial considerations (fixed income, underinsured); transportation (inability to travel to health care facilities); cultural/ethnic/religious practices (lifelong practices not part of mainstream medical care); and language barriers (e.g., among Hispanics and Asians). These factors may account for why elderly persons typically are diagnosed with advanced disease and why they do not participate in disease-prevention programs to the same degree as those younger in age. In addition, elders tend to have more chronic disease states, with signs and symptoms that can mask malignant conditions, thus preventing early detection and treatment while the cancer is still in a localized stage. The ability of elders to withstand the rigors of cancer treatment is further compromised by the deterioration of the immune system with increasing age. Thus it can be readily seen that this group has unique and challenging problems in relation to cancer development and cancer care.

### RACE

The rates of cancer incidence and death for both males and females are higher for African-Americans than for whites. The overall incidence and mortality rates for the former group are significantly higher in cancers of the lung, stomach, liver, uterine cervix, larynx, prostate, and esophagus. The 5-year survival rate for African-Americans diagnosed with cancer is only 38% compared with 54% for whites.[1]

Hispanic-Americans have lower incidence and mortality rates for cancer than do either black or white Americans. A survey for the American Cancer Society showed that Hispanic-Americans are not adequately aware of cancer warning signals and of ways to reduce cancer risk and they tend not to seek early detection or treatment.[1]

Cancer survival and sometimes even incidence also are related to socioeconomic factors such as poverty. The primary aspects of poverty that are known to affect the early detection, treatment, and survival for cancer are underemployment, inadequate education, substandard housing, chronic malnutrition, and the lack of access to medical care.[18]

### GEOGRAPHIC FACTORS

Differences in the geographic distribution of cancer occur. For example, primary cancer of the liver is common in Indonesia and parts of Africa and Asia but rare in other regions. Cancer of the breast is more common in the United States and Western Europe than it is in Japan. Ugandans, Nigerians, and South African blacks are at lowest risk for cancer of the lung, stomach, large intestine, uterus, and kidney. Genetic differences among populations may contribute to international variations but are not likely to be the only reason because migration from one country to another results in major changes in the cancer pattern.

### FACTORS AFFECTING PROGNOSIS

Trends are being evaluated to determine why the incidence of certain cancers has decreased, increased, or remained the same. There is reason to believe that the cure rate and the prognosis of cancer would improve substantially with earlier recognition and more complete reporting of early signs. Patients delay on average 3 months before seeking diagnosis for symptoms suggestive of cancer, thus reducing the chance of cure and long-term survival. Delay is related to the patient's perception of (1) the chance of having cancer, (2) the possibility of early detection and treatment, (3) the inconvenience of examination, (4) the need for relief of symptoms, and (5) the need for reassurance.

Success in treating many cancers awaits better and more sensitive diagnostic aids to detect lesions in their early stages. In some parts of the body, such as the skin and cervix, early recognition and prompt treatment often result in cure.

The prognosis also is affected by the intrinsic characteristics of the tumor, such as histologic type and grade, size, and rate of growth. Another important factor is age and general condition of the patient. The presence of debilitating conditions, such as infection, diabetes mellitus, or malnutrition, may adversely affect the outcome.

## PHYSIOLOGY

Basic to the understanding of cancer, its development, and subsequent treatment is a knowledge of normal cell kinetics. Much of what is now known about cancer cells is the result of research studies in which normal cells were transformed into malignant cells in a controlled laboratory setting. Cell transformation is recognized as a multistep process originating from a single proliferating cell. The transformed cell then has alterations in its ability to differentiate and proliferate normally.

### NORMAL CELLULAR PROLIFERATION

#### Characteristics of Normal Cells

Normal tissue contains large numbers of mature cells of uniform size and shape, each containing a nucleus of uniform size. Within each nucleus are the chromosomes, a specific number for the species, and within each chromosome is *deoxyribonucleic acid* (DNA). DNA is a giant molecule whose chemical composition controls the characteristics of *ribonucleic acid* (RNA), which is found in the nucleoli of cells and in the cytoplasm of the cell itself and which regulates cell growth and function. When ovum and sperm unite, the DNA and RNA within the chromosomes of each will govern the differentiation and future course of the trillions of cells that finally develop to form the adult organism. In the development of various organs and parts of the body, cells undergo differentiation in size, appearance, and arrangement; thus the histologist or the pathologist can look at a piece of prepared tissue through a microscope and know the portion of the body from which it came.

### Mitosis

Mitosis refers to the splitting of one cell into two cells. In the normal cell, multiplication takes place by an orderly process in response to a need such as trauma, surgery, or an inflammatory event. Once the need is met, cell multiplication stops. Normal cells recognize the presence of other cells near them by means of the process of *contact inhibition* through receptors located on the surface of the cell membrane. When cells are in close contact with other cells, they normally adhere closely together. This contact is responsible for inhibiting overlap of cells and disorganized growth. With normal cells these restraints on growth are controlled until the next need arises because of cell deaths. Some cell turnover rates are rapid, as occurs in the bone marrow, skin, and gastrointestinal tract. The need for cell replacement in these areas is greater than in slower-growing tissue.

### Cell Cycle Time

The concept of cell cycle time is pertinent to understanding normal cell replication and has implications for drug use in cancer therapy. Cell cycle time may be described as the interval from mitosis of a cell to its mitosis into daughter cells. Initially there is a stationary period ($G_O$) of apparent rest after mitosis takes place. The cells are not in the cycle but are viable and capable of undergoing mitosis if necessary. The cell cycle is divided into four phases (Figure 16-4): (1) a quiescent phase consisting of $G_1$ (G denotes a gap) in which RNA and protein synthesis begins; (2) $S_1$, a period of DNA synthesis; (3) $G_2$, further RNA and protein synthesis and the development of the mitotic spindle; and (4) mitosis (M).

## NORMAL ALTERATIONS IN CELL GROWTH

Some abnormal changes in cell growth are malignant growths (neoplasms). Other types of cellular growths are benign. **Hyperplasia** is an increase in cell number, whereas *hypertrophy* is an increase in cell size but not in number. Although many neoplasms are characterized by hyperplasia, many normal tissues also may undergo an increase in cell number. Wound healing, callus formation, and growth in embryonic tissue are all normal forms of hyperplasia.

**Metaplasia** is a reversible process in which one adult cell type in an organ is replaced by another adult cell type. The new cell type usually is not one normally seen in the area in which metaplasia occurs. The most common type of epithelial metaplasia is the change of columnar or pseudostratified columnar epithelium of the respiratory tract to squamous epithelium or squamous metaplasia. **Dysplasia** is an alteration in adult cells characterized by changes in their size, shape, and organization (Table 16-4).

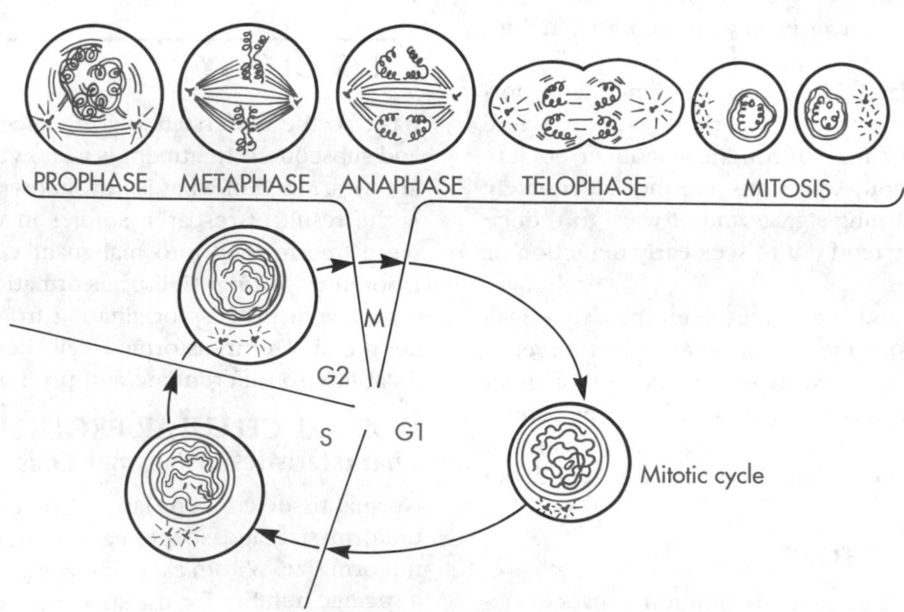


**FIGURE 16-4** Cell cycle. *G1,* RNA/protein synthesis, *S,* DNA synthesis; *G2,* RNA/protein synthesis and interphase; and *M,* mitosis. (Modified from Krakoff I: *Cancer chemotherapeutic agents* [American Cancer Society professional education publication], New York, 1977, American Cancer Society.)

## NORMAL CELL DIFFERENTIATION

All body tissue is derived from **stem cells,** which are immature cells with no specific cell lineage. These cells have the ability to proliferate rapidly to renew themselves as needed and to develop specialized functions as they grow and mature. The process, known as **cellular differentiation,** refers to the extent to which the cells resemble their normal forebears and thus have fully mature, specialized function and morphology. For example, all kidney cells are similar but are different from muscle cells, and each type has its specialized function. In malignant cells, changes in differentiation take place.

The method by which differentiation takes place is unknown. One current thought is that all cells carry the same genetic material but that selective repression of different genetic characteristics occurs because of buildup of different repressor substances in the cytoplasm. Different cells repress different genetic characteristics. Regardless of the process, cell differentiation, once begun, proceeds along a path toward specialized function and tissue line that cannot then revert to a previous immature state. Figure 16-5 shows the normal cellular differentiation process.

# PATHOPHYSIOLOGY

## CLASSIFYING AND NAMING NEOPLASMS

Tumors derive their names from the types of tissue involved (Table 16-5), but classification of malignant tumors is difficult because many contain several types of

**TABLE 16-4 Terms Denoting Cellular Changes**

| TYPE OF CELLULAR CHANGE | DEFINITION | EXAMPLE |
|---|---|---|
| Mitosis | Formation of new cell by cell division | Normal cell growth |
| Hyperplasia | Increase in cell number | Breast epithelium in pregnancy |
| Hypertrophy | Increase in cell size | Increase in muscle cell size with exercise |
| Atrophy | Decrease in cell size | Decrease in muscle cell size with disuse |
| Metaplasia | Replacement of one adult cell type by a different adult cell type | Replacement of columnar epithelium of respiratory tract by squamous epithelium |
| Dysplasia | Changes in cell size, shape, and organization | Changes in cervical epithelium in long-standing cervicitis |
| Anaplasia | Reverse cellular development to a more primitive cell type | Irreversible change accompanying cancer |
| Neoplasia | Abnormal cellular changes and growth of new tissues | Malignancies |

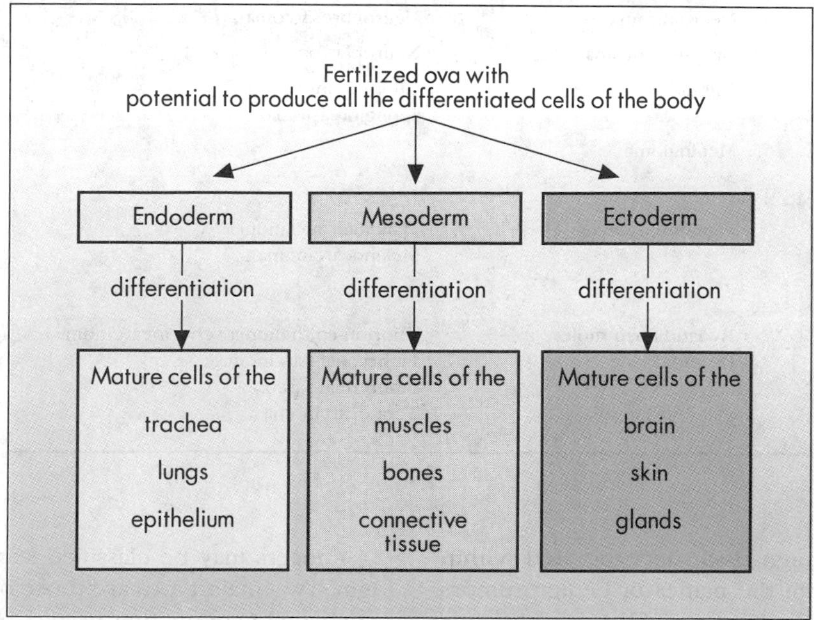


**FIGURE 16-5** Normal cellular differentiation. (From Lewis SM, Collier IC: *Medical-surgical nursing: assessment and management of clinical problems,* ed 3, St Louis, 1992, Mosby.)

**TABLE 16-5 Classification of Neoplasms**

| PARENT TISSUE | BENIGN TUMOR | MALIGNANT TUMOR |
|---|---|---|
| **EPITHELIUM** | | |
| Skin and mucous membrane | Papilloma<br>Polyp | Squamous cell carcinoma<br>Basal cell carcinoma<br>Transitional cell carcinoma |
| Glands | Adenoma<br>Cystadenoma | Adenocarcinoma |
| **ENDOTHELIUM** | | |
| Blood vessels | Hemangioma | Hemangiosarcoma<br>Angiosarcoma |
| Lymph vessels | Lymphangioma | Lymphangiosarcoma |
| Bone marrow | | Multiple myeloma<br>Ewing's sarcoma<br>Leukemia<br>Lymphosarcoma<br>Lymphangioendothelioma |
| Lymphoid tissue | | Reticular cell sarcoma (difficult to classify because of cell embryology)<br>Lymphatic leukemia<br>Malignant lymphoma |
| **CONNECTIVE TISSUE** | | |
| Embryonic fibrous tissue | Myxoma | Myxosarcoma |
| Fibrous tissue | Fibroma | Fibrosarcoma |
| Adipose tissue | Lipoma | Liposarcoma |
| Cartilage | Chondroma | Chondrosarcoma |
| Bone | Osteoma | Osteogenic sarcoma |
| Synovial membrane | Synovioma | Synovial sarcoma |
| **MUSCLE TISSUE** | | |
| Smooth muscle | Leiomyoma | Leiomyosarcoma |
| Striated muscle | Rhabdomyoma | Rhabdomyosarcoma |
| **NERVE TISSUE** | | |
| Nerve fibers and sheaths | Neuroma<br>Neurinoma (neurilemoma)<br>Neurofibroma | Neurogenic sarcoma<br><br>Neurofibrosarcoma |
| Ganglion cells | Ganglioneuroma | Neuroblastoma |
| Glial cells | Glioma | Glioblastoma<br>Spongioblastoma |
| Meninges | Meningioma | |
| **PIGMENTED NEOPLASMS** | | |
| Melanoblasts | Pigmented nevus | Malignant melanoma<br>Melanocarcinoma |
| **MISCELLANEOUS** | | |
| Placenta | Hydatidiform mole<br>Dermoid cyst | Chorion-epithelioma (choriocarcinoma)<br>Embryonal carcinoma<br>Embryonal sarcoma<br>Teratocarcinoma |

cells and may have benign tissue incorporated within them as well. In general, the names of benign tumors carry the suffix *-oma* after the name of the parent tissue, for example, neuroma or fibroma; there are some exceptions.

Cancers may be classified according to cell type or origin. Two main types are those of epithelial and of mesenchymal (connective tissue) origin. The term **carcinoma** denotes a malignant tumor of epithelial cells, and the term **sarcoma** denotes a malignant tumor of con-

**BOX 16-6 Classification of Malignant Lesions By Grade and Stage**

| GRADE | STAGE |
|---|---|
| **Grade 0**<br>Normal tissue | **Stage 0**<br>Cancer in situ |
| **Grade 1**<br>Well-differentiated, with minimal deviation from tissue of origin | **Stage I**<br>Tumor limited to tissue of origin |
| **Grade 2**<br>Moderately well-differentiated, with evidence of structural changes from normal tissue of origin | **Stage II**<br>Limited local spread |
| **Grade 3**<br>Poorly differentiated, with extensive structural changes from normal tissue of origin | **Stage III**<br>Extensive local and regional spread |
| **Grade 4**<br>Very anaplastic, with no resemblance to tissue of origin | **Stage IV**<br>Widespread metastasis |

**BOX 16-7 TNM Staging Classification System**

| | |
|---|---|
| **TUMOR** | |
| T0 | No evidence of primary tumor |
| TIS | Carcinoma in situ |
| T1, T2, T3, T4 | Ascending degrees of tumor size and involvement |
| **NODES** | |
| N0 | No evidence of disease in lymph nodes |
| N1a, N2a | Disease found in regional lymph nodes, metastasis not suspected |
| N1b, N2b, N3 | Disease found in regional lymph nodes; metastasis suspected |
| Nx | Regional nodes cannot be assessed clinically |
| **METASTASIS** | |
| M0 | No evidence of distant metastasis |
| M1, M2, M3 | Ascending degrees of metastatic involvement of the host, including distant nodes |

nective tissue cells. When a malignant tumor contains all three types of embryonal tissue, it is called a **teratoma.**

Tumors also are classified according to cellular maturity. When there is complete loss of identity with the tissue of origin, the tumor is called *undifferentiated* (anaplastic). Some tumors are known by the names of the scientists who first described them, for example, Hodgkin's disease and Wilms' tumor. Other tumors are named after the organ from which they arise, for example, hepatoma and thymoma.

## METHODS OF CLASSIFYING DEGREE OF MALIGNANCY

The degree of malignancy (grade) is based on the microscopic examination of the lesion. Tumors are graded by arabic numerals into four grades; the higher the grade, the worse the prognosis. A grade 1 tumor is the most differentiated (most like the tissue of origin) and therefore the least malignant, whereas grade 4 is the least differentiated (unlike the tissue of origin) and has a high degree of malignancy.

**Staging** is a form of classification describing the gross extent of the tumor and its spread (metastasis) rather than by histologic criteria (appearance). These classifications are useful to the physician in knowing whether the tumor may be expected to respond to treatment (Box 16-6).

Determination of the extent of the spread of cancer (staging) and the site of the original tumor is vital for planning therapy. The International Union Against Cancer has devised the TNM system of classification: *T,* tumor; *N,* regional lymph nodes; *M,* metastases. TNM is a uniform system used worldwide for describing the anatomic extent of cancer spread.

Adding a number to the letters (e.g., T1, T2, N1, N2) indicates the extent of the malignancy (Box 16-7). This system provides a type of "shorthand" notation to describe the particular tumor. The purpose of the TNM system is to define categories for all cases and also to allow subsequent and more detailed information to be added. A TNM classification has been identified for major cancer sites. It is important for treatment, planning, end-results reporting, communication, and the conduct of clinical trials.

## TYPES OF NEOPLASMS

### Benign Tumors

Benign (nonmalignant) tumors involve cellular proliferation of adult or mature cells growing slowly in an orderly manner in a capsule. These tumors do not invade surrounding tissue but may cause harm through pressure on vital structures within an enclosed structure such as the skull. Benign tumors remain localized, do not metastasize (spread), and do not recur once they are completely removed (Table 16-6).

### Malignant Tumors

A malignant cell is one in which the basic structure and activity have become deranged in a manner not fully understood. It is believed, however, that the basic process involves a disturbance in the regulatory functions of DNA. It is known that the DNA molecule is affected by radiation in certain instances, and it is speculated that it may be affected by other factors as well.

**TABLE 16-6 Differences Between Benign and Malignant Neoplasms**

| BENIGN | MALIGNANT |
|---|---|
| Limited growth potential | May proliferate rapidly or grow slowly |
| Localized | Spreads (metastasizes) throughout the body |
| Fibrous capsule | No enclosing capsule |
| Rarely recurs after removal | May recur even after treatment |
| Usually regular in shape | Irregular shape with poorly defined border |
| Cells similar to cell of parent tissue (well differentiated) | Cells much different from parent cells (poorly differentiated) |
| Expansive growth | Infiltrative growth |

In the neoplastic cell, normal restraints on growth are defective. It is believed that malignant neoplasms occur as the result of faulty mechanisms inside the cell nucleus. DNA, the permanent genetic material in nuclear chromosomes, contains information necessary for cell replication: the chemical code for cell growth and development. To convey this information, RNA serves as a messenger. Any small change in DNA (mutation) causes a distortion of biologic information, which results in the affected cells running wild. Malignant neoplasm is the result. The malignant cells lose the specialized function of the normal cell or may take on new characteristics and functions.

A characteristic of malignant cells that can be observed through a microscope is a loss of differentiation or likeness to the original cell (parent tissue) from which the tumor growth originated. Cancer cells may vary in their likeness to the tissue of origin. They may be well differentiated (very similar to the tissue of origin), moderately well differentiated (somewhat similar to the tissue of origin), or poorly differentiated (little similarity to the tissue of origin). Generally the cancer with more poorly differentiated cells has a poor prognosis because of a higher degree of malignancy.

The loss of differentiation is called **anaplasia.** Anaplasia is seen only in cancers and does not appear in benign neoplasms. In many cancer cells the chromosomes that carry genes are abnormal. They may be broken apart, have pieces missing or flipped over, or be shuffled among chromosomes. The terms ***translocation*** or ***deletion*** are used to describe the alteration in position or the absence of parts of chromosomes.

Other characteristics of malignant cells that can be seen through a microscope are the presence of (1) nuclei of various sizes, many of which contain unusually large amounts of chromatin (hyperchromatic cells), and (2) mitotic figures (cells in the process of division), which denote rapid and disorderly division of cells. (See Table 16-6 for characteristics of malignant cells.)

Tumor cells show less contact inhibition in vitro and therefore "pile up" in cultures, suggesting that surface properties of cancer cells are different from normal cells (Figure 16-6). The proportion of cancer cells actively proliferating in malignant tumors varies from multiplying at a rate equal to normal cells to a very rapid and indiscriminate rate.

Malignant tumors have no enclosing capsules; thus they invade adjacent and surrounding tissue, including lymph and blood vessels, through which they may spread to distant parts of the body.

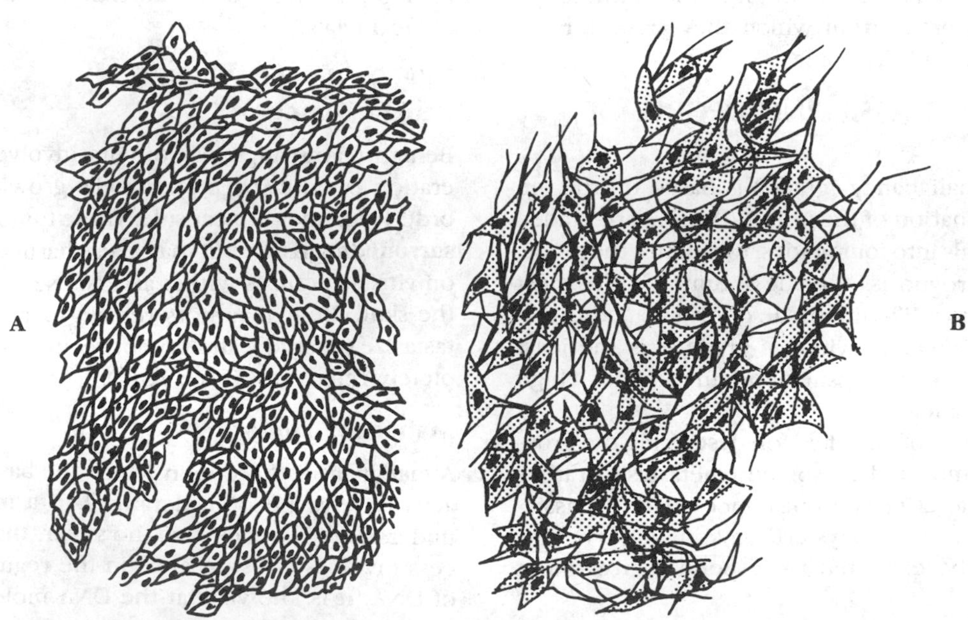


**FIGURE 16-6** **A,** Normal cell appearance. **B,** Abnormal cell appearance.

## CLINICAL MANIFESTATIONS OF CANCER

The clinical manifestations of cancer may be diverse and affect multiple systems, depending on the site and size of the tumor. Nurses need to be aware of these signs and symptoms to aid in early detection of cancer and to monitor the effects of therapy in relation to these manifestations.

Information obtained from the medical and nursing history will help to identify those persons with a familial tendency for cancer: a social history, marital and sex history, past medical history, and information about habits and occupation. These data may provide clues to identify the presence of cancer. Depending on the size and location of the tumor, many different signs and symptoms may be present.

### Local Effects

Benign tumors cause serious problems if they obstruct the lumen of tubular structures such as the ureter, trachea, or intestinal tract. Intraspinal and intracranial tumors cause problems because of the pressure they exert in a closed space. Tumors also may degenerate or by the pressure they exert cause atrophy and ulceration of overlying epithelium.

Malignant tumors may produce the same problems as benign tumors. In addition, because of their size and ability to infiltrate and destroy surrounding tissue, symptoms of obstruction, hemorrhage, ulceration, and secondary infection may be present.

### Systemic Effects

The term **paraneoplastic syndrome** is used to describe the systemic effects of cancer. These can be divided into the following categories: (1) hematologic, immunologic, and vascular abnormalities, (2) hormonal and endocrinologic effects, (3) neuromyopathies, (4) skin and connective tissue disorders, (5) gastrointestinal disorders, and (6) general and metabolic disorders. These effects do not occur in every patient but vary depending on the location and activity of the tumor (Table 16-7).

### Cachexia

**Cachexia** usually is a sign of advanced cancer. It was once thought to be the result of a progressive starvation of the patient. Although decreased food intake is a factor, it appears to be a complex derangement of the patient's metabolism. Clinical signs of cachexia are anorexia, early satiety, gradual or rapid weight loss, anemia, and asthenia (Table 16-8). In addition, other factors that may contribute to cachexia include immobilization, drugs, and reactive depression that often accompanies metastatic cancer. Along with this may be insomnia and a feeling of hopelessness, both of which contribute to anorexia and cachexia. There is an increased susceptibility to infection.

Therapy for the cachectic state is rarely successful unless the underlying cancer is treated. Glucose plus insulin, or androgens for males, may stimulate anabolism.

### Pain

It is estimated that as many as 75% of patients with cancer will experience pain sometime during their disease process. Pain is one of the most feared outcomes of the cancer event. The incidence and severity of the pain depends largely on the site of the cancer, the stage

**TABLE 16-7 Systemic Effects of Cancer**

| CATEGORY | PROBLEMS | CAUSE |
|---|---|---|
| Hematologic | Anemia, leukopenia, thrombocytopenia | Replacement of bone marrow by cancer cells |
| Immunologic | Infection | Deficiency of T and B cells |
| Vascular | Hemorrhage | Blood vessel erosion by tumor, disseminated intravascular coagulation (DIC) |
| Hormonal and endocrinologic | Syndromes such as Cushing's hyperthyroidism<br>Cachexia | Tumors of endocrine glands cause increased secretions; malignant lung tumors secrete trophic hormones<br>Hypermetabolism of tumors<br>Increased gluconeogenesis |
| Neuromuscular | Weakness, cerebellar disease, peripheral neuritis | Degenerative changes in CNS and peripheral nervous system |
| | Poor pulmonary respiration, stasis of secretions and pneumonia | Destruction of muscle protein, impaired cellular respiration, and failure of abdominal and intercostal muscles |
| | Urinary tract infection and constipation | Failure of smooth muscle in bladder and GI tract |
| Skin and connective tissue | Dermatomyositis | — |
| Gastrointestinal | Weakness, fatigue, weight loss | Malabsorption, chronic blood loss, impaired digestion |
| General disorders | Ascites<br>Pleural effusion | Metastatic implant in abdomen<br>Metastatic implant in pleural cavity |

**TABLE 16-8 Clinical Signs of Cachexia**

| SIGNS | CAUSE |
|---|---|
| Anorexia | Metabolites produced by cancer; food aversions caused by decreased taste and smell and by therapy |
| Early satiety and early filling | Cause unknown—patient is hungry but after a few bites feels full |
| Weight loss | Impaired digestion and absorption, hypermetabolism, negative nitrogen balance |
| Anemia | Decreased RBC production, increased RBC destruction or loss |
| Asthenia (marked feeling of muscle weakness, easily tired) | Biochemical alterations |

of the disease, and the presence and location of metastasis. The reaction to cancer pain depends on many factors, such as age, pain threshold, and experience with painful events. Cancer pain is discussed in more detail later in the chapter.

## Metastasis

**Metastasis** refers to the transplantation of tumor cells from one organ, or part, that is separated by distance from the original tumor location. Most deaths from cancer are the result of metastatic disease. A primary tumor or a metastatic site is defined by a lesion of approximately 1 cm in diameter, which contains a billion cells. The process of metastasis no longer is believed to be a random occurrence but a complex sequence of events. Even so, fewer than 0.01% of cancer cells survive the process to eventually establish a metastatic lesion.[16]

### Types of metastasis

Cancer spreads in several different ways (Figure 16-7). Cancer cells differ from normal cells in their unique ability to move without restraint into surrounding tissue. Tumor cells lack adhesiveness—the ability to stay in contact with other cells—so they can easily break away from the tumor mass of which they are a part and directly invade surrounding tissues. This is refered to as *local invasion.* Local spread involves infiltration into surrounding tissues and may involve hemorrhage, necrosis, ulceration, and fibrous replacement of the involved tissues. This produces the typical local effects of ulcerating, bulky, hemorrhagic masses or indurative, fibrosing lesions, with tissue fixation, distortion of the structure, and the dimpling of the skin that may be seen in some breast cancer. Infection may accompany this local infiltration. The cancer cells tend to spread along the path of least resistance—in tissue clefts, along blood vessels, or the perineural spaces. The fibrous capsule that covers some organs may limit growth. For example, primary tumors of the kidney, liver, or testes may increase the size of the organ without destroying the capsule. Local spread is not an orderly process but one that expands

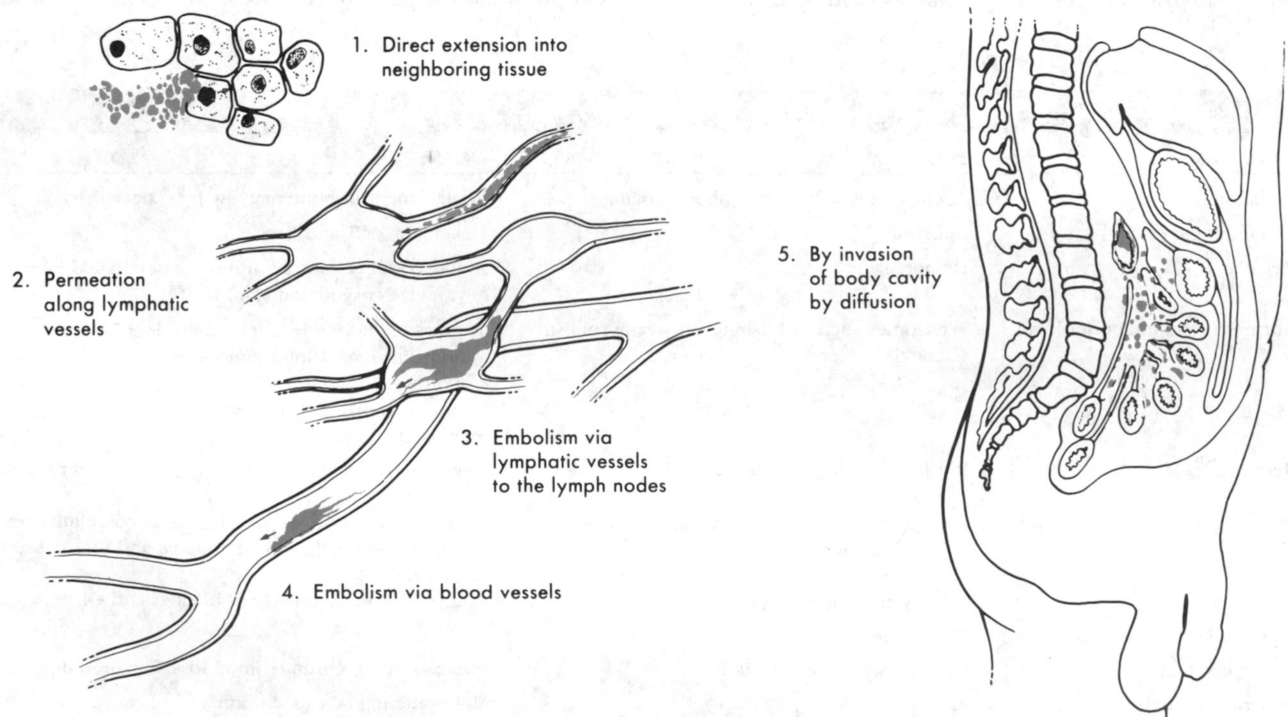


**FIGURE 16-7** Modes of dissemination of cancer.

unequally and haphazardly. Because of local spread, any cancer excision must include a margin of surrounding tissues to ensure removal of all malignant cells.

Cancer also spreads by *lymphatic permeation* and *embolization*. Once cells have invaded the lymph vessels, they then may detach and become emboli, which lodge in the lymph node, forming a metastatic lesion. Spread continues to the next group of nodes and into the other organs. The presence of cancer in the lymph nodes is certain evidence of spread, but even if lymph node metastasis does not occur, there still may be dissemination of malignant cells. The cell may pass through the lymph node without leaving a trace—to grow in other areas. This phenomenon is referred to as *skip metastasis*. Lymph nodes were once thought to be mechanical barriers completely separate from vascular dissemination of malignant disease. Research now demonstrates the presence of multiple lymphatic-venous interconnections throughout the body. Consequently, lymphatic and vascular dissemination takes place concurrently.[16] *Vascular* spread can result in more widely disseminated disease because of the ability of tumor cells to move freely through both the lymphatic and venous systems. Blood-borne cancer cells escape from the bloodstream by a process of attachment and invasion through endothelial cells lining the blood vessel (Figure 16-8).

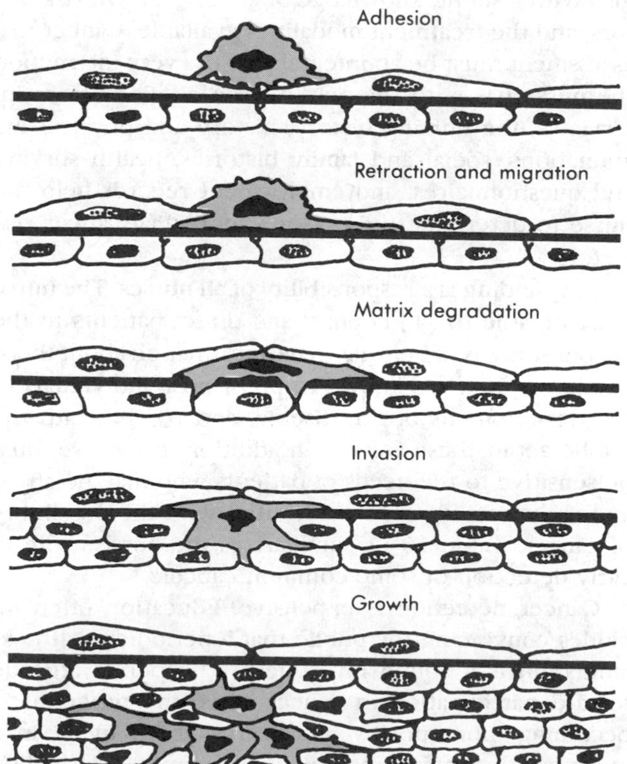


**FIGURE 16-8** Cancer cells exit from bloodstream. (Reprinted with permission from Rawls RL: In search of cancer control: understanding metastasis is crucial, *Chem Eng News* 63:11, 1985. Copyright © 1985 American Chemical Society.)

In *disseminative metastasis* (distant spread), there is almost always a high degree of histologic, cytologic, and functional similarity between the primary cancer and these metastases. Consequently, the type of cell and the probable site of the primary tumor can be identified from the morphologic features of the metastasis. In addition, metastases usually mimic the primary tumor in the formation of cell products and secretions.

Finally, cancer can spread by *diffusion*—the spread of clumps of cancer cells from the surface of the tumor by mechanical means. This type of spread is particularly prevalent in serous cavities such as the abdominal or the pleural cavity. In the peritoneal cavity, cells tend to gravitate to the pelvis. Cancer cells also can be implanted or "seeded" by the surgeon into the operative area, causing metastatic lesions. Metastasis may regress or disappear without apparent cause and may be dormant for many years, only to resume growth years later.

### Sites of metastases

The site of metastatic spread depends on the venous or lymphatic drainage of the organ involved, the type of cancer, and the tissue from which the cancer arises. Various body tissues seem to have different attraction for metastases, common sites being, in order, the liver, lungs, bone marrow, brain, and adrenal glands. Spleen, muscle, and skin rarely are involved. Table 16-9 shows organ distribution of metastases.

## PREVENTION

Nurses have a major responsibility in the prevention of cancer. Because of their knowledge about the disease and their contact with the public in inpatient and outpatient settings, in the home, and in various community activities, nurses have the opportunity and the obligation to teach about cancer and known risk factors.

A *risk factor* may be defined as something specific to an individual that increases his or her possibility of developing a malignancy. Risk factors must be identified and moderated. Three types of risk factors for cancer have been identified. *Life-style* factors are those over which the person has some control, especially tobacco use, diet, alcohol use, sunlight exposure, and sexual practices. *Environmental* factors include exposure to carcinogens and are at times beyond the individual's control. *Genetic* factors—conditions inherited at conception—are not usually controllable except through genetic counseling services. High-risk families, especially those at risk for breast, colorectal, and lung cancers, are being identified.

### PRIMARY PREVENTION

*Primary prevention* attempts to prevent a person's exposure to any known risk factor that might lead to disease. This is an insurmountable task in cancer prevention, inasmuch as all risk factors are not known or have

**TABLE 16-9 Organ Distribution of Metastases**

| TUMOR TYPE | METHOD OF DISSEMINATION | TARGET SITES |
|---|---|---|
| Sarcoma | Hematogenous via tumor venous drainage to pulmonary arteries | Lungs |
| Lung | Hematogenous and lymphatic direct access to arterial circulation from pulmonary vein | Liver, brain, lung, bone, nodes |
| Colorectal | Mesenteric lymphatics, lymphatic/hematogenous communications (thoracic duct) | Liver, intraperitoneal, lung |
| Prostate | Periprostatic venous plexus in communication with Batson's plexus of paravertebral veins | Bone |
| Testicular | Local lymphatic drainage, lymphatic/hematogenous communications to subclavian veins | Nodes, lung, brain |
| Head and neck | Local lymphatic drainage, lymphatic/hematogenous communications | Nodes, lung |
| Ovarian | Seeding to peritoneal surfaces, hematogenous and lymphatic communications | Intraperitoneal, liver, lung |
| Breast | Hematogenous and lymphatic mammary venous drainage communications with Batson's plexus | Nodes, lung, liver, bone, brain |

Kohn E, Liotta L. In Moosa AR: *Comprehensive textbook of oncology,* vol 1, ed 2, p. 136, Baltimore, 1991, Williams & Wilkins.

not been proved as factors in specific cancer development. There is, however, substantial evidence available that demonstrates a direct link between certain environmental and life-style factors and cancer development. Examples include smoking and lung cancer, excessive sun exposure and skin cancer, and low dietary fiber content and colon cancer. Nurses who have knowledge of these cancer risk factors must become more active in educating the public. This can be accomplished easily with the hospitalized patient or in the clinic setting where teaching and counseling are essential components of everyday practice. Participation in community health fairs where educational information and counseling are provided is an area in which all nurses can make meaningful contributions. Last, the nurse can act as a role model by not smoking, by using sun screen and not sunbathing to excess, by engaging in moderate exercise activities, and by eating a well-balanced diet.

## SECONDARY PREVENTION

*Secondary prevention* efforts are used mainly to prevent a fatal outcome when malignant tumors develop. Once the risk is known, definitive treatment is begun. For successful secondary prevention, there must be a stage in the natural history of the cancer when, if detected, it can be cured. In addition, there must be a means of detecting the cancer at an early stage. Nurses are more likely to be involved in secondary prevention efforts such as screening programs.

At present, early detection methods through health screening programs are not available for all cancers. The only screening tools that have enabled the detection of early asymptomatic cancers and are known to reduce cancer mortality are breast mammograms and cervical Pap tests. The use of chest x-ray films to screen for the presence of lung cancer has been largely unsuccessful because metastasis usually has developed by the time a lesion is large enough to appear on a roentgenogram. The American Cancer Society's guidelines for cancer-related checkups (Table 16-10) are not recommended for mass screening. They were developed so that the health care professional together with the patient can choose the most appropriate early-detection protocol that meets the risk potential.[31] The goal is to discover early cancer on an individual basis in persons who have no symptoms.

The nurse's role in screening and early detection begins with a sound knowledge of cancer, known risk factors, and the treatment modalities available. Cancer risk assessment must be an integral part of every interaction the nurse has with the public. Data obtained from interviews, the nursing history, history and physical examinations, social and family histories, health surveys and questionnaires, and employment records help the nurse to determine the person's individual cancer risk factors.

Case finding is a responsibility of all nurses. The nurse must be able to (1) counsel and direct patients to the proper sources of help, (2) have information about those conditions that are known to predispose individuals to the development of the disease, and (3) educate the public about these factors. In addition, the nurse must be sensitive to the needs of patients who may be afraid and embarrassed when confronted with the possibility of cancer. Table 16-11 summarizes the nurse's role in early detection of some common cancers.

Cancer detection is expensive. Education often includes convincing the public that a periodic health examination is a sound investment. The public attitude toward participation in cancer screening programs is becoming more positive. Concerns about living in a more healthy environment and maintaining healthy lifestyles are suggested as the reason for the change. People also are known to participate in screening programs if they perceive themselves to be at risk for cancer. Some cities have cancer detection centers where a complete

**TABLE 16-10 Guidelines for Cancer-Related Checkups***

| TEST OR EXAMINATION | GENDER | AGE (YEARS) | RECOMMENDATION |
|---|---|---|---|
| Papanicolaou test | Female | Over 20; under 20 if sexually active | Every 3 years after two initial negative tests 1 year apart |
| Pelvic examination | Female | 18-40<br>Over 40 or at menopause | Every 1-3 years with Pap test<br>Yearly |
| Endometrial tissue sample | Female | At menopause or women at high risk | High risk: history of infertility, obesity, failure of ovulation, abnormal uterine bleeding, estrogen therapy |
| Breast self-examination | Female | Over 20 | Monthly |
| Breast physical examination | Female | 20-40<br>Over 40 | Every 3 years<br>Yearly |
| Mammogram | Female | 35-40<br>40-49<br>Over 50 | One baseline mammogram<br>Every 1-2 years<br>Yearly |
| Stool guaiac slide test | Male and female | Over 50 | Yearly |
| Digital rectal examination | Male and female | Over 40 | Yearly |
| Sigmoidoscopic examination | Male and female | Over 50 | Every 3-5 years based on advice of physician |

*American Cancer Society recommendations.

physical examination, including chest radiograph, Pap smear, breast examination, proctoscopy, urinalysis, and blood cell count, is performed for a moderate fee. Nurses should be aware of clinics in their area where persons needing such resources may be referred.

## HEALTH TEACHING

Early detection of cancer can decrease mortality. The nurse must know and be able to explain the significance of the seven warning signs of cancer (Box 16-8), stressing that any of these signs should be reported immediately to a physician. It should be emphasized that any of these signs should be investigated medically but that their occurrence does not necessarily mean that the person has cancer.

All persons should know the most common sites of cancer. In women these are the breast, lung, gastrointestinal tract, and uterus (cervix) (see Figure 16-3). Women should be taught to examine their breasts each month immediately after the menstrual period or, after menopause, on a designated day each month. Even though the value of BSE in early detection is questioned, it should still be encouraged until all findings are in.

Women of all ages should know the importance of reporting any abnormal vaginal bleeding or other discharge occurring between menstrual periods or after menopause. (See Chapter 55 for details of early symptoms of cancer of the female reproductive system.)

Men should be made aware that their risk is greatest for cancer of the prostate, lung, and gastrointestinal tract. The incidence of testicular cancer overall is small; however, it is most prevalent in young men between the ages of 15 and 40 years. Testicular self-examination (TSE), like BSE in women, has not improved mortality rates but is still stressed for this high-risk age-group.

Elderly persons, as a group, require more individualized health teaching about cancer risk and detection methods. They are often more reluctant to voice their fears about cancer or to report physical complaints that could be signs of early malignant tumors. Some are reticent about seeking medical intervention because of their tenuous financial state or fears of becoming a burden on their family or just because they are uncomfortable in discussing their concerns. Still others simply are not aware of their increased risk as they age. All too frequently health care professionals do not encourage elders to participate in health education and screening programs even though it is clearly evident that cancer risk increases with age. The American Cancer Society's guidelines for cancer-related checkups (see Table 16-10) offer a guide related to a very broad age range and do not specifically address the needs of persons 65 years and older. Rather, the health care professional must

**BOX 16-8 Seven Warning Signs of Cancer**

1. Change in bowel and bladder habits
2. A sore that does not heal
3. Unusual bleeding or discharge
4. Thickening or a lump in the breast or elsewhere
5. Indigestion or difficulty in swallowing
6. Obvious change in a wart or mole
7. Nagging cough or hoarseness

**TABLE 16-11 Nurse's Role in Early Detection of Common Cancers**

| TYPE OF CANCER | RISK FACTORS | PREVENTION | NURSE'S ROLE |
|---|---|---|---|
| Skin | 1. Light complexion, red hair with freckles<br>2. Frequent exposure to sun or tanning parlors<br>3. Occupational exposure to chemicals, arsenicals, pesticides, coal tar products<br>4. Frequent exposure to ionizing radiation, x-rays, radioisotopes<br>5. Precancerous skin lesions<br>6. Genetic predisposition (xeroderma pigmentosum, albinism)<br>7. Change in mole (color, size, shape) | 1. Limit sun exposure between 10 AM-3 PM; do not exceed 15-30 min/day until tan is established<br>2. Cover exposed skin<br>3. Apply protective sunscreen (factor 15 or more)<br>4. Be aware of medications that increase photosensitivity (e.g., tetracycline)<br>5. Cleanse skin after use of chemical substances<br>6. In industry, wear protective clothing and, if exposed to chemicals, follow guidelines for cleansing skin | 1. Educate public to risk factors and behavior/life-style modification<br>2. Act as role model |
| Lung | 1. Habitual smoker (cigarettes, pipe, cigars)<br>2. Prolonged inhalation of side-stream smoke<br>3. Exposure to known occupational or environmental carcinogens (asbestos, hydrocarbons, radon)<br>4. Family history of lung cancer | 1. Do not smoke or if a smoker, stop<br>2. Monitor occupational and environmental exposure dosages/risks; wear protective clothing and masks<br>3. Have medical checkup if in high-risk group | 1. Lobby for smoke-free environment and employment setting<br>2. Participate in smoke-cessation programs<br>3. Educate youth to perils of smoking<br>4. Conduct research on smoking behavior/attitudes |
| Breast | 1. Family or personal history of breast, endometrial, ovarian cancer<br>2. Never married, no children, or first child after age 30<br>3. Early menarche and late menopause<br>4. History of fibrocystic disease<br>5. Triad of diabetes, obesity, and hypertension<br>6. High-fat diet | 1. Monthly BSE age 18 and older<br>2. Physical examination yearly<br>3. Baseline mammogram age 35-40 and yearly >age 50 or as directed by physician<br>4. Avoid high-fat diet and obesity | 1. Teach BSE<br>2. Educate women on risk factor–reduction strategies |
| Colorectal | 1. Black population<br>2. Age >40 years<br>3. Family history of colon cancer<br>4. Personal history of Crohn's disease, Gardner's syndrome, familial polyposis, ulcerative colitis >10 years' duration<br>5. Diet high in fat and alcohol | 1. Diet high in fiber, low in fat (<30% of total calories)<br>2. Avoid salt-cured or nitrite-cured foods<br>3. Avoid obesity<br>4. Annual occult stool examination >age 50 years<br>5. Yearly digital rectal examination >age 40 years<br>6. Sigmoidoscopy every 3-5 years >age 50 years | 1. Educate and counsel blacks and elders on benefits of screening programs and diet modifications<br>2. Participate in cancer prevention/detection programs<br>3. Identify cases of high-risk persons/family |
| Prostate | 1. Increasing age and blacks<br>2. Family history of prostate cancer<br>3. Exposure to cadmium, fertilizers; rubber-industry workers at risk<br>4. Sexual behavior (higher rates in hyperactive or promiscuous)<br>5. Change in bladder habits<br>6. Diet high in fat and alcohol | 1. Annual digital rectal examination >age 40 years<br>2. Test for prostate-specific antigen (PSA) and transrectal ultrasound show promise for early detection | 1. Educate elderly men, especially black males to risk factors<br>2. Promote and participate in screening programs |
| Testicular | 1. Young, white males (15-40)<br>2. Cryptorchidism<br>3. Testicular atrophy after viral infection (mumps)<br>4. Personal history of testicular cancer<br>5. Trauma<br>6. History of inguinal hernia<br>7. History of maternal ingestion of diethylstilbestrol during pregnancy | 1. Testicular self-examination monthly<br>2. Orchiopexy before age 2 years | 1. Educate and counsel value of self-examination<br>2. Encourage participation in screening program |

Modified from White L: *Semin Oncol Nurs* 1(3):184-190, 1986.

**TABLE 16-11 Nurse's Role in Early Detection of Common Cancers—cont'd**

| TYPE OF CANCER | RISK FACTORS | PREVENTION | NURSE'S ROLE |
|---|---|---|---|
| Cervical | 1. Early sexual activity, multiple partners<br>2. Genital infections (herpesviruses)<br>3. Dysplasia<br>4. Multiple pregnancies<br>5. Poor personal hygiene | 1. Barrier protection during coitis<br>2. Life-style modification<br>3. Annual pelvic examination and Pap test at age 20 or earlier if sexually active | 1. Educate to risk factors, especially teen-agers; distribute educational materials<br>2. Advocate American Cancer Society (ACS) guidelines<br>3. Participate in screening programs |
| Endometrial | 1. Increasing age<br>2. Triad of diabetes, hypertension, and obesity<br>3. Nulliparity<br>4. Early menarche and late menopause<br>5. History of hormonal therapy | 1. Annual pelvic examination and Pap test<br>2. Endometrial biopsy at menopause | 1. Same as with cervical above |

study each guideline for its appropriate application to this population subgroup. Table 16-12 is adapted from the ACS recommendations and addresses the specific early detection and checkup needs of elders.

Some elders may feel more confident and secure discussing their concerns about cancer with the nurse. The nurse must take advantage of all opportunities to teach elderly persons. Both the inpatient and clinic settings offer many occasions for assessing the cancer knowledge base of elders and any concerns they may express. In addition, nurses can use health fairs held at churches, nursing homes, and retirement communities to foster the elderly person's cancer education needs.

Two common misconceptions that lead the person to ignore symptoms should be corrected. The first is a belief that a disease as serious as cancer must be accompanied by weight loss. Weight loss usually is a late symptom of cancer. Another reason for neglect of cancer is the belief that absence of pain means that an indisposition is minor. It must be repeatedly emphasized to the public that pain is not an early sign of cancer and that cancer often is far advanced before pain occurs.

**TABLE 16-12 Early Detection and Cancer-Related Checkup Recommendations for Those 65 Years and Older**

| TEST | GENDER | RECOMMENDATION |
|---|---|---|
| Papanicolaou test and pelvic examination | F | Yearly after 3 consecutive negative test results; then every 1-3 years on advice of physician |
| Breast self-examination | F | Monthly |
| Breast physical examination and mammogram | F | Yearly |
| Digital rectal examination | M and F | Yearly |
| Stool occult test | M and F | Yearly |
| Sigmoidoscopic examination | M and F | Every 3-5 years based on advice of physician |

Modified from American Cancer Society recommendations.

## FACTORS THAT INTERFERE WITH HEALTH-SEEKING BEHAVIORS

Even though knowledge of cancer is more widespread than before, a more positive attitude toward the disease is essential if persons are to follow good health practices and seek help when warning signs of cancer are noted. Factors that may interfere with health-seeking behaviors include underestimation of the incidence of cancer and negative views about conventional therapies. The poor, minority groups, the less-educated, and men in general are less likely to have physical examinations on a regular basis.

Unfortunately, anxiety and fear may immobilize the individual. Despite all the public announcements that have been made in the past few decades, some people still think cancer must be hidden from others. This attitude stems partly from the fact that cancer in its terminal stages can be a painful and demoralizing disease. Some people fear cancer and shun persons who have the disease because they believe it is contagious. Scientific speculation on the possibility that a virus may be the cause has added to this fear. At this time, there is no conclusive evidence that cancer can be spread among human beings in a way similar to the spread of infectious diseases.

The positive aspects of cancer care should be emphasized. It is estimated that approximately one third of the persons for whom a diagnosis is made are cured by medical treatment. Another one third could perhaps be cured by medical treatment if the cancer were diagnosed

**BOX 16-9** ***Healthy People 2000*: Health Status Objectives by Year 2000 as Related to Cancer**

**REDUCTION IN DEATH RATES**

1. Reverse the rise in cancer deaths to achieve a rate of 130/100,000 persons.
2. Slow the rise in lung cancer deaths to a rate of no more than 42/100,000 persons.
3. Reduce breast cancer deaths to no more than 20.6/100,000 women.
4. Reduce deaths from cancer of the uterine cervix to no more than 1.3/100,000 women.
5. Reduce colorectal cancer deaths to no more than 13.2/100,000 persons.

**CANCER RISK REDUCTION**

1. Reduce cigarette smoking to a prevalence of no more than 15% among persons aged 20 or older.
2. Reduce dietary fat intake to an average of 30% of calories or less and average saturated fat intake to less than 10% of calories among persons aged 2 and older.
3. Increase complex carbohydrate and fiber-containing foods in the diets of adults to five or more daily servings for vegetables and fruits and to six or more daily servings for grain products.
4. Increase to 60% of the general population those who limit sun exposure, use sunscreens and protective clothing when exposed to sunlight, and avoid artificial sources of ultraviolet light (sun lamps, tanning booths).

**EARLY DETECTION GOALS**

1. Increase to 75% the proportion of care providers who routinely counsel patients about tobacco cessation, diet modification, and cancer screening recommendations.
2. Increase to 80% the proportion of women aged 40 and older who have received a clinical breast examination and mammogram, and to 60% of those aged 50 and older who have received them within the preceding 1 to 2 years.
3. Increase to 95% the proportion of women aged 18 and older with uterine cervix who have ever had a Pap test, and to 85% the number who had a Pap test within the preceding 1 to 3 years.
4. Increase to 50% the number of persons aged 50 and older who had fecal occult blood testing within the preceding 1 to 2 years and to 40% those who have ever had a proctosigmoidoscopic examination.
5. Increase to 40% the number of persons aged 50 and older visiting a primary care provider in the preceding year who had oral, skin, and digital rectal examinations during one such visit.

**SET SERVICE STANDARDS**

1. Ensure that Pap tests meet quality standards by monitoring and certifying all cytology laboratories.
2. Ensure that mammograms meet quality standards by monitoring and certifying at least 80% of mammography facilities.

From US Department of Health and Human Services. Public Health Service: *Healthy people 2000: Summary report,* Boston, 1992, Jones & Bartlett.

early enough. Only a third have cancer occurring in locations in which the disease has advanced beyond medical aid and before sufficient signs appeared to warn the patient of trouble. In spite of these facts, some persons think it is useless to report symptoms early because they believe that if they do have cancer, they cannot be cured. It can only be hoped that the recent publicity about well-known persons who have been treated for cancer will help overcome some of these attitudes. If nothing else, the open discussion in the media of cancer diagnosis and treatment should result in a better informed public than ever before. The health status objectives for the year 2000 as they relate to cancer are summarized in Box 16-9.

# MEDICAL MANAGEMENT

## DIAGNOSTIC PHASE

The word *cancer* has the ability to elicit a sense of fear and horror in most people. Almost everyone has personal knowledge of a relative or friend who has been diagnosed with a malignant tumor or has heard about the disabling and devastating effects of cancer and its treatment. It is small wonder that when a lump is discovered in the breast or when one experiences unexplained fatigue, weight loss, or changes in bowel or bladder habits, fear and dread become all-consuming. At other times a person who is feeling well undergoes a physical examination or routine chest x-ray examination, during which a suspicious lesion is discovered.

When a person has symptoms that cannot be explained away as the outcome of a benign physical process, the initial reaction is that cancer is the underlying cause. Consequently, the symptoms may be ignored or denied in the hopes that they will go away or endured until they become so severe that they require professional evaluation. Knowledge of cancer facts and risk factors does not always translate into rapid entry into the health care system and early diagnosis. Delay in seeking medical intervention has been attributed to increasing age, gender, personal finances, and social support available, as well as how one normally copes in stressful situations. Elderly persons constitute a high-risk group for cancer development. They are known to underreport their symptoms and therefore present with more advanced disease. They frequently are poor historians, some having several chronic illnesses with interrelated symptoms, and they often do not recognize that they belong to a cancer-prone group.[14] In addition, members of minority groups who have no health insurance or insufficient coverage also tend to delay seeking entry into the health care system.

Regardless of either early or late entry into the health care system, it is important that all health care professionals recognize the impact of a cancer diagnosis on the individual and entire family and refrain from placing blame directly or by inference.

## Diagnostic Studies

A wide variety of tests and procedures may be employed in the diagnosis of a malignant condition. Often it is the presenting signs and symptoms or the body system thought to be most prominently involved that will dictate the tests to be used. The discussion that follows is limited only to how the test relates to diagnosing malignant lesions.

### Laboratory tests

Cancer tumors produce hormones or proteins that may be detected by blood tests. Measurement of an enzyme, acid phosphatase, which is produced almost entirely by the prostate gland, gives evidence of the extent of prostatic disease. Another enzyme, alkaline phosphatase, is elevated in persons with bone metastases and sometimes in those with liver metastases. Blood in the stool, identified by the guaiac test, may be a sign of gastrointestinal cancer. Calcitonin increase has been shown to be a good indicator of thyroid and lung cancer.

**Cytology.** In 1942 Dr. George Papanicolaou demonstrated that the diagnosis of cancer can be made from the study of cells that have sloughed or exfoliated from a tumor. These cells are found in body secretions such as cervical discharges, sputum, gastric washings, pleural fluid, and urinary washings. The secretion is spread on a slide, stained, and examined by a pathologist, who can classify the tissue as benign, dysplastic ("suspicious"), or malignant. The main use of the Pap smear, as it is often called, is to diagnose cancer in a person who has no symptoms and to identify precancerous lesions or noninvasive cancer. If suspect cells are found, a biopsy must be performed to diagnose cancer. The Pap smear is most widley used in routine examination of cervical washings.

### Radiologic tests

**X-Ray and scanning procedures.** X-ray studies usually are ordered. The use of chest radiography is absolutely necessary if the patient is a smoker. Examination by means of gastrointestinal series, intravenous pyelogram, and mammography depends on areas where lesions are expected to be present.

The scanning technique, which permits the mapping of organs, plays an important part in the evaluation of the patient with cancer. Some of these procedures are described in Table 16-13.

**Radioisotope studies.** Various scanning procedures that involve the introduction of a radioactive substance into the body are used to detect primary or metastatic cancer. The radioisotope either concentrates in the tumor and shows up as a "hot spot" in the scan of the organ or the tumor does not concentrate the isotope and a "cold spot" surrounded by normal tissue that did concentrate the isotope is found. Radioisotopes used include the following:

1. Radioactive iodine: oral or by injection; used for diagnosis of thyroid disease
2. Radioactive iodine-tagged albumin: injected intravenously; used for locating brain tumors and to determine blood volume

**TABLE 16-13 X-ray and Scanning Procedures Used in Cancer Diagnosis**

| STUDY | PROCEDURE | COMMENT |
|---|---|---|
| Lymphangiography | Oil-based blue dye and procaine (Novocain) injected in skin of web between first and second toes or index and second fingers to show lymphatic drainage of extremities | Used in diagnosing lymph and metastatic cancer. Lymphomatous nodes have "foamy" or "lacy" structure. Metastatic nodes have "moth-eaten" appearance. Skin discoloration from dye may last 1 week |
| Xeroradiography | X-ray image on plate of selenium-coated metal | Provides picture of soft tissue |
| Tomography | X-ray image with ability to penetrate dense shadows | Provides picture of soft tissue |
| Thermography | Constructs photographic images of surface temperature | Identifies skin temperature elevations over inflammatory or malignant lesions |
| Computed tomography (CT) scan | X-ray beam and use of computer | Produces images of plane sections of body; identifies size and location of tumors |
| Magnetic resonance imaging (MRI) | Magnetic fields | Produces a cross-sectional image of the body; spares patient from x-ray exposure |
| Positron-emission tomography (PET) | Scanners that rotate around patient; image formed by positrons emitted by isotope injected into or inhaled by patient | Allows viewing of brain and body processes in three dimensions; gives a picture of biochemical and metabolic processes |

**Ultrasound.** Ultrasound probing, or *echography,* is performed by means of an electronic instrument that detects and records echoes of sound when they are reflected at the junction of tissue with different densities. The procedure is helpful in differentiating between cystic and solid tumors.

### Biopsy

Biopsy is the only definitive way that cancer can be diagnosed. *Incisional biopsy* is the surgical removal of a section of the neoplasm. If the tumor is small, the entire growth may be removed—a procedure called an *excisional biopsy.* When possible, an *aspiration biopsy* (needle biopsy)—removing a small plug of tumor by use of a needle or syringe—is used to avoid the larger incisional or excisional biopsy. Needle biopsy, although inexpensive and relatively simple to perform in an outpatient setting, has the potential of missing the malignant focus and "seeding" tumor cells along the needle track as it is inserted and withdrawn.

The biopsy specimen is examined under a microscope to obtain a histologic diagnosis as to the type of cancer. In some cases it may be possible to determine the degree of malignancy.

### Endoscopy

Hollow metal tubes equipped with a light are used to illuminate various body cavities, permitting visual inspection of the interior of the cavity being examined. These instruments are commonly referred to as *scopes* and are named for the organs they are to visualize. Thus a bronchoscope is used to examine the bronchus, a gastroscope is used to visualize the stomach, and a proctoscope is used to visualize the anus and sigmoid colon. A biopsy specimen of tissue or secretions usually is obtained during these endoscopic procedures. A local anesthetic that diminishes the gag reflex is used before bronchoscopic or gastroscopic examination. Usually no anesthetic is necessary for sigmoidoscopic examination. Peritonoscopy, which is used to examine the peritoneal cavity, is particularly helpful in visualizing peritoneal metastasis. A local anesthetic is used with this procedure.

### Other diagnostic methods

The search for a universal cancer marker that would indicate the presence of a malignant process regardless of tissue source has not been successful. However, "markers" have been determined for some specific cancers. Markers include secreted proteins, cell surface macromolecules, hormones, enzymes and isoenzymes, and components of the cytoplasm. It is now recognized that cancer cells resemble embryonic or fetal cells in appearance and in their ability to produce typically fetal cellular macromolecules. These macromolecules may be found in the cell, on the cell surface, or in body fluids. Their increased presence often is associated with a malignant process.[38] Table 16-14 notes some common cancer markers in use today.

**TABLE 16-14 Cancer Markers Used to Detect the Presence of Cancer**

| MARKER | TYPE OF CANCER |
|---|---|
| Carcinoembryonic antigen (CEA) | Lung and gastrointestinal |
| Alpha-fetoprotein (AFP) | Stomach, colon, and lung |
| Chorionic gonadotropin | Seminomas and choriocarcinomas |
| Ectopic hormone production | Lung, breast, and pancreas |
| Bence Jones protein | Multiple myeloma |
| Prostate-specific antigen (PSA) | Prostate |
| Genetic markers (chromosome translocation/rearrangements) | Chronic myelogenous leukemia (CML) |

## Medical Treatment Options

Often several physicians are involved in determining the appropriate treatment for cancer. The medical team chooses treatment on the basis of the biologic characteristics of the tumor, its clinical stage, and the condition of the patient. The tumor's histologic type is particularly important in determining the treatment to be used.

Therapy may be curative (removal of all traces of the disease from the body) or **palliative** (directed only toward relieving symptoms). At present four major forms of treatment are used: surgery, radiotherapy, chemotherapy, and biotherapy. The last is the newest form of treatment for cancer. Combinations of the four treatment modalities often are used to achieve the best results for each patient.

## SURGICAL INTERVENTION

Surgery, which is used to assist in the diagnosis of cancer, is the oldest known method of treatment. It can be employed to cure the disease or to palliate symptoms. The best treatment for cancer at present is complete surgical removal of all malignant tissue before metastasis occurs. Surgery must often be extensive and may require adjustments beyond that needed in many other conditions. The patient may not have sufficient time to become gradually accustomed to the idea of surgery and the effect it can have on one's body and life-style. The individual often faces the prospect of mutilating surgery with only the hope that it will cure the cancer and be lifesaving. Concern about what will happen to the family may be uppermost in the patient's mind. Obviously the individual and family need empathy and understanding as they attempt to accept the recommendations for immediate surgery.

Adjuvant surgical intervention is used principally to support other treatment modalities such as radiation and chemotherapy. Surgical placement of vascular access devices provides a means of administering chemotherapeutic agents directly into a tumor, organ system, or limb. Radiation therapy can be enhanced through the use of surgically implanted devices that house the radioactive material and provide concentrated therapy to a localized area.

Before surgery, careful assessment is required to evaluate the patient's ability to withstand the stress of the surgical procedure. Nutritional status and immunocompetence are vital to successful recovery and rehabilitation. Table 16-15 provides examples of surgical interventions now used in the treatment of cancer. The operative procedures used to treat various types of cancer are discussed in later chapters under the particular organ systems.

## NURSING MANAGEMENT

### ♦ ASSESSMENT

The assessment of the cancer patient who will undergo surgery is divided into the three areas around the surgical event: diagnostic phase, preoperative phase, and

#### Diagnostic Phase

During the diagnostic phase the nurse assesses the patient and family for the following:

1. Knowledge of the diagnostic process

**TABLE 16-15 Surgical Approaches to Cancer Care**

| INTERVENTION | EXAMPLE |
|---|---|
| Diagnosis | Breast biopsy |
| Staging | Staging laparotomy<br>Second-look laparotomy |
| Treatment of primary tumor | Curative resection (abdominal perineal resection) |
| Reconstruction, rehabilitation | Breast reconstruction<br>Continent urostomy or ileostomy |
| Palliative | Endocrine ablation<br>Pericardial window |
| Adjuvant | Paraaortic node dissection<br>Hickman line insertion |
| Complications of other methods | Excision of bowel stricture<br>Excision of radionecrotic tissue |
| Resection of metastases | Partial hepatectomy<br>Pulmonary resection |
| Cytoreductive | Abdominal soft tissue sarcomas<br>Ovarian peritoneal carcinoma |
| Emergencies | Obstruction<br>Hemorrhage |
| Cancer prevention | Colectomy (familial polyposis)<br>Orchidopexy (testicular tumors) |

From Havard CP, Topping AE: Surgical oncology. In Biard S, McCorkle R, Grant M, editors: *Cancer nursing: a comprehensive textbook*, Philadelphia, 1991, WB Saunders.

   a. Name of tests and procedures
   b. Rationale for tests/procedures
   c. What patient should know in preparation for test, during, and any special concerns afterward
   d. How tests/procedures will contribute to diagnosis
2. Physical status during previous 3 to 6 months
   a. Ability to perform normal activities
   b. Changes noted
      (1) Weight—stable, losing, gaining
      (2) Muscle mass and strength
      (3) Changes in appetite, sleep/rest, elimination
      (4) Comfort level
3. Emotional state
   a. Understanding need for diagnostic process
   b. Impact of hospitalization and possible diagnosis of cancer on
      (1) Patient's role in family, job security, finances
      (2) Family organization and function
      (3) Who provides emotional support to the patient
   c. Anxiety level
   d. Usual coping style in stressful situations

#### Preoperative Phase

During the preoperative phase, the nurse assesses the following:

1. Patient understanding and readiness to learn about the planned surgical intervention
   a. Role of surgery—cure, palliation, or other
   b. Name of surgical procedure and why it is planned
   c. Expected outcome of surgery and potential changes that may result in organ/body function or appearance
2. Prior surgical experiences
3. Capacity to make informed decision about planned surgery in terms of ability to retain and use factual information
4. Physical performance level and energy state
5. Nutritional status
   a. Weight-height ratio compared with ideal standard for age and gender
   b. Laboratory values: albumin, total protein, hemoglobin, hematocrit, lymphocyte count
   c. Ability to ingest and retain nourishment
   d. Food preferences and aversions
6. Understanding of the role of good nutrition to successful recovery and rehabilitation after surgery

#### Postoperative Phase

During the postoperative phase the nurse assesses the following:

1. Verbal and nonverbal responses that indicate fear of the surgical outcome

a. Increased tension, irritability, lack of concentration
b. Frequent questioning on same topic; dread about possible answer
2. Postoperative comfort level
a. Presence of pain
b. Location
c. Intensity and duration
d. Precipitating factors
3. Previous pain experience and successful coping strategies employed
4. Response to pain-relief strategies
5. Common signs and symptoms of postoperative infection
a. Fever and chills
b. Redness, swelling, odor, pain
c. Diaphoresis
d. Altered laboratory values, for example, blood cell counts, cultures
6. Risk factors for postoperative infection
a. Immunodeficiency secondary to disease process
b. Altered production of leukocytes or altered leukocyte response
c. Presence of invasive equipment or disruption of skin barrier
(1) Indwelling catheters
(2) Infusion lines
(3) Drains
(4) Incision
(5) Intubation
d. Environmental exposure
7. Signs of verbal or nonverbal cues concerning sexuality and sexual functioning
a. Inability to look at body (mastectomy scar/colostomy)
b. Statement of feeling no longer attractive; feminine; masculine
c. Feelings of low self-worth

## ♦ NURSING DIAGNOSES

Nursing diagnoses are determined from analysis of patient data. Nursing diagnoses for the patient undergoing diagnostic testing and surgical intervention may include but are not limited to the following:

| Diagnostic Title | Possible Etiologic Factors |
|---|---|
| Anxiety | Unknown diagnosis, threat of change in health status, change in role functioning |
| Coping, ineffective family | Inadequate information and understanding of diagnostic process, temporary family disorganization and role changes, inability to provide emotional and physical support to significant other |
| Knowledge deficit (related to surgery and its outcome) | Lack of interest or readiness to learn, lack of accurate information, cognitive limitations |
| Nutrition, altered: less than body requirements | Disease process (cancer cachexia), anorexia, taste changes, fatigue, diagnostic tests |
| Fear | Unknown surgical outcome, loss of body part or function, long-term illness |
| Pain | Surgical trauma, cancer metastasis |
| Infection, high risk for | Environmental exposure, decreased nutrition, decreased immune function, lack of personal hygiene |
| Sexual dysfunction | Altered body structure, physiologic limitations, lack of information, psychologic stress |

## ♦ EXPECTED PATIENT OUTCOMES

Expected patient outcomes for the person with cancer undergoing diagnostic testing and surgical intervention may include but are not limited to the following:

*Diagnostic phase*

1. Patient
a. Describes own anxieties and healthy ways to deal with them.
b. Describes purpose of diagnostic tests/procedures and how they will lead to a diagnosis.
c. Uses support persons and resources effectively.
2. Family members
a. Identify how they will deal with changes brought on by present situation.
b. Verbalize knowledge and understanding of diagnostic process.
c. Interact appropriately with patient and staff members, providing support and assistance as needed.

*Preoperative phase*

3. Patient's knowledge of procedure
a. Discusses and acknowledges deficit in knowledge of planned surgery.
b. Assumes responsibility for own learning by asking and listening to information provided.
c. Demonstrates knowledge of preoperative preparation measures and immediate postoperative care needs.
d. Verbalizes accurately the role of surgery and the expected outcomes.
4. Patient's knowledge of nutrition
a. Verbalizes understanding of factors causing nutritional deficits.
b. Discusses the role of nutrition for successful recovery from surgery.
c. Complies with nutritional support measures.

*Postoperative phase*

5. Outcome: Accepts results of surgical intervention and its outcome on the malignant condition.

6. Pain: Reports that pain is relieved and controlled.
7. Infection: Has no evidence of infection during postoperative period.
8. Patient's sexual role
   a. Expresses personal significance of lost body part and how limited functional capacity will affect sexuality and sexual functioning.
   b. Discusses concerns about sex role and self-concept and how it will affect partner.

## ♦ INTERVENTIONS

### Diagnostic Phase

The goal of all cancer therapy is to maximize the effects of therapy on the tumor while maintaining the patient's physiologic and emotional integrity. This is especially important to the patient who will undergo surgery, some of which is radical and mutilating in nature. The time of diagnosis is extremely stressful for both patient and loved ones. Although the word *cancer* may not be mentioned, it generally presents an overriding fear for all involved. This phase is not only emotionally draining but physically taxing for the patient. The signs of bodily wasting may already be present before medical intervention is sought and before a definitive cancer diagnosis is confirmed. Tests and procedures require the patient to go without usual nourishment while normal sleep and rest patterns are disrupted. Some tests cause discomfort, beginning with the preparation requirements: being immobilized in uncomfortable positions for lengthy intervals and being alone and isolated from family or familiar nursing staff members. Anxiety levels run high. The patient and family alternate between fearing the worst possible outcome—a cancer diagnosis—and hoping for a benign condition. Not only the patient is affected physically and emotionally during this phase; so too are all family members.

The nurse plays a pivotal role in the management of the patient's care during the diagnostic phase. Plans should be made to support the patient, as well as the entire family, at this critical time. Hospitalization of a family member and the fear of a cancer diagnosis can lead to changes in family roles that cause some members to assume responsibilities and tasks that are new and frightening to them. Adult children may need to take on the role of decision maker and caretaker and possibly provide needed financial assistance—all while taking care of their own families and job responsibilities. It is the spouse, however, who has the most significant role adjustment. At one time it was assumed that spouses of cancer patients were more or less passive observers instead of being actively involved in the cancer experience.[32] It is now recognized that spouses have the same needs as the patient: knowledge of the typical course of the disease, symptoms to expect, and the treatment options available. Husbands in particular have a difficult time providing emotional support because they are socialized to be providers and protectors in the family constellation and to suppress their fears. Consequently they may try to protect their wives from openly discussing their concerns about a cancer diagnosis at a time when communication of these fears is most needed.

Building a therapeutic relationship with both the patient and family will be best achieved by being open and honest in all communications—providing appropriate information about diagnostic tests and their rationale in the diagnostic process—and by maintaining in the patient a sense of realistic hope. Including the patient and family members in any decision making gives them a sense of personal control at a time when most are feeling helpless, powerless, and isolated in an unfamiliar environment. Table 16-16 summarizes family needs during the diagnostic phase and course of the illness.

### Preoperative Phase

When surgery is deemed to be the appropriate intervention, the patient will have questions and concerns regarding the type and the extent of the procedure. Many believe that they will be "cured" and consent to

**TABLE 16-16 Information Needed by Cancer Patients and Spouses Over the Course of Illness**

| DIAGNOSTIC PHASE | HOSPITAL PHASE | TREATMENT PHASE | ADAPTATION PHASE | RECURRENT PHASE |
|---|---|---|---|---|
| Type and purpose of diagnostic procedures to be performed<br>When test results can be expected<br>The person who is coordinating the care<br>The typical emotions that develop while awaiting diagnosis (e.g., anxiety, uncertainty) | Type of surgery planned<br>When pathology report will be available<br>Expected length of hospitalization<br>Role limitations to anticipate when patient is discharged<br>The effects of illness on other family members | Type and length of treatment planned<br>Anticipated side effects and when they may occur<br>Ways to minimize side effects<br>Likelihood of temporary role changes<br>Availability of cancer education and support groups | When follow-up exams or tests are necessary<br>The typical concerns during this phase (e.g., fear of recurrence)<br>Importance of balancing needs of patient and family members<br>Availability of cancer education and support groups | Type of treatment planned<br>Anticipated side effects and when they may occur<br>The typical feelings during this phase (e.g., uncertainty, sadness, fear)<br>Ways to maintain hope regardless of recurrence<br>Availability of support groups and community resources |

From Northouse LL, Peters-Golden H: *Semin Oncol Nurs* 9(3):77, 1993.

surgery with this thought in mind, refusing to believe any other outcome. For the patient and family to make informed decisions about treatment they need to know what role surgery will play in their particular situation. The role of surgery in cancer therapy has several aspects that must be communicated accurately and in detail. The initial role of surgery is *diagnosis and staging of disease.* The diagnosis and staging of some types of cancers require tissue biopsy obtainable only by surgical means. The type of surgical biopsy and its extent depend on the site and characteristics of the tumor. Some may require removing enlarged lymph nodes or obtaining tissue samples, such as during an abdominal laparotomy.

When definitive diagnosis of cancer has been made from tissue analysis, surgery may be the means employed for a "cure." The possibility of such a cure cannot always be predicted with certainty. The tumor mass will be excised with a wide margin of normal tissue surrounding it, but the possibility exists that micrometastasis or regional lymph node involvement, although not evident at the time of surgery, may be present.

Surgery as a *palliative* procedure is now a recognized and useful intervention for cancer patients with more advanced disease. Palliative surgery may be used to reduce the bulk of a growing, yet unresectable, tumor mass. Debulking some of the mass can relieve the discomfort from obstructions or nerve pain. Common palliative procedures that relieve colonic obstructions or spinal cord compression by laminectomy are major surgical procedures that increase the patient's quality of life. Surgical removal of hormone-producing organs has been used to curb the growth of tumors that depend on the hormone for growth. An example is removal of the ovaries (oophorectomy) for estrogen-dependent breast cancer. At other times, surgically implanted pumps and catheters provide chemotherapy directly into an organ or are used for regional perfusion. Last, surgery can be a method of *pain control* through a variety of surgical blocks.

Many variables are considered before surgery is attempted, and these must be conveyed openly to the patient. The first consideration is disease stage, location, and whether the mass can be successfully resected. The patient's emotional state will have considerable impact on the acceptance of a cancer diagnosis, as well as on postoperative recovery and rehabilitation. Elderly persons fear dying or becoming a burden to their families, physically and financially. Patients in early adulthood to middle age may be more physically able to withstand diagnostic testing and surgery, but they too have emotional concerns. These patients are in their most productive years in relation to career advancement, educational opportunities, and sexual activity. They may fear the loss of job security, financial independence, disfigurement, role adjustments within the family and community, and loss of reproductive capacity.

The health care team assesses several physical factors during the preoperative interval, which helps to predict how well the patient will withstand and recover from the surgery. These factors include age, nutritional status, performance status (Box 16-10), other active medical problems, and the results of blood cell count and chemistry studies. Although cancer affects all age-groups, its incidence is higher in those 65 years of age and older. This age-group has more chronic and disabling conditions that can complicate recovery. In addition the normal aging process, with resultant physiologic changes, affects the surgical outcome. Thus nursing management of the elderly patient offers many challenges. It is essential that the nurse have a basic understanding of the physiologic changes associated with normal aging. Preoperative assessment of age-related changes in each body system is a vital first step in facilitating a good surgical outcome and more rapid postoperative recovery. These assessment data provide baseline information on the patient's functional ability for each body system and a focus for specific preoperative teaching needs. In addition, a more comprehensive postsurgical plan of care can be devised that will alert the care team to the special needs of each elderly patient. (See Chapter 4 for a review of the common physiologic changes associated with normal aging.)

When surgery is not considered an emergency and time permits, the cancer patient will be nutritionally supported before surgery as necessary. Oral supplements, high in protein and calories, or total parenteral nutrition (TPN) if the patient cannot take and retain oral feedings, play a vital role in preoperative management. The nurse discusses with the patient and family the role of good nutrition in successful surgical outcome. Sound

**BOX 16-10 Karnofsky Performance Scale**

***A subjective assessment tool to assess and compare the patient's activity and performance ability***

| | |
|---|---|
| Normal; no complaints; no evidence of disease | 100 |
| Able to carry on normal activity; minor signs or symptoms of disease | 90 |
| Normal activity with effort; some signs or symptoms of disease | 80 |
| Cares for self; unable to carry on normal activity or to do active work | 70 |
| Requires occasional assistance but is able to care for most needs | 60 |
| Requires considerable assistance and frequent medical care | 50 |
| Disabled; requires special care and assistance | 40 |
| Severely disabled; hospitalization is indicated, although death is not imminent | 30 |
| Hospitalization is necessary; very sick; active supportive treatment necessary | 20 |
| Moribund; fatal processes progressing rapidly | 10 |
| Dead | 0 |

nutrition helps the patient heal more quickly and have more strength and energy and usually means a shortened recovery time and hospitalization. Compliance with nutritional repletion is encouraged. Family members are urged to take meals with the patient, bring in favorite foods from home, and support patient compliance. Blood or blood products will be administered on the basis of laboratory values. The nurse documents the patient's response to these interventions promptly and reports to the physician any difficulties encountered.

As with any surgical candidates, the preoperative teaching needs are addressed and any questions answered promptly. Discussion of any special equipment that may be needed during postoperative recovery occurs at this time, such as catheters, monitors, infusion lines, or chest tubes. The physician is required to provide all necessary information about the surgical procedure, risk factors, and possible complications as part of the patient's informed decision-making process. The nurse should attempt to be present when this discussion takes place, thus providing assistance in the decision process by clarifying information and dispelling misconceptions and fears. If the nurse cannot be present, follow-up questions can be helpful, for example, asking the patient to explain what he or she understands about the intended surgery and what it means personally, as well as answering any questions that may result.

### Postoperative Phase

One of the first questions heard from the patient on awakening from anesthesia after surgery may be "Was it cancer?" or "Did they get it all?" The family also may have the same questions. Fear that the findings were in fact malignant or that the tumor was unresectable is normal, and the nurse should anticipate it and be prepared to respond appropriately. Dealing honestly with these questions is essential to maintaining therapeutic communication and credibility. The nurse needs to be cognizant of what the surgeon has communicated so that information conveyed to the patient and family is consistent. The nurse will be able to clarify and explain what the surgery revealed. Early in the postoperative period only the preliminary pathology report is available because it may take several days to receive the final report. Until the final pathology report is received, the patient's concerns will be everpresent. Nursing care that provides physical and emotional comfort will help the patient during this waiting period. Being empathic and nonjudgmental regarding concerns is essential.

The physical care of the patient during the immediate postoperative phase of cancer surgery does not differ from the care needed by any patients undergoing a similar surgical procedure. Care includes comfort measures, skin and wound care, and careful assessment and monitoring of pulmonary, cardiovascular, urinary, and gastrointestinal function. Atelectasis and respiratory infection are two of the first complications encountered during the postoperative period. Good pulmonary toilet (turning, coughing, deep-breathing exercises) is especially important for the patient with cancer because many are already physically impaired and immunodeficient before surgery as a consequence of the disease process and the rigors of diagnosis and surgery. Thus these patients may not have the physical strength to ward off any type of infectious process. Sources of infection (e.g., indwelling catheters, infusion lines, drains) are numerous for the patient after surgery. The nurse must plan to scrutinize each potential source for the presence of infection; document findings; arrange for a culture of suspicious drainage; and notify the physician immediately. Maintenance of strict asepsis is of utmost importance in the immunocompromised patient. The nurse instructs the patient and other caregivers on the need for strict aseptic technique. Visitors with any infectious process should be advised to refrain from close contact with the patient during the critical period. Antibiotic therapy to cover a wide range of organisms may be prescribed. Teaching the patient and the support person the procedure for wound care and significant signs and symptoms of infection to report after hospitalization should be accomplished before discharge time. (See Chapter 25 for a more detailed discussion of the postoperative care of the patient.)

After surgery for cancer the patient must always face the prospect of a poor outcome and death, changes in life-style, and disruption of sexuality. Patients who have mastectomy for breast cancer or colostomy for colon cancer are especially concerned by body changes that make them feel less attractive and less lovable to their significant other. These reactions may be felt strongly but not verbalized to a caregiver or partner. Depression is a common outcome in 25% of patients who have undergone mastectomy and may manifest as mood disturbances and sexual dysfunction for as long as a year after surgery.[36] The patient who refuses to look at the mastectomy incision or the patient who lets others care for ostomy needs is indicating by this behavior that a serious problem may be present. It is the responsibility of health care professionals to explore patient feelings and concerns and how they believe the bodily change will affect sexual relationships with their partner. The nurse should encourage the inclusion of the partner in any discussion or information-sharing session related to the patient's sexuality or sexual dysfunction fears. Both the patient and partner need to know that because of the surgery, disease process, and decreased energy level in the postoperative and rehabilitation stage, sexual desire or the abilty to perform sexually may be diminished. Alternative methods of sexual expression (e.g., hugging, caressing, alternate positioning) can be suggested and information provided on available corrective measures such as breast reconstructive surgery or penile implants. Grieving a lost body part or function is natural, and the patient should be supported during this time.

In some instances the patient and partner may benefit by referral for sex counseling and education.

## ♦ EVALUATION

To evaluate the effectiveness of nursing interventions, compare patient behaviors with those stated in the expected patient outcomes. Successful achievement of patient outcomes for the cancer patient during the *diagnostic, preoperative, and postoperative phases* is indicated by the following:

*Diagnostic phase*

1. Patient
   a. Feels more relaxed, with anxiety at a manageable level.
   b. Describes the purpose of each diagnostic test and how it will help determine the diagnosis.
2. Family members
   a. Discuss strategies to deal with disruption of roles resulting from family member's illness.
   b. Appoint a liaison person who will communicate family concerns and desires to the health care team and will have input into decisions.

*Preoperative phase*

3. Knowledge of procedure
   a. Discusses and acknowledges a deficit in knowledge of planned surgery.
   b. Asks appropriate questions about intended surgery and expected outcome.
   c. Correctly names surgery to be performed.
   d. Correctly return demonstrates techniques for postoperative care (turning, coughing, breathing, and leg exercises).
4. Knowledge of nutrition
   a. States reasons for being nutritionally compromised or at risk for malnutrition.
   b. Cooperates by consuming diet and nutritional supplements.

*Postoperative phase*

5. Outcome: Able to verbally communicate fear about cancer and surgical outcome.
6. Pain
   a. Reports pain is relieved or controlled.
   b. Describes strategy providing the most effective pain relief.
   c. Uses relaxation technique to achieve pain relief.
7. Infection
   a. Has no evidence of infection during postoperative period.
   b. Able to name accurately the signs and symptoms of infection to report.
   c. Performs good personal hygiene measures.
8. Sexual role
   a. Verbalizes understanding of sexual change as a result of surgery.
   b. Discusses concerns about sex role, altered self-concept, and how this can affect the sex partner.
   c. Asks questions about alternative sexual practices and their techniques.

## RADIOTHERAPY

**Radiotherapy**, or the use of radiation in the treatment of disease, has been employed in the treatment of cancer since the discovery of x-rays in 1895 and radium in 1898. The principal radiation agents are (1) x-ray, which consists of electromagnetic radiation produced by waves of electrical energy traveling at a very high speed, (2) radium, which is a radioactive isotope occurring freely in nature, and (3) the artificially induced radioactive isotopes produced by bombarding the isotopes of elements with highly energized particles in a cyclotron. The most common sources of radiation for external beam therapy are the linear accelerator, the cobalt-60 teletherapy machines, and the betatron. The advantage of using these

### RESEARCH

Weintraub FN, Hogopian GA: The effect of nursing consultation on anxiety, side effects, and self-care of patients receiving radiation therapy, *Oncol Nurs Forum* 17(3) (Suppl):31-38, 1990.

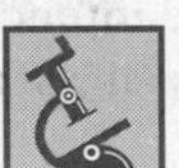

It is estimated that 60% of all patients with cancer will receive radiation therapy at some time during the course of the disease. Most of the treatments will be delivered on an outpatient basis, 5 days per week for an average of 4 to 6 weeks. Previous research findings indicate that anxiety does not decrease with treatment familiarity but tends to increase at the completion of therapy. This study, based on Orem's self-care model, explored the effect of weekly structured nursing consultation sessions on anxiety, severity of side effects experienced, and the number and effectiveness of self-care strategies used by 54 cancer patients undergoing radiation therapy. The experimental group was compared with a control group of cancer patients receiving radiation treatment who did not participate in the nursing consultation sessions and a third group of cancer patients who received standard care during therapy, as well as general health information provided by nurses on a weekly basis. The side effects profile (SEP) and Spielberger's State-Trait Anxiety Inventory (STAI) were used to collect data.

The outcome of this experimental study revealed no significant differences among the three groups in relation to severity of symptoms reported and the number of self-care strategies used. A limitation of this study was the lack of analysis of the presence or absence of differences among the three groups in the number and severity of side effects experienced, the number of self-care measures implemented, and the effectiveness of the self-care actions. The level of anxiety for the nursing consultation group, however, was consistently lower over time than the anxiety scores for the control and health-education groups. This study finding alone suggests that nursing interventions can have a positive effect on patient anxiety during radiation therapy.

high-energy x-ray beams lies in their ability to penetrate to a greater depth beneath the skin surface. Skin damage is kept to a minimum because only about 20% of the prescribed radiation dose is delivered to the skin. Orthovoltage or superficial x-ray beams deliver 100% of their dosage to the skin, creating greater integumentary side effects.[5] With high-energy beams, higher doses can be administered with fewer side effects.

Radiotherapy is effective in curing cancer in some instances; in other instances it controls the growth of cancer cells for a time. Because it may deter the growth of cancer cells, it may relieve pain even when extension of the disease is such that cure is impossible.

Radiation therapy is increasingly being used in lieu of surgery, particularly in patients with cancer of the larynx, prostate, and breast and in malignant melanoma of the eye. Research is directed toward modifying radiosensitivity and toward improving radiation therapy's effects on hypoxic tumor cells. See Research box, p. 396.

## Principle Underlying Radiotherapy

Radiation dose is prescribed in units called *grays* (Gy). In the past the dosage was measured by the amount of radiant energy absorbed by tissues and expressed in the unit *rad.* Both terms are used in radiation literature and often are referred to interchangeably (see Box 16-11). Ionizing radiation causes cell death either through direct damage to the double strands of DNA or as a consequence of biochemical changes that interfere with cellular repair and reproduction. Before radiation therapy is prescribed as a treatment modality, the radiosensitivity of the tissue targeted must be ascertained. *Radiosensitivity* is a measure of the potential susceptibility of cells to injury from ionizing radiation and the speed at which damage will occur. All body tissue has a known degree of radiosensitivity. The radiation oncologist must consider the maximal treatment dosage that can be administered safely without compromising th normal tissues surrounding the tumor. Other considerations include the patient's age, tumor size and stage, degree of spread, and the overall prognosis if radiation is used for treating the tumor. Table 16-17 lists selected organs with their sensitivity to radiation.

Cells that are in the mitosis (M) phase of the cell proliferative cycle are the most sensitive to the effects of radiation. However, damage also can occur during DNA synthesis (S) and during the resting phase ($G_0$).[23] Tissues that have high proliferative rates are most affected by radiation, such as the bone marrow, skin, and gastrointestinal tract. Tumor resistance to radiation is a major problem. Tissue hypoxia is one of the major factors contributing to radioresistance. Hypoxic cells are known to be *radioresistant* and require about three times as much radiation dosage as a well-oxygenated cell requires to achieve the same degree of cell kill. Cell kill refers to the number of tumor cells that are expected to be destroyed during the most sensitive phases of the cell cycle after a radiation treatment. Tumor cells become hypoxic when, because of tumor growth, they become more distanced from their nearest capillary blood supply. Oxygen is metabolized by and useful to only cells nearest to the capillary.

The mechanism of how hypoxia makes a cell radioresistant is not fully understood. It is believed, however, that oxygen present in a tumor cell makes the cell more radiosensitive by its ability to interact with free radicals and bind them into inorganic compounds, thus impairing cellular repair.[5]

A radiation treatment can range in time from 1 minute to a few minutes. The exact time depends on the dose to be delivered, the energy, the type of radiation beam, and the depth of the tumor. Frequency of treatment varies, with some patients being treated daily, five times per week.

In some cases patients may receive a "split course" of therapy by receiving part of the total dose followed by a rest of 1 to 2 weeks until the final high dose is achieved. Split course or fractionation is advantageous for several reasons. Normal cells that received a sublethal dose of radiation have time to repair the damage incurred. Tumor cells that were in a nonsensitive cycle phase may progress to a more radiosensitive phase; therefore a larger cell kill will be attained when treat-

**BOX 16-11 Terms Related to Radiation**

| Term | Definition |
|---|---|
| Roentgen | Amount of radiation exposure in the air |
| Rad | Amount of radiation absorbed per dose (1 rad = 100 ergs/g) |
| Gray (Gy) | International measure: 1 gray = 100 rad |
| Rem | Unit of measure used to express the biologic effect of one rad of x-rays |

**TABLE 16-17 Radiosensitivity of Selected Body Organs**

| ORGAN | RADIOSENSITIVITY |
|---|---|
| Bone marrow | High |
| Ovaries | |
| Testes | |
| Intestine | |
| Skin | Medium high |
| Oral cavity and esophagus | |
| Vagina, cervix | |
| Growing bone and cartilage | Medium |
| Fine vasculature | |
| Mature bone and cartilage | Medium low |
| Kidney | |
| Liver | |
| Thyroid | |
| Muscle | Low |
| Brain and spinal cord | |

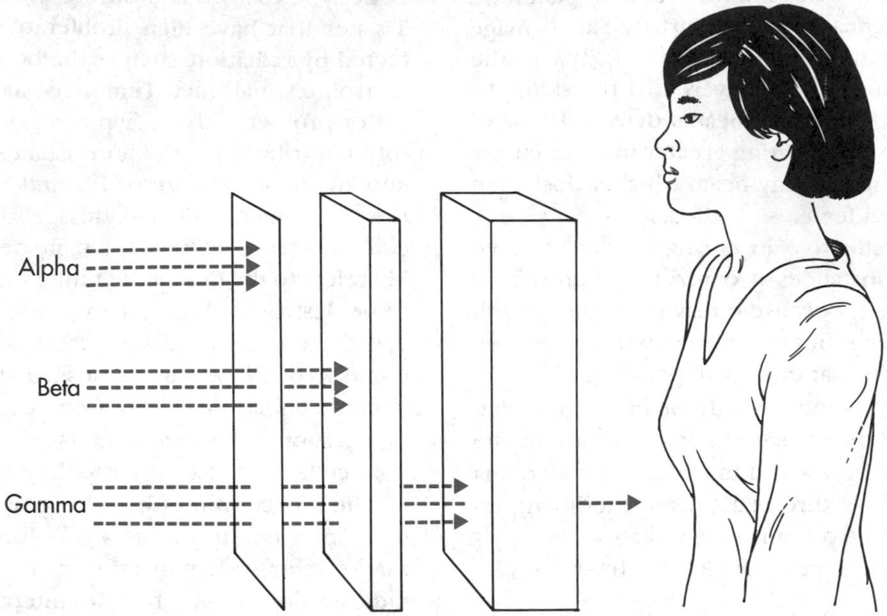


**FIGURE 16-9** Relative penetrating power of three types of radiation. (Modified from Bouchard-Kurtz R, Speese-Owens N: *Nursing care of the cancer patient,* ed 4, St Louis, 1981, Mosby.)

ment is resumed. Probably the most compelling reason to use fractionation is to provide time for reoxygenation of tumor cells, making them more sensitive to radiation effects.

The radiation used medically consists of alpha- ($\alpha$-), beta- ($\beta$-), and gamma- ($\gamma$-) rays (Figure 16-9). The $\alpha$- and $\beta$-rays cannot pass through the skin; $\gamma$-rays, however, have been found to penetrate several inches of lead, although lead shielding offers a considerable degree of protection. X-rays, which are similar to $\gamma$-rays, require lead protection.

Radiation can be delivered to the patient *externally* by exposure to rays, such as from an x-ray machine or from cobalt-60, or *internally,* either by placing radioactive material such as radium within the tissues or body cavity (sealed internal radiation) or by administering the materials intravenously or orally so that they are distributed throughout the body (unsealed internal radiation).

## EXTERNAL RADIOTHERAPY

Before any treatment is initiated, the patient will be thoroughly examined in the radiation oncology department and undergo a simulation phase. It is during simulation that the precise target area is defined and outlined with either ink markings or small permanent tatoo markings called *ports.* These outlines are essential so that only this small, defined area is within the radiation field.

Different ports may be used on different days, or the position may be changed at intervals during a daily treatment so that only a certain amount of radiation is given through each of several ports. When immobilizing or positioning devices are deemed necessary to help maintain proper positioning during the treatment, they are made specifically for the patient. The very young and elderly persons often require casts or molds, special boards, or safety belts. The need for organ-shielding devices also are determined during simulation. The pretreatment phase may require several sessions in the radiation oncology department. A picture of the patient in the exact position, with immobilizing devices and shields, is kept in the patient's treatment file. The photograph helps the technician responsible for administering the treatment to correctly position the patient. The technician must document the treatment number, the cumulative dose, patient positioning and immobilizing devices used, and any specific patient concerns or problems encountered.

External radiation therapy sometimes is used in conjunction with surgery, either for curative intent or for palliation of symptoms. Radiation therapy used alone can cure cancer of the skin, oral cavity, larynx, uterine cervix, prostate, pelvis, and Hodgkin's disease stages I, II, and IIIA. When radiation is used in conjunction with surgery, cancers of the head and neck, lung, breast, uterus, bladder, bone, and testes can be cured. When cure is the anticipated outcome of combined surgery and external radiation, the radiation may be administered preoperatively or postoperatively. The rationale for preoperative treatment is to decrease the tumor size and increase the potential for removal of all the tumor

**TABLE 16-18 Characteristics of Some Commonly Used Radioactive Agents**

| RADIATION SOURCE | HALF-LIFE (WHERE APPLICABLE) | RAYS EMITTED | APPEARANCE OR FORM | METHOD OF ADMINISTRATION |
|---|---|---|---|---|
| X-ray | — | γ | Invisible rays | X-ray machine |
| Radium | 1600 yr | α<br>β | In needles, plaques, molds | Interstitial (needles)<br>Intracavitary (plaques, mold) |
| Radon | 4 days | α<br>β<br>γ (low intensity) | In seeds, needles | Interstitial (seeds, needles) |
| Cesium ($^{137}Cs$) | 33 yr | β<br>γ | In needles, capsules | Interstitial (needles)<br>Intracavitary (capsules) |
| Cobalt ($^{60}Co$) | 5 yr | β<br>γ | External (cobalt unit)<br>Internal (needles, seeds, molds) | Machine (teletherapy)<br>Interstitial (needles, seeds) |
| Iodine ($^{131}I$) | 8 days | β<br>γ (low intensity) | Clear liquid | By mouth |
| Phosphorus ($^{32}P$) | 14 days | β | Clear liquid | By mouth, intracavitary, intravenous |
| Gold ($^{198}Au$) | 3 days | β<br>γ | Purple liquid | Intracavitary |
| Iridium ($^{198}Ir$) | 74 days | β<br>γ (low intensity) | In needles, wires, seeds | Interstitial |
| Yttrium ($^{90}Y$) | 3 days | β | Beads, needles | Interstitial |

during surgery, to eradicate subclinical disease that might be present beyond the intended surgical field, and to eradicate lymph nodes where disease could form or provide a mode for metastasis. The disadvantage of preoperative radiation concerns the delay in wound healing of normal tissues that were within the treatment field and thus damaged.

Postoperative radiation therapy usually is performed to eradicate any residual tumor and subclinical disease. Higher doses can be administered than could have been used before surgery. The most cited disadvantage of postoperative therapy is the delay in starting treatments until after wound healing is complete. Combination radiation therapy and chemotherapy are discussed in the chemotherapy section.

Patients receiving radiation therapy should know that they will be attended by radiotherapists who will be stationed outside the treatment room, observe the treatment on a television screen, and be in communication at all times. There is no pain associated with radiation therapy.

## Brachytherapy (Internal Radiation Therapy)

**Brachytherapy** is the placement of radioactive sources on or directly into a tumor. Internal radiation may be delivered by sealed or unsealed methods. In either type special precautions may be necessary, depending on the amount of radioactive material used, its location, and the kind of rays being emitted (Table 16-18). Special precautions may be taken if more than a tracer diagnostic dose has been given. Hospitals in which therapeutic doses of radioactive isotopes are administered are required to have a radiation safety officer. Quite often this person is a physicist. The radiation safety officer determines the precautions to be observed in each situation. Most hospitals have printed instruction sheets stating the precautions to be followed for each substance used. Personnel should be fully acquainted with all precautions and should be supervised in carrying them out. Generally, the patient will be placed in a private room while the radioactive substance is in place. A radiation precaution sign is placed on the door to the patient's room, and visitors are restricted.

### Sealed Internal Radiotherapy

Sealed internal radiotherapy is used to deliver a concentrated dose of radiation directly to the malignant lesion or tumor area. Usually this involves insertion of radioactive substances within hollow cavities or within tissues. The radioactive isotopes commonly used are cobalt-60, iridium-192, iodine-125, phosphorus-32, cesium-137, gold-198, and radium-226. These radioactive substances may be used in the form of molds, plaques, needles, wires, special applicators, or ribbons.

Placement of the sealed container may be carried out in the operating room, radiation department, or the treatment room. Exact positioning is essential so that radiation exposure to surrounding tissues and organs is minimized. X-ray films are taken to verify appropriate placement. The patient may then return to a private hospital room where the radioactive substance is inserted. This is called *afterloading* and is a technique

**TABLE 16-19 Cancers Treated With Brachytherapy**

| CANCER | TECHNIQUE | RADIOACTIVE SOURCE |
|---|---|---|
| Endometrial | Intracavitary | Radium, cesium |
| Cervical | Intracavitary | Radium, cesium |
| Prostate | Interstitial | Iodine, gold |
| Breast | Interstitial | Iridium |
| Ocular melanoma | Plaque therapy | Cobalt, iodine |
| Head and neck | Interstitial thermal | Iridium, cesium |
| Rectal | Interstitial | Cesium |
| Esophageal | Intraluminal | Cesium |
| Bronchogenic | Endobronchial | Iridium, iodine |

From Dow KH, Helderley LJ: *Nursing care in radiation oncology,* Philadelphia, 1992, WB Saunders.

used to prevent unnecessary exposure of staff members in various departments to the radiation source. The length of time the radiation material is left in place depends on the element used and the dose that has been prescribed. Time may range from a few hours to several days. Table 16-19 lists cancers treated with brachytherapy.

## Unsealed Internal Radiotherapy

Unsealed internal radiation is delivered to the patient by mouth as an "atomic cocktail" or as a liquid instilled into a body cavity. Exposure for persons caring for the patient can result from direct contact with emanations of the substance from the patient (external exposure) or from contact with the patient's discharges that contain the radioactive substances (internal exposure). It may be inhaled, ingested, or absorbed through the skin. The exposure varies with each of the substances used, and safety for the staff members caring for the patient depends on a thorough knowledge of the substance used and its action within the body. If only tracer doses (very small amounts) of radioactive substances are used, as for diagnostic purposes, no precautions are necessary.

Radioisotopes commonly used for unsealed brachytherapy include radioactive iodine ($^{131}I$), phosphorus ($^{32}P$), and gold ($^{198}Au$). These substances may be administered orally or intravenously or by direct instillation into a body cavity. Each isotope can be a source of radiation contamination to health care personnel. The mode of elimination from the body varies with the specific isotope, but generally traces may be found in urine, feces, vomitus, sputum, wound drainage, and perspiration. Specific instructions will be provided by radiation oncology personnel regarding precautions needed to protect staff members working with these patients.

## Protection of Health Care Professionals From Radiation Hazards

Radiation delivered externally (including x-rays) can harm persons working with the patient *only during* the time that the patient is being treated. This is true also

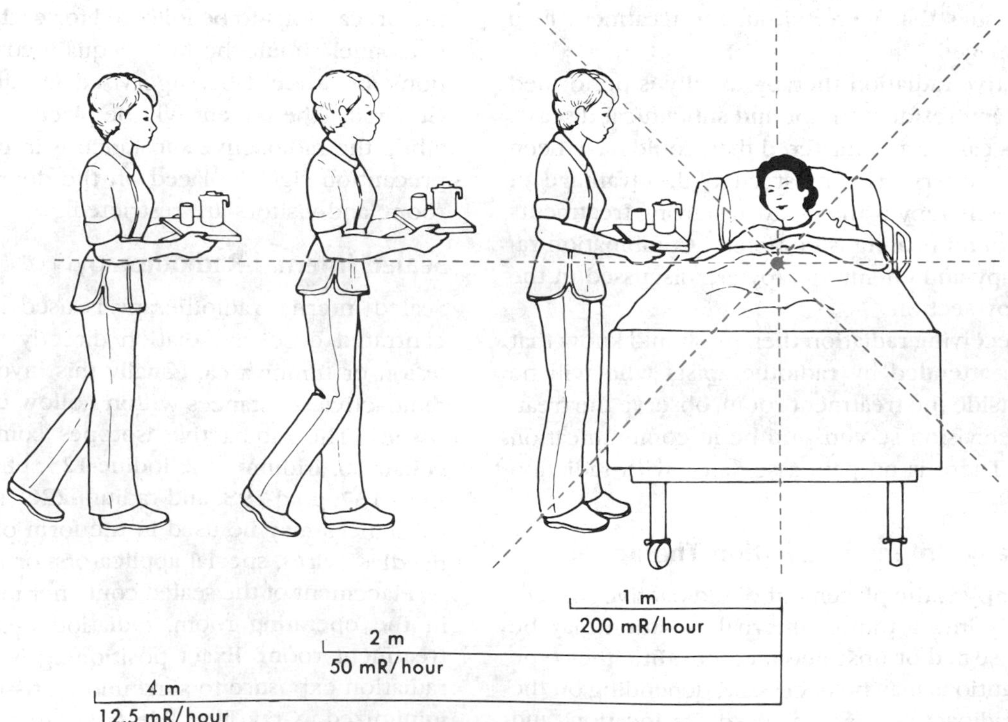


**FIGURE 16-10** Nurse nearest source of radioactivity (patient) is exposed to more radioactivity. (Modified from Bouchard-Kurtz R, Speese-Owens N: *Nursing care of the cancer patient,* ed 4, St Louis, 1981, Mosby.)

of the radiation from some radioactive substances used for other methods of treatment. Patients with internal radiation that emits γ-rays, however, may expose other persons to radiation for varying periods of time, and the time one can be exposed safely to the patient is important in planning care. The time interval required for the radioactive substance to be half dissipated is called its *half-life* (see Table 16-18). This period varies extremely widely, but as the end of the half-life is reached, danger from exposure decreases.

Exposure to radiation can be controlled in three ways: ***time, distance,*** and ***shielding.*** All emanations are subject to the physical law of inverse-square. For example, a person who stands 2 meters away from the source of radiation receives only one fourth as much exposure as when standing only 1 meter away. At 4 meters only one sixteenth of the exposure will be received. Therefore increasing the distance from the emanations decreases the exposure (Figure 16-10). ***Lead-lined gloves and a lead apron, which act as a shield to reduce exposure, should be worn by anyone who attends patients during x-ray treatment or during examination by fluoroscopy.***

High dose rate (HDR) brachytherapy is now being used for the treatment of inoperable lung cancer and for the palliation of cough, dyspnea, and hemoptysis. Therapy can be performed on an outpatient basis, because treatment time may be as little as a few minutes, and can be repeated in 2-week intervals. This treatment of lung cancer has only a local effect and no therapeutic effect on lymph nodes or metastatic disease.[24] The future role of this type of brachytherapy is not yet known.

## Side Effects of Radiation Therapy

When radiation therapy is used, some degree of radiation reaction may occur. The frequency and severity of reaction depend on the type of equipment used, the physician's treatment plan, and the patient's compliance with therapy. Early radiation reactions can be observed almost immediately after treatments begin. They generally are mild and last no more than several weeks. The side effects include both local (skin) and systemic sequelae such as fatigue, nausea, diarrhea, and bone marrow suppression. The damage is the result of radiation's effects on actively proliferating cells and the release of catabolic products as cells die. Intervention is of a supportive nature. If these self-limiting reactions become too disabling, their effects can be avoided or lessened by reducing the daily radiation dose.

Late radiation reactions can occur many months or years after therapy. The late effects are a progression of the earlier self-limiting reactions and are more localized than systemic. Debate as to the underlying cause of these late-occurring sequelae range from endarteritis of small vessels and proliferation of connective tissue damage to slowly proliferating cells.[33] Late effects usually are permanent.

Radiation therapy, although one of the major cancer treatment modalities, does have carcinogenic potential. The mechanism by which radiation induces cancer is not fully known at this time. It appears that cancers induced by radiation may be a combination of heredity and environmental factors that initiate or promote tumor growth.[8] It is known that secondary malignant conditions may develop in patients previously treated with radiation therapy. Leukemia or non-Hodgkin's lymphoma may develop in patients receiving irradiation for Hodgkin's disease, and breast cancer may develop in women who undergo multiple fluoroscopy.

Bone marrow suppression is almost always a side effect of radiation therapy. The recovery of bone marrow depends on the dose used and the tumor volume treated. When the total treatment dose exceeds 3000 cGy, the marrow is replaced by fatty and fibrous tissue.[33] Full bone marrow recovery is generally expected after chemotherapy, but full recovery may never be achieved after radiation therapy. (Table 16-20 indicates the early and late sequelae of radiation therapy; Table 16-21 presents a toxicity grading system used for evaluating radiation therapy's effects on specific tissues and organ systems.) It is important that patients be provided with information about the immediate and long-term side effects of therapy so that they can make informed decisions related to therapy.

# NURSING MANAGEMENT

## ♦ ASSESSMENT

The nurse working with the patient who is to receive radiation therapy should assess the following:

1. Understanding of the cancer diagnosis and the expected outcome of treatment with radiation (cure, palliation, adjunct)
2. Knowledge of the radiation treatment protocol
    a. Number of treatments
    b. Total dose in Grays (Gy) or rads
    c. Total length of treatment
    d. Area of body to be irradiated
3. Previous history of treatment with radiation therapy
4. Physical and emotional health, including skin integrity in treatment field
5. Knowledge of what to expect while receiving a radiation treatment
    a. Alone in room; monitored on TV screen and able to talk to technicians
    b. No sensation during treatment
    c. May be immobilized with special molds, casts, etc.
6. Knowledge of most common side effects of radiation treatment
7. Understanding of measures to prevent skin irritation and enhance activities of daily living during treatment

**TABLE 16-20 Possible Sequelae of Radiation Therapy**

| ANATOMIC SITE | ACUTE SEQUELAE (EARLY) | LATE SEQUELAE |
|---|---|---|
| Brain | Earache, headache, dizziness, hair loss, erythema | Hearing loss, damage to middle or inner ear, pituitary gland dysfunction, cataracts, and brain necrosis |
| Head and neck | Odynophagia, dysphagia, hoarseness, xerostomia, dysgeusia, weight loss | Subcutaneous fibrosis, skin ulceration, necrosis, thyroid dysfunction, dental decay, osteoradionecrosis of mandible, delayed wound healing, damage to middle and inner ear |
| Lung and mediastinum or esophagus | Odynophagia, dysphagia, cough, hoarseness, pneumonitis, carditis | Progressive fibrosis of lung, dyspnea, chronic cough; esophageal stricture<br>Rare: chronic pericarditis, myelopathy |
| Breast or chest wall | Odynophagia, dysphagia, hoarseness, cough; pneumonitis (asymptomatic); carditis; cytopenia | Fibrosis, retraction of breast; lung fibrosis; arm edema; chronic endocarditis, myocardial infarction<br>Rare: osteonecrosis of ribs |
| Abdomen or pelvis | Nausea, vomiting, abdominal pain, diarrhea; urinary frequency, dysuria, nocturia; cytopenia | Proctitis, sigmoiditis; rectal or sigmoid stricture; colonic perforation or obstruction; contracted bladder, urinary incontinence, hematuria, vesicovaginal fistula; rectovaginal fistula; leg edema; scrotal edema, sexual impotency; vaginal retraction or scarring; sterilization<br>Rare: damage to liver or kidneys |
| Extremities | Erythema, dry/moist desquamation | Subcutaneous fibrosis; ankylosis, edema; bone/soft tissue necrosis |

From Perez CA, Brady LW: *Principles and practices of radiation oncology,* ed 2, Philadelphia, 1992, JB Lippincott.

## ♦ NURSING DIAGNOSES

Nursing diagnoses are determined from analysis of patient data. Nursing diagnoses for the patient receiving radiation therapy may include but are not limited to the following:

| Diagnostic Title | Possible Etiologic Factors |
|---|---|
| Knowledge deficit (related to radiation therapy as cancer treatment) | Lack of information on how radiation affects cancer cells and the body; lack of information on expected outcome of therapy on disease process; lack of interest or readiness in learning about radiation therapy |
| Skin integrity, high risk for impaired (related to radiation therapy for cancer) | Radiation effects on skin, nutritional deficits, elderly age-group |

## ♦ EXPECTED PATIENT OUTCOMES

Expected patient outcomes for the patient *receiving radiation therapy for cancer treatment* may include but are not limited to the following:

1. Knowledge of radiotherapy procedure
   a. Describes why radiation therapy will be used to treat the cancer.
   b. Correctly describes the treatment plan for his or her particular disease process.
   c. Identifies the most common side effects to expect as a result of radiation treatment.
2. Knowledge of effects
   a. Identifies potential skin changes that may occur with radiation therapy.
   b. Demonstrates measures to prevent increasing skin impairment while undergoing radiation therapy.

## ♦ INTERVENTIONS

Radiation as a treatment modality for cancer can be a frightening prospect because of the many misconceptions and misinformation that surround it. Study of the needs of oncology patients who had undergone radiation therapy revealed that the need to receive correct information about radiation as a treatment method, its possible side effects, and treatment outcome was the number-one priority.[39]

Radiation has a "mysterious" mystique. Fear of radiation has been intensified because of media coverage of nuclear accidents in the United States at Three Mile Island and at Chernobyl in Russia. The general public has concerns about the potential lethal consequences of exposure to radiation. Some patients fear becoming "radioactive" and being a danger to anyone with whom they come in contact. The nurse can play a major role in dispelling patient and family fears of radiation therapy by assessing their understanding of how the treatment will be used; conveying correct information; and teaching about management strategies to employ during the course of therapy.

### Providing Patient Education

The nurse teaches the most common side effects that are anticipated: skin changes and the effects on the bone marrow. Patients must be informed that their body's reaction to radiation will depend on their age, nutritional status, stage and extent of the disease process, whether the tumor is radiosensitive, and whether the area has

**TABLE 16-21 Acute Radiation Toxicity Grading Scale for Specific Tissues and Organ Systems**

| ORGAN/TISSUE | 0 | GRADE 1 | GRADE 2 | GRADE 3 | GRADE 4 |
|---|---|---|---|---|---|
| Skin | No change over baseline | Follicular, faint or dull erythema, epilation, dry desquamation, decreased sweating | Tender erythema, epilation, dry desquamation, moderate edema | Moist desquamation other than skin folds, pitting edema | Ulceration hemorrhage, necrosis |
| Mucous membrane | No change over baseline | May experience mild pain not requiring analgesic | Patchy mucositis; may experience moderate pain requiring analgesic | Fibrinous mucositis; may include severe pain requiring narcotic | Ulceration, hemorrhage, or necrosis |
| Salivary gland | No change over baseline | Mild mouth dryness; slightly thickened saliva; slightly altered taste such as metallic | Moderate to complete dryness; thick, sticky saliva, markedly altered taste | — | Acute salivary gland necrosis |
| Pharynx and esophagus | No change over baseline | Mild dysphagia or odynophagia; may require topical anesthetic or nonnarcotic analgesics, soft diet | Moderate dysphagia or odynophagia; may require narcotic analgesics; puréed or liquid diet | Severe dysphagia or odynophagia with dehydration or weight loss >15% from pretreatment baseline requiring NG feeding tube, IV fluids, or hyperalimentation | Complete obstruction, ulceration, perforation, fistula |
| Upper GI | No change over baseline | Anorexia with <5% weight loss; nausea not requiring antiemetics; abdominal discomfort not requiring analgesics or parasympatholytic drugs | Anorexia with <15% weight loss; nausea or vomiting requiring antiemetics; abdominal pain requiring analgesics | Anorexia with >15% weight loss or requiring NG tube or parenteral support; nausea or vomiting requiring NG tube or parenteral support; abdominal pain (severe); hematemesis or melena; distention | Ileus, obstruction, perforation, GI bleeding; abdominal pain requiring tube decompression or bowel diversion |
| Lower GI including pelvis | No change over baseline | Increased frequency or change in bowel habits not requiring medication; rectal discomfort not requiring analgesics | Diarrhea requiring parasympatholytic drugs; mucous discharge; rectal or abdominal pain requiring analgesics | Diarrhea requiring parenteral support; severe mucous or blood discharge; abdominal distention | Obstruction, fistula or perforation, GI bleeding, abdominal pain or tenesmus requiring tube decompression or bowel diversion |
| Lung | No change over baseline | Mild symptoms—dry cough or dyspnea on exertion | Persistent cough requiring narcotic, antitussive agents; dyspnea with minimal effort but not at rest | Severe cough unresponsive to medications or dyspnea at rest; radiologic evidence of acute pneumonitis; oxygen or steroids required | Severe respiratory insufficiency; continuous oxygen or assisted ventilation |
| CNS | No change over baseline | Fully functional status with minor neurologic findings; no medication needed | Neurologic findings require home care; nursing assistance may be required; medication including steroids and antiseizure agents required | Neurologic findings require hospitalization | Serious neurologic impairment and may include paralysis, coma, or seizures; hospitalization required |

Modified from Perez CA, Brady LW: *Principles and practices of radiation oncology,* ed 2, Philadelphia, 1992, JB Lippincott.

*Continued.*

**TABLE 16-21 Acute Radiation Toxicity Grading Scale for Specific Tissues and Organ Systems—cont'd**

| ORGAN/TISSUE | 0 | GRADE 1 | GRADE 2 | GRADE 3 | GRADE 4 |
|---|---|---|---|---|---|
| Genitourinary | No change over baseline | Frequency or nocturia twice pretreatment habit; dysuria, urgency not requiring medication | Frequency or nocturia less frequent than every hour; dysuria, urgency, bladder spasm requiring local anesthetic | Frequency and nocturia hourly or more frequently; dysuria, pelvic pain, or bladder spasm requiring regular, frequent narcotic; gross hematuria | Hematuria requiring transfusion; acute bladder obstruction not secondary to clot, ulceration, or necrosis |

been previously irradiated. Careful assessment and history information will help provide these data, as well as furnish a beginning point for identifying teaching needs and allaying any psychologic concerns about the treatment. Age is more of a factor if the patient is older than 65 years. Cancer is a disease that increases in incidence as a person ages. In addition, immune system function declines with age, and regeneration of the bone marrow takes longer in elderly persons. The effects of fatigue are more pronounced, and skin is more fragile and more prone to breakdown.

The nurse provides information about the need for pretreatment consultation and simulation sessions. This will enable the patient and family to understand why treatments cannot be started immediately or why, for some tumors, not at all because of poor sensitivity to radiation. Full disclosure of what to expect during the treatment should substantially decrease anxiety levels.

## Promoting Skin Integrity

The anticipation of probable skin changes (erythema, pruritus) and decreased energy levels as a result of bone marrow depression provides the patient with knowledge of what to expect and some control in handling these outcomes. Maintaining good nutrition with a diet high in carbohydrate, protein, and calories supplies the needed energy requirements and facilitates a more tolerable activity level. Weight is checked weekly to determine if dietary measures are sufficient or if additional supplements are needed. Obtaining sufficient sleep and rest during the treatment phase also promotes the patient's ability to withstand and comply with the treatment plan. The patient should understand that results of laboratory studies (blood counts and chemistry evaluations) will be monitored at intervals to evaluate the effects of therapy on bone marrow production of essential cellular elements (WBC, RBC, platelet count).

The skin changes secondary to radiation are addressed before initiating therapy because changes in skin integrity begin with the first treatment. The slight erythema in the beginning may go unrecognized. The erythema is the result of the radiation effects on capillary blood flow and causes extracapillary cell injury. Vascular vasodilation and congestion occur in phases beginning within minutes of the first treatment, progress to frank erythema in 2 to 3 weeks, and then begin to fade. Long-term effects may occur months after irradiation is completed and are attributed to changes in endothelial permeability, edema, and increased skin temperature.[29]

Teaching skin care by demonstration–return demonstration and supplemented with verbal and written guidelines prevents unnecessary skin discomfort or alleviates existing problems. Measures the patient needs to know to prevent irritation to the radiation treatment field are addressed in the Guidelines box, below. In addition, the nurse should determine the patient's reading ability and comprehension before discharge; written instructions are important because most patients complete treatments on an outpatient basis.

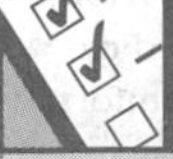

### Guidelines for Preventing Skin Irritation During Radiation Therapy

1. Cleanse radiation field (area within ink markings or inside tattoo outline) daily with mild soap and water. *Do not* erase ink markings if present (Figure 16-11).
2. Clean and keep dry skin folds that overlap and places where moisture collects (obese abdominal skin folds, under and between pendulous breasts, between buttocks or perineum).
3. Avoid use of perfumed soaps, lotions, or deodorant on involved skin surface.
4. Guard against irritation from belts, bras, rough clothing on treatment field. Cotton clothing is least irritating.
5. Do not use heating pads, hot water bottles, or ice packs on treated field.
6. Avoid exposure to sunlight. If unavoidable, use sunscreen for protection.
7. Do not swim in salt water or chlorinated swimming pools.
8. Use an electric razor only to shave within treatment area.
9. Do not scratch dry, itchy skin in treatment field.
10. Do not apply any lotions, powders, or ointments to treated area unless advised to do so by radiologist.

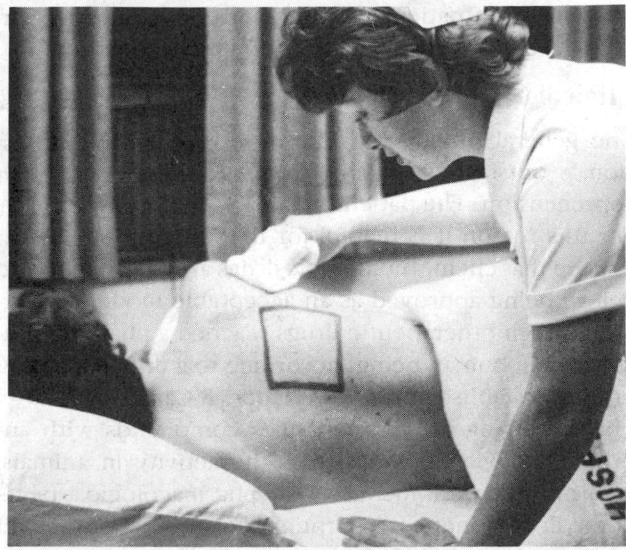

**FIGURE 16-11** When a bath is given, care must be taken not to remove skin markings used to guide the radiologist in giving x-ray treatments.

## ♦ EVALUATION

To evaluate the effectiveness of nursing interventions, compare patient behaviors with those stated in the expected patient outcomes. Successful achievement of patient outcomes for the patient receiving *radiation therapy for cancer* is indicated by the following:

1. Knowledge of radiotherapy procedure
   a. States that radiation therapy will be used to cure the cancerous condition—for example, Hodgkin's disease, prostate cancer, breast cancer.
   b. Correctly identifies the number of treatments and area to be irradiated and why completion of designated number of treatments is important.
   c. Describes correctly the most common side effects of radiation therapy: skin change and bone marrow depression.
2. Knowledge of effects
   a. Discusses why skin integrity may be compromised during radiation therapy.
   b. Demonstrates proper cleansing strategies for skin within treatment field.

## CHEMOTHERAPY

Advances in knowledge of cancer growth and chemotherapeutic agents have led to concomitant advances in cancer treatment. Improvement in overall survival and longer disease-free intervals can be directly ascribed to the use of chemotherapeutic agents, particularly in combination chemotherapy regimens and as adjuvant therapy.

**TABLE 16-22 Neoplastic Disease Response to Chemotherapy**

| RESPONSE | NEOPLASTIC DISEASE |
|---|---|
| Cures in advanced cancer | Gestational trophoblastic tumors<br>Acute lymphoblastic leukemia<br>Acute myeloblastic leukemia<br>Hodgkin's disease<br>Non-Hodgkin's lymphoma (children)<br>Diffuse histiocytic lymphoma<br>Burkitt's lymphoma<br>Testicular tumors |
| Cures with adjuvant chemotherapy | Wilms' tumor<br>Osteogenic sarcoma<br>Rhabdomyosarcoma |
| Minor responses with chemotherapy/adjuvant chemotherapy; no demonstrable prolongation of life | Non–small cell lung carcinoma<br>Head and neck cancer<br>Large bowel cancer<br>Liver cancer<br>Pancreatic cancer<br>Cervical cancer<br>Melanoma<br>Cancer of the adrenal cortex<br>Soft tissue sarcoma |
| Complete and partial remissions with uncertain prolongation of survival with chemotherapy/adjuvant chemotherapy | Multiple myeloma<br>Ovarian cancer<br>Endometrial cancer<br>Neuroblastoma |
| Complete remissions and increased survival with chemotherapy/adjuvant chemotherapy | Breast cancer<br>Small cell lung carcinoma<br>Acute myeloblastic leukemia<br>Non-Hodgkin's lymphoma, indolent<br>Prostate cancer<br>Chronic granulocytic leukemia |

Modified from Krakoff, IH: *CA,* 41:214-278, 1991.

Chemotherapy may be curative or palliative, or have negligible or uncertain effects depending on the type of cancer. Patients and families should be told that "incurable" does not mean untreatable or uncontrollable. Table 16-22 indicates neoplastic disease response to chemotherapy.

In the care of an individual patient with cancer, the expected benefit of chemotherapy (cure, control, or palliation) should be known by the physician, nurse, and patient. This allows for realistic goal setting by the caregivers, patient, and family. Such background also provides a perspective from which to view side effects. The potential for cure, prolonged disease-free survival, or reduction of symptoms is a benefit that most often outweighs the risk and discomfort of short-term toxicity and side effects. ***Conditions in which risk may outweigh benefits*** include overt or occult infections, bleeding dyscrasias, bone marrow depression, severe metabolic disturbances, renal or liver dysfunction, and pregnancy.

In addition, analogs of existing drugs have decreased the toxicity of some drugs. Carboplatin and iproplatin are "second generation" platinum compounds. Epirubicin and idarubicin are analogs of doxorubicin and daunorubicin and are thought to be less cardiotoxic. Many of these second-generation drugs are still in clinical trials.

*Adjuvant chemotherapy* refers to chemotherapy administered in conjunction with other surgery or radiation therapy. It is aimed at the destruction of micrometastases thought likely to be present but too small to be detected by current diagnostic techniques. Left untreated, the micrometastases have a high potential for tumor growth and cancer recurrence. With the use of chemotherapy at a time when the malignant cell population is small and likely to be susceptible, complete tumor cell eradication is possible. The goal is cure.

A feeling of well-being and knowledge that all diagnostic tests are negative for cancer understandably may cause the patient to question the need for adjuvant therapy. This is emphasized when side effects are experienced. A sensitivity to these feelings, coupled with the knowledge of the expected benefit of therapy, is the basis for both patient teaching and the supportive encouragement often needed for continued therapy.

## Clinical Trials

The general public and, at times, health care professionals outside of oncology view chemotherapy with apprehension. The patient may ask, "Am I a guinea pig?" For this reason it is helpful for the nurse to be able to explain that chemotherapeutic drugs are carefully tested before being approved as an acceptable mode of treatment. Chemotherapeutic drugs reached a phase of clinical trial in human beings according to a drug-screening process established by the National Cancer Institute. This screening process identifies compounds with antitumor activity, demonstrates the activity in animals, studies and determines all of the pharmacologic aspects of the drug (kinetics, absorption, dose, metabolism, and excretion), and defines toxicity. The drugs next go through the four phases of clinical trial outlined in Table 16-23. The effectiveness of the new agent is then compared with standard therapy to determine if the new drug is equal to or better than drugs currently used.

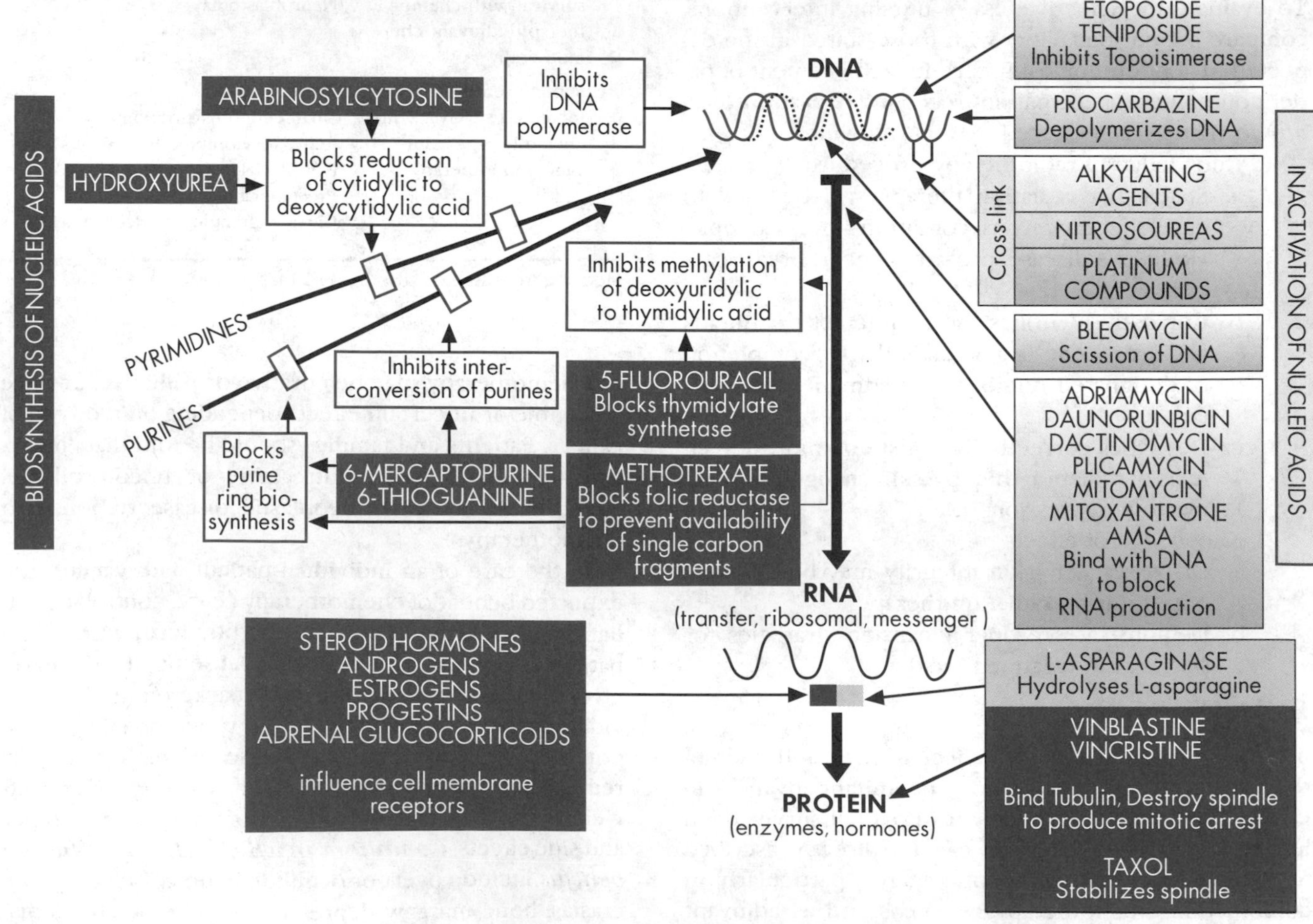


**FIGURE 16-12** Mechanism of action of chemotherapeutic agents in the cell cycle. (Modified from Krakoff IH: *CA* 41:268, 1991.)

**TABLE 16-23 Phases of Clinical Trials for Chemotherapeutic Drugs**

| PHASE | ACTION |
|---|---|
| I | Identify toxic reactions; determine optimal dose within safe limits and set schedule |
| II | Determine extent of antineoplastic activity |
| III | Compare action of new drug with standard antineoplastic drugs |
| IV | Determine effect on advanced cancer, effect of combined therapy with other antineoplastic drugs, and effect with adjuvant therapy |

## Principles of Chemotherapy

Normal and malignant cells progress through various phases in the cell cycle as they replicate (see Figure 16-4). Cancer chemotherapy is based on the actions of certain drugs, creating changes in the cell cycle phases. Figure 16-12 summarizes how some of the commonly used chemotherapeutic agents interrupt cell growth and replication. Drugs such as antimetabolites and vinca alkaloids that are effective during a particular point of the cell cycle are said to be *phase-specific drugs* (Figure 16-13). Drugs that are active throughout the cell cycle *(phase-nonspecific drugs)* include the alkylating agents, antibiotics, nitrosoureas, procarbazine, and dacarbazine (DTIC-Dome). Combinations of cycle-specific and cycle-nonspecific drugs have proved useful in constructing treatment regimens. One major factor that influences

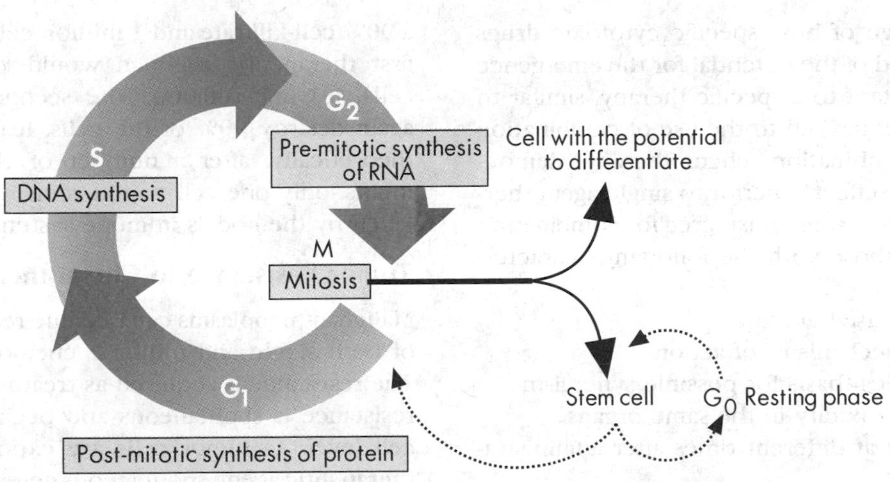


| Cell cycle phase-specific agents | Cell cycle phase-nonspecific agents |
|---|---|

**Cell cycle phase-specific agents**

**G1 Phase**
Asparaginase
Prednisone

**S Phase**
Antimetabolites
Cytarabine
5-Fluorouracil
Hydroxyurea
Methotrexate
Thioguanine

**G2 Phase**
Antibiotic
Bleomycin
Podophyllotoxin
Etoposide

**Mitosis**
Vinca Alkaloids
Vinblastine
Vincristine
Vindesine

**Cell cycle phase-nonspecific agents**

**Alkylating Agents**
Busulfan
Carboplatin
Chlorambucil
Cisplatin
Cyclophosphamide
Ifosfamide
Mechlorethamine
Melphalan

**Antibiotics**
Dactinomycin
Daunorubicin
Doxorubicin
Mitomycin

**Nitrosoureas**
Carmustine (BCNU)
Lomustine (CCNU)
Semustine (MeCCNU)

**Miscellaneous**
Dacarbazine
Procarbazine

**FIGURE 16-13** Common cancer chemotherapeutic agents and their activity within the cell cycle. (Modified from Makwell MB, Maher KE: *Semin Oncol Nurs* 8(2):117, 1992.)

the response of a cancer to chemotherapy is the fraction of tumor cells in replication at a given time, a percentage that varies among different tumors, among individual patients, and at different times in the same patient.

## Cell Population Growth

Chemotherapy is more effective when the tumor is small and growing rapidly, a time when a relatively high proportion of cells are undergoing division. At this time, tumor cells are more sensitive to chemotherapeutic agents that are toxic to dividing cells (phase-specific drugs). Larger, slower-growing tumors respond better to drugs that are effective regardless of whether a cell is dividing (phase-nonspecific drugs). Consequently the physician chooses the appropriate drug or combination of drugs, depending on tumor size and rate of growth.

### BOX 16-12 Principles of Chemotherapy Administration

1. Combination chemotherapy is far superior to single-agent chemotherapy.
2. Complete remission is the minimum requisite for cure and even increased survival.
3. First attempt at chemotherapy offers the best chance for significant benefit; therefore the initial therapy should be the type with maximum effectiveness.
4. Maximum doses of drugs are used to attain maximum tumor cell kill. Dose reduction to minimize toxicity has been called "killing patients with kindness."
5. *Neoadjuvant*, or induction chemotherapy, is always recommended for some specific cancers (breast).
6. Chemoprevention shows promise in prevention of some second primary cancers (head and neck).

## Combination Chemotherapy

Increased knowledge of how specific cytotoxic drugs exert their effect and of the potential for the emergence of tumor cells resistant to a specific therapy, similar to antibiotic resistance, has led to the use of combination chemotherapy. Combination chemotherapy demonstrates a therapeutic effect superior to single-agent therapy for many cancers. Drugs considered for combination chemotherapy are those with the following characteristics:

1. Are active when used alone
2. Have different mechanisms of action
3. Have a biochemical basis for possible synergism
4. Do not produce toxicity in the same organs
5. Produce toxicity at different times after administration

Repeated brief courses of drug therapy are given to reduce immunosuppressive effects. Principles of chemotherapy administration are listed in Box 16-12.

## Cell-Kill Hypothesis

The cell-kill hypothesis explains why patients must often have several or more courses of chemotherapy. Chemotherapy is thought to kill a fixed percentage of the total number of cancer cells. Theoretically, if a drug had a 90% cell-kill rate and 1 million cells were present, the first therapeutic regimen would kill 900,000 cancer cells, leaving 100,000. The second treatment would again destroy 90% of the cells, leaving 10,000. Again, theoretically, after a number of chemotherapy treatments, only one cell would remain and that would be killed by the body's immune system (Figure 16-14).

## Tumor Resistance to Chemotherapy

Malignant neoplasms can become resistant to the effects of both single and multiple chemotherapeutic agents. The resistance is acquired as treatment progresses. The resistance is spontaneous and begins at the individual cell level. As tumor cells are exposed to the chemotherapeutic agent, spontaneous genetic alterations occur such as mutations, translocations, and deletions that are then passed on as the cell divides. With each cell division the chance of developing drug resistance becomes greater. This phenomenon can be seen in the treatment of hematologic cancers such as acute leukemia and non-Hodgkin's lymphoma. At initial diagnosis 90% of patients with these conditions will respond effectively to a wide range of medications. When the disease relapses, the chemoresponse is less frequent and extends over a

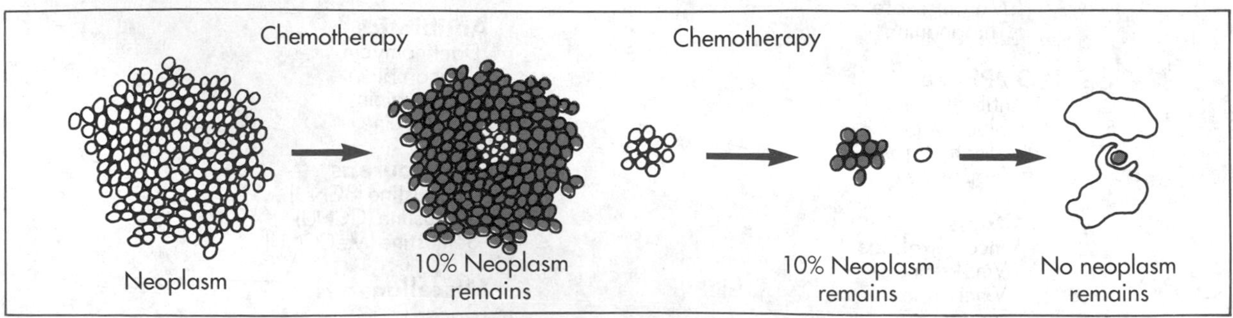


**FIGURE 16-14** Cell-kill theory. Chemotherapy destroys 90% of neoplasm; repeated chemotherapy repeats process until last neoplastic cell is killed by body's immune response. (Modified from *Cancer: chemotherapy and care,* Part I, Syracuse, NY, Bristol Laboratories.)

shorter period of time. The chance of a cure with use of the same drugs is therefore considerably reduced. As a consequence of this poor response to chemotherapy, the tumor burden (size) increases because cells are no longer sensitive to the chemotherapeutic agent and are not destroyed. Another example of drug resistance is seen in slow-growing tumors such as colon cancer in which fewer numbers of stem cells are present that are capable of self-renewal (differentiation). These tumors require more cell divisions to become the same size as fast-growing tumors (lymphomas). Therefore these types of malignant tumors also have an increased chance to develop drug resistance.[13]

Multiple-drug resistance (MDR) can occur when several agents are used in combination. MDR is achieved as described for single events even though their mechanism of action on the cell may occur at different phases of the cell cycle. Drugs that are known to become cross resistant include doxorubicin, daunorubicin, vinblastine, vincristine, Taxol, and etoposide.[13]

## Protection of Health Care Professionals from Chemotherapy Hazards

Some chemotherapeutic drugs are fetotoxic and carcinogenic. Health care workers who handle antineoplastic drugs can be exposed to low doses of the drug by direct contact, inhalation, and injection. Because the long-term effects of chronic exposure are not completely known

### Guidelines for Safety in Handling Chemotherapeutic Agents

A. Prevention of inhalation of aerosols
  1. Mix all drugs in an approved class II biologic safety cabinet (these contain a vertical laminar air-flow hood), wearing gloves at all times.
  2. Prime all IV bags containing drugs under the hood, if possible; use a maintenance bag of normal saline or D5W to prime the tubing and all the chemotherapy bags afterward.
  3. Use a needle with a hydrophobic filter to remove drugs from vials when in settings without a safety cabinet. Mix in a well-ventilated area with a pattern of air flow away from the drug preparer's face.
  4. Break ampules by wrapping a sterile gauze pad or alcohol wipe around the neck (decreases chance of droplet contamination).
  5. Vent vials with a hydrophobic filter needle (equalizes internal pressure).
  6. Do not clip needles, break syringes, or remove needles from syringes when disposing of them.
  7. Use a gauze pad when removing syringes and needles from IV injection ports or spikes from IV bags.

B. Prevention of drug absorption through the skin
  1. Wear surgical latex gloves and a gown made of low-permeability fabric with a closed front and cuffed long sleeves.
  2. Change gloves every 30 minutes if working consistently with drugs.
  3. Remove gloves immediately after spilling drug solution on them or puncturing or tearing them.
  4. Wash hands before putting on gloves and after removing them.
  5. Cover the work surface with a plastic-backed absorbent pad; change pad when cabinet is cleaned or after a spill.
  6. Clean all surfaces of the biologic safety cabinet before and after drug preparation: use 70% alcohol and a disposable towel. Discard towel in a leak-proof chemical-waste container.
  7. Use syringes and IV sets with Luer-Lok fittings.
  8. Place an absorbent pad under injection sites to catch accidental spillage.
  9. Label all antineoplastic drugs with a chemotherapy hazard label.
  10. Wash skin areas thoroughly with soap and water as soon as possible in the event of skin contact with drugs.
  11. Flush eyes with eye solution or clean water in the event of eye contact; seek medical attention.

C. Prevention of ingestion
  1. Do not eat, drink, chew gum, apply cosmetics, or smoke in drug-preparation areas.
  2. Keep all food and eating items away from the preparation area.
  3. Do not place food or drink in the same refrigerator with drugs.
  4. Wash hands before and after preparing or giving drugs.
  5. Avoid hand-to-mouth or hand-to-eye contact when handling the drugs.

D. Ensuring safe disposal
  1. Discard gowns and gloves after contamination in a waterproof container marked as contaminated waste.
  2. Discard and identify waste products in leak-proof, sealable plastic bags that are marked with a color, and label to indicate contents.
  3. Use puncture-proof containers for noncapped, nonclipped needles and sharp, breakable items.
  4. Keep waste containers in labeled, covered waste containers for disposal.
  5. Housekeeping personnel should be instructed in safe procedures and should wear surgical latex gloves and gowns.
  6. Place all drugs used in home chemotherapy in a leak-proof container; remove from home to a designated disposal area.

E. Prevention of contamination by body fluids
  1. Provide tight-fitting lid for urinals.
  2. Wear latex surgical gloves when handling body fluids.
  3. Place waterproof pad over toilet bowl before flushing to avoid splashing.
  4. Empty waste products into the toilet by pouring close to the water to avoid splashing. Close the lid and flush two to three times (in the home).
  5. Wear gloves and gown when handling linen soiled with body fluids; place in isolation linen bag for separate laundry.
  6. Place soiled linens in separate, washable pillow cases and wash twice, separately from other household linens (in the home).

Modified from Gullo SM: *Oncol Nurs Forum* 15:596-602, 1988.

**TABLE 16-24 Chemotherapeutic Agents by Classification, Route of Administration, and Side Effects**

| AGENTS | PRINCIPLE ROUTE OF ADMINISTRATION | NADIR* (DAYS) | ACUTE TOXIC SIGNS | MAJOR TOXIC MANIFESTATIONS |
|---|---|---|---|---|
| **ALKYLATING AGENTS** | | | | |
| Mechlorethamine ($HN_2$, Mustargen) | IV | 7-10 and 24-30 | N&V† | Therapeutic doses moderately depress peripheral blood cell count; excessive doses cause severe bone marrow depression with leukopenia, thrombocytopenia, and bleeding. Maximum toxicity may occur 2 or 3 weeks after last dose. Dosage, therefore, must be carefully controlled. Alopecia and hemorrhagic cystitis occur occasionally with cyclophosphamide and ifosfamide |
| Chlorambucil (Leukeran) | Oral | 7-14 | None | |
| Melphalan (Alkeran) | Oral | 7-14 | None | |
| Cyclophosphamide (Endoxan, Cytoxan) | IV<br>Oral | 7-14 | N&V | |
| Triethylthiophosphoramide (TSPA, Thio-TEPA) | IV | 14-28 | None | |
| Busulfan (Myleran) | Oral | 10-30 | None | |
| Mesna | IV | | | |
| **ANTIMETABOLITES** | | | | |
| Methotrexate | Oral<br>IV | 7-14 | None | Oral and digestive tract ulceration; bone marrow depression with leukopenia, thrombocytopenia and bleeding. Toxicity enhanced by impaired kidney function |
| 6-Mercaptopurine (6-MP, Purinethol) | Oral | 5-10 | None | Therapeutic doses usually well tolerated; excessive doses cause bone marrow depression |
| 6-Thioguanine (6-TG, Thioguan) | Oral | 8-14 | None | |
| 5-Fluorouracil (5-FU, Fluorouracil) | IV | 7-14 | None | Stomatitis, nausea, GI injury, bone marrow depression |
| Cytarabine (Ara-C, Cytosar-U) | IV | 7-14 | N&V | Bone marrow depression, megaloblastosis, leukopenia, thrombocytopenia |
| Floxuridine (FUDR) | IA | — | N&V | Stomatitis, GI injury, bone marrow depression, alopecia |
| **ANTIBIOTICS** | | | | |
| Doxorubicin (Adriamycin) | IV | 10-14 | N&V | Stomatitis, GI disturbances, alopecia, bone marrow depression. Cardiac toxicity at cumulative doses over 500 mg/$M^2$ *BSA* |
| Bleomycin (Blenoxane) | IV<br>SC | — | N&V, chills, fever | Mucocutaneous ulcerations, alopecia, pneumonitis and pulmonary fibrosis in cumulative doses over 400 μg |
| Dactinomycin (Cosmegen) | IV | 10-15 | N&V | Stomatitis, GI disturbances, alopecia, bone marrow depression |
| Daunorubicin (Cerubidine) | IV | 10-14 | N&V, fever | Bone marrow depression with leukopenia and thrombocytopenia, alopecia, stomatitis, cardiac toxicity at total lifetime dose of 600 mg/$M^2$ *BSA* |
| Plicamycin (mithramycin, Mithracin) | IV | 21-30 | N&V | Bone marrow depression, particularly thrombocytopenic bleeding, hypocalcemia, hepatic toxicity at large doses |
| Mitomycin C (Mutamycin) | IV | 21-28 | N&V | Bone marrow depression, GI injury, hypercalcemia, lung problems |
| Mitoxantrone (Novantrone) | IV | — | N&V | Bone marrow depression, alopecia, cardiac toxicity |
| **STEROID COMPOUNDS** | | | | |
| **Androgen** | | | | |
| Testosterone propionate | IM | — | None | Fluid retention, masculinization |
| Fluoxymesterone (Halotestin) | Oral | | | |
| Dromostanolone (Drolban) | IM | | | |
| Testolactone (Teslac) | Oral | | | |
| Methyltestosterone | Oral | | | |

Modified from Krakoff IH: *CA,* 41:270-276, 1991.

*Lowest point of leukocyte and thrombocyte count and greatest risk of infection and bleeding.

†Nausea and vomiting.

**TABLE 16-24 Chemotherapeutic Agents by Classification, Route of Administration, and Side Effects—cont'd**

| AGENTS | PRINCIPAL ROUTE OF ADMINISTRATION | NADIR* (DAYS) | ACUTE TOXIC SIGNS | MAJOR TOXIC MANIFESTATIONS |
|---|---|---|---|---|
| **Estrogen** | | | | |
| Diethylstilbestrol | Oral | — | Occasional N&V | Fluid retention, feminization<br>Uterine bleeding |
| Ethinyl estradiol (Estinyl) | Oral | | | |
| **Antiestrogen** | | | | |
| Tamoxifen citrate (Nolvadex) | Oral | — | N&V | Hot flashes |
| Leuprolide acetate (Lupron) | SC | | | |
| **Progestin** | | | | |
| Hydroxyprogesterone caproate (Prodrox) | IM | — | None | |
| Megestrol acetate (Megace) | Oral | | None | |
| Medroxyprogesterone acetate (Provera) | IM | | None | |
| Estramustine (Emcyt) | Oral | | N&V | |
| **Adrenal Cortical Compounds** | | | | |
| Cortisone acetate | Oral | — | None | Fluid retention, hypertension, diabetes, increased susceptibility to infection |
| Prednisone (Meticorten) | Oral | | | |
| Dexamethasone (Decadron) | Oral | | | |
| Methylprednisolone sodium succinate (Solu-Medrol) | IM<br>IV | | | |
| Hydrocortisone sodium succinate (Solu-Cortef) | IV | | | |
| **Antiadrenal** | | | | |
| Aminoglutethimide (Cytadren) | Oral | — | None | Adrenal insufficiency |
| **VINCA ALKALOIDS** | | | | |
| Vinblastine (Velban) | IV | 5-10 | N&V | Alopecia, areflexia, bone marrow depression |
| Vincristine (Oncovin) | IV | 3-5 | None | Areflexia, muscular weakness, peripheral neuritis, paralytic ileus, mild bone marrow depression |
| **MISCELLANEOUS DRUGS** | | | | |
| L-Asparaginase | IV | — | N&V, fever, hypersensitivity reactions | Anorexia, weight loss; somnolence, lethargy, confusion; hypoproteinemia, hypolipidemia, abnormal liver function tests; azotemia; granulocytopenia, lymphopenia, thrombocytopenia |
| Carmustine (BCNU) | IV | 12-14 and 26-32 | Fever, chills | Bone marrow depression |
| Lomustine (CCNU) | Oral | 12-20 and 35-45 | N&V | Bone marrow depression with leukopenia and thrombocytopenia; gonadal suppression |
| Streptozocin (Zanosar) | IV | — | N&V | Hypoglycemia |
| Mitotane (Lysodren) | Oral | — | N&V | Skin eruptions, diarrhea, mental depression, muscle tremors |
| Dacarbazine (DTIC-Dome) | IV | 14-25 | N&V | Bone marrow depression |
| Hydroxyurea (Hydrea) | Oral | 2-10 | None | Bone marrow depression, stomatitis, dysuria |
| Etoposide (VP-16) (Vepesid) | IV and oral | — | N&V | Alopecia |
| Cisplatin (Platinol) | IV | 7-14 | N&V | Bone marrow depression, renal tubular damage, deafness |
| Procarbazine (Matulane) | Oral | 20-35 | N&V | Bone marrow depression with leukopenia and thrombocytopenia, mental depression |

at this time, guidelines for safe handling of these agents have been established. The Occupational Safety and Health Administration (OSHA) of the U.S. Department of Labor and other health care institutions have proposed the guidelines summarized in the Guidelines box, on p. 409. It is essential that any health care provider working with chemotoxic drugs follow these guidelines to prevent injury to self and to others.

## Chemotherapeutic Agents

Drugs may be classified as alkylating agents, antimetabolites, plant (vinca) alkaloids, antibiotics, and steroids. Table 16-24 lists chemotherapeutic agents by classification, route of administration, and side effects.

### Alkylating agents

The alkylating agents are cell cycle nonspecific and act against already formed nucleic acids by cross-linking DNA strands, thereby preventing DNA replication and the transcription of RNA.

### Antimetabolites

The antimetabolites act by interfering with the synthesis of chromosomal nucleic acid. Antimetabolites are analogs of normal metabolites and block the enzyme necessary for synthesis of essential factors or are incorporated into the DNA or RNA and thus prevent replication. Most antimetabolites are pyrimidine analogs, purine analogs, or folic acid antagonists and are, in general, cycle specific.

### Vinca alkaloids

Vincristine sulfate and vinblastine sulfate are plant alkaloids that act as mitotic inhibitors. These agents exert their cytotoxic effect by binding to proteins within the cells, causing metaphase arrest. The vinca alkaloids are cell cycle specific. Although these two agents are similar in composition, mechanism of action, and metabolism, their antitumor spectrum, dose, and clinical toxicity differ.

### Antibiotics

Those antibiotics that demonstrate antitumor activity appear to affect either the function or synthesis of the nucleic acids. In addition, antimitotic and cell surface effects may be caused by these agents. The cytotoxic antibiotics are cell cycle nonspecific agents.

### Steroids

The corticosteroids are produced by the adrenal cortex and include mineralocorticoids and glucocorticoids. It is the glucocorticoids that, in addition to their use in numerous nonmalignant diseases, are effective in the treatment of many neoplastic disorders. In some malignant lesions (e.g., lymphomas, breast cancer, multiple myeloma, acute lymphocytic leukemia, and chronic lymphocytic leukemia) steroids exert a direct antitumor effect. Steroids also are able to reduce edema and inflammation around a tumor and therefore are useful for symptom relief. Many side effects are associated with long-term steroid use, most notably a compromised immunologic response to infection, osteoporosis, and a Cushingoid syndrome. Steroids in cancer treatment regimens often are given intermittently and for short periods and thus are not usually associated with the debilitating side effects associated with chronic, long-term use. Patients often describe an improved sense of well-being and an increased appetite while on prednisone therapy. With completion of a prescribed course of therapy, a brief period of fatigue, malaise, and emotional lability may be experienced.

Hormonal alteration may be a desired therapeutic goal when tumor growth is directly influenced by certain hormones. The mechanism whereby the steroid hormones stimulate or inhibit cellular growth is not clear; an important mechanism may be interference or alteration at the cell membrane.

Estrogen receptor assays are now routinely performed at the time of mastectomy for breast cancer. This technique has made it possible to evaluate the ability of a breast tumor to bind estrogen and thus project the probable sensitivity of the tumor to hormonal therapy.

## Common Side Effects of Chemotherapy

There is always some degree of injury to normal cells with treatment by cytotoxic drugs. The bone marrow, gastrointestinal epithelium, and hair follicles are most sensitive to chemotherapy because of their high rate of growth. Other side effects and toxicity include pulmonary toxicity, cardiac toxicity (congestive heart failure), genitourinary toxicity (cystitis, renal damage, sterility), neurotoxicity (numbness and tingling of the hands and feet, motor weakness), and hepatic toxicity. (Table 16-24 provides a review of toxicities for specific drugs.) Toxicities to the bone marrow, gastrointestinal tract, hair follicle, and reproductive system are addressed specifically in the following sections.

### Bone marrow effects

Chemotherapy is frequently toxic to the bone marrow and may produce neutropenia, thrombocytopenia, and anemia. Blood counts are obtained before administration and at regular intervals to identify nadir effect—the times that the blood count is lowest and the patient is most susceptible to infection and hemorrhage. Assessment is also made for signs and symptoms of other organ toxicity (Box 16-13).

*Infection* is a constant threat in the patient receiving chemotherapy. A cold or flu in a person with neutropenia may result in septicemic shock in a few hours. Intact skin and mucous membranes are first-line defenses against infection; thus care is directed to prevent breaks in skin integrity. Persons receiving chemotherapy are susceptible to middle-ear infections, sinusitis, and phar-

**BOX 16-13 Assessment of the Patient Receiving Chemotherapy**

IDENTIFICATION OF MARROW SUPPRESSION

1. WBC, platelet count, hemoglobin, hematocrit
2. Signs of bleeding (e.g., petechiae, ecchymosis)

IDENTIFICATION OF INFECTION

1. Inspect skin and mucous membranes daily (especially mouth, axillae, and perineum)
2. Auscultate respiratory tract
3. Monitor temperature, pulse, respiration
4. Most important: Monitor neutrophil count:
   a. A count of 500/mm$^3$ to 1000/mm$^3$ indicates moderate risk of infection
   b. A count of less than 500/mm$^3$ indicates severe risk of infection

IDENTIFICATION OF OTHER ORGAN TOXICITIES

1. Gastrointestinal toxicity
   a. Inspect mouth for white patches or ulcers
   b. Monitor weight, fluid, and electrolytes
   c. Assess for constipation, decreased bowel sounds
2. Liver toxicity: monitor liver enzymes
3. Cardiac toxicity
   a. Obtain baseline echocardiogram
   b. Check apical pulse for dysrhythmias
   c. Monitor for signs of congestive heart failure
4. Pulmonary toxicity
   a. Auscultate lungs
   b. Monitor for shortness of breath and cough (especially with bleomycin)
5. Urinary toxicity
   a. Monitor urine for blood
   b. Monitor for signs of cystitis (frequency with dysuria)
   c. Evaluate renal function by either serum creatinine or 24-hour urine for creatinine clearance
   d. Keep accurate intake and output
6. Neurotoxicity: assess for paresthesia and motor weakness

yngitis. Pneumonia is especially prevalent in patients with leukemia and in elderly persons.

In addition, signs of early infection may be absent and go unrecognized. A rise in body temperature of 1 to 2 degrees may be the only indication of a potentially dangerous situation. Localized inflammatory response may not occur in patients with severe leukopenia (<1000 cells/mm$^3$). The absence of granulocytes, also referred to as *polymorphonuclear leukocytes* (PMNs), prevents the formation of pus. Localized tenderness or pain may be the only sign of a skin or wound infection. Reverse isolation or "protective isolation" may be ordered to protect the patient from exposure to infection from caregivers, family members, and friends.

### Gastrointestinal effects

Changes in bowel habits commonly occur but usually do not require intervention. Alertness to the possibility of bleeding or ulceration must be part of the assessment of diarrhea or cramping. Vincristine may cause paralytic

**BOX 16-14 Drugs Causing Stomatitis**

Bleomycin (Blenozane)
Doxorubicin (Adriamycin)
Ara-C (Citarabine)
Cyclophosphamide (Cytoxan)
Daunorubicin (Cerubidine)
Methotrexate
5-Fluorouracil

ileus; therefore persons receiving this drug are specifically instructed to report constipation. Persons receiving narcotic-based pain medications may have constipation as a result, and a daily bowel regimen program may be indicated.

**Stomatitis.** *Stomatitis,* an inflammation of the oral mucous membranes, is a common side effect that may range from an erythema to mild or severe ulcerations. Guidelines for care of the person receiving chemotherapy (Guidelines box, p. 414) provides a summary of oral hygiene measures and treatments specific to stomatitis. Box 16-14 lists some drugs that can cause stomatitis.

**Nausea and vomiting.** Oncology nurses and patients often identify nausea and vomiting as the most uncomfortable and distressing side effects of chemotherapy. Four emetic syndromes have been identified in patients with cancer: (1) chemotherapy-induced emesis, (2) delayed emesis that occurs 1 to 4 days after treatment, (3) anticipatory emesis that occurs before the next scheduled therapy, and (4) emesis caused by factors other than chemotherapy, such as intestinal obstruction or other drug therapy (e.g., opiates). Depending on the type of emesis, different therapies are indicated. Relaxation techniques can be effective.

For the outpatient, nausea may interfere with the ability to continue daily work. Persistent vomiting may result in fluid and electrolyte imbalance, general weakness, and weight loss. Decline of nutritional status renders the person more susceptible to infection and perhaps less able to tolerate therapy. Such physiologic symptoms can accompany or precipitate psychologic responses that might include depression, withdrawal, and humiliation. The onset and duration of both nausea and vomiting vary greatly from patient to patient and with the drugs given.

### Alopecia

Alopecia can occur by two mechanisms. If the hair roots are atrophied, alopecia occurs readily and hair falls out either spontaneously or from combing, often in large clumps. If the hair shaft is constricted because of atrophy or necrosis, the hair will break off very near the scalp.

## Guidelines for Care of the Person Receiving Chemotherapy

1. Teaching the patient and significant others:
   a. Signs and symptoms of infection, thrombocytopenia
   b. How to read a thermometer (if appropriate) and when to notify the physician
   c. Good hygiene practices
      (1) Cleanse the perineum from front to back
      (2) Change underwear daily
      (3) Handwashing
   d. Information about prescribed drugs: name, dose, side effects, importance of taking as prescribed
   e. Use of antiemetics
   f. Importance of medical follow-up and blood studies
   g. Available support groups for chemotherapy patients
2. Preventing infection:
   a. Good hygiene, *especially handwashing* (patient, family, health professionals)
   b. Prevent exposure to people with known infection (other patients, staff, family, friends)
   c. Meticulous aseptic technique during intravenous infusions and dressing changes
      (1) Use povidone-iodine for skin preparation (Centers for Disease Control also considers alcohol, tincture of iodine, and chlorhexidine effective)
      (2) Use one tourniquet for patient's exclusive use
      (3) Use gloves for procedures
   d. No aspirin or acetaminophen (to prevent masking fever)
   e. Maintain intact skin and mucous membranes
      (1) Avoid bumping and breaking the skin
      (2) No injections
      (3) Keep fingernails short to prevent small skin breaks (nurse, patient, other caregivers)
      (4) Avoid anal intercourse
      (5) Avoid enemas, rectal medications, rectal thermometers
      (6) Avoid excessive friction and provide vaginal lubrication during sexual intercourse (use water-soluble jelly, if necessary)
   f. Maintain fastidious oral hygiene
      (1) Maintain teeth and gums in good condition; see dentist
      (2) Use mouth wash or oral irrigations (normal saline), mild peroxide solution (1 tablespoon in 240 ml water), sodium bicarbonate (1 teaspoon baking soda in 240 ml water)
      (3) Use mycostatin tablets or suspension, as necessary
      (4) Relieve dryness: drink water and other fluids
      (5) Use artificial saliva, as needed, in form of spray (Moi-Stir, Salivart, Ora-lub)
      (6) Stimulate saliva with gum, candies, buttermilk, yogurt
      (7) Brush teeth with soft toothbrush (small soft bristles) or use foam stick or swab
      (8) Brush teeth in short horizontal strokes at least 3 to 4 minutes, at least 3 times a day
      (9) Use fluoridated toothpaste or rinse, to prevent caries
      (10) Use Water Pik under low pressure or irrigation, if platelet count is low
   g. Use reverse isolation techniques as needed
   h. Maintain optimal respiratory function: turn, cough, and deep breathe patients confined to bed
3. Maintaining optimal gastrointestinal function:
   a. Give antidiarrheal medication as needed
   b. Plan daily bowel regimen for constipation, give stool softeners as prescribed
   c. Treat stomatitis
      (1) Oral nystatin (Mycostatin) or other antibiotics as prescribed
      (2) Milk of magnesia or Kaopectate to coat lesions
      (3) Dyclonine hydrochloride (Dyclone), Orabase, lidocaine (Xylocaine) viscous 2%, as local anesthetic before meals and as necessary
      (4) KY jelly, mineral oil, to coat lips and oral mucosa
      (5) Petrolatum (Vaseline) to coat lips (not if neutropenic)
      (6) Diphenhydramine hydrochloride (Benadryl) alone or in combination with Maalox and Kaopectate, as a rinse
      (7) Oral irrigations (see under infection) every 2 hours
      (8) Soft, bland foods, cold liquids tolerated by some persons
   d. Treat nausea and vomiting
      (1) Give antiemetics 30 to 45 min before chemotherapy; use large doses
      (2) Use auditory or diversional stimulation (music, slides, photographs)
      (3) Give antiemetics around the clock for severe nausea and vomiting
      (4) Use relaxation techniques, self-hypnosis, therapeutic touch
      (5) Eat foods that minimize nausea
4. Minimizing or preventing alopecia:
   a. Urge use of wigs, scarves, eyebrow pencil, false eyelashes
   b. Avoid frequent shampooing, combing, or brushing
   c. Use soft-bristle hair brush
   d. Advise against permanents and hair coloring (increase rate of hair loss)
5. Minimizing or preventing urinary effects—hemorrhagic cystitis, renal toxicity:
   a. Force fluids when taking cyclophosphamide
   b. Take cyclophosphamide early in the day
   c. Check serum creatinine or 24-hr urine for creatinine clearance before giving *cis*-platinum and streptozotocin
6. Minimizing effects of sterility:
   a. Provide birth control information and reproductive counseling
   b. Provide information about sperm banking before initiation of therapy for male patients

The root remains in the scalp, and a patchy thinning pattern of hair loss occurs.

After the initial diagnosis of cancer, alopecia may be the most traumatic psychologic side effect cancer patients may experience. It is a constant reminder of their disease, makes the illness visible to others, and may result in a significant change in body image.

### Sterility

Cancer chemotherapy has the capacity to affect most body organ systems to some degree. This is especially true in regard to the reproductive organs. Some chemotherapeutic drugs have the potential to cause genetic alterations, which in turn disrupt normal fetal development. In addition, some of the alkylating agents may cause transient or permanent sterility. Persons receiving chemotherapy need to be informed of the known and possible effects on fertility. After completion of chemotherapy, conception and the birth of normal, healthy children are possible for couples. It is customary to recommend that procreation be avoided until at least 2 years after completion of treatment.

## Dose Calculations

The dosage range for a particular drug is determined at the time of clinical trial and regimen development. Given these guidelines, the dosage for a specific individual must be calculated before starting therapy. Although some regimens may still prescribe milligrams per kilogram, drug doses usually are stated in terms of body surface area, and therefore the doses are given in milligrams per squared meter (mg/m$^2$). An individual's height and weight are used to determine body surface; therefore it is very important that height and weight are measured *accurately.*

## Methods of Administering Chemotherapeutic Agents

The route of administration is based on the metabolism and absorption of a given drug. The route of choice is that which will deliver the optimal amount of drug to the tumor. Chemotherapeutic agents are given orally, subcutaneously, intravenously, and intramuscularly.

Tumor cells in the central nervous system are difficult to access because many chemotherapeutic agents cannot pass through the blood-brain barrier. Use of the ***intrathecal*** route permits the introduction of high drug concentrations directly into the cerebrospinal fluid through a lumbar puncture or through a subcutaneous cerebrospinal reservoir (Ommaya reservoir) (Figure 16-15) without risk of the usual systemic side effects.[9] ***Intraarterial*** and ***intracavitary*** routes are also amenable to providing high-dose concentrations of a drug without undue systemic effects. These modes of drug administration may be used when a malignant organ or tissue tumor cannot be treated by surgical removal.

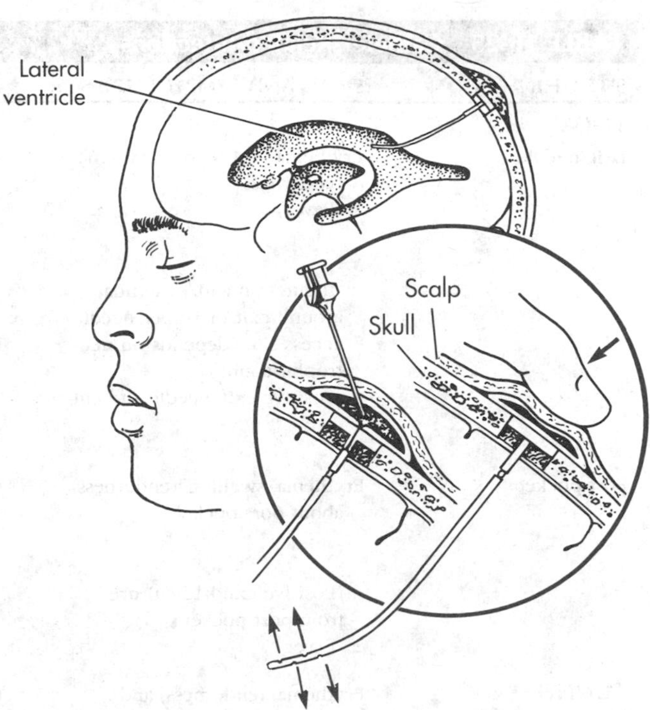


**FIGURE 16-15** Ommaya reservoir for administration of chemotherapeutic agents directly into the central nervous system (CNS). (Modified from Ratcheson RA, Ommaya AK: *N Engl J Med* 279:1025-1031, 1968.)

### Long-term drug delivery systems

The use of centrally placed venous access catheters and ports is now a common and accepted part of cancer chemotherapy. The kind used depends on the type of treatment, the mode of administration required, the frequency and need for access, and the patient's condition and preference if these can be accommodated. Centrally located catheters allow for intermittent or continuous administration of drugs, blood and blood products, antibiotics, and antiemetic and analgesic drugs, as well as total parenteral nutrition (TPN). These catheters come with single, double, and triple lumens for convenient multiple-drug administration.

The placement of central catheters must be performed under strict aseptic conditions in the clinic or operating room with use of either local or general anesthesia. Prevention of infection is of utmost importance when any central access device is used. Immunosuppression with neutropenia is a common side effect of many chemotherapeutic agents; therefore any infection can be life-threatening. The catheters generally are made of a silicone material and are radiopaque. These features permit easier placement through tissue and threading into the circulation, as well as visualization by x-ray or fluoroscopic examination to verify proper placement. The technique of "tunneling" the catheter beneath the skin aids in preventing bacterial entry and growth along the catheter tract. All tunneled catheters have a small "cuff" around which fibroblasts form and help secure the catheter in place. Figure 16-16 shows positioning of a Hickman/Broviac central catheter. The entry and exit sites of central catheters require sterile dressing changes two or three times a week until healing has occurred; then catheter care follows agency protocol. Table 16-25 provides an overview of central catheter infections and their management.[47]

Implanted venous access ports (VAP) are made of plastic, stainless steel, or titanium with resealable silicone septums and catheter (Figure 16-17). The placement of VAPs is similar to that described for "tunneled" catheters; however, the port itself is sutured into a "pocket" that appears as a small bump beneath the skin. Dressings may be necessary until the entry site is healed.

**TABLE 16-25 Catheter-Related Infections**

| SITE OF INFECTION | SIGNS AND SYMPTOMS | BASIS FOR DIAGNOSIS | MANAGEMENT |
|---|---|---|---|
| **LOCAL** | | | |
| Exit/needle | Erythema (>1.0 cm <2.0 cm), tenderness<br>± Fever | Clinical S&S<br>Exit/needle site culture | Local site care: ↑ frequency of skin care and dressing changes; alternative dressings; antimicrobial ointment |
| | ± Induration and/or exudate around exit or Huber needle access site (depends on neutrophil count) | | Oral antibiotics: nonneutropenic patient, limited inflammation |
| | + Positive exit/needle site culture | | IV antibiotics: neutropenic patient or progressive inflammation |
| Port pocket | Erythema, swelling, tenderness about port pocket | Clinical S&S<br>Aspiration and culture port pocket exudate (by physician) | IV antibiotics through port if cannulated; through peripheral vein if port not cannulated |
| | + Positive exudate culture from port pocket<br>± Fever | | Consider port removal |
| **TUNNEL** | Erythema, tenderness, and induration along SQ tract >2 cm from exit site<br>± Purulence/inflammation at exit site<br>± Positive culture from exit or insertion site<br>± Fever | Clinical S&S | IV antibiotics<br>Consider catheter removal |
| **SYSTEMIC** (septicemia) | | | |
| Thrombus-related | + S&S of SVC obstruction: neck-arm swelling; discomfort in neck, arm, chest, or back; increased superficial venous pattern<br>Fever and chills | Clinical S&S<br>Radiographic procedures: e.g., venogram, ultrasound<br>Catheter and peripheral blood culture (5-10 times increase in colony forming units catheter *v* peripheral) | IV antibiotics<br>Consider thrombolytic or anticoagulant therapy<br>Consider surgical resection of thrombus and affected vein<br>Consider catheter removal |
| Catheter colonization | Bacteremia or fungemia without catheter tract inflammation<br>Fever and chills | Clinical S&S<br>Catheter and peripheral blood culture (5-10 times increase in colony forming units catheter *v* peripheral)<br>Positive culture of catheter tip | Bacteremia—IV antibiotics<br>Fungemia—antifungal therapy<br>Consider catheter removal<br>? Antibiotic lock |

From Wickham R, Purl S, Welker D: *Semin Oncol Nurs* 8(2):138, 1992.
*S&S,* Signs and symptoms; ±, presence or absence of a sign or symptom; *SVC,* subclavian vein catheterization.

As with central catheters, VAP position is confirmed by x-ray or fluoroscopic examination.[9] Implantable access ports have less danger of becoming infected, occluded, or displaced compared with externally placed central catheters. The VAP can be used for bolus injections or short-term drug infusion. Special needles (Huber needles) must be used to prevent perforation or coring of the infusion port (Figure 16-18). A comparison of external catheters and implantable ports is presented in Table 16-26.

### Home Care and Chemotherapy Administration

The delivery of chemotherapy in the home or ambulatory care setting has been made practical with the advent of both *external* and *implantable pump systems.* The pumps have electronic internal power sources so that either intermittent or continuous drug administration is possible. The *external pumps* are small and lightweight and attach to either a belt or shoulder holster, thus permitting the patient free ambulation while the devices are in use. A major disadvantage of external pumps is

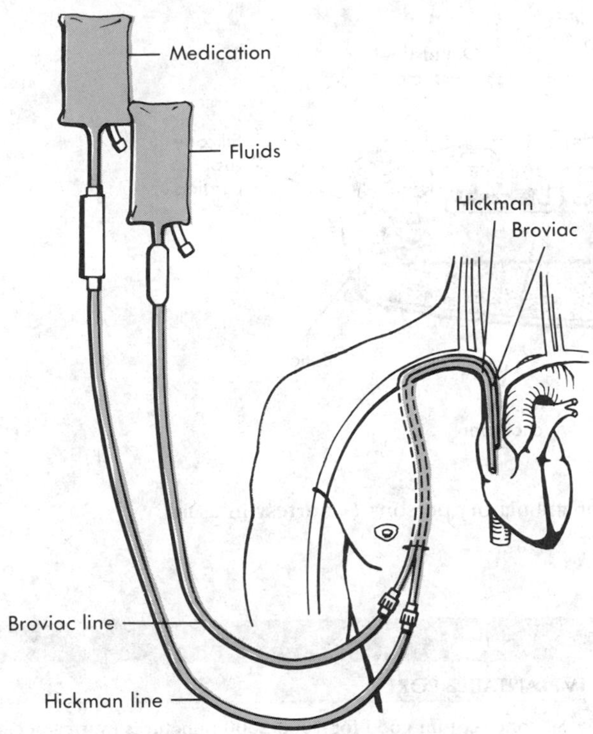


FIGURE 16-16 Double-lumen Hickman/Broviac catheters.

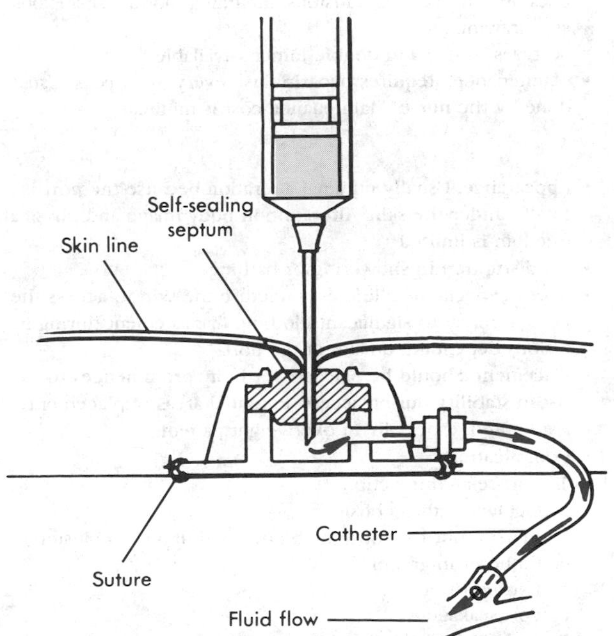


FIGURE 16-17 Drugs are administered through self-sealing infusion port.

the need for a family support person to receive instruction in their care and maintenance because the patient cannot be expected to manage the care alone.[9] An implantable drug-delivery system for ambulatory persons is seen in Figure 16-19.

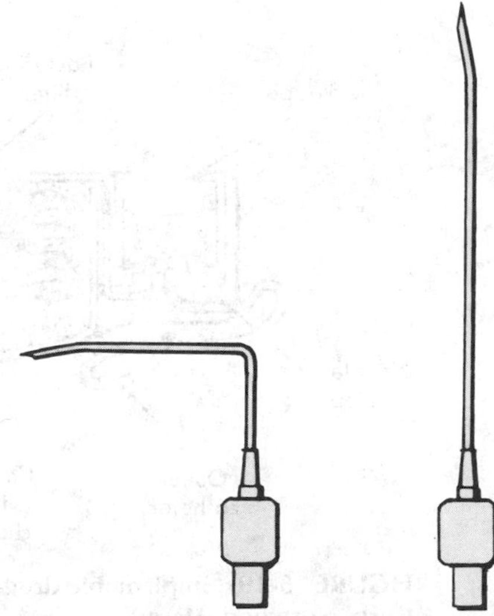

FIGURE 16-18 Special Huber needles used to inject medication through infusion port to prevent perforation of port.

The *implantable pumps* are inserted in the manner described for implanted ports (VAP). However, because these pumps generally are used for intraarterial chemotherapy for primary and metastatic liver carcinomas, they are situated in a pocket of the abdomen or infraclavicular fossa. The Silastic catheter is then threaded into the hepatic artery, superior vena cava, or subclavian vein. Other uses for implantable pumps now include administration of heparin and morphine.[9] Drugs are added percutaneously through a central inlet septum with a special needle. Drug refills usually are needed every 2 weeks.

The most common complication is development of a seroma over the pump pocket. This is an accumulation of sterile fluid that may be either aspirated by the physician or allowed to be absorbed by the body. Pump pocket infection is rare but may require removal of the pump. Patients are taught to resume activities as soon as the incision heals. Written instructions are given to the patient, including telephone numbers of health care professionals who can be consulted. The importance of keeping appointments for pump refilling is emphasized (Box 16-15).

## Bone Marrow Transplantation

Bone marrow transplantation (BMT) is used in patients with a variety of malignant hematologic and solid tumors. Conditions treated include acute and chronic leukemias, preleukemic states, lymphoma, multiple myeloma, neuroblastoma, and breast cancer. The patient's bone marrow is treated with high-dose chemotherapy or radiotherapy or a combination of both in preparation for receiving harvested marrow. The rationale for this intensive therapy is to eradicate the bone marrow and any malignant cells present and replace them with harvested marrow from either a human leukocyte antigen

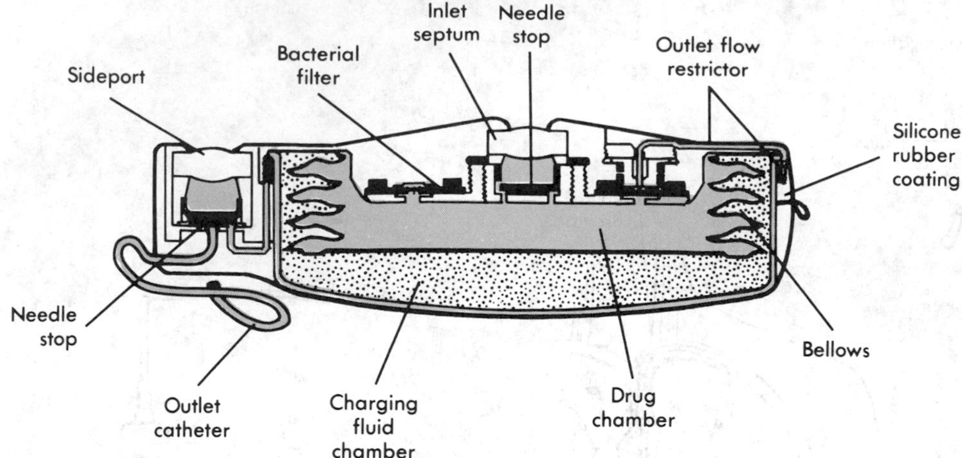


**FIGURE 16-19** Implantable drug-delivery system for ambulatory persons. (Courtesy Infusaid Corp, Norwood, Mass.)

**TABLE 16-26 Comparison of Venous Access Devices**

| EXTERNAL SILASTIC CATHETER | IMPLANTABLE PORTS |
|---|---|
| • May remain in place as long as trouble-free | • Silicone septum good for 1000-2000 punctures (varies per product and size needle used) |
| • Technically open system, though catheter closed by injection cap | • Completely closed system |
| • Barrier against infection: Dacron cuff | • Barrier against infection: skin |
| • Surgically inserted and removed | • Surgically inserted and removed |
| • Uses: All intravenous infusions, including transfusions and drawing | • Uses: All intravenous infusions, including blood transfusions and drawing |
| • Features: Single, double, and triple lumens available | • Features: Single and double lumens available |
| • Maintenance: Requires daily heparin flushes, regular dressing, and injection cap changes using aseptic techniques. Care is done by the patient or the family. Maintenance costs include heparin, syringes, needles, alcohol, dressing supplies, injection caps, etc. | • Maintenance: Requires heparin flush every 3-4 weeks. Usually done by the nurse. Maintenance cost is minimal |
| • Appearance: Alteration in body image and physical freedom. Changes are considerable with 4-5 inches of external catheter always present | • Appearance: Usually minimal alteration because the port is totally under the skin. Alteration in body image and physical freedom is limited |
| • Care must be taken with showering, bathing, and swimming | • No disruption in showering or bathing |
| • Access: Needle inserted into injection cap at the end of the external catheter. Some clothing displacement during infusions | • Access: Special needle must puncture the skin to access the port. Minimal to significant clothing displacement during infusions depending on site of the port. |
| • Placement: Can choose exit site for catheter | • Placement: Should be placed over bony prominences to assist in stability during access. Potential areas of placement are limited, especially in overweight patients |
| • Complications:<br>1. Catheter-related infections<br>2. Occlusion thrombosis<br>3. Infuses, but cannot draw blood (withdrawal occlusion)<br>4. Catheter damage, leakage, or dislodgement<br>5. Extravasation<br>6. Spontaneous blood backflow | • Complications:<br>1. Port-related infections<br>2. Occlusion thrombosis<br>3. Infuses, but cannot draw blood (withdrawal occlusion)<br>4. Catheter migration<br>5. Extravasation<br>6. Port leakage<br>7. Catheter-needle dislodgement |

From Burke MB et al: *Cancer chemotherapy: a nursing process approach,* Boston, 1991, Jones & Bartlett.

(HLA)–matched donor or the patient's own marrow. The goal is to achieve a more normal immune system after transplantation.

There are three types of tissue or bone marrow donors: allogeneic, usually from a sibling who has a close HLA match (see Chapter 72); syngeneic, from an identical twin; or the most recent type used, autologous bone marrow transplantation (ABMT) in which patients serve as their own donors. ABMT has been useful because it is frequently difficult to find a donor with a close HLA match.[37]

In ABMT the patient's marrow usually is disease-free

**BOX 16-15 Teaching the Patient Who Has an Implantable Infusion Pump**

1. Avoid contact sports or activities that may cause blunt trauma to the pump.
2. Avoid activities that cause an increase in body temperature (long, hot baths, saunas) or atmospheric pressure (stay in high-altitude areas): flow rate of pump may increase.
3. Keep appointments for pump refilling; catheter occlusion may occur because of complete emptying of pump reservoir (newer implantables have low-reservoir alarms).
4. Watch for infection, which is rare but may occur; the pump is a foreign body and chemotherapy-induced myelosuppression or sepsis predisposes to infection and inflammation.
5. Be alert for malfunction of pump: usually caused by motor failure, indicated by absence of backflow into a syringe or release of manual pressure after injection of 5 to 10 ml of fluid. In externally programmable pumps, failure is caused by computer operating system or microcomputer circuits.
6. Be alert for catheter occlusion; usually caused by drug incompatibility, resulting in precipitation in the drug chamber.

Modified from vonRoemeling E et al: *Oncol Nurs Forum* 13(2):17-24, 1986; Stewart CD: Nursing interventions in regional chemotherapy using surgical delivery systems. In *Nursing interventions in oncology, MD Anderson case reports and review,* Newton, Penn, 1989, Associations in Medical Marketing Co.

**BOX 16-16 Teaching the Bone Marrow Harvest Procedure to the Patient**

1. Explain that bone marrow forms special stem cells that produce all blood cells.
2. Discuss special preparation; for example, shower with antiseptic soap the evening before harvest.
3. Describe the harvest procedure:
   a. General or spinal anesthesia is used
   b. Needle is placed through skin in back side of hip bone
   c. If transplant is autologous, filtered bone marrow is frozen until needed
   d. If transplant is allogeneic or syngeneic, marrow is transferred to blood transfusion bag and given immediately through an intravenous line
4. Explain what happens after recovery.
   a. Pain in harvest sites can be relieved by medication
   b. Patient is out of bed the night of the harvest
   c. Pressure dressing is removed the day after harvest
   d. Surgical sites are kept clean and covered for 3 days; on each day clean the sites, apply Betadine ointment, and cover with adhesive bandage

or has been purged of tumor cells before reinfusion. The rationale for ABMT is based on the knowledge that higher doses of chemotherapy or radiation will increase the number of tumor cells killed in a logarithmic fashion; that is, doubling the dose may result in 10 times or more the number of tumor cells killed. Large doses of drugs can be given because ABMT provides a rescue for bone marrow depression.

Autologous bone marrow "harvest" (the term used for donating the bone marrow) is performed when the patient is in remission or when the tumor burden is small and bone marrow involvement cannot be microscopically identified. The purpose of the harvest is to collect enough stem cells (pluripotent cells) to reconstitute the hematopoietic system after therapy. (See Chapter 33 for discussion of the hematopoietic system.)

The marrow is obtained by multiple needle aspirations from the posterior iliac crest under general or spinal anesthesia, although the anterior iliac crest and sternum may also be used. The amount of marrow extracted ranges from 600 to 2500 ml for the average adult.

After processing, the marrow is given to the patient intravenously through a transfusion bag, or it can be frozen at − 140° C although − 196° C is preferred (cryopreservation). Marrow can be kept for a period of 3 years or more. Teaching the patient about bone marrow harvesting is described in Box 16-16.

It usually takes 10 to 28 days after infusion of the marrow before new growth of marrow cells (WBCs, RBCs, platelets) is seen within the peripheral circulation. It is during the first weeks after the BMT that the patient is most vulnerable to the effects of the induced pancytopenia. If allogeneic bone marrow is used, infection, hemorrhage, venoocclusive disease (VOD), and acute graft-versus-host disease (AGVHD) are the earliest and most hazardous side effects after transplantation. Any of these side effects, alone or in combination, can occur within the first 100 days after BMT. Infection must be avoided until granulocytes reach levels at which the body can defend against any type of bacteremia. Until this level is achieved, the patient is kept isolated in a private room and treated with prophylactic broad-spectrum antibiotics. Some patients are maintained in laminar air flow rooms for this purpose. Possible hemorrhage is treated with platelet transfusions and blood products. AGVHD may occur between 8 and 60 days after transplantation and may be *mild* (skin rash) to *severe* (involvement of skin, liver, intestine). Prophylaxis of AGVHD is achieved with the use of cyclosporine, methotrexate, and steroids, either alone or in combination.[12] The lungs and liver are the organs most often damaged by VOD within the first 4 weeks after transplantation. The incidence and severity may be lessened when the therapy for GVHD is included as part of the overall posttransplantation treatment regimen.

The FDA now approves the use of hematopoietic growth factors after BMT. Granulocyte colony-stimulating factor (GCSF) and granulocyte-macrophage colony-stimulating factor (GM-CSF) are glycoproteins that have the ability to stimulate bone marrow recovery through proliferation and maturation after myelosuppression. They also are becoming an important component of therapy for aplastic anemia, myelodysplastic syndrome, acquired immunodeficiency disease (AIDS), and bone marrow suppression after chemotherapy for cancer treatment.

Marrow grafting is costly because inpatient hospital stays may run from $50,000 to $120,000. The procedure often involves psychologic stress in patient, family, and nursing staff who may try to be positive about the outcome. It cannot be overemphasized that hope has a major role with BMT. The involvement of staff members and patient is intense in a BMT unit, and nurses may be placed in the paradoxic situation of providing hope to dying patients.[7] (See Chapter 10 for discussion of hope.)

## NURSING MANAGEMENT

### ♦ ASSESSMENT

The nurse working with the patient who is to receive chemotherapy should assess for the following:

1. Overall knowledge of the specific malignant tumor and the therapies available for treatment
2. Prior experience with chemotherapy or other cancer treatment modalities
3. Expected outcome on disease process from chemotherapy treatment
4. Knowledge of the chemotherapy drug protocol used
   a. Names of drugs
   b. Expected side effects
   c. Days of month receiving drugs
   d. Number of cycles
5. Status of venous system and need for other venous access devices
6. Attitude toward therapy and ability for compliance
7. Support persons and resources available

### ♦ NURSING DIAGNOSES

Nursing diagnoses for the cancer patient receiving chemotherapy may include but are not limited to the following:

| Diagnostic Title | Possible Etiologic Factors |
|---|---|
| Infection, high risk for | Disease entity, lack of knowledge, decreased nutrition, decreased immune response, chemotherapy effects on bone marrow |
| Fluid volume deficit, high risk for | Inadequate fluid intake, side effects of chemotherapy drugs (nausea, vomiting, diarrhea), anticipatory nausea and vomiting |
| Nutrition, altered: less than body requirements | Nausea and vomiting, anorexia, stomatitis, fatigue, weight loss >10% |
| Body image disturbance | Loss of body hair from chemotherapy, cancer cachexia |

### ♦ EXPECTED PATIENT OUTCOMES

Expected patient outcomes for the patient receiving chemotherapy for cancer may include but are not limited to the following:

1. Expresses knowledge of why chemotherapy will be used to treat cancer.
2. Displays a positive attitude toward receiving and complying with chemotherapy.
3. Can name each chemotherapeutic drug to be used and the major side effects to expect.
4. Recognizes why maintaining good nutrition and fluid balance is important while receiving chemotherapy.
5. Understands infection risk during course of chemotherapy.
6. Discusses potential for hair loss and coping mechanisms to deal with change in body appearance.

### ♦ INTERVENTIONS

Chemotherapy as a cancer treatment modality is employed for cure, palliation, or adjunct therapy. Its success depends on the type of malignant disease and its stage and extent. Patients facing chemotherapy for the first time usually know of another person who has received this form of therapy and can recite many of the "negative" aspects associated with it. They wonder if they will face the same discomforts, such as nausea and vomiting, weight loss, and hair loss to name but a few. The nurse working with the patient beginning chemotherapy must be open in acknowledging the side effects that can and do occur. However, the nurse also must be knowledgeable enough about therapy to be able to provide assurance that the side effects can be kept to a minimum and that the plan of care will strive to keep the patient as comfortable as possible.

The patient who enters treatment with a positive attitude about having chemotherapy and who has received both verbal and written information on how the drugs act, on side effects that are expected, and on how other medications and comfort measures will be used to alleviate symptoms is much more likely to accept this form of therapy and see it to its completion.

#### Preventing Infection

A large number of chemotherapeutic drugs can be expected to have some effect on the patient's bone marrow, gastrointestinal tract, and skin. The nurse will teach the patient and family the specific signs and symptoms that can be anticipated for each system. Teaching should include facts on the function of the bone marrow in relation to fighting infection (WBC/neutrophils), carrying oxygen and nutrients to body tissue (RBC), and blood clotting (platelets). When a chemotherapeutic drug affects the bone marrow, the body's ability to produce sufficient numbers of each cell type is compromised and cells that are produced may be of an immature type that cannot function normally. Therefore if insufficient numbers are produced or immature cells result, the patient will not have the ability to fight infections, will develop bleeding tendencies, and eventually will become anemic. Infection is one of the major causes of mortality in the cancer patient, especially the leukemic patient receiving chemotherapy.

Consequently, both patient and family members require instruction on the need and purpose of good personal hygiene, the need to avoid family, staff, or visitors who have an infectious process, and how to recognize the signs and symptoms of infection to report. The nurse will assess the patient closely for signs of infection from potential sources, such as wounds, indwelling catheter and tube sites, and areas of skin breakdown. Monitoring the vital signs, blood cell counts (CBC, Hgb, Hct, platelets), and blood chemistry tests will facilitate more rapid and timely intervention to counteract any infection process. For patients whose neutrophil count drops below normal acceptable levels (normal 4000-10,000/mm$^3$), the chemotherapy may be discontinued or the dose reduced to protect the person from overwhelming infection. The patient with leukemia is an exception to this strategy. Chemotherapy will be continued, and these patients will be placed in protective isolation. They may even have their food sterilized to prevent exposure to bacterial organisms that may be present.

## Maintaining Fluid Balance

The gastrointestinal tract is very sensitive to the effects of many chemotherapeutic agents. As a result, patients may lose their appetite (anorexia) and experience nausea and vomiting. Some will have diarrhea as well. The outcome is loss of body weight and fluid volume, which may result in dehydration. Nausea and vomiting are some of the more devastating side effects of chemotherapy. When nausea and vomiting are expected, the health care team focuses on either preventing or minimizing the incidence. Several methods have been successful: prophylaxis and continuous treatment. Treating nausea and vomiting prophylactically is based on the rationale that once vomiting occurs, it is difficult to stop. It is not easy to control the anxiety and fear that, in some patients, lead to anticipatory nausea and vomiting. If nausea and vomiting are known to occur, the patient usually will be prescribed antiemetic therapy before the chemotoxic drug is administered and then on an around-the-clock schedule. Antiemetic therapy only as needed still is used but is less advocated than in the past. If the nausea and vomiting and fluid loss are moderate to severe, the patient will receive rehydration with replacement parenteral fluids. Oral fluids are encouraged as tolerated; then normal fluid intake is resumed when side effects cease.

## Promoting Nutrition

Anorexia can be a direct result of the disease process, as well as an outcome of chemotherapy. It is important that the patient and family be aware that if the patient is able to eat and retain food and fluids, the consumption of a nourishing diet can help maintain energy level and meet body nutrient and repair needs. The patient needs encouragement to eat even when not hungry. When anorexia is accompanied by nausea and vomiting, an antiemetic is administered one-half hour before mealtime. The patient is taught to perform mouth care (brush teeth, rinse mouth thoroughly) so that foul taste and odor from vomiting can be eliminated. Resting in bed or in a comfortable chair before meals helps conserve energy reserves needed for eating. Patients often are more agreeable to eating breakfast than other meals, especially when they have had an uninterrupted night of sleep. When family members can join the patient at mealtime, it provides a more natural and positive feeling toward food, along with family togetherness. The nurse should caution against "filling up" on fluids such as coffee or tea, which have no caloric value but give a feeling of early satiety. Body weight is measured frequently so that nutritional interventions can be monitored. Enteral oral supplements or high-calorie between-meal snacks are commonly ordered. Total parenteral nutrition (TPN) is an option commonly used with the patient who is more severely malnourished. Anorexia is difficult for both the patient and the nurse. Constant vigilance, encouragement, and creativity are required of staff members to ensure that the patient meets nutritional needs.

## Promoting a Positive Body Image

Chemotherapeutic drugs can cause alopecia—loss of body hair—from thinning to total loss. Chemotherapeutic drugs act most efficiently on body cells that have a rapid mitotic cycle. The integumentary cells meet this criterion. Drugs that are most responsible for alopecia are alkylating agents, antimetabolites, and anticancer antibiotics. Box 16-17 lists the drugs most involved in causing hair loss.

Patients scheduled for chemotherapy that causes hair loss should be informed of this likelihood early in the course of therapy so that they can be prepared when the time of hair loss occurs. Some male patients shave their heads or cut the hair very short. Women also may cut their hair to minimize the psychologic distress that accompanies hair loss. The use of wigs, headscarves, or caps helps the patient maintain a sense of normalcy, hide the loss, and lessen the visible evidence of the loss. The patient should be informed that hair loss will cease when the offending drug is discontinued. Hair will regrow and

**BOX 16-17 Chemotherapeutic Drugs Most Responsible for Hair Loss**

| | |
|---|---|
| Bleomycin | 5-Fluorouracil |
| Cyclophosphamide | Hydroxyurea |
| Cytosine arabinoside | Methotrexate |
| Dactinomycin | Mitomycin-C |
| Daunorubicin | Mitoxantrone |
| Doxorubicin | Melphalan |
| Etoposide | Vincristine |

has been known to change shades and texture with regrowth. Hair loss generally begins within a week or two after the first dose and reaches its maximal loss in a month or two.

Patients often request the use of scalp tourniquets or hypothermia measures to avoid hair loss. Scalp tourniquets act by constricting blood flow to the scalp hair follicles, and hypothermia (ice packs) produces vasoconstriction of blood flow to the scalp. These techniques work in principle; however, they are not to be encouraged. Because chemotherapeutic drugs may not reach some cells of the scalp, the potential exists for cancer cells to find a sanctuary and continue to grow and spread. These mechanisms to prevent hair loss are contraindicated for patients with leukemia, lymphoma, sarcoma, mycosis fungoides, and cancer of the breast, lung, kidney, and stomach.[9]

Patients should be advised to avoid harsh shampoos, vigorous combing or brushing, and hot curling irons or rollers while receiving chemotherapy that results in hair loss, because these activities will cause increased breakage of the already fragile hair shaft. Although hair loss is one of the most obvious and emotionally painful aspects of chemotherapy, the patient can be well prepared to face the situation when it arises with strategies for coping, using resources such as those provided by the American Cancer Society concerning wigs, and reading materials about hair loss. (See Guidelines box, p. 414 for an overview of care guidelines.)

## ♦ EVALUATION

To evaluate the effectiveness of nursing interventions, compare patient behaviors with those stated in the expected patient outcomes. Successful achievement of patient outcomes for the patient receiving chemotherapy for cancer is indicated by the following:

1. States that chemotherapy is being used as an adjunctive treatment to follow surgery (e.g., mastectomy, colon resection).
2. States an intention to proceed with chemotherapy to enhance the chance of cancer cure.
3. Knowledge of drugs
   a. Correctly names each drug with its major side effects.
   b. Identifies a strategy to cope successfully with each side effect.
4. Knowledge of nutrition
   a. Consumes food items high in protein and carbohydrate at each meal first before drinking coffee or tea.
   b. Requests a milkshake or eggnog drink for between-meal snacks.
   c. Asks for antiemetic medication before meals when nauseated.
5. Knowledge of infection risk
   a. Washes hands after each trip to the bathroom; takes complete bath daily.
   b. Can describe signs and symptoms of infection to report.
   c. Asks family member with a cold to refrain from visiting.
6. Coping with hair loss
   a. Identifies chemotherapy drug that causes hair loss.
   b. Had partner purchase a wig to prepare for hair loss.
   c. Speaks of hair loss as a temporary problem that can be dealt with.

## IMMUNOTHERAPY

The role of immunotherapy in the prevention and treatment of cancer is being studied. Many scientists believe cancer occurs in the body more frequently than once in a lifetime; however, in most cases clinical evidence of the disease is not apparent. It is postulated that there is a natural immunity against the development of the disease and that cancer cells are destroyed almost as fast as they develop. Clinical malignancy may occur as a result of failure in the immunologic surveillance system of the body (see p. 366).

Studies of cancer in lower animals and in human beings show that when the normal cell becomes malignant, it often undergoes biochemical changes that result in information of new cellular antigens that cause an immune response.

This response has two major components. The first, or *cellular immune response* (see Chapter 13), produces lymphocytes capable of destroying tumor cells on contact. These lymphocytes (T cells) undergo division and are released into the bloodstream when stimulated by an antigen.

Another important cell, which collaborates with the T cell, is the macrophage. The macrophage, which is attracted to the immune lymphocyte, is immobilized in its vicinity and then activated by the lymphocyte. It is a relatively nonspecific cell that seems to have the ability to kill selectively malignant cells with which it comes in contact.

The second component of the immune response is *antibody production* that results from activation of lymphocytes (B cells). When stimulated by antigen, B cells proliferate and differentiate into plasma cells, which are the major source of antibody production.

In addition to B cells and T cells, a third immunologic component, natural killer (NK) cells, has been discovered.

The cells involved in the immune response interact and seem to exchange signals at both cellular and humoral levels. At present the immune response can handle only a limited number of tumor cells, up to 10 million. After a growth to 100 million tumor cells the immune response is not capable of preventing further growth. Once the cancer is large, it cannot be totally controlled by the immune system; thus immunotherapy cannot be

**TABLE 16-27 Immunotherapy/Biotherapy in Cancer Treatment**

| SPECIFICITY | ACTIVE | PASSIVE |
|---|---|---|
| Specific | Inactivated tumor vaccines (autologous, allogeneic)<br>Human tumor hybrids | Monoclonal antibodies<br>Human heterologous antiserum<br>T lymphocytes<br>Monoclonal lymphocytes<br>Bone marrow transplants |
| Nonspecific | Chemical immunostimulants<br>Biologic immunostimulants (such as BCG, *C. parvum*)<br>Cytokines (interferon, IL-2, TNF)<br>Chemotherapy | Lymphokine-activated killer cells (LAKC)<br>Activated macrophages |

From McDonald A. In Dow KH: *Nursing care in radiation oncology*, Philadelphia, 1992, WB Saunders.
*BCG*, Bacille Calmette-Guérin; *C. parvum, Corynebacterium parvum*; *TNF*, tumor necrosis factor.

the primary mode of cancer therapy. It is used after surgery, radiotherapy, and chemotherapy have removed the bulk of the tumor.

Immunologic treatment of cancer may involve active immunotherapy, either specific or nonspecific. Passive or adoptive immunotherapy may also be specific or nonspecific. Table 16-27 reviews immunotherapy/biotherapy in cancer treatment.

Nonspecific immunotherapy using the bacille Calmette-Guérin (BCG), *Corynebacterium parvum*, or specific allogeneic or autologous vaccines were the first attempts at immunotherapy in the 1960s. BCG is thought to be capable of enhancing the immune system's surveillance ability to detect malignant cells of melanoma and bladder cancer. However, this mechanism alone has had no long-term effects on a person's survival with these neoplasms.[28]

## BIOTHERAPY

Biologic research on the function of the immune system has spurred the development of the fourth cancer treatment modality, termed *biotherapy*. The focus of biotherapy is manipulation of the immune system through drugs, cells, and cell products that modify the body's response to cancer or cancer therapy.

## BIOLOGIC RESPONSE MODIFIERS

Biologic response modifiers (BRMs) can be classified into several categories: agents that restore, strengthen, or modify the immune system (such as *interferon* [INF]); cells that have direct antitumor activity (such as *tumor necrosis factor* [TNF] or *natural killer cells* [NK cells]); and agents that have other biologic effects (such as *growth factors* that can intervene in cellular growth and differentiation).

### Interferons

INFs comprise a group of glycoproteins (alpha, beta, gamma) produced by leukocytes in response to viral infections or other stimuli. All nucleated cells are capable of interferon production, which can be induced by natural or synthetic agents. INFs have the ability to alter cellular metabolism of both normal and cancer cells. INFs produce change in cellular enzymes required for cell growth and proliferation, therefore modifying the immune response. INFs also can activate NK cells, which are mediators that can identify and destroy some tumor cells. INF use in cancer therapy continues to be studied. At present INFs appears to be most effective when used with other agents such as TNF or some chemotherapeutic agents. INF may work synergistically with certain cancer drugs and radiation. INFs hold the most promise for patients whose immune system has not been weakened by previous treatment with chemotherapy or radiation. INFs are produced by recombinant DNA technology by the insertion of genes for an INF of each category into *Escherichia coli*. Table 16-28 reviews the common BRMs and their clinical applications. Table 16-29 details the most common side effects of biotherapy.

### Interleukins

Interleukins comprise a group of biologic factors that are capable of sending messages among cells of the immune system (lymphocytes, NK cells, macrophages, hematopoietic cells). They are produced by thymus cells and are involved in cell-mediated immunity. Of the nine interleukins known, IL-2 has been most thoroughly studied. The gene for IL-2 is produced by recombinant technology and is available for clinical use in the treatment of several cancers.

### Tumor Necrosis Factor

Tumor necrosis factor (TNF) is a lymphokine derived from activated monocytes and macrophages. TNF has direct cytotoxic effects on some tumor cells. Because of serious toxic effects, TNF is considered most effective when used in combination with other biologic agents.

### Growth Factors

Colony-stimulating factors (CSFs) are glycoproteins that are now available for clinical use in the development and activation of several hematopoietic cell lines. Human granulocyte CSF (G-CSF) stimulates the growth and activation of granulocyte precursor cells. As yet no evidence exists that G-CSF can stimulate myeloid and megakaryocyte cell lines. However, continued clinical application may reveal a broader range of activity than is presently known. *Granulocyte-macrophage* CSF (GM-CSF) stimulates myeloid precursor cells and is approved for use after both autologous and allogeneic bone mar-

**TABLE 16-28 Common Biologic Response Modifiers and Their Clinical Applications**

| BRM | SOURCE | ACTION | CLINICAL APPLICATION |
|---|---|---|---|
| Alpha INF | Non–T cell lymphocyte | Direct tumor cytotoxicity<br>Stimulates NK cells and lymphocytes<br>Stimulates differentiation of tumor cells | Hairy-cell leukemia, renal cell carcinoma, melanoma, Kaposi's sarcoma<br>Some response with chronic myelogenous leukemia and multiple myeloma |
| Beta INF | Fibroblasts | Similar to alfa INF | Limited data, but appears similar to alpha INF; no apparent advantage over alpha INF |
| Gamma INF | T lymphocytes and NK cells | Similar to alpha INF<br>Stimulates proliferation of macrophages and enhances monocyte activity | May have selective effect against chronic myeloid leukemia and non-Hodgkin's lymphoma |
| Interleukin (IL-2) | T cells in response to antigenic stimulus | Activates production of more IL-2 and cytotoxic T cells, NK cells, B cells; induces a killer cell called *lymphokine activated killer* (LAK) cell | Approved for use in renal cancer and melanoma alone or in combination with LAK |
| Tumor necrosis factor (TNF) | Activated by monocytes and macrophages | Attaches to specific receptor on tumor cell membrane; then is transported to cytoplasm where it affects lysosomes, interferes with lipoprotein lipase; stimulates intravascular clotting, causing damage to endothelial cells | Potential use is in combination with other biologic agents because of its severe vasoactive effects (vasodilation, thrombosis) |
| Growth factors (G-CSF) (GM-CSF) | Lymphokine (chemicals transmitted from lymphocytes) | G-CSF promotes growth of neutrophils<br>GM-CSF promotes differentiation of macrophages into monocytes/macrophages | G-CSF and GM-CSF use after BMT, aplastic anemia, AIDS, and after myelosuppression from chemotherapy and radiation therapy |
| Erythropoietin (EPO) | Kidney | Enhances erythrocyte growth and differentiation | End-stage renal disease |
| Monoclonal antibodies (MoAb) | Hybridoma technology using mice with live cancer cells<br>Clones produced specific to original cancer cell antigen | Attacks certain "target cells" using various radioactive substances and chemotherapy agents | Imaging tumors using radioisotope-labeled monoclones<br>Selectively purges bone marrow of cancer cells. Treats tumors by conjugating radioactive substances or chemotherapy agents that damage tumor cells by being close to the target or entering the tumor cell |

Modified from Casciato DA, Lowitz BB: *Manual of clinical oncology,* Boston, 1988, Little, Brown & Co.

row transplantation. Both G-CSF and GM-CSF have demonstrated ability to accelerate bone marrow recovery of neutrophil counts after myelosuppression.

*Erythropoietin* (EPO) is another recombinant growth factor that is approved for the treatment of anemia associated with end-stage renal disease and anemia resulting from chemosuppression of the bone marrow.

## Monoclonal Antibodies

Monoclonal antibodies (MoAbs) are produced by hybridoma techniques that involve immunizing animals (usually mice) with antigen, then fusing B cells from the mouse's spleen with tumor cells to make hybrid cells. MoAbs can be produced to bind with almost any antigen. They are effective in the serologic detection of tumors inasmuch as cells that have undergone malignant transformation often express antigens that are not found frequently on the surfaces of normal cells. These markers may be sensitive to detection of early cancer and can be used to monitor the progress of disease in patients undergoing therapy.

Cancer therapy with MoAbs is in its early trials. Some tumor responses have occurred, but MoAbs alone are not toxic enough to kill tumor cells. Anticancer drugs, radioisotopes, and other BRMs may be attached to MoAbs and targeted directly to tumor cells, thus bypassing normal cells.

Ongoing research efforts will no doubt provide new applications for BRMs in cancer diagnosis and therapy. The use of biotherapy is very expensive because of the

**TABLE 16-29 Common Side Effects of Biologic Response Modifiers and Their Frequency**

| SIDE EFFECT | INTERFERON | TNF | IL-2 | MoAbs | CSF |
|---|---|---|---|---|---|
| Mental status changes | F | F | F | N | N |
| Anxiety | F | F | F | N | N |
| Headaches | F | F | F | O | F |
| Dysrhythmias | F | F | F | N | N |
| Hypotension | F | F | F | N | O |
| Cardiac dysfunction | O | O | O | N | N |
| Angina | O | O | O | N | N |
| Fatigue | F | F | F | F | F |
| Fever | F | F | F | F | F |
| Chills | F | F | F | O | O |
| Respiratory distress | O | O | O | O | N |
| Weight gain/edema | F | O | F | O | O |
| Renal dysfunction | O | O | F | N | N |
| Hepatic dysfunction | O | F | F | O | O |
| Food/taste aversions | O | O | O | N | N |
| Anorexia | F | F | F | O | O |
| Nausea | F | F | F | O | O |
| Diarrhea | F | O | F | N | N |
| Rash/itching | F | F | F | F | F |
| Allergic symptoms | F | F | F | F | F |
| Anemia | O | O | F | N | N |
| Thrombocytopenia | O | O | O | N | N |
| Eosinophilia | O | O | F | N | N |
| Arthralgias | F | F | F | O | O |
| Myalgias | O | O | F | O | O |
| Bone pain | O | O | O | N | O |

From Shelton B, Belcher A. In Ashwanden P et al: *Oncology nursing: advances, treatments, and trends into the 21st century,* Rockville, Md, 1990, Aspen.
*TNF,* Tumor necrosis factor; *MoAbs,* monoclonal antibodies; *CSF,* colony-stimulating factors; *F,* frequently seen; *O,* occasionally seen; *N,* not seen.

advanced technology required to produce these products and the length of clinical trials needed to ascertain their effects on human subjects. Although approval has been given for the use of several of the BRMs (interferons and growth factors), third-party insurers are reluctant to provide coverage because of the experimental status of some of these products.

## NURSING MANAGEMENT

### ♦ ASSESSMENT

The nurse working with the cancer patient receiving biotherapy should assess for the following:

1. Understanding of the nature of biotherapy as a treatment modality and the goal for treatment outcome
2. Status of immune and neurologic systems
3. Knowledge of specific biotherapy protocols
   a. Names of agents in use
   b. Routes, sites, and frequency of administration
4. Knowledge of side effects and self-care strategies for symptom management

### ♦ NURSING DIAGNOSES

Nursing diagnoses are determined from analysis of patient data. Nursing diagnoses for the patient with cancer who is receiving biotherapy may include but are not limited to the following:

| Diagnostic Title | Possible Etiologic Factors |
|---|---|
| Knowledge deficit (related to receiving biotherapy) | Lack of exposure to or information about role in cancer treatment, ability and readiness to learn and retain information, misinformation and misconceptions |
| Self-care deficit (related to receiving biotherapy) | Lack of knowledge of expected side effects, lack of support systems |

### ♦ EXPECTED PATIENT OUTCOMES

Expected patient outcomes for the patient receiving biotherapy for cancer treatment may include but are not limited to the following:

1. States the rationale and goal of biotherapy in treating his or her cancer.
2. Discusses the role of own immune system in relation to biotherapy.
3. Describes the prescribed biotherapy protocol.
   a. Agents
   b. Frequency of administration
   c. Route and site for administration
4. Discusses side effects and self-care strategies for

symptom management and management of side effects.

## ♦ INTERVENTIONS

Biotherapy is the newest form of cancer therapy and is being used alone or as an adjunct therapy with chemotherapy. The cancer patient who is to receive biotherapy must have a basic understanding of his or her own malignant condition, how the immune system functions in relation to cancer, and why biotherapy is being prescribed. The rationale for using biotherapy in cancer treatment comes from the belief that if the immune system can be enhanced by specific biologic agents, tumor cells can be destroyed by the body's own defense system.

### RESEARCH

Stetz KM: Survival work: the experience of the patient and the spouse involved in experimental treatment for cancer, *Semin Oncol Nurs* 9(2):121-126, 1993.

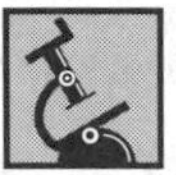

Twenty-four persons who had either advanced primary liver cancer or metastatic disease to the liver were studied in a 6-month longitudinal design study in which they and their spouses were interviewed before, during, and after receiving experimental cancer treatment. All were to be treated with chemoembolization for unresectable primary or metastatic liver cancer. The purpose of this study was to describe the experiences of patients and their spouses during experimental therapy, including their decision to enter a clinical trial and the processes that contributed to the patient's continuation of treatment. The study utilized grounded theory as the theoretic framework.

The primary psychosocial process that described the experiences of the person receiving experimental therapy was *survival work* (choosing life over death). Survival work was identified as having three phases. The first phase, *engaging,* included behavioral and social interactions and cognitions related to the decision to be treated. Engaging was further broken down into categories: (1) no other options, (2) fear of dying, (3) desire to survive, (4) need to do something, (5) belief that treatment will work, and (6) being offered the opportunity to try something. The second phase of survival work, *monitoring,* related to time: good time, bad or sick time, treatment time, couple time, travel time, and new discoveries. The third phase of survival, *carrying on,* reflected the patient's and spouse's life without hope that the treatment would curtail the cancer. Two nursing implications evolved from the study: (1) that nurses must have knowledge about the ethics of experimental protocols and their role in assisting the investigator in maintaining an unbiased approach in interacting with the experimental groups and (2) assessing and being aware of the experiences encountered by patients with advanced cancer undergoing experimental therapy, as well as the experiences of spouses. Only in this way can nurses provide meaningful assistance during the experimental treatment when many uncertainties are encountered.

### Providing Patient Education

The immune system is a complex system that protects the body by several mechanisms. The first function is *defense* against infection from microorganisms. The second function is *homeostasis* by the removal of damaged cells that result from normal cellular catabolism. The third function of the immune system is the mechanism of surveillance by which mutant cells are recognized as "not self" and removed from the body. When the immunosurveillance mechanism is functioning normally, it can eliminate these potential cancer cells, thus preventing them from growing and spreading within the body. When the surveillance mechanism is not functioning normally or becomes overwhelmed by numbers, the mutant cells result in tumor growth and cancer can develop.[19]

The practical application of biotherapy began with research in the 1970s on the antiproliferative effects of interferon on cancer cells. It was not until recombinant DNA technology became a reality that biologic response modifiers (BRMs) such as interferons, interleukins, myeloid growth factors, and monoclonal antibodies could be more thoroughly investigated and their potential in cancer therapy realized. The future application of BRMs looks promising, and use will expand as research and clinical trials continue. At present, however, some of the BRMs are considered experimental and others have only a limited range of usefulness. Although most investigations and clinical trials of BRMs were carried out at large research institutions such as the National Institutes of Health, patients are now able to receive them in small community hospitals, in outpatient departments, and in the home setting. As a result, it is the responsibility of nurses working with cancer patients to have knowledge of biotherapy and the side effects most commonly observed and to be able to teach the patient and family regarding the care needs and strategies for symptom management. The patient must be aware that biotherapy may have only a moderate effect on the tumor activity while producing side effects that are constitutionally debilitating and may last for several weeks after therapy has been discontinued.

The side effects for all BRMs are similar in nature, and the common ones are listed in Table 16-29. Not all side effects will be seen in each patient, but the patient should be informed that any of those listed can occur. The intensity of symptoms will depend on the biologic agent used, the dosage, and the route of administration. Each symptom can create significant discomfort when experienced alone, but when the patient must deal with the combined effects, care needs are significantly increased and the patient requires the assistance of supportive and knowledgeable persons. The side effects may occur shortly after administration and usually dissipate within 3 or 4 days; however, some symptoms may linger for several weeks.

### Promoting Self-Care

When the patient is to receive BRMs at home, either the patient or a support person will need instruction on the techniques of administration. Strategies for dealing with the side effects are of a supportive nature and include little in the way of pharmacologic interventions. The flulike symptoms are treated by keeping the patient in a quiet, calm environment and at rest. The use of relaxation and diversional activities should be encouraged. Fever and the discomfort from myalgia, arthralgias, headache, and bone pain can be alleviated by administration of acetaminophen. Aspirin and aspirin-containing products are to be avoided. Skin rashes should be reported to the physician if they persist beyond several days. Diphenhydramine (Benadryl) may be prescribed for pruritus, and the patient should be instructed not to scratch the area. Cold applications may be soothing and may be used as necessary. However, the patient and family should be told to protect the skin from direct contact with ice packs or wet applications that can cause frostbite or macerate the skin. Changes in mood with increasing anxiety and confusion often are encountered during therapy. Knowing that these symptoms may occur but will subside when treatment is over helps both the patient and family deal with them in a more positive way. The gastrointestinal symptoms are addressed by antiemetics, small, frequent meals, and good mouth care before and after meals and after vomiting. Fluid intake of sufficient amounts to prevent dehydration is necessary. Daily weigh-ins during the first several days of treatment when these side effects are most frequent will help the nurse or support person recognize nutritional deficits immediately.

It is easy for the patient receiving BRMs to become anxious, depressed, and angry. Outcomes cannot be predicted with certainty. The patient will already have been treated in most cases by one or a combination of the other cancer therapies and may become very discouraged and question continuing with therapy. The patient must be supported by sympathetic understanding of these feelings. False gestures of hope are avoided, but completion of the prescribed protocol may be the only way in which the physician can determine the effects of the BRMs on the tumor. Patients should know that they may withdraw from therapy at any time with the assurance that their care will not be affected by the decision.

## ♦ EVALUATION

To evaluate the effectiveness of nursing interventions, compare patient behaviors with those stated in the expected patient outcomes. Successful achievement of patient outcomes for the patient receiving biotherapy for cancer is indicated by the following:

1. Knowledge of biotherapy
   a. Correctly identifies the need to improve his or her own immune system so that it can be more effective in identifying cancer cells and eliminating them.
   b. States that biotherapy is still somewhat experimental as a cancer treatment, yet is willing to try it.
2. Correctly identifies the biologic agent(s) to be used and the proper dose and route of administration.
3. Describes the common side effects of biotherapy and strategies to manage symptoms.
4. Acknowledges need for physical and emotional support and accepts it readily when offered.

# OTHER CANCER TREATMENT MODALITIES

Even with advances in conventional cancer treatment modalities—surgery, radiation therapy, chemotherapy, and biotherapy—cancer remains the second leading cause of death in the United States. Therefore an urgent need exists for the development of new treatment modes or new ways in which existing treatment methods might be used in unique ways. Therapies such as hyperthermia and photodynamic therapy, although not exactly new, are again being scrutinized by means of a variety of clinical trials to ascertain their value in cancer treatment. See Research box, p. 426.

## HYPERTHERMIA

It has long been known that when normal and malignant cells are exposed to extremely high temperatures (40° to 42° C), they are destroyed. The mechanism by which this cytotoxicity occurs is not completely understood at present. Because many cancers recur after conventional cancer therapy at the local or regional level, it is thought that hyperthermia (HT) might be useful as an adjunctive therapy with radiation or chemotherapy. Clinical data seem to indicate a synergistic effect when hyperthermia is used concurrently or within a few hours of radiation treatment. Rationale for using hyperthermia and radiation therapy together comes from the knowledge that hyperthermia is most cytotoxic in the S phase of the cell cycle, whereas radiation therapy is known to be least effective in this phase. In addition, radiation therapy must have well-oxygenated cells to ensure sufficient cell kill, but the effectiveness of hyperthermia is not changed at all by cell hypoxia.[45] It is believed that hyperthermia might even increase blood flow to hypoxic tissue, making it less hypoxic and thus more vulnerable to radiation effects.

Four methods are used for local or regional hyperthermia: (1) ultrasonic (US) devices, (2) devices using electromagnetic waves, (3) devices that use alternating electromagnetic (EM) fields to heat by induction of electrical currents, and (4) devices using direct coupling of EM currents between needles or plates encompassing the tissue to be heated.

These methods may be either noninvasive (i.e., they do not use materials to enter the body) or invasive (e.g., by needle implants, interstitial seeds, and interstitial and intracavitary application of small antennae emitting EM waves). Whole body hyperthermia has been achieved by immersing the patient in liquid wax or circulating hot water or placing the patient in a heated cabinet.

Information to date on the efficacy of combined hyperthermia and radiation therapy is mixed at best. There is no general consensus on any advantage of combined therapy over radiation therapy alone. Some of the limitations and resistance to combined therapy is related to the patient's inability to tolerate the intensity of the treatment and length of time required at each session. Current clinical trials will help to determine the "thermal dose" necessary for specific tumors along with the length of treatment that can be tolerated by the human body.

### PHOTODYNAMIC THERAPY

Photodynamic therapy (PDT) is being studied as a possible therapy for deep-seated tumors. PDT requires the intravenous administration of a dye (sensitizer)—a specific mixture of hematoporphyrins—that localizes in malignant tissue. When the tissue is subjected to laser light by means of fiberoptic technology, a fluorescent flow can be seen. Once the malignant tissue is identified, it is believed that it can be destroyed by special drugs that are targeted directly to the tumor. PDT as a treatment modality is in the preliminary stage but appears to have value as a potential therapy in recurrent breast cancer, in head and neck tumors, and in bronchial, bladder, and early gynecologic cancer.[3]

## ONCOLOGIC EMERGENCIES

Oncologic emergencies may occur as a result of the disease process or its treatment. These emergencies include obstructions (increased intracranial pressure, spinal cord compression, superior vena cava syndrome, tracheal or bowel obstruction), metabolic syndromes (hypercalcemia, tumor lysis syndrome, syndrome of inappropriate antidiuretic hormone secretion, hyperviscosity, anaphylaxis, septic shock, disseminated intravascular coagulation, and cardiac toxicities (pericardial tamponade, cardiomyopathy with congestive heart failure) as described in Table 16-30. The oncology nurse is the health care professional frequently in a position to recognize these emergencies. A careful history and ongoing monitoring for signs and symptoms alert nurses to life-threatening conditions. During these crisis situations the patient may require transfer to an intensive care unit.

## CANCER PAIN

Pain is one of the most feared effects of cancer, although contrary to popular belief, it is frequently one of the last symptoms to appear. Pain is generally not a problem in the early, localized stage of disease. About 5% to 10% of patients with solid tumors have pain that interferes with activity or mood. When disease is in an advanced stage and metastasis has occurred, 60% to 90% of patients experience pain severe enough to require opioid drug therapy.[20]

Alleviation of pain is the responsibility and obligation of health care professionals. It is also generally mandated by the quality assurance policies of each health care institution that pain management strategies be carried out. The Oncology Nursing Society (ONS) developed a position paper on cancer pain in part because pain management is a significant clinical problem faced by the nurse caring for cancer patients and because the assessment and control of cancer pain has been poorly managed. The ONS statement legitimately places on the nurse the responsibility for identifying the problem of inadequate pain management and intervening to achieve optimal pain relief.

### STAGES

Three stages of cancer pain have been described: early, intermediate, and late. Early pain usually occurs after initial surgery for diagnosis or treatment and usually subsides after the third day; thus this pain is an acute episode that is short-term and temporary.

Intermediate-stage pain results from postoperative contraction of scars and nerve entrapment or from cancer recurrence or metastasis. This pain may subside or may be controlled by palliative therapy such as radiation, chemotherapy, neurosurgery, and analgesics. Therapy itself may initiate the pain.

Late-stage pain occurs in terminal cancer when therapy no longer controls the disease. This pain is chronic, may slowly increase in intensity, and at times may be intractable.

### CAUSES

Malignant neoplasms cause pain by five physiologic changes: bone destruction (the most frequent cause); obstruction of lumina (viscera or vessels); peripheral nerve involvement; pressure of growing tumors that cause ischemia, distention, and inflammation; and infection or necrosis of tissue. The pathophysiology of cancer pain is summarized in Table 16-31. The frequency and intensity of pain depend on the stage of the disease, its location, and the patient's age, gender, personality, pain perception, pain threshold, and previous pain experience.[17] The sources of pain associated with cancer treatment are summarized in Box 16-18.

The psychologic component of cancer pain is associated with the patient's perception of the threat and

**TABLE 16-30 Oncologic Emergencies**

| TYPE | PATHOPHYSIOLOGY | CLINICAL MANIFESTATIONS |
|---|---|---|
| **OBSTRUCTIVE** | | |
| Increased intracranial pressure | Increased brain mass from tumor, hemorrhage, or edema. Alteration in internal jugular vein flow caused by head/neck tumor or by surgical resection; results in alteration in function | Change in mental status, vomiting, headache, dizziness, seizures (see Chapter 57) |
| Spinal cord compression | Primary or metastatic lesions causing disruption of reflexes and motor function because of neuron impairment and interruption of motor or sensory nerve fibers. Symptoms depend on location | Flaccid paralysis, paresthesias, locomotion difficulties, respiratory impairment at C5 level (see Chapter 57) |
| Superior vena cava syndrome (SVC) | Obstruction of the SVC caused by primary (usually lung cancer) or metastatic tumors in the mediastinal or paratracheal nodes | Dyspnea, facial and neck swelling, chest pain, cough, dysphagia, ruddy edematous face |
| Tracheal obstruction | Reduction in lumen from tracheal stenosis, extrinsic compression, or mass in lumen | Signs and symptoms of inadequate gas exchange and respiratory function (see Chapter 37) |
| **METABOLIC** | | |
| Hypercalcemia | Bone disease or metastasis increases bone resorption with bone destruction and release of calcium in the extracellular fluid. It is believed the tumor may produce (1) a substance that enables bone resorption of calcium or (2) ectopic parathyroid hormone that increases serum calcium levels | N&V, constipation, muscle weakness, coma, dysrhythmias, polyruia, nephrolithiasis (see Chapter 20) |
| Tumor lysis syndrome (TLS) | Rapid tumor cell destruction after cytotoxic chemotherapy may result in release of intracellular electrolytes. May occur in cancers characterized by rapid cell growth (leukemia and lymphomas) | Hyperphosphatemia (oliguria, azotemia), hyperkalemia, hyperuricemia (N&V, lethargy, anuria, azotemia), hypocalcemia (see Chapter 20) |
| Syndrome of inappropriate antidiuretic hormone secretion (SIADH) | Increase in ADH seen in cancers such as lung carcinoma (especially oat cell), duodenal and pancreatic carcinoma, thymoma, lymphomas, uterine carcinoma, and CNS tumors. May also occur with some chemotherapeutic agents (cyclophosphamide, vincristine) | Fluid and electrolyte changes and neurologic changes (see Chapter 57) |
| Hyperviscosity | Increased blood viscosity from increase in cell number, loss of flexibility of cells, or overproduction of serum proteins. This causes increased resistance to blood flow | Bleeding from GI or urinary tracts or puncture sites; visual disturbance, headache, dizziness, weakness, dyspnea, distended neck veins |
| Anaphylaxis | Hypersensitivity responses (I, II, III, IV) caused by chemotherapeutic agents (asparaginase, cisplatin, neocarzinostatin, VM-26, doxorubicin, daunorubicin, bleomycin, cyclophosphamide, methotrexate, melphalan) | Signs of anaphylactic reactions (see Chapter 70) |
| Septic shock | Increased susceptibility to infection from impaired immune system or effect of immunosuppressive agents, leading to bacterial septicemia | Signs and symptoms of septic shock (see Chapter 22) |
| Disseminated intravascular coagulation (DIC) | Chronic bleeding consumes all clotting factors; may also result from sepsis | Thrombocytopenia, bleeding of mucous membranes and tissues (see Chapter 34) |
| **CARDIAC TOXICITIES** | | |
| Cardiac tamponade | Intrapericardial pressure increases from accumulation of fluid from direct tumor invasion, metastatic lesion, infection, or from pericardial thickening after radiation. Results in decreased diastolic ventricular filling and decreased stroke volume and cardiac output | Dyspnea, cough, chest pain, muffled heart sounds, cyanosis, edema, decreased systolic pressure, decreased central venous pressure (see Chapter 31) |
| Cardiomyopathy with congestive heart failure (CHF) | Chemotherapeutic drugs (such as anthracyclines, mithramycin, mitomycin, and cyclophosphamide) appear to damage cardiac myofibrils, causing sarcoplasmic reticular swelling that leads to destruction of the myofibril; hypertrophy of the heart muscle ensues with decreased function | Acute: tachycardia, dysrhythmias<br>Chronic: signs of CHF (see Chapter 31) |

**TABLE 16-31 Pathophysiology of Cancer Pain**

| CAUSE | TYPE OF PAIN |
|---|---|
| Bone destruction with infraction (fracture without displacement) | Increased sensitivity over area or sharp continuous pain |
| Obstruction of a viscus (gastrointestinal or genitourinary tract) | Severe, colicky, crampy type of pain; may be dull, diffuse, poorly localized |
| Obstruction of an artery, vein, or lymphatic | Dull, diffuse, aching (caused by arterial ischemia, venous engorgement, edema) |
| Infiltration, compression of peripheral nerves or nerve plexus | Continuous, sharp, or stabbing pain; sometimes hyperesthesia or paresthesia |
| Infiltration or distention of integument, fascia, or tissue (e.g., ascites) | Localized, dull aching pain |
| Inflammation, infection, and necrosis of tissue | Varied pain caused by pressure or ischemia |

stress of cancer and varies from individual to individual. Three categories of stressors have been identified: injury or threat of injury as a result of the cancer; loss or threat of loss (body part or death); and frustration of drives as a result of disabilities from the cancer or from the effect of therapies. Patients may respond with depression, decreased self-esteem, hostility, and irritability.

The sociologic effects include decreased interaction and participation in activities of daily living. Decreased productivity is characterized by absence from work, economic problems, and deterioration in family relationships. The spiritual effects of pain are evidenced by loss of hope and trust and an overwhelming feeling of despair, rejection, and sense of isolation. Figure 16-20 shows the multiple factors associated with pain.

Side effects of cancer pain include fatigue, sleeplessness, anorexia, and decreased movement, followed by the complications of immobility, namely muscle weakness, decubiti, contractures, and respiratory dysfunction.

## ASSESSMENT

Cancer pain may occupy the patient's entire attention and, unless treated vigorously, can demoralize the patient and interfere with all aspects of life. Pain tolerance is increased when the patient's energy is preserved for enjoyable activities. The nurse plays a vital role in assessing the patient's pain experience. Accurate documentation of the location (localized or radiating), intensity (mild, severe, dull, constant), what precipitates it (mobility, after eating, coughing), what provides comfort (repositioning, drugs) often influences the type of medical interventions prescribed. The patient's description of pain in a verbal or a written format (e.g., a pain diary) is helpful. Pointing out pain intensity on a pain scale is another method of assessing pain level and deciding on the most appropriate pain-relief strategy. For more information on pain assessment, see Chapter 17.

**BOX 16-18 Sources of Pain Associated With Cancer Treatment**

I. Diagnostic procedures
  A. Lumbar punctures
  B. Blood samples
  C. Angiography
  D. Endoscopy
  E. Biopsies
II. Surgery
  A. Acute postoperative pain
  B. Chronic postoperative pain
    1. Mastectomy
    2. Radical neck resection
    3. Lymphedema
    4. Thoracotomy
    5. Phantom-limb
III. Chemotherapy
  A. Acute
    1. Gastrointestinal distress
    2. Mucositis
    3. Myalgia
    4. Joint pain
    5. Cardiomyopathy
    6. Pancreatitis
    7. Extravasation
  B. Chronic
    1. Peripheral neuropathy
    2. Steroid pseudorheumatism
    3. Aseptic osteonecrosis
IV. Radiation
  A. Acute
    1. Skin burn
    2. Gastrointestinal cramping
    3. Proctitis
    4. Mucositis
    5. Itching
  B. Chronic
    1. Osteonecrosis
    2. Fibrosis
    3. Keratitis
    4. Demyelination
    5. Pneumonitis
    6. Bowel ulceration or obstruction
    7. Myelopathy
V. Other treatments and treatment complications

From Chapman CR, Kornell J, Syrjala KL. In McGuire D, Yarbro C, editors: *Cancer pain management,* Orlando, Fla, 1987, Grune & Stratton.

## MANAGEMENT

The ultimate goal of pain management is to provide pain relief and enable the patient to carry on with activities of daily living in as near to normal fashion as possible. Strategies may involve a combination of behavioral techniques such as relaxation or diversional activities, meditation, hypnosis, or imagery, in addition to the use of common nursing strategies. Interventions that may not

**BOX 16-19 Combination of Comfort Measures and Behavioral Techniques for Pain Relief**

1. Promote comfort:
   a. Meticulous hygiene
   b. Clean, dry, bed linen
   c. Control of odors
   d. Good body positioning such as with pillows, bed cradle, foot boards for the bedfast person
2. Maintain nutrition
3. Provide diversionary activities for distraction to decrease pain perception:
   a. Physical activities (e.g., working, walking, gardening, swimming)
   b. Mental relaxation activities (e.g., watching TV, reading, crafts, listening to music, comedy cassettes)
   c. Social (e.g., visits from family, friends)
4. Suggest and teach forms of noninvasive pain relief:
   a. Guided imagery
   b. Hypnosis
   c. Progressive muscle relaxation
   d. Transcendental meditation

always be thought of as pain-relief strategies include comfort measures that promote rest and sleep, good body positioning, nutrition, and patient teaching of how to decrease pain perception. Combinations of comfort and behavioral methods are provided in Box 16-19. At times conventional cancer therapies will themselves be used to achieve pain relief. Surgery may be used (1) to debulk a tumor, otherwise inoperable, when it is compressing a nerve or causing obstruction of a vessel and ischemic pain or (2) to repair pathologic fractures. Surgical procedures also may include simple nerve blocks such as to the brachial, sympathetic, intercostal, or epidural nerves. Radiation therapy frequently is used to treat bone pain caused by metastasis and the oncologic emergency of superior vena cava obstruction. Chemotherapy and hormonal therapies, although not used as often as radiation therapy and surgery, are believed to have a role in pain relief.

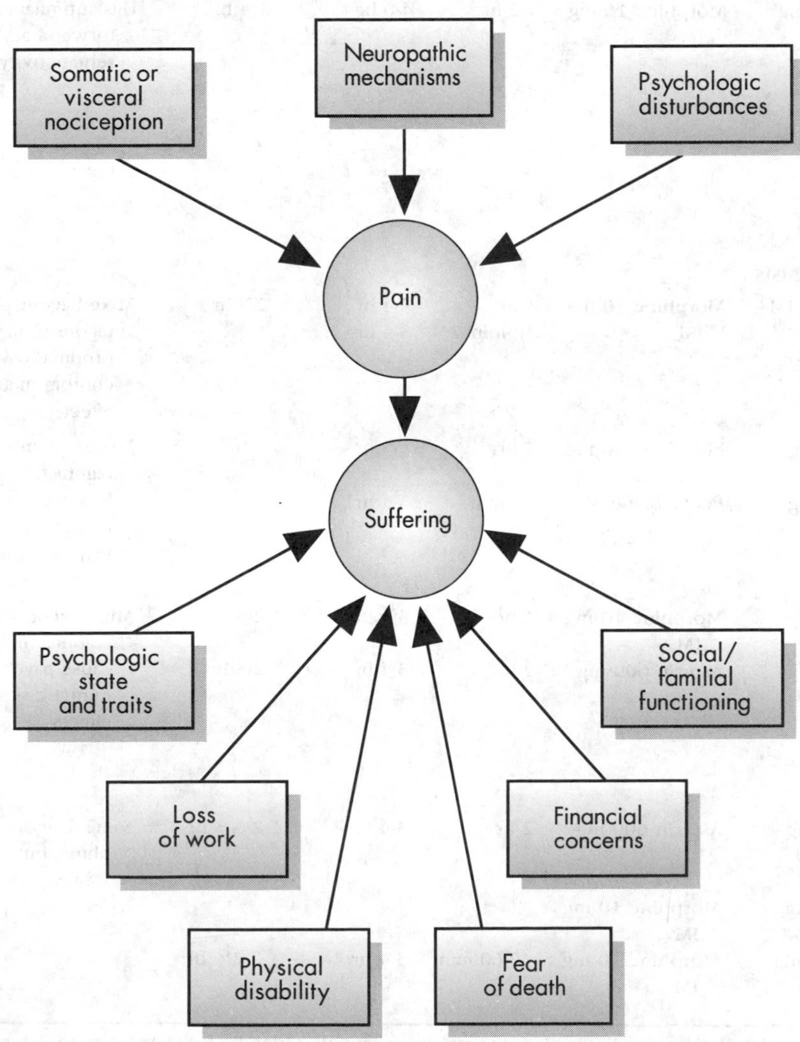


**FIGURE 16-20** Multiple factors associated with pain. (Modified from Portenoy RK: *CA* 138:332, 1988; and the American Cancer Society.)

**TABLE 16-32 An Equianalgesic Comparison of the Most Common Analgesics**

| GENERIC AND (TRADE) NAME | DOSE | EQUIVALENT TO* | PEAK EFFECT | DURATION | PLASMA HALF-LIFE | COMMENTS | PRECAUTIONS |
|---|---|---|---|---|---|---|---|
| **NON-NARCOTICS** | | | | | | | |
| Acetaminophen (Tylenol, Tempra, etc) | 600 mg PO | Aspirin 600 mg PO | 2 hr | 3-4 hr | 1-4 hr | Antipyretic and antiinflammatory action is weak | In large doses, may cause liver toxicity |
| | 600 mg rectal suppository | | Slower than oral | | | | |
| Acetylsalicylic acid (aspirin) | 600 mg PO | Morphine 2 mg IM | 2 hr | 3-4 hr | 15 min | Has antipyretic and antiinflammatory activity | Used with steroids, it may increase gastric bleeding |
| | 600 mg rectal suppository | | Slower than oral | | | | |
| Methotrimeprazine (Levoprome) | 20 mg IM | Morphine 10 mg IM | 1 hr | 4-6 hr | Unknown | A phenothiazine; recommend starting with 5 mg dose | May cause oversedation, orthostatic hypotension, liver toxicity |
| Zomepirac (Zomax) | 100 mg PO | Morphine 16 mg IM | 1-2 hr | 4-6 hr | 1-4 hr | Has antiinflammatory and antipyretic activity | Use with caution in patients with urinary tract infection, elevated BUN, creatinine, and in patients with aspirin sensitivity |
| **NARCOTICS** | | | | | | | |
| **Opioid Agonists/Antagonists** | | | | | | | |
| Butorphanol tartrate (Stadol) | 2 mg IM | Morphine 10 mg IM | 1 hr | 3-4 hr | 2.7 hr | Mixed agonist-antagonist; may produce psychotomimetic effect | May cause abstinence reaction in patients physically dependent on narcotics |
| | 2 mg IV | | 30 min | 3-4 hr | | | |
| Nalbuphine HCl (Nubain) | 10 mg IM | Morphine 10 mg IM | 1 hr | 4-5 hr | 5 hr | Mixed agonist-antagonist, but less psychotomimetic effect than pentazocine | Same precautions as with butorphanol |
| | 10 mg IV | Pentazocine 60 mg IM | 30 min | 3-4 hr | | | |
| Pentazocine HCl (Talwin) | 60 mg IM | Morphine 10 mg IM | 1 hr | 3-4 hr | 2-3 hr | Mixed agonist-antagonist, may cause psychotomimetic side effects | Same precautions as with butorphanol; use with caution in patients with cardiac abnormalities |
| | 30 mg PO | Aspirin 600 mg | 2 hr | 3-4 hr | 2-3 hr | | |
| **Opioid Agonists** | | | | | | | |
| Codeine sulfate | 30 mg PO | Aspirin 600 mg | 2 hr | 3-4 hr | 2½-3 hr | Same as morphine, but weaker | Not for IV use |
| | 200 mg PO | Morphine 10 mg IM | | | | | |
| | 120 mg IM | Morphine 10 mg IM | 30-60 min | 3-4 hr | 2-2½ hr | | |

From Catalano RB. In McGuire DB, Yarbro C, editors: *Cancer pain management,* Orlando, Fla, 1987, Grune & Stratton.

*The oral/parenteral efficacy ratio refers to the ratio of doses given by the two routes of administration necessary to produce equivalent "total" analgesic effect when both intensity and duration of effect are taken into account. If only maximal intensity or "peak" effect is considered, however, oral administration yields even less effective analgesia than parenteral administration. These studies were done on cancer patients. In other types of pain, equivalencies may not be the same.

## TABLE 16-32 An Equianalgesic Comparison of the Most Common Analgesics—cont'd

| GENERIC AND (TRADE) NAME | DOSE | EQUIVALENT TO* | PEAK EFFECT | DURATION | PLASMA HALF-LIFE | COMMENTS | PRECAUTIONS |
|---|---|---|---|---|---|---|---|
| **Opioid Agonists—cont'd** | | | | | | | |
| Hydromorphone HCl (Dilaudid) | 7.5 mg PO<br>3 mg rectal suppository | Morphine 10 mg IM<br>Hydromorphone 1.5 mg IM | 1 hr | 3-4 hr | 2-3 hr | Quick onset of action | Same precautions as with morphine |
| | 1.5 mg IM | Morphine 10 mg IM | 30 min | 3 hr | 2-3 hr | Has similar time effect as heroin; highly soluble | Same precautions as with morphine |
| | 1 mg IV | Morphine 10 mg IM | 15 min | 2-3 hr | | | |
| Levorphanol tartrate (Levo-Dromoran) | 4 mg PO | Morphine 10 mg IM<br>Levorphanol 2 mg IM | 2 hr | 4-5 hr | 15 hr | Same as morphine | Same precautions as with morphine |
| | 2 mg IM | Morphine 10 mg IM | 1 hr | 4-5 hr | | | |
| | 1 mg IV | Morphine 10 mg IM | 15-30 min | 3-4 hr | | | |
| Meperidine HCl (Demerol, Pethadol) | 50 mg PO<br>300 mg PO | Aspirin 600 mg<br>Morphine 10 mg IM<br>Meperidine 75 mg IM | 2 hr | 3-4 hr | 3 hr | Causes CNS excitation ranging from irritability to seizures | Not for chronic administration in patients with renal dysfunction |
| | 75 mg IM | Morphine 10 mg IM | 1 hr | 2-4 hr | | | |
| Methadone HCl | 20 mg PO | Morphine 10 mg IM<br>Methadone 10 mg IM | 2 hr | 4-5 hr | 15-22 hr | Same as morphine | Same precautions as with morphine |
| | 10 mg IM | Morphine 10 mg IM | 1 hr | 4-5 hr | | | |
| | 5 mg IV | Morphine 10 mg IM | 15-30 min | 3-4 hr | | | |
| Morphine sulfate | 30-60 mg PO | Morphine 10 mg IM | 2 hr | 4-5 hr | 2½-3 hr | May cause oversedation, confusion, visual disturbances, urinary retention | Contraindicated in patients with: impaired ventilation, asthma, elevated intracranial pressure, liver failure |
| | 10 mg IM | Morphine 10 mg IM | 1 hr | 4-5 hr | | | |
| | 5 mg IV | Morphine 10 mg IM | 15-30 min | 2-4 hr | | | |
| Oxycodone (with aspirin-Percodan; with acetaminophen-Percocet) | 5 mg PO<br>30 mg PO | Codeine 60 mg PO<br>Morphine 10 mg IM | 1 hr | 3-4 hr | 2-3 hr | Not available in IM or IV form | |
| Oxymorphone HCl (Numorphan) | 1 mg IM | Morphine 10 mg IM | 1 hr | 4-5 hr | Unknown | Highly soluble; not available orally | Same precautions as with morphine |
| | 0.5 mg IV | Morphine 10 mg IM | 15-30 min | 3-4 hr | | | |
| | 10 mg rectal suppository | Oxymorphone 1 mg IM | 2 hr | 6 hr | | | |
| Propoxyphene HCl (Darvon, Dolene) | 65 mg PO | Aspirin 600 mg | 2 hr | 3-4 hr | 12 hr | A "weak" narcotic; structurally related to methadone | Overdose can be complicated by convulsions |
| Propoxyphene napsylate (Darvon N) (with acetaminophen-Darvocet N) | 100 mg PO | Aspirin 600 mg | 2 hr | 3-4 hr | 12 hr | Same as propoxyphene HCl | |

## Pharmacologic Interventions

When medications are to be used to relieve pain, it is essential that the nurse understand how these agents can be best utilized, depending on the pattern of pain the patient is experiencing. When the pain is constant, it is most appropriate to administer analgesics on an around-the-clock schedule. This method of pain relief is used to prevent pain rather than to treat it after it has already occurred. This pattern of pain is amenable to long-acting analgesics or continuous infusions.

Even with the best scheduling to achieve pain relief, the patient may still experience *breakthrough pain.* Breakthrough pain is pain that occurs intermittently and spontaneously even with preventive scheduling. It may be related to certain activities (situational pain) such as walking, eating, or defecating. Breakthrough pain can be managed by supplementing the existing preventive mode with analgesics of rapid onset and of short duration. The use of patient-controlled analgesia (PCA) is one of the newest and most effective methods by which the patient can manage breakthrough pain. PCA allows the patient to administer a preset amount of medication at preset intervals. PCA has been found to be a means of giving the patient a feeling of control in cancer therapy, as well as providing freedom from pain. *Intermittent* pain is difficult to treat. It appears to respond most expeditiously to drugs of rapid and short duration given as needed or with the addition of PCA.

Administration of drugs as needed is not effective for chronic severe pain and contributes to tolerance and dependence. The patient loses confidence in the staff, and a vicious cycle of relief-pain-relief is set up.

Nonnarcotic agents are deemed most appropriate for the treatment of mild cancer pain. This category includes aspirin, acetaminophen, and nonsteroidal antiinflammatory drugs (NSAIDs). Aspirin is the most effective single analgesic for mild to moderate pain but is contraindicated if platelet counts are low. Nonnarcotic agents may have an additive and perhaps synergistic effect when used with narcotic analgesics and can therefore be effective in controlling more severe pain.

Narcotic analgesics (opioids) are reserved for moderate to severe cancer pain. They are divided into the categories of narcotic agonist or narcotic agonist-antagonist. Nurses must know the pharmacologic characteristics of the agents they are administering. Also of great importance is a knowledge of the equianalgesic effects of drugs used in pain relief. Table 16-31 compares the equianalgesic effects of common pain-relief medications.

Undertreatment of pain is an everpresent problem. There is always the underlying fear that the patient will become addicted to narcotics. *Addiction* refers to the uncontrolled dependence and craving of a substance so that the person cannot think of anything else but obtaining the drug. Addiction is not a realistic concern for the cancer patient. Cancer patients may, however, develop tolerance rather than addiction. Tolerance can occur at any time in anyone who is on a narcotics regimen and requires an increase in dosage to achieve the same analgesic relief. The nurse should anticipate the occurrence of tolerance in the patient whose tumor is not responding to therapy and continues to spread. Tolerance is not a reason to withhold medications for pain relief.

**TABLE 16-33 Adjuvant Drugs Useful in Cancer Pain Management**

| GENERIC NAME | TRADE NAME | CLASSIFICATION |
|---|---|---|
| Amitriptyline | Elavil, Emitrip, Enovil | Antidepressant |
| Carbamazepine | Tegretol | Anticonvulsant |
| Dexamethasone | Decadron | Corticosteroid |
| Dextroamphetamine | Dexedrine, Ferndex | Cerebral stimulant |
| Fluphenazine | Prolixin | Antipsychotic/neuroleptic |
| Haloperidol | Haldol | Antipsychotic/neuroleptic |
| Hydroxyzine | Vistaril, Atarax | Antianxiety |
| Methotrimeprazine | Levoprome | Neuroleptic |

Adjuvant analgesics frequently are used in combination with nonnarcotic and narcotic agents for relief of pain. Antidepressants, anticonvulsants for paroxysmal cutting-like pain, neuroleptics, and corticosteroids for bone pain from metastasis are commonly used medications. Table 16-33 notes examples of common adjuvant drugs used in the management of cancer pain.

Pain relief can be achieved by many different routes. Oral administration is preferred. Parenteral therapy produces higher initial serum and tissue levels, but the oral doses are as effective as parenteral doses in maintaining drug levels in the body. Intramuscular and subcutaneous injections are more difficult to administer and are painful to patients with marked muscle wasting. Tables 16-34 and 16-35 provide specific data on routes of administration and pharmacologic and nonpharmacologic pain intervention techniques. (See also Chapter 17 for an in-depth discussion of pain management.)

## HOME MANAGEMENT OF CANCER PAIN

Pain often is not effectively managed at home, resulting in the patient's decreased functional ability. Common reasons for not taking medications include misunderstanding dosages, feeling that pain cannot be controlled with the same degree of effectiveness as was achieved in the hospital, and inability to administer the medication accurately. This is a concern especially if the patient goes home with continuous subcutaneous infusion of an opioid or patient-controlled analgesia (PCA). Patients and families have fears similar to those of health care professionals concerning addiction and dependence on narcotics. It is therefore important that the patient and family be instructed about pain-control measures before discharge to home. The nurse must stress the need to follow the pain-relief protocol prescribed. If the patient can take medications orally, it should be emphasized that omitting doses or taking them on an as-needed basis can lead to breakthrough pain and unnecessary suffering. Subcutaneous infusions or PCAs are most useful for the patient who cannot take oral medications. There are, however, some disadvantages to these methods as the primary means of pain relief. Some patients feel overwhelmed by the technical aspects of these forms of pain management. Some fear the responsibility of self-medication. When the patient or family members indicate anxiety about using PCA, another form of pain relief should be considered. If a family member can take the responsibility of assisting with the PCA administration for the patient who is unwilling or unable to comply, all necessary teaching must be accomplished before the time of discharge. Subcutaneous continuous infusion requires the use of a small portable pump and a pediatric butterfly needle, but these do not appear to impede patient mobility and usually are acceptable to the patient and family. Names and telephone numbers should be provided for contacting persons who can assist in emergency situations or when pain relief cannot be maintained with the protocol in use.

Although complete freedom from pain is not always achieved, the patient can be kept comfortable in most cases. The use of behavioral interventions such as relaxation techniques, self-hypnosis, and meditation should be encouraged in combination with analgesics. In the home setting, surrounded by family members and a familiar environment, these combination strategies may provide a comfort level not equaled in the acute hospital setting. Nursing strategies for dealing more effectively with the cancer patient's pain are listed in the Guidelines box below.

**TABLE 16-34 Routes of Administration of Opioid Drugs**

| ROUTE | COMMENT |
|---|---|
| Oral | Preferred, if feasible |
| Buccal | Potentially effective if drug exposed to oral mucosa for prolonged period; not clinically available |
| Rectal | Morphine, oxymorphone, and hydromorphone available; very few studies, but generally believed to be equianalgesic to oral route |
| Subcutaneous: repetitive, continuous | Outpatient continuous infusion now possible with ambulatory pumps |
| Intramuscular | Limited role in chronic administration of opioids |
| Intravenous: repetitive, continuous, patient-controlled | Cost and need for manual dexterity and intact cognition may limit utility of patient-controlled pumps for many with cancer pain |
| Spinal: epidural (repetitive, continuous), intrathecal | Well-accepted, but many facets controversial including indications, best site of administration, appropriate timing of therapy, best technique for implantation, and best drug |
| Intraventricular | Effective, but should be considered experimental |

From Portenoy RK: *CA* 38:343, 1988.

## UNPROVED CANCER THERAPIES

An unproved therapy is defined as one that neither is based on scientific fact nor demonstrates any advantage in the clinical treatment of disease when reviewed by peer experts in the field. The general public use of unproved, unorthodox, or alternative treatment methods is not a recent phenomenon encountered by health care professionals. Dissatisfaction with the present mode of therapy, the fear of uncomfortable side effects of treatment and poor prognostic outcomes, and a perceived lack of responsiveness by health care professionals have prompted many patients to seek unconventional treatment modes. Nowhere today is this issue more pronounced than with the cancer patient. It is estimated that from 20% to 50% of those diagnosed with cancer will either try or contemplate trying an unproved therapy. It is interesting to note that cancer patients who solicit this type of therapy typically are well educated and informed on the success rate of current conventional therapies.[11]

Unproved therapies most frequently tried are metabolic therapy, which consists of special foods, minerals, and vitamins; diet treatment, megavitamins, mental imagery, spiritual or faith healing, and "immune" therapy.[11] Patients who seek out one of these alternative therapies, even while being treated with conventional therapy, are displaying an open disdain for medical therapy and ex-

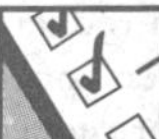

**Guidelines for Dealing Effectively With the Cancer Patient's Pain**

- Know the patient and the pattern of pain experienced. Document findings.
- Use an organized pain-assessment method that is easy to use and that provides sufficient data to assist in selecting the most appropriate intervention for relief.
- Understand the pharmacology of the drugs being used, including: classification, probable side effects, route of administration, expected outcomes in terms of when to expect pain relief to occur.
- Understand the difference between addiction, dependence, and tolerance.
- Use appropriate drug combinations.
- Become familiar with equianalgesic comparisons of common analgesics (see Table 16-31).
- Carry out patient and family teaching related to pain control; providing rationale and technical assistance.

**TABLE 16-35 Pharmacologic and Nonpharmacologic Interventions for Pain Relief**

| INTERVENTION* | TYPE OF EVIDENCE | COMMENTS |
|---|---|---|
| **PHARMACOLOGIC** | | |
| **Nonsteroidal Antiinflammatory Drugs (NSAIDs)** | | |
| Oral (alone) | Ib, IV | Effective for mild to moderate pain. Begin preoperatively. Relatively contraindicated in patients with renal disease and risk of or actual coagulopathy. May mask fever. |
| Oral (adjunct to opioid) | Ia, IV | Potentiating effect resulting in opioid sparing. Begin preoperatively. Cautions as above. |
| Parenteral (ketorolac) | Ib, IV | Effective for moderate to severe pain. Expensive. Useful where opioids contraindicated, especially to avoid respiratory depression and sedation. Advance to opioid. |
| **Opioids** | | |
| Oral | IV | As effective as parenteral in appropriate doses. Use as soon as oral medication tolerated. Route of choice. |
| Intramuscular | Ib, IV | Has been the standard parenteral route, but injections painful and absorption unreliable. Hence, avoid this route when possible. |
| Subcutaneous | Ib, IV | Preferable to intramuscular for low-volume continuous infusion. Injections painful and absorption unreliable. Avoid this route for long-term repetitive dosing. |
| Intravenous | Ib, IV | Parenteral route of choice after major surgery. Suitable for titrated bolus or continuous administration (including PCA), but requires monitoring. Significant risk of respiratory depression with inappropriate dosing. |
| PCA (systemic) | Ia, IV | Intravenous or subcutaneous routes recommended. Good, steady level of analgesia. Popular with patients but requires special infusion pumps and staff education. See cautions about opioids above. |
| Epidural and intrathecal | Ia, IV | When suitable, provides good analgesia. Significant risk of respiratory depression, sometimes delayed in onset. Requires careful monitoring. Use of infusion pumps requires additional equipment and staff education. |
| **Local Anesthetics** | | |
| Epidural and intrathecal | Ia, IV | Limited indications. Expensive if infusion pumps employed. Effective regional analgesia. Opioid sparing. Addition of opioid to local anesthetic may improve analgesia. Risks of hypotension, weakness, numbness. Use of infusion pump requires additional equipment and staff. |
| Peripheral nerve block | Ia, IV | Limited indications and duration of action. Effective regional analgesia. Opioid sparing. |
| **NONPHARMACOLOGIC** | | |
| **Simple Relaxation** (begin preoperatively) | | |
| Jaw relaxation<br>Progressive muscle relaxation<br>Simple imagery | Ia, IIa, IIb, IV | Effective in reducing mild to moderate pain and as an adjunct to analgesic drugs for severe pain. Use when patients express interest in relaxation. Requires 3-5 minutes of staff time for instructions. |
| Music | Ib, IIa, IV | Both patient-preferred and "easy listening" music are effective in reducing mild to moderate pain. |
| **Complex Relaxation** (begin preoperatively) | | |
| Biofeedback | Ib, IIa, Iv | Effective in reducing mild to moderate pain and operative-site muscle tension. Requires skilled personnel and special equipment. |
| Imagery | Ib, IIa, IIb, IV | Effective for reduction of mild to moderate pain. Requires skilled personnel. |
| **Education/Instruction** (begin preoperatively) | | |
| | Ia, IIa, IIb, IV | Effective for reduction of pain. Should include sensory and procedural information and instruction aimed at reducing activity-related pain. Requires 5-15 minutes of staff time. |
| **Transcutaneous Electrical Stimulation (TENS)** | | |
| | Ia, IIa, III, IV | Effective in reducing pain and improving physical function. Requires skilled personnel and special equipment. May be used as an adjunct to drug therapy. |

Modified from Acute Pain Management Guidelines Panel, Acute Pain Management in Adults: *Operative procedures: quick reference guide for clinicians,* Agency for Health Care Policy and Research (AHCPR) Pub No 92-0019, Rockville, Md., 1992, US Department of Health and Human Services.

*Insufficient scientific evidence is available to provide specific recommendations regarding the use of hypnosis, acupuncture, and other physical modalities for relief of postoperative pain.

*Ia,* Evidence obtained from meta-analysis of randomized controlled trials; *Ib,* evidence obtained from at least one randomized controlled trial; *IIa,* evidence obtained from at least one well-designed controlled study without randomization; *IIb,* evidence obtained from at least one other type of well-designed quasi-experimental study; *III,* evidence obtained from well-designed nonexperimental descriptive studies, such as comparative studies, correlational studies, and case studies; *IV,* evidence obtained from expert committee reports or opinions and/or clinical experience of respected authorities.

pressing a need to try and influence their disease outcome.

Health care professionals have a responsibility to know not only about current conventional treatment methods, but also about the unorthodox methods available to the public. When approached by the patient or family about "other" therapies, it is important to take time and discuss the potential advantages and disadvantages rather than to scoff at or show contempt for their comments. Attempting to discern "why" alternative therapy is being considered may lead to more open communication. Perhaps all that is needed is more time to discuss current treatment and expected outcomes. Encouraging more patient/family involvement in decision making about treatment or listening and acting on patient concerns and fears could make the difference between the patient following accepted and proved therapy versus unproved methods. Often it is possible to incorporate some of the unproved therapies into the current treatment regimen; for example, chemotherapy and relaxation or guided-imagery techniques used together may help the patient better handle side effects encountered. Discussion of the use of special, approved dietary supplements while the patient receives radiation might dissuade use of unproved dietary interventions. The patient also can be directed to the American Cancer Society for specific literature that addresses the outcomes of research on unproved therapies.

It is essential that the patient and family understand that not all cancers are curable with available treatment methods. The use of unorthodox therapies may in fact be more detrimental and toxic than conventional modes. Of vital importance are reassurance that the health care team is providing the best available treatment; will continue to support the patient and family with honesty and compassion; and will encourage self-care and patient involvement in treatment decisions.

When all efforts fail to dissuade the use of alternative therapy, health care professionals must recognize patients' rights in choosing how they want to be treated, and they should be supported in their decision. Should patients wish to return after attempting an unproved method, they need to know that they will be welcomed back and supported by the health care team.

## LIVING WITH CANCER

Rehabilitation is an essential component of cancer care and begins immediately after the diagnosis so that patients can maintain their highest level of physical, psychologic, spiritual, and social well-being.[15] With the advent of new and effective therapies for cancer, patients are recovering or living longer and in better health. Society's negative attitudes that must be overcome include the view of cancer as terminal rather than a curable or chronic disease. Emphasis should be on quality of life regardless of anticipated length of life.

Specific goals are established early in the disease process and are based on interdisciplinary team assessment, of which the patient and family are essential members. Comprehensive rehabilitation services, however, are often lacking for cancer patients.

Nurses are involved in prevention and health promotion as part of the rehabilitation process. The nurse's role in prevention consists of promoting new behaviors in the cancer survivor to reduce the risk factors for a second episode of malignant disease, as well as other preventable diseases. Health-promoting behaviors are those that sustain or increase the levels of well-being, self-actualization, and fulfillment of the individual—an approach to living that leads persons to their highest potential of well-being no matter what their diagnoses. Activities that are health promoting include exercise, interpersonal support, adequate nutrition, stress management, taking or assuming responsibility to identify activities to promote health, and finally achieving self-actualization through respect for accomplishments and worth along with a positive attitude.

Nurses must convince other nurses, the public, and other health care professionals that cancer is a chronic disease and that patients have rehabilitation needs. Some rehabilitation objectives and interventions are listed in Table 16-36. See Research box, p. 439.

## RESOURCES FOR CANCER EDUCATION, DETECTION, AND REHABILITATION

### FEDERAL ORGANIZATIONS

Federal recognition of the need to give intensive assistance to educational programs in cancer began in 1926 when Congress proclaimed April of each year as National Cancer Control Month. In 1937 the National Cancer Institute was created within the National Institutes of Health. This institute conducts an extensive program of research in the field of cancer.

Cancer patients also may obtain help from both Medicare and Medicaid. The Community Services Administration provides services through state agencies such as Welfare and Aging or by direct grants. The Rehabilitation Services Administration arranges and pays for services that help the cancer patient return to productive living. The passage of the National Cancer Act of 1971 provided impetus for the development of cancer clinical research centers. The goal was to translate research results into medical practice so that no one will be denied professional advice and care because of lack of facilities and knowledge. These centers combine research capability, demonstration of recent techniques and therapy, and community outreach programs.

Nurses can be articulate speakers for the cause of cancer care and cure, because they are intimately aware of the effects of cancer in threat to life and cost in dollars, disrupted lives, and human suffering. Nurses must as-

**TABLE 16-36 Interventions to Enhance Cancer Rehabilitation**

| OBJECTIVES | METHODS TO ACHIEVE GOALS |
|---|---|
| 1. Promote a positive attitude toward cancer rehabilitation. | 1. Emphasize that cancer is a chronic disease, not a terminal one.<br>2. Disseminate the improvements in cancer care and increased survival statistics in the lay literature. |
| 2. Promote the positive aspects in cancer care. | 1. Incorporate potential long-term and short-term rehabilitation needs as part of initial patient assessments in acute care settings and outpatient clinics.<br>2. Provide inservice programs for nurses and nonprofessional staff on prolonged survival and improved quality of life for cancer patients.<br>3. Increase the number and focus of publications reflecting the positive results in cancer care. |
| 3. Promote positive attitudes in nursing students toward cancer care. | 1. Arrange for student experiences with patients who have survived cancer.<br>2. Provide opportunities for students to have positive experiences helping patients manage side effects of cancer treatment.<br>3. Provide a balance of experiences with survivors of cancer and those in terminal stages. |
| 4. Promote positive self-care and independence of patients with cancer. | 1. Encourage participation in programs designed to help cope with cancer (e.g., I Can Cope, Living with Cancer).<br>2. Use referrals to other disciplines, (O.T., P.T., social work) as indicated for individual patients.<br>3. Inform patients regarding programs of American Cancer Society, such as Reach to Recovery, CanSurmount, Ostomy Rehabilitation Program. |
| 5. Promote successful integration in the workplace. | 1. Provide opportunities for patients to role-play how they will handle information about their diagnosis with co-workers.<br>2. Discuss patient's employment setting and routines to determine potential problems and solutions related to cancer-related disabilities. |

From Dudas S, Carlson S: *Oncol Nurs Forum* 15:187, 1988.

sertively express to their representatives in government the importance of a combined effort to eradicate cancer.

## AMERICAN CANCER SOCIETY

The American Cancer Society (ACS), a large national voluntary organization, has branches in all states and major cities. This huge organization, which is supported by voluntary gifts, has three main objectives: research, education, and services to cancer patients.

*Research* is a major focus, and the Society finances studies that seek the cause of cancer and the development of better methods of treatment. As part of its *educational* efforts, ACS publishes booklets and pamphlets for the use of health care providers, and it stimulates better preparation of professional persons in the care of patients with cancer by sponsoring institutes and other programs for these special groups. Information about available teaching materials may be obtained from the main office of the Society or from state or local offices.

In addition, ACS strives constantly to *educate* the public. It works intensively through magazines, radio, television, clubs, insurance companies, state departments of health, and medical and nursing organizations in an effort to reach all the population with the educational message of how cancer may be prevented and controlled. A large amount of literature for the lay person is prepared and distributed annually. Also, many excellent films for use in public education may be borrowed from the Society.

The Society also performs *services* for patients and their families. Branches in most communities provide assistance for cancer patients who cannot afford to pay for adequate care and for those who, although they can presently afford to pay, will eventually leave their families with too great a financial burden. Services may include dressings, transportation to and from clinics and physicians' offices, special drugs such as expensive hormones, blood, prostheses, and loan of equipment such as hospital beds. In some communities homemaking, visiting nurses, and rehabilitation services also are provided.

The Society also sponsors various patient groups organized to help people with the same disability. Lost Chord Clubs (laryngectomy patients), Reach to Recovery (mastectomy patients), and ostomy clubs have been formed in many cities. Individuals share what they have learned about coping with the problems resulting from therapy for their conditions. They visit patients either in the hospital or at home and hold regular group meetings. Patients and their families should know about the services of the Society before their own resources are

## RESEARCH

Mahon SM, Cella DF, Donovan MI: Psychosocial adjustment to recurrent cancer, *Oncol Nurs Forum* 17(3) (suppl): 47-54, 1990.

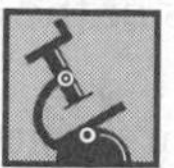

The ability to detect and treat cancer in its early stages has increased the number of persons who are alive 5 years after initial diagnosis. Inevitably some of these survivors will experience one or more cancer recurrences. Although considerable research efforts have been undertaken on the effect of the initial diagnosis of cancer on the individual, little has been directed toward the needs and psychosocial impact when cancer recurs. This descriptive study, using a convenience sample of 40 patients diagnosed with recurrent cancer, employed Lazarus and Folkman's theory of stress appraisal and coping as their research framework. Data from patient responses to the Impact of Events Scale (IES) and the Psychosocial Adjustment to Illness Scale—self-report (PAIS) were used to obtain information on the following questions: (1) How do patients describe the meaning of recurrence of cancer? (2) Do individuals perceive the diagnosis of recurrence and the initial diagnosis of cancer differently? and (3) What are the key psychosocial problems associated with recurrent cancer? The results of the study indicate that diagnosis of recurrence is more distressing than the initial diagnosis of cancer. The study further revealed that adjustment problems related to the patients' ability to manage their illness, work, domestic responsibilities, sexual relationships, social relationships and activities, and psychologic distress all require additional interventions to increase quality of life. Implications of this study are that nurses must be more aware of patient concerns and fears at the time of cancer recurrence and be ready to teach self-care strategies that can minimize the impact of these problems. The results of this study point out the need for longitudinal studies that examine responses from larger population samples regarding the impact of recurrent cancer on individuals and to determine more specifically the appropriate nursing strategies required to address these patient needs.

depleted, and local citizens should be urged to support the Society.

## OTHER ORGANIZATIONS

The following organizations can provide the cancer patient with educational materials and resources, usually free of charge, which are helpful in living with cancer.

American Cancer Society
1599 Clifton Road, N.E.
Atlanta, GA 30329

American Academy of Otolaryngology
Head and Neck Surgery, Inc.
1101 Vermont Avenue, N.W.
Suite 302
Washington, D.C. 20005

Breast Cancer Advisory Center
11426 Rockville Pike
Suite 406
Rockville, MD 20857

Leukemia Society of America, Inc.
733 Third Avenue
New York, NY 10017

Make Today Count
514 Tama Bldg.
P.O. Box 303
Burlington, IN 52601

National Cancer Information Clearinghouse
Room 10A18, Building 31
NCI/NIH
Bethesda, MD 20205

National Hospice Organization
1901 North Fort Myer Drive
Suite 307
Arlington, VA 22209

United Ostomy Association, Inc.
2001 West Beverly Blvd.
Los Angeles, CA 90057

## QUESTIONS TO CONSIDER

- What would you teach a person who knows nothing about the risk factors for cancer?
- What care for side effects would be needed for a patient receiving multiple toxic chemotherapeutic drugs?
- What would you teach a patient who states she wants to know how cancer spreads?
- How would you care for a patient who has advanced cancer to maintain hope and decrease helplessness and dependence?

## CRITICAL THINKING ACTIVITIES

- Marcus is a 54-year-old farmer. He extensively uses fertilizers in his farming operation. He and his family raise cattle, and their diet is typically high in animal fat. He thinks his father died of colon problems. Outline preventative measures that decreases Marcus' risk factors associated with cancer.
- Discuss the paradox associated with the use of chemotherapy for the treatment of cancer and the increased risk of developing cancer in response to chemotherapy.
- Larry is a 60-year-old with multiple myeloma. He is in the terminal stages of cancer and is experiencing severe pain. Discuss how you would address the problem and how you would go about deciding how to intervene.

## CHAPTER SUMMARY

### NATURE OF PROBLEM

- Delay in seeking treatment is the most important factor in a negative prognosis after a cancer diagnosis.
- Underestimation of the incidence of cancer and negative views about the therapy are two of the most important factors that inhibit health-seeking behaviors.

### ETIOLOGY, PHYSIOLOGY, AND PATHOPHYSIOLOGY

- Cancer research focuses on causes of abnormal cell growth (the role of chemicals and other pollutants, genetic factors, viruses) and therapies for cancer (surgical, drug, radiation, and immune system alteration).
- Changes in cells causing them to become malignant appear to be a disturbance in the regulatory functions of DNA, causing a loss of differentiation or likeness to the original cells.
- Tumor growth may be rapid or slow depending on factors such as immune surveillance, blood supply, hormones, number of cells proliferating, and the length of time in the cell cycle.
- Metastasis may occur through blood vessels, lymph vessels, direct extension, or by diffusion.
- Carcinogenesis is a combination of factors that include carcinogens, host susceptibility, environmental carcinogens, habits, customs, and viruses.
- Cancer has multiple local and systemic effects. Local effects result from obstruction, pressure, and destruction of surrounding tissue. Systemic effects may involve multiple organ systems and include cachexia, anorexia, pain, and various metabolic disorders.

### EPIDEMIOLOGY

- Cancer occurs most frequently in men and in persons older than 65 years of age.

### MEDICAL MANAGEMENT

- Diagnostic studies for cancer include laboratory blood tests, biopsy, and cytologic, radiologic, and endoscopic examination.
- Nursing care during the diagnostic phase includes assessment of psychologic and physiologic effects of cancer and interventions to help the patient and family cope. Multiple nursing diagnoses may be present pertaining to lack of knowledge, problems with coping, comfort, rest, nutrition, protective mechanisms, mobility, elimination, ventilation, sexuality, self-concept, roles, and spirituality.
- Medical management of cancer may include a combination of surgery, chemotherapy, radiation therapy, and biotherapy.
- Nurses teach patients about the expected outcomes of therapy and how to cope with side effects.
- Radiotherapy may be administered externally or internally. Side effects may compromise the GI system, the skin, or other systems.
- A combination of drugs usually is used in chemotherapy because many work in different phases of the cell cycle.
- Chemotherapeutic agents include alkylating agents, antimetabolites, antibiotics, steroids, vinca alkaloids, and various miscellaneous drugs.
- Drugs may be administered orally, subcutaneously, intravenously, intraarterially, intracavitary, or intrathecally.
- Nursing care during chemotherapy includes assessment, prevention and/or treatment of infection, gastrointestinal problems, alopecia, organ toxicities (liver, urinary or pulmonary, hematopoietic, genital, and systems).
- Biotherapy includes use of biologic response modifiers such as interferon, interleukin-2, and monoclonal antibodies.

### ONCOLOGIC EMERGENCIES

- Oncologic emergencies include obstructive, cardiac, and metabolic syndromes.

### CANCER PAIN

- Cancer pain results from physiologic and psychologic factors and usually can be controlled with the correct dose of drugs, administered consistently.

## REFERENCES

1. American Cancer Society: *1993 cancer facts and figures,* New York, 1993, The Society.
2. Anonymous: *Respiratory health effects of passive smoking: lung cancer and other disorders,* Environmental Protection Agency (EPA/600/6-90/006F), Washington, DC, 1990, Office of Health & Environmental Assessment.
3. Belcher A: New developments in treatment modalities. In Ashwanden P, editor: *Oncology nursing: advances, treatments, and trends into the 21st century,* Rockville, Md, 1990, Aspen Publishers.
4. Benito E, Giacosa A: *Public education on diet and cancer,* Dordrecht, Netherlands, 1991, Kluwer Academic Publishers.
5. Bogne F et al: Radiation therapy in cancer management: history and basic principles. In Moosa AR, editor: *Comprehensive textbook of oncology,* vol 1, ed 2, Philadelphia, 1990, JB Lippincott.
6. Bovbjirg D: Psychoneuroimmunology and cancer. In Holland JC, editor: *Handbook of psychooncology,* New York, 1990, Oxford University Press.
7. Brack G, LaClave L, Bliz S: The psychological aspects of bone marrow transplant, *Cancer Nurs* 11(3):221-229, 1988.
8. Bucholtz JD: Radiation carcinogenesis. In Dow KH, editor: *Nursing care in radiation oncology,* Philadelphia, 1992, WB Saunders.
9. Burke MB et al: *Cancer chemotherapy: a nursing process approach,* Boston, 1991, Jones & Bartlett.
10. Cartmel B et al: Professional and consumer concerns about

the environment, life style, and cancer, *Semin Oncol Nurs* 8(1):20-29, 1992.

11. Casseleth BR, Brown H: Unorthodox cancer medicine, *Cancer* 38(3):176-186, 1988.
12. Cleft RA, Petersen MD, Buckner CD: Marrow transplantation. In Moosa AR, editor: *Comprehensive textbook of oncology,* vol 1, Baltimore, 1991, Williams & Wilkins.
13. Dalton WS, Miller TP: Multidrug resistance, principles and practice of oncology, *PPO Updates* 5(7):1-13, 1991.
14. Dellefield ME: Informational needs and approaches for cancer detection in the elderly, *Semin Oncol Nurs* 4(3):156-168, 1988.
15. Dudas S, Carlson CE: Cancer rehabilitation, *Oncol Nurs Forum* 15(2):183-188, 1988.
16. Dudjak LA: Cancer metastasis, *Semin Oncol Nurs* 8(1):40-50, 1992.
17. Fanslow J: Pain management. In Baird SB, editor: *A cancer source book for nurses,* ed 6, 1991, American Cancer Society.
18. Freeman HP: Cancer in the socioeconomically disadvantaged, *CA* 39(5):266-288, 1989.
19. Grady C: Host defense mechanisms: an overview, *Semin Oncol Nurs* 4(2):86-94, 1988.
20. Gray G et al: A clinical data base for advanced cancer patients, *Cancer Nurs* 11(1):77-83, 1988.
21. Gullo SM: Safe handling of antineoplastic drugs: translating the recommendations into practice, *Oncol Nurs Forum* 15(4): 596-602, 1988.
22. Harley NH, Harley JH: Potential lung cancer risk from indoor radiation exposure, *CA* 40(5):265-275, 1990.
23. Hilderley LJ: Radiation oncology: historical background and principles of teletherapy. In Dow KH, editor: *Nursing care in radiation oncology,* Philadelphia, 1992, WB Saunders.
24. Jordan LN, Mantravadi VP: Nursing care of the patient receiving high dose brachytherapy, *Oncol Nurs Forum* 18(7):1167-1171, 1991.
25. Kritchevsky D: Diet and cancer, *CA* 41:328-333, 1991.
26. Kune G, Vitetta L: Alcohol consumption and the etiology of colorectal cancer: a review of the scientific evidence from 1957 to 1991, *Nutr Cancer* 18(2):97-111, 1992.
27. Kupchella CE: Environmental factors in cancer etiology, *Semin Oncol Nurs* 2(3):161-169, 1986.
28. Lotze MT, Rosenberg SA: The immunologic treatment of cancer, *CA* 38:68-94, 1988.
29. McDonald A: Altered protective mechanisms. In Dow KH, eidtor: *Nursing care in radiation oncology,* Philadelphia, 1992, WB Saunders.
30. McMillin S: Carcinogenesis, *Semin Oncol Nurs* 8(1):10-19, 1992.
31. Mettlin C: Research in cancer prevention and detection. In Hubbard SM: *Current Issues in Cancer Nursing Practice Updates* 1(4):1-10, 1992.
32. Northouse LL, Peters-Golden H: Cancer and the family: strategies to assist spouses, *Semin Oncol Nurs* 9(3):74-82, 1993.
33. Parker RG, Lowitz BB, Casciato DA: Principles of radiotherapy and chemotherapy. In Casciato DA, editor: *Manual of clinical oncology,* ed 2, Boston, 1988, Little, Brown & Co.
34. Penn I: Malignancies associated with immune deficiencies. In Moosa AR: *Comprehensive textbook of oncology,* vol 1, ed 2, Baltimore, 1991, Williams & Wilkins.
35. Purtello D: Genetic diseases, hamartomas, and familial occurrence of neoplasms. In Levine A, editor: *Cancer growth and prevention: etiology of cancer in man,* Dordrecht, Netherlands, 1989, Kluwer Academic Publishers.
36. Schain WS: Sexual and intimate consequences of breast cancer treatment, *CA* 38(3):154-161, 1988.
37. Schryber S, Lacasse CR, Barton-Burke C: Autologous bone marrow transplantation, *Oncol Nurs Forum* 14(4):74-80, 1987.
38. Sell S: Cancer markers. In Moosa AR, editor: *Comprehensive textbook of oncology,* vol 1, ed 2, Baltimore, 1991, Williams & Wilkins.
39. Sporkin E: Patient and family education. In Dow KH: *Nursing care in radiation oncology,* Philadelphia, 1992, WB Saunders.
40. Stewart CD: Nursing interventions in regional chemotherapy using surgical delivery systems. In *Nursing interventions in oncology, M.D. Anderson case reports and review,* Newton, Penn, 1989, Associations in Medical Marketing Co.
41. Theriault G: Cancer risks due to exposure in electromagnetic fields, In Brand P, editor: *Occupational cancer epidemiology,* New York, 1990, Springer Verlag.
42. Thomas DB: Epidemiology and prevention. In Moosa AR, editor: *Comprehensive textbook of oncology,* vol 1, ed 2, Baltimore, 1991, Williams & Wilkins.
43. Tomatis L: Prenatal carcinogenesis in cell differentiation, genes and cancer. In Kawkunoga T: *International Agency for Research on Cancer,* IARC Scientific Pub No 90, Lyon, France, 1988, The Agency.
44. US Department of Health and Human Services, Public Health Service: *Healthy people 2000: summary report,* Boston, 1992, Jones & Bartlett.
45. Voldagni R, Fei L, Knapp D: Important prognostic factors influencing outcome of combined radiation and hyperthermia, *Int J Radiat Oncol, Biol, Phys* 15:959-972, 1988.
46. von Roemeling E et al: Chemotherapy via implanted infusion pump: new perspectives for delivery of long-term continuous treatment, *Oncol Nurs Forum* 13(2):17-24, 1986.
47. Wickham R, Purl S, Welker D: Long-term central venous catheters: issues for care, *Semin Oncol Nurs* 8(2):133-147, 1992.
48. Willett WC, Stampfer ML, Colditz GA: Relation of meat, fat and fiber intake to the risk of colon cancer in a perspective study among women, *N Engl J Med* 323(11):1664-1672, 1990.
49. Yasko JW: Oncogenes and cancer suppression genes, *Semin Oncol Nurs* 8(1):30-39, 1992.

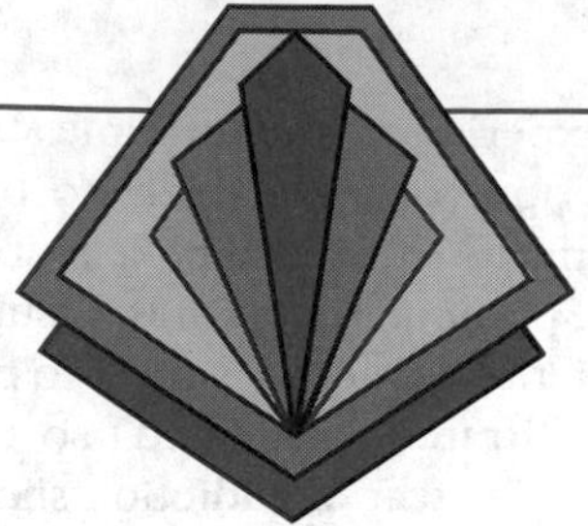

CHAPTER 17

# Pain

*Judith H. Watt-Watson*

## CHAPTER OBJECTIVES

***After studying this chapter, the learner should be able to do the following:***

1 Describe some common misbeliefs about pain management.
2 Describe the physiology of pain and related theories of pain transmission.
3 Compare factors that influence perception and response to pain.
4 Differentiate between acute and chronic pain assessment.
5 Compare assessment tools used in clinical practice.
6 Describe pharmacologic and nonpharmacologic approaches for pain management.
7 Identify five nursing implications for pain management.
8 Explain the purpose and methods of the team approach for chronic pain management.

## KEY TERMS

acupuncture
acute pain
autogenic training
behavior modification
biofeedback
causalgia
chronic pain
cordotomy
endorphins
gate control theory
guided imagery
hypnosis
intractable pain
intraspinal analgesic infusion
nerve block
neuralgia
nociceptors
nonopioid analgesics
nonsteroidal antiinflammatory drugs (NSAIDs)
opioid analgesics
pain detection threshold
pain tolerance
patient-controlled analgesia (PCA)
percutaneously inserted spinal cord electrical stimulator (PISCES)
phantom limb pain
psychogenic pain
referred pain
rhizotomy
somatic pain
sympathectomy
therapeutic touch
transcutaneous electrical nerve stimulator (TENS)
visceral pain

## NATURE OF THE PROBLEM

Pain relief is a management problem for many patients, their families, and the health professionals caring for them. Although pain is experienced by everyone to some degree, responses to it are unique for each person. Difficulties in recognizing and understanding someone else's pain are clinically well known. The International Association for the Study of Pain[18] has defined pain as an unpleasant sensory and emotional experience associated with actual or potential tissue damage or described in terms of such damage. Pain therefore is multidimensional and entirely subjective. Only the person experiencing the pain can describe or evaluate it. Pain can be evoked by a multiplicity of stimuli, but the reaction to it cannot be measured objectively. Pain is a learned experience that is influenced by the entire life situation of each person.

Pain accompanies many disorders, as well as some therapies. It is a sensation that is frequently feared by persons undergoing surgery. Although some persons with cancer do *not* experience it, pain is one of the major concerns people have about cancer.

Relief of pain and discomfort is a major nursing intervention and one that requires skill in both the art and science of nursing. It requires knowledge about concepts related to pain, data collection, and useful therapies. It also requires sensitivity and empathy—an effort on the part of the nurse to understand what the patient is experiencing and to communicate understanding and caring. It requires that the nurse use a systematic approach (nursing process) with the patient in pain. Too often management decisions are made without valid assessment and evaluation, including sufficient input from patients. This results in undermedication, overmedication, or medication when other interventions would be more effective.

## MISBELIEFS ABOUT PAIN

During the past 20 years research repeatedly has demonstrated that significant numbers of hospitalized patients experience moderate to severe pain unrelieved by treatment.* Inadequate knowledge and problematic attitudes of physicians and nurses have been well documented.[6,15-21] Although health professionals more recently have supported the principle of pain relief, this goal does not appear to have influenced practice. Health professionals either have not recognized unrelieved pain or have tolerated poor pain relief as the norm. Many patients have not been asked about their pain, or discrepancies have been documented between their pain ratings and those of health professionals.† This problematic communication is compounded if patients expect to have pain while hospitalized or are reluctant to ask staff members for help.[4,22,23,31,42] Some commonly held misbeliefs and incorrect beliefs guide our practice and may contribute to this ineffective pain management.[48] These misbeliefs are crucial to recognize and correct because they influence our approaches to both the assessment and management of pain.

Minimal or no pain should be the goal of pain management. A hospital admission should not automatically mean a pain experience for *any* patient, including elders, children, and infants. Patterns of pain intensity vary, and the diagnosis and/or type of surgery is *not* an effective primary basis for determining the amount of pain the person is experiencing or the analgesic required. Although not all pain can be removed, the use of multiple modalities usually can decrease it to at least the minimal range.

All pain tends to be assessed as acute pain. Chronic pain, however, differs from acute pain and needs to be assessed using different criteria (see p. 448). The basis of practice must be to believe that all pain is real and that malingerers (persons who deliberately lie about their pain) are rare (fewer than 1%). Patients in pain will not necessarily ask for help until they are in severe pain, and they may use words such as "pressure" or "soreness" instead of "pain." Patients may have concerns about being "a good patient" or fears about analgesics that interfere with their reporting pain.[39] Both children and elderly adults frequently experience unrelieved pain because health professionals incorrectly assume that their age precludes pain.[30] Careful observation, especially of facial expressions at rest and during movement, is particularly important with infants and with cognitively impaired elders.

*References 1, 4, 8, 23-25, 32, 34, 38, 43.
†References 3, 7, 15, 32, 38, 40.

Pain is a complex experience, and multiple strategies rather than only one approach are likely to be more successful in alleviating it. Incorrect beliefs about analgesic administration, particularly opioids, result in undermedication for patients.[2] Analgesics need to be given around the clock and titrated (regulated) so the pain levels are zero to mild. The fear of addiction should not prevent effective opioid doses, because addiction rarely occurs.

It is difficult to understand and recognize another person's pain. Therefore it is crucial to gain as much information about the patient as possible instead of making assumptions about what may be happening. Recognizing misbeliefs (incorrect beliefs) is an important step to more effective pain management.[46]

The nurse must be vigilant about personal expectations, biases, and factors that may interfere with the ability to deliver individualized nursing care. One research report discusses the effect of a patient's culture on the nurse's inference of suffering. See Research box below.

### RESEARCH

Davitz LL, Davitz JR: Culture and nurses' inferences of suffering. In Copp LA, editor: *Recent advances in nursing,* vol 11, New York, 1985, Churchill Livingstone.

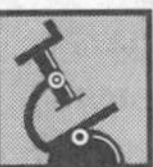

In the first part of this study, practicing nurses were asked to read a vignette describing a patient and injury and to rate the degree of physical pain and psychologic distress that they felt the patient was experiencing. The vignettes described patients from six backgrounds (Oriental, Mediterranean, African, Spanish, Anglo-Saxon/Germanic, and Jewish) and three levels of injury—mild, moderate, and severe. The study found that the background of the patient was a statistically significant factor that nurses used in determining the degree of suffering by these patients. In other words, when physical condition, age, and sex of the patient were controlled for, nurses judged patients of different backgrounds to have different degrees of suffering.

In the second part of the study, 1440 nurses from 13 countries rated 60 vignettes, with the research question asking: Do nurses from country X caring for a patient from country X with a certain medical problem assess the patient's degree of suffering the same as nurses from country Y might assess a patient from country Y with the same medical problem? The researchers found that nurses from different countries differ in their assessment of suffering.

These studies support the idea that nurses may generalize about the degree of suffering patients experience based on knowledge of the person's ethnic or cultural background and that nurses from different cultures may have different beliefs about the severity of pain experienced by patients. Nurses must examine their own beliefs about pain in order to be more objective in assessing the pain of others.

# PHYSIOLOGY OF PAIN

## PAIN RECEPTORS AND STIMULI

Pain receptors, called **nociceptors,** are free nerve endings of unmyelinated or lightly myelinated afferent neurons. Nociceptors are located extensively in the skin and mucosa and less frequently in selected deeper structures, such as viscera, joints, arterial walls, and bile ducts. Nociceptors respond to harmful or potentially harmful stimuli that may be chemical, thermal, or mechanical.[14] Chemical stimuli for pain include histamines, bradykinin, prostaglandins, and acids, some of which are released by damaged tissues. Anoxic tissue also releases chemicals that lead to pain. Tissue swelling may cause pain by creating pressure (mechanical stimulation) on nociceptors in adjoining tissues.

After tissue injury and in some pathologic conditions, pain receptors do not adapt to repeated stimulation and may become more sensitive.[19] As a result, pain sensitivity to a normally painful stimulus may be increased *(hyperalgesia)* or a normally nonpainful stimulus, such as touch, may be painful *(allodynia).*

## PAIN TRANSMISSION

Pain impulses are transmitted to the spinal cord by two types of fibers: thinly myelinated faster-conducting A-delta fibers and slower-conducting unmyelinated C fibers. Pain that may be described as "sharp" or "pricking" and that can be easily localized results from impulses transmitted by the *A-delta fibers.* An example of this type of pain is that felt by a needle prick. Pain that may be described as "burning," "dull," or "aching" and that is more diffuse results from impulses transmitted by the *C fibers.* Impulses transmitted on the larger diameter myelinated A-beta and A-alpha fibers have an inhibitory effect on those transmitted over A-delta and C fibers.

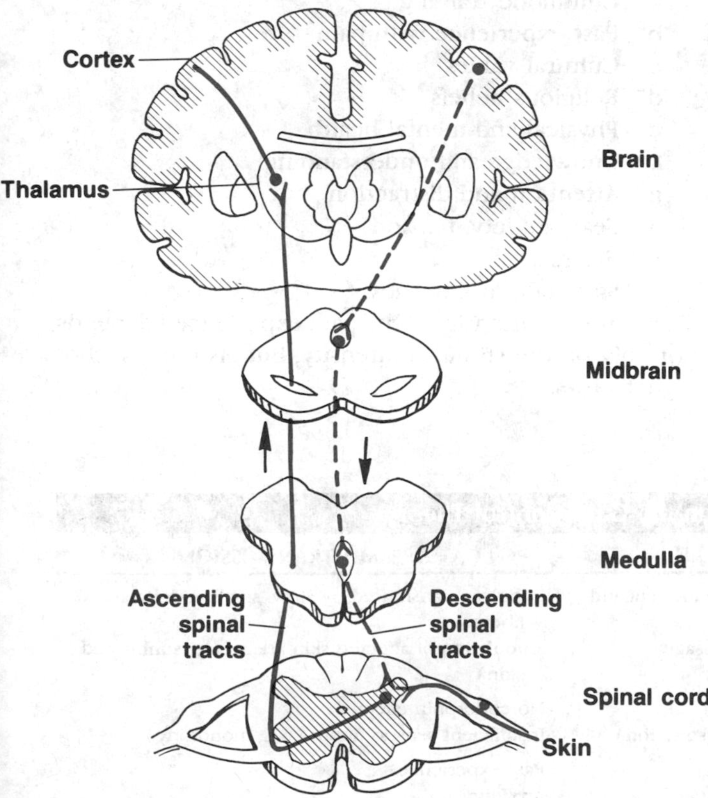


**FIGURE 17-1** Pathways of pain transmission to and from cortex.

The afferent nerve fibers enter the spinal cord through the dorsal root and synapse in the *dorsal horn* (Figure 17-1). The dorsal horn consists of several layers (laminae) with interconnections. Lamina II comprises an area called *substantia gelatinosa* (SG). Substance P is released at synapses in the SG and is thought to be a major neurotransmitter of the pain impulses.[9]

The pain impulses cross the spinal cord over interneurons and connect with *ascending spinal pathways.* The most important ascending pathways for nociceptive impulses located in the ventral half of the spinal cord are the spinothalamic tract (STT) and the spinoreticular tract (SRT). The STT is a discriminative system and conveys information about the nature and location of the stimulus to the thalamus and then to the cortex for interpretation. Impulses transmitted over the SRT (which goes to the brainstem and part of the thalamus) activate the autonomic and limbic (motivational-affective) responses.

## PAIN MODULATION

Discovery of receptors in the brain to which opiate compounds bind led to the discovery of two naturally occurring endogenous morphinelike pentapeptides (5-amino acid compounds), met-enkephalin and leu-enkephalin. These enkephalins are classified as **endorphins** (from the terms *endogenous* and *morphine*). Other endorphins, such as beta-endorphin, also have been identified. The endorphins are thought to suppress pain by (1) acting presynaptically to *inhibit release* of the neurotransmitter substance P or (2) acting postsynaptically to *inhibit conduction* of pain impulses.[15] The endorphins are found in high concentration in the basal ganglia of the brain, thalamus, midbrain, and dorsal horn of the spinal cord.

*Descending spinal pathways,* from the thalamus through the midbrain and medulla to the dorsal horns of the spinal cord, conduct nociceptive *inhibitory* impulses. Serotonin is one neurotransmitter that supports these inhibitory impulses. The endogenous descending pain–suppressive system is more effectively activated by nociceptive stimuli transmitted by A-delta fibers. Electrical stimulation by means of transcutaneous electrical nerve stimulators (TENS, p. 454) using low frequency and high intensity activates opiate analgesia. Acupuncture is also thought to use the opiate pathways.[15,17]

## THEORIES OF PAIN TRANSMISSION

Various theories of pain transmission have been proposed[21] (Box 17-1). The affect, specificity, and pat-

**BOX 17-1 Theories of Pain Transmission**

**AFFECT THEORY**

Pain is an emotion and its intensity depends on the meaning of the part involved; does not include physiologic aspects.

**SPECIFICITY THEORY**

Specific pain receptors project impulses over neural pain pathways to the brain; does not account for psychologic aspects of pain perception and variability of response.

**PATTERN THEORY**

Pain results from combined effects of stimulus intensity and summations of impules in the dorsal horn of the spinal cord; does not account for psychologic aspects.

**GATE CONTROL THEORY**

Pain impulses can be controlled by a gating mechanism in the dorsal horn of the spinal cord to permit or inhibit transmission. Gating factors include effect of impulses transmitted over fast or slow conducting nerve fibers and effects of descending impulses from the brainstem and cortex.

tern theories were early theories that led to the development of the gate control theory. Although the *gate control theory* does not fully explain pain transmission, it serves as a basis for understanding pain transmission.

The **gate control theory** was proposed by Melzack and Wall[29] in 1965. The theory proposes that the substantia gelatinosa (SG) in the spinal cord acts as a gating mechanism to permit or inhibit passage of pain impulses. The "gate" can be "closed" (so that the contact is not made, thus interrupting the pain impulse) by nerve impulses from the large non-nociceptive A-beta and A-alpha fibers or from the descending pathways. Impulses conducted over large fibers not only close the gate but also are sent immediately to the cortex for rapid identification, evaluation, and modification of the sensory inputs.[30] Impulses sent to the brainstem, the center for motivational-affective and sensory-discriminative actions, can influence cognition or evaluation in the cortex. Impulses are then sent from the cortex back to the SG via corticospinal pathways to inhibit or permit passage of pain impulses. Note in Table 17-1 the various factors that can open or close the gate.

## PAIN EXPERIENCE

The pain experience of each person includes the *perception of the pain* sensation and the *response* to this perception. Tolerance to the noxious stimulus influences both components.

### PAIN PERCEPTION

Perception of pain takes place in the cortex (cognitive-evaluative function) as a result of the stimuli transmitted up the spinothalamic and thalamocortical tracts. This *thinking-feeling component of pain is subjective,* highly complex, and individual; it is influenced by factors affecting stimulation of the nociceptors and transmission of the nociceptive impulse, as well as by cortical receptivity and interpretation:

1. Stimulation of nociceptors
   a. Increased number of stimuli
   b. Increased duration of the stimulus
2. Alteration of transmission
   a. Damage to nerve endings
   b. Inflammation, tumors, or injuries to spinal cord
3. Receptivity of cortex
   a. Inflammation; degenerative changes of brain
   b. Depression of brain function
   c. Anesthesia
4. Interpretation in cerebral cortex
   a. Childhood training
   b. Past experience with pain
   c. Cultural values
   d. Religious beliefs
   e. Physical and mental health
   f. Knowledge and understanding
   g. Attention and distraction
   h. Fear, anxiety, tension
   i. Fatigue
   j. State of consciousness

Therefore the intensity of the pain experienced depends not only on the stimulus intensity, but also on psychologic factors.[14]

**TABLE 17-1 Factors Affecting Pain Transmission Based on the Gate Control Theory**

| SITE | CLOSE GATE (BLOCK TRANSMISSION) | OPEN GATE (PERMIT TRANSMISSION) |
|---|---|---|
| Fibers | Impulses transmitted by large, fast, myelinated A-beta and A-alpha fibers<br>Stimulation of unaffected skin areas (e.g., massage) | Impulses transmitted by slow, small, A-delta and C fibers<br>Stimulation of affected skin areas (e.g., sunburned skin) |
| Brainstem (descending pathway) | Endorphin effect<br>Sufficient or maximum sensory input (e.g., distraction) | No endorphin effect<br>Insufficient sensory input (e.g., monotony) |
| Cortex | Past experiences<br>Feelings of pain control | Past experiences<br>Anxiety |

**BOX 17-2 Factors That Influence Pain Tolerance**

| INCREASE TOLERANCE | DECREASE TOLERANCE |
|---|---|
| Alcohol | Fatigue |
| Drugs | Anger |
| Hypnosis | Boredom |
| Warmth | Anxiety |
| Rubbing | Persistent pain |
| Distraction | Stress |
| Faith | |
| Strong beliefs | |

**BOX 17-3 Factors That Influence Responses to Pain**

Meaning of pain to individual person
Degree of pain perception
Past experience
Cultural values
Social expectations
Physical and mental health
Parental attitudes toward pain
Setting in which pain occurs
Fear, anxiety
Usual way of responding to stressors
Age
Preparation for pain context
Health professionals' responses

The intensity at which the noxious stimulus is subjectively judged as painful is called the **pain detection threshold.**[14] This sensory discrimination is relatively consistent within an individual and between different individuals, relative to the location and type of stimulus.

In contrast, **pain tolerance,** which is the maximum degree of pain intensity a person is willing to experience, is highly variable.[14] Numerous factors can increase or decrease pain tolerance (Box 17-2). Tolerance can vary between different individuals in the same situation and in the same individual in differing situations. For example, a woman with a tender breast lump may complain of more pain if her mother died of breast cancer. Individual persons can respond in many ways to any level of pain intensity, and pain tolerance is influenced by the meaning of the pain to the individual. It is important to remember that there is no right or wrong way to experience pain and *pain is whatever and whenever the patient says it is.*[26]

## THE MEANING OF PAIN

Pain has different meanings for each person and may differ for the same person at different times. In general, most persons view pain as a negative experience, although it also may have some positive aspects. Some examples of the meanings of pain include the following:

Harm or damage
Complication, such as infection
A new illness
Recurrence of illness
Fatal disease
Increasing disability
Loss of mobility
Aging
Healing
Necessary for cure
Punishment for sins
Challenge
Appreciation for suffering of others
Something to be tolerated
Release from unwanted responsibilities

Numerous factors influence the meaning of pain for an individual, including age, gender, sociocultural background, environment, and past or present experiences. For example, two women may be experiencing pain from a fractured leg. To the 75-year-old woman living alone with few social contacts, pain may be interpreted on the basis of fear of aging and inability to maintain her independent living status. The 28-year-old lawyer might interpret the pain as an expected nuisance, with the realization that healing will occur and she can get back to work soon.

## RESPONSE TO PAIN

People respond to pain in different ways, depending on their perception of the pain, including what it means to them. Some may be fearful, apprehensive, and anxious, whereas others are tolerant and optimistic. Some weep, moan, scream, beg for relief or help, threaten to destroy themselves, thrash about in bed, or move about aimlessly when in severe pain; others lie quietly in bed and may only close their eyes, grit their teeth, bite their lips, clench their hands, or perspire profusely when experiencing pain.

On the basis of their cultural beliefs some persons have been taught to endure severe pain without reacting outwardly, whereas others are taught to be very expressive when experiencing any degree of pain. People whose health beliefs and education emphasize prevention tend to accept pain as a warning to seek help. They expect that the cause of pain will be found and cured.

Numerous factors influence responses to pain (Box 17-3). One cannot predict how any given person will respond, and value judgments should not be made concerning how a patient responds. It is very important for health professionals to recognize misbeliefs about expected pain response that prevent effective pain management (see p. 444).

## LONGEVITY OF PAIN

There are two types of pain syndromes: acute and chronic. Unfortunately, many health care professionals provide care for the person experiencing chronic pain

**TABLE 17-2 Comparison of Acute and Chronic Pain**

| CHARACTERISTIC | ACUTE PAIN | CHRONIC PAIN |
|---|---|---|
| Onset | Usually sudden | May be sudden or develop insidiously |
| Duration | Transient (up to 3 months) | Prolonged (months to years) |
| Pain localization | Pain vs. nonpain areas generally well identified | Pain vs. nonpain areas less well identified; intensity becomes more difficult to evaluate (change in sensations) |
| Clinical signs | Signs of sympathetic overactivity (such as increased blood pressure) | Usually no change in vital signs (adaptation) |
| Purpose | Warning that something is wrong | Meaningless; no purpose |
| Pattern | Self-limiting or readily corrected | Continuous or intermittent; intensity may vary or remain constant |
| Prognosis | Likelihood of eventual complete relief | Complete relief usually not possible |

as though it were acute pain. There are many differences between acute and chronic pain (Table 17-2), and the approaches to pain relief are usually different, although some of the same techniques may be used.

## Acute Pain

**Acute pain** lasts no longer than 3 months. It is essentially a transient episode and informs the person that something is wrong. There is usually sudden onset from a perceived cause, and the painful areas can generally be well identified.

Sudden severe pain activates the autonomic nervous system, which may produce signs of sympathetic overactivity. These signs include tachycardia, increased blood pressure, pupillary dilation, diaphoresis, and stimulation of adrenal medullary secretion. In some situations, such as with severe visceral pain of sudden onset, vasodilation may occur with a subsequent fall in blood pressure and shock. Continuous painful stimulation can produce a steadily maintained reflex contraction of adjacent or distant muscles, such as abdominal rigidity in persons with intraabdominal pain.

Acute pain is commonly accompanied by increased muscle tension and anxiety, both of which may contribute to increased perception of pain (Figure 17-2). If the pain is moderate or severe, overt physiologic and behavioral signs facilitate assessment of the pain. The person usually seeks pain relief.

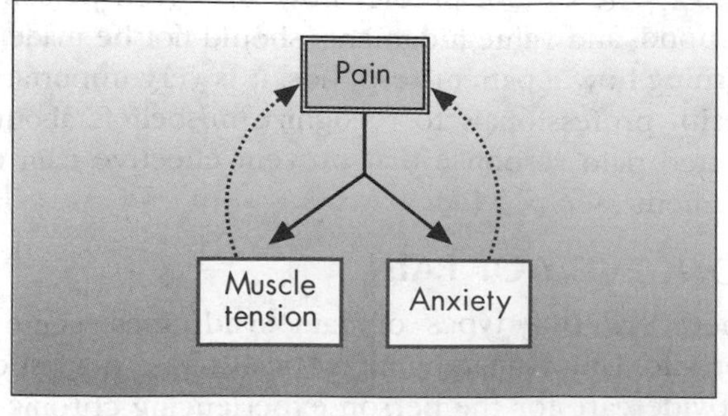


**FIGURE 17-2** Acute pain.

## Chronic Pain

Pain that persists longer than 3 months usually is classified as **chronic pain.** Either the source of pain is unknown or the pain cannot be eliminated. The pain sensation often becomes more diffuse, so that it is difficult for the person to identify a specific pain site. The pain originally may have been acute pain but persisted (e.g., full-thickness burns), or the onset may be so insidious that the person cannot state specifically when it was first experienced.

There are different types of chronic pain. *Intermittent* chronic pain occurs only at specific periods; at other times the person is pain free (migraine headaches). *Persistent* pain is always present, although there may be periods when pain is more or less intense (as occurs with low back pain). One form of persistent pain may increase in frequency because of the pathologic condition (pain from incurable cancer). (Cancer pain is discussed in Chapter 16.)

Chronic pain is characterized by irritability (often compounded by insomnia), which leads to decreasing interests and isolation from friends and family.[45] Added to this is the centering of the person's life on the pain experience, with increasing feelings of helplessness and hopelessness as the pain persists. Ultimately the person withdraws from social interactions (Figure 17-3).

The patient's world centers on ways to modify the pain experience. These patients experience tremendous disruptions in many aspects of their usual activities, including work, family roles, socialization, sleep, and leisure.[49] Some patients go from one physician to another seeking pain relief, which takes time, effort, and money. Even as they seek relief, they often lose faith in the ability of anyone to help them. The lack of continuity of care augments the problems. Physicians themselves may feel helpless when the patient continues to complain of pain. The development of pain clinics and inpatient pain teams has led to successful control of chronic pain for some (but not all) persons with chronic pain. Information about pain centers in the United States and Canada is presented in Box 17-4.

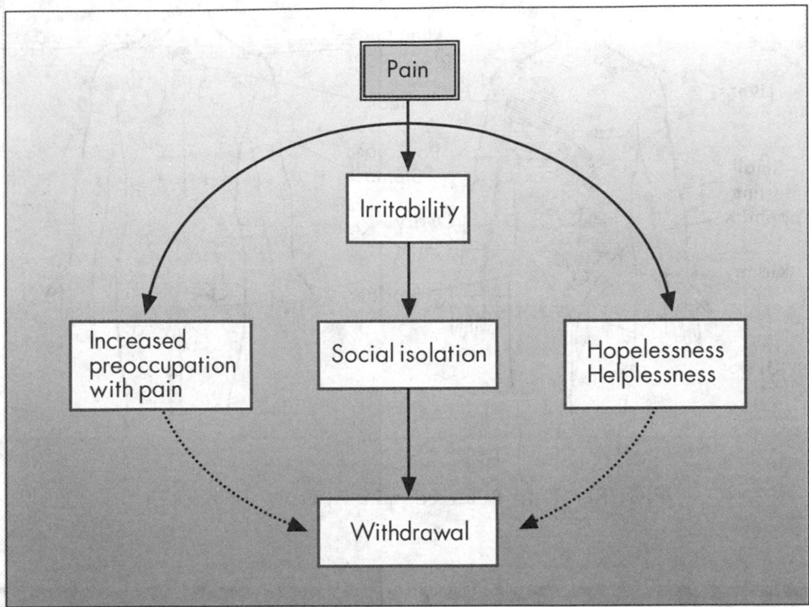


**FIGURE 17-3** Chronic pain.

**BOX 17-4 Organizations Providing Information About Pain-Relief Centers in the United States and Canada**

- American Chronic Pain Association, Box 850, Rockland, CA 95677; (916)632-0922
- National Chronic Pain Outreach Association, 7979 Old Georgetown Rd., Suite 100, Bethesda, MD 20814; (301)652-4948
- North American Chronic Pain Association of Canada (NAC-PAC), 6 Handel Court, Brampton, Ontario, Canada L6S 14; (416)793-5230
- International Association for the Study of Pain, 909 N.E. 43rd St., Suite 306, Seattle, WA 98105; (206)547-6409
- American Council for Headache Education, 875 Kings Highway, Suite 200, West Deptford, NJ 08096; (800)255-2243
- Migrane Foundation, 120 Carlton Ave., Toronto, Ontario, Canada M5A 4K2; (416)920-4916
- Commission for the Accreditation of Rehabilitative Facilities, 101 N. Wilmot Rd., Suite 500, Tucson, AZ 85711; written inquiries preferred

As a means of differentiating the acute and chronic types of pain, Crue has developed a taxonomy of pain, beginning with acute pain of short duration and ending with continuous intractable pain (unrelieved by therapeutic measures)[5]:

1. *Acute*—lasts a few days, is caused by tissue injury, and can be expected to end when source is removed
2. *Subacute*—similar to acute but persists days to weeks
3. *Recurrent acute pain*—exacerbations of chronic pain
4. *Ongoing cancer pain*—caused by progressive pathology
5. *Intractable benign pain* (adequate coping)—pain is continuous but persons are able to live productive lives
6. *Intractable benign pain* (inadequate coping)—person is completely disabled by the continuous pain

## SPECIFIC TYPES OF PAIN

### Somatic Versus Visceral Pain

Pain may originate in the skin and subcutaneous tissue, (superficial), in the muscles and bones (deep **somatic pain**), or in the body organs **(visceral pain).** Somatic and visceral pain differ in their characteristics, particularly in the quality of pain, localization, causes, and accompanying symptoms (Table 17-3).

### Referred Pain

**Referred pain** is felt in areas other than those stimulated. It may occur when stimulation is not perceived in the primary areas. For example, the person having a heart attack may complain only of pain radiating down the left arm when in fact the tissue damage is occurring in the myocardium.

Referred pain occurs most often with damage or injury to visceral organs, and the pain is referred to cutaneous surfaces (Figure 17-4). The origin of referred pain is complex and not clearly understood and may relate to one or more of the following[15]:

1. Referred pain usually occurs in structures that developed from the same embryonic dermatome.
2. Visceral and somatic nerves enter the nervous system at the same spinal level and share the same spinothalamic tracts.
3. Somatic pain is more common and the person has "learned" to interpret signals conducted on certain pathways as being somatic in origin.

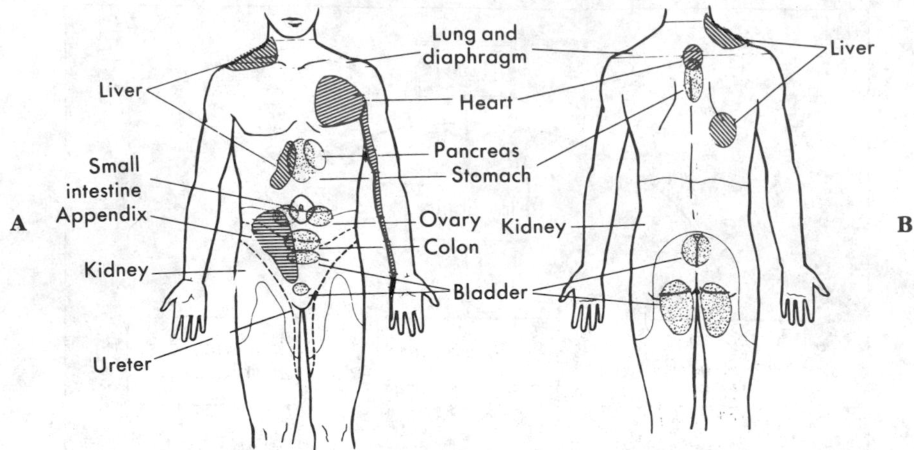


FIGURE 17-4 Referred pain. **A,** Front. **B,** Back.

**TABLE 17-3 Comparison of Somatic and Visceral Pain**

| | TYPE OF PAIN | | |
|---|---|---|---|
| | SUPERFICIAL | SOMATIC | |
| CHARACTERISTIC | Skin and Subcutaneous Tissue | Deep Muscles and Bones | Visceral (internal organs) |
| Quality | Sharp, pricking, burning | Sharp or dull and aching | Sharp, dull and aching, cramping |
| Localization | Good | Poor | Poor |
| Referred pain | No | No | Yes |
| Provoking stimuli | Cut, abrasion, excessive heat or cold, chemicals | Cut, pressure, heat, ischemia, displacement (bone) | Distention, ischemia, spasms, chemical irritants (no cutting) |
| Autonomic reactions | No | Yes | Yes |
| Reflex muscle contractions | No | Yes | Yes |

The cutaneous pattern of various referred pains is fairly constant and frequently seen in practice. The nurse should be able to recognize the possibility of visceral organ disease in patients who complain of cutaneous pain.

### Psychogenic Pain

The term **psychogenic pain** has been used to describe pain for which no pathologic condition has been found or in which the pain appears to have a greater psychologic basis than a physical one.[40] A caution here is that diagnostic tests are not definitive measures and may not be sophisticated enough to detect pathophysiologic changes. Distinguishing between physical and emotional components of pain is difficult, and it is important to remember that *all pain is real.*

### Neurologic Pain

Pain in the neurologic system occurs in different forms. **Neuralgia** is sharp, spasmlike pain along the course of one or more nerves. Two common areas of neuralgia are the trigeminal nerve in the face and the sciatic nerve in the lower trunk. **Causalgia,** a form of neuralgia, is severe burning pain associated with injury to a peripheral nerve in the extremities. The patient may go to great lengths to protect against irritating stimuli (which may be something as simple as the noise of a plane overhead).

**Phantom limb pain** is pain or discomfort perceived by the person to be occurring in an extremity that has been amputated. It is more likely to develop in those who had pain before amputation and may persist long after healing has occurred. The phenomenon of phantom limb pain has only recently been decreased postoperatively when patients are given preemptive (before surgery) analgesia.[20]

# MEDICAL MANAGEMENT

## PHARMACOLOGIC APPROACHES

### Analgesics

Two groups of analgesics, as well as adjuvant medications, are important components of effective pain management. **Opioid analgesics** (also called narcotics), such as morphine, act mainly on the central nervous system to alter the perception of pain. **Nonopioid analgesics,** such as aspirin, block impulses mainly in the

**TABLE 17-4 Dosing Data for Opioid Analgesics**

| DRUG | APPROXIMATE EQUIANALGESIC ORAL DOSE | APPROXIMATE EQUIANALGESIC PARENTERAL DOSE | RECOMMENDED STARTING DOSE (adults more than 50 kg body weight) | | RECOMMENDED STARTING DOSE (children and adults less than 50 kg body weight)'1 | |
|---|---|---|---|---|---|---|
| | | | ORAL | PARENTERAL | ORAL | PARENTERAL |
| **OPIOID AGONIST** | | | | | | |
| Morphine[2] | 30 mg q 3-4 hr (around-the-clock dosing)<br>60 mg q 3-4 hr (single dose or intermittent dosing) | 10 mg q 3-4 hr | 30 mg q 3-4 hr | 10 mg q 3-4 hr | 0.3 mg/kg q 3-4 hr | 0.1 mg/kg q 3-4 hr |
| Codeine[3] | 130 mg q 3-4 hr | 75 mg q 3-4 hr | 60 mg q 3-4 hr | 60 mg q 2 hr (intramuscular/subcutaneous) | 1 mg/kg 3-4 hr' | Not recommended |
| Hydromophone[2] (Dilaudid) | 7.5 mg q 3-4 hr | 1.5 mg q 3-4 hr | 6 mg q 3-4 hr | 1.5 mg q 3-4 hr | 0.06 mg/kg q 3-4 hr | 0.015 mg/kg q 3-4 hr |
| Hydrocodone (in Lorcet, Lortab, Vicodin, others) | 30 mg q 3-4 hr | Not available | 10 mg q 3-4 hr | Not available | 0.2 mg/kg q 3-4 hr[4] | Not available |
| Levorphanol (Levo-Dromoran) | 4 mg q 6-8 hr | 2 mg q 6-8 hr | 4 mg q 6-8 hr | 2 mg q 6-8 hr | 0.04 mg/kg q 6-8 hr | 0.02 mg/kg q 6-8 hr |
| Meperidine (Demerol) | 300 mg q 2-3 hr | 100 mg q 3 hr | Not recommended | 100 mg q 3 hr | Not recommended | 0.75 mg/kg q 2-3 hr |
| Methadone (Dolophine, others) | 20 mg q 6-8 hr | 10 mg q 6-8 hr | 20 mg q 6-8 hr | 10 mg q 6-8 hr | 0.2 mg/kg q 6-8 hr | 0.1 mg/kg q 6-8 hr |
| Oxycodone (Roxicodone, also in Percocet, Percodan, Tylox, others) | 30 mg q 3-4 hr | Not available | 10 mg q 3-4 hr | Not available | 0.2 mg/kg q 3-4 hr[4] | Not available |
| Oxymorphone[2] (Numorphan) | Not available | 1 mg q 3-4 hr | Not available | 1 mg q 3-4 hr | Not recommended | Not recommended |
| **OPIOID AGONIST-ANTAGONIST AND PARTIAL AGONIST** | | | | | | |
| Buprenorphine (Buprenex) | Not available | 0.3-0.4 mg q 6-8 hr | Not available | 0.4 mg q 6-8 hr | Not available | 0.004 mg/kg q 6-8 hr |
| Butorphanol (Stadol) | Not available | 2 mg q 3-4 hr | Not available | 2 mg q 3-4 hr | Not available | Not recommended |
| Nalbuphine (Nubain) | Not available | 10 mg q 3-4 hr | Not available | 10 mg q 3-4 hr | Not available | 0.1 mg/kg q 3-4 hr |
| Pentazocine (Talwin, others) | 150 mg q 3-4 hr | 60 mg q 3-4 hr | 50 mg q 4-6 hr | Not recommended | Not recommended | Not recommended |

From Acute Pain Management Guideline Panel: *Acute pain management: operative or medical procedures and trauma, Clinical Practice Guideline.* AHCPR Pub. No. 92-0032. Rockville, MD: Agency for Health Care Policy and Research, Public Health Service, U.S. Department of Health and Human Services. Feb. 1992.

**Note:** Published tables vary in the suggested doses that are equianalgesic to morphine. Clinical response is the criterion that must be applied for each patient; titration to clinical response is necessary. Because there is not complete cross tolerance among these drugs, it is usually necessary to use a lower than equianalgesic dose when changing drugs and to retitrate to response.

**Caution:** Recommended doses do not apply to patient with renal or hepatic insufficiency or other conditions affecting drug metabolism and kinetics.

[1]**Caution:** Doses listed for patients with body weight less than 50 kg cannot be used as initial starting doses in babies less than 6 months of age. Consult the *Clinical Practice Guideline for Acute Pain Management: Operative or Medical Procedures and Trauma* section on management of pain in neonates for recommendations.

[2]For morphine, hydromorphone, and oxymorphone, rectal administration is an alternate route for patients unable to take oral medications, but equianalgesic doses may differ from oral and parenteral doses because of pharmacokinetic differences.

[3]**Caution:** Codeine doses above 65 mg often are not appropriate due to diminishing incremental analgesia with increasing doses but continually increasing constipation and other side effects.

[4]**Caution:** Doses of aspirin and acetaminophen in combination opioid/NSAID preparations must also be adjusted to the patient's body weight.

periphery and decrease inflammatory-related pain by inhibiting the synthesis of prostaglandins. For some types of pain, such as with bone cancer, analgesics from both groups are necessary. Adjuvant medications such as diazepam (Valium) relieve pain—for example, muscle spasms—or decrease the side effects associated with some analgesics, particularly opioids.[33]

Nurses need to know the equianalgesic doses for both opioid and nonopioid analgesics. This means knowing the dose of any opioid that has the same strength (potency) as parenteral morphine 10 mg (Table 17-4).

Recognition of the widespread inadequacy of pain management has prompted recent corrective efforts within multiple health care disciplines, including surgery, anesthesiology, and nursing, as well as in pain management groups. These efforts are reflected in the *Clinical Practice Guideline: Acute Pain Management: Operative or Medical Procedures and Trauma* published by the Agency for Health Care Policy and Research (AHCPR) of the U.S. Department of Health and Human Services.[43] They list four major goals for the guideline. These are the following:

1. Reduce the incidence and severity of patients' acute postoperative or posttraumatic pain.
2. Educate patients about the need to communicate unrelieved pain so they can receive prompt evaluation and effective treatment.
3. Enhance patient comfort and satisfaction.
4. Contribute to fewer postoperative complications and, in some cases, shorter stays after surgical procedures.

### Opioid analgesics

Opioid analgesics are the most effective analgesics for relief of moderate to severe pain. They must be given around the clock to reach and maintain the steady blood levels necessary for pain relief. Side effects of opioids vary with the physiologic state of the patient. Constipation is the most common side effect, and laxatives should be given to any patient receiving opioids on a regular basis. Nausea and vomiting are experienced by some; these patients usually respond well to antiemetics. Sedation and drowsiness may occur for the first 48 to 72 hours, but one needs to consider that the patient may be catching up on sleep lost because of pain. Respiratory depression is rarely a problem with standardized doses and careful titration (slowly increasing the dose). Naloxone (Narcan) will reverse any depressive effect.

The oral route is preferred unless the patient is vomiting, unable or not permitted to swallow, or is in acute pain. Routes other than intramuscular or subcutaneous injection are rectal, intravenous, transdermal,[35] or epidural[42] (see Chapter 16). Slow-release preparations, such as MS Contin, are given every 8 to 12 hours, allowing less focus on the pain and better control with fewer side effects.[45]

**Concern about addiction.** Persons receiving opioids for pain relief very rarely develop addiction. The incidence of opioid addiction in hospitalized patients is less than 1%.[36] Patients are taking opioids for pain relief and not for the psychologic effect. Patients who are concerned about becoming addicted can be asked, "Would you take this medication if you were not in pain?" Unfortunately, health professionals are overly concerned about addiction, and opioids are underprescribed by physicians and underadministered by nurses.[2]

It is important to differentiate among tolerance, dependence, and addiction, as noted here:

| | |
|---|---|
| Tolerance | Larger doses are needed to produce desired effects |
| Dependence | Need to continue use of drug to prevent symptoms |
| Addiction | Behavioral pattern of compulsive drug use; drug used for psychologic effect |

*Drug tolerance* occurs with some patients and with some conditions, usually when the patient's pain is first being controlled and/or when the pain increases. This is a physiologic response and requires increasing the dose until pain relief is attained. There is no ceiling or maximum amount of opioid that can be given. *Physical dependency* (the appearance of physiologic withdrawal symptoms) *rarely happens* because as pain decreases, the dosage is gradually tapered and no symptoms are experienced. Physical dependency and drug tolerance are involuntary behaviors.

**Patient-controlled analgesia.** One method of providing more adequate pain control with opioids is the system of **patient-controlled analgesia (PCA).** The system consists of a syringe type of infusion pump that is filled with the prescribed opioid and is piggybacked into an intravenous injection port. PCA is activated when the patient pushes a button to release a set amount of opioid by bolus. A refractory time prevents delivery of another bolus before a preset time interval. The device also records the patient's attempts to receive the opioid in a given time period. The physician determines the opioid dosage and the refractory time interval.

Experience has demonstrated that persons using PCA tend to take less analgesia than those receiving the standard method of intramuscular injections.[19,21,37] PCA has been used for postoperative pain, for other types of acute pain such as sickle cell crisis, and for cancer pain.[13,19] Nursing activities related to PCA include maintaining the system, recording the number of times the patient activates the system, and monitoring the patient's pain relief.

**Intraspinal analgesic infusion.** Opioids (most commonly morphine) also can be administered through a catheter placed in the epidural or intrathecal space by the physician. An infusion device attached to the line provides a continuous supply of the opioid. This method—termed **intraspinal analgesic infusion**—relieves pain without diminishing CNS function. Patients with intractable pain can be well managed at home. The patient and family members need to know how to monitor the patient's response to the medication and how to care for the line. The reservoir usually holds a 2-week supply of opioid. It is refilled by a home health care provider.[28]

### Nonopioid analgesics

Mild to moderate pain generally can be controlled by nonopioid analgesics, most commonly nonsteroidal antiinflammatory agents, such as aspirin, and by acetaminophen.

*Acetaminophen* (Tylenol, Datril) is comparable to aspirin for analgesic effects but is not antiinflammatory. It causes less alteration in prothrombin level and has fewer side effects, but overdoses can cause severe liver damage. It is useful for persons who are allergic to aspirin and for whom aspirin is contraindicated, such as persons with a gastric ulcer.

**Nonsteroidal antiinflammatory drugs.** The **nonsteroidal antiinflammatory drugs (NSAIDs)** are the most widely used analgesics because of their general lack of serious side effects and their effectiveness in pain relief.[34] They act primarily by *inhibition of prostaglandin synthesis.* In lower doses these drugs have analgesic properties; in higher doses there is antiinflammatory action in addition to analgesia. The principal uses of NSAIDs are control of moderate pain of dysmenorrhea, arthritis and other musculoskeletal disorders, postoperative pain, and migraine headaches. They may be used for patients with bone cancer. NSAIDs commonly used for pain are listed in Table 17-5.

NSAIDs inhibit platelet aggregation, with resulting increased bleeding time. Common side effects include gastrointestinal disturbances, dizziness, tinnitus, and headache. Persons who are hypersensitive to aspirin also may be hypersensitive to NSAIDs. Acetylsalicylic acid (aspirin) is the most widely used NSAID analgesic for mild to moderate pain. Salicylates produce analgesia by blocking pain impulses peripherally or centrally, possibly in the hypothalamus, and by inhibiting synthesis of prostaglandins. Aspirin is a platelet aggregation inhibitor and a weak vitamin K antagonist. It produces an increased bleeding time and prolonged prothrombin time when given in large doses. Therefore it is contraindicated for persons receiving anticoagulant drugs.

Irritation of the gastric mucosa is a common side effect of NSAIDs, and these drugs should not be taken on an empty stomach. They are best taken with meals or with a snack such as a glass of milk, and persons with a history of peptic ulcer should avoid taking them. Aspirin should be avoided by children and teenagers because of the risk of Reye's syndrome.

### Other drugs for pain relief

Adjuvant drugs may be given along with analgesics to augment pain relief. They also may be an option for pain relief when other analgesics are not effective.

*Sedatives and antianxiety agents* sometimes are prescribed for persons with pain. These drugs do *not* have analgesic effect but may permit relaxation and decrease anxiety and thus prevent potentiation of pain. The drugs may permit the person to sleep and thus be better able to cope with the pain. In some persons sedatives and antianxiety agents may lead to disorientation and agitation, which can increase the pain and decrease the person's ability to cope. Treating pain with analgesics is the more effective and preferred method.

*Tricyclic antidepressants,* such as amitriptyline (Elavil), produce analgesia at doses lower than those used for depression. These drugs are useful in nerve injury pain, such as with postherpetic neuralgia (shingles).

*Anticonvulsants* such as phenytoin (Dilantin) and carbmazepine (Tegretol) are useful in nerve injury pain such as trigeminal neuralgia.

*Corticosteroids* such as dexamethasone (Decadron) are helpful in relieving pain from increased intracranial pressure, nerve compression, spinal cord compression, and bone metastases. These drugs have the positive effect of stimulating appetite and elevating mood.

*Counterirritants* are over-the-counter (OTC) drugs that relieve local pain by producing counterirritation (stimulation of the large A-beta fibers). Examples of counterirritants include ointments containing methyl salicylate (oil of wintergreen) or ethyl aminobenzoate and oil of cloves (for toothaches).

**TABLE 17-5 Nonsteroidal Antiinflammatory Drugs Commonly Used for Mild to Moderate Pain**

| GENERIC NAME | TRADE NAME | DOSAGE RANGE |
|---|---|---|
| Fenoprofen | Nalfon | 200 mg q 4-6 hr prn |
| Ibuprofen | Advil, Motrin | 400 mg q 4-6 hr prn |
| Mefenamic acid | Ponstel | 500 mg initially, then 250 mg q 6 hr prn (not to exceed 7 days) |
| Naproxen | Anaprox, Naprosyn | 550 mg initially, then 275 mg q 6-8 hr prn |
| Zomepirac | Zomax | 50-100 mg q 4-6 hr prn |

## NONPHARMACOLOGIC APPROACHES

Nonpharmacologic approaches should be considered along with analgesics for effective pain management. This type of intervention can alter pain transmission, modify the response to pain, and modify the pain stimulus.

### Altering Pain Transmission

#### Electrical stimulators

The purpose of electrical stimulators is to modify the pain stimulus by blocking or changing the painful stimulus with stimulation perceived as less painful. The success of this approach is thought to be explained by the gate control theory of pain transmission, that is, blockage of pain stimulus by stimulation of the large sensory fibers. Selected forms of electrical stimulation may activate the opiate or nonopiate descending pathways (Box 17-5).

The **transcutaneous electrical nerve stimulator (TENS)** is a battery-powered stimulator worn externally. It is a convenient, nonintrusive, nonaddictive type of pain therapy that can be learned easily by the patient. Success is variable, and it is usually used along with other pain therapies.

A number of TENS devices are on the market; all consist of a battery-powered portable pulse generator about the size of a pocket paging device. Control knobs on the generator permit adjustment of the impulse. The generator is connected by a pair of cables to electrically conductive tape electrodes placed at appropriate sites on the skin. The TENS delivers a balanced biphasic potential in a waveform.

TENS appears to be most useful for postoperative pain, posttraumatic pain, phantom limb pain, peripheral neuralgias, low back pain, and muscle pain.[11] It is less effective with cancer pain, inflammatory arthritis, and trigeminal neuralgia or in anxious or depressed persons.[38]

TENS electrodes should not be placed over hair, irritated skin, sutures, carotid sinus (may produce bradycardia), laryngeal or pharyngeal muscles (may trigger spasms), or the uterus of a pregnant woman.[10] A cardiac pacemaker may interfere with TENS effects. Suggested electrode placement may include (1) directly over the painful area, (2) at trigger points along the nerve pathways, or (3) at trigger points in the same dermatome as the pain.[38]

Routine skin care at the electrode sites includes the following:

1. Remove and clean electrodes at least once a day.
2. Wash skin with soap and water.
3. Allow skin to air dry.
4. Wipe skin with a prep pad before reapplying conductor pad.

If the skin becomes irritated, it may be cleaned with milk of magnesia, rinsed well, then air dried.[38]

Spinal cord stimulators are similar to TENS except that they are intrusive procedures. Instead of electrode placement on the skin, the electrodes are placed on or near the spinal cord. This is achieved either surgically over the ventral surface of the spinal cord or percutaneously through the back into the epidural space. Because the **percutaneously inserted spinal cord electrical stimulator (PISCES)** can be inserted under local anesthesia, it is preferred over surgical placement of the dorsal column stimulator electrodes (Figure 17-5). Postoperative care after dorsal column stimulator implantation includes the same care that follows laminectomy, with monitoring for infection and leakage of cerebrospinal fluid (see Chapter 58).

**BOX 17-5 Methods of Electrical Stimulation for Pain Control**

**TRANSCUTANEOUS ELECTRICAL NERVE STIMULATOR (TENS)**

Manually controlled stimulation of specific pain areas through externally placed electrodes

**PERCUTANEOUSLY INSERTED SPINAL CORD ELECTRICAL STIMULATOR (PISCES)**

Stimulation by an external transistorized receiver through leads inserted percutaneously in epidural space of spinal column

**DORSAL COLUMN STIMULATOR**

Stimulation by a transistorized receiver, implanted surgically in an infraclavicular or abdominal skin pouch, through electrodes surgically implanted on dorsum of spinal cord

#### Neurosurgical procedures

Constant relentless chronic pain that cannot be controlled by analgesics **(intractable pain)** may be reduced or eliminated by one of various neurosurgical procedures (Table 17-6 and Figure 17-6). Other forms of pain control usually are attempted before neurosurgical procedures.

Neurosurgical procedures do not play a major role in management of chronic pain. Major limitations include short duration of relief, occurrence of dysesthesia (pain induced by gentle touch of the skin), central pain syndrome (burning sensations in skin areas lacking sensation from surgical afferent interruptions), and possible further neurologic dysfunction.[46]

Neurectomy refers to the excision or resection of a nerve. It has limitations in that peripheral nerves may regenerate. Both rhizotomy and anterolateral cordotomy require laminectomy. A more commonly used procedure is percutaneous cordotomy, a closed stereotactic procedure in which the lesion is first located by using three-dimensional coordinates. The anterospinothalamic tracts are destroyed by electrodes inserted percutaneously. The patient is awake to provide feedback, thus providing more accurate site location and better pain relief. The effect usually lasts 18 to 24 months.[46]

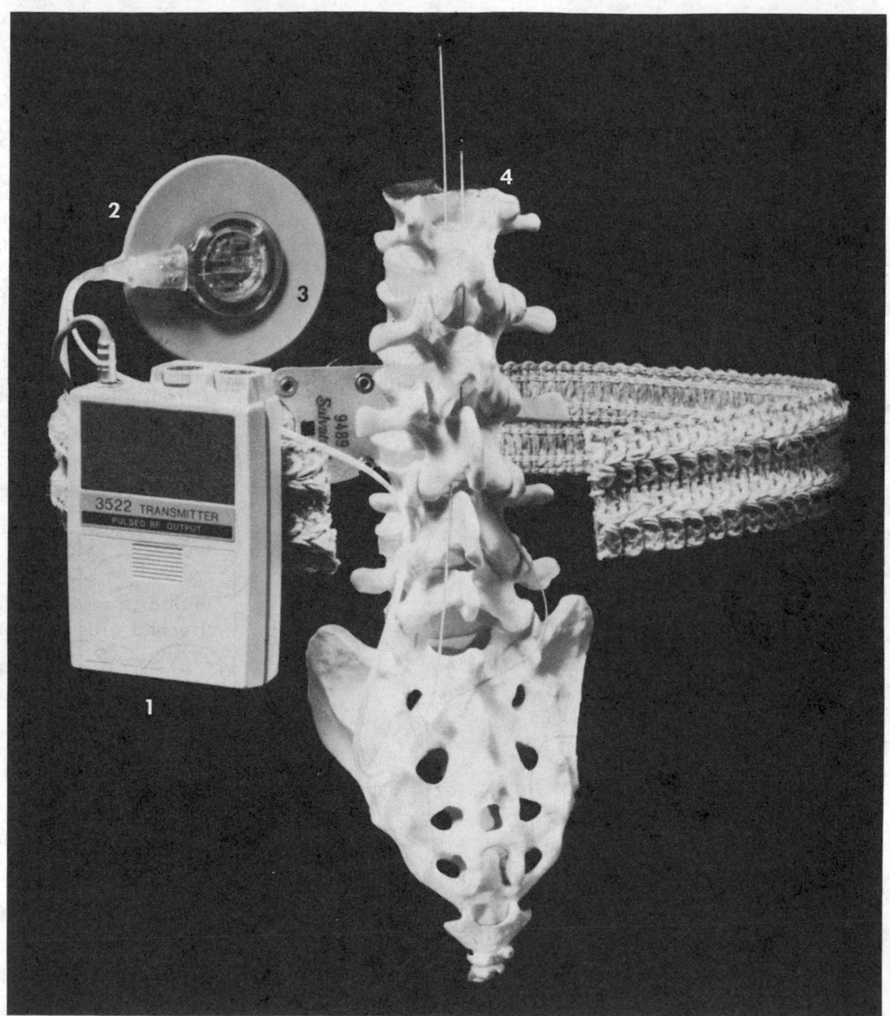


**FIGURE 17-5** Percutaneously inserted spinal cord electrical stimulator (PISCES). *1,* Stimulation transmitter. *2,* Receiver-extension. *3,* Antenna. *4,* Leads. (Courtesy Medtronic, Inc, Minneapolis, Minn.)

**TABLE 17-6 Neurosurgical Procedures for Pain Control**

| METHOD | USE |
|---|---|
| **NEURECTOMY** | |
| Severing of nerve fibers from the cell body | Trigeminal neuralgia (fifth nerve resection); incapacitating dysmenorrhea (presascral neurectomy) |
| **RHIZOTOMY** | |
| Resection of posterior nerve root before it enters spinal cord | Severe pain in upper trunk (e.g., lung cancer) |
| **CORDOTOMY** | |
| Severing of ascending anterolateral pain-conducting pathways of spinal cord | Severe pain of lower body (e.g., pelvic cancer) |
| **SYMPATHECTOMY** | |
| Excision or destruction of one or more sympathetic ganglia or nerves | Pain secondary to vascular insufficiency of extremities (e.g., Raynaud's disease) |

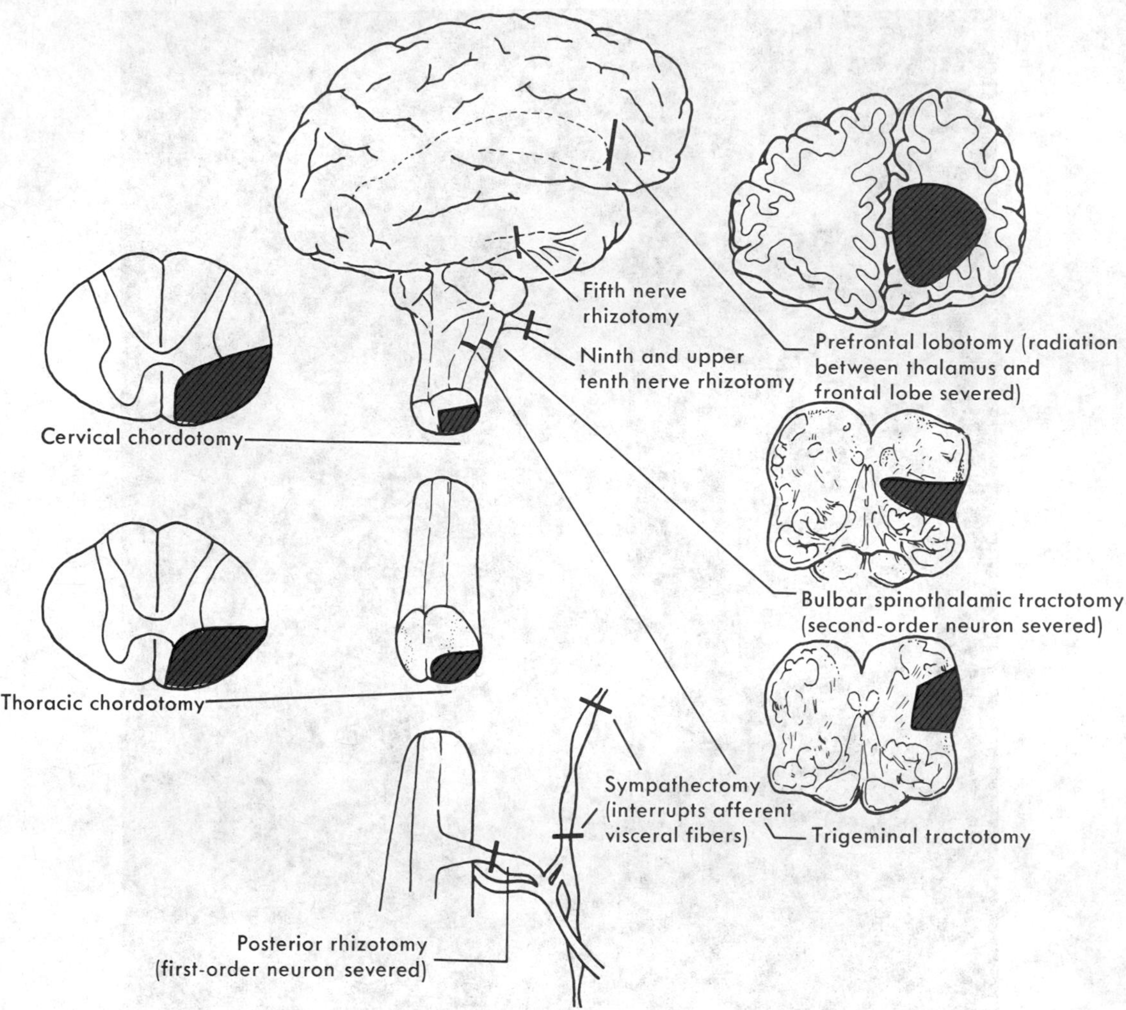


**FIGURE 17-6** Neurosurgical procedures for pain relief.

In a **rhizotomy** the posterior nerve root is resected before it enters the spinal cord. It interferes with the ability to perceive heat and cold; therefore, protection from extremes in temperatures is important for prevention of injury. The advantages of **cordotomy,** in which there is severing of the anterolateral pain-conducting pathways of the spinal cord, include a wide sense of analgesia below the surgical site while preserving other sensory and motor functions.[46] After surgery there may be temporary leg weakness and loss of bowel and bladder control from edema of the spinal cord; these usually disappear within 2 weeks. If quadriceps setting exercises are begun in the early postoperative period, walking will be less difficult.

Pain pathways in the brain also may be interrupted by stereotactic techniques (tractotomy, thalamotomy, lobotomy). These surgical procedures usually are reserved as a last resort for patients with intractable pain, usually from malignant invasion of cranial or facial structures. Lobotomy usually results in a change in personality.

### Nerve block

A **nerve block** involves the injection of substances such as local anesthetics or neurolytic agents (e.g., alcohol or phenol) close to nerves to block the conduction of impulses over the nerves. Nerve blocks frequently are used for the symptomatic relief of pain. They are used to treat chronic pain associated with peripheral vascular disease, trigeminal neuralgia, causalgia, and cancer.

### Acupuncture

**Acupuncture** is an ancient form of disease treatment that can be used for pain relief. Only recently has the method been used in Western countries. Small needles are skillfully inserted and manipulated at specific body points, depending on the type and location of pain. The gate control theory provides the best explanation for the success of acupuncture. The local stimulation of large-diameter fibers by the needles "closes the gate" to pain. It is not known to what extent the psyche and the power of suggestion contribute to the effectiveness of this therapy. Nursing intervention includes careful patient assessment and teaching.

## Modifying Pain Response

### Behavior modification

**Behavior modification** consists of a planned change in the way a person behaves by means of rewarding desired behavior and ignoring undesirable behavior. Forms of behavior modification are used unconsciously all the time: a young boy "throwing a tantrum" may be ignored, but as his behavior becomes more appropriate, his mother may reward him with her time and attention.

Behavior modification may be useful for persons with chronic pain. For example, one protocol for patients with chronic low back pain is to set a limit of 10 minutes daily for discussion of their pain experiences (with the exception of data-gathering interviews). Pain medications are given on a regular schedule to dissociate the feelings of pain with inappropriate use (reward) of analgesics or other unhealthy behaviors.

In using behavioral methods to alter pain-associated behavior or to encourage patient activities, success will occur only with a consistent approach on the part of the health care team. Although patients should always be praised for their efforts to comply or assist with treatment regimens, a true behavior modification program requires careful analysis of patient behavior and the development of a specific and comprehensive treatment plan.

### Biofeedback and autogenic training

Some persons are able to alter their body functions through mental concentration. In **biofeedback** training a machine that monitors brain wave activity (electroencephalograph [EEG]) is used. The individual concentrates on slowing his or her brain wave activity to rates at which pain and distress are unlikely to cause discomfort (i.e., complete relaxation). It may take many months of regular practice to achieve the desired level of control. The nurse should encourage and praise the person's efforts.

In **autogenic training** the same type of self-regulation is used to alter various autonomic nervous system functions, such as pulse, blood pressure, and muscle tension. Practiced use of transcendental meditation and other methods of concentration and self-control may achieve the same degree of autoregulation without the use of sophisticated physiologic monitoring equipment.

### Hypnosis

**Hypnosis** may be used in the treatment of various conditions, particularly when these conditions are aggravated by tension and stress. Patients are helped to alter their perception of pain through the acceptance of positive suggestions made to the subconscious. Many persons are able to learn self-hypnosis. Individual persons vary in their suggestibility and readiness to try this approach. The nurse's most helpful role may be to support the patient's desire to make hypnosis work.

# NURSING MANAGEMENT

## ♦ ASSESSMENT

Effective pain management can occur only when systematic and regular assessments take place. It is important to assess both *subjective* and *objective* data at least once a shift and sometimes more frequently when pain is anticipated.[12] Patient input is very important, and it is unfortunate that research has shown that health professionals document patients' pain differently than do patients themselves.* It is crucial to gather as much information from patients as possible to avoid making incorrect assumptions about what pain they are or are not experiencing. A variety of pain assessment tools are available.[7,25]

Unfortunately, many patients continue to have postoperative pain, and many will not ask for help.[32] For this reason it is best to use a rating scale to validate with patients the pain they are experiencing. The patient's rating of pain intensity is assessed and recorded both before and 1 hour after giving any analgesic. If the pain intensity does not decrease after the analgesic, such factors as the adequacy and timing of the dose and necessity for change in dose are assessed.

## Acute Pain

### Subjective data

Before pain occurs, it is useful to obtain data concerning the patient's expectation for pain relief. Many persons are unaware that they are expected to speak out when they have pain or discomfort. Some patients think they will be considered "complainers" or "bad patients" if they state that they are in pain.

It is distressing to note that most patients in several studies did not expect to have their pain relieved.[4,23,24,32] Patients need to be asked on admission about their expectations, knowledge, and concerns about pain. They should then be taught how and when to verbalize their discomfort and the various methods available for pain relief. As already mentioned, the best assessment of pain is the patient's own evaluation.

Data to be collected to assess the nature of the acute pain include the *location, intensity, quality, timing (onset, duration, frequency, cause),* and provoking and palliative factors. One approach for evaluating these characteristics is the use of the mnemonic PQRST[40]:

**P** Provoking factors: what makes the pain worse or relieves it

**Q** Quality: dull, sharp, crushing

*References 3, 8, 16, 39, 41, 43.

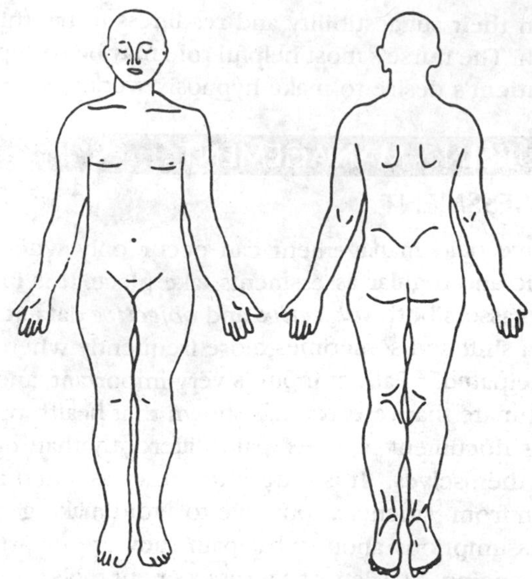

**FIGURE 17-7** Body diagrams for pointing out sites of pain. (From Watt-Watson JH, Donovan MI: *Pain management: nursing perspective,* St Louis, 1992, Mosby.)

**R** Region or radiation: site and radiation to other areas
**S** Severity or intensity
**T** Time: onset, duration, frequency, cause

Pain *intensity* can be determined by various means. Diagrams of the body can help patients point out the sites of their pain and its intensity (Figure 17-7). Pain intensity can be determined by various means. One way is to ask the patient to use a numerical rating to describe the pain or discomfort: 0 (no pain) to 10 (worst pain possible). Other scales to assess pain intensity are outlined in Box 17-6. The obtained data must be recorded. The pain scale score also can be recorded on a flow chart to provide ongoing assessment of progression of the pain (Figure 17-8). Another approach used mainly in research[27] is to ask the patient to mark an *X* on a visual analog scale (VAS). Pain intensity should be assessed at least once a shift or more often if the patient rated his or her pain high (7 to 10) and is receiving interventions for pain (such as analgesics, relaxation exercises, or TENS). When acute pain has subsided, further data can be collected about the *meaning* of pain for the person.

### Objective data

Objective data help the nurse identify possible pain or discomfort in a person who has not reported pain and can help to clarify the subjective response.

Objective signs of pain are of two types: physiologic and behavioral. Remember that *physiologic* signs of pain result from activation of the sympathetic nervous system (Box 17-7). With very severe acute pain, neurogenic shock may result from the stressful insult to the system. The *behavioral* signs are not specific to pain; therefore, if the observable data suggest that pain may be present, subjective data must be elicited to validate the assumption.

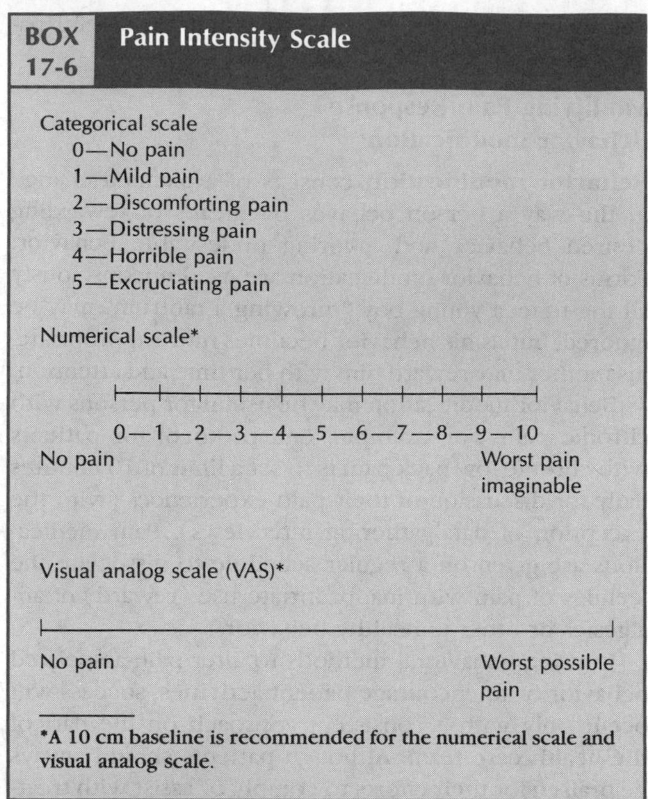

**BOX 17-6 Pain Intensity Scale**

Categorical scale
0—No pain
1—Mild pain
2—Discomforting pain
3—Distressing pain
4—Horrible pain
5—Excruciating pain

Numerical scale*

0—1—2—3—4—5—6—7—8—9—10
No pain — Worst pain imaginable

Visual analog scale (VAS)*

No pain — Worst possible pain

*A 10 cm baseline is recommended for the numerical scale and visual analog scale.

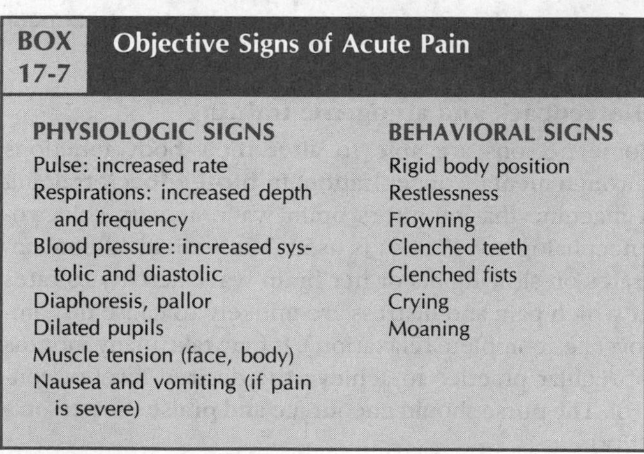

**BOX 17-7 Objective Signs of Acute Pain**

| PHYSIOLOGIC SIGNS | BEHAVIORAL SIGNS |
|---|---|
| Pulse: increased rate | Rigid body position |
| Respirations: increased depth and frequency | Restlessness |
| Blood pressure: increased systolic and diastolic | Frowning |
| Diaphoresis, pallor | Clenched teeth |
| Dilated pupils | Clenched fists |
| Muscle tension (face, body) | Crying |
| Nausea and vomiting (if pain is severe) | Moaning |

Specific objective data to be collected to assess the patient's pain include the following:

- Appearance (grimacing, gritting teeth, clenching fists, lying rigidly as if afraid to move)
- Motor behavior
- Affective and verbal responses
- Vital signs
- Skin: moisture, color
- Inspection and gentle palpation of painful area; identify trigger points that initiate pain, if present

Sometimes the patient's subjective response differs from the objective signs. For example, the patient may

## FLOW SHEET—PAIN

Patient ______________________________ Date ______________

*Pain rating scale used ______________________________

**Purpose: To evaluate the safety and effectiveness of the analgesic(s).**

Analgesic(s) ordered: ______________________________

| Time | Pain rating | Analgesic | R | P | BP | Level of arousal | ** Other | Plan and comments |
|---|---|---|---|---|---|---|---|---|
| | | | | | | | | |
| | | | | | | | | |
| | | | | | | | | |
| | | | | | | | | |
| | | | | | | | | |
| | | | | | | | | |
| | | | | | | | | |
| | | | | | | | | |
| | | | | | | | | |
| | | | | | | | | |
| | | | | | | | | |
| | | | | | | | | |
| | | | | | | | | |
| | | | | | | | | |
| | | | | | | | | |

* Pain rating: A number of different scales may be used. Indicate which scale is used and use the same one each time. Two common examples:
- 0 to 10 with 0 being no pain and 10 being as bad as it can be.
- Melzack's scale:
0 = no pain; 1 = mild; 2 = discomforting; 3 = distressing; 4 = horrible; 5 = excruciating
** Possibilities for other columns: bowel function, activities, nausea and vomiting, other pain relief measures. Identify the side effects of greatest concern to patient, family, physician, nurses, etc.

**FIGURE 17-8** Flow sheet for monitoring patient's response to pain. (May be duplicated for use in clinical practice.) (From McCaffery M, Beebe A: *Pain: clinical manual for nursing practice,* St Louis, 1989, Mosby.)

request an analgesic, a back rub, or other measure to relieve pain, but when the nurse arrives to carry out the request, the patient is found to be asleep. The patient may be exhausted from the pain and thus falls asleep. The patient who is sleeping or lying quietly is not necessarily pain free. He or she may be talking and joking with visitors in an attempt to distract himself or herself from pain. It is important to reiterate that pain is what the patient says it is, and although objective data may assist in confirming the existence of pain, the diagnosis must include both subjective and objective data.

## Chronic Pain

### Subjective data

Long-term pain requires a much more in-depth assessment of the pain syndrome. Hospitals or pain clinics that use a team approach in providing care to the person with chronic pain often develop their own pain history form or questionnaire (see references 27 and 47 for examples). This history may be collected by one or more health team members. Types of data to be collected to assess chronic pain include the following:

- Demographic data
- Sociocultural data
- History of the pain pattern from time of onset
- Factors perceived to increase or decrease the pain
- Effects of the pain on the person's life-style
- Meaning of the pain for the person
- Effects of the patient's pain on other family members or friends
- Measures used in the past and present for relief of pain

### Objective data

Physiologic signs of pain may be absent in the person with acute pain of 3 to 4 days' duration or with chronic pain because of the body's compensatory mechanisms. Although there is adaptation to the pain stimuli, the pain persists. The absence of physiologic signs, therefore, does not indicate absence of pain. Prolonged pain, however, may create changes in the person's appearance over time, perhaps as a result of decreased activity, decreased appetite, or lack of interest in appearance because of fatigue or depression.

Behavioral responses to chronic pain are varied and unique to the individual person. Here, also, there may be few overt signs to indicate the presence of pain. Changes usually occur in daily patterns related to sleeping, eating, socialization, and libido. If the person is extremely depressed because of the ongoing pain, withdrawal behaviors may be noted.

## ♦ NURSING DIAGNOSES

Nursing diagnoses are determined from analysis of patient data. Nursing diagnoses for the patient with pain may include but are not limited to the following:

| Diagnostic Title | Possible Etiologic Factors |
|---|---|
| Pain (acute, chronic) | Disease process (specify if possible): surgery, trauma, diagnostic studies, immobility, other causes |
| Knowledge deficit | Lack of previous instruction; misunderstanding |

Other nursing diagnoses may be appropriate after analysis of the subjective and objective data. Examples include but are not limited to the following:

- Activity intolerance, related to pain
- Anxiety, related to anticipation of pain or increasing pain
- Breathing pattern, ineffective, related to pain
- Mobility, impaired physical, related to pain
- Self-care deficit, related to pain
- Sexual dysfunction, related to pain
- Sleep-pattern disturbance, related to unrelieved pain

## ♦ EXPECTED PATIENT OUTCOMES

Expected patient outcomes for the patient experiencing pain may include but are not limited to the following:

1. States that pain is decreased by a lower rating on a scale of 0 to 10 (0, no pain; 10, most severe pain imaginable).
2. Demonstrates relaxed facial expression and body position and participates in activities.
3. Verbalizes factors that alter the pain and effective control measures.
4. If pain is present when patient is discharged, patient or significant other can
   a. Explain how, when, and for how long to apply heat or ice or to exercise to relieve pain.
   b. Explain prescribed medications (actions, dosages, frequency, side effects).
   c. Describe when to seek medical assistance if pain is not relieved as expected.
5. The person with *chronic pain* can
   a. State plans to participate in ongoing therapies.
   b. State plans for increasing independence in activities of daily living.
   c. Identify supports for encouragement and help.

## ♦ INTERVENTIONS

Pain is a complex experience involving sensory, affective, and behavioral components that require a multimodal treatment approach. Pain such as muscle spasms in the lower back may be relieved more effectively by heat and ultrasound than by medications. Strategies such as breathing exercises, muscle relaxation, imagery, and distraction do not replace analgesics for patients who need pharmacologic management. However, they can be useful adjuncts in reducing the dose required and in decreasing the pain while the patient waits for pain medication to work. Because pain is multidimensional, encouraging patients to use a broad range of pain relief methods will result in more effective pain management.

## Specific Interventions

Specific nursing interventions for pain relief include those related to preventing pain, modifying the stimulus, and modifying the response to pain as previously described. General guidelines for pain relief are listed here.

1. *Preparation for painful experiences.* Whenever possible, prepare patients for what to expect in terms of discomfort, measures of pain control, and management approaches *before* pain occurs (such as before painful tests or treatments). Intensity and duration of pain are decreased because of decreased anxiety and the patient's sense of control.
2. *Preventive approach.* Use pain relief measures *before* pain becomes moderate or severe. The more severe the pain, the less the possibility of relief.
3. *Placebo response.* Use methods such as your own positive attitude toward the patient as a placebo response—that is, some relief from discomfort not related specifically to the applied pain relief method. If the person expects relief from the pain, anxiety and muscle tension will decrease and decreased pain is experienced. This can be accomplished by suggestion ("This should help you feel better") or by using methods the patient believes will work.
4. *Patient's ability or will to participate.* Consider the patient's ability or will to be active or passive in using pain relief measures. Decreased ability results from severe pain, fatigue, sedation, depression, or unconsciousness. Decreased will occurs with some persons with chronic pain who have experienced numerous failures in pain relief.
5. *Varied pain relief measures.* Use more than one type of pain relief measure when appropriate. For example, give an analgesic, rub the patient's back, and then offer some distraction, or combine an analgesic with relaxation exercises and soft music of the patient's choice.
6. *Introduction of new pain relief measures.* Introduce a new method in combination with methods known to be effective. Some measures, such as distraction or relaxation, require practice and should not be discarded until after several tries.
7. *Use of analgesics*
   a. Assess and record the effectiveness of analgesics given.
   b. Ask the patient for a pain rating (0 to 10) before and 1 hour after each analgesic is given.
   c. Give analgesics to prevent or minimize pain.
   d. Give opioids on a regular basis rather than as needed (PRN) when acute pain is anticipated, such as after some surgical procedures.
   e. If the medications will be given "as needed," instruct patient to report the presence of developing or recurrent pain, and ask patient regularly for pain ratings.
   f. Determine which patients are at high risk for developing pain, and assess them frequently for presence of increasing pain.
   g. Use the oral route, when possible, if patient is not in acute pain, can swallow, and is not nauseated.
   h. Use the parenteral route in acute, intermittent pain to provide immediate, short-term relief.

## Modifying the Pain Stimulus

### Cutaneous stimulation

Cutaneous stimulation innervates the large A-beta fibers, closing the gate to impulses from the periphery. Methods of cutaneous stimulation include the following:

1. Lightly rubbing the affected area
2. Application of heat or cold to area
3. Whirlpool massage of area
4. Back rub

### Reducing additional physical stimuli

Although in many instances pain cannot be prevented, it is often possible to avoid additional pain when pain is already present. For example, when moving the body or an extremity, supporting the trunk or extremity will prevent increasing the pain by unilateral pulling on muscles, joints, and ligaments. Interventions include the following measures:

1. Use a turning sheet for patients with severe neck, back, or general trunk pain.
2. Place a pillow under a painful joint when helping a patient change position.
3. Support limbs at the joints rather than the muscle bellies when handling an extremity.
4. Use special beds (Stryker frame, Foster bed, CircOlectric bed) for patients with severe general or trunk pain.
5. Avoid bumping the bed or moving it suddenly.

### Reducing auditory and visual stimuli

The patient may experience sensory overload with subsequent potentiation of pain stimuli. If nurses could stand still for 5 minutes in the patient's environment and watch and listen, they might understand that some patients are almost continuously bombarded with noise and visual stimulation. If these are problems, it may be possible to change the environment. Changes include the following:

1. Move the patient to a quieter room away from the center of activity.
2. Dim bright lights; pull shades if sunlight is intense.
3. Keep verbal interactions at a minimum when pain is severe.
4. Encourage other patients to use headphones or keep television or radio at a reasonable level.
5. Control the number of persons entering the patient's room according to patient's wishes.

### Reducing social isolation

When external stimuli are decreased too much, the patient may lack distraction from the pain stimuli; thus pain perception is increased. Social isolation may occur for a variety of reasons. The serious nature of a patient's disease may necessitate being in a private room for an extended period; hospitalization far from home may mean few family members and friends can visit; extended periods of hospitalization may result in friends' losing interest in visiting; or the patient may complain so much that no one cares to visit to hear the monologue repeated.

Each of these causes of isolation may have a different solution. In any event, careful assessment may indicate that social isolation is a problem for the patient. Before determining the plan for addressing this problem, the patient should be consulted about the desire and need to alter the present situation. Possible nursing interventions include the following:

1. Place the patient with a compatible roommate.
2. Plan frequent contacts with health team members.
3. Facilitate visits by family and friends.
4. Help patient to be as comfortable (free of pain) as possible during visits by family or friends.

### Distraction and relaxation exercises

Patients can be taught to modify their sensory input to control pain by activities that promote distraction or relaxation.[27]

**Distraction.** Distraction interferes with the pain stimulus, thereby modifying the awareness of the pain. Mild or moderate pain can be modified by focusing on activity in the environment. A very quiet environment providing little or no sensory input actually can intensify the pain experience because the person has nothing to focus on but the painful stimulus.

Severe pain requires more active participation by the individual in an effort to block out the painful stimulus. This can be enhanced by involving two or more sensory modalities, such as vision, hearing, touch, or movement. The distractors must be powerful enough to involve the person's total interest without resulting in fatigue. Pain of long duration requires a variety of meaningful distractions such as the following:

1. Playing games, watching television
2. Talking with someone
3. Listening to favorite music
4. Rhythmic breathing
5. Focusing on an object

**Relaxation.** Full relaxation decreases muscle tension and fatigue that usually accompanies pain. It also helps to decrease anxiety, thereby preventing augmentation of the pain stimulus. In addition, relaxation techniques serve as a form of distraction.

Not all persons with severe pain are able to achieve sufficient relaxation to decrease the pain sensation. Relaxation exercises may be especially beneficial for persons with chronic pain to help reduce stress that exacerbates the pain and to help the person achieve a sense of control—of being better able to cope with the pain. There are numerous forms of relaxation techniques (see Chapter 7). Success with a relaxation technique requires practice and encouragement.

### Guided imagery

**Guided imagery** is the term used to describe the use of images to improve physiologic status, mental state, self-image, or behavior.[11] Relaxation exercises before the use of this approach facilitate the imaging process. Imagery techniques such as visualizing oneself in a favorite setting—for example, a quiet beach—are more effective with repeated use, thus indicating that some practice is necessary. This technique works best when the patient selects the image and how it is to be used.

### Therapeutic touch

A less traditional therapy, termed **therapeutic touch**, may be helpful to patients in pain.[51] The rationale for the success of therapeutic touch is not clearly understood. The nurse undergoes a brief period of meditation before coming in contact with the patient. During this period the nurse quiets his or her internal energy levels and then touches the patient and transmits the healing energies. Few nurses are trained in the use of therapeutic touch as described. It does seem to be helpful for some patients and some kinds of pain and is gaining respectability as an effective treatment.

## Modifying the Pain Response

### Explaining the problem

As a result of nursing assessment, it may become clear that the patient's response to pain is really the manifestation of a lack of knowledge about the cause of pain. Sometimes a simple explanation about what is causing the pain and how long it will last is all that is necessary. Understanding that pain or discomfort is to be expected may relieve anxiety or help the patient to alter expectations and be better prepared for what will happen. In all cases, an explanation that includes information about pain is given before each diagnostic test.

### Decreasing anxiety

Because anxiety increases pain, measures taken to decrease anxiety may help to decrease pain (see Chapter 7 for a discussion of stress). Interventions for the patient with pain and the family include the following:

1. Maintain a calm, quiet manner.
2. Help the patient explore concerns related to the pain (meaning of pain for the patient).
3. Respect the patient's response to pain, even if it differs considerably from what the nurse expects.
4. Hold the patient's hand, as appropriate.

5. Arrange for someone to be with the patient if the person fears being alone.
6. Talk with family or close friends and help them to allay their anxieties so that these are not transmitted to the patient.
7. Teach the family and close friends ways in which they can help the patient, such as massage, encouraging the patient to use distraction or relaxation techniques, or supporting painful parts when moving or changing the patient's position. People often feel helpless when observing a loved one in pain and may need help themselves to cope.

## Planning Care

The need to assess the person with pain is ongoing; yet the nurse must begin to plan an approach with the person in pain. Family members should be included when possible. The nurse is able to function independently with many interventions, but careful planning with other members of the health care team is necessary to ensure that all have the same patient outcomes or goals in mind.

One aspect of the treatment plan that often is forgotten or omitted is the incorporation of measures the patient thinks may help relieve the pain, even if these measures are different from those usually carried out in that institution. Without encouragement, the patient may hesitate to mention these possible remedies—for example, nonprescription liniments, special applications of heat and cold, unusual positioning, or favorite homemade foods or drinks. If there are no contraindications to the remedy the patient wishes to try, the health care team may consider using it before trying other relief measures.

Planning for the same health care team members to care for the patient regularly should result in a more consistent approach and plan of care. The small group of health care team members and the patient can develop a plan of care in which the patient's decisions are honored, and a daily routine can be developed that will reduce anxiety and frustration about constant changes. The plan should include, if appropriate, such items as specified hours for analgesic administration before uncomfortable procedures, specified blocks of time for rest or napping, and coordination between various departments, such as physical therapy and occupational therapy. For some patients fatigue is a great problem; thus regular visits to off-unit departments should be interspersed with rest periods; for other patients the most beneficial plan includes ensuring that they go directly from one department to the next so that time is not wasted getting in and out of bed or performing other painful maneuvers.

## Team Approach for Chronic Pain Control

In recent years knowledge of the nature of chronic pain and the need for coordinated efforts of different health care professionals have resulted in the establishment of pain clinics and inpatient pain teams for control of chronic pain.

### Pain clinics

Most pain clinics use a team approach that includes physicians (internists, dolorologists [pain specialists], surgeons, psychiatrists), nurses, physical and occupational therapists, social workers, psychologists, vocational rehabilitation counselors, and appropriate others. Each pain clinic is organized differently, and emphasis on different aspects of pain relief may vary from clinic to clinic. Usual approaches to pain relief include the following:

1. Behavior modification (with patient's approval)
2. Medications: opioids, NSAIDs, laxatives, tricyclic antidepressants
3. Exercise and activity prescriptions
4. Family training to support planned goals/activities

The responsibility of the nurse varies depending on the available team members and may include patient assessment, documentation of observations, creating and maintaining a therapeutic milieu, providing emotional support for patient and family, and patient teaching. Nurses who work in pain clinics must be skilled in nurse-patient interactions, be knowledgeable about the mechanisms of pain and the effectiveness of various treatment modalities, and possess patience and understanding as they assist patients in reaching their goals.

### Inpatient chronic pain teams

Persons with chronic persistent pain sometimes are admitted to a hospital for evaluation or initiation of treatment by a multidisciplinary health care team similar to that found in a pain clinic. One example is a team for evaluation and treatment of chronic back pain. Each team member evaluates the patient separately and shares his or her assessment in a team conference during which a specific treatment plan is developed.

Protocols are developed for the approach to be used in control of the chronic pain; all persons providing patient care during the hospitalization need to become familiar with the protocols so that a *consistent approach* is used. For example, protocols for control of chronic back pain in one large medical center include an initial immobilization phase in which patients are placed in pelvic traction and instructed to move as little as possible (e.g., eat in side-lying position). This phase is followed by a mobilization phase in which the patients are encouraged to be active (e.g., walk to physical therapy and to the cafeteria for meals and make their own beds). The type of nursing care is therefore different depending on which phase is being implemented.

Nursing responsibilities include patient assessment, documenting observations, carrying out phase-related activities, carrying out designated behavior modification modalities, and patient teaching.[44] The culmination of the hospitalization is a discharge conference with the patient and family members in which future treatment plans and recommendations are presented and discussed.

## ♦ EVALUATION

Evaluation is an important component that is often forgotten in the care of the patient with pain. Evaluation is vital to ensure that the effectiveness of the interventions continues or that the interventions be modified, replaced with another intervention, or discontinued. The essential questions to consider in regard to *acute* pain are as follows.

1. Does the patient still have pain?
2. If so, how does it compare with the pain experienced before the intervention—that is, the degree of pain relief?
3. If it is better but still present, should the same intervention(s) be continued unchanged or be modified?
4. Should new interventions be added?
5. If pain is not better, were sufficient data obtained in the initial assessment to determine the cause of pain?
6. Are there new data to indicate a different diagnosis?
7. What are the patient's thoughts about the continuing pain and the modes of intervention?

The essential questions to consider in regard to *chronic* pain are as follows:

1. To what extent is the patient participating in the planned therapeutic program?
2. What is the patient's assessment of present pain?

Pain teams often have special evaluation guidelines specific to their patient population and specific treatment goals for each patient.

## ✸ SPECIAL CONSIDERATIONS FOR CARE OF THE GERONTOLOGIC PATIENT

Opioids usually are well tolerated by elders as long as they are closely monitored for their response to the analgesic prescribed.[28] The following guidelines apply to the use of opioids in the elderly patient:

1. Height, weight, and body surface are not accurate measures in determining drug dosages in elders.
2. Analgesics usually last longer in elders because they are cleared more slowly from the body.
3. Age is not significant in determining dose, but it is important in determining frequency of dose.
4. Dose is based on the therapeutic response and undesirable side effects (confusion, untoward CNS effects, respiratory depression).
5. Patient may be hesitant in asking for pain relief. Monitor patient closely for nonverbal signs of pain. Stress of unrelieved pain leads to fatigue and anxiety, which are physically and psychologically debilitating.
6. Review other medications patient is taking to avoid drugs that may interact unfavorably with the analgesic.

Precautions to be observed with the use of NSAIDs in elders are as follows:

1. NSAIDs cause more perforated ulcers and bleeding episodes in elders than they do in younger adults.
2. Elders with renal impairment are at increased risk for liver and renal toxicity and are monitored closely for signs of toxicity, including serum levels of the NSAID.
3. Persons 70 years and older usually are started on one-half the adult dose and monitored closely for side effects; dose is increased slowly.

## QUESTIONS TO CONSIDER

- How does the assessment of acute pain differ from the assessment of chronic pain? Think about two patients for whom you have provided care—one with acute pain and one with chronic pain. In what ways did their responses to pain differ, and how did these responses influence different management approaches?
- What misbeliefs about pain are most prevalent in your areas of practice, and how have you tried to change them in relation to your practice and that of colleagues?
- Compare the equianalgesic doses and the duration of action for analgesics ordered for patients you are caring for.
- How do the following terms differ: *pain tolerance* and *pain threshold? pain tolerance* and *drug tolerance? drug dependence* and *drug addiction?*
- Interview three or four patients who are using a nonpharmacologic pain intervention. Compare and contrast the method, frequency of use, patient satisfaction, and effectiveness for pain relief. Were several modalities used, and was the combination of approaches successful?

## CRITICAL THINKING ACTIVITIES

- If you were a scientist who wanted to develop an ideal analgesic, what properties would you borrow from the opiods and the nonsteroidal antiinflammatory drugs if you could select only two properties from each? What side effects would you eliminate if you could eliminate one from each group? Why did you make the choices you made?
- Maria has just returned to her room from post anesthesia recovery. This morning she underwent a total hysterectomy. She is awake and complaining of severe pain. Select three pain modalities, other than medication that would be effective in reducing or controlling Mary's pain.

## CHAPTER SUMMARY

### NATURE OF THE PROBLEM

- Pain is a complex universal, yet individualized, experience.

### PHYSIOLOGY OF PAIN

- Nociceptors are pain receptors that respond to chemical, thermal, electrical, or mechanical stimuli. Chemical stimuli released by damaged tissues include histamines, bradykinins, prostaglandins, and acids.
- Pain impulses are transmitted over faster-conducting A-delta and slower-conducting C fibers to the substantia gelatinosa (SG) of the dorsal horn of the spinal cord. Ascending spinal pathways in the ventral spinal cord carry impulses to the thalamus and cortex.
- Some descending spinal pathways carry pain inhibitory impulses back to the SG. Pain impulses transmitted over A-beta fibers also have a suppressive effect on impulses over the A-delta and C fibers.
- Substance P is a neurotransmitter of pain impulses. Endorphins and serotonin are neurotransmitters of pain-inhibitory impulses.
- The gate control theory proposes that the SG is a gating mechanism that may modify the pain experience by "opening" or "closing" the gate to pain impulse transmission. The gating mechanism can be closed by impulses from A-beta and A-alpha fibers and from descending pathways from the brainstem and cortex.

### THE PAIN EXPERIENCE

- The pain experience is influenced by the individual person's pain perception and response.
- Pain perception is subjective, highly complex, and individual. It is influenced by characteristics of the pain stimuli and transmission and by receptivity and interpretation in the cerebral cortex.
- Pain detection threshold is the intensity of the stimulus necessary for the person to perceive pain.
- Pain tolerance is the maximum degree of pain intensity that the person is willing to endure before seeking relief. Pain tolerance may be enhanced by drugs, warmth, counterirritation, distraction, and strong beliefs; it may be decreased by fatigue, anxiety, boredom, continuous pain, or illness.
- Pain response is influenced by the degree of pain perception, past experiences, sociocultural values, health status, anxiety, and age.
- Acute pain is a sudden short-term event, usually with a known source, and is self-limiting or readily corrected. The typical clinical signs are usually present and pain areas generally well identified. Acute pain leads to action to relieve pain, with likelihood of eventual relief. Acute pain is characterized by anxiety and muscle tension.
- Chronic pain is a prolonged situation, often with no purpose. Pain areas are less easily defined. Pain may be continuous or intermittent and with few typical clinical signs. It leads to actions to modify the pain experience. Chronic pain is characterized by increased preoccupation with pain, hopelessness, and irritability, all leading to withdrawal.
- Superficial somatic pain is sharp and pricking, well localized, and usually not accompanied by autonomic reactions. Deep somatic and visceral pains are sharp or dull and aching, poorly localized, and usually accompanied by autonomic reactions.
- Referred pain is felt in areas other than those stimulated; it is usually visceral in origin.
- Phantom limb pain is perceived to be occurring in a limb that has been amputated.

### MEDICAL MANAGEMENT

- Opioids provide relief of moderate to severe pain. The oral route is preferred if possible. Constipation is the most serious side effect, and laxatives should be given to patients receiving opioids.
- Patient-controlled analgesia is a system of self-administration by means of an intravenous set-up whereby a prescribed preset bolus of opioid may be taken but not repeated until a prescribed refractory time has occurred.
- Acetaminophen and NSAIDs (such as aspirin) provide relief of mild to moderate pain.
- Electrical stimulators include TENS and spinal cord stimulators. TENS is a nonintrusive system, easily learned by the patient, and useful for postoperative, posttraumatic, peripheral neuralgia, and muscle and bone pain.
- Approaches to modify the person's pain response include behavior modification, biofeedback and autogenic training, hypnosis, careful explanations, and anxiety reduction.

### NURSING MANAGEMENT

- Subjective data for pain include the location, intensity, quality, timing (onset, duration, frequency, cause), and provoking or palliative factors.
- Objective data include facial expression, motor behavior, affective and verbal response, vital signs, skin color and moisture, and inspection and palpation of painful areas.
- Pain intensity can be determined by the use of pain scales or visual analog scales, in addition to asking the person to describe the pain.
- General nursing interventions for *pain relief* include preparing patients to rate their pain and to communicate when the pain begins to return, varying pain relief measures, trying new approaches, and giving analgesics as effectively as possible.
- Nursing interventions to *modify the pain* stimulus include preventing pain when possible; modifying the pain stimulus by cutaneous stimulation; reducing noise and visual stimuli; decreasing social isolation; using therapeutic touch, imagery, distraction, and relaxation exercises; and modifying the pain response by careful explanations and measures to decrease anxiety.

## REFERENCES


1. Abbott F et al: The prevalence of pain in hospitalized patients and resolution over six months, *Pain* 50:15-28, 1992.
2. Angell M: The quality of mercy, *N Engl J Med* 306(2):98-99, 1982.
3. Camp D: Comparison of nurses' recorded assessments of pain with perceptions of pain as described by cancer patients, *Cancer Nurs* 11:237-243, 1988.
4. Carr E: Postoperative pain: patients' expectations, *J Adv Nurs* 15:89-100, 1990.
5. Crue BL: The neurophysiology and taxonomy of pain. In Brena SF, Chapman SL, editors: *Management of patients with chronic pain,* New York, 1983, SP Medical and Scientific Books.
6. Diekmann J, Wassem R: A survey of nursing students' knowledge of cancer pain control, *Cancer Nurs* 14:314-320, 1991.
7. Donovan MI: A practical approach to pain assessment. In Watt-Watson JH, Donovan MI, editors: *Pain management: nursing perspective,* St Louis, 1992, Mosby.
8. Donovan M, Dillon P, McGuire L: The incidence and characteristics of pain in a sample of medical-surgical inpatients, *Pain* 30(1):69-78, 1987.
9. Dostrovsky J: Pathways of pain: update, *Perspect Pain Manag* 1(1):4-8, 1991.
10. Driscoll CE: Pain management, *Prim Care* 14(2):337-352, 1987.
11. Edgar L, Smith-Hanrahan C: Nonpharmacological pain management. In Watt-Watson JH, Donovan MI, editors: *Pain management: nursing perspective,* St Louis, 1992, Mosby.
12. Ferrell B, McCaffery M, Grant M: Clinical decision making and pain, *Cancer Nurs* 14:289-297, 1991.
13. Ferrell B, Nash C, Warfield C: The role of patient-controlled analgesia in the management of cancer pain, *J Pain Symptom Manage* 7:149-154, 1992.
14. Fields H: *Pain,* Toronto, 1987, McGraw-Hill.
15. Ganong WF: *Review of medical physiology,* ed 15, Norwalk, Conn, 1991, Appleton & Lange.
16. Grossman S et al: Correlation of patient and caregiver ratings of cancer pain, *J Pain Symptom Manag* 6:53-57, 1991.
17. Huhman M: Endogenous opiates and pain, *ANS* 4(4):62-71, 1982.
18. International Association for the Study of Pain (IASP): Pain terms: a list with definitions and usage, *Pain* 6:249-252, 1979.
19. Kane N et al: Use of patient-controlled analgesia in surgical oncology patients, *Oncol Nurs Forum* 15:29-32, 1988.
20. Katz J, Melzack R: Pain "memories" in phantom limbs: review and clinical observations, *Pain* 43:319-336, 1990.
21. Kim S: Pain: theory, research and nursing practice, *ANS* 2:43-59, 1980.
22. Kleiman RL et al: PCA vs regular IM injections for severe postop pain, *Am J Nurs* 87(11):1491-1492, 1987.
23. Kuhn S et al: Perceptions of pain relief after surgery, *Br Med J* 300:1687-1690, 1990.
24. Lavies N et al: Identification of patient, medical and nursing attitudes to postoperative opioid analgesia: stage 1 of a longitudinal study of postoperative analgesia, *Pain* 48:313-319, 1992.
25. Marks RM, Sachar EJ: Undertreatment of medical inpatients with narcotic analgesics, *Ann Intern Med* 78:173-181, 1973.
26. McCaffery M, Beebe A: *Pain: clinical manual for nursing practice,* St Louis, 1989, Mosby.
27. McGuire D: Comprehensive and multidimensional assessment and measurement of pain, *J Pain Symptom Manage* 7:312-319, 1992.
28. McKenry LM, Salerno E: *Mosby's pharmacology in nursing,* ed 18, St Louis, 1992, Mosby.
29. Melzack R, Wall PD: Pain mechanisms: new theory, *Science* 150:971-979, 1965.
30. Melzack R, Wall PD: *The challenge of pain,* New York, 1983, Basic Books.
31. Oberle K: Pain, anxiety and analgesics: a comparative study of elderly and younger surgical patients, *Can J Aging* 9(1):13-22, 1990.
32. Owen H, McMillan V, Rogowski D: Postoperative pain therapy: a survey of patients' expectations and their experiences, *Pain* 41(3):303-308, 1990.
33. Paice J: Pharmacological management. In Watt-Watson JH, Donovan MI, editors: *Pain management: nursing perspective,* St Louis, 1992, Mosby.
34. Paice J, Mahon S, Faut-Callahan M: Factors associated with adequate pain control in hospitalized postsurgical patients diagnosed with cancer, *Cancer Nurs* 14:298-305, 1991.
35. Payne R: Transdermal fentanyl: suggested recommendations for clinical use, *J Pain Symptom Manage* 7:540-544, 1992.
36. Porter J, Jick H: Addiction rare in patients treated with narcotics, *N Engl J Med* 303(2):123, 1980.
37. Royburn W et al: Patient-controlled analgesia for postcesarean section pain, *Obstet Gynecol* 72:136-139, 1988.
38. Rudy EF: *Advanced neurological and neurosurgical nursing,* St Louis, 1984, Mosby.
39. Seers K: Perceptions of pain, *Nurs Times* 2:37-42, 1987.
40. Sternbach RA: *The psychology of pain,* ed 2, New York, 1986, Raven Press.
41. Teske K, Daut R, Cleeland C: Relationships between nurses' observations and patients' self-reports of pain, *Pain* 16:289-296, 1983.
42. Turnage G, Clark L, Wild L: Spinal opioids: a nursing perspective, *J Pain Symptom Manage* 5:154-162, 1990.
43. US Department of Health and Human Services, Public Health Service: *Clinical practice guideline: Acute pain management: operative or medical procedures and trauma,* Rockville, Md, 1992, Agency for Health Care Policy and Research.
44. Vortherms R, Ryan P, Ward S: Knowledge of, attitudes toward, and barriers to pharmacologic management of cancer pain in a statewide random sample of nurses, *Res Nurs Health* 15(12):459-466, 1992.
45. Walker M, Wong DL: A battle plan for patients in pain, *Am J Nurs* 91(6):33-36, 1991.
46. Ward S et al: Patient-related barriers to management of cancer pain, *Pain* 52:319-324, 1993.
47. Warfield CA, Stein JM: Pain relief by electrical stimulation, *Hosp Pract* 18:207-218, 1983.
48. Watt-Watson JH: Nurses' knowledge of pain issues: a survey, *J Pain Symptom Manag* 2(4):207-211, 1987.
49. Watt-Watson JH: Neurological patient with chronic pain. In Baumann A, Dewis M, editors: *Decision making in neuroscience nursing,* St Louis, 1993, Mosby.
50. Watt-Watson JH, Evans R, Watson CP: Relationships among coping responses and perceptions of pain intensity, depression and family functioning, *Clin J Pain* 4(2):101-106, 1988.
51. Wright S: The use of therapeutic touch in the management of pain, *Nurs Clin North Am* 22(3):705-714, 1987.

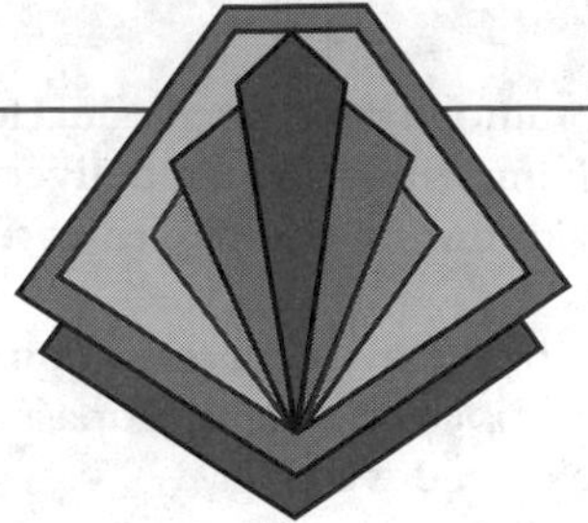

C H A P T E R 18

# Sleep Disorders

***Diane Broadbent Friedman***

## CHAPTER OBJECTIVES

***After studying this chapter, the learner should be able to do the following:***

1. Take a complete sleep history.
2. Describe the nature, pathophysiology, therapy, and teaching needs of persons with insomnia, narcolepsy, and sleep apnea.
3. Describe the relationship of sleep to chronobiology and the implications for nursing research.

## KEY TERMS

apnea
cataplexy
chronobiology
DIMS
episodic atonia
familial sleep paralysis
hypogognic hallucinations
hypopnea
insomnia
multiple sleep latency test (MSLT)
narcolepsy
parasomnia
pavor nocturnus
polysomnogram (PSG)
rapid eye movement (REM) sleep
sleep apnea
sleep hygiene
sleep paralysis
somnambulism

We usually divide our lives into two parts, waking and sleeping. We also commonly believe that our important activity occurs while we are awake and that sleep is a passive state initiated by simply closing our eyes. This belief contains the two most basic *misunderstandings* about sleep: sleep is not active or very important to life, and sleep is something that simply comes "naturally." These misunderstandings contribute to health professionals' and their patients' overlooking sleep problems and the role sleep plays in healing and health maintenance.

# INTRODUCTION TO SLEEP PROBLEMS

## ASPECTS OF NORMAL SLEEP

Sleep is difficult to define because as yet it is incompletely understood by researchers. From the sleeper's point of view, sleep is experienced as (1) being the deliberate initiation of a change or reduction in consciousness lasting an average of 8 hours, (2) commencing about the same time each 24-hour period, and (3) usually resulting in a feeling of restored physical, emotional, and intellectual energy. This definition contains three important concepts about normal sleep: *changes in consciousness, deliberate initiation of sleep,* and *timing of sleep.*

Although the sleeping person or observers may believe the sleeper is unconscious, the sleeping brain alternates among several active states during sleep, producing a series of predictable 90-minute sleep cycles. Unlike the unconsciousness produced by an anesthetic, the brain maintains all body systems during sleep, some of which are more active in sleep (such as secretion of growth hormone), and allows for restoration of alertness if required. Also, unlike animals, only humans can deliberately postpone the initiation of sleep. The record for sleep postponement is about 10 days.

Sleep commences about the same time each 24-hour period. The study of biologic rhythms places the study of sleep into a larger context. The timing for sleep is regulated by many subtle external factors (Box 18-1). Internal hormonal factors and neurologic activity maintain internal biologic clocks. These factors tend to occur

**BOX 18-1 External Factors Regulating Sleep**

- Sunrise, sunset, and length of day
- Ambient temperature
- Physical activity and rest
- Timing and composition of meals
- Timing of social/environmental cues, such as increased morning traffic noise

at the same time every 24 hours; therefore they help to "anchor" the onset and termination of sleep. Sleep research at the cellular level indicates that changes in the neuronal cell membrane and in the cell nucleus in several brain areas—including the suprachiasmatic nucleus of the hypothalamus, the pineal gland, and the pontine reticular formation of the brainstem—alter the cell's excitability in different stages of sleep.[9]

## NORMAL SLEEP FUNCTION

Sleep is usually initiated in the late evening about 8 hours before arising for morning work or daily routine. Some people require more or less than 8 hours to feel refreshed. Some people are "larks," falling asleep within moments of lying down and awakening alert and ready to go, whereas others are "owls," taking up to 30 minutes to fall asleep and feeling their most alert in the afternoon or early evening.

Sleep is initiated usually within 30 minutes of lying down. Sleep cycles of 90 minutes occur, initiated by very light stage I/II, followed by deep stage III/IV, and ending with lighter **rapid eye movement (REM)**/ dream sleep. If awakened from light stage I sleep, sleepers state that they were not asleep, whereas if awakened from other stages, they state that they were asleep or dreaming. Arousal can occur after each REM cycle. As the night progresses, the amount of time spent in stage III/IV shortens and the amount of REM lengthens. Thus more dreaming time occurs in the morning hours just before final awakening.

## NATURE OF SLEEP PROBLEMS

It is estimated that more than one half of all adults cite difficulties with sleeping at some time in their lives. These problems result in suffering; risk of accident; worry about loss of emotional, intellectual, or neurologic functioning; embarrassment; and exacerbation of other health problems. In 1983 the National Institutes of Mental Health (NIMH) determined that 35% of a nationally representative sample reported "trouble sleeping" in the previous year and that half of this group reported this as a "serious" problem. This means that approximately one of every three patients a nurse encounters may describe a sleep problem. Sleep problems have been historically overlooked, however, especially in the hospitalized patient when other circumstances appear more compelling.

Nurses can have a primary impact on helping persons with sleep problems and preventing sleep problems. The following instances of sleep problems highlight the need to detect sleep concerns or to prevent sleep problems from developing.

1. A 50-year-old woman describes a 10-year history of inability to stay asleep beyond 5 AM, dating from death of her husband.
2. A 65-year-old man comes to the emergency room for contusions after a minor traffic accident. He works the night shift, driving a newspaper delivery truck, and then stays awake during the day to care for his chronically ill wife.
3. A downcast young boy leaves the examining room after his mother describes how he must pass up summer camp because of bed-wetting.
4. An executive, whose head is immobilized in halo traction after a neck injury, describes sleeplessness at night, distorted conversations with physicians (probably related to medications), being awakened at night for procedures, and being disturbed by noises and vibrations amplified by the tongs.
5. A woman states that her husband falls asleep readily, even while sitting up in a chair, and that his skin color becomes bluish as he snorts and breathes irregularly.

Sleep problems can be categorized by the disruption in one or more of the aspects of normal sleep. Box 18-2 identifies different types of sleep problems. This chapter discusses only the most common types of sleep disorders:

**parasomnias** or disorders of arousal: dysfunctions associated with sleep, sleep stages, or arousal
**insomnia:** inability to initiate or maintain sleep
**narcolepsy:** sleep intrusion into wakefulness
**sleep apnea:** sleep problems involving other body systems

The last section of this chapter discusses research into sleep and circadian rhythms and its impact on nurses, both as researchers and as caregivers who must remain awake and alert at night. A source of additional information for professionals, patients, and families is the National Sleep Foundation.*

# PARASOMNIAS OR DISORDERS OF AROUSAL

Various types of parasomnias or disorders of arousal may occur (Table 18-1), especially in children, who often outgrow the dysfunction.

### SLEEPWALKING

Sleepwalking **(somnambulism)** usually occurs in children, although it may also be seen in adults. Children usually outgrow sleepwalking. It is characterized by sitting up or walking about during sleep. The sleepwalker's eyes are wide open, but the person appears in a daze, has purposeless movements, and may speak in short phrases, with no recollection in the morning. Twenty percent of somnambulists have a sleepwalking parent, and 5% to 15% of the population has sleepwalked at some time. Sleepwalking usually occurs in the first

*122 South Robertson Blvd., 3rd Floor, Los Angeles, CA 90048; phone: (310) 288-0466.

**BOX 18-2 Classification of Sleep and Arousal Disorders**

**DISORDERS OF INITIATING AND MAINTAINING SLEEP (DIMS)**

1. Psychophysiologic: transient and situational, persistent
2. Associated with:
   a. Psychiatric disorders: symptom and personality disorders, affective disorders, other functional psychoses
   b. Use of drugs and alcohol: tolerance to or withdrawal from central nervous system (CNS) depressants, sustained use of CNS stimulants, sustained use or withdrawal from other drugs, chronic alcoholism
   c. Sleep-induced respiratory impairment: sleep apnea DIMS syndrome, alveolar hypoventilation DIMS syndrome
   d. Sleep-related (nocturnal) myoclonus DIMS syndrome and/or "restless legs"
   e. Other medical, toxic, and environmental conditions
   f. Child-onset DIMS
   g. Other DIMS conditions: repeated REM interruptions, atypical polysomnographic features
   h. No DIMS abnormality: "short sleeper," subjective DIMS complaints without objective findings

**DISORDERS OF EXCESSIVE SOMNOLENCE (DOES)**

1. Psychophysiologic: transient and situational, persistent
2. Associated with:
   a. Psychiatric disorders: symptom and personality disorders, affective disorders, other functional psychoses
   b. Use of drugs and alcohol: tolerance to or withdrawal from CNS stimulants, sustained use of CNS depressants
   c. Sleep-induced respiratory impairment: sleep apnea DOES syndrome, alveolar hypoventilation DOES syndrome
   d. Sleep-related (nocturnal) myoclonus DOES syndrome and/or "restless legs"
   e. Other medical, toxic, and environmental conditions
   f. Other DOES conditions
   g. Intermittent DOES (periodic) syndromes: Kleine-Levin syndrome, menstrual-associated syndrome
   h. Insufficient sleep
   i. Sleep drunkenness
3. Narcolepsy
4. Idiopathic CNS hypersomnolence
5. No DOES abnormality: "short sleeper," subjective DOES complaints without objective findings

**DISORDERS OF THE SLEEP-WAKE SCHEDULE**

1. Transient: time-zone (jet lag) syndrome, work shift change in conventional sleep-wake schedule
2. Persistent: frequently changing sleep-wake schedule, delayed sleep phase syndrome, advanced sleep phase syndrome, non–24-hour sleep-wake syndrome, irregular sleep-wake pattern

**DYSFUNCTIONS ASSOCIATED WITH SLEEP, SLEEP STAGES, OR PARTIAL AROUSALS—PARASOMNIAS OR DISORDERS OF AROUSAL**

1. Sleepwalking (somnambulism)
2. Sleep terror (pavor nocturnus, incubus)
3. Sleep-related enuresis
4. Other dysfunctions
   a. Dream anxiety attacks (nightmares)
   b. Familial sleep paralysis
   c. Impaired sleep-related penile tumescence
   d. Sleep-related epileptic seizures, bruxism, head banging (jactatio capitis nocturna), painful erections, cluster headaches and chronic paroxysmal hemicrania, abnormal swallowing syndrome, asthma, cardiovascular symptoms, gastroesophageal reflux, hemolysis (paroxysmal nocturnal hemoglobinuria)
   e. Asymptomatic polysomnographic findings

Modified from Association of Sleep Disorder Centers and the Association for the Psychophysiological Study of Sleep, *Sleep* 2(1):21, 1979.

third of the night in stage III/IV sleep. Up to one half of all sleepwalkers either experience injury or narrowly avoid it.

Sleepwalkers should be led back to bed without being awakened. If the sleepwalker must be awakened, do not slap or shake the person or splash cold water on the face, but do say the person's name over and over. If the sleepwalker lies down to sleep on the floor, simply let the person stay there until awakening.

Protect the sleepwalker from injury. Place a bell at the bedside that will ring if the bedside is moved, or use a two-way radio in a child's room to awaken the parent when the child stirs. A protective gate or screen door may be placed across the entrance to the bedroom, but note that this blocks escape if there is a fire. Lock windows and doors to balconies. Imipramine, a tricyclic antidepressant, is sometimes prescribed for adult sleepwalkers who walk frequently and have been injured.

## SLEEP TERROR

Sleep terror **(pavor nocturnus)** usually occurs in children during the first part of the night in stage III/IV sleep. The child screams, arises from bed, wanders about in panic, and cannot be awakened or consoled. Autonomic changes (rapid pulse and respirations, sweating) can be noted. The child may be amnestic for the event. ***Sleep terror is often associated with sleepwalking.***

Interventions include planning sleep on a regular schedule. Do not try to awaken the child, because this may worsen the confusion. Usually the child will lie back on the pillow after several minutes, never having awakened. Benzodiazepines are sometimes given to patients

**TABLE 18-1 Parasomnias or Disorders of Arousal**

| TYPE OF DYSFUNCTION | COMMENTS |
|---|---|
| Sleepwalking | Walking while asleep |
| Sleep terror | Panic attack while asleep |
| Sleep-related enuresis | Bed-wetting; event begins in stage III/IV sleep, and enuresis occurs as sleep lightens |
| Dream anxiety attacks | Nightmares; REM phenomenon |
| Sleep-related epileptic seizures | Seizures occur more often during sleep; explains why sleep encouraged during short routine electroencephalograms (EEGs) |
| Sleep-related bruxism | Teeth grinding; dental assistance may be needed to preserve teeth |
| Sleep-related head banging (jactatio capitis nocturna) | Rhythmic head rocking and banging common in young children under age 5 years; occurs in stage I/II sleep |
| Familial sleep paralysis | Inability to move muscles when first awakening |
| Sleep-related cluster headaches | Associated with REM and relieved by indomethacin |
| Sleep-related abnormal swallowing syndrome | Inadequate swallowing of saliva during sleep |
| Sleep-related asthma | Early morning increase in bronchoconstriction; 46% of asthmatic attacks occur during last third of night |
| Sleep-related cardiovascular symptoms | Include paroxysmal nocturnal dyspnea, myocardial infarction (peak incidence, 4 AM to 6 AM), nocturnal angina, and premature ventricular contractions (more common in REM sleep) |
| Sleep-related gastroesophageal reflux | Caused more by posture than sleep |
| Sleep-related hemolysis | Probably related to combination of respiratory acidosis, change in acid-base balance, and renal clearance of defective red blood cells |
| Morning headaches | May be related to sleeping longer on weekends and delaying usual morning dose of caffeine |
| Impairment in penile erections | Changes in normal incidence of eretions; painful erections |

with severe episodes, because these suppress stage III/IV sleep.

## FAMILIAL SLEEP PARALYSIS

The person with familial **sleep paralysis** appears asleep but maintains consciousness. Occasionally, frighteningly vivid hallucinations may occur. The eyes may be open and can be moved, although the person is unable to move any other muscles. Although this is part of the tetrad of symptoms of narcolepsy, many normal people experience this. Intervention includes teaching family members to awaken the person by touch each day or allowing a pet dog or cat to awaken the person through touch.

## PENILE ERECTIONS

Men experience erections during REM sleep, regardless of sexual activity or dream content. If impairment of erections occurs during sleep, an underlying illness may be present, such as diabetes mellitus, or it may result from the effect of medications. *Painful erections* may occur during sleep, even though erections are not painful or difficult while awake. There may be a problem with the foreskin in uncircumcised men or a problem with the penile blood vessels. The man should be referred to a urologist for evaluation.

# INSOMNIA

## ETIOLOGY/EPIDEMIOLOGY

Insomnia is the difficulty with initiating or maintaining sleep. Epidemiologic studies estimate the number of Americans with insomnia to be in the millions. Insomnia is experienced by adults and children and affects males and females equally.

Insomnia can be caused by various factors:

1. Transient situations of emotional upset (such as loss of a job) or family needs (such as a child's illness)
2. Adoption of nonfunctional sleep habits
3. Psychiatric disorders, such as depression or psychoses
4. Use of drugs or alcohol
5. Respiratory impairment (see later section on sleep apnea)
6. Medical conditions associated with pain, anemia, fever, changes in nutritional status, or immobility
7. Attempting to sleep in nonconducive environmental conditions

It is important to remember that in many instances persons experience altered sleep patterns when the actual cause of the sleep changes may have been resolved long ago. For example, a woman may describe that she habitually arose at 5 AM to nurse her baby, and now several years later, she still awakens at that time and cannot go back to sleep. Another person may report inability to sleep after great anxiety associated with a job loss that has persisted, although the person has now been happily employed for several years.

## PATHOPHYSIOLOGY

Sleep onset can be delayed and arousal prolonged by active thought and worry, physical discomfort, or poor oxygenation. Worry and poor habits, such as sleeping with lights on or a TV or radio on, prolong sleep onset and cause arousals during light stage I sleep. Staying in bed longer than 8 hours or napping during the day fragments sleep; the person still sleeps 8 hours, but the total sleep time lengthens to fill 10 hours spent in bed. The person then believes the sleep is "poor."

Normally there is a clear boundary between and regular timing of sleep time and awake time. Meals and social and physical activities occur at predictable times during awake hours, and sleep occurs at night in a dark, quiet, comfortable, secure place. Biologic clocks are anchored in time by the regular occurrence of these events. For the person with insomnia, the distinction between waking/sleeping time is blurred by spending a prolonged time in bed, by not initiating the day's activities at a prompt time, or by staying up too late at night. These events cause a distortion in sleep and lead to a continuing cycle of poor sleep at the wrong time. Clinical manifestations of insomnia are discussed below.

The person may describe insomnia in many ways, depending on which aspect of sleeplessness is most troubling. Typical comments include the following: "I cannot go to sleep," "I am awake all night," and "I awaken early and can't go back to sleep." Persons with insomnia often monitor sleep by watching the clock. They may turn on the TV, read, or eat while waiting to feel sleepy. They may try to go to sleep earlier, stay in bed longer, take naps, use sleeping pills or alcohol to initiate sleep, or use caffeine to increase alertness during the day. They may also change their pattern of daily activities to compensate for a distorted sleep pattern by declining or omitting activities from the daily routine, saying "I'm just too tired." Some persons may not recognize a sleep problem at first because they have adapted to a changed sleep schedule over many years.

## PREVENTION

Prevention involves teaching persons and families about normal sleep and counseling them to be aware of events and activities that can enhance or detract from sleep. Often persons take steps to remedy a sleep problem, such as taking sleeping pills, taking naps, or drinking alcohol, which only exacerbate sleeping problems. Nurses must also teach persons that it is never too late to begin dealing with a sleep problem.

## MEDICAL MANAGEMENT

If the person has used sleeping pills or alcohol to help with sleep, supervised weaning from these substances is required. A schedule of reducing the dose of sleeping pills over a month or more, or a course of chlordiazepoxide hydrochloride (Librium) to assist with alcohol withdrawal, may be prescribed.

## DIAGNOSTIC TESTS

*Routine blood work,* such as a SMA 18 and complete blood count (CBC), is done to determine whether any hematologic, metabolic, cardiac, or respiratory diseases are contributing to sleeplessness. A thorough assessment, including questions to elicit signs of underlying depression or psychosis, should be done.

A **polysomnogram (PSG)** consists of an all-night sleep study conducted in a certified sleep laboratory. Sleep technicians monitor the following:

1. Sleep time and quality
2. Brain EEG activity to determine stages of sleep
3. Respiratory activity: intercostal muscle movement, air passage from nose and mouth, oxygen saturation using an ear lobe oximeter
4. Electrocardiogram (ECG) for monitoring cardiac rate
5. Electromyogram (EMG) monitoring of leg movement to detect abnormal movement of eye and face (to determine onset of REM sleep)
6. Occurrence of nightmares or "restless legs"

The PSG is performed when the person complains of insomnia and the physician is unable to make the diagnosis from a history and physical examination.

The **multiple sleep latency test (MSLT)** is a sleep study done in the sleep laboratory during the day to measure daytime sleepiness. At times it is needed to distinguish the sleepiness caused by poor nighttime sleep and sleepiness caused by narcolepsy.

# NURSING MANAGEMENT

## ♦ ASSESSMENT

A complete nursing assessment of sleep disorders is listed in Box 18-3. Never jump to a conclusion about a sleep problem without asking systematic questions about all sleep disorders, because one sleep problem can resemble another superficially. Keep in mind that many times insomnia begins as an understandable response to a stress—such as the loss of a spouse, illness of a family member, loss of a job—or after a difficult hospitalization or other stressful event. The person may come to terms with the stress or loss, but the new maladaptive sleep habits are now in place. The person may state that the sleep pattern began 5 years ago and that nothing is bothering him or her now to prevent sleep. This makes sense when one views *insomnia as a series of decisions that perpetuate a certain sleep pattern,* unfortunately a pattern that distresses instead of refreshes. The following data are important to highlight for a person with insomnia.

### Subjective Data

Data to be collected to assess the patient with insomnia include the following:

Beliefs about the sleep problems and ability to sleep restfully. Some people believe that they have inherited or developed a permanent mental change or disorder that will prevent regaining normal sleep.

Knowledge about normal sleep.

Sources of pleasure and difficulty in the person's life

## BOX 18-3 Sleep Interview

### GENERAL DATA

1. Statement of the sleep problem by patient, bed partner, or family: obtain a quantifiable answer about sleep, such as never sleeps, dozes off for an hour several times a night, or has trouble sleeping 5 nights out of 7, every other night, or on weekends only
2. Initiation of sleep problem: when possible, elicit cause
3. Factors that make it worse or better
4. Previous occurrences to patient or to other family member or friend
5. Modifications that need to be made for daytime activities or travel
6. Memories of frightening or upsetting incidences during sleep, such as sudden illness or death of a loved one or damage from storm, fire, or robbery
7. Occurrences of accidents or "near misses" as a result of sleep problems *(very important)*

### INSOMNIA DATA

(Remember that a complaint of insomnia may be caused by sleep apnea or other difficulties with sleep.)

1. Time person gets into bed and time person falls asleep
2. Number and times of awakenings at night
3. Interval before returning to sleep after each awakening
4. Time of final awakening, time of arising from bed, and what wakes the person up, such as noises, alarm clock, or treatment
5. Daytime naps: number, when, and how long
6. Dozing off briefly (same question as napping, but some persons answer this question differently)
7. Lying down to rest on couch or "resting eyes for a moment" (this counts as napping because person may be falling asleep)
8. Practices used to assist with sleep: type and regularity of use
9. Changes in sleep patterns because of sleep deficit
10. Places where sleep occurs more readily, such as somewhere else in the house or on vacation
11. Concerns that delay getting into bed or falling asleep
12. Amount of and recent changes in caffeine intake (coffee, tea, colas, other caffeinated beverages, caffeinated gum) and alcohol
13. Types of weekly exercise and recreational activities
14. Measures of coping with concerns
15. Recent illness or loss of relatives, friends, or pets
16. Activities of others in house or neighborhood that affect sleep, such as child who returns home late, spouse who leaves home early in morning, noise from a neighbor or dog, and noise from a nearby highway or airport

### SLEEP APNEA DATA

1. Description or reenactment by bed partner of the person's breathing pattern, including sound and volume of snoring, length of time that no air passes, and how the person starts to breathe again
2. Description by bed partner of differences in patient's breathing while on back, each side, and stomach and of changes in patient's skin color while asleep
3. Presence of morning headaches
4. Difficulty in awakening for the day
5. Number of pillows used; preference of sleeping in a certain chair
6. Degree of sleepiness during day; falling asleep at a movie, during a conversation, or while driving

### NARCOLEPSY-RELATED DATA

1. Presence of sudden irresistible urges to sleep; falling asleep and then awakening a few minutes later feeling refreshed
2. Experiences of a sudden loss of muscle tone, leading to drooping of the head or slumping to the floor, that occur during episodes of strong emotions (surprise, laughter, anger)
3. Experiences on awakening of feeling paralyzed until touched by another
4. Presence of visual, auditory, or tactile hallucinations at time of sleep initiation or awakening
5. Family history of unusual experiences in sleep

### SLEEP SCHEDULE DATA

1. Working hours
2. Experience of going to bed later each night
3. Daily scheduled activities, flexibility
4. Changes in sleep schedule as a result of changes in life schedule, such as retirement or hospitalization
5. Interruption of sleep because of family activities
6. Practice of sleeping through the day or staying up at night because of a specific purpose, such as fear that a calamity will befall during the night

### OTHER SLEEP-RELATED EVENTS

1. Uncomfortable feelings in legs when ready to fall asleep: location, type of sensations, duration, actions that make it better or worse, attempted remedies, and effect on sleep
2. Reports from bed partner of patient kicking or moving legs in sleep
3. Bed-wetting: frequency, time of occurrence, actions that make it better or worse, and reports of any nights of dryness
4. Dreams: upsetting recurring dreams, frightening nightmares, or sleep terrors
5. Sleepwalking: initiation, frequency, ability to be awakened easily or guided back to bed, experience of injury while sleepwalking, actions that make it better or worse, and steps taken to keep the person safe
6. Teeth grinding during sleep
7. Dysfunctions associated with sleep, such as chest pain, shortness of breath, heartburn/ulcer pain, morning headache, asthmatic attacks, frequent awakenings to urinate, hot flashes in menopausal woman, coughing, choking and gagging, and arthritic or other neuromuscular pain

and how the sleep problem has been affected by these.

Potential resources for life changes. For example, if a retired person has nothing to wake up for, can that person find transport to a senior citizens center, volunteer job, or activity group?

## Objective Data

Objective data include results from diagnostic tests and reports from a bed partner. A person may be asked to keep a *sleep diary, recording times of sleep initiation, arousals, naps,* and *time of awakening* in the morning.

## ♦ NURSING DIAGNOSES

Nursing diagnoses are determined from analyses of patient data. Nursing diagnoses for the patient with insomnia may include but are not limited to the following:

| Diagnostic Title | Possible Etiologic Factors |
|---|---|
| Sleep pattern disturbance | Adoption of counterproductive sleep habits |
| Knowledge deficit (about insomnia) | Incorrect self-monitoring and self-assessment of sleep |
| Fatigue | Reduced total sleep time |
| Fear | Personal concern about impossibility of ever sleeping well again |
| Diversional activity deficit | Immobility, depressed feelings, perceived loss of usefulness or of need for activity |
| Coping, ineffective (individual) | Habit of seeking sleep to avoid facing problems or of reviewing problems at sleep initiation |
| Injury, high risk for | Sleepiness during the day |

## ♦ EXPECTED PATIENT OUTCOMES

Expected patient outcomes for the patient with insomnia may include but are not limited to the following:

1. Patient/bed partner/family describe the basic aspects of normal sleep, with emphasis on factors that contribute to the patient's problem.
2. Is able to explain what is causing his or her sleep problem and how to improve sleep.
3. Patient/family carry out measures to reduce the insomnia and improve fatigue.
4. Has realistic expectations about the quality of sleep, and fear is reduced.
5. Identifies impediments to activity and develops and implements a plan for increasing diversional activity.
6. Participates in a plan to problem solve and cope with difficulties; does not think about problems at times of sleep.
7. Does not experience an injury because of sleepiness during normal awake period.

## ♦ INTERVENTIONS

### Facilitating Sleep

Encourage patient to talk about what interferes with his or her ability to fall asleep. Develop with patient a plan to improve sleep. Have patient keep a sleep diary listing activities undertaken before sleep, measures taken to improve sleep, and how successful the changes were in obtaining a good night's rest.

### Facilitating Learning

#### Promoting knowledge of normal sleep

Teach aspects of normal sleep to patient and family. Persons typically monitor their own sleep. This can contribute to the sleep problem, because the person may mistake a normal phenomenon for something abnormal or for a sign that the new sleep habits are not working.

#### Promoting sleep hygiene

A person with insomnia will benefit most from a reordering of sleep habits. Develop a plan for **sleep hygiene** with the patient and inform the physician of the plan, as appropriate. Physician advice may be required if intake patterns of alcohol, other drugs, or caffeine need to be changed. Patients must recognize that they must adhere to the plan faithfully every day, no matter what occurs. They are resetting their sleep-wake cycle, which takes several weeks to a month to accomplish. In developing the plan, choose from the elements listed here those which apply to the individual's sleep hygiene problem. Not all elements are appropriate for each person. The plan has *three important parts:* (1) *what the person does during the day* (use of time, naps, eating and drinking, exercise, diversion), (2) *what the person does to prepare for sleep,* and (3) *how the person interprets* his or her *sleep experience.*

The plan is to be followed faithfully for 1 month. If sleep is improved, adjustments can be made for one element at a time, such as resuming a reduced intake of alcohol or caffeine. Once the sleep pattern is established, however, only one element should be modified at a time. If the sleep pattern is weakened, the person can identify an element to which he or she is sensitive. Check with the person weekly to identify how the new plan is proceeding. Be generous with encouragement. Remember that a new way of sleeping is being taught to the person who is still partly convinced that he or she is one of the few persons in the world who never sleeps.

**Time spent in bed, sleep, and wake-up hours.** The person, in collaboration with the health professional, selects a sleep time and a wake-up time for a total time spent in bed of 7 to 8 hours, depending on how much sleep the patient thinks is needed. Ask what constraints the person has, such as time to get up for work or time arriving home from evening work, and what time the person likes to go to bed, based on time spent with family members or favorite late-night TV shows. The bed time and wake-up time should be followed faithfully, without alteration, for 1 month, so planning ahead for life-style preferences is important. This means the person will follow this schedule even if he or she is out late on Saturday nights or wants to sleep in on Sunday mornings. If the person does not sleep well one night, the schedule must be kept because it is an investment in a better night's sleep the next night.

**Napping.** No naps should be taken. This means not lying down during the day and not closing the eyes while sitting in the chair after dinner. If the person gets sleepy reading the paper, the paper should be read while standing up at the counter. If the person is tired an hour before the agreed-on sleep time, he or she should walk around, engage in an activity, or stand up while watching TV. This gives the body a firm message that all sleep will take place in bed during the nighttime hours only. Taking naps at other times fragments nighttime sleep. If, in following the schedule, the person does not sleep much the night before, taking a nap only hinders the possibility that sleep will come more easily the next night, which perpetuates the problem.

**Caffeine and alcohol.** The best and fastest change in sleep quality comes from the elimination of caffeine and alcohol from the diet during the start of this plan. However, persons who drink a lot of caffeine or even one alcoholic drink each day could experience withdrawal symptoms, so it is best to work with the physician on a safe plan for withdrawal. Also, the strength of this plan is to help the person experience improved sleep without experiencing uncomfortable symptoms that might lead the person to resume the previous, more comfortable patterns.

**Nutrition.** It is important to eat three meals a day composed of balanced nutrition at about the same time each day. On awakening in the morning, the person should wash, dress, and have some breakfast to give the body yet another message that it is time for the day to start. Breakfast may be large or simply toast and juice; the point is to give a regular nutritional time cue.

**Exercise.** Increasing activity gives the body another biologic message that the day is here. Even if the person is confined to bed, exercises can be developed to enhance a feeling of well-being. For persons who experience tension, stress, or worry or who face difficult problems, exercise can bring a respite from troubling thoughts or can be a time for thinking through problems instead of at bedtime. Any exercise, from active sports to walking to stationary exercise, is encouraged.

**Diversional activities.** It is important for the person to do something each day that brings enjoyment. It is equally important to have both something in life a person can look forward to and something that requires a person's special participation, creating a feeling of being needed. A person facing a continuing illness often experiences a curtailing of usual outlets for diversion and participation. Remember that what a person does with time during the day influences sleep time as well. An important part of a plan for better sleep is life-participating activity. Even if the person is confined to bed, a telephone is a link with others who could use the person's support and good will.

**Sleep environment.** Evening routines, such as checking door locks or letting the dog out, should be completed before the predetermined bedtime. By bedtime the person should be in night clothes and ready to get into bed. The bed covers should provide the proper comfort. Lights, TV, and radio should be off. The person should not read or eat in bed. Persons can be advised to turn the clock around so it cannot be checked during the night. The person needs to understand that awakening during the night is normal and sleep activity does not need to be monitored.

**Relaxation.** The final component of a sleep plan is the relearning of skills of relaxing when the person wants to go to sleep. A person can easily adopt the habit of postponing thoughts about troubling issues until in bed with the lights off. This is a habit and can be replaced by a more useful habit. A person cannot lie in bed "thinking about nothing" because the mind simply searches for something interesting to think about and usually selects some unfinished, compelling issues. Relaxation exercises can help persons regain and strengthen the ability to select something enjoyable to think about. If the person consciously selects something pleasant, the tendency to ruminate over troubles is weakened. Relaxation exercises must be practiced each night. If the person has difficulty mastering this task, a referral to a behavioral therapist may be appropriate.

#### Promoting realistic expectations of sleep

Reinforce that it is not realistic for the person to expect every night of sleep to be free of awakenings or disturbing thoughts and to be totally refreshing. The goal of the plan is to increase the number of nights that are restful. When this happens, fatigue and fear will be reduced, injury will be avoided, and the person will have the tools necessary to get back on track if problems with sleep occur in the future.

### ♦ EVALUATION

The person will monitor his or her own progress and record this daily. When the interventions just discussed are successful, no further follow-up will be necessary.

## NARCOLEPSY

Narcolepsy is a neurologic condition characterized by short, irresistible episodes of sleep intruding into wakefulness and recurring at frequent intervals. *Five abnormal sleep features* may be present: (1) *irresistible sleep attacks* with excessive *daytime sleepiness,* (2) *hypnogogic hallucinations,* (3) *cataplexy,* (4) *sleep-onset REM periods,* and (5) *sleep paralysis.* Any combination of the five features can be seen in narcolepsy, but at least two must be present to make a diagnosis.

Occasionally a person with normal sleep patterns may experience any one aspect of narcolepsy. The combination of symptoms, however, experienced consistently, sets narcolepsy apart.

## IRRESISTIBLE SLEEP ATTACKS AND EXCESSIVE DAYTIME SLEEPINESS

The sleep attacks, unpredictable and lasting a few moments to an hour, occur not only during monotonous sedentary activity, but also during mental or physical stimulation. The person may also feel unpleasantly drowsy throughout the day, resulting in poor performance of tasks.

## HYPNOGOGIC HALLUCINATIONS

This is the experience of vivid, troubling hallucinations, usually on awakening. The **hypnogogic hallucinations** are usually visual but can be auditory or tactile.

## CATAPLEXY

**Cataplexy** is an abrupt, reversible loss of muscle tone, usually brought on by strong emotions, such as fright, laughter, anger, or sudden increased stress. Cataplexy can be experienced variously from a feeling of slight weakness to a loss of strength in skeletal muscles to a complete loss of posture. Typically, the jaw sags, the head nods, the arms droop, and the legs buckle. Because attacks can be precipitated by listening to a funny joke or reexperiencing in memory a strongly unpleasant experience, persons suffering from cataplexy often try to restrict their emotional response to gain some control. *This atonia is similar to the atonia seen during REM sleep.*

## SLEEP-ONSET REM PERIODS

The normal sleeper passes through several stages of sleep and experiences REM sleep near the end of the 90-minute sleep cycle. In narcolepsy, when sleep occurs during the day in naps or during sleep attacks, the person goes into REM sleep within 5 minutes of going to sleep.

## SLEEP PARALYSIS

This frightening experience occurs just before falling asleep or on awakening. Sleepers find that, although they are completely awake, they cannot move the extremities, cannot speak, and may not even be able to breathe deeply. **Sleep paralysis** terminates spontaneously within several minutes but can be interrupted by being touched by someone. (One person plagued by sleep paralysis trained her dog to come and lick her hand each morning.) Often sleep paralysis is accompanied by hypnogogic hallucinations.

## ETIOLOGY

Two new research findings are fueling greater understanding of narcolepsy. First, several researchers have found a genetic link among persons with narcolepsy in which mild forms tend to cluster in some families, whereas more severe forms cluster in other families.[8] Some aspects of narcolepsy (cataplexy, excessive daytime sleepiness) are genetically transmitted in some breeds of dogs. Second, a genetic link has recently been discovered between narcolepsy and a class II antigen of the major histocompatibility complex known as DR2. Scientists theorize that narcolepsy may be a disease that links the involvement of the immune system and its response to severe psychologic stress with the development of disease in susceptible individuals.[1,8] This may help to explain the finding that in about one half of persons with narcolepsy, an abrupt change in the sleep-wake schedule and/or a major psychologic stress precede the first symptom.

## EPIDEMIOLOGY

Narcolepsy is not a rare condition. Its prevalence has been estimated at 0.05% to 0.06%, which indicates that about one of every 2500 people have this disorder, or 250,000 Americans.[1] Males are somewhat more affected than females. The age of onset varies from childhood to the 50s, with a peak incidence in the second decade of life, usually after puberty. Unrecognized and untreated, these irresistible, unwanted sleep attacks can be totally disabling. They interfere with the concentration required in school or at work and can result in accidents, leading to injury and death.

## PATHOPHYSIOLOGY

### Loss of Ability to Suppress Sleep

Normally the thalamus and cortical gray matter are highly active in wakefulness, resulting in general enhanced excitability of neurons, as well as selective inhibition of input. In drowsiness, reduction of synaptic transmissions occurs in the thalamus, despite an unchanged level of sensory input. It is unknown exactly which neurotransmitters and synaptic receptors relate to maintenance of alertness and initiation of sleep. Interestingly, the activity of the gray matter and thalamus in REM sleep closely resembles waking activity.

It is also unknown what neuronal changes occur with narcolepsy. Because this condition responds to stimulant drugs such as amphetamine, pemoline, and methylphenidate, however, it is hypothesized that some ratio of adrenergic/cholinergic neuronal activity is disrupted in sleep attacks and restored by these drugs.[8]

### Episodic Atonia

Normally, muscle tone is maintained during wakefulness and during all sleep stages *except REM* by activity in the cerebellum. In REM sleep, centers in the pons activate, producing active inhibition of muscle tone in all muscle groups except those of the eye, respiration, and penis. Usually this atonia is briefly interrupted or overcome by powerful excitatory inputs to muscle groups, resulting in the muscle twitches and jerks seen in REM sleep.

In cataplexy, sudden time-limited atonia is experienced, although no change occurs in consciousness. Because this disorder responds to monoamine oxidase (MAO) inhibitors and other tricyclic antidepressants, it is theorized that cataplectic attacks (as well as sleep paralysis and hypnogogic hallucinations) result from some malfunction of norepinephrine, dopamine, and serotonin neurotransmitters or receptors in the brainstem.

### Aspects of Dreaming Intruding Into Wakefulness

Dreaming usually occurs in REM sleep. REM sleep occurs at the end of each 90-minute sleep cycle, and longer periods of REM sleep occur at the end of the night. On awakening, all features of REM sleep (atonia and resulting paralysis of all muscle groups, except those for breathing and sight; dreaming) terminate. Less is known about the mechanisms of dreaming intruding into wakefulness. As just noted, however, because the person with narcolepsy responds to tricyclic antidepressants and MAO inhibitors, a disorder of neurotransmitters or receptors may exist somewhere in the brain.[1]

The clinical manifestations of narcolepsy are discussed below. The person with narcolepsy feels chronically drowsy, exhibits memory lapses and poor work performance, and may experience *microsleeps,* sleep periods of a few seconds that may appear as daydreaming. Night sleep can be frequently interrupted by frightening dreams and awakenings. Cataplexy may develop as long as 20 years after the more common symptom of sleep attacks and excessive daytime drowsiness. The paralysis may last from a few seconds to a few minutes. No known measures can terminate an attack, except to remove the emotional trigger so that another attack will not immediately follow recovery from the first.

## PREVENTION

As yet, no clear evidence exists concerning the prevention of narcolepsy. More effort is being directed toward the early recognition of the disorder, particularly in relatives of affected family members. If a parent has narcolepsy, there is a 1 in 50 chance that each child will have it.

## MEDICAL MANAGEMENT

The person who has sleep attacks and excessive daytime sleepiness is given CNS stimulants, such as amphetamine, pemoline (Cylert), or methylphenidate (Ritalin). Some side effects—such as irritability, tachycardia, and nocturnal sleep disturbances, as well as tolerance and drug dependence—may occur. Persons experiencing cataplexy, sleep paralysis, or hypnogogic hallucinations receive a tricyclic antidepressant, such as imipramine, protriptyline, or clomipramine. Doses are usually adjusted to achieve the best balance between improved daytime alertness and unwanted side effects. An experimental drug, gamma-hydroxybutyrate, shows some promise.

Daytime naps may also be prescribed to assist with daytime alertness. Three 15- to 20-minute naps spaced evenly throughout the day often help restore a feeling of alertness.

## DIAGNOSTIC TESTS

The PSG and MSLT (see p. 471) are the essential tests to distinguish narcolepsy from daytime sleepiness experienced by someone who simply sleeps poorly at night. The night sleep test (PSG) documents the night aspects of sleep. The MSLT, performed the next day, documents how readily the person falls asleep during a half-hour nap (four naps are observed during the next 8 hours after awakening from the PSG) and how quickly REM sleep occurs with each nap. A *normal* person may have one sleep-onset REM episode of four naps and may not be able to fall asleep for all the nap periods. A *sleepy* person may be able to fall asleep each time but does not have more than one sleep-onset REM period. A *narcoleptic* person falls asleep readily during each nap period and has more than one sleep-onset REM period. The physician may try to record a cataplectic attack if the patient reports a history of this with particular stressors.

## NURSING MANAGEMENT

### ♦ ASSESSMENT

A complete sleep history (see Box 18-3) is obtained from the person suspected of having narcolepsy. Data of particular importance include the following:

1. Understanding of narcolepsy and factors that increase or decrease symptoms
2. Experience with antinarcoleptic drugs and side effects (Are the drugs taken on holidays? Are doses self-adjusted?)
3. Safety practices and accident history, especially if the person drives
4. Family understanding and support
5. Problems and adjustments in employment or school performance

### ♦ NURSING DIAGNOSES

Nursing diagnoses are determined from analysis of patient data. Nursing diagnoses for the patient with narcolepsy may include but are not limited to the following:

| Diagnostic Title | Possible Etiologic Factors |
|---|---|
| Knowledge deficit (about narcolepsy) | Lack of information |
| Coping, ineffective (individual) | Purposeful emotional restriction and day-to-day difficulties |
| Fatigue | Excessive daytime sleepiness causing difficulty with treatment regimen and misunderstanding by family and employer or teacher |
| Injury, high risk for | Sleep attacks, cataplexy |

## ♦ EXPECTED PATIENT OUTCOMES

Expected patient outcomes for the patient with narcolepsy may include but are not limited to the following:

1. Describes the disorder and medication regimen and reports success with explaining narcolepsy to family or employer (or enlists the assistance of a person knowledgeable about narcolepsy).
2. Identifies purposeful avoidance of strong emotions as a way to cope with cataplectic attacks.
3. Describes a level of participation that satisfies family and work responsibilities.
4. Reports feeling less fatigue.
5. Reports improved job or school performance.
6. Demonstrates effective strategies for reducing exposure to risk factors in the environment; avoidable accidents and injuries do not occur.

## ♦ INTERVENTIONS

The major nursing strategies for the person with narcolepsy are teaching and support with effective ways of coping with the disorder. As control of sleepiness and cataplectic attacks is achieved, fatigue and job or school performance should improve and the potential for injury will decrease.

### Facilitating Learning

**Promoting understanding of narcolepsy**

Teach aspects of narcolepsy and rationale for the treatment plan. It is important that the person maintain close contact with the physician and nurse to monitor effectiveness of medications and treatment. Telephone follow-up may be used to maintain contact and support. Encourage the person and family to contact the American Narcolepsy Association,* which can provide information on local support networks. The association's newsletter contains up-to-date information on recent research findings and provides a forum for sharing ideas.

Assess and support the person's efforts to teach others about narcolepsy. Remind the person that it may take some practice before acquiring ease in teaching others.

**Promoting safety and personal risk assessment**

Teach the patient to consider carefully the risks of injury at home and at school or work. Rather than engage in denial or wishful thinking, the patient should consider problems caused by sleep attacks and cataplectic attacks. Some suggestions include the following:

1. Do not drive unless sleep attacks and cataplectic attacks are completely under control; then drive only for short distances during times of high wakefulness.
2. Do food preparation or self-grooming activities (handling knives, curling or clothes iron; cooking on stove) during quiet times (such as before others in the house awaken) to avoid times of surprise or emotion that can trigger an attack.
3. Learn to use the microwave oven for cooking to avoid burns from the stove.
4. If possible, live in a dwelling that has either no stairs or an enclosed staircase to minimize injury during falls.
5. Ask family members/co-workers to use a gentle aural signal before approaching to prevent triggering a sleep attack.

**Promoting participation in family life and work**

Encourage the person to meet with other persons with narcolepsy for mutual support or with the nurse in times of frustration, as well as success. Suggest that family members join a local narcolepsy support group to help deal with their own concerns. Narcolepsy can be a very difficult disorder to live with, but personal isolation and withdrawal will only make life more difficult.

# SLEEP APNEA

Sleep apnea is a sleep problem involving other body systems. A mutual relationship exists between sleep and other body systems; the sleep state affects the functioning of *all* body systems to some extent. In addition, the functioning of *any* body system affects the states of sleep. Many disease processes affect sleep or are affected by sleep, including asthma, gastroesophageal reflux, epilepsy, headache, fibrositis, myocardial instability, and chronic pain. This section focuses on sleep apnea and the mutual relationship between body systems and sleep.

## ETIOLOGY/EPIDEMIOLOGY

The gradual development of sleep apnea and its sequelae is incompletely understood. Although such factors as obesity and oropharyngeal architecture have been associated with this disorder, other neurologic and genetic factors may play a role even before any symptoms develop. Some researchers hypothesize that sleep apnea is a progressive illness resulting as a systemic response to years of decreased airway patency, reduced airflow, reduced ventilation,[8] stimulation of autonomic functioning, and disruption of reflexes required to maintain breathing during sleep. This produces a maladaptive response that results in a feedback loop of greater impairment.

Many unanswered questions remain concerning sleep apnea, including the following:

1. How much time does it take for sleep apnea syndrome to develop or for cardiac rhythm changes and hypertension to become severe?
2. How many sleepers who snore quietly and sporadically early in life will subsequently develop sleep apnea?
3. How can one predict who will develop milder or more severe forms of sleep apnea?

*P.O. Box 194025, San Francisco, CA 94119; (800)-222-6085 (in California, (800)-222-6086).

## PATHOPHYSIOLOGY

While reading the following discussion of normal and abnormal breathing during sleep, remember the following major points:

1. The understanding of breathing during sleep centers on the complex interrelationships and feedback loops between the neurologic and respiratory systems. These interrelationships have significant impact on the cardiovascular system and on sleep itself.
2. The two primary results of severely impaired breathing during sleep are (a) cardiac dysrhythmia, which can result in increased risk of cardiac fibrillation and death, and (b) excessive daytime sleepiness or reduction of daytime alertness, which can result in increased risk of accident, such as falling asleep while driving.

### Control of Breathing

Breathing is initiated by the respiratory center in the medulla. Breathing responds to body requirements through input from three sources: chemoreceptors in the carotid body, stretch/mechanical receptors located in the lung and chest wall, and input from other brain centers (see Chapter 35). In wakefulness, breathing is modified by conscious effort. In sleep, breathing patterns show clear differences between stage I, deeper, and REM (dreaming) sleep, indicating that brain centers controlling[9] sleep have a direct impact on breathing centers as well. In persons with sleep apnea, chemoreceptor responsiveness is reduced, possibly as a result of years of decreased oxygen saturation and increased carbon dioxide levels during sleep. It is not known if ventilatory compensation for resistive loading (stretch receptor responsiveness) is maintained in sleep. During sleep apnea, when many arousals occur in the night, the person becomes sleepier, leading to decreased arousability and longer apneas.

### Open Passageway to Lungs

The pharynx is the only nonrigid structure in the passageway to the lungs. The diameter is maintained by toned muscle in pharyngeal walls, allowing for closure only during swallowing, regurgitation, and speech. In non-REM sleep, this muscle tone is reduced; in REM sleep, it is greatly reduced. Only intercostal, diaphragmatic, and ocular muscles maintain tone in REM sleep. Some sleep experts theorize that the evidence of diminished upper airway tone with maintenance of diaphragmatic and intercostal muscle tone suggests separate neural control of these respiratory muscle groups.[8] The oropharynx of persons with sleep apnea may be anatomically small or may contain enlarged structures, or it may once have been large enough but now has a reduced diameter because of fat deposition in tissues.

### Response to Internal/External Stimuli

Breathing also depends on responsiveness to changed internal and external stimuli. In sleep, responsiveness to the following factors is reduced:

1. *Bronchial irritation.* Cough is reduced in REM and non-REM sleep and resumes only on arousal.
2. *Isocapnic hypoxia.* Partial oxygen pressure ($PO_2$) may fall as low as 70% of normal before sleepers are aroused. In REM sleep, arousal threshold is further reduced.
3. *Hypercapnia.* Most sleepers awaken before partial carbon dioxide pressure ($PCO_2$) rises to 15 mm Hg above wakefulness level. In REM sleep, arousal is further reduced.
4. *Alcohol and CNS depressants.* During sleep, these substances suppress upper airway tone, as well as arousal by medulla and higher cortical centers.

Responsiveness to all these factors is depressed further in a person whose sleep has been so fragmented as to lead to further depressed arousal thresholds. Moderate degrees of alcohol intoxication can decrease hypoxic and hypercapnic ventilatory responses to 50% of baseline values. Oxygen saturation of less than 80% of normal is considered severe.

### Apneas/Hypopneas

Different types of apneas occur (see Box 18-4 for definitions). Normal sleepers experience a few apneas/hypopneas each night; the apneas may be obstructive, central, or mixed. These apneas are fewer and shorter in duration than those in sleep apnea syndrome. The normal sleeper has a transient drop in oxygen saturation, transient bradycardia or tachycardia, and a transient rise in blood pressure; all return to normal levels when the apnea episode is over. The person with sleep apnea syndrome has decreased oxygen saturation (less than 80%) through the night that results in (1) maladaptive cardiovascular responses, (2) disrupted sleep, and (3) other difficulties, including morning headache, bed-wetting, and changes in mood, alertness, endurance, work per-

**BOX 18-4 Definitions of Apnea/Hypopnea**

| | |
|---|---|
| **Apnea** | Cessation of breathing for more than 10 seconds. |
| **Hypopnea** | Reduction, rather than complete elimination, of breathing. |
| **Obstructive apnea** | Breathing effort occurs with diaphragmatic and intercostal muscles, but no air passes through the mouth and nose. The pharynx collapses, producing obstruction. |
| **Central apnea** | No breathing effort is expended by thoracic muscles (message to breathe not received by lungs from medulla). |
| **Mixed apnea** | Begins as an absence of respiratory effort; when effort begins, however, obstruction results. |
| **Sleep apnea syndrome** | More than five apneic events per hour of sleep. |

formance, and intellectual and sexual functioning. The most serious life-threatening results are hypertension, cardiac dysrhythmias (bradycardia, tachycardia, premature ventricular contractions, second-degree atrioventricular block, prolonged sinus pauses, atrial fibrillation), and accidents from falling asleep while driving or doing other monotonous tasks.

The clinical manifestations of sleep apnea are described next. When sleep apnea is suspected, a sleeping partner is interviewed, as well as the sleeper. The bed partner may report most or all of the following details:

He falls asleep very easily in the chair or when he goes to bed for the night. Sometimes he is restless and dozes on and off for a while. He may begin snoring as soon as he falls asleep, or it may not start until later in the night. He used to snore only when he fell asleep on his back, but now he snores in any position. He snores very loudly, and you can hear him from other rooms in the house. Sometimes he stops breathing; after several moments, he snorts loudly, shudders or kicks his legs, then takes a deep breath and goes back to sleep. He may answer me if I speak to him, but he doesn't recall it in the morning. He does this all night long, but I think it happens more often in the early morning. He may get up frequently to urinate in the night, and sometimes he perspires heavily from all the moving around in bed. I hate to admit it, but sometimes I have to sleep in another room because the noise and his restlessness keep me awake. Yet, I am worried that he needs me there to wake him up if he goes too long without breathing. I think *I* am developing a sleep problem.

## PREVENTION

Because sleep apnea is not yet fully understood, steps to prevent its development are not completely known. In addition to encouraging normal weight and good pulmonary habits, it is advisable not to overlook or discount any reported symptoms of sleep apnea.

## MEDICAL MANAGEMENT

Medical management of the person with sleep apnea takes a graded approach to match the severity of the problem. For *mild* sleep apnea syndrome, the patient is advised to sleep on a side and to lose weight if obese. In addition, the patient should avoid all sleeping medication, CNS depressants, and alcohol. If these approaches do not provide improvement, drug therapy may be instituted. Medroxyprogesterone may be prescribed for those who also hypoventilate while awake. A trial of protriptyline is initiated for obese persons. Patients need to be followed closely, because the side effects of the drugs may work against the patient taking them faithfully.

For *moderate* sleep apnea syndrome, an oral surgeon or ear, nose, and throat (ENT) specialist may suggest removal of tonsils or realignment of the bite, either through jaw surgery or use of an appliance during sleep, if specific upper airway obstruction is found. In the absence of obstruction, a nasal *continuous positive airway pressure* (CPAP) system may be recommended. A CPAP system consists of an air pump connected to a mask worn over the nose during sleep. This air pump (to which supplemental oxygen may be added) delivers air to the oropharynx at a pressure sufficient to prevent collapse of the pharynx during sleep. For the first several nights, the CPAP system is worn while the patient sleeps in the laboratory, where sleep technicians adjust the air pressure in the mask to the amount required. When the CPAP system reduces apneic events, the sleeper will experience deeper and longer periods of sleep for the next several nights; arousal to breathe is unnecessary. Because increased REM sleep also means increased time during which the sleeper does not arouse as easily, the person needs to be observed for any difficulties. Wearing the mask takes some personal adjustment; however, most patients experience quick relief from their problems of daytime sleepiness and nighttime symptoms.

When a patient demonstrates pronounced oxygen desaturation or frequent cardiac dysrhythmias (*severe* sleep apnea syndrome), more extreme therapy is recommended. A *uvulopalatopharyngoplasty* (UPPP) may be performed by an ENT surgeon experienced with the treatment of sleep apnea patients. This procedure removes almost all the soft tissue at the back of the mouth to widen the pharynx. The patient must be cautioned, however, that in some people snoring will disappear but apnea can still be present. In addition, during the first 3 days postoperatively, regional edema can occlude the airway. A tracheostomy may be required to prevent sudden death. It may take a week to 10 days for the patient to swallow comfortably again. Special attention must be given to the obese person so that the airway will not occlude with supine sleeping postures.

## DIAGNOSTIC TESTS

The PSG (see p. 471) is the primary test. It should be performed at night because apneic episodes may be more frequent during REM sleep, and a sleeper may not have any REM sleep during afternoon naps. The test may be repeated after the patient undergoes treatment for sleep apnea to determine the degree of response.

Almost routinely the patient is sent for a consulting examination with an otolaryngologist or maxillofacial specialist to determine the extent to which oropharyngeal architecture impacts on the obstructed airway. Pulmonary function tests may also be ordered to detect any underlying contributing factors. The physician may request that much of the pulmonary testing be done with the patient in a supine position.

## NURSING MANAGEMENT

### ♦ ASSESSMENT

#### Subjective Data

Data to be collected to assess the patient with sleep apnea include the following:

- The patient's and family's understanding of the cause of the sleep apnea and the possible risks to health and life
- Understanding of how the cardiac and respiratory systems work

Awareness of contributing factors of obesity and alcohol intake
Sleep history, including use of sleeping pills; use of stimulants; and work, hobby, and accident history
Understanding of possible courses of action
Assessment of any emotional, social, or economic factors that may contribute to reluctance of patient and family to take part in treatment

### Objective Data

Data to be collected to assess the patient with sleep apnea include the following:

Blood pressure, respiratory assessment (including breath sounds, chest movement, presence of any thoracic deformities), degree of obesity, oropharyngeal assessment, level of awareness, skin color
Results of CBC, pulmonary, cardiac, and sleep studies
Presence of any other health problems

## ♦ NURSING DIAGNOSES

Nursing diagnoses are determined from analysis of patient data. Nursing diagnoses for the patient with sleep apnea may include but are not limited to the following:

| Diagnostic Title | Possible Etiologic Factors |
|---|---|
| Breathing pattern, ineffective | Airway obstruction or episodic loss of neurologic stimulus to breathe at night |
| Knowledge deficit (about sleep problem) | Lack of information |
| Fatigue | Altered sleep pattern; oxygen desaturation and frequent arousals at night |
| Injury, high risk for | Increased daytime sleepiness, fatigue, reduced vigilance and response time |

## ♦ EXPECTED PATIENT OUTCOMES

Expected patient outcomes for the person with sleep apnea may include but are not limited to the following:

1. Breathes easily at night.
2. Patient/family carry out a plan to remedy sleep apnea and will describe measures to take if sleep apnea does not respond to treatment.
3. Patient/bed partner/family can describe the effects of sleep apnea.
4. Sustains no injuries as a result of daytime sleepiness, fatigue, or decreased awareness.

## ♦ INTERVENTIONS

### Facilitating Learning

Nursing interventions consist primarily of patient/family teaching and counseling. As sleep apnea decreases with treatment, fatigue and potential for injuries also decrease.

It is important that both patient and bed partner/family understand normal breathing in sleep, the effects of sleep apnea, measures to take to prevent injury, and treatment regimen. Teaching includes the following:

1. Relationship between the pulmonary and cardiac systems
2. How sleep affects breathing
3. How uninterrupted sleep contributes to daytime functioning
4. How sleep apnea contributes to cardiac problems and leads to increased risk of accidents
5. Restrictions on operating machinery, including appliances and equipment at home, until risk of fatigue-related accidents subsides
6. Drug therapy regimen, side effects, expected time to determine efficacy, and who to contact if problems occur

The nurse may anticipate that the *patient* or *someone in the family* may *minimize the seriousness of sleep apnea* and may not be totally supportive of the means required to respond to the problem. It takes teaching and support to help a family come to the understanding that "plain old snoring" can indicate a serious health problem. In some sleep laboratories, the sleeper is videotaped throughout a night (with consent). If patients or family members doubt the seriousness of the problem, it can be instructive to let them see parts of the tape or sleep record to illustrate how long breathing does not occur or how often during the night the sleeper arouses.

### Promoting Effective Team Response

Successful treatment involves members of separate disciplines providing several modalities of therapy. A satisfactory therapeutic response from the family's point of view often hinges on one team member, such as the nurse, being willing to handle questions and concerns from family and other team members.

Obese patients need to lose weight. Successful participation in weight loss programs requires knowledgeable referral and supportive follow-up by a member of the treatment team. Surgical treatment requires input from many specialists, and patients and families benefit from someone who can handle questions and respond to concerns. A patient placed on CPAP will need information for the insurance company, as well as a 24-hour telephone number to call should problems with equipment occur in the middle of the night.

# CLINICAL CHRONOBIOLOGY: THE DEVELOPMENT OF A NEW AREA OF SCIENCE

The study of normal sleep and sleep problems falls within the broader area of inquiry known as **chronobiology,** or the study of biologic activities as they vary or oscillate predictably over time. Sleep is only one of many biologic events that occur at the same time every 24 hours. Other events that have predictable cyclic peaks and troughs every 24 hours include the following:

1. Core body temperature
2. Cell division
3. Production of red blood cells
4. Preferential migration of lymphocytes into spleen from the peripheral circulation
5. Production of hormones, such as cortisol and growth hormone
6. Muscle strength and alertness
7. Mental alertness[10]

Even more interesting, some of these events are apparently controlled by the action of internal pacemakers that are somewhat insulated from the activity of the environment, whereas other biologic rhythms depend much more on and are driven by environmental cues. For example, some biologic events depend on the person, turning out the lights and lapsing into sleep before they begin. Another compelling finding is that under circumstances of environmental change, such as changing time zones during airplane travel, working the night shift, or postponing sleep, some biologic rhythms are affected more than others and some take longer to readjust.[11] Therefore, not only does an individual rhythm lose its pattern transiently, but all rhythms that act on this one rhythm can also become asynchronous.

One focus of current sleep research is to determine how sleep changes as people age. Several researchers hypothesize that the circadian oscillators may lose some of their precise interrelatedness in aging, providing evidence for systematic age-related changes in the output of the circadian pacemakers.[4] Living in an institution with a reduction in exposure to bright outdoor illumination and social zeitgebers probably undermines the organization of sleep-wake rhythm.[2]

These findings are pertinent at the clinical level because the biologic rhythms of both patients and caregivers are affected by the patient's hospitalization. Regarding the patient, the following is only a partial list of factors at work when someone is hospitalized:

1. Pain, fatigue, uncertainty, and anxiety
2. Different bed and bedclothes in an unusual sleeping environment
3. Being awakened for procedures, vital signs, or medications
4. Reduced opportunity for exercise
5. Nutrient timing changes or food withheld
6. Medications depressing or accelerating different biologic functions
7. Lights being turned on or off during the sleep time
8. Living in an environmental temperature (too hot or too cold) that is not under patient control

It is not yet known to what degree, if any, a change in environmental conditions affects healing, recovery time, feelings of well-being, or response to treatment. All these environmental factors and more are being studied regarding how they affect sleep, response to treatment, and recovery time. What is most exciting for nursing research is that nurses make clinical decisions about many of these factors. (See Research box, at left.) Nursing research in the future will contribute to the determination of optimal timing for assessments and treatments and the creation of the chronobiologically most synchronous or most supportive environments for the patient.

Nurses must remember that their own biologic rhythms are also responding to the environment. Ongoing research has described the risks some workers face when they work and sleep at irregular hours[6,10] and effects on health and performance during day, evening, and night shifts. Some experts recommend that persons rotating from day to night shift make the best adjustment in sleep when the night shift is worked for a longer period. For example, rotating to the night shift for a month or more at a time is easier to adjust to than is rotating shifts every 1 or 2 weeks. Other research is focusing on the resetting of biologic clocks by exposure to very bright light at times of day that may exert the most influence on circadian oscillators.[3,7]

It would be interesting for further study to determine the effect of sleep interruption on the retention of information taught to patients and to determine the effect of hospital sleep interruption on home sleep patterns. It would be of further interest to determine whether such a nursing intervention as waiting until the person has finished an episode of REM sleep before waking her or him or timing nursing interventions to predicted com-

## RESEARCH

Gall K, Peterson T, Riesch SK: Night life: nocturnal behavior patterns among hospitalized elderly, *J Gerontol Nurs* 16(10):31-7, 1990.

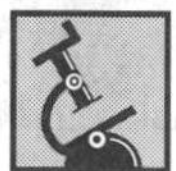

In an inpatient geriatric unit, 21 elderly people (ages 61 to 91; mean, 75.7 years) were visually observed at 30-minute intervals from 11 PM to 7 AM on the second, third, and fourth nights of hospitalization. These persons were not critically ill and not confused and did not have a preexisting sleep problem.

The investigators found that fewer subjects were sleeping at any given hour on the second night of study compared with the first night, and still fewer were sleeping on any given hour of the third night, as compared with the first or second nights. By night 3, less than 50% were asleep at any given hour. Treatments or medications interrupted sleep in three fourths of the subjects. Each time sleep was interrupted, it took at least 30 minutes for the person to fall back asleep. Sleep was particularly disrupted at 3 AM and between the hours of 5 and 6 AM.

| Study Night | 3 AM | 5 AM | 6 AM |
|---|---|---|---|
| 1 | 72% asleep | 80% | 40% |
| 2 | 56% | 55% | 20% |
| 3 | 47% | 40% | 30% |

pletion of 90-minute sleep cycles based on the time a particular patient fell asleep would improve sleep parameters, mood, memory, physical stamina, and other factors.

Florence Nightingale is often pictured with a lamp as she watches over wounded and sick soldiers through the night. No more apt picture could illustrate the growing body of knowledge concerning the interrelationships among biologic rhythms, especially sleep, as they are challenged in illness, modified because of professional commitment, and highlighted by new nursing contributions to this developing research area.

## QUESTIONS TO CONSIDER

- Taking into consideration the 90-minute sleep cycle, how could you best time the waking of a patient at night to take his or her vital signs?
- If a man with newly diagnosed sleep attacks caused by narcolepsy calls and states that his medication is not helping at all, what factors would you consider as you assess the situation?
- What assessment challenges might you expect as you assess a 70-year-old man whose spouse of 45 years has just mentioned that his snoring is a little louder than before, "but it's probably nothing"?
- What steps would you take to coordinate the care of a person having severe obstructive sleep apnea?

## CRITICAL THINKING ACTIVITIES

- You are caring for Sam, a patient suspected of having narcolepsy. One evening he calls you to his room and states that he is confused about information received from his doctor. His doctor explained that Sam's MSLT report was positive, but Sam does not understand the test or its results. How would you explain this finding to Sam? Considering all the interventions possible, which is of the highest priority?
- Chuck has been diagnosed with moderate sleep apnea syndrome. Upon examination he is found to have no specific upper airway obstruction; therefore the doctor orders a CPAP system for Chuck. When it arrives, Chuck asks you how and why it works. What is the best explanation regarding this treatment method?

## CHAPTER SUMMARY

### NATURE OF PROBLEM

- More than a half million adults have difficulty with sleeping at some time in their lives.
- Sleep disorders can be categorized by the type of disruption they cause including the following:
  *Parasomnia*—disorders of arousal
  *Insomnia*—inability to initiate or maintain sleep
  *Narcolepsy*—sleep intrusion into wakefulness that can challenge the pattern of daily living
  *Sleep apnea*—sleep problems that involve other body systems and can be life-threatening

### INSOMNIA

- Persons with insomnia must be taught not to take naps, sleeping pills, caffeine, or alcohol because these may exacerbate insomnia.
- Nurses need to understand the importance of a sleep schedule in treating sleep disorders.
- Problems of initiating or maintaining sleep may continue over many years, even when the precipitating factor has been resolved.
- Helping a patient master a problem with insomnia requires education about normal sleep and careful initiation of new sleep practices.

### SLEEP APNEA

- Loud snoring and breathing disturbances in sleep are symptoms of sleep apnea.

### GENERAL

- Nurses need to take special care with their own sleep habits, particularly when rotating from day to night shifts, because they may be at greater risk for accidents and slips in performance when deprived of sleep.

## REFERENCES

1. Bergstrom DL, Keller C: Narcolepsy: pathogenesis and nursing care, *J Neurosci Nurs* 24(3):153-157, 1992.
2. Bliwise DL: Sleep in normal aging and dementia, *Sleep* 16(1):40-81, 1993.
3. Czeisler CA et al: Exposure to bright light and darkness to treat physiologic maladaptation to night work, *N Engl J Med* 322:1253-1259, 1990.
4. Czeisler CA et al: Association of sleep-wake habits in older people with changes in output of circadian pacemaker, *Lancet* 340(8825):933-936, 1992.
5. Gall K, Petersen T, Riesch SK: Night life: nocturnal behavior patterns among hospitalized elderly, *J Gerontol Nurs* 16(10):31-37, 1990.
6. Gold DR et al: Rotating shift work, sleepiness and accidents related to sleepiness in hospital nurses, *Am J Public Health* 82(7):1011-1014, 1992.
7. Jewett ME, Kronauer RE, Czeisler CA: Light-induced suppression of endogenous circadian amplitude in humans, *Nature* 350:59-62, 1991.
8. Kryger MH, Roth R, Dement WB: *Principles and practice of sleep medicine,* Philadelphia, 1989, WB Saunders.
9. Lydic R, Biebuyck JF, editors: *Clinical physiology of sleep,* Bethesda, Md, 1988, American Physiological Society.
10. Moore-Ede MC, Sultzman FM, Fuller CE: *The clocks that time us: physiology of the circadian timing system,* Cambridge, Mass, 1982, Harvard University Press.
11. Whitehead DC, Thomas H, Slapper DR: A rational approach to shift work in emergency medicine, *Ann Emerg Med* 21:1250-1258, 1992.

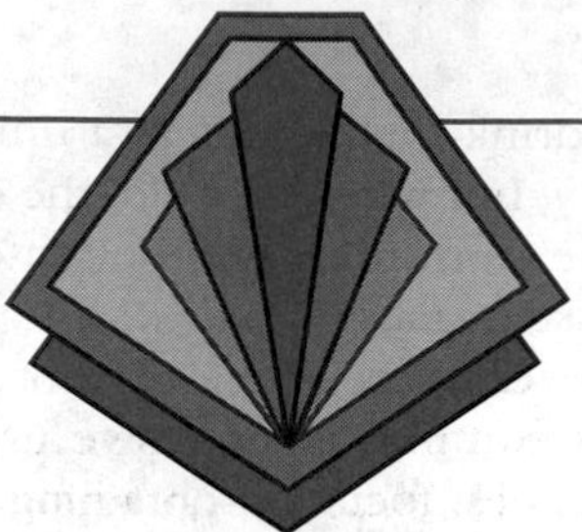

# CHAPTER 19

# Substance Abuse

***Elizabeth Anne Schenk***

## CHAPTER OBJECTIVES

***After studying this chapter, the learner should be able to do the following:***

1. Name at least three negative compulsions that are considered addictions.
2. Name one legal effort and one educational effort to prevent alcoholism and drug abuse.
3. Name five physical disorders often seen with alcoholism.
4. Discuss alcohol withdrawal and actions to treat the three different levels of withdrawal symptoms.
5. Name the six basic types of drugs, including how they are used, street names, effects, side effects, and symptoms of overdose.
6. Discuss why nurses are at increased risk for chemical dependency and codependency.
7. Differentiate between anorexia nervosa and bulimia.
8. Describe how the medical-surgical nurse can prepare the patient for entry into chemical dependency treatment.
9. Explain the reasoning behind self-help groups.

## KEY TERMS

addiction
alcoholism
anorexia nervosa
behavior modification
blood alcohol level
bulimia
chemical dependency
co-dependency
deliriant (inhalant)
delirium tremens (DTs)
dependence
depressant
detoxification
drug addiction
drug habituation
enabling behavior
ethyl alcohol
fetal alcohol syndrome
hallucinogen
intervention
intoxication
narcotic
physical dependence
psychologic dependence
relapse
stimulant
substance abuse
tolerance
Wernicke-Korsakoff syndrome
withdrawal

The subject of **substance abuse** is gaining increased attention. Treatment centers have emerged in many localities, and growing numbers of nurses are becoming involved in this specialty. There is a recognition that substance abuse entails a complex set of behaviors that are covered under the term **addiction.** The overriding characteristic of addiction is a preoccupation with obtaining the addictive substance, coupled with the inability to stop the associated behaviors, despite negative consequences. Persons may experience one or more addictions concurrently. An example is the alcoholic who also is a drug addict and a compulsive overeater.

## DEFINITION OF TERMS

Alcoholism and drug addiction are now commonly brought together under the term **chemical dependency.** This is in recognition that alcohol is a drug and that the person addicted to alcohol is also at great risk for addiction to other drugs.

Most modern definitions of **dependence** consist of two components—physical and psychologic dependence. **Physical dependence** refers to a physiologic state in which continuous and prolonged consumption of a drug or alcohol leads to the user's adapting to its

**BOX 19-1 Terms Used to Describe Responses to Drugs/Alcohol**

**Dependence** (also called *habituation* or *compulsive use*) Psychologic and/or physical need for a drug or alcohol
**Psychologic dependence** Needing a substance in order to reach a maximum level of functioning or feeling of well-being
**Physical dependence** Adaption of the body physiologically to chronic use of substance(s); symptoms of withdrawal occur when the substance is stopped or withdrawn
**Tolerance** Need for higher and higher doses of a substance to achieve the same results
**Cross-tolerance** Development of tolerance to one drug of a class leads to tolerance to drugs of the same class
**Withdrawal (abstinence syndrome)** Appearance of physiologic symptoms when use of a substance is stopped
**Drug abuse** Use of mind-altering substances in a way that differs from generally approved medical or social practices
**Metabolic tolerance** Substance is detoxified more quickly than normal
**Pharmacologic tolerance** Tissue reaction to substance is diminished

presence. **Tolerance** then develops. If use of the drug is interrupted, withdrawal symptoms occur. **Psychologic dependence** refers to craving for the drug. See Box 19-1 for a description of terms used to describe responses to drugs and alcohol.

The nurse can do much to encourage the treatment of alcoholism by first recognizing that many patients in the hospital may be alcohol- or drug-addicted, even when this is not listed as a diagnosis.

This chapter deals with four examples of substance abuse: *alcoholism, drug addiction, caffeine and tobacco dependency,* and *eating disorders.* In addition, two problems linked closely with substance abuse are discussed: *co-dependency* and the *impaired nurse.* Both have relevance to the medical-surgical nurse.

## ALCOHOLISM

**Alcoholism** is very common and may compound the problems of persons with other health disorders. Excessive alcohol intake may lead to coma or near death from acute alcohol poisoning, or if it occurs over a time, it may lead to numerous other health disorders. Alcoholism is recognized today as a treatable disease. Significant changes in the identification and treatment of alcoholism point toward advances that are having an important impact on this major health problem.

### ETIOLOGY

Alcohol abuse can become a problem over a variable period. The abuse of alcohol is often so episodic that it is difficult to identify. Some persons can drink large amounts for years without becoming alcoholic, whereas other persons become alcoholic after just a short period of heavy drinking. Some alcoholics drink only on weekends. Many may not drink for months at a time. Some drink only episodically, but when they do, the drinking is in a form of a binge, with the person often drinking to the point of unconsciousness.

In alcoholics, however, there is evidence of progression. Alcohol abusers continue compulsive use in the presence of consequences, focus on obtaining alcohol, and often have relapses after treatment. The alcoholic begins to develop an increasing physical dependence and tolerance for alcohol.[2] The drinking becomes uncontrollable and secretive. Blackouts (loss of memory from episodes of drinking) may start to occur. Feelings of guilt, shame, and remorse may occur, and the alcoholic drinks more to relieve these feelings. The alcoholic drinks to live and lives to drink.

### EPIDEMIOLOGY

Alcoholism is said to be the third major health problem in the United States. Conservative estimates are that about 90 million people use alcohol and at least 9 to 10 million persons are alcoholics or "problem drinkers." In addition, alcoholism adversely affects the mental health or functioning of another 30 million friends and relatives of alcohol abusers.

It has been estimated that 70% of alcoholics are male. The number of female alcoholics, however, is increasing.[16] Research has demonstrated that women are more likely to hide their problem drinking. In addition, women are not as likely as men to be involved in the three major systems that give external motivation for treatment (industrial programs, public intoxication and drunk driving laws, and the criminal justice intervention system).[22,25]

Alcohol is involved in nearly half of all deaths caused by motor vehicle accidents[23] and fatal intentional injuries, such as suicides and homicides. It has been found that victims are intoxicated in about one third of all homicides, drownings, and boating deaths. Almost half of all traffic fatalities are alcohol-related, and an estimated 40% of persons in the United States may be involved in an alcohol-related traffic crash sometime in their lives. Alcohol is involved in at least a quarter of all admissions to general hospitals. The costs of alcohol-related problems in the United States have been estimated to exceed $70 billion per year, with an additional $44 billion attributed to problems related to drug use.[25,27]

Included in the costs are medical expenses, lost wages, and fire loss. Also included are use and abuse of sick time, extended hospital stays, and increased medical and surgical complications.

#### Theories of the Cause of Alcoholism

Numerous theories have been advanced to explain the cause of alcoholism. Research is being done to expand the knowledge base about alcoholism. Thus far, no one theory can completely explain the syndrome.

Current theories can be divided into the following three categories:

1. Physiologic theories of the cause
2. Psychologic theories of the cause
3. Sociocultural-etiologic theories (also known as cultural-etiologic theories)

**Physiologic theories of etiology**

These theories operate on the belief that persons are predisposed to develop alcoholism because of some organic defect. Included are theories that suggest that there is a genetically determined biochemical defect in alcoholics, as well as theories that link alcoholism with a dysfunction of the endocrine system.

The incidence of alcoholism is high in families, and the risk of sons of impaired alcoholic men developing alcoholism over their lifetime is 30% to 50%. Studies of twins who have been adopted have also shown that the identical twins of an alcoholic will be alcoholic in 60% of the cases, whereas only 30% of the fraternal twins of an alcoholic will be alcoholic. Studies of children of alcoholic parents who were adopted shortly after birth and reared separately from the natural parents indicate that those who were adopted had a higher rate of alcoholism than did normal control subjects.

**Psychologic theories of etiology**

These theories are based on the assumption that some element in the personality structure and development leads to the development of alcoholism. Included among these theories are the *oral fixation theory* and the *behavioral learning theory.*

Although there has been a search for the "alcoholic personality," most studies have failed to find any specific personality traits that clearly differentiate alcoholics from normal drinkers. Common personality traits that have been identified as occurring in alcoholics include low stress tolerance, dependency, negative self-image, and feelings of insecurity and depression. It is not clear whether these traits precede alcoholism or are a result of it.

There is evidence that two types of personalities are particularly susceptible to alcohol abuse—the *antisocial personality,* found chiefly in men, and the *borderline personality,* found chiefly in women.

**Sociocultural or cultural theories of etiology**

These theories postulate a relationship between various groups in society and the incidence of alcohol use. For instance, Jews, Mormons, and Moslems have a very low rate of alcoholism, whereas the French have the highest rate. Individual attitudes toward alcohol and alcoholism to a large extent reflect the attitude of one's culture toward drinking. Another part of these theories is that stress factors in cultures may contribute to alcoholism.

One theory that is no longer recognized as valid is the moral etiologic theory. This theory held that alcoholism was either a moral fault or a sin of the alcoholic. Much of the early treatment of alcoholics was based on this theory, which is still subscribed to by some religious groups.

## PATHOPHYSIOLOGY

Alcohol is a central nervous system (CNS) depressant. It affects the brain by suppressing the activity of the neurotransmitter gamma aminobutyric acid (GABA). GABA is an inhibitory neurotransmitter. Thus alcohol inhibits the inhibitor. The so-called stimulating effects of alcohol occur because the first areas affected by the suppression of GABA are the higher centers of the brain governing self-control and judgment, which are inhibitory functions. Slowing the release of GABA to those areas results in a seemingly "stimulating" effect. As alcohol continues to accumulate in the brain, areas of the limbic system and brainstem become inhibited. **Intoxication** occurs and unconsciousness may set in. In fact, the brain may become so overwhelmed by alcohol that it can stop functioning permanently.

### Effects of Alcohol on Organ Systems

Alcohol affects every organ system in the body. The nurse working in a medical or surgical area is very likely to see an alcoholic patient with various pathologies secondary to alcohol abuse. Typical symptoms that may be seen include those listed in Table 19-1. The nurse needs to be aware that alcoholic patients may not admit to drinking excessively or that it is a problem for them. The presence of disease conditions associated with alcoholism should alert the nurse to gather more history about drinking patterns. It is also important for the nurse to assess the intoxicated patient for injuries, such as fractures or lacerations. These often occur when one is intoxicated.[21]

Cirrhosis of the liver is largely related to heavy alcohol consumption. It is the ninth leading cause of death in the United States. Rates of deaths for nonwhites are almost 70% higher than rates for whites,[29] and the rates for Native American males is triple that of white men.[28a] Table 19-2 compares normal function, pathophysiology, and clinical manifestations of alcoholism.

The active ingredient in alcoholic beverages is **ethyl alcohol** or ethanol. Most American beers contain 3% to 6% alcohol, wine contains 2% to 21% alcohol, and hard liquors contain 40% to 50% alcohol. A 12-ounce bottle of beer, a 4-ounce glass of wine, and 1½ ounces of hard liquor contain similar amounts of alcohol.

Alcohol does not require digestion and is absorbed in both the stomach and intestine. Absorption is accelerated by increased alcohol concentrations and an empty stomach. After absorption, alcohol is distributed equally throughout body fluids, passing across all mucous membranes. About 2% to 10% is lost through the lungs with respirations and through the kidneys with urination. About 90% of alcohol is disposed of

**TABLE 19-1 Effects of Alcohol on Organ Systems**

| BODY SYSTEM | EFFECTS | LATE EFFECTS |
|---|---|---|
| Central nervous system | Depression leading to loss of memory and ability to concentrate<br>Lessening of inhibitory functions<br>Self-control and judgment lessened | Unprovoked seizures<br>Wernicke-Korsakoff's syndrome<br>Brain atrophy<br>Sleep disturbances<br>Neuronal damage<br>Neuropathies |
| Cardiovascular system | Increased pulse rate<br>Vasomotor depression and vasodilation of cutaneous vessels with hypotension<br>Hypertension | Cardiomyopathy (irreversible)<br>Hyperlipidemia<br>Hyperuricemia<br>Coronary artery disease |
| Skeletal muscles | Lessening awareness of fatigue<br>Reduced muscular capacity for work | Skeletal myopathy |
| Immunologic system | Increased susceptibility to infection | Infections and communicable diseases |
| Gastrointestinal system | Stimulation of gastric secretions and gastric acid production<br>Irritation of GI mucosa<br>Constipation or diarrhea<br>Vomiting | Pancreatitis<br>Gastritis<br>Nutritional and vitamin deficiencies<br>Cancer of mouth and esophagus<br>Skin syndrome<br>Wernicke-Korsakoff's syndrome |
| Hepatic system | Few liver changes in acute ingestion | Cirrhosis of the liver<br>Cellular damage<br>Cell necrosis<br>Vitamin depletion (especially B complex vitamins)<br>Cell fibrosis<br>Liver failure<br>Interferes with clotting factors |
| Renal system | Diuretic effect from inhibition of antidiuretic hormone | |
| Pancreas | Epigastric pain: vomiting and rigidity of abdominal muscles | Pancreatitis |
| Hematologic system | | Anemia<br>Thrombocytopenia<br>Bone marrow depression<br>Prolonged clotting time |

**TABLE 19-2 Normal Function, Primary Pathophysiology, and Clinical Picture in Alcoholism**

| NORMAL FUNCTION | PRIMARY PATHOPHYSIOLOGY | CLINICAL MANIFESTATIONS |
|---|---|---|
| Gamma aminobutyric acid (GABA)—(neurotransmitter) | Activity of GABA is inhibited | Lessening of inhibitory functions; self-control and judgment lessened |
| Pancreas—synthesizes protein | Activation of proteolytic enzymes with autodigestion of pancreatic tissue | Epigastric pain; vomiting and rigidity of abdominal muscles |
| Liver—provides glucose during fasting; during carbohydrate ingestion removes glucose and stores it as glycogen | Infiltration of liver parenchymal cells with fat<br>Glucose broken down to acetaldehyde to acetic acid | Jaundice, enlarged liver, increased bleeding time, ascites, possible hepatic coma |
| Stomach and esophagus—normal food ingestion | Increased acid production; irritation of mucosa | Bleeding ulcers, gastritis; cancer of esophagus and mouth |
| Intestine—absorption of vitamins and minerals | Decreased absorption of thiamine, folic acid, and vitamin $B_{12}$ | Malabsorption syndrome, skin conditions, Wernicke-Korsakoff syndrome |
| Immunologic system—protection against infection | Increased susceptibility to infection | Infections and illness |
| Neuromuscular system—transmission of impulses | Abnormal transmission of impulses | Neuropathies and myopathies |

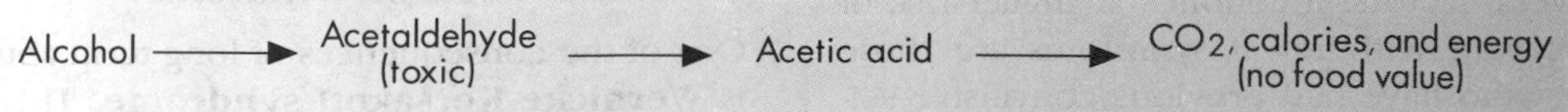


FIGURE 19-1 Metabolism of alcohol.

by metabolic processes that occur mainly in the liver (Fig. 19-1).

Alcohol has a diuretic effect, partly caused by the increased amounts of fluids ingested. Increased amounts of electrolytes—particularly potassium, magnesium, and zinc—may be excreted in the urine of heavy drinkers. Prolonged use of alcohol has a toxic effect on the intestinal mucosa, which results in decreased absorption of thiamine, folic acid, and vitamin $B_{12}$.

Because alcohol is not converted to glycogen, it cannot be stored, and it provides calories but no minerals or vitamins. One ounce of alcohol provides approximately 200 kcal. Most of the ingested alcohol is metabolized in the liver at a rate of 10 g/hr. The excess remains in the bloodstream, where it acts as a depressant and an anesthetic, which in turn slows down cellular metabolism. The anesthetic action of alcohol can have serious consequences. The margin of safety for the person anesthetized by alcohol is very small.

**Blood alcohol** levels depend on the amount ingested and the size of the individual. The amount of alcohol that is generally metabolized by the adult is 6 g of pure alcohol in 1 hour (the typical drink). The time from the last drink to maximal blood alcohol concentration (BAC) is usually 30 to 90 minutes.[27] Most states designate blood alcohol serum levels of 100 mg/100 ml (0.1%) as the legal limit for driving a motor vehicle. Some states such as California have lowered the legal limit for driving to 0.08%. Increasing blood alcohol levels have increasingly more serious side effects (Table 19-3).

The main symptom of alcoholism is that the usual

TABLE 19-3 Effects of Blood Alcohol Levels on Average-Sized Nontolerant Adult

| BLOOD ALCOHOL LEVELS (per 100 ml of Blood) | EFFECTS |
|---|---|
| 50-75 mg | Pleasant relaxed state, mild sedation, loosening of inhibitions |
| 100-200 mg | Overt signs of intoxication: loosening of tongue, clumsiness, beginning emotional changes |
| 200-400 mg | Severe intoxication: difficulty speaking, stumbling, emotional lability |
| 400-500 mg | Stupor, coma can result in person who is not a chronic alcoholic |
| Over 500 mg | Usually fatal |

drinking behaviors impair the individual's ability to function physically, psychologically, and socially. Usually alcoholism develops slowly, over a period of 10 to 20 years, until the person reaches a point where he "drinks to live and lives to drink."

Several clinical features have been found to occur with alcoholics:

1. Chronicity as a disease or disorder of behavior
2. Undue preoccupation with the intake of ethyl alcohol
3. Loss of control over the drinking pattern itself
4. Use of alcohol in a way that is dangerous to the drinker's physical health, interpersonal relationships, and/or economic functioning
5. Use of alcohol as a universal solution to problems
6. Incorporation of denial and other defense mechanisms as a necessary component of the disease
7. Loss of ability to express feelings

In addition, frequent intoxication affects multiple body systems.

## Fetal Alcohol Syndrome

Although fetal alcohol syndrome is not a focus of this text, it is mentioned briefly. Medical-surgical nurses may have the chance to educate patients and family members about the risk factors leading to this syndrome. Women who drink during pregnancy have a higher incidence of children with birth defects. The children of women who drink several times a day throughout pregnancy may be born with fetal alcohol syndrome. The syndrome can include the following:

1. Mental retardation
2. Microcephaly
3. Growth deficiencies
4. Facial abnormalities
5. Malformations of skeletal, urogenital, and cardiac systems

An increase in spontaneous abortions, stillbirths, and infant deaths is also associated with heavy drinking during pregnancy.[8,9] Even moderate drinking can result in the birth of children with significant lags in mental and motor development.[13] The reader is referred to a maternal-child text for further information.

## Alcohol Withdrawal

With continued drinking, a physiologic dependency on alcohol and tolerance for increasing amounts of it occur. Alcohol **withdrawal** affects motor control, mental status, and body functions. Symptoms range from mild tremors to severe agitation and hallucinations when alcohol is withheld. The type and severity of symptoms depend on several factors. Alcoholics at higher risk of experiencing severe withdrawal symptoms are those who are older, who have had previous convulsive seizures or **delirium tremens (DTs),** and who have coexisting acute illnesses or nutritional deficiencies.

It is important for the medical-surgical nurse to assess the severity of alcohol withdrawal. Proper medication given early in withdrawal can prevent the development of DTs, as well as possible seizures. The amount and frequency of medication varies, depending on the nature of the alcohol withdrawal. For this reason, the nurse should be familiar with the signs and symptoms of withdrawal.

*Mild alcohol withdrawal* is characterized by hand tremors, as well as mild restlessness and anxiety. Insomnia or restless sleep is often present. Anorexia and nausea are common. There is usually slight sweating with tachycardia and a normal or slightly elevated systolic blood pressure. The patient remains alert and oriented and generally does not experience seizures or hallucinations.

*Moderate alcohol withdrawal* is indicated by a worsening of many of the symptoms seen in mild withdrawal. The patient is visibly tremulous with restlessness and anxiety. There is marked insomnia, with nightmares. Vague, transient hallucinations may occur with variable confusion. Marked anorexia is accompanied by nausea and vomiting. Seizures may possibly be present. These seizures are generally not preceded by an aura, but are followed by a postictal stupor. The patient with moderate alcohol withdrawal is diaphoretic. The pulse rate is tachycardic to 100 to 120 beats/min, and the systolic blood pressure is elevated.[27]

*Severe alcohol withdrawal* may also be called delirium tremens, or DTs. This is an acute complication of alcohol withdrawal that is a *true emergency*. It is a pathologic state of consciousness resulting from interference with brain metabolism. The onset of DTs usually occurs 3 to 4 days after abstinence but may occur as long as a week after the last drink. DTs that are treated carry a 5% mortality rate, whereas untreated DTs have a 15% mortality rate. The symptoms of this severe withdrawal include uncontrollable shaking, extreme restlessness and agitation, and intense fear and anxiety. This is accompanied by marked confusion and disorientation, with often frightening visual and auditory hallucination. The patient is wakeful and often refuses all food and fluids. Dry heaves and vomiting may be present. The patient has marked hyperhidrosis (excessive sweating), and seizures are common. The pulse rate is elevated to 120 to 140 beats/min, and there is often marked elevation of the systolic and diastolic blood pressures.[27]

The medical-surgical nurse is responsible for monitoring the patient for symptoms of withdrawal and reporting those symptoms to the physician. A patient who is known to drink may have the initial presenting signs of irritability, a craving for alcohol, and a desire to leave the hospital. Timely and liberal use of PRN medications to prevent withdrawal may avert DTs.

### Wernicke-Korsakoff Syndrome

One of the consequences of long-term abuse of alcohol is **Wernicke-Korsakoff syndrome.** This can be seen in the medical-surgical areas, especially in elderly patients who may have drunk for a long period. The symptoms may also be seen in residents of nursing home facilities. With Wernicke-Korsakoff syndrome, the patient may recover from the initial illness, but amnesia and psychosis may continue. If the residual mental illness is severe, the person may require close supervision and intensive care.

Symptoms of Wernicke-Korsakoff syndrome include ocular disturbances, such as nystagmus and paralysis of the lateral rectus muscle of the eye. Ataxia is usually present, along with symptoms of disturbed mental functioning. The latter can include symptoms of DTs, as well as apathy, listlessness, psychosis, and severe confusion. Memory problems and confusion are commonly seen. At one time this syndrome was believed to be the result of neurologic damage from long-term alcohol use. It is now known, however, that *nutritional deficiency* is the causative factor. The specific nutritional deficiency is thiamine.

## PREVENTION

### Healthy People 2000

The report to the Surgeon General on health goals for the year 2000 contained several recommendations about alcohol and other drugs. These goals are linked with the prevention of alcohol and drug abuse, as well as problems related to these two areas. The goals include the following:

1. Reduce deaths caused by alcohol-related motor vehicle crashes to no more than 8.5 per 100,000 people from an age-adjusted baseline of 9.8 per 100,000 in 1987. Special target populations for this goal are presented in Table 19-4.[29]
2. Reduce cirrhosis deaths to no more than 6 per 100,000 people from an age-adjusted baseline of 9.1 per 100,000 in 1987.
3. Reduce drug-related deaths to no more than 3 per 100,000 people from an age-adjusted baseline of 3.8 in 1987.
4. Reduce drug abuse–related hospital emergency department visits by at least 20%. No baseline data were available at the time the report was published.

**TABLE 19-4 Alcohol-Related Motor Vehicle Crash Deaths per 100,000**

| | 1987 BASELINE | 2000 TARGET |
|---|---|---|
| American Indians/Alaskan men | 52.2% | 44.8% |
| People aged 15-24 | 21.5% | 18.0% |

From US Department of Health and Human Services, Public Health Service: *Healthy people 2000: national health promotion and disease prevention objectives,* Washington, DC, 1990, US Government Printing Office.

Risk reduction objectives related to alcohol and other drugs include the following:

1. Increase by at least 1 year the average age for first use of cigarettes, alcohol, and marijuana by adolescents aged 12 to 17. Baseline was age 11.6 for cigarettes, age 13.1 for alcohol, and age 13.4 for marijuana in 1988.
2. Reduce the proportion of high school seniors and college students engaging in heavy drinking of alcohol to no more than 28% of high school seniors and 32% of college students. Baseline was 33% of high school seniors and 41.7% of college students in 1989.
3. Reduce alcohol consumption by people aged 14 and older to an annual average of no more than 2 gallons of alcohol per person.
4. Increase the proportion of high school seniors who perceive social disapproval associated with the heavy use of alcohol, occasional use of marijuana, and experimentation with cocaine as shown in Table 19-5.
5. Increase the proportion of high school seniors who associate risk of physical or psychologic harm with heavy use of alcohol, regular use of marijuana, and experimentation with cocaine as shown in Table 19-6.

All 50 states have developed or are developing plans to meet these and other recommendations. It is evident that there is increased public awareness of the problems related to drug abuse. Organizations like Mothers Against Driving Drunk (MADD) and Students Against Driving Drunk (SADD) have been active in urging those who drink to designate as a driver someone who will abstain from drinking. They also have been effective in getting the drinking age raised to 21 in all 50 states and in lobbying for stronger laws against those who drive under the influence of alcohol or other drugs.

Nurses can play an important role in these goals being achieved through counseling and teaching of the public, especially of teenagers and young adults.

## Primary Prevention

Prevention of alcoholism is a complex issue. The goal of primary prevention is to stop involvement with drugs or alcohol before it ever occurs. Legally, efforts have been made to restrict the sale of alcohol to minors, as well as to institute fairly stringent legal consequences of use by minors. Current laws concerning drunk driving focus both on the need of the person to be educated about the disease and on the need to suffer the consequences of the actions caused by the alcoholism. Unfortunately, many of these efforts have not been very effective.

The key to prevention seems to be grounded in education. This education includes the teaching of fairly young children about the dangers of alcohol use and abuse. Many elementary schools now start these programs as early as the first or second grades. In addition, work may be done with children to increase their self-esteem, so that they may be better able to avoid peer pressure to drink as they become older.[7,28a]

Another attempt to educate persons involves families and employers of alcoholics. They are taught that alcoholism is a disease that needs treatment, but at the same time the person who is an alcoholic may need to suffer the consequences of the use so that help may be sought at an earlier time. This has sometimes been called "raising the bottom." Alcoholics usually are surrounded by persons who *enable* their use and abuse—for example, the wife who calls in to work for her drunk husband and tells the employer that he is sick with the flu. Without this **enabling behavior,** alcoholics might be forced to seek help earlier.

## Secondary Prevention

The importance of secondary prevention cannot be ignored. Prompt diagnosis and treatment can be important in assisting alcoholics to once again become productive members of society and thus save themselves and others from much heartache and expense.

It is often difficult to make the diagnosis of alcoholism or drug abuse without objective evidence. Some indications of problems include the following:

1. Frequent illnesses and related illnesses
2. Undue preoccupation with the intake of drugs or alcohol

**TABLE 19-5 Target Goals for High School Seniors Who Perceive Social Disapproval With Use of Drugs**

| BEHAVIOR | 1989 BASELINE | 2000 TARGET |
|---|---|---|
| Heavy use of alcohol | 56.4% | 70% |
| Occasional use of marijuana | 71.1% | 85% |
| Trying cocaine once or twice | 88.9% | 95% |

From US Department of Health and Human Services, Public Health Service: *Healthy people 2000: national health promotion and disease prevention objectives,* Washington, DC, 1990, US Government Printing Office.

**TABLE 19-6 Target Goals for High School Seniors Who Associate Physical or Psychologic Harm With Use of Drugs**

| BEHAVIOR | 1989 BASELINE | 2000 TARGET |
|---|---|---|
| Heavy use of alcohol | 44% | 70% |
| Regular use of marijuana | 71.5% | 90% |
| Trying cocaine once or twice | 54.9% | 80% |

From US Department of Health and Human Services, Public Health Service: *Healthy people 2000: national health promotion and disease prevention objectives,* Washington, DC, 1990, US Government Printing Office.

3. Mood swings
4. Violent or acting-out behavior
5. Denial about the use of substances
6. Financial difficulties
7. Loss of control over use
8. Use of alcohol or drugs in such a way as to endanger physical health, interpersonal relationships, and/or economic functioning
9. Use of substances as the universal answer to all problems
10. Loss of ability to express feelings
11. Use of defense mechanisms, including a strong denial of the problem that drugs or alcohol is causing

### Tertiary Prevention

The goal of tertiary prevention is to end the compulsive use of alcohol or other drugs or to minimize the negative effects of the use through treatment and rehabilitation. An example of tertiary prevention is the treatment of an alcoholic person in relapse with cirrhosis of the liver in a halfway house.

It is important to consider *tertiary prevention,* or the prevention of complications, for the patient with substance abuse. These complications occur not only because of the effects of the substance itself, but also because of the nutritional deficits that usually accompany the problem. These problems include *infections, neuropathy,* and *myopathies.* Complications for persons with drug addictions often occur as a result of disease acquired from dirty needles or equipment. Many alcoholics and drug addicts continue to drink or use despite the development of life-threatening complications. This fact is often difficult for health professionals to understand. Many patients with substance abuse will have to deal with these complications long after they have stopped the use of the substance.

## MEDICAL MANAGEMENT

The goal for discharge of patients with alcohol/drug detoxification without rehabilitation as determined by DRGs is 4 days. The nurse works collaboratively with the physician for implementation of prescribed medical therapy. Common medical therapy for management of detoxification follows.

Medical management of the alcoholic patient in acute withdrawal focuses on restoration of nutritional and metabolic equilibrium, prevention of seizures, and safe withdrawal from alcohol. Medication is used as needed, often in large doses because of the tolerance of the alcoholic for other mood-altering chemicals. These medications are discussed later in this chapter.

### Diagnostic Tests

Routine blood tests often reveal abnormalities that are directly related to alcoholism. These include elevated liver enzyme levels—that is, aspartate aminotransferase (AST/SGOT), alamine aminotransferase (ALT/SGPT), alkaline phosphatase, and bilirubin. Hypoglycemia may also be present if glycogen stores have been depleted. In addition, hypoalbuminemia and hyperglobulinemia are also present in patients with cirrhosis of the liver. Magnesium is often decreased in persons who are alcoholic, usually because of poor dietary intake. It is not uncommon to find anemias and other indicators of poor nutrition in alcoholic patients. Patients who are alcoholics often have an increased mean corpuscle volume (MCV) when the complete blood count (CBC) is done. This and an elevated gamma glutamyl transferase (GGT) are strong indicators of a possible diagnosis of alcoholism.

Other diagnostic tests demonstrate the concomitant diseases that usually accompany alcoholism. These tests include a urine toxicology screen to determine the use of other drugs. Patients are usually offered an HIV test. This is especially relevant for the patient who is abusing both drugs and alcohol. A urinalysis and urine culture are often done to rule out kidney pathologic conditions. A breathalizer test is often used to determine the blood alcohol level on admission.

### Medication

Medications used in the initial **detoxification** from alcohol include the following.

1. Chlordiazepoxide (Librium), diazepam (Valium), or similar drugs.
   a. These drugs are used in decreasing doses for their sedating and anticonvulsant effects during detoxification.
   b. See Box 19-2 for an example of a protocol to be used for alcohol withdrawal.
2. Anticonvulsant therapy, such as magnesium sulfate (2 ml of a 50% solution every 8 to 12 hours for several doses) (this medication is not used as frequently as it once was, but is commonly used in some institutions).
   a. Phenytoin (Dilantin) may be used for a longer period if the patient has a prior history of seizures or DTs.
3. Multivitamin supplement.
   a. Multivitamin supplements usually are given, at least for the first 3 to 5 days.
   b. Thiamine, 1 g every day is usually given, along with other B-complex vitamins.
   c. Patients may not have been eating a balanced diet for a long period and may have nervous system involvement.

**BOX 19-2 Protocol for Withdrawal From Alcohol Using Librium**

50 mg q 3 hr PRN for the first 24 hr
50 mg q 6 hr PRN for the next 24 hr
50 mg q 8 hr PRN for the next 24 hr

4. Antiemetics, such as Tigan or Phenergan, should be used PRN.
5. Antacids should be used for stomach discomfort as needed.
6. Antidiarrheals, such as Kaopectate or Lomotil (with serious diarrhea), should be used as needed.

The specific medication used may differ from setting to setting. However, one concept that is important for the nurse to remember is that many alcoholics need to receive medication for safe and effective detoxification. Medication should be given at the first sign of withdrawal symptoms.[26] There is no reason for alcoholics to suffer needlessly because health professionals may feel that they deserve to suffer or to be punished because "they did it to themselves." In actuality, detoxification can be dangerous and requires diligent observation by the nurse. Medication should be used freely in the first several days of treatment.

Treatment of DTs consists of the use of tranquilizing drugs, such as chlordiazepoxide or diazepam, and sedatives, such as paraldehyde given rectally, intramuscularly, or orally. High-caloric and high-vitamin diets may have to be given by nasogastric tube. The patient must be protected from physical injury and observed carefully for signs of cardiac failure. If at all possible, restraints should be avoided, because they increase agitation.

## Treatment

It is important for the medical-surgical nurse caring for the patient undergoing detoxification from drugs or alcohol to monitor the patient's vital signs as an indication of the level of withdrawal. Generally, vital signs are monitored every 2 to 4 hours for the first several days. A brief neurological assessment ("neuro checks") is done at the same time. Keeping accurate documentation of intake and output is important.

The nurse also provides a protective environment, especially for the first several days of detoxification. The patient is encouraged to begin participation in individual and group activities when able.

It is important for the nurse to be aware of safety needs of the alcoholic patient. Because of the effects of alcohol or other drugs, the person may become violent and attempt to hurt himself or herself or others. The behavior of the person may be erratic and unpredictable. In rare instances, restraints may have to be used until the person passes through the detoxification process. Side rails are also important to prevent the patient from falling out of bed. If the patient has a history of seizures, the side rails should be padded.

Because alcohol withdrawal may cause vivid and frightening visual or auditory hallucinations or other mental problems, it is important to remove items from the patient's area that could be harmful or destructive, including matches and sharp objects. The room of the patient should be adjacent to the nursing station for ease of observation.

## Diet

Many alcoholics enter treatment with a history of poor nutritional habits. They may have received as much as a third of their daily intake of calories from alcohol. They often have been too intoxicated to eat or have had no appetite for normal food. Also, alcohol is the most common cause of **acute gastritis,** which can result in severe vomiting, contributing to poor nutrition. Often, the person has consumed many calories from alcohol but has received no nutritional protein or other nutrients. In the initial detoxification period, diet is as tolerated, including encouraging liberal fluids. Intravenous fluids are usually not necessary. As the condition of the patient improves, appetite usually improves. The emphasis is on three well-balanced meals a day, with free access to snacks. Many patients find that they crave candy and other sources of sugar during this initial period. Usually this is not discouraged, because withdrawal from alcohol is the first priority.

Patients usually benefit from an assessment by a nutritionist or dietitian. Education about the importance of improved nutrition is essential.

If the patient has developed liver involvement with cirrhosis as a result of his or her alcoholism, dietary modification may be necessary. The reader is referred to Chapter 42 for further information about cirrhosis.

## Activity

The alcoholic patient is encouraged to be up as tolerated. In the first several days of withdrawal, stimulation may need to be minimized. It is important for the nurse to be aware of safety concerns of the alcoholic patient. The gait may be ataxic, leading to an increased risk of falls. Because of the risk of falls, side rails should be used while the patient is in bed. As the patient becomes stable, he or she is encouraged to be up most of the day and to take part in unit activities.

## Referral/Consultation

In some settings, the nurse assumes responsibility for making referrals to other services. Persons experiencing detoxification from drugs and alcohol are commonly referred to a psychologist, chemical dependency counselor, and dietitian. The physician and the nurse working in collaboration may recommend the consultation services of a neurologist and a psychiatrist. It is important to consider the importance of transferring the patient to a drug or alcohol treatment program. This may be on either an inpatient or outpatient basis and is discussed later in this chapter (see p. 508).

Critical pathways (also referred to as "collaborative care paths" or "care maps") have been developed in some inpatient and outpatient settings to guide both medical and nursing management. These critical pathways are collaboratively developed along time lines and include the information described previously for specific hours, days, or visits. Pertinent information about discharge planning and patient teaching to be implemented at specified times is also included. Because the nurse has a major role in these two aspects of care, these are discussed under Nursing Management (p. 498). A sample of the critical pathway for the patient undergoing detoxification from alcohol is included at the end of this chapter (see p. 514). A nursing care plan for this patient is also included on p. 516.

## Rehabilitation

The object of all treatment is to assist patients to stop drinking alcohol. When alcoholics do stop drinking, they can never take even a single drink without serious danger of relapsing. Studies have tried to demonstrate that alcoholics may be taught to control their drinking or to become so-called social drinkers, but this has not been substantiated. Alcoholics who are not currently drinking are never considered cured, only in recovery. Various methods of long-term treatment are used. These include the methods described below.

### Behavior modification

In the treatment of alcoholism, **behavior modification** methods may be attempted to discourage drinking behaviors. The best-known aversive agent used is disulfiram (Antabuse), which blocks the enzymatic action necessary to metabolize alcohol. Taken on a regular basis, the drug causes symptoms of nausea, vomiting, palpitations, and general prostration in the person who takes even a small sip of alcohol. The person is then conditioned to avoid alcohol. Disulfiram is usually used as an adjunct to other therapy. Sometimes it is also useful to provide a somewhat forced period of sobriety for an alcoholic who is unable to abstain in any other way.

### Group therapy

Much of the goal of group therapy with the alcoholic is to enable the person to see the relationship between the use of alcohol and the negative consequences that have occurred in his or her life. This in one sense is also a form of behavior modification. When the alcoholic becomes sober, he or she can see that many negative consequences and problems are no longer present.

Many alcoholics are socially isolated, and group therapy may assist the person to begin to relate to others in a caring and supportive environment. The group members can help the person look realistically at issues that are still a concern in recovery.

Associating with people who drink or use drugs should be discouraged for the newly recovering person. They may need assistance in planning ways of meeting new people with whom they can form more healthful relationships.

An important part of the treatment of the alcoholic is positive reinforcement. This usually occurs in the context of interpersonal relationships with the counselors and nurses, as well as with the other patients. Caring, emotional support and encouragement are very important. Because relapse in common, the dynamics of this relationship should be explored. Relapse and how to prevent it should be addressed by the patient's counselor or the nurse.

### Self-help groups

Alcoholics Anonymous (AA) is a group of self-acknowledged alcoholics whose aim is to stay sober and to help other alcoholics gain sobriety. There are AA groups that meet regularly in most communities. Meetings are of various types. Open meetings may be attended by anyone, not just the alcoholic. Closed meetings are limited to persons who are alcoholic. There are "lead" meetings, in which a recovering alcoholic tells his or her personal story of alcoholism, or meetings in which the members present discuss a topic. There are meetings in most communities for women only, men only, gay persons, young people, and, in larger communities, the deaf. There is no charge for attendance at the meetings—a free-will offering is usually taken.

Local groups are sometimes listed in the telephone directory, and larger communities publish directories of meetings for distribution. A phone call to AA (often the central office) will bring help in the form of telephone conversation, or an AA member will visit the alcoholic desiring help.

In some communities there is a reluctance on the part of AA members to have persons with other addictions attend meetings. This is partly because of lack of information about the disease of chemical dependence; it is also based partly on fear. With improved methods of diagnosing drug abuse and alcoholism, especially among younger persons, many AA groups are faced with younger people who have not suffered the same number or kind of consequences that the older members may have.

The AA philosophy focuses on the opportunity for the alcoholic to share personal experiences of alcohol abuse and control. Participation in AA may or may not be accompanied by the participation of the patient in other treatment modalities. AA has the highest success rate of any treatment program. The success of AA has led to the formation of other groups that share the same 12 step spiritual approach (see Box 19-3). These groups include Al-Anon, Families Anonymous, Narcotics Anonymous, Overeaters Anonymous, Emotions Anonymous, Cocaine Anonymous, and Gamblers Anonymous.

Many communities have alcohol clinics where medical and psychiatric help is available. In addition, many industries have employee assistance programs (EAPs) to aid impaired employees. Treatment centers that offer a variety of inpatient and outpatient programs are also more readily available now than ever before. Information on alcoholism and programs for alcoholics and others are available for interested individuals and groups.

**BOX 19-3 Twelve Steps of Alcoholics Anonymous**

1. We admitted we were powerless over alcohol—that our lives had become unmanageable.
2. Came to believe that a power greater than ourselves could restore us to sanity.
3. Made a decision to turn our will and our lives over to the care of God as we understood Him.
4. Made a searching and fearless moral inventory of ourselves.
5. Admitted to God, to ourselves, and to another human being the exact nature of our wrongs.
6. Were entirely ready to have God remove all these defects of character.
7. Humbly asked Him to remove our shortcomings.
8. Made a list of all persons we had harmed, and became willing to make amends to them all.
9. Made direct amends to such people whenever possible, except when to do so would injure them or others.
10. Continued to take personal inventory and when we were wrong promptly admitted it.
11. Sought through prayer and meditation to improve our conscious contact with God as we understood Him, praying only for knowledge of His will for us and the power to carry that out.
12. Having had a spiritual awakening as a result of these steps, we tried to carry this message to alcoholics, and to practice these principles in all our affairs.

From *Alcoholics Anonymous,* New York, 1976, Alcoholics Anonymous World Sources.

### Promoting Rehabilitation

Some persons still believe that it is only when alcoholic patients truly desire and seek help with their alcohol problem that treatment is useful. This is true in some cases, but, often by the time an alcoholic person seeks help, he or she has lost almost everything.[30] Recently, there has been emphasis on the use of a process called **intervention** to assist the alcoholic to receive help. Part of the reason for intervention is that the disease of alcoholism causes delusions or impairs judgment that keeps harmfully dependent persons locked into self-destructive patterns.

Interventions are *planned confrontations* by individuals who care about the person. It is important to realize that the intervention must be done by a person experienced in organizing and carrying out an intervention. Interventions can be problematic and even dangerous if carried out by someone who is not trained and experienced in this area. Rules for conducting interventions have been summarized as follows[14,29]:

1. Persons meaningful to the person must present the facts or data. The most meaningful person may be the employer or a family member.
2. The data presented should be specific and descriptive of events that have happened or conditions that exist.
3. The tone of the confrontation should not be judgmental.
4. The chief evidence should be tied directly to drinking, whenever possible.
5. The evidence of behavior should be presented in some detail and very explicitly.
6. The goal of the intervention is to have the alcoholic see and accept reality so that the need for help can be accepted.
7. The choices available for treatment should be offered. If possible, immediate treatment should be offered—for example, a bed in a treatment center can be reserved before the intervention, and the employer should stipulate that a condition to the employee's maintaining his or her job is immediate admission to the facility.

## NURSING MANAGEMENT

### ♦ ASSESSMENT

Both subjective and objective data are important to assess in the patient with alcoholism. The nurse gains information from interviewing and observing, as well as reviewing information from written sources, laboratory studies, and data from family or significant others. The nurse is reminded that two cardinal symptoms of the untreated alcoholic are denial and delusion. Therefore the information gathered from the patient may not always be accurate, and it is helpful to validate it with a family member or friend. It is often helpful for the nurse to verbalize the dangers of denying or minimizing drug/alcohol use.

The nurse should also be aware of her or his own attitude toward the alcoholic patient and any impact that may have on the interview. Despite a variety of symptoms and the tendency of the alcoholic to be vague about the amount of alcohol used, diagnosis by clinical interview is usually accurate.

### Subjective Data

Data to be collected to assess the patient with alcoholism include the following:

- Normal using or drinking patterns
- Date and time of last use or drink
- Substances used
- Quantity used
- Past history of blackouts, tremors, hallucinations, or DTs
- Past periods of abstinence/sobriety
- Normal dietary pattern
- Legal problems
- Family problems
- Occupational problems
- Family history of alcoholism
- Other medications used (mood altering and over the counter)
- Use of multiple physicians

The first five questions are important in all settings; the others may be asked at the discretion of the nurse.

## Objective Data

Data to be collected to assess the patient with alcoholism include the following:

- Abnormal response to preoperative medication, anesthetics, or sedatives
- Presence of tremors (usually worse in the morning)
- Nausea and/or vomiting, persistent complaints of GI distress
- Abnormal laboratory findings
- Symptoms of vitamin deficiency (pellagra or polyneuropathy)
- Body weight in relation to height
- Mental functioning
- Memory loss
- General behavior (e.g., may be argumentative and loud or depressed and withdrawn)
- Vital signs
- Presence of ascites
- Positive blood alcohol or urine alcohol level
- Petechiae

# ♦ NURSING DIAGNOSES

Nursing diagnoses are determined from analysis of patient data. Nursing diagnoses for the person with alcoholism may include but are not limited to the following:

| Diagnostic Title | Possible Etiologic Factors |
|---|---|
| Airway clearance, ineffective | Fatigue, infection, trauma, decreased consciousness |
| Breathing pattern, ineffective | Neuromuscular impairment |
| Thought processes, impaired | Alcohol- or drug-induced dementia |
| Injury, high risk for | Sensory deficits, lack of awareness of environmental hazards |
| Infection, high risk for | Decreased nutrition, decreased immune response |
| Fluid volume deficit, actual or high risk for | Decreased fluid intake, abnormal fluid loss |
| Temperature, high risk for altered body | Dehydration, sedation |
| Sleep pattern disturbance | Pain/discomfort related to withdrawal of substance being abused |
| Anxiety | Change in health status/role functioning |
| Activity intolerance | Generalized weakness |
| Mobility, impaired physical | Decreased strength and endurance, perceptual/cognitive impairment |
| Nutrition, altered; less than body requirements | Anorexia, inability to obtain food |
| Powerlessness | Inability to control alcoholism or drug addiction |
| Self-esteem disturbance | Inability to hold job, do necessary tasks; altered thought processes |
| Hopelessness | Loss of beliefs |
| Denial, ineffective | Unable to admit impact of alcoholism or drug abuse on life pattern |
| Grieving, anticipatory | Loss of use of alcohol or other drugs |
| Coping, ineffective (individual) | Maturational crises |
| Adjustment, impaired | Disability requiring change in life-style |
| Family processes, altered | Situational crisis of alcoholism or other drug abuse |
| Knowledge deficit | Lack of exposure/recall, cognitive limitation |
| Noncompliance | Alcoholic life patterns |
| Spiritual distress | Questioning of personal, spiritual values |
| Social isolation | Unaccepted social behaviors |

# ♦ EXPECTED PATIENT OUTCOMES

Expected patient outcomes for the patient with alcoholism may include but are not limited to the following:

1. Maintains a patent airway.
2. Maintains effective breathing pattern.
3. Improves thought process.
4. Avoids injury.
5. Remains free of infection.
6. Maintains adequate hydration.
7. Maintains normal body temperature.
8. Maintains normal sleep pattern.
9. Demonstrates decreased anxiety.
10. Demonstrates improved activity tolerance.
11. Achieves optimal mobility.
12. Maintains optimal nutrition.
13. Verbalizes powerlessness over drugs or alcohol.
14. Verbalizes improved self-esteem.
15. Verbalizes a sense of hope.
16. Admits the impact that alcohol or other drug abuse has on life pattern.
17. Verbalizes grief over not being able to drink.
18. Patient and family demonstrate improved and effective coping mechanisms.
19. Verbalizes knowledge of substances to avoid.
20. Patient and family verbalize plan to improve family processes.
21. Patient and family verbalize knowledge of disease and treatment.
22. Abstains from alcohol and other drugs.
23. Has decreased spiritual distress.
24. Demonstrates improved social interactions.

# ♦ INTERVENTIONS

## ➡ Managing Critical Care

The patient withdrawing from alcohol is acutely ill and should be placed in an area where he or she can receive intensive nursing care. Discussion of care for these patients follows.

### Maintaining a patent airway

The patient withdrawing from alcohol is prone to aspiration because of nausea and a decreased mental status and level of consciousness. The head of the bed should be elevated at least 30 degrees, and the patient should be encouraged to cough to clear the airway of secretions.

If the patient is unable to clear his or her own airway, suctioning will be necessary. A suction machine should be kept at the bedside or nearby. Fluids should not be offered by mouth until the patient is fully alert.

**Maintaining an effective breathing pattern**

Because the *effects of alcohol* can cause *respiratory depression,* the patient should be assessed for *apnea* or other *breathing difficulties.* Medications that will further compromise respirations, such as morphine, are not given. If narcotic use is suspected, Narcan may be administered. When Valium is used to control DTs, flumazenil (Romazicon) should be availble. The patient should also be encouraged to turn, cough, and breathe deeply at frequent intervals to prevent atelectasis.

**Improving thought processes**

The person experiencing alcohol withdrawal or DTs may have altered thought processes. This can manifest in such symptoms as disorientation, hallucinations, and paranoia. It is important to reorient the patient as needed and to reassure family members that mentation usually clears as the symptoms of withdrawal end. If this does not occur, the patient needs to be evaluated for Wernicke-Korsakoff's syndrome (see p. 488).

The nurse can assist in improving thought processes by medicating the patient liberally with Librium or a similar drug as ordered. The altered thought processes that occur in detoxification indicate the need for aggressive treatment. It may also be helpful to keep the patient from excessive stimulation, which can lead to increased confusion. Visitors are restricted. Lights are kept low, and every effort is made to keep the immediate environment as quiet as possible. Vitamin therapy is given to treat deficiencies, especially of the B vitamins.

**Preventing injury**

The alcoholic who has been drinking is at high risk for injury from trauma. Studies have shown that almost a third of all emergency trauma cases involve alcohol. Half of all traffic fatalities and victims of burns have been intoxicated. The cost of treatment of injuries related to the use of alcohol (both to the person, as well as innocent victims) runs into the billions.

In the initial withdrawal period, the alcoholic may be at risk for seizure activity. Seizure precautions should be taken, including keeping a padded tongue blade at the bedside. Medication is given as ordered to prevent DTs. Side rails should be padded and kept up. The patient is observed closely for signs of impending problems. See Chapter 57 for a more detailed discussion of seizures.

The nurse should also realize that the person experiencing DTs may become violent and inflict injury to himself or herself or others. If the person becomes so agitated as to pose a risk of harm to self or others, it may be necessary to place the person in leather restraints.

**Preventing infection**

As alcoholics continue to drink, their health deteriorates. They may suffer from a variety of infections, including tuberculosis. It is important to observe the patient for signs of infection and administer antibiotics as ordered. The patient experiencing detoxification should be encouraged to cough and breathe deeply to prevent atelectasis. The position of the patient who is unable to respond is changed frequently to prevent atelectasis and pressure sores.

Homeless alcohol abusers are at substantially increased risk of contracting tuberculosis. The nurse should monitor the patient for night sweats, late afternoon elevation of temperature, or other symptoms of tuberculosis. Unfortunately, patients with early tuberculosis are usually asymptomatic, and the disease is often well advanced before it is diagnosed.

Good nutrition and adequate hydration are essential parts of the treatment of all infections. If skin infections are present, appropriate treatment is begun. The nurse should also be aware that some alcoholics, especially the homeless, may have lice or scabies.

**Maintaining adequate hydration**

In the initial period of detoxification, the alcoholic patient may suffer from nausea and vomiting and may require intravenous fluids until nausea and vomiting cease. It may also be helpful to administer an antiemetic, such as Tigan. As the amount of alcohol in the body is reduced, the patient will be better able to tolerate fluids. The patient should be educated to drink water and juices, rather than caffeinated beverages or fluid that is high in sugar content, which will cause dehydration secondary to increased urination. Most treatment centers attempt to restrict the use of beverages containing caffeine, because of its stimulating effect.

**Maintaining normal body temperature**

Alcoholics, especially those who are homeless, are often victims of hypothermia. Alcohol ingestion makes the person unaware of temperature extremes, and in winter some alcoholics have frozen to death while sleeping on the street.

If a patient experiencing withdrawal from alcohol also has *hypothermia,* his or her temperature should be monitored frequently. The extremities should be checked for signs of frostbite and resulting ischemia. Extra blankets should be used to assist in warming the patient. If, on the other hand, the patient's temperature is elevated or the patient is diaphoretic, an assessment of the cause should be determined so that appropriate measures can be taken to maintain body temperature.

## Managing Rehabilitative Care

**Encouraging normal sleep pattern**

It is very common for the patient going through withdrawal to have insomnia. It may take several months for sleep to return to a normal pattern. Regular physical activity and establishment of a daily routine may help. What is most important is not to use sleeping medication, because the alcoholic is at risk of becoming dependent on the medication. Relaxation tapes and decreasing caffeine use may be helpful in inducing sleep.

**Decreasing anxiety**

Anxiety and depression are common in alcoholics. The patient is encouraged to share concerns and feelings and to learn to deal with anxious feelings. Generally, medications are not used to treat anxiety because of the risk of the person's developing cross-dependence on them. Relaxation exercises and techniques are taught and practiced.

Many persons benefit from a regular exercise program—such as walking, jogging, or swimming, which may help to relieve tension and decrease anxiety. The patient is encouraged to keep a "feeling log" that may be helpful in learning to identify specific feelings and what triggers them. Anxiety usually decreases as long-term sobriety is attained. If not, psychiatric help may be necessary.

**Promoting activity**

The person entering treatment may be weak because of poor nutrition, as well as because of complications of the alcoholism. As the withdrawal from alcohol occurs, strength improves. Many alcoholics will not have a regular program of physical exercise, and for this reason most inpatient treatment programs include daily periods of physical conditioning. Patients recovering from alcoholism are urged to maintain a regular exercise program after discharge.

**Promoting mobility**

As the patient's general condition improves and he or she grows stronger, emphasis can be given to improving mobility. Some will need assistance to develop an exercise program to strengthen specific muscle groups. A physical therapist can assist the patient with appropriate exercises to achieve this goal. The nurse needs to know what exercises have been recommended and the number of times they should be repeated daily, so that they can be incorporated into the patient's daily schedule.

**Promoting optimal nutrition**

Many alcoholics enter treatment with a history of poor nutrition. They may have received as much as a third of their daily intake of calories from alcohol. They often may have been too intoxicated to eat or have had no appetite for normal food. Also, alcohol is the most common cause of acute gastritis, which can result in severe vomiting, contributing to poor nutrition. Often addicted persons consume many "empty calories" and are malnourished. Some have chosen to use money for alcohol or drugs, rather than for food.

In the initial detoxification period, the diet is as tolerated, including liberal fluids. As the condition of the alcoholic improves, the appetite usually improves also. Then the emphasis is on three well-balanced meals a day, with free access to snacks. Many patients find that they crave sugar during this initial period, and it is not discouraged because withdrawal from alcohol is the first priority.

Patients usually benefit from assessment by a nutritionist or dietitian. Education about the importance of improved nutrition is essential. If the patient has liver involvement with cirrhosis, dietary restriction of protein is usually necesary. The reader is referred to the section on cirrhosis in Chapter 42 for further information.

**Accepting powerlessness**

The alcoholic person needs to accept that he or she is powerless over alcohol. This is the basis of almost all treatment approaches. It may be a difficult concept for alcoholics to understand—that through becoming powerless they achieve the ability to stay sober. Attendance at Alcoholics Anonymous meetings, group therapy, and discussions with other alcoholics all can help with this. Alcoholics need to understand that taking even one drink of alcohol can start them on the process of active drinking again. *Inherent in accepting this powerlessness is the realization that they have no control over alcohol, but that it controls them.*

**Increasing self-esteem**

It is important for these patients to build positive self-esteem, enabling them to acknowledge that they are worthwhile. This is important because many alcoholics continue to drink to cover their feelings of inadequacy and lack of self-worth. Positive self-esteem is important for continued recovery.

An important part of treatment of alcoholism leading to positive self-worth is positive reinforcement. This usually occurs in the context of interpersonal relationships with nurses and other staff, as well as with other patients. Caring, emotional support and encouragement are very important. This is demonstrated within the context of honesty and also by pointing out negative behaviors, defense mechanisms, and problems.

**Decreasing hopelessness**

Many alcoholics enter treatment with a great sense of hopelessness. They may have attempted treatment before without success. They may also feel that they will never be able to stop drinking, and that they will never achieve sobriety. In addition, many alcoholics drink to block their feelings of hopelessness, especially about the loss of family and friends and perhaps the loss of a job.

*Instilling hope* in the alcoholic patient *takes time.* Often, the most important treatment is the contact the person has with other recovering alcoholics. Listening to recovering persons "lead" a group meeting will help to instill a beginning sense of hope. Seeing other persons who once were worse off than they are now may help them to see the chance for recovery.

**Decreasing denial**

One of the real challenges in working with the alcoholic patient is facilitating the *breaking down of denial.* The patient characteristically is not aware of the havoc that his or her alcohol abuse has caused. Group therapy is used to enable the person to see the relationship between the use of alcohol and the negative consequences it has on his or her life. When the alcoholic becomes sober, many of the problems that have occurred in his or her life can be seen clearly for the first time.

Nurses working with these patients need to assist in pointing out areas of concern and consequences that the person has suffered as a result of alcoholism.

**Facilitating grieving**

Many alcoholics will actually go through a *grieving process for the loss of the alcohol.* For the recovering person, the loss and sadness over what has been given up (alcohol) can be quite intense. Practically all persons start drinking or using drugs because it is socially acceptable and fun. No one plans to become addicted and trapped by the compulsion to drink. For some, giving up alcohol may also mean the necessity of giving up their drinking friends. The alcoholic may be angry about the changes required and the realization that drinking is out of the question. *Grieving is a natural part of recovery because it implies an emotional response to loss.* The nurse can facilitate this grieving by encouraging the patient to talk about feelings and express the grief or anger. Letting the alcoholic know that this grief is normal and expected is helpful.

Depression may occur as the alcoholic recognizes and accepts the illness. Although the decision to stay sober will bring relief and assurance in the long run, alcoholics will have periods when the desire for a drink is very strong and they may become discouraged, even though they are able, with support, to resist the temptation to drink.

**Facilitating coping**

The patient will need assistance in learning to deal with life without the crutch of alcohol or drugs. This includes helping them to find a sense of spirituality and perhaps become reconnected with a religious organization or leader. Decision making may be difficult at first, and the person may require support to look at options. Just because the person becomes sober does not mean that all problems will be gone.

Allowing the person to vent emotions and responding with empathy (not sympathy) may assist him or her in letting go of anger or resentment. If indicated, the nurse may suggest professional counseling for the alcoholic.

It is not uncommon for alcoholics to have problems with intimacy and sexuality. They need to learn to trust others and to risk becoming vulnerable with another person. Marriage counseling may be necessary to help a couple regain a healthy marriage, especially if there has been a long history of problems as a result of alcoholism or drug addiction. Family therapy should be discussed and encouraged.

**Facilitating adjustment**

It is often difficult for the alcoholic person to adjust to the diagnosis of alcoholism, especially if alcoholism is seen as morally wrong. Denial that alcohol is a problem may be part of the difficulty. Denial is dicussed later in this chapter. The patient is encouraged to focus on one day at a time and to not consider having to stay sober forever. The patient is educated about the disease concept of alcoholism, which usually helps with adjustment. Attendance at *Alcoholics Anonymous (AA)* meetings is usually required as a part of both inpatient and outpatient treatment programs. Through daily assignments the person is helped to learn about himself or herself in relation to alcoholism.

Psychotherapy cannot help the patient who continues to drink. It can, however, be helpful as a part of the treatment program. Emotional problems that occur as part of the drinking do not automatically disappear when the person stops drinking. Some patients have problems that are unrelated to their drinking and need to gain insight about them. Therapy directed toward personal insight has been found to be effective only after the patient attains stable sobriety.

**Improving family processes**

As the alcoholic becomes more involved in the destructive process of the disease, the family also suffers. As a result, when an alcoholic family receives help, the family processes are usually in a state of dysfunction. Divorce may have occurred or is being discussed. Spouses, parents, and children have lost respect for and trust in the alcoholic. Other family members may also have become very enabling and codependent.[3]

It is unrealistic to think that family processes can be changed in a short period. Treatment of the family along with the alcoholic is important, not only to help the alcoholic recover, but also to allow the family to work through feelings of fear, distrust, and anger. Adult family members should be referred to Al-Anon, a 12-step support group for persons whose lives are affected by someone who is alcoholic. Children may be referred to Ala-Teen. Adult children of an alcoholic may benefit from referral to an ACA meeting.

The patient and family often need additional counseling to help them grow together and not apart. In spite of this, the divorce rate among couples where one member is an alcoholic is high, even after the alcoholic achieves sobriety.[3]

**Guidelines for Teaching the Alcoholic Patient**

- Disease concept of alcoholism
- Medical aspects of the disease, including complications
- Need for continued abstinence
- Importance of expressing feelings to stay sober
- Defense mechanisms
- Drugs to avoid
- Products that contain alcohol (for example, mouthwash and cough medicine)
- Importance of being honest with physician and dentist
- Signs and symptoms of impending relapse
- Importance of aftercare, including AA meetings

### Facilitating learning

Education about the disease of alcoholism is extremely important for the alcoholic and the family or significant others. See Guidelines box above for important topics that need to be covered. These persons also become sick in the midst of the alcoholic's becoming sicker and need understanding and education to help themselves and the alcoholic to recover.

Many over-the-counter drugs contain alcohol. Two examples of these are cough medicines and mouthwashes. The alcoholic also needs to know that the use of any mood-altering chemical may lead to relapse.

### Increasing compliance

The object of all treatment for alcoholism is to assist patients in achieving sobriety. When they do stop drinking, they are taught that they can never take one drink without the danger of relapse. In fact, the *most complicated and frustrating part of treatment is to prevent relapse.*

Some have suggested that alcoholics may be taught to become "social drinkers," but this has not been substantiated. Alcoholics who are currently not drinking are never considered cured, only recovering.

***Behavior modification may be used to discourage drinking behaviors.*** The best-known aversive agent is disulfiram (Antabuse), which blocks the enzymatic action necessary to metabolize alcohol. If the person drinks, Antabuse will cause nausea, vomiting, palpitations, and general ill feeling with even a small sip of alcohol. This conditions the person to avoid alcohol. Disulfiram is usually used with other therapy and may help the alcoholic attain a period of sobriety so that other therapy may be effective.

### Decreasing spiritual distress

Many alcoholics enter treatment spiritually bankrupt. Generally, they have been cut off from nurturing relationships with others, with self, and with a higher being. The person is forced, because of defense mechanisms, into a grandiose position of becoming a God of sorts. As the disease progresses, values decrease. Many persons may also see God as a punishing force who could never forgive the person for things done while he or she was drinking.

If the patient desires, the service of a chaplain should be offered. The patient should be educated about the difference in the spirituality talked about in AA and religion. As mentioned previously, some persons may have difficulty with the concept of a higher power or God. They can be encouraged to use a power of the group as a higher power until they are able to accept a sense of spirituality.

### Decreasing social isolation

The social isolation experienced by alcoholics can best be handled in a support group. The best-known group is *Alcoholics Anonymous (AA),* which is described in another part of this chapter. The AA philosophy focuses on the opportunity for the alcoholic to share personal experiences of abuse and control. Participation in AA may or may not be accompanied by the participation of the patient in other types of treatment. The success of AA has led to the formation of other groups that share the same 12-step approach.[1]

The chemically-dependent person may need to develop a completely different group of friends in order to stay sober and straight. This initially adds to the sense of isolation. As new group support is found, the social isolation usually improves. Also, it takes time for an alcoholic or drug addict to develop comfort in social situations without the substance he or she was using. This also improves with time.

## ✵ SPECIAL CONSIDERATIONS FOR CARE OF THE GERONTOLOGIC PATIENT

Alcoholism and drug abuse are problems in elderly persons. However, children or other concerned persons often are reluctant to help the elderly person seek assistance. The elderly person may have been a "closet drinker," hiding his or her use from others. Also, elderly persons may have abused drugs or alcohol for years, with the accumulated results of their use becoming evident as they age.[14,18]

Nurses working with elderly persons on medical-surgical nursing units should be aware of the possibility of substance abuse as a reason for confusion, falls, or other injuries. Other complications associated with alcohol abuse such as cirrhosis of the liver may be evident and be more severe than in the younger, healthier person.

The principles of treatment of substance abuse for the elderly person remain the same as for those younger in age. The issue of loneliness has been found to be a prime reason cited for the use of drugs and alcohol among elderly persons.

## ♦ EVALUATION

Evaluation of the patient with chemical dependency involves input from the patient, as well as family members or significant others. To evaluate the effectiveness of nursing interventions, compare patient behaviors with those stated in the expected patient outcomes. Successful achievement of patient outcomes for the patient with alcohol dependency is indicated by the following:

1. Able to clear own airway of secretions.
2. Has respiratory rate within normal range of 16-20/min.
3. Able to think more clearly.
4. Completes detoxification without incurring an injury.
5. Is free of infection.
6. Has good skin turgor, and mucous membranes are moist and pink.
7. Has body temperature that remains within normal range.
8. Able to sleep between 6 and 8 hours nightly and feels refreshed on awakening.
9. Able to sit or lie quietly without exhibiting nervousness.
10. Able to carry out own activities of daily living (ADLs) without assistance.
11. Has optimal mobility.
12. Eats a well-balanced diet, including foods from all groups in the food guide pyramid.
13. Abstains from alcohol and other drugs.
14. Demonstrates improved self-esteem by speaking positively about self.
15. Able to discuss plans for the future that reflect hopefulness.
16. Able to discuss his or her chemical dependency and plans to remain sober.
17. Able to verbalize grief about no longer being able to drink or use other drugs.
18. Demonstrates improved coping mechanisms, such as becoming less angry and frustrated when things do not go as planned.
19. Adjusts well to changes in life-style.
20. Patient and family verbalize that they were aware of problems in their interactions and are working to improve them.
21. Patient and family discuss chemical dependency and substances to be avoided.
22. Remains sober, attends aftercare meetings, and follows the 12-step program.
23. States that he or she is more comfortable acknowledging dependence on a greater power.
24. Interacts more comfortably with other persons.

# DRUG ABUSE

Because alcohol is in itself a drug, alcoholism and drug abuse are not mutually exclusive. There is an increasing tendency for persons who abuse substances to mix a variety of drugs and alcohol. Much of the information already covered in the section on alcoholism also pertains to drug abuse.

The history of nonmedical drug use is thousands of years old. As early as 5000 BC, the Sumerians referred to a "joy plant." This is believed to be a reference to the opium poppy plant. Since then, drugs have played a significant role in almost every culture. Even the results of historic events may have been altered, because the persons involved were under the influence of drugs. Different drugs have assumed importance in different periods of history. For instance, currently cocaine is more problematic than ever before. The newest problem drugs are the so-called designer drugs, many of which were unheard of several years ago.[6]

## ETIOLOGY/EPIDEMIOLOGY

In recent years, drug abuse has risen sharply. There are no reliable statistics on drug abusers, and experts disagree as to what actually constitutes drug abuse. Some include repeated use of any drug, whereas others limit it to those drugs that, used repeatedly, lead to habituation or addiction.[19]

Use of drugs has increased among adolescents and young adults. Drugs are readily available in most elementary and secondary schools and on most college campuses.

The terms *habituation* and *addiction* have been used to define the nature and extent of drug use. Drug **habituation** includes repeated use of a drug to a point where there is psychologic dependence. Drug **addiction** involves craving, psychologic dependence, and physical dependence. The latter includes development of *tolerance* for increasing dosages of the drug and the appearance of withdrawal symptoms on cessation of use of the drug. *Drug dependence* is another term that is used. This refers to a psychologic or physical dependence on a drug that is taken regularly.[22]

According to the Controlled Substance Act of 1971, there are five basic kinds of drugs:

1. Stimulants
2. Depressants
3. Hallucinogens
4. Narcotics
5. Cannabis

To this list could be added deliriants, such as glue and paint thinner. Examples of drugs in each of these classifications are presented in Table 19-7. Two drugs that are officially classed as stimulants are discussed separately. These are tobacco and caffeine.

## SPECIFIC DRUGS

### Stimulants

**Stimulants** are both natural and synthetic drugs that have a strong stimulating effect on the central nervous

**TABLE 19-7 Effects of Mood-Altering Drugs**

| DRUG | TOLERANCE | PHYSICAL DEPENDENCE | PSYCHOLOGIC DEPENDENCE |
|---|---|---|---|
| Narcotics | High | High | High |
| Barbiturates | Moderate | High | High |
| Methaqualone | Moderate | High | High |
| Tranquilizers | High | Moderate | High |
| Amphetamine | High | Low to moderate | High |
| Cocaine | Moderate | Low to moderate | High |
| Lysergic acid diethylamide (LSD) | Moderate | None | Moderate |
| Mescaline | Low | None | Moderate |
| Phencyclidine (PCP) | Low | None | Low |
| Marijuana | Low | None | Moderate |

system. They are accompanied by a feeling of alertness and self-confidence. Drugs included in this category are (1) amphetamines and (2) cocaine.

### Amphetamines

**Etiology/epidemiology.** Amphetamines and amphetamine-like drugs are synthetic psychoactive drugs that are available legally by prescription. They are available in both capsule and tablet forms. A powdered or crystalline-like form of amphetamine is methamphetamine, which must be injected. It is no longer legally produced in an injectable form.

Medical uses of amphetamines may include the treatment of narcolepsy, obesity, fatigue, and depression. Ritalin, an amphetamine-like drug, is used to treat children who are hyperactive. Common generic and brand names of amphetamines include dextroamphetamine (Dexedrine), methamphetamine (Methedrine), and amphetamine (Benzedrine).

Street names for amphetamines vary, but include the following:

**Street Names for Stimulants**

| | | |
|---|---|---|
| Pep pills | Ups | Meth |
| Dexies | Speed | Whites |
| Bennies | Crystal | |

**Pathophysiology.** Amphetamines are CNS stimulants. When swallowed or injected, they speed up the activity of the heart and brain. They dilate the pupil of the eye, increase the pulse rate, and elevate the blood pressure. The use of amphetamines also reduces fatigue, increases concentration, and decreases appetite. However, the feeling of alertness, often coupled with a sense of confidence and well-being, wears off, and the person experiences fatigue and depression, which may be extreme in nature.

Amphetamines have the potential to produce tolerance. The abrupt discontinuation of amphetamines usually does not produce physical withdrawal, although many persons have psychologic dependence on these drugs.

**BOX 19-4 Clinical Manifestations of the Use of Amphetamines**

1. Restlessness
2. Dizziness
3. Insomnia
4. Lack of appetite, dramatic weight loss
5. Diarrhea or constipation
6. Agitation and anxiety
7. Paranoia, paranoid psychosis
8. Cerebral hemorrhage
9. Myocardial infarction
10. Collapse from exhaustion

*Withdrawal often leads to profound depression and may lead to suicide.*

A summary of the clinical manifestations of amphetamine ingestion can be found in Box 19-4.

### Cocaine

**Etiology/epidemiology.** Cocaine is a psychoactive drug that comes from the leaves of the South American coca bush. Medical uses for cocaine include use as an anesthetic of choice for certain procedures and surgery involving the nose, throat, larynx, and lower respiratory passages. It may also be used as an ingredient in Brompton's solution, an oral medication that is used for terminal cancer patients.

Cocaine is used by sniffing, smoking, or injecting. When it is sniffed, or snorted, the effect of the drug is realized when the cocaine is absorbed through the mucous membranes of the nose. Cocaine may also be free-based. This is a process of heating the drug to separate it from whatever adulterants it may contain. When free base cocaine is injected, it produces a high that is more intense and more short-lived than when cocaine is smoked.

*Crack* is a mixture of cocaine and common baking soda and water. It is smoked, much like freebasing, and creates an intoxication more intense than cocaine alone.

Crack is a free base form of cocaine hydrochloride, so called because the cocaine has been separated from its hydrochloride base. It is called "crack" because of the characteristic crackling sound that is made when the crystals are heated. Cocaine powder is not smoked because heat destroys its effects. Crack is heat resistant and reaches the brain faster and in higher concentrations, producing a more intense euphoria within about 6 seconds.[12] The high is also more intense because crack contains as much as 90% pure cocaine, whereas cocaine hydrochloride may contain only 15% to 25% of pure cocaine. The feeling of exhilaration lasts a much shorter time, however—5 to 7 minutes in contrast with 30 minutes after using powdered cocaine. Crack is available

**BOX 19-5 Clinical Manifestations of the Use of Cocaine**

1. Stimulation of respiration and heart rate
2. Raising of blood pressure and blood sugar levels
3. Suppression of appetite
4. Dilation of the pupils
5. Constriction of certain blood vessels
6. Increase in levels of physical activity
7. Insomnia
8. Trembling
9. Sensations of extreme euphoria
10. Feelings of energy, power, confidence, and talkativeness

*There is a letdown effect of cocaine crash that occurs when the effect of the drug wears off.*

in crystal form and is considered to be even more addictive than other forms of cocaine.

Because it is usually less expensive than cocaine, crack has been readily available to less affluent persons. In addition, a recent trend is for heroin to be snorted with crack to prolong the high. The street names for cocaine are listed below.

**Street Names for Cocaine**

| | | |
|---|---|---|
| Blow | Flake | Superblow |
| Coke | Nose candy | Toot |
| Crack | Rock | White |
| Dust | Snow | White girl |

**Pathophysiology.** Cocaine acts as a CNS stimulant. It blocks the uptake or reabsorption mechanism of the neurotransmitters, thus prolonging the effects of norepinephrine and dopamine on the brain and peripheral nerves. It also breaks down neurotransmitters. The habitual use of cocaine eventually depletes the brain's supply of dopamine and norepinephrine.[12]

Because of the stimulation of the brain by cocaine, there is a surge in the systolic blood pressure with its use. This surge in blood pressure has been linked with sudden neurologic insults, including *subarachnoid hemorrhage. Cocaine use in high doses can precipitate fatal ventricular dysrhythmias, as well as seizures.*[5]

The use of cocaine during pregnancy causes constriction of the uterine blood vessels, leading to deprivation of oxygen and nutrients to the developing fetus. This increases the risk of spontaneous abortion during the first trimester and can cause premature delivery and premature separation of the placenta. It can also slow fetal growth and cause congenital abnormalities. Use during the first trimester of pregnancy can interfere with the formation of neurologic pathways of the brain of the fetus.[12] Cocaine has also been found to lead to in-utero brain hemorrhage and stroke.[5] Clinical manifestations resulting from the use of cocaine are listed in Box 19-5.

Chronic sniffing of cocaine can destroy the nasal tis-

**RESEARCH**

Lillie-Blanton M, Anthony J, Schuster C: Probing the meaning of racial/ethnic group comparisons in crack cocaine smoking, *JAMA* 269(8):993-997, 1993.

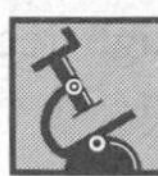

This study probed the meaning of reported racial and ethnic differences in the prevalence of crack cocaine smoking. It also attempted to estimate the degree to which crack cocaine smoking was associated with personal factors specific to race/ethnicity. 8814 individuals who resided within households in the United States were interviewed. Subjects were selected using a multistage area probability sampling of all residents aged 12 years and older. The findings provided evidence that, given similar social and environmental conditions, crack use does *not* strongly depend on race-specific (e.g, biologic) personal factors. The study also provided evidence that prevalence estimates unadjusted for social environmental risk factors may lead to misunderstanding about the role of race or ethnicity in the epidemiology of crack use.[20]

sues. Smoking it can cause lesions in the lungs. Tolerance and psychologic dependence can develop, and an overdose can cause convulsions, respiratory paralysis, and death. A cocaine psychosis that is characterized by a loss of pleasure, loss of orientation, hallucinations, insomnia, concern with minor details, stereotyped behavior, and an increased potential for violence occurs in some persons. Treatment with an antipsychotic medication may be necessary to relieve the symptoms.

Abrupt withdrawal from cocaine can lead to physical symptoms of withdrawal, especially if the cocaine was used on a daily basis. These symptoms include irritability, sleep disturbances, and cravings. See Research box above.

## Depressants

**Depressants** are synthetic drugs that have a depressant action on the CNS. Drugs included in this category are the following:

1. Sedatives and methaqualone
2. Barbiturates
3. Tranquilizers

### Sedatives and methaqualone

**Etiology/epidemiology.** Methaqualone is a nonbarbiturate sedative-hypnotic. It is the active ingredient in the drugs Quaalude and Mequin. It is available as a prescription drug but has also become a common and popular street drug. It is taken orally. Because of its nonsoluble nature, it cannot be injected.

**Common Street Names for Methaqualone**

| | |
|---|---|
| Ludes | Love drug |
| Soaps, soapers, or sopes | Wallbangers |
| 714s | Lemons |

Methaqualone was first made in the early 1950s as a treatment for malaria in India. In the 1960s it was used as a sedative in Europe; 1965 saw it manufactured in the United States. It was at first thought not to be addicting. Its use as a street drug began in the 1960s and 1970s. This drug is no longer available through legitimate channels, but it is available on the street.

**Pathophysiology.** Methaqualone is a CNS depressant that is unrelated to other sedatives or barbiturates. It slows the CNS and impairs coordination, walking, and talking. It also possesses anticonvulsant, anesthetic, and cough-suppressant effects. Its primary effect is drowsiness. If the user resists the sleep-inducing effects of the drug, he or she experiences a relaxed, mellow sense of well-being.

The repeated use of methaqualone produces tolerance, as well as physical and psychologic dependence. Withdrawal from the drug produces headache, fatigue, dizziness, nausea, anxiety, skin problems, abdominal cramps, seizures, and vomiting if the withdrawal is not medically supervised.

Overdoses occur when the CNS-depressing effects of the drug slow down the person's rate of breathing to the extent that consciousness is not possible. Most overdoses occur when the drug is combined with other drugs, such as alcohol, that potentiate its action. Symptoms of overdose include delirium, coma, restlessness, convulsions, and vomiting.[17]

Withdrawal from methaqualone requires the use of medication, which may include diazepam or phenobarbital.

### Barbiturates

**Etiology/epidemiology.** Barbiturates are synthetic drugs that are classified as "sedative hypnotics." They arise from barbituric acid. They are used medically to treat epilepsy and insomnia and to sedate patients before and during surgery. Barbiturates are also commonly used street drugs.

Barbiturates are taken by mouth (capsule or elixir), used as a suppository, or injected. They were first synthesized in the early 1900s by two German scientists. Currently about 10 derivatives of barbituric acid are in use.

There are many common names for barbiturates. The names usually refer to the drug type, the drug effect, the drug name, or the color of the particular capsule. The names are listed below.

**Common Street Names for Barbiturates**

| | |
|---|---|
| Yellow jacket (pentobarbital) | Barbs |
| Red devil (secobarbital) | Downs or downers |
| Phennie (phenobarbital) | Rainbows |
| Blue heaven or blue devil (amobarbital) | Blues |
| | Goof balls |

**BOX 19-6 Clinical Manifestations of the Use of Barbiturates**

1. Feeling of well-being
2. Euphoria
3. Relief from anxiety
4. Side effects, including difficulty in breathing, lethargy, allergic reactions, nausea, and dizziness

**Pathophysiology.** Barbiturates cause depression of the CNS, including slowing of physical and mental reflexes. The continued use of these drugs can cause physical and psychologic dependence, as well as tolerance.

Clinical manifestations of the use of barbiturates are listed in Box 19-6. Alcohol and other CNS depressants tend to potentiate the effects of barbiturates and can be very dangerous when used with them. Accidental overdoses are common. A person who is physically dependent on barbiturates will experience various withdrawal symptoms. Mild withdrawal includes irritability, restlessness, anxiety, and sleep disturbances. An extreme form of barbiturate withdrawal can be life threatening and includes symptoms of convulsions, delirium, and hyperpraxia. Detoxification includes appropriate medication, which may be a long-acting barbiturate given in diminishing dosages.

### Tranquilizers

**Etiology/epidemiology.** Minor tranquilizers are psychoactive drugs that are taken to reduce anxiety. They may also be used as a muscle relaxant. *They are the most commonly prescribed drugs in the world today.* Tranquilizers are available in prescription form in capsule, tablet, and liquid forms. Illicitly, they are sometimes injected. Common types of tranquilizers are those found in the benzodiazepine family and include the following:

1. Chlordiazepoxide
2. Diazepam (Valium)
3. Prazepam (Antrax or Vestran)
4. Oxazepam (Serax)
5. Lorazepam (Ativan)
6. Clorazepate (Tranxene)
7. Alprazolam (Xanax)

These drugs are relatively new; the first tranquilizer was developed in 1950. Diazepam was first marketed in 1963.

**Pathophysiology.** Minor tranquilizers slow the activities of the CNS. They also have anticonvulsant and muscle-relaxant properties and produce a sense of relaxed well-being. When the effects of the drug wear off, however, users frequently experience an increased level of anxiety. Tranquilizers cause physical and psychologic dependence, and tolerance to them can develop. Clinical

**BOX 19-7 Clinical Manifestations of the Use of Tranquilizers**

**SIDE EFFECTS INCLUDE THE FOLLOWING:**

1. Skin rash
2. Headache
3. Nausea
4. Impairment of sexual function
5. Dizziness
6. Light-headedness

**SIGNS OF OVERDOSE INCLUDE THE FOLLOWING:**

1. Sleepiness
2. Confusion
3. Loss of consciousness
4. Diminished reflexes

manifestations of the use of tranquilizers are listed in Box 19-7.

Withdrawal symptoms from minor tranquilizers often appear within 12 to 24 hours, especially if the use has been heavy and prolonged. These symptoms include anxiety, sweating, insomnia, vomiting, tremors, delirium, and seizures. The patient must be detoxified with a regimen of medication that is gradually decreased over time.

### Hallucinogens

**Hallucinogens** are natural and synthetic drugs that affect the mind and produce changes in perception and thinking. Included in this category is phencyclidine (PCP), which is discussed separately from the hallucinogens.

**Etiology/epidemiology.** Hallucinogens include lysergic acid diethylamide (LSD), mescaline, psilocybin, and 3,4-methylene-dioxyamphetamine (MDA). They are found on the streets in a wide range of forms, including powder, peyote buttons, mushrooms, capsules, and tablets. LSD may be found as tablets, pellets, blotter paper, chips, and sheets of paper containing tattoos or stamp-like pictures of cartoon figures. Hallucinogens are taken orally, although MDA can be sniffed and injected. They may be put on sugar cubes or mixed in other food.

Common street names for these drugs are found below.

**Common Street Names of Hallucinogens**

| | |
|---|---|
| LSD | Acid, barrels, blotter, domes, microdots, purple haze, windowpane |
| Mescaline | Buttons, cactus, mesc, mescal buttons |
| MDA | Love drug, mellow drug of America |
| Psilocybin | Magic mushroom, shroom |

Psilocybin and mescaline have been used in religious rites by cultures in the Western hemisphere for centuries. MDA was first synthesized in the 1930s and used as an appetite suppressant. LSD was first synthesized in 1938, and the first "trip" that was documented occurred in 1943 when the drug was accidently absorbed through the skin.

**BOX 19-8 Clinical Manifestations of the Use of Hallucinogens**

1. Stimulation at first and then depression
2. Anxiety
3. Depressed appetite
4. Increased body temperature
5. Increased heart rate
6. Increased respiration
7. Dilated pupils; with psilocybin, dizziness, numbness of face, and shivering may also occur
8. Altered sensory awareness
9. Senses become more acute
10. User thinks that colors can be heard and sounds seen
11. Fantasies and illusions
12. Hallucination-like happenings
13. User may not be aware that hallucinations are not real
14. Past and present experiences meld together, leading to feeling of oneness, compassion, and love for all things

**Pathophysiology.** Most of the effects of hallucinogens are psychologic, although nausea and vomiting are not uncommon possible reactions. Clinical manifestations of the use of hallucinogens are listed in Box 19-8. Tolerance to these drugs occurs rather quickly (usually after 3 days of use), and there is cross-tolerance among the four drugs.

Hallucinogens have a profound psychologic effect on most people. The effect has been described as a process of amplifications, with the drug being a catalyst. Hallucinogens amplify and distort the users' experience of the environment and put them in touch with thoughts and feelings. In low doses, MDA produces a peaceful euphoria. With higher doses, it mimics LSD experiences without the hallucinations.

The feelings brought on by MDA, mescaline, and psilocybin lasts from 6 to 8 hours, whereas those of LSD usually last 8 to 12 hours. Toward the end of the "trip," the person will gradually reenter reality. A person's attempts to resist the effects of the drug seem to increase the chances of a negative experience, or a "bad trip."

Flashbacks may occur with use of the hallucinogens. In these, the user reexperiences the effects of the drug without having taken it. Bad trips are described as being characterized by tremendous confusion, unpleasant sensory images, and extreme panic. These bad trips often center on a feeling of impending danger or feelings of being threatened. Paranoid behavior is common, as well as psychotic breaks from reality during the bad trip. If the drug has precipitated psychotic breaks, some persons never return to a "normal" or previous state of consciousness.

Care during these situations includes getting the person into a nonstimulating environment and staying with the person until the effects of the trip wear off. Reassurance of the fact that the person is experiencing a drug trip is helpful. Some experts recommend giving niacin (500 mg) as a way to bring the person down from a bad trip.

Although there have been no reports of deaths from LSD, there have been documented instances in which the person died as a result of trying to do something impossible while on a trip. An example is trying to fly—that is, the person actually believes he or she will be able to fly and leaps from a window or rooftop in an attempt to do so.

### Phencyclidine

Phencyclidine (PCP) is a synthetic drug that is generally described as an anesthetic-hallucinogen. However, it is chemically unrelated to hallucinogens such as LSD and mescaline.

**Etiology/epidemiology.** PCP was first synthesized in 1957 and tested as a general anesthetic for humans. Testing stopped in the mid-1960s because of side effects of agitation and delirium. It presently is available as an anesthetic agent used by veterinarians. In the late 1960s and 1970s the drug became available as a street drug. It was banned from legal manufacture for use in humans in 1978 but is still produced illegally.

PCP, produced as a white or yellowish-white powder, has a variety of forms, including tablets and capsules. As angel dust, it is sprinkled on tobacco or marijuana and smoked. It may also be snorted or injected. Common street names for PCP are listed below.

| Common Street Names for PCP | |
|---|---|
| Angel dust | Embalming fluid |
| Animal tranquilizer | KJ killer |
| Crystal | Peace pill |
| Dust | Synthetic marijuana |
| Hog | |

**Pathophysiology.** Different doses of PCP produce different physical effects. These can be found in Box 19-9.

Psychologic effects of PCP ingestion last from 1 to 6 hours, with 24 hours needed to return to baseline. Research seems to indicate that the bad trip rate of PCP is five times that of other drugs. Chronic users may experience flashbacks. The dose of PCP may indicate the nature of the effects. These are found in Box 19-10.

Although there is disagreement about whether PCP is physically addicting, there is wide agreement that it is psychologically habit-forming.

PCP overdoses are dangerous, because the person may die as a result of respiratory or cardiac arrest. Symptoms of PCP intoxication include a variable response. These include the following:

1. Violent or combative to nearly unconscious
2. Little or no pain response
3. Inability to speak
4. Elevated blood pressure and pulse rate with slight fever[22]

**BOX 19-9 Dose-Related Physical Manifestations of the Use of PCP**

| DOSE | EFFECTS |
|---|---|
| 5 mg | Physical sedation<br>Numbness of extremities<br>Loss of muscle coordination<br>Dizziness<br>Constricted pupils, blurred or double vision, and involuntary eye movements<br>Flushing and profuse sweating<br>Nausea and vomiting<br>Increase in blood pressure, heart rate, and respiratory rate (breathing is shallow) |
| 5 to 10 mg | Marked drop in blood pressure, breathing, and heart rates<br>Shivering, increased salivation, and watering of the eyes<br>Loss of balance, dizziness, and rigidity of muscles<br>In some cases, repetitive movements, such as rocking<br>Analgesic and anesthetic properties apparent |
| Over 10 mg | Extreme agitation, followed by seizures or coma<br>Symptoms similar to mental confusion and delusion of schizophrenia |

From Scott L: *PCP* (pamphlet), Charlotte, NC, 1981, Charlotte Drug Educational Center.

**BOX 19-10 Dose-Related Psychologic Manifestations of the Use of PCP**

| DOSE | EFFECTS |
|---|---|
| Low | Euphoria and sense of alcohol-like intoxication<br>Changes in body image<br>Mood swings from ecstasy to panic<br>Hallucinations and confusion about time and space<br>In final stage in some cases, a sense of despair and emotional isolation, possibly leading to a feeling of paranoia and a sense of impending death |
| Moderate | Increase in effects felt at low dose<br>Loss of sense of contact with environment |
| High | Symptoms of mental and emotional confusion similar to schizophrenia |

From Scott L: *PCP* (pamphlet), Charlotte, NC, 1981, Charlotte Drug Educational Center.

The person intoxicated by PCP becomes more agitated by noise, bright lights, and talking.

PCP use may result in psychosis that lasts from several days to 2 weeks. It is often mistaken for acute schizophrenia. Individuals may be actively suicidal and become depressed when the acute psychosis has passed.

### Narcotics

**Narcotics** are drugs that are derived from the opium poppy or produced synthetically. The use of these has been recorded far back in history. Synthetic production of narcotics has occurred in the past 30 to 50 years. In general, narcotics lower the perception of pain.

**Etiology/epidemiology.** Heroin is one narcotic that is abused to a large extent. There has been a shift toward younger addicts and an increase in the percentage of whites using heroin. On the streets, heroin is known as "H," horse, junk, hard stuff, smack, or scag.

There are several different forms of narcotics. See Table 19-8 for a listing of these drugs, their medical use, and route of administration.

**Pathophysiology.** Heroin and morphine are alkaloids of opium that depress the central nervous system. The clinical manifestions of their use and that of other narcotics appear in Box 19-11. A major concern about heroin users is that they commonly inject the drug with contaminated needles, which places them at high risk of acquiring HIV, hepatitis, and other infections, such as septicemia. Narcotic addicts develop both tolerance and physical and psychologic addiction. Withdrawal may be painful and should be under medical supervision. Clonidine (Catepres) is often used for purposes of detoxification from narcotics. The heavier the use, the longer detoxification may take. Symptoms of withdrawal may include nausea, cramps, chills, sweating, watery eyes, running nose, and restlessness.[22]

**TABLE 19-8 Narcotics**

| NAME | MEDICAL USE | ROUTE OF ADMINISTRATION |
|---|---|---|
| Heroin | None in the United States | By injection or sniffing |
| Morphine | Ease pain | By mouth, smoking, or injection |
| Opium | Ease pain, treat diarrhea, and suppress cough | By mouth or smoking |
| Codeine | Suppress cough and reduce pain | By mouth or injection |
| Meperidine | Relieve pain | By mouth or injection |
| Methadone | Ease pain and to help those dependent on heroin | By mouth or injection |

From O'Brien R, Cohen S: *The encyclopedia of drug abuse,* New York, 1984, Facts on File.

Heroin is an expensive habit, and many addicts resort to crime to support it.

**Methadone maintenance.** One approach to the treatment of narcotic addiction is the methadone maintenance program. The drug is given legally as a part of a rehabilitation program. The drug reduces the severity of the heroin withdrawal but must itself be tapered off. There are many controversies surrounding methadone programs, and many professionals discourage its use, recommending instead detoxification leading to abstinence.

### Cannabis

**Etiology/epidemiology.** Cannabis, or marijuana, comes from the Indian hemp plant. It can grow wild or is fairly easily cultivated. Marijuana is usually smoked as a cigarette (joint, reefer) or in a pipe. Other paraphernalia may be used, including water-filled pipes known as "bongs." There are many slang terms for marijuana, including the following: dope, grass, herb, joint, pot, reefer, roach, smoke, stuff, and weed.

Marijuana has been used as both a medical and nonmedical drug for more than 3000 years. It has been used since the 1850s in the United States. Its popularity as a street drug began to occur in the twentieth century. It is still one of the most popular and commonly abused drugs, especially among young people.

Hashish, or hash, is a resinous extract of the leaves and flowering part of the marijuana plant. It is more concentrated than marijuana and has more intense effects.

Marijuana is used increasingly to reduce eye pressure in glaucoma patients and to control side effects of cancer chemotherapy.

**Pathophysiology.** Marijuana and other forms of cannabis seem to act as CNS depressants. They depress higher brain centers and consequently release lower centers from inhibitory influences. The physical mani-

**BOX 19-11 Clinical Manifestations of the Use of Narcotics**

1. Relief of pain and feeling of well-being
2. Shallow breathing
3. Reduced hunger and thirst
4. Reduced sexual drive
5. Drowsiness
6. Euphoria
7. Lethargy
8. Heaviness of limbs
9. Apathy
10. Loss of ability to concentrate
11. Loss of judgment and self-control
12. Overdoses can cause coma, convulsions, respiratory arrest, and death

**BOX 19-12 Physical Manifestations of the Use of Marijuana**

1. Drying of the eyes and mouth
2. Increase in appetite and food consumption
3. Can produce glucose intolerance, leading to hyperglycemia, which can be a problem in those with diabetes
4. Reddening of eyes
5. Impairment of short-term memory
6. Increased heart rate and blood pressure
7. Decreased body temperature
8. Impairment of coordination

**BOX 19-13 Psychologic Manifestations of the Use of Marijuana**

1. Altering of perception (e.g., altering of sight, sound, touch, sense of time, and taste)
2. Feeling of well-being and intoxication, although depression and panic may occur
3. Confusion and distortion of reality may occur

**BOX 19-14 Clinical Manifestations of the Use of Inhalants**

1. Slurred speech
2. Blurred vision, bloodshot eyes
3. Inflamed mucous membranes, nosebleeds
4. Bad breath
5. Light-headedness
6. Ringing in the ears
7. Watering eyes
8. Loss of coordination
9. Excessive nasal secretions
10. Loss of consciousness or seizures lasting 20 to 45 minutes with large doses

festations of marijuana use appear in Box 19-12. Research indicates that marijuana may affect chromosome segregation during cell division. Because marijuana is a fat-soluble molecule, parts of it may be stored in the body for 30 days or more.

In addition to its physical effects, marijuana has important psychologic effects, including distortion of time (Box 19-13). A classic description of the time distortion is that "seconds seem like minutes, minutes seem like hours, and hours seem like days."

Psychologic addiction develops in users. Crisis situations may occur in the form of an anxiety reaction to the marijuana high. A calming and reassuring approach has been found to be helpful.

### Deliriants

**Etiology/epidemiology. Deliriants** are any chemicals that give off fumes or vapors that, when inhaled, produce symptoms similar to intoxication. They may also be called inhalants. Vasodilators—such as amyl nitrate and butyl nitrite, which are used medically—are also considered inhalants.

The fumes or vapors from inhalants are sniffed through the nose, or the vapors are put into a bag or captured in a balloon to increase the concentration of the inhaled fumes.

The history of the use of inhalants is traced back to ancient Greece. Sniffing commercial products and solvents was first documented in the 1950s. No medical use exists for commercially-prepared inhalants. Of course, the vasodilators and anesthetic agents have a legitimate medical purpose.

Deliriants or inhalants have a psychoactive or mood-altering effect when the vapors are inhaled or sniffed. Most fall into one of three categories:

1. Solvents (tuleo, glue, gasoline)
2. Aerosol sprays
3. Anesthetics

Solvents include commercial products that are not commonly thought of as drugs. These include glue, gasoline, kerosene, lighter fluid, paint products, lacquer thinner, spot remover, and nail polish remover. Such products as hair spray, deodorant, insecticides, and cookware coating sprays are examples of aerosols. Anesthetics that are used recreationally include ether, chloroform, and nitrous oxide.

Typically, persons using solvents and aerosols are among the youngest drug users, with most being teenagers.

**Pathophysiology.** Almost all inhalants are CNS depressants that slow the user's heart rate, brain activity, and breathing. The clinical manifestations of the use of inhalants can be found in Box 19-14.

The prolonged use of inhalants may lead to liver, kidney, blood, and bone marrow damage. The sniffing of toluene, found in gasoline and commercial cleaners, has been demonstrated to cause irreversible brain damage. This may be demonstrated as forgetfulness, inability to think clearly, depression, irritability, hostility, and paranoia.

Deliriants also have an impact on the peripheral nervous system and produce symptoms similar to those of multiple sclerosis. These include poor coordination, inability to walk, poor bladder control, decreased mobility, and decreased ability to perform ADLs and to meet basic needs.

Some inhalants cause tolerance. Physical dependency is a possibility. Symptoms of withdrawal include chills, hallucinations, headaches, stomach pains, cramps, and DTs.

The psychologic effects of deliriants include a feeling

of stimulation and energy. At higher doses, the user may feel intoxicated. The development of psychologic dependence is a real possibility.

Use of large amounts of aerosols or solvents can cause death as a result of cardiac arrest after dysrhythmias. Death from inhalants is usually caused by suffocation because of the displacement of oxygen in the lungs. Sniffing inhalants from a bag or balloon increases the risk of suffocation. Misuse of commercial aerosol products used to chill food have been reported to cause death by freezing the lungs of the user.

The CNS effects of inhalants are potentiated by other CNS depressants, thus increasing the chances of overdose.

## OTHER DEPENDENCIES

### CAFFEINE

#### Etiology/Epidemiology

Caffeine is the most accepted and used psychoactive substance in the United States. Many beverages and other products contain caffeine. Because of its availability and widespread use, most persons do not view caffeine as a drug.

The use of tea leaves in China dates back at least 4000 years. In the 1200s the Arabians used coffee. Caffeine was first isolated from coffee in 1820. In its pure state, caffeine is a white powder or white needle-shaped crystals. It has been used as an additive in carbonated beverages since the early 1900s.

Medically, caffeine is present in many headache remedies, cold medications, diuretics, diet aids, and other prescriptions. (See Box 19-15 for the amount of caffeine in commonly used beverages.)

#### Pathophysiology

Caffeine stimulates the CNS, as well as the digestive system and the kidneys. The clinical manifestations of this stimulation appear in Box 19-16. Physical dependence occurs with regular intake of 350 mg for an adult. The withdrawal symptoms include severe headaches, irritability, and tiredness.

Caffeine makes most people feel energetic and alert. Too much caffeine can precipitate an anxiety attack. Long-term involvement can lead to depression, persistent anxiety, low-grade fever, nausea, ringing in the ears, and chronic insomnia. A fatal dose of caffeine is considered to be about 10 g, or 10,000 mg.

Research seems to indicate that excessive use of caffeine may contribute to the development of heart disease, as well as to bladder cancer.

**BOX 19-15 Caffeine Content of Products**

| Product | Caffeine |
|---|---|
| Coffee | |
| Brewed, per cup | 75 to 155 mg |
| Instant | 60 to 90 mg |
| Decaffeinated | 2 to 4 mg |
| Tea, per cup | 25 to 75 mg |
| Carbonated sodas (all colas [except those labeled caffeine-free], Dr. Pepper, Mountain Dew, Sunkist Orange) | 30 to 70 mg |
| Chocolate | |
| Hot cocoa | 30 to 70 mg |
| Candy (1 oz) | 6 mg |
| Over-the-counter drugs | |
| Anacin, Excedrin, Vanquish, Doan's Pills | 16 to 65 mg |
| No-Doz, Vivarin | 100 to 200 mg |
| APC tablets | 30 to 100 mg |
| Diet Aids | |
| AYDS, Dexatrim, Prolamine | 140 to 200 mg |

**BOX 19-16 Clinical Manifestations of the Use of Caffeine**

1. Increased blood pressure
2. Increased urination
3. Stomach distress (acidity)
4. Tachycardia (with large doses)
5. Headaches (with large doses)
6. Nervousness (with large doses)
7. Insomnia (with large doses)

### NICOTINE

#### Etiology/Epidemiology

Over 50 million Americans smoke more than 600 billion cigarettes yearly. It is one of the most physically damaging and addictive habits in which a large number of people engage. Smoking has been linked to heart and blood vessel disease, chronic bronchitis and emphysema, and cancer of the lungs, larynx, mouth, esophagus, bladder, pancreas, and kidneys. It is far easier to become addicted to cigarettes than to alcohol or other drugs.

Tobacco is used by smoking, chewing, or inhaling. Snuff is usually placed between the gums and the cheek.

#### Pathophysiology

The nicotine in tobacco acts as a stimulant to the CNS. Nicotine is present in the brain within a few seconds of the beginning of smoking. Smokers claim that smoking produces relaxation; however, smoking releases epinephrine, which may create physiologic stress. Nicotine acts as an appetite suppressant. In large doses it produces tremors, decreased urine output, and a rapid respiratory rate.

Withdrawal symptoms occur with the stoppage of cigarette smoking. These include the following:

1. Decreased heart rate
2. Weight gain
3. Impairment of psychomotor performance

4. Nervousness and anxiety
5. Headaches
6. Fatigue
7. Insomnia
8. Constipation or diarrhea

The craving for a cigarette often continues for an extended period. Nicotine addiction has implications for the medical-surgical patient. This may include management of respiratory status after surgery or the management of the person who has developed chronic pulmonary disease as the result of years of smoking.

## NURSING MANAGEMENT

### ♦ ASSESSMENT

Most early indications of drug use are covered in the preceding description of individual classes of drugs. The reader is also referred to the assessment section under the section on alcoholism on p. 493. Breaks in the skin are an objective sign that must be noted when assessing for drug addiction. If the person has been "mainlining" (that is, injecting the drug directly into the vein), needle marks, scars, or small scabs can be seen on the hands and forearms or instep. However, many other veins are used as points of entry to conceal addiction, including the dorsal vein of the penis, sublingual blood vessels, or the conjunctival artery of the eyelid.

The reader is referred to the section on assessment of the alcoholic (p. 493) for other relevant subjective and objective data, nursing diagnoses, and specific outcomes.

Because of the expense involved, users often sell their belongings, steal, or become prostitutes to get money to supply their drug habit. Each day abuse of drugs costs the American economy millions of dollars.

It is important for the nurse caring for the drug-addicted person to examine her or his attitudes about caring for the patient. Attitudes that include negativity, moral superiority, anger, indifference, or sympathy are seldom, if ever, helpful. The nurse should also realize that punishment and/or deprivation of the person is also counterproductive. In addition, attempts to control the person are usually counterproductive. Instead, efforts should focus on controlling environmental factors. Finally, the nurse should realize that substances can be and often are brought into the hospital by visitors. The person needs to be observed for signs of recurrent drug use, because many drug- and alcohol-addicted persons are very resourceful in securing substances and in covering up their use.

Medical-surgical nurses often have questions about pain control when dealing with drug-addicted and alcoholic patients. They often undermedicate the patient, fearing that the drug use will lead to addiction. It is important to realize that not keeping the patient comfortable may actually predispose the patient to a relapse of the addiction. The patient should receive the pain medication for only as long as he or she requires it, in the view of the nurse or other professional who knows the patient. It is common for the drug-addicted patient, in particular, to require higher doses of pain medication than the average person. It is also important to realize that addiction tends to increase the amount of drug required to produce anesthesia. Thus these persons will require a longer time to recover from the anesthesic.

### ♦ INTERVENTIONS

The treatment of withdrawal from drug abuse is discussed in each section under the specific drugs. (See Table 19-9 for more detail on acute intoxication and withdrawal.) General rehabilitation follows the guidelines for treatment of the alcoholic. This can be found in the section on alcoholism (p. 495). Today, most treatment centers treat alcoholics and drug addicts side-by-side. In fact the majority of persons receiving treatment for chemical dependency today have a history of abuse of both alcohol and drugs.

One difference between drugs and alcohol is that in most cases the possession and use of drugs are illegal. In the United States the addiction to narcotics has been considered a crime ever since the passage of the Harrison Narcotic Act of 1914. Education is making the public more aware of the primary nature of the disease of drug addiction.

Evaluation of the patient with drug abuse is the same as that for the person with alcoholism (p. 499).

## OTHER ADDICTIVE BEHAVIOR PATTERNS

### EATING DISORDERS

Eating disorders, such as anorexia nervosa and bulimia nervosa, have been known since ancient times, when they were described as "nervous consumption" and "anorexia hysteria."[10] Compulsive overeating is also considered an eating disorder, but it is not discussed in this chapter.

#### Etiology/Epidemiology

The incidence of eating disorders, especially anorexia and bulimia, is high in certain subpopulations where maintenance of excessively low weights is required. These include models, ballet dancers, and flight attendants. Adolescent girls often have a preoccupation with losing weight. It is estimated that from 5% to 15% of this group meet the criteria for bulimia. Although the incidence of eating disorders is much higher in females, some males also experience anorexia and/or bulimia.

#### Prevention

Prevention of eating disorders is difficult. It is generally recognized that they provide a way of coping with stress and relieving tension; aiding the young person to develop a healthy self-concept and positive ways to express

**TABLE 19-9 Clinical Manifestations and Treatment of Acute Intoxication and Withdrawal of Mind-Altering Drugs**

| DRUG GROUP | ACUTE INTOXICATION: CLINICAL MANIFESTATIONS | ACUTE INTOXICATION: TREATMENT | CLINICAL MANIFESTATIONS OF WITHDRAWAL |
|---|---|---|---|
| Narcotics | Respiratory depression, bradycardia, hypotension, cold clammy skin, decreased body temperature; deep sleep, stupor, or coma; pin-point pupils | Maintain ventilation, provide oxygen<br>Give narcotic antagonist: naloxone (Narcan) 0.4 mg IV<br>Monitor vital signs every 15-30 min until patient is conscious<br>Treat for shock | (Not life-threatening)<br>Early: restlessness, irritability, drug craving, yawning, lacrimation, diaphoresis, rhinorrhea, followed by "yen" sleep (intense desire to sleep; sleeps restlessly)<br>Later: awakens with more severe symptoms, nausea, vomiting, anorexia, abdominal cramps, bone and muscle pain, tremors, piloerection (gooseflesh) |
| Other CNS depressants | Same as narcotics (above) | Lavage if recent oral ingestion with possible activated charcoal treatment<br>Maintain ventilation, provide oxygen<br>Monitor vital signs every 15-30 min until patient is conscious<br>Position patient side-lying or prone, not supine<br>Treat for shock<br>Hemodialysis for renal shutdown | (May be life-threatening)<br>Insomnia, restlessness, tremors, anorexia, followed by convulsion, and symptoms similar to DTs (confusion, visual and auditory hallucinations), fever, dehydration |
| CNS stimulants | Labile cardiovascular symptoms (flushing or pallor, pulse and blood pressure changes, dysrhythmias), hyperpyrexia, mental disturbances (agitation, paranoia, hallucinations), convulsions, circulatory collapse | Give chlorpromazine, 25-50 mg IM<br>Provide a quiet environment<br>Orient patient to reality<br>Monitor vital signs until stable | (Withdrawal is not severe)<br>Somnolence, apathy, irritability, depression, fatigue |
| Hallucinogens | Physiologic toxicity low at doses that produce strong psychologic effects<br>Acute panic reaction (bad trip) may lead to suicide<br>"Flashback" episodes<br>Prolonged psychotic disorders (paranoia, depression)<br>Phencyclidine: CNS depression or stimulation may lead to death | Provide quiet, supportive environment and constant attention<br>Give diazepam (Valium), 2-10 mg IM and/or major tranquilizers (thorazine IM) for severe anxiety | No evidence of withdrawal symptoms |
| Cannabis | Adverse reactions infrequent<br>Simple depression, paranoid ideation, confusion, disorientation, hallucinations | Provide support and reassurance<br>Give tranquilizer for agitation | (Withdrawal symptoms rare)<br>Insomnia, anorexia |
| Deliriants | Slowing of heart rate, brain activity, and breathing<br>Slurred speech, blurred vision, inflamed mucous membranes, excessive tearing, and nasal secretions<br>With high doses, loss of consciousness and seizures may occur<br>Brain damage may occur (memory loss, depression, paranoia, hostility)<br>Feeling of stimulation and energy<br>Death may occur from suffocation or cardiac arrest | Maintain airway<br>Maintain respirations<br>Provide quiet environment and provide support<br>Monitor vital signs<br>Orient patient to reality | Chills, hallucinations, headaches, stomach pains, cramps, DTs |

tension and stress may help. The reader is referred to the discussion on prevention in the section of this chapter referring to alcoholism (p. 488).

Currently, eating disorders are more promptly recognized by both health professionals and the general public. Teachers in high schools and colleges may also play a significant role in diagnosis of this condition.

## Pathophysiology

The pathophysiology occurring with **bulimia** is related to the constant purging of the gastrointestinal system. If laxatives are used in large amounts, the individual may experience a loss of rectal tone and the loss of great amounts of minerals with diarrhea. If the person purges by vomiting, loss of enamel on the teeth is common, leading to decay and to infection of the mouth and gums. Gastrointestinal bleeding may also occur, along with gastritis or esophagitis, from the contact of the mucosa with stomach acids during vomiting. Malnutrition is common.

With **anorexia,** the patient suffers from frank malnutrition, leading to depletion of muscle mass, skin lesions, loss of hair, neuromuscular abnormalities, and cessation of menses in females.

Bulimia or anorexia becomes a way to "anesthetize" intense feelings and to cope with stress and relieve tension. The person, who does not have adequate coping skills, attempts to deny difficult events, minimize distress, and rationalize stress. When tension builds to high levels, food (or lack of food) serves as a coping mechanism.

Control is a recurring theme for persons suffering from anorexia or bulimia. They fear losing control and being spontaneous. These fears cause them to set up rules and regulations (ritualistic behaviors) for everything they do. Restrictive eating and purging are attempts made by the bulimic to control the body, especially after an eating binge. Restrictive eating often functions as evidence of willpower and control over the body. Purging is seen as a way to bring the body back under control. There is a vicious cycle of bingeing and purging in many of these persons. Clinical manifestations of bulimia and anorexia are listed in Box 19-17.

**BOX 19-17 Clinical Manifestations of Bulimia and Anorexia**

1. Loss of tooth enamel
2. Tooth decay
3. Infection of the mouth
4. Gastrointestinal bleeding
5. Gastritis or esophagitis

(Items 1–5: associated with vomiting of food and gastric acid)

6. Malnutrition
7. Loss of rectal tone
8. Loss of minerals and bone mass
9. Diarrhea

(Items 7–9: associated with purging)

10. Amenorrhea
11. Hyperactivity without fatigue
12. Agitated behavior
13. Disorganized thinking
14. Excessive weight loss
15. Sleep disorder
16. Epigastric pain

### Anorexia nervosa

With anorexia nervosa, weight loss leads to a body weight of at least 15% less than the expected norm based on age and height. The person is intensely fearful of becoming obese, and the menstrual cycle usually is absent. The person experiences low self-esteem and a distortion of body image and feels fat even when emaciated.

### Bulimia

Bulimic patients present with episodes of binge eating during which they feel a lack of control. This has been defined as at least two bingeing episodes a week for at least 3 months. The patient attempts to prevent weight gain through regular self-induced vomiting or the use of laxatives, restrictive dieting, fasting, and increasingly vigorous exercise. The patient shows an excessive concern with body shape and weight.[10]

## Medical Management

The medical management of the patient with anorexia or bulimia often centers around nutritional management. Intravenous therapy, hyperalimentation, or tube feedings may be necessary to sustain life. Supplemental vitamins are usually administered, and infections are treated if present. It is not helpful to use psychoactive drugs with these patients. They need to regain coping abilities without the use of medications. Psychotherapy is often imperative to enable the person to face the truth of his or her behavior, to improve self-esteem, and to curb the need to be in control at all times.

# NURSING MANAGEMENT

## ♦ ASSESSMENT

Both subjective and objective data are important to assess in the patient with bulimia or anorexia. These patients are similar to the alcoholic patient in that they may manifest a strong sense of denial of their problem. Information should be validated with a family member if possible.

## Subjective Data

Data to be collected to assess the patient with bulimia or anorexia include the following:

- Typical eating patterns
- History of bingeing or purging
- Laxatives used—type and quantity
- Patient's perception of weight and body image
- Family history of eating disorders
- Family problems
- Past problems with eating disorders

Average weight
Use of drugs or alcohol
Complaints of problems, especially gastrointestinal problems
Exercise pattern
Sleep disturbances
Amenorrhea

### Objective Data

Data to be collected to assess the patient with bulimia or anorexia include the following:

Presence of low weight in relation to height
Evidence of loss of tooth enamel
Hyperactivity or agitated behavior

## ♦ NURSING DIAGNOSES

Nursing diagnoses are determined from analysis of patient data. Nursing diagnoses for the patient with bulimia or anorexia may include but are not limited to the following:

| Diagnostic Title | Possible Etiologic Factors |
|---|---|
| Nutrition, altered: less than body requirements | Limited intake, vomiting, purging |
| Fluid volume deficit | Decreased fluid intake, abnormal fluid loss |
| Infection, high risk for | Malnutrition |
| Activity intolerance | Generalized weakness |
| Body image disturbance | Perceives self as being grossly overweight |
| Self-esteem, chronic low | Altered thought processes: sees self as overweight |
| Anxiety | Change in health status/role functioning |
| Coping, ineffective (individual) | Maturational crises |
| Denial, ineffective | Unable to admit impact of disease on life pattern |
| Noncompliance | Person's value system (health belief, cultural and social influences) |
| Knowledge deficit | Lack of interest in learning |
| Social isolation | Unaccepted social behavior |

## ♦ EXPECTED PATIENT OUTCOMES

Expected patient outcomes for the patient with bulimia or anorexia may include but are not limited to the following:

1. Maintains optimal nutrition.
2. Maintains adequate hydration.
3. Remains free of infection.
4. Demonstrates improved activity tolerance.
5. Maintains positive body image.
6. Verbalizes improved self-esteem.
7. Demonstrates improved management of anxiety.
8. Demonstrates improved and effective coping mechanisms.
9. Admits that bulimia or anorexia is a problem in her or his life.
10. Verbalizes a plan to carry out desired health-related behavior.
11. Verbalizes knowledge of disease and treatment.
12. Demonstrates increased ability to cope with interpersonal encounters and social isolation.

## ♦ INTERVENTIONS

### ➠ Managing Critical Care

A teenage girl with bulimia or anorexia may be admitted to the hospital because of severe malnutrition and dehydration. She will require intensive therapy to improve her life-threatening condition.

#### Maintaining optimal nutrition and hydration

Efforts must be made to support the nutritional status of the patient until a more normal eating pattern is restored. If needed, tube feedings, intravenous feedings, or hyperalimentation may be prescribed. The nurse must be aware that the patient may try to sabotage efforts to restore nutrition. The patient is weighed at frequent intervals to determine the success of the plan of care. The goal of nutritional therapy is to assist the patient in learning to eat a well-balanced diet with an adequate caloric count. A consultation with the dietitian is usual. The patient is given extra support before, during, and after meals.

Positive reinforcement by members of the staff is important as the patient makes even the smallest improvement in eating. After the patient's condition is stabilized, a written contract with the patient may be used to aid in behavioral change. When the patient is no longer critically ill, attention is given to the following interventions.

#### Preventing infection

Persons with bulimia or anorexia are malnourished, and as a result, their defense mechanisms (immune system) are impaired. They are at risk of developing infections, such as tuberculosis. They should be tested for tuberculosis and, if they test positive, should be started on preventive chemotherapy (see Chapter 37).

Persons with upper respiratory infections should not be allowed to visit the patient. Patients should be given basic instructions in proper hygiene (good handwashing, appropriate skin care).

#### Improving activity tolerance

Persons who are severely malnourished are usually weak and not able to be as active as usual. Early in the course of their disease, some persons engage in considerable exercise in an attempt to lose weight. If it is confirmed that this has been their pattern, they should be counseled about appropriate amounts of exercise.

#### Improving body image

It is important to assess the patients' perceptions and feelings about their body image. Even though they may appear extremely thin to others, they perceive themselves as being overweight. Cultural influences often play an important role in these diseases. As mentioned earlier, bulimia and anorexia are very common among ballerinas, airline attendants, and fashion models, where a premium is placed on a lean appearance. If preteen and teenage girls use them as their role models, they will probably be resistant to suggestions that they need to eat more. Patients with bulimia and anorexia often require psychiatric therapy to work through their deep-seated negative feelings about themselves and their appearance.

It is helpful if all persons working with the patient meet together to decide the best approach to the patient and develop a treatment plan for the patient. It is very important that all health care providers use a consistent approach. Failure to do so gives the patient the opportunity to play one caregiver off against another.

Patients may require months of therapy before they can accept the need to change their body image by eating an adequate amount and gaining weight.

#### Improving self-esteem

Because the patient with bulimia or anorexia is suffering from low self-esteem, it is important that the nurse convey unconditional acceptance of the patient as a person. This does not mean that inappropriate behavior is ignored or allowed. It is usually helpful to have patients identify their strengths and potentials. They should also be encouraged to participate in planning and directing their own care. It is helpful to have them set short-term goals that are achievable. For example, a goal for the week might be eating all of the food offered on at least 3 of 7 days.

It is important that caregivers observe interactions between the patient and family to determine how the family may be affecting the patient's self-esteem. It may be necessary for the nurse to discuss with family members how their interactions are affecting the patient's perception of self. Counseling for family members is often necessary and helpful.

In some situations the patient should be taught assertive communication skills. It may be helpful if the patient is taught to become aware of the harmful effects of negative self-talk and to explore ways to cope best with negative criticism from others.

#### Decreasing anxiety

Patients are encouraged to share concerns and feelings and to learn to deal with anxious feelings. Anxiety may decrease if patients are involved in planning their daily schedules so that they feel more in control. It is also helpful to maintain a calm environment in which patients feel safe.

Encouraging patients to keep a "feeling log" may help them to identify situations that cause anxiety. Reassurance and support from caregivers usually make the person less anxious. Teaching patients relaxation exercises and assisting them to practice them several times daily usually helps to decrease anxiety.

#### Facilitating coping

Most persons with bulimia or anorexia started their eating practices as they approached puberty. Similar to persons with other addictions, they may have a problem with intimacy and sexuality. They need to learn to trust others and to feel more positive about themselves as persons worthy of being loved. Considerable therapy may be necessary for the individual to work through her or his feelings about her or his own sexuality.

Providing a supportive environment in which the person feels free to vent emotions may assist in getting rid of underlying anger or resentment. As mentioned earlier, the nurse needs to be nonjudgmental about the patient's behavior and provide positive feedback, support, and encouragement.

#### Increasing compliance

Persons with bulimia or anorexia may have had their disease for a long time before they reach medical attention. Recovery will not occur rapidly, and much patience is required of nurses as they assist the patient to achieve the goal of eating a balanced diet. A nonjudgmental attitude by the nurse is essential to developing rapport. As mentioned previously, positive reinforcement with even the smallest improvement in eating or gaining weight is important. Many patients will require psychiatric therapy to assist them in their recovery.

#### Decreasing denial

The patient with bulimia or anorexia is often very well defended psychologically and is not ready to confront her or his denial. When this is so, the patient's behavior is supported and the patient is not confronted about the denial. A major nursing goal is to develop a trusting relationship with the patient. It is also important to provide a calm environment in which the patient can feel safe.

#### Guidelines for Teaching the Patient With an Eating Disorder

Educating the patient about the eating disorder is important. Elements of the teaching include the following:

1. Disease concept of eating disorders
2. Medical aspects of the disease
3. The need for an adequate and prudent diet
4. The importance of finding healthy ways to cope with life
5. The awareness of an increased tendency to transfer obsessions
6. Signs and symptoms of relapse
7. Importance of aftercare
8. Importance of a stable support system

With time and effective treatment (including psychotherapy), the patient is able to discuss the effect that bulimia or anorexia has on her or his life.

**Facilitating learning**

Both the patient and family or other persons significant to the patient need to be educated about bulimia or anorexia. They need to understand the negative effects that restricting food intake or bingeing and purging has on the body. They also need to understand that the patient may have relapses, and it may take some time before full recovery is achieved.

Patients will need to examine how they dealt with stress in the past and how they might deal with it in the future. The Guidelines box, p. 512, lists the topics to be covered when teaching these patients.

**Decreasing social isolation**

Because these patients are often socially isolated, they need to be encouraged to socialize with and begin to trust others. The patient should be referred to *Overeater's Anonymous (OA),* which can serve the same purpose for these patients as AA does for those addicted to alcohol or drugs.

### Evaluation

To evaluate the effectiveness of nursing interventions, compare patient behaviors with those stated in the expected patient outcomes. Successful achievement of patient outcomes for the patient with anorexia or bulimia is indicated by the following:

1. Sustains weight gain.
2. Has good skin turgor with moist and pink mucous membranes.
3. Does not have nosocomial infection.
4. Able to be up and about without assistance and able to do own activities of daily living (ADL).
5. Speaks positively about own body image, and exhibits pleasure at change in appearance.
6. Demonstrates improved self-esteem by speaking positively about self.
7. Appears less anxious and sits or lies quietly without exhibiting nervousness.
8. Demonstrates improved coping mechanisms by being less angry and frustrated and not withdrawing when things do not go as planned.
9. Verbalizes that bulimia or anorexia is a problem that is affecting her or his life and needs to be addressed.
10. Discusses how to maintain weight at desired level, participates in moderate exercise, and attends OA meetings regularly.
11. Discusses her or his disease, how to care for self, how to avoid complications, and the need for regular follow-up.
12. Interacts more comfortably with a variety of persons.

## CO-DEPENDENCE

Another example of addictive behavior that is often encountered by the medical-surgical nurse is **co-dependence.** An overview of this problem is included here because the co-dependent person's approach to the substance abuser can have an effect on the care provided by the nurse. In addition, nurses themselves are often drawn into negative patterns of behavior, which are thought to be a chief cause of "burn-out." Nurses who give too much to others without taking care of themselves often become depleted. In addition, they are at high risk for developing alcoholism or drug dependence themselves.

Co-dependence has often been used to describe a person who is emotionally involved with a chemically dependent person. The co-dependent is someone who develops an unhealthy pattern of coping as a reaction to someone else's drug or alcohol use. Recently, however, the definition of co-dependence has been expanded. It is now seen as a disease entity with a definable onset, a set of physical and psychologic symptoms, and a predictable medical course.

Definitions of co-dependence vary, but there is agreement that the persons manifest dysfunctional responses to life and they derive their self-esteem from their ability to control themselves and others.

Characteristics of co-dependence include the following[4,11,31]:

1. Perfectionism
2. Denial
3. Poor communication
4. Caretaking
5. Inability to identify, express, and manage feelings
6. Difficulty forming and maintaining close relationships
7. Feeling responsible for others' behavior or feelings
8. Constantly seeking approval from others
9. Feelings of powerlessness
10. Feeling morally superior
11. Difficulty in setting limits
12. Feeling "super responsible" or "super irresponsible"
13. Martyrdom
14. Need to control
15. Any addictive behavior
16. Stress-related illness

Recovery from co-dependence starts with the person learning to care for himself or herself. The use of a journal to record feelings may be helpful. Breaking through the denial of the co-dependent person is often difficult. The person also requires help to learn to set appropriate boundaries, grieve past losses, and acquire the skill of reparenting. Daily affirmations may be used to reinforce the self-worth of the person.

# NURSING CARE PLAN

## PERSON EXPERIENCING WITHDRAWAL FROM ALCOHOL

**DATA:** Mrs. B. is a 67-year-old retired school teacher who has lived alone since the death of her husband 5 years ago. She retired from teaching 2 years ago. She has three children, but they all live out of town and she sees them infrequently. Her health has been good, except for some aches and pains that she has treated with "a stiff drink." Before her husband died, she had been a social drinker, having one or two drinks a week. Her alcohol consumption has now increased to at least half a fifth per day. She admits to using alcohol to ease her loneliness and to help her sleep. She does not see her drinking as a problem. She was seen in the emergency room for a fall that resulted in a severely sprained ankle. Her breathalyzer result was 0.189. Laboratory tests indicated elevated liver function studies, prolonged clotting times, and anemia.

The nursing history was obtained from a close friend who brought her to the hospital. The friend identified the following:

- She had suffered from at least three falls in the past 6 months.
- She had lost 10 pounds in the past year and eats sporadically.
- She has stopped seeing most of her friends because she believes that they are too busy for her.

Mrs. B. was admitted to the hospital with a diagnosis of alcoholism and need for detoxification. Collaborative nursing activities include those to assess (1) Mrs. B.'s potential for alcohol withdrawal and (2) the presence of any complications associated with her alcoholism. Nursing actions include the following:

- Monitoring vital signs frequently
- Assessing neurologic function, along with vital signs
- Monitoring intake and output
- Encouraging the intake of fluids as tolerated
- Administering prescribed medications to treat the withdrawal
- Allowing Mrs. B. to express her feelings about her drinking
- Administering vitamins, including thiamine and other B complex vitamins
- Assessing for signs and symptoms of alcohol withdrawal

### ■ NURSING DIAGNOSIS

High risk for injury related to lack of awareness of environmental hazards, decreased cognitive status, and decreased coordination/equilibrium

| Expected Patient Outcome | Nursing Interventions | Rationale |
|---|---|---|
| Mrs. B. completes detoxification without injury. | Medicate as ordered with Librium on a regular basis (50 mg q 3-4 hr). | Alcoholics may require large amounts of medication to prevent dangerous withdrawal symptoms. |
| | Keep side rails up while in bed. | Side rails may prevent falling from bed. |
| | Observe for seizure activity. Keep seizure equipment at bedside. | Seizure activity may occur with moderate or severe withdrawal. |
| | Minimize stimulation to reduce noise in patient's room. | Excessive stimulation may increase chance of hallucinations. |
| | Keep lighting at a low level. | |
| | Speak softly when addressing the patient. | |
| | Observe for signs of increasing tremors or confusion. | Tremors and confusion that are increasing may herald impending DTs. |
| | Measure vital signs q 2-4 hr. | The pulse rate correlates with the level of withdrawal. |

### ■ NURSING DIAGNOSIS

Altered nutrition: less than body requirements related to anorexia and excessive drinking

| Expected Patient Outcome | Nursing Interventions | Rationale |
|---|---|---|
| Mrs. B. begins to receive adequate food and fluid. | Record intake and output q 8 hr. | Recording intake and output will give an indication of hydration. |
| | Provide intravenous fluids if unable to drink without nausea/vomiting. | Gastritis may prevent drinking or eating. |
| | Give antiemetics as ordered. | Nausea and vomiting are common with withdrawal. |
| | Give antacids as ordered. | Antacids neutralize HCl acid and decrease gastric symptoms. |
| | When person is able, provide small, frequent meals. | Appetite usually improves as withdrawal progresses. |
| | Force fluids when nausea has resolved. | Dehydration is often a problem. |

## NURSING CARE PLAN

### PERSON EXPERIENCING WITHDRAWAL FROM ALCOHOL—cont'd

**■ NURSING DIAGNOSIS**

Sleep pattern disturbance related to withdrawal from alcohol

| Expected Patient Outcome | Nursing Interventions | Rationale |
|---|---|---|
| Mrs. B. sleeps at least 6 hr per night. | Keep stimulation to a minimum. | Quiet environment will help induce sleep. |
| | Use relaxation measures as appropriate. | Relaxation facilitates rest to promote healing, thus decreasing pain. |
| | Avoid use of sleeping medications. | Patient may develop dependence on sleeping medications. |

**■ NURSING DIAGNOSIS**

Knowledge deficit of alcoholism as a disease related to lack of exposure to information and denial

| Expected Patient Outcome | Nursing Interventions | Rationale |
|---|---|---|
| Mrs. B. verbalizes nature of alcoholism and need for treatment. | Teach about disease and problems associated with drinking. | Education will help diminish shame and guilt. |
| | Consult chemical dependence counselor. | Counseling can facilitate treatment and intervention if drinking continues. |
| | Arrange for AA contact. | AA contact can help patient learn from others, diminish sense of isolation, and give her someone to call when she feels a need to have a drink. |
| | Arrange for sharing of information with treatment source, if person agrees. | Sharing of information can facilitate treatment. |

## IMPAIRED NURSES

The issue of the impaired nurse is important to nurses in many different settings. This includes the medical-surgical areas of nursing. It has been estimated that one of every six or seven nurses will develop an addiction to drugs or alcohol before she or he leaves nursing. A nurse will rarely spend time working in a hospital or other health care setting without having to confront the issue of an impaired nurse.[28]

Over the past several years, many states have developed programs to assist the nurse who is impaired by either alcoholism or drug addiction. One of the main reasons for the establishment of these programs is that the rate of chemical dependence in nurses or other health professionals is greater than in the general public, principally because these persons have greater access to mood-altering substances. For instance, nurses may handle narcotics every day and may succumb to the temptation to use them. Before the inception of peer assistance programs (through either the state boards of nursing or state nursing associations), the nurse often was fired and then was free to migrate to another facility, where the cycle might start over again.

In March 1978, nurses from several states attended a meeting held in Manhattan to discuss the problem of the alcoholic nurse. By 1980 two organizations of nurses interested in alcoholism were active in encouraging help. These were the Drug and Alcohol Nursing Association (DANA) and the National Nurses Society on Addiction (NNSA). In 1981 the American Nurses Association (ANA) created a Task Force on Addiction and Psychological Disturbance to formulate guidelines for state nursing associations to develop programs to help the impaired nurse. At their 1982 convention, the American Nurses Association adopted a resolution that recognized its responsibility to assist nurses who are impaired.

In 1980 two states, Maryland and Ohio, had peer assistance programs in place. This effort has grown so that almost every state now has a program.[28]

The peer assistance programs have several goals: (1) to assist the nurse who is impaired to receive treatment; (2) to protect the public from the untreated nurse; (3) to help the recovering nurse reenter nursing in a

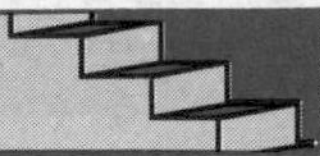

## CRITICAL PATHWAY Alcohol/Drug Detoxification Without Inpatient Rehabilitation

**DRG#: 435 Expected LOS: 4**

| | Day of Admission Day 1 | Day 2 | Day 3 | Day of Discharge Day 4 |
|---|---|---|---|---|
| **Diagnostic Tests** | CBC, UA, SMA/18,* drug screen | | | |
| **Medications** | Librium 10 mg PO q4hr PRN agitation; antiemetic q4hr PRN; antacid PRN; vitamins daily ($B_{12}$, thiamine 100 mg) | Librium 10 mg PO q4hr PRN agitation; antiemetic q4hr PRN; antacid PRN; vitamins daily (thiamine 100 mg) | Librium 10 mg q4hr PRN agitation; antiemetic q4hr PRN; antacid PRN; vitamins daily | Vitamins daily |
| **Treatments** | VS q2hr; I & O q8hr; neurochecks q2hr; provide protective environment | VS q2hr; I & O q8hr; neurochecks q2hr; participates in individual and group activities | VS q4hr; discontinue I & O; neurochecks q4hr; participates in individual and group activities and counseling | VS q8hr; participates in outpatient individual or group counseling |
| **Diet** | Clear liquids; advance diet as tolerated; force fluids | Regular diet; force fluids | Regular diet; force fluids | Regular diet |
| **Activity** | Up as tolerated; protect from falls if unstable; minimize stimulation | Up as tolerated; protect from falls if unstable; minimize stimulation | Up ad lib | Up ad lib |
| **Consultations** | Chemical dependence (CD) counselor; neurologist; psychiatrist | CD counselor | CD counselor | |

*Serum calcium, phosphorus, triglycerides, uric acid, creatinine, BUN, total bilirubin, alkaline phosphate, aspartate aminotransferase (AST) (formerly serum glutamic oxaloacetic transaminase [SGOT]), alanine aminotransferase (ALT) (formerly serum glutamic pyruvic transaminase [SGPT], lactic dehydrogenase (LDH), total protein, albumin, sodium, potassium, chloride, total $CO_2$, glucose.

systematic, planned, and safe way; and (4) to assist in monitoring the continued recovery of the nurse for a period of time. The reentry of the nurse may include a restriction from handling controlled drugs for a period of time.

The basis of these programs is one nurse helping another. Many volunteers in these programs are nurses who are themselves recovering or who are working in the field of chemical dependence.

## QUESTIONS TO CONSIDER

- What factors make the diagnosis of chemical dependence or substance abuse difficult to establish?
- Why do alcoholics and drug addicts fail to stay sober?
- What common factors do all addictive behaviors share, and what treatment modalities do they have in common?
- A nurse is caring for a patient who is withdrawing from alcohol. The blood alcohol level on admission was 0.200. The patient's pulse is 122 beats/min and the blood pressure is 182/98. What other symptoms and signs should the nurse assess?
- What factor do genetics play in the diagnosis of alcoholism?

## QUESTIONS TO CONSIDER—cont'd

- What responsibility does the nurse have in reporting a co-worker who is stealing drugs?
- You admit Mr. S. to a medical-surgical unit with diagnosis of a fractured leg secondary to a fall. During the interview, he admits that he drinks heavily but asks you not to tell anyone. What would you do?
- Why are 12-step programs effective in the treatment of dependent people?
- What actions can a nurse take to prevent becoming co-dependent?

## CRITICAL THINKING ACTIVITIES

- Dean, 39, is admitted to the hospital for acute pancreatitis. He is having severe pain, rated as a 12 on a scale of 1-10. He is a known abuser of narcotics and is requesting pain medication q 1-2 hours. How would you go about problem-solving and making a decision regarding the treatment of Dean's pain?
- Carrie, 19, is addicted to barbiturates. She frequently takes pentobarbital and secobarbital in combination with alcohol. On any given day Carrie is euphoric and calm. Today she is experiencing difficulty breathing, lethargy, and nausea. What classification of drug do barbiturates represent? Distinguish between the expected clinical manifestations of barbiturates and side effects that Carrie is experiencing.

## CHAPTER SUMMARY

### INTRODUCTION

- Examples of addictions include alcoholism, drug addiction, and eating disorders (anorexia nervosa and bulimia nervosa).
- Alcoholism and drug addiction are considered diseases and are commonly referred to as chemical dependencies.
- Dependence includes physical and psychologic dependence and is defined as the need to continue use of the substance to prevent withdrawal symptoms.
- Tolerance, a decreased susceptibility to the effects of a substance, develops with increased use of alcohol or drugs.
- Enabling behavior by family, friends, or co-workers enables the alcoholic or drug addict to continue the use of the substance.

### ALCOHOLISM

- Alcoholism is the third major health problem in the United States and affects more than 10 million persons.
- An estimated 7% of the adult population suffer from the disease of chemical dependence.
- Theories concerning the cause of alcoholism include physiologic, psychologic, and sociocultural theories.
- Alcohol is a central nervous system depressant that affects the brain by suppressing the activity of the neurotransmitter gamma aminobutyric acid (GABA).
- The so-called stimulating effects of alcohol occur because the first areas of the brain affected by its depressant properties are the higher centers that affect judgment and self-control.
- Ninety percent of alcohol is metabolized in the liver.
- The amount of alcohol in the blood at any one time is called the blood alcohol level.
- Alcohol withdrawal includes symptoms ranging from mild tremors to severe agitation and hallucinations.
- Delirium tremens (DTs) are an acute complication of alcohol withdrawal that requires aggressive therapy to prevent mortality and morbidity.
- Medication used in the initial period of detoxification includes chlordiazepoxide (Librium), diazepam (Valium), phenytoin (Dilantin), magnesium sulfate, and multivitamins.
- Wernicke-Korsakoff syndrome is a complication of alcoholism that includes symptoms of psychosis, amnesia, and apathy.
- Alcoholics Anonymous (AA) is a group of self-acknowledged alcoholics whose aim is to stay sober and to help other alcoholics gain sobriety.

### DRUG ABUSE

- Drug habituation is the repeated use of a drug to the point of psychologic dependence.
- Drug addiction includes craving, psychologic dependence, and physical dependence.
- The basic categories of drugs of abuse include stimulants, depressants, hallucinogens, narcotics, cannabis, and deliriants.
- Caffeine is the most accepted and widely used psychoactive substance in the United States and is found in many beverages and health products.
- Drug addicts who use drugs intravenously are at increased risk for the development of AIDS and hepatitis.
- It is not unusual for persons with chemical dependence to also experience symptoms of a psychiatric disorder.
- A co-dependent is a person who has let someone else's behavior affect him or her and is obsessed with controlling other people's behavior.

### OTHER ADDICTIVE BEHAVIOR PATTERNS

- The diagnosis of eating disorders includes anorexia nervosa, bulimia nervosa, and compulsive overeating.

### IMPAIRED NURSE

- Nurses and other health professionals are at increased risk for the development of chemical dependence.

## REFERENCES

1. *Alcoholics anonymous,* New York, 1976, Alcoholic World Service.
2. American Psychiatric Association: *Diagnostic and statistical manual of mental disorders,* ed 3, Washington, DC, 1987, The Association.
3. Captain C: Family recovery from alcoholism: mediating family factors, *Nurs Clin North Am* 24(1):55-64, 1989.
4. Covello B: Codependency taints nursing's goals, *RN* 54(4):132-135, 1991.
5. Dubiel S: Action stat! Cocaine overdose, *Nursing '90* 20(3):33-36, 1990.
6. Dubiel S: Drug abuse: designer drugs, *Adv Clin Care* 6(5):22, 1991.
7. Eels M: Strategies for promotion of avoiding harmful substances, *Nurs Clin North Am* 26(4):915, 1991.
8. Felblinger D: Substance abuse in women: a growing challenge for nurses, *Med Surg Nurs Q* 1(1):101-109, 1992.
9. Flandermeyer A et al: Nursing care of women who abuse alcohol, *Med Surg Nurs Q* 1(1):122-139, 1992.
10. Flood M: Addictive eating disorders, *Nurs Clin North Am* 24(1):45-54, 1989.
11. Hall S, Wray L: Codependency: nurses who give too much, *Am J Nurs* 89(11):1456, 1989.
12. House M: Cocaine, *Am J Nurs* 90(4):40, 1990.
13. Jacques J, Snyder M: Newborn victims of addiction, *RN* 54(4):47, 1991.
14. Johnson L: How to diagnose and treat chemical dependency in the elderly, *J Gerontol Nurs* 15(12):22-26, 38-39, 1989.
15. Johnson V: *Intervention,* Minneapolis, 1987, Hazelden Foundation.
16. Joyce C: The woman alcoholic, *Am J Nurs* 89(10):1314-1318, 1989.
17. Kinney J: *Clinical management of substance abuse,* St Louis, 1991, Mosby.
18. Krach P: Discovering the secret: nursing assessment of elderly alcoholics in the home, *J Gerontol Nurs* 16(11):32, 1990.
19. Levy G, Hickey J: Fighting the battle against drugs, *RN* 54(4):44, 1991.
20. Lillie-Blanton M, Anthony J, Schuster C: Probing the meaning of racial/ethnic group comparisons in crack cocaine smoking, *JAMA* 269(8):993-997, 1993.

21. Mitiguy J: Alcohol and head trauma, *Addict Nurs Network* 3(2):52, 1991.
22. *Mosby's medical, nursing, and allied health dictionary,* ed 4, St Louis, 1994, Mosby.
23. Perrine M et al: Epidemiological perspectives on drunk driving. In Surgeon General's workshop on drunk driving: background papers, Washington, DC, 1989, US Department of Health and Human Service.
24. Deleted in proofs.
25. Rice D et al: *The economic costs of alcohol and drug abuse and mental illness,* San Francisco, 1990, Institute for Health and Aging.
26. Rich J: Action stat! Acute alcohol intoxication, *Nursing '89* 19(9):33, 1989.
27. Sommers M: Alcohol intoxication and multiple trauma: a catastrophic combination, *Med Surg Nurs Q* 1(1):110-121, 1992.
28. Sullivan E: *Nursing and health care: the supplement: chemical dependency in the nursing profession* NLN Pub No 41-2365, 1990.
28a. US Department of Health and Human Services, Public Health Service: *Health United States 1989 and prevention profile,* Washington, DC, 1990, US Government Printing Office.
29. US Department of Health and Human Services, Public Health Service: *Healthy people 2000: national health promotion and disease prevention objectives,* Washington, DC, 1990, US Government Printing Office.
30. Williams E: Strategies for intervention, *Nurs Clin North Am* 24(1):95, 1989.
31. Zerwekh J, Michaels B: Co-dependency: assessment and recovery, *Nurs Clin North Am* 24(1):109, 1989.

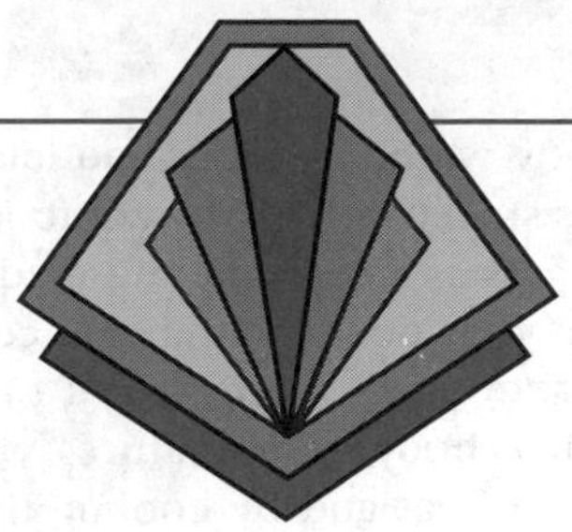

C H A P T E R 20

# Fluid and Electrolyte Imbalance

***Mary Kay Lehman***

## CHAPTER OBJECTIVES

***After studying this chapter, the learner should be able to do the following:***

1 Describe the mechanisms for maintaining fluid and electrolyte balance.
2 Describe the mechanisms and effects of fluid deficit and excess.
3 Describe the mechanisms and effects of deficits and excesses of sodium, potassium, calcium, and magnesium.
4 Identify data indicating fluid and electrolyte imbalances.
5 Develop a nursing care plan for a patient with a fluid and electrolyte imbalance.

## KEY TERMS

| | | |
|---|---|---|
| antidiuretic hormone (ADH) | hypermagnesemia | osmolality |
| Chvostek's sign | hypernatremia | osmolarity |
| colloid osmotic pressure | hyperosmolar | osmosis |
| diffusion | hypocalcemia | osmotic diuresis |
| edema | hypokalemia | pulmonary edema |
| electrolyte | hyposmolar | tetany |
| extracellular fluids | hyponatremia | third-spacing of fluids |
| hydrostatic pressure | hypomagnesemia | transcellular fluid |
| hypercalcemia | interstitial fluid | Trousseau's sign |
| hyperkalemia | intravascular fluid | water intoxication |

The body fluids of human beings have been described as "a sea within." Like sea water, these fluids are composed of water that contains dissolved electrolytes and other substances. The amount and location of the water and its constituents are constantly changing; that is, they are being taken in, used, shifted among compartments, and excreted but ever maintained in the delicate balance dictated by nature, a dynamic equilibrium. When diseases and their medical or surgical treatments interrupt this healthful state, fluid and electrolyte imbalances occur. These imbalances manifest as excesses, deficits, or abnormal shifts among body compartments.

This chapter reviews normal fluid and electrolyte balance and describes the causes, prevention, assessment, and management of imbalances of body fluids, sodium, potassium, calcium, magnesium, and hydrogen ions. Each imbalance is discussed separately, although in most instances a disturbance in the balance of one is accompanied by a disturbance in the balance of one or more of the others.

Although a physician prescribes medical therapy to prevent and treat imbalances, nurses must carry out the following vital functions:

1. Recognizing situations that are likely to cause imbalances
2. Intervening to prevent imbalances
3. Carrying out preventive and therapeutic measures prescribed by the physician and monitoring patients' responses to these measures
4. Recognizing signs and symptoms of fluid and electrolyte disturbances
5. Monitoring patients to prevent and recognize imbalances related to their specific conditions or treatments
6. Alleviating the effects of disturbances on the comfort and safety of patients

# MAINTENANCE OF FLUID AND ELECTROLYTE BALANCE

## BODY FLUID AND ELECTROLYTE COMPARTMENTS, DISTRIBUTION, AND FUNCTIONS

### Body Fluids

Fluid and electrolytes are found in the body either within the cell *(intracellular)* or outside the cell *(extracellular)*. The **extracellular fluid** (ECF) is contained in two compartments: the **interstitial fluid** (fluid between the cells) and **intravascular fluid** (fluid in the blood vessels). A third type of fluid, transcellular, denotes fluid separated by a layer of epithelial cells from other ECF.[6] **Transcellular fluid** includes digestive juices; water and solutes in the renal tubules and bladder; intraocular fluid; and cerebrospinal fluid. Some authorities consider this to be a part of the extracellular compartment, and others consider it to be a separate compartment. Transcellular fluid makes up 1% to 3% of body weight.

Body water is the largest single constituent of the body, representing 45% to 75% of body weight. The volume and distribution of body water vary with age and gender (Figure 20-1). In the newborn infant, almost three fourths of the body weight is water, with the greatest percentage found in the extracellular compartment. The volume and distribution change over time, and by adulthood in the young male only 60% of body weight is water, and two thirds of this is in the intracellular compartment. In the average young female only approximately 50% of body weight is water. This difference between men and women is caused by an increased amount of fat in women. Fat is essentially water-free.

Body water has multiple functions. The extracellular water maintains blood volume and serves as the body's transport system to and from cells. Intracellular fluid (ICF) provides the internal aqueous medium for cellular chemical function. Body water cushions and lubricates, helps give the body its structure, hydrolyzes food in the digestive system, and acts as a reactant and medium for the chemical reactions that occur within the cell. Adequate body water balance is also necessary (1) for the maintenance of normal body temperature, which is achieved by distributing heat and by cooling the body via evaporation from the skin, (2) for the elimination of waste products, and (3) for making possible all transportation within the body.

### Electrolytes

All body fluids contain *electrolytes,* which are chemical compounds in solution that have the ability to conduct an electrical current. In solution, electrolytes break into charged particles called *ions.* Positively charged ions are called *cations,* and negatively charged ions are called *anions.* Electrolytes are distributed in different concentrations in the intracellular, intravascular, and interstitial compartments (Table 20-1).

The electrolyte quantities given in Table 20-1 are in milliequivalents per liter. A *milliequivalent* is a unit of measurement of chemical activity. It is important to remember that 1 mEq of any specific ion is chemically equal to 1 mEq of any other ion. When electrolytes are measured in milliequivalents, the number of cations equals the number of anions. Electrolytes also can be measured in terms of weight such as in milligrams per 100 ml. When the electrolytes are measured in this way, the number of cations does not equal the number of anions, because the weights are not the same. For example, 1 mEq of hydrogen equals 1 mg of hydrogen, whereas 1 mEq of chloride equals 35.5 mg of chloride; 1 mEq of hydrogen has the same chemical activity as 1 mEq of chloride, but the weights (in milligrams) are different. At times nurses need to be able to make conversions between the two systems of measurement. Box

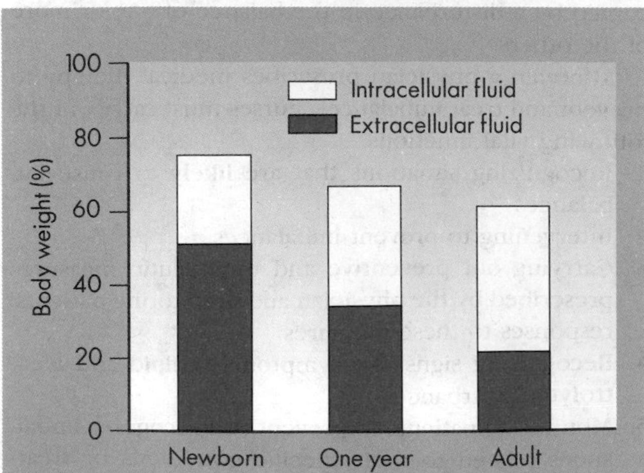


**FIGURE 20-1** In newborn infant more than half of total body fluid is extracellular. As child grows, proportions gradually approximate adult levels.

**TABLE 20-1 Normal Electrolyte Content of Body Fluids***

| ELECTROLYTES (ANIONS AND CATIONS) | EXTRACELLULAR: INTRAVASCULAR (mEq/L) | EXTRACELLULAR: INTERSTITIAL (mEq/L) | INTRACELLULAR (mEq/L) |
|---|---|---|---|
| Sodium ($Na^+$) | 142 | 146 | 15 |
| Potassium ($K^+$) | 5 | 5 | 150 |
| Calcium ($Ca^{++}$) | 5 | 3 | 2 |
| Magnesium ($Mg^{++}$) | 2 | 1 | 27 |
| Chloride ($Cl^-$) | 102 | 114 | 1 |
| Bicarbonate ($HCO_3^-$) | 27 | 30 | 10 |
| Protein ($Prot^-$) | 16 | 1 | 63 |
| Phosphate ($HPO_4^=$) | 2 | 2 | 100 |
| Sulfate ($SO_4^=$) | 1 | 1 | 20 |
| Organic acids | 5 | 8 | 0 |

*Note that the electrolyte level of the intravascular and interstitial fluids (ECFs) is approximately the same and that sodium and chloride contents are markedly higher in these fluids, whereas potassium, phosphate, and protein contents are markedly higher in ICF.

20-1 gives the formulas for these conversions.

Transcellular fluids have very distinct patterns of electrolyte concentration. For example, gastric secretions have a high hydrogen ion concentration, pancreatic secretions have a high bicarbonate concentration, and renal tubular and bladder fluids vary on a daily basis. Gastric, pancreatic, and intestinal juices and bile all contain high concentrations of sodium. Although the concentration of electrolytes varies, electrical neutrality is maintained in all fluid compartments; that is, the solution contains equal quantities in terms of chemical activity (milliequivalents per liter) of anions and cations.

Each electrolyte has specific functions. The general functions of all electrolytes are to (1) promote neuromuscular irritability, (2) maintain body fluid volume and osmolality, (3) distribute body water between fluid compartments, and (4) regulate acid-base balance.

### Osmolality/Osmolarity

Before normal fluid and electrolyte balance are discussed, the terms *osmolality* and *osmolarity* need to be defined, although they are frequently used interchangeably in a discussion of body fluids. **Osmolality** is an expression of the concentration of solution in terms of 1000 g of *water*. Neither the temperature (which can affect volume) nor the amount of solute has an effect on the osmolality of a solution. A 1-osmole solution is made by adding 1 g mole of solute to exactly 1000 g of water. The volume of the solution is then greater than 1 L.

**Osmolarity** is an expression of concentration in terms of 1000 ml of *solution*. Temperature and the amount of solute affect the amount of water in 1000 ml of solution. A 1-osmolar solution is made by placing 1 g mole of solute in a container and then adding water sufficient to make exactly 1 L of solution.

From the preceding, it can be seen that 1-osmolar solution and 1-osmole solution are not exactly the same. However, if the concentration of solute is small and the temperature is within normal body temperature range, the difference is negligible. This is why the difference between osmolarity and osmolality is negligible in normal body fluids.

**BOX 20-1 Formulas for Calculating Milliequivalent Quantity of an Ion and of a Salt From Weight (in Milligrams) and Conversion Between Milliequivalents per Liter and Milligrams per 100 Milliliters**

**CALCULATION OF MILLIEQUIVALENT QUANTITY OF AN ION**

$$\text{mEq} = \frac{\text{Atomic weight of ion}}{\text{Valence}}$$

**CALCULATION OF MILLIEQUIVALENT QUANTITY OF A SALT FROM WEIGHT IN MILLIGRAMS**

$$\text{mEq} = \frac{\text{Weight in milligrams}}{\text{Atomic weight}} \times \text{Valence}$$

Example: 0.5 g of NaCl = 500 mg; molecular weight of NaCl = 23 (atomic weight of $Na^+$) + 35.5 (atomic weight of $Cl^-$) = 58.5; valence = 1

$$\text{Thus } \frac{500}{58.5} \times 1 = 8.5\text{, or 500 mg of NaCl} = 8.5 \text{ mEq of NaCl}$$

**CONVERSION OF MILLIEQUIVALENTS PER LITER TO MILLIGRAMS PER 100 ML**

$$\text{mg/100 ml} = \frac{\text{mEq/L} \times \text{Atomic weight}}{10 \times \text{Valence}}$$

**CONVERSION OF MILLIGRAMS PER 100 ML TO MILLIEQUIVALENTS PER LITER**

$$\text{mEq/L} = \frac{\text{mg/100 ml} \times 10 \times \text{Valence}}{\text{Atomic weight}}$$

## NORMAL EXCHANGE OF FLUID AND ELECTROLYTES

In the healthy human being, body fluids (water and electrolytes) are constantly being lost and must be replaced to maintain normal processes. The fluid that is lost is not pure water but always contains some electrolytes; thus both water and electrolytes must be replaced daily. By knowing the concentration of fluid and electrolytes in the various compartments, the nurse can anticipate which fluid and electrolyte imbalance most probably will occur if abnormal losses occur from any particular site.

In a state of health, body fluids are lost daily from the kidneys, lungs, gastrointestinal tract, and skin, with negligible amounts being lost in saliva and tears. Two processes demand continual expenditure of water: control of body heat and excretion of metabolic waste products. The volume of fluid used in these processes depends on such things as external temperature, humidity, metabolic rate, and physical activities. In normal fluid balance the output of fluid equals the intake of fluid. In addition, a balanced diet provides excess amounts of electrolytes; the excess is excreted, and electrolyte balance is maintained. This balance is regulated primarily by the function of the kidney tubules.

Table 20-2 summarizes the normal routes of gains and losses of fluid in an adult consuming approximately 2500 calories per day. It should be noted that approximately two fifths of the normal fluid intake is obtained from water in food, or "preformed water." Solid foods such as meat and vegetables are 60% to 90% water. The fact that a large quantity of water is obtained from food has important implications if a person's food intake decreases substantially.

Approximately two fifths of the fluid lost daily is lost through the insensible route (skin, lungs, and gastrointestinal tract). These losses are not perceptible. Insensible loss through the skin refers to invisible perspiration. When visible perspiration occurs, such as that after

**TABLE 20-2 Normal Fluid Intake and Loss in an Adult Consuming 2500 Calories per Day (Approximate Figures)**

| INTAKE | | OUTPUT | |
|---|---|---|---|
| ROUTE | AMOUNT OF GAIN (ml) | ROUTE | AMOUNT OF LOSS (ml) |
| Water in food | 1000 | Skin | 500 |
| Water from oxidation | 300 | Lungs | 350 |
| Water as liquid | 1200 | Feces | 150 |
| | | Kidneys | 1500 |
| TOTAL | 2500 | TOTAL | 2500 |

heavy physical activities or with shock, the loss of water through the skin is greater than the normal 500 ml. Fecal loss increases in the presence of diarrhea or watery stools. Persons with certain pulmonary problems lose more than the normal amount of fluid (350 ml) from the lungs. Increased loss of fluids through these insensible routes also results in the loss of electrolytes. An increase in respiratory rate and/or body temperature results in an increase in insensible losses.

## INTERNAL REGULATION OF BODY WATER AND ELECTROLYTES

Fluid and electrolyte balance depends on an adequate intake and output. This means that the intake must equal the output. The control of intake and output is regulated by various internal mechanisms. In this section the regulation of body water and major electrolytes is discussed. The reader is referred to physiology texts for a more in-depth review.

### Sodium and Water

#### Thirst

The major control of actual fluid intake is thirst. The thirst center is located in the ventromedial nucleus of the hypothalamus. Impulses from this center can stimulate the cerebral cortex, which interprets this stimulation as the perception of thirst. The thirst center is stimulated by hypertonic body fluid, isoosmotic contraction, decreased blood pressure, decreased cardiac output, dryness of the mouth, and angiotensin (p. 523). How these factors cause the thirst center to be stimulated is not fully understood. It is thought that the dehydration (shrinkage) of cells in the thirst center causes stimulation of the neurons, which transmit the impulse to the cerebral cortex, which translates the sensation to that of thirst. Most of the time thirst is not thought of as a control of water intake, because social and cultural habits greatly influence the quantity of liquid human beings drink. Persons who depend on others to supply their intake of fluid or persons who have a sudden increase in fluid loss (bleeding, increased sweating) will complain of being thirsty. Some evidence suggests that human beings also have a salt appetite, which may be important in times of extreme sodium depletion such as with prolonged heat exposure and perspiration.

#### Kidney

The major organ controlling output is the kidney, which is under the influence of several control mechanisms. The kidney is responsible for regulating the volume and osmolality of body fluids. The osmolality of body fluids depends predominantly on sodium and its associate anions. The maintenance of water and sodium balance depends on glomerular filtration rate (GFR), antidiuretic hormone (ADH), and the aldosterone-renin-angiotensin system.

Glomerular filtration in the kidney is an involved topic (see Chapter 48). Three factors determine glomerular filtration: glomerular capillary blood pressure, the hydrostatic pressure of Bowman's capsule, and plasma protein concentration. Many factors and pathophysiologic states can affect these three factors and thus change glomerular filtration. Conditions such as shock and hypertension change glomerular capillary blood pressure. Changes in the pressure of Bowman's capsule can be caused by urinary obstruction. A decrease in plasma protein concentration can occur with increased loss, decreased intake, or decreased production of proteins. Damage to the basement membrane of the capsule, as in glomerular nephritis, will decrease filtration from the glomeruli.

#### Antidiuretic hormone

**Antidiuretic hormone (ADH)** is a hormone produced by the supraoptic and paraventricular nuclei of the hypothalamus and released from the posterior pituitary gland. The neurons in the hypothalamus receive input from volume receptors in the left atrium and great veins and from osmoreceptors in the hypothalamus. Volume receptors are stimulated by changes in atrial blood volume or blood pressure. Impulses from the volume receptors are transmitted by afferent nerve fibers to the hypothalamus. Increased blood volume or increased blood pressure increases the firing of the volume receptors, stimulates the hypothalamus, and inhibits ADH production. Conversely, decreased blood volume or blood pressure decreases the firing of the volume receptors and increases ADH production.

Osmoreceptors are stimulated by changes in cell size. The addition of pure water to the body fluids increases the size of the cells in the osmoreceptors and leads to the inhibition of ADH production. A loss of pure water causes the cells to shrink and stimulates the secretion of ADH. ADH secretion also is stimulated by angiotensin, narcotics, stress, heat, nicotine, antineoplastic agents, and anesthetic agents. Figure 20-2 depicts the factors and mechanisms involved in ADH production and the results of ADH production.

ADH acts on the kidney cells by stimulating 3′5′-cyclic adenosine monophosphate (AMP) release, and the

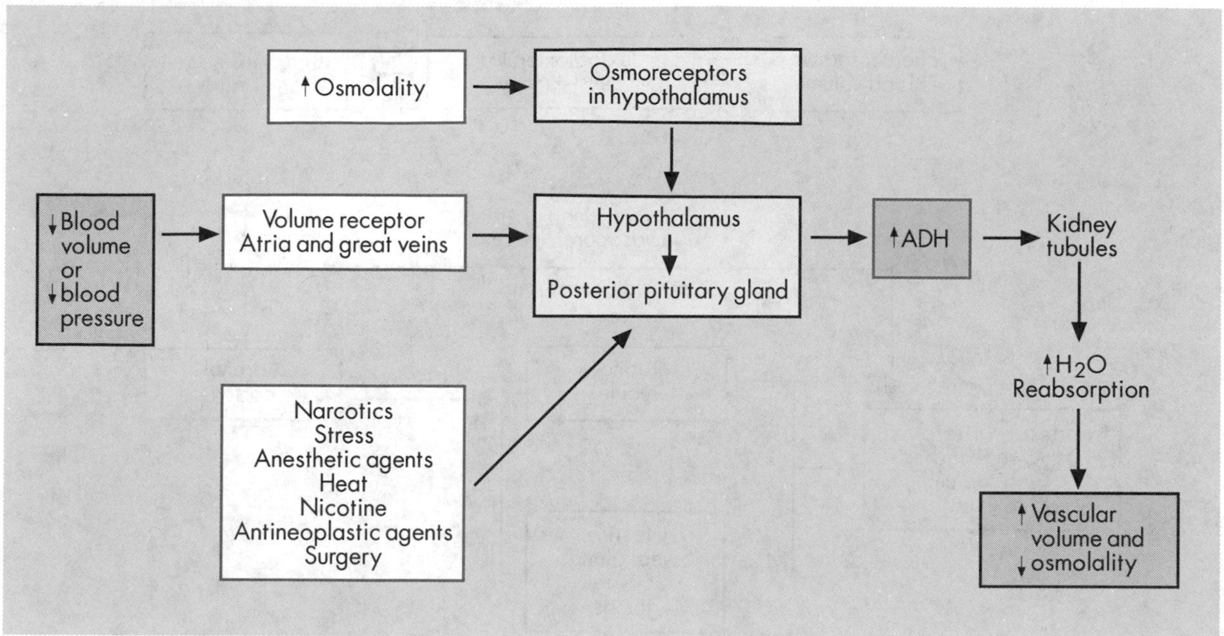


**FIGURE 20-2** Factors and mechanisms involved in antidiuretic hormone (ADH) production, and effect of ADH.

cyclic AMP causes appropriate cellular metabolism. In the kidney, ADH causes increased water reabsorption in the distal convoluted tubules and collecting ducts. It also may stimulate the pumping of sodium in the loop of Henle and regulate the rate of blood perfusion, both of which would lead to increased water reabsorption. In the presence of ADH, the kidney can concentrate urine to 1200 mOsm/kg $H_2O$.

The conservation of water increases blood volume and blood pressure and decreases osmolality. Because ADH can be secreted in response to factors other than a deficit of water (narcotics, anesthetic agents, stressors), fluid overload can occur. Patients who are at high risk of inappropriate ADH secretion need to be monitored closely by the nurse. This includes postoperative patients (see Chapter 25), as well as psychiatric patients who have been treated for 10 to 15 years, usually for schizophrenia. The condition is known as the *syndrome of inappropriate secretion of ADH (SIADH)*. It also may occur in those with closed head injury, and nurses caring for such patients should assess their patients' intake and output with this in mind. SIADH may be life-threatening if unrecognized and is usually self-limiting.

### Aldosterone-renin-angiotensin system

Aldosterone is a hormone produced by the zona glomerulosa of the adrenal cortex. It increases the kidney's reabsorption of sodium and thus water in the proximal tubules and the distal convoluted tubules. In the complete absence of aldosterone a person may excrete 25 g of sodium per day, whereas if large quantities of aldosterone are present, no sodium will be excreted.

The major stimulus for aldosterone production is a reflex initiated by the kidney. Cells in the kidney monitor sodium levels and blood volume. When the serum sodium level or the blood volume decreases, the juxtaglomerular cells in the kidney secrete a protein, *renin.* Renin acts on *angiotensinogen,* a plasma protein formed in the liver, to form *angiotensin I.* Angiotensin I is converted to *angiotensin II* by another enzyme. Angiotensin II stimulates the adrenal cortex to secrete aldosterone. Aldosterone causes the retention of sodium by the kidneys, intestines, and sweat and salivary glands. In addition, angiotensin II causes vasoconstriction of arterial smooth muscles, thus decreasing the GFR. It also causes systemic vasoconstriction, resulting in hypertension.

Some aldosterone may be secreted in response to adrenocorticotropic hormone (ACTH). Another important fact is that aldosterone is catabolized by the liver, and with liver failure, because of ineffective catabolism, inappropriate amounts of aldosterone may lead to sodium and water retention. Figure 20-3 depicts the factors and mechanisms involved in aldosterone production and the effects of aldosterone production.

### Third factor

Glomerular filtration, ADH, and the aldosterone-renin-angiotensin system do not explain the kidney's complete control of sodium and water reabsorption and excretion. It is hypothesized that a third factor is involved in the control of sodium and water balance.[9] The term *third factor* is used because little is known about this mechanism. Three other factors seem to assist in the control of sodium and water: (1) a natriuretic hormone, (2) intrarenal physical factors, and (3) redistribution of blood flow. Research is ongoing in these areas.

## Potassium

Potassium ($K^+$) is the major intracellular cation and regulates *intracellular* osmolality. Potassium is very im-

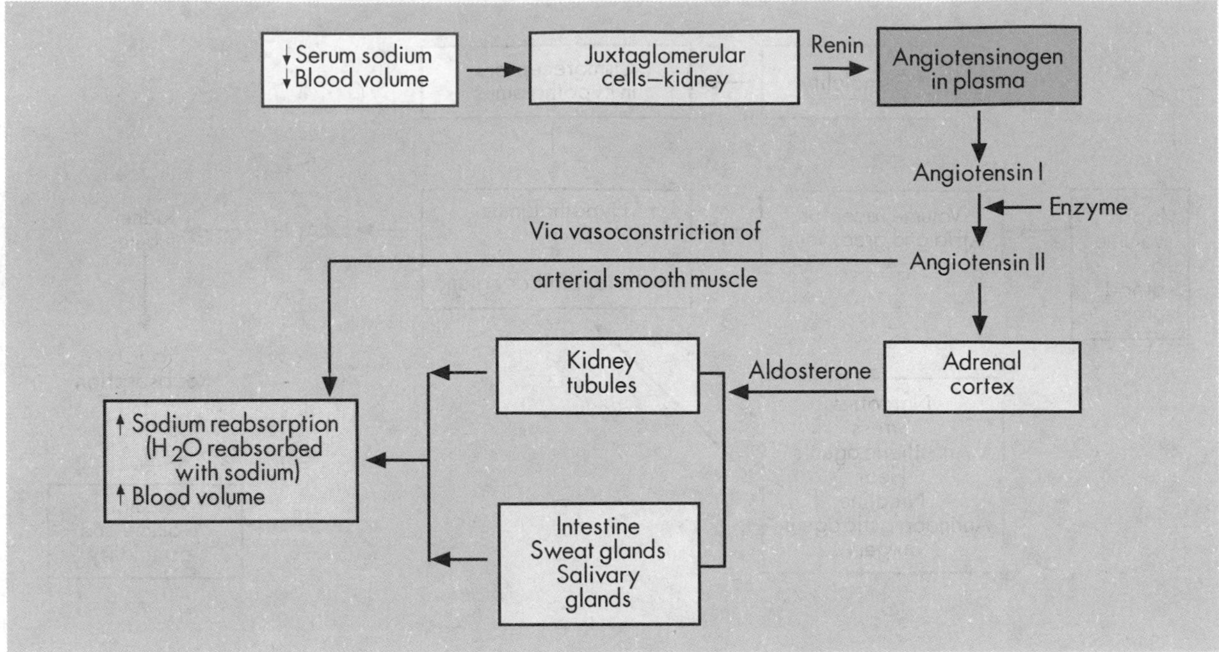


**FIGURE 20-3** Factors and mechanisms involved in aldosterone production and effects of aldosterone production.

portant in the conduction of nerve impulses and promotion of proper skeletal and cardiac muscle activity. Because of potassium's role in the excitability of nerves and muscles, it is important that the extracellular concentration of potassium be maintained within the narrow, normal range. (Review potassium values in Table 20-1.)

The major excretion site of excess potassium is the kidney. Most of excess potassium (80% to 90%) is excreted in the urine, and the remainder is excreted by the gastrointestinal tract. Potassium is completely filtered by the kidney, but most of the filtered potassium is reabsorbed in the proximal tubules and the loop of Henle. Glomerular filtration of potassium plays only a minimal role in normal potassium excretion. The control of renal excretion of potassium resides in the ability of the distal tubular cells to secrete potassium into tubular fluid. As extracellular potassium levels rise, more potassium moves into all cells, including the distal tubular cells. This higher concentration in the cells facilitates potassium secretion into tubular fluid because of the gradient difference between the distal tubular cells and the fluid in the tubular lumen. Conversely, if potassium intake is low or if there is increased loss of potassium through the gastrointestinal tract, the potassium level in the distal tubular cells is decreased. This causes a decrease in the gradient, and less potassium is secreted.

Even though glomerular filtration plays only a minimal role in the amount of potassium excreted in the urine, it is an important point to remember. Certain situations interfere with the reabsorption of the filtered potassium in the proximal tubules, and this can lead to an increased loss of potassium. Osmotic diuretics and disease states that produce osmotic diuresis are examples of situations in which there is interference with the reabsorption of potassium in the proximal tubules. Tubular diuretics, such as hydrochlorothiazide and furosemide, also enhance the loss of potassium.

Aldosterone can increase the amount of potassium secreted by the distal tubules. The aldosterone-secreting cells of the adrenal cortex are sensitive to the extracellular concentration of potassium. If the extracellular concentration of potassium increases, aldosterone is secreted and stimulates the distal tubular cells to secrete more potassium. The renin-angiotensin system is not involved in this stimulation of aldosterone.

It is apparent that a conflict arises when potassium and sodium levels are high, because these changes stimulate aldosterone production to move in different ways. What happens in such a situation is unknown. This is not the only conflict that can arise between different electrolytes. Hydrogen ion concentration affects potassium levels. The existence of a low hydrogen ion concentration increases potassium excretion and leads to potassium depletion (hypokalemia). The presence of a high hydrogen ion concentration (acidosis) decreases potassium excretion and can cause potassium excess (hyperkalemia).

## Calcium

### Factors influencing distribution

Calcium ($Ca^{++}$) plays a major role in the promotion of neuromuscular irritability and muscular contractions. Calcium and phosphorus are found primarily in the bones and teeth (99%) and dissolved in the blood (1%). The amounts of dissolved calcium and phosphorus are in an inverse relationship. As one increases, the other decreases. The inverse relationship must be maintained because if both are elevated at the same time, they form an insoluble precipitate. The dissolved portion of calcium is carried in the blood in two forms: bound to protein, particularly albumin, and ionized. The serum levels that usually are reported are measures of total dissolved calcium (both bound and ionized). The ionized fraction can be measured separately, but this is a more expensive test and is not routinely performed. Only the ionized fraction is involved in the promotion of neuromuscular activity.

The ionized portion must be maintained within fine limits because a decrease in ionized calcium has profound effects on the body, for example, *tetany* (p. 540). In a person with normal serum protein and albumin levels and a normal calcium level, the ionized fraction is usually a little greater than 50% of the total dissolved level. Because part of the dissolved calcium is bound to protein, the concentration of serum calcium varies as the protein level varies. If the total protein and albumin levels fall, the total serum calcium level will fall. Persons with serum calcium levels below normal resulting from a decrease in protein or albumin may exhibit no symptoms of *hypocalcemia* because, although their total calcium level is low, the ionized fraction may still be within normal limits.

The ratio between the dissolved calcium that is bound and the ionized fraction is affected by the acid-base status. Acidosis causes more calcium to be ionized, whereas alkalosis causes more of the ionized fraction to become bound. These changes are probably not detrimental to persons with a normal serum calcium level, but alkalosis in a person who already has a low serum calcium level can lead to tetany. Calcium also binds to other agents such as citrate, which normally is metabolized by the liver. Because citrate is commonly used as an anticoagulant in stored blood, persons receiving a large number of transfusions rapidly should be watched carefully for signs of hypocalcemia. Some authorities recommend that for every 3 to 4 units of blood given rapidly, the patient should receive 10 ml of calcium gluconate.[2]

#### Control of calcium levels

The level of calcium depends on three hormones: parathormone, vitamin D, and calcitonin. *Parathormone* is a hormone produced by the parathyroid gland, and decreased calcium levels stimulate its production. Parathormone causes increased movement of calcium from the bone, increased absorption of calcium from the gastrointestinal tract, and increased reabsorption of calcium in the renal tubules, all of which lead to an increase in serum calcium levels. Parathormone also increases the excretion of phosphorus by the kidneys.

*Vitamin D* is a hormone that is formed by the action of sunlight on a provitamin that is present in the skin or is obtained from dietary sources. Vitamin D is hydroxylated by reactions in the liver and kidney to its active form. Vitamin D is essential for the absorption of calcium from the gastrointestinal tract. Parathormone cannot increase the absorption of calcium from the gastrointestinal tract unless activated vitamin D is present. Vitamin D significantly increases the effectiveness of parathormone in bone resorption. In addition, vitamin D and parathormone are interlinked in another way. The major control point for the blood concentration of active vitamin D is the hydroxylation step in the kidney, which is stimulated by parathormone. Therefore a low calcium level stimulates the secretion of parathormone, which then activates vitamin D; both then increase the absorption of calcium from the gastrointestinal tract and the resorption of calcium from the bone.

*Calcitonin,* a hormone produced by the thyroid gland, decreases calcium levels by preventing bone resorption of calcium. It opposes the effects of parathormone and vitamin D on bones. High calcium levels stimulate the thyroid gland to release calcitonin, which inhibits the release of calcium from the bone and thus lowers serum calcium levels.

## MOVEMENT OF FLUIDS BETWEEN COMPARTMENTS

The preceding discussion has referred to the fact that water and solutes are in various compartments. The water and solutes in these compartments are not static but are constantly moving between compartments. Movement of water and solutes is how needed materials are carried to and waste products removed from the cells.

### Fluid and Solute Transport Between Extracellular and Intracellular Compartments

Fluids and electrolytes flow between the extracellular and intracellular compartments by passive or facilitated diffusion, osmosis, and active transport. Some electrolytes and other solutes flow between the two compartments with a concentration gradient by the process of passive or facilitated **diffusion.** For other solutes to move into the cell, they must flow against a concentration gradient by *active transport.* Active transport is not well understood, but it implies that solutes are moving against a concentration gradient or an electrical potential gradient. The mechanism involves the expenditure of energy. It has been shown that with the expenditure of one high-energy phosphate bond from adenosine triphosphate (ATP), three sodium ions move out of the cell, and two potassium ions move into the cell. Active transport uses a large percentage of the energy formed each day, because sodium is constantly diffusing into the cell and potassium is constantly diffusing out of the cell. Active transport is required to keep the concentration of the two electrolytes in the appropriate amounts within the cell.

Water, like solutes, moves between the extracellular compartment and the intracellular compartment. The movement of water is controlled by the osmolality of the two compartments. Sodium is the main regulator of extracellular osmolality, and potassium is the main regulator of intracellular osmolality.

Water moves from an area of high concentration of water (low concentration of solutes) to an area of low concentration of water (high concentration of solutes). This process is called **osmosis.** The movement of water will continue until the osmolality between the two compartments is approximately equal. Therefore if the water content increases in the extracellular compartment or the solute concentration decreases in the extracellular compartment, water moves into the cells to equalize the osmolality. Likewise, if the water content decreases in the extracellular compartment or the solute concentration increases in the extracellular compartment, water moves from the cells to equalize osmolality. Solutes move back and forth between the two compartments, but the cell membrane is more permeable to water than it is to solutes.

The mechanisms that control water and sodium levels control osmolality and thus the movement of fluid between the extracellular compartment and the intracellular compartment. Various disease states can change the osmolality and membrane permeability and cause cellular edema or cellular dehydration.

## Fluid Transport Between Vascular and Interstitial Spaces

The control of fluid movement between the vascular and interstitial spaces is governed by Starling's law of the capillaries. Two different types of pressure influence the flow of fluid between the vascular space and the interstitial space. These are hydrostatic pressure and colloid osmotic pressure (oncotic pressure). **Hydrostatic pressure** is that pressure caused by the blood pressing against the walls of the blood vessels. Hydrostatic pressure also exists in the tissue but is minimal (5 torr or less), and some authorities believe that the hydrostatic pressure in the tissue is actually a negative pressure.[4] Hydrostatic pressure effectively pushes fluid out of the vascular bed into the interstitial space.

**Colloid osmotic pressure** is the pressure needed to overcome the pull of the proteins, especially albumin, in the blood. The proteins do not pass freely through the walls of the capillaries because of their size. A few proteins are present in the interstitial space, but a much larger concentration is in the vascular space. The colloid osmotic pressure within the vascular space serves as a force to ***pull*** or ***absorb*** fluid from the interstitial space.

The difference between the vascular hydrostatic pressure and the vascular colloid osmotic pressure determines the movement of fluid between the vascular and interstitial spaces. For example, in Figure 20-4, the tissue hydrostatic pressure and tissue colloid osmotic pressure would be zero. The hydrostatic pressure at the arteriole end of the capillary (approximately 40 torr) is greater than the hydrostatic pressure at the venule end of the capillary (approximately 10 torr). The colloid osmotic pressure stays approximately the same throughout the vascular bed and equals about 25 torr.

The difference between the hydrostatic pressure and colloid osmotic pressure at the arteriole end of the capillary is +15 torr (40 torr − 25 torr = 15 torr) and favors the movements of fluid out of the vascular compartment. The difference between the hydrostatic pressure and colloid osmotic pressure at the venule end of the capillary is −15 torr (10 torr − 25 torr = −15 torr) and favors the movement of fluid into the vascular compartment (see Figure 20-4).

Overall, this system allows fluids high in nutrients and oxygen to diffuse out of the vascular bed at the arteriole end of the capillary and fluids containing waste products to move back into the vascular bed at the venule end

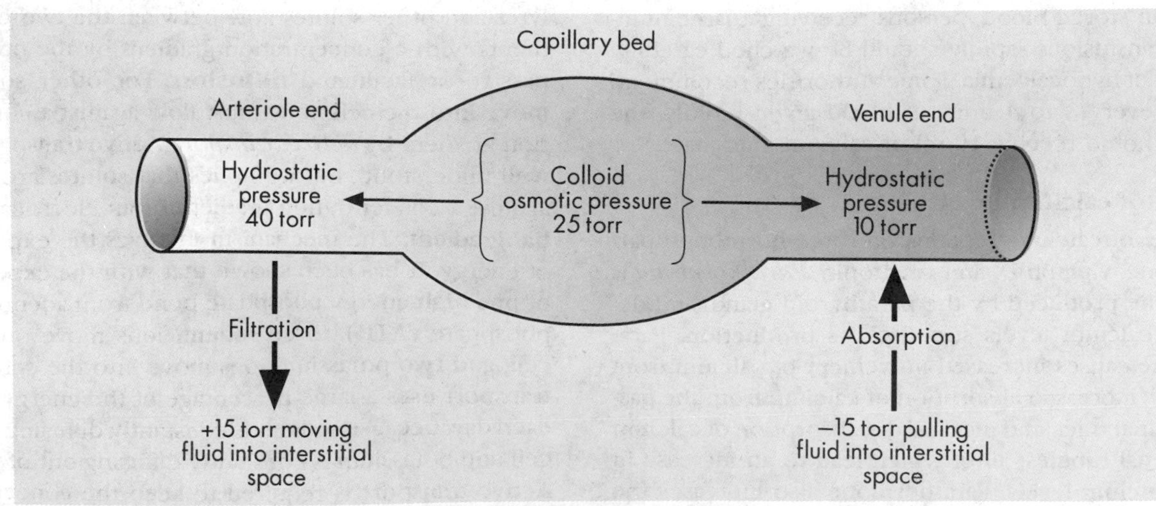


**FIGURE 20-4** Pressure difference across capillary provides for movement of fluid, nutrients, and waste between interstitial and vascular spaces.

of the capillaries. The system is not perfect, however, and some excess fluid is left in the interstitial space. In addition, some proteins may escape from the vascular bed and, if allowed to accumulate, act as a force to pull even more fluids from the vascular bed. The lymphatic system picks up the excess fluid and the escaped proteins and returns them to the vascular space.

Multiple factors affect the hydrostatic pressure. At the arteriole end of the capillary, the hydrostatic pressure depends on the volume of blood, viscosity of the blood, force of the heart, and resistance of the blood vessels. Hydrostatic pressure at the venous end depends on the venous pressure. The venous pressure in turn depends on the condition of the veins, respiration, and skeletal muscle contractions. The colloid osmotic pressure depends on the protein level, which depends on the dietary intake, the liver's ability to produce proteins, and the fact that excess proteins are not lost from the body. Various disease states can interfere with any of these multiple factors and result in edema. Damage to the lymphatic system can also cause edema.

## FLUID IMBALANCE

As previously noted, the osmolality of the ECF varies proportionally with its sodium concentration. Sodium and its anions (chloride and bicarbonate) make up 90% to 95% of the total solute in the ECF. When a change occurs in the sodium-to-water ratio, a disturbance in osmolality results; that is, the ECF becomes more dilute **(hyposmolar)** or more concentrated **(hyperosmolar)** than normal. A considerable change in the concentration of solutes other than sodium in the ECF also can cause osmolar disturbances.

Hyposmolality of the ECF causes water to move into body cells by osmosis to equalize the concentration of fluid on both sides of the cell membrane. Hyperosmolality of the ECF causes water to move out of the cells to dilute the ECF and to equalize the concentration of solutes in both compartments.

**TABLE 20-3 Water and Sodium Imbalances**

| TYPE OF IMBALANCE | WATER IMBALANCE | SODIUM IMBALANCE |
|---|---|---|
| Hyperosmolar | Water ↓ in relation to sodium and other solutes | Sodium or other solutes ↑ in relation to water |
| Hyposmolar | Water ↑ in relation to sodium and other solutes | Sodium ↓ in relation to water |
| Isotonic volume excess | Water ↑ proportionally with sodium | Sodium ↑ proportionally with water |
| Isotonic volume deficit | Water ↓ proportionally with sodium | Sodium ↓ proportionally with water |

When there are changes in the volume of ECF but no change in osmolality, an *isotonic* volume disturbance results. There is no significant change in the sodium-to-water ratio; sodium deficits or excesses are accompanied by proportional water deficits or excesses. There is no appreciable movement of water between the ICF and ECF compartments, and the imbalance is essentially restricted to the ECF compartment. Table 20-3 shows the types of fluid imbalances that are likely to occur.

## HYPEROSMOLAR IMBALANCE: EXTRACELLULAR WATER DEFICIT AND SOLUTE EXCESS

An extracellular water deficit occurs when the amount of water in the extracellular compartment is diminished in proportion to the solutes contained therein. An increase in solutes in proportion to water produces the same imbalance, known as hyperosmolar or hypertonic imbalance, in which the serum osmolality is above the normal 275 to 290 mOsm/kg. Dehydration often is used to describe any type of volume depletion; however, the precise definition of dehydration is water loss without electrolyte loss.

### Etiology

Imbalances may originate in either the fluid or the solute portion of the ECF. There may be (1) decreased intake of water, (2) excess loss of water without proportional loss of solutes, (3) increased solute intake without sufficient water, and (4) excess accumulation of solutes secondary to a particular disease condition.

Any person who does not have fluids available to drink, who cannot take fluids independently, or who does not respond to thirst is likely to develop a water deficit.

In a disaster such as a flood or an earthquake, a supply of drinkable water or fluids may not be available and would lead to a water deficit in residents. Patients who are unable to ask for fluids, to identify their need for fluid, or to swallow easily may develop a fluid deficit. Thus a patient with a cerebrovascular accident and aphasia may not be able to communicate a desire for fluids or may have difficulty swallowing fluids that are offered. A confused or disoriented patient may not be aware of thirst. Patients who are comatose, weak, or catatonic also may develop fluid deficits because of the inability to ask for fluids, swallow, or respond to thirst. Note that these problems are most likely to occur in very young or elderly persons.

Although loss of body water usually is accompanied by loss of electrolytes, there are a number of conditions in which water is lost in excess of electrolytes. These include increased loss through the lungs in hyperventilation or in secretions from a tracheostomy, through the skin with a high fever, through the gastrointestinal tract when there is watery diarrhea, or in urine when the kidneys fail to concentrate solutes.

## Pathophysiology

When solutes are taken in without sufficient water (such as occurs with intake of tube-feeding solutions that are high in protein, dextrose, and electrolytes), hyperosmolality results. The excess of solutes causes an **osmotic diuresis,** that is, the body's attempt to excrete a solute load through the kidneys by excreting a large volume of urine. Formation of the urine in this process requires the use of a great deal of water, interferes with the normal water conservation mechanisms, and results in a water deficit.

Several conditions lead to endogenous (internal) addition of excess solutes—large amounts of glucose can accumulate in the blood in diabetes mellitus, and glucose and ketone bodies can accumulate in the blood in diabetic ketoacidosis (see Chapter 43). A large volume of nitrogenous waste products results from metabolism of a high-protein diet. All of these solute excesses cause large water losses from osmotic diuresis.

When an extracellular water deficit occurs, water moves out of the cells to replace water lost from the extracellular compartment, thus maintaining an adequate circulating blood volume. If the water deficit is not corrected, the cells eventually become unable to compensate for extracellular losses; cellular dehydration ensues, and circulation begins to fail. As both ICFs and ECFs decrease, cell function is impaired because food, oxygen, and waste products are diffused inadequately. Brain cells are particularly sensitive to these changes, and a disruption of brain cell function develops that manifests as mental changes in the patient.

Thirst and weight loss are early symptoms of water deficit and become more pronounced as the deficit increases. Body temperature begins to rise as less water is available for temperature regulation. When cells are unable to continue providing water to replace ECF losses, signs of collapse of the circulatory system appear. A dry mouth and throat cause difficulty with speech. Signs and symptoms of water deficit are shown in Table 20-4.

**TABLE 20-4 Signs and Symptoms of Water Deficit**

| | MODERATE DEFICIT | SEVERE DEFICIT |
|---|---|---|
| Skin | Flushed, dry | Cold, clammy |
| Mouth | Dry mucous membranes | Dry, cracked tongue |
| Eyes | Decrease in tears | Soft, sunken eyeballs |
| Cardiovascular system | — | Tachycardia, low blood pressure, rapid respirations |
| Central nervous system | Apprehension, restlessness | Lethargy, coma |
| Blood | — | Hemoconcentration, increase in hematocrit, BUN, electrolytes |
| Urine | High specific gravity, scant amount (except with osmotic diuresis) | Oliguria, highly colored urine |
| Other | Thirst, weight loss | Thirst, weight loss, fever |

## Prevention

Prevention is crucial in the nursing care of patients who are at risk of developing a water deficit. The nurse is alert to those patients who may not be receiving adequate fluid intake, monitors their intake and output, and plans a schedule for offering fluids to them. Patients who are hyperventilating for long periods of time, regardless of the reason, should have their fluid intake increased somewhat, because they are losing more fluid than usual through the lungs. Those receiving high-protein tube feedings need sufficient water to prevent osmotic diuresis and water deficit.

## anagement

therapy are to treat the underlying causes to urther water loss and to replace lost fluid. ıysician can use several methods, such as those based on serum sodium concentration or change in the patient's weight, to calculate the volume of water loss.[3] For instance, if a patient has lost 4 kg of body weight, the fluid deficit equals 4 L (1 kg weighs 1 L). Therapy will require replacement of the volume lost plus about 1.5 L of fluid to supply current daily need. Often the replacement is administered over a period of several days, because too rapid infusion of fluid may cause sudden intercompartmental shifts of water and pulmonary edema as a result of cardiac overload.

When the water deficit is not severe, fluids can be replaced orally if the patient is able to drink fluids. Otherwise, intravenous fluids are given.

Intravenous glucose and water usually are given first to replace the water loss and increase urinary flow. Urinary output must be adequate so that electrolytes in excess of body needs can be excreted. Solutions that contain electrolytes are therefore not given until renal function is established. Normal saline or half-strength saline (0.45%) can be given with other ions—potassium, calcium, and lactate—as needed.

In addition to providing fluids and participating in the treatment of conditions underlying water loss, nurses use measures to decrease discomfort and ensure patient safety. *Mouth care* is especially important to relieve dryness of mucous membranes and remove debris on lips and teeth. Safety measures such as side rails on beds are necessary for patients who have developed restlessness, confusion, lethargy, or other mental changes as a result of water deficit. Monitoring intake and output and changes in the patient's weight and vital signs will indicate whether the patient's condition is improving or deteriorating.

A state of adequate hydration is evidenced by mental alertness, moist mucous membranes, and urinary output that is approximately equal to fluid intake.

## HYPOSMOLAR IMBALANCE: WATER EXCESS OR WATER INTOXICATION

When there is an excess of water in relation to solutes in the ECF, a hyposmolar (hypotonic) imbalance known as **water excess** or **water intoxication** (cellular edema) exists. Although this imbalance is not common, it can develop when water intake exceeds the ability of the kidneys to excrete it. Usually there is a concomitant increase in secretion of ADH, which promotes water retention and aggravates the water excess.

Under normal conditions, a decrease in osmotic pressure suppresses ADH production and permits free water to be excreted by the kidneys.

### Etiology

One or more of the following conditions exists when water intoxication develops: (1) excess intake of electrolyte-free fluid, (2) increased secretion of ADH, or (3) decreased or inadequate output of urine.

Water excess can be caused by ingestion of large amounts of tap water, a behavior called *psychogenic polydipsia.* The ingestion of frequent sips of tap water by one who is not able to tolerate food or other fluids because of illness also can lead to water excess. Some treatments that lead to excessive water intake are multiple tap water enemas and absorption of water from irrigating solutions during transurethral resection of the prostate gland.

Excess or inappropriate secretion of ADH occurs in response to stressors, drugs, and anesthetics. It also can accompany inflammatory conditions of the lung (tuberculosis, pneumonia) and brain (encephalitis, meningitis), endocrine disturbances, and tumors in the lungs (especially oat cell carcinoma), pancreas, duodenum, and other body organs.[2] Inadequate kidney function or renal failure potentiates the development of water excess.

A low serum sodium or sodium deficit also can produce a hyposmolar imbalance (see discussion of sodium deficit, p. 534).

### Pathophysiology

When water intoxication occurs, hyposmolar water excess in the extracellular compartment quickly becomes an *intracellular water excess.* A lesser concentration of solutes is present in the ECF as compared with that in the ICF; therefore water moves into the cells to equalize concentration on both sides of the cell membranes, causing the cells to swell.

Because brain cells are particularly sensitive to the increase in intracellular water, the most common signs are manifestations of changes in the patient's *mental status.*

In acute water intoxication, there is swelling of the cells, which may develop rapidly and dramatically. Signs of water intoxication are listed in Box 20-2.

**BOX 20-2 Signs of Acute Water Intoxication**

- Changes in behavior: confusion, incoordination, convulsions
- Hyperventilation
- Sudden weight gain
- Warm, moist skin
- Increased intracranial pressure: slow bounding pulse with an increase in systolic and decrease in diastolic blood pressures
- Peripheral edema, usually not marked

When the condition develops more slowly, there may be apathy, sleepiness, anorexia, nausea, and vomiting. A low serum sodium concentration is a usual finding.

### Prevention

Water intoxication can be anticipated by identifying patients with one or more risk factors. Daily weights and careful monitoring of intake and output will help to detect the problem before it becomes severe.

### Management

The primary intervention for water intoxication is water restriction. In severe cases of hyposmolarity, when the serum sodium is critically depressed (<116 mEq/L), administration of furosemide (Lasix) and infusion of 3% to 5% hypertonic saline may be used. The saline raises the sodium level while the diuretic causes water loss. Administration of saline without diuretics does not maintain the sodium level because sodium will continue to be excreted by the kidneys. Furosemide inhibits some of this urinary sodium excretion and assists in preventing hypervolemia.

During treatment, hourly intake and output measurements are necessary. Infusions should be given by use of a controlled infusion device to prevent too rapid administration. Daily body weight, breath sounds, serum sodium levels, and neurologic status also are assessed.

Providing for the safety of patients with this imbalance is a priority nursing function because of the confusion and other mental changes that occur. Any patient who is receiving a large amount of water orally, rectally, or intravenously should be monitored carefully for signs of water intoxication, especially if a condition of excess ADH prevails. Coherent patients who may be at risk for this problem should be instructed to report any new tightness of rings and/or shoes.

## ISOTONIC VOLUME DEFICIT: EXTRACELLULAR FLUID DEFICIT

Conditions that cause a loss of water together with a loss of electrolytes lead to *isotonic volume deficit,* also known as *ECF depletion.*

**TABLE 20-5 Fluid Composition of Total Internal Secretions***

| | APPROXIMATE ml OF FLUID (DAILY) |
|---|---|
| Saliva | 1500 |
| Gastric juice | 2500 |
| Intestinal juice | 2000 |
| Pancreatic juice | 1500 |
| Bile | 500 |
| TOTAL | 8000 ml/24 hr |

*Note that approximately 8 L of fluid are used daily for digestive purposes. Normally, most of this fluid is reabsorbed. Some of each of the ions found in blood plasma is present in each of the fluids listed, but the individual concentration varies with each fluid.

## Etiology

Water and electrolytes are lost in hemorrhage and profuse sweating. About 8 L of fluid circulate through the gastrointestinal tract per day (Table 20-5). These fluids are derived from the ECF; therefore vomiting, diarrhea, draining intestinal fistulas, and surgical openings such as ileostomy and cecostomy result in ECF loss. Severe losses can deplete the extracellular compartment rapidly.

## Pathophysiology

In isotonic volume deficit, the extracellular osmolality does not change, because sodium, the chief contributor to extracellular osmolality, is lost along with water. Consequently, water content of the cells is not affected immediately, and the deficit remains restricted to the extracellular compartment. If the loss of ECF continues, ICF will move into the ECF, resulting in intracellular dehydration. Fluid movement is from the extracellular compartment to outside the body, depleting vascular and interstitial volumes. Signs of ECF depletion are listed in Box 20-3.

## Prevention

Nurses are responsible for identifying and monitoring patients at risk of developing isotonic fluid deficit. Taking postural vital signs is one method used to detect this deficit before cardiovascular symptoms develop. *Postural vital signs* are the comparison of a person's blood pressure and pulse measured from a lying position to a sitting or standing position. A drop in blood pressure of 10 torr or more with an increase in pulse rate indicates postural hypotension and signals a state of isotonic fluid depletion.

The healthy person who is perspiring profusely needs extra dietary salt and should drink extra fluids. Patients on low-sodium diets and those with draining gastrointestinal fistulas are prone to develop sodium depletion. They should always be taught to increase their salt intake slightly whenever they perspire profusely. Patients who have hot packs applied to large areas of the body also lose sodium and water, although the loss may not be as readily noticeable as perspiration. Attention to ingesting more salt and water than usual in situations of excessive heat may prevent heat exhaustion.

**BOX 20-3 Signs of Extracellular Fluid Depletion**

Skin: poor turgor
Mouth: dry mucous membranes
Cardiovascular: postural hypotension (early), low blood pressure, tachycardia, increased respiration, decreased vein filling
Weight: loss
Urine: low output, increased specific gravity

## Management

Treatment consists of identifying and correcting the underlying cause to prevent further fluid and electrolyte loss and of replacing those fluids and electrolytes that have been lost. Hemorrhage must be controlled. Vomiting may be treated with antiemetics such as trimethobenzamide hydrochloride (Tigan), prochlorperazine (Compazine), or promethazine hydrochloride (Phenergan) and diarrhea with antidiarrheal drugs, that is, dephenoxylate (Lomotil), paregoric, and kaolin and pectin (Kaopectate).

Any patient who is losing body fluids through perspiration, fever, or loss of gastrointestinal fluid should be given salty fluids to drink. Meticulous mouth care relieves the discomfort of dry mucous membranes.

As blood volume decreases, postural hypotension develops, and the patient's safety may be threatened by the resultant weakness, dizziness, or fainting on standing upright. Loss of fluid through a tracheostomy can be minimized with humidity therapy.

# ISOTONIC VOLUME EXCESS: EXTRACELLULAR FLUID EXCESS AND EDEMA

If there is an excess of body water with a concomitant increase in sodium, the excess fluid will be retained in the *extracellular* compartments and lead to the formation of edema. **Edema** is the accumulation of fluid in the interstitial spaces.

## Etiology

Edema can be produced by any of the following: increase in capillary fluid pressure, decrease in capillary oncotic pressure, increase in interstitial oncotic pressure, and any condition that increases the amount of aldosterone circulating in the blood. Causes of edema with clinical examples are shown in Table 20-6.

**TABLE 20-6 Causes of Edema According to Underlying Physiologic Mechanism**

| FLUID PRESSURE | ONCOTIC PRESSURE |
|---|---|
| **INCREASED CAPILLARY FLUID PRESSURE** | **DECREASED CAPILLARY ONCOTIC PRESSURE** |
| **Increased Venous Pressure** | **Loss of Serum Protein** |
| Vein obstruction | Burns, draining wounds, fistulas |
| Varicose veins | Hemorrhage |
| Thrombophlebitis | Nephrotic syndrome |
| Pressure on veins from casts, tight bandages, or garters | Chronic diarrhea |
| Increased total volume with decreased cardiac output | |
| Congestive heart failure | **Decreased Intake of Protein** |
| Fluid overloading | Malnutrition |
| | Kwashiorkor |
| **Sodium and Water Retention, Increased Aldosterone** | |
| | **Decreased Production of Albumin** |
| Decreased renal blood flow | Liver disease |
| Congestive heart failure | |
| Renal failure | **INCREASED INTERSTITIAL ONCOTIC PRESSURE** |
| Increased production of aldosterone | **Increased Capillary Permeability to Protein** |
| Cushing's syndrome | Burns |
| Aldosterone added to system | Inflammatory reactions |
| Corticosteroid therapy | Trauma |
| Inability to destroy aldosterone | Infections |
| Cirrhosis of liver | Allergic reactions (hives) |
| | **Blocked Lymphatics: Decreased Removal of Tissue Fluid and Protein** |
| | Malignant diseases |
| | Surgical removal of lymph nodes |
| | Elephantiasis |

## Pathophysiology

According to Starling's law of the capillaries (p. 526), an equilibrium exists between the forces filtering fluid out of the capillary and the forces absorbing fluid back into the capillary (see Figure 20-4). Three changes that can alter this equilibrium and lead to increased interstitial fluid (edema) are (1) an increase in capillary fluid pressure, (2) a decrease in capillary colloid osmotic (oncotic) pressure, and (3) an increase in interstitial oncotic pressure.

### Increased capillary fluid pressure

Increase in capillary fluid pressure results from the overloading of the vascular compartment. The high pressure pushes fluid out of the vessels into the surrounding interstitial tissues. More important, if the increase in hydrostatic pressure is great enough, large amounts of fluid will be pushed across the alveolocapillary membrane into the alveoli of the lungs. **Pulmonary edema** can occur unless this process is reversed.

Overloading of the vascular system may be caused by giving too much fluid within a short period of time to a person who, because of circulatory or renal disease, cannot dispose of the surplus. Elderly persons tolerate increases in blood volume very poorly, because with inelastic vessels only relatively small increases in volume are needed to markedly increase the hydrostatic pressure. Monitoring the central venous pressure (see Chapter 29) is one method used to determine if overloading is occurring. Retention of sodium and water, which occurs in cardiac and renal dysfunction, is one of the most common causes of increased vascular volume and results in high capillary fluid pressure and edema.

Overloading of the vascular system also may be caused by giving solutions high in proteins so rapidly that the body cannot dispose of protein that is in excess of its need. This overloading causes fluids to be pulled into the intravascular compartment from other body fluid compartments. The blood volume increases rapidly, neutralizing the oncotic pressure but increasing the hydrostatic pressure of the vascular system. Fluid is then pushed back into the tissues. Overloading the vascular system is a risk when fluids such as plasma, plasma expanders, albumin, blood, or total parenteral nutrition are given to any person regardless of age or state of health.

### Decreased capillary oncotic pressure

Proteins in the blood (particularly albumin) are necessary to create the oncotic pressure that holds fluids in the vessels. When the capillary oncotic pressure is decreased, fluid moves out of the vascular compartment into the interstitial spaces. When serum proteins are low because of inadequate intake (severe malnutrition), excess loss from burns or renal disease, or decreased production in the liver, edema results.

**Increased interstitial oncotic pressure**

An increase in interstitial oncotic pressure increases the pull of fluid from the vascular compartment into the interstitial spaces. Proteins may leak out of blood vessels because of increased capillary permeability such as occurs in inflammatory or allergic reactions. In the healthy person, edema does not develop immediately after the initial movement of fluid into the interstitial spaces because of the body's compensatory mechanisms, which include the existing low interstitial fluid pressure and the lymph system, which removes excess fluids and proteins.

**Fluid collection in potential fluid spaces**

The same mechanisms that create edema in the interstitial spaces can create fluid collection in potential fluid spaces—that is, in spaces between two membranes that normally contain only traces of fluid (Table 20-7). **Third spacing of fluids** is defined as the shift of fluid from the vascular space to an area of the body where it is unavailable for functional use. The symptoms of fluid collection in these spaces are caused by the pressure of the collected fluid on adjoining organs or walls. Large amounts of fluid may be sequestered in an operative site and in tissues surrounding an injury. An accumulation of fluid in all body tissues is called generalized edema, or *anasarca*.

## Prevention

The possibility of overhydration is considered whenever intravenous fluids are being given and during planning of "forced fluid" regimens. Overhydration can easily occur in persons with renal or circulatory impairment. Usually such persons must restrict fluid and sodium intake.

Patients on a low-sodium diet need to know which foods to avoid. They should read labels on all prepared foods, because many contain large amounts of sodium, and they may need assistance in planning ways to adhere to fluid restriction. When medications are prescribed to be taken at home, patients are taught the purpose of each drug and its usual side effects. If nonprescription medications may be used, the patient should be instructed to avoid those containing sodium. Patients also should record the fluid taken with medications, monitor their weight daily, and notify the physician if there is a significant change.

**TABLE 20-7 Fluid Collection in Potential Fluid Spaces**

| POTENTIAL FLUID SPACE | LOCATION | FLUID |
|---|---|---|
| Intrapleural | Between lung and chest wall | Pleural effusion |
| Pericardial | Between heart and pericardial sac | Pericardial effusion |
| Peritoneal | Between intestines and abdominal wall | Ascites |

## Management

### Assessment

In general, ***weight gain*** is the best indicator of an extracellular volume excess, because several liters of fluid can be retained without visible evidence of edema. Inasmuch as hydrostatic pressure in the capillaries is greatest in the lower parts of the body, edema collects in these areas. This is called *dependent* edema. When one is standing or sitting with feet on the floor, edema develops in the ankles and feet; when one is in a supine position, edema fluid collects in the sacral area of the back.

If a finger is pressed over an edematous area, the indentation made by the finger will remain briefly as the fluid is pushed to another area; this is called *pitting edema*. Fluid refills the interstitial place in the "pit" area gradually. A subjective measure is sometimes used to describe pitting edema on a scale from "one plus" (+) to "four plus" (++++), with the latter indicating severe pitting edema because it takes longer for displaced fluid to move back into the pit area. Skin over parts of the body with marked edema usually is tight, smooth, and shiny. It is cool and pale because of poor circulation. If edema is very severe, fluid will leak out of pores when the skin is pressed. This is called *weeping* edema.

Overhydration causes neck vein engorgement, so that these veins appear distended even when the patient is in an upright position (see Figure 29-12). Clothing and shoes begin to feel tight and uncomfortable.

**Determining cause**

The treatment of edema depends on the condition that has caused it. Congestive heart failure usually is treated with digitalis, diuretics, and sodium and fluid restriction. Cirrhosis of the liver also is treated with sodium and fluid restriction and possibly mild diuretics, especially spironolactone (Aldactone). Renal failure requires severe restrictions of water and electrolytes or their removal by dialysis.

Reducing sodium intake alone may reduce edema because the supply of body sodium is reduced and that which remains appears to be needed to maintain isotonicity of the blood.

Malnutritional edema responds to adequate dietary intake, especially to the addition of protein to the diet, unless the condition is far advanced, as occurs in starving children and adults in famine areas where kwashiorkor is a common cause of death. Edema associated with infections and burns resolves over time as the underlying cause responds to treatment.

Excess fluid in the tissues results in poor cellular nutrition as cells are pushed further apart and away from capillaries. Normal exchange of nutrients and wastes is interrupted. Edematous tissues therefore are poorly nourished, are susceptible to trauma and infection, and heal poorly. Caution must be taken to protect edematous parts of the body from prolonged pressure, injury, and extremes of heat and cold. Skin over these parts should be kept well lubricated to prevent dryness. If edematous areas are exposed to extensive moisture from incontinence or perspiration, they should be washed and dried frequently to prevent maceration.

When edema is caused by venous stasis, elevating dependent body parts and applying supportive stockings to the legs help promote venous return. Extremities that become edematous as a result of surgery or trauma also should be elevated and supported.

Great care must be taken if intravenous fluids are being administered to a person with edema. The use of an intravenous administration pump will add a margin of safety to the control of solution flow rate.

### Diuretics

Edema often is treated with diuretics that act on the kidneys. Thiazide diuretics, the most commonly used, inhibit reabsorption of sodium and chloride in the proximal renal tubules and thus promote excretion of sodium and water, or *diuresis*. Potassium usually is lost along with sodium and water unless a potassium-sparing diuretic is used. Fluid and electrolyte imbalances are undesirable but rather common side effects of diuretic therapy. Hypokalemia may be prevented by increasing intake of foods high in potassium: orange juice, bananas, raisins, and dates. When diuretics are given, a large amount of fluid is lost from the vascular compartment, decreasing its hydrostatic pressure and causing fluid to be pulled back into it from the interstitial compartment.

Before excess fluid in the interstitial spaces can be excreted, it must be moved back into the vascular compartment; otherwise, diuresis causes serious vascular depletion. Table 20-8 shows some diuretics and their effects.

**TABLE 20-8 Common Diuretics and Their Effect on Fluid and Electrolyte Balance**

| GENERIC NAME | TRADE NAME | METHOD OF ADMINISTRATION | PEAK EFFECT | PROBABLE EFFECTS ON FLUID AND ELECTROLYTE BALANCE |
|---|---|---|---|---|
| Thiazides | | | | |
| Chlorothiazide | Diuril | Oral | 4 hr | Hyponatremia<br>Hypokalemia<br>↓ ECF volume<br>Hyperglycemia<br>Hyperuricemia |
| Hydrochlorothiazide | Esidrix<br>HydroDiuril | Oral | 3-4 hr | Hypomagnesemia |
| Loop diuretics (act mainly on ascending loop of Henle) | | | | |
| Furosemide | Lasix | IM or IV<br>Oral | ½ hr<br>2-4 hr | Hypokalemia<br>Hyperuricemia<br>↓ ECF volume |
| Ethacrynic acid | Edecrin | Oral<br>IV | 2-4 hr<br>½ hr | Hyponatremia |
| Bumetanide | Bumex | Oral<br><br>IM<br><br>IV | ½-1 hr<br><br>40 min<br><br>5 min | Hypokalemia<br>Hypouricemia<br>Hyponatremia<br>Hypocalcemia<br>Hypochloremia |
| Aldosterone antagonist (opposes potassium-losing action of aldosterone) | | | | |
| Spironolactone | Aldactone | Oral | 72 hr | Hyperkalemia<br>Hyponatremia |
| Potassium-conserving action | | | | |
| Triamterene | Dyrenium | Oral | 4-8 hr | Hyperkalemia |
| Osmotic agent | | | | |
| Mannitol | Osmitrol | IV infused over 24-hr period | — | Hyponatremia<br>Hypochloremia<br>↑ ECF volume |

# ELECTROLYTE IMBALANCE

As noted earlier, sodium, potassium, calcium, and magnesium are the principal cations in the body. Chloride, bicarbonate, and phosphate are the principal anions. Although these electrolytes make up less than 5% of the total body weight, life cannot be sustained unless body fluids contain exactly the right amount of each in the right concentration within each of the fluid compartments.[8] In addition, no single electrolyte can be out of balance without causing other electrolytes to be out of balance also.

Sodium, potassium, and calcium are all essential for the passage of nerve impulses. Whenever the concentration of any of these cations is increased or decreased in body fluids, the increase or decrease is reflected in the stimulation of muscles by nerves. The muscles may become weak and atonic because of inadequate stimulation, or they may become somewhat spastic because of excess stimulation.

## SODIUM

The normal concentration of sodium in the blood is 138 to 145 mEq/L. Sodium is the most prevalent cation in the ECF and controls the osmotic pressure of this compartment. It is essential for neuromuscular functioning, for many intracellular chemical reactions, and for helping to maintain acid-base balance in the body. The sodium gradient theory states that sodium must be present for glucose to be transported into cells.

As previously mentioned, aldosterone causes reabsorption of sodium in the kidney tubules (p. 523). When the sodium supply becomes low, renal loss of sodium drops to zero. Aldosterone does not greatly influence sodium *concentration,* however, because as sodium is reabsorbed, water also is reabsorbed in equal proportions.

### Sodium Deficit

A low sodium level in the blood, **hyponatremia,** can result from either a sodium loss or a water excess (dilutional hyponatremia) (p. 529).

#### Etiology

The treatment of cardiac conditions and hypertension with diuretics and restricted sodium intake is a frequent cause of hyponatremia. The minimum daily requirement for sodium is 2 g/day. Sodium depletion also results from loss of gastrointestinal or biliary drainage and draining fistulas. Diseases interfering with aldosterone secretion, such as Addison's disease, result in excessive losses of sodium and water.

Sodium depletion also can occur in the shifting of body fluids so that the sodium and water are "trapped" in certain body areas and are not accessible for use. This can occur in massive edema, ascites, burns, or small bowel obstruction.

**TABLE 20-9 Comparison of Serum Sodium Levels With Total Body Sodium***

| CONDITION | SERUM SODIUM | TOTAL BODY SODIUM |
|---|---|---|
| Prolonged sweating | Low (hyponatremia) | Low |
| Diuretics and low-sodium diets | Low | Low |
| Addison's disease | Low | Low |
| Edema (cardiac, renal hepatic disease) | Low or normal | High |
| Excretion of dilute urine, early stages of gastrointestinal sodium loss | Normal | Low |
| Excess oral or IV sodium intake | High (hypernatremia) | High |
| Water and sodium loss with water loss > sodium loss | High | Low |

*Note that a low or high serum level does not necessarily correspond with total body sodium.

Anyone who is perspiring profusely because of climate, exercise, or fever is losing large amounts of both sodium and water. A form of chronic renal disease, "salt-wasting nephritis," also causes large daily losses of sodium ions. Sodium depletion caused by any of the aforementioned conditions is aggravated by a low-sodium diet.

#### Pathophysiology

Sodium loss from the intravascular compartment causes fluid from the blood to diffuse into the interstitial spaces. As a result, the sodium in the interstitial fluid is diluted. In response to this reduction in sodium concentration in the ECF, potassium moves out of the ICF. Therefore the patient with a sodium imbalance is also likely to have a potassium imbalance.

The decreased osmolality of ECF that exists with sodium loss creates a condition similar to water excess; that is, water moves into the cells by osmosis and leaves the extracellular compartment depleted. It differs from water intoxication because there is not an excess of total body water but an intercompartmental movement of water and depletion of the extracellular compartment.

The laboratory test for plasma sodium does not always give an accurate indication of total body sodium. Some clinical conditions in which the level of serum sodium is not an accurate indicator of total body sodium can be seen in Table 20-9. Sodium readily combines with bicarbonate or chloride to help maintain acid-base balance. Signs and symptoms of hyponatremia are listed in Box 20-4.

**BOX 20-4 Signs and Symptoms of Hyponatremia**

Headache
Muscle weakness
Fatigue and apathy
Postural hypotension
Anorexia, nausea, and vomiting
Abdominal cramps
Weight loss

**SEVERE**

Mental confusion
Delirium
Shock
Coma

### Prevention

Athletes and persons who work in very hot environments are advised to ingest fluids that contain sodium and to add some salty foods to their diets. If salt is not replaced along with water—that is, if thirst is quenched by drinking large amounts of tap water alone—water intoxication (p. 529) can occur. Salt tablets can be taken during the period of adaptation to an exceptionally hot environment; however, increased dietary sodium is the treatment of choice. Diuretics such as the thiazides eventually may cause sodium depletion; therefore the patient who is receiving extensive diuretic treatment should be observed for symptoms of sodium depletion. Because many patients receiving diuretics are at home, they should be taught to report symptoms of sodium depletion to the physician. These patients should not be on severely restricted sodium diets.

When a nasogastric tube needs to be irrigated, normal saline should be used in preference to water. Plain water irrigation washes sodium out of the stomach and leads to hyponatremia.

### Management

Treatment of shock, if present, is the first concern. Saline solution, usually 0.9% sodium chloride, is given intravenously at a rapid rate. Plasma expanders also may be infused.

If other electrolytes (potassium, calcium, bicarbonate) have been depleted, these also need to be replaced. Treatment that alleviates the underlying cause will prevent further sodium loss. Salt or salty foods are added to the diet for sodium depletion, which develops slowly or follows profuse perspiration (diaphoresis) or vomiting. (See Chapter 22 for a more detailed description of the treatment.)

Safety measures, such as the use of side rails on the bed, supervision of ambulation, and frequent observation, are necessary if the patient becomes weak or confused or experiences marked hypotension.

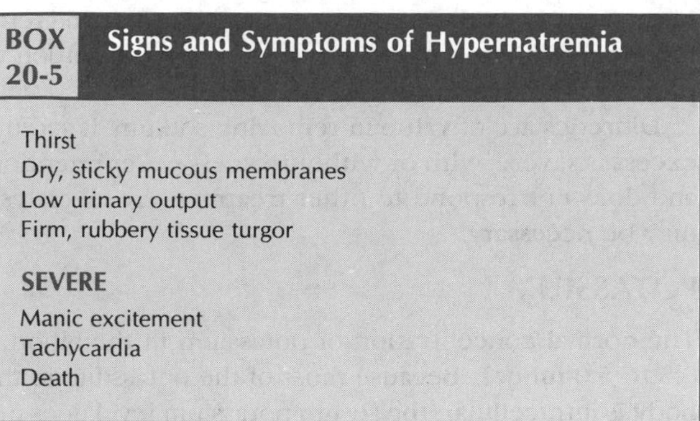
**BOX 20-5 Signs and Symptoms of Hypernatremia**

Thirst
Dry, sticky mucous membranes
Low urinary output
Firm, rubbery tissue turgor

**SEVERE**

Manic excitement
Tachycardia
Death

## Sodium Excess

A serum sodium level greater than 145 mEq/L is known as **hypernatremia.** There are actually two kinds of sodium excess, edema and hypernatremia. When there is a sodium and water excess, edema exists; when there is an excess of sodium in relation to water in the extracellular compartment, hypernatremia exists. As seen in Table 20-9 hypernatremia does not necessarily indicate an excess of total body sodium.

### Etiology

Hypernatremia occurs when more water than sodium is lost from the body and sodium concentration in the blood rises. It can also result from an abnormally large oral intake of sodium such as when a child accidentally eats many salt tablets or when intravenous saline is infused so rapidly that the body cannot excrete the amount not needed.

### Pathophysiology

If sodium becomes concentrated in ECF, osmolality rises, water leaves the cell by osmosis and enters the extracellular compartment to dilute fluids there, and the cells are water-depleted. The presence of hypernatremia suppresses aldosterone secretion, and sodium is excreted in the urine. Signs and symptoms of hypernatremia are listed in Box 20-5.

### Prevention

Sodium excess can be prevented in persons whose ability to excrete it is impaired. Persons with kidney failure, congestive heart failure, or increased aldosterone production need to have sodium intake restricted. Whenever intravenous electrolyte solutions are being given, the urinary output must be adequate so that portions of the electrolytes not needed by the body can be excreted. This usually means that fluid intake should not exceed urinary output.

### Management

Water alone is given to treat sodium excess. If cardiac and renal function are normal, a liberal amount of water is administered orally, or 5% dextrose in water is given intravenously. In the absence of normal cardiac and renal function, hydration must be carried out with caution to prevent fluid overloading in the patient.

Diuretics are of value in removing sodium. If sodium excess is severe, with or without excess water retention, and does not respond to other treatment, renal dialysis may be necessary.

## POTASSIUM

The normal concentration of potassium in the blood is 3.5 to 5.0 mEq/L. Because most of the potassium in the body is intracellular, the serum potassium level does not necessarily indicate the total body potassium content. Maintenance of serum potassium within normal range, however, is vital to normal body functions.

Potassium has a direct effect on the excitability of nerves and muscles, contributes most to the intracellular osmotic pressure, and helps maintain acid-base balance and normal kidney function. A potassium deficit is associated with excess alkalinity (alkalosis) of the body fluids, and a potassium excess accompanies an excess of acid (acidosis). These conditions are discussed in Chapter 21.

Potassium is the major cation of the cells. During the formation of new tissues (anabolism) or when glucose is converted to glycogen, potassium enters the cell. With tissue breakdown (catabolism) such as occurs with trauma, dehydration, or starvation, potassium leaves the cell. The body conserves potassium less effectively than it conserves sodium, and the kidneys excrete potassium even when the body needs it. Normally about 5% of the total body potassium is excreted each day.

### Potassium Deficit

A low level of serum potassium, below 3.5 mEq/L, is known as **hypokalemia.**

#### Etiology

The patient who has food withheld for several days, is dehydrated, or is given large amounts of parenteral fluids with no replacement of potassium develops potassium depletion. The parenteral administration of 5% dextrose in water without the addition of potassium tends to dilute the potassium in the extracellular fluids. This dilution, in addition to the lack of a balanced diet and to potassium loss caused by catabolism of body proteins, accounts for many instances of electrolyte imbalance in the postoperative patient. Persons who eat an inadequate diet, who take no food for an extended period of time, or who are losing large amounts of fluid from the

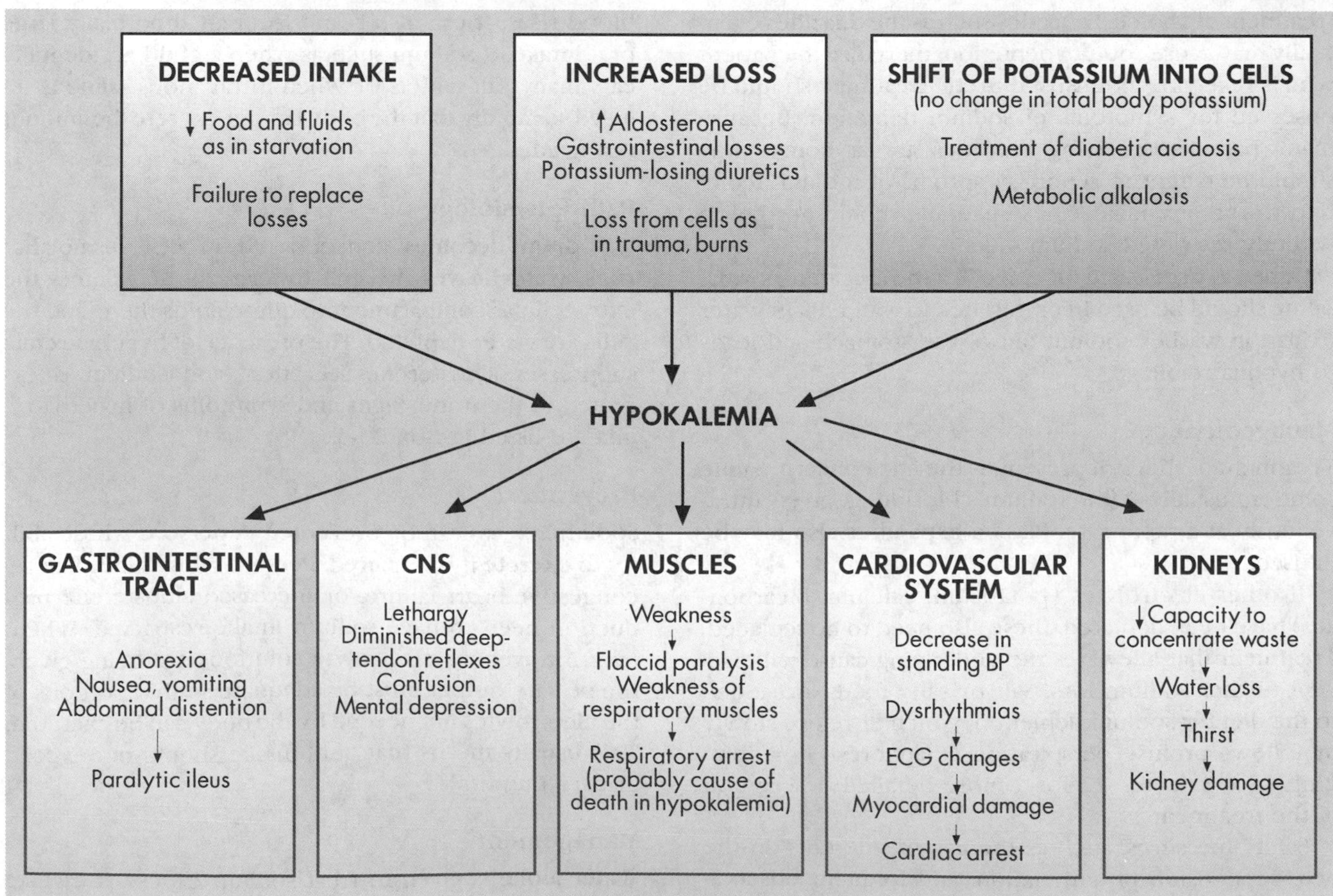


**FIGURE 20-5** Causes and effects of hypokalemia.

gastrointestinal tract through vomiting, diarrhea, or a draining fistula usually are given intravenous solutions that contain potassium.

The practice of giving multiple enemas is becoming much less common, because it is now known that some of the enema fluid is absorbed though the bowel wall and dilutes the potassium in the interstitial compartment. Hypertonic enema solutions may damage cells in the bowel mucosa, causing potassium loss. Figure 20-5 summarizes the causes and effects of hypokalemia.

The patient with potassium deficit shows characteristic electrocardiographic changes—flattened or inverted T waves with prolonged QT segments and prominence of a U wave. (See Chapter 29 for discussion of a normal ECG.) The most striking symptom of hypokalemia is muscle weakness. Other symptoms are apathy, abdominal distention, anorexia, vomiting, and paralytic ileus.

Digitalis toxicity can occur in persons taking digitalis if they develop hypokalemia. Persistent potassium deficit may cause kidney and heart damage. (See Chapter 31 for detailed discussion of digitalis toxicity.)

### Pathophysiology

Movement of sodium (inward) and potassium (outward) across the cell membrane causes depolarization of the membrane and initiates an action potential—this creates nerve and muscle activity. When extracellular potassium is low, the resting membrane potential increases (hyperpolarization), and the cell becomes less excitable. For this reason the major symptoms of hypokalemia are muscle weakness and atony.

Potassium is involved in acid-base balance inasmuch as it moves out of the cells when hydrogen ions move into the intracellular compartment in acidosis; therefore hyperkalemia accompanies acidosis. As the acidosis is treated, potassium moves back into the cells, and hypokalemia may develop. In alkalosis, hypokalemia usually develops because of movement of potassium into cells and also because potassium is excreted by the kidneys while hydrogen ions are being retained.

Whenever sodium is retained in the body through reabsorption by the kidney tubules, potassium is excreted. Thus whenever aldosterone secretion is increased, such as during the stress response, potassium is excreted. Potassium also may be lost in the urine when there is considerable urinary output and as a result of certain diuretics (the thiazides, furosemide) and the corticosteroids.

### Prevention

Hypokalemia can be prevented by being alert to the conditions that cause potassium depletion (vomiting, diarrhea, and diuretics) and by monitoring the patient for early warning signs. If there is an order for enemas until results are clear, the nurse should not give more than three enemas to a patient without consulting the physician, because this treatment may result in water intoxication and potassium loss.

### Management

With severe hypokalemia the patient may die unless potassium is administered promptly. The safest way to administer potassium is orally. When potassium is given intravenously, the rate of flow must be monitored closely to prevent hyperkalemia and atrial arrest. The usual rate of infusion should not exceed 20 mEq/L of potassium per hour. Because potassium is irritating to the veins, it is given very diluted, usually 20 to 40 mEq/L of intravenous solution. In some instances potassium is given at a greater concentration (40 mEq/100 ml) over a 4-hour period. When potassium is administered in this concentration, it should be delivered by a controlled infusion pump such as an IVAC or IMED pump. Because of the potential cardiovascular complications that can occur with this concentration of potassium, a cardiac monitor can be used so that changes in the patient's cardiac status will be identified immediately.

Persons who are receiving potassium-losing diuretics should be instructed to include foods high in potassium in their diet (Table 20-10). If low serum potassium levels are shown to result from diuretic therapy, a potassium supplement may be prescribed, usually in the form of potassium chloride (elixir of potassium chloride), or a potassium-sparing diuretic such as triamterene (Dyrenium) may be used. Persons taking diuretics at home should be taught to recognize symptoms of potassium depletion, such as muscle weakness, anorexia, nausea, and vomiting and to report these symptoms to the physician. Because potassium supplements are irritating to the gastrointestinal tract, they should be given with at least one half glass of water.

## Potassium Excess

A serum potassium level greater than 5 mEq/L is termed **hyperkalemia.** This condition does not occur as frequently as hypokalemia, especially if renal function is normal.

### Etiology

Hyperkalemia is caused by the movement of potassium out of the cells, an increased intake of potassium, and the decreased excretion of potassium. Movement of potassium out of the cells occurs whenever severe tissue damage is present as in sepsis, fever, trauma, or surgery. This movement also occurs in metabolic acidosis and insulin deficiency/hyperglycemia.

Shock, which often accompanies tissue damage, reduces renal function, thus promoting hyperkalemia. Great danger exists in giving extra potassium to any patient with poor renal function. If the patient is dehydrated or has lost vascular fluid, glucose and water or plasma expanders usually are given until renal function returns. Untreated adrenal insufficiency also is a con-

**TABLE 20-10 Foods High in Potassium**

| FOOD SOURCE | AMOUNT | mEq |
|---|---|---|
| Fruits | | |
| Apricots | | |
| Canned | ½ c | 6.0 |
| Dried | 4 halves | 5.0 |
| Fresh | 3 small | 8.0 |
| Banana | 1 small | 9.6 |
| Strawberries | 1 c | 6.3 |
| Grapefruit sections | ¾ c | 5.1 |
| Melon | | |
| Cantaloupe | ½ small | 13.0 |
| Honeydew | ¼ medium | 13.0 |
| Watermelon | ½ slice | 5.0 |
| Nectarine | 1 medium | 6.0 |
| Orange | 1 medium | 5.1 |
| Orange juice | ½ c | 5.7 |
| Peach | | |
| Dried | 2 halves | 5.0 |
| Fresh | 1 medium | 6.2 |
| Protein foods | | |
| Beef | 3 oz | 8.4 |
| Chicken | 3 oz | 9.0 |
| Frankfurters | 1 | 3.0 |
| Liver | 3 oz | 9.6 |
| Pork | 3 oz | 9.0 |
| Veal | 3 oz | 11.4 |
| Scallops | 1 large | 6.0 |
| Turkey | 3 oz | 8.4 |
| Milk | | |
| Whole | 1 c | 8.8 |
| Powdered, whole | ¼ c | 10.0 |
| Buttermilk | 1 c | 8.5 |
| Skim | 1 c | 8.8 |
| Powdered, skim | ¼ c | 13.5 |
| Vegetables* | | |
| Asparagus | | |
| Fresh | ½ c | 4.7 |
| Frozen | ½ c | 5.5 |
| Beans | | |
| Dried, cooked | ½ c | 10.0 |
| Lima | ½ c | 9.5 |
| Beet greens | ½ c | 8.5 |
| Broccoli | ½ c | 7.0 |
| Cabbage, raw | 1 c | 6.0 |
| Carrots, raw | 1 large | 8.8 |
| Celery, raw | 1 c | 9.0 |
| Collards | ½ c | 6.0 |
| Mushrooms, raw | 4 large | 10.6 |
| Mustard greens | ½ c | 5.5 |
| Peas, dried | ½ c | 6.8 |
| Potato | | |
| Baked, white | ½ c | 13.0 |
| Boiled, white | ½ c | 7.3 |
| Baked, sweet | ½ c | 8.0 |
| Spinach | ½ c | 8.5 |
| Tomatoes | ½ c | 6.5 |
| Brussels sprouts | ⅔ c | 7.6 |
| Squash, winter, baked | ½ c | 12.0 |
| Miscellaneous | | |
| Peanut butter | 2 tbsp | 5.0 |
| Nuts, unsalted | 25 | 4.5 |
| Beverages that contain large amounts of cocoa, cola drinks, and dry, instant coffee and tea. | | |

* Most raw vegetables contain potassium, much of which is lost during cooking.

traindication for giving potassium inasmuch as these patients have increased potassium levels because of an aldosterone deficiency. If the patient with potassium intoxication needs a blood transfusion, fresh blood must be used. Cells in blood that has been kept for several days tend to release potassium during storage. Administration of stored blood may increase the person's blood potassium level still further. Figure 20-6 shows the causes and effects of hyperkalemia.

Time is an important factor in the development of hyperkalemia. A rise of serum potassium of only 1 to 3 mEq/L that occurs rapidly can be lethal. On the other hand, some persons with renal failure develop severe hyperkalemia slowly and seem to be able to adjust to the potassium excess with few symptoms. Because there are huge stores of potassium inside the cells, the kidney's efficient excretion of potassium is a safety factor that reduces hyperkalemia when a rapid shift of potassium into the extracellular compartment occurs and the excess becomes dangerous.

The person with potassium intoxication develops spasticity of muscles because of their overstimulation by nerve impulses. Nausea, colic, diarrhea, and skeletal muscle spasms are common. The muscles later become weak because (1) overstimulation produces an accumulation of lactic acid and (2) potassium is lost from the muscle cells.

If the condition is not controlled, overstimulation of the cardiac muscle will cause the heartbeat to become irregular and eventually stop. Electrocardiographic evidence of potassium elevation includes tall, peaked, symmetric, or tented T waves with a short QT segment. As the blood potassium level increases further, the QRS complex spreads, and atrial arrest occurs.[6]

### Pathophysiology

Hyperkalemia in ECF has the opposite effect from hypokalemia on the resting cell membrane. The membrane potential is decreased (partially depolarized), and the cell becomes more excitable. Potassium excess therefore causes nerve and muscle irritability. Severe hyperkalemia, however, soon leads to muscle weakness and flaccid paralysis, and the patient may die of cardiac failure. Cardiac monitoring should be provided for patients experiencing hyperkalemia.

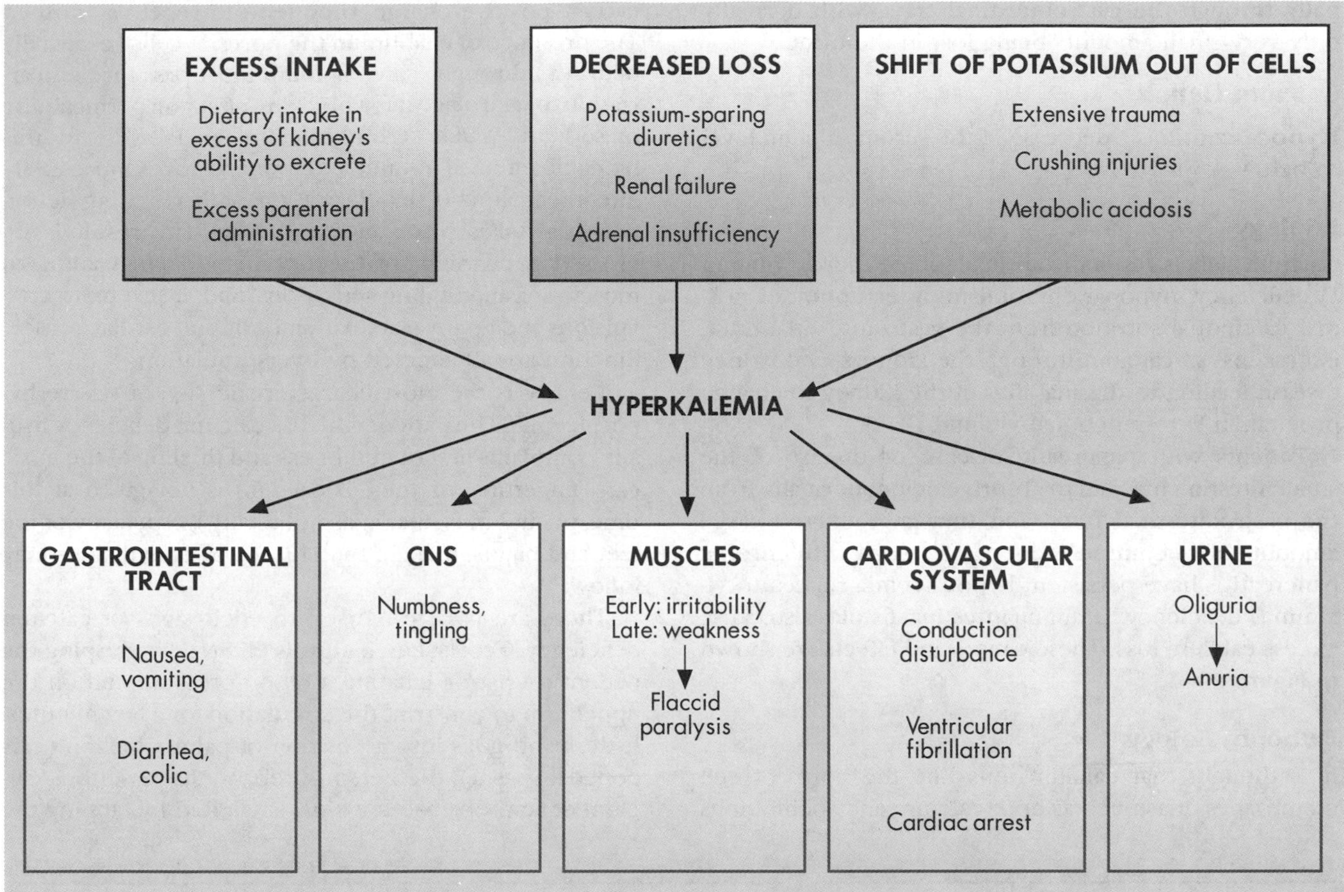


**FIGURE 20-6** Causes and effects of hyperkalemia.

### Prevention

Hyperkalemia can be anticipated and prevented in persons who for any reason have a significant decrease in urinary output, especially if they are receiving oral or intravenous potassium preparations.

### Management

When potassium intoxication occurs, the person is allowed nothing orally, and an infusion of 10% glucose with regular insulin may be given to induce transfer of potassium from the serum to ICF. If the patient has acidosis, correction of the acidosis will result in movement of potassium back into the cell (p. 524). A cation exchange resin such as polystyrene sulfonate (Kayexalate) also may be given. It works by exchanging other cations in the resin for potassium in the intestine. The potassium is then excreted in the stool. Good bowel function must be maintained if this therapy is to be effective. If the patient is in acute renal failure, dialysis is necessary. Calcium given intravenously antagonizes the effect of potassium on the heart. Patients with hyperkalemia should be most carefully prevented from undergoing any undue cellular catabolism because the process, regardless of cause, results in dumping more potassium into body fluids. Gastrointestinal bleeding with retention of blood cells in the intestines is a rich source of potassium.

Persons with potassium intoxication are placed on bed rest and receive complete nursing care until the potassium blood level returns to normal. Those persons who retain potassium secondary to renal failure or to a decrease in aldosterone will need instruction in restricting foods high in potassium (see Table 20-10). If salt substitutes are being used, patients need to be aware that these usually contain potassium as a substitute for sodium.

## CALCIUM

The normal calcium level in the blood is 4.5 to 5.8 mEq/L. Calcium in the blood is in two forms: ionized and bound to plasma proteins. Free, ionized calcium is needed for (1) blood coagulation, (2) smooth, skeletal, and cardiac muscle function, (3) nerve functions, and (4) bone and teeth formation. Only the ionized calcium is physiologically active.

Both vitamin D and parathyroid hormone must be present for calcium to be absorbed from the gastrointestinal tract (p. 525). Parathyroid hormone maintains the serum calcium level within normal limits by mobilizing calcium from bone. Calcium is excreted principally through the gastrointestinal tract, with normally only very small amounts being lost in the urine.

## Calcium Deficit

**Hypocalcemia** is a decrease of the serum calcium level to below 4.5 mEq/L.

### Etiology

Calcium deficit results from inadequate intake, vitamin D deficiency, hypoparathyroidism, interruption of normal calcium absorption from the gastrointestinal tract, excess loss of calcium through the kidneys, and kidney disease leading to the inability of the kidney to change provitamin D to functional vitamin D.

Patients with pancreatic disease or disease of the small intestine may fail to absorb calcium normally from the gastrointestinal tract, and they may excrete large amounts of calcium in the feces. Persons with chronic pancreatitis have persistent hypocalcemia related to vitamin D deficiency. Draining intestinal fistulas also cause excess calcium loss. These causes and effects are shown in Figure 20-7.

### Pathophysiology

It is thought that calcium ions line the pores of cell membranes. Inasmuch as both calcium and sodium ions carry a positive charge, they tend to repel each other. The presence of calcium in the pores of cells (especially neurons) through which sodium must pass for depolarization to take place has a blocking effect on permeability of sodium. When serum calcium levels are low, this blocking effect is minimized, sodium moves more easily into the cell, and depolarization with resulting action potential takes place more readily.[4] The result is increased excitability of the nervous system leading to muscle spasm, tingling sensations, and, if severe, to convulsions and tetany. Skeletal, smooth, and cardiac muscle function are all affected by overstimulation.

**Tetany** is the most characteristic sign of severe hypocalcemia. The patient who has calcium deficiency usually complains first of numbness and tingling of the nose, ears, fingertips, or toes. If calcium is not given at this time, painful muscular spasms (tetany), especially of the feet and hands, muscle twitching, and convulsions may follow.

There are two tests used to elicit signs of calcium deficiency. **Trousseau's sign** is elicited by grasping the patient's wrist or inflating a blood pressure cuff on the upper arm to constrict the circulation for a few minutes. If the hand goes into a position of palmar flexion (carpopedal spasm), the person probably has a serious calcium deficit. **Chvostek's sign** is elicited by tapping the

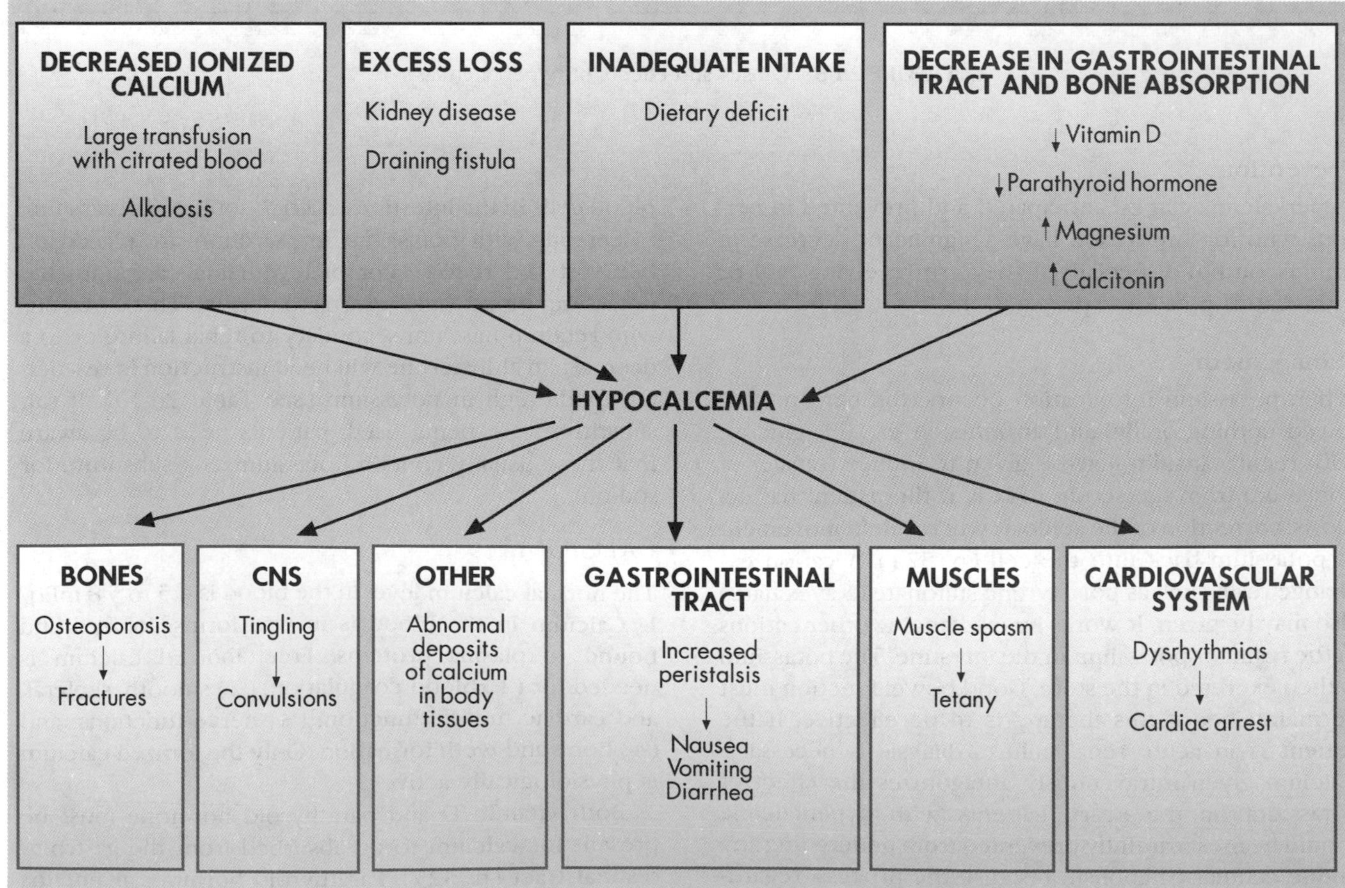


**FIGURE 20-7** Causes and effects of hypocalcemia.

patient's face lightly over the facial nerve (just below the temple). A calcium deficit is probably present if the facial muscles twitch.

### Prevention

Calcium deficiency can be prevented by alertness to conditions of inadequate intake, excess calcium loss, or vitamin D deficiency. Patients who are on extremely poor diets or who have calcium-depleting conditions should be monitored for signs of hypocalcemia. Teaching persons with a low intake of calcium and vitamin D to include more of these nutrients in the diet is an important nursing action.

### Management

The drug of choice in treating calcium deficiency is a 10% intravenous solution of calcium gluconate given slowly.[2] In milder cases a high-calcium diet or oral calcium salts may be sufficient. When decreased parathyroid hormone or vitamin D is the causative factor, these substances must be supplied. When the serum phosphorus level rises, the calcium level falls; aluminum hydroxide gel can be given to lower a high serum phosphorus concentration.

Patients with thyroid surgery must be watched closely for symptoms of calcium deficiency (tetany), because of the possibility that parathyroid glands may have been inadvertently removed with the thyroid tissue or may be temporarily suppressed by local edema.

Because chronic hypocalcemia can result in loss of calcium from bone to replenish low serum calcium, persons with this condition must be carefully moved, turned, or ambulated to prevent fractures of the demineralized bone. Calcium preparations must be given with caution to cardiac patients, because calcium has an effect on the heart similar to that of digitalis. Calcium gluconate should always be available for emergency use.

### Osteoporosis

In recent years a great deal of interest and information has been generated regarding osteoporosis, a condition prevalent in postmenopausal women (see Chapter 51).

Normally in young persons the constant processes of bone formation and resorption are in equilibrium, but after age 40 resorption becomes greater, causing structural weakness of bones and increased risk of fracture. The problem is compounded because calcium intake and absorption in the intestine decrease with age, creating a negative calcium balance over time. To correct the deficit, calcium is released from bone to make it available for vital nerve and muscle function. If there is a long-term deficiency, the calcium-depleted bones become porous and brittle.

To prevent osteoporosis, young women are advised to have an adequate daily intake of calcium and vitamin D, to exercise regularly, to avoid smoking, and to decrease phosphorus and caffeine intake. After menopause the usual recommended daily allowance of 1000 mg of calcium should be increased to 1500 mg.[8] Vitamin D, which increases calcium absorption, also may need to be added to the daily regimen of postmenopausal women.

It should be noted that *disuse osteoporosis* can occur in persons of either gender or age. It results from immobility over a period of time and may lead to bone fractures from moving the patient in bed. This may be prevented by passive exercise, performed regularly with the patient in a wheelchair or elevated to an upright position on a tilt table.

Long-term therapy with corticosteroids is another cause of osteoporosis, because the corticosteroids promote calcium mobilization from bones and inhibit calcium absorption.

## Calcium Excess

A serum calcium level above 5.8 mEq/L is called **hypercalcemia.**

### Etiology

Hypercalcemia can result from excessive intake of calcium, especially in milk and absorbable calcium-containing antacids (milk-alkali syndrome), from excessive vitamin D intake, and from conditions that promote release of calcium from the bones into ECF. These causes and their effects are shown in Figure 20-8.

### Pathophysiology

The blocking effect of calcium on cell membrane permeability is accentuated in the presence of high serum calcium levels. Nerve and muscle activity is depressed. The activity of cardiac muscle is depressed, gastrointestinal motility decreases, and skeletal and smooth muscles become fatigued. Deep tendon reflexes are decreased or absent.[6]

When a person is immobilized for any reason, calcium leaves the bone and concentrates in ECF. Normal retention of calcium in the bones is believed to be caused by the pressure exerted on bones by active movement or exercise. When a large amount of calcium accumulates in ECF and passes through the kidneys, calcium can precipitate and form stones (calculi), a not infrequent complication of immobilization.

Calcium precipitates more readily in alkaline solution. This can be a problem in a urinary tract infection, which increases the alkalinity of the urine, because renal calculi are more likely to be formed. Metastatic carcinoma, multiple myeloma, hyperparathyroidism, and other diseases with extensive bone involvement also produce marked hypercalcemia.

The person with hypercalcemia commonly complains of polyuria and severe thirst. Gastrointestinal symptoms, including anorexia, nausea, vomiting, and constipation,

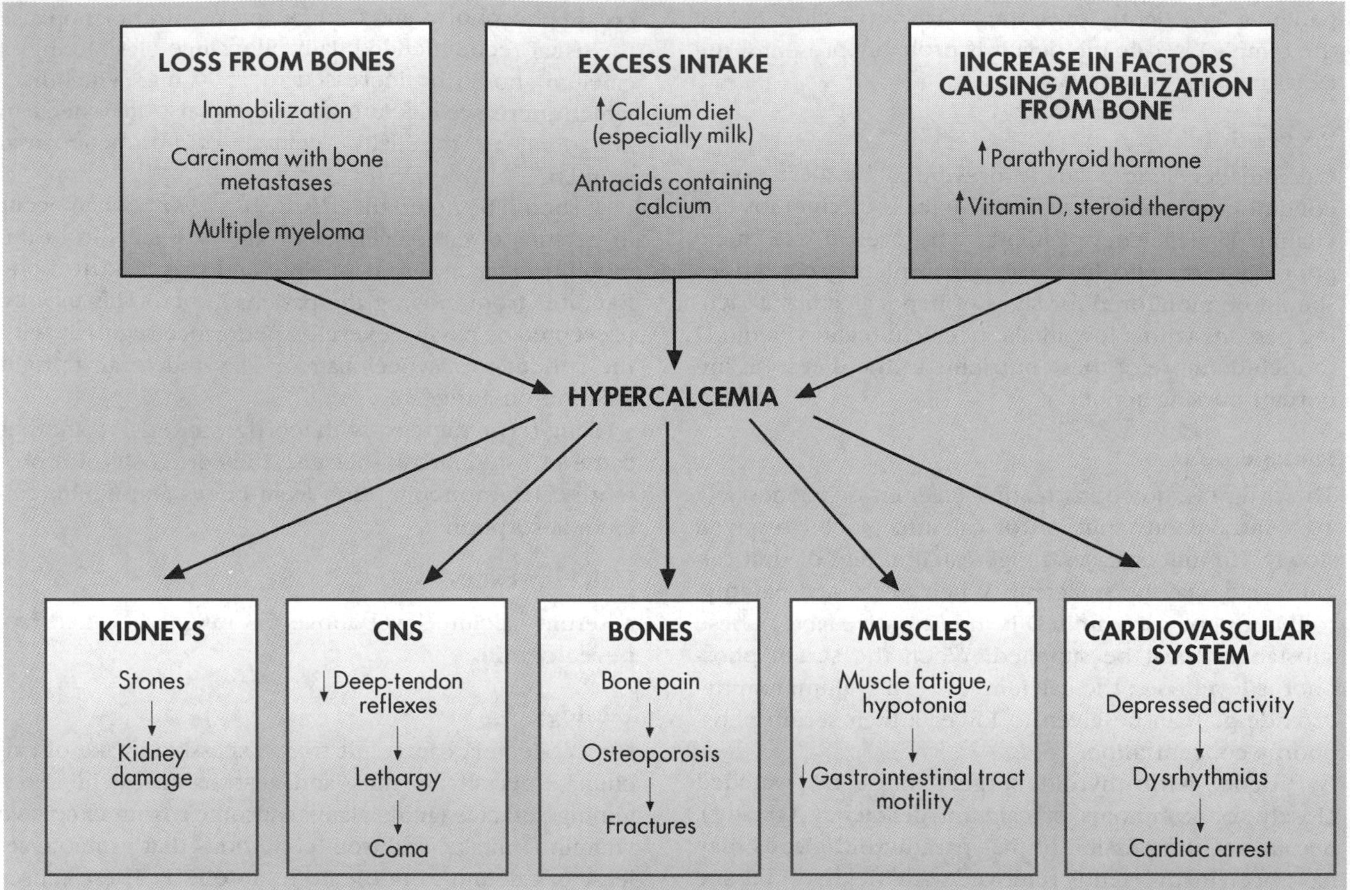


**FIGURE 20-8** Causes and effects of hypercalcemia.

also may develop. Without treatment the patient may become lethargic, confused, and comatose. Deep bone pain and radiographic evidence of bone cavitation may be present.

Hypercalcemic crisis is an emergency condition that is signaled by intractable nausea and vomiting, dehydration, stupor, coma, and azotemia.[7]

One treatable cause of hypercalcemia is hyperparathyroidism secondary to a secretory adenoma of the parathyroids. It usually is benign and can be removed surgically, which permits the body's calcium content to return to normal.

### Prevention

Hypercalcemia can be alleviated in persons who are immobilized by helping them to exercise muscles in uninvolved parts of the body. A tilt table may be used to put a patient who is unable to stand unassisted in an upright, weight-bearing position so as to provide pressure on the bones. Patients who are immobilized in a back-lying position should be encouraged to use a trapeze bar, and all patients who are able should move about as much as possible and, with the use of side rails and other means, engage in activities that require muscle action.

### Management

The only definitive treatment is removal of the cause. Because calcium excretion is promoted by excretion of sodium, hypercalcemia is treated with intravenous saline and a diuretic (furosemide). If this treatment fails, inorganic phosphate preparations given orally or intravenously may be effective. Mithramycin (Mithracin), a potent antitumor drug, has been used successfully to reduce serum calcium. If the hypercalcemia is caused by multiple myeloma or other cancers, glucocorticoids may be effective in reducing hypercalcemia, either because they decrease the size of the tumor or because the effect of the tumor on bone is reduced.

Because persons with marked hypercalcemia often are losing calcium from their bones or have malignant involvement of bone, special care should be taken to prevent pathologic fractures. Even the pressure used in giving a back rub sometimes must be avoided.

Careful attention must be directed to the prevention of calcium stone formation in the kidneys. Acid-ash fruit juices, cranberry and prune juice, or ascorbic acid can be given to promote urinary acidification and discourage stone formation. Urinary tract infections must be avoided. Good perineal care and meticulous technique in caring for Foley catheters are mandatory.

Unless a contraindication exists, persons with hypercalcemia are encouraged to drink 3000 to 4000 ml of fluids per day to reduce the possibility of renal calculi and to overcome the thirst that accompanies hypercalcemia.

## MAGNESIUM

The normal serum magnesium level is within the range of 1.5 to 2.5 mEq/L. About 50% of magnesium is located in bones, 5% in ECF, and the remaining 45% in the intracellular compartment. It functions in the activation of enzymatic reactions, especially in carbohydrate metabolism. Magnesium has a sedative effect on the central nervous system similar to that of calcium. It has been used successfully to prevent convulsions in toxemia of pregnancy. High serum levels result in vasodilation with lowering of blood pressure.

### Magnesium Deficit

**Hypomagnesemia** is a serum magnesium level below 1.5 mEq/L.

#### Etiology

Hypomagnesemia is most frequently caused by disturbances in the gastrointestinal and renal systems (Figure 20-9). Chronic alcoholism usually is accompanied by a severe magnesium deficit that is caused by a decreased dietary intake of magnesium, increased gastrointestinal losses, and intestinal malabsorption.

Magnesium levels decrease with the following conditions:

1. Loss of intestinal fluids through draining fistulas, diarrhea, steatorrhea, and gastrointestinal suction
2. Prolonged malnutrition
3. Renal disorders
4. Drug therapy with aminoglycosides and loop diuretics
5. Endocrine disorders such as increased secretion of ADH, aldosterone, and thyroid hormone

#### Pathophysiology

A low serum magnesium level leads to increased neuromuscular irritability by increasing acetylcholine release, increasing the sensitivity of the myoneural junction to acetylcholine, diminishing the threshold of excitation of the motor nerve, and enhancing the force of contraction of the myofibril.[7]

In the presence of a large amount of calcium in the gastrointestinal tract, calcium is absorbed in preference to magnesium, and the magnesium is excreted. Conversely, low calcium levels increase magnesium absorption. The kidneys effectively conserve magnesium when

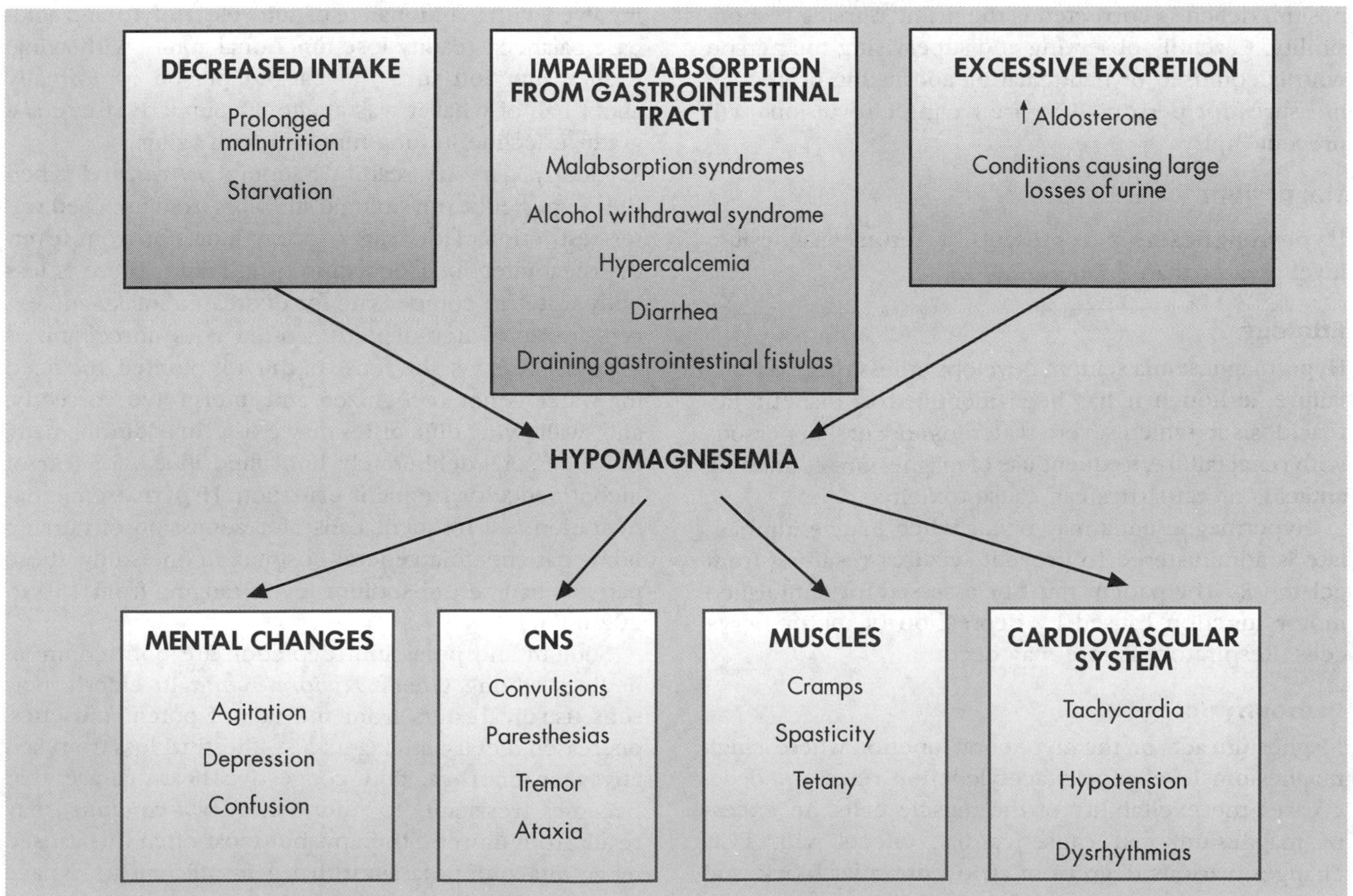


**FIGURE 20-9** Causes and effects of hypomagnesemia.

intake is low. Hypocalcemia and hypokalemia that are unresponsive to therapy may indicate hypomagnesemia.

Metabolically, magnesium is closely interrelated with both calcium and potassium. Magnesium inhibits transport of parathyroid hormone from the glands, causing a decrease in the amount of calcium being released from bone, resulting in a calcium deficit. Hypomagnesemia potentiates the action of digitalis, leading to toxicity.[7] Hypomagnesemia usually manifests by behavioral and neurologic symptoms such as confusion, hallucinations, convulsions, increased reflexes, tremors, muscle spasms, and parathesias.

#### Prevention

Dietary teaching and management can help prevent magnesium deficit, especially in persons with magnesium-depleting conditions. Fruits, green vegetables, whole-grain cereals, milk, meats, and nuts are good dietary sources of magnesium.

#### Management

The treatment of magnesium deficit consists of the correction of the underlying cause and of the administration of magnesium salts orally or parenterally. Oral magnesium sometimes causes diarrhea; therefore it is often replaced by intravenous or deep intramuscular injection.

Providing for the safety of the patient until the magnesium deficit is corrected is the prime nursing responsibility. Carefully observing and supervising the person who is confused or hallucinating and taking protective measures for persons who are having convulsions will prevent injury.

### Magnesium Excess

**Hypermagnesemia** represents a serum magnesium level greater than 2.5 mEq/L.

#### Etiology

Hypermagnesemia seldom develops unless there is renal failure, although it has been identified in diabetic ketoacidosis in which severe water loss occurs. In persons with renal failure, frequent use of magnesium-containing antacids or cathartics can cause toxicity.

Hypermagnesemia may occur when magnesium sulfate is administered to prevent seizures resulting from eclampsia. The patient must be assessed for diminished motor function caused by depression of motor nerve cells. Respiratory failure may occur.

#### Pathophysiology

Magnesium acts on the myoneural junction where a high magnesium level blocks acetylcholine release and decreases the excitability of the muscle cells. An excess of magnesium can cause cardiac effects with ECG changes, various degrees of atrioventricular block, and premature ventricular contractions.[2]

The vasodilating effect of magnesium is accentuated in hypermagnesemia and can lead to hypotension because of peripheral vasodilation. The person may experience a sense of heat, thirst, nausea, and vomiting with mild hypermagnesemia. If the excess becomes greater, drowsiness, loss of deep tendon reflexes, and respiratory depression occur. Severe hypermagnesemia, at a level as high as 15 to 20 mEq/L, will lead to coma and death as a result of cardiac arrest.[2]

#### Management

Correction of the underlying cause corrects the magnesium excess. If renal failure occurs, dialysis is necessary. Intravenous calcium gluconate may be a useful temporary treatment because calcium has an antagonistic effect on magnesium.

## ✸ SPECIAL CONSIDERATIONS FOR CARE OF THE GERONTOLOGIC PATIENT

Elderly persons are particularly vulnerable to fluid and electrolyte disorders because of the following changes:

1. Less total body water as a result of less lean body mass, more fat
2. Decline in function of vital regulatory organs
3. High incidence of chronic illnesses
4. Diminished ability to reestablish homeostasis when an imbalance has occurred

The kidneys and lungs, which are the organs most involved with maintenance of fluid, electrolyte, and acid-base balance, steadily lose functional ability with aging. Kidney function in a 90-year-old person is normally about half of what it was at age 30. Similarly, there is a gradual decline in lung function with aging.

Elderly persons readily become *dehydrated* when they experience physiologic stressors from imposed water restrictions (for tests or x-ray films) or from fever, diarrhea, infections, and diuretic therapy. There is less body water to compensate for decreased intake and excess losses. Water depletion often goes unrecognized for many reasons: the sense of thirst is blunted, the need for water is not recognized and interpreted correctly, and swallowing difficulties may exist.[1] In addition, many older persons deliberately limit fluid intake for fear of incontinence or frequent urination. Hypernatremic dehydration is a frequent cause for admission of nursing home patients to a general hospital. In one study, these patients had serum sodium levels ranging from 150 to 202 mEq/L.[5]

Sodium and potassium depletion are both common findings among elders. *Hyponatremia* in elderly persons usually results from the use of potent diuretics, decreased dietary intake, excess intestinal loss from laxatives or diarrhea, and congestive heart failure that becomes resistant to diuretics. *Hypokalemia* may result from diuretic therapy, but most often it is caused by an intake of potassium that is insufficient to replace daily losses. Frequent enemas, which are common among older persons, also produce hypokalemia. Some symptoms of hypokalemia, such as apathy, confusion, and weakness, all too often are mistakenly attributed to old age.

## ASSESSMENT OF FLUID AND ELECTROLYTE IMBALANCE

The nurse needs to recognize the symptoms of fluid and electrolyte imbalance and make ongoing physical assessments of those patients who have a potential for fluid and electrolyte imbalances (Table 20-11). For subjective data such as headache, thirst, nausea, or dyspnea, time of onset and extent of symptoms are ascertained. Objective data can be compared with baseline assessments made at the time of the patient's entry into the health care system.

Data of particular importance in assessing fluid and electrolyte imbalance are comparison of fluid intake to output and changes in the patient's weight. Acutely ill medical patients and patients undergoing major surgery should have their fluid intake and output and daily weight closely monitored. If patients and families are given explanations, they can participate, when appropriate, in measuring and recording the intake and output. Totaling the fluid intake and output every hour, every 8 hours, or every 24 hours gives the nurse and physician additional data to determine if the patient may have a fluid imbalance.

Because symptoms of fluid and electrolyte imbalance are sometimes not very specific, a good rule is to be alert for any changes in behavior, level of consciousness, vital signs, skin turgor, muscle strength, and condition of mucous membranes. Baseline observations made during the first encounter with a patient are essential for comparison with subsequent observations to be able to detect changes.

## INTAKE AND OUTPUT MONITORING

### Intake Record

The intake record should show the type and amount of all fluids the patient has received and the route by which these were administered. This includes fluids given orally, parenterally, rectally, or by tubes. A record of solid food intake is sometimes necessary, especially with very young children. Foods that are eaten in a semisolid state but that are basically liquid such as gelatin or ice cream are recorded as fluids. Ice chips are recorded by dividing the amount of chips by one half (60 ml of chips would equal 30 ml of water). Patients may receive a considerable amount of fluid intake through the frequent sucking of ice chips.

### Urinary Output

Urinary output is recorded by recording time and amount of each voiding. If renal function is a major concern, as in a severely burned patient, an indwelling catheter is used so that the amount of urinary drainage can be recorded every hour and fluid intake regulated accordingly. It has been said that nothing is more difficult to obtain in a modern hospital than an accurate record of urinary output, and unfortunately this statement is often true. Conspicuous signs posted on the patient's chart and in the utility room and bathrooms help to prevent the discarding of urine before it is measured. Flow sheets kept close to the patient's room facilitate recording of intake and output and other patient data.

Specific gravity of urine, normally 1.010 to 1.025, is an indicator of fluid balance. A high specific gravity is indicative of fluid depletion, and a low specific gravity accompanies fluid excess. Oliguria, a urine output of less than 20 ml/hr, also signals a fluid-depleted state. If measurement of intake and output is delegated to a para-

**TABLE 20-11 Assessment of Fluid and Electrolyte Imbalance**

| | FLUID EXCESS | FLUID LOSS/ELECTROLYTE IMBALANCE |
|---|---|---|
| Behavior | Tires easily; change in behavior, confusion, apathy | Change in behavior, confusion, apathy |
| Head, neck | Facial edema, distended neck veins | Headache, thirst, dry mucous membranes |
| Upper gastrointestinal tract | Anorexia, nausea, vomiting | Anorexia, nausea, vomiting |
| Skin | Warm, moist, taut, cool feeling where edematous | Dry, decreased turgor |
| Respiration | Dyspnea, orthopnea, productive cough, moist breath sounds | Changes in rate and depth of breathing |
| Circulation | Loss of sensation in edematous areas, pallor,* bounding pulse, ↑ blood pressure | Pulse rate changes, dysrhythmias, postural hypotension |
| Abdomen | Increased girth, fluid wave | Distention, abdominal cramps |
| Elimination | Constipation | Diarrhea, constipation |
| Extremities | Dependent edema, "pitting," discomfort from weight of bedclothes | Muscle weakness, tingling, tetany |

*Pallor: edema decreases the intensity of skin color by increasing the distance between the skin surface and the pigmented or vascular areas. In the dark-skinned person, pallor is observed by absence of underlying red tones that give brown and black skin "glow." The brown skin appears more yellow-brown, and the black skin appears more ashen gray.

professional, the nurse must supervise closely and evaluate records for accuracy.

### Wound Drainage

All drainage from body orifices or artificial openings should be measured. This would include such drainage as that from an ileostomy, for a T tube after exploration of the common bile duct, or from any catheter draining a surgical area. If there is excessive drainage from a wound, it may be necessary to weigh the dressings. Fluid loss is the difference between the wet weight and the dry weight of the dressing.

### Gastrointestinal Output

Vomitus, gastrointestinal drainage, and liquid stools are measured as accurately as possible and are described by color, content, and odor. Gastric secretions are watery and pale yellow-green; they usually have a sour odor. However, if the acid-base balance has been upset, gastric secretions may have a fruity odor because of the presence of ketone bodies (acetone). Bile is somewhat thicker than gastric juice and may vary from bright yellow to dark green in color. It has a bitter taste and acrid odor. Intestinal contents vary from dark green to brown, are likely to be quite thick, and have a fecal odor. The amount of fluid retained during irrigation of nasogastric tubes is added to "intake" and needs to be subtracted from total drainage before it is recorded.

It is difficult to determine accurately the amount of water lost in the stools, but a description of their consistency and a record of the number of stools passed gives a good estimate. The color of stools also is recorded.

### Other Output

Fluid aspirated from any body cavity such as the abdomen (paracentesis) or pleural spaces (thoracentesis) must be measured. The fluid contains not only electrolytes and water but also proteins. Blood loss from any part of the body is measured carefully.

Diaphoresis is difficult to measure without special laboratory equipment; however, it may be important to estimate the loss of fluid by this route in some patients. Careful note of excessive perspiration and its duration is made. If the clothing and linen become saturated, dry and wet weights may be taken. Accurate recording of body temperature helps the physician determine how much fluid should be replaced inasmuch as fluid loss through the skin and lungs increases as temperature rises. A patient who has a high fever and is breathing rapidly can lose as much as 2500 ml/day through the lungs.[2]

## DAILY WEIGHT

The daily weight record is often the best way to determine the onset of dehydration or the accumulation of fluid either as generalized edema or as "hidden" fluid in body cavities. An increase of 1 kg in weight is equal to the retention of 1 L (1000 ml) of fluid in the edematous patient. If the weight record is to be accurate, the patient must be weighed on the same scale and at the same hour each day and must be wearing the same amount of clothing. Circumstances that may affect the weight should be kept as nearly identical as possible from day to day. Usually weights are taken in the early morning before the patient has eaten or defecated but after voiding. When extremely accurate measurements are needed, all clothing and even wound dressings are removed before the patient is weighed. A person maintained on intravenous fluids alone can be expected to lose approximately 0.2 to 0.5 kg/day.

## LABORATORY VALUES

Laboratory determinations of serum levels of the specific electrolytes help in making decisions concerning electrolyte excesses or deficits. When there is water excess, hemodilution occurs and the hematocrit, hemoglobin, blood urea nitrogen (BUN), and electrolyte levels are decreased. With excessive fluid loss hemoconcentration occurs, and the hematocrit, hemoglobin, BUN, and electrolyte levels are increased.

## LUNG AUSCULTATION

Regular auscultation of the lungs helps identify states of fluid excess. Moist breath sounds (crackles) that do not clear when the person coughs indicate a collection of fluid in the alveoli.

# REPLACEMENT AND MAINTENANCE OF WATER AND ELECTROLYTES

## GENERAL PRINCIPLES

Replacement of the water and electrolyte losses from the body and the necessary daily intake of these substances and other nutrients usually are accomplished by one of the following methods: (1) oral intake, (2) tube feeding (gavage), (3) intravenous infusion, and (4) total parenteral nutrition.

The best way to administer water, electrolytes, and nutrients is to give them orally. When fluids can be tolerated by the stomach but cannot be swallowed, a nasogastric tube may be passed, and fluids containing all the essentials of a balanced diet may be given through it. Normal saline solution or plain water also may be given by slow drip through the tube to replace fluid loss and provide for daily fluid needs.

If it is not possible for a patient to take food or fluid through the alimentary tract, the most common method of replacement is by intravenous infusion. A vein in an extremity or the neck is commonly used. An intravenous infusion may be given by introducing a needle or intracatheter into a vein and taping it in place or by making an incision (cutdown) and threading a polyethylene catheter (intracatheter) into the vein. The intracatheter is the method of choice for total parenteral nutrition (TPN) in which a concentrated nutrient solution is infused into the superior vena cava. (For further information on TPN, see Chapter 45.)

Fluids given by any route should be spaced throughout the 24-hour period. Not only does this practice help to maintain normal body fluid levels, but it also provides for better regulation of the electrolyte balance by the kidneys and prevents the end products of metabolism and toxic materials from being excreted in concentrated form. In this way the danger of renal damage, formation of calculi, and irritation of the lower urinary tract is reduced. In addition, fluid spacing prevents overloading of the circulation, which may result in dilution of body fluids, with resultant fluid and electrolyte shifts, the most serious of which causes pulmonary edema (Chapter 31).

Concentrated solutions of sugar or protein should always be given slowly and in small amounts at a time, because they require body fluids for dilution. Hypertonic saline solution may cause fluid to diffuse from the tissues to equalize the concentration of salt in the vascular compartment; therefore it too should be given slowly and in small amounts. Because of the rapid dilution by the larger amounts of blood at the superior vena cava, it is the preferred site for infusions of hypertonic solutions given by parenteral hyperalimentation.

Giving concentrated solutions rapidly and in large amounts into the alimentary tract causes a rapid shift of fluid from the vascular compartment into the intestinal lumen and a resultant decrease in blood volume, which can lead to shock. The "dumping syndrome," which sometimes occurs after a gastric resection, is caused by this abnormal shift of fluid. Concentrated solutions sometimes are given intentionally to reduce cerebral edema. Giving large amounts of fluid either orally or parenterally is potentially dangerous even in a healthy person, and therefore fluids of any kind should never be replaced faster than they are lost.

The size of the patient should be considered in administering fluids. The small adult normally has less fluid in each body compartment, especially in the intravascular system. This person therefore becomes seriously dehydrated more quickly than a larger adult and needs to have fluid losses replaced more promptly. Persons with small or inelastic vascular systems also become overhydrated easily. It is important to remember that the vascular system of a person who has had a large portion of the body such as a limb removed either by surgery or through trauma is not the same size as previously.

## ORAL INTAKE

Adults who have no circulatory or renal malfunction usually are given between 2500 and 3000 ml/day. Precautions should be taken so that the overzealous patient does not drink too much fluid in a day or does not take too much (3 to 4 glasses) at one time. Excessive water intake may cause water intoxication.

When they are ill, many persons find it difficult to eat or drink even though they are allowed to do so. There are many ways that the nurse can help the patient take adequate food and fluids orally and thus avoid the need for parenteral fluids. Fruit drinks, tea, coffee, ginger ale, or other soft drinks may be substituted for part of the water. Soup, bouillon, milk, eggnog, and cocoa provide both fluid and nutrients. Juicy fruits and other semisolid foods with a high fluid and nutrient content such as custard, ice cream, or gelatin may be more palatable than regular meals and tap water. Popsicles are an effective means of offering fluids, especially to children. Care must be taken, of course, that any substitutions are allowed on the diet prescribed for the patient. If a fluid record is needed, the amount of fluid given in semisolid form is estimated and recorded.

The methods used in presenting food and fluids to patients may influence their consumption; often a small amount of either food or fluid offered at frequent intervals is more acceptable than is a large amount presented less often. Serving foods that the patient likes may improve appetite. For example, carbonated beverages may be better tolerated by patients who are nauseated. Consideration should always be given to the cultural and aesthetic aspects of eating.

Vomiting and diarrhea are common symptoms of many illnesses, and most people suffer from them from time to time. Sodium and some potassium are lost in vomiting and diarrhea, whereas chloride is lost only in vomitus. As soon as fluids are tolerated, the patient who has vomiting or diarrhea should be served salty broth and tea or another fluid high in potassium (see Table 20-10) to replace the losses. These liquids are much higher in sodium than they are in potassium. Orange juice is the liquid of choice for replenishing potassium. This measure often helps the patient feel less weak and exhausted. Dry soda crackers often are tolerated when fluids are not and can be used to replace sodium.

A patient with a draining fistula from any portion of the gastrointestinal tract loses sodium, calcium, and potassium, and dietary supplements are necessary. Extra milk will replace all the losses, and the patient is instructed to increase milk intake somewhat above normal levels. For the body to use the calcium, vitamin D also must be available, but most milk is now fortified with vitamin D. Persons with a permanent fistulous opening, such as an ileostomy, need to be especially careful to supplement sodium and potassium when vomiting, diarrhea, or fever add to their already unusually large loss of electrolytes.

The nurse needs to know which foods contain large and small amounts of various essential nutrients, minerals, and vitamins (see Chapter 6). When losses must be restored, the patient needs more than is required in the usual adequate diet. It is especially important to know which foods and fluids are high or low in potassium and sodium and which foods are complete proteins. Bananas, citrus fruits, all fruit juices, many fresh vegetables, coffee, and tea are relatively high in potassium and low in sodium content. Salty broths and tomato juice provide extra sodium but have a high potassium content. Meat, milk, and eggs are all complete protein foods and contain relatively large quantities of both sodium and potassium. Current nutrition literature and the dietitian or nutritionist should be consulted as necessary.

The nurse frequently has an order to "force fluids." Because the amount required depends on the size of the patient, the amount of fluid loss, and the patient's circulatory and renal status, no standard amount can be given. The nurse must therefore make a judgment as to the desirable amount and inform members of the nursing team or family members who will care for the patient. If there is any question, the physician is consulted.

If an elderly person living at home complains of pronounced weakness without apparent cause, the nurse should ask whether cathartics or enemas have been taken. If so, stopping this procedure, eating foods with high sodium and potassium content, and increasing the fluid intake may relieve the symptoms. Methods to combat constipation without purging should be taught.

Any patient with renal or circulatory impairment, as may occur in shock, cardiac decompensation, or constriction of blood vessels because of disease, may develop electrolyte imbalance. Sodium and water may be held in the tissues, the potassium level of the blood may rise, acidosis may develop from inadequate tissue oxygenation, or the kidneys may be unable to excrete waste products properly. Patients with cardiac and renal impairment are instructed to avoid taking too much food that contains sodium, potassium, or bicarbonate.

## GAVAGE (TUBE FEEDING)

Water, a physiologic solution of sodium chloride, high-protein liquids, or a regular diet that has been passed through a blender and diluted is often given by gavage to older children and adults (see Chapter 45). As previously mentioned, high-protein tube feeding can cause water deficit through osmotic diuresis. A need to increase water intake along with the tube feeding should be considered when (1) the patient complains of thirst, (2) protein content of the tube feeding is high, (3) the patient has a fever, (4) urinary output is decreased or very concentrated, and (5) signs of water deficit develop.

## PARENTERAL FLUIDS

### Types of Solutions

The nurse needs to know the common solutions used parenterally (Table 20-12). A hypotonic solution of 5% dextrose in distilled water often is used to maintain fluid intake or to reestablish water volume. Ascorbic acid and vitamin B (Solu-B) frequently are added. Dextrose, 5%, in saline solution may be given depending on the serum levels of sodium and the vascular volume, and potassium chloride may be added to meet normal intake needs of potassium and to replace losses. A physiologic solution of sodium chloride is given primarily when sodium chloride has been lost in large amounts such as in loss of gastrointestinal fluids or in burns and when patients have vascular volume deficits. A one-sixth molar lactate solution may be ordered when sodium, but not chloride, needs replacement; ammonium chloride solution may be used to replace chlorides when added sodium is undesirable. Balanced solutions that contain several electrolytes may be used to replace fluid loss in surgical patients. Ringer's solution and lactated Ringer's solution are examples.

**TABLE 20-12 Solutions for Intravenous Use**

| | CONTENTS OF SOLUTIONS | | | | | | | | |
|---|---|---|---|---|---|---|---|---|---|
| | CATIONS (mEq/L) | | | | ANIONS (mEq/L) | | | | |
| TYPE OF SOLUTION | $Na^+$ | $K^+$ | $Ca^{++}$ | $Mg^{++}$ | $NH_4^+$ | $Cl^-$ | $HCO_3^-$ LACTATE | $PO_4^-$ | GLUCOSE (g/L) |
| 5% dextrose in water | | | | | | | | | 50 |
| 10% dextrose in water | | | | | | | | | 100 |
| Normal saline (0.9%) | 154 | | | | | 154 | | | |
| 3% saline | 513 | | | | | 513 | | | |
| Ringer's solution | 147 | 4 | 4 | | | 155 | | | |
| 5% dextrose in Ringer's lactate | 130 | 4 | 3 | | | 109 | 28 | | 50 |
| Ringer's lactate | 130 | 4 | 3 | | | 109 | 28 | | |
| Ammonium chloride (0.9%) | | | | | 170 | 170 | | | |
| Sodium lactate ⅙ molar | 167 | | | | | | 167 | | |
| 5% dextrose in 0.2% saline | 34 | | | | | 34 | | | 50 |
| 5% dextrose in 0.45% saline | 77 | | | | | 77 | | | 50 |

Body needs for carbohydrates may be partially met by giving fructose or 10% or 20% glucose in distilled water, but these solutions are hypertonic and require additional water for excretion.

Amino acid preparations (Aminosol) seldom are given by standard intravenous methods. Whole blood is the fluid of choice to replace blood loss, but plasma, 25% salt-poor albumin, or plasma volume expanders can be given to substitute for blood protein loss and are used to reestablish normal blood volume and prevent shock. Dextran is the most generally accepted plasma volume expander. It increases the oncotic pressure of the blood, thus increasing the reabsorption of fluid from interstitial spaces and increasing plasma volume. Low-molecular-weight dextran decreases the viscosity of the blood, allowing greater flow of blood through the capillaries; thus it is useful in treating cardiogenic, hemorrhagic, or septic shock (see Chapter 22). It may cause a prolonged bleeding time and is contraindicated in patients with renal failure, severe bleeding disorders, and severe congestive heart failure.[7]

## Management

Intravenous fluids that contain electrolytes should be run slowly to allow the body to regulate their use. The patient is watched carefully for untoward signs (excess of fluids or electrolytes). Increased serum potassium (hyperkalemia) can be particularly dangerous because it may cause cardiac arrest. When solutions that contain electrolytes are given, the nurse monitors the urinary output carefully and reports any marked decrease in the amount to the physician. Because the kidneys select the ions needed and excrete surplus ones, a normal output is essential. If the nurse is planning the sequence of intravenous fluids, hydrating fluids such as one-half strength physiologic solution of sodium chloride or glucose in water solution should be given first if the patient primarily has a water deficit. Renal failure and untreated adrenal insufficiency are contraindications for the use of potassium. If these conditions are known or suspected to exist, the nurse should verify orders for its administration. Many physicians do not start intravenous therapy for the day until blood chemistry results have been reported.

Usually the rate of administration of fluids is ordered by the physician and depends on the patient's illness, the kind of fluid given, and the patient's age. An infusion is rarely run at a rate faster than 4 ml/min. If it is given continuously or if it is given when there is impaired renal function or impaired cardiac function, it is rarely run faster than 2 ml/min. The usual rate for replacement of fluid loss is 3 ml/min. This rate allows time for the fluid to diffuse into ECF compartments and avoids overloading the circulation or raising the blood volume high enough to produce a diuretic effect. The equipment used for fluid administration may have varying numbers of drops per milliliter, and the nurse needs to check the equipment used to determine the rate of delivery, because it is not the drops per minute but the milliliters per minute that are important.

Nurses should question the advisability of the rather common practice of speeding up the rate of flow of solutions given intravenously primarily to complete the treatment at a specified time. Every nurse should recognize the initial signs of pulmonary edema (bounding pulse, engorged peripheral veins, hoarseness, dyspnea, cough, or pulmonary rales) and should watch closely for them in those patients who are receiving concentrated solutions, those who must be given any intravenous solution rapidly, and those whose age or physical condition places them at special risk. At the first signs of increased blood volume, the rate of flow of the infusion should be reduced to a "keep open" rate or barely running at 5 to 6 drops/min, and the physician notified. Special care needs to be taken in giving fluids to infants, elderly patients with circulatory impairment, patients whose hearts are decompensated, those with renal impairment, those who have had plasma shifts such as

**TABLE 20-13 Complications of Intravenous Fluid Therapy**

| OBSERVATIONS | NURSING ACTIONS |
|---|---|
| **CIRCULATORY OVERLOAD** | |
| Bounding pulse, venous distention, hoarseness, dyspnea, cough, pulmonary rales, restlessness | Notify physician<br>Reduce flow to "keep open" rate<br>Raise head of bed to facilitate breathing |
| **LOCAL INFILTRATION** | |
| Decreased rate or cessation of fluid flow<br>Tissue around needle or catheter site cold, pale, swollen, hard<br>Complaint of local pain | Stop infusion<br>Arrange to restart infusion at another site<br>Apply moist heat<br>Elevate lower arm |
| **THROMBOPHLEBITIS** | |
| Pain, redness, warmth, edema along vein | Same as for local infiltration<br>Cold compresses may be applied initially |
| **PYROGENIC REACTION** | |
| Fever, chills, general malaise, nausea, and vomiting 30 min after infusion started<br>Hypotension (if severe) | Switch to another infusion solution and run at "keep open" rate<br>Notify physician<br>Monitor vital signs<br>Save infusion fluid for culture |
| **ANAPHYLACTIC REACTION (WITH PROTEINS)** | |
| Apprehension, dyspnea, wheezing, tightness of chest, itching, hypotension | Switch infusion to nonprotein solution and run at "keep open" rate<br>Notify physician<br>Monitor vital signs |

burned patients, and those with extensive tissue trauma from other causes. Patients whose plasma has shifted need to be watched especially carefully because after a few days the plasma tends to shift back suddenly from the interstitial tissue to the blood, potentially producing an increase in blood volume with resulting pulmonary edema.

It is imperative that the nurse check the labels of fluid bottles carefully for correctness of content and record accurately the fluids given. (For details of equipment and nursing techniques needed in parenteral fluid administration, refer to a textbook on fundamentals of nursing.)

Patients who are receiving fluids intravenously are observed frequently so that symptoms indicating the need to slow down, speed up, or stop the infusion may be noted (Table 20-13). The tissue at the site of the inserted needle or catheter is checked at intervals for signs of infiltration or inflammatory reaction. If infiltration occurs, the infusion should be stopped at once and plans made to restart it. Solutions that contain potassium are very irritating, and extravasation may cause tissue necrosis. When dextran or other protein solutions are being given, the patient is observed for signs of anaphylactic reaction (apprehension, dyspnea, wheezing respirations, tightness of chest, itching, hypotension) (see Chapter 70).

## RELIEF OF SYMPTOMS

Persons with fluid and electrolyte imbalance often have extreme thirst, nausea, and vomiting. These symptoms are distressing, and the nurse should know measures that can be used to give the patient relief.

### THIRST

Thirst, the first and most insistent sign of dehydration, sometimes causes the patient more misery than surgery or the symptoms of a disease. It may develop even when fluids have been withheld only for a number of hours. If fluids are being withheld intentionally, thirst often is made more bearable by explaining to the patient why the fluids are being withheld and when they will be reinstituted.

Usually thirst is relieved readily by taking fluids. When fluids cannot be taken orally, the administration of fluids parenterally usually gives relief. It is often helpful to explain this to the patient. Mouth care will allay some of the discomfort from thirst. This care includes cleansing the tongue, teeth, and mucous membranes lining the oral cavity. It may be necessary to repeat the procedure every hour. Solutions that contain glycerine or alcohol should be avoided because of their drying effect. A mixture of hydrogen peroxide and saline is effective in removing dried secretions.

When fluids are not permitted, the water pitcher at the bedside is removed, and if the patient cannot be relied on not to get up and drink at a water tap, special provisions such as insistence on bed rest may be necessary. Thirst sometimes compels the patient to obtain water in any way possible.

Pronounced and continued thirst despite the administration of fluids is not normal and should be reported. In the immediate postoperative period, this kind of thirst suggests internal hemorrhage, elevation of temperature, or some other untoward development. In the chronically ill patient it may indicate the onset of disease such as diabetes mellitus in which extra water is used by the kidneys to eliminate glucose in the urine. It is also a symptom of hypercalcemia.

### NAUSEA AND VOMITING

Fluid and electrolyte imbalances may cause nausea and vomiting. Vomiting in turn frequently leads to further fluid and electrolyte imbalances as a result of the loss of gastric secretions. A vicious cycle may be set up:

Vomiting → Losses → Vomiting → (and so on)

Treatment of severe nausea and vomiting consists of replacing the fluids and electrolytes by parenteral methods and the use of antiemetic medications. The care of the person experiencing nausea and vomiting is described in Chapter 45.

## QUESTIONS TO CONSIDER

- What measures would you recommend to young women to prevent osteoporosis?
- How would you explain a low potassium diet to an elderly patient with a hearing deficit?
- Explain the relationship between vitamin D, parathyroid hormone, and calcium absorption.
- Why are elderly persons at particular risk of dehydration?
- What is the best method to administer water, electrolytes, and nutrients? Why?

## CRITICAL THINKING ACTIVITIES

- Mrs. Green is a patient on your unit with a diagnosis of dehydration. The physician has ordered "force fluids." You must make a judgment as to the desirable amount, since there is no "standard" or specific amount prescribed. Identify additional data that are necessary for you to make a prudent nursing decision.
- Al, 55, has advanced cancer of the lung. He has been nauseated for several weeks following chemotherapy and has become malnourished. An SMA-12 (chemistry profile) indicates a serum albumin of 2.2 mg/dl. Identify the data relevant for assessing calcium balance/imbalance and data needed to confirm your conclusions about the patient's electrolyte status.

## CHAPTER SUMMARY

### MAINTENANCE OF FLUID AND ELECTROLYTE BALANCE

- Concepts of fluid and electrolyte and acid-base balance reviewed in Chapters 20 and 21 provide the basis for understanding the care of patients with disorders of the cardiovascular, respiratory, endocrine, renal, and digestive systems, as well as the care of those with burns.
- Internal regulation of sodium and water is controlled by thirst, the kidney, ADH, the aldosterone-renin-angiotensin system, and third factor.

### FLUID IMBALANCE

- When a change in the sodium-to-water ratio occurs, a disturbance in osmolality results; that is, the ECF becomes dilute (hyposmolar) or more concentrated (hyperosmolar) than normal.

### ELECTROLYTE IMBALANCE

- When the concentration of sodium, potassium, or calcium is increased or decreased in body fluids, the increase or decrease is reflected in the stimulation of muscles by nerves.
- Losses of fluid and electrolytes occur through the skin by diaphoresis and oozing from severe wounds or burns; from gastrointestinal drainage and enemas; from the kidneys because of diuretic use and polyuria; from hemorrhage; and through the trapping of fluids by wound swelling, edema, ascites, and intestinal obstruction.

### SPECIAL CONSIDERATIONS FOR CARE OF THE GERONTOLOGIC PATIENT

- Elderly persons are particularly vulnerable to fluid and electrolyte disorders because of the following changes: (1) less total body water, (2) declines in the function of vital regulatory organs, (3) the high incidence of chronic illness, and (4) a diminished ability to reestablish homeostasis when an imbalance has occurred.

### ASSESSMENT OF FLUID AND ELECTROLYTE IMBALANCE

- Assessment of fluid and electrolyte balance includes the monitoring of laboratory values, fluid intake, fluid output (urinary output, wound drainage, gastrointestinal drainage, fluid from any body cavity, diaphoresis), daily weight, and urine specific gravity.

## REFERENCES

1. Brocklehurst JC, Allen S: *Geriatric medicine for students,* ed 3, New York, 1987, Churchill Livingstone.
2. Goldberger E. *A primer of water, electrolyte and acid-base syndromes,* ed 7, Philadelphia, 1986, Lea & Febiger.
3. Groer MW, Shekleton ME: *Basic pathophysiology: a holistic approach,* ed 3, St Louis, 1989, Mosby.
4. Guyton A: *Textbook of medical physiology,* ed 8, Philadelphia, 1990, WB Saunders.
5. Himmelstein DV et al: Hypernatremic dehydration in nursing home patients, *J Am Geriatr Soc* 31:466-471, 1983.
6. Horne M, Heitz UE, Swearingen PL: *Fluid, electrolyte, and acid-base balance: a case study approach,* St Louis, 1991, Mosby.
7. Metheny NM: *Fluid and electrolyte balance—nursing considerations,* ed 2, Philadelphia, 1992, JB Lippincott.
8. Symposium on fluid, electrolytes, and acid-base balance, *Nurs Clin North Am* 22(4):749-872, 1987.
9. Vander AJ, Luciano DS: *Human physiology: mechanisms of body functioning,* ed 5, New York, 1990, McGraw-Hill.

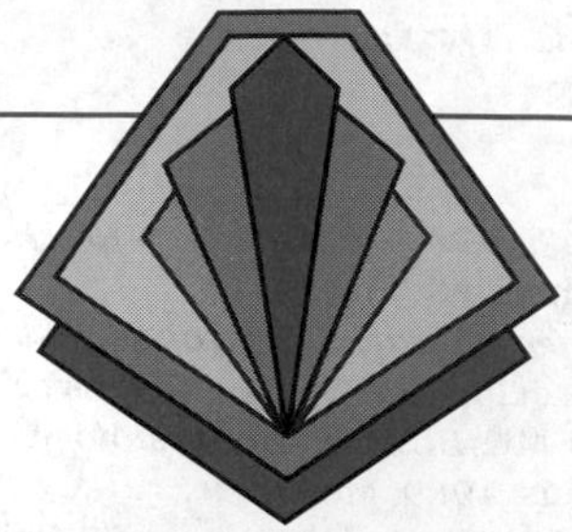

CHAPTER 21

# Acid-Base Imbalance

***Mary Kay Lehman***

## CHAPTER OBJECTIVES

***After studying this chapter, the learner should be able to do the following:***

1 Describe the mechanisms that maintain acid-base balance.
2 Differentiate between metabolic and respiratory acidosis and alkalosis.
3 Describe the causes and effects of each type of acid-base imbalance.
4 Identify data indicating acid-base imbalances.
5 Describe the management of patients with acid-base imbalances.

## KEY TERMS

acidosis
acid-base balance
alkalosis
bicarbonate
buffer
carbonic acid
compensation
metabolic acidosis
metabolic alkalosis
pH
respiratory acidosis
respiratory alkalosis

This chapter reviews the regulation of normal acid-base balance. Mechanisms that regulate acid-base balance—including chemical buffer systems, the respiratory system, and the kidneys—are explored. Causes, prevention, clinical manifestations, and interventions for acid-base imbalances are discussed.

Although the prescription of medical therapy to prevent and treat imbalances is the responsibility of the physician, nurses must carry out the following vital functions:

1. Recognizing situations likely to cause imbalances
2. Intervening to prevent imbalances
3. Carrying out preventive and therapeutic measures prescribed by the physician and monitoring patients' responses to these measures
4. Recognizing signs and symptoms of acid-base disturbances
5. Monitoring patients to prevent and recognize imbalances related to their specific conditions or treatments
6. Alleviating the effects of disturbances on the comfort and safety of patients.

## REGULATION OF ACID-BASE BALANCE

Hydrogen ions are vital to life and health. A stable concentration of hydrogen ions in body fluids results in **acid-base balance.** The concentration of hydrogen in the body is less than that of other ions (0.00004 mEq/L). Hydrogen ion concentration is expressed as **pH.** The negative logarithm of the hydrogen ion concentration is the pH value; thus pH has an inverse relationship with the hydrogen ion concentration.

Normal arterial body pH is 7.35 to 7.45. A value of less than 7.35 is present in **acidosis** (excess accumulation of hydrogen ions), and a value of greater than 7.45 is present in **alkalosis** (reduction of hydrogen ions). Limits of pH compatible with life are 7 to 7.8.

Hydrogen circulates throughout the body fluids in two forms: the volatile hydrogen of carbonic acid and the nonvolatile form of hydrogen in organic acids, such as sulfuric, pyruvic, phosphoric, and lactic acids. In a day's time, many acids are produced as the end products of metabolism. In the normal person, the lungs excrete 13,000 to 30,000 mEq/day of the volatile hydrogen in carbonic acid ($H_2CO_3$) as $CO_2$, and the kidneys excrete approximately 50 mEq/day of nonvolatile acids.

Mechanisms that regulate acid-base balance include chemical buffer systems, the respiratory system, and the kidneys (Table 21-1).

### CHEMICAL BUFFER SYSTEMS

The body cells are very sensitive to changes in the pH value, which is kept relatively constant by the buffer systems in the body. A **buffer** is a substance that can act as a chemical sponge, by either soaking up or releasing hydrogen ions so that the pH value remains sta-

**TABLE 21-1 Mechanisms Regulating Acid-Base Balance**

| ACTION TIME | EFFECT |
|---|---|
| **CHEMICAL BUFFERS IN CELLS AND ECF** | |
| Instantaneous | Combine with acids or bases added to the system to prevent marked changes in pH |
| **RESPIRATORY SYSTEM** | |
| Minutes to hours | Controls $CO_2$ concentration in ECF by changes in rate and depth of respiration |
| **KIDNEYS** | |
| Hours to days | Increases or decreases quantity of $NaHCO_3$ in ECF<br>Combines $HCO_3^-$ or $H^+$ with other substances and excretes them in urine |

ble. The main buffer systems of the body are the carbonic acid–bicarbonate system, the phosphate system, and protein. The carbonic acid–bicarbonate buffer system is the system that is monitored clinically. If this buffer system is stable, the other buffer systems are stable.

## Carbonic Acid–Bicarbonate Buffer System

The carbonic acid–bicarbonate system is present in extracellular fluid (ECF). **Carbonic acid** is formed by the combination of carbon dioxide and water: $CO_2 + H_2O \leftrightarrows H_2CO_3$. When a strong base is added to the body fluids, it is buffered by carbonic acid to a **bicarbonate** salt and water: $H_2CO_3 + NaOH \rightarrow NaHCO_3 + H_2O$. When a strong acid is added to the system, the bicarbonate buffer changes it to a salt and carbonic acid: $HCl + NaHCO_3 \rightarrow NaCl + H_2CO_3$. This carbonic acid then dissociates into carbon dioxide and water and can be excreted by the lungs and kidneys.

The ability to maintain a stable pH relies essentially on maintenance of the normal ratio of 20 parts bicarbonate to 1 part carbonic acid. The normal serum bicarbonate level is 22 to 26 mEq/L. The carbonic acid level is determined by taking the $P_{CO_2}$ level (normally 40 mm Hg) and multiplying it by the constant 0.03, the dissolvability factor of $CO_2$. This computation gives an approximate figure of 1.2. From these figures it can be seen that the normal bicarbonate–carbonic acid ratio is 20:1 (Figure 21-1).

This ratio of 20:1 is maintained by the lungs and the kidneys. The carbonic acid concentration is controlled by excretion by the lungs of the gas carbon dioxide. The depth and rate of respiration change in response to changes in carbon dioxide. The bicarbonate concentration is controlled by the kidneys, which selectively retain or excrete bicarbonate in response to the body's needs.

## Phosphate Buffer System

The phosphate buffer system is present in cells and ECF; it is especially active in the kidneys. Like bicarbonate, phosphate can "mop up" spare hydrogen ions. Conversely, one molecule of phosphoric acid can donate up to three hydrogen ions to make up for any hydrogen ion deficits. Phosphate groups may occur free in plasma or bound to certain organic compounds. Even when bound, phosphate can exert some buffering influence.[2]

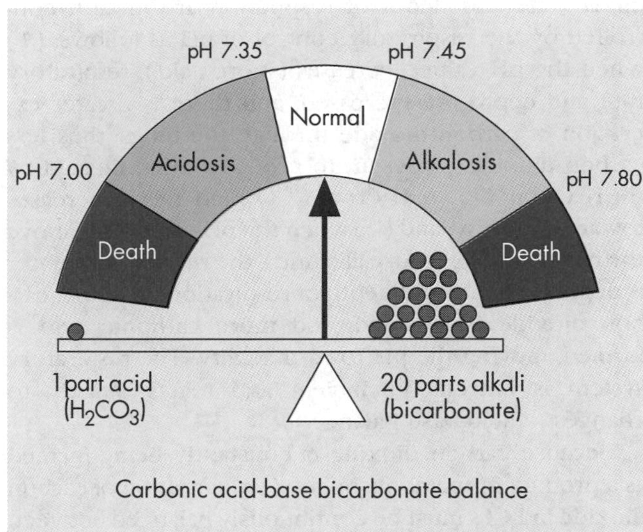


**FIGURE 21-1** Note that relationship of 1 part carbonic acid to 20 parts bicarbonate maintains hydrogen ion concentration (pH) within normal limits. Increase in $H_2CO_3$ or decrease in $HCO_3^-$ causes acidosis; similarly, decrease in $H_2CO_3$ or increase in $HCO_3^-$ causes alkalosis. (Redrawn from Abbott Laboratories: *Fluid and electrolytes,* North Chicago, 1970, Abbott Laboratories.)

The phosphate system is composed of sodium and other cations in combination with $H_2PO_4^-$ and $HPO_4^=$. When a strong acid is present, the following action takes place: $Na_2HPO_4 + HCl \rightarrow NaCl + NaH_2PO_4$. A hydrogen ion is excreted via the urine in the $NaH_2PO_4$. A strong base is buffered in the following reaction: $NaOH + NaH_2PO_4 \rightarrow Na_2HPO_4 + H_2O$. $Na_2HPO_4$ is a weak base and minimizes the pH change.[1]

## Protein Buffer System

The protein buffer system is located in the plasma and inside cells; the protein hemoglobin in red blood cells is one of the proteins involved. Although most protein buffers are intracellular, they assist in buffering ECF. Some of the amino acids in proteins contain free acid radicals, —COOH, which can dissociate into $CO_2$ + H, thus adding a hydrogen ion. Other proteins have basic radicals, $—NH_3OH$, which can dissociate into $NH_3^+$ and $OH^-$; the $OH^-$ combines with a hydrogen ion to form water, thus removing one hydrogen ion from body fluid. The protein buffer system is the most plentiful chemical buffer system in the body.[1]

# RESPIRATORY CONTROL OF pH

The respiratory control center in the brain responds to increases of carbon dioxide and hydrogen ions in body fluids. Rate and depth of respiration are in turn controlled by the respiratory control of pH as follows: (1) when the pH value decreases (more acid), respiratory rate and depth are increased, and there is greater excretion of carbon dioxide through the lungs; thus less carbon dioxide is present to produce carbonic acid by the reaction: $CO_2 + H_2O \leftrightarrows H_2CO_3$, and the pH increases toward alkalinity; and (2) when the pH value rises above the normal range (more alkaline), the respiratory center is depressed, rate and depth of respiration decrease, carbon dioxide is retained, and more carbonic acid is formed, moving the pH toward acidity. The respiratory system is extremely efficient and reacts quickly to changes in acid-base balance.

Because carbon dioxide is constantly being formed as a product of metabolism, the concentration of carbon dioxide in ECFs must be continuously balanced between the rate of metabolism and the rate of pulmonary excretion. The buffering capacity of the respiratory system is more than double that of all the chemical buffers combined.

## RENAL REGULATION OF pH

Both chemical buffers and respiratory regulation have limited ability to make complete adjustments in the pH level, and it remains for the kidneys to make permanent adjustments in the pH level of body fluids. The renal regulation of the pH level is affected by control of the retention or excretion of bicarbonate and hydrogen ions. The kidneys usually excrete an acid urine because of the excess of acid metabolic products (nonvolatile acids), which must be eliminated by the renal route. Normally, almost all of the bicarbonate formed by the kidneys is retained.

Hydrogen ions secreted by kidney tubule cells and bicarbonate filtered into the glomerular filtrate combine in the kidney tubules to form carbon dioxide and water, which is excreted through exhalation ($CO_2$) and in urine ($H_2O$). In acidosis, excess hydrogen ions are secreted into the kidney tubules, where they combine with buffers and are excreted in the urine. In alkalosis, bicarbonate ions enter the tubules, where there exists a lack of the hydrogen ions with which they normally combine to form carbonic acid; the bicarbonate ions combine instead with sodium or other cations and are excreted in the urine. Hydrogen ions can be exchanged for sodium and potassium ions in the kidney tubules; therefore excretion or conservation of hydrogen ions can result in imbalances of sodium and potassium.

## COMPENSATION

The kidneys and lungs serve a compensatory function in relation to maintaining acid-base balance. In a disease state that leads to an acid-base imbalance, the normal bicarbonate–carbonic acid ratio of 20:1 is lost. In **compensation**, the kidneys attempt to compensate for changes in blood $CO_2$ by making a corresponding change in blood *bicarbonate,* and the lungs attempt to compensate for abnormal changes in blood bicarbonate by making corresponding changes in blood $CO_2$. Compensation is an effort to maintain the normal 20:1 ratio. Figure 21-2 illustrates what happens in metabolic acidosis and how compensation of acid-base imbalance can occur.

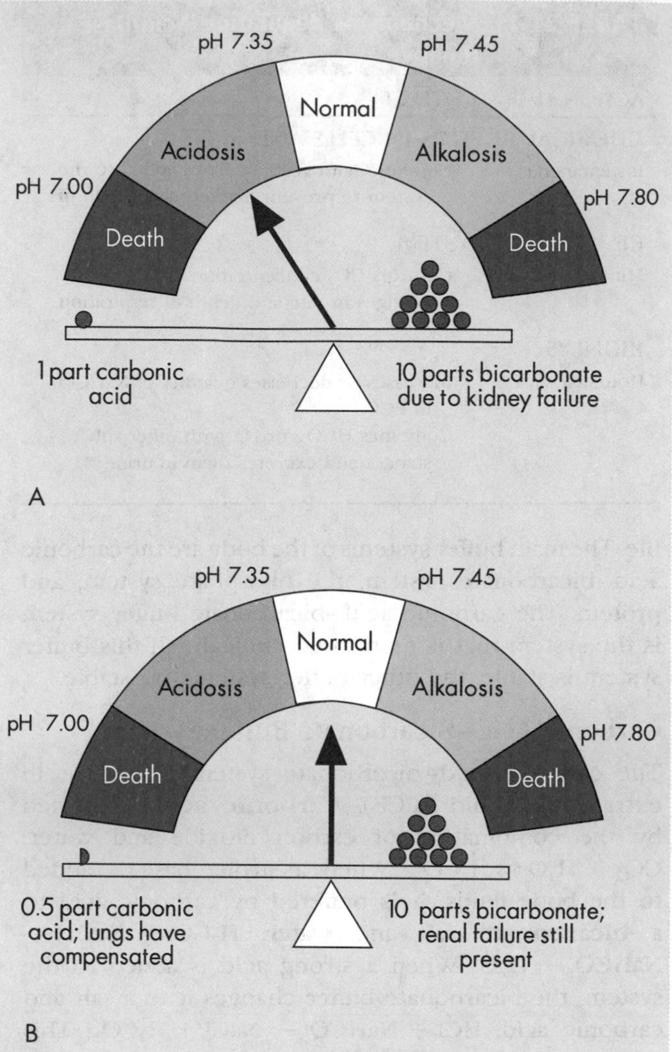


**FIGURE 21-2** **A,** Example of metabolic acidosis. Bicarbonate is decreased because of renal failure. Carbonic acid to bicarbonate ratio is 10:1; acidosis is present. **B,** Example of compensation. Note that bicarbonate is still decreased, but now carbonic acid is also decreased. Ratio returned to 20:1; pH level is normal.

Another compensatory mechanism that can be used by the body in the presence of acid-base problems is *shifting of hydrogen ions from the extracellular to the intracellular compartment or vice versa.* When there is an increased level of hydrogen ions (metabolic acidosis), these ions can be shifted into the intracellular compartment in exchange for *potassium.* This shift alone increases the pH level of the blood. In addition, because the hydrogen ion concentration is now higher in the renal tubule cells, hydrogen is excreted in exchange for the reabsorbed sodium. In *metabolic alka-*

**TABLE 21-2 Types of Acid-Base Disturbances and Compensatory Mechanisms**

| PHYSIOLOGIC CAUSES | METHOD OF COMPENSATION |
|---|---|
| **RESPIRATORY ACIDOSIS** | |
| Carbonic acid excess: lungs not removing sufficient $CO_2$ (hypoventilation) | Bicarbonate production by kidneys increased; bicarbonate retained and chloride excreted instead by kidneys; secretion and excretion of hydrogen ions in urine increased |
| **RESPIRATORY ALKALOSIS** | |
| Carbonic acid deficit: lungs removing too much $CO_2$ (hyperventilation) | Kidneys increase excretion of bicarbonate ions |
| **METABOLIC ACIDOSIS** | |
| Bicarbonate deficit: retention of acid metabolites, diabetic ketoacidosis, excess acid intake (salicylate poisoning), hyperkalemia, or loss of bicarbonate | Increased rate and depth of respiration cause increased excretion of $CO_2$ by lungs; formation of bicarbonate ions in the kidneys increased |
| **METABOLIC ALKALOSIS** | |
| Bicarbonate excess: excess intake (sodium bicarbonate, carbonated drinks) or retention of bicarbonate, potassium depletion, loss of acid | Rate and depth of respiration decreased; lungs retain more $CO_2$; kidneys excrete bicarbonate |

**TABLE 21-3 Laboratory Values in Uncompensated and Partially Compensated Acid-Base Disturbances**

| | pH | $P_{CO_2}$ | HCO |
|---|---|---|---|
| **RESPIRATORY ACIDOSIS** | | | |
| Uncompensated | Below 7.35 | ↑ | Normal |
| Partially compensated | Move toward normal, but still ↓ | ↑ | ↑ |
| **RESPIRATORY ALKALOSIS** | | | |
| Uncompensated | Above 7.45 | ↓ | Normal |
| Partially compensated | Move toward normal, but still ↑ | ↓ | ↓ |
| **METABOLIC ACIDOSIS** | | | |
| Uncompensated | Below 7.35 | Normal | ↓ |
| Partially compensated | Move toward normal, but still ↓ | ↓ | ↓ |
| **METABOLIC ALKALOSIS** | | | |
| Uncompensated | Above 7.45 | Normal | ↑ |
| Partially compensated | Move toward normal, but still ↑ | ↑ | ↑ |

*losis,* hydrogen ions are pulled from the intracellular compartment, and potassium ions are shifted into the intracellular compartment. Again, this shift alone helps to lower the pH level. Also, because potassium ion concentration is now higher in the renal tubule cells, potassium is excreted for the conserved sodium, and hydrogen ions are also conserved. These compensatory mechanisms can lead to hyperkalemia when acidosis is present and hypokalemia when alkalosis is present.

It must be remembered that the buffer systems and the compensatory mechanisms provide for only temporary adjustment, and the underlying cause of the disturbance must be identified and corrected. However, the kidneys can make permanent adjustments, as seen in persons who have respiratory acidosis as a result of chronic obstructive pulmonary disease (see Chapter 37).

## TYPES OF ACID-BASE DISTURBANCES

There are two types of acidosis (respiratory and metabolic) and two types of alkalosis (respiratory and metabolic). Table 21-2 shows the four types that occur, their physiologic causes, and their compensatory mechanisms. The major effect of acidosis is depression of the central nervous system, as evidenced by disorientation followed by coma. Alkalosis is characterized by overexcitability of the nervous system, and the muscles may go into a state of tetany and convulsions. Acid-base imbalance always produces an imbalance of the body's other cations as well; therefore symptoms of these imbalances also occur.

## LABORATORY TESTS

The following laboratory values are used in diagnosing and monitoring acid-base disturbance:

pH (normal): 7.35 to 7.45

$P_{CO_2}$ (normal): 35 to 45 mm Hg

Plasma bicarbonate (normal): 22 to 26 mEq/L

Both pH and $P_{CO_2}$ are determined from a sample of arterial blood, a blood gas analysis.

Table 21-3 shows whether laboratory values characteristic of the four types of acid-base disturbances are increased or decreased and the results of the body's compensatory efforts when partial compensation occurs.

## RESPIRATORY ACIDOSIS: CARBONIC ACID EXCESS

Any factor that decreases the rate of pulmonary ventilation increases the concentration of dissolved carbon dioxide, carbonic acid, and hydrogen ions and results in **respiratory acidosis.** An excess of carbon dioxide (hypercapnia) can cause carbon dioxide narcosis. In this condition, carbon dioxide levels are so high that they no longer stimulate respirations but depress them. Associated with the decreased respiratory rate are lack of

**BOX 21-1 Causes of Respiratory Acidosis**

Damage to respiratory center in medulla
Depression of respiratory center by drugs (narcotics)
Obstruction of respiratory passages: pneumonia, chronic bronchitis
Loss of lung surface for ventilation
- Atelectasis
- Pneumothorax
- Emphysema
- Pulmonary fibrosis

Weakness of respiratory muscles
- Poliomyelitis
- Hypokalemia

oxygen and hypoxia. During respiratory acidosis, potassium moves out of the cells, producing hyperkalemia. Ventricular fibrillation may occur if the blood potassium level is greatly increased.

## ETIOLOGY

Respiratory acidosis can result from a number of pathologic conditions: (1) damage to the respiratory center in the medulla, (2) obstruction of respiratory passages—for example, pneumonia, chronic bronchitis, (3) loss of lung surface for ventilation—for example, atelectasis, pneumothorax, emphysema, pulmonary fibrosis, (4) weakness of respiratory muscles—for example, poliomyelitis, hypokalemia, and (5) severe depression of respirations—for example, as a result of overdose of respiratory depressant drugs. Chronic obstructive pulmonary disease (COPD) is the most common cause of respiratory acidosis. Causes of respiratory acidosis are summarized in Box 21-1. See Table 21-4 for major signs and symptoms.

## PREVENTION

Persons with diseases that limit lung excursion and therefore limit gaseous exchange, such as emphysema, should not take carbonated beverages or bicarbonate of soda. These substances tend to make the blood more alkaline than normal, and respirations are depressed in an effort to correct this imbalance. Depression of respirations is highly undesirable for these patients. Persons with $CO_2$ retention should be advised to avoid sedatives, tranquilizers, alcohol, and cough medications that contain narcotics.

Any person with symptoms of inadequate oxygenation or carbon dioxide retention requires medical treatment. Early recognition and treatment of the primary condition often prevent its becoming complicated by acid-base imbalance. Therefore any person with symptoms suggestive of anemia, cardiac insufficiency, or chronic bronchitis, emphysema, asthma, or other obstructive diseases of the bronchioles should receive medical attention. These conditions are discussed in detail in later chapters of the book.

**TABLE 21-4 Major Signs and Symptoms and Therapy for Acid-Base Imbalances**

| SIGNS AND SYMPTOMS | THERAPY |
|---|---|
| **RESPIRATORY ACIDOSIS** | |
| Hyperpnea | Bronchodilators |
| Visual disturbances | Postural drainage |
| Headache | Chest clapping |
| Late: confusion, drowsiness, coma | Mechanical ventilation |
| Potassium excess | |
| **RESPIRATORY ALKALOSIS** | |
| Lightheadedness | Treatment of underlying condition |
| Numbness or tingling of fingers or toes | |
| Late: tetany, convulsions | |
| Potassium deficit | |
| **METABOLIC ACIDOSIS** | |
| Headache and mental dullness | Treatment of underlying condition |
| | Sodium bicarbonate (IV) |
| Kussmaul's respirations | Fluid and electrolyte replacement |
| Late: disorientation, coma | |
| Potassium excess | |
| **METABOLIC ALKALOSIS** | |
| Confusion, dizziness | Treatment of underlying condition |
| Numbness or tingling of fingers or toes | Diuretic: acetazolamide (Diamox) |
| | Fluid and electrolyte replacement |
| Late: tetany, convulsions | |
| Potassium deficit | |

## MANAGEMENT

Treatment is aimed at increasing the alveolar ventilation rate to improve the exchange of carbon dioxide and oxygen. This objective is accomplished by identifying and treating the cause of the inadequate ventilation. Bronchodilators may be used to reduce bronchial spasm. Respiratory infections may be treated with antibiotics. Postural drainage and chest clapping are necessary in persons with obstruction of respiratory passages. Adequate hydration is also important to assist in removal of secretions. Supplemental oxygen may be used as necessary.

Because the respiratory center is narcotized by the increased amounts of carbon dioxide, the lowered oxygen tension of the blood is the stimulus for respiration. If a patient whose respiratory drive is dependent on a low $Po_2$ level is given large amounts of oxygen, the stimulus for breathing is removed, and respirations will cease. For this reason, uncontrolled oxygen delivery is never used with patients with carbon dioxide narcosis.

Low-flow oxygen (1 to 3 L/min) is given to a patient with COPD who maintains a chronically high $PCO_2$ level. Respiratory treatments are usually given using compressed air or room air instead of oxygen in these situations. If signs of ventilatory failure are present, the $PCO_2$ level is greater than 50 to 60 mm Hg, and the $PO_2$ level is less than 50 mm Hg, the patient may require intubation and mechanical ventilation.[2]

The major nursing responsibility is to recognize patients who have the potential for developing respiratory acidosis because of conditions that interfere with normal respiratory gas exchange. A patient whose airway is compromised by the presence of secretions must be encouraged to cough frequently or may need to undergo nasopharyngeal or tracheal suctioning. Pulmonary hygiene measures may be used to promote removal of secretions.

## Respiratory Alkalosis: Carbonic Acid Deficit

### ETIOLOGY

Excessive pulmonary ventilation decreases hydrogen ion concentration and thus causes **respiratory alkalosis.** A common cause of respiratory alkalosis is *hyperventilation.* A person who hyperventilates blows off large amounts of carbon dioxide. Hyperventilation may be caused by anxiety, pain, hypoxia, or lesions affecting the respiratory center in the medulla (brain tumor, encephalitis). Other causes of respiratory alkalosis are conditions that greatly increase metabolism (hyperthyroidism) and the overventilation of patients with mechanical respirators. Causes of respiratory alkalosis are summarized in Box 21-2. See Table 21-4 for major signs and symptoms.

### PATHOPHYSIOLOGY

Carbonic acid deficit causes vasoconstriction of cerebral blood vessels, which results in cerebral hypoxia. This decrease in cerebral blood flow contributes to the lightheadedness and confusion present in respiratory alkalosis. If the alkalosis becomes more severe, tetany and convulsions may be present. These manifestations are due to an increase in binding of serum calcium and a decrease in ionized calcium. Serum potassium levels will be decreased because the kidneys retain hydrogen ions and excrete potassium instead.

### PREVENTION

Respiratory alkalosis can be prevented in a person who is hyperventilating from anxiety or pain by administering a few whiffs of carbon dioxide or by having the person breathe into a paper bag and then rebreathe the exhaled carbon dioxide. Care should be taken in adjusting mechanical respirators so that the patient is not being forced to take breaths too deeply or rapidly. Correction of hypoxia prevents respiratory alkalosis in these situations.

**BOX 21-2 Causes of Respiratory Alkalosis**

- Hyperventilation syndrome (caused by anxiety, hysteria)
- Hyperventilation caused by the following:
  - Fever
  - Hypoxia
- Pulmonary disorders
- Lesions affecting the respiratory center in the medulla
  - Brain tumor
  - Encephalitis
- Excess assisted ventilation
- Hyperthyroidism

### MANAGEMENT

Treating the underlying condition usually effectively resolves the respiratory alkalosis. Respiratory alkalosis becomes especially dangerous when it leads to cardiac dysrhythmias caused partly by a decreased serum potassium level. If a patient who is receiving assisted ventilation complains of dizziness or shows any signs of muscle irritability, it is likely that the depth of respiration is too great, and the respiratory rate of the machine should be decreased. If tetany is present, calcium gluconate is given intravenously (Chapter 20). Renal function must be maintained to promote renal compensation of the disturbance.

## Metabolic Acidosis: Bicarbonate Deficit

When excess organic acids are added to the body fluids or when bicarbonate is lost, a **metabolic acidosis** or nonrespiratory acidosis results.

### ETIOLOGY

In such conditions as uncontrolled diabetes mellitus or starvation, glucose either cannot be used or is not available for oxidation. The body compensates for this by the use of body fat for energy, producing abnormal amounts of ketone bodies in the process. In an effort to neutralize the ketones and maintain the acid-base balance of the body, plasma bicarbonate is exhausted. The resultant acid-base imbalance is called metabolic acidosis or *ketoacidosis.* This condition can develop in anyone who does not eat an adequate diet and whose body fat must be burned for energy. It is the reason that extremely low-carbohydrate or high-protein–no carbohydrate reduction diets are criticized by nutrition experts.

Metabolic acidosis can also develop whenever excessive amounts of lactic acid are produced, such as in prolonged strenuous muscle exercise or when oxidation takes place in cells without adequate oxygen, such as occurs in heart failure and shock. Loss of large amounts of alkaline intestinal secretions, such as in severe diar-

**BOX 21-3 Causes of Metabolic Acidosis**

Increased acid production
- Ketoacidosis (uncontrolled diabetes mellitus, starvation)
- Uremic acidosis (renal failure)
- Lactic acidosis (shock, respiratory or cardiac arrest)

Increased acid ingestion
- Salicylates, ethanol, ethylene glycol

Loss of bicarbonate
- Severe diarrhea
- Intestinal fistulas

**BOX 21-4 Causes of Metabolic Alkalosis**

Loss of stomach acid
- Gastric suctioning
- Persistent vomiting

Excess alkali intake

Loss of potassium

Intestinal fistulas

rhea or through fistulas, can also create a bicarbonate deficit.

The normal functioning kidney excretes an excess of hydrogen ions in conditions of acidosis and, in so doing, retains potassium so that hyperkalemia, as well as acidosis, is present. In kidney failure, metabolic acids accumulate in the bloodstream. Causes of metabolic acidosis are listed in Box 21-3.

Headache and mental dullness are early signs of acidosis. The patient in acidosis is hyperpneic and has deep respirations (Kussmaul's respirations). This breathing pattern represents an attempt to blow off carbon dioxide, thus compensating for the acidosis. If the condition is untreated, disorientation, stupor, coma, and death occur.

Hyperkalemia results from the movement of potassium out of the cells as hydrogen ions move in and from the retention of potassium by the kidneys. Aside from laboratory evidence, there may be few indications of the acidosis until the pH level falls to 7.1 or lower. See Table 21-4 for major signs and symptoms of metabolic acidosis.

### PREVENTION

Metabolic acidosis can be prevented by careful medical management or, when possible, by prevention of the conditions that lead to acidosis.

### MANAGEMENT

Treatment of acidosis is directed toward the underlying cause and restoration of electrolyte balance. If the acidosis is severe, intravenous sodium bicarbonate is sometimes given. Bicarbonate preparations must be administered with caution, because they can induce a metabolic alkalosis and lead to tetany and convulsions. When acidosis is caused by renal failure, renal dialysis is necessary.

As the acidosis is corrected, potassium moves back into cells, and hypokalemia develops. If a patient being treated for acidosis needs to receive potassium, it is given after the acidosis has been partially corrected and as the pH level is returning to normal. It is important to bear in mind that even though acidosis is accompanied by hyperkalemia, the patient may be potassium-depleted. The potassium leaves the cells in exchange for the hydrogen ions, and much of it is excreted.

Maintenance of good respiratory function in a patient with metabolic acidosis facilitates the excretion of carbon dioxide. If the kidneys are functioning well, they can help correct the acidosis by producing more bicarbonate. Because some conditions that lead to metabolic acidosis cause a hyperosmolar state as well, osmotic diuresis will take place, and the patient will need fluid replacement along with careful monitoring of intake and output. If changes in the sensorium have resulted, safety precautions are instituted.

## METABOLIC ALKALOSIS: BICARBONATE EXCESS

When excessive amounts of acid substance and hydrogen ions are lost from the body or when large amounts of bicarbonate or lactate are added orally or intravenously, the result is an imbalance in which there is an excess of base elements, called **metabolic alkalosis.** This type of imbalance does not occur as often as does metabolic acidosis. In alkalosis, potassium enters the cells and hypokalemia results. A potassium loss causes a metabolic alkalosis, whereas an alkalosis causes hypokalemia.[2] An excess of bicarbonate in distal tubular fluid causes obligatory potassium loss.

### ETIOLOGY

Metabolic alkalosis can occur in the following conditions: (1) loss of hydrochloric acid from the stomach caused by vomiting or gastric drainage from a nasogastric tube (loss of chloride leaves more sodium to combine with and retain bicarbonate in the kidneys), (2) loss of potassium ions through intestinal fistulas or diarrhea or in the urine, (3) ingestion of large amounts of sodium bicarbonate or other systemic antacids to treat indigestion or ulcers, (4) infusion of excessive amounts of bicarbonate or lactate intravenously, (5) diuretic therapy, and (6) excessive mineralocorticoids. Causes of metabolic alkalosis are listed in Box 21-4.

In metabolic alkalosis, breathing becomes depressed in an effort to conserve carbon dioxide for combination with water in the blood to raise the blood level of carbonic acid. Symptoms that can occur are mental confusion, dizziness, numbness and tingling in extremities, muscle twitching, and later, tetany and convulsions. Electrocardiographic changes consistent with hypokalemia may be present (see Chapter 20). See Table 21-4 for major signs and symptoms of metabolic alkalosis.

### PREVENTION

Persons must be cautioned against the excessive use of sodium bicarbonate to alleviate indigestion. Controlling the conditions that can cause metabolic alkalosis can prevent this imbalance from developing. If drug therapy is causing the alkalosis, these drugs should be discontinued and others substituted where possible.

### MANAGEMENT

Treatment is aimed at correcting the cause of the metabolic alkalosis. Sodium chloride or ammonium chloride may be given orally or intravenously. If the condition is associated with loss of sodium chloride, potassium must be restored because it is lost with the sodium. It is given in the form of potassium chloride. A diuretic that acts as a carbonic anhydrase inhibitor (Diamox) may help relieve the alkalosis by increasing excretion of bicarbonate by the kidneys.

The nurse assists in maintenance of good respiratory function so that compensation can take place through this mechanism. Careful monitoring of the patient for adequate renal function and safety precautions are important in the nursing care of patients with metabolic alkalosis. Because convulsions may occur, precautions are taken for the patient's protection.

## QUESTIONS TO CONSIDER

- Why is low-flow oxygen (1 to 3 L/min) given to patients with obstructive pulmonary disease?
- Explain one common method of preventing respiratory alkalosis.
- Which acid-base imbalance occurs frequently in persons with diabetes mellitus? Why?
- What is the role of potassium in acid-base balance?
- Kussmaul's respirations are an indication of which acid-base imbalance? What does this breathing pattern indicate?

## CRITICAL THINKING ACTIVITIES

- A 50-year-old man is admitted to the hospital with a hernia. He admits to frequent laxative use and occasional diarrhea. He undergoes a hernia repair and postoperatively develops a paralytic ileus. Analyze this clinical situation, and determine what acid-base imbalance would the patient be at greatest risk of developing.

## CHAPTER SUMMARY

### REGULATION OF ACID-BASE BALANCE

- Mechanisms that regulate acid-base balance include chemical buffer systems, the respiratory system, and the kidneys.
- The respiratory control center in the brain responds to increases of carbon dioxide and hydrogen ions in body fluids by changing the rate and depth of respiration.
- The renal regulation of the pH level is effected by control of the retention or excretion of bicarbonate and hydrogen ions.

### TYPES OF ACID-BASE DISTURBANCES

- The major effect of acidosis is depression of the central nervous system, as evidenced by disorientation followed by coma.
- Alkalosis is characterized by overexcitability of the nervous system, and the muscles may go into a state of tetany and convulsions.
- Any factor that decreases the rate of pulmonary ventilation increases the concentration of dissolved carbon dioxide, carbonic acid, and hydrogen ions and results in respiratory acidosis.
- Excess pulmonary ventilation decreases hydrogen ion concentration and thus causes respiratory alkalosis.
- When excess organic acids are added to the body fluids or when bicarbonate is lost, metabolic acidosis results.
- When excessive amounts of organic acid substance and hydrogen ions are lost from the body or when large amounts of bicarbonate or lactate are added, the result is an imbalance in which there is an excess of base elements, or metabolic alkalosis.

## REFERENCES

1. Guyton A: *Textbook of medical physiology,* ed 8, Philadelphia, 1990, WB Saunders.
2. Horne M, Heitz U, Swearingen P: *Fluid, electrolyte, and acid-base balance*—a case study approach, St Louis, 1991, Mosby.
3. Taylor DL: Respiratory alkalosis: pathophysiology, signs, and symptoms, *Nursing '90* 20(8):60–61, 1990.

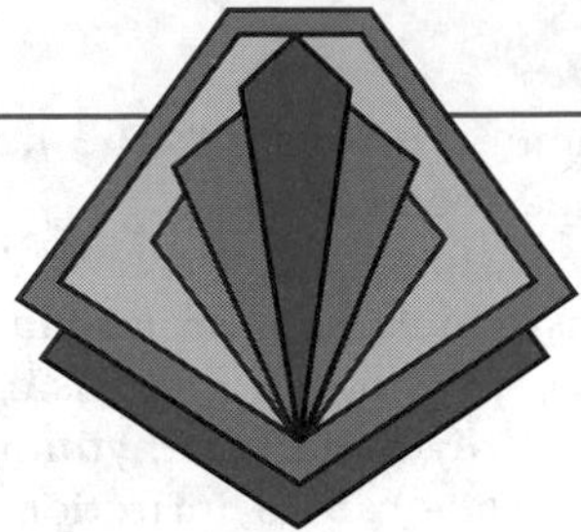

C H A P T E R 22

# Shock

***Martha L. Allen***

## CHAPTER OBJECTIVES

***After studying this chapter, the learner should be able to do the following:***

1 Contrast three major types of shock.
2 Describe early and late pathophysiologic changes that occur with shock.
3 Describe organ damage that may occur with shock.
4 Describe different methods of monitoring for shock.
5 Describe methods of fluid replacement during shock.
6 Identify effects of pharmacologic agents used to treat shock and nursing measures for patients receiving drug therapy.
7 Describe therapeutic measures for shock other than fluids and drug therapy.

## KEY TERMS

adult respiratory distress syndrome (ARDS)
anaphylactic shock
arterial oxygen pressure ($Pa_{O_2}$)
arterial oxygen saturation ($Sa_{O_2}$)
autotransfusion
cardiogenic shock
central venous pressure (CVP)
colloid solutions
crystalloid solutions
distributive shock
fluid challenge
intraarterial monitoring
hypovolemic shock
hypoxemia
military antishock trousers (MAST)
mixed venous oxygen saturation ($Sv_{O_2}$)
myocardial depressant factor
neurogenic shock
pulmonary artery pressure (PAP)
pulmonary capillary wedge pressure (PCWP)
septic shock
systemic vascular resistance (SVR)
thermistor
third spacing of fluids

## NATURE OF THE PROBLEM

Shock is a syndrome characterized by hypoperfusion of body tissues and results in a lack of oxygen to cells. Any condition that prevents cells from receiving adequate blood and oxygen supplies can interfere with their metabolism and produce shock.

Blood flow depends on pressure changes within the vascular compartment. Blood flows from areas of greater pressure to areas of lesser pressure. In the systemic circulation, the mean pressure is highest in the aorta, where the blood leaves the left ventricle, and lowest in the right atrium. For the necessary pressure gradients to exist so that blood can flow, the following three factors are necessary:

1. An adequate amount of blood for the heart to pump around the body
2. Ability of the heart to pump blood
3. Blood vessels with good tone, able to constrict and dilate to maintain normal pressure

Shock results from the disruption of one or more of these factors.

## ETIOLOGY

Shock may be classified as hypovolemic, cardiogenic, or distributive (Box 22-1).

### HYPOVOLEMIC SHOCK

Hypovolemic shock is the most common type of shock. Any condition that reduces the *volume* within the vascular compartment by 15% to 25% can result in hypovolemic shock. Characteristically, the signs and symptoms of hypovolemic shock progress in direct proportion to the percentage of blood loss from the intravascular spaces (Table 22-1). Common causes of hypovolemic shock include the following:

1. Excessive blood loss: trauma (most common cause), gastrointestinal (GI) bleeding, coagulation disorders, surgery
2. Loss of body fluids other than blood: excessive diuresis (diabetic ketoacidosis or other hyperosmolar states), plasma loss from excessive vomiting or diarrhea
3. Movement of fluid from the vascular compartment

**BOX 22-1 Types of Shock**

| | |
|---|---|
| **Hypovolemic** | Shock from loss of fluid from vascular system (through blood loss or fluid loss) |
| **Cardiogenic** | Shock from inability of heart to pump blood to tissues (decreased cardiac output) |
| **Distributive** | Shock from massive vasodilation (from interference with sympathetic nervous system or effects of histamine or toxins) |

to a body compartment that does not usually contain a large amount of fluid, such as the gastrointestinal tract, peritoneal cavity or the interstitial space; for example, 5 to 10 L of fluid may collect in the bowel with bowel obstruction. Peritonitis may result in the accumulation of 4 to 6 L of fluid in the peritoneal cavity within 24 hours. The collection of a large amount of fluid in a body compartment other than the vessels or the cells is referred to as **third spacing of fluid.**

## CARDIOGENIC SHOCK

Cardiogenic shock results from the inability of the heart to pump sufficient blood to perfuse the cells of the body. Because cardiac output is the product of stroke volume and heart rate, the body compensates for decreased stroke volume by increasing heart rate. Initially this will maintain cardiac output. Tachycardia, however, can have a deleterious effect on the heart. Oxygen consumption is increased, and because the coronary arteries fill during diastole, the filling time is decreased. The heart thus needs more oxygen and receives less.

Although cardiogenic shock may be caused by various cardiac conditions—including cardiac tamponade, restrictive pericarditis, pulmonary embolism, severe valvular disease, or dysrhythmias (arrhythmias), the most common cause is myocardial infarction. Studies have shown that in most patients who die from cardiogenic shock, at least 40% of the left ventricle was damaged by a recent infarction or by a recent infarction plus a previous scar. Despite improvements in managing cardiogenic shock, the mortality still remains greater than 80%.

## DISTRIBUTIVE SHOCK

Distributive shock is caused by massive dilation of the blood vessels, resulting in disproportion between the size of the vascular space and the amount of circulating blood. As vessels dilate, blood pressure falls and blood pools in dilated vessels, resulting in a decrease in venous return to the heart and a fall in cardiac output.

Types of distributive shock include neurogenic, anaphylactic, and septic. It may also occur with vasodilator drugs or acute renal insufficiency. **Neurogenic shock** results from interference with the sympathetic nervous system, which helps maintain vasomotor tone. Spinal cord injury, spinal anesthesia, and rarely, brain damage are among the causes. **Anaphylactic shock,** which is a type of allergic reaction, (see Chapter 70) may occur when a sensitized person has contact with an antigen. Vasoactive substances—including histamine, kinins, and prostaglandins—are released and cause massive vasodilation in the body. The endothelial cells that line the

**TABLE 22-1 Clinical Manifestations of Hypovolemic Shock**

| PARAMETER (FOR A 70-kg MALE) | CLASS I EARLY | CLASS II MODERATE | CLASS III MAJOR OR PROGRESSIVE | CLASS IV SEVERE OR PROFOUND |
|---|---|---|---|---|
| Approximate blood volume loss (ml) | Up to 750 | 750-1500 | 1500-2000 | 2000 or more |
| % of blood volume | Up to 15% | 15%-30% | 30%-40% | 40% or more |
| Neurologic/behavioral status | Slightly anxious | Mildly anxious, restless; muscle fatigue and weakness evident | Agitated, confused; progressive decrease in activity; progressive thirst evident | Stuporous, lethargic, unconscious; dilated pupils may be evident |
| Heart rate | <100 | >100 Mild tachycardia | >120 Tachycardia | 140 or higher Irregular pulse, decreased pulse amplitude |
| Blood pressure | Normal | Normal | Decreased | Severe hypotension |
| Pulse pressure (mm Hg) | Normal or increased | Decreased | Decreased | Decreased |
| Respirations | 14-20, normal | 20-30, normal | 30-40, hyperpnea | >35, shallow, irregular |
| Urine output (ml/hr) | 30 or more | 20-30 | 5-15 | Negligible |
| Capillary blanch test | Normal | Slight delay | Defined delay | No refilling observed |
| Skin | Pale flushed, slightly cool | Slightly cold, pale | Cold and moist | Cold and cyanotic, mottled |

From McQuillian KA, Wiles CE: Initial management of traumatic shock. In Cardona DV et al: *Trauma nursing from resuscitation through rehabilitation,* Philadelphia, 1988, WB Saunders.

capillaries separate and expose the basement membrane, which is permeable to fluid and plasma proteins. Large quantities of fluid may leak out of the capillaries, causing severe hypovolemia.[6]

### Septic Shock

**Septic shock** is another form of distributive shock that may result from various infections, including those caused by both gram-positive and gram-negative bacteria, viruses, and fungi. Gram-negative bacteria—including *Escherichia coli, Klebsiella-Enterobacter-Serratia* (KES), *Pseudomonas,* and *Proteus*—are the most frequent causative organisms in septic shock. Infections anywhere in the body can result in septic shock. The most common sites of infections leading to septic shock are the urinary tract, respiratory tract, and blood. Some gram-negative organisms that may cause sepsis and septic shock are normal flora of the intestinal tract. As long as they remain in the intestinal tract, they do no harm and are even beneficial. However, if these organisms enter the bloodstream, they are lysed by leukocytes and release an endotoxin. Septic shock may result. Septic shock can be viewed as part of the continuum from infection to sepsis to septic shock to multiple organ dysfunction syndrome.[1]

Conditions that predispose to septic shock include the following:

1. Extremes of age (very young, very old)
2. Immunosuppressive and steroid therapy
3. Chronic illness affecting the immune system (e.g., AIDS)
4. Surgery, especially urologic and gastrointestinal
5. Poor nutritional status
6. All forms of instrumentation (e.g., intravenous lines, indwelling catheters)

Elderly men with benign prostatic hypertrophy are particularly susceptible to septic shock, because they have a high incidence of urinary tract infections and are often subjected to invasive urologic procedures.

The mechanism by which septic shock occurs is not completely understood. Some believe that early in sepsis, fluid leaks out of the vascular system and the resultant shock is simply a form of hypovolemic shock.[15] Others see the primary cause as faulty cellular metabolism from the direct effect of the toxins.[30]

The release of the endotoxin from the gram-negative organism into the bloodstream causes the release of numerous vasoactive substances within the body, including histamine, prostaglandins, serotonin, bradykinin, and endorphins. Some cause massive vasodilation, others cause selective vasoconstriction, and some cause an increase in capillary permeability. The result is major fluid shifts and maldistribution of blood within the body. The massive vasodilation results in hypotension despite the cardiac output usually being very high in the early stages. The high cardiac output (hyperdynamic state) is thought to cause the warm, flushed skin in early septic shock. As septic shock progresses, cardiac output falls and the clinical picture resembles that of other types of shock.

Septic shock is of particular importance, because it has a high mortality rate and is likely to have resulted from a hospital-acquired infection. It has been estimated that 1 in every 100 persons admitted to hospitals in the United States acquires gram-negative sepsis, and of these, 40% will go on to develop septic shock.[21]

# PHYSIOLOGY

## MAINTENANCE OF NORMAL BLOOD FLOW

As previously noted, shock results from the catastrophic disruption in one or more components of the cardiovascular system. When the functional integrity of this system remains intact and the demand for oxygen and nutrients keeps pace with supplies, cells and tissues function normally.

To assess normal functioning, oxygen use must be determined. This is done by assessing two key parameters—oxygen delivery ($DO_2$) and oxygen consumption ($SvO_2$). $DO_2$ is the product of cardiac output multiplied by saturation and hemoglobin level. $SvO_2$ is the product of cardiac output multiplied by hemoglobin level and the difference in arterial and venous saturation.[29]

Oxygen use is directly affected by the adequacy of the blood supply, the pumping effectiveness of the heart, and the functional integrity of the vascular system. These three essential components of the cardiovascular system sustain the balance between the blood added to the arterial system with each heartbeat and the blood flowing through arteries to the vascular beds through precapillary arterioles.

Functional control of the cardiovascular system is designed to maintain effective arterial pressure and to sustain adequate blood flow to vital organs. It does this by regulating control of both blood pressure and blood volume. The neural hormonal responses of the autonomic nervous system regulate this control by four mechanisms: neural regulators, circulating mediators, autoregulation, and local mediation.[4]

*Neural regulation* of arteriolar muscles is by the sympathetic component of the autonomic system. Stimulation of α-adrenergic receptors causes vasoconstriction, and stimulation of β-adrenergic receptors causes vasodilatation. *Circulating mediators* are the bloodborne hormones, such as glucocorticoids, that can be activated in times of stress. These hormones increase sensitivity of muscle cells to catecholamines, which directly affect vasomotor tone.

*Autoregulation* is accomplished by myogenic reflexes that allow regulation of the vascular bed blood flow by automatically altering vascular resistance with changes in arterial pressure. This maintains pressure and volume in individual organ systems, especially the brain. *Local mediators* (e.g., lactic acid, carbon dioxide, potassium), which are products of metabolism generated by tissues adjacent to arterioles, affect arterial pressure by vasodilation. During periods of high metabolic demand, this mechanism significantly increases blood flow to local areas of need.[27]

When shock occurs, these same mechanisms play key roles in survival of cells and vital organ systems. When they fail or are overwhelmed by the extent of the stress, there may be a drop in blood pressure and maldistribution of blood flow, which is directly related to hypoxia, oxygen debt, shock, and shock-related organ failure.[25]

# PATHOPHYSIOLOGY

## EARLY STAGE

In the early stage of shock, the body responds to hypoperfusion as it would to any other stressor. Many changes that occur are mediated through the sympathetic nervous system. Stimulation of the sympathetic nervous system results in secretion of norepinephrine from the sympathetic fibers and epinephrine and norepinephrine by the adrenal medulla. Both α- and β-adrenergic receptors are stimulated throughout the body. α-Receptors respond by causing vasoconstriction; β-receptors respond by causing vasodilation ($\beta_1$) and increasing rate and strength of contraction of the heart ($\beta_2$). Other organs with $\beta_2$-receptors are also stimulated (respiratory system). The skin and the abdominal organs, which are rich in α-receptors, receive a decreased blood supply because of vasconstriction. The heart and skeletal muscles, which are rich in β-receptors, receive an increased blood supply because of vasodilation. The heart beats faster and harder, and the respiratory rate increases in response to β-stimulation, thereby increasing oxygen delivery to the tissues. All the compensatory responses mediated through the sympathetic nervous system occur rapidly.

The overall effect of the sympathetic nervous system response in hypovolemic and cardiogenic shock is an increase in **systemic vascular resistance (SVR)** (the resistance in the vascular system against which the heart must eject). The widespread vasodilation characteristic of septic shock negates the effect of norepinephrine, resulting in a decreased SVR.

Another compensatory response, mediated through the renin-angiotensin system, occurs more slowly. As cardiac output falls, the blood flow to the kidneys decreases. The juxtaglomerular cells respond by secreting renin, which acts on a plasma protein, converting it to angiotensin I. This is converted to angiotensin II in the lungs and has two major effects: It causes vasoconstriction and causes the adrenal cortex to secrete aldosterone. Aldosterone causes the kidneys to retain sodium and water and secrete potassium, resulting in an increased blood volume. The secretion of potassium may result in *hypokalemia* during this stage of shock. In addition, decreased cardiac output results in decreased hydrostatic pressure in the capillaries, causing fluid to shift from the interstitial space into the capillaries. This also improves blood volume.

For a short period the compensatory mechanisms have a beneficial effect. The most vital organs, the heart and the brain, receive an adequate blood supply at the expense of the less vital organs, such as the kidneys, and other abdominal organs. This allows time for the underlying cause of shock to be corrected. However, if the underlying problem is not or cannot be corrected, the

**TABLE 22-2 Major Pathophysiologic Changes in Shock**

| CHANGE | EFFECT |
|---|---|
| **EARLY STAGE (COMPENSATORY/NONPROGRESSIVE)[11]** | |
| Increased epinephrine and norepinephrine | Increased cardiac output to increase blood flow to tissues |
| α- and β-adrenergic-receptors stimulated | |
| Alpha effects: skin and most viscera | Vasoconstriction and decreased blood supply |
| Beta effects: heart and skeletal muscles | Vasodilation and increased blood supply and heart rate |
| Renin-angiotensin response | Vasoconstriction and secretion of aldosterone; sodium and water retention; potassium loss |
| Increased glucocorticoids and mineralocorticoids | Sodium and water retention to increase intravascular volume; potassium loss |
| Hypoxemia | Hyperventilation; provides more oxygen to tissues; may cause respiratory alkalosis |
| Decreased hydrostatic fluid pressure | Fluid shifts from interstitial space to intravascular space to increase vascular volume |
| **LATE STAGE (NONCOMPENSATORY/PROGRESSIVE)[11]** | |
| Decreased blood flow to heart | Impaired cardiac pumping ability (decreased cardiac output); blood pressure decreases |
| Anaerobic metabolism | Acidosis; decreased adenosine triphosphate; failure of cellular sodium-potassium pump (potassium leaves cell; sodium and water enter cell); cellular damage |
| Arteriolar dilation and venule constriction | Fluid shift from intravascular to interstitial space |
| Decreased blood flow to kidney | Decreased kidney function (oliguria or anuria, retention of nitrogenous waste products and potassium) |
| Decreased blood flow to pancreas | Production of myocardial depressant factor (MDF) |

compensatory mechanisms will not be able to continue to perfuse vital organs sufficiently, and the mechanisms themselves will have a deleterious effect on the body. Shock will then progress to a later stage.

There are few signs of shock in the early stage; the patient may be restless, and the pulse and respiratory rates may be increased. In distributive shock, the extremities are warm and flushed because of vasodilation; this is often called "warm shock." Signs in the later stage of any type of shock include cool, clammy skin; decreased blood pressure; and lethargy or unconsciousness; this is called "cold shock" or late shock. Table 22-2 summarizes the pathophysiologic changes in early and late shock. The signs and symptoms of shock are reviewed in Table 22-3.

## LATE STAGE

As shock progresses, blood flow to all body tissues becomes impaired. Cells in vasoconstricted organs receive insufficient oxygen, and aerobic metabolism is replaced by anaerobic metabolism. Energy in the form of adenosine triphosphate (ATP) is produced very inefficiently. Only 2 mol of ATP are produced for each mole of glucose metabolized, in contrast to 38 mol in aerobic metabolism. In addition, lactic acid is formed and cannot be further metabolized in the absence of oxygen. Acidosis and energy deficiency result. Without enough energy, the sodium-potassium pump fails. Potassium leaves the cells, and sodium and water enter, damaging various organelles. Lysosomes, which have an important role in phagocytosis, contain digestive enzymes that are ordinarily contained within a wall. When the lysosome is damaged, the digestive enzymes spill into the rest of the cell and destroy it. As these enzymes come in contact with adjacent cells, these cells also are destroyed and release their digestive enzymes. Cellular death results in organ death.

Acid metabolites cause dilation at the arteriole end of the capillaries (precapillary sphincter) and constriction at the venule end (postcapillary sphincter). Increased hydrostatic pressure within the capillary results and causes fluid to shift from the capillary into the interstitial space; the blood volume is decreased even further. In addition to the increase in pressure within the capillaries, increased capillary permeability may occur. This is most likely to occur in *septic shock* because of the release of large amounts of histamine and serotonin in response to the presence of gram-negative toxins. Proteins are able to leak through the capillary walls, increasing the osmotic pressure in the interstitium. This causes a further shift of fluid out of the capillaries. Longstanding hypoxemia of the capillaries also can result in increased capillary permeability, so that in the late stages of *cardiogenic* and *hypovolemic shock*, this type of fluid shift also may occur. Decreased blood supply to the kidneys results in oliguria or anuria. The serum creatinine and the blood urea nitrogen (BUN) levels increase. The kidneys are not able to excrete the increasing amounts of potassium that are accumulating in the blood as a result of cellular damage, and hyperkalemia results, which is worsened by the acidosis. *Hyperkalemia* depresses the conduction and contractility of the heart.

Vasoconstriction of the splanchnic vessels in response to sympathetic stimulation causes ischemia of the ab-

**TABLE 22-3 Comparison of Signs and Symptoms in Early and Late Shock by Body System**

| | EARLY SHOCK | LATE SHOCK |
|---|---|---|
| **Respiratory system** | Hyperventilation; ↑ minute volume; ↓ $Paco_2$; normal $Pao_2$* | Respirations shallow; breath sounds may suggest congestion; ↑ $Paco_2$; ↓ $Pao_2$* |
| **Cardiovascular system** | Blood pressure normal to slightly lowered; ↑ diastolic pressure; ↓ pulse pressure; tachycardia; cardiac output normal in hypovolemic shock, slightly decreased in cardiogenic shock, and increased in septic shock; mild vasoconstriction in hypovolemic and cardiogenic shock; vasodilation in septic shock | ↓ Blood pressure; ↓ cardiac output; tachycardia continues; vasoconstriction worsens in hypovolemic, cardiogenic, and septic shock |
| **Renal system** | Decreased urine output; ↑ urine osmolality; ↓ urine sodium concentration; hypokalemia | Oliguria or complete renal shutdown; hyperkalemia; buildup of waste products |
| **Acid-base balance** | Respiratory alkalosis | Metabolic acidosis; respiratory acidosis |
| **Vascular compartment** | Fluid shift from interstitial space to intravascular compartment; thirst | Fluid shift from intravascular space to interstitial and intracellular spaces, causing edema |
| **Skin** | Minimal to no changes in hypovolemic and cardiogenic shock; warm, flushed skin in septic shock | Cool, clammy skin in hypovolemic, cardiogenic, and septic shock; cool, mottled skin in neurogenic and vasogenic shock |
| **Hematologic system** | Release of red blood cells (RBCs) from bone marrow to increase vascular volume; platelet aggregation | Disseminated intravascular coagulation (DIC) |
| **Mental-neurologic system** | Restless; alert; confused | Lethargy; unconsciousness |
| **GI-hepatic system** | No obvious changes | Perfusion decreases; bowel sounds possibly diminished |

*$Paco_2$, Carbon dioxide pressure; $Pao_2$, oxygen pressure.

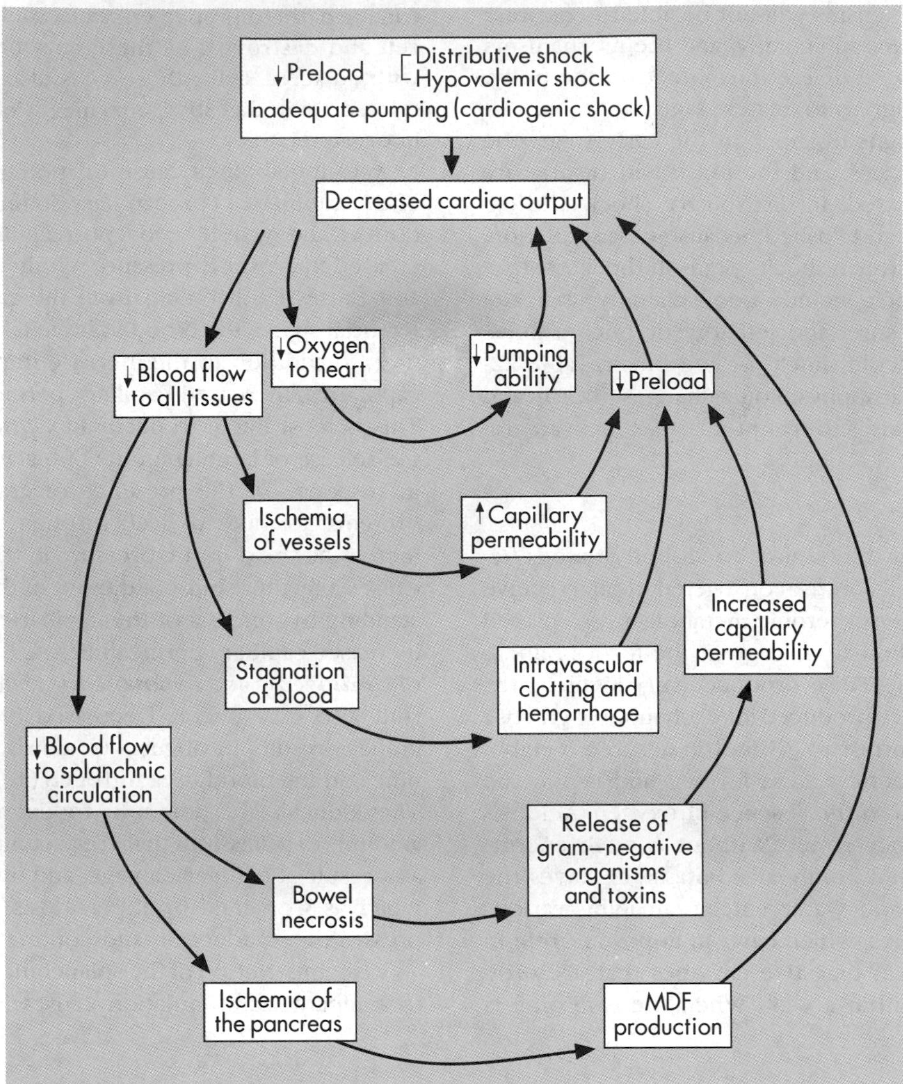


**FIGURE 22-1** Shock causes shock.

dominal organs. Of particular importance is the pancreas. In response to hypoxemia, the pancreas forms and secretes a substance called **myocardial depressant factor** (MDF), which depresses the contractility of the heart. As this enzyme is initially released in the bloodstream, it alters the overall efficiency of cardiac muscle function. Although cardiac function may be sustained initially by the compensating tachycardia that occurs, a lowered stroke volume reflective of left ventricular failure occurs.[28] Eventually cardiac output falls and the heart itself, despite the compensatory mechanisms, receives an inadequate blood supply. This further impairs its electrical and mechanical activity.

Shock is a dynamic process, *with shock itself causing shock*[8] (Figure 22-1). At some point a cycle begins that cannot be interrupted, and an irreversible stage of shock develops. Even if the primary problem is corrected and good supportive care is given, the patient will die. However, the exact point at which shock becomes irreversible is not known. Regardless of the symptoms, all efforts should be made to reverse the progression of shock to prevent damage to vital organs.

## ORGAN DAMAGE

### Brain

Blood flow to the brain is under the control of local influences rather than the autonomic nervous system. In response to decreased blood flow, the vessels dilate so that the brain, as with the heart, is preferentially perfused. As shock progresses, the local control mechanisms are inadequate and decreased perfusion of the brain occurs. Cerebral *hypoxia* results in *lethargy* and eventually *coma.* The accumulation of toxic substances and acidosis may compound the signs of hypoxia.

### Heart

Although deterioration of cardiac function is a primary problem only in cardiogenic shock, the heart eventually is affected in all types of shock. As cited previously, in the early stage of most types of shock, the heart is unimpaired. As shock worsens, the pumping ability of the heart is affected and cardiac output decreases. As the heart muscle becomes increasingly hypoxic, it begins to show disturbances of electrical activity. Dysrhythmias have a detrimental effect on cardiac output, and some may be fatal. In the later stages of shock, deterioration of myocardial function is probably the most important factor in the further progression of shock.[8]

## Lungs

The effect of shock on the lungs has been determined only recently. During the Vietnam War, many victims of shock after trauma survived the early complications because of the use of massive blood transfusions and renal dialysis. The effect of shock on the lungs surfaced as a later complication. The pulmonary condition that results from hypoperfusion of the lungs has been known by various names, including shock lung, white lung, and Da Nang lung. It is now generally known as **adult respiratory distress syndrome (ARDS)** (see Chapter 37).

ARDS can result from any condition that causes hypoperfusion of the lungs but is seen most often as a consequence of hemorrhagic, traumatic, anaphylactic, or septic shock.[19,29a] It is characterized by increased permeability of the pulmonary capillaries to proteins and water, resulting in noncardiac pulmonary edema. Type 2 pneumocytes are destroyed, impairing the production of surfactant that normally prevents collapse of the alveoli. Alveoli either become filled with fluid or collapse, and lungs become stiff.

In the early stages, **hypoxemia** (decreased oxygen in the blood) results from impaired gas exchange, and hyperventilation occurs, resulting in hypocapnia and respiratory alkalosis. Platelet aggregation in the pulmonary capillaries further damages the lungs. Hypoxemia persists despite administration of increasing amounts of oxygen. As shock progresses, ventilation is impaired, and carbon dioxide is retained. Respiratory acidosis results. As hypoxemia increases, platelet aggregation increases, and a destructive cycle is initiated.

## Gastrointestinal Tract

Sympathetic stimulation, which occurs early in shock, causes redistribution of blood flow to vital organs. This results in decreased blood flow to the GI tract. Bowel function decreases, and paralytic ileus may result. If the blood supply is severely impaired for a time, necrosis of the intestinal mucosa may occur. Microorganisms that are normally found in the bowel lyse and release endotoxins when they are attacked by the leukocytes in the blood. Shock, from whatever cause, will now also have a septic component. The gastric mucosa commonly ulcerates when it becomes ischemic, which may result in occult bleeding or massive hemorrhage.

## Kidneys

The kidneys contain about 2.4 million nephrons, each of which is capable of forming urine. Each nephron is composed of a glomerulus that is made up of capillaries and collecting tubules (see Chapter 48). Under normal conditions the pressure within the glomerulus is sufficiently high to force fluid out of the capillaries into the collecting chamber. When the systolic pressure falls below 70 mm Hg, glomerular filtration ceases, and the body is unable to rid itself of fluid and nitrogenous wastes. Urinary output is decreased in both the early and the late stages of shock. In the early stage, low output is caused by sympathetic stimulation of the $\alpha$-receptors in the kidneys, resulting in vasoconstriction and a fall of pressure within the glomeruli. Decreased pressure causes a drop in the glomerular filtration rate. Also, the secretion of aldosterone and ADH causes sodium and water reabsorption.

As shock progresses, the tubules—which are perfused by the peritubular capillaries—begin to suffer from a lack of oxygen and nutrients, and acute *tubular necrosis* develops. The tubular epithelial cells slough and block the tubules, causing loss of nephron function.

## Liver

Sympathetic stimulation causes vasoconstriction in the liver. In the early stages of shock, this can be beneficial. Normally the liver is capable of storing large amounts of blood in its veins. With vasoconstriction it can release up to 350 ml of blood into the general circulation, resulting in improved cardiac output. With continued sympathetic stimulation and decreased blood flow, liver tissue is affected. In septic shock there is an increase in oxygen uptake and a decrease in energy production in the liver. All types of shock affect the metabolic functions of the liver, including the excretion of bile and cholesterol, gluconeogenesis, detoxification, and protein and cholesterol synthesis.[12]

The sinusoids of the liver are lined with Kupffer cells, which are part of the mononuclear phagocyte system (MPS). These cells are very powerful phagocytes and destroy the many bacteria from the colon that reach the liver by way of the portal system. Normally, only a very few bacteria get past the MPS. With the destruction of the MPS, bacteria enter the general circulation and produce toxins, which under normal circumstances would be detoxified by the liver. The liver can no longer perform this function, and overwhelming infection and toxicity result.

## Blood

Disseminated intravascular coagulation (DIC) (see Chapter 34) can cause or result from shock. It is characterized by intravascular clotting, resulting in the formation of microthrombi in the capillaries. Clotting factors in the blood may be activated by acidosis, stagnation, and procoagulation substances. Acidosis and

**BOX 22-2 Parameters for Assessing Status of the Patient in Shock**

**HEMODYNAMIC MONITORING**
- Blood pressure (cuff and/or intraarterial)
- Pulse
- Central venous pressure
- Pulmonary artery pressure
- Pulmonary capillary wedge pressure
- Cardiac output
- Electrocardiogram
- Pulse pressure
- Systemic vascular resistance

**RESPIRATORY MONITORING**
- Respiratory rate, depth
- Breath sounds
- Blood gas levels
  - pH
  - $Pao_2$
  - $Paco_2$
- Percent $O_2$ saturation
- Mixed venous return ($Svo_2$)

**FLUID AND ELECTROLYTE MONITORING**
- Serum electrolyte levels
- Blood lactate and pyruvate levels
- Intake
  - By mouth
  - Intravenous
  - Nasogastric
  - Irrigation solutions
  - Solution in medications
- Output
  - Urinary
  - GI tract
  - Sweating
  - Dressings
- Weight
- Serum creatinine level
- BUN level
- Serum and urine osmolality
- Urine specific gravity

**NEUROLOGIC MONITORING**
- Alertness
- Orientation
- Confusion

**HEMATOLOGIC MONITORING**
- Erythrocytes
- Hematocrit and hemoglobin levels
- Leukocytes
- Platelets
- Prothrombin and partial thromboplastin times
- Clotting time
- Fibrin degradation factor

**OTHER MONITORING**
- Bowel sounds
- Skin temperature

stagnation are common in all forms of shock. Therefore DIC may occur with all types of shock. In septic shock, however, the bacterial toxins and the prostaglandins that are released enhance coagulation and make DIC even more likely.[25a] Clotting in the capillaries causes a depletion of clotting factors in the rest of the body. Hemorrhage may then occur from surgical incisions, injection sites, intravenous insertion sites, or the GI tract. Intravascular clotting results in a further decrease in tissue perfusion and acidosis, and a vicious cycle ensues. The hemorrhage caused by DIC decreases the cardiac output even further and worsens tissue perfusion. The mortality in patients with DIC in association with infection and shock is very high.

# MEDICAL MANAGEMENT

Medical management is determined by the stage of shock and the patient's signs and symptoms. The details of treatment are included under the intervention section later in this chapter.

# NURSING MANAGEMENT

## ◆ ASSESSMENT

There are few signs in the early stages; the patient may be restless and complain of feeling weak. Pulse and respiratory rates may be increased. Cool, clammy skin; decreased blood pressure; and lethargy or unconsciousness are signs of well-advanced, late shock.

To identify and treat shock before it reaches the late phase, one should monitor certain key parameters. The various methods for monitoring shock and the parameters used in assessing shock appear in Box 22-2 and are then discussed in more detail.

### Hemodynamic Assessment

Hemodynamic alterations are often the first sign of the onset of shock. The patient's hemodynamic status can be assessed at various levels (Figure 22-2).[24a]

#### Vital signs

Vital signs are assessed frequently. In the early stages of shock, the pulse is usually increased. As shock progresses, the pulse becomes quite rapid and difficult to palpate. Irregularities in the pulse may develop as cardiac dysrhythmias occur.

Early in shock the blood pressure may be normal, slightly decreased, or even elevated because of compensatory vasoconstriction. Blood pressure can be heard without difficulty at this stage. As shock progresses, the blood pressure may be difficult to auscultate, and it may be possible to obtain the systolic pressure only by palpation. If intraarterial pressure monitoring is not instituted, Doppler ultrasound may be helpful in obtaining the blood pressure.

Venous pulsation in the neck is noted. Both the external and the internal jugular veins should be examined. Generally the external jugular vein is easier to see, but the internal jugular is more reliable as a sign of elevated right-atrial pressure. Normally, venous pulsations are visible when the patient is lying flat but not when the head is elevated to 45 degrees (Figure 22-3). Neck veins that are not visible when the patient is in the horizontal position may indicate an abnormally low intravascular volume. This may be seen in both hypovolemic and

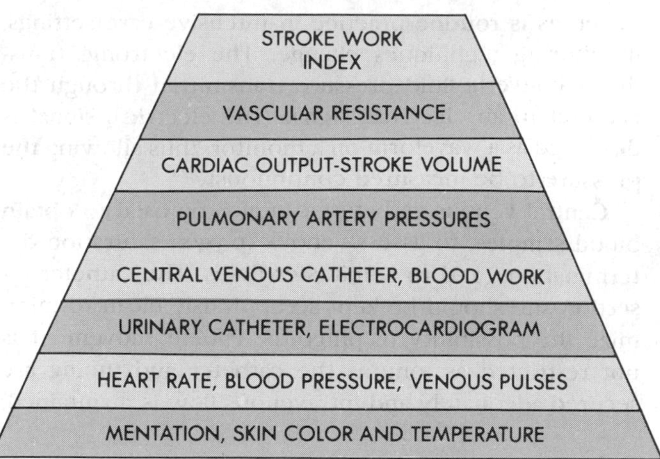


**FIGURE 22-2** Levels of hemodynamic monitoring. (From Ellerbe S: ***Fluid and blood component therapy in the critically ill and injured,*** New York, 1981, Churchill Livingstone.)

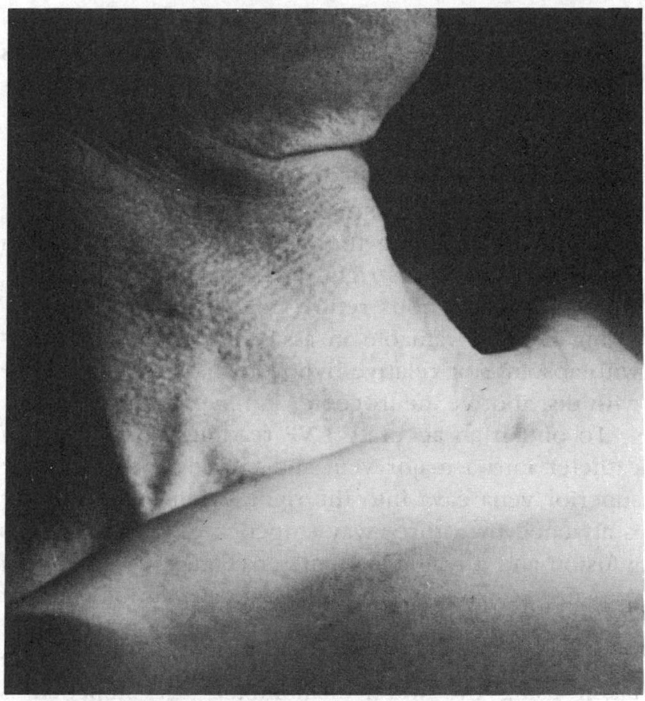

**FIGURE 22-3** Distended external jugular neck vein of the patient with failure of the right side of the heart. (From Daily EK, Schroeder J: ***Techniques in bedside hemodynamic monitoring,*** ed 5, St Louis, 1994, Mosby.)

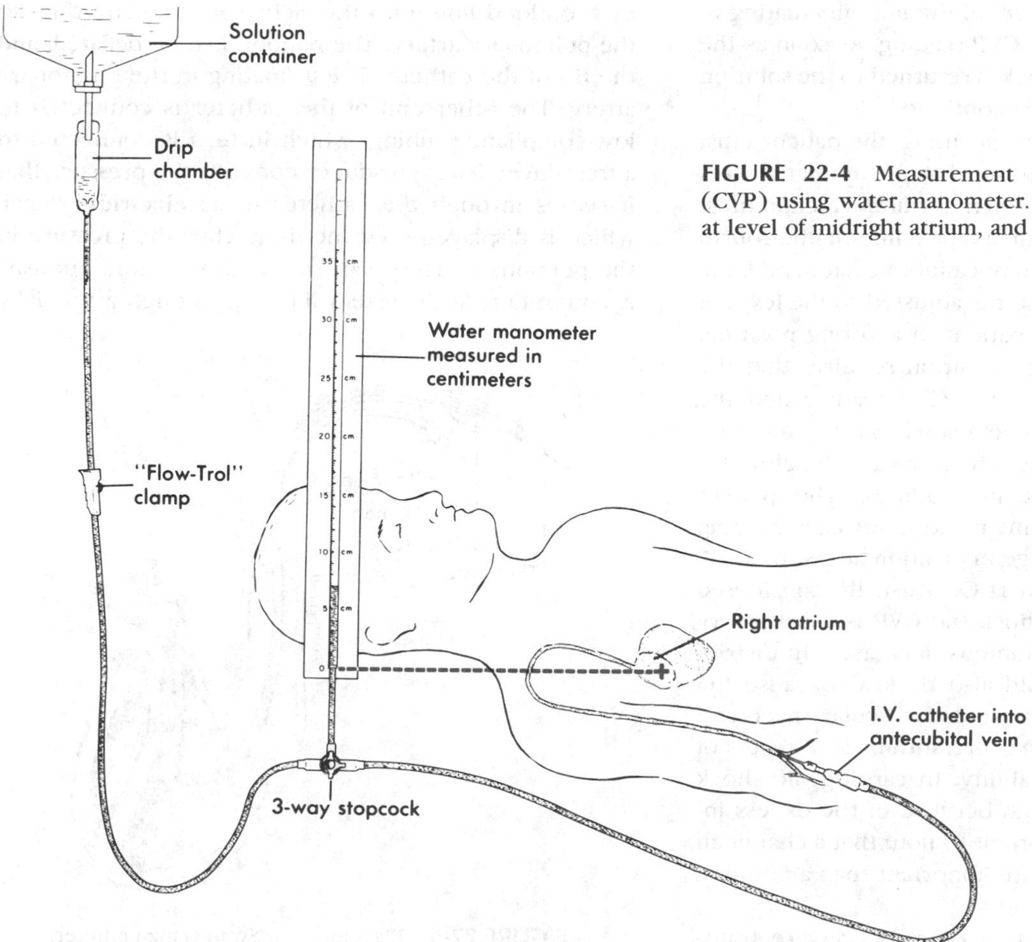


**FIGURE 22-4** Measurement of central venous pressure (CVP) using water manometer. Zero point on manometer is at level of midright atrium, and CVP reading is 7 cm $H_2O$.

distributive shock. In cardiogenic shock the neck veins are often distended, even when the head of the patient's bed is elevated more than 45 degrees. This indicates excessive fluid volume.

### Central venous pressure

**Central venous pressure (CVP)** is a more accurate means of determining the fluid status of a patient in shock. CVP measures right-ventricular filling pressure, which reflects venous return to the heart. CVP monitoring is most valuable in assessing status in patients with absolute or relative hypovolemia, including those with distributive, neurogenic, and hypovolemic shock.

To obtain an accurate CVP reading,[18] one inserts a catheter into a major vein and threads it through the superior vena cava into the right atrium. The catheter is attached by a three-way stopcock to an intravenous infusion and a water manometer (Figure 22-4) or to a pressure transducer. The intravenous solution (usually 5% glucose in water) is allowed to drip slowly into the vein to keep the vein open. When a reading is to be taken using the water manometer, the stopcock is opened to the manometer, and the manometer is filled with the intravenous solution. The stopcock is then turned to the venous opening of the patient. The fluid level in the manometer should fluctuate with each respiration. The fluid is allowed to stabilize before a reading is taken, and the highest level of the fluid fluctuating in the column is used for the CVP reading. As soon as the reading is taken, the stopcock is returned to the solution position, and the infusion is continued.

For the CVP reading to be accurate, the patient must be relaxed, and the zero point of the manometer must always be at the level of the right atrium, which in most people is level with the midaxillary line at the fourth intercostal space. If the patient cannot lie flat in bed, the zero point on the manometer is adjusted to the level of the right atrium with the patient in a sitting position. Any change in the patient's position requires that the zero point be reset. The initial CVP reading and the position that the patient was in when it was taken should be recorded, because these will serve as a baseline for comparison with subsequent readings. The patient should be placed in the same position for each reading because even a slight change in position alters the CVP.

A range of 5 to 15 cm $H_2O$ is usually considered normal. In hypovolemic shock the CVP is usually very low because the blood volume is decreased. In distributive shock the CVP would also be low, because the blood has pooled in the expanded vascular space and fluid has been lost into the interstitium as a result of increased capillary permeability. In cardiogenic shock the CVP is likely to be high because of the excess intravascular fluid. It is important to note that a change in the trend of the CVP is more important than a numeric reading.

When the catheter is attached to a pressure transducer, as is routine practice in intensive care settings, monitoring techniques change. The electronic transducer converts fluid pressure transmitted through the catheter to an electrical signal. The electrical signal is displayed as a waveform on a monitor, thus allowing the pressure to be measured continuously.[24]

Central venous catheters can also be used to obtain blood samples, to assess venous oxygen saturation determinations, and to administer fluids. The catheter insertion site should be kept scrupulously clean to minimize the possibility of phlebitis. Patient movement is not restricted as long as the catheter and tubing are secured adequately and intravenous flow is maintained.

### Pulmonary artery pressures

The status of the left side of the heart can best be evaluated by the measurement of **pulmonary artery pressure (PAP)** and **pulmonary capillary wedge pressure (PCWP).** A mean PAP of less than 10 mm Hg may indicate decreased blood volume, resulting in decreased preload in the left ventricle. A mean PAP of more than 20 mm Hg may indicate poor myocardial contractility and left-ventricular overload.

These pressures are measured with a special balloon-tipped (Swan-Ganz) catheter (Figure 22-5). The catheter is inserted into a vein, usually the subclavian, and advanced to the atrium. The balloon is inflated and carried by the blood flow into the right ventricle and then to the pulmonary artery. The balloon is then deflated, and the tip of the catheter is left floating in the pulmonary artery. The other end of the catheter is connected to low-compliance tubing, which in turn is connected to a transducer. The transducer converts the pressure that it senses through the catheter to an electrical signal, which is displayed on a monitor. Thus the pressure in the pulmonary artery can be monitored continuously. A continuous flush system infusing through a specially

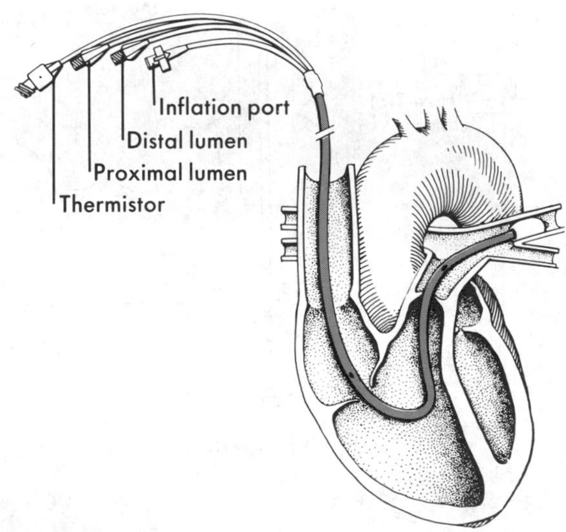


**FIGURE 22-5** Placement of Swan-Ganz catheter.

designated small-bore, rigid intravenous tubing usually is used to maintain patency of the catheter and quality of the waveform.

In individuals without lung or pulmonary vascular disease, PAP is a good indicator of how well the left side of the heart is functioning. Pressure changes in the left ventricle are reflected in the left atrium and back to the pulmonary artery. However, if any disease exists in the lungs, as frequently occurs in shock, the PAP does not accurately reflect left-ventricular pressure. In this case the PCWP should be obtained. By inflating the balloon, which is near the tip of the catheter, the pulmonary artery can be occluded. This blocks communication between the pulmonary artery and the lumen of the catheter, allowing for pressure that is ahead of the occluded artery to be transmitted through the catheter. The PCWP is *identical* to the *left-atrial pressure.*

The nurse caring for the patient with PAP monitoring must be aware of the common complications that can occur with this type of invasive monitoring (Table 22-4). The appearance of either a *right-ventricular* or *PCWP waveform* on the monitor can have serious consequences for the patient. Dislodgement of the tip of the catheter from the pulmonary artery into the right ventricle can result in the occurrence of *premature ventricular beats* (PVBs) or even *ventricular tachycardia.* Progression of the catheter into a small vessel in the pulmonary vasculature can occlude the vessel and result in *pulmonary infarction.* Prolonged inflation of the balloon can have the same effect. The nurse must be able to distinguish the normal PAP waveform from both right-ventricular and PCWP waveforms (Figure 22-6). It is essential that sterile technique be maintained during insertion of the PAP catheter and during dressing changes.

### Intraarterial monitoring

**Intraarterial monitoring** is usually instituted along with PAP monitoring. A catheter is inserted into a radial, brachial, or femoral artery and attached to a transducer in much the same way as the pulmonary artery catheter (Figure 22-7).

As was the case with the pulmonary artery catheter, a continuous flush system infusing through a small-bore, rigid intravenous tubing maintains the patency of the catheter and the quality of the waveform. Because hemorrhage is a possible complication, the insertion and connections in the system must be monitored frequently. The extremity distal to the insertion site must be monitored for signs of arterial occlusion (color, tem-

**TABLE 22-4 Complications of Pulmonary Artery Pressure (PAP) Monitoring**

| COMPLICATION | INDICATIONS | INTERVENTIONS |
|---|---|---|
| Infection | Chills<br>Headache<br>Malaise<br>Generalized aching<br>Flushed face<br>Warm skin<br>Elevated temperature | 1. Notify physician immediately.<br>2. Prepare for removal of catheter.<br>3. Administer antibiotics as ordered.<br>4. Provide symptomatic relief. |
| Ventricular dysrhythmias: premature ventricular beats (PVBs), or short runs of ventricular tachycardia | "Skipped heartbeats"<br>Irregular pulse<br>PVBs noted on cardiac monitor | 1. Notify physician immediately.<br>2. Prepare for repositioning of catheter.<br>3. Administer antidysrhythmic drugs if problem persists after repositioning. |
| Sustained ventricular tachycardia or ventricular fibrillation | Lightheadedness, progressing to loss of consciousness<br>Loss of consciousness<br>Pulselessness<br>Dysrhythmia noted on cardiac monitor<br>Respiratory arrest | 1. Notify physician immediately.<br>2. Prepare for repositioning of catheter.<br>3. Defibrillate. |
| Pulmonary infarction | Chest pain<br>Hemoptysis<br>Fever<br>Friction rub<br>Elevated lactate dehydrogenase (LDH)<br>Area of opacity on chest roentgenogram<br>Decreased $PaO_2$ | 1. Notify physician immediately.<br>2. Administer oxygen.<br>3. Prepare for repositioning or removal of catheter.<br>4. Provide symptomatic relief. |
| Valvular damage | Depends on extent of damage<br>Patient may be asymptomatic or may develop symptoms of congestive heart failure or new murmur | 1. Notify physician of development of new murmur or new symptoms. |

From Asheervath J, Blevins D: *Handbook of clinical nursing practice,* Norwalk, Conn, 1986, Appleton-Century-Crofts.

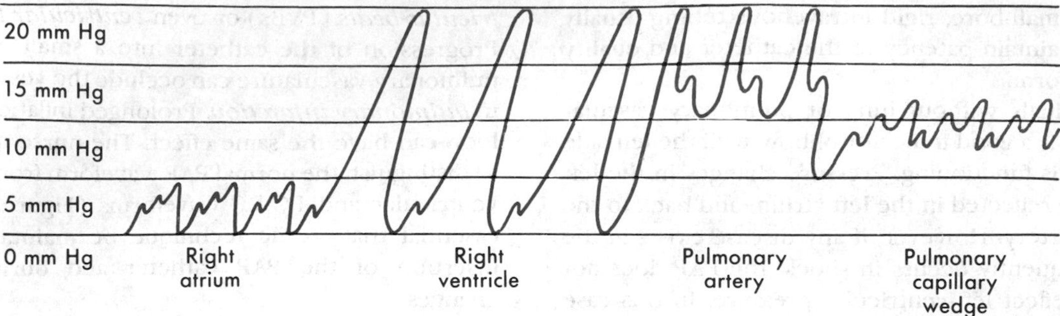


**FIGURE 22-6** Characteristic waveforms of pulmonary artery pressure (PAP) monitoring. (From Asheervath J, Blevins D: *Handbook of clinical nursing practice,* 1986, Norwalk, Conn, Appleton-Century-Crofts.)

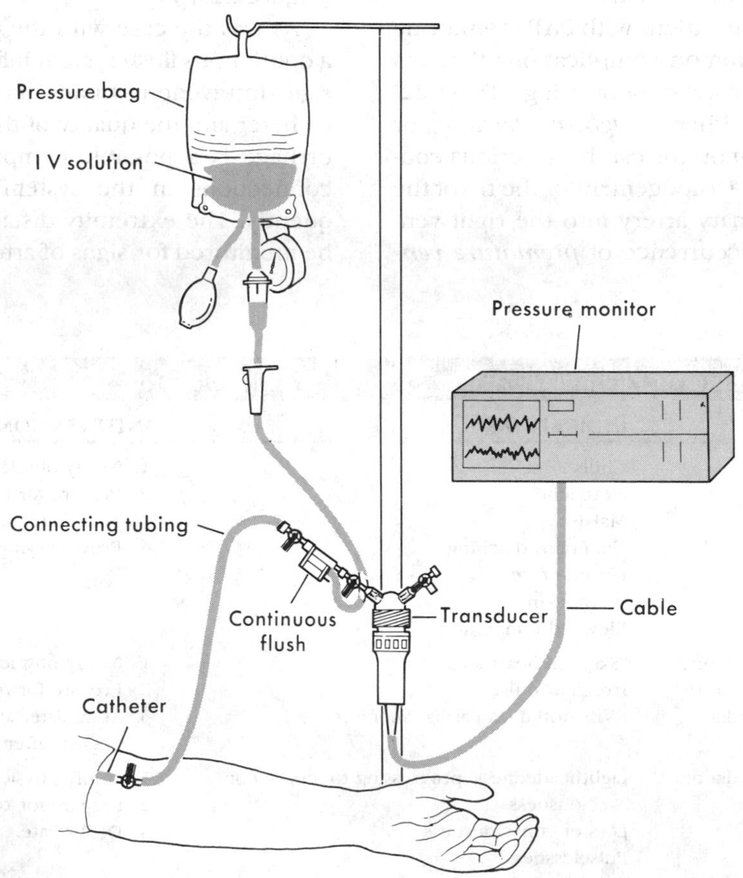


**FIGURE 22-7** Connections between intraarterial catheter, transducer, monitor, and fluid. (From Daily EK, Schroeder J: *Techniques in bedside hemodynamic monitoring,* ed 5, St Louis, 1994, Mosby.)

perature, movement, presence or absence of pulses, pain) (Table 22-5). It is essential that sterile technique be maintained during insertion of the catheter and during dressing changes. A patient who is ill enough to require hemodynamic monitoring has little reserve to fight infection.

### Cardiac output and cardiac index monitoring

Pulmonary artery catheters allow for cardiac output and cardiac index to be monitored at the bedside. Such catheters have a port through which fluid can be injected into the right atrium. A **thermistor** (sensor to measure temperature) is located at the tip of the catheter and

**TABLE 22-5 Complications of Intraarterial Pressure Monitoring**

| COMPLICATION | INDICATIONS | INTERVENTION |
|---|---|---|
| Hemorrhage | Obvious excessive bleeding<br>Tachycardia<br>Hypotension<br>Pallor<br>Diaphoresis<br>Tachypnea<br>Restlessness<br>Dizziness<br>Headache | 1. Control bleeding<br>a. If bleeding is occurring at the puncture site, apply pressure.<br>b. If part of the system has become disconnected, immediately turn the stopcocks to stop bleeding.<br>2. Attach a syringe containing sterile saline until contaminated parts of the system are replaced with sterile parts.<br>3. Notify the physician if a large amount of blood has been lost.<br>4. Prepare the patient for blood replacement if loss has been large. |
| Thrombus or embolus | Pallor, loss of pulse, and coolness of skin distal to the site of the thrombus<br>Pain | 1. Notify the physician immediately.<br>2. Instruct patient to lie quietly.<br>3. Prepare to administer $O_2$. |
| Infection of catheter site | Redness and warmth at the site<br>Possible fever | 1. Notify the physician.<br>2. Prepare for removal of the catheter.<br>3. Send the catheter tip for culture. |
| Bacteremia | High fever<br>Chills | 1. Notify the physician.<br>2. Prepare for removal of the catheter. |

Modified from Asheervath J, Blevins D: *Handbook of clinical nursing practice,* Norwalk, Conn, 1986, Appleton-Century-Crofts.

attached to a wire that runs through the catheter and is attached to a cardiac output computer. Iced or room-temperature saline solution is injected into the right atrium. The solution travels with the blood into the pulmonary artery. The thermistor senses the extent of temperature change, and from these data the computer is able to calculate cardiac output. In addition to its use in determining cardiac output and cardiac index, the thermistor can be used to monitor central or core body temperature.

The data from the pulmonary artery catheters can be used to measure systemic vascular resistance (SVR). As SVR increases, cardiac output falls.

### Oxygen utilization monitoring

In all types of shock a discrepancy exists between the amount of oxygen delivered to the cells and the amount they need. Oxygen delivery is affected by cardiac output, serum hemoglobin concentration, and the amount of oxygen in the blood (measured by **arterial oxygen pressure,** or **$Pao_2$**). If any of these decreases, the cells normally compensate by extracting more oxygen than normal from the blood as it passes by them. Blood in the veins then has a lower-than-normal oxygen content. By sampling blood that is a mixture of venous blood from the entire body, oxygen utilization by the body can be determined. Blood in the pulmonary artery is used for this purpose. The difference between the **oxygen saturation of arterial blood ($Sao_2$)** and the **oxygen saturation of the mixed venous blood ($Svo_2$)** reflects cellular utilization of oxygen. In both hypovolemic shock and cardiogenic shock, the fall in cardiac output causes the cells to extract more oxygen, with a resultant decrease in $Svo_2$. In septic shock, however, especially in the early stages, this is not the case. The $Svo_2$ may be abnormally high, despite the cells apparently not receiving enough oxygen. This may be a result of the high cardiac output seen in early shock. Other possible reasons include inability of the cells to extract oxygen because of the effects of endotoxins on them and the passage of blood through some organs, with little gas exchange occurring because of clogged capillaries.

The $Svo_2$ can be measured by withdrawing blood from a pulmonary artery catheter. However, the preferred way is to monitor the $Svo_2$ by use of a fiberoptic pulmonary artery catheter, which will display a continuous value on a monitor.

Table 22-6 lists the hemodynamic parameters found in various types of changes in shock.

## Respiratory Assessment

As cited earlier, hypoperfusion of the lungs, which frequently occurs in shock, may result in ARDS. This may be suspected very early in the course of the disease from changes in the patient's mentation, as caused by hypoxemia. The patient is observed for *cough* and *dyspnea,* which develop as ARDS progresses. Changes in respiratory rate and in the color of the mucous membranes and skin are important indicators of pulmonary status. Breath sounds are auscultated. Early in the course of the disease the lungs may be clear, but as ARDS progresses, crackles and gurgles may be heard.

If the patient is receiving mechanical ventilation, the amount of pressure required to deliver a specific tidal volume is noted. As the lungs become increasingly stiff, the pressure required to deliver the volume increases.

**TABLE 22-6 Hemodynamic Parameters in Various Types of Shock**

| | HYPO-VOLEMIC | CARDIO-GENIC | DISTRIBUTIVE* |
|---|---|---|---|
| Cardiac output | Low | Low | High |
| Pulmonary capillary wedge pressure (PCWP) | Low | High | Low |
| Mixed venous oxygen saturation ($Svo_2$) | Low | Low | High |
| Systemic vascular resistance (SVR) | High | High | Low |

* In the late stage of septic shock, severely depressed cardiac function results in a clinical picture similar to that of cardiogenic shock.

With ARDS, the PAP may rise, although the PCWP remains normal.[19]

Arterial blood gas levels may provide valuable information and are monitored as indicated, depending on the patient's condition. Characteristically with ARDS, the $Pao_2$ level falls, in spite of ventilation with increasing amounts of oxygen, because of physiologic shunting of blood through the lungs to the left side of the heart. Physiologic *shunting* occurs because many alveoli are either collapsed or filled with fluid, and diffusion cannot occur because of an increase in the distance between the air and blood across the capillary alveolar membrane. In the earlier stages of ARDS, when a sufficient number of alveoli are functioning, the arterial carbon dioxide pressure ($Paco_2$) is usually normal or more likely low because of the rapid diffusion of carbon dioxide and the hyperventilation that results from hypoxia.

However, as ARDS progresses and the lungs become increasingly stiff, an acute restrictive condition occurs and ventilation and diffusion are impaired. In this stage, the $Paco_2$—as well as the $Pao_2$—are affected. The $Paco_2$, which was decreasing as a result of hyperventilation, begins to increase as a result of hypoventilation.

Arterial blood gas determinations are also used to assess the acid-base balance of the patient. In the early stages of shock, mild respiratory alkalosis typically occurs from the hyperventilation that is part of the stress response. As shock progresses and tissue becomes progressively hypoxemic, anaerobic metabolism takes place and metabolic acidosis occurs. In the advanced stages of shock, as respiratory compensation decreases and ARDS becomes progressively worse, respiratory acidosis may also develop.

## Fluid and Electrolyte Assessment

The urinary output and the CVP most accurately reflect fluid status. An indwelling urinary catheter is usually inserted, and the urine output is measured hourly. Other output—such as GI drainage, wound exudate, or perspiration—is measured or estimated as accurately as possible. Body weight often gives a more accurate assessment of fluid changes than does the measurement of intake and output; however, this can be an inaccurate determinant of intravascular volume when third spacing of fluid occurs. Noting the presence of edema, auscultating the chest for the presence of fluid, and measuring the abdominal girth for the development of ascites are means of assessing fluid collection in the third space.

In the early stages of shock, the serum potassium concentration may be abnormally low as a result of increased levels of aldosterone because of the stress response. However, as shock progresses, the serum potassium level may become abnormally high as damaged cells release potassium. As urinary output falls, the body is unable to eliminate the excess amounts of potassium accumulating in the serum. If potassium is administered in the early stage of shock, it is extremely important that the urinary output and serum electrolytes be monitored frequently.

The concentration of other serum electrolytes may be abnormal as a result of acid-base abnormalities, altered renal function, or fluid therapy. Serum enzyme levels may be elevated because of ischemia and damage to the heart, liver, and pancreas.

## Neurologic Assessment

In shock the brain may be adversely affected by hypoxia, acid-base imbalance, or toxins. Often, subtle changes in mentation are the earliest signs of cerebral hypoxia. The patient is observed for increasing restlessness. Sedation should not be given until the patient's status has been assessed further and it has been determined that the restlessness does not have an organic cause. In the late stages, when perfusion of the brain is severely impaired, loss of consciousness occurs. Vital signs and arterial blood gas determinations can aid in assessing the cause of subtle neurologic changes.

## Hematologic Assessment

The hemoglobin and hematocrit levels are valuable tools for assessing blood loss in hypovolemic shock secondary to hemorrhage. It must be remembered, however, that the hemoglobin and hematocrit levels do not drop immediately with loss of an excessive amount of blood, because plasma is lost along with the blood cells. The blood that remains in the intravascular compartment initially will have a normal concentration of RBCs. Within a few hours after a blood loss, the hemoglobin and hematocrit levels begin to decrease as the kidneys retain water and electrolytes in response to low perfusion.

An increase in hemoglobin and hematocrit levels may be seen in some types of shock. Increased capillary permeability, which occurs primarily in septic and anaphylactic shock, permits water and electrolytes to move out of the capillaries, leaving behind blood with a high concentration of cells. Hematocrit levels also are relative to fluid volume and may be decreased due to fluid replacement.

Patients in shock are assessed for the development of DIC. The nurse may be the first to observe that the patient is bleeding for an excessively long time after a venipuncture or that blood is oozing from an incision. If DIC is suspected, laboratory studies are initiated; clotting factors (including fibrinogen and platelet counts) are decreased, prothrombin time (PT) and partial thromboplastin time (PTT) are prolonged, and fibrin degradation products are increased.

### Abdominal Assessment

Decreased blood flow to the intestines may result in decreased peristalsis or paralytic ileus (see Chapter 47). Decreased or absent bowel sounds are noted. Assessment of gastric drainage and stools for occult blood is necessary because of the high incidence of GI tract bleeding with shock.

## ♦ NURSING DIAGNOSES

Nursing diagnoses are determined from analysis of patient data. Nursing diagnoses for the person with shock may include but are not limited to the following:

| Diagnostic Title | Possible Etiologic Factors |
|---|---|
| Airway clearance, ineffective | Decreased energy, endotracheal intubation |
| Gas exchange, impaired | Decreased lung compliance, interstitial edema |
| Breathing pattern, ineffective | Inadequate perfusion of respiratory muscles |
| Cardiac output, decreased | Myocardial hypoxia, myocardial depressant factor |
| Tissue perfusion, altered (cardiopulmonary) | Hypovolemia, decreased cardiac output |
| Fluid volume deficit (2) | Blood loss, increased capillary permeability, vasodilation |
| Injury, high risk for | Confusion from hypovolemia |
| Infection, high risk for | Invasive monitoring, indwelling catheter, decreased immune response |
| Anxiety | Threat of death |
| Pain, high risk for | Invasive lines, endotracheal tube, immobility |
| Activity intolerance | Imbalance between oxygen supply and demand |

## ♦ EXPECTED PATIENT OUTCOMES

Expected patient outcomes for the person with shock may include but are not limited to the following:

1. Airway remains free from secretions.
2. Blood gas levels ($Paco_2$ and $Pao_2$) are within normal limits.
3. Respiratory rate and tidal volume are within normal limits.
4. Intravascular volume, as noted by hemoglobin and hematocrit levels and hemodynamic values, returns to normal limits.
5. Urinary output and hemodynamic values are within normal limits.
6. No injury or infection occurs.
7. Offers statements of feeling relaxed; shows no physical signs of anxiety.
8. Offers statements of feeling comfortable.
9. Tolerates activity and care without an increase in pulse rate of more than 20 per minute.

## ♦ INTERVENTIONS

Treatment of shock varies to some extent, depending on the cause of the shock, the organ systems affected, and the preexisting condition of the patient. In the early, acute phase of shock, the major role of the nurse is continuous assessment of the patient's clinical status and assisting with administration of therapies necessary to stabilize the patient's condition.

Fundamentally, the same priorities that exist for treating any life-threatening emergency hold true for shock. The priorities for shock management are as follows:

1. **Airway:** A patent airway must be maintained to maximize oxygen uptake and carbon dioxide removal. To accomplish this, a nasal or oral airway may be inserted. When respiratory failure is a high potential, the airway is secured with an endotracheal tube.
2. **Breathing:** Oxygen is administered immediately at the level ordered. This may include preparations to ventilate the patient by mechanical ventilation. These measures support breathing and enhance ventilation and gas exchange between the airway and the circulation.
3. **Circulation:** The pump (the heart) is supported by the administration of fluids—including blood—to increase blood volume, improve cardiac output, and maximize oxygen transport to the cells. Vasoactive and cardiogenic drugs may also be prescribed to enhance cardiovascular functioning and oxygen transport to the cells.
4. **Diagnosis:** Shock can be treated most effectively if the underlying cause can be determined and treated. For example, if the cause of shock is hypovolemia secondary to massive bleeding, efforts will be made to find the site of the bleeding and stop it, if possible. Blood and fluids will be used to improve intravascular volume and cardiac output. This will then improve exchange of oxygen and carbon dioxide at the cellular level. If the cause of shock is sepsis, antibiotics, antiviral agents, or antifungal agents will be administered intravenously, and if the cause is anaphylaxis, epinephrine is given.

### Promoting Fluid Balance and Cardiac Output

#### Fluid replacement

The need to administer fluids to the patient with hypovolemic shock is obvious. At times, fluid replacement

**TABLE 22-7 Fluids Used for Replacement Therapy in Shock**

| TYPE | USES/INDICATIONS | ADVANTAGES | DISADVANTAGES | SPECIAL CONSIDERATIONS |
|---|---|---|---|---|
| **BLOOD AND BLOOD PRODUCTS** | | | | |
| Whole blood | Replace blood volume and maintain hemoglobin (Hb) level at 12-14 g/100 ml | Provides intravascular volume<br>Increases oxygen-carrying capacity of blood | Potential associated risks of hepatitis, HIV infection, and allergic reactions<br>Delayed administration because of necessary typing and cross-matching<br>Possibility of type and cross-match errors | Whole blood should be stored at 0°-10° C (32°-50° F), but warmed at least 20-30 min before administration (*never* infuse cold blood).<br>Use *fresh* whole blood whenever possible to avoid adverse metabolic changes related to stored blood. |
| RBCs (packed, concentrate)<br>Fresh, frozen (also called leukocyte-poor) | Increase hematocrit to minimum level of 30%<br>Correct RBC deficiency and improve oxygen-carrying capacity of blood | Concentrated form helps prevent excess fluid administration in patients with cardiogenic shock (increases oxygen-carrying capacity with less volume loading)<br>Associated with fewer risks of metabolic complications when compared with stored whole blood (decreased amount of transfused antibodies, electrolytes, and so on)<br>Provides economic use of blood as a resource; frees other blood components, such as platelets and clotting factors to be concentrated and stored | Same as above for whole blood<br>Slow infusion rate because of increased viscosity<br>Decreased content of plasma proteins and coagulation factors when compared with whole blood<br>Inadequate (alone) for volume replacement and correction of hypovolemia<br>Altered blood clotting with administration of more than 20 units; for every 4 units of RBCs over 20, 1 unit of fresh frozen plasma should be administered to replenish clotting factors<br>High cost of frozen (thawed) RBCs | Administer via Y-connector tubing with normal saline to increase infusion flow rate.<br>Washed RBCs (resuspended in saline) can be given in shock to decrease red cell adhesiveness (washing decreases cell's fibrinogen coating). |
| Human plasma (fresh, frozen, or dried) | Restore plasma volume in hypovolemic shock without increasing the hematocrit level<br>Restore clotting factors (except platelets) | Effective for rapid volume replacement<br>Contains clotting factors | Expensive<br>Deficient of RBCs | Human plasma carries risk of hepatitis, HIV infection, and allergic reactions.<br>Administer fresh frozen plasma promptly after thawing to prevent deterioration of clotting factors V and VIII. |
| **COLLOID SOLUTIONS** | | | | |
| Plasma protein fraction (Plasmanate, Plasma-Plex) | Expand plasma volume in hypovolemic shock (while cross-matching being completed)<br>Increase the serum colloid osmotic pressure | Can be used interchangeably with 5% human serum albumin<br>Osmotically equivalent to plasma<br>Associated with low risk of hepatitis | Expensive<br>Deficient of clotting factors<br>Associated with larger number of side effects, such as hypotension and hypersensitivity, than those reported with 5% albumin (because of presence of globulins) | Plasma protein fraction is prepared from pooled plasma heated to 60° C (140° F) for 10 hr.<br>This procedure reduces risk of transmission of hepatitis viruses. |

From Rice V: *Shock: a clinical syndrome, the clinical continuum of septic shock, shock management,* Secaucus, NJ, 1985, Critical Care Nurse/Hospitals Publications.

**TABLE 22-7 Fluids Used for Replacement Therapy in Shock—cont'd**

| TYPE | USES/INDICATIONS | ADVANTAGES | DISADVANTAGES | SPECIAL CONSIDERATIONS |
|---|---|---|---|---|
| Plasma protein fraction—cont'd | | | Hypotension induced by rapid intravenous administration (greater than 10 ml/min)<br>Associated with risk of HIV infection | Rapid administration of large dosages can alter blood coagulation.<br>This solution should be used cautiously in patients with congestive heart failure (caused by added fluid and rapid plasma volume expansion) and in patients with renal failure (caused by added proteins). |
| Albumin<br>5%<br>25% (salt poor) | Increase plasma colloid osmotic pressure<br>Rapidly expand plasma volume | Rare allergic reactions (less than 0.01% in all albumin solutions combined)<br>Rare transmission of hepatitis virus | Potential leakage from capillaries in shock states associated with increased capillary permeability<br>Possible precipitation of congestive heart failure after rapid infusion in patients with circulatory overload and compromised cardiovascular function | Albumin does not contain preservatives; therefore each opened bottle should be used at once.<br>Rate of administration of 5% albumin should not exceed 2-4 ml/min.<br>Rate of administration of 25% albumin should not exceed 1 ml/min.<br>25% albumin is reserved for use in patients with pulmonary or peripheral edema and hypoproteinemia.<br>Administer with a diuretic to ensure diuresis. |
| **PLASMA EXPANDERS** | | | | |
| Dextran<br>Low-molecular-weight dextran (LMWD) (dextran 40, Rheomacrodex, Gentran 40)<br>High-molecular-weight dextran (HMWD) (dextran 70, Gentran 70 and 75, Macrodex) | Rapidly expand plasma volume | All dextrans: associated with low incidence of anaphylactic reactions; less expensive than protein solutions<br>LMWD: associated with fewer allergic reactions than HMWD; facilitates blood flow by decreasing RBC adhesiveness<br>HMWD: leaks from the capillaries less readily than LMWD; can effectively increase plasma volume for up to 24 hr | LMWD: 70% excreted unchanged in urine, so urine osmolality and specific gravity are altered; potential osmotic nephrosis and renal tubular shutdown; possible bleeding from raw surfaces caused by decreased platelet adhesiveness; side effects include decreased levels of hemoglobin, hematocrit, fibrinogen, and clotting factors V, VIII, and IX<br>HMWD: 50% excreted unchanged in the urine, so urine osmolality and specific gravity altered; higher incidence of allergic reac- | Avoid use of dextran in patients with active hemorrhage, hemorrhagic shock, coagulation disorders, and thrombocytopenia.<br>Bleeding times can be prolonged when the correct dose of dextran 70 (1.2 g/kg/day) or dextran 40 (2 g/kg/day) are exceeded.<br>Administer dextran in dextrose solutions to patients with sodium restriction. |

*Continued.*

**TABLE 22-7 Fluids Used for Replacement Therapy in Shock—cont'd**

| TYPE | USES/INDICATIONS | ADVANTAGES | DISADVANTAGES | SPECIAL CONSIDERATIONS |
|---|---|---|---|---|
| Dextran—cont'd | | | tions when compared with LMWD; increases blood viscosity and platelet adhesiveness | |
| Hetastarch (Hespan, Volex) | Expand plasma volume | Same volume expansion characteristics of albumin but with a longer duration of action (up to 36 hr)<br>Associated with low risk of allergic and anaphylactic reactions (0.085%)<br>Cost of hetastarch is about one half that of plasma protein fraction and albumin<br>Nonantigenic<br>No danger of transmission of hepatitis virus | Potential dilution of plasma proteins and decreased plasma colloid osmotic pressure<br>Potential dilution of clotting factors with resultant coagulation changes<br>Potential circulatory overload in patients with severe congestive heart failure and compromised renal function<br>Increased serum amylase level (>200 mg/100 ml), peaking within 1 hr of intravenous administration of hetastarch and persisting for 3-4 days (caused by action of amylase in hetastarch degradation) | Do not use if solution is cloudy or deep brown or if it contains crystals.<br>Monitor clotting studies and platelet counts, observing for prolonged PT and PTT and thrombocytopenia.<br>Safety and compatibility of additives with hetastarch have not been established; manufacturer recommends infusing hetastarch through separate line, when possible, or piggy-backing second drug.<br>Maximum infusion rate in acute hemorrhagic shock is 20 ml/kg/hr.<br>Monitor serum albumin level; if it falls below 2 g/100 ml, consider substituting albumin for hetastarch. |
| Mannitol (Osmitrol) | Raise intravascular volume<br>Reduces interstitial and intracellular edema<br>Promote osmotic diuresis | Reduces intracellular swelling<br>Increases urinary output | Potential circulatory overload in patients with congestive heart failure, pulmonary congestion, and renal dysfunction | |
| **CRYSTALLOID SOLUTIONS (ISOTONIC)** | | | | |
| Normal saline | Raise plasma volume when RBC mass is adequate<br>Replace body fluid | Considered by some to be most important salt for maintaining and replacing extracellular fluid<br>Increases plasma volume without altering normal sodium concentration or serum osmolality | Potential fluid retention and circulatory overload caused by sodium content | |
| Lactated Ringer's solution (Hartmann's solution) | Replace body fluid<br>Buffer acidosis | Lactate converted to bicarbonate in liver, which buffers acidosis<br>Lactate replaces bicarbonate, preventing precipitation of calcium bicarbonate and calcium carbonate | Increased lactic acidosis in shock caused by lactate<br>Fluid retention and circulatory overload caused by sodium content | Lactate conversion requires aerobic metabolism; therefore it should be used cautiously in shock and other hypoperfusion states. |

**TABLE 22-7 Fluids Used for Replacement Therapy in Shock—cont'd**

| TYPE | USES/INDICATIONS | ADVANTAGES | DISADVANTAGES | SPECIAL CONSIDERATIONS |
|---|---|---|---|---|
| Lactated Ringers solution—cont'd | | Lactate more stable than bicarbonate and more compatible with ions present in solution | | |
| Ringer's solution | Replace body fluid<br>Provide additional potassium and calcium | Does not contain lactate, so can be given to patients with hypoperfusion | Potential hyperchloremic metabolic acidosis caused by high chloride concentration<br>Potential fluid retention and circulatory overload caused by sodium content | |
| **CRYSTALLOID SOLUTIONS (HYPOTONIC)** | | | | |
| One-half normal saline | Raise total body fluid volume | | Potential interstitial and intracellular edema caused by rapid movement of this fluid from vascular space<br>Dilution of plasma proteins and electrolytes | |
| 5% dextrose in water (D5W) | Raise total body fluid volume<br>Provide calories for energy (200/1000 ml) | Distributed evenly in every body compartment (acts as free water)<br>Reverses dehydration<br>Prevents hyperosmolar state<br>Maintains adequate renal tubular flow (facilitates water excretion) | Dilution of plasma proteins and electrolytes caused by rapid metabolism of glucose and resultant free water | |

is the only therapy needed in this type of shock. Distributive and septic shock are accompanied by hypovolemia because fluid is leaking out of the capillaries and because the vascular space has increased with the vasodilation. Fluids are always part of the treatment. However, patients with cardiogenic shock also *may* require fluid therapy, although many may require fluid *restriction* or removal of fluid. Before fluid therapy is instituted for cardiogenic shock, a pulmonary artery catheter is inserted, and the pulmonary end-diastolic pressure measured. If the pressure is less than 20 mm Hg, fluid therapy may be beneficial.[14,22]

Current therapies for cardiogenic shock focus on improving tissue perfusion by enhancing oxygen delivery to vital organs during shock. Two means of accomplishing this are by increasing hemoglobin levels and/or by increasing cardiac output. Hemoglobin levels and oxygen-carrying capacity of blood can be improved by infusing packed RBCs. Cardiac output from the left side of the heart can be impaired because of low circulating volume in some instances. **Fluid challenges,** limited controlled intravenous infusions of **crystolloids** or **colloids,** can be given to improve circulation and thus oxygen delivery. Such fluid challenges tend to be no greater than 200 ml and rarely are given without exact continuous monitoring of cardiac function using the pulmonary artery catheter.[2,21,24]

Various fluids may be given to the patient in shock. It is generally agreed that the patient who has sustained a large blood loss will require whole blood replacement. Much disagreement surrounds what other types of fluids should be used to treat shock. Both advantages and disadvantages exist to all types of resuscitative fluids, including blood.

Table 22-7 lists fluids used for replacement therapy in shock.

**Whole blood.** The administration of whole blood for shock is controversial. It has the obvious advantage of increasing the oxygen-carrying capacity of the blood. It also has many disadvantages (transmission of diseases, transfusion reactions, cost). If massive transfusions are given, additional problems may result. Because blood for transfusion contains an anticoagulant to prevent it from clotting while it is being stored, the patient who receives large amounts of blood may develop clotting defects. Stored blood is also deficient in platelets and other clotting factors. Massive transfusions of cold blood can result in hypothermia, which can cause cardiac dysrhythmias.

Stored blood also contains some debris resulting from the aggregation of platelets, leukocytes, and fibrin. It is believed that some of this debris is able to pass through standard blood filters and is eventually filtered out of the blood by the pulmonary capillaries. This probably causes little difficulty in the patient who receives only a few units of blood, but it is likely to cause a problem for the patient who receives massive transfusions. It is recommended by some that microfilters be used when large quantities of blood are transfused.[16]

The pH value of stored blood is lower than that of normal blood. The added anticoagulant makes the blood more acid. Also, because blood is stored in an airtight bag, the metabolism that continues is anaerobic, and the end products are lactic and pyruvic acid. Despite all the disadvantages, until a blood substitute is available for general use, blood must be given to maintain relatively normal hemoglobin and hematocrit levels.[10]

Some patients who are losing large amounts of blood may be given transfusions with their own blood, which has been collected from the bleeding site with special equipment. **Autotransfusion** has been used in patients bleeding massively from an uncontaminated wound, as well as in patients who bleed excessively during surgery. Although it does eliminate transfusion reactions, HIV infection, and viral hepatitis, it is not without risks. The most common complication of autotransfusion is hemolysis resulting in renal failure, coagulopathy, embolization of debris, and sepsis.[15,16] Its main use is in patients who are bleeding so rapidly that the supply of stored blood is becoming depleted.

**Other types of fluid therapy.** Fluids generally are classified as either crystalloid or colloid solutions (see Table 22-7). Controversy over which of these is better for the treatment of shock has existed since the 1960s. In theory, colloids would seem to be superior because they should have the ability to hold fluid within the vascular compartment. However, when shock results in increased capillary permeability, the colloidal particle may leak into the interstitium and be followed by water. Another important consideration is cost. Colloids are generally much more expensive than crystalloids and therefore should be used only if their effect can be shown to be clearly superior to that of crystalloids.[9,30]

Regardless of the type of fluid that the patient receives, the nurse must carefully monitor the rate at which it is administered. The patient is assessed fre-

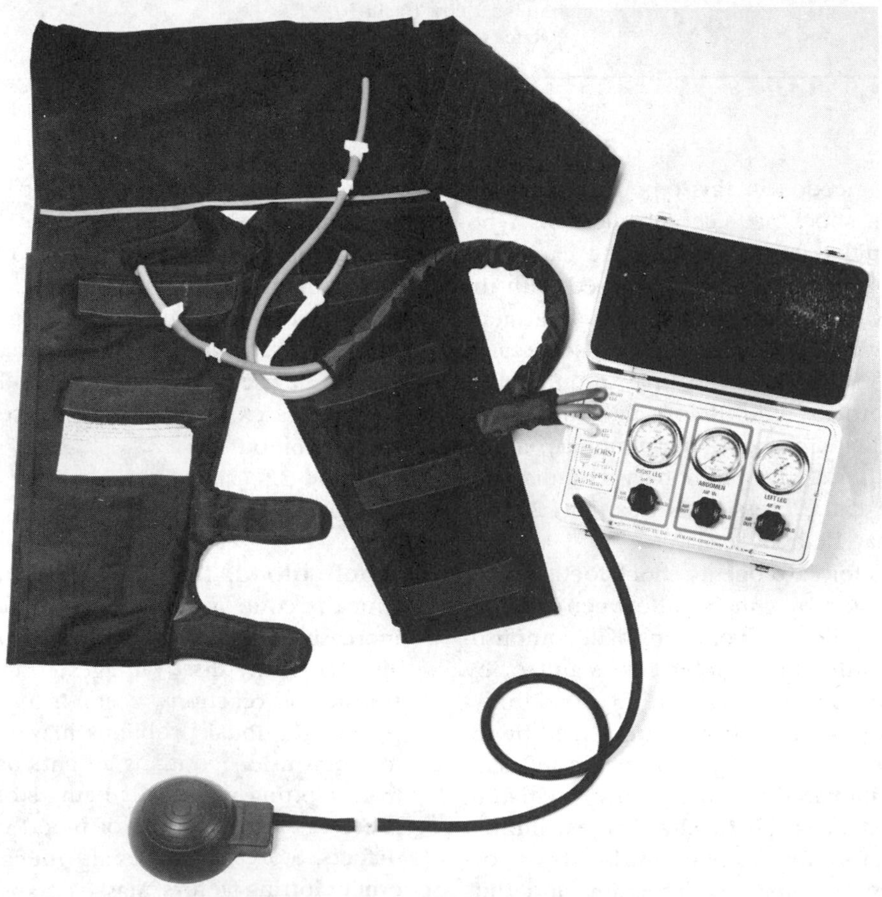

**FIGURE 22-8** Military antishock trousers (MAST) with inflation device and manometers. (Courtesy The Jobst Institute, Toledo, Ohio.)

quently for signs of hypovolemia, fluid overload, or adverse reactions to the type of fluid being administered (see Chapter 20). Neck veins are observed for distention, and lungs are auscultated for signs of fluid (crackles, gurgles) and signs of reaction (e.g., rash, swelling).

#### Fluid redistribution

Another way in which fluid resuscitation may be accomplished is by the use of **military antishock trousers (MAST).** The suit consists of three inflatable parts, one for each leg and one for the abdomen (Figure 22-8). When they are inflated, the trousers autotransfuse the upper circulation with up to 2 L of blood from the lower extremities, redirecting blood to the heart, lungs, and brain.[17] The trousers also increase peripheral resistance, which helps compensate for decreased blood volume. If bleeding in the lower extremities is present, the MAST helps to control bleeding by tamponade (counterpressure). The suit is used as a temporary measure until adequate fluid can be administered. When the suit is to be removed, it must be deflated gradually to prevent a sudden fall in peripheral resistance and a return of shock.

#### Medications

If fluid therapy alone is not sufficient to reverse the shock state, vasoactive drugs may be given. Most vasoactive drugs are catecholamines, which stimulate α- or β-adrenergic-receptors in the body. Generally, stimulation of α-adrenergic-receptors causes vasoconstriction, and stimulation of β-adrenergic-receptors causes vasodilation. Stimulation of β-adrenergic-receptors also causes the heart to increase its rate *(chronotropic effect)* and strength of contraction *(inotropic effect)*. The abdominal viscera, skin, and muscles respond primarily to the alpha effects of the catecholamines. (See Chapter 7 for review of effects of stimulation of adrenergic receptors.)

Mixed α- and β-adrenergic drugs are used most often (Table 22-8). In the very early stage of shock, particularly shock characterized by vasodilation, the patient may benefit from drug therapy that results in vasoconstriction. This would enhance the body's normal compensatory mechanisms and increase the blood supply to the brain and the heart, allowing time for the primary problem to be corrected. However, if the primary problem is not or cannot be corrected, compensatory vasoconstriction itself can harm the body. Vasoconstrictive drugs, if used after the early stages of shock, may harm the kidneys and result in renal failure. They may also cause ischemia of the bowel, resulting in bowel necrosis and sepsis, and ischemia of the pancreas, resulting in the release of MDF.

Vasodilatory drugs may be effective in counteracting the adverse effects of the body's compensatory mechanisms. They also decrease the pressure against which the failing heart has to pump, thereby decreasing the oxygen needs of the heart. However, they are not without danger. They may cause a fall in an already low arterial pressure, reducing coronary artery filling and making the heart even more hypoxic. Fluid therapy must be given with vasodilator drugs to maintain cardiac output. *Dopamine,* the most frequently used drug in the treatment of shock, has a variable effect depending on the dose administered. In certain dosage ranges it *increases cardiac output* by an *inotropic effect* on the heart and at the same time ***selectively dilates the renal and mesenteric vessels, increasing perfusion of the kidneys and the abdominal viscera.*** Selecting the proper drug depends to some extent on the cause of shock and how far it has progressed.

A combination of drugs may be given. Dopamine and nitroprusside may be given together to increase cardiac output by combining the inotropic effect of dopamine with the decreased peripheral resistance effected by nitroprusside. Low-dose dopamine may be given for its effect on renal and mesenteric perfusion along with dobutamine for its inotropic effect.

Patients receiving vasoactive drugs require very careful monitoring. Ideally, intraarterial and pulmonary pressure monitoring should be instituted. If the blood pressure is being measured by both cuff and intraarterial line, the two readings may vary. It is imperative that everyone working with the patient use the same measurements in adjusting the rate of drug infusion.

*Steroids* are often administered to patients in shock; however, ***their use is controversial.*** Many benefits from their use have been suggested, the most important being stabilization of lysosomal membranes, thereby preventing the leak of destructive enzymes.[12] There is a significant debate among physicians, however, about whether steroids enhance survival chances from shock. Studies have consistently failed to show any increase in patient survival after use of steroids in the treatment of shock, such as septic shock.[21,23]

Many drugs are being used experimentally in the treatment of shock, particularly in septic shock. These include naloxone, calcium channel blockers, prostaglandin inhibitors, nonsteroidal antiinflammatory drugs, endotoxin antibodies, and other agents.*

Care of patients receiving vasoactive drugs is summarized in the Guidelines box, p. 583.

### Assisting With Cardiac Support

When the left ventricle becomes severely impaired, as in cardiogenic shock or in the late stages of any type of shock, its function may be augmented by the use of the intraaortic balloon pump[18] (see Chapter 31). A balloon-tipped catheter is inserted into the aorta by way of the femoral artery. The catheter is attached to a machine that inflates and deflates the balloon in synchrony with the patient's cardiac cycle. During systole the balloon is deflated as the heart pumps blood into the aorta. During diastole the balloon inflates, enhancing blood flow to the

*References 3, 5, 7, 10a, 13, 26.

## TABLE 22-8 Vasoactive Drugs Frequently Used to Treat Shock

| | EFFECT | ADVANTAGES | DISADVANTAGES |
|---|---|---|---|
| **MIXED α- AND β-ADRENERGIC DRUGS** | | | |
| Norepinephrine (levarterenol) | $β_1$: Pronounced effect in low doses<br>Positive inotropic and chronotropic effects | May improve cardiac output by increasing rate and stroke volume. | Increases $O_2$ need of heart |
| | $β_2$: Weak effect<br>Dilation of coronary arteries | May improve blood flow to heart | |
| | α: Pronounced effect, especially in higher doses<br>Vasoconstriction | May improve oxygenation of heart by increasing coronary artery perfusion pressure, especially in presence of hypotension | May decrease cardiac output by increasing afterload<br>Increases $O_2$ need of heart |
| Epinephrine | $β_1$: Pronounced effect<br>Positive inotropic and chronotropic effect | May improve cardiac output by increasing stroke volume and rate | Increases $O_2$ need of heart |
| | $β_2$: Pronounced effect, especially in lower doses<br>Dilates coronary arteries and vessels in skeletal muscles | May increase blood supply to heart | May shunt blood away from vital organs because of dilation of vessels in skeletal muscles |
| | α: Pronounced effect in higher doses | May improve oxygenation of heart by increasing coronary perfusion pressure | May decrease cardiac output by increasing afterload<br>Increases $O_2$ need of heart |
| Dopamine | Dopaminergic receptors: pronounced effect in low (2-5 μg/kg/min) and moderate doses (5-10 μg/kg/min); α effect in high doses (>10 μg/kg/min) | Improves perfusion of kidneys and abdominal viscera | |
| | $β_1$: Pronounced effect in moderate dose range<br>Positive inotropic and chronotropic effect | Improves cardiac output | Increases $O_2$ need of heart |
| | $β_2$: Moderate effect<br>Dilates coronary arteries | Increased blood supply to heart | |
| | α: Pronounced in high doses<br>Offsets dopaminergic and beta effects<br>Vasoconstriction | May improve oxygenation of heart by increasing coronary perfusion pressure | May decrease cardiac output by increasing afterload<br>Increases $O_2$ need of heart |
| Dobutamine | $β_1$: Pronounced effect<br>Positive inotropic effect<br>Minimal chronotropic effect | Improves cardiac output by increasing stroke volume<br>Lack of rate increase allows more coronary filling time than other inotropic drugs | Increases $O_2$ need of heart |
| | $β_2$: Weak effect<br>Some dilation of coronary arteries | May improve coronary artery blood flow | |
| | α: Minimal effect | | |
| **β-ADRENERGIC DRUGS** | | | |
| Isoproterenol | $β_1$: Very pronounced effect<br>Strong positive inotropic and chronotropic effects | Increases cardiac output by increasing stroke volume and rate | Pronounced increase in $O_2$ need of heart<br>Cardiac dysrhythmias |
| | $β_2$: Very pronounced effect<br>Dilates coronary arteries and vessels in skeletal muscles<br>Lowers peripheral resistance | May increase blood supply to heart<br>May improve cardiac output by decreasing afterload | Decreased blood pressure may decrease coronary artery perfusion pressure |
| **NON-CATECHOLAMINE AGENT** | | | |
| Amrinone | Acts directly on cardiac cells | Increases myocardial contractility<br>Increases cardiac output | Decreases blood pressure by vasodilation |
| **VASODILATORS** | | | |
| Nitroprusside | Acts directly on smooth muscle, dilating both veins and arterioles | Decreases $O_2$ need of heart by decreasing both preload and afterload<br>Decreases pulmonary congestion by decreasing preload<br>Increases cardiac output by decreasing afterload | Decreases in peripheral resistance can decrease coronary artery perfusion pressure |
| Nitroglycerine | Acts directly on smooth muscle<br>Effect on veins—pronounced<br>Effect on arterioles—weak | Decreases $O_2$ need of heart by decreasing both preload and, to a lesser extent, afterload | Decrease in preload can decrease cardiac output and coronary artery perfusion pressure |

### Guidelines for Care of Patients Receiving Vasoactive Drugs

1. Monitor blood pressure every 5 to 15 minutes at the beginning of the infusion and every 15 minutes thereafter to maintain a *mean* blood pressure at prescribed level, usually 80 mm Hg.
2. Drug must be diluted in a compatible solution and administered slowly by intravenous pump (for control).
3. Observe peripheral site of infusion (if used) frequently for signs of infiltration; necrosis and sloughing of tissues may occur with infiltration.
4. If infiltration occurs, infiltrate area around site with norepinephrine blockers (phentolamine [Regitine]) as prescribed.
5. Monitor urinary output.
6. When discontinuing drug infusion, taper infusion slowly while continuing to monitor blood pressure every 15 minutes.

heart, which is perfused during diastole, and to the rest of the body. During the next period of systole the balloon deflates again, leaving a space in the aorta that must be filled. This causes a reduction in resistance, which allows the heart to eject a larger quantity of blood with less effort than would normally be required.

Complications may occur with use of the balloon pump, the most common being vascular insufficiency of the extremity distal to the insertion site. Frequent assessments are made of the pulses, color, temperature, movement, and sensation of the extremity, and any abnormality is reported immediately. Infection may occur with this procedure, as with any invasive procedure; therefore the patient's temperature is also monitored.

The use of tne intraaortic balloon pump is a temporary measure intended to enhance cardiac output only until the heart is able to function adequately on its own.

## Assisting With Respiratory Support

Most patients in shock have some degree of hypoxemia. Oxygen is usually administered because tissues are already suffering from oxygen deprivation caused by decreased blood flow. Because the energy system of the body is impaired, the muscles used in ventilation may not function adequately, and breathing may have to be assisted. If symptoms of ARDS develop, positive end-expiratory pressure (PEEP) may have to be used. Positive pressure at the end of expiration prevents surfactant-deficient alveoli from collapsing, resulting in atelectasis. Coughing and deep breathing are important. If the patient is too weak to cough or if an endotracheal tube is in place, suctioning is necessary to keep the airway free of excessive secretions. Meticulous mouth care is necessary while the endotracheal tube is in place, because the mouth remains open and swallowing may be difficult. The patient with an endotracheal tube in place is unable to talk; therefore a nonverbal form of communication, such as a magic slate, is necessary.

## Preventing Injury and Infection

In the early stages of shock the patient may exhibit restlessness, which may then progress to confusion. During this time, injury is likely to occur if preventive measures are not taken. If the patient attempts to remove or disconnect life-saving equipment, soft restraints may have to be applied.

Infections occur often in patients with shock because of the many invasive procedures that are performed and the depression of the immune system associated with the stress response. Some potential sources of infection are indwelling catheters, arterial lines, pulmonary artery catheters, intravenous lines, endotracheal tubes, surgical incisions, and traumatic wounds. Meticulous sterile technique must be used with endotracheal suctioning, dressing changes, tubing changes, and urinary catheter care. Patients who are receiving steroids or who have experienced excessive blood loss are at even greater risk for developing infection.

Complications of immobility must be prevented. The patient in shock may remain in one position for an extended period because of hypotension from loss of intravascular fluid, the limitation of movement from invasive technologies, and the constant activity occurring at the bedside. Such immobility can predispose the patient to complications, such as thrombi, pneumonia, and pressure ulcers.

Daily, detailed skin assessment is essential. Frequent turning (when clinically possible) and maintenance of clean, intact skin aid in prevention of ischemic skin and pressure ulcers. If immobility is prolonged or hypoperfusion severe, the use of therapeutic mattresses and beds should be considered.

## Promoting Comfort and Rest

The patient should be kept as comfortable as possible. Patients in shock should remain flat, with the legs elevated if necessary. If a patient in shock has difficulty breathing, a small pillow may be used to elevate the head slightly.

Rest is important. All nonessential activities should be eliminated because activity increases the body's need for oxygen and nutrients, substances already deficient in the cells of the patient in shock.

Ambient temperature should be kept at a comfortable level. Excessive warmth increases the metabolic rate of the tissues, thereby increasing their oxygen need. Excessive coolness may cause the blood to flow even more sluggishly through the microcirculation, enhancing the formation of microthrombi. Patients with an endotracheal tube in place or who are very lethargic may not be able to express how they feel. Covers should be used according to the room temperature.

Both the conscious patient and the family will probably experience considerable anxiety. The nurse should remain calm and explain all interventions whenever possible. It may be necessary to repeat explanations frequently to both patient and family, because anxiety can interfere with their ability to comprehend and to remember.

## ♦ EVALUATION

To evaluate the effectiveness of nursing interventions, compare patient behaviors with those stated in the expected patient outcomes. Successful achievement of patient outcomes for the patient in shock is indicated by the following:

1. Airway is clear of secretions.
2. Arterial blood gas levels are within normal limits (pH of 7.35 to 7.45; $Paco_2$ of 35 to 45 mm Hg; $Pao_2$ of 80 to 100 mm Hg).
3. Respiratory rate is 16 to 20/min, with a normal tidal volume.
4. Intravascular volume is normal, as evidenced by Hct level of 42% to 52% for men and 37% to 47% for women (levels above 32% may be acceptable); Hgb level of 14 to 18 g/dl for men and 12 to 16 g/dl for women; CVP, PAP, PCWP, etc. measurements are within normal limits.
5. Urinary output is at least 50 ml/hr.
6. Experiences no injuries or infection.
7. Offers statements of feeling relaxed; demonstrates no physical signs of anxiety; makes needs known.
8. Offers statements of feeling comfortable and free of pain.
9. Tolerates activity without an increase in pulse rate of more than 20 beats/min.

## QUESTIONS TO CONSIDER

- How would you expect your assessment findings of a patient in cardiogenic shock to differ from those of a patient in hypovolemic shock?
- What would you include in your assessment to determine whether a patient was receiving adequate fluid replacement?
- How would you assess the comfort of a patient with an endotracheal tube?
- How would you assess the effect of vasoactive drugs on your patient?

## CRITICAL THINKING ACTIVITIES

- During report the nurse from the previous shift tells you that she suspects that Mr. Cane's myocardial contractility is compromised. When you ask about Mr. Cane's data that may suggest decreased myocardial function, the nurse replies that his mean PAP is above 10. How would you respond when given this information?
- While assessing the 48-hour IV flow rates on a patient receiving a vasoactive drug, you note that each shift has been running the drug at a different rate. What are some of the possibile explanations for a variation in flow rate?

## CHAPTER SUMMARY

### NATURE OF PROBLEM

- Shock is a syndrome characterized by hypoperfusion of body tissues and tissue hypoxia.

### ETIOLOGY

- The major classifications of shock are hypovolemic, cardiogenic, and distributive shock.

### PHYSIOLOGY

- Shock results in a derangement of cellular metabolism; if shock advances, it can affect all body systems.

### PATHOPHYSIOLOGY

- The early stage of shock is characterized by a stress response.
- At some point in the progress of untreated shock, the process becomes irreversible and results in death.

### NURSING MANAGEMENT

- The management of shock includes the following:
  a. Fluid therapy—blood and blood products, plasma expanders, colloids, crystalloids
  b. Drug therapy—vasodilators, vasoconstrictors, inotropes
  c. Supportive care—cardiac support, respiratory support, prevention of injuries and infections, promotion of comfort

## REFERENCES

1. Ackerman MH: The systemic inflammatory response, sepsis, and multiple organ disfunction: new definitions for an old problem, *Crit Care Nurs Clin North Am* 6(2):243-250, 1994.
1a. Asheervath J, Blevins D: *Handbook of clinical nursing practice,* Norwalk, Conn, 1986, Appleton-Century-Crofts.
2. Barone JE: Treatment strategies in shock: use of oxygen transport measurements, *Heart Lung* 20(1):81-86, 1991.
3. Bone RC: A critical evaluation of new agents for the treatment of sepsis, *JAMA* 266(12):1686-1691, 1991.
4. Boyle J: Cardiovascular physiology. In Bullock J, Boyle J, Wang MB: *Physiology,* Media, Pa, 1991, Harwal Publishing.
5. Calandra T et al: Treatment of gram-negative septic shock with human IgG antibody to *Escherichia coli* J5: a prospective double-blind, randomized trial, *J Infect Dis* 158(2):312-319, 1988.
6. Dickerson M: Anaphylaxis and anaphylactic shock, *Crit Care Nurs Q* 11(1):68-74, 1988.
7. Gorelick K et al: Randomized placebo-controlled study of E5 monoclonical antitoxin antibody. In Larrick J, Borrebaeck C, eds: *Therapeutic monoclonical antibodies,* New York, 1990, Stockton Press.
8. Guyton AC: *Textbook of medical physiology,* ed 8, Philadelphia, 1990, WB Saunders.
9. Hancock BG, Eberhard NK: The pharmacological management of shock, *Crit Care Nurs Q* 11(1):19-29, 1988.
10. Hardaway RM: *Shock: the reversible stage of dying,* Littleton, Mass, 1986, PSG Publishing.
10a. Hazinski MF: Mediator-specific therapies for the systemic inflammatory response syndrome, sepsis, severe sepsis, and septic shock: present and future approaches, *Crit Care Nurs Clin North Am* 6(2):309-319, 1994.

11. Houston MC: Pathophysiology of shock, *Crit Care Nurs Clin North Am* 2(2):143-149, 1990.
12. Jurkovich GJ, Moore EE, Eiseman B: The liver in shock. In Hardaway RM: *Shock: the reversible stage of dying,* Littleton, Mass, 1986, PSG Publishing.
13. Littleton MT: Prostaglandins and leukotrienes as mediators of shock and trauma, *Crit Care Nurs Q* 11(2):11-20, 1988.
14. MacLean LD: Shock, *Br Med Bull* 44(2):437-452, 1988.
15. Martin E et al: Autotransfusion systems, *Crit Care Nurs* 9(7):65–72, 1989.
16. McQuillan KA, Wiles CE: Initial management of traumatic shock. In Cardona DV et al: *Trauma nursing from resuscitation through rehabilitation,* Philadelphia, 1988, WB Saunders.
17. McSwain NE: Pneumatic anti-shock garment: state of the art, 1988, *Ann Emerg Med* 17(5):506-526, 1988.
18. Millar S: *AACN procedure manual for critical care,* Philadelphia, 1985, WB Saunders.
19. Perry AG: Shock complications: recognition and management, *Crit Care Nurse Q* 11(1):1-8, 1988.
20. Rice V: *Shock: a clinical syndrome, the clinical continuum of septic shock, shock management,* Secaucus, NJ, 1985, Crit Care Nurs/Hospitals Publications.
21. Rice V: Shock, a clinical syndrome: an update. I. An overview of shock, *Crit Care Nurs* 11(4):20-27, 1991.
22. Rice V: Shock, a clinical syndrome: an update. III. Therapeutic management, *Crit Care Nurs* 11(6):41-43, 1991.
23. Schumer W: Corticosteroids in the treatment of shock, *Prog Clin Biol Res* 236B:249-259, 1987.
24. Shoemaker WC: Monitoring and management of acute circulatory problems: the expanded role of the physiologically oriented critical care nurse, *Am J Crit Care* 1(1):38-53, 1992.
24a. Shoemaker WC: Pathophysiology, monitoring, and therapy of acute circulatory problems, *Crit Care Nurs Clin North Am* 6(2):295-307, 1994.
25. Shoemaker WC et al: Hemodynamic and oxygen transport monitoring to titrate therapy in shock, *New Horizons* 1(1):145-157, 1993.
25a. Shelton BK: Disorders of hemostasis in sepsis, *Crit Care Nurs Clin North Am* 6(2):373-388, 1994.
26. Soulioti AM: Naloxone for septic shock, *Lancet* 2(8620):1133-1134, 1988.
27. Suhl J: Patients with shock. In Clochlsey J et al, eds: *Critcal care nursing,* Phildelphia, 1993, WB Saunders.
28. Tuchschmidt J, Daniels O, Jeffery CF: Oxygen consumption in sepsis and septic shock, *Crit Care Med* 19(5):664-671, 1991.
29. Vincent JL et al: Oxygen uptake/supply dependency, *Am Rev Resp Dis* 142:2-7, 1990.
29a. Vollman KM: Adult respiratory distress syndrome: mediators on the run, *Crit Care Nurs Clin North Am* 6(2):341-358, 1994.
30. Weil MH, Rackow EC: Colloidal osmotic pressure and its implications for the fluid management of patients in shock. In Hardaway RM: *Shock: the reversible stage of dying,* Littleton, Mass, 1986, PSG Publishing.

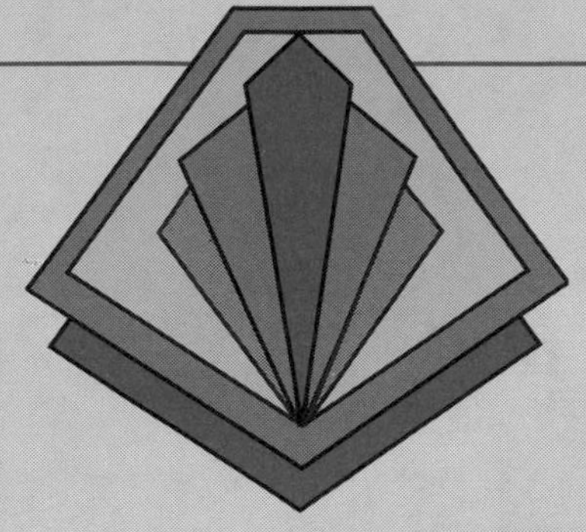

UNIT IV

# Surgery: Perioperative Nursing

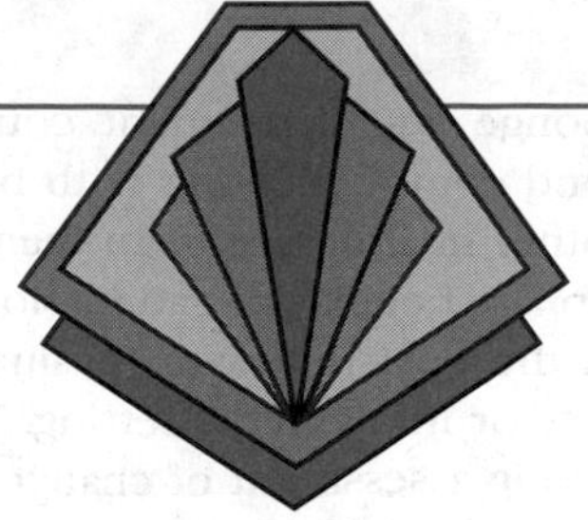

CHAPTER 23

# Preoperative Nursing

*Arlene W. Keeling*
*Grace A. Muro*
*Barbara C. Long*

## CHAPTER OBJECTIVES

***After studying this chapter, the learner should be able to do the following:***

1 Identify the major influences on the emergence of operating room nursing.
2 Describe the preoperative phase as a component of the surgical experience.
3 Identify different types of surgeries.
4 Identify the biopsychosocial responses of patients to surgery.
5 Discuss preoperative patient assessment.
6 Identify nursing diagnoses for the preoperative patient.
7 List risk factors for potential postoperative complications.
8 Discuss desired nursing outcomes for the preoperative phase.
9 Discuss nursing interventions in the preoperative phase.
10 Explain the concept of *informed consent.*
11 Discuss final preparations for the preoperative patient.

## KEY TERMS

ambulatory surgery
cosmetic surgery
curative surgery
diagnostic surgery
deep breathing exercises
emancipated minor
external surgery
informed consent
major surgery
minor surgery
internal surgery
palliative surgery
postoperative leg exercises
premedication
preoperative phase
psychologic preparation
restorative surgery
same-day surgery

# OVERVIEW

## HISTORY OF SURGERY

Surgery emerged as a medical specialty in the mid-nineteenth century. At that time concepts about antisepsis were vague and surgery resulted in a mortality rate of 70% to 90%. Surgery was performed as a last resort. Superficial tumor removal, drainage of infection, traumatic surgery, stone removal, and head and face operations were the extent of surgical attempts. Performing surgery in street clothes, washing hands only after surgery, not wearing gloves, and using the same instruments on patient after patient were commonplace. Surgeons believed that sepsis was the result of the patient's inability to withstand the procedure.

It was not until the latter half of the nineteenth century that discoveries in antiseptic techniques and anesthesia changed the course of surgery. In 1847, Semmelweiss' work on the importance of handwashing before and after procedures greatly reduced the incidence of postoperative infections and puerperal fever after childbirth. In 1865, Lister proposed that germs should be prevented from entering the surgical wound. Lister's germ theory of disease opened the door to the development of antiseptic techniques in surgery. As a result, Joseph Lister became known as the father of antiseptic surgery. Today, providing a safe, therapeutic environment for the surgical patient through the practice of aseptic techniques is a result of his work.

As anatomic knowledge and surgical techniques improved, the search for safer methods of analgesia during surgery became imperative. Beginning with a demonstration of the use of nitrous oxide during a tooth extraction in 1846, great strides were made in the use of anesthesia during a variety of surgical, obstetric, and diagnostic procedures. Over time, surgery was performed to improve and prolong life rather than as a last-resort measure. With the knowledge explosion in science and technology in the twentieth century, advances in this specialty have been enormous.

## PERIOPERATIVE NURSING: PAST AND PRESENT

The presence of nurses in the surgical arena was not recognized as important during the early years of surgery. Nurses accompanied patients from the wards to the operating room, performed technical tasks to assist the surgeons, and then returned with the patients to the ward. With the advances in surgery, surgeons gradually recognized the importance of nurses in the operating room. Operating room nursing education began in the late nineteenth century at Massachusetts General Hospital when student nurses were first allowed in the operating room for clinical instruction. By the early 1900s, student nurses entered operating rooms daily for clinical experience. There they learned duties relating to the sterilization of instruments, the preparation of dressings and supplies, and their role as assistants during surgery.

Perioperative nursing, as we know it today, is an outgrowth of operating room nursing as it was practiced in its early years. Unlike the earlier focus, however, contemporary perioperative nursing practice is patient-centered rather than task-oriented. *Perioperative nursing practice* is defined as the activities performed by the professional nurse during the preoperative, intraoperative, and postoperative phases of the patient's surgical experience. Each phase of the role begins and ends at an appointed time in the chain of events involved in surgical intervention, and each includes a variety of nursing activities that are performed in terms of the nursing process.

The **preoperative phase** begins when the decision for surgical intervention is made. The scope of nursing activities includes but is not limited to preoperative assessment of the patient's physical, psychologic, and social states, the planning of nursing care that is required to prepare the patient for surgery, and the implementation of nursing interventions. This phase ends when the patient is safely transported to the operating room and transferred to the operating room nurse for care.

The intraoperative phase begins with the receiving of the patient in the operating room and ends when the patient is transferred to the postanesthesia care unit (PACU). During this phase nursing responsibilities focus on the continuing assessment of the patient's physiologic and psychologic states and the planning and implementation of effective nursing interventions to promote safety and privacy, as well as prevent wound infection and promote healing. Specific nursing activities include providing emotional support to the patient during induction of anesthesia and throughout the procedure, establishing and maintaining functional positioning, being vigilant of the aseptic environment, protecting the patient from electrical hazards, assisting in fluid balance, ensuring accurate sponge and instrument counts, assisting the surgeon, and communicating with both the patient's family and other health care team members.

The postoperative phase begins with admission to the PACU and ends with the final follow-up evaluation of the patient in the home or in a clinical setting. Nursing activities include ongoing assessment of changes in the physical and psychologic status of the patient, along with appropriate planning and implementation of care. Activities include frequent monitoring of airway patency, vital signs, and neurologic status, as well as providing intravenous fluids and blood, accurately assessing output from all drains, and providing a thorough summary report of the patient's status to the nurse receiving the patient on the unit and to the patient's family or friends.

## TYPES OF SURGERY

Most surgical procedures are given names that describe the site of the surgery and the type of surgery performed. For example, appendectomy refers to removal *(-ectomy)* of the appendix. Common surgical suffixes are listed in Box 23-1. Some surgeries carry the name of the surgeon who developed the technique, such as the Billroth procedures (partial gastrectomies). Surgeries may be classified according to the extent, purpose, or body site of the surgery or the timing or physical setting.

### EXTENT

Surgeries may be classified as minor or major procedures. **Minor surgery** is simple surgery that presents little risk to life. It may be performed in a surgeon's office, clinic, ambulatory setting or in an inpatient surgical suite. Many minor surgeries are performed with the use of local anesthesia although general anesthesia may be used (see Chapter 24). Although the operation is termed "minor," it is rarely viewed as a minor episode by the patient and may evoke fears and concerns. *Major surgery* is performed in a surgical suite, usually in a hospital setting, although in selected instances (such as for hernia repair) it may take place in ambulatory surgical centers. **Major surgery** usually is performed with use of general or regional anesthesia. It is more serious than minor surgery and may involve risk of life.

**BOX 23-1 Common Surgical Suffixes**

-ectomy: removal of an organ or gland
-rrhaphy: repairing
-ostomy: providing an opening (stoma)
-otomy: cutting into
-plasty: formation or plastic repair
-scopy: looking into

## PURPOSE

Surgery may be classified according to the reasons for which it is performed:

1. **Diagnostic**—determines cause of symptoms (i.e., biopsy, exploratory laparotomy)
2. **Curative** (also known as *ablative*)—removes diseased part (e.g., appendectomy)
3. **Restorative** (also known as reconstructive)—strengthens weakened area (e.g., herniorrhaphy), rejoins disconnected or injured area (e.g., bone pinning), or corrects deformities (e.g., mitral valve replacement)
4. **Palliative**—relieves symptoms without curing disease (e.g., sympathectomy)
5. **Cosmetic**—improves appearance (e.g., face lifting)

## BODY SITE

Surgery may be performed externally or internally. In **external surgery** the skin or underlying tissues are readily accessible to the surgeon. Plastic surgery is an example of external surgery. **Internal surgery** involves deep penetration of the body, such as surgery of organs, major blood vessels, or bone structure. Surgery also may be classified by location of body parts or systems, such as cardiovascular surgery, chest surgery, intestinal surgery, or neurologic surgery. Information specific to these types of surgery can be found in appropriate chapters elsewhere in the text.

## TIMING OR PHYSICAL SETTING

Surgery may be planned or unplanned. An example of unplanned surgery is *emergency surgery,* such as that which follows major trauma or hemorrhage of internal organs. Although the same principles related to preoperative care apply in both planned and unplanned surgery, modifications must be made for emergency surgery because of the limited preoperative time period.

**Ambulatory surgery** is that which does not require overnight hospital admission. The patient is admitted to the surgical center (either in a hospital or ambulatory surgical center) on the day of surgery, remains there for postoperative care, and is discharged before the end of the day.

In the past all patients were admitted to the hospital for preparation one or more days before major surgery. The most recent trend, in response to the national mandate to reduce health care costs, is **same-day surgery.** The patient is admitted on the same day of the planned surgery to a regular inpatient unit or to a special same-day surgery unit. Nurses on the special unit may be involved in patient assessment and preoperative teaching that is carried out on an outpatient basis before the hospital admission. Patients are responsible for their own physical preparation for surgery; therefore these patients must receive the necessary preoperative teaching and counseling well before admission. On the patient's arrival at the surgical admission suite (SAS), final preparations for surgery are completed.

# BIOPSYCHOSOCIAL RESPONSES IN THE PREOPERATIVE PHASE

Surgery is a unique experience for each patient, depending on the underlying psychosocial and physiologic factors present. Thus no two persons respond alike to the same operation, nor does one person respond in like manner to different surgeries. Although some operations are considered minor procedures by hospital personnel, surgery is always a major experience for the patient and family. Surgery is a stressor that produces both physiologic stress reactions (neuroendocrine responses) and psychologic stress reactions (anxiety, fear). Surgery is also a social stressor, requiring family adaptation to temporary or lasting role changes.

## THE BIOLOGIC RESPONSE: NEUROENDOCRINE

The stress that results from either impending elective surgery or emergency surgery causes a physiologic stress reaction in the body. Most of the signs and symptoms result from stimulation of the sympathetic nervous system. On the patient's admission, therefore, blood pressure and heart rate may be elevated. The patient may experience anorexia. Other signs may be related to increased adrenocortical activity. Because of the increased production of aldosterone and glucocorticoids, the patient may retain fluid and have an increase in blood glucose levels.

## THE PSYCHOLOGIC RESPONSE

**Anxiety** is a normal adaptive response to the stress of surgery. Anxiety occurs in the preoperative phase as the patient anticipates the surgery or postoperative problems such as pain and discomfort, changes in body image or function, increased dependency, loss of control, family concerns, or potential changes in life-style. Anxiety may be decreased if the patient perceives the surgery as having positive results, such as curing disease, relieving discomfort, or creating a more attractive physical appearance. On the other hand, anxiety usually is increased when the underlying pathologic condition is, or is believed to be, malignant or life-threatening (e.g., open heart surgery).

Surgery that is performed on body areas that are visible to others may leave scars that are perceived by the patient or significant others as disfiguring. Surgery of vital organs such as the heart, lungs, and kidneys may be threatening to the patient in terms of survival. Surgery of the mouth or throat may create temporary breathing problems that can be perceived as threatening. Surgery of the extremities or surgery such as a colostomy may result in permanent changes in life-style, especially in

**BOX 23-2 Fears Related to Surgery**

**GENERAL**

Fear of unknown
Loss of control
Loss of love from significant others
Threat to sexuality

**SPECIFIC**

Diagnosis of malignancy
Anesthesia
Dying
Pain
Disfigurement
Permanent limitations

activities of daily living (eating, bathing, dressing, walking). Surgery on body areas that have special meaning to the person such as the breast, genitalia, or reproductive organs will have differing effects and responses.

Psychologic responses are not directly related to the extent of the surgery, because they are influenced by the patient's past experiences, perceptions of what the surgery means to self-image, and possible changes in life-style. The patient who has had previous experience with surgery may respond either positively or negatively to the present surgery. A previous negative experience can be transferred to the present experience and increase anxiety. On the other hand, a previous negative experience is sometimes viewed by the patient as an entirely separate event that happened under different circumstances and thus may not influence the present experience.

Having major surgery involves putting one's life under the control of others and subjecting oneself to intrusion into the body and possible pain. It also may involve permanent changes of life-style. Some of the fears underlying preoperative anxiety are elusive, and the patient may not be able to identify their causes. Others are more specific (Box 23-2). Fear of the unknown is the most common. If the diagnosis is uncertain, fear of a malignant condition is common. Fears concerning anesthesia usually are related to dying. Fears concerning pain, disfigurement, or permanent disability may be realistic or may be influenced by myths, lack of information, or stories recited by friends.

Some surgeons will cancel surgery for a patient who is extremely anxious. Patients with anxiety levels so high that they cannot cope with their anxiety before surgery frequently experience difficulty in the postoperative period. This is also true of patients who express no emotion in the preoperative phase. These patients are more apt to be angry, resentful, confused, or depressed in the postoperative period. They are also more vulnerable to psychotic reactions than are patients with lower levels of anxiety.

In contrast, patients with a moderate amount of anxiety who can identify and begin to cope with their feelings in the preoperative phase may experience a smoother postoperative course. Thus patients should be given every opportunity to verbalize their fears and concerns during the preoperative period.

## THE SOCIOLOGIC RESPONSE

The patient hospitalized for surgery, even if only for one day, experiences a disruption in his or her usual role. This disruption inevitably causes role adaptation on the part of other family members and friends as they help with transportation of the patient to and from the hospital, psychologic support of the patient, child care, and other family responsibilities. Inability to work also may be a problem to both the patient and the family. Job security may be threatened, and financial stress may result.

Families and friends may be anxious for a variety of reasons. They may be concerned about the final outcome of the surgery and changes in life-style or routines that may result. They may also experience the stresses of providing emotional support for the patient at a time when they themselves are stressed. When the patient is admitted to the hospital, family and friends may find themselves in an unfamiliar, highly technical medical environment. This unfamiliar setting can be stressful in and of itself. In addition, family and friends also may have their own previous experiences with surgery—memories and unpleasant associations. As a result they may be under a great deal of stress and exhibit behaviors that could be misunderstood by health care workers. Because of this possibility, a careful assessment of the family situation and needs should be completed.

## NURSING MANAGEMENT

### ♦ ASSESSMENT

Assessment of the patient during the preoperative phase begins with the initial contact between patient and nurse and is ongoing throughout the period. Assessment should be holistic, reflecting the physiologic, psychologic, spiritual, and social needs of the patient and the family or significant others. Assessment of the patient is an interdisciplinary activity. Responsibilities for the assessment extend to all members of the health care team.

#### Physiologic

Patients should be in the best possible physical condition before surgery. A thorough review of systems should be performed to assess neurologic, respiratory, cardiovascular, endocrine, gastrointestinal, renal, skin, and musculoskeletal status. Some operative and postoperative complications can be prevented or ameliorated if patients who are at high risk of developing complications are identified early and preventive measures are taken. Much of the data needed by the nurse to make a thor-

**BOX 23-3 Preoperative Allergy Assessment by Nurse**

*Possible allergens*
- Soaps and cleansing solutions
- Iodine and dyes
- Medications
- Adhesive tape

ough physiologic assessment can be obtained in collaboration with the physician.

The nurse collects physiologic data in the preoperative phase for two reasons: (1) to obtain baseline data for comparison during the intraoperative and postoperative phases and (2) to identify potential problems that may require preventive nursing interventions before surgery. If the patient has been hospitalized, the admission history and physical assessment should contain much of the pertinent data that can serve as baseline data for surgery. Recording of the data is important for comparison when changes occur during the perioperative period and for planning nursing care.

Of particular importance is information about any allergies the patient has to medications, soap, or adhesive tape (Box 23-3). This information is needed by members of the surgical team who will be using various cleansing solutions to prepare the skin. They also will be applying dressings and administering medications to the patient.

### Persons at average surgical risk

A complete preoperative assessment of the patient's neurologic status, as well as accurate documentation of that status, is imperative so that changes that might occur during surgery can be accurately assessed and interventions taken. Such factors as level of consciousness, orientation to time and place, equality of strength in hand grips, and gait must all be noted. Any deficiencies, such as weakness on one side from a preexisting condition, must be documented. If any severe neurologic problems exist, appropriate interventions should be initiated to correct these before surgery. Particular attention should be given to sensory deficits and problems such as difficulties with vision or hearing. This baseline information needs to be communicated to other members of the surgical team. Baseline data on the patient's muscle strength and ability to move the extremities and to ambulate are also important for the care of the patient in the operating room and after surgery. Any limitations should be carefully recorded.

A complete preoperative assessment of the patient's respiratory status is also necessary. A chest x-ray examination may be ordered to aid in the diagnosis of lung disease. If interference with pulmonary function is suspected, additional tests will be ordered, such as vital capacity tests, pulmonary function tests, and arterial blood gas studies. If signs of upper respiratory infection

**TABLE 23-1 Risk Factors for the Development of Postoperative Pulmonary Complications**

| CONDITION | EFFECT |
|---|---|
| **INCREASED RESPIRATORY SECRETIONS** | |
| **Risk Factors** | |
| Smoking | Irritation of lining of bronchial passages |
| Chronic lung disease | Decreased ciliary action to remove secretions |
| Respiratory infection | Secretions will block bronchial passages or alveoli |
| **DECREASED THORAX EXPANSION** | |
| **Risk Factors** | |
| Obesity<br>Age (elderly)<br>Skeletal deformities (e.g., scoliosis) | Lung does not expand fully, resulting in hypoventilation |

are present (rhinitis, pharyngitis, fever, cough), surgery will be postponed, if possible, until the symptoms abate.

Interference with ventilation as a result of anesthetics or pooled respiratory secretions, or both, is a common postoperative occurrence that may lead to the complications of atelectasis and pneumonia. A preoperative baseline assessment of the person's ventilatory status is important for early identification of whether the patient is at high risk for the development of postoperative respiratory complications. Early identification of these patients is essential for their care. Patients at high risk include (1) those scheduled for upper abdominal or thoracic surgery, (2) those who will receive inhalant anesthesia, (3) the obese, (4) smokers, (5) patients suffering from chronic lung disease, and (6) elderly persons. Table 23-1 summarizes the major risk factors for postoperative pulmonary complications.

Preoperative assessment of the patient's cardiovascular status is essential for the identification of signs of heart disease that need correction before surgery. Vital signs are obtained. An electrocardiogram (ECG) to detect signs of cardiac dysrhythmias or heart damage often is ordered for persons older than 40 years of age. Central venous pressure or pulmonary arterial pressure measurements may be obtained if the patient has known or suspected heart disease and fluid volume overload is a potential problem. If surgery is to be performed on major blood vessels or on the extremities, the presence and strength of peripheral pulses are recorded. Comparison of preoperative and postoperative findings helps determine adequacy of circulation.

Routine blood work (CBC and electrolyte levels) is done on all patients to detect blood dyscrasias, infection, liver disease, or electrolyte imbalances. It also serves as baseline data for identifying postoperative differences. If the patient has a low hematocrit or blood hemoglobin level or if major surgery that may involve considerable blood loss is planned, blood typing and cross-matching is done so that blood will be available for transfusion if necessary. In the case of elective surgery, patients may want to donate their own blood several weeks to months before surgery so that they may receive it back (autologous transfusion). This decreases the risk of the patient's contracting HIV or hepatitis B from blood transfusion.

Assessment of the patient's renal status is also important preoperatively. Adequate renal function is necessary to maintain fluid and electrolyte balance during the perioperative period. A preoperative urinalysis is therefore routinely ordered to assess renal status. Abnormalities in the urinalysis must be noted. Presence of albumin or a low specific gravity may indicate the possibility of kidney disease, and further evaluation may be necessary before surgery can safely be performed. Acetone in the urine may indicate diabetes mellitis or malnutrition. Bacteriuria, fever, and patient report of urgency, frequency, or burning on voiding may all be indicative of urinary tract infection (UTI). Urinary tract infection usually is treated with antibiotics before surgery is attempted.

The patient's endocrine status is also important. Metabolic tests for glycosuria and blood glucose levels are obtained before surgery to check for signs of diabetes mellitus. Preoperative thyroid tests also may be indicated. Postoperative complications can be minimized if this existing medical condition is treated or controlled before surgery.

Both *nutritional status* and *hydration status* must be assessed for all patients during the preoperative phase. Malnourished persons with nutritional deficits or excesses are poorer surgical risks than the well-nourished, and postoperative complications are more likely to develop. Ideally, the patient's nutritional status should be optimal before surgery. If not, deficiencies will be corrected if possible. All patients are weighed before surgery. A recorded weight is used as baseline data for the anesthetist to calculate medication dosages. It also is used to assess postoperative fluid retention. In addition to nutritional status, the hydration of the patient should be assessed before surgery. If the patient has an acute fluid volume deficit resulting from trauma with blood loss, blood and intravenous fluids must be replaced preoperatively. Dehydration from other causes, such as chronic diarrhea, also must be treated before surgery. Signs of dehydration include decreased skin turgor, dry mucous membranes, high hematocrit level, decreased blood pressure, and increased pulse rate. Table 23-2 identifies other critical assessment data that should be obtained and recorded in the preoperative period, and Table 23-3 identifies the effects of common medications on surgery and anesthesia.

### Persons at high risk for surgical/anesthesic complications

No two persons respond to surgery in exactly the same way. A number of variables influence physiologic and psychologic responses throughout the entire surgical experience. These include age, the presence of chronic diseases or disabilities, and impaired nutritional status. Careful nursing assessment and preoperative medical and nursing intervention may be required to decrease the risk of surgery and postoperative complications in these persons.

*Elderly patients* are at high risk for developing complications in surgery from the surgery itself or from the anesthesia. Surgery can be performed on persons of any age, from the newborn to the very elderly. Persons at the extremes of age are less able to tolerate stress such as tissue trauma (surgery) or infection. (Consult a pediatrics textbook for the effects of surgery on an infant or child.) The ability of the elderly patient to tolerate surgery depends on the extent of the physiologic changes that have occurred with the aging process, the duration of the surgical procedure, and the presence of one or more chronic diseases. Elderly persons vary

**TABLE 23-2 Additional Assessment Information by System**

| SYSTEM | ASSESSMENT FACTOR |
|---|---|
| Neurologic/psychologic | Alcohol use<br>Psychotropic drugs |
| Respiratory | Allergies<br>Smoking |
| Cardiovascular | Pacemaker<br>Automatic implanted cardiac defibrillator (AICD) |
| Musculoskeletal | Artificial limbs<br>Metal implants (spinal fusion, joint replacements) |

**TABLE 23-3 Medications That Can Adversely Affect Anesthesia or Surgery**

| MEDICATION | EFFECT |
|---|---|
| Antibiotics | Potentiate muscle relaxants |
| Anticoagulants | Increase bleeding and hemorrhage |
| Antihypertensives | Affect anesthesia and compensatory ability (hypotension may occur) |
| Aspirin | ↓ Platelet aggregation<br>Potentiates effect of anticoagulants |
| Diuretics (thiazides) | Possible potassium imbalance |
| Steroids | ↓ Neuroendocrine response<br>Antiinflammatory effect; may delay wound healing |
| Tranquilizers | Potentiate effect of narcotics and barbiturates<br>Hypotension |

greatly in the extent to which physiologic changes occur. Very elderly persons (older than 80 years of age) generally have a greater number of changes than those in their 60s or 70s. The changes that affect responses to surgery involve all of the body systems. The greater the number of changes, the greater the potential for the patient to develop a postoperative complication. Table 23-4 outlines the physiologic changes of aging that may adversely affect surgery.

Patients with *chronic diseases* are also at high risk for developing complications in surgery from the surgery itself or from the anesthesia. The existence of one or more chronic diseases does not necessarily increase surgical risk. The nature and extent of the disease or diseases and the degree to which they are under control are the important variables. Nursing assessment and documentation of these conditions are critical in the preoperative period.

*Pulmonary disease,* such as chronic obstructive pulmonary disease (COPD), may affect the person's response to the anesthetic and ability to cope with respiratory problems after surgery. In preparation for surgery the pulmonary status of persons with COPD will be carefully evaluated and measures will be instituted to improve ventilation/perfusion. In persons with a history of recent respiratory infection, surgery will be delayed until they are in optimal condition. Most surgeons prefer that persons who are heavy smokers decrease their smoking for a few days before surgery inasmuch as smoke irritates the tracheobronchial tree, resulting in increased secretions that impinge on the airway and decrease ventilation.

Persons with chronic pulmonary problems must be monitored very carefully during surgery and in the early postoperative period. Atelectasis, respiratory insufficiency, and respiratory acidosis are common occurrences.

*Cardiovascular disease* can affect the individual's response to surgery. A heart that pumps effectively and blood vessels that constrict effectively are necessary for the prevention of shock and fluid imbalances. Body responses to hemorrhage and inflammation depend on an adequate supply of red and white blood cells. Surgery usually is postponed if the patient's cardiovascular functioning is not at its optimal level. Measures are initiated to improve the cardiovascular status and reduce the risk of surgery. Careful monitoring for potential cardiac problems is done by both physicians and nurses during the intraoperative and postoperative phases.

*Renal insufficiency* can increase the risk of surgery

**TABLE 23-4 Physiologic Changes Related to the Aging Process That Can Affect Surgery**

| PHYSIOLOGIC CHANGES | EFFECTS | POTENTIAL POSTOPERATIVE COMPLICATIONS |
|---|---|---|
| **CARDIOVASCULAR** | | |
| ↓ Elasticity of blood vessels<br>↓ Cardiac output<br>↓ Peripheral circulation | ↓ Circulation to vital organs<br>Slower blood flow | Shock (hypotension), thrombosis with pulmonary emboli, delayed wound healing, postoperative confusion, hypervolemia, decreased response to stress |
| **RESPIRATORY** | | |
| ↓ Elasticity of lungs and chest wall<br>↑ Residual lung volume<br>↓ Forced expiratory volume<br>↓ Ciliary action<br>Fewer alveolar capillaries | ↓ Vital capacity<br>↓ Alveolar volume<br>↓ Gas exchange<br>↓ Cough reflex | Atelectasis, pneumonia, postoperative confusion |
| **URINARY** | | |
| ↓ Glomerular filtration rate<br>↓ Bladder muscle tone<br>Weakened perineal muscles | ↓ Kidney function<br>Stasis of urine in bladder<br>Loss of urinary control | Prolonged response to anesthesia and drugs, overhydration with IV fluids, hyperkalemia, urinary tract infection, urinary incontinence |
| **MUSCULOSKELETAL** | | |
| ↓ Muscle strength<br>Limitation of motion | ↓ Activity | Atelectasis, pneumonia, thrombophlebitis, constipation or fecal impaction |
| **GASTROINTESTINAL** | | |
| ↓ Intestinal motility | Retention of feces | Constipation or fecal impaction |
| **METABOLIC** | | |
| ↓ Gamma globulin level<br>↓ Plasma proteins | ↓ Inflammatory response | Delayed wound healing, wound dehiscence or evisceration |
| **IMMUNE SYSTEM** | | |
| Fewer killer T cells<br>↓ Response to foreign antigens | ↓ Ability to protect against invasion by pathogenic microorganisms | Wound infection, wound dehiscence, pneumonia, urinary tract infection |

because of difficulty in removing increased amounts of electrolytes, especially potassium, and waste products from catabolism. Persons with renal disease are at high risk for the development of fluid overload problems during surgery because of the amounts of parenteral fluids administered in the setting of their reduced output.

*Endocrine diseases* that are influenced by hormonal changes occurring with the stress response can affect the patient's response to surgery. Diabetes mellitus should be well controlled before surgery and monitored closely both during and after surgery. Glucocorticoid activity and potassium changes after surgery can influence insulin utilization. If the wound is in an area where the patient has impaired circulation, such as legs and feet, healing may be delayed. In persons who have increased levels of adrenocortical hormones, such as occurs in pituitary or adrenocortical disease or for those receiving exogenous hormones, healing may be delayed because of an antiinflammatory response. In contrast, persons with Addison's disease (hypofunction of the adrenal cortex) or patients receiving hormonal replacement will require additional replacement therapy because of the stress of surgery.

Patients with *impaired nutritional status* are at high risk for developing complications from surgery or anesthesia. Patients most likely to have nutritional deficiencies are those who are elderly and those who are chronically ill, particularly persons with gastrointestinal tract conditions or malignant tumors. The person who is emaciated or cachectic or who has lost considerable weight below an acceptable level usually has a prolonged postoperative recovery.

The *undernourished* person already has diminished reserves of carbohydrates and fats. Body proteins will be utilized to provide the necessary energy requirement to maintain metabolic functioning of cells. Nitrogen imbalances will be greater than normal, and less protein will be available for healing. Collagen, the connective tissue that is the substance of scar tissue, is a protein. Wound healing therefore becomes considerably delayed, and wound separation and infection may occur.

If the surgery is not an emergency and can be delayed for several weeks, the undernourished patient is placed preoperatively on a high-protein, high-carbohydrate diet. In the preoperative or postoperative period total parenteral nutrition (TPN) may be given until the patient is able to tolerate a high-protein, high-carbohydrate diet by mouth. High protein intake will not result in increased body protein unless there is sufficient carbohydrate to provide the necessary energy. Activity or exercise also is required for protein synthesis.

Nutritionally depleted patients usually have a deficiency of vitamins. Vitamins $B_1$, C, and K are necessary for wound healing and clot formation, and supplemental vitamins may be prescribed. Box 23-4 summarizes the common causes of both preoperative and postoperative malnutrition.

**BOX 23-4 Persons at High Risk for Delayed Postoperative Recovery Resulting from Malnutrition**

**PREOPERATIVE MALNUTRITION**

Chronic infection
Inflammatory bowel disorders
Chronic pancreatitis
Carcinoma of stomach or colon
Liver disease
Renal disease
Congestive heart failure
Weight loss (10% of body weight in 3 months before surgery)

**POSTOPERATIVE MALNUTRITION**

Abdominal trauma
Severe multiple trauma (especially pelvic, hip, and leg fracture)
Major burns
Wound sepsis
Acute pancreatitis
Small bowel fistulas
Severe peritonitis

The *obese* patient presents several risk factors for surgery, including enlarged organs such as heart, kidneys, and liver. During surgery, fluctuations of vital signs are more common in the obese person, resulting from the excessive demands on the cardiovascular system. The surgeon incising through layers of fatty tissue has to exert more traction on the tissues to expose the surgical site; this increases trauma to the tissues. Incisional hernias may occur at a later date. During the immediate postoperative period these patients often require more assistance with turning, coughing, and deep breathing. Excess fat deposits often limit movement of the diaphragm, thereby decreasing ventilation. It is also more difficult for obese persons to move about, and they may require additional assistance. Both decreased activity and decreased diaphragm expansion are contributing factors to development of postoperative pulmonary complications. Decreased activity also causes predisposition to thrombophlebitis. Although weight reduction usually cannot be accomplished preoperatively, it is important for the nurse to identify obesity as a risk factor and make appropriate plans for postoperative management.

## Psychologic

Preoperative assessment of the psychologic reaction of the patient includes the collection of both subjective and objective data. Much of the data concerning knowledge and perceptions of the coming event will be obtained directly from the patient (Box 23-5). It is necessary to know the level of the patient's understanding of the surgical event before any teaching can take place. Because persons respond on the basis of their perceptions, it is important to find out exactly how the surgery

**BOX 23-5 Assessment of Preoperative Anxiety**

**SUBJECTIVE DATA**

1. Understanding of proposed surgery
   - Site
   - Type of surgery to be done
   - Information from surgeon regarding extent of hospitalization, postoperative limitations
   - Preoperative routines
   - Postoperative routines
   - Tests
2. Previous surgical experiences
   - Type, nature
   - Time interval
3. Any specific concerns or feelings about present surgery
4. Religion, meaning for patient
5. Significant others
   - Geographic distance
   - Perception as source of support
6. Changes in sleep patterns

**OBJECTIVE DATA**

1. Speech patterns
   - Repetition of themes
   - Change of topic
   - Avoidance of topics related to feelings
2. Degree of interaction with others
3. Physical
   - Increased pulse and respiratory rates
   - Increased hand movements and perspiration
   - Increased activity level
   - Increased voiding frequency

**RESEARCH**

Friedman S, Badere B, Fitzpatrick S: The effects of television viewing on preoperative anxiety, *J Post Anesth Nurs* 7(4):243-250, 1992.

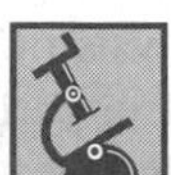

Previous studies have looked at the relationship between preoperative anxiety and postoperative course. However, few studies have looked at methods to decrease preoperative anxiety. To investigate preoperative anxiety and possible anxiety reduction strategies, the investigators devised a clinical study to examine the effects of television viewing on preoperative anxiety. The study compared patients who were not able to watch television in the preoperative setting with those who were. The investigators hypothesized that television viewing in the preoperative setting would decrease preoperative anxiety. A purposive sampling method was chosen so that the study population could be selected using certain criteria. The sample consisted of adult patients 18 to 77 years old who were admitted to the preoperative area at least 2 hours before surgery. A total of 76 subjects participated in the study. However, due to incomplete data on seven of the questionnaires, 7 of the subjects were rejected. Of the remaining 69 subjects, 39 had no television access and the remaining 30 did. Statistical comparisons of the two groups suggest that there was a significant difference in the anxiety levels of the two groups. As hoped, the hypothesis was proven correct: Those subjects who watched television in the preoperative area had significantly lower levels of anxiety than those who did not.



is perceived. Patients may not be able to identify specific concerns, and further exploration may be indicated. If the nurse has identified cues on which conclusions are drawn, these conclusions should be validated with the patient.

Signs of anxiety in the presurgical patient are no different from those in other persons. Signs vary from person to person and can be observed in a number of ways. Highly anxious persons may talk rapidly, ask many questions without waiting for answers, repeat the same questions, or change topics frequently during the interaction. They may deny that they have any worries or fears, but their actions belie this. Some patients will not talk about the forthcoming surgery, responding only in monosyllables, whereas others cry and display anger; both behaviors are overt signs of anxiety. Physical signs include increased pulse and respiratory rate, moist palms, constant hand movements, and restlessness. Changes in sleep patterns also provide clues about increased anxiety. Major causes of insomnia are worry, fear, and concerns about the future.

Knowledge of the meaning of religion for the patient can help the nurse identify a possible source of support. The effect of family members or significant others on the patient's level of anxiety needs to be determined. Some significant others increase the patient's anxiety by transmission of their own anxiety by hovering over the patient, displaying anxious behaviors, or by offering false reassurances. Others are calm, and it is observed that the patient's anxiety is reduced when they are present. See Research box above.

## Social Factors/Family

Assessing the social situation of the patient and family is particularly important if the nurse is incorporating the family as client in the preoperative period. The financial situation of the patient may have considerable implications for both the immediate surgical intervention and the follow-up care. Appropriate referrals to social workers should be made early in the preoperative phase so that discharge planning may be initiated. The social network of support for the patient and family also should be assessed during the preoperative phase. If the family is large, the members should be encouraged to appoint a spokesperson or family liasion, so that not all members are contacting the physician or nurse for information. Specific needs of the family may include lodging if they are from out of town (such as at a tertiary care treatment center). Most communities have a hospitality house to which the family members can be referred for sustenance, support, and lodging during this stressful period.

## ♦ NURSING DIAGNOSES

Nursing diagnoses are determined from analysis of patient data. Nursing diagnoses for the preoperative patient may include but are not limited to the following:

| Diagnostic Title | Possible Etiologic Factors |
|---|---|
| Anxiety | Lack of information about surgery<br>Body image changes<br>Change in health status |
| Nutrition, altered: less than body requirements | NPO Status<br>Chronic diarrhea |
| High risk for altered respiratory function | Anesthesia/sedation, pooled secretions, surgical procedure |
| High risk for potential complication: deep vein thrombosis | Venous stasis, dehydration, increased coagulability of blood |
| Infection, high risk for | Inadequate skin preparation |
| Sleep-pattern disturbance | Anxiety, environment |

See Research box below.

## ♦ EXPECTED PATIENT OUTCOMES

Expected patient outcomes for the patient during the preoperative phase may include but are not limited to the following:

1. Relates an increase in psychologic and physiologic comfort.
2. Experiences adequate nutrition and hydration.
3. Complications of atelectasis or pneumonia are minimized.
4. Complication of deep vein thrombosis are minimized.
5. Complication of postoperative wound infection are minimized.
6. Has adequate rest in the preoperative period.

### RESEARCH

Dennison P, Keeling A: Clinical support for eliminating the nursing diagnosis of knowledge deficit, *Image* 21(3):142-44, 1989.

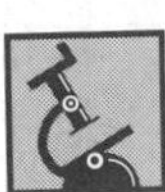

In this study, content analysis of notes accompanying the diagnostic label of "knowledge deficit" revealed that nurses focused their attention on promoting knowledge as an entity in itself rather than addressing a specific behavior (e.g., anxiety or self-care deficit) that related to the patient's lack of information. In reality, knowledge is but one aspect of the factors that determine human behavior, and the nurse's role encompasses more than that of educator. Rather than providing information alone, the nurse's role is to provide assistance to patients with the interpretation of their illness experience and the integration of that experience and its implications into their life-styles. Nurses are not primarily teachers. Eliminating the label "knowledge deficit" would force the nurse to focus on the human response to actual or potential health problems that the nurse is capable of diagnosing and likely to treat.

## ♦ NURSING INTERVENTIONS

Having identified the patient's specific needs and formulated nursing diagnoses, the nurse must collaborate with other health care professionals to implement the plan for treatments, teaching, and emotional support for the patient. A major focus of nursing intervention during this period is **psychologic preparation** of the patient for surgery.

### Preoperative Patient Education

#### Promoting psychologic and physiologic comfort

The purpose of preoperative teaching is to help decrease patient anxiety that might result from lack of information about the surgery. Preoperative teaching prepares the patient for what to expect of surgical procedures or routines and what sensations may be experienced. It also provides the patient with methods for decreasing anxiety and with strategies for enhancing postoperative recovery.

Considerable nursing research has focused on preoperative patient teaching. In general, research has demonstrated that preoperative teaching is effective in (1) decreasing patient anxiety, (2) altering unfavorable attitudes, (3) influencing postoperative recovery, and (4) promoting satisfaction with care.[4,6-8]

Much preoperative teaching focuses on information or activities that may help to decrease patient anxiety. Additional teaching includes activities that enhance physiologic healing by preventing postoperative complications. Because of short postoperative hospital stays, discharge teaching must be initiated during the preoperative period.

Anxiety and fear experienced before surgery may be decreased by different approaches: explanations about what will occur during the expected surgery *(procedural),* what the patient may experience during the perioperative period *(sensory),* and what actions may help to decrease the anxiety *(psychologic).* Fear of the unknown may be partly relieved by knowing what to expect. Procedural information generally has a positive effect by changing the unknown to the known. If the patient is highly anxious, however, too much information may serve only to increase the anxiety.

The amount of information to give preoperatively depends on the background, interest, and stress level of the patient. A good way to decide is to ask patients what they would like to know about the forthcoming surgery and to base responses on the types of questions asked. Persons under considerable stress, such as those in moderate to severe pain, cannot cope with much added stimuli and simple explanations are indicated. A highly anxious person has a narrow perceptual field and may not assimilate concurrent events and information. It is also important to remember that giving someone information does not necessarily mean that the information has been perceived or understood.

The preoperative information helpful to most patients relates to preoperative tests and activities, events related to the surgery, and expectations about what will happen postoperatively. Most patients are less anxious and participate more effectively if they know the reasons for tests and preoperative activities.

Patients experiencing high anxiety may benefit from learning about *situations* that may be experienced during the perioperative period, such as drowsiness after premedication, coldness in the surgical suite (blankets will be applied), absence of discomfort before general anesthesia (except for the needle prick from the IV line through which the initial anesthesia probably will be given), and discomfort in the early postoperative period (medication will be given). It may be helpful to explain the expected pain relief routines so that the patient knows to ask for medication *before* pain becomes severe (see Chapter 17).

Preoperative teaching is done as early in the preoperative period as possible to permit time for the patient to learn. *Preadmission* teaching has been found to be effective for patient learning, and it requires less admission teaching time. Booklets and pamphlets have proved very useful for reinforcing the information. Preadmission teaching has been used recently to address patients' informational needs in preparation for ambulatory surgery or same-day admission. Teaching during the 24 hours before surgery has been demonstrated to be less effective than teaching initiated at an earlier date. This finding is related to high anxiety levels in patients immediately before surgery. Review or reinforcement of previously learned materials, however, is effective immediately before surgery. See Research box above.

**RESEARCH**

Kratz A: Preoperative education: preparing patients for a positive experience, *J Post Anesth Nurs* 8(4):270-275, 1990.

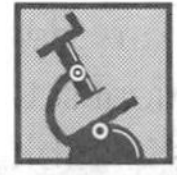

Education can be lost amid the fast pace of advanced technology, decreased financial reimbursement, and increased volume of ambulatory surgery. Preoperative education is important to the patient, family, physicians, and nurses, and it can be provided in many ways. This article describes a preoperative registration education program developed at Hartford Memorial Hospital (Hartford, Wis). Hartford's experience has shown that the program facilitated decreased anxiety and earlier patient discharge, with resultant decrease in cost of hospitalization. Other institutions can tailor this patient-focused education program to their needs. Preoperative education is both an important and rewarding area of nursing and should not be lost in the fast-paced health care environment.

### Providing emotional support

Demonstrating a caring attitude is essential in providing emotional support for patients and families during the stressful time before surgery. The opportunity to talk with a supportive, knowledgeable person will help patients begin to identify the reasons for their anxiety and to marshal coping responses. It is helpful for the nurse to plan for a quiet, unhurried time to sit down with the patient and provide an opportunity to ask questions and talk about concerns. Thus, spending time with the patient is one aspect of demonstrating caring. Touch is another form of communication that sends the message, "I care." Some patients will talk more readily while receiving a back rub. Just knowing that a nurse is interested and cares helps to reduce anxiety. Knowing that anxiety is a normal reaction to the threat of surgery may help to remove the often self-imposed expectation, "I shouldn't be nervous." Preoperative visits by the operating room nurse are helpful in many instances, especially in those situations that provoke a great deal of anxiety, such as heart surgery. The visit promotes the feeling that "someone in surgery knows me as an individual and will look after me." If it is known that the patient will be in intensive care for a period of time after surgery, a visit by a nurse from the intensive care unit also may help to allay anxiety.

Empowering patients by increasing their sense of control before surgery is essential for decreasing patient anxiety. Loss of control is one of the fears associated with surgery. Allowing patients to participate in decision making concerning care when that is a realistic option helps to meet the need for the patient to maintain some control over the events. Patients also may be taught activities that help to decrease anxiety and to gain a sense of control over their reactions. The most common approaches are deep breathing, relaxation exercises, music therapy, and guided imagery.

Supporting family and friends is a third component of providing emotional support in the preoperative phase. The patient's family members or close friends are frequently as anxious as the patient in the time before surgery. This anxiety can be transmitted to patients, increasing their anxiety levels. The same principles described in exploring concerns and giving information to the patient hold true for significant others. Listening is especially important. Some of the family members' needs are quite different from the patient's. They may simply need to know where to wait during surgery, what time the surgery will be done and where to find food, bathrooms, elevators, telephones, parking, or a place to stay the night. All this information should be given in a calm, timely manner. See Research box, p. 600.

**RESEARCH**

Sheperd S: Helping ambulatory surgery patients cope with emotions, *J Post Anesth Nurs* 5(2):103-105, 1990.

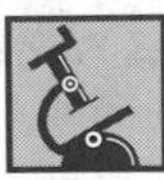

Ambulatory surgical settings often are described as "happier places" than inpatient settings. However, ambulatory patients exhibit strong emotions, including fear, confusion, embarrassment, anger, sadness, and sometimes full-blown panic, despair, and helplessness. Nurses in these centers must guard against being lulled into a false sense of ease about emotional issues. There is no "recipe" for dealing with difficult, abstract, emotional situations. A common mistake helpers make is that of trying to talk people out of their feelings. Active listening is important. Being in touch with ourselves and sharing with patients is essential to being present with the patient in his or her experience.

### Use of medications

Not infrequently, the anxious preoperative patient may require medication to relieve anxiety. Among those drugs most commonly used are Midazolam (Versed), Lorazepam (Ativan), and Diazepam (Valium). Other medications that may be administered include hypnotics (such as chloral hydrate, flurazepam), narcotics, anticholinergics, and/or histamine receptor antagonists (cimetidine and ranitidine). The nurse should be aware that any of these medications may be needed and should not hesitate to ensure that the patient is made comfortable during this stressful time. Table 23-5 lists the dosages and routes of administration for commonly used antianxiety agents.

### Promoting adequate nutrition/hydration

On the day before surgery there is usually no change in the patient's diet. (One exception is bowel surgery, in which case patients may be placed preoperatively on a low-residue or clear-liquid diet). If general anesthesia is planned, food and fluids usually are not permitted for 4 to 8 hours before surgery. The presence of food or fluids in the stomach increases the possibility of aspiration of gastric contents should the patient vomit while under anesthesia. Such vomiting with aspiration can lead to aspiration pneumonia. If it should be discovered that the patient has consumed food or fluids when "nothing by mouth" (NPO) has been ordered, the surgeon is notified. This finding may require rescheduling of the surgical procedure. If local or spinal anesthesia is planned, a light meal or clear liquids may be permitted.

Patients who are dehydrated will have parenteral fluids initiated before surgery. If it is anticipated that the patient may have decreased peristalsis after surgery (such as after gastrointestinal surgery), a nasogastric tube may be inserted before surgery.

**TABLE 23-5 Commonly Ordered Antianxiety Medications**

| MEDICATION | DOSAGE (MG) | ROUTE |
|---|---|---|
| Midazolam (Versed) | 1-4 | IM, IV |
| Lorazepam (Ativan) | 0.5-2 | PO, IM |
| Diazepam (Valium) | 5-15 | PO, IM, IV |

### Minimizing the potential for atelectasis or pneumonia

Teaching the patient about the necessity of deep breathing and coughing after surgery is a common component of preoperative education. Deep breathing facilitates oxygenation and removal of residual inhalant anesthetics. It also prevents alveolar collapse that leads to atelectasis. Coughing removes secretions that may block the airways. All patients potentially at risk for postoperative pulmonary complications are taught deep breathing and coughing exercises before surgery. Waiting to do so until the patient is awakening from anesthesia decreases the possibility that these exercises will be carried out effectively; anesthesia and postoperative pain decrease the ability to retain information.

All patients need to know how to perform correct diaphragmatic breathing because it increases lung expansion by permitting the diaphragm to descend fully (Box 23-6). Many men normally breathe diaphragmatically, whereas few females do. With diaphragmatic breathing, the *abdomen rises with inspiration and falls with expiration.* The nurse assesses the patient's normal breathing pattern by placing a hand lightly on the patient's abdomen and asking the patient to take a deep breath. If diaphragmatic breathing does not occur naturally, the patient can be taught to inspire deeply while pushing the abdomen up against the hand. It is important for the patient to hold the breath for 3 seconds for most effective alveolar expansion. If there is difficulty with a deep cough, encourage the patient to do a "huff" cough. Repeated huff coughs often stimulate a deep cough. The patient also is shown how to splint an incision with a pillow, towel, or hands to help decrease pain while coughing. See Research box, p. 601.

### Minimizing the potential for deep vein thrombosis

Preoperative teaching about essential leg exercises is important to minimize the patient's potential for postoperative deep vein thrombosis (DVT). Venous stasis in the postoperative period may lead to thrombophlebitis (blood clot). This in turn could lead to a pulmonary embolism. Patients at high risk for the development of DVT include those who (1) will have decreased mobility after surgery, (2) have a history of decreased peripheral circulation, or (3) experience cardiovascular or pelvic surgery. These patients will need to perform exercises

**BOX 23-6 Deep Breathing and Coughing Exercises**

**DEEP BREATHING**
1. Lie in semi-Fowler's or high Fowler's position with knees flexed to relax abdomen and allow full chest expansion.
2. Place a hand lightly on the abdomen.
3. Breathe in slowly through nose, letting chest expand and feeling abdomen rise against hand.
4. Hold breath for 3 seconds.
5. Exhale slowly through pursed lips (abdomen contracts).
6. Repeat deep breathing three times, then cough (see below).

**COUGHING**
1. Breathe in as described above.
2. Count to 3.
3. On "3," cough *deeply* three times.
4. If unable to cough deeply, do repeated "huff" coughs (forced expiration with glottis open).

postoperatively to prevent venous stasis in the legs. Leg exercises help to prevent venous congestion by "pumping" the blood along the veins. Valves in the veins prevent backflow of blood.

Moving and turning in bed help to prevent pulmonary and circulatory complications, prevent decubiti, stimulate peristalsis, and decrease pain. During the postoperative period, patients can be taught how to use the side rails effectively for turning and how to sit up on the side of the bed with the least amount of pull on the incision.

*To turn to right side:*
1. Slide hips to left side of bed.
2. Support incision with right hand.
3. Flex left knee.
4. Grasp right side rail with left hand.
5. Pull with left hand while pushing with left leg to turn.

*To sit up on side of bed before ambulation:*
1. Move to edge of bed.
2. Raise head of bed to high Fowler's position.
3. Drop feet over side of bed.
4. Push up to sitting position with hand closest to edge of bed (other hand can support the incision).

### Minimizing the potential for postoperative wound infection

**Bowel preparation.** Cleansing the bowel preoperatively by means of enemas is not a routine procedure. The surgeon makes the decision on the basis of the surgical site and type of surgery to be performed. Preoperative enemas may be ordered before gastrointestinal tract surgery or surgery on the pelvic, perineal, or perianal areas. The purpose of the preoperative enema is to prevent injury to the colon and to provide better visualization of the surgical area. Enemas should be given if a patient has had x-ray studies involving barium immediately before surgery, because barium remaining in the intestinal tract may cause predisposition to postoperative fecal impactions. Enemas given preoperatively should be effective.

If enemas are to be given until the returns are clear, it is important to remember that fluid excess and potassium deficits can occur with repeated enemas. It is common practice to check with the physician if returns are not clear after the third enema. One method is to give up to three enemas the evening before surgery and then, if the returns are still not clear, to repeat the enemas the following morning. Repeated enemas are very tiring to the patient and may irritate rectal and bowel mucosa.

Controversy exists regarding the benefits of antibiotic

**RESEARCH**

Yount S, Schoessler M: A description of patient and nurse perceptions of preoperative teaching, *J Post Anesth Nurs* 6(1):17-25, 1991.

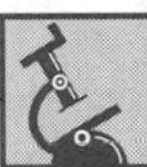

While research has shown preoperative teaching to be an essential nursing activity, it has become increasingly difficult to accomplish. Increased outpatient surgery and morning admission on the day of surgery have reduced time available for assessment and preparation activities, including teaching. In this study, 116 postsurgical patients and 159 hospital-employed nurses completed an investigator-developed questionnaire. The statements were written to operationalize the five dimensions of preoperative teaching: psychosocial support, situational information, patient role, sensation-discomfort, and skills training. For each of the questionnaire statements, subjects were asked to (1) rate the importance on a 5-point Likert type of scale ranging from "not important" to "very important" and (2) indicate the preferred timing for teaching to occur: before admission to the hospital, between admission and surgery, or at the time of the event. Patients also indicated whether they received the teaching from a nurse. Mean ratings of importance for both groups ranged from moderately important to important, with the nurses reporting the wider range of importance. Analysis showed a discrepancy between nurse and patient rank orderings as determined by mean ratings of importance. Patients rated the order or importance as listed above, which is parallel to the reported frequency of receiving instruction. The two groups differ in the ordering only in the placement of skills training. Nurses placed skills training second; patients placed it last. Both groups preferred delivering and receiving teaching between admission to the hospital and surgery. Independent *t* test results indicated nurses assigned more importance to psychosocial support and skills training than did patients; patients assigned more importance to sensation-discomfort than did nurses.

enemas, because of the disturbance of the ecology of the bowel flora. If antibiotic enemas are ordered, synthesis of vitamin K by intestinal bacteria may be inhibited; supplementary vitamin K may therefore be given to prevent increased bleeding after surgery.

**Skin preparation.** The recommended practices developed by the Association of Operating Room Nurses (AORN) Recommended Practices subcommittee provide a guideline for preoperative skin preparation of the operative site.[1] The goal of this skin preparation is to reduce the risk of postoperative wound infection by (1) removing soil and transient microbes from the skin, (2) reducing the resident microbial count to subpathogenic amounts in a short period of time and with the least amount of tissue irritation, and (3) inhibiting rapid rebound growth of microbes.

*Recommended practice No. 1:* "The area surrounding the operative site should be clean."[1] Cleansing of the skin can be accomplished by patient showers (with such solutions as Hibiclens) and by washing the operative site either on the patient unit or immediately before applying the antimicrobial agent in the operating room. The operative area skin should be assessed for skin integrity before cleansing. Traumatized skin may require saline irrigation as the cleansing agent. Hair should remain at the operative site unless it interferes with the surgical procedure (e.g., craniotomy). Shaving should be done only when other methods of hair removal are not available or when time does not permit their use. Shaving should be done as close to the time of the operative procedure as possible. The wet method of shaving is desirable.

**RESEARCH**

Jepsen OB, Bruttomesso KA: The effectiveness of preoperative skin preparations: an integrative review of the literature, *AORN J* 58(3):477-484, 1993.

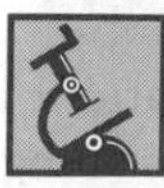

This article reviews several studies, including preoperative whole-body disinfections, operative site skin preparations, and hair-removal techniques. The clinical studies strongly support preoperative skin preparation using antimicrobial agents during repeated (two) showers, using showers rather than baths for reducing skin flora, using chlorhexidine to reduce the incidence of postoperative wound infections, using alcohol to enhance drape adherence to skin, using either 70% isopropyl alcohol or iodophor-in-alcohol solution for 1 minute before applying antimicrobial adhesive wound drapes. Studies also support that a clippers or a depilatory cream should be used to remove hair. Preoperative skin preparation profoundly influences how well wounds heal after surgery, and researchers should continue to develop new techniques for skin disinfection.

*Recommended practice No. 2:* "The skin of the operative site and surrounding area should be prepared with an antimicrobial agent before the incision."[1] The agent used should have broad-spectrum antimicrobial action, be nontoxic, and provide long-acting antimicrobial protection. See Research box below.

In the case of ambulatory surgery or same day admission, patients are responsible for their own shower and general cleansing. Further skin preparation will be done in the operating room.

### Promoting rest and sleep

Because surgery is traumatic and therefore stressful, energy is required for coping. Sleep and rest conserve energy and thus are important before surgery. A sedative usually is ordered for the night before surgery to ensure a good night's rest. If additional sedation or medication for pain is given during the night, it must be given at least 4 hours before the preoperative medication.

The preadmitted patient should be allowed to sleep on the morning of surgery for as long as possible and to rest undisturbed until shortly before administration of the preanesthetic medication. Many patients therefore prefer to take their bath or shower the evening before surgery rather than in the morning. The patient who has bathed the night before is given an opportunity to wash hands and face and to perform mouth care. The patient is reminded not to swallow any water if fluids by mouth are not permitted. A hospital gown is worn to surgery.

Comfort implies readiness for surgery and ability to marshal effective coping mechanisms. The patient should have an opportunity to have last-minute questions answered. Explanations for last-minute routines are given if this was not done previously. If the surgery is to be delayed even for a short time, both the patient and family should be informed.

### Final preparations for surgery

**Informed consent.** Before surgery the patient is asked to sign a statement indicating consent to have the operative procedure performed. The consent implies that the patient has been given the information necessary to understand the nature of the procedure, as well as the known and possible consequences of the procedure. The physician has the responsibility to provide the patient with sufficient information to weigh the risks and benefits of the proposed surgery (disclosure duty). The information usually includes the nature of the surgery with its benefits and risks, alternatives to the surgery and those benefits and risks, and prognosis if treatment is withheld. Risks include bodily harm or death, but not the common possible postoperative complications such as infection. Legal responsibility for obtaining informed consent from the patient, therefore, resides with the physician. Verbal consent is as binding as written consent.

Signing of the official consent form primarily provides

evidence that the consent process has occurred and that the patient is aware of the concept of informed consent. The signature of a member of the health care staff (as required by specific states or hospitals) merely provides witness to the signature of the patient or family member. The nurse's signature does not reflect the substance of the informed consent process.

The role of the nurse in this process is one of patient advocate. The nurse should verify that the patient has discussed with the physician the risks and benefits of the surgery and the alternatives. If this discussion has not taken place, the nurse should consult with the physician. To clarify any misconceptions and to facilitate the decision-making process the nurse also should assess the patient's understanding of what is to occur in surgery and afterward. Patients may decide to refuse surgery, and it is their right to do so. Nurses have the responsibility to see that the decision is an informed one. It is imperative that this process occur before the patient receives any sedation.

If an adult is incapable of giving informed consent, consent must be obtained from the next of kin. The order of kin relationship for an adult, as determined from legal intestate succession, is usually spouse, adult child, parent, sibling. A parent or legal guardian usually provides consent for a minor child. "Emancipated minors," that is, minors who are married or earning their own livelihood and retaining the earnings, can sign their own permit. The signature of the husband or wife of a married minor is also acceptable.

In an emergency situation, the surgeon may operate without written permission of the patient or family, although every effort is made to contact a family member or guardian if time permits. Consent in the form of a telephone call is permissible in this situation. The call must be witnessed.

**Safeguarding personal belongings.** Objects such as eyeglasses or prostheses sent to the operating room with the patient may become lost or damaged. For this reason, prostheses such as dentures and prosthetic limbs or eyes usually are removed, labeled, and placed in safekeeping. Patients who want to take religious medals to the operating room should be advised that in many instances paper emblems can be obtained from their clergy. All money and jewelry, including wedding rings, should be sent home with the family or removed from the bedside and sent to the hospital safe.

**Premedication.** Before the patient is transferred to the operating room, a routine checklist (Box 23-7) is completed to ensure that the patient has been properly prepared for surgery. Before any premedication is given, it is imperative that a check is made to ascertain that a consent form has been completed and placed at the front of the chart. After premedication has been given, the

**BOX 23-7 Sample Preoperative Checklist**

| | YES | NO | N/A |
|---|---|---|---|
| Identaband checked (correct name and number) | | | |
| Blood identification band in place | | | |
| NPO since ________ | | | |
| Patient properly attired for surgery: | | | |
| • hospital gown | | | |
| • jewelry removed | | | |
| • dentures removed | | | |
| • other prostheses removed | | | |
| • chewing gum removed | | | |
| • lipstick and makeup removed | | | |
| • all nail polish removed | | | |
| • hair pins and clips removed | | | |
| Patient voided or catheterized—time: ________ | | | |
| Premedication given and charted—time: ________ | | | |
| Preoperative BP: ____ P ____ R ____ T ____ | | | |
| Operative permit signed and in chart | | | |
| Blood permit signed and in chart | | | |
| Old chart attached | | | |
| Addressograph plate or preprinted labels in chart | | | |
| Clinical laboratory reports in chart | | | |
| Interim summary in chart | | | |
| Scheduled medications placed on "hold" | | | |
| Isolation—type: ____ | | | |
| Remarks: | | | |

Date: Signed: ____________________

**BOX 23-8 Premedications Frequently Used**

Antianxiety agents:
- Midazolam (Versed)
- Diazepam (Valium)
- Lorazepam (Ativan)

Narcotics:
- Meperidine (Demerol)
- Morphine
- Fentanyl

Anticholinergics:
- Atropine
- Glycopyrrolate (Robinul)

patient will be too sleepy to ensure that he or she understands the purpose and risks of the surgery and gives consent. The purposes of **premedication** are (1) to decrease anxiety and provide sedation (sedatives, hypnotics), (2) to decrease secretion of saliva and gastric juices (anticholinergics), and (3) to relieve pain and discomfort (narcotics). These medications frequently are given "on call to the OR" but also may be given just before anesthesia induction in the operating room suite (Box 23-8). Premedications may be omitted altogether, depending on the preference of the anesthesiologist. The use of premedication is particularly important if airway clearance problems are anticipated (anticholinergics are used) and before major surgery such as heart surgery when the patient is particularly anxious. Once premedications have been administered, it is essential that the patient be kept in bed with the side rails up to ensure safety.

**Preoperative checklist.** A final set of preoperative vital signs should be taken at this time. These provide a baseline for identification of significant changes during the intraoperative and postoperative phases. It is normal for the pulse rate and systolic blood pressure to be increased from baseline levels as a result of the immediacy of the stressful situation; however, significant changes are reported to the surgeon. Other data to be reported are temperature elevation (possible infection) or expressions of a new or different type of pain.

The patient's identification band is checked for accuracy, legibility, and firmness of attachment. The band will also be checked by the nurse in the operating room suite. This action protects the patient from undergoing surgery designated for another person.

The patient usually is placed on a stretcher, covered carefully with a blanket, and transported to the operating suite. The nurse should accompany the patient to the operating room if the person is critically ill, medically unstable, or extremely anxious. It is essential that the patient's old chart and current chart accompany the patient. Well-documented, accurate preoperative information serves as a reference for the surgical team, as well as providing a concise evaluation of all preoperative care.

## EVALUATION: THE PREOPERATIVE DOCUMENTATION

The nursing report, both oral and written, serves as a concise evaluation of the care given during the preoperative phase. Biopsychosocial assessment data are recorded and any important findings reported to the operating room nurse. Any preoperative teaching and the patient's response to that teaching also should be recorded. In addition, any relevant social factors that need to be considered while the patient is in surgery should be reported. Preoperative medications and laboratory results also should be mentioned to the operating room nurse.

## QUESTIONS TO CONSIDER

- What strategies could a nurse implement to ensure that preoperative patient teaching can occur in a fast-paced ambulatory surgical clinic?
- What is the purpose of preoperative skin preparation?
- Discuss the risk for the development of deep vein thrombosis for the following patients: (1) a 32-year-old, obese woman with diabetes who is scheduled for total abdominal hysterectomy, (2) a young, previously healthy male who is scheduled for emergency appendectomy, and (3) a 75-year-old man who is scheduled for open heart surgery.
- Why is it important to teach deep breathing and coughing exercises to patients in the preoperative phase?

## CRITICAL THINKING ACTIVITIES

- Mrs. Todd, 68, is scheduled for a bowel resection in the morning. It is known that there is a tumor present that is producing a partial obstruction. It is not known whether the tumor is malignant. Mrs. Todd is very concerned about the outcome of her surgery. What signs and symptoms would you observe for in order to assess her physiologic status? Psychologic status?
- Give at least one fear that may be expressed by patients undergoing each of the following types of surgery in addition to fear of the surgery itself or anesthesia: emergency; diagnostic; cosmetic; palliative; curative.

## CHAPTER SUMMARY

### INTRODUCTION

- Contemporary perioperative nursing practice is patient-centered rather than task-oriented.
- Perioperative nursing practice is defined as the activities performed by the professional nurse during the preoperative, intraoperative, and postoperative phases of the patient's surgical experience.

- The preoperative phase begins when the decision for surgical intervention is made.

### TYPES OF SURGERY

- Surgery may be classified by extent, purpose, body site, timing, or physical setting.

### BIOPSYCHOSOCIAL RESPONSES IN THE PREOPERATIVE PHASE

- Surgery is a unique experience for each patient. Surgery is a stressor that produces both physiologic stress reactions and psychologic reactions. It is also a social stressor, requiring family adaptation to temporary or lasting role changes.

### NURSING MANAGEMENT

- Nursing management of the preoperative patient includes physiologic, psychologic, and family assessment.
- Populations at high risk for surgical/anesthetic complications include elderly patients, patients with chronic diseases, and patients with impaired nutritional status.
- Nursing diagnoses for the preoperative patient include anxiety, related to lack of information, body image changes, or change in health status; nutrition, alteration in; high risk for potential complication, respiratory; high risk for nosocomial infections; and sleep pattern disturbance.
- Desired nursing outcomes in the preoperative phase include the following: (1) the patient will relate an increase in psychologic and physiologic comfort; (2) the patient will experience adequate nutrition and hydration; (3) complications of atelectasis or pneumonia will be minimized; (4) the complications of deep vein thrombosis and postoperative wound infection will be minimized; and (5) the patient will have adequate rest in the preoperative period.
- Nursing interventions to decrease anxiety include preoperative teaching, emotional support, relaxation, diversion, and medications.
- The nurse should promote adequate nutrition and hydration.
- Preoperative teaching about coughing and deep breathing is essential.
- Preoperative teaching about the importance of mobility in the postoperative phase is essential.
- Hypnotic agents may be required to promote sleep.
- Final preparations for surgery include completing the physical care documented on the preoperative checklist, safeguarding belongings, obtaining informed consent, and transporting the patient to the operating room.

## REFERENCES


1. Association of Operating Room Nurses Recommended Practices subcommittee: Recommended practices for preoperative skin preparation of patients, Part 3. In *AORN standards and recommended practices for perioperative nursing,* Denver, 1993, The Associated Press.
2. Dennison P, Keeling A: Clinical support for eliminating the nursing diagnosis of knowledge deficit, *Image* 21(3):142-144, 1989.
3. Friedman S, Badere B, Fitzpatrick S: The effects of television viewing on preoperative anxiety, *J Post Anesth Nurs* 7(4):243-250, 1992.
4. Kratz A: Preoperative education: preparing patients for a positive experience, *J Post Anesth Nurs* 8(4):270-275, 1993.
5. Jepsen OB, Bruttomesso KA: The effectiveness of preoperative skin preparations, *AORN J* 58(3):477-484, 1993.
6. Sheperd S: Helping ambulatory surgery patients cope with emotions, *J Post Anesth Nurs* 5(2):103-105, 1990.
7. Wong C: Preoperative patient preparation, *J Post Anesth Nurs* 5(3):149-156, 1990.
8. Yount S, Schoessler M: A description of patient and nurse perceptions of preoperative teaching, *J Post Anesth Nurs* 6(1):17-25, 1991.

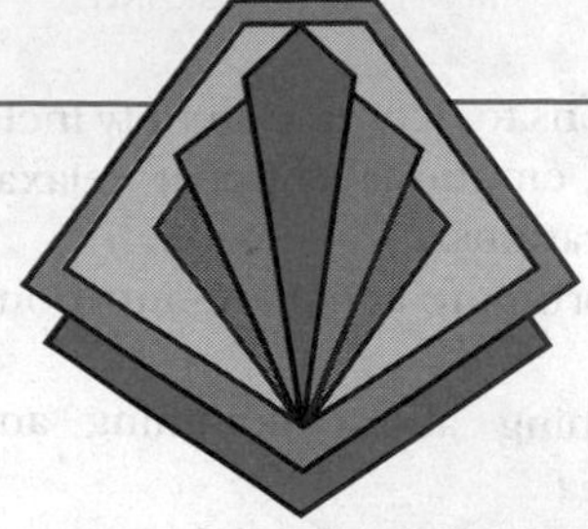

CHAPTER 24

# Intraoperative Nursing

*Grace A. Muro*
*Arlene W. Keeling*
*Barbara C. Long*

## CHAPTER OBJECTIVES

***After studying this chapter, the learner should be able to do the following:***

1. Describe the intraoperative phase as a component of the surgical experience.
2. Identify the subspecialties in surgery.
3. Identify the members of the surgical health care team.
4. Discuss the significance of aseptic technique maintenance.
5. Identify appropriate attire for wear in the surgical suite.
6. Describe the different types of anesthesia.
7. Identify the physiologic stress responses to anesthesia and surgery.
8. Discuss intraoperative patient assessment.
9. Identify intraoperative nursing diagnoses.
10. Identify the areas of high risk for patients in the intraoperative phase.
11. Identify desired patient outcomes for the intraoperative phase.
12. Discuss nursing interventions to minimize intraoperative risks.
13. Discuss the importance of evaluation of nursing care interventions.

## KEY TERMS

anesthesiologist
aseptic technique
barbiturates
circulating nurse
general anesthesia
induced hypothermia
induction phase
inhalation anesthesia
intraoperative phase
local anesthesia
maintenance phase
malignant hyperthermia
narcotics
nerve block anesthesia
nurse anesthetist
operating surgeon
preinduction phase
regional anesthesia
reversal/extubation phase
scrub nurse
skeletal muscle relaxant
spinal anesthesia
surgical assistant
universal precautions

The arrival of the patient in the operating room initiates the **intraoperative phase.** This phase continues until the patient is transferred to the postanesthesia receiving unit. Patient assessments begun in the preoperative phase are continued by the surgical health care team. Assessment of physical, emotional, and psychologic status is performed by both the anesthesiologist and the perioperative nurse to determine the patient's readiness for surgery. Intraoperative activities of the health care team are directed toward efficient facilitation and completion of the surgical procedure, maintenance of homeostasis, ensurance of patient safety, and support of the patient's psychosocial needs.

## TYPES OF SURGERY

The types of operations performed in a hospital or other facility vary according to the expertise of the surgeons on the staff, the community in which the facility is located, and the equipment available. Surgeons' training typically focuses on one subspecialty. Each subspecialty involves procedures performed in a specific system or anatomic region (Box 24-1).

## THE SURGICAL HEALTH CARE TEAM

During the intraoperative phase, the surgical patient is surrounded and closely monitored by individuals as-

**BOX 24-1 Procedures of Surgical Subspecialties**

**GENERAL SURGERY**
Digestive system structures, abdominal wall, thyroid, and breast—e.g., mastectomy, bowel resection, ventral herniorrhaphy

**GYNECOLOGY AND OBSTETRICS**
Female reproductive system—e.g., hysterectomy, cesarean section

**GENITOURINARY SURGERY**
Male reproductive system, male and female renal system—e.g., prostatectomy, cystoscopy

**ORTHOPEDIC SURGERY**
Musculoskeletal system—e.g., knee reconstruction, fracture repair, spinal fusion

**NEUROSURGERY**
Brain, spinal cord, and nerves—e.g., cerebral aneurysm clipping, laminectomy

**THORACIC AND CARDIOVASCULAR SURGERY**
Pulmonary structures, heart, great vessels, and peripheral vascular system—e.g., lung resection, femoral-popliteal vein bypass graft, mitral or aortic valve repair

**OPHTHALMIC SURGERY**
Eye structures—e.g., corneal transplantation, vitrectomy, cataract removal

**OTORHINOLARYNGOLOGY, HEAD, AND NECK SURGERY**
Ear, nose, throat, trachea, and esophagus—e.g., stapedectomy, laryngectomy, tracheostomy

**PLASTIC AND RECONSTRUCTIVE SURGERY**
Congenital or trauma-induced abnormalities or disfigurement, cosmetic corrections—e.g., skin grafting, cleft palate repair, face lift

signed specific duties. These persons make up the surgical health care team. The team works collaboratively to maintain homeostasis and to achieve a successful outcome for the surgical patient. The team comprises a surgeon, surgical assistants, an anesthesiologist or nurse anesthetist, a circulating nurse, and a scrub nurse (Figure 24-1).

The **operating surgeon** possesses the ability to perform the intended operation and the knowledge and judgment to diagnose and manage the patient before, during, and after the surgical intervention. The surgeon may be assisted by a surgical resident, an intern, a physician's assistant, or a perioperative nurse. The **surgical assistant** facilitates the efficient completion of the procedure by providing wound retraction and assisting with hemostasis, suturing, or other tasks requested by the surgeon.

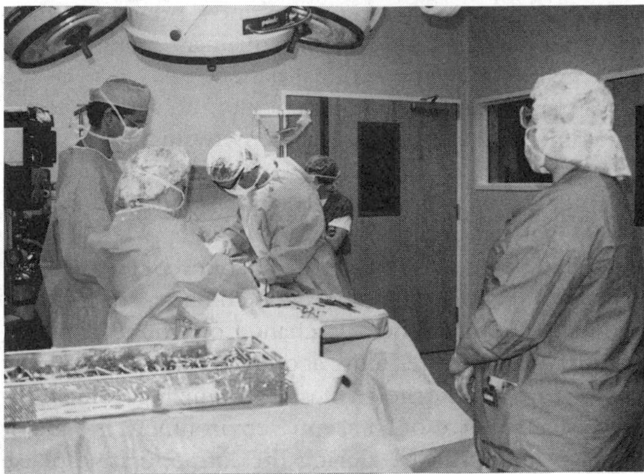

**FIGURE 24-1** The surgical team: surgeon, assistant, scrub nurse, and perioperative nurse.

The **anesthesiologist** is a physician who specializes in the administration of anesthetic agents and monitoring of patients' responses to these agents. The anesthesiologist maintains the overall well-being of the patient during and immediately after a surgical intervention. The **nurse anesthetist** is an advanced registered nurse practitioner who, after additional training and certification in anesthesia, may administer an anesthetic and monitor a patient under the supervision of an anesthesiologist.

The **circulating nurse** is a registered professional nurse who coordinates the overall patient care activities and environment of the operating room. This person is vital to the effective flow of patient care before, during, and after the surgical procedure and for this reason is called a *perioperative nurse.*[2] The circulating nurse has the overall picture of patient care needs and serves as a patient advocate throughout the surgical experience. Further discussion of perioperative nursing activities may be found in the section on nursing management of the intraoperative patient (pp. 617-628).

The **scrub nurse** may be either a nurse or a surgical technician. This person is responsible for the preparation of sterile supplies and instrumentation for the procedure, the delivery of requested items to the surgeon and assistants, and the return of these items at the end of the procedure.

A number of allied personnel also contribute to meeting the needs of the surgical patient. These persons include clerical personnel, blood bank employees, laboratory technicians, pharmacists, central service employees, radiologists, pathologists, and nursing assistants.

## ASEPTIC TECHNIQUE MAINTENANCE

Postoperative wound infection is a serious, potentially fatal complication. Because most wound infections are acquired in the operating room, most preventive measures are directed toward three primary areas:

1. Preparation of the surgical patient
2. Technical and aseptic practice of the surgical team
3. Maintenance of the surgical environment

Preparation of the surgical patient is discussed in Chapter 23. Intraoperatively, strict standards for environmental control, proper attire, and appropriate surgical hand scrub, as well as strict adherence to **aseptic technique** and good operative technique, are aimed at reducing the incidence or chance of wound contamination. All personnel must acquire the knowledge necessary to perform their role in minimizing contamination. Maintenance of an aseptic environment is a major focus of nursing care during the intraoperative phase and is discussed later in the implementation of nursing care activities. Any break in technique exposes the patient to a risk that could have been prevented. Concern for asepsis carries over into the postoperative period and remains a major focus of nursing care.

## SURGICAL SUITE DESIGN

The activities that occur in a surgical suite have one common goal: to provide a safe, therapeutic environment for the patient. The purposes of a modern surgical suite are as follows:

- To ensure geographic isolation from unauthorized persons
- To centralize equipment, supplies, and personnel
- To obtain bacteriologic isolation through specific practices, attire, delivery, and disposal systems

The floor plan of a surgical suite is divided into three zones: unrestricted, semirestricted, and restricted. The *unrestricted area* provides an entrance to and exit from the surgical suite. The holding/admission area and postanesthesia care unit may be found in this zone, along with dressing rooms, lounges, offices, and storage areas. Street clothes are permitted in this area. The *semirestricted area* provides access to the procedure rooms and peripheral support areas within the surgical suite. Proper operating room attire is required to be worn by all personnel in this area. Peripheral support areas consist of storage areas for clean and sterile supplies, a sterile processing area and corridors leading to procedure rooms, and substerile utility areas. The *restricted area* includes the procedure room in which surgery is performed and adjacent substerile areas where the scrub sinks and autoclaves are located. In addition to proper operating room attire, a surgical mask is required to be worn by all personnel in this area for maximum protection from possible contamination.

An effective communication system is a vital link within a surgical suite, which by design must have distinct separate and closed areas. An intercom system that links a procedure room with other procedure rooms, admission areas, blood bank, radiology department, and postanesthesia unit assists in relaying appropriate information among all members of the health care team. Call light systems are effective in summoning personnel for emergent or routine assistance.

## PROTECTIVE BARRIERS (ATTIRE)[6]

Known sources of contamination in the surgical suite are people (skin, hair, and nasopharynx), contaminated inanimate objects, air, and human error (aseptic technique breaks). Efforts are made to reduce or eliminate these sources through the following:

- Appropriate operating room attire for personnel
- Effective barrier fabrics for patients and personnel for use in the sterile field
- Strict housekeeping protocols
- Efficient air-handling systems
- Meticulous adherence to aseptic technique by the surgical team

Operating room attire worn by health care workers within the operating room lessens the risk of infection for the patient. Each item of attire serves as a means of protection against potential sources of environmental contamination. Apparel includes scrub suit, hat or hood, shoe covers, and face mask (Figure 24-2).

***Scrub suits*** are one- or two-piece pantsuits. Cover jackets or gowns may be worn to maximize skin coverage. Material should be lint-free, cool, and comfortable.

***Head coverings*** (caps and hoods) are used because hair attracts, harbors, and sheds bacteria. Hoods are nec-

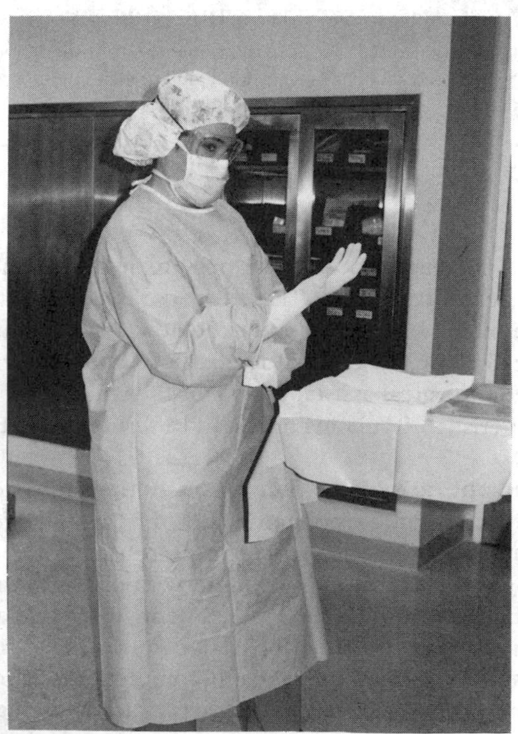

**FIGURE 24-2** Operating room attire.

essary for coverage of beards. All possible head and facial hair, including sideburns and neckline, should be completely covered before other attire is donned. This prevents the possibility of bacteria being shed onto the scrub suit.

*Shoe coverings* should be worn by all persons entering the restricted areas of the surgical suite. When the same shoe covers are worn in the operating room for successive operations, they will have a very high bacterial count, with the potential for cross-infection. The shoe covers are removed when personnel leave restricted areas, and clean ones are reapplied on their return. This prevents cross-contamination with other areas of the hospital. In the interest of safety, clogs, sandals, and canvas shoes should not be worn in the operating room. Clogs can be a hazard when a person tries to move quickly, and if sharp objects are accidentally dropped, sandals and canvas shoes provide little protection.

*Masks* worn by personnel in restricted areas of the surgical suite prevent droplets from the oropharynx or nasopharynx from being expelled into the surgical environment. Disposable high-filtration masks should completely cover the mouth and nose and be secured to prevent venting from occurring at the sides.

Masks should be worn either completely on or completely off. They should not be draped loosely around the neck. If this is done, bacteria that have been filtered onto the mask will become dry and airborne. When masks are removed, only the strings are touched to reduce contamination of the hands from the nasopharyngeal area. Masks are changed between cases and more often if they become moist during a long case.

An additional consideration of operating room attire includes jewelry. Dangling necklaces and earrings may fall into the sterile field. Rings with stones should not be worn because they interfere with good handwashing. In addition, they could possibly injure a patient's skin during transfers.

*Lead aprons* and *thyroid shields* are protective attire worn to protect operating room personnel from radiologic exposure. These items are worn when personnel must be present during fluoroscopy procedures or when x-ray use is necessary during any surgical procedure.

No operating attire—including surgical uniforms, head coverings, and shoe covers—should be worn outside the surgical suite, because this creates a two-way hazard. Any contaminants that come in contact with the operating room team members can become airborne and find susceptible hosts outside the surgical suite. Conversely, bacteria present outside the suite may be carried back to the surgical suite on the operating room attire. If changing clothes is not feasible, head and shoe coverings are removed and the scrub clothes are covered by a clean cover gown with a back closure when a person leaves the operating suite. Ideally the scrub suit should be changed when the person returns, because the cover gown is not an effective barrier to potential external contaminants.

## PROTECTIVE BARRIERS FOR MAINTAINING STERILE FIELD

Personnel who work within the sterile field must don a sterile gown and sterile surgical gloves before touching any object within the sterile field. The gowns and gloves prevent microorganisms on hands and clothing from contaminating the wound during surgery and also protect the personnel from microorganisms present in the patient.

To create and maintain a barrier, draping materials that minimize the passage of microorganisms between sterile and nonsterile areas are selected. The patient and the operating bed are covered with sterile drapes, exposing only the prepared site of incision. Instrument tables are covered with sterile drapes. To be effective, materials used for drapes must be resistant to blood and other fluid, lint-free, and meet or exceed National Fire Protection Agency standards.

## UNIVERSAL PRECAUTIONS

A discussion of aseptic technique maintenance is not complete without mention of universal precautions. Uncontained blood and body fluids—an inevitable part of surgery—present a great hazard to operating room personnel. Because routine medical history and examination cannot identify all patients with HIV, hepatitis, or other blood-borne pathogens, universal precautions are used for all patients. The Centers for Disease Control and Prevention (CDC) has outlined these precautions, and the Occupational Safety and Health Administration (OSHA) has adopted these universal procedures as part of their requirements for maintenance of a safe working environment. The **universal precautions** are summarized in Box 24-2.

*Eyewear* protects the mucous membranes of the eyes. Goggles with enclosed sides offer better protection than eyeglasses. All personnel who will be in close proximity to the operative site or in attendance throughout the surgical procedure should wear protective eyewear.

*Double gloving* is recommended for personnel when donning sterile attire to enter the sterile field. Nonsterile *latex* or *vinyl gloves* are worn during contact with patients, handling contaminated items, or for any decontamination or housekeeping procedure.

## ENVIRONMENTAL CONTROLS

*Temperature and humidity* are important design factors. High relative humidity should be maintained; moisture provides a relatively conductive medium, allowing static to leak to earth as fast as it is generated. Temperature is purposely kept cool to deter bacterial growth. Most pathogenic bacteria metabolize and reproduce at or near normal body temperature, and bacterial growth may be inhibited by keeping room temperature below

**BOX 24-2 Universal Precautions**

1. All health care workers should use appropriate barrier precautions to prevent skin and mucous membrane exposure when contact with blood or other body fluids of any patient is anticipated. Gloves should be worn for touching blood and body fluids, mucous membranes, or non-intact skin of all patients, for handling items or surfaces soiled with blood or body fluids, and for performing venipuncture and other vascular access procedures. Gloves should be changed after contact with each patient. Masks and protective eye wear or face shields should be worn during procedures that are likely to generate droplets of blood or other body fluids to prevent exposure of mucous membranes of the nose, mouth, and eyes. Gowns or aprons should be worn during procedures that are likely to generate splashes of blood or other body fluids.
2. Hands and other skin surfaces should be washed immediately and thoroughly if contaminated with blood or other body fluids. Hands should be washed immediately after gloves are removed.
3. All health care workers should take precautions to prevent injuries caused by needles, scalpels, and other sharp instruments or devices during procedures; when cleaning used instruments; during disposal of used needles; and when handling sharp instruments after procedures. To prevent needlestick injuries, needles should not be recapped, purposely bent or broken by hand, removed from disposable syringes, or otherwise manipulated by hand. After they are used, disposable syringes and needles, scalpel blades, and other sharp items should be placed in puncture-resistant containers for disposal; the puncture-resistant containers should be located as close as practical to the use area. Large-bore reusable needles should be placed in a puncture-resistant container for transport to the reprocessing area.
4. Although saliva has not been implicated in HIV transmission, to minimize the need for emergency mouth-to-mouth resuscitation, mouthpieces, resuscitation bags, or other ventilation devices should be available for use in areas in which the need for resuscitation is predictable.
5. Health care workers who have exudative lesions or weeping dermatitis should refrain from all direct patient care and room handling of patient-care equipment until the condition resolves.
6. Spills of blood or body fluids should be wiped up as soon as possible with a fresh 10% bleach solution or other antimicrobial solution known to be effective against blood-borne pathogens, such as Staphene.

From Occupational Safety and Health Association, Department of Labor: Federal Register 56:64175-64180, 1991.

body temperature. Recommended temperatures are between 68° and 72° F, and recommended humidity levels are between 50% and 55%.[18] The combination of increased humidity and decreased temperature is also desirable to minimize drying of the patient's exposed tissue.

*Airborne contamination* is controlled in the operating room by keeping air currents and movement to a minimum. Microorganisms in the air settle on horizontal surfaces. Proper cleaning of these surfaces between cases and at the end of the day aids in the control of this contamination. Housekeeping protocols for room and furniture cleaning between procedures and at the end of each day's operating schedule are meticulously followed.

Conventional operating room ventilation systems use high-efficiency particulate air filters to reduce particles in the room air. Inlet air is dispersed from vents in the ceiling and exhausted through vents at floor level. Slightly less air is exhausted than is introduced to create a positive pressure gradient within the room. The positive pressure prevents potentially contaminated air from entering the room when a door is opened briefly. Therefore doors to the procedure rooms must remain closed at all times.

Traffic in and out of the operating suite is kept to a minimum. Only essential personnel are allowed inside the operating room. As the number of persons increases, potential contamination from bacterial shedding and air turbulence increases.

## STERILIZATION OF SUPPLIES

Microorganisms that do not normally invade healthy tissue are capable of causing infection if introduced directly into the body. For this reason it is imperative that all supplies and instruments used for the surgical procedure be adequately sterilized. Sterilization renders items safe for contact with tissue without transmission of infection as long as their sterility is maintained. The sterilization of products for use in the surgical suite must be performed according to guidelines established by the regulatory agencies that conduct research and set guidelines for the methods, products, and equipment used in sterilization processes. These agencies include the Centers for Disease Control and Prevention (CDC), the Occupational Safety and Health Administration (OSHA), the Association of Operating Room Nurses (AORN), the Food and Drug Administration (FDA), and the American Association for Medical Instrumentation (AAMI).

## SURGICAL HAND SCRUB[5]

All members of the surgical team perform a surgical hand scrub before donning sterile gown and gloves. Hands are a major source of pathogenic bacteria, and gloves may become punctured or torn during the procedure, exposing the patient to microbial contamination. The major objective of the surgical scrub is to reduce the microbial skin count as much as possible and to leave an antimicrobial residue on the skin to prevent regrowth. This is achieved by the following measures:

- Mechanical removal of soil and transient microbes

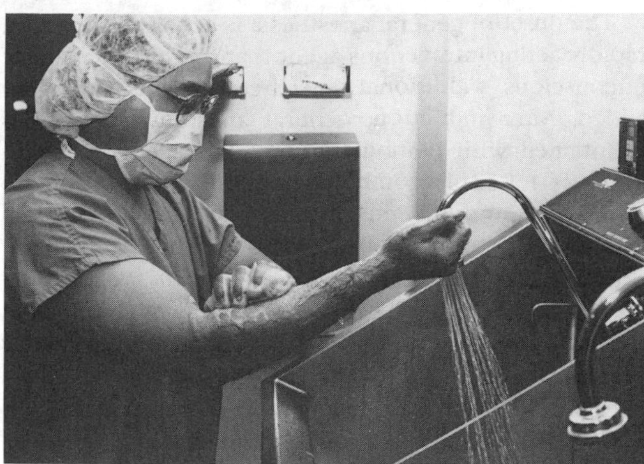

**FIGURE 24-3** Surgical hand scrub.

from the hands and forearms (methodical scrub procedure)

- Chemical reduction of the resident microbial count to as low a level as possible (use of antimicrobial solution)

The hand scrub procedure should include the following:

- Remove jewelry.
- Clean nails and nailbeds with a file under running water.
- Scrub fingers, hands, and forearms in that order, keeping hands and arms upward at all times (Figure 24-3).
- Treat each finger, hand, and forearm like a four-sided peg to ensure complete anatomic coverage with scrub brush.
- Rinse and lather both hands thoroughly; rinse.
- Enter operating room, with hands and forearms remaining angled upward, to don sterile gown and gloves.

## SURGICAL INCISION SITE PREPARATION[1]

The purpose of preoperative skin preparation is to establish an operative site as free as possible from dirt, skin oils, and transient microbes, as well as to reduce the resident microbial count as much as possible. This should be accomplished with the least amount of tissue irritation. Hair removal may be performed before the patient arrives at the operating room or in the operating room immediately before surgery. Hair removal should be performed as close as possible to the surgery start.

The operative site is prepared with an antimicrobial agent (or agents). Criteria used in selection of the agent include broad-spectrum activity, speed of action, potential for skin irritation and sensitivity, and flammability characteristics. Povidone-iodine (Betadine) and chlorhexidines (Hibiclens and Bactoshield) are some examples of antimicrobial agents used for both the surgical hand scrub and the patient operative site scrub. The surgical site scrub begins at the incision line and proceeds to the periphery of the area involved. A soiled sponge is never brought back over a previously scrubbed area. Open wounds and body orifices are prepared last, even when these areas are the proposed incision line.

**BOX 24-3 American Society of Anesthesiology (ASA) Classification for Anesthesia Risk Evaluation**

**ASA I**

A normal, healthy patient

**ASA II**

A patient with a mild systemic disease (e.g., mild diabetes, controlled hypertension, anemia)

**ASA III**

A patient with severe systemic disease that limits activity (e.g., angina, prior myocardial infarction)

**ASA IV**

A patient with an incapacitating disease that is a constant threat to life (e.g., heart failure, renal failure)

**ASA V**

A moribund patient not expected to survive 24 hours (e.g., ruptured aneurysm, head trauma with increasing intracranial pressure)

**ASA VI**

A patient declared legally dead according to state definition, whose organs are to be removed and prepared for donation

**CLASS E**

A patient in any classification that requires emergent surgery and a full evaluation is not possible (e.g. ASA IE).

# ANESTHESIA

Anesthesia renders the patient insensitive to pain in one area of the body or the body as a whole. The objectives of anesthesia are to produce analgesia and amnesia, to induce muscle relaxation, and to control the autonomic nervous system reflexes. Anesthetics are given by an experienced person who has been trained in the administration of anesthetic agents.

Many different types of anesthetic agents are available, and the choice of these agents, as well as the method of administration, is based on many factors. The physical condition and age of the patient, the presence of coexisting diseases, the type, site, and duration of the operation, and the patient's preference are all considered by the anesthesiologist in evaluating a patient. The American Society of Anesthesiology developed a classification system (Box 24-3) to identify the risk factors based on the patient's health status. As part of the preoperative evaluation, the anesthesiologist places the patient in a class according to physical status.[11]

## PREOPERATIVE MEDICATIONS

Preoperative medications may be given to reduce preoperative anxiety (sedatives, hypnotics), to minimize secretions in the respiratory tract and mouth (anticholinergics), to relieve pain (narcotics), and to decrease metabolism so that less anesthetic agent is necessary. Medications are selected on the basis of the preoperative assessment findings and the demands of the intended surgical procedures.

Preoperative medication may be given in the unit before transport to the operating room suite or in the holding area after arrival in the operating suite. Patients are observed closely for signs of untoward reactions, which include vomiting, hypotension, and cardiac and sensory changes.[14]

## GENERAL ANESTHESIA

**General anesthesia** is produced by inhalation or by injection of anesthetic drugs in the bloodstream, or a combination of both. General anesthesia is accomplished in four phases. The phases are preinduction, induction, maintenance, and reversal. The **preinduction phase** begins as soon as the patient is brought into the procedure room and ends immediately before the induction of anesthesia. The **induction phase** begins with the introduction of anesthetic agents and ends with intubation and stabilization of the patient. Induction involves putting the patient safely to sleep. A patent airway and adequate ventilation must be ensured. The **maintenance phase** starts when stabilization is accomplished and ends when reversal of anesthesia is initiated near the procedure's end. The **reversal/extubation phase** begins with closure of the wounds and ends before patient transport to the postoperative unit. Potential problems during this phase include laryngospasm, vomiting, slow spontaneous respirations, and uncontrolled reflex movement.

The onset of general anesthesia is accomplished by a rapidly acting intravenous agent that renders the patient unconscious. Additional anesthetic agents are then added. After induction, general anesthesia usually is maintained with combinations of the agents listed in Table 24-1. Use of a combination of inhalation anesthetic agents—along with muscle relaxants, narcotic analgesics, barbiturates, and other neuroleptic and antiemetic drugs—is referred to as *balanced anesthesia.*[12]

**Inhalation anesthesia** is produced by having the patient inhale the vapors of certain volatile liquids or gases. Oxygen is always given before, along with, and after these anesthetic agents are administered. Inhalation agents are eliminated through ventilation of the lungs with oxygen. The gas mixture may be administered by mask or into the lungs through an endotracheal tube inserted into the trachea through the nose or the mouth. The use of endotracheal intubation ensures that an airway can be maintained when the chest wall is open. The endotracheal tube may have a balloon that is inflated after insertion; the balloon fills the tracheal space, lessening the chance of aspiration of gastric contents. Regardless of the skill of the anesthesiologist, an endotracheal tube may cause some irritation to the trachea and subsequent edema. It is not uncommon for the patient to complain postoperatively of a sore, irritated throat. Some of the more common inhalation anesthetics in use are described in Table 24-1.

Several measures are used during inhalation anesthesia to promote the safety of both patient and health care workers. Oxygen is administered throughout the procedure, and a method of continuous analysis of the percentage of oxygen in the patient's bloodstream is used. A pulse oximeter is the recommended standard equipment to provide this analysis. A scavenging method for waste anesthetics (carbon dioxide absorber) must be used to avoid unnecessary exposure to health care per-

**TABLE 24-1 Inhalation Anesthetic Agents in Common Use**

| AGENT | ADVANTAGES | DISADVANTAGES |
|---|---|---|
| ENFLURANE (ETHRANE) | Rapid induction and recovery; some muscle relaxation on its own | Circulatory/respiratory depression (dose-dependent); shivering with emergence |
| HALOTHANE (FLUOTHANE) | Rapid induction; low incidence of postoperative nausea/vomiting; nonirritating | Shivering with emergence; circulatory/respiratory depression; reduces urinary output; hepatic toxicity; associated with hyperpyrexia |
| ISOFLURANE (FORANE) | Smooth, rapid induction; good muscle relaxation; nonirritating; cardiovascular stability; low incidence of nausea and vomiting | Shivering with emergence; strong odor; respiratory irritant |
| NITROUS OXIDE | Rapid induction and recovery; nonirritating; potentiator for other inhalation agents—"carrier of gases" | Possible hypoxia with excessive amounts |

sonnel. In addition, breathing circuits, masks, endotracheal tubes, and reservoir bags are all disposable, providing a clean circuit for each patient, thus avoiding potential cross-contamination.

*Intravenous medications* frequently are administered as an adjunct to inhalation agents and provide a reversible, safe state of anesthesia. Intravenous agents are metabolized and excreted by the kidneys independent of ventilatory function. They are administered by bolus dose or continuous drip infusion.

Barbiturates, narcotics, and muscle relaxants are the three main categories of intravenous drugs. **Barbiturates** act directly on the central nervous system and produce sedation and sleep. **Narcotics** eliminate pain. **Skeletal muscle relaxants** *(neuromuscular blocking agents)*, which are frequently employed in combination with anesthetics, have the following uses[12]:

- Facilitating endotracheal intubation
- Preventing laryngospasm
- Producing adequate muscle relaxation during anesthesia to facilitate surgery
- Reducing the amount of general anesthetic needed

Muscle relaxants completely relax skeletal muscles, facilitate the passage of endotracheal tubes, and diminish tissue trauma. During induction, sufficient relaxation is necessary for endotracheal intubation. The muscle relaxation that occurs during general anesthesia results from depression of neuromuscular transmission and loss of skeletal muscle tone. In many surgeries, full muscle relaxation is required to facilitate the surgeon's handling of an anatomic part for surgical correction (e.g., intraabdominal or thoracic surgery).

Muscle relaxants cause respiratory depression or paralysis; thus the patient is observed closely for signs of respiratory distress during and after administration of the drug. If respiratory problems develop, patients will require intubation and mechanical ventilatory assistance. Some of the intravenous anesthetic agents in common use are described in Table 24-2.

## REGIONAL ANESTHESIA

When general anesthesia is not desirable or is contraindicated, **regional anesthesia** may be used alone or in conjunction with conscious sedation. Major advantages of regional anesthesia are as follows[17]:

- It has less systemic effect on body functions.
- It is safer than general anesthesia
  —for use in elderly persons

**TABLE 24-2 Intravenous Anesthetic Agents in Common Use**

| AGENT/CLASS | ADVANTAGES | DISADVANTAGES |
|---|---|---|
| **DROPERIDOL (INAPSINE)** | | |
| Intravenous tranquilizer | Potentiates narcotics and strong antiemetic barbiturates | Hypotension, tachycardia |
| **MIDAZOLAM (VERSED)** | | |
| Intravenous tranquilizer | Induction achieved within narrow dose range and short period; high incidence of partial or complete impairment of recall for several hours | Depresses respiration and causes fluctuation of vital signs |
| **SUFENTANIL CITRATE (SUFENTA)** | | |
| Intravenous narcotic | Rapid onset producing hypnosis and anesthesia without use of additional agents; inhibits sympathetic response to surgical stress | Respiratory depression and skeletal muscle rigidity |
| **THIOPENTAL SODIUM (PENTOTHAL SODIUM)** | | |
| Intravenous or rectal (for children) barbiturate | Rapid, smooth induction and recovery | Laryngospasm with stimulation of larynx; respiratory depression with high doses; sudden drop in blood pressure |
| **FENTANYL CITRATE (SUBLIMAZE)** | | |
| Intravenous or intramuscular narcotic | Abolition of stress response; very potent analgesic | Respiratory depression; muscle rigidity and bradycardia may occur |
| **ALFENTANIL (ALFENTA)** | | |
| Intravenous narcotic | Very brief duration of action | Elimination is slow, and repeated doses exert more prolonged effect |

—when cardiac and/or respiratory dysfunction exist
—if there has been recent food intake
—when surgery is superficial

There are several techniques for regional anesthesia, and the choice depends on the type and duration of surgery, the preferences of the anesthesiologist and surgeon, and, if possible, the preference of the patient.

**Spinal anesthesia** provides regions of anesthesia from the abdomen to the toes. A spinal (subarachnoid block) or an epidural block is used. Spinal anesthesia is not used for surgery of the upper part of the body because it causes paralysis of the diaphragm and the intercostal muscles used in respiration. With spinal anesthesia the patient may be conscious of pulling sensations during the operation but experiences no pain. Occasionally a feeling of faintness and nausea may result from these sensations. Because of the sympathetic blockade, hypotension may occur with both spinal and epidural anesthesia.

**Nerve block anesthesia** involves injection of the anesthetic agent into and around a nerve group. Major blocks involve multiple nerves, whereas minor blocks involve a single nerve. For example, a brachial plexus or an axillary nerve block would anesthetize the arm.

## LOCAL ANESTHESIA

**Local anesthesia** (infiltration) blocks depolarization by interfering with sodium-potassium exchange across the nerve cell membrane, preventing conduction of pain impulses from their site of origin. The agent is injected into a specific area at the operative site and interferes with impulses from the central nervous system to the operative site while tissues are being manipulated.[19] Intravenous sedation often is given as an adjunct to relieve anxiety and to produce amnesia. Local anesthesia usually is used when the surgery to be performed involves superficial tissues such as simple suturing, skin biopsies, or removal of superficial cysts. If an anesthesiologist is present, the anesthesia technique is known as *monitored anesthesia care.* If an anesthesiologist is not present, monitoring responsibilities belong to the perioperative nurse.

When regional or local anesthesia is used, the patient is awake during the procedure although a preoperative medication or an intravenous adjunct agent may decrease awareness of the surroundings. A screen often is used to restrict the patient's vision of the surgical area. The conversation and activities of the members of the operating room staff should be carried on with the patient's consciousness in mind. Local anesthetics in common use are listed in Table 24-3.

**TABLE 24-3 Local Anesthetics in Common Use**

| USAGE | ADVANTAGES | DISADVANTAGES |
|---|---|---|
| **LIDOCAINE* (XYLOCAINE)** | | |
| Topical<br>Local infiltration<br>Epidural<br>Spinal | Rapid onset<br>Lack of local irritant effect | Short duration |
| **BUPIVACAINE (MARCAINE)** | | |
| Local infiltration<br>Epidural<br>Spinal<br>Nerve blocks | Long duration (2-3 times longer than lidocaine)<br>High potency<br>Prolonged pain relief after procedure | Onset is slow |
| **TETRACAINE (PONTOCAINE)** | | |
| Epidural<br>Spinal | Longer duration than most other drugs | Onset is slow<br>Slow rate of destruction: greater systemic toxicity |

*Most widely used.

## OTHER TYPES OF ANESTHESIA

**Induced hypothermia** may be used as an adjunct to other anesthetic agents. Hypothermia refers to the reduction of body temperature below normal to reduce oxygen and metabolic requirements. Extracorporeal cooling, a method of bloodstream cooling, consists of removing the blood from a major vessel, circulating it through coils immersed in a refrigerant, and returning it to the body through another vessel. Bloodstream cooling is the fastest method for producing hypothermia and is used primarily for patients undergoing open-heart surgery.

## ANESTHESIA COMPLICATIONS

The anesthetics-related operative mortality rate is relatively low. For a healthy person the risk is about 0.01%. Some of the more common complications of anesthesia are related to the untoward reactions to the anesthetic agents. The major complication is cardiac arrest. Laryngospasm and inhalation of gastric contents are serious potential complications that may occur during the emergence phase of general anesthesia.[14] Some less critical complications may occur, such as shivering during the reversal stage in the operating room, and extra warmth is provided before the patient is transferred to the postanesthesia unit. Common postoperative complications and interventions used to prevent or treat them are discussed in Chapter 25.

Both general and regional anesthesia cause a dilation of peripheral blood vessels and a drop in blood pressure. Venous blood pools in dependent areas, reducing blood return to the heart and lungs for oxygenation and redistribution. General anesthesia depresses the medulla, which maintains cardiac output and peripheral vascular constriction. Muscle relaxants reduce the milking action of normal muscles that assist in venous return. Spinal or epidural anesthesia blocks autonomic output, causing vasodilation and venous pooling. Peripheral vascular injury can occur with occlusion of the vessels. The anesthesiologist constantly monitors the patient and is prepared to compensate for complications of these changes when they occur. The perioperative nurse, knowledgeable about anesthesia methods, patient risk factors, complications, and preventive interventions, is able to provide efficient and appropriate assistance to the anesthesiology team members.

**Malignant hyperthermia** is a life-threatening complication of general anesthesia. Halogenated inhalation agents (e.g., halothane) are all suspect for triggering a malignant hyperthermia crisis, as are depolarizing neuromuscular relaxants, particularly succinylcholine. Patients who have an inherited defect in the membrane of the skeletal muscle or who have a family history of a malignant hyperthermia crisis are at greatest risk. The defect is believed to be present in the sarcoplasmic reticulum where the triggering agent sets off the release of calcium. Intracellular calcium ion levels increase with muscle contraction but fail to decrease. The reasons for this are unclear. The high intracellular calcium level of the muscle cells accelerates their metabolic rate dramatically. A number of resultant chemical changes take place and, if not controlled, may lead to renal failure, neurologic damage, heart failure, and disseminated intravascular coagulation (DIC). The physical signs of malignant hyperthermia commonly include unexplained tachycardia, unstable blood pressure, tachypnea, muscle rigidity, cyanotic skin mottling, and rapidly rising body temperature.[20]

# PHYSIOLOGIC STRESS RESPONSES TO SURGERY AND ANESTHESIA

Surgery and anesthesia affect all body systems. The organ systems are interdependent, and when one system is affected, to a certain extent all the systems are affected. A thorough understanding of how the various organ systems can be affected by anesthesia and surgery is essential to establish a scientific basis for intraoperative caregiving by the health care team.

## NEUROENDOCRINE RESPONSES

Neuroendocrine responses play a major role in the reaction of a patient to the stress of surgery. The responses include stimulation of the autonomic nervous system (primarily the sympathetic nervous system) and stimulation of selected hormones (primarily aldosterone and glucocorticoid hormones from the adrenal cortex and antidiuretic hormone from the posterior pituitary). Table 24-4 summarizes the effects of endocrine changes on the patient.

Stimulation of the *sympathetic nervous system* serves to protect the body from further damage. Vasoconstriction of peripheral blood vessels enables the body to compensate for blood loss and redirect blood flow to critical areas such as the heart and brain. Increased cardiac output also helps to maintain blood flow. Severe trauma or excessive blood loss, however, will overwhelm the compensatory mechanisms, and blood pressure will fall. Certain types of anesthetics or high spinal anesthesia also may interfere with the compensatory vasoconstriction, producing hypotension.

One aspect of the sympathetic response that may produce undesirable effects is the decrease in gastrointestinal activity. Psychologic stress in the preoperative period may lead to anorexia and constipation. After the trauma of surgery, the patient may experience anorexia, gas pains, and constipation from diminished peristalsis in the gastrointestinal tract. Peristalsis may cease completely after abdominal surgery involving manipulation of abdominal organs.

**TABLE 24-4 Effects of Endocrine Changes Associated With Surgery**

| PHYSIOLOGIC CHANGES | RESULTS | OBSERVED EFFECT |
|---|---|---|
| ↑ Norepinephrine secretion | Peripheral vasoconstriction | Helps maintain blood pressure when circulating volume is decreased |
| | ↓ Gastrointestinal activity | May lead to anorexia or constipation |
| ↑ Aldosterone secretion | Sodium retention | Maintains circulating blood volume<br>Increases susceptibility to fluid overload<br>Decreases urinary output |
| ↑ Glucocorticoid secretion | Gluconeogenesis<br>↑ Protein catabolism<br>Ketogenic effect<br>Antiinflammatory effect<br>↑ Platelet production | Provides energy to meet stress of surgery<br>Provides an additional energy source<br>Provides amino acids for cell synthesis after tissue destruction<br>Provides fat as an energy source<br>Increases susceptibility to infection<br>Promotes clotting to prevent bleeding<br>Contributes to development of thrombophlebitis |
| ↑ Antidiuretic hormone (ADH) secretion | Water reabsorption in the kidney tubules | Maintains circulating blood volume<br>Increases susceptibility to fluid overload<br>Decreases urinary output |

*Adrenocortical activity* is increased in response to the trauma of surgery, producing greater amounts of aldosterone and glucocorticoid. Aldosterone enhances sodium reabsorption by the kidney. This serves to retain fluid to compensate for fluid lost through blood loss, diaphoresis, and respirations. When sodium is reabsorbed by the kidneys, potassium is excreted; thus after surgery there is a loss of potassium.

In addition to the increase in aldosterone secretion, there is also an increase in antidiuretic hormone (ADH) by the posterior pituitary gland during the first 24 to 48 hours after surgery. Water is reabsorbed by the kidney, and renal output is decreased. After surgery the increased production of aldosterone and ADH is evidenced by a decreased urinary output as compared with fluid intake. Spontaneous diuresis occurs as the amount of ADH is decreased, usually in about 24 to 48 hours.

The increase in the amount of glucocorticoid from the adrenal cortex is thought to mobilize cellular stores of fats and amino acids for energy and protein synthesis. Healing tissues require protein. Glucose is released for energy, with resultant hyperglycemia and glycosuria. Patients who have diabetes must be carefully monitored for signs of ketosis.

## METABOLIC RESPONSES

After surgery the patient is in a relative state of starvation; metabolism is increased, and nutrient intake is decreased. *Carbohydrate metabolism* increases as a result of the increased production of glucocorticoid hormones. With major surgery, there are periods when the patient is not permitted to eat and receives dextrose by intravenous fluids. This fluid replacement is not adequate to meet the body's energy needs. Anorexia also may occur as part of the stress response, thus adding to the problem of inadequate carbohydrate intake even if food is permitted by mouth. The body must supply its glucose needs by the breakdown of stored liver glycogen or by the synthesis of glucose from noncarbohydrate sources.

*Fat metabolism* increases to allow the mobilization of fat from the cells so that it is available as an energy source. With the decreased intake of carbohydrates and fats after surgery, body fats are metabolized for energy and the patient loses weight.

*Protein metabolism* is increased after surgery to supply essential amino acids necessary for tissue healing. Body proteins consist of combinations of amino acids, of which nitrogen is an essential component. When tissues break down during catabolism after surgery, some of the nitrogen is lost. As new tissue is formed, essential amino acids are needed. If none of these amino acids is taken in, the body will continue to break down existing tissue proteins to obtain the amino acids that it needs for healing. The "leftover" amino acids not used at that time are broken down to nitrogen end products such as urea and are excreted. A negative nitrogen balance results; nitrogen loss exceeds nitrogen intake.

## ORGAN SYSTEM RESPONSES

The stressors of surgery and anesthesia have several effects on the *cardiovascular system.* Each surgical position has an effect on the circulatory system (see section on patient positioning, p. 619). In addition, all anesthetic agents affect cardiac function. Inhalation agents depress myocardial contractility and alter heart rate, preload, and afterload. Both general and regional anesthesia cause a dilation of peripheral blood vessels and a drop in blood pressure. Venous blood pools in dependent areas, reducing blood return to the heart and lungs for oxygenation and redistribution.

Several surgical events (e.g., manipulations of structures in the abdomen) initiate sympathetic responses that increase heart rate and arterial blood pressure. Laryngoscopy and intubation can increase the heart rate and systolic pressures as a result of sympathetic system activation.

The physiologic changes in the cardiovascular system in the aging heart make elderly persons more susceptible to the complications of surgery and anesthesia. There is a change in muscle fibers, reduced efficiency in contractions, a decreased irritability of the myocardium, and less elasticity in the arteries.

The *respiratory system* is also directly affected by each surgical position (see p. 619). Preoperative medications depress respiratory function. Spinal block anesthesia depresses respirations. Regional anesthesia, however, has much less effect than general anesthesia on respiratory functions. Surgical procedures can have a direct effect on respirations. Upper abdominal and thoracic procedures have the greatest influence on respiratory function. Tidal volume, vital capacity, and functional residual capacity are among the functions most adversely affected. This reduced function continues postoperatively during the first 24 to 48 hours.

Several preoperative factors increase the risk of pulmonary complications during a surgical procedure. Preexisting respiratory dysfunction or disease impairs the mechanical function of the chest. Obesity may promote hypoxemia and respiratory acidosis by decreasing respiratory muscle efficiency. Smoking depresses the mucociliary activity that moves sputum and foreign particles from the lower airways, increases bronchospasm, and causes bronchial constriction. With advanced age, vital capacity, forced expiratory volumes, and maximum breathing capacity decrease while residual volume and functional residual capacity increase. Also, in elderly persons, laryngeal, pharyngeal, and other airway reflexes are less effective, increasing the risk of pulmonary aspiration. Interference with adequate ventilation can lead to a true medical emergency and requires immediate intervention. Continual intraoperative assessment must be performed by both the anesthesiologist and the perioperative nurse.

*Renal function* is altered by surgery and anesthesia. Because the patient receives nothing by mouth and has inadequate fluid replacements, underfunction results. Hypotension from blood loss limits the nutrients to the kidneys, and blood is not filtered efficiently. A systemic response may be initiated because of an accumulation of wastes. Certain agents, such as contrast media, may have a direct toxic effect on the kidneys. Increases in aldosterone and ADH secretion decrease urinary output (see section on neuroendocrine responses). The aging kidney loses some of its ability to filter and clear medication and anesthesia from its system. The older person is thus more prone to kidney and bladder infections during invasive procedures.

The *integumentary system* is under great stress from pressure created by surgical positions and lengths of procedures. Pressure sore development can result if extensive care and preventive methods are not used. In addition, the skin plays an important role in conserving heat. During open surgical procedures, loss of body heat is accelerated and may be a cause of hypothermia. Metabolic rate increases approximately 13% for every 1° C heat loss.[13] In patients with compromised cardiopulmonary function, especially pediatric and elderly patients, the heat loss creates additional strain and increases both morbidity and mortality. Major skin changes occur in the elderly patient population. In addition to a general thinning of the skin, there is a decrease in the collagen, which leads to decreased elasticity. The skin is more fragile and friable.

## NURSING MANAGEMENT

The unique nature of the intraoperative environment creates an inevitable focus on the many technical activities required to facilitate the surgical procedure and maintain patient safety. However, the perioperative nurse is also responsible for meeting the patient's psychosocial needs. Nursing practice in the operating room includes assessment, planning, implementing, and evaluating nursing activities to meet individual needs of patients who require a surgical intervention.

### ♦ ASSESSMENT

When patients are admitted to the operating room suite, the perioperative nurse must assess the patient's physical and emotional status, paying particular attention to any factors that would increase surgical risk. A preoperative interview should take place on the patient's arrival to the operating room admission suite (Figure 24-4). Astute interviewing skills and communication of a caring attitude are important for a thorough assessment of both physical and emotional status of the patient.

Preoperative data to be collected to assess the patient undergoing surgery include the following:

- Subjective data from the patient
- The patient's history and physical examination
- Significant laboratory findings
- Results of diagnostic studies
- Documentation from health care professionals in the clinic, physician's office, preadmission unit, surgical admission suite, hospital unit

In addition to a thorough assessment of the patient's subjective and objective data before surgery, it is imperative that the perioperative nurse understand the effects that surgery and anesthesia may have on each patient (see section on anesthesia complications and physiologic stress responses to surgery and anesthesia). A

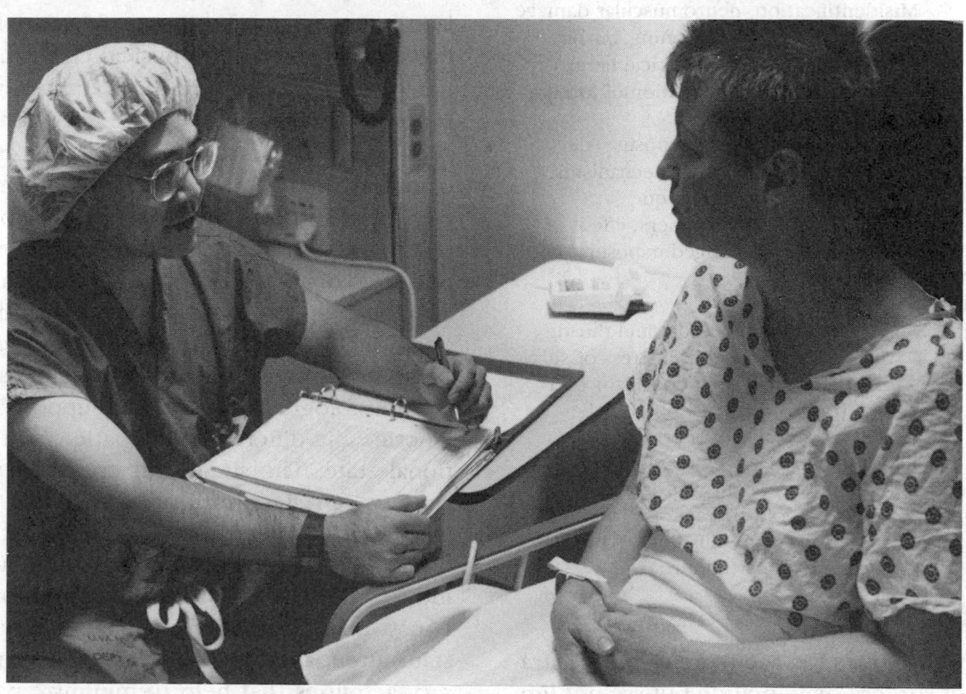

**FIGURE 24-4** Preoperative interview.

combination of this knowledge and collected preoperative data enables the perioperative nurse to identify factors that can increase risks for individual patients. In particular, special considerations must be made for the care of elderly persons. Because of the normal aging process, these patients may face higher risks. Specifics about additional risks for elders are discussed on p. 595. After a review of the information accumulated during assessment activities, nursing diagnoses, expected patient outcomes, and an intraoperative plan of care are formulated. Assessment continues during the patient's transfer into the operating room, positioning on the operating room table, induction of anesthesia, and during and immediately after the surgical procedure so that the patient's status can be compared with preoperative factors and expected postoperative outcomes.

## ♦ NURSING DIAGNOSES

Nursing diagnoses provide guides for the nursing activities of the perioperative nurse immediately before, during, and after surgical procedures. The nursing diagnoses discussed in this chapter focus on high-incidence problem areas for patients during a surgical intervention.

Nursing diagnoses for the patient in the intraoperative phase of surgery may include but are not limited to the following:

| Diagnostic Title | Possible Etiologic Factors |
|---|---|
| Anxiety, high risk for elevated | Unfamiliar environment, fear of impending surgery/anesthesia, intraoperative diagnosis |
| Skin integrity, high risk for impaired | Immobility, improper positioning, obesity or emaciation, pooling of preparation solutions |
| Injury (trauma), high risk for | Misidentification, neuromuscular damage from improper positioning, burns from chemical or electrical hazards, physical hazards, retention of foreign objects |
| Infection, high risk for postoperative wound | Excessive body cavity exposure, decreased body defense mechanisms, break in aseptic technique |
| Thermoregulation, ineffective (high risk for alteration in normothermia) | Cool operative environment, effect of anesthetics, prolonged exposure, cool solutions |
| Fluid volume deficit, high risk for | Rapid loss of blood/body fluid during the surgical procedure, stress of surgical intervention, anticoagulant therapy, trauma, preexisting disorders (e.g., bleeding disorders) |
| Fluid volume excess, high risk for | Rapid intake of excessive fluid or sodium, stress of surgical intervention, corticosteroid therapy, preexisting conditions (e.g., Cushing's syndrome, congestive heart failure) |

## ♦ EXPECTED PATIENT OUTCOMES

Expected patient outcomes for the patient in the intraoperative phase of surgery may include but are not limited to the following:

1. Shows little or moderate subjective or objective evidence of anxiety.
2. Remains free of signs of skin breakdown after surgery.
3. Remains free from injury/trauma related to electrical, chemical, physical factors.
4. Remains free of postoperative wound infection.
5. Is normothermic on admission to the postanesthesia receiving unit.
6. Maintains an adequate fluid volume.

## ♦ INTERVENTIONS

Having identified the patient's specific needs and formulated nursing diagnoses, the nurse must collaborate with other members of the health care team to implement the plan for patient care during the intraoperative phase of the surgical experience. As discussed previously, anesthesia and all the components of the surgical experience place great stress on the body and may result in postoperative complications for the patient. The major focus of nursing intervention during this period is maintenance of patient safety and prevention of postoperative complications.

### Minimizing Anxiety

Most patients experience some anxiety when facing a surgical intervention. As discussed in Chapter 23, an important part of preoperative nursing intervention is helping the patient to cope with this anxiety. Perioperative events such as the disclosure of possible complications, anesthesia, intraoperative diagnosis, or postoperative pain may trigger an increase in anxiety level immediately before surgery. The perioperative nurse usually can identify anticipatory anxiety in the patient on admission to the operative suite because the patient is likely to exhibit signs of anxiety when the surgery is imminent. Interventions at this time focus on providing support by gentle physical contact, maintenance of personal dignity, a quiet and unhurried surgical environment, attentiveness to the needs of the patient, and provision of comfort accessories such as a warm blanket or pillow. In addition, providing information about the environment and what to expect before performing a nursing action decreases the patient's fear of the unfamiliar environment. Soothing words and an empathic attitude help promote a nurturing atmosphere in the operating room's high-technology environment. By communicating an overall attitude of caring and providing physiologic and emotional support, nurses can make a noticeable difference in a patient's preoperative emotional state. The successful use of methods to reduce anxiety can significantly enhance the effectiveness of preoperative medications, can permit a reduction in dosage, or can even eliminate their need. During the induction phase of anesthesia, provision of physical security, maintenance of personal dignity, and close, constant attendance by the perioperative nurse are necessary activities that help to minimize patient's fears and thereby facilitate the induction of anesthesia. See Research box, p. 619.

**RESEARCH**

Parsons EC, Kee CC, Gray P: Perioperative nurse caring behaviors, *AORN J* 57(5):1106-1114, 1993.

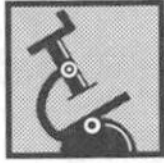

The purpose of this study was to identify perioperative nurse behaviors perceived as caring by surgical patients and to determine if certain behaviors are perceived as more important than others. Provision of a relaxed atmosphere, teamwork, and a professional demeanor were three behaviors identified by the surgical patients studied. Patients who perceive that their nurses are concerned with their well-being may be better prepared to deal with the stress of surgical intervention. Caring is an inherent part of perioperative nursing practice.

## Minimizing Risks for Impairment of Skin Integrity

A breakdown in skin integrity may occur from improper positioning. Prolonged pressure on the bony prominences, pressure on the peripheral nervous or vascular systems, or shearing force of sheets and drapes during patient movement may be responsible for areas of skin breakdown. Irritation or burning from solutions used in skin preparations, as well as burning from misuse of electrical equipment, also can result in postoperative skin breakdown. Nursing responsibilities for the prevention of these complications are discussed in the following section.

## Minimizing Risks for Injury and Trauma

### Patient positioning

The patient may be placed in a variety of positions for the surgical procedure. Each has its own unique risks for the patient. Figure 24-5 illustrates common surgical positions and indicates the associated pressure points. The perioperative nurse must understand the basic components of safe positioning and participate in the teamwork necessary to assess, plan, implement, and evaluate the care necessary to keep the patient free from injury/trauma resulting from complications of positioning. A thorough knowledge of the physiologic consequences of positioning, patient limitations, positioning equipment, and procedures is necessary to facilitate coordination among all members of the health care team. The preoperative interview provides an opportunity for the nurse to identify patients at risk for potential problems with an intended surgical position. Influencing factors that may potentiate complications from positioning include preexisting conditions such as arthritis, diabetes, obesity, nerve dysfunction, age (very young or elderly persons), decreased muscle tone, and compromised cardiopulmonary status.

Anesthetic agents increase the risks associated with positioning because of their effect on body systems (see discussion of anesthesia complications). Physiologic changes during positioning affect the respiratory, circulatory, nervous, skeletal, and integumentary systems. Coupled with the effects of anesthesia and surgery on body systems, positioning can become a potential great danger for all surgical patients.[8]

The *respiratory system* is influenced greatly by positioning. The respiratory system is most vulnerable to the prone and the lithotomy positions. The thoracic cage normally expands in all directions except posteriorly. In these positions there is mechanical restriction of lung expansion at the ribs or sternum and the reduced ability of the diaphragm to push down against abdominal muscles. Respiratory function is impaired because of interference with normal movements. Lung tissue compliance is decreased, thereby reducing the volume of air that can be inspired for rapid exchange. In addition, a change in position alters the pulmonary capillary blood flow volume, thereby affecting the amount of blood available for oxygenation.

In elderly persons, anatomic and functional changes occur in the respiratory system. Lungs lose elasticity, and muscles responsible for inhalation and exhalation may be weakened, contributing to a minimal tidal exchange for these patients. These changes increase the risk for pulmonary complications.

Several changes in the *cardiovascular system* that occur with positioning also may result in complications. Pressure or obstruction of a vessel, or both, cause the greatest amount of damage to the cardiovascular system. A tight restraint, crossed legs, or limb hyperextension can compromise blood flow by compression of a vessel against a bony structure. The volume of blood returned to the heart and lungs can be reduced, affecting oxygenation and distribution of oxygenated blood. Rapid movements during changes in positioning may cause sudden hypotension. An example of this occurs when legs are lowered quickly from the lithotomy position. The lithotomy position also may lead to circulatory pooling in the lumbar region and compression of abdominal contents on the inferior vena cava and abdominal aorta. In both situations, there is a decrease in venous return. This in turn affects cardiac output.

Most of the problems associated with the *neurologic system* are not discovered until recovery from anesthesia is complete.

Postoperative sedation may mask symptoms of peripheral nerve damage for days. Most postoperative palsies result from an inappropriate position on the operating table. Damage to peripheral nerves usually is the result of direct mechanical pressure. Ischemia and insufficient blood supply caused by stretching or compression are chief factors in nerve injuries. The lithotomy position is especially likely to cause injury to the saphenous and common perineal nerves. These injuries result from either misplaced stirrups or acute flexion of the thighs. In all positions in which the arms are extended on armboards, hyperextension of the arms may cause damage to the brachial plexus.[10]

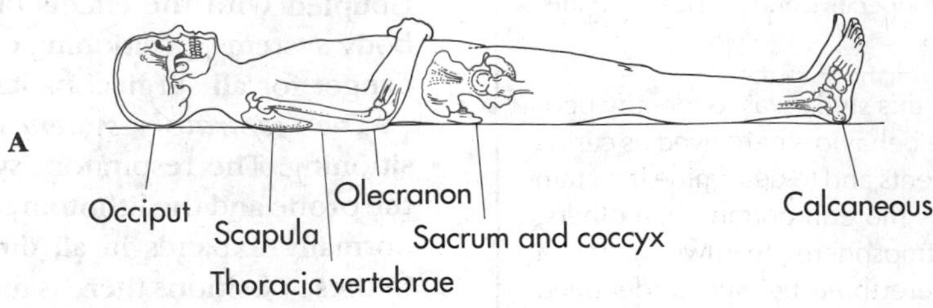


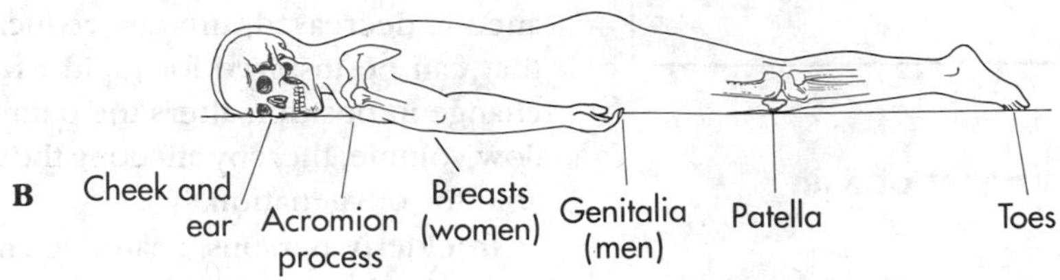


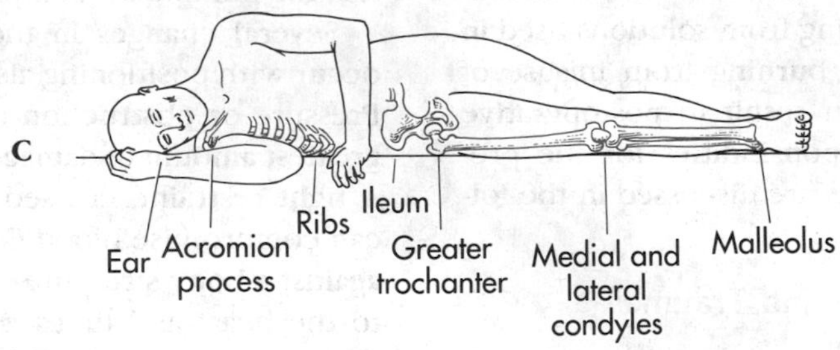


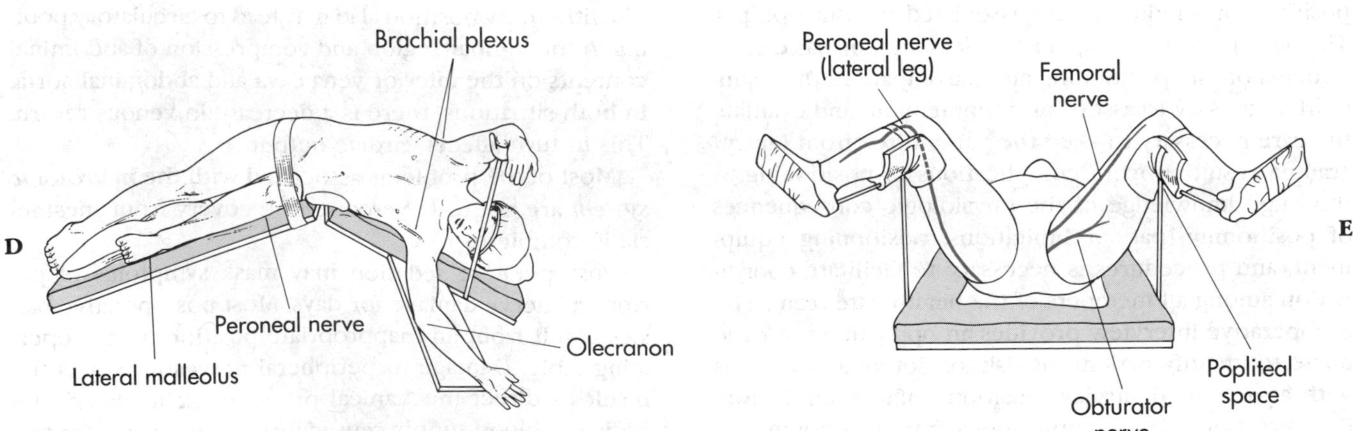


**FIGURE 24-5** Examples of common surgical positions and their associated potential pressure points. **A,** Supine (dorsal recumbent) position. **B,** Prone position. **C,** Lateral position. **D,** Lateral (kidney) position. **E,** Lithotomy position.

Preserving the *integumentary system* is a major nursing responsibility in the operating room. Poor positioning can result in the development of decubitus ulcers. Tissue perfusion is a critical factor in the prevention of pressure sores. Compression of vessels, external pressure, uneven body weight distribution, and constant pressure on bony prominences can result in pressure sores. Patients in debilitated states, such as those with peripheral vascular disease, hypotension, diabetes, or paralysis, are at greater risk for pressure sore development. Elderly persons are prone to shearing force skin tears when being moved across the operating table and placed into position. Elders also are vulnerable to pressure injury because aged skin loses elasticity and subcutaneous fat. Commonly used operative patient positions are described in Table 24-5 and pictured in Figure 24-5.

**TABLE 24-5 Commonly Used Operative Patient Positions**

| DESCRIPTION | COMMENTS |
|---|---|
| **SUPINE** | |
| Flat on back with arms at side, palms down, legs straight with feet slightly separated | Most commonly used position; venous pooling in the legs may result from a reduction of venous pressure |
| **PRONE** | |
| Patient lies on abdomen with face turned to one side, arms at sides with palms pronated, elbows slightly flexed; feet elevated on pillow to prevent plantar flexion | Patient is anesthetized in supine position and then placed prone; respiratory excursion is decreased; risk for facial nerve, genitalia, and breast injury |
| **TRENDELENBURG** | |
| Patient supine; head and body are lowered into a head-down position; knees are flexed by "breaking" table | Respiratory excursion is decreased from upward movement of abdominal viscera; cerebral edema or venous thrombosis may occur because of congestion of the cerebral vessels |
| **LITHOTOMY** | |
| Patient lies on back with buttocks to edge of table; thighs and legs are placed in stirrups simultaneously to prevent muscle injury; head and arms are secured to prevent injury | Elastic wraps or antiembolitic stockings may be used on legs to prevent thrombus formation; risk for vein compression in legs, increased intraabdominal pressure, injury to obturator and femoral nerves because of flexion of thighs; risk for acute hypotension when legs are lowered |
| **LATERAL** | |
| Patient lies on side; table may be bent in middle | Risk for injury to dependent brachial plexus, pressure sore development over the dependent greater trochanter of femur; potential interference with cardiac action because of possible shift in heart position |

Many interventions can be initiated to minimize the complications in patient positioning.[8] Distribution of body weight should be as even as possible, and the patient should be maintained in correct alignment. Positioning of extremities must not exceed a 90-degree angle to the body. Bony prominences such as heels, elbows, and sacrum are vulnerable pressure points and should be well padded. Special full-length flotation mattresses such as gel pads should be used for lengthy procedures. The safety strap should be applied 2 inches above the knees to avoid pressure on the popliteal nerve. Compression of the popliteal nerve from stirrups or knee braces also should be avoided. Antiembolic stockings should be used to decrease venous pooling in the lower extremities. Changing positions gradually is important to prevent drastic shifts in blood volume from one area of the body to another. Foam-filled cushions in a variety of sizes and shapes are used to maintain adequate respiratory excursion and to prevent pressure on the chest, breasts, genitalia, and abdominal structures. Guidelines related to patient positioning are summarized in the Guidelines box below.

A detailed procedure for each surgical position should be written and available for operating room personnel who are responsible for or assist with positioning of patients. Detailed documentation by the perioperative nurse should include the type of position, any changes in positioning made intraoperatively, placement of extremities, type and placement of positioning aids and supplemental padding, and the site of placement of the electrosurgical conduction pad.

### Electrical, chemical, and physical hazards

Many perioperative nursing activities are focused on the protection of the patient from electrical, chemical, and physical hazards. The use of electricity introduces haz-

**Guidelines for the Prevention of Complications of Surgical Positioning**

- Maintain patient in correct alignment, and distribute body weight equally.
- Pad all bony prominences well with foam-filled cushions, gel pads, or full-length flotation mattresses as needed.
- Use antiembolic hose to decrease venous pooling.
- Change patient positions gradually to avoid drastic shifts in blood volume.
- Avoid local compression from safety straps, knee braces, or stirrups.
- Position extremities at no more than a 90-degree angle to the body.

ards of electric shock, power failure, and fire to patients. Faulty wiring, inadequately maintained equipment, and a lack of regard for precautionary measures can cause a spark, resulting in a fire. If a voltage exists between any two electrical conductors touching the patient, the flow of current can result in electric shock or electrocution. If the voltage is high enough, ventricular fibrillation and sudden death may result. The operating room is an area containing many potential life-threatening and mechanically injurious situations related to electrical shock, burn, fire, and explosions. It is imperative that all members of the surgical health care team have current knowledge of the equipment and supplies most often involved in such incidents. The most significant hazards are inadequately trained personnel, malfunctioning equipment as a result of improper maintenance, inappropriate design of operating room suites, and inappropriate surveillance by team members.[7]

Federal regulations govern the marketing and safety standards of electronic devices used in operating rooms, and the Joint Commission on Accreditation of Healthcare Organizations also has standards that must be met. Policy and procedure regarding the in-servicing, operation, and maintenance of electrical equipment should be written and followed. When electrical equipment is in use, hazards can be minimized or prevented by the following perioperative nursing interventions:

- Use only electrical equipment designed for operating room use.
- Use cords of adequate length.
- Ground the patient correctly.
- Test equipment before use.
- Establish and follow sound clinical engineering testing and maintenance programs.
- Participate in in-service sessions for new equipment, and maintain an adequate knowledge base for correct use of all electrical equipment.
- Verify that correct attachments for a piece of equipment are being used.
- Report faulty equipment immediately.
- Maintain humidity levels at 50% or higher to minimize static electricity.
- Prevent the pooling of fluids under the patient.

*Chemical hazards* in the operating room include exposure to solutions used for cleaning, cementing bone, gas sterilization of instruments, and skin preparation. Iodine and iodophors are bactericidal agents used frequently in skin preparations. These are two of the most effective solutions for preoperative skin scrubbing but are irritants to the skin if the concentration is too high. In addition, alcohol, which sometimes is used in incision site preparation, is flammable. Precautions necessary for prevention of injury from any hazardous chemicals are many. As patient advocates, the nursing personnel must ensure proper labeling to comply with the National Fire Protection Association standards. Safe storage for hazardous chemicals away from immediate patient areas must be provided for and maintained. All personnel must be aware of and follow safe chemical usage recommendations set by the hospital's safety department and the manufacturing company. It is imperative that the perioperative nurse determine or verify any patient allergies that may increase risk of injury from certain solutions intended for use during the surgical procedure. Prevention of pooling under the patient of all solutions used in skin preparation is necessary to prevent unnecessary irritation to the skin or provide a focus for an electrical shock or burn.

Because of the anesthetic's effect, patients may be unable to respond to stimuli, be unaware of environmental hazards, and be unable to control movement; yet they are exposed to *physical hazards* such as falls and bodily injury. It is the responsibility of the perioperative nurse, along with other members of the surgical health care team, to protect the patient from injury that physical hazards are capable of causing. Prevention of injury includes careful movement into and out of positions, appropriate positioning methods (refer to patient positioning), and the maintenance of protective devices—for example, side rails up on stretcher and use of operating table safety straps. Transfer of the patient onto the operating table and postoperatively onto the unit bed or stretcher must be accomplished with adherence to safety measures. Safety can be promoted by ensuring that sufficient support help is obtained for the transfer, that all tubes are visible and protected from inadvertent removal, and that the movement is coordinated among all team members.

To ensure that injury does not occur from *misidentification* of the patient or the correct operative site, it is mandatory that the perioperative nurse verify the patient's identity and operative site. This should be done verbally (unless not possible), by patient identification band, and by chart documentation. Absolutely no discrepancy should exist between operative consent information and what the patient states. The perioperative nurse must bring any discrepancy or concerns to the attention of the surgeon, anesthesiologist, patient, and when necessary, the hospital administrator. Surgery should be delayed until there is appropriate resolution to any issue about accurate information, patient identity, or patient consent.

### Prevention of foreign object retention

Because of the high level of risk to the patient related to foreign object retention in the surgical wound, counting materials used during a surgical procedure is an important intraoperative nursing intervention. Sponges, sharps, and instruments are counted before the start of surgery and again at closure to ensure a safe outcome. Policy and procedure must be written with specific guidelines to be followed for the counting of items dur-

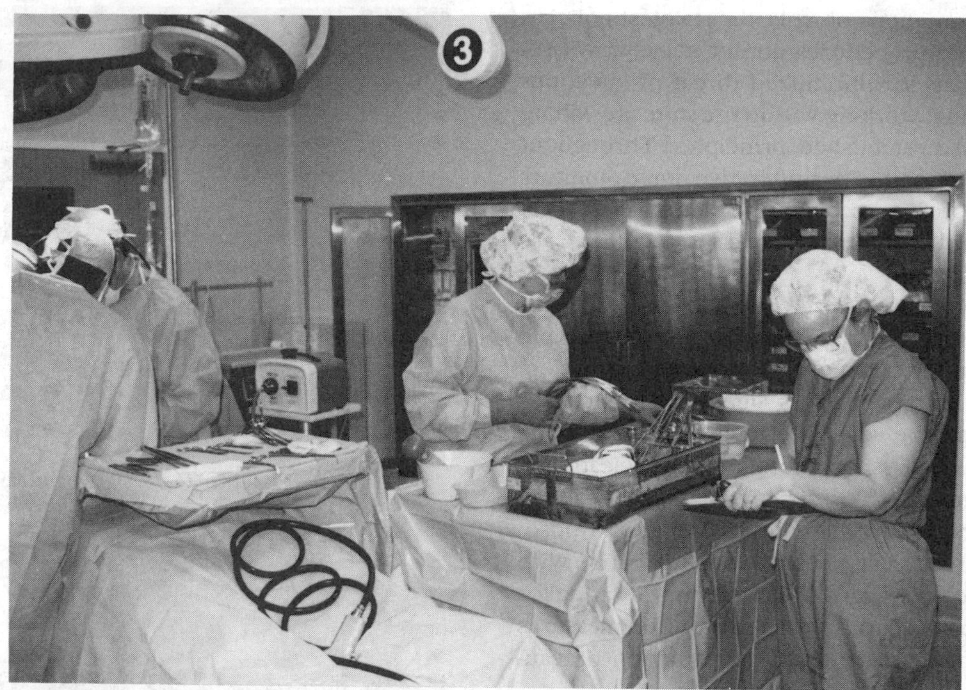

**FIGURE 24-6** The surgical count procedure.

ing each surgical procedure. It is imperative that all nursing personnel adhere to the appropriate count procedure (Figure 24-6).

Sponges and other products (e.g., vessel loops) used intraoperatively to facilitate attainment of the goals of the surgical procedure contain a radiopaque strip that is identifiable by radiologic examination. In the event of an incorrect count, arrangements are made for an x-ray film to be obtained to confirm the presence or absence of the missing item in the patient. If an item is identified by the film to be present in the operative site, the surgeon will reenter the site to retrieve the item. A recount is performed immediately to confirm the correct number of the item in question.

As with all other nursing interventions, documentation must be thorough in regard to the count procedure. After items are counted, the results and a list of responsible personnel must be recorded. Any corrective action taken in the event of a discrepancy and the resultant outcome are also recorded.

## Minimizing Risks for Postoperative Wound Infection

All patients who undergo surgery have the potential to acquire an infection. Surgical intervention breaks down some of the body's primary defenses against infection. Infection can have a negative effect on the outcome of surgery and even endanger the life of a patient. Protecting the patient from infection is a major goal of intraoperative nursing interventions. During the preoperative assessment, the nurse identifies host factors that increase the risk for infection (e.g., nutritional status, age, and underlying disease). Nursing interventions during the intraoperative period cannot change these factors; however, the goal is to control the number and types of microorganisms present during surgery. Many of the activities that are directed toward achieving this goal are related to monitoring and controlling the environment. The most important measure in preventing postoperative wound infection is adherence to meticulous aseptic technique principles and to CDC's universal precautions. The entire surgical team has a responsibility to uphold principles of aseptic technique and follow the policies and procedures established to ensure that the surgical suite is protected from unnecessary, additional risks resulting from increases in microbial population.[3]

*Creating and maintaining the sterile field* is the responsibility of the perioperative nurse. The standards and recommended practices for perioperative nursing[2] provide guidelines in areas related to the maintenance of a sterile field. These areas include basic aseptic technique, traffic patterns in the surgical suite, environmental controls, operating room attire, sterilization, barrier materials, surgical hand scrub, and preoperative skin preparation of patients. Information about these areas—crucial to aseptic technique maintenance—is discussed earlier in this chapter. Optimal patient care requires the acquisition of knowledge about each of the aforementioned areas, self-discipline, and fulfillment of the responsibility to be diligent in the maintenance of an aseptic environment for all patients. Operating room suites with ideal environmental controls, the strictest policies, and most thorough procedures do not necessarily provide ideal situations for minimized threat of infections unless the personnel working within the suite are willing to adhere to these established principles. Throughout the surgical procedure, the perioperative nurse monitors adherence to aseptic technique principles by all surgical team members and ensures that breaks in technique are corrected.

Intraoperatively, *compliance with isolation precautions* in providing care for patients with a communicable disease helps stop the chain of transmission. In addition, situations occur in which gross signs of infection are discovered during the surgery. Documentation of the appropriate wound classification (i.e., clean, clean-contaminated, contaminated, or dirty) will assist the infection control nurse with follow-up planning and nosocomial wound infection reporting. Communication with the postoperative unit ensures that the nurses caring for the patient will be prepared to use prevention measures such as observing "wound and skin" isolation precautions.

Etiologic factors in a wound infection and wound healing are many and may be environmental, host, or pathogenic. (Wound healing is discussed in Chapter 25.) One factor, attended to intraoperatively by the surgeon, that can facilitate healing is appropriate closure and drainage of a dead space when necessary. Closure of an incision with minimal trauma is facilitated by placing sutures in close approximation to achieve an anatomically secure wound. Wound edges will not heal readily if not in close contact. A dead space may occur from separation of wound edges or by air trapped between layers of tissue. Serum, blood, or other fluid may accumulate in a dead space and prevent healing.

## Drains

If it is anticipated that fluid may collect in a body area near the wound after surgery, the surgeon usually inserts a tube or drain to permit the fluid to escape. One end of the tube or drain is placed in or near the organ or cavity to be drained, and the other end is passed through the body wall, usually through a separate small incision near the operative site. Drains are usually made of latex or silicone. In some cases, drainage is by gravity through a tube—for example, a T-tube (Figure 24-7) or Penrose drain. In most cases a self-contained closed suction system is used for wound drainage. These suction drains create a negative pressure in a reservoir. The negative pressure gently suctions fluid from the wound into the attached reservoir. The Hemovac and Jackson-Pratt drains (Figures 24-8 and 24-9) are examples of closed-suction drainage systems. Closed drains also may be attached to wall or portable suction devices for a greater range of suction capacity. The level of suction is based on the amount and area to be evacuated and is set by the surgeon.

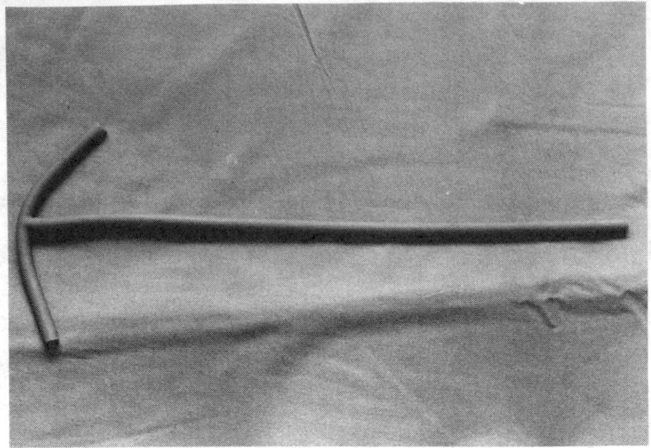

**FIGURE 24-7** T tube drain.

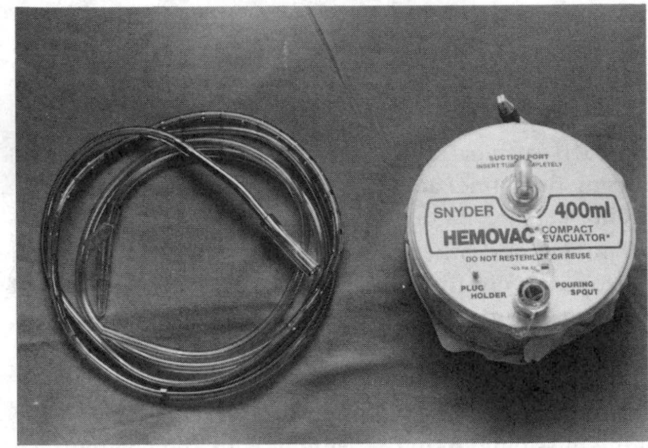


**FIGURE 24-8** Hemovac drain.

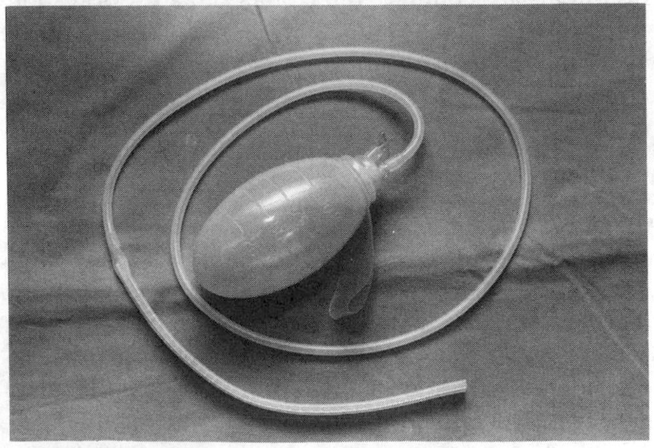

**FIGURE 24-9** Jackson-Pratt drain.

*Chest tubes* are inserted for drainage of the pleural cavity after chest procedures. The purpose of the chest tube is to evacuate air or fluid that has accumulated within the pleural space to ensure the postoperative expansion of lungs. One or more chest tubes are inserted intraoperatively and are connected to a closed collection unit. Water in the collection unit seals off the outside air to maintain a negative pressure within the pleural cavity. Air from the chest bubbles through the water and escapes through an outlet tube. Fluid drainage is collected in a reservoir where it can be accurately measured. (For further discussion, see Chapter 37.)

Nursing interventions related to drains focus on the preparation of the drainage system components, assessment of patency and drainage, and accurate documentation for postoperative nurses. After the tubing is placed by the surgeon, the sterile connection is attached to the evacuator or suction source using universal adapters and strict aseptic technique. Assessment of the patency of the system and the amount, type, color, and consistency of the drainage is performed. The type, location, and drainage assessment is thoroughly recorded and included in verbal reporting to the nurse in the postoperative receiving unit.

### Dressings

Protection of incision sites from contamination is a means of minimizing risk for postoperative wound infection. After surgery is completed, a sterile dressing is applied to the wound and secured. Dressings also serve to absorb drainage, protect the incision from trauma, and give support to the incision and surrounding skin. The perioperative nurse is responsible for ensuring dressing security and documenting the condition of the dressing before transfer of the patient to the postoperative unit.

## Minimizing the Risks for Alteration in Normothermia

### Hypothermia

Normally, body heat is maintained by activity, wearing clothing, or covering with blankets. Cool ambient air, prolonged exposure, the use of cool fluids, and immobility of the patient in the operating room all interfere with normal body temperature maintenance. Anesthetic agents may affect temperature-regulating mechanisms, decrease metabolism, cause vasodilation, or reduce patient sensitivity to cold (see anesthesia section). Factors that put patients at risk for alterations in body temperature are trauma (because of exposure), advanced age (because of limited cardiovascular reserve, loss of fat and subcutaneous tissue, degenerative changes in thermoregulating mechanism), malnutrition (causes a decrease in metabolism), prolonged preoperative inactivity, and sedation. These factors can be determined during the preoperative assessment. The greatest heat loss occurs in the first hour of surgery; therefore heat conservation methods should be initiated early by the perioperative nurse.[13] See Research box above.

**RESEARCH**

Blansett MT: The effects of rewarming hypothermic postanesthesia patients using Thermadrape covering, heat lamps, and warmed cotton blankets, *J Post Anesth Nurs* 5(2):80-84, 1990.

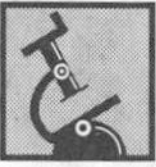

This article includes a brief review of hypothermia and describes contributing factors that cause hypothermia in the operating room, as well as the methods used to rewarm patients in the postanesthesia care unit (PACU). Thermadrape coverings (OR Concepts, Inc, Roanoke, Tex) were studied to determine if they were effective in maintaining body temperature within a normothermic range. Of 55 patients evaluated in the PACU, the 18 (32%) who received Thermadrape coverings in the perioperative period remained normothermic. The methods used to rewarm postanesthesia patients included three combinations: Thermadrape and warmed cotton blankets, warmed cotton blankets and heat lamps, and warmed cotton blankets alone.

An intervention that can be initiated immediately after admission to the operating room is the application of warm blankets. Before surgery begins, the patient should remain covered as much as possible. This necessitates that an ample supply of blankets be available in warming cabinets at all times. Another intervention that is used successfully during preoperative preparations is a radiant lamp. The application of thermal coverings, especially a covering for the head, is recommended to reduce radiant heat loss. During surgery the use of an automatic thermal blanket under the patient is a common intervention. During most surgical procedures a large amount of fluid is administered intravenously for replacement and topically for wound irrigation before closure. The perioperative nurse ensures that all fluids presented to the anesthesiologist or added to the surgical field are warm. In the immediate postoperative period, warm blankets are applied as soon as surgical patient drapes are removed.

### Hyperthermia

Hyperthermia may occur in the surgical patient. Risk factors include dehydration, illness resulting in fever, vasoconstriction from medication, endocrine disorders such as thyroid disease, intracranial infection or injury to the hypothalamus, and a history of the anesthetic complication of malignant hyperthermia[20] (see p. 636).

During surgery nursing interventions for cooling include removing excessive drapes, applying alcohol or cool water to the patient's skin, assisting with the monitoring of vital signs, use of an automatic cooling blanket, and assisting with the preparation and administration of cool intravenous fluids and emergency medications. A

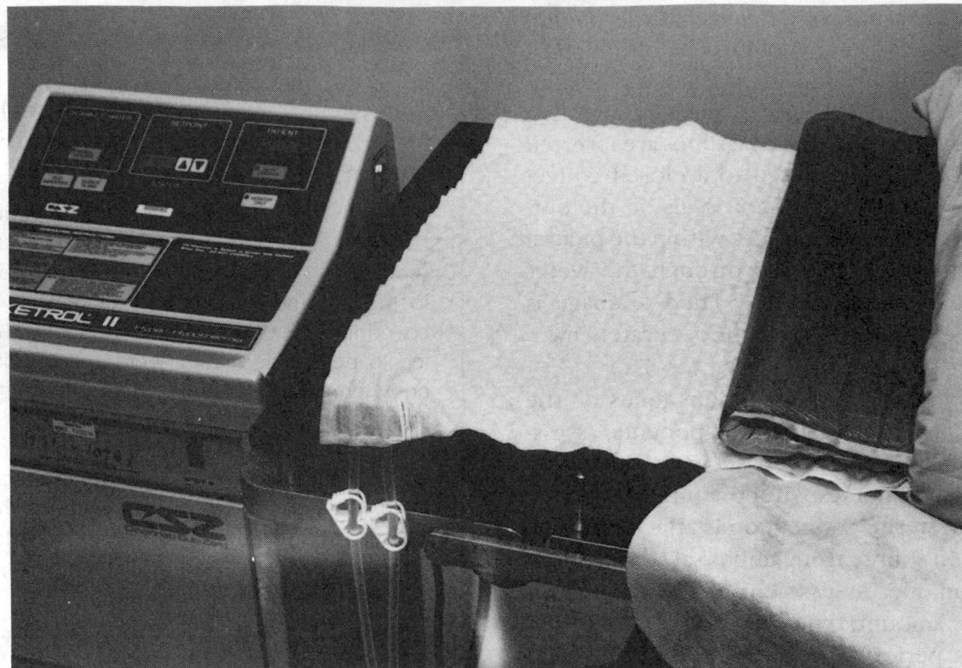

**FIGURE 24-10** Hypothermia/hyperthermia mattress.

baseline temperature for all patients should be recorded preoperatively. Before all surgical procedures, preparation is necessary to guarantee that supplies are available for all nursing interventions to minimize risks for any alteration in normothermia. In addition, the perioperative nurse must be knowledgeable about the causes of heat loss, nursing interventions to minimize heat loss, risk factors in patients, and appropriate operation of the automatic hyperthermia/hypothermia unit and mattress (Figure 24-10). The proper functioning of the automatic unit must be ascertained before use.

As with all nursing interventions, thorough documentation should include all measures taken, equipment used (including serial numbers and temperature settings), and any changes noted. Communication with the postoperative receiving unit is imperative for the continuity of patient care. This is especially important in cases in which an alteration in normothermia resulted in an emergent situation. The occurrence of a patient emergency intraoperatively may warrant a special arrangement for an intensive care unit bed that was not planned for originally.

## Minimizing Risks for Fluid Volume Deficit or Excess

Intraoperative monitoring of fluid loss and adequate replacement is a responsibility of high priority throughout the procedure for both anesthesiologist and perioperative nurse. The perioperative nurse assists the anesthesiologist in monitoring the patient during surgery. The nurse who has a working knowledge of fluid and electrolyte imbalances and how to assess for them, as well as how to prevent or correct them, can anticipate problems and offer greater assistance to the anesthesiologist. During procedures in which intravenous conscious sedation is used, the perioperative nurse assumes total responsibility for monitoring duties.

A thorough preoperative assessment will reveal risk factors for fluid volume deficit in patients, which include trauma, preexisting bleeding disorders, the presence of fluid deficit, recent intake of anticoagulant medications, impaired renal function, and age (the very young and the elderly person are subject to fluid imbalances more readily because of immature or impaired body functions). A deficit in fluid volume occurs more commonly in patients who are receiving nothing by mouth, who have intraoperative blood and body fluid losses, who have age-associated decreases in total body water and plasma volumes, or who experience neuroendocrine responses to surgery and anesthesia. Hypovolemia usually occurs when intraoperative bleeding is not controlled and can result in hypovolemic shock.

Risk factors for fluid volume excess include a rapid intake of fluid or sodium, the presence of chronic renal failure or congestive heart failure, neuroendocrine responses to surgery and anesthesia, and corticosteroid therapy (results in sodium retention). Excess intake of intravenous fluid causes hypervolemia and can result in congestive heart failure and edema.

Nursing interventions to minimize fluid volume deficit or excess begin with an accurate preoperative assessment of patients to determine risk factors. The perioperative nurse assists with the preparation and administration of intravenous fluids, ensuring an adequate

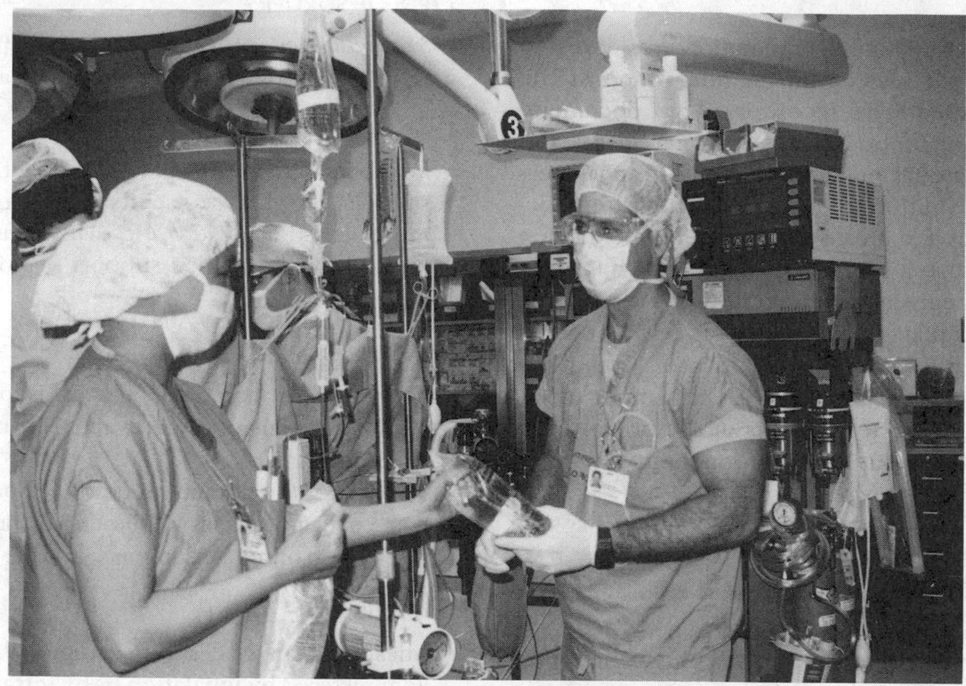

**FIGURE 24-11** Providing intraoperative fluids.

supply at all times (Figure 24-11). In addition, the nurse facilitates the preparation and sending of blood specimens to the laboratory. Indwelling Foley catheters are inserted before the start of surgery if the patient is at risk for alteration in normal fluid volume balances, if the surgery is expected to be lengthy, or if the anticipated blood loss may be great. Urine output is recorded hourly. Blood loss is monitored by keeping accurate record of the fluids administered into the wound, the amount of fluid suctioned from the operative cavity, and the amount of saturation of all sponges (sponges may be weighed for a thorough estimation). Assessment of the available blood and/or ordering of additional blood must be performed continuously to remain ahead of anticipated needs.

The anesthesiologist records all blood products given, the amount of solutions used by the surgeon, the estimated blood loss, and all intraoperative events concerning fluid imbalances. The perioperative nurse records this information during local procedures when an anesthesiologist is not present. The anesthesiologist and perioperative nurse communicate to the caregiver on the receiving unit collaboratively.

## ♦ EVALUATION

Evaluation of perioperative patient care is achieved by comparing the patient's responses to interventions with the expected outcomes. Through evaluation, the extent of goal attainment and the effectiveness of the nursing interventions can be determined. Evaluation is ongoing throughout the surgical intervention, in the immediate postoperative period before transfer to the receiving unit, after transfer to the receiving unit, and—in the case of the ambulatory surgery patient—after the patient's arrival back home.

### Observation

Goal attainment can be assessed by observation of both subjective and physiologic data. Observations that indicate attainment of expected outcomes include the following:

1. Shows little subjective or objective evidence of anxiety.
2. Exhibits no discolored or broken skin.
3. Shows no signs of injury/trauma from physical, chemical, or electrical trauma.
4. Exhibits no swelling or redness at the incision site.
5. Is normothermic.
6. Maintains stable vital signs without evidence of hypovolemia or cardiac overload.

It is necessary for the perioperative nurse to be astute in assessment techniques to pick up subtle condition changes, as well as obvious ones.

Postoperative visits to the patient are greatly encouraged and provide an opportunity for the perioperative nurse to further evaluate intraoperative interventions. Feedback about postoperative findings from nursing peers on patient care units can supply valuable information for evaluation and should be encouraged. In ambulatory surgery settings, a follow-up telephone call to the patient at home should be made by nursing personnel. This can be useful in obtaining feedback about the nursing care received during the surgical intervention.

## Documentation

Specific details of nursing documentation are addressed in the individual sections of nursing interventions. The intraoperative patient care record is a legal document, provides protection for both patients and caregivers, and should clearly state all nursing interventions and measured results. In addition to its legal value, written documentation serves as a means for evaluating the nursing care rendered and as a valuable communication tool for postoperative caregivers. Continuing with or changing components in a plan of care can be decided on the basis of documented patient observations. Communication of important data about the patient among members of the health care team assists in the provision of continuity of care for that patient throughout the entire surgical experience.

## QUESTIONS TO CONSIDER

- Discuss the components of the perioperative nurse's role that enhance his or her ability to serve as patient advocate throughout the surgical experience.
- Discuss the relationship of (a) operating room suite design and (b) surgical attire to infection control for patients.
- Why are combinations of anesthetic agents often necessary and beneficial to patients throughout the surgical experience?
- Describe the role of the nurse in care of patients experiencing anesthetic complications.
- Discuss the relationship of thorough preoperative assessments and patient outcomes during and after surgery.
- Discuss the risk factors in surgical positioning for (a) the elderly patient and (b) the diabetic patient.

## CRITICAL THINKING ACTIVITIES

- Numerous surgeries are scheduled for the following day, and the work load in sterile services is heavy. When a technician calls in ill, the nursing supervisor decides to send a nursing assistant to sterile services to help prepare supplies and instruments for the next day's surgeries. If you were the supervisor, would you have made the same or a different decision?
- While scrubbed on a major surgical case, another nurse points out to you that you appeared to contaminate your glove. You are fairly sure that you did not. What is the best way to approach this difference of opinion?

## CHAPTER SUMMARY

- The intraoperative phase of the surgical experience begins with the patient's arrival in the operating room suite and continues until the patient is transferred to the postanesthesia unit.

### TYPES OF SURGERY

- Subspecialties of surgery involve procedures performed in a specific body system or anatomic region.

### THE SURGICAL HEALTH CARE TEAM

- Members of the surgical health care team include the surgeon, surgical assistants, the anesthesiologist or nurse anesthetist, the circulating nurse, the scrub nurse, and other allied support personnel.

### ASEPTIC TECHNIQUE MAINTENANCE

- Postoperative wound infection is a potentially fatal complication: maintenance of an aseptic environment is a major focus of nursing care during the intraoperative phase.
- Wearing of the correct operating room attire (scrubs, hair covering, masks) is essential for decreasing the risk of personnel serving as a source of infection.

### ANESTHESIA

- Anesthesia may be general, regional, or local and is administered by inhalation or by intravenous injection or is localized by regional block, field block, or spinal, epidural, topical, or infiltrative means.

### PHYSIOLOGIC STRESS RESPONSES TO SURGERY AND ANESTHESIA

- An understanding of how the body systems are affected by anesthesia and surgery is essential to establish a scientific basis for intraoperative caregiving by the health care team.

### NURSING MANAGEMENT

- Nursing practice in the operating room includes assessment, planning, implementation, and evaluation of nursing activities to meet individual needs of patients requiring a surgical intervention.
- Nursing diagnoses for the intraoperative patient include high risk for elevated anxiety, impairment of skin integrity, injury/trauma (caused by misidentification, improper positioning, or hazards—chemical, electrical, physical, or retention of foreign objects), postoperative wound infection, alteration in normothermia, and fluid volume deficit or excess.
- Desired patient outcomes include the following: the patient (1) will show little evidence of anxiety, (2) will be free of signs of skin breakdown, (3) will be free from injury/trauma, (4) will be free of signs of postoperative wound infection, (5) will be normothermic, and (6) will maintain adequate fluid volume.
- The perioperative nurse can be instrumental in reducing patient anxiety by providing physiologic and emotional support and communicating an overall attitude of caring.
- A major focus of nursing interventions during the intraoperative phase is maintenance of patient safety and prevention of postoperative complications.

- Evaluation of patient care is achieved by comparing the patient's responses to interventions with the expected outcomes.
- Postoperative feedback is obtained by postoperative patient visits, patient surveys, findings from nursing peers on other units, and postoperative telephone calls.
- Documentation of intraoperative interventions and patient responses must be thorough. This is a means of providing continuity of care for the patient throughout the surgical experience.

## REFERENCES


1. Association of Operating Room Nurses: Recommended practices: skin preparation, *AORN J* 55(2):555-562, 1992.
2. Association of Operating Room Nurses: A model for perioperative nursing practice. In *Standards and recommended practices,* Denver, 1993, The Association.
3. Association of Operating Room Nurses: Recommended practices: aseptic technique. In *Standards and recommended practices,* Denver, 1993, The Association.
4. Association of Operating Room Nurses: Recommended practices: surgical attire. In *Standards and recommended practices,* Denver, 1993, The Association.
5. Association of Operating Room Nurses: Recommended practices: surgical hand scrub. In *Standards and recommended practices,* Denver, 1993, The Association.
6. Association of Operating Room Nurses: Recommended practices: universal precautions in the perioperative setting, *AORN J* 57(2):554-558, 1993.
7. Bailey SL: Electrical injuries: considerations for the perioperative nurse, *AORN J* 49(3):773-778, 1989.
8. Biddle C, Cannady JJ: Surgical positions: their effect on cardiovascular, respiratory systems, *AORN J* 52(2):350-359, 1990.
9. Blansett MT: The effects of rewarming hypothermic postanesthesia patients using Thermadrape covering, heat lamps, and warmed cotton blankets, *J Post Anesth Nurs* 5(2):80-84, 1990.
10. Cooper DE et al: The prevention of injuries of the brachial plexus secondary to malposition of the patient during surgery, *Clin Orthop* 228:33-41, 1988.
11. Ferrari A: Anesthesia and perioperative nursing implication. In Fairchild SS: *Perioperative nursing principles and practice,* Boston, 1993, Jones & Bartlett.
12. Garrett N: Anesthesia pharmacology for general endotracheal anesthesia, *Semin Periop Nurs* 2(2):8-12, 1993.
13. Kneedler JA, Dodge GH: *Perioperative patient care,* ed 2, Boston, 1991, Jones & Bartlett.
14. Lord EV: General anesthesia: what the perioperative nurse needs to know, *Semin Periop Nurs* 2(2):6-8, 1993.
15. Occupational Safety and Health Association, Department of Labor: Occupational exposure to bloodborne pathogens; final rule, *Federal Register* 56:64175-64180, 1991.
16. Parsons EC, Kee CC, Gray P: Perioperative nurse caring behaviors, *AORN J* 57(5):1106-1114, 1993.
17. Schiffer DH: Regional anesthesia: considerations for the perioperative nurse, *Semin Periop Nurs* 2(2):23-32, 1993.
18. Sword SL: The surgical setting. In Fairchild SS: *Perioperative nursing principles and practice,* Boston, 1993, Jones & Bartlett
19. Watson DS: Safe nursing practices involving the patient receiving local anesthesia, *AORN J* 53(4):1055, 1058-1059, 1991.
20. Wlody GS: Malignant hyperthermia, *Crit Care Nurs Clin North Am* 3(1):129-134, 1991.

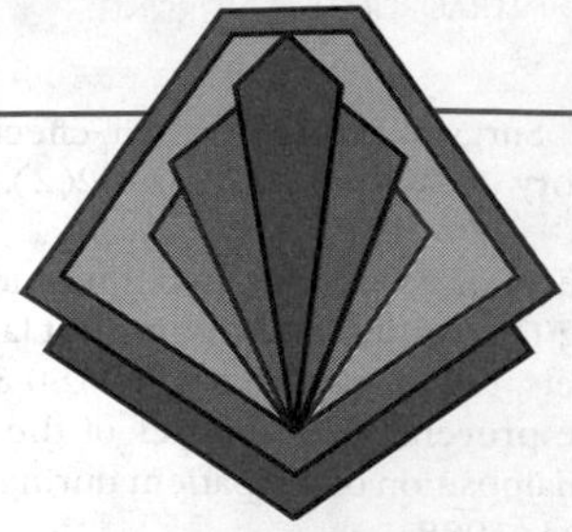

C H A P T E R 25

# Postoperative Nursing

**Grace A. Muro**
**Arlene W. Keeling**
**Barbara C. Long**

## CHAPTER OBJECTIVES

***After studying this chapter, the learner should be able to do the following:***

1. Describe the postoperative phase as a component of the surgical experience.
2. Identify postoperative complications that may compromise a patient's safety and stability after anesthesia and surgical intervention.
3. Discuss the patient's risk factors for potential postoperative complication.
4. Discuss postoperative patient assessment.
5. Identify postoperative nursing diagnoses.
6. Identify desired patient outcomes for the postoperative phase.
7. Discuss nursing interventions to prevent and/or treat postoperative complications.
8. Discuss the interventions to minimize anxiety in patients and their families during the postoperative course.
9. Discuss the relevance of evaluation and documentation of nursing care interventions.
10. Identify the benefits of follow-up communication and referrals for the patient's later postoperative recovery.

## KEY TERMS

dehiscence
distention
evisceration
hypothermia
postanesthesia care unit (PACU)
pulse oximetry
urinary retention
wound healing by primary intention
wound healing by secondary intention
wound healing by tertiary intention

The postoperative phase begins with the transfer of the patient from the operating room to the appropriate postoperative unit. It ends with the discharge of the patient from the surgical facility or the hospital. The goal of the postoperative phase is the patient's return, as quickly as possible, to an optimal level of functioning. Wound healing should be promoted, and postoperative complications should be prevented. This chapter discusses the nursing role during the postoperative recovery period.

## THE IMMEDIATE POSTANESTHESIA PHASE

In most hospitals, any patient who has received general or regional anesthesia is admitted to a **postanesthesia care unit (PACU).** Postanesthesia care assists the patient through the physiologic transition from intraoperative to postoperative progression. The immediate postanesthesia phase presents multifaceted challenges in patient care. Anesthesia and surgical interventions place great stress on all body systems (see Chapter 24). It is necessary for the postanesthesia nurse to understand the patient's risks for postoperative complications in body system functioning, alterations in comfort and skin integrity, and the biopsychosocial responses that may occur. Special clinical expertise is required to deliver maximal patient care when complications, often of an emergent nature, arise. In addition, expertise is needed to ensure the patient's return to a state of physiologic homeostasis that is the same or improved over the preoperative state.

To meet the criteria for transfer from the PACU to the clinical unit or to the home, the patient must be stable and free from symptoms of complications. The potential for the development of postoperative complications, however, continues beyond the immediate postoperative phase. Ongoing thorough nursing assessment is essential to providing care after the patient is transferred to a specific clinical unit. Nursing interventions focus on minimizing the potential for postoperative complications and promoting partnership with the patient in planning and implementing recovery. Effective preoperative patient teaching (see Chapter 23) prepares the patient for a role in facilitating the recovery course. In the postoperative phase the nurse reinforces this information. In addition, the nurse continues planning for the patient's discharge. A goal of the postoperative phase is to ensure that both patient and family have an opportunity for adequate understanding of the postsurgical plan of care.

In the present era of health care reform, more and more patients are being discharged the same day of surgery or the following day. In addition to economic incentives, improvements in surgical techniques and new anesthesia developments have made ambulatory and short-stay surgery both safe and feasible. The time that the patient remains at the health care facility has been greatly reduced. As a result, increased responsibility has been placed on the patient and significant others to follow through with observations and treatments after they return home. For this reason, assessing the patient's needs and providing assessment-based informational support before discharge are crucial tasks for nurses who care for these patients in the early postoperative period. Although the importance of these educational needs is recognized, this chapter focuses on the immediate phase of the postoperative recovery course during which nursing interventions are directed toward maintaining patient stability, promoting safety, and preventing later postoperative complications.

## NURSING MANAGEMENT

### ♦ ASSESSMENT

Assessment is a continuous process, leading to nursing diagnoses and implementation of appropriate nursing interventions. Assessing, planning, and implementing care for the postoperative patient require that preoperative information be ascertained and compared with postoperative data.

The PACU nurse receives a report on the patient's condition from members of the operating room team before assuming responsibility for patient care. The following patient data should be obtained:

Current medical diagnosis
Surgical procedure performed
Known allergies
Agents administered
Complications during surgery
Blood and intravenous fluids received
Estimated blood loss (EBL)
Pertinent preoperative problems

**BOX 25-1 Postoperative Patient Assessment**

**RESPIRATORY STATUS**
Patency of airway
Respirations: depth, rate, character
Breath sounds: presence, character
Chest expansion
Patient position to facilitate ventilation
Ability to deep breathe and cough

**NEUROLOGIC STATUS**
Level of consciousness
Ability to follow commands
Sensation and ability to move extremities after regional anesthesia

**CARDIAC STATUS**
Blood pressure
Pulse rate, strength (presence distal to limb surgery)
Skin color and temperature
Capillary filling
Monitoring systems—connected and functioning

**TEMPERATURE**
Skin color
Body temperature

**SURGICAL SITE DRESSINGS AND DRAINS**
Dressings: frank bleeding
Drainage systems—connected and functioning

**GASTROINTESTINAL STATUS**
Nausea/vomiting
Nasogastric tube patency; amount and character of drainage

**BODY FLUIDS**
Intravenous fluids—rate, amount in bag, patency of tubing
Urine output >30 ml/hr

**SKIN INTEGRITY**
Reddened areas, skin breaks

**COMFORT AND SAFETY**
Pain—presence, character, severity
Patient position
Necessity for side rails
Call cord within reach

**ANXIETY—PATIENT AND FAMILY**
Emotional status—anxiety, restlessness, family whereabouts, communication

After receiving this report, the nurse completes a thorough patient assessment. Box 25-1 describes areas of assessment and corresponding observations.

### Respiratory Status

Assessing respiratory status is of primary importance during the immediate postoperative period. Both a patent airway and adequate respiratory function should be ascertained. The postoperative patient has experienced some interference with the respiratory system. As a re-

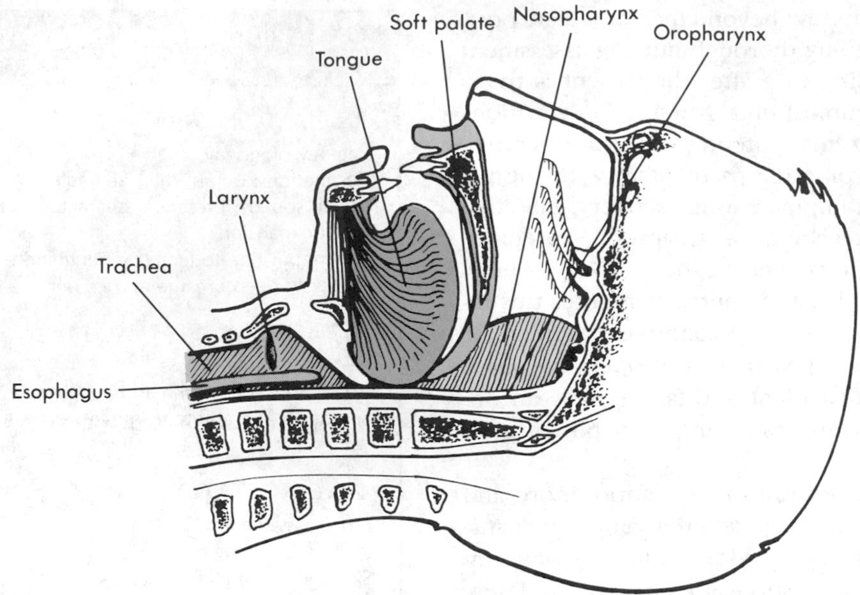


**FIGURE 25-1** Obstruction of airway by tongue blocking oropharynx in unconscious person lying in supine position.

sult, maintaining a patent airway is crucial. Respiratory changes can occur at any point, from the time a preoperative medication is given until several days after the surgical intervention. The leading cause of postoperative morbidity and mortality is respiratory complication. Immediate respiratory complications that may occur include airway obstruction, hypoventilation, aspiration, and laryngospasm.

### Airway obstruction

In assessing respiratory status, the nurse first checks for airway patency. Airway obstruction most frequently occurs as a result of the tongue—relaxed from anesthesia—falling back against the pharynx (Figure 25-1) or secretions or other fluids collecting in the pharynx, trachea, or bronchial tree. All noisy breathing (e.g., snoring, gurgling, wheezing, crowing) indicates some type of airway obstruction. Obstruction can occur, however, without being accompanied by noise.

Assessment of the rate and depth of respirations, symmetry of chest expansion and excursion, bilateral presence of breath sounds, and type of breath sounds is completed. Total absence of breath sounds on one side may signal the presence of a pneumothorax, an obstruction, or fluid or blood within the pleural space.

### Hypoventilation

Hypoventilation diminishes the exchange of oxygen between the alveoli and the atmosphere. Tissue hypoxemia is the result of decreased oxygen delivery. The following factors can place the patient at high risk for inadequate respiratory function:

- Narcotics (respiratory center depression)
- Insufficient reversal of neuromuscular blocking drugs (residual muscle paralysis)
- Increased tissue resistance (emphysema, infections)
- Decreased lung and chest wall compliance (pneumonia, restrictive diseases)
- Obesity; gastric and abdominal distention
- Constrictive dressings
- Incision site close to the diaphragm
- General rather than regional anesthesia
- Postoperative pain

Hypoventilation may lead to atelectasis in the later postoperative period.

### Aspiration

Aspiration is the inhalation of gastric contents or blood into the tracheobronchial system. Aspiration usually is caused by regurgitation; however, aspiration of blood may result from trauma or surgical manipulation (e.g., after tonsillectomy). Aspiration of gastric contents can cause chemical irritation, pneumonitis, destruction of tracheobronchial mucosa, and an increased risk of secondary infection. Patients at risk for aspiration are those who have undergone surgery of the oropharynx, have suffered facial trauma, have stomach contents but are in need of emergent surgery, or have a history of hiatal hernia. In addition, the obese patient has an increased incidence of esophageal reflux, and the pregnant patient tends to have an increase in gastric fluid volume.

### Laryngospasm

Laryngospasm is a spasm of laryngeal muscle tissue. It may manifest as complete or partial closure of the vocal cords and result in obstruction of the respiratory tract.

If not treated, laryngospasm can cause hypoxia, cerebral damage, and death. Therefore laryngospasm is a potential emergency in the immediate postoperative period. Patients at risk for laryngospasm are those who have been exposed to airway irritation. Irritation can be caused by certain anesthetic agents, laryngoscope blades used in intubation, endotracheal tube placement, or surgical stimulation (e.g., bronchoscope passage). In the PACU, repeated suctioning and irritation by the endotracheal tube or artificial airway can cause laryngospasm. Dyspnea, crowing sounds, hypoxemia, and hypercapnia are symptoms of laryngospasm.

## Neurologic Status

On the patient's arrival in the PACU level of consciousness can vary from unconscious to wakeful, depending on the type of anesthetic agent used during the surgery. Patients who have received general anesthesia usually are unconscious but arousable. Generally they can breathe without the assistance of an Ambu (breathing) bag or mechanical ventilation. Most patients return to an oriented state in approximately 1 hour, with a tendency to fall asleep when left alone. However, these patients are arousable by either verbal or tactile stimulation.

Neurologic status is ascertained by observing the patient's level of consciousness. Response to verbal or noxious stimuli is noted. Pupils are assessed for responsiveness to light and equality. Equality and strength of hand grip also are assessed. A hand grip sustained for 5 seconds is an indication that neuromuscular function is returning. The ability to move all extremities also is assessed and noted.

### Complications of general anesthesia

Prolonged somnolence and muscle weakness are major nervous system complications that may occur immediately after general anesthesia. Failure to awaken promptly or completely is usually the result of the anesthetic's residual effect. Other causes of stupor include severe hypoxia, hypothermia, metabolic imbalances, hyponatremia, hyperglycemia, and severe hypercapnia. Muscle weakness usually results from prolonged effects of muscle relaxants. Renal failure and electrolyte imbalances can delay recovery from muscle relaxants. Emergence delirium is another alteration in level of consciousness that may occur during the immediate postanesthesia phase. In this short-lived state the patient demonstrates increased motor activity, disorientation, and vocalizations.

### Complications of regional anesthesia

Complications, although rare, can occur if a patient has received spinal anesthesia. These complications are the result of neurologic injury caused by local anesthetic toxicity, needle trauma, or cord ischemia. Symptoms can include hypoxemia, agitation, hypotension, and nausea.

Spinal anesthesia interferes with innervation of the bladder. The abdomen is palpated to assess for bladder distention (see section on urinary retention).

## Cardiovascular Status

Surgery and anesthetic agents predispose patients to complications of the cardiovascular system. Hypotension and cardiac dysrhythmias are the most commonly encountered cardiovascular complications in the immediate postanesthesia period. Later complications include venous thrombosis and pulmonary embolism. Early recognition and management of cardiovascular complications before they become serious are critical.

The pulse is assessed for rate and quality. The pulse rate may be increased or decreased. A weak, thready pulse with a significant drop in blood pressure can indicate hemorrhage or circulatory failure. The presence and strength of peripheral pulses distal to an operative site or cast on an extremity are used to measure adequacy of circulation.

Adequate circulation is important in the postoperative period to provide adequate oxygenation to all tissues, especially to the traumatized tissue for commencement of wound healing. Pallor in light-skinned patients and a dullness or decrease in red tones in dark-skinned patients indicates decreased circulation to the skin. Pallor in dark-skinned patients may be more easily assessed by examining the mucous membranes of the mouth. Vasoconstriction may result from cold temperatures or a decrease in the amount of circulating blood as a result of blood loss or from the neuroendocrine response to stress. The nail beds are checked for capillary return. If circulation is adequate, pinkness should return to the nail after it is "flicked" by the examiner's finger.

### Hypotension

A number of factors in the early postoperative period cause circulatory changes that may result in lowering the blood pressure. A mild decrease in blood pressure from the normal preoperative range is not uncommon during the early postoperative period. It is usually well tolerated in healthy patients and does not require treatment. Shock, however, must be prevented because the brain, heart, kidneys, and other vital organs do not tolerate long periods of hypoxemia. A weak, thready pulse with a significant drop in blood pressure may indicate hemorrhage or circulatory failure. Possible causes of postoperative hypotension are summarized in Box 25-2.

Blood pressure is monitored carefully in the early postoperative period. Changes in blood pressure readings are more significant than consistently high or low readings. An increase in systolic pressure may be related to anxiety or pain. Hypotensive changes can be caused by shock, although other signs of shock usually appear before changes in blood pressure occur.

Hemorrhagic shock occurs when there is a loss of

**BOX 25-2 Possible Causes of Postoperative Hypotension**

Moving patient from operating room table to bed
Jarring of patient's bed during transport
Drugs, anesthesia
Loss of blood and other body fluids
Cardiac dysrhythmias
Cardiac failure
Inadequate ventilation
Pain
Residual sympathectomy from conductive anesthesia
Pooling of blood in the extremities

circulatory blood volume and subsequent insufficient transport of oxygen to the cells. Shock must be prevented because the brain, heart, kidneys, and other vital organs do not tolerate long periods of hypoxemia. Hypotension, hypoxemia, and hypovolemia compromise the supply of oxygen to the cardiac muscle and can place patients at higher risk for myocardial infarction. Identification of the following risk factors during assessment will assist the health care team members in planning preventive and treatment measures:

- Preexisting coronary artery disease
- Diabetes
- Obesity
- Debilitated status

#### Cardiac dysrhythmias

Hypoxemia and hypercapnia are common causes of postoperative cardiac dysrhythmias, especially premature beats and sinus tachycardia. These dysrhythmias often can be corrected by adequate ventilation. Other common causes of postoperative cardiac dysrhythmias include pain, hypovolemia, gastric distention, acidosis, and occasionally acute myocardial infarction.

Early detection depends on careful monitoring of heart rate, rhythm, and blood pressure. Heart rate and rhythm must be accurately assessed. These parameters should initially be obtained at least every 15 minutes in the postanesthesia recovery phase. Continuous cardiac and blood pressure monitoring by means of invasive or noninvasive devices may be necessary.

#### Venous thrombosis

The formation of clots in the veins of the pelvis and the lower extremities, which impairs circulation, is a fairly common and potentially serious postoperative complication. Blood clots develop because of a roughness in the vessel wall such as occurs from trauma, venous stasis (slowing of blood flow), and hypercoagulability. Platelets adhere to the vessel wall, and the resulting inflammatory response stimulates blood coagulation and fibrin development, resulting in a blood clot on the vessel wall (thrombophlebitis). Postoperative clots often form in a vein of the foot, calf, thigh, or pelvis. The clot grows, usually in the direction of the slow-moving blood. It can occur in either a deep or superficial vein (Figure 25-2).

Venous stasis occurs postoperatively for a number of reasons. A major contribution to venous stasis is inactivity of the legs. Every time the leg is moved, the muscle compresses the vein, pushing the blood toward the heart (venous pump); valves prevent the blood from moving backward. Exercise therefore promotes return of venous blood to the heart and prevention of venous stasis.

The development of postoperative venous thrombosis may be attributed to several risk factors. Intrinsic factors include older age, obesity, malnutrition, and contraceptive use. Pathologic conditions that increase risk are malignant conditions, congestive heart failure, history of previous deep vein thrombosis, and polycythemia. Patients who undergo pelvic, abdominal, or thoracic surgery or who have had fracture of the hip or lower extremities are at greater risk. In addition, prolonged sitting with the legs dependent, decreased mobility, intestinal distention, pressure on the popliteal area, anesthetic effects, and tight dressings or casts on lower extremities also contribute to the potential for the development of venous thrombosis. A venous blood clot may develop without any local symptoms (phlebothrombosis). Homans' sign (pain on dorsiflexion of the foot) indicates a phlebothrombosis, but this sign may not always be present. Pain and local tenderness in the leg are signs of thrombophlebitis. The first indication of difficulty may be a pulmonary embolism.

**Pulmonary embolism.** A clot or portion of a clot may break away and flow through the heart into the pulmonary circulation until it occludes a pulmonary vessel (pulmonary embolism). Emboli alter the pulmonary circulation and decrease the function of the right and left sides of the heart. Dyspnea is the most common patient complaint. Other symptoms include tachypnea, chest pain, anxiety, diaphoresis, syncope, rales in the affected lung, tachycardia, and cyanosis. Signs of a *pulmonary embolism* depend on the size of the blood vessel that has been occluded. In some patients, pulmonary embolism causes sudden death. Any complaints of sudden sharp thoracic or upper abdominal pain or dyspnea, as well as any signs of shock, should be reported immediately to the physician.

### Thermoregulation

Premedications, anesthesia, and the stress of surgery interact in a complex fashion to disrupt normal thermoregulation (see Chapter 24). Both hypothermia (temperature below 35° C) and hyperthermia (temperature above 39° C) are associated with physiologic alterations that may interfere with recovery. Patients at the age extremes and those who are extremely debilitated are at even greater risk for the development of postoperative temperature abnormalities.

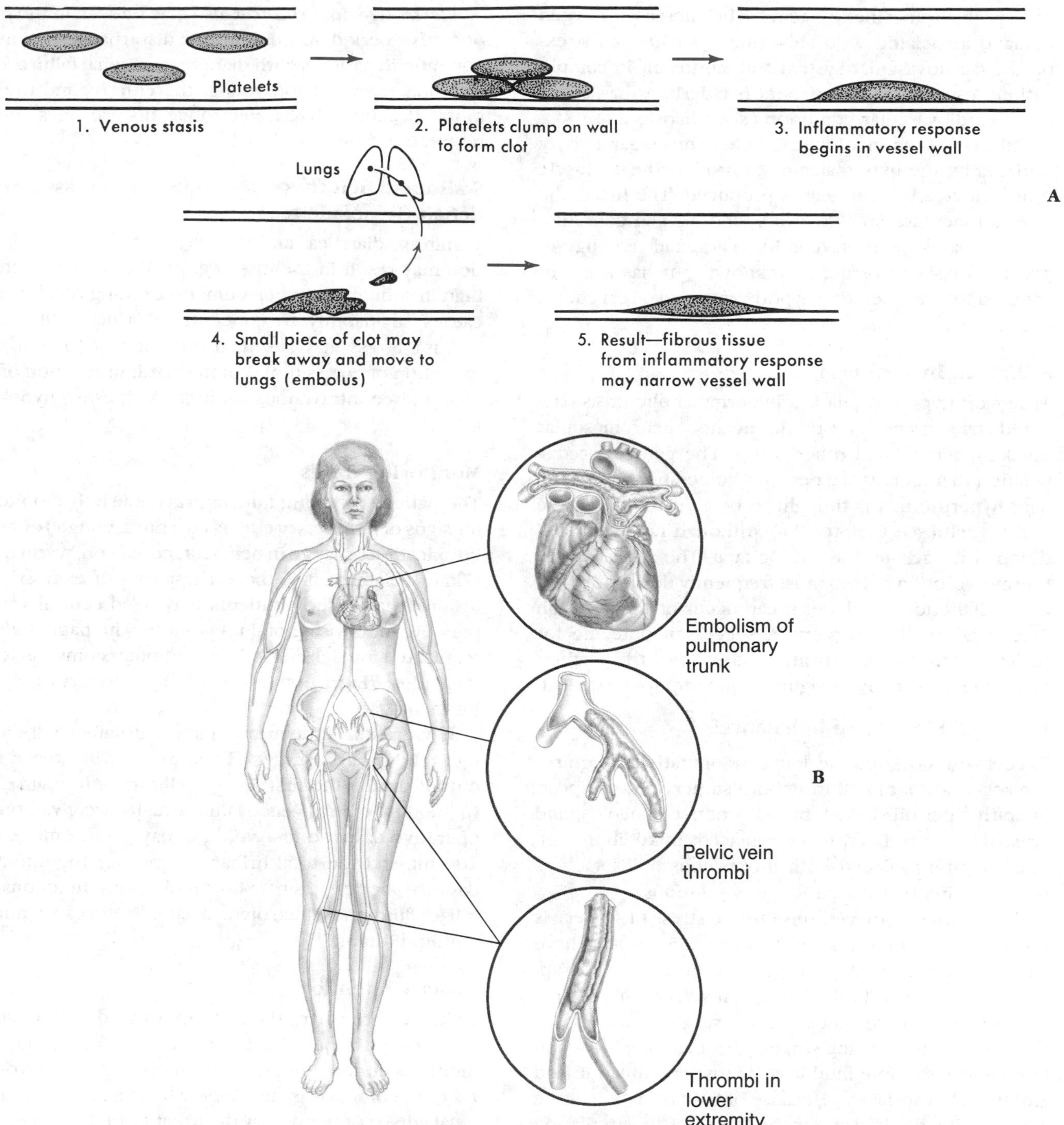


**FIGURE 25-2** **A,** Diagram illustrating the formation of thrombus on wall of vein after venous stasis, resulting in narrowing of blood vessel. **B,** Common locations of venous thrombi. (**B** from Canobbio MM: *Cardiovascular disorders,* St Louis, 1990, Mosby.)

## Hypothermia

General anesthesia depresses the body's temperature-regulation center in the brain. Narcotics and muscle relaxants suppress shivering, which normally helps the body generate heat. Cool air temperatures in the operating room, cool intravenous infusions administered during surgery, and open wounds combine to contribute to the development of a state of postoperative **hypothermia.** Hypothermia produces vasoconstriction, increases heart rate, increases blood pressure, and eventually increases cardiac workload.

**Postanesthesia shivering.** Postanesthesia shivering is a potential complication for any surgical patient who has received anesthetic agents. The increased oxygen demand associated with shivering places added stress on the cardiovascular system and can result in complications, especially if the patient is elderly or has an existing cardiovascular condition (see Chapter 24).

Shivering is an involuntary skeletal muscular activity initiated by the hypothalamus to produce heat. Muscle tone is increased and heat is produced. The metabolic rate can increase 50% to 100%, and oxygen consumption increases up to sevenfold.[3] The exact etiology of postanesthesia shivering is unknown but has been attributed to intraoperative hypothermia and direct effects of anesthetic agents.

#### Malignant hyperthermia

Malignant hyperthermia is a hypermetabolic crisis triggered by certain anesthetic agents, neuromuscular blocking agents, and other drugs. The genetic predisposition that increases a person's vulnerability to malignant hyperthermia is thought to be a defect within the muscle cell (see Chapter 24). Although rare, this condition is dangerous and can be fatal. The actual hyperthermic reaction occurs most frequently during the general anesthetic period, but it can occur or recur within 2 to 3 hours after surgery. A successful outcome for patients with the complication of malignant hyperthermia depends on early recognition and prompt treatment.

### Fluid and Electrolyte Imbalances

Excessive blood volume lost intraoperatively requires replacement therapy during both surgery and the postoperative period. Blood, blood products, colloids, and crystalloids may need to be replaced. In addition, volume may be replaced with intravenous fluids such as normal saline or lactated Ringer's solutions.

The normal body response to the stress of surgery is renal retention of water and sodium. Patients often have abnormal avenues of postoperative fluid loss. Postoperative parenteral fluid requirements vary with the patient's preoperative status and the surgical procedure.

Fluids are lost during surgery through blood loss and increased insensible fluid loss (by hyperventilation and exposed skin surfaces). Because of fluid retention at the surgical site, fluids also may be "lost" to the circulation after major surgery in which tissue dissection was extensive.

For at least 24 to 48 hours after surgery, fluids are retained by the body because of the stimulation of antidiuretic hormone (ADH) as part of the stress response to trauma and the effect of anesthesia. During surgery renal vasoconstriction and increased aldosterone activity also occur, leading to increased sodium retention with subsequent water retention. *Overhydration* can occur with vigorous fluid replacement, especially in the small elderly patient. Both water intoxication and pulmonary edema can occur depending on the type and amount of fluids given.

*Electrolyte disturbances* also may be seen in the postoperative period. Although these disturbances are more common in patients with diabetes and renal failure, they also may occur in the young, the elderly, and the debilitated patient. Such electrolyte disturbances should be treated promptly.

#### Sodium deficit (hyponatremia) and potassium deficit (hypokalemia)

Vomiting, diarrhea, and prolonged nasogastric intubation may result in the loss of gastrointestinal secretions high in sodium and potassium. Preexisting renal disease causes an inability to concentrate urine, with loss of sodium. Stress may result in retention of sodium with excretion of potassium. Prolonged administration of potassium-free intravenous solutions will cause hypokalemia.

#### Monitoring fluids

The patient receiving fluids intravenously is monitored for signs of pulmonary edema (dyspnea, cough) or water intoxication (change in behavior, confusion, warm moist skin). Weight gain is the earliest sign of excessive infusion. Small elderly patients may need central venous pressure monitoring of fluid volume. The patient also is monitored for signs of sodium and potassium deficit and for acidosis. Extra potassium may be necessary to replace losses by gastric secretion.

If hydration is adequate, a patient usually voids within 6 to 8 hours after surgery. Fluid intake will exceed fluid output during the first 24 to 48 hours. Although 2000 to 3000 ml of intravenous fluid usually are given on the operative day, the first voiding may not be more than 200 ml, and the total urinary output for the operative day may be less than 1500 ml. As body functions stabilize, fluid and electrolyte balance returns to normal within 48 hours.

#### Urinary retention

**Urinary retention,** the inability to void, may occur in the early postoperative period. Urinary retention commonly occurs after spinal anesthesia or surgery of the rectum, colon, or gynecologic structures as a result of local edema or temporary disturbance of the innervation of the bladder musculature.

Urinary retention is characterized by the voiding of little or no urine over a 6- to 8-hour period. Light palpation of the bladder over the lower portion of the abdomen just above the symphysis pubis usually elicits discomfort, and distention may be observed. Occasionally the overdistended bladder expels just enough urine to relieve the pressure within it temporarily and the patient voids frequently in small amounts but without discomfort. This pattern is called *retention with overflow.* Box 25-3 summarizes common causes of postoperative urinary retention.

*Urinary tract infections* may occur in patients who

**BOX 25-3 Causes of Urinary Retention**

- Recumbent position
- Nervous tension
- Effects of anesthetics that interfere with bladder sensation and the ability to void
- Pain caused by movement
- Pain at the surgical site after bladder or urethral surgery

have indwelling catheters inserted after surgery, particularly after pelvic surgery. Prolonged bed rest leading to urinary stasis also may be a contributing factor. Signs of urinary tract infection include frequency with dysuria; fever also may be present. These symptoms usually are observed 24 to 48 hours after surgery.

## Skin Integrity

During surgery, patients are at high risk for skin breakdown as a result of a prolonged surgical position, immobility, and preexisting risk factors (see Chapter 24). The postoperative caregiver must be aware of these risks and inspect for affected or potentially affected sites. Immobility in the immediate postoperative phase and exposure to moisture from body fluid drainage and/or vomitus place the patient at further risk for an alteration in skin integrity.

## Gastrointestinal Disturbance

### Nausea and vomiting

*Nausea and vomiting* are distressing postoperative side effects. These side effects may be related to a number of factors: effect of certain anesthetics on the stomach, decreased peristalsis producing a collection of fluid and gas in the stomach, drinking fluids before peristalsis returns, psychologic factors in patients who anticipate postoperative vomiting, drug idiosyncrasies, pain, disturbances in electrolyte balance, and a history of motion sickness.

Persistent postoperative vomiting is usually a symptom of pyloric obstruction, intestinal obstruction, or peritonitis. Vomiting tires the patient, puts a strain on the incision, and causes excessive loss of fluids and electrolytes. Choking while vomiting may lead to aspiration pneumonia.

### Hiccoughs

*Hiccoughs* interfere with eating and sleeping and are among the most exhausting postoperative complications. The exact cause of postoperative hiccoughs is not known, but it is known that dilation of the stomach, irritation of the diaphragm, peritonitis, and uremia cause either reflex or central nervous system stimulation of the phrenic nerve. Fortunately, hiccoughs usually disappear within a few hours and are not a common postoperative complaint.

### Abdominal distention and gas pains

Postoperative **distention** is a result of an accumulation of nonabsorbable gas in the intestines caused by a reaction to the handling of the bowel during surgery, by swallowing of air during recovery from anesthesia, and by passing of gases from the bloodstream to the atonic portion of the bowel. Distention will persist until the tone of the bowel returns to normal and peristalsis resumes. Most patients experience distention to some degree after abdominal and renal surgery.

Patients with abdominal distention complain of diffuse abdominal pain. High distention may cause dyspnea by pressure on the diaphragm and may lead to atelectasis. Abdominal girth is increased because of the collection of gas; this can be measured with a tape measure to determine progress. Percussion produces a drumlike (tympanic) sound as compared with a dull sound occurring with ascites or obesity. Acute gastric dilation may produce signs of shock (restlessness; rapid, weak, thready pulse; hypotension) and overflow vomiting. Gas pains in the intestinal tract usually occur as peristalsis is beginning to return, and these can be extremely painful. Bowel sounds usually are audible on auscultation. The return of peristalsis may not occur for 24 hours or more.

## Pain

Pain is a common occurrence after nearly all types of surgical procedures. Pain results from cutting, pulling, and manipulating tissues and organs. Postoperative pain is most severe after intrathoracic, intraabdominal, and major orthopedic surgeries. It may result from stimulation of nerve endings by chemical substances released at the time of surgery or from tissue ischemia caused by interference of blood supply to tissue. Reduced blood supply may be caused by pressure, muscle spasm, or edema. Trauma to the nerve fibers in the skin produces sharp localized pain. Extensive dissection and prolonged retraction of muscle and fascia produce deep, long-lasting pain. Pain originating in the visceral organ may be referred to a distant portion of the body surface or deep within a different area. It usually is characterized as a deep, aching pain. A hollow, visceral organ such as the ureter or bile duct can develop muscle spasms characterized as cramping pain (see Chapter 17).

After surgery, other factors can add to the pain sensation: pressure from tissue edema, infections, distention, muscle spasms surrounding the incisional area, and tight dressings or casts. Postoperative pain usually lasts 24 to 48 hours but may continue longer depending on the extent of the surgery, the pain threshold of the patient, and response to pain. The presence of pain can prolong convalescence because it can interfere with return to activity.

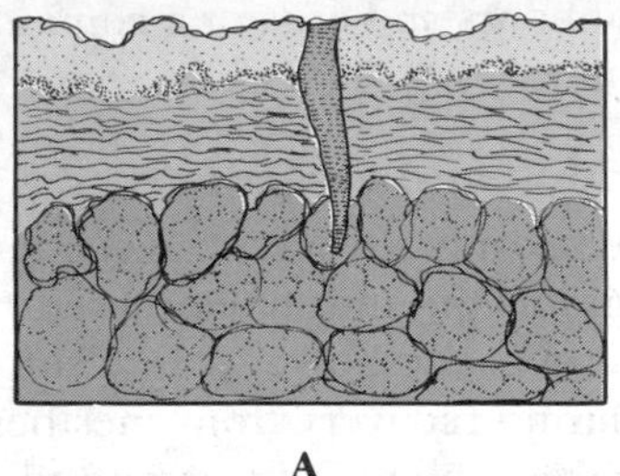
A

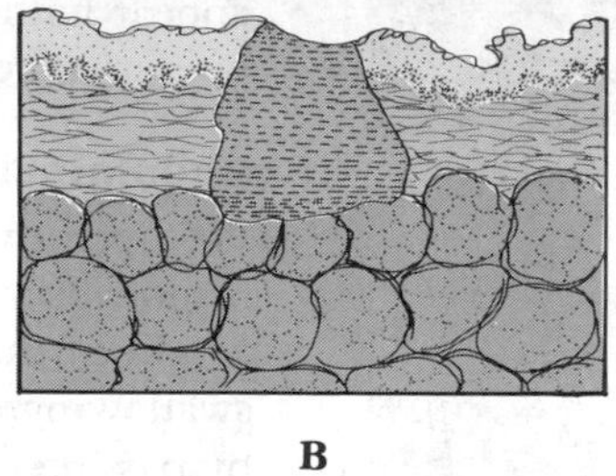
B

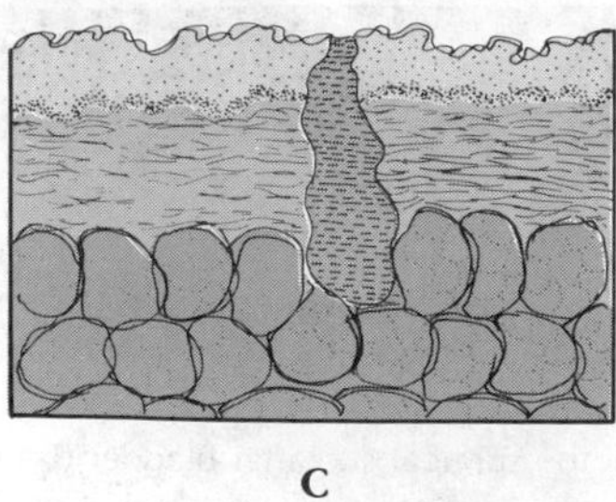
C

**FIGURE 25-3** Types of wound healing. **A,** Primary. **B,** Secondary. **C,** Tertiary.

When the patient complains of pain in the postoperative period, it should not be assumed that the pain is incisional in nature. It is important to try to ascertain the possible cause of the pain. It is important to remember that pain is a subjective experience and occurs when the patient says it does. Patients should be told before surgery that measures will be taken to reduce any postoperative discomfort they experience.

## Wounds

### Wound healing process

Tissues may heal by one of three ways: primary, secondary, or tertiary intention. **Wound healing by primary intention** occurs in most surgical incisions. The incision is a clean straight line with all layers of the wound (muscle, subcutaneous tissue, and epithelial tissue) well approximated by suturing. If these wounds remain free of infection and do not separate, healing is quick with minimal scarring (Figure 25-3).

**Wound healing by secondary intention** is seen in wounds such as ulcers with edges that cannot be approximated. Healing occurs by a filling in of the wound by granulation tissue over a larger area. These wounds have a greater possibility for infection.

**Wound healing by tertiary intention** occurs when there is a delay between injury and suturing. The time period permits more microorganisms to penetrate the wound; therefore there will be a greater inflammatory reaction.

**Influencing factors.** Major factors that can delay wound healing are age, nutrition (lack of sufficient vitamin C or protein), circulation (provides blood components and nutrients at the site), corticosteroids (suppression of inflammation), presence of foreign bodies, infection, dead space, and irradiation (affects fibroblastic activity). Enzymatic activity in wounds is highest during the early stages of wound healing; therefore new wounds are more sensitive to factors that delay healing.

Wounds in children normally heal more rapidly than those in adults because of increased metabolism and good circulation. Wounds in elderly persons often heal more slowly because of decreased fibroblastic activity and impaired circulation.

Obese persons have excessive subcutaneous tissue that is poorly supplied with blood vessels, and therefore wounds may heal more slowly. Persons with peripheral vascular disease have impaired circulation to the legs, which can cause delayed healing of leg ulcers.

### Wound infection

After surgery the patient remains at risk for wound infection. Excessive body cavity exposure and decreased body defense mechanisms are among the contributing factors to postoperative wound infection (see Chapter 24). Wound infection is a major type of nosocomial infections. A wound may become infected as a result of factors intrinsic to the patient, factors that can delay healing, and the effectiveness of aseptic technique used by health care personnel. Objective signs of infection include fever, swelling, erythema, purulent discharge, and increased white blood cell count. These signs usually occur after the immediate postoperative period, but prevention begins preoperatively and continues throughout the perioperative experience. Understanding the principles of universal precautions, isolation, wound healing, and wound care is imperative for the postanesthesia care nurse.

A contaminated wound usually becomes infected. A wound that is infected will not heal until the infection is eliminated. The greater the number of bacteria or amount of necrotic tissue present, the longer healing will be delayed.

### Hemorrhage

Hemorrhage is most likely to occur within 48 hours after surgery. Hemorrhage may be caused by the slipping of a ligature (suture) or the dislodging of a clot. During surgery small vessels may go unnoticed because of decreased blood pressure or use of a tourniquet. Hemorrhage may occur with the reestablishment of blood flow. Careful assessment of wound dressings and drainage systems is required.

### Wound dehiscence and evisceration

Wound disruption or **dehiscence** is a partial to complete separation of the wound edges. Wound **evisceration** is protrusion of abdominal viscera through the

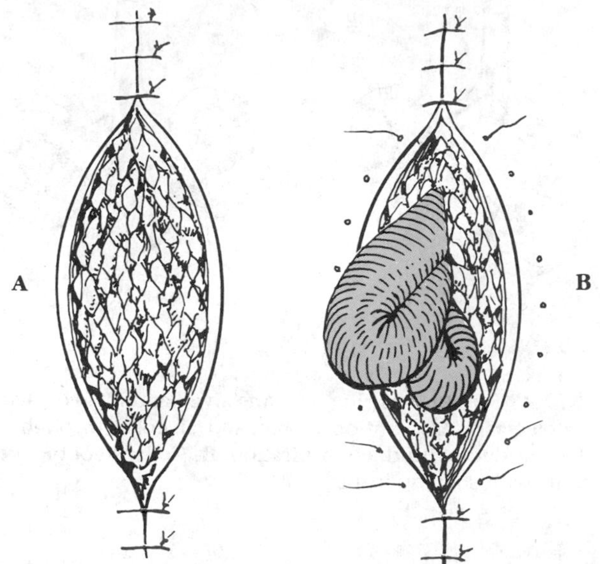


FIGURE 25-4 **A,** Wound dehiscence. **B,** Wound evisceration.

incision and onto the abdominal wall (Figure 25-4). Wound separation that occurs during the first 3 days usually is related to technical factors such as the suturing. After the early postoperative period, dehiscence usually is associated with postoperative complications such as distention, vomiting, excessive coughing, dehydration, or infection. Many of these complications can be prevented by careful assessment and continued monitoring, as well as the institution of vigorous preventive measures (ventilatory exercises, ambulation, adequate fluid intake, aseptic technique), on the part of the nurse. Factors such as cachexia, hypoproteinemia, avitaminosis, increased age, decreased resistance to infection, malignant tumor, multiple trauma, or hypothermia also can cause wound separation.

On a subjective level, the patient may report a "giving" sensation at the incision or a feeling of wetness. If evisceration has occurred and if a loop of bowel is obstructed, the patient will complain of severe localized pain at the incision. The dressing will be saturated with clear pink drainage. The wound edges may be partially or entirely separated, and loops of intestine may be lying on the abdominal wall. Signs of shock may occur.

## Psychologic Aspects

The immediate postanesthesia period is often a frightening time for the patient. Psychologic support is imperative for physical and emotional well-being. Immediately after surgery, most patients are somnolent. As the patient awakens, anxiety is often a major concern.

### Anxiety

Some of the concerns that were present in the preoperative period (see Chapter 23) may continue into the postoperative period. These concerns generally focus on the performed surgery, the results of the surgery, and the temporary or permanent effects that may change a patient's life-style. Anxieties are expressed in many different ways. It must be remembered that expressions such as anger, resentfulness, crying, excessive joking, inappropriate laughter, or withdrawal may all be signs of anxiety and often are seen in the postoperative period. Some of these feelings may be projected against the surgeon, nurse, housekeeping aide, food, and so forth.

Frequently fears exist relating to prognosis. Is the surgery really going to correct the original problem? Am I going to die? Will the problem recur? Will there be more pain? What permanent effects will occur? How will my life change?

#### Concerns specific to the surgery performed

Sometimes patients doubt the accuracy of information they have been given. They may wonder if surgery was really needed. They may still worry that they have cancer but that nobody is telling them the truth. If they do have cancer, they may think that it is more extensive than they are being told.

#### Concerns over loss of a body part

Surgery frequently means removal of tissue. If an organ such as the uterus or part of the colon is removed or if part of a limb, breast, or face is removed, patients are faced with a change in self-image. They may experience grief over the lost part. For complete recovery the patient needs to identify feelings and cope with the perceived changes.

#### Concerns about the future

The patient may have concerns about changes in roles, return to work, life-style, emotional status, economic implications of the surgery, or prognosis. An overriding concern may actually be the patient's inability to predict and control the future. Dealing with uncertainty becomes a major theme.

## ♦ NURSING DIAGNOSES

Nursing diagnoses are determined from postoperative analysis of patient assessment data. Nursing diagnoses for the postanesthesia patient may include but are not limited to the following:

| Diagnostic Title | Possible Etiologic Factors |
|---|---|
| Airway clearance, ineffective | Secretions from anesthesia, tongue blocking airway, improper positioning |
| Gas exchange, impaired | Drug effects, incisional pain, constrictive dressings |
| Aspiration, high risk for | Decreased consciousness, suppressed protective reflexes |
| Cardiac output, decreased | Hypotension, preexisting cardiac problems |
| Injury (trauma), high risk for | Sensorimotor deficits, residual anesthesia effects, disorientation, venous stasis |
| Fluid volume excess/deficit, high risk for | Excess/insufficient intravenous fluids, stress on renal/endocrine systems |

| Diagnostic Title | Possible Etiologic Factors |
|---|---|
| Thermoregulation, ineffective | Cold environment, prolonged exposure during surgery, anesthetic agents, excessive warming methods, infection |
| Pain, acute | Surgical incision |
| Urinary retention | Anesthesia and drug effects |
| Skin integrity, high risk for impaired | Improper positioning, shearing forces, pressure against body, advanced age |
| High risk for alteration in comfort: nausea, vomiting, hiccoughs | Effects of anesthetic agents, pain, movement in the immediate postoperative period; anxiety |
| Infection, high risk for (in postoperative wound) | Break in sterile technique, nonadherence to universal precautions, intrinsic factors |
| Anxiety, high risk for | Pain, strange environment, possible change in health status |

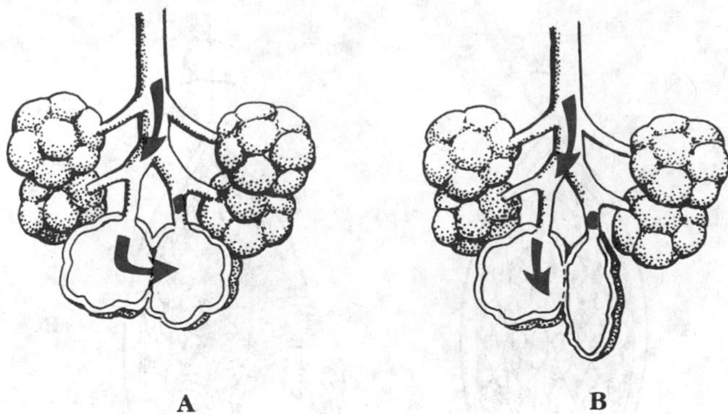


FIGURE 25-5 Mucous plug blocking alveolar duct in obstructive atelectasis. **A,** Aeration of blocked alveolus through intraalveolar duct with deep inspiration. **B,** Collapse of blocked alveolus with shallow inspiration.

## ♦ EXPECTED PATIENT OUTCOMES

Expected patient outcomes for the postanesthesia patient may include but are not limited to the following:

1. Respiratory function
   a. Will maintain a patent airway with lungs clear to auscultation.
   b. Will maintain normal baseline arterial blood gas values and have oxygen saturation level at 96% or above.
   c. Will successfully eliminate blood, mucus, or vomitus through the mouth and not experience aspiration.
2. Will have preoperative values for pulse and blood pressure.
3. Injury
   a. Will not experience injury related to falls, pressure, or improper positioning.
   b. Will return to a state of wakefulness and/or demonstrate the ability to move all extremities.
   c. Will experience adequate venous return and avoid deep vein thrombosis and pulmonary embolism.
4. Will maintain a normal fluid balance and avoid signs and symptoms of dehydration or overhydration.
5. Will maintain a body temperature within normal range.
6. Will not show signs of severe pain (facial grimacing, crying and holding the painful area, diaphoresis).
7. Will successfully empty the bladder within 8-10 hours after surgery.
8. Will maintain skin integrity.
9. Will not have uncontrolled nausea and vomiting or hiccoughs.
10. Will not exhibit redness or swelling at the wound site during hospitalization.
11. Will demonstrate the ability to cope with fears, frustrations, and concerns over surgical events.

## ♦ NURSING INTERVENTIONS

### Promoting Optimal Respiratory Function

The goal of respiratory care for the postanesthesia patient is to maintain pulmonary ventilation that is adequate to prevent hypoxemia (a deficiency of oxygen in the blood) and hypercapnia (an excess of carbon dioxide in the blood). Nursing management plays a critical role in the prevention of respiratory complications. In the immediate postanesthesia period, two of the most common causes of inadequate pulmonary exchange are airway obstruction (ineffective airway clearance) and hypoventilation (impaired gas exchange).

#### Maintaining airway patency

Excessive secretions from the nasopharynx or tracheobronchial mucosa can lead to partial or complete airway obstruction (Figure 25-5). When secretions pool in the lower airway as a result of shallow breathing and immobility after surgery, pulmonary infection may occur. Removal of these secretions in the early postoperative period can prevent obstruction and the occurrence of infection. Unless the patient can manage these secretions by coughing them up and expectorating them, they must be removed by suctioning. Pharyngeal suctioning often is all that is required. If endotracheal suctioning is necessary, the patient should receive hyperventilation with 100% oxygen before and after each introduction of the catheter into the trachea. When thick secretions are a problem, the humidity of the air breathed is increased to keep secretions as thin as possible and to prevent dry air from further irritating the respiratory passages. Blockages can be prevented by keeping secretions moist, taking deep breaths, and coughing up the secretions.

The patient may arrive in the recovery room with an airway in place, either pharyngeal (mouth or nose to pharynx) or endotracheal (mouth or nose to just above

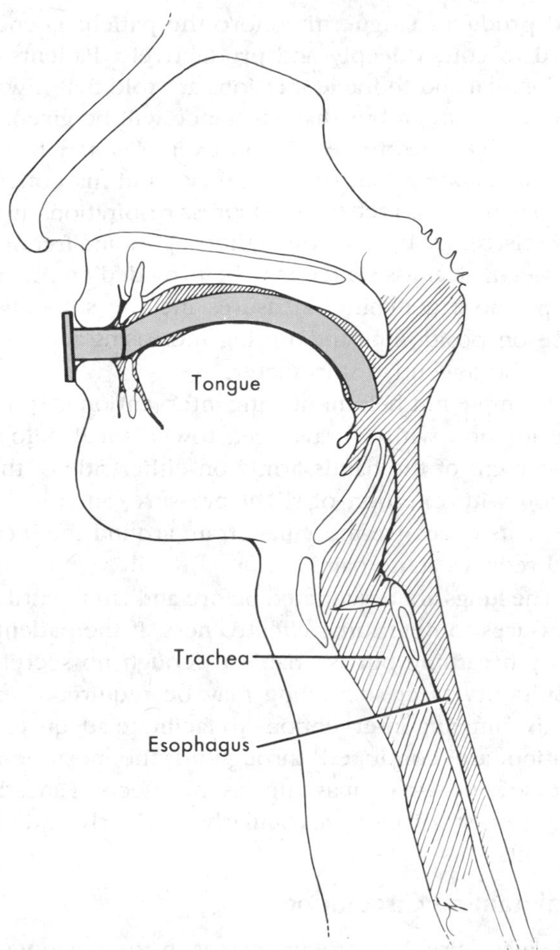


**FIGURE 25-6** Pharyngeal airway in place to prevent tongue from blocking oropharynx.

the bifurcation of the trachea). The *pharyngeal* airway (Figure 25-6) is most commonly used. It keeps the air passage open and the tongue forward until the pharyngeal reflexes have returned. It is removed as soon as the patient begins to awaken and has regained cough and swallowing reflexes. After this time the presence of an airway can be irritating and can stimulate vomiting or laryngospasm.

The *endotracheal* airway not only prevents the tongue from falling back but also prevents airway obstruction resulting from laryngospasm. The endotracheal tube is removed when the patient is awake and able to maintain the airway, as evidenced by the patient's ability to raise the head and grip a hand, as well as by normal blood gas levels.

### Promoting gas exchange

Gas exchange is promoted by the delivery of oxygen, by encouraging deep breathing, yawning, and coughing, by proper positioning, and by administering pharmacologic agents to reverse the effects of anesthetic agents.

## RESEARCH

Berels DJ, Marz MS: $Sao_2$ monitoring in the postanesthesia care unit, *J Post Anesth Nurs* 6(6):394-401, 1991.

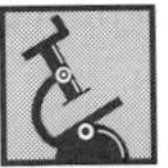

Airway management is of primary concern to the PACU nurse. One of the most obvious complications is hypoxemia. The introduction of pulse oximetry provided an objective way of determining the patient's respiratory status. The purpose of this study was to accurately and objectively assess patients' respiratory status on discharge by comparing subjective information with $Sao_2$ levels; 10% of the PACU's monthly volume was studied for 3 months. While subjective scores indicated that patients were ready for discharge, $Sao_2$ levels were unsatisfactory, contraindicating discharge from the PACU for the patients studied. As a result of this study, anesthesiologists at the investigators' institution have established pulse oximetry as a standard of care in the postanesthesia care unit.

Oxgyen is given postoperatively to almost all patients because anesthesia decreases pulmonary expansion and leads to areas of atelectasis in the lungs. The net result can be hypoxemia. Ventilation is promoted in the postanesthesia phase by oxygen therapy, breathing exercises, and other therapies. Oxygen is administered by nasal prongs or disposable face mask or through the endotracheal or tracheostomy tube if one is in place.

How long postoperative oxygen therapy should be continued depends on the individual patient. As a general rule, all patients should receive oxygen at least until they are conscious and able to take deep breaths on command. Prolonged use of oxygen therapy is guided by arterial blood gas determinations. Patients with thoracic or upper abdominal incisions or with preexisting pulmonary disease may be given oxygen for several hours, perhaps until the next day. Special care must be taken in administering oxygen to patients with chronic obstructive pulmonary disease so that hypoxemia, which is their stimulus to breathe, is not entirely corrected. Any patient experiencing shivering, which dramatically increases oxygen consumption, should receive oxygen therapy until the shivering ceases.

Continuous monitoring of oxygen saturation ($Sao_2$) level is a necessary postoperative intervention and can be easily accomplished by use of a pulse oximeter. Portable $Sao_2$ monitoring or pulse oximetry detects hypoxemia. **Pulse oximetry** is a less expensive, less painful, and noninvasive way to monitor a patient's $Sao_2$ level as compared with obtaining arterial blood gas values. A plastic clip is applied to the patient's finger and is connected by cable to the pulse oximeter monitor. Use of pulse oximetry has proved useful in the early detection of decreased oxygen delivery. See Research box above.

To help maintain normal levels of arterial blood gases

and to counteract hypoventilation, all patients need to be encouraged to breathe deeply at frequent intervals. Taking deep breaths or yawning also can prevent atelectasis. If the patient is unconscious or will not breathe deeply when stimulated, the lungs can be hyperventilated passively with a breathing bag and mask.

### Positioning to support ventilation and prevent aspiration

The most desirable position to ensure maintenance of a patent airway depends on the size and condition of the patient, the anesthesia used, the surgery performed, and the amount of experienced nursing care available. Ideally the patient should be in a position to breathe normally with full expansion of all portions of the lungs. Positioning also attempts to facilitate drainage and removal of blood, secretions, or vomitus and to prevent aspiration.

Until protective reflexes have returned, the best position for most patients is *side lying* or *semiprone,* with the head tilted back and the jaw supported forward. Aspiration can occur unless the *whole body* is turned. Turning the patient's head when the chest and shoulders remain in the back-lying position is useless. The disadvantages related to diminished chest expansion in the side-lying position can be reduced by turning the patient frequently and by raising the flexed upper arm and placing it on a pillow.

The supine position with head hyperextended permits fullest expansion of the lungs, but it is potentially dangerous in the immediate postanesthesia period because of the potential for aspiration of obstruction from secretions. If the supine position must be used, suctioning equipment must be available at the bedside and the patient should be monitored frequently.

### Facilitating drug reversal

The effects of anesthetic agents may have to be reversed. Anesthesia may paralyze the natural physiologic response for proper ventilation. Barbiturates, narcotics, muscle relaxants, and inhalation anesthetic agents depress respirations. The nurse and physician must determine if it is necessary to administer drugs that can reverse these effects. Examples include naloxone (Narcan) for reversal of narcotics and atropine or glycopyrrolate (Robinol) with neostigmine for reversal of muscle relaxants.

### Promoting coughing

All of the ventilatory measures used to ensure adequate postsurgical ventilation are followed by *deep coughing* to remove any secretions that have been loosened. Coughing may be contraindicated in a few instances, such as after brain, spinal, or eye surgery, because of the increased intracranial or intraocular pressure that can result.

A shallow cough is ineffective in mobilizing secretions and produces fatigue; therefore the patient is encouraged to cough deeply and productively. Patients with abdominal and thoracic incisions are told that it will be painful to cough but that assistance will be given. Narcotics given before ventilation exercises may facilitate patient cooperation; on the other hand, narcotics decrease the cough reflex and depress respirations and the exercises must be performed thoroughly and frequently.

Mechanical assistance may be provided by the nurse to promote coughing. Measures include splinting the incision, positioning and turning, increasing activity, and use of an incentive spirometer.

A simple but helpful nursing intervention is splinting the incision with a drawsheet, towel, small pillow, or placement of the hands firmly on either side of the incision with exertion of slight pressure. Such splinting prevents excessive muscular strain around the incision and reduces acute pain.

The lungs are auscultated before and after ventilatory measures to determine effectiveness. If the patient has noisy breathing but is unable to cough up secretions, respiratory tract suctioning may be required. Postoperative nursing interventions to facilitate adequate ventilation are continued throughout the postoperative course as necessary inasmuch as the effects of anesthesia may persist for days, particularly in elderly and obese patients.

## Maintaining Circulation

Adequate circulation is important in the postoperative period to provide adequate oxygenation to all tissues, especially to the traumatized tissue in the incisional area to support initial wound healing. A dressing that appears too tight should be loosened, if permissible, or the condition should be reported at once to the physician. Positioning should not constrict circulation. Pressure on the legs, particularly the popliteal space, must be avoided.

Significant changes from baseline data in pulse, blood pressure, or bleeding status are reported to the physician. A weak, thready pulse with a significant drop in blood pressure may indicate hemorrhage or circulatory failure. The surgeon or anesthesiologist, or both, are notified at once if any of these signs occur, especially if the skin becomes cold, moist, pale, or cyanotic or if the patient suddenly becomes restless or apprehensive. Oxygen therapy is initiated to increase the oxygen saturation of the circulating blood. Other therapies to treat shock also are initiated. These may include Trendelenburg's position, rapid infusion of intravenous fluids, and the administration of various drugs.

### Treating cardiac dysrhythmias

When a cardiac dysrhythmia is detected, it is important to ascertain if the patient has a history of such a disturbance. Dysrhythmias unchanged from those that existed preoperatively usually do not require treatment.

Hypoxemia and hypercapnia are common causes of postoperative cardiac dysrhythmias, especially premature beats and sinus tachycardia. These dysrhythmias often can be successfully suppressed by improving ventilation. Oxygen is started while the physician is being notified. A patient with poor gas exchange should receive ventilatory assistance with a bag and mask.

Frequent premature beats of ventricular origin that are not decreased by oxygen therapy usually are treated immediately with intravenously administered antidysrhythmic agents. If the dysrhythmia is caused by a perioperative myocardial infarction, appropriate steps, including the administration of thrombolytic agents, may be initiated. Sinus bradycardia is countered by the administration of atropine intravenously. *In the event of a life-threatening dysrhythmia, such as ventricular fibrillation or cardiac asystole, resuscitation efforts are started immediately.*

## Preventing Injury

The nurse who provides postanesthesia care must place great emphasis on patient safety until the person is fully awake or has complete return of sensations after regional blocks. The unconscious patient must be protected from falling and from injury as a result of improper positioning. Side rails should be maintained in the upright position. The patient should be turned frequently and placed in a good body alignment to prevent nerve damage from pressure and to prevent muscle and joint strain caused by lying in one position for a long time.

If emergence delirium should occur, the muscle activity and increased movement may result in injury to the patient. Preventive measures such as use of padded side rails should be taken.

Both unconscious patients and patients who have had spinal or epidural anesthesia have a loss of sensation and thus are unresponsive to sensory stimuli. Warming blankets, heat lamps, or cast driers must be used with great care to prevent burns. In addition, pressure to anesthetized extremities must be avoided and care must be taken during positioning of extremities.

### Promoting neurologic recovery from anesthesia

It is important to continuously attempt to arouse patients, encourage deep breathing, and check level of consciousness. Over the course of an hour most patients return to an oriented state with a tendency to fall back to sleep. However, they are arousable by verbal and tactile stimulation. Maintenance of pulmonary and circulatory function helps to eliminate most residual anesthetic agents and facilitates the patient's return to an awake state.

Nursing interventions for complications of spinal anesthesia (hypoxemia, agitation, hypotension, and nausea) focus on improving cardiac output and blood pressure and are collaborative with the anesthesiologist. Oxygen therapy is initiated, and fluids usually are increased. Medications to increase blood pressure may be used for treatment of hypotension. Ephedrine and phenylephrine are examples.

Fluids must be administered carefully after spinal anesthesia. If bladder distention is detected, urinary catheterization frequently is required. Patients who are discharged on the same day of their surgery should be required to void before they leave.

### Facilitating venous return

Antiembolic stockings frequently are applied preoperatively to facilitate blood return from the lower extremities to the heart. These remain in place until the patient is ambulatory.

Postoperative thrombophlebitis often can be prevented by nursing management. No pressure should be permitted on the popliteal area. If legs are supported on pillows, pressure should be equally distributed along the entire leg. Because of the danger of dislodging a clot, *the muscle portion of a patient's leg should not be massaged postoperatively.* A patient who is observed rubbing a leg should be questioned about discomfort.

Nursing interventions to recognize and prevent deep vein thrombosis also may prevent pulmonary embolism from occurring. Symptoms must be reported to the patient's physician immediately.

*Intermittent external pneumatic compression* to the legs may be prescribed. This consists of a pneumatic cuff that extends from the feet to below the knee or to the upper portion of the thighs. The cuff is inflated rapidly to 40 to 50 mm Hg pressure, held for 10 to 12 seconds, and then deflated for 45 seconds. The procedure is not uncomfortable and has demonstrated marked effectiveness in patients at high risk. See Research box, p. 644, left.

## Maintaining Fluid and Electrolyte Balance

Fluid volume deficits require fluid replacement after major surgery. Most patients receive intravenous fluids to maintain fluid and electrolyte balance. The exact amount and type of fluid administered depend on the surgical procedure, as well as the patient's age, weight, body surface area, preoperative status, intraoperative course, and individual response to stress. A solution of 5% dextrose in 0.95% sodium chloride commonly is given. Lactated Ringer's solution may be given for prolonged periods to supply the necessary electrolytes. Potassium may be added to an intravenous solution after the first 24 postoperative hours. Careful monitoring of the patient's intravenous fluid administration is essential to ensure adequacy of replacement and prevention of fluid overload.

The intravenous site should be checked to ensure that the needle or cannula remains in the vein and that no extravasation has occurred. The arm should be positioned to facilitate the flow of intravenous fluids. Careful attention should be paid to avoid kinking of the tubing.

**RESEARCH**

Hull et al: Effectiveness of intermittent pneumatic leg compression for preventing deep vein thrombosis after total hip replacement, *JAMA* 263:2313-1317, 1990.

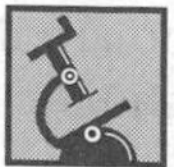

A randomized trial was performed in consecutive patients undergoing total hip replacement to evaluate the effectiveness of sequential intermittent calf and thigh compression for preventing venous thrombosis compared with a control group given no prophylaxis. Both groups underwent case finding for deep vein thrombosis using combined fibrinogen I-125 leg scanning, impedance plethysmography, and venography. Venograms showed the presence of deep vein thrombosis in 77 (49%) of 158 control patients compared with 36 (24%) of 152 patients given intermittent compression. Results of combined impedance plethysmography and leg scanning were insensitive in this patient group (sensitivity, 46%); the use of venography was required to detect more than half the patients with venous thrombosis. Sequential intermittent leg compression clinically and statistically significantly reduced the frequency of both proximal vein and calf vein thrombosis. Case finding resulted in early detection and treatment of patients with venous thrombosis.

The oral administration of fluid is begun as soon as the patient can tolerate this method of fluid replacement. Sips of water are offered first. Some persons cannot tolerate iced fluids but are able to suck on ice chips. Ice is recorded as intake (2 parts ice equal 1 part water). Quantities of fluids are restricted until active bowel sounds are present.

## Maintaining Normothermia

Body temperature is monitored frequently during the postoperative period. The patient may have mild hypothermia on arrival in the clinical unit. Rewarming interventions can protect the patient from the development of cardiac dysrhythmias and further complications. Fever (indicated by temperature over 38.5° C) should be reported promptly to the surgeon. Slight elevations in temperature are common on the night of surgery. They usually respond promptly to improved pulmonary ventilation and an increased fluid intake.

Body temperature is obtained on admission to the PACU and monitored continually. Axillary, rectal, and oral temperature measures indicate shell (skin) temperature. Tympanic and esophageal temperatures are accurate measures of core temperature. Esophageal temperature is measured with a sensor attached to an esophageal stethoscope. A limitation of the esophageal method is that it is invasive and typically can be used only when patients are under general anesthesia. Tympanic temperature measurement is obtained by a probe placed in the external auditory mucosa. The tympanic method is fast, accurate, and noninvasive and presents little discomfort to the patient.

**RESEARCH**

Summers S: Axillary, tympanic, and esophageal temperature measurement: descriptive comparisons in postanesthesia patients, *J Post Anesth Nurs* 6(6):420-425, 1991.

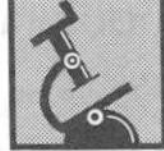

Data in this study support the reviewed literature indicating that core temperature or measures of cranial, thoracic, and abdominal cavities are more accurately obtained by esophageal and tympanic thermometers than by the axillary method. The tympanic temperature measurement was found to be accurate, noninvasive, and convenient to use.

### Treating hypothermia

Interventions for hypothermia include constant body temperature monitoring, administration of warm intravenous solutions, and the use of warm blankets, hydrothermia mattresses, warm air blankets, and warming lights (radiant heat). In addition, the nurse may increase room temperature or apply head/body coverings.

### Treating malignant hyperthermia

The actual malignant hyperthermic reaction occurs most frequently during the general anesthesia period. It can, however, occur or recur during the recovery period within 2 to 3 hours of anesthesia administration. Nurses should be familiar with the condition and be able to respond quickly and appropriately if it occurs. The anesthesiologist is notified of any significant change in body temperature. Treatment includes the following measures:

- Administration of oxygen
- *Immediate* intravenous administration of dantrolene sodium, per order
- Initiation of hypothermic measures such as cooling blankets, cooled intravenous solutions, cold nasogastric lavage, and ice packs
- Continuous monitoring of the patient in an intensive care unit for 48 hours

If not promptly and successfully reversed, the condition can be fatal. See Research box above.

## Promoting Comfort

From the patient's point of view the distress of postoperative pain is probably the most significant postoperative problem. Adequate and prompt pain relief is a critical nursing intervention. Effective management of pain begins with a trusting nurse-patient relationship. The offer of support, objectivity, and reassurance assists in pain relief and increases the patient's ability to relax.

In the immediate postanesthesia period, narcotic analgesics are given for pain when warranted, with the realization that pronounced depression of the respiratory, circulatory, or central nervous system may follow. Because the patient generally has not completely recovered from the effects of anesthesia, the first postoperative dose of a narcotic usually is reduced to about one half the dose to be received after full recovery from anesthesia. The goal is to keep the patient fairly comfortable without overmedication. It is usually necessary to administer narcotics during the first 12 hours after major surgery. If severe pain is expected, medication should be offered to the patient at regular intervals around the clock to maintain effective blood levels.

Analgesics have greater effect if they are administered before pain becomes severe. One method to determine the severity of pain that a patient is experiencing is to use a pain-rating scale in which the patient rates pain level on a scale from one to ten.

Analgesics may be given by several methods. The intramuscular route may be used for patients with stable circulatory functions. If circulation is decreased, as with shock, medication given intramuscularly may remain in the tissue and then be absorbed suddenly when circulation is restored, leading to overdosage. The intravenous route is safer and faster and often is preferred.

One intravenous method that is widely used today is the administration of narcotics by patient-controlled analgesia (PCA). The patient receives a predetermined bolus of narcotic intravenously by activating a hand control when pain relief is desired. The effective use of PCA is based on the assumption that patients can best evaluate and manage their own pain. The mechanism is set to prevent repeated dosage at too frequent intervals. Usually 10 minutes is required before another dose can be given. Persons using PCA usually take lower dosages because they control their pain relief. Assessing and documenting the patient's response to the PCA therapy are nursing responsibilities. The nurse may need to remind or assist the patient in this process during the early postoperative period when the person is groggy.

Another method of administering postoperative narcotics is the delivery of the drugs directly into the epidural or subarachnoid space. The catheter is inserted by an anesthesiologist. Epidural analgesia blocks pain transmission at the spinal cord level. Evidence is accumulating that epidural analgesia is the treatment of choice for controlling many types of pain, including postoperative pain. Epidural narcotics produce analgesia for 15 to 16 hours without significant respiratory depression or sympathetic, motor, or sensory disturbances. Epidural analgesia is highly effective for major orthopedic surgery of the lower extremities. Epidural catheters should be well secured with tape. To prevent dislodgment of the epidural catheter, great care must be taken in moving patients.

The amount of analgesic medication required by patients varies according to age and type of surgery. Numerous individual variables relate to pain perception and reaction. In general, after the first 48 to 72 hours following surgery, pain usually decreases in severity and may be controlled by a less potent analgesic. Physicians frequently write "prn" orders for different analgesics and doses, thus permitting the nurse to select the combination that best meets the patient's immediate needs.

Morphine sulfate and meperidine are the more commonly used narcotics. An alternative to narcotic analgesics is the use of nonsteroidal antiinflammatory drugs (NSAIDs) to relieve postoperative pain. These drugs, including ketorolac tromethamine (Toradol) (see Research box above) and diclofenac sodium (Voltaren), have the advantage over narcotics in not suppressing the cough center. In addition, NSAIDs do not affect the rate or depth of respirations.

## RESEARCH

Kenny GNC, Ketorolac tromethamine—a new nonopioid analgesic, *Br J Anaesth* 65:445-447, 1990.

The problem of inadequate relief of postoperative pain has been recognized for many years and has been the subject of considerable research. Ketorolac tromethamine is a new nonsteroidal antiinflammatory drug (NSAID) that exhibits potent analgesia. It has been investigated extensively for use in postoperative analgesia both as the sole agent and as a supplement to opioid analgesics. The quality of analgesia achieved may be better when ketorolac is administered regularly in addition to an opioid, with the probability of decreased frequency of adverse effects such as respiratory depression.

### Promoting Urinary Elimination

Urinary output is closely monitored after surgery until normal urinary function is reestablished. A urinary output of at least 30 ml/hr is required to maintain adequate kidney function, but 50 ml/hr is desirable. Urinary output typically is less than fluid intake during the first 24 hours because of the fluid shifts that occur in response to the stress of surgery. In addition, the specific gravity of the urine will be high. The bladder is palpated for distention when output is low to identify possible urinary retention.

Initial postoperative voiding may be facilitated by measures such as offering fluids, getting the patient up to the bathroom or commode as permitted, running water in the bathroom, pouring water over the perineum, and ensuring the patient time and privacy.

If these measures are not effective, urinary catheterization may be required. An indwelling catheter may be necessary if the inability to void persists. Indwelling catheters are inserted at the time of surgery after certain procedures, such as pelvic surgery, that frequently are complicated by pelvic edema and urinary retention. Meticulous catheter care is imperative. Fluids by mouth are encouraged as soon as they can be tolerated. Increasing the patient's fluid volume aids in "flushing" the bladder.

## Maintaining Skin Integrity

Maintaining skin integrity is another nursing responsibility in the postoperative period. Interventions focus on the treatment for any reddened or affected areas reported by the perioperative nurse, as well as the prevention of unnecessary pressure on vulnerable points of the body.

Suspicious or reddened areas must be monitored and treated. Gentle massage of these areas facilitates circulation and alleviates or reduces the potential for further breakdown. Positioning the body in proper alignment, padding bony prominences, and avoiding weight or pressure on extremities are effective interventions. Turning a patient frequently in the early postoperative period until the person is able to turn independently also is important.

Linens should be changed as often as necessary to avoid the problem of having skin exposed to moisture for prolonged periods. Skin exposed to moisture from blood or body fluid drainage should be cleansed and dried as quickly as possible. Dressings should be reinforced to contain drainage.

Special attention should be given to the elderly patient, who is extremely vulnerable to skin breakdown as a result of loss of skin elasticity and diminished subcutaneous fat. Pressure against or weight on any area of the body and shearing forces against the skin during movement should be avoided.

## Relieving Nausea and Vomiting

To prevent possible aspiration, the patient who is vomiting should be positioned in a side-lying position. Fluids are omitted for several hours, and the patient is advised to lie quietly in bed. The emesis basin and soiled linen are cleaned and changed. Frequent oral care is provided. When vomiting has subsided, and unless contraindicated, sucking on ice chips, taking sips of ginger ale or hot tea, or eating small amounts of dry solid food may relieve the patient's nausea. Antiemetics such as trimethobenzamide hydrochloride (Tigan) or prochlorperazine dimaleate (Compazine) may be administered by injection. Research is ongoing concerning the effectiveness of the newer antiemetic ondansetron (Zofran) for postoperative relief. Because vomiting can be a sign of drug idiosyncrasy, the presence of other side effects should be carefully assessed and the pattern of vomiting in relation to the administration of drugs noted. Accurate recording of intake and output of fluids and electrolyte balance is important.

### Relieving hiccoughs

Hiccoughs may be relieved by such a simple measure as having the patient rebreathe carbon dioxide at 5-minute intervals by inhaling and exhaling into a paper bag held tightly over the nose and mouth. Aspiration of the stomach will stop hiccoughs caused by gastric dilation. Chlorpromazine hydrochloride is used to treat mild cases of hiccoughs and is theorized to reduce hypersensitivity of the phrenic nerve.

### Relieving abdominal distention

Ambulation is one of the most effective means for stimulating peristalsis and expulsion of flatus. Ambulation usually is begun and encouraged very early in the postoperative course. Dilation of the stomach can be relieved by aspiration of fluid or gas with a nasogastric tube. Hot or cold liquids tend to cause gas build-up and thus should be avoided when peristalsis is sluggish; ice chips do not have the same effect because the water warms before it reaches the stomach.

## Preventing Wound Infection

Observance of universal precautions, adherence to isolation principles, when necessary, and meticulous wound care are major components of nursing interventions to prevent infection. Adherence to universal precautions (see Chapter 24) is imperative in caring for all patients. Observing principles of isolation precautions, when necessary, helps prevent cross-contamination among patients. Communication of necessary precautions to other health care personnel ensures continuity of care for the patient throughout the postoperative course. Explanation of these precautions to both patient and family members usually results in good compliance as well as prevention of unnecessary contamination.

Interventions to prevent wound infection are necessary throughout the postoperative course. An expected outcome is that wounds will remain clean, dry, and intact. Frequent assessment of dressings and accurate recording of findings are vital in the immediate postoperative period. The surgeon must be notified immediately if signs of complications are noted.

### Caring for the wound

Meticulous care of the surgical incision is an important nursing measure that facilitates wound healing. When a surgical wound site is redressed or treated, strict aseptic technique must be scrupulously followed. Gloves and masks should be worn when dressings are changed or an open wound is treated.

The nurse must ensure complete connection of drains to drainage bags or suction ports. The primary purpose of catheters, tubes, or drains is to permit the escape of body fluids that may be harmful to a patient if allowed to accumulate within a body cavity. Fluids are removed by either gravity or mechanical means. All drains from the surgical site or nearby body cavity should be observed frequently in the early postoperative period. Accurate recording of output from drains is critical. Excess drainage should be reported to the surgeon immediately.

(Commonly used drains are discussed in Chapter 24.)

Antibiotics frequently are ordered by the physician for the prophylactic prevention of infection. Administration of these antibiotics must take place at the scheduled times to maintain adequate blood levels.

Hemorrhage can interfere with wound healing. The best intervention for hemorrhage is early detection. When bleeding is noted on a dressing, the amount can be outlined with a pen and rechecked at 10- to 15-minute intervals for signs of change. If there is bleeding from a tube into a container, the drainage is marked with the time and the amount so that the rapidity of bleeding can be determined at frequent intervals. If bleeding is profuse, measures to control it are instituted. For example, a pressure dressing can be applied over an existing dressing. In addition, constant monitoring of vital signs is required.

A patient who is bleeding internally or in profuse amounts usually is returned immediately to surgery where the incision is opened and the bleeding vessel is ligated.

### Treating wound dehiscence and evisceration

A wound dehiscence or evisceration will disrupt healing. If either of these occurs, the surgeon is notified immediately, the patient is placed in a low Fowler's position, kept quiet, and instructed not to cough. Protruding viscera are covered, preferably with a warm, sterile saline dressing. Interventions to treat shock are initiated if signs and symptoms of shock are present. A minor wound dehiscence may be either resutured or allowed to remain open and heal by secondary intention. In the presence of infection or drainage, the wound usually is left open. The treatment for evisceration is immediate closure of the wound using local or general anesthesia.

## Relieving Anxiety

On awakening from anesthesia, the patient needs frequent orientation to place and reassurance of not being alone. The patient also needs to know that the operation is over and that recovery from anesthesia is satisfactory. Reassurance should be offered that loved ones have been notified of the patient's safe arrival in the recovery room. Careful explanations of procedures should be given even when it appears that the patient is not alert. The need for privacy should be considered at all times. The patient who receives this type of support frequently recovers from anesthesia faster, with fewer complications, and with less incisional pain. The patient who has had regional anesthesia needs the same considerations and reassurance that sensation and movement in the extremities will return.

The environment of a postanesthesia unit is usually hectic. Patient care needs change swiftly and sometimes dramatically. Among the many challenges for the postanesthesia nurse is the incorporation of caring practices into planning. A balance of caring and technologic skills provides a safe and supportive approach to patient care. Choosing to share positive information, using nonstressful words and touch, and promoting comfort can help relieve patient anxiety. See Research box above.

**RESEARCH**

Iacono MV: Precious moments of caring, *J Post Anesth Nurs* 8:26-27, 1993.

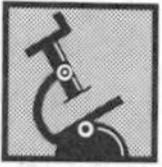

Postanesthesia nursing provides a unique opportunity to develop caring attitudes and promote caring practice. The fear and anxiety of waking up alone, confused, and in unfamiliar surroundings are lessened when the nurse provides time to attend to the patient's need for nurturing. Precious moments can be used for interaction and connection with the patient. Family members can be greatly relieved by calm and respectful treatment of their loved one.

The gerontologic patient has special needs that must be considered. The coping responses of the older patient frequently are threatened by physiologic, psychologic, and social stresses. A hurried, unfamiliar environment can be distressing to the older patient.

Older patients whose intellectual function is intact should not be treated as though they are incapable of decision making or understanding. However, declining sensory function and increased time needed for processing new information may alter the patient's processing ability. Thus elders need adequate time to cope with an overall slowness of many physical and mental responses.

A caring attitude helps the elderly patient maintain self-esteem. This caring behavior facilitates the patient's participation in the plan of care and therefore promotes a positive patient outcome.

### Supporting exploration of concerns

Later in the recovery period, taking the time to sit down with the surgical patient and discuss the person's concerns is just as important a nursing action in many instances as any of the interventions for physical care. Time must be allotted for this practice. If a specific concern is expected, the topic may have to be introduced by the nurse who has established rapport with the patient—letting the patient know that it is permissible to talk about this topic.

With the trend toward ambulatory surgery and early hospital discharge, place and time constraints exist on the opportunities for effective nurse-patient interaction in addressing some issues. Recent nursing research studies have dealt with concerns of surgical patients who are coping with the stresses of early discharge. See Research box, p. 648, left.

**RESEARCH**

Caldwell LM: Surgical outpatient concerns: what every perioperative nurse should know, *AORN J* 53:761-767, 1991.

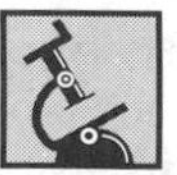

Outpatient surgery has been a growing phenomenon in the health care field for nearly two decades. In this study, 76 adult patients were surveyed by interviews and questionnaires to determine what patients find stressful about outpatient surgery. Concerns included fear of the unknown, fear of being discharged too early, fear of pain and complications after discharge, and uncertainty about the availability and continuity of care after discharge. Nursing interventions include emotional and informational support, specifically helping patients identify resources available to them in both the surgical center and their own community.

**RESEARCH**

Noonan AT et al: Family-centered nursing in the postanesthesia care unit: the evaluation of practice, *J Post Anesth Nurs* 6:13-16, 1991.

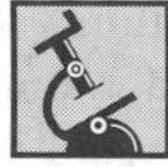

The specific focus of this study was the evaluation of the patients and families who participated in the experience of open visitation in the PACU. A questionnaire was developed to assess several dimensions of the experience. Results showed that 89% of the patients and 96% of the families involved felt that the open visitation policy was beneficial. Data also were collected from the PACU nurses who participated, and two thirds stated a perceived benefit to patients and family members.

### Including the family

Family needs also must be considered. The family is kept informed of the patient's postoperative progress. Information that can be shared with family members helps to lessen their anxiety.

For several decades, researchers have investigated the value of involving parents in their child's perioperative care. Family and patient stress in pediatric populations is reduced by family visitation in the postanesthesia unit. The level of anxiety also can be reduced in postoperative adult patients by allowing family visitation. Family visitation early in the postoperative period can alleviate fears, enhance communication between health care personnel and family members, and prepare family members about what to expect on discharge to another unit or to home. Patient and family responses to early visitation have been positive. See Research box above, right.

Most surgeons discuss the results of the operation with the family immediately after the surgery and also visit the patient, briefly telling what was found and providing reassurance. Family members frequently are highly anxious about the patient's condition and may not perceive or understand all that the surgeon tells them. Patients often experience periods of amnesia during the hours when they first regain consciousness and may not remember what they have been told. To provide satisfactory answers to the patient and family's questions, the nurse needs to know what information was given. The family also needs to know what to expect when the patient returns to the unit or when the patient is ready for discharge.

It is important for the nurse to recognize that the patient who is discharged directly to home after surgery may be unable to absorb a great deal of information. Therefore a follow-up telephone call should be made by nursing personnel to complete both the education and evaluation. During this call the nurse can provide information and reinforce predischarge teaching. The nurse also can provide emotional support and referral if necessary. Usually an appointment is made for a follow-up examination in the surgeon's office or clinic within 1 to 2 weeks after discharge. Referrals to home health nurses, rehabilitation programs, support groups, and other health professionals also should be made on the basis of individual patient needs.

## ♦ EVALUATION

Evaluation of nursing interventions is the fourth step in the nursing process. The results of evaluation either support maintaining the nursing interventions or identify the need for making alterations in the plan of care. The emphasis is always on the expected patient outcomes. Assessment of the patient's responses to interventions is ongoing throughout the entire postoperative phase. Therefore evaluation also must be ongoing.

To evaluate the effectiveness of nursing interventions, compare patient behaviors with those stated in the expected patient outcomes. Successful achievement of patient outcomes for the surgical patient in the postoperative phase is indicated by the following:

1. Respiratory function
   a. Maintains patent airway, with lungs clear to auscultation.
   b. Maintains blood gases within normal limits and oxygen saturation 96% or above.
2. Maintains regular pulse and stable blood pressure at preoperative levels.
3. Injury
   a. Has no injuries or falls.
   b. Is oriented to time, place, and person.
   c. Is able to move all extremities.
4. Has urine output >30 ml/hr and no observable swelling or edema.
5. Maintains normal body temperature.

6. States that pain level is acceptable and shows no evidence of facial grimacing or guarding.
7. Voids spontaneously within 8 to 10 hours after surgery.
8. Shows no redness or skin breakdown.
9. Has no nausea or vomiting and tolerates oral fluids.
10. Shows wound healing without evidence of dehiscence or infection.
11. States that anxiety is relieved and indicates that patient and caregivers are confident they can provide needed care after discharge.

Many institutions have developed surveys that ask patients to evaluate the care and attention they received while they were undergoing care. These postoperative surveys can be a valuable quality improvement tool. Feedback obtained from the surveys has been used to modify standards of patient care.

### Documentation

The postanesthesia patient care record is a legal document and should be clear and concise. Standards of care or critical pathways for care should be written and implemented. A written care plan reflecting the nursing process ensures that the attainment of outcomes and goals for patient care can be determined by the nursing team. Implementations or variations from the standard of care should be thoroughly recorded. Complete documentation portrays accountability for the care delivered to the patient.

Written information about the patient from one health care worker to another helps to maintain continuity of care. Records can be used to identify what actually happened during a patient's surgical experience if a question arises at a later time. In addition, records may be utilized by researchers to collect retrospective data for a study. For these reasons, accurate documentation is extremely important.

## QUESTIONS TO CONSIDER

- Identify three nursing interventions that may be implemented to promote patient safety and stability after general anesthesia.
- Your PACU patient demonstrates the following signs and symptoms: tachycardia, temperature increase, increase in blood pressure, tachypnea, mottled skin, and muscle rigidity. What nursing interventions should be initiated?
- List several causes of airway obstruction during the immediate postoperative recovery period.
- You note the following changes in vital signs in a 46-year-old male patient admitted to the PACU after thoracic surgery: pulse 124 beats/min, BP 90/60 mm Hg, respirations 32/min and labored. Identify and discuss the nursing interventions that should be initiated.

## CRITICAL THINKING ACTIVITIES

- Placing a warm blanket, hyperthermia pad, or warming light on the patient is a nursing intervention specific to the immediate postoperative period. What complication is this directed at preventing, and what is the rationale?
- Mr. Walker, 82, has just been returned to your unit from the recovery room. He had a skin graft for a decubitus ulcer and is diabetic. What advantage or disadvantage does Mr. Walker have regarding his wound healing potential?

## CHAPTER SUMMARY

### THE IMMEDIATE POSTANESTHESIA PHASE

- The postoperative phase of the surgical experience begins with the patient's arrival in the postanesthesia unit and continues until the patient is returned home.
- The goal of the postoperative phase is the patient's return to physiologic homeostasis that is the same as or improved over the preoperative state.
- The postanesthesia care nurse must understand the patient's risks for postoperative complications and be prepared to intervene when they occur.

### NURSING MANAGEMENT

- To assess, plan, and implement care of the postoperative patient, preoperative information must be ascertained and compared with postoperative data.
- Assessing respiratory status is crucial during the immediate postoperative period. Both a patent airway and adequate respiratory function should be ascertained.
- Continuous monitoring of oxygen saturation level is a necessary postoperative intervention and can be easily achieved by the use of pulse oximetry.
- Prolonged somnolence and muscle weakness are major nervous system complications that may occur in the immediate postoperative period. Prevention of injury is foremost at this time.
- Hypotension and the occurrence of cardiac dysrhythmias are the most commonly encountered cardiovascular complications in the immediate postanesthesia period.
- Excessive blood volume and body fluid loss during surgery requires postoperative intravenous replacement.
- Tympanic temperature measurement is an accurate indication of core body temperature. It is fast and noninvasive and presents little discomfort to the patient.
- Special attention should be given to elderly persons, who are especially vulnerable to alteration in skin integrity and at high risk for many of the potential postoperative complications.

- Meticulous care of the surgical incision is an important nursing intervention that facilitates wound healing.
- Effective management of pain begins with a trusting nurse-patient relationship. Providing adequate postoperative pain relief is essential. Narcotics or NSAIDs may be used.
- Among the many challenges for the postanesthesia nurse is the implementation of caring practices into a busy environment. A balance of caring and technologic skills provides a safe and supportive approach to patient care.
- Family needs must be considered. Family members should be kept informed of the patient's postoperative progress.
- Evaluation compares the expected outcomes and patient goals established during assessment with the patient's current status. Goal attainment can be assessed by observations of both subjective and physiologic data.

## REFERENCES


1. Berels DJ, Marz MS: $Sao_2$ monitoring in the postanesthesia care unit, *J Post Anesth Nurs* 6(6):394-401, 1991.
2. Caldwell LM: Surgical outpatient concerns: what every perioperative nurse should know, *AORN J* 53:761-767, 1991.
3. Heffline MS: A comparative study of pharmacologic versus nursing interventions in the treatment of postanesthesia shivering, *J Post Anesth Nurs* 6:311-320, 1991.
4. Hull RD et al: Effectiveness of intermittent pneumatic leg compression for preventing deep vein thrombosis after total hip replacement, *JAMA* 263:2313-2317, 1990.
5. Iacono MV: Precious moments of caring, *J Post Anesth Nurs* 8:26-27, 1993.
6. Kenny GNC: Ketorolac tromethamine—a new nonopioid analgesic, *Br J Anaesth* 65:8-25, 1990.
7. Noonan AT et al: Family-centered nursing in the postanesthesia care unit: the evaluation of practice, *J Post Anesth Nurs* 6:13-16, 1991.
8. Summers T: Axillary, tympanic, and esophageal temperature measurement: descriptive comparisons in postanesthesia patients, *J Post Anesth Nurs* 6(6):420-425, 1991.

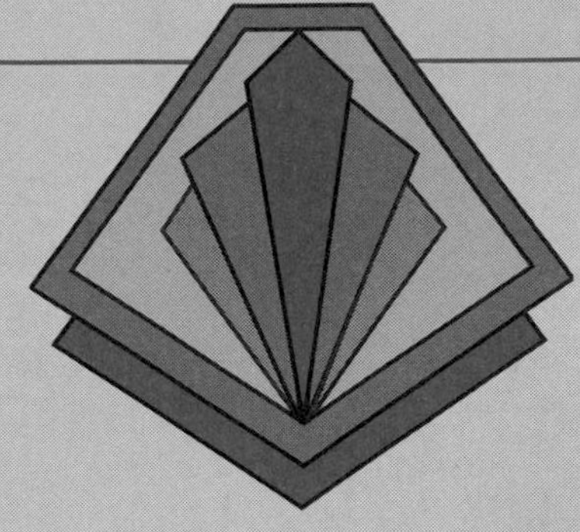

UNIT V

# Special Environments of Care

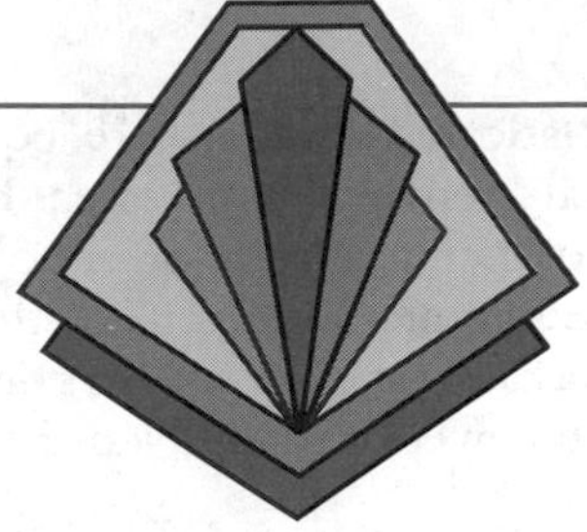

# CHAPTER 26

# Critical Care Environment

*Maj. Deborah J. Kenny**
*Maura A. Hopkins*

## CHAPTER OBJECTIVES

***After studying this chapter, the learner should be able to do the following:***

1 Describe the physical and psychologic environment of critical care units.
2 Identify the types of data needed for the care of critically ill patients.
3 Describe interventions to alleviate physiologic stressors that are specific to the critical care setting.
4 Describe interventions to prevent and alleviate psychologic stressors for the critically ill patient, the family, and the nurse.

## KEY TERMS

adult respiratory distress syndrome (ARDS)
baseline systems assessment
cardiac monitoring
continuous arteriovenous hemofiltration (CAVH)
critical care environment
hemodynamic monitoring
intraaortic balloon pump (IABP)
intraarterial monitoring
intracranial pressure (ICP)
invasive technique
mechanical ventilation
positive end-expiratory pressure (PEEP)
pulmonary artery monitoring
Stevens-Johnson syndrome
Swan-Ganz catheter
total parenteral nutrition (TPN)
toxic epidermal necrolysis
ventricular assist device (VAD)

The critical care unit is a unique environment in which the most sophisticated medical, nursing, and technical interventions can be integrated to combat life-threatening illness. Since nursing's earliest days the concept of locating the sickest patients together and nearest the nurses' station has underlined the importance of frequent assessment and rapid intervention. From postoperative wards to polio centers to the evolution of the coronary care unit, the concentration of highly specialized caregivers with access to unique technology has remained the nucleus of the development of **critical care environments.** The units for patient care are referred to as intensive care units (ICU), critical care units, coronary care units (CCU), and other names that identify the type and the intensity of patient care.

The role of the nurse in the care of the critically ill patient has remained the focal point of the success of the critical care unit. Through the vigilant observation of a patient's ever-changing condition, the critical care nurse is able to monitor the complex treatment regimens, quickly identify problems and initiate appropriate therapies, and intervene to prevent or correct life-threatening situations. The critical care setting varies from the multipurpose ICU to units specially designed for patients with a common type of problem, such as medical, surgical, coronary, cardiothoracic (open heart), neurologic/neurosurgical, pediatric, pulmonary, renal/dialysis, neonatal, burn, organ transplantation, and shock/trauma units.

In any critical care setting the goal of nursing remains the same: to provide continuous, optimal nursing care to patients in life-threatening situations, remaining alert to the physiologic, psychologic, and social needs of the patient as an integrated being. This chapter provides an overview of some of the common aspects of critical care nursing and the critical care environment. Effects of the critical care environment on patient, family, and staff are discussed. Assessment of the critically ill patient is described, followed by interventions designed to alleviate physiologic, physical, psychologic, and social stressors experienced by critically ill patients.

*Views expressed are those of the author and not the United States Army.

# ENVIRONMENT IN THE CRITICAL CARE UNIT

## PHYSICAL ENVIRONMENT

The critical care unit is designed, equipped, and staffed to meet the anticipated needs of patients in life-threatening situations. The physical layout is frequently a modified circular design around a central nurses' station, allowing for direct visualization of all patients at all times. Patients may be separated into individual cubicles or situated in a large open area with curtains for partitions. The advantage of direct nurse-patient visualization may accompany the disadvantages of limited privacy and patient exposure to frequent crisis interventions. The central nurses' station contains monitoring equipment so that nurses can provide continuous surveillance of vital data whether they are at the bedside or at the nurses' station.

Supplies and equipment in critical care areas are highly sophisticated and must be readily accessible for all patients (Box 26-1). Certain pieces of equipment are in constant use at each bedside (e.g., cardiac monitor, oxygen, hemodynamic monitoring equipment, and suction equipment), whereas others must be available within seconds (defibrillator, ventilator, 12-lead electrocardiogram [ECG] machine, emergency medications). In older institutions existing hospital space has often been converted to critical care use, and as the need for more specialized and sophisticated critical care equipment grows the critical care environment often becomes overcrowded. The use of centralized power columns—with all monitoring equipment, oxygen, suction, electrical outlets, and a work area at each patient's bedside—has become popular in newer or remodeled critical care environments.

**BOX 26-1 Equipment Commonly Available Within or Near the Critical Care Unit**

**MONITORS**
- Cardiac
- Hemodynamic (intraarterial, pulmonary artery, central venous)
- Intracranial pressure
- Respiratory
- Temperature
- External arterial pressure

**GENERAL EQUIPMENT**
- Emergency medications
- ECG machine
- Defibrillator/cardioverter
- Pacemaker
- Oxygen therapy equipment
- Intubation equipment
- Intravenous equipment
- Ventilator
- Arterial blood gas analyzer
- Fluoroscopy
- Doppler flow detection device
- Hyperthermia/hypothermia machine
- Bed scale
- Flush setups for pressure monitoring

**BEDSIDE EQUIPMENT**
- Bed with removable headboard
- Oxygen and manual ventilation bag
- Compressed air source
- Suction
- Resuscitation backboard
- Intravenous infusion controller/pump
- Overhead lighting
- Multiple electrical outlets

**SUPPORTIVE SERVICES**
- Pharmacy
- Laboratory
- Respiratory therapy
- Radiology
- Dialysis

## PSYCHOLOGIC ENVIRONMENT—STRESS ON PATIENT AND STAFF

The critical care environment confronts patients with advanced forms of medical and nursing therapies. Although the patient and family are partially aware of the dynamics of critical care, their attention primarily focuses on the appearance of this special environment: flashing lights, buzzing machines; painful procedures; and a noisy, brightly lit, crowded, hyperactive environment. The stressors on the patient and family are immense, heightened by those treatment modalities that may prove lifesaving.

The stress on the nursing staff in the critical care area stems partially from very high expectations: advanced knowledge of physiology related to all body systems, astute observational and physical assessment skills, abil-

**BOX 26-2 Stressors on Patients, Families, and Staff in the Critical Care Environments**

**PATIENT/FAMILY**
- Unfamiliar environment, new faces
- Noise, light levels
- Sensory deprivation/overload
- Interruption of sleep/wake cycles
- Inaccessibility of family, friends
- Lack of privacy
- Lack of information/understanding of prognosis, care plan
- Lack of information/understanding of policies, procedures
- Anticipation of painful interventions
- Confusion/disorientation related to physiologic factors
- Impaired communication related to intubation
- Observation of crisis intervention in other patients
- Fear related to diagnosis
- Fear of death
- Conflict between patient/family goals and staff goals

**STAFF**
- Expectations of self
- Expectations of peers, clinical supervisors, other health care team members, hospital administrators
- Intricate machinery and techniques
- Closed, crowded work area
- Constant contact with seriously ill, dying patients
- Continual vigilance over multiple patients
- Constant emergency readiness
- Sustained high activity level
- Limited breaks away from the high-stress unit
- Limited communication with many patients related to intubation or altered level of consciousness
- Limited opportunity to communicate with some families
- Isolation from other nurses in the hospital
- Ethical conflicts related to issues of resuscitation and use of life-maintenance equipment

ity to quickly prioritize and make decisions regarding patient care, and technical proficiency in operating the highly sophisticated equipment. In addition, nurses are increasingly faced with complex ethical issues that demand their time and emotional energy. In addition, the constant vigilance and emergency-ready attitude may promote an uneasy sense of impending crisis. Critical care nurses require excellent communication skills in dealing with the patient and family's psychologic and social needs, continually incorporating interventions that the nurse might be tempted to assign a lower priority in a critical situation.

Both the patient and the nurse are bombarded by continuous, varied stressors in the critical care environment (Box 26-2). Low-level stress can be challenging and stimulating and may help enhance creativity, production, and performance in any area. However, continuous high-level stress can be devastating, both physically and psychologically. (Review Chapter 7 on stress, stressors, and stress management.) It is important for the critical care nurse to understand how stressors and stress affect both the patient and family and to implement the appropriate interventions to optimize their situation. In addition, nurses must be aware of their own stressors, including positive and negative effects. They must safeguard their own physical and psychologic health and recognize how insufficient or ineffective coping mechanisms can lead to burnout. The critical care environment is a powerful milieu that must be well understood by nurses who wish to use it advantageously.

## Assessment of the Critically Ill Patient

The nursing process is the same in critical care situations as it is in any other patient setting. Management of critically ill patients requires establishing a data base, identifying actual and potential nursing diagnoses, delineating priorities, defining outcome criteria, executing the planned intervention, and modifying future outcomes and plans on the basis of current outcomes. Management of critically ill patients differs from management of other patients because of an ever-changing data base; a larger number of complex, interrelated problems; frequent priority reorganization; and time limitations imposed by the rapidly changing condition of the patient.

The assessment process for the critically ill patient differs from the assessment of other patients only in reference to the types of technical devices available to assist in data collection. The cardiac monitor, hemodynamic monitoring lines, and laboratory analyses provide data that must be incorporated into the total patient assessment. They are adjuncts to the direct observational data that the nurse gathers through careful history taking and physical examination. Monitored data are useless unless correlated with physical findings and integrated into meaningful analysis by the critical care nurse.

### NURSING HISTORY

There are three main routes by which critically ill patients come to a critical care unit: direct admission, usually through the emergency department, transfer from another patient care division in the same or a different hospital, and postoperative admission after certain operations. The patient admitted directly to the critical care unit (e.g., in the case of a myocardial infarction) often is accompanied by family or friends. The patient and family members are sources for obtaining a thorough and accurate history of the current illness and past illnesses or hospitalizations, as well as a patient profile, social information, and usual coping strategies. Although emphasis is placed on alleviating physiologic problems at the time of admission, one member of the health care team may concurrently interview family members so that crucial facts about the patient's history can be used immediately in patient care. Even in the critical care setting, an accurate and thorough patient history is a vital part of intelligent, individualized care planning and intervention.

When the patient is transferred from another nursing division—directly, after surgery, or from another hospital—consultation between the transferring and receiving nursing staffs is essential. The critical care nurses benefit from the care plan developed by nurses who have had an opportunity to interact with the patient and family at an earlier time. Communication of pertinent history, patient preferences, coping mechanisms, and family dynamics expedite interventions by the critical care nurse to reduce the initial stress of the unfamiliar critical care environment.

### PHYSICAL EXAMINATION

As with the assessment of any patient, history taking is followed by physical examination. Inspection, palpation, percussion, and auscultation are used to elicit directly observed patient data. As in any other setting, an explanation of the procedures is given even if the patient's comprehension is questionable, and the cooperation of the patient is sought. (Refer to a physical assessment textbook for a thorough explanation of the use of these techniques.)

### MONITORED DATA

Nurses in all clinical settings utilize tools for discrete data collection from patients, such as stethoscopes, sphygmomanometers, thermometers, and scales. Critical care nurses have the additional advantage of access to tools that are capable of continuous data collection, such as cardiac monitors, hemodynamic pressure lines, and intracranial pressure monitoring devices. The explosion in critical care technology since the 1970s is providing the critical care nurse with amazing quantities of objective data with minimal time spent in system operations. Computerized monitoring systems are available that occupy less space and provide more capabilities than ever before. The most sophisticated of the patient data management systems takes information from all the continuously monitored parameters (ECG, dysrhythmias, respirations, intraarterial pressure, pulmonary artery pressure, venous oxygen saturation [$Svo_2$], central venous pressure, intracranial pressure, and body temperature), combines it with manually entered data (such as body weight, height, intake and output, and times of drug administration), and prepares a wide array of hemodynamic calculations and patient response trends for analysis by critical care practitioners.

In the 1990s, as critical care moves into the next century, information systems will go further than data collection and analysis by moving directly into clinical intervention. For example, computerized intravenous medication administration systems now exist that can titrate the administration of vasoactive drugs by adjusting infusion pump flow rates in response to continuously measured intraarterial pressure. The parameters are set by the clinician, but the execution is determined by the computer within the pump. At this time, certain types of continuous monitoring devices are used in all critical care environments. Also, computers aid the physician in deciding the course of treatment on the basis of input data and treatment paths. As technology takes on an increasingly larger role in the treatment of critically ill patients, basic physical assessment skills become more important in determining appropriate treatment.

## Cardiac Monitoring

**Cardiac monitoring** consists of placing conductive electrodes on the patient's chest that recognize the electrical activity of the heart and relay it to a video display screen. Both the patient's ECG and a digital count of the heart rate are displayed at the bedside. Alarm limits are individually set by the nurse so that if the patient's heart rate rises or falls beyond a safe range, a tone will sound to alert the nurse. In monitoring systems with computerized dysrhythmia analysis, the monitor also recognizes specific rhythm abnormalities, such as single or paired premature ventricular contractions, bigeminal rhythms, runs of ventricular tachycardia, ventricular fibrillation, or asystole (see Chapter 30). Variations in the audio or visual display of the alarm can alert the nurse to the relative seriousness of the dysrhythmia, even from a distance. Respiratory rate often can be monitored through the same set of chest electrodes, measuring chest wall movement or impedance. Cardiac/respiratory monitoring is a noninvasive procedure that poses minimal risk to the patient.

## Hemodynamic Monitoring

**Hemodynamic monitoring** is a term that refers to invasive monitoring of the arterial or venous vascular system by means of a continuous electronic monitoring device. Table 26-1 lists the normal values and definitions of cardiovascular pressures, many of which can be measured at the patient's bedside.

**TABLE 26-1 Hemodynamic Pressures: Definitions and Normal Values**

| HEMODYNAMIC PRESSURE | DEFINITION AND EXPLANATION | NORMAL VALUES |
|---|---|---|
| Mean arterial pressure (MAP) | Average perfusion pressure created by arterial blood pressure during the complete cardiac cycle. The normal cardiac cycle is one-third systole and two-thirds diastole. These three components are divided by 3 to obtain the average perfusion pressure for the whole cardiac cycle. $\text{MAP} = \frac{(2 \times \text{diastolic}) + \text{systolic}}{3}$ | 70-100 mm Hg |
| Central venous pressure (CVP) | Pressure created by volume in the right side of the heart. When the tricuspid valve is open, the CVP reflects filling pressures in the right ventricle. Clinically, the CVP is often used as a guide to overall fluid balance. | 2-4 mm Hg<br>3-8 cm water ($H_2O$) |
| Left atrial pressure (LAP) | Pressure created by volume in the left side of the heart. When the mitral valve is open, the LAP reflects filling pressures in the left ventricle. Clinically, the LAP is used after cardiac surgery to determine how well the left ventricle is ejecting its volume. In general, the higher the LAP, the lower the ejection fraction from the left ventricle. | 5-12 mm Hg |
| Pulmonary artery pressure (PAP) (systolic, diastolic, mean) (PA systolic [PAS], PA diastolic [PAD], PAP mean [$PAP_M$]) | Pulsatile pressure in the pulmonary artery, measured by an indwelling catheter. | PAS 20-30 mm Hg<br>PAD 5-10 mm Hg<br>$PAP_M$ 10-15 mm Hg |
| Pulmonary capillary wedge pressure or pulmonary artery wedge pressure (PCW or PCWP or PAWP) | Pressure created by volume in the left side of the heart. When the mitral valve is open, the PAWP reflects filling pressures in the pulmonary vasculature, and pressures in the left side of the heart are transmitted back to the catheter "wedged" into a small pulmonary arteriole. | 5-12 mm Hg |

Modified from Thelan LA et al: *Critical care nursing: diagnosis and management,* ed 2, St Louis, 1994, Mosby.

### Intraarterial Monitoring

**Intraarterial monitoring** involves inserting a catheter into an artery, usually the radial or the femoral artery. The catheter is connected to a high-pressure flush system normally filled with heparinized saline solution. A pressurized automatic flush device delivers an average of 1 to 3 ml solution per hour through the catheter to maintain patency. When an electronic transducer is connected to the system and attached to the bedside monitor, a waveform appears on the monitor that represents the fluctuation of the patient's blood pressure in the catheterized artery. A numeric display of the arterial pressure also appears on the monitor; in most patients this direct intraarterial pressure correlates very closely with external cuff pressure measurements.

Intraarterial pressure monitoring also provides direct access to arterial blood, which can then be easily obtained without further needle punctures for various laboratory tests, including arterial blood gas analysis. Intraarterial catheters with fiberoptic tips are capable of continuous bedside monitoring of arterial pH, carbon dioxide pressure ($PCO_2$), and oxygen pressure ($PO_2$). However, intraarterial cannulation is not without its complications (Box 26-3). Nursing responsibilities include setup and safe, aseptic maintenance of the flush system and catheter insertion site; maintenance of a patent catheter with accurate waveform and pressure readings; and continuous patient observation to prevent the immediate life-threatening complication of hemorrhage.

### Pulmonary Artery Monitoring

**Pulmonary artery (PA) monitoring** with a **Swan-Ganz catheter** (see Figure 22-5) is used to monitor cardiovascular function in critically ill patients. The catheter, which has several openings along its length, is inserted into the superior vena cava via the subclavian or internal jugular vein. A balloon at the distal tip is filled with approximately 1 ml of air, and the catheter is floated through the right side of the heart until the tip lies in the PA (see Figure 22-5). The balloon is then deflated. PA, central venous pressure (CVP), and pulmonary capillary wedge pressures (PCWP) can be obtained from the catheter once it is connected to a pressurized flush device and transducer-monitor system. In addition, cardiac output measurements can be obtained. The PA catheter is useful in providing data about left and right ventricular failure and in evaluating the effectiveness of vasopressor drugs. It is a significant tool in the management of severe cardiac failure and cardiogenic shock (see Chapter 31). (Table 26-2 lists the hemodynamic indexes that can be computed from monitored data.) In addition, the catheter serves as a central venous access line for the infusion of fluids and potent medications. PA catheters are replacing single-purpose CVP lines because the information they provide on left-sided heart function (wedge pressure, cardiac output) cannot be obtained from a single right-sided heart catheter (CVP line).

In many critical care units a more advanced form of the pulmonary catheter is being used. This newest catheter has a fiberoptic light that, with use of reflection spectrophotometry, measures mixed venous oxygen saturation ($SvO_2$). Minute-by-minute changes in the systemic oxygen saturation can be monitored, reducing the frequent sampling of arterial blood gas while rapidly demonstrating the effects of various clinical interventions on systemic oxygenation. This catheter has the capability of measuring the same parameters obtained by means of the conventional PA catheter. As with intraarterial pressure monitoring, PA monitoring also is not without risk (Box 26-4). Nursing responsibilities are similar to those for arterial catheters, with the addition of continuous waveform observation to detect catheter-tip migration.

### Intracranial Pressure Monitoring

**Intracranial pressure (ICP)** is frequently monitored in critically ill patients who have or are suspected of having intracranial disease or secondary increases in intracranial pressure. A catheter placed through the skull into either the subarachnoid space or the cerebral ventricle allows changes in pressure within the cranial cavity to be monitored directly by means of a transducer and tubing system. ICP monitoring allows continuous observation of the patient's response to therapies aimed at lowering ICP and shows immediately the patient's tolerance of nursing measures, such as turning, suctioning, and changes in bed position, that can cause an unsafe rise in ICP. Cerebrospinal fluid also can be aspirated for analysis, culture, or relief of elevated ICP unresponsive to other therapies. Nurses are responsible for obtaining

**BOX 26-3 Complications of Intraarterial Monitoring**

Bleeding
Distal obstruction of the artery/ischemia
Air embolism
Inflammation/infiltration
Infection
Thrombosis
Paresthesias

**BOX 26-4 Complications of Pulmonary Artery Monitoring**

Infection
Dysrhythmias
Pulmonary infarction
Pulmonary artery rupture
Balloon rupture with air embolism
Intracardiac knotting
Thrombophlebitis
Air embolism

**TABLE 26-2 Normal Hemodynamic Indexes, Definitions, Formulas, and Normal Values**

| MEASUREMENT | DEFINITION AND EXPLANATION | FORMULA | NORMAL VALUE |
|---|---|---|---|
| Cardiac output (CO) | The amount of blood pumped out by a ventricle. Clinically, it can be measured using the thermodilution CO method, which calculates CO in liters per minute (L/min). | Heart rate × Stroke volume | 4-6 L/min (at rest) |
| Cardiac index (CI) | CO divided by body surface area (BSA), tailoring the CO to individual body size. A BSA conversion chart is necessary to calculate CI, which is considered more accurate than CO because it is individualized to height and weight. CI is measured in liters per minute per square meter BSA (L/min/m$^2$). | $\frac{\text{Cardiac output}}{\text{Body surface area}}$ | 2.2-4.0 L/min/m$^2$ |
| Stroke volume (SV) | Amount of blood ejected by the ventricle with each heartbeat. Hemodynamic monitoring systems calculate SV by dividing cardiac output (CO in L/min) by the heart rate (HR) then multiplying the answer by 1000 to change liters to milliliters (ml). | $\frac{\text{Cardiac output}}{\text{Heart rate}}$ | 60-70 ml |
| Stroke volume index (SI) | SV indexed to BSA. | $\frac{\text{Stroke volume}}{\text{Body surface area}}$ | 40-50 ml/beat/m$^2$ |
| Systemic vascular resistance (SVR) | Mean pressure difference across the systemic vascular bed, divided by blood flow. Clinically, SVR represents the resistance against which the left ventricle must pump to eject its volume. This resistance is created by the systemic arteries and arterioles. As SVR increases, CO falls. SVR is measured in either units or dynes/sec/cm$^{-5}$. If the number of units is multiplied by 80, the value is converted to dynes/sec/cm$^{-5}$. | $\frac{\text{MAP-CVP (mm Hg)} \times 80}{\text{Cardiac output}}$ | 10-18 units or 800-1400 dynes/sec/cm$^{-5}$ |
| Systemic vascular resistance index (SVRI) | SVR indexed to BSA. | — | 2000-2400 dynes/sec/cm$^{-5}$/m$^2$ |
| Pulmonary vascular resistance (PVR) | Mean pressure difference across pulmonary vascular bed, divided by blood flow. Clinically, PVR represents the resistance against which the right ventricle must pump to eject its volume. This resistance is created by the pulmonary arteries and arterioles. As PVR increases, the output from the right ventricle decreases. PVR is measured in either units or dynes/sec/cm$^{-5}$. PVR is normally one sixth of SVR. | $\frac{\text{Mean PAP} - \text{Mean PCWP}}{\text{Cardiac output}}$ | 1.2-3.0 units or 100-250 dynes/sec/cm$^{-5}$ |
| Pulmonary vascular resistance index (PVRI) | PVR indexed to BSA. | — | 225-315 dynes/sec/cm$^{-5}$/m$^2$ |
| Left cardiac work index (LCWI) | Amount of work the left ventricle does *each minute* when ejecting blood. The hemodynamic formula represents pressure generated (MAP) multiplied by volume pumped (CO). A conversion factor is used to change mm Hg to kilogram-meter (kg-m). LCWI is always represented as an indexed volume (BSA chart). LCWI increases or decreases because of changes in either pressure (MAP) or volume pumped (CO). | — | 3.4-4.2 kg-m/m$^2$ |
| Left ventricular stroke work index (LVSWI) | Amount of work the left ventricle performs with *each heartbeat.* The hemodynamic formula represents pressure generated (MAP) multiplied by volume pumped (SV). A conversion factor is used to change ml/mm Hg to gram-meter (g-m). LVSWI is always represented as an indexed volume. LVSWI increases or decreases because of changes in either pressure (MAP) or volume pumped (SV). | — | 50-62 g-m/m$^2$ |

Modified from Thelan LA et al: *Critical care nursing: diagnosis and management,* ed 2, St Louis, 1994, Mosby.

**TABLE 26-2 Normal Hemodynamic Indexes, Definitions, Formulas, and Normal Values—cont'd**

| MEASUREMENT | DEFINITION AND EXPLANATION | FORMULA | NORMAL VALUE |
|---|---|---|---|
| Right cardiac work index (RCWI) | Amount of work the right ventricle performs *each minute* when ejecting blood. The hemodynamic formula represents pressure generated (PAP mean) multiplied by volume pumped (CO). A conversion factor is used to change mm Hg to kilogram-meter (kg-m). RCWI is always represented as an indexed value (BSA chart). Similar to LCWI, the RCWI increases or decreases because of changes in either pressure (PAP mean) or volume pumped (CO). | — | 0.54-0.66 kg-m/$m^2$ |
| Right ventricular stroke work index (RVSWI) | Amount of work the right ventricle performs with *each heartbeat.* The hemodynamic formula represents pressure generated (PAP mean) multiplied by volume pumped (SV). A conversion factor is used to change mm Hg to gram-meter (g-m). RVSWI is always represented as an indexed value (BSA chart). Similar to LVSWI, the RVSWI increases or decreases because of changes in either pressure (PAP mean) or volume pumped (SV). | — | 7.9-9.7 g-m/$m^2$ |

**TABLE 26-3 Types of Intracranial Pressure Monitoring Devices**

| DEVICE/PLACEMENT | ADVANTAGES/USES | DISADVANTAGES |
|---|---|---|
| **INTRAVENTRICULAR CANNULA** | | |
| Lateral ventricle in nondominant hemisphere through burr hole | CSF measurement<br>CSF drainage<br>Drug administration<br>Compliance testing | Rapid CSF drainage can result in collapsed ventricles or subdural hematoma<br>Cannula tip may catch on ventricular wall<br>Risk of intracerebral bleeding and infection<br>May become plugged with debris<br>Possible difficult insertion due to shifting or collapse of ventricle |
| **SUBARACHNOID SCREW** | | |
| Subarachnoid space through twist drill hole | Pressure monitoring<br>Less risk of infection than cannula<br>Useful with small ventricles<br>Does not penetrate brain | Compliance testing may be unreliable<br>No CSF drainage<br>Some risk of infection<br>Risk of hemorrhage or hematoma during insertion<br>Brain may herniate into bolt, making recording unreliable |
| **EPIDURAL SENSOR** | | |
| Epidural space<br>Burr hole<br>Fiberoptic sensor | Lowest risk of infection<br>Easy to insert<br>Dura not penetrated | No direct measurement of CSF<br>No CSF drainage<br>Inability to recalibrate to zero<br>Cannot measure compliance |
| **INTRAPARENCHYMAL** | | |
| Intraparenchymal *via* twist drill<br>Fiberoptic sensor | Easy to insert<br>Direct pressure<br>Compliance testing<br>One-time zero and calibration | Risk of intracerebral bleeding and infection<br>No CSF drainage |

From Swearingen PL, Keen JH: *Manual of critical care: applying nursing diagnoses to adult critical illness,* St Louis, 1991, Mosby.
*CSF,* Cerebrospinal fluid.

accurate pressure measurements, analyzing trends and patient response to interventions, and preventing complications of monitoring. Scrupulous sterile technique is essential in handling the catheter or screw insertion site and all connections in the monitoring tubing system because microorganisms have a direct pathway to enter the cerebrospinal fluid. (See Table 26-3 for a description of the different types of intracranial pressure monitoring devices.)

A new type of fiberoptic intracranial catheter is able to read ICPs directly at the tip of the catheter. The sensed pressures are converted into a waveform and digital value that can be displayed on the bedside monitor. Although entry into the subarachnoid or intraventricular space to measure ICP is still necessary, this catheter does not require the use of a fluid-filled pressure tubing/transducer system and therefore eliminates one source of potential contamination.

## Summary of Monitoring

The preceding items represent a few of the invasive monitoring techniques available to the critical care nurse for data collection. In all cases the nurse must be knowledgeable about maintaining these lines: the normal appearance of the waveform associated with each line, the usual procedures necessary to prevent complications, and the signs and symptoms of actual complications. The risk to the patient from invasive monitoring lines is significantly reduced when the lines are handled and cared for by knowledgeable personnel. In addition to the invasive lines used for the various types of monitoring, nurses in critical care also must be familiar with and able to maintain central lines used for medication. A new type of central line—a peripherally inserted central venous catheter (PICC)—is inserted and maintained by nurses. These lines may become more common than the conventional central lines, at least for medications. See Research box above.

### RESEARCH

Abi-Nader JA: Peripherally inserted central venous catheters in critical care patients, *Heart Lung* 22(5):428-434, 1993.

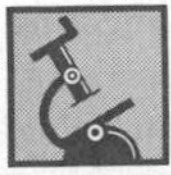

Increasing use of long-term intravenous therapy has required the development of catheters that can be inserted peripherally into central veins. Peripherally inserted central venous catheters (PICCs) are inserted into the antecubital fossa by nurses to provide access sites for long-term antibiotic, chemotherapeutic, or parenteral nutrition therapy. In this study 92 patients receiving PICCs for intravenous therapy were studied to determine clinical outcomes and cost. Findings indicated that of the 92 PICC insertions there were five cases of phlebitis and one case of catheter-related sepsis. The author believes that with training, nurses can safely insert and maintain PICCs with minimal complications and that PICCs offer a cost-effective alternative to conventional jugular or subclavian central venous catheters.

## BASELINE ASSESSMENT

The complete history and physical examination provide the necessary foundation for further ongoing data collection in the critical care setting, and the importance of accurate and thorough initial information cannot be overemphasized. However, the multiple sources of data and the continually fluctuating stability of critically ill patients make constant priority reorganization a necessity. On the basis of continual patient observation, the critical care nurse updates the data base to reformulate short-term goals and interventions.

Patient assessment must be thorough, yet rapid. The physical and psychologic reactions of an entire organism under stress must be taken into account and not be limited by the usual or the expected. Patient assessment also must be organized and repetitive so that small alterations or deviations from previous findings will be noticed. Finally, the assessment must be individualized, with time and attention given to particularly significant aspects.

Many critical care units utilize some form of a systems approach to patient assessment. Frequently a complete head-to-toe systems review at the beginning of the shift takes place, at which time the nurse gathers an initial data base (Figure 26-1). More time and depth are spent on the systems that present the greatest real or potential threat to the patient. When completed and documented, the **baseline systems assessment** presents an accurate status report on the patient's condition. Throughout the rest of the shift, the nurse notes all the changes as the patient's condition improves or deteriorates from the baseline, keeping track of vital parameters on an ongoing flow sheet (Figure 26-2).

Once initial patient assessment is completed, nursing diagnoses are established and nursing care plans formulated. Nursing interventions for critically ill patients are based on these care plans.

Throughout this text, nursing interventions have been described for care of the patient with a particular type of physiologic impairment. These are interventions intended to improve the patient's physiologic functioning before the impairment reaches the critical stage. In some critically ill patients, many of these interventions have already been utilized without success, and the patient's physiologic condition deteriorates to the critical level, necessitating acute life-sustaining interventions. For other patients, the first presentation of the illness is critical (such as acute myocardial infarction or severe trauma), and interventions are immediately necessary to sustain life.

The remaining three sections of this chapter focus on the physiologic, psychologic, and social interventions

*Text continued on p. 668.*

**ASSESSMENT** Time Care Plan Reviewed ____________ Pertinent Patient Problem # ____________
Shift: ____________ Assessment Time: ____________ Name: ____________

**NEUROLOGICAL**
Alert Lethargic Agitated
Confused Coma Cough Gag
Orientation ____________
Person Place Time
Hallucinations / Delusions
Neuromuscular Blockers c̄ s̄
Speech: Cleared Slurred
Dysphasic Intubated
Spinal / C-spine:
Immobilization
Hearing: Good Hard of Hearing Deaf
Ventriculostomy Site ____________
Face: Symmetrical Nonsymmetrical

**SAFETY**
Level A B C
Side Rails UP R/L Call Light in Reach □
ID Band Checked □
Restraints=check q̄ □
UE LE Soft Leather
Reason - ____________
Allergy Band ____________
Isolation Type ____________

**SKIN AND MUCOUS MEMBRANES**
Skin Color: ____________
Cyanotic Pale
Jaundiced: Sclera Skin
Turgor: Normal Poor Taut
Temperature: Warm Cool Cold
Dry Diaphoretic Flaking Mottled
Decubitus: Location & Description ____________
____________
____________
Mucous Membrane: Moist Dry Cracked
Color ____________
Lesions: Type ____________
Peripheral Edema
Location ____________
Pitting ____________
Dependent ____________
Stoma: Color ____________
Location ____________
Drainage ____________
Protruding ____________

**WOUNDS/LARGE DRESSING/INCISION**
Site #1 ____________
#2 ____________
#3 ____________
#4 ____________
Color/Drainage #1 ____________
#2 ____________
#3 ____________
#4 ____________
Time/Type drsg change #1 ____________
#2 ____________
#3 ____________
#4 ____________
Additional ____________
____________
____________
____________

**NUTRITION**
Enteral
Rate ____________ Solution ____________
Tube ____________
Parenteral
Oral Diet ____________ NPO
Tolerated ____________
Caloric Count ____________

**CARDIOVASCULAR**
Cap Refill(secs) ____________
Periphery: Warm Cool Cold
Neck Veins: Distended Flat
A-line:
Allens Test ____________
Correlates with cuff ____________
Swan-Ganz: Waveform-dampened
normal site ____________
Calibrated and Zeroed
A-Line Swan-Ganz CVP
IV ____________
Swelling Redness Tenderness
c̄ or s̄
Hep Lock Blood Return + or –
Swelling Redness Tenderness
c̄ or s̄
Alarm Limits: Time ____________
HR ___ ___ BP ___ ___ On

**GASTROINTESTINAL**
Bowel Sounds: Regular Hypoactive
Hyperactive Absent
Abdomen: Soft Firm Hard Distended
Non-distended Non-tender Tender
Impaction
Nasogastric: Placement Check □
Suction: Cont Intermittent
Clamped
Drainage Color: ____________
Other: ____________
____________
Gastrostomy: Clamped TF
Red Robinson: Clamped DD
Abdominal Girth :cm ____________
Emesis:
Color ____________

**GENITOURINARY**
Void Straight Cath
Continent Incontinent
Foley External Catheter
Type: Cloudy Clear Clots
Sediment
Color: ____________
Genitalia: Appearance ____________
____________
Drainage: ____________

**SEE DIAGRAM FOR LOCATION OF ABRASIONS, BRUISES, BURNS ECT.**

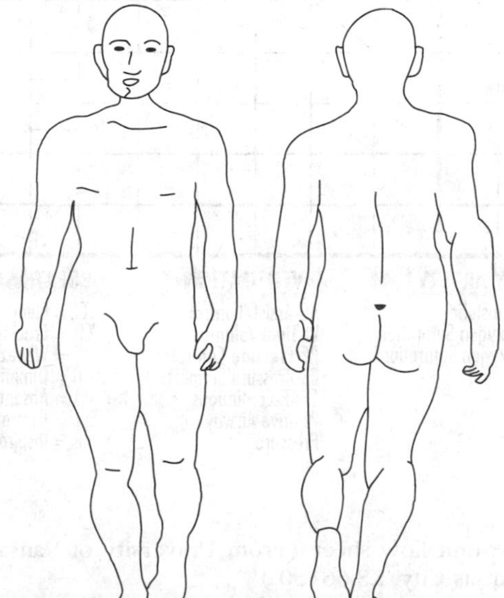

**RESPIRATORY**
Intubation date ____________
ET Tube Position ____________ cm
Size ____________ Route ET NT
Trach Site Appearance ____________
____________
Size/Type ____________
Airway Type ____________
Use of Accessory Muscle □
Chest Excursion: Symmetrical
Asymmetrical Flail
Cough:
Sputum: Color ____________
Consistency: ____________
Amount: ____________
Odor: ____________

**PLEURAL CHEST TUBES**
Site/Drainage Type Air Leak
#1 ____________ c̄ s̄
#2 ____________ c̄ s̄
#3 ____________ c̄ s̄

| | #1 | #2 | #3 |
|---|---|---|---|
| Suction | □ | □ | □ |
| H2O Seal | □ | □ | □ |

Subcutaneous Emphysema c̄ or s̄
Location: ____________
I.S. ____ cc greatest volume

**DRAINS/LOCATION/DRAINAGE**
(Color, Consistency, Odor)
Hemovac: R/L ____________
Drainage: ____________
Jackson Pratt:R/L ____________
Drainage: ____________
Shirley Drains:R/L ____________
Drainage: ____________
Other:R/L ____________
Drainage: ____________
Other:R/L ____________
Drainage: ____________
____________

**DISCHARGE PLANNING/FAMILY PATIENT TEACHING** ____________
____________
____________
____________
____________
____________

**FIGURE 26-1** Sample critical care assessment form, which is completed with each change of personnel. (From University of Kansas Medical Center, 3901 Rainbow Boulevard, Kansas City, KS 66160.)

OPER. PROCEDURE/DIAGNOSIS ______________________ DATE OF OPER. ________

Date: __________ Admission/Hospital Day # ______________ Physician/# ______________

Unit ______________ Bed # ______________

| CARDIOVASCULAR | | | | | | | PULMONARY ARTERY | | | | | | | | RESPIRATORY | | | | | | | | |
|---|---|---|---|---|---|---|---|---|---|---|---|---|---|---|---|---|---|---|---|---|---|---|---|
| Time | Temp O/A/R | HEART RATE | CARDIAC RHYTHM | BP A.LINE | BP CUFF | MAP | S/D | $\overline{PA}$ / PCW | RA CVP | | $SaO_2$ | $SvO_2$ | CO / CI | SVR | RATE | CHARACTER | BREATH SOUNDS | SPUTUM | $F_1O_2$ | TYPE VENT | VENTILATION AC | IMV | VT |
| 0000 | | | | | | | | | | | | | | | | | | | | | | | |
| 0100 | | | | | | | | | | | | | | | | | | | | | | | |
| 0200 | | | | | | | | | | | | | | | | | | | | | | | |
| 0300 | | | | | | | | | | | | | | | | | | | | | | | |
| 0400 | | | | | | | | | | | | | | | | | | | | | | | |
| 0500 | | | | | | | | | | | | | | | | | | | | | | | |
| 0600 | | | | | | | | | | | | | | | | | | | | | | | |
| 0700 | | | | | | | | | | | | | | | | | | | | | | | |
| 8HR. Total | | | | | | | | | | | | | | | | | | | | | | | |
| 0800 | | | | | | | | | | | | | | | | | | | | | | | |
| 0900 | | | | | | | | | | | | | | | | | | | | | | | |
| 1000 | | | | | | | | | | | | | | | | | | | | | | | |
| 1100 | | | | | | | | | | | | | | | | | | | | | | | |
| 1200 | | | | | | | | | | | | | | | | | | | | | | | |
| 1300 | | | | | | | | | | | | | | | | | | | | | | | |
| 1400 | | | | | | | | | | | | | | | | | | | | | | | |
| 1500 | | | | | | | | | | | | | | | | | | | | | | | |
| 8HR. Total | | | | | | | | | | | | | | | | | | | | | | | |
| 1600 | | | | | | | | | | | | | | | | | | | | | | | |
| 1700 | | | | | | | | | | | | | | | | | | | | | | | |
| 1800 | | | | | | | | | | | | | | | | | | | | | | | |
| 1900 | | | | | | | | | | | | | | | | | | | | | | | |
| 2000 | | | | | | | | | | | | | | | | | | | | | | | |
| 2100 | | | | | | | | | | | | | | | | | | | | | | | |
| 2200 | | | | | | | | | | | | | | | | | | | | | | | |
| 2300 | | | | | | | | | | | | | | | | | | | | | | | |
| 8HR. Total | | | | | | | | | | | | | | | | | | | | | | | |
| 24HR. Total | | | | | | | | | | | | | | | | | | | | | | | |

**CARDIOVASCULAR**

TEMP O-ORAL

A. Line-Arterial Line

**PULMONARY ARTERY**

S/D Systolic/Diastolic
$SaO_2$ Arterial Oxygen Saturation
$SvO_2$ Venous Oxygen Saturation
CO Cardiac Output

**VENTILATION**

AC-Assist/Control
Vt-Tidal Volume
PC-Pressure Control
PS-Pressure Support
CPAP-Continuous Positive Airway Pressure

**BREATH SOUNDS**

CL = Clear
CR = Crackles
W = Wheezes
D = Diminished
A = Absent
Exp = Expiratory
Ins = Inspiratory

**SPUTUM**

C = Cough
PC = Productive Cough
T = Tenacious
RS = Requires Suction
M = Moderate
C = Copious
BT = Blood Tinged

**PULSES**

R = Radial
PT = Post Tibial
DP = Dorsalis Pedis
B = Brachial
4+ = Bounding
3+ = Easily felt
2+ = Barely palpable
1+ = Present with DOPPLER
0 = Absent

**FIGURE 26-2** Sample intensive care unit flow sheet. (From University of Kansas Medical Center, 3901 Rainbow Boulevard, Kansas City, KS 66160.)

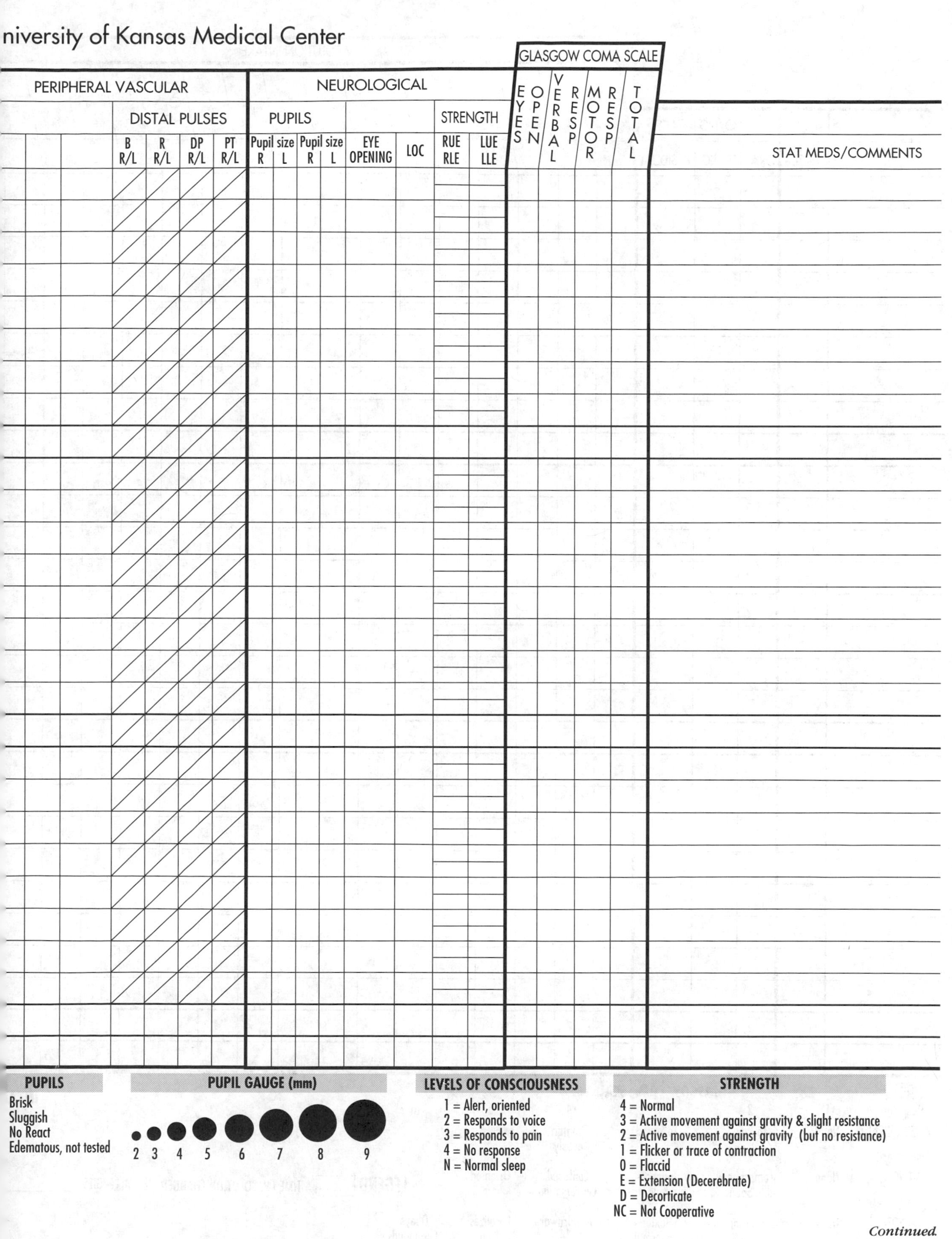

niversity of Kansas Medical Center

| PERIPHERAL VASCULAR | | | | | | | NEUROLOGICAL | | | | | | | | GLASGOW COMA SCALE | | | | | | STAT MEDS/COMMENTS |
|---|---|---|---|---|---|---|---|---|---|---|---|---|---|---|---|---|---|---|---|---|---|
| | | DISTAL PULSES | | | | | PUPILS | | | | | | STRENGTH | | | | | | | | |
| | | B R/L | R R/L | DP R/L | PT R/L | | Pupil size R | Pupil size L | Pupil size R | Pupil size L | EYE OPENING | LOC | RUE RLE | LUE LLE | EYES OPEN | VERBAL RESP | MOTOR RESP | TOTAL | | | |

**PUPILS**

Brisk
Sluggish
No React
Edematous, not tested

**PUPIL GAUGE (mm)**

2 3 4 5 6 7 8 9

**LEVELS OF CONSCIOUSNESS**

1 = Alert, oriented
2 = Responds to voice
3 = Responds to pain
4 = No response
N = Normal sleep

**STRENGTH**

4 = Normal
3 = Active movement against gravity & slight resistance
2 = Active movement against gravity (but no resistance)
1 = Flicker or trace of contraction
0 = Flaccid
E = Extension (Decerebrate)
D = Decorticate
NC = Not Cooperative

*Continued.*

| | Finger Stick | PO/NG INTAKE | | | IV SOLUTION INTAKE | | | | | | | | | | | | | | | | |
|---|---|---|---|---|---|---|---|---|---|---|---|---|---|---|---|---|---|---|---|---|---|
| | | ORAL | TF/NG | RESIDUAL | | | | | | | | | | | | | C.O. Flush | Heparin Flush | PCA | | |

GRAND INTA

**GLASGOW COMA SCALE**

| Responds | 1 | 2 | 3 | 4 | 5 | 6 |
|---|---|---|---|---|---|---|
| EYES OPEN | None | To Pain | To Sound | Spontaneously | | |
| VERBAL | None | Incomprehensible Sound | Inappropriate Words | Confused Conversation | Oriented | |
| MOTOR | None | Extension | Flexion Abnormal | Withdrawal | Localizes Pain | Obeys Commands |

LEGEND ☐ = TIME I.V. SOLUTION CHANGED

ALLERGIES ______

**FIGURE 26-2, cont'd** Sample intensive care unit flow sheet.

| Initials | Signature | Initials | Signature |
|---|---|---|---|
| | | | |
| | | | |
| | | | |

BLOOD PRODUCTS

OUTPUT

| | CHEST TUBES #1 | #2 | | U.O. | SP. GR. | | | JACKSON PRATT | HEMOVAC | | NG | NG PH | BOWEL SOUNDS | EMESIS | STOOLS HEMATEST | Time |
|---|---|---|---|---|---|---|---|---|---|---|---|---|---|---|---|---|
| | | | | | | | | | | | | | | | | 0000 |
| | | | | | | | | | | | | | | | | 0100 |
| | | | | | | | | | | | | | | | | 0200 |
| | | | | | | | | | | | | | | | | 0300 |
| | | | | | | | | | | | | | | | | 0400 |
| | | | | | | | | | | | | | | | | 0500 |
| | | | | | | | | | | | | | | | | 0600 |
| | | | | | | | | | | | | | | | | 0700 |
| | | | | | | | | | | | | | | | | 8HR. Total |
| | | | | | | | | | | | | | | | | 0800 |
| | | | | | | | | | | | | | | | | 0900 |
| | | | | | | | | | | | | | | | | 1000 |
| | | | | | | | | | | | | | | | | 1100 |
| | | | | | | | | | | | | | | | | 1200 |
| | | | | | | | | | | | | | | | | 1300 |
| | | | | | | | | | | | | | | | | 1400 |
| | | | | | | | | | | | | | | | | 1500 |
| | | | | | | | | | | | | | | | | 8HR. Total |
| | | | | | | | | | | | | | | | | 1600 |
| | | | | | | | | | | | | | | | | 1700 |
| | | | | | | | | | | | | | | | | 1800 |
| | | | | | | | | | | | | | | | | 1900 |
| | | | | | | | | | | | | | | | | 2000 |
| | | | | | | | | | | | | | | | | 2100 |
| | | | | | | | | | | | | | | | | 2200 |
| | | | | | | | | | | | | | | | | 2300 |
| | | | | | | | | | | | | | | | | 8HR. Total |
| | | | | | | | | | | | | | | | | 24HR. Total |

U.O.- Urine Output

**24 HOUR INTAKE & OUTPUT**

| | Yesterday | Today |
|---|---|---|
| Intake | | |
| Output | | |

| | | |
|---|---|---|
| Weight | | |
| Dialysis | | |
| | Pre | Post |

**GRAND TOTAL OUTPUT** ______

DATE ______

*Continued.*

| LAB | 00 | 01 | 02 | 03 | 04 | 05 | 06 | 07 | 08 | 09 | 10 | 11 | 12 | 13 | 14 | 15 | 16 | 17 | 18 | 19 | 20 | 21 | 22 | 23 |
|---|---|---|---|---|---|---|---|---|---|---|---|---|---|---|---|---|---|---|---|---|---|---|---|---|
| pH (7.35-7.45) | | | | | | | | | | | | | | | | | | | | | | | | |
| $PCO_2$(35-45) | | | | | | | | | | | | | | | | | | | | | | | | |
| $PaO_2$(80-100) | | | | | | | | | | | | | | | | | | | | | | | | |
| $F_IO_2$ | | | | | | | | | | | | | | | | | | | | | | | | |
| | | | | | | | | | | | | | | | | | | | | | | | | |
| RBC(4.2-6.1) | | | | | | | | | | | | | | | | | | | | | | | | |
| HgB(12-18) | | | | | | | | | | | | | | | | | | | | | | | | |
| Hematocrit(42-52) | | | | | | | | | | | | | | | | | | | | | | | | |
| Platelet Ct.(150-400) | | | | | | | | | | | | | | | | | | | | | | | | |
| WBC(5000-10,000) | | | | | | | | | | | | | | | | | | | | | | | | |
| Lymph (20%-40%) | | | | | | | | | | | | | | | | | | | | | | | | |
| Mono(2%-8%) | | | | | | | | | | | | | | | | | | | | | | | | |
| Segs(55%-70%) | | | | | | | | | | | | | | | | | | | | | | | | |
| Bands (0-6%) | | | | | | | | | | | | | | | | | | | | | | | | |
| Myelo (0%) | | | | | | | | | | | | | | | | | | | | | | | | |
| | | | | | | | | | | | | | | | | | | | | | | | | |
| Protime:(11-12.5) | | | | | | | | | | | | | | | | | | | | | | | | |
| PTT(30-40) | | | | | | | | | | | | | | | | | | | | | | | | |
| Fibrinogen(200-400) | | | | | | | | | | | | | | | | | | | | | | | | |
| FDP<10μg | | | | | | | | | | | | | | | | | | | | | | | | |
| | | | | | | | | | | | | | | | | | | | | | | | | |
| | | | | | | | | | | | | | | | | | | | | | | | | |
| Na(136-145) | | | | | | | | | | | | | | | | | | | | | | | | |
| K+(3.5-5.0) | | | | | | | | | | | | | | | | | | | | | | | | |
| Cl(90-110) | | | | | | | | | | | | | | | | | | | | | | | | |
| $CO_2$(23-30) | | | | | | | | | | | | | | | | | | | | | | | | |
| GLU(70-115) | | | | | | | | | | | | | | | | | | | | | | | | |
| BUN(5-20) | | | | | | | | | | | | | | | | | | | | | | | | |
| Creat.(0.7-1.5) | | | | | | | | | | | | | | | | | | | | | | | | |
| CA (9-10.5) | | | | | | | | | | | | | | | | | | | | | | | | |
| $Po_4$(2.5-4.5) | | | | | | | | | | | | | | | | | | | | | | | | |
| MG(1.6-3) | | | | | | | | | | | | | | | | | | | | | | | | |
| Uric Acid (2-8.5) | | | | | | | | | | | | | | | | | | | | | | | | |
| T Prot(6-8) | | | | | | | | | | | | | | | | | | | | | | | | |
| Albumin(3.2-4.5) | | | | | | | | | | | | | | | | | | | | | | | | |
| T Bili (0.1-1) | | | | | | | | | | | | | | | | | | | | | | | | |
| Alk Phos(30-85) | | | | | | | | | | | | | | | | | | | | | | | | |
| AST (5-40) | | | | | | | | | | | | | | | | | | | | | | | | |
| Direct Bili 0.1-0.3 | | | | | | | | | | | | | | | | | | | | | | | | |
| Amylase (59-190) | | | | | | | | | | | | | | | | | | | | | | | | |
| Serum Osmo (275-300) | | | | | | | | | | | | | | | | | | | | | | | | |
| | | | | | | | | | | | | | | | | | | | | | | | | |
| Myoglobin (6-65) | | | | | | | | | | | | | | | | | | | | | | | | |
| CPK Total 5-75 | | | | | | | | | | | | | | | | | | | | | | | | |
| MB% <5% | | | | | | | | | | | | | | | | | | | | | | | | |
| LDH 90-200 | | | | | | | | | | | | | | | | | | | | | | | | |
| | | | | | | | | | | | | | | | | | | | | | | | | |
| **DRUG LEVELS** | | | | | | | | | | | | | | | | | | | | | | | | |
| | | | | | | | | | | | | | | | | | | | | | | | | |
| Antibiotics: Peak/Trough | | | | | | | | | | | | | | | | | | | | | | | | |
| | | | | | | | | | | | | | | | | | | | | | | | | |
| | | | | | | | | | | | | | | | | | | | | | | | | |
| | | | | | | | | | | | | | | | | | | | | | | | | |
| | 00 | 01 | 02 | 03 | 04 | 05 | 06 | 07 | 08 | 09 | 10 | 11 | 12 | 13 | 14 | 15 | 16 | 17 | 18 | 19 | 20 | 21 | 22 | 23 |

**FIGURE 26-2, cont'd** Sample intensive care unit flow sheet.

| TREATMENTS | 2300-0700 | 0700-1500 | 1500-2300 |
|---|---|---|---|
| **Activity** | | | |
| ROM Self=S Active=A UPPER | | | |
| Passive=P LOWER | | | |
| Chair/Dangle: frequency/duration | | | |
| Turn & Reposition (side & time) | | | |
| Splints | | | |
| Support Stockings off 20 minutes | | | |
| | | | |
| **Hygiene** | | | |
| Bed/Bath | | | |
| Eye Care | | | |
| Mouth Care | | | |
| Skin Care/Shave | | | |
| Foley/Perineal Care | | | |
| | | | |
| **Drains** | | | |
| Nasogastric Tube | | | |
| Anti Reflux Valve | | | |
| Chest Tube: Milk or Strip | | | |
| Foley Catheter | | | |
| Fecal Bag/Pezzar | | | |
| Ostomy Bag | | | |
| **Respiratory** | | | |
| Cough & /Deep Breath | | | |
| Trach Care/ET Care | | | |
| Spirometer Device | | | |
| | | | |
| **Equipment** | | | |
| Special Mattress | | | |
| Special Bed | | | |
| Enteral Feeding Bag Δ q24 | | | |
| Enteral Pump | | | |
| IV Pump | | | |
| PCA Pump | | | |
| Hypo/Hyperthermia Blanket | | | |
| Aqua K pad/Air mattress | | | |
| Commode | | | |
| Bunnyboot/heel protectors | | | |
| **Musculo-Skeletal Devices** | | | |
| Cervical Collar | | | |
| Traction | | | |
| Foot Board | | | |
| External Fixator | | | |
| Cast | | | |
| Pin Care | | | |
| | | | |
| **Tubing/Drsg (T/D)** | | | |
| Art. Line-site | | | |
| Central-site | | | |
| | | | |
| Swan-Ganz-site | | | |
| Peripheral-site | | | |
| | | | |
| | | | |
| Flush System | | | |
| | | | |
| Initial/Signature | | | |

| Patient Response to Treatment |
|---|
| |

| CULTURE REPORTS | | Date Culture Taken |
|---|---|---|
| | | |

| OTHER TESTS | | | | |
|---|---|---|---|---|
| Time | EKG Area | X-Ray Area | CT-Scan | Other |
| | | | | |

| INVASIVE LINE INSERTION | | | | | |
|---|---|---|---|---|---|
| Time | New Site (N) or J Wired (J) | Type of Catheter | Site | X-Ray Placement Checked | # of Attempts |
| | | | | | |

necessary for the critically ill patient regardless of the initial underlying pathophysiology.

## ALLEVIATION AND PREVENTION OF PHYSIOLOGIC AND PHYSICAL STRESSORS

The ultimate goal of nursing intervention for any patient, regardless of the nature of the illness, is to promote, sustain, and restore optimal levels of physiologic, psychologic, and social functioning. However, in a critical care setting, the immediate goal of ensuring a patient's survival initially determines the priorities for intervention; physiologic problems must be addressed first. Once life-threatening stressors have been alleviated, priorities are reorganized and other problems can be addressed.

Physiologic priorities are determined by the degree of threat to the person's survival. Certain body systems are more prone to disorders requiring intensive therapeutic interventions and are frequently encountered in the critical care unit. These disorders are listed by system, along with the specific critical care interventions employed and additional interventions necessary to prevent complications of therapy.

### RESPIRATORY SYSTEM

The highest priority in caring for a critically ill patient is the maintenance of a patent airway and adequate ventilation.

#### Acute Respiratory Failure

Acute respiratory failure (see Chapter 37) may occur as a primary pulmonary deficit or as the result of a large number of other disorders that can affect the adequacy of ventilation or respiration. Crushing chest injuries, high-level spinal cord injury, neuromuscular diseases, extensive thoracic surgery, end-stage chronic obstructive pulmonary disease (COPD), sepsis, severe pneumonia, severe pulmonary edema, adult respiratory distress syndrome (ARDS), pulmonary embolus, congestive heart failure, sleep apnea, and shock are some of the conditions that may be exhibited by patients in respiratory failure requiring critical care. Interventions in respiratory failure are first directed at establishing an unimpeded airway, through endotracheal intubation via the nose or the mouth or through a tracheostomy. Assisted ventilation may then be provided by a manual resuscitation device (Ambu or anesthesia bag), followed by placement of the patient on continuous mechanical ventilation. **Mechanical ventilation** may be classified by the method through which air enters the lungs, that is, pressure-cycled, volume-cycled, or negative pressure. Ventilatory support mandates observation of the proper functioning of the equipment, as well as assessment of the impact of the mechanical support on the patient's respiratory status. The goal of mechanical ventilation is to provide a sufficient volume of appropriately oxygenated air to maintain serum pH, arterial carbon dioxide pressure ($PaCO_2$), arterial oxygen pressure ($PaO_2$), and arterial oxygen saturation ($SaO_2$) within normal limits for the patient. Adequate ventilation is achieved through careful mechanical manipulation of the respiratory rate, tidal volume, fractional inspired oxygen concentration ($FiO_2$ or percent of 100% oxygen delivered), inspiratory to expiratory time ratio, and peak airway pressure. (See Box 26-5 for modes of ventilation.)

In some disease states, such as neuromuscular conditions, ventilator settings closely approximate normal ventilation, and the respirator accomplishes the work that the weakened chest muscles cannot achieve. In other situations the ventilator settings are manipulated to create a specific mechanical effect, as with high-frequency jet ventilation in bronchopleural fistula. In this condition large tidal volumes are contraindicated because their delivery under pressure would maintain the patency of the fistula. Instead, very small tidal volumes (50 to 400 ml) are delivered through a specially designed endotracheal tube at a rapid rate (100 to 200 cycles per minute). Minute ventilation (total amount of air delivered in 1 minute) may remain normal, but the unusual breathing pattern reduces stress on the fistula and enhances healing. Unilateral pulmonary problems such as bronchopleural fistula also may be treated

**BOX 26-5 Common Modes of Ventilation**

**CONTROLLED MECHANICAL VENTILATION (CMV)**
Preset tidal volume at preset rate. Patient does not breathe spontaneously. Used for patients with drug-induced paralysis, CNS depression, and neuromuscular dysfunction.

**INTERMITTENT MANDATORY VENTILATION (IMV)**
Preset tidal volume at preset rate. Patient may breathe spontaneously between breaths given by ventilator.

**SYNCHRONIZED INTERMITTENT MANDATORY VENTILATION (SIMV)**
Breath initiated by patient; ventilator senses effort and assists by delivering a preset volume. Number of assists per minute is preset; therefore not every breath is assisted.

**ASSIST-CONTROL VENTILATION (ACV)**
Breath initiated by patient; ventilator senses effort and delivers a preset volume with every breath.

**PRESSURE-SUPPORT VENTILATION (PSV)**
Breath initiated by patient; ventilator senses effort, and preset positive pressure is used to augment patient's effort. Patient controls rate and volume. Used to decrease the work of breathing while increasing the inspired volume.

**POSITIVE END-EXPIRATORY PRESSURE (PEEP)**
Constant baseline pressure remains even after expiration. Used to maintain open alveolar airways.

through the use of a double-lumen endotracheal tube that separates the right from the left main-stem bronchus and allows two ventilators to deliver appropriately different modes of asynchronous mechanical ventilation to each lung.

Mechanical ventilation is a complex therapy that poses major risks for the critically ill patient, including pneumothorax, atelectasis, decreased cardiac output (especially if positive end-expiratory pressure is used), gastrointestinal bleeding from a stress ulcer, fluid imbalance, and infection. Preventive nursing interventions for all patients receiving mechanical ventilation include frequent assessment of all body systems and laboratory work, position changes in bed, suctioning to remove secretions, intermittent deep ventilation (bagging or sighing), administration of antacids via nasogastric or gastrostomy tube, and scrupulous sterile technique in airway management to prevent respiratory tract infection.

### Adult Respiratory Distress Syndrome

A particularly threatening respiratory complication that occasionally develops in critically ill patients is the **adult respiratory distress syndrome (ARDS)** (see Chapter 37). ARDS was previously known as shock lung, wet lung, or postpump lung. This condition has various predisposing factors, including a number of disorders seen in the critically ill: shock, trauma, disseminated intravascular coagulation (DIC), fat embolism, cardiopulmonary bypass, sepsis, cardiac arrest, and multiple blood transfusions. Damage to the alveolocapillary membrane and increased capillary permeability lead to pulmonary edema and diffuse microatelectasis. ARDS is characterized by severe dyspnea and hypoxemia that is refractory (nonresponsive) to oxygen therapy, diminished lung compliance, and a significant ventilation-perfusion defect.

The goals for management of ARDS are to maintain tissue oxygenation ($Pao_2 \geq 60$ mm Hg) with the lowest $Fio_2$ level possible, to reduce pulmonary edema, to maintain cardiac output, and to prevent further complications. The primary intervention for ARDS is mechanical ventilation with the addition of **positive end-expiratory pressure (PEEP).** The use of PEEP aids in reexpanding alveoli and preventing further alveolar collapse, thus improving oxygen transport. Nursing interventions for the patient with ARDS are the same as those for any patient with respiratory failure who is receiving mechanical ventilation.

In rare severe cases of ARDS an extreme intervention sometimes is used to maintain systemic oxygenation while giving the lungs a chance to heal.[3] Extracorporeal membrane oxygenation (ECMO) provides a temporary pulmonary bypass. Although minimal respiration takes place in the lungs, mechanical ventilation with PEEP is continued to prevent further fibrosis and consolidation of lung tissue. Improved lung function is facilitated by postural drainage, chest physiotherapy, and tracheobronchial suctioning. Once initiated, ECMO therapy may be used for several days, during which time the most proficient nursing care is required to monitor the patient's progress and prevent the critical complications of disconnection, bleeding, embolus, decreased tissue perfusion, and infection.

## CARDIOVASCULAR SYSTEM

Cardiovascular problems requiring intensive patient care are so frequently encountered that many institutions have specific critical care units designed for the care of these patients (coronary care unit, postoperative cardiothoracic unit). After support of ventilation, maintenance of cardiac function and systemic circulation is the highest priority in life-threatening situations. Disorders of the cardiovascular system that frequently require intensive observation and intervention include acute myocardial infarction, cardiogenic shock, congestive heart failure, severe dysrhythmias, open heart surgery, and major vascular surgery.

*Drug therapy* is frequently used first for severe cardiovascular disorders and may be continued until more definitive measures can be employed. Various cardioactive and vasoactive drugs are administered solely in critical care settings where their dosage and effects can be very closely monitored and titrated as necessary. Such interventions include inotropic agents (Table 26-4) used in an attempt to maintain cardiac output and hemodynamic parameters at stable levels. Other interventions may include fibrinolytic therapy in the form of tissue plasminogen activator (TPA). The early administration of TPA causes the breakdown of thrombi in the coronary arteries, stopping the progressive evolution of a myocardial infarction (see Chapter 30). Highly potent medications often have a very small margin between therapeutic and toxic dosage levels, and the critical care nurse must ensure the correct dose and delivery route while monitoring its effect on the patient.

When drug therapy is insufficient to significantly or lastingly improve the patient's condition, certain **invasive techniques** may be beneficial. *Temporary transvenous pacing* may restore or enhance cardiac function until a permanent pacemaker can be implanted. In emergency situations, external pacing may be initiated while a decision is made on further intervention. For patients with recurrent, refractory, or lethal dysrhythmias an *automatic implantable cardioverter-defibrillator* (AICD) may be surgically implanted (see Chapter 30). This device recognizes ventricular tachycardia and ventricular fibrillation and automatically shocks the heart when life-threatening dysrhythmia is detected. The AICD is used successfully to avert sudden cardiac death in specific patient populations.

An **intraaortic balloon pump (IABP)** may be necessary for the patient who requires a temporary decrease in the workload of the myocardium. A catheter is

**TABLE 26-4 Inotropic Agents Used in the Intensive Care Unit**

| DRUG | USE | PRIMARY ACTION |
|---|---|---|
| Digitalis | Congestive heart failure<br>Tachydysrhythmias | Increased myocardial contractility through inhibition of sodium-potassium pump; prolonged AV conduction |
| Dopamine | Cardiogenic shock<br>Septic shock<br>Decreased urine output | Dose:<br>0.5-2.0 μg/kg/min: increased renal blood flow, diuresis<br>2.0-7.5 μg/kg/min: increased renal blood flow, increased cardiac output<br>7.5-20.0 μg/kg/min: increased afterload (vasoconstriction); May decrease cardiac output<br>>20.0 μg/kg/min: increased afterload, decreased cardiac output |
| Dobutamine | Severe congestive heart failure<br>Cardiogenic shock | Increased myocardial contractility through stimulation of beta receptors in heart |
| Amrinone | Congestive heart failure<br>Cardiogenic shock | Increased myocardial contractility through inhibition of phosphodiesterase; vasodilation and decreased afterload |

threaded into the aorta from a femoral artery. The distal 40-ml balloon inflates during ventricular diastole to increase coronary artery filling and deflates just before ventricular systole to decrease afterload and improve left ventricular ejection (see Figure 31-11). Indications for IABP are listed in Box 26-6. Nursing care includes critical minute-by-minute assessment of the patient's physiologic response to IABP therapy and intervention to prevent complications.

The **ventricular assist device (VAD)** is most often used to assist patients who have left-sided heart failure and cannot be weaned from cardiopulmonary bypass surgery and for patients with a severely damaged myocardium. The VAD is a temporary assist device in which catheters are implanted into the left atrium or left ventricle to divert oxygenated blood into a roller pump located outside the body. The pump bypasses the left ventricle and returns the blood directly to the aorta, thus decreasing myocardial workload by reducing preload. Right ventricular assist also can be provided for patients with severe right-sided heart failure; with this the cannula bypasses the right ventricle. The nurse continually assesses the patient's response to therapy through evaluation of hemodynamic data. Proper mechanical function of the device is also critical because occlusion or disconnection could cause rapid death.

**BOX 26-6 Indications and Complications of Intraaortic Balloon Pump Therapy**

| INDICATIONS | COMPLICATIONS |
|---|---|
| Cardiogenic shock with a reversible component | Ischemia of the catheterized leg |
| Low cardiac output states | Thrombus formation with eventual embolization |
| Patients difficult to remove from cardiopulmonary bypass support | Infection |
| Acute myocardial infarction | Aortic damage (aortic wall dissection, intimal laceration) |
| Unstable angina | Balloon rupture with gas embolus (rare) |
| Drug-resistant lethal dysrhythmias with ischemic cause | |

**BOX 26-7 Measures to Reduce Myocardial Workload**

**ENHANCE OXYGENATION**

Supplemental oxygen
Assisted ventilation
Semi-Fowler's position
Vasodilators
Antidysrhythmics

**DECREASE PHYSICAL EXERTION**

Bed rest
Passive range of motion exercises
Stool softeners, laxatives

**DECREASE SYMPATHETIC STIMULATION**

Reduce environmental stimuli (noise, lights)
Limit visitors to supportive persons
Inform and reassure patient and family
Provide continuity in caregivers
Individualize interventions to reduce specific anxieties

As mentioned previously, the use of a VAD is a temporary intervention. If the heart is unable to recover sufficient contractile strength, the patient may be evaluated for cardiac transplantation. During the wait for transplantation, cardiac function may be supplied by a ***total artificial heart*** (TAH). After years of research the TAH has been developed into a bichambered, pneumatically driven design. After the patient's heart is removed, the TAH is attached to the atria remnant, pulmonary artery, and aorta. After pneumatic drive tubing is inserted through the chest and attached to a large-drive console, which controls heart function and cardiac output, the chest is closed. Research continues with both the VAD and TAH in which the ultimate goal is that both devices could become completely implantable.

Prevention of physiologic stressors to the cardiovascular system is a continual priority for care of all critical care patients. Most preventive measures are aimed at myocardial workload reduction and include all measures that enhance oxygenation, decrease physical exertion, and decrease sympathetic stimulation (Box 26-7).

Finally, in addition to decreasing myocardial workload, the myocardium must be protected from a unique hazard of the critical care environment: ***electrical microshock***. The invasive monitoring and therapeutic interventions utilized with critically ill patients often create a direct pathway to the heart (central venous pressure lines, pulmonary artery catheters, temporary pacemakers). Direct contact with stray or leaked current could prove fatal, particularly in critically ill patients whose resistance may be further decreased through other breaks in skin integrity and through electrolyte imbalances. Critical care nurses are responsible for the safe and proper use of electrical equipment, as well as for the implementation of appropriate electrical safety precautions.

## NEUROLOGIC SYSTEM

A number of neurological disorders, most often either the result of trauma, intracranial neoplasms, or infections, may necessitate critical care during an acute phase of illness. These include subdural and subarachnoid hemorrhage, direct head injuries, spinal cord injury, massive cerebrovascular accident, intracranial aneurysm rupture, and preoperative and postoperative care of certain patients undergoing craniotomy for surgical repair of a structural defect.

Specialized neurologic interventions for critically ill patients are aimed at maintaining a homeokinetic state of brain metabolism and controlling elevations in intracranial pressure (ICP) (see Chapter 57). ICP monitoring (see p. 657) may be used to assess the extent of potentially dangerous rises in ICP.

Removal of cerebrospinal fluid is one method of controlling rising ICP. Other interventions include osmotic diuresis to remove excess fluid from brain tissue, steroids to reduce cerebral edema by stabilizing the cell membrane, and controlled mechanical hyperventilation to maintain adequate oxygenation and to artificially reduce circulating carbon dioxide levels (decrease $PaCO_2$). Lowered $PaCO_2$ will trigger cerebral vasoconstriction, reducing the potential for progressive interstitial cerebral edema.

Efforts to lower the overall metabolism of the brain will reduce the brain's requirements for its natural substrates, oxygen and glucose. This is especially important when transport of these elements is impaired. Interventions to reduce brain metabolism include generalized hypothermia by use of a cooling mattress and induction of barbiturate coma. Caring for the artificially comatose patient requires the same attentive observations and extensive nursing interventions to prevent complications as are employed for the naturally comatose patient, with the addition of mechanical ventilation (see Chapter 57). In addition, complete neurologic assessment of the patient must be thoroughly performed when the sedation is reduced or withdrawn. Any level of unconsciousness necessitates sensitive communication, even though the patient's comprehension may not be apparent.

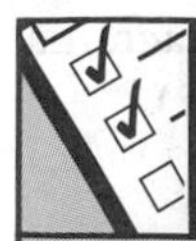

### Guidelines for Preventing Increased Intracranial Pressure in the Critically Ill Person

- Maintain patent airway
- Minimize arterial blood gas changes
  - Oxygenate patient before and after suctioning
  - Limit suctioning to 15 seconds
- Maintain mechanical hyperventilation
- Elevate head of bed 30 degrees (facilitates venous drainage without impeding arterial supply)
- Maintain head and neck in straight alignment
- Prevent overtight tracheostomy ties
- Prevent Valsalva's maneuver (increases ICP)
  - Assist patient in turning
  - Prevent coughing, sneezing, constipation
- Monitor hydration status, intake, and output

Spinal cord injury can manifest in various ways depending on the type and location of the lesion. Injury above the C4 level may result in respiratory failure because of paralysis of the diaphragm and intercostal muscles. Autonomic dysreflexia is a life-threatening condition seen in cervical and high thoracic injuries. It is caused by sudden neurovascular dysfunction below the cord injury level. It results from an exaggerated sympathetic nervous system response to a stimulus such as bladder distention, temperature extremes, or even tight sheets. The patient experiences pounding headache, sweating above the level of injury, hypertension, and bradycardia. Goals in the management of spinal cord injuries are to preserve remaining function, prevent further neurologic deficits, and prevent complications and deformities. Interventions include immobilization, management of actual or potential respiratory problems, urinary catheterization, and use of drugs such as steroids to stabilize the neuromembrane, antacids, stool softeners, and antihypertensives.

In addition to neurosurgical disorders and spinal cord injuries, patients with a variety of neurologic diseases may be seen in the critical care unit during acute exacerbations or at the end stages of progressively debilitating conditions that sometimes necessitate mechanical ventilation. These diseases include amyotrophic lateral sclerosis, Guillain-Barré syndrome, myasthenia gravis, and sometimes multiple sclerosis. All four of these degenerative disorders are either known or suspected to be mediated by autoantibodies or circulating immune complexes. Therapeutic plasmapheresis may be performed to temporarily cleanse the blood of the antigenic agents.

Nursing interventions to prevent physiologic stressors to the neurologic system are aimed at supporting diminished neurologic capacity, preventing injury and infection, reducing pain, and preventing intracranial pressure elevations (see Guidelines box, p. 671).

## RENAL SYSTEM

Acute renal failure in the critically ill patient may result from a primary intrarenal cause, such as acute glomerulonephritis or acute cortical necrosis, or from a structural defect. It may be the result of directly nephrotoxic agents as in heavy metal poisoning or pharmacologic agents, such as aminoglycoside antibodies. Most often, however, acute renal failure in critically ill patients is the secondary result of any disorder that severely reduces cardiac output and renal perfusion, including cardiac arrest, left ventricular failure, or hemorrhage.

Interventions for the patient who has renal failure are intended to provide the regulatory functions that the kidneys can no longer maintain. The nurse keeps accurate daily weights and intake/output records so that only the exact amounts of body fluids lost plus a percentage for insensible losses are replaced. Laboratory values are monitored carefully, with electrolyte intake being limited and pharmacologic drugs—for example, sodium polystyrene sulfonate (Kayexalate)—being used as necessary for electrolyte removal. Diuretics are given to increase marginal renal function. Nutrition is altered through restricted protein intake inasmuch as the body cannot appropriately excrete the nitrogen that is produced by amino acid breakdown. The nurse evaluates acid base balance, anticipating metabolic acidosis from the build-up of acid metabolic wastes (ketones and lactic acid). All other body systems are affected by the progression of acute renal failure, and continuous interventions are necessary to prevent altered acid base and electrolyte levels from impairing cardiovascular, respiratory, and neurologic function. Therefore the nurse is alert for such factors as ECG changes indicative of increased myocardial irritability and altered contractility, electrolyte imbalances, changes in ventilatory pattern such as Kussmaul's breathing, presence of crackles, acidotic breath, and decreased level of consciousness or altered mentation or behavior.

When renal failure has reached a level that is unresponsive to medical intervention, dialysis becomes necessary to mechanically remove the waste products of body metabolism (see Chapter 50). Intermittent hemodialysis or peritoneal dialysis (Box 26-8) may be initiated for the critically ill patient and may be performed for several hours a day, 3 to 5 days per week. Box 26-8 presents the advantages and disadvantages of the various methods to control fluid and electrolytes in persons with renal failure.

An alternate method of continuous ultrafiltration, also known as **continuous arteriovenous hemofiltration (CAVH)**, may be used to remove excess fluid from patients with acute renal failure. Arterial blood is removed from the body and passed through a semipermeable membrane that removes water and dissolved solutes but returns blood cells and plasma proteins to the body via a venous line. The filtration is accomplished by a pressure gradient established primarily by the patient's mean arterial pressure and is thus a slow and consistent process that may be better tolerated by critically ill patients. Some patients also may require intermittent hemodialysis to further clear uremic toxins, or dialysate can be added to the CAVH system (CAVH-D) and slow continuous dialysis can be accomplished. Nursing responsibilities center on hemodynamic monitoring and prevention of potential complications such as disconnection, clotting embolus formation, electrolyte imbalance, clotting abnormalities, and infection.

### BOX 26-8 Advantages/Disadvantages of Hemodialysis, Peritoneal Dialysis, and Continuous Ultrafiltration

| HEMODIALYSIS | PERITONEAL DIALYSIS |
|---|---|
| Rapid, efficient correction of severe serum abnormalities | Well tolerated by even very unstable patients |
| Short time period for actual dialysis | Inexpensive procedure |
| Expensive procedure | Technologically simple procedure |
| Requires highly technical equipment | Must be performed over several hours or days |
| Poorly tolerated by very unstable patients | Cannot be performed on patients with recent abdominal surgery |
| Risk of hemorrhage | Risk of peritonitis |

**CONTINUOUS ULTRAFILTRATION**

- Highly effective if fluid removal is primary goal
- Well tolerated by critically ill patients
- Slow correction of severe electrolyte abnormalities
- Relatively inexpensive procedure
- Must be performed over several hours or days
- Greater risk of hemorrhage because of length of procedure

## GASTROINTESTINAL SYSTEM

The most common gastrointestinal problem seen in the critical care setting is *acute gastrointestinal bleeding.* This may be the medical diagnosis in a newly admitted patient, or it may be a complication, such as a stress ulcer, in an already critically ill person. Interventions such as gastric lavage with iced saline and administration of agents that inhibit gastric acid secretion are intended to control bleeding until its cause and extent are determined. Various drugs, as well as a Sengstaken-Blakemore tube, may be used to control bleeding from esophageal varices (see Chapter 42). Administration of blood components and crystalloid fluids is initiated to reverse the hypovolemia of acute hemorrhage. Vasopressor medications cannot be administered to raise systemic blood pressure until the hypovolemic state is corrected. Once the patient's condition has stabilized sufficiently and the site of bleeding has been identified, surgery may be performed to repair the affected area.

The primary function of the gastrointestinal system is to ingest and digest liquid and solid nutrients. For many critically ill patients this process is interrupted for a lengthy period in which either enteral or **total parenteral nutrition (TPN)** may be substituted (see Chapter 45). TPN solutions contain the essential protein, carbohydrate, and fat necessary to establish a catabolic state in which positive nitrogen balance is maintained. The critical care nurse assesses the adequacy of hydration and electrolyte balance as well as caloric intake. In addition, the nurse takes active measures to prevent infection, the primary complication of TPN.

Prevention of gastrointestinal complications such as stress ulcers (see Chapter 45) in critically ill patients requires active nursing interventions. Patients at highest risk include those who are receiving no oral intake, who are undergoing mechanical ventilation, who have liver dysfunction, who are receiving anticoagulants, and who have undergone any severe physiologic stress. In addition to the administration of local antacids, systemic histamine inhibitory agents (such as ranitidine) and agents to increase gastric motility (such as metoclopramide), specific interventions are required to reduce the psychologic stress inherent in the critical care environment.

## MUSCULOSKELETAL/INTEGUMENTARY SYSTEMS

Hypersensitivity reactions to various agents may be so severe that life-threatening illness may develop. Two disorders that can cause critical illness are **Stevens-Johnson syndrome** and **toxic epidermal necrolysis.** Both disorders are severe inflammatory syndromes characterized by epidermal slough, mucosal inflammation, and ulceration. Clinical symptoms include fever, systemic toxicity, and erythema multiforme lesions. The syndromes are precipitated by a major physiologic stressor such as a drug reaction, mycoplasmic pneumonia, herpes simplex infection, collagen vascular disorder, or pregnancy. Despite intensive medical and nursing interventions, mortality can be as high as 65%.

Although few primary musculoskeletal problems necessitate critical care, most critically ill patients have severe restrictions placed on their mobility. Bed rest, weakness, and pain, as well as attachment to numerous therapeutic and monitoring devices, significantly limit normal motion. Preserving function of weight-bearing muscles, maintaining joint mobility, and preserving continuous skin integrity are significant challenges to critical care nurses. All of the preventive and supportive nursing care techniques used with any patient who has restricted mobility are appropriate in the ICU. The progression of the ICU patient to the highest level of activity facilitates improvement in physiologic function and reassures the patient of an improving condition. See Chapter 67 for information on prevention of pressure ulcers.

One of the most serious potential complications of immobility is development of a deep vein thrombus, which can embolize and travel to the lungs. Pulmonary emboli are found in up to 60% of all persons after an autopsy is performed. Signs and symptoms of pulmonary embolism include dyspnea, pleuritic chest pain, fever, hemoptysis, tachycardia, and pleural friction rub. Preventive interventions can be instrumental in reducing the risk of these serious complications (see Guidelines box above).

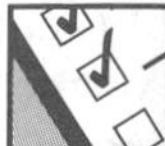

### Guidelines for Preventing Pulmonary Embolus

Elevation of lower extremities
Use of antiembolism stockings
Hourly active foot dorsiflexion
Active/resistive range of motion exercises
Observation of Homans' sign
Coughing and deep breathing exercises
Administration of low-dose heparin as ordered
Inspection of intravenous sites with routine needle changes

## REPRODUCTIVE SYSTEM

Although preeclampsia (proteinuria, edema, and hypertension) complicates approximately 5% of all pregnancies, most patients with these conditions are successfully managed outside the critical care environment. In a few cases, however, complications may require invasive monitoring and aggressive intervention. A syndrome of hemolysis, elevated liver enzymes, and low platelet count (HELLP) is potentially fatal and may be identified late in pregnancy or within the first 48 hours after delivery.

The management of severe pregnancy-induced hypertension is becoming more common as high-risk mothers are transferred to the critical care unit immediately after delivery for continuous monitoring and treatment with nitroprusside or other antihypertensive drugs administered intravenously. High-risk mothers may be admitted to the critical care unit for optimal health care management. Close consultation with obstetricians and obstetric nurses is required to maintain an optimal environment for the fetus and mother. Therapy is aimed at stabilizing the mother's condition by reducing hypertension, moderating coagulopathies, maximizing ventilation and hydration, and preventing preterm labor. Emergency cesarean section delivery may be performed in the critical care unit for severe maternal or fetal distess. In some tertiary centers, obstetric mini-critical care units are being established to maximize care for both the fetus and mother.

## IMMUNOLOGY/ORGAN TRANSPLANTATION

Many medical practitioners believe that gaining knowledge and control over the body's immune response is the ultimate key to the health care of the future (see Chapters 13 and 69 through 72 for discussions of the immune system). All critically ill patients are compromised hosts, facing the physiologic stress to the immune system caused by severe illness. The severely immunocompromised patient presents some of the greatest challenges in critical care. Whether the immunosuppression is induced (immunosuppressive drugs, chemotherapy, radiation therapy) or acquired (AIDS, severe combined immunodeficiency diseases, severe systemic lupus erythematosis), life-threatening sepsis and shock may develop from the patient's inability to resist infection. Nursing care focuses on interventions for current infections, protection from futher infections, and optimization of natural defenses through maintenance of skin integrity, cleanliness, hydration, and nutrition.

The combination of immunosuppressive therapy and increasingly sophisticated surgical techniques has allowed organ transplantation to move from the realm of the experimental to the commonplace. Both natural and artificial organs have been implanted with varying degrees of success. Development of cross-species xenograft has advanced from the well-accepted porcine cardiac valve implant to the experimental baboon liver transplant. The decades-old practice of transfusing living blood cells has blossomed into the development of synthetic blood substitutes, as well as bone marrow transplantation to generate new blood tissue. Transplantation of heart, heart-lung, kidney, liver, and pancreas or islet cells is now performed at medical centers throughout the country.

The critical care nurse may be actively involved in the transplantation process in two very different ways. The nurse may care for posttransplant patients, using the latest technology and most advanced clinical skills to expedite a successful recovery and facilitate a return to healthy life. Or the nurse may care for the transplant donor, completing meticulous pretransplant tasks while providing emotional care to the anguished family in an often sudden and tragic situation. In either case, the critical care nurse has the privilege of providing care to those in need and of knowing the dramatic difference one's care can make in someone else's life.

## ALLEVIATION AND PREVENTION OF PSYCHOLOGIC STRESSORS

Despite the continuous attention the critical care nurse must devote to the assessment of and the intervention in physiologic derangements, the nurse also must focus attention on recognizing the psychologic stressors that confront the patient and family. The emotional discomfort and distress that the patient and family endure not only affect psychologic health but also have a direct impact on physical recovery.

The initial step in preventing or alleviating psychologic stress is to identify the patient's and family's perception of the critical event. Their perceptions will be affected by their individual personalities, current psychologic health, general understanding of the current situation and its projected outcome, tolerance of ambiguity, and normal patterns of coping. Initial perceptions are often significantly affected by previous exposure to similar events, either positive or negative, and general level of familiarity with medical interventions and the hospital environment. Six specific interventions nurses can utilize in any setting to reduce the psychologic stress of illness are detailed in the following discussion.

### ACKNOWLEDGING, ACCEPTING, AND ENCOURAGING PATIENT/FAMILY TO AIR THEIR FEELINGS

Because the critically ill person is alienated from familiar surroundings and daily living patterns and is dependent on others to meet the most basic needs of survival, the patient becomes partially or totally isolated from usual support systems.

Feelings of helplessness, powerlessness, loneliness, and depersonalization, as well as disturbances in body image, are common. Modes of expressing and therefore relieving the frustration, anger, hostility, fear, and depression generated by these feelings are limited by the physical constraints of the critical care environment. Whether a primary nursing approach or other delivery model is used, consistently assigned caregivers are essential to developing a physiologically and psychologically therapeutic bond with the patient and family.

An atmosphere of openness and acceptance that encourages expression of feelings can help provide patients with a means of coping. Talking with patients openly and honestly decreases feelings of depersonalization and prevents isolation and alienation. Anger and hostility are often indicative of fear and anxiety. Depression and withdrawal may be signs of hopelessness, loneliness, powerlessness, or loss and are normal and expected. Encouraging expression of feelings helps the patient identify the reasons for feeling or behaving in a way that may seem strange or wrong. At the same time it provides protection and permission to feel and act that way. Nurses or other health care team members who are helping a patient to talk about feelings must be ready to accept whatever emotionally laden information might be expressed. Nonjudgmental recognition and acceptance of the patient's feelings help to reinforce the patient's right to the feelings.

Patients undergoing intubation are unable to express their feelings freely even when alert and oriented and are therefore particularly vulnerable to psychologic stressors. It is a natural tendency to communicate less with those who cannot talk easily and the nurse must guard against this. Keeping a letterboard, paper and pencil, or a "magic slate" within the patient's reach and providing assistance when the patient desires it will help to reduce the sense of isolation. However, such methods are not convenient for the expression of personal feelings or involved concerns. The nurse can recognize clues to the patient's emotional state by appearance and behavior and by knowing the types of concerns the patient is most likely to have. The nurse can verbalize the potential concerns, allowing the patient to validate them as appropriate. Expressing empathy for the patient and family conveys acceptance and understanding.

## PROVIDING INFORMATION/CLARIFYING MISCONCEPTIONS ABOUT PHYSICAL STATUS, GOALS OF TREATMENT, AND INTERVENTIONS

It is the patient's *perception* of stressors and not the stressor itself that determines the patient's reaction to stressors, the illness, and the environment. It is essential that the patient and family receive adequate information and simple explanations. Without explanations the critical care environment presents a mysterious and threatening array of noxious stimuli, which may be perceived as extremely unnatural and even magical. The highly sophisticated equipment increases the patient's feelings of vulnerability, and the patient may worry that the cardiac monitor is actually keeping the heart beating, that a blood transfusion indicates hemorrhaging, or that chest physiotherapy signifies pneumonia. A very common misconception of patients after coronary artery bypass surgery is that "open heart" surgery involved cutting the heart wide open and sewing it back together again. Such a perception can lead to a drastic alteration in body image.

Much of what patients learn about their health problems depends on what is taught, both directly and indirectly, by the health care team. Patient teaching in critical care requires short-term goals. Pain, discomfort, weakness, anxiety, and transient confusion are some of the obstacles to learning that these patients experience. Despite these obstacles, patients and families need simple, repetitive explanations of all procedures and the purpose of each intervention, as well as an introduction to rehabilitation plans and health maintenance strategies. Patients may not understand or believe what they are told the first time, or anxiety and denial may prevent accurate recollection. Reinterpretation and reiteration of diagnosis, prognosis, goals of treatment, types of interventions, and expectations of the patient and family may be continually necessary during the entire critical care stay. Explanations should be given by the same few caregivers to encourage a bond of continuity and to minimize the confusion of differing approaches and wording. If the patient and family are apprised of the patient's current status, as well as of changes in plans, the situation is perceived accurately and the future is planned realistically, thus ensuring their cooperation by making them members of the health care team.

## ENCOURAGING AND SUPPORTING THE INVOLVEMENT OF PATIENT/FAMILY IN DECISION MAKING AND CARE

The essence of crisis intervention is to help persons cope with a major life crisis that a critical illness may precipitate. Critical care nursing is far broader in scope and more future oriented than crisis intervention alone, but specific situations within the critical care setting may require the immediacy and limited focus of crisis intervention. At that time the patient and family are directed in establishing short-term goals and are given limited choice in acceptable responses. As the crisis situation stabilizes, even though it may be no less critical, the patient and family are given additional information and further responsibility in estabishing mutual goals and choosing alternate responses. When the patient and family are knowledgeable about the goals of therapy and understand the patient's diagnosis, current status, and prognosis, they can then be involved in many aspects of care planning and can make decisions consistent with the treatment regimen.

Involvement of the persons who represent the patient's significant support system decreases feelings of powerlessness, frustration, and anxiety. In addition, when these emotionally important figures, whether family or friends, understand and support the treatment goals and are involved in the patient's care, they are better able to sustain and expand this behavior after the patient leaves the critical care unit and hospital. Even when a patient is unconscious, visits by key support figures who talk to and touch the patient may have positive, if unmeasurable, effects on the patient while helping to decrease the family's feelings of helplessness.

An alert patient can be directly involved in care planning and establishing goals of treatment. One specific mechanism to increase the patient's feeling of personal control is to encourage involvement in structuring the daily schedule of activities. The knowledge that the preferences of the patient are important to the nursing staff and that the patient is viewed as capable of making decisions reinforces the centrality of the patient's role in recovery.

The environment of the critical care unit is a major stressor with which both the patient and family must cope. (The many external stressors are outlined in the first section of this chapter.) In addition, disturbed thought processes and perceptual distortions are often likely to be seen in patients who are given narcotics and sedatives, are highly anxious, have multiple interrelated debilitating physical problems, have disturbed metabolic and respiratory function, are deprived of sleep, and are older. Reality reinforcement on a continuing basis is necessary for these persons. Although some environmental factors cannot be altered, specific interventions can be implemented by the nurse to provide a sensory-regulated environment. Interventions designed to help create a balance between sensory deprivation and sen-

### Guidelines for Minimizing Sensory Deprivation/Overload

**REDUCE NOISE LEVEL**

Avoid excessive conversation.
Avoid raising voice to talk to persons outside conversational range.
Utilize carpeting as feasible.
Avoid continuous playing of radio or TV; turn on/off at appropriate intervals.
Locate nursing lounge away from patient care area.

**MAINTAIN DAY/NIGHT ORIENTATION**

Dim lights at night.
Raise/lower shades or open/close window curtains in normal day/night pattern.
Reinforce progression of day in relation to specific events, such as meals.

**MAINTAIN TIME ORIENTATION**

Position large-numeral clocks in easy view.
Provide wall calendars.
Allow wrist watches for certain patients.
Provide frequent reorientation to person, place, time.

**PROMOTE REST AND SLEEP**

Schedule most exerting activities so that rest period may follow.
Coordinate health care team activities to provide periods of uninterrupted sleep.
Minimize routine cleaning or stocking at night.

**PROVIDE POSITIVE TACTILE STIMULI**

Touch/hold patient's hand during conversation.
Use soothing physical contact as able (back rubs, face cleansing, etc.).
Encourage family to touch patient, hold hands despite dressings, etc.

**MAINTAIN PERSONAL/SOCIAL INTEGRITY**

Address patient by name; identify self by name.
Provide full and complete information, explanations, and instructions.
Avoid discussion over the patient; include the patient in rounds.
Establish flexible visiting hours.
Encourage visits by family, significant others.
Make visiting rule exceptions for children and even pets when special circumstances arise.
Allow important personal belongings at bedside.

**REDUCE PAIN AND DISCOMFORT**

Administer analgesics appropriately to relieve pain.
Reposition immobile patients q 2 hr.
Prepare patients for all potentially uncomfortable or painful procedures.

**MAINTAIN FUTURE ORIENTATION**

Discuss transfer plans early with both patient and family.
Initiate teaching regarding rehabilitation and health maintenance strategies as appropriate.

sory overload in the critical care setting are listed in the Guidelines box at left.

## PREPARING PATIENT/FAMILY FOR TRANSFER FROM CRITICAL CARE UNIT

Transfer from the critical care unit to another setting may cause significant stress for some patients and their families. The critical care area represents security and protection with its sophisticated electronic equipment and attentive, highly skilled staff members. Patients know that transfer means moving to an area where there are fewer nursing personnel per patient, less direct contact with nursing personnel, no automatic or obvious monitoring devices, and no direct observation of the patient from the nurses' station. Greater independence and higher levels of activity will be expected of patients on the transfer unit, and the support of familiar nursing staff members will be lost. Patients may have conflicting feelings about the transfer as an indicator of physical improvement if they do not feel as well or as independent as they anticipated at the time of transfer.

The anxiety precipitated by the transfer can be prevented or reduced if the patient and family are taught to interpret the meaning of particular signs and symptoms and are helped to understand the true purpose of equipment and routines. Signs that indicate progress need to be pointed out continuously, beginning when they first appear. Initiating the discussion of transfer plans with the patient and family as soon as the patient's condition begins to stabilize in the critical care unit will help them adjust to and prepare for the relocation. Along with the projected date of transfer, patient and family need to know what to expect on the new unit and what will be expected of them. Ideally, a nurse from the receiving unit should meet the patient and family before transfer. After transfer, visits from the critical care staff are helpful in conveying continued concern for the patient's welfare, as well as in providing objective validation of continued progress. With careful planning and execution, transfer from the critical care unit can be a triumphant rather than a traumatic event.

## PROVIDING SUPPORT IN ETHICAL DECISION MAKING

In many ways, the major technologic advances currently available in hospitals have moved beyond society's ability to understand and keep pace with the associated ethical dilemmas. Life can be prolonged in ways and in clinical conditions that were previously impossible. Not infrequently, life can be maintained past all known hope of recovery. Tremendous emotional, financial, legal, and societal ramifications exist as patients are stabilized into conditions for which long-term health care options are very limited. For example, few families and even fewer skilled care facilities have the resources to care for a patient who requires continuous mechanical ventilation.

With the advent of advance directives, it has largely fallen on nurses' shoulders to gather information as to patients' wishes in making decisions about the extent of their care or treatment. Often a patient has no advance directive or is incompetent to render such a decision, leaving the family or significant others to determine the kind of medical care the patient would or would not want in this situation. Critical care nurses frequently assist families with these highly emotional decisions related to foregoing resuscitation or withdrawing life support systems. Assisting families with these decisions is painfully complex. See Research box at right.

As with all health care professionals, the critical care nurse must examine his or her own beliefs about life and death, termination of life, organ/tissue donations, and use of limited resources. Education and support for the nurse are available from formal classes, support groups, peers, and hospital ethics committees. Ethics committees are available to patients, families, and staff members who wish consultation and support in difficult or divisive situations.

Biomedical advances at times seem to challenge the compassionate aspects of ethical issues. The critical care nurse is the professional caregiver qualified to play a pivotal role in identifying and promoting the patient's wishes.

**RESEARCH**

Jezewski MA et al: Consenting to DNR: critical care nurses' interactions with patients and family members, *Am J Crit Care* 2(4):301-309, 1993.

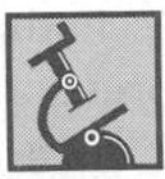

The use of high technology in critical care units allows sicker patients to be kept alive longer. As a consequence critical care nurses face many complex ethical issues. A study of 22 experienced critical care nurses involved in the do not resuscitate (DNR) process revealed that assisting patients and families in making DNR decisions can be painfully complex. Conflicts over the meaning of DNR are common, and critical care nurses must fully explain the process to patients and family. The main concern among the nurses in the study was whether DNR patients should be maintained in the ICU at high cost. The nurses believed that DNR patients should be moved to a medical or surgical unit, freeing beds for patients who were expected to survive. The authors recommend that studies of this kind be conducted in units other than ICUs to help contribute to a better understanding of the DNR process.

## Prevention and Alleviation of Social Stressors for Patient/Family

In the critical care setting the patient's physiologic needs often assume priority over psychologic needs, and the patient's needs as a social being may be virtually ignored. Limited visiting hours, the strange technical environment, and the aura of danger in the critical care unit isolate patients from their supportive family and friends and prevent them from assuming their usual social roles. For the most part, a person who is critically ill is viewed by staff members primarily in the patient role. The more significant roles of spouse, parent, child, lover, sibling, friend, or provider may go virtually unrecognized unless staff members initiate interventions to provide continuity in these relationships.

Such continuity is fostered through some of the same types of interventions that were utilized to reduce psychologic stress: increased visiting between patient and family; inclusion of family into discussions of disease process, prognosis, and plans of care; and reporting by family of events and activities occurring in the other significant spheres of the patient's life. Relaying telephone messages between the patient and distant friends is one way to maintain contact with the patient's external world.

One of the most effective and important ways to prevent disruption in relationships is to prepare family or friends for their first visit with the patient in the critical care unit. The patient's physical appearance and the critical care environment should be explained thoroughly before the visitor enters. Visitors need to understand the patient's level of consciousness, as well as ability to communicate and comprehend communication. They need to be made aware of the importance of their presence to the patient and the patient's need for their support. When visitors approach the bedside, a staff member should remain with them to facilitate their initial interaction with the patient. At each subsequent visit the nurse caring for the patient meets with the significant others to answer questions and apprise them of the patient's progress.

In addition to supporting the maintenance of the patient's current roles and relationships, the critical care nurse also must recognize the inevitability of actual role change for some patients and families during a critical illness. Roles of provider, decision maker, employer, employee, and leader may be altered, reversed, or eliminated. At this point some of the responsibilities of the patient need to be assumed by family and friends.

During the critical phase of illness the family members will be attempting to cope with significant role changes and may need assistance in working through problems that arise as family members and friends assume or fail to assume these additional responsibilities. The nurse needs to be aware of this problematic time and is in a position to provide the family with professional guidance, such as from a social worker, to assist in reorganizing themselves and their resources. The nurse may help the family appoint a temporary leader from among their ranks, one who knows and is able to represent the wishes of the family as a whole and who could be contacted in the event of an emergency. The nurse also may help the family to plan visiting schedules that will meet the patient's needs without preventing the family members from maintaining their own responsibilities. It is a period of great emotional stress for both patient and family.

That emotional stress eventually may climax in the death of the critically ill patient. (See Chapter 10 for a complete discussion of dying and death.) The following are suggestions for the critical care nurse caring for a dying patient:

1. Examine your own feelings about death.
2. Listen attentively to assess the needs of the patient and family.
3. Remain available; be physically and emotionally present.
4. Use touch in caring for the patient and family.
5. Provide reassurance of the patient's continued care, even if the patient is not to be resuscitated. Provide information.
6. Attempt to remain nonjudgmental about family or hospital issues.
7. Respect the person-family relationship, which existed long before the patient-hospital relationship.
8. Include the family in care.
9. Provide for patient and family privacy.
10. Provide the opportunity for the family to exercise religious or cultural traditions.

Providing comprehensive care to critically ill patients and their families is a demanding task. The critical care nurse combines the technologic sophistication of this unique setting with a personal, individualized care approach to maximize the potential outcomes for the patient.

## QUESTIONS TO CONSIDER

- Who should or should not be admitted to a critical care unit? What factors would a list of admission criteria include?
- How does mechanical ventilation differ for patients with varying causes of respiratory failure?
- What are the major infection control problems in critical care units?
- If the family of a critically ill patient with a terminal disease asked your opinions of withdrawal of life support, how would you respond?

## CRITICAL THINKING ACTIVITIES

- As part of your job you are required to cross train in the critical care unit. How will you function differently in critical care as compared with a regular medical or surgical unit?
- You are caring for two patients in the critical care unit. Jack is to receive a demand transvenous pacemaker, and Bob has just had an automatic implantable cardioverter-defibrillator implanted. In what ways are these patients similar? Different?
- You are the nurse caring for Mrs. Tucker in a critical care unit in which visiting hours are strictly enforced. You recognize that Mrs. Tucker is critically ill and most likely will not survive the night. The family wishes to stay with her during her final hours. How would you handle this situation?

## CHAPTER SUMMARY

### ENVIRONMENT IN THE CRITICAL CARE UNIT

- Numerous types of critical care units exist. They are designed, equipped, and staffed to meet the anticipated needs of patients in life-threatening situations.
- Inherent in the critical care environment are multiple stressors for the patient, the family, and the nurse. Identification and amelioration of these physiologic, psychologic, and social stressors are the goals of critical care nursing.

### ASSESSMENT OF THE CRITICALLY ILL PATIENT

- Critical care nurses build on clinical knowledge from all specialties. Any organ system dysfunction may result in critical illness, requiring invasive or specialized equipment for assessment and intervention.
- The nursing process is the same in critical care situations as in other patient care settings. The nurse establishes a data base, identifies actual and potential nursing diagnoses, defines outcome criteria, and executes the planned interventions based on clinical priorities. Evaluating the results and modifying the plan are ongoing processes.
- The assessment of the patient in a critical care environment incorporates data from cardiac monitoring and hemodynamic monitoring.

### ALLEVIATION AND PREVENTION OF PHYSIOLOGIC AND PHYSICAL STRESSORS

- The highest priority in care of the critically ill person is the respiratory system.
- Many patients with critical illness will have acute respiratory failure and require ventilator support.
- Adult respiratory distress syndrome (ARDS) following multiple insults like shock, DIC, emboli, cardiopulmonary bypass, sepsis, and so forth is due to alevolocapillary membrane damage, increased capillary permeability, and diffuse microatelectasis.

- ARDS results in severe hypoxemia nonresponsive to oxygen therapy.
- Many of the disease pathologies affecting the cardiovascular system result in critical situations requiring care within critical care units.
- Most patients with critical cardiovascular problems will require drug therapy; additionally, patients may require use of IABP and VAD.
- Specialized neurological interventions designed to monitor and control ICP will be required for patients with various types of critical neurological problems.
- Renal failure often is part of the clinical picture of the critically ill patient and will require the usual interventions including hemodialysis, peritoneal dialysis, or ultrafiltration.
- Acute gastrointestinal bleeding is the most common gastrointestinal problem seen in the critical care setting.
- Total parenteral nutrition will be required by many critically ill patients.
- Hypersensitivity reactions (e.g., Stevens-Johnson syndrome and toxic epidermal necrolysis following a drug reaction, mycoplasmic pneumonia and so forth) result in critical care problems.
- Deep vein thrombus and pulmonary emboli are two of the major complications that can result from immobility.
- Pregnancy induced hypertension and HELLP syndrome are two problems of pregnancy that are now being treated in critical care units.
- The immunosuppression associated with organ transplantation, diseases such as AIDS, and drugs can result in sepsis, pulmonary infections, and other complications that require critical care.

### ALLEVIATION AND PREVENTION OF PSYCHOLOGIC STRESSORS

- The critical care environment results in separation of patients from their families. Nurses, more than ever, must be providing care to the family as well as to the patient.
- The nurse must keep the patient and the family informed of goals and interventions and involve the patient and family in decision making.
- Controlling sensory overload or sensory deprivation is a major focus of care in critical care settings to decrease psychological stressors.
- Although stressful, the critical care environment provides a feeling of security; patients and family need to be prepared for transfer from the critical care environment.
- The advancement of medical technology has made the prolongation of life possible in ways never before experienced. Careful attention to the ethical, social, and financial implications of critical care technology is necessary to maintain focus on the patient's quality of life.

## REFERENCES

1. Abi-Nader JA: Peripherally inserted central venous catheters in critical care patients, *Heart Lung* 22(5):428-434, 1993.
2. Jezewski MA et al: Consenting to DNR: critical care nurses' interactions with patients and family members, *Am J Crit Care* 2(4):302-309, 1993.
3. Stillwell SB: *Mosby's critical care nursing reference,* St Louis, 1992, Mosby.
4. Swearingen PL, Keen JH: *Manual of critical care: applying nursing diagnoses to adult critical illness,* St Louis, 1991, Mosby.
5. Thelan LA et al: *Critical care nursing: diagnosis and management,* ed 2, St Louis, 1994, Mosby.

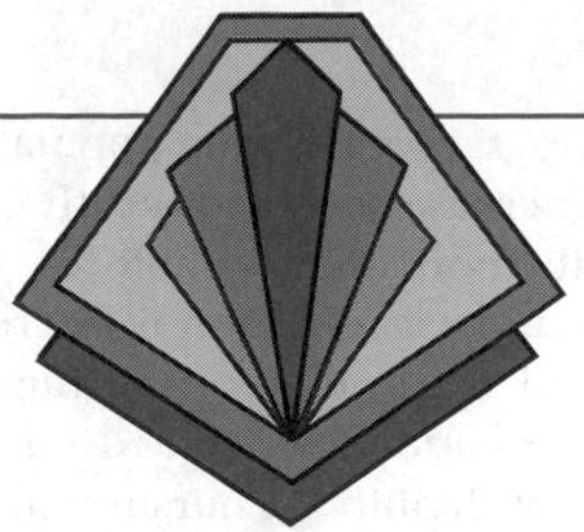

C H A P T E R 27

# Home Care Environment

***Carol E. Smith***

## CHAPTER OBJECTIVES

***After studying this chapter, the learner should be able to do the following:***

1 Describe the trends in health care leading to expansion of home care for medical-surgical patients.
2 Discuss the skills used in managing the transition from acute to home care.
3 Use the nursing process with home care patients and their families.
4 Discuss the home residence as the environment for providing nursing care.
5 Explain the continuous quality improvement process as applied to home care.
6 Identify issues pertinent to home health care.

## KEY TERMS

case-managed care
discharge planning
evaluation
family assessment
family education
home care
home health care nurse
home intravenous antibiotic therapy (HIAT)
learning
medication assessment
nutrition assessment
primary caregiver
quality improvement
transitional care
transition specialist
translocation syndrome

This chapter assists the learner with home care of the medical-surgical patient. Forecasters of health care indicate that hospital closings will continue, whereas home care services will increase by as much as 31% annually throughout the 1990s. In 1991, $181 million was spent on home intravenous therapy alone.[9] Medical-surgical home nursing care will be necessary for a wide range of adults. Patients may require one or two home visits or around-the-clock nursing care. The nursing process in home care will include expanded assessment of the individual and the home environment, development of nursing diagnoses based on family data, generation of expected outcomes negotiated with the patient, and evaluation of effectiveness of care in relation to withdrawing or terminating care. Nurses involved in home health will use many skills to provide care to their medical-surgical patients. These skills and the issues that challenge nurses in home care are discussed in this chapter. The nursing process is presented to illustrate the unique aspects of assessing, planning, implementing, and evaluating nursing care in the home.

## DEFINITIONS AND TRENDS IN HOME CARE

**Home care** is the provision of nursing care in the person's residence. Continuity of care can be defined as the effective and efficient transition of the patient from hospital to home; it is essential to successful home care. Continuity of care from acute care settings to home management helps ensure an easy transition for the patient and family. This definition connotes the preparation of the patient for discharge from one health care setting to another, as well as coordination of appropriate resources. Congruence between patient and family needs for health care at different stages of illness, together with the nursing care provided, will ensure continuity of care. Continuity of care implies that assistance from health care professionals in acute or home care settings focuses on the ultimate goal of self-care: well-educated, highly motivated patients and families who know what to expect when the patient is discharged to home, can manage as much self-care as possible, can progress toward the highest level of functioning, and can accept help from available resources.

The home care nurse's caseload routinely includes patients with complex multiple illnesses such as cardiac disease, respiratory disease, diabetes, cancer, and neurologic problems. The **home health care nurse** may provide or direct nursing services to assist with activities of daily living (ADLs), to manage wound care, and as the examples in this chapter illustrate, to teach families about the technologic aspects of care.

Home care reimbursement from Medicare and most

third-party payers provides for teaching, assessment of unstable conditions, and provision of direct care. Several principles differentiate home care from medical-surgical care in institutions. The first principle is that home care is continuous (versus episodic) in perspective. In other words, the interrelatedness of the illness to the patient's life-style is considered. The nurse also emphasizes the comprehensive impact of the patient's situation on the whole family. Concern for the effect of environmental factors on the family and patient are apparent in home care practice.

The promotion of patient and family involvement in care is fundamental as the home care nurse recognizes that self-care may be the only option when insurance and other benefits are depleted. For example, intravenous administration of an antibiotic at home by a visiting nurse was uncommon 15 years ago, whereas today, nurses teach family members to perform this procedure independently. The realities of the economic health care dilemmas dictate that the home care nurse advocate efficient use of professional and family resources.

Trends in health care today have led to an expansion of home care services. Economic trends in health care, technologic innovations, and population demographics have resulted in increasing numbers of adult patients who require medical-surgical care in the home setting. Home care, as an alternative to expensive institutional care, obtained consumer support in the 1970s. Home care has been documented as cost effective in financial analysis studies conducted by insurance companies, health care professionals, pharmaceutical laboratories, and federal regulatory agencies.[6] The projected insolvency of Medicare and Medicaid, along with the increasing number of older persons in our society, provides the imperative for continued development of home health care delivery systems. Community health organizations, such as the Visiting Nurse Association and other agencies, have established innovative and cost-effective programs of home health care. However, more funding for services of these home care agencies is needed. Home care nursing services often are augmented by private companies that supply both equipment and specialists for the vast array of technologic care being provided in the home.

Technologic progress has influenced home care greatly. Patients can now be monitored at home through computer linkages to sophisticated diagnostic systems. Technologic innovations such as small, easily programmed intravenous infusion pumps have made parenteral home therapies safe and affordable. A variety of respiratory therapies, ranging from oxygen compression tanks to mechanical ventilators, are widely used today with elders or patients with multiple chronic illnesses. Infusion of blood, home defibrillators, and home monitoring of patients at risk for cardiac dysrhythmias are common today. The continued use of technology and future advances will increase the population of patients dependent on such care at home.

The changing demographics of our population also have influenced the increase in home health care. The number of elders will more than double by the year 2030, whereas the younger generation is decreasing in numbers. With reduced governmental programs for the aged, limitations on the amount of skilled nursing services, and decreased availability of nursing home facilities, more elderly persons will need home care. The needs of elders may vary significantly—from medical patients dependent on technology to surgical patients who require short-term home rehabilitation before returning to work. Many persons can benefit from home care. The combined influences of the patient's physical and psychologic characteristics and the social and economic support available to the family affect the outcome of care provided in the home. In each family, different factors will influence the outcomes of home care. Repeated assessment of these factors is necessary for modifying the home care plan as patient, family, and environmental factors change over time. The home as the environment for nursing care offers a particular challenge to those involved in home care. Nurses will need to develop special skills in working with families in their homes to manage the transition from acute to home care.

## TRANSITION FROM ACUTE CARE TO HOME CARE

In their work with patients in the home, nurses frequently use special skills, including gaining access to the home, discharge planning, transitional care, family education, and case-managed care. These skills are discussed here.

### GAINING ACCESS TO THE HOME

Health care professionals can readily list reasons for patients to have home care. However, patients and families may view the home care nurse as an added expense and invasion of privacy. One essential skill is the ability to gain entry into the home. Providing nursing care in a person's home cannot be undertaken without developing a successful approach or introduction to home care services. It is hoped that the nurse and other professionals in the acute care setting initiate discharge planning and that the family accepts the need for the home care nurse and possibly other professionals in their home.

Ideally the first visit with the patient and family should be conducted in the hospital before discharge, but often the first visit is to the home. Therefore the initial contact with the patient by the home care nurse is almost always by telephone. When telephoning, identify yourself as a nurse, and the agency from which you are calling. You may need to remind family members that they were referred to your agency by either the hospital discharge team or their physician. Explain that the purpose of the call is to set up an initial home visit. Establish that the purpose of the initial visit is to discuss the patient and family's home health care needs. Set the time of the visit at the patient's convenience, and state the amount of time it will take. Ask how the family wishes you to enter the home: through front door or back door, possibly with a hidden key. Repeat your name, and have them write down a telephone number where they can reach you. Remember that your tone of voice and the manner in which you conduct the telephone conversation establishes your respect for the patient. Closing with the comment, "I look forward to working with you," accentuates the participatory partnership the nurse will seek to develop.

For the home visit itself, the nurse must obtain the address and check directions to the location. At the first visit the patient's needs are assessed and available home care options are discussed. The nurse must be prepared with all essentials needed for assessment (e.g., history-taking forms, stethoscope, other equipment) and supplies necessary for already prescribed treatments (e.g., teaching materials, bandages for wound dressing). Typically the home care nurse will carry a bag that contains essential equipment but will need to check the contents and add anything necessary for a particular patient. Also, carry your charting materials, whether paper, nursing note forms, or tape recorder for dictation. It is best to tell the family you will be taking notes to document the patient's progress during home care. Your bag also should contain printed teaching materials that can be discussed and then left with the patient and family. The printed materials are selected based on the family's needs for teaching about illness, direct patient care, or other services available.

Information also should be available on the costs of home care services, insurance reimbursement, and other economic details that the family will need. Options to reduce home care expenditures safely, such as family members providing wound dressing changes 3 days a week or the nurse reducing visits to twice weekly, should be explored. Family members may desire 100% professional care or, on the other hand, may believe they can manage all the care themselves. The nurse must analyze each situation and suggest the best options. The nurse assesses the family's caregiving abilities in light of the patient's condition. The nurse should note that most insurers have restrictions on the lifetime amount the patient can be reimbursed for home care. Insurers also have limits on what they will pay for selected patient conditions. Discussing the economics of the health care situation with families can be difficult, but understanding that cost-effective use of their insurance will maintain coverage for them at a later date is essential.

At the first home visit, expect the family to welcome you in a social way, by introducing you to others present, asking you to sit down or have coffee, and so on, just as they would any visitor. Share with the family your pleasure at meeting them and then reiterate the purpose of the visit and the time limits previously set. State simply that you would like to hear how they are managing at home and to check the patient's condition. In this way, you communicate your desire to hear their concerns and also establish that the patient will be examined. Families often are unsure of the nurse's role in the home and need to be able to predict what will happen at each visit. Because the nurse is a guest entering the home, normal social protocol should be followed. For example, if you will be late, telephone the family as to when they can expect you. Do not automatically ask to go to the patient's bedroom. Explain each of the steps of your examination and services provided. Acceptance of home care services is essential if the continuity of care is to be maintained. If discharge planning in the hospital was used to initiate continuity of care, entry into the home usually is readily gained.

## DISCHARGE PLANNING

The term **discharge planning** has been used to describe the process of assisting patients and families with their health care needs as they move from one health care setting to another. The overall purpose of discharge planning is to provide continuity of care. Discharge planning includes many activities, from projecting patient needs at discharge to coordinating professionals and volunteers involved in follow-up care. In the mid-1970s, the American Nurses Association published guidelines for discharge planning for hospitals and community health agencies. In many hospitals and in other situations, the community health nurse meets with the patient before discharge. In other situations, discharge planning is provided by the nurse caring for the patient in the hospital. Hospital discharge planning often uses rating scales designed to identify patients with complex needs that necessitate home care.

The discharge planning process encompasses the assessment of the family's needs for teaching, counseling, and nursing care after discharge from the acute care setting. An important component of discharge planning is determining the resources within and external to the family that will be available when the patient returns home. The nurse accomplishes discharge planning by matching the patient and family's abilities to provide self-care with appropriate and acceptable community and family resources. Resources range from home health nursing care to equipment rental. Discharge planning may or may not include a referral to a home care agency. If the patient and family are able to meet their own needs after discharge, they may not require any further assistance at home. However, medical-surgical patients have many complex problems, and even if they are able at discharge to meet their own needs, a short-term post-discharge nursing visit can be used to evaluate the patient and praise the family on their self-management. Family members may underestimate the difficulties they will face when caregiving is necessary 24 hours a day. Assisting families in accepting outside help is a valuable but sometimes difficult task. For some patients a telephone call after discharge can be used to evaluate self-care status and provide continuity of care. The telephone call should be organized to ask specifically about the patient's condition and caregiver fatigue so that follow-up care can be instituted as necessary.

Discharge planning can be either a group process or conducted by one nurse or a social worker. The group process takes place in a team conference, where personnel from various disciplines and the patient and family discuss the patient's discharge. When the nurse plans discharge, he or she also includes the patient, family, and other professionals, but usually not in a formal meeting.

The key to either the formal group or the informal discharge planning process is communication with the patient and family. The nurse coordinates the communication and documents the discharge plan on the health care record. Documentation should include both short- and long-term discharge planning goals, as in the following example:

Ho Chung, a 57-year-old man of Chinese descent, is hospitalized for neurologic complications of Lyme disease (an infection from a tick bite). The short-range goals for Mr. Chung include being able to eat and bathe with assistance as his neurologic function improves. His long-range goals for discharge include being able to perform his ADLs with assistance from a home health aide three times a week and his family on the other days. At home his long-term goal is to resume independent ADLs as he works with nursing, occupational, and physical therapy.

The written plan should include how each goal will be accomplished. What the patient is doing in physical and occupational therapy should be documented, with the nursing staff reinforcing these activities on the unit. Who is responsible for a goal or the specific activity related to that goal also should be documented. The date of evaluation should be written so that the nursing staff can reassess progress. Discharge planning allows for continuity of care as the patient moves from the acute care setting to home. For discharge planning to be effective, it begins well before discharge and identifies patients needing home care. Characteristics of patients and various aspects of their medical-surgical treatment that influence their need for home care are listed in Box 27-1. These are not the only criteria, but they are the most common ones. The nurse must be alert for others. Remember that patients may not have any of the characteristics that indicate they will need home care, yet they still need discharge planning. Discharge planning begins at hospital admission and is an ongoing process. Although the critical elements of discharge planning and teaching are known, these elements are not always met. The Research box, p. 685, summarizes findings from a review of 10 published teaching plans for patients receiving home intravenous antibiotic therapy.

At the very least, discharge planning should provide the patient and family with (1) instruction in appropriate self-care, (2) identification of family and community resources, (3) awareness of procedures to follow for emergencies, (4) knowledge of follow-up care, and (5) family teaching specific to the patient's concerns. If home care is needed, explanation of home care services, telephone numbers, and, when possible, introductions to home care personnel become part of discharge planning. During hospitalization, as the patient progresses, the nurse collects data or modifies preexisting data, reflecting the change in the patient's health status and ability to function. Discharge planning builds on the patient's strengths and abilities.

**BOX 27-1 Characteristics of Patients That Influence the Need for Home Care**

1. Patients who cannot manage nursing care on their own
   a. Comatose or semicomatose patients
   b. Disoriented, confused, or forgetful patients
   c. Frail elderly persons
   d. Patients who live alone
   e. Patients who do not live alone, but persons at home cannot care for patients adequately
   f. Patients who have no home, or those whose present home is no longer adequate
2. Patients who need dressings and wound care
   a. Patients who have complicated dressings
   b. Patients who cannot do the dressing themselves
   c. Patients who will probably not do the dressing unless supervised
3. Patients who need equipment and transportation (function shared with social services)
4. Patients with medication schedules
   a. Patients with complex schedules or injections
   b. Patients who are noncompliant
5. Patients with ostomies (for example, colostomy, ileostomy)
6. Patients with special teaching needs (for example, new diabetic, complex diet, injections)
7. Patients who are terminally ill
8. Patients receiving therapy (occupational, physical, speech)
9. Patients with tubes (Foley, gastrostomy, suprapubic, nasogastric, tracheostomy)
10. Patients being transferred
    a. From another hospital or nursing home
    b. To another hospital or nursing home (e.g., Veterans Administration hospital)

The typical patients who need referrals are those with chronic illness, such as arthritis, cancer, cerebrovascular accident, chronic renal failure, congestive heart failure, diabetes mellitus, emphysema, hypertension, or myocardial infarction, and those who are respirator dependent.

Modified from Rasmusen L: *Nurs Management* 15(5):39-43, 1984.

## Determining Discharge Planning Needs

The initial interview before the patient's discharge includes an assessment of the patient's needs, that is, biologic, psychologic, social, and spiritual needs. The nurse assesses the home environment by asking several questions. Who does the patient live with? What are the living arrangements? Does the patient live in a house or

**RESEARCH**

Hileman J, Rebeck S, Smith C: *Literature review of discharge teaching plans of home antibiotic infusion,* Unpublished paper, Sept, 1993, University of Kansas Medical Center, Kansas City, Kan.

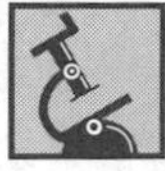

Ten published discharge teaching plans were reviewed to establish consistencies among them. The following summary provides the results.

All 10 programs provided discharge teaching in the hospital, and all were coordinated or taught by nurses. Only six programs, however, provided in-home teaching or involved a family member or significant other. Only one program provided teaching through the physician's office.

Average length of antibiotic treatment ranged from 15.5 to 22.9 days, although only one program reported making telephone calls to the patient. Eight programs gave a 24-hour telephone number to patients.

Educational methods varied and included films, written procedures lists, one-on-one demonstration, and lectures. Only three of the programs required return demonstration by the patient.

Initiation of teaching and the length of educational services varied. Charges for the services were not addressed.

apartment? Are there stairs to the house or building or stairs within the premises? Are all essential rooms on the same floor, such as the bathroom, bedroom, and kitchen? Is the living environment adequate to meet the patient's needs at the time of discharge? Adequacy can include basics such as running water or indoor plumbing, heat or cooling, and cleanliness. The nurse also asks specific questions pertaining to the patient's medical-surgical care. For example, does the patient receiving intravenous antibiotics have refrigeration storage for the medication? Do patients undergoing peritoneal dialysis have a clean area where they can work with their equipment?

The nurse also should assess the patient's and family's support systems. Who will be available to the patient when discharged? This includes immediate family members or significant others living with the patient. Ask what extended family members, children, friends, or neighbors are part of the patient's support system. In what group activities has the patient previously engaged to meet social needs? Will the patient be able to interact with these groups on discharge? What sources of spiritual support does the patient have? Can religious or other groups assist with care or prevent social isolation by visiting or telephoning regularly?

The nurse needs to determine if the patient and family have adequate coping mechanisms to manage the illness and the common stressors of home care. Ask the patient and family what they do to get along during difficult times. Will these coping strategies work for them now, or will they require assistance in developing new coping strategies because of a change in the patient's condition and its subsequent impact on the family? What learning needs will the patient and family have? Can these be adequately met before discharge, or will they require ongoing teaching? Finally, discuss the family's feelings about taking the patient home. Are they fearful of the patient's condition, worried about the extra responsibilities, or overly optimistic about their ability to care for the patient? The more realistic the expectations that the family has about home care, the more likely they are to adjust successfully.

### Financial Assessment

Financial assessment must be undertaken before discharge and throughout the home care visits. Financial assistance may be needed because home health care can be expensive and may not be reimbursable. If the home care is reimbursable, there often are extra expenses not covered by insurance or governmental programs. For example, utility bills may increase because of equipment necessary for care. Special services from a pharmacist or supplies such as enteral feeding products may be essential, costly, and reimbursable only on a limited basis. Caring for the patient in the home also may have caused a family member to quit or reduce employment hours, thus reducing income.

Financial assessment is often difficult for nurses to undertake. It may seem an invasion of privacy to be asking about available financial resources, especially in the person's own home. Nurses need financial data about patients to ensure they receive the full benefits for which they are eligible under government or private insurance. Nurses need to understand the services that are reimbursed by different insurers; unfortunately, patients can run out of medications or supplies before insurance reimbursement is completed. In today's economic climate, with the high costs of health care, even middle-income families may need assistance because they may be ineligible for governmental programs or other assistance. Also, identifying the resources currently used by the family allows the nurse to identify other possible sources of financial assistance. Box 27-2 lists financial resources that may be available to patients requiring home care. Referral to a social worker or financial discharge planner who is aware of the current eligibility and reimbursement criteria is essential, especially for elders.

Some states allow a Medicaid waiver that will pay for supportive home care for elders if the costs are less and the person qualifies for admission to a nursing home.

Last, during the initial assessment the nurse determines if the family is currently using any community resources to meet their needs. If so, how many, and how frequently? If the patient and family are using community resources that are satisfactory, the nurse will want to

**BOX 27-2 Financial Resources Screening Checklist**

1. Check the governmental or private resources available to the patient (benefits vary with each plan):

| | |
|---|---|
| ______ Medicaid | ______ Financial help from family |
| ______ Medicare A (home care services) | ______ Disability payments |
| ______ Medicare B (home care equipment) | ______ Retirement pensions |
| ______ Health insurance including HMOs and PPOs | ______ Welfare programs |
| ______ Employer insurance | ______ Meals on Wheels |
| ______ Social Security | ______ United Way agencies |
| ______ American Cancer Society (free bandages, equipment) | ______ Private insurance |
| ______ Multiple Sclerosis Society (wheelchair loans) | ______ Savings accounts |
| ______ Volunteer or charitable organization resources | ______ Veterans Administration |
| ______ Old-age assistance | ______ Military retirement |
| ______ Supplemental Security Income | |

2. Do you think that your total income for this year was enough to meet your (the patient and other family members) usual monthly expenses and bills?

   ______ Yes ______ No

3. In the past 6 months, has money been spent on the patient's physician, hospital, nursing home, or medication bills that has not been reimbursed by insurance?

   ______ Yes ______ No

consider these when making a referral, if one is necessary. If possible, the nurse in the acute care setting calls on the skills of the *transition specialist* to help with discharge planning. The *role of the transition specialist* is discussed next.

## TRANSITIONAL CARE

The concept of **transitional care** was developed by Brooten and colleagues.[3] The transitional period is the time from discharge planning to physiologic recovery. A nurse educated as a **transition specialist** can make a difference in both the quality and the cost of care at home. The transition specialist meets with the family while the patient is still in acute care to begin discharge planning. In addition, the transition specialist makes home visits before the patient's discharge to assess the home environment. The transition specialist is then available to the family after discharge. The study of Brooten and co-workers revealed that interventions instituted by transition specialists, including patient education, counseling, home visits, and telephone availability, were successful in terms of quality care.[2] An average cost saving of 25% was realized when discharge planning and home nursing services were used versus longer hospitalization.

To manage transition from hospital to home, patients and family members must manage activities ranging from use of sterile technique to assessment of the adult's psychologic status. To manage home care, the family members must acquire new knowledge and skills, be motivated to help the patient, and adapt to the change created in the roles of family members. The problems typically reported by families who provide home care include the burden of providing daily physical care, financial strain, and difficulty coping with individual role and schedule disruptions.[13] Other problems include the stress of learning the nursing care, unavailability of resources, the difficulty of accepting help from others, and observing any negative changes in the patient such as infection or malnutrition. Further problems noted in long-term home care include equipment failure, the need for home remodeling, and social isolation.[15]

In addition to dealing with these general problems, the nurse transition specialist reviews the literature to identify concerns shared by populations of patients they discharge. The key to providing successful transitional care lies in designing the nursing interventions specifically for each family. The interventions for the family of the patient being monitored for cardiac dysrhythmias in the home compared with the patient needing enteral feeding are very different. For example, the problems reported by patients receiving intravenous antibiotic therapy include difficulty in manipulating syringes and maintaining sterile technique.

Several problems experienced by home patients have been documented, including difficulties with finances, body image and sexual relations, social stigma, changes in each person's role within the family, and environmental issues such as how to arrange the living quarters for safety. These problems have been reported to recur depending on the patient's condition and factors such as the ability to return to work, length of time on ventilator each day, and availability of family support and external resources.

Stiller,[16] in a study of patients at home receiving various types of "high-tech care," suggested that family success with home care was inhibited by psychosocial factors, not the type of technology. Family coping ability, patient prognosis, and role disruption were worse in the families who were unsuccessful with home care. In addition, mental or emotional problems of patient or family members and caregiver fatigue were the problems experienced by these families. Stiller also observed that female patients had more frequent rehospitalizations from home care because their spouses had difficulty in managing the caregiver role. This information can be used by the transition specialist to prevent family crises. One of the key skills used by the transition specialist is family education.

## FAMILY EDUCATION

The term **family education** is used to emphasize that the teaching skills employed in home health care involve the entire family or all significant others. A large part of home care nursing is teaching the patient and the significant other. In this context the nurse's skill in assessing readiness to learn, providing information, and evaluating outcomes of teaching must be carried out with a group.[11] The home, as the environment for learning, also influences the teaching strategies used. Individual family members often have varying expectations and roles in the education process. The male patient may be interested in learning about the technical aspects of his care but might ask his wife to manage all his medications. In addition, a daughter might be called on to learn about the financial aspects of insurance, equipment loans, or Medicare benefits. The nurse assists the family in their decisions about who should learn what and may even be involved in resolving conflicts between family members who believe other members learned incorrectly. The steps for teaching the family are similar to those for individual patient teaching. Family education, therefore, begins with assessment and diagnosis of learning needs. The final steps include implementing and then evaluating the teaching.

The expected outcome of teaching is learning. **Learning** is considered to have taken place when behavior has changed so that the patient and the nurse agree that the person's health is enhanced. Thus teaching is not just imparting information but also ensuring that a *change in behavior* occurs. To assist family members to manage home care, they may need to change routines in daily schedules and responsibilities for household duties. The nurse may need to provide counseling, as well as external resources, to support these changes in behavior.

### Assessing Learning Needs

Assessing the patient and family's understanding of the illness and its treatment establishes a baseline for teaching. Box 27-3 provides sample interview questions to determine what patients already know about their health care. The nurse can link new knowledge to information the family already has and reinforce behavior change. Any barriers to learning that the patient and family may have, such as reading difficulties or lack of desire to learn, need to be assessed. Learning is influenced by attitudes, beliefs, and values. Attitude or desire to learn will vary greatly for each person through the various stages of home health care. Desire to learn is affected by the grieving process as well as by beliefs and values. Patients and families who are in a stage of denial will have difficulty learning. For those who are in denial and unable to learn a procedure such as intravenous antibiotic therapy, the nurse may need to do the procedure and gradually shift the family to self-care as the individuals are able to cope. Another situation that presents a learning difficulty is the family that needs to change a wound dressing but does not have money to buy bandages. In this situation, before teaching, the home care nurse would obtain dressings from the American Cancer Society, local church organization, or other organization. The Guidelines box, p. 689, identifies interventions the nurse may use for improving patients' willingness or motivation to learn the necessary home care instruction.

The nurse also must assess the information that family members desire. In addition to information about the patient's biologic condition, family members have personal knowledge and skills needs. The biologic condition and family members' personal skill and knowledge needs identified by home care nurses in one study are shown in Figures 27-1 to 27-3. The nursing interventions or skills needed to manage home care are related to each patient's biologic or pathophysiologic condition. Home care nurses indicated in this study that family members needed to know the skills of lifting, turning, and moving a patient, in addition to learning how to perform such tasks as neurologic checks (see Figure 27-1). Along with these personal learning needs, home care nurses recognized the family members' need for knowledge of

**BOX 27-3 Sample Interview Questions in Assessing Patients' Knowledge About Their Health Care**

1. Can you tell me what you have learned about your illness?
2. You have had surgery before. Can you tell me what you remember from that experience?
3. When you spoke with your physician/pharmacist, what did he or she tell you was important to know about your medications?
4. Have you heard about your therapy from anyone else who has had your health problem?
5. Have you read or heard reports about the treatments your physician wants you to undergo?

For patients who have physical limitations, careful assessment of their abilities should be done before determining the type of teaching plans and evaluation to use. For instance, some stroke patients' perception and knowledge can be evaluated by using picture boards to assist them to identify frequently used articles.

Modified from Smith CE: *Patient education: nurses in partnership with other health care professionals* (p. 62), New York, 1987, Grune & Stratton.

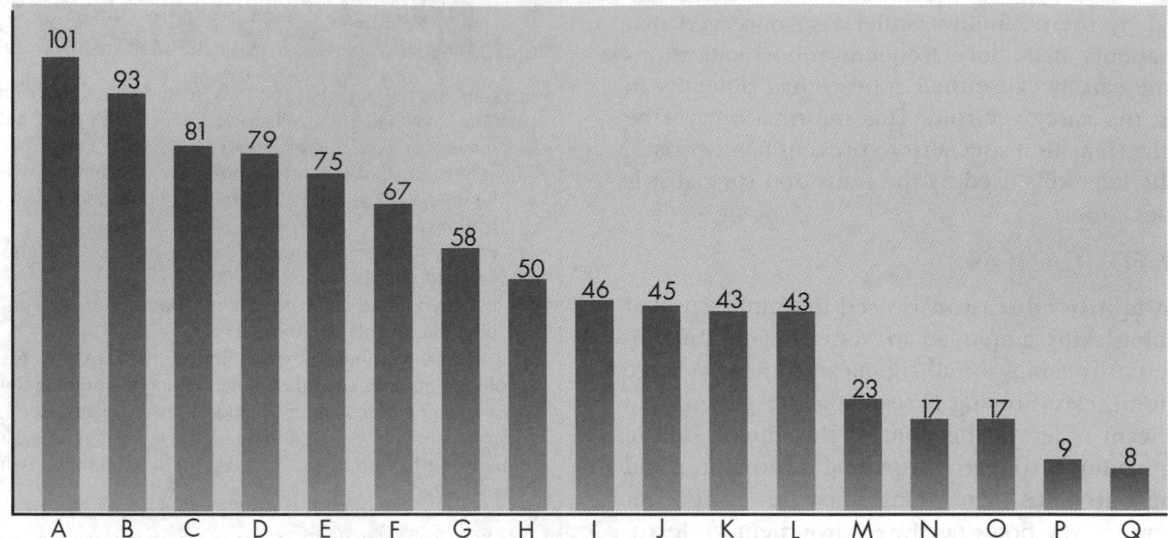


**FIGURE 27-1** Family members' biologic skill needs for providing home care: as prioritized by registered nurse respondents (figure represents number who indicated first-priority rating). *A,* Lifting, turning, moving; *B,* cardiopulmonary resuscitation; *C,* range of motion; *D,* gastrointestinal—nausea/vomiting; *E,* cardiovascular—apical pulse measurement; *F,* drug side effects; *G,* injections; *H,* sterile dressings; *I,* constipation; *J,* diarrhea; *K,* blood pressure measurement; *L,* respiratory; *M,* genitourinary—catheter care; *N,* eyes, ears, nose, throat—sensory-perceptual changes; *O,* neuro-temperature; *P,* charting; *Q,* neurologic checks. (From Quiring JD: RN perspective of home health care needs of family members, *Kans Nurse* 59[3]:10, 1985.)

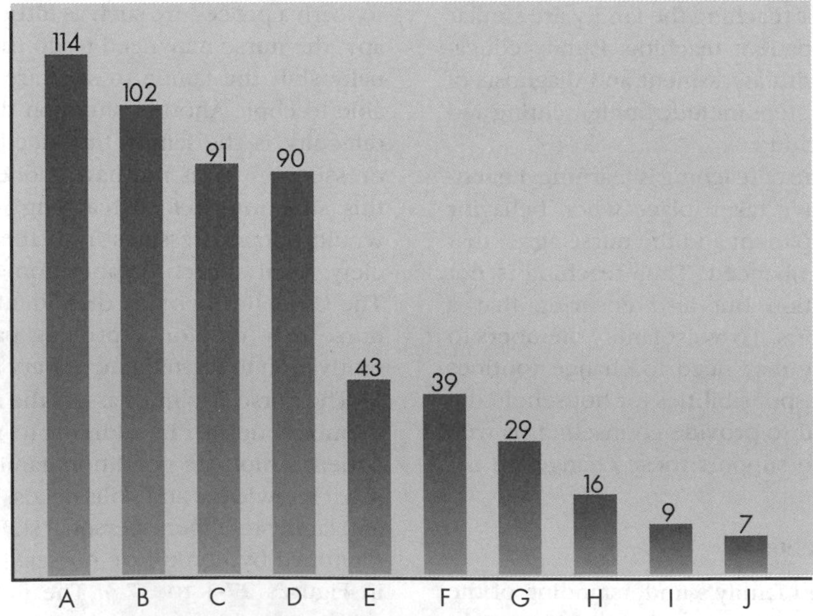


**FIGURE 27-2** Family members' personal skill needs for providing home care: as prioritized by registered nurse respondents (number indicates first-priority rating). *A,* Art of listening; *B,* promotion of independence/self-care; *C,* attitude toward seriously ill; *D,* establish rapport; *E,* confidentiality/privacy; *F,* promotion of health; *G,* interview; *H,* facilitating development of special abilities; *I,* life histories; *J,* avoiding patient abuse. (From Quiring JD: RN perspective of home health care needs of family members, *Kans Nurse* 59[3]:10, 1985.)

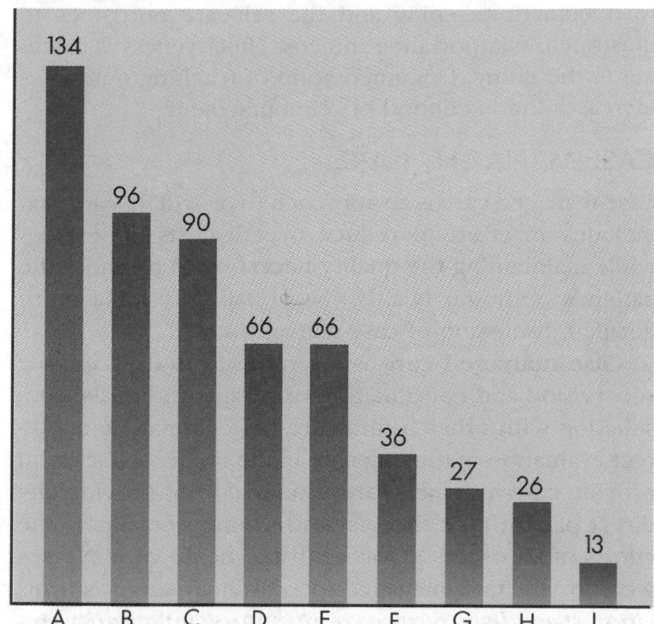


**FIGURE 27-3** Family members' personal knowledge needs for providing home care: as prioritized by registered nurse respondents (number indicates first-priority rating). *A,* Meaning/purpose; *B,* depression; *C,* hope; *D,* dying; *E,* grief; *F,* loneliness; *G,* fulfillment; *H,* bereavement; *I,* sexuality. (From Quiring JD: RN perspective of home health care needs of family members, *Kans Nurse* 59[3]:10, 1985.)

### Guidelines for Enhancing Willingness or Motivation to Learn

1. Provide counseling to reduce patient or family anxieties.
2. Explore past teaching experiences that created negative attitudes toward learning.
3. Compliment individuals and groups on information already learned.
4. Determine what the person wants to learn and teach this first.
5. Take steps to overcome deficiencies in perceptual skills, such as vision limitations and memory loss.
6. Complete discharge planning so that financial, housing, or other needed assistance can be found to decrease patient's worries.

Modified from Smith CE: *Patient education: nurses in partnership with other health care professionals* (p. 66), New York, 1987, Grune & Stratton.

depression, grief, and other potential psychologic problems that occur in home care (see Figure 27-3).

After assessment is completed, the data collected must be analyzed to determine nursing diagnoses that clearly indicate the patient's and family's problems or strengths. For example, the nursing diagnosis of *Coping, family: (potential for growth related to learned management of home care treatments)* identifies the family's strengths. Nursing diagnoses that illustrate problems with learning are described in the section on *knowledge deficits* later in this chapter.

## Planning and Implementing Family Education

Planning patient teaching in the home care setting is based on three major objectives for the patient: (1) comprehension of the illness and its treatment(s), (2) accepting the impact of illness and treatment(s) on life-style, and (3) demonstrating management of treatment procedures and home care. Understanding the patient and family's life-style will help the nurse to plan with them about how to adapt changes with the least disruption. When a medical regimen causes minimal disruptions in life-style, the patient is more likely to comply with it. Teaching is more effective when it includes not only knowledge of treatment but also counseling about scheduling so the patient and family can incorporate home care into their daily routines. The nurse also must plan learning objectives related to symptom control, management of exacerbations, treatment protocols, problem solving, and financial difficulties.

Implementation of teaching plans can take many forms in home health care. The use of computer-assisted instruction and videotapes in the home has been successful. Particularly useful is the technique of videotaping the teaching session in the patient's home and leaving the tape there for future viewing. Videotapes illustrating problems that arise in home care, such as contamination of intravenous antibiotic injection ports, slipping of an occlusive dressing, and even signs and symptoms of infection, can be portrayed. The key is that solutions to these problems also are modeled on the videotape for the patient and family members to review. One-to-one demonstration of technical procedures also is effective—as is describing methods of care over the telephone. Many and varied methods of teaching that incorporate the whole family and emphasize the need to change behavior are most likely to have positive results. Using praise and reinforcement and providing an opportunity to ask questions and to evaluate learning effectiveness are important parts of implementation.

Research review of patient education was undertaken to determine what effect patient teaching had on chronic illnesses.[7,8] Behaviorally oriented education programs that emphasized changing the environment in which patients care for themselves so that home care is easily managed were the most successful in improving the clinical course of chronic diseases. An example of modifying the home environment might include rearranging furniture so that it is in the field of vision of the patient who is rehabilitating from a cerebrovascular accident (CVA) and has residual hemianopsia. Requiring modification of the environment actively enlists the patient in changing behavior toward desired objectives.

Establishing cues as reminders of the new behavior required by patients increases adjustment to home care.

For example, encouraging patients with many treatments to try and schedule these with meals or other regular activities helps them remember to perform the activities.

### Evaluating Outcomes and Identifying Barriers to Home Teaching

The goal of teaching is to have patients and families incorporate necessary changes in behavior to adapt to illness and its resulting impact. Learning takes place in areas of *knowledge, attitude,* and *behavior*. Evaluation, the last step of the nursing process, is essential to patient education. **Evaluation** is based on what the patient and family believe they need to learn, as well as the learning objectives designed by the home care nurses. *Learning objectives* are stated outcomes that are *measurable* and *realistic*. Through the evaluation of the objectives, the nurse helps the patient and family to recognize needs for future learning and identifies success with past learning.

Questioning or listening to patient answers is a common method of evaluating learning. The *method of evaluation used should be acceptable and nonthreatening to the patient and family.* In addition to verbal questioning, the nurse should observe for evidence that the patient understands how to incorporate changes brought on by the illness. For instance, key questions could include how the patient plans to balance rest and activity during the day or plans meals and snacks to meet altered caloric and nutrient needs.

There are barriers to teaching in the home that nurses must be prepared to address. The nurse must remember to bring teaching materials for the home visit even if the patient has received handouts before discharge. Duplication of materials and information reinforces previous teaching.

Family members may make statements such as, "We are being taught something different now than what the hospital nurse or doctor instructed." The nurse must coordinate patient teaching and clarify consistency of information for the family. Often it is only the terminology or differences in language that cause confusion. The nurse builds on teaching materials already given to the patient so that it does not appear that only new content is being taught. Also, duplication of teaching efforts must be avoided. For example, the nurse and physical therapist should decide who will be responsible for teaching range-of-motion exercises, thus reducing the cost of education.

Another difficulty for home teaching is the wide age variation in patients and families. The home care nurse must consider the developmental, cognitive, and potential learning challenges for children and elders in the family.

Instruction is incorporated into patient care activities, allowing return demonstration and involving the patient and family in evaluating the outcomes. It is also essential to document teaching and the self-care outcomes to illustrate the importance and cost effectiveness of teaching in the home. Documentation of teaching outcomes increases the likelihood of reimbursement.

## CASE-MANAGED CARE

Case-managed care is an approach to providing care that includes an effort to reduce overall costs of services while maintaining the quality necessary to promote the patient's optimum health. (See Chapter 1 for a more detailed discussion of case management.)

**Case-managed care** is a term used to describe the supervision and coordination of paraprofessionals, consultation with other health care professionals, and a direct evaluation of nursing care in the home. Nurses who provide case-managed care usually do not provide any direct patient care themselves but may coordinate the efforts of all others involved in the home care. Nurses who provide case-managed care also may serve as *transition specialists, service coordinators,* and *quality improvement advocates.* The case manager conducts a detailed assessment of the patient's needs, discusses options with the patient and family, arranges for selected services to be coordinated with the home care agency staff, and then ensures quality care by evaluating patient outcomes on a periodic basis. In the case-managed situation, the nurse may have a caseload of 40 to 50 families.[4]

The nurse who provides case-managed care must develop many skills, must understand the patient's physical condition, and must be well-versed in the complexity of the patient's insurance or other financial coverage. The case manager needs skill in motivating families toward self-care, recognizing fragmentation of care, facilitating delivery of services on behalf of the family, and advocating for continuing resources when necessary. Arranging long-term services that match the patient's changing acuity level is a key element of case-managed care. Case managers do much of their work by telephone; thus they must be skilled in communication.

Case-managed care is supported by private industries and the federal government as a means of reducing insurance costs and making early hospital discharge to the home safe and less expensive. The nurse in case-managed care can be employed by a home health agency, hospital, health maintenance organization (HMO) discharge program, or an insurance company. Some nurse entrepreneurs have established their own companies that provide case-managed services for Blue Cross/Blue Shield or for the employees of large corporations. These nurses have become skilled in matching the patients' needs with the most cost-effective resources available.

The nurse who provides direct care to patients in the home is involved in case management instead of being a case manager. This nurse has a varying caseload of five to seven families daily. The total number of families managed depends on geographic location, amount of time spent with each family, and the frequency of visits necessary.

The skills needed by the nurse providing direct care to families are similar to those of the nurse acting as a case manager. Both nurses provide teaching and counseling and encourage self-care. The nurse managing the case in the home provides direct surveillance and monitors the patient's condition. The nurse providing direct care discusses the patient's needs with the case manager, who can assist with resource allocation and help anticipate any problems. Communication with the family is the key element in the success of case management. Other special skills used in the home are discussed in detail in the next section.

## NURSING MANAGEMENT

The ultimate goal of home care is to assist the patient and family to their maximal level of everyday functioning. In some cases the highest level of function may be the patient's complete recovery and return to work. In other situations the maximal function may be the family's ability to manage the patient's care in the home without professional assistance. In either case the implementation of nursing interventions will vary greatly, depending on the family and patient.

During data analysis the nurse develops nursing diagnoses based on the assessment data from the family. Along with these actual nursing diagnoses, the nurse determines potential diagnoses based on common discharge planning issues seen in home care. From the actual data-based nursing diagnoses and discharge planning process, several expected outcomes are generated specific to each family. The implementation of nursing interventions are directed by the nursing diagnoses and concomitant expected outcomes. Direct care is provided in the home by means of nursing interventions such as skin care, ambulation, or wound management.

Expected outcomes and implementation of specific interventions appropriate for the technologically dependent patient at home are described here. The examples given to illustrate the use of the nursing process in home care are based on clinical experiences with technologically dependent adult patients. Growing numbers of patients and their families successfully manage home care with mechanical ventilators, parenteral nutrition infusions, home hemodialysis, intravenous antibiotics or chemotherapy, and other life-sustaining interventions. Using the nursing process with these families supports their adaptive responses to the impact of technologic dependency. A priority for nursing research announced by the National Center for Nursing Research of the National Institutes of Health is to develop an understanding of patients' technologic dependence across the life span.

The discussion that follows outlines the steps of the nursing process employed in the management of adult medical-surgical patients who require various technical therapies at home. The implementation of highly technical home therapies has been well researched in the adult patient with no disease *complications*. Additional interventions may be necessary when the patient or family experiences confounding factors such as multiple illnesses, living alone, lack of a suitable home environment, or inability to accept dependency on technology.

The ***human-machine interface,*** which occurs when patients depend on technologically complex equipment, is a challenge that nurses can address through the use of the nursing process. Home care, even in the face of machines or technologic dependency, allows families to exert control over their lives, continue their self-actualization, and maintain their highest level of wellness and functioning. Nurses facilitate home care by advocating patients' independent living, educating families about technologic care, and providing them with resources.

Several researchers have verified the efficacy and cost effectiveness of home care for technologically dependent patients.[14] Advantages of home care over institutional care for the patient include *decreased nosocomial infection* and *improved nutritional status*. Home care allows for the resumption of more normal interactions and routines. More normal daily living follows adaptation to the noise of the machine and worry about machine failure. Even with these worries, greater sense of control and morale have been reported by both patients receiving home care and their families.

Finally, financial benefits of home care versus institutional care have been well documented. In-home use of technology costs approximately one-third as much as hospital care and even less when skilled services are not needed 24 hours a day. However, costs of any technologically involved care provided at home are not always fully covered. Considering the significance of such advantages, many institutions in the United States have reported discharge preparation protocols for home care of patients dependent on "high-tech" therapy.

The combined influences of the physical and psychologic environments of the home continuously affect the outcomes of care provided. Repeated assessment of these influences is necessary for modifying the care plan as patient and family environmental factors change over time. The home as the environment for nursing care offers a particular challenge to those involved. Nurses who work with families in their homes will need to develop special skills.

### ♦ ASSESSMENT

#### The Home

The family home is a unique environment for providing nursing care to the adult patient. Both psychologic and physical aspects need to be taken into account in developing the nursing care plan. The physical environment of the home must be assessed for safety, accessibility, and appropriate areas to provide care.

The psychologic factors affecting care in the home are many, varied, and rapidly changing. They have an impact on the patient's adaptation to home care and include motivational as well as financial particulars, patient and family expectations, and developmental, social, and community influences.

### Psychologic environment

The patient's attitude toward discharge to home, family members' reactions to the caregiver role, and the family's ability to accept help from the home care team all influence the outcome of care. Before discharge, the patient and family's attitudes toward home care are determined. The patient's motivation to return home and the family's willingness to provide and accept home care are important determinants of successful home management. The patient and family's perceptions and concerns about recovery will influence acceptance of home care. In addition, the importance of autonomy and privacy may influence acceptance.

The availability, expense, and type of services considered for home care should be discussed. A *backup plan* needs to be negotiated when services become too intrusive or expensive or when friends or others assisting in the home become ill or unavailable.

**Financial influences.** Home health care can be a financial burden for families. Cost analyses indicate that home care expenses vary in relation to the type, intensity, and length of services needed. Medicare, Blue Cross/Blue Shield, and an increasing number of private insurance companies pay for acute, posthospital home care services to reduce the length of hospital stay. For such coverage, however, the care required must be defined as intermittent rather than ongoing. Medicaid and a few insurers will pay for longer-term home care services for those whose condition is chronic. Supplemental coverage can be obtained in some cases from agencies that provide old-age assistance, workers' compensation, disability, Medicaid, or other financial aid programs. Regardless, the family must pay deductibles and only a percentage is covered; thus most persons pay some out-of-pocket costs.

Each of these financial resources varies in the requirements the patient must meet, the length of time benefits are allowed, and the types of equipment or supplies provided. Typically the complete description of the therapies, equipment, and services covered are included in manuals available from each financial group.

Even with these financial benefits, families will incur costs that are not covered. Some uncovered costs can be reduced through the use of volunteer, charity, community, or religious resources. For example, the local American Cancer Society will provide bandages and other supplies free of charge, and some church or volunteer groups provide transportation for clinic appointments. The family member who provides care for the adult at home may have time lost from work, thus increasing the financial burden. The nurse's role is to assess the psychologic impact of the financial situation on the family, coordinate the use of available resources, and refer the family to social workers, case managers, or insurance experts.

**Patient and family expectations.** Both the patient's and the family's willingness and motivation for home care must be assessed in light of their expectations of home care. Ask the family to describe what they expect home care will entail. Listen carefully to what the family expects the professionals to do in daily care. Does the family desire around-the-clock service or only availability of a nurse by telephone? Does the patient desire physical care from family members and medication or equipment monitoring from professionals? Do family members recognize the possible changes in their daily schedule that providing home care may bring?

How have the family members reacted to having outside persons coming into their private residence? Can the family obtain support from extended-family members, friends, and religious or community resources? Other long-range expectations of home care, such as the patient or family members becoming self-sufficient so that home services can be terminated or the feasibility of the patient's return to work, can be assessed on a continuing basis. The nurse must realize that as home care continues, the resources, motivation, and emotional reactions of the family and patient will change and must be taken into account in revising the home care plan.

**Developmental, social, and community influences.** The nurse must take into account other factors in assessing the psychologic environment of the home as the setting for care. One important factor is the family's developmental level. Individuals and families at different developmental levels will have different needs, skills, and resources to use in home care management. Family developmental stages and the major tasks associated with each are depicted in Table 27-1.[5]

These stages vary in length, may repeat, may overlap, and may not be sequential. Other tasks may be of prime concern depending on the family, its life-style, and available social and community supports.

Homebound patients often are concerned about other developmental tasks, such as obtaining child care or caring for grandparents. The nurse who assists the family in finding affordable day-care for children or live-in help for grandparents can then assist the family to focus on care of the patient at home.

Social and community support for home care also influences the psychologic environment and thus the outcomes of care in the residence. Social support is made up of actions from various sources that assist the person

**TABLE 27-1 Stages of Family Development**

| STAGE OF DEVELOPMENT | TASK |
|---|---|
| 1. Married couple | Establishing a mutually satisfying marriage<br>Fitting into the extended family network |
| 2. Childbearing families | Adjusting to parenthood<br>Encouraging the development of infants<br>Establishing a satisfying home for both parents and infant(s) |
| 3. Families with preschool-aged children | Adapting to the critical needs and interests of preschool children in stimulating, growth-promoting ways<br>Coping with energy depletion and lack of privacy as parents |
| 4. Families with school-aged children | Fitting constructively into the community of families with school-aged children<br>Encouraging children's educational achievement |
| 5. Families with adolescent children | Balancing freedom with responsibility as adolescents mature<br>Establishing postparental interests and careers as growing parents |
| 6. Families as "launching center" | Releasing young adults into work, military service, college, marriage, and so on with appropriate rituals and assistance<br>Maintaining a supportive home base |
| 7. Middle-aged parents | Rebuilding the marriage relationship<br>Maintaining kin ties with older and younger generations |
| 8. Aging family members | Coping with bereavement and living alone<br>Closing the family home or adapting it to aging<br>Adjusting to retirement |

Modified from Duvall E: *Marriage and family development,* Philadelphia, 1977, JB Lippincott.

to meet his or her personal goals or manage the demands of a particular situation. Social support has been identified in health care research as possibly affecting a person's adjustment to illness and ability to manage acute or chronic health problems. In terms of home care, ***social support refers to the tangible and intangible help received from others.*** Tangible help ranges from assistance with physical care to telephone visitations, whereas intangible help encompasses emotional support through encouragement or feedback. Social support most often is received from the persons in the immediate or extended family.

The nurse will find that communities also have resources that can be mobilized to provide the patient and family with social support as part of their home care. Religious denominations, neighborhood associations, community centers, voluntary service groups, and professionally led support groups can all be sources of social support. These groups can be used so that the patient or family caregiver does not become isolated and overburdened with care. Studies have indicated that social and community support also can lessen the depression of the caregiver that may result from the demands and changes brought on by home care.

### Physical environment

The home is the physical environment for delivery of nursing care. Any physical environment used for patient care requires assessment in terms of safety, accessibility, and appropriateness for care. The criteria used to assess the safety of the home depend to some extent on the patient's abilities and needs. The home of a patient who is discharged with equipment for hemodialysis may require alterations in the home to provide a safe environment for care. Modifications in the home environment for safety also may be based on the patient's disabilities or physical condition, such as the need for high-rise toilet seats, grab bars in the bathroom, or changing a living room into a bedroom.

Guidelines for assessing the physical environment should always include basic information about the home within that community. The location of the residence in relation to necessary home care services, durable medical equipment companies, and care sites for emergencies are important. Some rural residents may be willing and motivated to have home care but are 50 miles away from the closest home health care provider. Even urban dwellers may find out that their metropolitan area does not have an agency that provides necessary equipment, such as mechanical ventilators. Often an assessment of the community in such situations will uncover resources that will allow home care to take place safely.

A recent national survey[13] revealed that 25% of the persons who received total parenteral nutrition at home live in rural areas, and the family members of these patients provide more hours of care per day on the average compared with their urban counterparts. Fortunately, more assistance from neighbors and friends was reported available to these rural families.

The home health care nurse needs to help the family identify helpful resources and accept help to prevent caregiver burnout. Possibly a retired nurse in the rural community can be asked to provide care until family members have managed the transition from the hospital discharge. In the urban setting, a hospital-based pulmonary nurse specialist might provide periodic home visits to a ventilator-dependent patient. Another factor related to location of the residence is the availability of transportation to and from needed resources. Arrangements for trips to the grocery, pharmacy, and clinic are part of the safety of home management. Finding and training community resources to ensure safety of care are frequent challenges for the home care nurse.

The physical environment of the home should always be assessed for basic factors that affect the patient's health and adjustment to home care. Adequacy of heating, cooling, electrical outlets, plumbing, and refrigeration, as well as access to a telephone, should be determined. Lack of these resources does not preclude home care unless these are necessary for safety. Some antibiotics that are infused intravenously may require refrigeration. Proper storage would have to be found for the family whose home lacks refrigeration facilities. Plumbing and toilet facilities also need to be assessed in relation to the patient's nursing care needs. Another basic factor that affects the patient's adjustment to home care and is influenced by the physical environment is an area in which the patient can rest. The patient may be bedridden, unable to climb stairs, or restricted to one area because of medical equipment. Problem solving must be employed to ensure that family members can use the space in their home the way they desire and that the medical equipment does not cause too much noise or interference.

## The Patient

### Physical assessment

Assessment of the adult patient in the home encompasses many of the same data collection procedures appropriate in the acute care setting. In the acute care setting the patient is assessed by staff members around the clock. ***In the home setting, the patient and family members are the primary data collectors who monitor and provide care.*** Thus assessment in the home setting begins with exploring the patient and family's self-management. The patient and primary family caregivers should be asked to describe the patient's condition and discuss any concerns. The nurse providing home care may not have seen the patient for a few days and will depend on the family's observations or monitoring of specific data. The nurse's questions should illustrate to the patient and family that their information is important.

Assessment in the home proceeds in an orderly fashion. The nurse starts by asking the patient and family about their own concerns. The patient and caregiver are asked specific questions about the priority nursing diagnoses, medical problems, or signs and symptoms that the patient is experiencing. A man being seen at home for a wound infection may have reported his incision sore and tender but that the throbbing pain seemed to be decreased. The nurse would follow up by asking if anything had alleviated the tenderness, such as the warm, moist soaks used twice daily for cleansing the area. The patient also would be asked if anything aggravated the tenderness or made the symptoms worse, such as wound drainage. If drainage was reported, the nurse asks about the quantity or amount. It helps to obtain specific information by asking the family to describe the size of the drainage area. The type of drainage in terms of color, odor, and presence of blood or exudate should be observed by the nurse to obtain objective data. The nurse would determine if any signs or symptoms were associated with the subjective tenderness, such as swelling or elevated body temperature. These signs or symptoms are measurable and can be documented as objective data. Thus, with each problem area, the nurse gathers data from the patient and family that provide detailed characteristics for comparison. The detailed characteristics are used to analyze the symptoms being described. By comparing the characteristics from one visit to the next, the nurse monitors the patient's symptoms. The assessment concludes with questions about any other concerns. New nursing diagnoses may emerge over time while other diagnoses are being resolved.

### Psychologic assessment

Another essential assessment component is determining the patient and family's psychologic response to each problem. One man with a wound infection may react to the reduced tenderness and swelling as good news, whereas another believes he has a serious condition. The patient's psychologic response is influenced by many factors, such as length of illness, presence of multiple symptoms, and reaction of family members.

The primary caregiver's psychologic reactions also should be assessed. The **primary caregiver** is the person who provides the most physical or daily care for the patient. The primary caregiver may be a spouse, sibling, significant other, or grown child. Many persons may be involved in home care. In the case of one patient at home with an indwelling epidural catheter for infusion of analgesics, the husband was the primary caregiver. The home care nurse had assessed his ability to manage the infusions, distinguish untoward effects (respiratory depression) from side effects (nausea, pruritus) and obtain assistance from other family members. The responsibility of providing care for a loved one with physical pain can be psychologically demanding; thus the home care nurse asked the grown children to telephone and visit to provide respite and support for their father.

## Treatment Plan

The treatment plan includes health care professionals' prescriptions for medication, diet, exercise, and physical or psychologic care. The nurse discusses with the patient the specific therapy he or she was given and exactly how it is being carried out. In addition, the nurse asks the patient and family about any difficulties with treatments, obtains their opinions about the benefits or drawbacks of the therapy, and discusses these issues with them. Also important is the possible use of a health aide to assist the patient and give the family member time to rest inasmuch as the caregiver too may have chronic illness.

The treatment plan or therapy prescriptions provided by the patient's health care professional will influence the general care the patient needs. The treatment plan also will dictate any special skills the patient and family must master. Overall assessment of the patient's treatment plan should include questioning about general care, medications, nutrition, home environment, emergency procedures, specific patient needs, and equipment checks. General care assessment includes needs for assistance with hygiene, elimination, communication, rest and activity schedules, transportation, socialization, and continued contact with health care professionals.

**Medication assessment** is used to determine if the patient and caregiver know the purpose of medications and how to give them. To obtain a firsthand view of their knowledge, have the patient or family caregiver responsible for giving medications show you the medicines. In the home setting, patients and families must be alert not only to untoward effects and side effects but also to indications that medications are ineffective. They must anticipate dosage and schedules so they do not run out of medications at times when pharmacies are not open. Assessing actual dose taken versus prescribed dose is critical because there may be various reasons why patients and families change the dosage, including finances or forgetfulness. They do not want to be labeled as "bad patients"; thus they may state the prescribed dose as the actual dose. Confusion over multiple medications is a frequent problem. It also is common for patients to resume medications they took before hospitalization but that no longer are prescribed. Therefore the nurse asks about what is taken daily and when taken and requests that the patient count the remaining number of pills in the prescription to determine how many were taken and if that number is correct according to the new prescription.

**Nutrition assessment** includes collection of subjective data that the patient is tolerating foods or special diets, as well as objective data such as weight and calorie counts. Ability to follow through on diet prescription commonly is affected by costs of foods and lifelong eating habits. In determining nutritional status, the nurse also should assess the patient's hydration. Family members may have difficulty forcing fluids or restricting intake, if this is necessary. The home health care nurse can support the caregiver in these efforts.

*Assessment of knowledge of emergency procedures* is necessary with each family. Each family should demonstrate its ability to use the community's emergency telephone system and to call the home health care nurse for less serious situations. Family members can be taught cardiopulmonary resuscitation (CPR) if they desire or need this information. Equipment checks are a very specific and important part of home care assessment. Typically, each piece of equipment comes with written material that outlines the safety checks, cleaning procedures, and routine maintenance. The family must understand the manuals and incorporate safety checks into everyday schedules. The Guidelines box above lists guidelines a home health care nurse can use to assess the ability of the patient and family to manage intravenous antibiotic therapy safely at home.

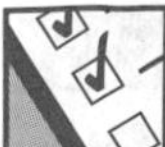

### Guidelines for Intravenous Antibiotic Therapy Equipment/Infusion

Supplies and teaching materials are based on the location of the intravenous site, whether that be peripheral or central access. Check each of the following:

1. Insertion site appearance of inflammation or phlebitis
2. Intravenous insertion catheter condition
3. Infusion tubing, filter set, pole for hanging solution bag
4. Alcohol, povidone-iodine (Betadine), antibiotic ointment for changing dressing on insertion site
5. Gloves and masks for use while cleansing site
6. Tape, transparent dressing
7. Antibiotic medication
8. Needles, syringes, disposable container for used needles
9. Anaphylaxis kit for allergic reactions and identification band or bracelet for known allergies

Assessment of specific emergency procedures, home environment, and special patient needs are all based on the patient's particular treatment plan. The nurse observes the family and patient's handling of procedures to assess their abilities to provide the care correctly. After assessing the patient's specific care needs, as dictated by the treatment plan, the nurse turns to data gathering and resources available to the family.

## The Family

**Family assessment** is essential because the success of home care depends on the ability of family members or significant others to draw on and use internal and external resources. *Internal resources* include the family's or individual's positive attitude toward home care, ability to problem solve or seek advice, and willingness to accept help or assistance from *external resources.* Accepting help from friends, neighbors, and church or community groups often is difficult for families because of the strong value of independence in our culture. The home health care nurse can determine the availability of these and other external resources and then assess the family's willingness to accept such help.

Each family member's reactions to the role he or she carries out in relation to home care influences the family's internal resources. A grown child working full time

## RESEARCH

Smith CE, Holcroft C: *Situational depression in long-term home care of technologically-dependent patients and their family caregivers*, Unpublished paper, 1992, University of Kansas Medical Center, Kansas City, Kan.

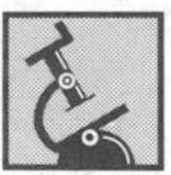

Reports have indicated that situation-based depression (nonpsychiatric depression) is a common problem affecting long-term therapy. The purpose of this study was to measure level (mild to severe), frequency, and factors associated with situation-based depression as part of a larger study on quality of life in long-term TPN patients and caregivers. Hypotheses were that patients and caregivers differ in their frequency and experiences of depressive episodes. Questionnaires were returned from 116 patients (m = 52 years of age) and 121 caregivers (m = 52.5 years of age) who were randomly selected from academic, hospital, and infusion agencies across the United States. Patients (m = 52 years of age) had Crohn's disease, ischemic bowel or radiation enteritis, or nonterminal cancer; the average length of TPN therapy was 4.6 years.

Methods included use of the Center for Epidermiologic Studies—Depression Scale (CES-D) (a 20-item scale developed by the National Institute of Mental Health to rate symptoms of situational depression). Subjects were instructed to write about things that made them feel "unhappy, sad, gloomy, depressed, blue, hopeless, or discouraged" on an investigator-generated instrument consisting of six topics known to be related to depression ("TPN complications, family members aren't being helpful, disease gets worse, miss out on activities, financial strain, and miss my friends"). The CES-D scores of patients ranged from no depression to severe depression (m = 16.1), whereas caregivers appeared to have lower levels of depression (m = 12.0). Both patients and caregivers reported situation-based depression from *never* to *daily*, with an average frequency of weekly. Handwritten responses were coded by means of content analysis. Patient responses indicated that depression was associated most frequently with complications (infection), missing out on activities, and expense, whereas caregivers indicated expense, TPN complications, and the disease becoming worse. Mild situational depression occurred frequently, and severe depression occurred in 16 patients and 6 caregivers. Helping patients and families to anticipate the various factors associated with depression and to learn coping behaviors may lessen the frequency and severity of situation-based depression.

might not be able to help with the patient's daily physical care but might contribute grocery shopping. The home care nurse may need to assess periodically family members' role responsibilities in home care inasmuch as these change over time. Also, individual reactions to responsibilities and the energy required to carry them out vary with the length of time that caregiving continues. Situational depression in both patients and caregivers is not uncommon in cases in which home care requires technologic equipment, such as that needed for total parenteral nutrition (TPN). (See Research box at left.) Families also react to changes, whether improvement, decline, or stabilization, in the patient's condition during home care. Interview questions that can be used to assess caregiver roles and reactions are listed in Box 27-4. Many times negative reactions to caregiving can be improved by obtaining relief such as *respite care* or financial assistance for the family.

### BOX 27-4 Caregiver Role Assessment

1. How have the responsibilities of the members of the family changed since the patient has been at home?
2. How do you and other family members feel about these changes in responsibility?
3. Has your health changed since you have been caring for the patient at home? If so, describe how.
4. Family members tell us they have emotional reactions to the changes in the person they are caring for. What has your experience been with these emotional reactions?
5. Family members often state that responsibilities of home care can be overwhelming and difficult. Do you find this true or not true?
6. Family members also have found they have gained strengths or a sense that they are successful in caring for the patient at home. Do you find this to be true or not true?
   Tell me about when you have not felt successful.
   Tell me the successes you have experienced.

## ♦ NURSING DIAGNOSES

Nursing diagnoses are based on the assessment data collected in the home and on the data gathered from discharge planning. These data are analyzed to identify the patient and family's responses to the pathologic condition, medical regimen, treatment plan, and home nursing care. The nursing diagnoses should reflect each family's actual and potential problems and strengths. By diagnosing strengths, the nurse identifies abilities family members can use in dealing with the actual and potential problems they will face. Analyzing the data to determine the coping skills, external resources, and other family strengths is essential because most eventually must manage the home care alone.

The patient and family may be experiencing translocation syndrome related to moving from the acute care setting into the home. **Translocation syndrome** is a stress reaction to leaving an environment that is perceived as highly protective and safe. The stress response to transferring from one health care setting to another has been measured in several studies. Elevated levels of catecholamines were found in the urine of patients transferring to medical floors after being in coronary care units. Relocation of elderly persons into nursing homes has been associated with increases in death rates. Nurses have found that when patients are prepared for transfer well before the relocation takes place, less stress is experienced. In preparing for discharge to the home, the nurse must anticipate the stress or anxiety the patient or family members may experience when they leave the environment of the acute care setting, where health care professionals are readily available. Extensive preparation—through teaching and involvement of the patient and family in coordinating resources that are readily accessible and economically feasible—lessens translocation stress.

The following nursing diagnoses also may be seen in family members who manage home care. The nursing diagnoses presented in this section are based on information from experienced home care nurses, nursing research studies, and data from studies of adults in the home. These diagnoses have been categorized into problem areas of ***resource management, family dysfunction,*** and ***knowledge deficits.***

Resource management is the ability to obtain and effectively use resources both inside and outside the family for the patient's home care. Resources may include people, equipment, and monies. Resource management is discussed in more depth in the implementation section.

## Nursing Diagnoses Based on Resource Management

### Home maintenance management, impaired

Insufficient financial resources are a common problem reported by families at home. Reimbursements from insurance companies or Medicare vary widely and are constantly changing. The home care nurse must be skilled in understanding governmental regulations and advocating for the patient's eligibility for coverage. The nurse may enlist the help of a social worker familiar with home care coverage codes and regulations to ensure that information on the costs of home care covered by insurers is made available to the family. In addition, the nurse (with the assistance of the social worker) needs to identify any voluntary sources of financial support for families. Some private agencies, such as the American Cancer Society, may provide bandages, equipment, or other care services free or at a nominal charge.

The nurse also must be concerned about specialty services available to the family. In some instances, the technical support services needed by the patient may be at such a distance that safety is a concern. When this occurs, the nurse must ensure that the family recognizes and can readily manage emergencies such as equipment failure or lack of supplies. Should home care no longer be needed because the family has learned to manage on its own, the nurse must document this change.

### Self-care deficit: bathing/hygiene, dressing/grooming, feeding, toileting

In many instances the patient requires daily physical care such as feeding, bathing, or assistance with grooming or toileting. Also, technical care, including tracheal suctioning, wound irrigation, or intravenous fluid administration, may be required. Family members provide a wide variety of physical care at home for patients undergoing chemotherapy, those debilitated with Alzheimer's disease, or those recovering from a cerebrovascular accident (CVA).

Family members' fatigue and stress are problems the home care nurse must address. Another complicating factor is the lack of acceptance of help from outside the family. The family may be a closed system that does not desire help from the outside or feels shame when members cannot provide care by themselves. The nurse may need to use values-clarification strategies to assist the family with this issue. The nurse will employ problem solving and several other counseling techniques with psychologically related nursing diagnoses.

### Decisional conflict related to constraints imposed by long-term home care

Dealing with the patient's chronic disability and the home care management creates constraints on family members' daily schedules and use of the home for activities. The family must make many decisions each day about the patient's home care. These decisions may result in conflicts between family members. The patient and family members have direct responsibility for managing such conflicts. Patients and families experiencing chronic illness must live with the constraints imposed by the disease and the home care. Therefore the nurse may use ***conflict-resolution strategies*** to help ensure that an equitable decision-making process is used.

### Diversional activity deficit

Patients with chronic disease, visible disabilities, or equipment as part of their treatment report experiences of negative ***social stigma.*** Friends may fear that activities are too much of a physical strain for the patient with a chronic illness. Extended family members may believe that visiting the home causes the family more grief over the patient's disability. Employers may believe that the presence of medical equipment such as oxygen tubing will make the workplace unappealing to customers. Many people feel uncomfortable around visible changes in the patient and environment and avoid visiting. Potential visitors may feel vulnerable: "If it happens to her, it can happen to me." The patient and family need assistance to anticipate these problems and suggestions on how to deal with such reactions. Being homebound may impose an additional stigma on the patient who is striving for or needs diversional activity.

## Nursing Diagnoses Based on Family Dysfunction

When data from home care assessment are analyzed, nursing diagnoses related to family dysfunction may be apparent. Home care places many demands on families. Meeting these demands can cause physical fatigue of

## RESEARCH

Smith C, Prouty D: *Caring for the caregiver*, Unpublished paper, June 1993, University of Kansas Medical Center, Kansas City, Kan.

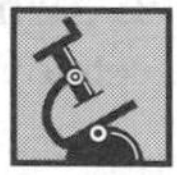

Caregivers of chronically ill persons in the home have a formidable and often overwhelming task. Nurses must be sensitive to the needs of both the patient and the caregiver. As part of the initial and ongoing assessment, nurses should assess motivational styles of caregivers to promote continuity and effective delivery of patient care.

In this study predominant motivational styles of caregivers to chronic patients in the home setting were determined by means of C. Daniel Batson's criteria.* These styles and suggested nursing interventions are described here.

Caregivers may have one style of motivation at one time and another when circumstances change. Thus nursing assessment of caregiver motivational style must be ongoing and nursing interventions flexible.

**REWARD SEEKING**

To feel deserving of the anticipated reward, the caregiver motivated by rewards, such as praise, recognition, or money, must personally help the patient. Therefore the reward-seeking person may suffer burnout. Nurses need to assess such caregivers for rewards they value and provide praise and support for accomplishments. Teaching this caregiver how to be efficient may prevent burnout.

**PUNISHMENT AVOIDANCE**

The goal for the person who wishes to avoid punishment is to behave in a manner that prevents shame, social disapproval, or any other event perceived as punishment. Promotion of positive feedback from other family members to the caregiver, referral to respite care, and freedom to express anger without judgment may help the punishment avoider sustain patient care activities.

**AROUSAL REDUCTION**

The caregiver who finds the patient's pain difficult or impossible to bear will not be able to continue caring for the patient unless his or her own anxiety is reduced. Sources of anxiety for the caregiver require nursing assessment. Personal, family, and community resources—when identified and used—may be helpful to this caregiver. The nurse can provide positive reinforcement for effective caregiving behaviors. Patients who assume responsibility for their own care may help relieve the caregiver's anxiety.

**ALTRUISM**

Caregivers who are altruistic seek to understand the needs of the patient and act so that those needs can be met. Help offered is consistent with the wishes of the patient. Most caregivers are altruistic to some degree. Secondary motivational styles may be present and should be assessed. The nurse may discover that sharing assessment findings with the caregiver leads to effective caregiver interventions.

*Batson CD et al: *J Personality and Social Psychology* 45:706-718, 1983.

individual members and a variety of psychologic dysfunctions within the family.

### Adjustment, impaired

Caring for a family member in the home may alter individual members' everyday activities, interactions, and pattern of social contacts. Participation in religious, leisure, and school activities may be affected. Shifting of household responsibilities may make some family members feel overworked. These changes in life-style may be permanent or temporary, depending on the patient's situation and the resources available to the family. The nurse can assist family members to predict the disruptions that home care might create and support them in adjusting to these disruptions.[12]

### Coping, family: compromised

The length of home care affects coping within the family. The longer that home care is required, the more the family's coping skills can become depleted. More situational crises arise during prolonged home care, which also challenges the family's coping abilities. Other contributing factors include past experiences and realistic expectations of home care. The family with positive past experiences that can accurately predict the length of home care and that has realistic expectations about the daily schedule is better able to cope with prolonged home care.

### Family processes, altered

Home care generally disorganizes a family, at least temporarily. Communication patterns will be altered. Meaningful interactions such as confidential talks, teasing, or humorous exchanges and physical comforting by hugs may decrease. Until the feeling of disruption ebbs and a sense of predictability returns, family processes will be disrupted. The nurse can ask family members to describe how home care has changed family function. Their own description will help clarify the alterations in communications and personal exchanges they are missing. Steps to rekindle these helpful family processes should be instituted.

### Role performance, disturbance in

A spouse as the home caregiver may have to drastically change the role previously assumed (e.g., from noncook to cook, yard work only to housekeeper). The designated caregiver may perceive home care as an overwhelming burden. The studies of caregiver burden indicate that it is the *perceived* burden more than the actual physical or financial drain that predicts role performance problems.[1] Caregivers vary in their motivation to help (see Research box at left). Interventions for altered role performance include teaching about new responsibilities and social support. *Social support* in the form of helping with everyday care, contacts with a network of peers, acceptance of caregiving by family members, and provision of emotional concern or praise seems to ease the perception of burden in a caregiver who welcomes these gestures.

## Nursing Diagnoses Based on Knowledge Deficits[11]

Nursing diagnoses based on knowledge deficits frequently are seen in home health care. Subjective and objective data from the patient and family must be scrutinized to determine the specific cause of the knowledge deficit. Several common causes are discussed here.

### Knowledge deficit related to transfer of learning into the home setting

Patients and families often state that carrying out procedures they were taught or observed in the hospital seems more complicated at home. A common concern is the confusion caused by medical terminology that is difficult to understand and that may vary between hospital and home care nurses. Using the patient's own words is best. Another concern is that at home, health care personnel are not immediately available, which may decrease the person's confidence. Also, adaptations in procedures may be necessary in the home. Such adaptations may be difficult for family members or patients to devise. Also, the complexity of scheduling the total care, including bathing, feeding, and technical treatments, may be difficult. The varied aspects of transferring learning into the home need to be discussed with the family before the patient's discharge. An emphasis on problem solving that incorporates the patient and family environment, including daily routines, will prove helpful. The nurse should make sure family members realize they can contact the home health agency if they have questions between visits.

### Knowledge deficit related to psychologic state (anxiety)

Another personal factor that can make a difference in the patient and family's learning is their mental or psychologic state. Much has been written about how anxiety affects perceptions and behavior. It generally is accepted that persons who have moderate to severe anxiety may be able to focus only on their immediate concerns. Consequently, the information given when the patient is moderately anxious may be so distorted that the person may not learn what is intended. Hospitalization may increase a person's anxiety level. Nurses may need to employ methods to reduce anxiety so that the patient and family can attend to learning. For some patients, complex equipment may be overwhelming and create increased anxiety. The nurse initially may need to perform the technical care and gradually teach self-care as the patient or family is able to manage it.

### Knowledge deficit related to the patient's physiologic state

Physical factors play a significant part in the patient's knowledge deficit. These factors may include the presence of acute illness or pain, fluid and electrolyte imbalance, altered nutritional states, lack of endurance, or medications, each of which can alter mental alertness. Other physical factors related to treatments also may interfere with motor abilities and learning.

Certain electrolyte and nutritional states alter the patient's cognitive functioning. The patient may be confused or hallucinatory or simply may be too weak to devote the necessary energy to learning. After the electrolyte imbalance has been corrected, the patient will be better able to concentrate and learn. Patients may lack the physical energy to perform a psychomotor task, such as a dressing change, or they may lack the mental energy to concentrate on learning. Arthritic problems with advancing age may make fingers less functional for fine motor tasks. The tactile perception in elders also may be reduced so that manipulation of small objects, such as needles and syringes, can be frustrating. Nurses must determine any physical changes that might hamper learning and take steps to alleviate these barriers when teaching patients and families.

### Knowledge deficit related to cultural and socioeconomic factors

Cultural and socioeconomic factors can influence the patient's response to teaching. These factors can include a language barrier, cultural background as related to health practices, or lack of finances to purchase necessary home care equipment. The following patient example is used to illustrate how several of these factors affect learning.

A patient from a middle-Eastern culture had a transverse colostomy and recovered very well. She needed home care because she showed no interest in the colostomy or in performing any of the needed care. In her culture it was taboo to allow a member of her family to touch her body; yet she could not afford home care services and was uninsured. Through an interpreter who interviewed the patient, it was determined that a neighbor, also of her culture, was willing to learn colostomy care and eventually teach the patient self-care. Once the nurse learned about the taboo and the woman's lack of interest, the nurse turned her attention to teaching the neighbor, who in turn could instruct the patient at home.

This situation illustrates how important it is to consider all factors that affect patient teaching.

### Knowledge deficit related to health beliefs

People are more likely to behave in a certain way if they believe that the behavior fosters good health and that they are at risk for a complication or if they recognize a benefit from the learned behavior. For example, a young woman at home receiving intravenous antibiotic therapy is more likely to refrigerate the intravenous solutions as required when she understands the potential risk of contamination. If the woman does not perceive that this activity will be of some benefit or if she does not feel threatened by the possibility of developing an infection, she may not follow the teaching.

Folkways about health practices also affect home care, and nurses may include these remedies (when safe) in their teaching. It is always good practice to ask patients what they believe will add to their success in home care management and try to incorporate folk remedies the family feels necessary. Because the patient controls his or her own care, folkways may be used and the health care professional may be unaware of it.

**Knowledge deficit related to illiteracy**

Literacy reports suggest that less than 20% of the adult population reads above the fifth-grade level and that in the United States the median literacy is approximately at the tenth-grade level. Many times the educational materials distributed are above the patient's reading levels. A mismatch of written material and the patient's reading ability can account for unsuccessful learning.

Not only should the printed word be at an appropriate level for the patient, but also the vocabulary used by the nurse. Results of patient education studies indicated that common "medical words" are not understood by patients. Words such as "hematoma," "secretions," and "post-op" were incorrectly defined by a large number of those surveyed. How often do nurses use those words in their teaching and assume that the patient understands what they mean? Even for functionally literate patients, the stress associated with illness may reduce their comprehension of spoken words, written materials, and even visual teaching resources. Teaching and reteaching, with opportunities for patients to ask about terms and ideas they do not understand, are important aspects of treating knowledge deficits. Because reteaching patients may not be reimbursed, further education may be included in other care or be charged to the family.

## ♦ EXPECTED PATIENT OUTCOMES

Planning is directed by the outcomes expected to result from home health care. Statements are made of expected outcomes so that the patient, family, and home health care nurse agree that the outcomes are realistic and measurable. Expected outcomes are based on the patient's condition as reflected in nursing diagnoses, standards of nursing practice, and results from clinical research studies. The following section contains examples of planning home care.

## ♦ INTERVENTIONS

Interventions for the adult patient in the home are based on discharge planning, assessment data, nursing diagnoses, and expected patient outcomes *negotiated with* the patient or the family. The critical nursing interventions of resource management, counseling, and teaching are implemented with every family. *Resource management includes coordination of services, products, and personnel necessary for cost-effective home care.* The interventions implemented by the home care nurse will depend on the internal and external resources available to the family. Coordinating the resources, counseling, and providing information are essential aspects of the nurse's role in home care implementation.

### Planning and Implementing Home Care

**Home intravenous antibiotic therapy**

Numerous clinical studies have established **home intravenous antibiotic therapy (HIAT)** as a safe approach for many adult patients. The frequency with which patients dependent on intravenous therapy are discharged to home care has increased dramatically. Patients are discharged from the hospital when the signs and symptoms of acute infection are under control. Then, when the patient shows the following characteristics, the patient is ready for home teaching.

1. Patient and family agree to manage HIAT.
2. Patient has peripheral vein or central line catheter in place.
3. Family has created a suitable environment in the home for infusion therapy.

**BOX 27-5 Family and Patient Learning Needs for Home Intravenous Antibiotic Therapy**

**EMERGENCY PROCEDURES**

How to stop bleeding if venous access device is detached
How to seal puncture or fracture of intravenous line
How to perform emergency withdrawal of angiocatheter that has become displaced from hub
What to do if an electrical power failure occurs (if pump is used)
How to recognize allergic reaction and treat anaphylaxis
What to do if an equipment failure occurs
How to reach home-care 24-hour services (emergency telephone numbers)
How to store medication in the home
How to notify fire department and emergency services, if needed

**HOME ENVIRONMENT**

How to rearrange or remodel home to accommodate safe storage of supplies
How to notify pharmacy and establish appropriate delivery of medicine and supplies
How to reach the home care equipment company
How to set up a patient call system
How to order and obtain supplies
How to operate and care for special medical equipment (infusion pumps, needles, medication systems)

**SPECIAL PATIENT NEEDS**

How to monitor for signs of infection
How to provide diversional activities (hobbies, pastimes, recreation)
How to identify signs of an insertion-site infection
How to submit insurance papers or obtain other sources of funds
How to travel with the intravenous access device
How to make arrangements for care from other person if primary caregiver is ill

4. Arrangements for supplies, medication, laboratory blood studies, and emergency care have been made.

When met, these expected outcomes ensure that the resources necessary for successful HIAT are available to the patient. The first expected outcome of eliciting the patient and family's agreement to manage HIAT is essential. If the family is not motivated to undertake this complicated therapy, difficulties will arise with home care. Family members need to know emergency procedures, how to manage the home environment, and how to handle the patient's special needs. (See Box 27-5 for a listing of learning needs for patients on HIAT and their families.)

Patients receive HIAT to treat many infections—for example, osteomyelitis, endocarditis, urinary tract infections, septic arthritis, cellulitis, pyelonephritis, pelvic inflammatory disease, prostatitis, and complications from medical devices inserted into the body. The incidence of infections, coupled with physician and industry efforts to secure Medicare funding for home antibiotic therapy, are likely to increase the numbers of patients receiving HIAT.

Researchers had documented not only the efficacy, safety, and cost savings of infusions in the home but also the effectiveness of teaching patients and families to manage intravenous antibiotics in the home. Nursing interventions can be determined on the basis of nursing diagnoses and expected patient outcomes (Table 27-2).

It is helpful to have more than one expected outcome for each diagnosis to provide more than one objective criterion for measuring the results of nursing interventions. The data that need to be gathered to evaluate the results should be readily available and inexpensive. White blood cell (WBC) counts or wound culture laboratory tests may be the most definitive way of determining acute exacerbation of infection, but they are expensive and relatively difficult to obtain and would not be used unless other data (high fever and so forth) indicate that the expected outcomes have not been met. *Expected outcomes used in home care must be simple to use and analyze.* The patient and family must collect most of the data needed to judge if expected outcomes are met because they monitor their own home care. If the data to be collected are difficult for the patient to obtain (e.g., unable to read small markings on a thermometer or unable to determine color changes on the chemical strips used to check nitrates indicating urinary tract infection), another person in the home must be taught to gather this information.

**Procedures in implementing HIAT.** The overall expected outcome with HIAT is that the patient's infection will be eliminated. However, because HIAT requires complicated technical care, expected outcomes that reflect the patient and family member's ability to undertake each aspect of HIAT must be carefully written. (See Guidelines box, p. 702, for the 18 procedural steps typically used for infusing antibiotics.) It is clear from these steps that the terminology the patient must learn just to read these directions can be overwhelming. It is important that instructions not be initiated before the patient accepts the idea of self-administration and learns some of the common terms.

Before patients can undertake administering infusions, they need clear understanding of the reasons for the therapy and why it will take place in the home. The presence of an intravenous needle often signifies to the family that the person is very ill and that the connection to the tubing means the patient should be bedridden with restricted activities. Families may experience anxiety over the patient's condition and ineffective coping related to wanting the patient home yet being afraid to manage HIAT. These problems can be treated by providing information and counseling strategies to build family members' confidence in giving care. Patients and families need reassurance that continued intravenous therapy can be safely conducted in the home. They need to understand that any patient has a potential for an acute exacerbation of infection and may require rehospitalization. The signs of acute infection are listed for them so that they feel confident in deciding when to call for help. The advantages of being mobile and returning to work and household activities are presented to them. The teaching/evaluation tool (Table 27-3) can be used to enter dates on which information was given. The nurse indicates the relevant teaching and evaluation activities by initialing the appropriate column on the tool.

**TABLE 27-2 Nursing Diagnoses and Expected Outcomes for the Person Receiving Home Intravenous Antibiotic Therapy**

| NURSING DIAGNOSES | EXPECTED OUTCOMES |
|---|---|
| Coping, family: compromised, related to ambivalence toward HIAT | Patient/family member (1) state rationale for HIAT, (2) demonstrate readiness to learn by handling equipment or asking questions, and (3) state they agree to undertake HIAT. |
| Infection, high risk for acute exacerbation | Patient remains free of high-grade fever and other signs of infection specific to the patient (e.g., cough, sputum for pneumonia; painful joints for osteomyelitis). |
| Knowledge deficit: management of HIAT related to new treatment | Patient/family member demonstrate each step of HIAT, using safe, aseptic technique. |

### Guidelines for the Person Receiving Home Intravenous Antibiotic Therapy

1. Each morning, review the scheduled times for your medication, and plan your activities to allow enough time for the infusion
   a. One-half hour before the scheduled infusion, check your temperature and compare this on the graph to the previous day's level. Check the insertion site of your intravenous (IV) catheter (teach patients to look for signs for infection, skin irritation, and stability of catheter in the vein). If problems exist with the catheter, telephone the home care nurse, who may be able to provide appropriate instructions.
   b. Draw up antibiotic medication in syringe. (If premixed solutions are not available, several other steps specific to mixing are added here.)
2. Remove the bag of IV solution from the refrigerator 15 minutes before administration to allow it to warm up.
3. Check the expiration date and dosage of any premixed solutions.
4. Draw heparin-saline solution into a syringe if premixed solution is not available, and replace the cover on the needle.
5. Hang the IV bag on a hanger above your arm.
6. Squeeze the drip chamber, and purge all air from the tubing, making sure there is fluid in the drip chamber.
7. Cleanse the rubber stopper of your IV catheter with an alcohol swab for 1 minute.
8. Remove the cap from the needle at the end of the IV tubing.
9. Insert needle into the gummed rubber stopper of your IV catheter.
10. Establish a flow rate by adjusting the flow-control clamp so that solution in the ___ml bag will take ___minutes to infuse. That means that ___drops of solution must fall into the drip chamber every 30 seconds. (Blanks are filled in by nurse.)
11. Check flow rate periodically. When the infusion is completed, remove the needle from the gummed rubber stopper.
12. Replace the cap over the needle.
13. Wipe off the gummed rubber stopper again with an alcohol swab.
14. Remove the cap from the syringe containing the heparin-saline solution, and inject it into the gummed rubber stopper.
15. Remove the needle of the syringe from the gummed rubber stopper, and replace the cap over the needle.
16. Carefully dispose of all your needles so that no one will accidentally be injured (use a coffee can with cover; this may be brought to the hospital pharmacy later for proper disposal).
17. Record on your monitoring sheet that infusion was completed and that IV insertion site looks normal.
18. If you have any questions, call the hospital and ask the pharmacist or IV nurse for assistance.

## ♦ EVALUATION

The last step of the nursing process is evaluation. Evaluation consists of making a judgment as to whether home care has been successful. This judgment depends on comparison of the patient and family's status with the expected outcomes of home care.

### BOX 27-6 Required Patient Data for Quality Improvement Process in Home Health Care

1. Types and length of nursing and other home services
2. Nursing and medical diagnoses
3. Age, gender, income level, and other demographic data
4. Age and relationship of family members providing care to the patient
5. Source of the patient's referral
6. Source of payment for home care services

If expected outcomes have not been achieved, the reasons for this are ascertained. If the patient's physical function falls short of the expected outcomes, the nurse must identify factors contributing to this problem. The nurse may see signs that the patient's pathophysiologic condition is worsening. Referral to the physician or arrangements for transportation to a medical facility may be necessary. Evaluation might reveal that the expected outcomes have not been achieved because of factors other than the patient's physical condition. The patient may have misunderstood what he or she was taught, the resources arranged at discharge may not have been obtained, or the family members may have found home care overwhelming. Another reason expected outcomes are not met is that they may have been unrealistic in terms of the allotted time. The nurse reassesses the situation and establishes new outcomes in conjunction with the patient and family.

Evaluation also reveals many instances in which patients have achieved their expected outcomes. The nurse should acknowledge this with the patient and family. When families are given recognition for their achievements, they feel supported in their efforts. Evaluation data, whether indicative of achievement or not, must be documented, with the rationale related to the outcomes. Evaluation data may be used for justification for reimbursement of extended home care or for the involvement of other home care resources. For the patient to continue to receive Medicare home health care benefits beyond the 2 to 3 weeks of intermittent care allowable, "exceptional circumstances" must be proved. Many patients may qualify for up to 2 months of home care reimbursement when the nurse provides data that document the need for continued home care.

### Continuous Quality Improvement

Quality improvement is another aspect of evaluation (see Chapter 1 for a more detailed discussion of quality assessment and improvement processes). **Quality improvement** is a formal process of aggregating data to form a basis for evaluating groups of patients and various aspects of care. Examples of data obtained about groups of patients necessary for the quality improvement process are listed in Box 27-6.

**TABLE 27-3 Teaching Evaluation Tool: Peripheral Intravenous Therapy (Enter Dates and Initials)**

| KNOWLEDGE/SKILLS | INFORMATION GIVEN/ DEMONSTRATED | | RECITES INFORMATION/ RETURN DEMO | | COMMENTS |
|---|---|---|---|---|---|
| | Client | Other | Client | Other | |
| Purpose of therapy | | | | | |
| Potential complications | | | | | |
| Tx of complications | | | | | |
| Emergency plan | | | | | |
| Obtaining supplies | | | | | |
| Tubing flushes | | | | | |
| Dressing changes | | | | | |
| Prep med/solution | | | | | |
| Initiate infusion | | | | | |
| Control infusion | | | | | |
| D/C infusion | | | | | |
| Other: | | | | | |
| | | | | | |
| | | | | | |

Nurse's initials/signature ____________________

Used by permission of Kristine Williams, RN, MS, School of Nursing, University of Kansas Medical Center, Kansas City, Kans.

These data can be used to project trends in home care services for a particular group of patients. Data that reflect nursing care hours and types of home services used can help identify personnel needed in home health care. Medical and nursing diagnoses help establish appropriate case management. Financial data can be used to plan future services, budget for weekend services, recruit specific types of personnel needed in a home care agency, and justify needed programs to policymakers.

One of the most interesting aspects of quality improvement is the use of patient outcome data from several families to evaluate nursing care. The case records or charts of several patients can be reviewed to determine if specific nursing interventions were successful or if the amount of resources used were adequate to meet the expected patient outcomes. Using quality improvement processes, nurses in home care can establish *cost-effective interventions.* Nurses can be leaders in developing home care programs that promote the highest possible level of health and function for a specific adult population.

Quality improvement processes and evaluation of individual families also can be used to identify issues pertinent to home care, some of which are discussed next.

## Issues in Home Care

Many issues affect the practice of home care nursing. These include factors that affect delivery of care such as the cost of nursing services, availability of services and community resources, and patient or family responses to home care. Also, competition between home care delivery services often occurs. Reimbursement for professional nurses versus home health aides may influence who provides care. Scarcity of services for patients dependent on technologically complex equipment may limit care in some locales. Communities with few resources (free clinics, volunteer agencies, self-care groups) may be unable to provide support for families caring for adults in the home. Home care nurses can bring the issues of affordable home care, national health insurance, and development of resources for in-home care of elders to legislative or community groups for resolution.

Many issues arise in the everyday care of patients in the home. As with nursing of adults in any setting, an individual may elect not to follow prescribed regimens. Families may refuse the medical and nursing care available to them. The nurse in home care advises, but ultimately the patient and family decide whether to follow through. Third-party reimbursement may not pay for professional nursing services. Nurses may observe or suspect abuse or neglect of the patient as family caregivers become overwhelmed with the patient's care. Also, there may be sociocultural or religious conflicts between the family's and the health care professional's approaches to the patient's care. The home care nurse must identify such conflicts and other issues and discuss these with the patient, family, or other health care professionals.

Caring for various groups of patients highlights issues particular to each group. Caregiver fatigue, social isolation, and role change are problematic in many cases. The need for custodial or respite care also may be apparent. Care of dying patients in the home has increased significantly with the success of the hospice movement. The family's coping skills and a focus on palliative care become issues in long-term terminal care. Home care nurses must be open to discussion of spiritual concerns, life review, and reconciliation.

Another challenge comes from patients at home who require rehabilitative care. Persons with neuromuscular diseases, CVAs, or spinal cord injuries may require the assistance of physical and occupational therapists. Safety in the home also includes checking the environment for areas that have the potential to cause accidents. Patients with Alzheimer's disease may benefit from mental health or gerontology specialists. Other specialists also may need to be available to patients in their home, such as speech or respiratory therapists. Transportation to clinics and rehabilitation centers may need to be arranged. Services that enhance persons' abilities to manage their own care will increase costs but are essential to self-care. The issue of providing the needed services for home care in the most cost-effective manner will continue to be a challenging issue.

## QUESTIONS TO CONSIDER

- What are the major determinants of whether intravenous antibiotic therapy can be implemented at home?
- What approaches would you consider for a patient who needs daily physical care in the home but has no insurance and an elderly spouse?
- What criteria are used to determine needs for home care after early discharge from the hospital?
- What advantages do transitional care and case-managed care offer for home care?
- How do the skills needed for family education in the home differ from individual patient teaching in the hospital?

## CRITICAL THINKING ACTIVITIES

- Edward, 55, has chronic pancreatitis requiring antibiotic therapy every 6 hours and TPN therapy at night. His wife works part-time, his son Marvin is an auto mechanic and lives nearby, and his daughter Jane is a nurse's aide who works at night and lives 20 minutes away. Edward's care includes administration of the antibiotics and TPN via an Abbott pump, and Groshong care. In addition, he is no longer able to assume his responsibilities around the house, such as lawn care and home maintenance tasks. Analyze this situation and discuss possible considerations in teaching family members to assume responsibility for various aspects of Edward's care at home. Discuss alternatives for who should learn which aspects of care.
- Brad, 75, has severe coronary artery disease, a history of myocardial infarction, and hypertension. He is on multiple medications and frequently forgets to take them. Provide creative techniques that may assist Brad to improve compliance to his medication regimen.

## CHAPTER SUMMARY

### DEFINITIONS AND TRENDS IN HOME CARE

- Providing nursing care to the ill adult in the home will be an increasing challenge in the decades ahead. Forecasters of health care indicate that hospital closings will continue, whereas home care services will increase. Medical-surgical nursing care in the home will be necessary for a wide range of adults.
- The trends responsible for the increasing need for home care nursing include the emphasis on continuity of care, promotion of family involvement in care, economic limitations on expenses in health care, and the demographics of an aging population.

### TRANSITION FROM ACUTE CARE TO HOME CARE

- Skills to manage the patient's transition from acute to home care range from establishing a relationship on entering the home to case-managed care, which incorporates supervision of many families and advocating cost reductions in health care services.
- Discharge planning, family education, and transitional care are the major skills used in home care nursing. Discharge planning includes resource management, coordination of hospital and community services, and adequate preparation for home care. Family education is based on research that supports the use of patient instruction, with the added dimension of teaching a group, the family. Transitional care incorporates the skills of discharge planning and family education, with emphasis on continuity and self-managed care in the home.
- The acuity level of persons who require care in their homes will continue to rise, and the technologic aspects of care, including use of mechanical equipment or invasive procedures such as intravenous therapies, will increase in home care. These factors, coupled with shorter hospital stays, will require increasing sophistication in the area of transitional care, starting with discharge planning.

- The uniqueness of the residence as the environment for care must be taken into account with an adult who requires home care. The nurse uses special skills: entering the patient's home, teaching families, planning discharge, providing transitional care, and assuming case management.

NURSING MANAGEMENT

- Patients may require one or two home visits or around-the-clock nursing care. The nursing management of persons in home care includes expanded assessment of the patient and the home environment, development of nursing diagnoses based on family data, generation of expected outcomes negotiated with the patient and family, implementation of appropriate care, and extensive evaluation of the effectiveness of care.
- The nursing process in home care is an expansion of that used with hospitalized patients. Assessment is broadened to include recognition of environmental, financial, social, and community influences on care. The assessment of the patient's condition, psychologic status, and response to treatment is undertaken in light of family analysis.
- Data analysis from assessment in home care has resulted in identification of common nursing problems. These nursing problems can be stated as nursing diagnoses such as self-care deficits, ineffective family coping, and knowledge deficits.
- Expected patient outcomes and implementation in home care can be readily illustrated through the example of patients at home receiving intravenous antibiotic therapy. The patient dependent on technologically complex equipment exemplifies the needs of those with acute conditions, complicated teaching requirements, and family coping challenges. Research suggests these needs can be met in a cost-effective manner with high-quality home nursing care.
- Evaluation of home nursing care is a complicated process that includes continuous quality improvement and identification of issues related to home management. Specific data are needed to evaluate groups of patients managed at home. Availability of resources and national health insurance are some of the issues affecting home nursing care today.

## REFERENCES


1. Archbold P et al: Mutuality and preparedness as predictors of caregiver role strain, *Res Nurs Health* 13:375-384, 1990.
2. Brooten D et al: A randomized clinical trial of early hospital discharge and home follow-up of very-low-birth-weight infants, *N Engl J Med* 315:934-938, 1986.
3. Brooten D et al: Early discharge and specialist transitional care, *Image: J Nurs Sch* 20(2):64-88, 1988.
4. Cronin C, Maklebust J: Case-managed care: capitalizing on the CNS, *Nurs Manage* 20(3):38-47, 1989.
5. Duvall, E: *Marriage and family development,* Philadelphia, 1977, JB Lippincott.
6. Harris M: The changing scene in community health nursing, *Nurs Clin North Am* 23(3):559-568, 1988.
7. Lindeman C: Patient education. In Fitzpatrick JJ, Taunton RL, Benoliel JQ, editors: *Annual review of nursing research,* New York, 1988, Springer.
8. Lindeman C: Patient education, Part II. In Fitzpatrick JJ, Taunton RL, Benoliel JQ, editors: *Annual review of nursing research,* New York, 1989, Springer.
9. National Association for Home Care: *Basic statistics about home,* 1992, Washington DC, Author.
10. Rooney A: A Joint Commission perspective on home infusion therapy III. *Hospital-Home-Health* 8(8):104-106, 1991.
11. Smith CE: *Patient education: nurses in partnership with other health care professionals,* New York, 1987, Grune & Stratton.
12. Smith CE: Technology and home care. In Fitzpatrick JJ, Jacox AK, Stevenson J, editors: *Annual review of nursing research,* New York, Springer (in press).
13. Smith CE, Giefer CK, Bieker L: Technological dependency: a preliminary model and pilot of home total parenteral nutrition, *J Community Health Nurs* 8(4):245-254, 1991.
14. Smith CE et al: Financial and technological costs of high technology home care, *Nurs Econ* 10(5):369-373, 1992.
15. Smith CE et al: Responsibilities and reactions of family caregivers of patients dependent on total parenteral nutrition at home, *Public Health Nurs* 10(2):122-128, 1993.
16. Stiller SB: Success and difficulty in high-tech home care, *Public Health Nurs* 5(2):68-74, 1988.

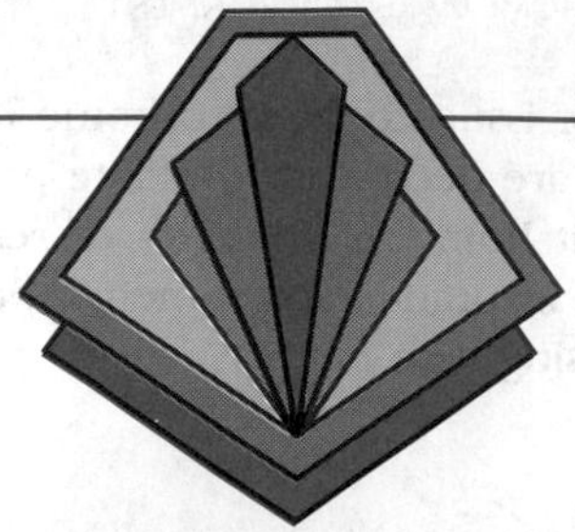

# CHAPTER 28

# Emergency Care Environment

*Nancy K. Barr*

## CHAPTER OBJECTIVES

***After studying this chapter, the learner should be able to do the following:***

1. Articulate the evolution of the body of knowledge for emergency nursing.
2. Identify nursing interventions that will increase safety in the emergency department environment.
3. Describe the parameters and guidelines for conducting an initial assessment of a trauma patient.
4. Identify principles of management and care of persons suffering multiple trauma.
5. Identify assessment guidelines and principles of emergency management for patients with selected cardiovascular, respiratory, integumentary, musculoskeletal, environmental, toxicologic, and gastrointestinal emergencies.
6. Describe the care of a person who was sexually assaulted.
7. Describe the nurse's role in caring for victims of domestic violence.

## KEY TERMS

blunt abdominal trauma
cardiac tamponade
compartment syndrome
deep frostbite
dry drowning
flail chest
Good Samaritan statute
heat cramps
heat exhaustion
heat stroke
immersion syndrome
incipient frostbite
multiple trauma
near-drowning
penetrating trauma
peritoneal lavage
pneumothorax
postimmersion syndrome
pressure points
primary survey
rape trauma syndrome
secondary survey
superficial frostbite
tension pneumothorax
trauma
trauma centers
triage
urgent care
wet drowning

During the past 10 years the demands on emergency nursing have been increasing because of the changing health care needs of society. The rising incidence of street and domestic violence, the lack of adequate insurance, and the unavailability of access to primary care are the major reasons for increased use of health care in emergency centers. Because of the current health care crisis (lack of health insurance), one of every three persons seeking care in the emergency department is seeking primary care.[13,14] The increased use of emergency centers and the fact that many nurses are called on to provide emergency care in the community support the need for all nurses to know the basics of nursing interventions, standards of care, and expectations for emergency nursing.

Before specific emergency problems are detailed, emergency nursing in general and concepts such as triage, critical pathways, communication, environmental factors, and information regarding mandatory reporting and preservation of the chain of evidence when working with situations that have any question regarding legal consequences are discussed.

## SCOPE OF PRACTICE FOR EMERGENCY NURSING

The Emergency Nursing Scope of Practice was approved by its association in 1988.[9] It uses the same framework as the American Nurses Association's social policy statement: core, dimensions, boundaries, and intersection. Emergency nursing crosses body systems, disease processes, problems, care settings, age-groups, and populations. Nursing practice in the emergency department requires knowledge of the person throughout the life span.[9] To be completely proficient in trauma care, the nurse should take a trauma nursing course designed according to the guidelines of the Emergency Nurses Association.[22]

Emergency nursing activities occur in a sequential arrangement or flow pattern based on the acuity of the person's condition. Emergency nursing includes provision of care to persons whose problems range from nonacute to life-threatening. In fact, most persons who request emergency department service typically are ambulatory and have nonacute conditions; therefore there is a trend for emergency departments to add a specific care area for these persons. Some hospitals use the terms "fast track" or **urgent care** to identify a designated area in or near the emergency department for persons with nonacute conditions. These areas may be open only after their physicians' offices have closed, or they may provide quick service 24 hours a day. Fast track or urgent care areas have been developed because these care environments are less expensive treatment areas. The persons treated at these areas require less time with the health care staff because of the nature of their signs and symptoms. Regardless of whether emergency departments are designed to separate the nonacute from the acute case and regardless of ability to pay, every person requesting care must be evaluated on arrival.[6,15]

## TRIAGE

Because the needs of patients seeking care in emergency departments vary greatly, triage systems have been implemented within emergency departments. This assessment usually is completed by an emergency department nurse who performs the triage for the department. **Triage** is a continuous and highly visible process in the emergency department today. Triage comes from a French word meaning "choice."[24] The triage system is used to identify those patients whose condition is most seriously compromised so that they are the first to receive medical intervention. The choosing, sorting out, and placing of priorities on care have been practiced since patient care began and have been used extensively in disasters and wars. A standardized four-color-coded triage system quietly communicates to all health care providers the priority of treatment (Box 28-1). However, triage as a systematic method to be employed by health care personnel in both prehospital situations and emergency departments has come into its own.

The nurse performing the triage function completes an assessment on the patient in a timely manner that determines the category of care the person requires. The categorization of patients in prehospital situations and in emergency departments is based on a time frame—just as for disasters. Persons who need to be seen immediately have an *emergent* or life-threatening situation; persons who need to be seen as soon as possible have an *urgent* condition that has the potential of becoming a life-threatening situation; and persons who can be seen as time allows have *nonurgent* conditions, with no life-threatening symptoms at the time of presentation and no symptoms that typically become life-threatening. This system of prioritization of patients and these labels are used by the Emergency Medical System (EMS). The use of these common terms provides for understanding of the situation and more uniform prehospital and in-hospital communication and care. Fast track or urgent care areas handle persons with urgent or nonurgent conditions. Persons with emergent conditions are seen in the usual emergency department area. Box 28-2 presents a listing of the typical emergent, urgent, and nonurgent complaints of persons seeking care at a level II trauma center in a community hospital over a 24-hour period.

### BOX 28-1 Four-Color Coded Triage System

**0—BLACK: DEAD**

**1—RED: CRITICAL OR LIFE-THREATENING**

These victims have a reasonable chance of survival only if they receive immediate treatment. Emergency treatment is initiated immediately and continued during transportation. This category includes victims with respiratory insufficiency, cardiac arrest, hemorrhage, and severe abdominal injury.

**2—YELLOW: SERIOUS**

These victims can wait for transportation after they receive initial emergency treatment. They include victims with immobilized closed fractures, soft-tissue injuries without hemorrhage, and burns on less than 40% of the body.

**3—GREEN: MINIMAL**

Victims in this category are ambulatory, have minor tissue injuries, and may be dazed. They can be treated by nonprofessionals and held for observation if necessary.

From Baker II FJ: *Top Emerg Med* 1(1):149-157, 1979.

## CRITICAL PATHWAYS IN EMERGENCY DEPARTMENTS

Time tracking of patients in the emergency department is essential for many reasons, such as to ensure quality of care practice, to track and trend work load activity, and to have appropriate staffing to match workload. A system that many hospitals are using to achieve this is with critical pathways. Use of critical pathways in the emergency department incorporates time frames to achieve specific outcomes or to complete specific interventions.[19]

For example, a person with an arm injury and signs of a fracture will have an x-ray examination to determine the type of fracture. A critical pathway for this type of patient identifies the x-ray examination as the major diagnostic activity to be accomplished and a time frame for completion, such as 20 minutes after the assessment and evaluation by the emergency department physician and the emergency department nurse. Once mutually identified interventions, outcomes, and times are deter-

**BOX 28-2 Presenting Complaints of Persons Seeking Emergent, Urgent, or Nonurgent Care at a Community Hospital Over a 24-Hour Period**

Abdominal pain
Abdominal problem
Back pain
Behavioral problem
Cardiopulmonary arrest
Cardiovascular problem (chest pain)
Cough
Diarrhea
Difficulty breathing
Dizziness
Earache
Environmental injury (heat stroke)
Eye injury
Eye problem (blurred vision)
Eye problem (infection)
Eye problem (conjunctivitis/pink eye)
Fever
Genital problem (sore and discharge)
GI bleeding (black stools)
GI bleeding (bloody stools)
GI bleeding (vomiting blood)
Head injury
Head wound (cut/scrape)
Headache
Head/neck problem (stiff neck)
Insect bite
Joint pain
Lower extremity injury (sprain/strain)
Lower extremity problem (swelling, no history of injury)
Lower extremity wound (cut)
Multiple injuries (auto accident)
Multiple problems (achy, dizzy, tired)
Multiple wounds (cuts/scrapes from fall)
Nausea/vomiting
Neck injury
Neck wound
Neurologic problem (confusion)
Neurologic problem (weak one side, unable to walk)
Nosebleed
Overdose
Palpitations (heart racing, skipping beats)
Pregnancy problem (abdominal pain)
Pregnancy problem (bleeding)
Rash
Respiratory problem (drowning)
Sick (feel bad, tired, irritable)
Trunk injury
Trunk wound
Upper extremity injury
Upper extremity problem (swelling, inflammation)
Upper extremity wound (cut)
Urinary problem (burning, pain, frequency, blood in urine)
Vaginal bleeding (nonpregnant)
Weakness
Wheezing

mined for a particular patient population or diagnosis, the nurse can assume that the interventions and outcomes should be completed within the time period and there will be no need to make additional telephone calls to ascertain why an activity has not been completed. Although critical pathways are tools and guidelines, they provide standardization of care, consistency with interventions, and a means to evaluate effectiveness of care. Thus critical pathways promote quality of care, increase effectiveness of care, increase staff communication, and increase staff and patient satisfaction. Refer to Chapter 1 for more information on critical pathways.

## COMMUNICATION

Maintaining effective communication in any clinical setting is a challenge. However, in the emergency department the challenge is compounded because of the number of health care personnel involved in the care of the patient and because of the emergent situation. What is being said may not be heard because of the anxious state of the patient or the patient's family. Because of the flurry of activity in the emergent situation, perceptions come into play. It is important for the emergency department nurse to know the impact perceptions have on communication and to understand the consequences if perceptions are not clarified and dealt with.

Regardless of the type or location of the emergent incident, one extremely important communication need is the ability to access emergency help. All agencies and communities that provide health care have a code or system that activates a call for help within an extremely short period of time. Most communities in the United States (but not all) now have a 911 access number for activating the emergency medical system. The single emergency-number concept was first established in 1968.[15] However, some areas still do not have this universal system. The nurse must know the code for activating or summoning help in these settings.

The importance of calling for help is reaffirmed by the algorithms of the American Heart Association. The 1992 algorithms mandate that if only one person responds to an emergency involving an adult, the first action after ascertaining unresponsiveness is to call for help.[8] If the victim is an infant, an attempt to provide assistance after assessment is the first response; then a call for help is placed. In each situation after calling for help, the nurse implements or continues lifesaving or supportive measures. Activation of the emergency system is imperative to allow for early provision of definitive care.

The chain of survival—early access, early cardiopulmonary resuscitation (CPR), early defibrillation, and early advanced care—is the principle that must be used in part or in whole for all emergent events.[8] Implementing this chain of survival requires excellent communication skills to elicit the appropriate emergency medical personnel, vehicle, and equipment and to direct care in a clear, concise manner.

Excellent communication skills are essential in dealing with the increasing occurrence of violence. Application of communication techniques to deescalate a pattern of violent behavior before it is out of control is a mandatory nursing behavior. Appropriate techniques to deescalate such a situation include a calm and interested demeanor, a lowered and controlled voice, and a willingness to avoid interrupting the verbal responses of those involved. If a nurse finds it impossible to apply these communication skills in a particular situation, another nurse must be asked to take over or assist.[10]

Other communicaton principles to apply in an environment of uncontrolled behavior include the following[10]:

1. Keep communication on the here and now, and make no promises.
2. Keep hands at waist level and open toward the other person to demonstrate nonverbally that you are hiding nothing.
3. Use the rule of five, that is, no more than five words in a sentence with all words less than five letters. For example, "Stand still now."
4. Communicate only requests that are achievable.
5. Avoid commands that include "should not" and "cannot" statements.

Consistent use of these principles can decrease the potential for uncontrolled behavior and improve communication.

## ENVIRONMENT

The nurse working in the emergency arena must focus on controlling environmental factors that can infringe on quality care. Noise is a major environmental factor and a significant stressor in the emergency department.[16] Nurses must make an effort to work quietly and to identify this approach (quiet work) as a standard for the emergency department. As new emergency departments are being constructed, soundproofing is being included wherever possible. However, many other noise-controlling behaviors can be implemented, including the following:

1. Setting all telephones on soft ring
2. Equipping all dispatch radios with telecommunication devices that limit the broadcast to one person (e.g., earphones, telephones)
3. Setting alarms on monitors as low as safely possible
4. Closing doors quietly and as appropriate

The implementation of these few activities will greatly enhance the quality of the caregiving environment.

Another group of factors that should be of concern to nurses in emergency departments are environmental characteristics that contribute to violence: long waiting times, unpleasant waiting areas, lack of access to refreshments, insufficient and uncomfortable seating, and no feedback to patients and significant others regarding a patient's condition or progress. Attention to these environmental details deescalates the potential for violent behavior and provides a safer working environment.

Nurses need to evaluate the care provided in emergency departments to identify ways to decrease waiting times, a period that seems endless to persons waiting. Nurses are among the primary communicators with patients and significant others. They keep patients and significant others informed of planned treatments and other updates with care. In addition, the emergency department nurse's involvement with constructing a new emergency department or remodeling the existing department is paramount. The nurse provides input to the building committee, architects, and administrators about the needs of the emergency department patient treatment area to enhance care and the design of the patient and family waiting areas.

## LEGAL CONSIDERATIONS

Nurses must be aware of emergency department cases that require reporting as mandated by local and state jurisdictions, for example, suspected child and elder abuse, accidental deaths, suicides. Each emergency department will have written policies and procedures to assist nurses and other health care givers in making appropriate reports.

The chain of evidence (e.g., securing of clothing and specimens from rape victims, security of evidence from victims of violent acts) must be preserved at all times. Security of evidence is mandated by local and state laws for any reportable situation. The evidence usually requires constant vigilance by the emergency department staff (usually the RN) until it is officially turned over to the local or state authorities. Each emergency department will have written policies and procedures to assure staff obtain, label, and secure specimens according to regulations to maintain chain of evidence.

# TRAUMA

The systems (e.g., emergency medical alert and communication networks, transportation vehicles, fire and police resources, trauma centers) that support a person who has been involved in a traumatic situation have become more sophisticated within the past 20 years. Familiarity with the trauma system in the community, awareness of the cost of trauma to the community, and dissemination of information about the impact of trauma on the nation's problems are part of the responsibility of nurses involved in trauma care.

**Trauma,** which is the most common cause of death in persons younger than 40 years, is the leading killer of one of the nation's most valued resources—young people.[4] It is the fourth leading cause of death in persons of all age-groups; more than 60 million injuries occur

**TABLE 28-1 Year 2000 National Health Objectives for Unintentional Injuries**

| CATEGORY | TARGET RATE | 1987 RATE |
|---|---|---|
| **DEATHS (PER 100,000)** | | |
| All unintentional injuries | <29.3 | 34.5 |
| Motor vehicle crashes | <16.8 | 18.8 |
| Fall or fall-related injuries | <2.3 | 2.7 |
| Drowning | <1.3 | 2.1 |
| Residential fires | <1.2 | 1.5 |
| **HOSPITALIZATIONS (PER 100,000)** | | |
| Hip fractures (age 65+) | <607 | 714 |
| Nonfatal poisoning | <88 | 103 |
| Nonfatal head injuries | <106 | 125 |
| Nonfatal spinal cord injuries | <5 | 5.9 |
| **RISK-REDUCTION OBJECTIVES** | | |
| Use of occupant protection systems (seat belts, inflatable safety restraints, child safety seats) | >85% | 42% |
| Use of helmets | | |
| Motorcyclists | >80% | 60% |
| Bicyclists | >50% | 8% |

From the US Department of Health and Human Services, Public Health Service: *Healthy people 2000: national health promotion and disease prevention objectives,* Washington, DC, 1990, US Government Printing Office.

**BOX 28-3 Measures to Increase Home Safety**

**FLOORS**

Anchor large rugs and carpets.
Use nonskid backing on small rugs.
Avoid floor wax unless nonskid.

**STAIRS**

Ensure uniform height.
Use nonskid treads.
Mark risers with contrasting color.
Have strong hand rails at appropriate heights.
Have adequate lighting.

**BATHROOM**

Have hand rails in tub or shower.
Use skidproof bath mats.
Apply treads in tub or shower floor.
Have shower seat for elderly or unstable persons.

annually in this country. Unintentional injuries are a major source of morbidity and mortality in the United States; therefore accident prevention is a major public health goal.[29] The U.S. Public Health Service and the American Public Health Association actively promote accident prevention. National health care objectives for the year 2000, derived under the direction of the Department of Health and Human Services and the Public Health Service, are listed in Table 28-1. Suggestions for achieving these goals include the following:

1. Enacting laws
   a. Requiring use of vehicle safety belts and motorcycle helmets
   b. Requiring that handguns be designed to minimize the likelihood of accidental discharge, especially by children
   c. Requiring installation of sprinkler systems in residences where fire hazards exist
2. Increasing functional smoke detectors to at least one per floor of every residence
3. Teaching injury prevention and control in all schools
4. Requiring use of effective head, face, eye, and mouth protection for sports that pose risk of injury
5. Improving signs, signals, markings, and lighting of roads for increased visibility

This discussion on care of the trauma patient first focuses on prevention of trauma in general. Then principles of out-of-hospital care are presented. Finally, an overview of general care of the trauma patient in the emergency department is detailed.

## PREVENTION OF TRAUMA

Accidents are the underlying cause of trauma. Although there is no single cause of accidents, human error is a predominant factor. Onset of illness such as a cerebrovascular accident or myocardial infarction accounts for only a small percentage of accidents. More than one half of all accidents that involve motor vehicles are the result of improper driving practices or human error. A much smaller percentage of accidents are caused by vehicle defect or poor road conditions. Alcohol is a factor in approximately 50% to 75% of fatal motor vehicle crashes.[4] Illegal drugs, as well as many legally prescribed medications, can cause a slowing of reaction time, thus contributing to the occurrence of accidents.

The home is a dangerous place. Accidents that occurred in and around the home have resulted in tens of thousands of deaths and millions of disabling injuries.[27] Falls, which accounted for about one half of the deaths as a result of trauma in the home, usually are preventable. Falls frequently occur as persons, particularly those who are elderly, walk from room to room. Some falls are caused by heavily waxed floors, loose rugs, poor lighting, scattered toys, and other conditions that could have been corrected (Box 28-3). People fall from roofs, windows, high ladders, and steps, often because they have not used proper equipment or precautions.

Burns and other injuries result from improper use of solvents and cleansing agents. The number of electrical appliances used in the home has increased the danger of electrical shock and fire from overloaded circuits. Many persons die in fires caused by burning cigarette ashes dropped on furniture or rugs or discarded in waste containers and by cigarettes that are dropped when the smoker falls asleep. Homeowners with older heating systems need to be taught to have these systems checked for gas leaks or other unsafe features. Members of a household should hold fire drills and know what to do if a fire occurs. Smoke alarms in kitchens, bedrooms, hallways, and basements should be considered essential.

Children are the victims of most accidental poisonings, although adults also are at risk. All poisonous substances should be kept in original containers, tightly capped, and *never* placed in containers such as soft-drink containers, drinking glasses, or cups. Medications should never be removed from the source bottle and placed in an unmarked bottle. Likewise, medications should never be taken from unmarked or poorly marked containers.

Nurses working in home health care can assess the safety of the home during home visits and teach accident-prevention measures.

Criminal violence, including child abuse and domestic violence, and injuries from bullets, bombs, and sporting injuries—although representing a smaller portion of the total number of deaths or cases requiring hospitalization—are among the major causes of traumatic accidents. These causes also are preventable.

Nurses should alert the public to the importance of accident prevention. As participants in legislative activities, community committees, and community education, nurses must continually emphasize the role of human error and violence in trauma. In all activities the need is for emphasis on prevention as the primary method for decreasing the effects and related costs of trauma to society.

## GOOD SAMARITAN STATUTE

Nurses potentially encounter trauma situations as bystanders or because of trauma to family members. When an off-duty nurse happens on an accident, there is an ethical and moral, if not a legal, duty to stop and render assistance. To encourage professionals to help accident victims, the legislatures of all states have passed statutes that grant health care professionals immunity from liability for negligent acts. These statutes, named after the biblical "Good Samaritan," state that a health care professional who stops and aids accident victims without compensation will not be liable for untoward results related to his/her acts.

There is, of course, an exception to the **Good Samaritan statute.** The law does not exempt a nurse from acts that constitute gross negligence. The statute states that if care was rendered in good faith and an emergency existed, the nurse will be free from liability. If, however, the nurse acts willfully, with gross negligence, a judgment of liability is possible.

## TRAUMA CENTERS

**Trauma centers** are classified according to national designations that are implemented by state rules and regulations. Facilities are classified as level I, level II, or level III trauma centers. Level I–designated facilities are usually tertiary referral centers located in large metropolitan areas and have a strong commitment to manage all types of trauma and emergencies. To offset the cost of the trauma service, as well as to ensure that clinical skills are maintained at a high level, at least 1000 trauma patients per year are treated. The immediate availability of specialists and clinicians 24 hours a day is mandatory for a level I trauma care facility.[4] Level II trauma facilities have similar characteristics, with the exception of in-house availability of specialists. Specialists are on call and must be available within an established time frame, usually 20 to 30 minutes.[4] Level III facilities are most often located in smaller institutions in communities in which a level I or II facility is unavailable. Level III centers have a commitment to adequately stabilize trauma patients and clear and concise protocols for transfer to level I or II facilities.[6] Facilities may elect to have a non-trauma emergency department. This designation needs to be clearly communicated to the local community and emergency medical systems.

**BOX 28-4 First-Aid Principles for Use at Scene of Accident or Injury**

1. Remove the patient from a hazard only when the risk (e.g., fire) outweighs the danger of moving the patient.
2. Call for help.
3. Establish an airway, usually by elevating the jaw (see Chapter 30).
4. Initiate cardiopulmonary resuscitation (CPR) as indicated (see Chapter 30).
5. Control obvious hemorrhage, usually with direct pressure.
6. Splint spine and extremity injuries.
7. Transport as soon as possible.

## TRAUMA CARE

### Assessment, Analysis, and Action

In trauma care the nurse must be familiar with first-aid principles at the scene of an accident or injury. These principles are summarized in Box 28-4 in order of priority. They demonstrate the continual interaction among assessment, analysis, and action. To apply these principles at the scene of an accident, the nurse or other trauma health care professionals conduct what is called a **primary survey:** airway, breathing, circulation, hemorrhage, neurologic status, and behavior. This primary survey usually is conducted in the prehospital system and is repeated on arrival in the emergency department. These assessments are executed very rapidly and always are performed in a systematic way.[15] A secondary survey is completed in the field when help arrives and is repeated on arrival at the emergency department. A **secondary survey** is conducted to detect problems that do not pose an immediate threat to life but that can become more serious or life-threatening if not treated.

## TRAUMA FLOW RECORD

PATIENT'S NAME ____________________

MEDICAL RECORD NUMBER ____________________

| DATE | TIME ARRIVED | BROUGHT BY | LAST TETANUS |
|---|---|---|---|
| AGE | SEX | WEIGHT | ALLERGIES |
| Hx OF TRAUMA | | | |
| | | | TEAM ACTIVATION ___ Y ___ N |

| | TEAM | TRAUMA SURGEON | ANESTHESIA/MD | CRNA | ORTHOPEDIST | NEUROSURGEON | OR CREW |
|---|---|---|---|---|---|---|---|
| NAME | XXXXXXXXX | | | | | | |
| TIME CALLED | | | | | | | |
| TIME ARRIVED | XXXXXXXXX | | | | | | |

**ON ARRIVAL**

MAST PANTS _____ ON _____ NONE
RIGHT LEG INFLATED _____ Y _____ N
LEFT LEG INFLATED _____ Y _____ N
ABDOMEN INFLATED _____ Y _____ N
NECK IMMOBILIZED _____ Y _____ N
ON SPINE BOARD _____ Y _____ N
SPLINT ____________________
IV'S – SITE _____ FLUID _____ INFUSED ____________
SITE _____ FLUID _____ INFUSED ____________
_____ –TOTAL FLUID INFUSED PREHOSPITAL
CARDIAC MONITOR _____ Y _____ N
AIRWAY _____ ORAL _____ NASAL _____ MASK _____ EOA
_____ CANNULA _____ ET _____ NT( _____ Rt. _____ Lt.)
NASOGASTRIC TUBE _____ Y _____ N (_____ Rt. _____ Lt.)
FOLEY _____ Y _____ N
OTHER ____________________

1. ABRASION
2. AVULSION
3. BURN
4. CONTUSION
5. CREPITUS
6. ECCHYMOSIS
7. PENETRATION
8. HEMATOMA
9. LACERATION
10. OPEN FRACTURE
11. DEFORMITY
12. PAIN

**PRIMARY**

AIRWAY _____ OPEN _____ OBSTRUCTED _____ INTUBATED — FIRST M.D. EXAMINER ____________ TIME ______
C-COLLAR ON _____ YES _____ NO
BREATHING _____ NORMAL _____ LABORED _____ NOT BREATHING _____ ETOH ON BREATH
CIRCULATION _____ PULSES PRESENT _____ PULSES NOT PALPATED _____ CARDIAC RHYTHM PRESENT
HEMORRHAGE _____ GROSS (AREA ____________________ ) _____ NONE
NEURO STATUS _____ ORIENTED & CONVERSES _____ DISORIENTED & CONVERSES _____ INAPPROPRIATE WORDS
_____ INCOMPREHENSIBLE SOUNDS _____ MOVEMENT TO PAIN ONLY _____ NO RESPONSE
– BEHAVIOR _____ COOPERATIVE _____ UNCOOPERATIVE _____ COMBATIVE _____ OTHER ( ____________ )

**SECONDARY SURVEY**

HEAD _____ NO EVIDENCE OF INJURY _____ LACERATIONS _____ ABRASIONS _____ CONTUSIONS _____ SWELLING
EYES _____ OPEN SPONTANEOUSLY _____ TO VERBAL STIMULI _____ TO PAIN _____ DO NOT OPEN _____ UNABLE TO ASSESS
LEFT PUPIL _____ REACTIVE _____ CONSTRICTED _____ FIXED/SMALL _____ FIXED/MID _____ FIXED/DILATED _____ NOT ASSESSED
RIGHT PUPIL _____ REACTIVE _____ CONSTRICTED _____ FIXED/SMALL _____ FIXED/MID _____ FIXED/DILATED _____ NOT ASSESSED
NECK _____ NORMAL _____ ABRASIONS _____ LACERATIONS _____ SWELLING _____ VEINS DILATED _____ TRACHEA DEVIATED
CHEST – Rt. _____ CLEAR _____ LACERATIONS _____ PENETRATING WOUNDS _____ FLAIL _____ HEMOPNEUMOTHORAX
Lt. _____ CLEAR _____ LACERATIONS _____ PENETRATION WOUNDS _____ FLAIL _____ HEMOPNEUMOTHORAX
HEART _____ NORMAL SOUNDS/RHYTHM _____ SOUNDS MUFFLED _____ RHYTHM IRREGULAR _____ NO SOUNDS
ABDOMEN _____ SOFT _____ RIGID _____ TENDER – _____ RUQ _____ LUQ _____ RLQ _____ LLQ _____ LACERATIONS _____ CONTUSIONS _____ ABRASION
PELVIS _____ SOLID _____ TENDER/UNSTABLE
EXTREMITIES – LEFT ARM _____ NORMAL _____ ABRASIONS _____ LACERATIONS _____ DEFORMITIES _____ SWELLING _____ OPEN Fx.
RIGHT ARM _____ NORMAL _____ ABRASIONS _____ LACERATIONS _____ DEFORMITIES _____ SWELLING _____ OPEN Fx.
LEFT LEG _____ NORMAL _____ ABRASIONS _____ LACERATIONS _____ DEFORMITIES _____ SWELLING _____ OPEN Fx.
RIGHT LEG _____ NORMAL _____ ABRASIONS _____ LACERATIONS _____ DEFORMITIES _____ SWELLING _____ OPEN Fx.
PULSES PRESENT – LEFT ARM _____ Y _____ N RIGHT ARM _____ Y _____ N LEFT LEG _____ Y _____ N RIGHT LEG _____ Y _____ N
BACK/SPINE _____ NORMAL _____ ABRASIONS _____ LACERATIONS _____ CONTUSIONS _____ DEFORMITIES _____ TENDERNESS
SKIN _____ WARM _____ COOL _____ CLAMMY _____ DRY _____ DIAPHORETIC _____ PALE _____ FLUSHED _____ CYANOTIC/MOTTLED
OTHER ____________________

**FIGURE 28-1** Trauma flow record. (Modified from St. Joseph Health Center, Kansas City, Mo.)

PATIENT'S NAME ______________________

MEDICAL RECORD NUMBER ______________________

| TIME | BP/Rt. | BP/Lt. | P | R | T. | TIMES DONE OR INSERTED | | | | | | | | | | | | | | | | COMMENTS |
|---|---|---|---|---|---|---|---|---|---|---|---|---|---|---|---|---|---|---|---|---|---|---|
| | | | | | | NG | FOLEY | URINE | DIPSTICK | DPL | ABG | Lab. | BLOOD | AVAILABLE | CERVICAL | SPINE | CXR | PELVIS | TO CT SCAN | FROM CT SCAN | OTHERS | XRAY | |
| | | | | | | | | | | | | | | | | | | | | | | |

| REVISED TRAUMA SCORE | | | ADM | 1HR | DIS |
|---|---|---|---|---|---|
| RESPIRATORY RATE/MIN | 10-29 | 4 | | | |
| | >29 | 3 | | | |
| | 6-9 | 2 | | | |
| | 1-5 | 1 | | | |
| | 0 | 0 | | | |
| SYSTOLIC BLOOD PRESSURE | >89 | 4 | | | |
| | 76-89 | 3 | | | |
| | 50-75 | 2 | | | |
| | 1-49 | 1 | | | |
| | 0 | 0 | | | |
| REVISED T S | SUBTOTAL | | | | |

| GLASGOW COMA SCALE | | | ADM | 1HR | DIS |
|---|---|---|---|---|---|
| EYE OPENING | SPONTANEOUS | 4 | | | |
| | TO VOICE | 3 | | | |
| | TO PAIN | 2 | | | |
| | NONE | 1 | | | |
| VERBAL RESPONSE | ORIENTED | 5 | | | |
| | CONFUSED | 4 | | | |
| | INAPPROPRIATE WORDS | 3 | | | |
| | INCOMPREHENSIBLE WORDS | 2 | | | |
| | NONE | 1 | | | |
| MOTOR RESPONSE | OBEYS COMMANDS | 6 | | | |
| | PURPOSEFUL | 5 | | | |
| | WITHDRAWS | 4 | | | |
| | FLEXION | 3 | | | |
| | EXTENSION | 2 | | | |
| | NONE | 1 | | | |
| GLASGOW COMA SCALE TOTAL | | | | | |

| TOTAL GCS POINTS 13-15=4, 9-12=3, 6-8=2, 4-5=1 | | ADM | 1HR | DIS |
|---|---|---|---|---|
| GLASGOW COMA SCALE POINTS | | | | |
| TOTAL TRAUMA SCORE (REVISED T S + GCS PTS) | | | | |
| RIGHT PUPIL | SIZE RESPONSE | | | |
| LEFT PUPIL | SIZE RESPONSE | | | |

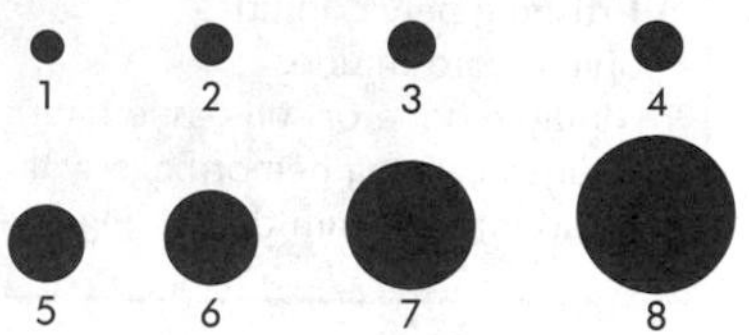


**FIGURE 28-2** Ongoing trauma flow record. (Modified from St. Joseph Health Center, Kansas City, Mo.)

Figure 28-1 presents information on complete primary and secondary surveys.

The primary and secondary surveys begin the initial cycle of trauma care[6]:

1. Cycle I, field stabilization and resuscitation
2. Cycle II, in-house resuscitation and operative phase
3. Cycle III, critical care
4. Cycle IV, intermediate care
5. Cycle V, rehabilitation.

After primary and secondary surveys are completed in the field, a determination is made regarding additional interventions and transport to the most appropriate facility.

Assessment of the trauma patient is a priority intervention for the nurse in a trauma situation. The primary and secondary surveys (Figure 28-1), as well as the continuous assessment (Figure 28-2), which require the nurse to be extremely proficient, are accomplished by use of techniques of auscultation, palpation, and observation.

Assessment, analysis, and action are ongoing in the trauma situation. Figure 28-2 depicts another portion of a trauma flow record, which reveals ongoing data that are recorded and reflects how some of the data from the primary and secondary survey are combined to identify a trauma score. Other information being collected and recorded includes fluids, medications, and blood or blood components that are administered and the response of the patient; urine, blood, nasogastric, and other secretion loss; and cardiac rate and rhythm strips.

Analysis of data occurs concurrently with data collection. Some of the major judgments demanded of the nurse caring for the patient who has experienced trauma are presented next.

### Multiple trauma

Many trauma patients sustain **multiple trauma** or injury to two or more body systems (Box 28-5). Motor vehicle crashes and falls, two major causes of trauma, may involve injury to the head or neck, an extremity, or chest/abdominal area. Penetrating wounds to the chest wall may also affect the abdomen.

Persons with severe injuries require intravenous fluids initiated as soon as possible to prevent or control shock. In the field or emergency room, two or three large-bore intravenous catheters are placed for administration of fluids and drugs. A central line may be inserted. An indwelling bladder catheter is inserted to monitor urinary output, as well as core body temperature.

In multiple trauma, the trauma team focuses on the highest priority problem of the particular patient first and then moves to the next problem. Some problems such as penetrating wounds of the heart and aorta require immediate surgery. At other times, if bleeding is controlled, surgery can be delayed while the team focuses on additional problems. Although the trauma team has priorities, the needs of the total patient must be kept in focus.

The trauma team must always consider that treatment of one system may add to the problems of another injured system. For example, large amounts of fluid given to prevent or alter renal problems may compromise an inadequate ventilatory system, leading to failure of both systems. Assessment, analysis, and action in trauma require focusing on these multiple-system problems.

**BOX 28-5 Severe Injuries Often Seen in Multiple Trauma**

Crushing and penetrating chest injuries
Crushing pelvic injuries
Spinal cord injuries
Multiple bone or soft tissue injuries
Injuries causing hemorrhage with shock
Head injuries with decreasing level of consciousness

### Respirations

The rate, depth, and character of respirations provide clues to the presence of ventilatory, CNS, or metabolic problems. Most trauma victims breathe a little faster than normal (18 to 24/min). In the presence of abnormal respiratory effort (nasal flaring; suprasternal, intercostal, or substernal retractions), the airway may be partially obstructed. The type of noise accompanying respirations may indicate the degree and location of a partial obstruction. The following findings suggest specific emergency care problems:

1. Rate
   a. Slow (below 10/min): ventilatory or CNS problems
   b. Rapid (above 26/min): hypoxia, acidosis, shock
2. Depth
   a. Shallow: shock, chest pain, chest injuries
   b. Deep: hypoxia, hypoglycemia, metabolic acidosis
3. Sounds
   a. Inspiratory stridor: upper airway obstruction (above tracheal bifurcation)
   b. Expiratory wheezes or stridor: lower airway obstruction
4. Frothy, blood-tinged sputum: lung injury, pulmonary edema, pulmonary embolus

### Circulation

Persons who sustain major trauma or a major stressor to the body usually develop shock (hypovolemic, neurogenic, multisystem failure shock). Signs of shock vary depending on the type or severity of shock. Clinical findings associated with shock include changes in cardiac rate and rhythm (tachycardia and dysrhythmias) and decrease in blood pressure. Most hemodynamic measurements (cardiac output, cardiac index, systemic vascular resistance, pulmonary artery pressure, pulmonary artery wedge pressure, central venous pressure, cardiac work index, stroke volume index, and stroke work index) are abnormal. The exact changes vary with the type of shock (see Chapter 22). Pulmonary congestion with changes in arterial blood gases can be present if respiratory contusion has occurred. Urinary output is decreased and can result in increases in blood urea nitrogen and serum creatinine levels. Skin temperature may be warm in neurogenic shock or cool in hypovolemic or multisystem failure shock. Skin color may change. Neurologic function usually is altered regardless of type of shock. Shock—its presentation and its treatment—is discussed in detail in Chapter 22.

### Level of consciousness

Level of consciousness usually is altered in trauma. But alterations in level of consciousness have many causes (Box 28-6).

When *shock* or *respiratory insufficiency* occurs, decreased oxygenation of the brain is present, either because of an insufficient amount of blood to carry the oxygen or decreased intake of oxygen. These conditions can lead to loss of consciousness. The *pupils will be equal and may be dilated.* (Normally, 20% of the population has slight differences in pupil size but both pupils react equally to light.)

When unconsciousness occurs because of the effect of *drugs* or *chemicals,* the pupils are *equal* and may be *constricted* or *dilated,* depending on the effect of the specific drug. Information from relatives may elicit data concerning history of diabetes, liver or kidney disease, and medication taken by the victim. Suggestive data such as an empty pill container can be useful in the identification of unconsciousness caused by drug overdose.

If there has been *trauma to the brain,* it is important to ascertain level of consciousness at different times. Temporary loss of consciousness followed by alertness and *equal pupils* usually indicates a *concussion.* If there is no skull fracture present, the patient simply is observed for 24 hours. Alertness after injury followed by increasing loss of consciousness usually indicates an *intracranial hematoma.* The pupils usually are *unequal.* Medical attention is urgent if an intracranial hematoma is suspected. The pupils *also may be unequal* if the patient has had a *cerebrovascular accident* (stroke). All assessment of level of consciousness includes the Glasgow coma scale (see Figure 28-2).

An unconscious person should be placed in a position that facilitates patency of the airway (side-lying position, also known as the *position of recovery,* is preferred unless contraindicated), and the respiratory status should be constantly monitored.

**BOX 28-6 Possible Causes of Changes in Level of Consciousness**

1. Hypoxia (decreased oxygen to brain)
   a. Respiratory insufficiency
      (1) Airway obstruction from foreign body, secretions
      (2) Pneumothorax
      (3) Spinal cord injury
   b. Shock
      (1) Cardiogenic cardiac arrest
      (2) Hypovolemic hemorrhage
      (3) Multisystem failure shock
2. Metabolic (chemical brain depressants)
   a. Extrinsic
      (1) Drugs: alcohol, narcotics, barbiturates, antihistamines, tranquilizers
      (2) Poisons: carbon monoxide, carbon tetrachloride, hydrocarbons, methane gas
   b. Intrinsic
      (1) Ketones: diabetic ketoacidosis, starvation
      (2) Glucose: hypoglycemia, hyperglycemia
      (3) Ammonia: liver failure
      (4) Urea: kidney failure
      (5) Hormonal hypofunction: hypothyroidism, adrenocortical insufficiency
      (6) Electrolyte imbalance: sodium, potassium, calcium, hydrogen ions
3. Brain pathologic conditions
   a. Trauma: concussion, brainstem contusion, intracranial hematoma
   b. Seizures: epilepsy, tumors, idiopathology
   c. Cerebrovascular accident: cerebral hemorrhage, thrombosis
   d. Tumors: benign, malignant
   e. Infections: meningitis, encephalitis

### Sensation

Trauma may cause *pain* if there is soft tissue injury, fracture, or visceral damage. Pain also may occur with tissue anoxia such as with obstruction of blood vessels or frostbite. Data are obtained from the patient concerning pain location (region), severity, quality, onset, duration, and provoking factors. One suggested approach for evaluating these parameters is the use of the mnemonic *PQRST*[23]:

**P** Provoking factors: what makes the pain worse or relieves it
**Q** Quality: dull, sharp, crushing, etc.
**R** Region or radiation: site and radiation to other areas
**S** Severity (on a scale of 1 to 10, where 1 is no pain and 10 is the worst imaginable pain)
**T** Time: onset, duration, constancy

For a further discussion of pain, see Chapter 17.

*Loss of sensation* may result from injury to peripheral nerves or nerves in the CNS. Peripheral nerve injuries may occur with fractures, lacerations, penetrating wounds, or dislocations. Loss of sensation concurrent with loss of movement and absence of local tissue or bone injury indicates CNS injury, such as spinal cord injury or cerebral hemorrhage.

### General Interventions in Trauma

Some general principles of management when accidental injuries or sudden illnesses occur serve as guidelines in giving first aid:

1. Remain calm and think before acting.
2. Identify yourself as a nurse to victim and bystanders.
3. Do a primary survey for *priority* data (cessation of breathing or heartbeat, interference with breathing, hemorrhage, coma).
4. Carry out measures as indicated by the primary survey (see Box 28-4).
5. Do a secondary survey.
6. Keep the victim lying down or in the position in which he or she is found (unless CPR is necessary), protected from dampness or cold. Position in a way that supports airway management and some degree of comfort.
7. Avoid unnecessary handling or moving of the victim; move the victim only if danger is present.
8. If the victim is conscious, explain what is occurring and provide assurance that help will be given.
9. Do not give oral fluids if there is a possibility of abdominal injury or if anesthesia will be necessary within a short time.
10. Do not transport the victim until all first-aid measures (e.g., immobilizing the spine) have been carried out and appropriate transportation is available.
11. Establish two peripheral intravenous lines with large-bore needles.

Lifesaving measures are implemented when the primary survey indicates the presence of breathing or circulatory difficulties. After breathing has been reestablished and excessive bleeding controlled, other interventions are carried out when the secondary survey is completed.

The victim is kept in a supine or sitting position, depending on symptoms, until all necessary interventions are carried out. Wounds are covered and fractures splinted before the victim is transported. Because shock is a possibility when major trauma occurs, the victim should be protected from chilling. On a cold day, protection may be needed underneath the victim, with sufficient covering to prevent loss of body heat but not cause vasodilation. Oral fluids are rarely given and then only to a conscious person showing signs of shock if there will be a considerable delay before medical care can be obtained and if abdominal injury is not present.

Trauma produces anxiety. It may be perceived by the victim as life-threatening and a source of pain and disability. The person may be unsure of what is happening, leading to a fear of the unknown. There may be concern about economic problems such as the cost of medical care and loss of time from work. In addition, many persons have been found to have already been experiencing some other temporary anxiety and were under stress immediately before the time of the accident.

The very nature of the experiences after the emergency contributes additional anxieties. The victim is transported, perhaps by strangers, in an ambulance to a hospital emergency department. Significant others are relegated to a waiting room, sometimes with little information provided. Victims may see or hear other persons who are upset. They may be alone. They may wait for long periods for medical attention and results of tests or treatment, whereas higher priority victims are receiving care. Small incidents become blown out of proportion, and a casual remark may be misinterpreted. Five minutes can seem like an hour.

Health personnel who work with trauma victims from the primary point of input into the health care system until the emergency is over are prepared to meet the physical life-threatening needs. Because these needs assume priority, it is easy to overlook the psychologic needs of the victim and significant others. A calm, interested approach that conveys concern to the victim as a person is helpful. Giving information frequently during all phases of emergency care to both patient and significant others will help them understand what is occurring and that help is being provided, thus decreasing some of the anxiety.

Varying levels of tolerance to stress are found in different individuals. Highly anxious persons may need someone to stay with them. At the scene of an accident a calm bystander can be helpful. Some hospitals provide selected volunteers for that purpose. All health personnel need to evaluate frequently their own effectiveness in assessing anxiety and in conveying understanding and emotional support to the victim and significant others during an emergency.

# CARE OF SELECTED EMERGENT CONDITIONS

## CARDIOVASCULAR SYSTEM

### Myocardial Infarction

The need for emergent care for myocardial infarction or for a cerebrovascular incident usually is identified from the primary survey. If the person's condition is not stable, basic life support or advanced cardiac life support measures are instituted. (See the American Heart Association's algorithms in Chapter 30). Once the person's condition is stabilized, measures to prevent further tissue damage are instituted. Myocardial infarction must be considered in a person who experiences sudden onset of chest pain without precipitating factors. The quality of substernal chest pain varies among individuals but usually is described as "squeezing," "crushing," or "heavy" and may radiate to the arms, jaw, or neck. The pain may be mild and described as "indigestion." The pain of myocardial infarction is not relieved by rest or nitroglycerin. The person may be apprehensive and experience diaphoresis, nausea and vomiting, lightheadedness, and dyspnea.

More than half of the deaths caused by myocardial infarction occur before the person is admitted to the hospital and within two hours after onset of symptoms.[4] Some communities have established mobile coronary care units that respond immediately in these situations with advanced life-support systems. After any emergency care, measures to maintain stabilization are implemented. These include the continued use of monitoring, fluid and pharmacologic support, and oxygen, if required. The conscious person may be more comfortable in a well-supported sitting position. A calm atmosphere is of utmost importance, and the person should never be left alone. Fear adds an additional stress to the already overburdened heart. (Myocardial infarction is discussed in Chapter 30.)

## Cardiac Tamponade

**Cardiac tamponade** is a compression of the heart resulting from leakage of blood into the pericardial sac. The accumulating blood cannot escape and exerts pressure against the heart, interfering with cardiac pumping. Pericardial lacerations from stab wounds tend to seal and cause tamponade, whereas gunshot wounds produce a larger opening with bleeding into the chest cavity. Symptoms of cardiac tamponade include neck vein distention from increased venous pressure, a paradoxical pulse (weaker during inspiration), dyspnea, and Kussmaul's respiration. The person is placed in high Fowler's position and transported to the hospital. Treatment consists of pericardiocentesis.

## Vascular Emergencies

### Aneurysms

Undiagnosed aneurysms are vascular emergencies because their potential to rupture is unknown. Aneurysms are outpouchings of arteries caused by a combination of congenital defects in the vascular wall and degenerative changes. When aneurysms rupture, several things happen: first, there is acute, severe pain; second, the patient can bleed to death immediately if it is an abdominal vessel; and third, flow to that part of the body is lost and can result in tissue damage or system failure. Aneurysms typically occur at bifurcation sites of major vessels such as the circle of Willis in the cerebrum or the abdominal aorta in the abdomen. The latter is commonly referred to as a "Triple A"—abdominal aortic aneurysm. Initial interventions for the emergent situation are establishment of two peripheral lines for volume replacement or pharmacologic access. High-flow oxygen via a mask or cannula is initiated, and pain control is necessary if the patient is hemodynamically stable and if the level of consciousness will not be compromised. A CT scan will be done immediately to confirm the presence of an aneurysm and to provide some clues on how to proceed.

Cerebral aneurysms may or may not be treated immediately with surgery. Persons with cerebral aneurysms need the institution of measures to prevent or decrease elevations in intracranial pressures (ICPs). Neurologic monitoring is implemented to identify any changes associated with increased ICP or rebleeding. Respiratory support with a ventilator may be necessary. After initiating hemodynamic and respiratory support measures and doing appropriate diagnostic tests, this patient is transferred to an ICU for the needed continual care (see Chapter 57 for discussion of cerebral aneurysms).

Abdominal aneurysms produce pain in the low back, abdomen, or groin. Acute pain and hypotension occur when the aneurysm ruptures. Abdominal aneurysms can rupture, and death occurs almost instantaneously. These aneurysms can dissect or leak, resulting in severe hemorrhage, instability of other organs or systems, and pain. In these situations, volume replacement and respiratory support are essential until the patient can be taken for emergency surgery. A CT scan may be done if time permits. The single most important intervention for a person who has a leaking or dissecting abdominal aneurysm is immediate surgery.

### Occlusions

Occlusions of portions of the vascular system because of thrombi or emboli are emergent situations. The thrombi or emboli can lodge or occlude an area of the peripheral venous system (venous thrombosis or thrombophlebitis) or pulmonary vasculature or the arterial system (coronary, cerebral, or peripheral). Occlusion of the arterial system is more dangerous, and the sequelae may not be as repairable as with the venous occlusion. A thrombus in its simplest form is a blood clot that occludes a vessel and remains in place. A thrombus becomes an embolus when it is dislodged from one vascular area and lodges in another vascular area causing an occlusion of blood flow distal to the area. Other particles such as air, fat, and intravenous catheter tubing also can act as emboli.

In patients coming to the emergency department, one of the most common occlusions seen is that of the coronary vessels. The patient usually presents with severe chest pain and other signs and symptoms of an acute myocardial infarction (AMI). Emergency management for the person with suspected MI is discussed on page 716.

Another type of emergent occlusion is an occlusion of a peripheral artery. This occlusion requires immediate attention, because circulation may be severely compromised with acute peripheral arterial occlusion. Often there are no pulses present; the use of an amplifying device for detecting a brachial or femoral pulse is required. The patient's history is extremely important and should focus on the onset of the problem and the time the extremity began to feel cool. History has a paramount role in the development of a differential diagnosis and in determining the underlying cause and therefore the appropriate intervention for a peripheral occlusion. The affected extremity needs to be treated very carefully because it can be easily traumatized. Pain is severe. Immediate surgery will be necessary if an occlusion is present (see Chapter 32 for the discussion of peripheral vascular system).

Disruption of the cerebral vascular flow commonly is caused by cerebral occlusions. However, cerebral hemorrhage also occurs. Patients entering with cerebral occlusion or hemorrhage may have various presenting complaints including unconsciousness, headache, or focal neurologic deficits. A detailed history is the most significant noninvasive diagnostic tool for differentiating a diagnosis of a cerebral thrombosis, cerebral embolism, or cerebral hemorrhage.

Cerebral thrombosis is the formation of an obstructing clot (thrombus) within one of the cerebral vessels. It usually occurs in persons 50 years of age and older. The history often includes the presence of atherosclerosis or transient ischemic attacks (TIAs). Acute and gradual onset of the symptoms is common. The patient may, in fact, experience temporary improvement. Signs and symptoms include mild headache, rare stiff neck, and, typically, difficulty in speech and weakness of an arm or leg.[3] Most thrombotic strokes occur following a period when the circulation is quiet. Thus most ischemic attacks from thrombosis occur between the hours of 8 AM and 12 noon.

*Cerebral embolism* is the obstruction of a cerebral artery by a clot formed elsewhere in the body that breaks loose and floats free. Cerebral emboli usually occur in middle-aged adults. The history frequently includes one or more of the following: rheumatic heart disease, cardiac dysrhythmias, anterior myocardial infarction (AMI), oral contraceptive use, sickle cell disease, and TIAs. Cerebral emboli often develop during physical activity and produce a neurologic deficit that is maximum at onset. There is an acute, very abrupt onset, moderate headache, and a rare stiff neck.[5]

*Cerebral hemorrhage* is bleeding into brain tissue caused by a rupture of a cerebral artery. The incidence of cerebral hemorrhage increases with age. There usually is a history of hypertension and an acute precipitous onset, such as severe headache, stiff neck, rapid loss of consciousness, and abnormal breathing.[5] See Chapters 56 and 57 for detailed discussion of assessment of the neurologic system and intervention for persons with cerebral thrombi, emboli, or hemorrhage.

## RESPIRATORY SYSTEM

### Chest Injuries

Injuries to the chest, either from penetrating or blunt trauma, may result in chest wounds, causing open or tension pneumothorax, hemothorax, flail chest, cardiac tamponade, or rib fractures (Table 28-2). These conditions are described in more detail in Chapter 37.

Persons with chest trauma are considered to have sustained serious injury until proved otherwise. Primary consideration in emergency management is maintenance of an open airway, breathing, and circulation. *Oxygen* is administered. Rapid transport after initial emergency measures is essential.

#### Open chest wounds

Chest wounds create a problem if there is intrusion into the pleural space. Air is drawn into the pleural space

**TABLE 28-2 Some Major Injuries Affecting Chest Wall and Pleural Cavity**

| INJURY | CAUSATIVE FACTORS | SIGNS AND SYMPTOMS | INITIAL EMERGENCY CARE |
|---|---|---|---|
| Rib fracture | Blow to chest | Pain on inspiration; local tenderness | Transport |
| Flail chest | Ribs fractured in more than one place; chest wall becomes unstable | Paradoxical respirations; respiratory distress; chest pain | Apply external pressure: sandbags, pillow, hand; give oxygen; transport with flail side down |
| Open pneumothorax (open sucking wound) | Penetrating trauma to chest; loss of subatmospheric intrathoracic pressure as air moves in and out of wound | Sucking sound on chest wall during inspirations; tracheal deviation | Cover wound with occlusive dressing; give oxygen |
| Simple pneumothorax | Laceration of pleurae, hyperinflation (blast injuries, driving accidents), loss of subatmospheric intrathoracic pressure | Sudden onset of chest pain: decreased breath sounds of affected area; dyspnea, tachypnea | Semi-Fowler's or Fowler's position; give oxygen |
| Tension pneumothorax | Complication of other types of pneumothorax; air enters pleural cavity but cannot escape | Respiratory distress; paradoxical chest movements; neck vein distention; tracheal deviation to unaffected side | Maintain airway and breathing; give oxygen; needle thoracotomy by trained person |
| Hemothorax | Blunt and penetrating chest injuries; injuries to major blood vessels and heart; blood collects in pleural cavity | Decreased breath sounds; dyspnea; cyanosis and signs of shock if severe | Treat for shock; give oxygen |

because of the existing subatmospheric pressure. The resultant increased pressure causes **pneumothorax** (collapse of the lung) (see Chapter 37). A sucking noise is heard as the air is drawn into the pleural space, and respirations are impaired. The opening should be covered immediately. A nonporous material may be used because air can pass through a standard dressing or material. Plastic wrap, which is not only nonporous but tends to cling to the skin, is excellent. If a porous dressing is used, it must be covered with petrolatum to create an air barrier. After the chest wound has been sealed, a pressure dressing is applied. Continual monitoring of respirations is indicated. If a nonporous dressing is applied the patient must be monitored for **tension pneumothroax.** With tension pneumothorax air enters the pleural cavity through a leak in the visceral pleurae with inspiration but cannot escape during expiration. Positive pressure builds up in the pleural space and causes a shift in mediastinal structures away from the affected side. This results in compression of the unaffected lung and decreased venous return to the heart (Figure 28-3).

### Flail chest

**Flail chest** results when multiple adjacent ribs are fractured in two places. The chest wall becomes unstable and responds paradoxically during inspiration; that is, the affected side falls with inspiration as the unaffected side rises. The opposite effect occurs with expiration. If ventilation becomes inadequate, atelectasis, hypercapnia, hypoxia, accumulation of secretions, and ineffective

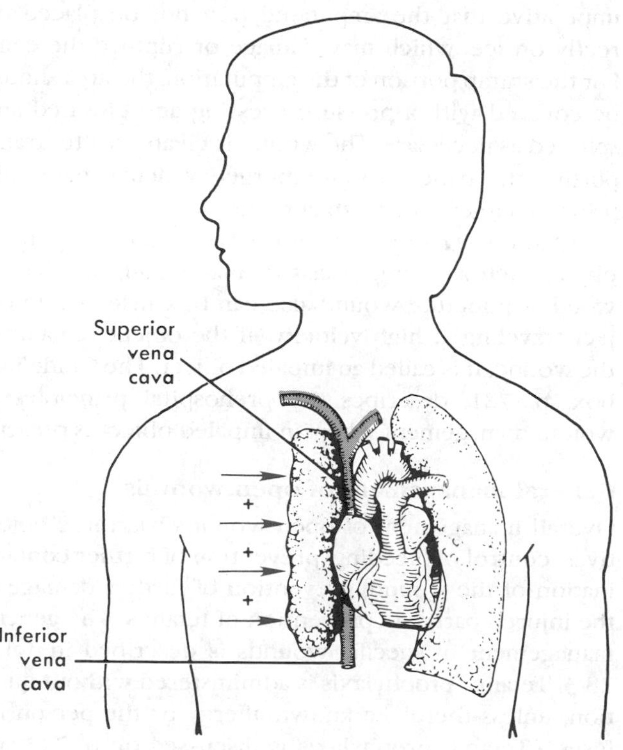


**FIGURE 28-3** Tension pneumothorax.

cough occur. Ventilatory assistance may be necessary (see Chapter 37).

### Near-drowning (immersion syndrome)

Drowning is a leading cause of accidental death in the United States. Many of these drownings occur in home swimming pools. **Near-drowning** is the term that refers to asphyxiation or partial asphyxiation from a fluid medium, with the person either recovering spontaneously or resuscitated at least temporarily. There are two types of drowning.[23,24] **Wet drowning** is the most common type and refers to *asphyxiation* from the aspiration of fluid into the lungs, inhaled as the person panics and gasps for breath. **Dry drowning** refers to asphyxiation from laryngospasm that prevents both air and water from entering the lungs.

The effect of water aspirated into the lungs depends on the amount and type of water. Salt water produces more severe changes than does fresh water. Fresh water is rapidly absorbed into the circulation, causing temporary hypervolemia, hemodilution, and intravascular hemolysis. Salt water, because of its hypertonicity, pulls fluids into the alveoli, causing persistent hypovolemia with hemoconcentration and pulmonary edema. Asphyxiation results in arterial hypoxemia and metabolic acidosis (from excess lactic acid formation). Neurologic damage may result from prolonged hypoxemia, and kidney damage may result from intravascular hemolysis.

If the victim of near-drowning has ceased breathing, artificial ventilation (see Chapter 37) is initiated as soon as possible, even before the victim has been completely removed from the water. If the carotid pulse is absent, cardiac resuscitation is started immediately. Time should not be wasted trying to remove water from the lungs. Persons who have experienced near-drowning need close observation for at least 24 hours, even if they indicate that they feel all right. Pulmonary edema resulting in severe respiratory distress can develop several hours later.[23,24]

**Postimmersion syndrome** is defined as death after submersion in very cold water. It is thought to be caused from dysrhythmias resulting from vagal stimulation.[23,24]

## INTEGUMENTARY SYSTEM
### Wounds

Wounds commonly are of two types: closed soft tissue injury and open (Table 28-3), with categories for each type of wound. *Closed soft tissue injury* is one in which there is damage to tissues beneath the skin but no break in the skin surface itself. Closed soft tissue injuries are termed *contusions* and *hematomas.* Both have discoloration (called *ecchymosis*) and usually are caused by a blunt force crushing the tissue and vessels beneath the skin. If there is no swelling, the injury is a *contusion.* If there is a lump or swelling, it is known as a *hematoma.* Basic interventions for these injuries are pressure dressings, ice, and elevation.

**TABLE 28-3 Types of Wounds**

| TYPE | DESCRIPTION | THERAPY |
|---|---|---|
| **CLOSED WOUND** | | |
| Contusion (bruise) | Injury by blunt object; blood vessels rupture, and blood seeps into tissue; edema from trauma to injured cells | Apply ice or cold compresses for 72 hours; analgesics for pain; elevate and rest injured part |
| **OPEN WOUNDS** | | |
| Abrasion | Scraping of skin surface (brush burn) | Wash well with soap and water; keep clean; no covering necessary* |
| Laceration | Jagged cut through skin and underlying tissue | Wash well with soap and water; edges approximated by "butterfly" adhesive or by suturing* |
| Incision | Straight cut through skin and underlying tissue by sharp knife | Same as for laceration |
| Avulsion | Skin or skin and underlying tissue torn loose but remain attached to the skin | Place skin over underlying tissue; cover with dressing; in emergency department the area is cleansed thoroughly and sutured* |
| Amputation | Skin or other body part torn from the body | See text* |
| Puncture | Penetration of skin and underlying tissue by sharp-pointed object; skin quickly seals over when object is removed | Soak wound; encourage bleeding in small wound to wash out bacteria; monitor for signs of infection* |
| Stab | Form of puncture wound by large object such as a knife, stick, or piece of glass | Do not remove object; stabilize object to prevent further damage; control bleeding; seek immediate medical attention* |

*Tetanus prophylaxis is given.

*Open wounds* are of four general types (Table 28-3): abrasions, lacerations, avulsion, and puncture wounds. Any open wounds should be assessed for the need for tetanus prophylaxis. If swelling exists, ice and elevation may also be used to treat these wounds. *Abrasions* are superficial and are caused by rubbing or scraping off the skin surface. They are typically painful and embedded with dirt, gravel, or other foreign materials.

*Lacerations* are cuts made with a sharp object such as a knife or piece of glass. They often are jagged, which distinguishes them from incisions, which are clean, smooth cuts. Lacerations can be superficial, involving only the skin itself, or may involve subcutaneous tissue, nerves, blood vessels, muscle, and even internal organs.

An *avulsion* occurs if the skin itself or the skin and underlying tissue are torn loose from the body and hang as a flap. As long as the skin remains attached to the body, it is an avulsion. When parts of the skin or body are torn away from the body, it is an *amputation.* All amputated tissue should be kept and brought with the patient; the potential for reattachment exists if prompt surgery or microsurgery is undertaken. The amputated part should be kept cool. The amputated part should be rinsed with sterile normal saline to free it of any contamination and wrapped in a sterile gauze dressing or clean material that has been soaked with sterile cool saline or lactated Ringer's.[12] If there is no access to these solutions, cool water will do until replacement with saline or lactated Ringer's is accomplished. The gauze-covered amputated part should be placed in a plastic bag or container of sterile saline and kept on ice. It is imperative that the amputated part not be placed directly on ice, which may damage or rupture the cells. For the stump portion of the amputation, the area should be covered with a pressure dressing and elevated and splinted as necessary. The wound is cleansed after transporting the patient to an emergency department, and prior to surgery for reattachment.

A *puncture wound* is a stab wound made by a pointed object such as a knife, scissors blade, nail, or sliver of wood. A puncture wound also can be caused by an object traveling at high velocity. If the object remains in the wound, it is called an impaled object. The Guidelines box, p. 721, describes the prehospital principles of wound management when an impaled object is present.

### General management of open wounds

Overall management of open wounds has three objectives: control of bleeding, prevention of further contamination of the wound, prevention of further damage of the injured part, and prevention of tetanus. The general management of specific wounds is described in Table 28-3. Tetanus prophylaxis is administered without question, unless there is a known allergy or the person refuses. (Tetanus prophylaxis is discussed on p. 722 and in Table 28-4.) Control of bleeding is described next.

## Guidelines for Prehospital Wound Management for Impaled Foreign Body

1. Do not remove the impaled object.
2. Control hemorrhage by direct pressure.
3. Do not apply pressure over the impaled object itself or over tissue that lies behind the cutting edge.
4. Stabilize the impaled object in place with a bulky dressing; do not shorten the impaled object.
5. Transport the patient without delay.

**TABLE 28-4 Tetanus Prophylaxis After Injury**

| PREVIOUS TETANUS TOXOID INJECTIONS | TYPE OF WOUND | PROPHYLAXIS |
|---|---|---|
| 3 or more | Clean, minor | <10 yr: none<br>>10 yr: tetanus toxoid |
| | All other | <5 yr: none<br>>5 yr: tetanus toxoid |
| Less than 3 or none | Clean, minor | Tetanus toxoid |
| | All other | Tetanus toxoid and tetanus immune globulin (TIG) |

From Diphtheria, tetanus, and pertussis guidelines for vaccine prophylaxis and other measures, *MMWR* 34:405-425, 1985.

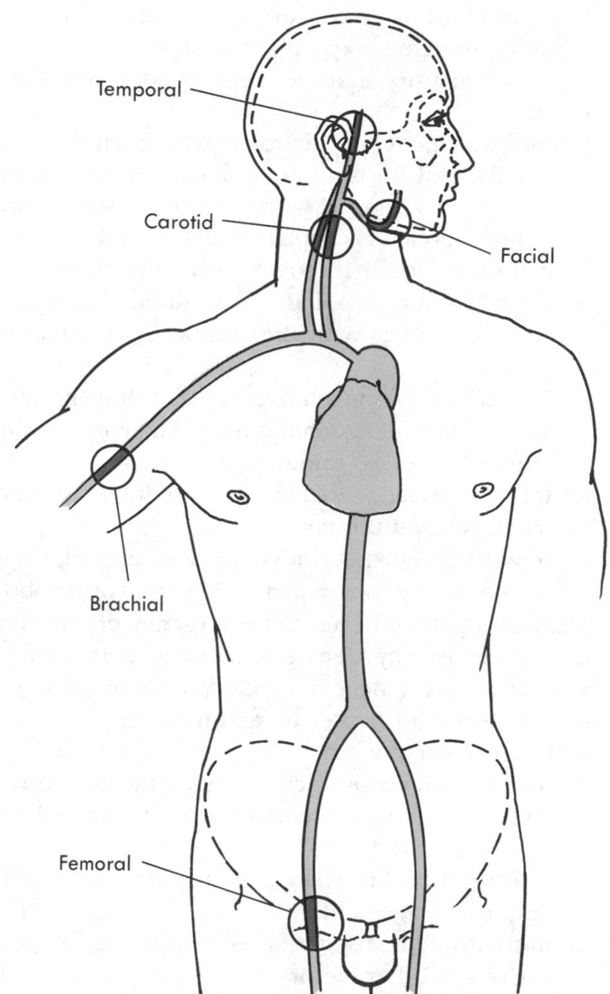


**FIGURE 28-4** Pressure points: location at which large blood vessels may be compressed against bone to help control hemorrhage.

**Control of bleeding.** Control of bleeding is achieved through application of direct pressure at **pressure points** (points where large vessels may be compressed against the bone). Initially it may be done manually and then with a pressure dressing. With severe bleeding from an extremity wound, the extremity should be splinted with some type of device that provides immobilization and a pressure dressing applied. Splinting devices may be anything available as long as immobilization is provided. If the bleeding cannot be controlled by the manual pressure or pressure dressing, point control should be tried. Point control is applied by hand pressure on the proximal artery above the injury (Figure 28-4). The use of a tourniquet is a last resort.

**Wound cleansing.** Research results indicate that the single most important factor for healing and prevention of wound infections is *cleansing.* This may be done by using irrigation techniques with copious amounts of normal saline. This intervention is usually initiated and completed in the emergency department. Some patients, however, need surgical intervention, and wound cleansing is continued in the operating room. Wound cleansing may include some type of bacteriostatic cleanser and, if so, the wound is then rinsed with normal saline.[2,25]

## Burns

Burns constitute the major cause of trauma to the integumentary system. Burns are caused by extremes of temperature, caustic chemicals, electrical current, or radiation. Thermal burns cause injury to 2 million persons every year. Approximately 100,000 victims are hospitalized, and 12,000 persons die.[12] The most common victims are children and elderly persons.

Appropriate care of persons with burns requires prompt, accurate first aid and emergency care. The initial care for burns at the site of injury includes the following measures:

1. Remove victim from source of burn.
2. With an electrical burn, if the victim is still in contact with the electrical source, do not touch the victim. Remove electrical source with a dry, nonconductive object.
3. After removal of the victim from the source of the

burn, establish a patent airway and assess for inhalation injury. Give oxygen if available.

4. Check circulatory status and ensure adequacy of circulation.
5. Initiate treatment specific for type of burn
   a. For thermal burn, remove nonadherent clothing and jewelry; cover with dressings (sterile preferred but clean acceptable) dampened with normal saline and then cover with a dry cover.
   b. If scald injury, cool the skin surface with cool solution. Cover with dressing as for thermal injuries.
   c. If chemical burn, remove any clothing and flush area with copious amounts of water for a minimum of 20 to 30 minutes.
   d. If tar or asphalt, cool tar with cool liquids. Do not try to peel off the tar.
   e. If radiation burns, remove contaminated clothing; be sure not to contaminate other areas of the body.
6. Transport patient to nearest emergency department.

In the emergency department, rapid and accurate care is necessary. The emergent care of burns is discussed in detail in Chapter 68 and includes:

1. Establish airway.
2. Initiate intravenous access; two large-bore catheters should be inserted. Frequently a central line will be inserted.
3. Insert indwelling Foley catheter for hourly urine output management.
4. Initiate fluid resuscitation as indicated by burn severity and other factors.
5. Insert nasogastric tube if appropriate.
6. Initiate pain management with intravenous morphine sulfate.
7. Provide tetanus prophylaxis (see below).
8. Transport or transfer to burn unit for wound care and continuous management of fluids, pain, etc.

### Tetanus Prophylaxis

Tetanus prophylaxis is a potential part of the intervention protocol for all open wounds regardless of the cause. The Centers for Disease Control and Prevention (CDC) in Atlanta has public education brochures available for distribution.[28] The current guidelines are described in Table 28-4. Tetanus toxoid is administered without question, unless there is a known allergy or the person refuses. Tetanus toxoid injection is administered to pregnant women without question; reassurance and pertinent information must be addressed. The determination to administer tetanus toxoid alone or as a combination of tetanus and diphtheria toxoid (dT 0.5 ml) is based on the history of the patient and current community practice. The most common practice is the combination prophylaxis. If there is a question about the contamination of the wound or if the history of the person indicates a questionable history about previous tetanus immunization, tetanus immune globulin (TIG) is administered with the tetanus toxoid (see Table 28-4).

## ENVIRONMENTAL INJURIES

### Heat-Related Injuries

In addition to burns, three common types of emergencies result from exposure to heat.

#### Heat cramps

**Heat cramps** are sudden muscle pains caused by loss of sodium chloride in perspiration and worsened by the dilution of serum sodium as a result of the person's drinking large quantities of water during strenuous exercise in hot weather. The best treatment is prevention by taking extra salt and water or drinking a balanced salt-containing fluid such as Gatorade when severe exertion is anticipated. The immediate treatment consists of salty fluids and foods by mouth, extra water, and rest for a few hours in a cooler environment.

#### Heat exhaustion

**Heat exhaustion** is vasomotor collapse caused by the inability of the body to supply the peripheral vessels adequately with sufficient fluids to produce the perspiration needed for cooling and yet meet vital tissue requirements. The condition usually follows an extended period of vigorous exercise in hot weather, particularly when a person has not had a period of acclimatization. Persons taking diuretics or experiencing diarrhea, particularly the elderly, are also at risk. The symptoms are faintness, weakness, headache, and sometimes nausea and vomiting. The skin is pale and moist. Body temperature can range from slightly above normal to very high. Heat exhaustion often can be prevented. "Extra Salt" was often used in athlete training in past years. Currently this practice is discouraged. Increased oral fluids is the first-line intervention; then salt is emphasized during very hot weather. Emergency care consists of treating for shock and transporting the victim to a medical center. Fluids, preferably containing salt, should be given.

#### Heat stroke

**Heat stroke** (sunstroke) is a serious condition in which excessive body heat is retained. It requires *immediate emergency treatment.* It is caused by a failure of the perspiration-regulating mechanism in the hypothalamus. Contributing factors include cardiovascular disease, alcoholism, obesity,[23] old age, prior febrile illness, and selected drugs (diuretics, sedatives, antipsychotics, and anticholinergics). Heat stroke typically is seen during a heat wave and may occur in healthy young persons who exercise vigorously in hot weather. The person undergoing vigorous exercise in intense heat may perspire profusely for some time and then become dehydrated and fail to produce sufficient perspiration to maintain normal body temperature. The skin is dry, hot, and flushed in contrast to the pale, moist skin of the person suffering from heat exhaustion. The victim becomes confused, dizzy, and faint and may quickly lose consciousness. Body temperature is usually above 41° C (106° F).

Without treatment most victims of heat stroke will die, but with prompt and vigorous treatment almost all will recover. Treatment consists of actions to reduce the body temperature immediately while transporting the victim to an emergency department. The victim should be placed in a cool place such as an air-conditioned room while awaiting transportation. The person should be wrapped in a wet sheet, and a fan should be used to increase evaporation. These measures are continued during transportation.

If the elevated temperature is allowed to persist, serious permanent damage to the brain and the entire nervous system can occur. Treatment is continued until the core (rectal) temperature has been lowered to at least 39° C (102° F), and the temperature must then be checked carefully for several hours for a sudden rise. The patient should respond when the temperature lowers. Failure to respond may indicate that brain damage has occurred. Persons do not recover from heat stroke as quickly as from heat exhaustion. Often there is faulty heat regulation for days and a lowered tolerance to heat for years and sometimes for life. The person who has had a heat stroke should be advised to plan activities so that repeated long exposures to heat are avoided.

## Cold-Related Injuries

### Accidental hypothermia

Hypothermia is a condition in which the core body temperature drops below 35° C (95° F). The extent of the cooling effect that occurs with exposure to extreme cold depends on the temperature and exposure time, the thermal conductivity of the environment, and the amount of air current present. Moisture is a good conductor; air is not. Wet clothing therefore contributes to increased cooling of the body. Several light layers of clothing to provide air insulation will keep a person warmer than one heavy layer. Air movement contributes to heat loss; thus lower environmental temperatures can be tolerated better in the absence of wind (wind-chill factor).

When the body is exposed to cold, shivering occurs to produce heat by increased metabolism. As the cold increases, shivering ceases and heat loss exceeds heat production. The person becomes listless, apathetic, and sleepy and may become indifferent to the surroundings and not seek adequate protection. Pulse and respirations become slower as metabolism decreases. Freezing of the extremities, unconsciousness, and finally death will result if help is not received.

The victim needs to be kept warm while being transferred to a medical facility. Wet clothing is removed immediately and warmed blankets applied. Rubbing the skin is to be avoided because this action can cause skin damage. Warm liquids may be given if the victim is conscious.

Core rewarming is the priority care given when the patient enters the health care setting. Core rewarming is achieved by blowing warm, humidified oxygen into the lungs.[23] The person suffering hypothermia should be monitored closely during rewarming. Hypovolemic shock can occur from vasodilation if peripheral areas are rewarmed faster than the core. Therefore fluid warming is mandated for persons who are hypothermic to prevent peripheral vasodilation. If intravenous fluids are given, overloading the circulation is a potential complication. Vital signs are monitored for sudden changes. Cardiac monitoring also may be indicated during the rewarming period to observe for signs of cardiac irritability, including ventricular fibrillation and cardiac arrest.

### Frostbite

Cellular injury occurs with exposure to extreme cold. Cell water freezes, and the resulting ice crystals damage the cell. The degree of injury depends on the depth of freezing. Frostbite occurs most frequently in exposed areas such as the nose, cheeks, ears, and fingers and can be prevented by adequate covering with loose-fitting dry clothing. Toes also are susceptible because of dampness and tight pressure from shoes or boots. Persons with circulatory problems are more prone to develop frostbite.

Frostbite can be classified as incipient, superficial, or deep. **Incipient frostbite** often goes unnoticed and is evidenced by paleness or loss of color of the skin. Removing the victim to a warm room, cupping the injured part with the hands, or placing fingers in the armpit for warmth may be all that is needed. Tingling occurs with warming.

**Superficial frostbite** may develop if incipient frostbite is not noticed. Freezing extends into the superficial tissue below the skin. The frozen part is soft, and white skin does not redden with pressure. Dark skin has a dull ashen shade. The frozen part may be warmed by covering. Heat is not applied because it may damage the injured tissue, but the frozen part may be immersed gently in warm water (43° C [110° F]) or warm soaks may be applied. Contrary to popular belief, the frozen part should never be rubbed with snow because this action increases the trauma to the injured tissue.

**Deep frostbite** is evidenced by hardness of the frozen tissue as a result of injury to deep subcutaneous tissue. After thawing, the skin becomes hyperemic and edematous with blister formation. The edema subsides in 24 to 48 hours, and tissue breakdown with necrosis results. The frozen part should be covered to warm it, and the victim should be taken to a medical center as soon as possible. The care is then similar to that for vascular disease of the extremities (see Chapter 32). Efforts are made to decrease the oxygen needs of the tissues while healing takes place, to improve blood supply by the use of drugs, and to prevent infection of open lesions. Necrotic tissue may have to be débrided for healing to occur.

## Bites

Animal bites constitute about 1% of emergency department visits. The most common perpetrators are dogs and cats (about 95%); however, rat bites and other types of animal bites are seen as well. Animal bites may result in puncture wounds, lacerations, and avulsions if the client pulls away from the animal while the animal's teeth are clenched. Dog bites crush the skin and underlying tissue or produce avulsion if the victim pulls away, whereas cat bites produce puncture wounds. Systemic manifestations of animal bites include hemorrhagic shock and death, cat-scratch fever, rat-bite fever, and tularemia. Additional information regarding signs and symptoms and care of persons with these diseases may be obtained from public health textbooks. Flushing the area with copious amounts of normal saline under high pressure, if in the emergency department, or with clean water if the incident occurs in the field, is the initial treatment of any animal bite. The bite is then treated with débridement and dressed with fluffy absorbent dressings. With any animal bite the potential for the person acquiring rabies must be considered. The safest and most pain-free way for determining the need for rabies therapy is impounding the animal for a 10-day observation period. If this is not possible, a decision concerning intervention must be made on the basis of the history of the bite. Tetanus prophylaxis should be administered.

### Spider bites

In the United States three types of spider bites prompt visits to the emergency department, the black widow spider, the brown recluse spider, and the tarantula.[12] Bites of the black widow spider and the brown recluse spider produce specific sequelae and require intervention. The tarantula bite, which produces a local reaction with rare systemic consequences, causes the most panic because of the appearance of the insect.

The black widow spider bite is difficult to find and usually produces a systemic reaction, sometimes involving a muscular response. The bite has a very specific appearance—two very tiny puncture wounds, with a halo appearing around the wound site. The initial treatment is to gently clean the area with soap and water, splint the site if an extremity is involved, and transport the person to the hospital. Splinting the limb prevents movement of the extremity, which diminishes absorption of the venom and it also alleviates pain. The specific intervention for this bite is to administer antivenom serum.

The brown recluse spider bite is classic and produces a textbook picture. Initially the bite is painless, but within a few hours blebs or purpura form and a local tingling or painful sensation starts. The area is very irregular in appearance, and blanching occurs as the area widens. There is eventually necrosis and sloughing, leaving a depressed scar. Systemic responses cause feelings of nausea or weakness. These symptoms often occur within the first 24 hours of the bite. The area must be cleansed gently, and application of a dry dressing is warranted. Additional treatment is based on individual symptoms and may include rest, antibiotics, and antiinflammatory medicines for muscle aches. Tetanus prophylaxis should be administered.

### Snake and fish bites

Snake and fish bites are considered emergency situations and must be treated specifically. Because these bites usually are confined to specific geographic regions of the country, it is wise to consult the state or region's poison control center for specific information about signs and symptoms and therapeutic interventions.

### Insect bites

Insect bites are common reasons for persons to seek emergency care. The most common perpetrators are fleas, lice, chiggers, mosquitos, wasps, bees, and ticks. The most important intervention for these bites is to obtain a detailed history from the person seeking attention. General questions include a description of the insect and outdoor activities. Questions regarding living conditions and pets in the house might be asked if the flea is considered the source of the bite. If lice are suspected, questions about hats, hairbrushes, and bed linen may be asked. If pubic lice are noted, questions about sexual activity are appropriate. The history provides the appropriate intervention strategies.

The most common insect bites that can produce severe reactions are those of wasps and bees. Death can occur either because of the number of bites (especially in young children) or from anaphylactic shock (see Chapter 70) if the victim is allergic to the protein in the venom. The reaction may be slow in developing or sudden and acute. Sensitized persons should avoid areas where bees and wasps are found and should have epinephrine (Adrenalin) available for immediate parenteral use if anaphylaxis occurs. The wearing of a Medic-Alert tag facilitates emergency care if the victim is unconscious.

When a person is stung by a bee, the stinger with the venom bag is left in the skin. The stinger should be removed immediately because venom continues to be pumped into the skin from the bag. Removal of the stinger by grasping and pulling is to be avoided inasmuch as this action pushes more venom into the skin. The stinger is removed by a scraping motion. Ice can be applied to prevent absorption of the venom (heat should be avoided). A paste of sodium bicarbonate and water or a weak solution of ammonia may help by counteracting the formic acid present in the venom. Adolph's meat tenderizer, containing papain, digests the protein in the venom. Individuals who severely react to bees and wasps should consider desensitization.

Tick bites can cause tick fever by transmission of a toxin, a virus as in Colorado tick fever, or rickettsiae as in Rocky Mountain spotted fever. Sudden removal of a tick will result in its mouthpiece remaining. Applying gasoline or turpentine to the head of a tick or applying the hot end of a previously lighted match to the body will cause the tick to drop off within 10 minutes. Care must be taken with any of these methods, since they might kill the tick but leave the head imbedded. Ice can be applied to reduce absorption of toxin.

Tick bites also may cause Lyme disease, seen mostly in the Northeast, Midwest, and West Coast of the United States, in some parts of Europe, and in Australia. The initial lesion begins with a reddened area that expands slowly with central clearing; it often is found in the groin, axilla, or thigh.[21,23] Flulike symptoms occur in about half the cases. Late symptoms include arthritic pains and chronic synovitis that may result in permanent disability. Tetracycline relieves early symptoms and may prevent late manifestations. Arthritis is treated with intravenous penicillin and refractory cases with ceftriaxone (a cephalosporin).

### Human bites

Human bites account for 0.2% of all emergency department visits.[12] The degree of injury is directly related to the force applied when the insult occurs. The oral hygiene of the assailant must be considered in developing intervention strategies for a human bite. Sequelae of a human bite include localized infections, the potential for a systemic response in the form of toxic shock syndrome (see Chapter 15), hepatitis (see Chapter 42), and infection with the human immunodeficiency virus (HIV) (Chapter 71). These systemic responses typically occur as the wound is healing or after it has healed. Care includes careful cleaning and vigorous irrigation of the wound. The decision to suture the wound requires judgment based on the time the incident occurred and the location of the wound.

Insect and human bite wounds require the same precautions for tetanus immunization as previously described on p. 722.

## MUSCULOSKELETAL SYSTEM

### Injuries of the Extremities

In evaluating persons with musculoskeletal injuries, a consistent and disciplined thought process for the assessment is imperative. The area *must always be visualized;* therefore all clothing must be cut away from the area that is injured. Any jewelry that might constrict circulation must be removed. Three major points must be addressed during the assessment phase: *history, signs of musculoskeletal injury, and signs of complications.*[9]

History includes the mechanism of injury, what forces were applied and in what direction, the presence of pain, the location of the pain, what sensations the patient experienced with the injury (hearing a snap, crackle, or pop), and presence of tenderness, numbness, or tingling in the injured area. Signs of musculoskeletal injury include deformity, unnatural motion, shortening of the extremity, swelling, redness or ecchymosis, painful or absent motion, grating of bone ends, or protrusion of bone ends from the wound. Signs of complications include absent distal pulses, absent sensation or motion distal to the injury, and signs of shock.

Injuries occurring to the musculoskeletal system usually are not life-threatening injuries with the exception of traumatic amputation with significant blood loss. However, shock, tachycardia, and hypotension may be present and require aggressive fluid resuscitation. Musculoskeletal injuries are managed after other injuries with higher priority have been evaluated and treated. The basic principle of care for a person who has a musculoskeletal injury is to splint the site. Immobilization by splinting accomplishes several objectives; it alleviates pain, prevents secondary injury, prevents a closed injury from becoming an open injury, and reduces local hemorrhage and swelling (see Guidelines box, p. 726). The amputated part should always be brought in with the patient for possible reattachment. (See p. 720 for management of the amputated part.)

Techniques of splinting include covering all open wounds with sterile dressings before splinting. All fractures that are angulated should be gently pulled into straight alignment (force should never be used). The examiner should not attempt to push exposed bone ends back beneath the skin. The site should be immobilized above and below the injury firmly enough to prevent movement but not so firmly to occlude circulation. Neurovascular integrity must be assessed before and after immobilization. Capillary refill and distal pulses must be evaluated after splinting. Distal pulses must be present, and capillary refill should be less than 2 seconds. The presence of diminished sensation of dullness and sharpness above and below the injured site must be addressed.

Splinting should be accomplished before moving any patient with a musculoskeletal injury. Types of splints used for immobilization are rigid, soft, and traction. After the area is immobilized with an appropriate splint, a cold pack should be applied to the injured area, which should be elevated above the level of the heart, if possible.

Other common musculoskeletal injuries include degloving, amputation (discussed in the section above), crushing injuries, compartment syndrome, and fat embolism syndrome. Degloving occurs in motor vehicle crashes (MVCs) or industrial accidents when shearing forces separate the skin from the underlying fascia. The result is disruption of circulation and tissue necrosis. The area involved must be cleansed and irrigated and prepared for extensive débridement and skin grafting.

Crushing injuries usually involve cellular destruction.

## Guidelines for Management of Fractures

1. Do not move patient before splinting a fracture (unless there is danger of fire, explosion, or radiation).
2. Cover open wound before splinting.
3. Support fractured bone and move it as little as possible while splinting.
4. Splint fracture in the position it is found.
5. In *severely angulated* fractures of the *shaft* of the extremity bone decrease muscle spasm and prevent damage to blood vessels by straightening severe angulation of bone shaft with the following procedure:
   a. Place one hand just below fracture and other hand farther down extremity
   b. Apply gentle traction to straighten extremity
   c. Maintain traction until extremity is splinted. Caution must be taken to prevent contaminated tissue from being pulled into the wound with this maneuver if an open fracture is present.
6. *Never* straighten deformities of a *joint* (shoulder, elbow, wrist, knee).
7. Apply splints to include joint above and below fracture.
8. Pad rigid splints (boards) for comfort.
9. Reinforce soft splints (pillows) with a rigid material such as a magazine or board.
10. If using air splint:
    a. Inflate only by mouth to a point where the thumb leaves a slight dent
    b. Keep fingers and toes free for assessment of circulation
11. Handle fractured part gently to prevent pain and shock.

Damage to the vascular network and nerve structures distal to the injury makes crushing injuries difficult to treat. Depending on the extent and severity of the crush injury, crush syndrome may follow. Hemorrhage from the damaged tissue, destruction of muscle and bone tissue, fluid loss possibly resulting in hypovolemic shock, and myoglobinuria resulting in renal failure, coma, and death are the possible complications associated with crush injuries.

The area of injury must be gently cleansed, active bleeding must be controlled, and the injured extremity must be elevated above the level of the heart to reduce swelling and pain. Hemodynamic status of the patient is supported with administration of blood, blood products, plasma expanders, colloids, or crystalloids and vasoactive medication as appropriate based on continual monitoring (see Chapter 22).

**Compartment syndrome** occurs as pressure—either from an internal source such as hemorrhage or edema or from an external source such as casts or medical antishock trousers (MAST)—and begins to increase inside the osteofascial space (compartment) of the forearm or lower leg. Compartment syndrome occurs in the distal portion of the upper and lower extremities. Compression of nerves, vasculature, and muscle tissue results. Symptoms associated with compartment syndrome include ischemic pain that cannot be controlled with pain medication and increased pain when the extremity is elevated above the level of the heart. In compartment syndrome the injured extremity must be elevated, but it must not be higher than the heart. If the extremity is higher than the level of the heart, arterial flow is compromsed, and decreased perfusion to the compromised extremity may occur. A pressure device is used to determine the compartment pressure: 20 mm Hg or less is normal, 21 to 40 mm Hg indicates decreased tissue perfusion, and 41 mm Hg or above indicates ischemia.[12] A fasciotomy (surgical incision of the tissue and muscle to relieve pressure) may be required to decrease the pressure and to prevent further tissue damage and the loss of the extremity. Compartment syndrome usually presents itself within 24 to 48 hours of injury.

Fat embolism most commonly occurs as a complication in a person with a fracture of the long bone or pelvis. A fat embolism is the result of fatty tissue being dislodged because of the fracture and moving into blood vessels that have been severed as a result of the injury. As the fat droplets are too large to pass through capillaries in the pulmonary system, they occlude a vessel in the pulmonary vascular system. The individual exhibits symptoms of tachypnea and hypoxia as seen with any pulmonary emboli. Petechiae also are seen (see Chapter 37). Interventions include high-flow oxygen and preparation for ventilatory support as needed. The extremity must be immobilized and provisions made for minimal movement of the extremity to prevent more displacement of the fatty tissue. Musculoskeletal injuries are discussed in detail in Chapter 64.

### Fracture of the Spine

Any questionable injury to the head, neck, or back is treated as a fracture of the spine. The victim should not be moved when being examined for fracture of the spine (neck or back). The examiner slides a hand under the victim and checks for point tenderness along the length of the spine. Bruises on the head may indicate that a force has been exerted that could cause a neck fracture. Bruises on the shoulder, back, or abdomen frequently are seen with back fractures, but a spinal fracture can be present in the absence of any bruises. If the spinal cord has been damaged, there may be loss of movement or sensation to the extremities. X-ray films of the neck/cervical area are obtained to determine any fractures when cervical trauma is suspected.

Two problems can occur from a fractured spine: damage to the spinal cord and neurogenic shock. If the cervical spine is fractured, there may be interference with respiration. Respiratory status must be continually monitored. The victim may use diaphragmatic breathing for a short period but be unable to sustain this. Artificial ventilation is more difficult in that the neck cannot be hyperextended because this movement can cause further injury to the spinal cord. The head can be extended by gentle traction and the jaw pulled forward to open the airway. Traction must be maintained until the neck can be supported in this position. *The neck should never be flexed, twisted, or hyperextended if a fracture is suspected.* If the victim is not having difficulty with respiration, the neck can be splinted in the position in which it was found.

The person with a potential spine fracture must be transported on a firm base, preferably a back board. *Forward or backward flexion of the spine is to be avoided* to prevent further trauma to the spinal cord. The victim should be slid, not rolled, in straight alignment onto the back board. It takes several persons working together to move the victim safely. The victim remains on the back board during the initial diagnostic tests in the emergency department.

Neurogenic shock is caused by a loss of sympathetic stimulation resulting in the body's inability to vasoconstrict. Resulting symptoms are usually tachycardia, hypotension, and lack of perfusion to vital organs; depressed cerebral, respiratory, and cardiac function is seen. Treatment is based on symptoms. Neurogenic shock and its treatment are discussed in Chapter 22.

## TOXICOLOGIC EMERGENCIES

A poison is a chemical agent capable of producing harmful effects on a biologic system. With excessive exposure, any chemical can become a poison. All toxicologic emergencies may be reported to the nearest poison control center, and in some states hospital licensing rules and regulations require that all toxicologic emergencies be reported.[17]

Poisoning, either unintentional or deliberate, remains a major cause of accidental deaths. On average there are 4000 deaths from poisoning in the United States each year.[29] Morbidity is higher in children than in adults. Poisoning in adults commonly occurs from not checking medication labels (overdose or wrong medication), from lack of knowledge (e.g., taking alcohol and sedatives together), from taking an excess amount in an attempt to obtain a desired effect, or from a suicide attempt.

### Common Accidental Poisoning Prevention

Education of the public is directed toward increasing awareness of safety hazards in the home, particularly in homes with children. Nonpotable liquids should be kept tightly capped in their original containers in places that are not easily accessible to children and should *never* be placed in a soft-drink bottle, drinking glass, or cup.

Patient teaching includes the following:

1. Read labels on *all* medication containers (prescription or over-the-counter drugs) before taking medication.
2. Read labels on all over-the-counter drugs to identify possible hazards.
3. Take all medications in the prescribed doses, following the prescribed directions.
4. Do not increase dosage outside of stated limits in an effort to increase a desired effect.

### Assessment

A *rapid* assessment is made to determine whether poisoning or overdose has occurred so that immediate action can be taken to prevent or diminish the effects of the poison or drug. Poisoning is suspected when there is a sudden onset of symptoms, especially in a young child. Symptoms vary, depending on the cause of the poisoning, but may include nausea and vomiting, abdominal pain, convulsions, change in level of consciousness, and decreased pulse and respiratory rates. The most common pattern of drug poisoning is coma with flaccid muscles and hypotension; this may be confused with head injury or metabolic states. Table 28-5 depicts common complications associated with drug intoxication, along with the causes.

If poisoning is suspected, the lips and mouth are examined for signs of burns, excessive salivation, or difficulty in swallowing. The breath is noted for an odor such as that from petroleum products or cleaning compounds. Care should be taken by emergency department staff to protect themselves (gloves, masks) from contamination, including blood and other body fluids, and chemicals. Pupillary changes may be noted with selected drugs (Box 28-7); some drugs such as the phenothiazines may cause either constricted or dilated pupils. Time should not be wasted looking for needle marks.

An accurate history regarding the incident needs to be obtained. Data are collected to identify (1) clues that poisoning is a possibility, (2) the type and quantity of the agent, and (3) how long ago the event occurred. A conscious victim is questioned for information concerning what and how much was taken. If the person is unconscious, identification of the poison or drug can be facilitated by asking others to look for clues while examining the victim. Empty containers, spilled fluids, open medication bottles, or syringes may provide needed information. *All* potential agents in their original containers should be gathered and taken to the hospital with the victim. The physician may need to know the

**BOX 28-7 Pupillary Changes With Selected Drugs**

| DILATED | CONSTRICTED |
|---|---|
| Anticholinergics | Opioids |
| Tricyclic antidepressants | Propoxyphene (Darvon) |
| Amphetamines | Organophosphate insecticides |
| Phenothiazines | Phenothiazines |
| Glutethimide (Doriden) | |
| Cocaine | |
| Hallucinogens | |

**TABLE 28-5 Complications of drug intoxication**

| FINDING | COMMON CAUSES* | FINDING | COMMON CAUSES* |
|---|---|---|---|
| Aspiration | Petroleum distillates/hydrocarbons | Hyperthermia | Phenothiazines |
| | Organophosphates | | CNS stimulants |
| | CNS depressants (chloral hydrate) | | Anticholinergics |
| | Antidepressants | | Salicylates |
| Behavioral disturbances | Anticholinergics | | Antidepressants |
| | Hallucinogens | Hypothermia | CNS depressants (barbiturates) |
| | Psychotropic drugs | | Alcohols (ethanol) |
| | Organic solvents | | Opiates |
| | CNS stimulants | Ileus | Narcotic analgesics |
| Bradycardia | Cardiac glycosides (digoxin) | | Anticholinergics |
| | Beta-adrenergic blockers (propranolol) | | Antidepressants |
| | | | Meprobamate |
| | Organophosphates | | |
| | Calcium channel blockers (nifedipine, verapamil) | Metabolic acidosis | Salicylates |
| | | | Alcohols (methanol, ethylene glycol) |
| Cardiac dysrhythmias | CNS stimulants (cocaine) | Nystagmus | Anticonvulsants |
| | Cardiovascular drugs | | CNS depressants |
| | Antidepressants | | Phencyclidine |
| | Theophylline | Pulmonary edema | Organophosphates |
| | Propoxyphene | | Salicylates |
| Coma, hyperreflexia, tachycardia, mydriasis | Antidepressants | | CNS depressants (ethchlorvynol) |
| | Anticholinergics/antihistamines | | Opiates |
| | Phenothiazines | | Antidepressants |
| Coma, hypotension, flaccidity | CNS depressants (barbiturates, benzodiazepines) | Restlessness, pyrexia, hyperreflexia | Anticholinergics |
| | | | Strychnine |
| | Ethanol | | Phencyclidine |
| | Opiates | | Amphetamines |
| Hallucinations | Antihistamines/anticholinergics | Seizures/hyperreflexia | CNS stimulants (cocaine) |
| | CNS stimulants | | Organophosphates |
| | Organic solvents | | Phencyclidine |
| | Hallucinogens (PCP, LSD) | | Propoxyphene |
| Hepatic failure | Acetaminophen | | Antidepressants |
| | Carbon tetrachloride | | Theophylline |
| | *Amanita* mushrooms | | Salicylates |
| | Isoniazid | | Hypoglycemic agents |
| Hyperpnea | CNS stimulants | Tachycardia | CNS stimulants |
| | Carbon monoxide | | Antihistamines/anticholinergics |
| | Salicylates | | Antidepressants |
| | Alcohols (methanol) | | Theophylline |

From Bauer RL, Watson WA: Clinical toxicology. In Stein JH, editor: *Internal Medicine,* ed 4, St Louis, 1994, Mosby.
*Substances in parentheses are common examples. CNS, central nervous system; PCP, phencyclidine hydrochloride; LSD, lysergic acid diethylamide.

ingredients of the agent for those situations in which an antidote is indicated.

### Interventions

Immediate action is necessary if poisoning is suspected; in some instances delay of a few minutes may make a difference between life and death. An *unconscious* victim must be transported *without delay* to the nearest medical facility, and the emergency medical system (EMS) should be employed (call 911).

If the victim is *conscious,* have someone call a physician immediately if possible. If a private physician is not available, a *poison control center* can give rapid and accurate information. Most large cities have poison control centers that maintain an extensive file on the most common substances and drugs. The telephone number usually is easily obtained from a list of emergency numbers in the front of the telephone directory.

Management consists of stopping absorption of the poisonous substances or drug and initiating supportive care. (see Guidelines box, p. 729). Poisonous substances can be inhaled, absorbed from the skin or mucous membranes, ingested, or injected. The type of intervention depends on the method by which the poison entered the system.

**Inhaled poison.** Persons who have inhaled a toxic gas first need to be removed from the site to fresh air and

### Guidelines to Stop Absorption of Poisons

**INHALED POISON**

1. Remove victim from source of toxic gas.
2. Assess cardiopulmonary status and give artificial ventilation if possible.
3. Give oxygen, if available.

**CONTACT POISON**

1. Rinse skin with copious amount of water.
2. Remove garments and rinse skin again.

**INGESTED POISON**

1. If person is conscious:
   a. Call physician or poison control center for assistance.
   b. Substances other than caustics or hydrocarbons:
      (1) Induce emesis by giving 15 to 30 ml syrup of ipecac; follow with full glass of warm water.
      (2) Inactivate poison by giving activated charcoal (especially after drug ingestion).
   c. Caustics or hydrocarbons (petroleum products):
      (1) Give nothing by mouth.
      (2) Seek immediate medical attention.
      (3) Do not induce emesis.
2. If person is unconscious, transport without delay to medical facility.

given oxygen if available. As in any emergency, cardiopulmonary status is assessed and resuscitation started if indicated. The victim is transported immediately to a medical center.

*Carbon monoxide* is one of the more common toxic gases. It is odorless and occurs as a result of incomplete combustion such as that which occurs during fires or from automobile exhaust. It cannot be filtered by the use of a cloth face mask. Toxicity occurs because of the higher affinity of hemoglobin for carbon monoxide than for oxygen. The victim becomes profoundly hypoxic and loses consciousness. Carboxyhemoglobin has a deep red color that is seen in the mucous membranes of all victims. It may also be noted on the skin of white or light-colored persons.

**Contact poison.** Poisonous substances absorbed through the skin or mucous membranes should be *rinsed* off immediately with *copious amounts of water* without taking time to remove garments. Then the garments that contain the substance are removed, and the skin is rinsed again. The person is placed in a shower if the body is involved.

**Ingested poison.** The most common form of poisoning is by ingestion of a poisonous substance or an excessive amount of a drug. Ingestion of drugs can affect almost every system of the body (see Table 28-5). Absorption of the agent can be prevented by inducing vomiting, by using lavage to eliminate the agent, and by giving a substance that will make the poisonous agent inert.

***Elimination of ingested poison.*** The first treatment objective is removal of the ingested poison (except with ingestion of caustics or hydrocarbons). *Vomiting* is the best method because gastric lavage does not remove substances in stomach pouches that are inaccessible to lavage. Lavage with a cuffed endotracheal tube to prevent aspiration is indicated for unconscious persons.

The recommended method of inducing vomiting is by the oral administration of 30 ml (15 ml for children) of *syrup of ipecac.* The dose may be repeated once in 20 minutes if necessary. The victim is encouraged to drink a glass of water 3 to 5 minutes after administration of the syrup of ipecac to promote complete emptying of the stomach. Mechanically induced vomiting, such as tickling the back of the throat, usually is ineffective because only a small amount is vomited.

*Caustic* substances such as lye erode the esophagus as they are ingested and frequently result in esophageal perforation and subsequent esophageal stenosis. Drinking acidic substances such as vinegar water or citrus juices to counteract the basic property of lye is *not* recommended because it may result in an exothermic reaction, causing additional pain and burning.[20] *Hydrocarbons,* which are found in all petroleum products, produce a severe pneumonia from direct aspiration into the lungs during ingestion. Emergency care for caustic or hydrocarbon ingestion consists in giving nothing by mouth and seeking immediate medical attention.

***Inactivation.*** Activated charcoal is an efficient method of inactivation of selected drugs, particularly analgesics (especially aspirin), barbiturates and other hypnotics, amphetamines, and tricyclic antidepressants. Activated charcoal will absorb a drug and prevent it from being absorbed by the gastrointestinal tract. It should be administered within 30 minutes of poisoning to achieve maximal effect but can be given later with good results. It is given *after* (neither before nor concurrently with) ipecac. Activated charcoal can be purchased at a drugstore (Nuchar A, Norit A, or Activated Charcoal by Merck). The adult dose is 50 to 100 g. It is often mixed with sorbitol. Saline laxatives are then given to remove the adsorbed poison because the absorption capacity of activated charcoal is reversible.[20]

***Antidotes.*** If it is known exactly what poisonous substance or drug has been ingested, a specific antidote may be given in some cases by the physician. See Table 28-6 for listing of antidotes for particular poisons. The use of a "universal antidote" has not proved to be effective.

**Injected poison.** Toxic substances can be injected through the skin such as by insect bites or needle injection. Drugs most commonly injected are heroin, barbiturates, and amphetamines. Stimulants such as the am-

**TABLE 28-6 Specific Antidotes**

| | ANTIDOTE | DOSAGES |
|---|---|---|
| Opiates (heroin, meperidine, propoxyphene, pentazocine, diphenoxylate) | Naloxone | Loading dose: From 0.4 to 2.0 mg iv; repeat in 2-5 min as necessary<br>Maintenance dose: sufficient to maintain desired level of consciousness |
| Organophosphates | Atropine | Loading dose: 2 mg iv or im every 2-5 min until hypersalivation is controlled<br>Maintenance dose: sufficient to suppress hypersalivation |
| Organophosphates | Pralidoxime | Loading dose: 1-2 g iv<br>Maintenance dose: 1-2 g after 2-3 hr |
| Methanol, ethylene glycol | Ethanol | Loading dose: 0.6-0.7 g/kg<br>Maintenance dose: sufficient EtOH* to maintain serum alcohol level at 100 mg/dl (approximately 125 mg/kg/hr) until methanol, ethylene glycol concentration <10 mg/dl |
| Cyanide | Amyl nitrite<br>Sodium nitrite<br>Sodium thiosulfate | Amyl nitrite ampuls inhaled every 2-3 min; monitor blood pressure; then 10 ml 3% sodium nitrite iv over 5 min; then 50 ml 25% sodium thiosulfate over 10 min |
| Iron salts | Deferoxamine | Hypotensive patients: 10 mg/kg/hr iv for 4 hr; then 5 mg/kg/hr iv for 8 hr, then 2-5 mg/kg/hr/iv until serum iron level is less than 100 μ/dl<br>Normotensive patients: 40 mg/kg im every 4-12 hr (total dose should not exceed 6 g/24 hr) |
| Acetaminophen | *N*-Acetylcysteine | 140 mg/kg po then 70 mg/kg every 4 hr po for 17 doses |
| Carbon monoxide | Oxygen | 100% by face mask or hyperbaric |
| Benzodiazepines | Flumazenil | Loading dose: 1-5 mg iv<br>Maintenance dose: sufficient to maintain desired level of consciousness |

From Bauer RL, Watson WA: Clinical toxicology. In Stein JH, editor: *Internal medicine,* ed 4, St Louis, 1994, Mosby.
*EtOH, ethylalcohol or ethanol.

phetamines produce hyperactivity and "uncooperative" behavior. Overdose may produce tachycardia, chills, and collapse. Depressants such as heroin or barbiturates produce respiratory depression, resulting in coma and death. Overdose often occurs because the victim is unaware of the potency of the drug purchased illegally. Substance abuse is discussed in Chapter 19.

### Supportive care

Nursing care of the acutely poisoned patient may make the difference between a favorable and a fatal outcome. Vital signs and mental status are the critical assessment factors. Keep the person warm enough to prevent chilling, and monitor closely for changes in physical signs such as rapid thready pulse, respiratory distress, cyanosis, diaphoresis, and other signs of vascular collapse, vasogenic shock, or impending death. Monitor vital signs at least every 15 minutes for several hours, and report changes to the physician immediately. Record symptoms of nausea, vomiting, and abdominal pain, and monitor all vomitus for signs of blood. Observe stools and urine for abnormal constituents such as blood. Maintain prescribed intravenous fluids.

Interventions for life-threatening conditions, such as airway maintenance and maintenance of blood pressure, are critical elements. If respirations are depressed, give prescribed oxygen, and suction as needed. Mechanical ventilation may be necessary. Turn unconscious patients frequently to provide drainage from each bronchus.

If the poisoning was a suicide attempt, institute safety precautions. Several major tranquilizers (especially tricyclic antidepressants) are extremely dangerous. Patients overdosing with these medicines require cardiac monitoring, other appropriate treatments, and continued medical follow-up. Psychiatric consultation often is recommended, and a psychiatric clinical nurse specialist can be a helpful resource. Monitor for withdrawal symptoms all persons addicted to heroin or morphine derivatives who have overdosed. Symptoms usually appear within 12 to 18 hours and include yawning, sweating, shaking, vomiting, diarrhea, lacrimation, runny nose, abdominal pain, backache, and other flulike symptoms (see Chapter 19).

## Food Poisoning

A number of toxicants occur in plants and animals that are ingested as food. Some toxicants are introduced by mistake as pesticides during plant growth, as food additives, or as part of food packaging. Commercially packaged foods are monitored closely, and products are withdrawn from the market if contamination is suspected.

### Bacteria

**Etiology.** Food poisoning occurs more frequently than is reported because most persons recover quickly without treatment. The incidence of food poisoning from commercially prepared foods has become relatively uncommon in the United States, but food poisoning from home-cooked foods or improper handling of foods still occurs.

**TABLE 28-7 Bacterial Food Poisoning**

| ORGANISM | VOMITING | DIARRHEA | FEVER | ONSET | DURATION | SOURCES |
|---|---|---|---|---|---|---|
| *Staphylococcus aureus* | Severe | Occasionally | — | 1-8 hr | 8-24 hr | Meat, poultry, fish, cream-filled foods, mayonnaise |
| *Salmonella* | Occasionally | + | + | 8-48 hr | 2-5 days | Poultry, eggs, meat |
| *Shigella* | Occasionally | + | + | 24-72 hr | 3-7 days | Salads, seafood |
| *Escherichia coli* | Rare | + | — | 24-72 hr | 1-3 days | Uncooked foods, contaminated water |
| *Campylobacter jejuni* | — | Severe | + | 1-10 days | 2-7 days | Meat, poultry, fish, mushrooms, contaminated water |
| *Clostridium perfringens* | Occasionally | Severe | — | 8-16 hr | 1-4 days | Rewarmed foods |
| *Clostridium botulinum* | Occasionally (diplopia, dysphagia, respiratory failure) | Rare | — | 24-96 hr | High mortality | Improperly canned foods |

Bacteria act in different ways in the intestines. Some organisms such as *Shigella, Salmonella,* and *Clostridium jejuni* (Table 28-7) multiply in the intestines, causing infection. Bacteria such as *Staphylococcus aureus* and *Escherichia coli* produce a toxin in the intestines (enterotoxins). Bacteria such as the clostridia produce a toxin in foods (exotoxin) that acts on the intestines when ingested. Food poisoning is not caused by food that has spoiled or decomposed unless the food contains disease-causing bacteria. Many food poisonings are caused by *S. aureus.*

**Prevention.** Acute food poisoning can be prevented (Box 28-8). Rigid control of slaughterhouse practices has decreased the incidence of food poisoning. Pasteurization of milk destroys salmonellae. Rigorous enforcement of sanitary practices by food handlers can decrease food poisoning by *Staphylococcus, E. coli,* and *Salmonella* organisms. Food handlers should not be allowed to work if they have even minor infections on their hands or do not adhere to the requirements for handwashing after using the toilet. Toilets should not be adjacent to kitchens.

**BOX 28-8 Prevention of Food Poisoning**

1. Keep meats, fish, poultry, mayonnaise, and cream-filled foods refrigerated.
2. Avoid slow cooling of meat and poultry.
3. Use a meat thermometer when cooking large pieces of meat, especially pork.
4. Stuff poultry immediately before roasting (warm stuffing is a good medium for bacterial growth).
5. Can low-acid foods (foods other than tomatoes or fruits) under pressure to prevent botulism.
6. Discard any can that bulges.
7. Cook all meats and poultry thoroughly.

Health teaching should include the proper handling and cooling of foods. Home canning is still practiced, but many persons are unaware of the need to process low-acid foods under pressure to prevent botulism. The U.S. Department of Agriculture, state agricultural departments, the home economics departments of schools, and newspapers usually have booklets available on home canning methods.

**Interventions.** If symptoms are very mild, no interventions are indicated. If fluid loss is severe, fluid balance should be restored, and bed rest may be indicated. Fluids such as tea or broth may be well tolerated. If severe dehydration occurs, intravenous fluids may be necessary.

There is no emergency first-aid treatment suitable for *Clostridium botulinum* poisoning. The victim should be taken to a hospital for medical care. Data are obtained concerning the source of the poisoning, and any other persons who might have eaten the contaminated food are contacted immediately. Medical treatment consists of supportive therapy and the administration of botulinum antitoxin. Antitoxin cannot undo damage that has already occurred but can prevent further damage. Approximately 65% of these patients die within 3 to 16 days after onset of symptoms. Fortunately this type of poisoning is now quite rare. The local health department should be notified of any possibility of food poisoning.

**Plants**

Poisoning from plants is usually not a problem, because people have learned to identify poisonous foods. Mushroom poisoning still occurs, however, when people eat uncultivated mushrooms thinking that they are of a safe variety. Two types of mushroom poisoning can occur. One type contains the alkaloid muscarine, which has a *parasympathetic effect.* Symptoms develop immediately after eating and are characterized by sweating, lacrimation, salivation, dyspnea, vomiting, and muscle tremors. Respiratory and circulatory depression may occur. The second type of mushroom poisoning has an *atropine-like effect.* Symptoms occur 6 to 24 hours after ingestion and are characterized by nausea and vomiting, bloody diarrhea, dehydration, and muscle weakness. Circulatory system collapse and central nervous system (CNS) involvement may occur.

First-aid treatment for mushroom poisoning is the same as for drug poisoning: induce vomiting with syrup of ipecac, give fluids, and then give activated charcoal. After the ipecac, give 30 mg of magnesium sulfate (Epsom salts) in water by mouth to hasten evacuation. Medical care should be obtained. When in doubt, contact the poison control center.

## ABDOMINAL EMERGENCIES

Three types of abdomen-related emergencies are commonly seen in emergency departments: abdominal trauma with disruption to the liver, spleen, bladder, and intestines; gastrointestional bleeding; and abdominal pain. The first two problems are discussed in this section. Abdominal pain is discussed as part of the discussion of pain management.

### Abdominal Trauma

Abdominal organs can be injured by blunt trauma or penetrating trauma. **Blunt abdominal trauma** results when energy from a force to the abdomen is diffused into the abdominal cavity. Causes of blunt trauma include motor vehicle accidents, falls, contact sports, and physical abuse.[23] **Penetrating trauma** can result from many types of injuries, such as falls onto objects that become impaled. Two major causes are gunshot wounds and, to a much lesser extent, stab wounds.

The principles of care for persons who have experienced abdominal trauma are the same as for all trauma patients. That is, airway patency and adequacy of respiratory effort should be ensured. Supplemental oxygen should be provided. External bleeding is controlled, two large-bore intravenous lines are inserted, blood pressure is controlled with fluids, and the spine should be protected. A gastric tube and urinary catheter should be inserted.

**Blunt trauma**

Blunt abdominal trauma should be considered whenever there has been an application of force in the area from the fourth rib to the hips.[23] General signs and symptoms of blunt trauma include pain and rigidity of the abdomen, presence of palpable masses, and signs and symptoms of shock. Bruises and abrasion of the abdomen may be present.

If the patient's hemodynamic status is unstable in the presence of fluid replacement and in the absence of external bleeding, blunt trauma should be considered as a very probable condition.

Blunt trauma is diagnosed on the basis of diagnostic **peritoneal lavage** and abdominal computed tomography (CT). Additional organ-specific studies such as angiograms, cystograms, and intravenous pyelograms may be conducted. Laboratory studies of renal and liver function and hematologic studies (red blood cells, hematocrit, hemoglobin, white blood cells, platelets) also will be undertaken.

A major decision that needs to be made is whether the patient requires emergency abdominal surgery.[23] Emergency abdominal surgery will be necessary if the patient's hemodynamic status deteriorates and all other potential causes are controlled. Additional indications for exploratory surgery are (1) progressive drops in hemoglobin or hematocrit values, (2) abnormal results on peritoneal lavage or CT scan, (3) evidence of perforation or free air in the abdomen, (4) evidence of peritonitis, and (5) increasing tenderness and rigidity.

**Penetrating trauma**

Penetrating injuries from gunshot wounds require emergency surgery more frequently than do stab wounds, which require surgery only about one third of the time.[23] With penetrating injuries, evisceration can occur. Evisceration is treated by covering the affected area with a wet, sterile dressing until definitive treatment is possible.

**Specific organ damage with abdominal trauma**

Although all organs of the abdomen can be damaged with blunt or penetrating trauma, some organs are more frequently damaged.

**Stomach.** Stomach injuries most commonly occur with penetrating trauma. Stomach trauma is diagnosed by the presence of blood on gastric aspirate in the peritoneal lavage specimen, or free air on an abdominal x-ray film.

**Liver.** The liver, being the largest solid organ of the body, with its anterior location is prone to both blunt and penetrating injuries. Because the liver is highly vascular, hemodynamic instability occurs rapidly. Liver damage may be diagnosed with CT scan or on exploratory laparotomy. Small lacerations of the liver often will heal by themselves, but large lacerations require surgical repair.

**Spleen.** Injury of the normal spleen occurs almost one half of the time with blunt trauma of the abdomen. However, if the spleen is enlarged—as might be true with portal hypertension and some lymphadenopathy or hematologic conditions—the chance of injury increases greatly. Characteristics of a ruptured spleen include *Kehr's sign,* which is referred pain to the left shoulder, abdominal tenderness and rigidity, and of course hemodynamic instability (tachycardia, increased respiratory rate, decreased blood pressure, decreased alertness and responsiveness, and diaphoresis). Serum laboratory data may reveal decreased hemoglobin and hematocrit levels and elevated white blood cell count.[11] Results of an abdominal CT scan provide definitive diagnosis.

Treatment focuses on repairing and salvaging the spleen. Splenectomy is performed only if the spleen is not salvageable, because persons without spleens are at greater risk for developing subsequent pneumococcal infections.[23]

**Pancreas.** Pancreatic injury in abdominal trauma usually is the result of a penetrating trauma. Because the pancreas is positioned behind the liver and stomach in the retroperitoneal space, pancreatic damage does not appear on peritoneal lavage. Serum amylase elevation supports the diagnosis of pancreatic damage. The patient is provided supportive care with repair of the organ.

**Kidneys.** The kidneys lie retroperitoneally and can be contused or fractured (lacerated) with blunt trauma. Penetrating wounds also can occur. Diagnosis is made by CT scan or with intravenous pyelogram.[23] Suspicion of an injury may be substantiated by examination of the urine. Although some kidney damage can be repaired, sometimes partial or complete removal of the kidney is necessary.

**Bladder.** An empty bladder is not injured by blunt trauma, but if the bladder is distended, it may rupture. Findings of gross blood on urinalysis or cystogram results support the presence of bladder injuries. Bladder injuries may be surgically repaired or treated conservatively with suprapubic catheter placement.[23]

Bladder trauma is one of the types of injuries that can result from the wearing of a seat belt in motor vehicle accidents.[24] Of importance is that a shoulder harness–seat belt combination spreads the force of impact over a larger area and decreases the chance of bladder damage. It is important to remember that although safety belts may cause problems, the injuries that result when safety belts are not worn far outweigh the risk of bladder injury or other trauma that might result from wearing safety belts.

**Intestines.** The intestines frequently are injured with blunt or penetrating trauma because of their (1) anterior location, (2) lack of protective structures, (3) vascularity, and (4) extent or size. Diagnosis is based on the results of peritoneal lavage and CT scan, although definitive diagnosis requires surgical exploration. Surgery is performed to repair the disruption, to control bleeding, and to remove intestinal contents that may have leaked into the peritoneal cavity. The care of these patients incorporates the same measures needed by persons with peritonitis and requiring intestinal surgery (see Chapter 47).

**Abdominal vascular organs.** The abdominal aorta, hepatic veins, and inferior vena cava are major vessels in the abdomen that may be damaged with blunt or penetrating abdominal trauma. Small areas of bleeding may be apparent only on peritoneal lavage or CT scan. Frequently, however, the loss of blood is so severe that the resultant hemodynamic instability is very severe and leads to a high index of suspicion.[24] Emergency surgical repair is required, and blood volume replacement must be initiated.

## Gastrointestinal Bleeding

Throughout most of the gastrointestinal (GI) tract, the lumen of the gut is separated from the capillary blood supply by only a layer of epithelial cells. Any degree of injury to the epithelium therefore may cause bleeding. Blood loss can range in severity from chronic, intermittent, or nearly inconsequential bleeding to sudden massive hemorrhage that may be life-threatening or fatal.

### Etiology

Acute upper gastrointestinal bleeding is a common emergency situation that costs about 1 billion dollars a year.[26] Despite a number of recent advancements in diagnosis and treatment, the overall mortality rate associated with GI bleeding has remained 10% for the past 50 years. Most patients with moderate to severe upper GI bleeding, regardless of whether their condition is clinically stable at the time of initial presentation, are admitted to the critical care unit for observation, evaluation, and treatment. Mortality is lower among patients with lower GI bleeding. Major causes of GI bleeding in the United States are summarized in Box 28-9.

### Intervention

The primary care objectives for persons with GI bleeding are to replace fluid volume, identify the cause of bleeding, and control bleeding. The first goal is met by initiation of at least two large-bore intravenous catheters for provision of access for fluid and blood infusion. History has a significant role in determining the cause of bleeding and interventions for persons with GI bleeding. The presence of pain is diagnostic and should be thoroughly investigated during the history. The patient's responses to the following questions regarding the presence of pain help to establish the differential diagnosis: (1) the location and type of pain, (2) its radiation or extent, (3) the quality of the discomfort, (4) its quantity or frequency, (5) factors that alleviate or aggravate the

**BOX 28-9 Major Causes of Gastrointestinal Hemorrhage**

**UPPER GASTROINTESTINAL BLEEDING**

Duodenal ulcer
Erosive gastritis
Gastric ulcer
Esophageal varices
Mallory-Weiss tears
Esophagitis
Duodenitis

**LOWER GASTROINTESTINAL BLEEDING**

Carcinoma of left portion of colon
Diverticular disease
Inflammatory bowel disease
Polyps
Carcinoma of right portion of colon
Angiodysplasia of right portion of colon

distress, (6) its timing and patterns, and (7) the setting in which it occurs.[26]

Palpation is an important assessment tool. The liver is the only abdominal organ of the GI tract in which palpation can determine normality according to specific parameters. If the liver is enlarged, it is likely that the spleen will be enlarged also. If the spleen can be palpated, it is probably two to three times its normal size. An increase in spleen size is an indicator of portal hypertension and a typical response in persons with hepatomegaly. An enlarged spleen is not a life-threatening emergency unless there is associated abdominal trauma.

While assessment of the abdomen is being completed and decisions about definitive care are being made, hemodynamic monitoring is initiated and continued every 15 minutes until the patient is stabilized and transferred. A nasogastric tube usually is inserted, which allows for gavage of the upper gastrointestinal tract. Endoscopic evaluations are performed to determine the exact cause of the GI bleeding. These may be done in the emergency department by the endoscopic team, or the patient may be transferred to the gastrointestinal laboratory. The patient will be transferred to the critical care unit as soon as the initial care and assessment are completed. (See Chapters 42, 45, and 47 for a complete discussion of care of persons with gastrointestinal bleeding and bleeding from varices.)

## MANAGEMENT OF PAIN

The presence of pain is a frequent non–life threatening reason that people seek emergency care. Pain management is required for a variety of reasons. Persons who decide they can no longer tolerate pain will seek help. Typically the pain is acute and related to a well-known or well-defined cause, follows a predictable course, and is self-limiting and correctable. Some of the most common sources of pain include abdominal pain, migraine pain, tooth pain, gallbladder colic, and kidney stone pain. The most significant nursing function in these instances is to obtain an accurate history. Pain assessment can be accomplished by determining where the pain is, what the pain feels like, how the pain changes with time, and how strong the pain is. When the person believes the pain can no longer be tolerated, pain control becomes an emergency. The PQRST system referenced on p. 715 may also help with pain assessment. It is important for the patient to describe the type of pain being experienced on a 0 to 10 scale basis—for example, extremely severe pain, 10; moderate pain, 5; mild pain, 2. Whatever the patient says regarding the interpretation of pain is what the pain is, and wherever the patient says the pain is located is where the pain is. Documentation of the patient's vital signs, affect, behavior, energy level, past experiences with pain, and the meaning of pain to the patient and to the family is very important.

The next function is to identify the cause of the pain. A variety of diagnostic invasive and noninvasive tests are used to determine the cause. While the tests are in progress, the next priority intervention is the relief of pain.

Pain management principles guide this last intervention. After the appropriate pain management medication is administered, an assessment of the pain relief must occur at specified intervals. These assessment intervals are based on nursing judgment as a result of the history, the type of pain medication administered, and the stability of the patient's vital signs and mental status. (See Chapter 17 for a detailed discussion of pain.)

## SEXUAL ASSAULT: RAPE

Rape is one of the violent crimes for which an increasing number of persons, primarily women, are seeking help. Despite the increasing number of rapes reported, it is estimated that the incidence of unreported rape is from 200% to 300% higher.

It is difficult to obtain statistics concerning the sociologic variables relating to rape because of the large number of unreported cases. There are many misconceptions concerning rape; some *facts* include the following:

1. Rape occurs among persons of all social classes.
2. Rape occurs mostly between persons of the same race.
3. Most rapes are committed by someone the victim knows.
4. Males, especially young boys, may be rape victims; the attacker usually is another heterosexual male.

Rape is a major problem in prisons in the United States. Some prison reform groups are actively addressing this problem, with the major emphasis on protecting the young and vulnerable from attack.

## RAPE CRISIS CENTERS

Rape crisis centers are available in many large cities. These centers differ in their functions but usually provide one or more of the following:

1. Direct service to the rape victim
2. Service to professional agencies (health, law)
3. Community education

Service to health professionals and education of the community are efforts to help change the system for the rape victim.

Many victim services are staffed by volunteers, some of whom have been raped themselves, who serve as victim advocates throughout the medical examination and police interview. Some form of follow-up service, such as counseling, may be available. Some rape crisis centers have volunteer attorneys who can offer the victim legal advice or representation.

## RAPE TRAUMA SYNDROME

Rape is a traumatic event for the victim physically, psychologically, and socially. **Rape trauma syndrome** refers to all the trauma and the effects experienced by the rape victim. *Physical* force often is used. A weapon may be used either to threaten or injure the victim, or the hands or fists may be used to beat the victim or threaten choking. Injury also can occur as the victim is attempting self-defense or is struggling on the ground or floor. The vagina and perineum may be injured by force used during the sexual attack, and the rectum also may be lacerated if anal sex has been attempted. Sexually transmitted diseases, including human immunodeficiency virus (HIV) infection, may be contracted.

*Psychologic* trauma usually is severe; the rape victim is in a state of crisis. Fear is a dominant theme because the victim perceives the event as life-threatening. Other feelings expressed by victims are depersonalization, shame, degradation, defilement, violation, guilt, humiliation, and anger. The victim not only has been under threat of harm but also has been subjected in many instances to multiple sexual assaults by one or more persons. Fellatio (oral sex) frequently is demanded, and some rapists will urinate on the victim before leaving. There is also the fear of contracting HIV infection.

The person who has been raped goes through the same phases as any person facing a crisis situation. The initial phase is one of shock and disbelief. After the initial acute phase, there is a period of pseudoequilibrium when the victim rationalizes the event or attempts to suppress thoughts concerning the rape. Later there are periods of depression, phobic reactions, and nightmares.

The rape victim also experiences *sociologic* crisis. If the victim is married, the marital relationship may be affected. If he/she is single, he/she often fears repeated occurrences and may feel the need to move, especially if the attack occurred in his/her home or apartment. Decisions must be made concerning whom to tell about the incident, because loss of needed support of family and friends may occur. Job security or relationships with co-workers may be threatened. Sociologic problems take considerable time to resolve, but concerns related to these potential problems may occur during the initial emergency period.

## PREVENTION

All persons need to know the measures they can take to help prevent rape from occurring (Box 28-10). It would also be helpful if everyone learned methods of self-defense. Some communities introduce both issues of rape and self-defense into secondary school curricula. Many YWCAs teach classes in self-defense. Rape crisis centers and police stations may provide information on availability of classes in the community.

Persons who are raped may seek medical help directly or call the police, who will then take the victim to the appropriate facility for medical examination. Some victims fear reprisal by the rapist or are unwilling to let others know about the rape and therefore do not seek medical attention. Victims need to be encouraged to report the incident.

Most hospitals have developed protocols for care of the rape victim in the emergency department, including the following measures:

1. High priority in triage
2. Provision for privacy without leaving the victim alone
3. Provision of a victim advocate (such as a worker from the rape crisis center)

### BOX 28-10 Rape Prevention Measures

#### PREVENTION OF ATTACK

Set house lights to go on and off by timer.
Keep light on at all entrances.
Place safety locks on windows and doors.
Have key ready before reaching door of house or car.
Look in car before entering.
Insist on identification before letting a stranger in house; check identification with agency if suspicious.
Do not list first name on mailbox or in telephone directory.
Be alert when walking in street; walk in lighted areas.
Walk down center of street if possible.
Avoid lonely or enclosed areas.

#### IF ATTACKED

Run toward a lighted house; yell "Fire!"
Spit in rapist's face; act bizarre; vomit.
Rip off rapist's glasses.
Step hard on rapist's foot (instep).
Aim at eyes; try to gouge eyes, scrape face.
Hit throat at Adam's apple (larynx).
Use fighting and screaming with caution; this may scare some rapists, encourage others.
Try talking to avoid rape.
Make close observations about rapist, car, location.

4. Routines to ensure protection and comfort of the victim:
   a. Person(s) designated to have primary contact with the victim
   b. Authority of the primary contact person to make the decision for the victim's readiness for medical examination or police interview (if no life-threatening injury is present).
   c. Ensure "chain for evidence" for specimens is maintained. This means there is clear documentation of injuries and specimens are collected and stored according to protocols.

## NURSING MANAGEMENT

### ♦ ASSESSMENT

#### Subjective Data

The victim will be asked many questions by the examiner to identify the type of assault and potential for injury. If the victim has been threatened, she may have succumbed through fear, and this needs to be elicited. Victims often talk freely to the nurse about their feelings: their fears concerning injury, mutilation, or death at the time of assault or present fears concerning pregnancy or sexually transmitted disease. Other feelings of degradation, feeling "dirty," shame, feeling guilty, and so forth, may be expressed. Anger may be directed at the assailant or projected toward medical care personnel.

Data are collected related to pain or discomfort, whether localized or generalized and diffused. The victim may complain of a sore throat if choking occurred or if oral sex was involved. Nausea also may be present.

#### Objective Data

Objective behavioral signs are noted. Some victims respond emotionally and cry, shake, laugh inappropriately, or are extremely restless. Other victims appear overtly calm and subdued; the effect of the experience may hit them later.

A head-to-toe assessment for signs of physical trauma usually is conducted by the physician. The clothing will be inspected and described and often is requested or impounded by the police for evidence. Clothing should not be washed or discarded. Other data needed by the police include samples of the assailant's hair from combing of pubic hair and fingernail deposits for samples of the assailant's tissue.

#### Diagnostic Tests

Papanicolaou smears of the vagina, mouth, or rectum and saline suspensions are obtained to test for the presence of sperm. An acid phosphate test determines recency of intercourse. Test results will be inconclusive if the victim has bathed or douched since the rape. Tests for sexually transmitted disease are completed at the initial visit to obtain baseline information for future comparison.

A pregnancy test is done initially and repeated if the next menses is missed. Tests for HIV antibody are performed and repeated in 2 to 4 months. Tests for other sexually transmitted diseases are conducted and repeated at appropriate intervals.

### ♦ INTERVENTION

#### Emotional Support

Most victims need to talk with someone who cares about what is happening to them and who is nonjudgmental. The nurse uses crisis intervention theory to decide how best to help the victim. Many hospitals have contacts with the rape crisis center, and the victim is given the choice of having a victim advocate from the center to be present during the entire examination period, both medical and legal. Medical examinations or interviews by the police are not begun until the volunteer arrives.

Preparation for the physical examination is carried out in advance. Having a pelvic examination after a sexual assault can be a traumatic experience, especially if the victim has never had a pelvic examination.

#### Sexuality

The victim has many concerns related to his/her sexuality. Time is needed to work through these concerns, and long-term counseling is helpful to many victims.

Concern about possible *pregnancy* depends on the circumstances: whether the woman is in the childbearing years, whether birth control is in effect at the time of sexual assault, and at what point in the menstrual period the rape occurs. If pregnancy is a possibility, postcoital hormone contraceptive therapy usually is initiated immediately.

Concern about *sexually transmitted diseases* (STD), including HIV, is common. Ceftriazone is given intramuscularly and tetracycline is given orally after the initial examination as a preventive measure. The person needs to know that medical follow-up is important and that he/she should be retested for STD, including HIV, at appropriate intervals. In addition, the woman may experience vaginal discharge, itching, and a burning sensation caused by an acute vaginal infection (vaginitis).

### DISCHARGE PLANS

Clean clothes need to be provided, and no victim of sexual assault should ever be sent home alone. A list of battered women's houses is a must for the emergency department. Social workers may be contacted to help determine a safe place of residence for the victim. Frequently the victim goes to the police station to follow up with the police report after medical care is completed. The victim needs to know about the availability of follow-up medical services and counseling services. Some medical centers have psychiatrists who are especially interested in counseling rape victims.

## Domestic Violence

Recent focus on the number of individuals (usually women) physically abused and the subsequent deaths demands review. It is estimated that 2 million women are physically assaulted every year in the United States—usually by their husband or boyfriend, and 1400 women die from the injuries.[18] This translates into a woman being beaten at the rate of one every 15 seconds. It also is estimated that 25% to 33% of all women seeking care in emergency departments come because of physical injury from domestic violence. Thus the emergency department staff must be alert to this problem. There are several key issues for the emergency department staff to consider when caring for patients suspicious of sustaining physical abuse. First, incorporate questions and observations into the initial assessment when there is a suspicion of domestic violence; historical questions and examination techniques may elicit information or evidence about domestic abuse. Victims may not readily share this information if it is not solicited. However, if given the opportunity, the victim will often share the information. Second, staff must know the resources that are available for victims of domestic violence. For example, easily accessible financial help and "safe-housing." Victims, once placed in safe-environments, must be helped to use the legal system to maintain their safety. Long-term counseling, vocational rehabilitation, and other support will be necessary to promote total health. Last, the emergency department staff must have clear procedures on how to handle cases of domestic violence and must define the process used for notification of local legal authorities.

## Questions to Consider

- How does triage impact care for patients in emergency departments?
- What type of emergency department visits are totally preventable?
- What are some ways to heighten staff members' awareness of the noise in the emergency department and the stress of waiting in a waiting room of the department?
- If you came upon four people injured in a multiple car accident and the initial review shows the following, what would you do?
  a. A man standing dazed by a car
  b. A woman on the ground, apparently thrown from a car, with her right leg bent underneath her; she is conscious
  c. A man in the driver's seat, conscious, with blood on his face
  d. An unconscious woman sitting by the man with blood on her face

## Critical Thinking Activities

- While skating on her new roller blades, Debi was hit by a cyclist. You are the first to arrive at the scene of the accident. Debi is sitting up, crying, alert, but anxious. What should you do?
- Ted suffered heat stroke and was taken to a rural hospital. Upon arrival at the ED, the nurse wrapped Ted in wet sheets and turned a fan toward him since cooling blankets were not readily available. Ted's temperature was assessed on an hourly basis, and the sheets were removed when his temperature reached 101.6° F. Critique the actions of the ED nurse, and state possible consequences if the nurse's actions are incorrect.
- Todd, 28, fell off a roof while working. He has a wrist fracture, several small lacerations, and a swollen ankle. You are the triage nurse in a busy ED. To what category will you assign Todd when presented for care? Provide rationales for your decision.

## Chapter Summary

### Emergency Nursing Scope of Practice

- Emergency nursing has grown as a nursing specialty during the past 25 years as indicated by (1) development of a scope of nursing practice, (2) a certification offering, and (3) publication of a professional journal.
- Changes in health care needs of society, caused by such events as the rising incidence of social and domestic violence and the lack of adequate health insurance have increased visits to the emergency department.
- Triage is the process in the emergency department to ensure that the patient who needs the care the most, gets it.
- The use of critical pathways for patient care in the emergency department provides a system of checks and balances that promote quality and efficiency.
- Excellent communication skills have a key role in emergency nursing.
- Control of the emergency department environment, particularly decreasing noise and modifying potential violence, is a key nursing goal.

### Trauma

- Trauma is the leading cause of death of one of the nation's most valued resources—young people.
- The single most important factor in the cause of accidents is human error.

- Trauma centers, which are designated as level I, II, or III centers by national standards, are governed by specific rules and regulations of the state in which the trauma center is located.
- Primary and secondary surveys are key tools in the assessment of a person who has undergone traumatic injury. These surveys begin cycle I of trauma care.
- Statutes protect health care givers who render assistance with good faith and without gross negligence when they are off duty.
- The principles of intervention for use at the scene of an accident or injury are to (1) remove the patient from a hazard only when the risk (e.g., fire) outweighs the danger of moving the patient, (2) call for help, (3) establish an airway, usually by elevating the jaw, (4) initiate cardiopulmonary resuscitation as indicated, (5) control obvious hemorrhage, usually with direct pressure, (6) splint spine and extremity injuries, and (7) transport as soon as possible.
- The person who suffers multiple trauma will need immediate insertion of intravenous lines to allow for fluid and drug administration, management of shock (see Chapter 22), management of depressed level of consciousness, respiratory support, and control of pain.
- Signs of respiratory distress seen in trauma patients are rapid, shallow respirations, abnormal breath sounds, changes in sputum, sinus tachycardia, high or low blood pressure, poor oxygenation, and anxiety or confusion.
- Signs of hypovolemic shock related to trauma include sinus tachycardia, decreased blood pressure (systolic blood pressure below 90 mm Hg), weak peripheral pulses, lungs clear, decreased urinary output, skin cool and moist, no edema, and variable neurologic changes.
- Level of consciousness is altered in trauma for a variety of reasons.
- Changes in level of consciousness are the first indicator of hypoxia or brain injury.
- General interventions in trauma include remaining calm and thinking before acting, identifying oneself as a nurse to the victim and bystanders, conducting a rapid assessment, carrying out lifesaving measures as indicated by the primary survey, performing a secondary survey, and, finally, initiating first aid measure.

## CARE OF SELECTED EMERGENT CONDITIONS

### CARDIOVASCULAR SYSTEM

- The person with a suspected myocardial infarction who is breathing should be placed in a comfortable, well-supported sitting position, given oxygen (if available), cared for calmly to minimize anxiety, and transported to a hospital as soon as possible.
- The patient with a suspected AMI is assessed rapidly, and oxygen and drugs are initiated to limit necrosis.
- Cardiac tamponade is compression of the heart from blood accumulation in the pericardial sac, resulting in extreme depression of cardiac output.
- Vascular emergencies are usually aneurysms or occlusions.
- Obtaining a patient's history is one of the single most important interventions for differentiating among cerebral thrombosis, embolism, and hemorrhage.
- The common sites of aneurysms are abdominal and cerebral.
- The major sites of occlusion are coronary arteries, cerebral arteries, and peripheral arteries.
- Regardless of the site, disruption of vascular flow is an emergency.

### RESPIRATORY SYSTEM

- Patients with open chest wounds need to be monitored for tension pneumothorax if the wound is closed at the site of injury.
- Flail chest frequently accompanies rib fractures and can severely compromise the function of respiration.
- Death from drowning can be wet or dry or can occur as a postimmersion syndrome.

### INTEGUMENTARY SYSTEM

- Open wounds are of four general types: abrasions, lacerations, avulsion, and punctures.
- Wound management has three general objectives: control of bleeding, prevention of further contamination of the wound, and prevention of further damage to the injured part.
- One of the most important interventions that prevents wound infection is irrigation with normal saline, using a 30 ml syringe and a number 18 plastic needle. This produces the pressure required to remove foreign material from most wounds but does not destroy tissue.
- The major pulse points for control of bleeding are the temporal, the carotid, the facial, the brachial, and the femoral arteries.
- Burns are the major trauma to the integumentary system.
- At the site of the burn, the victim must be removed from the source of the fire, airway established, oxygen given, circulation assessed and supported, and emergency treatment of the burn initiated (the emergent care of burns is discussed in Chapter 68).
- Tetanus prophylaxis is required for all wound management.

### ENVIRONMENTAL INJURIES

- Heat-related injuries are preventable.
- Treatment of heat-related injuries includes cooling the person and treating the shock and sodium and water deficit.
- Hypothermia occurs when the body temperature is below 35° C. Shivering will help protect the body at first, but then all body processes slow. Freezing of extremities and loss of consciousness precede death.
- In rewarming, the core body temperature must be increased first; rubbing of the skin is to be avoided.
- Frostbite occurs with exposure to extreme cold; the

water in cells freezes, and the ice crystals damage the cells.

- Frostbite ranges from incipient to deep. Frostbite can be prevented.
- The oxygen needs of the tissue need to be decreased while the area recovers after frostbite.
- Tetanus prophylaxis is a critical part of the intervention for tissue damage.
- Animal bites are usually from cats and dogs and cause damage by puncture wound, lacerations, and avulsions.
- Controlling hemorrhage and cleansing the site are the focus of nursing care for animal bites. Appropriate tetanus prophylaxis is necessary.
- History regarding the animal's immunization is critical; if immunization history is vague or unknown, instructions by the nurse must include the need to impound the animal immediately, for observation for 10 days to observe for rabies.
- Spider bites are a common cause of emergency visits.
- The bites of black widow spiders require antivenom therapy.
- The bites of brown recluse spiders require cleansing, antibiotics, rest of the extremity, and treatment of systemic symptoms.
- Wasp and bee stings can result in anaphylactic shock. Treatment for anaphylactic shock is described in Chapter 70.
- Tick bites cause various types of problems; the most serious is Lyme disease.
- Human bites are one of the most dangerous bites and can result in toxic shock syndrome, hepatitis, and HIV infection.

## MUSCULOSKELETAL INJURIES

- Evaluation of a person with musculoskeletal injuries includes the possession of a disciplined thought process for assessment and the ability to ascertain how the injury happened, what forces were applied and in what direction, the presence of pain, and location, what sensations the person experienced with the injury, and the presence of tenderness, numbness, or tingling in the injured area.
- Musculoskeletal injuries of the extremities require appropriate splinting of fractures, control of hemorrhage, and monitoring of compartment syndrome and fat embolism symptoms.
- Any injury to head, neck, or back should be treated as a possible vertebral fracture, including not moving the person before applying appropriate traction and support and never flexing or extending the neck.
- The major life-threatening emergencies with fracture of the spine are spinal core damage resulting in respiratory depression if at fifth cervical vertebra or above and neurogenic shock (see Chapter 22).

## TOXICOLOGIC EMERGENCIES

- A key principle in caring for a person who exhibits the signs and symptoms of a toxicologic emergency is that with excessive exposure, any chemical can become a poison.
- Prevention of accidental poisoning is a primary focus of care.
- Rapid assessment that allows for interventions to diminish the effects of the poison is necessary.
- The history must help identify the agents so appropriate therapy can be instituted.
- The priority of interventions for a person with toxicologic emergencies is to transport as quickly as possible, stop absorption of the poison, deactivate the poison, or give appropriate antidotes.
- Supportive care of the respiratory and cardiovascular systems is critical in accidental poisoning.
- Food poisoning can result from *Shigella, Salmonella, Clostridium jejuni, Staphylococcus aureus,* and *Escherichia coli* and can be prevented.
- Dehydration is the major complication of food poisoning.
- *Clostridium botulinum* poisoning can be controlled somewhat by an antitoxin. However, the antitoxin does not undo the damage that has occurred and the mortality is high.

## ABDOMINAL EMERGENCIES

- Blunt and penetrating abdominal injuries can result from trauma and disrupt the integrity of the liver, spleen, pancreas, kidneys, intestines, abdominal vascular organs, stomach, and bladder. The liver and the spleen are the most frequently damaged organs.
- Peritoneal lavage and abdominal CT scan are the major diagnostic tools in abdominal trauma.
- Management of abdominal trauma follows the basic trauma interventions of airway maintenance, establishing intravenous lines, etc.
- In the absence of external bleeding, abdominal trauma should be suspected as a cause of hemodynamic instability unresponsive to fluids.

## GASTROINTESTINAL BLEEDING

- Major causes of upper and lower gastrointestinal hemorrhage in the United States are duodenal ulcers, erosive gastritis ulcers, esophageal varices, Mallory-Weiss tears, esophagitis, duodenitis, carcinoma of left and right aspects of the colon, diverticular disease, inflammatory bowel disease, polyps, and angiodysplasia of the right aspect of the colon.
- A major focus of care in GI bleeding is to identify the cause, to institute measure to maintain vascular volume, and to control bleeding.

## MANAGEMENT OF PAIN

- Pain causes many persons to seek emergency care.
- Pain may result from a variety of causes, requiring excellent assessment.
- Pain assessment may be enhanced by use of the PQRST system and a visual analogue scale. The effects of the pain on the total person must be assessed on a regular basis. Reassessment of pain is also imperative.

## SEXUAL ASSAULT: RAPE

- Rape crisis centers have three main functions: victim service, service to professional agencies, and community education.
- A rape victim suffers psychologic, sociologic, and physiologic trauma.
- Rape victims require high-priority triage, a need to have someone in constant attendance, and a need for protocols to be followed exactly, especially notifying the local authorities and ensuring the "chain of evidence" with all specimens is maintained.
- Nursing interventions for rape victims include emotional support, knowledge about STD testing and care, including testing for HIV infection, knowledge about pregnancy prevention, and knowledge about resources to deal with sexuality related concerns.
- Rape victims should never be sent home alone.

## DOMESTIC VIOLENCE

- An estimated 2 million women are physically assaulted every year in the United States, usually by their husband or boyfriend, and 1400 women annually die from the injuries.
- The emergency department must have clear protocols on how to handle victims of domestic violence and the reporting process to the local legal authorities and system.

# REFERENCES


1. Bauer RL, Watson WA: Clinical toxicology. In Stein JH, editor: *Internal medicine,* ed 4, St. Louis, 1994, Mosby.
2. Cantrill SV: Facial trauma. In Rosen P et al, editors: Vol I. *Emergency medicine: concepts and clinical practice,* ed 3, St. Louis, 1992, Mosby.
3. Caplin LR: Cerebrovascular disease (stroke). In Stein JH, editor: *Internal medicine,* ed 4, St. Louis, 1994, Mosby.
4. Cardona V et al: *Trauma nursing from resuscitation through rehabilitation,* Philadelphia, 1988, WB Saunders.
5. Caroline N: *Emergency medical treatment: a text for EMT-As and EMT-intermediates,* Boston, 1991, Little, Brown
6. Derlet R, Nishio D: Refusing emergency care to patients who present to an emergency department, *Ann Emerg Med* 19(3):262-267, 1990.
7. *Diphtheria, tetanus, and pertussis: guidelines for vaccine prophylaxis and other measures, MMWR* 34:405-425, 1985.
8. Emergency Cardiac Care Committee and Subcommittees of the American Heart Association: Guidelines for cardiopulmonary resuscitation and emergency cardiac care. I. Introduction, *JAMA* 268(16):2289-2295, 1992.
9. Emergency Nurses Association: Emergency nursing: scope of practice, *J Emerg Nurs* 5(4):361-364, 1989.
10. Fazio J: *Violence in the emergency department: strategies for survival,* Course presented at the Emergency Nurses Association Scientific Assembly, Seattle, 1993.
11. Greenberg L: Fast action for splenic rupture, *Am J Nurs* 94(2):51, 1994.
12. Harwood-Nuss A et al: *The clinical practice of emergency medicine,* Philadelphia, 1991, JB Lippincott.
13. Headlines: *Am J Nurs* 93(8):9, 1993.
14. Health Security Act, 1993: United States of America, Washington, DC, 1993, US Government Printing Office.
15. Lamros N: *Assessment and intervention in emergency nursing,* ed 3, Norwalk, Conn, 1992, Appleton & Lange.
16. Lenahan G: ED noise: a legitimate patient care and staff stress issue . . . emergency department, *J Emerg Nurs* 19(3): 181-182, 1993.
17. Missouri Department of Health: Hospital licensing rules and regulations. In *Proposed rules and regulations for hospital emergency services,* Jefferson City, Mo, 1993, The Department.
18. Namuth T: When did he stop beating his wife? *Newsweek,* Vol CXXIII(26):21, 1994.
19. Nelson M: Critical pathways in the emergency department, *J Emer Nurs* 19(2):110-114, 1993.
20. Nicholson DP: The immediate management of overdose, *Med Clin North Am* 67:1279-1291, 1983.
21. Paparone P: The summer scourge: Lyme disease, *Am J Nurs* 90(6):44-47, 1990.
22. Rea R: *Trauma nursing core course,* ed 3, Chicago, 1991, Emergency Nurses Association.
23. Sheehy SB: *Emergency nursing: principles and practice,* ed 3, St Louis, 1992, Mosby.
24. Sheehy SB, Marvin JA, Jimmerson CL: *Manual of clinical trauma care: the first hour,* ed 2, St Louis, 1994, Mosby.
25. Simon B: Principles of wound management. In Rosen P et al, editors: Vol I. *Emergency medicine: concepts and clinical practice,* ed 3, St. Louis, 1992, Mosby.
26. Thelan LA et al: *Critical care nursing: diagnosis and management,* ed 2, St Louis, 1994, Mosby.
27. US Bureau of the Census: *Statistical abstracts of the United States,* ed 108, Washington DC, 1988, US Government Printing Office.
28. US Department of Health and Human Services, Public Health Service: *Diphtheria, tetanus and pertussis: what you need to know.* Atlanta, 1992, Centers for Disease Control.
29. US Department of Health and Human Services, Public Health Service: *Healthy People 2000: national health promotion and disease prevention objectives,* Washington DC, 1990, US Government Printing Office.

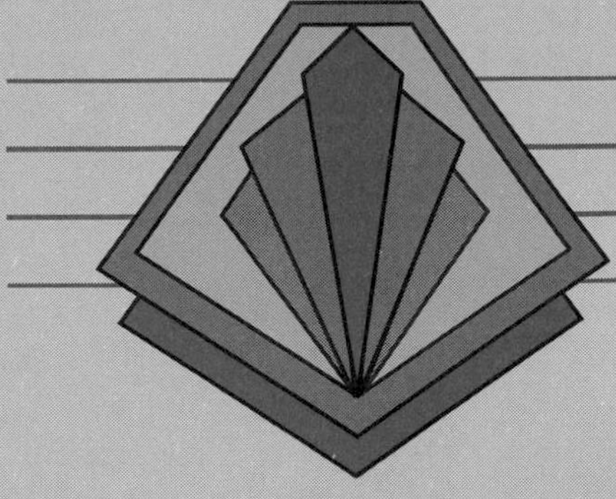

P A R T   T W O

# Alterations in Human Functioning

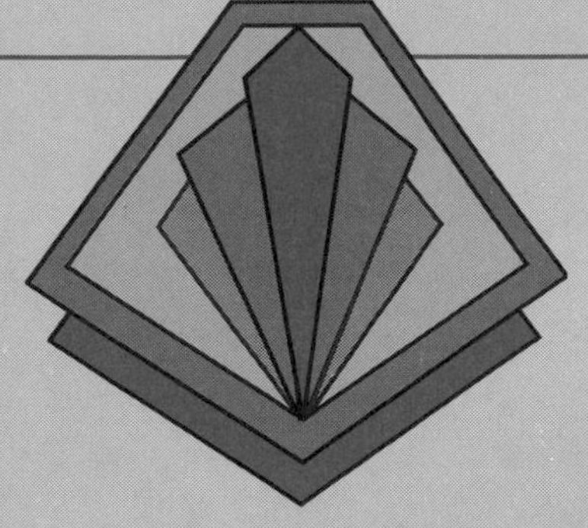

UNIT VI

# Alterations in Fluid and Gas Transport

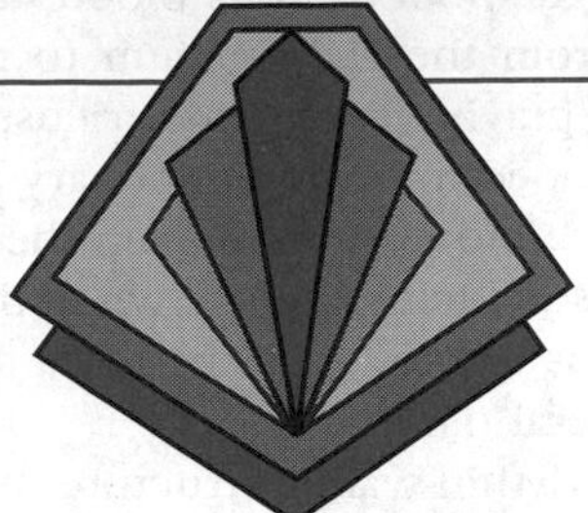

CHAPTER 29

# Assessment of the Cardiovascular System

*Terri Abraham*

## CHAPTER OBJECTIVES

***After studying this chapter, the learner should be able to do the following:***

1 Describe the basic structure and function of the heart.
2 Describe the conduction system of the heart in relation to the cardiac cycle.
3 Identify factors that affect cardiac output.
4 Describe physiologic changes that occur in the cardiovascular system with aging.
5 Identify common manifestations of altered cardiac functioning.
6 Identify diagnostic tests used to assess cardiac functioning and the significance of each.
7 Describe nursing care of a patient undergoing cardiac catheterization and electrophysiologic study.

## KEY TERMS

action potential
afterload
aortic diastolic pressure
atrial diastolic gallop
atrial systole
atrionodal junction
atrioventricular (AV) node
atrioventricular (AV) valves
automaticity
bundle of His
cardiac catheterization
cardiac cycle
cardiac index
cardiac output
central venous pressure (CVP)
circumflex coronary artery (CCA)
conductivity
contractility
coronary arteriography
depolarization
diastole
echocardiography
electrophysiologic (EP) study
excitability
heart sound
Holter monitor
isovolumetric ventricular contraction
isovolumetric ventricular relaxation
left anterior descending (LAD) artery
left coronary artery (LCA)
left ventricular end-diastolic pressure (LVEDP)
maximal ventricular ejection
multiple gated acquisition (MUGA) scanning
murmurs
myocardial imaging
palpitation
pericardial friction rub
phonocardiography
point of maximal impulse (PMI)
positron emission tomography (PET)
preload
pulmonary artery end-diastolic pressure (PAEDP)
pulmonary artery pressure (PAP)
pulmonary capillary wedge pressure (PCWP)
pulsus alternans
pulsus paradoxus
Purkinje's fibers
pyrophosphate scan
reduced ventricular ejection
refractory period
repolarization
resting membrane potential
semilunar valves
sinoatrial (SA) node
stress testing
stroke volume
syncope
systole
thallium imaging
transesophageal echocardiography (TEE)
ventricular angiography
ventricular diastolic gallop

Heart disease continues to be the leading cause of death in America. In 1989, cardiac and vascular disease claimed nearly 1 million American lives. More than 6 million people alive today have a history of myocardial infarction, or angina pectoris, or both.

In 1992 it was estimated that 1.5 million Americans sustained a myocardial infarction and that 500,000 of them died. Of those deaths, 300,000 persons died before reaching the hospital. In essence, more than half of cardiac deaths occur within 2 hours of the onset of symptoms. These statistics strongly support the need for educating the public to recognize cardiac emergencies and to employ basic cardiac life-support measures as soon as possible.

During the past 15 years the death rate for cardiovascular disease has decreased significantly. Major contributing factors to this decline include reduction of risk factors and changes in life-style. Major modifiable risk factors include hypertension, hypercholesterolemia, and cigarette smoking. Thrombolytic agents, advanced technology, improved surgical techniques, and more effective medical management further contributed to this reduced mortality.[6]

This chapter is the first of three chapters that focus primarily on the heart. A review of anatomy and physiology of the heart, physiologic changes with aging, and cardiac assessment, including diagnostic tests, are included in this chapter. Cardiac dysrhythmias and cardiac disorders are discussed in Chapters 30 and 31.

# ANATOMY AND PHYSIOLOGY

## BASIC STRUCTURE

The heart is a relatively small organ that weighs 300 g and is approximately the size of a fist. It is located in the middle of the mediastinum, where the lungs partially overlap it. This pulsatile four-chambered pump beats approximately 72 times per minute, pumping more than 5 L of blood each minute, or about 2000 gallons per day. It continually propels oxygenated blood into the arterial system and receives poorly oxygenated blood from the venous system. The heart muscle rests on the diaphragm and is tilted forward and to the left so that the apex of the heart is rotated anteriorly.

The heart is enclosed by the *pericardium,* which consists of two layers: the inner layer (visceral pericardium) and the outer layer (parietal pericardium). The two pericardial surfaces are separated by a pericardial space that normally contains approximately 10 to 20 ml of thin, clear pericardial fluid. This lubricating fluid moistens the contacting surfaces of the pericardial layers and serves to reduce the friction produced by the pumping action of the heart. The visceral pericardium actually encases the heart and extends several centimeters onto each of the great vessels. The parietal pericardium is attached anteriorly to the manubrium and xiphoid process of the sternum, posteriorly to the vertebral column, and inferiorly to the diaphragm.

There are three layers of cardiac tissue: *epicardium*—the outer layer of the heart, which is the same structure as the visceral pericardium; *myocardium*—the middle layer of the heart, which is composed of striated muscle fibers and is responsible for the heart's contractile force; and *endocardium*—the innermost layer of the heart, which consists of endothelial tissue. The endocardium lines the inside of the heart's chambers and covers the heart valves.

## CHAMBERS

The heart is divided into two halves by a muscular wall *(septum)* (Figure 29-1). Each half has an upper collecting chamber *(atrium)* and a lower pumping chamber *(ventricle).* Oxygen-poor venous blood enters the right atrium, flows from the right atrium to the right ventricle (mainly by gravity) when the tricuspid valve is opened, and is pumped into the pulmonary artery to the lungs. Oxygen-rich blood returns from the lungs to the left atrium, enters the left ventricle when the mitral valve is opened, and is ejected into the aorta for distribution to the peripheral tissues.

The *right atrium* is a thin-walled structure that serves as a reservoir for venous blood returning to the heart. Venous blood returns to the heart via the superior and inferior venae cavae and the coronary sinus, which drains venous blood from the heart muscle. Blood is temporarily stored in the right atrium during right ventricular systole (contraction). During ventricular diastole (filling), approximately 80% of the venous return to the right atrium flows by gravity into the ventricle through the tricuspid valve. The remaining 20% of the venous return is delivered to the ventricles during atrial systole. This additional 15% to 20% of the venous return, which is actively propelled into the ventricles, is called the "atrial kick."

The *right ventricle* is normally the most anterior structure of the heart and is situated immediately beneath the sternum. The right ventricle receives venous blood from the right atrium during ventricular diastole. During ventricular diastole this blood is propelled through the pulmonic valve into the pulmonary artery and then to the lungs. Because the pulmonary system is a low-pressure system, the overall workload of the right ventricle is much lighter than that of the left ventricle. The right ventricle has a crescent-shaped chamber and a thin outer wall that is 4 to 5 mm thick. This thin structure is suitable for right ventricular systole, because the right ventricle contracts against low resistance.

The thin-walled *left atrium* receives oxygenated blood from the four pulmonary veins and serves as a reservoir during left ventricular systole. Blood flows by gravity from the left atrium into the left ventricle through the opened mitral valve during ventricular diastole. Left atrial contraction then propels the remaining 20% of the venous return and provides a significant increment of blood volume to the left ventricle. This atrial kick serves to stretch the ventricle and prime it for ventricular ejection.

The *left ventricle* receives blood from the left atrium through the opened mitral valve during ventricular diastole. Blood is then ejected through the aortic valve into the systemic arterial circulation during ventricular systole. The left ventricle must contract against a high-pressure systemic circulation to deliver blood flow to the peripheral tissues. Therefore the left ventricular chamber is surrounded by 8 to 15 mm of thick musculature, which is approximately two to three times the thickness of the right ventricle. The thick musculature and ellipsoidal-sphere shape contribute to the powerful expulsive ability of the left ventricular chamber during systole.

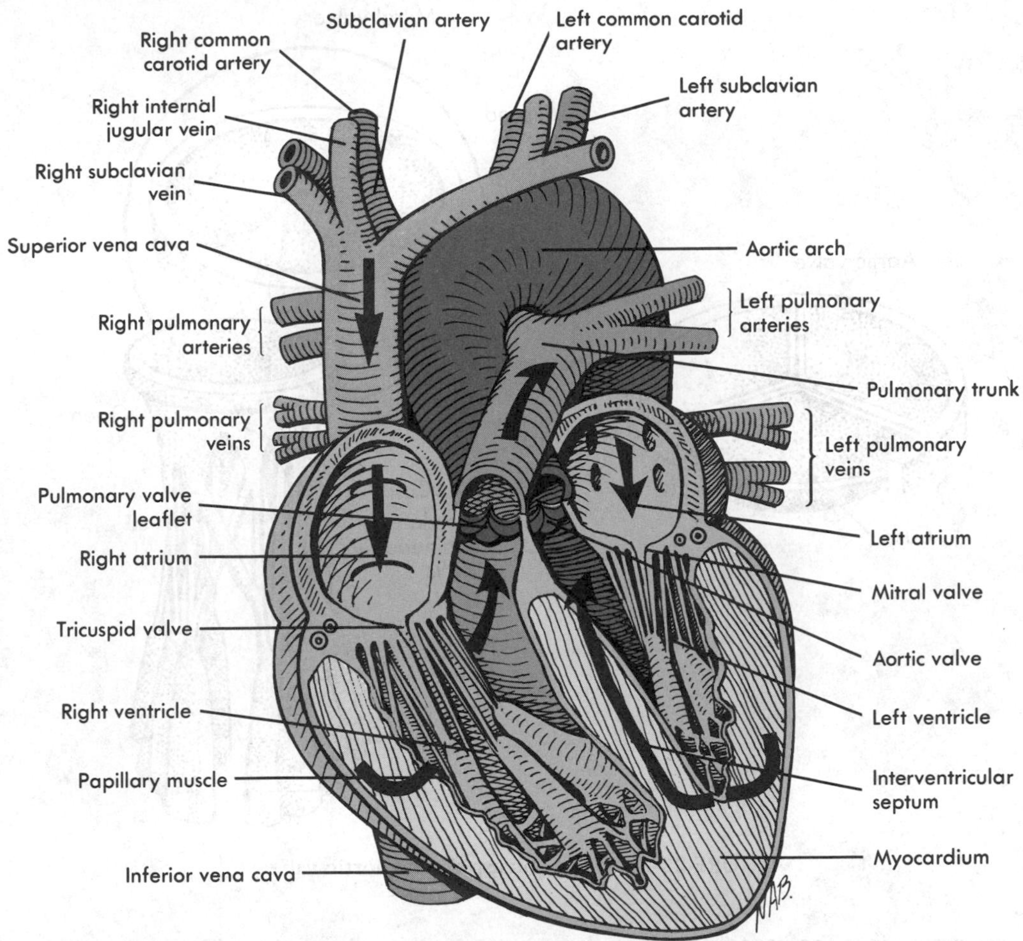


**FIGURE 29-1** Heart in frontal section; course of blood through the chambers.

## VALVES

The four cardiac valves are flaplike structures that function to maintain unidirectional (forward) blood flow through the heart chambers. These valves open and close in response to pressure and volume changes within the cardiac chambers. The cardiac valves can be classified into two types: the **atrioventricular (AV) valves,** which separate the atria from the ventricles; and the **semilunar valves,** which separate the pulmonary artery and the aorta from their respective ventricles.

### Atrioventricular Valves

The AV valves are the *tricuspid* valve, located between the right atrium and the right ventricle, and the *bicuspid* (or *mitral*) valve, located between the left atrium and left ventricle. The tricuspid valve contains three leaflets held in place by fibrous cords called the *chorda tendineae cordis,* which in turn are anchored to the ventricular wall by the papillary muscles. The mitral valve on the left side of the heart is a bicuspid valve with two valve cusps or leaflets. It also is attached to chorda tendineae cordis, which extend to the papillary muscles (Figure 29-2). The chorda tendineae cordis are extremely important because they support the AV valves during ventricular systole to prevent valvular prolapse into the atrium. Some leaflet overlapping occurs during closure of the AV valves, which helps to prevent the backward flow of blood. Damage to the chorda tendineae cordis or to the papillary muscles would permit valvular regurgitation of blood back into the atrium during ventricular systole. During diastole the AV valves serve as a type of funnel inasmuch as they allow blood to flow from the atria to the ventricles. The diameter of the AV cusps is almost double that of the orifice they occlude. In general, the AV valves are structurally much more complex than the semilunar valves.

### Semilunar Valves

The semilunar valves include the *aortic* and *pulmonic* valves. The structural design of the semilunar valves is quite different from the AV valves; each consists of three cuplike cusps (see Figure 29-2). The pulmonic valve lies between the right ventricle and the pulmonary artery. The aortic valve lies between the left ventricle and the aorta. These valves are open during ventricular systole (contraction) to permit blood flow into the aorta and the pulmonary artery. They are closed during diastole (relaxation) to prevent retrograde flow from the aorta

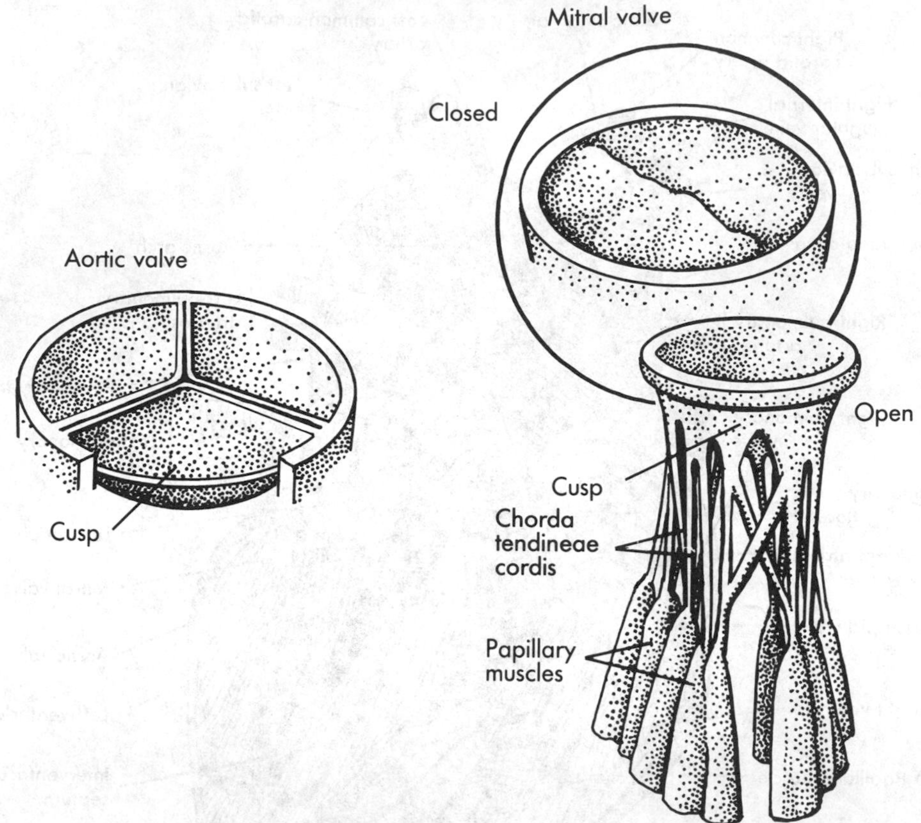


**FIGURE 29-2** Mitral (bicuspid) and aortic valves.

and the pulmonary artery into the ventricles when they are relaxed.

## CORONARY ARTERIES

The coronary arteries arise from the aorta (just behind the cusps of the aortic valve) in an area known as *Valsalva's sinus.* The function of the coronary artery system is to provide an adequate blood supply to the myocardium. Despite scientific advances in the field of cardiology, coronary artery disease and its complications remain the leading cause of death in the United States (see Chapter 31).

There are two main coronary arteries, the *left* and the *right* (Figure 29-3). The **left coronary artery (LCA)** divides into two branches: the **left anterior descending (LAD) artery** and the **circumflex coronary artery (CCA).** The LAD branch supplies the left ventricular myocardium, the septum, the anterior papillary muscle, and portions of the right ventricle. In addition, the LAD artery usually supplies the anterior apex as well as some portion of the posterior apex. The CCA typically emerges at a sharp 90-degee angle from the LCA and is then directed toward the lateral left ventricle and apex. The CCA and its branches supply most of the left atrium, the lateral wall of the left ventricle, and part of the posterior wall of the left ventricle. Diagonal branches arise between the LAD artery and the CCA and are distributed along the free wall of the left ventricle.

Two important external landmarks are used in tracing coronary circulation. These anatomic landmarks are sulci or grooves and include the following: the *atrioventricular groove,* which encircles the heart between the atria and the ventricles; and the *interventricular groove,* which divides the right and left ventricles. The meeting of the two anatomic grooves on the posterior side of the heart is known as the *crux* of the heart. The location of the crux is significant because this is where the AV node is located. The phrases "dominant left" circulation and "dominant right" circulation refer to whether the right or the left coronary artery turns at the crux of the heart and supplies the posterior interventricular groove. Therefore, if the CCA extends as far as the posterior interventricular groove, the circulation is considered to be dominant left. This condition occurs in only 10% to 15% of all human beings.

The right main coronary artery (RCA) arises from the right Valsalva's sinus off the aorta and courses around the right AV groove. Its branches supply the right ventricle, a portion of the septum, and in more than 50% of all humans, the sinoatrial (SA) node. In approximately 67% of all humans, the RCA turns at the crux of the heart and descends in the posterior interventicular groove. The hearts of these persons are classified as "right dominant." The posterior descending branch of the RCA then supplies the posterior aspect of the septum and the posterior left papillary muscle before terminating in several branches to the left ventricular wall.

Great variation exists in the branching pattern of

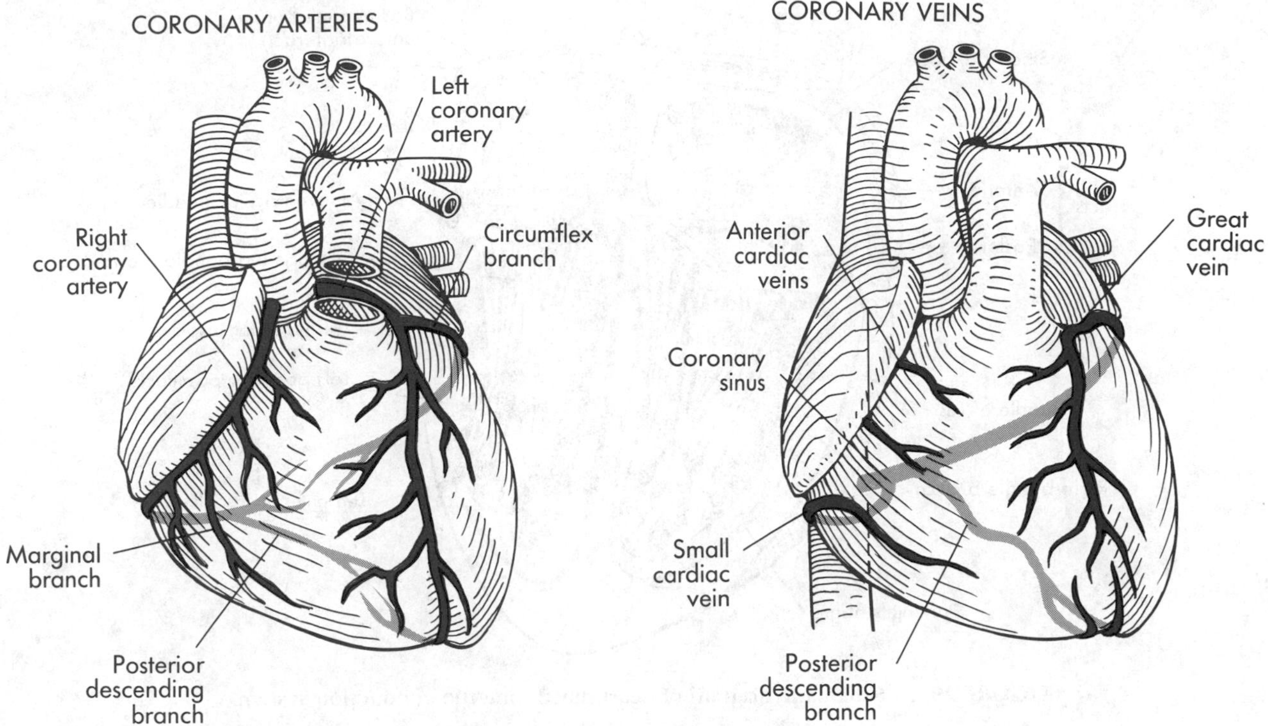


**FIGURE 29-3** Coronary blood vessels.

the coronary arteries. In approximately 18% of the population, the CCA also reaches the crux of the heart with the RCA; this is the so-called balanced coronary artery pattern. In the remaining persons, no true posterior interventricular branch exists; rather, many branches from either main coronary artery supply the posterior septum.

Coronary artery blood flow to the myocardium occurs almost exclusively during *diastole,* when coronary vascular resistance is diminished. During *systole,* coronary vascular resistance is increased because of the increased ventricular wall tension produced by ventricular contraction. During diastole, blood enters the coronary arteries at the pressure that exists at the moment in the aortic arch. This particular pressure is termed **aortic diastolic pressure.**

Coronary venous drainage is accomplished via three subdivisions of the heart's venous system: (1) the thebesian veins drain a portion of the right atrial and right ventricular myocardium; (2) the anterior cardiac veins drain a large portion of the right ventricle; and (3) the coronary sinus and its branches drain the left ventricle and most myocardial venous return.

## CONDUCTION SYSTEM

### Properties of Cardiac Muscle

The mechanical contraction of the heart is the product of a stimulus-response process. The following properties are integral components of the electromechanical events in the heart.

#### Automaticity

The ability of the heart to initiate impulses regularly and spontaneously is known as **automaticity,** or rhythmicity. Although most cardiac cells have this ability, it is the prominent property of the SA node, making it the dominant pacemaker in the normal heart. Pacemaker cells are known to have lower resting membrane potentials than other myocardial cells and exhibit *spontaneous* depolarization.

#### Excitability

The ability of cardiac cells to respond to a stimulus by initiating a cardiac impulse is known as **excitability.** It should be noted that excitatory cells differ from pacemaker cells in that pacemaker cells do not require a stimulus to initiate an impulse.

#### Conductivity

The ability of cardiac cells to respond to a cardiac impulse by transmitting the impulse along cell membranes is referred to as **conductivity.** Cells specialized in this function are found in the conduction system. The arrangement of cells outside the conduction system ensures rapid conduction through intercalated disks joining adjacent cells.

#### Contractility

The ability of cardiac cells to respond to an impulse by contracting is known as **contractility.** Contractile cells compose the largest mass of the myocardium.

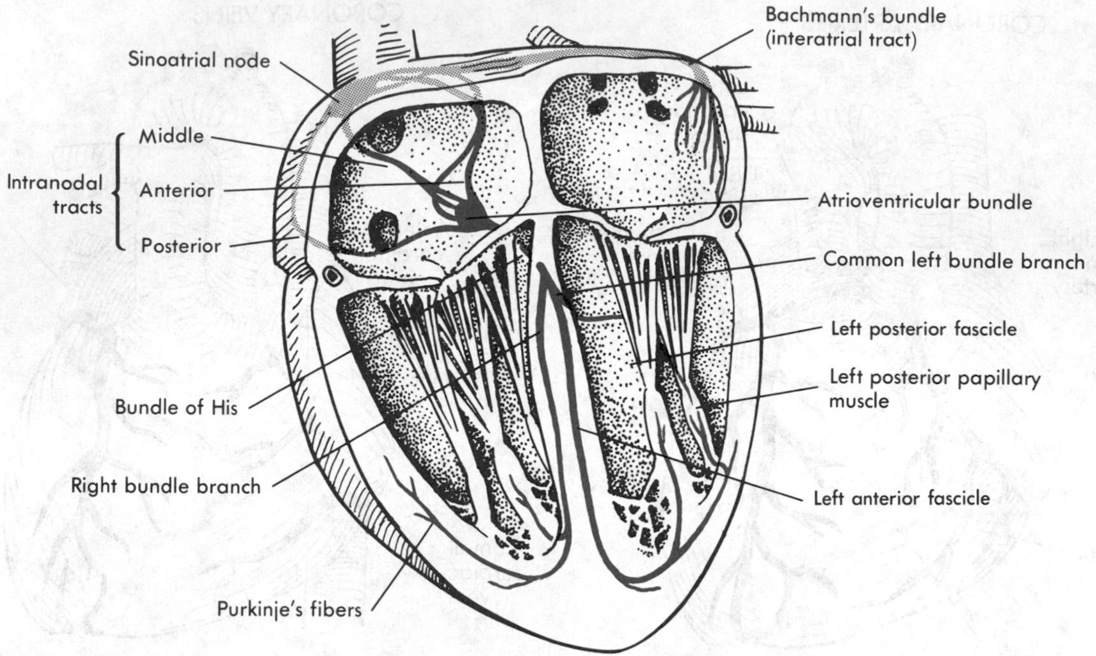


**FIGURE 29-4** Schematic diagram of heart illustrating the conduction system.

## Anatomy of Conduction System

The pacemaking center of the normal heart is the **sinoatrial (SA) node** or "sinus," node (Figure 29-4). It is composed of a group of highly specialized tissues located in the right atrium adjacent to the superior vena cava. Automatically and at regular intervals, an electrical impulse is emitted from the SA node at a rate of 60 to 100 beats per minute. The atria are then depolarized, and the impulse travels to the AV node via three tracts designated as anterior, middle, and posterior *internodal tracts.* A fourth tract, called *Bachmann's bundle,* branches off the anterior nodal tract and transmits the impulse to the left atrium.

The three internodal tracts meet at the **atrionodal junction.** The junctional area refers to the region where atrial and ventricular tissues merge. This junction contains the AV node. The junctional cells above and below the AV node are capable of pacemaking activity under many circumstances (e.g., failure of the SA node to fire).

The **atrioventricular (AV) node** itself is located on the right side of the interatrial septum. These cells lack the ability to initiate electrical impulses (i.e., automaticity), but they are uniquely responsible for a brief physiologic delay in the conduction of the impulse to the ventricles.

The **bundle of His** begins anatomically as the "tail" of the AV node. It is a short, thick cable of fibers separated by collagen septa that bifurcate into the right bundle branch (RBB) and the left bundle branch (LBB).

The RBB extends down the right side of the interventricular septum and is covered by a connective tissue sheath. It extends to reach the anterior papillary muscle of the right ventricle, where it merges with the Purkinje system. It lies close to the septal surface for much of its length, and therefore its functional ability is vulnerable to right ventricular pressure changes.

The LBB bifurcates into anterior and posterior fascicles. The anterior fascicle extends anteriorly down the left side of the interventricular septum to reach the anterior papillary muscle. The posterior fascicle is shorter and thicker and extends to the posterior papillary muscle of the left ventricle. Both fascicles connect with the Purkinje system and equally share in the spread of the impulse to the left ventricle.

**Purkinje's fibers** lie as a network on the endocardial surface and penetrate the myocardium of both ventricles. They are responsible for the transmission of the impulse to both ventricular free walls. Purkinje's cells are elongated and contain intercalated disks, which contribute to the superiority of conductivity in myocardial tissue.

Cells outside the conduction system also play a role in the conduction of an impulse. A surface membrane, the sarcolemma, surrounds each cell and acts as a selectively permeable barrier to sodium and potassium ions. Adjacent myocardial cells are connected end to end by a thickened portion of the sarcolemma known as an *intercalated disk.* These disks act as low-resistance pathways to the transmission of an impulse between cells.

## Sequence of Cardiac Activation

Depolarization (activation of the cardiac muscle) is initiated by an impulse from the SA node. The impulse first spreads through the right atrium and then activates the left atrium. Atrial activation normally is accomplished in 0.11 second or less.

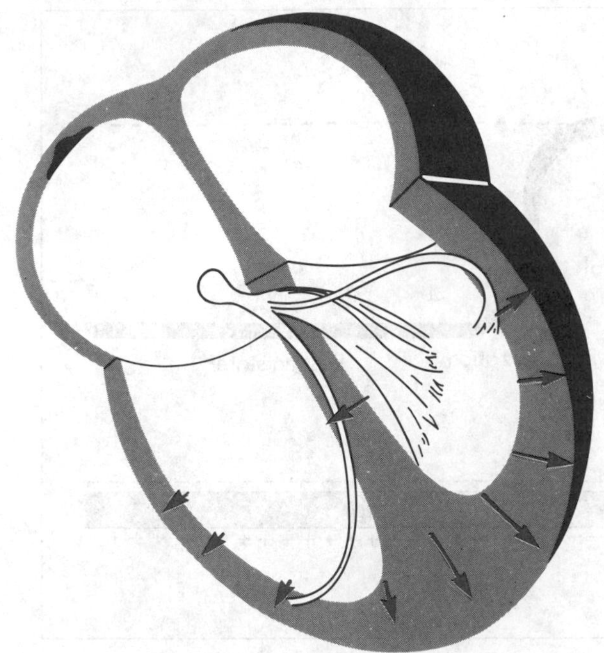

FIGURE 29-5 Sequence of electrical activation in the heart. (From Conover MB: *Understanding electrocardiography: arrhythmias and the 12-lead ECG,* ed 6, St Louis, 1992, Mosby.)

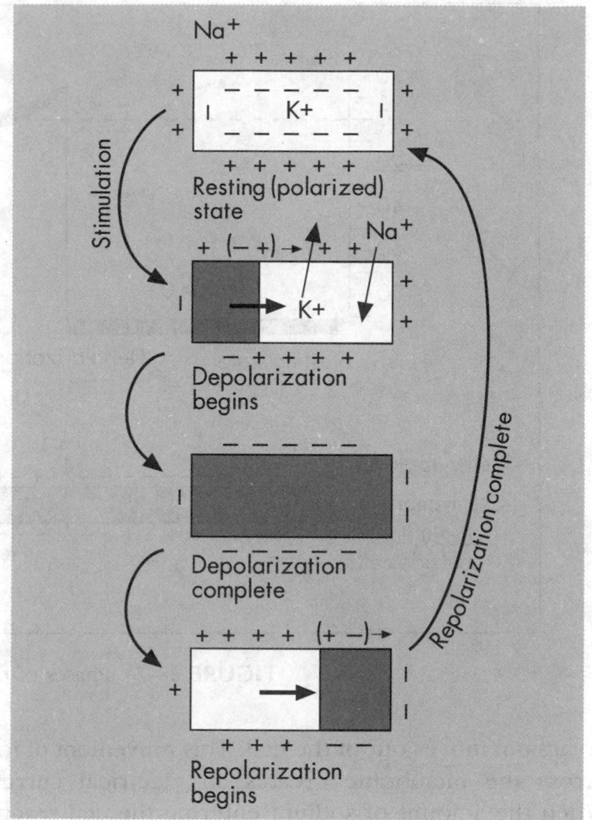


FIGURE 29-6 Schematic diagram illustrating process of depolarization and repolarization.

Shortly after the impulse reaches the left atrium, it also activates the junctional region and subsequently the AV node. The AV node delays the impulse about 0.1 second before the impulse enters the bundle of His.

On reaching the bundle of His, the impulse is transmitted along to the bundle branches. Within the ventricles, the first structure to be activated is the ventricular septum. The septum is activated by the impulse traveling from the left side to the right side (Figure 29-5).

The impulse then continues down the remaining length of the bundle branches and into the Purkinje network, thus activating the ventricular walls almost simultaneously. Activation of the ventricular muscle then proceeds from the apex back toward the base of the heart to complete the process.

Depolarization of cardiac musculature proceeds from endocardium to epicardium. Repolarization in the atria follows this same pathway. In contrast, repolarization of ventricular musculature proceeds from epicardium to endocardium. Knowledge of the sequence of activation is fundamental to analysis of the electrocardiogram (ECG).

### Action potential

The resting myocardial cell has a membrane potential (i.e., an electrical charge) as a result of the relative distribution of sodium and potassium ions extracellularly. Whenever the cell is stimulated, the membrane potential undergoes a change. A graphic record of this change forms the basis for an ECG. The change in electrical potential in response to a stimulus is known as the **action potential.** The two components of the action potential are depolarization and repolarization.

### Resting membrane potential

In the resting state the inside of the cell is negative with respect to the outside (Figure 29-6). Initiation and conduction of cardiac impulses depend on the cell's ability to maintain an electrical potential gradient when the cell is at rest. The main factor that contributes to the −90 mV resting membrane potential is the cell's permeability to potassium and not to sodium. The sodium-potassium exchange pump is responsible for actively transporting sodium out of the cell and potassium into the cell. The hydrolysis of the high-energy phosphate adenosine triphosphate (ATP) provides the energy for the functioning of this pump. Because more sodium is pumped out of the cell than potassium is moved in, a net outward current of positive ions further enhances the cell's negativity during the resting phase.

### Depolarization

The initiation of a cardiac impulse begins with the process of **depolarization.** Depolarization indicates the rapid reversal of the resting membrane potential, which results from the following sequence of events: (1) the cell membrane permeability to sodium increases spontaneously (as in pacemaking cells) or in response to a stimulus; (2) a rapid influx of sodium occurs; and (3)

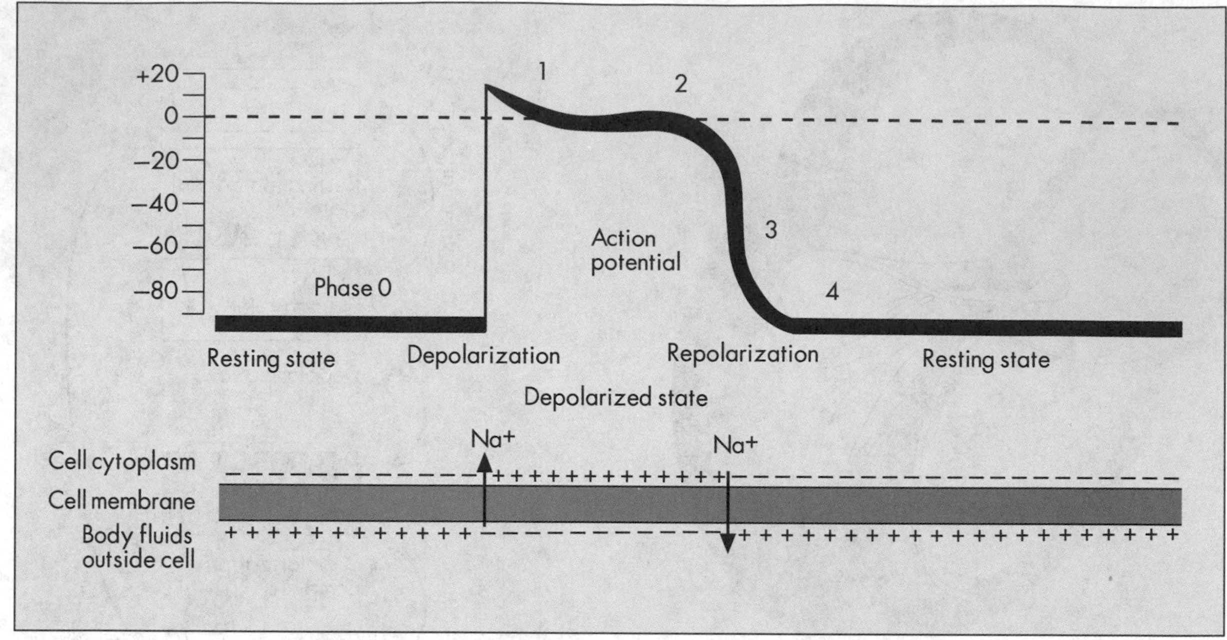


**FIGURE 29-7** Phases of the action potential of cardiac muscle.

potassium moves out of the cell. This movement of ions across the membrane creates an electrical current. When the amount of sodium entering the cell reaches a critical level, an electrical impulse is generated. The impulse may spread as a wave of depolarization to adjacent cells.

## Repolarization

**Repolarization** is the process by which the cell is returned to the resting state. The following sequence occurs: (1) the cell membrane permeability to sodium decreases and (2) sodium leaves the cell, whereas potassium returns through an active ion transport system.

### Phases of action potential

**Phase 0.** Phase 0 is the tall upstroke of the action potential that occurs when the cell is stimulated, causing the cell membrane to become permeable to sodium ions. Fast sodium channels open to allow sodium to rush into the cell, creating a positive intracellular membrane potential of 0 to +20 mV (Figure 29-7).

**Phase 1.** Phase 1 represents a brief period of rapid repolarization secondary to an outward positive current carried mainly by potassium ions. Further, sodium influx is abruptly terminated as soon as the cell depolarizes. These two factors cause a slight decline in intracellular positivity.

**Phase 2.** Phase 2 of the action potential is often referred to as the *plateau phase.* It is sustained by an influx of positive ions, primarily calcium, through the slow calcium channels into the cell (Figure 29-8). This inward current results in prolonged refractory by maintaining the cell in a depolarized state, allowing time for completion of muscular contraction. This channel supplies the cell with calcium necessary for contraction. The effects of calcium channel blocker drugs on myocardial contractility and conduction are discussed in Chapters 30 and 31.

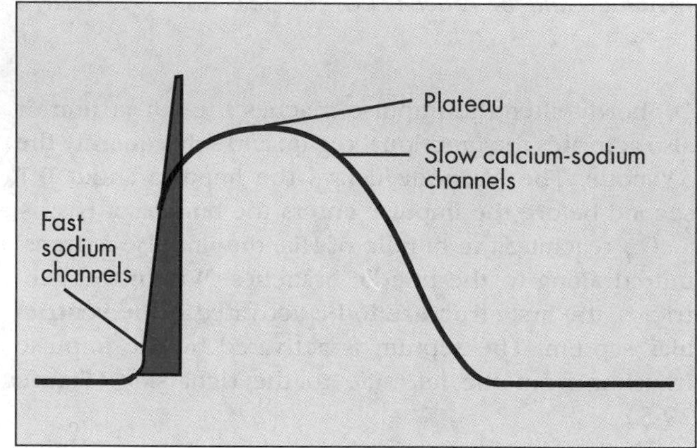


**FIGURE 29-8** The differing effects of the fast sodium channels and the slow calcium-sodium channels on the action potential. The flow of sodium throughout the fast sodium channels initiates the action potential, and then these channels close *(shaded area).* The flow of current through the slow calcium channels is responsible for the plateau and duration of the action potential. (From Conover MB: *Understanding electrocardiography: arrhythmias and the 12-lead ECG,* ed 6, St Louis, 1992, Mosby.)

**Phase 3.** During phase 3 the sodium pump, along with the increased loss of intracellular potassium, causes a rapid restoration of negativity to the cell.

**Phase 4.** Phase 4 is the return of the cell to the resting membrane potential.

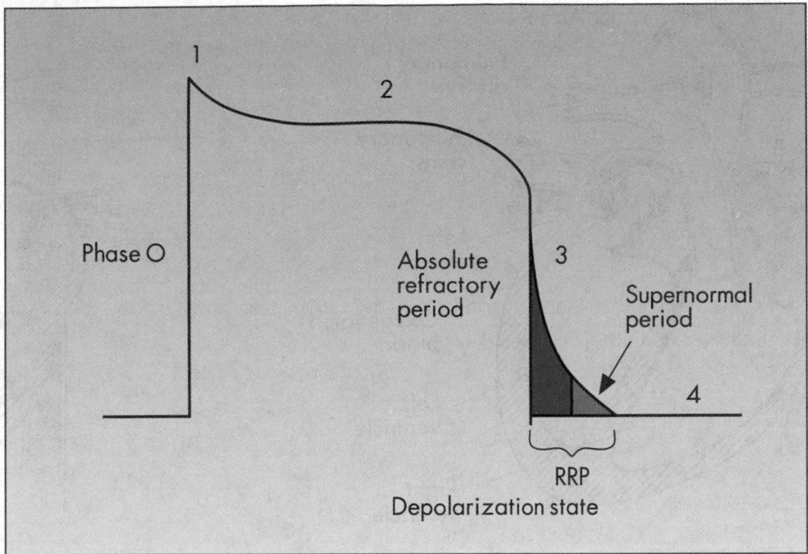


**FIGURE 29-9** Schematic of the action potential showing the absolute and relative refractory period *(RRP)*. A strong stimulus will produce a response in the first part of the RRP and a mild stimulus in the latter part *(supernormal period)*.

### Refractoriness

The inability of cardiac cells to respond to successive stimuli is known as *refractoriness*. During the *absolute refractory period*, no stimulus will produce a response. This period begins with depolarization and extends through a portion of the repolarization period until the sodium ion carrier sites are again free to transport the sodium ions necessary for depolarization (Figure 29-9).

Refractoriness progressively diminishes in the *relative refractory period*, which occurs in the final stage of repolarization. During this interval a stimulus of sufficient strength will produce a response. When the resting state is attained, the cell is no longer refractory. During the latter period, a mild stimulus will initiate a cardiac impulse. This is known as the *supernormal period*.

## Cardiac Cycle

The action potential itself does not cause the myofibrils to contract. The electrical stimulation initiates muscular contraction by stimulating the release of calcium ions in the sarcoplasmic reticulum of the muscle. Calcium ions then catalyze the chemical reaction that promotes the interdigitating and sliding of the actin and myosin filaments along each other, producing muscle contraction (see Chapter 63).

The **cardiac cycle** has two phases, diastole and systole. Relaxation and filling of both atria and then both ventricles take place during **diastole.** Contraction and emptying of both atria and then both ventricles occur during **systole.**

### Diastole

The diastolic phase of the cardiac cycle is subdivided into the following phases: (1) isovolumetric ventricular relaxation, (2) rapid ventricular filling, (3) slow ventricular filling, and (4) atrial systole (Table 29-1 and Figure 29-10, *A*).

The initial phase of **isovolumetric ventricular relaxation** begins as soon as the aortic valve and pulmonic valve close. During this time the myocardial muscle relaxes, and ventricular pressure falls. However, the falling ventricular pressure is still higher than atrial pressure; therefore the AV valves remain closed. Because these valves remain closed, a large amount of blood collects in the atria. As ventricular pressure begins to drop more rapidly to its low diastolic level, the higher pressure in the atria pushes the AV valves open and allows blood to flow rapidly into the ventricular cavity. This second phase of diastole, *rapid ventricular filling*, lasts for approximately the first third of diastole and causes intraventricular pressures to rise. As ventricular pressure increases, it impedes further rapid filling, and the resultant slowing of ventricular filling marks the third phase of diastole. This phase of *slow ventricular filling* is referred to as *diastasis*. Both the atrial and the ventricular chambers are relaxed, and blood entering the atria flows passively into the ventricles. During the phase of **atrial systole,** electrical depolarization spreads through the atria and pauses at the AV node for 0.10 second. The atrial musculature then contracts, propelling an additional 20% to 30% of blood into the ventricle before ventricular contraction.

### Systole

The ventricular systolic phase of the cardiac cycle is subdivided into phases of isovolumetric ventricular contraction, maximal ventricular ejection, and reduced ventricular ejection (see Table 29-1 and Figure 29-10, *B*).

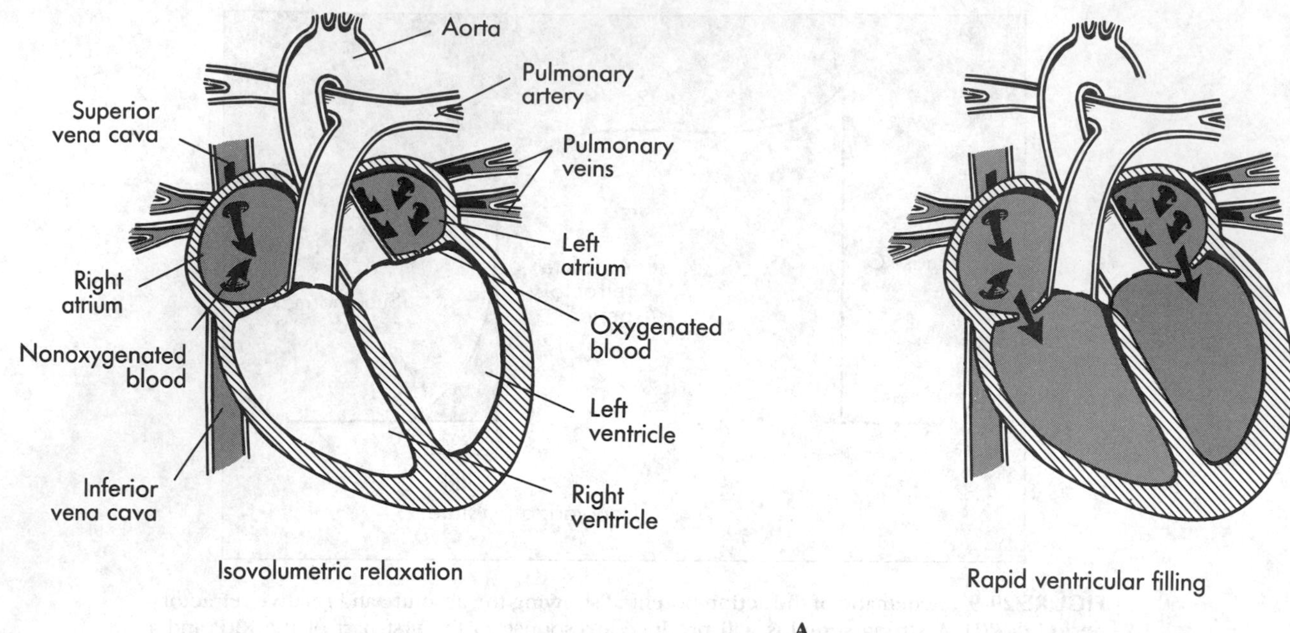


**FIGURE 29-10** Events during the cardiac cycle. **A,** Diastole. **B,** Systole.

**TABLE 29-1 Events During the Cardiac Cycle**

| PHASE | VALVES: PULMONARY AND AORTIC | VALVES: MITRAL AND TRICUSPID | ACTIONS | PRESSURE (P) CHANGES |
|---|---|---|---|---|
| **DIASTOLE** | | | | |
| Isovolumetric relaxation | Closed | Closed | Blood collects in atria. | Atrial P increases until greater than ventricular P. |
| Rapid ventricular filling | Closed | Open | Blood flows rapidly into ventricles from pressure differential. | Atrial P decreases; ventricular P increases. |
| Slow ventricular filling | Closed | Open | Blood flows passively into ventricles. | Same as for rapid filling. |
| Atrial systole | Closed | Open, then close | Atrial contraction pushes additional blood into ventricles. | Ventricular P becomes greater than atrial P. |
| **SYSTOLE** | | | | |
| Isovolumetric contraction | Closed | Closed | Myocardial tension increases. | Ventricular P increases; aortic P decreases until ventricular P greater than aortic P. |
| Maximal ventricular ejection | Open | Closed | Blood is pumped from ventricles into pulmonary artery and aorta. | Ventricular P decreases. |
| Reduced ventricular ejection | Open, then close | Closed | Some blood ejected. | Ventricular pressure decreases rapidly when ventricles relax. |

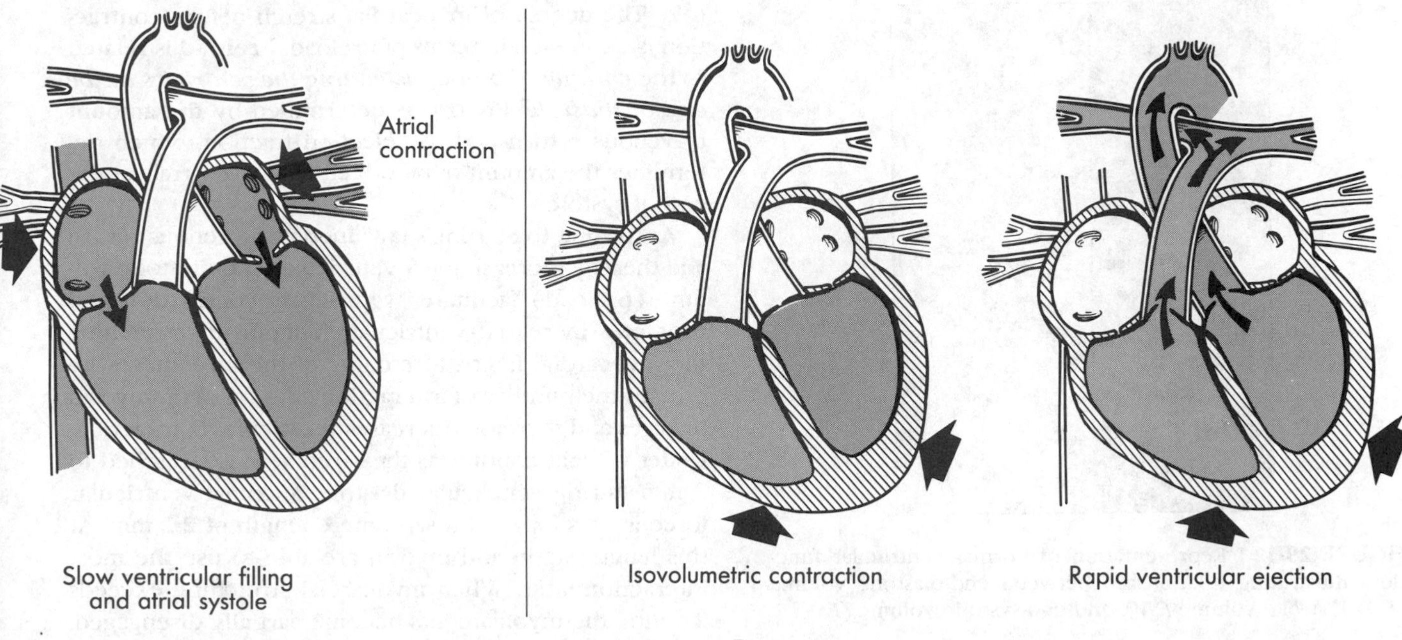


During the **isovolumetric ventricular contraction** phase, myocardial tension and intraventricular pressure increase, whereas no change occurs in blood volume or muscle fiber length. At this time the aortic valve is closed because pressure in the aortic root exceeds left ventricular pressure. The higher pressure in the aortic root is the result of a previous systole that has just ejected blood into the aorta. As this aortic blood is distributed to the periphery, aortic pressure falls slowly. At the same time, intraventricular pressure and tension are increasing. When intraventricular pressure exceeds aortic root pressure, the aortic valve opens and **maximal ventricular ejection** begins. Blood from the ventricles is pumped into the pulmonic and systemic circulations. As the ejection rate starts to slow, the phase of **reduced ventricular ejection,** or *protodiastole,* begins. The ventricles remain contracted, but little blood is being ejected from the ventricle into the aorta. Ventricular pressure actually falls slightly below aortic root pressure, but some blood is still being ejected simply because of the momentum built up by the contraction. At the end of systole, ventricular relaxation begins suddenly, and a rapid decrease in intraventricular pressure occurs. The higher pressure in the large arteries and in the aortic root immediately pushes blood back toward the ventricles, thus snapping shut the semilunar valves.

## Cardiac Output

The *amount of blood ejected from the left ventricle into the aorta per minute* is called the **cardiac output.** Although the right ventricle ejects an equivalent amount of blood into the pulmonary artery, it is not included in the measurement of total cardiac output. Rather, cardiac output (CO) is equivalent to **stroke volume** (SV) (volume of blood ejected from the left ventricle with each contraction) times heart rate (HR) (number of heartbeats per minute):

$$CO = SV \times HR$$

The average cardiac output is 5.6 L/min in the average man. However, during periods of strenuous exercise, the cardiac output may reach 20 to 25 L/min. Because cardiac requirements vary according to individual body sizes, a more accurate means of assessing tissue perfusion is to compute the cardiac index. The **cardiac index** is obtained by dividing the cardiac output by the patient's total body surface area:

$$\text{Cardiac index} = \frac{\text{CO (L/min)}}{\text{Body surface area (m}^2\text{)}}$$

Therefore the cardiac index represents the cardiac output in terms of liters per minute per square meter of body surface. This corrects an individual's cardiac output to match body size. The normal range for cardiac index is 2.4 to 4.0 L/min. The cadiac output is based solely on the amount of blood ejected by the left ventricle into the systemic circulation. The average 70-kg man has an approximate cardiac index of 3 L/min.

### Stroke volume

**Stroke volume** is the *amount of blood ejected by the left ventricle into the aorta per beat.* At the completion of each filling phase, or diastole, the ventricle contains approximately 120 ml of blood (end-diastolic volume [EDV]) (Figure 29-11). Under normal circumstances, the

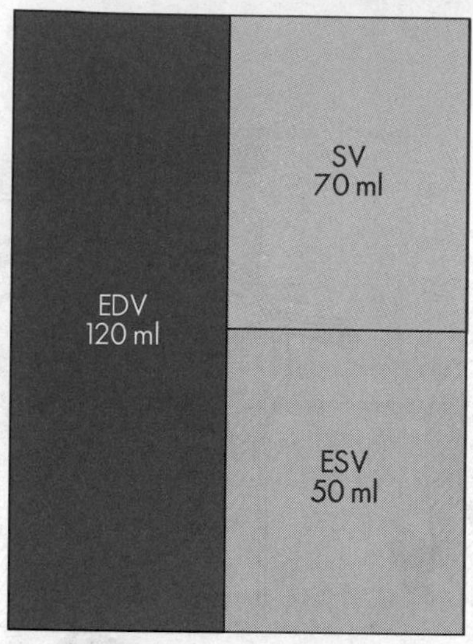


**FIGURE 29-11** Representation of normal ventricular function, illustrating relationship between end-diastolic volume *(EDV),* stroke volume *(SV),* and end-systolic volume *(ESV).*

heart ejects approximately two thirds of the EDV. The blood that is ejected is termed the *ejection fraction.* The volume of residual blood in the ventricle at the end of systole is known as the end-systolic volume (ESV). Therefore stroke volume can be defined as the difference between the volume of blood contained in the ventricle at the end of diastole and the volume of blood remaining at the end of systole:

$$SV = EDV - ESV$$

### Control of cardiac output

Cardiac output depends on the relationship between two important variables—stroke volume and heart rate. Despite fluctuations in one of these two variables, cardiac output can be maintained at relatively constant levels by compensatory adjustments made in the other variable. For example, if the heart rate slows, the time for ventricular filling (diastole) is lengthened. This lengthened period allows for an increase in preload and a subsequent increase in stroke volume. Conversely, if the stroke volume falls, the heart rate can increase to compensate temporarily and maintain cardiac output. Therefore the actual determinants of cardiac output are the mechanisms regulating stroke volume and heart rate.

**Control of stroke volume.** Three significant factors affecting stroke volume and thus cardiac output are preload, contractility, and afterload.

***Preload.*** Starling's law of the heart states that myocardial fiber responds with a more forceful contraction when it is stretched. An example of this phenomenon is that of increasing the stretch of a rubber band to obtain a more forceful recoil when the rubber band is released. Myocardial fibers can be stretched by increasing the volume of blood delivered to the ventricles during diastole. The degree of myocardial stretch before contraction is expressed in terms of preload. **Preload** is related to the *volume of blood distending the ventricles at the end of diastole.* Preload is determined by the amount of venous return and the ejection fraction, which determines the amount of blood left in the ventricle at the end of systole.

According to Starling's law, increasing venous return and thereby increasing left ventricular end-diastolic volume (preload) facilitates ventricular contraction and promotes increased ventricular function by stretching the myocardial fibers. Stretching of the sarcomeres increases the number of interaction sites for actin-myosin linkages and therefore increases ventricular contraction. Under normal conditions the sarcomere is stretched to 2 mm during ventricular diastole. Maximal ventricular force is developed at a sarcomere length of 2.2 mm. At this length, actin and myosin are able to use the most interaction sites. When myocardial stretching exceeds 2.4 mm, the myofilaments become partially disengaged, and fewer contractile sites are activated. Because Starling's length-tension relationship is functional only within physiologic limits, it is important to note that prolonged, excessive stretching of the myocardial fibers eventually will lead to a decrease in cardiac output by reducing the stroke volume (as in ventricular hypertrophy).

***Contractility.*** Contractility is another major mechanism involved in the control of stroke volume. By definition, contractility refers only to *a change in the inotropic state of the muscle without a change in myocardial fiber length or preload.* Increased contractility (inotropism) is a function of the increased intensity of interaction at the actin-myosin linkages. Contractility can be increased by sympathetic stimulation or by the administration of substances such as calcium or epinephrine. Increased contractility improves ventricular emptying during systole, thereby increasing the stroke volume.

***Afterload.*** Another factor involved in the control of stroke volume is afterload. **Afterload** is defined as the *amount of tension the ventricle must develop during contraction to eject blood from the left ventricle into the aorta.* The major impedance against which the left ventricle must pump is determined primarily by peripheral vascular resistance. Increase in pressure resulting from hypertension or vasoconstriction produces an increased resistance to pumping and will necessitate an increase in ventricular tension to eject blood. The afterload on the heart is affected not only by the amount of aortic pressure but also by the size of the heart. This relationship between ventricular tension, arterial pressure, and ventricular size is known as Laplace's law:

$$\text{Ventricular tension} = \text{Arterial pressure} \times \text{Ventricular radius}$$

As this simplified version of Laplace's law indicates, both hypertension and dilation of the ventricular chamber increase ventricular tension (increase afterload). Therefore, if arterial pressure increases, the ventricle must pump against higher resistance to empty adequately. Also, if ventricular radius increases, ventricular volume will increase. Thus at the same level of aortic pressure, the afterload against which an enlarged or dilated left ventricle must work is higher than that encountered by a normal-sized ventricle.

Excessive elevation of the afterload may impair ventricular emptying, thereby reducing stroke volume and cardiac output.

**Control of heart rate.** The autonomic nervous system (ANS) regulates the heart through two distinctly opposing sets of nerves, the sympathetic and the parasympathetic nervous systems. Afferent fibers accompany the efferent fibers of both these systems.

The sympathetic fibers arise from the thoracic spinal cord and reach the entire atria and ventricles as well as the SA and the AV nodes. The control of the ANS on the heart is mediated by neurotransmitters. The sympathetic nervous system neurotransmitter is norepinephrine. The *sympathetic fibers* have both *positive chronotropic* (increase rate) and *inotropic* (increase force) effects. Therefore with an increase in sympathetic stimulation, the neurotransmitter norepinephrine is released from the nerve endings and produces the following effects: increase in heart rate, increase in atrial and ventricular contractility, and increase in the speed of electrical conduction through the AV node.

The parasympathetic fibers originate in the medulla and have their innervation primarily in the atrial musculature and in the SA and AV nodes; however, parasympathetic stimulation has been shown to reach the ventricles. The *parasympathetic fibers* have a *negative chronotropic* effect and may exert a slightly negative inotropic effect; however, in the healthy circulatory system, this negative inotropic effect is compensated for by the increased filling that occurs as a result of a lengthened diastole. Stimulation of the parasympathetic system causes the release of the neurotransmitter acetylcholine at the vagal nerve endings and has basically the opposite effect of norepinephrine. Parasympathetic stimulation causes a decrease in the rate of discharge of the SA node, a decrease in the rate of conduction from the atria to the ventricles, and a decrease in the force of atrial contraction and probably also of ventricular contraction. The final effect of ANS control on the heart is the balance between these two opposing nervous systems at any one time. It is thought that the heart is normally under the control of vagal inhibition and maintains a resting heart rate of 65 to 75 beats/min.

The effects of the ANS can be greatly influenced by several additional factors, such as the central nervous system (CNS) and pressoreceptor reflexes. Impulses from the cerebral cortex can have a significant effect on the heart rate. Pain, fear, anger, and excitement can cause substantial increases in the heart rate. Also, reflex changes caused by stimulation of the pressoreceptors can influence heart rate. The *baroreceptor reflex,* with afferent branches in the aortic arch, carotid sinus, and other pressoreceptor zones, functions as a negative feedback mechanism to regulate pressure in the arteries and regulate the resistance of vessels in the vasculature. Consequently, an episode of hypotension would cause a sudden drop of blood pressure in the aorta or carotid sinus and would stimulate the pressoreceptors less intensely. The cardiac inhibitory center would then be stimulated less, and the result would be a reflex increase in the heart rate.

Many other important factors are involved in the control of heart rate, including body temperature, medication, catecholamines, arterial blood gas tensions, hormones other than epinephrine, and plasma electrolyte concentrations.

In summary, ventricular function and thus cardiac output are influenced by heart rate and stroke volume. Heart rate is primarily controlled by the ANS, and stroke volume depends on the three distinct variables of preload, contractility, and afterload.

## PHYSIOLOGIC CHANGES WITH AGING

The number one cause of death in persons who are 65 years or older is cardiovascular disease. Age-related changes take place in the chemical composition, cells, and tissues of the heart and blood vessels and influence many aspects of cardiovascular functioning. However, despite the physiologic changes of aging, the heart is able to meet the day-to-day demands and function adequately. It is only under unusual circumstances or increased stress that the deteriorating function of the heart is most apparent. For instance, asymptomatic ischemia may cause significant functional impairment. Not only is coronary atherosclerosis more prevalent in elders, but it also frequently manifests as an occult (hidden) disease. It is crucial to detect the occult form of this disease to determine necessary interventions such as pharmacotherapy and alterations in life-style.

With advancing age, life-styles often change with regard to eating, drinking, smoking, and physical activity. A sedentary life-style versus habitual exercise can produce a significant difference in cardiac output (see box, p. 758).

### Heart

Progressive left ventricular hypertrophy that occurs with aging is accompanied by a rise in arterial systolic blood pressure. Of interest is that heart weight increases in women but not in men. Ventricular septal thickness and the circumference of all four cardiac valves increase. By age 40 years the circumference of the aortic valve generally surpasses that of the pulmonic valve. In both genders the leaflet thickness and calcification of the mitral and aortic valves increase progressively and signif-

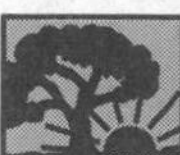

## GERONTOLOGIC PATIENT CONSIDERATIONS

### ASSESSMENT

Count the pulse for a full minute at rest and after exertion. The pulse is often slower and may be irregular because elders are more prone to decreased cardiac output and dysrhythmias.

Monitor changes in blood pressure:

- Systolic blood pressure in elders may normally be as high as 160 mm Hg (as compared with 140 mm Hg in younger adults). A widened pulse pressure also may be observed.
- Check blood pressure in a lying, sitting, and standing position to detect postural hypotension because vasomotor control is decreased in the elders.

When assessing the heart, note that the apical impulse may be harder to locate. Murmurs are common from thickening and calcification of the valves.

Monitor for signs of mental confusion, lethargy, indigestion, and weakness in the elderly person; these may be early signs of cardiac disease. Angina is commonly noted with ischemic heart disease.

Assess elderly patient with myocardial infarction for signs of congestive heart failure, a common complication.

### INTERVENTION

Prevent falls in elders that may be associated with bradycardia, postural hypotension, or myocardial infarction.

- Teach elders to move and stand slowly to prevent falling because of hypotension (drop attacks).
- Teach the patient who is taking diuretics or antihypertensives to move slowly and cautiously.
- Teach elders to avoid standing for long periods (blood pooling), especially over a hot stove or in the shower (heat causes vasodilation, thus lowering blood pressure).

Teach foot pumping exercises, which are performed before rising from bed or chair to increase venous return.

Teach patient and significant others to seek early medical attention for unexplained illness, unrelieved indigestion, or sudden changes in behavior.

### COMMON DISORDERS IN ELDERS

Congestive heart failure
Angina pectoris
Myocardial infarction
Dysrhythmias

**TABLE 29-2 Physiologic Changes of Cardiovascular System With Aging**

| CHANGES | POSSIBLE OUTCOME |
|---|---|
| **HEART** | |
| Increased subendocardial fat<br>Increased deposition of lipofuscin pigment in cardiac cells<br>Increased amounts of connective tissue and changes in properties of connective tissue | Decreased cardiac output<br>Decreased compliance<br>Less efficient pump |
| **VALVES** | |
| Thickening, calcification, and fibrosis, particularly in aortic and mitral valves | Systolic murmurs (usually ejection)<br>Possible disturbance in blood flow to coronary arteries |
| **RATE AND RHYTHM** | |
| Increased amounts of connective tissue in SA nodes, internodal tracts, AV nodes, and bundle branches<br>Atrial atrophy | High rate response to exercise/stress is less effective and takes longer to return to normal<br>Sinus dysrhythmias, atrial flutter, extrasystoles |
| **ARTERIES** | |
| Thickening of intima<br>Thinning and fragmentation of elastin, leading to arterial stiffening<br>Increase in absolute number of collagen fibers | Reduced compliance of blood vessels and peripheral vascular resistance (PVR)<br>Increased pulse wave velocity<br>Less effective baroreceptor response<br>Slight increase in blood pressure; increase in systolic and slower rate of increase in diastolic |

icantly with advancing age. These rigid valves can lead to audible systolic murmurs, usually of an ejection nature.

An increase in average myocyte (muscle cell) size primarily explains the increase in heart mass; however, the simultaneous change in the amount and functional properties of myocardial collagen plays a key role in causing physiologic cardiovascular abnormalities of aging. The increased connective tissue contributes to myocardial stiffness and decreased cardiac compliance. The amount of subendocardial fat also increases, and the endocardium undergoes fibrosis, thickening, and sclerosis (Table 29-2).

A decreased peak-systolic left ventricular wall stress occurs with aging. Increasing left ventricular wall thickness and increasing body surface area with age are presumed to be contributing factors. The isovolumetric relaxation period also is prolonged, resulting in incomplete relaxation during early diastolic filling. However, enhanced ventricular filling occurs later in diastole as a result of a compensatory, augmented atrial contribution to ventricular filling.

## Arteries

Both the aorta and its branches and the large pulmonary arteries and their branches undergo progressive dilation and elongation with age. Because the enlargement is both transverse and longitudinal, the aorta tends to become tortuous. The large pulmonary arteries, however, appear to be too short with too low a pressure to dilate longitudinally. These alterations are caused by fragmentation, degeneration, and reduction in the amount of elastic tissue, as well as by increased collagen amount and structural changes. Because of decreased vascular distensibility, arterial pulse pressure increases as a result of increased systolic pressure (with less change in diastolic pressure). A larger portion of forward blood flow is imposed on the left ventricle because of decreased aortic size during diastole, resulting in increased impedance to blood flow and decreased cardiac output. The generalized loss of elasticity in the arterial system can lead to a sluggish baroreceptor response. The baroreceptors are then less able to modulate blood pressure, particularly during rapid postural change.

### Conduction system

Prolonged atrioventricular (AV) conduction with disturbances in cardiac rate and rhythm occur in aging healthy persons as a result of fibrosis and fatty infiltration.[3] Fibrotic changes occur predominantly in the ventricular system, whereas fatty deposits tend to occur in the SA and AV nodes, as well as in the atria.

### Exercise and cardiovascular response

As stated earlier, age-related changes in the cardiovascular system are significantly more pronounced in response to exercise. The overall increase in heart rate during vigorous exercise is less in elderly persons. Older persons without significant coronary artery disease may demonstrate increases in stroke volume greater than in younger adults to compensate for the lesser increases in heart rate. Persons of all ages exhibit comparable increases in left ventricular end-diastolic volume during upright exercise at low workloads. At higher workloads, in older persons whose heart rate increase is less, increases in left ventricular volume and stroke volume may continue throughout physical exercise. In contrast, younger persons at higher workloads tend to exhibit accelerated heart rates and decreased end-diastolic and end-systolic volumes.

Left ventricular ejection fraction has been shown to decrease, or fail to increase, with more exercise in persons with coronary artery disease. Similarly, reductions in left ventricular ejection fraction from rest to exercise also could be attributed to aging.

## Purpose of Cardiac Assessment

Systematic cardiac assessment provides the nurse with baseline data useful for identifying the physiologic and psychosocial needs of the patient and for planning appropriate nursing interventions to meet these needs. The nurse is in a unique position of ongoing patient monitoring and thus is able to take immediate action when signs occur that indicate alterations of cardiac function.

## Subjective Data

Subjective data obtained by means of a detailed patient history may be as diagnostically significant as laboratory data and ECG recordings in the assessment of the patient with suspected cardiac disease. Accurate assessment data are necessary to identify cardiac risk factors pertinent to the individual, as well as to determine the psychodynamic family relationships that must be addressed throughout the diagnostic, treatment, and follow-up phases.

The cardinal symptoms of heart disease include *dyspnea, chest pain* or discomfort, *edema, syncope, palpitations,* and excessive *fatigue.* Cyanosis is usually a sign rather than a symptom, but it also may be an important feature of the patient's history, particularly in patients with congenital heart disease. An important principle of cardiovascular evaluation is that cardiovascular function, which may be adequate at rest, may be insufficient during exercise or exertion. Therefore careful attention should be directed to the effects of activity on the patient's symptoms.

## DYSPNEA

*Dyspnea,* one of the most common and distressing symptoms of cardiopulmonary disease, is described as an abnormally uncomfortable awareness of breathing. The patient complains of shortness of breath. Because dyspnea is associated with a variety of diseases, as well as with anxiety, the history is a necessary tool in evaluating the etiologic factors.

Different types of dyspnea exist; therefore the history must include factors that precipitate and relieve dyspnea and data regarding the patient's body position when dyspnea occurs.

*Dyspnea on exertion* is a common symptom of cardiac dysfunction. In the early stages of heart failure, dyspnea usually is provoked only by effort and is relieved promptly by rest. It is important to identify the amount of exertion necessary to produce dyspnea, because the less the cardiac reserve (heart's ability to adjust and adapt to increased demands), the less effort is required to precipitate dyspnea.

*Orthopnea* refers to dyspnea in the recumbent position. It is usually a symptom of more advanced heart failure than is exertional dyspnea. Patients relate that they may use two or more pillows to sleep restfully in a semiupright position. When the person assumes the recumbent position, gravitational forces redistribute blood from the lower extremities and splanchnic bed, increasing venous return. The augmentation of intrathoracic blood volume elevates pulmonary venous and capillary pressures, resulting in a transient pulmonary congestion. Orthopnea usually is relieved in less than 5 minutes after the patient sits upright.

*Paroxysmal nocturnal dyspnea,* also known as cardiac asthma, is characterized by severe attacks of shortness of breath that generally occur 2 to 5 hours after the onset of sleep. This condition frequently is associated with sweating and wheezing and wakens the patient from sleep. These frightening attacks are precipitated by an increased blood volume caused by the reabsorption of edema that was pooled in dependent portions of the body during the day. When the patient lies in a recumbent position, there is a redistribution of the increased intravascular volume with a specific rise in intrathoracic blood volume. The diseased heart is unable to compensate for this increase in blood volume and unable to pump extra fluid into the circulatory system; therefore pulmonary congestion results. Paroxysmal nocturnal dyspnea is relieved by having the patient sit on the side of the bed or even get out of bed. However, unlike simple orthopnea, 20 minutes or more may be required for the patient with paroxysmal nocturnal dyspnea to obtain relief.

## CHEST PAIN

Although pain or discomfort in the chest is one of the cardinal symptoms of cardiac disorders, it is essential to recognize that chest pain can be precipitated by various conditions. For example, chest pain may be caused by ischemic heart disease, acute dissection of the aorta, or acute pericarditis, or it may occur in pulmonary disorders (e.g., pleurisy and pulmonary embolism).

A common cause of chest pain, however, is not associated with cardiovascular disease, but rather with anxiety. Therefore, to evaluate chest pain correctly, the following list of characteristic symptoms should be addressed during a thorough history:

| | |
|---|---|
| 1. Onset | When was chest pain first noticed? |
| 2. Manner of onset | Did the pain or discomfort start suddenly or gradually? |
| 3. Duration | How long did the pain last? |
| 4. Precipitating factors | Ask patient to describe possible precipitating factors (e.g., exertion, food, anxiety, emotions). |
| 5. Location | Where did the pain originate? Did it radiate? To what area? |
| 6. Quality | Ask patient to describe how symptoms feel (e.g., sharp, dull). |
| 7. Intensity | Ask patient to describe severity of the pain (e.g., if pain interfered with any activities). |
| 8. Chronology and frequency | Has this pain occurred in the past? If so, how often? |
| 9. Associated symptoms | Do any other signs or symptoms occur at the same time? |
| 10. Aggravating factors | What makes the pain worse? |
| 11. Relaxing factors | What makes symptoms less intense? |

## EDEMA

Edema is defined as an accumulation of excess fluid in the interstitial spaces. The retention of considerable amounts of extracellular fluid may occur without associated edema. In fact, weight gains of up to 7 kg of water can occur before the abnormality is detected. Because early manifestations of edema may be subtle, careful comparison of daily weights is required to determine weight gains resulting from fluid retention. Normally, basal body weight varies little from day to day; therefore subtle weight gains resulting from fluid retention are readily detectable.

The numerous causes of edema include congestive heart failure, fluid overload, and obstruction of venous drainage. Therefore, depending on the specific cause of the edema, it may be localized to one particular body part, organ, or tissue; or it may have a generalized distribution. (For a more in-depth discussion of edema, see Chapter 20.)

## SYNCOPE

Syncope is defined as a generalized muscle weakness with an inability to stand upright, accompanied by loss of consciousness. The most common cause of syncope is decreased perfusion to the brain. Any condition that results in a sudden reduction of cardiac output and therefore reduced cerebral blood flow could potentially cause a syncopal episode. In patients with cardiovascular disorders, conditions such as orthostatic hypotension, hypovolemia, or a variety of dysrhythmias (e.g., heart block and severe ventricular dysrhythmias) may precipitate syncope.

## PALPITATIONS

**Palpitation** is a common subjective phenomenon defined as an unpleasant awareness of the heartbeat. It may be precipitated by a change in cardiac rate or rhythm or by an increase in myocardial contractility. Patients may describe their heartbeat as "pounding," "racing," or "skipping." Palpitations that occur either during or after strenuous activity are considered physiologic and represent an awareness of the overactivity of the heart. Palpitations that occur during mild exertion may suggest the presence of heart failure, anemia, or thyrotoxicosis. Other noncardiac factors that may precipitate palpitations include the following: nervousness, heavy meals, lack of sleep, and a large intake of coffee, tea, alcohol, or tobacco.

## FATIGUE

Fatigue and lassitude have many causes, and therefore these symptoms are not diagnostic of cardiovascular disorders. However, fatigue as a symptom associated with heart failure may result from such states as nocturia, insomnia, and nocturnal dyspnea. In addition, fatigue may be a direct consequence of the heart failure itself. The exact physiologic mechanism responsible for fatigue related to heart failure is not known, but it is probably a consequence of an inadequate cardiac output. Such fatigue can occur during effort or at rest and generally worsens as the day progresses. Fatigue that occurs after mild exertion may indicate a low cardiac reserve if the heart is unable to meet even small increases in metabolic demands.

# OBJECTIVE DATA

Physical examination of the cardiovascular system includes the use of inspection, palpation, percussion, and

**BOX 29-1 Physical Inspection for Assessment of Cardiac Function**

- Skin color
- Neck vein distention
- Respiratory rate and character
- Location of point of maximal impulse (PMI)
- Presence of edema
- Nail clubbing
- Capillary filling

auscultation. The following is a description of the essential components in cardiovascular assessment. For a detailed description of the techniques involved, the reader is referred to a physical assessment textbook.

## INSPECTION

### Skin Color

The color of the patient's skin and mucous membranes should be noted (Box 29-1). A person's "normal" color depends on race, ethnic background, and life-style and is an indication of adequate cardiac output and circulation. Pallor may indicate anemia, hypoxia, or peripheral vasoconstriction. *Cyanosis,* a bluish discoloration of the skin, is most easily observed by examining the earlobes, oral mucosa at the base of the tongue, the lips, and the nailbeds.

There are two types of cyanosis, central and peripheral. In central cyanosis the tongue is characteristically cyanotic. This form of cyanosis is caused by low arterial oxygen saturation and generally is seen in patients who have congenital heart defects with left-to-right shunts or in those with pulmonary diseases that interfere with ventilation or diffusion.

Peripheral cyanosis results from low cardiac output and generally is accompanied by decreased skin temperature and mottling. In contrast to central cyanosis, no cyanosis of the tongue is present. (For further information on skin color, see Chapter 66.)

### Neck Vein Distention

A general estimate of venous pressure can be obtained by observation of the neck veins (Figure 29-12). Normally, when a person is in a supine position, the neck veins are distended. However, when the head of the bed is elevated at a 45-degree angle, the neck veins are collapsed. The jugular veins reflect venous tone, blood volume, and right atrial pressure. Therefore distended neck veins suggest increased venous pressure, which may be caused by right-sided heart failure, circulatory volume overload, superior vena caval obstruction, or tricuspid valve regurgitation.

### Respirations

Next, the rate and character of the patient's respirations are assessed. Normally, an adult breathes comfortably at a rate of 12 to 20 times per minute. Particular attention is paid to the ease or difficulty in breathing and the patient's general demeanor.

### Point of Maximal Impulse

Inspection of the anterior chest is best accomplished with the patient lying in a supine position, either flat or with the head slightly elevated. Observe and palpate the precordium for the **point of maximal impulse (PMI),** which is a faint heaving of the chest wall caused by the forward thrusting of the ventricles during systole. The location of the PMI helps to locate the apex of the heart, which lies approximately 0.5 cm to the left of the PMI. The PMI normally is located in the left fifth intercostal space in the midclavicular line, or 8 to 10 cm to the left of the midsternal line. Any pulsation noted below the third intercostal space on the left precordium is known

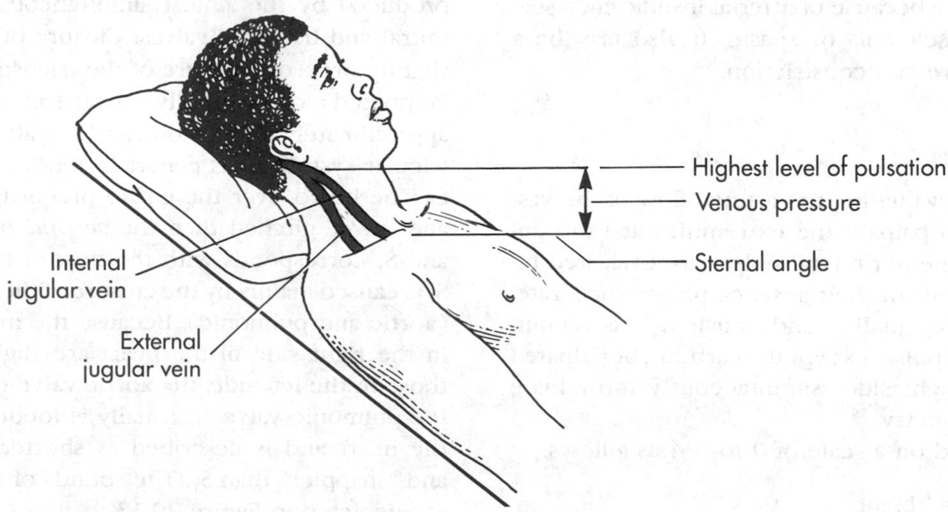


**FIGURE 29-12** Position of internal and external jugular veins used in measuring venous pressure.

as the *PMI;* any pulsation above the third intercostal space generally is not related to the heart but rather to the great vessels. The PMI is not always visible, but it usually is palpable.

### Peripheral Edema

An important indicator of cardiovascular function is the presence or absence of peripheral edema, especially in the feet, ankles, legs, and sacrum. Edema that disappears on elevation of the body part may be caused by gravity flow or by interruption of the venous return to the heart as a result of constricting clothing or pressure on the veins of the lower extremities.

In contrast, ***pitting edema*** does not disappear with elevation of the extremity or body part, and it may indicate fluid overload or a pathologic condition (e.g., congestive heart failure) when cardiac pumping efficiency is impaired. Edema is identified by inspection and palpation. Pitting edema is present if an indentation is left in the skin after a thumb or finger has been used to apply gentle pressure (see Chapter 20).

Nutritional deficiencies caused by decreased circulation can produce dry skin, thickened nails, brittle hair, and occasional hair loss in an extremity (characteristic of peripheral vascular disease).

The nails also must be assessed for clubbing and capillary refill. The exact cause of ***clubbing*** is not known at present; however, clubbing of the fingers is typical of congenital heart defects and pulmonary arteriovenous (A-V) fistulas with right-to-left shunting. *Capillary filling,* usually called ***blanching,*** is an indicator of peripheral circulation to the fingers and toes and can be tested in all nailbeds. The examiner presses a thumbnail against the edge of a patient's fingernail or toenail and then quickly releases it. The normal response is whitening (blanching) of the area when pressure is applied and brisk return of color when pressure is released. Lack of the blanching response may indicate lack of circulation to the finger or toe because of arterial insufficiency secondary to atherosclerosis or spasm. It also may be a reflection of severe vasoconstriction.

## PALPATION

### Peripheral Pulses

One method for evaluating the arterial flow of the vascular system is to palpate the extremities and the peripheral pulses. The peripheral pulses are evaluated bilaterally on the basis of their absence or presence, rate, rhythm, amplitude, quality, and equality. It is recommended that each pulse, except the carotids, be palpated on the left and right sides simultaneously to evaluate contralateral symmetry.

Pulses are rated on a scale of 0 to +4 as follows:

0 = Absent
\+ = Palpable, but diminished
++ = Normal, or average
+++ = Full and brisk
++++ = Full and bounding, often visible

### Apical Impulse

Normally, the apical impulse is felt as a single, light tap. The presence of anything other than a single, light tap may suggest a myocardial pathologic condition and should be reported to the physician. A thrill, or palpable murmur, indicates the presence of significant turbulent blood flow across an intracardiac shunt or a severely stenotic valve. A thrill has been described as a vibration similar to that of a cat's purr. A thrill is more readily palpated after the patient exhales forcefully. Frequently, having the patient in a left lateral position or leaning forward will accentuate the vibration.

## PERCUSSION

The use of percussion for detecting cardiac enlargement generally has been replaced by the more accurate use of palpation. Therefore the use of percussion in the cardiovascular examination is considered to be somewhat limited. Usually only the left border of cardiac dullness can be determined, inasmuch as this is located near the PMI, or within the midclavicular line. Cardiac dullness noted below the fifth intercostal space, beyond the left midclavicular line, or to the right of the sternum is characteristic of cardiac hypertrophy. Unfortunately, mild to moderate degrees of cardiac hypertrophy or dilation usually are not detectable by percussion.

## AUSCULTATION

Auscultation of heart sounds enables a nurse to establish baseline data for identifying current and future cardiac problems that require nursing intervention. Cardiac auscultation also assists the nurse in evaluating a patient's progress (e.g., effect of activity on heart rate) or in monitoring responses to medications (e.g., quinidine or digitalis preparations).

### Heart Sounds

The ***first* heart sound** ($S_1$) generally is thought to be produced by the almost simultaneous closures of the mitral and tricuspid valves. Closure of the mitral valve slightly precedes closure of the tricuspid valve, but the combined closure usually is heard as one sound. $S_1$ lasts approximately 0.10 second and signals the onset of ventricular systole. $S_1$ is generally loudest at the apex but can be heard over the entire precordium. $S_1$ is longer and lower pitched than the *second heart sound* ($S_2$), and $S_1$ corresponds with the beat of the carotid pulse. $S_2$ is caused mainly by the closure of the semilunar valves (aortic and pulmonic). Because the mechanical events in the right side of the heart are slightly slower than those in the left side, the aortic valve closes just before the pulmonic valve. $S_2$ usually is loudest at the base of the heart and is described as shorter, higher-pitched, and "snappier" than $S_1$. The sounds of the cardiac cycle are depicted in Figure 29-13.

The diaphragm chest piece is most useful in listening to high-pitched sounds and murmurs. These include such sounds as $S_1$, $S_2$, and ejection sounds and clicks.

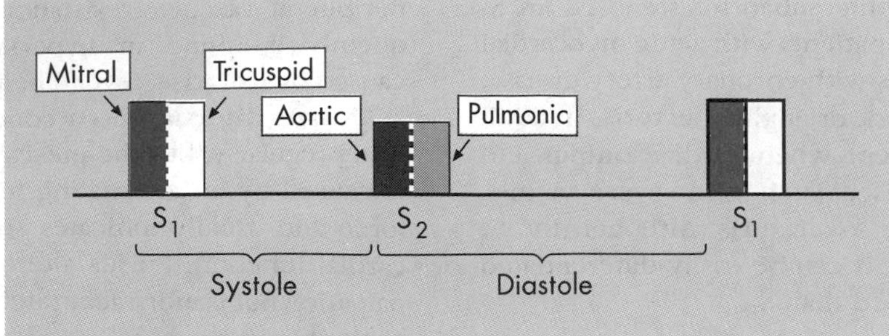


**FIGURE 29-13** Heart sound $S_1$ is the closure of mitral and tricuspid valves; $S_2$ is the closure of the aortic and pulmonic valves. Systole is the interval between $S_1$ and the start of $S_2$; diastole is $S_2$ to the start of $S_1$. Diastole is longer than systole.

The diaphragm should be placed firmly on the chest wall so that when it is removed, an indentation is present on the patient's skin. The bell chest piece is most useful in detecting low-pitched sounds and murmurs. These include the third heart sound ($S_3$), the fourth heart sound ($S_4$), and mitral and tricuspid diastolic rumbles. The bell should be placed lightly on the chest wall, barely creating an airtight seal. If the bell is placed firmly on the skin, it will act as a diaphragm.

### Splitting of $S_1$ and $S_2$

The two main components of $S_1$ (closure of the mitral and tricuspid valves) are asynchronous, because left ventricular contraction usually occurs slightly ahead of right ventricular systole. The $S_1$ may be split in persons who have right bundle branch (RBB) block, left-sided mechanical defects (e.g., mitral stenosis) or tricuspid valve dysfunction associated with pulmonary hypertension.

Because left ventricular contraction slightly precedes right ventricular contraction, the aortic valve normally closes slightly before the pulmonic valve. On inspiration, intrathoracic pressure decreases and facilitates an increase in venous blood return to the right side of the heart. This increased blood return delays the closure of the pulmonic valve and results in a normal physiologic, split $S_2$. On expiration, closure of the aortic and pulmonic valves occurs almost simultaneously and therefore is heard only as a single sound. In conditions of increased blood flow or increased right ventricular pressure (atrial septal defect or pulmonary artery stenosis), there may be a "fixed" splitting of $S_2$; that is, both components of $S_2$ are heard in both inspiration and expiration. A fixed split is considered abnormal and may occur in RBB block, pulmonary hypertension, and right ventricular failure related to atrial or ventricular septal defects.

### Extra heart sounds

Extra heart sounds include ejection sounds (systolic clicks), opening snaps, and $S_3$ and $S_4$. Of these sounds, the two that occur most frequently and are discussed here are $S_3$ and $S_4$ (Figure 29-14).

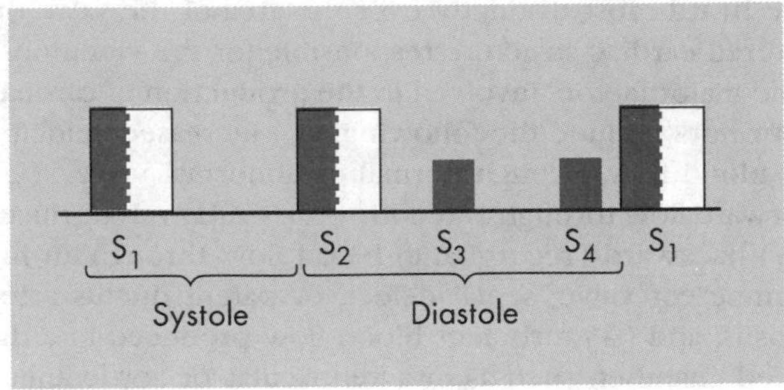


**FIGURE 29-14** Location of extra heart sounds during cardiac cycle.

**Ventricular diastolic gallop,** or $S_3$, is a faint, low-pitched sound produced by rapid ventricular filling in early diastole. This occurs when the volume of early filling is increased or a decrease occurs in ventricular compliance. Ventricular "gallop" describes the canter of a horse, which frequently is mimicked at heart rates greater than 100. When this sound is present in healthy children and young adults, it is almost always a normal condition and is referred to as a ***physiologic*** $S_3$. A physiologic $S_3$ results from the transition from rapid to slow filling in a healthy compliant ventricle. An $S_3$ heard in an older person usually is a pathologic sign and frequently is one of the first signs of serious heart disease or cardiac decompensation, as seen in congestive heart failure. An audible $S_3$ is associated with elevated mid-diastolic left ventricular filling pressures. $S_3$ is typically present in such states as left-to-right shunts, mitral regurgitation, congestive heart failure, and constrictive pericarditis.

**Atrial diastolic gallop,** or $S_4$, is a low-frequency sound that occurs under circumstances of altered ventricular compliance, either left or right. $S_4$ occurs late in diastole when atrial systole ejects blood into a noncompliant ventricle. Because the presence of an audible $S_4$ is related to a decrease in left ventricular compliance and an increase in left ventricular end-diastolic pressure, it is often heard in hypertensive cardiovascular disease and idiopathic hypertrophic subaortic stenosis. An $S_4$ frequently is identified in patients with acute myocardial infarctions and in patients with coronary artery disease, especially during an attack of angina pectoris. In addition, an $S_4$ may be present when cardiac output and stroke volume are increased, such as in severe anemia, thyrotoxicosis, and large A-V fistulas. Although the $S_4$ sound occurs close to $S_1$, it can be easily differentiated because $S_4$ is lower-pitched than $S_1$.

### Murmurs

**Murmurs** are audible vibrations of the heart and great vessels that occur because of turbulent blood flow. Turbulent blood flow may be produced by hemodynamic events or by structural alterations occurring in the heart or in the walls of the great vessels. In general, murmurs are heard most distinctly over the area of the valve or altered cardiac structure responsible for the vibrations. The major factors involved in the production of cardiac murmurs include the following: (1) increased velocity of blood flow through normal or abnormal valves, (2) forward flow through a stenotic or irregular valve orifice, (3) backward (regurgitant) blood flow through an incompetent valve, septal defect, or patent ductus arteriosus, and (4) turbulent blood flow produced in a dilated chamber, such as in a ventricular or aortic aneurysm.

Murmurs generally are characterized according to timing (position in the cardiac cycle), intensity, quality, pitch, location, and direction of radiation. These characteristics provide data concerning the location and nature of the cardiac abnormality.

### Pericardial Friction Rub

A **pericardial friction rub** is an extra heart sound originating from the pericardial sac. This rub may be a sign of inflammation, infection, or infiltration. It occurs as the heart moves. Pericardial friction rubs may have specific subcomponents (different sounds), each associated with a particular cardiac movement. The heart moves with atrial and ventricular systole and with ventricular diastole. Each of the sound components of a pericardial friction rub corresponds to a movement of the cardiac cycle and is described as a short, high-pitched, scratchy sound.

## ABNORMAL PULSES

A *hypokinetic* (weak) pulse signifies a narrowed pulse pressure, that is, decreased difference between systolic and diastolic pressures. It usually is produced by a low cardiac output and is associated with increased peripheral vascular resistance. This type of pulse may be palpable in such conditions as severe left ventricular failure, hypovolemia, or mitral and aortic valve stenosis.

A *hyperkinetic* (bounding) pulse represents a widened pulse pressure. It usually is associated with an increased left ventricular stroke volume and a decrease in peripheral vascular resistance. This type of pulse frequently is found in hyperkinetic circulatory states caused by exercise, fever, anemia, and hyperthyroidism.

**Pulsus alternans** is a condition in which the heart beats regularly, but the pulses alternate in amplitude. It is caused by an alternating left ventricular contractile force and usually indicates severe depression of myocardial function. Pulsus alternans may be detected by palpation but is more accurately assessed by auscultation of the blood pressure.

**Pulsus paradoxus** signifies a reduction in the amplitude of the arterial pulse during inspiration. Variations in pulse strength can be palpated, but a paradoxic pulse is most readily detected by sphygmomanometry. The difference between the peak systolic pressures at which sounds are audible *only* during expiration and later when sounds are audible during both inspiration and expiration is a measure of the magnitude of the paradoxic pulse. Normally the difference between these two pressures should not exceed 8 mm Hg.

Pulsus paradoxus is an accentuation of the normal decrease in systolic arterial pressure with inspiration. This is a result of decreased left ventricular stroke volume and the transmission of negative intrathoracic pressure to the aorta. Pulsus paradoxus may occur in conditions such as cardiac tamponade and constrictive pericarditis, but it also may occur in patients with chronic obstructive airway disease who have wide swings of intrapleural pressure during respiration.

# DIAGNOSTIC TESTS

Cardiovascular diseases usually are diagnosed by correlating laboratory test results with findings from the patient interview and the physical examination. The laboratory tests ordered most frequently in patients with heart disease or suspected heart disease include the following: blood tests, urinalysis, electrocardiography (see Chapter 30), invasive hemodynamic monitoring, sonic studies, dynamic studies, radiography, scintigraphic studies, and angiography.

The nurse may be directly or indirectly involved in these tests and procedures and should understand why a particular test or examination is being performed and what it will contribute to the patient's diagnosis. This information enables the nurse to prepare the patient adequately before any diagnostic procedure and to observe and record signs and symptoms while caring for the patient.

## LABORATORY TESTS

A complete blood cell count (CBC) is ordered for all patients with documented or suspected heart disease for evaluation of the overall health status. Data concerning red and white blood cells (RBCs and WBCs) are helpful in diagnosing infectious heart diseases and myocardial infarctions (Table 29-3). RBCs may be elevated

**TABLE 29-3 Selected Laboratory Tests for Cardiovascular Disorders**

| TEST | NORMAL VALUES | SIGNIFICANCE IN HEART DISORDERS |
|---|---|---|
| Serum RBC | Men: 4.7-6.1 million/mm$^3$<br>Women: 4.2-5.4 million/mm$^3$ | Decreased in subacute endocarditis<br>Increased with inadequate tissue oxygenation<br>Decreased in some congenital heart disease with right-to-left shunt |
| Serum WBC | 5000-10,000/mm$^3$ | Increased in acute and chronic heart inflammations and in acute myocardial infarction |
| Erythrocyte sedimentation rate (ESR) | Men: up to 15 mm/hr<br>Women: up to 20 mm/hr | Increased in acute myocardial infarction and infectious heart disease |
| Prothrombin time (PT) | 11-12.5 sec<br>100% compared to control | Indicates rapidity of blood clotting; used to monitor anticoagulant therapy with Coumadin (warfarin sodium) |
| Activated partial thromboplastin time (APTT) | 30-40 sec | More sensitive than PT; used to monitor heparin therapy |
| Blood urea nitrogen (BUN) | 5-20 mg/100 ml | Increased with decreased cardiac output |
| Serum proteins | 6-8 g/100 ml | Levels below 5 g/100 ml seen with edema |

as a physiologic response to inadequate tissue oxygenation. The *erythrocyte sedimentation rate* (ESR) is a measurement of the rate at which RBCs "settle out" of anticoagulated blood in an hour. The rate of RBC settling is increased if the proportion of globulin to albumin increases or if fibrinogen levels are excessively increased. Nonspecific increases in globulin and fibrinogen levels occur when the body responds to injury or inflammation, as seen with infectious heart disorders or myocardial infarction.

*Blood coagulation tests,* including prothrombin time (PT) and activated partial thromboplastin time (APTT), indicate the rapidity of blood clotting. These tests are useful during anticoagulation therapy (see Table 29-3). A *blood urea nitrogen* (BUN) determination is primarily useful as an indicator of renal function. Decreased cardiac output leading to a low renal blood supply and reduction in glomerular filtration rate will elevate the BUN.

## Blood Lipids

The blood (plasma) lipids are composed mainly of cholesterol, triglyceride, phospholipid, and free fatty acids, all of which are insoluble in water and require a "carrier" to transport them. The carriers for plasma lipids are the proteins to which they are bound, thus the name *lipoproteins.* There are four major classes of lipoproteins: chylomicrons, very low–density lipoproteins, low-density lipoproteins, and high-density lipoproteins, all of which contain varying levels of cholesterol, triglycerides, and phospholipids.

*Chylomicrons* are composed mainly of triglycerides and originate in the intestine after the absorption of dietary fat. Chylomicrons should not be found in the plasma after 12 to 14 hours of fasting. Studies to date have not shown elevated chylomicron levels to be associated with premature coronary artery disease.

*Very low–density lipoproteins* (VLDLs) are composed primarily of triglycerides and are synthesized in the liver. Sustained elevations of VLDLs sometimes have been associated with atherosclerosis; however, the exact relationship of triglycerides to coronary heart disease is not yet clear.

*Low-density lipoproteins* (LDLs) are composed of approximately 50% cholesterol and are thought to have the greatest correlation with coronary artery disease. According to the insudation theory of atherogenesis, LDLs can enter the arterial intima and produce arterial endothelial injury, which can lead to progressive atherosclerotic plaque formation and eventually produce clinical manifestations, including ischemic heart disease. Lipoprotein (a) (LP[a]) is a protein associated with LDL. High plasma levels of LP(a) have been correlated with an increased risk for atherothrombotic cardiovascular disease. LP(a) structurally is similar to plasminogen, which explains its ability to interfere with the processes involved in plasmin generation and clot lysis.[5]

*High-density lipoproteins* (HDLs) are composed of mostly protein with a modest amount of cholesterol and a considerable amount of phospholipids. This lipoprotein appears to have the lowest atherogenic potential. In fact, studies have demonstrated that HDLs are inversely associated with coronary heart disease. In vivo tests indicate that HDLs may carry cholesterol away from tissues, including atheromatous plaques. It appears that HDLs may even provide protection against coronary heart disease.

Before blood tests are performed for the detection of elevated lipids, the patient must fast for 12 hours. No alcoholic beverages or lipid-influencing drugs (e.g., estrogens, oral contraceptives, steroids, salicylates) may be taken. If the patient is under stress or has any acute illness, the tests should be postponed. Because lipid levels may fluctuate greatly from day to day, repeated blood samples are obtained before a definitive diagnosis of hyperlipidemia is assigned. Disorders of lipid metabolism are classified according to their lipoprotein pattern and are discussed in Chapter 31.

### Blood Cultures

Blood culture tests are crucial in the diagnosis of infectious diseases of the heart such as endocarditis. Blood cultures are obtained by venipuncture, and special care should be taken not to contaminate the cultures. Results of these blood cultures will identify the organism responsible for the infective process and the organism's sensitivity to various antibiotics. This information will aid the physician in planning an effective course of antibiotic therapy.

### Enzyme Studies

Enzymes, which are located in all tissues, catalyze the biochemical reactions of the body. When cell membranes are damaged, such as in myocardial infarction, enzymes leak out of the damaged myocardial cell and escape into the serum. The serum enzyme measurements that are used to detect myocardial necrosis are serum aspartate aminotransferase (AST) (formerly serum glutamic oxaloacetic transaminase [SGOT]), creatine kinase (CK), lactic dehydrogenase (LDH), and hydroxybutyrate dehydrogenase (HBD). Because these enzymes are located in various body tissues, numerous conditions other than myocardial damage may produce enzyme elevations; for example, the brain, pancreas, and liver are all rich sources of AST. If a person were to develop chest pain concurrently with pancreatic or liver disease, an elevated AST level may be mistaken for myocardial necrosis. Fortunately, two of the enzymes, CK and LDH, have isoenzymes that are thought to be present almost exclusively in myocardial muscle.

The CK molecule has two subunits, which have been identified as follows: M, associated with muscle; and B, associated with brain. The brain and gastrointestinal tract contain modest amounts of the BB dimer, and skeletal muscle contains large amounts of the MM form. Heart muscle contains huge quantities of MM, but it also contains the MB hybrid form of CK. Because $CK_{MB}$ is not found in any other tissue, its presence in the serum is a sensitive indicator of myocardial damage.

Of the five LDH isoenzymes, $LDH_1$ has been found to be the most sensitive indicator of myocardial damage. Specifically, the $LDH_1/LDH_2$ ratio is very helpful in distinguishing myocardial infarction from other causes of chest pain or vascular instability. Normally the $LDH_1$ value is less than $LDH_2$; however, in the presence of acute myocardial infarction, $LDH_1$ is not only elevated but also exceeds $LDH_2$. (For further discussion of cardiac enzymes, see Chapter 31.)

### Urinalysis

A routine urinalysis is performed to determine the effects of cardiovascular disease on renal function and the existence of concurrent renal or systemic diseases, such as glomerulonephritis, hypertension, or diabetes. Mild to moderate proteinuria (usually albuminuria) can be seen in patients with malignant hypertension and venous congestion of the kidneys secondary to congestive heart failure or constrictive pericarditis. The presence of RBCs in the urine may indicate infective endocarditis or an embolic kidney disease.

Recently the detection of myoglobin in the urine (myoglobinuria) has been useful in the diagnosis of myocardial infarction. At present, clinical experience with this test remains limited; however, it may prove to be a sensitive indicator of myocardial damage. Destruction of infarction of striated muscle liberates myoglobin, and because of its small size, the molecule filters through the glomerulus and is excreted in the urine.

### Serologic Tests

Syphilis can play an important role in the development of aortic disorders. The patient may have aortic insufficiency, aortic aneurysms, or disease of the orifices of the coronary arteries. Because of the relationship between syphilis and heart disease, a routine VDRL (Venereal Disease Research Laboratories) test is performed on all cardiac patients.

## INVASIVE HEMODYNAMIC MONITORING

Invasive monitoring techniques used to evaluate the hemodynamic status of the critically ill patient have greatly increased the data base on which health professionals can plan and evaluate therapeutic modalities. Numerous devices are used in hemodynamic monitoring. (For a detailed description of this particular aspect of care, see reference 2.)

### Central Venous Pressure

**Central venous pressure (CVP)** measurements reflect the pressures in the right atrium and provide information regarding changes in right ventricular pressure. For many years it was thought that CVP accurately reflected changes in left ventricular function. However, it has now been documented that although the CVP may provide information about left-sided heart pressures, the CVP is not as accurate as other methods in reflecting rapid changes in cardiovascular status.

The primary factors affecting CVP are the circulating blood volume, right-sided pump function, and the degree of peripheral vasoconstriction. Therefore the CVP is best utilized in *monitoring blood volume and adequacy of the venous return to the heart.* Because the CVP reflects the pressure in the great veins as blood returns to the right side of the heart, a low (or falling) reading may indicate an inadequate blood volume (hypovolemia), and fluid replacement may be necessary. A high (or rising) CVP usually is secondary to left-sided pump failure. This decrease in cardiac contractility may lead to congestive heart failure and pulmonary edema. Unfortunately, the patient's hemodynamic status may be severely altered before representative changes in the CVP are evident.

The normal values for CVP will vary with the use of different equipment; however, a range of 5 to 15 cm of water is acceptable. It is important to note that a change or a trend in the CVP is more important than the actual numeric value. For example, if the CVP of a patient who has had a myocardial infarction should change from 5 to 10 cm in a 30-minute period, the physician should be notified. Even though both 5 cm and 10 cm are "normal" values, it is crucial to monitor the trend of a rising CVP. (For additional information on CVP, see Chapter 22.)

## Intraarterial Blood Pressure Measurement

In the critically ill patient, the stroke volume and thus the cardiac output may be decreased to such an extent that cuff blood pressure readings may be inaccurate. As the stroke volume falls, Korotkoff's sounds become increasingly more difficult to auscultate and blood pressure readings have been found to be in error by as much as 25 mm Hg. In this particular patient population, invasive arterial blood pressure monitoring will more accurately reflect actual blood pressure.

Arterial catheters may be placed in various arteries; however, the radial, brachial, and axillary arteries are used most often. Normally the arterial catheter is attached to a transducer, which converts the mechanical pressure of the pulses to electrical impulses and can be viewed as waveforms on an oscilloscope. Generally the arterial line also is used to obtain blood samples for arterial blood gas determinations. Catheter patency is maintained with the use of an arterial flush system.

The patient with an arterial line requires frequent observation. It is essential that the extremity with the arterial line be kept uncovered so that the site can be monitored for bleeding caused by loose connections in the system. Also, the pulse, color, and temperature of the extremity distal to the catheter should be assessed every 2 hours so that early signs of circulatory compromise or thrombosis may be detected.

## Pulmonary Artery and Pulmonary Capillary Wedge Pressures

To obtain essential information regarding left ventricular function, a balloon-tipped catheter (Swan-Ganz catheter) may be introduced into the pulmonary artery. The pulmonary artery catheter permits the measurement of the **pulmonary artery end-diastolic pressure (PAEDP)** and the **pulmonary capillary wedge pressure (PCWP)** (Table 29-4).

The best indicator of left ventricular function is the **left ventricular end-diastolic pressure (LVEDP).** Because a direct relationship exists among the PAEDP, the PCWP, and the LVEDP, an elevated PAEDP or PCWP reflects an elevated LVEDP. Elevations in LVEDP result from impaired left ventricular contractility, which does not permit adequate emptying of the ventricles.

**TABLE 29-4 Pulmonary Artery and Capillary Wedge Pressures**

| TYPE | COMMON ABBREVIATION | NORMAL VALUES |
|---|---|---|
| Left ventricular end-diastolic pressure | LVEDP | 12-15 mm Hg |
| Pulmonary artery end-diastolic pressure | PAEDP | 4-12 mm Hg |
| Pulmonary capillary wedge pressure | PCWP | 4-12 mm Hg |

In the healthy person the PAEDP and the PCWP will be similar. However, in the presence of increased peripheral vascular resistance such as that found in pulmonary embolism, the PAEDP will rise while the PCWP remains normal. Therefore, to evaluate the true LVEDP accurately, the PCWP must be monitored. The PCWP is a critical factor affecting the transudation of fluid from the vascular space to the interstitial and alveolar spaces in the lungs. Normally the PCWP ranges from 4 to 12 mm Hg. PCWP exceeding 25 mm Hg suggests imminent pulmonary edema.

Insertion of the pulmonary artery catheter often is accomplished through a small incision (cutdown) made in an antecubital vein. The catheter is threaded into the vein, through the superior vena cava, through the tricuspid valve, and into the pulmonary artery. One of the lumens of the pulmonary artery catheter is attached to a monitor that usually presents a numeric reading and a display of waveforms that indicate the location (capillary bed, pulmonary artery, or right ventricle) of the catheter. The balloon is then inflated so that it wedges the catheter in a distal branch of the pulmonary artery (Figure 29-15). Once the balloon is inflated, it occludes the pressure produced by the right side of the heart. The reading (or measurement) obtained when the balloon is inflated is the PCWP and reflects pressures in the pulmonary capillary bed and left-sided heart function. The balloon must be deflated quickly and should never be left inflated for more than a few seconds so that damage to the pulmonary circulation does not occur. The nurse usually obtains measurements of the PCWP every few hours or more frequently if the patient's condition is unstable or if pharmacologic modifications of preload and afterload are being used.

The type of pulmonary artery catheter used will determine what hemodynamic measurements other than PAEDP and PCWP can be obtained. Some catheters have a third lumen that contains a thermistor. This is used to determine cardiac output by the thermodilution technique. A fourth (proximal) lumen ends at the level of the right atrium and is used to monitor CVP and to obtain blood samples. A four-lumen thermodilution catheter is illustrated in Figure 29-16.

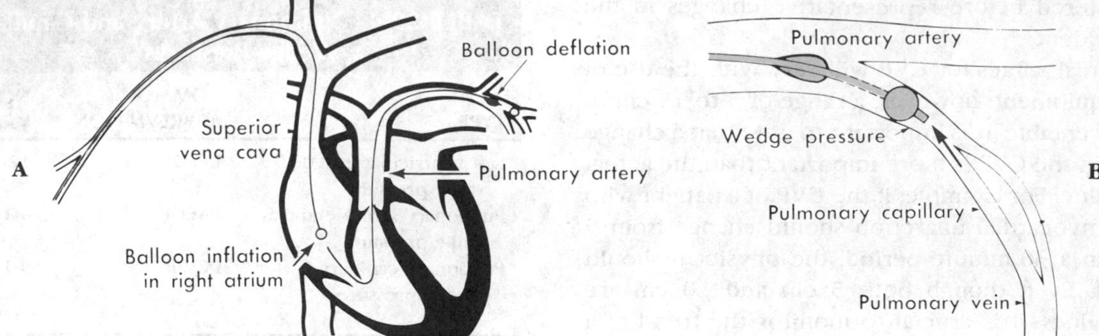


**FIGURE 29-15** **A,** Flow-directed, balloon-tipped catheter showing inflation of balloon in right atrium and consequent "floating" of catheter throughout right ventricle and out to distal pulmonary artery branch. Balloon is deflated, advanced slightly, and reinflated slightly to obtain pulmonary capillary wedge pressure (PCWP). **B,** During the initial positioning of the balloon-tipped catheter in pulmonary artery, balloon is deflated. Catheter is then advanced and balloon is reinflated just enough to obtain PCWP. (From Daily EK, Schroeder JS: *Techniques in bedside hemodynamic monitoring,* ed 5, St Louis, 1994, Mosby.)

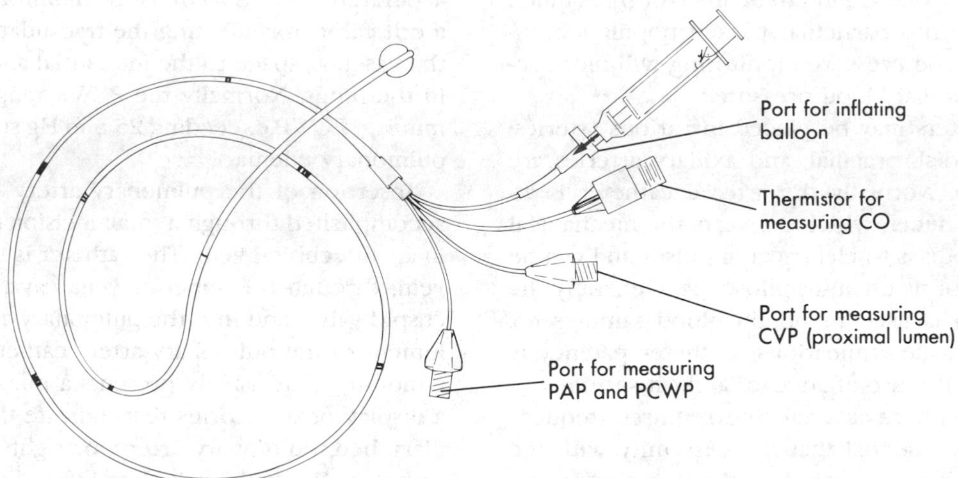


**FIGURE 29-16** Four-lumen thermodilution pulmonary artery catheter for measuring cardiac output *(CO),* central venous pressure *(CVP),* pulmonary artery pressure *(PAP),* and pulmonary capillary wedge pressure *(PCWP).*

## SONIC STUDIES

### Echocardiography

Echocardiography uses ultrasound to provide a method for assessing cardiac structure and mobility in a noninvasive manner. A small transducer usually is placed on the patient's chest at the level of the third or fourth intercostal space near the left lower sternal border. The technician then angles the transducer in varying directions to visualize specific areas of the heart. The transducer transmits high-frequency sound waves and then receives these waves back from the patient as they are reflected off different structures. The ultrasonic beam, which is reflected back from the patient's heart, produces "echoes" that are viewed as lines and spaces on an oscilloscope. These lines and spaces represent bone, cardiac chambers and valves, the septum, and muscle. A copy of the echocardiogram is recorded on paper and becomes a permanent graphic record of the findings.

Because echocardiography is a noninvasive procedure, it is safer than cardiac catheterization; thus whenever possible, echocardiography is completed first and then followed with cardiac catheterization as necessary. There are virtually no contraindications to performing an echocardiogram. In fact, for the critically ill patient, portable echocardiography can be performed at the bedside. No special preparation is necessary for the test; the patient can eat and take medications as usual. Patient teaching regarding the echocardiogram should include not only the purpose of the test but also the fact that it is painless and takes approximately 30 to 60 minutes to

**BOX 29-2 Conditions Detected or Evaluated by Echocardiography**

- Abnormal pericardial fluid
- Valvular disorders, including prosthetic valves
- Ventricular aneurysms
- Cardiac tumors, such as atrial myxomas
- Some forms of congenital heart disease, such as atrial septal defects
- Cardiac chamber size
- Stroke volume and cardiac output
- Some myocardial abnormalities, such as idiopathic hypertrophic subaortic stenosis (IHSS)

**BOX 29-3 Clinical Indications for Transesophageal Echocardiography**

- Aortic dissection/aneurysm
- Mitral valve prosthetic dysfunction
- Mitral valve regurgitation
- Infective endocarditis
- Congenital heart disease
- Intracardial thrombi (especially left atrium and left atrial appendage)
- Cardiac tumor
- Intraoperative assessment: LV function, adequacy of valve repair/replacement

complete. During the procedure the patient will have to lie quietly. The position assumed for the test is lying supine, turned slightly onto the left side with the head elevated 15 to 20 degrees. Inasmuch as no adverse or untoward effects occur from echocardiography, the patient may resume normal activities as soon as the examination is completed. Numerous conditions can be detected or evaluated by echocardiography (Box 29-2).

## Transesophageal Echocardiography

Because ultrasound waves do not trace through air, patients who are receiving mechanical ventilation or have chronic pulmonary disease are poor candidates for echocardiography. Anatomic considerations such as thoracic cage deformity also can restrict its usefulness. In addition, it is difficult to visualize the posterior location of the left atrium from the precordium. The esophageal approach to cardiac imaging is an effective alternative for overcoming some of these limitations.

**Transesophageal echocardiography (TEE)** allows high-restriction ultrasonic imaging of the cardiac structures and great vessels via the esophagus. TEE uses a transducer affixed to the tip of a modified, flexible endoscope that is advanced into the esophagus and manipulated to produce clear posterior images of the heart. Anatomic structures easily visualized with TEE include the left atrium, the left atrial appendage, and the aortic and mitral valves.

Indications for TEE (Box 29-3) are expanding significantly. This procedure can be performed at the bedside without contrast dye. One major limitation of TEE is failure to visualize the aortic arch and arch vessels.

### Nursing care of patient undergoing transesophageal echocardiography

Any history of esophageal surgery, dysfunction, or malignancy must be ascertained, as well as any history of allergic reactions to topical anesthetics or sedatives. If the procedure is to be performed on an outpatient basis, the patient should arrange for transportation because of the effects of sedation. The patient is given nothing by mouth for at least 4 to 6 hours before the procedure.

Vascular access is established with an intravenous line or intermittent venous access device. The patient is encouraged to void before the procedure. Dentures and other oral prosthetics must be removed. Intravenously administered sedatives are prescribed to decrease anxiety.

Suction and resuscitation equipment should be readily available. Cardiac rhythm, vital signs, and oxygen saturation ($Sao_2$) are monitored throughout the procedure. The patient is given a topical anesthetic by spray or gargle to reduce coughing or gagging during probe insertion. Additional sedation, usually diazepam (Valium) or midazolam (Versed), may be given.

The procedure consists of placing the patient in a chin-to-chest position to facilitate passage of the endoscope through the oropharynx. A bite block may be used to prevent damage to the teeth and probe. The scope is advanced 30 to 35 cm to allow posterior visualization of the left atrium by the transducer. To view the left ventricle, the scope is advanced into the stomach and flexed upward for an inferior view. The procedure usually takes about 5 to 20 minutes.

After TEE, to prevent tracheal aspiration, the patient should receive nothing by mouth until the gag reflex returns. The patient is assisted to sit up or is positioned on the side and encouraged to cough. Throat lozenges or rinses can be used to ease throat soreness.

### Complications of transesophageal echocardiography

The potential for esophageal perforation exists, especially if preexisting esophageal disorders such as carcinoma are present. Complications associated with probe insertion include pharyngeal bleeding, cardiac dysrhythmia, vasovagal reaction, and transient hypoxemia.

## Phonocardiography

**Phonocardiography** involves the use of electrically recorded amplified cardiac sounds. Special microphones attached to the patient's chest pick up cardiac sounds produced by pressure changes in the heart and great vessels. The sounds are graphically recorded on special phonograph paper so that a permanent record is available. Phonocardiography can be helpful in determining the exact timing and characteristics of murmurs and extra heart sounds. Frequently phonocardiograms are used in conjunction with echocardiograms so that a comparison can be made between sound *(phono)* and motion *(echo)*. Patient preparation is similar to that described for the echocardiogram.

## DYNAMIC STUDIES

### Holter Monitor

Resting ECGs supply much valuable information about a person's cardiovascular status. However, for some patients who experience cardiovascular symptoms (chest pain, palpitations) only during exertion or while performing daily activities, a more dynamic method for studying the ECG is necessary.

The **Holter monitor** is used to obtain a continuous graphic tracing of a patient's pulse while the person performs daily activities. The Holter monitor is a small, portable ECG monitor about the size of a large transistor radio. The patient is attached to the monitor by a precordial lead system, and the monitor itself can be carried with the use of a shoulder strap. Generally the patient is attached to the Holter monitor for approximately 24 hours. During this time the patient is required to keep a log or diary of daily activities. The log should include the time, present activity, any medication taken, and any unusual sensations the person experiences while attached to the monitor. When the monitoring period is completed, the physician compares the ECG with the patient's log to determine if any correlations exist between the ECG and the patient's activities. The Holter monitor is helpful in documenting transient or episodic dysrhythmias and sometimes is used to evaluate patients for pacemaker therapy.

### Stress Testing

**Stress testing** (ECG during exercise) or exercise testing is a noninvasive test to evaluate cardiovascular response to a progressively graded workload. Stress testing may be performed for a variety of reasons (Box 29-4).

> **BOX 29-4 Indications for Performing a Stress Test**
>
> - Evaluation of the patient with symptoms suggestive of coronary artery disease
> - Determination of the patient's physical work capacity and aerobic capacity
> - Determination of the patient's functional capacity after a myocardial infarction and as an aid in planning an exercise rehabilitation program
> - Evaluation of exercise-induced dysrhythmias
> - Evaluation of the symptom-free person older than 40 years of age who is at risk for coronary artery disease
> - Evaluation of pharmacologic interventions for dysrhythmias, angina, or ischemia

The exercise test can be performed with a bicycle ergometer (stationary bicycle with adjustable resistance to pedaling) or a treadmill (moving belt that can be adjusted so that the person either walks or runs on a gradient). The patient's blood pressure and ECG are monitored closely during and after the stress test. Because the stress test is designed to progressively increase myocardial oxygen demand, some patients may experience untoward effects and the test may need to be terminated. Conditions that necessitate termination include the following: (1) ventricular tachycardia, (2) fall in peak systolic blood pressure and/or fall in heart rate despite increased workload, (3) vertigo, (4) frequent premature ventricular beats, (5) chest pain (angina), (6) severe dyspnea, (7) severe anxiety, and (8) diagnostic ST segment depression (see Chapter 30).

Manifestations of an abnormal reaction to the stress test reflect an imbalance between supply and demand for myocardial oxygen caused by myocardial ischemia. Many criteria exist for evaluating a stress test result as positive and may vary with individual patients. The most common criteria are listed in Table 29-5.

Adequate preparation for stress testing is extremely important. Although the procedure is not considered painful, it can be extremely fatiguing; patients may become anxious because they will be exercising at a level that might produce such cardiovascular symptoms as dyspnea, palpitations, and chest pain. After reviewing the purpose and method of stress testing, the patient should be advised to do the following:

1. Get adequate rest the night before the test.
2. Avoid coffee, tea, and alcohol the day of the test.
3. Avoid smoking and taking nitroglycerin during the 2 hours immediately before the test.
4. Eat a light breakfast or lunch at least 2 hours before the test.
5. Wear comfortable, loose-fitting clothes. (Women should be advised to wear a bra for support.)
6. Wear sturdy, comfortable walking shoes.
7. Consult with the physician about taking medications before the test. (Digoxin, propranolol, and vasodilators may affect the results of the stress test.)
8. Inform the physician if any unusual sensations develop during the test (e.g., chest pain, dizziness).
9. Rest after the test. (Do *not* take a hot shower; a bath in warm water 1 to 2 hours after the test is permitted.)

## RADIOLOGIC TESTS

### Chest Roentgenograms

A roentgenogram (x-ray film) of the chest may be taken to determine overall size and configuration of the heart, as well as individual cardiac chamber size. Most abnor-

**TABLE 29-5 Criteria for Evaluating a Stress Test**

| ASSESSMENT PARAMETER | POSSIBLE INDICATORS OF POSITIVE STRESS TEST RESULT |
|---|---|
| ECG | ST segment depressions 1 mm or more are generally regarded as indicative of ischemia.<br>Dysrhythmias: exercise-induced premature ventricular beats in the healthy person are of little prognostic significance unless they occur in conjunction with ST segment depression; persons with both exercise-induced ventricular dysrhythmias and significant ST depression are likely to have severe coronary artery disease. |
| Hemodynamics | An exercise-induced, sustained reduction of peak systolic blood pressure of 10 mm Hg or more may be an inappropriate blood pressure response to stress testing and is a highly specific sign of multivessel coronary artery disease.<br>An inappropriate heart rate response to exercise may correlate with impaired left ventricular function. |
| Symptoms | Typical anginal pain induced by exertion is a reliable symptom of coronary artery disease. |
| Cardiac auscultation | Development of $S_3$ suggests advanced coronary artery disease and myocardial dysfunction.<br>Development of transient $S_4$ after stress testing may result from increased turbulence and volume of blood flow.<br>Development of systolic murmurs often is caused by papillary muscle dysfunction, which suggests coronary artery disease. |

malities of heart size can be detected with a standard posteroanterior and lateral view of the chest. Calcifications in the pericardium, heart muscle, valves, or large blood vessels also can be visualized in such a cardiovascular film.

## Cardiac Fluoroscopy

Cardiac fluoroscopy facilitates observation of the heart from varying views while the heart is in motion. Fluoroscopy can be used to detect ventricular aneurysms, which appear as a paradoxical bulging during systole. In addition, fluoroscopy is used to monitor prosthetic valve movement and to assess the position of cardiac calcifications during the cardiac cycle. Because of the increased risk of exposure to radiation during fluoroscopy, many institutions no longer use this diagnostic technique; rather, procedures such as echocardiograms and phonocardiograms are used more frequently.

# SCINTIGRAPHIC STUDIES

## Myocardial Imaging

**Myocardial imaging** is used to identify myocardial infarctions, evaluate myocardial perfusion, and assess left ventricular function. This technique can provide invaluable information in the presence of conflicting data. For example, if a patient has recently undergone coronary artery bypass surgery, the cardiac enzymes may already be elevated and may complicate the diagnosis of a new infarction. Also, certain ECG abnormalities (e.g., left bundle branch [LBB] block, pacer-induced beats) may complicate the usual ECG indicators of a new infarction. Unfortunately, at times a patient is either unable to supply a history or furnishes conflicting data about a cardiovascular episode. In all these examples, myocardial imaging can provide a relatively safe and noninvasive technique for evaluating myocardial function.

### Static myocardial imaging

Techniques that are used to produce a static picture of a myocardial image include stannous pyrophosphate scan, thallium imaging, pharmacologic myocardial perfusion imaging, and technetium 99m sestamibi myocardial perfusion SPECT imaging.

**Stannous pyrophosphate scan.** The **pyrophosphate scan** referred to as "hot spot" imaging, typically uses the agent technetium 99m stannous pyrophosphate. A minute dose of the radioisotope is injected into an antecubital vein. The patient then waits approximately 2 hours while the renal system clears the unbound technetium so that the heart can be visualized. In the healthy myocardium there will be a homogeneous tracer distribution of the radiopharmaceutic agent. In the damaged heart, however, the uptake of the radioactive material will increase. A gamma (γ)-scintillator camera is used to identify the area of increased uptake (hot spot). This type of scanning plays a less significant role in imaging acute myocardial infarction because of technical difficulties. For example, false-positive results can occur if the scan is performed too early because the isotope failed to clear the intravascular volume. This problem is magnified if the patient also has renal failure. The test is best performed 1 to 3 days after the infarction. Because such a minute isotope amount is administered during the examination, no toxic or allergic reactions have been noted, and it is considered radioactively safe for both patient and staff members.

**Thallium imaging. Thallium imaging** can be referred to as "cold spot" imaging because the isotope is taken up by healthy myocardial tissue and not by the infarction area; thus this area remains a "cold spot." A γ-scintillator is used to detect the distribution of the radioisotope. Thallium imaging, which most often is used with exercise testing, can provide valuable information regarding myocardial infarction. Because the radioisotope is a potassium analog, it behaves as an intracellular monovalent cation. The isotope is actively transported across healthy myocardial cells, where extraction by these cells is significantly high. With ischemia, blood supply is diminished and thus a lesser amount of the isotope is delivered to such areas. Therefore an area of diminished thallium uptake (cold spot) surrounded by an area of normal myocardial uptake results. Cellular release of the isotope exceeds its accumulation after the initial uptake, resulting in washout of the tracer from the perfused areas, with redistribution of the isotope to the ischemic areas. Ischemic and infarcted tissue can then be differentiated because the infarcted myocardium is unable to take up the redistributed tracer.

Thallium scanning can be helpful in quantifying the amount of myocardium at risk during acute infarction by use of two resting scans to localize the affected area. The resting scan is obtained in the very early phase, whereas a redistribution scan is obtained 3 to 4 hours later. The total area of ischemia and infarction is visible on the initial scan. During the period before the redistribution scan, a border zone area has an opportunity to extract the isotope. Thus a smaller cold spot is visible when redistribution occurs. This technique is useful in assessing the efficacy of therapeutic interventions, such as thrombolytic therapy, as well as providing direction for further treatment based on the degree of myocardium still in jeopardy.

Because the amount of thallium used is small, the risk is considered to be minimal.

**Pharmacologic myocardial perfusion imaging.** *Dipyridamole* is a potent coronary vasodilator. By blocking cellular re-uptake of adenosine, dipyridamole acts to increase blood and tissue concentrations of adenosine, which in turn promotes optimal coronary vasodilation. In normal coronary arteries, dipyridamole increases flow three to four times that of baseline values. In arteries with stenosis of less than 50%, the increase in flow will be proportionately less. In arteries with more severe stenosis (greater than 70%), flow increases are more significantly reduced or may not increase at all. Variation of low coronary vascular reserve in stenotic versus normal arteries provides the scientific rationale for using imaging agents that are distributed according to coronary blood flow.

*Adenosine* perfusion imaging has been proposed as an alternative to dipyridamole perfusion imaging. Adenosine has a substantially shorter half-life (2 to 10 seconds) than does dipyridamole, whose half-life is several minutes. Furthermore, adenosine elicits more consistent maximal coronary vasodilation over a shorter period than does dipyridamole. Side effects, which occur frequently during adenosine administration, most commonly are headache, dyspnea, chest pain, and facial flushing. Side effects generally disappear within 1 to 2 minutes, rarely requiring the administration of aminophylline as an antagonist.

**Technetium 99m ($^{99m}$Tc) sestamibi myocardial perfusion SPECT imaging.** Tc-sestamibi is a new nonredistributing radionuclide agent being used in the evaluation of effectiveness of thrombolytic and other interventional therapy in the treatment of acute myocardial infarction. Typically Tc-sestamibi (Cardiolite) is administered in the emergency department, followed by thrombolytic or interventional therapy. Once hemodynamic stability has been established, patients are transported to the radiology department for perfusion imaging. Because minimal redistribution occurs with this agent, late images still delineate the initially nonperfused myocardial region at risk. Improvements in scintigraphy after reinjection and delayed imaging provide an assessment of salvaged myocardium.

### Dynamic myocardial imaging

Static scans do not give any information about the systolic or diastolic performance of the infarcted heart. A second way of imaging myocardial function is the use of a *dynamic* scan to assess cardiac wall motion and global left and right ventricular function. The easiest method for performing this type of imaging is the multiple gated acquisition cardiac blood pool imaging.

**Multiple gated acquisition scanning. Multiple gated acquisition (MUGA) scanning** has the capability of demonstrating cardiac wall motion to enable assessment of injury as well as capacity of cardiac function. The technique lends itself well to the portable imaging techniques required to scan myocardial infarction in acutely ill patients.

Gated blood pool imaging is a noninvasive radionuclide method. ECG leads are attached to the patient, and the ECG is then synchronized to a computer and a γ-camera. A small amount of technetium 99m (attached to either human serum albumin or to autologous RBCs) is injected intravenously. After the radioactivity reaches a state of equilibrium (approximately 3 to 5 minutes), the patient is placed in a supine position with the γ-camera positioned over the precordium. The computer then constructs an average cardiac cycle that represents the summation of several hundred heartbeats. Enough data are generated so that an outline of the left side of the heart in all phases of the cardiac cycle can be seen.

Gated blood pool imaging offers several advantages in assessment of patients with myocardial infarction in addition to assessment of ventricular and segmental wall function. Because all RBCs are tagged, their counts reflect blood volume. Thus, if the heart can be positioned on the scan so that the left ventricle is isolated from the other chambers, left ventricular ejection function can be determined from left ventricular counts. The ejection fraction, calculated from the computer-reconstructed image of end diastole and end systole, may provide an early indicator of deteriorating cardiovascular functioning in patients with congestive heart failure or low cardiac output and in those who are at risk of developing cardiotoxicity caused by high doses of doxorubicin

(Adriamycin). Right ventricular ejection fraction also can be determined, but it is less accurate because of difficulty in separating right atrial counts.

Mild injury of the cardiac wall is reflected in MUGA scanning as hypokinesia or mild depression of myocardial contraction versus a more severe disturbance that produces akinesia or dyskinesia. Clinical interventions are determined according to improvement or deterioration of global function and wall motion segments. Other important information, such as recognition of right ventricular infarction and aneurysm formation, can be easily recognized. In addition, the effects of pharmacotherapeutics (e.g., nitroglycerin, vasodilators) on ventricular function can be evaluated.

Stress-testing ventriculography also can be performed to evaluate the ejection fraction during exercise. Some patients with coronary artery disease demonstrate a normal resting ejection value. However, under maximal stress, the ejection fraction may decrease, or an abnormality in a specific region of the heart may become apparent.

### Positron Emission Tomography

**Positron emission tomography (PET)** represents a radionuclide-based imaging technique that uses short-lived radionuclides as tracers to report both perfusion and metabolic events. These tracers generally are given by intravenous injection or inhalation and only occasionally by intraarterial injection. Myocardial uptake is proportional to the quantity of tracer delivered by the amount of blood flow, by the fractional extraction, and by the loss of tracer through decay, metabolism, and flow. The tracer elements readily pass through the tissues and are simultaneously detected by counters placed on opposite sides of the body, a process known as *annihilation coincidence detection.*

Under normal circumstances the well-perfused, aerobically metabolizing myocardium prefers free fatty acids for energy production from oxidative metabolism. When ischemia is present, more glucose and less fatty acid tend to be utilized. PET is particularly useful in demonstrating this process by incorporating radioisotopes into biochemically relevant components (such as C palmitate or F-2-fluoro-2-deoxyglucose) used in the study and by demonstrating myocardial flow deficits in patients with coronary disease. PET also provides the basis for vigorous medical management of asymptomatic coronary atherosclerosis. In addition, it is useful in evaluating the effectiveness of interventions such as thrombolysis, cholesterol reduction, bypass surgery, and percutaneous transluminal coronary angioplasty (PTCA).

## CARDIAC CATHETERIZATION

**Cardiac catheterization** is an extremely valuable diagnostic tool for obtaining detailed information about the structure and function of the cardiac chambers, valves, and great vessels. Cardiac catheterization may include studies of the right side of the heart, the left side of the heart, and coronary arteries. Studies of the coronary arteries are performed to detect the presence and extent of coronary artery disease and to evaluate the effects of medical and surgical treatment of the disease. There are many indications for performing a cardiac catherization (Box 29-5). Often, persons will have undergone several other diagnostic procedures before being evaluated by catheterization.

**BOX 29-5 Reasons for Performing Cardiac Catheterization**

- Confirmation of the presence of suspected heart disease, including congenital heart disease, valvular disease, and myocardial disease
- Determination of the location and severity of the disease process
- Preoperative assessment to determine if cardiac surgery is indicated
- Evaluation of ventricular function after surgical revascularization
- Evaluation of the effect of medical treatment modalities on cardiovascular function
- Performing specialized cardiac techniques such as the placement of an internal pacemaker

### Right-Sided Heart Catheterization

Right-sided heart catheterization is performed when congenital heart disease is suspected or to evaluate certain acquired conditions, such as tricuspid stenosis or valvular incompetence. Blood samples and blood pressure readings are taken, ECG studies are obtained, and cineradiographs of the right chambers of the heart and the pulmonary arterial circulation are made.

To perform a catheterization of the right side of the heart, a catheter is inserted via cutdown into a large vein (e.g., the medial cubital or brachial vein). The catheter is then threaded with the use of fluoroscopy into the superior vena cava, the right atrium, the right ventricle, the pulmonary artery, and pulmonary capillaries. As the catheter is passed through the various chambers and vessels, blood samples are obtained to determine the oxygen content and saturation. In the presence of a left-to-right atrial shunt, blood samples would indicate a higher oxygen content in the right atrium than in the superior or inferior vena cava. Blood pressure measurements also are recorded (Figure 29-17). Normal blood pressures in the heart vary among the chambers. The pressure is highest in the left ventricle because of the stronger ventricular contractions. Normally the **pulmonary artery pressure (PAP)** is approximately 25/10 mm Hg or approximately one fifth of the systemic blood pressure. Elevations in chamber pressures such as an elevated left atrial pressure can indicate mitral stenosis or insufficiency and possibly left ventricular failure.

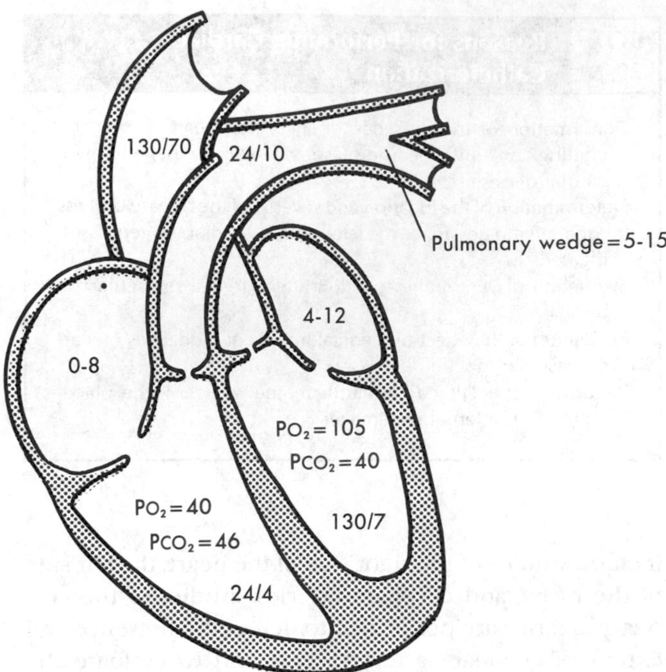


**FIGURE 29-17** Pressure readings and blood gases in millimeters of mercury (mm Hg) in chambers of heart and major blood vessels.

## Left-Sided Heart Catheterization

Left-sided heart catheterization is performed to evaluate pressures of the left side of the heart, valvular competency, and left ventricular function. A catheter is passed into the aorta from either the brachial or the femoral artery with the use of fluoroscopic visualization. After the catheter reaches the aorta, it is manipulated around the aortic arch, down the ascending aorta, and through the aortic valve into the left ventricle. Pressure-gradient measurements are obtained to detect pressure changes across the valves. In the presence of a stenotic valve, the chamber pressure proximal to the stenosis will be significantly higher than the pressure in the distal chamber. Pressure gradients are recorded by taking continuous pressure measurements while simultaneously pulling the catheter back through a valve. Normally a pressure gradient exists across the mitral and tricuspid valves (see Figure 29-17). Therefore a decrease in the gradient is indicative of stenosis. Conversely, no pressure gradient exists across the aortic and pulmonic valves; therefore, if a gradient is present, it is of diagnostic importance.

## Ventricular Angiography

**Ventricular angiography** may be performed during the left-sided heart catheterization. This procedure involves the injection of contrast material into the ventricle while concomitant roentgenograms are taken. Information about contractility, aneurysm formation, valvular disorders (e.g., mitral regurgitation), and the ejection fraction can be obtained.

## Coronary Arteriography

Selective coronary arteriography also may be completed during the left-sided heart catheterization. A catheter is introduced into the arterial system through either a femoral or a brachial arteriotomy. The catheter is threaded (using fluoroscopy) to the aortic root; the tip of the catheter is then advanced into the right and left coronary ostia. Approximately 2 to 5 ml of contrast medium is injected into each coronary artery, and cineangiographic films are taken to monitor the progression of the dye. The contrast medium outlines the entire coronary circulation and enables the examiner to evaluate the anatomy of the coronary arteries, as well as stenotic segments and collateral vessels.

The introduction of contrast material into the coronary arteries may produce transient chest pain or discomfort. The presence of the dye may temporarily displace coronary artery blood flow, producing transient ischemia. Sublingual nitroglycerin frequently is administered to relieve the anginal discomfort. In addition, medications such as isosorbide (Isordil) may be given to dilate vessels so that greater visualization of the coronary arteries may be achieved. Occasionally the injection of contrast material into the right coronary artery may suppress the SA node, producing bradydysrhythmias, and intravenous atropine may be required.

## Patient Preparation

Preparation for cardiac catheterization is extremely important. Even after careful explanations, most patients are somewhat apprehensive. It is important to include the family in the instructions to alleviate their anxiety; this will facilitate their support of the patient. The patient may be concerned about both the procedure and the results. Preparation should include information about the procedure and the more common sensations that may be experienced during the catheterization.

Instruction should include a brief description of the room environment during cardiac catheterization. The information is presented to provide reassurance and ensure that the patient understands the various sensations that can be expected. The patient is questioned concerning any history of drug allergy, especially to contrast media. A recent study by Verderber et al.[7] illustrated a positive correlation between a combination of modeling cognitive-behavioral skills and coping techniques and reduction of patient anxiety after cardiac catheterization.

Usually the meal before the procedure is withheld. If the procedure is scheduled for later in the day, the patient may be permitted a clear liquid breakfast. A mild sedative may be given before the procedure, and an antibiotic may be ordered as a prophylactic measure.

For adults, a local anesthetic is injected over the vein

to be used and a small cutdown is performed. Relatively little discomfort is involved in a right-sided heart catheterization, although the patient may feel pressure in the femoral or antecubital area. During a left-sided heart catheterization with ventricular angiography, the patient may experience a warm, flushing sensation as the contrast medium is injected. This flushing sensation lasts for approximately 30 seconds. The patient also may experience nausea and "fluttering" sensations produced by ectopic beats from catheter manipulation or from catheter advancement as it is threaded through the heart. The small amount of contrast material injected into the coronary arteries during coronary arteriography does not produce the warm, flushing sensation noted in ventriculography, although the patient may experience some pain or tightness in the chest.

If chest discomfort or alterations in blood pressure occur, the patient is instructed to cough as fast and as hard as possible. This coughing maneuver facilitates the clearing of the contrast material from the coronary arteries and also acts as a mechanical stimulus to the heart if ectopic beats occur. In addition, coughing appears to help alleviate the feelings of lightheadedness and nausea that might result after injection of the dye.

The body's physiologic responses to cardiac catheterization are numerous and vary with each person. It is therefore essential that the patient understand the importance of alerting the physician to any unexpected or unusual sensations that might arise during the catheterization.

### Nursing Care After Catheterization

Regardless of the type of cardiac angiographic study performed, the postprocedure nursing care will be the same. These procedures generally last from 1 to 3 hours and can be tiring for the patient. After the examination many patients like to rest or sleep, but they may resume usual activities as soon as their vital signs are stable.

The patient's *pulse* (on the operative side) and *blood pressure* (on the opposite side) are monitored every 15 minutes for 1 hour and then every 30 minutes for 3 hours. It is essential to check the pulses distal to the catheter insertion site to determine the patency of the cannulated artery. Occasionally the amplitude of the pulse may be slightly diminished for approximately 24 hours because of arterial spasm or edema at the site. At times thrombus formation may totally obliterate the distal pulse, and surgery may be necessary to correct impaired circulation. The cutdown site should be closely monitored for signs of bleeding, inflammation, tenderness, or swelling (hematoma).

If a *femoral* approach was used, the patient is kept on bed rest for 12 to 24 hours. Frequently the patient will return from the catheterization with either a weight, sandbag, or ice applied to the femoral site. The patient should not have the head of the bed elevated more than 30 degrees and should avoid flexing the femoral area. If the *brachial* site is used, the arm is kept straight for several hours (with the use of an armboard), but the patient can be up in the room as soon as vital signs are stable. If any bleeding occurs from the cutdown site, firm pressure is applied directly over the site and the physician is notified. For the first 24 hours after catheterization, intake and output are monitored.

Hypotension may develop as a result of the sometimes profound diuretic effect of the contrast material used during angiography. Complications during cardiac catheterization are infrequent; however, cardiac dysrhythmias, including ventricular fibrillation, can occur. After the procedure, the development of tachycardia or any other dysrhythmia is reported to the physician immediately.

To reduce stress for the patient, many cardiac catheterization laboratories now permit patients to wear their glasses, dentures, and watches during the procedures. They also may have piped-in music or allow patients to bring a radio or favorite records with them.

## ELECTROPHYSIOLOGIC STUDY

The **electrophysiologic (EP) study** is a technique that systematically assesses the electrical stability of the heart. The degree of invasiveness depends on which area of the heart is to be studied. This procedure requires electrode catheter placement within the heart to record intracardiac electrical activity. More detailed information about the heart's electrical activity can be obtained with the EP study than with the surface ECG because of the proximity of the catheters to the cardiac conduction system. Examples of information that can be gained include exact sequence of atrial and ventricular activation, localization of areas of conduction disturbances (such as accessory pathways, areas of ischemia and infarction, dysrhythmia focuses), and effectiveness of antidysrhythmic management. Although EP studies are used more frequently than in the past for diagnostic purposes, the EP study is not routinely ordered. Use is currently reserved for persons not responding to treatment.

Similar to cardiac catheterization, an EP study is performed under laboratory conditions with fluoroscopy used to guide the pacing electrodes into position. Vascular sites most frequently used for catheter placement are the femoral, brachial, and basilic veins. Subclavian and jugular veins rarely are used, whereas arterial cannulation is performed only when left ventricular stimulation is necessary.

For the initial EP study especially, antidysrhythmic drugs usually are discontinued for approximately five half-lives to prevent pharmacologic interference with the study. Drugs typically tested include amiodarone, encainide, flecainide, tocainide, mexiletine, quinidine, bretylium, lidocaine, procainamide, disopyramide, propranolol, and phenytoin. Three to six intracardiac pacing catheters connected to a multichanneled electrogram may be used depending on the information to be obtained. A surface ECG usually is recorded simultaneously for comparison and evaluation. Atrial and bundle of His electrograms are typically recorded, as well as various measures of the conduction system. When indicated, dysrhythmias may be initiated by applying a series of programmed extra stimuli to areas of the heart. Pacing also may be used to terminate a tachycardia by inhibiting impulse transmission in conduction pathways.

The EP study usually lasts 2 to 4 hours. At the completion of testing, catheters are removed and pressure is applied at the insertion site for at least 10 minutes, followed by application of antiseptic ointment and a dry, sterile pressure dressing. Depending on the severity of dysrhythmia, patients must be continuously monitored in a telemetry or intensive care unit, where they can be closely observed and have rapidly accessible emergency equipment.

An EP study may be performed intraoperatively, which requires placement of electrodes directly on the endocardium. This technique sometimes is used for the patient with a ventricular aneurysm to facilitate localization of the dysrhythmia substrate, which can be removed along with the aneurysm. Another use is localization of an accessory pathway before surgical removal.

Complications of EP studies are similar to those of cardiac catheterization and include hemorrhage, perforation, hematoma, pulmonary emboli, deep vein thrombus, pneumothorax, phlebitis, infection, cerebrovascular accident (stroke), angina with resultant ischemia or infarction, dysrhythmia, and death. The few published reports of death associated with EP studies are estimated at less than 0.01%.[4]

The many nursing responsibilities for these patients are challenging. Patients referred for EP studies may experience fear, anxiety, frustration, and depression. For some the EP study may be perceived as experimental, especially if various antidysrhythmic medication regimens were unsuccessful. Others have survived sudden cardiac death, perhaps more than once. In essence, each patients' psychoemotional needs are unique and frequently complex. A thorough nursing history and physical assessment are important in establishing a data base so that a comprehensive plan of care can be formulated.

Nurses play a key role in preparing patients for the EP study. Reinforcing physician information about the indications for the test, the procedure itself, rationale, and risks may allay anxiety for the patient as well as the family. A description of the equipment used and the room's appearance also may be helpful. It is important to inform patients that they will be awake throughout the procedure, thus providing the opportunity to ask questions and follow the instructions of the EP team.

Postprocedural observations for complications include assessment and documentation of vital signs; peripheral pulses; insertion site; and color, warmth, and sensation of extremities. Initially these observations are performed every 15 minutes and gradually increased to every 4 hours. The extremity used for the study is immobilized, and the patient is placed on bed rest for 4 to 6 hours if venous access was used or 6 to 12 hours for arterial access. Observations for signs and symptoms of drug toxicity and allergy are critically important, especially if new antidysrhythmic drugs are prescribed. The nurse must be aware of the drug protocol, as well as potential drug interactions and incompatibilities. Documentation of stability or changes in rhythm and frequency of ectopy is essential.

Discharge planning includes a review of medications, indications for use, directions for administration, and side effects, as well as signs and symptoms associated with the medical condition and dysrhythmia. The family and patient are instructed to contact the physician if the patient experiences new or increased chest pain, syncope, dyspnea, diaphoresis, or palpitations.

## CRITICAL THINKING ACTIVITIES

- JoAnn is a practicing cardiovascular nurse practitioner in a rural community. She is interviewing and performing a physical assessment on Mr. Young, 36, and Mr. Hull, 69. Discuss how JoAnn's interview and physical assessment would differ between the two individuals.
- Mr. Knorr, 52, is scheduled for a coronary arteriography (cardiac cath). For 2 weeks he has been complaining of chest pain on exertion, relieved by rest. The nurse is preparing to teach Mr. Knorr about the procedure. She realizes that Mr. Knorr and his wife are extremely anxious. Discuss how the nurse should approach patient teaching to diminish their anxiety. Include specific statements that demonstrate your communication techniques.

## CHAPTER SUMMARY

### ANATOMY AND PHYSIOLOGY

- Electrophysiologic properties of the heart include automaticity, excitability, conductivity, and contractility.
- The action potential has two components, depolarization and repolarization. The main ions involved in this process include sodium, potassium, and calcium.
- Phases of the cardiac cycle include diastole (isovolumetric relaxation, rapid and slow ventricular filling, atrial systole) and systole (isovolumetric contraction, maximal and reduced ventricular ejection).
- Determinants of stroke volume include preload, afterload, contractility, and heart rate.
- Physiologic changes of the cardiovascular system with aging include increased amounts of fat and connective tissue, as well as calcification and fibrosis of valves, leading to possible decreased cardiac output and reduced vascular compliance.

- Cardiovascular disease is the number one cause of death in persons 65 years or older

### SUBJECTIVE DATA

- The cardinal symptoms of heart disease include dyspnea, chest pain or discomfort, edema, syncope, palpitations, and excess fatigue.

### DIAGNOSTIC TESTS

- Methods to assess cardiovascular functioning include laboratory tests, invasive hemodynamic monitoring, sonic studies, dynamic studies, radiologic tests, scintigraphic studies, cardiac catheterization, and electrophysiologic studies.

## REFERENCES

1. American Heart Association: *Heart facts,* Dallas, 1992, The Association.
2. Darovic GO: *Hemodynamic monitoring: invasive and noninvasive clinical application,* ed 2, Philadelphia, 1993, WB Saunders.
3. Fleg JL et al: Age-associated changes in the components of atrial ventricular conduction in apparently healthy volunteers, *J Gerontol* 45(3):M95-100, 1990.
4. Mercer ME: The electrophysiology study: a nursing concern, *Crit Care Nurse* 7(2):58-65, 1987.
5. Scaner AM: Lipoprotein(a): a genetic risk factor for premature coronary heart disease, *JAMA* 267(24):3326-3329, 1992.
6. US Department of Health and Human Services, Public Health Service: *Healthy people 2000: national health promotion and disease prevention objectives,* Washington, DC, 1990, US Government Printing Office.
7. Verderber A et al: Preparation for cardiac catheterization, *J Cardiovasc Nurs* 7(1):75-77, 1992.

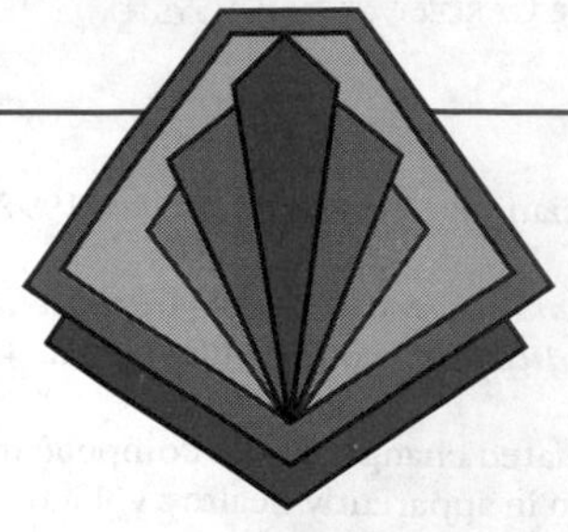

C H A P T E R 30

# Management of Persons With Dysrhythmias and Coronary Artery Disease

***Terri Abraham***

## CHAPTER OBJECTIVES

***After studying this chapter, the learner should be able to do the following:***

1 Recognize common dysrhythmias associated with the cardiac conduction system, as obtained from electrocardiogram or electrocardiographic signal averaging.
2 Describe treatment modalities for patients with cardiac dysrhythmias.
3 Identify teaching needs of patients receiving antiarrhythmic therapy.
4 Plan nursing interventions for patients requiring pacemakers, cardioversion, or defibrillation.
5 Describe the technique of basic life support.
6 Identify risk factors for coronary heart disease.
7 Explain medical and nursing management for angina pectoris and myocardial infarction.
8 Describe cardiac rehabilitation after myocardial infarction.

## KEY TERMS

altered automaticity
angina pectoris
arrhythmia
artificial ventilation
atrial fibrillation
atrial flutter
atrial tachycardia
atrioventricular (AV) block
augmented unipolar limb leads
basic life support
bundle branch block (BBB)
cardiac arrest
cardiac rehabilitation
cardiogenic shock
cardiopulmonary resuscitation
cardioversion
chylomicrons
coronary artery bypass graft (CABG)
coronary artery disease (CAD)
coronary atherosclerotic heart disease (CAHD)
creatine kinase (CK)
defibrillation
dysrhythmia
electrocardiogram (ECG)
electrocardiographic signal averaging
external cardiac compression
high-density lipoproteins (HDL)
hyperlipoproteinemia
idioventricular rhythm
intermediate-density lipoproteins (IDL)
intravascular stenting
junctional escape rhythm
junctional tachycardia
lactic acid dehydrogenase (LDH)
low-density lipoproteins (LDL)
myocardial infarction (MI)
normal sinus rhythm
P wave
pacemaker
paroxysmal atrial tachycardia (PAT)
percutaneous transluminal coronary angioplasty (PTCA)
postmyocardial infarction syndrome
PR interval
precordial unipolar leads
premature atrial beat (PAB)
premature junctional beat (PJB)
premature ventricular beat (PVB)
pulse generator
QRS complex
QT interval
reentry
serum aspartate aminotransferase (AST)
sick sinus syndrome (SSS)
sinus bradycardia
sinus dysrhythmia
sinus tachycardia
standard limb leads
ST segment
supraventricular tachycardia (SVT)
T wave
telemetry
unstable angina
U wave
ventricular fibrillation (VF)
ventricular standstill
ventricular tachycardia (VT)
very low–density lipoproteins (VLDL)

# CARDIAC DYSRHYTHMIAS

Persons with heart disease or with conditions that can affect heart function may experience cardiac dysrhythmias, which in certain situations may lead to cardiac arrest. Although the term *dysrhythmia* is preferred to denote a disturbance or variation from normal heart rhythm, the term *arrhythmia* can be used interchangeably with dysrhythmia.

At present, various pharmacologic agents, cardiac pacemakers, and electrical stimulation techniques are useful in the control of dysrhythmias. These methods and salient features of the common dysrhythmias are presented here. Because the care of persons with cardiac dysrhythmias is complex, the review that follows is not sufficient for the nurse with primary responsibility for monitoring patients in an intensive care setting. For further study, the reader is referred to more specialized texts.

## DETECTION OF CARDIAC RHYTHM

### Electrocardiogram

The **electrocardiogram (ECG)** is a graphic representation of the electrical forces produced within the heart (see Chapter 29). It is a necessary component in the assessment of cardiovascular status, but it is important to remember that this tool has limitations. For example, a resting ECG may be normal, even in the presence of heart disease. Conversely, abnormal variances may be seen in the ECG of a normal heart. It is therefore essential that the ECG be used in conjunction with data obtained from the patient history, physical assessment, and laboratory tests.

There are numerous indications for obtaining an ECG (Box 30-1). Continuous electrocardiographic monitoring for dysrhythmia detection is possible in the inpatient setting.

It is important to prepare the patient before any type of electrocardiographic procedure. Those patients who are unfamiliar with the procedure may fear receiving a shock or being electrocuted. The patient should be informed of the step-by-step procedure and assured of its safe, painless nature. Once the ECG is taken, the correct interpretation is based on knowledge of the electromechanical system of the heart, as well as the significance of each portion of the ECG tracing.

**BOX 30-1 Most Common Examples of ECG Use**

- Evaluation of tachycardia, bradycardia, or dysrhythmias
- Evaluation of sudden onset of dyspnea
- Evaluation of pain occurring in the upper portion of the trunk and in the extremities
- Evaluation of syncopal episodes
- Evaluation of shock state or coma
- Preoperative evaluation
- Evaluation of postoperative hypotension
- Evaluation of hypertension, murmurs, or cardiomegaly
- Evaluation of artificial pacemaker function

#### Standard 12-lead ECG

The electrocardiographic tracing represents the net electrical activity or electrical potential variations of the atria and ventricles as each depolarizes and repolarizes. The electrical currents passing through the heart are subsequently conducted to the body surface. These currents can be detected by electrodes and then measured when they reach the surface.

Basically the ECG machine is a galvanometer designed to measure the electrical potential difference between two locations on the body surface. The conventional 12-lead system uses several electrode sites to record potential differences at the body surface. A pair of electrodes, consisting of a positive and a negative terminal, constitutes an ECG lead. Representative tracings obtained from the 12 leads are shown in Figure 30-1.

The patient is first attached to the ECG machine as the examiner places self-adhesive electrode patches, electrode plates, or suction cup electrodes on the upper and lower extremities. These are designated as right arm (RA), left arm (LA), right leg (RL), and left leg (LL). The chest (or precordial) electrode is placed and moved across the chest wall six times during the latter portion of the ECG. Newer ECG machines are equipped with all six precordial leads, which are applied at the same time. These 10 sites are combined in pairs through a switching network connected to the lead selector switch. The operator of the ECG machine need only select the desired lead with the selector switch.

Effective contact between the skin and the electrode is facilitated by the use of electrode jelly, which contains electrolytes and an abrasive to interrupt the waterproof layer of the skin. In addition, the position of the patient should be uniformly flat if possible. Assuming a sitting or side-lying position severely alters the position of the heart relative to the electrodes. The discussions that follow clarify the individual leads and their respective electrode sites.

**Standard limb leads.** The **standard limb leads,** designated by Roman numerals I, II, and III, consist of electrodes applied to the right arm (RA), left arm (LA), and left leg (LL) (Figure 30-2). The right leg (RL) electrode acts only as a grounding electrode. The limb leads are termed *bipolar leads* because each registers the electrical potential difference between two anatomic sites.

*Lead I* records the difference between the RA and LA potentials. The LA electrode is positive. (The importance of the positive electrode is more apparent in later discussions.)

*Lead II* records the difference between the RA and LL potentials. The LL electrode is positive.

*Lead III* records the difference between the LA and LL potentials. The LL electrode is positive.

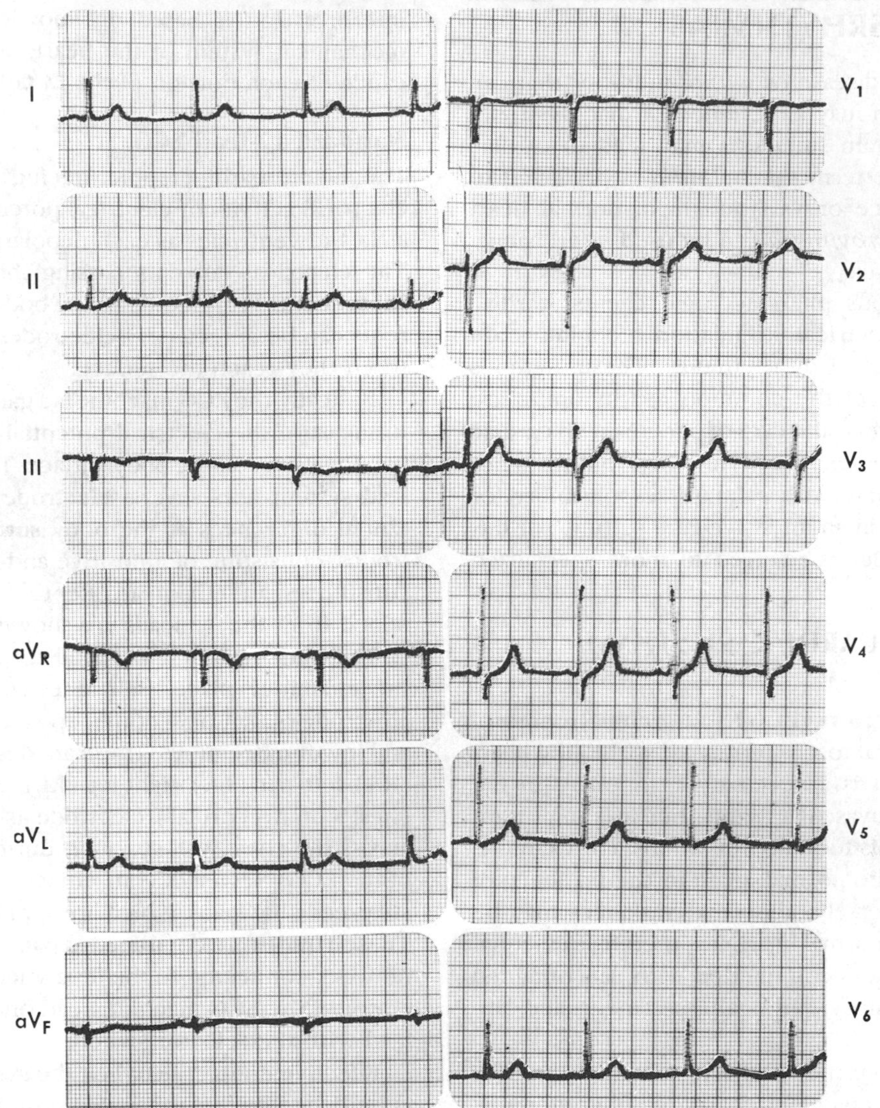


**FIGURE 30-1** Twelve-lead ECG showing normal sinus rhythm. (From Kinney MR et al: *Comprehensive cardiac care,* ed 7, St. Louis, 1991, Mosby.)

**Augmented unipolar limb leads.** The **augmented unipolar limb leads** are designated by the abbreviated forms aVR, aVL, and aVF (*a* represents augmented; *V* represents unipolar). For these leads the right arm (*R*), left arm (*L*), and left leg (*F*) become the respective positive electrodes (Figure 30-3).

The negative (central) terminal is formed by electrically joining the remaining two limb electrodes. Such a connection essentially nullifies any potential variation at the negative terminal. The electrical potential variation is recorded only by the positive electrode, thus the term *unipolar lead.* For clinical purposes the amplitude of the recordings from these electrodes is augmented by approximately 50% to produce a tracing that is easier to interpret. Together, the augmented and standard limb leads provide the six frontal plane leads.

**Precordial unipolar leads.** There are six precordial or chest leads designated by the symbols $V_1$ through $V_6$ (Figure 30-4). *V* designates the unipolar design of these leads, which register the electrical variations of the heart in the horizontal plane (Figure 30-5). The negative (central) terminal of each V lead is formed by the joining of the three limb lead electrodes. The positive electrode is an electrode that is placed on six different sites across the chest. As in the case of the limb leads, these connections are made automatically when the lead selector is turned to "V."

### Monitoring

To perform continuous cardiac monitoring and to provide for patient mobility during hospitalization, the conventional ECG leads have been modified to eliminate

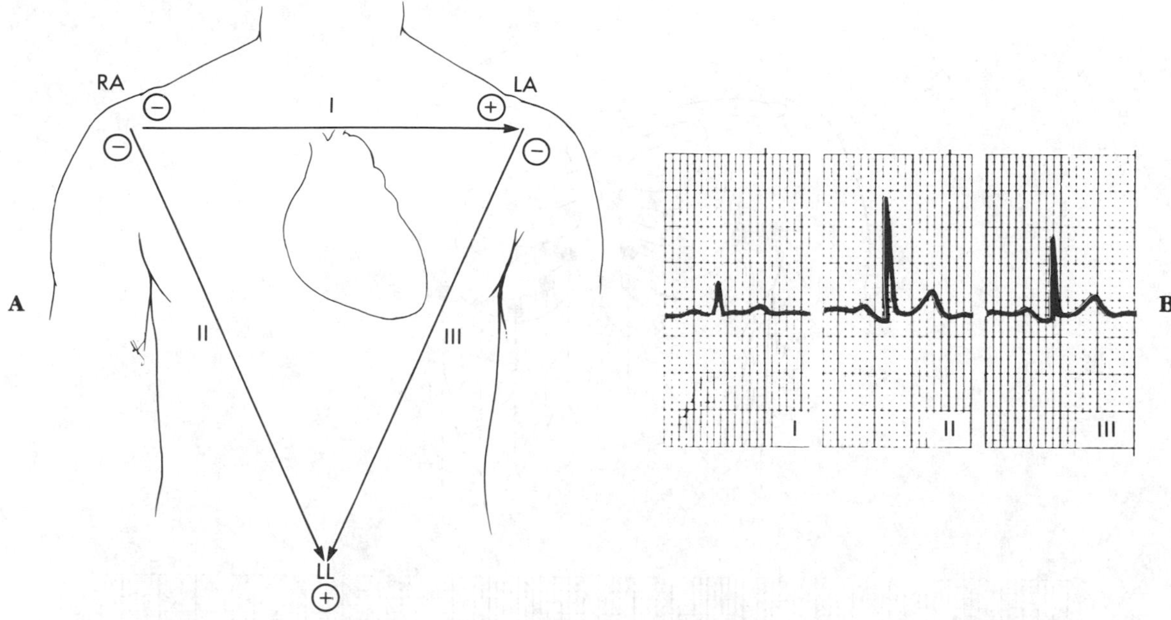


**FIGURE 30-2** Schematic representation of standard limb lead system. (**B** from Kinney MR et al: *Comprehensive cardiac care,* ed 7, St Louis, 1991, Mosby.)

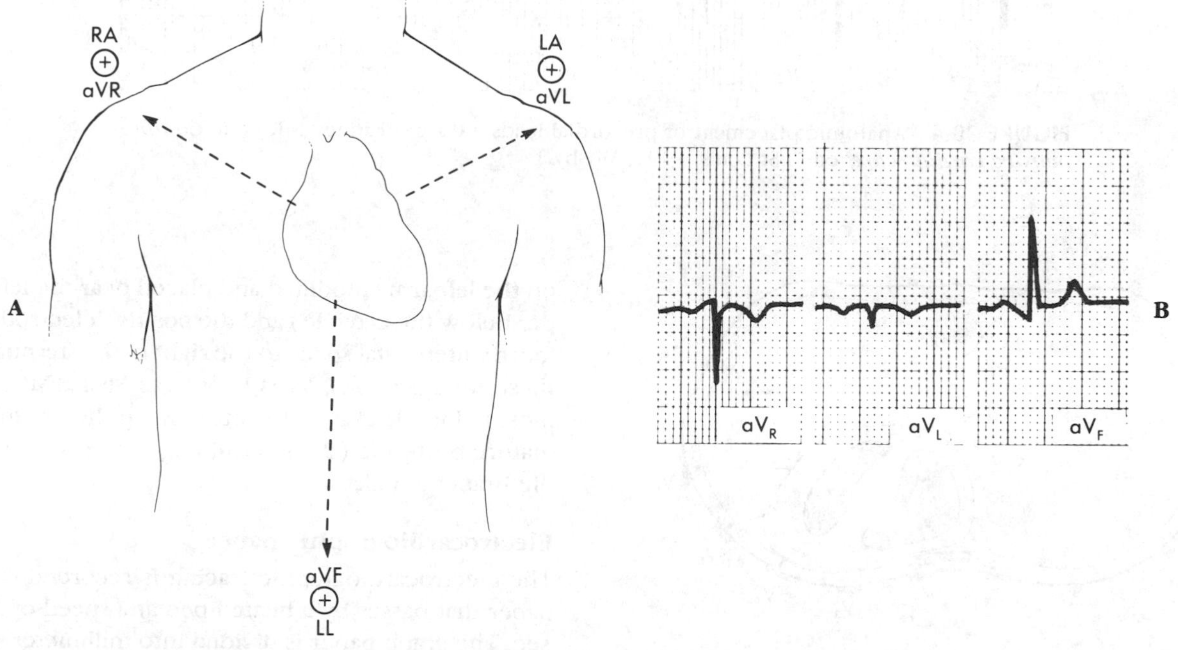


**FIGURE 30-3** Schematic representation of augmented unipolar limb lead system. (**B** from Kinney MR et al: *Comprehensive cardiac care,* ed 7, St Louis, 1991, Mosby.)

cumbersome wiring. The most popular leads for continuous dysrhythmia monitoring are lead II and lead $V_1$ ($MCL_1$: *M* for modified; *CL* for bipolar hookup [not chest lead]).

During the monitoring period the patient wears two, three, or five electrodes; each consists of a conducting gel pad surrounded by an adhesive. These electrodes are attached by small lead wires to a cable connected to a wall-mounted monitor. The monitor consists chiefly of an oscilloscope screen (for the ECG tracing display), a lead selector switch, and a heart rate indicator. This is sometimes known as a "hardwire" monitor.

An alternative type of continuous monitoring is known as **telemetry.** The telemetry system requires no

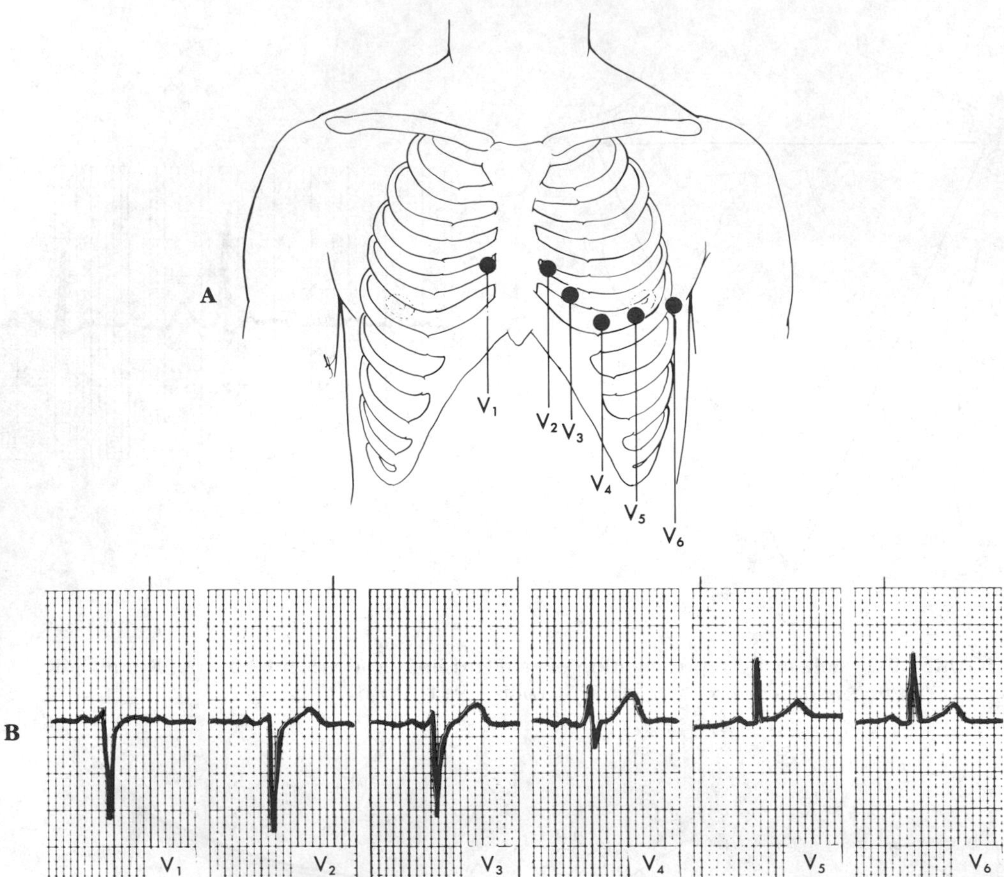


**FIGURE 30-4** Anatomic placement of precordial leads. (**B** from Kinney MR et al: *Comprehensive cardiac care,* ed 7, St Louis, 1991, Mosby.)

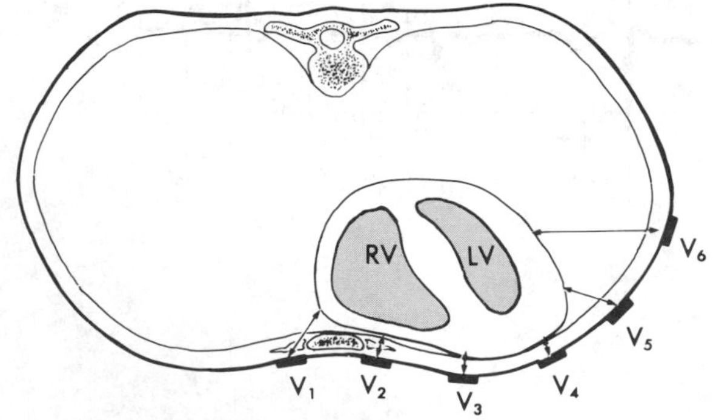


**FIGURE 30-5** Cross section of heart showing precordial leads $V_1$ through $V_6$ in a horizontal plane.

cables that would restrict patient mobility; instead, electrical impulses are transmitted by antennae to an oscilloscope at the nurses' station or at the bedside.

Lead II is produced by placing the negative electrode on the right arm (modified and placed near the right shoulder below the clavicle) and the positive electrode on the lower left rib cage (eighth intercostal space).

Lead $V_1$ is produced by placing the negative electrode on the left arm (modified and placed near the left shoulder below the clavicle) and the positive electrode at the fourth intercostal space to the right of the sternum. With these modifications, $V_1$ is known as $MCL_1$. $MCL_1$ is the most helpful lead for (1) determining the origin of premature beats and (2) determining the presence of bundle branch blocks.

### Electrocardiographic paper

The electrocardiographic tracing is recorded on graph paper that passes by a heated pen at a speed of 25 mm/sec. The graph paper is divided into millimeter squares. The millimeter squares are grouped and divided into larger squares by thick lines occurring every fifth square (Figure 30-6).

Horizontally, each millimeter square represents 0.04 second of time elapsed. Each thick line denotes the passage of 0.20 second. Fifteen hundred (1500) small, or 300 large, squares represent 1 minute. With this information, one can measure the duration of any complex or interval by determining the number of small squares and multiplying by 0.04 second.

Heart rate may be measured or estimated quickly by any of the following three methods:

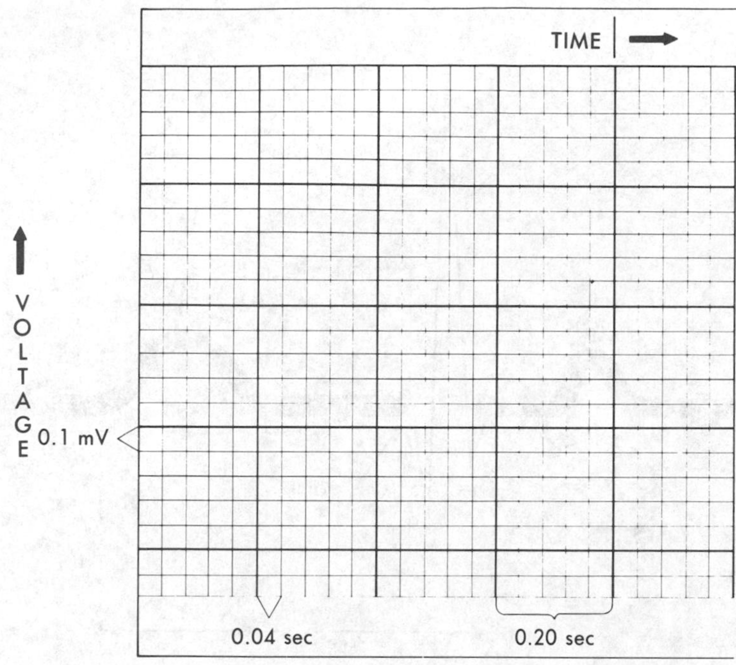


**FIGURE 30-6** Components of ECG paper.

1. Measure the interval between consecutive QRS complexes, determine the number of small squares, and divide 1500 by that number.
2. Measure the interval between consecutive QRS complexes, determine the number of large squares, and divide 300 by that number. As with method 1, this approach is used only when the heart rhythm is regular.
3. Determine the number of R-R intervals within 6 seconds and multiply by 10. (The ECG paper is conveniently marked at the top with slashes that represent 3-second intervals). This is a most helpful method when the heart rhythm is irregular. If it is *very* irregular, a longer period (30-60 seconds) should be used.

Vertically, each small square is 1 mm in height and represents 0.1 mV of voltage. Thus each large square represents 5 mm or 0.5 mV. The ECG machine is calibrated before use so that 1 mV produces a 10-mm deflection.

The voltage or amplitude of a wave or complex in a given lead indirectly indicates the electrical activity of the muscle below the exploring or positive electrode. For example, hypertrophied myocardium will produce abnormally high voltage in some leads, whereas infarcted myocardium could produce no voltage or low-voltage waves. The reader is referred to a coronary care text for a more detailed discussion of the significance of voltage.

### Waves, complexes, and intervals

The waves recorded electrocardiographically have been arbitrarily designated by the letters *P, Q, R, S, T,* and *U* (Figure 30-7). A discussion of each wave follows an explanation of the basic concept of wave generation.

The baseline of the ECG tracing is known as the *isoelectric line* (Figure 30-8). Waves are deflections, either above (positive) or below (negative) the isoelectric line. The direction of deflection is determined by the following: (1) the direction in which the electrical impulse flows, (2) the distance between the source of the impulse and the exploring electrode, and (3) the site of the electrode. As a rule, when the flow of electrical current is directed toward the positive or exploring electrode, the deflection will be positive. Conversely, when the flow of electrical current is directed away from the positive electrode, the deflection will be negative. When the flow of electrical current is directed perpendicular to a line between the negative (or central) terminal and the positive electrode, either no deflection or a biphasic deflection occurs.

**P wave.** The **P wave** represents the depolarization of the atria (Table 30-1). Normally the P wave is gently rounded, does not exceed 2 to 3 mm in amplitude, and is 0.11 second or less in duration. It is normally positive in leads I, II, aVF, and $V_4$ to $V_6$. It is negative in aVR and variable in all other leads. A P wave that does not comply with these criteria may be diagnostic of atrial enlargement or hypertrophy or may denote the presence of a pacemaker other than the sinoatrial (SA) node. Repolarization of the atria also produces a wave, but it generally is hidden within the QRS complex.

**PR interval.** The **PR interval** is a measurement of the

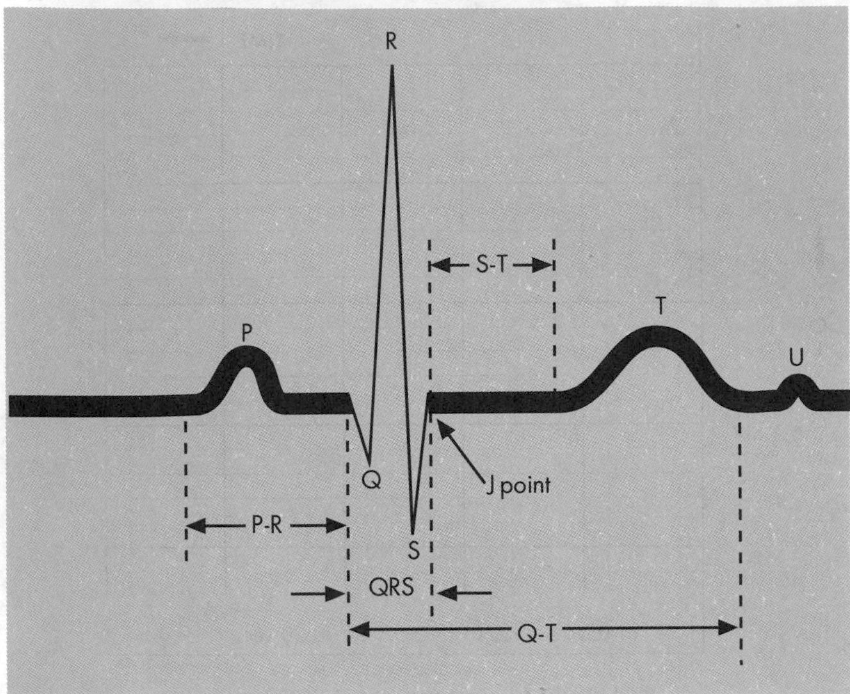


**FIGURE 30-7** Schematic drawing of ECG waves produced by the cardiac cycle.

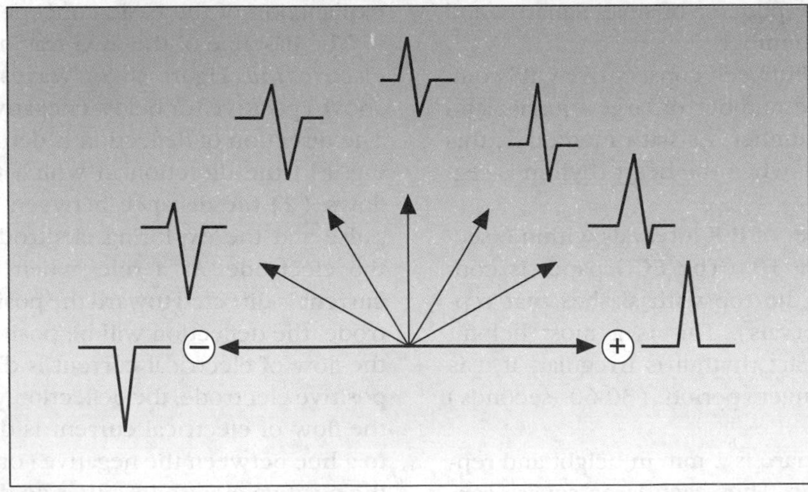

**FIGURE 30-8** Several mean vectors and their resultant ECG complex. Especially note the following: (1) a mean current perpendicular to the lead axis produces an equiphasic deflection, and (2) a mean current parallel to the lead axis results in the tallest complex possible if the current flows toward the positive electrode and the deepest complex possible if the current flows toward the negative electrode. (From Conover MB: *Understanding electrocardiography: arrhythmias and the 12-lead ECG,* ed 6, St Louis, 1992, Mosby.)

amount of time taken for the impulse to travel from the SA node to the ventricular musculature. It includes the normal physiologic delay of impulse conduction by the atrioventricular (AV) node. The interval is measured from the beginning of the P wave to the beginning of the QRS complex. Normally the PR interval measures from 0.12 to 0.20 second.

**QRS complex.** The **QRS complex** represents depolarization of the ventricles and thus is often the most significant portion of the ECG. It is important to note that the Q, R, and S waves are separate waves and must be named correctly. If the first deflection from the isoelectric line is negative, it is a Q wave (Q waves are not always present). The first positive deflection from the

**TABLE 30-1 Electrical Activity of the Heart and Resultant ECG Findings**

| ELECTRICAL ACTIVITY OF HEART | ECG EVENTS |
|---|---|
| SA node fires | Not recorded |
| Wave of depolarization spreads through atria | P wave |
| Slight pause at AV node | Isoelectric baseline between P wave and QRS complex |
| Atrial repolarization | Not recorded; overpowered by electrical activity of ventricles |
| Ventricular depolarization | QRS complex |
| Ventricular repolarization | T wave |

isoelectric line is an R wave. The negative deflection following an R wave is an S wave. A small Q wave of less than 0.04-second duration is a normal finding in leads I, II, III, aVL, aVF, and $V_4$ to $V_6$. The full duration of the QRS complex is measured from the first deflection from the isoelectric line (whether it is a Q or an R wave) to the junction point (J-point). The *J-point* is where the QRS complex ends and the ST segment begins. The normal QRS complex is 0.05 to 0.10 second.

**ST segment.** The **ST segment** represents the plateau (phase 2) of the action potential. It is normally isoelectric because no difference exists in electrical potential among the action potentials of the heart. No current flow occurs because all cells are at zero potential. Normally there may be slight elevation not greater than 1 mm or subtle depression not greater than 0.5 mm. Abnormal elevations or depressions of the ST segment can occur as a result of derangement in the action potential. Some causes include myocardial muscle injury, conduction disturbances, preexcitation, hypertrophy, tachycardia, and digitalis effect.

**T wave.** The **T wave** represents phase 3 of the action potential, when the ventricles are being rapidly repolarized. It is normally rounded, slightly asymmetric, and of the same polarity as the QRS complex. The height of the T wave should not exceed 5 mm in a limb lead or 10 mm in a precordial lead. It is normally a positive wave in leads I, II, and $V_3$ to $V_6$. The T wave is a negative deflection in lead aVR and variable in all other leads.

The effective refractory period is present during the beginning of the T wave. At the peak of the T wave, more of the fast sodium channels have recovered and therefore a stronger-than-normal stimulus can produce a successful action potential. However, some fibers are still unresponsive, and conduction velocity is very slow. Electrical chaos and subsequent ventricular fibrillation may occur. The approximate location of this vulnerable period is illustrated in Figure 30-9. Some causes of T

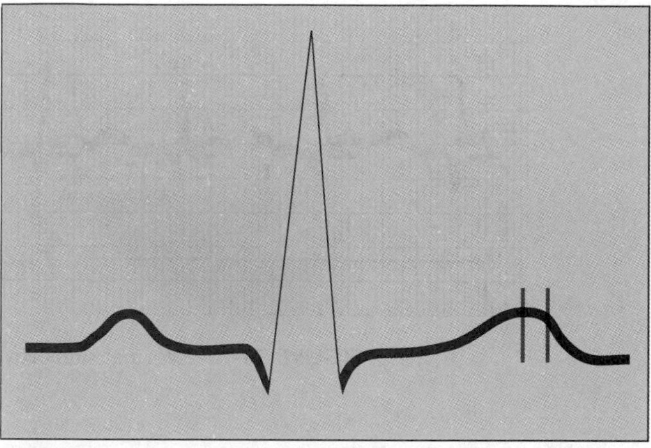

**FIGURE 30-9** Approximate location of the vulnerable period. (From Conover MB: *Understanding electrocardiography: arrhythmias and the 12-lead ECG,* ed 6, St Louis, 1992, Mosby.)

wave abnormality include ischemia, ventricular hypertrophy, quinidine therapy, digitalis therapy, acid-base imbalance, hyperkalemia, and ventricular extrasystoles.

**QT interval.** The **QT interval** is measured from the beginning of the QRS complex to the end of the T wave. It represents the entire duration of ventricular depolarization and repolarization. The normal QT value varies with age, gender, and heart rate. As a rule, however, the QT interval should be less than half the preceding R-R interval. Because the actual termination of the T wave is sometimes difficult to determine, measuring the QT interval accurately is not always easy. It is important, however, to be aware of any change in the QT interval because an abnormality in this measurement may indicate drug and electrolyte imbalances.

**U wave.** The **U wave** is a small wave sometimes seen after the T wave. It usually deflects in the same direction as the T wave and is best seen in lead $V_3$. It has been suggested that the U wave represents late repolarization of papillary muscle. The U wave is affected by many drugs and conditions but is best known for its prominence in hypokalemia.

### Normal sinus rhythm

The term **normal sinus rhythm (NSR)** implies that cardiac electrical activity is within normal limits as indicated by the following criteria (Figure 30-10):

1. P waves present and regular. If the SA node is initiating electrical activity in a rhythmic manner, atrial depolarization should occur in a rhythmic manner.
2. Atrial rate (P waves) between 60 and 100 beats/min. This represents the range of normal rates for the SA node.

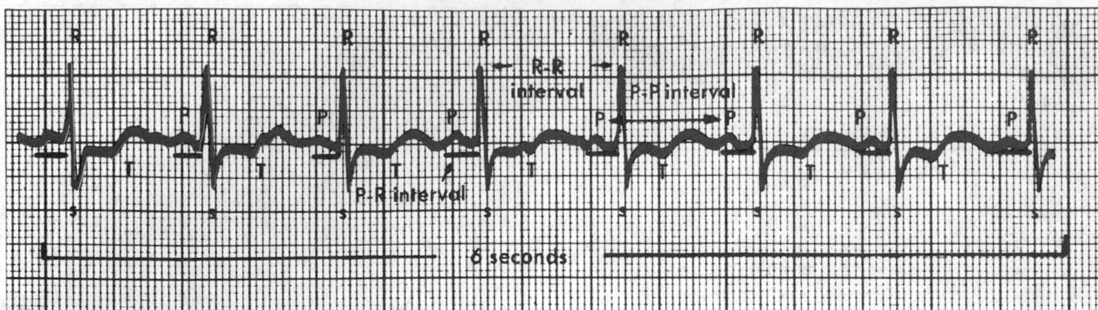


**FIGURE 30-10** Normal sinus rhythm showing R-R, P-P, and PR intervals.

3. Each P wave is followed by a QRS complex. This verifies conduction of the impulse initiated by the SA node into the ventricles and implies that the heart rhythm is regular and the heart rate is also between 60 and 100 beats/min.
4. In addition, normal PR interval and QRS duration indicate normal functioning of all components of the conduction system.

**Electrocardiogram and aging**

As described in Chapter 29, degenerative changes occur in the conduction system with aging. The ECG consequently is affected. The components most notably affected are the duration of the PR and QT intervals, the duration and morphology (shape) of the atrial and ventricular complexes, and aspects of ventricular repolarization such as ST segment and T wave changes.

## Electrocardiographic Signal Averaging

**Electrocardiographic signal averaging** of the surface QRS complex is used to detect low-amplitude, high-frequency signals in the terminal portion of the QRS complex or in the early ST segment. It is a noninvasive, computerized method of analyzing standard ECGs that identifies patients at risk for ventricular tachycardia. Sustained ventricular tachycardia (see p. 796) can be a precursor of sudden cardiac death. It is important to accurately determine which patients are at high risk so that appropriate medical and nursing interventions can be implemented. Although late potentials have been reported in patients with ventricular tachycardia, the independent role of quantitative, signal-averaged variables alone or in combination with other diagnostic predictors of arrhythmogenesis has yet to be established.

Electrocardiographic signal averaging involves amplification of electrical signals from the heart that have a voltage too small to be recorded by a standard ECG. Ischemia and infarction can cause the extreme slowing of conduction that results in this delayed activity. Typically, approximately 200 identical QRS complexes are grouped and averaged, resulting in a waveform that appears smooth and continuous. Signal averaging minimizes the level of noise that contaminates the ECG signal and thereby exposes signals of a microvolt level normally hidden within noise, such as skeletal muscle noise, especially from respiratory muscles, and noise from electrical equipment, amplifiers, and electrodes.[19]

Equipment necessary to perform signal averaging includes ECG leads, an amplifier, an analog-digital converter, and a personal computer with software to average the QRS waveforms and store data. Patient interface with the electrodes is of primary importance to obtain and analyze data. Cleansing and mildly abrading the skin are necessary before attachment of the electrodes.

Probably the most significant contribution of the signal-averaged ECG is in the management of patients after acute myocardial infarction (see Chapter 31). Other indications for use include unexplained syncope, nonischemic congestive cardiomyopathy, and evaluation of antiarrhythmic drug therapy. The rate of postinfarction sudden death precipitated by ventricular tachycardia that degenerates into ventricular fibrillation is approximately 10% to 15%; these deaths usually occur within 2 years after the myocardial infarction. Antiarrhythmic therapy for all patients after infarction is unwarranted and may be harmful. Thus identification of those patients who will need treatment is critical for overall management.

# TYPES OF CARDIAC DYSRHYTHMIAS

The term **dysrhythmia** (also called **arrhythmia**) refers to the presence of a heart rate and rhythm other than normal sinus rhythm (NSR). There are many types of dysrhythmias (Table 30-2), which are grouped in the following discussion according to anatomic origins. Abbreviations typically used to name specific dysrhythmias are listed in Box 30-2. The mechanisms that underlie the dysrhythmias are discussed before the specific dysrhythmias.

## Arrhythmogenic Mechanisms

Most dysrhythmias are believed to be caused by (1) abnormalities in *impulse formation* because of (a) altered automaticity (enhanced or abnormal automaticity) or (b) triggered activity (early or delayed afterdepolarizations), (2) abnormalities of *conduction* caused

**BOX 30-2 Abbreviations Denoting Cardiac Dysrhythmias**

| | |
|---|---|
| SSS | Sick sinus syndrome |
| PAB | Premature atrial beat |
| PAT | Paroxysmal atrial tachycardia |
| PJB | Premature junctional beat |
| SVT | Supraventricular tachycardia |
| PVB | Premature ventricular beat |
| VT | Ventricular tachycardia |
| RBBB | Right bundle branch block |
| LBBB | Left bundle branch block |
| LAH | Left anterior hemiblock |
| LPH | Left posterior hemiblock |

by a block or reentry, or (3) a combination of these. The following is a brief discussion of these mechanisms.

### Altered automaticity

**Altered automaticity** may occur in both pacemaker and nonpacemaker cells. Automaticity (the ability to depolarize spontaneously without external stimulation) is a property that normally is confined to the cells of the SA node. The SA node usually depolarizes at a faster rate than other potential pacemaker cells (sometimes called *latent pacemakers*) and thus controls the electrical activity of the heart. A variety of conditions can alter the automaticity of the SA node and produce faster or slower than usual heart rates. If the rate of the SA node falls below the rate of latent pacemaker cells, *escape rhythms* may ensue.

If the rate of phase 4 depolarization in latent pacemaker cells found in the AV node or ventricular conduction system increases, *enhanced automaticity* is said to exist. The results of this may be premature beats or tachycardias. Some causes for this enhanced automaticity are hypoxia, catecholamines, hypokalemia, hypocalcemia, atropine, heat, trauma, and digitalis toxicity.

Even cells that do not normally have automaticity may develop *abnormal automaticity* if the resting membrane potential is reduced sufficiently (usually −60 mV). This may be a consequence of ischemia, infarction, hypokalemia, hypocalcemia, or cardiomyopathy. This abnormal automaticity is not easily suppressed by the activity of faster pacemakers.

### Triggered activity (late potentials)

Triggered activity refers to repetitive ectopic firing, which is the result of afterdepolarizations. These afterdepolarizations occur either during or after repolarization; thus they are not the same as altered automaticity and are not sustained by a reentry circuit. It is only when the afterdepolarization achieves threshold potential that triggered activity results. The afterdepolarization may reach threshold because of a shortening of the cycle length or increased levels of catecholamines. Researchers have demonstrated not only that a relationship exists between this delayed activation and ventricular dysrhythmias but also that this delayed activation represents the substrate for reentry ventricular tachycardia.[4,18] A frequent cause of afterdepolarizations is digitalis toxicity.

### Reentry

**Reentry** occurs when an impulse is delayed long enough within a pathway of slow conduction that it is still viable when the remaining myocardium repolarizes. The impulse then reenters surrounding tissue and produces another impulse. The initiating impulse may be either normal sinus or ectopic (Figure 30-11). One-way conduction is necessary because without it the impulse would cancel itself out within the area of slow conduction. Any condition that decreases the amplitude of the action potential, such as ischemia, hypercalcemia, or calcification of the conducting fibers, can cause cardiac conduction disturbance, resulting in either heart block or a reentry rhythm.

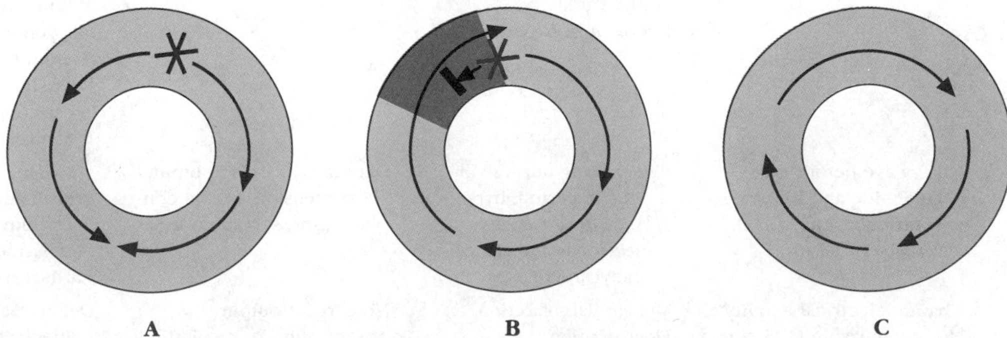


**FIGURE 30-11** Mechanism of reentry. **A,** Impulses travel from the stimulus in opposite directions around the ring to meet and cancel each other out. **B,** Pressure has been applied at the shaded area in the ring, at which point the impulse is blocked and travels only in the opposite direction. Pressure is then removed, and the impulse continues around and around **(C)** on its one-way journey as long as refractory tissue is not encountered. (From Marriott HJL, Conover MB: *Advanced concepts in arrhythmias,* ed 2, St Louis, 1989, Mosby.)

**TABLE 30-2 Comparison of Selected Cardiac Dysrhythmias**

| DYSRHYTHMIA | DESCRIPTION | ETIOLOGY | SYMPTOMS/ CONSEQUENCES | TREATMENT |
|---|---|---|---|---|
| **DYSRHYTHMIAS OF SINUS NODE** | | | | |
| Sinus dysrhythmia | Phasic shortening then lengthening of P-P and R-R interval | Respiratory variation in impulse initiation by SA node | Usually none | Usually none |
| Sinus tachycardia | P waves present followed by QRS<br>Rhythm regular<br>Heart rate 100-150 beats/min | Increased metabolic demands<br>Decreased oxygen delivery, congestive heart failure, shock, hemorrhage, anemia | May produce palpitations<br>Prolonged episodes may lead to decreased cardiac output | Treat underlying cause<br>Occasionally sedatives |
| Sinus bradycardia | P waves present followed by QRS<br>Rhythm regular<br>Heart rate <60 | Physical fitness<br>Parasympathetic stimulation (sleep)<br>Brain lesions<br>Sinus dysfunction<br>Digitalis excess | Very low rates may cause decreased cardiac output: lightheadedness, faintness, chest pain | Atropine if cardiac output is decreased<br>Pacemaker<br>Treat underlying cause if necessary |
| **ATRIAL DYSRHYTHMIAS** | | | | |
| Premature atrial beats | Early P wave<br>QRS may or may not be normal<br>Rhythm irregular | Stress, ischemia, atrial enlargement, caffeine, nicotine | May produce palpitations<br>Frequent episodes may decrease cardiac output<br>Is sign of chamber irritability | Sedation<br>Quinidine<br>May require no treatment |
| Atrial tachycardia | P wave present (may merge into previous T wave), QRS usually normal, rapid heart rate usually >150/min | Sympathetic stimulation, chemical stimuli (caffeine, nicotine), drug toxicity | Palpitations<br>Possible anxiety | Usually none<br>Prolonged episodes may require carotid sinus pressure, vagal stimulation, verapamil, digitalis, or beta blockers |
| Atrial fibrillation | Rapid, irregular P waves (>350/min)<br>Ventricular rhythm irregularly irregular<br>Ventricular rate varies, may increase to 120-150/min if untreated | Rheumatic heart disease<br>Mitral stenosis<br>Atrial infarction<br>Coronary atherosclerotic heart disease<br>Hypertensive heart disease<br>Thyrotoxicosis | Pulse deficit<br>Decreased cardiac output if rate is rapid<br>Promotes thrombus formation in atria | Digitalis<br>Quinidine<br>Cardioversion |
| **VENTRICULAR DYSRHYTHMIAS** | | | | |
| Premature ventricular beats (PVBs) | Early wide bizarre QRS, not associated with a P wave<br>Rhythm irregular | Stress, acidosis, ventricular enlargement<br>Electrolyte imbalance<br>Myocardial infarction<br>Digitalis toxicity<br>Hypoxemia, hypercapnia | Same as for premature atrial beats | Procainamide<br>Quinidine<br>Disopyramide (Norpace)<br>Lidocaine<br>Mexiletine<br>Oxygen<br>Sodium bicarbonate<br>Potassium<br>Treat congestive heart failure |
| Ventricular tachycardia | No P wave before QRS; QRS wide and bizarre; ventricular rate >100, usually 140-240 | PVB striking during vulnerable period; hypoxemia; drug toxicity; electrolyte imbalance; bradycardia | Decreased cardiac output, hypotension, loss of consciousness, respiratory arrest | Lidocaine<br>Procainamide<br>Bretylium<br>Mexiletine<br>Cardioversion |
| Ventricular fibrillation | Chaotic electrical activity<br>No recognizable QRS complex | Myocardial infarction<br>Electrocution<br>Freshwater drowning<br>Drug toxicity | No cardiac output<br>Absent pulse or respiration<br>Cardiac arrest | Defibrillation<br>Epinephrine<br>Sodium bicarbonate<br>Bretylium<br>CPR |

**TABLE 30-2 Comparison of Selected Cardiac Dysrhythmias—cont'd**

| DYSRHYTHMIA | DESCRIPTION | ETIOLOGY | SYMPTOMS/ CONSEQUENCES | TREATMENT |
|---|---|---|---|---|
| **VENTRICULAR DYSRHYTHMIAS—cont'd** | | | | |
| Ventricular standstill | Can be distinguished from ventricular fibrillation only by ECG<br>P waves *may* be present<br>No QRS<br>"Straight line" | Myocardial infarction<br>Chronic diseases of conducting system | Same as for ventricular fibrillation | CPR<br>Pacemaker<br>Intracardiac epinephrine<br>Isoproterenol |
| **IMPULSE CONDUCTION DEFICITS** | | | | |
| First-degree atrioventricular (AV) block | PR interval prolonged, >0.20 sec | Rheumatic fever<br>Digitalis toxicity<br>Degenerative changes of coronary atherosclerotic heart disease<br>Infections<br>Decreased oxygen in AV node | Warns of impaired conduction | Usually none as long as it occurs as an isolated deficit |
| Bundle branch block | Same as normal sinus rhythm (NSR) except QRS duration >0.10 | Hypoxia, acute myocardial infarction, congestive heart failure, coronary atherosclerotic heart disease, pulmonary embolus, hypertension | Same as first-degree AV block | Usually none unless severe blockage of left posterior division (see text) |
| Second-degree AV blocks | P waves usually occur regularly at rates consistent with SA node initiation. (Not all P waves followed by QRS; PR interval may lengthen before nonconducted P wave or may be consistent; QRS may be widened.) | Acute myocardial infarction | Serious dysrhythmia that may lead to decreased heart rate and cardiac output | May require temporary pacemaker |
| Complete third-degree AV block | Atria and ventricles beat independently<br>P waves have no relation to QRS<br>Ventricular rate may be as low as 20-40/min | Digitalis toxicity<br>Infectious disease<br>Coronary artery disease<br>Myocardial infarction | Very low rates may cause decreased cardiac output: lightheadedness, faintness, chest pain | Pacemaker<br>Isoproterenol to increase heart rate<br>Epinephrine if isoproterenol ineffective |

## Dysrhythmias Originating in Sinoatrial Node

### Sinus dysrhythmia

Because of the varying influence of sympathetic and parasympathetic stimulation on the SA node, it is rare for sinus rhythm to be absolutely regular. Minor variations in P-P intervals are normal. In fact, the absence of these variations in patients who have had acute myocardial infarctions has been associated with an increased incidence of mortality.[11,14] However, when P-P intervals vary by more than 0.16 seconds, the term **sinus dysrhythmia** is applied. The P waves have a constant morphology, and the PR interval and QRS duration are within normal limits. Changes in P-P intervals are accompanied by changes in R-R intervals (Figure 30-12).

Sinus dysrhythmia is the most frequently noted dysrhythmia. It is typically found in young adults and elderly persons. In one type of sinus dysrhythmia the cyclic pattern of changing P-P or R-R intervals correlates with the patterns of inspiration and expiration. During inspiration the intervals shorten as the heart rate increases. Conversely, the intervals lengthen during expiration. This phenomenon results from a reflex inhibition of vagal tone or an enhancement of sympathetic tone, or both. Its occurrence is favored by slower heart rates and ingestion of drugs, such as digitalis, that enhance vagal tone.

Sinus dysrhythmia is not treated unless the bradycardiac phase is marked, causing symptoms. With slower heart rates, some patients may experience palpitations or dizziness if the P-P intervals are unusually long. Absence of sinus dysrhythmia in acute myocardial infarction may indicate a need for diuretics.

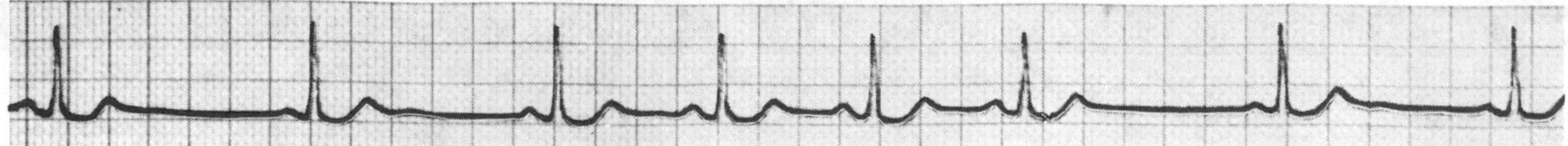

**FIGURE 30-12** Sinus dysrhythmia. Lead II showing phasic variations in P-P interval of more than 0.16 second; irregular rhythm; PR interval, 0.16 second; and QRS complex, 0.06 second. (From Kinney MR et al: *Comprehensive cardiac care,* ed 7, St Louis, 1991, Mosby.)

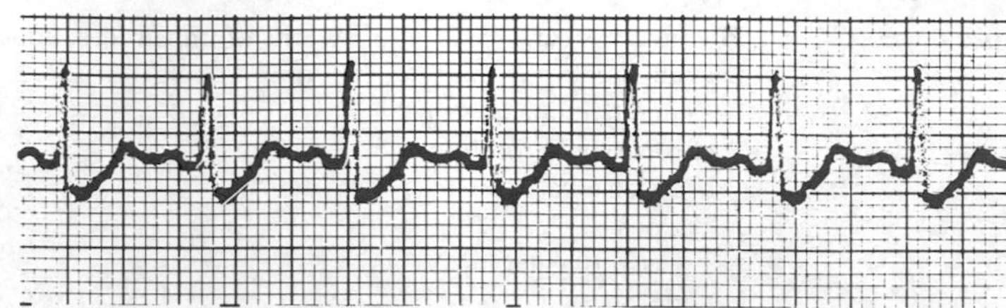

**FIGURE 30-13** Sinus tachycardia. Lead II showing heart rate of 115 beats/min, regular rhythm, normal PR interval, and normal QRS duration.

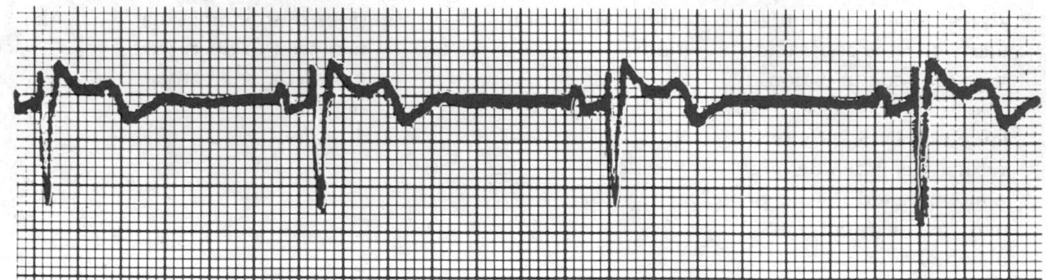

**FIGURE 30-14** Sinus bradycardia. Lead $V_1$ showing heart rate of approximately 44 beats/min, regular rhythm, normal PR interval, and normal QRS duration.

### Sinus tachycardia

**Sinus tachycardia** (Figure 30-13) is characterized by an atrial and ventricular rate of 100 beats/min or more. Generally the upper limit with sinus tachycardia is 160/min, but the rate may increase to 200 under extreme exertion. The mechanism underlying sinus tachycardia is enchanced automaticity.

The P waves are sinus in origin, but they may appear more peaked than usual with very high rates. Intervals and complexes are within normal limits. The onset of sinus tachycardia usually is gradual inasmuch as the sinus node rate increases in response to higher metabolic needs.

Sinus tachycardia is associated with the ingestion of alcohol, tea, coffee, or tobacco. It is a normal physiologic response to exertion, fever, fear, excitement, or any condition that requires a higher basal metabolism. Clinically it is a short-term compensatory mechanism associated with heart failure, hypovolemia, and hypotension. It is also often seen with hyperthyroidism and may be produced by drugs such as atropine, epinephrine, and isoproterenol.

Generally, sinus tachycardia is a benign rhythm. The patient may complain of palpitations or have no symptoms. In the patient with a compromised myocardium, the tachycardia may cause a decrease in cardiac output with resultant lightheadedness, chest pain, and heart failure. In the presence of acute myocardial ischemia, higher heart rates may trigger ventricular dysrhythmias.

### Sinus bradycardia

**Sinus bradycardia** (Figure 30-14) is characterized by atrial and ventricular rates of less than 60 beats/min. It should be noted that some researchers use a rate of 50 or below as an indication of bradycardia. In all other respects, sinus bradycardia has the normal parameters for sinus rhythm. It may develop gradually or occur suddenly for a brief period.

Bradycardia generally results from increased vagal tone or decreased symphathetic tone. It is frequently

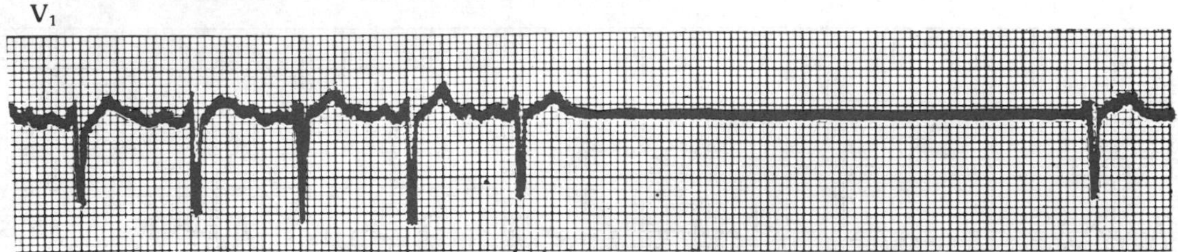


FIGURE 30-15 Sick sinus syndrome (SSS) in the form of tachycardia/bradycardia. (From Marriott HJL, Conover MB: *Advanced concepts in arrhythmias,* ed 2, St Louis, 1989, Mosby.)

seen in elderly persons and in athletes and also may be associated with sleep, vomiting, eye surgery, intracranial tumors, and myocardial infarction. Carotid sinus stimulation and parasympathomimetic drugs induce sinus bradycardia in many patients.

Generally, sinus bradycardia is a benign rhythm. In association with myocardial infarction, it may be a beneficial rhythm because it reduces myocardial oxygen demand. If the heart rate is too slow to maintain adequate cardiac output, the patient may be predisposed to syncope and congestive heart failure. Administration of atropine or isoproterenol usually is effective in increasing the heart rate. The patient with refractory bradycardia who has symptoms may require a permanent implantable pacemaker (see p. 803).

### Sick sinus syndrome

**Sick sinus syndrome (SSS)** is a term describing several clinical disorders of SA node function caused by cellular physiologic abnormalities that interfere with impulse formation, transmission, and conduction. The SA node dysfunction often is accompanied by depressed automaticity of lower pacemakers (e.g., AV junction), as well as conduction disturbances in the atria, AV node, bundle branches, or ventricles.

The *tachycardia-bradycardia syndrome* is the most common type of SSS (Figure 30-15). Typically, it is characterized by the presence of a sinus bradycardia with intermittent episodes of atrial tachydysrhythmias. The episode of tachydysrhythmia often is followed by a long pause before returning to sinus bradycardia. Complications of this inefficient rhythm include congestive heart failure and cerebrovascular accidents resulting from thromboembolisms. In addition, cerebral blood flow may be decreased, producing symptoms similar to confusion in the elderly person.

Some patients may remain free of symptoms or may complain only of palpitations. For the patient with severe symptoms, the heart rhythm should be stabilized by the use of a permanent implantable pacemaker.

## Dysrhythmias Originating in the Atria

### Premature atrial beat

The **premature atrial beat (PAB)** is initiated by an ectopic focus in the atria (Figure 30-16). It is characterized by a premature P wave with a contour different from that of a sinus P wave. This premature P wave sometimes is called a P′ (P prime) wave. The location of the ectopic focus within the atria determines its shape. The QRS complex may or may not be normal, and the PAB is followed by a pause approximately equal to the sinus cycle (measured R to R). The atrial impulse may be nonconducted (blocked) because of refractoriness of the ventricles at the time the impulse arrives. The nonconducted atrial beat (blocked PAB) is the most common cause of irregularities in the heart rhythm.

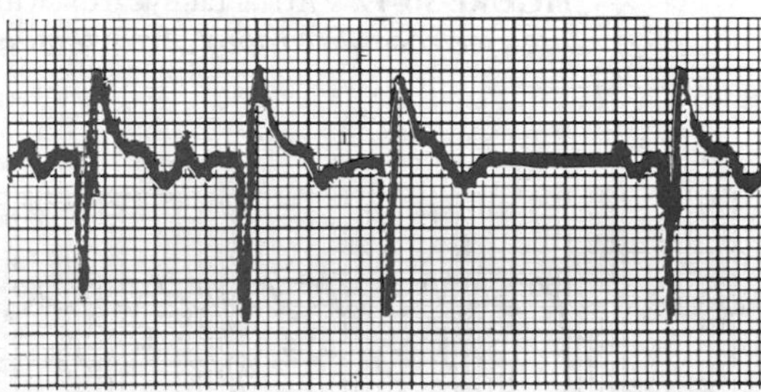

FIGURE 30-16 Premature atrial beat (PAB). Lead V, showing third beat is PAB with abnormal early P wave followed by normal QRS complex.

The PAB may be associated with stress or the use of caffeine or tobacco products. It also is seen in the clinical setting with infection, inflammation, and myocardial ischemia. Frequent PABs may warn of impending atrial fibrillation or tachycardia.

In the absence of organic disease, no treatment is required. Often the omission of caffeine and tobacco will suppress the atrial focus. If symptoms are present or organic disease is known, PABs may be suppressed by digitalis, quinidine, or procainamide.

### Atrial tachycardia

In **atrial tachycardia** the atrial rate is approximately 150 to 250 beats/min. In contrast to atrial flutter or fibrillation, P waves are present but may be hidden in the T waves of the preceding beats when the ventricular rate is high. The QRS complex generally is normal, and the ventricular rhythm is regular.

When atrial tachycardia occurs suddenly, it is called

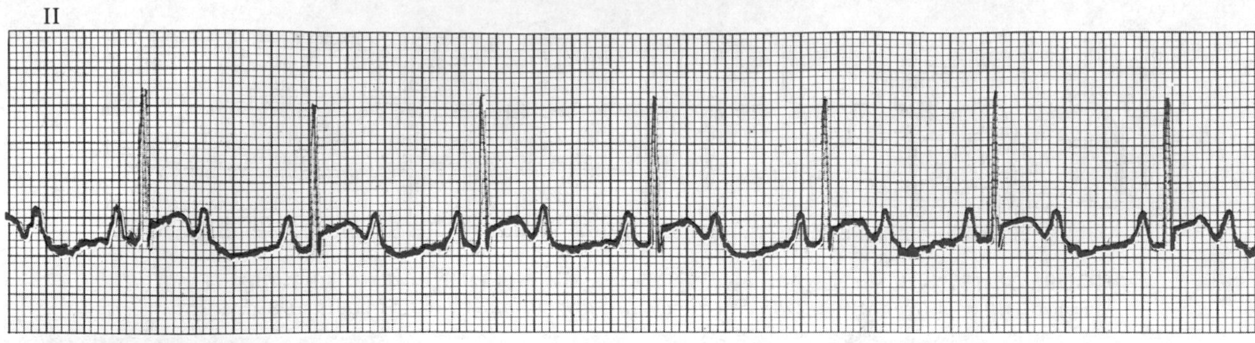


**FIGURE 30-17** Atrial tachycardia with 2:1 AV conduction. (From Conover MB: *Understanding electrocardiography: Arrhythmias and the 12-lead ECG,* ed 6, St Louis, 1992, Mosby.)

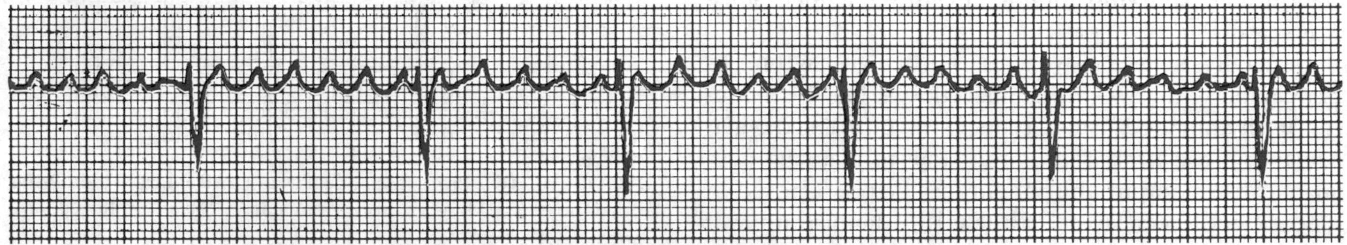

**FIGURE 30-18** Atrial flutter (lead $V_1$). Rate of atrial flutter waves is 300 beats/min. Ventricular rate is 50 to 75/min.

**paroxysmal atrial tachycardia (PAT).** Transient episodes of PAT may occur in children and young adults in the absence of heart disease. When underlying disease is present, it usually is rheumatic heart disease.

The patient may complain of palpitations and experience anxiety during a tachycardic episode. Short, infrequent episodes require no treatment. Generally, hemodynamic changes are not severe unless the episode is persistent, the rate is greater than 200/min, or underlying disease exists. Lengthy paroxysms may require carotid sinus pressure, vagal stimulation, or intravenous administration of verapamil, digitalis, or beta blockers to slow the rate or restore sinus rhythm. Some patients may benefit from receiving instruction in the performance of Valsalva's maneuver to cause slowing of the rate. Digitalis and propranolol are the drugs of choice if vagal stimulation is unsuccessful. Should hypotension or congestive heart failure (CHF) complicate the dysrhythmia, cardioversion is indicated.

Atrial tachycardia *with block* is characterized by the same rapid atrial rate, but some impulses are not conducted into the ventricles (i.e., are "blocked"). The AV nodal conduction ratio is usually 2:1, producing a ventricular rate of 75 to 125/min (Figure 30-17). This dysrhythmia is associated with organic heart disease. Digitalis toxicity and potassium depletion in the patient receiving digitalis are two conditions that also favor its development. The treatment depends on the clinical picture and often is aimed at correcting the underlying cause.

When atrial tachycardia is caused by digitalis toxicity, failure to discontinue the medication may result in death. Treatment includes bed rest, continuous cardiac and hemodynamic monitoring, and restriction of sympathetic stimulation. In severe cases of hemodynamic compromise, phenytoin or digitalis antibody is indicated.

### Atrial flutter

In **atrial flutter** the atria depolarize at a rate of 250 to 350 beats/min. This mechanism of atrial flutter is a single reentry circuit within the right atrium. The atrial depolarizations produce flutter (F) waves that give the baseline a sawtooth appearance (Figure 30-18). The QRS configurations are normal. There is no measurable PR interval because it is often difficult to determine electrocardiographically which atrial impulse actually is conducted to the ventricles. With rapid atrial rates, the AV node physiologically prevents conduction of each atrial impulse to the ventricles. In hyperthyroidism, however, increased conduction may occur. Despite this protective mechanism the ventricular rate is often greater than 150/min if untreated (2:1 conduction).

Atrial flutter is seen less often than atrial fibrillation but usually indicates underlying disease. It is associated most frequently with coronary atherosclerotic heart dis-

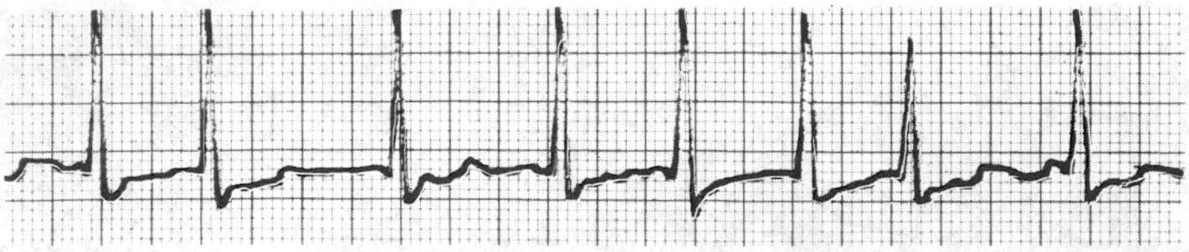

FIGURE 30-19 Atrial fibrillation (lead II). Atrial rate is rapid with varying conduction to ventricles, irregular rhythm, normal QRS complex, no definite P waves visible, and PR interval not measurable.

ease (CAHD), pulmonary embolism, mitral valve disease, and thoracic surgical procedures.

The potentially rapid ventricular rate of atrial flutter may result in a decrease in cardiac output. The major goal of treatment is conversion to sinus rhythm or control of the ventricular rate. To protect an already compensated myocardium from the metabolic demands of rapid contractions, direct current cardioversion (see p. 807) is the treatment of choice in the patient with an acute myocardial infarction.

Cardioversion is highly successful in converting atrial flutter to sinus rhythm, often with 50 watt-seconds (joules) or less. If cardioversion is unsuccessful or if atrial flutter is recurrent, digitalis usually succeeds in slowing the ventricular rate by lengthening AV nodal conduction time. In some cases the addition of quinidine, procainamide, or propranolol to digitalis therapy may result in conversion to sinus rhythm. Atrial pacing may be used in patients for whom pharmacologic and external cardioversion methods have been unsuccessful.

#### Atrial fibrillation

**Atrial fibrillation** (Figure 30-19) is the most rapid of atrial dysrhythmias. It is generated and perpetuated by one or more rapidly firing ectopic foci. The atria depolarize chaotically at rates of 350 to 600 beats/min. The baseline is characteristically composed of irregular undulations without definable P waves. The QRS complex usually is normal, but the ventricular rhythm is irregularly irregular. If untreated, the ventricular rate will generally be 100 to 180/min.

Atrial fibrillation may be paroxysmal and transient, or it may be chronic. The latter generally indicates underlying heart disease. It is typically associated with pericarditis, thyrotoxicosis, cardiomyopathy, CAHD, hypertensive heart disease, and rheumatic mitral valve disease. Its development also is related to atrial infarction.

Because of ventricular rhythm irregularity and the loss of synchronous atrial contractions *(atrial kick)*, cardiac output is decreased and a pulse deficit often exists. In the presence of mitral stenosis, thrombi may form in the atria and cause embolisms, which may lodge in the pulmonary or peripheral blood vessels. The goal of therapy is to prevent these complications through the control of the ventricular rate and the use of anticoagulants in certain patients.

The treatment for atrial fibrillation depends on the circumstances. Often, correction of the underlying condition will convert the rhythm to sinus rhythm. If the patient's hemodynamic condition deteriorates, with symptoms of CHF and hypotension, immediate intervention with cardioversion is highly successful. Cardioverison is contraindicated in several conditions, including digitalis toxicity, severe AV block, and SSS.[5]

Drugs commonly used to control the ventricular rate include digitalis, beta blockers, and calcium antagonists. After the ventricular rate has been slowed, drugs for conversion to sinus rhythm include quinidine, disopyramide, procainamide, propafenone, encainide, flecainide, and amiodarone. The goal is to attain a resting ventricular heart rate of 60 to 80 beats/min or to restore sinus rhythm. The patient must be monitored for heart rate and blood pressure until stable.

### Dysrhythmias Originating in the Atrioventricular Junction

#### Premature junctional beats

The **premature junctional beat (PJB)** arises from an ectopic focus either (1) at the junction of atrial and AV nodal tissue or (2) at the junction of AV nodal tissue and the bundle of His. The causative mechanisms may be triggered activity caused by digitalis toxicity or altered automaticity resulting from ischemia. If the PJB arises from the first junction, the P wave will be inverted and premature and will precede the QRS complex. In the second case, the P wave either is hidden in the QRS or is inverted and follows the QRS (Figure 30-20). The abnormal timing and the inversion of the P wave are caused by depolarization of the atria in a retrograde fashion. The QRS is normal, but the PR or RP (when P waves follow the QRS) interval is less than 0.12 second.

PJBs may occur in the normal heart. They also may result from digitalis toxicity, ischemia, hypoxia, or electrolyte imbalance. Treatment, when needed, is directed toward correcting the underlying cause. Quinidine, propranolol, and procainamide may suppress PJBs. Phenytoin (Dilantin) is particularly useful in the suppression of the PJBs secondary to digitalis toxicity.

#### Junctional rhythms

When the SA node fires at a rate less than 40 to 60 beats/min, the automatic cells in the AV junction may initiate

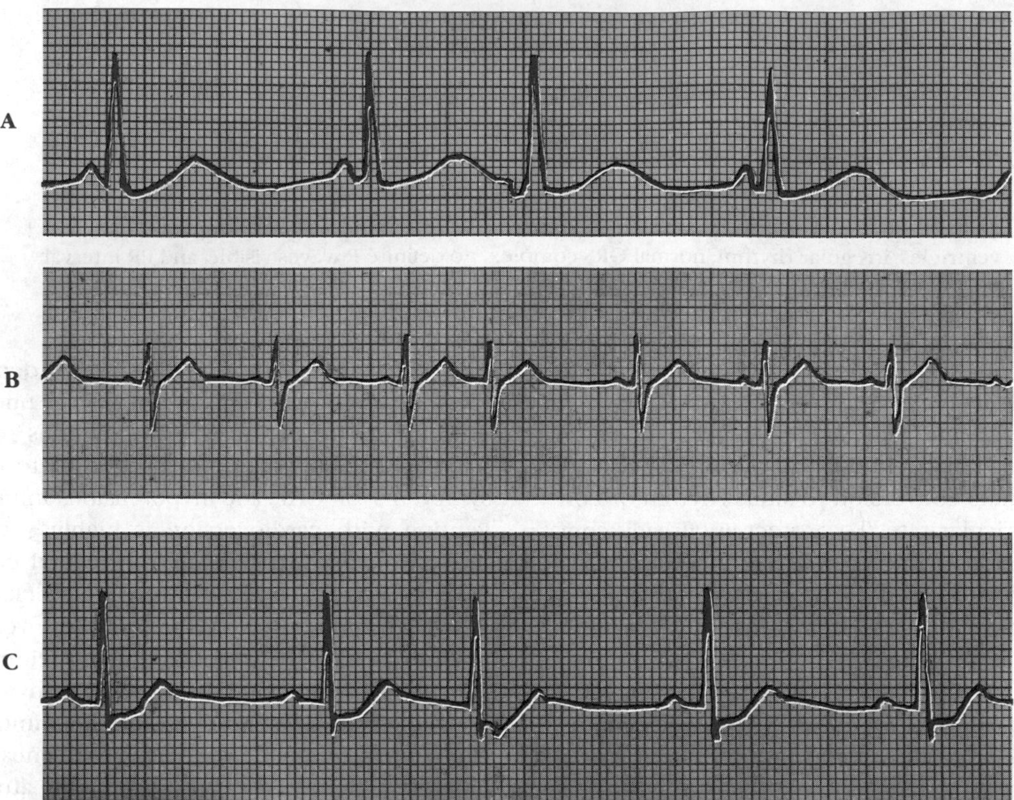


**FIGURE 30-20** Premature junctional beats (PJBs). **A,** Inverted P wave (third QRS complex). **B,** P wave hidden in fourth QRS complex. **C,** P wave follows third QRS complex. (From Conover MB: *Understanding electrocardiography: arrhythmias and the 12-lead ECG,* ed 6, St Louis, 1992, Mosby.)

impulses (escape beats) to stabilize the rhythm. If a single junctional escape beat occurs, the cycle length is longer than the longest sinus cycle. A succession of beats from the junction is a **junctional escape rhythm.**

The P waves may occur before, during, or after the QRS. The QRS is normal, and the ventricular rhythm is regular. Junctional escape rhythm occasionally is found in the well-trained athlete with sinus bradycardia. It also occurs when sinus bradycardia complicates an acute inferior wall myocardial infarction. Junctional escape rhythm generally is not treated unless the loss of atrial kick produces symptoms of low cardiac output. In such a case the patient may require artificial pacing.

When the automaticity of a junctional pacemaker increases to a rate greater than 60/min, it may usurp the SA node as the pacemaker of the heart. At a rate of 60 to 100/min, the rhythm is called *accelerated* junctional rhythm.

A **junctional tachycardia** exists when the rate exceeds 100/min. Junctional tachycardia is associated with digitalis toxicity, acute inferior myocardial infarction, acute rheumatic fever, and open heart surgical procedures. Digitalis is the drug of choice to slow the ven-cular rate. If digitalis toxicity is present, phenytoin or ranolol is effective.

Junctional tachycardia may occur paroxysmally. Because of the rate, it is often difficult to distinguish it from paroxysmal atrial tachycardia (PAT). Both junctional tachycardia and PAT often are referred to as **supraventricular tachycardia (SVT),** indicating that the rhythm originates above the ventricles (Figure 30-21).

## Dysrhythmias Originating in the Ventricles

### Premature ventricular beats

The **premature ventricular beat (PVB)** arises from an ectopic focus in the ventricles. The characteristic wide, bizarre QRS (usually greater than 0.12 second) makes the PVB readily identifiable on the ECG tracing (Figure 30-22). There is no associated P wave preceding the QRS complex, and the T wave is in the opposite direction from the main QRS deflection. Approximately 50% of PVBs are followed by a compensatory pause so that the interval from the beat preceding to the beat following the PVB is equal to two sinus cycles. The other 50% of the PVB beats result in retrograde conduction to the atria, causing the next sinus P wave to be early, and a less than full compensatory pause occurs.

If several PVBs of different configuration are noted in an ECG tracing, they are said to be *multiform.* This indicates the presence of more than one ectopic focus

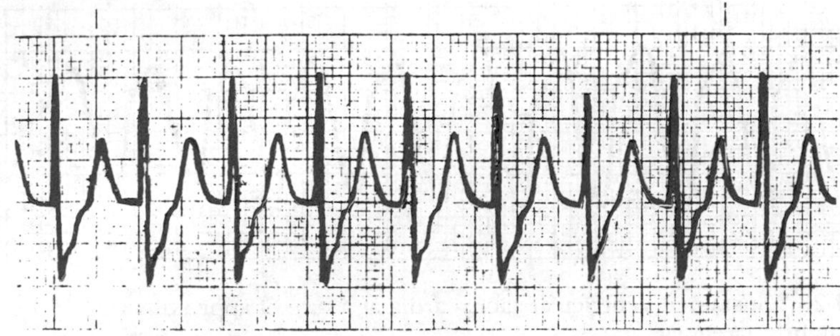

**FIGURE 30-21** Supraventricular tachycardia (SVT). Origin is atrial or junctional. If P waves are present, they are not visualized; they may be present in preceding T wave.

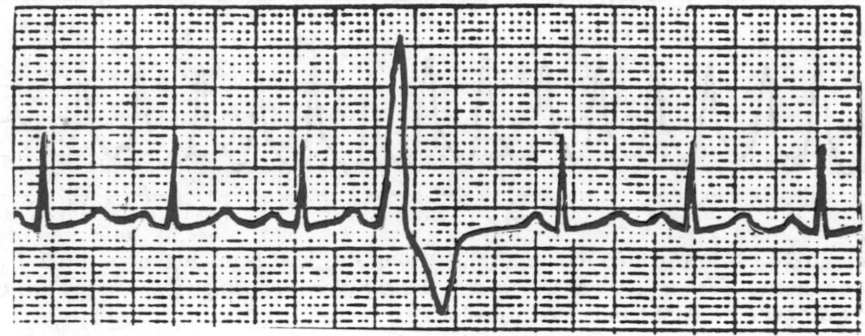

**FIGURE 30-22** Premature ventricular beat (PVB). Lead II showing fourth beat is a PVB with wide early QRS complex; no P wave associated with beat.

in the ventricles or one ectopic focus but multiple reentry pathways within the ventricle, thus producing complexes of differing forms. PVBs also may have various degrees of prematurity. It is important to note the relationship of the PVB to the Q, R, S, and T waves of the preceding beat. Remember that an electrical impulse of any kind that stimulates the heart near the peak of the T wave (vulnerable period; see Figure 30-9) may precipitate a more dangerous or lethal dysrhythmia.

Even in the absence of heart disease, PVBs occur often and increase in number with a person's age. The incidence and frequency of occurrence are higher, however, for the population with heart disease. The patient with an acute myocardial infarction must be monitored closely for the presence of PVBs. Clinically, PVBs also are associated with CHF, digitalis toxicity, and electrolyte imbalances. In the latter cases treatment of the underlying cause may abolish the dysrhythmia. Pharmacologic suppression of the PVBs most often is accomplished with lidocaine, procainamide, quinidine, or disopyramide.

PVBs occurring in conjunction with an acute myocardial infarction may lead to more serious dysrhythmias and must be suppressed. Lidocaine is an intravenous preparation that is a first-line choice for immediate suppression of ventricular irritability. Most authors agree that in the face of an acute myocardial infarction, PVBs should be treated if they (1) occur more frequently than 5/min, (2) fall in the vulnerable period (known as the R-on-T phenomenon), (3) are multiform, (4) occur in pairs or multiples, or (5) are accompanied by a history of ventricular tachycardia or fibrillation.[1] After initial suppression, PVBs may be controlled on a long-term basis with oral antiarrhythmic agents.

### Ventricular rhythms and tachycardia

If the SA node and AV junction fail to initiate impulses, a ventricular pacemaking cell will automatically begin to initiate impulses at an inherent rate of 20 to 40 beats/min. This is known as **idioventricular rhythm.**

If the rate of the ventricular-initiated rhythm increases to 40 to 100/min, it is known as an *accelerated* idioventricular rhythm (a common misnomer is *slow ventricular tachycardia*). It may be seen in digitalis toxicity, as a complication of an acute myocardial infarction, and as a reperfusion dysrhythmia after thrombolytic therapy (see p. 825). Generally, neither of these rhythms is treated except to correct underlying abnormalities. Suppression of the heart's dominant and perhaps only rhythm could be hazardous. If the cardiac output is low and symptoms of CHF, syncope, or hypotension develop, the patient may require temporary or permanent arti-

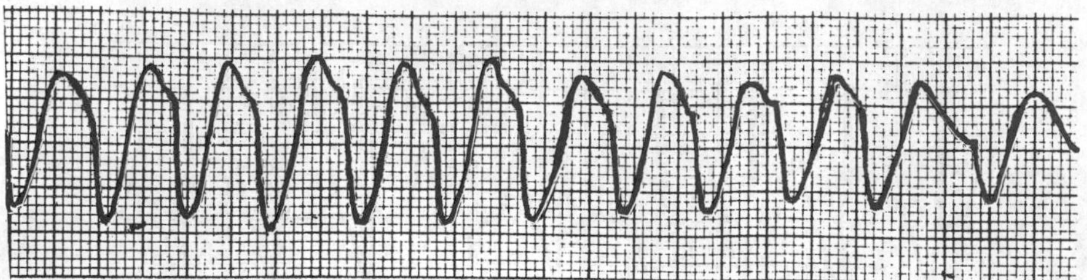

**FIGURE 30-23** Sustained ventricular tachycardia at a rate of approximately 150 beats/min; rhythm is slightly irregular.

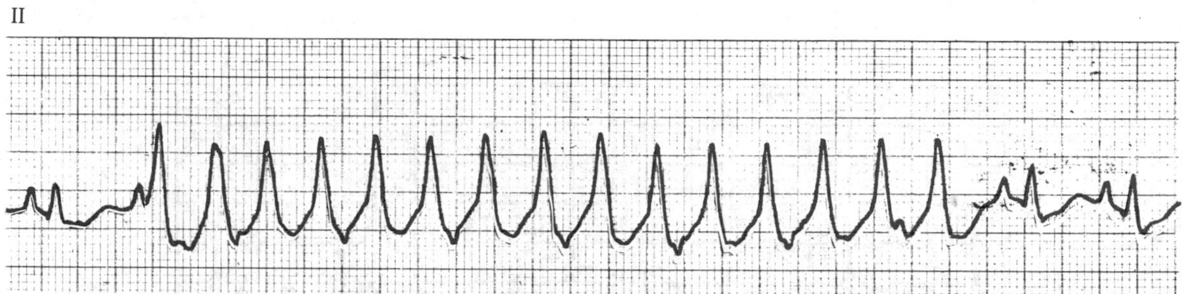


**FIGURE 30-24** Nonsustained monomorphic VT. In this lead II tracing, note the 2:1 retrograde conduction. (From Conover MB: *Understanding electrocardiography: arrhythmias and the 12-lead ECG,* ed 6, St Louis, 1992, Mosby.)

ficial pacing. Atropine also may be helpful in stimulating the return of SA node activity.

By definition, three or more successive PVBs constitute **ventricular tachycardia (VT)** (Figure 30-23). The ventricular rate is greater than 100/min and usually is 140 to 240. The rhythm is regular or slightly irregular. P waves may be present but are not associated with the QRS complexes. VT may complicate any form of heart disease and may be a direct result of a PVB striking during the heart's vulnerable period. Conditions that favor its occurrence include hypoxemia, drug toxicity, electrolyte imbalance, and bradycardia.

VT is classified as *sustained* (lasting more than 30 seconds) or *nonsustained.* Most instances of sustained VT occur as a result of reentry and are associated with coronary artery disease, myocardial infarction, and dilated cardiomyopathy. A less common mechanism is triggered activity as a result of early or delayed afterdepolarizations. Digitalis intoxication or excessive catecholamine levels are contributing factors when triggered activity is the underlying mechanism. Abnormal automaticity may occur in the postinfarction period as a result of the loss of fast sodium channels, contributing to the development of VT.

Nonsustained VT (Figure 30-24) may occur in patients with or without cardiac disease and may be associated with palpitations or recurrent syncope. In the absence of severe ventricular dysfunction, nonsustained VT may be a precursor of sustained VT and sudden death. Repeated and more prolonged episodes of nonsustained VT in the second week after myocardial infarction may be a forewarning of ventricular fibrillation and require aggressive evaluation and treatment.

Intravenously administered procainamide frequently is the drug of choice because it prolongs the refractory period and slows conduction in the ventricle. Lidocaine is used only if acute myocardial ischemia/infarction is considered to be the cause of VT. If pharmacologic measures are unsuccessful, the alternative is cardioversion. Ongoing VT suppression is obtained with oral antiarrhythmic medications.

### Ventricular fibrillation and standstill

In **ventricular fibrillation (VF)** the ventricles twitch chaotically, much as the atria do in atrial fibrillation. The most frequent cause is coronary artery disease. Frequently VF is the terminal event in sudden cardiac death. It may occur without warning after reperfusion. The ECG tracing consists of a bumpy line of unidentifiable waves (Figure 30-25). The fibrillatory waves may be coarse (as pictured) or fine (smooth).

In **ventricular standstill** (asystole) the ECG tracing is a flat line. No electrical activity is noted; all pacemaking cells have failed. Clinically, VF and standstill cannot be differentiated without the ECG. Both are fatal dysrhythmias that require immediate measures. The patient has no blood pressure, pulse, or audible heartbeat; respirations quickly cease. CPR must be instituted im-

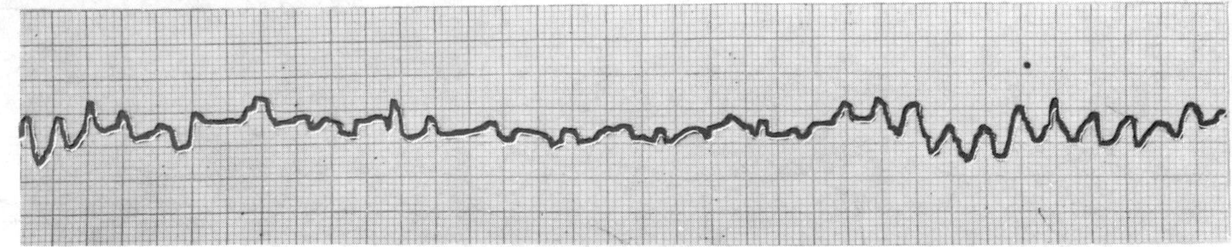

**FIGURE 30-25** Ventricular fibrillation (lead II). No QRS complexes, and no definite P waves visible. Tracing shows electrical chaos in myocardium.

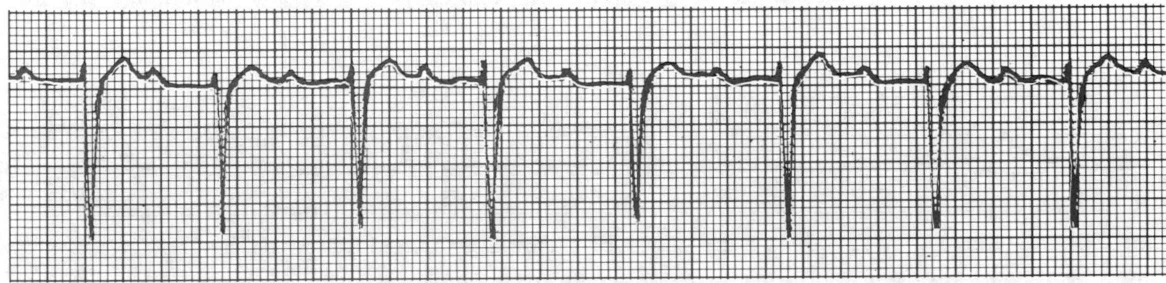

**FIGURE 30-26** First-degree AV block. PR interval is an overlong 0.33 second. (From Conover MB: *Cardiac arrhythmias,* ed 2, St Louis, 1978, Mosby.)

mediately and defibrillation performed within 1 minute to prevent biochemical derangements that further compromise the patient's condition.

Defibrillation is nonsynchronized cardioversion (see p. 807) that is indicated when QRS complexes and T waves are not discernible. It also is indicated if the rhythm appears to be asystole because, depending on the recorded ECG lead, both fine and coarse VF may mimic asystole.

## Conduction Abnormalities

### Atrioventricular block

A block to conduction of an impulse may occur at any point along the conduction pathways. One common area of block is the atrioventricular junction. The severity of the block is identified by degrees; first-, second-, or third-degree **atrioventricular (AV) block.**

*First-degree AV block* is present when the PR interval is prolonged to greater than 0.20 second, indicating a conduction delay in the AV node (Figure 30-26). It usually is found in association with rheumatic fever, digitalis toxicity, acute myocardial infarction, and the degenerative changes of CAHD in the conducting tissue. When a first-degree AV block occurs in isolation, no treatment is necessary.

An increase in the incidence of first-degree AV block is known to accompany older age. In a study by Felg et al.,[6] six of seven men with first-degree block were older than 65 years. When first-degree AV block occurs in isolation, it is not always associated with clinical heart disease nor does it affect prognosis. Persons with first-degree AV block, however, may be more susceptible to digitalis toxicity.

*Second-degree AV block* may be divided into two categories. Type I (Wenckebach or Mobitz I) is characterized by a PR interval that progressively lengthens until a P wave is not followed by a QRS complex (Figure 30-27). The nonconducted beat is the result of the arrival of the impulse during the refractory period of the AV node. The ratio of P waves to QRS complexes may be 5:4, 4:3, 3:2, or 2:1. Any drug that slows AV conduction may cause a type I block, but such blocks are most often seen in the patient with an acute inferior wall myocardial infarction, digitalis toxicity, or acute myocarditis or after cardiac surgery. Type I blocks often are transient and reversible. Generally no treatment is required unless symptoms occur because of the slow ventricular rate induced by 2:1 conduction.

Type II (Mobitz II) second-degree AV block is less common but more serious than type I. A type II block is characterized by nonconducted sinus impulses despite constant PR intervals (Figure 30-28). Usually the QRS complexes are widened because of a bundle branch block. The dropped beat represents a form of intermittent blockage of both bundle branches. The defect is found in either the bundle branches or the bundle of His. Type II blocks, which occur most often in the patient with an acute anterior septal wall myocardial infarction, are a warning of an impending third-degree block. Type II blocks also may occur in chronic fibrotic

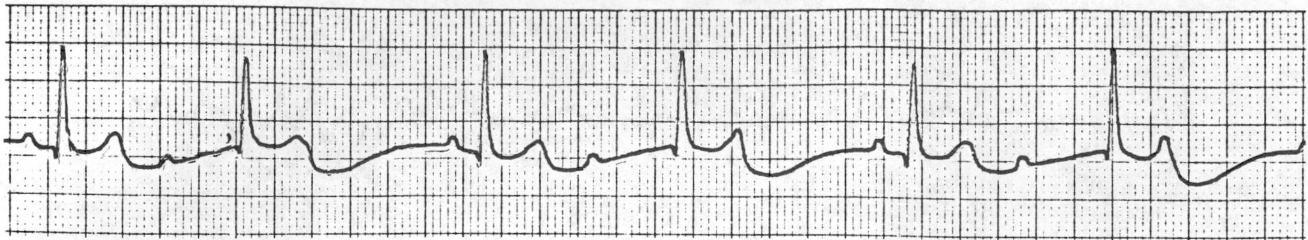

**FIGURE 30-27** Second-degree AV block, type I (Wenckebach). Every third P wave is hidden in preceding T wave; conduction is 3:2. Note progressive lengthening of PR interval before dropped QRS complex.

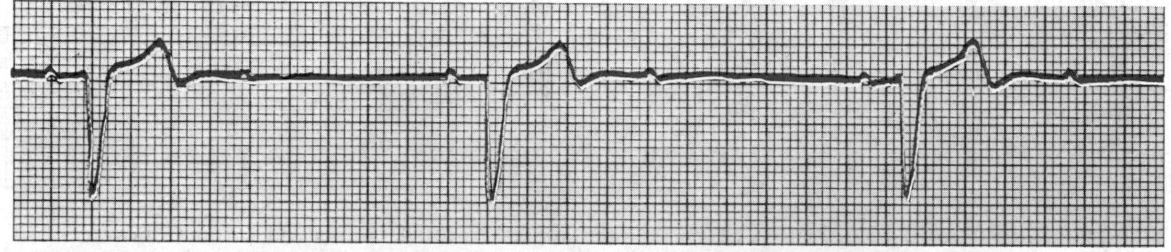

**FIGURE 30-28** Second-degree AV block, type II with 2:1 conduction (From Conover MB: *Understanding electrocardiography: arrhythmias and the 12-lead ECG,* ed 6, St Louis, 1992, Mosby.)

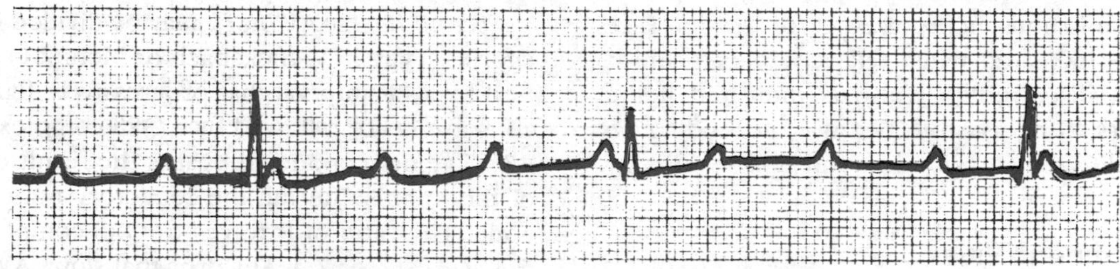

**FIGURE 30-29** Third-degree (complete) AV block. Atrial rate is 105 beats/min, and PR intervals vary. Narrow QRS complex indicates origin above ventricles.

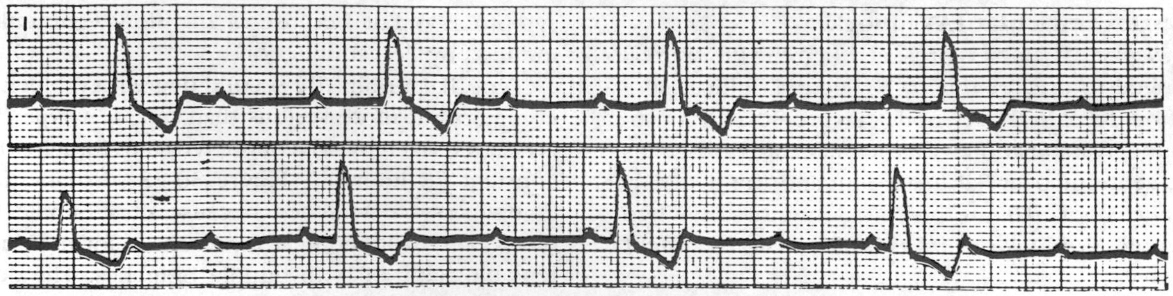


**FIGURE 30-30** Complete (third-degree) AV block. The strips are continuous. In the presence of sinus tachycardia (rate, 108/min), an independent idioventricular rhythm occurs (rate, 36/min). Note that the ventricular rhythm is absolutely regular, whereas the P-to-R relationship is constantly changing. (From Marriott HJL, Conover MB: *Advanced concepts in arrhythmias,* ed 2, St Louis, 1989, Mosby.)

disease of the conduction system. A temporary pacemaker usually is inserted prophylactically until the conduction stabilizes. If the block is persistent, the patient will benefit from a permanent implantable pacemaker.

In *third-degree AV block* (complete heart block) all the sinus or atrial impulses are blocked, and the atria and ventricles are forced to beat independently. The ventricles are driven by either a junctional or a ventricular pacemaker cell. The usual lesion is in the bundle of His or the bundle branches but may also be AV nodal. The rate and dependability of the ventricular rhythm are related to the level of the lesion. If a junctional pacemaker drives the ventricles, the ventricular rate will be at least 40 to 60 beats/min, indicating that the block is located above the bifurcation of the bundle of His. The QRS complexes are typically narrow (Figure 30-29). This block may be a transient complication of inferior posterior myocardial infarction or digitalis toxicity. Atropine is useful in restoring conduction.

If a ventricular pacemaker drives the ventricles, the rate will be 20 to 40 beats/min, and the patient may experience syncope, CHF, altered mentation, or angina. The QRS complex is abnormally wide, indicating that the block lies below the AV node (Figure 30-30). The prognosis is more serious if complete heart block accompanies anterior myocardial infarction. Generally the patient will require a permanent artificial pacemaker. Epinephrine or isoproterenol administered intravenously may increase the ventricular rate temporarily until artificial pacing can be instituted.

### Bundle branch block

A **bundle branch block (BBB)** occurs as a permanent defect or as a transient block secondary to tachycardia, CHF, acute myocardial infarction, pulmonary embolus, hypoxia, or metabolic derangements. In all these cases, the electrical impulse spreads from one ventricle to the other by abnormal pathways, thus producing distinct ECG tracings, which usually are alterations in the normal appearance and width of the QRS complex.

The *right bundle branch* is the more delicate structure of the two bundles and has a longer refractory period in some persons. In the younger patient right bundle branch block (RBBB) often results from right ventricular hypertrophy, whereas CAHD usually is the cause in the older patient. The QRS complex is widened to 0.10 second or greater. Among the most classic ECG changes is the M-shaped QRS in $V_1$ and $V_2$. In the absence of other conduction defects, no intervention is necessary.

The *left bundle branch* has a main trunk that bifurcates into the left anterior and left posterior divisions. A block may occur in the main trunk or in either of the divisions. A block in the main trunk produces a complete left bundle branch block (LBBB) resulting in a QRS greater than 0.12-second duration, large R waves in $V_5$ and $V_6$, and deep wide S waves in $V_1$ through $V_3$. LBBB is associated with severe CAHD, valvular disease, hypertensive disease, cardiomegaly, and acute anterior wall myocardial infarction. It also may occur as a result of degenerative changes in the conduction system.

Blocks of the anterior or posterior division are known as *left anterior hemiblock* or *left posterior hemiblock*, respectively. Because the left posterior division is the sturdier, its blockage carries a poor prognosis. It is important to determine *all* blocks to conduction that may coexist. Whenever sufficient blockage is present to leave the heart dependent on one fascicle for conduction to the ventricles, the patient is a candidate for a permanent artificial pacemaker.

## NURSING MANAGEMENT

### ♦ ASSESSMENT

Depending on the person's physical condition and the severity of the dysrhythmia, varying clinical effects may be experienced. Careful data collection is essential to assess the overall impact produced by a disorder of the heartbeat. A heart rhythm that is benign to one person may be life-threatening to another. The key lies in recognizing the many factors that may be pertinent to the occurrence of a dysrhythmia. Although dysrhythmias most frequently occur in persons with underlying heart disease, some are noted in the absence of disease.

A careful history, physical assessment, and dysrhythmia interpretation provide the optimal evaluation of potentially dangerous cardiac events.

### Subjective Data

Subjective data obtained by means of a detailed patient history (see Chapter 29) are as diagnostically important as laboratory data and ECG recordings in the assessment of the person with a cardiac dysrhythmia. A history should include the following:

1. Subjective complaints or symptoms
2. Activities or situations that may have precipitated or preceded the symptoms
3. Onset of the dysrhythmia (gradual versus sudden)
4. Current medications
5. History of the six cardinal symptoms of altered cardiovascular status: dyspnea, chest pain or discomfort, palpitations, edema, syncope, and excessive fatigue
6. Concerns or anxious feelings

### Objective Data

Objective data consist of monitoring the patient in addition to monitoring ECG tracings and include the following:

1. Circulatory changes
   a. Changes in cardiac rhythm; irregular heartbeat
   b. Abnormal pulses
   c. Murmurs or extra heart sounds
   d. Blood pressure changes

**BOX 30-3 One Approach for Systematic Interpretation of ECG Tracing**

1. Rate (atrial and ventricular)
2. Rhythm (atrial and ventricular)
3. Presence or absence of P waves
4. PR interval
5. QRS complex
6. Relationship of QRS to P wave
7. QT interval
8. Interpretation

NOTE: A normal sinus rhythm has an atrial (P) and ventricular (QRS) rate of 60 to 100 beats/min, a regular rhythm (constant P-P and R-R intervals), and a P wave before every QRS.

   e. Delayed capillary refill
   f. Cyanosis
   g. Edema
2. Respiratory changes
   a. Respiratory rate
   b. Respiratory effort with activity
   c. Breath sounds: presence of crackles or wheezes
3. Neurologic: change in level of consciousness
4. Body temperature; diaphoresis
5. Electrolyte imbalances
6. State of hydration
7. Behavior, appearance
8. ECG tracing: changes in impulse initiation and/or conduction (Box 30-3 suggests one approach to reading the ECG tracing).

## ♦ NURSING DIAGNOSES

Nursing diagnoses are determined from analysis of patient data. Nursing diagnoses for the patient with cardiac dysrhythmias may include but are not limited to the following:

| Diagnostic Title | Possible Etiologic Factors |
|---|---|
| Cardiac output, decreased | Bradycardia, tachycardia, heart block, CHF, shock, reduced stroke volume |
| Activity intolerance | Generalized weakness, imbalance between myocardial oxygen supply and demand, immobility, bed rest |
| Tissue perfusion, altered cardiovascular | Decreased cardiac output, coronary artery disease, myocardial infarction, angina, CHF, pulmonary edema |
| Pain | Coronary artery occlusion or vasopasm, hypoxia, overactivity, diagnostic tests, immobilty/improper positioning |
| Anxiety | Threat of death, threat/change in health status/socioeconomic status/role, threat to self-concept |
| Knowledge deficit (cardiovascular disease process and treatment) | Lack of exposure/recall, information misinterpretation, cognitive limitation, unfamiliarity with information sources |

## ♦ EXPECTED PATIENT OUTCOMES

Expected patient outcomes for the person with cardiac dysrhythmias may include but are not limited to the following:

1. Identifies factors that increase cardiac workload.
2. Demonstrates cardiac tolerance to increased activity (stable pulse and blood pressure).
3. Identifies factors that reduce activity intolerance.
4. Progresses to highest level of mobility possible.
5. Demonstrates improved peripheral circulation (decreased chest pain, dyspnea, and light-headedness).
6. Uses effective coping mechanisms in managing anxiety.
7. Describes underlying disease process, as well as purpose, rationale, and preparation for diagnostic testing.
8. Assesses pulse rate and rhythm accurately.
9. Describes events that may precipitate dysrhythmias.
10. Describes the medication regimen for managing the dysrhythmia.
11. Indicates plans for medical follow-up.

## ♦ INTERVENTIONS

Certain nursing interventions are appropriate for most persons with a cardiac dysrhythmia. These measures are discussed here. Some persons, however, may require artificial pacemakers to control the dysrhythmia. When the dysrhythmia leads to an unstable condition, cardioversion or defibrillation may be required for conversion to a hemodynamically stable rhythm.

### Promoting Adequate Cardiac Output

The following interventions are directed toward ongoing monitoring of the status of the dysrhythmia, its effect on the patient's cardiac output, and the effectiveness of therapy:

1. Monitor for dysrhythmias on ECG tracings.
2. Assess vital signs for changes; document rate and rhythm of pulse.
3. Monitor effects of daily activities on cardiac status, occurrence of dysrhythmias, and need for oxygen.
4. Monitor for signs of fluid overload and electrolyte imbalance.

**TABLE 30-3 Antidysrhythmic Agents***

| CLASS | ELECTROPHYSIOLOGIC EFFECTS AND USES | AGENTS | ADDITIONAL COMMENTS |
|---|---|---|---|
| I | All drugs in this class are characterized by inhibition of $Na^+$ influx during phase 0 depolarization; the class has been divided into 3 subcategories (A, B, and C) | | |
| IA | Moderate decrease in $Na^+$ influx; prolong action potential and ERP<br>Used mostly for ventricular dysrhythmias; quinidine and disopyramide also used for atrial fibrillation and flutter, SVT | Disopyramide (Norpace) | Has significant anticholingergic and negative inotropic SE<br>Contraindicated in severe CHF and 2nd or 3rd degree heart block |
| | | Procainamide (Pronestyl, Procan) | IV administration can cause hypotension<br>Has an active metabolite (NAPA) with class III properties |
| | | Quinidine (Quinaglute, Duraquin) | May increase AV conduction in atrial tachydysrhythmias; digoxin should be given first<br>Has mild vagolytic SE |
| IB | Minimal decrease in $Na^+$ influx; shorten repolarization and action potential<br>Depress ventricular automaticity and interrupt reentry circuits<br>Used for ventricular dysrhythmias<br>Can be used in combination with other dysrhythmic agents | Lidocaine (Xylocaine) | SE mild and dose-related<br>Available only as IV preparation<br>Contraindicated in severe liver or renal disease |
| | | Mexiletine (Mexitil) | Often used in combination with IA agents |
| | | Phenytoin (Dilantin) | Often used for digitalis-induced dysrhythmias |
| | | Tocainide (Tonocard) | Effective orally; suitable for long-term therapy |
| IC | Marked decrease in $Na^+$ influx; slight prolongation of refractory period but little effect on action potential duration; no effect on SA node<br>Slow conduction through His/purkinje system<br>Most potent of class I agents<br>Used for life-threatening ventricular dysrhythmias | Flecainide (Tambocor) | Can worsen ventricular dysrhythmias<br>Significant negative inotropic SE |
| | | Indecainide (Decabid) | SE similar to flecainide<br>Contraindicated in 2nd or 3rd degree heart block |
| | | Propafenone (Rhythmol) | SE similar to other drugs in class<br>Also has slight beta-adrenergic blocking activity. |
| II | Beta-adrenergic blocking agents (See Table 30-4) | | |
| III | Prolong action potential and refractory period<br>Depress SA automaticity and conduction in AV node, ventricular conduction system, and ventricular myocardium<br>Used for ventricular dysrhythmias<br>Amiodarone also used for SVT and atrial tachydysrhythmias refractory to other therapy | Amiodarone (Cordarone) | May cause bradycardia and sinus arrest<br>Time needed to achieve steady serum levels may be considerable |
| | | Bretylium tosylate (Bretylol) | May cause severe hypotension<br>Available only in parenteral preparations |
| IV | Calcium channel blocking agents (See Table 30-4) | | |

**Note:* Dosages are revised continually; consult the most currently available pharmaeceutic reference for specific information and side effects.
*ERP,* Effective refractory period; *SE,* side effects; *SVT,* supraventricular tachycardia.

5. Administer prescribed pharmacotherapy (Tables 30-3 and 30-4).
6. Encourage appropriate increases in activity and ambulation to prevent overwhelming increases in cardiac workload.

## Promoting Activity and Rest

Enhance the patient's activity tolerance by encouraging slower activity or shorter periods of activity with more rest periods. The pulse increases by approximately 50 beats/min with strenuous activity. This rate is safe provided it returns to the resting pulse within 3 minutes. Plan nursing strategies to promote rest and minimize unnecessary disturbances.

## Promoting Tissue Perfusion

Instruct the patient to avoid becoming overly fatigued and to stop activity immediately in the presence of chest pain, dyspnea, lightheadedness, or faintness, which indicate insufficient oxygen reaching the tissues because of decreased cardiac function. Decreased tissue perfusion causes cellular hypoxia with subsequent ischemia, cellular swelling, and cellular death.

## Promoting Comfort

Chest pain results from inadequate circulation to the heart muscle. The degree of pain perception and tolerance can be influenced by psychologic as well as physical factors (see Chapter 17). Assess for causes of de-

**TABLE 30-4 Agents in Other Classes With Antidysrhythmic Uses***

| CLASS | ELECTROPHYSIOLOGIC EFFECTS AND USES | AGENTS |
|---|---|---|
| Beta-adrenergic blocking agents (Class I antidysrhythmics) | Interfere with $Na^+$ influx; depress automaticity and prolong ERP of AV node<br>Limit response to sympathetic stimulation<br>Used for tachydysrhythmias (especially digitalis- or catecholamine-induced) | Acebutolol (Sectral) S<br>Esmolol HCl (Brevibloc) S<br>Propranalol (Inderal) NS<br>Sotalol HCl (Betapace) NS |
| Calcium channel blocking agents (Class IV antidysrhythmics) | Increase ERP in AV node and slow rate of SA node<br>IV preparations used for SVTs and control of ventricular rate in atrial flutter and atrial fibrillation | Diltiazem (Cardizem)<br>Verapamil (Calan, Isoptin) |
| Cholinergic blocking agents | Minimize effects of increased vagal tone<br>Increase rate of SA node and conduction in AV node<br>Used for severe sinus bradycardia (especially that caused by hypersensitive carotid sinus syndrome) | Atropine sulfate |
| Sympathomimetic agents | Stimulate both $beta_1$ and $beta_2$ receptors<br>Used in cardiac emergencies (cardiac standstill) and heart block | Epinephrine (Adrenalin)<br>Isoproterenol (Isuprel) |
| Cardiac glycoside | Slow conduction through the AV node<br>Used to control ventricular rate in atrial flutter and atrial fibrillation but can cause heart block and ventricular dysrhythmias | Digoxin (Lanoxin) |
| Miscellaneous | Depress SA node and AV node activity<br>Inhibit effects of stimulation by catecholamines<br>In WPW, interrupt and reroute reentry pathways through the AV node<br>IV preparation used for SVT | Adenosine (Adenocard) |

**Note:* Refer to most currently available pharmaceutical reference for specific information on dosage and side effects.
*NS,* Nonselective beta-adrenergic blocking activity; *S,* $beta_1$ selective blocking activity; *SVT,* supraventricular tachycardia; *WPW,* Wolff-Parkinson-White syndrome.

creased pain tolerance, such as lack of knowledge, fear, or fatigue. Reduce or eradicate factors contributing to increased discomfort. All pain is authentic regardless of cause. Provide a calm environment to decrease stress and anxiety, and provide rest periods if fatigue is present during physical activities. Evaluate effects of pain intervention measures (including prescribed pharmacologic agents).

## Promoting Relief of Anxiety and Feeling of Well-Being

Facilitate a reduction in the patient's present level of anxiety. Anxiety varies in intensity depending on the severity of the threat as perceived by the patient, as well as the person's success in coping. Measures to reduce anxiety and stress are discussed in Chapter 7.

## Facilitating Learning

Delay teaching until the person is ready. The patient needs to be relatively free of pain and excessive anxiety to learn. Teaching includes the following:

1. Nature of the dysrhythmia in terms of the patient's level of understanding
2. How to assess pulse rate and rhythm
3. Nature and treatment regimen of underlying disease process
4. Life-style modifications, coping strategies, and support networks
5. Symptoms requiring medical intervention and precipitating factors
6. Medication regimen
7. Need for medical follow-up

# ♦ EVALUATION

To evaluate the effectiveness of nursing interventions, compare patient behaviors with those stated in the expected patient outcomes. Successful achievement of patient outcomes for the patient with cardiac dysrhythmias is indicated by the following:

1. States factors that increase cardiac workload.
2. Has stable pulse and blood pressure with increased activity.
3. States factors that reduce activity intolerance.
4. Progresses to highest level of mobility possible.
5. Has decreased chest pain, dyspnea, and lightheadedness.
6. Shows effective coping mechanisms in managing anxiety.
7. Correctly describes underlying disease process and diagnostic tests.
8. Accurately assesses pulse rate and rhythm.
9. Correctly describes events that may precipitate dysrhythmias.
10. Correctly describes medication regimen for managing the dysrhythmia.
11. Explains planned medical follow-up.

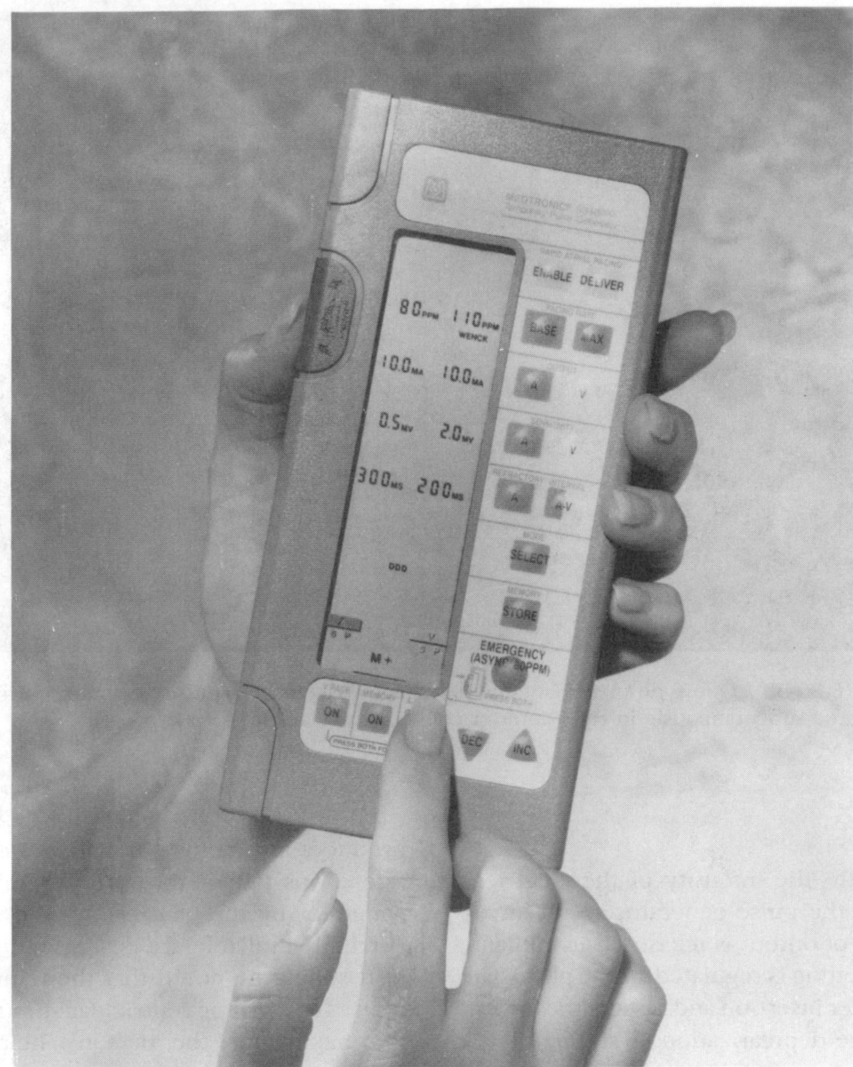


**FIGURE 30-31** Temporary (external) pacemaker. Pulse generator is powered by a 9-volt alkaline battery. Electrode is passed into heart before being attached to pulse generator. (Courtesy Medtronic, Inc., Minneapolis, MN 55432-3576.)

## PACEMAKERS

### Indications for Use

The artificial **pacemaker** has become a leading modality in the control of potentially dangerous dysrhythmias. Pacemakers may be temporary (Figure 30-31) or permanent (Figure 30-32). Indications for artificial pacemakers are summarized in Box 30-4. Some of these conditions require only temporary pacing. Permanent pacing is an option when the condition is recurrent or persistent.

The artificial pacing system consists of a pulse generator and a pacing wire that delivers the stimulus to the heart to control heart rate. The pacing unit initiates and maintains the heart rate when the natural pacemakers of the heart are unable to do so.

### Pulse Generator

The **pulse generator** is powered by battery cells. Technologic advances have occurred in both power sources and electronic circuitry, and currently lithium batteries lasting 6 years or more are used in most pacemakers. Research is directed toward power sources that may function for extended periods. For example, nuclear-powered pacemakers (plutonium-238 source) can last 20 years or more. Other pacemakers can have their batteries recharged externally.[15] For most pacemakers in which lithium or the older mercury-zinc battery is used, battery exhaustion is inevitable. When the generator battery fails, the implantable unit that contains the batteries must be replaced surgically.

The pulse generator has several controls, including energy output, heart rate, and mode of pacing. In a temporary pacemaker system, these controls can be easily regulated, and because of technologic advances in permanent pacers, selected persons are supplied with "programmable" pacers that can be controlled from outside the body.

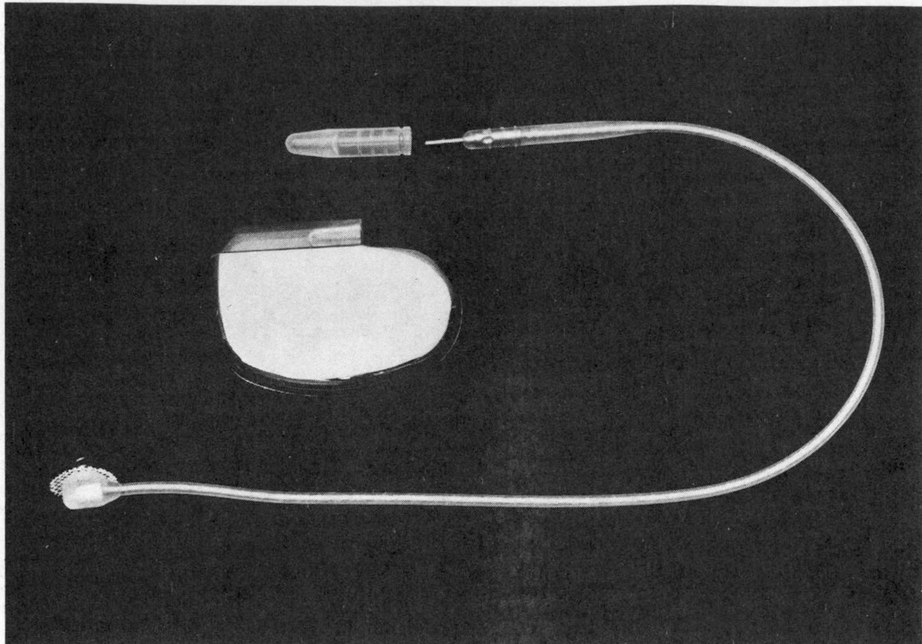

**FIGURE 30-32** One type of implantable permanent pacemaker (pulse generator), usually implanted subcutaneously in right anterior chest below clavicle.

### Energy output

Energy output refers to the intensity of the electrical impulse delivered by the pulse generator to the myocardium. The amount of output is measured in milliamperes (mA). The mA setting is regulated by the physician at the time of pacemaker insertion and is set at the lowest level that will produce depolarization. A setting of 1.5 mA usually is sufficient to cause depolarization. However, depending on the condition of the patient and the placement of the pacer wire, a higher mA setting may be necessary.

### Heart rate

Heart rate is set according to the desired therapeutic aim and the clinical condition of the patient. With few exceptions the heart rate usually is set between 70 and 80 beats/min. If the purpose of inserting a pacemaker is to suppress dysrhythmias, the rate usually is set higher, often 100 to 120 beats/min.

### Mode of pacing

There are two basic modes of artificial pacing: fixed rate (asynchronous) and demand mode. In the *fixed-rate mode* the pacemaker fires electrical stimuli at a preset rate regardless of the person's inherent rhythm. Because of the hazards of a pacing stimulus falling within the vulnerable period, asynchronous pacing rarely is used today.

The most popular mode is the *demand* or *standby mode*. An electrode at the tip of the pacing wire is able to sense the person's own heartbeats. The pacemaker produces a stimulus only when the person's own heart rate drops below the rate per minute preset on the generator by the physician. Some types of pacemakers currently available are described in Box 30-5.

It should be noted that the temporary pacemaker is limited to atrial or ventricular stimulation. The potential for maximizing the person's hemodynamic status is much greater with the various types of permanent pacemakers.

If a person has a functioning conduction system below the atrium but has difficulty in impulse formation from the SA node, a pacing catheter may be placed in the atrium. Atrial pacing has been somewhat difficult to achieve; however, it more closely approximates the normal electrical activity of the heart (Figure 30-33). Ventricular pacing results in a retrograde depolarization, which does not mimic the normal conduction system. Despite this retrograde stimulation and depolarization, most persons achieve a cardiac output sufficient for their physiologic needs.

## Complications of Pacemaker Therapy

The use of artificial pacemakers is not without potential complications. Complications usually arise because of improper pacer functioning and the presence of the pacemaker wires as a foreign object in the body.

### Infection

For the person with a temporary pacemaker, local infection or hematoma formation may occur at the venous cutdown site. With a permanent pacemaker, local infec-

**BOX 30-4 Indications for Artificial Pacemakers**

1. Adams-Stokes attack (syncope secondary to third-degree AV block)
2. Third-degree AV block with slow ventricular rate
3. Acute myocardial infarction (MI) with Mobitz II AV block
4. Right bundle branch block plus left anterior hemiblock or left posterior hemiblock (particularly with acute MI)
5. New left bundle branch block associated with acute MI
6. Symptomatic sinus bradycardia unresponsive to medical therapy
7. Atrial fibrillation with slow ventricular rate in the patient who requires digitalis therapy
8. Carotid sinus syncope
9. Suppression of dysrhythmias (atrial or ventricular tachydysrhythmias)
10. Dysrhythmias occurring during or after cardiac surgery
11. Sick sinus syndrome
12. Prophylaxis before anesthesia and surgery in patients with history of cardiac arrest or AV blocks

**BOX 30-5 Types of Pacemakers**

1. Stimulation of ventricles only
   a. QRS-inhibited (demand) pacing
   b. P wave–triggered ventricular pacing (SA node still determines heart rate and atrial kick is maintained)
2. Stimulation of atria only (requires the presence of a normal conduction system below the atria)
3. Stimulation of both atria and ventricles (simulates the normal impulse formation and conduction; has artificial PR interval to maintain synchronous contraction of the cardiac chambers)

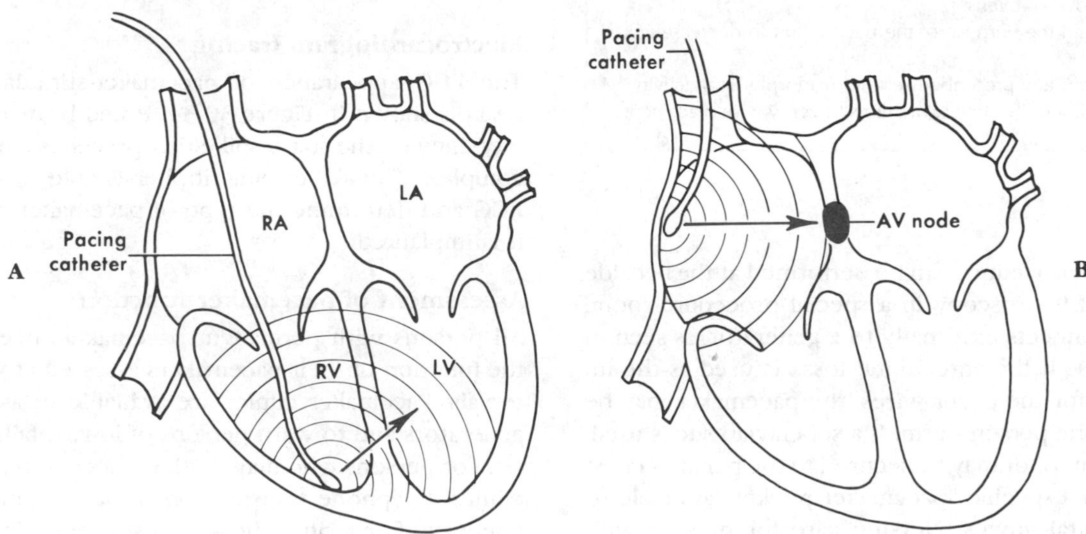


**FIGURE 30-33** **A,** Ventricular pacing. Impulses are initiated in ventricle. **B,** Atrial pacing. Impulses are initiated in atrium and travel to ventricles by normal conduction system.

tion at the suture line or sepsis may occur. The person is monitored daily for any signs of inflammation or infection.

### Dysrhythmias

The pacemaker wire and electrode can irritate the ventricular wall, producing ectopic activity. Less frequently the pacer electrode may dislodge and move about, producing electrical stimulation and potential dysrhythmias. The most common causes of pacemaker failure are displacement of the pacing wire electrode and battery failure. Both these situations require minor surgery to make repairs.

### Electrical interference

Interference from electrical sources is a particular area of concern for the person with an external (temporary) pacemaker. The person must be careful to avoid contact with any electrical machinery that is not properly grounded, as well as magnetic fields and microwave ovens. A small electrical charge passing via the pacer wire directly into the heart could initiate lethal dysrhythmias.

## Temporary Pacemakers

For temporary pacing the pacer wire usually is passed transvenously to the right atrium or ventricle (see Figure

## Guidelines for Care of the Person With a Temporary Pacemaker

1. Monitor pacemaker performance:
   a. Assess heart rate to ensure that it has not fallen below preset level. *If heart rate is below preset level, notify physician.*
   b. Using an ECG tracing or cardiac monitor, note the presence of pacing stimulus "pacer spikes" and whether a P wave or QRS complex follows each stimulus.
   c. Assess the person for signs of pacemaker malfunction, such as weakness, dizziness, hypotension, or fainting.
2. Maintain pacemaker system integrity:
   a. Ensure that catheter terminals are securely connected to the pulse generator.
   b. Ensure that the pulse generator is adequately secured to the person so that accidental dislodgment of the system is avoided.
3. Assess patient safety and comfort:
   a. Monitor for signs of inflammation or infection at the catheter insertion site.
   b. If clinically permitted, assist the person with range of motion exercises for the involved extremity.
   c. Ensure that the person avoids contact with any improperly grounded electrical equipment, magnetic fields, and microwave ovens.
   d. Explain the purpose of the pacing unit to decrease anxiety.
   e. Explain any prescribed restrictions in physical activity.
   f. Monitor daily chest x-ray films to verify wire placement.

30-33). This procedure can be performed at the bedside or by use of fluoroscopy in a special procedure room. The wire connects externally to a generator, as seen in Figure 30-31. If the antecubital fossa is used as the insertion site for the pacer wires, the pacemaker may be secured to the person's arm. If a subclavian site is used, the pulse generator may be secured to the person's chest or placed in a specific "pacemaker pocket" available or cut in hospital gowns. Nursing care for persons with temporary external pacemakers is summarized in the Guidelines box above.

## Permanent Pacemakers

The same pacemaker system exists for permanent pacing, except that the generator itself is more compact and may be implanted subcutaneously (see Figure 30-32). The permanent pacing generator may be implanted in the right or left subclavicular areas, and the pacing wire is passed through the major veins to the right side of the heart (transvenous or endocardiac). Alternatively, the generator may be implanted subcutaneously in the abdomen, with the pacing wire passed upward and sutured to the left ventricle (epicardial).

Permanent pacemakers are inserted in the operating room or in a special procedure room. The transvenous approach to insertion does not require general anesthesia, which greatly decreases the risk of this procedure. In epicardial pacing, however, the electrode is passed transthoracically to the myocardium, where it is sutured in place. This procedure requires geneal anesthesia because a thoracotomy is required to provide access to the heart.

### Immediate nursing care

Immediate nursing care for the person with a permanent pacemaker includes connecting the person to a cardiac monitor or ECG machine to assess pacemaker function. An intravenous line is maintained should the person require fluids or medications, including antiarrhythmic drugs. Data about the person's pacemaker should be clearly identified in the patient's chart, with the type and model of pacemaker, its location, the milliampere setting, rate, and mode of pacing included.

The incision site is covered by a pressure dressing and is monitored for bleeding and infection. Safe nursing care also includes ensuring that only electrically safe equipment is used on or near the person with a pacemaker.

### Electrocardiogram tracing

The ECG appearance of pacemaker-stimulated heartbeats is shown in Figure 30-34. Paced beats are readily identified by the sharp spike that precedes a paced ECG complex. The skilled practitioner is able to analyze an ECG and determine the type of pacemaker and where it is implanted.

### Assessment of pacemaker function

All persons with permanent pacemakers need to have the function of their pacemakers assessed at varying intervals. Pacemaker clinics are available to assess pulse generators and to warn persons of low or failing batteries. For persons who may not have access to pacemaker clinics, telephone transmission of pacer functioning is one way of ensuring follow-up assessment. By means of special equipment, the sound tone of a pacemaker can be transmitted over the telephone to special recording equipment. The pacemaker tone is electronically converted into a signal that is recorded on an ECG strip. With a brief telephone call, the pacemaker rate and other data concerning pacemaker function can be assessed.

### Patient teaching

The following instructions concerning pacemaker function and care should be given to the patient:

1. Check pulse daily for 1 full minute at relatively the same time.
2. Report any sudden slowing or increase in pulse rate.
3. Notify physician of any pain or redness over incision site.
4. Wear loose-fitting clothing around the pacemaker area for increased comfort.

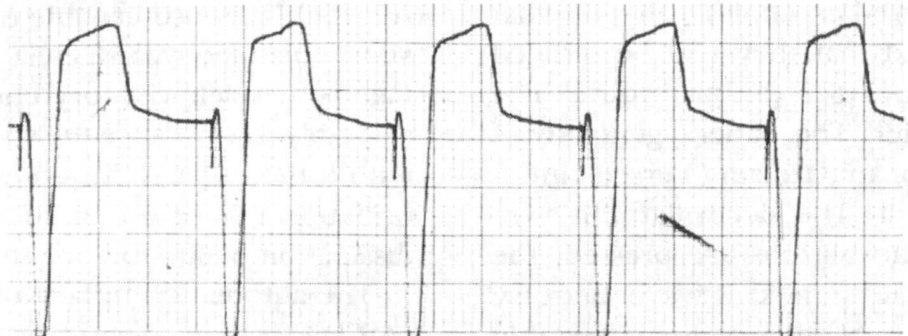

**FIGURE 30-34** Pacemaker ECG (lead $V_1$). Rate is 78, rhythm regular, QRS complex wide, and no P waves visible. Pacing stimulus (spike) precedes each QRS.

5. Have pacemaker function checked at special centers (in person or by telephone) at instructed intervals.
6. Carry an identification card or an emergency alert identification tag specifying the type of pacemaker, name of manufacturer, settings, name of hospital where implanted, and name of physician; keep duplicate card at home.
7. Show the identification card to airport employees at the safety detection station so that a hand scanner can be used rather than conventional detectors.
8. Avoid closeness to magnetic fields or microwave ovens.

### External Transcutaneous Pacemakers

External pacemakers were first introduced in the 1950s. The device was refined since its invention and was generally successful in restoring cardiac rhythm, but the external stimulation was often painful. Thus it was largely replaced by the internal pacemaker in 1959. In the 1980s, external pacemakers and pads were improved to ensure cardiac stimulation at lower current levels. They are now being used again, particularly in emergency situations.

External pacing, as a temporary treatment modality, can correct the same dysrhythmias as endocardial pacemakers. Examples of indications for use include (1) overdrive suppression of ventricular tachydysrhythmias, (2) restoration or acceleration of rhythm when asystole or bradycardia occurs because of drug effect, myocardial infarction, or heart block, (3) in the presence of thrombocytopenia or leukopenia when endocardial pacing is contraindicated, (4) during emergencies when there is a time constraint against inserting a pacemaker wire, and (5) as a prophylaxis during invasive procedures, such as pulmonary artery line insertion, cardioversion, or electrophysiologic studies.

Pacing usually is achieved by application of two electrodes to the chest wall, one over the cardiac apex and the other on the back beneath the left scapula. An electrical current is delivered between the electrodes via an output pulse delivered in milliamperes controlled by the operator. Most devices function in the demand mode and are equipped with a built-in oscilloscope to allow monitoring of pacer activity.

## CARDIOVERSION AND DEFIBRILLATION

**Cardioversion** is the use of electrical energy to convert a cardiac dysrhythmia (other than ventricular fibrillation) to one that is more hemodynamically stable, preferably a sinus rhythm. **Defibrillation** generally applies to unsynchronized electrical countershock during a ventricular fibrillation emergency. Cardioversion differs from defibrillation in that the electrical discharge is synchronized with the R wave to avoid triggering ventricular fibrillation by accidental discharge during the ventricular vulnerable period.

Electrophysiologically, the electrical countershock produces a simultaneous depolarization of a critical mass of cardiac fibers, thus halting the asynchronous chaos of a fibrillation or the rapid firing of a tachycardia. In some cases, especially in elective cardioversion, the shock will be delivered more than once until the correct level of voltage is reached. Once the heart is fully depolarized, the SA node is better able to resume control of the heart.

For emergency defibrillation, the paddles from the defibrillator are placed at the third intercostal space to the right of the sternum and the fifth intercostal space on the left midaxillary line. Either conducting gel or saline pads must be applied between the paddles and the skin to ensure conductance and to minimize skin burning. The button on each paddle is depressed simultaneously to release 200 to 360 watt-seconds (joules) to the patient. Defibrillation must be performed rapidly for ventricular fibrillation and most cases of ventricular tachycardia.

When the cardioversion is elective (e.g., conversion of atrial flutter, atrial fibrillation, or paroxysmal atrial tachycardia), the procedure differs slightly. The patient should have nothing by mouth for 8 hours in advance. In many cases the daily digitalis dose may be withheld that day or for several days in advance. Selected patients who are receiving anticoagulants should continue to receive this therapy. Oral antiarrhythmics (see Tables 30-3 and 30-4) are also frequently given in advance.

Patients should be prepared psychologically for what to expect and be reassured that they will be sedated and probably will not remember the procedure. The atmosphere should be quiet. The patient generally is given diazepam (Valium) or midazolam (Versed) intravenously for amnesic effect. The defibrillator is synchronized so that when the buttons are pressed, the impulse is not initiated until the next R wave. Because of this precaution, the danger of entering the vulnerable period is eliminated. For most elective procedures, the amount of watt-seconds or joules required for conversion is lower than that required for defibrillation. The patient is monitored after cardioversion until vital signs are stable.

## Recent Advances in Defibrillation

### Current-based defibrillation

Recent studies have shown that current is a better descriptor of defibrillation than energy is, thus favoring the use of a current-based approach.[9] The higher the energy level or frequency of shocks, the greater is the amount of myocardial damage that can occur. If transthoracic impedance could be accurately determined before defibrillation or cardioversion, inappropriately high or low energies could be avoided in patients with high transthoracic impedance. Some defibrillators have been modified to allow advanced prediction of transthoracic impedance. Once impedance is determined, the defibrillator automatically selects the energy necessary to provide the specified current. Although still under investigation, this approach to defibrillation and cardioversion may develop as the safest and most effective method to restore rhythm and hemodynamic stability with reduced risk of profound myocardial damage and deterioration.

### Automatic implantable cardioverter defibrillator

More than half of the deaths from coronary artery disease in the United States each year are sudden deaths occurring within 24 hours of the onset of symptoms and frequently before the patient reaches the hospital. The pathophysiology of sudden cardiac death remains obscure. Numerous studies have shown that pathologic evidence of acute myocardial infarction or fresh thrombi is often absent. Furthermore, the severity of the coronary artery disease present in patients who die suddenly is sometimes less than that in patients who survive longer or equal to that found in patients dying of other causes. Many researchers conclude that the cause of sudden cardiac death is not occlusive thrombosis or myocardial damage but a derangement in the heart's electrical stability, most often deteriorating into ventricular fibrillation.

The first permanent implantation of an automatic defibrillator was performed in 1980. This device automatically senses ventricular fibrillation and, within approximately 15 to 20 seconds, delivers an electrical countershock. It is also capable of identifying and correcting ventricular tachycardia via cardioversion. One advantage is that defibrillatory energy requirements are considerably less because the shock is being applied directly within the heart. With conventional transthoracic defibrillation, a large amount of energy is necessary because dissipation occurs before the charge reaches the heart.

The automatic implantable cardioverter defibrillator (AICD) system consists of a pulse generator and two lead or sensing systems that continuously monitor heart activity and automatically deliver a countershock to correct a dysrhythmia as necessary. The device is implanted surgically, usually through a median sternotomy or lateral thoracotomy approach. The AICD has been approved by the Food and Drug Administration (FDA) for two categories of patients: (1) those who have survived one or more episodes of sudden cardiac death resulting from ventricular tachycardia or ventricular fibrillation, with episodes not associated with acute myocardial infarction and (2) those who have experienced recurrent, refractory, life-threatening ventricular dysrhythmias that can induce sustained hypotensive ventricular tachycardia or ventricular fibrillation, or both, despite conventional antiarrhythmic drug therapy. In the future, it is conceivable that selection criteria may be broadened.

# CARDIOPULMONARY RESUSCITATION

Myocardial infarction (heart attack) is the leading cause of death in America. The American Heart Association estimates an incidence of 1.5 million victims per year, of whom approximately one third will die. Of these deaths, 350,000 take place outside the hospital and usually occur within 2 hours after the onset of symptoms.[1] Thus sudden death from ischemic heart disease is the most serious and most important medical emergency today. It seems reasonable to assume that many of these deaths might be prevented by prompt and appropriate interventions that provide either rapid entry into the emergency medical system (see Chapter 28) or cardiopulmonary support by means of **cardiopulmonary resuscitation (CPR).**

Cardiopulmonary arrest is recognized by the cessation of breathing and circulation and signifies a state of clinical death. Immediate and definitive action must be instituted within 4 to 6 minutes after the arrest or biologic death will occur.

The person who has suffered a **cardiac arrest** appears clinically dead. Unresponsiveness, cessation of respiration, development of pallor and cyanosis, absence of heart sounds and blood pressure, loss of palpable pulse, and dilation of the pupils are present. (Pupillary response can be misleading in patients who are receiving drugs such as atropine or opium derivatives or in the presence of corneal pathologic conditions.) Absence of ventilation can be determined by auscultation, feeling for movement of air from the mouth or nostrils, and assessing chest expansion. The presence of a pulse should be assessed by palpation of the carotid or femoral artery. If a hospitalized patient is being monitored by means of an ECG machine or cardiac monitor, the ECG pattern of *ventricular fibrillation* or, less often, *ventricular asystole* will appear.

## TECHNIQUES OF BASIC LIFE SUPPORT

**Basic life support** is an emergency procedure that consists of recognizing an arrest and initiating proper CPR techniques to maintain life until the victim either recovers or is transported to a medical facility where advanced life-support measures are available or the rescuer is too exhausted to continue (Table 30-5).

### Step I—Assess Level of Consciousness

Persons may appear to be unconscious when in fact they are either asleep, deaf, or possibly intoxicated. Unconsciousness is confirmed by shaking the victim's shoulders and shouting, "Are you OK?" If the person does not respond, help is summoned and the victim is placed in the supine position on a *firm* surface.

### Step II—Open the Airway

The tongue is the most common cause of respiratory obstruction in the unconscious person. The head tilt–chin lift (Figure 30-35) and the jaw thrust (Figure 30-36) are the two recommended methods for opening and maintaining the airway.[8] Jaw thrust (without head tilt)

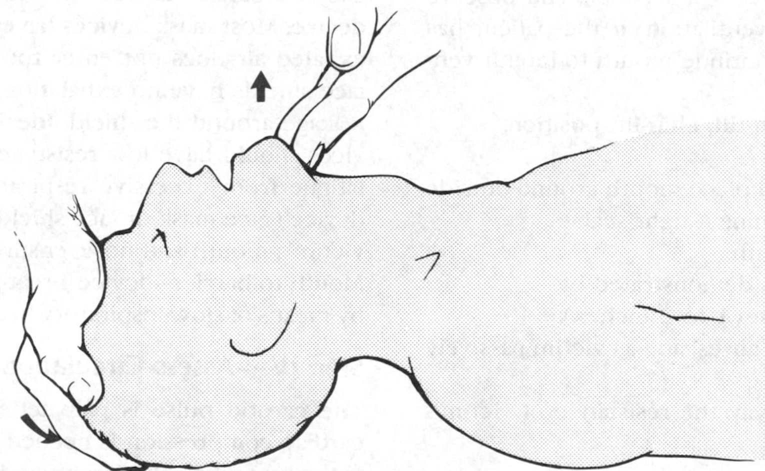

**FIGURE 30-35** Head tilt–chin lift maneuver for opening airway. Place one hand on forehead, and place tips of fingers of other hand under lower jaw near chin. Bring chin forward while pressing forehead down.

**TABLE 30-5 Sequence of Cardiopulmonary Resuscitation (CPR)**

| FINDINGS | ACTION | ABCs OF ACTION |
|---|---|---|
| No response | | |
| Absence of respirations; cyanosis, dilated pupils | Open airway | A—Open *airway* |
| Respirations still absent | Initiate artificial ventilation | B—Restore *breathing* |
| Carotid pulse not palpable | Initiate external cardiac compressions | C—Restore *circulation* |
| ECG; ventricular fibrillation | Drug therapy; defibrillation | D—Provide *definitive* treatment |

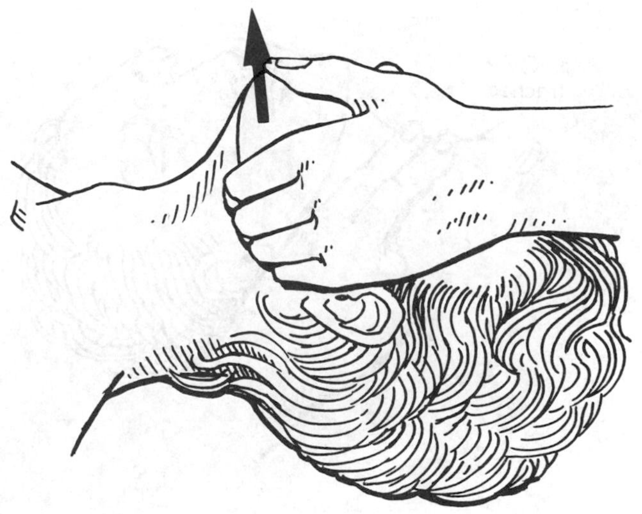

**FIGURE 30-36** Jaw thrust maneuver for opening airway.

is the safest first approach to opening the airway of a victim with a suspected neck injury. The head must be carefully supported to avoid turning from side to side or tilting it backward. While maintaining an open airway, the rescuer should take 3 to 5 seconds to *look, listen,* and *feel* for spontaneous breathing. The rescuer places an ear over the victim's nose and mouth while looking at the victim's chest. The rescuer looks to see if the chest moves with respiration, listens for air escaping during exhalation, and feels for air movement against the face.

## Step III—Initiate Artificial Ventilation

### Mouth-to-mouth ventilation

To initiate **artificial ventilation** if the victim is not breathing, give two mouth-to-mouth breaths (as described below) lasting 1½ to 2 seconds, and observe the person for adequate ventilation. If the patient has not resumed breathing, continue mouth-to-mouth ventilation:

1. Maintain victim in head-tilt, chin-lift position.
2. Pinch nostrils.
3. Take a deep breath and place mouth around outside of victim's mouth, forming a tight seal.
4. Blow into victim's mouth.
5. Adequate ventilation is demonstrated by
   a. Rise and fall of chest (1 to 2 inches).
   b. Hearing and feeling air escape as victim passively exhales.
   c. Feeling in own airway the resistance of victim's lungs expanding.

### Mouth-to-nose ventilation

Mouth-to-nose ventilation is indicated when it is impossible to open the victim's airway, if the mouth is seriously injured, or if a tight seal cannot be established around the mouth. The rescuer places one hand on the forehead to tilt the head back and uses the other hand to lift the lower jaw and close the mouth. After taking a deep breath, the rescuer seals the mouth around the victim's nose and begins blowing until the lungs expand. Occasionally, when mouth-to-nose ventilation is used, it may become necessary to open the victim's mouth or lips to allow air to escape on exhalation because the soft palate may produce nasopharyngeal obstruction.

### Mouth-to-stoma ventilation

Direct mouth-to-stoma artificial ventilation should be performed for the laryngectomy patient. For the patient with a temporary tracheostomy tube, mouth-to-tube ventilation should be initiated after the cuff is inflated.

### Mouth-to-barrier ventilation

An alternative to direct mouth-to-mouth ventilation is use of a barrier device such as a face shield and mask device. Most mask devices have a one-way valve so that exhaled air does not enter the rescuer's mouth; many face shields have no exhalation valves, which cause air leakage around the shield. Ideally, mouth-to-barrier devices should have low resistance to gas flow to reduce fatigue from excessive respiratory effort.[2] The barrier device (face mask or face shield) is positioned over the victim's mouth and nose, ensuring an adequate air seal. Mouth-to-barrier–device breathing should be initiated by means of slow inspiratory breaths (1½ to 2 seconds).

## Step IV—Assess Circulation

The carotid pulse is palpated rapidly to determine if cardiac compression is needed. The carotid pulse is located by finding the larynx and then sliding the fingers laterally into the groove between the trachea and the sternocleidomastoid muscle (Figure 30-37). If the carotid pulse is not palpable in 5 to 10 seconds, help is again summoned and cardiac compressions are initiated. The carotid pulse is palpated because the rescuer will already be at the victim's head and generally no clothing

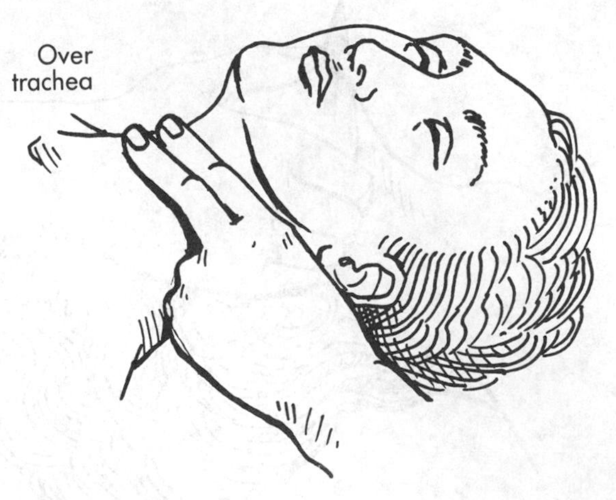


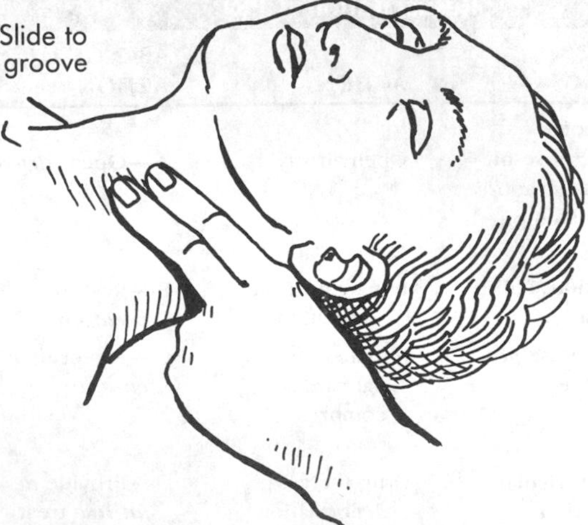


**FIGURE 30-37** Locating carotid artery.

has to be removed to assess the pulse. In addition, the carotid arteries are central, and sometimes these pulses will persist when more peripheral pulses have diminished and are no longer palpable. If a pulse is palpable but breathing is absent, rescue breathing should be initiated at a rate of 12 times per minute after the initial two breaths of 1½ to 2 seconds each. If the pulse is absent, cardiac arrest is confirmed and external chest compression must be initiated after the initial two breaths.

## Step V—Initiate External Cardiac Compression

**External cardiac compression** (sometimes called *external cardiac massage*) is the rhythmic compression of the heart between the lower half of the sternum and the thoracic vertebral column. This intermittent pressure compresses the heart, raises intrathoracic pressure, and produces an artificial pulsatile circulation. Correctly performed cardiac compressions can produce a peak systolic blood pressure of more than 100 mm Hg, but the diastolic pressure is close to zero and the mean blood

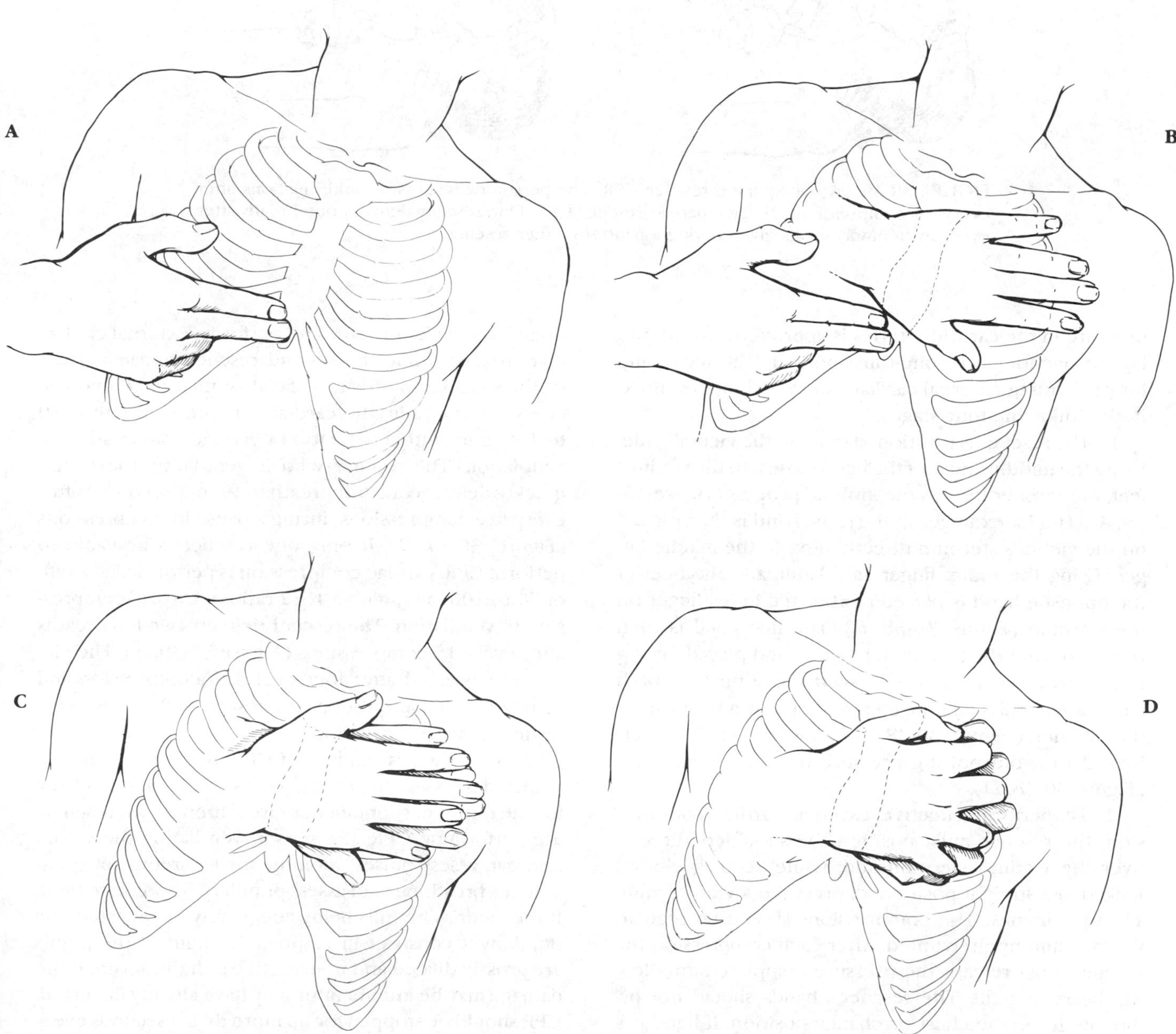


**FIGURE 30-38** Positioning of hands on sternum in external cardiac compression. **A,** Middle finger locates xiphoid process; index finger is positioned next to middle finger. **B,** Heel of opposite hand is placed on sternum next to index finger. **C,** First hand is removed from landmark position and placed on top of other hand so heels of both hands are parallel and fingers point away. **D,** Fingers may be interlocked to avoid pressure on ribs.

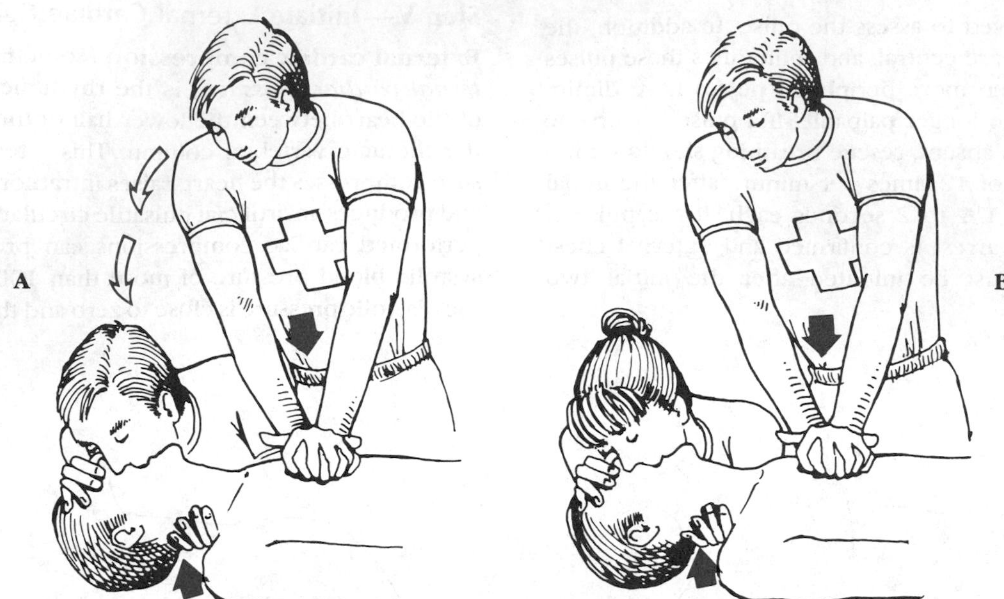


**FIGURE 30-39** **A,** One-person rescuer CPR. The person delivers two rapid inflations after every 15 compressions. **B,** Two-person rescuer CPR. One rescuer delivers one breath after every five compressions given during a pause by other rescuer.

pressure in the carotid arteries is approximately 40 mm Hg, or one-fourth to one-third normal. The technique for performing external cardiac compression is outlined in the following four stages:

1. The rescuer is positioned close to the victim's side. Using the middle finger of the hand closest to the victim's feet, the rescuer locates the xiphoid process (Figure 30-38, *A*). The index finger of the same hand is then placed on the victim's sternum directly next to the middle finger. Using the index finger as a landmark, the heel of the opposite hand is placed next to the index finger on the sternum (Figure 30-38, *B*). The first hand is then removed from the landmark position and placed on top of the hand on the sternum, so that the heels of both hands are parallel and the fingers are pointing away from the rescuer (Figure 30-38, *C*). Fingers may be interlocked to avoid putting pressure on the patient's ribs (Figure 30-38, *D*).

2. To perform effective external cardiac compression, the rescuer must position the shoulders directly over the victim's sternum and, while keeping elbows locked in a straight position, depress the lower sternum 1½ to 2 inches. The compressions should be regular, smooth, and uninterrupted. After each compression the rescuer must release the pressure completely to allow the heart to refill. The rescuer's hands should not ordinarily leave the chest or change position. If hand position must be changed to ventilate or move the victim, proper hand position must be relocated using the technique described.

3. Artificial circulation must always be accompanied by artificial ventilation. It is hoped that two rescuers will be available to administer CPR. One rescuer is positioned at the victim's side and performs external cardiac compression while the second rescuer remains at the victim's head to perform artificial ventilation. If two rescuers are available, the cardiac compression rate is 80 to 100/min, with a 5:1 ratio of cardiac compression to ventilation. The rescuer who is ventilating the victim quickly delivers one full breath (1½ to 2 seconds) after every five compressions during a pause in compressions (Figure, 30-39, *B*). If only one rescuer is available to perform CPR, cardiac compression is performed at a rate of 80 to 100/min, with a 15:2 ratio of cardiac compression to ventilation. The rescuer delivers two full breaths after every 15 compressions (Figure 30-39, *A*). The victim is reassessed after four cycles of compression and ventilation. If the pulse is still absent, CPR is resumed, beginning with ventilation.

4. After the first minute of CPR, the carotid pulse is palpated to assess the effectiveness of CPR and to check for the return of spontaneous circulation. If two rescuers are performing CPR, the person ventilating the victim also can assess pulses, monitor for the return of spontaneous breathing, and assess pupillary response to light. If the victim's brain is being adequately oxygenated, the pupils will constrict in response to light. If the pupils are grossly dilated and nonreactive to light, severe brain damage may be imminent or may have already occurred. CPR should be stopped for no more than 7 seconds every 4 to 5 minutes to assess the return of spontaneous pulse and respiration. Rescuers should continue to perform CPR until one of the following takes place:

a. Spontaneous circulation and ventilation return.
b. Another rescuer takes over basic life support.
c. Victim is transported to an emergency facility

**TABLE 30-6 Drugs Commonly Used in Cardiac Resuscitation**

| DRUG | ROUTE AND DOSAGE | ACTIONS AND INDICATIONS |
|---|---|---|
| Atropine sulfate | 0.5-1 mg by IV bolus; may be repeated at 3-5 min intervals up to a total of 0.04 mg/kg | Reduces vagal tone; enhances AV conduction; accelerates heart rate in cases of pronounced sinus bradycardia |
| Bretylium tosylate (Bretylol) | 5 mg/kg IV bolus followed by defibrillation; may be increased to 10 mg/kg and repeated at 15-30 min intervals until maximal dose of 30 mg/kg has been given | For ventricular fibrillation and tachycardias that have not responded to other forms of therapy |
| Calcium chloride, 10% solution | 2-4 mg/kg by IV bolus; may repeat at 10 min intervals | To increase myocardial contractile function; no significant beneficial effect during CPR; use during resuscitation limited to treat calcium channel blocker toxicity and acute hyperkalemia or hypocalcemia |
| Dobutamine hydrochloride (Dobutrex) | 2.5-20 μg*/kg/min by IV | Used to treat refractory pump failure; direct receptor stimulating agent; increases myocardial contractility |
| Dopamine hydrochloride (Intropin) | 5 μg/kg/min by IV drip; may be increased up to 20 μg/kg/min; add norepinephrine if dopamine is >20 μg/kg/min | Actions depend on dosage; 2-10 μg/kg/min generally has β-receptor–stimulating action on heart, with resultant increase in cardiac output; >10 μg/kg/min has α-receptor–stimulating action, with resultant peripheral vasoconstriction |
| Epinephrine hydrochloride (Adrenalin), 1:10,000 solution | Recommended 1.0 mg IV push; repeat q 3-5 min as needed; if used endotracheally, use full 1 mg<br>Intermediate: 2-5 mg IV push, q 3-5 min<br>High: 0.1 mg/kg IV push, q 3-5 min | Positive inotropic and chronotropic action; peripheral vasoconstrictor; causes ventricular fibrillation<br>Pulseless ventricular tachycardia more amenable to defibrillation; increases perfusion pressure of cardiac compressions |
| Isoproterenol hydrochloride (Isuprel) | 2-10 μg/min by IV bolus or intracardiac; dosage should be titrated to heart rate and blood pressure response<br>Should be used, if at all, with *extreme* caution | Potent inotropic and chronotropic agent; may induce or exacerbate myocardial ischemia caused by greatly increased myocardial oxygen requirements; no appreciable effect in cardiac arrest from asystole or electromechanical dissociation; recommended only in hemodynamically significant and atropine-refractory bradycardia on temporary basis until pacemaker can be implanted |
| Norepinephrine bitartrate (Levophed) | 0.5-1 μg/min as initial dose; average adult dose, 2-12 μg/min; should be titrated to blood pressure response; patients with refractory shock may require 8-30 μg/min | Potent vasopressor and positive inotropic effects; increases peripheral resistance; used in severe hypotension with low total peripheral resistance |
| Sodium bicarbonate (50 mEq) | 1 mEq/kg by IV bolus; may repeat maximum of one half this dose; further doses governed by arterial blood gas and pH determinations | To counteract metabolic acidosis |
| Lidocaine hydrochloride (Xylocaine) | Initial bolus 1-1.5 mg/kg; additional boluses of 0.5 mg/kg may be given at 3-5 min intervals up to total of 3 mg/kg if needed | Antiarrhythmic; shortens refractory period and suppresses automaticity of ectopic foci; useful in treatment of both ventricular tachycardia and fibrillation |
| Magnesium sulfate | 1-2 g IV over 15 min, then 1 g IM q 4-6 hr | Torsades de pointes, suspected hypomagnesemic state, or severe refractory ventricular fibrillation |
| Procainamide | 20-30 mg/min (maximum 17 mg/kg) | Refractory ventricular fibrillation |
| Nitroglycerine | 10-20 μg/min IV (if blood pressure >100 mm Hg) | Myocardial ischemia, hypotension/shock, acute pulmonary edema |
| Nitroprusside | 0.1-5.0 μg/kg/min IV (if blood pressure >100 mm Hg) | Hypotensive agent |

* μg (Micrograms) sometimes is written *mcg.*

where qualified personnel assume the responsibility for CPR.

d. Victim is pronounced dead by a physician.
e. Rescuer is exhausted and unable to continue.

## IN-HOSPITAL CARDIAC ARRESTS

Many hospitals have prepared teams of personnel, including physicians, nurses, anesthesiologists, and technicians, who can be called to give immediate and complete care in the event of a cardiac arrest. Most hospitals are equipped with a cardiac arrest tray or have access to a specially equipped cart on which all necessary emergency items are available. Equipment needed includes an ECG machine, a suction device, oxygen, defibrillator, airway and Ambu or other breathing bag, laryngoscope, a variety of endotracheal tubes, cutdown set, intravenous fluids, and tracheostomy set.

Medications usually administered during a cardiac arrest generally are available on the emergency cart. Some of these medications are described in Table 30-6.

For a more detailed discussion of basic life support and for information on advanced life support, see reference 2.

### COMPLICATIONS OF CARDIOPULMONARY RESUSCITATION

The most common complication of external cardiac compression is fracture of the ribs. This may occur in some persons even though the technique of external cardiac compression was performed correctly. Other possible complications despite correct CPR technique include fractured sternum, costochondral separation, and lung contusions. If medications were injected into the heart during the resuscitative effort, the patient is monitored carefully for signs of hemothorax, pneumothorax, or pericardial tamponade. Any indication of labored respiration, paradoxical pulse, muffled heart sounds, tachycardia, decreased breath sounds, or drop in blood pressure is reported to the physician immediately. Laceration of the liver also may occur as a result of compressions performed over the xiphoid process.

### INTERNAL CARDIAC COMPRESSION

In this seldom-used method of cardiac massage, a thoracotomy is performed and the heart is massaged with the hands or stimulated with an electric current. In most cases, open heart compression will not succeed when proper external compressions coupled with appropriate drug therapy and ventilation have failed. Internal compression is necessary in some instances or conditions, such as in cardiac tamponade, in crushing or penetrating chest injuries, and in the presence of an anatomic chest deformity that precludes adequate and effective compression by external cardiac massage.

## CORONARY ARTERY DISEASE: CORONARY ATHEROSCLEROTIC HEART DISEASE

The term **coronary artery disease (CAD)** is a generic designation for many different conditions that involve obstructed blood flow through the coronary arteries. Some texts refer to coronary artery disease as coronary heart disease (CHD) and/or ischemic heart disease (IHD); however, these terms are not specific and are gradually being abandoned. **Coronary atherosclerotic heart disease (CAHD)**, the most common type of coronary artery disease, is discussed in this text. For a discussion of the more unusual nonatherosclerotic forms of coronary artery disease, the reader is referred to specialized texts.

### EPIDEMIOLOGY

Coronary atherosclerosis is recognized as the leading cause of death in the industrialized Western world. In the United States, CAHD (angina, sudden death, myocardial infarction) has reached epidemic proportions. Each year approximately 1 million Americans die of the disease and another 2.5 million are disabled by it. The annual economic cost is overwhelming, averaging tens of billions of dollars.

The increased incidence of CAHD in the last 60 years has been causally linked to affluence and prosperity. There are many factors involved in this increase, however, such as increased longevity and improved recognition of the disease.

Epidemiologic studies have shown that the incidence of coronary atherosclerosis is much higher in men than in women of childbearing age, in older persons, and in the affluent. Nutrition has become a key factor in epidemiologic studies, forming the link between affluence and an increased rate of coronary atherosclerosis. In such countries as the United States and Finland, where diets are high in calories, total fat, cholesterol, and refined carbohydrates, the incidence of coronary atherosclerosis is extremely high, whereas in a country such as Japan, where the diet is low in calories, total fat, and cholesterol, coronary atherosclerosis is infrequent or rare.

#### BOX 30-6 Risk Factors for Developing Coronary Atherosclerotic Heart Disease

**NONMODIFIABLE RISK FACTORS**

1. Age
2. Gender
3. Race
4. Family history

**MODIFIABLE RISK FACTORS**

**Major Risk Factors**

1. Elevated serum lipid levels (hyperlipoproteinemia)
2. Habitual diet high in calories, total fats, cholesterol, refined carbohydrates, sodium
3. Hypertension
4. Obesity
5. Glucose intolerance
6. Cigarette smoking

**Minor Risk Factors**

1. Personality type
2. Sedentary living
3. Psychologic stress
4. Oral contraceptive use

### Risk Factors: General Considerations

Although a tremendous amount of research (both epidemiologic and experimental) is being conducted to learn the cause of CAHD, the exact cause remains unknown. Certain characteristics, however, have been singled out as being common in persons who have or are at risk of developing coronary atherosclerosis (Box 30-6 and Figure 30-40). These common characteristics or risk factors have evolved from many different types of

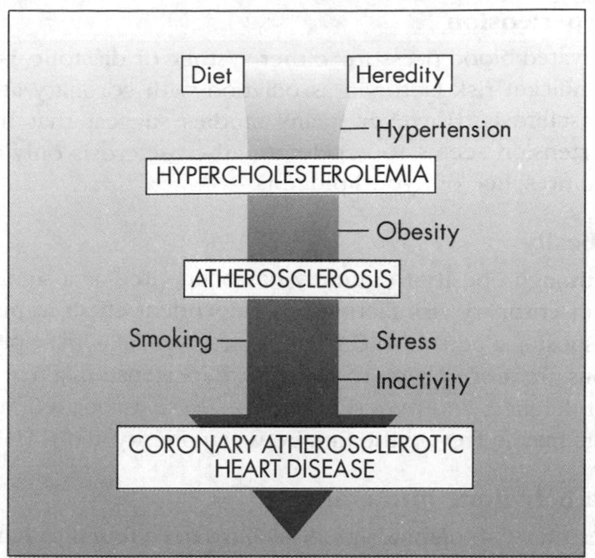


**FIGURE 30-40** Predisposing factors in the development of coronary atherosclerotic heart disease (CAHD).

research studies and therefore require special interpretation.

Although risk factors help to screen persons who are at high risk for developing CAHD, the presence of a risk factor does not definitively indicate the presence or severity of coronary atherosclerosis. Conversely, the absence of risk factors for CAHD does not mean that person necessarily will be free from coronary atherosclerosis. At present there is strong evidence supporting a prudent approach to the prevention of coronary atherosclerosis. It is believed that the three major risk factors in CAHD are high blood pressure, hypercholesterolemia, and cigarette smoking. Cessation of smoking, a lowering of blood lipids by diet, and a reduction in blood pressure can reduce the risk of CAHD. Prevention efforts require identification of risk factors and efforts to correct or alter those risk factors that can be modified.

## Nonmodifiable Risk Factors

### Age and gender

Clinical evidence of coronary atherosclerosis may occur in the second and third decades of life. Although women seem somewhat immune until after menopause, the disease is already a major cause of death for men aged 35 to 44 years. The mortality in CAHD rapidly increases with age, so that by age 55 to 64, 40% of all deaths among men are caused by this single disease. Although there seems to be a strong and constant relationship between age and the onset of CAHD, this may simply reflect prolonged exposure to other atherogenic factors.

### Race

Before 1968, nonwhites tended to have lower mortality rates from CAHD than whites. Since that time there has been a higher mortality rate in nonwhites who are younger than 65 years of age. The fact that African-Americans have a 45% greater chance of developing hypertension may play a significant part in these statistics.[1]

### Family history

A family history of CAHD occurring in parents or siblings (before the age of 50) increases the risk of developing premature atherosclerosis. This familial disposition is thought to be related to both genetic and environmental factors. It is not clear to what extent genetic elements act in combination with environmental factors such as nutrition, socioeconomic status, and other risk factors. In addition, other mechanisms of genetic transmission are not yet known.

## Major Modifiable Risk Factors

### Hyperlipoproteinemia

Strong evidence indicates that an elevation in serum lipid levels **(hyperlipidemia)** is a major risk factor in the development of atherosclerosis. Cholesterol and triglycerides, the major serum lipids, are transported in the blood bound to specific proteins. Defects in the metabolism of these lipid-protein complexes comprise a group of disorders known as **hyperlipoproteinemias.** Some of these disorders are also highly related to the premature development of atherosclerosis.

Five types of lipoproteins have been identified: **chylomicrons, very low–density lipoproteins (VLDL), low-density lipoproteins (LDL), intermediate-density lipoproteins (IDL),** and **high-density lipoproteins (HDL)** (see Chapter 29). LDL, or β-lipoprotein, is most directly associated with CAHD. As a molecule LDL is approximately 50% cholesterol by weight. Other lipoproteins contain cholesterol but in lesser amounts. Unlike LDL, HDL is inversely related to CAHD risk. In fact, HDL may serve to remove cholesterol from tissues.

The hyperlipoproteinemias have been classified on the basis of clinical and laboratory data into five types with recommendations for therapy (Table 30-7). The conditions may be primary (familial) or secondary to some other condition or process. The goal of therapy for most patients is reduction of the rate of development of atherosclerosis. Many physicians are urging that blood lipid testing be done periodically and that preventive therapy begin early in childhood.

Cholesterol and LDL have been found to have a higher associative and predictive value for CAHD than do triglycerides. Cholesterol in the body comes from two sources: it can be taken into the body directly in food, or it can be manufactured by the liver and intestine. Approximately 0.8 g of cholesterol is manufactured by the liver each day. Cholesterol is involved in lipid transport and is excreted with bile salts into the intestine to participate in the digestion and absorption of fats. The complex process by which cholesterol is manufactured, distributed, and eliminated is not very well understood,

**TABLE 30-7 Types of Hyperlipoproteinemias**

| TYPE | ABNORMALITY | CLINICAL FEATURES OF ELEVATED LEVELS |
|---|---|---|
| I | ↑ Chylomicrons | Eruptive xanthoma, pancreatitis, organomegaly |
| IIa | ↑ LDL | Premature atherosclerosis, corneal arcus, tendinous and tuberous xanthomas |
| IIb | ↑ LDL and VLDL | |
| III | ↑ IDL | Glucose intolerance, hyperuricemia, premature atherosclerosis |
| IV | ↑ VLDL | Glucose intolerance, hyperuricemia |
| V | ↑ VLDL and chylomicrons | Hepatosplenomegaly, eruptive xanthoma, glucose intolerance |

although it is widely believed that the inherited endocrine system plays a definite part because of its effect on the metabolic processes. Studies have shown that when a large amount of saturated fat is eaten, the cholesterol level in the blood tends to rise. When the saturated fats are replaced by polyunsaturated fats, the blood cholesterol level tends to fall.

Persons with serum cholesterol levels greater than 300 mg/dl have been found to have four times more risk of CAHD than those with levels less than 200 mg/dl. It would therefore appear prudent to take measures to decrease or maintain serum cholesterol levels below 200 mg/dl. The upper limit of normal for serum cholesterol is 220 to 240 mg/dl.

### Dietary patterns

The contemporary American diet, rich in total calories, total and saturated fats, cholesterols, refined sugars, and salt, is a significant coronary risk factor. The national dietary average for fat consumption is still very high in the United States, with approximately 50% of our dietary calories being derived from fats. Studies indicate that populations that consume low-fat diets generally have been found to have lower serum cholesterol levels than those consuming high-fat diets. In addition, populations consuming diets reduced in calories, total fats, saturated fats, and cholesterol not only have a lower cholesterol level but also have a lower incidence of and mortality from CAHD.

The American Heart Association[1] has endorsed a policy recommending some modification in diet for everyone: reducing the fat content of the diet, substituting polyunsaturated fat for saturated fat, and maintaining body weight at normal levels. Some sources of polyunsaturated fat are corn, cottonseed, soy, and safflower oils and margarines incorporating these oils in liquid form. Oils that have been hydrogenated contain more saturated fat, as do coconut oil, butterfat, and animal fats.

### Hypertension

Elevated blood pressure, either systolic or diastolic, is a significant risk factor in association with coronary atherosclerosis. However, many studies suggest that hypertension seems to accelerate atherosclerosis only in the presence of hyperlipidemia.

### Obesity

Although obesity frequently has been cited as a significant coronary risk factor, its independent effect in predisposing a person to CAHD is controversial. Obese persons are more prone to diabetes, hypertension, glucose intolerance, and hyperlipidemias. These associated factors may in fact be the link between obesity and CAHD.

### Carbohydrate intolerance

Persons with diabetes mellitus have been found to have a greater prevalence and severity of coronary atherosclerosis. However, it is difficult to isolate diabetes mellitus as a single factor because it is well established that hypertension, obesity, and hyperlipidemia also are frequent in persons with impaired carbohydrate tolerance.[10]

### Cigarette smoking

In general, the risk of death from CAHD is two to six times higher in smokers than in nonsmokers, and the risk is proportional to the number of cigarettes smoked per day. Fortunately, persons who stop smoking have a lesser risk of developing CAHD than those who continue to smoke. Pipe and cigar smokers have been found to have only a slightly increased risk of cardiovascular death and morbidity.

The relationship between cigarette smoking and CAHD is not totally clear, but is has been suggested that the adverse effects of cigarette smoking on the heart and blood vessels involve the effects of nicotine and carbon monoxide. Specific changes include increased myocardial oxygen demand induced by nicotine, interference with oxygen supply by carboxyhemoglobin, and adhesion of platelets. In addition, cigarette smoking has itself been associated with decreased levels of HDL compared with levels for nonsmokers and ex-smokers.[3]

## Psychosocial Influences

There is significant evidence of behavioral and other psychosocial influences on the course of atherosclerosis and CAHD. Furthermore, smoking behavior and diet patterns notably change depending on the degree of stress an individual perceives is being experienced.

Low socioeconomic status was assigned highest priority by Tyroler and associates.[17] There is an inverse relationship between morbidity and mortality associated with CAHD and socioeconomic status. This process is not completely understood, but one possibility is that it could be linked to other risk factors. For example, it is known that persons in lower socioeconomic positions are more obese, smoke more heavily, and have higher blood pressures and serum cholesterol levels when compared with persons in higher socioeconomic positions. Social support systems and level of education also may affect this variable. Minimal social resources, as well as occupations with low autonomy and high demand, are associated with increased risk of CAHD. The stress response appears to play a focal role between physical and behavioral components.

Increased plasma levels of circulating cortisol and catecholamines have been associated with the development of hypertension and atherosclerosis. Catecholamines have known effects on platelet aggregation and lipid metabolism, both of which are involved in the genesis of CAHD. Cortisol enhances the sensitivity of arterioles to catecholamines, influences cholesterol and triglyceride levels, and affects sodium retention.

The association between behavioral patterns and the incidence of CAHD has been made. In early studies, persons with type A personality characteristics were found to have twice the risk of developing CAHD compared with the type B personality, which has totally opposite characteristics. However, several recent prospective studies fail to confirm these earlier findings. In fact, it now appears that not only is the global type A behavior pattern not a reliable indicator of subsequent development of CAHD but it actually may even represent a positive and healthy coping pattern.[7]

## PATHOPHYSIOLOGY

The exact cause of atherosclerosis is still unknown. Coronary atherosclerosis involves the localized accumulation of lipid and fibrous tissue within the coronary arteries, resulting in arterial narrowing and possible occlusion. As the atherosclerosis progresses, the narrowing of the lumen is accompanied by vascular changes that affect the functional ability of the coronary arteries to dilate. The result of this atherosclerotic process is a variable reduction of blood flow to the myocardium.

Manifestations of coronary atherosclerosis are the result of an imbalance between myocardial oxygen supply and myocardial oxygen demand. These manifestations, such as angina or coronary insufficiency, generally do not appear until the atherosclerotic process is well advanced. Despite alterations in vessel architecture and function, often greater than 75% of the coronary vessel is occluded before myocardial ischemia or dysfunction is produced. Coronary ischemia implies a relative deficit in myocardial oxygen to supply the normal aerobic metabolism of a functioning myocardium. The balance between myocardial oxygen supply and demand may be altered by a number of factors, as illustrated in Figure 30-41.

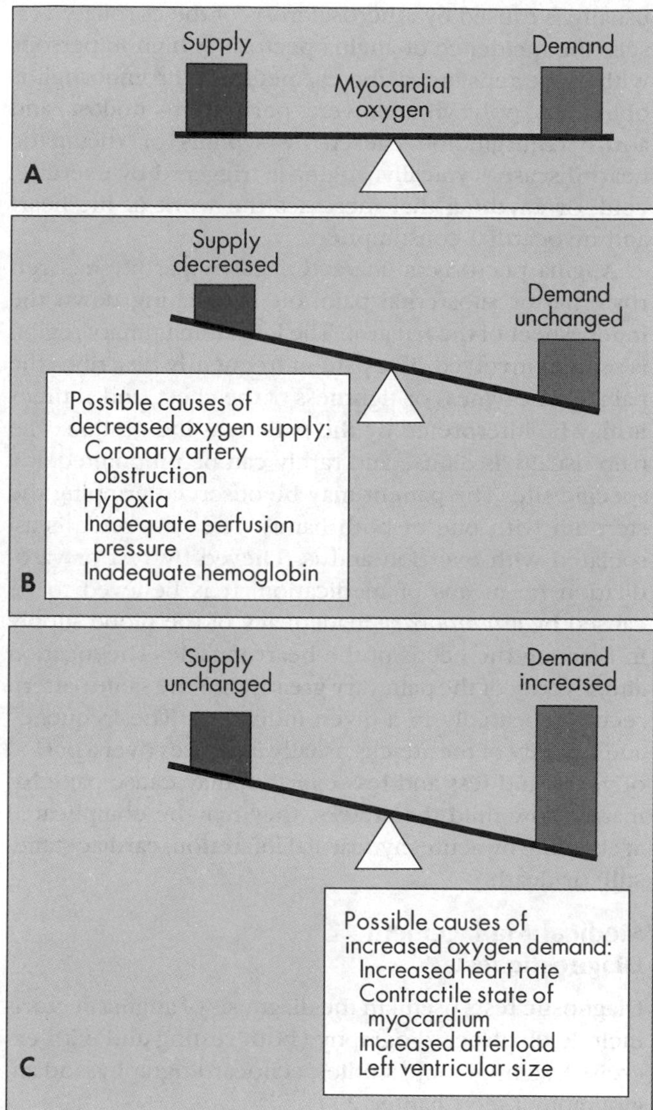


**FIGURE 30-41** Balance between myocardial oxygen supply and myocardial oxygen demand ($MVO_2$). **A,** Normal balance. **B,** Imbalance: supply is decreased, while demand remains unchanged. **C,** Imbalance: supply unchanged, but demand is increased. Atherosclerotic coronary vessels are limited in ability to increase oxygen supply.

Atherosclerotic lesions usually occur near the origin and bifurcation of the main coronary vessels in the epicardial segment of the coronary artery. These lesions tend to be localized and focal; however, in advanced coronary atherosclerosis, diffuse involvement of the coronary arteries can be seen.

Therefore the primary significance of coronary atherosclerosis is that the lesion, either alone or in conjunction with coronary occlusion, causes *myocardial ischemia.* Myocardial ischemia is then responsible for producing the clinical manifestations of CAHD: (1) *angina pectoris,* (2) *acute myocardial infarction,* and (3) *sudden cardiac death.*

## ANGINA PECTORIS

### Etiology

**Angina pectoris** occurs when myocardial oxygen demand exceeds myocardial oxygen supply. Although it usually is caused by atherosclerosis of the coronary vessels, the incidence of angina pectoris is high in persons with hypertension, diabetes mellitus, thromboangiitis obliterans, polycythemia vera, periarteritis nodosa, and aortic regurgitation caused by syphilis or rheumatic heart disease. Typically, angina is triggered by exercise, cold, or anything that increases the work of the heart and myocardial consumption.

Angina pectoris is characterized by paroxysmal retrosternal or substernal pain, often radiating down the inner aspect of the left arm. The left submammary region is seldom involved. The patient frequently describes the pain as a heaviness or tightness of the chest, and at times it may be interpreted by the patient as indigestion. The pain usually is diffuse and rarely can be pinpointed at a specific site. The patient may be observed gripping the sternum with one or both hands. The pain often is associated with exertion and is relieved by rest or vasodilation by means of medication. It is believed to be caused by a *temporary* inadequacy of the blood supply in meeting the needs of the heart muscle. The location and severity of the pain vary greatly, but the same pattern recurs repeatedly in a given individual. The frequency and severity of the attacks usually increases over a period of years, and less and less exertion may cause pain. No matter how mild the attacks, they may be complicated at any time by acute myocardial infarction, cardiac standstill, or death.

## Medical Management

### Diagnostic tests

Diagnostic tests useful in the diagnosis of angina pectoris include electrocardiography (both resting and with exercise), scintigraphic studies, echocardiography, and angiography (see Chapter 29).

### Medication

Drug therapy consists of vasodilators (nitrates, especially nitroglycerin), beta-adrenergic blocking agents, and calcium channel blockers (Table 30-8). The calcium channel blockers inhibit the movement of calcium ions across cell membranes via the calcium channel. Under normal circumstances, ions cannot penetrate the lipid membrane of either heart or smooth muscle cells. However, with appropriate electrical or chemical stimulation, molecular channels are formed that permit ion passage into the cell through a gating mechanism. Unlike the rapid sodium ion channel that permits inward depolarization, the calcium ion channel is much slower and ionic current is much smaller, hence the term *slow* channel. The exact mechanism by which these drugs block the calcium channel pathway is not yet clear, but inotropic and chronotropic activity are depressed. By reducing the cardiac activity, a balance can be achieved between myocardial oxygen supply and demand. Decreasing the heart rate also allows for prolonged diastole, which augments perfusion of the coronary arteries. Another benefit of calcium blockers is their potent vasodilatory effects. Exaggerated release of substances such as catecholamines and prostaglandins is known to produce vasoconstriction. Calcium channel blockers interfere with vasoconstriction and have been shown to be effective in reducing coronary vasospasm.

### Treatment

**Percutaneous transluminal coronary angioplasty.** An alternative approach to coronary bypass surgery for selected persons with single-vessel coronary artery disease is **percutaneous transluminal coronary angioplasty (PTCA).** The procedure consists of mechanically dilating the coronary vessel wall by compressing the atheromatous plaque. During PTCA, a specially designed balloon-tipped catheter is inserted under fluoroscopic guidance (similar to cardiac catheterization) and advanced to the site of the coronary obstruction. Once in position, the balloon on the catheter is inflated to provide compression and rupture the atheromatous plaque.

The complications associated with PTCA include sudden occlusion of the coronary artery through spasm, clot, or collapse. Arterial dissection or rupture may occur, and there is always the possibility of myocardial infarction. About 5% to 10% of persons undergoing

**TABLE 30-8 Drugs Commonly Used to Treat Angina Pectoris**

| TYPE | AGENTS | EFFECT |
|---|---|---|
| Vasodilator | Nitroglycerin<br>Amyl nitrate<br>Isosorbide (Sorbitrate) | Peripheral vasodilation to decrease peripheral resistance, decrease systolic blood pressure, produce venous pooling, and decrease preload; coronary vasodilation to redistribute myocardial blood flow more efficiently |
| Beta-adrenergic blocking agents | Propanolol (Inderal)<br>Metoprolol (Lopressor)<br>Nadolol (Corgard)<br>Atenolol (Tenormin)<br>Esmolol (Brevibloc) | Decrease myocardial oxygen demands to decrease heart rate, blood pressure, myocardial contractility, and calcium output |
| Calcium channel blockers | Verapamil (Calan, Isoptin)<br>Nifedipine (Procardia)<br>Diltiazem (Cardizem) | Inhibit calcium ion transportation into myocardial cells to depress inotropic and chronotropic activity, decreasing cardiac workload; also have vasodilatory effects |

PTCA require emergency coronary bypass surgery because of coronary occlusion; therefore preparation is similar to preparation for coronary bypass surgery.

After a successful PTCA most patients are hospitalized for 2 to 4 days in either a cardiology unit or an intensive care unit. Anticoagulants are administered prophylactically to prevent thrombosis, and ECG monitoring is maintained for the first 24 hours to monitor any signs of myocardial ischemia or arrhythmias.

**Intravascular stenting.** Restenosis persists as the single greatest limitation of percutaneous transluminal coronary angioplasty. Despite acceptable short-term rates of successful vein graft dilation, stenosis recurs in 30% to 60% of patients, depending on the location of dilation within the graft. A recent approach to solving the dilemma of restenosis has been to seek ways of "stenting" or maintaining the cylindric lumen produced by the balloon. Two techniques currently are being investigated. The first is to produce a "biologic stent" during balloon dilation through coagulation of collagen, elastin, and other tissues in the vessel wall by *laser photocoagulation* or *radio frequency–induced heat.* Preliminary results with the laser technique appear most encouraging.

The second technique has been to develop *prosthetic intravascular cylindric stents* capable of maintaining good luminal geometry after balloon deflation and withdrawal. To date, this approach has had the widest clinical application, both in preventing acute closure and limiting late restenosis.

**Laser therapy for cardiovascular disease.** Light is a form of electromagnetic energy that lasers use under controlled conditions. During the past few years a number of percutaneous devices for use in peripheral and coronary arteries have undergone clinical trials. As laser light interacts with tissue, it is transmitted, scattered, reflected, or absorbed. A thermal reaction occurs when target tissue absorbs the laser light. This thermal reaction produces necrosis, hemostasis, coagulation, evaporation of tissue, cutting, or vaporization, depending on the time of application, power density, and focusing of spot size.

Each medium produces a specific wavelength and affects a different tissue response to laser radiation. The *carbon dioxide* laser is absorbed by water, causing intracellular water temperature elevation to the boiling point. The *argon* laser is large and bulky, requiring higher voltage than ordinary electrical outlets provide. Areas of current research in the treatment of cardiovascular disease include transluminal and percutaneous laser angioplasty, myocardial revascularization, and percutaneous resection of an aberrant conduction pathway, valvular calcium, or hypertrophic myocardium.

Nursing care after laser angioplasty is similar to postcatheterization care. It is important to heighten the patient's awareness of the value of risk-factor reduction to prevent the advance of coronary artery disease.

### Diet

It is especially important for persons with angina to follow a recommended low-fat diet: saturated fats <10% of calories, monounsaturated fats 10% to 15%, polyunsaturated fats <10%, and cholesterol <300 mg/day (see Chapter 6).

### Activity

No restrictions are placed on activity within the patient's limitations.

## Surgical Management

### Coronary artery bypass surgery

Because surgical intervention does not alter the atherosclerotic process, the choice between medical or sur-

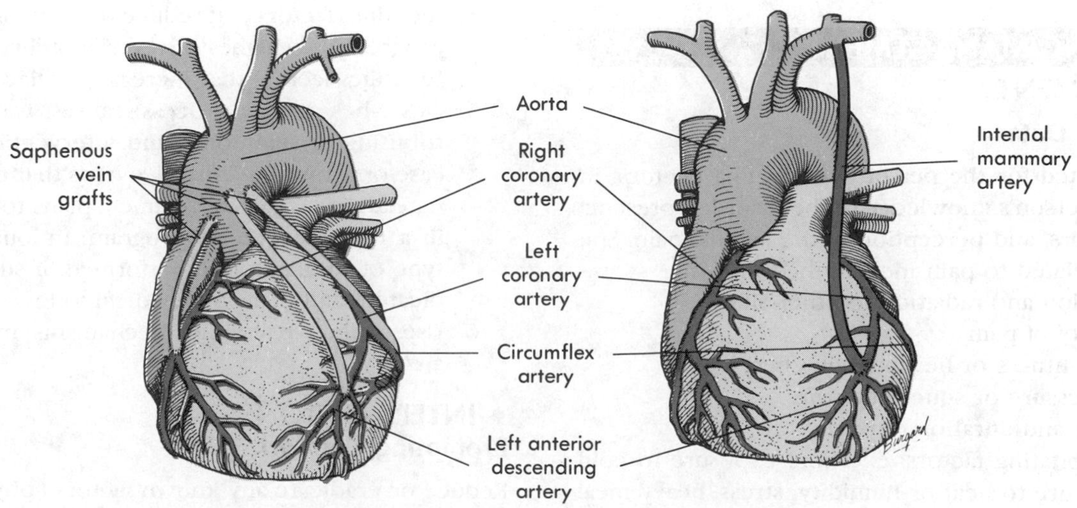


FIGURE 30-42 Coronary artery bypass grafts.

gical management for CAHD is sometimes controversial. Generally, drug therapy is effective in the earlier phases of CAHD. It can decrease anginal pain and decrease the workload of the heart while at the same time increasing the oxygen and blood supply to the myocardium.

Surgical intervention in the form of **coronary artery bypass graft (CABG)** may not prolong life or reduce the occurrence of myocardial infarction, but it does reduce angina and improve activity tolerance. Therefore, as CAHD progresses, many patients and physicians will choose bypass surgery to improve the quality of life. Coronary artery bypass surgery is a dramatically effective treatment for severe coronary disease. If severe narrowing of one or more branches of the coronary arteries exists, as indicated by coronary arteriography, a CABG may be recommended as a prophylactic measure.

The purpose of coronary artery bypass (jump graft) surgery is to increase blood flow to the myocardium (myocardial revascularization). Many persons show marked improvement after this surgery and usually do not require nitrates to maintain relief of symptoms.

The surgical technique varies somewhat among surgeons, and some surgeons routinely use cardiopulmonary bypass during the operation, whereas others do not. When the saphenous vein is used for the graft, one end is sutured to the aorta and the other end is sutured to the coronary artery distal to the occlusion (Figure 30-42). When an internal mammary artery is used, the distal end of this vessel is freed from the anterior chest wall and sutured in place distal to the occlusion in the coronary artery. Coronary bypass surgery is performed on the right coronary artery (RCA), the left anterior descending (LAD) artery, and the circumflex coronary artery (CCA) and their major branches. The care of the person undergoing coronary artery surgery is similar to that of those having other cardiac surgery (see Chapter 31).

# NURSING MANAGEMENT

## ♦ ASSESSMENT

### Subjective Data

Data collected for the person with angina pectoris include the person's knowledge of the disorder, presence of risk factors, and perception of the anginal pain. Specific data related to pain include the following:

1. Location and radiation to other sites
2. Quality of pain
   a. Tightness or heaviness in chest
   b. Pressure or squeezing pain
3. Onset and duration of pain
4. Precipitating factors: exertion, exposure to cold, exposure to heat or humidity, stress, heavy meal
5. Relieving factors: rest, nitroglycerin

### Objective Data

When anginal pain is present, data are collected regarding the person's behavior, increases in vital signs, and changes in cardiac rhythm. During an anginal attack, the person may become apprehensive and press the hands against the chest.

## ♦ NURSING DIAGNOSIS

Nursing diagnoses are determined from analysis of patient data. Nursing diagnoses for the patient with angina pectoris may include but are not limited to the following:

| Diagnostic Title | Possible Etiologic Factors |
|---|---|
| Pain/discomfort | Coronary artery occlusion, vasospasm, decreased coronary blood flow, hypoxia, diagnostic tests, overactivity |
| Tissue perfusion, altered: cardiovascular | Hypertension, angina, coronary artery occlusion |
| Activity intolerance | Sedentary life-style, generalized weakness, imbalance between oxygen supply and demand, bed rest, immobility, pain, fatigue |
| Knowledge deficit: disease process, prognosis, treatment | Lack of exposure/recall, information misinterpretation, language differences, unfamiliarity with information sources, lack of interest, cognitive limitation |
| Anxiety | Threat of or actual change in health status, role functioning, socioeconomic status; threat to self-concept; threat of death |

## ♦ EXPECTED PATIENT OUTCOMES

Expected patient outcomes for the person with angina pectoris may include but are not limited to the following:

1. States feeling more comfortable.
2. Demonstrates cardiac tolerance to increased activity (stable pulse and blood pressure).
3. Identifies factors that reduce activity tolerance and progresses to highest level of mobility possible.
4. Identifies factors that increase cardiac workload.
5. Describes disease process, causes, variables contributing to symptoms, and interventions for disease or symptom control; events that may precipitate attacks; medical regimen; plans to participate in a regular exercise program; rationale for and type of surgery to be performed, if surgery is indicated; and plans for medical follow-up.
6. Uses effective coping mechanisms in managing anxiety.

## ♦ INTERVENTIONS

### Promoting Comfort

Reduce or eradicate any known factors (physiologic or psychologic) that are contributing to increase in pain.

Assess for causes of decreased pain tolerance, such as fatigue, lack of knowledge, or anxiety. Fatigue from increased oxygen demands with a decreased oxygen supply increases pain perception; therefore take measures to reduce fatigue, such as providing rest periods if fatigue is present during physical activities. Provide a calm environment to decrease stress and anxiety that can increase the pain experience.

*Nitroglycerin* remains the drug of choice for treatment of pain from acute ischemic attacks. A nitroglycerin tablet placed sublingually and allowed to dissolve in the saliva often will relieve the pain of angina within 1 to 2 minutes. The person should experience a burning sensation on the tongue and may experience a throbbing sensation in the head. Some persons frequently experience flushing and headache from the vasodilation properties of nitroglycerin. Fortunately, these side effects diminish as the person develops a tolerance for the drug. If the pain does not subside after three doses of nitroglycerin are given 5 minutes apart, the person is instructed to call the physician or go to the nearest medical center. Nitroglycerin sprays are no more effective than tablets and may well be less effective. The sprays are more costly, and there is no conclusive evidence that they act faster.

Long-acting forms of nitrates are being used more commonly to diminish attacks and increase exercise capacity. Nitroglycerin ointment can be applied to any surface of the body that is not hairy. This cream is prescribed in doses of one half to several inches and is spread on cellophane-like paper and placed on the person's chest or another part of the body. The cream is absorbed slowly through the skin over many hours. The site of application is changed daily. An easier method of application is by means of a commercially prepared transdermal patch system. The date and time of application are noted on the transdermal unit, and the unit is changed every 24 hours. Tolerance develops with all organic nitrates during therapy, especially when dosing schedules are prescribed to provide therapeutic effects throughout 24 hours.

A variety of medium- and long-acting beta-adrenergic blocking agents are currently in use in the management of angina pectoris (see Table 30-8). Beta blockers prevent angina by reducing myocardial oxygen requirements during stress or exertion. Intravenous beta blockers such as esmolol hydrochloride (Brevibloc) are ultra short–acting and also cardioselective. Brevibloc is administered as a continuous infusion. Beta blockade is abolished within minutes of terminating the infusion, as a result of rapid degradation of the drug by tissue and serum enzymes.

## Promoting Tissue Perfusion

Instruct the patient to avoid becoming overly fatigued and to stop activity immediately in the presence of chest pain, dyspnea, lightheadedness, or faintness, indicating low tissue perfusion. Decreased tissue perfusion causes cellular hypoxia with subsequent ischemia, cellular swelling, and cellular death.

## Promoting Activity and Rest

Enhance the patient's activity tolerance by encouraging slower activity or shorter periods of activity with more rest periods. Pulse increases of 50 beats/min occur with strenuous activity; this rate is safe provided it returns to the resting pulse rate within 3 minutes. Most persons with angina pectoris can tolerate mild exercise such as walking and playing golf, but exertion such as running, climbing hills or stairs rapidly, and lifting heavy objects causes pain. Anginal pain is likely to be evoked more easily in cold weather, because the vessels normally constrict to conserve body heat. When persons with angina pectoris must be exposed to the cold, they should err on the side of being too warmly clothed. It is unwise to sleep in a cold room, and walking against the wind and uphill should be avoided because these activities increase the workload of the heart and cause pain.

If possible, the person should participate in a regularly

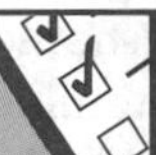

### Guidelines for Teaching the Person With Angina

1. Rationale for symptoms and prevention of anginal pain
   a. Avoid excessive activity in cold weather, especially activity against resistance
   b. Avoid overeating
   c. Sleep in a warm room
   d. Minimize exposure to stressful situations when possible
   e. Use stress-reducing activities such as relaxation exercises when stress is present
2. Medications
   a. Nitroglycerin tablets
      (1) Carry tablets for immediate use if necessary
      (2) Keep tablets in original container tightly closed
      (3) Store tablets in a cool, dry place
      (4) Inspect expiration date and have replacement available
   b. β-Adrenergic agents and calcium channel blockers
      (1) Monitor pulse and report to physician a pulse rate less than 50/min
      (2) Take β-adrenergics with food
      (3) Take calcium channel blockers 1 hour before or 2 hours after meals
      (4) Check with physician before omitting medication
      (5) Avoid driving if dizziness is present
3. Activity
   a. Plan for a regular activity program
   b. Increase extent of exercises gradually
   c. Avoid overexertion
   d. If necessary, take nitroglycerin before exercise if pain is anticipated
   e. Space exercise with rest periods
4. Medical follow-up
   a. Continue medical follow-up as instructed
   b. Report to physician if anginal pain increases

scheduled exercise program, spacing exercise periods with rest periods. A conditioned person experiences less of a rise in blood pressure and pulse rate on exertion. The result is a decrease in myocardial oxygen demand and an increase in the amount of exercise or work the person can do before an imbalance occurs between myocardial oxygen supply and demand. Some persons may have to take nitroglycerin prophylactically before they engage in exercise, but the key to healthful activity is to avoid overexertion.

### Facilitating Learning

Delay teaching until the person is ready. To be able to learn the patient needs to be relatively free of pain and excessive anxiety. Promote a positive attitude and active participation of the patient and family to encourage compliance. Points to be included in the teaching are listed in the Guidelines box, p. 821.

### Promoting Relief of Anxiety and Feeling of Well-Being

Facilitate a reduction in the patient's present level of anxiety. Because excessive emotional strain also causes vasoconstriction by releasing epinephrine into the circulation, emotional outbursts, worry, and tension should be minimized. Persons with angina may need continuing help in accepting situations as they find them. The family, the spiritual adviser, business associates, and friends can sometimes help. An optimistic outlook helps to relieve the work of the heart. Many persons who learn to live within their limitations live out their expected life span despite the disease.

## ♦ EVALUATION

To evaluate effectiveness of nursing interventions, compare patient behaviors with those stated in the expected patient outcomes. Successful achievement of patient outcomes for the person with angina pectoris is indicated by the following:

1. States that anginal pain has lessened or is absent.
2. Demonstrates hemodynamic stability (stable pulse and blood pressure) to increased activity (such as with showering or walking).
3. Identifies stressful activities that precipitate symptoms of activity intolerance and avoids them.
4. Articulates factors that precipitate symptoms of angina.
5. Articulates the nature of angina, events that precipitate attacks, medical regimen, plans for participation in a regular exercise program, and plans for medical follow-up.
6. Demonstrates effective management of anxiety and physical symptoms through correct use of established coping mechanisms.

## UNSTABLE ANGINA

**Unstable angina** frequently is referred to as preinfarction angina, crescendo angina, or intermittent coronary syndrome. Unstable angina is characterized by an increase in the frequency, severity, or duration of symptoms or prolonged ischemic pain without infarction. Most patients with unstable angina have severe diffuse disease and need to be closely monitored in the coronary care unit. Therapy includes bed rest, sedation, supplemental oxygen, nitrates, and beta blockers. Intraaortic balloon pumping (see Chapter 31) may be indicated for the patient with symptoms whose condition is severely compromised. Coronary arteriography is indicated, and depending on the results of the procedure or the patient's response to medical treatment, coronary bypass surgery is considered. Specific guidelines for the management of persons with unstable angina have recently been published by the Agency for Health Care Policy and Research (AHCPR). A guide for patients with this condition and their families is also available.[18]

Theoretically, severe coronary artery stenosis produces turbulent flow and stasis, which may increase platelet aggregation. Aspirin and heparin are two agents frequently used to prevent reductions in coronary blood flow and distal coronary perfusion pressure caused by platelet accumulation at the site of stenosis. Cigarette smoking is a known risk factor for coronary disease. Platelet aggregation may be increased by nicotine stimulation of catecholamine secretion.

As with unstable angina before infarction, recurrent angina shortly after infarction is due either to a transient decrease of myocardial oxygen supply or to a transient increase of myocardial oxygen demand under the condition of a fixed coronary reserve. Decreased myocardial oxygen supply can be due to transient thromboses or platelet aggregation in severely diseased vessels, as well as excessive constriction of arteries proximal to the site of atherosclerotic narrowing. Factors that may increase myocardial demand include tachydysrhythmias, hypermetabolic states, hypertension or hypotension, anemia, drugs, hypervolemia, or hypovolemia, mitral regurgitation, ventricular aneurysm, ventricular septal defect, and severe left ventricular failure.

## MYOCARDIAL INFARCTION

### Etiology

Acute **myocardial infarction (MI)** is caused by sudden blockage of one of the branches of a coronary artery. It may be extensive enough to interfere with cardiac function and cause immediate death, or it may cause necrosis of a portion of the myocardium, with subsequent healing by scar formation or fibrosis. *Coronary occlusion* is a general term for blockage of a coronary artery. The blockage may be caused by formation of a thrombus in the coronary artery *(coronary thrombosis),* sudden progression of atherosclerotic changes, or prolonged constriction of the arteries.

### Pathophysiology

Infarction is not immediately total and complete; rather, ischemic injury evolves over several hours toward com-

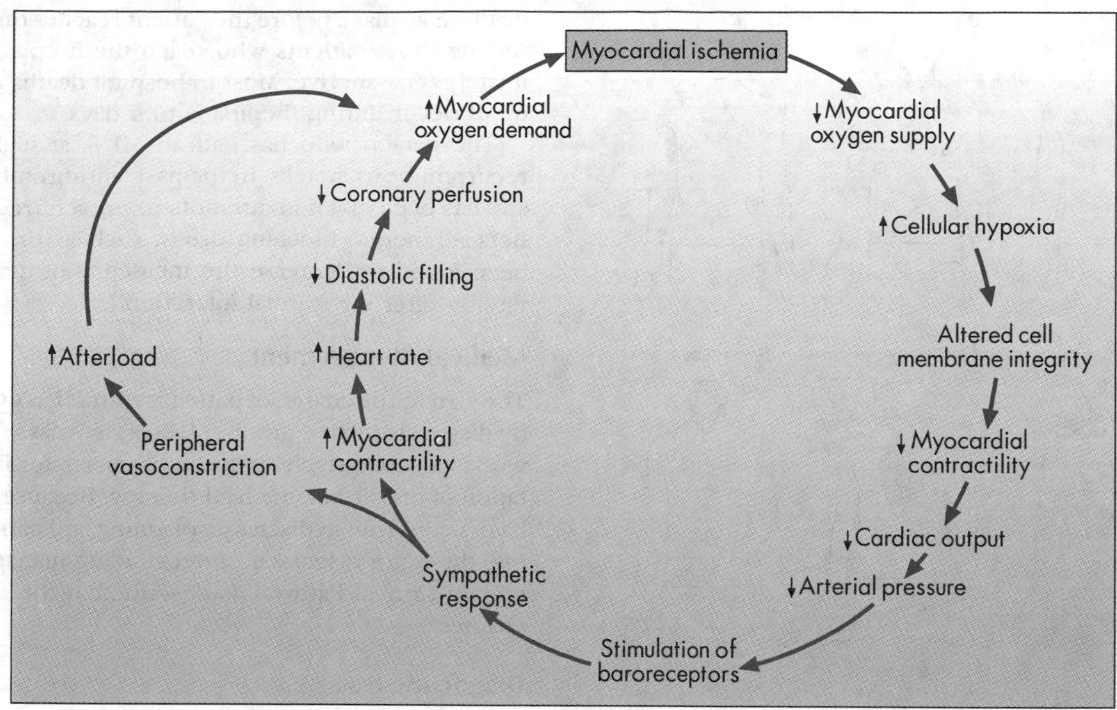


**FIGURE 30-43** Effects of prolonged myocardial ischemia.

plete necrosis and infarction. During an acute ischemic process, the subendocardial layer of the myocardium is most susceptible to hypoxia, and cellular ischemia usually manifests in this area before it involves the full thickness of the ventricular myocardium. Ischemia almost immediately alters the integrity and the permeability of the cell membrane to vital electrolytes, thereby producing depressed myocardial contractility. The autonomic nervous system attempts to compensate for the depressed cardiac performance, resulting in a further imbalance between myocardial oxygen supply and demand (Figure 30-43).

Prolonged ischemia lasting more than 35 to 45 minutes produces irreversible cellular damage and necrosis of cardiac muscle. Contractile function in the necrotic area ceases permanently. The infarcted or necrotic area is surrounded by a zone of ischemia, made up of potentially viable tissues. The final size of the infarct depends on whether the marginal area in the ischemic zone succumbs to prolonged ischemia or is able to develop and maintain collateral circulation. The prognosis after an acute MI reflects the degree of functional impairment of the heart.

The clinical features of acute MI are determined by both the anatomic location and the extent of occlusive coronary disease. Knowledge of the anatomic location of the MI enables one to anticipate whether arrhythmias, conduction disturbances, and congestive heart failure are likely to occur. The location of the infarct is, of course, directly related to the disease in a particular region of the coronary circulation. An *anterior wall myocardial infarction* results from lesions in the left anterior descending (LAD) branch of the left main coronary artery (see Chapter 29). Because the LAD branch supplies most of the left ventricle, an anterior infarct often is associated with a substantial loss of left ventricular muscle mass and can result in severe hemodynamic disturbances. An *inferior wall myocardial infarction* most often is caused by occlusion of the right coronary artery (RCA). Because the RCA is often proximal to the origin of both the AV node and the SA node arteries, it frequently is accompanied by ischemia of the AV node, the proximal bundle of His, and the SA node as well. Abnormalities of impulse conduction and formation caused by ischemia or infarction are primary factors contributing to the development of serious arrhythmias early in the course of inferior infarction.[3] *Lateral wall* infarcts usually are caused by occlusion of the left circumflex coronary artery and may be complicated by the hemodynamic changes similar to an anterior infarction when a large mass of myocardium is disrupted.

Pain is the most frequent complaint of the patient with an MI. The person typically complains of sudden, severe, crushing, or viselike pain in the substernal region. This pain may radiate into the left and sometimes the right arm and up the sides of the neck (Figure 30-44). At other times it may simulate indigestion or a gallbladder attack with abdominal pain and vomiting. Persons often become restless and fear that they are dying. They may become short of breath and cyanotic and show signs of severe shock. On ausculation, crackles or wheezes may be audible. The pulse usually is rapid, and it may be barely perceptible. The blood pressure usually falls, and the patient may collapse. $S_1$ and $S_2$ heart

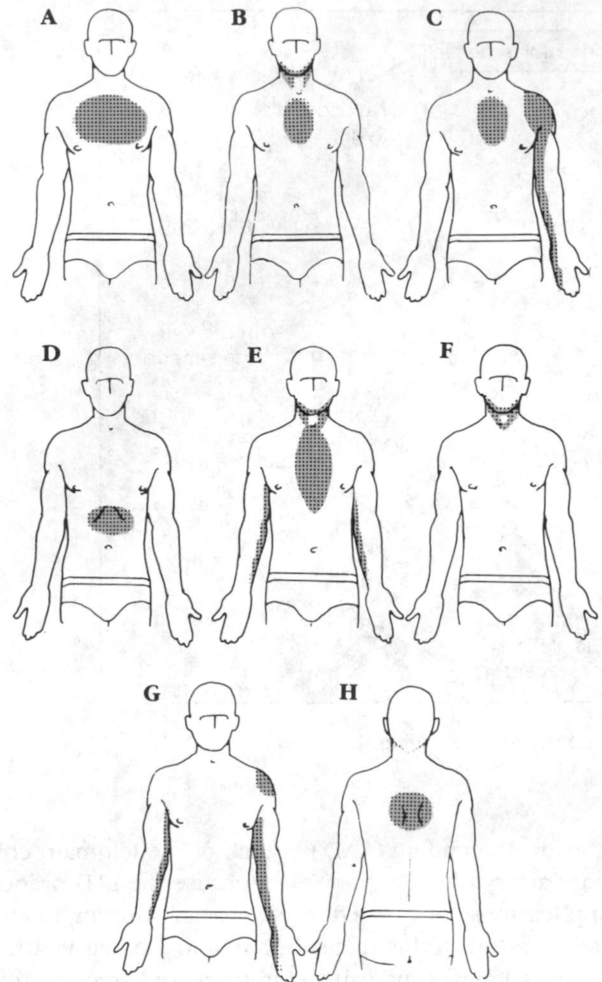


**FIGURE 30-44** Sites where ischemic myocardial pain may be referred. **A,** Upper chest. **B,** Beneath sternum radiating to neck and jaw. **C,** Beneath sternum radiating down left arm. **D,** Epigastric. **E,** Epigastric radiating to neck, jaw, and arms. **F,** Neck and jaw. **G,** Left shoulder, inner aspect of both arms. **H,** Intrascapular.

sounds often are faint; $S_4$ can often be heard; and at times an $S_3$ (gallop rhythm), which indicates left ventricular failure, may be evident. A soft systolic murmur may be heard at the apex. The symptoms of cardiogenic shock (see Chapter 22) occur as a result of inadequate cardiac output from decreased myocardial contractility and ineffective pumping.

Although pain is the most common initial complaint, it is not necessarily present. Approximately 15% to 20% of myocardial infarcts may be painless. The incidence of painless infarcts increases with age, and in elders, the chief complaint may be sudden shortness of breath. Other less common presenting symptoms include confusion, sudden dysrhythmias, unexplained drop in blood pressure, or sudden loss of consciousness.

## Prognosis

Mortality in persons with acute MI is high, ranging from 30% to 40%; however, a substantial number of these deaths take place before the patient reaches the hospital. Among those patients who reach the hospital, approximately 80% survive. Most in-hospital deaths as a result of MI occur during the first 3 to 4 days.

The person who has had an MI is at high risk for recurrent heart attacks. In the past, antithrombotic therapy has been given in attempts to prevent recurrences. Beta-adrenergic blocking drugs, such as timolol, have been found to decrease the incidence of death in the months after myocardial infarction.[3]

## Medical Management

The goal for discharge of patients with MI as determined by diagnosis-related groups (DRGs) is 7 days. The nurse works collaboratively with the physician for implementation of prescribed medical therapy. Because the nurse has a major role in discharge planning and patient teaching, these are discussed under nursing management. A sample Critical Pathway is described at the end of the chapter.

### Diagnostic tests

Laboratory tests used in diagnosing the presence of an MI can be divided into three categories: nonspecific indicators of tissue necrosis and inflammation, ECG, and serum enzymes. Other diagnostic procedures include myocardial scintigraphy, myocardial perfusion imaging, and gated pool imaging (see Chapter 29).

**Nonspecific indicators.** The nonspecific reaction to myocardial injury is a *leukocytosis* that begins within a few hours after the onset of pain as an inflammatory response to the injured cardiac tissue. This leukocytosis often reaches 12,000 to 15,000/$mm^3$ and lasts for approximately 3 to 7 days. In general, high white blood cell (WBC) counts are associated with larger infarcts. The *erythrocyte sedimentation rate* (ESR), another nonspecific indicator, rises during the first week after infarction and remains elevated for several weeks.

**Electrocardiogram.** The term *transmural myocardial infarction* denotes that the full thickness of the wall of the myocardium has been involved. *Pronounced Q waves, ST-segment elevation, and T-wave abnormalities* are often evident during acute transmural infarction. These ECG changes are apparent in the leads overlying the area of myocardial necrosis. If an infarct does not involve the entire thickness of the myocardium, it is termed *nontransmural* or *subendocardial.* In this situation there are no Q waves present and the characteristic ECG changes are limited to the ST segment and the T wave. It must be emphasized that the ECG does not always provide definitive evidence of the ischemic process.

**Serum enzymes.** When cardiac muscle cells die, certain enzymes are released into the bloodstream via the coronary lymphatic drainage. These enzymes include

**creatine kinase (CK), serum aspartate aminotransferase (AST)** (formerly termed serum glutamic-oxaloacetic transaminase [SGOT]), and **lactic acid dehydrogenase (LDH).**

A pattern of enzyme elevations after an acute MI is a valuable diagnostic indicator. However, enzyme interpretation is somewhat limited in that enzyme elevations are not solely specific to myocardial damage. For example, AST is found mainly in heart muscle, but it also is present in the liver and to some extent in the skeletal muscle. LDH is found in the heart, liver, kidney, brain, skeletal muscle, and erythrocytes. CK occurs in the heart, skeletal muscle, and brain cells. Because of the lack of specificity of these enzymes, coexisting processes such as cirrhosis of the liver may produce misleading enzyme elevations.

To increase the specificity of these enzymes, measurements of the enzyme fractions or isoenzymes are taken. Fractionating the CK enzyme into isoenzymes is the most specific enzymatic indication of MI. $CK_1$ (BB) is found in brain, lungs, bladder, and bowel; $CK_2$ (MB) is found almost exclusively in the myocardium; and $CK_3$ (MM) is found in the serum of all patients for 48 hours after a transmural infarction, but it also may be elevated in the person with crescendo, or unstable angina, even in the absence of true infarction. The total CK value is elevated within 3 to 6 hours after an acute MI, peaks in 12 to 18 hours, and returns to normal in 3 to 4 days (Figure 30-45).

Because of the extensive tissue distribution of LDH, it can be elevated in a variety of disorders. Fractionating LDH into its five isoenzymes allows for greater specificity. Normally, $LDH_2$ is most prominent in the serum. The myocardium is especially rich in $LDH_1$, so that when an infarction occurs, the serum level of $LDH_1$ becomes higher than that of $LDH_2$ and the LDH pattern is said to be "flipped."

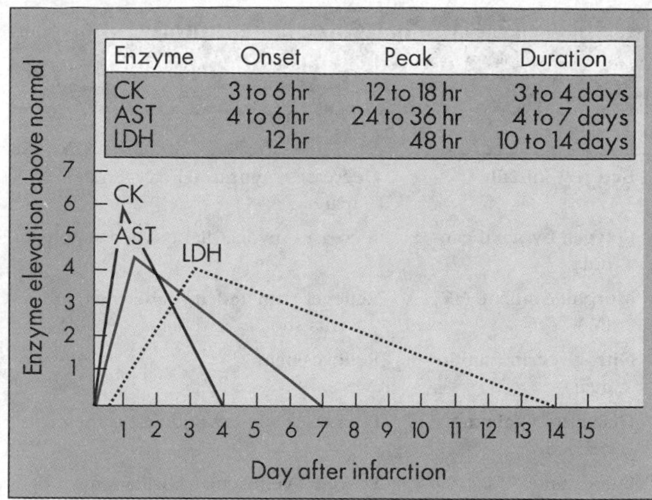


**FIGURE 30-45** Patterns of serum enzyme levels after myocardial infarction.

## Medication

**Analgesics.** Analgesic drugs are given for relief of pain. During the acute phase, intravenously administered morphine or lidocaine may be prescribed. Nitroglycerin also is effective.

**Thrombolytic therapy.** Thrombolytic agents such as streptokinase, urokinase, and tissue plasminogen activator (TPA) activate fibrinolytic processes to lyse the clot.[12] The value of thrombolytic therapy is its ability to be administered within the crucial period between coronary artery occlusion and actual myocardial tissue necrosis. This period can range between 3 to 6 hours after the initial infarction has occurred. Nursing implications of the use of any thrombolytic agent begin with accurate identification of candidates and prompt implementation of treatment. A thorough nursing history and assessment should be performed, focusing on actual or potential bleeding problems or tendencies. Assessments for signs of bleeding must be continued throughout the infusion.

Additional assessment during intravenous thrombolytic therapy includes noninvasive markers of reperfusion. Recognition of these markers is especially important for documenting the patient's response to intravenous thrombolytic therapy. For instance, rapid resolution of ST-segment elevation signals recanalization of the infarcted artery; thus the choice of a monitoring lead that demonstrates ST-segment elevation is recommended.

Observation for occult bleeding is crucial during and after thrombolysis. The patient must be continuously assessed for changes in neurologic status, evidence of gastrointestinal bleeding, or signs and symptoms of cardiac tamponade. If these occur, the physician must be notified because a decision to discontinue thrombolytic therapy, reverse anticoagulation, or administer blood products must be reached quickly to avoid life-threatening complications.

The primary goal during the immediate postthrombolytic period is to maintain arterial patency. Anticoagulants, antiplatelet medications, and mechanical interventions have been used to achieve this end.

**Other medication.** *Beta-adrenergic blocking agents* may be prescribed to reestablish the balance between myocardial oxygen supply and demand. They reduce the duration of ischemic pain and the incidence of ventricular fibrillation. *Anticoagulants* may be given for patients on a regimen of bed rest or limited activity.

## Treatment

Goals for treatment include prevention of further tissue injury and limitation of infarct size (Table 30-9). Interventions are aimed at maximizing myocardial tissue perfusion and reducing myocardial tissue demands. Myocardial tissue oxygenation can be improved with supplemental oxygen. When relaxation occurs with pain

**TABLE 30-9 Summary of Medical Interventions for Acute Phase of Myocardial Infarction**

| ACTIONS | RATIONALE |
|---|---|
| Bed rest initially | Decreases myocardial oxygen demand |
| Oxygen by nasal cannula | Increases myocardial oxygen supply |
| Morphine sulfate (IV, IM) | Relieves pain and apprehension; prevents shock |
| Nitroglycerin (sublingual) | Relieves pain |
| Diazepam (Valium) as needed | Decreases anxiety and restlessness |
| Lidocaine | Prevents ventricular fibrillation |
| Beta blockers | Decrease heart rate and force of contraction, decreasing oxygen requirements of the heart |
| Thrombolytic therapy | Activates fibrinolysis to lyse clot |
| Heparin (IV) (may be omitted for mild cases) | Prevents thromboembolic events |

relief and with improved tissue oxygenation, cardiac workload is thereby reduced. Cardiac monitoring is used to detect occurrence of dysrhythmias. Percutaneous transluminal coronary angioplasty (PTCA) (see p. 818) may be performed to reopen an occluded artery. Reperfusion of the myocardium also can be achieved by coronary artery bypass grafts (see p. 819).

### Diet

A low-cholesterol, low-salt diet usually is prescribed.

### Activity

Bed rest usually is prescribed for 24 to 48 hours to decrease oxygen demand. Progressive ambulation is then started unless complications (see p. 830) have occurred.

# NURSING MANAGEMENT

## ♦ ASSESSMENT

### Subjective Data

During the acute phase of MI, pertinent subjective data include the patient's perception of the cardiac pain and both the patient's and family's feelings about the patient's condition.

1. Patient's perception of pain
   a. Location and radiation to other sites
   b. Quality of the pain
   c. Onset and duration
   d. Associated factors: exertion, stress, at rest
   e. Relieving factors
2. Presence of associated symptoms: dyspnea, nausea, dizziness, weakness, sleep disturbances
3. Feelings of patient and family
   a. Uneasiness or feelings of impending doom
   b. Fear of death
   c. Possible denial or depression

### Objective Data

Monitoring objective data of the patient's response to the MI both physically and psychologically, as well as signs of complications, is an important part of the nursing care of the person with MI. The patient is monitored constantly for *dysrhythmias*. One of the most serious threats to the person during the acute phase is ventricular fibrillation (see p. 796), often heralded by premature ventricular beats (PVBs). Other objective data include the following:

1. Behavior: signs of anxiety
2. Changes in vital signs: increased pulse rate, decreased blood pressure
3. Associated signs: diaphoresis, vomiting, sudden dysrhythmias
4. Breath sounds: presence of crackles or wheezes
5. Serum enzyme levels (see p. 824).

## ♦ NURSING DIAGNOSES

Nursing diagnoses are determined from analysis of patient data. Nursing diagnoses of the patient with MI may include but are not limited to the following:

| Diagnostic Title | Possible Etiologic Factors |
|---|---|
| Tissue perfusion, altered: cardiovascular | Decreased cardiac output, pulmonary edema, CHF, angina, coronary artery disease, vasospasm or vasoconstriction |
| Cardiac output, decreased | Reduced stroke volume, CHF, cardiogenic shock, valvular stenosis/insufficiency, bradycardia, tachycardia, heart block |
| Pain/discomfort | Coronary artery vasospasm or occlusion, hypoxia, immobility, overactivity, diagnostic tests, improper positioning |
| Activity intolerance | Dysrhythmias, CHF, angina, electrolyte imbalance, sedentary life-style, decreased mobility |
| Anxiety | Threat of death; threat/change in health status, socioeconomic status/role; threat to self-concept |
| Knowledge deficit (disease process, prognosis, treatment) | Lack of exposure/recall, information, misinterpretation, ineffective coping patterns |

### Guidelines for Care of the Person During the Acute Phase of Myocardial Infarction

Monitor for cardiac dysrhythmias, notify physician if increased ventricular irritability (coupling of premature ventricular beats [PVBs]) is present.
Monitor vital signs for signs of cardiogenic shock (hypotension, weak thready pulse, cold clammy skin, mental confusion).
Monitor breath sounds for signs of respiratory congestion (crackles, wheezes).
Administer prescribed medications: intravenous morphine, intravenous lidocaine, anticoagulants, thrombolytics, tranquilizers, or sedatives.
Administer supplemental oxygen as needed; maintain oxygen therapy in the presence of persistent pain, hypotension, dyspnea, or dysrhythmias.
Position patient in semi-Fowler's position to enhance oxygenation.
Maintain patient on prescribed bed rest for 24 to 48 hours; encourage progressive ambulation when permitted.
Maintain patient on prescribed low-cholesterol, low-salt diet; avoid extremes of hot or cold foods.
Administer stool softener to prevent constipation from effects of opiates and decreased mobility and to prevent Valsalva's maneuver.
Start patient teaching as described on p. 828.

## ♦ EXPECTED PATIENT OUTCOMES

Expected patient outcomes for the person with MI may include but are not limited to the following:

1. Demonstrates cardiac tolerance to increased activity (stable pulse and blood pressure).
2. States breathing is easier and fatigue is decreased.
3. Identifies factors that increase cardiac workload.
4. States feeling more comfortable.
5. Identifies factors that reduce activity tolerance and progresses to highest level of mobility possible.
6. Participates in a program of progressive activity.
7. Uses effective coping mechanisms in management of anxiety.
8. Describes the nature of MI and how the healing process relates to the treatment regimen, variables contributing to symptoms and interventions for disease or symptom control, risk factors that can be modified and plans to alter life-style (if appropriate), plans to participate in a regular exercise program, rationale for and type of surgery if surgery is indicated, any dietary restrictions, and plans for ongoing medical care.

## ♦ INTERVENTIONS

The patient is admitted to the coronary care unit (CCU), which is equipped with special systems for monitoring cardiac rhythms and vital signs (see Chapter 26). The unit is staffed by nurses with expertise in cardiovascular nursing. Guidelines for care of the person with an MI are listed in the Guidelines box above). A critical care pathway for the patient with MI without complications is described on p. 832.

**TABLE 30-10 Interpretation of Changes in Vital Signs During an Acute Myocardial Infarction**

| VITAL SIGN | CHANGE | INTERPRETATION |
|---|---|---|
| Blood pressure | High | Increased myocardial oxygen demand |
| | Low (>80 mm Hg) | Decreased coronary perfusion with further myocardial ischemia |
| Heart rate | Increased | Possible shock |
| Heart rhythm | Irregular | Potential life-threatening dysrhythmia |
| Respirations | Slow | Possible morphine toxicity |
| | Crackles (rales) | Pulmonary edema |

### Promoting Oxygenation/Tissue Perfusion

Instruct the patient to avoid becoming overly fatigued and to stop activity immediately in the presence of chest pain, dyspnea, lightheadedness, or faintness. Decreased tissue perfusion causes cellular hypoxia with subsequent ischemia, cellular swelling, and cellular death. Oxygen is administered by nasal cannula for the first 24 to 48 hours and longer if persistent pain, hypotension, dyspnea, or dysrhythmias occur. Monitor vital signs carefully for changes indicating possible complications (Table 30-10). Position the patient in semi-Fowler's position to permit greater diaphragm expansion, thus improving lung expansion and better $CO_2/O_2$ exchange.

### Promoting Adequate Cardiac Output

1. Monitor the patient for the following parameters:
   a. Dysrhythmias on ECG tracings
   b. Vital signs
   c. Effects of daily activities on cardiac status, as evidenced by occurrence of dysrhythmias and need for oxygen
   d. Signs of fluid overload and electrolyte imbalance
2. Document rate and rhythm of pulse.
3. Administer pharmacotherapy as prescribed.
4. Plan nursing strategies to promote rest and minimize unnecessary disturbances.

### Promoting Comfort

The amount of pain and discomfort a patient will experience is highly variable. Some persons experience severe pain, and others have minimal discomfort. After an intravenous route is established, the patient is given morphine sulfate to relieve pain and apprehension and also to produce vasodilation. Continued episodes of chest pain may be related to the size of the infarction, the relative lack of collateral circulation, and an increased myocardial oxygen demand. Control of this pain is essential to provide comfort and rest and also to decrease sympathetic stimulation, which increases myocardial oxygen demands.

## Providing Rest

To limit the size of the infarction and to prevent any complications, the patient usually is placed on a regimen of bed rest with commode privileges for 24 to 48 hours. Assistance with activities of daily living (ADL) is given during this period. Sedation with diazepam (Valium) or an equivalent drug may be prescribed to relieve anxiety and restlessness in the crisis situation and to promote sleep. Rest and reassurance are essential. Patients are assured that the most dangerous stage of the MI has passed and that the purpose of the CCU is for continued monitoring and safety during the early recovery period. The nurse plays an integral role in providing support not only to the patient but also to the family. Calmness and competence can be extremely reassuring.

## Promoting Activity

After the first 24 to 48 hours, patients usually are encouraged to increase their activity gradually depending on the extent of the infarction. The patient usually first sits on a chair for increasing periods of time and then begins ambulation by the fourth or fifth day. During this period the person is continually monitored for signs of dysrhythmias, presence of cardiac pain, and changes in vital signs.

## Promoting Nutrition and Elimination

Fluids are provided initially, followed by resumption of solid foods according to the patient's needs. Extremely hot or cold foods are avoided initially, and small frequent feedings may be better tolerated. Salt restrictions may be prescribed, particularly for those persons with signs of heart failure, and low-calorie, low-cholesterol diets often are prescribed.

A stool softener is prescribed from the beginning because constipation is common from the effects of narcotics and decreased activity. Use of bedpans and straining should be avoided because the Valsalva maneuver causes changes in blood pressure and heart rate, which may trigger ischemia, dysrhythmias, pulmonary embolus, or cardiac arrest.

## Promoting Relief of Anxiety and Feeling of Well-Being

Anxiety varies in intensity and depends on the patient's perception of the severity of the threat, as well as the person's success in coping. Provide the patient and family with opportunities to explore their concerns and to explore alternative methods of coping, if appropriate.

## Facilitating Learning

Teaching is delayed until the patient is ready. The patient needs to be relatively free of pain and excessive anxiety to learn. Promote a positive attitude and active participation of the patient and family. Both patient and significant others need to know the nature of myocardial infarction, risk factors, variables contributing to symptoms, and the interventions for disease or symptom control. The initial teaching is similar to that for angina (see Guidelines box, p. 821). Additional teaching during the rehabilitative phase is listed in the Guidelines box above.

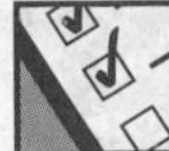

### Guidelines for Teaching the Person With a Myocardial Infarction

1. Effect of myocardial infarction and healing process
2. Prevention of further risks
   a. Discontinue smoking
   b. Correct existing hypertension with continued medical follow-up
   c. Eat a diet low in calories, saturated fats, and cholesterol; decrease salt, if hypertensive
   d. Participate in a weight-reduction program, if appropriate
   e. Take prescribed prophylactic medications (beta blockers)
3. Effect of activity on heart and participation in planned program of increased activity under medical supervision
4. Resumption of sexual activity (if appropriate)
   a. Abstention from sexual intercourse as directed, usually for 4 to 6 weeks
   b. Reporting to physician the following symptoms occurring during or following intercourse
      (1) Dyspnea or increased heart rate continuing for more than 15 minutes after intercourse
      (2) Extreme fatigue
      (3) Chest pain during intercourse
      (4) Palpitations for more than 15 minutes after intercourse
      (5) Insomnia after intercourse
5. Effect of stressors on the heart and benefits of stress management techniques (e.g., relaxation exercises)
6. Benefits of participation in group-counseling sessions for both patient and spouse
7. Benefits of return to usual home activities and relationships as soon as possible
8. Benefits of return to work at earliest opportunity as prescribed specifically by physician

# ♦ EVALUATION

To evaluate the effectiveness of nursing interventions, compare patient behaviors with those stated in the expected patient outcomes. Successful achievement of patient outcomes for the patient with MI is indicated by the following:

1. Demonstrates hemodynamic stability (stable pulse and blood pressure) to increased activity (such as with showering or walking).
2. Is free of dyspnea and fatigue with increased activity.
3. Articulates factors that precipitate symptoms.
4. States that symptoms of discomfort have lessened or are absent.
5. Identifies stressful activities that reduce activity tolerance and avoids them.

6. Participates in a program of progressive activity.
7. Demonstrates effective management of anxiety and physical symptoms through appropriate use of established coping mechanisms.
8. Articulates the nature of MI, variables contributing to symptoms, modifiable risk factors, plans to participate in regular exercise program, dietary restrictions, and plans for ongoing medical care.

## SPECIAL CONSIDERATIONS FOR CARE OF THE GERONTOLOGIC PATIENT

The prevalence of coronary disease has been shown to increase with advancing age. (Changes of the cardiovascular system seen in elderly persons are described in Chapter 29). Older patients are more likely to suffer an MI during sleep. Chest pain may be diminished despite substantial tissue damage; Mueller et al.[13] demonstrated that chest pain was absent in 75% of their patients 85 years of age and older. The pain also may be atypical. Decreased arterial compliance and decreased left ventricular performance may be present, which raises the tendency for cardiac output to decrease in response to a decrease in venous return. Adverse drug reactions are common in elders. Reactions may be the result of increased sensitivity to drug action, altered pattern of drug distribution, or the effect of aging and disease on organ function.

## HOME CARE CONSIDERATIONS

### Cardiac Rehabilitation

**Cardiac rehabilitation** is a process by which a person is restored to and maintains optimal physiologic, psychosocial, vocational, and recreational status. This process of rehabilitation involves progressive activity and exercise and education of the patient and family. Rehabilitation of the person who has suffered myocardial infarction begins the moment the person is admitted to the hospital for emergency care and may continue for months and even years after discharge from the hospital.

### Progressive Activity

During the 1960s, 2 to 3 weeks of bed rest were recommended for the person who had an MI. Today the hazards of prolonged bed rest are well documented, and patients with uncomplicated MIs (no evidence of severe dysrhythmias, congestive heart failure, or shock) progress rapidly through a supervised program of increased activity. Activity progression is based on the metabolic equivalent of the task (MET), a term used to describe the energy expenditure for various activities. METs can be assigned to activities regardless of a person's weight. One MET represents the energy expenditure of a person at rest; it equals approximately 3.5 ml/$O_2$/kg of weight per minute.

A patient hospitalized with MI usually is limited to activities with low MET levels (i.e., 1 to 3 METs). For example, using a bedside commode requires 3 METs and using a bedpan requires 4 METs. Champion athletes can perform at equal to or greater than 20 METs, whereas the average middle-aged man after an uncomplicated MI is capable of performing at a level of 8 to 9 METs.

More than 50% of all MIs are uncomplicated, and these patients will be discharged from the hospital in approximately 7 days. Because most patients will need to do 3 to 4-MET level activities when they return home, in-hospital activities should be geared toward reaching this level. In some institutions it is the physical therapist who supervises the exercise program, working closely with both the medical and nursing personnel to coordinate activities. During the first few days after an uncomplicated MI, the patient is instructed and encouraged to perform lying or sitting exercises (arms, legs, and trunk) at low MET levels. Then exercises progress to standing and slow walking in the hall. Patients are supervised constantly during these activities, and their vital signs and heart rhythms are constantly monitored.

Patients are taught early in the exercise program how to check their own pulses. This enables them to become familiar with the normal rate, rhythm, and response to exercise. Normally, patients can expect to have an increase in heart rate and systolic blood pressure with exercise. An exercise session is terminated if any of the following abnormal responses occur during exercise:

1. Cyanosis, cold sweat, faintness, extreme fatigue, severe dyspnea, marked pallor, ataxia, chest pain
2. Resting heart rate greater than 100 or an increase in heart rate greater than 20 over resting pulse; decrease or no change in heart rate despite exercise
3. Dysrhythmias, frequent PVBs, supraventricular tachycardia, various AV blocks, tachycardia greater than 120
4. Resting blood pressure greater than 160/95 mm Hg or an increase in systolic blood pressure of more than 40 mm Hg; decrease or no change in systolic pressure despite exercise

Progressive exercise is continued throughout the hospitalization. The nurse may be an integral member of the interdisciplinary team involved in instructing and supervising the program. Patients should exercise twice a day for approximately 20 minutes. Patients who will need to climb stairs at home gradually progress so that they can climb stairs in the supervised hospital environment. There are many psychologic as well as physiologic benefits to early and progressive activity. Most patients feel that activity is a positive sign and that they are making progress and are recovering from their infarction. Exercise also gives the patients a sense of control over their bodies and tends to decrease anxiety and depression during the convalescent period.

### Home Exercise Program

During the posthospitalization convalescent period, many patients are encouraged to begin a 2- to 12-week walking program. This is a structured program designed to have the patient walk 2 miles in less than 60 minutes by the end of the 12 weeks. Persons are encouraged to work through this program at their own rate until they have achieved a pace just below a slow jog and their heart rate is below the prescribed rate set by the cardiologist.

After completion of the walking program, some persons will progress to a supervised outpatient exercise training program. Physical conditioning improves the maximal oxygen uptake ($Vo_2$ max), which is a measure of the maximal rate at which oxygen can be delivered to the tissues. Unfortunately, not all postinfarction patients are physiologically capable of participating in a rigorous exercise program. Eventually, most patients are encouraged to participate in a maintenance (lifetime), unsupervised, home-based exercise program designed specifically for them.

### Teaching and Counseling

Education of the patient and family members enables them to assume a more active role in their own health care. A great deal of anxiety and apprehension can be allayed by providing information about the cardiac condition and its management. Although teaching methods and the amount of information presented may vary, several key concepts need to be presented (see Guidelines box, p. 828; Research box at right).

The patients and their partners may need teaching and reassurance regarding resumption of *sexual activity.* Many feel that after MI their sex life is over, fearing a second MI during intercourse. Approximately 80% of all postcoronary patients will be able to resume sexual activity without serious risk. The other 20% need not totally abstain, but their sexual activity should be limited according to their cardiac capacity. Once patients with an uncomplicated MI are capable of walking two flights of stairs without difficulty, they generally are able to perform sexual intercourse safely. In many hospitals, exercise stress tests are given to help the physician determine the patient's cardiac capacity and when sexual activity can be resumed. Coital positions that require less effort on the part of the person after MI can be suggested. Persons can be encouraged to participate in sexual closeness (such as cuddling) until intercourse is permitted. The person should report adverse signs occurring during intercourse to the physician.

During the hospitalization period many patients experience denial, depression, and anxiety. Generally, patients tend to become more anxious on the second day of hospitalization, after the immediate threat of death from the infarction has passed. Depression may begin several days later and may continue after the person is discharged. About 50% of persons continue to experience irritability and tension up to 1 year after an MI.[16] If the spouse is either overprotective or overcritical of the patient's behavior or of changes in the marriage roles and functions during the recovery period, the marriage may deteriorate. The spouse is therefore included in teaching and counseling sessions, and both patients and families are encouraged to talk about their feelings and concerns. Often in group sessions, a feeling of camaraderie develops as several persons face similar problems.

Physical symptoms may persist during the year after an MI and include excessive fatigue, chest pain, or dyspnea. Persons experiencing these symptoms often learn how to manage their symptoms and resume normal activities. More than 85% of all patients with uncomplicated MI are able to return to work, and this, along with resuming normal sexual functioning and usual activities, aids tremendously in the adjustment period.

**RESEARCH**

McCance KL et al: Preventing coronary heart disease in high-risk families, *Res Nurs Health* 8:413-420, 1985.

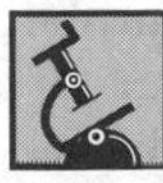

This experimental study examined the effects of preventive nursing intervention to reduce risk of coronary heart disease (CHD). The sample consisted of 58 relatives (spouses, siblings, parents, and children) of 19 victims (aged 30 to 55 years) of sudden death from coronary occlusion. The experimental groups were visited in their homes 3 to 5 months later. Interventions consisted of education/information about cardiovascular risk factors and methods of decreasing risk (blood pressure control, smoking effects, and dietary control of cholesterol, alcohol, and sodium) provided on an individualized supportive approach. The control group received questionnaires on the same time frame; information for blood pressure and cholesterol screening was attached to the first questionnaire. Reduction of CHD risk was measured at 7 months by reported changes in high-risk CHD behaviors, changes in health beliefs, and reported participation in blood pressure and serum cholesterol screenings.

No overall main effects of nursing interventions were demonstrated for health beliefs between the experimental or control groups except for sibling groups. There were greater decreases of alcohol and high-fat meat intake and higher rates for blood pressure and serum cholesterol screening by the experimental group receiving nursing intervention.

## COMPLICATIONS OF MYOCARDIAL INFARCTION

The more common complications of MI are dysrhythmias, cardiogenic shock, and congestive heart failure (see Chapter 31). Other complications include ventricular aneurysm, postmyocardial infarction syndrome, pericarditis (see Chapter 31), and embolism (see Chapter 32).

## Dysrhythmias

Dysrhythmias that may occur with an MI include sinus bradycardia and tachycardia, atrial fibrillation, ventricular dysrhythmias (PVBs, ventricular tachycardia, ventricular fibrillation), and all degrees of atrioventricular block. These dysrhythmias are discussed earlier in this chapter.

## Cardiogenic Shock

**Cardiogenic shock** is a shock state of primary cardiac origin. It is most frequently caused by MI, but it also may be the result of severe valvular dysfunction, intractable dysrhythmias, ruptured aortic aneurysm, obstruction to flow between cardiac chambers (atrial myxoma), severe congestive heart failure, massive pulmonary embolism, or cardiac tamponade.

### Pathophysiology

Shock occurs in approximately 15% of all patients hospitalized with the diagnosis of acute MI. When cardiogenic shock follows an MI, it is the result of severe left ventricular failure. So much myocardium has been damaged (usually more than 40% of the left ventricle) that inadequate systemic perfusion occurs secondary to low cardiac output. As the shock state progresses, there is decreased coronary artery perfusion, leading to the development of extended areas of cardiac muscle ischemia and necrosis throughout both ventricles. This progressive ischemia and infarction lead to further deterioration of left ventricular function, and if unchecked, to death. The mortality for cardiogenic shock is very high; 80% to 90% do not survive.

Severe organ hypoperfusion is characterized by metabolic acidosis (caused by anaerobic metabolism and lactate production), hypotension with a systolic blood pressure less than 90 mm Hg, tachycardia, urinary output less than 20 ml/hr, cold clammy skin, and mental confusion or lethargy.

### Management

Cardiogenic shock is a medical emergency that requires immediate intervention and constant attention to prevent irreversible cell damage and death. Therapy is aimed at correcting factors that contribute to decreased tissue perfusion, such as cardiac dysrhythmias, hypoxemia, and pain. Lactic acidosis may be partially compensated for through use of hyperventilation and buffering agents such as sodium bicarbonate. Invasive monitoring systems include catheters in the pulmonary artery, systemic artery, and urinary bladder. The left ventricular end-diastolic pressure is reflected in the pulmonary capillary wedge pressure, which is used as a guide to fluid therapy. Hypovolemia must be corrected carefully to avoid inducing a fluid overload—a situation that could result in acute pulmonary edema.

Vasopressors and cardiotonic agents are chosen to raise the systemic arterial pressure without increasing the workload (and therefore the oxygen requirements) of the myocardium. Dopamine and norepinephrine frequently are used to raise the systemic arterial pressure and cardiac output. Nitroprusside may be added in small amounts to decrease afterload and to reduce systemic vascular resistance. Every effort is made to maintain systemic arterial pressure at an absolute minimum of 60 mm Hg, preferably 90 mm Hg; total coronary artery collapse occurs at approximately 40 mm Hg.

Unless the shock state can be reversed with reinstatement of adequate cardiac output and tissue oxygenation, the patient will continue to deteriorate and death will ensue. Patients who require extensive pharmacologic support and in whom it is believed sufficient myocardium remains undamaged to allow for eventual recovery may benefit from initiation of intraaortic balloon counterpulsation (see Chapter 31).

## Ventricular Aneurysm

Aneurysms of the ventricular myocardium are predominantly a result of transmural MIs. Traumatically induced or congenitally formed aneurysms are rare. In 12% to 15% of persons sustaining MIs, the resultant myocardial necrosis and scar formation lead to a weakened ventricular wall. During systole the high pressures within the ventricle cause the weakened myocardium to bulge outward. Blood collects in the aneurysm or outpouched area and is a potential source of emobli. Cardiac output may be compromised. If symptoms develop, the patient usually has congestive heart failure and recurring dysrhythmias. Symptoms usually occur when 20% or more of the ventricle has been involved. Most ventricular aneurysms occur in the apex and anterior part of the heart.

Diagnosis usually is made in the presence of a ventricular gallop, persistent ST elevations after an MI, a chest x-ray film showing an enlarged left ventricle, and a paradoxical expansion of the aneurysmal sac during systole, which can be seen on fluoroscopy.

Treatment consists of a ventricular aneurysmectomy in which the aneurysm sac is excised and the ventricle sutured together. If the area excised includes part of a coronary artery, bypass surgery is performed simultaneously. Operative mortality is less than 5%.

## Postmyocardial Infarction Syndrome (Dressler's Syndrome)

A few patients develop a **postmyocardial infarction syndrome** approximately 1 to 6 weeks after an acute MI, characterized by pleural pain, joint pains, and fever. It is thought to be due to an autoimmune reaction to the myocardial necrosis. Aspirin usually is effective for the discomfort, and more severe symptoms usually respond quickly to a short intensive course of corticosteroids.

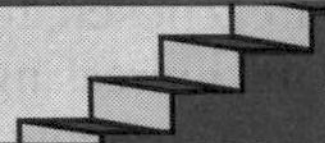

## CRITICAL PATHWAY Myocardial Infarction Without Complications

**DRG #: 122 Expected LOS: 7**

| | Admit to ICU<br>Day of Admission<br>Day 1 | Day 2 | Move Out of ICU<br>Day 3 |
|---|---|---|---|
| **Diagnostic Tests** | CBC, UA, SMA/18,* cardiac enzymes with isoenzymes q8hr × 3, PT/PTT, ECG, chest x-ray film | PT/PTT, ECG | CBC, PT/PTT, SMA/6,† ECG |
| **Medications** | IV, Heparin, IV analgesic; cardiac drugs (beta blocker, Ca++ blocker, nitrates, antiarrhythmics, diuretics, BP control); aspirin, stool softener, Rx for anxiety/sleep | IV, heparin, IV/PO analgesic; titrate cardiac drugs; aspirin, stool softener, Rx for anxiety/sleep | IV to saline lock, heparin, PO analgesic; titrate cardiac drugs; aspirin, stool softener, Rx for anxiety/sleep |
| **Treatments** | Cardiac monitor, $O_2$, I & O q8hr, VS and cardiopulmonary assessment q4hr, wt, ELS, Stat ECG with chest pain anytime | Cardiac monitor, $O_2$, I & O q8hr, VS and cardiopulmonary assessment q4hr, wt, ELS | Telemetry; titrate $O_2$, I & O q8hr, VS and cardiopulmonary assessment q8hr; wt, ELS |
| **Diet** | Low sodium, fat, and cholesterol; decaf drinks | Low sodium, fat, and cholesterol; decaf drinks | Low sodium, fat, and cholesterol; decaf drinks |
| **Activity** | Bed rest; bedside commode with help | Bed rest; to BR with help | Bed rest; up to BR; up in chair × 2 with help |
| **Consultations** | | Cardiac rehab | Cardiac rehab, ETT |

*Ca++*, Calcium channel; *CC*, cardiac catheterization; *disc*, discontinue; *ECHO*, echocardiography; *ELS*, elastic leg stockings; *ETT*, exercise thallium test; *PT*, prothrombin time; *PTT*, partial thromboplastin time; *SMA*, sequential multiple analysis; *UA*, urinalysis; *VS*, vital signs.

## QUESTIONS TO CONSIDER

- How do the described dysrhythmias differ in terms of ECG findings and therapy?
- How do the principles of automaticity and excitability relate to cardioversion/defibrillation?
- What is being done in your community to increase the public's awareness of risk factors for coronary atherosclerotic heart disease; how would you go about teaching the lay public about the health problem?
- Examine the chart of a patient who has had a myocardial infarction. What ECG changes did you note? What changes occurred in the serum enzyme levels? How do the changes you noted compare with the usual pattern for MI? What significance do these changes have for nursing interventions?
- You are called by your neighbor to come over because she thinks her husband should go to the doctor, but he says it is not necessary because he only has indigestion. You find him sitting up in a chair looking pale and sweating; pulse is 98/min. He says that he has a viselike pain in the upper abdomen. His wife says she wants to take him to an emergency care center. What decisions should you make concerning his care?

## CRITICAL THINKING ACTIVITIES

- Mr. Bradshaw, 80, is under your care on a general medical-surgical unit. He is in the hospital for diabetes and pneumonia. You know he has a history of sick sinus syndrome. Several hours into your shift you note that he is becoming more confused. How do you go about differentiating senility from tachycardia-bradycardia syndrome?
- You are caring for two men in room 526. Mr. Cole, 52, recently had an MI, and the cardiac monitor indicates he is having occasional PVCs. Mr. Rogers, 73, recovering from insertion of a pacemaker, is having occasional PVCs. Analyze the significance of each dysrhythmia in these two patients.

## CHAPTER SUMMARY

### CARDIAC DYSRHYTHMIAS

- An ECG is a graphic record of the electrical activity of the heart muscle. It is recorded on a grid that allows measurement of time and voltage.
- A normal cardiac complex consists of a P wave, a QRS

| Day 4 | Day 5 | Day 6 | Day of Discharge Day 7 |
|---|---|---|---|
| Room air oximetry, Holter | ETT, ECHO as indicated, PT/PTT | CC as indicated, PT/PTT | PT |
| IV saline lock, disc heparin, PO analgesic; titrate cardiac drugs; aspirin, stool softener, Rx for anxiety/sleep | IV saline lock, PO analgesic; titrate cardiac drugs; aspirin, stool softener, Rx for anxiety/sleep | Disc saline lock; adjust cardiac drugs for home; aspirin, stool softener, Rx for anxiety/sleep *Pre-CC:* Rx to reduce anxiety as indicated; IVs after CC | Adjust cardiac drugs for home; aspirin, stool softener, Rx for anxiety/sleep, disc IV |
| Telemetry, disc $O_2$; I & O q8hr, VS and cardiopulmonary assessment q8hr, ELS | Telemetry, I & O q8hr, VS and cardiopulmonary assessment q8hr, ELS | Disc telemetry, disc I & O, VS q12hr, wt; assess cardiopulmonary systems q12hr; ELS *Post CC:* assess drainage, VS, and neurocirculatory systems q 15 min × 4, q 30 × 4, q hr × 4, q4hr; pressure dressing and pack to CC site for 4 hr | VS q12hr; assess cardiopulmonary systems q12hr; remove ELS |
| Low sodium, fat, and cholesterol; decaf drinks | NPO for treadmill; low sodium, fat, and cholesterol; decaf drinks; NPO p̄ MN for CC except for Rxs | NPO for CC; continue with previous diet post nausea; force fluids | Low sodium, cholesterol |
| Up in room; walk in hallway with help × 2 | Up in room; walk in hallway with help × 4 | Bed rest post CC for 8 hr (lie supine, affected leg flat) | Ambulate in hallway; up ad lib |
| Cardiac rehab, dietary, social service | Cardiac rehab | Cardiac rehab | Cardiac rehab |

*Serum calcium, phosphorus, triglycerides, uric acid, creatinine, BUN, total bilirubin, alkaline phosphate, aspartate aminotransferase (AST) (formerly serum glutamic-oxaloacetic transaminase [SGOT]), alanine aminotransferase (ALT) (formerly serum glutamate pyruvate transaminase [SGPT]), lactic dehydrogenase (LDH), total protein, albumin, sodium, potassium, chloride, total $CO_2$, glucose.
†Serum sodium, potassium, chloride, total $CO_2$, glucose, BUN.

complex, and a T wave. The exact configuration varies according to the lead being recorded.

- Electrocardiographic signal averaging is a noninvasive, computerized method of analyzing standard ECGs.
- The mechanisms responsible for the genesis of dysrhythmias include altered automaticity, triggered activity, and reentry.
- Dysrhythmias originating in the sinoatrial node include sinus dysrhythmias, sinus tachycardia, sinus bradycardia, and sick sinus syndrome.
- Dysrhythmias originating in the atria include premature atrial beat, atrial tachycardia, atrial flutter, and atrial fibrillation.
- Dysrhythmias originating in the atrioventricular (AV) junction include premature junctional beat and junctional rhythms.
- Dysrhythmias originating in the ventricle include premature ventricular beat, ventricular rhythms and tachycardia, and ventricular fibrillation and standstill.
- Conduction abnormalities include AV block and bundle branch block.
- Treatment for cardiac dysrhythmias involves identification and elimination of the cause (if possible), drugs or electrical suppression of ectopic impulse initiation, and modalities to regulate heart rate (drugs, regulation of oxygen demand, artificial pacemakers).
- General nursing interventions for persons with dysrhythmias include promoting adequate cardiac output, activity and rest, tissue perfusion, comfort, relief of anxiety and a feeling of well-being, and patient/family learning.
- Artificial pacing may be by temporary or permanent pacemakers; the basic modes of pacing include fixed-rate mode and demand or standby mode. Complications include infection, dysrhythmias, and electrical interferences.
- Cardioversion and defibrillation are two methods for using electrical energy to convert a cardiac dysrhythmia to one that is more hemodynamically stable. Defibrillation is unsynchronized electrical countershock, whereas cardioversion synchronizes with the R wave to prevent accidental discharge during the ventricular vulnerable period.
- The automatic implantable cardioverter defibrillator (AICD) is an implanted device that automatically de-

livers a countershock upon sensing ventricular fibrillation.

### CARDIOPULMONARY RESUSCITATION

- Two life-threatening dysrhythmias are ventricular fibrillation and ventricular standstill; CPR must be initiated and maintained until definitive treatment is effective.
- Steps of basic life support include assessment of level of consciousness, opening of airway, initiation of artificial ventilation, assessment of circulation, and initiation of external cardiac compressions.

### CORONARY ARTERY DISEASE: CORONARY ATHEROSCLEROTIC HEART DISEASE

- Nonmodifiable risk factors for CAHD include advancing age, gender (males), race, and a positive family history of CAHD.
- Major modifiable risk factors for CAHD include hyperlipoproteinemia, hypertension, diabetes mellitus, and cigarette smoking; a diet high in cholesterol and saturated fats contributes to the risk.
- Behavioral and psychosocial influences are strongly correlated with the occurrence of CAHD.

### ANGINA PECTORIS

- Angina pectoris is chest pain caused by reversible myocardial ischemia. Treatment involves increasing myocardial blood and oxygen supply (with medications or surgery) and reducing myocardial oxygen demands. The most commonly used drugs for treating angina pectoris are vasodilators, beta-adrenergic blocking agents, and calcium channel blockers.
- Coronary artery bypass graft (CABG) consists of circumventing a coronary occlusion using a saphenous vein or internal mammary artery graft.
- An alternative to CABG for selected persons is percutaneous transluminal coronary angioplasty (PTCA). A balloon-tipped catheter is inserted into the coronary artery, and the balloon is inflated to rupture the atheromatous plaque.
- Intravascular stenting consists of maintaining the cylindric lumen of the coronary artery (after PTCA) by laser photocoagulation or radio frequency–induced heat.

### MYOCARDIAL INFARCTION

- Myocardial infarction is the result of prolonged myocardial ischemia, which causes irreversible cellular damage. The clinical consequences depend on the location of the coronary artery occlusion and the extent of necrosis.
- Diagnosis of MI is based primarily on the clinical picture, ECG findings, and elevation of serum enzyme levels. Medical interventions include promotion of improved coronary circulation and tissue oxygenation, relief of pain, and prevention of further tissue damage and complications.
- Thrombolytic agents to activate fibrinolytic processes to lyse the clot must be given within 3 to 6 hours of the initial infarction.
- Nursing interventions for MI include promoting oxygenation, tissue perfusion, adequate cardiac output, comfort, activity, nutrition, and elimination; providing rest; promoting relief of anxiety; and patient teaching. During cardiac rehabilitation, patients are encouraged to participate in a planned activity program.
- Complications of MI include dysrhythmias, cardiogenic shock, CHF, ventricular aneurysm, postmyocardial infarction syndrome, pericarditis, and embolism.

## REFERENCES

1. American Heart Association: *Heart facts,* Dallas, 1992, The Association.
2. American Heart Association: *Textbook of advanced cardiac life support,* Dallas, 1993, The Association.
3. Braunwald E: *Heart disease: a textbook of cardiovascular medicine,* ed 3, Philadelphia, 1988, WB Saunders.
4. Breithardt G, Borggrefe M: Recent advances in the identification of patients at risk of ventricular tachyarrhythmias: role of ventricular late potentials, *Circulation* 75:1091-1096, 1987.
5. Cox JL: Evolving applications of the maze procedure for atrial fibrillation, *Ann Thorac Surg* 55:578-580, 1993.
6. Fleg JL et al: Age-associated changes in the components of atrioventricular conduction in apparently healthy volunteers, *J Gerontol* 45(3):M95-M100, 1990.
7. Groer MW, Shekleton ME: *Basic pathophysiology: a holistic approach,* ed 4, St Louis, 1994, Mosby.
8. Guidelines for cardiopulmonary resuscitation and emergency cardiac care, *JAMA* 268(16):2184-2198, 1992.
9. Hopson JR, Hopson RC, Kerber RE: The role of energy and current successful defibrillation and cardioversion: C16 arrhythmias and conduction disturbances, *Cardiol Board Rev* 6(5):31-45, 1989.
10. Hurst JW: *The heart,* ed 6, New York, 1986, McGraw-Hill.
11. Kleiger ER et al: Decreased heart rate variability and its association with increased mortality after acute myocardial infarction, *Am J Cardiol* 59:256-262, 1987.
12. Misenski M: Pathophysiology of acute myocardial infarction: a rationale for thrombolytic therapy, *Heart Lung* 17:743-750, 1988.
13. Mueller RT et al: Painless myocardial infarction in the elderly, *Am Heart J* 119(1):202-204, 1990.
14. Pipilis A et al: Heart rate variability in acute myocardial infarction and its association with infarct site and clinical course, *Am J Cardiol* 67:1137-1139, 1991.
15. Purcell JA, Burrows SG: A pacemaker primer, *Am J Nurs* 85:553-568, 1985.
16. Runions J: A program for psychological and social enhancement during rehabilitation after myocardial infarction, *Heart Lung* 14:117-125, 1985.
17. Tyroler HA et al: Task force: environmental risk factors in coronary heart disease, *Circulation* 76(suppl I):1139-1144, 1987.
18. US Department of Health and Human Services, Public Health Service, Agency for Health Care Policy and Research: Clinical practice guideline: diagnosing and managing unstable angina, Rockville, Md, 1994.
19. Vatterott PJ et al: Signal-averaged electrocardiography: a new noninvasive test to identify patients at risk for ventricular arrhythmias, *Mayo Clin Proc* 63:931-942, 1988.

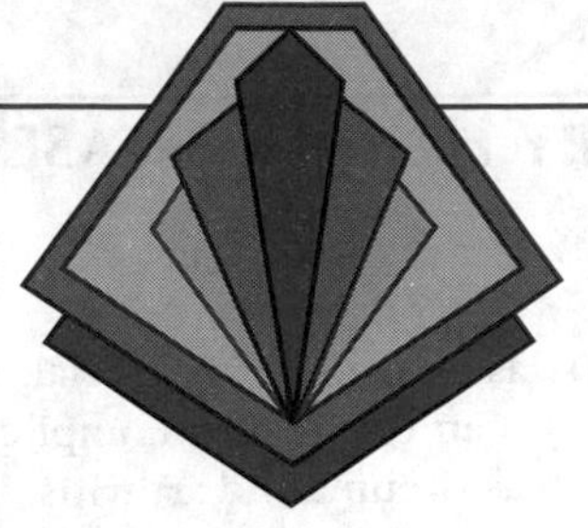

C H A P T E R 31

# Management of Persons With Valvular and Inflammatory Heart Disease and Congestive Heart Failure

*Terri Abraham*

## CHAPTER OBJECTIVES

***After studying this chapter, the learner should be able to do the following:***

1 Differentiate among the different inflammatory and valvular heart diseases.
2 Explain the pathophysiology and medical and nursing management of inflammatory heart diseases, valvular heart diseases, and congestive heart failure.
3 Plan care for a patient with congestive heart failure.
4 Develop a teaching plan for a patient undergoing cardiac surgery.
5 Describe the method and purpose for cardiopulmonary bypass used during some cardiac surgeries.
6 Describe preoperative and postoperative nursing care for the person undergoing cardiovascular surgery.

## KEY TERMS

acute pulmonary edema
alcoholic cardiomyopathy
annuloplasty
aortic regurgitation
aortic stenosis
backward heart failure
caged ball prosthetic valve
caged disk prosthetic valve
cardiac tamponade
cardiac transplantation
cardiogenic shock
cardiopulmonary bypass
cold cardioplegia
commissurotomy
digitalis
endocarditis
forward heart failure
heart failure
high output heart failure
intraaortic balloon pump (IABP)
left ventricular failure
low-output heart failure
mediastinitis
mitral regurgitation
mitral stenosis
mitral valve prolapse
myocarditis
percutaneous aortic balloon valvuloplasty
pericardial friction rub
pericardiocentesis
pericarditis
pulmonary regurgitation
pulmonary stenosis
rheumatic heart disease
right ventricular failure
stenting allograft
subacute bacterial endocarditis (SBE)
syphilitic cardiovascular disease
tilting disk prosthetic valve
tricuspid regurgitation
tricuspid stenosis
valve replacement
valvuloplasty
ventricular assist devices
xenograft

## EPIDEMIOLOGY OF HEART DISEASE

In the United States cardiovascular disorders cause more deaths than all other diseases combined. Nearly 66 million Americans (more than one in four persons) have some form of cardiovascular disease. In 1990, almost 1 million Americans died of heart and blood vessel disease. This figure represents almost as many deaths as from cancer, influenza, accidents, chronic obstructive pulmonary disease, and all other causes combined.[1]

The type of cardiovascular disorder that causes death varies with age. In the United States, congenital heart disease and closely related vascular disorders are responsible for disabling 25,000 newborn infants each year. The most common cause of death from heart disease after the age of 25 years is coronary atherosclerotic heart disease (CAHD).

Other cardiovascular disorders that cause substantial morbidity and mortality include hypertensive heart disease, rheumatic heart disease, and cerebrovascular disease. Fortunately, despite the discouraging statistics related to the incidence of cardiovascular disorders, there has been a steady reduction in mortality from cardiovascular disease. In the United States the past decade has witnessed a tremendous expansion in cardiovascular research and much progress has been made in preventing and treating cardiovascular disease. This reduction in mortality suggests an effective application of increased knowledge regarding the causes, diagnosis, treatment, and, most significantly, the prevention of heart disease.[3]

Although the exact pathogeneses of many types of heart diseases are not yet known, extensive epidemiologic studies are in progress in an attempt to delineate further preventive measures. Observational epidemiologic studies have identified numerous risk factors for cardiovascular disease. The implication is that with pharmacologic interventions and behavior modification, especially in regard to changes in life-style, the manifestations of cardiovascular disease may be decreased, delayed, or even eliminated.[7] Further definitive research protocols are now being developed to study the validity of these implications. At present it is believed that screening and public education can effect a significant reduction in the morbidity and mortality from cardiovascular disorders.

## CLASSIFICATION OF HEART DISEASE

Heart disease can be divided into two general groups, congenital and acquired. *Congenital* heart disease is caused by error in the embryologic development of the heart's structures. In *acquired* heart disease heart damage may occur because of inflammation, infection, chemical agents, or diminished blood supply. Onset may be sudden or gradual. For example, inflammation may cause scarring of heart valves, muscle, or outer coverings that can impair the heart's function. Any changes in the coronary vessels that supply the heart muscle can decrease its efficiency.

Heart disease can be classified according to a specific cause such as rheumatic fever, infective endocarditis, or hypertension. It also is classified according to anatomic changes such as valvular scarring. Progression of any of these diseases can lead to cardiac failure and cardiac dysrhythmias. These complications cause many of the symptoms commonly associated with heart disease, but with early diagnosis and treatment, these problems may be prevented or controlled.

## INFLAMMATORY HEART DISEASES

### PERICARDITIS

#### Etiology

Pericarditis can occur as a result of bacterial, viral, or fungal infection. It also can occur as a complication of a systemic disease such as rheumatoid arthritis, systemic lupus erythematosus, scleroderma, uremia, or myocardial infarction or as a result of trauma.

#### Pathophysiology

**Pericarditis** is an inflammatory process of the visceral and/or parietal pericardium. It can be acute or chronic and can spread from or to the myocardium. *Acute pericarditis* is further classified as fibrinous or exudative. The exudate that accompanies acute pericarditis may be serous, purulent, or hemorrhagic. When fluid accumulates in the pericardial sac, **cardiac tamponade** (compression of the heart) may occur, causing a decrease in venous return to the heart and a decrease in ventricular emptying, which can lead to cardiac failure. If not diagnosed and treated promptly, cardiac tamponade may result in shock and death. *Chronic pericarditis* can be constrictive or adhesive. If a constrictive band surrounds the heart, cardiac tamponade occurs.

#### Acute Pericarditis

A predominant clinical manifestation of acute pericarditis is a **pericardial friction rub** along with severe precordial chest pain, which may closely resemble that of acute myocardial infarction. The patient may complain of pain over the left shoulder (left trapezial ridge), which may radiate to the neck and down the left arm; it is intensified when the person is lying supine and is relieved by sitting. The pain also may intensify when the patient coughs, swallows, or breathes deeply. Dysphagia is commonly experienced.

Typically, the temperature is elevated and a leukocytosis of $10,000/mm^3$ to $20,000/mm^3$ is present. In the exudative form of acute pericarditis, the electrocardiogram (ECG) may show a bradycardia with low-voltage QRS complexes caused by attenuation of the pericardial fluid or an atrial fibrillation or flutter.

Symptoms of cardiac tamponade are listed in Box 31-1. Radiographs may show a pericardial effusion, although results of an echocardiogram are more diagnostic. If the

**BOX 31-1 Symptoms of Cardiac Tamponade**

- Diminished or absent point of maximal impulse
- Diminished heart sounds
- Tachycardia
- Paradoxical pulse
- Narrowed pulse pressure
- Distended neck veins (increased central venous pressure)

accumulation of pericardial fluid is gradual, the patient may notice little pain. As much as 1 L of clear or serosanguineous fluid may accumulate.

## Medical Management

If the underlying cause of the pericarditis is known, it is treated specifically, such as with antibiotics. Otherwise clinical symptoms of fever, malaise, and pain are treated.

If the pericardial effusion is small or absent, therapy for pericarditis is supportive, with administration of nonsteroidal antiinflammatory agents, including indomethacin. One of the main complications is recurrence after cessation of antiinflammatory drug therapy.

If the effusion is large, the physician may perform a **pericardiocentesis** (pericardial tap) to remove excess fluid. An approach below the sternum with resection of the xiphoid or a small anterolateral thoracotomy may be used. Occasionally, after removal of the fluid the physician will instill antibiotics directly into the pericardial sac. A pericardial fenestration (pericardial window) may be performed to provide continuous drainage of pericardial fluid. Complications include atelectasis and introduction of infectious agents. Corticosteroids may be administered to reduce inflammation.

## Chronic Pericarditis

Chronic constrictive pericarditis may result from fibrosis of the pericardial sac secondary to trauma or neoplastic disease. The thick fibrous pericardium tightens around the heart and decreases its efficiency as a pump.

Chronic constrictive pericarditis is three times more prevalent in men than in women. Patients may complain of dyspnea and fatigue and exhibit symptoms of congestive heart failure as a result of the diminished ability of the heart to function as a pump.

Removal of the pericardium (pericardiectomy) may be necessary to restore cardiac function. A median sternotomy (open) approach usually is performed, which provides good access to the pericardium, as well as to most cardiac structures in the event of unexpected problems. Postoperative care is similar to that for other heart surgery (see p. 861). Other measures to restore more efficient pumping include digitalization, diuretic therapy, and a low-sodium diet.

## Nursing Management

Monitor pulses and heart sounds for changes that suggest cardiac tamponade. Provide prescribed analgesics as appropriate. Give supportive care if fever and malaise are present. Teach patient and family members about the nature of the disease, medication regimen, and signs and symptoms of recurrent pericarditis.

# MYOCARDITIS

## Etiology/Pathophysiology

**Myocarditis** is an inflammatory disease of the myocardium that causes an infiltrate in the myocardial interstitium and injury to adjacent myocardial cells atypical of infarction. Myocarditis may be primary with an unknown etiology or secondary from an identifiable cause such as drug hypersensitivity or toxicity and infection. Very often this inflammatory process develops secondary to acute endocarditis or pericarditis. Myocarditis may be classified as acute (benign or fulminant) or chronic.

Infection can result in one of three ways: invasion of the myocardial tissue by organisms, production of toxins (diphtheria), or an autoimmune reaction (rheumatic fever, systemic lupus erythematosus). Worldwide the most frequent infectious agents are rickettsiae, bacteria, protozoans, and metazoans. In North America infection most often is caused by a virus. The most frequently implicated viral agent is picornavirus. Coxsackievirus B accounts for nearly 50% of the cases, and coxsackievirus A, echovirus, and poliovirus account for most of the remainder. Other viruses include influenza A and B, rubella, mumps, rabies, Epstein-Barr, and hepatitis. Myocarditis can be caused by several other infections, as well as by noninfectious agents. Recently the association of myocarditis with acquired immunodeficiency syndrome (AIDS) has been demonstrated; possible mechanisms include opportunistic viral infection or the human immunodeficiency virus (HIV) itself.

Symptom manifestation can be divided into two distinct phases: an acute viral phase and a chronic phase with symptoms unrelated to the viral infection. During the acute phase symptoms are flulike and include fever, lymphadenopathy, pharyngitis, myalgias, and gastrointestinal complaints. Hepatitis, encephalitis, nephritis, and orchitis also can occur.

The most common cardiac symptom during the acute phase is pericardial pain, which may be associated with a friction rub because the pericardium is so inflamed. Other cardiac manifestations include signs of congestive heart failure, syncope, pericardial effusion, and ischemia. ECG changes include ST-segment elevation, T-wave flattening or inversion, appearance of Q waves, and QT-interval prolongation. Ventricular ectopy can include multiple forms of premature ventricular beats and ventricular tachycardia. ECG abnormalities may disappear after recovery or persist for several years.

Preliminary laboratory findings are nonspecific, including elevation of the erythrocyte sedimentation rate, viral titers, and levels of various enzymes (such as lactic dehydrogenase, creatine kinase, and the transaminases). Mild to moderate leukocytosis with atypical lymphocytes may be seen. Chest radiographs may show the heart size normal or enlarged. In the fulminant form of acute myocarditis, pulmonary crackles may be auscultated. Although the diagnosis of myocarditis may be suspected clinically, it must be confirmed histologically by endomyocardial biopsy at a time when lymphocytic infiltration and myocyte damage are present (within 6 weeks of the acute illness).

### Medical Management

Patients with myocarditis often are treated with bed rest and digitalis to prevent heart failure and cardiogenic shock. Immunosuppression may be beneficial in reducing myocardial inflammation and in preventing irreversible myocardial damage. Medical therapy also involves treatment of the underlying disease with antibiotics, conventional therapy for congestive heart failure, and management of dysrhythmias.

### Nursing Management

Nursing care includes assessment of clinical function to determine baseline performance, followed by assessment for stabilization, improvement, or deterioration, which also may include concurrent congestive heart failure. Nurses participate in prebiopsy and postbiopsy care of patients. An important nursing diagnosis is anxiety as it relates to the sudden onset of heart disease and the fear of the biopsy itself. Providing emotional support and encouraging verbalization of feelings are important at this time.

Postbiopsy nursing diagnoses focus on the potential for injury that can occur during the procedure, such as hematoma or bleeding at the cannulation site, cardiac tamponade, or pneumothorax. A pressure dressing applied to the cannulation site remains in place for at least 24 hours. The site is inspected for bleeding, ecchymosis, or swelling. Shortness of breath, changes in breath sounds, dyspnea, and alterations in respiratory rate and pattern of breathing must be reported to a physician. A chest x-ray film may be obtained to rule out pneumothorax. Vital signs should be monitored closely to assess for continued hemodynamic stability.

Monitoring for congestive heart failure (see p. 875) is an important nursing consideration. Measures to decrease cardiac workload include frequent rest periods, provisions for a quiet environment, and the use of semi-Fowler's position. The nurse may administer medications to increase contractility and decrease preload and afterload.

If immunosuppressive therapy is administered, the patient is at higher risk for infection; modified protective isolation may be used. Aseptic technique must be adhered to during the care of the patient's indwelling lines and during dressing changes.

## ALCOHOLIC CARDIOMYOPATHY

### Etiology

When any form of ethanol (the chief substance in alcoholic beverages) is consumed in large quantities for more than 5 years, it has a direct toxic effect on cardiac tissue. Additives in alcoholic beverages also can create their own toxic effects. Persons with **alcoholic cardiomyopathy** usually are well-nourished; only 15% of these patients have thiamine deficiency, which is seen in many alcohol-dependent persons.

### Pathophysiology

The onset of alcoholic cardiomyopathy usually is gradual with nonspecific fatigue and dyspnea on exertion. Physical examination may reveal pulmonary crackles, cardiac murmur, edema, and increasing blood pressure and central venous pressure (CVP). ECG changes may show low-voltage QRS complexes and ST-segment abnormalities. Conduction defects and dysrhythmias also may occur. Symptoms progress to congestive heart failure and thromboemboli, but liver enlargement is not usually present.

Electron microscopic studies of heart tissue may show fatty degeneration of myocardial cells, and the heart itself may become flabby.[3] Chest radiographs show an enlarged heart with hypertrophic left ventricle and general pulmonary congestion.

### Management

Medical treatment is primarily symptomatic. Vasodilator therapy may be helpful to reduce oxygen demand on the heart, and prolonged bed rest is thought by some to reduce the size of the enlarged heart.

More than 10% of the adult population is involved in "heavy" alcohol consumption. It is therefore not surprising that alcoholic cardiomyopathy is such a major health problem. Nurses have an important role in stressing the need for moderation in ethanol intake and in teaching patients that complete abstention from alcohol may halt the progression or even reverse alcoholic cardiomyopathy. Nursing management is similar to that for myocarditis.

## INFECTIVE ENDOCARDITIS

Infective **endocarditis** is an infection of the endocardium and most often of the heart valves. The disease has commonly been classified in the past on the degree of acuteness. *Acute endocarditis* occurs rapidly, often on normal heart valves, and if untreated may cause death within days to weeks. Even with treatment the mortality is high.[3] **Subacute bacterial endocarditis (SBE)** develops more gradually, usually on previously damaged heart valves, and responds well to treatment.

### Etiology

The more recent method of classification of infective endocarditis is on the basis of the causative organism. The hemolytic streptococci are the major causative organisms, especially in the subacute form. Other major infective agents include staphylococci, such as *Staphylococcus aureus* and *S. epidermidis,* and enterococci. Major causes of underlying cardiac pathologic conditions include rheumatic valvular disease, congenital heart disease, and degenerative heart disease. In some cases, endocarditis is preceded by intrusive procedures such as dental procedures, minor surgery, gynecologic examinations, and insertion of indwelling urinary catheters or renal shunts. Other persons at high risk include those who "mainline" street drugs (inject drugs directly into the veins), because of the possibility of bacteremia from contaminated needles and syringes.

### Pathophysiology

A previously damaged cardiac valve or a ventricular septal defect produces turbulent blood flow, allowing bacteria to settle on the low-pressure side of a stenotic valve or a ventricular septal defect. The hallmark of endocarditis is the platelet-fibrin-bacteria mass on the valve constituting a vegetation. The organisms bombard the heart valves, become embedded in the valve matrix, and result in vegetative growths that may scar and perforate the leaflets. Endocarditis will develop in 1% to 4% of persons who have artificial heart valve implants.

Further risk results if the vegetative growths break free of the valves, enter the bloodstream, and cause emboli. If the vegetative emboli enter such organs as the spleen and kidney, abscesses may form.

The onset of SBE is gradual, and the patient reports malaise and general achiness. Low-grade fever is usually present, although a high fever usually occurs if *S. aureus* is the causative organism. Other frequently reported symptoms include arthralgias, arthritis, low back pain, myalgias, tenosynovitis, anorexia, weight loss, chest pain, and occasional hemoptysis. Physical examination may reveal splenomegaly, clubbing of the fingers, the presence of Osler's nodes (small, raised, tender, bluish areas) on fingers or toe pads, and small capillary hemorrhages (petechiae) in the conjunctiva, mouth, and extremities. On auscultation, murmurs may be audible over the cardiac valves. A normocytic normochromic anemia (see Chapter 34) is usually present.

### Prevention

*Primary prevention* includes correction of any underlying cardiac defect, if possible; measures to prevent bacteremia; good oral hygiene; and avoidance of intraarterial or intravenous catheters in persons with underlying cardiac disease. *Secondary prevention* includes early and vigorous treatment of any infections, especially streptococcal, and use of prophylactic antibiotics when persons with underlying cardiac disease undergo dental treatment or surgical procedure.

### Medical Management

#### Diagnostic tests

Blood cultures are essential to guide antibiotic therapy. Chest x-ray films are obtained to identify any cardiac abnormalities. Echocardiography demonstrates valvular vegetations greater than 3 to 4 mm in size. Cardiac catheterization may be performed to evaluate ventricular and valvular function.

#### Medication

In infective endocarditis the affected areas have impaired cellular or humoral host defenses; therefore the major aim of therapy is to eliminate all microorganisms from the vegetative growths and to prevent the development of complications. If symptoms go untreated for weeks or months, the incidence of embolic complications and progressive involvement of the heart valves are greatly increased. Therefore, after several specimens have been obtained for blood cultures and the infecting organism is identified, intravenous antibiotic therapy is initiated. It is important that antibiotic therapy be continued *for a prolonged time,* even after symptoms abate, to eradicate all organisms.

#### Treatment

When necessary, deteriorated heart valves are surgically replaced with prostheses (see p. 849).

## NURSING MANAGEMENT

### ♦ ASSESSMENT

### Subjective Data

Data to be collected to assess the patient with infective endocarditis include the following:

Feelings of general malaise, headache or fatigue
Anorexia
History of fever, weight loss, or night sweats
Pain in joints, back, or chest

### Objective Data

Objective data to be collected to assess the patient with infective endocarditis include the following:

Temperature elevation
Small capillary hemorrhages (petechiae) in conjunctiva, mouth, and extremities
Audible murmur over cardiac valves
Adventitious breath sounds and use of accessory muscles

### ♦ NURSING DIAGNOSES

Nursing diagnoses are determined from analysis of patient data. Nursing diagnoses for the patient with infective endocarditis may include but are not limited to the following:

| Diagnostic Title | Possible Etiologic Factors |
|---|---|
| Cardiac output, decreased | Valvular insufficiency |
| Tissue perfusion, altered: decreased | Decreased blood flow |
| Activity intolerance | Imbalance between oxygen supply/demand |
| Infection, high risk for | Decreased immune response |
| Knowledge deficit: self-management | Lack of exposure/recall |

### ♦ EXPECTED PATIENT OUTCOMES

Expected patient outcomes for the patient with infective endocarditis may include but are not limited to the following:

1. States that fatigue is decreased.
2. Demonstrates cardiac tolerance to increased activity (stable pulse and blood pressure).
3. Avoids becoming overly fatigued and stops activity when experiencing chest pain, dyspnea, lightheadedness, or faintness.
4. Avoids additional infection.
5. Practices preventive behaviors to minimize future episodes of endocarditis.

## INTERVENTIONS

### ♦ Promoting Cardiac Output

Continue monitoring for onset of systolic or diastolic murmurs, adventitious breath sounds, and use of accessory muscles. Crackles are associated with left-sided heart failure, and use of accessory muscles increases with worsening failure. Provide oxygen therapy as prescribed.

### Promoting Tissue Perfusion

Instruct patient to avoid becoming overly fatigued and to stop activity immediately in the presence of chest pain, dyspnea, and lightheadedness or faintness, which indicate decreased tissue perfusion. Blood pressure and pulse are assessed at rest, during activity, and immediately after activity to assess tolerance.

### Promoting Activity and Rest

Encourage active range of motion as tolerated, but provide passive range of motion at least twice daily. Rest periods of 30 to 60 minutes should be provided between all activities.

### Preventing Infection

Peak and trough drug levels are determined as prescribed to ensure therapeutic outcomes of antibiotic administration and to avoid potential negative outcomes. Renal function is assessed by monitoring BUN and creatinine levels, because many antibiotic agents have nephrotoxic effects. Patients should avoid others with infections.

### Facilitating Learning

Teach patient and family members to inform all physicians and dentists regarding the history of infective endocarditis so that appropriate antibiotic therapy can be given before intrusive procedures. Teach the patient to brush with a soft-bristled toothbrush and to floss appropriately to protect the gums and prevent caries. Good dental hygiene is of utmost importance to decrease the risk of a recurrent endocarditis.

## ♦ EVALUATION

To evaluate the effectiveness of nursing interventions, compare patient behaviors with those stated in the expected patient outcomes. Successful achievement of patient outcomes for the patient with infective endocarditis is indicated by the following:

1. States that fatigue is decreased.
2. Has stable pulse and blood pressure.
3. Stops activity when chest pain, dyspnea, lightheadedness, or fatigue occurs.
4. Has no additional infection.
5. Practices preventive behaviors to minimize future episodes of endocarditis.

## RHEUMATIC HEART DISEASE

**Rheumatic heart disease** is an acute inflammatory reaction. It may involve (1) the lining of the heart or endocardium (endocarditis), including the valves, resulting in scarring, distortion, and stenosis of the valves, (2) the heart muscle (myocarditis), or (3) the outer covering of the heart (pericarditis) where it may cause adhesions to surrounding tissues. The development of symptoms of chronic rheumatic heart disease in later life depends on the location and severity of the damage and other factors. Somewhat fewer than 10% of persons with rheumatic fever develop rheumatic heart disease, and about one half of those with rheumatic heart disease have *mitral stenosis* (see p. 841). It is possible for rheumatic fever and rheumatic heart disease with mild symptoms to go undiagnosed, or the disease may be subclinical with no noticeable symptoms. Thus the discovery of rheumatic heart disease is made years later. Careful recall of illness in childhood may include a recollection of "growing pains," confirming the likelihood that the patient had rheumatic fever during childhood.

Prophylactic penicillin is prescribed during acute episodes of rheumatic fever and for several years thereafter. Continuous antibiotic prophylaxis for life may be necessary for those persons with significant rheumatic heart disease. In persons with significant carditis during acute rheumatic fever, corticosteroids may be prescribed to decrease the cardiac inflammation. If congestive heart failure occurs during this period, bed rest, sodium and fluid restrictions, diuretics, and digoxin usually are prescribed. (For more information on rheumatic disease, see Chapter 65.)

## SYPHILITIC CARDIOVASCULAR DISEASE

### Epidemiology

**Syphilitic cardiovascular disease** usually occurs from 10 to 20 years after the primary syphilitic infection. Because the highest incidence of primary syphilis is among persons in their early 20s, persons with symptoms of syphilitic heart disease usually are older than 30 to 50 years of age.

### Pathophysiology

In cardiovascular syphilis the spirochetes attack the aorta, the aortic valve, and the heart muscle. The portion of the aorta nearest the heart usually is affected, and the elastic wall of the aorta becomes weakened and bulges. This bulge is known as an *aneurysm.* As the aneurysm grows, it may press on neighboring structures such as the intercostal nerves and cause pain. Aneurysms also may be present without symptoms. Evidence may be discovered on radiographic examination. There is a possibility that the aneurysm may rupture as it increases in size, and the person is encouraged to avoid strenuous activities that might cause a sudden increase in the pressure exerted against the bulging vessel. Surgical resection of the aneurysm sometimes is possible (see Chapter 32).

Syphilis also may attack the aorta more diffusely, causing *aortitis.* The aorta becomes dilated, and small plaques that contain calcium are laid down. There may be complaints of substernal pain associated with exertion caused by constriction at the orifices of the coronary arteries. Thrombi may develop along the aorta, and emboli may occur, resulting in severe complications such as myocardial infarction or cerebral emboli.

Spirochetes may attack the aortic valve, causing it to become scarred. This causes *aortic insufficiency,* and the person may have a bounding pulse and a high systolic blood pressure because of the extra effort demanded of the ventricles to pump blood into the systemic circulation. Heart failure eventually occurs.

### Prevention

It is the aim of health organizations and medical personnel to treat all persons with syphilis before they develop cardiovascular disease or any of the other complications of late syphilis. Primary syphilis can be arrested; however, once syphilis has affected the aorta and the valves of the heart, little can be done except to treat the patient symptomatically.

### Management

The use of penicillin in the treatment of the patient with cardiovascular syphilis is thought to possibly prolong life, because penicillin destroys any active organisms and permits healing to occur. Treatment at this stage, however, will not restore damaged aortic tissue or damaged aortic valves, and extensive scarring may occur. The person with syphilitic heart disease should be given guidance in planning activities of daily living and in selecting work that places the least possible burden on the damaged heart and aorta. In certain cases of aortic insufficiency, surgery is possible.

## CARDIOVASCULAR EFFECTS OF COCAINE ABUSE

Despite the widespread use of cocaine, medical investigation of its systemic effects in humans is sparse and frequently controversial. Cocaine is classified as a local anesthetic (see Chapter 24) and a sympathomimetic drug. It is a tropane alkaloid of the evergreen shrub, *Erythroxylon coca,* which is cultivated extensively in Bolivia and Peru. Crack cocaine is a heat-stable, freebase form of cocaine that is suitable for smoking and that causes an almost immediate, often intense, response.

Cocaine is metabolized rapidly in the liver by hepatic enzymes and in the bloodstream by plasma cholinesterase. Persons with impaired liver function are subject to the prolonged effects.[11] Depending on the urine acidity (enhanced excretion occurs with a decreased urine pH), 10% to 20% of the drug is excreted unchanged. Cocaine toxicity is characterized by generalized stimulation, including hyperthermia, acute agitation, tachycardia, hypertension, diaphoresis, and acidosis. Fatal pulmonary edema has been associated with cocaine intoxication, as well as seizure activity, cardiac dysrhythmias, and respiratory arrest with doses approaching 1 g.

Cardiovascular collapse is secondary to a combination of hyperthermia, hypoxia, acidosis, and CNS stimulation. Myocardial ischemia and infarction have been associated with cocaine use. The pathogenesis remains uncertain; hypotheses include coronary artery thrombosis, embolus, or spasms; increased thrombogenicity; and increased myocardial oxygen demand. Treatment options include beta blockers for ventricular dysrhythmias, nitrates and calcium channel blockers if coronary artery pathogenesis is suspected, and aspirin or other thrombolytic agents for acute ischemic events. (For further discussion on substance abuse and nursing implications, see Chapter 19.)

# VALVULAR HEART DISEASE

## PATHOPHYSIOLOGY

Healthy and competent heart valves facilitate unidirectional blood flow through the heart. The atrioventricular valves (AV) (mitral and tricuspid) prevent blood from flowing back into the atria from the ventricles during systole. During diastole, blood flows through the AV openings and passively opens the AV valves. During systole, the intense ventricular contractions force the valve flaps back into a closed position. Simultaneous contraction of the papillary muscles and the resultant tension on the chorda tendineae cordis prevent the valve flaps from being forced back into the atria (see Figure 29-1). The semilunar valves (SV) (aortic and pulmonic) prevent blood from flowing back into the ventricles from the aorta and pulmonary artery during diastole.

When the AV or SV valves become diseased, they may become stenosed and obstruct the normal flow of blood through the heart, or they may become insufficient and cause regurgitation or backflow of blood into the cardiac chamber from which the blood was previously propelled (Figure 31-1). Initially, the heart can compensate for the stenosed or insufficient valves through gradual hypertrophy of the myocardium. Medical treatment can facilitate a more effective compensation for the dysfunctional valve for years. However, if the stenosis or insufficiency worsens, congestive heart failure eventually will ensue, and valve replacement or repair is indicated.

## TYPES OF VALVULAR DISEASES

### Mitral Stenosis

#### Etiology

Two thirds of all persons with mitral stenosis are women. **Mitral stenosis,** the most common disease of the mitral

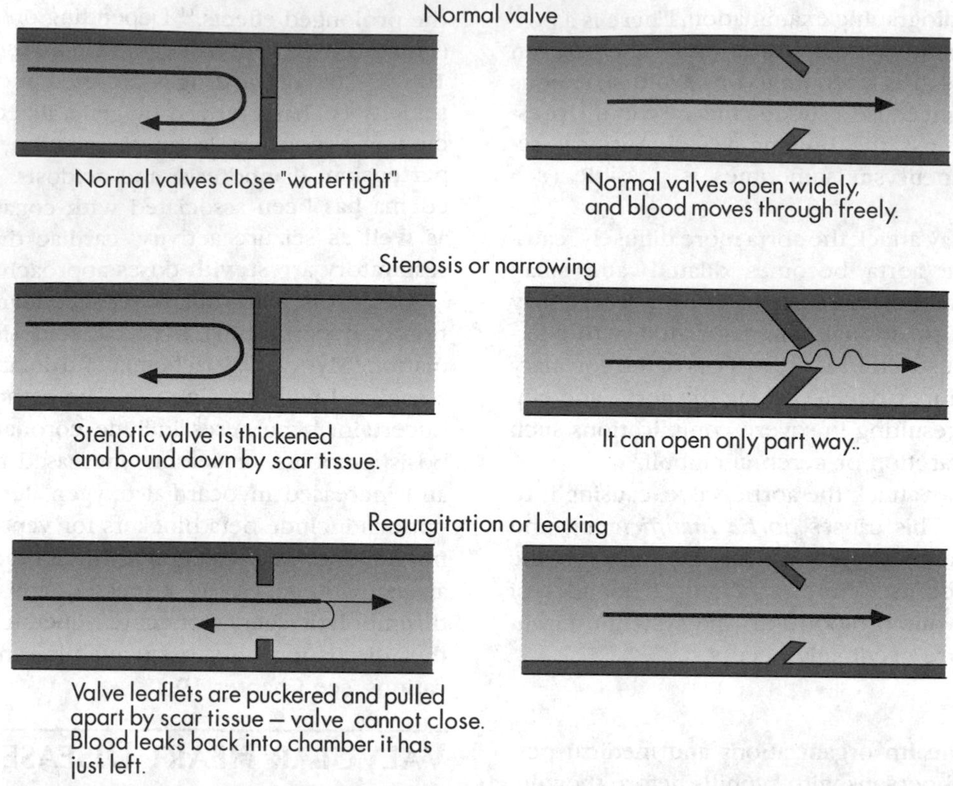


**FIGURE 31-1** Diseases of heart valves.

valve, is predominantly an acquired disease. Rheumatic fever, which is the primary cause of mitral stenosis, causes adhesions or fibrosis of the chorda tendineae cordis or commissures. Nonrheumatic causes include atrial myxomas, bacterial vegetation, thrombus formation, or calcification of the mitral annulus.

### Pathophysiology

Rheumatic fever can cause valve thickening by calcification and fibrous tissue formation. The valve leaflets or commissures are fused together and become stiffened, resulting in a progressively narrowed and immobile valve. The chorda tendineae cordis also will shorten and thicken, and the mitral orifice may decrease in size from its normal 4 to 6 $cm^2$ to less than 1 $cm^2$.[8] Progressive stenosis of the mitral aperture causes increasingly elevated left atrial pressures as a result of the additional trapped blood in the left atrium (Figure 31-2).

Hypertrophy of the left atrium develops as the heart compensates for the increased contractile strength needed to propel the blood through the stenosed valve. The elevated left atrial pressure causes pulmonary hypertension and congestion. As the stenosis becomes more severe, higher pulmonary artery pressures impede right ventricular function and precipitate right-sided heart failure. The left ventricle receives insufficient end-diastolic blood volumes, leading to a decrease in the cardiac output and eventual left ventricular atrophy.

To complicate further the hemodynamic status from inadequate left ventricular filling and pulmonary congestion, atrial fibrillation develops in 50% of persons with mitral stenosis. When the atria fibrillate, the normal end-diastolic "kick" from a unified atrial contraction is eliminated and again, less blood fills the ventricles for systole. Without an effective atrial contraction, blood may pool and stagnate in the atria, resulting in thrombus formation and possible arterial embolization to the brain, kidneys, spleen, and extremities.

Many persons with mitral stenosis remain symptom-free for approximately 20 years after the initial attack of rheumatic carditis. Symptoms may occur gradually or abruptly depending on the severity of the stenosis (Box 31-2). When acute symptoms develop, a rapid progression of the disease to death usually occurs between 5 to 10 years unless relieved by surgical intervention.

The principal symptom of mitral stenosis is *dyspnea*, which is largely the result of reduced compliance of the lungs. *Dyspnea on exertion* (DOE), *paroxysmal nocturnal dyspnea* (PND), and *orthopnea* occur as a result of pulmonary hypertension. These symptoms may be precipitated by emotional stress, respiratory infection, sexual intercourse, or atrial fibrillation with a rapid ventricular response. Some persons experience a dry cough, dysphagia, or bronchitis because of bronchial irritation as a result of an enlarged left atrium. Pressure exerted on the laryngeal nerve by an enlarged pulmonary artery

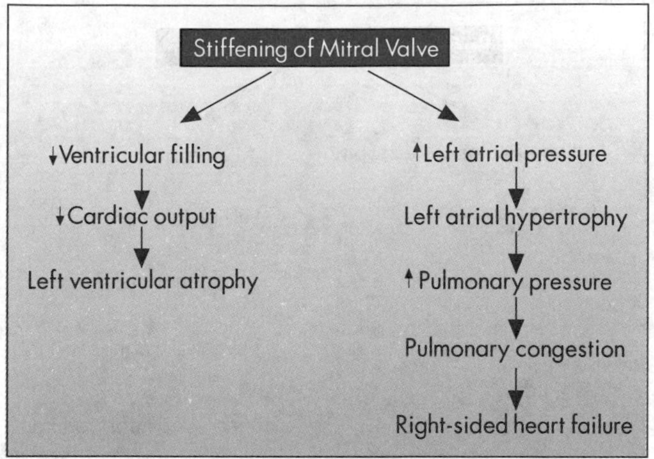


**FIGURE 31-2** Pathophysiology of mitral stenosis.

**BOX 31-2 Effect of Mitral Orifice Size on Emergence of Symptoms**

| | |
|---|---|
| >2.6 sq cm | No symptoms with exertion |
| 2.1-2.5 sq cm | Symptoms with extreme exertion |
| 1.6-2.0 sq cm | Symptoms with moderate exertion |
| <1.5 sq cm | Symptoms with minimal exertion |

From Hurst JW, editor: *The heart,* ed 7, New York, 1990, McGraw-Hill.

**TABLE 31-1 Findings in Valvular Heart Disorders**

| DISORDER | CHEST RADIOGRAPH | ELECTROCARDIOGRAM | ECHOCARDIOGRAM | CARDIAC CATHETERIZATION |
|---|---|---|---|---|
| Mitral stenosis | Left atrial enlargement<br>Mitral valve calcification<br>Right ventricular enlargement<br>Prominence of pulmonary artery | Left atrial hypertrophy<br>Right ventricular hypertrophy<br>Atrial fibrillation | Thickened mitral valve<br>Left atrial enlargement | Increased pressure gradient across valve<br>Increased left atrial pressure<br>Increased PCWP<br>increased right heart pressure<br>Decreased CO |
| Mitral regurgitation | Left atrial enlargement<br>Left ventricular enlargement | Left atrial hypertrophy<br>Left ventricular hypertrophy<br>Atrial fibrillation<br>Sinus tachycardia | Abnormal mitral valve movement<br>Left atrial enlargement | Mitral regurgitation<br>Increased atrial pressure<br>Increased LVEDP<br>Increased PCWP<br>Decreased CO |
| Aortic stenosis | Left ventricular enlargement<br>Aortic valve calcification<br>May have enlargement of left atrium, pulmonary artery, right ventricle, right atrium | Left ventricular hypertrophy | Thickened aortic valve<br>Thickened ventricular wall<br>Abnormal movement of aortic leaflets | Increased pressure gradient across valve<br>Increased LVEDP |
| Aortic regurgitation | Left ventricular enlargement | Left ventricular hypertrophy<br>Tall R waves<br>Sinus tachycardia | Left ventricular enlargement<br>Abnormal mitral valve movement<br>Increased movement of ventricular wall | Aortic regurgitation<br>Increased LVEDP<br>Decreased arterial diastolic pressure |
| Tricuspid stenosis | Right atrial enlargement<br>Prominence of superior vena cava | Right atrial hypertrophy<br>Tall peaked P waves<br>Atrial fibrillation | Abnormal valvular leaflets<br>Right atrial enlargement | Increased pressure gradient across valve<br>Increased right atrial pressure<br>Decreased CO |
| Tricuspid regurgitation | Right atrial enlargement<br>Right ventricular enlargement | Right ventricular hypertrophy<br>Atrial fibrillation | Prolapse of tricuspid valve<br>Right atrial enlargement | Increased atrial pressure<br>Tricuspid regurgitation<br>Decreased CO |

*CO,* Cardiac output; *LVEDP,* left ventricular end-diastolic pressure; *PCWP,* pulmonary capillary wedge pressure.

causes hoarseness. Excessive fatigue and weakness occur as a result of decreased cardiac output. Other symptoms include peripheral and facial cyanosis. Hemoptysis, usually a late sign, is due to the rupture of a bronchial vein. Eventual right-sided heart failure will lead to jugular vein distention, pitting edema, and hepatomegaly.

Diagnosis of mitral stenosis is established by clinical symptoms, such as an opening snap (OS), created by the forceful opening of the mitral valve, followed by a diastolic rumbling. This diastolic rumbling or murmur results from increased velocity of blood flow that narrows after left ventricular contraction. However, with a severely calcified valve, the diastolic murmur is absent. ECG changes indicate right ventricular hypertrophy, and chest x-ray films show left atrial enlargement. Mitral stenosis also can be diagnosed with a cardiac catheterization (see Chapter 29) to determine the extent of stenosis. The catheterization will provide information on the cardiac output, valve leaflet function, and elevated pulmonary artery pressures (Table 31-1). The most sensitive and noninvasive diagnostic indicator is the echocardiogram, which will show an impedance of flow, fusion of valve leaflets, and poor leaflet separation during diastole.

## Mitral Regurgitation

### Etiology

**Mitral regurgitation** occurs more commonly in men than in women. It also is the most prevalent lesion in patients who have heart failure with active rheumatic carditis. Similar to mitral stenosis, rheumatic heart disease is the predominant cause of mitral regurgitation, but there are many other factors, both acquired and congenital, that contribute to its cause. **Mitral valve prolapse** is a form of mitral insufficiency seen most often in thin, young women; it often is symptomless.[9] Weakness, rupture, or fibrosis of a papillary muscle secondary to ischemic coronary artery disease, ventricular aneurysm, or myocardial infarction can cause mitral regurgitation. Papillary muscle dysfunction allows the valve leaflets to flop in the direction of the left atrium during systole, and the blood flows backward. Other acquired factors include trauma and dysfunction of a prosthetic mitral valve. A person with idiopathic hypertrophic subaortic stenosis (IHSS) can develop mitral regurgitation as a result of displacement of the anterior leaflet of the mitral valve during systole. Bacterial endocarditis may cause erosion of the cusps or chorda tendineae cordis, resulting in mitral regurgitation.

### Pathophysiology

In chronic mitral insufficiency or regurgitation a variable amount of blood from the left ventricle is shunted back through the mitral orifice to the left atrium. This backflow of blood will cause both the left atrium and left ventricle to dilate and hypertrophy. In response to increasing preload and left atrial pressure, the pulmonary venous and arteriolar pressures also rise and eventually cause right-sided heart failure (Figure 31-3). As the ventricle hypertrophies, it becomes dysfunctional and the cardiac output decreases. Concurrently, the left atrium is often fibrillating, diminishing the cardiac output even further.

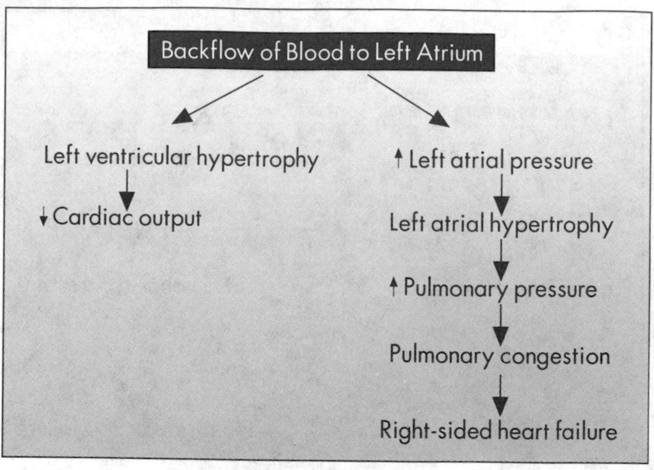


**FIGURE 31-3** Pathophysiology of mitral regurgitation.

In persons with mitral regurgitation, *fatigue* and *weakness* related to a decreased cardiac output are the predominant complaints. Right-sided heart failure with its sequelae of hepatic congestion, edema, ascites, and distended neck veins occurs in severe mitral regurgitation. Some persons experience palpitations (from atrial fibrillation) or paroxysmal nocturnal dyspnea.

In *acute* mitral regurgitation, progressive *dyspnea on exertion* and frequent *pulmonary edema* from an elevated left atrial pressure are the primary symptoms. The atrial pressure is transmitted immediately to the pulmonary veins, causing the congestive symptoms. Because the ventricle has not yet hypertrophied, the cardiac output remains sufficient and the fatigue is not a problem. Although persons with mitral regurgitation commonly have atrial fibrillation, thrombus formation in the atria is less common than with mitral stenosis because of backflow and resultant turbulence of blood.

The diagnosis of mitral regurgitation is made by the presence of clinical symptoms and auscultation of a blowing, high-pitched systolic murmur and third heart sound. The first heart sound ($S_1$) may not be heard, depending on the severity of regurgitation. A chest x-ray film reveals left atrial enlargement and occasional left ventricular dilation. ECG tracings show left ventricular hypertrophy and, less commonly, right ventricular hypertrophy (see Table 31-1). The echocardiogram may identify mitral valve cusp prolapse, ruptured chorda tendineae cordis, and enlargement of the left atrium and left ventricle. A vectorcardiogram indicates left ventricular hypertrophy. Definitive diagnosis is made by a cardiac catheterization (see Chapter 29) or left ventricular angiography, which will assess left ventricular function and the degree of regurgitation.

## Aortic Stenosis

### Etiology

Aortic valvular disease is less common than mitral disease and occurs in about 25% of all persons with chronic valvular heart disease. Eighty percent of adults with aortic stenosis are men.

**Aortic stenosis** can be rheumatic in origin inasmuch as myocarditis invades the valve, causing edema, inflammation, formation of granulation tissue, scarring, and, finally, fusion of the leaflets. Rheumatic aortic stenosis is almost always concomitant with rheumatic disease of the mitral valve. Calcium deposits in aortic valves of elderly persons also cause aortic stenosis and is called idiopathic calcific aortic stenosis.

Congenital valvular disease or malformation is the predominant etiologic factor in aortic stenosis. A congenitally deformed valve may remain symptomless for several years; however, it is more susceptible to bacterial endocarditis, rheumatic fever, and calcification.

### Pathophysiology

When the aortic valve becomes stenosed, thus obstructing left ventricular outflow during systole, left ventricular hypertrophy develops as a compensatory mechanism to continue pumping the same blood volume through the narrowed opening. As the stenosis progresses and compensatory mechanisms are no longer effective, cardiac output decreases. The left atrium cannot empty adequately, and thus the pulmonary system becomes congested. The hypertrophied left ventricle elevates myocardial oxygen needs and at the same time compresses the coronary arteries at a pressure exceeding coronary perfusion pressure. Thus myocardial oxygen needs increase and the supply decreases. This phenomenon gives rise to the myocardial ischemia and angina that are characteristic of more severe aortic stenosis. Eventually, right-sided heart failure will ensue (Figure 31-4).

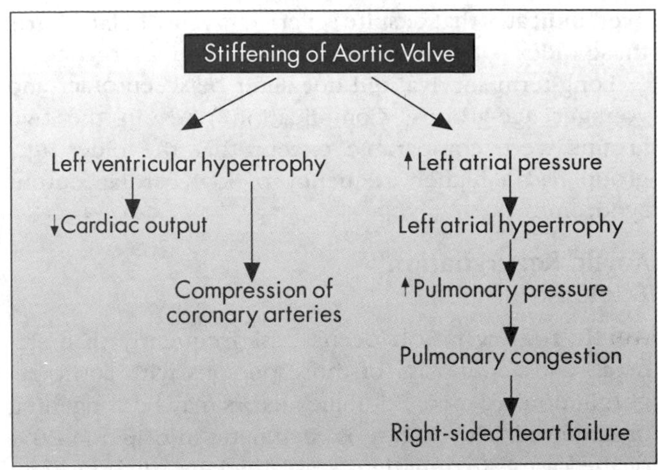


**FIGURE 31-4** Pathophysiology of aortic stenosis.

Aortic stenosis rarely becomes significantly debilitating until the aortic orifice is about one third its normal size.[8] Symptoms occur late in the disease even with severe stenosis, because the hypertrophied left ventricle is able to generate pressures strong enough to maintain an adequate cardiac output and because the mitral valve prevents the high intraventricular pressures from affecting the atrium and pulmonary vasculature. When the mitral valve also is diseased, the onset of symptoms may be more rapid and may be compounded.

Gradually increasing obstruction without clinical symptoms usually occurs until 40 to 50 years of age in most persons. There are three characteristic symptoms of aortic stenosis: *exertional dyspnea, angina pectoris,* and *exertional syncope.* Exertional dyspnea results from diminished cardiac reserve and elevation of the pulmonary capillary pressures. Angina pectoris (see Chapter 30) is secondary to diminished coronary perfusion and increased myocardial oxygen needs. Exertional syncope is caused by a decline in arterial pressure secondary to vasodilation in exercising muscles and a fixed cardiac output.

Other symptoms that occur only in the late stages of the disease include fatigue, weakness, orthopnea, paroxysmal nocturnal dyspnea, and pulmonary edema. Symptoms of right-sided heart failure (i.e., hepatomegaly, atrial fibrillation, systemic venous hypertension) usually are end-stage symptoms. If aortic stenosis goes untreated, the survival rate is 1.5 to 3 years.

Aortic stenosis is diagnosed by a harsh, rough, midsystolic murmur and a systolic thrill over the aortic area, by clinical symptoms, and by cardiac catheterization and angiography (see Table 31-1).

### Aortic stenosis in elders

Degenerative aortic stenosis is the most common valve disorder in adults. The incidence of aortic valve stenosis appears to be increasing in correlation with the increasing average age of the population. In the past decade there has been an increase in the number of cardiac operations performed on patients 70 years of age and older despite the higher but acceptable perioperative mortality and morbidity in this population.

A study by Olsson et al[13] indicated that despite the poorer preoperative condition of patients older than 80 years who undergo aortic valve replacement for aortic stenosis, a favorable postoperative course, similar to that of younger age-groups, can be expected. The total mortality rate was higher in the older group because of a large number of early deaths, which could reflect the poorer preoperative condition of this group mainly because of more advanced heart failure. Patients in the older age category tend to be offered surgery at a later stage of their disease. The postoperative outcome, however, indicates that despite severe left ventricular failure, these older patients benefited from surgical treatment.

Long-term survival did not differ between older and younger age-groups. Complication rates in the two groups were comparable except that the older age-group had a higher frequency of low cardiac output syndrome.

## Aortic Regurgitation

### Etiology

**Aortic regurgitation** occurs less frequently than stenosis, and about 75% of those persons with aortic regurgitation are men. Etiologic factors may be congenital or acquired. The disease is rheumatic in origin in 80% of the cases. Rheumatic disease thickens, deforms, and contracts the valve leaflets. Dilation of the annulus also may occur and produce insufficiency. In persons with isolated aortic regurgitation (i.e., without associated mitral disease) rheumatic heart disease does not play such a prominent causal role.

Syphilis is a rarely seen cause of dilation of the annulus and widening of the commissures. Fewer than 5% of the cases of aortic insufficiency in the United States are related to syphilis. Bacterial endocarditis can cause bacterial vegetation on valve leaflets, which initiates the inflammatory response and can cause erosion of the valve.

Marfan's syndrome is another etiologic factor related to aortic regurgitation. As a generalized, systemic disease of connective tissue, it can cause necrosis of the aorta, dilation of the aortic ring, and aneurysm formation, thus causing insufficiency. Another cause is congenital malformation, which, as with aortic stenosis, renders the aortic valve more susceptible to endocarditis and rheumatic fever and can thus cause aortic insufficiency.

### Pathophysiology

When the aortic valve is deformed congenitally or by infectious processes, the leaflets may not close properly and the annulus may be dilated, loose, or deformed. This allows a regurgitation of blood from the aorta back into the left ventricle during diastole. The ventricle dilates and hypertrophies with this greater volume of blood and thus compensates with a more forceful and rapid ejection (Figure 31-5).

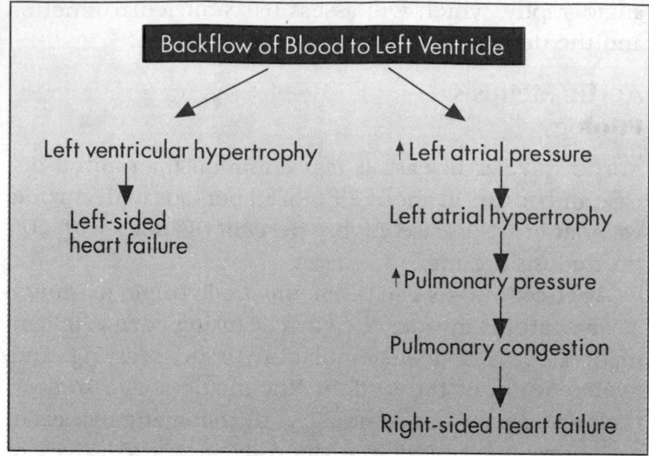


**FIGURE 31-5** Pathophysiology of aortic regurgitation.

Studies have indicated that more than 50% of the left ventricular ejection volume must reflux into the left ventricle before a person has symptoms. Because of this cardiac compensation, symptoms in uncomplicated aortic insufficiency are rare until left ventricular failure is imminent.

Persons with aortic regurgitation remain symptom-free for years because of the myocardium's ability to hypertrophy. Symptoms usually begin with an awareness of the heartbeat, which is uncomfortable and more prominent on the left side-lying position. *Sinus tachycardia* may occur with exertion or stimulation, and *premature ventricular beats* occur. Exertional dyspnea secondary to cardiac decompensation, orthopnea, paroxysmal nocturnal dyspnea, and diaphoresis always indicate impending left-sided heart failure. Angina may develop at rest or with exertion secondary to myocardial ischemia or pounding on the chest wall by the heart. End-stage disease is indicated by hepatomegaly, ankle edema, and ascites.

Diagnosis is made from clinical findings of a soft, blowing aortic diastolic murmur and a widened pulse pressure. The ECG will indicate left ventricular hypertrophy with ST-segment depression and T-wave inversion. Cardiac catheterization will determine the severity of the valve disease (see Table 31-1). Echocardiogram indicates the amount of ventricular volume overload, the stroke volume, and ejection fraction. Angiography may be used to determine the severity of coronary artery disease.

## Tricuspid Stenosis

### Etiology

**Tricuspid stenosis** is a more uncommon valvular disease that occurs four to five times more frequently in women than in men. This lesion rarely is isolated and usually occurs with mitral stenosis or aortic stenosis but generally not with mitral regurgitation. Rheumatic heart disease is the usual cause of tricuspid stenosis.

### Pathophysiology

The fusion of the commissures and shortened and fused chorda tendineae cordis cause the tricuspid orifice to narrow. Blood is blocked returning to the heart. The systemic pressure is increased as a result of the obstruction, and there is a reduced right ventricular output.

Symptoms of right-sided heart failure in the patient with tricuspid stenosis include *hepatomegaly* and *jugular vein distention,* as well as *cardiac cirrhosis* and resulting jaundice. The decrease in blood volume returned to the heart results in decreased cardiac output and causes fatigue, weight loss, and hypotension.

### Tricuspid Regurgitation

**Tricuspid regurgitation** is uncommon because normal valve leaflets are very small and valve closure is primarily reliant on the contraction of the valvular ring. Consequently, tricuspid insufficiency caused by rheumatic, carcinoid, or bacterial destruction of the leaflets is rare. Right ventricular dilation from any cause may dilate the tricuspid ring or displace the papillary muscles and cause regurgitation. An insufficient tricuspid valve allows blood to flow back into the right atrium, causing venous engorgement and diminishing right ventricular output (see Table 31-1).

### Pulmonary Stenosis

**Pulmonary stenosis** is a rare valvular disease that usually is congenital in origin, although it may be caused by cancer or rheumatic fever. In pulmonary stenosis the pulmonic valve narrows, causing less blood to flow forward. As a result, blood flows back into the right ventricle and right atrium. Both the right ventricle and atrium hypertrophy to compensate for the volume of blood received. Symptoms of pulmonary stenosis include a harsh systolic murmur, fatigue, and dyspnea on exertion. As the condition worsens, the patient will have symptoms of right-sided heart failure (p. 872) (hepatomegaly, ascites, and edema).

### Pulmonary Regurgitation

**Pulmonary regurgitation** also is a rare condition caused by infective endocarditis, tumors, or rheumatic fever. The pulmonic valve leaflets become incompetent and fail to close. Blood flows back into the right ventricle during systole. The right ventricle and right atrium hypertrophy. The patient will exhibit symptoms of right-sided heart failure similar to those of pulmonary stenosis.

## MEDICAL MANAGEMENT

### Diagnostic Tests

Diagnostic tests for valvular diseases are described in the previous sections under each type of valve dysfunction and also are summarized in Table 31-1.

### Medication

Signs of heart failure are treated with diuretics (see p. 874) and vasodilator therapy, including angiotensin converting enzyme (ACE) inhibitors. Symptomatic improvement usually is only temporary. Digitalis therapy is given when atrial fibrillation occurs. Antibiotic therapy with intramuscular benzathine penicillin G is prescribed if endocarditis is present. Salicylates are recommended for symptomatic relief of arthralgia, arthritis, or severe pericardial pain. Nitroglycerin relieves concurrent angina. Administration of steroids is not advisable because of potential tissue friability, which makes surgery more difficult. Anticoagulant therapy usually is not necessary until end-stage heart disease; it may be given then to prevent emboli from blood turbulence.

### Treatment

Medical therapy is primarily pharmacologic. Oxygen is prescribed when cardiac output is diminished.

For a narrowed aortic valve orifice **percutaneous aortic balloon valvuloplasty** may be performed. It is indicated for patients with critical aortic stenosis who are high-risk surgical candidates (pulmonary disease, renal insufficiency, coronary artery disease, and advanced age). The procedure consists of insertion of a vensus sheath through the femoral artery up to the heart with use of cardiac catheterization techniques (see Chapter 29). The sheath is advanced across the stenotic aortic valve to the ventricle. For balloon dilation an exchange guidewire is advanced through the catheter to the ventricle. The dilation balloon catheter is then advanced over the wire and across the aortic valve. The balloon is repeatedly inflated with a combined solution of contrast medium and saline until the "waist" produced in the balloon by the calcified aorta disappears. After the final balloon inflation, the balloon catheter is removed.

Measurements of cardiac output, aortic valve gradient, and resting right and left heart hemodynamics are taken throughout the procedure. After the procedure, direct pressure must be applied for 15 to 30 minutes, followed by application of a pressure dressing or sandbags over the arterial site to prevent hemorrhage or hematoma. Continuing bed rest, mobilizing the affected limbs, and encouraging deep breathing to prevent atelectasis are important, especially for elderly persons. Volume depletion is a significant concern because of blood loss from the catheter and fluid restriction before the procedure. In addition, a diuretic effect can occur because of the dye, which creates increased left ventricular function and cardiac output. Most patients remain in the intensive care unit 24 to 48 hours after aortic balloon valvuloplasty.

### Diet

Because most patients with valvular disease eventually show symptoms of congestive heart failure, a sodium-restricted diet is prescribed (see p. 881).

### Activity

Physical activities that produce fatigue are restricted. With advanced disease, bed rest or sitting position can help to increase oxygen supply and facilitate breathing.

## SURGICAL MANAGEMENT

When physical limitations become significant despite appropriate medical therapy, surgical intervention is inevitable. Cardiac valves may be *repaired* or *replaced* depending on the severity and type of valvular dysfunction.

**BOX 31-3 Types of Valve Repair**

**ANNULOPLASTY**
Repair of ring or annulus of incompetent or diseased valve

**VALVULOPLASTY**
Repair of valve, suturing of torn leaflets

**COMMISSUROTOMY**
Dilation of valve; repair of a leaflet or commissure, fibrous bond or ring

## Valve Repair

Cardiac valves can be repaired by annuloplasty, commissurotomy, or valvuloplasty (Box 31-3).

### Annuloplasty

**Annuloplasty** is a procedure to reduce an enlarged annulus (fibrous ring surrounding the valve). The procedure involves the use of a prosthetic ring that is sutured into the circumference of the mitral or tricuspid annulus. The stitches are pulled together toward the prosthesis, reducing the size of the valve orifice.

### Valvuloplasty

**Valvuloplasty** is direct suture repair of torn leaflets or clefts by open heart surgery in which cardiopulmonary bypass is performed. The advantages of operative valve repair over valve replacement include (1) higher survival rates, (2) fewer cardiac complications (especially thromboembolism), (3) lower operative mortality and morbidity, (4) potential improvement in left ventricular function, (5) reduced need for anticoagulation, and (6) lower cost. Mitral valvuloplasty has gained increasing acceptance as the surgery of choice for mitral regurgitation, including cases of rheumatic etiology. A different form of valvuloplasty is *percutaneous aortic balloon valvuloplasty* (see p. 847), a nonsurgical procedure for aortic valve repair.

### Commissurotomy

*Mitral* **commissurotomy** is the separation or incision of the stenosed valve leaflets at their borders or commissures. Two techniques are used for a commissurotomy—open or closed. Controversy exists over the two methods, with an open commissurotomy being the procedure of choice.

An *open* commissurotomy usually is performed through a median sternotomy or a right anterolateral thoracotomy incision. This allows for proper visualization of the mitral valve. Cardiopulmonary bypass is used, and after the incision of the left atrium, the valve is inspected and the atrial thrombus removed.

The commissures are then incised with a scalpel, and new mobilized leaflets are attached to the chorda tendineae cordis. Disadvantages of this approach include those associated with open heart surgery, that is, difficult cannulation during cardiopulmonary bypass and clotting problems. The advantages include fewer thrombotic and embolic complications and fewer atrial tears with resultant hemorrhage. If the valve disease appears to be so advanced that replacement is indicated, the heart is already open.

A *closed* commissurotomy (without bypass) is performed through a left posterolateral thoracotomy. The fifth rib is removed to prepare for a closed or open operation. Some closed commissurotomies are performed in the fourth and fifth interspace with a transection of a rib, if necessary. After the incision is made, the atrium is palpated to detect any thrombi. If a thrombus is present, the procedure is converted to an open procedure to remove the clot. Otherwise, the surgeon inserts a finger through a small incision, dividing the papillary muscle longitudinally from the apex toward the base. The atrium is digitally examined for thrombi, and the valve is examined for calcium particles. Some surgeons may digitally open the fused commissures and use a dilator to open the valve and relieve the stenosis. The advantages of the closed approach include a shorter operating time, greater simplicity, and less blood replacement. Systemic emboli, atrial wall tears, inadequate alleviation of the stenosis, and mitral regurgitation are risks of this method of commissurotomy.

One major advantage of mitral valve repair over a mitral replacement is the mortality rate. The operative mortality for a commissurotomy is 1% to 2%, compared with 10% for a mitral valve replacement.[5]

## Valve Replacement

### Replacement procedures

**Valve replacement** is considered when the valve is so stenosed and calcified that repair would not achieve long-term relief of obstruction. Variables that affect the results of the valve replacement include the patient's general clinical condition and level of myocardial functioning before surgery and the type of valve used.

The heart usually is approached by a median sternotomy. Cardiopulmonary bypass (see p. 857) is used in an open procedure. The diseased valve leaflets are excised at the annulus, and the remaining annuli are sized with an obturator. The loose chordae are excised to avoid their becoming tangled in the new valve, and the prosthetic valve is sutured into the new annulus. Although the mortality rate with an aortic valve replacement is less than 5%, it is greater for the mitral valve. Risk factors include physiologic and chronologic age, chronicity, types of valvular lesion, and left ventricular function. Valvular replacement surgery increases mortality in persons older than 70 years of age.[12] (See Research box, p. 849.)

Recently, surgical treatment for atrial fibrillation has

## RESEARCH

Nair CK et al: Ten years experience with mitral valve replacement in the elderly, *Am Heart J* 124:154-159, 1992.

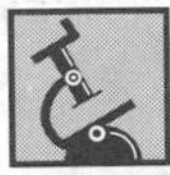

In this study of mitral valve replacement in elders, multivariate analysis of the data revealed a perioperative mortality rate of 15% for the sample of 126 patients and 12% when emergency surgery was excluded. For the purpose of this study, the term *elderly* was designated as 70 years or more. The data also revealed a higher perioperative mortality rate when compared in general with younger patients. Predictors of perioperative mortality in elders included coronary artery disease, female gender, elevated mean pulmonary artery pressure, and prolonged time on cardiopulmonary bypass in the presence of aortic calcification. During a 4-year follow-up, mortality was significantly higher for elders than for younger patients, especially during the first 2 years. After 2 years, mortality in elders stabilized and the incidence was similar to that of the younger group. Further inquiry is required to compare mitral valve replacement in elders with alternate procedures (valve repair and percutaneous valvuloplasty), especially in high-risk groups.

been performed simultaneously with mitral valve replacement by use of a modified *maze procedure.* This involves an incision that completely encircles the orifices of the pulmonary veins, isolating them from the rest of the heart to prevent the formation of pathways to other areas of the conduction system. Cox's procedure involves placing a single incision between the pulmonary veins rather than around them, thus reducing extra aortic cross-clamp time.[6] Although the maze procedure is still being tested, it may offer promise for successful outcomes to otherwise high-risk cases.

The *Ross procedure* is the preferred method of aortic valve replacement. It uses the patient's own pulmonary valve, which has all the characteristics inherent in the patient's aortic valve, most notably similarity of leaflet endothelium and fibroblasts capable of maintaining leaflet structure self-repair. This procedure is specifically indicated for young patients in whom a long life span is indicated. Primary indications include isolated aortic valve disease, congested or acquired severe aortic stenosis, and severe aortic regurgitation with or without dilation of the aortic root. Contraindications include dissection of the aorta, Marfan's syndrome, and other diseases that cause significant aortic root enlargement. A routine midline sternotomy is performed, with cannulation of the ascending aorta and right atrium, followed by cardiopulmonary bypass. Extreme care must be taken in removing the pulmonary valve to avoid damage to the left main coronary artery. The pulmonary valve is kept immersed in blood in the pericardial cavity for preservation before implantation. A homograft valve

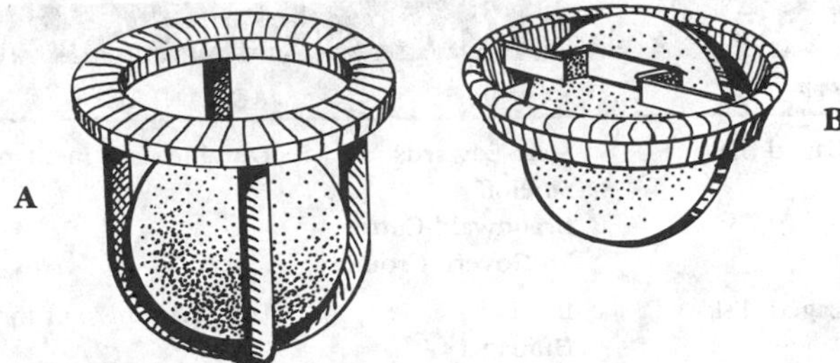


**FIGURE 31-6** Heart valve prosthesis. **A,** Caged ball valve. **B,** Tilting-disk valve.

(human transplant) is carefully inserted into the pulmonary position. The patient's removed pulmonary valve is trimmed of excess fat and muscle and inserted into the aortic root and sutured in place.

Care of the patient undergoing heart surgery is discussed on p. 852.

### Types of valves

The ideal valve used for replacement should include the following characteristics: durable, hemodynamic accuracy, nonhemolytic, nonthrombogenic, easily inserted, anatomically suitable, and a low incidence of endocarditis.[15] There are a wide variety of prosthetic valves available. The advantages and disadvantages of each valve type are listed in Table 31-2.

**Caged-ball prosthetic valves** consist of a metal cage with a synthetic, freely moving ball inside; the cage is attached to a sewing ring (Figure 31-6, *A*). The ring and struts of the cage are covered by a synthetic cloth. The cloth-covered ring is sutured carefully into the existing valve annulus. Within 2 to 3 months, tissue covers the cloth and the incidence of thromboembolism decreases. Caged-ball valves come in various sizes and slightly varying designs and materials.

**Caged-disk prosthetic valves** occupy less space in the ventricles than do other valves and require less force to move the occluding disk. This type of valve creates more obstruction to blood flow than do other types of valves. If the disk "sticks" in the cage, causing total obstruction of blood flow, hemodynamics are seriously compromised.

**Tilting-disk prosthetic valves** have occluders that tilt or pivot within a ring rather than balls or disks that pop back and forth in a cage (Figure 31-6, *B*). This type of valve produces nearly central blood flow through its orifice, providing more normal blood flow. However, the valve may develop areas under the pivoting points where thrombi can form as a result of the blood stasis.

**Stenting allografts** are human heart valves that are supported or "stented" by an underlying frame. Allografts provide relatively normal hemodynamic characteristics with central flow, no thromboemboli, and little hemolysis. Allografts are difficult to procure in quantity, however.

**TABLE 31-2 Types of Prosthetic Cardiac Valves**

| TYPE | EXAMPLES | ADVANTAGES | DISADVANTAGES |
|---|---|---|---|
| Caged ball | Starr-Edwards<br>Smeloff<br>Braunwald-Cutter<br>McGovern-Cromie | Durable, low incidence of endocarditis | Large size that may create obstruction to blood flow |
| Caged disk | Beall<br>Hufnagel<br>Cross-Jones<br>Kay-Shiley | Low incidence of thromboemboli | Disk may stick, causing severe obstruction of blood flow |
| Tilting disk | Bjork-Shiley<br>Wada-Cutter<br>St. Jude<br>Lillehei-Kaste | Central blood flow, low incidence of hemolysis | Higher incidence of thrombus |
| Stenting allograft | — | Central blood flow, low incidence of hemolysis, no thromboemboli | High incidence of regurgitation |
| Xenograft | Porcine | Silent valves, low incidence of thromboembolism or hemolysis | High incidence of calcification over time |

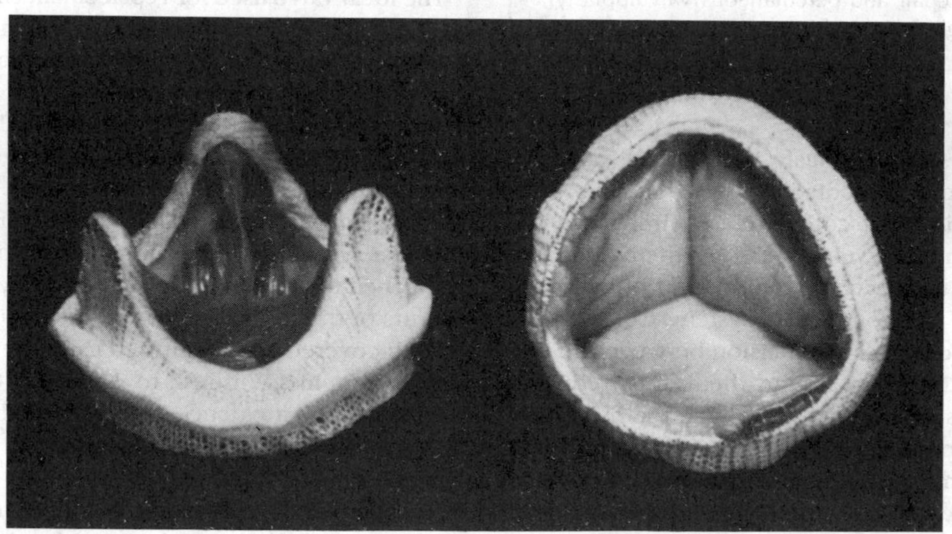

**FIGURE 31-7** Porcine valve prostheses (two views).

**Xenograft** bioprosthetic valves are composed of valves from species other than human, are more easily available than other valves, and can be obtained in all sizes. *Porcine* xenograft valves (Figure 31-7) are most frequently used. The hemodynamic performance has been similar to that of human heart valves. Many patients with this type of valve may not require anticoagulants. Approximately 70% to 80% of patients older than 35 years of age are free of primary tissue failure at 10 years. After 10 to 12 years, the process will accelerate calcification on the valve.[15] Because of a higher incidence of calcification over a long period, porcine valves are now used less often in young persons or in patients with renal failure who require dialysis.

## Anticoagulation

Patients with mechanical or bioprosthetic valves are at a high risk for systemic emboli. Antithrombotic agents are used to decrease the incidence of thrombi developing. A major risk to patients receiving antithrombotic agents is bleeding. Warfarin (Coumadin) is the most common antithrombotic medication used with both kinds of valves. Maintenance of warfarin is based on the prothrombin time (PT); a therapeutic PT is 1.2 to 1.5 of the control time. If bleeding occurs while the patient is taking warfarin, the dosage may be lowered or other medications added. Dipyridamole (Persantine) is another type of antithrombotic agent. It inhibits platelet aggregation while not affecting the PT. Dipyridamole may be used in conjunction with warfarin to prevent embolization. The normal dose to reduce platelet aggregation is 225 to 400 mg/day; orthostatic hypotension may occur.

## NURSING MANAGEMENT

### ♦ ASSESSMENT

Many of the symptoms of valvular heart disease are related to decreased cardiac output. Therefore the assessment data that the nurse obtains are essentially the same for any person with valvular heart disease.

#### Subjective Data

Persons with different types of valvular disease exhibit different symptoms. Data to be collected to assess the patient with valvular heart disease include the following:

- Fatigue and weakness: in severe valvular disease the fatigue may be overwhelming
- Dysnea: occurrence, type
- Many persons experience DOE, orthopnea, or PND, depending on the extent of ventricular involvement and failure
- Angina: occurrence, location, quality, and measures to relieve pain
- Palpitations: occurrence, precipitating condition or events, such as lack of sleep, dietary intake of caffeine
- Syncope: occurrence
- Peripheral edema: site, extent, time of day, alleviating factors
- Concerns about health status

#### Objective Data

Objective data are collected by inspection, auscultation, and palpation.

- Observation/inspection
  - Body posture/position and comfort level
  - Character and rate of respirations, flaring of nostrils
  - Use of supplemental oxygen
  - Skin color and temperature, including presence of cyanosis, mottling, petechiae, and other skin discolorations
  - Nailbed color and capillary refill
  - Neck vein engorgement
  - Myocardial heaves (can be observed in severe left ventricular hypertrophy)
  - Diaphoresis
- Auscultation
  - Cardiac rate and rhythm
  - Heart sounds (murmurs, $S_3$, $S_4$) (Table 31-3)
  - Breath sounds, comparing contralaterally
  - Presence of adventitious sounds (crackles, wheezes)
- Palpation
  - Temperature of extremities
  - Pulse rate and rhythm: irregular, fast pulse is often palpable in persons with mitral stenosis who experience atrial fibrillation
  - Equality and symmetry of pulses; pulse deficit or pulsus alternans, widened pulse pressure
  - Presence of edema, pitting or nonpitting
  - Signs of phlebitis (increased calf diameter, positive Homans' sign)

**TABLE 31-3 Auscultatory Difference in Valvular Heart Disease**

| VALVULAR DISORDER | GENERAL FINDINGS | MURMURS |
|---|---|---|
| Mitral stenosis | $S_1$ snapping, louder<br>Palpable thrill at apex | Soft, low-pitched, rumbling<br>Diastolic |
| Mitral regurgitation | $S_1$ soft or absent<br>$S_3$ present<br>Palpable thrill at apex | High-pitched, blowing<br>Pansystolic |
| Aortic stenosis | $S_2$ soft<br>Left-sided $S_4$<br>Systolic thrill at heart base | Low-pitched, harsh, rasping<br>Midsystolic |
| Aortic regurgitation | $S_3$ present<br>Systolic thrill over aortic area | High-pitched, blowing<br>Diastolic |
| Tricuspid regurgitation | Systolic thrill at lower left sternal border | High-pitched, blowing<br>Pansystolic |

### ♦ NURSING DIAGNOSES

Nursing diagnoses are determined from analysis of patient data. Nursing diagnoses for the patient with valvular heart disease may include but are not limited to the following:

| Diagnostic Title | Possible Etiologic Factors |
|---|---|
| Anxiety | Threat to health status |
| Fatigue | Decreased cardiac output |
| Activity intolerance | Weakness, imbalance between oxygen supply/demand |
| Fluid volume excess | Decreased cardiac output |
| Knowledge deficit | Lack of exposure/recall |

### ♦ EXPECTED PATIENT OUTCOMES

Expected patient outcomes for the person with valvular heart disease during the medical phase of treatment may include but are not limited to the following:

1. States feeling comfortable, with decreased signs of anxiety.
2. States that breathing is easier and fatigue occurs less frequently with activity.
3. Rests between activities.
4. Shows no weight increase from fluid retention.

5. Is able to:
   a. Explain the nature of the valvular disease
   b. State the name, purpose, dosage, frequency, and side effects of any medication therapy
   c. Explain any prescribed dietary sodium modifications
   d. Describe a work, rest, and activity program to conserve energy and decrease exertional dyspnea
   e. Describe the rationale for and the type of surgery to be performed, if surgery is indicated
   f. State plans for continued medical therapy

## ♦ INTERVENTIONS

Because heart failure may be present, the care of the person with valvular heart disease who is receiving medical therapy may be similar to that for heart failure (see p. 878).

### Decreasing Anxiety

Valvular diseases lead to decreased cardiac functioning; this poses a threat to life and therefore is anxiety-provoking. Measures to decrease anxiety through stress-reducing approaches (see Chapter 7) are especially helpful. Telling the patient and family what to expect with diagnostic tests and surgery can help reduce the anxiety level.

### Promoting Activity/Rest Balance

Fatigue is a major discomfort because of the decreased cardiac output with subsequent oxygen imbalance. Assist the patient to plan for rest periods between activities. Monitor pulse before and after activities. The pulse should return to baseline within 10 minutes after activity; a longer period denotes that activity must be decreased. Additional signs of excessive activity include labored breathing or patient reports of dyspnea on exertion.

### Promoting Fluid Balance

Observe for signs of fluid excess by continued monitoring of daily weights, intake and output, inspection of neck veins, and auscultation of heart and breath sounds. Observe the skin for changes in appearance, capillary perfusion, and the presence and extent of edema.

### Facilitating Learning

Patient teaching includes the following:

1. General anatomy of the heart and the function and purpose of the cardiac valves
2. Effect of medications: diuretics, cardiac glycosides, anticoagulants, and antibiotics
3. Prophylactic use of antibiotics before and after dental work and surgical procedures, if there is a prior history of rheumatic fever
4. Effect of a sodium- or fluid-restricted diet on cardiac function, if prescribed
5. Assessment of fluid formation in the extremities
6. Need to plan for a work, rest, and activity program to conserve energy and to identify intolerance to activity (DOE, fatigue, pulse that does not return to baseline within 10 minutes after activity)
7. Purpose and procedures for diagnostic tests in preparation for surgery, if appropriate
8. Purpose and nature of surgical intervention, if appropriate

## ♦ EVALUATION

To evaluate the effectiveness of nursing interventions, compare patient behaviors with those stated in the expected patient outcomes. Successful achievement of patient outcomes for the patient with valvular heart disease is indicated by the following:

1. States feeling more comfortable and has decreased signs of anxiety.
2. Breathes more easily and has less fatigue with activity.
3. Rests between activities.
4. Has stable weight.
5. Correctly describes nature of the disease, medication regimen, sodium modifications, rest/activity program, and plans for continued medical or surgical therapy.

# NURSING MANAGEMENT: The Patient Undergoing Heart Surgery

In the third decade of this century, the first heart surgery procedure was performed on a human patient in England. It consisted of a closed repair of a stenosed mitral valve, or mitral commissurotomy. Since that time great progress has been made in a variety of heart surgery procedures, including valve repairs and replacements, structural defect and congenital anomaly repairs, coronary artery bypass grafting, and total heart transplants (Table 31-4). Currently, research is being done to implant and test prosthetic heart chambers and total prosthetic hearts. Today's surgeon has the advantage of a highly sophisticated technology to aid in performing these extremely delicate yet vital procedures, a technology advanced enough to allow many Americans to undergo heart surgery each year.

One term frequently used to describe heart surgery is also commonly misused; the term *open heart surgery* often is used in referring to any surgical procedure performed on the heart. In the strict sense, however, open heart procedures are those in which the heart muscle itself is incised and the internal heart structures are directly visualized. A coronary artery bypass procedure is not, therefore, a true open heart procedure. True open heart procedures always involve the use of cardiopulmonary bypass. It is perhaps best to avoid the term *open heart surgery* entirely and instead to refer specifically to the actual procedure being performed, particularly when one speaks with the patient and family. It is not

**TABLE 31-4 Types of Cardiac Surgery**

| ACTION | SURGICAL PROCEDURES | USE OF CARDIOPULMONARY BYPASS |
|---|---|---|
| Repair or replacement | Correction of congenital defects; valve replacements; valvuloplasty; thoracic aortic aneurysm repair | Yes |
| Vascular bypass | Coronary artery bypass | Yes |
| Release of constriction | Pericardial fenestration; pericardiectomy; closed mitral commissurotomy | No |
| Replacement of diseased heart with healthy heart | Transplantation | Yes |

uncommon to find patients scheduled for coronary artery bypass grafting who believe that their heart will be opened during the procedure.

## PREOPERATIVE CARE

All of the preparations necessary for a person about to undergo a surgical procedure (see Chapter 23) apply to the patient being prepared for heart surgery. In addition, there are a number of specific considerations that are pertinent to the cardiac surgical patient.

### History

Persons being admitted for cardiac surgery may have exhibited cardiac and pulmonary symptoms for months or years before this admission. They will have undergone extensive testing to establish the underlying pathologic condition and to delineate the severity of the condition. Testing may have included chest x-ray films, cardiac catheterization, coronary angiography, echocardiography, phonocardiography, nuclear cardiac studies, electrocardiogram, stress testing, and blood serum analyses.

It is necessary for the nurse caring for the heart surgery patient to understand each patient's pertinent medical history to individualize care appropriately. It is necessary to know the underlying nature of the heart condition, how long it has been diagnosed, and the particular surgical procedure chosen to correct it. The relative degree of cardiac impairment will be demonstrated in the patient's limitations in life-style. The current manifestations of the illness may range from no symptoms to intermittent pain to debilitating heart failure. It is important to be aware of past cardiopulmonary or circulatory conditions or disorders, such as myocardial infarction, bacterial endocarditis, pulmonary embolus, blood clotting abnormalities, and a history of smoking, that might place the patient at higher risk for developing postoperative complications.

The patient's current medical regimen is very important, and medications or therapeutic measures that the patient was using before admission must be noted. It may be necessary to modify some of these measures once the patient is hospitalized, and all such changes in medication, diet, activity, and other areas must be carefully explained. Without an adequate explanation, the patient or family may feel that such changes during hospitalization are an indictment of the care provided at home, rather than seeing them as necessary preoperative preparations.

### Physiologic Preparation

Despite the fact that the person scheduled for heart surgery may have suffered from the cardiac condition for years, it is desirable to have the person in the best physical condition possible at the time of surgery. This is one goal of patient care during the preoperative period, however short or long that may be. Efforts will have been made to help the overweight patient reach a safe body weight, to assist the patient who smokes to stop or nearly stop, to eliminate or reduce edema and establish body fluids and electrolytes in normal balance, to correct or control cardiac dysrhythmias, to eliminate any signs of infection—in short, to achieve the healthiest state possible in light of the severity of the illness and the urgency of the surgery.

Therefore, along with a thorough knowledge of the patient's history, as already mentioned, it is necessary to obtain a complete data baseline to document the patient's condition just before surgery. Although many of the preoperative tests and preparations may have been performed in the days or weeks before the scheduled surgery, the person usually is admitted to the hospital at least 1 or 2 days before the planned procedure. At this time, a chest x-ray film, an ECG, and full laboratory screening will be performed. For selected patients, arterial blood gas analyses and even pulmonary function studies may be obtained to help establish a baseline of respiratory status and to plan appropriate and aggressive preoperative, intraoperative, and postoperative pulmonary care. Baseline vital signs (including apical and radial heart rates and bilateral arm blood pressures), integrity of all pulses (both proximal and distal), neurologic status, height, weight, nutritional status, elimination patterns, and psychologic status are carefully assessed and recorded in the immediate preoperative period.

### Facilitating Learning

In the past several years preoperative teaching programs for heart surgery patients have become well established.

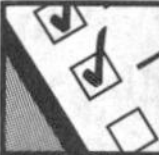

## Guidelines for Preoperative Teaching for the Person Undergoing Cardiac Surgery

1. General information
   a. Places of care during hospitalization
      (1) CCU or ICU after surgery
      (2) Return to general patient care division in 2 to 3 days
   b. Visiting hours and location of waiting rooms
2. Description of surgery
   a. Simple explanation of anatomy of heart and effect of the patient's cardiovascular disorder (e.g., incompetent valve, obstructed coronary artery)
   b. Explanation of surgical procedure
   c. Definition of any unfamiliar terms: bypass, extracorporeal
   d. Length of time in surgery: 2 to 4 hours
   e. Length of time until able to see family (usually 1½ to 2 hours after surgery)
3. Preparation for surgery
   a. Shower or bath night before surgery with special antimicrobial soap
   b. Surgical shave: shaving of entire chest and abdomen, neck to groin and left midaxillary line to right
   c. Legs shaved if saphenous vein grafts will be used
   d. Preoperative medication
4. Explanation of monitors
   a. Round patches on chest connected to a cardiac monitor that records patient's heartbeats
   b. Monitor makes beeping sound all the time
5. Explanation of lines
   a. Intravenous routes for fluid and medications
   b. Central venous line in neck or chest to monitor fluid status
   c. Pulmonary artery catheter in chest or neck to measure pulmonary pressures and monitor fluid status
   d. Plastic connector line to obtain blood samples without a needle stick
6. Explanation of drainage tubes
   a. Indwelling urinary catheter
   b. Chest tube: bloody drainage is expected
7. Explanation of breathing tube
   a. Tube in windpipe connected to machine called ventilator
   b. Unable to speak with tube in place but can mouth words and communicate in writing
   c. Tube is removed when patient is fully awake and stable
   d. Secretions in lungs or tube removed by nurse using a suction catheter
   e. Food and oral fluids not permitted until breathing tube is removed
8. Explanation and demonstration of activities and exercises
   a. Purpose of activity is to promote circulation, keep lungs clear, and prevent infection
   b. Activity includes:
      (1) Turning from side to side in bed
      (2) Sitting on edge of bed
      (3) Sitting in chair the night of or the morning after surgery
   c. Range-of-motion exercises
   d. Deep breathing using sustained maximal inspiration
   e. Tubes and lines will restrict movement somewhat, but nurse will assist patient
9. Relief of pain
   a. Some pain will be experienced, but it will not be excruciating (different pain than original angina if this was present)
   b. Frequent pain medication will be given to help relieve the pain, but patient should always tell nurse when pain is present

These fairly structured approaches still allow the nurse to individualize a teaching plan for any particular patient and yet ensure that all necessary topics are covered in a consistent manner for all patients (see Guidelines box, above).

### General information

Although most persons admitted for heart surgery have undergone previous hospitalizations, there will be significant differences in this particular stay, and an initial overview of general information is helpful to most patients and families. Frequently, the family will be requested to identify one spokesperson who will be told where to meet the surgeon after the operation and who will be allowed to call the intensive care unit (ICU) nurses for information. This serves to enhance the consistency and thoroughness of information given to the family while reducing the interruptions from multiple sources.

### Information concerning the intensive care unit

Many patients and family members benefit from a tour of the ICU, both to familiarize them with the equipment and to locate important areas such as waiting rooms and restrooms. Such a tour should always be conducted by ICU personnel who can accurately yet reassuringly describe the myriad sights and sounds that assail the untrained observer. Timing of the tour must be convenient for the ICU personnel, who should greet the patient and family members when they arrive, without appearing so rushed that the patient and family feel that they are imposing.

At times a tour may be omitted depending on the acuity of the ICU patients and the level of critical activity in the unit. If there is any possibility that a tour might prove distressing or unusually anxiety-provoking to the patient or family, it should be replaced with a general description of the sights, sounds, and activities that the patient is likely to encounter. It is important that all discussions of the stay in the ICU center about the unique attention and in-depth care that the patient will receive from specially qualified nurses.

### Description of surgery

Specific instruction must be given concerning the particular type of heart surgery the patient will undergo. Simple diagrams or plastic heart models can be used to illustrate what type of cardiac problem the patient has

**TABLE 31-5 Techniques and Equipment Commonly Used After Cardiac Surgery**

| TECHNIQUE/EQUIPMENT | PURPOSE |
|---|---|
| Intubation; ventilator for 12-24 hr | Maintain open airway and ventilation |
| Cardiac monitoring | Identify dysrhythmias |
| Chest tubes (one to four) | Drain blood and air from chest |
| Intravenous lines | Replace fluids; monitor CVP |
| Intraarterial lines | Monitor blood pressure; obtain arterial blood samples |
| Pulmonary artery line (Swan-Ganz) | Monitor pulmonary artery and capillary wedge pressure; monitor cardiac output |
| Indwelling urinary catheter (Foley) | Monitor urinary output for signs of impaired renal function |

and how the surgery will correct it. The type of chest incision to be made should be described: most commonly, a median sternotomy is performed for all bypasses and some valve procedures, whereas a left anterior axillary chest approach is used for certain selected repair procedures. In addition, the internal thigh incision for obtaining vein grafts is described for selected coronary artery bypass patients.

### Explanation of preoperative and postoperative procedures

It is important to describe the types of interventions and equipment that are made necessary by the intricacy of heart surgery. Specific aspects of the equipment and techniques that will be of special significance to the patient are described (Table 31-5).

Explain that the patient will receive continuous observation in the ICU and may at times be awakened to receive necessary nursing care, such as taking vital signs, obtaining blood specimens, taking x-ray films, turning, coughing, and deep breathing. Demonstrate the types of exercises in which the patient will be expected to participate actively. Document the patient's preoperative ability to cough and use assistive breathing devices for later comparison and encouragement postoperatively.

### Teaching approaches

Initial assessment of the patient's knowledge and ability to learn is essential to planning a thorough, individualized teaching plan. Continued reassessment of the patient's readiness to learn and retention ability is important throughout the preparative education period. Teaching sessions should be conducted at planned times and in a quiet area. The pace should be adapted to the patient's interest and ability to master the information presented. Opportunities should be allowed for the patient to demonstrate understanding of concepts and techniques. Adjunctive printed information should be given to all patients to reinforce what has been taught verbally (see Nursing Care Plan, p. 856).

## Psychologic Preparation

Patients scheduled to undergo heart surgery are usually aware that they are facing a potentially life-threatening situation; however, no two patients will manifest this awareness in the same way. A complete psychosocial evaluation is becoming a routine part of the preparative care of heart surgery patients in medical centers throughout the country. This evaluation is one part of the multidisciplinary team approach, which usually consists of the medical referral physician, cardiac surgeon, psychologist, clinical nurse specialist or practitioner, social worker, and dietitian.

The psychosocial evaluation looks at patients and significant others in relation to the presence of support mechanisms, the use of defense mechanisms (longstanding versus situational), and established methods of adaptation. Combined with an assessment of patients' basic levels of understanding of the experience they are about to undergo, a sound plan can be developed to enhance patients' preoperative and postoperative psychologic well-being.

It has been established that a small amount of anxiety enhances learning, whereas too much anxiety blocks learning. The highly anxious person may benefit from limited and carefully worded preoperative teaching, with an emphasis on a simple understanding of the surgical procedure. Highly fearful or anxious patients are most prone to serious misconceptions about their illness, the surgical procedure itself, and the anticipated outcome. It is important to include significant others in the preoperative teaching plan when the patient is unusually worried or appears to have significant misconceptions. It also is important to address patients' fears very seriously, no matter how unusual they might sound. Patients must be given frequent opportunity to vent their concerns to supportive, understanding staff members.

Patients who consistently reject the offer of information about their illness and impending surgery also need a supportive environment in which they feel safe. Information should not be pressed on those who truly do not wish to hear it; for them, such defense mechanisms may be tremendously important. Rather, a complete psychosocial evaluation may point out ways in which staff members and significant others can assist in maintaining the psychologic well-being both before and after surgery. Conversely, it also may reveal that for some patients, highly restricted visiting and family contact may be desirable for a few days postoperatively.

Finally, as more and more patients have relatives and friends who have undergone heart surgery, they may be

# NURSING CARE PLAN

## PREOPERATIVE CARE FOR PERSON UNDERGOING CARDIAC SURGERY

**DATA:** Ms. P. is a 40-year-old stockbroker who was admitted to the hospital for a mitral valve repair. She has a history of rheumatic fever as a child and mitral stenosis. Six months ago, Ms. P. was admitted to the hospital for chest pain, dyspnea, and tachydysrhythmia (atrial fibrillation). A cardiac catheterization revealed a narrowed orifice of the mitral valve (2.2 cm sq). A loading dose of digoxin was given, with a maintenance dose of 0.125 mg daily. Ms. P. was an avid runner, averaging 3 miles/day before this hospitalization.

Over the course of the past 6 months, Ms. P. has been unable to maintain any activity level and has complained of severe dyspnea and fatigue. During this hospital admission, tests revealed the mitral orifice now to be 2.0 $cm^2$. It was decided that surgery was warranted.

The nursing history identified the following:

- Ms. P. has a limited understanding of the surgical procedure and of invasive lines.
- She states she is willing to undergo the procedure but is concerned because she has a low pain threshold.

Nursing activities include monitoring the following:

- Heart rhythm and rate: opening snap, $S_3$
- Breath sounds
- Intake and output
- Serum electrolytes: potassium, calcium
- Activity tolerance

### ■ NURSING DIAGNOSIS

Knowledge deficit related to the surgical procedure and invasive lines

| Expected Patient Outcomes | Nursing Interventions | Rationale |
|---|---|---|
| Describes the anatomy of the heart and valve repair. | Describe the anatomy of the heart and valve repair in simple terms using a model. | Use of models can facilitate learning. |
| Describes events pertaining to the surgery. | Discuss events related to the surgery: | |
| | 1. Shower night before surgery | Knowing what to expect helps to decrease preoperative anxiety. |
| | 2. Preoperative medication | Preoperative medication is given before line insertion. |
| | 3. Length of surgery (2-4 hours) | |
| | 4. Family visitation (2 hours after surgery) | Early family visitation decreases patient's anxiety. |
| | 5. Length of ICU stay (1-2 days) | |
| | 6. Patches placed on chest | Patches will monitor heart rate and rhythm. |
| Describes purpose of lines. | Explain purpose of lines: | Because of the many lines in place postoperatively, advance knowledge will help decrease postoperative anxiety. |
| | 1. IV for fluids and medications | |
| | 2. Line in neck or chest to monitor fluid status (CVP) and pulmonary pressures (PAP) | |
| | 3. Arterial line to measure blood pressure and obtain blood samples without a needle stick | |
| | 4. Epicardial pacing wires placed before closure of chest (may require pacing postbypass) | Wires are used to improve conduction and cardiac output. |
| Describes events related to breathing tube. | Explain events related to breathing tube: | Awakening to find a ventilator tube in place can be frightening unless advance knowledge is given. |
| | 1. Tube in windpipe connected to a ventilator | |
| | 2. Patient unable to talk | |
| | 3. No food or drink given before tube removal | This will prevent aspiration. |
| | 4. Tube removed when patient is fully awake (about 14-16 hours after surgery) | |
| | 5. Secretions are removed using a suction catheter | |
| Describes drainage tubes. | Describe drainage tubes: | |
| | 1. NG tube placed in nose to remove gastric contents | NG tube prevents gastric reflux during ventilation. |
| | 2. Indwelling urinary catheter | Indwelling urinary catheter will accurately measure fluid output. |
| | 3. Chest tubes | Chest tubes remove bloody drainage. |

## NURSING CARE PLAN

### PREOPERATIVE CARE FOR PERSON UNDERGOING CARDIAC SURGERY—cont'd

■ **NURSING DIAGNOSIS**

Anxiety related to ability to tolerate postoperative pain

| Expected Patient Outcome | Nursing Interventions | Rationale |
|---|---|---|
| Expresses less concern about postoperative pain. | Describe postoperative pain: will become apparent after the anesthetic wears off and will be different from original pain | Knowledge of what to expect can decrease anxiety. |
| | Describe measures to reduce pain:<br>1. Tell nurse about the pain before it becomes severe<br>2. Medication will be given frequently during the first 2 days, then when necessary<br>3. Relaxation will help to decrease pain and help breathing | Knowing what to expect about the pain and measures that can be taken for pain relief can decrease anxiety and perception of postoperative pain.<br>Pain will cause patient to splint chest, affecting breathing and pulse (tachycardia). |

concerned about postoperative psychologic problems that they have observed. The health professional will exercise judgment in introducing this topic in preoperative teaching, but when it appears indicated or if the topic arises, an explanation should be given of the factors that may precipitate a postoperative or ICU psychosis: sleep deprivation, stress, and sensory overload from continuous environmental stimuli. Patients who develop the psychosis may complain of depression, inability to sleep, or of having "bad dreams" when they do sleep. These symptoms usually disappear after the patient's condition allows a few lengthy intervals of undisturbed sleep. For some patients, preoperative awareness of the effects of such stressors may prevent the patients from fearing that they are "losing their minds" if such symptoms arise. A sedative may be given the night before surgery to aid the patient in maintaining a calm state and obtaining a restful night's sleep despite a normal amount of apprehension.

## INTRAOPERATIVE PERIOD

Preoperative medications frequently include a narcotic analgesic, a sedative, an anticholinergic agent, and sometimes an antibiotic. The patient's skin often is prepared in a specially designated area adjacent to the operating room. A light analgesic is given first, followed by insertion of various intravenous and intraarterial lines. The patient is monitored during the insertion of the lines. When the patient is fully anesthetized, intubation and mechanical ventilation are begun.

If the cardiac surgery to be performed is a coronary artery bypass, either autologous superficial saphenous vein segments or an internal mammary artery is used for grafts, which are "harvested." With saphenous veins, portions of the veins are removed from one leg by use of longitudinal, interrupted incisions. The internal mammary artery (IMA) is retrieved by retracting the sternum and entering the pleural space. The tissue is dissected to obtain the IMA (Figure 31-8). Studies have shown that 40% to 50% of saphenous vein grafts close within 10 years, whereas 90% of IMA grafts remain patent 10 years after the operation.

The heart is exposed through either a midline sternotomy or an anterolateral thoracotomy incision, and retractors are used to hold the chest open.

### Cardiopulmonary Bypass

Some heart surgery procedures can be performed without artificial ventilation and circulation, but most procedures require either partial or total **cardiopulmonary bypass.** In *partial,* or left heart, bypass, blood is drained from the left atrium and ventricle and is passed through a pulsatile pump or roller pump, which returns the blood to the common femoral artery or the descending aorta. In this type of bypass, the pulmonary circulation is not interrupted.

In *total* cardiopulmonary bypass both oxygenation and circulation of the blood are performed by the bypass machine. Venous blood is removed from the body via cannulas placed in either the right atrium or the inferior and superior venae cavae (Figure 31-9). The blood passes through the oxygenating mechanism of the bypass machine, is oxygenated, and is then pumped back into the arterial circulation of the body through cannulas placed either in the ascending aorta (most common) or in the femoral artery. A venting tube usually is introduced through the apex of the left ventricle or left atrium and is connected to the pump to aspirate intracardiac blood and maintain decompression.

The bypass pump circuits must be primed before use

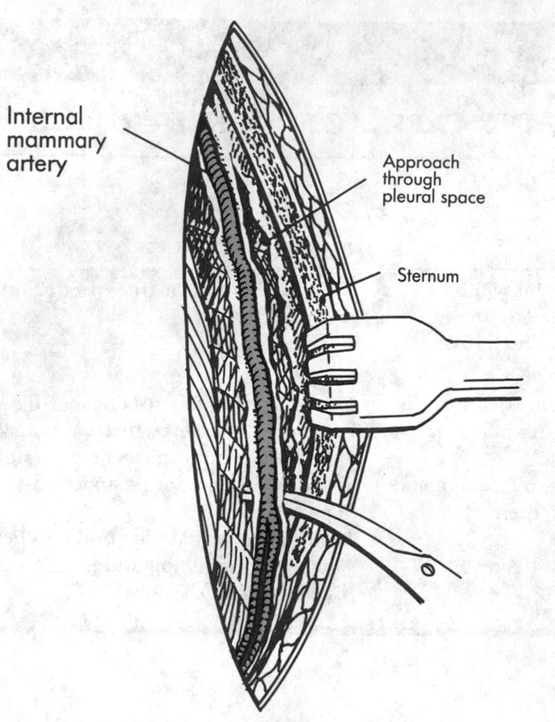


**FIGURE 31-8** The internal mammary artery (IMA) is resected from the inner chest wall.

with a fluid volume of approximately 2500 ml. In the past a large portion of that volume was composed of crossmatched type-specific whole blood. Currently, more centers are using an entirely blood-free hemodilution primer consisting mainly of lactated Ringer's solution. The advantages of the nonblood primer include decreased viscosity, limited hemolysis, and no risk of transfusion reaction and hepatitis from the primer solution. The main concern in using a nonblood primer is maintenance of an adequate hematocrit value. This can be achieved by intermittent additions of blood to the system during the cardiopulmonary bypass process.

In addition to performing blood oxygenating and circulating functions for the body, the bypass machine has two other distinct functions. It can act as a source for the direct administration of medications into the systemic circulation. It also is able to provide systemic hypothermia by cooling the perfusate to temperatures that range from mildly (30° to 34° C) to profoundly (15° C) below body temperatures. Hypothermia decreases the tissues' metabolic needs, thereby lowering the body's overall oxygen consumption. A reduced need for oxygen enhances myocardial tissue preservation during times such as when the aorta is clamped.

### Cold cardioplegia

Myocardial tissue preservation is of primary concern in all cardiac surgery procedures and especially in surgery for ischemic heart disease. In recent years a clearer understanding of the principles involved in myocardial tis-

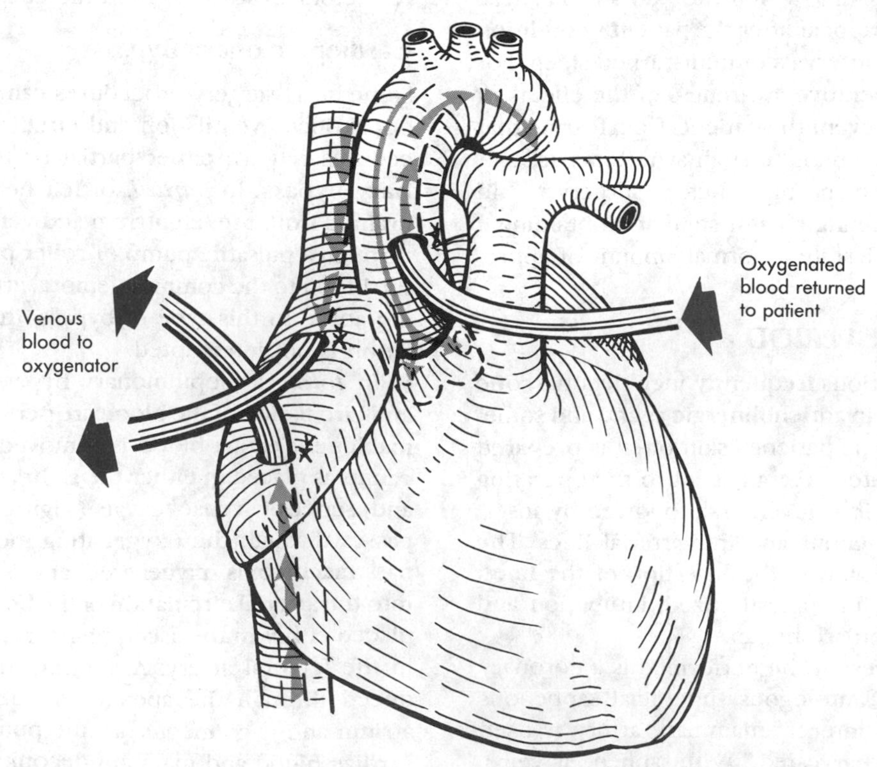


**FIGURE 31-9** Cardiopulmonary bypass.

sue preservation has resulted in the widespread use of cold cardioplegia solutions.

**Cold cardioplegia** consists of infusing an alkaline hyperosmotic solution that contains potassium, calcium chloride, mannitol, and other substances into the aortic root. It usually is infused for a few minutes immediately after aortic cross-clamping and again after about 30 to 45 minutes or when myocardial temperatures rise above 19° C. External cardiac cooling is achieved by a continuous infusion of lactated Ringer's solution at about 4° C into the pericardium. Several variations of the cold cardioplegia technique are in use, and it appears that this development has significantly improved myocardial tissue preservation in the intraoperative phase by supercooling the myocardium and drastically reducing its oxygen requirements.

### Termination of procedure

Once the surgical repair has been executed, the cardioplegia infusion is terminated. The blood in the bypass pump is slowly rewarmed, and the patient's body temperature is brought back to near normal. If the aorta was cross-clamped, it is unclamped at this time and the heart, which had been stopped during hypothermia, is restarted (see Chapter 30). The lungs are reexpanded, and when the cardiac rhythm is good, weaning from the bypass machine is begun. Blood volume is given back to the patient from the bypass machine, and the patient remains on decreasing amounts of partial bypass until weaning is complete. Systemic heparinization, which was done to promote blood flow during bypass and to prevent blood from clotting quickly in the operative field, is reversed with protamine.

Epicardial pacing wires may be attached directly to the right ventricular wall, the right atrial wall, or the internal chest wall and are then brought through the incision to the chest surface. There they may be used for temporary cardiac pacing if needed during the postoperative period. Chest tubes are inserted as indicated for blood drainage and air evacuation, if necessary. The incisions are closed and dressed, and the patient is taken to the recovery room.

### Side effects of cardiopulmonary bypass

Although cardiopulmonary bypass has been the most significant advance in the rapidly growing area of safe and effective cardiac procedures, it has a number of specific, potentially deleterious side effects. It creates a shocklike state, in which there is a functionally low hematocrit value (produced by hemodilution), decreased platelets (shearing forces during bypass), decreased systemic arterial pressures, and decreased perfusion to major organs (Figure 31-10). A prolonged decrease in blood pressure may result in neurologic changes, such as encephalopathy or cerebral anoxia. Decreased perfusion to the vital organs also can contribute to neu-

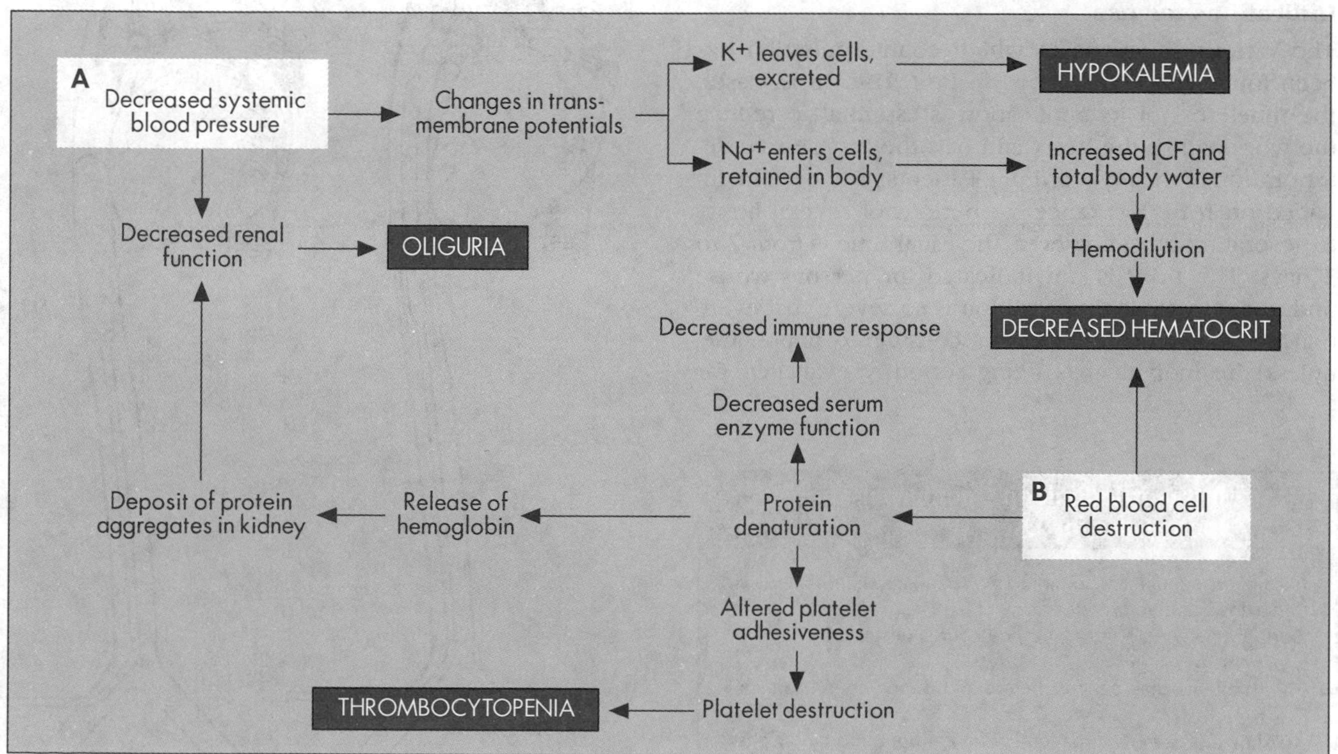


**FIGURE 31-10** Some effects of the shocklike state **(A)**, and red blood cell destruction **(B)**, that may occur with cardiopulmonary bypass. Clinical signs are indicated in boxes. *ICF,* Intracellular fluid.

rologic changes or renal ischemia, leading to acute renal failure. In addition, red blood cell destruction occurs during cardiopulmonary bypass.

Some patients may experience difficulties in being weaned from extracorporeal circulation. These persons may require circulatory assistance such as the intraaortic balloon pump to temporarily augment their circulatory system.

## Interventions for the Person With Intraaortic Balloon Counterpulsation

A counterpulsation device is one that assists the circulation of blood through the body by pumping when the heart is in ventricular diastole. The hemodynamic result of this action is to augment intraaortic blood pressure during diastole. The physiologic effects of counterpulsation are therefore an increase in coronary artery perfusion, a decrease in preload (the degree to which the myocardium is stretched before contracting), and a decrease in afterload (the resistance against which blood is expelled).

The two primary goals in the use of circulatory assist devices are to provide temporary assistance to the patient's circulation until the pathophysiologic condition is corrected and to afford optimal conditions for repair or resting of the heart until it can provide adequate circulation unaided. The **intraaortic balloon pump (IABP)** is a counterpulsation device capable of achieving these goals in selected patients.

### Indications for use

The various situations in which counterpulsation has been found useful are listed in Box 31-4. In all cases, the timeliness of its application is essential to reduce the workload of the heart and halt the progressive deterioration of the myocardium. Patients have been maintained on IABP assistance for periods of several hours to several months; however, the usual time is from 2 to 3 days. The IABP is not indicated for persons whose underlying pathologic condition is so severe that eventual weaning from the IABP is considered impossible, unless the individual is being seriously evaluated for heart transplantation. Absolute contraindications are few; the two primary ones are aortic valve incompetence and aortic aneurysm.

### Technique

The intraaortic balloon is inserted percutaneously or by cutdown into the right or left femoral artery. It is advanced into the thoracic aorta and is sutured into place at the insertion site after the balloon tip has been correctly positioned just distal to the left subclavian artery. The end of the balloon catheter is attached to a pump console, which alternately inflates and deflates the balloon with carbon dioxide gas.

The timing of the inflation-deflation sequence is of the utmost importance in obtaining maximal counterpulsation effect. By means of the ECG to trigger the pumping mechanism and the arterial waveform to determine effectiveness of the counterpulsation, the balloon is timed to inflate just at the beginning of ventricular diastole, immediately after closure of the aortic valve. The balloon remains inflated during diastole and

**BOX 31-4 Intraaortic Balloon Counterpulsation: Indications for Use**

- Cardiogenic shock secondary to acute myocardial infarction
- Other low cardiac output states
- During emergency diagnostic procedures on unstable cardiac patients
- In unstable cardiac patients before and during open heart surgery
- Assistance in removing patients from cardiopulmonary bypass postoperatively
- Drug-resistant, life-threatening dysrhythmias
- Unstable angina pectoris
- Severe acute myocardial infarction

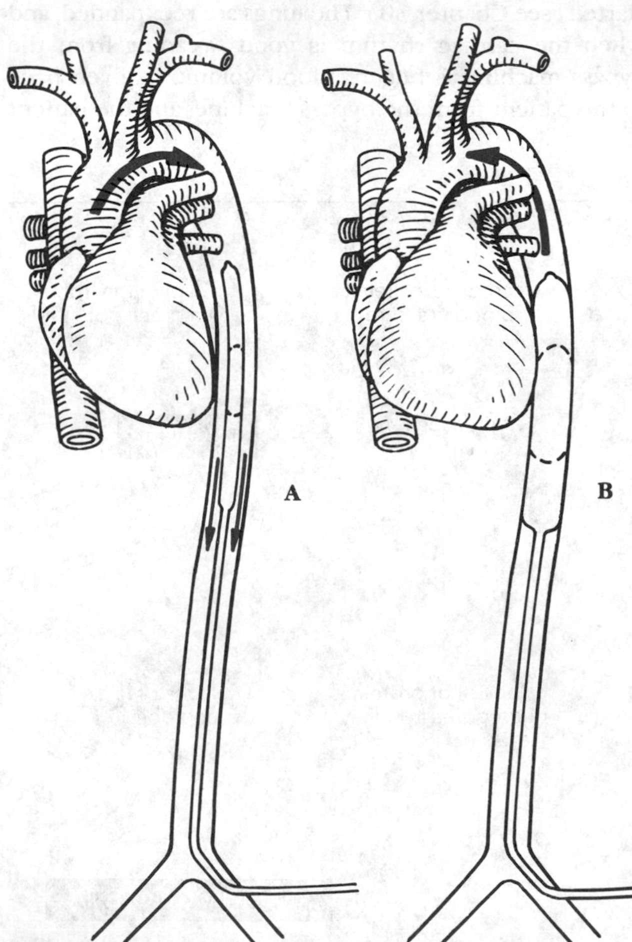


**FIGURE 31-11** Representation of intraaortic balloon positioned just distal to left subclavian artery. **A,** Balloon is deflated, allowing forward blood flow during systole. **B,** Balloon is inflated to increase coronary perfusion during diastole.

is then timed to deflate immediately before the next ventricular systolic ejection or just before the aortic valve reopens (Figure 31-11). Improper balloon timing not only defeats the purpose of counterpulsation but also could directly damage the myocardium, particularly in early inflation or late deflation in which the heart would be ejecting blood against a partially inflated balloon.

When the balloon is inflated during diastole, it causes an intraaortic pressure rise known as *diastolic augmentation.* This heightened diastolic pressure caused by balloon inflation forces blood in the aortic arch to flow in a retrograde fashion and provides increased coronary artery filling. This process achieves the goal of improving oxygen delivery to the myocardium.

When the balloon deflates at the end of diastole, it reduces pressure in the aorta, causing blood in the aortic arch to move from an area of higher pressure to one of lower pressure and to fill the space previously occupied by the balloon. This decreases the pressure in the aortic arch, reducing the resistance that the left ventricle must overcome to eject blood during systole; hence afterload is reduced. A sustained reduction in afterload will allow the left ventricle to eject more of its stroke volume during each contraction, thus leaving more space for ventricular filling. This usually results in a secondary decrease in preload as the left ventricle becomes and remains more efficient.

#### Nursing management for the person undergoing intraaortic balloon counterpulsation

The patient undergoing IAB counterpulsation requires intensive nursing observation and care. All vital signs and indexes of cardiac function must be observed continually and recorded; frequently the patient will be receiving vasopressor and antidysrhythmic drugs, and it is the nurse's responsibility to titrate these for the desired effects. Intubation and ventilatory support may be in place. All such factors require meticulous nursing intervention.

In addition, the patient with an IABP in place requires specific observation and care to prevent possible complications, such as circulatory insufficiency in the catheterized leg, aortic damage, and infection. Circulation checks of all pulses in both lower extremities are performed before insertion and hourly thereafter until the balloon is removed. No hip flexion is allowed on the catheterized side; well-padded leg restraints must be used if the patient is unable to cooperate. The head of the bed is not elevated more than 30 degrees to prevent balloon migration upward in the aorta. The patient should be tilted and carefully positioned on alternate sides every 2 hours to prevent skin breakdown and other consequences of limited mobility. The dressing on the balloon insertion site must be kept clean and dry and should be changed every 24 to 72 hours with use of sterile technique.

Considerable psychologic support is necessary for the patient and family during such critical therapy. The physical size and noise of the pump console are not only intimidating but the pump's presence only reinforces everyone's awareness of the frailty of the patient's heart and uncertainty about the future. Careful but simple explanations of the pump's action are necesary for those patients who are alert enough to understand; it is important that they not get the mistaken idea that the pump is working instead of their heart. Some patients with this type of misunderstanding fear that they will die if the pump stops even momentarily. Such intense fear makes them anxious and restless and further increases the body's demand for oxygen. Continuous reassurance and repeated simple explanations are essential; some patients may benefit from mild sedation.

### Ventricular Assist Devices

An alternative approach for patients in ventricular failure is left or right **ventricular assist devices** (LVAD or RVAD). These devices provide rest for the ventricles while artificially replacing systemic pumping.[3] They generally are indicated for profound intraoperative myocardial depression with failure to wean from the cardiopulmonary bypass. Patients requiring this type of assistance are critically ill and require care in an intensive care unit. (For further information see Chapter 26.)

## POSTOPERATIVE CARE

### ➡ Managing Critical Care

After the conclusion of the heart surgery, patients are transferred to the postanesthesia recovery area or taken directly to a cardiovascular or surgical ICU where typically they will remain for 1 to 2 days. During this time the patient will need continuous observation and professional nursing care to promote optimal recovery and prevent complications, which are most serious in the first 48 hours after surgery (see Guidelines box, p. 864). A sample Critical Pathway for coronary artery bypass graft surgery without complications is found on pp. 862-863.

Complete observation, thorough assessment, careful planning, and knowledgeable intervention may be organized through a systems approach to care.

### Cardiovascular System

One of the major goals of patient care in the immediate postoperative period is to promote cardiovascular function, adequate tissue perfusion, and stabilization of vital signs. To evaluate cardiovascular function thoroughly, the patient will have an intraarterial line and a pulmonary artery catheter (Swan-Ganz), each connected to a pressure transducer and continuous monitor; a CVP line connected to a pressure transducer and monitor; and a continuous electrocardiograph monitor.

#### Promoting cardiac function

***Blood pressure*** and ***heart rate*** are monitored continuously and are recorded every 15 minutes until stable,

## CRITICAL PATHWAY Coronary Artery Bypass Graft Without Complications

**DRG #: 107 Expected LOS: 9**

| | Day of Admission Day 1 | To ICU After Surgery Day 2 | Day 3 | Transfer Out of ICU Day 4 |
|---|---|---|---|---|
| **Diagnostic Tests** | CBC, UA, SMA/18,* PT/PTT, T & X, ABGs, chest film, ECG | CBC, SMA/6,† Mg++, PT/PTT, ABGs, ECG, chest film | CBC, SMA/6,† PT/PTT, ABGs, ECG, chest film after removal of PCT | CBC, SMA/6,† PT/PTT |
| **Medications** | Home medications, no aspirin | IVs (filling pressure maintained) IV antibiotic, KCl replacement, IV analgesic, nitroglycerine | IVs, IV analgesic, IV antibiotic, aspirin 5 gr daily, stool softener | IV to saline lock, IV or PO analgesic, IV antibiotic, aspirin 5 gr daily, iron tab daily, stool softener |
| **Treatments** | Wt and ht, VS q8hr, I & O q8hr, elastic leg stockings, pHisoHex shower | Monitor I & O q2hr (including NG, Foley, chest tube), VS q1hr; intubated on ventilator with $O_2$; thigh-high elastic leg stockings on unaffected leg; wt | Monitor I & O q4hr (NG, Foley, PCT removed), VS q4hr; nasal $O_2$; after extubation inspiratory spirometer; thigh-high elastic leg stockings on unaffected leg; wt | Telemetry, I & O q8hr, VS q6hr; dressings changed chest and leg; inspiratory spirometer, elastic leg stockings, wt |
| **Diet** | As at home | NPO | Clear liquids to full liquids, fluid restriction | Diet as tolerated, low sodium, fat, and cholesterol; fluid restriction |
| **Activity** | Up as tolerated | Bed rest, HOB elevated 30 degrees; T q1hr | Bed rest, dangle and up in chair with assistance × 2; T, C, & DB q2hr | Bed rest, up in chair × 3, brief walk in hall with assistance; T, C, & DB q2hr |
| **Consultations** | Respiratory therapist, perioperative nurse, primary nurse, anesthesiologist | | | Cardiac rehabilitation (dietary, exercise therapist, counselor on stress reduction) |

*ABGs,* Arterial blood gases; *CBC,* complete blood cell count; *T, C, & DB,* turn, cough, and deep breathe; *disc,* discontinue; *PCT,* pleural chest tube; *PT,* prothrombin time; *PTT,* partial thromboplastin time; *SMA,* sequential multiple analysis; *T & X,* type and crossmatch; *UA,* urinalysis; *VS,* vital signs.

then every hour thereafter. *CVP, pulmonary artery pressure, pulmonary capillary wedge pressure,* and *cardiac output* measurements are obtained every 2 to 4 hours as indicated by changes in the patient's condition. The radial pulse is checked for rate, rhythm, and volume, with bilateral comparisons made. The apical and radial pulses are checked simultaneously for any differences (pulse deficit), which could be indicative of such complications as atrial fibrillation. Distal peripheral pulses, either posterior tibial or dorsalis pedis, are checked for strength and bilateral equality.

The *cardiac pattern* is monitored continuously for the first several postoperative days, and the ECG pattern is compared with the preoperative baseline to detect any changes. Cardiac dysrhythmias are common in the immediate postoperative period; they may be the result of operative trauma from incision of the left ventricle, prolonged use of anesthesia, extracorporeal circulation, alterations in potassium levels, hypotension, hypovolemia, or hypoxia.

The treatment for dysrhythmias depends on the cause and the type of dysrhythmia produced. Treatment modalities include antidysrhythmic drugs such as lidocaine and procainamide (Pronestyl), cardiotonics such as digoxin, potassium replacement, and temporary pacing.

**Temporary atrial pacing.** *Temporary atrial pacing* is used in the management of four general cardiac disorders: supraventricular dysrhythmias, bradydysrhythmias, ventricular dysrhythmias (see Chapter 30), and low cardiac output.

*Supraventricular dysrhythmias* commonly occur after cardiac surgery because of edema or inflammation of atrial tissue. The tachycardia resulting from enhanced automaticity or circus movement reentry can produce hemodynamic deterioration as a result of decreased left ventricular diastolic filling. Atrial pacing is effective by overdriving or suppressing rapid atrial stimulation, converting the dysrhythmia to normal sinus rhythm or interrupting reentry pathways through the atria by introducing properly timed electrical stimuli.

*Bradydysrhythmias* after cardiac surgery usually are transient but may be associated with low cardiac output, which predisposes patients to dizziness and syncope.

| Day 5 | Day 6 | Day 7 | Day 8 | Day of Discharge Day 9 |
|---|---|---|---|---|
| | CBC, SMA/6† | ECG, chest film after removal of pacing wire | | |
| IV saline lock, PO analgesic, IV antibiotic, aspirin 5 gr daily, iron tab daily, stool softener | IV saline lock, PO analgesic; disc antibiotic; aspirin 5 gr daily, iron tab daily, stool softener | Disc saline lock; PO analgesic; aspirin 5 gr daily, iron tab daily, stool softener | PO analgesic, aspirin 5 gr daily, iron tab daily, stool softener | PO analgesic, aspirin 5 gr daily, iron tab daily, stool softener |
| Telemetry, I & O q8hr, VS q6hr; disc all dressings; inspiratory spirometer; elastic leg stockings, wt | Telemetry, I & O q8hr, VS q6hr, elastic leg stockings, wt | Disc pacing wire (VS q 30 min after removal × 4); disc telemetry; I & O q8hr, VS q6hr, elastic leg stockings | Disc I & O; VS q8hr, elastic leg stockings, wt | Staples removed, VS q8hr, elastic leg stockings |
| Regular diet, low sodium, fat, and cholesterol; fluid restriction | Regular diet, low sodium, fat, and cholesterol; fluid restriction | Regular diet, low sodium, fat, and cholesterol | Regular diet, low sodium, fat, and cholesterol | Regular diet, low sodium, fat, and cholesterol |
| Up walking in room × 4, walk in hallway with assistance × 1; T, C, & DB q2hr | Up walking in room × 4, walk in hallway with assistance × 2; T, C, & DB q2hr | Up walking in room × 4, walk in hallway with assistance × 3; C & DB q2hr | Up walking in room × 4, walk in hallway × 4; C & DB q2hr | Up walking ad lib |

*Serum calcium, phosphorus, triglycerides, uric acid, creatinine, BUN, total bilirubin, alkaline phosphate, aspartate aminotransferase (AST) (formerly serum glutamic-oxaloacetic transaminase [SGOT]), alanine aminotransferase (ALT) (formerly serum glutamate pyruvate transaminase [SGPT]), lactic dehydrogenase (LDH), total protein, albumin, sodium, potassium, chloride, total $CO_2$, glucose.
†Serum sodium, potassium, chloride, total $CO_2$, glucose, BUN.

Atrial pacing can be used to control slow sinus rates caused by drugs such as beta blockers or calcium channel blockers administered before surgery.

Treatment of choice for *ventricular tachycardia* is intravenously administered lidocaine, electric cardioversion, or rapid ventricular pacing. In some cases ventricular tachycardia can be indirectly interrupted with rapid atrial pacing, leading to ventricular capture. The atria are paced at a rate faster than the intrinsic rate of the ventricular tachycardia. Once the ventricular rhythm is overridden, atrial pacing may be abruptly stopped or progressively slowed until satisfactory heart rate is sustained.

Postoperative temporary pacing frequently is required to augment cardiac output by increasing heart rate. Slow junctional rhythms (see Chapter 30), a frequent cause of low cardiac output immediately after cardiac surgery, is highly responsive to atrial pacing. Furthermore atrial pacing is preferred over ventricular pacing because atrial contraction is preserved, enhancing stroke volume.

Precautions must be taken with atrial wires. A rapid atrial pacemaker generator (see Chapter 30) capable of pacing 400 to 800 beats/min should not be connected to a ventricular wire, which could result in ventricular fibrillation. Epicardial pacing wires are a potential source for lethal ventricular dysrhythmias if they come in contact with a ground current. These electrodes, when not in use, must be electrically isolated by securing them beneath nonconductor tape or with a rubber finger cot to the chest wall.

Daily care of wires to prevent infection is important. Removal of the electrodes is achieved by use of a slow, steady, but firm pull on the wires. After removal of the wires, the site is covered with an occlusive gauze dressing for 48 hours while the patient is monitored for signs and symptoms of cardiac tamponade.

With the increasing use of computerized monitoring systems, the nurse has a highly sophisticated adjunct to help obtain, store, and analyze ECG information when it is most vital. If the ECG status remains somewhat uncertain as recovery progresses, the patient may be

## Guidelines for Nursing Care of the Person After Cardiac Surgery

I. Monitoring
   A. Cardiovascular
      1. Blood pressure and pulse (rate, pulse deficit)
      2. Pulmonary artery pressure (PAP), pulmonary capillary wedge pressure (PCWP), cardiac output (CO), central venous pressure (CVP), left atrial pressure (LAP)
      3. ECG for signs of dysrhythmias
      4. Body temperature
      5. Skin color, temperature, capillary filling
      6. Signs of hypovolemic shock (decreased CVP, decreased LAP, decreased PCWP, decreased cardiac output)
      7. Signs of cardiac tamponade (cessation of chest drainage, restlessness, decreased blood pressure, increased CVP, increased PAP, increased LAP)
   B. Respiratory
      1. Respirations: rate, depth, quality
      2. Breath sounds
      3. Chest tubes for patency and drainage
      4. Autotransfuse chest tube drainage
   C. Neurologic
      1. Level of consciousness
      2. Pupillary size and reaction
      3. Orientation
      4. Movement and sensation of extremities
   D. Gastrointestinal
      1. Nausea
      2. Anorexia
   E. Urinary
      1. Output (amount)
      2. Color
      3. pH and specific gravity
   F. Fluid and electrolyte balance
      1. Intake/output balance
      2. Daily weights
      3. Serum potassium and calcium levels
   G. Presence of discomfort: pain, fatigue
   H. Ability to sleep
   I. Behavior: depression, fear, disorientation, hallucinations

II. Promoting oxygen/carbon dioxide exchange
   A. Preoxygenation and suction during intubation; suction as necessary after extubation
   B. Position with head only slightly elevated; turn side to side
   C. Encourage breathing exercises
   D. Give analgesics before breathing and coughing exercises
   E. Encourage range-of-motion exercises and progressive activity

III. Promoting fluid and electrolyte balance
   A. Record accurate intake and output
   B. Maintain prescribed flow rates of parenteral fluids
   C. Give prescribed supplemental IV potassium chloride

IV. Promoting comfort
   A. Give narcotic analgesics every 3 hours during the first 24 hours, then as needed
   B. Give frequent mouth care
   C. Control environment for comfort
   D. Change bed linens when diaphoresis is present (assure person that this is common)
   E. Plan activities to permit periods of sleep
   F. Provide back rubs for backache
   G. Splint incision during coughing
   H. Encourage patient to share feelings and experiences

V. Promoting activity
   A. Provide for passive then active range-of-motion exercises
   B. Encourage ambulation when permitted

VI. Teaching
   A. Progressive return to physical activity as recommended by the physician
   B. Rehabilitation exercise program
   C. Sexual activity usually permitted in 3 to 4 weeks
   D. Signs of overexertion include fatigue, dyspnea, pain
   E. Eat a balanced diet with any prescribed modifications (such as no added salt or low cholesterol)
   F. Medications
      1. Name, dosage, schedule, action, and side effects of prescribed medications
      2. Use of prescribed medications as needed
   G. Signs that may persist: dyspnea, pain, night sweats
   H. Signs requiring medical attention (fever, increasing dyspnea, or chest pain with minimal exertion)
   I. Need for ongoing medical care

transferred from the ICU to a cardiac step-down unit or telemetry unit for several days so that the ECG pattern may continue to be monitored closely.

### Preventing hypothermia

Although patients are rewarmed before termination of bypass, they frequently experience temperature drops of 2° to 5° C after separation from bypass. This temperature afterdrop usually occurs over a 60- to 90-minute period, causing patients to be mildly hypothermic on arrival to the intensive care unit. The temperature of patients who undergo cardiac surgery can be measured by the following routes: tympanic, nasopharyngeal, pulmonary artery, urinary bladder, esophageal, rectal, and skin.

Shivering as a means of heat production is *not* desirable after cardiac surgery because it creates increased myocardial work, carbon dioxide and lactic acid production, and cutaneous vasoconstriction. Therefore rewarming the patient is important. Measures to facilitate patient rewarming include (1) vasodilation with nitroprusside (creates more effective heat distribution than do blankets), (2) application of perfusion blankets above and below the patient,[14] (3) fluid-filled thermal blankets (less effective when peripheral vasoconstriction is present),[14] and (4) plastic covering or blankets around the patient's head. Once the body temperature has warmed, cool or diaphoretic skin may be an indication of shock.

As with skin temperature, *skin color* indicates the patient's perfusion state. The nailbeds should be pale pink, blanch easily, and return to pink color quickly, indicating good capillary refill. Cyanosis, either central or peripheral, can reflect poor perfusion or poor oxygenation, or both. The causative agent must be quickly differentiated and eliminated. Although cyanosis usually is not an early or reliable indicator of blood oxygen concentration, it can develop rapidly in the acutely ill patient and must be immediately reversed.

### Maintaining blood volume and chest drainage

A major concern of both the public and the health care community has been the potential risks (hepatitis, cytomegalovirus infection, toxoplasmosis, transfusion reactions) associated with the use of homologous (banked blood) transfusions. The Davol *autotransfusion* system is a waterless chest drainage system used routinely for collection of postoperative mediastinal drainage. The system easily converts from a drainage to a collection system. Controlled suction of −20 cm water is applied to the system. Sodium citrate solution is added as an anticoagulant preservative. When the desired volume of blood has been collected, the autotransfusion bottle is removed and replaced with another bottle. The collected bottle is then reinfused into the patient by means of filtered tubing.

Blood loss directly affects the systemic perfusion status, and both the chest incision and the chest tubes must be observed frequently for signs of unusually profuse drainage. Chest tube drainage, which should be slow and fairly consistent, usually does not exceed 100 ml/hr after the first 2 postoperative hours. The patient is routinely turned from side to side every 2 hours to assist in proper chest drainage. The total blood drainage during the first 24 hours usually averages 500 ml.

A change in chest drainage color to a very bright red from a dark red, a sustained hemorrhage that lasts for over 1 minute, or a sudden cessation of chest drainage are abnormal findings that must be reported immediately. Cessation of chest drainage within the first few postoperative hours usually indicates clotting of the chest tube within the mediastinum. This could predispose the patient to *cardiac tamponade,* a life-threatening emergency (see p. 836). Tamponade indicates a compression of the heart caused by excessive amounts of blood or blood clots collecting between the heart and the anterior chest wall. The return of venous blood to the right atrium and the cardiac output can be significantly impaired. Other signs of cardiac tamponade, in addition to minimal or no chest tube drainage, include sudden increase in bleeding from the midline incision, restlessness, decreased blood pressure, increased CVP and pulmonary artery pressure (PAP), and decreased urinary output. The physician must be notified at once, and cardiac decompression by needle aspiration or other methods will be undertaken.

### Maintaining blood pressure

Maintenance of a stable systemic blood pressure in the postoperative period may be difficult in some patients. *High* blood pressure must be controlled so that the weakened heart muscle does not have to work excessively hard to maintain an adequate cardiac output. Excessive myocardial workload increases myocardial oxygen demands, which may not be met. Pharmacologic intervention may be necessary in the form of vasodilators, such as sodium nitroprusside, which reduce vascular resistance and decrease afterload, thereby decreasing myocardial workload and oxygen demands.

More difficult to control and potentially more life-threatening is the *unstable low* blood pressure, which could indicate hypovolemia or shock. Hypovolemia is not uncommon after cardiac surgery and usually is corrected with blood or plasma transfusions or plasma volume expanders (e.g., low–molecular weight Albumisol and Hespan) rather than with large-volume noncolloidal solutions. "Fluid pushes" rarely are used to increase systemic blood pressure, because of the sudden extra workload created for the heart.

A postoperative shock state not caused by hypovolemia may be cardiogenic in nature. **Cardiogenic shock** (see Chapter 30) is caused by an impairment of the pumping action of the heart muscle and results in inadequate cardiac output and tissue perfusion. Specific impairments may include myocardial depression as a result of anesthetics and hypothermia, trauma of surgery, mechanical impedance to contraction caused by an implanted prosthetic valve, decreased compliance of the ventricle because of scar tissue or hypertrophy, preexisting heart disease not corrected by surgery, or dysrhythmias associated with an inadequate stroke volume.

Therapy for cardiogenic shock is directed toward improvement in myocardial contractility. Correction of any specific underlying cause will be attempted, as in eliminating cardiac dysrhythmias. Pharmacologic support may include vasoconstrictors such as dopamine hydrochloride to raise arterial pressure, although care must be taken not to increase undue blood return to the heart and peripheral resistance unless cardiac output is increased. Sympathetic agents such as epinephrine may be used for their cardiotonic effects. Isoproterenol is a preferred catecholamine because it combines inotropic with chronotropic effects and decreases peripheral and pulmonary vascular resistance. Frequently a combination of medication will be used to achieve the desired result of improving cardiac output with a minimum of side effects. Drug dosage administration is individually titrated to obtain desired effects. Whenever cardiac and vasopressor medications are given by continuous intravenous infusion, careful cardiac and blood pressure monitoring must be maintained, and the medications should always be administered via intravenous infusion pumps.

If pharmacologic support is inadequate in reversing or minimizing cardiogenic shock, a temporary mechanical assistive device may be employed to reduce the cardiac workload. *Intraaortic balloon counterpulsation* (see p. 860) may be used for several hours or several days and may be inserted at any time that its use is indicated in the preoperative, intraoperative, or postoperative period. Circulatory assistance also can be obtained through the use of *left ventricular assist devices* (see p. 861).

### Prophylaxis

Some patients receive prophylactic medications in the postoperative period. Antibiotics may be initiated just before surgery and continued postoperatively for 3 to 5 days to help prevent infection from numerous potential sources in the perioperative period. Anticoagulants will be given, starting about the third postoperative day, to patients receiving prosthetic mechanical valve implantations. The anticoagulation is necessary to prevent embolus formation on the surface of the valves and will be continued after the patient's discharge.

## Respiratory System

All patients receiving general anesthetics, especially those having undergone cardiopulmonary bypass, require meticulous attention to maintaining a clear and patent airway. Removal of excess pulmonary secretions, proper aeration of lungs and oxygenation of blood, and maintenance of chest tube patency are essential.

The rate, depth, and quality of respirations are monitored and recorded, and the patient's breath sounds are assessed through chest auscultation. During the intubation period, preoxygenation and suctioning should be administered as frequently as necessary to clear the patient's secretions (see Chapter 36). The patient is turned from side to side every 2 hours; positioning is used to help loosen and mobilize secretions. Arterial blood samples for blood gas analysis or oxygen saturation measurements by pulse oximetry are obtained to document the status of the patient's systemic oxygenation. Drainage and patency of chest tubes are noted, particularly when there is a known pleural leak. Daily chest x-ray films are obtained as ordered or more frequently if a sudden change is noted. During the intubation period the lungs are auscultated frequently to detect any shift in endotracheal tube placement.

After extubation it is important to observe the patient for any signs of respiratory distress. The patient is helped to splint the incision and encouraged to cough and deep breathe at least every 2 hours while awake. Administering medication for pain before the patient coughs may help increase the effort to cough, but some patients may require nasotracheal suctioning even after extubation. Preoperative instructions that were given regarding incentive spirometry or nebulization devices should be reinforced as the patient is assisted in using them. Aggressive pulmonary hygiene must be maintained for the first postoperative week.

## Neurologic System

After surgery the patient's neurologic status must be carefully assessed, including level of consciousness, pupil size and reaction, orientation, and movement and sensation of extremities.

Patients usually begin to awaken within 1 to 2 hours after surgery. Failure to awaken may be the result of unusually deep anesthesia or of embolization of air, calcium fat, or thrombotic particles to the brain. A return of consciousness that seems sluggish and in which the patient does not seem to regain full alertness after a day or two may have been caused by poor cerebral perfusion or microembolization during cardiopulmonary bypass.

Pupil size, equality, and reaction to light are checked frequently in the immediate postoperative period. Pupil dilation may be caused by excessive carbon dioxide in the blood or by such cardiac medications as atropine. Constricted pupils may be caused by dopamine. Disorientation and restlessness may be signs of hypoxia or embolization to the brain in addition to being symptoms of fatigue, fear, or sensory overload. Impaired sensation or muscular control of any portion of the body after surgery indicates a neurologic deficit that requires careful observation and complete evaluation by specialists.

## Renal System

Careful observation of hourly urinary output, as well as urine color, pH, and specific gravity, provides essential information about renal function. Adequate urinary output is at least 20 to 30 ml/hr. It is common for increased sugar and acetone to be found in the urine for the first several hours after cardiopulmonary bypass. This evaluation usually is not treated unless it coincides with sustained elevated serum glucose levels. Specific gravity may be elevated because of oliguria or the presence of red blood cells as a result of extracorporeal circulation.

Renal insufficiency in the patient after heart surgery is caused by complications of cardiopulmonary bypass. The destruction of red blood cells can cause sludging in the kidneys. If low-perfusion states occurred during the surgical procedure, the kidneys themselves may have been damaged, resulting in acute tubular necrosis. This is marked by oliguria with increased blood urea nitrogen and serum creatinine levels. If the acute tubular necrosis is severe and prolonged, temporary renal replacement therapy or hemodialysis (see Chapter 50) is initiated to sustain the patient through the acute phase. Return of kidney function after acute tubular necrosis usually is gradual but complete. Up to 25% of patients may encounter some form of renal failure after bypass.

## Gastrointestinal System

Gastrointestinal symptoms, such as anorexia and nausea, may occur after cardiac surgery. Contributing factors include drug therapy, prolonged perfusion time, preexisting GI disease, vasopressors, perioperative hypoperfusion/hypotension, systemic hypothermia, stress, and anxiety. Although anorexia occurs more commonly than nausea,[2] the latter is more distressing. Procainamide can affect appetite. Comfort measures to decrease nausea are instituted. Small amounts of food, when permitted, may be more palatable than a large plateful.

## Maintaining Fluid and Electrolyte Balance

The patient receives necessary blood products after heart surgery to maintain a stable hematocrit volume. Hemoglobin and hematocrit values and prothrombin time are obtained daily to assess the extent of blood loss and the effect of replacement therapy. Plasma and plasma expanders are given to avoid hypovolemia and to maintain a normal osmotic gradient. Crystalloid intravenous solutions are administered to ensure adequate circulating volume.

*Accurate recording of intake and output* is essential for the first few postoperative days. Fluids are limited to reduce the chance of fluid overload and increased cardiac workload. Intravenous fluids are carefully titrated by intravenous infusion pumps. Daily weights are obtained, and diuretics are administered if fluid retention occurs.

Serum electrolyte levels are obtained several times during the first 24 hours and at least daily thereafter. Initially the serum glucose level may be grossly elevated; this is transient. Serum potassium levels are monitored; supplemental intravenous potassium chloride usually is given in the immediate postoperative period, particularly in conjunction with diuretic use.

## Promoting Comfort, Rest, and Sleep

Alleviation of pain is important in the postoperative period, and patients should be kept as comfortable as possible (see Chapter 25). This not only adds to a sense of security but reduces the stress on the heart, decreases the need for oxygen, and promotes healing. Other comfort measures are routinely employed, such as positioning in bed, controlling environmental temperature, and giving frequent oral hygiene.

After cardiac surgery the patient is weak and tires from activity very quickly. Activity periods should be organized so that rest periods are frequent (even if brief) and uninterrupted.

## Promoting Psychologic Adaptation

The psychologic ramifications of heart surgery, sleep deprivation, and sensory overload can be overwhelming. Some persons experience a period of depression or disorientation after surgery, whereas others may become unreasonably fearful or experience hallucinations. The disorientation may even progress to panic. The nurse should be alert to subtle behavioral changes and reassure the person and family that these reactions are common and do not mean that the patient is "losing his mind." At the same time, physiologic causes of the behavior must be ruled out.

It is very helpful to the patient and family if the nursing staff attempt to personalize the patient's experience as much as possible. It is rather easy to lose sight of the person behind the monitoring equipment in an ICU. Calling the patient by name, using frequent physical contact with orienting the patient to time and place, and including the patient in any discussions that are held at the bedside help to decrease the sense of isolation.

## Promoting Activity

Passive arm exercises are started shortly after surgery, followed by active exercises as the person gains strength. Mobilization of the person depends on the operation and the status of the heart.

Persons who have had surgery for patent ductus arteriosus and mitral stenosis may be kept in Fowler's position postoperatively and are encouraged to move their arms and legs. Backache from lying flat on the back, even for short periods, is common.

The time of ambulation for each patient depends on the patient's progress and condition, but (other than the aforementioned exceptions) it usually proceeds as follows. The first day the feet are dangled over the side of the bed for 15 minutes in the morning and afternoon, and the person is allowed to sit in a chair at the side of the bed for 15 minutes in the afternoon and evening. Walking around the room is permitted by the third postoperative day. The fourth day the patient is allowed to walk around the room and to sit in the chair for gradually increasing periods of time. By the fifth day walking longer distances is encouraged. During ambulation, close supervision is necessary, and activity that causes excessive fatigue, dyspnea, or an increased pulse or respiratory rate is discontinued. If any of these symptoms appear, the patient is returned to bed, and the physician is consulted before further activity is attempted.

## Facilitating Learning

Definite instructions must be provided regarding when the person may attempt to climb stairs. The activity should be done slowly. Only two or three steps should be attempted the first time, after which the number of steps is gradually increased. The patient should rest two or three times while climbing one flight of stairs.

The person and family need to be told that no marked improvement will be noticed after the operation—that it will be at least 3 to 6 months before the full result of the surgery can be ascertained. It is essential that all persons be given this information so that they will not be depressed by dyspnea or pain that may still be present postoperatively.

In preparation for discharge from the hospital, the person is asked to make a list of normal daily activities. This list is discussed with the physician to determine the activities that are appropriate. Sexual intercourse usually is permitted within 3 to 4 weeks after surgery. Patients usually are advised to start activities slowly and progress gradually to more energy-consuming tasks. The physician will want the patient to return for frequent medical follow-up examinations, at which time advice will be given regarding additional activities. The person is allowed to do anything that does not cause fatigue or pain but must be kept from attempting too much too soon.

The family should be aware of how much the person may be encouraged to do. Because the patient may have been an invalid before surgery, the family may be as fearful as is the person about an increase in activity. Persons are encouraged to return to work as soon as permitted. To prevent misunderstandings, physicians need to give the person specific directions regarding return to work.

## MEDIASTINITIS AFTER CARDIAC SURGERY

During any surgical procedure, bacteria from exogenous and endogenous sources can lead to an infection. The negative inspiratory force with the normal physiologic act of inspiration may be enough to cause bacteria on the suture line to be drawn into the soft tissue of the sternal wound. Chest drainage systems that create negative pressure on the mediastinal space also can draw bacteria into soft tissue from the suture line. Sternal osteomyelitis causes instability and abscess formation within the bone.

Patients who recover from **mediastinitis** have a reasonable outlook for leading a productive life without impairment. Some residual loss in upper extremity strength may occur from deconditioning, anterior chest wall instability subsequent to significant removal of portions of the sternum and costochondral joints, and effects of prolonged hospitalization.

Organisms responsible for mediastinitis include gram-positive organisms such as *Staphylococcus epidermidis* and *S. aureus* and gram-negative organisms such as *Candida albicans* and *Pseudomonas, Klebsiella, Enterbacter,* and *Aspergillus.* Exogenous sources of the infecting organisms include shedding from the surgical team and the environment of the intensive care unit. Endogenous sources include any pathogenic organism that has infected the patient at other body sites, as well as the patient's normal flora.

Major preoperative risk factors include the presence of a serious noncardiac illness, malnutrition, obesity, chronic obstructive pulmonary disease (COPD), alcohol dependence, and diabetes. Other factors include preoperative use of steroids, presence of a preoperative infection (such as pneumonia or a dental abscess), age because of associated decrease in the efficiency of the immune system, and a history of previous sternotomy.

Risk of perioperative infection increases with use of the internal mammary arteries versus saphenous veins because of the necessity for more extensive dissection, with associated bleeding and a decrease in blood supply to the sternum. Multiple valve replacement can result in increased rate of infection because of the more prolonged and complex nature of the procedure.

Postoperative risk factors include the following: cardiopulmonary bypass time greater than 3 hours, prolonged operative time (greater than 3 hours), postoperative hemorrhage and hematoma formation, low cardiac output, postoperative invasive lines, and the intensive care environment.

### Signs and Symptoms

Excessive pain that begins on postoperative days 3 to 4 should cause suspicion, as well as progressive erythema around the incision and any drainage from the sternal wound (clear or purulent). Audible or palpable evidence of bone instability can occur with osteomyelitis of the sternum. Sternal separation can occur with coughing and deep breathing. Bubbling from the incision on expiration or suction of air into the wound on inspiration is possible. The patient may exhibit signs and symptoms of septicemia with or without positive blood cultures. Advanced stages of sternal infection can result in wound dehiscence. Fever can occur 48 to 72 hours after surgery, ranging from 38.3° to 39.4° C (101° to 103° F). White blood cell counts also may be elevated above $11{,}000/mm^3$.

### Medical Management

#### Prophylaxis

During the preoperative period, prevention includes prophylactic antibiotics and iodine showers or scrubs. During surgery, thorough hemostasis, stable mechanical closure of the sternum, and antibiotics contribute to reduced risk. After surgery, *early* removal of invasive lines, judicious use of antibiotics, and use of low levels of positive end-expiratory pressure to act as internal tamponade for hemostasis may prevent sternal infection.

#### Treatment

Medical treatment of mediastinal infections and sternal wounds varies according to the extent of the infectious process. Superficial infections are treated by wound incision and drainage, with application of a dressing. When the sternum is infected, the sternum must be débrided, including removal of bone wax and sternal wires. Continuous irrigation with antibiotic/antiseptic solutions and wound drainage should occur for 7 to 10 days.

When mediastinitis is present, the sternum must be extensively débrided. Generally the wound is left open to heal by secondary intention and granulation. If costal chondritis is present, diseased cartilage is removed. Muscle or omental flaps are used to revascularize the area and eliminate dead space. Muscles frequently used include pectoralis major, latissimus dorsi, serratus anterior, rectus abdominis, and external oblique.

### Nursing Management

Nursing measures directed at identification of patients at risk, as well as early detection of wound infection, can help to reduce preoperative incidence of infection and mortality. Operating room nurses must be alert concerning laminar flow, blood loss during surgery, number of personnel in the operating room, and number of door openings during procedure. Postoperative nursing measures in the intensive care unit must be directed at infection control.

## CARDIAC TRANSPLANTATION

Cardiac transplantation is the most effective therapeutic modality to significantly prolong life in patients with end-stage heart disease. Despite the positive outcomes of cardiac transplantation, donor availability and complications from infection, rejection, and immunosuppressive drug therapy continue to be serious problems (see Chapter 72). At least half of all cardiac transplantations are performed for dilated cardiomyopathy and most of the remainder for end-stage heart disease caused by extensive coronary artery disease.[4] Ventricular dilation and poor systolic ejection lead to myocardial failure. The clinical presentation of end-stage heart disease varies. Symptoms include those of cardiac failure and dysrhythmias, altered mental status resulting from inadequate perfusion, and dyspnea from increased respiratory effort.

**Cardiac transplantation** involves excision of the recipient's diseased heart, with subsequent replacement with the donor human heart. After a median sternotomy, initiation of cardiopulmonary bypass, and dissection, the recipient's heart is removed. Cardiectomy requires transection of the main pulmonary artery and aorta and partial resection of the atria, leaving the posterior walls intact. These portions serve for surgical attachment to the donor heart and also retain their systemic and pulmonary venous connections.

The donor cardiectomy differs from that of the recipient in that the heart is removed in toto, although slight surgical modifications must be made before reimplantation. The organ is trimmed to fit the recipient's atria and great vessels. Anastomoses are made between the recipient left atria, septum, right atria, the aortas, and the pulmonary arteries (Figure 31-12).

Overall condition of the donor heart, ischemic time, myocardial preservation techniques, and pharmacotherapy ultimately influence the integrity of the donor heart's newly independent mechanical and electrical responses. The new heart's initial postperfusion electrical response is slow and chaotic. QRS complexes frequently are wide, reflecting a ventricular escape rhythm. This idioven-

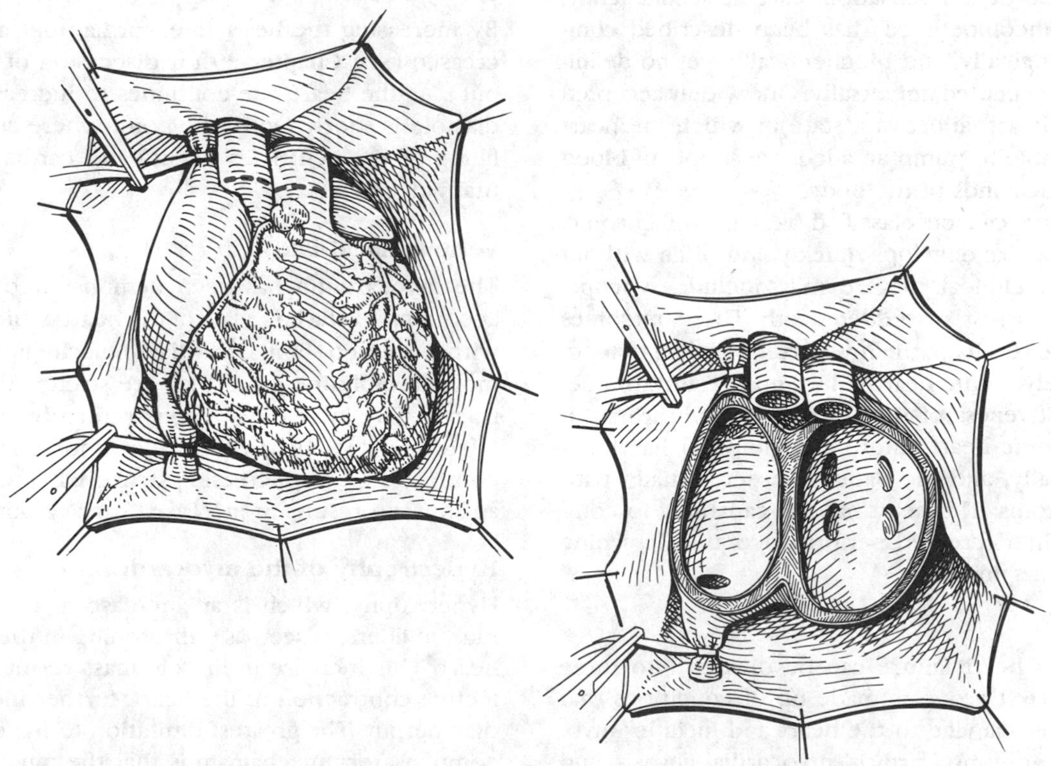

**FIGURE 31-12** Heart transplantation. The diseased heart is removed, leaving the posterior walls of the atria. The new heart is then anastomosed to the atrial walls and great vessels.

tricular rhythm eventually is replaced by a faster and more stable sinus rhythm. During the immediate post-implantation period, the myocardium must adapt to the absence of autonomic enervation. Frequently it is necessary to augment its inotropic and chronotropic function with intravenous catecholamines, such as dopamine and isoproterenol, until hemodynamic parameters stabilize.

Postoperative care of the person with a transplanted heart is the same as that for other heart surgery. Radionuclear imaging and right cardiac catheterization may be performed weekly for the first 4 weeks to assess graft viability. A low-cholesterol, low-sodium diet is prescribed. For additional information on organ transplantation, see Chapter 72.

# HYPERTENSIVE HEART DISEASE

Hypertensive heart disease refers to changes in the heart from prolonged sustained hypertension, which increases afterload. The heart enlarges (as seen on radiographic examination) in an attempt to compensate for the increased cardiac workload. If the underlying hypertension is untreated, cardiac failure results. Hypertension is discussed in Chapter 32.

# CONGESTIVE HEART FAILURE

**Heart failure** (also known as *congestive heart failure [CHF],* cardiac decompensation, cardiac insufficiency, and cardiac incompetence) has been described clinically, physiologically, and biochemically; yet no definition has been accepted universally. One widely accepted definition of heart failure is a state in which the heart no longer is able to pump an adequate supply of blood to meet the demands of the body.

Heart failure can be classified as acute or chronic. *Acute* heart failure develops quickly and often without warning. The clinical picture may include syncope, shock, cardiac arrest, or sudden death. These outcomes are clearly the results of the myocardium failing to function adequately. Acute heart failure may result from decreased effectiveness of the heart after myocardial infarction. *Chronic* heart failure, on the other hand, develops gradually, and the patient is seen initially with milder symptoms. The heart has the capability to compensate for the decreased performance, thus lessening the severity of symptoms.

## ETIOLOGY

The causes of heart failure can be divided into three groups. The *first* group is made up of conditions that result in direct damage to the heart and includes myocardial infarction, myocarditis, myocardial fibrosis, and ventricular aneurysm.

The *second* is made up of conditions that result in ventricular overload (see Chapter 29). Overload can be described in two subgroups:

1. *Preload.* Preload is the ventricular blood volume at end-diastole, the maximal ventricular blood volume for the beat of the heart. According to Starling's law, once the preload has reached a given limit, the effectiveness of the contraction diminishes, resulting in heart failure. Increased preload can result from mitral or aortic regurgitation, atrial or ventricular septal defects, or rapid infusion of intravenous solutions.

2. *Afterload.* Afterload is the force that the ventricle must develop to eject blood into the circulatory system. This is the pressure against which the heart must work. Increased afterload may develop from aortic or pulmonary valve stenosis, systemic hypertension, or pulmonary hypertension.

The *third* group of conditions that can lead to heart failure are those resulting in constriction of the ventricle, which limits ventricular filling and thus decreases stroke volume. Constriction can result from cardiac tamponade, constrictive cardiomyopathies, and pericarditis.

## PATHOPHYSIOLOGY

### Cardiac Compensatory Mechanisms

Three mechanisms of compensation that enable the weakened heart to continue to meet the metabolic demands of the body are tachycardia, ventricular dilation, and hypertrophy of the myocardium.

#### Tachycardia

By increasing the heart rate, cardiac output also is increased (see Chapter 29 for discussion of cardiac output). As the heart rate continues to increase, however, diastole is shortened to the point where an inadequate filling of the ventricles occurs and cardiac output actually decreases.

#### Ventricular dilation

The myocardium has been demonstrated to function according to Starling's law of the heart, which states that within certain limits, cardiac muscle fibers contract more forcibly the more they are stretched before contraction. By increasing venous return to the heart, the fibers are stretched, which allows for a more forceful contraction, thus increasing stroke volume. This mechanism then results in increased cardiac output.

#### Hypertrophy of the myocardium

Hypertrophy, which is an increase in the diameter of muscle fibers, is seen as a thickening in the walls of the heart. This increase in muscle mass results in more effective contraction of the heart, further increasing cardiac output. The greatest limitation to hypertrophy as a compensatory mechanism is that the muscle mass outgrows the coronary artery supply, resulting in hypoxia and decreased effectiveness.

## Homeostatic Compensatory Mechanisms

When cardiac compensatory mechanisms become inadequate to continue to meet the metabolic needs of the body, homeostatic compensatory mechanisms are activated. Knowledge of these physiologic responses is essential in understanding the treatment modalities for congestive heart failure.

### Vascular system

As the circulating blood volume is decreased, sympathetic stimulation and release of norepinephrine result in generalized vasoconstriction. Both arterial circulation and venous circulation are affected.

### Kidneys

Vasoconstriction and low cardiac output have a profound effect on renal perfusion. When cardiac output falls to one half to two thirds of normal, complete anuria can occur. As arterial pressure in the kidneys is diminished, glomerular filtration is reduced, resulting in retention of sodium and water. Aldosterone secretion by the adrenal cortex is stimulated, resulting in further reabsorption of sodium by the renal tubules. Osmotic pressure is increased by the rising sodium concentration, leading to release of antidiuretic hormone by the hypothalamus. The end result is increased tubular reabsorption of water, leading to fluid overload and edema (Figure 31-13).

### Liver

The venous volume increases to such an extent that hepatic congestion develops, resulting in decreased effectiveness of all hepatic functions. The liver normally metabolizes aldosterone and antidiuretic hormone. Because the congested liver has a reduced ability to metabolize these substances, hepatic congestion serves to further compound heart failure.

## Classifications of Heart Failure

Heart failure has been classified into three main categories. These include backward versus forward, low-output versus high-output heart failure, and left versus right.

### Backward versus forward heart failure

**Backward heart failure** is said to be the result of damming up of blood in the vessels proximal to the heart. **Forward heart failure,** conversely, is the result of the inability of the heart to maintain cardiac output. It should be emphasized that because the heart is part of a closed system, forward failure and backward failure always are associated with each other.

### Low- versus high-output heart failure

With the development of diagnostic tools that allow the measurement of cardiac output (cardiac catheterization), heart failure can be classified by the effectiveness of the heart as a pump. When cardiac output remains normal or above normal but the metabolic needs of the body are not met, the condition is termed **high output heart failure.** Causes of high-output failure include hyperthyroidism, anemia, Paget's disease, and arteriovenous fistula. When cardiac output falls below normal, the results are termed **low-output heart failure** and

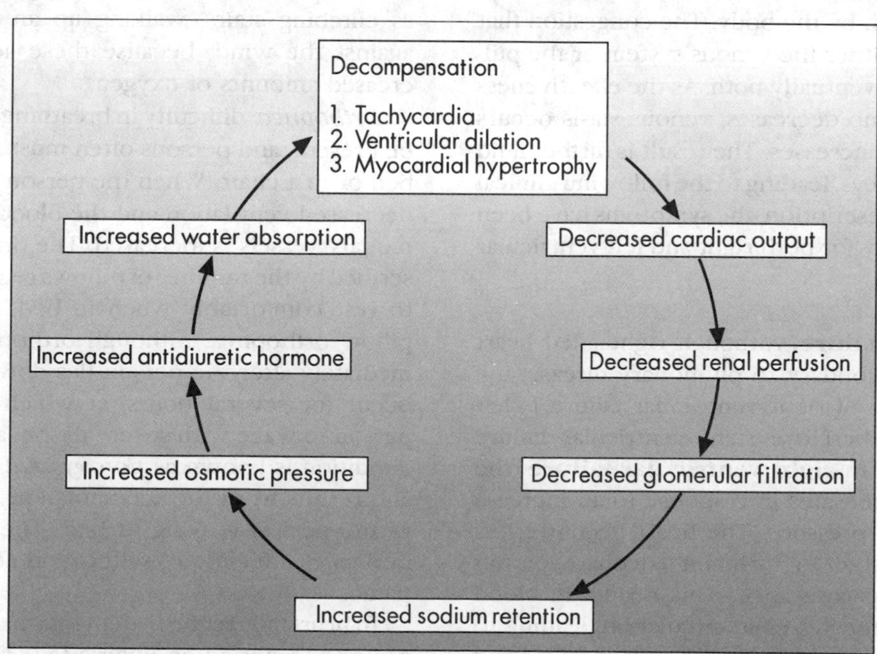


**FIGURE 31-13** Sequelae compounding decompensation in chronic heart failure.

**BOX 31-5 Signs and Symptoms of Congestive Heart Failure**

**RIGHT VENTRICULAR FAILURE**
- Peripheral edema (pitting)
- Liver enlargement with right upper quadrant pain
- Ascites
- Distended neck veins

**LEFT VENTRICULAR FAILURE**
- Dyspnea
- Orthopnea
- Paroxysmal nocturnal dyspnea (PND)
- Cheyne-Stokes respirations
- Fatigue
- Auscultatory crackles

can result from arteriosclerosis, hypertension, myocardial infarction, and valvular disorder.

### Left- versus right-sided heart failure

The most common event would be for one ventricle to fail before the other. Because the left ventricle is most often affected by coronary atherosclerosis and hypertension, heart failure usually begins there. Left ventricular failure usually is signaled by pulmonary congestion and edema. Right ventricular failure most often is triggered by left ventricular failure. Right ventricular failure usually leads to systemic venous congestion and peripheral edema. However, when the patient seeks health care, signs and symptoms of both right- and left-sided heart failure usually are present.

The symptoms of heart failure are the result of excessive fluid retention by the body. The congestion that results can involve either the venous system or the pulmonary system and eventually both. As the effectiveness of the heart as a pump decreases, venous stasis occurs and venous pressure increases. The result is further fluid retention by the kidneys, leading to the following clinical picture. For ease of description, the symptoms have been described individually for both right and left ventricular failure (Box 31-5).

**Right ventricular failure.** Although right-sided heart failure can occur secondary to pulmonary disease, the most common cause of right ventricular failure is left ventricular failure; therefore right ventricular failure rarely is seen alone. In **right ventricular failure,** the right ventricle compensates in response to an increase in pulmonary artery pressure. The heart becomes less effective and is unable to maintain adequate output against the increased resistance. This results in blood damming back into the systemic circulation, leading to peripheral edema. This *edema* is of the *pitting* type and is nontender. It also is known as *dependent edema* because it occurs in dependent parts of the body such as the legs or sacrum. As the edema becomes more pronounced, it progresses up the legs into the thighs, external genitalia, and lower portion of the trunk. As the tissue becomes extremely engorged, the skin cracks and fluid may "weep" from the tissues.

The *liver* also can become engorged with intravascular fluid, resulting in *enlargement* and tenderness in the right upper quadrant of the abdomen. As the venous stasis increases, pressure within the portal system becomes so great that fluid is forced through the blood vessels into the abdominal cavity. The collection of fluid *within the abdomen,* known as *ascites,* can reach volumes of more than 10 L. This great volume of fluid can displace the diaphragm, resulting in severe respiratory distress. A paracentesis (see Chapter 41) may be required to relieve the pressure on the diaphragm. *Distended neck veins* as a result of the increased systemic venous pressure usually are observed when the patient is in a sitting position (see Figure 29-16).

**Left ventricular failure.** In **left ventricular failure,** the left ventricle cannot pump oxygenated blood coming from the lungs at a volume necessary to meet the demands of the body. Symptoms are the result of congestion of the lungs with fluid that is forced from the pulmonary circulation into the pulmonary tissues, causing pulmonary edema and pleural effusion. Fluid may be present in the interstitial tissues, alveoli, bronchioles, or pleural space.

***Respiratory signs and symptoms.*** *Dyspnea,* labored breathing, is an early symptom of left ventricular failure. It is caused by interference with gas exchange as a result of the fluid in the alveoli. Dyspnea may occur or may become worse only on physical exertion, such as climbing stairs, walking up an incline, or walking against the wind, because these activities require increased amounts of oxygen.

*Orthopnea,* difficulty in breathing when lying flat, may be present, and persons often must sleep propped up in bed or in a chair. When the person is lying flat, there is decreased ventilation and the blood volume in the pulmonary vessels is increased. The orthopnea often is described by the number of pillows required for the patient to rest comfortably when in bed, for example, three-pillow orthopnea. Although orthopnea may occur immediately after the person lies down, it often does not occur for several hours, at which time it causes the person to wake with severe dyspnea and coughing. This condition is known as *paroxysmal nocturnal dyspnea* and results from the accumulation of fluid in the lungs as the person is lying in bed. The patient usually experiences a feeling of suffocation and often awakens in panic.

In heart failure the patient may experience alternating periods of *apnea* or *hyperpnea* (Cheyne-Stokes respirations). Often because of respiratory insufficiency, an inadequate amount of oxygen is delivered to the brain.

The decrease in oxygen makes the respiratory center in the brain insensitive to the amounts of carbon dioxide in the arterial blood, and respirations cease either until the carbon dioxide content in the arterial blood increases enough to stimulate the respiratory center or until the oxygen level in the blood drops to a level that is low enough to stimulate the respiratory center. This results in hyperpnea. These periods of overbreathing result in greater than normal decreases in carbon dioxide content of arterial blood, producing another period of apnea. Periodic overbreathing often begins as the patient goes to sleep and decreases as sleep deepens and ventilation decreases. High concentrations of oxygen generally are contraindicated because this measure would prevent the reflex stimulus to respiration caused by low oxygen content in the blood.

A persistent hacking *cough* often is a symptom of left-sided heart failure. The cough usually is productive of large quantities of frothy sputum, which occasionally is blood-tinged. Coughing results from congestion of trapped fluid, which is irritating to the mucosal lining of the lungs and bronchi. On auscultation, *crackles* can be heard. Crackles are the moist popping and crackling sounds heard most often at the end of inspiration.

***Fatigue.*** Persons with heart failure commonly note fatigue after activities that ordinarily are not tiring. The fatigue results from impaired blood circulation to tissues as a result of the decreased cardiac output. The reduction in tissue oxygen decreases the aerobic production of adenosine triphosphate (ATP), the immediate energy source for muscle contractions. Also, the impaired circulation decreases removal of metabolic waste products, resulting in further decreased muscle function.

***Pain.*** Cardiac pain is *not* a typical symptom of heart failure; however, angina pectoris can occur from the decrease in cardiac output. Cardiac pain associated with congestive heart failure is most likely to occur in patients with coronary artery disease. Coronary artery disease increases the patient's sensitivity to a deficiency in the oxygen content in the circulating blood. As heart failure develops, the blood is less effectively oxygenated and angina occurs. As the fluid overload state is corrected, the chest pain resolves.

## MEDICAL MANAGEMENT

### Diagnostic Tests

The most common diagnostic tests for the person experiencing congestive heart failure include a chest roentgenogram, ECG, echocardiogram, and cardiac catheterization (see Chapter 29).

### Medication

#### Digitalis therapy

**Digitalis** is the major therapeutic approach in the treatment of congestive heart failure. Digitalis and its derivatives usually are effective in improving myocardial function in persons with congestive heart failure. The positive inotropic action of digitalis preparations enhances mechanical performance by strengthening the force of myocardial contraction. This leads to increased cardiac output and increased blood flow to the kidneys. Digitalis preparations also decrease heart rate (automaticity) and cardiac conduction velocity, which permits the ventricles to relax more, allowing time for better filling of the ventricles with blood.

When acute congestive heart failure occurs, the physician usually orders an *optimal therapeutic dose* of a digitalis preparation to slow the ventricular rate and decrease symptoms. This larger dose given over a short period of time is called a *loading,* or *digitalizing,* dose. In some instances the dose may approach the toxic level, and the person is observed carefully for signs and symptoms of toxicity (Box 31-6). The full effect of the digitalizing drug is realized when the heart and circulation return to normal under treatment, and the symptoms of toxicity are more evident at this time. Because digitalis preparations have a *cumulative effect* and are slowly eliminated, early recognition of toxic symptoms and discontinuance of the drug will decrease their severity. After the optimal therapeutic dose has been determined, the person is given a daily maintenance dose of digitalis.

Several factors predispose the person to digitalis toxicity. One of the most common is hypokalemia, which potentiates the effects of digitalis. When potassium is depleted in the body or myocardium, the heart becomes more excitable and dysrhythmias may occur. Decrease in potassium levels below the normal range of 4.0 to 5.4 mEq/L can occur whenever excess potassium is lost from the body such as occurs in vomiting and diarrhea or induced diuresis. Most of the diuretics used to treat congestive heart failure result in the loss of potassium along with sodium and water. To replace the potassium lost through diuresis, persons often are given a supplemental form of potassium such as potassium chloride. Some diuretics have potassium added to them, but many physicians prefer to order the diuretics and potassium separately. In addition, foods such as orange juice or

**BOX 31-6 Signs and Symptoms of Digitalis Toxicity**

**CARDIOVASCULAR EFFECTS**
- Bradycardia
- Tachycardia
- Bigeminy
- Ectopic beats
- Pulse deficit

**GASTROINTESTINAL EFFECTS**
- Anorexia
- Nausea and vomiting
- Abdominal pain
- Diarrhea

**NEUROLOGIC EFFECTS**
- Headache
- Double vision
- Blurred or colored vision
- Drowsiness, confusion
- Restlessness, irritability
- Muscle weakness

**TABLE 31-6 Digitalis Preparations**

| | DIGOXIN (LANOXIN) | G-STROPHANTHIN (OUABAIN) |
|---|---|---|
| Digitalizing dose | 1.25-1.5 mg (oral)<br>0.75-1.5 mg (IV)<br>(in divided doses) | 0.25-0.5 mg IV<br>(over 12-24 hr) |
| Maintenance dose | 0.125-0.5 mg (oral) | — |
| Onset | Oral: 1-2 hr<br>IV: 15-20 min | IV: 3-10 min |
| Peak | Oral: 6-8 hr<br>IV: 1-5 hr | IV: 30-120 min |
| Duration | 6 days | 1-3 days |

bananas, which are high in potassium and low in sodium content, are encouraged.

Other predisposing factors to digitalis toxicity include severe liver and kidney disease—because the liver inactivates the drug and the kidney excretes it—and primary myocardial disease, which makes the myocardium more sensitive to the drug. Increased toxicity also occurs with alkalosis, hypercalcemia, hypomagnesemia, and hypothyroidism. If digitalis toxicity occurs, the medication is stopped at once and other therapy instituted as necessary.

Digoxin (Lanoxin) is the drug of choice for congestive heart failure (Table 31-6). If given intramuscularly, digoxin should be injected deeply and the area massaged after injection because the drug is a tissue irritant. Before a digitalis preparation is given, the apical pulse rate is taken. If this rate is below 60 the medication should be withheld until the physician has been consulted. The pulse also is evaluated for changes in rhythm. The pulse rate of persons with irregular rhythm should always be taken for a full minute for accuracy. Response to digitalis is evaluated on the basis of relief of symptoms, that is, decreased edema, loss of weight, fluid output greater than fluid intake, and no dyspnea or cyanosis.

### Diuretic therapy

Diuretic therapy is not a substitute for digitalis therapy, which has a direct action on the myocardium. Diuretics are potentially dangerous medications, and their use is instituted only after symptoms of heart failure persist after digitalization and sodium restriction. The purpose of diuretic therapy is to decrease cardiac workload by reducing circulating volume and thus reduce preload.

Essential to proper initiation of diuretic therapy is determining how much fluid should be removed from the patient by establishing a "dry weight," or edema-free weight. This can be accomplished by gradually removing fluid by use of diuretics and assessing the patient's blood pressure. When the patient becomes hypotensive, particularly orthostatic, this signals the physician that too much fluid has been removed. The patient is then permitted to reaccumulate a small amount of fluid until hypotension no longer occurs. The weight at which this occurs is then considered the patient's dry weight. This determination can be accomplished solely by adjusting the dose of diuretics. Adjustments in diuretic therapy can best be achieved while the patient is hospitalized; however, changes in dry weight when the patient is discharged will affect the equilibrium obtained during hospitalization.

Diuretics function by increasing the urinary output, which decreases blood volume, thereby reducing cardiac workload. This is accomplished primarily by inhibiting the reabsorption of sodium by the kidneys. Mercurial diuretics affect the proximal tubules; furosemide and ethacrynic acid affect the ascending loop of Henle; thiazides and triamterene affect the distal tubule; and spironolactone exerts its effect on the collecting duct. Dosages and side effects of these diuretics are listed in Table 31-7.

At present, the *thiazides* are the diuretics of choice in the treatment of heart failure. The thiazides are inexpensive, easy to take, and effective when taken over a long period. Because these patent drugs can lead to electrolyte imbalance, serum chemistry levels should be observed closely, particularly at the onset of therapy. The major complication is hypokalemia, which can be prevented by the intake of foods high in potassium or by potassium supplements.

If thiazides are ineffective, an oral aldosterone antagonist, such as spironolactone (Aldactone) or triamterene (Dyrenium), may be given with the thiazide. These drugs work by competitive inhibition of aldosterone, resulting in retention of potassium and excretion of sodium and water.

The most potent diuretics currently available are furosemide (Lasix), bumetanide (Bumex), and ethacrynic acid (Edecrin). These medications are reserved for severe congestive heart failure or when other forms of treatment are ineffective in relieving symptoms. These agents also increase renal blood flow and therefore may prove effective in treating heart failure when renal function also is impaired. Therapy is best initiated in the hospital setting so that electrolyte and acid-base balance may be monitored.

### Other medication

*Vasodilators* may be used to decrease afterload by decreasing resistance to ventricular emptying. The more commonly used agents are nitroprusside, hydralazine (Apresoline), and prozosin (Minipress). Nifedipine, a calcium channel blocker, also has vasodilator effects. Captopril (Capoten), a drug with antihypertensive properties, also is a vasodilator and blocks sodium retention by suppressing aldosterone. Vasodilators are more effective in the treatment of acute rather than chronic heart failure. Medications given to increase cardiac con-

**TABLE 31-7 Diuretics Used in the Treatment of Heart Failure**

| TYPE | EXAMPLE | ONSET/PEAK/DURATION | DOSE | SIDE EFFECTS |
|---|---|---|---|---|
| Thiazide | Chlorothiazide (Diuril) | 2 hr/4 hr/6-12 hr | 0.5-1.0 g once or twice a day | Gastrointestinal upsets (can be minimized by taking medication with meals); hypokalemia; hyperglycemia |
| | Hydrochlorothiazide (Esidrix, HydroDiuril) | 2 hr/4 hr/6-12 hr | 25-100 mg/day | |
| Loop | Furosemide (Lasix) | 1 hr/1-2 hr/6-8 hr | 20-80 mg/day orally (may be given intravenously in doses up to 600 mg in 24 hr to treat pulmonary edema) | Similar to thiazide diuretics; also ototoxicity and blood dyscrasias |
| | Bumetanide (Bumex) | Oral: 30-60 min/1-2 hr/4-6 hr<br>IV: within minutes/15-30 min | Oral 0.5-2 mg qd<br>IV/IM 0.5-1 mg (may be repeated at 2-3 hr intervals ×2; maximum 10 mg qd) | |
| | Ethacrynic acid (Edecrin) | 30 min/2 hr/6-8 hr | Oral 50-200 mg qd<br>IV 0.5-1.0 mg/kg body weight | |
| Potassium sparing | Spironolactone (Aldactone) | Gradual/3 days/2-3 days after therapy discontinued | 25-50 mg four times a day | Gastrointestinal irritation; hyperkalemia |
| | Triamterene (Dyrenium) | Rapid/7-9 hr/12-16 hr | 150-200 mg qd | |

tractility, in addition to digitalis, include *sympathomimetics* such as dopamine and dobutamine and *phosphodiesterase inhibitors* such as amrinone (Inocor).

## Treatment

The goal of medical management is to improve cardiac output without increasing cardiac workload. In addition to medications, prescribed activity, and diet, oxygen therapy is given. Hemodynamic monitoring with a pulmonary artery catheter may be used to evaluate left ventricular function and the patient's response to therapy.

## Diet

A sodium-restricted diet is prescribed to prevent fluid excess.

## Activity

The patient is placed on a balanced program of activity and rest.

# NURSING MANAGEMENT

## ♦ ASSESSMENT

### Subjective Data

Data to be collected to assess the patient with congestive heart failure concern the person's perception of breathing ability, fluid retention, response to activity, and knowledge of and response to the cardiac failure, including the following:

Shortness of breath and presence of cough
Presence of orthopnea (number of pillows needed for sleep)
Recent weight gain
Edema, especially pedal
Dizziness or confusion
Fatigue
Exercise or heat intolerance
Discomfort: anginal or abdominal pain
Appetite
Usual bowel patterns
Concerns, anxieties
Knowledge of condition
Usual coping skills

### Objective Data

Objective data focus primarily on signs of fluid retention and include the following:

Respiratory distress, increased effort, and respiratory rate
Neck vein distention: presence, degree
Adventitious breath sounds
Heart sounds: presence of $S_3$ or gallop rhythm
Edema: site and degree of pitting
Coolness of extremities
Pulse changes
Abdominal distention
Daily weights
Level of consciousness
Character of stools

# NURSING CARE PLAN

## PERSON WITH CONGESTIVE HEART FAILURE

**DATA:** Mr. A. is a 65-year-old white man with congestive heart failure who was admitted to the hospital with increased fluid retention. He has a history of hypertension and atherosclerotic heart disease. He has felt tired for several weeks and has experienced increased dyspnea on exertion, vertigo, and syncope. He has had two myocardial infarctions, the most recent being 6 months before admission. A cardiac catheterization performed several months previously revealed triple vessel disease, decreased left ventricular function with an ejection fraction of 25%, and poorly developed collaterals. He has been on a regimen of antianginal medications that have kept him pain-free, although he has been cognizant of progressive intolerance to exertion and increasing peripheral edema. On admission, his medication included bumetanide 20 mg bid, captopril 25 mg tid, digoxin 0.25 mg qd, diltiazem 90 mg q 6 hr, and nitroglycerine ointment 2% in a 2-inch patch q 6 hr.

The nursing history identified the following:

- Mr. A. has very little understanding of his medications and his low-sodium, low-cholesterol diet.
- The episodes of dyspnea have been increasingly anxiety-provoking.
- Mr. A. does not understand the need to take his medication, especially when he does not feel sick.
- Mr. A. has had increasing weight gain, approximately 10 pounds before admission.

Collaborative nursing activities include those to assess Mr. A.'s response to current therapeutic regimen and those to assess the presence of any complications associated with the regimen. Nursing actions include monitoring the following:

- Daily weights and intake/output
- Vital signs
- Breath sounds
- Response to exertion
- Heart rate and rhythm
- Serum electrolytes

### ■ NURSING DIAGNOSIS

Decreased cardiac output, related to reduced stroke volume, resulting in a compromised state

| Expected Patient Outcomes | Nursing Interventions | Rationale |
|---|---|---|
| Maintains pulse and respirations within normal limits. | Organize care to provide scheduled periods for rest and to minimize unnecessary disturbances. | Exercise and physical activity increase cardiac output, heart rate, and blood pressure. |
| Identifies factors that increase cardiac workload. | Explain and encourage increases in activity and ambulation to prevent a sudden increase in cardiac workload. | Regular exercise makes the heart more efficient so that stroke volume increases and heart rate is not appreciably altered. |
| | Monitor respirations q 4 hr for increased effort, pulse for tachycardia. | |
| | Monitor heart sounds q 4 hr for presence of gallop rhythm. | |
| | Teach Mr. A. to avoid Valsalva's maneuver. | Surge of blood to heart after intrathoracic pressure decreases causes increase in cardiac workload. |

### ■ NURSING DIAGNOSIS

Altered tissue perfusion, related to decreased blood flow to tissues and edema

| Expected Patient Outcomes | Nursing Interventions | Rationale |
|---|---|---|
| Has fewer episodes of syncope and vertigo. | Encourage movement and activity as tolerated. | Movement promotes circulation to tissues. |
| | Assess neck vein distention, edema of extremities and coolness of skin q 4 hr; weigh daily. | Assessment will provide information on fluid overload. |
| Experiences no skin breakdown. | Eliminate or reduce pressure points by changing position frequently, use of pressure mattress, etc. | Excess interstitial fluid interferes with diffusion of oxygen to cells. Cellular nutrition and respiration depend on adequate blood flow. Hypoxia causes cellular swelling and injury. |
| | Give diuretics and sodium-restricted diet as prescribed. | |

NURSING CARE PLAN

## PERSON WITH CONGESTIVE HEART FAILURE—cont'd

### ■ NURSING DIAGNOSIS

Activity intolerance related to imbalance between oxygen supply and demand

| Expected Patient Outcomes | Nursing Interventions | Rationale |
|---|---|---|
| Progresses to highest level of mobility possible with less fatigue and dyspnea. | Encourage rest periods according to daily schedule and during the first hour after meals. | Any factor that compromises cardiovascular function reduces tolerance to activity. |
| Identifies factors that reduce his activity intolerance. | Assess Mr. A.'s response to activity (pulse, blood pressure, respirations). | |
| | Increase Mr. A.'s tolerance for activity by having him perform activity more slowly or for a shorter period of time with more rest periods. | Pacing of activity decreases myocardial oxygen demand. |
| | Explain the effects of increased oxygen demand with decreased oxygen supply. | |

### ■ NURSING DIAGNOSIS

Knowledge deficit (pathophysiology of heart failure, rationale for therapy) related to lack of recall, poor understanding

| Expected Patient Outcome | Nursing Interventions | Rationale |
|---|---|---|
| Describes the pathophysiology, symptoms, and rationale for therapy of CHF. | Discuss with Mr. A.:<br>1. Basis of the symptoms and rationale for therapy<br>2. Self-monitoring for recurring signs of CHF<br>3. How to be active yet avoid fatigue<br>4. Management of prescribed sodium-restriction diet<br>5. Need for follow-up care | If Mr. A. understands reasons for the symptoms and how therapy will modify the symptoms, he will be more ready to learn about his care and to follow through with prescribed care. |
| | Examine Mr. A.'s health beliefs and past experiences related to illness and assess the impact on his desire/ability to learn. | Learning is influenced by values, beliefs, and previous experiences. |

## ♦ NURSING DIAGNOSES

Nursing diagnoses are determined from analysis of patient data. Nursing diagnoses for the patient with congestive heart failure may include but are not limited to the following:

| Diagnostic Title | Possible Etiologic Factors |
|---|---|
| Gas exchange, impaired | Ventilation/perfusion imbalance |
| Cardiac output, decreased | Reduced stroke volume, cardiogenic shock, valvular insufficiency, hypertension |
| Activity intolerance | Imbalance between oxygen supply/demand |
| Anxiety | Threat of death; threat/change in health status, socioeconomic status |
| Fluid volume excess | Impaired myocardial contractility |
| Tissue perfusion, altered: decreased | Decreased blood flow, hypervolemia, immobility, pulmonary edema |
| Nutrition, altered: less than body requirements | Anorexia, sodium imbalance |
| Constipation | Inactivity, GI edema |
| Knowledge deficit | Lack of exposure/recall |

## ♦ EXPECTED PATIENT OUTCOMES

Expected patient outcomes for the person with congestive heart failure may include but are not limited to the following:

1. Achieves normal respiratory rate without use of supplemental oxygen; states breathing is easier, confusion is decreased.

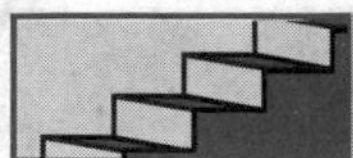

## CRITICAL PATHWAY Congestive Heart Failure Without Complications

**DGR #: 127 Expected LOS: 6**

| | Day of Admission Day 1 | Day 2 | Day 3 |
|---|---|---|---|
| **Diagnostic Tests** | CBC, UA, SMA/18,* ABGs, PT/PTT, chest film, ECG | SMA/6,† PT/PTT, echocardiogram | SMA/6,† PT/PTT, chest film, ABGs |
| **Medications** | IV @ TKO rate; digitalis, diuretic, low-dosage anticoagulant, vasodilator, bronchodilator, antidysrhythmic; Rx for rest/anxiety | IV @ TKO rate; digitalis, diuretic, low-dosage anticoagulant, vasodilator, bronchodilator, antidysrhythmic; Rx for rest; stool softener | IV @ TKO rate; digitalis, diuretic, low-dosage anticoagulant, vasodilator, bronchodilator, antidysrhythmic; Rx for rest; stool softener |
| **Treatments** | I & O q8hr; wt; $O_2$; VS q4hr; cardiac monitor; assess cardiopulmonary system q4hr; assess skin and give special care q2hr; elastic leg stockings | I & O q8hr; wt; $O_2$; VS q4hr; cardiac monitor; assess cardiopulmonary system q4hr; assess skin and give special care q2hr; elastic leg stockings | I & O q8hr; wt; $O_2$; VS q6hr; cardiac monitor; assess cardiopulmonary system q6hr; assess skin and give special care q6hr; elastic leg stockings |
| **Diet** | Full liquids, low sodium; restrict fluids | Soft, low sodium; provide 6 small meals/day | Soft, low sodium; provide 6 small meals/day |
| **Activity** | Bed rest, HOB elevated 30 degrees | Bed rest, HOB elevated 30 degrees; to BR with assistance | Up in chair with assistance × 4; HOB elevated 30 degrees while in bed |
| **Consultations** | Cardiology | Home health, dietary | |

*ABGs,* Arterial blood gases; *BR,* bathroom; *CBC,* complete blood cell count; *disc,* discontinue; *HOB,* head of bed; *PT,* prothrombin time; *PTT,* partial thromboplastin time; *SMA,* sequential multiple analysis; *TKO,* to keep open; *UA,* urinalysis; *VS,* vital signs.

2. Demonstrates cardiac tolerance to increased activity (pulse and blood pressure are stable).
3. Performs ADL without undue fatigue.
4. Uses effective coping mechanisms in managing anxiety.
5. Maintains stable weight within established parameters.
6. Maintains intact skin.
7. Eats prescribed sodium restricted diet.
8. Maintains soft and formed stools.
9. Describes the nature of the disease, signs and symptoms requiring medical care, medication therapy, diet and activity prescriptions, and plans for follow-up care.

## ♦ INTERVENTIONS

At many acute care hospitals, patients with acute congestive heart failure are admitted to medical or cardiac intensive care units. Occasionally the physician may elect to place the patient in the usual room accommodations where the environment is less stressful and where family members can visit more routinely. The decision about room placement is made on the basis of degree of failure and specific responses of the patient to the acute situation.

Care of the person with congestive heart failure is summarized in the Guidelines box, p. 880. A sample critical pathway and a nursing care plan for the person with congestive heart failure without complications are found on pp. 876-879.

### Providing Oxygenation

In heart failure the oxygen content of the bloodstream may be markedly reduced because of the less effective oxygenation of the blood as it passes through the congested lungs. The patient may be more comfortable and better able to rest while receiving oxygen because it helps in reducing dyspnea and fatigue. Oxygen usually is administered by nasal cannula at 2 to 6 L/min. Baseline arterial blood gas levels are obtained at initiation of oxygen therapy and intermittently during therapy to assess effectiveness of the treatment. Breathing often is made easier by maintaining the patient in semi-Fowler's or high Fowler's position. These positions maximize oxygenation by permitting greater lung expansion.

### Promoting Rest and Activity

Reducing the requirements of the body for oxygen can best be effected by providing the patient with the degree of activity that does not compromise myocardial function, as demonstrated by the presence of symptoms. If the degree of heart failure is mild, with only edema of the legs or minimal pulmonary congestion, the patient may be treated on an ambulatory basis with only a regimen of less strenuous activity and more rest than usual.

If the degree of heart failure is severe, a program of

| Day 4 | Day 5 | Day of Discharge Day 6 |
|---|---|---|
| ECG | SMA/6,† PT/PTT, chest film, ABGs | PT/PTT |
| IV saline lock; adjust drugs for home use; Rx for rest; stool softener | IV saline lock; adjust drugs for home use; Rx for rest; stool softener | Disc IV saline lock; adjust drugs for home use |
| I & O q8hr; wt; $O_2$; VS q8hr; cardiac monitor; assess cardiopulmonary system q8hr; assess skin and give special care q8hr; elastic leg stockings | I & O q8hr; wt; disc $O_2$; VS q8hr; disc cardiac monitor; assess cardiopulmonary system q8hr; elastic leg stockings | Wt; disc I & O; VS q8hr; assess cardiopulmonary system q8hr; elastic leg stockings |
| Soft, low sodium; provide 6 small meals/day | Soft, low sodium; provide 6 small meals/day | Soft, low sodium; provide 6 small meals/day |
| Up walking in hallway with assistance × 2, up in chair × 4; HOB elevated 30 degrees while in bed | Up walking in hallway with assistance × 2, up in chair × 4; HOB elevated 30 degrees while in bed | Up walking in hallway |

*Serum calcium, phosphorus, triglycerides, uric acid, creatinine, BUN, total bilirubin, alkaline phosphate, aspartate aminotransferase (AST) (formerly serum glutamic-oxaloacetic transaminase [SGOT]), alanine aminotransferase (ALT) (formerly serum glutamate pyruvate transaminase [SGPT]), lactic dehydrogenase (LDH), total protein, albumin, sodium, potassium, chloride, total $CO_2$, glucose.
†Serum sodium, potassium, chloride, total $CO_2$, glucose, BUN.

bed rest or limited activity may be necessary until symptoms abate. The amount of activity permitted each person is based on the extent of the symptoms such as dyspnea and fatigue. A careful assessment must be made each day to determine to what extent the person can perform ADL such as eating and bathing. Most patients prefer to maximize their independence, and this is encouraged within the limitations of their symptoms.

The patient often is orthopneic and tends to be more comfortable sitting than lying in bed. If the patient is placed in a chair, the feet are elevated to reduce pooling of fluid in the dependent limbs. When the patient is placed on bed rest, the high Fowler's position often is most comfortable. A pillow may be placed lengthwise behind the shoulders and back in such a manner that full expansion of the rib cage is possible. A foot block can be used to keep the patient from slipping toward the foot of the bed. The arms also may be supported on pillows to reduce the pull on the shoulder muscles (Figure 31-14). An over-the-bed table may be placed close to the patient to allow resting the head and arms.

Sedation is used judiciously for patients with heart failure inasmuch as oversedation may mask symptoms of increasing failure. In addition, immobility increases the risk of venous thrombosis and embolus. Patients with heart failure often are apprehensive and may have difficulty relaxing; thus diazepam (Valium), 2 to 10 mg three to four times a day, may be prescribed. Chloral hydrate may be used if the person is unable to sleep despite nursing measures to promote rest.

### Ambulation

Ambulation is started slowly to avoid overloading the heart and to determine how much activity the heart can tolerate without again showing signs of failure. The regimen varies depending on individual patient response. When a patient has been on restricted bed rest, activities progress slowly through stages of dangling, sitting up in a chair, and then walking increased distances under close supervision. The patient is assessed for signs indicating that activity cannot be tolerated, including dyspnea, fatigue, and increased pulse rate that does not stabilize readily. If these signs or symptoms occur, the person is returned to bed. If dyspnea is present, the head of the bed is elevated and oxygen is administered by nasal cannula at a low flow of 1 to 3 L/min. The physician is consulted before further ambulation is attempted.

The plan for increased activity is explained to the patient and family members. They should understand that if activity tires the person excessively, it may be curtailed. Overactivity can produce physical and mental setbacks that delay ultimate recovery. In the early stages of ambulation, it is important to begin stressing the importance of the rate of activity; that is, the demand on the heart is decreased when a normal activity is performed more slowly than before.

### Guidelines for Care of the Person With Congestive Heart Failure

1. Provide oxygenation
   a. Administer oxygen by nasal cannula at 2-6 L/min as prescribed
   b. Give oxygen as needed for dyspnea
   c. Patient should be well supported in semi-Fowler's or high Fowler's position
2. Provide rest and activity
   a. Reinforce importance of conservation of energy and planning for activities that avoid fatigue
   b. Encourage activity within prescribed restrictions; monitor for intolerance to activity (dyspnea, fatigue, increased pulse rate that does not stabilize)
   c. Assist with ADL as necessary; encourage independence within patient's limitations
   d. Provide diversional activity that will assist in conservation of energy
3. Monitor for signs of fluid and potassium imbalance; record daily weights
4. Provide skin care, particularly over edematous areas; use prophylactic measures to prevent skin breakdown
5. Assist in maintaining an adequate nutritional intake while observing prescribed dietary modifications (sodium restrictions)
6. Monitor for constipation; give prescribed stool softeners
7. Give prescribed medications
   a. Digitalis (take apical pulse before administration)
   b. Diuretics (assess for hypokalemia)
   c. Vasodilators
   d. Drugs to reduce anxiety and promote sleep
8. Provide patient/family opportunities to discuss their concerns
9. Teach patient about the disorder and self-care (see Guidelines box, p. 882)

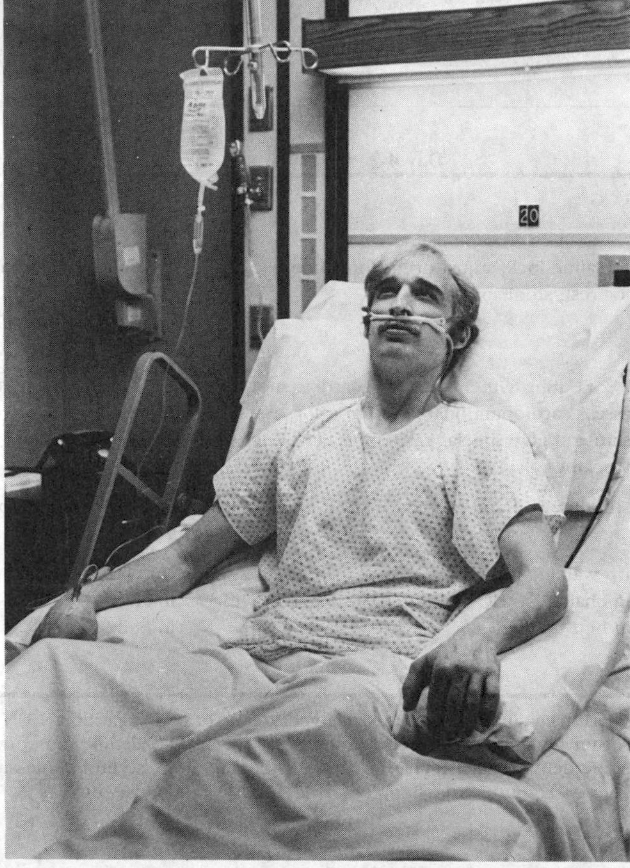


**FIGURE 31-14** Patient sitting upright with pillows under head and each arm to promote chest expansion and comfort.

## Decreasing Anxiety

Most persons are aware of the importance of an effective functioning heart to maintain life, and they also are acquainted with symptoms that indicate a failing heart. Therefore anxiety usually occurs when symptoms of heart failure are present. Anxiety can cause increased breathlessness, which is then interpreted by the patient as an increase in the severity of the heart failure, and this in turn increases the anxiety.

The goal of intervention is to help break the anxiety–increased symptoms–anxiety circle by helping the patient (1) identify feelings and the content related to those feelings, (2) identify strengths that can be used for coping, and (3) learn what can be done to decrease the anxiety. Learning about measures to control heart failure and measures to reduce stress may be helpful. Working with family members in the same manner also is helpful to decrease their anxiety so that they can be of greater support to the patient.

## Facilitating Fluid Balance

Fluid restriction is less commonly instituted than in the past as long as the person is on a sodium-controlled diet and is receiving diuretics or digitalis, or both. When sodium intake is controlled, patients usually do not experience thirst and will control their own fluid intake. The kidneys also remove water from the body to maintain proper sodium concentration. If fluids are restricted, the amount of fluid permitted is prescribed by the physician and a plan is made, in conjunction with the patient if possible, to space the fluids over the day depending on patient preferences. Usually one half of the fluids are planned for meals and the other half for between meals. If thirst does present a problem, frequent mouth care may add to patient comfort.

Although careful records of intake and output are kept on most patients with cardiac failure, the best method to estimate progress and response to prescribed diet, medications, and other forms of treatment is daily monitoring of the patient's weight. Weight gain indicates fluid retention; 1 kg of weight gain represents 1 L of fluid retention. The weight is carefully recorded on admission and then daily while the patient is hospitalized.

The patient with severe heart failure is weighed on a litter scale, which contains a stretcher to minimize exertion. The patient should be weighed at the same time of day with the same amount of clothing. A good practice is to weigh the patient each morning after the bladder has been emptied and before breakfast is eaten. The patient also is encouraged to continue to take his or her weight daily after being discharged to provide weight gain information for the health care provider.

## Providing Skin Care

Edematous skin is poorly nourished and very susceptible to breakdown. Edema of the sacrum is prevalent in patients with heart failure restricted to bed rest, and decubiti can develop quickly. The patient is carefully positioned and turned frequently to minimize breakdown. Measures to prevent skin breakdown are instituted early because prevention is more cost-effective for both patient and care provider, in addition to promoting patient comfort, both physical and mental. Inflatable mattresses are of assistance in preventing decubiti, but they do not eliminate the need for turning the patient.

## Promoting Nutrition

During the acute stage of congestive heart failure the diet should be bland, low-calorie, and low-residue, with vitamin supplement. Anorexia often occurs because of edema in the gastrointestinal tract, dyspnea, fatigue, and the effect of medications. Frequent small feedings minimize exertion and reduce gastrointestinal blood requirements, which can tax the failing heart. Care must be taken in providing a diet that meets the metabolic demands of the body so that body wasting does not occur.

### Sodium intake

Edema often is effectively controlled in patients with heart failure by restriction of sodium intake. The degree of restriction depends on the severity of the failure and the extent of diuretic therapy. A severely restricted sodium diet rarely is prescribed because the diet is unpalatable and expensive, resulting in poor patient compliance.

The amount of sodium in the normal diet is 3 to 10 g/day. Sodium restriction in persons receiving diuretics may not be dropped below 3 g/day because of the dangers of hyponatremia from removal of sodium, as well as water, by the action of the diuretic on the kidneys. In mild cardiac failure a "no added salt" (NAS) diet is prescribed and is essentially a normal diet except that no extra salt is added to prepared foods, and obviously salted foods such as potato chips are omitted. For moderate or severe heart failure, the amount of sodium permitted is specifically prescribed. Vitamin supplements usually are required when severely restricted sodium diets are prescribed.

Low-sodium diets can be made more appealing by adding salt substitutes to food in place of table salt. Because many salt substitutes contain potassium, the patient's need for potassium must be assessed. Often the increased intake of potassium is beneficial when the patient is receiving diuretic therapy. The use of herbs, such as basal, dill, bay leaves, garlic (powder not salt), and tarragon, often makes the food more appetizing.

### Nutrition education of patients and family

The rationale for dietary and fluid restrictions must be explained to both the patient and the family. Family members must understand the necessity for these restrictions so they do not present the patient with food or fluids that are unacceptable. The patient needs to learn early about the food and fluid restrictions to be followed after discharge. This allows time for answering questions and planning menus. The ambulatory patient may need frequent interactions with the dietitian or nurse before being able to follow the diet adequately.

## Promoting Elimination

It is advisable for the person with cardiac disease to avoid straining at defecation, which places an extra burden on the heart. During straining against a closed glottis (Valsalva's maneuver), venous return to the heart is decreased as a result of increased intrathoracic pressure. When this pressure is released after straining, a large amount of venous return creates an increased workload on the heart.

The feces can be kept soft by giving a mild cathartic such as milk of magnesia, a mild bulk cathartic such as psyllium (Metamucil), or a stool-softening agent such as sodium docusate (Colace). If an enema becomes necessary, it should be of low volume and given with a small rectal tube inserted only 3 to 4 inches.

The use of a bedpan often is uncomfortable and does not facilitate bowel evacuation. The necessity for use of a bedpan often creates anxiety in the patient. For these reasons the patient usually is permitted to use a bedside commode. The patient should be assisted to and from the commode.

## Facilitating Learning

Teaching is initiated early in the person's hospitalization to permit time for learning and asking questions. Many episodes of recurring congestive heart failure might be prevented if patients were able to follow the prescribed drug therapy, avoid dietary indiscretions, avoid excessive physical activity, and recognize and report recurring symptoms to their physician. Repeated episodes of congestive heart failure can lead to serious consequences such as liver cirrhosis, pulmonary fibrosis, and enlargement of the spleen and kidneys. (See Guidelines box, p. 882, for patient teaching.)

# ♦ EVALUATION

To evaluate the effectiveness of nursing interventions, compare patient behaviors with those stated in the expected patient outcomes. Successful achievement of patient outcomes for the patient with congestive heart disease is indicated by the following:

**Guidelines for Teaching the Person With Congestive Heart Failure**

1. Monitor for signs and symptoms of recurring congestive heart failure and report these signs and symptoms to the physician or clinic:
   a. Weight gain of 1-1.5 kg (2-3 lb) over a short period of time (about 2 days)
   b. Loss of appetite
   c. Shortness of breath
   d. Orthopnea
   e. Swelling of ankles, feet, or abdomen
   f. Persistent cough
   g. Frequent nighttime urination
2. Avoid fatigue and plan activity to allow for rest periods
3. Plan and eat meals within prescribed sodium restrictions
   a. Avoid salty foods
   b. Avoid drugs with high sodium content (e.g., some laxatives and antacids, Alka-Seltzer)—read the labels
   c. Eat several small meals rather than three large meals per day
4. Take prescribed medications
   a. If several medications are prescribed, develop a method to facilitate accurate administration
   b. Digitalis: check own pulse rate daily; report a rate of less than 60/min to physician and signs and symptoms of toxicity
   c. Diuretics
      (1) Weigh self daily at same time of day
      (2) Report weight gain to physician
      (3) Eat foods high in potassium and low in sodium (such as oranges, bananas)
   d. Vasodilators
      (1) Report signs of hypotension (lightheadedness, rapid pulse, syncope) to physician
      (2) Avoid alcohol when taking vasodilators
5. Report to physician for follow-up as directed

1. Has normal respiratory rate without use of supplemental oxygen, breathes more easily, and is not confused.
2. Demonstrates tolerance of activities that reflect increased cardiac workload.
3. States that ADLs are performed without fatigue.
4. Uses effective coping mechanisms in managing anxiety.
5. Maintains stable weight within established parameters.
6. Manifests intact skin.
7. Eats prescribed sodium-restricted diet.
8. Has stools that are soft and formed.
9. Appropriately describes nature of the disease, signs and symptoms requiring medical care, medication therapy, diet and activity prescriptions, and plans for follow-up care.

## ACUTE PULMONARY EDEMA

### Etiology

**Acute pulmonary edema** is a medical emergency arising from severe left ventricular failure. It usually results from prolonged strain on a diseased heart. It also may result from inhalation of irritating gases or from too rapid administration of plasma, serum albumin, whole blood, or intravenous fluids; or it may be associated with barbiturate or opiate poisoning.

### Pathophysiology

In pulmonary edema caused by heart failure, cardiac output is decreased, resulting in an increase in left atrial pressure. This results in an increase in pulmonary vein and capillary pressure. As the pulmonary capillary pressure exceeds the intravascular osmotic pressure, serous fluid is rapidly forced into the alveoli. Fluid rapidly reaches the bronchioles and bronchi, and patients literally begin to drown in their own secretions.

Signs and symptoms of pulmonary edema include restlessness and vague uneasiness at the onset. As pulmonary edema progresses, profound dyspnea, pallor, cough productive of large quantities of blood-tinged frothy sputum, audible wheezing, and cyanosis develop. Tachycardia often is present.

### Medical Management

The goals in the treatment of acute pulmonary edema include physical and mental relaxation, relief of hypoxemia, retardation of venous return, and improvement of cardiovascular function.

The patient with acute pulmonary edema is placed in bed in *high Fowler's position,* and the physician is summoned immediately. Treatment usually is begun by administering *morphine sulfate,* 10 to 15 mg intravenously. The intravenous route is preferred because vascular collapse may hinder its absorption from subcutaneous tissues. Anxiety is relieved by morphine, which increases venous capacitance and lowers left atrial pressure and which may decrease ventilation.

To relieve hypoxemia, the physician often orders *oxygen* at 40% to 70% to be delivered by face mask. Humidification is desirable to keep secretions moist and to facilitate mobilization of these secretions. Occasionally the patient with severe pulmonary embarrassment requires intubation to deliver adequate tidal volumes and oxygen concentration. Intubation also aids in removing secretions by suctioning. Extubation often is possible within hours of the initiation of therapy. In the treatment of pulmonary edema, *aminophylline* also may be administered intravenously to dilate the bronchi, increase urinary output, and increase cardiac output.

The treatments described earlier for congestive heart failure also are implemented for pulmonary edema, including (1) rapid *digitalization,* (2) institution of diuretic therapy with *furosemide* or *bumetanide, (3) vasodilators,* and (4) administration of *dopamine* or *dobutamine.* Serum potassium levels are obtained immediately because these patients have significant diuresis and lose large amounts of potassium.

Two more radical and controversial treatments that

may be used when the preceding regimens fail include phlebotomy and rotating tourniquets. The purpose of phlebotomy is to decrease the amount of circulating blood to decrease pulmonary engorgement; however, this process removes hemoglobin that may further contribute to hypoxemia.

The purpose of rotating tourniquets is to pool blood in the extremities, thus reducing cardiac overload. As much as 1 L of blood may be trapped in the extremities when tourniquets are used. The tourniquets are placed on three extremities at one time. Every 15 minutes in clockwise or counterclockwise order, one tourniquet is placed on the extremity that has no tourniquet and one tourniquet is removed. Thus each extremity is occluded for 45 minutes. A rotating tourniquet machine uses blood pressure cuffs as tourniquets and automatically pumps and deflates the cuffs to obtain the desired effect. Because the purpose of this therapy is to occlude venous blood, the tourniquets should not obliterate arterial pulses in the extremity. If an extremity does not return readily to normal color on release of a tourniquet, the physician is informed. When the procedure is terminated, the tourniquets are released, one every 15 minutes to prevent a sudden increase in venous return and recurrence of pulmonary edema.

### Nursing Management

Nursing interventions for the patient with pulmonary edema are similar to those for acute congestive heart failure. Emphasis is placed on relieving anxiety, monitoring respiratory status and response to oxygen therapy, positioning the patient to facilitate breathing, and giving the prescribed medications.

## QUESTIONS TO CONSIDER

- How would you explain to a patient the difference between congestive heart failure and myocardial infarction?
- Why do dysfunctions of the mitral and aortic valves, which are on the left side of the heart, lead to right-sided heart failure?
- How do valve repair and valve replacement differ? What are the differences among the three types of valve repair?
- What would you tell a patient who asks you what will happen after cardiac surgery?
- Examine the chart of a patient who has congestive heart failure. How do the patient's symptoms compare with the usual symptoms? Did the patient have left- or right-sided failure, or both? What data would indicate improvement in the pumping capabilities of this patient's heart? What are the specific learning needs of this patient relative to the heart failure?

## CRITICAL THINKING ACTIVITIES

- Katy has cardiomyopathy and is awaiting a cardiac transplant. When notified that a donor has been found, Katy experiences both joy and sorrow about obtaining an organ. Why might Katy be having mixed feelings about her transplant?
- You are caring for Mrs. Block, 74, who has acute congestive heart failure. How will your knowledge of the cardiogenic shock patient assist you in caring for Mrs. Block? Or will it be of no value to you, since these are different conditions?
- While caring for Mr. Ball, who has congestive heart failure, you note that he is becoming restless and irritable. Upon further assessment you note that he is also pale with audible wheezing. His heart rate is 140, and he is gasping for air. How should you respond? What is the probable cause of the patient's reaction?

## CHAPTER SUMMARY

### INFLAMMATORY HEART DISEASE

- All layers of the heart (pericardium, myocardium, and endocardium) may become inflamed. Patients with these conditions have the usual signs of inflammation and also may develop heart failure. Measures to prevent further episodes are important aspects of the treatment regimen.

### VALVULAR HEART DISEASE

- Mitral and aortic valvular disease occur more frequently than do pulmonic and tricuspid valvular disease. Rheumatic fever is a common precursor. The two basic problems that compromise normal functioning of the valves are stenosis and regurgitation (insufficiency). Stenosis causes a narrowing of the valvular orifice and impedes the forward flow of blood. Regurgitation causes incomplete closure of the valve and allows blood to flow backward.
- Cardiac murmurs are a common physical finding in patients with valvular heart disease. Depending on the severity of the disease, the patient may develop such clinical symptoms as those associated with heart failure.
- Treatment of valvular disease involves management of clinical symptoms. Surgical repair of the valve or replacement of the valve with an artificial valve may be necessary.

### NURSING MANAGEMENT OF THE PATIENT WITH HEART SURGERY

- Types of heart surgery include repair or replacement of valves, repair of ventricular aneurysms, coronary artery bypass, release of constriction, or heart transplantation.

- Teaching is a major preoperative nursing intervention for cardiovascular surgery and includes information about the ICU, surgery, and preoperative and postoperative procedures.
- In total cardiopulmonary bypass, both the oxygenation and circulation of the blood are bypassed and performed by the bypass machine, thus permitting the heart to be incised and opened for surgery. The machine also permits administration of medications and can provide systemic hypothermia. Side effects of the procedure include hemodilution, decreased platelets, shock, and decreased perfusion to major organs.
- Intraaortic balloon counterpulsation is a method by which a balloon is inserted into the thoracic aorta as temporary assistance for circulation. When inflated, the balloon forces blood retrograde to increase coronary filling; when deflated, it decreases pressure in the aortic arch, thus facilitating afterload.
- Postoperative nursing care after cardiovascular surgery includes monitoring cardiovascular, respiratory, neurologic, and urinary systems; monitoring and promoting fluid and electrolyte balance and oxygen/carbon dioxide exchange; promoting patient comfort and activity; and patient teaching.

## CONGESTIVE HEART FAILURE

- Congestive heart failure (CHF) refers to a state of circulatory congestion resulting from heart failure and its compensatory mechanisms. Symptoms may involve the pulmonary circulation, the systemic venous circulation, or both.
- Medical therapy for CHF consists of reducing oxygen requirements through oxygen therapy and rest, optimizing cardiac output with medications (digitalis, diuretics, vasodilators), and providing a sodium-restricted diet plan.
- Nursing interventions for CHF consist of providing oxygenation; promoting rest and activity, nutrition, and elimination; providing skin care and emotional support; and patient teaching.
- Pulmonary edema represents the most severe form of congestion resulting from left ventricular failure; it requires immediate medical and nursing intervention.

## REFERENCES


1. American Heart Association: *Textbook of advanced cardiac life support,* Dallas, 1993, The Association.
2. Ball GB, Grap MJ: Postoperative GI symptoms in cardiac surgery patients, *Crit Care Nurse* 12(1):56-62, 1992.
3. Braunwald E: *Heart disease: a textbook of cardiovascular medicine,* ed 3, Philadelphia, 1988, WB Saunders.
4. Copeland J et al: Selection of patients for cardiac transplantation, *Circulation* 75:2-9, 1987.
5. Cosgrove E et al: Results of mitral valve reconstruction, *Circulation* 74(suppl 1):182-187, 1986.
6. Cox JL: Evolving applications of the maze procedure for atrial fibrillation, *Ann Thorac Surg* 55:578-580, 1993.
7. Groer MW, Shekleton ME: *Basic pathophysiology: a holistic approach,* ed 4, St Louis, 1994, Mosby.
8. Hurst JW: *The heart,* ed 6, New York, 1986, McGraw-Hill.
9. Hurst AH: Mitral valve prolapse: physical assessment, complications, and management, *Nurs Pract* 10(4):15-17, 1985.
10. King KB et al: Coronary artery bypass graft surgery in older women and men, *Am J Crit Care* 1(2):28-35, 1992.
11. McAllister RG: Age-related changes in drug handling in men, *Am Cardiol* 57:59C-62D, 1986.
12. Nair CK et al: Ten years' experience with mitral valve replacement in the elderly, *Am Heart J* 124:154-159, 1992.
13. Olsson M et al: Aortic valve replacement in octogenarians with aortic stenosis: a case-control study, *J Am Coll Cardiol* 20(7):1512-1516, 1992.
14. Reitzband Ream AK: Uses of hypothermia in cardiovascular surgery. In Nreane AK, Fogdall R: *Acute cardiovascular management,* Philadelphia, 1982, JB Lippincott.
15. Whitman G: Prosthetic cardiac valves, *Prog Cardiovasc Nurs* 2:116-123, 1987.

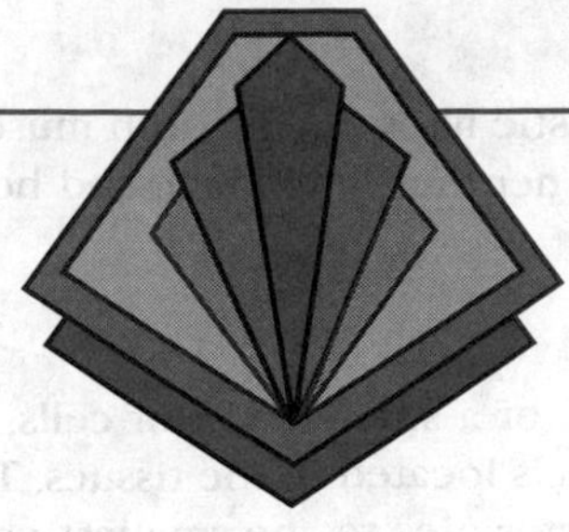

# CHAPTER 32

# Management of Persons With Vascular Problems

**M. Eileen Walsh**

## CHAPTER OBJECTIVES

***After studying this chapter, the learner should be able to do the following:***

1 Identify risk factors associated with the development of vascular disease.
2 Compare nursing interventions for patients with arterial embolism and deep vein thrombosis.
3 Differentiate between superficial thrombophlebitis and deep vein thrombosis.
4 Describe nursing care of patients undergoing arterial or venous surgery.
5 Explain the pathophysiologic basis for lymphedema.
6 Identify nursing interventions for patients with hypertension.

## KEY TERMS

aneurysm (aortic, abdominal)
anticoagulants
arterial embolism
arterial occlusive disease
arterial ulcer
arteriovenous fistula
atherectomy
balloon angioplasty
deep vein thrombosis (DVT)
digital subtraction angiography
duplex ultrasonography
embolectomy
endarterectomy
essential hypertension
hypertension (HTN)
hypertensive crisis
impedance plethysmography
intermittent claudication
laser angioplasty
lymphangiography
lymphedema
malignant hypertension
phantom limb pain
primary Raynaud's disease
prosthesis
Raynaud's phenomenon
renin-angiotensin system
secondary hypertension
thrombectomy
thromboangiitis obliterans
thrombolytics
thrombophlebitis
Trendelenburg's test
Unna paste boot
varicose veins
venography
venous ulcer

Problems of the vascular system refer to conditions that disrupt blood flow through the arteries and veins, excluding the coronary arteries (see Chapter 31) and cerebral vessels (see Chapter 57). The following vascular diseases are discussed in this chapter:

1. Arterial: arterial occlusive disease, thromboangiitis obliterans, Raynaud's phenomenon, aneurysm, and arterial embolism
2. Venous: superficial thrombophlebitis, deep vein thrombosis, varicose veins
3. Arterial and venous: arteriovenous fistula, leg ulcers
4. Lymphedema
5. Hypertension

This chapter includes lymphedema because the lymphatic system complements the function of the vascular system. A section on hypertension also is included because it is a major risk factor for vascular disorders.

## THE VASCULAR SYSTEM

To fully understand the pathophysiologic changes that occur in vascular disorders, it is important to know the normal structures and functions of the vascular system; a brief review follows.

### STRUCTURE AND FUNCTION

Body cells depend on an intact and functioning vascular system. This vascular system is a closed circuit consisting of the systemic and pulmonary circulations. Blood circulates from the left side of the heart to the tissues and back to the right side of the heart. It then flows through the lungs and back to the left side of the heart. The main components of the vascular system are the arteries, capillaries, and veins.

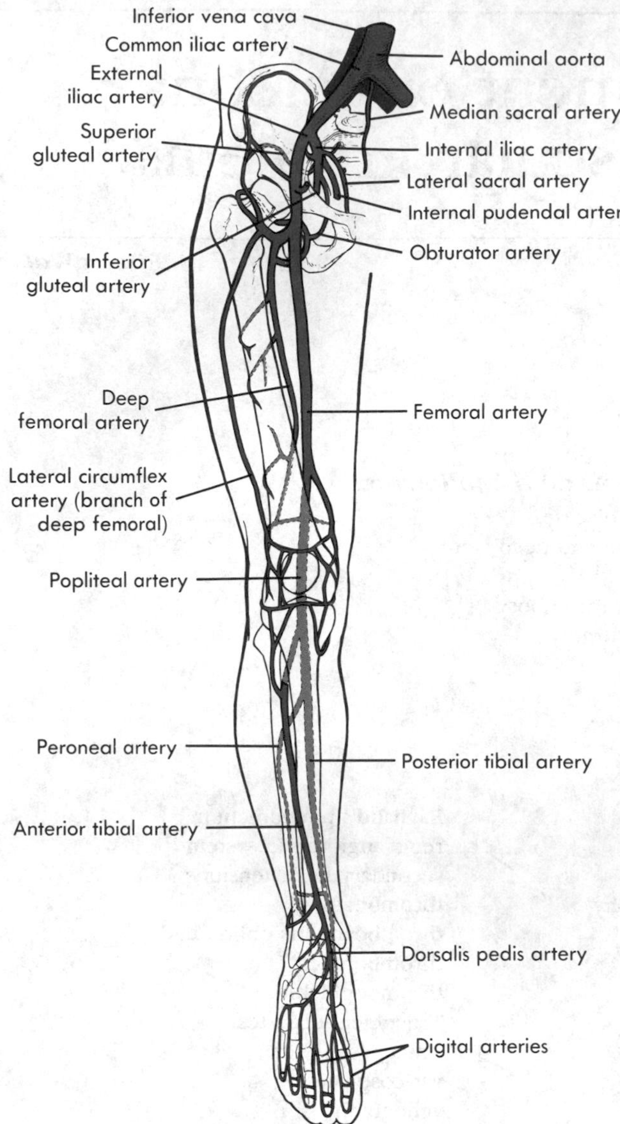


**FIGURE 32-1** Major arteries of lower limb. (From Seeley RR, Stephens TD, Tate P: *Anatomy and physiology,* ed 2, St Louis, 1992, Mosby.)

## Arteries

Arteries are thick-walled vessels transporting oxygen and blood via the aorta from the heart to the tissues. As the arteries approach the tissues, they branch into smaller vessels called *arterioles* (Figure 32-1). Arteries are composed of three tissue layers:

1. Inner layer of endothelium (intima)
2. Middle layer of connective tissue, smooth muscle, or elastic fibers (media)
3. Outer layer of connective tissue (adventitia)

The media forms the major portion of the vessel wall. In the large arteries the media is composed primarily of elastic and connective tissue enabling the artery to respond to alteration of blood volume while maintaining a constant flow. In the smaller arteries and arterioles there is much less elastic fiber; the smooth muscle contracts and relaxes by nervous, chemical, and hormonal factors.

## Capillaries

Capillaries, composed of a single layer of cells, are minute, thin-walled vessels located in the tissues. The capillaries connect the arterioles to the smallest veins and venules, allowing for the exchange of essential cellular products. Nutrients, oxygen, and regulatory substances move into the cells, whereas waste products, carbon dioxide, and cellular secretions move from the cells into the blood.

## Veins

Veins are thin-walled vessels transporting deoxygenated blood from the capillaries back to the right side of the heart. Veins are composed of three layers: intima, media, and adventitia. These layers differ from arterial walls, however, as there is little smooth muscle and connective tissue. This makes the veins distensible, enabling the accumulation of large volumes of blood. The sympathetic nervous system innervates the veins, causing venoconstriction, decreased venous volume, and increased circulating blood volume. Major veins, particularly those in the lower extremities, have one-way valves that allow blood flow against gravity (Figure 32-2).

# PATHOPHYSIOLOGY

All peripheral vascular disorders are characterized by a reduction in blood flow and hence oxygen through the peripheral vessels. As the tissue oxygen needs exceed the supply, areas of ischemia and ultimately necrosis will develop. It is the extent to which the tissues are deprived of oxygen that gives rise to the manifestations of symptoms. Furthermore, the inherent ability of the vascular system to develop collateral circulation, or alternate circulatory pathways, affects this process.

Several factors can contribute to the development of peripheral vascular disease. Pathologic changes within the blood vessels, including atherosclerotic changes, thrombus formation, and embolization, are the most common causes. Other factors such as increased coagulability of blood, blood pressure changes, and inflammatory processes can affect circulation. Heart failure also impedes peripheral blood flow from a reduction in cardiac output with resultant systemic venous congestion. Mechanical or chemical trauma may contribute to vascular disorders.

# PHYSIOLOGIC CHANGES WITH AGING

Degenerative changes occur in the vascular system as part of normal aging. These changes affect the walls of the blood vessels causing problems in the transport of blood and nutrients to the tissues. Increased thickness in the intimal wall results from fibrosis and is further affected by the accumulation of collagen and calcium.

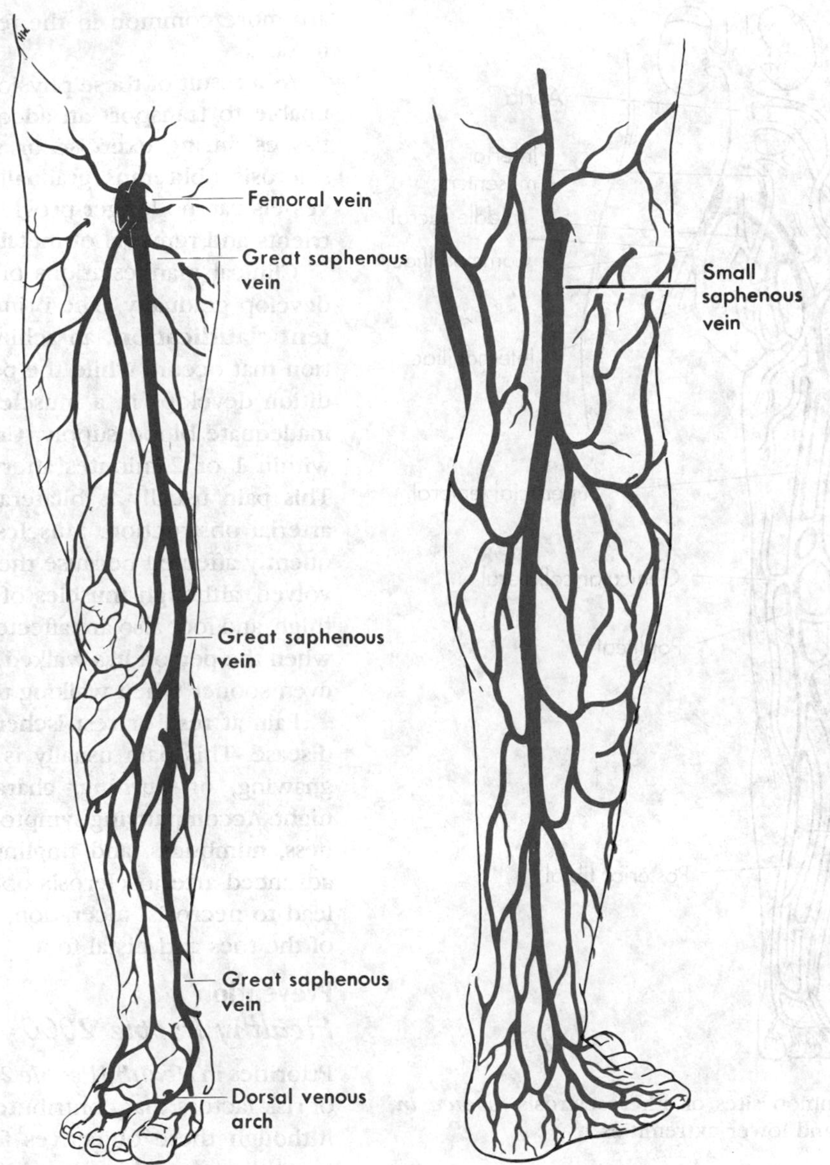


**FIGURE 32-2** Superficial veins of the leg and foot. (From Anthony CJ, Thibodeau GA: *Textbook of anatomy and physiology,* ed 13, St Louis, 1990, Mosby.)

The elastic fibers of the media become thin and calcified, greatly decreasing the elasticity and flexibility of the vessels and increasing peripheral vascular resistance. The result is a rise in blood pressure and less flow through the vessels, leading to a decreased supply of oxygen and nutrients to the tissues coupled with an accumulation in the tissues of cellular secretions, waste products, and carbon dioxide.

# ARTERIAL DISORDERS

Any disturbance in the structure of the arteries interferes with transport of blood from the heart to the tissues. The symptoms of arterial disease are not caused by the degree of obstruction or narrowing but by the degree to which the involved body part is deprived of circulation. This in turn is affected by such factors as blood pressure and presence or absence of collateral circulation. The following arterial diseases are discussed: arterial occlusive disease, thromboangiitis obliterans, Raynaud's phenomenon, aneurysm, and arterial embolism.

## ARTERIAL OCCLUSIVE DISEASE

### Etiology

**Arterial occlusive disease** most often is caused by arteriosclerosis obliterans, a disease of segmental arteriosclerotic narrowing or obstruction within the intima of the arteries. The lower extremities are more commonly involved (Figure 32-3). The superficial femoral artery, iliac arteries, and popliteal arteries are the most

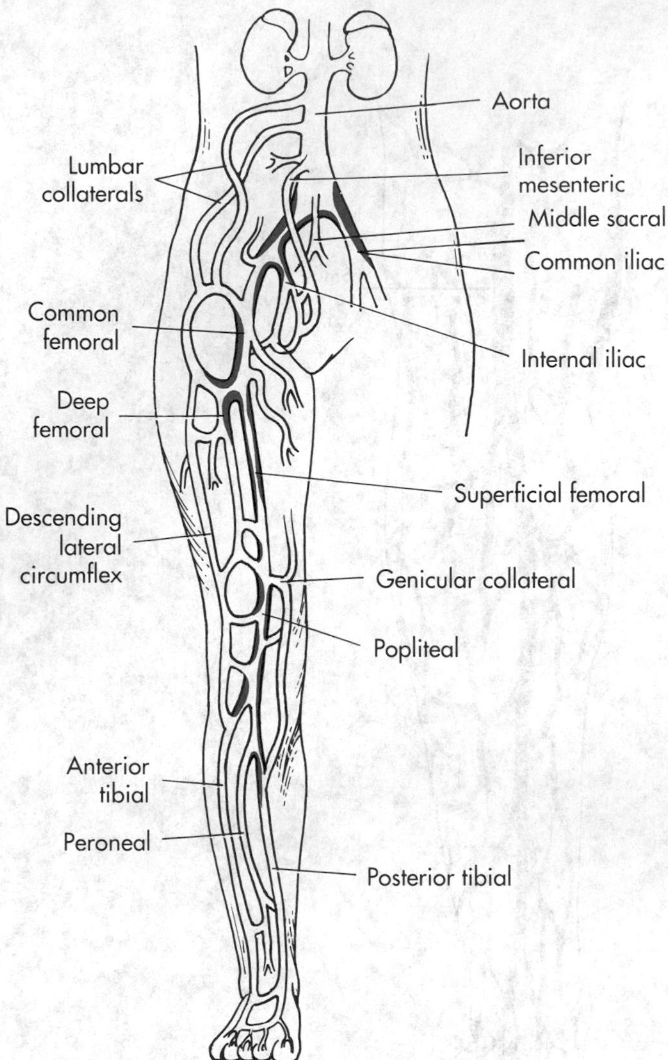


**FIGURE 32-3** Common sites of atherosclerosis *(shown in color)* in the aorta and lower extremities.

frequent sites of involvement. Atherosclerotic plaque typically develops at points of branching, bifurcation, or vessel narrowing.

## Epidemiology

Arterial occlusive disease is more prevalent in men, but symptoms typically do not occur until 50 to 70 years of age. In persons with diabetes mellitus, arteriosclerosis obliterans is more progressive, affecting the smaller distal vessels below the knee.

## Pathophysiology

The primary lesion of arteriosclerosis obliterans is atheromatous plaque formation in the intima causing partial or complete occlusion. In addition, there is usually calcification of the media and a gradual loss of elasticity that further weakens the arterial walls and predisposes to aneurysm dilation or thrombus formation. Aneurysms are more common in the femoral artery and popliteal fossa.

As a result of these physiologic changes, the artery is unable to transport an adequate blood volume to the tissues during exercise or rest. Symptoms of arteriosclerosis obliterans gradually appear when the blood vessels can no longer provide tissues with required nutrients and removal of metabolic wastes.

Clinical manifestations of arteriosclerosis obliterans develop gradually. The primary symptom is **intermittent claudication,** an aching pain or cramping sensation that occurs while the person is walking. This condition develops in a muscle that is exercised with an inadequate blood supply. Cramping usually disappears within 1 or 2 minutes after cessation of the exercise. This pain usually is bilateral and distal to the site of arterial obstruction. Muscles of the calf are more frequently affected because the femoral artery often is involved, although muscles of the lower back, buttocks, thigh, and foot also are affected. Symptoms usually occur when the person has walked one half to two blocks and even sooner when walking up a grade.

Pain at rest, or rest ischemia, is indicative of severe disease. This pain usually is described as dull, aching, gnawing, or burning, characteristically occurring at night. Accompanying symptoms such as feelings of coldness, numbness, and tingling also may be present. In advanced arteriosclerosis obliterans, rest ischemia may lead to necrosis, ulceration, and gangrene, particularly of the toes and distal foot.

## Prevention

### *Healthy People 2000*

Priorities in *Healthy People 2000*[5] include the alteration of risk factors that contribute to cardiovascular disease. Although these objectives focus more specifically on heart disease and stroke, they are applicable to arterial occlusive disease because atherosclerosis has the same etiologic factors. The detection, evaluation, and management of high blood pressure and high blood cholesterol level are important. Control of other risk factors such as smoking, obesity, and physical inactivity also are included in *Healthy People 2000.* The following risk-reduction objectives are significant to arterial occlusive disease:

- Increase to at least 50% the proportion of persons with high blood pressure whose blood pressure is under control. (Baseline: 11% controlled among persons aged 18 through 74 in 1976-1980; an estimated 24% for persons aged 18 and older in 1982-1984)
- Increase to at least 90% the proportion of persons with high blood pressure who are taking action to help control their blood pressure. (Baseline: 79% of aware hypertensive persons aged 18 and older were taking action to control their blood pressure in 1985)
- Reduce the mean serum cholesterol level among adults to no more than 200 mg/dl. (Baseline: 213 mg/

dl among persons aged 20 through 74 in 1976-1980, 211 mg/dl for men and 215 mg/dl for women)

- Reduce the prevalence of blood cholesterol levels of 240 mg/dl or greater to no more than 20% among adults. (Baseline: 27% for persons aged 20 through 74 years in 1976 to 1980, 29% for women and 25% for men)
- Increase to at least 60% the proportion of adults with high blood cholesterol who are aware of their condition and are taking action to reduce their blood cholesterol to recommended levels. (Baseline: 11% of all persons aged 18 and older, and thus an estimated 30% of persons with high blood cholesterol, were aware that their blood cholesterol level was high in 1988)
- Reduce dietary fat intake to an average of 30% of calories or less and average saturated fat intake to less than 10% of calories among persons aged 2 and older. (Baseline: 36% of calories from total fat and 13% from saturated fat for persons aged 20 through 74 in 1976-1980; 36% and 13% for women aged 19 through 50 in 1985)
- Reduce overweight to a prevalence of no more than 20% among persons aged 20 and older and no more than 15% among adolescents aged 12 through 19. (Baseline: 26% for persons aged 20 through 74 in 1976-1980, 24% for men and 27% for women; 15% for adolescents aged 12 through 19 in 1976-1980)
- Increase to at least 30% the proportion of persons aged 6 and older who engage regularly, preferably daily, in light to moderate physical activity for at least 30 minutes per day. (Baseline: 22% of persons aged 18 and older were active for at least 30 minutes five or more times per week, and 12% were active seven or more times per week in 1985)
- Reduce cigarette smoking to a prevalence of no more than 15% among persons aged 20 and older. (Baseline: 29% in 1987, 32% for men and 27% for women)

### Primary prevention

Primary prevention is an extremely important means of reducing the incidence of peripheral vascular disease. Nurses in all clinical settings can provide health education about the risk factors that affect development of arteriosclerotic disease contributing to peripheral vascular disease (Box 32-1). Inasmuch as these disorders normally develop with advancing age, older adults in particular can benefit from this information.

**BOX 32-1 Risk Factors for Peripheral Vascular Disease**

| | |
|---|---|
| Age (elderly) | Obesity |
| Sex (male) | Lack of exercise |
| Cigarette smoking | Emotional stress |
| Hypertension | Diabetes mellitus |
| Hyperlipidemia | Family history of atherosclerosis |
| Presence of coronary artery disease | |

*Cigarette smoking* is a major contributory factor in the development of peripheral vascular problems. Nicotine causes vasoconstriction and spasms of the arteries, thus reducing circulation to the extremities. The carbon dioxide inhaled in cigarette smoke reduces oxygen transport to the tissues.

*Hypertension* causes the elastic tissue in the arteries to be replaced by fibrous collagen tissue. This makes the arterial wall less distensible and increases the resistance to blood flow (see p. 920).

*Hyperlipidemia* refers to the elevation of lipid levels, such as cholesterol and triglycerides, within the blood. Cholesterol and triglycerides contribute to the development of atherosclerotic plaque in the vessels (see Chapter 31). Most patients with arterial occlusive disease also may have coronary artery disease.

*Obesity,* or excess body weight in relation to height (see Chapter 6), places an added burden on the heart and blood vessels. Excess fat compromises blood vessels and contributes to increased venous congestion. Obese persons also are more prone to physical inactivity, diabetes, hypertension, and hyperlipidemia.

Physical activity promotes muscle contraction and relaxation. It improves the return of venous blood to the heart by the pumping of muscle on the veins and aids in the development of collateral circulation, which is useful for venous return when veins are blocked. *Physical inactivity,* therefore, may compromise circulation.

*Emotional stress* stimulates the sympathetic nervous system and causes peripheral vasoconstriction. Stress also can cause increased cholesterol and platelet levels, decreased clotting time, and sustained high blood pressure.

The exact mechanism by which *diabetes mellitus* contributes to the development of peripheral vascular disease is unknown, although smaller-caliber vessels are more frequently affected. Changes in glucose and fat metabolism are thought to affect the atherosclerotic processes.

### Secondary prevention

Secondary prevention is important because peripheral vascular diseases can become chronic and potentially disabling. Most affected persons are subject to periods of exacerbation and complications such as infection, injury, thrombosis, and amputation. Those with early symptoms are encouraged to seek medical care. Increasing one's knowledge of specific disorders and preventing future occurrences are essential.

### Tertiary prevention

A vascular rehabilitation program is a new and important concept in the management of patients with vascular disease, particularly arterial occlusive disease. Patients

**TABLE 32-1 Diagnostic Tests for Arterial Disorders**

| PURPOSE | PROCEDURE | COMMENTS |
|---|---|---|
| **CONTINUOUS WAVE (CW) DOPPLER ULTRASONOGRAPHY** | | |
| Evaluate arteries and veins<br>Determine blood flow direction<br>Calculate ankle/brachial indexes (ABI) | High-frequency sound waves directed to artery or veins through hand-held transducer moved across skin surface; audible tone produced proportional to blood velocity | Noninvasive<br>Portable for bedside examination |
| **DUPLEX ULTRASONOGRAPHY** | | |
| Evaluate arteries and veins<br>Measure blood velocity<br>Monitor patency of bypass grafts<br>Provide bypass graft surveillance<br>Determine blood flow direction | Computer interfaces, high-frequency sound waves directed to artery via hand-held transducer moved across the skin surface<br>Combination of Doppler (audio) and B-mode (video) ultrasonography<br>Produces a video (anatomic) and audio (blood flow) representation of the vascular network | No discomfort experienced<br>Noninvasive<br>Color flow capability |
| **VELOCITY WAVEFORM/SEGMENTAL LIMB PRESSURE** | | |
| Evaluate arterial stenosis and occlusion | Systolic pressure readings from each limb segment obtained by pneumatic pressure cuffs and Doppler probe; pressure readings and waveforms compared | Noninvasive |
| **PULSE VOLUME WAVEFORM/SEGMENTAL LIMB PRESSURE** | | |
| Evaluate arterial stenosis and occlusion | Pneumatic pressure cuffs attached to extremities; pressure changes recorded by pressure transducer as waveforms during cuff inflation and deflation<br>Pressure readings and pulse volume waves are compared | Noninvasive |
| **EXERCISE TESTING** | | |
| Determine amount of exercise that produces initial claudication and absolute claudication<br>Calculate ankle-brachial indexes (ABI) | Ankle pressure, pulse volume, and blood pressure measured before and after person walks on treadmill at specific speed and grade | Exercise should be stopped at onset of pain<br>Patient with cardiac history may need physician consultation |
| **RADIONUCLIDE SCAN** | | |
| Visualize vascular system and detect changes in blood vessels<br>Assess arterial blood flow; determine perfusion pressure<br>Identify arterial obstruction or vascular abnormality<br>Determine patency of bypass graft | Injection of radionuclide followed by scanning of area at predetermined intervals to determine accumulation of radionuclide | Explain to patient that radiation dose is usually less than that received from diagnostic x-rays |
| **ARTERIOGRAPHY (ANGIOGRAPHY)** | | |
| Visualize arterial system and detect vascular changes<br>Assess arterial blood flow<br>Identify arterial obstruction, vascular abnormality, or aneurysm | Dye inserted through catheter inserted into femoral or brachial artery, followed by x-ray films | Transient flushing and burning sensation felt when dye is inserted<br>Assess injection site for bleeding and hematoma<br>Assess peripheral pulses distal to site q hr for 4-8 hr<br>Assess sensation distal to site<br>Monitor for allergic reaction to dye (dyspnea, flushing, hives, nausea, vomiting)<br>Monitor blood creatinine<br>Encourage fluids to facilitate excretion of dye |
| **DIGITAL SUBTRACTION ANGIOGRAPHY** | | |
| Visualize vascular system<br>Determine presence and extent of occlusion | Dye injected through catheter inserted into blood vessel; x-ray signals are digitized | Same as for arteriography |

**TABLE 32-1 Diagnostic Tests for Arterial Disorders—cont'd**

| PURPOSE | PROCEDURE | COMMENTS |
|---|---|---|
| **TRANSCUTANEOUS OXIMETRY** | | |
| Evaluate severity of limb ischemia<br>Assess healing of ulcers<br>Determine level of amputation | Sensors placed on skin to measure oxygen diffusion gradient between electrode and capillaries | Explain to patient that measurements may be taken in several positions |
| **MAGNETIC RESONANCE IMAGING (MRI)** | | |
| Evaluate vascular network (arteries, veins)<br>Measure blood flow velocities<br>Assess stages of vascular disease | Radiofrequency pulses excite protons, which give a signal creating an image | Explain to patient that the space is very tight<br>Noise level may be high; ear plugs provided |

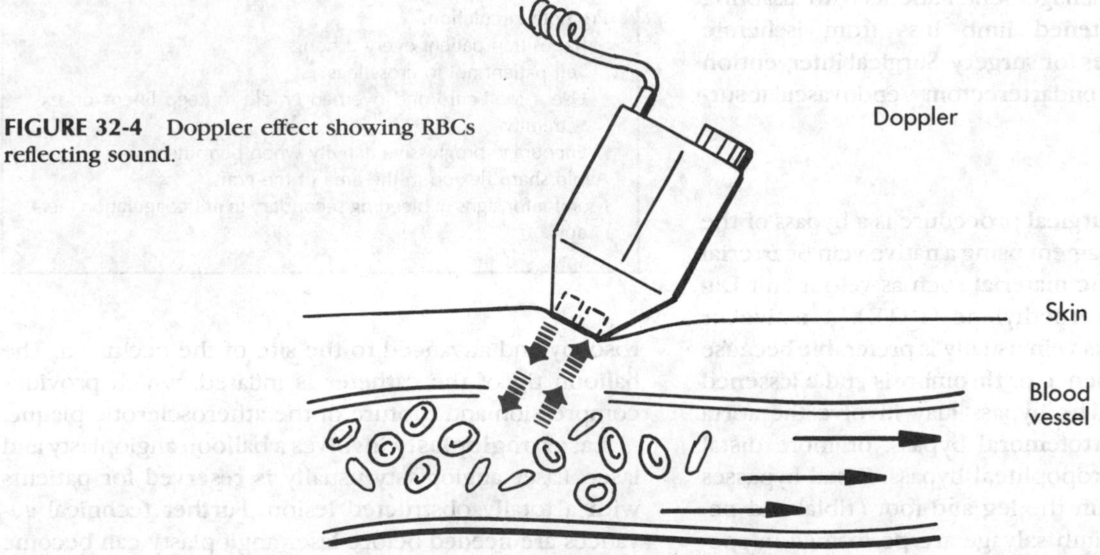


**FIGURE 32-4** Doppler effect showing RBCs reflecting sound.

with intermittent claudication can be assisted to improve their functional ability by increasing walking distance and time. Overall aerobic conditioning and improvement in collateral circulation also are evident. Those persons who have undergone surgical interventions, such as bypass grafts and amputations, benefit from improved aerobic conditioning, collateral blood flow, and muscle strengthening.

## Medical Management

The goal for discharge of patients with arterial occlusive disease as determined by DRGs is 7 to 10 days. The nurse works collaboratively with the physician for implementation of prescribed medical therapy. Because the nurse has a major role in discharge planning and patient teaching, these are discussed under nursing management.

### Diagnostic tests

Several tests may be appropriate in the diagnosis of arterial occlusive disorders (Table 32-1). Noninvasive techniques include ultrasonography (Figure 32-4), segmental limb pressure, pulse volume recordings, and exercise testing. Invasive procedures such as arteriography also can aid in the diagnosis.

### Medication

Pharmacologic therapy with vasodilators, although of questionable merit, may benefit some patients. If hyperlipidemia is a factor, a lipid-lowering medication may be prescribed. Diabetic persons with arterial occlusive disease receive careful regulation on a regimen of oral hypoglycemic agents or insulin.

### Treatment

Cessation of cigarette smoking is of primary importance, as are management of underlying lipoprotein abnormalities and meticulous attention to skin and foot care.

### Diet

No special diet is recommended unless the person has an associated disease such as hyperlipidemia, in which case a low-fat, low-cholesterol diet is advocated. For persons with diabetes a calorie-restricted diabetic diet is indicated.

#### Activity

A daily walking program is strongly advised. Patients also should be encouraged to participate in a vascular rehabilitation program.

#### Referral/Consultation

In some settings the nurse assumes responsibility for making referrals to other services. The nurse may refer the patient to a vascular rehabilitation program.

### Surgical Management

Surgical management is indicated for the patient unresponsive to medical management. Patients with disabling symptoms or threatened limb loss from ischemic changes are candidates for surgery. Surgical intervention includes bypass graft, endarterectomy, endovascular surgery, and amputation.

#### Bypass graft

The most common surgical procedure is a bypass of the obstructed arterial segment using a native vein or arterial segment or a synthetic material such as velour-knit Dacron or polytetrafluroroethylene (PTFE). A native or autogenous saphenous vein usually is preferable because there is a lower incidence of thrombosis and a lessened risk of graft failure. The bypass may involve the aorta itself, as with an aortofemoral bypass, or more distal vessels such as femoropopliteal bypass. Distal bypasses of the small arteries in the leg and foot (tibial and peroneal arteries) for limb salvage are performed in specialized institutions. Nursing management of the patient after bypass graft surgery is described in the Guidelines box, above.

**Guidelines for Nursing Care of the Person After Bypass Graft Surgery**

Monitor skin color and temperature distal to the graft site every hour.
Assess sensation and movement in the distal limb.
Assess peripheral pulses in the involved limb (see Figure 32-5).
- Sudden absence of pulse may indicate thrombosis.
- Mark location of peripheral pulse with a pen to facilitate frequent assessment.
- Use Doppler ultrasonography if pulses are difficult to palpate.
- Compare pulses of involved limb with pulses of noninvolved limb.

Monitor extremity for edema.
Check incision for redness, swelling, and drainage.
Monitor and immediately report signs of complication, such as increasing pain, fever, changes in drainage, absent or weakening pulse, change in skin color, limitation of movement, or paresthesia.
Promote circulation.
- Reposition patient every 2 hours.
- Tell patient not to cross legs.
- Use a footboard and overbed cradle to keep linens off extremity.
- Encourage progressive activity when permitted.

Avoid sharp flexion in the area of the graft.
Monitor for signs of bleeding secondary to anticoagulation therapy.

#### Endarterectomy

An **endarterectomy** is the stripping and removal of atherosclerotic plaque along the intima and inner medial arterial wall by use of a specially designed catheter.

#### Endovascular surgery

Endovascular surgery is an evolving experimental specialty in which a catheter-based system serves as an adjunct or replacement for traditional vascular reconstructive procedures. These procedures include balloon angioplasty, laser angioplasty, atherectomy, and stents. **Balloon angioplasty** can be used as the primary treatment—percutaneous balloon angioplasty—in patients with single-level disease. Intraoperative balloon angioplasty is used in patients with more severe and advanced disease as an adjunct to surgery.[1] Intraoperative balloon angioplasty is most often used to improve iliac artery blood flow before a more distal arterial operation. A specially designed catheter is inserted by means of fluoroscopy and advanced to the site of the occlusion. The balloon tip of the catheter is inflated, which provides compression and rupture of the atherosclerotic plaque.

**Laser angioplasty** involves a balloon angioplasty and laser. Laser angioplasty usually is reserved for patients with a totally obstructed lesion. Further technical advances are needed before laser angioplasty can become a more widely used treatment option.[6]

**Atherectomy** is a new alternative to balloon angioplasty. A special catheter is used to strip away the atherosclerotic plaque. Further work needs to be undertaken before it is accepted as a routine vascular procedure.[4]

Intravascular stents provide a rigid yet flexible structure to maintain the integrity of the vascular wall and patency of the artery. Stents have been placed after inadequate results from balloon angioplasty. The most successful placement has occurred in the iliac arteries.

#### Amputation

Amputation is a necesary treatment in patients with severely advanced arterial occlusive disease and gangrene. Most patients undergoing amputations have diabetes. The toes are more frequently amputated than any other body part.

The level of amputation is determined by the extent of the disease process, ease of the stump to be fitted with a functional prosthesis, and the level of an adequate blood supply to provide wound healing. If possible a below-the-knee (BK) amputation is performed inasmuch as this maintains knee function, allows for greater stability with a prosthesis, and requires a lower increase in energy expenditure for ambulation. A BK amputation usually is made at the lower third of the leg, leaving a 12- to 18-cm stump. An above-the-knee (AK) amputation can be made at any level, although frequently it is below the midthigh to maintain an adequate stump for prosthetic attachment. Sometimes an AK amputation is required after an unsuccessful BK amputation.

Nursing management of the patient after an amputation is discussed in the next section.

## NURSING MANAGEMENT

### ♦ ASSESSMENT

#### Subjective Data

Subjective data to be collected to assess the patient with arterial occlusive disease include the following:

- Intermittent claudication
  - Presence of limp during exercise, particularly walking
  - Aching pain or cramping sensation in calf, lower back, buttock, thigh, or foot, which develops with walking
  - Relief of symptoms on cessation of walking or short rest period
  - Effect of medications such as vasodilators on symptom relief
- Limb-threatening ischemia
  - Presence of pain at rest
  - Sudden onset of pain
  - Feeling of numbness, tingling in feet or leg

#### Objective Data

Objective data to be collected to assess the patient with arterial occlusive disease include the following:

- Intermittent claudication
  - Ankle-brachial index (ABI) between 0.9 and 0.5 or a change from rest to exercise
  - Strength of peripheral pulses; graded as 0, pulse cannot be felt; 1+, pulse present but definitely diminished; or 4+, abnormally strong (2+ and 3+ are normal intensities) (Figure 32-5)
  - Difference in strength of peripheral pulses bilaterally
  - Presence of risk factors (see Box 32-1)
- Limb-threatening ischemia
  - ABI $<0.4$
  - Strength of peripheral pulses; graded as above
  - Prolonged ($>3$ sec) or absent capillary refill
  - Changes in skin color
  - Presence of ulcers or gangrene, especially heel and between toes
  - Change in temperature of extremities—cool or cold to touch
  - Tissue changes of thickened nails, dry skin, loss of hair
  - Loss of muscle tone
  - Presence of risk factors (see Box 32-1)
  - Postural color change of feet from marked pallor on elevation to delayed color return or dependent rubor with dangling

#### Diagnostic Test Findings

Several tests may be used to diagnose arterial occlusive disease. These tests are outlined in Table 32-1. Specific diagnostic tests for intermittent claudication include exercise testing. The initial claudication distance and absolute claudication distance are recorded. The ABI will show a change from rest to after exercise. The normal ABI is 1.0 or $>0.9$, which indicates that the ratio of ankle systolic pressure to brachial systolic pressure is equal. An ABI between 0.9 and 0.5 usually is seen in patients with claudication. An ABI of 0.4 occurs in limb-threatening ischemia or rest ischemia. Test results for limb-threatening ischemia show the area of arterial stenosis or obstruction and the extent of collateral circulation.

### ♦ NURSING DIAGNOSES

Nursing diagnoses are determined from analysis of patient data. Nursing diagnoses for the patient with arterial occlusive disease may include but are not limited to the following:

| Diagnostic Title | Possible Etiologic Factors |
|---|---|
| Tissue perfusion, altered (lower extremity) | Decreased arterial blood flow |
| Skin integrity, high risk for impaired | Ischemia, immobility |
| Infection, high risk for | Lack of knowledge, ulcers, gangrene |
| Activity intolerance | Immobility, imbalance between oxygen supply/demand |
| Injury (trauma), high risk for | Sensorimotor deficit, lack of awareness of environmental hazards |
| Knowledge deficit: disease, diagnostic tests, therapeutic management | Lack of exposure/recall, unfamiliarity with information sources |

### ♦ EXPECTED PATIENT OUTCOMES

Expected patient outcomes for the patient with arterial occlusive disease may include but are not limited to the following:

1. Describes measures to promote tissue perfusion.
2. States measures to maintain skin integrity.
3. States measures to decrease risk of infection.
4. Discusses plans to participate in a regular exercise program or activity.
5. Uses preventive strategies to avoid injury.
6. Describes the diseases accurately, how signs and symptoms relate to the disease, and how the disease will alter daily living; describes the purpose of each diagnostic test and any special preparation;

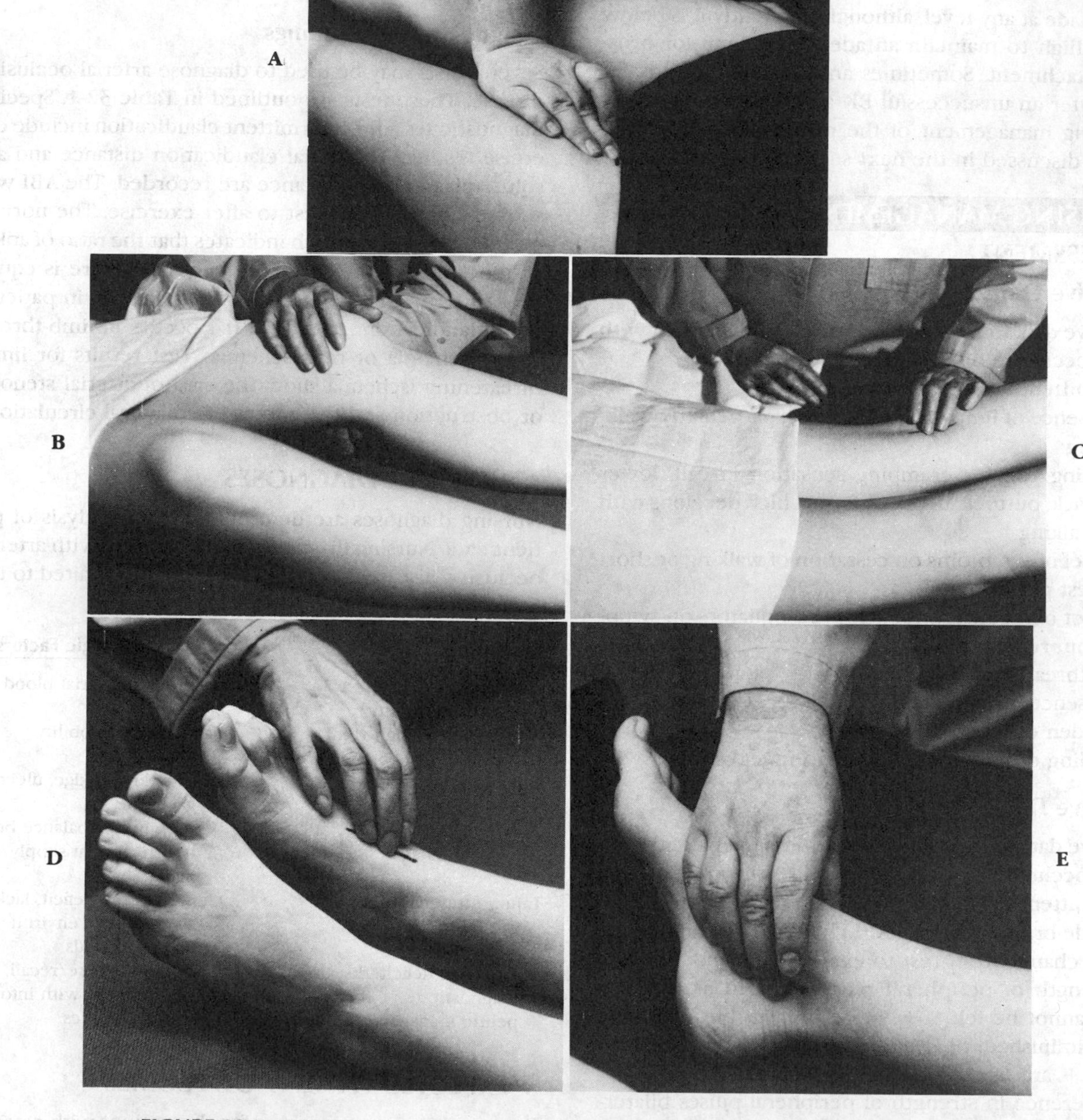


**FIGURE 32-5** **A,** Palpation of femoral pulse. **B,** Palpation of popliteal pulse with patient in the dorsal recumbent position. **C,** Palpation of popliteal pulse with patient in the prone position. **D,** Palpation of dorsal pedal pulse. **E,** Palpation of posterior tibial pulse. (From Malasanos L et al: *Health assessment,* ed 4, St Louis, 1990, Mosby.)

and explains measures to relieve symptoms and plans for follow-up care.

## ♦ INTERVENTIONS

### Promoting Tissue Perfusion

Nursing interventions are directed toward activities that promote tissue oxygenation and include the following:

1. Maintain a warm environmental temperature of about 21° C (70° F).
2. Places legs in *slight dependency* (uses gravity to enhance tissue perfusion), and avoid elevating legs, which impedes arterial flow.
3. Avoid pressure on affected extremity; use padding for severe ischemia.

4. Avoid vigorous massage of extremities (may promote embolus formation).
5. Teach patients to carry out above activities in addition to the following:
   a. Avoid chilling (causes vasoconstriction) and exposure to cold; layer clothing in cold weather.
   b. Avoid constrictive clothing that impedes circulation: rolled garters, socks with tight banding, girdles, tight waistbands, and tight shoelaces.
   c. Avoid crossing legs at knees (places pressure on arteries of legs).
   d. Quit smoking (nicotine causes vasoconstriction and vasospasms; inhaled carbon dioxide reduces oxygen-carrying capacity of blood).

## Maintaining Skin Integrity and Preventing Infection

Because of decreased tissue oxygenation from impaired circulation, the skin is at high risk for breaking down with subsequent infections. Nursing activities include examining the skin on a daily basis when the patient is hospitalized and encouraging the patient to be as mobile as possible. If redness or other signs of infection are present, notify the physician. Teach the patient to assess and protect the skin:

1. Assess skin on a daily basis for intactness, dryness, redness, and lesions; use mirror to inspect areas that are difficult to see, such as heels and plantar surface of toes.
2. Take a daily bath in tepid water (three times per week if skin is very dry).
   a. Use a neutral soap to prevent skin irritation.
   b. Wash gently; avoid scratching and vigorous rubbing.
   c. Dry skin gently.
   d. Lubricate skin with moisturizing agent; avoid using alcohol (dries skin).
3. Take meticulous care of feet.
   a. Bathe each toe and dry well.
   b. Use only prescribed foot powders.
   c. Wear clean cotton socks, and change socks daily to prevent moisture build up and potential irritation.
4. Avoid wearing shoes that do not "breathe"; those made of synthetic materials prevent evaporation and contribute to fungal infections.
5. Avoid application of direct heat, including hot water.
6. Contact health care professional at onset of skin breakdown such as abrasions, lesions, or ulcerations.

## Promoting Activity

Activity improves circulation through muscle contraction and relaxation. Exercise also stimulates collateral circulation that increases blood flow to the ischemic area. Teach the patient to carry out general and specific exercises and to allow adequate time for rest between vigorous activities.

### General exercises

1. Engage in a regular aerobic exercise program that includes activities such as walking, swimming, jogging, or bicycling (see Chapter 6).
2. Do 30 to 45 minutes of activity with warm-up and cool-down activities on 3 alternate days.
3. Walk at a slow pace on a daily basis.
4. Participate in a vascular rehabilitation program.

### Special exercises

1. Perform the following Buerger-Allen exercises on a daily basis:
   a. Lie flat with legs elevated above heart level for 2 to 3 minutes.
   b. Sit for 2 to 3 minutes with legs relaxed and slightly dependent.
   c. Flex, extend, invert, and evert feet for 30 seconds in each position.
   d. End by lying flat with legs at heart level, and cover with warm blanket for 5 minutes.
2. Perform other exercises such as ankle rotations, ankle pumps, and knee extension on a daily basis.

## Preventing Injury

With decreased circulation to the extremities, sensation may decrease. Injuries may include cuts or abrasions, burns, and excessive pressure (leading to further ischemia). Teach the patient to carry out the following activities:

1. Wear comfortable protective shoes at all times (do not go barefoot); alternate shoes on a daily basis to allow for airing.
2. Trim nails carefully: Cut at regular intervals, soak in warm water to soften nails, use straight nail clippers, and avoid using scissors to prevent cutting skin.
3. Avoid scratching and rubbing feet to prevent abrasions.
4. Check water temperature carefully (ability to sense temperature may be decreased).
5. Seek medical advice for thickened or deformed nails, blisters, corns, calluses, and ulcerations (self-treatment may cause infection).

## Addressing Problems of Amputation

Amputation involves loss of a body part; therefore feelings of grief usually are experienced. (For further discussion on loss and grief see Chapter 10.) Before and after surgery the patient should exercise to strengthen arm and leg muscles; this promotes circulation and helps prevent knee and hip contractures.

After surgery about 10% of patients experience uncomfortable sensations—**phantom limb pain;** this is similar to pain experienced before amputation. It also is described as a cramp or uncomfortable sensation. In most instances this discomfort disappears with time; however, in some persons the pain may become chronic. Even though the limb is removed, the pain is a real sensation and should not be dismissed as illusionary.

A **prosthesis** may be used immediately or within 5 weeks of surgery. A cast also may be applied over the dressing to allow for attachment of a metal pylon prosthesis (Figure 32-6). A permanent prosthesis is made months after surgery to allow for stump shrinkage and molding. Postoperative nursing management is described in the Guidelines box, p. 897.

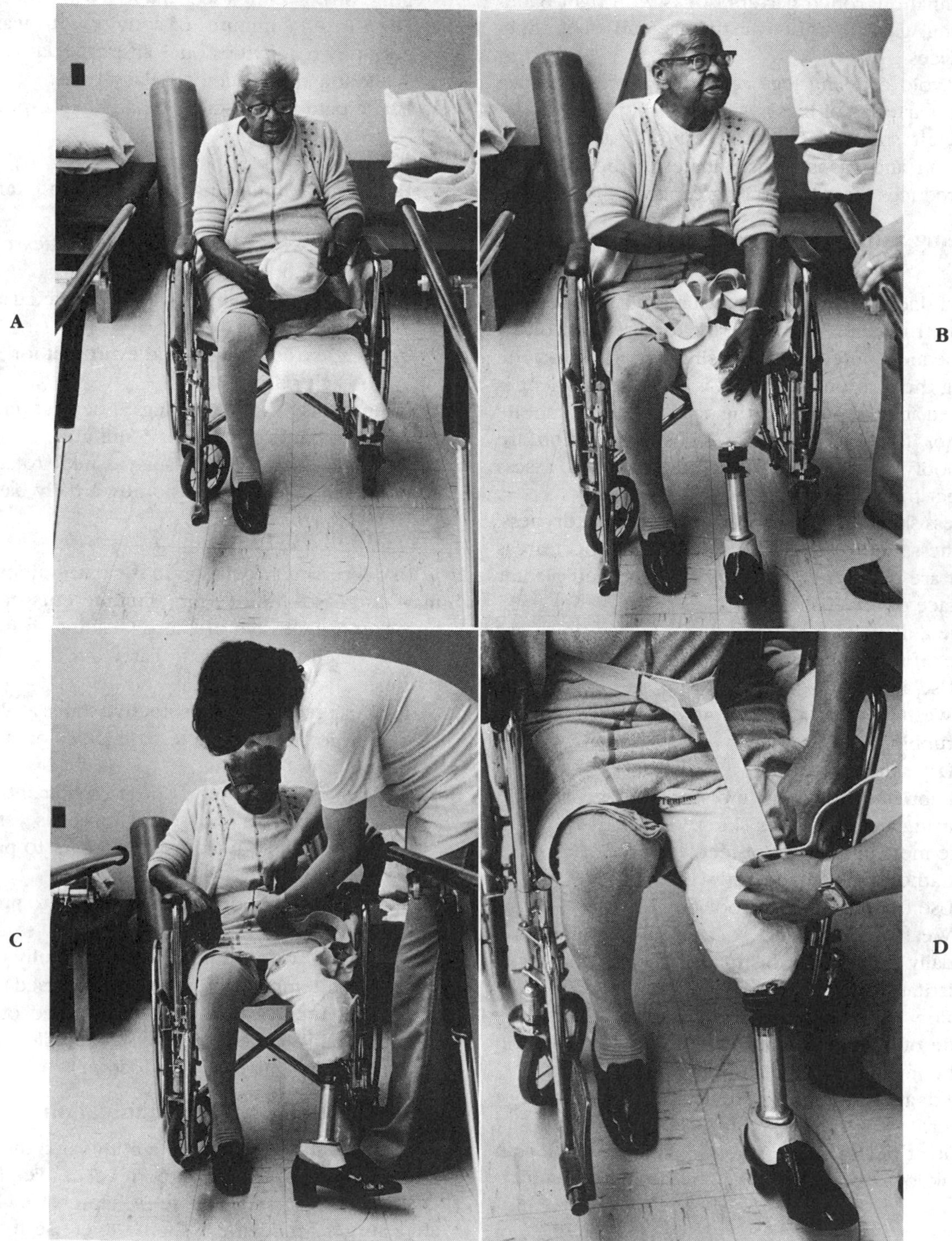

**FIGURE 32-6** **A,** Patient uses care in putting on stump sock. **B,** Prosthesis is slipped over sock. **C,** Belt is secured around waist. **D,** Length of strap is adjusted.

## Guidelines for Nursing Care of the Person After an Amputation

Assess stump and monitor catheter drainage for color and amount; report signs of increased drainage.
Position patient with no flexion at hip or knee to avoid contractures; encourage prone position.
Maintain patient in low-Fowler's or flat position after AK amputation.
Support stump with pillow for first 24 hours (according to physician preference and avoiding flexion); place rolled bath blanket along outer aspect to prevent outward rotation.
Encourage exercises to prevent thromboembolism:
- Active ROM of unaffected leg, ankle rotations and pumps
- Use of overhead trapeze when moving in bed
- Push-ups from sitting position in bed
- Quadriceps sets (see Chapter 25)
- Lifting stump and buttocks off bed while lying flat on back to strengthen abdominal muscles

Teach care of stump.
- Inspect for redness, blister, and abrasions.
- Wash stump with mild soap, rinse with water, and pat dry.
- Avoid use of alcohol, oils, and creams.
- Remove stump bandage or stump sock and reapply as needed; use firm smooth figure-of-8 Ace wrapping (Figure 32-7) to reduce swelling and shape stump (if rigid dressing not used).

Encourage patient to ambulate using correct crutch-walking technique.
- Keep elbows extended; limit elbow flexion to 30 degrees or less.
- Avoid pressure on axilla.
- Bear weight on palms of hands, not on axilla.
- Maintain upright posture (head up, chest up, abdomen in, pelvis in, foot straight).

Monitor patient's ability to use a prosthesis (see Figure 32-6).

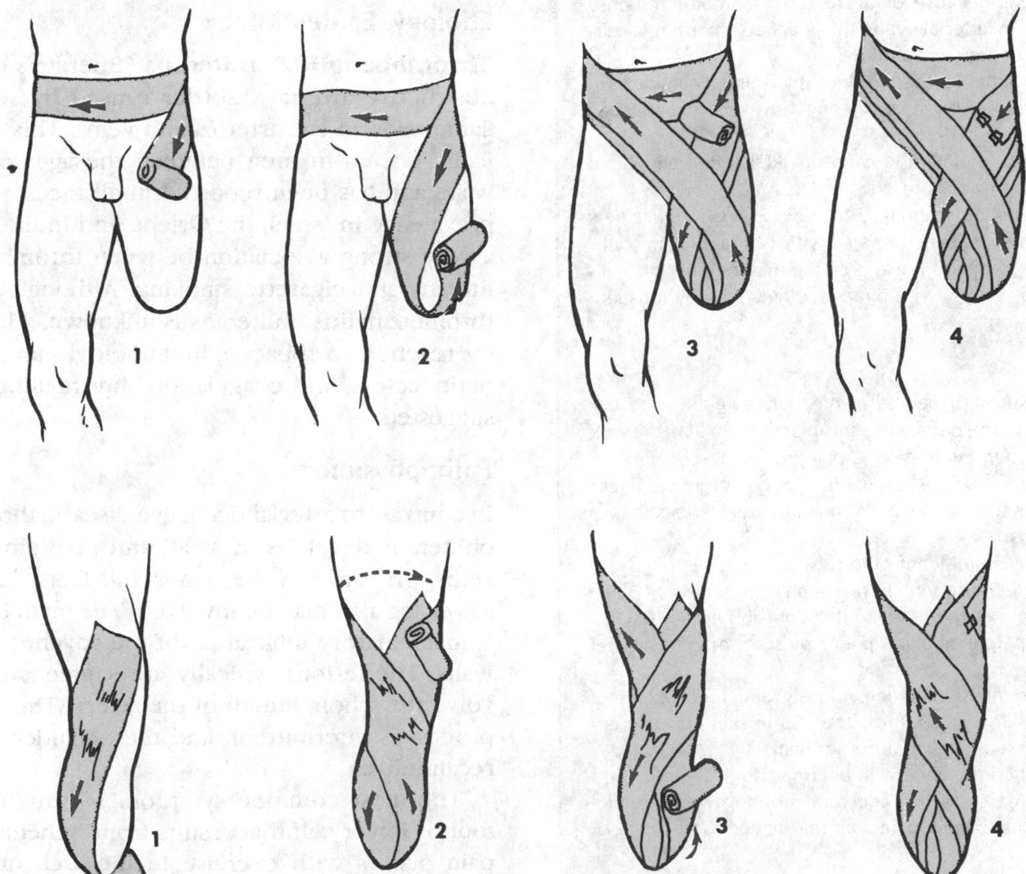


**FIGURE 32-7** *Top,* Correct method for bandaging midthigh amputation stump. Note that bandage must be anchored around patient's waist. *Bottom,* Correct method for bandaging midcalf amputation stump. Note that bandage need not be anchored around the waist.

## ♦ EVALUATION

To evaluate the effectiveness of nursing interventions, compare patient behaviors with those stated in the expected patient outcomes. Successful achievement of patient outcomes for the patient with arterial occlusive disease is indicated by the following:

1. Correctly describes measures to promote tissue perfusion.
2. Correctly describes measures to maintain skin integrity.
3. Correctly describes measures to decrease risk of infection.
4. Participates in regular exercise program or activity.
5. Correctly demonstrates preventive strategies to avoid injury.
6. Correctly describes disease, diagnostic tests, measures to relieve symptoms, and plans for follow-up care.

## ✹ SPECIAL CONSIDERATIONS FOR CARE OF THE GERONTOLOGIC PATIENT

Because degenerative changes occur in the vascular system as part of the normal aging process, special considerations are required in the care of elders (see the accompanying box, below, left).

### Complications

Complications of arterial occlusive disease include restenosis of an arterial segment after surgical intervention, thrombus formation at the graft sites, and graft infection. Careful postoperative follow-up through graft surveillance is essential in preventing these complications. Graft surveillance by means of arterial duplex scan is recommended at 1 week, 6 months, and 1 year after surgery.

Complications of amputation include nonhealing or infection of the stump, thromboembolism, and flexion contractures.

### GERONTOLOGIC PATIENT CONSIDERATIONS

**ASSESSMENT**

Assess peripheral pulses and skin of lower extremities of all elderly persons because of decreased vasomotor response and changes in arterial walls that decrease peripheral circulation and tissue oxygenation.

Assess extent of activities that produce intermittent claudication and occurrence at night; symptoms are more pronounced with age.

Assess ability to ambulate and carry out ADL when peripheral vascular problems are present.

Assess blood pressure. Normal systolic blood pressure in elders may be 160 mm Hg (as compared with 140 mm Hg in younger adults). A widened pulse pressure may be present.

Assess ability to comply with pharmacologic therapy if patient has hypertension.

**INTERVENTION**

Carry out measures to decrease infection potential; the decreased immune response of elders places them at higher risk of infection when circulation is compromised.

Use measures to increase circulation to compromised area: lower the legs for arterial problems and elevate legs for venous problems.

Teach patient and significant other:

- Foot care to decrease infection potential; if necessary place lamb's wool between toes to prevent rubbing.
- Location and palpation of peripheral pulses to monitor arterial circulation.
- Need to examine skin of legs closely and report signs of decreased skin temperature, changes in skin appearance, and cuts or scratches that do not heal.

Facilitate patient compliance with pharmacologic hypertension therapy. Decreased vision and remembering when to take medications are common factors that affect compliance of the elders.

**COMMON DISORDERS IN ELDERS**

Arteriosclerosis obliterans
Leg ulcers from chronic deep vein insufficiency
Hypertension

## THROMBOANGIITIS OBLITERANS

### Etiology/Epidemiology

**Thromboangiitis obliterans** (Buerger's disease) is an obstructive arterial disorder caused by segmented inflammation in the arteries and veins. This disorder typically occurs in men between the ages of 20 and 40 years and has been reported in all races, with a higher prevalence in Israel, the Orient, and India. There is also a very strong association between thromboangiitis obliterans and cigarette smoking. Although the cause of thromboangiitis obliterans is unknown, a hypersensitivity reaction to tobacco, immunologic mechanisms, genetic factors, and coagulation abnormalities have been suggested.

### Pathophysiology

In contrast to arterial occlusive disease, thromboangiitis obliterans develops in small and medium arteries and veins, primarily in the hands and feet. The wrists and lower leg also may be involved. The main characteristic is inflammatory infiltration of the adventitia and medial walls. The lesions typically are segmental but may involve the whole length of the artery. The inflammatory process is intermittent, and the occluded arteries may recannulize.

The most common symptom is claudication of the foot or lower calf that results from ischemic changes. If pain occurs with exercise in the arch of the foot or instep, claudication may be present. Claudication may extend proximally as the disease progresses; however, it rarely occurs in the aortoiliac segment.

With involvement of the hands the pain usually is bilateral and symmetric. Changes in skin color or temperature, sensitivity to cold, and ulcers or gangrene of the digits may be present. Superficial thrombophlebitis may coexist.

Diagnostic tests usually include angiography of the involved vessels, **digital subtraction angiography, duplex ultrasonography,** and exercise testing (see Table 32-1).

### Medical Management

The goal of medical management is to halt further progression of the disease. A major effect is directed toward complete abstinence from cigarette smoking. Pharmacologic therapy with calcium channel blockers and antiplatelet agents is controversial. A sympathectomy—removal of sympathetic ganglia and nervous tissues to eliminate vasospasms—may be successful if performed in the early stage. In advanced stages amputation of ulcerated fingers and toes may be necessary.

### Nursing Management

Nursing management of persons with thromboangiitis obliterans is similar to care of patients with other types of arterial disorders. This includes preventing injury, patient teaching to promote activity, and promoting tissue perfusion and comfort. In addition, the patient is taught to recognize signs of thrombophlebitis (redness, heat) and arterial obstruction (pallor, coldness).

## RAYNAUD'S PHENOMENON AND PRIMARY RAYNAUD'S DISEASE

### Etiology/Epidemiology

**Raynaud's phenomenon** is one type of vasospastic disease characterized by episodic arterial spasm of the extremities, predominantly of the hands. Raynaud's phenomenon may be caused by drugs, connective tissue diseases, constant trauma from occupational hazards, nerve or blood vessel compression, obstructive arterial diseases, increased blood viscosity, or endocrine disorders.

**Primary Raynaud's disease** develops more frequently in young women before 45 years of age and is more prevalent during the winter months. A higher incidence has been found in places with a cool damp climate. The exact cause of primary Raynaud's disease is unknown, although an alteration in sympathetic innervation, emotional stress, and hypersensitivity of the digital arteries to cold have been postulated.

### Pathophysiology

Few pathologic changes occur in the early stages. With greater severity of the disease, there is intimal hyperplasia. Persons with Raynaud's disease typically complain of chronically cold hands and feet, especially during the winter months. Spasm of the digital arteries and arterioles causes pallor of the distal extremity, followed by cyanosis. After the spasms the involved area becomes intensively reddened, with tingling and a throbbing pain. Severe pain is a rare finding. Most spasms resolve within 15 minutes. Many patients do not have the classic tricolor changes; some experience only pallor or cyanosis. With longstanding Raynaud's disease, ulcerations may develop on the fingertips and toes.

A cold stimulation test is used to diagnose Raynaud's phenomenon. Skin temperature changes are recorded by a thermistor attached to each finger. The patient's hand is submerged in an ice-water bath for 20 seconds, and ongoing temperature recordings are obtained. A comparison is then made with baseline values. Angiography of the hand or foot may be of help in visualizing the digital arteries.

### Medical Management

Medical management is primarily aimed at conservative measures. The person is advised to protect against exposure to cold and to quit smoking. Pharmacologic therapy with calcium channel blockers, vascular smooth muscle relaxants, and vasodilators may be prescribed to promote circulation and reduce pain. Biofeedback techniques to increase skin temperature and thereby prevent spasms have been beneficial in some cases. A sympathectomy may be indicated to relieve vasospastic symptoms. An upper extremity sympathectomy has provided patients with only temporary relief, whereas a lumbar sympathectomy has a higher level of success.

If ulcerations and gangrene occur, the involved area may need to be amputated. In addition, medical management of Raynaud's phenomenon is directed at identification of underlying cause.

### Nursing Management

Nursing management of persons with Raynaud's phenomenon or disease is similar to that for patients with other arterial disorders. Data collection includes the effect of associated factors, such as emotional stress, exposure to cold, cigarette smoking, and the effect of relieving factors such as warmth. In addition to preventing injury and promoting tissue perfusion, the following interventions are emphasized:

1. Teach effects of smoking on arterial flow, that is, nicotine causes vasoconstriction; recommend smoking-cessation techniques such as behavior modification, stimulus control, biofeedback, nicotine gum, nicotine patch, and hypnosis.
2. Discuss ways to avoid exposure to cold.
   a. Wear adequate clothing to promote warmth.
   b. Layer clothes as needed.
   c. Wear gloves and socks during winter months.
   d. Use caution when cleaning refrigerator and freezer.
   e. Wear gloves when handling frozen foods.
3. Avoid occupations that require constant exposure to cold or use of vibrating tools.
4. Discuss importance of decreasing emotional stress.

5. Avoid drugs that will cause vasoconstriction, such as birth control pills, beta-adrenergic blockers, and ergotamines.
6. Suggest antiinflammatory analgesics to promote comfort.

## ANEURYSM

### Etiology

An **aneurysm** is a localized dilation of an artery extending the vessel at least 1.5 times its normal size. Causes of aneurysms include congenital abnormalities, trauma, infection, aortitis, and connective tissue disorders. The etiologic relationship of atherosclerosis to aneurysm disease has recently been questioned. The term *nonspecific* is now used to identify all other causes of aneurysm disease.

### Epidemiology

During the past few decades there has been an increased frequency of diagnosed aortic aneurysm disease, a result of the increased age of the population and improved diagnostic capabilities. Aneurysm disease is the thirteenth leading cause of death in the United States. This disease is more common in men between 50 and 70 years of age than in other adults. Cigarette smoking and hypertension are strongly associated with aneurysm disease. There also is a genetic predisposition for aneurysm development.

### Pathophysiology

Pathophysiologic changes cause weakness of the arterial wall, resulting in dilation and potential rupture. The intimal wall is destroyed and the media is damaged, with a marked loss of elastin. Inflammation, biochemical changes in the proteolytic enzyme elastase, and genetic factors may contribute to nonspecific aneurysm disease. The extent of arterial damage and clinical manifestations depend on the size, type, and location of aneurysm.

Types of aneurysms are fusiform, saccular, and dissecting (Figure 32-8). A fusiform aneurysm, the most common type, takes the shape of a spindle around the circumference of the vessel. The saccular aneurysm appears as a sac or outpouching on the side of the vessel. A dissecting aneurysm develops from an intimal tear leading to the accumulation of blood in a newly formed cavity between the intima and media. A dissecting aneurysm is further classified by the site of the intimal tear and the extent of the dissecting hematoma. Arterial hypotension and medial wall degeneration are associated with dissecting aneurysms.

Although an aneurysm can develop in any artery, the aorta is the most frequently affected. The popliteal and femoral arteries also are sites of aneurysm formation. Of these the popliteal artery is the more common site; however, there is an increasing incidence of femoral aneurysms from its frequent use for graft anastomoses.

Aortic aneurysms occur in both the thoracoabdominal aorta and the abdominal aorta. Thoracoabdominal aortic aneurysms develop in the ascending, transverse, and descending aorta (Figure 32-9). Patients usually have no symptoms until the aneurysm compresses adjacent structures such as the trachea and bronchus. Pain in the chest, abdomen, flank, or back may occur. Other symptoms include dyspnea, cough, and wheezing. The infrarenal aorta, just below the renal arteries and above the iliac bifurcation, is the most common location for an abdominal aortic aneurysm. This aneurysm is lined with a clot or has an ulcerated area of plaque. These patients usually have no symptoms, and the aneurysm usually is detected accidentally on a routine chest or abdominal film. Abdominal or back pain may be signs of enlargement. A pulsatile mass in the abdomen may be palpated depending on the size of the aneurysm.

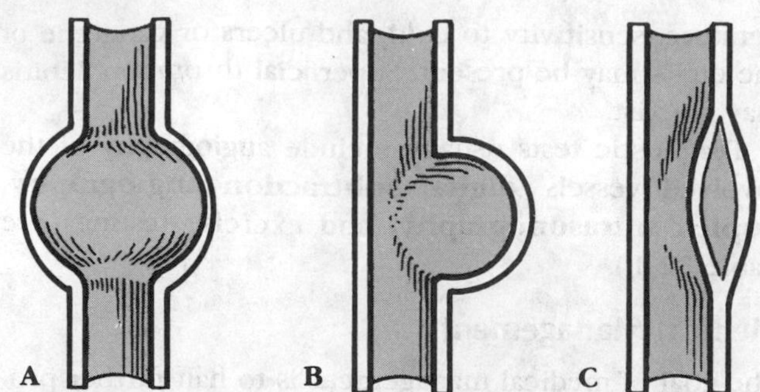


**FIGURE 32-8** Types of aneurysms. **A,** Fusiform. **B,** Saccular. **C,** Dissecting.

### Prevention

#### Primary prevention

Primary prevention includes teaching patients about the close association of cigarette smoking and hypertension with aneurysm disease. Patients should be encouraged to quit smoking. Hypertension should be carefully controlled.

#### Secondary prevention

Because a familial tendency exists, first-degree relatives of patients with known aneurysm disease should undergo ultrasound screening to detect the presence of an aneurysm. Patients with known hypertension who smoke should have a careful physical examination to check for aneurysm disease.

### Medical Management

A symptom-free patient with a small aneurysm—less than 4.0 cm—usually is managed medically, with follow-up physicians' appointments and repeat diagnostic testing at 6-month or 1-year intervals. Aneurysms between 4 and 6 cm are carefully managed. Those larger than 6 cm are treated surgically inasmuch as the risk of rupture (70% to 80%) exceeds the risk of operative morbidity and mortality (up to 5%). Depending on the

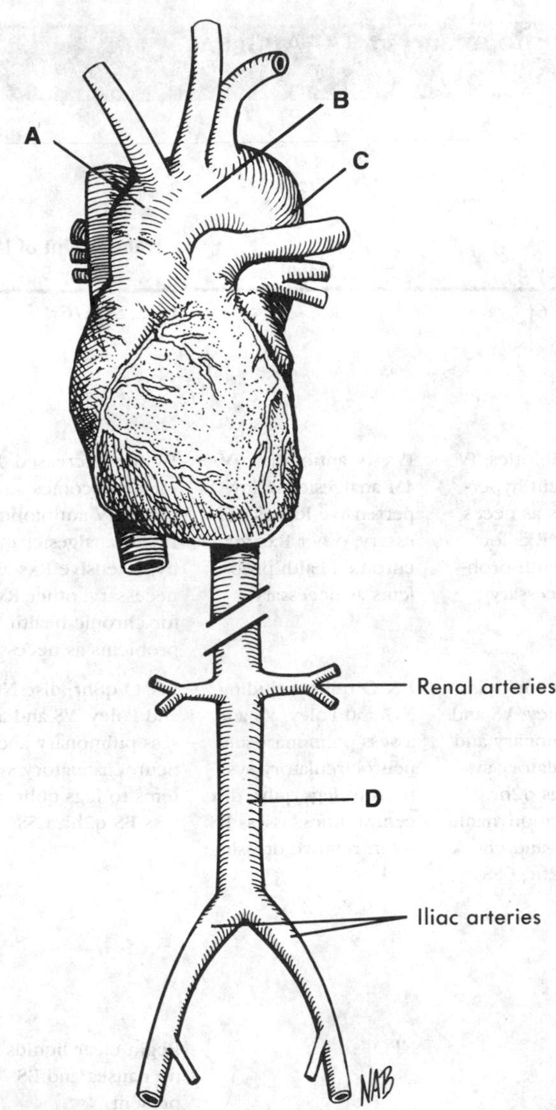


**FIGURE 32-9** Common sites of aortic aneurysms. **A,** Ascending aorta. **B,** Transverse aorta. **C,** Descending aorta. **D,** Abdominal aorta.

growth rate, presence of symptoms, and physiologic age of the patient, surgery may be the best treatment option. Aneurysm growth is typically at a rate of 0.5 cm per year.

The goal for discharge of patients with abdominal aortic aneurysm disease as determined by DRGs is 7 to 10 days. The nurse works collaboratively with the physician for implementation of prescribed medical therapy. Because the nurse has a major role in discharge planning and patient teaching, these are discussed under nursing management.

### Diagnostic tests

Ultrasonography is useful in determining the size, shape, and location of the aneurysm. Special conducting gel is applied to the skin, and a Doppler probe is then placed on the skin. Computed tomography (CT) scanning uses ionizing radiation to obtain cross-sectional images of the aorta. Contrast-enhanced CT is helpful in detecting retroperitoneal hematoma, which indicates rupture and the relationship of the aneurysm to the renal arteries. Aortography can assist in defining the extent of the aneurysm, especially those with suprarenal and iliac involvement. Radiopaque dye is injected and the aorta is visualized. Magnetic resonance imaging (MRI) uses radiofrequency energy and a magnetic field to produce images.

### Medication

No special medication is given to treat aneurysm disease. However, hypertension should be well controlled with antihypertensive agents.

### Treatment

There is no special treatment for the patient with an aneurysm whose condition is medically managed. Treatment is discussed under surgical and nursing management.

### Activity

There are no activity limitations for the person with an aneurysm.

### Referral/Consultation

In some settings the nurse assumes responsibility for making referrals to other services. In collaboration with the primary physician the nurse may refer the patient to a vascular surgeon for consultation. Referrals generally are not necessary unless the patient requires surgery. Critical pathways have been developed in some inpatient and outpatient settings to guide both medical and nursing management. These critical pathways are collaboratively developed along time lines and include the information already described for specific days. Pertinent information about discharge planning and patient teaching to be implemented at specified times also is included. Because the nurse has a major role in these two aspects of care, these are discussed under Nursing Management. A sample of a critical pathway for the six areas of care discussed in this medical management section is presented on pp. 902-903.

## Surgical Management

Elective surgery is the treatment of choice in patients with an aneurysm greater than 4 cm. Emergency surgery of a ruptured or dissecting aneurysm is critical for patient survival. Surgery consists of aortic aneurysm repair by use of a synthetic graft material of Dacron or Gortex to replace the diseased aorta. A standard transperitoneal or retroperitoneal approach can be used. The retroperitoneal approach is indicated when the abdomen needs to be protected from entry. Repair of thoracoabdominal aneurysms may require shunting or cardiopulmonary

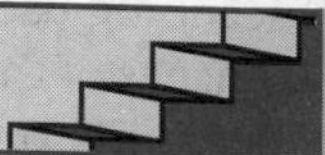

## CRITICAL PATHWAY Abdominal Aortic Aneurysm (AAA) Below Level of Kidney

**DRG #: 108 Expected LOS: 7 to 10**

| | Day of Admission Day 1 | Day of Surgery (to ICU from OR) Day 2 | Day 3 | Day 4 | Transfer Out of ICU Day 5 |
|---|---|---|---|---|---|
| **Diagnostic Tests** | CBC, UA, SMA/18,* PT/PTT, T & X, Chest and abdominal x-ray films, CT chest and abdomen, ECG | CBC, SMA/6,† ABGs | CBC, SMA/6† | | CBC, SMA/6† |
| **Medications** | IVs, IV antibiotics, IM/PO analgesic; antihypertensive Rxs as necessary; other Rxs for chronic health problems as necessary | IVs, IV antibiotics, IV analgesic; antihypertensive Rxs as necessary; other Rxs for chronic health problems as necessary | IVs, IV antibiotics, IV analgesic; antihypertensive Rxs as necessary; other Rxs for chronic health problems as necessary | IVs, IV antibiotics, IV/IM analgesic; antihypertensive Rxs as necessary; other Rxs for chronic health problems as necessary | IV rate decreased, PO intake becomes adequate; IV antibiotic. IV/IM analgesic; antihypertensive Rxs as necessary; other Rxs for chronic health problems as necessary |
| **Treatments** | I & O q8hr; VS q4hr; CSS | I & O (including Foley and NG) q hr × 12, then q2hr × 12; VS and assess pulmonary and neurocirculatory systems to legs q hr × 12, then q2hr × 12; monitor hemodynamic parameters and check dressing q hr; CSS; intubated on ventilator with $O_2$ (extubate when appropriate) | I & O q4hr including NG and Foley; VS and assess pulmonary and neurocirculatory systems to legs q2hr; monitor hemodynamic parameters and check dressing q2hr; CSS | I & O q8hr including NG and Foley; VS and assess pulmonary and neurocirculatory systems to legs q4hr; disc central lines; assess BS q2hr; remove dressing; CSS | I & O q8hr; disc NG and Foley; VS and assess pulmonary and neurocirculatory systems to legs q6hr; assess BS q2hr; CSS |
| **Diet** | Clear liquids if no nausea, NPO p̄ MN | NPO | NPO | NPO | Begin clear liquids if no nausea and BS present |
| **Activity** | Bed rest, DB q2hr; keep HOB <30 degrees | Bed rest; keep bed flat without sharp flexion of hip/knee; DB q2hr | Bed rest; keep bed flat without sharp flexion of hip/knee; T & DB q2hr | Bed rest; keep HOB <30 degrees; up walking in room with help × 4; T & DB q2hr | Bed rest; keep HOB <30 degrees; up walking in room with help × 4; T & DB q2hr |
| **Consultations** | RT, perioperative nurse, primary nurse, other specialist as needed for other medical problems; anesthesiologist | RT | RT | RT | Social service |

*BS,* Bowel sounds; *CBC,* complete blood cell count; *CSS,* compression support stocking; *CT,* computed tomography; *DB,* deep breathe; *disc,* discontinue; *HOB,* head of bed; *p̄ MN;* after midnight; *PT,* prothrombin time; *PTT,* partial thromboplastin time; *RT,* respiratory therapist; *SMA,* sequential multiple analysis; *T & DB,* turn and deep breathe; *TKO,* to keep open; *T & X,* type and crossmatch; *UA,* urinalysis.

| Day 6 | Day 7 | Day 8 | Day 9 | Day of Discharge Day 10 |
|---|---|---|---|---|
| | CBC, SMA/6† | CBC, SMA/18* | | |
| IV rate decreased as PO intake becomes adequate; IV antibiotics, IM/PO analgesic; antihypertensive Rxs as necessary; other Rxs for chronic health problems as necessary | IV @ TKO rate; IV antibiotics, IM/PO analgesic; antihypertensive Rxs as necessary; other Rxs for chronic health problems as necessary | IV to saline lock; PO analgesic; antihypertensive Rxs as necessary; other Rxs for chronic health problems as necessary | Disc saline lock; PO analgesic; antihypertensive Rxs as necessary; other Rxs for chronic health problems as necessary | PO analgesic; adjust Rxs for home use |
| I & O q8hr; VS and assess pulmonary and neurocirculatory systems to legs q6hr; assess BS q2hr; CSS | I & O q8hr; VS and assess pulmonary and neurocirculatory systems to legs q6hr; assess BS q2hr; CSS | I & O q8hr; VS and assess pulmonary and neurocirculatory systems to legs q8hr; CSS | Disc I & O; VS and assess pulmonary and neurocirculatory systems to legs q8hr; CSS | VS and assess pulmonary and neurocirculatory systems to legs q8hr; CSS |
| Clear liquids; advance to full liquids or soft diet | Full liquids or soft diet | Regular diet | Regular diet | Regular diet |
| Up walking in room with help × 6; T & DB q2hr | Up walking in hallway with help × 2; up ad lib in room | Up walking in hallway with help × 6; up ad lib in room | Up walking in hallway with help × 6; up ad lib | Up ad lib |

*Serum calcium, phosphorus, triglycerides, uric acid, creatinine, BUN, total bilirubin, alkaline phosphate, aspartate aminotransferase (AST) (formerly serum glutamic-oxaloacetic transaminase [SGOT], alanine aminotransferase (ALT) (formerly serum glutamate pyruvate transaminase [SGPT]), lactic dehydrogenase (LDH), total protein, albumin, sodium, potassium, chloride, total $CO_2$, glucose.
†Serum sodium, potassium, chloride, total $CO_2$, glucose, BUN.

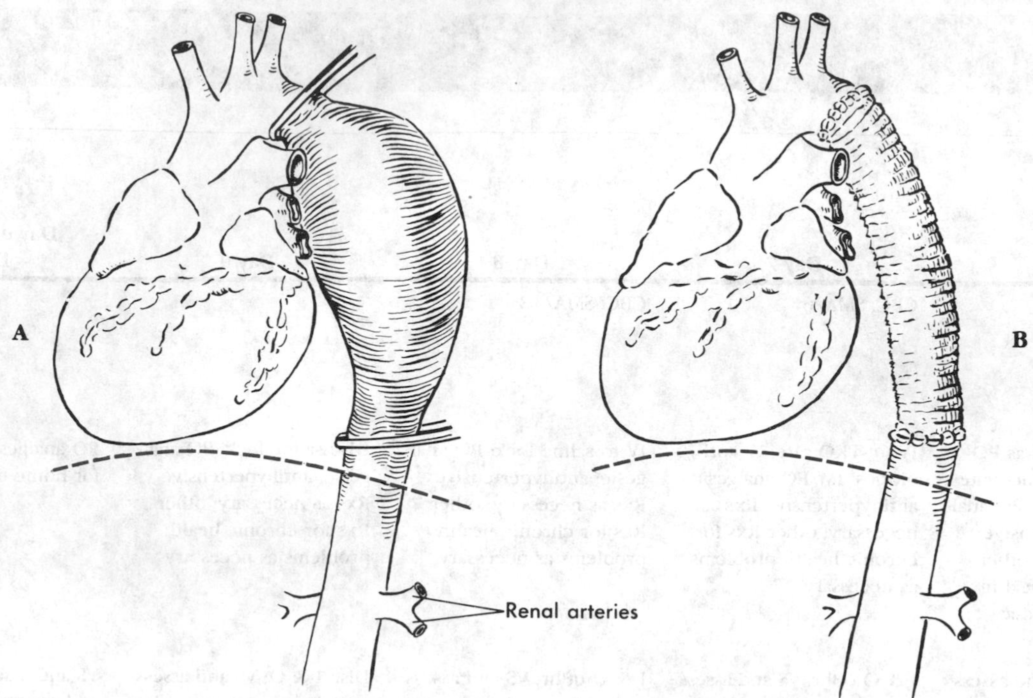


**FIGURE 32-10** Aneurysm of descending thoracic artery. **A,** Resection of thoracic aorta with cardiovascular clamps in place. **B,** Permanent replacement graft after resection of aneurysm.

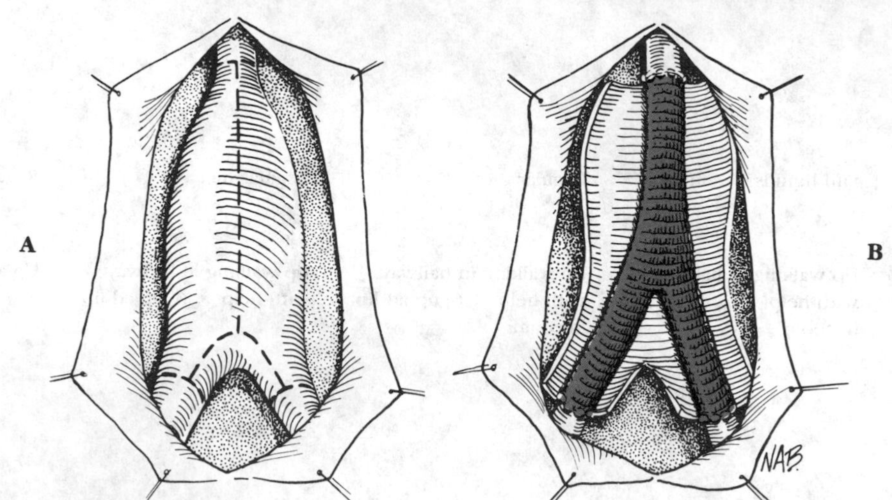


**FIGURE 32-11** **A,** Abdominal aneurysm of aorta and iliac arteries. **B,** Bifurcation graft used to replace excised aneurysm.

bypass. Clot and debris are removed from the aneurysm, and the graft is anastomosed proximally and distally. Oftentimes an aortobifemoral bypass graft is used because of significant disease in the iliac and femoral arteries. Once the graft is attached, the remaining arterial wall is sutured over the graft (Figures 32-10 and 32-11). Complications of surgery include hemorrhage, myocardial infarction, injury to adjacent bowel or ureters, renal failure, stroke, graft infection, and death. Endovascular surgery is an emerging technique to repair the aneurysm through the vessel itself.[3]

## NURSING MANAGEMENT

### ♦ ASSESSMENT

#### Subjective Data

Subjective data to be collected to assess the patient with an aneurysm include the presence of symptoms such as abdominal pain or back pain, dyspnea, coughing, and wheezing.

### Objective Data

Objective data to be collected to assess the patient with an aneurysm include the palpation of a pulsatile mass in the abdomen, abdominal tenderness, and the presence of wheezing.

### Diagnostic Test Findings

Diagnostic test findings include the presence of abdominal aortic aneurysm on ultrasound, CT scan, aortogram, or MRI.

## ♦ NURSING DIAGNOSES

Nursing diagnoses are determined from analysis of patient data. Nursing diagnoses for the patient with abdominal aortic aneurysm may include but are not limited to the following:

| Diagnostic Title | Possible Etiologic Factors |
|---|---|
| Tissue perfusion, altered (renal, bowel, lower extremity) | Decreased arterial blood flow, immobility, graft thrombosis, distal embolization |
| Fluid volume deficit | Abnormal fluid loss from hemorrhage or hematoma |

## ♦ EXPECTED PATIENT OUTCOMES

Expected patient outcomes for the person having abdominal aortic aneurysm surgery may include but are not limited to the following:

1. Maintains tissue perfusion as evidenced by:
   a. BUN and creatinine levels within normal limits.
   b. Urine output of 25 to 30 ml/hr.
   c. Presence of distal pulses, posterior tibial and anterior tibial.
   d. Absence of abdominal distention or postoperative ileus.
2. Exhibits signs of adequate fluid volume:
   a. Vital signs and hemodynamic variables within normal range for patient.
   b. Minimal to absent wound drainage.
   c. Absence of abdominal pain or back pain.
   d. Hemoglobin and hematocrit values within normal range for patient.

## ♦ INTERVENTIONS

### Maintaining Tissue Perfusion

1. Monitor vital signs and hemodynamic variables (if present): central venous pressure (CVP), pulmonary artery pressure (PAP), pulmonary capillary wedge pressure (PCWP).
2. Measure urinary output and monitor for hematuria. Check BUN and creatinine levels.
3. Assess bowel sounds and passage of gas; maintain nasogastric tube (NG) to relieve distention; monitor output.
4. Check peripheral pulses; note presence and quality.

### Promoting Fluid Volume

1. Monitor vital signs and hemodynamic variables (if present).
2. Check dressing for excessive drainage.
3. Assess for abdominal pain or back pain, which may be related to retroperitoneal hemorrhage.
4. Check hemoglobin and hematocrit values.

## ♦ EVALUATION

To evaluate effectiveness of nursing interventions, compare patient behaviors with those stated in the expected patient outcomes. Successful achievement of patient outcomes for the person with aneurysm is indicated by the following:

1. Manifests adequate tissue perfusion as evidenced by:
   a. BUN 5 to 20 mg/dl and creatinine levels 0.7 to 1.5 mg/dl.
   b. Urine output of 25 to 30 ml/hr.
   c. Presence of distal pulses.
   d. Absence of abdominal distention or postoperative ileus.
2. Demonstrates signs of adequate fluid volume:
   a. Vital signs and hemodynamic variables within normal range for patient.
   b. Wound drainage minimal or absent.
   c. Abdominal and back pain absent.
   d. Hemoglobin and hematocrit values within normal range for the patient.

## ARTERIAL EMBOLISM

### Etiology/Epidemiology

An **arterial embolism** is a common cause of occlusion of both large and small arteries. Macroembolic episodes involve the superficial femoral, aortic, popliteal, iliac, and common femoral arteries. These emboli most commonly originate in the heart as a result of atrial fibrillation, myocardial infarction, prosthetic heart valve, and cardiomyopathy. Emboli have been associated with immobility, anemia, and cardiomyopathy.

### Pathophysiology

An embolus originally develops as a blood clot or thrombus from breakdown and ulceration of atherosclerotic plaque. Once the thrombus becomes detached from its site of origin, it becomes an embolus. Emboli tend to lodge in areas of bifurcation, especially the femoral or popliteal arteries, hence obstructing blood flow and causing ischemia.

The clinical manifestations of an arterial embolism depend on the size of the embolus, presence of collateral circulation, and the proximity to a major organ. There is an abrupt onset of severe pain from the sudden cessation of circulation. Distal pulses are absent, and the extremity becomes cold and pale. Paresthesia and numbness develop as the peripheral nerves become affected by ischemia. Irreversible ischemic changes or sensory

**TABLE 32-2 Anticoagulants Used in Treatment of Vascular Disorders**

| ACTION | DOSAGE | SIDE EFFECTS |
|---|---|---|
| **HEPARIN** | | |
| Forms complex with antithrombin III, which inhibits thrombin action<br>Intravenous route produces immediate action; duration is 2 hr<br>Subcutaneous route used for maintenance and prophylaxis | Intravenous:<br>Bolus 5000-10,000 U<br>Continuous drip: 20,000-30,000 U/day at 0.5 U/kg/min in 5% dextrose or NS<br>Subcutaneous:<br>5000 U 2 hr before surgery and every 8-12 hr thereafter<br>NOTE: dosage adjusted to maintain APTT at 1.5-2 times laboratory control<br>Normal APTT = 33-45 sec<br>Prolonged APTT = 60-100 sec<br>Acute arterial embolism: 100,000 U<br>Deep vein thrombosis: bolus 5000-10,000 U (1000 U/hr) | Hemorrhage, spontaneous bleeding, epistaxis, bleeding gums, hematoma, GI bleeding with black tarry stools |
| **WARFARIN SODIUM (COUMADIN, PANWARFIN)** | | |
| Inhibits vitamin K–dependent clotting factor synthesis (factors II, VII, IX, and X)<br>Depresses prothrombin activity<br>Peaks in 36-72 hr<br>Duration is 2-5 days | Oral:<br>10 to 15 mg/day until prothrombin time within therapeutic range<br>Then 2 to 10 mg/day<br>NOTE: dosage adjusted to maintain PT at 2.0-2.5 times laboratory control<br>Normal PT = 11-12 sec<br>Prolonged PT = 17-19 sec | Same as for heparin |

*APTT,* Activated partial thromboplastin time; *PT,* prothrombin time.

**TABLE 32-3 Thrombolytics Used in Treatment of Deep Vein Thrombosis (DVT) and Arterial Emboli**

| ACTION | DOSAGE | SIDE EFFECTS |
|---|---|---|
| **STREPTOKINASE (STREPTASE, KABIKINASE)** | | |
| Synthetic protein derived from streptococcal bacteria<br>Activates plasminogen by forming streptokinase-plasminogen complex | IV: Loading dose 250,000 IU over 30 min<br>Then 100,000 IU/hr for 24-72 hr (arterial thrombosis) or 72 hr (DVT) | Bleeding, bronchospasm, rash, urticaria |
| **UROKINASE (ABBOKINASE, BREOKINASE, WIN-KINASE)** | | |
| Human proteolytic enzyme derived from cultured kidney cells<br>Directly converts circulating plasminogen to plasmin | DVT bolus: 4400 IU/kg over 10 min<br>Then 4400 IU/kg/hr<br>Arterial: 4000 IU/min with heparin | Same as for streptokinase |
| **TISSUE PLASMINOGEN ACTIVATOR (TPA)** | | |
| Naturally occurring enzyme made by recombinant DNA<br>Directly converts circulating plasminogen to plasmin | IV: Loading dose 50 mg over 2 hr; then 30-50 mg for 4-6 hr (0.1 IU/kg/hr) | Same as for streptokinase |

loss and muscle paralysis may result if reperfusion is delayed.

## Medical Management

Medical management for acute arterial embolism includes bed rest, drug therapy, and possibly surgery. **Anticoagulants** (heparin and warfarin sodium) (Table 32-2) prolong the clotting time and prevent clot extension and new clot formation. Rapid anticoagulation with a bolus of heparin is followed by continuous heparin infusion. **Thrombolytics** (Table 32-3) are useful for dissolving existing thrombi when rapid dissolution of the clot is required to preserve organ and limb function before neurologic damage occurs. Streptokinase, urokinase, and tissue plasminogen activator (tPA) impair coagulation by increasing fibrinolytic activity. After the

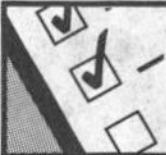

## Guidelines for Care of the Person Receiving Anticoagulant or Thrombolytic Therapy

1. Monitor the infusion accurately; maintain desired therapeutic rate of units per minute or hour.
2. Assess skin for signs of bleeding: bleeding gums, nosebleeds, petechiae (pinpoint red areas on skin), ecchymosis (bruising), hematoma formation, and venipuncture sites.
3. Monitor urine, stool, emesis, and gastric secretions for blood.
4. Avoid administration of medications by intramuscular route to prevent bleeding.
5. Avoid unnecessary bleeding.
   a. Use a soft toothbrush and brush teeth gently.
   b. Use an electric razor rather than razor blade for shaving.
   c. Avoid use of rectal thermometers (may cause mucosal bleeding).
6. Special care with *anticoagulant therapy:*
   a. Give heparin by deep subcutaneous injection; use a fine-gauge needle at a 90-degree angle; do not aspirate nor massage site after injection (can result in bleeding); rotate sites on a regular basis.
   b. Administer protamine sulfate, if necessary, as a heparin antagonist to reverse anticoagulant effects.
   c. Hold pressure for 3 to 5 minutes on venipuncture sites.
   d. Monitor results of blood work: a partial thromboplastin time should be 2 to 3 times normal level (normal APTT is 33 to 45 seconds); a prothrombin time (PT) should be 1.2 to 1.5 times normal level (normal PT is 11 to 12 seconds).
   e. Avoid use of aspirin; aspirin inhibits platelet adhesion, thus having an anticoagulant effect.
7. Special care with *thrombolytic therapy:*
   a. Assess patient for signs of intracranial bleeding—headache, vomiting, disorientation, mental confusion.
   b. Assess patient for signs of retroperitoneal bleeding—low back pain, muscle weakness, or numbness in lower extremity.
   c. Assess patient for allergic reaction—chill, bronchospasm, rash, malaise; an IV steroid may be given to counteract potential allergic reaction.
   d. Avoid insertion of unnecessary venous and arterial lines; insert before initiation of therapy if necessary.
   e. Hold pressure on all venipuncture and other bleeding sites for 20 to 30 minutes to allow blood to clot.
   f. Give medication to avoid GI ulceration or bleeding.

infusion the patient is started on heparin and oral anticoagulants. Blood products may be given to counteract effects of thrombolytics if hemorrhage occurs. Aminocaproic acid, a fibrinolysis inhibitor, may be necessary.

An **embolectomy,** surgical removal of a blood clot, is the main form of therapy when large arteries are obstructed. Success of the embolectomy depends on the length of time the extremity was ischemic; surgery must be performed within 6 to 10 hours to prevent muscle necrosis and limb loss.

Diagnostic studies such as an arteriogram or duplex ultrasonography can be helpful in identifying the causative factor and planning surgical approach (see Table 32-1). These studies are completed only if there is no delay in revascularization.

### Nursing Management

Monitor the patient during the acute phase for changes in skin color and temperature of the extremity distal to the embolus. Increasing pallor, cyanosis, or coldness of the skin indicates vessel occlusion. Keep the extremity warm but do not apply heat; avoid chilling. Monitor peripheral pulses for presence, quality, and bilateral symmetry.

Keep the patient on complete bed rest to prevent potential progression of the embolism. Keep the affected extremity flat or in a slightly dependent position to promote circulation, as indicated by the physician. Do not use knee gatch or apply restraints to affected extremity. Use an overbed cradle to protect the affected extremity from the pressure of bed linens. Monitor effects of anticoagulant and thrombolytic therapy. Assess for local or systemic bleeding (see Guidelines box, above). After embolectomy, assess for compartment syndrome, which can occur with reperfusion after prolonged ischemia.

Patient teaching after the acute phase of arterial embolism includes information about measures to prevent further arterial problems. Teaching about oral anticoagulant therapy is essential (see Guidelines box, above).

## Guidelines for Teaching the Person Receiving Oral Anticoagulant Therapy

Know general action, dosage, and side effects of oral anticoagulants; avoid medications containing aspirin, which also has an anticoagulant effect.

Take oral anticoagulant at same time every day; do not stop taking unless advised by physician.

Inspect for signs of bleeding: bleeding gums, nosebleeds, bruising, red areas on skin, cuts that do not stop bleeding with direct pressure, blood in urine or stool; report these signs promptly to health care professional.

Wear a Medic Alert bracelet or carry an identification card containing drug name, dosage, physician name and phone number in case of emergency.

Complete blood tests (APTT, PT) as scheduled to monitor and adjust drug dosage.

Carefully monitor intake of dark green and yellow vegetables, which are sources of vitamin K that counteracts anticoagulant effects of warfarin (Coumadin).

Restrict alcohol intake, because it increases anticoagulant effect.

# VENOUS DISORDERS

Problems with veins arise when there is alteration in the transport of blood from capillary beds back to the heart.

Changes in smooth muscle and connective tissue make the veins less distensible and limit recoil capacity. Valves in the veins may malfunction, causing backflow of blood. The major venous diseases are thrombophlebitis of the superficial and deep veins and varicose veins.

## SUPERFICIAL THROMBOPHLEBITIS

### Etiology/Epidemiology

Superficial **thrombophlebitis** most often involves the greater or lesser saphenous veins of the lower extremity (see Figure 32-2). In the upper extremity, superficial thrombophlebitis is rare, primarily caused by prolonged administration of intravenous solutions. Superficial thrombophlebitis is more commonly seen in women, especially during pregnancy, and in elders. There is an increased incidence in the postoperative period and in patients with varicose veins.

### Pathophysiology

Superficial thrombophlebitis results from both venous thrombosis and inflammation in a superficial vein. Because the superficial veins are close to the surface of the skin, inflammation may be easily seen by inspection. Patients with superficial thrombophlebitis have pain, tenderness, redness, and a palpable induration along the course of the vein. Edema is not a characteristic finding.

### Medical Management

Superficial thrombophlebitis usually is treated conservatively. Patients may continue to ambulate with use of compression support stockings. If the thrombophlebitis is more diffuse and involves the thigh, bed rest with leg elevation and use of local moist heat is indicated. Anticoagulation is not necessary; however, administration of oral nonnarcotic analgesics or nonsteroidal antiinflammatory drugs may help to alleviate pain and decrease inflammation. If the thrombophlebitis ascends to the saphenofemoral junction, surgical intervention is required to prevent extension into the deep femoral system.

### Nursing Management

Nursing management of the patient with superficial thrombophlebitis is primarily teaching; most patients are not hospitalized. Patients should watch for signs of ascending thrombophlebitis: extending pain, tenderness, and redness, which they should report promptly to their physician. It also is important to tell patients that although extremely rare, deep vein thrombosis or pulmonary embolization can develop. Proper application and use of compression support stockings is discussed in the Guidelines box, above.

Other important topics for teaching are measures to increase tissue perfusion by preventing venous stasis (and thereby preventing pain) and measures to prevent recurrences:

1. Prevention of venous stasis
   a. Avoid prolonged sitting or standing.
   b. Elevate legs when sitting.
   c. Avoid crossing the legs at the knee.
   d. Wear compression support stockings.
   e. Avoid constriction on leg veins by tight bands (socks and garters).
   f. Carry out daily exercises and physical activity to promote blood flow by contraction of leg muscles.
      (1) Practice dorsiflexion of feet while sitting or lying down.
      (2) Walk daily; increase distance as tolerated.
      (3) Swim several times weekly if possible.
      (4) Use stationary bicycle.
2. Prevent recurrence
   a. Maintain desired weight for height.
   b. Modify life-style at work and at home to prevent long periods of standing or sitting.
   c. Follow daily activity program.
   d. Take special precautions if pregnant (because of increased pressure on veins) or for any surgical procedure (especially orthopedic or major abdominal surgery).

**Guidelines for Teaching About Compression Support Stockings**

Measure calf at largest circumference; measure leg length from bottom of heel to bend of knee.
Wear correct size with appropriate pressure gradient.
Apply stocking before getting out of bed.
Turn all but foot of stocking inside out, slide foot into stocking, and pull stocking over leg to ease application.
Remove stocking at bedtime if desired; if leg aches at night, stocking may be of benefit if worn in bed.
Keep a second stocking on hand for use when the other is being laundered.

## DEEP VEIN THROMBOSIS

### Etiology

The main factors that lead to the development of **deep vein thrombosis (DVT)** are venous stasis, vessel wall injury, and hypercoagulability of the blood (Figure 32-12). Stasis of blood can occur with incompetent valves or inactive muscles. Familial deficiencies of anticlotting factors such as antithrombin III, protein C, protein S, and heparin cofactor II contribute to hypercoagulation states.

### Epidemiology

DVT develops in a significant number of hospitalized patients. It is estimated that 50,000 to 100,000 deaths occur annually from its major consequence, pulmonary embolization. DVT is more common in women and is not race-specific. Risk factors associated with DVT are listed in Box 32-2.

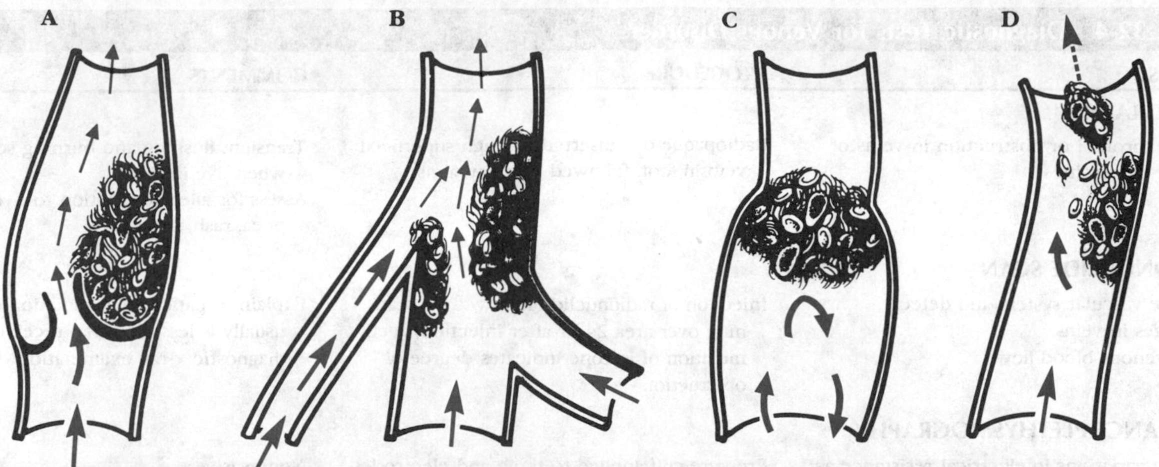


**FIGURE 32-12** Development of deep vein thrombosis with arrows indicating direction of blood flow. **A,** Thrombus in a valve pocket of a deep vein with blood flowing beside thrombus. **B,** Thrombi tend to form at bifurcations of deep veins with some slowing of blood flow. **C,** Complete occlusion of the vein by a thrombus forcing backflow of blood. **D,** An embolus that has broken off from a thrombus and is floating in the bloodstream could migrate to the lungs and cause pulmonary embolus.

**BOX 32-2 Risk Factors for Deep Vein Thrombosis**

- Age over 40 years
- Prior history of DVT
- Coagulation abnormalities
- Surgeries
  - Major abdominal or pelvic surgeries
  - Orthopedic procedures involving lower extremity
- Postthrombotic syndrome
- Estrogen and oral contraceptive use
- Pregnancy
- Obesity
- Heart disease
- Advanced neoplasms
- Limb trauma

## Pathophysiology

Thrombi form as red cells, platelets, and fibrin accumulate and attach to one end of the vein wall. The more proximal end of the thrombus freely floats in the lumen, readily able to break apart and migrate as an embolism. DVT more commonly develops in the veins of the lower extremity: the small calf veins and the popliteal and femoral veins. Thrombus usually originates in the soleal vein valvular sinuses of the calf muscle, extending into the deep calf veins and the posterior tibial and peroneal veins. A small percentage of these thrombi further extend into the popliteal, femoral, or iliac veins.

Clinical manifestations of DVT depend on the location of the affected vein, size of the thrombus, and presence of collateral circulation. More than 50% of patients with DVT are symptom-free. Calf pain, edema, and increased calf circumference may be present with calf or popliteal vein thrombosis. Venous thrombosis at the level of the iliac and femoral veins causes pain with extensive swelling of the entire limb. Some patients do not have any symptoms until a pulmonary embolism occurs.

## Prevention

*Primary prevention* of DVT is directed at education of the public, especially those older than 40 years of age. In particular women who are pregnant and those taking birth control pills or estrogen supplementation should be aware of the potential risk of developing DVT. Measures to promote tissue perfusion and prevent venous stasis are listed on p. 908.

*Secondary prevention* includes the identification of patients at risk for developing DVT. Most surgical patients older than 40 years of age—particularly those with heart disease who are undergoing major abdominal, pelvic, or orthopedic surgery—require prophylaxsis. This usually consists of low-dose heparin before and after surgery. Other medication prophylaxis may include ergotamine, which alters the coagulability of the blood, or low molecular–weight dextran. External periodic calf compression devices also have been effective in the postoperative period.

## Medical Management

DVT is an acute, potentially life-threatening condition that necessitates hospitalization. The current standard of care for treatment is anticoagulation with heparin followed by long-term oral anticoagulation. This measure prevents thrombus propagation and inhibits new thrombus formation.

The goal for discharge of patients with DVT as de-

**TABLE 32-4 Diagnostic Tests for Venous Disorders**

| PURPOSE | PROCEDURE | COMMENTS |
|---|---|---|
| **VENOGRAPHY** | | |
| Identify thrombi or obstruction in veins of lower extremities | Radiopaque dye inserted through superficial vein in foot, followed by x-ray films | Transient flushing and burning sensations when dye injected<br>Assess for allergic reaction to dye (dyspnea, rash, urticaria) |
| **RADIONUCLIDE SCAN** | | |
| Visualize vascular system and detect changes in veins<br>Assess venous blood flow | Injection of radionuclide followed by scanning over area 24 hr after injection; accumulation of isotope indicates degree of obstruction | Explain to patient that radiation dose usually is less than that received from diagnostic x-ray examination |
| **IMPEDANCE PLETHYSMOGRAPHY** | | |
| Measure variations in electrical resistance as a result of changes in blood volume in deep vein thrombophlebitis | Pressure cuff applied to thigh and electrodes applied to calf; measurements taken during inflation and deflation | Noninvasive |
| **DUPLEX ULTRASONOGRAPHY** | | |
| (See Table 32-1) | | |

termined by DRGs is 7 to 10 days. The nurse works collaboratively with the physician for implementation of prescribed medical therapy. Because the nurse has a major role in discharge planning and patient teaching, these are discussed under nursing management.

### Diagnostic tests

A venous duplex ultrasonogram provides the most accurate anatomic and physiologic information for DVT diagnosis. A venogram also may be ordered to assist with the diagnosis. Other diagnostic tests include the use of **impedance plethysmography**—although it is less accurate than venography in detecting calf vein thrombi—and radionuclide **venography** and radioisotope-labeled fibrinogen, which are more useful in detecting thrombosis of the calf (Table 32-4).

### Medication

Initial anticoagulation consists of intravenous heparin and then warfarin (Coumadin) (see Table 32-2). Thrombolysis with fibrinolytic agents, such as streptokinase, urokinase, or tissue plasminogen activator, may be used (see Table 32-3).

### Diet

The patient with DVT requires no special diet. A regimen of Coumadin, however, requires that foods high in vitamin K be carefully monitored because vitamin K can counteract the effects of Coumadin.

### Activity

Patients with DVT that does not involve the calf are restricted to bed rest for 5 to 7 days to allow time for the clot to adhere to the vessel wall. The affected leg is elevated to promote venous return and prevent edema. Patients can ambulate with support stockings, and they are fitted for compression support stockings of either thigh- or knee-length depending on physician preference. Standing still and sitting are avoided.

### Referral/Consultation

In some settings the nurse assumes responsibility for making referrals to other services. The nurse may initiate contact with the stocking fitter for accurate measurement of compression support stockings. Other potential referrals may include physical therapy for ambulation after complete bed rest, social services for home care needs, and a nutritionist for dietary guidelines.

## Surgical Management

A **thrombectomy** is indicated only in patients with impending tissue loss or venous gangrene. A vena cava interruption device such as a Greenfield vena cava filter (Figure 32-13) is used when anticoagulation is contrain-

**Guidelines for Nursing Care of the Person Requiring Surgery for Vena Caval Interruption**

- Assess insertion site; if there are signs of bleeding or hematoma, apply pressure over site and notify surgeon.
- Keep patient on bed rest for first 24 hours; encourage ROM exercises to promote venous return.
- Assist patient in ambulation when permitted; elevate legs when sitting or lying to promote circulation.
- Keep elastic bandage snug and without wrinkles to maintain even pressure on leg veins.
- Medicate with prescribed analgesics and antiinflammatory agents to promote comfort.

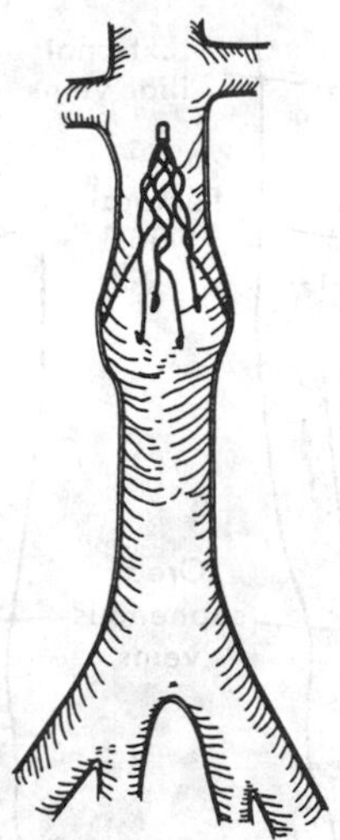

FIGURE 32-13 Greenfield vena cava filter. (Courtesy Meditech Division, Boston Scientific Corp, Watertown, Mass.)

dicated or recurrent thromboembolism develops despite anticoagulation. It can be used as mechanical protection in patients after pulmonary embolectomy. Nursing care after surgery for vena caval interruption is described in the Guidelines box, p. 910.

## NURSING MANAGEMENT

### ♦ ASSESSMENT

#### Subjective Data

Subjective data to be collected to assess the patient with DVT include the following:

- Pain in calf muscle at rest or during exercise
- Pain in thigh
- Tenderness over calf or thigh to palpation
- Previous history of DVT; presence of other associated risk factors
- Sudden onset of chest pain, dyspnea, or rapid breathing, which may indicate pulmonary embolism

#### Objective Data

Objective data to be collected to assess the patient with DVT include the following:

- Presence of ankle edema
- Calf circumference difference of 1.2 cm in women or 1.4 cm in men
- Increased resistance or pain on voluntary dorsiflexion of foot
- Rapid swelling of entire limb with iliofemoral DVT
- Engorged collateral veins in the thigh
- Increased skin temperature

#### Diagnostic Test Findings

A positive result of venous duplex scan or noncompressibility of veins is indicative of thrombus. A bedside Doppler study can detect abnormal blood flow or no flow in the area of the thrombosed vein. Impedance plethysmography detects changes in electrical impedance of the tissues. A filling defect or sharp cutoff on a venogram indicates thrombosis.

### ♦ NURSING DIAGNOSES

Nursing diagnoses are determined from analysis of patient data. Nursing diagnoses for the patient with DVT may include but are not limited to the following:

| Diagnostic Title | Possible Etiologic Factors |
|---|---|
| Tissue perfusion, altered peripheral | Decreased venous blood flow, immobility |
| Pain: leg | Inflammation, edema, venous stasis |
| Knowledge deficit: pharmacotherapy, support stockings, surgery | Lack of exposure/recall unfamiliarity with information sources |

### ♦ EXPECTED PATIENT OUTCOMES

Expected patient outcomes for the patient with DVT may include but are not limited to the following:

1. Has adequate circulation to lower extremity: palpable distal pulses and warm, pink extremity.
2. Shows signs of decreased pain: states feeling more comfortable and has less edema.
3. Explains need for medical therapy: understands major action and side effects of anticoagulants and thrombolytics, complies with restriction to bed rest, wears support stockings, avoids sitting and standing still, and explains signs and symptoms of pulmonary embolism.

### ♦ INTERVENTIONS

#### Maintaining Tissue Perfusion

1. Keep patient with noncalf DVT on bed rest for 5 to 7 days (or as indicated).
2. Apply compression support stockings, usually below knee with 30 to 40 mm Hg gradient pressure (see Guidelines box, p. 908).
3. Ambulate as soon as able.
4. Avoid standing still and sitting.
5. Check pulses distal to site of thrombosis.
6. Assess presence of edema.
7. Keep affected extremity elevated.
8. Monitor calf circumference.
9. Maintain anticoagulant or thrombolytic therapy (see Tables 32-2 and 32-3).
10. Monitor for signs of pulmonary embolus, sudden onset of chest pain, dyspnea, rapid breathing, tachycardia.

#### Promoting Comfort

1. Medicate with analgesics to alleviate pain and discomfort.
2. Provide nonsteroidal antiinflammatory medications to reduce edema.

### Teaching

1. Discuss with patient and family the major action and side effects of anticoagulants and thrombolytics.
2. Emphasize need to assess for bleeding and to take measures to prevent bleeding.
3. Discuss importance of bed rest.
4. Explain rationale for use of compression support stockings and importance of correct usage.
5. Discuss long-term management with Coumadin for 3 months to 1 year and need for periodic blood work.
6. Explain need to continue to wear compression support stockings.

## ♦ EVALUATION

To evaluate the effectiveness of nursing interventions, compare patient behaviors with those stated in the expected patient outcomes. Successful achievement of patient outcomes for the patient with DVT is indicated by the following:

1. Has adequate circulation to lower extremity as indicated by palpable distal pulses and warm pink extremity.
2. States that pain is decreased and has less edema.
3. Correctly explains medications, complies with bed rest, wears support stockings, avoids sitting and standing still, and explains signs and symptoms of pulmonary embolism.

## VARICOSE VEINS

### Etiology/Epidemiology

**Varicose veins** are prominent, abnormally dilated veins developing most often in the lower extremities because of the effects of gravity on venous pressure. At least 20% of the adult population is affected. The highest incidence is in women between 30 and 50 years of age. Varicose veins can develop from the congenital absence of a valve or acquired incompetence of the valve. They often occur as a result of thrombophlebitis or external pressure on the veins from pregnancy, ascites, or abdominal tumors. Other associated factors are prolonged standing, constrictive clothing, and marked obesity. Varicose veins also can occur as a result of sustained elevations in venous pressure from chronic diseases such as heart disease and cirrhosis. Spider veins, venous stars, or telangiectasias often are mistaken as varicose veins. These are simply small, dilated cutaneous veins that appear as a blemish. They are more commonly seen in the medial, posterior, and lateral aspects of the thigh and typically do not require surgical intervention.

### Pathophysiology

The greater and small saphenous veins are most often involved (Figure 32-14). The vein wall is weakened from a deficiency in elastin or collagen, and it does not withstand normal pressure. The vessel dilates with pooling of blood and the valves become stretched and incompetent.

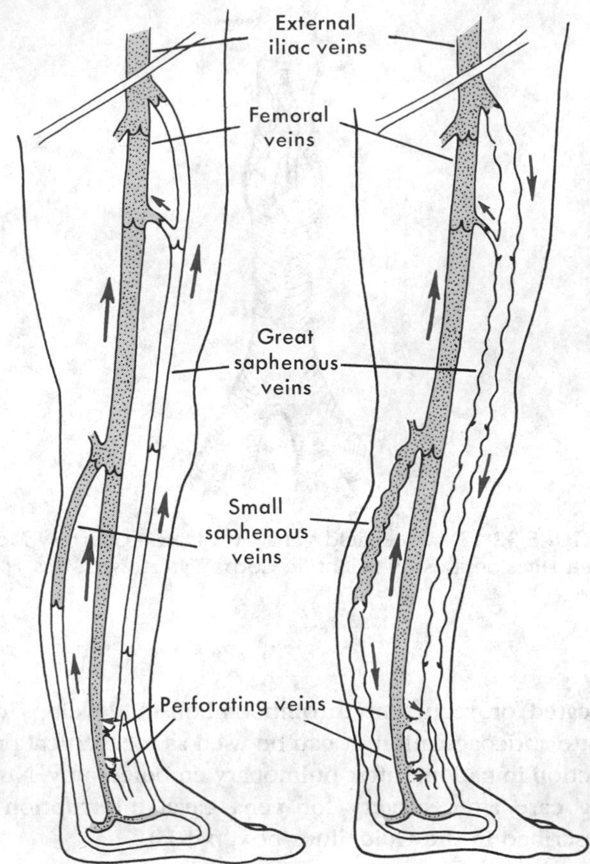


**FIGURE 32-14** Varicose veins. *Left,* Venous flow in normal veins. *Right,* Venous flow in varicose veins.

Varicose veins can be classified as primary or secondary. *Primary varicose veins* have a gradual onset and affect the superficial veins. Often there are no accompanying symptoms except the appearance of darkened tortuous veins. Clinical manifestations include dull aches, muscle cramps, pressure, heaviness, and fatigue. *Secondary varicose veins* affect the deep veins as a result of chronic venous insufficiency or deep vein thrombosis. Symptoms of marked edema, pain, changes in skin color, and ulceration may be present.

**Trendelenburg's test,** a simple noninvasive diagnostic tool, assesses the competency of the venous filling time. The patient lies down with the affected leg raised to allow for venous emptying. A tourniquet is then applied above the knee, and the patient stands. The direction and filling time are recorded both before and after the tourniquet is removed. Incompetent valves are evident when the veins fill rapidly from backward blood flow.

A venous duplex scan is ordered to assess anatomic and physiologic changes in veins (see Table 32-1).

### Medical Management

Many varicose veins can be treated by conservative medical therapy. This includes elevation of affected limb,

**TABLE 32-5 Characteristics of Arterial and Venous Diseases**

| ARTERIAL DISEASE | VENOUS DISEASE |
|---|---|
| **SKIN** | |
| Cool or cold; hairless, dry, shiny; pallor on elevation and rubor on dangling | Warm; tough, thickened; mottled, pigmented areas |
| **PAIN** | |
| Sharp, stabbing; worsens with activity and walking; lowering feet may relieve pain | Aching, cramping; activity and walking sometimes help; elevating feet relieves pain |
| **ULCERS** | |
| Severely painful; pale, gray base; found on heel, lateral malleolus, toes, and dorsum of foot | Moderately painful; pink base, with irregular, pigmented skin edge; found on medial aspect of ankle |
| **PULSES** | |
| Often absent or diminished | Usually present |
| **EDEMA** | |
| Infrequent | Frequent, especially at end of day and in areas of ulceration |

compression with support stockings, maintenance of an exercise program, and use of pneumatic compression pumps. Sclerotherapy, an outpatient approach to treatment of small varicose veins or large telangiectases, involves the injection of a sclerosing agent into the varicose vein. Compression bandages are applied for 4 days; bruising is common after removal. Hyperpigmentation of the skin may develop in 1 to 2 weeks and persist for 6 to 8 months.

### Surgical Management

Surgical intervention that employs vein ligation and stripping is indicated for more advanced cases to relieve pain, reduce swelling, or provide cosmetic results. The greater saphenous vein is ligated at the saphenofemoral junction. Several small incisions at the groin, knee, and ankle are made to strip the saphenous vein. Perforator veins are ligated. Sterile dressings are placed over incisions, and an elastic bandage is wrapped from foot to the groin for compression.

### Nursing Management

Persons with varicose veins, especially those with a family history, should wear elastic stockings during activities requiring long periods of standing or when pregnant. Moderate exercise and elevation of the legs during sitting help to prevent venous congestion. No continual pressure should be applied to the veins.

Nursing care of the patient after vein ligation and stripping includes teaching the patient to watch for the following:

1. Bleeding: elevate the leg, apply pressure over the wound, and notify the vascular surgeon.
2. Elevate leg to promote venous return when lying or sitting.
3. Take prescribed analgesics as necessary and 30 minutes before ambulation.
4. Keep elastic bandage snug and wrinkle-free to maintain even pressure on veins; do not remove bandage for daily care.
5. Return for follow-up appointment with vascular surgeon.
6. Know that bruising is common when bandages are removed.
7. Watch for skin color changes.

## ARTERIAL/VENOUS DISORDERS

Disorders of the vascular system generally interfere with circulation to the tissues, leading to characteristic clinical manifestations. With *arterial* insufficiency, there is decreased blood flow to the tissues, producing *ischemia*. Pulses usually are diminished or absent, and sharp, stabbing pain occurs because of the ischemia, particularly with activity. There is interference with nutrients arriving to the tissues, leading to ischemic ulcers and changes in the skin (Table 32-5). In *venous* insufficiency, blood reaches the tissue but blood return to the heart is diminished, leading to venous *congestion* and *stasis*. Pulses are present. The venous congestion leads to edema, skin changes, and stasis ulcers.

## ARTERIOVENOUS FISTULAS

### Etiology/Epidemiology

An **arteriovenous fistula** is an abnormal direct communication between an artery and vein caused by a congenital anomaly or an acquired disorder. Congenital fistulas,which are often multiple, affect circulation to an entire region or area such as the arm or leg. Most acquired arteriovenous fistulas are caused by penetrating injuries from trauma. A single arteriovenous fistula is rare. More often, multiple fistulas affect circulation to an entire region or area such as the arm or leg.

### Pathophysiology

In an arteriovenous fistula, the high arterial blood flow bypasses the capillary network and goes into the veins. This causes an increase in venous pressure that predisposes to venous engorgement, dilation, and aneurysm development. The veins become thickened as the artery thins and loses its elastic and muscular properties.

Clinical manifestations of arteriovenous fistulas may include pain at the site of a fistula; edema and asymmetry of an extremity; tortuous, dilated superficial veins; and venous pulsations. Venous bruit and thrill may be present from turbulent blood flow. Testing includes use of arteriography and Doppler ultrasonography.

### Medical Management

Small peripheral arteriovenous fistulas may not require intervention. Surgical intervention may be indicated when ulceration, bleeding, or severe arterial or venous insufficiency occurs. The most common procedure is closure of the fistula with embolic material such as Gelfoam, glass beads, or muscle. Large fistulas may be repaired or resected with ligation of involved artery.

### Nursing Management

Nursing management is primarily related to teaching and support. Compression support stockings can help prevent discomfort and edema. Postoperative care includes assessing skin color, temperature, and pulses in the limb distal to the surgery.

Teaching includes information about the underlying disease and measures to prevent symptoms of venous insufficiency and promote venous return.

## LEG ULCERS

### Etiology

Most leg ulcers result from chronic venous insufficiency or postthrombotic syndrome and severe varicose veins. Less commonly, they develop from arterial obstruction. Other causes include burns, leg trauma, and neurogenic disorders.

### Epidemiology

Chronic venous insufficiency is estimated to affect 3.5% of the adult population. Persons with diabetes mellitus are at high risk for development of leg ulcers because of vascular insufficiency.

### Pathophysiology

A leg ulcer is an open necrotic lesion that results from inadequate exchange of oxygen and other nutrients to the tissues because of decreased circulation. The same underlying pathophysiologic changes that contribute to the development of chronic venous or arterial insufficiency are involved. Secondary bacterial infection frequently occurs, delaying healing.

Clinical manifestations vary, depending on the underlying problem. A **venous ulcer** or stasis ulcer is usually moderately painful and located on the medial aspect of the ankle. Edema and pigmentation changes are common around the area of ulceration. An **arterial ulcer** or ischemic ulcer is usually more painful with necrotic, pale-gray base; it frequently develops on the heel, lateral malleolus, toes, and dorsum of the foot. Pale or mottled skin is common around the base of the ulcer. Edema occurs infrequently, and peripheral pulses are diminished or absent.

### Medical Management

#### Diagnostic tests

Commonly performed tests include a venous duplex scan and photoplethysmography. A photoplethysmogram may show ankle venous refill time of less than 22 seconds, indicating venous insufficiency.

#### Medication

Topical and systemic antibiotics may be prescribed to prevent infection; systemic antibiotic therapy is the most effective route. Periodic culture of wound drainage may be ordered to monitor effectiveness of the antibiotics. Diuretics may be ordered for severe edema.

#### Treatment

Necrotic tissue is débrided by mechanical, chemical, or surgical means. A wet-to-dry dressing may be applied to débride the wound *mechanically.* The dressing is applied damp and removed when dry, pulling off the debris that has adhered to the dressing. *Chemical* beads or enzyme ointments such as fibrinolysins may be placed over the ulcer to break down the debris. Other dressings with hydrophilic properties or hydrocolloid action create a moist environment and can be directly applied to the ulcer. Necrotic tissue also can be cut away with the aid of *surgical* instruments, usually a scalpel.

An **Unna paste boot** may be applied to cover small, newly formed ulcers in ambulatory persons (Figure 32-15). This boot protects the ulcer and provides constant even support. The boot is made of a special type of gauze impregnated with glycerin, sorbitol, gelatin, magnesium aluminum salicylate, zinc oxide, and calamine that hardens around the patient's leg.

The Unna boot is generally changed twice per week, although it may be changed more often if copious drainage occurs. Compulan, a low-stretch elastic bandage, may be applied to the leg after the ulcer has healed.

To promote venous return the patient wears compression stockings with 30 to 40 mm Hg pressure except when sleeping. The stockings can be ready-wear or custom-made. Intermittent pneumatic compression can be used to increase venous flow and to promote extracellular fluid clearance. Various types of segmental

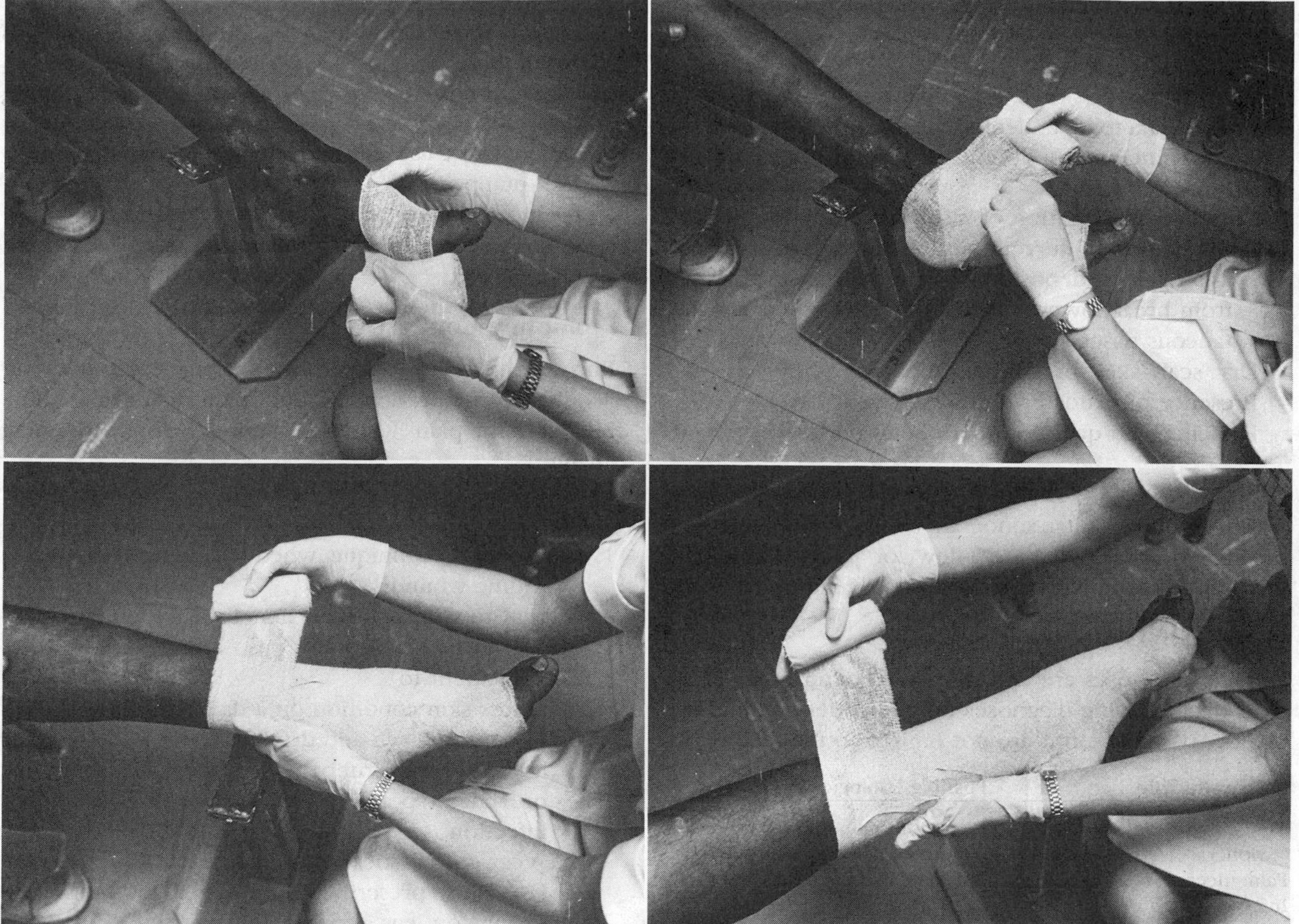

**FIGURE 32-15** Nurse applying Unna paste boot using specially impregnated gauze. Note ulcers on inferior aspect of patient's foot.

gradient pumps can be ordered for use at home. The amount of pressure and length of time are prescribed by the physician. Whirpool therapy may be of help in treating some ulcers.

### Diet

Although essential vitamins and minerals are important to promote wound healing, no specific diet is required.

### Activity

With severe lower-extremity edema, bed rest with leg elevation above the level of the heart is indicated; otherwise activity and ambulation are encouraged.

### Referral/Consultation

In some settings the nurse assumes responsibility for making referrals to other services. A vascular surgeon may be consulted for severe venous ulcers. A vascular clinical nurse specialist or nurse expert in wound management may be consulted for wound care management and homegoing needs such as compression pump and compression support stockings.

### Surgical Management

Recurrent venous ulcers and nonhealing arterial ulcers may require surgical intervention. Ligation of incompetent veins may be necessary. Arterial bypass and reconstruction can be used to revascularize the artery and restore circulation. Amputation may be required if less aggressive means are unsuccessful.

## NURSING MANAGEMENT

## ♦ ASSESSMENT

### Subjective Data

Subjective data to be collected to assess the patient with a leg ulcer include the following:

- Pain at medial malleolus (venous); more discomfort when standing
- Painful areas on heel; lateral aspect of ankle, toes, or dorsum of foot (arterial)
- Swelling of leg
- Limitation in mobility or activity
- History of chronic venous insufficiency or postthrom-

botic syndrome, varicose veins, diabetes, arterial obstruction

### Objective Data

Objective data to be collected to assess the patient with a leg ulcer include the following:

Presence of edema
Presence and location of ulcer
Pigmentation of surrounding skin, which is brawny as a result of deposits of hemosiderin, a byproduct from breakdown of red blood cells, in the subcutaneous tissue
Dry, scaly skin surrounding the ulcer
Presence of exudate from ulcer, necrotic base
Presence and quality of peripheral pulses

### Diagnostic Test Findings

A venous duplex ultra-sonogram shows valvular incompetence by reversed blood flow, or photoplethysmogram indicates impaired ankle venous refill time.

## ♦ NURSING DIAGNOSES

Nursing diagnoses are determined from analysis of patient data. Nursing diagnoses for the patient with a leg ulcer may include but are not limited to the following:

| Diagnostic Title | Possible Etiologic Factors |
|---|---|
| Tissue perfusion, altered peripheral | Decreased blood flow (venous or arterial) |
| Pain: ulcer | Inflammation, necrosis |
| Infection, high risk for | Lack of knowledge, decreased cellular nutrition |
| Knowledge deficit: ulcer care, prevention | Lack of exposure/recall, misinterpretation of information |

## ♦ EXPECTED PATIENT OUTCOMES

Expected patient outcomes for the patient with a leg ulcer may include but are not limited to the following:

1. Shows signs of ulcer healing: absence of further breakdown, beefy-pink tissues, absence of exudate, and lack of necrotic tissue.
2. States pain is lessened.
3. Describes measures to prevent infection.
4. Demonstrates care of the ulcer.

## ♦ INTERVENTIONS

### Promoting Tissue Perfusion

1. Maintain proper body positioning to improve circulation by gravity:
   a. Elevate head of bed on 3- to 6-inch blocks for an *arterial* ulcer.
   b. Elevate lower extremities above heart level to decrease edema for a *venous* ulcer.
2. Use overbed cradle to protect leg from pressure of bed linens.
3. Use cotton between toes to prevent pressure on a toe ulcer.
4. Change dressing using prescribed therapy.
5. Apply topical antibiotics or administer intravenous antibiotics.
6. Put on compression support stockings before getting out of bed.
7. Demonstrate use of intermittent pneumatic compression pump.
8. Promote activity and ambulation.
9. Encourage participation in routine aerobic exercise program.

### Promoting Comfort

Encourage the use of prescribed analgesics and antiinflammatory medication to reduce pain and inflammation. Medicate for pain 30 to 45 minutes before a dressing change.

### Preventing Infection

1. Use aseptic technique when changing dressing or débriding wound.
2. Administer antibiotics on time to maintain therapeutic blood level.
3. Teach patient to
   a. Assess skin condition on a daily basis.
   b. Keep skin clean and dry.
   c. Avoid wearing rubber-soled shoes because they prevent evaporation and thus contribute to foot infection.
   d. Wear cotton socks and change daily.
   e. Use only prescribed ointments and antibiotic creams on legs and feet.
   f. Keep pathways in home free of clutter to avoid possible injury to legs and subsequent infection.
   g. Contact health care professional at onset of skin breakdown.

### Facilitating Learning

Teaching includes prevention of infection, maintenance of skin integrity, and compliance with measures to increase peripheral tissue perfusion. Teach the patient the correct method of dressing changes, and discuss resources in the community for obtaining necessary supplies.

## ♦ EVALUATION

To evaluate effectiveness of nursing interventions, compare patient behaviors with those stated in the expected patient outcomes. Successful achievement of patient outcomes for the patient with a leg ulcer is indicated by the following:

1. Manifests ulcer healing as indicated by absence of further breakdown, beefy-pink tissues, absence of exudate, and lack of necrotic tissue.
2. Indicates pain has lessened.
3. Correctly describes measures to prevent infection.
4. Correctly demonstrates care of the ulcer.

## ✷ SPECIAL CONSIDERATIONS FOR CARE OF THE GERONTOLOGIC PATIENT

Because many of the patients with leg ulcers are elderly, it is important to know whether the patient can perform the dressing change unassisted. Some elderly patients have difficulty seeing the ulcer area and positioning themselves to change a dressing despite the use of a mirror. Sometimes a spouse or neighbor is needed to assist with this task. Some patients may require a home health nurse. Other factors to consider include the availability and cost of dressing supplies inasmuch as many elders are on a fixed budget. The cost of compression support stockings and a pneumatic compression pump also must be considered.

# LYMPHEDEMA

## ETIOLOGY

**Lymphedema** is an abnormal accumulation of lymph within the tissues caused by an obstruction in flow. Lymphedema can be classified as primary or secondary. Primary lymphedema results from hypoplastic, aplastic, or hyperplastic development of the lymphatic vessels. Symptoms may manifest at birth, during puberty, or in middle age. Secondary or acquired lymphedema most often develops from trauma to the lymph nodes. Frequent causes include surgical removal of lymph nodes, radiation-induced fibrosis, inflammation, lymphomas, and parasitic infections.

## EPIDEMIOLOGY

Primary lymphedema affects women more frequently than men. Filarial infections, prevalent in tropical climates, are the most common worldwide cause of secondary lymphedema.

## PATHOPHYSIOLOGY

The lymphatic vessels carry lymph from the tissues back into the venous circulation. This system is made up of small thin vessels that are found throughout the body in close proximity to the veins. The lymphatics begin as capillaries that drain the tissues of lymph (a fluid similar to plasma) and tissue fluid that contains cells, cellular debris, and proteins. The lymph flows through oval bodies called *lymph nodes,* which remove noxious agents such as bacteria and toxins. The flow then drains into the thoracic duct and the right lymphatic duct, which empty into the junction of the internal jugular vein and subclavian vein (Figure 32-16).

Pathophysiologic changes may include (1) roughening of the surface of the lymphatic vessel, (2) dilation of some lymph channels with thickening and edema of the lymphatic tissue, and (3) fibrosis and separation of elastic fibers that may be present in inflammatory states. Recurrent episodes of lymphedema may cause fibrosis and hyperplasia of lymph vessels, leading to a severe enlargement of the extremity, called elephantiasis.

Lymphedema of the lower extremities begins with mild swelling at the ankle, which gradually extends to the entire limb. Initially, the edema is soft and pitting but then progresses to firm, rubbery, nonpitting edema. Left leg swelling is more common than right leg swelling. This condition is aggravated by prolonged standing, pregnancy, obesity, warm weather, and menstruation.

## PREVENTION

*Primary prevention* may include health teaching about lymphedema, especially to women. Travelers to the tropics should be aware of the potential risk of parasitic infestation from filaria.

Types of *secondary prevention* involve measures to protect patients from extensive surgical lymph node dissection or removal (such as with a mastectomy) and from radiation of lymph nodes whenever possible.

## MEDICAL MANAGEMENT

### Diagnostic Tests

Diagnostic tests include the use of **lymphangiography,** the injection of a contrast medium directly into the lymphatic vessels to detect lymph node defects and lymph node involvement in metastatic cancer. An x-ray film is taken after injection of a radiopaque dye and again in 24 hours. Periodic roentgenograms are effective for up to 6 months inasmuch as the dye remains in the lymph system. Radioisotope lymphography involves injection into the foot, with subsequent scanning. A CT scan may show a honeycomb pattern in the subcutaneous compartment.

### Medication

Diuretics can be prescribed to temporarily decrease size of limb. Benzopyrones, which break down protein by activating macrophages, may decrease viscosity and facilitate lymph flow. Long-term antibiotic therapy may be indicated to control recurrent cellulitis and infection.

### Treatment

Treatment consists of elevation of the foot of the bed on blocks at a height of 8 inches, wearing of compression support stockings, and use of an intermittent pneumatic compression device.

### Diet

There is no special diet to treat lymphedema; however, the patient receiving diuretic therapy requires adequate potassium. Salty and spicy foods that cause a predisposition to fluid retention and edema should be avoided.

### Activity

Standing still for long periods of time is contraindicated. If infection is present, activity is restricted to bed rest with leg elevation.

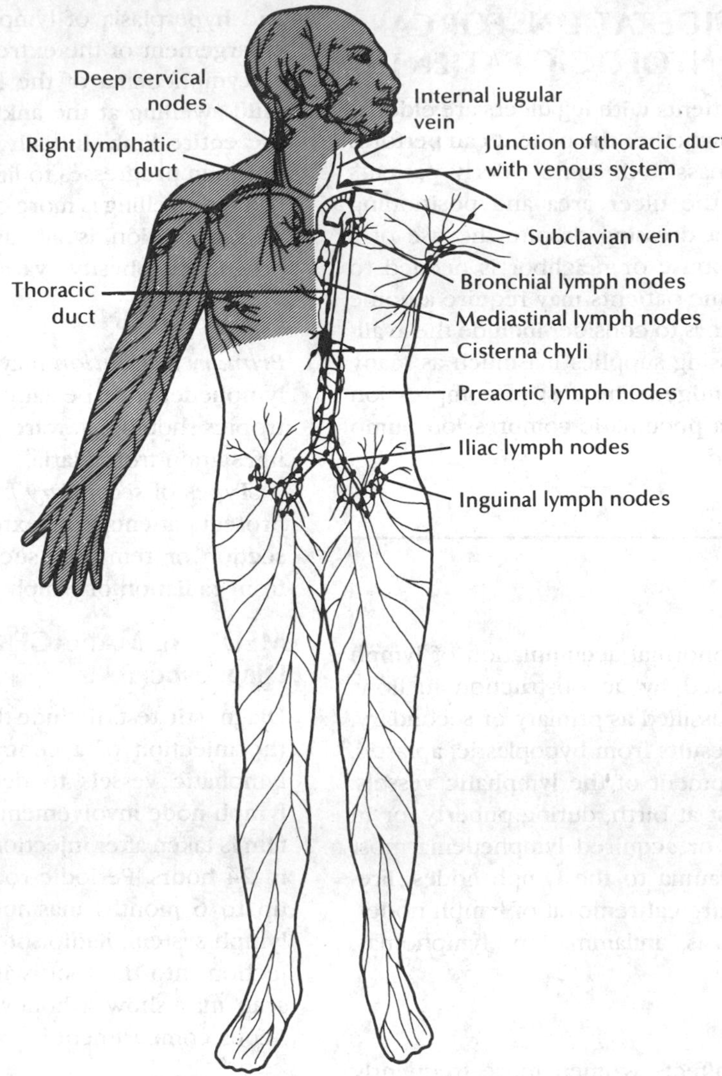


**FIGURE 32-16** Lymph pathways of the lower limb drain into the subclavian vein. (From Hamilton WJ: *Textbook of human anatomy,* ed 2, St Louis, 1976, Mosby.)

### Referral/Consultation

In some settings the nurse assumes responsibility for making referrals to other services. A physical therapy consultation may be appropriate if the patient needs additional assistance with mobility. A wound care specialist may be of help if infection is present, and referral may be indicated for measurement for compression support stockings and an intermittent pneumatic compression device.

## SURGICAL MANAGEMENT

Surgery is restricted to severe cases of lymphedema that are unsuccessfully treated by medical management. The most frequent reason is to reduce the size and bulk of the limb. Surgery also may be used to decrease the incidence of recurrent infections and to improve the cosmetic appearance of the involved limb. The surgical approaches are varied. In general, surgery is directed at restoring lymphatic function or improving the patient's symptoms. Microsurgery involving vein grafting to small lymph vessels has been successful.

## NURSING MANAGEMENT

### ♦ ASSESSMENT

### Subjective Data

Subjective data to be collected to assess the patient with lymphedema include the following:

Onset of swelling in affected limb

History of surgical removal of lymph nodes, radiation therapy, recurrent inflammation, parasitic infection

Functional limitation of swelling

Effectiveness of current therapy to decrease swelling

### Objective Data

Objective data to be collected to assess the patient with lymphedema include the following:

Presence of edema, pitting or nonpitting
Location of edema—more common in left leg
Comparison in size of extremities
Texture of skin: firm, rubbery
Association with prolonged standing, pregnancy, obesity, warm weather, and menstruation

### Diagnostic Test Findings

Lymphangiography shows the type and site of lymphatic involvement. A radioisotope lymphogram shows reduced uptake of isotope by the lymph vessels. A CT scan indicates the number and size of lymph nodes.

## ♦ NURSING DIAGNOSES

Nursing diagnoses are determined from analysis of patient data. Nursing diagnoses for the patient with lymphedema may include but are not limited to the following:

| Diagnostic Title | Possible Etiologic Factors |
|---|---|
| Infection, high risk for | Lack of knowledge |
| Body image disturbance | Change in body appearance |
| Knowledge deficit | Lack of exposure/recall |

## ♦ EXPECTED PATIENT OUTCOMES

Expected patient outcomes for the person with lymphedema may include but are not limited to the following:

1. Describes measures to prevent infection.
2. Expresses acceptance of body image changes.
3. States measures to improve lymph circulation.

## ♦ INTERVENTIONS

### Preventing Infection

1. Assess skin daily for intactness, swelling, redness, and lesions.
2. Provide meticulous care to skin, especially feet.
3. Complete entire course of prescribed antibiotics.
4. Avoid application of nonprescribed topical ointments and creams.

### Promoting a Positive Body Image

1. Encourage expression of concerns regarding swelling of affected limb.
2. Discuss alteration in clothing and shoes to accommodate swelling.
3. Teach importance of adherence to measures that decrease edema.

### Facilitating Learning

1. Perform passive and active exercise of involved limb.
2. Elevate affected extremity.
3. Avoid standing still for long periods.
4. Wear compression support stockings.
5. Avoid constrictive clothing.
6. Exercise on a regular basis.
7. Place foot of bed up on 8-inch blocks.
8. Use pneumatic external compression pump as ordered.
9. Take medications as prescribed.
10. Adhere to dietary restrictions as indicated.

## ♦ EVALUATION

To evaluate effectiveness of nursing interventions, compare patient behaviors with those stated in the expected patient outcomes. Successful achievement of patient outcomes for the patient with lymphedema is indicated by the following:

1. Correctly describes measures to prevent infection.
2. Correctly expresses acceptance of body image change.
3. Correctly describes measures to improve lymph circulation.

# Hypertension

Hypertension is discussed here because it is a major risk factor for vascular disease. **Hypertension (HTN)** is defined as a consistent systolic blood pressure ≥140 mm Hg and/or a consistent diastolic blood pressure ≥90 mm Hg. A more complete classification of blood pressure developed by a national task force to establish a consistent diagnosis of hypertension is listed in Table 32-6. This categoric classification is based on the average of two or more blood pressure readings, not on a single elevated reading.

## ETIOLOGY

There are two types of HTN: essential (primary or idiopathic) and secondary. **Essential hypertension** accounts for more than 90% of all types of HTN. Although there is no generally accepted cause of essential hypertension, several theories have been postulated, including arteriolar changes, alterations in sympathetic tone, hormonal influences, and genetic factors. **Secondary hypertension** develops as a consequence of an underlying

**TABLE 32-6 Classification of Hypertension***

| | CHARACTERISTICS | |
|---|---|---|
| STAGE | SYSTOLIC (mm Hg) | DIASTOLIC (mm Hg) |
| 1 | 140-159 | 90-99 |
| 2 | 160-179 | 100-109 |
| 3 | 180-209 | 110-119 |
| 4 | ≥210 | ≥120 |

From Report of the Joint National Committee on Detection, Evaluation and Treatment of High Blood Pressure, US Department of Health and Human Services, Public Health Services, NIH Publication, Bethesda, Md, 1992, National Institutes of Health.
*Age 18 or older.

**TABLE 32-7 Causes of Secondary Hypertension**

| DISORDER/CONDITION | MECHANISM |
|---|---|
| *Kidney* | |
| Renal parenchymal disease (glomerulonephritis, renal failure) | Most often cause a renin- or sodium-dependent HTN; physiologic changes relate to type of disease and severity of renal insufficiency |
| Renovascular disease | Decrease in renal perfusion from atherosclerotic or fibrotic narrowing of renal arteries; causes marked increase in peripheral vascular resistance and cardiac output |
| *Adrenal cortex* | |
| Cushing's syndrome | Increase in blood volume |
| Primary aldosteronism | Increase in aldosterone, causing sodium and water retention that increase blood volume |
| Pheochromocytoma | Excess secretion of catecholamines (norepinephrine increases peripheral vascular resistance) |
| *Coarctation of aorta* | Causes marked elevated blood pressure in upper extremities with decreased perfusion in lower extremities |
| *Head trauma or cranial tumor* | Increased intracranial pressure reduces cerebral blood flow; resultant ischemia stimulates medullary vasomotor center to raise blood pressure |
| *Pregnancy-induced HTN* | Cause unknown; generalized vasospasm may be a contributing factor |

disease or condition (Table 32-7). In most instances hypertension subsides when the disease is treated or controlled.

## EPIDEMIOLOGY

The incidence of hypertension increases with age and varies considerably among different groups. In the United States, HTN occurs more often in men than in women (although the rate increases in women after menopause) and is nearly twice as prevalent among black persons than among whites. HTN in blacks is usually more severe. There is increased incidence and severity of HTN in African-Americans living in the southeastern United States compared with those residing in other areas. (See Box 32-3 for a summary of risk factors in essential hypertension.) In addition, it is estimated that another 50% of adults in the United States have undiagnosed HTN. The exact number, however, is unknown because most persons with elevated blood pressure are symptom-free and others avoid pursuing treatment.

**BOX 32-3 Risk Factors in Essential Hypertension**

Age: advancing
Sex: male
Race: black
Family history: hypertension
Obesity: associated with increased intravascular volume
Atherosclerosis: narrowing of arteries increases blood pressure
Smoking: nicotine constricts blood vessels
High-salt diet: sodium causes water retention, increasing blood volume
Alcohol: increases plasma catecholamines
Emotional stress: stimulates sympathetic nervous system

## PATHOPHYSIOLOGY

Blood pressure is the pressure exerted by the blood on the vessels through which it flows. Systolic pressure is the pressure during ventricular contraction; diastolic pressure is pressure during ventricular relaxation. Blood pressure is regulated by two factors: blood flow and peripheral vascular resistance. Factors that determine blood flow are the volume of blood ejected from the left ventricle with each contraction (stroke volume) and the heart rate (see Chapter 31). Peripheral vascular resistance is affected primarily by the diameter of the blood vessel and to a lesser degree by the viscosity of the blood. Increased peripheral vascular resistance from narrowing of the arterioles is the most common characteristic in HTN.

Dilation and constriction of the peripheral arterioles are controlled by several mechanisms, primarily the sympathetic nervous system and the renin-angiotensin system. The vasomotor center in the medulla can be stimulated by the baroreceptors (Figure 32-17) or by psychogenic stress. Impulses are then carried through the sympathetic nervous system, causing the release of catecholamines such as norepinephrine and epinephrine. Norepinephrine is released from the postganglionic nerve fibers, causing blood vessel constriction and increased peripheral resistance. Epinephrine is secreted by the adrenal medulla, causing vasoconstriction. Epinephrine also increases ventricular contraction force and increased cardiac output.

Renal regulation is an essential component of blood pressure control (Figure 32-18). Activation of the **renin-angiotensin system** occurs with reduced blood flow to the kidneys. Renin leads to the formation of angiotensin, a potent vasoconstrictor, that stimulates secretion of aldosterone to promote retention of sodium and water.

In the kidneys the renal vessels thicken and perfusion diminishes, depriving the glomerulus of its blood supply.

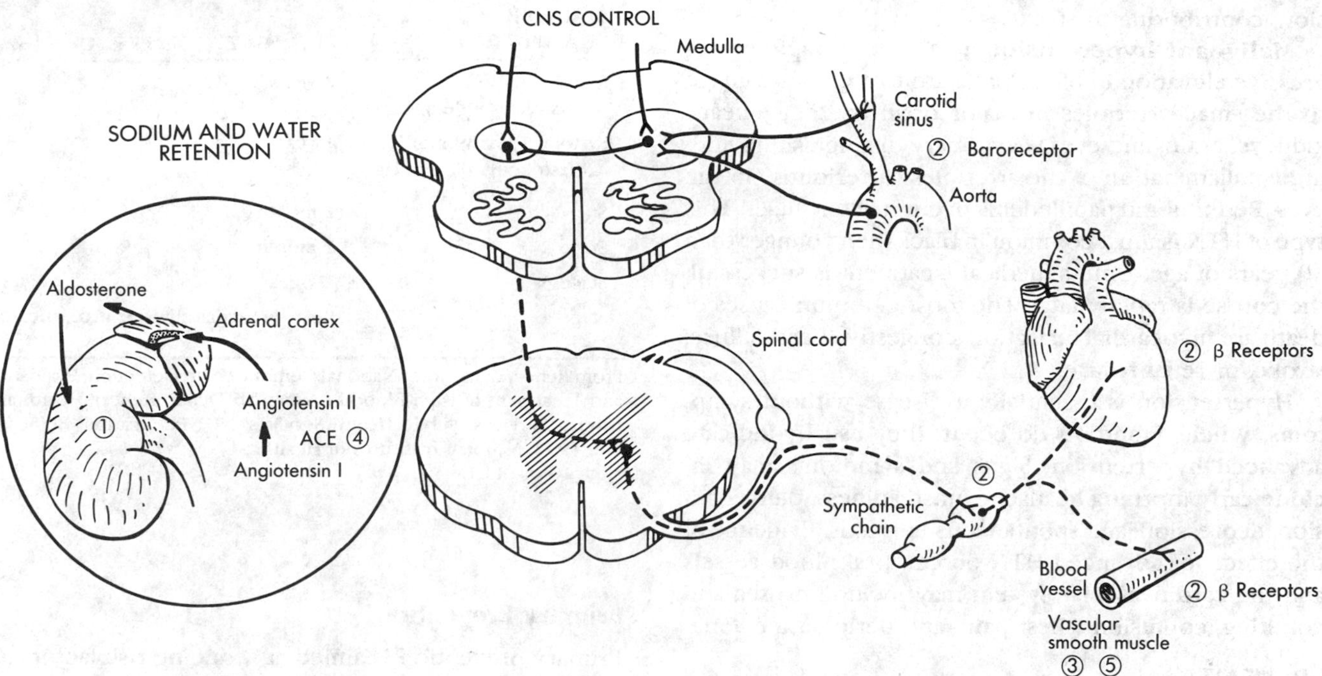


**FIGURE 32-17** Sites of blood pressure regulation and action of antihypertensive drugs. 1, Diurectics. 2, Adrenergic inhibitors. 3, Vasodilators. 4, ACE inhibitors. 5, Calcium antagonist. *ACE,* Angiotensin converting enzyme.

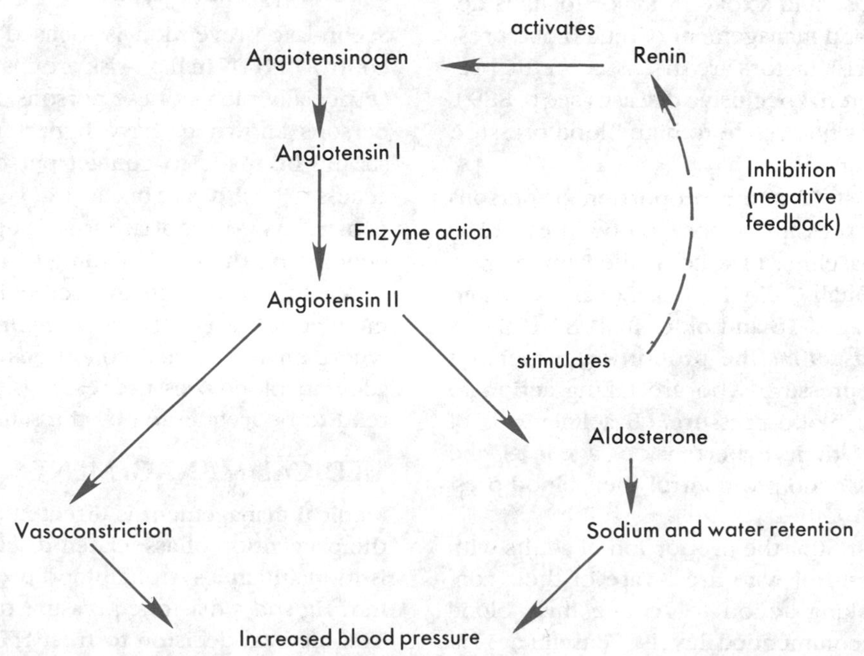


**FIGURE 32-18** Diagram of the effect of the renin-angiotensin system on blood pressure.

Permanent renal damage and possible renal failure may result. Cerebral ischemia and arteriosclerosis can develop as a result of the progressive effects of hypertension, contributing to stroke.

**Malignant hypertension** is a severe, rapidly progressive elevation in blood pressure that causes damage to the small arterioles in major organ systems (heart, kidneys, brain, and eyes). A primary distinguishing finding is inflammation of the arterioles (arteriolitis) in the eyes. Retinitis and papilledema occur in later stages. This type of HTN is most common in black men younger than 40 years of age. Unless medical treatment is successful, the course is rapidly fatal. The most common causes of death are myocardial infarction, congestive heart failure, stroke, or renal failure.

Hypertension is essentially a disease without symptoms. When symptoms do occur, they usually indicate advanced hypertension. Signs and symptoms may include early morning headache, unsteadiness, blurred vision, depression, and spontaneous epistaxis. Evidence of the effects of advanced HTN on cerebral blood vessels and the cardiovascular system may include nausea and vomiting, confusion, chest pain, and peripheral edema.

## PREVENTION

Hypertension contributes not only to vascular disorders but also to cardiac, renal, and cerebral vascular diseases. Thus it is important to control HTN through prevention.

### Healthy People 2000

A priority in *Healthy People 2000*[5] is to reduce incidence of heart disease and stroke. A major focus is detection, evaluation, and management of high blood pressure. Other related risk factors are discussed in the prevention section of arterial occlusive disease (see p. 889).

Specific objectives that relate to high blood pressure include the following:

- Increase to at least 50% the proportion of persons with high blood pressure whose blood pressure is under control. (Baseline: 11% controlled among persons aged 18 through 74 in 1976-1980; an estimated 24% for persons aged 18 and older in 1982-1984)
- Increase to at least 90% the proportion of persons with high blood pressure who are taking action to help control their blood pressure. (Baseline: 79% of persons aware of their hypertension, aged 18 and older, were taking action to control their blood pressure in 1985)
- Increase to at least 60% the proportion of adults with high blood cholesterol who are aware of their condition and are taking action to reduce their blood cholesterol to recommended levels. (Baseline: 11% of all persons aged 18 and older, and thus an estimated 30% of persons with high blood cholesterol, were aware that their blood cholesterol level was high in 1988)

**TABLE 32-8 Recommendations for Follow-Up of Initial Blood Pressure Measurements***

| STAGE/BP MEASUREMENT | RECHECK BLOOD PRESSURE |
|---|---|
| Systolic <130 mm Hg, diastolic <85 mm Hg | 2 years |
| Systolic 130-139 mm Hg, diastolic 85-89 mm Hg | 1 year |
| Stage 1 | 2 months |
| Stage 2 | 1 month |
| Stage 3 | 1 week |
| Stage 4 | Refer immediately to source of care |

From Report of the Joint National Committee on Detection, Evaluation and Treatment of High Blood Pressure, US Department of Health and Human Services, Public Health Services, NIH Publication, Bethesda, Md, 1992, National Institutes of Health.
*Age 18 or older.

### Primary Prevention

Primary prevention is aimed at reducing risk factors associated with hypertension (see Box 32-3). Health education programs include teaching about moderate sodium intake, a decreased saturated fat diet, maintenance of optimal body weight for height, cessation of cigarette smoking, moderate consumption of alcohol, and the use of effective coping strategies to minimize stress.

### Secondary Prevention

Secondary prevention is focused on identification and control of HTN in high-risk groups, such as black persons (especially men), obese persons, and blood relatives of persons known to have hypertension. A major effort should be made to contact persons who have limited access to health care because of geographic or economic constraints. Appropriate follow-up should be made depending on the initial finding (Table 32-8).

Mass blood pressure screenings are not recommended at present. These screenings typically take place where environmental conditions may contribute to inaccurate blood pressure readings. In addition, these sites tend to be frequented by the same people.

## MEDICAL MANAGEMENT

Medical management is directed at control of HTN and the prevention of associated diseases. The primary goal is to maintain a systolic blood pressure of less than 140 mm Hg and a diastolic pressure of less than 90 mm Hg. The medical decision to treat HTN is based on the degree of blood pressure elevation, the presence of risk factors, and the extent of damage to associated organ systems. In most instances both nonpharmacologic and pharmacologic measures are needed.

**TABLE 32-9 Oral Medications for Treatment of Hypertension**

| DRUG | ACTION* | SIDE EFFECTS* |
|---|---|---|
| **DIURETICS** | | |
| **Thiazide/Thiazide-Like Diuretics** | | |
| Bendroflumethiazide (Naturetin)<br>Benzthiazide (Aquatag, Exna)<br>Chlorothiazide (Diuril)<br>Chlorthalidone (Hygroton)<br>Cyclothiazide (Fluidil)<br>Hydrochlorothiazide (Esidrix, Hydrodiuril)<br>Hydroflumethiazide (Saluron)<br>Indapamide (Lozol)<br>Methyclothiazide (Enduron)<br>Metolazone (Zaroxolyn)<br>Polythiazide (Renese)<br>Quinethazone (Hydromox)<br>Trichlormethiazide (Diurese, Metahydrin) | Block sodium reabsorption in cortical portion of ascending tubule; water excreted with sodium, producing decreased blood volume.<br>NOTE: thiazides ineffective in renal failure | Increased levels of BUN, uric acid, blood glucose, calcium, cholesterol, and triglycerides<br>Decreased potassium<br>Possible postural hypotension in summer from sodium loss.<br>GI upset, dry mouth, thirst weakness, muscle aches, fatigue, tachycardia<br>Sexual dysfunction<br>May cause increased blood levels of lithium |
| **Loop Diuretics** | | |
| Bumetanide (Bumex)<br>Ethacrynic acid (Edecrin)<br>Furosemide (Lasix) | Block sodium and water reabsorption in medullary portion of ascending tubule; causes rapid volume depletion | Decreased potassium<br>Thirst, skin rash, postural hypotension, nausea, vomiting |
| **Potassium-Sparing Diuretics** | | |
| Amiloride (Midamor)<br>Spironolactone (Aldactone)<br>Triamterene (Dyrenium) | Inhibit aldosterone; sodium excreted in exchange for potassium | Drowsiness, confusion<br>Increased potassium levels<br>Diarrhea<br>Gynecomastia with Aldactone |
| **ADRENERGIC INHIBITORS** | | |
| **Beta-Adrenergic Blockers** | | |
| Acebutolol (Sectral)<br>Atenolol (Tenormin)<br>Betaxolol (Kerlone)<br>Carteolol (Cartrol)<br>Metoprolol (Lopressor)<br>Nadolol (Corgard)<br>Penbutolol (Levatol)<br>Pindolol (Visken)<br>Propranolol (Inderal)<br>Timolol (Blocadren) | Block beta-adrenergic receptors of sympathetic nervous system, decreasing heart rate and blood pressure.<br>NOTE: beta blockers should not be used in patients with asthma, COPD, CHF, and heart block; use with caution in diabetes and peripheral vascular disease | Bronchospasms<br>Bradycardia, fatigue, insomnia<br>Sexual dysfunction<br>Peripheral vascular insufficiency<br>Increased triglycerides |
| **Centrally Acting Alpha Blockers** | | |
| Clonidine (Catapres)<br>Guanabenz (Wytensin)<br>Guanfacine (Tenex)<br>Methyldopa (Aldomet) | Activate central receptors that suppress vasomotor and cardiac centers, causing a decrease in peripheral resistance. NOTE: rebound hypertension may occur with abrupt discontinuation of drug (except with Aldomet) | Drowsiness, sedation<br>Dry mouth<br>Fatigue<br>Sexual dysfunction<br>Orthostatic hypotension<br>Positive Coomb's test with Aldomet |
| **Peripheral-Acting Adrenergic Antagonists** | | |
| Guanadrel (Hylorel)<br>Guanethidine (Ismelin)<br>Rauwolfia serpentina (Raudixin)<br>Reserpine (Serpasil) | Deplete catecholamines in peripheral sympathetic postganglionic fibers<br>Block norepinephrine release from adrenergic nerve endings | Orthostatic hypotension<br>Lethargy, depression<br>Sexual dysfunction<br>Nasal congestion (with Raudixin and Serpasil) |

*COPD,* Chronic obstructive pulmonary disease; *CHF,* congestive heart failure.
*Primary actions and most common side effects are included and are related to entire drug category; consult a drug reference or drug package insert for more specific information.

*Continued*

**TABLE 32-9 Oral Medications for Treatment of Hypertension—cont'd**

| DRUG | ACTION* | SIDE EFFECTS* |
|---|---|---|
| **ADRENERGIC INHIBITORS—cont'd** | | |
| **Alpha$_1$-Adrenergic Blockers** | | |
| Doxazosin mesylate (Cardura)<br>Prazosin (Minipress)<br>Terazosin (Vasocard, Hytrin) | Block synaptic receptors that regulate vasomotor tone; reduce peripheral resistance by dilating arterioles and venules | "First dose" syncope, orthostatic hypotension, weakness, palpitations, decreased low density lipoproteins |
| **Combined Alpha- and Beta-Adrenergic Blockers** | | |
| Labetalol (Normodyne, Trandate) | Same as for beta blockers | Bronchospasm, orthostatic hypotension, peripheral vascular insufficiency |
| **VASODILATORS** | | |
| Hydralazine (Apresoline)<br>Minoxidil (Loniten) | Dilate peripheral blood vessels by directly relaxing vascular smooth muscle<br>NOTE: usually used in combination with other antihypertensives as they increase sodium and fluid retention and can cause reflex cardiac stimulation | Headache, dizziness<br>Tachycardia, palpitations, fatigue, edema |
| **ACE INHIBITORS** | | |
| Benazepril (Lotensin)<br>Captopril (Capoten), captopril/HCTZ (Capozide)<br>Enalapril (Vasotec), enalapril/HCTZ (Vaseretic)<br>Fosinopril (Monopril)<br>Lisinopril (Prinivil, Zestril), lisinopril/HCTZ (Prinzide, Zestoretic)<br>Ramipril (Altace)<br>Quinapril (Accupril) | Inhibit conversion of angiotensin to angiotensin II, thus blocking the release of aldosterone, thereby reducing sodium and water retention | "First dose" hypotension, headache, dizziness, fatigue<br>Increased potassium<br>Cough, skin reactions |
| **CALCIUM ANTAGONISTS** | | |
| Amlodipine besylate (Norvasc)<br>Diltiazem (Cardizem)<br>Diltiazem XR (Dilacor)<br>Felodipine (Plendil)<br>Isradipine (DynaCirc)<br>Nifedipine (Procardia), nifedipine XR (Adalat)<br>Nitrendipine<br>Verapamil (Calan, Isoptin)<br>Verapamil SR | Inhibit influx of calcium into muscle cells; act on vascular smooth muscles (primary arteries) to reduce spasms and promote vasodilation | Dizziness, fatigue, nausea, headache, edema |

## Diagnostic Tests

Diagnostic tests used to determine the possible cause of HTN and the extent of the disease on other organ systems, or to provide baseline information, may include the following:

1. Serum levels of sodium, potassium, calcium, BUN, and creatinine, as well as hemoglobin and hematocrit values (severity and possible causes)
2. Urinalysis and renal function studies (effect on kidneys and as baseline for drug therapy)
3. ECG, chest x-ray film, and possibly an echocardiogram to determine extent of left ventricular hypertrophy or aortic calcification
4. Intravenous pyelogram (IVP) (extent of renal damage)

## Medication

Antihypertensive medications have a protective effect against damage to the heart, kidneys, and brain, as well as renal failure, in patients with mild hypertension. Drug treatment has been shown to successfully lower a consistent diastolic blood pressure of 94 mm Hg and greater. An individual decision is made to treat patients with diastolic blood pressure readings between 90 and 94 mm Hg.

Many medications are available to treat HTN (Table 32-9). Drug selection is determined by use of a step-care approach. Therapy is started with a small dose of a less potent drug (diuretic, beta blocker). Additions of drugs, substitutions, and dosage adjustments are based on the patient's response. The step-care approach follows:

**TABLE 32-10 Medication for Treatment of Hypertensive Emergencies**

| DRUG | ACTION* | SIDE EFFECTS* |
|---|---|---|
| **VASODILATORS** | | |
| Sodium nitroprusside (Nipride, Nitropress)<br>Nitroglycerine<br>Diazoxide (Hyperstat)<br>Hydralazine (Apresoline) | Dilate peripheral blood vessels by relaxing vascular smooth muscle | Headache, dizziness<br>Tachycardia, palpitations, fatigue, nausea, edema<br>NOTE: thiocyanate toxicity may occur with sodium nitroprusside |
| **ADRENERGIC INHIBITORS** | | |
| Phentolamine (Regitine)<br>Trimethaphan camsylate (Arfonad)<br>Labetalol (Normodyne, Trandate)<br>Methyldopa (Aldomet) | Block adrenergic receptors of sympathetic nervous system, thereby dilating peripheral blood vessels and reducing peripheral vascular resistance | Tachycardia, orthostatic hypotension |

*Primary action and common side effects are included and are related to entire drug category; consult drug reference or drug package insert for more specific information.

1. Use a diuretic, beta blocker, calcium antagonist, or angiotensin converting enzyme (ACE) inhibitor.
2. If ineffective after 1 to 3 months, increase dosage of drug, add a second drug of a different class, or substitute another drug.
3. Add a third drug of a different class or substitute a second drug.
4. Add a fourth drug of a different class or substitute a third drug; evaluate further and refer to a specialist if ineffective.

After 1 year of satisfactory blood pressure control, a stepdown approach may be effective in patients also adhering to nonpharmacologic measures.

### Treatment

Life-style modifications to aid in lowering blood pressure without use of drugs include the following:

1. Weight control
2. Diet: restriction of sodium and saturated fats
3. Cessation of cigarette smoking
4. Restriction of alcoholic beverages
5. Activity: maintenance of a regular aerobic exercise program
6. Referral/consultation: smoking cessation, biofeedback

## COMPLICATIONS

With prolonged hypertension the elastic tissue in the arterioles is replaced by fibrous collagen tissue. The thickened arteriole wall becomes less distensible, creating even greater resistance to blood flow. This process can lead to decreased tissue perfusion, especially in the target organs: heart, kidneys, and brain.

In the heart, decreased coronary perfusion may cause angina or myocardial infarction. As the heart is forced to work against a consistently elevated aortic pressure, left ventricular hypertrophy and congestive heart failure may result.

## HYPERTENSIVE CRISIS

**Hypertensive crisis** refers to a situation that requires immediate blood pressure lowering. Although such cases are relatively uncommon, prompt recognition and management are essential to prevent organ dysfunction. Clinical conditions that may precipitate a hypertensive crisis include hypertensive encephalopathy, intracranial hemorrhage, left ventricular heart failure, dissecting aortic aneurysm, severe hypertension of pregnancy, head trauma, extensive burns, unstable angina, or acute myocardial infarction. It also may occur in patients with poor hypertension control and in those who abruptly discontinue their medications. Parenteral drug administration through IV and IM routes is used to quickly lower markedly elevated blood pressure. Intravenous medications are administered by drip and titrated according to the patient's response. Common drugs used in the treatment of hypertensive emergencies are listed in Table 32-10.

## NURSING MANAGEMENT

### ♦ ASSESSMENT

### Subjective Data

Subjective data to be collected to assess the patient with HTN include the following:

1. Presence of early morning headache, blurred vision, confusion, exertion dyspnea
2. Presence of risk factors
3. Course and compliance with therapy for previously diagnosed HTN
4. Current knowledge of HTN: definition, meaning of systolic and diastolic readings, and effects of high blood pressure on heart, kidneys, and brain

## Objective Data

Objective data to be collected to assess the patient with HTN include the following:

1. Two or more blood pressure measurements taken in both arms with the patient in supine and sitting positions
2. Height and weight
3. Examination of neck and abdomen for bruits
4. Auscultation of heart for abnormal heart sounds: $S_3$, $S_4$, murmurs—evidence of left ventricular hypertrophy
5. Palpation of peripheral pulses: rate, amplitude, quality, bilateral symmetry
6. Funduscopic eye examination by trained clinician for presence of arteriolar narrowing or hemorrhage

## ♦ NURSING DIAGNOSES

Nursing diagnoses are determined from analysis of patient data. Nursing diagnoses for the patient with HTN may include but are not limited to the following:

| Diagnostic Title | Possible Etiologic Factors |
|---|---|
| Knowledge deficit: HTN risk factors, medications | Lack of exposure/recall, misinterpretation, unfamiliarity with information sources |
| Noncompliance drug regimen, ongoing care | Patient value system, treatment side effects |
| Sexual dysfunction | Lack of knowledge of effects of medication |

## ♦ EXPECTED PATIENT OUTCOMES

Expected patient outcomes for the patient with HTN may include but are not limited to the following:

1. Defines HTN.
2. Explains meaning of systolic and diastolic blood pressure.
3. Explains effects of HTN on heart, kidneys, and brain.
4. Demonstrates correct procedures for self-management and recording of blood pressure.
5. Maintains blood pressure within desirable range.
6. Describes therapeutic regimen.
7. Describes plan to participate in other measures to promote desirable blood pressure (dietary changes, exercises, stress reduction).
8. Explains the effects of prescribed antihypertensives on sexual function (as appropriate).
9. Takes antihypertensive medications as prescribed.

## ♦ INTERVENTIONS

Nursing interventions for the person with HTN are focused primarily on patient teaching and counseling. Teaching is directed toward increasing knowledge about HTN, risk factors, associated disases, and the treatment regimen. Other efforts are intended to assist the person in making behavioral changes to further reduce, control, or maintain blood pressure within desirable range.

### Teaching About Hypertension

The patient needs to understand the concepts of blood pressure and hypertension. Use simple terms to define systolic and diastolic blood pressure. Explain the effects of HTN on the heart, kidneys, and brain. Teach self-monitoring of blood pressure using a reliable instrument. Discourage use of coin-operated machines inasmuch as they are often inaccurate. Encourage the patient to keep a written record of blood pressures, including date and pertinent information if elevated or lowered.

### Teaching About Risk Factors

Explain that excess salt intake contributes to fluid retention; increased fluid increases blood pressure. Teaching should include the following:

1. Avoid adding salt to foods during preparation and at the table and substitute herbs.
2. Avoid highly salted foods, such as potato chips, pretzels, nuts, canned soups, and packaged luncheon meats.
3. Minimize eating in fast food restaurants.
4. Reduce intake of saturated fats to maintain body weight and control atherosclerotic changes.
5. Use moderation in alcohol consumption; alcohol may potentiate certain antihypertensive medications in addition to raising blood pressure.

Other factors to discuss include cessation of smoking, engaging in exercise, and reducing stress:

1. Explain the effects of *nicotine* on blood vessels.
2. Suggest use of behavior modification, group therapy, or hypnosis as means of stopping smoking.
3. Discuss need to participate in a regular *aerobic exercise program* three times a week, consisting of 20 to 45 minutes of activity with warm-up and cool-down procedures.
4. Identify sources of *stress.*
5. Demonstrate relaxation techniques such as deep breathing, progressive muscle relaxation, and imagery that can help lower blood pressure.

### Teaching About Medication

Patients who take prescribed medications to control blood pressure should know the name and type of drug, general action, dosage, and administration schedule. Provide the patient with written information, if possible. Common side effects include potassium depletion and orthostatic hypotension. *Potassium depletion,* seen mostly with use of diuretics, can be avoided by eating foods high in potassium or taking a multivitamin that contains potassium or a potassium supplement. *Orthostatic hypotention* is a common side effect of antihypertensive therapy. It is often worse in the mornings (when blood pressure is normally lower), after alcohol ingestion (vasodilator), and with immobility following exercise. Orthostatic hypotension may be avoided by the following measures:

1. Rise slowly from a lying or sitting position to standing.

2. Sit down immediately if feeling faint; lower head.
3. Avoid long periods of standing (blood pools in legs, temporarily causing hypovolemia).
4. Avoid very hot showers or baths (cause vasodilation, temporarily decreasing blood pressure).
5. Take medication at bedtime if drug can cause "first dose" hypotension or syncope. Discuss use of once-a-day medication if possible.
6. Suggest participation in an exercise program; join with a friend.
7. Include family and significant others in the teaching process to provide support and promote adherence to therapeutic regimen.
8. Explain reason for regular health care follow-up inasmuch as HTN is a chronic condition.
9. Contact patients who consistently cancel follow-up appointments.

### Preventing Noncompliance

Noncompliance with the therapeutic regimen is a major reason for inadequate HTN control. One cause of noncompliance is the absence of symptoms until advanced stages; hence the person may not perceive a need to adhere to therapy. A second factor is the experience of unpleasant medication side effects and hesitancy to seek professional follow-up. If several medications are prescribed, it is sometimes difficult to remember to take the medications correctly.

Measures to help increase compliance with therapy include the following:

1. Be sure patient understands that absence of symptoms does not indicate control of blood pressure; remind patient that symptoms do not occur until advanced stages of the disease.
2. Advise patient against abrupt withdrawal of medication; rebound hypertension can occur.
3. Encourage patient to discuss unpleasant side effects of medication and other nonpharmacologic therapies with a health care professional.
4. If remembering to take the medications is a problem, discuss alternate ways to remember, such as taking medications with meals or by placing medications in separate containers labeled with time of day.

### Maintaining Sexual Function

Sexual dysfunction is a potential side effect of adrenergic inhibitors. In general, beta-adrenergic blockers and alpha blockers decrease ejaculation ability. Beta blockers also depress libido. Specific drugs such as clonidine interfere with erection. The nurse must discuss these adverse effects that may contribute to noncompliance. Define terms of sexual dysfunction such as libido, erection, and ejaculation in simple terms. Encourage patient to report promptly any problems to a health care professional. Include patient's sexual partner in the teaching if possible. Suggest that patients consult with physician if alternate medication is needed.

## ♦ EVALUATION

To evaluate the effectiveness of nursing interventions, compare patient behaviors with those stated in the expected patient outcomes. Successful achievement of patient outcomes for the person with HTN is indicated by the following:

1. Correctly defines HTN.
2. Correctly explains the meaning of systolic and diastolic blood pressure.
3. Correctly explains the effects of HTN on heart, kidneys, and brain.
4. Correctly demonstrates procedure for self-management and recording of blood pressure.
5. Maintains blood pressure within desirable range.
6. Correctly describes therapeutic regimen.
7. Participates in other measures to promote desirable blood pressure (dietary changes, exercise, stress reduction).
8. Correctly explains the effects of prescribed antihypertensives on sexual function (as appropriate).
9. Takes antihypertensive medications as prescribed.

## QUESTIONS TO CONSIDER

- What are the similarities and differences in patient teaching for persons with arterial and venous disorders?
- How would you position the leg of a person with an arterial problem? Does this positioning differ from that for a venous problem? What is the physiologic basis for the positioning?
- How would your nursing care be altered for the patient undergoing a below-knee amputation if the patient were 40 years old versus age 75?
- What approaches might you use to assist an elderly patient with hypertension who is noncompliant in taking prescribed medications?
- What important preventive nursing measures should be implemented for the patient receiving thrombolytic therapy?

## CRITICAL THINKING ACTIVITIES

- Maria, 62, is recovering from a recent myocardial infarction. She is in atrial fibrillation. She suddenly complains of a severe pain in her left leg. The nurse notes that pulses are absent and the leg is cool to touch. Upon further questioning, Maria states that her leg feels somewhat numb. Hypothesize about the possible problem and cause.
- How would you differentiate between a venous and arterial disorder and lymphedema?

## CHAPTER SUMMARY

### ARTERIAL DISORDERS

- Risk factors associated with the development of vascular problems include cigarette smoking, hypertension, hyperlipidemia, obesity, physical inactivity, emotional stress, diabetes mellitus, and a family history of atherosclerosis.
- Primary prevention through health education about risk factors is an important means to reduce the incidence of vascular disorders.
- Arterial disorders develop from any disturbance in the structure of the arteries, causing diminished blood flow and decreased oxygen and nutrients to reach the tissues.
- Clinical manifestations of arterial disorders are caused not by the degree of obstruction but rather by the extent to which the affected tissues are deprived of circulation.
- Medical therapy for patients with arterial occlusive disease incudes smoking cessation, a diet low in saturated fats, weight reduction, regular exercise, and control of associated diseases (diabetes, HTN).
- Intermittent claudication is a cramplike muscle pain that develops during exercise and ceases 1 to 2 minutes after stopping the exercise. It usually is unilateral, affects primarily the calf muscles, and indicates arterial occlusive disease.
- Peripheral pulses may not be felt (0), or they may be diminished (1+) or abnormally strong (4+) in patients with arterial disorders.
- Anticoagulants such as heparin and warfarin sodium (Coumadin) prolong clotting time, prevent extension of an existing clot, and inhibit further clot formation. Anticoagulants do not dissolve an existing clot.
- A teaching plan for a patient receiving Coumadin must include the prevention of bleeding.
- Protamin sulfate is a heparin antagonist, and vitamin K counteracts the effects of Coumadin.
- Thrombolytics such as streptokinase and urokinase dissolve existing thrombi.
- Nursing interventions for the patient undergoing arterial bypass surgery include frequent assessment of peripheral pulses and the graft site, avoidance of flexion in the area of the graft, and position changes to promote circulation.
- Positioning a patient with an arterial disorder may include placement of the extremity flat in bed or in a slightly dependent (15-degree) position to promote circulation. Elevation is contraindicated in arterial disorders.
- An important nursing intervention for the patient after an amputation is to avoid flexion of the hip or knee, thus preventing contractures.
- A teaching plan for a patient with arterial problems includes measures to prevent infection and injury, maintain skin integrity, and increase peripheral tissue perfusion, as well as methods to alter risk factors.
- An aneurysm is a local or diffuse dilation of an artery. Depending on location and size of the aneurysm, surgical resection may be necessary. A synthetic graft is used to replace the diseased segment.

### VENOUS DISORDERS

- Thrombophlebitis can affect the superficial or deep veins. Thrombophlebitis in a deep vein can lead to a pulmonary embolus.
- Noncal+, deep vein thrombosis is treated by bed rest with periodic elevation of the affected extremity above the heart level to prevent venous stasis and reduce edema.
- Patients with chronic venous disorders such as varicose veins should be taught measures to increase peripheral perfusion. These include avoiding constrictive clothing, never crossing legs at the knee, and avoiding long periods of sitting or standing. Elevating legs when sitting and wearing compression support stockings are important.

### ARTERIAL/VENOUS DISORDERS

- An arteriovenous fistula is an abnormal direct connection between an artery and a vein that can lead to arterial or venous insufficiency.
- Leg ulcers can develop secondary to arterial or venous disorders. The primary treatment goal is to promote wound healing and prevent infection.
- Wet-to-dry dressings and débriding chemicals remove necrotic tissue from leg ulcers. A special protective boot (Unna paste boot) may be applied over ulcers for ambulatory patients. Arterial bypass surgery endovascular techniques, or an amputation may be necessary for nonhealing chronic ulcers.

### LYMPHEDEMA

- Lymphedema results from interference with the drainage of interstitial fluid from the tissues through the lymph system; the affected extremity becomes edematous.
- Teaching the patient with lymphedema includes elevating the affected extremity, wearing compression support stockings, taking prescribed diuretics as ordered, and avoiding an excess intake of high-sodium foods.

### HYPERTENSION

- Hypertension is defined as a consistent systolic pressure >140 mm Hg and/or a consistent diastolic pressure >90 mm Hg. Hypertension is a major cause of coronary artery disease, cardiac failure, strokes, and renal failure.
- Drugs to control hypertension include diuretics (especially thiazides), peripheral and central acting adrenergics, beta blockers, vasodilators, ACE inhibitors,

and calcium antagonists. Medications are added in steps, as necessary, to control the blood pressure within desirable range.

- Persons with hypertension should monitor their own blood pressure, take prescribed medications, exercise, avoid salty foods, stop smoking, and continue with follow-up care.

## REFERENCES


1. Bergan JJ, Yao JST: *Venous disorders,* Philadelphia, 1991, WB Saunders.
2. Lovell MB, Harris KA: Abdominal aortic aneurysms, *J Vasc Nurs* 9:2-6, 1991.
3. Moore WS: *Vascular surgery: a comprehensive review,* ed 3, Philadelphia, 1991, WB Saunders.
4. Payne JS: Alternative for revascularization: peripheral atherectomy devices, *J Vasc Nurs* 10(3):8-13, 1992.
5. Report of the Joint National Committee on Detection, Evaluation and Treatment of High Blood Pressure, US Department of Health and Human Services, Public Health Services, Bethesda, Md, 1992, National Institutes of Health.
6. Young JR, Graor RA, Olin JW, Bartholomew JR: Peripheral vascular diseases, St. Louis, 1991, Mosby.

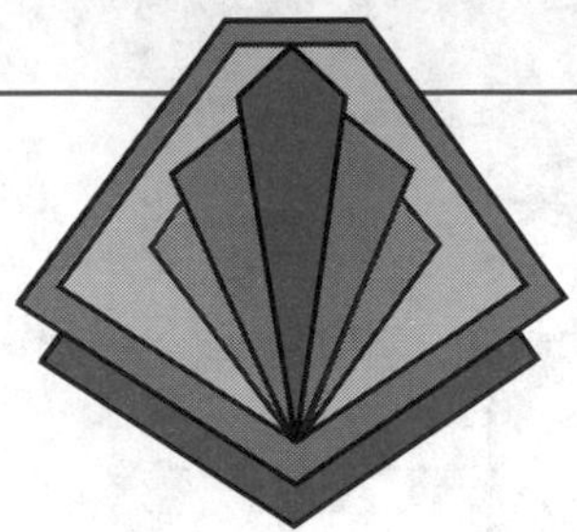

CHAPTER 33

# Assessment of the Hematologic System

***Marilyn S. Lottman***
***Kathryn Sabo Thompson***

## CHAPTER OBJECTIVES

***After studying this chapter, the learner should be able to do the following:***

1 Assess persons with suspected hematologic disorders.
2 Analyze components of the hematopoietic system and explain the scheme of stem cell differentiation.
3 Collect and assess subjective and objective data gathered during a hematologic assessment of patients with suspected hematologic disorders.
4 Apply diagnostic studies results of the hemoglobin and hematocrit levels, red blood cell indexes, and peripheral smear results to the hematologic system assessment.
5 Review bone marrow examination results to further patients' understanding of a hematologic diagnosis.

## KEY TERMS

anisocytosis
basophils
bone marrow
bone marrow aspiration
bone marrow biopsy
eosinophils
erythrocytes
erythropoiesis
erythropoietin
granular leukocytes
hematopoiesis
Kupffer's cells
leukocytes
lymphocytes
macrocytic
macrophages
mean corpuscular hemoglobin (MCH)
mean corpuscular hemoglobin concentration (MCHC)
mean corpuscular volume (MCV)
microcytic
monocytes
neutrophils
nongranular leukocytes
normochromic
normocytic
peripheral blood smear
phagocytosis
platelets
poikilocytosis
polymorphonuclear leukocytes (PMN)
reticuloendothelial system (RES)
stem cell
thrombocytes

## ANATOMY AND PHYSIOLOGY

Diseases associated with the reticuloendothelial system (RES) are diverse in their underlying pathologic manifestations, disease course, and response to treatment. Most often the accompanying symptoms result from interference with the normal development and function of the blood components: **erythrocytes** (red blood cells [RBCs]), **platelets,** (thrombocytes), **leukocytes** (white blood cells [WBCs]), and altered **hematopoiesis** (blood cell production). Normally, homeostasis is maintained through a balance between the rate of production of normal blood cells and the rate of destruction. Disorders of the blood occur when this balance is lost. Disturbances in the coagulation mechanism also result in blood disorders.

### COMPONENTS OF THE HEMATOPOIETIC SYSTEM

The hematopoietic system includes blood and its components and bone marrow, as well as the RES, which is located throughout the body. Its function is phagocytizing foreign materials and lysing (breaking down) RBCs.

#### Blood

Blood is an aqueous solution (plasma) that contains water, proteins, electrolytes, and inorganic and organic

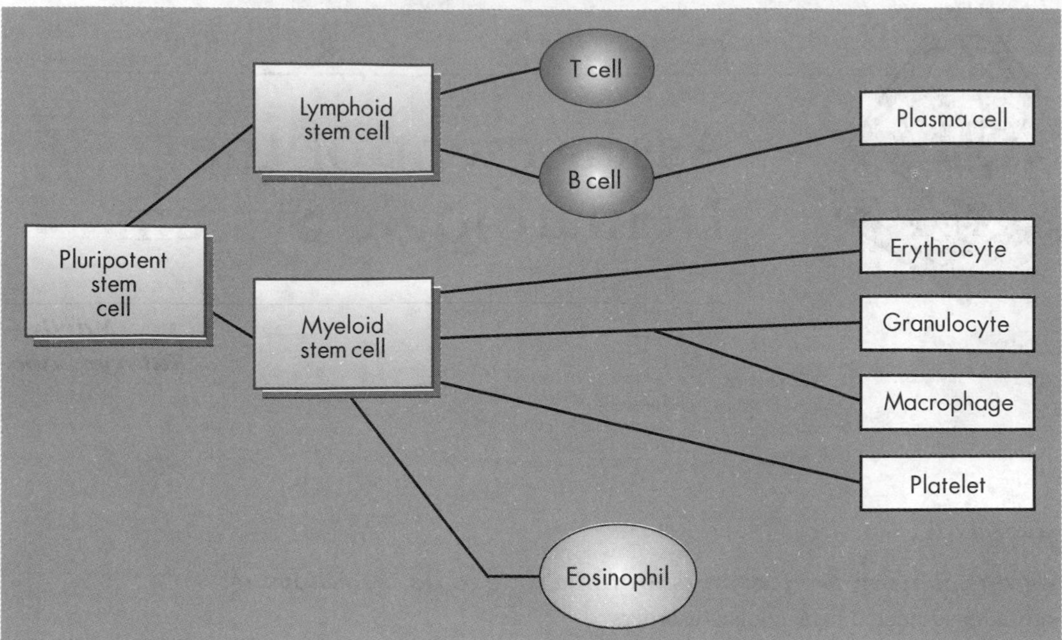


**FIGURE 33-1** Scheme of stem cell differentiation showing typical progenitor cell for erythrocytes, granulocytes, and platelets.

constituents. Cells make up 7% to 9% of the blood.

The cell components of blood include erythrocytes, leukocytes, and thrombocytes or platelets. All normal cells are derived from a single **stem cell** that can divide into lymphoid and blood stem cells. These stem cells can in turn become progenitor cells that divide along a specific single pathway (Figure 33-1). This process is known as *hematopoiesis* and takes place in the *bone marrow* of the skull, vertebrae, pelvis, sternum, ribs, and proximal epiphysis of long bones. Production may occur in all the long bones during periods of increased demand, such as with hemorrhage or during cell destruction (hemolysis).

### Red blood cells (erythrocytes)

An RBC is a nonnucleated biconcave disk that is soft and pliable. These characteristics enable the RBC to change its shape during passage through the microcirculation. The RBCs major component is hemoglobin (Hgb), a protein that transports oxygen and carbon dioxide and maintains normal pH through a series of intracellular buffers (see Chapter 21). The Hgb molecule contains globin (two pairs of polypeptide chains) and four heme groups, each one containing an atom of ferrous iron. Thus each Hgb molecule can unite with four oxygen molecules to form oxyhemoglobin (a reversible reaction). Carbon dioxide is carried by the globin portion of the Hgb molecule.

Maturation of RBCs in the bone marrow requires adequate amounts and use of vitamin $B_{12}$, folic acid, proteins, enzymes, and minerals (iron, copper). **Erythropoiesis** (RBC formation) can be greatly stimulated by the secretion of a hormone **erythropoietin** from the kidneys; this occurs when RBCs decrease in number below normal (such as with severe blood loss) or when demand for oxygen increases (tissue hypoxia). RBCs circulate for 120 days and are then destroyed by the macrophages of the RES. Most of the iron is removed from the heme and can be used to form new heme groups. Small amounts of iron lost daily in urine and feces and through menstrual flow must be replaced by iron ingestion (see Chapter 34). The remainder of the heme is broken down to form bilirubin and is secreted into the bile. Energy in the form of adenosine triphosphate (ATP) is required to maintain cell membrane integrity and the relatively low sodium and high potassium content of the RBC.

### White blood cells (leukocytes)

WBCs may be classified into two groups as follows: **granular leukocytes** (also called granulocytes or **polymorphonuclear leukocytes [PMN]**), consisting of neutrophils, eosinophils, and basophils; and **nongranular leukocytes,** consisting of monocytes and lymphocytes. The granulocytes contain enzymes that kill and digest bacteria with degranulation of the bacteria. Once activated, circulating WBCs remain in circulation for an average of 6 to 8 hours. The specific cascade of WBC formation is in response to several different stimulants.

**Neutrophils** are present in the circulation or along the capillary walls (the margination pool). They move into the tissues and mucous membranes and serve as the body's primary defense against bacterial infection through the process of phagocytosis (see Chapter 13). **Eosinophils** are involved in allergic responses and destruction of parasitic worms. The response of **basophils** is similar to that of mast cells in immunologic reactions.

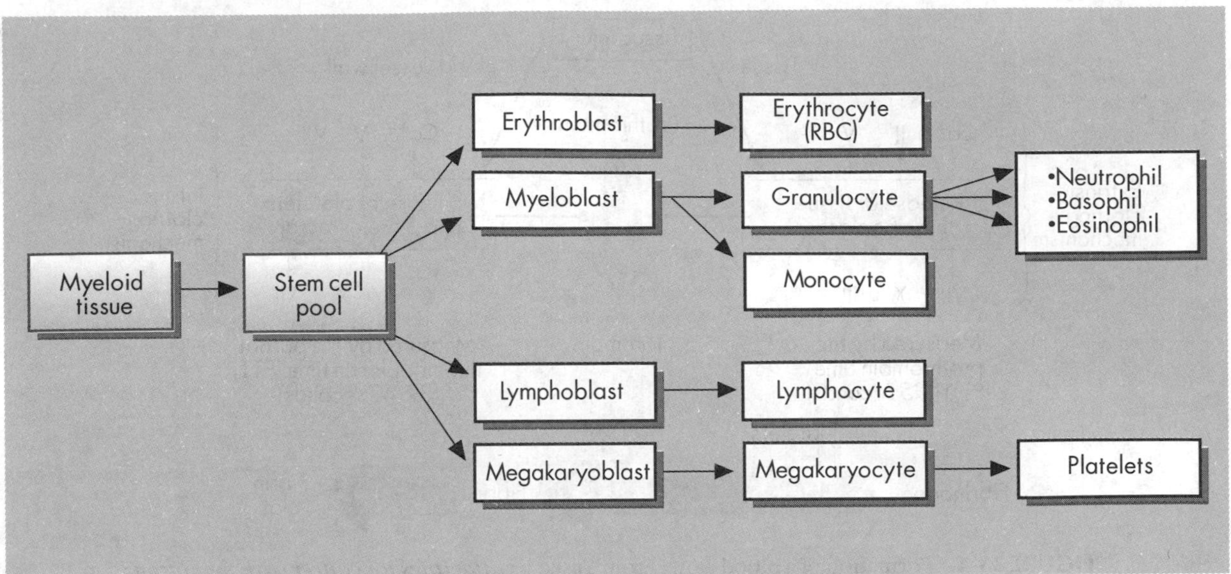


**FIGURE 33-2** Formation of blood cells from myeloid tissue. (From Yasko J: *Guidelines for cancer care: symptom management,* Reston, Va, 1983, Reston Publishing.)

**Monocytes** are larger than neutrophils and have one large folded or kidney-shaped nucleus. They leave the circulation and become tissue **macrophages,** which also have phagocytic action, removing dead and injured cells, cell fragments, and microorganisms.

**Lymphocytes** are mononuclear with a round or an oval nucleus. They originate primarily in lymphoid tissue (lymph nodes) but also in the bone marrow. There are two types of lymphocytes, the long-lived circulating T lymphocytes (from the thymus) and short-lived noncirculating B lymphocytes. T lymphocytes initiate the cellular immune response, whereas B lymphocytes (immunoglobulins) initiate the humoral immune response (see Chapter 13).

### Platelets

Platelets **(thrombocytes)** are not cells but granular, disk-shaped, nonnucleated cell fragments. Approximately two thirds of all platelets are within the circulatory system, and the remainder are present in the spleen as a reserve pool. Platelet life span is approximately 6 to 10 days. Platelets also derive from the stem cells and are essential to hemostasis and coagulation (Figure 33-2). Hemostasis results from the adhesion and aggregation capabilities of platelets to plug small breaks in blood vessels. Platelets also release thromboplastin (factor III), which, in the presence of calcium ions, converts prothrombin into thrombin in the first step of the coagulation mechanism (Figure 33-3). In the second step of the coagulation mechanism, thrombin promotes the conversion of fibrinogen (a soluble plasma protein) into fibrin (an insoluble strand) (Figure 33-4). Step one requires coagulation factors IV, V, VIII, IX, X, XI, and XII, whereas step two requires factors IV and XIII (Box 33-1). (For further discussion on hemostasis, see Chapter 34.)

STEP 1
PROTHROMBIN — Thromboplastin / Calcium ions and other factors → THROMBIN

STEP 2
FIBRINOGEN — Thrombin / Calcium ions and factor XIII → FIBRIN

**FIGURE 33-3** Basic steps in the coagulation process.

**BOX 33-1 Coagulation Factors**

| | |
|---|---|
| Factor I | Fibrinogen |
| Factor II | Prothrombin |
| Factor III | Thromboplastin, tissue thromboplastin |
| Factor IV | Calcium |
| Factor V | Proaccelerin, labile factor |
| Factor VII | Serum prothrombin conversion accelerator (SPCA) |
| Factor VIII | Antihemophilic globulin (AHG)<br>Antihemophilic factor (AHF) |
| Factor IX | Plasma thromboplastin component (PTC), Christmas factor |
| Factor X | Stuart-Prower factor |
| Factor XI | Plasma thromboplastin antecedent (PTA) |
| Factor XII | Hageman factor, contact factor |
| Factor XIII | Fibrin-stabilizing factor, fibrinase |

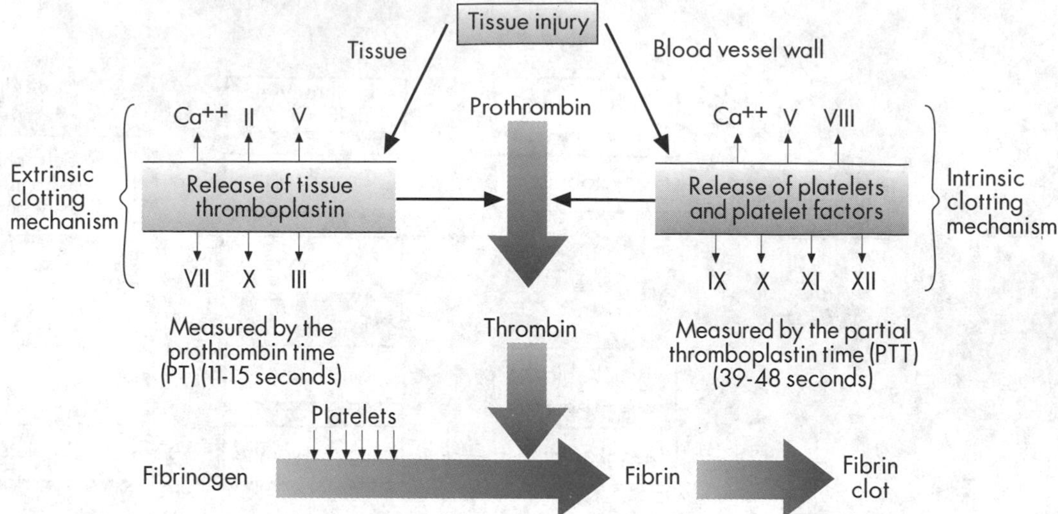


**FIGURE 33-4** Formation of a blood clot. (From Yasko J: *Guidelines for cancer care: symptom management,* Reston, Va, 1983, Reston Publishing.)

### Reticuloendothelial System

The **reticuloendothelial system (RES),** also called the *mononuclear phagocyte system* or *macrophage system,* includes circulating monocytes and their precursor cells in the bone marrow. It also includes more or less fixed mononuclear phagocytic cells (also called *macrophages*) found in blood channels in the spleen and liver **(Kupffer's cells),** in the lymphatic system, in serosal cavities of the body, in the lungs, in general connective tissue, and in the bone marrow (see Chapter 13).

The RES is responsible for **phagocytosis,** the process of engulfing and removing "wasted" white blood cells. In addition to phagocytosis, the RES processes the Hgb of RBCs that have reached the end of their life span, splitting Hgb into an iron-containing substance and bilirubin.

## PHYSIOLOGIC CHANGES WITH AGING

The effect of aging on hematopoiesis is still being studied, with findings that are sometimes ambiguous or of questionable clinical significance. Evidence from studies of mouse marrow show that stem cells have a limited capacity to proliferate. Findings from animal studies suggest that changes related to aging do not have clinical significance.[1] The cellularity of human marrow decreases with age, but this may be the result of an increase in fat from osteoporosis rather than a decrease in hematopoietic cells.

In human beings the total number of leukocytes and differential counts shows no variation through middle age and no gross changes in old age. In general the leukocyte count does not rise as high in response to infection, and studies suggest that elderly persons have a diminished marrow granulocyte reserve.

The Hgb level decreases after middle age, although the decrease in women seems to be relatively less than that in men. Unexplained anemia in elders has been noted, but iron absorption is not impaired; however, use of orally administered iron is reduced because of the side effect of constipation. This anemia does not appear to be related solely to age.[1] Serum iron and iron-binding capacity decrease in elders, and low serum vitamin $B_{12}$ and folic acid levels occur in a significant number of elderly persons—but without anemia.

No age-related changes in platelets have been reported. Some of the plasma coagulation factors have been reported to increase with age (factors I, V, VII, and IX). Partial thromboplastin time (PTT) may be shortened.[1] RBC sedimentation rate increases significantly, but this rate is of limited value in detecting disease in elders. (See box, p. 935, for special considerations for elderly persons with hematologic problems.)

# SUBJECTIVE DATA

A variety of disorders affect the hematopoietic system. In addition to primary hematologic disorders, secondary effects from disease of another body system may manifest in abnormal hematologic findings. For example, the anemia associated with renal insufficiency is the consequence of disease outside the hematopoietic system.

The cause of any hematologic abnormality must be assiduously pursued. The importance of accurate diagnosis, combined with the very diverse and frequently nonspecific signs and symptoms, makes it likely that the person will become involved in an arduous diagnostic

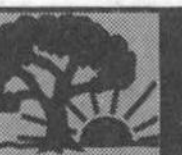

## GERONTOLOGIC PATIENT CONSIDERATIONS

### ASSESSMENT

Assess adequacy of iron and folic acid intake.
Assess presence and extent of fatigue and ability to carry out ADL.

### INTERVENTION

Help patient with nutritional deficiency anemia plan diet that includes food rich in iron and folic acid, as appropriate.
Help patient plan for rest periods when fatigue is present.
Teach patient and significant others:
- Importance of prescribed replacement therapy and ways to facilitate compliance.
- Need to report signs of increasing fatigue to physician.
- Measures to prevent infection with leukemia. Elderly persons have the added risk factor of decreased immune response and are highly susceptible to pneumonia.

### COMMON DISORDERS IN ELDERS

Nutritional deficiency anemia
Leukemia (acute nonlymphocytic leukemia [ANLL], chronic lymphocytic leukemia [CLL])
Lymphoma

## RESEARCH

Haberman M et al: Quality of life of adult long-term survivors of bone marrow transplantation: a qualitative analysis of narrative data, *Oncol Nurs Forum* 20:1545-1553, 1993.

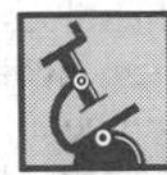

The purpose of this study was to gather information on the quality of life after bone marrow transplantation (BMT). The method consisted of content analysis of an eight-item, open-ended questionnaire covering topics of post-BMT demands, coping strategies with BMT, current health problems, quality of life, and concerns for the future. Most long-term survivors perceived themselves as cured and leading meaningful lives despite lingering side effects. Nursing implications include providing timely information on known long-range side effects of BMT, providing hope for a meaningful life after BMT, and promoting self-care activities.

process. At the time of initial contact the patient already is experiencing the stress of sudden onset of illness or the gnawing fear or suspicion that all is not well. The explanations offered and the time allowed for verbalization and questions are means of providing a positive foundation for the long-term care that may follow. This is vital if future therapy involves bone marrow transplantation (BMT). See Research box, above, right.

A thorough history includes detailed information about the person's symptoms and a thorough review of systems. In the history taking of a person with suspected hematologic disease, other key points to include are family history, drug history, exposure to chemicals, and general nonspecific complaints offered by the patient.

## FAMILY HISTORY

The existence of inherited hematologic disorders, such as sickle cell disease and malignant tumors, requires a detailed family history. Questions regarding disease or presence of symptoms among relatives should include reference to parents and siblings. More specific disorders, such as hemophilia, may involve questions to grandfathers, uncles, and nephews. For other disorders, female relatives need to be considered. Questions should explore instances of severe or prolonged bleeding after minor trauma, dental extractions, or surgery. The occurrence of jaundice or anemia in relatives also should be ascertained.

## DRUGS AND CHEMICALS

Drugs may induce or potentiate hematologic disease (Box 33-2). Most notable are the hematologic effects of the cytotoxic drugs used in cancer chemotherapy and the neutropenia associated with chloramphenicol. A thorough history of drugs ingested by a person is a crucial part of assessment. Many persons regularly ingest "something to help me sleep," "something to calm me down," or "just aspirin." Analgesics, tranquilizers, laxatives, and sedatives often are overlooked by persons when asked about drugs. Specific, often rephrased questioning is necessary to obtain a complete drug history.

Certain chemicals may exert a potentially harmful effect on the hematopoietic system. To obtain a history of exposure to chemicals, an occupational history is useful.

## FEVER

Fever is a common manifestation of many of the hematologic disorders and is an important question to be asked during the history. Fever typically occurs in lymphoma, primarily Hodgkin's disease and leukemia. Severe chills may accompany hemolytic disorders. Night sweats frequently are associated with both lymphoma and leukemia.

## FATIGUE AND MALAISE

Fatigue and malaise are difficult symptoms to evaluate because they frequently accompany many physical and emotional disorders. Information regarding the occurrence of these symptoms should be included in the history. When combined with physical and laboratory findings, they are of some diagnostic value. In addition, the person's subjective description of such symptoms lends some insight into perception of the illness, the extent to which the illness is affecting daily living, and the ability to adapt.

**BOX 33-2 Some Drugs Implicated in Hematopoietic Suppression***

Acetophenetidin (1, 3)
Acetylsalicylic acid (aspirin) (1, 2, 3)
Acetyl sulfisoxazole (3)
Aminosalicylic acid (3, 4)
Ammonium thioglycolate (3)
Amodiaquin HCl (3)
Arsenicals (1, 2, 3, 4)
Arsphenamine (1, 2)
Atabrine (1, 2)
γ-Benzene hexachloride (1, 3)
Benzene (1, 2, 3, 4)
Bishydroxycoumarin (3, 4)
Carbamide (2)
Carbon tetrachloride (1)
Carbutamide (Orabetic) (2)
Chloramphenicol (1, 2, 3, 4)
Chlordane (1)
Chlorophenothane (DDT) (1, 2)
Chlorothiazide (3)
Chlorpheniramine maleate (3)
Chlorpromazine (Thorazine) (3)
Chlorpropamide (2)
Chlortetracyline (1, 3)
Cinophen (3)
Coldricine (2, 3)
Cycloheximide (3)
Dextromethorphan HBr (2)
Diethylstilbestrol (2)
Diphenylhydantoin (Dilantin) (4)
Dipyrrone (3)
Ethinamate (2)
Fumagillin (3)
Hair lacquer (3)
Imipramine HCl (3)
Iproniazid (1)
Isoniazid (1, 3, 4)
Lead (1)
Lithium carbonate (1)
Mephenytoin (Mesantoin) (1, 2)
Meprobamate (1, 2, 3)
Methaminodiazepoxide (Librium) (3)
Methapyrilene HCl (4)
Methylpromazine (3)
Mezapine (2)
β-Naphthoxyacetic acid (2)
Nitrofurantoin (4)
Novobiocin (4)
Nystatin (2)
Oxyphenabutazone (2)
Para-aminosalicylic acid (3, 4)
Penicillin (1, 2, 3, 4)
Phenobarbital (1, 2, 3, 4)
Phenylbutazone (Butazolidin) (1, 2, 3)
Pipamazine (1)
Primidone (1)
Prochlorperazine (Compazine) (2, 3)
Pyrimethamine (Daraprim) (1, 2, 3)
Quinidine (2)
Quinine (2, 3)
Reserpine (2)
Stibophen (2)
Streptomycin (1, 2, 3)
Sulfamethoxypyridazine (Kynex) (2, 3, 4)
Tetracycline (3)
Thenalidine tartrate (3)
Thioridazine HCl (3)
Tolazoline HCl (1, 2)
Tolbutamide (1, 2, 3)
Tolbutamide (Orinase) (2)
Trifluoperazine (1, 3)
Trifluoperazine (Stelazine) (3)
Trimethadione (Tridione) (1, 2)

From Miale J: *Laboratory medicine: hematology,* ed 6, St Louis, 1982, Mosby.
*More than 500 are listed in the latest report of the American Medical Association subcommittee on blood dyscrasias. The drugs listed in this table are those that have produced dyscrasias when given alone. *1,* Pancytopenia; *2,* thrombocytopenia; *3,* leukopenia; *4,* anemia.

# OBJECTIVE DATA

A thorough physical examination is performed in the assessment of a person with a hematologic disorder. It is useful to recognize target organs and alterations that may reflect hematologic disease.

## SKIN

Skin manifestations of hematologic disease are often readily visible. *Petechiae, ecchymoses,* and *purpura* are associated with decreased platelets (thrombocytopenia) and other bleeding disorders. *Jaundice,* when observed, may be associated with pernicious anemia, hemolytic disease, or primary liver dysfunction. *Pallor* is typically associated by the layperson with disorders of the blood. Pallor as a criterion for assessment may be deceptive because many healthy persons have pale complexions, whereas some severely anemic patients may have ruddy complexions.

*Changes in skin texture* also may be observed. Except in severe cases, the patient most likely will not observe such changes. With iron deficiency anemia the patient may notice dry skin, dry hair, and brittle nails. Severe itching, especially on the palms, often is associated with Hodgkin's disease and also may occur with polycythemia vera, especially after bathing. In persons with leukemia and lymphoma, infiltrative lesions of the skin may be observed on any portion of the body.

## HEAD AND NECK

The sclerae of the eyes are examined for jaundice and the conjunctivae for pallor. Retinal hemorrhages may occur in persons with severe anemia and thrombocytopenia. Questions also may elicit a history of visual disturbances.

The oral mucosa is observed for pallor, bleeding tendency, and ulceration. The tongue may be very smooth in association with both pernicious anemia and nutritional deficiencies.

The neck is observed primarily for evaluation of lymph nodes. Nodes may be so large as to be visible. A "lump" on the neck often is the reason for seeking medical attention. Enlarged tumors may obstruct breathing or elicit coughing or difficulty in swallowing.

## CHEST

Firm pressure with the fingertips is exerted along the sternum and ribs to elicit any tenderness that may be present. Such tenderness may reflect a leukemic process or multiple myeloma. Lung sounds are assessed for signs of pneumonia, another common occurrence with leukemia or multiple myeloma.

### ABDOMEN

The abdomen is percussed and palpated with special attention to the liver and spleen. Both organs are prone to enlargement in association with hematologic disease.

### BACK AND EXTREMITIES

The skeletal system is evaluated primarily for pain, joint deformity, and arthritis. Bone pain may be associated with malignant conditions of hematologic origin. In persons with hemolytic processes and in some hematologic malignancies, there is increased uric acid production and a corresponding increase in the incidence of gout. Joint deformities are associated with bleeding disorders and pathologic fractures with other disorders.

### LYMPH NODES

Lymph nodes are widely distributed in the body and are routinely examined by palpation of the body part being examined. In the healthy adult the only palpable nodes are in the inguinal region and less often in the axilla. With disease the cervical and supraclavicular nodes may become palpable. Further evaluation of lymph nodes requires x-ray examination, lymphangiography, and biopsy. It is important to recognize that any enlarged lymph node may reflect a disease process and should be evaluated thoroughly. Enlarged lymph nodes may be painful if they infringe on other organs.

### NERVOUS SYSTEM

Many neurologic abnormalities may develop in persons with hematologic disorders. These catastrophic complications are caused by bleeding or infection within the central nervous system. Infiltration of malignant leukemic or lymphomatous cells may produce signs and symptoms of cerebral tumor. In addition, some of the lymphomas, especially Hodgkin's disease, may produce a dementia as a remote effect. Initial physical examination should therefore include assessment of mental status, cranial nerve function, sensory function (pain, touch, position, vibratory sensation), and motor function (strength, reflexes, plantar response).

## DIAGNOSTIC TESTS

Extensive blood examinations are performed as part of the diagnostic work-up of a person suspected of having a hematologic disorder (Table 33-1). The most frequent laboratory tests are Hgb and hematocrit (Hct) levels, red blood cell indexes, and peripheral smear, which includes WBC counts and differential. The information obtained from such studies provides important clues as to the pathology of the disorder. In addition to their diagnostic value, blood studies are used to monitor a patient's progress and response to treatment. The confirmation of a hematologic disease often depends on an examination of a peripheral blood smear and results of the bone marrow examination.

**TABLE 33-1 Laboratory Tests for Hematologic Assessment**

| BLOOD CELL | FUNCTION | DIAGNOSTIC TEST |
|---|---|---|
| ERYTHROCYTES (RBCs) | To mediate the exchange of oxygen and carbon dioxide between lungs and tissue, the transportation of oxygen, and excretion of carbon dioxide | RBC, hemoglobin (Hgb), hematocrit (Hct), reticulocyte count<br>Blood indexes: Hgb, mean corpuscular hemoglobin concentration (MCHC), mean corpuscular hemoglobin (MCH)<br>Red cell fragility<br>Morphologic description in stained smear |
| PLATELETS (THROMBOCYTES) | To produce platelet plug; to promote thrombin production<br>To provide factor IV to neutralize the action of heparin | Platelet aggregation<br>Platelet count<br>Bleeding time |
| LEUKOCYTES (WBCs) | | WBC with differential |
| Granulocytes | | Skin tests for anergy |
| Neutrophils (PMN, SEGs) | To initiate phagocytosis | Immunoelectrophoresis<br>Radial immunodiffusion |
| Eosinophils | To reverse allergic responses, parasitic infestations | |
| Basophils | To mediate hypersensitivity reactions | |
| Lymphocytes | To form immunoglobulins, humoral (B lymphocytes), cellular (T lymphocytes), immune responses | |
| Monocytes | To initiate phagocytosis | |

*SEGs,* Segmented neutrophils.

### HEMOGLOBIN AND HEMATOCRIT

A Hgb test measures the amount of Hgb in circulation. The packed red blood cell volume, or Hct, is the ratio of RBC volume to the whole blood volume (Table 33-2).

### RED BLOOD CELL INDEXES

The RBC indexes consist of the **mean corpuscular volume (MCV), mean corpuscular hemoglobin**

**TABLE 33-2 Normal Values of Cellular Blood Components**

| TYPE | NORMAL VALUES | |
|---|---|---|
| RBCs | Male: 4.6-6.1 million/mm³<br>Female: 4.0-5.4 million/mm³ | |
| Hematocrit (Hct) | Male: 45%-52%<br>Female: 37%-48% | |
| Hemoglobin (Hgb) | Male: 13-18 g/100 ml<br>Female: 12-16 g/100 ml | |
| Mean corpuscular volume (MCV) | 80-95 μm³ | |
| Mean corpuscular Hgb concentration (MCHC) | 32%-36% | |
| WBCs | 5000-10,000/mm³ | |
| Neutrophils | 55%-70% | Differential blood cell count—totals 100% |
| Eosinophils | 1%-4% | |
| Basophils | 0%-1% | |
| Monocytes | 2%-6% | |
| Lymphocytes | 25%-40% | |
| Platelets | 150,000/mm³ | |

**BOX 33-3 Descriptive Cell Characteristics in Anemia**

**SIZE**

**Macrocytic** (large)
**Normocytic**
**Microcytic** (small)

**HEMOGLOBIN**

**Normochromic**
**Hypochromic** (decreased)

**(MCH),** and the **mean corpuscular hemoglobin concentration (MCHC).** The MCV estimates the average size of the RBC. Both the MCH and the MCHC measure the content of the Hgb in RBCs. The MCHC is considered more accurate than the MCH because it measures the entire blood volume of Hgb rather than just from a single cell. The RBC indexes provide a differential diagnosis of the type of anemia. Normal values are indicated in Table 33-2.

## PERIPHERAL BLOOD SMEAR

Each blood cell possesses microscopic features that identify and set the cell apart from other cell types. Examination of the **peripheral blood smear** provides information concerning the etiology of an anemia. The size and shape of the RBC is observed (Box 33-3). Alteration in the size of the RBC is classified as **anisocytosis;** alteration in shape of the RBC is noted as **poikilocytosis.** The WBC may be examined to provide

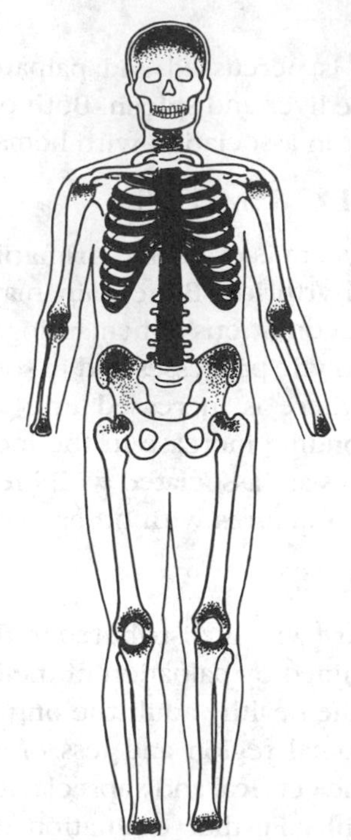

**FIGURE 33-5** Sites of active bone marrow *(shaded areas).* (From Yasko J: *Guidelines for cancer care: symptom management,* Reston, Va, 1983, Reston Publishing.)

information about adequate bone marrow production. Platelet count may indicate a tendency for bleeding. Often this information, when combined with data from the history, physical examination, and other laboratory tests, determines the medical diagnosis.

## BONE MARROW EXAMINATION

An adjunct to the peripheral blood smear is the bone marrow examination. Generally the bone marrow is examined when the diagnosis is not clearly established from the peripheral blood smear or when further information is needed. A bone marrow specimen is obtained by **bone marrow aspiration** or **bone marrow biopsy.** (Figure 33-5 illustrates sites of active bone marrow.)

### Bone Marrow Aspiration

Aspiration is the most common procedure for obtaining a bone marrow sample. The procedure is possible because normal **bone marrow** is soft and semifluid and can therefore be removed by aspiration through a needle. Bone marrow aspiration is most likely to be performed in persons with severe anemia, neutropenia (decreased number of WBCs), acute leukemia, and thrombocytopenia (decreased number of platelets).

#### Procedure

The skin surrounding the puncture site (Figure 33-6) is shaved, if necessary, and cleansed with an antiseptic such as povidone-iodine complex (Betadine). Sterile towels are placed around the site. The skin and periosteum are anesthetized to decrease pain. First, the most superficial layer of the skin is infiltrated with procaine. After a few seconds the needle is further advanced until bone is touched. Procaine is then injected to anesthetize the periosteum.

The marrow aspiration needle is inserted; when the marrow cavity is entered, the marrow stylet is removed from the needle, and a sterile syringe is attached. The syringe plunger is drawn back until marrow appears in the syringe. As the plunger is drawn back, the person will experience a brief, sharp pain, sometimes described as a burning sensation. The pain is caused by the suction exerted as the plunger is pulled back. At this point the nurse's hands placed gently on the person's shoulder and a calm warning coupled with a reminder to lie still serve well to prevent a sudden jerk or movement by the patient.

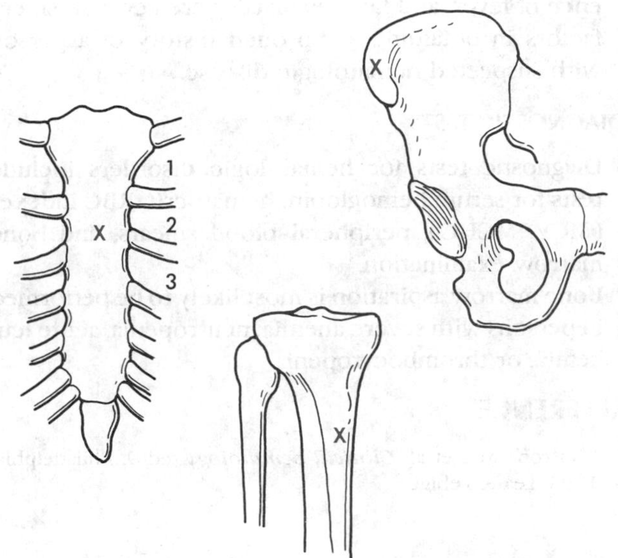


**FIGURE 33-6** Sites for bone marrow aspiration: sternum, iliac crest (most common), and tibia.

After the needle is removed, a pressure dressing is applied over the aspiration site to arrest the minimal bleeding that occurs. If the patient has thrombocytopenia, pressure is applied for 3 to 5 minutes.

Some persons may complain of tenderness at the aspiration site for a few days. Most often, no pain or discomfort is experienced after the procedure.

## Bone Marrow Biopsy

A **bone marrow biopsy** is indicated when a large sample of bone marrow is needed. Persons most likely to undergo a bone marrow biopsy are those with pancytopenia (more than one altered cell type), myelofibrosis, metastatic tumor, lymphoma, and multiple myeloma. The most common site for bone marrow biopsy is the posterosuperior iliac spine. (The sternum also is used.) The initial steps in the biopsy procedure are similar to those outlined for bone marrow aspiration. The use of a Jamshidi needle allows for a core of marrow to be collected (Figure 33-7).

After a bone marrow aspirate or biopsy, patients are

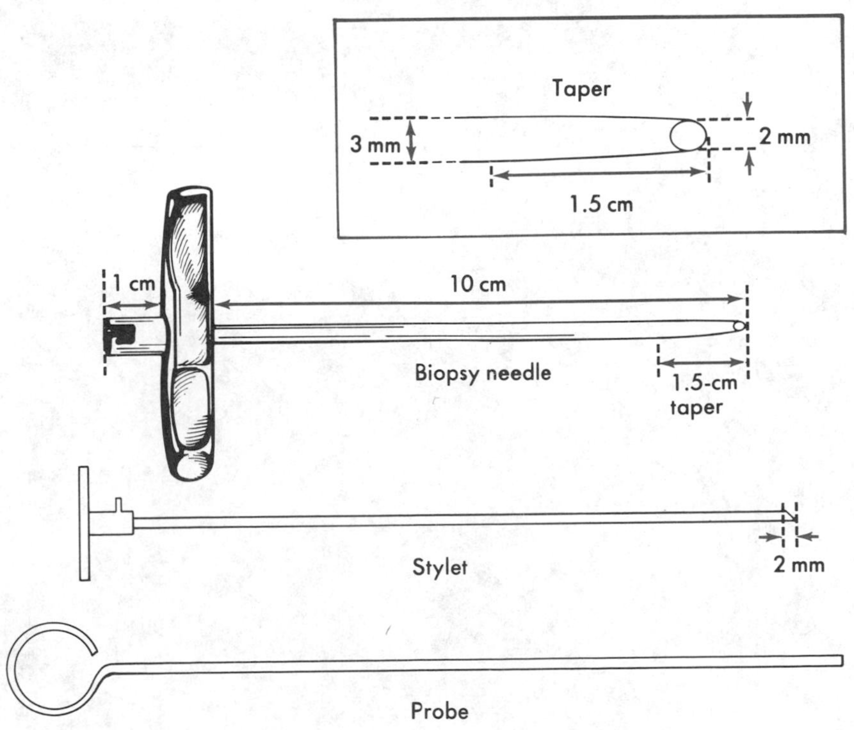


**FIGURE 33-7** Bone marrow biopsy needle showing shape and size.

assessed for bleeding from the site. Other comfort measures, such as assisting the person to freshen up, often are needed to help the person relax and rest comfortably.

From microscopic examination of the bone marrow, iron stores can be determined, as can the morphology of the progenitor cell (see Figure 33-1). Large immature cell changes may be observed; infiltration with leukemic cells and absence of cells, as in aplastic anemia, can be determined.

Other diagnostic tests are discussed throughout the text along with the specific disorder to which they pertain.

## CRITICAL THINKING ACTIVITIES

- How would you describe to patients the results of their blood laboratory work-up in terms they could understand?
- What special considerations would you keep in mind if you were assessing an elderly patient with a hematologic disorder as compared with a younger person?
- How would you prepare a patient who is going to have a bone marrow examination performed for the first time?

## CHAPTER SUMMARY

### ANATOMY AND PHYSIOLOGY

- The hematopoietic system is made up of the blood (erythrocytes, leukocytes, platelets) and the reticuloendothelial system.

### SUBJECTIVE DATA

- Family history, drug use and chemical exposure, presence of fever, and fatigue/malaise are key assessment factors in obtaining a thorough history of a person with suspected hematologic disease.

### DIAGNOSTIC TESTS

- Diagnostic tests for hematologic disorders include tests for serum hemoglobin, hematocrit, RBC indexes (MCV, MCHC), peripheral blood smears, and bone marrow examination.
- Bone marrow aspiration is most likely to be performed in persons with severe anemia, neutropenia, acute leukemia, or thrombocytopenia.

## REFERENCE

1. Wintrobe MM et al: *Clinical hematology,* ed 9, Philadelphia, 1993, Lea & Febiger.

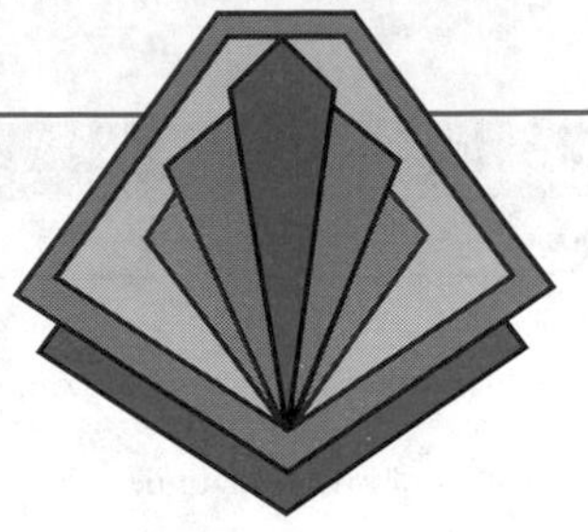

CHAPTER 34

# Management of Persons With Hematologic Problems

*Marilyn S. Lottman*
*Kathryn Sabo Thompson*

## CHAPTER OBJECTIVES

***After studying this chapter, the learner should be able to do the following:***

1 Compare and contrast different types of anemias in terms of pathophysiology, assessment, and interventions.
2 Analyze the genetic factors of sickle cell disease and describe the nature of and nursing care for patients with sickle cell crisis.
3 Compare and contrast disorders of hemostasis, platelets, and coagulation (thombocytopenia, thrombocytosis, hemophilia, vitamin K deficiency, and disseminated intravascular coagulation) and describe nursing interventions.
4 Analyze nursing interventions and therapeutic modalities in four types of leukemia.
5 Differentiate between Hodgkin's disease and non-Hodgkin's lymphoma, and describe related interventions.

## KEY TERMS

acute lymphocytic leukemia (ALL)
acute myelogenous leukemia (AML)
anemia
aplastic anemia
autoimmune hemolytic anemia
bone marrow transplantation
chronic lymphocytic leukemia (CLL)
chronic myelogenous leukemia (CML)
disseminated intravascular coagulation (DIC)
enzyme deficiency anemia
erythrocytosis
folic acid deficiency
genetic counselor
hemoglobinopathy
hemolytic anemia
hemophilia
hereditary spherocytosis
Hodgkin's disease
hypoprothrombinemia
idiopathic thrombocytopenic purpura (ITP)
iron deficiency anemia
leukemia
lymphangiography
megaloblastic anemia
neutropenia
neutrophilia
non-Hodgkin's lymphomas
polycythemia vera
sickle cell anemia
sickle cell crisis
sickle cell disease (Hb SS)
sickle cell trait
sickling syndromes
stress erythropoiesis
thalassemia
thrombocytopenia
thrombocytosis

Management of persons with hematologic problems can be challenging because of the diversity and subtlety of symptoms. The symptoms are related to one or more malfunctions within the blood components, and thorough management must be ensured after a complete assessment is obtained. Each nursing intervention for hematologic symptoms must be constantly evaluated. Subtle changes in a patient's reticuloendothelial system can cause a change in the plan of care. To obtain the most optimal health for a patient with a hematologic disorder, the nurse must be prepared with information to address the related problems.

## DISORDERS ASSOCIATED WITH ERYTHROCYTES

The major health problems associated with erythrocytes are the anemias (including hemoglobinopathies) and erythrocytosis (polycythemia).

### ANEMIA

**Anemia** refers to a deficiency of RBCs, as reflected in a decreased Hgb level, packed cell volume (Hct), and RBC count. Anemias may be divided into those that are the result of blood loss, impaired production of RBCs, in-

**TABLE 34-1 Types of Anemia and Clinical Manifestations**

| TYPE | CAUSES | CLINICAL MANIFESTATIONS |
|---|---|---|
| **SECONDARY TO BLOOD LOSS** | | |
| Acute | Hemorrhage | Early: weakness, cool moist skin, tachycardia, hypotension; late: decreased Hgb and Hct |
| Chronic | Gastrointestinal or other malignancy, bleeding ulcers, bleeding hemorrhoids, menorrhagia | Decreased RBCs, Hgb, Hct, MCV, and MCHC; fatigue |
| **SECONDARY TO IMPAIRED PRODUCTION OF RBCs** | | |
| Aplastic anemia | Drugs, chemicals, radiation, chemotherapy, virus, congenital, autoimmune mechanism | Pallor of skin and mucous membranes, fatigue, palpitations, exertional dyspnea, pancytopenia, bleeding tendency, infections |
| Chronic anemia | Chronic illness, renal disease | Decreased serum iron concentration, fatigue |
| **HEMOLYTIC ANEMIAS** | | |
| Hereditary spherocytosis | Genetic: inherited as autosomal dominant trait | Spherocytes and increased reticulocytes on peripheral blood smear; fatigue, exertional dyspnea |
| Thalassemia | Genetic: decreased synthesis of one of globin chains of Hgb | Microcytosis, hypochromic RBCs, decreased growth at pubescence, eventual cardiac failure |
| Sickle cell disease | Genetic hemoglobinopathy | Painful episodes; vasoocclusive crises; chronic leg ulcers, chronic renal and ocular problems; sickled cells on peripheral blood smears |
| Enzyme deficiency anemia | Genetic: deficiency of glucose-6-phosphate dehydrogenase (G6PD) | Episodic hemolytic episodes, decreased levels of G6PD |
| Acquired hemolytic anemia | Drug-induced or autoimmune response | Presence of RBC antibody on antiglobin or Coombs' test |
| **NUTRITIONAL ANEMIAS** | | |
| Iron deficiency anemia | Chronic blood loss, inadequate intake | Fatigue, exertional dyspnea; microcytosis; low serum iron concentration |
| Megaloblastic anemia | Deficiency in vitamin $B_{12}$ or folic acid | Macrocytosis; glossitis and neurologic abnormalities with vitamin $B_{12}$ deficiency |

*MCHC,* Mean corpuscular hemoglobin concentration; *MCV,* mean corpuscular volume.

creased destruction of RBCs, or nutritional deficiency. The anemias are summarized in Table 34-1.

Anemia also may be differentiated by examining the size of red cells and the amount of Hgb contained. The suffix *-cytic* refers to RBC size, and *-chromic* refers to amount of Hgb (see Box 33-4).

## Prevention

### Primary prevention

Some types of anemia, such as aplastic anemia and nutritional anemias, can be prevented by health teaching. Exposure to certain chemicals and drugs places human beings at high risk for aplastic anemia. Occupational health nurses provide information to workers about health risks in the environment and ways in which risk factors can be decreased. Nurses in all settings teach about dietary needs for iron and vitamins. Persons with low income can be taught to identify inexpensive food sources of the vitamins and minerals necessary for hematologic health. Nurses also can become politically active to ensure adequate governmental funding for low-cost nutritonal programs for persons with marginal incomes.

Women who have long-term blood loss because of heavy menstrual bleeding also are at risk for anemias, as are other persons with long-term, slow blood loss. These persons need to know of the risks and the need for continued monitoring of their RBC indexes.

### Secondary prevention

Occupational health nurses are involved in identifying industrial chemicals or processes that place workers in danger and in screening employees as pertinent. Screening for anemias in any setting occurs during routine physical examinations with blood tests.

Diseases such as sickle cell anemia and the thalassemias are hereditary; therefore marriage between carriers of defective genes may result in children with the disease. One of the most difficult and sensitive roles for nurses is that of **genetic counselor,** communicating to persons with hereditary problems the risk factors involved and the possibility of having children with severe hematopoietic disease. With this knowledge the couples then can make their own informed decisions.

## Anemia Caused by Blood Loss

### Etiology and pathophysiology

**Acute blood loss.** The anemia associated with acute blood loss is the direct result of the decrease in circulating RBCs. The adult of average build has a total blood volume of approximately 6000 ml. Usually an adult can lose 500 ml of blood without serious or lasting effects. If the loss reaches 1000 ml or more, serious acute consequences may result.

Signs and symptoms include those associated with hypovolemia and hypoxemia (see Table 34-1). Weakness, stupor, irritability, and cool, moist skin may be observed. Vital signs demonstrate hypotension and tachycardia. Decreased Hgb and Hct levels may not be evident until several hours after the blood loss has occurred. The severity of the patient's symptoms correlates with the severity of the blood loss.

**Chronic blood loss.** The body has remarkable adaptive powers and may adjust fairly well to a severe reduction in RBCs and Hgb, provided the condition develops gradually. A person may remain free of symptoms even though the total RBC count may drop to almost half its normal amount. With chronic anemia, determinations of RBC counts, Hgb and Hct levels, mean corpuscular volume (MCV), and mean corpuscular hemoglobin concentration (MCHC) are important diagnostic tests. All indexes usually are below normal (see Table 33-2 for normal values).

Chronic blood loss is the most common cause of iron deficiency anemia. When blood loss is continuous and moderate in amount, the bone marrow may be able to keep up with the losses by increasing the production of RBCs. Eventually, if the cause of chronic blood loss is not found and corrected, the bone marrow will not be able to keep pace with the loss, and symptoms of anemia appear (see Table 34-1).

#### Medical management

Successful treatment for anemia caused by blood loss requires immediate identification of the source of the loss and institution of appropriate treatment. In addition, transfusion therapy or iron supplements may be needed.

*Transfusion therapy* usually is not indicated in symptom-free persons with chronic anemia because it unnecessarily exposes the person to risks associated with transfusion (see Chapter 70). Transfusion of erythrocytes is reserved for those patients whose cardiovascular system is compromised by the anemia and in whom rapid correction by other means is not possible.

Transfusion of whole blood may be used in the treatment of anemia caused by acute blood loss. For virtually all other anemias, packed red blood cells rather than whole blood are used in transfusions because the total blood volume generally is normal and administration of whole blood may produce circulatory overload and pulmonary edema.

*Iron supplements* may be needed by the person with anemia from chronic blood loss because of depletion of iron stores. The iron usually is given in the form of ferrous sulfate (see p. 954).

#### Nursing management

Nursing interventions for acute blood loss are the same as those for hypovolemic shock (see Chapter 22). The person receiving blood transfusions is monitored for signs of transfusion reactions.

If the Hgb count is very low, weakness and fatigue may be present. Nursing interventions include scheduling of activities to promote rest and to optimize use of limited energy levels.

## Aplastic Anemia

#### Etiology

**Aplastic anemia** (anemia as a result of impaired erythrocyte production) affects all age-groups and both genders. The incidence is 1:100,000 of the population. In approximately one half of patients with aplastic anemia in the United States, no etiologic agent is identifiable. Predictable bone marrow depression occurs with antineoplastic drugs. Aplastic anemia may follow exposure to certain drugs, including chloramphenicol, sulfonamides, phenylbutazone (Butazolidin), and anticonvulsant agents such as mephenytoin (Mesantoin). Insecticides such as DDT and chemicals, particularly benzene, also are thought to cause aplastic anemia. Infections associated with the pathogenesis of aplastic anemia include hepatitis (types B and non-A, non-B), Epstein-Barr virus, cytomegalovirus, and miliary tuberculosis. The defect leading to aplastic anemia is most likely injury or destruction of a common stem cell (see Figure 33-1), which affects all subsequent cell populations. Aplastic anemia also may be congenital.

#### Pathophysiology

Aplastic anemia usually is characterized by depression or cessation of activity of all blood-producing elements. There is a decrease in WBCs (leukopenia), a decrease in platelets (thrombocytopenia), and a decrease in the formation of RBCs, which leads to an anemia (Table 34-2). The process may be chronic or acute depending on the causative factor of the anemia.

Symptoms of aplastic anemia usually develop gradually over weeks or months but may appear suddenly. Pallor of the skin and mucous membranes is characteristic, in addition to fatigue, palpitations, and exertional dyspnea. Infections of the skin and mucous membranes occur with severe granulocytopenia; hemorrhagic symptoms (bleeding into the skin and mucous membranes and spontaneous bleeding from the nose, gums, vagina, and rectum) occur with severe thrombocytopenia. Results of a physical examination often are normal. The hemogram characteristically reveals a pancytopenia (a marked decrease in the numbers of all cell types). The reticulocyte count is low. Definitive diagnosis is made by bone marrow examination. Attempts at bone marrow aspiration may yield a "dry tap" because of hypocellularity and a decrease in active marrow. Bone marrow biopsy often is necessary for diagnosis of aplastic anemia.

**Medical management**

The immediate treatment for aplastic anemia is the removal of the causative agent, if known. In the past, treatment for aplastic anemia was aimed mainly at stimulating hematopoiesis through the administration of steroids and androgen therapy. These agents have been shown to be of limited value and can produce toxic side effects. In recent years, **bone marrow transplantation** from a donor with identical human leukocyte antigen (HLA) has emerged as the treatment of choice for persons younger than age 40 years with severe aplastic anemia. The remainder of persons are treated with immunosuppressive therapy. Transplantation centers are reporting survival rates of 60% to 80%.[2]

The prognosis for aplastic anemia depends primarily on the severity of the anemia, method of treatment, and general supportive care. In addition, a higher treatment success rate occurs in patients who receive transplantation early and have not received blood products, especially from the potential bone marrow donor. Patients who have undergone transfusion have a higher mortality from development of graft-versus-host disease. If transfusions are essential, then leukocyte-poor RBCs and platelets should be used (see Chapter 70). Patients who are not successfully treated often die of complications associated with repeated hemorrhage and infection.

## NURSING MANAGEMENT

### ♦ ASSESSMENT

Subjective data to be collected to assess the patient with aplastic anemia include a history of exposure to chemicals (insecticides, benzene) and drugs, in addition to a family history of aplastic anemia. The person is questioned about the ability to carry out activities of daily living (ADLs) without dyspnea and fatigue. Physical examination includes monitoring for signs of infection (from the leukopenia) and bleeding (from the thrombocytopenia).

### ♦ NURSING DIAGNOSES

Nursing diagnoses are determined from analysis of patient data. Nursing diagnoses for the patient with aplastic anemia may include but are not limited to the following:

| Diagnostic Title | Possible Etiologic Factors |
|---|---|
| Infection, high risk for | Decreased immune response, decreased neutrophil production |
| Injury (trauma), high risk for (bleeding, falls) | Lack of awareness of environmental hazards, tissue hypoxia, syncope associated with anemia and weakness |
| Fatigue | Imbalance between oxygen supply and demand |
| Knowledge deficit | Lack of exposure/recall |

### ♦ EXPECTED PATIENT OUTCOMES

Expected patient outcomes for the person with aplastic anemia may include but are not limited to the following:

1. Does not develop infection.
2. Does not fall.
3. Has no signs of bleeding (any bleeding is quickly controlled).
4. Feels rested and has adjusted ADLs to limited energy levels.
5. Explains measures to prevent infection, hemorrhage, and fatigue.

### ♦ INTERVENTIONS

Nursing care depends on the severity of symptoms. The patient may be critically ill. Prevention of infection and bleeding is the focus of nursing care.

#### Preventing Infection

The following activities may be carried out for the hospitalized patient:

1. Place patient in private room; avoid contact with visitors or staff members who have infection.
2. Place patient in protective isolation or laminar air flow room (see Chapter 16) if necessary.
3. Provide meticulous hygiene, including daily bath, careful oral hygiene, and perineal care; use antiseptic creams.
4. Avoid catheterization.
5. Use povidone-iodine skin cleansing 1 minute before parenteral injections (or other prescribed preparations).
6. Maintain a clean environment.
7. Stress careful handwashing by all caregivers.
8. Provide emotional support for anxiety when infection occurs.

#### Preventing Hemorrhage

Excessive bleeding may be prevented by the following actions:

1. Monitor all sites for potential bleeding.
2. Test urine (Hemastix) and stool (guaiac) for blood.
3. Keep venipuncture and intramuscular injections to a minimum.
4. Apply pressure to venipuncture for 5 minutes, arterial puncture for 10 minutes.
5. Use soft toothbrush or swab for mouth care.
6. Keep mouth clean and free of debris with normal saline rinse if bleeding occurs.
7. Avoid taking rectal temperatures, administering rectal medications, or giving enemas.
8. Avoid invasive procedures.

#### Preventing Fatigue

Decreased oxygen-carrying capacity of the blood decreases oxygen supply to the tissues, leading to fatigue with activity. Measures to prevent fatigue include providing frequent rest periods, avoiding fatigue-producing activities, and monitoring the patient for signs of excessive fatigue or shortness of breath with activities.

**TABLE 34-2 Normal Function, Primary Pathophysiology, and Clinical Manifestations in Aplastic Anemia**

| NORMAL FUNCTION | PATHOPHYSIOLOGY | CLINICAL MANIFESTATIONS |
|---|---|---|
| **RED BLOOD CELLS** | | |
| Major component is Hgb, which provides transportation of oxygen and carbon dioxide to cells | Reduction or depletion of hematopoietic stem cells, with decreased production of erythrocytes, platelets, and leukocytes<br>Decreased tissue oxygenation | Pallor of skin and mucous membrane; fatigue and exertional dyspnea<br>Low Hgb and Hct levels |
| **PLATELETS** | | |
| Adhesion and aggregation capabilities to plug small breaks in small blood vessels<br>Release of thromboplastin, which, in presence of calcium ions, converts prothrombin into thrombin in initial step of coagulation process | Fewer platelets available for blood coagulation | Bleeding tendency, as evidenced by ecchymosis, purpura, and petechiae<br>Bleeding from nose, mouth, vagina, and rectum<br>Low platelet count |
| **WHITE BLOOD CELLS** | | |
| *Neutrophils* serve as primary defense against bacterial infection through phagocytosis<br>*Monocytes* remove dead and injured cells, cell fragments, and microorganisms<br>*Lymphocytes* participate in cellular immune response (T cell) and humoral immune response (B cell) | Fewer WBCs make a person more susceptible to infection (decreased phagocytosis, decreased immune response) | Complaints of many infections, frequent sick days<br>Low WBC count |

## Facilitating Learning

All persons with aplastic anemia need to know how to protect themselves from infection and excessive bleeding. Points to emphasize are listed in the Guidelines box at right.

## ♦ EVALUATION

To evaluate the effectiveness of nursing interventions, compare patient's behaviors with those stated in the expected patient outcomes. Successful achievement of patient outcomes for the patient with aplastic anemia are indicated by the following:

1. Shows no signs of infection.
2. Does not fall.
3. Shows no signs of bleeding (e.g., petechiae, hemorrhage) (any bleeding is quickly controlled).
4. Feels rested and has no fatigue with ADLs.
5. Correctly explains measures to prevent infection, hemorrhage, and fatigue.

## Hemolytic Anemia

**Hemolytic anemia** (anemia caused by increased erythrocyte destruction) results when the RBCs are destroyed at such a rapid rate that the bone marrow is unable to compensate for the loss. The severity of the anemia is determined by the degree of lag between the rate of erythrocyte destruction (hemolysis) and the rate of bone marrow production of RBCs (erythropoiesis).

Hemolytic anemia is divided into congenital and ac-

### Guidelines for Teaching the Person With Aplastic Anemia

1. Prevent infection
   a. Use good handwashing technique.
   b. Avoid contact with those who have infections.
   c. Avoid sharing eating utensils and bath linens.
   d. Take a bath every day (or every other day if skin is dry); keep perineal area clean.
   e. Use good oral hygiene.
   f. Eliminate intake of raw meats, fruits, or vegetables.
   g. Report signs of infection immediately to physician.
2. Prevent hemorrhage
   a. Observe for signs such as bloody urine, stool, and petechiae, and report these to physician.
   b. Use a soft toothbrush or swab for mouth care.
   c. Keep mouth clean and free of debris.
   d. Avoid enemas or other rectal insertions.
   e. Avoid picking or blowing the nose forcefully.
   f. Avoid trauma, falls, bumps, and cuts; avoid contact sports.
   g. Avoid use of aspirin or aspirin preparations (anticoagulant effect).
   h. Use an electric razor.
   i. Use adequate lubrication and gentleness during sexual intercourse.
3. Prevent fatigue
   a. Take frequent rest periods between ADLs and activity.
   b. Avoid excessive workload or heavy lifting, and ask for assistance with strenuous activity.
   c. Increase time necessary for routine care.
   d. Decrease activity if shortness of breath, dizziness, or sensation of heaviness in extremities occurs.
   e. Report signs of increased fatigue with activity to physician.

quired. *Congenital hemolytic anemias* includes hereditary spherocytosis, the hemoglobinopathies, thalassemia, and enzyme deficiency anemia. **Hereditary spherocytosis,** inherited as an autosomal dominant trait, is characterized by a membrane abnormality that leads to osmotic swelling of the RBC and susceptibility to destruction by the spleen. It usually is detected in childhood but may appear initially in adulthood.

Diagnosis depends on observation of spherocytes on the peripheral blood smear and by laboratory demonstration of increased osmotic fragility of the RBCs. The reticulocyte count usually is elevated, as is the serum bilirubin level. Bilirubin is derived from the breakdown of the hemoglobin released by the destroyed RBCs. Occasionally, red cell survival time will need to be determined. This is accomplished by labeling the cells with radioactive chromium and measuring the rate of decrease of radioactivity for 1 to 2 weeks (chromium survival). Symptoms include those typically associated with anemia (pallor, fatigue, exertional dyspnea), jaundice from the increased serum bilirubin level, and an enlarged spleen from the increased RBC destruction.

Hereditary spherocytosis is almost invariably corrected by splenectomy.

## Thalassemia

### Etiology/Pathophysiology

**Thalassemia** is an inherited disorder affecting primarily Italians, Greeks, Chinese, Southeast Asians, and black persons. It is characterized by a decreased synthesis of one of the globin chains of hemoglobin. The beta (β) chain is most often affected (β-thalassemia). As a result, there is decreased synthesis of hemoglobin and an accumulation of the alpha globin chain in the erythrocyte. These alterations result in decreased RBC production and a chronic hemolytic anemia.

There are two presentations of thalassemia (Table 34-3). The heterozygous state, *thalassemia minor,* is associated with a mild anemia that usually is symptomless; no therapy is required. The homozygous condition, *thalassemia major,* is characterized by a severe anemia. The RBCs are characteristically hypochromic (low MCH) and microcytic (low MCV). Hemoglobin electrophoresis is diagnostic. Growth failure begins about ages 10 to 12 years. Eventually, cardiac failure develops and death usually occurs between ages 17 and 30.[7]

**TABLE 34-3 Types of Thalassemia**

| TYPE | STATE | SYMPTOMS | THERAPY |
|---|---|---|---|
| Thalassemia minor | Heterozygous | Mild anemia, usually symptomless | None required |
| Thalassemia major | Homozygous | Severe anemia<br>Low MCH<br>Low MCV | Transfusion |

### Medical management

At present, the only treatment available for thalassemia is transfusion therapy. Transfusions may be administered either to alleviate severe symptoms or to maintain the Hgb at a near-normal level continuously to allow for a more normal life-style. The latter approach incurs the risk of producing iron overload from frequent transfusions, a problem that can be ameliorated by the use of an iron-chelating agent such as deferoxamine.

### Nursing management

The nurse must be familiar with transfusion therapy (see Chapter 70) and sensitive to the emotional needs of patients receiving frequent transfusions. Because the average age at which death occurs is 17 to 30 years, the nurse should be aware of the hopelessness and depression that may occur in this population.

## Enzyme Deficiency Anemia

### Etiology/Pathophysiology

Deficiency of enzymes in the pathways that metabolize glucose and generate ATP (Embden-Meyerhof and pentose phosphate shunt pathways) frequently leads to premature RBC destruction **(enzyme deficiency anemia).** The most common clinically significant enzyme abnormality is that of *glucose-6-phosphate dehydrogenase* (G6PD). This disorder often occurs in a mild form among African-Americans. It occurs in a more severe form in certain population groups in the Mediterranean area and may cause a chronic hemolytic anemia.

Anemia generally occurs in G6PD deficiency only when the patient is exposed to an oxidant drug (aspirin, sulfonamides, antimalarial drugs) after infection or during the newborn period. Acute hemolysis of varying severity, which generally is self-limiting, results. The patient may experience back pain, jaundice, and hemoglobinuria as evidence of the hemolytic process. Diagnosis is established by assay for the enzyme.

### Management

Treatment is recognition of the disorder and cessation of the offending drug. Nursing care involves teaching the patient to avoid oxidant drugs.

## Sickle Cell Disease: A Hemoglobinopathy

Normal Hgb is composed of heme (red) and globin (protein component). The globin portion comprises two pairs of polypeptide chains, α and β. There is a specific amino acid sequence and number for each of the polypeptide chains. Any deviation in the normal number or sequence of essential amino acids results in abnormal Hgb synthesis.

Disorders of hemoglobin synthesis are categorized as **hemoglobinopathies.** They result from abnormalities in one or both of the polypeptide chains (α or β) or in any one of the more than 500 amino acids. One of the most common hemoglobinopathies is Hb S disease (sickle cell anemia). Abnormalities in Hgb are diagnosed through serum electrophoresis (see Chapter 70).

### Etiology/Epidemiology

Sickle cell anemia is the most common genetic disorder in the United States. **Sickle cell disease (Hb SS)** is homozygous recessive (Table 34-4 and Figure 34-1) and is characterized by a chronic hemolytic anemia.

Sickle cell anemia occurs predominantly in the black population. It is estimated that 1 in 12 African-Americans is a sickle cell carrier and that 1 in 65 develops sickle cell anemia. To a lesser extent, sickle cell disease also occurs in persons from Asia Minor, India, the Mediterranean area, and the Caribbean area.

### Pathophysiology

The basic abnormality lies within the globin fraction of the Hgb, where a single amino acid (valine) is substituted for another (glutamic acid) in the sixth position of the β chain. This single amino acid substitution profoundly alters the properties of the Hgb molecule (Table 34-5). Because of the intermolecular rearrangement, Hb S is formed instead of normal Hb A. Hb S has normal oxygen-carrying capacity.

However, when the oxygen tension of RBCs decreases, Hb S polymerizes, causing the Hgb to distort and realign the RBC into a sickle shape (Figure 34-2). The sickle cell in circulation leads to increased blood viscosity, which prolongs circulation time. This decrease in circulation time causes an increase in the hypoxic time of the cell, promoting further sickling. The development of sickle cells leads to plugging of the small circulation, further decreasing cellular pH and oxygen tension (Figure 34-3).[2] Anaerobic metabolism is occurring, and the tissue ischemia can occur in any organ. This vicious cycle leads to further hypoxia, infarction of organs, and painful crisis. The affected cells have a shortened life span of 7 to 20 days, as compared to the normal 105 to 120 days.

**TABLE 34-4 Phenotypes for Sickle Cell**

| GENETIC RELATIONSHIP | HEMOGLOBIN ALLELES | SICKLE CELL DISEASE |
|---|---|---|
| Homozygous dominant | Hb A, Hb A | No disease |
| Heterozygous | Hb A, Hb S | Sickle cell trait |
| Homozygous recessive | Hb S, Hb S | Sickle cell anemia |

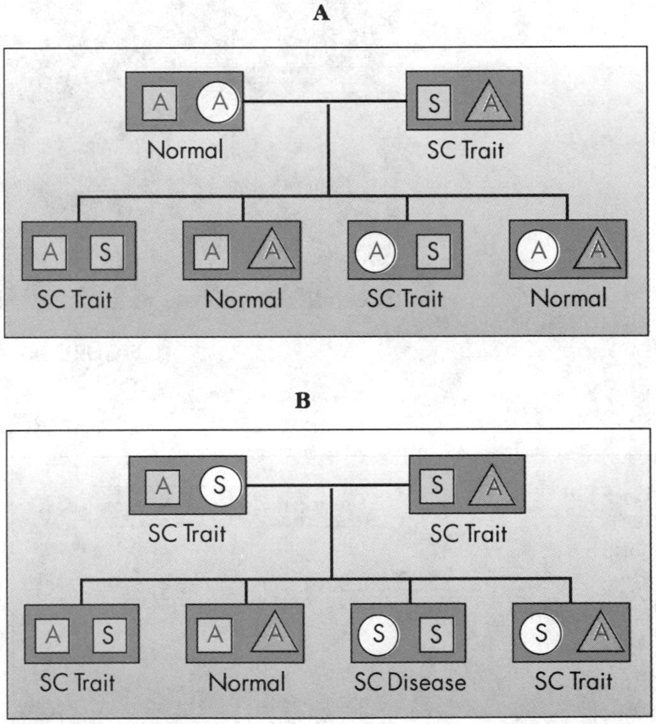

**A**



**B**



**FIGURE 34-1** **A,** When one parent has sickle cell trait (Hb SA) and the other does not (Hb AA), a 50% probability (2/4) exists that a child will have sickle cell trait. **B,** When both parents have sickle cell trait, there is a 25% probability (1/4) that a child will have sickle cell disease and a 50% probability of sickle cell trait.

**TABLE 34-5 Normal Function, Primary Pathophysiology, and Clinical Manifestations in Sickle Cell Disease**

| NORMAL FUNCTION OF HEMOGLOBIN | PATHOPHYSIOLOGY | CLINICAL MANIFESTATIONS |
|---|---|---|
| Hgb A is major Hgb fraction in adults and consists of two α- and two β-chains, which form a smooth, round shape | Inheritance of homozygous Hgb S interferes with function and structural integrity of Hgb molecule | Chronic hemolytic anemia classified as normochromic and normocytic; peripheral blood smears demonstrate sickled RBCs |
| Carries oxygen to tissues and carbon dioxide from tissues to be expelled by lungs | When cellular oxygen tension decreases, RBC distorts itself into sickle shape | |
| | Sickled cells increase viscosity of the blood, slowing circulation and causing increased cellular hypoxia and plugging of circulation to the organs; infarcts can occur in central nervous system, eyes, lungs, liver, spleen, kidney, joints, and bone | Vasoocclusive or "painful" crisis, cerebrovascular accident (CVA), retinal hemorrhage, pulmonary infarct, hepatomegaly, autosplenectomy, renal failure, enlarged heart, bone and joint abnormalities, leg ulcers |

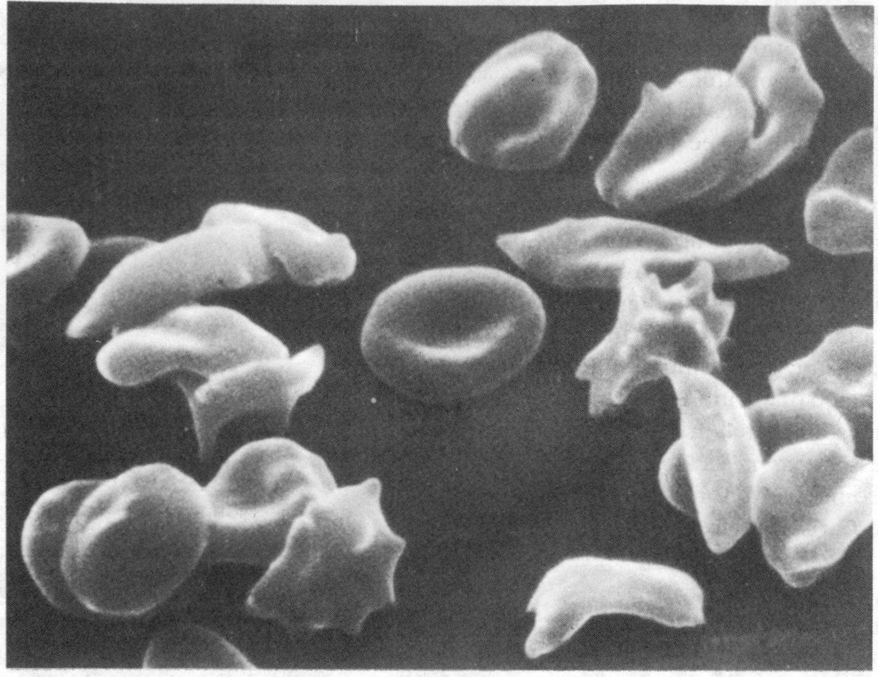

**FIGURE 34-2** Sickled red cells.

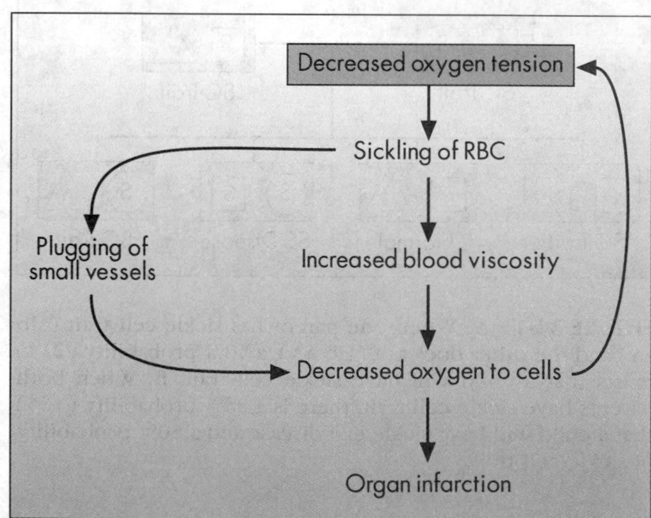


**FIGURE 34-3** Physiologic effects of RBC sickling.

**TABLE 34-6 Types of Sickle Cell Disorders**

| TERM | CHARACTERISTIC | HEMOGLOBIN MOLECULE |
|---|---|---|
| Sickle cell trait | Carrier of Hb S<br>Persons are symptom-free | Hb SA |
| Sickle cell disease | Presence of sickling with associated symptoms | Hb SS |
| Sickle cell syndromes | Diseases associated with presence of Hb S | Hb SC (sickle cell Hb C)<br>Hb SD (sickle cell Hb D)<br>Hb Sβ (sickle cell thalassemia) |

Different terminologies are used with discussions of sickle cell anemia (Table 34-6). Only the homozygous condition of Hb SS describes the classic form of the disease called **sickle cell anemia.** The heterozygous state, Hb SA, refers to the often asymptomatic condition called **sickle cell trait.** In addition, a category of sickling disorders, called **sickling syndromes,** is associated with the presence of Hb S.

Sickle cell disease often is diagnosed in early childhood. This form of the disease often is fatal by middle age. The gradations of sickling and symptoms vary both in occurrence and intensity. The complexity of this disorder and the problems that can arise from it make sickle cell disease a major health problem.

Anemia usually is severe, chronic, and hemolytic. When encountered in the health care setting, the person has one of many complications inherent in sickle cell disease (Box 34-1).

The painful vasoocclusive episode is the most common event in sickle cell disease. The pain is a manifestation of localized bone marrow necrosis affecting the juxtaarticular areas of the long bones, spine, pelvis, ribs,

**BOX 34-1 Clinical Manifestations of Sickle Cell Disease**

**ACUTE EPISODES**

Pain: usually in back, chest, or extremities; may be localized, migratory, or generalized

Fever: low grade, 1 to 2 days after onset of pain

Vasoocclusive crises: occlusion of blood vessels by the sickled cells; may occur in areas such as the brain (CVA), chest, liver, or penis (priapism)

**CHRONIC PROBLEMS**

Leg ulcers: usually of the medial malleolus

Renal problems: renal insufficiency from repeated infarctions

Ocular problems: microinfarctions of the peripheral retina leading to retinal detachment and blindness

and sternum. Usually it is the event on which sickle cell patients and medical personnel focus their attention and concern.[3] The frequency of painful episodes varies greatly. Some patients experience one or two episodes per month, whereas others only have one or two a year. The duration of the episode also varies and may last from 1 to 10 days. Physical and probably emotional factors (stress) precipitate a painful episode. Physical factors include events that cause dehydration or change the oxygen tension in the body, such as infection, overexertion, weather changes (cold), high Hgb levels, ingestion of alcohol, and smoking.[3]

Bacterial infection is a major cause of morbidity and mortality in patients with sickle cell disease. Persons with other hemoglobinopathies, such as Hb SC and Hb S, seem to be at lower risk for infection. Persons with sickle cell disease are particularly susceptible, primarily because most experience functional asplenia (no spleen function). Meningitis, sepsis, pneumonia, and urinary tract infections are potential risks for the person with sickle cell disease.

#### Healthy person with sickle cell disease

Persons with severe complications increasingly represent a relatively small number of all patients with sickle cell disease.[4] This is because of management of symptoms during an episodic presentation of the disease and prevention of a crisis by early intervention. Many sickle cell patients are quite healthy, seldom experience severe pain, and live nearly normal life spans. For the adult with sickle cell disease, it is hoped that issues of employment, insurability, and positive self-image will be improved through increased recognition of the healthy person with sickle cell disease.

#### Sickle cell crisis

The sudden exacerbation of sickling can bring about a condition known as **sickle cell crisis.** Sickle cell crisis may be thrombotic, aplastic, megaloblastic, or splenic sequestration. *Vasoocclusive,* or *thrombotic, crisis* is the most common type and is caused by occlusion of blood vessels by the sickled cells. Pain is the primary symptom in thrombotic crisis. *Aplastic crisis* is most often secondary to infection and a temporary decrease in erythropoiesis resulting from the continuous stimulus for production of new RBCs. Because of the shortened RBC survival, the anemia rapidly worsens. Diagnosis may be made by bone marrow examination. Megaloblastic crisis appears in some cases to be caused by the depletion of bone marrow stores of folic acid. In such cases the crisis may be treated or prevented by administration of folic acid. Splenic sequestration crisis occurs when the spleen suddenly increases in size, leading to pooling of blood in the spleen and subsequent hypovolemia. Signs of shock are present.

#### Medical management

No specific therapy is available to treat sickle cell disease. Transfusion therapy may be given; the blood products generally used are packed RBCs. The goal of transfusion therapy depends on the specific condition: replacing RBCs for anemia, lowering the percentage of Hb S in an infarction, and increasing the amount of circulating Hgb and thus oxygen in overwhelming infections, leg ulcers, and pregnancy.

Analgesics, oxygen, and adequate hydration are given for vasoocclusive episodes. Pneumococcal vaccine may be given to prevent pneumococcal infections. Therapeutic apheresis also may be initiated.

## NURSING MANAGEMENT

### ♦ ASSESSMENT

#### Subjective Data

Data to be collected concern the person's knowledge and feelings about the disease and factors that appear to precipitate crisis or exacerbate symptoms. Fatigue may be reported when anemia is severe. Data pertaining to pain characteristics are appropriate when pain is present.

#### Objective Data

Objective data to be collected include vital signs, presence of blood in the urine, and overt signs of pain and restlessness.

### ♦ NURSING DIAGNOSES

Nursing diagnoses are determined from analysis of patient data. Prioritizing of nursing diagnoses depends on patient status and main concerns. Nursing diagnoses for the patient with sickle cell disease may include but are not limited to the following:

| Diagnostic Title | Possible Etiologic Factors |
|---|---|
| Pain | Imbalance between oxygen supply and demand |

| Diagnostic Title | Possible Etiologic Factors |
|---|---|
| Fluid volume deficit | Infection, over-exertion, weather changes, high Hgb levels, alcohol, smoking |
| Infection, high risk for | Decreased immune response |
| Tissue perfusion, altered | Decreased blood flow |
| Gas exchange, impaired | Ventilation/perfusion imbalance |
| Activity intolerance | Imbalance between oxygen supply and demand |
| Coping, ineffective (individual); coping, family: compromised | Crisis, prolonged disability |
| Knowledge deficit | Unfamiliarity with information |

## ♦ EXPECTED PATIENT OUTCOMES

Expected patient outcomes for the person with sickle cell disease may include but are not limited to the following:

1. Feels more comfortable and rested.
2. Has moist skin and mucous membranes.
3. Does not develop infection.
4. Has warm skin; reports no tissue pain.
5. Breathes easily and regularly.
6. Does not complain of fatigue or shortness of breath with activity.
7. Makes informed decisions with partner about family planning.
8. Describes the basis of the anemia, availability of genetic and regular counseling, measures to prevent infection, and events that may cause crisis.

## ♦ INTERVENTIONS

### Promoting Comfort and Oxygenation

The person who experiences weakness and fatigue from the anemia is assisted in planning daily activities to include rest periods. Oxygen is given for dyspnea or excessive fatigue with exertion.

Nursing care for painful episodes involves all the principles of pain management (see Chapter 17). The goal is to relieve the pain but not overmedicate. This usually involves the use of both narcotic and nonnarcotic analgesics. Astute evaluation of the effectiveness of pain medication is most important. Trends in managing pain in sickle cell crisis may include the use of patient-controlled analgesia by means of an infusion device through either a peripheral intravenous, CVP or VAD site.

### Promoting Hydration

The vasoocclusive nature of painful episodes requires adequate hydration to decrease blood viscosity. Patients who are supposedly in a steady state of their disease are advised to drink 4 to 6 quarts daily; this requirement increases to 6 to 8 quarts daily during a painful episode. If intravenous hydration is necessary, careful attention must be given to venous access, with avoidance of multiple punctures and infiltration. Use of a small-bore (No. 23) needle is recommended[3] because fewer needle sticks should be necessary to start the IV.

### Preventing Infection

Because patients with sickle cell disease have a high risk for infection, monitoring for early signs is important. Sites where infection is most likely to occur include intravenous insertion sites and CVP/VAD sites. Early signs of respiratory infection (cough, abnormal breath sounds) are reported to the physician.

### Promoting Tissue Perfusion

The patient is monitored for signs of pain that indicate blood vessel occlusion. Changes in pain or mental status are reported to the physician.

### Promoting Activity Tolerance

Persons who are trying to maintain independence with ADLs are encouraged to take regular rest periods. Increased time may be needed for daily care because of the patient's fatigue or dyspnea.

### Facilitating Family Planning and Genetic Counseling

Many people are now deciding when or if they want to have children. This is increasingly true for persons with genetic disorders such as sickle cell disease. Some forms of birth control, such as the intrauterine device (IUD), are not as highly recommended as other forms, such as the diaphragm or spermicides, for persons with sickle cell disorders. An IUD has a higher incidence of infection than the diaphragm or spermicides. To make a wise decision about contraception, a couple must be provided with accurate information about side effects, risks, and options (see Chapter 52). Such family counseling must be performed by persons who are well versed and knowledgeable about the options.

Family planning for persons with sickle cell disease can be a most difficult issue. The fact that a person carries a gene for the disorder makes it possible that this gene will be carried into the next generation. Although moral and ethical arguments can be made, it is ultimately the personal decision of the involved couple. Information about local services can be obtained from the National Association of Sickle Cell Disease.*

### Facilitating General Counseling

Sickle cell patients may sometimes be labeled as malingerers because some of them demonstrate difficult behavior patterns that are influenced by anxiety over their chronic illness. Counseling and the use of support groups are encouraged to minimize behavioral dependency. In caring for this patient population, it is also helpful to maintain a sense of respect and consideration for persons who experience frequent crises and yet continue to try to live as normal a life as possible.

*3345 Wilshire Blvd, Suite 1106, Los Angeles, CA 90010-1880.

# NURSING CARE PLAN

## PERSON WITH SICKLE CELL CRISIS

**DATA:** Mr. S. is a 24-year-old, married, African-American mail carrier, who is father of one child. He was diagnosed at age 10 years as having sickle cell disease but had been largely symptom-free until 2 years before this admission. When he was admitted with symptoms of sickle cell crisis, he had severe joint pain in upper and lower extremities, moderate fever (38.1° C), and shortness of breath.

**PHYSICAL EXAMINATION:** Coarse rales in both lower lobes, cyanosis of lips and nailbeds, dry scaly skin on both legs, 2+ pitting edema with a small (2 cm) reddened area over each medial malleolus. No hair was visible on toes. His Hgb was 9 g/dl.

**PHYSICIAN ORDERS:** Oxygen by nasal cannula, 4L/min, bed rest with bathroom privileges, morphine sulfate 15 mg IM q 3-4 hr prn. He was given two units of packed cells to be followed by IV fluids. Sickle cell crisis with congestive heart failure was diagnosed.

The nursing history identified the following:

- Mr. S. is very "worried" about the outcome of the hospitalization and his ability to "catch his breath."
- He expresses concern about his ability to support his family and be a "father" to his son and especially to take part in athletic events: "I'm hardly a man." His wife has assumed responsibility for some of the yard work, formerly his responsibility.
- He continues to exercise and jogs several times a week. He smokes one pack of cigarettes per day and states he has never been "a big fluid drinker," although he does have a beer a day. He states that he does not know what brings on the crisis.
- He is concerned about his sexual relationship with his wife because of his general fatigue. They had one child before he was aware of the genetic nature of the disease and expresses concern about having other children who might inherit the disease.

Collaborative nursing actions include those to maintain fluid and electrolyte balance, as well as peripheral and pulmonary oxygen/carbon dioxide balance, and to prevent further vascular occlusion.

Nursing actions include monitoring for the following:

- Signs of infection: hyperthermia, abnormal fluid, positive blood and sputum cultures, tachycardia, tachypnea.
- Signs of increased fluid/electrolyte imbalance, CHF and renal failure: hematocrit, electrolyte levels, intake and output, skin turgor; respiratory status (rate, depth of respiration, presence of crackles or wheezes, skin color, level of consciousness), renal function (creatinine, blood urea nitrogen).

### ■ NURSING DIAGNOSIS

Anxiety related to threat to self-concept, health status and role functioning

| Expected Patient Outcome | Nursing Interventions | Rationale |
|---|---|---|
| Shows decreased signs of anxiety. | Give Mr. S. opportunities to explore concerns about the effects of the disorder. | Making the unknown known may decrease anxiety. |
| | Assess his knowledge of sickle cell anemia and correct misunderstandings. | |
| | Teach relaxation measures. | Relaxation decreases the psychomotor responses to anxiety. |

### ■ NURSING DIAGNOSIS

High risk for infection related to spleen dysfunction, inadequate primary defense (broken skin), and inadequate secondary defenses (decreased hemoglobin)

| Expected Patient Outcome | Nursing Interventions | Rationale |
|---|---|---|
| Is free of infection. | Use good medical asepsis. | Aseptic technique decreases patient's contact with pathogenic organisms; infection is predicated on type and number of organisms to which patient is exposed, as well as patient resistance to infection. |
| | Restrict persons (staff members/visitors) with any type of infection. | Restricting persons with infection decreases patient's contact with infectious agents. |

# NURSING CARE PLAN

## PERSON WITH SICKLE CELL CRISIS—cont'd

### ■ NURSING DIAGNOSIS

Pain in joints and chest related to poor pain management techniques, lack of knowledge

| Expected Patient Outcome | Nursing Interventions | Rationale |
|---|---|---|
| States that he feels comfortable. | Give prescribed analgesics on a regular basis, and evaluate effectiveness of medication: obtain orders for increased doses if necessary. | Pain of sickle cell crisis is excruciating, and large doses of medication may be required. |
| | Identify measures Mr. S. has found helpful and include these measures in the care. | Patients often have the most accurate information for their pain control. |
| | Support joints gently when assisting patient to do ROM exercises. | Improper support increases stress on joints and increases pain. |
| | Use moist heat or massage, if helpful. | Heat dilates blood vessels and increases circulation to the area. Massage may increase circulation and relax tense muscles. |
| | Use other pain-relieving measures; person with frequent crises may benefit from learning special techniques such as biofeedback or self-hypnosis. | Biofeedback and self-hypnosis decrease the physiologic responses to pain (muscle spasm, increased pulse). |

### ■ NURSING DIAGNOSIS

Activity intolerance related to decreased oxygen transport

| Expected Patient Outcome | Nursing Interventions | Rationale |
|---|---|---|
| Has no dyspnea with activity and feels rested. | Provide prescribed oxygen as needed. | High concentration of $O_2$ in alveoli increases diffusion across membranes. |
| | Limit activities and provide periods of rest. | Decreased activity decreases $O_2$ needs of body. |
| | Administer prescribed transfusion (packed red cells). | Packed cells increase the number of RBCs available to carry $O_2$ to tissue cells in the anemic person. |

### ■ NURSING DIAGNOSIS

Sexual dysfunction related to fatigue, pain, fear of pregnancy

| Expected Patient Outcome | Nursing Interventions | Rationale |
|---|---|---|
| States that the sexual relationship is satisfying. | Discuss coital positions that require less energy for the person who becomes tired easily. | Coitus requires energy and involves neuromuscular activity; side lying or male-inferior position is less demanding for male patient. |
| | Suggest coitus at times of day when Mr. S. is less fatigued (morning, afternoon). | Fatigue increases with continued daily activities and demand on cardiovascular system. |
| | Discuss genetic counseling and contraceptive methods. | Knowledge of and use of reliable methods to prevent pregnancy reduce fear that may cause sexual dysfunction. |

# NURSING CARE PLAN

## PERSON WITH SICKLE CELL CRISIS—cont'd

### ■ NURSING DIAGNOSIS

Self-esteem disturbance related to loss of body function, change in life-style and masculine role

| Expected Patient Outcome | Nursing Interventions | Rationale |
|---|---|---|
| States satisfaction with life and self. | Provide opportunities for Mr. S. to discuss feelings about inability to fulfill expected roles. | Verbalization of concerns decreases their impact and assists in problem solving. |
| | Assist Mr. S. to identify personal strengths. | Focusing on strengths and positive factors provides a basis for personal growth. |
| | Assist Mr. S. to explore alternative ways to meet role expectations. | Concern over losses may immobilize patient; providing assistance in exploring alternatives fulfills a nurse's therapeutic role. |
| | Suggest joining a support group or obtaining counseling to minimize dependency behaviors. | Research shows that increased social support from family and groups increases recovery from disease and disability and facilitates rehabilitation. |

### ■ NURSING DIAGNOSIS

Knowledge deficit related to lack of exposure/recall and unfamiliarity with information sources

| Expected Patient Outcome | Nursing Interventions | Rationale |
|---|---|---|
| Describes the nature of the disorder and care requirements. | Review with Mr. S. the basis of sickle cell disease and genetic effects. | Knowledge of causes of disease is *one* factor in ensuring patient compliance with medical regimen and adherence to preventive measures. |
| | Provide resources for family planning and genetic counseling. | Persons and groups with in-depth knowledge of family planning methods help patients identify a family planning method that conforms to the patient's cultural and religious values. |
| | Encourage Mr. S. to avoid situations that cause crises (see text). | (See first rationale.) |
| | Teach Mr. S. to drink 4 to 6 quarts fluid daily. | Dehydration is a primary cause of RBC sickling. |

## Facilitating Learning

Teaching for the person with sickle cell disease includes the following:

1. Knowledge of the disease
2. Avoidance of situations that cause crisis (infection, overexertion, emotional stress, alcohol, cigarette smoking)
3. Importance of adequate fluid intake
4. Availability of psychologic support services and social resources
5. Need for medical follow-up

A nursing care plan for the patient with sickle cell disease is presented on p. 951.

## ♦ EVALUATION

To evaluate the effectiveness of nursing interventions, compare patient behaviors with those stated in the expected patient outcomes. Successful achievement of patient outcomes for the patient with sickle cell anemia are indicated by the following:

1. Feels more comfortable and rested.
2. Has moist skin and mucous membranes.
3. Has no infection.
4. Has warm skin and no tissue pain.
5. Breathes easily and regularly.
6. Has no complaints of fatigue or shortness of breath with activity.

7. Has made informed decisions with partner about family planning.
8. Correctly describes the basis of the anemia, availability of genetic and regular counseling, measures to prevent infection, and events that may cause crisis.

## Acquired Hemolytic Anemia

### Etiology/Pathophysiology

Acquired hemolytic anemia is most often drug-induced or is caused by an autoimmune disorder. In the latter case an antibody develops that is directed against an antigen on the individual's own erythrocytes. The antibody-coated RBCs are destroyed prematurely by reticuloendothelial cells, particularly in the spleen. **Autoimmune hemolytic anemia** may result from lymphocytic lymphomas or chronic lymphocytic leukemia, in the course of certain connective tissue disorders or idiopathically. Diagnosis is confirmed by demonstrating the presence of the antibody on the RBCs (antiglobin or Coombs' test) (see Chapter 70).

Drugs produce hemolysis in various ways. Methyldopa (Aldomet) is associated with production of an autoantibody and a positive Coombs' test result in approximately 20% of patients and a hemolytic anemia indistinguishable from an idiopathic autoimmune hemolytic anemia in 1%. More rarely, high-dose penicillin produces hemolysis through production of an antibody that requires the presence of penicillin on the RBC membrane for its effects to occur.

### Medical management

Medical therapy for autoimmune hemolytic anemia includes administration of corticosteroids, which are beneficial in approximately 50% of patients, or danazol (Danocrine), a gonadotropin inhibitor. Splenectomy is performed for those patients not sufficiently responsive to steroids or danazol and often is successful in controlling or ameliorating the disease. Transfusions may be given cautiously for life-threatening anemia, but this may be difficult and dangerous because of the autoantibody reacting not only with the patient's RBCs, but also with all donor cells.

### Nursing management

Nursing management consists of teaching the patient about the drug therapy, preparing the patient for surgery if indicated, and helping the patient and family to cope with the illness.

## Iron Deficiency Anemia

### Etiology/Pathophysiology

Iron is a fundamental part of the Hgb molecule, and its deficiency leads to production of RBCs with a decreased amount of Hgb and ultimately to fewer RBCs. The average adult body contains approximately 4 g of iron, 3 g of which are in Hgb, 500 mg to 1 g in iron stores in the liver and bone marrow, and the rest in certain tissues and enzyme systems. Average daily loss of iron by the body is approximately 1.5 mg, which is compensated for by absorption from the diet of approximately that amount of iron daily. This tenuous balance may be compromised by chronic blood loss, which may be physiologic, such as in menstruation, or pathologic, as in gastrointestinal (GI) or other bleeding. This compromise results in **iron deficiency anemia.**

Gradual development of iron deficiency anemia may permit adaptation with few clinical signs of anemia. Some persons may develop fatigue and exertional dyspnea (Box 34-2). With severe iron deficiency anemia, the nails become brittle and spoon-shaped (concave) and develop longitudinal ridges. The papillae of the tongue atrophy, and the tongue has a smooth, shiny, bright-red appearance. The corners of the mouth may crack and become red and painful (cheilosis). The anemia, which is characteristically hypochromic and microcytic, may be detected by observation of the peripheral blood smear and/or by blood cell indexes. Diagnosis may be confirmed by a low serum iron level and elevated serum iron–binding capacity or by a low serum ferritin level or absent iron stores in the bone marrow.

### Medical management

The first step in medical therapy is to determine and correct the cause. Repletion of iron stores in the body may then be accomplished by the administration of iron. Oral iron supplement usually is given in the form of ferrous sulfate.

### Nursing management

Patient teaching is the major nursing intervention, especially with a patient newly diagnosed with iron deficiency anemia. Because ferrous sulfate may be irritating to the GI tract, it should be taken after meals and with orange juice or vitamin C to increase the iron absorption. The person is told that the stools will be black and that symptoms of diarrhea or nausea should be reported to the physician. Constipation is a major side effect of iron supplementation, and a stool softener may be needed. When the patient cannot tolerate oral iron preparations or is unable to absorb iron properly, parenteral iron

**BOX 34-2 Clinical Manifestations of Iron Deficiency Anemia**

**MILD**

Fatigue and exertional dyspnea

**SEVERE**

Brittle, spoon-shaped nails with longitudinal ridges
Smooth, shiny tongue
Cheilosis

therapy is used. It is administered by deep intramuscular injection by use of the Z-track method.

Poor diet rarely is the sole cause of iron deficiency anemia but may be a contributing factor. The nurse assesses these patients for their knowledge and intake of a well-balanced diet and refers persons with insufficient financial means for food, medication, or medical attention to available community resources, including dietitian, social worker, or such resources as Meals on Wheels.

## Megaloblastic Anemia

**Megaloblastic anemia** refers to anemias with characteristic morphologic changes caused by defective deoxyribonucleic acid (DNA) synthesis and abnormal RBC maturation. On the peripheral blood smear, macrocytic RBCs and hypersegmented neutrophils (increased number of nuclei) are present. In the bone marrow, erythroid precursors can be found that are two to three times larger than normal, with nuclei that are immature relative to their cytoplasmic development.

### Etiology/Pathophysiology

Most megaloblastic anemias are caused by deficiency of either *vitamin $B_{12}$* or *folic acid* (see the following discussion). Both are essential in the synthesis of DNA, and their deficiency leads to impaired nuclear development in cells throughout the body. Deficiency of either leads to anemia and often leukopenia and thrombocytopenia. Administration of medication that interferes with DNA metabolism, such as chemotherapeutic agents and anticonvulsants, also can cause megaloblastic anemias.

### Vitamin $B_{12}$ deficiency

Vitamin $B_{12}$, obtained from dietary sources, combines with intrinsic factor in the stomach and is carried to the ileum, where it is absorbed and transported by a carrier protein to the tissues of the body.

**Pathophysiology.** Diagnosis of $B_{12}$ deficiency is made by demonstration of a low serum vitamin $B_{12}$ level in a patient with macrocytic anemia and megaloblastic bone marrow. In addition to the general symptoms associated with anemia, patients with $B_{12}$ deficiency may manifest neurologic abnormalities; in particular, they may develop a *peripheral neuropathy* and a *loss of balance* resulting from an abnormality of the posterior and lateral columns of the spinal cord (subacute combined degeneration).

A deficiency of vitamin $B_{12}$ may be the result of dietary deficiency, surgical removal of the stomach, malabsorption syndromes, or pernicious anemia. *Pernicious anemia* (PA) is caused by the absence of intrinsic factor. Dietary vitamin $B_{12}$ therefore cannot be absorbed. Diagnosis of PA is confirmed by an abnormal Schilling test result, which demonstrates the inability to absorb vitamin $B_{12}$ unless intrinsic factor also is administered.

**Medical management.** Treatment of vitamin $B_{12}$ deficiency consists of parenteral administration of vitamin $B_{12}$, usually once a month by nurses in an outpatient setting. The most common cause of relapse in persons with PA is their reluctance to continue therapy for life.

**Nursing management.** Patient teaching is a focus of nursing care and discharge planning. The patient must be assisted to understand the nature of the illness and the absolute necessity for continued treatment.

### Folic acid deficiency

**Folic acid deficiency** anemia may be caused by dietary deficiency, often in association with chronic alcoholism, overcooking of vegetables, malabsorption syndromes, and medications that inhibit the enzyme involved in normal folate absorption through the intestinal wall.[5]

Signs and symptoms are associated with the underlying disease and anemia in general. Laboratory findings include macrocytic anemia, megaloblastic changes in the bone marrow, and a low serum folate level.

**Management.** Most persons respond promptly to oral folic acid and a well-balanced diet. Return visits to nurse clinics and community health nurse home visits will help the person incorporate dietary modifications into daily life. Patients who drink alcohol excessively may be referred to Alcoholics Anonymous. Patients with financial limitations are referred to appropriate community resources.

# ERYTHROCYTOSIS

**Erythrocytosis** refers to an abnormal increase in erythrocytes. It may be caused secondarily by hypoxia (from high altitudes or from pulmonary and cardiac disease), by certain erythropoietin-producing tumors, or as a primary disorder (polycythemia vera). With hypoxia, RBCs increase as a compensatory mechanism to carry additional oxygen. Principal laboratory tests to determine the nature of erythrocytosis include determination of the arterial oxygen concentration, RBC volume, and plasma volume.

## Stress Erythropoiesis

Elevation of the Hgb and Hct levels may occur when the total RBC mass volume is normal but the plasma volume is decreased, leading to a contraction of the plasma volume. This **stress erythropoiesis** occurs predominantly in middle-aged men who are obese, hypertensive, and smokers. It is self-limiting and requires no therapy.

## Polycythemia Vera

### Pathophysiology

**Polycythemia vera** (primary polycythemia) is a bone marrow disorder characterized by erythrocytosis, usually with a simultaneous leukocytosis and thrombocy-

**BOX 34-3 Clinical Manifestations of Polycythemia Vera**

**EARLY STAGE**
No symptoms

**MODERATE STAGE**
Headaches, vertigo, tinnitus, blurred vision

**LATE STAGE**
Thrombosis, embolization
Nose bleeds, ecchymoses, GI bleeding

tosis. Hypervolemia, increased blood viscosity from the increased RBC mass, and platelet dysfunction occur. The etiology is unknown.

Symptoms frequently are absent in the early stages. As hypervolemia develops, symptoms include headaches, vertigo, tinnitus, and blurred vision. Thromboses with embolization may result from the increased blood viscosity, and the skin may develop a more reddened appearance. Platelet dysfunction may lead to nosebleeds, ecchymoses, and GI bleeding (Box 34-3). Thromboembolic events occur frequently and generally account for the early mortality rate.

Splenomegaly typically is found in polycythemia vera on physical examination, but it is not common in other types of erythrocytosis. Laboratory tests demonstrate an increased total RBC volume and a plasma volume that is either increased or normal. The Hct at sea level is greater than 53%. Arterial oxygen concentration is usually normal.

**Medical management.** Usual treatment is periodic phlebotomy aimed at maintaining the Hct and Hgb at a normal level. In some patients who need phlebotomy too frequently, other modes of therapy may be required, such as the use of radioactive phosphorus ($^{32}P$) or an alkylating agent such as busulfan. There is an increased incidence of other hematologic disorders arising in the course of polycythemia vera, especially acute leukemia, and this has been accentuated with the use of alkylating agents in the treatment regimen.

**Nursing management.** Teaching for the person with polycythemia vera includes the following:

1. Nature of the disorder
2. Importance of continued medical care, blood tests, and phlebotomy
3. Name, dosage, frequency, desired action, and side effects of prescribed medications
4. Signs of extremity thromboses (swelling, redness, pain) requiring immediate medical attention
5. Maintenance of hydration to decrease blood viscosity

# DISORDERS OF HEMOSTASIS, PLATELETS, AND COAGULATION

## PATHOPHYSIOLOGY

Normal hemostatic functioning is an intricate system that requires vascular integrity, normal numbers and functioning of platelets, and normal clotting factors. Although each of the essential components arises separately and is independently regulated, the balanced interplay among these components is necessary to protect the body from excessive bleeding or excessive thrombi formation.

Primary hemostasis involves the formation of a platelet plug over a damaged area of endothelial cells lining a blood vessel. Primary hemostasis is completed with the formation of the platelet plug. Secondary hemostasis is the formation of a fibrin clot overlying the platelet plug. This process requires the sequential activation in the cascade of clotting factors (Figure 34-4). The major steps are the formation of thrombin from prothrombin leading to the formation of fibrin from fibrinogen. (Coagulation factors are listed in Box 33-1.)

A *fibrinolytic* mechanism exists to balance clot formation and leads to *clot lysis.* Two enzymes are involved in clot lysis, plasminogen and plasmin. Plasminogen is the inactive form that circulates in the blood. It is converted to plasmin by the action of active Hageman factor in addition to other factors. Plasmin then degrades and dissolves the clot. Streptokinase is an enzyme that is fibrinolytic.

Another balance to clot formation are substances called *anticoagulants.* A naturally occuring anticoagulant is heparin, which acts by interferring with activation of several coagulation factors, including activation of thrombin. Coumarin derivatives interfere with synthesis of coagulation factors II, VII, IX, and X in the liver by interfering with vitamin K. Heparin interferes with the intrinsic mechanisim whereas coumadin interferes with the extrinsic mechanism.

Disorders of platelets and coagulation are listed in Box 34-4.

## THROMBOCYTOPENIA

### Etiology

**Thrombocytopenia** is defined as a lower-than-normal number of circulating platelets. Laboratory values for a normal adult platelet count range from 150,000 to 400,000/mm³. The many types of thrombocytopenia may result from (1) decreased platelet production, (2) decreased platelet survival, (3) increased platelet destruction (most common form), or (4) sequestration of blood in the spleen.

The most common cause of increased destruction of platelets is **idiopathic thrombocytopenic purpura (ITP).** ITP occurs most often in the second and third decades of life and is caused by production of an autoantibody (IgG) directed against a platelet antigen. It

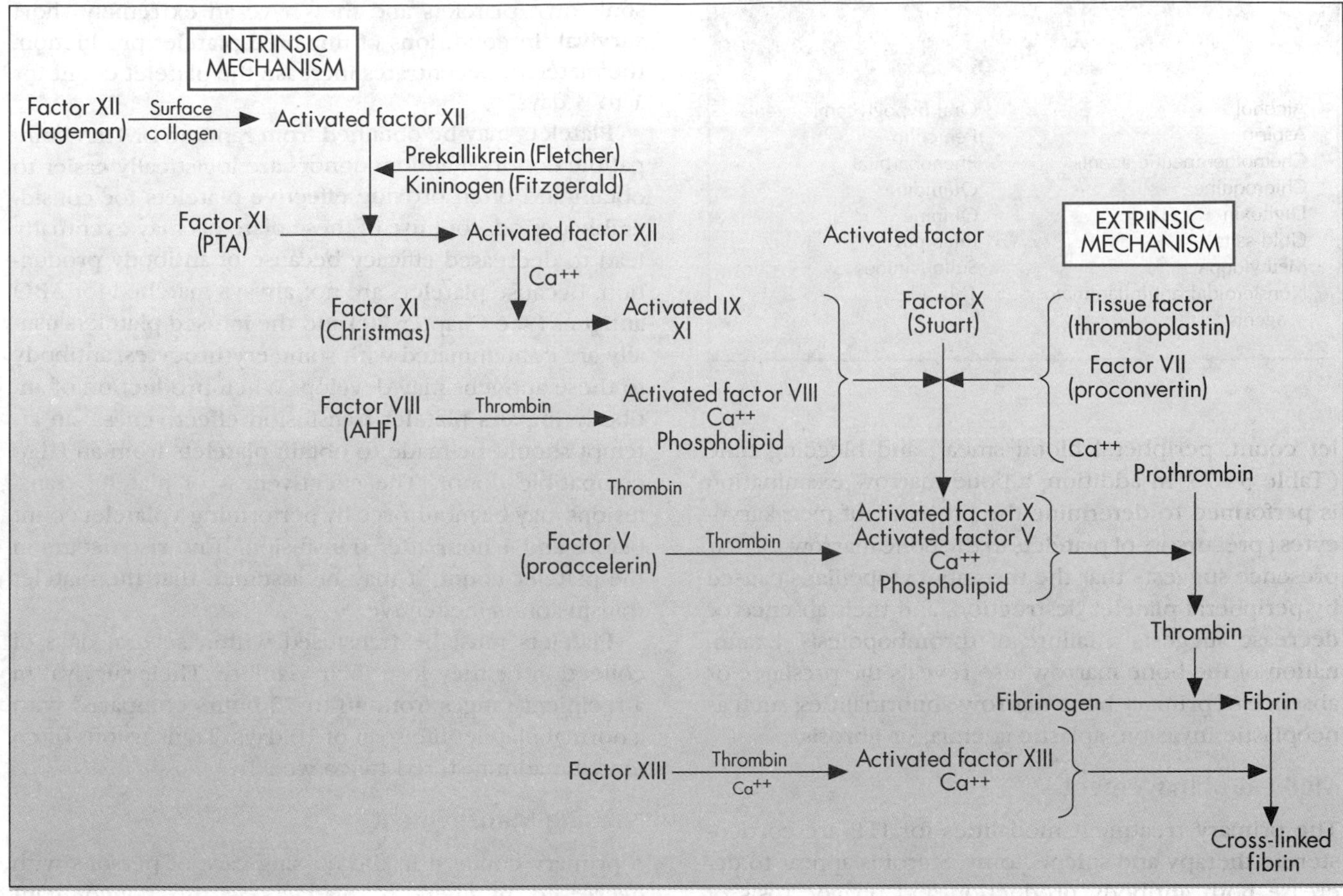


**FIGURE 34-4** Mechanisms of blood coagulation.

**BOX 34-4 Disorders Associated With Platelets and Coagulation**

| | |
|---|---|
| **PLATELETS** | |
| Thrombocytopenia | Decreased number of platelets |
| Thrombocytosis | Increased number of platelets |
| Bleeding syndromes | Disorders of platelet function |
| **COAGULATION** | |
| **Congenital** | |
| Hemophilia A | Decrease of factor VIII |
| Hemophilia B | Decrease of factor IX |
| von Willebrand's disease | Decrease of factor VIII and defective platelet aggregation |
| **Acquired** | |
| Vitamin K deficiency | Decrease of factors II, VII, IX, and X |
| Disseminated intravascular coagulation | Stimulates first the clotting process, then the fibrinolytic process |

has thus been suggested that this disorder be named *autoimmune* thrombocytopenia purpura (ATP).[7]

Platelet destruction also may be drug-induced. Approximately 70 drugs (some of which are listed in Box 34-5) have been shown to induce thrombocytopenia.[7] Platelet counts generally return to normal within 1 to 2 weeks after the drug is withdrawn; some drugs such as gold salts may require several months.

Secondary thrombocytopenia may result from aplastic anemia, acute leukemia, and conditions causing splenomegaly (such as cirrhosis or lymphomas) that lead to sequestration of blood in the spleen.

## Pathophysiology

The major signs of thrombocytopenia observable by physical examination are *petechiae, ecchymoses,* and *purpura* on the skin. Petechiae occur only in platelet disorders. The person may give a history of menorrhagia, epistaxis, and gingival bleeding. The patient is questioned about recent viral infections, which may produce a transient thrombocytopenia; drugs in current use; and extent of alcohol ingestion.

Diagnostic tests include complete laboratory studies to ascertain the status of all blood components. The most frequently used tests for assessment of platelets are plate-

**BOX 34-5 Selected Drugs Typically Causing Thrombocytopenia**

| | |
|---|---|
| Alcohol | Oral hypoglycemic agents |
| Aspirin | Penicillin |
| Chemotherapeutic agents | Phenobarbital |
| Chloroquine | Quinidine |
| Digitoxin | Quinine |
| Gold salts | Rifampin |
| Methyldopa | Sulfonamides |
| Nonsteroidal antiinflammatory agents | Thiazides |

let count, peripheral blood smear, and bleeding time (Table 34-7). In addition, a bone marrow examination is performed to determine the presence of megakaryocytes (precursors of platelets in the bone marrow). Their presence suggests that the thrombocytopenia is caused by peripheral platelet destruction, and their absence or decrease suggests a failure of thrombopoiesis. Examination of the bone marrow also reveals the presence or absence of primary bone marrow abnormalities, such as neoplastic invasion, aplastic anemia, or fibrosis.

## Medical Management

The primary treatment modalities for ITP are corticosteroid therapy and splenectomy. Steroids appear to decrease both antibody production and phagocytosis of the antibody-coated platelets. Splenectomy removes the principal organ involved in destruction of the antibody-coated platelets. Other therapeutic modalities include danazol, γ-globulin, or immunosuppressive drugs. Plasma exchange, a form of experimental therapy, may have some efficacy in acute ITP.

### Platelet transfusion

Transfusion with platelet concentrates may be used in persons with thrombocytopenic bleeding. It is not usually helpful for ITP because the transfused platelets are rapidly destroyed by the same mechanism as the person's own platelets and they have an extremely short survival. In conditions of impaired platelet production, the platelet concentrates increase the platelet count for 1 to 3 days.

Platelets may be obtained from random or HLA-compatible donors. Random donors are logistically easier to obtain and often provide effective platelets for considerable periods, but use of these platelets may eventually lead to decreased efficacy because of antibody production. Because platelets are not always matched for ABO antigens (see Chapter 70) and the infused platelets usually are contaminated with some erythrocytes, antibody to these antigens may develop. When production of antibody impairs platelet transfusion effectiveness, an attempt should be made to obtain platelets from an HLA-compatible donor. The effectiveness of platelet transfusions may be monitored by performing a platelet count before and 1 hour after transfusion. If no rise occurs in the platelet count, it may be assumed that the platelet transfusion is ineffective.

Platelets must be transfused within several days of collection or they lose their viability. Their survival in a recipient ranges from 48 to 72 hours compared with a normal platelet life span of 10 days. Transfusions often must be administered twice weekly.

## Nursing Management

A primary concern in the nursing care of persons with decreased numbers of platelets is the concomitant bleeding tendency. Bleeding associated with trauma is likely with a platelet count less than 60,000/mm$^3$. Spontaneous hemorrhage may be a life-threatening possibility when the platelet count is less than 20,000/mm$^3$.

Ongoing nursing assessment of the patient is essential and includes alertness for increased ecchymoses, petechiae, bleeding from other sites, and any change in mental status. The need for avoidance of trauma is obvious. Bleeding precautions to institute for persons with counts below 20,000/mm$^3$ include the following:

1. Test all urine and stools for blood (guaiac).
2. Avoid rectal temperatures.

**TABLE 34-7 Common Bleeding/Coagulation Blood Tests**

| TEST | DESCRIPTION | NORMAL VALUE |
|---|---|---|
| Bleeding time | Evaluation of vascular and platelet factors—the time it takes for a small stab wound to stop bleeding | 2-9 min |
| Clotting time | Time required for solid clot to form (less sensitive test than PTT) | 5-10 min |
| Prothrombin time (PT) | Indicates rapidity of blood clotting (indicative of adequacy of extrinsic coagulation pathway; factors I, II, V, VII, X) | 11-16 sec; 100% as compared with control levels |
| Partial thromboplastin time (PTT) | More sensitive test than PT to evaluate adequacy of intrinsic coagulation pathway (fibrin clot formation) | 60-70 sec |
| Activated partial thromboplastin time (APTT) | Modified PTT; more sensitive; quicker to perform; frequently used to monitor heparin therapy and hemophilia | 30-45 sec |

3. Avoid intramuscular injections.
4. Apply pressure to all venipuncture sites for 5 minutes and to all arterial puncture sites for 10 minutes.

Patient teaching is an important component of patient care. Points to be included in the teaching are listed in the Guidelines box below.

## THROMBOCYTOSIS

**Thrombocytosis** is defined as the presence of an abnormally high number of platelets in the circulating blood. It may be seen in association with polycythemia vera, myelofibrosis, splenectomy, iron deficiency anemia, or chronic inflammatory diseases; or it may occur as a separate neoplastic disorder, hemorrhagic thrombocythemia.

The major problems incurred by persons with thrombocytosis are thrombosis or increased bleeding tendencies. Medical and nursing management is similar to that described for persons receiving anticoagulation therapy (see Chapter 32).

## DISORDERS OF PLATELET FUNCTION

Mild bleeding syndromes may be caused by quantitatively normal but functionally defective platelets. The most common cause of such platelet abnormalities is drugs, particularly aspirin. Aspirin inhibits the release of intrinsic platelet adenosine diphosphate (ADP) and produces a defect in platelet aggregation. The defect remains for the life span of the platelet. A variety of familial and nonfamilial platelet disorders also have been described, and defective platelet function typically occurs in persons with uremia. The abnormality may be detected by a test of bleeding time or, more sensitively, by platelet aggregation tests. Disorders of platelet function have clinical manifestations and patient care needs similar to those of thrombocytopenia, although the bleeding abnormality usually is mild.

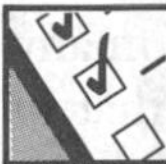

### Guidelines for Teaching the Person With Thrombocytopenia

1. Nature of the disorder
2. Signs of decreased platelets (petechiae, ecchymoses, gingival bleeding, hematuria, menorrhagia)
3. Name, dosage, frequency, and side effects of prescribed medications (corticosteroids) and importance of not stopping corticosteroid medications suddenly
4. Measures to prevent injury
   a. Use a soft toothbrush or swab for mouth care.
   b. Keep mouth clean and free of debris.
   c. Avoid intrusions into rectum (e.g., rectal medications, enemas).
   d. Use electric shaver.
   e. Apply direct pressure for 5 to 10 minutes if any bleeding occurs.
   f. Avoid contact sports, elective surgery, and tooth extraction.
   g. Avoid blood thinning drugs, such as aspirin, that decrease sticking ability of platelet.
5. Need for follow-up medical care

## HEMOPHILIA

### Etiology/Epidemiology

**Hemophilia** is a hereditary coagulation disorder. Both hemophilia A (factor VIII deficiency) and hemophilia B (factor IX deficiency) are inherited as sex-linked recessive disorders and are therefore almost exclusively limited to males. An example of the inheritance pattern of hemophilia is shown in Figure 34-5. The incidence of hemophilia A is 1:10,000, and for hemophilia B, 1:100,000 of the male population.

### Pathophysiology

The diagnosis of hemophilia usually is made in infancy or early childhood. The clinical history is one of lifelong bleeding tendency. A history of excessive bleeding after circumcision or dental extractions frequently is obtained. Persons with hemophilia may give a history of bleeding into any part of the body—spontaneously or after trauma (Box 34-6).

A diagnosis of hemophilia is made by specific assays for factors VIII and IX. The partial thromboplastin time (PTT), which reflects the intrinsic pathway of coagulation, is prolonged in both hemophilia A and hemophilia B. The platelet count and prothrombin time (PT) are normal.

Complications associated with hemophilia are the direct result of the bleeding tendency. Frequently the person experiences repeated episodes of spontaneous bleeding into the joints, resulting in several joint deformities. Bleeding that is life-threatening involves retroperitoneal, intracranial, and paratracheal soft tissue hemorrhages.

### Medical Management

Treatment consists of replacement of the deficient coagulation factor when bleeding episodes do not respond to local treatment (ice bags, manual pressure or dressings, immobilization, elevation, topical coagulants such as fibrin foam and thrombin). Because the deficient factors are contained in plasma, the treatment used for many years was fresh plasma and blood or fresh frozen plasma. In major hemorrhages, adequate blood levels

**BOX 34-6 Clinical Manifestations of Hemophilia**

- History of lifelong bleeding tendency
- Repeated episodes of spontaneous bleeding into joints
- Excessive bleeding after dental extractions
- Life-threatening hemorrhages: retroperitoneal, intracranial, paratracheal

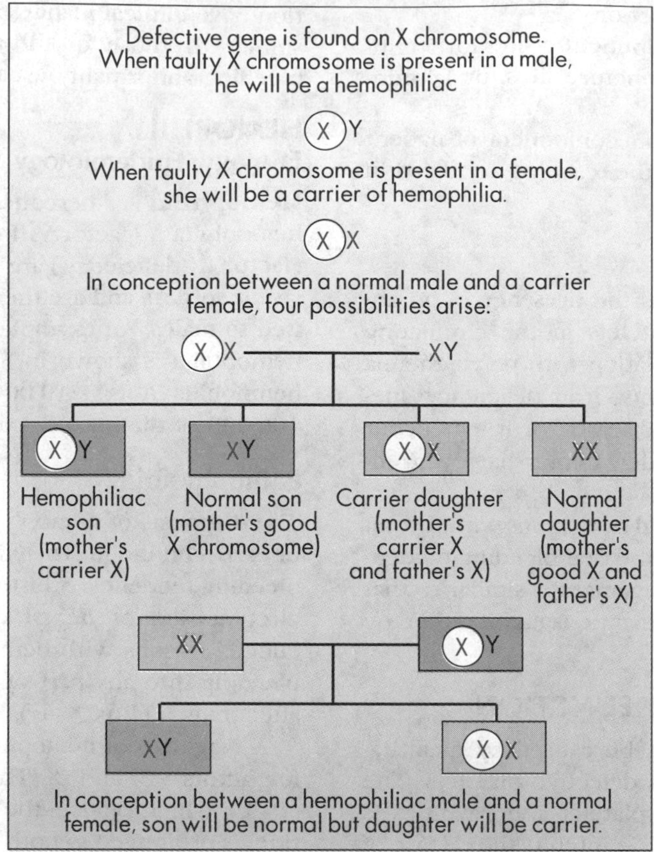


**FIGURE 34-5** Pattern of inheritance of hemophilia.

were difficult to maintain without overloading the person's circulation with large volumes of blood and plasma. The discovery of cryoprecipitate in 1964 led the way to the development of commercially prepared concentrated preparations such as fibrinogen, factor VIII, and a concentrate containing the four vitamin K–dependent factors (prothrombin and factors VII, IX, and X). Concentrates avoid the problem of circulatory overload and produce fewer adverse effects (e.g., urticarial or febrile reactions) in some patients. High cost and possible contamination with the virus of serum hepatitis or acquired immunodeficiency syndrome (AIDS) have been drawbacks, however, to the use of some of the concentrates from pooled blood.

A number of persons with hemophilia A have developed AIDS from transfusions of factor VIII concentrate. This problem has been corrected with the testing of blood donors for evidence of the human immunodeficiency virus (HIV) virus and with heat treatment of the factor VIII concentrates that kills the AIDS virus.

In classic hemophilia the treatment of choice for an acute bleeding episode is infusion of concentrates of the antihemophilic factor (factor VIII). One such concentrate is cryoprecipitate. This concentrate is extracted and concentrated by slowly thawing previously frozen plasma at refrigerator temperature. Most of the factor VIII remains as a gel and can be separated from the rest of the plasma by centrifugation. The gel is reconstituted by the addition of saline solution. After the antihemophilic factor is extracted, the remaining plasma may be used for other purposes. This process results in a concentration of factor VIII as high as 15 to 40 times that of normal plasma. It can be produced and stored in any well-equipped blood bank at a cost well below that of other concentrates. Treatment with cryoprecipitate is conducted in ambulatory care centers. Home infusion programs also control bleeding episodes effectively, thereby decreasing the need for hospitalization and absence from school or work.

DDAVP (D-amino-8-D-arginine vasopressin) has been demonstrated to increase the factor VIII level in persons with von Willebrand's disease and mild hemophilia A. It is given intravenously and has been associated with few side effects. It does not carry the risk of transmitting hepatitis, AIDS, or other disorders and should play an increasingly significant role in the treatment of these disorders.

The outlook for the person with hemophilia has been greatly improved by the availability of transfusion therapy. In the past, many persons with factor VIII deficiency died in infancy or in the first 5 years of life. Surgical procedures can now be performed and joint deformity prevented, thus increasing quality of life. Today many persons with moderate or mild hemophilia can live normal, productive lives.

### Nursing Management

Adults with hemophilia generally are knowledgeable about their disease. They must be aware of the possibility of hemorrhage after dental extraction, injury, or surgery. Persons who have hemophilia should carry a card or wear a Medic-Alert tag that includes their name, blood type, physician's name, and their disorder so that medical treatment will not be delayed if they should accidentally sustain injury and lose consciousness.

Pain control and the threat of spontaneous bleeding episodes are ongoing stressors the person must confront. Those persons who are able to meet the demands of their illness and adapt their life-styles accordingly are able to live productive lives as individuals, spouses, parents, and employees. Genetic counseling, aimed at explaining the pattern of inheritance of hemophilia, may be of great value to adults contemplating parenthood. Such counseling can serve to assist potential parents to evaluate realistically their ability to raise a child afflicted with hemophilia and to anticipate ways to meet the demands placed on both them and the child.

The National Hemophilia Foundation* is an organization established for persons with hemophilia and their families. There are 45 chapters across the United States. The basic function of the national organization is hemophilia research. In addition, it establishes standards for chapters, publishes literature, produces films, and promotes health care legislation in Washington, DC. Local chapter services include special camps for children with hemophilia; parent, child, and adult counseling; group therapy sessions for parents; and a newsletter that reports on advances in hemophilic care. A chapter may function as a liaison agent between hospitals and families with insurmountable bills for blood.

## VITAMIN K DEFICIENCY

### Etiology

Vitamin K, a fat-soluble vitamin, is a cofactor in the synthesis of clotting factors II, VII, IX, and X. Approximately 50% of required vitamin K is obtained from a normal diet, and 50% is produced by intestinal bacteria. Deficiencies in vitamin K can be anticipated in persons who have a decreased intake and who are given broad-spectrum antibiotics (such as neomycin sulfate) that decrease the growth of intestinal bacteria. Interference with vitamin K absorption occurs with primary intestinal disease (e.g., ulcerative colitis, Crohn's disease), biliary disease, and malabsorption syndromes. Drugs such as coumarin derivatives and large doses of salicylates, quinine, and barbiturates interfere with vitamin K function.

*110 Greene St, Suite 303, New York, NY 10012.

### Pathophysiology

Symptoms are those of **hypoprothrombinemia** superimposed on the underlying disease. Bleeding is similar to other coagulation disorders—that is, bleeding of the mucous membranes and into the tissues. Postoperative hemorrhage may be observed. In severe cases GI bleeding may be massive. The PT is prolonged.

### Medical Management

Treatment consists of therapy for the underlying disorder and cessation of causative drugs. For mild disorders a water-soluble vitamin K preparation (menadione) is given orally or parenterally. In severe disorders a fat-soluble vitamin K preparation (phytonadione) may be given. Fresh frozen plasma will partially correct the disorder immediately, whereas vitamin K therapy takes 6 to 24 hours to be effective but does not have the complications of fresh frozen plasma.

### Nursing Management

Nursing management includes monitoring of vital signs and patient teaching regarding safety precautions to prevent bruising or bleeding episodes (avoid trauma, use soft toothbrush, avoid intramuscular injections, and apply direct pressure immediately on any bleeding sites).

## DISSEMINATED INTRAVASCULAR COAGULATION

**Disseminated intravascular coagulation (DIC)** is a response of the body's hemostatic mechanisms to a variety of diseases or injury. DIC is a complicated and potentially fatal process that is characterized initially by clotting and secondarily by hemorrhage. It almost always occurs in response to a primary disease.

### Etiology

DIC is essentially an imbalance between the processes of coagulation and anticoagulation. Many disease states may alter the normal balance of clotting and fibrinolytic factors, which under normal conditions prevent bleeding while maintaining the fluidity of the blood. DIC may be directly or indirectly initiated by conditions that trigger at least one of three mechanisms: factor XII formation, activation of factors II and X, and tissue thromboplastin release[2] (Box 34-7). Stimuli such as sepsis, anoxia, or burns most likely cause activation of the intrinsic clotting system by the release of factor XII after endothelial cell wall damage and platelet aggregation. DIC may be caused by factor VII activation from massive trauma or the release of tissue thromboplastin from an amniotic fluid embolus entering the maternal circulation. Proteolytic enzymes in snake venom can cause direct activation of factors II and X.

### Pathophysiology

The primary disease causes the initiation of the clotting process. This response is generalized and occurs

**BOX 34-7 Precipitating Conditions Associated With Disseminated Intravascular Coagulation**

**ENDOTHELIAL CELL WALL DAMAGE: FACTOR XII FORMATION**

| | |
|---|---|
| Anaphylaxis | Vasculitis |
| Systemic lupus erythematosus | Anoxia |
| Transfusion reaction | Acidosis |
| Sepsis | Liver disease |
| Burns | |

**TISSUE THROMBOPLASTIN RELEASE: FACTOR VII ACTIVATION**

| | |
|---|---|
| Carcinoma | Extracorporeal circulation |
| Leukemia | Abruptio placentae |
| Blunt trauma | Amniotic fluid embolus |
| Hemolytic anemia | Retained dead fetus |
| Sepsis | |

**ACTIVATION OF FACTORS II AND X**

| | |
|---|---|
| Snake venom | Pancreatitis |
| Liver disease | |

Modified from Williams I, Earles AN, Pack B: *Nurs Clin North Am* 18(1):215-229, 1983.

throughout the vascular system, creating a state of *hypercoagulability.* The fibrinolytic processes, which normally operate to limit clot extension and dissolve clots, are then stimulated (Figure 34-6). As clotting factors are depleted and fibrinolysis continues, a state of *hypocoagulability* develops.

The most common sequela of DIC is hemorrhage. This paradox is caused by (1) decreased platelets, (2) depletion of clotting factors II, V, VIII, and fibrinogen in the clotting process, and (3) the production of fibrin degradation products (FDPs) through fibrinolysis. The FDPs act as anticoagulants, which increase the hemorrhagic tendency.

Laboratory findings may be the only indications of DIC in the early stages and usually include thrombocytopenia, low levels of fibrinogen, and prolonged PT and PTT (Table 34-8). In addition, low levels of factors V and VIII are present, and abnormal RBCs may be found on peripheral smear. Characteristically, there is evidence of fibrinolysis, which is reflected in increased fibrin split products, D-dimers, and prolonged thrombin time. As the disorder progresses, clinical manifestations may include *bleeding of the mucous membranes and tissues* (petechiae, ecchymoses). Oral, vaginal, gastrointestinal, and rectal bleeding and bleeding after injections and venipunctures may occur.

## Medical Management

The management of DIC must always begin with treatment of the primary disease. Once this has been initiated, the goal is to control the bleeding and restore normal levels of clotting factors. Blood products such as fresh frozen plasma, platelet packs, cryoprecipitate, and fresh whole blood may be administered to replace the depleted factors. Heparin has been used to inhibit the underlying thrombotic process; however, it too often promotes rather than decreases bleeding, and its use is controversial.

## Nursing Management

Nursing intervention in the care of the patient with DIC is extremely challenging. The person who develops DIC

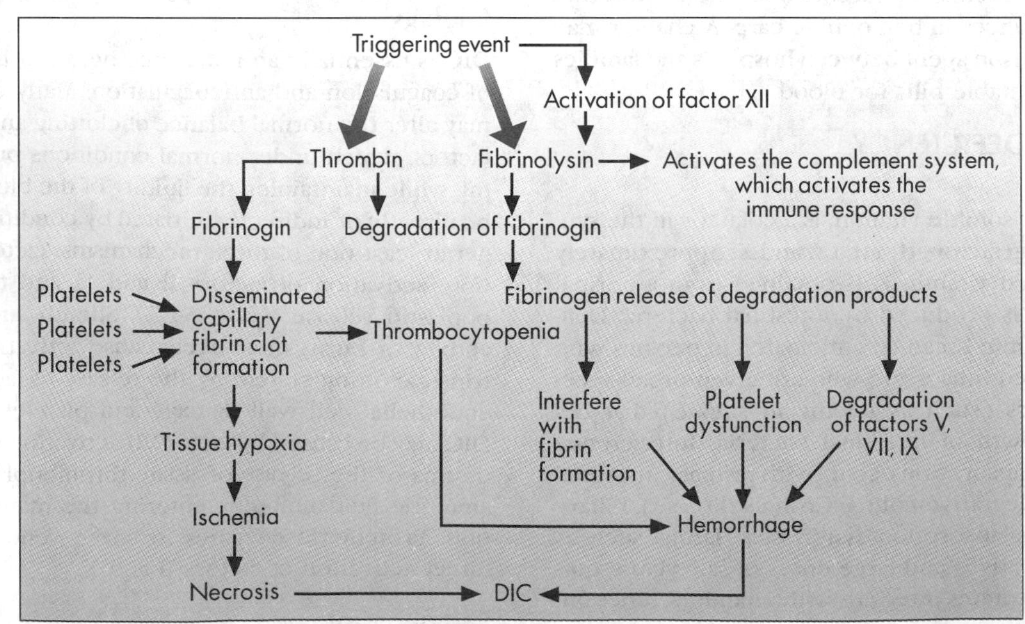


**FIGURE 34-6** Pathophysiology of disseminated intravascular coagulation. (From Yasko JM: *Guidelines for cancer care: symptom management,* Reston Va, 1983, Reston Publishing.)

**TABLE 34-8 Laboratory Profile of Disseminated Intravascular Coagulation**

| DIAGNOSTIC TEST | NORMAL VALUE | EXPECTED VALUE IN DIC |
|---|---|---|
| Prothrombin time (PT) | 11-15 sec | Prolonged |
| Partial thromboplastin time (PTT) | 60-70 sec | Usually prolonged |
| Thrombin time | 10-13 sec | Usually prolonged |
| Fibrinogen level | 200-400 mg/100 ml | Decreased |
| Platelet level | 150,000-400,000/mm$^3$ | Decreased |
| Factor assay (II, V, VII, VIII, IX, X, XI, XII) | | Decreased levels of factors V, VIII, and IX |
| Fibrinogin/fibrin degradation products (FDP) | <10 | Increased |
| Protamine sulfate test (soluble fibrin monomer) | Negative | Strongly positive |
| Antithrombin III levels (AT-III) (used to monitor response to therapy) | 89%-120% | Decreased |

From Yasko JM: *Guidelines for cancer care: symptom management,* Reston, Va, 1983, Reston Publishing.

is critically ill and frequently has numerous sites of bleeding. The amount and nature of drainage from chest and nasogastric tubes, oozing from surgical incisions, or progressive discoloration of the skin should be noted and recorded.

Continual observation for new bleeding sites and for an increase or decrease in bleeding is an integral part of the nursing plan, especially if heparin therapy is being used. The susceptibility of these persons to bleeding presents special problems; medications should be given orally or intravenously if at all possible, and small-gauge needles should be used when other injections are necessary. The precautions previously described for thrombocytopenia are applicable to the patient with DIC (see Guidelines box, p. 959).

Maintaining fluid balance assumes great importance. Persons with DIC usually lose large quantities of blood and receive frequent transfusions and other fluid replacement. In addition to monitoring blood infusion rates carefully, the nurse must be alert to signs of fluid overload such as slow, bounding pulse and increasing central venous pressure. Hourly urine output is recorded not only as another indication of cardiac function but also because of the possibility of renal thrombi formation and subsequent renal failure.

Frequently the patient is comatose, and the presence of purpura, numerous intravenous lines, and drainage tubes makes the patient's appearance especially upsetting to the family. Most of the primary conditions associated with DIC are of a sudden nature, and the family requires preparation and help in understanding this catastrophic occurrence and support during the long period of treatment.

# DISORDERS ASSOCIATED WITH WHITE BLOOD CELLS

The WBC (leukocyte) system is composed of neutrophils, lymphocytes, monocytes, basophils, and eosinophils. All but the lymphocytes are derived from a common stem cell. The primary function of WBCs is to provide for humoral and cellular response to infection. Neutrophils are primarily responsible for phagocytosis and the destruction of bacteria and other infectious organisms. Lymphocytes are the principal cells involved in immunity, which is responsible for the development of delayed hypersensitivity and the production of antibodies (see Chapter 13). Any compromise in the integrity of the WBC system renders a person susceptible to infection.

## NEUTROPENIA

### Etiology/Pathophysiology

**Neutropenia** is defined as a neutrophil count of less than 2000/mm$^3$. Neutropenia may occur as a primary hematologic disorder, but more often it is seen in association with other disorders, including malignant diseases of the bone marrow, aplastic anemia, megaloblastic anemia, use of chemotherapeutic agents, and hypersplenism. The degree of susceptibility to infection is in direct proportion to the degree of neutropenia. Persons with severe neutropenia are at risk of contracting a life-threatening infection.

### Medical Management

Severe neutropenia, sometimes referred to as *agranulocytosis,* occurs as a reaction to a variety of drugs and chemicals, including sulfonamides, propylthiouracil, and chloramphenicol. Specific treatment consists of removing the offending agent.

Granulocyte transfusion may be used for the patient with severe neutropenia whose condition is life threatening—for example, with the development of an infection.[7]

### Nursing Management

A person with a compromised WBC system is highly susceptible to life-threatening infections. Nursing care is directed toward protecting the patient from potential sources of infection and assiduous monitoring to detect the earliest signs of infection so that prompt therapy may be instituted. Likewise, patients and family members must be taught to recognize early signs of infection. The patient wears a mask when going from the unit for a test or x-ray examination. Meticulous washing of the hands by medical and nursing personnel and strict asepsis are mandatory. The environment should be kept scrupulously clean and dustless, and no person with any type of infection should be allowed in contact with the patient. Family members and hospital personnel need frequent reminders of this. Mild colds and respiratory tract infections, taken for granted in daily life, are serious threats to patients with decreased numbers of WBCs.

Patients should be in private rooms with posted isolation signs. When this is not possible, cautious screening of roommates for a potential source of infection is mandatory. To decrease exposure to bacteria, fresh fruits, vegetables, and flowers are not permitted.

(Further discussion of nursing care of patients with neutropenia is contained in Chapter 16.)

## NEUTROPHILIA

**Neutrophilia** is defined as a neutrophil count greater than 10,000/mm$^3$. Such an increase is a normal response to infections, primarily bacterial infections. Prolonged elevation of the neutrophil count, especially in the absence of an apparent cause, demands a diligent search for the underlying cause. Persistent elevated neutrophil counts are associated with leukemia, polycythemia vera, myeloid metaplasia, and various systemic and inflammatory disorders.

## LEUKEMIA

### Etiology

**Leukemia** is a malignant disorder of the hematopoietic system involving the bone marrow and lymph nodes; it is characterized by uncontrolled proliferation of leukocytes and their precursors. With rare exceptions, the bone marrow is involved at the onset, with infrequent manifestations in other hematopoietic organs that lead to organ enlargement (splenomegaly, hepatomegaly). The proliferation of one type of cell often interferes with the normal production of other hematopoietic cells, resulting in the development of immature cells, thrombocytopenia, and anemia. The immaturity of the WBCs leads to decreased immunocompetence and increased susceptibility to infections. The cause of leukemia is unknown.

Although the causative factors that lead to the development of acute leukemia in most patients have not been identified, some predisposing relationships have been discovered. Persons with specific chromosomal aberrations, such as occurs with Down syndrome, von Recklinghausen's neurofibromatosis, and Fanconi's anemia, have an increased incidence of acute leukemia. Chronic exposure to chemicals, such as benzene; drugs that cause aplastic anemia; and radiation exposure have been associated with an increased incidence of the disease. An increased risk for development of acute leukemia has been noted after cytotoxic therapy for Hodgkin's disease, non-Hodgkin's lymphoma, multiple myeloma, polycythemia vera, and breast, lung, and testicular cancers.

The leukemias are classified as acute or chronic and are further subdivided according to cell type or maturity. *Acute* leukemias involve immature cells and are categorized according to the predominant cell in the bone marrow. They are subclassified as acute lymphocytic leukemia (ALL) or acute nonlymphocytic leukemia (ANLL) according to the specific morphology of the leukemic cell. ANLL is further classified as acute myelogenous (AML), promyelocytic, monocytic, and other varieties according to cell type. Distinguishing among the various subclassifications of ANLL is difficult, but it is important to do so because newer chemotherapeutic agents appear to have more success against some types and almost none against others. *Chronic* leukemias may be lymphocytic, as in chronic lymphocytic leukemia (CLL), or granulocytic, as in chronic granulocytic or myelogenous leukemia (CML) (Table 34-9).

### Pathophysiology

Acute leukemias have a rapid onset and a short course ending in death if untreated. The paucity of normal WBCs leads to numerous infections such as pneumonia and septicemia. Early symptoms include fever, lymphadenopathy, pallor and fatigue from anemia, and ecchymoses. WBC count may be normal, decreased, or increased.

Chronic leukemias have a more insidious onset. Median survival of patients with CML is 3 to 4 years and with CLL, 2 to 10 years, depending on the stage at diagnosis. Early signs include fatigue, weakness, anorexia, and weight loss characteristic of a hypermetabolic state. An enlarged spleen and liver usually can be palpated. The WBC count usually is considerably elevated.

### Acute Lymphocytic Leukemia

#### Epidemiology

Of persons with **acute lymphocytic leukemia (ALL)**, 80% are children, with a peak incidence between 2 and 4 years and an extreme decrease after age 10.

#### Pathophysiology

ALL is a malignant disorder arising from a single lymphoid stem cell (see Figures 33-1 and 33-2), with impaired maturation and accumulation of the malignant cells in the bone marrow. Diagnosis is confirmed by bone marrow aspiration or biopsy, which typically shows different stages of lymphoid development, from very immature to almost normal cells. The degree of immaturity is a guide to the prognosis: the greater the number of immature cells (increased percentage of lymphocytes and presence of blast cells on a peripheral smear and bone marrow aspiration), the poorer the prognosis.

Signs and symptoms of ALL include anemia, bleeding,

**TABLE 34-9 Clinical Manifestations and Common Chemotherapeutic Agents Used in Different Leukemias**

| LEUKEMIA | PEAK AGE (YR) | CHARACTERISTIC SYMPTOMS | WBC LEVEL | BONE MARROW CELL PREDOMINANCE | COMMON CHEMOTHERAPEUTIC AGENTS |
|---|---|---|---|---|---|
| Acute lymphocytic leukemia (ALL) | 2-4 | Fever, infections of respiratory tract, anemia, bleeding of mucous membranes, ecchymoses, lymphadenopathy | Decreased, normal, or increased | Lymphoblasts | Regimens with vincristine and prednisone, 6-mercaptopurine, methotrexate |
| Acute myelogenous leukemia (AML) | 12-20, after 55 | Same as ALL except less lymphadenopathy | Normal, decreased, or increased | Myeloblasts | Cytarabine, 6-thioguanine, doxorubicin (Adriamycin), daunomycin |
| Chronic lymphocytic leukemia (CLL) | 50-70 | Weakness, fatigue, lymphadenopathy, pruritic vesicular skin lesions, thrombocytopenia, anemia, splenomegaly | Increased (20,000-100,000) | Lymphocytes | Alkylating agents (e.g., chlorambucil), glucocorticoids |
| Chronic myelogenous leukemia (CML) | 30-50 | Weakness, fatigue, anorexia, weight loss, splenomegaly | Increased (15,000-500,000) | Granulocytes | Busulfan |

lymphadenopathy, and a predisposition to infection. A blood smear may show immature lymphoblasts. The platelet count and Hct level are reduced in most patients.

### Medical management

Perhaps more dramatically than in any other malignant disorder, chemotherapy has improved the prognosis of children with ALL. Untreated patients have a median survival time (MST) of 4 to 6 months. With current chemotherapy the MST is close to 5 years, and approximately 50% of children with ALL can now be cured.

Complete remissions are obtained in more than 90% of patients treated with chemotherapeutic regimens, most of which include vincristine and prednisone. Maintenance of remission is accomplished with a combination of drugs, usually including the antimetabolites 6-mercaptopurine and methotrexate. In most regimens, vincristine and prednisone are administered intermittently during the maintenance program. Appropriate duration of therapy in patients who continue free of disease remains unsettled, but in most centers it is approximately 3 years. The use of "prophylactic" treatment of the central nervous system (i.e., intrathecal administration of methotrexate with or without craniospinal radiation) has greatly diminished recurrences. Because the blood-brain barrier does not allow parenteral infusion of chemotherapy to reach the leukemic cells, the central nervous system acts as a sanctuary for the leukemia. Intrathecal administration of chemotherapy or craniospinal radiation, or both, eradicates the leukemic cells.

## Acute Myelogenous Leukemia

### Epidemiology

**Acute myelogenous leukemia (AML)** can occur at any age but occurs more often at adolescence and after age 55.

### Pathophysiology

AML arises from a single myeloid stem cell and is characterized by the development of immature myeloblasts in the bone marrow. Clinical manifestations are the same as for ALL (see Table 34-9). The WBC count may be low, normal, or high. Bone marrow aspiration reveals a marked increase in myeloblasts.

### Medical management

In the untreated patient or in one who is nonresponsive to therapy, the MST is approximately 2 to 3 months. Current therapy includes the use of cytarabine, 6-thioguanine, and doxorubicin or daunomycin. Complete remission occurs in 50% to 75% of treated patients, and the MST is approximately 2 to 3 years. Approximately 20% of patients are in complete remission at 5 years and are capable of prolonged disease-free periods (remission). Although patients in remission clearly have an improved quality of life, induction of therapy is arduous, often requiring weeks in the hospital with the need for intensive supportive care (blood component replacement and antibiotic therapy). Bone marrow transplantation (see p. 967) with the use of HLA-identical allogenic bone marrow is being used with increasing frequency. Transplanting the patient's own (autologous) bone marrow obtained after a remission with chemotherapy or radiation therapy is another option.

## Chronic Lymphocytic Leukemia

### Epidemiology

**Chronic lymphocytic leukemia (CLL)** occurs at any age but is found mainly between ages 50 and 70. It is three times more common in men.

### Pathophysiology

CLL is characterized by a proliferation of small, abnormal, mature B lymphocytes, often leading to decreased synthesis of immunoglobulins and depressed antibody response. The accumulation of abnormal lymphocytes begins in the lymph nodes, then spreads to other lymphatic tissues and the spleen. The number of mature lymphocytes in the peripheral blood smear and bone marrow is greatly increased.

The onset is insidious with weakness, fatigue, and lymphadenopathy. Symptoms include pruritic vesicular skin lesions, anemia, thrombocytopenia, and an enlarged spleen (see Table 34-9). The WBC count is elevated to a level between 20,000 and 100,000; this increases blood viscosity, and a clotting episode may be the first warning. Bone marrow biopsy shows infiltration of lymphocytes.

### Medical management

The MST of persons with CLL is 4½ to 5½ years. As a general rule, persons are treated only when symptoms, particularly anemia, thrombocytopenia, or enlarged lymph nodes and spleen, appear. Chemotherapeutic agents used in the treatment of CLL are most often one of the alkylating agents, such as chlorambucil, and the glucocorticoids (see Chapter 16).

## Chronic Myelogenous Leukemia

### Epidemiology

**Chronic myelogenous leukemia (CML)** occurs at any age but primarily from ages 30 to 50. The incidence is slightly higher in men.

### Pathophysiology

The primary defect in CML is an abnormal stem cell leading to an uncontrolled proliferation of the granulocytic cells. As a result of this proliferation, there is a marked increase in the number of circulating granulocytes. In most cases a characteristic chromosomal abnormality, the *Philadelphia chromosome,* is present, involving deletion of a portion of one of the arms of chromosome 21 and its addition to another chromosome.

Characteristic symptoms of chronic leukemia occur: fatigue, weakness, anorexia, weight loss, and splenomegaly (see Table 34-9). Diagnosis of CML is made on the basis of an elevated WBC count (15,000 to 500,000), granulocytes on the peripheral blood smear that range in maturity from blast cells to mature neutrophils, and granulocytic hyperplasia in the bone marrow. The Philadelphia chromosome is present in 80% of patients.

CML frequently changes from a chronic indolent phase into an accelerated phase that progresses rapidly into a fulminant neoplastic process sometimes indistinguishable from an acute leukemia. The accelerated phase of the disease (blastic phase) is characterized by increasing numbers of granulocytes in the peripheral blood. Often there is a corresponding anemia and thrombocytopenia. Fever and adenopathy also may develop. Of patients with CML, 50% to 60% progress to the blastic phase. Once the CML enters the blastic phase, the treatment is the same as chemotherapy for AML.

### Medical management

Busulfan (Myleran), an alkylating agent, and hydroxyurea, both oral agents, are the most common drugs used. They often are effective in decreasing symptoms but have minimal impact on survival. Additional approaches include allogenic bone marrow transplantation in the chronic phase and autologous transplantation (see p. 967) in the acute blastic phase.

### Nursing management

Leukemia, by its nature, is a diverse illness. The varied courses and response or lack of response to treatment also add to the diversity. Nursing diagnoses, expected patient outcomes, and nursing interventions for persons with malignancies can be found in Chapter 16.

In acute phases of the disease and during aggressive chemotherapy, nursing care is aimed toward the prevention of complications and supportive therapy. Decreased WBC and platelet counts render the person vulnerable to *severe infections* and *bleeding* episodes. Frequent transfusions of both whole blood and component therapy (platelets, WBC) often are necessary.[6,7] Many patients require the insertion of an indwelling central venous catheter for the administration of chemotherapy and/or total parenteral nutrition and for diagnostic blood work.

Many focuses of nursing care are beyond those found in the life-threatening situations. Each person with leukemia responds in a different way. It cannot be predicted for certain if an individual will respond to a prescribed treatment or how long a remission will last. Likewise, how the individual incorporates the illness into life is also unique to each person. Nursing has a key role in patient education. Before discharge from the hospital, the person should possess basic knowledge of the disease process and the importance of continued medical follow-up. Knowledge of specific drug therapy and anticipated side effects is also a component of the teaching plan. Of utmost importance in learning is the ability of the person to identify the body's signals that blood abnormalities exist. Petechiae, ecchymoses, and gingival bleeding (indicating infection) are again the warning

**Guidelines for Teaching the Person With Leukemia**

Nature of the disease process and its effects
Prevention of infection
Drug regimen: name, side effects (see Chapter 16)
Method of arranging for chemotherapy administration and periodic blood counts
Symptoms requiring immediate medical attention (fever, bleeding)
Available community resources (American Cancer Society, Leukemia Society*)
Need for continual medical follow-up
Meticulous oral care to prevent stomatitis

*600 Third Ave, New York, NY 10016.

signs to seek prompt medical attention. Bone pain, often severe, may signal blastic crisis (acute proliferation of immature cells).

Persons whose illness runs the course of several months to years often become highly knowledgeable about their disease, blood components, related symptoms, and specific chemotherapeutic drugs. These persons sometimes discuss their progress in terms of changes in their blood counts. Over time many patients become attuned to how such changes affect them. For example, they often can predict their count by how they feel. Many such persons respond well to being included in their plan of care during hospitalization and in preparation for discharge.

Time set aside for patient teaching (see Guidelines box above) also allows for a sharing time with the individual. This time may provide the foundation for an honest nurse-patient relationship from which emotional support may be given the person as attempts are made to adapt to the many stressors associated with leukemia.

### Bone Marrow Transplantation

Bone marrow may be removed from one person and given intravenously to another person or withdrawn at one time and given to the same person at another time. It is being used increasingly in several hematologic malignant conditions after large doses of chemotherapy or radiation therapy. The amount of chemotherapy or radiation therapy that can ordinarily be administered is limited by toxicity to the bone marrow. By transplanting bone marrow after these therapeutic modes, much larger therapeutic doses can be administered.

Bone marrow transplantation generally is used (1) in children with ALL who have relapsed and have been reinduced into a second complete remission with chemotherapy, (2) in younger patients with ANLL in either a first or second remission, and (3) in persons with CML in the chronic phase who have either a syngeneic or allogeneic donor.

Among nonmalignant diseases, bone marrow transplantation has had its greatest impact with aplastic anemia. For additional information on bone marrow transplantation and care of the transplant patient, see Chapter 72.

# DISORDERS ASSOCIATED WITH THE LYMPH SYSTEM

## ASSESSMENT OF LYMPH NODES

The normal lymph node consists of connective tissue encapsulating a fine mesh of reticular cells. The reticuloendothelial cells function chiefly in the phagocytosis of cellular debris. The chief function of lymphocytes, which are the main cells comprising the lymph nodes, is to provide an immune response to antigens presented to the node from the structure being drained by the node.

Lymph node enlargement results from an increase in the number and size of lymphoid follicles with proliferation of lymphocytes and reticuloendothelial cells. Lymphadenopathy also may occur when the node is invaded by cells normally not present (leukemic cells, cancer cells). In the lymphomas the actual nodal structure is destroyed by the malignant cells.

Normally lymph nodes are not palpable. With disease and the consequent increase in size, the nodes become palpable. In a routine physical examination the lymph nodes are examined by palpation.

**Lymphangiography** is a radiologic technique used for evaluation of lymph nodes to detect the presence of disease. This procedure is especially valuable in the assessment of those nodes that are anatomically too deep in the abdomen to allow for evaluation by palpation (paraaortic). For this procedure a small incision is made on the dorsal surface of each foot so that the small lymph channels are made accessible, and dye is instilled. All lymph chains and nodes fill with dye and are then visible on roentgenograms. X-ray films usually are obtained immediately after the dye is absorbed and again at intervals of 24 and 48 hours after the procedure. In addition, because the dye remains in the lymph nodes for as long as 6 months after the initial study, disease status and response to therapy can be periodically evaluated with routine abdominal roentgenograms.

Computed tomography (CT scan) also is used to assess abdominal lymph nodes. The CT scan is used as a monitoring tool to evaluate the patient's disease process, remission during chemotherapy, and after treatment. Assessment by periodic CT scans (every 6 to 12 months) helps to evaluate the remission or to detect a relapse.

## HODGKIN'S DISEASE

### Etiology/Pathophysiology

**Hodgkin's disease** is a malignant disorder of lymph nodes. The etiology is unknown. Diagnosis requires biopsy and pathologic examination of the suspicious node. The presence of the Reed-Sternberg cell remains the pathologic hallmark of the disorder, but four pathologic variants of Hodgkin's disease have been recognized: *lymphocyte predominant, nodular sclerosis, mixed cellularity,* and *lymphocyte depletion.* The lymphocyte predominant and nodular sclerosis types have the best prognosis, and lymphocyte depletion has the worst. The most important prognostic indicator is the stage of the disease at the time of diagnosis. Accurate staging is crucial to the subsequent treatment regimen. The diagnostic work-up is often arduous and difficult, and explanation of the many facets of the complex diagnostic procedures helps provide the emotional support so often needed during this time.

Systemic symptoms that may be associated with Hodgkin's disease include *fatigue, weakness, anorexia, unexplained* fever, *night sweats,* and *generalized pruritus.* Physical examination may show enlargement of lymph nodes, liver, and spleen. A chest roentgenogram may identify the presence of a mediastinal mass. A bone marrow biopsy is performed to determine if there is marrow involvement. The liver and spleen are evaluated by radionuclide scanning or by CT scan. Lymphangiography is performed to evaluate the intraabdominal nodes. A *staging laparotomy* is performed in some circumstances to obtain a biopsy specimen of retroperitoneal lymph nodes and both lobes of the liver and to remove the spleen. The rationale for this procedure is the limitations of nonsurgical diagnosis of liver, spleen, and intraabdominal node involvement.

The classification into stages allows for comparison of persons with similar disease involvement and their response to a given treatment regimen. Over time such comparisons have identified the treatment course most appropriate for a described disease. The revised Ann Arbor staging classification for Hodgkin's disease is shown in Box 34-8.

**BOX 34-8 Ann Arbor Clinical Staging Classification of Hodgkin's Disease**

**STAGE I**

Involvement of a single lymph node region (I) or of a single extralymphatic organ or site ($I_E$)

**STAGE II**

Involvement of two or more lymph node regions on the same side of the diaphragm (II) or localized involvement of an extralymphatic organ or site and of one or more lymph node regions on the same side of the diaphragm ($II_E$)

**STAGE III**

Involvement of lymph node regions on both sides of the diaphragm (III), which also may be accompanied by involvement of the spleen ($III_S$) or by localized involvement of an extralymphatic organ or site ($III_E$) or both ($III_{SE}$)

**STAGE IV**

Diffuse or disseminated involvement of one or more extralymphatic organs or tissues, with or without associated lymph node involvement

The presence or absence of fever, night sweats, or unexplained loss of 10% or more of body weight in the 6 months preceding admission are denoted by the suffix letters B and A, respectively. Biopsy-documented involvement of stage IV sites also is denoted by letter suffixes: M, marrow; L, lung; H, liver; P, pleura; O, bone; D, skin and subcutaneous tissue.

## Medical Management

Radiation therapy (Figure 34-7) is used for stages IA, IB, IIA, and IIB. This treatment yields a cure rate of approximately 90% for stage I and 80% for stage II. Combination chemotherapy is the treatment of choice for stages IIIB and IV. Therapy of stage IIIA is controversial and involves chemotherapy, radiation, or a combination of these therapies. The most frequently used combination is the MOPP regimen, which consists of mechlorethamine (nitrogen mustard), Oncovin (vincristine), procarbazine, and prednisone (Table 34-10). This regimen is administered in a 2-week course each month with prednisone added during the first and fourth course. The drugs are administered for at least 6 months or for two or three courses after the attainment of complete remission. Complete remissions are achieved in approximately 80% of these patients; long-term, disease-free remissions and probable cures occur in half of this group. Continuing chemotherapy beyond the attainment of complete remission has not been shown to improve survival. Combinations such as ABVD (Table 34-10) are likely to be added to the treatment regimen if relapse occurs, and complete remission can again be attained. Initial use of alternating courses of MOPP and ABVD has increased response rates. (See p. 971 for nursing management.)

# NON-HODGKIN'S LYMPHOMAS

## Etiology/Pathophysiology

The **non-Hodgkin's lymphomas** include a broad spectrum of lymphoid malignant diseases with different histopathologies, disease courses, and responses to therapy. The cause is unknown, although viruses have been implicated. Accurate identification of the histopathology is crucial to the determination of the treatment plan. The classifications are reviewed here only briefly so that familiarity with terminology will allow the reader to review charts and treatment plans. Also, recognition of the diversity of the disease course, prognosis, and the importance of an extensive diagnostic work-up is useful to the nurse for patient and family teaching.

One classification separates the non-Hodgkin's lymphomas into *lymphocytic, histiocytic,* or *mixed cell types,* each of which may appear as nodular or diffuse on microscopic examination. These have been subdivided into "favorable" and "unfavorable" histology (Box 34-9). In general a nodular pattern of cell structures

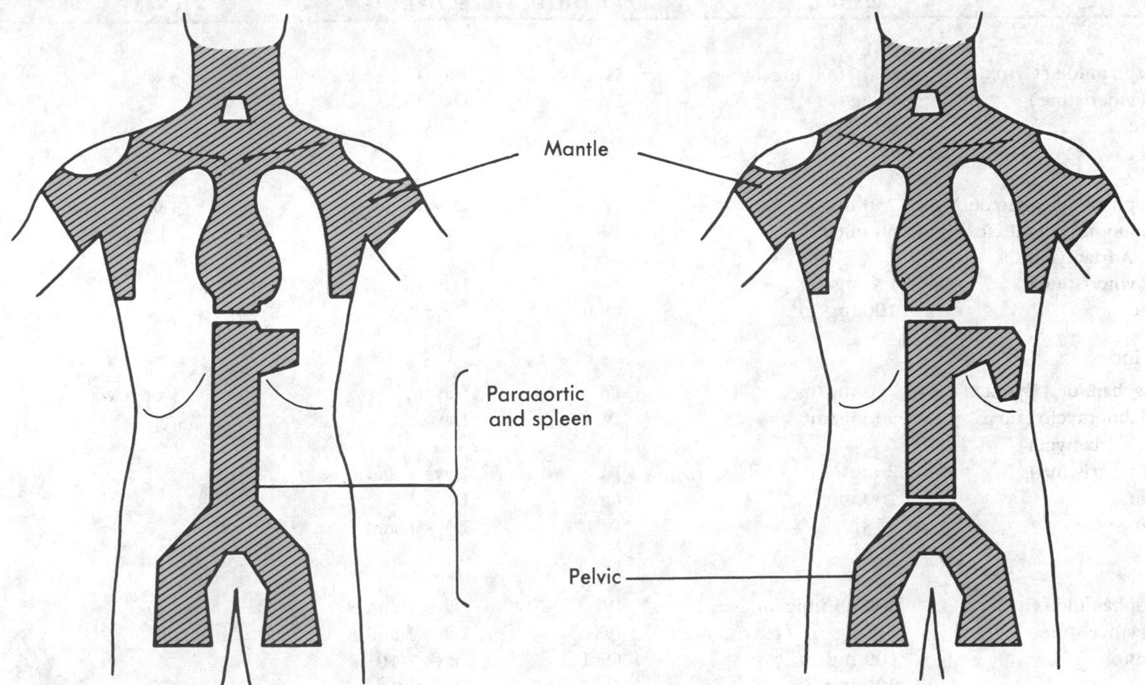


**FIGURE 34-7** Diagram of mantle and inverted Y fields used in total lymphoid radiotherapy of Hodgkin's disease. (From Rosenberg SA, Kaplan HS: *Calif Med* 113:23, 1970.)

**TABLE 34-10 Chemotherapeutic Regimens for Treatment of Hodgkin's Disease**

| NAME | DRUGS | DOSAGE | METHOD | SCHEDULE | CYCLE |
|---|---|---|---|---|---|
| MOPP | Mechlorethamine (nitrogen mustard) | 6 mg/m² | IV | Days 1 and 8 | 2 wk with 2-wk rest period |
| | Oncovin (vincristine) | 1.4 mg/m² | IV | Days 1 and 8 | |
| | Prednisone | 20 mg/m² | Oral | Days 1-14 | |
| | Procarbazine | 100 mg/m² | Oral | Days 1-14 | |
| ABVD | Adriamycin (doxorubicin) | 25 mg/m² | IV | Days 1 and 15 | 2 wk with 2-wk rest period |
| | Bleomycin | 10 mg/m² | IV | Days 1 and 15 | |
| | Vinblastine (Velban) | 6 mg/m² | IV | Days 1 and 15 | |
| | Dacarbazine (DTIC-Dome) | 150 mg/m² | IV | Days 1-5 | |

conveys a more favorable prognosis than a diffuse pattern. A lymphocytic cytology is more favorable than a histiocytic one, and a mixed cellularity–histiocytic is intermediate in its prognosis.

Characteristically, patients with non-Hodgkin's lymphoma have a median age of 50 to 60 years. Patients most often have *nontender peripheral lymphadenopathy* that may appear bulky. The *liver and spleen may be moderately enlarged.* Other symptoms that may occur include unexplained *fever, night sweats,* and *weight loss.*

The diagnosis of non-Hodgkin's lymphoma is made by examination of pathologic lymph node tissue. Accurate histologic classification is of importance, and often slides are sent to major cancer centers for consul-

**BOX 34-9 Non-Hodgkin's Lymphomas**

**"FAVORABLE" HISTOLOGY**

Nodular poorly differentiated lymphocytic lymphoma (NLPD)
Nodular mixed lymphocytic and histiocytic lymphoma (NML)
Well-differentiated lymphocytic lymphomas of the nodular (NLWD) or diffuse (DLWD) type

**"UNFAVORABLE" HISTOLOGY**

Nodular histiocytic (NHL)
Diffuse poorly differentiated lymphocytic (DPDL)
Diffuse histiocytic lymphoma (DHL)
Diffuse mixed lymphoma (DML)
Diffuse undifferentiated lymphoma (DUL)

## TABLE 34-11 Chemotherapeutic Regimens for Treatment of Non-Hodgkin's Lymphomas

| DRUGS | DOSAGE | METHOD | SCHEDULE | CYCLE |
|---|---|---|---|---|
| **COP** | | | | |
| Cyclophosphamide (Cytoxan) | 800-1000 $mg/m^2$ | IV | Day 1 | 3 wk |
| Oncovin (vincristine) | 2 mg | IV | Day 1 | |
| Prednisone | 60 $mg/m^2$ | Oral | Days 1-5 | |
| **CHOP** | | | | |
| Cyclophosphamide (Cytoxan) | 750 $mg/m^2$ | IV | Day 1 | 3 wk |
| Hydroxydaunomycin (doxorubicin, Adriamycin) | 50 $mg/m^2$ | IV | Day 1 | |
| Oncovin (vincristine) | 1.4 $mg/m^2$ | IV | Day 1 | |
| Prednisone | 100 $mg/m^2$ | Oral | Days 1-5 | |
| **CHOP-Bleo** | | | | |
| Cyclophosphamide (Cytoxan) | 750 $mg/m^2$ | IV | Day 1 | 3 or 4 wk |
| Hydroxydaunomycin (doxorubicin, Adriamycin) | 50 $mg/m^2$ | IV | Day 1 | |
| Oncovin (vincristine) | 2 mg | IV | Days 1 and 5 | |
| Prednisone | 100 mg | Oral | Days 1-5 | |
| Bleomycin | 15 U | IV | Days 1 and 5 | |
| **COPP** | | | | |
| Cyclophosphamide (Cytoxan) | 400-650 $mg/m^2$ | IV | Days 1 and 8 | 4 wk |
| Oncovin (vincristine) | 1.4 $mg/m^2$ (max, 2 mg) | IV | Days 1 and 8 | |
| Procarbazine | 100 $mg/m^2$ | Oral | Days 1-10 | |
| Prednisone | 40 $mg/m^2$ | Oral | Days 1-14 | |
| **BACOP** | | | | |
| Bleomycin | 5 $U/m^2$ | IV | Days 15 and 22 | 4 wk |
| Adriamycin (doxorubicin) | 25 $mg/m^2$ | IV | Days 1 and 8 | |
| Cyclophosphamide (Cytoxan) | 650 $mg/m^2$ | IV | Days 1 and 8 | |
| Oncovin (vincristine) | 1.4 $mg/m^2$ (max, 2 mg) | IV | Days 1 and 8 | |
| Prednisone | 60 $mg/m^2$ | Oral | Days 15-28 | |
| **Pro-MACE** | | | | |
| Prednisone | 60 $mg/m^2$ | Oral | Days 1 to 14 | 4 wk |
| Methotrexate | 1.5 $g/m^2$ | IV | | |
| Adriamycin (doxorubicin) | 25 $mg/m^2$ | IV | Days 1 and 8 | Follow with MOPP regimen (see Table 30-10); then restart Pro-MACE |
| Cyclophosphamide | 650 $mg/m^2$ | IV | Days 1 and 8 | |
| Etoposide (VP 16) | 120 $mg/m^2$ | IV | Days 1 and 8 | |
| Leucovorin | 50 $mg/m^2$ | IV | q 6 hr for 5 days | |
| **M-BACOD** | | | | |
| Methotrexate | 200 $mg/m^2$ | IV | Days 8 and 15 | Repeat cycles every 3 wk |
| Bleomycin | 4 $units/m^2$ | IV | Days 1 and 21 | |
| Adriamycin (doxorubicin) | 45 $mg/m^2$ | IV | Days 1 and 21 | |
| Cyclophosphamide | 600 $mg/m^2$ | IV | Days 1 and 21 | |
| Oncovin (vincristine) | 1 $mg/m^2$ | IV | Days 1 and 21 | |
| Dexamethasone | 6 $mg/m^2$ | Oral | Days 1-5 and 21-25 | |
| Leucovorin rescue | 10 $mg/m^2$ | Oral | q 6 hr for 8 doses, beginning 24 hr after each methotrexate dose | |
| **MACOP-B** | | | | |
| Methotrexate | 100 $mg/m^2$, then 300 $mg/m^2$ | IV<br>IV/4 hr | Wk 2, 6, 10<br>Wk 2, 6, 10 | Cycles may be repeated |
| Leucovorin rescue | 15 mg | Oral | q 6 hr for 6 doses beginning 24 hr after methotrexate | |
| Adriamycin (doxorubicin) | 50 $mg/m^2$ | IV | Wk 1, 3, 5, 7, 9, 11 | |
| Cyclophosphamide | 350 $mg/m^2$ | IV | Wk 1, 3, 5, 7, 9, 11 | |
| Oncovin (vincristine) | 1.4 $mg/m^2$ | IV | Wk 2, 4, 8, 10, 12 | |
| Prednisone | 75 mg | Oral | Daily doses tapered over last 15 days | |
| Bleomycin | 10 $U/m^2$ | IV | Wk 4, 8, 12 | |
| NOTE: CNS prophylaxis also given to patients with bone marrow involvement after bone marrow remission | | | | |
| Methotrexate | 12 mg | Intrathecal (IT) | Wk 6-8 | |
| Cytarabine | 30 $mg/m^2$ | IT | Wk 6-8 | |

tation regarding the classification. Once the diagnosis is made, the extent of the disease (staging) must be determined. As with Hodgkin's disease, accurate staging is a crucial factor required to determine the treatment regimen. The staging work-up is similar to that for Hodgkin's disease, except that staging laparotomies are less often needed. Explanations of the extensive work-up and its importance in determining the treatment plan are an important focus of patient teaching during the diagnostic period.

### Medical Management

The complexity of the disease and the array of treatment regimens used encourages nurse-physician discussion of the treatment plan. It is especially important that the goals of therapy be shared, whether curative or only local or systemic palliation.

In general, radiotherapy is the initial treatment when the disease has a localized presentation. Local field radiation is used. Total nodal radiation is reserved for patients whose disease is more widespread. Chemotherapy is the mainstay of treatment of non-Hodgkin's lymphomas that are not localized (Table 34-11).

*Nodular poorly differentiated lymphocytic lymphoma* is the most frequently occurring non-Hodgkin's lymphoma. In some patients, observation is reasonable until the disease shows signs of progression. Treatment with a single alkylating agent, most often chlorambucil, is effective in that it produces a response rate that extends survival. Combination chemotherapy, however, produces higher response rates, including complete remissions, but is not yet shown to be curative. Median survival time (MST) is 7 to 10 years.

In *diffuse histiocytic lymphoma,* which includes most of the cases previously designated as reticulum cell sarcoma, combination chemotherapy has been superior to single-agent therapy. Survival is significantly prolonged in those who demonstrate a complete response, and a significant minority of this group are cured. Chemotherapy regimens produce complete responses in 40% to 60% or more of patients, whose MST is well over 3 years.

In *nodular histiocytic* and *nodular mixed histiolymphocytic* types, complete responses have been achieved with single agents, and 50% to 70% of those treated with COP, COPP, MOPP, and other combinations have shown a MST of 55 months for those who attained a complete response and 13 months for those in whom only a partial response was attained.

## NURSING MANAGEMENT

### ♦ ASSESSMENT

*Subjective* data include (1) knowledge of the disorder, (2) effect of fatigue on the ability to carry out ADLs, (3) appetite and present nutritional status, and (4) discomfort from night sweats or pruritus. *Objective* data specifically include condition of the skin (such as excoriations from scratching), weight, lymphadenopathy, and liver/spleen size.

### ♦ NURSING DIAGNOSES

Nursing diagnoses are determined from analysis of patient data. Nursing diagnoses for the patient with lymphoma may include but are not limited to the following:

| Diagnostic Title | Possible Etiologic Factors |
|---|---|
| Knowledge deficit | Unfamiliarity with information |
| Activity intolerance | Generalized weakness, imbalance between oxygen supply and demand |
| Comfort, alteration in | Pruritus, night sweats |

Other nursing diagnoses may be identified on the basis of effects of chemotherapy or radiation therapy (see Chapter 16).

### ♦ EXPECTED PATIENT OUTCOMES

Expected patient outcomes for the patient with lymphoma may include but are not limited to the following:

1. Describes the nature of the disorder, therapeutic regimen, need for continued medical follow-up, and community resources.
2. Decreases activity level when fatigued or short of breath with exertion or states alterations in ADL to adapt to physical changes.
3. Feels more comfortable; describes measures to diminish pruritus and has minimal skin breakdown from scratching.

### ♦ INTERVENTIONS

#### Facilitating Counseling and Learning

Hodgkin's and non-Hodgkins diseases most often affect young adults; therefore special attention needs to be given to minimizing the impact of the illness and its treatment on their lives, not only during the treatment period, but later as well. Before the initiation of treatment, therapy-induced sterility should be discussed. For young women receiving radiation therapy alone, surgical relocation of the ovaries outside the field of radiation may be performed. Sterility frequently occurs in association with chemotherapy (see Chapter 16). For women, this is often temporary, and the ability to conceive and bear normal children often returns after therapy is completed. For men, sterility is more frequently permanent. For this reason the option of sperm banking should be discussed before beginning either radiation therapy or chemotherapy.

To allow for work and career development, every effort should be made to schedule treatment at those times and days of the week that least interfere with work and other important events in the person's life. The nurse has a crucial role in assisting patients to develop a realistic approach to the illness and to meet successfully the demands and limitations imposed by the illness and its treatment.

Persons with lymphomas have periods of remission and recurrence. Such peaks and valleys are stressful and disruptive. Many patients describe subsequent courses of treatment after a recurrence as more stressful than the initial treatment. Comments include "Is it worth it? I don't have the same faith." Other patients, realistially encouraged by the initial response to treatment, are able to express an optimistic outlook, "It worked the first time. It will work again." Recognition of the stress involved in therapy requires that support systems be available to the patient. The health care tèam can provide some of the needed support and guidance as the person learns to incorporate the illness into daily life.

*Patient teaching* includes the following:

1. Knowledge of the disorder, its treatment, and prognosis
2. Name, dosage, frequency, and side effects of medications
3. Arrangements for chemotherapy or radiation treatments and for periodic blood cell counts
4. Symptoms requiring immediate medical attention (fever, bleeding)
5. Need for continued medical follow-up
6. Resources available in the community: financial assistance and local support groups (American Cancer Society)

### Promoting Activity Tolerance

Generalized weakness and shortness of breath with exertion are indications to the patient dealing with lymphoma that a change in level of activity must occur. The change in activity may be related to side effects of chemotherapy or radiation therapy (see Chapter 16) or to the disease process itself. The nurse assists the patient to balance rest with activity and to identify ways to decrease the activity level. Emotional support and active listening are essential to assist the patient through loss of independence.

### Promoting Comfort

Fever, pruritus, and profuse night sweats may lead to general discomfort. Measures to ease pruritus and prevent excoriations of the skin are instituted (see Chapter 67). Frequent changes of night clothing or bed linens may be necessary. A high fluid intake is encouraged to replace the lost fluid from night sweats and fever.

## ♦ EVALUATION

To evaluate effectiveness of nursing interventions, compare patient behaviors with those stated in the expected patient outcomes. Successful achievement of patient outcomes for the patient with lymphoma is indicated by the following:

1. Correctly describes the nature of the disorder, the therapeutic regimen needed for continued medical follow-up, and community resources.
2. Limits activity and takes rest periods; correctly states ways to adapt ADL to physical changes.
3. Feels more comfortable; correctly describes measures to decrease pruritus and has no flaky skin or skin breakdown indicative of scratching.

# Infectious Mononucleosis

## ETIOLOGY/EPIDEMIOLOGY

Infectious mononucleosis is an acute disease caused by a herpeslike virus, the Epstein-Barr virus. It occurs more often in young persons, the highest incidence occurring between 15 and 30 years of age.

Signs and symptoms of infectious mononucleosis are varied (Box 34-10). It is a benign disease with a good prognosis. Onset may be subtle, appearing almost as flulike symptoms. Malaise is a frequent early complaint, and it is often accompanied by fever, enlargement of lymph nodes, sore throat, headache, generalized aches and pains resembling those of influenza, and moderate enlargement of the liver and spleen. Rupture of the spleen and encephalitis are rare complications. Diagnosis is established by the heterophil agglutination or Monospot blood test. This test is based on a certain substance being present in the blood of a person with infectious mononucleosis that causes clumping, or agglutination, of the washed erythrocytes (antigen) of another animal. The test result is almost always positive after 10 to 14 days of the illness. Other laboratory findings are a great increase in the number of mononuclear leukocytes, which lends the name to the disease, and an increase in atypical lymphocytes. At the height of the disease the WBCs may range between 10,000 and 20,000 cells/$mm^3$.

## MEDICAL MANAGEMENT

Infectious mononucleosis is self-limiting, and with rest affected persons usually recover spontaneously within a few weeks. The patient is advised to avoid heavy lifting or contact sports when splenomegaly is present. Most persons can return to activities that do not require heavy exertion in 1 to 2 weeks and to normal activities in 4 to 6 weeks. Some persons have persistent fatigue for several months.

**BOX 34-10 Clinical Manifestation of Infectious Mononucleosis**

**MILD**

Fever, malaise

**MODERATE**

Enlarged lymph nodes, sore throat, headache, generalized aches, moderate enlargement of liver and spleen

**SEVERE (RARE)**

Rupture of spleen, encephalitis

## NURSING MANAGEMENT

**Nursing care is aimed at relief of symptoms and promotion of rest and comfort.**

## QUESTIONS TO CONSIDER

- How would your care differ if the patient with aplastic anemia said, "I feel so lonely and frightened when everyone has to wear masks and gloves when they come in to see me"?
- What approaches might you consider for teaching a person with hemophilia how to administer clotting factors at home?
- How would your care differ if the patient with Hodgkin's disease said, "When I go home, I'm not going to take this chemotherapy"?
- What approaches might you consider for teaching a person at risk measures to prevent infection and bleeding?

## CRITICAL THINKING ACTIVITIES

- You are administering platelets to one patient and whole blood to another patient. Will your procedure for, or monitoring of, the administering of these two products vary? If so, why?
- You are working on a hematology unit and caring for patients with differing types of anemia. Lydia has iron deficiency anemia, John has hereditary spherocytosis, and Ryan has aplastic anemia. How will the nursing care for these three patients compare? What can you infer about the care of all patients with anemia based on your care of these three patients?
- You are caring for Sarah, a teenager who has sickle cell anemia. When teaching Sarah about thrombotic crisis, what information needs to be included?

# CHAPTER SUMMARY

- Major health problems of the hematopoietic system include RBC disorders (anemias, erythrocytosis); disorders of hemostasis, platelets, and coagulation; WBC disorders (neutropenia, neutrophilia, leukemia); disorders of the lymph system (lymphomas); and infectious mononucleosis.

### DISORDERS ASSOCIATED WITH ERYTHROCYTES

- Anemias may be caused by blood loss, impaired RBC production, increased RBC destruction, or nutritional deficiencies.
- Weakness and fatigue are major signs of anemia as a result of decreased oxygenation from lack of Hgb and increased energy needs required by increased RBC production.
- Aplastic anemia is anemia that results from impaired RBC production and is characterized by pancytopenia. Treatment is by bone marrow transplantation or immunosuppressive therapy. Nursing interventions include preventing infection and hemorrhage.
- Sickle cell anemia is a hemolytic anemia with a genetic basis. A sickle cell crisis occurs when the RBCs become deoxygenated and sickle-shaped, causing plugging of small vessels, leading to organ infarction and necrosis.
- Nursing interventions for sickle cell disease include promoting comfort and hydration, counseling, and teaching.
- Ingestion of iron compounds is part of the therapy for iron deficiency anemia only; it will not help the other types of anemias.
- Megaloblastic anemia is a macrocytic anemia from defective DNA synthesis and abnormal RBC maturation; causes include vitamin $B_{12}$ and folic acid deficiencies and administration of chemotherapeutic and anticonvulsant drugs.
- Erythrocytosis is an abnormal increase in RBCs, as seen with polycythemia vera.

### DISORDERS OF HEMOSTASIS, PLATELETS, AND COAGULATION

- Thrombocytopenia is a decrease in the number of circulating platelets and leads to bleeding; persons with thrombocytopenia need to learn how to prevent injury and hemorrhage.
- Hemophilia is a hereditary coagulation disorder; hemophilia A is a lack of coagulation factor VIII, and hemophilia B is a lack of factor IX; maintenance therapy consists of blood factor replacement therapy and prevention of injury.
- Disseminated intravascular coagulation (DIC) is a coagulation disorder characterized initially by clotting and secondarily by hemorrhage, resulting from an alteration in the balance between clotting factors and fibrinolytic factors; the person usually is critically ill.

### DISORDERS ASSOCIATED WITH WHITE BLOOD CELLS

- Persons with alteration of WBCs are at a high risk of infection because leukocytes are a major factor in the body's defense against invading microorganisms.
- The leukemias are malignant disorders characterized by uncontrolled proliferation of WBCs and their precursors; the cause is unknown.
- Leukemias may be acute or chronic, lymphocytic or nonlymphocytic (primarily myelogenous). Acute leukemias have a rapid onset and a short course if untreated; chronic leukemias have a more insidious onset and longer course. The major therapies for leukemias are chemotherapy and bone marrow transplantation.

### DISORDERS ASSOCIATED WITH THE LYMPH SYSTEM

- Lymphomas (Hodgkin's disease and non-Hodgkin's lymphomas) are malignant disorders of the lymph system; radiotherapy and chemotherapy are the major medical treatments.

## REFERENCES

1. Carnevali D, Reiner A: *The cancer experience: nursing diagnosis and management,* Philadelphia, 1990, JB Lippincott.
2. Harmening DM: *Clinical hematology and fundamentals of hemostasis,* ed 2, Philadelphia, 1992, FA Davis.
3. Rozell MS, Hijazi M, Pack B: The painful episode in sickle cell disease, *Nurs Clin North Am* 18(1):185-199, 1983.
4. Williams I, Earles AN, Pack B: Psychological considerations in sickle cell disease, *Nurs Clin North Am* 18(1):215-229, 1983.
5. Williams SR: *Nutrition and diet therapy,* ed 7, St Louis, 1993, Mosby.
6. Wintrobe MM et al: *Clinical hematology,* ed 7, Philadelphia, 1989, Lea & Febiger.
7. Wyngaarden JB, Smith LH: *Cecil textbook of medicine,* ed 19, Philadelphia, 1992, WB Saunders.

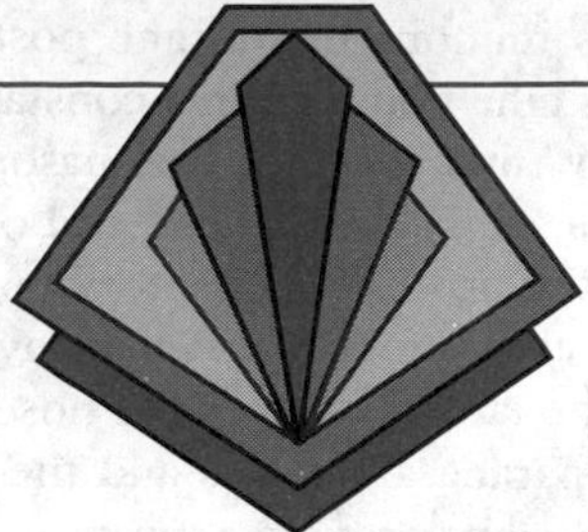

CHAPTER 35

# Assessment of the Respiratory System

***Josephine Jacobs Brucia***
***Mary Kay Lehman***

## CHAPTER OBJECTIVES

***After studying this chapter, the learner should be able to do the following:***

1 Define selected terms.
2 Identify structural components of the upper and lower airways and their primary functions.
3 Describe the mechanisms of pulmonary ventilation, gas exchange, pulmonary circulation, and control of respiration.
4 Identify physiologic changes that occur in the respiratory system with aging.
5 Identify data to collect in a nursing history for the patient experiencing a pulmonary dysfunction.
6 Recognize major symptoms associated with respiratory disease and the significance of each.
7 Describe the technique of physical examination of the respiratory system.
8 Describe diagnostic tests used to diagnose problems of the respiratory system and nursing responsibility associated with each test.
9 Differentiate between respiratory acidosis and alkalosis.

## KEY TERMS

adventitious sound
arterial blood gases
bronchoscopy
compliance
crackles (rales)
diffusion
dyspnea
fremitus
hemoptysis
hyperventilation
hypoventilation
mucociliary system
$Pa_{O_2}$
$Pa_{CO_2}$
phonation
pleural friction rub
pulmonary function test
pulmonary resistance
respiration
respiratory acidosis
respiratory alkalosis
rhinitis
$Sa_{O_2}$
thoracentesis
thoracoscopy
ventilation
ventilation-perfusion ($\dot{V}/\dot{Q}$)ratio
wheezes (rhonchi)

Breathing is an activity that most of us rarely think about throughout our daily lives. However, the ease or discomfort with which we breathe has a major impact on the quality of our daily activities.

The act of breathing involves the two interrelated processes of ventilation and respiration. **Ventilation** is the mass movement of air from outside the body through the conducting system to the alveoli. The conducting system includes both the upper and lower airways. **Respiration** consists of the dual processes of oxygen uptake and carbon dioxide elimination between the body and its environment. The only place respiration can occur is at the alveolar-capillary membrane, where oxygen (from air) and carbon dioxide (from cellular waste) can move in and out of the body.

To effectively intervene with patients' pulmonary problems, nurses must be knowledgeable about the structure and function of the upper and lower airways, the major pulmonary signs and symptoms, and the implications of data gathered in the assessment process.

# ANATOMY AND PHYSIOLOGY

## UPPER AIRWAY

The upper airway consists of the nose and sinuses, the pharynx and tonsils, and the larynx and laryngopharynx.

### Nose and Sinuses

The nose is supported by the nasal bones, the nasal processes of the maxillary bones, the cartilaginous and bony parts of the septum, and the upper and lower nasal cartilages. Air enters the nose through the two nostrils (nares), which are separated by the septum. The septum, which is usually straight and thin in the child, is rarely straight in adults, because in many cases it has been injured.

The nasal cavities are located between the roof of the mouth and the frontal, ethmoid, and sphenoid bones. Three projections, lined with mucous membrane and called the turbinate bones, are located on the lateral walls of each nasal cavity (Figure 35-1). The turbinates provide a large surface area with a rich blood supply that warms and humidifies ambient air as it passes through this area. Large particles are filtered out of inhaled air by precipitation or by stimulation of mechanical receptors located in the nasopharynx, which results in the sneeze reflex.[3]

The vestibule of the nose is the anterior part of the nose. The vestibule extends posteriorly a short distance to a point at which its lining changes from skin to mucous membrane. This mucous membrane posterior to the vestibule contains cilia that beat in a constant wave-like motion to carry mucus into the nasopharynx. Trapped in the mucus are bacteria, dust, and other foreign matter entering the nose. The olfactory epithelium is located in a small area superiorly and provides the end-organ of smell. The lateral walls of the nose contain the openings for the paranasal sinuses and the nasolacrimal ducts. These openings provide a means of aeration of and mucus drainage from the sinuses. The blood supply to the nose comes from both the external and internal carotid systems.

Four sets of paranasal sinuses are located on either side of the head (Figure 35-2). These sinuses are air-filled spaces in the skull that serve to lighten the head. They drain into the nasal cavities through the openings behind the turbinates. The maxillary sinuses are the largest and most accessible. The sinuses are lined with mucous membrane that is continuous with that of the nose. The functions of the nose and nasal sinuses are to warm, moisten, and filter air in preparation for the lungs; to house receptors for olfaction; and to promote vocal resonance.

### Upper Throat: Pharynx and Tonsils

The pharynx is the space behind the oral cavity that extends from the base of the skull to the larynx. The

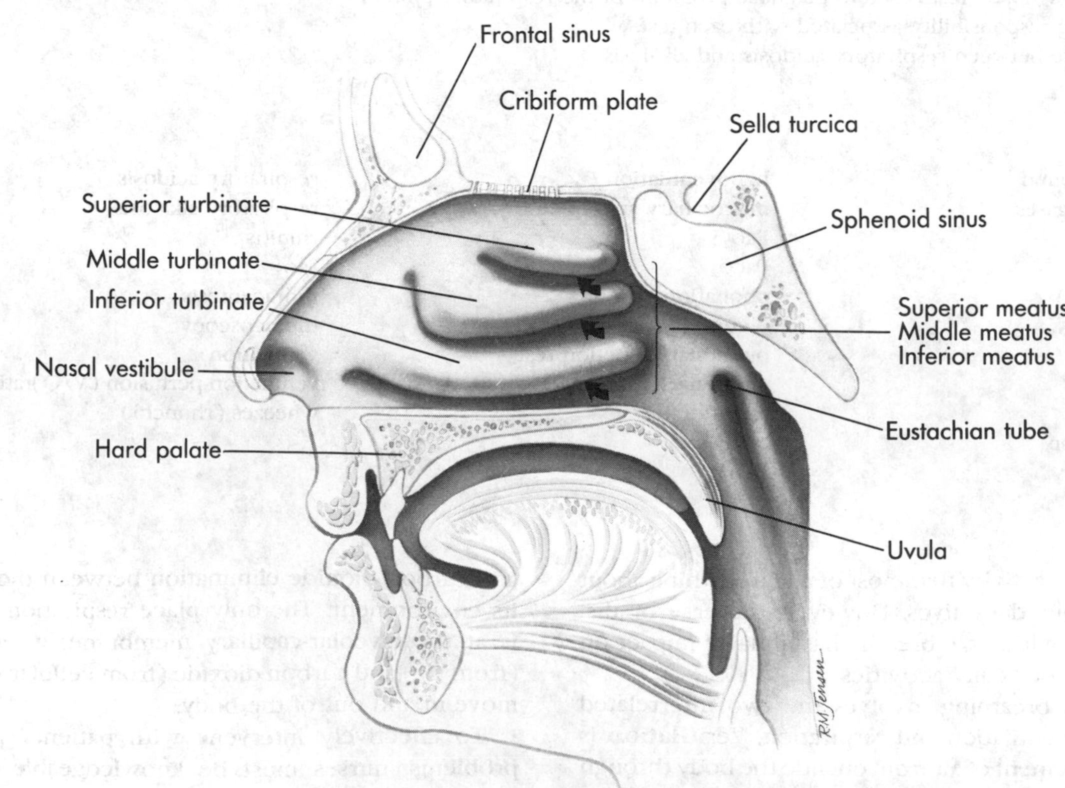


**FIGURE 35-1** Lateral wall of nose, showing superior, middle, and inferior turbinates. (From DeWeese DD, et al: *Otolaryngology—head and neck surgery,* ed 7, St Louis, 1988, Mosby.)

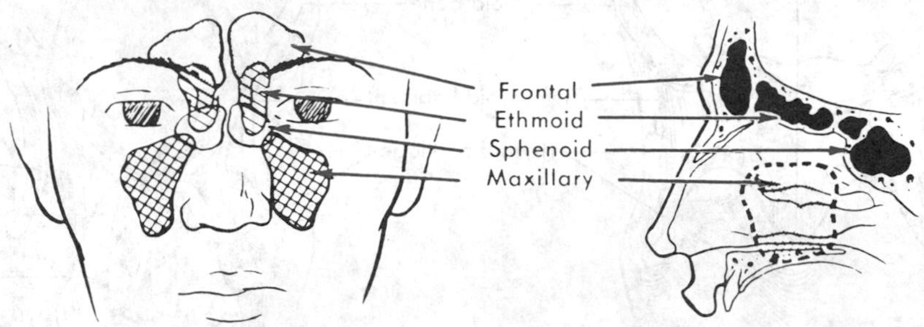


**FIGURE 35-2** Location of sinuses.

pharynx can be considered in three parts: the nasopharynx, the oropharynx, and the laryngopharynx (Figure 35-3). It is lined with mucous membrane.

The adenoids are located in the nasopharynx, the palatine tonsils anterior to the oropharynx, and the lingual tonsils in the hypopharynx. The adenoids and tonsils are made up of lymphoid tissue that helps to filter the circulating lymph of bacteria or other foreign matter that penetrate the body, especially by way of the nose and mouth.

## Lower Throat: Larynx and Laryngopharynx

The larynx forms the upper extremity of the trachea. The framework of the larynx is made up of several cartilages held together by muscle and ligaments (Figure 35-4). The cartilaginous framework of the larynx protects the vocal cords and affords a stiffness that permits an airway. The thyroid cartilage, commonly termed the *Adam's apple,* is the largest cartilaginous element in the larynx and serves to protect the inner structures. The hyoid bone lies just above the thyroid cartilage and forms an attachment for the larynx and tongue. The cricoid cartilage lies just below the thyroid cartilage and articulates with the arytenoid cartilages, which swing in and out to open and close the vocal cords by opening and closing the glottis (the opening formed between the vocal cords). The larynx is lined with mucosa continuous with that of the laryngopharynx and trachea. The vagus nerve innervates the larynx by means of the recurrent laryngeal nerve.

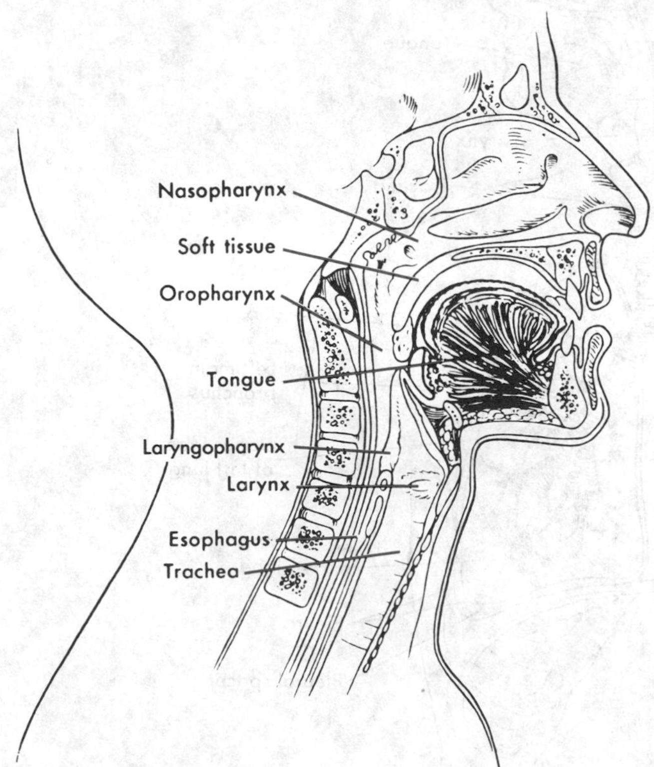


**FIGURE 35-3** Sagittal section of head showing pharynx and larynx.

The chief function of the larynx is to serve as an airway between the pharynx and trachea. A leaf-shaped lid of fibrocartilage (epiglottis) protects the glottis by covering the entrance to the larynx during swallowing to prevent aspiration of food or fluids. The closing of the glottis also allows for an increase of intrathoracic pressure, which is needed, for example, in coughing or lifting. This increased pressure gives added advantage to the use of the muscles of the shoulder and thorax. The cough reflex, like the sneeze reflex, helps remove inhaled particles from the respiratory tract. An additional function of the larynx is **phonation.** The larynx creates sounds as a result of vocal cord vibrations that are formed into speech patterns by the movement of the pharynx, palate, tongue, teeth, and lips.

# LOWER AIRWAY

## Structure and Function of Respiratory Tract

The *conducting airways* (trachea, right and left mainstem bronchi, and bronchioles), which terminate into *respiratory units* (respiratory bronchioles, alveolar ducts, and alveoli), make up the lower airways (Figures 35-5 and 35-6).

In addition to providing a passageway for air, the conducting airways serve three functions: filtering, warming, and humidifying air. Air inspired through an intact respiratory tree is cleansed of all particles larger than 2 μm in diameter before reaching the alveoli. The removal of particulate matter, such as dust and bacteria, preserves the sterility of the alveoli and is accomplished

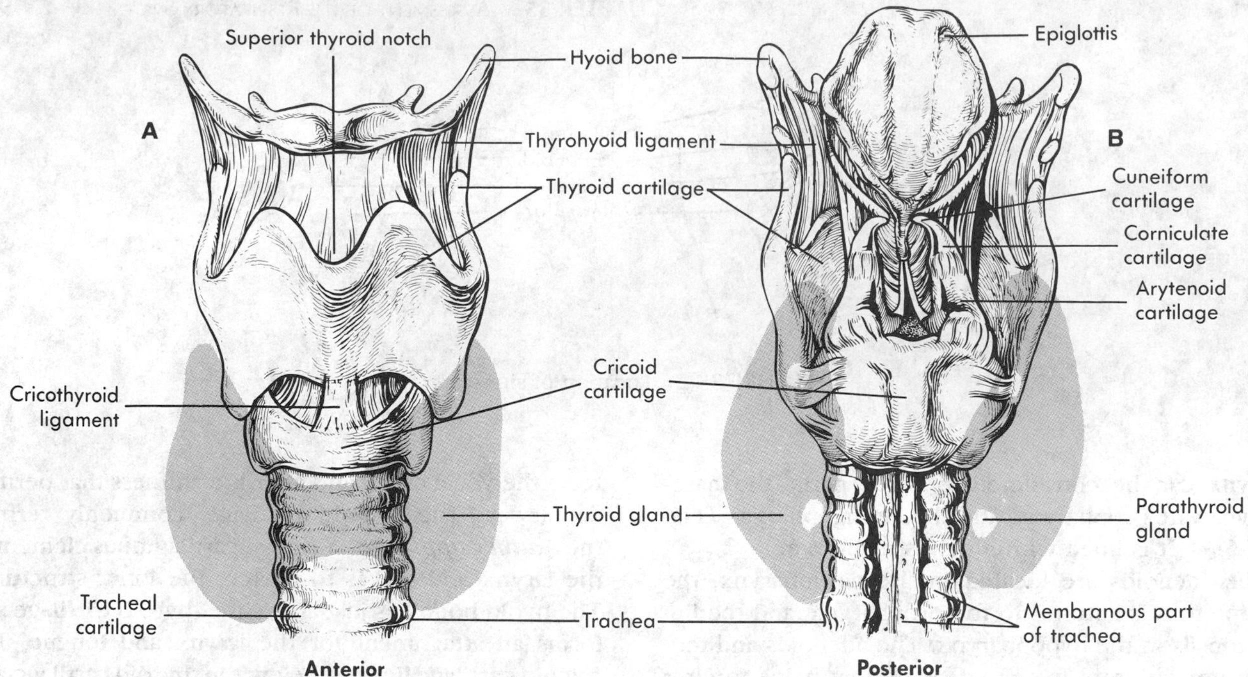


**FIGURE 35-4** Anterior aspect of larynx. (From Francis CC: *Introduction to human anatomy,* ed 6, St Louis, 1975, Mosby.)

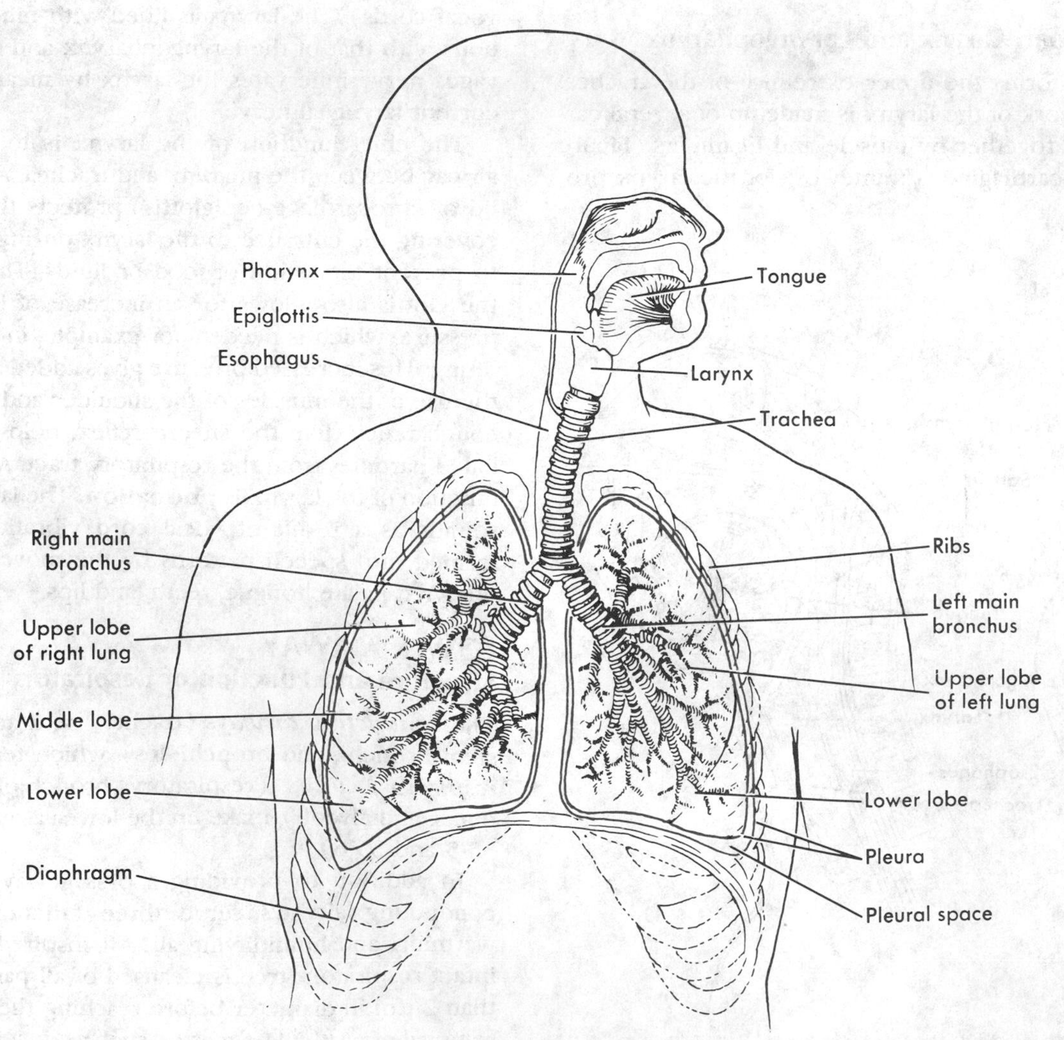


**FIGURE 35-5** Anatomy of the thorax and lungs.

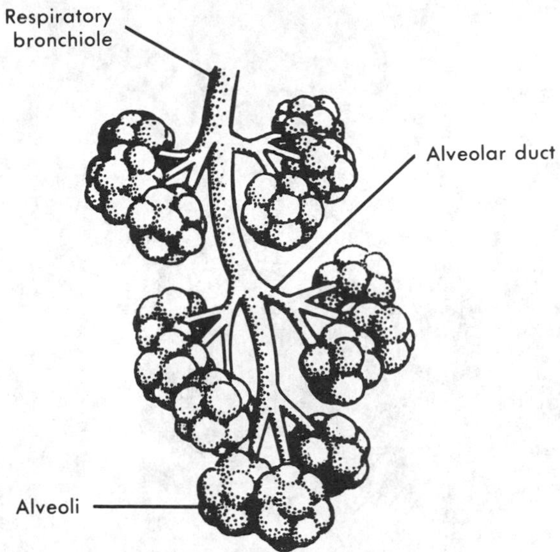


**FIGURE 35-6** Respiratory unit.

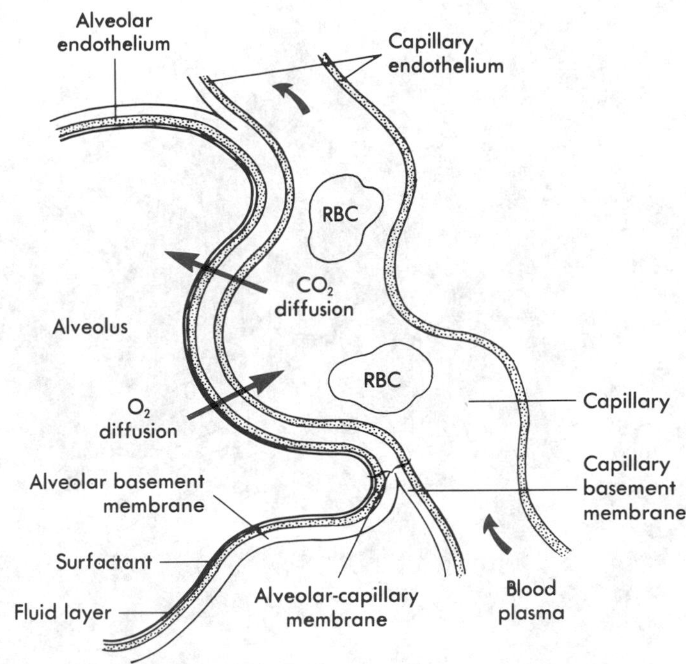


**FIGURE 35-7** Alveolar-capillary membrane.

by the **mucociliary system,** one of the lung's primary defense mechanisms. The mucociliary system consists of *cilia,* which line the respiratory tract from the laryngopharynx through the terminal bronchioles, and a dual-layered *fluid lining* secreted by *goblet cells* and *subendothelial glands.* The fluid lining that lies on top of the cilia consists of a lower serous and upper mucopolysaccharide (mucous) layer. Inhaled particles are trapped in the mucous layer and are propelled upward toward the pharynx by the continuous rapid beating of the cilia. After reaching the pharynx, mucus and particles are removed from the airways by swallowing, coughing, or sneezing. The process of particle removal by the mucociliary system is often referred to as the *mucociliary escalator.*

The warming and humidifying functions are made possible by the rich capillary blood supply in the submucosal layer of the airways. During inspiration, air is heated to body temperature, and up to 1000 ml/day of water is used to raise the humidity of the inspired air to at least 80%. On expiration, some of this water is reabsorbed, thus conserving fluid; an average of 300 ml/day is lost in normal respiration.

As mentioned earlier, respiration occurs only at the alveolar-capillary membrane. *Alveoli,* which number 300 million in adults, are minute sacs that arise from the walls of the respiratory bronchioles and alveolar ducts. The alveolus itself is composed of a single layer of squamous epithelium and an elastic basement membrane. These two layers, together with the interstitium and the endothelial and basement layers of the adjacent capillary, form the alveolar-capillary membrane or interface. It is across this membrane, a distance of less than 1 μm, that **diffusion** *of carbon dioxide and oxygen occurs* (Figure 35-7). The spherical interconnected structure of the millions of alveoli provides a large (50 to 100 m) surface area for gaseous diffusion to occur.

In addition to their respiratory function, the alveoli prevent lung collapse by producing *surfactant,* a phospholipid that decreases surface tension and prevents interstitial fluid from traversing into the lung space. Any foreign matter that deposits in healthy alveoli is engulfed by macrophages and disposed of through the circulatory system.

## Lungs and Thoracic Cavity

The lungs themselves are subdivided into lobes. The right lung has three lobes: upper, middle, and lower. The left lung has only two lobes: upper and lower. Air is conducted to each lobe through lobar bronchi that branch off the main stem bronchi. An important difference between the right and left lungs is the size of the airways leading to them. The right bronchus is significantly wider and shorter and extends at a straighter angle from the trachea, making it the more likely lodging point of aspirated material. The left bronchus is narrower and extends at more of a right angle off the trachea, making it more difficult to suction secretions from the left lung.

The thoracic cavity is lined with a continuous *serous* membrane known as the pleura. One surface of it lines the inside of the rib cage (parietal pleura), and the other surface (visceral pleura) covers the lungs. The space between the two surfaces is known as a *potential space.* It normally contains a few milliliters of serous fluid that prevents friction rub when the two surfaces come together.

The lungs lie in and are protected by the thoracic

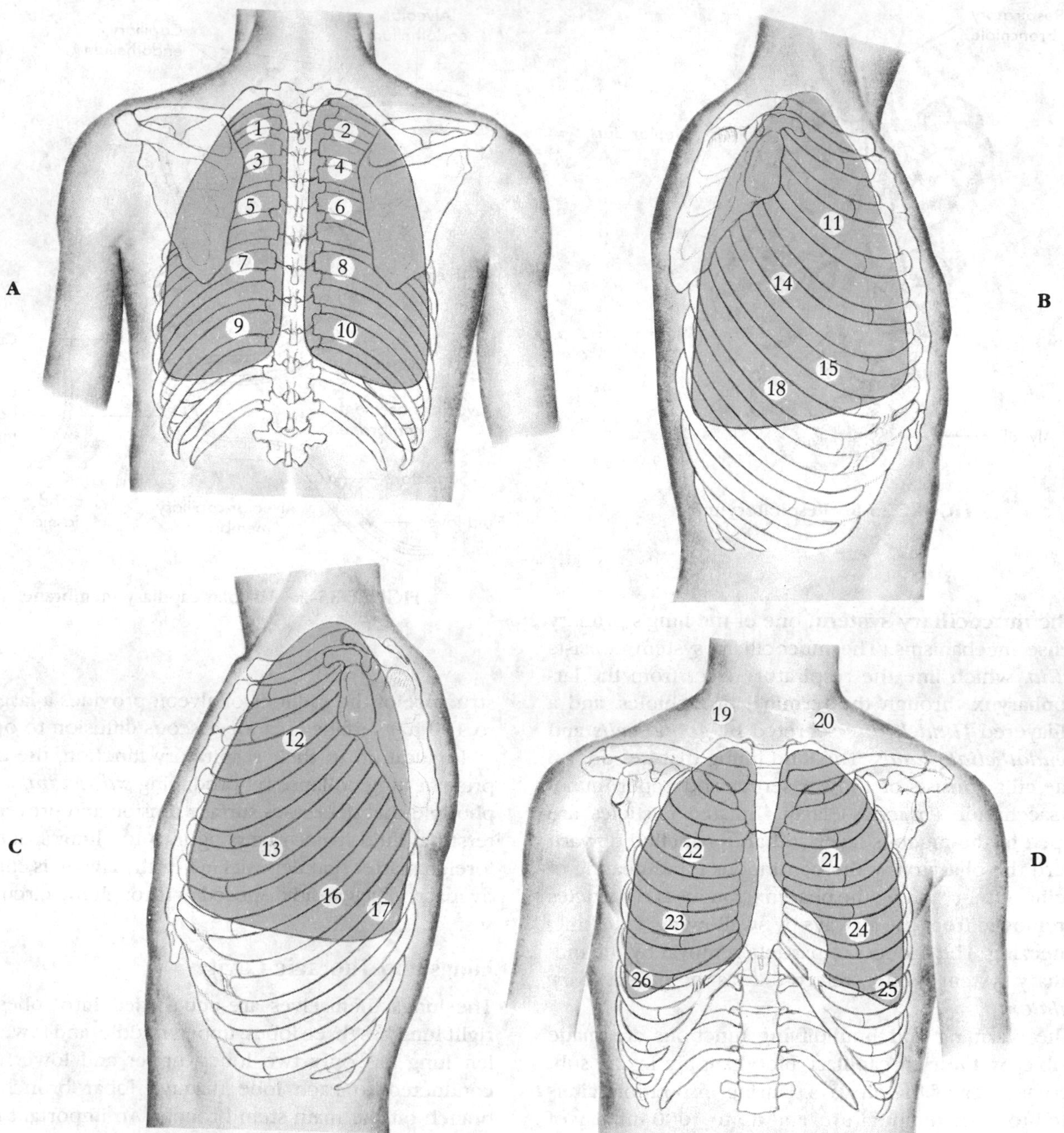


**FIGURE 35-8** Numbers indicate a recommended sequence for percussion and auscultation during a routine screening examination. **A,** Posterior thorax, **B,** Right lateral thorax. **C,** Left lateral thorax. **D,** Anterior thorax. (From Seidel H et al: *Mosby's guide to physical examination,* ed 3, St Louis, 1995, Mosby.)

cavity. This bony cage is composed of the sternum and ribs anteriorly and the ribs, scapulae, and vertebral column posteriorly. The lungs extend from the apices (just above the clavicles) to the bases (the eleventh or twelfth rib). Figure 35-8 illustrates the borders of each lobe.

## Respiratory Muscles

The major function of the respiratory muscles is to pump air in and out of the lungs. This is essential for maintaining arterial blood gas levels within acceptable limits.[6]

The primary muscles of *inspiration* include the *diaphragm,* the *external intercostals,* the *internal parasternal intercostals,* and the *scalene muscles.* The major inspiratory muscle is the diaphragm, which is innervated by the phrenic nerve.

Although normal quiet expiration does not require active muscle contraction, relaxation of the abdominal muscles at the far end of inspiration allows passive descent of the diaphragm during expiration. When expiration is active—for example, as a result of exercise—the *internal intercostal* and *abdominal muscles* contract to assist expiration of air out of the lungs.

*Accessory muscles* that are used when breathing is labored include the *sternocleidomastoids, pectoralis major and minor, trapezii,* and *laryngeal muscles.* The scalene muscles were formerly thought to be accessory muscles, but recent research has demonstrated that the contraction of these muscles during inspiration is necessary for diaphragmatic descent to occur.[6]

## Mechanisms of Pulmonary Ventilation

Air moves in and out of the lungs as a result of the principle of gas flow; that is, movement is from an area of greater pressure to an area of lesser pressure. At the start of inspiration, the atmospheric air pressure is greater than alveolar pressure; therefore air moves through the respiratory passageway into the alveoli. When the alveolar pressure exceeds atmospheric pressure, expiration occurs, and air moves out of the lungs into the atmosphere.

The pressure gradient between the alveoli and the atmosphere is established by changes in the size of the thoracic cavity. As the size of the thorax increases, pressure decreases, and air flows into the lung. Thoracic size is increased by contraction of the diaphragm and the external intercostal muscles. The diaphragm descends as it contracts and flattens, increasing the longitudinal diameter of the thorax. The external intercostals, parasternal internal intercostal, and the scalene muscles pull the ribs up and out, elevating the sternum and increasing both the anteroposterior and lateral diameters of the chest.

As the thorax expands, it pulls the lungs with it because of cohesion between the moist surfaces of the lungs and chest wall. Expiration is normally a passive process that results from the elastic recoil of the lungs and thoracic muscles. It is this ability of the lungs to stretch and recoil that is evaluated by **pulmonary function testing** (see Table 35-9, *A* and *B*). The ability of the lungs to stretch is measured in terms of compliance. **Compliance** is the volume increase in lungs for every unit increase in intraalveolar pressure. This relationship is defined by the following formula:

$$\text{Compliance} = \text{Change in volume}/\text{Change in pressure}$$

Thus lungs with increased (high) compliance have a larger increase in volume for each unit of pressure. Lungs with increased compliance characterize a group of pulmonary disorders known as obstructive diseases. Lungs with decreased (low) compliance have a decreased volume for each unit of pressure. Decreased lung compliance characterizes lung disorders called restrictive diseases (see Chapter 37).

The other property that affects the ability of the lungs to ventilate is pulmonary resistance. This property is evaluated by measuring lung volume and airflow over time (see Table 35-9, *C*). **Pulmonary resistance** *is made up of tissue resistance and airway resistance.* Tissue resistance results from the friction created as tissues move against each other during lung expansion. Airway resistance results from friction encountered by air passing through the airways. The major factor affecting pulmonary resistance is the radius of the airways. The following factors reduce airway radius: (1) bronchial innervation of the smooth muscle of the bronchus (bronchoconstriction) (e.g., bronchospasm), (2) external compression (e.g., thoracic tumor), and (3) internal obstruction (e.g., mucus).

## Gas Exchange

In the alveoli, oxygen diffuses across the alveolar-capillary membrane from the alveoli into the blood because the partial pressure of oxygen (oxygen tension, $PO_2$) of *alveolar air* (100 mm Hg) is greater than the $PO_2$ of venous blood (40 mm Hg). Carbon dioxide diffuses in the opposite direction, because the $PCO_2$ of *venous blood* (46 mm Hg) is greater than the $PCO_2$ of alveolar air (40 mm Hg). The pulmonary diffusion capacity for carbon dioxide is much greater than that for oxygen, and thus carbon dioxide diffuses more readily.

Diffusion of oxygen is *decreased* by the following factors: (1) decreased atmospheric oxygen, (2) decreased alveolar ventilation, (3) decreased alveolar-capillary surface area, and (4) increased alveolar-capillary membrane thickness.

## Lung Circulation

The lungs receive blood from both pulmonary and bronchial circulation. *Bronchial circulation* provides blood flow to the tissues of the tracheobronchial tree. *Pulmonary circulation* is made up of the entire blood volume received from the right ventricle of the heart. The deoxygenated blood from the right ventricle is carried through the main pulmonary artery to successively branching vessels that follow the bronchi to the respiratory units. Within the alveolar walls, the branching capillaries form a dense network that has been described as a sheet of blood. Thus the circulatory system matches the vast surface created by the alveoli to provide for the rapid efficient exchange of oxygen and carbon dioxide. Newly oxygenated blood then travels via the *four pulmonary veins* back to the left atrium, where it is circulated throughout the body via the aorta.

## Ventilation-Perfusion Relationships

Exchange of oxygen and carbon dioxide between alveolar air and pulmonary capillary blood occurs by gaseous *diffusion.* It is imperative that lung *ventilation (air flow)* and *perfusion (blood flow)* are relatively evenly matched so that adequate oxygen and carbon dioxide exchange can occur. Both air flow to the alveoli and blood flow to the pulmonary capillaries have volumes of 4 to 6 L/min. A normal *ventilation-perfusion* ratio (usually depicted as $\dot{V}/\dot{Q}$) ranges from 0.8 to 1.2. A low ventilation-to-perfusion ratio exists when alveoli cannot receive ambient air. Blood flowing through the capillaries in contact with the occluded alveoli would have low oxygen and high carbon dioxide levels (see Figure 35-15). A clinical situation that can cause low ventilation-to-perfusion ratios is when secretions block bronchioles leading to alveoli. A high ventilation-to-perfusion ratio exists when a pulmonary capillary is blocked. In this situation, oxygen and carbon dioxide levels in the alveoli remain the same as those of ambient air. A clinical situation that can cause high ventilation-to-perfusion ratios is pulmonary emboli.

## Control of Respiration

Breathing is an automatic loop process by which multiple sensors (chemoreceptors) continually feed data to a central processor (medulla oblongata and pons), which then directs respiratory muscles that adjust ventilation to maintain homeostasis (Figure 35-9). In addition, humans are equipped with an override feature (cerebral cortex), so that ventilatory patterns can be consciously altered.

The major sensors are the central and peripheral chemoreceptors. *Central chemoreceptors,* located near the medulla, are *sensitive to pH* and *carbon dioxide level changes* in the cerebral spinal fluid. The response can be summarized as follows:

Increased carbon dioxide = Decreased pH
= Increased respiration

Decreased carbon dioxide = Increased pH
= Decreased respiration

In healthy individuals, ventilation is regulated by the central chemoreceptor response to levels of $CO_2$. It is important to remember that after a few days of exposure to elevated carbon dioxide levels, the central chemoreceptor becomes ineffective ($CO_2$ narcosis).

*Peripheral chemoreceptors,* located in the carotid body and aortic arch, respond to low arterial blood oxygen levels. The peripheral sensor mechanism is believed to be a built-in backup mechanism, and it does not function under normal physiologic conditions (Figure 35-9).

When the central chemoreceptor is not functioning because of elevated carbon dioxide levels of more than a few days' duration, the person's peripheral chemoreceptor response to a decreased oxygen level maintains respiration. Elevating the oxygen level without simultaneous lowering of the carbon dioxide level will result in apnea and death.

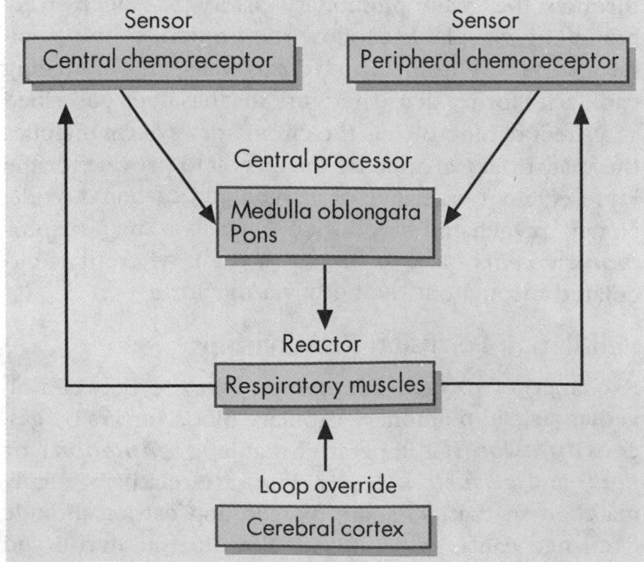


**FIGURE 35-9** Respiratory control loop.

## PHYSIOLOGIC CHANGES WITH AGING

The nurse assessing the older adult's respiratory system will observe normal variations in clinical findings that are the result of anatomic and physiologic changes associated with aging.

The thorax becomes more rigid with diminished rib movement from cartilage calcification and partial muscle contraction.[12] Kyphosis (hunchback) results in an increased anteroposterior diameter. Muscle atrophy of the pharynx and larynx decreases the ability to cough and clear airways effectively. Lung elasticity is diminished, resulting in decreased pulmonary compliance. Airway resistance increases and blood flow to the pulmonary-capillary membranes decreases, resulting in increased mismatch of air ventilation ($\dot{V}$) and blood perfusion ($\dot{Q}$).

An individual with these changes will present a clinical picture of *decreased vital capacity, decreased residual volume,* and *decreased forced expiratory volume.*[8] (See Table 35-8.) The patient can be observed to have a slight increase in resting respiratory rate with a simultaneous decrease in tidal volume. Although arterial carbon dioxide tension does not change, arterial oxygen tension will be lower. The other classic variant resulting from pulmonary structural changes is that a larger interval will be required for return to resting respiratory rate after exertion. Assessment, interventions, and common disorders found in elderly persons are listed in the Gerontologic Patient Considerations box, p. 983.

# SUBJECTIVE DATA

## UPPER AIRWAY

Before the physical examination, the nurse elicits information specific to the upper airways. A detailed symptom analysis is required whenever the patient indicates a positive history for upper airway dysfunction (for specific symptom analysis refer to a basic nursing text).

### Nose and Sinuses

Data relevant to assessment of the nose and sinuses can be obtained by asking questions about the following:

## GERONTOLOGIC PATIENT CONSIDERATIONS

### ASSESSMENT

Assess lung sounds; diminished lung sounds are common in elderly persons because of thickened alveoli and decreased rib cage expansion (thorax stiffening).

Assess respiratory status with activity; dyspnea with exertion may occur from decreased pulmonary oxygen diffusion.

Monitor effects of drugs that may interfere with breathing, such as narcotics and hypnotics. Elderly persons may have decreased drug clearance from decreased glomerular filtration rate (GFR) and nephron activity or from decreased hepatic function.

Monitor for signs of pneumonia, to which older persons are highly susceptible. Elderly patients may present with symptoms of mental confusion, tachycardia, or dyspnea, rather than the customary signs of cough, fever, and rales (crackles).

### INTERVENTION

Encourage as much activity as the person can tolerate to promote ventilation, such as paced walking.

Suggest that patient sit upright for meals and for 20 to 30 minutes after meals to prevent pulmonary aspiration during eating.

Encourage pneumococcal and influenza vaccine prophylaxis.

Teach patient the importance of oral care to help prevent pneumonia.

For the elderly patient with pneumonia, maintain good hydration (with close monitoring to prevent fluid imbalances) and assist with respiratory therapy and position changes.

### COMMON DISORDERS IN ELDERS

Pneumonia
Lung cancer
COPD

1. Obstruction of nares
   a. History of mouth-breathing (time of day or night, duration, and frequency)
   b. History of nasal surgery or injury to nose
   c. Use of nasal drops or spray (type, amount, frequency, and duration of use)
2. Nasal discharge
   a. Color, amount, and consistency of discharge
   b. Nasal bleeding (epistaxis)—one or both nares
   c. Presence of nasal crusting or pain
3. History of sinusitis
   a. Headaches (location and severity)
   b. Relationship of sinusitis to certain seasons or types of weather

## Upper Throat: Pharynx and Tonsils

Data relevant to dysfunction of the pharynx and tonsils can be obtained by asking questions about the following if the patient has a dry or sore throat:

1. Work or home environment (e.g., exposure to recent illness, inhalation of fumes or dust, or low humidity level)
2. Pain on swallowing (dysphagia)
3. History of alcohol use

## BOX 35-1 Cough Descriptors

### TIMING

1. Chronic
2. Acute
3. Paroxysmal (periodic forceful episodes that are difficult to control)

### QUALITY

1. Productive-nonproductive
2. Dry-moist
3. Barking
4. Hoarse
5. Hacking

## Lower Throat: Larynx and Laryngopharynx

Questions related to dysfunction of the larynx and laryngopharynx in a patient experiencing a change in voice (hoarseness) include the following:

1. Acute or chronic
2. Frequency
3. Smoking and alcohol use history
4. Excessive use of voice (i.e., excessive speaking or shouting)

# LOWER AIRWAY

Before the physical examination is performed, a nursing history is obtained. Elements critical to assessment of respiratory status are the following:

1. Exposure to known risk factors, such as cigarette smoke
2. Presence of common pulmonary symptoms
3. Impact of respiratory illness on functional capacity
4. Current medications and treatments, including prescription, nonprescription, and "folk" remedies
5. Acceptable level of health the patient hopes to attain

The major symptoms associated with respiratory disease are *cough, dyspnea, chest pain, sputum production, hemoptysis,* and *wheezing.* Whenever the patient indicates the presence of pulmonary symptoms, a full analysis of the symptoms is completed. Analysis of these symptoms is discussed next.

## Cough

*Coughing,* the explosive expulsion of air from the lungs, has two main functions. *It protects the lungs from aspiration, and it helps propel foreign matter and excess mucus up through the airways.* Coughing is also the most common symptom of respiratory disease. Box 35-1 lists terminology used to describe the types of cough.

One aspect of chronic cough that is difficult to assess is the actual time of onset. The individual is often not aware of its onset or attributes its presence to identifiable causes, such as smoking or sinusitis. A family member or close associate might be able to more accurately iden-

## RESEARCH

Janson-Bjerklie S, Carrieri VK, Hudes M: The sensations of pulmonary dyspnea, *Nurs Res* 35(3):154-159, 1986.

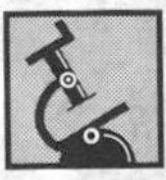

The study of a convenience sample of 68 subjects with a variety of pulmonary diseases compared recalled physical and emotional sensations during episodes of acute dyspnea. Although frequency of sensations were found to be similar across disease categories, some differences in magnitude and character of the dyspnea experience were found among disease groups. Physical sensations experienced during episodes of dyspnea clustered into categories of suffocation, tightness, and congestion.

tify actual time of onset. It is important to identify those factors the patient (and spouse or friend) believes contribute to the cough. Areas to explore include these factors commonly associated with *cough: activity, body position, environmental irritants, vocalization (normal speech, shouting, singing, whispering), weather, anxiety,* and *infection.*

## Dyspnea

Dyspnea is a subjective perception of being short of breath. Dyspnea involves both a physiologic and cognitive component. First, awareness of breathing must occur; then it must be interpreted as inadequate for the degree of activity. A retrospective descriptive study of people's sensations of dyspnea is presented in the Research box above.

The physiologic component is not fully understood, but it appears that dyspnea is related more to the ventilatory component of breathing than to respiration.[9] Dyspnea associated with respiratory disease results from pathologic changes that increase airway resistance, decrease pulmonary compliance, alter the pulmonary vascular system, or weaken the respiratory muscles. Although dyspnea is associated with many underlying cardiopulmonary diseases, two common mediating processes that are present, regardless of underlying pathology, are *increased respiratory muscle activity* and *respiratory muscle weakness.*

Box 35-2 presents those aspects of the patient's dyspnea that are important to assess.

Because of its insidious nature, the actual onset of chronic dyspnea is difficult to identify. Relatives or close associates of the person might be able to help in identifying the time of onset. Often it is helpful to offer suggestions, such as having the person associate past birthdays or holidays with the presence of dyspnea. When assessing the severity of dyspnea, subjective terms—such as mild, moderate, or severe—should be avoided. A number of tools in the literature provide a means for the clinician to quantify the person's experience of dyspnea.[1,4,5,11] Many of these instruments provide a systematic magnitude estimate using the dyspneic person's verbal report; thus they are amenable to clinical assessment without requiring special equipment. The instruments often focus on the person's perception of dyspnea related to activities of daily living (ADLs). An example of one of the magnitude scales is a scale developed by the American Thoracic Society (Table 35-1).

### BOX 35-2 Dyspnea Descriptors

**TIMING**

1. Chronic or acute
2. Episodic or paroxysmal
3. Onset
4. Duration
5. Frequency

**CHARACTERISTICS**

1. Perceived severity
2. Phase of respiratory cycle when occurs
   a. Inspiratory
   b. Expiratory
   c. Throughout entire cycle
3. Other symptoms related to dyspnea
4. Associated factors
   a. Time of day
   b. Seasonal or weather changes
   c. Environmental irritants
   d. Anxiety
   e. Body position
      (1) Paroxysmal nocturnal dyspnea (PND): sudden onset while sleeping in recumbent position
      (2) Orthopnea: breathlessness on assuming recumbent position

## Chest Pain

Chest pain of pulmonary origin can derive from the chest wall, parietal pleura, visceral pleura, or the lung parenchyma itself. Table 35-2 summarizes the types of chest pain related to pulmonary conditions.

Whenever the patient indicates the presence of chest pain, the symptom requires detailed investigation. (Chapter 17 includes specific guidelines for pain assessment.)

## Sputum Production

The lung *goblet cells* and *mucous glands* secrete mucus that coats the interior lung surface. Mucus is constantly propelled upward toward the pharynx by the lung cilia. Sputum—composed of mucus, cellular debris, microorganisms, blood, pus, and foreign particles—is the substance ejected from the lungs by coughing or clearing the throat.

It is important to clarify whether the patient is describing saliva or sputum. To accurately assess the type and amount of sputum production, specimen collection

**TABLE 35-1 American Thoracic Society/Five-level Scale of Breathlessness, Graded 1 to 5**

| GRADE | DESCRIPTION |
|---|---|
| 1 | Are you troubled by shortness of breath during walking on the level or walking up a slight hill? Yes ____ No ____ |
| 2 | Do you have to walk slower than people of your age on the level because of breathlessness? Yes ____ No ____ |
| 3 | Do you ever have to stop for breath when walking at your own pace on the level? Yes ____ No ____ |
| 4 | Do you ever have to stop for breath after walking about 100 yards or after a few minutes walking on the level? Yes ____ No ____ |
| 5 | Are you too breathless to leave the house or breathless on dressing or undressing? Yes ____ No ____ |

**TABLE 35-2 Thoracic-Pulmonary Chest Pain**

| ORIGIN | CHARACTERISTICS | POSSIBLE CAUSE |
|---|---|---|
| Chest wall | Well-localized constant ache increasing with movement | Trauma, cough, herpes zoster |
| Pleura | Sharp, abrupt onset increasing with inspiration or with sudden ventilatory effort (cough, sneeze), unilateral | Pleural inflammation (pleurisy), pulmonary infarction, pneumothorax, tumors |
| Lung parenchyma | Dull, constant ache, poorly localized | Benign pulmonary tumors<br>Carcinoma<br>Pneumothorax |

might be required (see p. 994). The patient's sputum production should be analyzed for onset, pattern of occurrence, exposure to risk factors, associated illnesses, consistency, odor, color, and amount. Common descriptors for sputum are presented in Box 35-3.

### Hemoptysis

**Hemoptysis** *is the coughing up of blood or bloody or blood-tinged sputum.* The source of bleeding might be from anywhere in the upper or lower airways or from the lung parenchyma. The patient usually perceives hemoptysis as an indicator of serious illness and will often appear anxious or afraid. If hemoptysis is present, a description of onset, duration, amount, and color (for example, bright red or frothy) is obtained. As with any symptom, a full analysis is appropriate. *It is important to differentiate between hemoptysis and hematemesis.* This can be difficult if the patient has swallowed bloody sputum or, conversely, aspirated bloody vomitus. If a specimen has been saved, it might be possible to assess its origin by criteria noted in Box 35-4.

**BOX 35-3 Sputum Descriptors**

**AMOUNT**

1. Scant (few teaspoons)
2. Copious

**CONSISTENCY**

1. Thick
2. Viscous (gelatinous)
3. Tenacious (sticky)
4. Frothy
5. Mucoid (clear, thin to moderately thick)
6. Watery
7. Mucopurulent (thick, viscous; color: cream, yellow, or green)
8. Casts (from bronchioles, rubbery)

**BOX 35-4 Bedside Assessment of Hemoptysis and Hematemesis**

| HEMOPTYSIS | HEMATEMESIS |
|---|---|
| Usually frothy | Never frothy |
| pH (of blood) alkaline | pH (of blood) acidic |

### Wheezing

Wheezing is a continuous sound produced when air passes through the smaller bronchi or bronchioles where there is increased airway resistance. Airway resistance is increased by bronchoconstriction or an increase of mucus in the bronchi. Audible wheezing can be heard throughout the respiratory cycle or only during inspiration or expiration. When bronchoconstriction is present, wheezing will be greater on expiration. If wheezing is present, a full analysis of it is completed.

## PULMONARY RISK FACTORS

Major risk factors associated with pulmonary disease are *smoking, history of previous pulmonary disorders, environmental irritants,* and *genetic predisposition.*

### Smoking

Smoking has been implicated as a major cause of lung disease. There is a strong relationship between smoking and the development or exacerbation of chronic bronchitis, emphysema, asthma, lung carcinoma, and respiratory infections.*

*The reader is referred to the Jan. 6, 1989, issue of the *Journal of the American Medical Association*, which is devoted entirely to the subject of the effects of smoking.

*Passive smoking* has been implicated as increasing the *nonsmoker's risk of developing carcinoma.* Maternal smoking is known to increase the incidence of respiratory illness in children and may be related to increased lung cancer risk in later life.[13] The known acute effects of cigarette smoking include increased airway resistance, increased mucus in small airways and later increased secretions in large airways, reduced lung recoil, vascular changes, and respiratory bronchiolitis.[2]

The patient's current or past history of smoking behaviors must be determined. The type of smoking material (tobacco, marijuana) and the mode of smoking (pipe, cigarette, or cigar) should be identified. *It is also important to explore the use of smokeless tobacco, particularly in the younger male population, because of its relationship to upper airway disorders.* Variable effects of smoking that should be assessed include an estimate of depth of inhalation, number of puffs per cigarette, use of a filter, brand of cigarette smoked, and presence of other risk factors.[10]

Questions relevant to smoking history are as follows:

1. How long?
2. How much in pack-years? (see the following formula)
3. Is smoke inhaled?
4. How much of the cigarette (cigar, pipe) is smoked?
5. Have attempts been made to quit?
6. Is there a desire to quit?

The nurse can determine how much tobacco is smoked by the following equation (cigarettes are determined by "pack-years"; cigars, pipes, marijuana, and smokeless tobacco are determined as amount used per day):

"Pack-year" = Number of years smoked × Number of packs smoked per day (for example, 20 years of 2 packs/day = 40 pack-years)

### History of Previous Pulmonary Disorders

The patient should be asked about the following illnesses:

1. Childhood allergies and frequent pulmonary infections
2. History of influenza (especially *Haemophilus influenzae*), chronic sinusitis, frequent colds, pneumonia, and pleurisy
3. Chest surgery
4. Tuberculosis
5. Adult-onset allergies

### Environmental Irritants

This category includes atmospheric pollutants (dust, fungal spores, vapor, fumes, and gases), occupational contaminants (chemical fumes, coal dust, and molds), and environmental factors.

The following areas should be addressed during the nursing history:

1. Residence or work in heavy industry areas
2. Residence or work in area of heavy automobile traffic
3. Known high-risk occupations (for example, mining, foundry work, welding, textile, quarry work, wood and paper mills, farming, and chemical manufacturing)
4. Exposure to bird droppings in an enclosed space (e.g., chicken house, old buildings being remodeled)
5. Travel and residential history, where person has lived or visited (certain pulmonary disorders, such as histoplasmosis or "farmer's lung" related to geographic areas) (see Chapter 37)

### Genetic Disorders

A genetically predetermined deficiency in the proteinase inhibitors $\alpha_1$-antitrypsin and $\alpha_2$-macroglobulin is associated with a high risk of developing emphysema. To identify the possible presence of this risk, inquiry into the following areas is helpful:

1. Does the patient or any family member have a documented history of enzyme deficiency?
2. Is there a strong family history of chronic obstructive pulmonary disease (COPD)?
3. Has either the patient or any family member developed respiratory symptoms at an early age?
4. Does either the patient or any family member have a history of liver disease? NOTE: There is also a correlation between liver disease and $\alpha_1$-antitrypsin deficiency.

## ASSESSMENT OF FUNCTIONAL ABILITY

Individuals experiencing pulmonary dysfunction tend to perceive their illness in terms of its impact on their ability to carry out activities of daily living (ADLs). One study of persons with COPD found that participants would describe symptoms such as "weakness," "tiredness," or "loss of libido"; but in retrospect it is believed that these were the onset of COPD-related dyspnea. An example of a nursing assessment tool that asks questions about the functional areas of locomotion, biofunctional activities, and vocalization is presented in Box 35-5.

## MEDICATION AND TREATMENT

In addition to obtaining information about all prescription and nonprescription medications and treatments, it is also important to ask about any additional methods used by the patient to treat illness. Patients are often unwilling to share folk remedies at their initial interview for fear of disapproval by caregivers. Patients must be approached in a nonjudgmental manner. A neutral inquiry such as, "Is there anything you have found that seems to help you feel better?" conveys receptiveness on the part of the interviewer.

## ESTABLISHING THE PATIENT'S HEALTH GOAL

Because pulmonary disorders run the spectrum from total cure without residual damage to chronic terminal illness, the patient's goals for health will be highly individualized. A functional approach to defining the pa-

**BOX 35-5 Nursing Assessment of Activities of Daily Living**

| Do any of the following make you short of breath? | YES | NO |
|---|---|---|
| a. Walking fast on flat ground (l) | ____ | ____ |
| b. Walking uphill (l) | ____ | ____ |
| c. Climbing stairs (l) | ____ | ____ |
| d. Bending over to do something, such as tying shoes or picking up an object (l) | ____ | ____ |
| e. Any work requiring arms raised above chest, such as combing your hair (l) | ____ | ____ |
| f. Talking (v) | ____ | ____ |
| g. Yelling (v) | ____ | ____ |
| h. Laughing (v) | ____ | ____ |
| i. Sleeping (b) | ____ | ____ |
| j. Eating (b) | ____ | ____ |
| k. Bowel movements (b) | ____ | ____ |
| l. Sexual activity (b) | ____ | ____ |
| m. Any other activity | ____ | ____ |

From Brucia J: Unpublished master's thesis, 1982, p. 104.
*b*, Biofunctional; *l*, locomotion; *v*, vocalization.

tient's health goals will provide visible meaningful goals for both caregivers and the patient. An example of a functional goal would be, "I want to be able to cook my meals."

# OBJECTIVE DATA

## UPPER AIRWAY

In addition to the interview, physical examination provides objective data necessary to identify specific upper airway disorders.

### Nose and Sinuses

Inspection of the nose includes looking for deformities, asymmetry, and inflammation. The nasal mucosa is normally redder than oral mucosa. The inferior and middle turbinates are observed for color, edema, exudate, or polyps. The nasal septum is observed for deviation, bleeding, or perforation. Some septal deviation (Figure 35-10) is common in most adults and is usually asymptomatic, although it can produce nasal obstruction. Abnormal findings in assessing the nose include any excessive redness, edema, exudate, or bleeding, as well as the presence of any furuncles. Red, swollen nasal mucous membranes accompanied by watery to mucopurulent nasal discharge indicate *acute* **rhinitis.** Nasal mucosa that is swollen, pale, boggy, and usually gray to dull red is seen in persons with *allergic rhinitis.* Soft pale gray mobile structures found in the middle meatus are polyps that can develop in persons with allergic rhinitis.

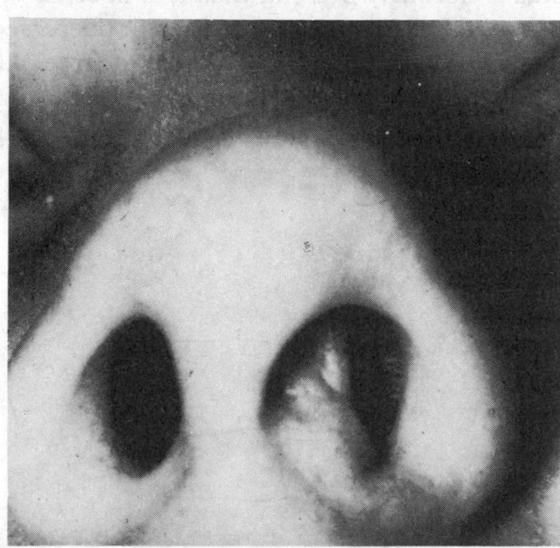

**FIGURE 35-10** Septal deviation. Anterior end of septal cartilage is dislocated and projects into nasal vestibule. (From Saunders WH et al: *Nursing care in eye, ear, nose, and throat disorders,* ed 4, St Louis, 1979, Mosby.)

The sinuses are palpated for signs of tenderness of the frontal and maxillary areas when inspecting the nose. The normal frontal and maxillary sinuses can be visualized by illuminating them in a dark room with a specially shaped, lighted bulb or a lighted transillumination tip. This examination is referred to as *transillumination.* If disease is present, the light will not penetrate the sinuses, or it will reveal fluid levels indicative of obstruction to drainage of the sinuses. Roentgenologic examination of the sinuses can help establish the diagnosis of sinusitis. No physical preparation is necessary, and usually no contrast medium is used, because the normal sinus is filled with air, which in itself casts a shadow in contrast to surrounding structures.

### Pharynx and Tonsils

The oropharynx, that portion of the pharynx directly posterior to the oral cavity bounded by the nasopharynx above and laryngopharynx below, is examined with a tongue blade and a mirror. The anterior and posterior tonsillar pillars, the uvula, the tonsils, and the posterior pharynx are inspected for color, symmetry, evidence of exudate, edema, ulcerations, and tonsillar enlargement. Redness and swelling of the tonsils, pillars, and uvula with white or yellow exudate on the tonsils might indicate streptococcal infection. Tonsils can be enlarged without being infected.

### Larynx and Laryngopharynx

The larynx can be examined by an *indirect laryngoscopy;* the person being examined sits in a chair with the head tilted back and is asked to stick out the tongue. The examiner then grasps it with a gauze sponge and pulls it forward and down. A warmed laryngeal mirror is introduced into the back of the throat until the larynx is visualized. It is examined at rest and during attempts to speak (phonation). If the gag reflex is very sensitive, the pharyngeal wall can be sprayed with a topical anesthetic, such as 2% cocaine or 2% tetracaine (Pontocaine). Tetracaine is preferred by some physicians because it is less toxic than cocaine. A *direct laryngoscopy* is performed on children, on adults who are unable to cooperate for an indirect examination, and on all persons with suspicious lesions of the larynx.[7]

## LOWER AIRWAY

Physical examination of the chest provides objective data that, along with information obtained during the interview, form the data base necessary to formulate nursing diagnoses appropriate to the individual. The pulmonary examination should be conducted with the person sitting upright on the edge of the bed, if possible. Adequate lighting and a relaxed, quiet environment are essential to obtain maximum information.

Detailed instruction on the techniques for performing the chest examination are beyond the scope of this book. The reader is referred to a textbook of physical assessment for in-depth information on the techniques of pulmonary physical assessment.

### Inspection

The patient is observed for general appearance, respiratory rate and pattern, and thoracic configuration (Figure 35-11). It is important to take adequate time to thoroughly observe the patient before moving to the "hands on" component of the examination. By observing general appearance, respiratory rate and pattern, the presence and character of the person's cough, and sputum production, the nurse can determine which components of the pulmonary examination are appropriate for assessing the patient's current respiratory status. Table 35-3 indicates the normal and abnormal findings for each component of inspection.

### Palpation

The chest is palpated to evaluate skin and chest wall status. Palpation of the chest and spinal column is a general screening technique to identify the presence of underlying abnormalities, such as inflammation. The chest is also palpated for **fremitus,** which are vibrations felt on the chest surface when sound passes through underlying tissue and air- or fluid-filled space. Fremitus can be caused by secretions in the large airways, a pleural friction rub, or lung consolidation. Vocal (tactile) fremitus is normally present; thus it is necessary to determine whether fremitus is increased or decreased. The chest is also palpated for symmetry and degree of lateral chest expansion from maximal exhalation to maximal inhalation. Possible normal and abnormal findings are presented in Table 35-4.

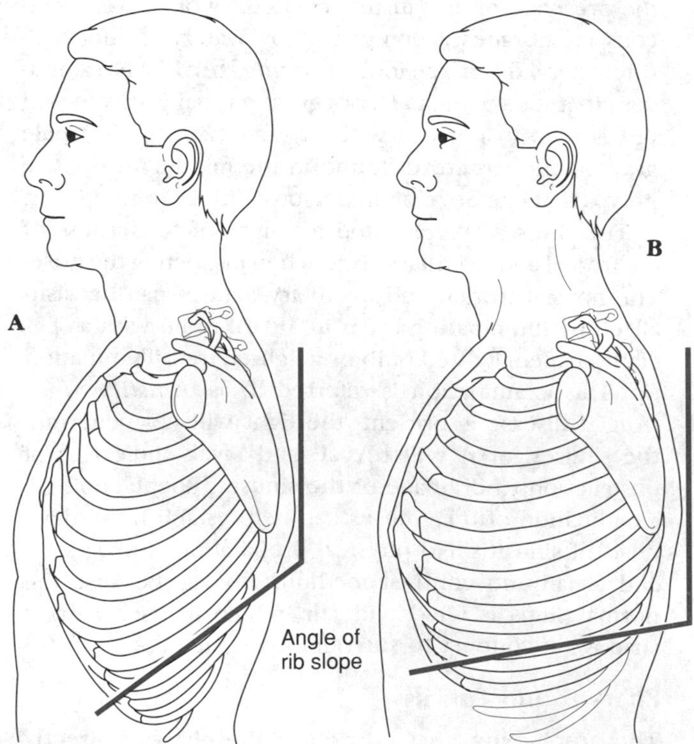


**FIGURE 35-11** **A,** Normal thorax configuration. **B,** Increased anteroposterior diameter. Note contrast in the angle of the slope of the ribs. (From Barkauskas VH et al: *Health and physical assessment,* St Louis, 1994, Mosby.)

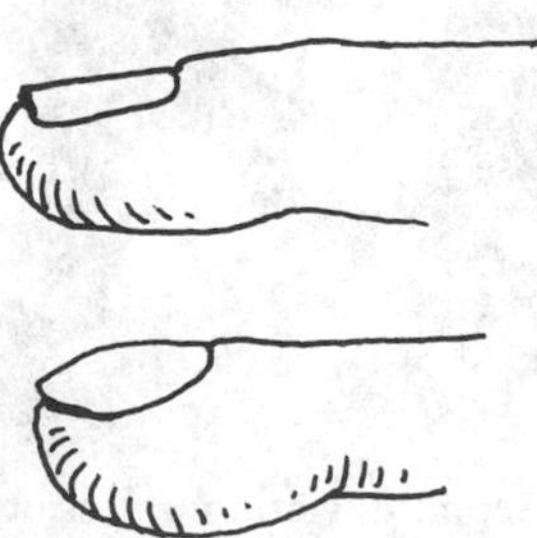

**FIGURE 35-12** Comparison of normal nail *(top)* and digital clubbing *(bottom).*

**TABLE 35-3 Possible Findings by Inspection in a Pulmonary Examination**

| OBSERVE | NORMAL | ABNORMAL |
|---|---|---|
| General appearance | Quiet respiration<br>Sitting or reclining without difficulty<br>Skin translucent, appears dry<br>Nailbeds pink<br>Mucous membranes pink and moist*<br>Cyanosis or pallor assessed by establishing an early individual baseline | Lips puckered when exhaling<br>Restless and apprehensive<br>Leans forward with hands or elbows on knees<br>Skin: diaphoretic, dull pale, or ruddy<br>Cyanosis: skin or mucous membranes have bluish cast<br>Central cyanosis: results from decreased oxygenation of blood†<br>Peripheral cyanosis: result of local vasoconstriction or decreased cardiac output<br>Nail clubbing: painless enlargement of terminal phalanges related to chronic tissue hypoxia (Figure 35-12) |
| Trachea | Midline in neck | Tracheal deviation; displacement either lateral, anterior, or posterior<br>Jugular venous distension (see Chapter 28)<br>Cough: strong or weak, dry or wet, productive or nonproductive<br>Sputum production: amount, color, odor, consistency (p. 985) |
| Rate | Eupnea: 12 to 20 | Tachypnea: rate >20 breaths/min<br>Bradypnea: rate <10 breaths/min |
| Breathing pattern | Minimal effort with inspiration: passive, quiet expiration<br>Inspiration/expiration ratio: 1:2<br>Male: diaphragmatic breathing<br>Female: thoracic breathing | Hyperpnea: increased breathing depth<br>Accessory muscle breathing<br>Apnea: total absence of breathing<br>Biots: irregular rhythm with periods of apnea<br>Cheyne-Stokes: cyclical deeper and shallower breaths, followed by periods of apnea<br>Kussmaul's: deep, rapid, and regular breathing<br>Paradoxical: portion of chest wall moves in during inhalation and out during exhalation<br>Stridorous: audible, loud, low-pitched sound with inhalation and exhalation |
| Thoracic configuration | Symmetric appearance<br><br>Anteroposterior diameter (AP) less than transverse diameter<br>Spine straight<br><br>Scapulae on same horizontal plane | Chest expands unevenly<br>Muscular development asymmetric<br>Barrel chest: AP diameter increased in relation to transverse diameter (Figure 35-13)<br>Kyphosis: increased thoracic curvature<br>Scoliosis: increased lateral curvature<br>Scapular placement asymmetric |

*Dark-skinned people might have normal bluish-pigmented mucous membranes.
†Central cyanosis is relevant to respiratory status. Observe nailbeds, mucous membrane, and lips.

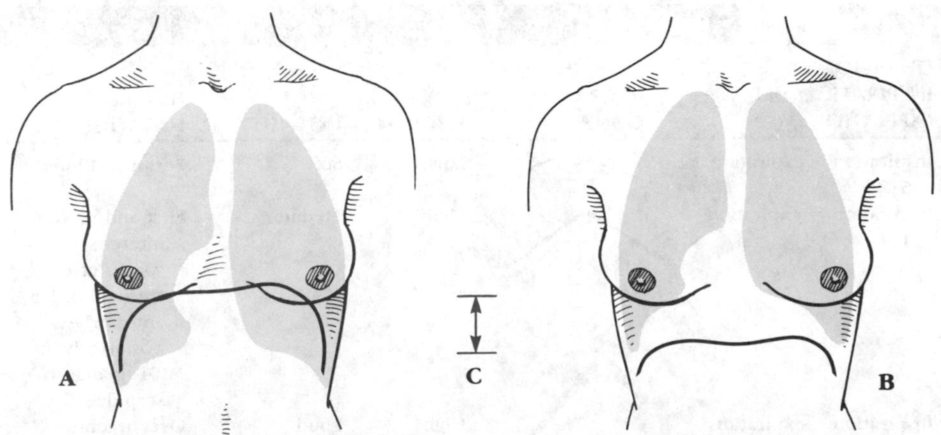


**FIGURE 35-13** Diaphragmatic excursion. **A,** Position of diaphragm at full-end expiration. **B,** Position of diaphragm at full-end inspiration. **C,** Range of diaphragmatic movement—distance from expiration to inspiration.

**TABLE 35-4 Possible Findings by Palpation in a Pulmonary Examination**

| PALPATE | NORMAL | ABNORMAL |
|---|---|---|
| Skin and chest wall | Skin nontender, smooth, warm, and dry | Skin moist or exceedingly dry<br>Crepitation—"crackling" when skin palpated—caused by air leak from lung into subcutaneous tissue |
| | Spine and ribs nontender | Localized tenderness |
| Fremitus* | Symmetric, mild vibrations felt on chest wall during vocalization | Increased fremitus—a result of vibration through more solid medium, such as lung tumors<br>Decreased fremitus—a result of vibration through increased space in the chest, such as pneumothorax or obesity<br>Asymmetric fremitus is always abnormal |
| Lateral chest expansion | Symmetric 3 to 8 cm expansion† | Expansion less than 3 cm, painful or asymmetric† |

*Normal fremitus varies from person to person. An individual's baseline must be established.
†Reduced expansion can result from either an overexpanded chest (barrel chest) or from a restricted chest.

**TABLE 35-5 Possible Findings by Percussion in a Pulmonary Examination**

| PERCUSSION | NORMAL | ABNORMAL |
|---|---|---|
| Lung fields | Resonant, low-pitched, hollow, easily heard sounds; equal quality bilaterally | Hyperresonant: heard with air trapping or pneumothorax<br>Dull or flat: results from decreased air in lungs (tumor, fluid) |
| Diaphragm position and movement | Resting diaphragm at 10th thoracic vertebra<br>Each hemidiaphragm moves 3-6 cm (see Figure 35-13) | High position—stomach distension or phrenic nerve damage<br>Decreased or no movement in either hemidiaphragm* |

*Decreased excursion can result from hyperinflated lungs pushing down on diaphragm, diaphragmatic disorders, or loss of diaphragmatic innervation.

**TABLE 35-6 Characteristics of Breath Sounds**

| SOUND | DURATION OF INSPIRATION and EXPIRATION | DIAGRAM OF SOUND | PITCH | INTENSITY | NORMAL LOCATION | ABNORMAL LOCATION |
|---|---|---|---|---|---|---|
| Vesicular | Inspiration > expiration 5:2 | | Low | Soft | Peripheral lung | Not applicable |
| Bronchovesicular | Inspiration = expiration 1:1 | | Medium | Medium | First and second intercostal spaces at the sternal border anteriorly; posteriorly at T4 medial to scapulae | Peripheral lung |
| Bronchial (tubular) | Inspiration < expiration 1:2 | | High | Loud | Over trachea | Lung area |

From Malasanos L et al: *Health assessment,* ed 4. St Louis, 1990, Mosby.

**TABLE 35-7 Abnormal (Adventious) Lung Sounds**

| TYPE | PHYSIOLOGY | AUSCULTATION | SOUND | PATHOLOGY |
|---|---|---|---|---|
| **CRACKLES (RALES)** | | | | |
| Fine | Air passing through secretions in alveoli | Heard at end of inspiration | Several hairs rubbed together between fingertips | Pneumonia, heart failure (may occur normally in elderly bedridden persons) |
| Medium | Air passing through secretions in bronchioles or bronchi | Heard midway during inspiration | Fizzing of carbonated drink | Later stages of pneumonia, heart failure, pulmonary edema |
| Coarse | Air passing through secretions in large airways, especially trachea | Heard at beginning of inspiration | Rough gurgling | Persons with repressed cough reflexes, unable to clear own secretions |
| **WHEEZES (RONCHI)** | Air passing through narrow passages | Heard mostly during expiration, but may also occur with inspiration | Loud musical gurgling | Obstructive lung disease |
| **PLEURAL FRICTION RUB** | Rubbing of inflamed pleura | May occur throughout respiratory cycle, heard best at base of lung at end of expiration | Scratching, grating, rubbing | Inflamed pleura |

## Percussion

Percussion is used to assess the lung fields and the position and movement of the diaphragm (excursion). Percussion notes are produced from vibration created by tapping the chest wall. The quality of the percussion note depends on the density of underlying tissue and the amount of air through which the vibration passes. Table 35-5 identifies common normal and abnormal percussion findings.

## Auscultation

Airway and lung status can be assessed by auscultating breath and voice sounds transmitted through the chest wall. The origin of breath sounds is unclear.

To hear breath sounds throughout all lung spaces, one must instruct the patient to take slow, moderate to deep breaths through the mouth. Breath sounds are assessed during both inspiration and expiration. The duration of inspiratory time to expiratory time, intensity, and pitch of breath sounds are assessed. Except for normally diminished breath sounds in the left upper lobe, breath sounds should be approximately symmetric in intensity and character when comparing the two lungs.

*Changes in breath sounds that may indicate underlying pathology include decreased or absent breath sounds, increased breath sounds, and superimposed breath sounds, also known as* **adventitious sounds.** Increased breath sounds are heard when such conditions as atelectasis and pneumonia increase lung tissue density. Decreased or absent breath sounds occur whenever transmission of sound waves through the lung tissue or chest wall is reduced. Conditions that decrease sound transmission include lung hyperinflation, air or fluid in the pleural space, shallow breathing, or increased chest wall thickness. Adventitious breath sounds can be caused by a variety of underlying pathologies that cause excess mucus or fluid, tissue inflammation, bronchospasm, or airway obstruction. Tables 35-6, 7, and 8 present normal and abnormal sounds that may be heard during auscultation.

**TABLE 35-8 Voice Sounds***

| TYPE | INSTRUCTION TO PATIENT | NORMAL SOUND | ABNORMAL (indicates consolidation) |
|---|---|---|---|
| **Egophony** | Say prolonged "e" | Muffled "e" | "a" |
| **Whispered pectoriloquy** | Whispered "1, 2, 3" | Muffled "1, 2, 3" | Loud, 'ear "1, 2, 3" |
| **Bronchophony** | Say "1, 2, 3" | Muffled "1, 2, 3" | Loud, clear "1, 2, 3" |

*Examiner auscultates for characteristics changes when voice sounds are transmitted through chest wall

## CLINICAL APPLICATION OF PULMONARY NURSING ASSESSMENT

The process of nursing assessment must be highly individualized (see Guidelines box, p. 992). In view of the patient's current respiratory status, the nurse tailors the interview and physical examination to maximize data gathering without increasing respiratory distress.

After initial assessment of the current respiratory status, the nurse selects components of the pulmonary examination appropriate to the patient's level of respira-

**BOX 35-6 Components of Pulmonary Examination for Respiratory Distress**

| | |
|---|---|
| Acute respiratory distress | Inspection: all components<br>Auscultation: breath sounds, abnormal sounds |
| Moderate respiratory distress | Interview: as tolerated; divide into several brief sessions<br>Inspection: all components<br>Palpation: thoracic expansion<br>Percussion: to assess resonance<br>Auscultation: breath sounds, abnormal sounds |
| Mild respiratory distress | All components of pulmonary examination |

tory distress. Components of the pulmonary examination that should be included for each of the three respiratory distress categories previously identified are presented in Box 35-6.

# DIAGNOSTIC TESTS

## RADIOLOGIC EXAMINATION OF THE THORAX AND LUNGS

Patients are usually familiar with the roentgenologic examination. In recent years, there has been an increase in consumer awareness of the danger of excessive exposure to radiation. The patient should have a full explanation of the type of test to be performed and the benefits (knowledge gained) in relation to risk from radiation exposure.

Chest film studies are indicated for the following reasons:

1. To detect alterations of the lung caused by pathologic processes, such as tumors, inflammation, fractures, fluid or air accumulation
2. To determine appropriate therapy
3. To evaluate effectiveness of treatment
4. To determine position of tubes and catheters
5. To provide a way of following the progression of lung disease

### Chest Films

Chest film studies are best performed in the radiology department. However, if the patient is acutely ill, the test can be completed at the bedside with a portable x-ray camera. The x-ray camera moves from the front to the back of the body—that is, anteroposterior (AP). Standard chest x-ray films are preferably taken with the patient in the standing position, although the sitting or supine position can be used. The standard views are as follows:

1. Posteroanterior (PA)—x-rays pass through the back to the front of the body
2. Lateral—x-rays pass through the side of the body (usually left side)

**Guidelines for Clinical Assessment**

*Initial nursing assessment*

Goal: to quickly determine the patient's respiratory status

Initial assessment components used include the following:

1. Determine chief complaint
2. Rapid inspection of the following:
   a. General appearance
   b. Respiratory rate/pattern
   c. Thoracic configuration

On the basis of clinical signs observed during the initial assessment, the patient's respiratory status might be categorized as one of the following:

1. *Acute respiratory distress*
   a. General appearance
      (1) Extremely apprehensive, restless, or lethargic
      (2) Might verbalize, "Help, I can't get my air," or may be unable to speak
      (3) Skin diaphoretic, grayish, bluish, or a deep ruddy color
   b. Respiratory rate/pattern
      (1) Rate increased >20 or decreased <12
      (2) Shallow and gasping
      (3) Might be any of abnormal patterns listed in Table 35-7
      (4) Inspiratory/expiratory (I:E) ratio prolonged
   c. Thoracic configuration
      (1) Accessory muscle breathing with noticeable clavicular lift, retracting intercostal muscles
      (2) Chest might appear asymmetric at rest or on expansion
2. *Moderate respiratory distress*
   a. General appearance
      (1) Somewhat apprehensive, restless, or might try to minimize respiratory distress
      (2) Skin might be diaphoretic, ruddy, or grayish in appearance
   b. Respiratory rate/pattern
      (1) Respiratory rate mildly elevated
      (2) Inspiratory/expiratory ratio might be slightly prolonged
   c. Thoracic configuration
      (1) Slight clavicular lift
3. *Mild respiratory distress*
   a. General appearance
      (1) Relaxed
      (2) Can verbalize detailed chief complaint
      (3) Skin translucent, color within normal limits
   b. Respiratory rate/pattern
      (1) Normal or slightly increased
   c. Thoracic configuration
      (1) Thoracic or diaphragmatic breathing
      (2) Chest expansion is symmetric

Special views might be required to visualize specific parts of the chest. The special views include the following:

1. Oblique—x-ray films slanted at specific angles
2. Lordotic—x-ray films slanted at 45-degree angle from below to visualize lung apices
3. Decubitus—x-ray films taken with patient lying on either side to visualize free fluid in chest

See Guidelines box, p. 993 for preparation procedure.

### Guidelines for Preparing the Person for Radiographic Examination

1. Explain specific procedure.
2. Instruct patient to remove all clothing above the waist and wear a gown open in the back. The patient must remove metal objects above the waist because metal restricts x-rays from passing through the body.
3. The procedure is noninvasive and should cause no discomfort.
4. Patient will probably be alone in the room, but someone is nearby and always has voice contact.
5. Patient will probably be asked to take a deep breath and hold it.
6. If it is necessary for persons to be in the room while x-ray is being taken, they will wear lead apron to protect them from radiation exposure.

## Tomography

Tomography is a special technique that permits better visualization of a single layer or plane of the lungs. It is used to study cavities, neoplasms, and lung densities. The patient is required to lie still while an x-ray tube is rapidly moved over the lung at approximately 1-cm intervals. The procedure takes approximately 15 minutes.

## Computed Tomography

Computed tomography (CT) is rapidly replacing standard tomographic examination. Conventional tomography resulted in a blurred film, except for the one plane being observed. CT scanning uses computer programming to enhance and process the x-ray film "slices" to produce a clear picture of the chest cavity structures.

## Fluoroscopic Examination

When dynamic information about the chest—such as diaphragmatic movement, lung expansion and contraction, or cardiac action—is required, fluoroscopy is the preferred examination.

## Ultrasound (Echogram)

In an ultrasound examination, harmless, high-frequency sound waves are emitted and penetrate the thorax. These sound waves bounce back and are converted by a transducer to a pictorial image of the area being studied. Ultrasound of the thorax can provide information about pleural effusion or opacities in the lung.

# RADIOLOGIC EXAMINATION OF VENTILATION AND PERFUSION

## Lung Scan (Pulmonary Scintiphotography)

Lung scan procedures involve the use of a scanning device that records the pattern of pulmonary radioactivity after the inhalation or intravenous injection of gamma ray–emitting radionucleotides, thus providing a visual image of the distribution of ventilation or blood flow in the lungs. These studies provide valuable information about ventilation-perfusion patterns and aid in the diagnosis of parenchymal lung disease and vascular disorders, such as pulmonary embolism. See Guidelines box above for preparation procedure.

### Guidelines for Preparing the Person for Lung Scan or Pulmonary Angiography

Radiopaque iodine is the radionucleotide usually used for both pulmonary angiography and lung scan. Always carry out the following activities:
1. Check patient for iodine allergy.
2. Obtain an order (often a standing order) to administer 10 drops of Lugol's solution several hours before the test to block thyroid uptake of radioactive iodine.

In a *perfusion scan, radiopaque iodine is injected intravenously.* The lungs are then scanned, and the pattern of particle distribution in the lung vasculature is recorded. Areas of poor radionucleotide uptake are suggestive of pulmonary vascular disorders. In a *ventilation scan, the radioactive gas is inhaled, and the lungs are scanned to detect abnormal diffusion of the gas throughout the lungs.*

## Pulmonary Angiography

Pulmonary angiography is used to detect pulmonary emboli and a variety of congenital and acquired lesions of the pulmonary vessels. A radiopaque material is injected via a catheter into a systemic vein, the right chambers of the heart, or the pulmonary artery, and the distribution of this material is recorded on film.

## Positron Emission Tomography (PET)

PET uses the capability of computerization to study regional pulmonary perfusion and ventilation-perfusion relationships. A radioisotope that releases positrons (positively charged particles with the same mass as an electron) is inhaled by or injected into the individual. As the short-lived radioisotope decays, it releases gamma rays that are recorded by the computerized scanner.

# EXAMINATION OF THE SPUTUM

## Sputum Analysis

Examinations of sputum are usually required when chest disease is suspected. The mucous membrane of the respiratory tract responds to inflammation by an increased flow of secretions that often contain causative organisms. The volume, consistency, color, and odor of the sputum are observed and recorded (Box 35-7).

Sputum examination includes the following tests:

1. *Gram stain* usually gives enough information about organisms and cells present to give a presumptive diagnosis.

**BOX 35-7 Sputum Color Analysis**

1. Colorless or clear mucoid: noninfectious process
2. Creamy yellow: staphylococcal pneumonia
3. Green: *Pseudomonas* pneumonia
4. "Currant jelly": *Klebsiella* pneumonia
5. Rusty: pneumococcal pneumonia
6. Pink frothy: pulmonary edema

2. ***Culture*** identifies specific organisms to enable making a definitive diagnosis. It should be collected before initiation of antibiotic therapy and thereafter to monitor effectiveness of antibiotic therapy.
3. ***Sensitivity*** serves as a guide to antimicrobial therapy by identifying antibiotics that prevent growth of the organism present in the sputum. It is collected before initiation of antibiotic therapy. Culture and sensitivity (C & S) are usually ordered together.
4. ***Acid-fast bacilli*** (AFB) determines the presence of mycobacterium tuberculosis, which—after taking up a dye—is not decolorized by acid alcohol.
5. ***Cytology*** assists in identification of lung carcinoma. Sputum contains sloughed cells from the tracheobronchial tree; thus malignant cells might be present. Although the presence of malignant cells indicates carcinoma, the absence of cells might indicate that either there is no tumor or that the tumor is not shedding cells.
6. ***Quantitative test*** is the collection of sputum over a period of 24 to 72 hours.

## Sputum Collection

Tests to be performed on sputum are explained to the patient so that a suitable specimen will be obtained. The patient is instructed to collect only sputum that has come from deep in the lungs. When not instructed adequately, patients often expectorate saliva rather than sputum. They are likely to exhaust themselves unnecessarily by shallow, frequent coughing that yields no sputum suitable for study and that affords them little relief from discomfort. ***The first sputum raised in the morning is usually the most productive of organisms.*** During the night, secretions accumulate in the bronchi, and just a few deep coughs will bring them to the back of the throat. If patients do not know this fact, on awakening they may almost unconsciously cough, clear their throats, and swallow or expectorate before attempting to produce the specimen.

The patient should be supplied with a wide-mouthed container and instructed to expectorate directly into it. Because the sight of sputum is often objectionable to the patient and to others, the outside of the glass container is covered with paper or other suitable covering. Usually 4 ml of sputum is sufficient for laboratory tests and examinations. Nursing implications for sputum collection include the following:

1. Patients who have difficulty producing sputum or who have very tenacious sputum might be dehydrated. Encourage fluid intake.
2. Collect specimen before meals to avoid possible emesis from coughing.
3. Instruct patient to rinse mouth with water before collecting specimen to decrease sputum contamination.
4. Instruct patient to notify staff as soon as specimen is collected so that it can be sent to the laboratory as soon as possible.

Occasionally patients have difficulty producing sputum for examination. Inhalation of a hypertonic solution, such as 10% saline in distilled water, is used to stimulate sputum production. Other methods to collect sputum include the following: (1) endotracheal aspiration with a suction catheter and special sputum collection container, (2) transtracheal aspiration (insertion of a needle with a catheter through the cricothyroid cartilage), and (3) fiberoptic bronchoscopy (pp. 999-1000).

## Gastric Washings

Gastric aspiration is occasionally used to collect gastric contents, which may contain swallowed sputum. It is usually performed when the diagnosis or suspected diagnosis is tuberculosis. Because most patients swallow sputum when coughing in the morning and during sleep, an examination of gastric contents can reveal causative organisms.

The procedure requires the following steps:

1. Breakfast is withheld before aspiration.
2. A nasogastric tube is passed into the stomach.
3. A large syringe is connected to the nasogastric tube, and a specimen of stomach contents is gently withdrawn.
4. The specimen is placed in a covered container.
5. The nasogastric tube is withdrawn.

# SKIN TESTING

For various pulmonary disorders, the skin is tested for an antigen-antibody reaction to the proteins of the infectious agent. This cell-mediated or delayed hypersensitivity reaction is manifested by induration caused by cellular infiltration at the site of the injection in persons who have been sensitized to the proteins of the infectious agent. Skin testing for *Mycobacterium tuberculosis* with either tuberculin-purified protein derivative (PPD) or old tuberculin (OT) is the most common type of test. However, skin testing also can be conducted for ***mycobacteria other than the tubercule bacilli*** and for ***fungal infections*** resulting from ***coccidioidin, histoplasmin,*** and ***blastomycin.*** The primary purpose of skin testing is to detect individuals who are infected with the suspect organism but who are not necessarily diseased.

### Guidelines for Administering the Mantoux Test

1. Draw up 0.1 ml of PPD, OT, atypical (tuberculin), or fungal antigen, using a tuberculin syringe and ½-inch, 24- to 26-gauge needle.
2. Cleanse the site (dorsal surface of forearm).
3. Keeping skin slightly taut, insert the needle (bevel upward) just beneath the skin surface.
4. Inject the solution, creating a 6- to 10-mm wheal.
5. Read the test site with a millimeter ruler 48 to 72 hours after injection. The site should be lightly palpated to determine the presence or absence of induration. The largest diameter of induration should be measured and recorded in millimeters. Any erythema at the site should also be noted.
6. Interpretation of induration:
   a. 10 mm or more = highly significant for past or present infection.
   b. 5 mm through 9 mm = doubtful reaction.
   c. 0 through 4 mm = little or no sensitivity; however, if patient's history indicates exposure, the test should be repeated.

In this capacity, skin testing is primarily a screening device. Skin antigens can also be used for presumptive diagnosis; however, a positive skin test reaction must be substantiated with other diagnostic evidence before active disease can be confirmed. Skin testing can produce false-positive and false-negative results (usually in immunosuppressed, older, or newly infected people).

### Skin Test Administration

Skin tests can be administered by intracutaneous injection (Mantoux method), jet gun, or multiple puncture tests (tine, mono-vacc, and heaf-type). The *Mantoux test is the only method used for diagnosis.* The jet gun or multiple puncture methods are used *only* for screening tests. (See Guidelines box above for administration procedure.)

## PULMONARY FUNCTION TESTS

Pulmonary function testing is a noninvasive method of assessing the functional capacity of the lungs. These tests cannot be used by themselves to diagnose specific diseases, but they are an integral part of the diagnostic process. Pulmonary function tests (PFTs) are used for the following purposes:

1. Screening for the presence of pulmonary disease
2. Preoperative evaluation
3. Evaluating the patient's condition for weaning from a ventilator
4. Researching pulmonary physiology
5. Documenting the progression of pulmonary disease or effects of therapy
6. Studying the effects of exercise on respiratory physiology

### Assessment of Lung Properties

The functional ability of the lungs is assessed by measuring properties that affect (1) ventilation and (2) respiration.

1. Ventilation
   a. Static properties focus on lung distensibility—that is, on the bellows action of the thorax and lungs. Static properties are assessed through measurement of lung volumes and functional capacities (Table 35-9, *A* and *B*).
   b. Dynamic properties are those aspects of lung mechanics that affect the resistance within the airways. These properties are assessed by pulmonary function tests that measure volume/time relationships (Table 35-9, *C*).
2. Respiration
   a. Diffusion properties are those aspects of lung function that affect the ability of gas to move across the alveolar-capillary membrane (Table 35-9, *D*).
   b. Perfusion properties affect the supply of blood to the lungs (Table 35-9, *D*).

Normal values for pulmonary function tests are calculated by taking into consideration the following variables for each individual being evaluated: (1) age, (2) gender, (3) height and weight, and (4) individual effort in performing each test.

### Measurement of Ventilation

Ventilatory studies are performed by having the patient breathe through a mouthpiece connected to a spirometer that measures the air moving through the apparatus. The spirometer is connected to a recording device that documents air volume, usually in liter measurements. Some measurements, such as the residual volume, cannot be measured directly and are calculated mathematically. The interrelationship of lung volumes and capacities that measure *static properties* is shown in Figure 35-14. The volumes and capacities are defined, and clinical implications of each measurement are given in Table 35-9.

Spirometric measurement of lung *dynamic properties* are of particular clinical significance, because they relate the volume of air expired to the time required for expiration. One of the most meaningful clinical measurements is the forced expiratory volume (FEV). The FEV measures the amount of air in liters forcefully expired over 1, 2, or 3 seconds after a full inspiration. The FEV is an accurate indicator for obstructive diseases, because airway obstruction becomes worse on expiration and particularly when expiration is forceful and rapid. The FEV at 1 second is the most clinically accurate of the three measurements and is particularly useful when expressed as a percentage of the forced vital capacity (FVC). An $FEV_1/FVC$ of 80% or greater is considered normal.

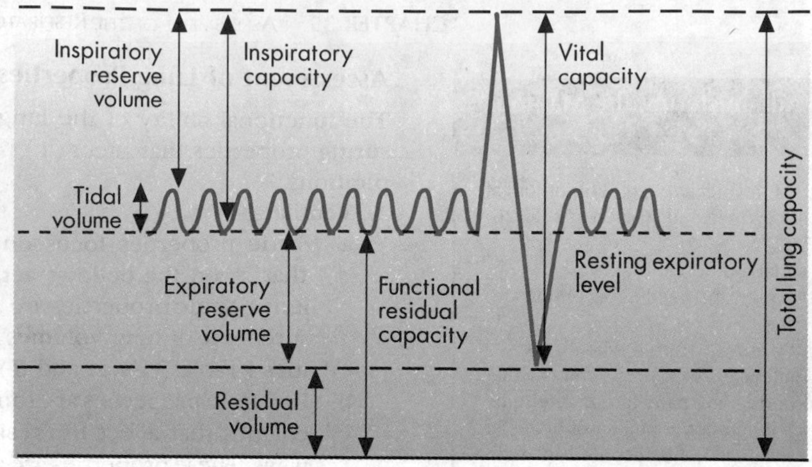


**FIGURE 35-14** Lung volumes and capacities illustrated by spirography tracing. (Adapted from Wade JF: *Respiratory nursing care,* ed 2, St Louis, 1977, Mosby.)

**TABLE 35-9 Definitions and Implications of Pulmonary Function Tests**

| DEFINITIONS | | CLINICAL IMPLICATIONS: OBSTRUCTIVE DISEASES | CLINICAL IMPLICATIONS: RESTRICTIVE DISEASES |
|---|---|---|---|
| **A. LUNG VOLUME (NONOVERLAPPING MEASURES)** | | | |
| Tidal volume (TV) | Volume of gas inspired and expired with a normal breath | General measure of ventilatory ability | |
| Inspiratory reserve volume (IRV) | Maximal volume that can be inspired from the end of a normal inspiration | ↓ | ↓ |
| Expiratory reserve volume (ERV) | Maximal volume than can be exhaled by forced expiration after a normal expiration | Clinically useful when combined with RV-FRC | |
| Residual volume (RV) | Volume of gas left in lung after maximal expiration | ↑ | ↓ |
| **B. LUNG CAPACITIES (COMBINATIONS OF VARIOUS VOLUMES)** | | | |
| Inspiratory capacity (IC) | Maximal amount of air than can be inspired after a normal expiration (TV + IRV) | ↓ | ↓ |
| Functional residual capacity (FRC) | Amount of air left in lungs after a normal expiration (ERV + RV) | ↑ | ↓ |
| Vital capacity (VC) | Maximal amount of air that can be expired after a maximal inspiration (TV + IRV + ERV) | ↓ | ↓ |
| Forced vital capacity (FVC) | Maximal amount of air that can be expelled with a maximal effort after a maximal inspiration | ↓ | ↓ |
| Total lung capacity (TLC) | Total amount of air in lungs after maximal inspiration (TV + IRV + ERV + RV) | ↑ | ↓ |
| **C. VOLUME/TIME RELATIONSHIPS** | | | |
| Minute volume (MV) | Volume inspired and expired in 1 min of normal breathing | ↑ | ↓ |
| Forced expiratory volume in 1 sec ($FEV_1$) | Amount of air expelled in the first second of the forced vital capacity maneuver | ↓ | — |
| $FEV_1$/VC ratio | Amount of air forcefully expelled in 1 sec compared with total amount forcefully expelled | ↓ | — |
| Maximal voluntary ventilation (MVV), also termed maximal breathing capacity (MBC) | Amount of air exchanged per minute with maximal rate and depth of respiration | ↓ | — |
| **D. DIFFUSION/PERFUSION MEASUREMENTS** | | | |
| Diffusing capacity ($D_x$) | Assesses ability of gas molecules to cross alveolar-capillary membrane | ↓ | ↓ |
| Nitrogen washout ($N_2$) | Measurement of amount of nitrogen in lungs at end expiration; indicates uniformity of gaseous distribution in lungs | ↓ | ↓ |

### Measurement of Respiration

It is best to measure efficiency of respiration by both PFTs and other parameters, such as arterial blood gas measurements. Two variables affecting respiration that PFTs can measure are the ability of gas to diffuse across the alveolar-capillary membrane and the ratio of ventilated alveoli to perfused capillaries.

### Alveolar-Capillary Diffusion

The ability of gas to diffuse across the alveolar-capillary membrane is measured by a test called *diffusing capacity* ($D_x$). The patient breathes a measured amount of carbon monoxide from a closed system. The rate of carbon monoxide removal from the closed system indicates the status of the alveolar-capillary membrane.

### Ventilation-Perfusion Relationship

For the lung to perform gas exchange efficiently, the ventilation-perfusion ratio (V/Q ratio) must be balanced. That is, areas that receive ventilation should be well perfused with blood, and areas that receive blood flow should be capable of ventilation (Figure 35-15). Although in the normal lung—with its many millions of gas exchange units—some imbalance in ventilation and perfusion exists, this has little effect on overall gas exchange function. In fact, adaptive mechanisms appear to exist that divert blood flow to the best ventilated regions of the lungs or redirect ventilation away from nonperfused areas in order to maintain a normal ratio in the range of 0.8 to 1.2. Alteration in ventilation-perfusion relationships (either overall or in circumscribed areas of lung tissue) is largely responsible for the *hypoxemia* or *hypercapnia* seen in clinical practice. The nitrogen washout test measures ventilation-perfusion relationships. Ambient air, and thus air in the lungs, is known to contain 80% nitrogen. The nitrogen washout test requires the patient to breathe 100% oxygen to wash out all the nitrogen from the lungs. After a measured time, the patient's expired air is measured for nitrogen content. Unevenly ventilated alveoli that receive less of the inspired oxygen will take longer to wash out lung nitrogen.

For pulmonary function testing, patients are required to breathe into a mouthpiece while wearing a noseclip; thus they often fear smothering or having a dyspneic episode. Thorough preparation for the test includes an explanation of the procedure to decrease the patient's apprehension.

## ARTERIAL BLOOD GASES

Arterial blood gas analysis provides objective determination of the following: (1) arterial blood oxygenation, (2) gas exchange, (3) alveolar ventilation, and (4) acid-base balance. The arterial blood gas parameters that assess function of the respiratory system are shown in Table 35-10. A blood sample is obtained from a radial, brachial, or femoral artery with a preheparinized syringe

**TABLE 35-10 Arterial Blood Gases**

| RESPIRATORY FUNCTION | MEASUREMENTS | NORMAL VALUE |
|---|---|---|
| Acid-base balance | pH: hydrogen ion concentration | 7.35-7.45 |
| Oxygenation | $PaO_2$: partial pressure of dissolved $O_2$ in blood | 80-100 mm Hg |
| | $SaO_2$: percentage of $O_2$ bound to hemoglobin | 95%-98% |
| Ventilation | $PaCO_2$: partial pressure of $CO_2$ dissolved in blood | 38-45 mm Hg |

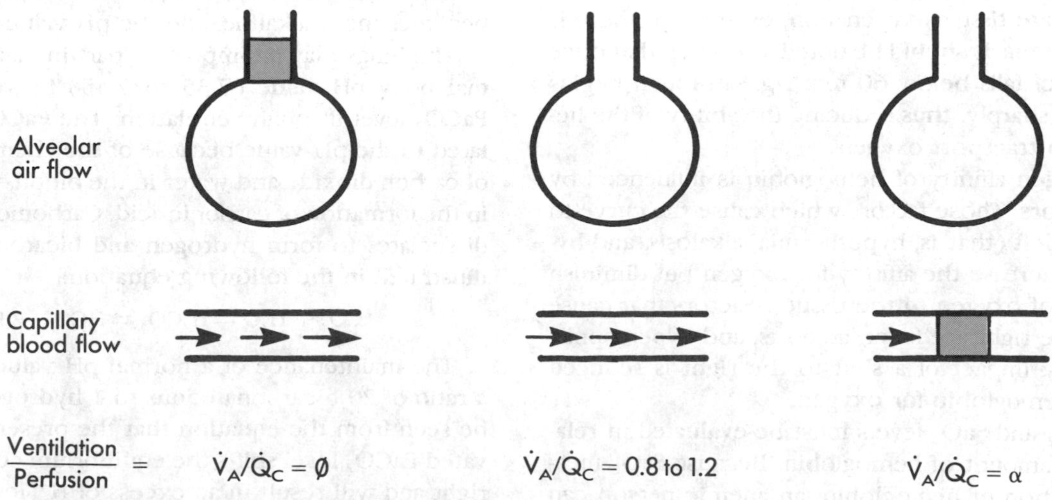


**FIGURE 35-15** Range of ventilation to perfusion ratios from zero to infinity. (Adapted from West JB: *Ventilation, blood flow and gas exchange,* ed 3, Oxford, 1977, Blackwell.)

to prevent clotting. The syringe is capped after obtaining the blood sample to prevent contact with air and is placed in an ice-water container until analyzed. Pressure is maintained over the puncture site for at least 5 mintues after needle withdrawal to prevent bleeding.

Patients with blood-clotting abnormalities may require that pressure be applied to the sample site for longer than 5 minutes. Nursing implications include assessing the site periodically and applying pressure for as long as necessary to prevent hematoma formation or bruising.

## Measurement of Oxygenation

Both **$PaO_2$** and **$SaO_2$** levels are measured to determine the adequacy of arterial blood oxygenation. The $PaO_2$ level measures oxygen dissolved in the blood; however, the amount of oxygen carried in the blood in this form is small. Most oxygen is transported in chemical combination with hemoglobin. The $SaO_2$ level measures the oxyhemoglobin saturation or that percentage of the hemoglobin which is combined with oxygen. More than 90% of the oxygen-carrying capacity of blood is accounted for by oxyhemoglobin, with the partial pressure of oxygen acting as the driving force for this chemical combination.

The relationship of $PaO_2$ to $SaO_2$ is demonstrated in the oxyhemoglobin dissociation curve. This relationship is not directly linear; many factors affect the affinity of the heme molecule for oxygen. The sigmoid curve represents the saturation percentages that occur at various $PaO_2$ levels. As can be seen in the oxyhemoglobin dissociation curve (Figure 35-16), in the upper portion of the curve, hemoglobin has an increased affinity for oxygen, so that large changes in $PO_2$ levels can be tolerated without significantly changing the saturation. For example, at a $PO_2$ level of 100 mm Hg, hemoglobin saturation is almost total—97%; even if the $PO_2$ level should fall to 70 mm Hg, the saturation would only decrease to 94%. This serves as a protective mechanism that ensures adequate tissue oxygenation, even when there is mild hypoxemia. It should be noted, however, that once the $PO_2$ level falls below 60 mm Hg, saturation begins to decrease sharply, thus reducing the ability of the hemoglobin to transport oxygen.

The oxygen affinity of hemoglobin is influenced by various factors. Those factors which cause the curve to shift to the left (that is, hypothermia, alkalosis, and hypocapnia) increase the affinity for oxygen but diminish the release of oxygen to the tissues. Factors that cause a shift to the right are fever, acidosis, and hypercapnia. The primary impact of a shift to the right is reduced affinity of hemoglobin for oxygen.

The $PaO_2$ and $SaO_2$ levels must be evaluated in relation to the amount of hemoglobin. Because $SaO_2$ measures saturation of hemoglobin, an anemic person can have a normal saturation but still be inadequately oxygenated.

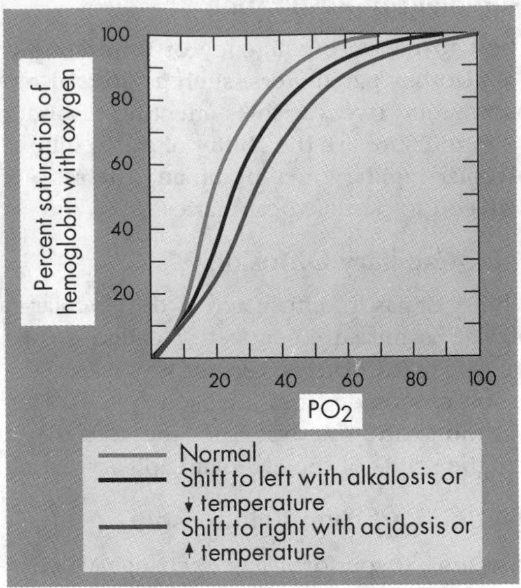


**FIGURE 35-16** Oxyhemoglobin dissociation curve. (Reproduced with permission from Comroe JH Jr: *Physiology of respiration,* ed 2, St Louis, 1974, Mosby.)

## Assessment of Ventilation

The **$PaCO_2$** level is measured to determine the adequacy of ventilation and depends on the amount of carbon dioxide produced by the body and the ability of the lungs to eliminate it. **Hypoventilation** is shown by an elevated $PaCO_2$ level, and **hyperventilation** is indicated by a decrease in $PaCO_2$ to below normal levels.

## Measurement of Acid-Base Balance

Arterial blood pH is a measurement of hydrogen ion concentration. Because pH is expressed as a negative logarithm, as the hydrogen ion concentration increases and blood becomes more acid, the pH value falls. When the hydrogen ion concentration decreases, the blood becomes more alkaline, and the pH value rises.

The lungs play an important part in maintaining normal body pH value (7.35 to 7.45) by regulating the $PaCO_2$ level through ventilation. The $PaCO_2$ level is related to the pH value because of the chemical reaction of carbon dioxide and water in the blood, which results in the formation of carbonic acid. Carbonic acid, in turn, dissociates to form hydrogen and bicarbonate ions, as illustrated in the following equation:

$$CO_2 + H_2O \rightleftarrows H_2CO_3 \rightleftarrows HCO_3^- + H^+$$

The maintenance of a normal pH value depends on a ratio of 20 bicarbonate ions to 1 hydrogen ion. It can be seen from the equation that the presence of an elevated $PaCO_2$ level shifts the equilibrium equation to the right and will result in an excess of $H^+$ ions. When this occurs, the pH falls and the patient is said to be in **respiratory acidosis.** Conversely, when the $PaCO_2$

level is decreased, the equation shifts to the left, resulting in an increased pH and **respiratory alkalosis.**

## ENDOSCOPIC EXAMINATION

### Laryngoscopy

Direct laryngoscopy is usually performed after the patient is administered a local anesthesic of 10% cocaine or a general anesthetic. A sedative (for example, secobarbital, meperidine, or another narcotic) and atropine sulfate are given 1 hour before the examination. Atropine is essential before administering both local and general anesthetics, because it reduces the volume of secretions. For direct laryngoscopy, the person is placed in a reclining position, with the head in a head holder. If no head holder is available, the head is extended over the edge of the table and manually supported by a physician or nurse. In some cases, a suspension device can be applied to the laryngoscope so that the physician's hands are free for instrumentation or manipulation of the focus of the microscope. *Microlaryngoscopy* using an operating microscope is becoming more widely used. This method provides magnification and binocular vision.

The laryngoscope—a hollow, metal tube with a handle at the proximal end and a light at the distal end—is introduced by a physician through the mouth into the laryngopharynx, elevating the epiglottis, and making the interior of the larynx easily visible. Minor surgical procedures, such as a biopsy or the removal of a small benign tumor, can be performed by looking through this instrument.

The interior of the larynx can also be visualized by x-ray films and tomography. Radiopaque contrast material is instilled into the larynx. These x-ray films are less commonly used than laryngoscopy. Xerography is also used to evaluate the larynx.

Nursing management after a laryngoscopy includes the following:

1. Patient is NPO until gag reflex returns (approximately 2 hours).
2. Check for gag reflex by gently touching back of throat with tongue blade.
3. If gag reflex is present, have patient try drinking water before other fluids or food is given to prevent accidental aspiration.

### Bronchoscopy

A bronchoscopic examination is performed by passing a bronchoscope into the trachea and bronchi (Figure 35-17). By use of either a rigid bronchoscope or a flexible fiberoptic bronchoscope, the larynx, trachea, and bronchi can be visualized. Diagnostic bronchoscopic examination includes observation of the tracheobronchial tree for abnormalities, tissue biopsy, and aspiration of sputum for testing.

Bronchoscopy is used to aid in the diagnosis of carcinoma of the lung. Bronchial biopsy, bronchial brush-

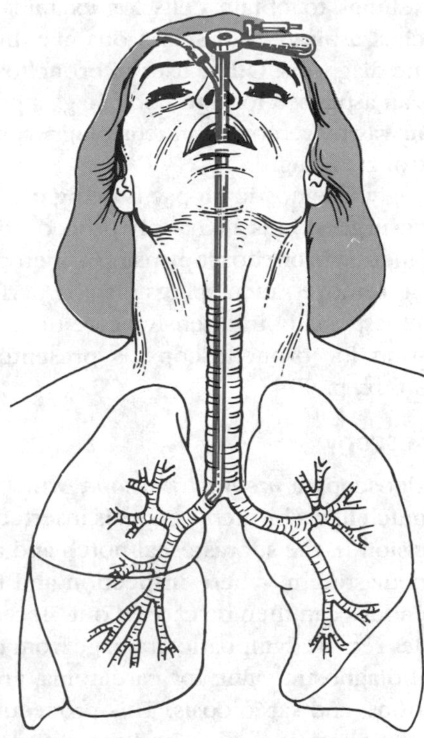

**FIGURE 35-17** Bronchoscope inserted through trachea into bronchus. (From DeWeese DD, Saunders WH: *Textbook of otolaryngology,* ed 7, St Louis, 1988, Mosby.)

**Guidelines for Preparing the Person for Bronchoscopy**

**PREBRONCHOSCOPY**

1. Instruct patient to brush and floss teeth and rinse with antiseptic mouthwash night and morning before procedure.
2. Instruct patient not to eat or drink for 8 hours before procedure.
3. Instruct patient to remove dentures before procedure and to report any loose teeth to physician or nurse before procedure begins.
4. Reassure patient as necessary. Most patients are anxious both about the bronchoscopy and about what the results might indicate, such as carcinoma of the lung.
5. Explain to patient that a short-acting sedative will be given in the operating room before the procedure and that a local anesthetic (usually lidocaine) will be applied to the throat.

**POSTBRONCHOSCOPY**

1. Patient is NPO until gag reflex returns. Give sips of water after reflex returns to be sure patient is able to swallow without difficulty.
2. Patient is positioned in semi-Fowler's position or on either side to facilitate removal of secretions, unless surgeon specifies a different position.
3. Patient is monitored for laryngeal edema or laryngospasm, such as stridor, or increasing shortness of breath.
4. If bronchoscopy is performed in ambulatory surgery, patient is kept until gag reflex returns and patient is able to swallow water with ease.
5. If tissue biopsy specimen was obtained, explain to patient that sputum may be blood streaked for a few days.

ings or washings to obtain cells for examination, and transbronchial aspiration of secretions may be used to establish the diagnosis. Other uses of bronchoscopy are to remove an aspirated foreign body (e.g., a peanut), to clear the airway by removing mucus plugs with suction, or to control bleeding.

Increasingly, diagnostic biopsy is being performed in ambulatory surgery or as a day-only procedure in a hospital. Therapeutic bronchoscopy using a fiberoptic bronchoscope to remove mucus plugs may be performed at the bedside, especially in intensive care units.

Preparation for bronchoscopy is presented in the Guidelines box, p. 999.

### Mediastinoscopy

In mediastinoscopy a *mediastinoscope,* which is an instrument much like a bronchoscope, is inserted through a small incision in the suprasternal notch and advanced into the mediastinum, where inspection and biopsy of the lymph nodes can then be carried out. Because these lymph nodes receive lymphatic drainage from the lungs, they are of diagnostic value for carcinoma, granulomatous infections, and sarcoidosis. This procedure is performed in the operating room, and the patient receives a general anesthetic.

### Thoracoscopy

Recently thoracoscopy is being used to perform many procedures formerly requiring an open thoracotomy. Thoracoscopy allows visualization of intrathoracic contents by means of transthoracic instrumentation. Although local anesthesia can be used, most surgeons prefer general anesthesia because it permits optimal patient comfort, improves surgical accessibility, and avoids the potential problems of pneumothorax that may occur when the patient is awake.[7a]

A simple fiberoptic mediastinoscopy, a rigid bronchoscope, a flexible bronchoscope, or newer video-assisted laparoscopic instrumentation may be used to perform thoracoscopy.[7a] Single lung ventilation in which the lung on the operative side is allowed to collapse is desirable because it permits a more panoramic view of the intrathoracic structures and permits the surgeon to perform the desired procedures without being limited by the inflated lung. During the procedure the patient is monitored by periodic arterial blood gas analysis, pulse oximetry, and end-tidal carbon dioxide measurements. The lung on the operative side is inflated by the anesthesiologist at the end of the procedure.

Thoracoscopy can be used to obtain a pleural biopsy specimen to aid in the diagnosis of pleural disease, stage malignancies, resect tumors, perform esophageal operations, resect pericardium, and perform many other thoracic surgical procedures.

Intrapleural adhesions, the inability of the patient to tolerate single-lung anesthesia, or instrument failure can prevent successful performance of the procedure. The preferred position of the patient in the operating room is the lateral decubitus, which also permits easy conversion to thoracotomy should a complication arise.[7a]

## THORACENTESIS

**Thoracentesis** involves the insertion of a needle into the pleural space. Indications for a thoracentesis include the following:

1. Removal of pleural fluid for diagnostic purposes
   a. The pleural fluid can be examined for specific gravity, white blood cell count, differential cell count, red blood cell count, and protein, glucose, and amylase concentrations.
   b. The fluid can be cultured and checked for the presence of bacteria and abnormal or malignant cells.
   c. The gross appearance of the fluid, the quantity obtained, and the location of the site of the thoracentesis should be recorded.
2. Biopsy of the pleura
3. Removal of pleural fluid when it is a threat to patient safety or comfort
4. Instillation of antibiotics or other medications into the pleural space

The Guidelines box below presents care of a patient undergoing thoracentesis.

### Guidelines for Care of the Person Undergoing Thoracentesis

1. Explain procedure. Emphasize the importance of not moving, breathing quietly, and not coughing during the procedure to avoid damage to the pleura. Although a local anesthetic is used, discomfort might be felt when the needle enters the pleura.
2. Patient's respiratory status and vital signs are assessed before the procedure to collect baseline data.
3. If possible, the patient sits on the edge of the bed with feet supported on a chair. With the use of an elevated overbed table, the patient is helped to maintain a position with the head resting upon folded arms. Patients who are unable to sit up should be turned to the unaffected side with the head of the bed elevated 30 degrees.
4. Reassure and provide physical support, such as holding patient's hand, as needed.
5. Monitor vital signs, general appearance, and respiratory status throughout the procedure. No more than 1500 ml of pleural fluid should be removed within a 30-minute period because of the risk of intravascular fluid shift with resultant pulmonary edema.
6. After the needle is withdrawn, a sterile occlusive dressing and pressure is applied to the site.
7. After thoracentesis, the patient is positioned on the unaffected side with the insertion site up.
8. Monitor respiratory status, vital signs, and puncture site. Observe for signs of the following complications:
   a. Intravascular shift: hypotension, a rapid thready pulse, and increasing shortness of breath.
   b. Lung trauma: coughing paroxysms, bloody sputum, or tracheal deviation.

## CRITICAL THINKING ACTIVITIES

- ► Compare and contrast the physiologic differences between the right and left bronchi. Discuss how this knowledge would be beneficial in caring for an elderly patient with left lower lobe pneumonia, increased secretions, and dysphagia.
- ► In the past, emergency practice included the routine administration of sodium bicarbonate to treat acidosis associated with cardiac shock. Thinking in terms of the oxyhemoglobin dissociation curve, explain why this practice is currently discouraged.

# CHAPTER SUMMARY

### ANATOMY AND PHYSIOLOGY

- Breathing includes the movement of air in and out of the lungs (ventilation) and exchange of oxygen and carbon dioxide between capillary blood and alveolar air across the alveolar-capillary membrane (respiration).
- Although normal changes associated with aging decrease lung function, the lungs have a large reserve capacity.

### SUBJECTIVE DATA

- A nursing history of the person with pulmonary problems includes information about risk factors, pulmonary symptoms, functional capacity, current treatment, and the person's desired level of health.
- The major pulmonary symptoms are cough, dyspnea, chest pain, sputum production, hemoptysis, and wheezing.

### OBJECTIVE DATA

- Pulmonary physical assessment includes inspection of the chest and breathing patterns, palpation of the chest wall for fremitus, percussion of lung fields and diaphragm movement, and auscultation of breath and voice sounds.
- Pulmonary assessment must be tailored to accommodate the person's level of respiratory distress.

### DIAGNOSTIC TESTS

- Diagnostic testing is performed to assess the origin of pulmonary symptoms and to assess the ventilatory and respiratory capacity of the lungs.

## REFERENCES


1. American Thoracic Society: Recommended respiratory disease questionnaire for use with adults and children in epidemiological research, *Am Rev Respir Dis* 118(1):7-53, 1978.
2. Bates B: *A guide to physical examination,* ed 3, Philadelphia, 1987, JB Lippincott.
3. Bates D: *Respiratory function in disease,* ed 3, Philadelphia, 1989, WB Saunders.
4. Borg G: Psychophysical bases of perceived exertion, *Med Sci Sports Exerc* 14:377-381, 1982.
5. Borg G: Physical performance and perceived exertion, *Studia Psychol Paedagog* 11:1-64, 1962.
6. De Troyer A, Estenne M: Functional anatomy of the respiratory muscles, *Clin Chest Med* 9(2):175-193, 1988.
7. DeWeese D, Saunders W: *Textbook of otolaryngology,* ed 5, St Louis, 1977, Mosby.

7a. Douglas JM: Diagnostic thoracostomy. In Sabiston DC, Lyerly HK: *Sabiston essentials of surgery,* ed 2, Philadelphia, 1994, WB Saunders.

8. Ebersole P, Hess P: *Toward healthy aging,* ed 4, St Louis, 1994, Mosby.
9. Edlund B, Wheeler E: Adaptation to breathlessness, *Topics Clin Nurs* 2(3):11-25, 1980.
10. Killian KJ: The objective measurement of breathlessness, *Chest* 88(2):84S-90S, 1985.
11. McCaffrey TV, Kern EB: Clinical evaluation for nasal obstruction: a study of 1000 patients, *Arch Otolaryngol* 105:542-545, 1979.
12. Roach L: Skin changes: the subtle and the obvious. In *Assessing vital functions accurately,* Horsham, Pa, 1978, Intermed Communications.
13. Westia B: Assessment under pressure: when your patient says "I can't breathe," *Nurs '84* 14(5):34-40, 1984.

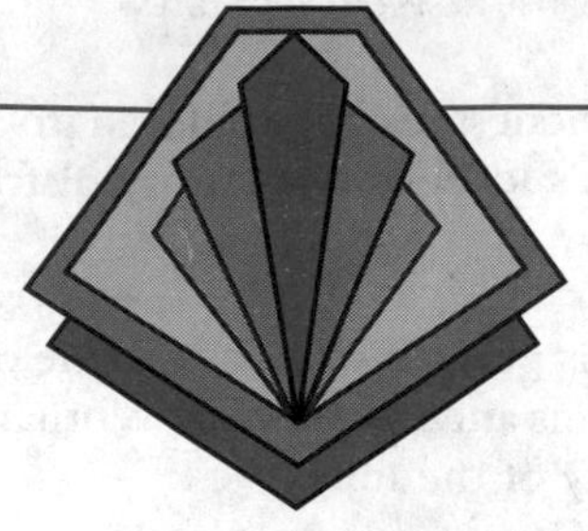

# CHAPTER 36

# Management of Persons With Problems of the Upper Airway

*Wilma J. Phipps*

## CHAPTER OBJECTIVES

***After studying this chapter, the learner should be able to do the following:***

1 Describe the etiology, pathophysiology, clinical manifestations, and management of the patient with rhinitis and sinusitis.
2 Compare acute pharyngitis with acute follicular tonsillitis and peritonsillar abscess in relation to etiology, clinical manifestations, and management.
3 Describe the nursing care of the patient after nasal surgery.
4 Identify conditions that cause obstructions of the upper airway and their management.
5 Describe nursing care for the patient who has an endotracheal tube or tracheostomy.
6 Discuss the precautions to be observed when feeding the patient who is intubated.
7 Describe clinical manifestations and management of the patient experiencing epistaxis and malignancies of the upper airway.
8 Describe the nursing care of the patient after a partial laryngectomy and after a total laryngectomy with radical neck dissection.
9 Describe speech methods used by patients after a total laryngectomy.

## KEY TERMS

acute follicular tonsillitis
acute laryngeal edema
acute rhinitis
allergic rhinitis
anosmia
antral irrigation
arytenoidectomy
Caldwell-Luc procedure
cavernous sinus thrombosis
chronic laryngitis
chronic rhinitis
composite resection
conservative neck dissection
cuffed tube
deviated septum
electronic artificial larynx
endoscopic sinus surgery (ESS)
endotracheal tube
esophageal speech
ethmoidectomy
free flaps
functional endoscopic sinus surgery (FESS)
functional neck dissection
group A beta-hemolytic streptococci (GABHS)
hemilaryngectomy
hypertrophied turbinates
laryngeal paralysis
modified neck dissection
mucocele
myocutaneous flaps
nasal polyps
nasoseptoplasty
osteoplastic flap operation
partial laryngectomy
rhinitis
simple acute laryngitis
sinusitis
sphenoid sinus
subtotal laryngectomy
supraglottic laryngectomy
thyroplasty
total laryngectomy
tracheoesophageal puncture (TEP)
tracheostomy
transnasal approach
vertical partial laryngectomy

Mary Lynn Droughton, MSN, RN, assisted in the revision of this chapter.

The upper airway includes the nose and sinuses, upper throat (nasopharynx, oropharynx, and tonsils), and lower throat (laryngopharynx and larynx). Disorders of the upper airway are very common, and patients often ask nurses to give them advice about these kinds of problems.

Disorders that affect the nose or olfactory nerve may lead to **anosmia,** or loss of the sense of smell. Anosmia may result from (1) nasal obstruction, which prevents air currents from reaching the olfactory epithelium; (2) skull fracture across the cribriform plate at the roof of the nose where part of the olfactory nerve enters the nose; (3) viral infections, which affect the olfactory nerve; or (4) some meningiomas, which may form in the olfactory area. A perverted sense of smell, called *parosmia,* may also be present during sinusitis or an upper respiratory tract infection.

# INFECTIONS OF THE NOSE AND SINUSES

The skin around the external nose is easily irritated during acute attacks of rhinitis or sinusitis. Furunculosis (boils) and cellulitis (see Chapter 67) occasionally develop. Infections around the nose are extremely dangerous because the venous blood supply from this area drains directly into the cerebral venous sinuses. Septicemia therefore can occur easily. No pimple or lesion in the area should ever be squeezed or "picked"; hot packs may be used. If any infection in or around the nose persists or shows even a slight tendency to spread or increase in severity, a physician should be consulted.

## RHINITIS

### Etiology/Epidemiology

**Rhinitis** refers to inflammation of the mucous membrane of the nose. It may be acute or chronic.

**Acute rhinitis** (coryza, common cold) is an inflammatory condition of the mucous membranes of the nose and accessory sinuses caused by a filtrable virus. It affects almost everyone at some time and occurs most often in the winter, with additional high incidences in early fall and spring. Some of the known causes of the common cold are 100 serotypes of rhinoviruses, coronoviruses, adenoviruses, echoviruses, influenza and parainfluenza viruses, and coxsackievirus. The common cold is spread by droplet nuclei from sneezing, and the condition is contagious for the first 2 to 3 days. Secondary invasion by bacteria may complicate the cold, causing pneumonia, bronchitis, sinusitis, and otitis media.

**Allergic rhinitis** (hay fever) can be acute and seasonal when caused by the pollens of grasses and flowers, or it may be chronic and perennial when associated with numerous allergens, such as house dust, animal dander, wool, and certain foods.

**Chronic rhinitis** is a chronic inflammation of the mucous membrane caused by repeated acute infections, by an allergy, or by *vasomotor rhinitis.* The cause of vasomotor rhinitis is unclear, but this condition may result from an instability of the autonomic nervous system caused by stress, tension, or some endocrine disorder. Often it is mistaken for nasal allergy, but an allergen cannot be identified. There is an increased formation of nasal mucus. Rhinitis can also be caused by the overuse of nose drops *(rhinitis medicamentosa);* a rebound phenomenon occurs after the immediate effect of the nose drops with the return to congestion. Discontinuing use of the nose drops usually clears up this condition within a week or two.

### Pathophysiology

All forms of rhinitis cause sneezing, nasal discharge with nasal obstruction, and headache, but the form of these symptoms varies with the different types of rhinitis (Table 36-1). Acute rhinitis also includes signs of acute inflammation (early chilliness followed by "feverishness" and malaise). A painful throat is not always associated with a cold. However, the pharynx may feel sore because of early dryness followed by irritation from postnasal drainage. If uncomplicated, the cold is usually self-limiting and lasts for about 1 week.

In chronic rhinitis, acute symptoms are absent. The chief complaint is nasal obstruction accompanied by a feeling of stuffiness and pressure in the nose. Polyp formation (p. 1018) may occur, and vertigo may be present.

### Medical Management

No specific treatment exists for the common cold. The goals of treatment are to (1) relieve symptoms, (2) inhibit spread of the infection, and (3) reduce the risk of bacterial complications such as sinusitis and otitis media. Studies have indicated that oral antihistamines are not effective in treating viral upper respiratory infections. They are helpful, however, in treating allergic rhinitis. The recommended treatment for relieving nasal conges-

**TABLE 36-1 Symptoms of Rhinitis**

| | ACUTE RHINITIS | ALLERGIC RHINITIS | CHRONIC RHINITIS |
|---|---|---|---|
| Nasal discharge | Initially watery, then mucoid | Thin, watery | Serous, mucopurulent, or purulent |
| Eyes | Tearing during early phase | Tearing, itching | No tearing |
| Turbinates | Edematous | Pale, edematous, mucoid | Enlarged |
| Nasal polyps | No | Sometimes | Sometimes |
| Headache | Generalized | Generalized | Generalized |

## Guidelines for Correct Administration of Nose Drops

1. Wash hands.
2. Assume a position that will facilitate flow of medication:
   a. Sit in chair and tip head well backward, or
   b. Lie down with head extended over edge of bed, or
   c. Lie down with pillow under shoulders and head tipped backward.
3. Turn head to side that will receive the drops.
4. Place no more than 3 drops of solution into each nostril at one time (unless otherwise prescribed).
5. Remain in position with head tilted backward for 3 to 5 minutes to permit solution to reach posterior nares.
6. If marked congestion is still present 10 minutes after nose drop insertion, another drop or two of solution may be administered (nasal constriction from first insertion may facilitate additional drops reaching posterior nares).

tion and enhancing eustachian tube function is decongestants (sympathomimetic amines). The decongestants are administered as nasal drops or sprays two or three times for no more than 3 days[5] (see Guidelines box above). Two commonly prescribed decongestants are oxymetazolin (Afrin 0.05%) and xylometazoline (Otrivin 0.1%). The side effects of sympathomimetic amines include rebound nasal congestion (with chronic use), nervousness, and transient increases in blood pressure. Sympathomimetic amines are contraindicated in patients receiving tricyclic antidepressants or monoamine oxidase (MAO) inhibitors. Room humidifiers are helpful in liquefying nasal secretions.[5]

For allergic rhinitis the treatment consists of maintaining an allergen-free environment (see Chapter 70). Hyposensitization or desensitization (administering the allergen in gradually increasing doses to establish an "immunity") may be helpful. Antihistamines give relief to most persons, but their effectiveness often decreases as the "hay fever season" continues.

For chronic rhinitis a careful medical follow-up is indicated. When nasal obstruction persists, surgery may be necessary to remove polyps (polypectomy) or to remove tissue obstruction (septoplasty) (see p. 1017).

If the nasal passages are dry, a nasal spray of normal saline can be purchased in a drug store or it can be made by mixing 1 teaspoon of salt in 1 quart of water. The homemade solution should be made fresh daily. The solution is best administered from a spray bottle with both nostrils open.

### Nursing Management

Nursing management is directed toward patient teachings. See Guidelines box above, right.

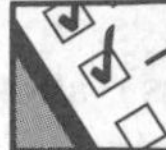

## Guidelines for Teaching the Person with Rhinitis

1. Obtain additional rest.
2. Drink at least 2 to 3 L of fluid daily.
3. Medications: use nasal spray or nose drops two or three times/day as ordered (see Box 36-2).
4. Prevention of further infection:
   a. Blow nose with both nostrils open to prevent infected matter from being forced into eustachian tube.
   b. Cover mouth with disposable tissues when coughing and sneezing to prevent droplet nuclei from contaminating the air.
   c. Dispose of used tissues carefully.
   d. Avoid exposure when possible (i.e., avoid crowds, people with colds, specific allergens). Elderly persons and those with chronic lung disease are particularly vulnerable and should have a flu shot yearly.
   e. Wash hands frequently and especially after coughing, sneezing, and so on. Evidence suggests that many colds are transmitted from person to person by hand contact and from touching objects handled by a person with a cold.
   f. Seek medical attention if the following are present:
      (1) High fever, severe chest pain, earache.
      (2) Symptoms lasting longer than 2 weeks.
      (3) Recurrent colds.

## BOX 36-1 Microbial Causes of Sinusitis

**ACUTE**

Viral
Rhinovirus
Influenza
Parainfluenza
Adenovirus

**BACTERIAL**

*Streptococcus pneumoniae*
*Haemophilus influenzae*
*Moraxella catarrhalis*

**CHRONIC**

*Staphylococcus aureus*
*Haemophilus influenzae*
Anaerobic organisms

Adapted from Leach JL, Schaeffer S: Sinusitis. In Rakel RE: *Conn's current therapy 1993,* Philadelphia, 1993, WB Saunders.

## SINUSITIS

### Etiology/Epidemiology

The sinuses are air-filled cavities lined with mucous membranes. Any inflammation of the mucous membranes of the sinuses is called **sinusitis.** This is a frequent disorder, although it is less common since the advent of antibiotics. Often patients who complain of sinusitis do not have a sinus infection but some other disorder.

Sinusitis may be acute or chronic. The most common types of acute sinusitis are allergic and viral. It is often difficult to distinguish between these two types, although the patient's history may be helpful. *Allergic*

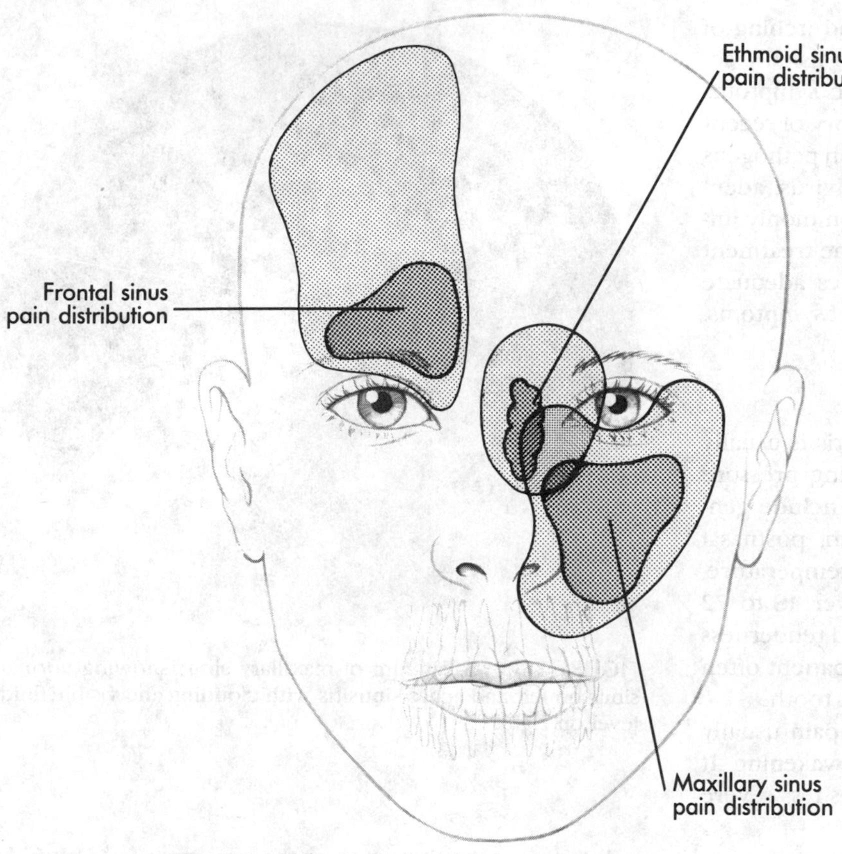


**FIGURE 36-1** Sinus pain: area of local tenderness and pain referral. Maxillary sinus pain frequently is referred to teeth. Frontal pain is generally localized to supraorbital area. Ethmoid pain is generally deep to eye. (From DeWeese DD et al: *Otolaryngology—head and neck surgery,* ed 7, St Louis, 1988, Mosby.)

**TABLE 36-2 Location of Pain With Sinusitis**

| SINUS | PAIN LOCATION |
|---|---|
| Maxillary | Over cheek and upper teeth (Figure 36-1) |
| Frontal | Above the eyebrow (Figure 36-1) |
| Ethmoid | Medial and deep in the eye (Figure 36-2) |
| Sphenoid | Deep behind the eye, over the occiput, or top of head |

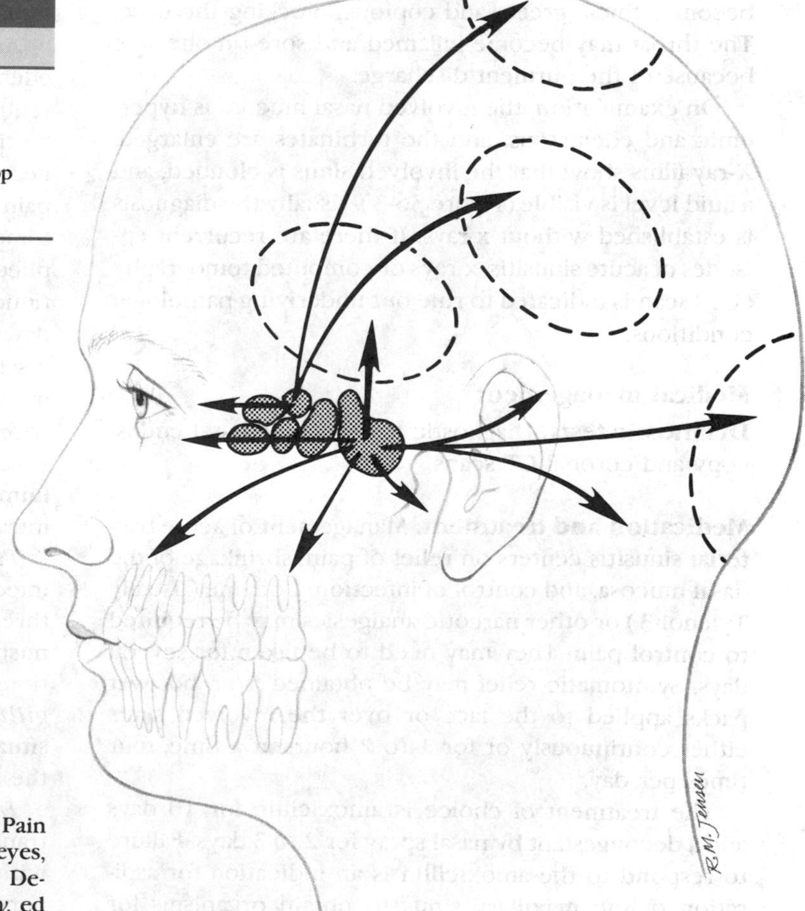

**FIGURE 36-2** Pain from anterior ethmoid deep to eye. Pain from posterior ethmoid cells and sphenoid refers to the eyes, teeth, ears, or the temporal area of the occiput. (From DeWeese DD et al: *Otolaryngology—head and neck surgery,* ed 7, St Louis, 1988, Mosby.)

*rhinitis* is usually seasonal, and redness and itching of the eyes may be present. *Viral sinusitis* is usually accompanied by fever, malaise, and systemic symptoms such as "achiness." There may also be a history of recent exposure to an infected person. The common pathogens found in sinusitis are rhinovirus, influenza virus, adenovirus, and parainfluenza virus. The most commonly implicated organisms are listed in Box 36-1. The treatment of rhinosinusitis is nonspecific and includes adequate fluid intake and reporting of any worsening of symptoms.

## Acute Bacterial Sinusitis

### Pathophysiology

The first symptom of acute bacterial sinusitis is usually a stuffy nose followed by slowly developing pressure over the involved sinus. Other symptoms include general malaise and toxicity, persistent cough, postnasal drip, headache, slightly elevated or normal temperature, and mild leukopenia. Symptoms worsen over 48 to 72 hours until there is severe localized pain and tenderness over the involved sinus (Table 36-2). The patient often believes that the pain is due to an infected tooth.

In acute frontal and maxillary sinusitis, pain usually does not appear until 1 to 2 hours after awakening. It increases for 3 to 4 hours and then becomes less severe in the afternoon and evening.

There may be bloody or blood-tinged discharge from the nose in the first 24 to 48 hours. The discharge rapidly becomes thick, green, and copious, blocking the nose. The throat may become inflamed and sore on one side because of the purulent discharge.

On examination, the involved nasal mucosa is hyperemic and edematous, and the turbinates are enlarged. X-ray films show that the involved sinus is clouded, and a fluid level is visible (Figure 36-3). Usually the diagnosis is established without x-rays. If there are recurrent episodes of acute sinusitis, x-rays or computed tomography (CT) scan is indicated to rule out underlying pathologic conditions.

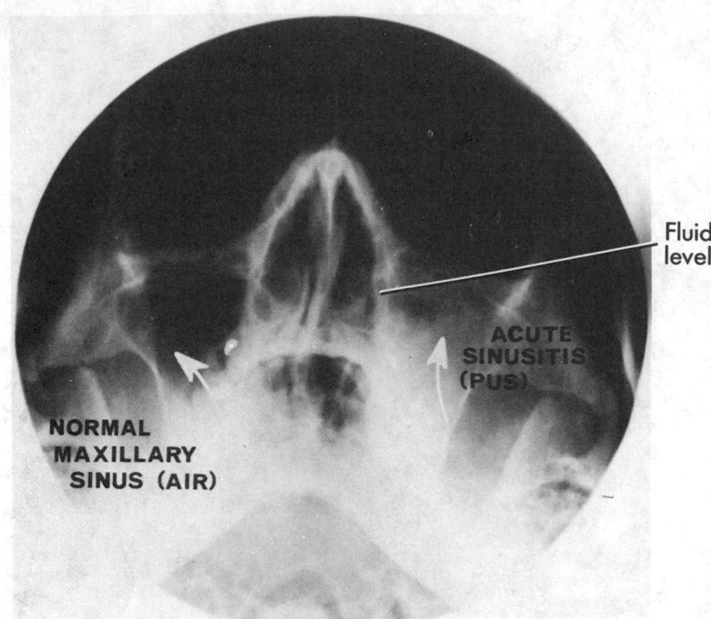


**FIGURE 36-3** X-ray film of maxillary sinus showing normal sinus on left and acute sinusitis with clouding and visible fluid level on right.

### Medical management

**Diagnostic tests.** Diagnostic tests include nasal endoscopy and coronal CT scans.

**Medication and treatment.** Management of acute bacterial sinusitis centers on relief of pain, shrinkage of the nasal mucosa, and control of infection. Codeine (usually Tylenol-3) or other narcotic analgesics may be required to control pain. They may need to be taken for several days. Symtomatic relief may be obtained from hot wet packs applied to the face or over the involved sinus either continuously or for 1 to 2 hours at a time, four times per day.

The treatment of choice is amoxicillin for 10 days and a decongestant by nasal spray for 2 to 3 days. Failure to respond to the amoxicillin is an indication for aspiration of the maxillary sinus to obtain organisms for culture and sensitivity. Other therapy includes a humidifier and saline irrigations to improve mucociliary function.[12]

*Acute frontal sinusitis* with pain, tenderness, and edema of the anterior cortex of the frontal sinus usually requires hospitalization. High-dose intravenous antibiotics and nasal decongestants by spray are usually ordered. Codeine may be given as Tylenol-3 to control pain. It may need to be taken for several days. Symptomatic relief may be obtained from hot wet packs applied to the face or over the involved sinus either continuously or for 1 to 2 hours at a time, four times per day. When the infection has subsided the patient can be discharged on an oral antibiotic. In some cases, osteomyelitis of the frontal bone will occur, and *Staphylococcus aureus* is the most common organism responsible. Osteomyelitis is diagnosed by technetium and gallium scans and is treated with a prolonged course of intravenous antistaphylococcal antibiotics.[12]

*Fungal sinusitis* infections can range from mild infections resembling chronic sinusitis to severe life-threatening invasive infections. Noninvasive fungal sinusitis is often found in patients following other infections or prolonged administration of antibiotics. *Aspergillus* and *Candida* species are commonly found in these situations. Treatment may require surgical drainage of the sinuses.

*Invasive fungal sinusitis* is most likely to occur in transplant patients, patients on chemotherapy, patients with acquired immunodeficiency syndrome (AIDS), or persons with poorly controlled diabetes. *Aspergillus* and

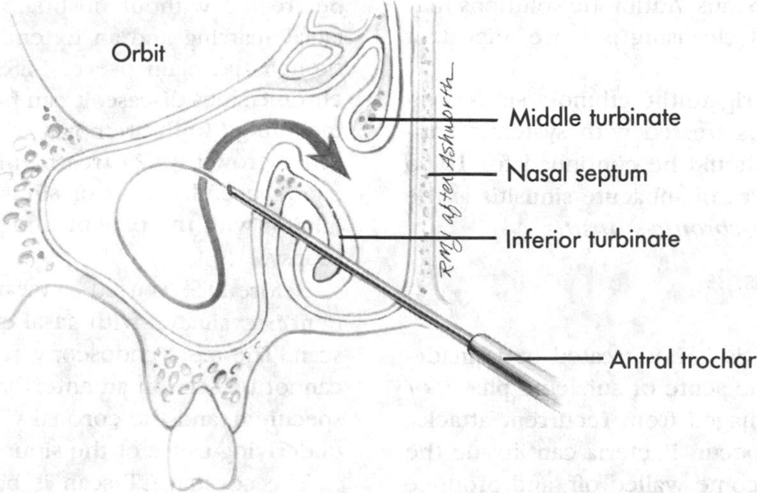


**FIGURE 36-4** Trochar inserted under the inferior turbinate (through the medial wall of the antrum). Contents of the sinus are washed into the nose through the natural ostium. (From DeWeese DD et al: *Otolaryngology—head and neck surgery,* ed 7, St Louis, 1988, Mosby.)

*Mucor* are two types of fungi most prone to cause invasive disease. Symptoms include facial fullness, cranial neuropathies, and pain. Proptosis of the eye, facial swelling, and blood-tinged nasal discharge may be present. On examination the nasal mucosa appears gray or black. The diagnosis is confirmed by biopsy of the affected membranes. These patients should be hospitalized. Treatment is with amphotericin B intravenously, aggressive surgical management, and attempts to correct the underlying immunodeficiency. Despite treatment, many patients will not survive.[12]

**Diet.** Diet is as desired by the patient with emphasis on increased fluid intake.

**Activity.** Activity is as desired by the patient.

**Referral/Consultation.** No referrals are necessary.

## Subacute Bacterial Sinusitis

### Pathophysiology

The measures described above cure more than 90% of patients with acute bacterial sinusitis. A subacute infection persists in the remaining 10%. Persistent purulent discharge is the only constant symptom. An x-ray or CT scan is indicated to determine whether one or more sinuses are involved. Because it is uncommon for acute sinusitis to persist, the causative organism may be unusual.[2] Special culture techniques may be necessary and antibiotic sensitivity studies are essential. The most commonly isolated organisms are *H. influenzae, S. aureus, S. pneumoniae,* and *Branhamella catarrhalis. B. catarrhalis* is not sensitive to penicillin or amoxicillin, and treatment requires systemic sulfonamide therapy or erythromycin with a sulfonamide.

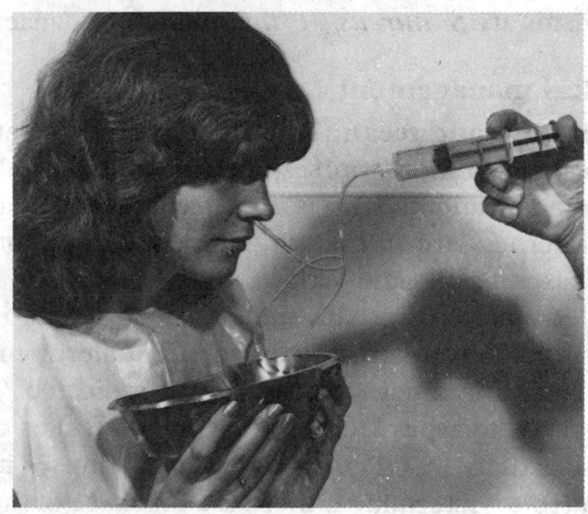

**FIGURE 36-5** Irrigation of the maxillary sinus. With the head tipped forward, solution returns via the natural ostium and out the anterior portion of the nose for examination and/or culture. (From DeWeese DD et al: *Otolaryngology—head and neck surgery,* ed 7, St Louis, 1988, Mosby.)

### Medical management

**Medication and treatment.** Treatment consists of vasoconstriction of nasal mucosa, moist heat, and irrigation of the involved sinus. Pain is not severe and requires no medication.

**Antral irrigation,** in which the anterior wall of the maxillary sinus is punctured, is the preferred treatment for subacute sinusitis. Anesthesia is obtained with an injection of 2 to 3 ml of 1% lidocaine (Xylocaine) with 1:100,000 epinephrine under the upper lip. A 16-gauge needle (with stylet in place) is rotated through the soft tissue and bone (Figures 36-4 and 36-5). When proper placement of the needle is assured, saline solution is instilled to wash out the sinus. Antibiotic solutions may be used, but mechanical cleansing is more important than the solution used.[2]

It is not possible to irrigate the ethmoid sinuses directly, and *ethmoiditis* is treated with systemic antibiotics. The antibiotics should be continued for 10 to 14 days.[2] Proper treatment of subacute sinusitis is the best means of preventing *chronic sinusitis.*

## Chronic Bacterial Sinusitis

### Pathophysiology

When suppurative sinusitis is not treated or is inadequately treated during the acute or subacute phase, or when the mucosa is damaged from recurrent attacks, permanent change may occur. Bacteria can invade the tissue of the sinuses, become walled off, and produce chronic inflammation. With prolonged infection of soft tissue, pathologic change may become irreversible and the patient has *chronic sinusitis.*[2] The major symptom is congestion and thick, green, purulent nasal discharge that lasts for weeks or months. Fever or facial pain, or both, may be present. The most commonly involved organisms are *S. aureus, H. influenzae,* and anaerobes.

### Medical management

**Medication and treatment.** The usual treatment is decongestants in short courses, antibiotics, and nasal saline irrigations. Patients who do not have fever, facial pain, or tenderness are *not* usually helped by antibiotics. In such cases, nasal saline irrigations, adequate oral intake, and decongestants usually are sufficient. When patients do not respond to treatment, surgery, allergy management, or an immunologic workup is indicated. The sinuses may be aspirated to obtain organisms for culture and sensitivity. A CT scan of the nasal sinuses may be indicated to determine if there is a blockage of the nasal sinus drainage system, polyps, mucoperiosteal thickening, or other findings that would require endoscopic sinus surgery, which is discussed below.[12]

### Surgical management

Treatment of *chronic sinusitis* involves surgery to remove all diseased soft tissue and bone, adequate postoperative drainage, and obliteration of the sinus cavity when necessary. The goal of surgery is to eradicate infection and leave contiguous structures normal.

**Functional endoscopic sinus surgery (FESS).** In functional endoscopic sinus surgery (FESS), also known as **endoscopic sinus surgery (ESS),** a fiberoptic endoscope that illuminates and magnifies is used to enter the sinus. This procedure requires advanced training of the surgeon, and in some institutions, it is becoming the standard practice.

Endoscopic sinus surgery has revolutionized the diagnosis and treatment of patients with sinus disorders. It has made it possible for patients with sinus disease to be treated without hospitalization and has prevented facial scarring and an extended recovery period.[12] Although the main use of FESS is to treat recurrent or chronic sinus disease, it can be used for other purposes, including (1) the removal of polyps, foreign bodies, or other growths; (2) treatment of recurrent or chronic pain caused by nasal or sinus blockage; and (3) examination with the patient under anesthesia, usually with biopsy.

Before FESS is used to treat chronic sinusitis, the patient is evaluated with nasal endoscopy and coronal CT scan. The nasal endoscopy reveals subtle changes that cannot be seen in an anterior rhinoscopy using a nasal speculum, and the coronal CT scan can determine the underlying cause of the sinusitis.

The coronal CT scan is best performed after acute inflammation has subsided and medical treatment attempted.

The purpose of FESS is to reestablish sinus ventilation and mucociliary clearance by removal of tissue from the osteomeatal complex (the area of the anterior ethmoids and middle meatus).

The surgical goals of FESS include removing diseased tissue, promoting sinus drainage, improving sinus ventilation, removing objects or masses, and alleviating pain. The procedure can be performed with the patient under local or general anesthesia. If local anesthesia is used, the procedure is performed in an ambulatory surgery center where the patient is kept for 2 to 3 hours postoperatively and then discharged.

Functional endoscopic sinus surgery is performed as follows: Small nasal endoscopes are used to dissect the diseased tissue. The surgeon uses the CT scan as a guide to nasal anatomy and to locate diseased tissue.[17] In early sinus disease the cells are opened to allow for ventilation and drainage. In advanced disease the cells may need to be removed. A major advantage of fiberoptic endoscopy is that it allows the surgeon to remove all the diseased tissue while preserving more healthy tissue and thus preserving more of the function of the sinus.[13]

### Nursing management

Because this is an outpatient procedure, the patient has preadmission tests and preoperative teaching scheduled a few days before surgery. Postoperatively the nurse assesses the patient by telephone within 24 hours of discharge.[13] Teaching of the patient is crucial, and essential points are listed in the Guidelines box on p. 1009.

If inflammation or infection is noted during the surgery, antibiotics will be administered and continued for a total of 10 to 14 days. Some surgeons also order a *steroid nasal spray* for a few days. To maintain moisture to mucosa all patients will begin normal saline sprays after packing is removed. Saline irrigations may be necessary for those with considerable nasal crusting.

***Complications.*** Functional endoscopic sinus surgery in the hands of an experienced surgeon has few

## Guidelines for Teaching Home Care to the Person Having Endoscopic Sinus Surgery

1. Pain.
   a. There will be some discomfort after surgery, but it is more of an ache and pressure from the packing in the nose than actual pain.
   b. The pain may increase during the week after surgery because of swelling and secretions in the sinus.
   c. Most patients obtain relief by taking acetaminophen. If your physician expects you will have more pain, a pain medication will be prescribed.
   d. Never take aspirin or any product containing aspirin because aspirin can cause bleeding.
2. Drainage.
   a. There will be an increase in drainage after surgery.
   b. A small amount of bright red bleeding is normal and may continue for a week.
   c. Old blood that accumulated during the surgery is reddish brown, and it will drain for a week or more. It is of no concern.
   d. A small dressing (dry pad) will be placed beneath your nose to absorb any drainage.
   e. You may need to change the pad several times each day, depending on the amount of drainage. The drainage pad can be discontinued when the drainage stops.
   f. After drainage stops, a thicker, yellowish green drainage may continue for several weeks.
3. Breathing.
   a. Your head may feel stuffy, and the mucous membranes of your nose may swell. This is normal and expected.
   b. This will increase during the first week after surgery and then decrease over the next couple of weeks.
   c. After this, breathing through your nose should improve.
   d. Keeping your head elevated and sleeping with an extra pillow will help make you more comfortable. In this position there will be less swelling and better drainage of nasal secretions.
   e. A cool mist humidifier at the bedside will help loosen secretions and prevent crusting of the nose. *Be sure to follow* the manufacturer's *directions for cleaning the unit so that bacteria will not grow,* be dispersed into the air, and infect you or others.
   f. At your first postoperative visit, the packing will be removed and you will be given instructions for cleaning your nose.
4. Precautions during the first week.
   a. Do not blow your nose until after your first office visit, usually 3 to 5 days after surgery.
   b. Blowing your nose puts too much pressure on the surgical site.
   c. If you feel fluid or congestion in your nose, gently sniff back the fluid and expectorate it from your mouth.
   d. Try not to sneeze, because this will put too much pressure on the surgical site.
   e. If you must sneeze, keep your mouth open and sneeze through your mouth.
   f. Do not bend over and do not lift heavy objects; both put too much pressure on surgery site.
5. Rest and activity.
   a. Your body needs extra rest to heal.
   b. Take it easy the first week, and then return to normal activities.
   c. Usual time to be off work or school is 5 to 7 days unless you work in a dusty or dirty environment.
   d. After 1 week you may swim, jog, or do other exercise. If bright red bleeding occurs, stop activity until bleeding stops, and then gradually resume activity.

complications. Complications that can occur are nasal bleeding, orbital hematoma, injury to the optic nerve, blindness, and cerebrospinal fluid rhinorrhea.[17]

**Caldwell-Luc surgery.** The **Caldwell-Luc procedure** is the generally accepted operative procedure for chronic maxillary sinusitis that cannot be cured with antibiotics and other medical therapy. It is also called a *radical antrum* operation. Local or general anesthesia may be used.

The procedure is performed through an incision under the upper lip (Figure 36-6). Part of the anterior bony wall of the antrum is removed, producing a permanent window (Figure 36-7). All of the diseased mucosa and periosteum is removed through the window. The bone of the lateral wall of the nose in the inferior meatus, which divides the nose from the antrum, is removed.[2] The mucous membrane and periosteum of the lateral wall of the nose are preserved and fashioned into a hinged flap.

The antrum may be packed to prevent bleeding. Packing is removed through the nose 24 to 48 hours post-

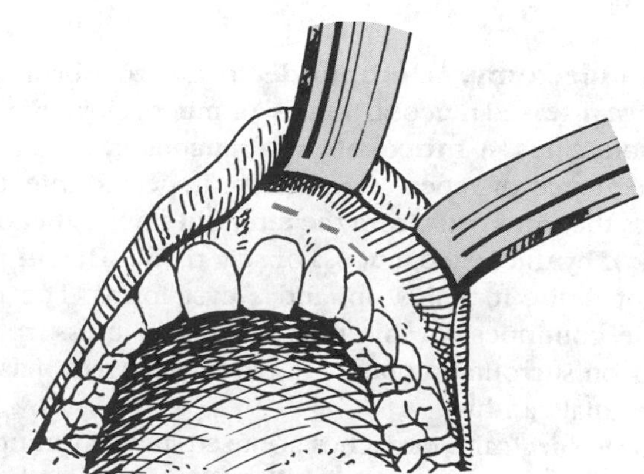

**FIGURE 36-6** The incision into the maxillary sinus (Caldwell-Luc surgery) is made under the upper lip.

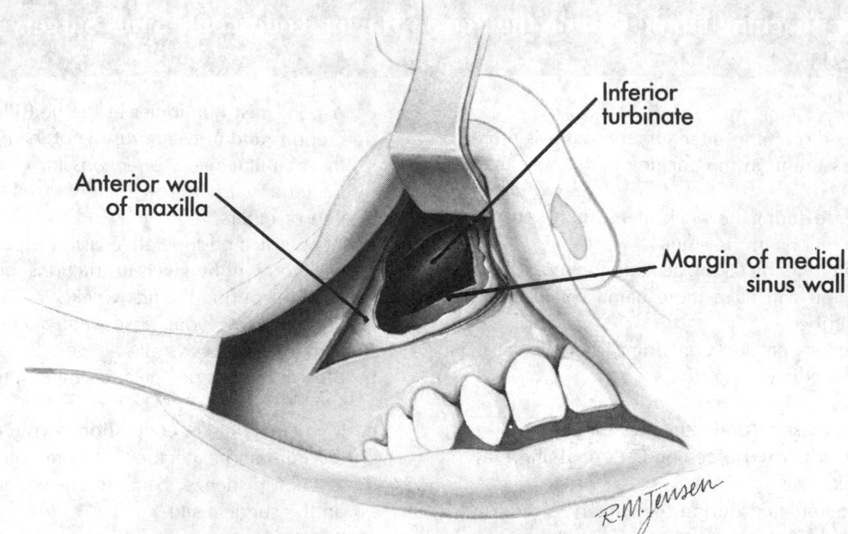


**FIGURE 36-7** Caldwell-Luc surgery. After removal of the sinus mucosa or polypoid tissue, a window is made into the nose along its floor, allowing dependent drainage from the maxillary sinus. Incision is closed with absorbable sutures. (From DeWeese DD et al: *Otolaryngology—head and neck surgery,* ed 7, St Louis, 1988, Mosby.)

operatively. As the maxillary sinus heals, the exposed bone is covered by mucosa. Numbness of the upper lip and upper teeth may be present for several months after a Caldwell-Luc operation, because some nerves to these structures pass through the site of the incision. Interference with eating will occur initially. Only liquids will be given for at least 24 hours, followed by a soft diet for several days.

***Nursing management.*** In addition to general care of the patient following sinus surgery, patient teaching specific to Caldwell-Luc surgery includes the following:

1. Do not chew on affected side until incision heals.
2. Use caution with oral hygiene to avoid injury to the incision.
3. Avoid wearing dentures for about 10 days.
4. Avoid blowing nose for about 2 weeks after packing has been removed.
5. Avoid sneezing; if you must sneeze, keep mouth open.

**Ethmoidectomy.** An **ethmoidectomy** is performed to remove diseased mucosa, polyps, or mucoceles from the ethmoid sinus. A **mucocele** is a mucous cyst that is a consequence of repeated infection. Repeated infection causes the sinus ostia from the ethmoid sinus to become blocked by thickened mucosa or scar tissue. Thus mucus cannot drain, it builds up, and a cyst forms. The mucocele continues to enlarge, resulting in pressure necrosis on surrounding bone. It can be seen as a mass at the medial canthus.

Three surgical approaches are used in performing an ethmoidectomy: (1) transnasally, (2) transantrally, or (3) externally. General or local anesthesia with sedation may be used. Ethmoidectomy is commonly used to remove nasal polyps arising in the ethmoid sinus. Ethmoid cells are removed, creating a single large cavity that is packed for 24 to 48 hours. Usually steroids are given intranasally to prevent nasal polyps from recurring.

In the **transnasal approach** the surgery is performed using a headlight and operating microscopes or endoscopes. This approach is technically difficult, and complications to the orbit can cause cerebrospinal fluid rhinorrhea.

In a *transantral ethomoidectomy* a Caldwell-Luc incision is used (see Figures 36-6 and 36-7). The ethmoid cells are removed from below. It is difficult to remove anterior ethmoid cells using this approach, and a combined intranasal and transantral approach may be necessary. Complications of the transantral approach can be damage to the infraorbital nerve causing numbness of the lip or upper teeth.

The *external approach* is preferred for ethmoid surgery because it allows better visualization and reduces the risks of complications such as damage to the optic nerve and cerebrospinal fluid leak. An ethmoidectomy entails removal of ethmoid air cells (Table 36-3). The incision is made in the inner half to the eyebrow downward along the side of the nose (Figure 36-8). Ethmoidectomy is performed to remove nasal polyps (which frequently originate in the ethmoid cells) and to remove diseased mucosa or mucoceles. A pressure dressing is usually applied over the eye to prevent postoperative edema.

**Sphenoid sinus surgery.** Surgery of the **sphenoid sinus** can be accomplished using an endoscopic technique, through an external or transantral ethmoidectomy approach, or through a transseptal approach (see

**TABLE 36-3 Types of Sinus Surgery**

| PROCEDURE | USE |
|---|---|
| **FUNCTIONAL ENDOSCOPIC SINUS SURGERY (FESS)** | |
| Sinus endoscope enters sinus and removes diseased mucosa and opens sinus ostia | Chronic sinusitis<br>Removal of polyps |
| **CALDWELL-LUC (RADICAL ANTRUM OPERATION)** | |
| Clearing out of maxillary sinus through incision under upper lip | Chronic maxillary sinusitis |
| **TRANSNASAL, EXTERNAL, OR TRANSANTRAL ETHMOIDECTOMY** | |
| Various approaches used to excise infected ethmoid or sphenoid cells | Chronic ethmoid or sphenoid sinusitis |
| **FRONTAL SINUS SURGERY** | |
| Complete removal of diseased mucosa of both frontal sinuses; space packed with subcutaneous fat from abdomen | Chronic frontal sinusitis |
| **SPHENOID SINUS SURGERY** | |
| Ethmoid sinus removed and anterior wall of sphenoid sinus opened | Chronic sphenoid sinusitis |

Table 36-3). The ethmoid sinus is usually removed and the anterior wall of the sphenoid sinus opened. Diseased tissue is removed along with the mucous membrane lining the sinus. To facilitate drainage directly into the nasopharynx, the sinus ostium is opened wide.[17]

**Frontal sinus surgery.** The advent of the **osteoplastic flap operation** makes frontal sinus surgery different from that performed on the other sinuses. Surgery of the other sinuses basically provides for an open, well-drained cavity, which in the past proved inadequate for the frontal sinuses because recurrence of disease was common. The osteoplastic flap operation allows for complete removal of diseased mucosa of the frontal sinus and for obliteration of the sinus so that it is no longer functional or continuous with the inner nose.

The osteoplastic flap procedure is performed through a "gull-wing" or "cross-bow" incision.[6] In men the incision extends along the eyebrows and connects along the bridge of the nose. In women, where baldness is not a problem in later life, the incision connects both temporal areas a few centimeters posterior to the hairline. Both incisions give excellent postoperative cosmesis and are extended to the periosteum of the bone overlying the frontal sinus.

The skin overlying the sinus is reflected, and a radiograph of the frontal sinus (obtained preoperatively) is used as a template for sawing the lateral and superior borders of the anterior frontal bone. The anterior bone

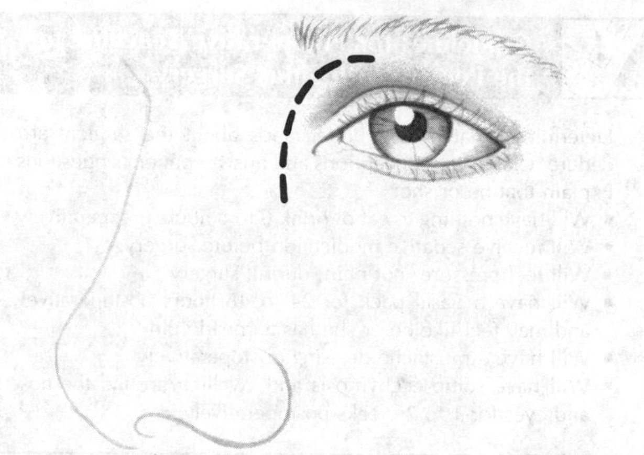

**FIGURE 36-8** Medial canthal incision for external ethmoidectomy. (From DeWeese DD et al: *Otolaryngology—head and neck surgery,* ed 7, St Louis, 1988, Mosby.)

is then reflected inferiorly, thus exposing the entire contents of the frontal sinus. The mucosa is removed under direct vision, and an operating microscope is used to ensure that all fragments of mucosa are removed. An incision is then made in the left lower abdominal quadrant, and subcutaneous fat is obtained for adipose obliteration of the sinus. The bony flap and skin are then repositioned, and a pressure dressing is applied to minimize postoperative swelling.

Postoperatively, pain in the frontal area is not significant after 24 hours. Pain in the abdominal area, however, often lasts several days and serous drainage from this area is common after the drain is removed. Sutures are removed about the fifth postoperative day. Because nasal packs are not used, special oral hygiene care is not needed. Preoperative and postoperative teaching for patients having sinus surgery can be found in the Guidelines boxes on p. 1012.

## NURSING MANAGEMENT

### ♦ ASSESSMENT

#### Subjective Data

- Obstruction of nares
  - History of mouth breathing—time of day or night, duration, and frequency
  - History of change in or loss of smell or taste
  - History of nasal surgery or injury to nose
  - Use of nasal drops or spray—type, amount, frequency, and duration of use
- Nasal discharge
  - Color, amount, and consistency of discharge
  - Blood/drainage—one or both nares
  - Presence of nasal crusting or pain
- History of sinusitis
  - Pain—location and severity
  - Cough, postnasal drip
  - Relationship of sinusitis to certain seasons or types of weather

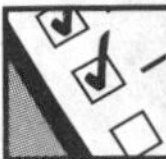

### Guidelines for Preoperative Teaching for the Person With Sinus Surgery

Determine what patient understands about the surgical procedure. Clarify misconceptions and answer patient's questions. Explain that he or she:

- Will have nothing to eat or drink 6 to 8 hours preoperatively.
- Will receive sedative medication before surgery.
- Will feel pressure, not pain, during surgery.
- Will have a nasal pack for 24 to 48 hours postoperatively and may feel like he or she has a "head cold."
- Will have a mustache dressing postoperatively.
- Will have some ecchymosis and swelling around the nose and eyes for 1 to 2 weeks postoperatively.

History of smoking
Other general symptoms such as malaise

## Objective Data

Elevated temperature and drainage from nasal cavity (serous, mucopurulent, purulent)
Polyps (pale, soft, edematous outpouching of nasal or sinal mucosa) may be present and are usually bilateral in inflammation of the nose and sinuses
Redness and edema of mucous membrane

## ♦ NURSING DIAGNOSES

Nursing diagnoses are determined from assessment of patient data. Possible nursing diagnoses for the person with sinusitis may include but are not limited to the following:

| Diagnostic Title | Possible Etiologic Factors |
|---|---|
| Airway clearance, ineffective | Infection or obstruction (nasal polyps) |
| Pain (headache and facial) | Infection in nose and sinuses |
| Sensory/perceptual alteration (related to change in sense of smell and taste) | Infection in sinuses, destruction of sinus cells, changes in mucosa; nasal drainage of green, foul-smelling material |
| Knowledge deficit (related to condition and treatment) | Lack of knowledge about factors that lead to infection of sinuses and how to prevent recurrent infection |

## ♦ EXPECTED PATIENT OUTCOMES

Expected patient outcomes for the person with sinusitis may include but are not limited to the following:

1. Nasal drainage is improved; drainage is thin and clear.
2. Nasal edema and edema of face are reduced.
3. Pain is improved, and patient rates it from 0 to 2 on visual pain scale (0 to 10).
4. Patient states that sense of taste is slightly improved.
5. Patient who has lost sense of smell can state precautions to take such as installing gas detectors, observing food for spoilage, and installing smoke detectors and changing their batteries routinely.
6. The patient can state ways to prevent further attacks by:
   a. Avoiding crowds during periods of high incidence of infection
   b. Getting adequate rest
   c. Eating a well-balanced diet
   d. Limiting milk products, which increase mucus
   e. Avoiding smoking and secondhand smoke
   f. Limiting alcohol intake (dehydrating effect)
7. The patient demonstrates the correct use of nose drops.
8. The patient knows how to use prescribed medi-

### Guidelines for Postoperative Care for the Person With Sinus Surgery

1. After general anesthesia, position patient well onto the side to prevent swelling or aspiration of bloody drainage.
2. Administer cool mist via face tent or collar, or provide humidifier.
3. When the patient is awake, remind him or her to expectorate secretions and not swallow them.
4. Encourage mid-Fowler's position when fully awake to promote drainage and decrease edema.
5. Apply ice compresses over nose (or ice bag over maxillary or frontal sinuses) in the early postoperative period.
6. Monitor the patient for:
   a. Excessive bleeding from nose (may be evidenced by repeated swallowing).
   b. Decreased visual acuity, especially *diplopia,* indicating damage to optic nerve or muscles of globe of eye.
   c. Complaints of pain over the involved sinus, which may indicate infection or inadequate drainage.
   d. Fever—take temperature rectally.
7. Give frequent mouth care using a soft toothbrush. If there is an oral incision, mouth care is given before meals to improve appetite and after meals to decrease danger of infection.
8. Change nasal pad when it is soiled.
9. Apply ice compresses to ecchymotic areas to constrict blood vessels, decrease oozing and edema, and help relieve pain.
10. Encourage liberal fluid intake. Patient may be very thirsty because of dry mouth from breathing.
11. Teach patient to:
    a. Avoid blowing nose for at least 48 hours after packing is removed to prevent bleeding.
    b. Avoid sneezing; if patient must sneeze, he or she should keep mouth open.
    c. Avoid lifting heavy objects.
    d. Report signs of infection (fever, purulent discharge) to surgeon.
    e. Expect tarry stools from swallowed blood for a few days.
    f. Avoid constipation (Valsalva's maneuver can cause bleeding).
    g. Expect that ecchymosis of nose and eyes will begin to change color over next 1 to 2 weeks.
    h. Take prophylactic antibiotics as prescribed; do not stop until all medication is taken.

cations and knows what over-the-counter medications to avoid.
9. The patient states plans for follow-up care.

## ♦ INTERVENTIONS

Preoperative teaching and postoperative teaching for the patient having sinus surgery are outlined in the Guidelines boxes on p. 1012.

The major nursing strategy for the patient with sinusitis who is *not* having surgery is teaching. Important points in teaching include the following:

1. Avoid factors that contribute to the sinusitis.
   a. Avoid chilling and cold, damp atmospheres.
   b. Avoid air conditioning when outside air is warm and moist, if this precipitates sinus irritation.
   c. Avoid smoking and being around smokers (further irritates damaged mucous membranes).
   d. Avoid fatigue.
   e. Try to avoid persons with upper respiratory infections.
   f. Protect nose during swimming; avoid diving.
   g. Inform dentist of chronic sinus condition before tooth extraction.
2. Maximize treatment of sinusitis.
   a. Use acetaminophen rather than aspirin for pain relief; apply moist heat over sinus.
   b. During an acute sinus infection, get additional rest and drink 2 to 3 L of fluids per day.
   c. Take antibiotic for prescribed time period, even if symptoms abate.
   d. Keep room temperature constant (changes in room temperature aggravate sinusitis).
   e. Increase humidity with bedside humidifier and nasal sprays.
   f. If allergens are a contributing factor, prepare an environmentally controlled bedroom (see Chapter 70).

## ♦ EVALUATION

Nasal airway is patent, temperature is normal, and nasal discharge is clear; patient has no headache. Patient can distinguish common smells.[17]

### Complications of Sinusitis

Complications of sinusitis usually are the result of inadequate therapy during the acute stage or a delay in treatment.

According to DeWeese et al.[2] signs and symptoms of complications include the following:

1. Generalized persistent headache
2. Vomiting
3. Convulsions
4. Chills or high fever
5. Edema or increasing swelling of the forehead or eyelids
6. Blurring of vision, diplopia, or persistent retro-ocular pain
7. Signs of increased intracranial pressure
8. Personality changes or dulling of the sensorium
9. Increase in white cell count above 20,000

Other complications include the following[17]:

1. Orbital or periorbital cellulitis
2. Orbital or periorbital abscess
3. Cavernous sinus thrombosis
4. Bacteremia or septicemia
5. Osteomyelitis

Some of these complications are discussed below.

#### Orbital complications

Most orbital infections (75%) are caused by extension from paranasal sinusitis. Most frequently the ethmoid sinuses are involved. *Orbital complications* include ***inflammatory edema, orbital cellulitis, subperiosteal abscess, orbital abscess,*** and ***cavernous sinus thrombosis.*** Complications are treated vigorously with intravenous antibiotics and, in case of abscess, incision and drainage.

**Cavernous sinus thrombosis** occurs when there is extension of infection through the venous pathways (usually the angular vein) to the cavernous sinus. The patient is very ill, with chills and a temperature as high as 41° C (106° F). There is pain deep behind the eye, and the patient becomes toxic and may become semicomatose. Cavernous sinus thrombosis is a very serious complication of sinusitis that can cause death in 48 to 72 hours if untreated. More than 25% of patients who develop this complication will die even when adequately treated. The primary treatment is with intravenous antibiotics.

# INFECTIONS OF THE PHARYNX AND LARYNX

## ACUTE PHARYNGITIS

### Etiology/Epidemiology

Acute pharyngitis is the most common throat inflammation. It may be caused by hemolytic streptococci, staphylococci, other bacteria, filtrable viruses, or fungi. **Group A beta-hemolytic streptococci (GABHS)** are the cause of 15% to 20% of the cases of acute pharyngitis. The most common cause, however, is viruses, which account for 70% of the cases of acute pharyngitis.[14] There is also increased evidence of gonococcal pharyngitis caused by the gram-negative diplococcus. *Neisseria gonorrhoeae.* The disease is increasingly found in both men and women. When gonorrhea is suspected, a throat culture is indicated. A severe form of acute pharyngitis often is referred to as *strep throat* because of the frequency of streptococci as the causative organisms.

### Pathophysiology

Dryness of the throat is a common complaint. The throat appears red, and soreness may range from slight scratch-

**TABLE 36-4 Types of Pharyngitis, Pathophysiology, and Clinical Manifestations[15]**

| PATHOPHYSIOLOGY | CLINICAL MANIFESTATIONS |
|---|---|
| **GROUP A BETA-HEMOLYTIC STREPTOCOCCAL (GABHS)** | |
| Uniform infection of pharyngeal walls | Sore throat, slightly elevated temperature, malaise |
| Purulent exudate, edema of lymphoid tissue of palate, tonsils, uvula | |
| **GONOCOCCAL OR VIRAL** | |
| Vesicles may be present on pharyngeal walls and tonsils | Minimal discomfort<br>Fever, diffuse sore throat |
| **INFECTIOUS MONONUCLEOSIS (EPSTEIN-BARR VIRUS)** | |
| Exudate on pharyngeal walls and tonsils | Sore throat, cervical lymphadenopathy, and fever |
| Spleen may be enlarged | |
| **FUNGAL (ESPECIALLY CANDIDIASIS [THRUSH])** | |
| Develops in patient who is immunosuppressed and on prolonged antibiotics | Pus, dysphagia, white plaques in mouth or on pharyngeal walls |

iness to severe pain with difficulty in swallowing. A hacking cough may be present. Children often develop a very high fever, whereas adults may have only a mild elevation of temperature. Symptoms usually precede or occur simultaneously with the onset of acute rhinitis or acute sinusitis. Pharyngitis can occur after the tonsils have been removed because the remaining mucous membrane can become infected. Pharyngitis is also a common manifestation of infectious mononucleosis (Table 36-4).

### Medical Management

Acute pharyngitis usually is relieved by hot saline throat gargles. An ice collar may make the person feel more comfortable. For adults acetylsalicylic acid administered orally as a gargle or in Aspergum may be prescribed. Lozenges containing a mild anesthetic may help relieve the local soreness. Moist inhalations may help relieve the dryness of the throat. A liquid diet usually is better tolerated, and fluids to at least 2.5 L per day are encouraged. Oral hygiene may prevent drying and cracking of the lips and usually refreshes the mouth. If the temperature is elevated, the patient should remain in bed and, even if ambulatory and afebrile, should have extra rest.

A throat culture is necessary to identify the offending organism. If beta-hemolytic streptococcus is identified, the drug of choice is penicillin. For the person allergic to penicillin, erythromycin or another antibiotic will be prescribed. As with other infections treated with antibiotics, the patient must understand the need to take

**Guidelines for Patient Teaching for the Person With Pharyngitis or Tonsillitis**

1. Comfort measures: use warm saline gargles, ice collars, moist inhalations, mouth care
2. Need for fluid intake of at least 2 to 3 L/day
3. Symptoms of recurrence requiring medical attention: fever, excessive pain, pus, dysphagia
4. Rationale for prophylactic antibiotic therapy for pharyngitis in patients with a history of rheumatic fever or infective endocarditis to prevent reinfection

the prescribed antibiotic until the course is completed. This will vary from 7 to 12 days, depending on the organism and the severity of infection. Patients must understand that they should continue therapy for the prescribed number of days, even if they are symptom-free.

Persons with a history of bacterial endocarditis or rheumatic fever are usually given penicillin prophylactically.

### Nursing Management

The major role of the nurse is patient teaching, which is presented in the Guidelines box above.

## ACUTE FOLLICULAR TONSILLITIS

### Etiology/Epidemiology

**Acute follicular tonsillitis** is an acute inflammation of the tonsils and their crypts. It is usually caused by the *Streptococcus* organism. It is more likely to occur when the person's resistance is low and is very common in children.

### Pathophysiology

The onset is almost always sudden, and symptoms include sore throat, pain on swallowing, fever, chills, general muscle aching, and malaise. These symptoms often last for 2 to 3 days. The pharynx and tonsils appear red, and the peritonsillar tissues are swollen. Sometimes a yellowish exudate drains from crypts in the tonsils. A throat culture usually is taken to identify the offending organism.

### Medical and Nursing Management

The patient with acute tonsillitis is encouraged to rest and take generous amounts of fluids orally. Warm saline throat irrigation may be ordered, and antibiotics are given for streptococcal pharyngitis. Acetominophen (Tylenol) and sometimes codeine sulfate may be ordered for pain and discomfort. An ice collar applied to the neck may relieve discomfort.

### Complications

Complications of untreated tonsillitis include heart and kidney damage, chorea, and pneumonia. Incidence of these complications is decreasing with the widespread use of penicillin and early diagnosis. Most physicians believe that persons who have recurrent attacks of tonsillitis should have a tonsillectomy. This procedure is usually performed from 4 to 6 weeks after an acute attack has subsided (see p. 1019).

Because the person with acute tonsillitis is usually cared for at home, the nurse should help in teaching the general public the care that is needed (see Guidelines box, p. 1014). The office nurse, the clinical nurse, the nurse in industry, the school nurse, and the community health nurse have many opportunities to do this teaching.

### Peritonsillar Abscess

A peritonsillar abscess is an uncommon local complication of acute follicular tonsillitis in which infection extends from the tonsil to form an abscess in the surrounding tissues. The presence of pus behind the tonsil causes difficulty in swallowing, talking, and opening the mouth; and the person may be unable to swallow. Pain is severe and may extend to the ear on the affected side.

#### Medical and nursing management

If antibiotics to which the offending organism is sensitive are administered early, infection subsides. If the peritonsillar abscess is caused by anaerobic organisms, hydrogen peroxide (an oxidizing agent) in the form of a mouthwash may help relieve symptoms. Acute streptococcal or staphylococcal tonsillitis may also cause a peritonsillar abscess to form. If an abscess forms, it will be incised and drained. During the operation, the patient's head usually is lowered, and suction is applied as soon as the incision is made to prevent the patient from aspirating the drainage. Warm saline irrigations, an ice collar, or narcotics may relieve discomfort. If acute follicular tonsillitis is treated adequately, peritonsillar abscess is not likely to occur.

## LARYNGITIS

### Simple Acute Laryngitis

#### Etiology/Pathophysiology

**Simple acute laryngitis** is an inflammation of the mucous membrane lining the larynx accompanied by edema of the vocal cords. It may be caused by a cold, by sudden changes in temperature, or by irritating fumes. Symptoms vary from a slight huskiness to complete loss of voice. The throat may be painful and feel scratchy, and a cough may be present.

#### Medical management

Laryngitis in adults usually requires only symptomatic treatment. The person is advised to remain indoors in an even temperature and to avoid talking for several days or weeks, depending on the severity of the inflammation. Steam inhalations may be soothing and cough syrups or home remedies for coughs provide relief to some patients. Smoking or being near others who are smoking should be avoided. Additional fluids by mouth help to prevent dehydration and drying of the throat.

#### Nursing management

The nursing role is mainly patient teaching, which would include the following:

1. Need to take antibiotics as prescribed (not to stop antibiotics when feeling better)
2. Need to increase fluid intake
3. For smoker, need to stop smoking and, for both smokers and nonsmokers, need to avoid smoky environments (secondhand smoke)
4. Referral to a support group for persons wanting to stop smoking
5. Precautions in using steam inhalations

### Chronic Laryngitis

#### Etiology

Some people who use their voices excessively, who smoke a great deal, or who work continuously where there are irritating fumes develop a **chronic laryngitis.** Hoarseness usually is worse in the early morning and in the evening. There may be a dry, harsh cough and a persistent need to clear the throat. All persons with persistent hoarseness should be examined by laryngoscopy to rule out cancer of the larynx.

#### Medical management

Treatment may consist of removal of irritants, voice rest, correction of faulty voice habits, steam inhalations, and cough medications. Additional fluids by mouth are encouraged to prevent dehydration and drying of the throat.

# OBSTRUCTIONS OF THE NOSE AND THROAT

## PATHOPHYSIOLOGY

The upper airway may become partly obstructed, leading to interference with breathing. Obstructions may occur at the base of the tongue (tumor), in the nose (deviated septum, hypertrophied turbinates, or nasal polyps), pharynx (enlarged tonsils and adenoids), or larynx (laryngeal paralysis or edema, cervical esophageal tumor).

The signs and symptoms of upper airway obstruction include difficulty in breathing through the nose, dry mucosa, postnasal drip, nasal discharge, bleeding from the nose, and loss of sense of smell.

## MEDICAL MANAGEMENT

Management is mainly surgical. The types of surgery are discussed under each of the obstructions.

## NURSING MANAGEMENT

### ♦ ASSESSMENT

#### Subjective Data

Symptoms of nasal obstruction include presence or absence of and duration of the following:

- Noisy, difficult breathing
- Dry mucosa
- Postnasal drip
- Nasal discharge
- Nasal crusting
- Anosmia (loss of sense of smell)
- Bleeding from nose

If nasal trauma is present, additional symptoms include displacement of the bones, cosmetic deformity, pain, and ecchymosis around the eyes or jaw.

#### Objective Data

- Inspection for deformity or asymmetry
- Some septal deviation is common in adults (Figure 36-9) and is asymptomatic
- Check for abnormal findings in nose
  - Excessive redness
  - Edema
  - Exudate
  - Bleeding

### ♦ NURSING DIAGNOSES

Nursing diagnoses are determined from an analysis of patient data. Possible nursing diagnoses for the person with obstruction of the nose and throat may include, but are not limited to, the following:

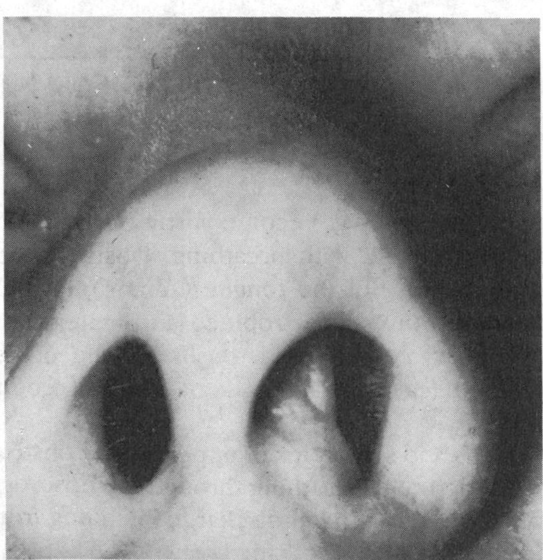

**FIGURE 36-9** Septal deviation. Anterior end of septal cartilage is dislocated and projects into nasal vestibule. (From Saunders WH et al: *Nursing care in eye, ear, nose, and throat disorders,* ed 4, St Louis, 1979, Mosby.)

| Diagnostic Title | Possible Etiologic Factors |
|---|---|
| Body image disturbance | Severe trauma/disfiguring surgery |
| Knowledge deficit (related to condition and its treatment) | Lack of exposure to information |
| Pain | Trauma/obstruction |
| Sensory/perceptual alterations (olfactory) | Trauma/surgery |

### ♦ EXPECTED PATIENT OUTCOMES

Expected patient outcomes for the person with an obstruction of the nose or throat may include, but are not limited to, the following:

1. Patient states he or she is comfortable.
2. Patient can state care required after surgery and discharge from hospital.
3. Patient knows how to prevent nosebleeds or to treat them if they occur.

## DEVIATED SEPTUM

### Etiology/Epidemiology

**Deviated septum** is a common cause of nasal obstruction in older children and adults. It may be congenital but usually is the result of an injury.

### Pathophysiology

The nasal septum, which is normally thin and straight, may be deviated from the midline and protrude more to one side of the nasal passage than to the other (see Figure 36-9). The deviation may cause a *nasal obstruction that increases when infection or allergic reaction occurs* and that is evidenced by marked, noisy, and difficult breathing. There may be a postnasal drip, or the mucosa may become so dry that crusts form. A broken nose can lead to chronic sinusitis if not treated, even though it may cause no immediate problem. Some persons may have a deviated septum that does not cause obstruction, and thus surgery is not necessary.

### Surgical Management

Surgery is performed when obstruction occurs and consists of a nasoseptoplasty (Box 36-2).

**BOX 36-2 Surgeries to Relieve Nasal Obstruction or Trauma**

**NASOSEPTOPLASTY**
Reconstruction of nasal septum

**RHINOPLASTY**
Reconstruction of external nose after trauma or for cosmetic reasons

**NASAL POLYPECTOMY**
Removal of polyps from nose

### Nasoseptoplasty

**Nasoseptoplasty,** which involves reconstruction of the nasal septum, is widely used to treat a deviated septum. In this procedure an incision is made through the mucosa at the caudal end of the septal cartilage. The septal mucous membranes are elevated, and the septal cartilage is separated from its bony attachments and straightened. The septal mucous membranes are then approximated to prevent bleeding.

Nasal septal splints made of plastic or Silastic are inserted into the nose to prevent *synechiae* (a type of scar tissue) and to keep the septum in place. The nose may be packed for 24 to 48 hours to prevent a hematoma from forming between the septal flaps and to hold the septum in place.[17] The patient is usually given antibiotics until the packing is removed. The splints and nasal packing are removed by the surgeon. Reconstruction of the external nose (rhinoplasty) is often combined with septoplasty.

### Rhinoplasty

Reconstructive surgery of the nose can be used either to correct an anatomic problem or for cosmetic reasons. Bone and cartilage may be removed from the nose if it is irregular, or they may be inserted if a defect such as a saddle nose is being corrected (Figure 36-10). Most rhinoplasties are performed with the patient under local anesthesia. The incision is usually made at the end of the nose inside the nostril so that it is not conspicuous.

The nose is usually protected with a plaster-of-Paris splint, adhesive tape dressing, or plastic mold following a plastic procedure on the nasal bones. Firm healing develops on about the tenth day. There will be *ecchymosis* and *swelling* around the eyes and nose for 10 to 14 days after surgery. Iced compresses and an ice bag are commonly used to hasten fluid reabsorption from the surgical site. The patient needs to know that it will be several weeks before the final result of the surgery will be evident.

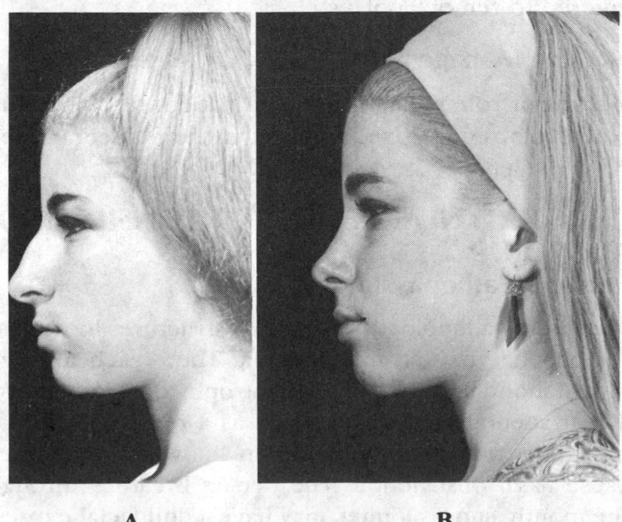


**FIGURE 36-10** **A,** Preoperative appearance of 16-year-old girl. **B,** Postoperative appearance 1 year after rhinoplasty. (From Peck GC: Surgery of the nasal tip. In Masters FW, Lewis JR, Jr, editors: *Symposium on aesthetic surgery of the nose, ears, and chin,* vol 6, St Louis, 1973, Mosby.)

## Nursing Management

After nasal surgery the patient is placed in mid-Fowler's position to decrease local edema, and cool mist is given via collar or face tent, and iced compresses are usually applied to the nose to lessen the discoloration, bleeding, and discomfort. Patients can usually apply their own iced compresses.

The patient is monitored for signs of hemorrhage (see Guidelines box, p. 1018). Some oozing on the dressing below the nose (Figure 36-11) is expected, and this dressing may be changed as necessary. If bleeding becomes pronounced, the surgeon is notified and material for repacking the nose is prepared. This material consists of a hemostatic tray containing gauze packing, umbilical tape for posterior packing, a few small gauze sponges, small catheter (used for inserting a postnasal plug), packing forceps, tongue blades, and scissors. The surgeon may require a head mirror, good light, epinephrine 1:1000 or other vasoconstrictor, 4% topical lidocaine (Xylocaine) or 4% cocaine solution, applicators, nasal speculum, and suction.

Because packing blocks the passage of air through the nose, a partial vacuum is created during swallowing, and the person may complain of a sucking action when attempting to drink. Postnasal drainage, the presence of old blood in the mouth, dryness of the mouth from mouth breathing, and loss of the ability to smell often lead to anorexia. Frequent mouth care is important. Pa-

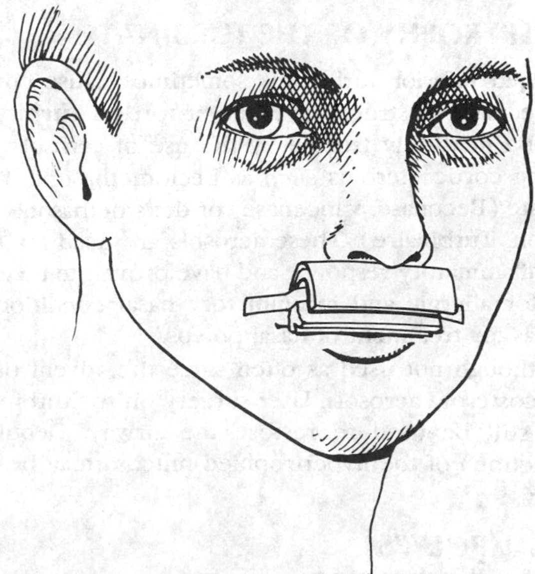

**FIGURE 36-11** Dressing placed under the nose to catch nasal drainage. Also called a *mustache dressing* or a *drip pad.*

**Guidelines for Care of the Person After Nasal Surgery**

1. Assessment.
   a. Monitor for hemorrhage.
      (1) Excessive blood on nasal dressing.
      (2) Bright red vomitus.
      (3) Repeated swallowing (check back of throat with penlight for blood running down throat).
      (4) Rapid pulse.
      (5) Restlessness.
   b. Monitor for infection: fever, elevated white blood cell count (WBC).
2. Discomfort.
   a. Mid-Fowler's position to decrease local edema.
   b. Cool mist via collar or face tent.
   c. Ice compresses over nose for 24 hours PRN.
   d. Support and sedation for patient apprehension because of difficulty in breathing caused by blockage of nasal passages.
   e. Frequent oral care.
   f. Change dressing under nose PRN.
3. Nutrition.
   a. Food as tolerated.
   b. Encourage increased fluid intake.
4. Patient teaching.
   a. Avoid blowing nose for 48 hours after packing removed.
   b. Avoid constipation (Valsalva's maneuver) and vigorous coughing until healing occurs (can initiate bleeding).
   c. Expect stools to be tarry for several days.
   d. Expect face to be discolored around eyes and nose for several days.
   e. Cosmetic effect from nasal surgery cannot be judged for 6 to 12 months (time for tissue to return to normal and for scar resolution).

**tient teaching is described in Guidelines box (above) on postoperative care.**

## HYPERTROPHY OF THE TURBINATES

Enlarged inferior turbinates sometimes cause considerable nasal obstruction. **Hypertrophied turbinates** may be medically treated by the use of aerosols containing corticosteroids such as beclomethasone dipropionate (Beconase, Vancenase) or dexamethasone (Decadron, Turbinaire). These aerosols are used for their antiinflammatory response and have proven to be effective for allergic and inflammatory nasal conditions as well as for treatment of nasal polyps.

Although not used as often since the advent of the corticosteroid aerosols, laser surgery on the turbinates, may still be used to restore the airway. Debulking (resection) of the hypertrophied mucosa may be necessary.

## NASAL POLYPS

### Etiology/Epidemiology

**Nasal polyps** are grapelike growths of the mucous membranes of the sinus mucosa into the cavities of the nose and paranasal sinuses. The exact cause of nasal polyposis is unknown, but some believe it is related to the inflammatory response. Supporting this theory is the fact that persons with chronic viral or bacterial infections have a higher incidence of nasal polyps. Nasal polyps are common and affect men twice as often as women. They are frequently associated with allergies, cystic fibrosis, asthma, disorders of ciliary motility, chronic rhinitis, and chronic sinusitis.

### Pathophysiology

Approximately 8% of patients with nasal polyps also have symptoms of asthma and intolerance to aspirin, indomethacin, and the nonsteroidal antiinflammatory drugs (NSAIDs). The cause of the triad of nasal polyps, asthma, and aspirin sensitivity is unknown, but the patient may have an acute asthmatic attack in response to infection, anesthesia, surgery, or the administration of aspirin. All of the above could be considered stressors for the hyperresponsive airway of the person with asthma.

### Medical Management

#### Medication and treatment

Nasal polyps can be treated by corticosteroid sprays or by local injection of a steroid into the polyp. Steroid sprays are used for long-term reduction of size of polyps, to prevent recurrence, and to reduce the inflammatory response, thus reducing swelling.

Antibiotics such as amoxicillin or erythromycin are prescribed when infection is present. Persistent polyps may require a nasal polypectomy to remove the polyps; a functional endoscopic sinus surgery (FESS), in which polyps are removed (see p. 1008); or a Caldwell-Luc operation (see p. 1009), in which the maxillary sinus is entered to remove polyps.

### Nursing Management

The major role of the nurse is in patient teaching. The points to be emphasized are listed in the Guidelines box, p. 1019 (left).

## CHRONIC ENLARGEMENT OF TONSILS AND ADENOIDS

### Etiology/Pathophysiology

Tonsils and adenoids are lymphoid structures located in the oropharynx and nasopharynx. They reach full size in childhood and then begin to atrophy during puberty. When adenoids enlarge, usually as a result of chronic infections but sometimes for no known reason, they cause nasal obstruction. The person breathes through the mouth, snores loudly, may have a dull facial expression, and may have reduced appetite, because the blocked nasopharynx can interfere with swallowing. Hypertrophy of the tonsils does not usually block the oropharynx but may affect speech and swallowing and cause mouth breathing.

### Guidelines for Teaching the Person With Nasal Polyposis

1. Elevate head of bed to decrease nasal edema and improve breathing through nose.
2. Increase humidity to thin secretions and reduce dryness of nose. Use central humidifier on furnace or use room humidifier. Increase fluid intake, and use saline nasal spray.
3. Prevent respiratory infections by avoiding persons with upper respiratory infections and avoiding crowds. Notify physician at first sign of infection so appropriate therapy can be started.
4. Seek prompt medical attention if signs of recurrence of polyp(s).
5. Take medications as ordered. Be aware of side effects such as drowsiness if antihistamines are prescribed.

## Surgical Management

The tonsils and adenoids are removed when they become enlarged and cause symptoms of obstruction, when they are chronically infected, when the person has repeated attacks of tonsillitis, or after repeated peritonsillar abscesses. Chronic infections of these structures usually do not respond to antibiotics and may become foci of infection by spreading organisms to other parts of the body such as the heart.

### Tonsillectomy

Tonsillectomy in adults may be performed with the patient under either general or local anesthesia. After the tonsils are removed, pressure is applied to stop superficial bleeding. Bleeding vessels are tied off with sutures or by electrocoagulation. The person is monitored carefully for hemorrhage (see Guidelines box at right), especially when sleeping, because a very large amount of blood may be lost without any external evidence of bleeding. The physician may be able to control minor postoperative bleeding by applying a sponge soaked in a solution of epinephrine to the site. The person who is bleeding excessively often is returned to the operating room for surgical treatment to stop the hemorrhage.

If sutures are used, the person will have more pain and discomfort than that occurring after a simple tonsillectomy and may be unable to take solid foods for several days. Some otolaryngologists prescribe acetaminophen instead of aspirin for pain after tonsillectomy because aspirin increases the tendency for bleeding.

The tough, yellow, fibrous membrane that forms over the operative site begins to break away between the fourth and eighth postoperative days, and hemorrhage may occur. The separation of the membrane accounts for the throat being more painful at this time. Pink granulation tissues soon become apparent, and by the end of the third postoperative week the area is covered with mucous membrane of normal appearance. Postoperative care is outlined in the Guidelines box above, right.

### Guidelines for Care of the Person After Tonsillectomy

1. Position patient on side until fully awake after general anesthesia or in mid-Fowler's position when awake.
2. Monitor for hemorrhage.
   a. Frequent swallowing (inspect throat).
   b. Bright red vomitus.
   c. Rapid pulse.
   d. Restlessness.
3. Comfort.
   a. Give 30% cool mist via collar.
   b. Apply ice collar to neck (will also reduce bleeding by vasoconstriction).
   c. Use acetaminophen in place of aspirin.
4. Food and fluids.
   a. Give ice-cold fluids and bland foods during initial period (e.g., ice chips, Popsicles, Jello).
   b. Milk is usually not given, because it may increase mucus and cause the patient to clear throat.
   c. Advance to normal diet as soon as possible.
5. Patient teaching.
   a. Avoid attempting to clear throat immediately after surgery (may initiate bleeding).
   b. Avoid coughing, sneezing, vigorous nose blowing, and vigorous exercise for 1 to 2 weeks.
   c. Drink fluids (2 to 3 L/day) until mouth odor disappears.
   d. Avoid hard scratchy foods, such as pretzels or popcorn, until throat is healed.
   e. Report signs of bleeding to physician immediately.
   f. Expect more throat discomfort between fourth and eighth postoperative days because of membrane separation.
   g. Expect stool to be black or dark for a few days because of swallowed blood.
   h. Resume normal activity immediately, as long as it is not stressful or requires straining.

# LARYNGEAL PARALYSIS

## Etiology

**Laryngeal paralysis** may result from disease or injury of either the laryngeal nerves or the vagus nerve. Some causes include aortic aneurysm, mitral stenosis, laryngeal cancer, subglottic or cervical esophageal tumors, bronchial carcinoma, neck injuries, severing or stretching of the recurrent laryngeal nerve during thyroidectomy, and prolonged intubation of patients in intensive care units. The major diagnostic method is laryngoscopy.

## Pathophysiology

Either one or both vocal cords may be paralyzed. If only one cord is affected, the airway is adequate and only the voice may be affected.[2] Efforts to improve the voice in persons with unilateral cord paralysis have been accomplished by injecting a small quantity of Gelfoam or Teflon into the paralyzed cord. This swells the cord and pushes it toward the midline where the other cord can approximate it better during phonation.

Bilateral paralysis causes a *poor airway* that results in *incapacitating dyspnea, stridor on exertion,* and a

**TABLE 36-5 Diagnostic Tests and Purposes**

| TEST | PURPOSE |
|---|---|
| Indirect laryngoscopy | To diagnose vocal cord abnormality |
| Videostroboscopy (observe vocal cord vibration during phonation): fiberoptic laryngoscope is attached to a videotape to record actual cord motion | To diagnose abnormal vibrations of cord |
| Electromyography | To determine innervation and thus movement of vocal cord(s) |
| Computed tomography (CT) scan | To determine cause of vocal cord pareses or paralysis such as tumor or aneurysm along course of recurrent laryngeal nerve |

Adapted from Sigler BA, Schuring LT: *Ear, nose and throat disorders,* St Louis, 1993, Mosby.

*weak voice.* A sudden bilateral vocal cord paralysis is uncommon and is usually a result of a massive cerebrovascular accident or blunt trauma, both of which are usually incompatible with life. Treatment of bilateral cord paralysis is aimed at restoration of the airway, not at improvement of the voice. Airway management is discussed under Laryngeal Edema.

## Medical Management

### Diagnostic tests

Diagnostic tests and their purposes are listed in Table 36-5.

### Medication

Depending on the patient's symptoms one or more of the following medications may be prescribed. If the patient is experiencing *gastroesophageal reflux,* antacids, which neutralize gastric acid, or $H_2$ inhibitors, which reduce the amount of gastric acid produced, may be ordered.

If the patient has signs and symptoms of an infection, appropriate antibiotics will be prescribed. For patients with swelling of the vocal cords systemic steroids are often ordered and for those with spastic movements of the cords botulinum may be injected.

## Surgical Management

A tracheostomy may be necessary to maintain the airway. Tracheostomy is discussed below (see p. 1021). Treatment of cord paralysis may involve excision of nodules or polyps, or a **thyroplasty**, in which a stent is inserted to reapproximate the vocal cords, may be performed.

Other possible procedures include an **arytenoidectomy,** in which a portion of one of the arytenoid cartilages is resected, thus increasing the diameter of the posterior portion of the glottis sufficiently to improve breathing.[16]

# LARYNGEAL EDEMA

**Acute laryngeal edema** is a medical emergency. It may be caused by anaphylaxis, urticaria, acute laryngitis, serious inflammatory disease of the throat, or edema after intubation. Acute laryngeal edema causes the airway to narrow or close and requires restoration of the airway. Treatment of acute laryngeal edema consists of administration of an adrenal corticosteroid or epinephrine. A tracheostomy or intubation may be necessary (see p. 1021). Edema of the larynx may be chronic because of irradiation treatment of the larynx or tumors of the neck, thus requiring a tracheostomy.

## Airway Management

An airway may be partially or completely obstructed as mentioned above. In partial airway obstruction the individual displays respiratory distress and produces sounds such as gurgling, snoring, or stridorous ventilations. When the airway is completely obstructed, the conscious person will have no breath sounds and will display signs of severe respiratory distress progressing to respiratory arrest. Airway obstruction is confirmed in the unconscious person when attempts to ventilate the person do not produce chest movement and no expiratory air passes from the individual's airway.

The type of intervention used to reestablish and maintain airway patency depends on the individual's level of consciousness, respiratory status, and the cause of airway obstruction. The conscious person with an obstructed airway must be assessed for adequacy of air exchange. If the individual can talk and cough, air exchange is adequate and interventions can be focused on the underlying cause. The conscious person with a completely obstructed airway will not be able to speak or cough and will soon lose consciousness if the obstruction is not relieved. Special maneuvers such as chest or abdominal thrusts and back blows are administered if the obstruction is caused by a foreign object blocking the airway. Organizations such as the American Heart Association and the American Red Cross offer training programs to certify proficiency in these basic lifesaving techniques.

In the unconscious individual the tongue falls back, covering the glottis. By simply lifting the chin, the tongue is moved forward, opening the airway. An alternative position to keep the tongue from obstructing the unconscious person's glottis is to place the individual in a side-lying position.

When a person has a mechanical obstruction of the airway and is expected to be unconscious for some time, it may be necessary to use an artificial airway.

## Artifical Airways

### Oral airways

The simplest type of artificial airway is an oropharyngeal airway. The oropharyngeal airway keeps the tongue from falling back over the glottis. This type of airway is never used in a conscious individual, because it may cause vomiting or laryngospasm. An oropharyngeal airway must be inserted correctly to avoid pushing the tongue back against the glottis.

The esophageal gastric airway consists of a face mask with two ports. The lower port is for the esophageal tube, which is introduced into the esophagus to prevent gastric contents reflux. The upper port is used for ventilation. The esophageal gastric tube airway is never inserted into a conscious person.

### Endotracheal and tracheostomy tubes

When a person is no longer able to maintain his or her own airway, an **endotracheal tube** or **tracheostomy** is necessary. An endotracheal tube is usually chosen initially as a means of providing the airway; tracheostomy is only performed if airway maintenance is necessary for a prolonged period of time or if trauma to the airway prevents the use of an endotracheal tube. Although the tracheostomy has the *disadvantage* of a higher risk of infection, it is often elected for airway management because it is *much more comfortable than an endotracheal tube and allows the person to eat.*

In endotracheal intubation a tube is passed through either the nose or mouth into the trachea, whereas in a tracheostomy an artificial opening is made in the trachea into which a tube is inserted (Figure 36-12). These procedures are used (1) to establish and maintain a patent airway, (2) to prevent aspiration by sealing off the trachea from the digestive tract in the unconscious or paralyzed person, (3) to permit removal of tracheobronchial secretions in the person who cannot cough adequately, and (4) to treat the patient who requires positive pressure ventilation that cannot be given effectively by mask. Whether an intubation or a tracheostomy is performed initially depends on the facilities available and the wishes of the physician. Most physicians consider it safer to do an emergency endotracheal intubation and then perform a tracheostomy as a nonemergency procedure in the operating room if prolonged support of the airway is needed. In this instance the endotracheal tube is not removed until after the tracheostomy opening is made.

A tracheostomy is necessary when an endotracheal tube cannot be inserted or when it is contraindicated, as in severe burns or *larygneal obstruction* caused by *tumor, infection,* or *vocal cord paralysis.* Once the airway is secured, either by intubation or tracheostomy, secretions are aspirated, and well-humidified oxygen is usually given. If the patient is unable to sustain respiration, a mechanical ventilator (see Chapter 37) is attached to either the endotracheal tube or the tracheostomy tube. When mechanical ventilation is required, a cuffed tube is used. Usually an endotracheal tube is not left in place longer than 10 to 14 days. If the patient is unable to maintain a patent airway after this period of time, a tracheostomy is performed.

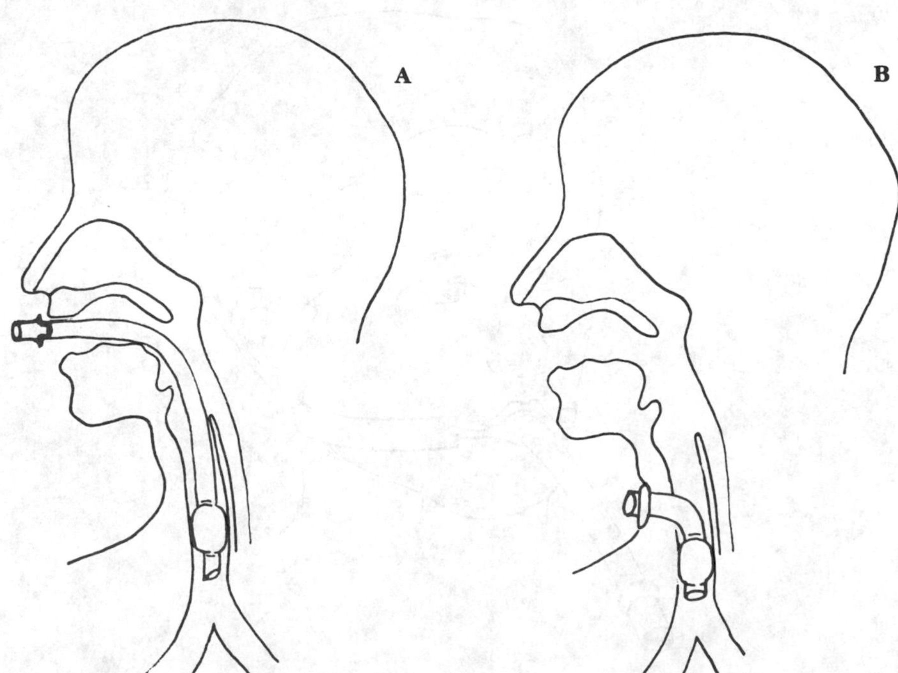


**FIGURE 36-12** **A,** Position of endotracheal tube. **B,** Position of tracheostomy tube.

The endotracheal tube is made of plastic with an inflatable cuff so that a closed system with the ventilator may be maintained (Figure 36-13). The tube is inserted via the mouth or nose through the larynx into the trachea. If an oral endotracheal tube is used, a rubber airway or bite block is often necessary to prevent the patient from biting down on the tube and obstructing the airway.

Two potentially fatal complications can occur in patients with endotracheal tubes. These are *accidental extubation* and *displacement of the endotracheal tube.* Tips of endotracheal tubes have been shown to shift as

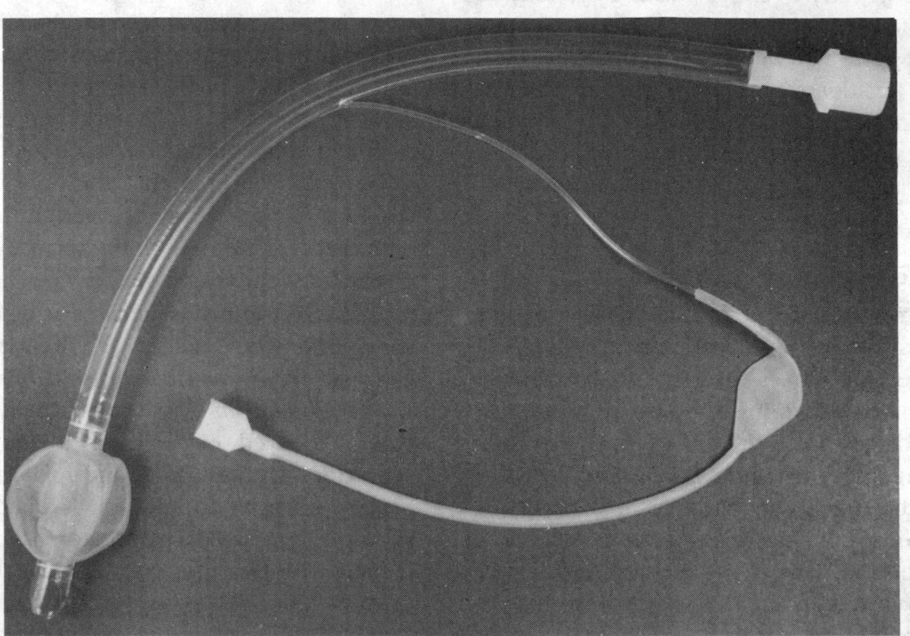

**FIGURE 36-13** Forregar high-volume, low-pressure cuffed endotracheal tube. Cuff shown here is not inflated. Low-pressure cuff is preferred, because it is less likely to cause tracheal damage.

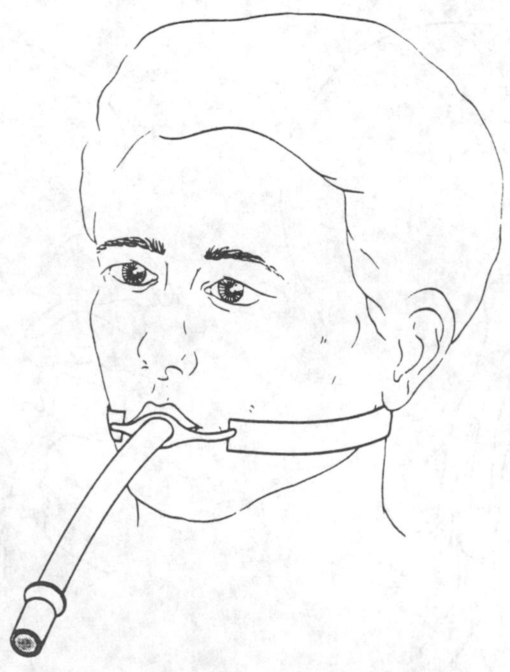

**FIGURE 36-14** Comfit endotracheal tube holder. (From Kaplow R, Bookbinder M: *Heart Lung 23*(1):59-66, 1994.)

much as 2 cm in the trachea when patients flex or extend their necks or laterally tip their heads. Usually the endotracheal tube is affixed to the patient's face with waterproof tape above and below the lips and around the endotracheal tube to keep it in place. This method can cause facial skin breakdown, especially in patients with leukemia or who are immunosuppressed. For this reason, commercially available endotracheal tube holders that use no tape are available[10] (Figures 36-14 to 36-16). A recent research study compared these holders with the tape method known as the Lillihei harness after the surgeon who designed it (see Research box below).

Tracheostomy tubes are usually made of metal or plastic. They may have only a single lumen or may have both an inner and outer cannula (Figure 36-17). All

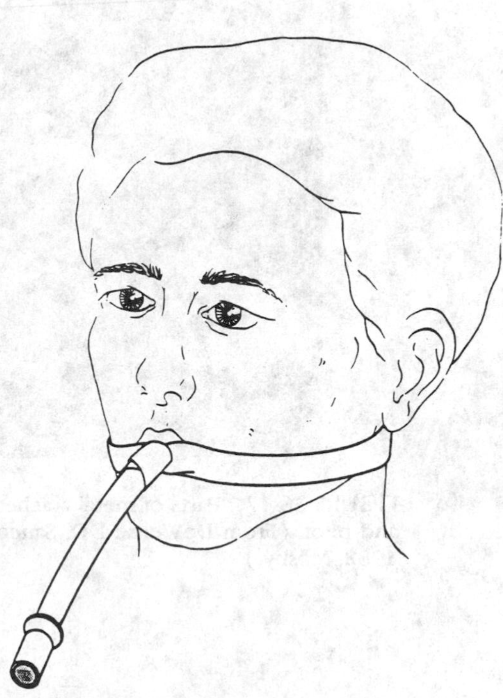

FIGURE 36-15 Dale endotracheal tube holder. (From Kaplow R, Bookbinder M: *Heart Lung 23*(1):59-66, 1994.)

## RESEARCH

**Kaplow R, Bookbinder M: A comparison of four endotracheal tube holders, *Heart Lung* 23(1):59-66, 1994.**

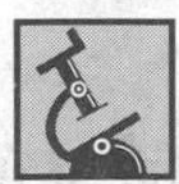

The purpose of this study was to compare four methods (Lillihei harness, Comfit, Dale, and SecureEasy) of securing endotracheal tubes in orally intubated adult patients in one intensive care unit.

The sample consisted of 121 patients. Subjects were evaluated every 12 hours for stabilization of the endotracheal tube and integrity of facial skin. The facial skin of those on the Lillihei method was only examined once after the tube was removed, because removal of tape every 12 hours would increase the risk of skin breakdown. Patients had to meet the following criteria to be included in the study: (1) at least 18 years of age, (2) orally intubated within the last 8 hours, and (3) facial skin intact. The instrument used to collect the data was adapted from a four-part questionnaire developed by Tasota for a study of endotracheal tube holders in a surgical intensive care unit.

Part II of the questionnaire contained 20 items related to patient care issues and was completed every 12 hours by the primary nurse. Part III consisted of six questions on facial skin integrity also completed by the primary nurse. Part IV consisted of four questions about comfort that could be answered "yes" or "no" by the patient after extubation. The study found the SecureEasy holder to be the most secure. Of the variables that affect extubation, prolonged coughing and gagging had the greatest impact. The fewest incidents of skin breakdown occurred with the SecureEasy and Dale holders. Patients' answers about comfort showed that discomfort with turning was least with the Lillihei harness. Nurses expressed most satisfaction with the SecureEasy holder.

This study suggested that the SecureEasy holder is the preferred alternative when the Lillihei method should not be used because of the potential for skin breakdown when tape is used on the face.

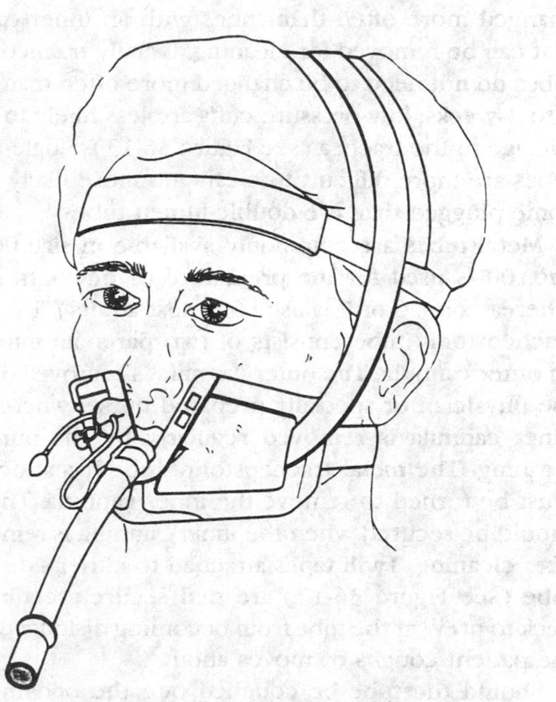

FIGURE 36-16 SecureEasy endotracheal tube holder. (From Kaplow R, Bookbinder M: *Heart Lung 23*(1):59-66, 1994.)

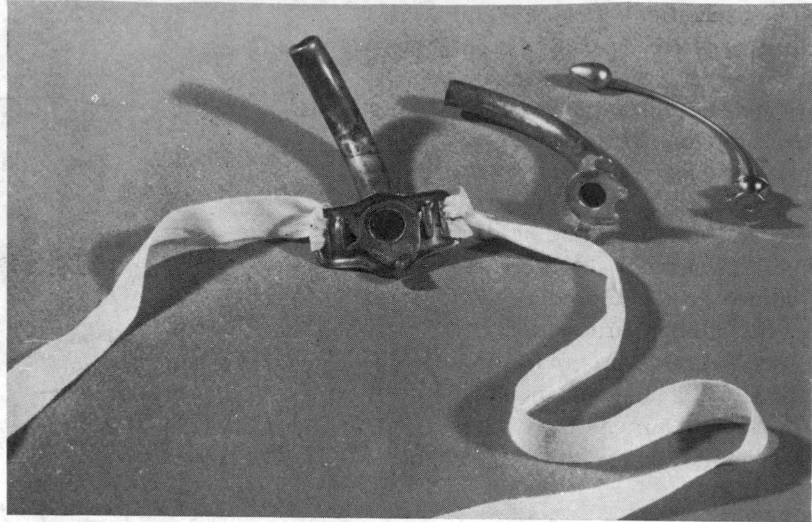

**FIGURE 36-17** Parts of metal tracheostomy tube: outer tube with ties attached, inner tube, and pilot. (From DeWeese DD, Saunders WH: *Textbook of otolaryngology,* ed 6, St Louis, 1982, Mosby.)

adult-sized plastic tubes have a cuff that is inflated with air to fill the space between the outside of the tube and the trachea when a sealed airway is required for mechanical ventilation. Single-lumen tubes may need to be changed more often than tubes with an inner cannula that can be removed for cleaning. Usually tracheostomy tubes do not need to be changed more often than every 2 to 3 weeks; low-pressure cuffs are less likely to cause damage to the trachea (see Figure 36-13). Single-lumen tubes are more difficult to clean and more likely to become plugged than are double-lumen tubes.

Metal tubes are commonly available in size 00 to 8 (no. 00 is used for the premature or newborn infant, whereas a no. 6 or 7 is used for most adults). The metal tracheostomy tube consists of two parts, an inner and an outer cannula. The outer cannula is removed only by the physician or specially prepared nurse, whereas the inner cannula is removed regularly by the nurse for cleaning. The metal tracheostomy tube has a lock that must be turned to remove the inner cannula. The lock should be secured when the inner cannula is reinserted after cleaning. Twill tapes attached to either side of the tube (see Figure 36-17) are tied securely behind the neck to prevent the tube from becoming dislodged when the patient coughs or moves about.

Should the tube be coughed out, the opening may close, and the patient will be unable to breathe. Therefore a tracheal dilator or curved hemostat is always kept at the bedside so that the opening can be held open if the tube is dislodged. Some surgeons prefer to place a retention suture on each side of the tracheostomy opening and tape the end of the suture to the skin. If the opening shows signs of closing, tension can be placed on the sutures to widen the opening.

The operative wound may be sealed with a plastic spray, or a small dressing may be placed around the tracheostomy tube. Although drainage should be minimal, the wound is inspected frequently for bleeding during the immediate postoperative period. The dressings are changed as they become soiled with mucous drainage. Occasionally, young children require elbow restraints to prevent them from removing the tube or putting objects into it.

Depending on the patient's condition, a tracheostomy can be either temporary or permanent; the person who has a laryngectomy (see p. 1036) will have a permanent tracheostomy. Any patient who has had a tracheostomy is apprehensive and is often fearful of choking. Thus when feasible, the procedure is thoroughly explained to the patient before surgery. Both *patient* and *family* need to *understand* that the *patient will be unable to speak* and that *constant attendance will be provided until the patient can manage his or her own airway safely.*

A fenestrated tracheostomy tube has an opening on the upper surface of the outer cannula that allows air inspired through the nose and mouth to pass through the tube. When the external opening is plugged, air can pass over the vocal cords, allowing the individual to talk. If ventilatory assistance is required, the inner cannula can be inserted so that the patient can be connected to a ventilator.

## PROCEDURE FOR CRITICAL CARE

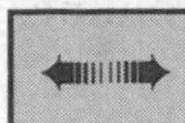

### PERFORMING ENDOTRACHEAL OR TRACHEOSTOMY TUBE SUCTIONING

1. All persons with tubes require suctioning and should be suctioned as often as necessary. The frequency of suctioning is determined by auscultation. Much of the ability to produce an effective cough is lost, because it is impossible for the person who is intubated to build up the pressure needed to create an expulsive cough.
2. The mouth and oropharynx above the cuff are suctioned first. This catheter is discarded, and a *sterile catheter* is used to suction the trachea. It is not necessary to deflate the cuff each time the patient is suctioned. The nurse may wish to deflate the cuff once per shift to remove secretions pooled on top of the cuff and to ensure that it is properly sealed. Deflation should be performed when the nurse is ready to suction the trachea.
3. Suction as deeply as possible. In an adult a catheter can be introduced through an endotracheal tube approximately 45 to 55 cm (18 to 22 in). The recommended depth through the tracheostomy tube is 20 to 30 cm (8 to 12 in). The catheter should be approximately one half the diameter of the tube.
4. A fenestrated catheter with a whistle tip is attached to the suction outlet. The catheter is always inserted without suction. Once the catheter is in place, suction is applied by placing the thumb over the fenestration in the catheter.
5. Before beginning suctioning, the patient is hyperoxygenated with 100% oxygen. An Ambu, anesthesia, or Laerdal bag is used to deliver 6 to 10 breaths of 100% oxygen. Preoxygenation with 100% oxygen is necessary, because oxygen will be removed during suctioning.
6. The suction catheter is lubricated with sterile water or a water-soluble lubricant. In the person with a tracheostomy, suctioning usually stimulates coughing. If the patient coughs, the catheter is removed, because its presence obstructs the trachea and the patient must exert extra pressure to cough around it. As coughing occurs, the nurse or the patient should have tissues ready to receive mucus, which may be ejected with force.
7. If mucus is tenacious and difficult to remove, sterile saline solution may be instilled into the tube just before suctioning. From 5 to 15 ml is commonly used.
8. Although some clinicians recommend that the patient's head and shoulders be turned to the right when suctioning the left bronchus and vice versa, there is no objective evidence that this technique improves suctioning the desired bronchus. In most people the right main-stem bronchus is easier to enter anatomically and thus is suctioned more often than the left bronchus. The catheter is rotated as it is withdrawn with the suction on.
9. To prevent hypoxia, the patient must **not** be suctioned longer than 10 to 15 seconds at a time and should rest 1 to 3 minutes between aspirations, and 100% oxygen should be administered between suctioning. If secretions are interfering with breathing, suctioning may have to be more frequent.
10. The patient is monitored for signs of hypoxia such as tachycardia, bradycardia, or ectopic beats.

## Managing Critical Care
## Care of the Person who is Intubated

**An endotracheal or tracheostomy tube provides a direct route for introduction of pathogens into the lower airway, increasing the risk of infection. It is essential that the following preventive nursing interventions be consistently implemented.**

**1. Minimize infection risk**
   **a. Endotracheal airways irritate the trachea, resulting in increased mucous production. Assess the patient regularly for excess secretions, and suction as often as necessary to maintain a patent airway. See Critical Care Procedure (above) for sterile suctioning procedure.**
   **b. Provide constant airway humidification. Endotracheal airways bypass the upper airway that normally humidifies and warms inspired air. An external source of warmed, humidified air must be provided to avoid thickening and crusting of bronchial secretions.**
   **c. All respiratory therapy equipment should be changed every 24 hours. In addition:**
      **(1) Replace any equipment that touches the floor.**
      **(2) Remove water that condenses in equipment tubing. Do not pour condensed water back into humidifier reservoir, because it may contain pathogens.**
   **d. Provide frequent mouth care. Secretions tend to pool in the mouth and in the pharynx, particularly if the cuff of the tube is inflated. There is an increased risk of ulceration or abrasion of the lips and oropharynx when an endotracheal tube or oral airway is present.**
      **(1) Gently suction oropharynx as needed.**
      **(2) Inspect the lips, tongue, and oral cavity regularly.**
      **(3) Clean the oral cavity with swabs soaked in saline.**
      **(4) Apply moisturizing agent to cracked lips.**
   **e. Maintain adequate nutritional levels.**
      **(1) The person with an endotracheal tube is allowed nothing by mouth. Nourishment will be given parenterally or by gastroin-**

### Guidelines for Care of the Intubated Person Receiving Gastrointestinal Feedings

1. Assess for the presence of bowel sounds.
2. Elevate the head of the bed at least 30 degrees.
3. Inflate the tube cuff.
4. Administer the gastrointestinal feeding to which methylene blue dye has been added.
5. Assess at regular intervals for aspiration. The presence of methylene blue in secretions indicates aspiration.
6. Regularly assess for tube placement and residual stomach contents.

testinal feedings. Gastrointestinal supplemental feedings pose less infection risk and are more economical. See box (above) for guidelines for administering gastrointestinal feedings to the intubated patient.

(2) The patient with a tracheostomy tube is usually able to swallow and have a normal oral intake. Some experts prefer that the cuff on the tracheostomy tube be inflated while the patient is eating to prevent aspiration. Others believe that the inflated cuff bulges into the esophagus and makes swallowing more difficult, and they therefore prefer that the cuff be deflated. Nursing assessment will determine which technique to use. Methylene blue dye can be swallowed before each feeding or mixed with the tube feeding. If the dye does not appear in tracheal secretions, it is safe to proceed with the meal.

2. Ensure adequate ventilation and oxygenation.
   a. Assess lung sounds regularly. Unless the individual's underlying lung pathologic condition alters lung ventilation, breath sounds should be heard bilaterally, and chest expansion should be symmetric. If a **cuffed tube** is inserted too far, it will slip into one of the main-stem bronchi (usually the right) and occlude the opposite bronchus and lung, resulting in *atelectasis* on the *obstructed side.* Even if the tube is still in the trachea, airway obstruction will result if the end of the tube is located on the carina (area at lower end of trachea at point of bifurcation of main-stem bronchi). This will result in dry secretions that obstruct both bronchi. Although these complications are more common with the use of an endotracheal tube, they can occur with a tracheostomy tube, especially in a small person with a short neck. In either case the tube is pulled back until it is positioned below the larynx and above the carina. The tube is then fastened securely in place.
   b. Turn and reposition the patient every 2 hours for maximum ventilation and lung perfusion.
   c. Assess respiratory frequency, tidal volume, and vital capacity.
   d. Perform postural drainage, cupping (clapping), and vibrating as appropriate.
3. Provide safety and comfort.
   a. Most endotracheal and tracheostomy tubes have cuffs for the following reasons:
      (1) To provide a sealed airway for positive pressure ventilation
      (2) To prevent aspiration in the unconscious person, during meals or during tube feedings
      (3) To exert pressure on bleeding sites following throat or neck surgery
   b. Assess tube placement at regular intervals.
      (1) The tube is secured around neck with tape or specially designed ties.
      (2) The endotracheal tube is marked to establish a landmark for position comparison and to measure and document the length of tube that extends beyond the patient's lips.
   c. Change tapes or ties whenever soiled to decrease skin irritation.
   d. Always keep a spare tube at the bedside.
   e. Minimize sensory deprivation.
      (1) Patients with endotracheal tubes or tracheostomy tubes with the cuff inflated cannot talk. Therefore an acceptable communication mode must be established.
         (a) Organize questions so that the patient can use a simple "yes" or "no" response, nodding head, using hand signals, or squeezing the nurse's hand.
         (b) The patient may be able to use an erasable board or note pad to communicate.
         (c) Always talk to the patient and explain all procedures.
         (d) Reorient the patient frequently.
         (e) Encourage family and friends to talk with the patient.
         (f) Keep call light (or tap bell) within patient's reach.
         (g) Reinforce that the ability to speak will return when the tube is removed.
4. Observe special considerations during immediate extubation period.
   a. Monitor for signs such as increased respiratory distress, increased hoarseness, and laryngeal stridor, indicating upper airway obstruction secondary to laryngeal edema.
   b. Assess for adequacy of cough and gag reflex.
   c. After removal of a tracheostomy tube there is a temporary air leak at the incision site.

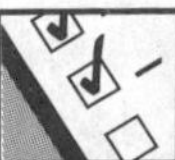

**Guidelines for Inflating an Endotracheal or Tracheostomy Cuff**

The cuff should be inflated to a volume that provides adequate occlusion around the tube without increasing the risk of tracheomalacia, tracheal stenosis, tracheoesophageal fistula, or erosion through a major blood vessel. Many experts recommend the "minimal leak technique," which follows.

1. Using a 10- or 20-ml syringe, slowly inject air into cuff.
2. As air is introduced, assess for air leak around tube. This is determined (1) by ability of patient to talk or make sounds, and (2) by nurse being able to feel air coming from patient's nose or mouth.
3. When the airway is sealed and no passage of air around the tube can be detected, remove 0.5 ml of air. This creates a "minimal leak" and assures that the lowest possible pressure is being exerted on the tracheal wall.
4. Auscultate over the trachea while ventilating the patient with either an Ambu bag or mechanical ventilator. A small amount of air should be heard gurgling past the cuff.
5. If an adequate seal cannot be obtained with 25 ml of air, notify the physician.
6. The exact pressure in the cuff can be measured by connecting the pilot balloon to a hand-held meter. To do this, the balloon is inflated with a syringe, in the normal fashion, until a seal is obtained. The syringe is removed and the meter attached. The meter reading, in cm $H_2O$, is then recorded, and the pressure in the cuff is checked each shift to ensure consistency.

d. The stoma can be suctioned. However, frequent use of the stoma for suctioning can delay closure and healing of the tracheostomy incision.

Although the low-pressure cuffs used today reduce the risk of tracheal wall damage, it is important to inflate the cuff with the correct amount of air (see the Guidelines box above).

## Care of the Person with a Tracheostomy

Although nursing care of persons with either endotracheal or tracheostomy tubes is similar, patients with tracheostomies have additional nursing care needs. Analgesics and sedatives are given judiciously so as not to depress the respiratory center. The patient is suctioned as often as necessary, possibly every 5 minutes during the first few postoperative hours. The need for suctioning can be determined by the sound of the air coming from the tracheostomy tube, especially after the patient takes a deep breath. When respirations are noisy and pulse and respiratory rates are increased, the patient needs to be suctioned. Patients who are conscious can usually indicate when they need to be suctioned. With any sign of respiratory distress, such as an increase in pulse or respirations, the tube should be suctioned. If mucus is blocking the inner cannula of a silver tube and cannot be removed by suction, the inner cannula is removed to open the airway. When the mucus is thick, the inner cannula should be cleaned and replaced at once because the outer tube may also become blocked. If, despite these measures, the patient becomes cyanotic, the physician should be summoned at once. A patient who is able to cough up his or her own secretions probably will require suctioning less frequently. The amount of mucus subsides gradually, and the patient eventually may go for several hours without being suctioned. However, even when secretions are minimal, the patient is apprehensive and needs constant attendance. Critical care procedure describes routine tracheostomy care.

See Critical Care Procedure below for the details of suctioning a person with an endotracheal or tracheostomy tube.

### Maintaining air humidification

Because the insertion of the endotracheal or tracheostomy tube bypasses the upper airway, the patient's ability to humidify and warm inspired air is lost. Therefore, whether the patient is on or off the ventilator, the inspired air should be heated and humidified to prevent mucosal irritation and drying of secretions. *Large-bore* tubing is needed to provide this mist because water

**PROCEDURE FOR CRITICAL CARE**

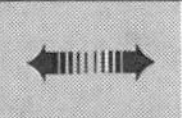

**PERFORMING TRACHEOSTOMY CARE**

*Materials:* Sterile suction catheter, cleansing solutions (usually hydrogen peroxide and saline), tracheostomy care kit or two sterile basins, sterile applicators, sterile gloves, tracheostomy dressing (must be a nonshredding material), twill tape, disposable bag, and antibiotic ointment.

1. Wash hands, put on nonsterile gloves and protective face shield or goggles.
2. Explain procedure.
3. Suction mouth or oropharynx if needed.
4. Prepare sterile work field.
5. Remove soiled tracheostomy dressing and discard in disposable bag.
6. Discard nonsterile gloves, wash hands, and put on *sterile gloves.* If tracheostomy has inner cannula, remove and clean it in hydrogen peroxide solution. Rinse with saline solution.
7. Inspect inner cannula lumen for patency before reinserting it.
8. Replace tracheostomy ties if soiled. Always hold tracheostomy in place with one hand while ties are being changed. If possible, a second nurse can assist to ensure that tube is not accidentally dislodged.
9. Tie end of twill tapes in a square knot on one side of neck.
10. Using sterile technique, clean tracheostomy incision. Apply antibiotic ointment.
11. Apply sterile tracheostomy dressing.

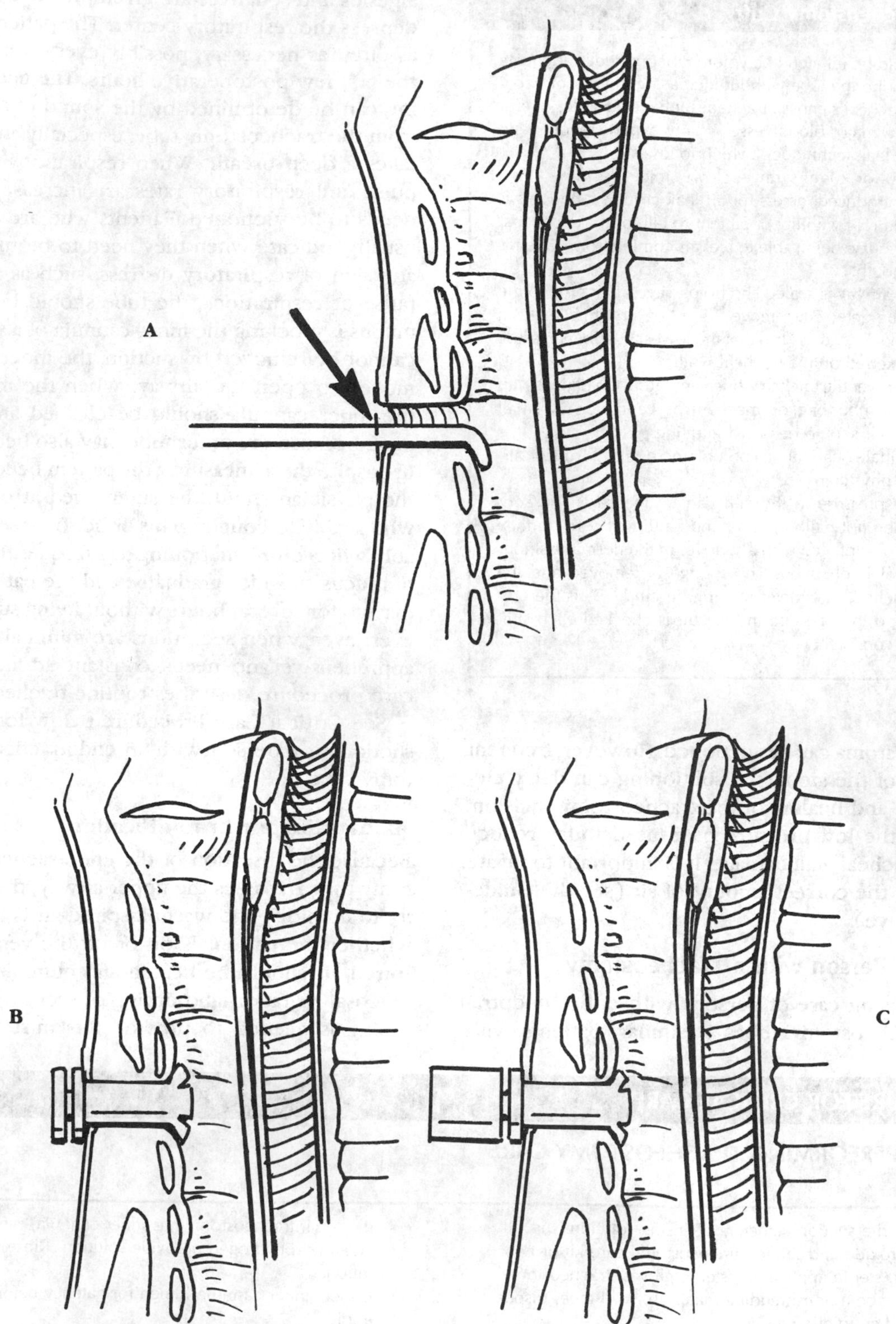


**FIGURE 36-18** Tracheal button. **A,** Inserting bent pipe cleaner into stoma to measure stoma depth. Pipe cleaner gently pulled back to hook on the anterior tracheal wall. Distance from pipe cleaner bend to skin surface determines length of tracheostomy button. **B,** Solid plug inserted into tracheostomy button prevents button from being coughed out and allows patient to breath through upper airway. **C,** Hollow tube adaptor replaces stoma plug to allow for suctioning or assisted ventilation with Ambu-bag.

particles condense in *small-bore* tubing. A noticeable difference in the viscosity of secretions is evident in patients who do not receive mist for even as short a period as 30 minutes. Other important nursing care measures and observations vary with the route of intubation—via the larynx or from below the larynx. The patient who has an endotracheal tube in place usually has an increased volume of oropharyngeal secretions because of irritation from the tube. The patient also has great difficulty in swallowing (especially if an oral tube is used), necessitating frequent oropharyngeal suctioning.

### Providing nourishment

The patient with an endotracheal tube is allowed nothing by mouth. Nourishment is given intravenously or by nasogastric tube feedings. The patient with a tracheostomy tube in place is usually able to swallow and have a normal oral intake. As mentioned earlier, some experts prefer that the cuff on the tracheostomy tube be inflated while the patient is eating to prevent aspiration. Others believe that the inflated cuff bulges into the esophagus and makes swallowing more difficult, and therefore they prefer the cuff to be deflated. Nursing assessment determines which technique to use. In determining if the patient aspirates food, it is often helpful to feed the patient red gelatin. The consistency of gelatin makes it easier to swallow than water, and the red color makes it easy to detect if aspirated into the lower airway.

### Weaning from tracheostomy tube

Patients who have had tracheostomies for a period of time may require progressive weaning before the tracheostomy tube can be safely removed (decannulation). One method of weaning involves the use of a tracheal button.[7] A tracheal button is a hollow Teflon tube with a serrated distal end that is inserted into the tracheal stoma where the end fits against the anterior tracheal wall (Figure 36-18). When the button is in place, a solid plug is inserted to spread the distal end flanges, which secures the tube in place. The button keeps the stoma tract open and allows the patient to breathe and clear secretions through the upper airway.

If the patient has difficulty breathing, the solid plug can be removed and the patient can be ventilated with an Ambu bag fitted with an adaptor. Routine suctioning through the tracheal button is discouraged, because the suction catheter tends to hit the posterior wall of the trachea, causing ulceration and bleeding. If the tracheostomy tube must be reinserted after several hours or days, it can be easily reinserted because the stoma has been kept open with the button.[7]

Some patients will have a permanent tracheostomy. A discussion of their home care follows.

### Guidelines for Discharge Instructions for the Person With a Tracheostomy or Laryngectomy

The nose normally filters and warms the air that we breathe. This function is lost with a tracheostomy or stoma; therefore extra humidity is necessary to moisten the air you breathe. Measures that you can take to *increase humidity* include the following:

1. Use a cool mist humidifier in the room where you spend most of your time. Also, use it in your bedroom at night.
2. Cover the stoma during the day with a dampened stoma cover and remoisten it when it dries.
3. Wash stoma with a washcloth and warm water and soap daily.
4. You can use a syringe or eyedropper to instill 3-5 ml of normal saline in your tracheostomy tube, laryngectomy vent, or stoma. This will loosen mucous plugs before suctioning. Normal saline can be made by boiling 1 tsp of table salt in 1 qt of tap water for 20 minutes, cooling the solution, and placing it in a clean bottle with a lid. Make new solution every 2 days, because it does not contain a preservative.
5. Keep stoma covered when you go outside to prevent cold air, dust, or pollens from getting in the tube or stoma. Use a scarf, bib, crocheted cover, or shirt that buttons at the neck.

*Other precautions include the following:*

6. You can bathe in a tub or take a shower, being careful to keep soap and water from entering the tube or stoma. A stoma shower guard or a hand-held shower can be used.
7. You can shampoo as long as you keep shampoo and water out of the tube or stoma. You may need someone to help you shampoo.
8. Men can shave using an electric or a manual razor. Be sure to cover stoma so that lather and particles do not fall into the opening.
9. You may *not* swim, because water would enter your lungs.
10. Drink at least 8-10 glasses of fluid daily. More fluid is needed during hot weather or when home heating is in use.
11. Avoid persons who have colds or the flu or are not feeling well.
12. Call your physician immediately if you feel like you are getting a cold or other respiratory infection.
13. You can use antihistamines or decongestants but be aware that they dry secretions; take extra fluids and increase humidity if taking them.
14. Increasing your activity will help thin secretions and make them easier to cough or suction up.
15. Wear a medical identification bracelet or carry a card that states you are a neck breather. Emergency cards stating "I am a total neck breather" can be obtained from your local branch of the American Cancer Society.
16. Persons with a tracheostomy or laryngectomy often have dry mouth and bad breath. Pay special attention to brushing and flossing your teeth at least two times daily. Keep mouth clean and fresh by using baking soda and salt gargle (1 tsp of salt, 1 tsp of baking soda, and 1 qt of water).

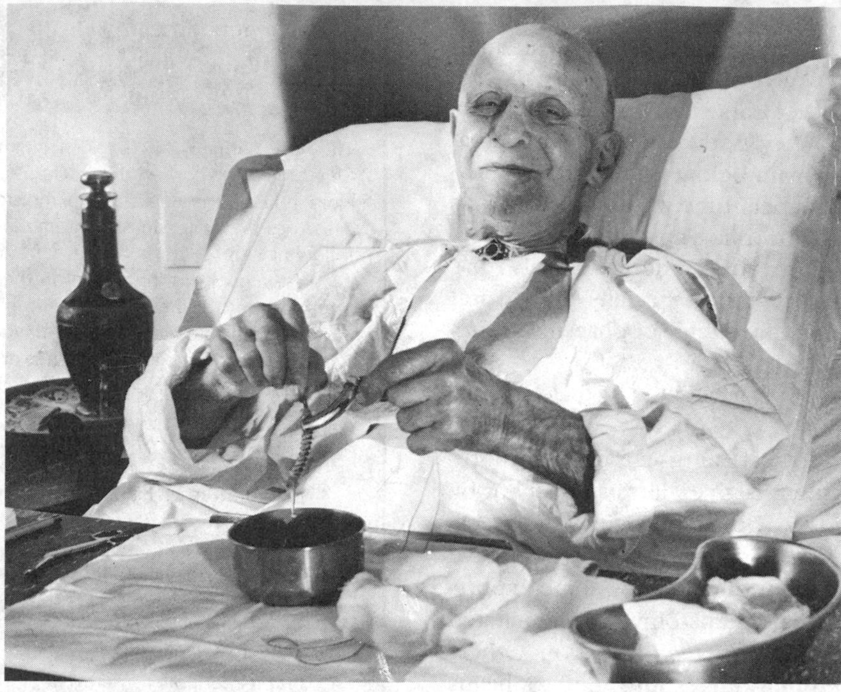

**FIGURE 36-19** This 82-year-old man cares for his own tracheostomy tube. He is about to clean inner tube with small tube brush.

## ❦ HOME CARE CONSIDERATIONS

### Care of the Tube

Persons to be discharged with a tube in place are taught to care for and change the tube while in the hospital (Figure 36-19). A mirror will be necessary to perform this procedure, which may begin a few days after surgery.

Patients who go home with the tracheostomy tube in place must be provided with necessary supplies or with instructions as to where to secure them. They should have suction equipment, which can be rented for home use or obtained in many communities through the local chapter of the American Cancer Society. Suction can be provided by attaching a suction hose to a faucet. Many hardware stores carry the necessary equipment. The amount of suction is controlled by the stream of water.

The patient should be given written instructions about how to care for the tube and the instructions should be reviewed with the patient and significant other before discharge. Points to be included in the written instructions are listed in the Guidelines box, p. 1029.

# TRAUMA OF THE UPPER AIRWAY

## FRACTURES OF NASAL BONES AND SEPTUM

Fractures of the nasal bones and septum commonly occur from relatively minor injuries, such as falls, or from more severe injuries, such as automobile accidents or fights. If there is no displacement of the bone, no obstruction to the airway, and no cosmetic deformity, treatment is not needed. When airway obstruction or bone displacement occurs (Figure 36-20), simple reduction is performed. Most simple nasal fractures can be reduced by applying firm pressure on the convex side of the nose. Nasal fractures should be reduced within the first 24 hours if at all possible. Local anesthesia is used. After 24

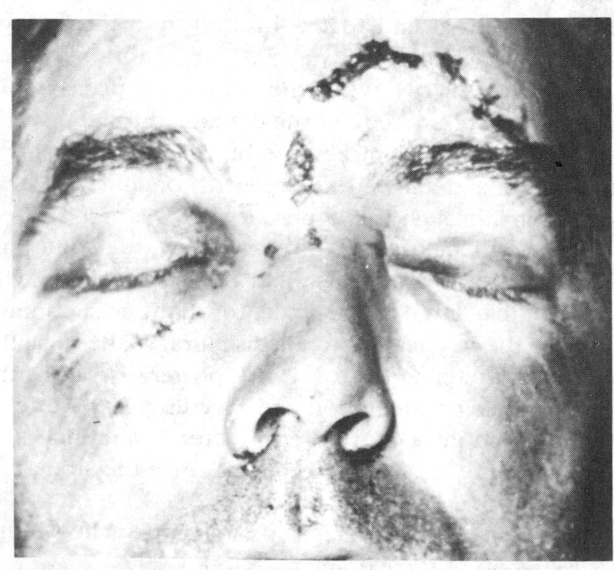

**FIGURE 36-20** Laterally displaced fracture of nose secondary to trauma. Pressure on convex side will restore alignment.

hours the reduction becomes more difficult and may require general anesthesia.

## FRACTURES OF THE MAXILLARY AND ZYGOMATIC BONES

Fractures of the maxillary and zygomatic bones are seen after automobile accidents and fights.[9] These fractures are generally reduced with the patient under anesthesia. Patients may also require wiring of the teeth with all the attendant problems of that procedure.

## EPISTAXIS

### Etiology/Pathophysiology

Epistaxis (nosebleed) usually originates from the tiny blood vessels in the anterior part of the septum. Bleeding from the posterior part is more common in elderly persons and is more likely to be severe. In adults, nosebleeds are more common in men than in women.

The most common cause of epistaxis is trauma to the nasal mucosa from damage by a foreign object.[8] Other causes include picking the nose, local irritation of the mucous membrame from lack of humidity in the air, chronic infection, violent sneezing, or blowing of the nose. Systemic causes include coagulation defects such as hemophilia, leukemia, and purpura.

Although persons with hypertension do not have more nosebleeds that normotensive persons, they tend to bleed more profusely when they do have a nosebleed.

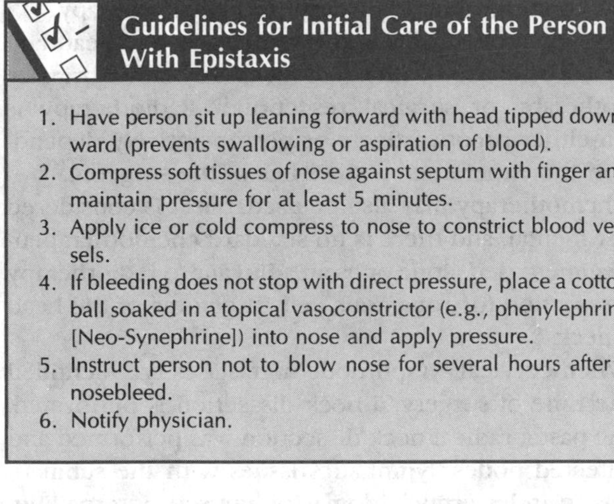

**Guidelines for Initial Care of the Person With Epistaxis**

1. Have person sit up leaning forward with head tipped downward (prevents swallowing or aspiration of blood).
2. Compress soft tissues of nose against septum with finger and maintain pressure for at least 5 minutes.
3. Apply ice or cold compress to nose to constrict blood vessels.
4. If bleeding does not stop with direct pressure, place a cotton ball soaked in a topical vasoconstrictor (e.g., phenylephrine [Neo-Synephrine]) into nose and apply pressure.
5. Instruct person not to blow nose for several hours after a nosebleed.
6. Notify physician.

Nosebleed is usually unilateral, and some persons are more prone to nosebleed than are others. Persons with frequent nosebleeds should have a complete physical examination to see if a cause can be determined.

### Medical Management

Most nosebleeds can be controlled with simple measures (see the Guidelines box below). If these measures are ineffective, medical intervention should be obtained. After identifying the site of the bleeding, the physician cauterizes the bleeding point with a silver nitrate stick or electrocautery. If the bleeding point cannot be seen, a *postnasal pack* may be inserted (Figure 36-21). Because this procedure is extremely painful and may cause complications, patients should be admitted to the hospital. For example, the pressure of the postnasal pack may stimulate the sinopulmonary reflex, causing the patient to stop breathing. In this situation the pack must be removed immediately. If no problems occur, the pack is left in place 3 to 5 days and then removed very gently. Medical management includes adequate oxygenation, humidification, analgesia, bedrest, blood transfusions, intravenous fluids, systemic antibiotics, and sedation. If the posterior pack fails to control the bleeding, another pack may be placed and the patient may be taken to surgery for ligation of the internal maxillary artery or to the x-ray department for embolization of the bleeding vessels.

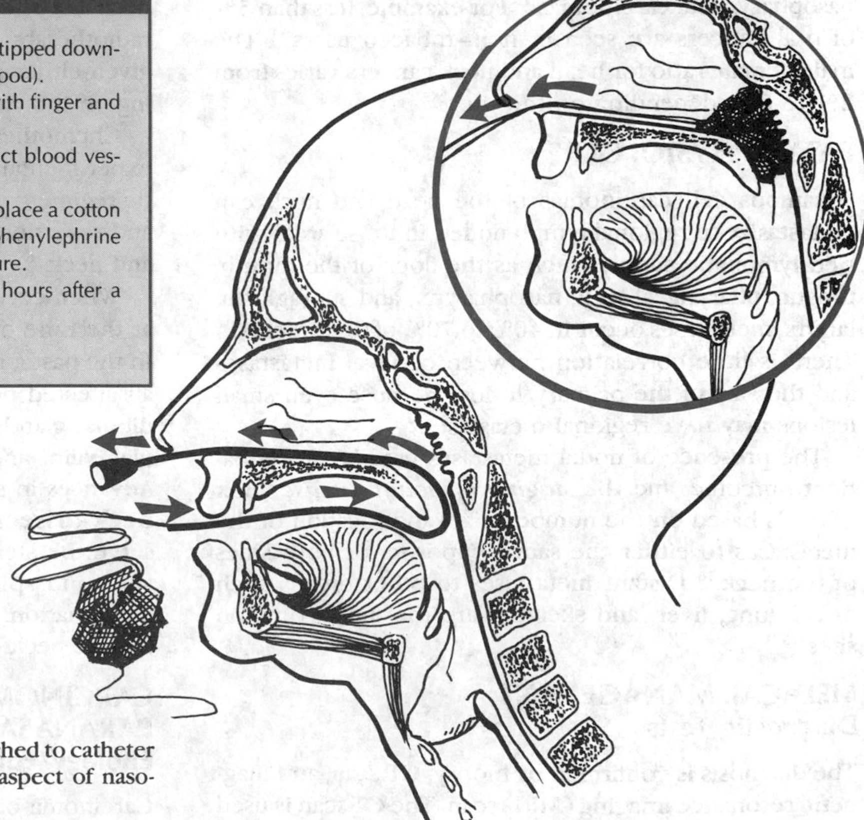

**FIGURE 36-21** Postnasal packing. Pack is attached to catheter and then pulled through mouth to posterior aspect of nasopharynx.

### Nursing Management

Severe epistaxis can cause apprehension because of the profuse bleeding not only from the nose but also flowing into the throat. The person is kept in mid-Fowler's position and is urged not to swallow blood, because it may cause nausea and vomiting. The position of the postnasal pack must be checked frequently by viewing the posterior oropharynx for bleeding or slippage. Nasal packs may slip out of place and cause airway obstruction. The patient is monitored for signs of complications (confusion, agitation, increased lethargy, and changes in vital signs, especially in respirations and pulse). Nasal packs also make eating and swallowing difficult; a liquid diet is usually more tolerable.

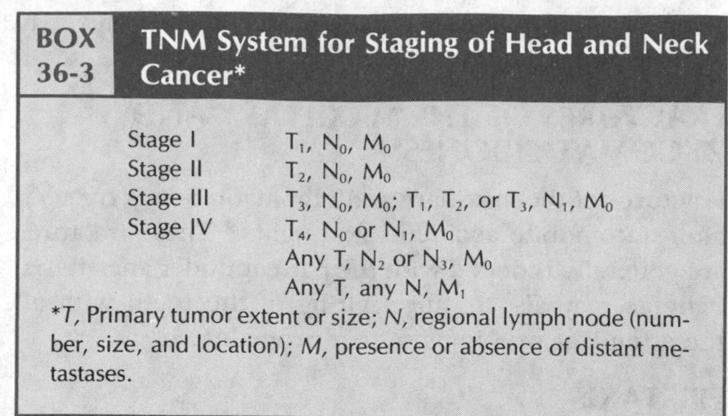

**BOX 36-3 TNM System for Staging of Head and Neck Cancer***

| | |
|---|---|
| Stage I | $T_1$, $N_0$, $M_0$ |
| Stage II | $T_2$, $N_0$, $M_0$ |
| Stage III | $T_3$, $N_0$, $M_0$; $T_1$, $T_2$, or $T_3$, $N_1$, $M_0$ |
| Stage IV | $T_4$, $N_0$ or $N_1$, $M_0$ |
| | Any T, $N_2$ or $N_3$, $M_0$ |
| | Any T, any N, $M_1$ |

**T*, Primary tumor extent or size; *N*, regional lymph node (number, size, and location); *M*, presence or absence of distant metastases.

## MALIGNANCIES OF THE UPPER AIRWAY

Malignancies of the head and neck can occur in several sites, including (1) lip and oral cavity; (2) pharynx: nasopharynx, oropharynx, and laryngapharynx; (3) larynx; (4) paranasal sinuses; (5) salivary gland; and (6) thyroid gland.[11]

### ETIOLOGY/EPIDEMIOLOGY

Ninety percent of cancers of the head and neck are squamous cell carcinoma.

The exact mechanism for the development of the malignant phenotype is not understood. *Heavy alcohol use* and *tobacco abuse* are considered to be definite etiologic factors with the exception of sinonasal and nasopharyngeal carcinomas.[16] For example, less than 5% of oral cancers are seen in non–tobacco users.[11] The male/female ratio for head and neck cancers varies from 2:1 to 8:1, depending on the site.

### PATHOPHYSIOLOGY

Squamous cell carcinomas of the head and neck can metastasize to regional lymph nodes. In those areas with rich lymphatic supply, such as the floor of the mouth, tongue, pharyngeal wall, nasopharynx, and supraglottic larynx, metastases occur in 40% to 70% of the patients.[16] There is little correlation between cervical metastases and the size of the primary lesion, because even small lesions may have regional metastases.

The presence of nodal metastases greatly affects patient outcome, and the *staging of nodal disease* (Box 36-3) is based on the number, size, and location of the metastases to either the same, opposite, or both sides of the neck.[16] Distant metastases to other organs such as the lung, liver, and skeleton are the most common sites.[16]

### MEDICAL MANAGEMENT

#### Diagnostic Tests

The diagnosis is confirmed by biopsy, CT scan, and magnetic resonance imaging (MRI) scan. The CT scan is used to differentiate between benign and malignant lesions and to determine how far the tumor has extended. It also identifies the presence of any bony destruction. The MRI scan with gadolinium enhances tumor imaging in soft tissues and shows tumor extension and tumor secretions. The radiolucency of the tumor and its secretions are different, which is why both can be identified on MRI with gadolinium.

#### Treatment

Treatment of squamous cell carcinomas of the head and neck depends on the size of the primary tumor and the presence of nodal metastasis. The usual TNM system for staging head and neck cancer is shown in Box 36-3. Persons with stages III and IV are automatically placed in the advanced stage category requiring combined therapy with radiotherapy, surgery, and chemotherapy.

Persons with stage I and II cancers of the head and neck can be treated with equal success by either primary radiotherapy or surgical resection.[16] Radiotherapy is given either preoperatively or postoperatively depending on the experience and wishes of the surgeon.

Chemotherapy may also be used, but it is considered experimental, and there is no standard chemotherapeutic regimen used alone or as an adjuvant to radiotherapy and resection for squamous cell carcinoma of the head and neck.[16]

When cervical lymph node metastases are identified at the time of surgery, a neck dissection is performed. In the past a radical neck dissection was performed and all affected nodes, lymphatic tissues with the submandibular gland, sternocleidomastoid muscle, internal jugular vein, and spinal accessory nerve were removed. Advances in surgical techniques have led to **modified neck dissection** in which an attempt is made to preserve the sternocleidomastoid muscle, internal jugular vein, and spinal accessory nerve by themselves or in combination. Most patients receive radiotherapy following the neck dissection.[16]

### CARCINOMA OF THE NASAL CAVITY AND PARANASAL SINUSES

#### Etiology/Epidemiology

Carcinoma of the nasal cavity has its highest incidence in men between 60 and 70 years of age. Exposure to

**BOX 36-4 Clinical Manifestations of Carcinoma of Nasal Cavity and Paranasal Sinuses**

**MAXILLARY SINUS**

Bump on hard palate; nasal obstruction and bleeding as the tumor breaks into the nasal cavity; swelling of cheek with pain; swelling of the gums may cause toothache or result in ill-fitting dentures; if the tumor impinges on the infraorbital nerve there may be numbness of the cheek, increased lacrimation, exophthalmos, and diplopia; more advanced tumors may result in displacement of the eye, extraocular muscle palsy, hyperesthesia of the cheek, and inability to open the mouth

**FRONTAL SINUS**

Patients frequently present with swelling and frontal pain that mimic a sinus headache; pain occurs when the tumor invades bone and causes bony destruction; if tumor invades the ethmoids and orbit, the eye on that side will be displaced, resulting in double vision (diplopia)

**SPHENOID SINUS**

Major complaint is steady, deep-seated temporoparietal headaches; because of its close proximity to the cavernous sinus, a tumor extending into this area causes compression of the third, fourth, and sixth cranial nerves, causing diplopia

**ETHMOID SINUS**

These tumors cause medial orbital swelling, puffiness of the face, decreased vision, excessive tearing (epiphora), and olfactory complaints; death is caused by direct extension of the tumor into the vital areas of the skull

**Guidelines for Care of the Person After Paranasal Surgery**

1. Routine tracheostomy care (see p. 1040).
2. Nasogastric tube or gastroscopy tube for feeding (see Chapter 45).
3. Monitor patient for signs of meningitis: fever, headache, stiff neck, neck rigidity.
4. Mouth care.
   a. A gentle spray or oral irrigation may be indicated.
   b. Oral irrigating solutions include saline and hydrogen peroxide, weak sodium bicarbonate, or antibiotic solution.
   c. Know where suture line is to prevent damage to it when irrigating mouth.
   d. Because the person may have difficulty in swallowing, it may be necessary to aspirate the irrigating solution from the mouth; care must be taken to prevent trauma to the sutures by the suction. Management of saliva may also be a problem because of the swallowing difficulty.
5. Adjustment to prosthesis may be a problem because of a poor fit.
   a. Prosthesis causes pressure, leading to pain.
   b. Eating may cause nasal regurgitation.
6. Long-term follow-up after discharge.
   a. Seen weekly for at least 6 weeks.
   b. If receiving radiation therapy postoperatively will be seen for several more weeks.
7. Eye prosthesis.
   a. Have to complete radiotherapy before being fitted for prosthesis.
   b. After radiotherapy it may take 4 to 6 months for healing to occur and the patient to be ready for the eye prosthesis.

certain substances has been implicated in some malignancies of the nasal cavity. These substances include wood dust and leather dust (inhaled by furniture workers) and exposure to nickel compounds, chromate compounds, hydrocarbons, nitrosamines, and dioxane. Risk is higher also among snuff users, workers in the shoe industry, and textile and asbestos workers.[16]

When questioned about exposure to the substances just mentioned, the majority of persons give no history of exposure. Most, however, have signs and symptoms of a long-standing chronic sinusitis. Common complaints include a stuffy nose, sinus headache, and facial pain.

Clinical manifestations of malignancies of the nasal cavity and paranasal sinuses are listed in Box 36-4.

## Medical Management

*Chemotherapy* has become very useful in the management of carcinoma of the sinus and is used in conjunction with *radiation* and *surgery.*

Surgery for maxillary sinus and palate tumors often consists of removal of the entire upper jaw *(maxillectomy),* removal of the entire palate (hard and soft), and removal of one eye *(orbital exenteration).* Split-thickness skin grafts are usually applied to the operative area. Postoperatively, the deformity of the jaw is managed with a dental prosthesis that closes off the defect in the mouth (Figure 36-22). Radical surgery is required because of the danger of recurrence. Meningitis is a potential postoperative complication, and prophylactic antibiotics are usually prescribed.

Maintenance of an airway postoperatively is critical for these patients, and sometimes a tracheostomy is performed. A gastrostomy tube is inserted to ensure adequate liquid and caloric intake, because eating is difficult until the prosthesis is fitted. Several different prostheses are usually needed before a final one fits because of shrinking of the cavity as healing progresses. Often they need to be changed weekly.

## Nursing Management

Postoperative care is outlined in the Guidelines box above.

Persons who undergo radical surgery of this type have a number of emotional adjustments to make. Alteration in their physical appearance is readily visible; the person feels conspicuous and different. In addition to disfigurement, these patients have all the normal fears of surgery and of cancer. Fear, anger, and grief are normal reactions to the situation. Fear is focused on concerns about the future, the ability to live normally, and being rejected. Anger and grief are common responses to the loss and the helplessness to control the loss. Oral communication also may be a problem immediately after surgery, and every effort is made to allow the person to express needs

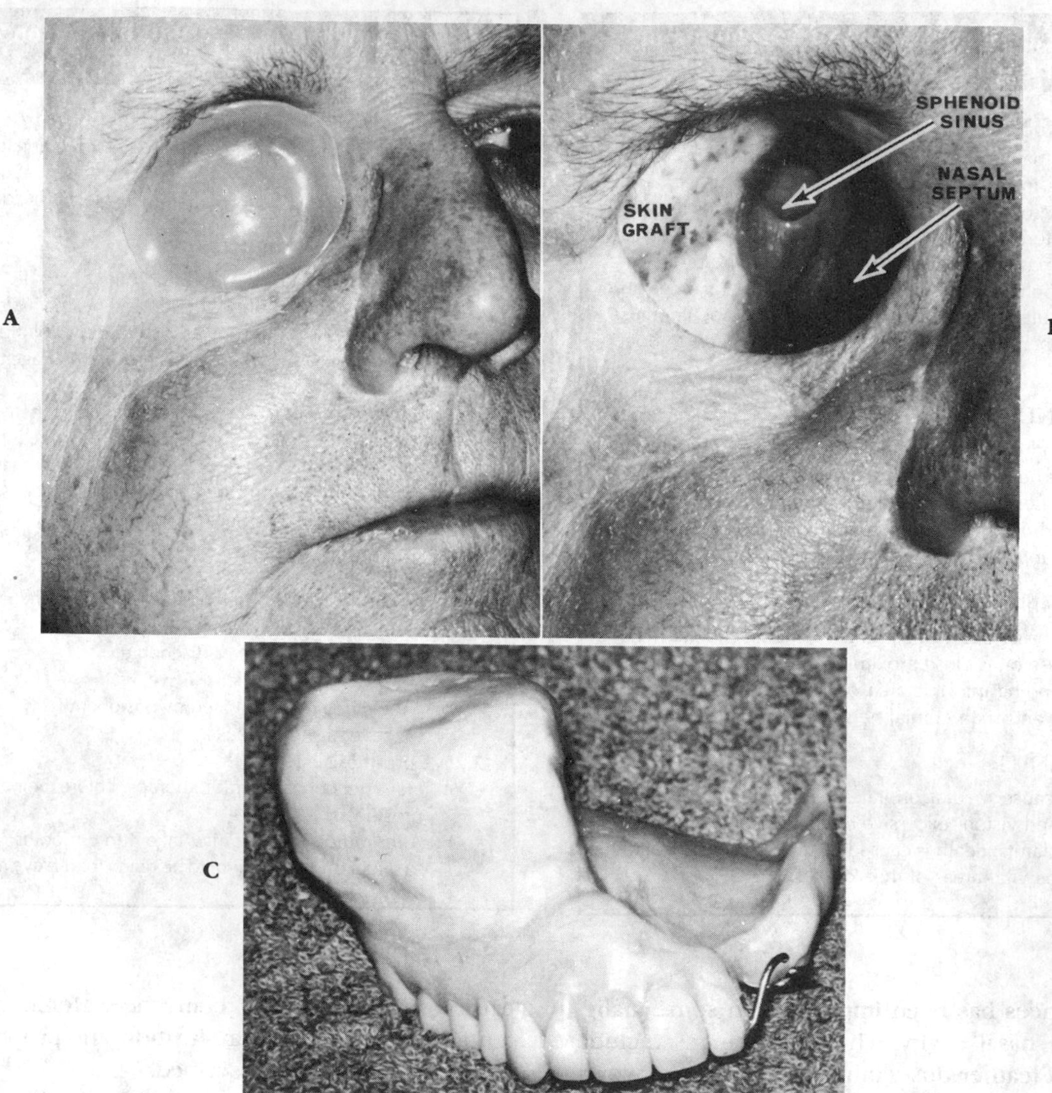


**FIGURE 36-22** Patient after maxillectomy and orbital exenteration. **A,** Orbital prosthesis in place. Eyeglasses worn over this further improves appearance. **B,** Defect in orbit with skin graft lining upper and lateral wall of orbital-maxillary cavity. **C,** Upper denture worn with large obturator to fill in defect created by maxillectomy.

and feelings by writing if necessary. Conveying compassion and concern to the person is important.

## CARCINOMA OF THE OROPHARYNX

### Etiology/Epidemiology

Carcinoma of the oropharynx is second only to malignancy of the larynx in malignancies of the upper respiratory tract. Ninety to ninety-five percent of the tumors are squamous cell carcinoma. At the time of diagnosis, nodes are involved in more than 60% of the cases and in 23% there is bilateral nodal involvement. When metastasis occurs it is to the lung, bone, and liver in that order of frequency.[4] Cancer of the oropharynx is more common in persons between 50 and 70 years of age. The male/female ratio is 5:1. The clinical manifestations of malignancies of the oropharynx are listed in Box 36-5.

**BOX 36-5 Clinical Manifestations of Malignancies of the Oropharynx**

- History of prolonged sore throat is most common symptom.
- With a tumor in the palatine arch, ulceration and pain are early symptoms.
- Tumors at base of tongue ulcerate later, have fewer nerve fibers, and tend to be discovered later.
- Otalgia (deep-seated earache) is a common complaint as pain is referred along the ninth cranial nerve.
- Speech difficulties and nasal regurgitation are late symptoms.
- Asymptomatic mass in the neck is the first sign of a malignancy in 25% of persons.

### Medical Management

Radiotherapy and surgical excision are the treatments for oropharyngeal cancers. Early stage lesions may be managed with excision or radiotherapy alone.[16] Advanced stage tumors are treated with radiotherapy and extensive resection requiring reconstruction with skin grafts, local musculocutaneous flaps, distant pedicled musculocutaneous flaps, or microvascular free tissue transfer.[16]

### Nursing Management

Following extensive surgery for an oropharyngeal malignancy, the emphasis is on maintaining respiration and nutrition, taking proper care of the graft or flap, and maintaining communication.

#### Maintaining the airway

Edema of the oral cavity or oropharynx causes airway obstruction, and a tracheostomy is commonly performed. Tracheostomy care is discussed earlier in this chapter (see p. 1021).

#### Maintaining nutrition

A feeding tube is necessary to maintain nutrition, because the patient cannot swallow properly because of swelling in the mouth, inability to move the tongue, inability to swallow saliva, and weakness.[17]

#### Maintaining the skin flaps and graft site

Proper care of the skin flap and of the skin graft donor site is essential to a successful outcome for the patient. Each is discussed below.

**Skin flap care.** To prevent the formation of a hematoma or seroma, Jackson-Pratt or Hemovac drains are inserted in the incision at the time of surgery.[17] Continuous suction needs to be maintained postoperatively. This means that the drains may need to be aspirated periodically using sterile technique to remove clots in the catheters that would interfere with the suctioning.[17] Pressure on the flap from dressings, tracheostomy ties, and so on needs to be avoided so that circulation to the flap is not compromised.

**Skin flap donor site care.** The site is covered with a protective dressing. The outer dressing is removed after 24 hours. The inner dressing usually remains in place for 7 to 10 days. The donor site is soaked in the bathtub to remove the dressing so that healing of the site will not be disturbed.

If the donor site has not dried, a heat lamp may be used to assist in drying. Pressure on the donor site by bed covers and pajama bottoms is avoided to decrease discomfort.

#### Maintaining communication

Because of tracheostomy the patient is unable to speak. In the immediate postoperative period the patient may be asked to signify "yes" or "no" to questions by squeezing the nurse's hand, raising a finger, or so on. As the patient recovers, alternative methods, including having the patient write notes, may be used.

## CARCINOMA OF THE LARYNX

### Etiology/Epidemiology

Squamous cell carcinoma of the larynx is increasing in frequency. It is estimated that in the United States over 12,600 new cases and over 3800 deaths occur every year.[1] Cancer of the larynx limited to the true vocal cords grows slowy because of the limited lymphatic supply. Elsewhere in the larynx (epiglottis, false vocal cords, and pyriform sinuses) lymphatic vessels are abundant, and cancer of these tissues often spreads rapidly and metastasizes early to the deep lymph nodes of the neck.

Cancer of the larynx is five times more common in men than in women, and it occurs most often in persons over 60 years of age. There appears to be a relationship between cancer of the larynx and heavy smoking, heavy alcohol intake, chronic laryngitis, vocal abuse, and family predisposition to cancer. Because of an increase in the number of women who are heavy smokers, the incidence of carcinoma of the larynx among this group is increasing. Carcinoma of the larynx may invade deeper structures and cause vocal cord paralysis or metastasis to the neck.

### Pathophysiology

Squamous cell carcinoma can arise from any part of the laryngeal mucous membrane. It is often preceded by leukoplakia.

The most common presenting symptom is *persistent hoarseness,* often associated with *otalgia* and *dysphagia.* Tumors confined to the true vocal cords rarely metastasize to the cervical lymph nodes, whereas tumors of supraglottic and infraglottic portions of the larynx have a 35% to 40% incidence of metastasis to mid- to low-jugular nodes. Diagnosis of laryngeal carcinoma is usually made by flexible fiberoptic laryngoscopy. If a laryngeal ulceration or mass is found, a biopsy of the lesion is taken for pathologic confirmation of the diagnosis.

Anyone, but especially any smoker, who becomes progressively hoarse or is hoarse for longer than 2 weeks should be urged to seek medical attention at once. If treatment is given when hoarseness first appears (caused by the tumor's preventing the complete approximation of the vocal cord), a cure usually is possible. Signs of metastases of cancer to other parts of the larynx include a sensation of a lump in the throat, pain in the Adam's apple that radiates to the ear, dyspnea, dysphagia, enlarged cervical nodes, and cough.

### Medical Management

The expected length of stay for patients with carcinoma of the larynx as determined by DRG is 7 days. Common therapy for the person with carcinoma of the larynx includes the following.

**TABLE 36-6 Laryngectomy Surgery for Cancer**

| TYPE | DESCRIPTION | VOICE RESULT |
|---|---|---|
| **PARTIAL LARYNGECTOMY** | | |
| Hemilaryngectomy | Opening into larynx through thyroid cartilage with removal of diseased false cord, arytenoid, and one side of thyroid cartilage | Hoarse voice |
| Supraglottic partial laryngectomy | Horizontal incision passes above true cords (left intact) with removal of epiglottis and diseased tissue | Normal voice |
| **TOTAL LARYNGECTOMY** | Removal of epiglottis, thyroid cartilage, and 3 or 4 tracheal rings; closure of pharynx with trachea; permanent tracheostomy | No voice |

### Diagnostic tests

Diagnostic tests include direct and indirect fiberoptic laryngoscopy; chest x-ray of lung to determine if there is metastasis to the lung, a second primary tumor, or chronic obstructive pulmonary disease; barium swallow to rule out metastases to the esophagus; and CT scan to determine if there is metastasis to lymph nodes or adjacent structures.

### Medication

No medications are prescribed except continuance of medications patient was on before admission (e.g., digitalis preparations, diuretics).

### Treatment

The primary therapy is surgical excision or primary radiotherapy. Patients with early-stage lesion ($T_1$ or $T_2$) that are localized to the glottis have an 85% to a 90% cure rate when treated either with primary radiotherapy or surgical resection.[16] Surgery is accomplished with endoscopic laser excision or **partial laryngectomy**[16] (Table 36-6).

Patients with more extensive tumors ($T_3$ or $T_4$) require a combined approach of surgical resection with postoperative radiotherapy. Newer treatment regimens add chemotherapy with cisplatinum and 5-fluorouracil along with radiotherapy in an attempt to preserve the larynx.[16]

If the regimen just described fails, or the tumor recurs after therapy, or there are extensive tumors with cartilaginous invasion, a **total laryngectomy** is usually required.[16] Some patients will also require a modified neck dissection. A discussion of each of these procedures follows.

Wound complications with laryngectomy include hematoma, seroma, infection, dehiscence, and carotid artery rupture (blowout).

**Hemilaryngectomy.** In **hemilaryngectomy,** which is also called a **vertical partial laryngectomy,** one half of the larynx is removed (Figure 36-23). This procedure is usually well tolerated; difficulty in swallowing is not a long-term problem, but the patient is not allowed to swallow for 7 to 10 days postoperatively. The quality of the voice is adequate for communication.

Removal of more than one half of the larynx or a portion of the second vocal cord is called a **subtotal laryngectomy.** If more of the second cord is removed the patient will have more difficulty in swallowing. Thin liquids are the most difficult to swallow, and thickened liquids and soft foods are recommended. The speech pathologist works with patients on their swallowing postoperatively.[2]

**Supraglottic laryngectomy.** When the supraglottis is invaded by cancer, a **supraglottic laryngectomy** (horizontal partial laryngectomy) is performed. The procedure usually involves the removal of endolaryngeal structures from the tip of the epiglottis down to and including the laryngeal vertical[2] (Figure 36-24). Because the true vocal cords are preserved, the patient's voice quality is excellent. The major postoperative problem is the danger of aspiration because of difficulty in swallowing. Aspiration may occur because the major reflex arc that causes closure of the larynx is initiated by sensory receptors in the supraglottic larynx, which has been removed. These patients will need special swallowing training postoperatively. Although patients take variable amounts of time to learn to swallow safely, most will be able to take feedings by mouth.

After partial laryngectomy, a temporary tracheostomy tube is inserted and removed when edema in the surrounding tissues subsides. The person is not on absolute voice rest but is not permitted to use the voice until the surgeon gives specific approval (usually 3 days postoperatively). In the past whispering was allowed, but it is now believed that whispering can further damage the voice. This problem is currently under study. The person usually adjusts quite readily to relatively minor limitations of speech. The main problems encountered by persons undergoing partial laryngectomy are those of swallowing and aspiration, which are discussed above.

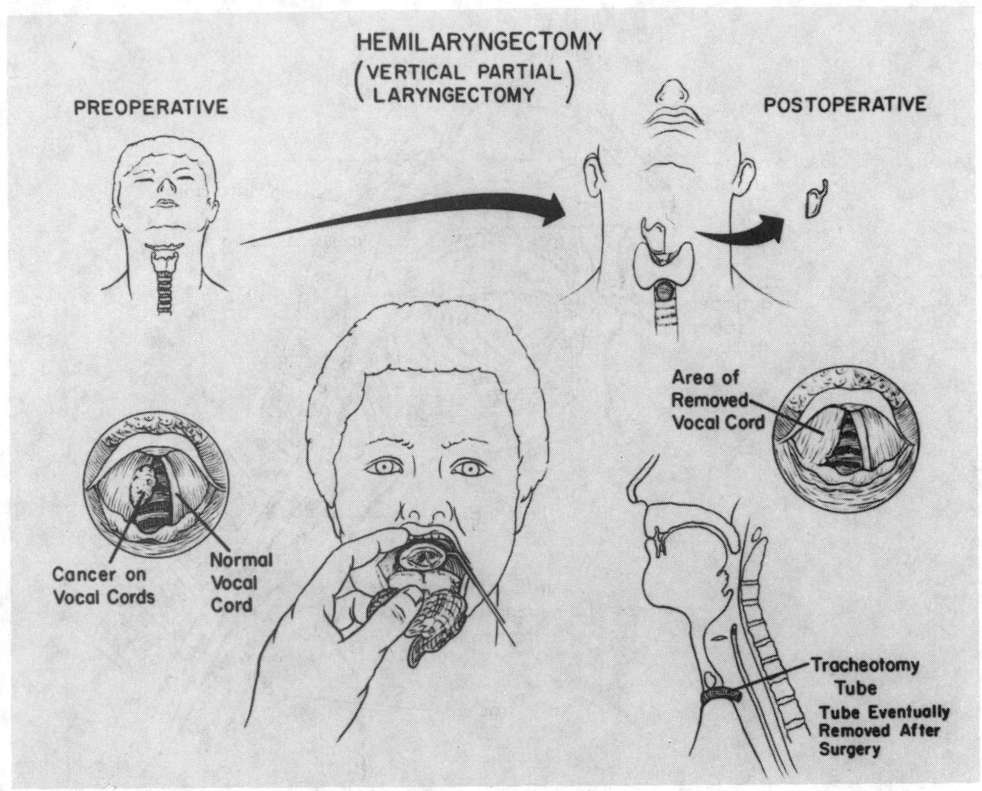


**FIGURE 36-23** The technique of vertical partial laryngectomy. (From DeWeese DD et al: *Otolaryngology—head and neck surgery,* ed 7, St Louis, 1988, Mosby.)

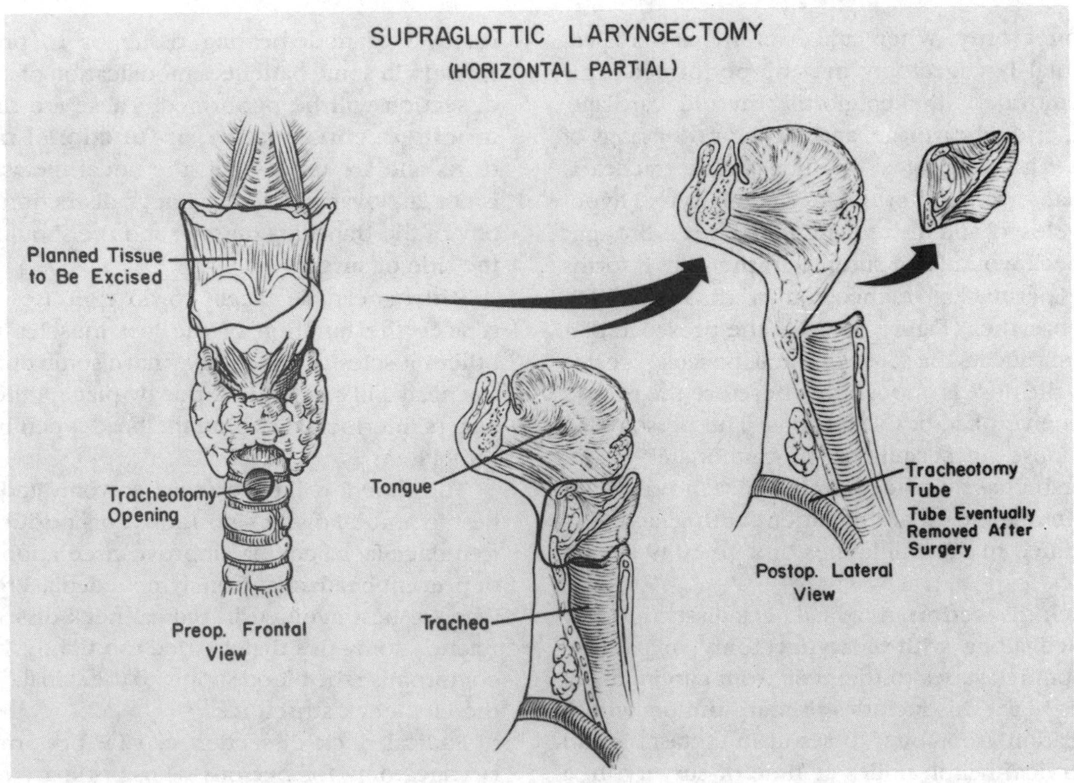


**FIGURE 36-24** The technique of supraglottic laryngectomy. Removal of the endolaryngeal structures from tip of epiglottis down to laryngeal vertical. (From DeWeese DD et al: *Otolaryngology—head and neck surgery,* ed 7, St Louis, 1988, Mosby.)

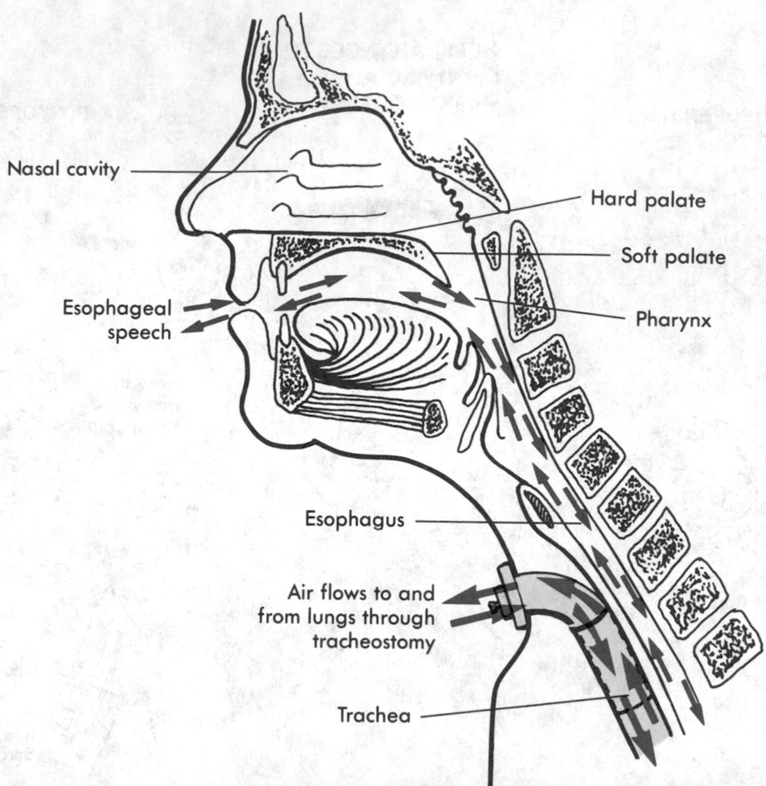


**FIGURE 36-25** Permanent tracheostomy: no connection exists between trachea and esophagus.

**Total laryngectomy.** When cancer of the larynx is advanced, a total laryngectomy may be performed. This includes removal of the epiglottis, thyroid cartilage, hyoid bone, cricoid cartilage, and three or four rings of the trachea. The pharyngeal opening to the trachea is closed, the anterior wall of the laryngopharynx (hypopharynx) is closed, and the remaining trachea is brought out to the neck wound and sutured to the skin. It forms an opening (permanent tracheostomy)[2] through which the patient breathes (Figure 36-25). The presence of a tracheal stoma affects the sense of smell, because breathing through the nose is impossible; therefore the person does not receive olfactory sensations. The person also has a runny nose, because he or she cannot sniff in and out. The person has no voice because of removal of the larynx. The nursing care of the patient with a laryngectomy is outlined in the Guidelines box, p. 1039 (left).

**Radical neck dissection.** A radical neck dissection may be performed along with a laryngectomy in patients whose risk of metastases to the neck from carcinoma of the larynx is high. This includes primary tumors whose size and location are known to result in metastasis and palpable cervical lymph nodes at time of surgery. In a radical neck dissection the submandibular salivary gland, sternocleidomastoid muscle, internal jugular vein, and spinal accessory nerve are removed to ensure complete removal of node-bearing tissue or to prevent nodal spread.[2] In some patients a modification of a radical neck dissection will be performed. These are referred to as **modified, conservative,** or **functional neck dissections** and are used when the nodal metastatic disease is not far advanced. Radical neck dissection causes atrophy of the trapezius muscle, and the shoulder drops on the side of surgery.

Patients can be taught to do exercises to gradually replace the function of the lost muscles with that of other muscles. A patient may have some difficulty lifting the head and can achieve this by placing the hands with fingers interlocked behind the head when lifting it from the pillow.

The patient will have a tracheostomy and can breathe best in a mid-Fowler's position. This position also helps to reduce facial edema, improve circulation, and reduce or prevent headaches from lymphedema. Pressure dressings are best avoided in radical neck dissection, as are tracheostomy ties that are tied too tightly, because they compromise the blood supply to the skin flaps protecting the vital neck structures.[11]

Radical neck dissection can be performed without laryngectomy for persons whose primary malignant lesion is in the oral cavity, oropharynx, or parasinuses. Often the procedure accompanies other procedures and is termed a **composite resection.** Composite resec-

### Guidelines for Care of the Person After a Laryngectomy

Elevate head of bed 45 degrees.
Encourage coughing, deep breathing every 4 hours. Maintain oxygen to tracheostomy collar.
Incentive spirometry if ordered.
Assess airway patency every shift and PRN.
Vital signs.
Quality and rate of respiration.
Skin color (pallor, cyanosis).
Auscultation of lungs every shift and PRN.
Monitor hydration and ensure adequate fluid intake to maintain healthy oral mucosa; provide mouth care at least three times per day.
Record intake and output every shift.
Weigh daily at the same time and in same amount of clothing.
Provide stoma and stoma vent care every shift and PRN.
Ambulate TID and PRN.
Begin teaching laryngectomy care.
Assess anxiety level and provide emotional support.
Assist patient in communicating.
Provide patient with writing materials, picture board.
Use questions that can be answered yes or no.
Reinforce use of artificial speech device and encourage its use.
Assess suture line and stoma site every 4 hours.
Report erythema, purulent drainage, hematoma.
Care for suture line and stoma site as ordered by surgeon.
Monitor drain function and output.
Maintain suction to drain at level ordered.
Milk tubing every 1-2 hours for 24 hours; and then every 4 hours and PRN.
Report changes in amount and color of drainage or air leak.
Administer enteral feedings per order.
Assess patient's tolerance of feedings.
Assess bowel sounds every shift and PRN.
Report intolerance to feedings (nausea, fullness, inability to tolerate prescribed amount of feedings).
Record amount, consistency, and frequency of stools.
Assess swallowing ability and provide support when oral diet resumes.
Monitor patient's reaction to change in body image.
Be sensitive to patient's reactions to changes in appearance.
Provide time to listen to patient.
Encourage use of Lost Chord Club.
Prepare patient for discharge.
Monitor ability of patient or significant other to perform airway management care.
Provide patient with list of supplies necessary for home care.
Provide information about soft diet.
Review written instructions in home-going booklet.
Refer to home nursing staff to assess patient's ability to perform self-care at home.

**tions may include either radical neck dissection in addition to the removal of the mandible; removal of the mandible and resection of the floor of the mouth; or removal of the mandible, floor of the mouth, and the tongue. The nursing care for these patients is outlined in the Guidelines box at right. Emotional reactions to this type of radical surgery may be profound. Disfigurement is readily visible, and reactions to the change in body image are marked. In addition to the usual fears**

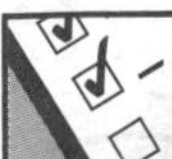

### Guidelines for Care of the Person After Radical Neck Dissection

Elevate head of bed 30 degrees.
Maintain oxygen mist therapy if ordered.
Encourage coughing, deep breathing, and use of incentive spirometer.
Assess airway for signs and symptoms of increasing airway obstruction (stridor, dyspnea, increased pulse and respiratory rate).
Keep tracheostomy set at bedside.
Monitor vital signs every 4 hours.
Assess for early signs and symptoms of bleeding (potential for carotid hemorrhage).
Ensure blood availability with blood bank.
Maintain venous access with large-bore needle.
If hemorrhage occurs: STAT page physician, apply direct pressure, suction airway, reassure patient.
Care for suture line as ordered.
Maintain drainage function and output.
Maintain suction to drain.
Milk tubing every 1-2 hours for 24 hours; and then q 4 hr PRN.
Assess output and document every shift.
Check for air leak.
Assess for signs and symptoms of infection of suture line (erythema, pus, elevated temperature).
Assess skin flap every shift for signs and symptoms of poor drain patency or infection: swelling, bleeding, oozing of suture line.
Monitor intake and output and record every shift.
Monitor for evidence of chylous fistula (lymphatic leak from thoracic duct into neck wound).
Opaque or milky drainage from wound.
Observe color and amount of drainage and report any change to physician.
Place on lactose-free diet.
Monitor shoulder droop secondary to loss of nerve supply to trapezius muscle.
Inability to raise hand over head.
Reinforce need to do shoulder strengthening exercise tid.
Consult physical therapist with concerns about patient's exercises.
Monitor patient's ability to ingest optimal caloric intake.
Observe swallowing attempts and assess for aspiration.
Report inability to comply with recommended intake to physician and dietitian.
Provide emotional support during eating.
Monitor depression, which is not uncommon following disfiguring surgery; also in persons who are alcoholic and suffering from withdrawal (DTs).
Identify patient support system and involve them and patient in planning and giving care.
Plan for specific time to provide emotional support.
Help patient verbalize feelings about having cancer, changes in body image, and life-style.
Encourage adequate caloric intake.
May have difficulty in swallowing related to postoperative swelling and radiation preoperatively.
Weigh daily at same time and with same amount of clothing.
Monitor attempts to swallow and check for aspiration.
Consult with dietitian and physician if desired caloric intake cannot be met.
Teach patient about role of diet in wound healing.
Refer to home care nursing staff to assess patient's ability to care for self at home.

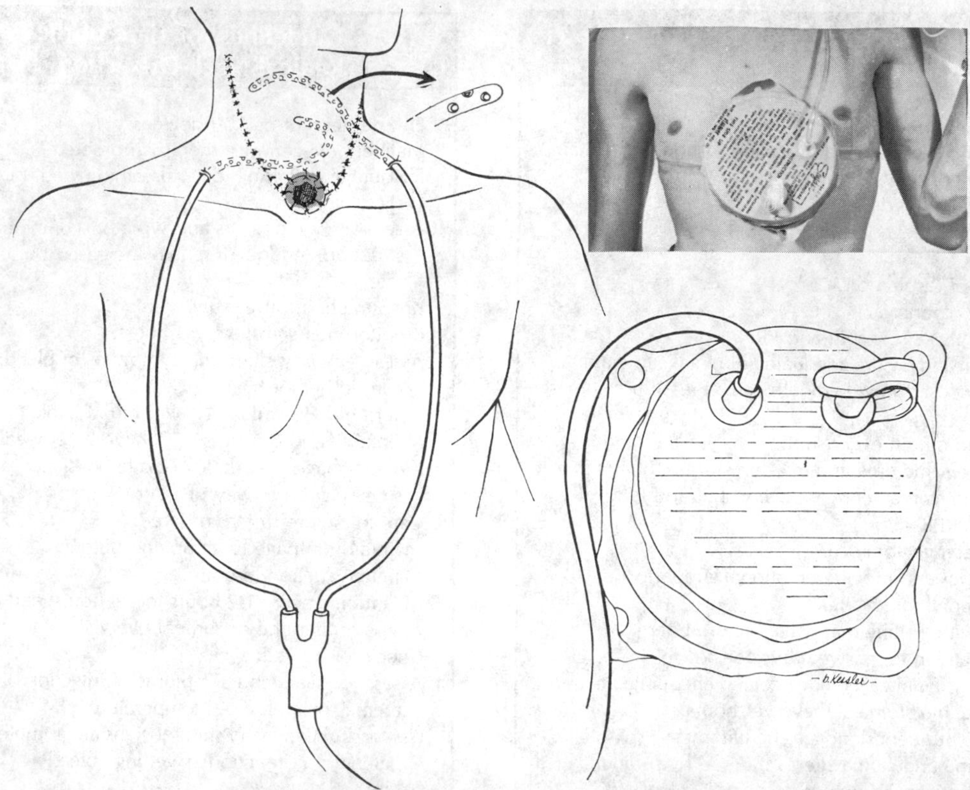

**FIGURE 36-26** Hemovac apparatus for constant closed suction. In this system of wound drainage, suction is maintained by plastic container with spring inside that tries to force apart lids and thereby produces suction that is transmitted through plastic tubing. Neck skin is pulled down tight, and no external dressing is required. Container serves as both suction source and receptacle for blood. It is emptied as required, and drainage tubes are left in neck for 3 days. (From DeWeese DD et al: *Otolaryngology—head and neck surgery,* ed 7, St Louis, 1988, Mosby.)

of surgery and cancer, the patient having a composite resection may have fears of rejection and fears concerning the future.

Often a Hemovac (Figure 36-26) or another suction device is placed in the incision in the operating room. Its purpose is to maintain constant drainage from the neck wound and prevent pressure on the skin flaps. The drain is checked regularly to see that it is working properly and there is no edema, which might indicate that a hematoma is developing. The tubing is milked every 1 to 2 hours for the first 24 hours postoperatively and then every 4 hours and as needed. Changes in the amount or color of drainage should be reported to the surgeon.

#### Diet

Diet includes tube feedings postoperatively progressing to soft diet.

#### Activity

The patient is up in a chair on the first postoperative day and walks in the hall every 4 hours beginning the second postoperative day.

#### Referral/Consultation

In some settings the nurse assumes responsibility for making referrals to other services. Common referrals for persons with laryngectomy include social work, speech pathology, respiratory therapy, and physical therapy.

## Nursing Management of the Patient with Laryngeal Surgery

### Preoperative care

The person who is to have a laryngectomy is told by the physician that breathing will occur through a permanent opening made in the neck and that normal speech will not be possible. This is often depressing to the patient, because it may threaten economic status as well as life. In some instances it is helpful to receive a visit from another person who has made a good recovery from laryngectomy and who has undergone rehabilitation successfully. In other instances the visit may depress the patient further. Careful assessment must be made to determine if the person will benefit from such a visit and whether the visit should be made preoperatively, immediately after surgery, or later in the recovery period.

In some medical centers the visit is planned for 5 to 7 days postoperatively. Even though the patient and significant other are hesitant about allowing the visit, they often indicate that the visit was helpful and improved their outlook about the patient's future.

Often no one else can give a person reassurance that speech can be regained as well as a fellow patient. Many large cities have a Lost Chord Club or a New Voice Club, and the members are willing to visit hospitalized patients. Information regarding these clubs may be obtained by writing to the International Association of Laryngectomees.* Local speech rehabilitation centers may supply instructive films and other resources. The local chapter of the American Cancer Society and the local health department also have information available. If possible, the family also should learn about the method of esophageal speech that the person will learn to use.

## Managing Critical Care

### Immediate postoperative care

Most patients undergoing head and neck surgery will be placed in an intensive care unit because of their need for (1) hemodynamic monitoring, (2) airway monitoring, and (3) wound and flap monitoring.[11]

**Maintaining proper positioning.** To minimize venous and arterial pressure in the neck, which would increase the risk of swelling and hemorrhage, the head of the bed is elevated 30 to 45 degrees. The neck is maintained in a slightly flexed position to minimize tension on the suture lines. Some patients will require greater neck flexion or rotation to minimize tension or flexion of the flaps used for reconstruction. The patient is usually up in the chair on the first postoperative day and can walk in the hall with assistance on the second day.[11]

**Maintaining a patent airway.** Some degree of airway obstruction is common in head and neck patients, either from tumor, edema from preoperative radiotherapy, or surgery close to the airway.

To prevent emergency airway situations, a tracheostomy is performed at the time of surgery. A cuffed tube is used for the following reasons: (1) to allow ventilation postoperatively when the patient is late in waking up, (2) to prevent blood from the surgical site entering the tracheobronchial tree, and (3) to prevent pharyngeal and gastric secretions from soiling the bronchial tree.[11]

The cuff is kept inflated until the morning after surgery or until the patient can manage his or her secretions. Even with low-pressure cuffs, the cuff is deflated at least every 8 hours to prevent damage to the tracheal wall. To prevent aspiration of secretions accumulated above the cuff, the patient is suctioned after the cuff is deflated (see p. 1025). The patient is suctioned every 2 to 4 hours to prevent the buildup of secretions in the tracheobronchial tree or in the tracheostomy tube. It may be necessary to instill 3 to 5 ml of sterile saline in the tube to soften and dislodge thickened secretions.

Patients receive cool mist therapy with a T-tube or cervical mask. They also receive intermittent positive-pressure breathing (IPPB) treatments, forced inspiration, chest physiotherapy (see Chapter 37), and if necessary aerosol and systemic bronchodilators.

When a cuffed tube is no longer necessary, which is not earlier than 3 days postoperatively, an uncuffed tube is inserted. Cuffless tubes are less harmful to the trachea, interfere less with swallowing, and minimize aspiration. Because there is no cuff, secretions cannot accumulate above it. Also, it allows the patient to occlude the tube with a finger (when the airway is not obstructed) and to speak, which is a big psychologic boost to the patient. As the patient is able to expectorate secretions and has an adequate airway, the tube will be plugged for increasing periods of time (see p. 1029). The goal is to remove the tube and allow the opening to close by secondary intention before discharge from the hospital in 7 days. Some patients' tubes are removed as early as 3 days postoperatively when most patients leave the ICU and move to the step-down unit.

Exceptions to some of the above are patients who have a total laryngectomy who have a permanent tracheotomy. Because the trachea is permanently separated from the digestive tract, oropharyngeal secretions cannot be aspirated into the tracheobronchial tree unless a pharyngocutaneous fistula develops, which is a possible complication of total laryngectomy. The other exception is the patient who has a tracheoesophageal fistula created for voice restoration after laryngectomy. Most of these patients have a regular nasogastric tube, and therefore aspiration is insignificant.[11]

**Managing the wound.** Because of the nature of head and neck surgery, complications are always a threat. The reasons for this are extensive undermining of subcutaneous tissues to elevate the skin flaps, contamination at the time of surgery when the upper aerodigestive tract is entered, and the poor quality of tissue in persons who receive preoperative radiotherapy. Complications that can occur include hematoma, wound dehiscence, tissue loss, pharyngocutaneous fistula, and carotid artery rupture.[11]

Assessment of the operative wound is of crucial importance. The surgical site is closed either with interrupted or running sutures and in some centers most often with skin staples. The site is left exposed (no dressing). The absence of a dressing makes it easier to monitor the wound site. The persons caring for the patient need to be familiar with the initial appearance of the wound so that any changes are readily apparent. The viability of the skin flaps is assessed by noting *color, temperature,*

*American Cancer Society, Inc., 1599 Clifton Road NE, Atlanta, Ga.

***capillary refill,*** and ***induration.*** Slight erythema and induration of the skin flaps are normal in the early postoperative period. It is important that the incision lines be kept free of crusting and exudates.

The suture line is assessed for signs of approximation, edema, color, and drainage. The incision is cleansed with half strength hydrogen peroxide solution using sterile technique. Cotton swabs are used to remove scabs. Antibiotic ointment is applied to the wound to seal the suture line. Patients who receive radiotherapy preoperatively are more prone to wound dehiscence or the development of a pharyngocutaneous fistula. Drain exit sites and the tracheostomy incision receive the same care as the suture line. A minimal amount of bleeding from skin edges is normal in the immediate postoperative period. A more diffuse ooze of darker red blood along with swelling of the wound is an indication that hematoma is developing and the surgeon is notified immediately. See p. 1036 for a listing of wound complications.

**Monitoring the closed drainage system.** A closed drainage with continuous suction is used to eliminate dead space and prevent accumulation of blood, serum, and other secretions under the skin flaps. Many drainage systems are available (Davol, Hemovac, Jackson-Pratt), and all provide a continuous negative pressure of 80 to 120 mm Hg. They are monitored for function, presence of air leaks, and type and amount of drainage. If the drainage system is not functioning properly, a ***massive hematoma under tension*** can develop. This requires that the patient return to surgery for exploration, control of bleeding, and restoration of the drainage system.[11]

If air continuously seeps into the drainage system, negative pressure will not be maintained. Air leaks should be corrected immediately. If the air leak is through the suture line, the problem can be solved by adding sutures or applying thick antibiotic ointment to the incision. In some situations a circular dressing is applied to the neck if no reconstruction flap is involved. If the leak is minimal, the drain can be connected to wall suction. When a massive air leak occurs, the drain may need to be removed. In some situations the patient will return to surgery for closure of the leak and proper drain replacement.[11]

The tubing is milked every hour for the first 24 hours and then every 4 hours and as needed to check for patency. The wound is examined at these times to determine if fluid is accumulating under the flaps.

The type and amount of drainage are recorded every 8 hours. The amount of drainage in the first 16 hours can vary from less than 100 ml to 300 ml. Initially the drainage is sanguineous to serosanguineous. The drains are pulled when the drainage is less than 30 ml/24 hr. Purulent or granular serous drainage mixed with air (with an odor to it) indicates a probable pharyngocutaneous fistula.[11]

#### Ongoing postoperative care

Postoperative care of the person with a laryngectomy is essentially the same as that described for tracheostomy (see p. 1025) except that these persons will have a laryngectomy tube in place—a tube that is shorter and wider in diameter than a tracheostomy tube. Some patients may not have a tube in the stoma after the operation because the stoma is a permanent one kept open initially by the sutures and because their surgeon believes that there is less tissue reaction and a better stoma if no tube is used. If a laryngectomy tube is used, it remains until the wound is healed and a permanent fistula has formed—usually in 2 to 3 weeks.

The nasogastric tube (inserted during the surgical procedure) is used for the instillation of food and fluids at regular intervals postoperatively (Figure 36-27). The use of the tube to give food is thought to minimize contamination of the pharyngeal and esophageal suture lines and to prevent fluid from leaking through the wound into the trachea before healing occurs. The nasogastric tube is removed as soon as the person can safely swallow. Ability to tolerate a soft diet is a prerequisite for discharge. The person then needs careful attention in the first attempts to swallow. Aspiration cannot occur because the trachea no longer communicates with the esophagus.[11]

The sense of smell is affected after laryngectomy because breathing through the nose is impossible; therefore the patient does not receive normal olfactory sensations. Some patients report that they are able to smell, and most have drainage from the nose for a period of time. See Guidelines boxes (p. 1039) for a summary of postoperative care of the patient with a laryngectomy and for postoperative care of the patient with a neck dissection.

Some alteration of appearance is readily visible, which may cause the person to feel somewhat conspicuous. Anger, grief, or denial may be part of the normal response to the change in body image. (For further information on psychologic support, refer to Chapter 9.)

### Speech Rehabilitation

Until recently **esophageal speech** was the primary speech method after laryngectomy. Although this method of speech was successful for many laryngectomees, others could never learn to use it. In addition, the increased use of radiotherapy after laryngectomy causes fibrous tissue to form, making esophageal speech less possible.

#### Tracheoesophageal puncture

For a number of years, surgeons had been working to develop other forms of speech after laryngectomy. In 1980 the first successful procedure using surgical-prosthetic voice restoration was introduced. In this procedure a **tracheoesophageal puncture (TEP)** is made

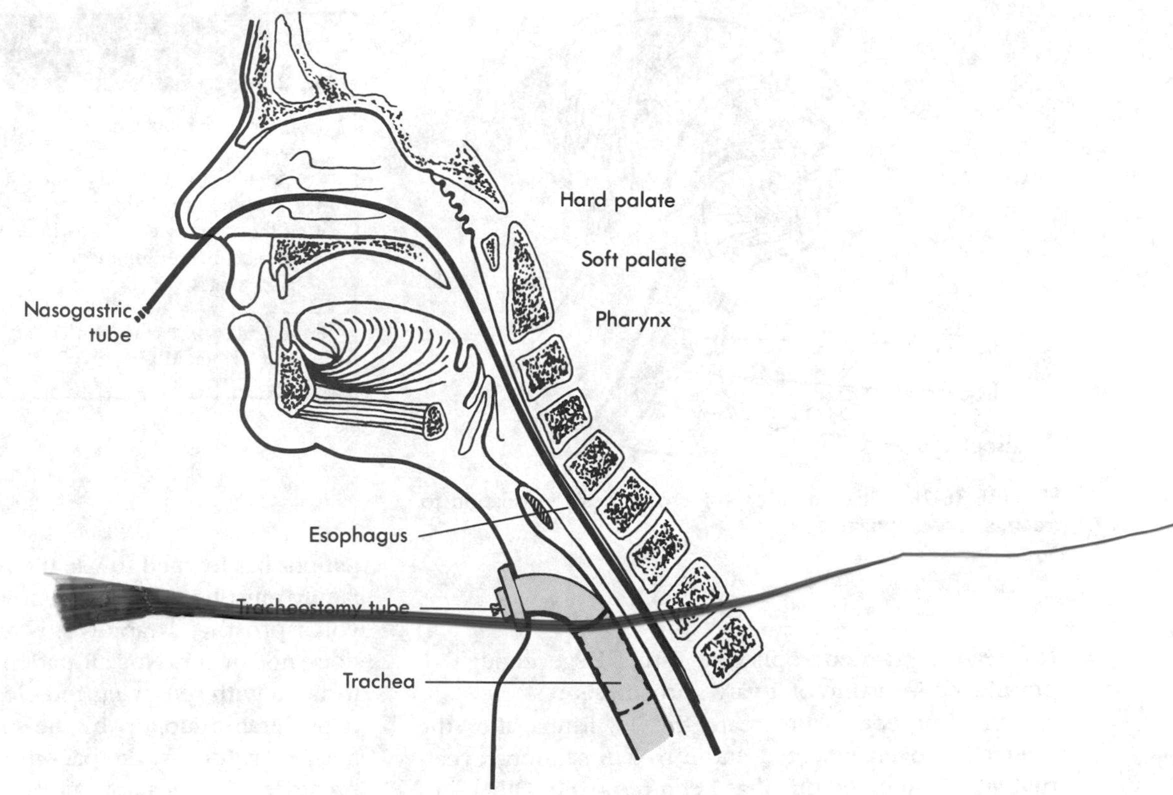


**FIGURE 36-27** Position of tracheostomy tube and nasogastric tube after total laryngectomy.

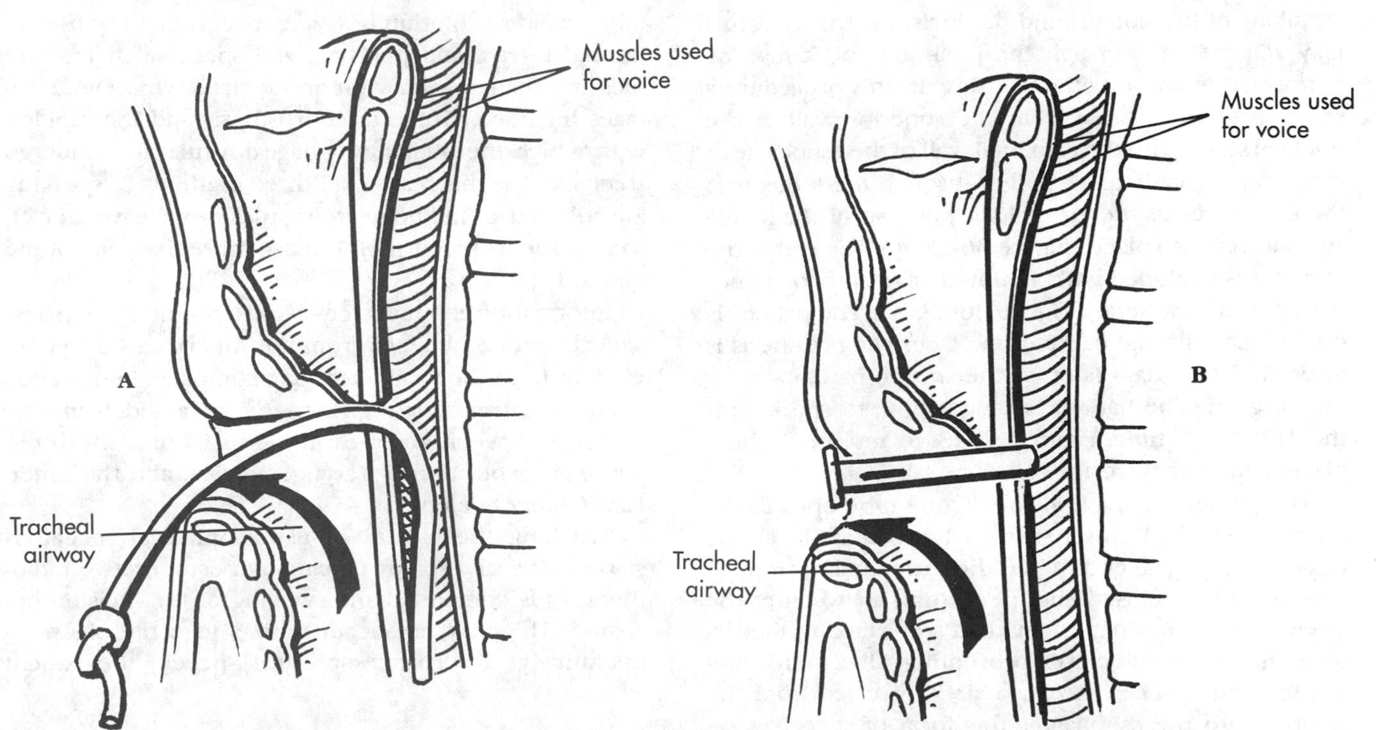


**FIGURE 36-28** Trachoesophageal puncture (TEP). **A,** Placement of red rubber catheter into TEP. Note knot in end of catheter to prevent passage of stomach contents. **B,** Placement of voice prosthesis into TEP.

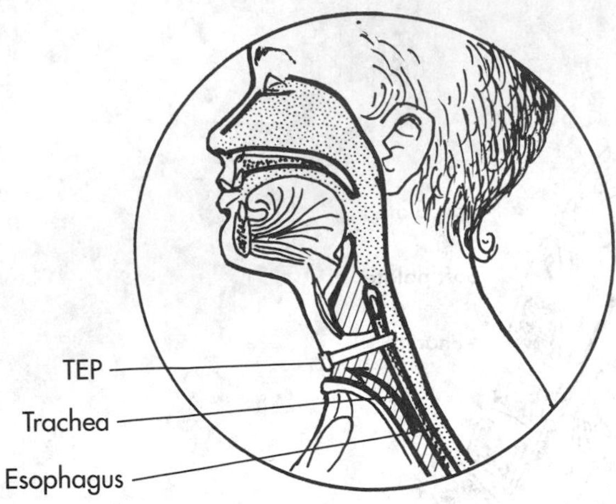


**FIGURE 36-29** Placement of voice prosthesis in relation to trachea and esophagus.

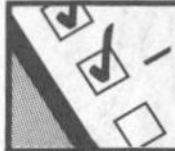

## Guidelines for What to Do if Prosthesis Comes Out

1. Insert red rubber catheter approximately 6-8 inches into fistula.
2. Tie a knot in the end of the catheter (see Figure 36-30).
3. Tape end of catheter to chest.
4. If the catheter cannot be inserted, contact your surgeon or speech therapist immediately. This may indicate that fistula is closing.

From Sigler BA, Schuring LT: *Ear, nose and throat disorders,* St Louis, 1993, Mosby, p 267.

to create a tracheoesophageal fistula large enough to permit the insertion of a valve prosthesis.

Some surgeons will create the TE fistula after the larynx has been resected and a frozen section reveals that all of the carcinoma has been removed. Other surgeons prefer to wait until the patient has completed postoperative radiotherapy. This may be as long as 3 to 6 months after surgery. The reason for deferring TE fistula to this time is that this allows time for edema of the incision to abate. Also, radiotherapy may cause shrinking of the skin around the incision. The TE fistula may require an overnight hospital stay, or it may be performed in an outpatient setting. In this procedure a small fistula is created from the superior wall of the tracheal stoma into the proximal wall of the esophagus.[11] A red rubber catheter is pulled through the fistula into the esophagus at the 12 o'clock position of the stoma and sutured into place (Figure 36-28, *A*). The end of the catheter is occluded with an umbilical clamp, or a knot is tied in the catheter (Figure 36-28, *A*). The patient is discharged with the catheter in place. The prosthesis is inserted 5 to 7 days later by the speech pathologist or the surgeon. The patient is taught how to speak with the TEP at this time. Figures 36-28, *B,* and 36-29 show placement of the prosthesis.

The prosthesis is a hollow silicone tube open at the tracheal end and closed with a horizontal slit at the laryngopharyngeal end. When the patient talks, air pressure opens the closed end, permitting air to enter the laryngopharynx. When the patient stops talking, the laryngopharyngeal end closes, preventing saliva from draining into the trachea. Because air is diverted from the trachea into the esophagus, this form of speech is referred to as *tracheoesophageal speech.*

The stoma must be occluded during speech, either by placing a finger over the opening of the valve or by using a special tracheostomal valve inserted after the patient has learned to use the prosthesis. The patient or family must be taught to remove, clean, and reinsert the voice prosthesis rapidly so that stenosis of the fistula does not occur. Not all patients and families are comfortable with removing and cleaning the prosthesis, and considerable support by the speech pathologist may be necessary. Ideally, the patient should be able to use the prosthesis for speaking and be able to clean and reinsert it before discharge from the hospital.

The patient and significant other need to be taught what to do if the prosthesis comes out. See Guidelines box above.

Advantages of tracheoesophageal speech include more rapid restoration of voice, speech that is closer to normal in rate and phrasing, and speech that is more pleasing than speech with an electrolarynx. Disadvantages include reliance on a prosthesis and the rapidity with which the tracheoesophageal fistula may undergo stenosis.[2] For this reason, all three methods of speaking are still in use, and none are mutually exclusive. In fact, some patients find it useful to use more than one of the methods (Box 36-6).

Information about devices used to produce electronic speech can be obtained from the American Cancer Society or from the local telephone company. Information about esophageal speech can be obtained from the American Speech and Hearing Association,* the International Association of Laryngectomies, and the American Cancer Society.

Teaching the patient to use esophageal speech is started after all therapy (including postoperative radiotherapy) is completed and swelling of the incision has abated. This may not occur until 3 to 6 months postoperatively. To learn esophageal speech, the patient

*American Speech and Hearing Association, 10801 Rockville Pike, Rockville, MD 20852.

**BOX 36-6 Speech Methods After Total Laryngectomy**

**TRACHEOESOPHAGEAL PROSTHESIS**
Formation of a tracheoesophageal fistula with insertion of a silicone prosthesis that produces a sound in the esophagus (Figure 36-28, *B*)

**ESOPHAGEAL SPEECH**
Speech produced by expelling swallowed air (burping) across constricted tissue in the pharyngoesophageal segment

**EXTERNAL SPEECH AIDS**
Mechanical devices, such as a vibrator or electronic artificial larynx, used externally (Figure 36-30)

must first practice burping. This provides the moving column of air needed for sound, while folds of tissue at the opening of the esophagus act as the vibrating surface. The patient must learn to coordinate articulation with esophageal vocalization made possible by aspirating air into the esophagus. The new voice sounds are natural, although somewhat hoarse. The qualitites of speech provided by the use of the nasopharynx are still present. The patient may have digestive difficulty while learning to speak; this is caused by swallowing air during practice, by unusual strain on abdominal muscles, and by nervous tension. Digestive difficulties usually abate with proficiency in speaking.

Most patients learn esophageal speech best at a special clinic. Although some individuals may need to go to a nearby city for this instruction, they usually must remain away from home for only 1 or 2 weeks. Motivation and persistent effort are essential in learning this kind of speech; encouragement and support from the professional staff and the patient's significant others are important to the patient's morale. About 75% of all patients who have their larynx removed master some sort of speech, and the average person can return to work 1 or 2 months after leaving the hospital.

If a person is unable to learn esophageal speech in 60 to 90 days after surgery, a *speech aid* such as a vibrator or an **electronic artificial larynx** (Figure 36-30) may be prescribed. Various mechanical devices are available, and the new ones permit a natural type of speech, providing pitch inflections and volume control. The local chapter of the American Cancer Society or the local telephone company can provide information about the purchase of these devices.

## Reconstructive Surgery

Because of the extensive surgery required to treat malignancies of the head and neck, reconstructive surgery has become common practice. In the past, skin grafts and pedicle or rotation skin flaps were used for reconstruction. Today myocutaneous flaps or free flaps are the major reconstructive flaps used after radical neck dissection and traumatic defects of the head and neck.[3]

### Myocutaneous flaps

**Myocutaneous flaps** use the axial blood supply that supplies muscle mass, as well as cutaneous and subcutaneous tissue. The inclusion of muscle with its blood supply when transferring the skin allows for a much greater range of rotation of the flap. The *pectoralis ma-*

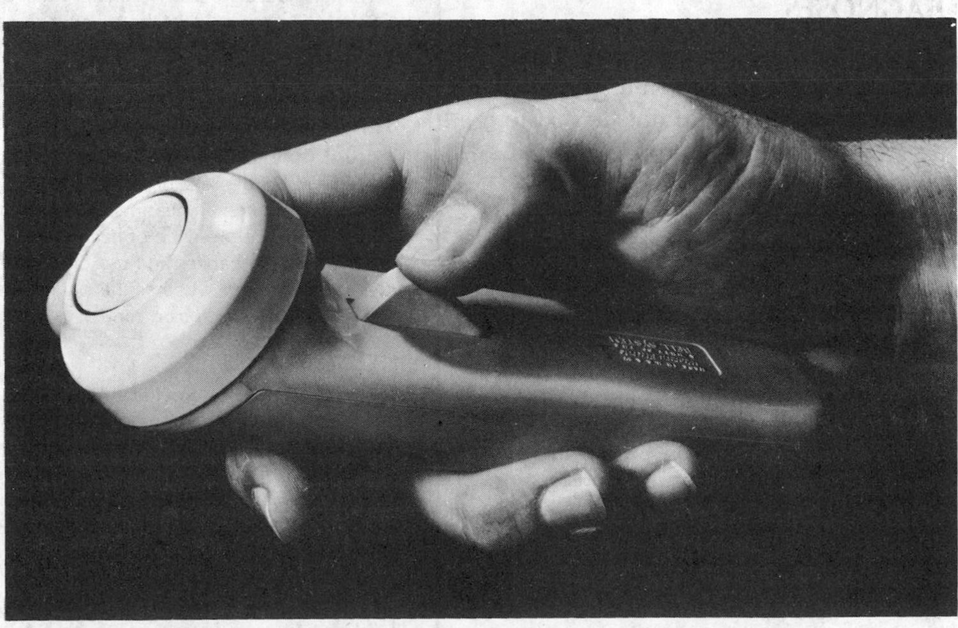

**FIGURE 36-30** Battery-powered electronic artificial larynx for patient who has total laryngectomy. (Courtesy Illinois Bell Telephone Co.)

*jor,* the *latissimus dorsi,* the *trapezius,* and the *sternocleidomastoid* muscles can be used for *myocutaneous flaps.*

### Free flaps

**Free flaps** consist of harvested tissue separated from the donor site with the vein and artery. The vein and artery are anastomosed to recipient vessels close to the defect (microvascular anastomosis). It is also possible to harvest flaps containing soft tissue and bone to reconstruct the mandible after mandibulectomy.

Close postoperative monitoring of any type of skin flap is essential. Monitoring includes the following:

1. Direct observation, unless the wound is completely covered with a dressing: some surgeons exteriorize (bring to the outside) a small segment of buried flaps for monitoring purposes.
2. Doppler is used to monitor for patency of the anastomoses. The surgeon indicates the area where the Doppler is to be applied. Hourly assessments are made for at least the first 24 hours.

To prevent clot formation in the recipient graft, the hematocrit is kept below 30 and sometimes as low as 25 before considering blood replacement. Some surgeons order low-dose aspirin or even heparin to prevent clot formation. It should be remembered that persons with a below-normal hematocrit fatigue easily because the oxygen-carrying capacity of the blood is reduced.

## NURSING MANAGEMENT: The Patient Undergoing Total Laryngectomy

### ♦ NURSING DIAGNOSES

Nursing diagnoses are determined from analysis of patient data. Nursing diagnoses for the person undergoing total laryngectomy may include but are not limited to the following:

| Diagnostic Title | Possible Etiologic Factors |
|---|---|
| Airway clearance, ineffective | Presence of laryngectomy tube, increased tracheobronchial secretions, crusts, mucus, serosanguineous plugs |
| Anxiety | Threat to self-concept, inability to speak, threat to socioeconomic status, alcohol withdrawal |
| Skin integrity, impaired | Surgical incision, preoperative radiotherapy, malnourished state |
| Infection, high risk | Surgical incision, fistula |
| Communication, impaired verbal | Laryngectomy |
| Pain, acute postoperative | Surgery |
| Nutrition, altered: less than body requirements | Swallowing difficulty, malnourished because of alcoholism |
| Body image disturbance | Disfiguring surgery |

### ♦ EXPECTED PATIENT OUTCOMES

Expected patient outcomes for a person undergoing a total laryngectomy may include but are not limited to the following:

1. Has a patent airway.
2. Does not exhibit signs of anxiety (restlessness, increased pulse, respirations, blood pressure).
3. Surgical incision is healed and is free of infection and dehiscence.
4. Does not develop an infection in suture line.
5. Communicates effectively.
6. Is comfortable, appears relaxed, and is able to sleep.
7. Does not lose more than 5 lb during hospitalization.
8. Begins to acknowledge feelings about change in body image.

### ♦ INTERVENTIONS

Nursing interventions can be found in the Nursing Care Plan, pp. 1047-1049.

### ♦ EVALUATION

To evaluate the effectiveness of nursing interventions, compare patient behavior with those stated in the ex-

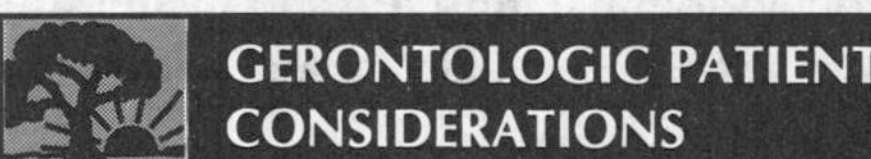

### GERONTOLOGIC PATIENT CONSIDERATIONS

#### ASSESSMENT

Assess nutritional status because many of these patients have a history of alcohol abuse.

Assess for signs and symptoms of alcohol withdrawal:
- Tremors: occurs 6-48 hours after alcohol withdrawal
- Seizures: occurs 12-24 hours after last drink; usually are *grand mal* seizures and not preceded by an aura
- Delirium tremens (DTs): acute complication of alcohol withdrawal; signs and symptoms include restlessness and irritability, headache, nausea, insomnia, and nightmares; usually treated with chlordiazepoxide (Librium) or another CNS depressant

Assess for diminution in hearing and use of hearing aids. Inform all personnel of presence of hearing aid.

Assess for visual changes and use of eyeglasses.

Assess mobility and whether the patient uses an ambulatory assistive device such as a cane.

#### INTERVENTIONS

Work with dietitian to provide a high-calorie, high-protein diet with extra snacks to improve nutritional status.

Monitor mental status to determine if patient is exhibiting signs of alcohol withdrawal.

Discuss patient's symptoms of alcohol withdrawal with surgeon to determine if surgery will be postponed.

#### COMMON DISORDERS IN ELDERS

Alcoholism
Malignancies
Pneumonia

# NURSING CARE PLAN

## PERSON WITH LARYNGECTOMY

**DATA:** Mr. K., a 68-year-old man, had noted progressive hoarseness for several months. Indirect laryngoscopy and biopsy confirmed cancer of the larynx, and he was admitted for a total laryngectomy. His wife accompanied him to the hospital and planned to be with him as much as possible during his hospitalization. She was attentive and supportive.

The following pertinent data were identified on admission:

- He was visibly apprehensive (pacing the floor, restless, asking repeated questions).
- His major concerns centered on the extent of the cancer and on communication problems postoperatively.
- Height 175 cm (5 ft 10 in), weight 68 kg (150 lb).
- He wears glasses; near vision is poor without glasses.

Before surgery, Mr. K.'s primary nurse spent time with him, encouraging him to explore his concerns and providing information about what to expect in the postoperative period and care that would be provided. After the interaction, Mr. K.'s restlessness decreased and he was observed talking quietly with his wife and watching TV.

During surgery, the larynx was removed; a permanent tracheostomy was performed with insertion of a temporary laryngectomy tube. A nasogastric tube was inserted, to be removed after Mr. K. was swallowing well. During the first postoperative day, Mr. K. again appeared apprehensive (restlessness, pointing frequently to his tracheostomy, pulling on wife's hand, and pointing to call cord to call the nurse). Breath sounds in the upper lobes were clear but were absent in the lower lobes. Codeine and acetaminophen were prescribed for pain.

### ■ NURSING DIAGNOSIS

Ineffective airway clearance related to secretions in upper airway and laryngectomy tube

| Expected Patient Outcomes | Nursing Interventions | Rationale |
|---|---|---|
| Respirations effortless, quiet, and at baseline rate | Place patient in semi-Fowler's position. | Uses gravity to help expand thorax and decrease pressure on lower lobes. |
| Breath sounds clear at all lobes | Suction laryngectomy tube as often as needed as evidenced by noisy respirations, increased pulse and respiratory rate, and restlessness (may be every 5 minutes initially). | Air blowing through secretions produces noisy respirations; pulse and respirations are increased when oxygen intake is decreased; restlessness may indicate decreased oxygenation. |
| | Provide tracheostomy care. | Keeping tube open will facilitate air exchange. |
| | Provide air humidification. | Humidity will help keep secretions liquid for easier removal and prevent mucous plugs. |
| | Encourage deep breathing and coughing. | Deep breathing will help aerate lower lobes; coughing will help expel the secretions. |

### ■ NURSING DIAGNOSIS

Anxiety related to breathing difficulties and inability to communicate

| Expected Patient Outcome | Nursing Interventions | Rationale |
|---|---|---|
| Patient rests quietly, does not call frequently for suctioning | Explain to patient and carry out regular suctioning of tracheostomy. | If patient knows tube will be suctioned frequently, fear of possible asphyxiation should decrease. |
| | Develop a means of communication (e.g., cards with needs printed clearly or paper for writing). Be sure patient wears his glasses. | If patient can communicate needs, anxiety should decrease. His glasses are needed for visual communication. |
| | After initial period, and if wife is willing and able, teach her to help with suctioning tracheostomy. | Participating in husband's care may assist wife to feel she is helping, thus decreasing her anxiety (anxiety can be transmitted to patient). |
| | Encourage patient to care for own tracheostomy when feasible. | Self-care enhances feelings of control of situation. |

*Continued.*

# NURSING CARE PLAN

## PERSON WITH LARYNGECTOMY—cont'd

### ■ NURSING DIAGNOSIS
Pain related to surgery

| Expected Patient Outcome | Nursing Interventions | Rationale |
|---|---|---|
| Is relaxed and signals feeling comfortable. | Give prescribed analgesic to prevent pain from becoming severe. | Analgesics will decrease transmission and interpretation of pain stimuli. |
| | Encourage other pain-relieving measures such as relaxation exercises or distraction. | Help to minimize pain perception. |
| | Provide nose and mouth care while nasogastric tube is in place. | Tube may irritate nose; mouth becomes dry and uncomfortable from open mouth breathing and decreased lubrication (unable to swallow fluids); also may cause earache. |

### ■ NURSING DIAGNOSIS
Nutrition, altered: less than body requirements (related to difficulty swallowing)

| Expected Patient Outcome | Nursing Interventions | Rationale |
|---|---|---|
| Weight is not less than 5 lb from baseline. | Give prescribed tube feedings via nasogastric tube until patient can swallow well. | Tube feedings provide more adequate nutrients than IV fluids; swallowing is impaired initially from postoperative edema of lower pharynx. |
| | When nasogastric tube is removed, give fluids until patient is swallowing well. | Fluids are easier to swallow initially past the edematous area. |
| | Explain anatomic changes to patient (no connection between esophagus and tracheostomy). | This may help to decrease patient's concern of choking. |
| | Stay with patient during initial eating of semisolid and solid foods. | He may fear choking and not be willing to swallow initially; encouragement by nurse with assurance of suctioning if necessary may give patient more confidence. |
| | Use measures to encourage eating as necessary (tray for wife so they can eat together, selection of desired foods, etc.). | Return to usual eating patterns may encourage patient to eat. |
| | Encourage him to monitor weight two to three times per week until baseline weight is regained. | Participating in own weight monitoring may motivate him to eat. |

### ■ NURSING DIAGNOSIS
Impaired verbal communication related to surgery

| Expected Patient Outcomes | Nursing Interventions | Rationale |
|---|---|---|
| Communicates with others. | Encourage him to communicate via an established system (e.g., hand signals, writing) during initial period. | With larynx removal, sounds cannot be made by previous method of vibrating vocal cords. |
| Begins speech rehabilitation using electronic larynx. | Support activities of speech therapist:<br>1. Encourage practice with device.<br>2. Discuss availability of mechanical devices for speech or telephone use.<br>3. Discuss TEP that is scheduled for 2 weeks after completion of radiotherapy. | Until he has tracheoesophageal puncture (TEP) in about 8 weeks, device will help him communicate. Ability to communicate raises self-confidence. |

## NURSING CARE PLAN

### PERSON WITH LARYNGECTOMY—cont'd

**■ NURSING DIAGNOSIS**

Impaired skin integrity related to surgery, malnourished state

| Expected Patient Outcome | Nursing Interventions | Rationale |
|---|---|---|
| Surgical incision is healing; no evidence of hematoma or dehiscence. | Clean incision using sterile technique. Monitor drainage device for patency. Milk tubing as prescribed and PRN.<br>Check appearance of wound and report changes promptly. | Keeping incision clean promotes healing. Keeping drain patent prevents formation of hematoma under tension. Hematoma places pressure on suture line, interfering with approximation of skin edges and possible wound dehiscence. |

**■ NURSING DIAGNOSIS**

High risk for infection related to surgery and poor nutritional status

| Expected Patient Outcome | Nursing Interventions | Rationale |
|---|---|---|
| Does not develop an infection in suture line. | Clean suture line every 4 hours and PRN using sterile technique; monitor negative drainage system for patency.<br>Milk tube as necessary to prevent hematoma. | Keeping suture line clean helps to prevent infection. Preventing hematoma formation reduces opportunity for bacteria to grow in hematoma, which is an excellent culture medium. |

**■ NURSING DIAGNOSIS**

Knowledge deficit related to lack of exposure/recall

| Expected Patient Outcome | Nursing Interventions | Rationale |
|---|---|---|
| Describes self-care. | Teach patient:<br>1. Description of anatomic changes<br>2. Care of stoma, including self-suctioning<br>3. Methods to protect stoma<br>4. Availability of community resources<br>5. Recommended soft diet for 2 weeks after discharge | Providing own care will give him self-confidence; care is needed to keep the tracheostomy open for air exchange.<br>He may be interested in the Lost Chord Club for sharing of experiences.<br>This helps patient develop confidence in eating a variety of foods. |

pected patient outcomes. Successful achievement of patient outcomes for the patient with a total laryngectomy is indicated by the following:

1. Arterial blood gases (ABGs) and pulse oximetry are within normal limits; respirations are quiet and 16 per minute; breath sounds are clear. Patient has an effective cough and is not short of breath.
2. Patient appears relaxed, is able to rest at appropriate intervals, and is able to fall asleep without medication.
3. Edges of skin wound are clean and approximated well; no drainage from incision; temperature is normal, white blood cell count (WBC) is not elevated. There is no evidence of a fistula.
4. There is no evidence of infection in surgical incision; suture line has no discharge.
5. Patient communicates effectively with electronic speech device.
6. Patient is able to do more of own activities of daily living (ADL) and is able to control discomfort with oral analgesic.
7. Patient is able to swallow, is able to eat a soft diet with snacks, and is beginning to gain weight.
8. Patient mixes with other patients in a support group, talks about changes in appearances, and appears to be coping well.

## ✸ SPECIAL CONSIDERATIONS FOR CARE OF THE GERONTOLOGIC PATIENT

Special considerations for care of the elderly can be found in the box on page 1046.

## HOME CARE CONSIDERATIONS

Home care considerations for the person who had a laryngectomy are presented in the Guidelines box, p. 1039. In addition, the patient will be seen by a nurse from home care nursing who will visit the patient and evaluate progress. The nurse will also reinforce teaching and assess how well the patient and significant other are coping with the patient's surgery and diagnosis. The patient will have outpatient appointments with a physical therapist for neck exercises and with a speech pathologist for assistance with communicating.

## QUESTIONS TO CONSIDER

- What actions can you take to prevent spreading a cold to your patients?
- Discuss the postoperative care of a person having sinus surgery or nasal surgery.
- After a laryngectomy, how would you monitor the patient? Why?
- What resources are available in your community to assist the person who is unable to speak after a total laryngectomy?

## CRITICAL THINKING ACTIVITIES

- Compare and contrast the nursing care of a 45-year-old patient who is post partial laryngectomy with that of a 56-year-old patient who is post total laryngectomy with radical neck dissection.
- Debate the advantages and disadvantages of various vocal restoration methods used for individuals after a total laryngectomy.
- What specific behavior might indicate that an individual after radical neck surgery or permanent laryngectomy is not adjusting to changes in appearance?

## CHAPTER SUMMARY

### INFECTIONS OF THE NOSE AND SINUSES

- The major infections of the nose and sinuses are rhinitis (common cold), allergic rhinitis (hay fever), chronic rhinitis secondary to repeated infections, or allergy; sinusitis caused by a bacteria or virus.
- Persons with allergic rhinitis (hay fever) are usually sensitive to pollen of grasses such as ragweed (see Chapter 70).
- It is important for persons who are allergic to know which allergens they are allergic to and to avoid these allergens if at all possible. For this reason they need to know how to prepare an environmentally controlled bedroom (see Chapter 70).
- Persons with acute sinusitis usually have a severe headache and pain over the infected area. Fever is common and is related to the amount of sinus obstruction. If the sinus is abscessed, fever may be as high at 40° C (104° F).
- Subjective assessment of the person with a nose or sinus problem includes a careful history of previous infections, how they were treated, and self-treatment by the person, including the use of over-the-counter medications.
- Acetaminophen is recommended instead of aspirin in persons with nasal problems, because aspirin may be associated with nasal polyposis.
- Functional endoscopic sinus surgery (FESS) is being used more often to treat chronic sinusitis. Other procedures include Caldwell-Luc, ethmoidectomy, sphenoid sinus surgery, and frontal sinus surgery.
- Postoperative care for persons having sinus surgery includes the following:
  1. Place patient in side-lying position until reacted from anesthesia and then mid-Fowler's position.
  2. Administer cool mist by face tent or collar.
  3. Apply ice compresses over nose or ice bag over maxillary or frontal sinuses.
  4. Monitor for bleeding and for decreased visual acuity, such as diplopia, which indicates damage to the optic nerve.
  5. Provide frequent mouth care using a soft toothbrush.
  6. Change nasal pad when soiled.
  7. Teach patient not to blow nose for at least 48 hours after packing is removed.
  8. Instruct patient to avoid constipation because Valsalva maneuver can cause bleeding.
  9. Instruct patient to avoid sneezing or sneeze with mouth open.
  10. Instruct patient to avoid lifting heavy objects or bending over.

### INFECTIONS OF THE PHARYNX AND LARYNX

- The most common throat inflammation is acute pharyngitis. Group A beta-hemolytic streptococci (GABHS), staphylococci, and other bacteria and viruses may be sources of infection. Pharyngitis caused by *Neisseria gonorrhoeae* is being seen more commonly in both men and women.
- A throat culture is taken to obtain material for culture and sensitivity so that appropriate antibiotic therapy can be determined.
- Prophylactic antibiotics are often prescribed for persons with pharyngitis who have a history of rheumatic fever or bacterial endocarditis.

### OBSTRUCTIONS OF THE NOSE AND THROAT

- Obstructions of the nose, such as deviated septum, are treated surgically by nasoseptoplasty.
- Rhinoplasty can be used to correct an anatomic problem or for cosmetic reasons.
- Postoperative care after nasal surgery includes the following:

1. Monitor for hemorrhage.
2. Place patient in mid-Fowler's position to decrease local edema.
3. Apply ice compresses over the nose for 24 hours, as needed. Give cool mist via collar or face tent.
4. Offer food and fluids as tolerated.
5. Provide frequent oral care.
6. Change dressing under nose, as needed.
7. Teach patient to avoid blowing nose for 48 hours after packing is removed to prevent bleeding.
8. Teach patient to avoid constipation and vigorous coughing until healing occurs because coughing and Valsalva maneuver may initiate bleeding.
9. Explain that stools may be tarry for several days.
10. Cosmetic effects cannot be judged for 6 to 12 months.

- Nasal polyps are common and affect men twice as often as women. They are treated with corticosteroid sprays or injection of steroid into the polyps. The patient is taught the following:
  1. Elevate head of bed to decrease nasal edema and improve breathing.
  2. Increase humidity and increase fluid intake.
  3. Prevent respiratory infections by avoiding persons with an upper respiratory infection and crowds.
  4. Take medications as ordered.
- Tonsils and adenoids are removed surgically when they cause symptoms of obstruction or are chronically infected.
- Postoperative care after tonsillectomy includes the following:
  1. Position on side until awake and then in mid-Fowler's position.
  2. Monitor for hemorrhage.
  3. Give 30% cool mist by collar.
  4. Apply ice collar to neck.
  5. Use acetaminophen in place of aspirin for discomfort.
  6. Give ice-cold fluids and bland foods. Avoid milk because it increases mucus and causes patient to clear throat.
  7. Teach patient not to clear throat (may cause bleeding) and to avoid coughing, sneezing, vigorous nose blowing, and vigorous exercise.
  8. Expect more throat discomfort between fourth and eighth postoperative days (membrane separation).
- Laryngeal paralysis is caused by disease or injury of the laryngeal nerves or the vagus nerve. It is diagnosed by laryngoscopy. It can be treated medically but may require surgery.
- Acute laryngeal edema is a medical emergency that is treated with a corticosteroid or epinephrine. If severe it is treated with endotracheal intubation or tracheostomy because of airway obstruction.
- When a patient cannot maintain his or her own airway, intubation with an endotracheal or tracheostomy tube may be necessary. Endotracheal tubes are used for short periods of time. If longer intubation is required, a tracheostomy performed in the operating room is the treatment of choice.
- General care of the person with an endotracheal or tracheostomy tube includes measures to minimize infection, including proper suctioning technique, humidification of the airway, proper care of respiratory therapy equipment, frequent mouth care, and adequate nutrition.
- To ensure adequate ventilation and oxygenation, the patient's lung sounds are assessed frequently. Turning and repositioning every 2 hours, assessing respiratory frequency, tidal volume and vital capacity, and providing chest physiotherapy including clapping, vibrating, and postural drainage are essential.
- Precautions pertaining to endotracheal or tracheostomy tubes include assessing tube placement at regular intervals, keeping a spare tube on hand for emergencies, minimizing sensory deprivation by developing a method of communication, talking directly to the patient and explaining all procedures, reorienting the patient frequently, encouraging family and friends to talk with the patient, keeping call light within reach, and reinforcing that the patient will be able to speak after extubation.
- Precautions to be observed after extubation include frequent monitoring for respiratory distress, adequacy of cough and gag reflex, and care of stoma incision.
- Patients who are being discharged with an endotracheal or tracheostomy tube in place will need to be taught how to care for their own tubes before discharge. The home will need to be visited before discharge to be sure that the patient and equipment can be accommodated. Community sources for equipment and supplies will need to be determined before discharge.
- The patient discharged with a tracheostomy or laryngectomy is given home-going instructions that include increasing humidity with a cool mist humidifier, covering stoma with a dampened stoma cover; washing stoma daily with washcloth and warm water and soap; suctioning stoma or tube; keeping stoma covered when going outside; precautions when bathing, shampooing, and shaving; and wearing a medical identification bracelet or carrying a card saying "I am a total neck breather."

## MALIGNANCIES OF THE HEAD AND NECK

- Heavy alcohol use and tobacco abuse are etiologic factors in persons with head and neck cancers.
- Postoperative care after paranasal surgery includes gentle mouth care with an oral irrigating solution of saline and hydrogen peroxide, weak sodium bicarbonate, or antibiotic solution.
- Oropharyngeal cancers are treated with radiotherapy and surgical exicsion. With extensive resection, reconstructive surgery with skin grafts or flaps will be

necessary. A suction device will be placed in the incision and will require careful monitoring to ensure that it is draining properly.

- Progressive or persistent hoarseness that lasts longer than 2 weeks requires medical evaluation for cancer of the larynx.
- Carcinoma of the larynx is treated with surgery or radiotherapy.
- Partial laryngectomy may be achieved by hemilaryngectomy, or supraglottic partial laryngectomy, after which the person will be able to speak.
- Total laryngectomy is necessary when cancer of the larynx is far advanced. Persons with total laryngectomy are unable to speak normally but will be able to have some form of speech.
- The three major forms of speech following laryngectomy are esophageal, tracheoesophageal, and external speech aid. Tracheoesophageal speech requires the formation of a fistula after all the carcinoma has been removed. This procedure is called a tracheoesophageal puncture (TEP).
- A radical neck dissection is commonly performed along with total laryngectomy because of the risk of metastasis in the neck in some patients.
  1. Postoperatively the person will have a laryngectomy tube and a nasogastric tube in place.
  2. Communication is impaired because of the loss of ability to speak and the person will require speech rehabilitation.
- Patients undergoing laryngectomy may benefit from a visit from a member of the Lost Chord or New Voice club who has undergone laryngectomy and is successfully rehabilitated.
- Postoperative care following laryngectomy includes the following:
  1. Proper positioning: head elevated 30 to 45 degrees.
  2. Maintaining patent airway including proper suctioning of trachesostomy.
  3. Managing the wound by assessing viability of skin flaps (color, temperature, capillary refill, and induration).
  4. Suture line assessment (approximation, edema, color, and drainage) and suture line care to remove scabs and keep suture line clean.
  5. Monitoring closed drainage system to keep tube patent and avoid a massive hematoma under tension. Monitoring includes milking tubing, recording type and amount of drainage, checking for air leaks.
  6. A nasogastric tube is inserted during surgery and removed as soon as person can swallow. The patient must be able to tolerate a soft diet before discharge, which is on the seventh day (DRG requirement).
  7. Assisting patient in communicating.
  8. Being sensitive to patient's reaction to changes in appearance.
  9. Preparing patient for discharge.
- Postoperative care of a patient with a neck dissection is similar to that for a patient with a laryngectomy and includes the following:
  1. Elevating head of bed 30 degrees
  2. Monitoring for airway obstruction
  3. Caring for suture line and assessing skin flaps
  4. Maintaining drainage system
  5. Monitoring shoulder droop
  6. Monitoring ability to ingest optimal calories
  7. Monitoring for depression
- Myocutaneous and free flaps are the major reconstructive flaps used after radical neck dissection.

## REFERENCES


1. American Cancer Society: *Cancer facts and figures 1993*, Atlanta, 1993, The Society.
2. DeWeese DD, Saunders WH: *Otolaryngology—head and neck surgery,* ed 7, St Louis, 1987, Mosby.
3. Drougton ML, Krech RL: Head and neck cancer resection and reconstruction: from past to present, *Today's OR Nurse* 14(9):25-34, 1992.
4. Goodman MS: Head and neck malignancies. In Groenwald SL, editor: *Cancer nursing: principles and practices,* Boston, 1987, Jones & Bartlette.
5. Groothius JR: Viral respiratory infections. In Rakel RE: *Conn's current therapy 1993,* Philadelphia, 1993, WB Saunders Co.
6. Hassard AD, Holness RO: The "cross-bow" incision and nasal flap: its blood supply on clinical application. *Head Neck Surg* 7:135-138, 1984.
7. Heffner JE, Sahn SA: The technique of weaning from tracheostomy, *J Crit Illness* 2(6):74-78, 1987.
8. Hirsch JE: Ear, nose and throat. In Thompson JM et al: *Mosby's manual of clinical nursing,* ed 2, St Louis, 1989, Mosby.
9. Holt JE: Orbital blowout fracture, *Ear Nose Throat J* 62:346-351, 1983.
10. Kaplow R, Bookbinder M: A comparison of four endotracheal tube holders, *Heart Lung* 23(1):59-66, 1994.
11. Lavertu P, Droughton ML: Postoperative management following head and neck surgery. In Sviak E, Higgins D, Scivers A, editors: *The high risk patient: management of the critically ill,* Philadelphia, Lea & Febiger. (In press.)
12. Leach JL, Schaeffer S: Sinusitis. In Rakel RE: *Conn's current therapy 1993,* Philadelphia, 1993, WB Saunders Co.
13. Miller WE: The role of the outpatient nurse in endoscopic sinus surgery, *ORL Head Neck Nurs* 10(3):20-24, 1992.
14. Mulgrew B, Dropkin ML: Coping with craniofacial resection: a cases study, *The Journal,* pp 8-27, Summer 1991.
15. Pichichero ME: Streptoccal pharyngitis. In Rakel RE: *Conn's current therapy 1993,* Philadelphia, 1993, WB Saunders Co.
16. Scher RL, Richtsmeier WJ: Otolaryngology: head and neck surgery. In Sabiston DC, Jr, Lyerly KH, *Sabiston: Essentials of surgery*, ed 2, Philadelphia, 1994, WB Saunders Co.
17. Sigler BA, Schuring LT: *Ear, nose and throat disorders,* St Louis, 1993, Mosby.
18. Yonkers AJ: Sinusitis: inspecting the causes and treatment, *Ear, Nose Throat J* 71(6):258-262, 1991.

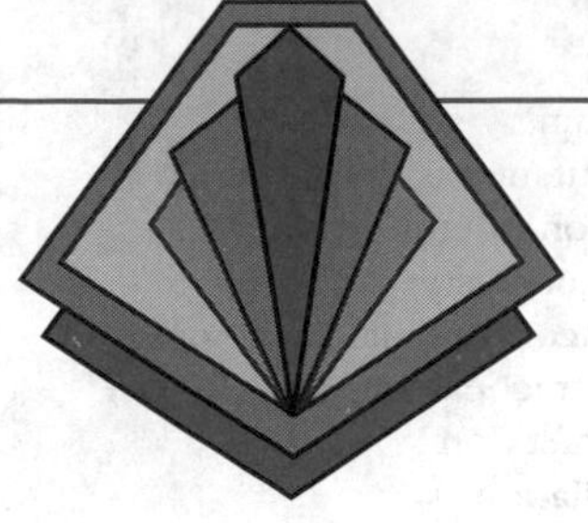

C H A P T E R 37

# Management of Persons With Problems of the Lower Airway

*Wilma J. Phipps*
*Josephine Jacobs Brucia*

## CHAPTER OBJECTIVES

***After studying this chapter, the learner should be able to do the following:***

1 Describe primary and secondary prevention of respiratory problems.
2 Differentiate between restrictive and obstructive pulmonary disorders.
3 Describe the nature of viral respiratory infections and methods of assisting effective coughing.
4 Compare community-acquired and hospital-acquired pneumonias.
5 Describe incidence, preventive measures, and treatment of tuberculosis.
6 Compare fungal infections of the respiratory tract.
7 Explain the pathophysiology of adult respiratory distress syndrome (ARDS).
8 Describe incidence, prevention, and therapy for lung cancer.
9 Discuss the points to include in a teaching plan for the patient who is to have resectional surgery of the lung.
10 List five precautions to be observed in care of chest tubes and a closed drainage system, and give the rationale for each.
11 Differentiate between a closed, open, and tension pneumothorax in terms of clinical manifestations and nursing management.
12 Describe the treatment for each type of pneumothorax.
13 Explain the pathophysiology of and interventions for chronic bronchitis, pulmonary emphysema, and asthma.
14 Describe how you would teach the patient with chronic obstructive pulmonary disease (COPD) to use a metered-dose inhaler and an inhaler with a spacer.
15 Discuss the clinical manifestations of cystic fibrosis (CF) in adults.
16 Describe the nature of respiratory failure and the care of the patient with an artificial airway and mechanical ventilation.
17 Differentiate between a pressure-cycled and a volume-cycled ventilator.
18 Describe the methods used in weaning the patient from the ventilator.

## KEY TERMS

adult respiratory disease syndrome (ARDS)
apnea
alveolocapillary membrane
aspiration pneumonia
atypical pneumonia
bilobectomy
biphasic airway pressure
blastomycosis
blunt injury
breathing exercise
bronchopleural fistula (BPF)
caseation necrosis
chronic bronchitis
chronic obstructive pulmonary disease (COPD)
clapping
closed pneumothorax
coccidioidomycosis
community-acquired pneumonia (CAP)
continuous positive airway pressure (CPAP)
cystic fibrosis
decortication
diffusion
directly observed therapy (DOT)
exploratory thoracotomy
flail chest
fractured ribs
hemothorax
histoplasmosis
hospital-acquired pneumonia
hypoventilation hypoxemia
liquefaction necrosis
lobectomy
mechanical ventilation
mycobacterium other than TB (MOTT)
nasal cannula
nosocomial pneumonia

open pneumothorax
paradoxical breathing
penetrating injury
perfusion
pneumonectomy
pneumothorax
positive-end expiratory pressure (PEEP)
pressure-support ventilation (PSV)
primary TB complex
pulmonary contusion
pulmonary embolism (PE)
pulmonary emphysema
reactivation tuberculosis
respiratory acidosis
respiratory failure
respiratory insufficiency
sarcoidosis
segmental postural drainage
segmental resection (segmentectomy)
sleeve lobectomy
spontaneous pneumothorax
sputum
subcutaneous emphysema
tension pneumothorax
thoracoplasty
tracheobronchial suctioning
transtracheal catheter
TB infection
ventilation
vibrating
volume-cycled ventilator
wedge resection

Many diseases affect the respiratory system, including both acute (short-term) and chronic (long-term) diseases. Substantial changes in the relative incidence of diseases affecting the respiratory system have occurred in the past few decades. Although chronic infectious disorders, such as tuberculosis, lung abscess, and bronchiectasis, have decreased, persons with chronic bronchitis and emphysema now survive longer and constitute an increasing number of persons with chronic respiratory disease, along with those with environmental lung disease. In addition, modern intercontinental travel has increased the incidence of parasitic lung infestations in the western world. Also, the reduction of immunologic competence that occurs with cancer chemotherapy, immunosuppressant medications administered after organ transplantation, or with acquired immune deficiency syndrome (AIDS) has resulted in an increased incidence of opportunistic infections of the lungs with a variety of microorganisms that were rarely pathogenic in the past.

The most significant pulmonary diseases are those that are chronic and have increased dramatically in recent years. Current statistics indicate that 17 million Americans have emphysema, asthma, and chronic bronchitis. This number can be expected to increase yearly as the number of elderly persons in our society increases. Because most diseases of the respiratory tract are not reportable, the full extent of both acute and chronic illness is difficult to estimate. However, known facts about disability from chronic pulmonary diseases indicate that they are a major health problem and that they cause tremendous losses in productivity in the United States. The Social Security Administration reports that disability payments to persons with chronic pulmonary problems are second only to payments to persons with heart problems. Whereas mortality from tuberculosis has declined, mortality from bronchitis, emphysema, and lung cancer has continued to rise yearly.

## PULMONARY DISEASE PREVENTION

The objectives of health education in relation to pulmonary diseases are the same as for other diseases. Prevention, early diagnosis, prompt and often continued treatment, limitation of disability, and rehabilitation should be emphasized for all persons. Early symptoms of respiratory diseases are probably those most often ignored by the general population. With the exception of acute pulmonary disorders, the major factor preventing early diagnosis and treatment of pulmonary diseases is the insidious nature of their signs and symptoms. Nurses should encourage individuals and families to seek proper medical attention if they have symptoms such as *cough, difficulty breathing, production of sputum, shortness of breath,* and *nose and throat irritation* that do not subside within 2 weeks. These symptoms are suggestive of respiratory diseases and should be investigated.

Tobacco use is the leading cause of preventable death in the United States. Several organizations, most notably the American Lung Association (ALA), the American Cancer Society (ACS), and the American Heart Association (AHA), along with the federal government have launched campaigns to reduce tobacco use in the United States. The stated objective of the U.S. government was to reduce the proportion of smokers in the national population to 25% by 1990. This figure was not reached, however, and the figures for 1991 (25.6%) and 1992 (26.5%) indicate that slightly more than the desired 25% of adults over age 18 were smokers. The figures also indicate differences in rates by gender, age-groups, race and ethnicity, educational level, and socioeconomic status. Table 37-1 provides more information.

Efforts are also underway to decrease smoking among young people. Two reports by the Centers for Disease Control and Prevention (CDC) published in 1994 attest to the problem of tobacco use among youth and describes plans to prevent young persons from beginning to use tobacco.[9,11]

In a report to the surgeon general from the Office of Smoking and Health, the foreword points out that this is the first report to focus on young people alone, and it underscores the seriousness of tobacco use, its relationship to other adolescent problem behaviors, and the responsibility of all citizens to protect our children's health. The use of tobacco, particularly cigarette smoking, has not declined over the past decade, and 28% of

**TABLE 37-1 Percentage of Adults Age 18 and Over Who Were Current Cigarette Smokers by Gender, Age-Group, Racial Ethnicity, Level of Education, and Socioeconomic Status**

| CHARACTERISTIC | 1991 | 1992 |
|---|---|---|
| **GENDER** | | |
| Men | 28.1 | 28.6 |
| Women | 23.5 | 24.6 |
| **AGE-GROUP** | | |
| 18-24 | 22.9 | 26.4 |
| 25-44 | 30.4 | 30.8 |
| 45-64 | 26.8 | 27.3 |
| >65 | 13.3 | 14.0 |
| **RACE/ETHNICITY** | | |
| White | 26.0 | 27.2 |
| Black | 29.4 | 27.8 |
| Hispanic | 20.1 | 20.7 |
| Native American/Native Alaskan | 31.9 | 39.4 |
| Asian/Pacific Islander | 15.9 | 15.2 |
| **EDUCATIONAL LEVEL (YEARS)** | | |
| <12 | 32.0 | 31.8 |
| 12 | 39.9 | 31.1 |
| 13-15 | 23.4 | 24.1 |
| >16 | 13.6 | 15.5 |
| **SOCIOECONOMIC STATUS** | | |
| At/above poverty level | 24.7 | 25.4 |
| Below poverty level | 33.1 | 34.9 |
| Unknown | 26.0 | 26.9 |
| TOTAL | 25.6 | 26.5 |

From Centers for Disease Control and Prevention: United States National Health Survey, 1991 and 1992, *MMWR* 43(19):342-346, 1994.

high-school seniors are currently cigarette smokers.[11] The committee who worked on the report reached six major conclusions:

1. Nearly all first use of tobacco occurs before high-school graduation; this finding suggests that if adolescents can be kept tobacco free, most will never start using tobacco.
2. Most adolescent smokers are addicted to nicotine and report that they want to quit but are unable to do so; they experience relapse rates and withdrawal symptoms similar to those reported by adults.
3. Tobacco is often the first drug used by those young people who use alcohol, marijuana, and other drugs.
4. Adolescents with lower levels of school achievement, with fewer skills to resist pervasive influences to use tobacco, with friends who use tobacco, and with lower self-image are more likely than their peers to use tobacco.
5. Cigarette advertising appears to increase young people's risk of smoking by affecting their perceptions of the pervasiveness, image, and function of smoking.
6. Community-wide efforts that include tobacco tax increases, enforcement of minors' access laws, youth-oriented mass media campaigns, and school-based tobacco-use prevention programs are successful in reducing adolescent use of tobacco.

In the United States, most daily smokers (82%) began smoking before age 18, and more than 3000 young persons begin smoking each day.[11] Attempting to reduce tobacco use among this group, the CDC published "Guidelines for School Health Programs To Prevent Tobacco Use and Addiction." The guidelines offer recommendations for school health problems for students from the kindergarten through the 12th grade. The seven recommendations below summarize strategies that are effective in preventing tobacco use among youth. To ensure the greatest impact, schools should implement all seven recommendations.

1. Develop and enforce a school policy on tobacco use.
2. Provide instruction about the short-term and long-term negative physiologic and social consequences of tobacco use, social influences on tobacco use, peer norms regarding tobacco use, and refusal skills.
3. Provide tobacco-use prevention education in kindergarten through 12th grade; this instruction should be especially intensive in junior high or middle school and should be reinforced in high school.
4. Provide program-specific training for teachers.
5. Involve parents or families in support of school-based programs to prevent tobacco use.
6. Support cessation efforts among students and all school staff who use tobacco.
7. Assess the tobacco-use prevention program at regular intervals.

Along with the campaign to decrease smoking, there has been increased emphasis on reducing pollution in the environment, which has resulted in legislation such as the Clean Air Act. With the resurgent use of wood stoves, particularly in urban areas, wood smoke has become the major source of pollutants, suspected to be potent carcinogens (polycyclic organic matter) in the United States. Under the auspices of the Clean Air Act, the U.S. Environmental Protection Agency has taken action to implement a nationwide emissions control program for wood stoves. Some of the measures taken to reduce pollution are presently threatened, since some believe they are too costly for the benefits achieved. This issue will be at the forefront through the 1990s, and nurses, as health professionals and concerned citizens, will need to keep themselves informed about proposed changes and their effects on health.

Nurses seeking current information about respiratory

diseases and their treatment are referred to the ALA and its local branches for information. The American Thoracic Society, the medical section of the ALA, publishes a journal* that is an excellent source of current information on all acute and chronic respiratory diseases. The ALA also publishes the *Bulletin,* many booklets and pamphlets, and newsletters that aid nurses in educating the public and in teaching patients.

## CLASSIFICATION OF PULMONARY DISORDERS

One way to classify lung diseases is to differentiate the various pulmonary disorders on the basis of how they affect ventilation. This system divides pulmonary disorders into either restrictive or obstructive ventilatory defects. A third category of pulmonary disorders consists of those that affect the pulmonary vascular system and thus alter the ability of the lung to carry out respiration.

Although it is convenient to classify pulmonary disorders according to these categories, pulmonary diseases rarely fall exclusively into one of the three groupings. Of the three categories, *obstructive airway disease* (OAD) has been most criticized as being inaccurate and misleading because it implies that the primary pathology of diseases falling within this category is obstruction of the airways. For example, emphysema, a major OAD, causes limitation to expiratory airflow by enlargement of alveolar air space through tissue destruction, rather than by primary airway obstruction. Pulmonary experts have recommended that diseases resulting in diminished expiratory airflow be identified as syndromes of *chronic airflow limitation.* In the clinical setting, however, *OAD* or **chronic obstructive pulmonary disease (COPD)** continues to be the most common terminology used to describe this group of pulmonary disorders.

Communication among health professionals is hampered by both the many terms used to label chronic airflow limitation and by inconsistent definition. Thus pulmonary diseases fall under the classification umbrella of chronic airflow limitation, OAD, or COPD.

**American Review of Respiratory Diseases,* published by the American Lung Association, 1740 Broadway, New York, NY.

### RESTRICTIVE LUNG DISEASE

In restrictive lung disease, there is a limitation to full expansion of the lungs. Static lung volumes are diminished as a result of decreased lung or thoracic compliance (Table 37-2).

Patients with a restrictive disorder may demonstrate respiratory alkalosis caused by a compensatory increase in respiratory frequency (rate) to offset diminished lung volumes. When the increased respiratory rate no longer adequately compensates for the diminished lung volumes, *hypoxemia* (low arterial blood oxygen) occurs. Clinically, persons with restrictive disorders exhibit some degree of dyspnea. Often they will become dyspneic only on exertion. As the restrictive disease progresses, however, persons will become dyspneic at rest. Additionally, persons with restrictive disorders often have a dry, hacking cough. Table 37-3 lists major disorders that result in primarily restrictive ventilatory defects.

### OBSTRUCTIVE AIRWAY DISEASE

Obstructive airway disease includes any process that limits airflow on expiration. Both lung compliance (lung expansibility) and airway resistance are increased. These pathophysiologic changes alter the ability to move air out of the lungs, which results in characteristic changes in both static and dynamic lung volume measurement (see Table 37-2). Clinically, persons with OAD may exhibit a prolonged expiration time, increased anteroposterior thorax diameter, and hyperresonance on percussion. Persons with pulmonary disorders characterized by the preceding description have been identified as having COPD, which has classically included any mixture of *emphysema, chronic bronchitis,* and *asthma,* although some experts believe that asthma should not be included. The ongoing controversy over what should or should not be included under COPD lends support

**TABLE 37-2 Comparison of Pulmonary Function Test Results in Restrictive and Obstructive Disease**

| TEST | RESTRICTIVE | OBSTRUCTIVE |
|---|---|---|
| FVC | Decreased | Decreased or normal |
| RV | Decreased | Increased |
| TLC | Decreased | Normal or increased |
| RV/TLC | Normal or increased | Significantly increased |
| $FEV_{1.0}/FVC$ | Normal or increased | Decreased |
| $FEV_{3.0}/FVC$ | Normal or increased | Decreased |

FVC, Forced vital capacity; RV, residual volume; TLC, total lung capacity; FEV, forced expiratory volume (in 1, 3 seconds).

**TABLE 37-3 Restrictive Pulmonary Diseases**

| ALTERATION | DISEASE EXAMPLE |
|---|---|
| Parenchymal inflammation | Pneumonia, adult respiratory distress syndrome |
| Space-occupying lesions | Tumors, malignancies |
| Diffuse pulmonary disease | Silicosis, fibrosis |
| Pleural disease | Pleural effusion |
| Lung collapse | Pneumothorax, atelectasis |
| Resectional surgery | Pneumonectomy |
| Neuromuscular disorders | Poliomyelitis, Guillain-Barré syndrome |
| Central nervous system (CNS) depression | Narcotics, cerebral edema |

to those who argue that the classic subdivisions of COPD be abandoned and that all be classified as *chronic airflow limitation*. However, because COPD is the most frequently used terminology in the clinical setting, discussion of COPD in this chapter includes these three conditions.

The third category of pulmonary disorders considered in this chapter is those identified as resulting in *pulmonary vascular disease*. Pulmonary vascular diseases include any process that results in the narrowing or occlusion of pulmonary blood vessels. In pulmonary vascular disease, efficiency of pulmonary respiration is compromised, usually resulting in hypoxemia. Clinically, patients have *dyspnea, increased respiratory frequency, digital clubbing, atelectasis,* and *chest pain*. Pulmonary vascular disease may result from primary pulmonary hypertension or as a sequela of either circulatory or lung disease. Only pulmonary vascular disease related to pulmonary emboli and pulmonary infarction is discussed here. This chapter presents restrictive diseases first, beginning with the infectious diseases. Obstructive lung diseases and pulmonary vascular diseases are discussed later in the chapter.

# INFECTIOUS DISEASES OF THE RESPIRATORY TRACT

The respiratory tract is in contact with the environment via inhalation of ambient air. Fortunately, the lung has a variety of defense mechanisms to prevent contamination of the respiratory tract with infectious agents (Box 37-1).

## VIRAL INFECTIONS

Many acute respiratory disorders are caused by viral pathogens. Presently, more than 100 viruses have been found to be directly related to respiratory infections. Some diseases may be caused by one virus, or different viruses may cause the same symptoms. Although viral respiratory infections such as the common cold tend to be self-limiting, certain viral strains can induce life-threatening illness by themselves or as a result of secondary bacterial infections.

### Common Cold, Influenza

#### Etiology

The specific virus causing the common cold is unknown. Influenza is usually caused by one of three myxoviruses that are categorized as influenza types A, B, or C. Type A influenza virus has a greater tendency to mutate than the other viral types; thus it is more often the strain that causes worldwide epidemics.

#### Epidemiology

Few persons escape upper respiratory tract infections (URIs). The average among the general population is three colds per person each year. Indeed, Americans spend more than 380 million days in bed each year because of colds and influenza.

Respiratory diseases, primarily virus infections, are responsible for 30% to 50% of time lost from work by adults and from 60% to 80% of time lost by children from school. The frequency of their occurrence, the number of people affected, the resulting economic loss, and the possibility that URI may lead to more serious diseases are reasons why colds and influenza merit serious attention.

#### Prevention

Colds and influenza are communicable diseases spread by droplet nuclei. The only known way to totally prevent spread of URIs from one individual to another is to isolate the infected person, which is extremely difficult in our society. However, there are several ways to minimize the spread of infection. Persons with colds should avoid crowded places such as theaters. The individual should particularly avoid contact with, and therefore exposure of, infants and young children, persons who have chronic lung diseases such as bronchitis and emphysema, those who have recently had an anesthetic, and elderly people. Covering the nose and mouth when sneezing and coughing prevents the contamination of the air breathed by others. Frequent *washing of hands, covering of coughs and sneezes,* and *careful disposal of waste tissues* are *protective health measures* that are advisable for everyone; however, they become increasingly important when known respiratory tract infection exists. Because colds and influenza are communicable diseases, the principles for protection of oneself and others should be practiced.

The CDC[13] recommends that the following populations at risk for influenza-related complications receive influenza vaccine every fall:

- Persons 65 years of age or older
- Residents of nursing homes and other chronic-care facilities that house persons of any age with chronic medical conditions
- Adults and children with chronic disorders of the pulmonary or cardiovascular systems, including children with asthma
- Adults and children who have required regular medical follow-up or hospitalization during the preceding year because of chronic metabolic diseases (including diabetes mellitus), renal dysfunction, hemoglobinopathies, or immunosuppression (including immunosuppression caused by medications)
- Children and teenagers (6 months to 18 years of age) who are receiving long-term aspirin therapy and therefore may be at risk for developing Reye syndrome after influenza

The CDC[13] also recommends vaccinations for caregivers and others who could transmit the influenza virus to vulnerable patients:

## BOX 37-1 Lung Defense Mechanisms

### UPPER AIRWAY DEFENSES AGAINST PULMONARY INFECTION

#### Removing Particulate Matter From Inspired Air

Particles greater than 20 μm settle back on surfaces
Particles 5-10 μm deposited in nose
Particles 0.1-10 μm remain suspended in air for long periods and are then inhaled
Particles 1-5 μm deposited in tracheobronchial tree
- Droplet nuclei 2-4 μm (dried particles from sneezing, coughing, talking)
- May contain viruses or bacteria
- Spread organisms from person to person

#### Minimizing Microbial Population on Membranes of Upper Respiratory Tract

Mucocillary transport
- Posterior two thirds of nasal cavity, sinuses, and nasopharynx lined by *ciliated epithelium* covered with thin layer of mucus
- Dense concentration of small blood vessels present beneath ciliated epithelium and mucous layers
- Mucus and fluid produced = 1000 ml/24 hr in normal persons
- Mucus and fluid carried at rate of 5-10 mm/min back into hypopharynx by beating action of cilia
- Substances in secretions inhibit microbial growth and prevent organisms from sticking to mucous membranes
  - Immunoglobulins (secretory IgA)
  - Lysozyme
  - Complement

#### Minimizing Possibility of Aspiration

Motor function of upper airway
- Laryngeal mechanism—closes glottis when swallowing to protect larynx
  - Gag reflex also closes glottis
  - Clearing throat/spitting clear upper airway

Contamination of lower respiratory tract
- Impaired clearance of particles in upper airway = spread of bacteria
- Accumulation of debris and microbes → penetration of tissues = sinusitis, otitis media
- Accumulation of debris and microbes → aspiration into trachea; lung abscess caused by anaerobic bacteria secondary to severe gingival disease
- Intoxication or distraction → aspiration
- Normal sleep → minor aspiration
- Aspiration of pharyngeal contents → lung → bacterial pneumonia

### LOWER RESPIRATORY TRACT CLEARANCE MECHANISMS

#### Pulmonary Reflex

Cough—involuntary reflex elicited by stimulation of irritant receptors in subepithelium of hypopharynx, larynx, and tracheobronchial tree: mediated by vagus nerve
- Facilitator of mucociliary clearance
- Aids in dealing with gross contamination from above larynx

Bronchoconstriction—reflex response to airway irritants
- Decreased size of bronchus and forced expiration and cough propel debris toward mouth
- Excessive bronchoconstriction (asthma) = decreased expiratory airflow, air trapped in lung, difficulty with effective cough

#### Mucociliary Clearance

Mucus secreted by epithelial goblet cells from submucosal glands; 0.10-100 ml passes up trachea into hypopharynx and is swallowed; amount and nature of mucus secreted are controlled, in part, by parasympathetic nervous system affected by neurohumoral stimulation (adrenergic or cholinergic) and by direct mucosal irritation

Cilia (200 cilia/each cell surface) beat rhythmically 1200 beats/min mouthward beginning at terminal bronchioles → larynx; beating of cilia → overlying mucous layer → mouthward at rate of 0.5 mm/min in small airways to about 10 mm/min in major bronchi

Clearance increased by:
- Bronchodilator drugs
  - Beta-adrenergic agents (ephedrine) stimulate transport of water and salt into mucus = ↓ viscosity of mucus
  - Methylxanthines (aminophylline) → ↑ mucus production and ciliary activity

Ciliary function depressed by:
- Chronic exposure to airway irritants—cigarette smoke and other irritants
- Pharmacologic agents—100% $O_2$, anticholinergic agents, alcohol
- Infection such as viral bronchitis

Mucus production increased by:
- Chronic irritation of respiratory tract → increase in number of mucus-secreting goblet cells = ↑ mucus
- Inflammatory response to irritation → ↑ numbers of phagocytic cells and amount of cellular debris in mucus (especially DNA) = ↑ viscosity of mucus, which is less readily moved along by ciliary action

Immotile cilia—congenital impairment
- *Kartagener's syndrome*—sinusitis, recurrent lung infection, and sinus inversus
- *Cystic fibrosis*—infection, chronic inflammatory increases in respiratory mucus volume and viscosity = impaired lung clearance and progressive lung damage

### INTRAPULMONARY DETOXIFICATION MECHANISM

#### Phagocytes

Alveolar macrophage
- Phagocytosis of particles—inhaled particulate debris, bacteria, or cell constituents
- Kills most microbes

Polymorphonuclear neutrophil present in blood (normally only small number in lung)
- Avid phagocyte—kills microbes
- Defends against established infectious processes
- Infection—products of inflammation attract neutrophils to site of infection (chemotaxis)

Factors interfering with phagocytosis
- Inhibition of alveolar macrophage function
  - Cigarette smoke
  - Other inhaled pollutants—ozone, nitrogen dioxide, oxygen
  - Drugs—corticosteroids, antineoplastic and antiinflammatory cytoxic agents, ethanol (alcohol)
  - Metabolic derangements—uremia, hyperglycemia of diabetes mellitus
  - Acquired granulocytopenia—bone marrow depression from cytoxic drugs

**BOX 37-1 Lung Defense Mechanisms—cont'd**

**Immunoglobulins**

IgA and IgG—most important for lung defense; present in secretions of respiratory tract as well as in blood
- IgA antibodies—specific for viral antigens; neutralize viruses and prevent infection
- IgG predominates in terminal lung units; antigen-specific IgG contributes to local defense against bacterial infections (important in neutralizing highly pathogenic encapsulated bacteria [especially *Streptococcus pneumoniae* and *Haemophilus influenzae*], which are resistant to phagocytosis)

**Cell-Mediated Immunity (CMI)**

One half of lymphocytes in and around airways are thymus-derived lymphocytes, or *T cells*
- Found in lymphoid aggregates adjacent to bronchi (bronchus-associated lymphoid tissues, or BALT)

T cells important in:
- Resistance to some viral infections
- Resistance to most fungal infections
- Infections by organisms that survive and multiply inside host cells: *Mycobacterium tuberculosis, Brucella, Listeria monocytogenes, Pneumocystis carinii*

Impaired CMI = ↑ susceptibility to infection
- Deficient T-cell function (anergy) associated with:
  - Neoplasms—lymphoma
  - Cytotoxic or corticosteroid therapy
  - Systemic diseases—sarcoidosis, malnutrition
- Some lung infections occur almost exclusively with severely impaired CMI—pneumonia caused by cytomegalovirus, herpes zoster, *Aspergillus* species, or *Pneumocystis carinii*

- Physicians, nurses, and other personnel in both hospital and outpatient care settings
- Employees of nursing homes and chronic-care facilities who have contact with patients or residents
- Providers of home care to persons at high risk (e.g., visiting nurses, volunteer workers)
- Household members (including children) of persons in high-risk groups

### Pathophysiology

Symptoms of either a cold or influenza usually appear suddenly, and the infection may be full-blown within 48 hours. Box 37-2 presents the signs and symptoms associated with a URI.

The infected individual is contagious for 2 to 3 days after onset of symptoms. The course of a URI is variable but ordinarily lasts from 7 to 14 days. It is difficult to determine when a cold or influenza ends and when complications appear. Tracheobronchitis is a complication usually caused by a secondary bacterial infection. Acute sinusitis and otitis media may also follow a URI.

### Medical and nursing management

Treatment of colds and influenza is directed toward relief of symptoms and control of complications. Persons considered to be at higher risk, such as those with chronic lung disease or those who are immunologically compromised, should be encouraged to seek medical assistance. Additionally, persons who display a continued temperature elevation, headache, or muscular aches should seek the advice of a physician. The Guidelines box below outlines general treatment of URI symptoms.

Additionally, influenza vaccine should be given yearly to all persons at high risk for developing complications of influenza. The vaccine is recommended for all persons with chronic heart or lung disease unless they are allergic to eggs or egg products or have had a previous reaction to the vaccine. It is also recommended for all persons age 65 or older because they are at high risk of developing complications from influenza.

**BOX 37-2 Signs and Symptoms of Upper Respiratory Tract Infection**

| SIGNS | SYMPTOMS |
|---|---|
| Cough | General malaise |
| Nasal discharge | Rhinitis |
| Erythematous pharynx | Sore throat |
| Conjunctivitis | Watery eyes |
| Laryngitis | |
| Low-grade temperature | |

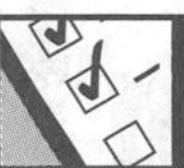

**Guidelines for Managing Upper Respiratory Tract Infection**

Increased fluid intake (3 to 4 L/day)
Frequent rest periods
Medications
- Antipyretics/analgesics: acetylsalicylic acid, acetaminophen
- Oral decongestants: pseudephedrine
- Nasal decongestants: ephedrine, 0.5% to 2%
  - NOTE: use of nasal decongestants should be time limited to avoid increasing severity of nasal symptoms
- Cough suppressants if cough is nonproductive

## Acute Bronchitis

### Etiology

Bronchitis can be acute or chronic (chronic bronchitis is discussed later in this chapter). Acute bronchitis is an inflammation of the bronchi and usually the trachea (tracheobronchitis).

### Epidemiology

Although acute bronchitis occurs most often in persons with chronic lung disease, it also occurs as an extension of a URI in persons without underlying lung disease and is therefore communicable. It also may be caused by physical or chemical agents such as dust, smoke, or volatile fumes. As air pollution increases, the incidence of acute bronchitis increases. Acute bronchitis is typically viral in origin, but bacterial pathogens such as *Streptococcus pneumoniae* and *Haemophilus influenzae* may also cause bronchitis either as a primary or secondary infection (Box 37-3).

### Pathophysiology

As part of the inflammatory process, there is increased blood flow to the affected area causing an increase in pulmonary secretions. A painful cough with sputum production, low-grade fever, and malaise are common symptoms. The patient may have pain beneath the sternum caused by inflammation of the tracheal wall. Bronchitis without tracheitis is never seen, and the term *tracheobronchitis* would be more appropriate for this condition.[39] Symptoms usually last 1 to 2 weeks but may continue for 3 to 4 weeks. Rhonchi and wheezes are heard on chest examination. If symptoms worsen and there is a high fever, shortness of breath, pleuritic chest pain (pain on inspiration), rapid respirations, and rales or signs of consolidation on physical examination of the chest, pneumonia is suspected.

**BOX 37-3 Infectious Causes of Acute Bronchitis**

**VIRUSES**

Rhinovirus
Adenovirus
Influenza A and B
Parainfluenza virus
Respiratory syncytial virus (RSV)

**BACTERIA**

*Streptococcus pneumoniae*
*Haemophilus influenzae*
*Moraxella catarrhalis*
*Bordetella pertussis*
*Mycoplasma pneumoniae*
*Chlamydia pneumoniae* (TWAR strain)

From Rich EA, Ellner JJ: Acute bronchitis. In Rakel RE, editor: *Conn's current therapy,* Philadelphia, 1993, Saunders.

### Medical management

Treatment of acute bronchitis is mainly supportive and includes the following:

1. Codeine or dextromorphan is prescribed if cough is bothering the patient and increasing pain. It is only prescribed if the patient has little sputum. If the patient has a productive cough, it would not be given because cough is a protective mechanism to clear airway of secretions.
2. Decongestants and antihistamines are used sparingly, if at all, because they tend to dry secretions and make them more difficult to remove.
3. Encourage oral fluid intake, 2 to 3 L/day, if there is no contraindication to increasing fluid intake.
4. Aspirin helps reduce fever and alleviate some of the symptoms of inflammation.
5. Rest is encouraged to give the body a chance to heal.
6. Amantadine (Symmetrel), 100 to 200 mg daily until symptoms have subsided, is used to prevent or shorten the course of influenza A. It must be started within 24 to 48 hours after onset of symptoms.
7. Bronchodilator therapy is prescribed for patients who are wheezing and for those whose peak expiratory flow rate is prolonged.[37] An inhaled beta ($\beta$-)-agonist such as metaproterenol (Alupent), 2 puffs/day alone or with a theophylline preparation, is usually prescribed.
8. Patients who are smokers are urged to quit.
9. Antibiotics are usually not prescribed unless there is evidence of a bacterial infection. Exceptions would include a protracted course of more than 2 weeks in persons with underlying chronic disease such as diabetes mellitus, cirrhosis, congestive heart failure, or chronic obstructive pulmonary disease (COPD), as well as elderly persons in general.[39] All these persons are at a higher risk for pneumonia.

### Nursing management

Nursing care is also supportive and is directed toward helping the patient meet the prescribed therapy and avoid future infection.

**Assisting with coughing.** Help the patient cough effectively. Coughing is normally a mechanism that aids in the removal of inhaled foreign materials. When an infection is present, the throat becomes dry and irritated, and mucus production increases as part of the lungs' defense mechanisms.

Receptors for the cough reflex are located in the tracheal and bronchial mucosa, with the largest concentration of them found in the larynx, carina, and bifurcations of the large and medium-sized bronchi. When these receptors are stimulated, impulses are transmitted primarily via the afferent nervous pathways (vagus, phrenic, spinal motor nerves) to expiratory musculature (larynx, tracheobronchial tree, diaphragm, abdominal wall).

To produce an effective cough, a deep inspiration must be followed by maximal expiratory effort against a closed glottis. This results in a tremendous increase in intrathoracic pressure. As the glottis opens, mucus and inhaled particles are forced out of the airways at a high velocity.

Persistent coughing can be very annoying and tiring to the patient and those around him or her. Complications of persistent coughing include insomnia, exhaustion, vomiting, urinary incontinence, rib or muscle trauma, pneumothorax, or fainting. If cough is present, give medication, if prescribed. Table 37-4 lists frequently used medications and their desired effects.

Assist with coughing as necessary by supporting chest (front and back) with an open palm as the patient coughs. Teach the patient to cough effectively to maintain a clear airway, and collect required specimens. Tell the patient to take a deep breath, force the air out down to residual volume, contract the diaphragm, exhale forcefully, and then cough. Successful airway clearance and an effective breathing pattern should help return vital signs to prebronchitis levels.

Additional assistance in achieving therapeutic goals includes the following:

1. Provide for good drainage of tracheobronchial secretion.
2. If antibiotics are prescribed, give on time to maintain therapeutic blood levels.
3. If steam vaporization is prescribed, use precautions described on p. 1069.
4. If a bronchodilator is ordered, teach patient how to use an inhaler with a spacer (see p. 1127).
5. Offer fluids frequently to ensure an intake of 2 to 3 L daily.

**TABLE 37-4 Medications Used To Treat Cough**

| DESIRED EFFECT | MEDICATIONS PRESCRIBED |
|---|---|
| ↑ Secretions | Expectorants |
| | Ammonium chloride |
| | Ammonium carbonate |
| | Sodium iodide |
| | Potassium iodide (saturated solution, SSKI) |
| | Terpin hydrate |
| ↓ Secretions | Anticholinergic agents |
| | Atropine |
| Thin secretions | Mucolytic agents |
| | Acetylcysteine (Mucomyst) |
| | Desoxyribonuclease (Dornavac) |
| Depress cough reflex | Antitussives |
| | Narcotic |
| | Codeine |
| | Nonnarcotic agents |
| | Benzonatate (Tessalon) |
| | Noscapine (Nectadon) |
| | Dextromethorphan hydrobromide (Romilar) |
| | Carbetapentane citrate (Toclase) |
| | Levopropoxyphene napsylate (Novrod) |
| | Chlophedianol hydrochloride (Ulo) |

**Assisting with comfort and activities of daily living (ADL)**

1. Place the patient in position of comfort; semi-Fowler's or high-Fowler's position should improve the patient's ability to breathe.
2. Assist with ADL as necessary during acute phase of illness.

**Facilitating learning.** The patient should be taught to avoid persons with URIs. If URI does occur, the patient should seek medical attention.

If the patient smokes cigarettes, he or she should be encouraged to quit smoking. Group programs are helpful to some persons, and the local branches of the ALA, ACS, or AHA can supply the names of local programs to help persons stop smoking.

## BACTERIAL INFECTIONS

### Pneumonia

#### Etiology

Pneumonia is an acute inflammation of lung tissue resulting from inhalation or transport via the bloodstream of infectious agents or noxious fumes or from radiation treatment.

#### Epidemiology

Of all the infectious diseases, pneumonia is the leading cause of death in the United States. More than 3 million cases of pneumonia occur in the United States yearly. Table 37-5 includes risk factors typically associated with the incidence of various types of pneumonia. Most pneumonias are communicable diseases; the mode of transmission depends on the infecting organism. Pneumonia is classified according to the offending organism rather than the anatomic location (lobar or bronchial), as was the practice in the past.

Within the past decade, there have been significant changes in pathogens causing bacterial pneumonia and dramatic shifts in antimicrobial resistance patterns. Many new antimicrobial agents have been developed in response to pathogen resistance. These include β-lactamase inhibitors, fluoroquinolones, macrolides, and azalides. The nurse must keep up-to-date about these changes because drugs now in use may become ineffective in the future. A newer way to classify the pathogens is to divide bacterial pneumonia into **community-acquired pneumonia (CAP)** (Table 37-5) and **hospital-acquired pneumonia.** Table 37-6 shows the prevalence of specific pathogens in these pneumonias. This classification is used in the following discussion.

**TABLE 37-5 Community-Acquired Pneumonia (CAP)**

| ORGANISMS | EPIDEMIOLOGY | THERAPY |
|---|---|---|
| *Streptococcus pneumoniae* | Cause of 50% to 80% of CAP in young adults and 20% to 50% in elderly and debilitated persons | High-dose penicillin G for those requiring hospitalization; are Pen-VK orally for those treated as outpatients |
| Streptococci other than *pneumoniae* species | Cause of 1% to 2% of CAP in healthy adults and 5% to 12% in elderly and debilitated persons (cerebrovascular accidents dementia, esophageal disease) | High-dose penicillin G or ampicillin; erythromycin, clindamycin, or vancomycin for those allergic to penicillin |
| Staphylococci *(S. aureus, S. epidermidis)* | Implicated in 3% to 9% of CAP; risk factors: residence in nursing homes or chronic-care facilities, IV drug abuse, Hickman catheters, hemodialysis, diabetes mellitus, renal failure, influenza epidemics | Resistant to penicillin G and ampicillin; synthetic penicillin effective (oxacillin, nafcillin, methicillin), or cefazolin for most cases because incidence of methicillin-resistant *S. aureus* (MRSA) in community is low; when MRSA confirmed, vancomycin preferred agent |
| *Haemophilus influenzae* | Second leading cause of CAP in United States after *S. pneumoniae*; cause of 8% to 20% of CAP; risk factors: elderly persons, those with COPD or other preexisting disease(s); Mortality may be as high as 20% to 30% among bacteremic patients; lower in healthy adults | Resistant to penicillin G; 15% to 20% of strains produce β-lactamase and are resistant to ampicillin; drugs of choice: cefuroxime (Zinacef), amoxicillin-clavulanate (Augmentin), ampicillin-sulbactam (Unasyn) |
| Gram-negative bacilli (primarily Enterobacteriaceae) | Rare in healthy adults; accounts for 4% to 12% of CAP; risk factors: old age, residence in nursing homes or chronic-care facilities, diabetes mellitus, COPD, heart failure, ethanol abuse, neurologic impairment, malnutrition, or any associated disease that overcomes host defenses and colonizes oropharynx and lower respiratory tract | Resistant to penicillin, ampicillin, erythromycin, and tetracyclines; cefuroxime or cefotetan (second-generation cephalosporins), ceftriaxone (Rocephin, third-generation cephalosporin), and fluoroquinolones—ciprofloxacin (Cipro) effective in treating gram-negative pneumonia |
| Aspiration pneumonias<br>Anaerobic organisms of the upper airway | Implicated in 5% to 15% of CAP; risk factors: preexisting neurologic or esophageal disease; aspiration of oropharyngeal bacilli may occur in esophageal or neurologic impairments; difficulty swallowing, ethanol or drug abuse, and impaired mental status may cause acute pneumonitis, chronic necrotizing pneumonia, lung abscess, or empyema | Erythromycin, tetracycline, or doxycycline effective; 14- to 21-day course of therapy recommended to prevent relapse |
| Atypical pneumonia *(Chlamydia, Mycoplasma, Legionella* species)<br>***Chlamydia pneumoniae*** (TWAR strain—named after first two isolates: TN-138 for *Taiwan* and AR-39 for *acute respiratory*) | Responsible for 2% to 6% of CAP; *C. pneumoniae* first recognized as source of pneumonia in 1985; risk factor: overcrowding in living and sleeping quarters (barracks, college dormitories, homeless shelters, etc.) | Treatment of choice: tetracycline for 7 to 10 days; erythromycin may be used; doxycycline, 100 mg 2 times daily, when course of disease protracted |
| *Mycoplasma pneumoniae* | Accounts for 20% to 30% of CAP in adults under age 35; 3% to 10% in those ages 35 to 60; 3% in those over 60; most older adults have serum antibodies to *M. pneumoniae* | Erythromycin, 4 times daily; tetracycline, 4 times daily; or doxycycline, 2 times daily |
| *Legionella pneumophila* (first described as cause of pneumonia in 1976) | Accounts for 2% to 14% of CAP; virulent and may account for 30% of CAP in acute respiratory failure; fatality rates of 10% to 30%; *Legionella pneumophila* more severe than other "atypical" pathogens; hyponatremia in 30% to 50% of cases; *Legionella* organisms are gram-negative rods difficult to visualize on smear; specialized culture media may be required | IV erythromycin, 1 g q 6 hr; may be reduced to 500 mg q 6 hr (IV or PO) when clinical improvement; because of relapse with short-term therapy, drug given for full 21 days; doxycycline, 100 mg twice daily, used when erythromycin not tolerated |

Modified from Rich EA, Ellner JJ: Acute bronchitis. In Rakel RE, editor: *Conn's current therapy,* Philadelphia, 1993, Saunders.

**TABLE 37-6 Prevalence of Specific Pathogens in Community-Acquired and Hospital-Acquired Pneumonias**

| | PREVALENCE (%) | |
|---|---|---|
| PATHOGEN | COMMUNITY ACQUIRED | HOSPITAL ACQUIRED |
| *Streptococcus pneumoniae* | 30-70 | 3-8 |
| *Staphylococcus aureus* | 3-9 | 10-20 |
| *Haemophilus influenzae* | 8-20 | 1-8 |
| *Enterobacteriaceae* | 4-12 | 30-50 |
| *Pseudomonas aeruginosa* | <2 | 15-20 |
| *Legionella pneumophila* | 2-8 | <4 |
| *Mycoplasma pneumoniae* | 2-15 | Rare |
| *Chlamydia pneumoniae* | 2-6 | Rare |
| Anaerobic bacteria | 5-15 | 2-20 |

From Lynch JP: Bacterial pneumonia. In Rakel RE, editor: *Conn's current therapy,* Philadelphia, 1993, Saunders.

**BOX 37-4 Different Clinical Presentations of Community-Acquired Pneumonia***

| PRESENTATION 1 | PRESENTATION 2 | PRESENTATION 3 |
|---|---|---|
| Abrupt onset | Indolent onset | (Mimics influenza) |
| High fever | Low-grade fever developing over days | Nausea |
| Pleuritic chest pain | Malaise | Vomiting |
| Rigors | Fatigue | Headache |
| Purulent sputum | | Myalgias |

From Lynch JP: Bacterial pneumonia. In Rakel RE, editor: *Conn's current therapy,* Philadelphia, 1993, Saunders.
*Another presentation may be seen in elderly or debilitated persons. This presentation is characterized by lethargy, confusion, malaise, and anorexia. Fever and leukocytosis may be absent in 25% of this group.

**Community-acquired pneumonia.** CAP is responsible for more than 800,000 hospitalizations and 50,000 deaths annually in the United States. CAP may infect healthy individuals, but more than 70% of the cases occur in persons with preexisting disease (e.g., COPD, coronary artery disease, diabetes mellitus, malignancy, alcohol abuse) or impairments in host defenses. Mortality for persons with CAP who require hospitalization ranges from 5% to 15%, with even higher rates in the elderly and debilitated populations. The incidence of specific pathogens varies among specific patient populations and is dictated by host and environmental factors. *Streptococcus pneumoniae* is the most common cause of CAP in all age-groups, but its prevalence has declined. *Haemophilus influenzae* and aerobic enteric gram-negative bacilli have increased and now cause 15% to 30% of CAPs. *Mycoplasma pneumoniae* primarily affects adolescents and young adults, but it can cause severe pneumonia in older and debilitated persons. *Legionella pneumophila* accounts for less than 6% of CAP but has been associated with a disproportionately high rate of respiratory failure and death.[33] Box 37-4 lists clinical manifestations of CAP.

**Atypical pneumonia.** *Chlamydia, Mycoplasma,* and *Legionella* species and *viruses* are the cause of **atypical pneumonia.** Persons with atypical pneumonia do not have the classic features of acute bacillary pneumonia, such as pleuritic chest pain, blood-tinged sputum, and rigors. Instead, they have a nonproductive cough and patchy bronchopneumonia or interstitial infiltrates and symptoms such as sore throat, headache, arthritis, myalgias, gastrointestinal (GI) symptoms, and viral prodromal symptoms.[33]

**Hospital-acquired pneumonia.** The pathogens causing pneumonia in the hospital setting are different from those causing CAP. From 0.5% to 1% of patients develop pneumonia while hospitalized. However, the mortality rate for these patients is 30% to 50% because of coexisting diseases and the high prevalence of gram-negative bacteria (GNB) that are resistant to many antibiotics. When gram-positive bacilli are involved, the mortality rate decreases to 5% to 20%.[33]

From 75% to 85% of **nosocomial pneumonias** are caused by GNB. The remaining cases result from gram-positive bacteria (*Staphylococcus aureus* and *Streptococcus* species). *Pseudomonas aeruginosa* causes 20% to 30% of nosocomial pneumonias and is the most common pathogen found in these patients.

The second most common pathogen responsible for nosocomial pneumonia is *S. auerus,* which occurs when there are impairments in host defenses or other risk factors (e.g., indwelling central venous catheters, chronic renal failure, residence in a neurosurgical intensive care unit [ICU], coma, recent surgery, arteriovenous shunts or fistulas).[33] *Enterobacter* species are the third most common cause of nosocomial pneumonia. Several factors put hospitalized patients at risk for nosocomial pneumonia (Box 37-5).

Nosocomial pneumonia occurs with aspiration of endogenous oropharyngeal bacteria into the lower respiratory tract. Oropharyngeal and tracheal colonization with GNB often occurs when patients have impaired defenses or serious underlying disease. Colonization of the stomach may lead to subsequent colonization of the airway and lower respiratory tract. Agents that increase gastric pH (e.g., antacids, $H_2$ antagonists) have been associated with higher rates of nosocomial pneumonia in critically ill patients being mechanically ventilated.[33]

Environmental factors implicated in the transmission of bacteria are contaminated ventilator tubing and inadequate handwashing by medical staff. Nosocomial pneumonia can also be spread hematogenously to the

**BOX 37-5 Risk Factors for Development of Nosocomial Pneumonia**

Residence in an ICU
Mechanical ventilation (those requiring 48 hours or more of ventilation in an ICU have a 10% to 20% chance of developing pneumonia)
Endotracheal intubation or tracheostomy
Recent surgery
Debilitation or malnutrition
Invasive devices
Neuromuscular disease
Depressed level of alertness
Aspiration
Antacid use
Age 60 or older
Prolonged hospital stay
Any serious underlying disease

From Lynch JP: Bacterial pneumonia. In Rakel RE, editor: *Conn's current therapy,* Philadelphia, 1993, Saunders.

lung from infections in wounds, soft tissue, or the urinary tract.

### Pathophysiology

Pneumonia results in inflammation of lung tissue. Depending on the particular pathogen and the host's physical status, the inflammatory process may involve different anatomic areas of the lung parenchyma and the pleurae. Table 37-7 lists the normal function, primary pathophysiology, and clinical manifestations of pneumonia.

### Prevention

#### *Healthy People 2000*

*Healthy People 2000* has three recommendations about pneumonia.

1. Reduce epidemic-related pneumonia and influenza deaths among people aged 65 and older to no more than 7.3 per 100,000 (baseline: 9.1 per 100,000 during 1980 to 1987).*[40]

*NOTE: Epidemic-related pneumonia and influenza deaths are those that occur above and beyond the normal yearly fluctuations of mortality. Because of the extreme variability in epidemic-related deaths from year to year, the target is a 3-year average.

**TABLE 37-7 Normal Function, Primary Pathophysiology, and Clinical Manifestations of Pneumonia**

| NORMAL FUNCTION | PATHOPHYSIOLOGY | CLINICAL MANIFESTATIONS |
|---|---|---|
| **MUCOCILIARY SYSTEM** | | |
| Cleanses inhaled air by trapping particles | Hypertrophy of mucous membrane lining lung, resulting in hypersecretion | Increased sputum production and cough<br>Anaerobic—foul-smelling sputum<br>*Klebsiella*—currant jelly color<br>*Staphylococcus*—creamy yellow<br>*Pseudomonas*—green<br>Viral/mucopurulent |
| | Bronchospasm from increased secretions | Localized or diffuse wheezing, dyspnea |
| **ALVEOLOCAPILLARY MEMBRANE** | | |
| Oxygen/carbon dioxide exchange | Increased capillary permeability resulting in excess fluid in interstitial spaces | Chest x-ray films: consolidation: localized/bacterial; diffuse/viral |
| | Decreased surface area for gas exchange | Hypoxemia |
| **PLEURA** | | |
| Maintains close approximation of lungs and chest wall; minimizes friction during lung expansion and contraction | Inflammation of pleurae | Chest pain<br>Pleural effusion<br>Dullness on percussion<br>Decreased breath sounds<br>Decreased vocal fremitus |
| **RESPIRATORY MUSCLE** | | |
| Expands and contracts chest wall and thus pleura and lungs | Hypoventilation<br>Respiratory acidosis (in presence of underlying disease) | Decreased chest expansion<br>Hypercapnia and low arterial blood pH |
| **LUNG DEFENSE SYSTEM** | | |
| Protects normally sterile lung from invasion by pathogens | Bacteremia | Elevated white blood count: leukocytes (15,000 to 25,000/mm$^3$)<br>Neutrophilia<br>Tachypnea, fever |

Approximately 80% to 90% of all influenza-associated deaths in the United States occur in people aged 65 and older, the fastest growing age-group of the population. During six influenza epidemics from 1972 to 1982, the incidence of influenza-associated deaths in this age-group was 34 to 104 times greater than in younger people. Reduction of deaths in this age-group has been hindered by relatively low vaccine use, partial antigenic mismatches of vaccine strain and circulating strain because of the continual emergence of new virus strains, and decreased immune response to vaccine with increasing age of recipients. A combination of approaches is desired: (1) increase vaccine use from the current level of approximately 20% to 60% to 80% of people aged 65 and older, with a special emphasis on promoting vaccine in the highest-risk groups, particularly those with chronic cardiopulmonary disease; (2) improve the match between vaccine and circulating strains by more aggressive surveillance for new variants in the Pacific Basin region and by streamlining vaccine production and quality control techniques to reduce the lag between recognition of variants and incorporation in vaccine; and (3) develop and introduce inactivated vaccines of higher immunogenicity in elderly persons (e.g., conjugated or adjuvant vaccines) or supplemental live/attenuated vaccines capable of inducing local immunity. Pending these improvements, use of antiviral prophylaxis with influenza vaccination in influenza outbreaks is recommended.

2. Reduce pneumonia-related days of restricted activity to 38 for people aged 65 and older (per 100 people) from a 1987 baseline of 45 days.

Pneumonia and other lower respiratory infections are a major cause of illness in the United States, primarily in older adults. *S. pneumoniae* and influenza virus are the most important respiratory pathogens that cause disease in elderly persons. Effective pneumococcal and influenza vaccines are now available for use by older adults.

Achieving these objectives depends on increased use of current vaccines, the availability of new vaccines, better diagnostic methods, and earlier treatment. Immunization of older adults with influenza and pneumococcal vaccine will reduce the number of days of restricted activity caused by respiratory illness. Federal, state, and local health departments, organizations of health professionals, and primary care physicians should all help in the promotion and delivery of vaccines to persons recommended for immunization. Third-party payors of health care can also do more to promote recommended immunizations.[40]

3. Increase to at least 90% the proportion of public health departments that provide adult immunization for influenza, pneumococcal disease, hepatitis B, tetanus, and diphtheria.

Appropriate public support for the purchase and delivery of vaccines against influenza, pneumococcal disease, and hepatitis B is likely to lead to higher coverage through the private sector involvement as well. Achievement of this objective can be enhanced if the current level of public support for childhood vaccines is maintained (i.e., the same number of doses are purchased regardless of prices; and state and local health departments maintain the same level of commitment). New resources will be required to cover purchase and delivery of adult immunization. Some local health departments will have to remove other barriers to immunizations, such as requiring physical examinations, physician referrals, or enrollment in another health department program before services are rendered.[40]

**Primary prevention.** Pneumococcal vaccine is available and is mentioned in all three *Healthy People 2000* objectives.

**Secondary prevention.** The nurse's role in secondary prevention primarily involves teaching the public about the need for early diagnosis and treatment of respiratory infections. This is especially so for elderly persons living in their own homes who may not be receiving regular medical care. Even those receiving medical care may believe that their symptoms are not serious enough for them to seek medical attention. They need to understand that because of their age, they become more ill more rapidly than they did when they were younger.

**Tertiary prevention.** Nursing care for those that are hospitalized with pneumonia should be directed at assisting the person to recover as soon as possible so as to avoid the debility associated with prolonged bedrest and inactivity.

Table 37-8 summarizes methods used to prevent various types of pneumonia.

### Medical management

Not all patients with CAP have to be hospitalized. In general, persons aged 55 and younger who are in good health and have no serious preexisting condition (e.g., COPD, ethanol abuse, congestive heart failure, renal failure, liver disease, cerebrovascular accidents [CVAs], malignancy, debilitation) can be treated on an outpatient basis as long as they respond well to oral therapy. Persons who develop systemic toxicity, prostration, respiratory failure, or hypoxemia have to be hospitalized. Parenteral antibiotics for 2 to 3 days often improve the patient's condition sufficiently that oral antibiotics can be substituted and treatment continued on an outpatient basis.

The expected length of stay of patients with pneumonia as determined by diagnosis-related groups (DRGs) is 5.1 days. Common medical therapy for management of pneumonia is discussed next.

**TABLE 37-8 Methods Used to Prevent Pneumonia**

| TYPE OF PNEUMONIA | METHODS |
|---|---|
| Streptococcal | Pneumonia polysaccharide vaccine for those at high risk, effective 3 to 5 years against multiple strains of pneumococcal polysaccharides |
| Gram negative, gram positive | Frequent handwashing<br>Adequate ventilation<br>Every 24 hours:<br>Changing open container solutions<br>Changing respiratory equipment<br>Tracheostomy and endotracheal airways treated with sterile technique<br>Sterile technique when suctioning<br>Turning and repositioning every 2 hours<br>Necessity of not draining condensation in ventilator equipment back into liquid reservoir |
| Aspiration | Positioning patients with decreased consciousness to facilitate drainage of secretions<br>Inflating endotracheal or tracheostomy cuff before feeding<br>Ensuring proper placement of nasogastric tube before giving tube feeding<br>Always checking for gag reflex before feeding patient with decreased consciousness |
| Viral, *M. pneumoniae* | Prompt treatment of unresolved URI or acute bronchitis<br>Limiting contact with people who have viral infections<br>Maintaining optimal nutrition |

**Diagnostic tests**

1. Chest x-ray film to confirm lung consolidation and distribution, pleural effusion
2. Sputum studies for culture and sensitivity; if unable to obtain specimen by usual means, may use:
   a. Transtracheal aspiration
   b. Bronchoscopy with aspiration, biopsy, or bronchial brushing
3. Arterial blood gas (ABG) studies
4. Hematology
   a. White blood cell (WBC) count for bacterial pneumonia
   b. Cold agglutinins and complement fixation for viral studies
5. Thoracentesis to obtain pleural fluid specimen if pleural effusion present

**Medications.** Unless the clinical findings and Gram's stain are classic for a specific organism, initial treatment of CAP is with a broad-spectrum antimicrobial. Therapy is then modified when more culture data are available.[33] Table 37-5 lists effective antimicrobials for specific pathogens.

Nosocomial pneumonia requires very aggressive therapy because of the high mortality associated with this type of pneumonia. Box 37-6 lists treatment for hospital-acquired pneumonia.

**Treatments.** Oxygen should be given at 6L/min per nasal cannula. Turning, coughing, and deep breathing are performed regularly.

**Diet.** The patient should have a high-calorie, high-protein diet with frequent small feedings.

**Activity.** The patient should be on bedrest but may be out of bed to use the toilet or commode chair.

**Referral/Consultation.** In some settings the nurse assumes responsibility for making referrals to other services. Common referrals for the patient with CAP requiring hospitalization include a dietitian, physical therapist, and social services professional.

Critical pathways (also referred to as "collaborative care paths" or "care maps") have been developed in some inpatient and outpatient settings to guide both medical and nursing management. These critical pathways are collaboratively developed along time lines and include the information previously described for specific hours, days, or visits. Pertinent information about discharge planning and patient teaching to be implemented

**BOX 37-6 Empiric Antimicrobial Therapy for Hospital-Acquired Pneumonia**

**FOR PATIENTS ON MECHANICAL VENTILATION OR RESIDING IN ICU**

Ceftazidime (Fortaz, Tazidime, Tazicef), ticarcillin-clavulanate (Timentin), or imipenem-cilastatin (Primaxin)
plus
Aminoglycoside (gentamicin or tobramycin)

**OUTSIDE ICU**

Ceftriaxone (Rocephin), cefotaxime (Claforan), ticarcillin-clavulanate, or piperacillin (Pipracil)
plus
Aminoglycoside

**OPTIONS FOR PATIENTS ALLERGIC TO PENICILLIN**

Ciprofloxacin (Cipro) plus aminoglycoside
Aztreonam (Azactam) plus vancomycin (Vancocin)
Clindamycin (Cleocin) plus aztreonam
Vancomycin plus metronidazole (Flagyl) plus aztreonam

From Lynch JP: Bacterial pneumonia. In Rakel RE, editor: *Conn's current therapy,* Philadelphia, 1993, Saunders.

at specified times also is included. Becase the nurse has a major role in these two aspects of care, these are discussed under Nursing Management.

## NURSING MANAGEMENT

### ♦ ASSESSMENT

#### Subjective Data

Data to be collected to assess the patient with pneumonia include the following:

History and character of onset and duration of cough, fever, shaking chills, chest pain, sputum production (amount, color, consistency)

Self-care modalities used to treat symptoms

History of exposure to persons with infection, pulmonary irritants

#### Objective Data

Data to be collected to assess the patient with pneumonia include the following:

Signs of other chronic diseases and general debilitation

Vital signs: elevated temperature (39° C to 40° C [102.2° F to 104° F]) or low-grade temperature elevation; tachycardia/tachypnea

Pulmonary examination

Inspection: accessory muscle retraction, central cyanosis, respiratory grunting on expiration, restricted chest movement

Palpation: decreased expansion on affected side of chest, increased tactile femitus

Percussion: dullness

Auscultation: bronchial breath sounds, inspiratory crackles (rales), decreased vocal fremitus (pleural effusion), egophony (consolidation)

Laboratory findings

Chest x-ray film: diffuse involvement—atypical pneumonia; lobar involvement—typical pneumonia

Hematology: WBC—elevated 15,000 to 25,000/$mm^3$; cold agglutinins—complement fixation/viral or *M. pneumoniae*

ABG studies: hypoxemia/respiratory alkalosis; if underlying chronic disease, respiratory acidosis

### ♦ NURSING DIAGNOSES

Nursing diagnoses are determined from analysis of patient data. Nursing diagnoses for the person with pneumonia may include but are not limited to the following:

| Diagnostic Title | Possible Etiologic Factors |
|---|---|
| Airway clearance, ineffective | Decreased energy, fatigue, tracheobronchial inflammation |
| Gas exchange, impaired | Alveolocapillary membrane changes, altered oxygen delivery |
| Pain | Pleural inflammation, coughing paroxysms |
| Infection, high risk for | Compromised lung defense system |
| Knowledge deficit: conditions, treatments | Lack of exposure to or unfamiliarity with information |
| Nutrition, altered: less than body requirements | Increased metabolic needs<br>Anorexia from infectious process, sputum production |

### ♦ EXPECTED PATIENT OUTCOMES

Expected patient outcomes for the person with pneumonia may include but are not limited to the following:

1. Demonstrates effective cough with adequate sputum production. (Both cough and sputum production decreased within 72 hours of treatment initiation. Patient with chronic lung disease returns to prepneumonia status.)
2. Demonstrates improved ventilation and adequate oxygenation of tissues. pH returns within normal limits. Oxygen tension ($Po_2$) during active disease: 60 to 80 mm Hg; after resolution of disease, arterial $Po_2$ ($Pao_2$) is within normal limits.
3. Reports absence of chest pain.
4. Does not develop a superinfection.
5. States when influenza and pneumonia vaccines should be taken.
6. Knows the signs and symptoms that should be reported to the physician.
7. Describes the cause and factors contributing to the occurrence of pneumonia and names common symptoms indicating pneumonia.
8. Has improved appetite, and weight gain returns weight to near preillness level.

### ♦ INTERVENTIONS

#### Administering Medications and Treatments

1. Before beginning administration of prescribed antibiotic, collect sputum for culture. If blood culture is ordered, also draw blood before therapy is begun.
2. Monitor antibiotic blood levels by giving antibiotics at scheduled times. (Table 37-5 lists the antibiotic therapy currently employed in treating pneumonia.)
3. Give medication prescribed to relieve pain. Codeine may be prescribed because it is less likely to inhibit the cough reflex than more potent narcotics.
4. Begin oxygen therapy.

#### Administering Oxygen Therapy

Oxygen by mask or cannula (Figures 37-1 and 37-2) is usually ordered when $Po_2$ is less than 60 mm Hg. When supplemental oxygen is necessary, it may be administered by nasal prongs or by mask. The method used depends on the patient's condition and the concentration of oxygen required. The nurse should be familiar with the various devices used to administer oxygen, and when oxygen is in use, the nurse should check the equipment frequently to ensure it is working properly.

When the patient is having difficulty exchanging oxygen and carbon dioxide, such as occurs in pulmonary edema, oxygen may be given under positive pressure. In some situations, such as COPD, low-flow rates of oxygen are indicated. The use of low-flow oxygen is discussed on p. 1134. ***In all situations, the nurse should remember that the patient with hypoxemia may not be breathless or cyanotic because cyanosis does not occur until there is 5 g or more of deoxygenated hemoglobin.*** In persons with anemia, all the available heme is completely saturated with oxygen, and thus they are never cyanotic even though they may be hypoxemic. ***For this reason, an increase in the pulse rate may be the first indication that the patient is experiencing hypoxemia.*** Patients receiving oxygen therapy are monitored with ABGs.

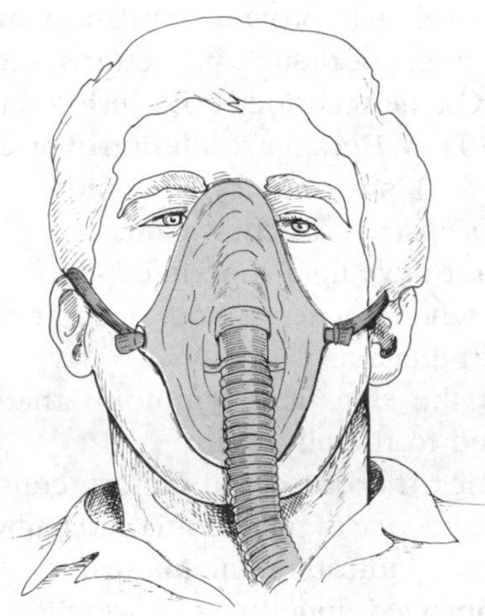

**FIGURE 37-1** Simple face mask. (From Abels LF: *Mosby's manual of critical care,* St Louis, 1979, Mosby.)

## Facilitating Breathing

Help the patient breathe deeply and expand the chest to increase ventilation.

1. Place patient in position to facilitate breathing, usually upright or semi-upright position (Figure 37-3).
2. A pillow may be placed lengthwise at the patient's back to provide support and thrust thorax slightly forward, allowing freer use of the diaphragm.
3. The patient who must be upright to breathe may find it restful to put head and arms on a pillow placed on an overbed table (Figure 37-4).
4. For the patient with severe hypoxemia, side rails should be in place. The patient can use them to assist in moving about in bed.
5. Some patients may breathe best when sitting up in a large armchair while leaning on a smaller chair placed in front of them. This chair is blocked to prevent it from slipping.

## Maintaining Ventilation, Humidity, and Comfortable Temperature

1. Most patients are most comfortable if air is cool and not too humid. An air-conditioned room may make the patient more comfortable.
2. If patient has nose, throat, or bronchial irritation, warm moist air from a humidifier or vaporizer may be helpful.
3. Because of concern about cross-infection from room humidifiers, follow the recommendations provided by the Centers for Disease Control and Prevention (CDC) (Box 37-7).

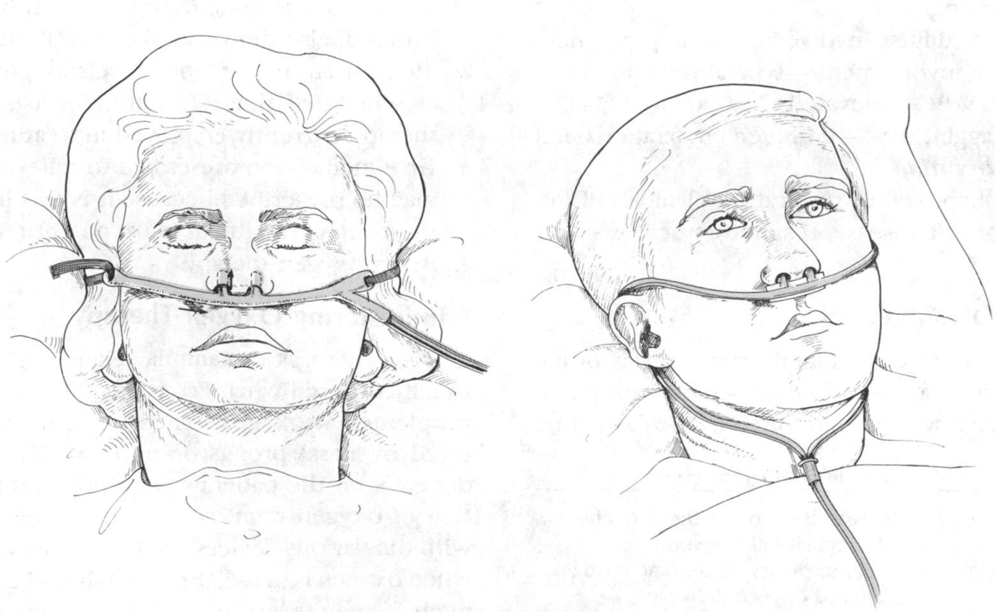

**FIGURE 37-2** Two types of nasal cannulas. (From Abels LF: *Mosby's manual of critical care,* St Louis, 1979, Mosby.)

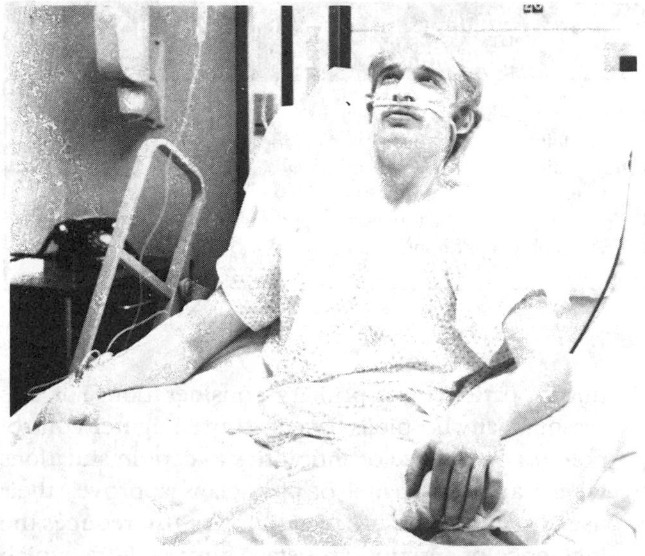

**FIGURE 37-3** Patient sitting upright with pillow under head and each arm to promote chest expansion and comfort.

**BOX 37-7 CDC Recommendations When Using a Humidifier**

1. Use only a direct-heated humidifier or a nebulizer with a bacterial filter. Cold vapor or cool-mist humidifiers are not recommended because they cannot withstand daily sterilization.
2. Use only sterile water in the humidifier, and drain remaining water each time the humidifier is refilled, or at least every 24 hours. Tap water is not safe to use because it is frequently contaminated with *Pseudomonas, Flavobacterium, Actinetobacter,* or other organisms.
3. Establish a routine maintenance schedule.
4. Set medical guidelines to determine which patients should receive humidification and which should not. It may not be advisable to use humidifiers for immunosuppressed patients.
5. Do not send humidifying unit home with patients because of the concern about transporting highly resistant hospital organisms into the community.

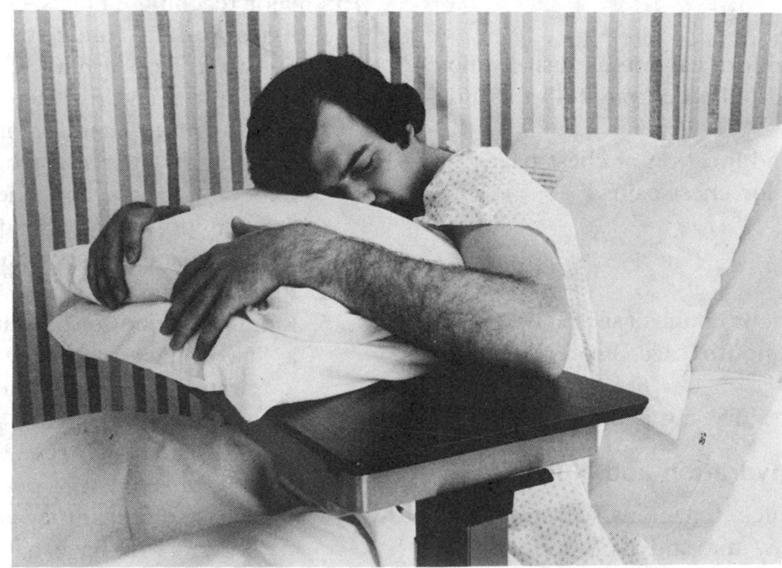

**FIGURE 37-4** Pillows placed on overbed table provide comfortable support for patient who must sleep in upright position.

**Vaporizers**

Small electric vaporizers can be purchased at most local drugstores. However, when a patient cannot afford to purchase one, the nurse can assist in improvising equipment for inhalation and proper humidity. An empty coffee can or a shallow pie tin can be filled with distilled water and placed on an electric plate in the person's room to increase humidity. If the inhalation is to be directed, an ordinary steam kettle or a tea kettle with a longer improvised paper spout may be used. The paper should be changed frequently. A few drops of menthol or oil of eucalyptus can be put into the water. Benzoin causes corrosion in the kettle, which is exceedingly difficult to remove. The kettle and electric plate should be placed a safe distance from the face so that the medicated steam can be breathed freely but the person cannot be burned by accidently tipping the kettle or by touching the hot plate. After the 25- to 30-minute treatment, equipment should be removed from the bedside.

## Maintaining Effective Airway Clearance

1. Monitor for increased respiratory distress.
2. Assist patient to cough effectively.

3. If unable to clear own airway, suction airway using sterile technique (see Chapter 36).
4. Assist with nebulizer therapy.
5. Administer bronchodilators as ordered. Monitor for side effects and response to therapy.
6. Change position frequently to assist in mobilizing secretions.
7. Ensure fluid intake adequate to thin secretions.
8. Assist with ADL, pacing activities to prevent fatigue and respiratory distress.

### Maintaining Adequate Gas Exchange

1. Monitor ABG results, and assess respiratory status for signs of hypoxemia and hypoventilation.
2. Encourage patient to be as active as possible without increasing respiratory distress. If comatose, turn and reposition every 2 hours, with passive range of motion (ROM) every 4 hours.
3. Encourage deep breathing every 1 to 2 hours.
   a. Incentive spirometer
   b. Slow inhalation, hold for few seconds, slow exhalation

### Promoting Comfort

1. Place in position of comfort; patients are usually most comfortable with head of bed elevated 45 to 90 degrees.
2. Assess for character and location of chest pain.
3. Administer analgesics for chest pain:
   a. Acetylsalicylic acid
   b. Acetaminophen
   c. Codeine
4. Splint chest when patient coughs (see p. 1099).
5. Administer frequent mouth care. Protect lips and nares with lubricant.
6. Keep patient warm and dry and avoid chilling.

### Promoting Adequate Hydration and Nutrition

Dehydration results in thick, tenacious secretions. The best liquefying agent is water, and it is preferable to hydrate the patient adequately rather than attempt to loosen secretions with mist therapy. If the patient does not have cardiovascular disease requiring fluid restriction, a fluid intake of 3 to 4 L/day should be provided.

1. Encourage oral fluids. If patient is receiving intravenous (IV) fluids, monitor rate. Observe for signs of fluid volume deficit or excess.
2. Offer small, frequent feedings. Encourage high-carbohydrate and high-protein foods.

### Preventing Spread of Infection

1. When universal precautions are used, respiratory isolation is unnecessary.
2. Handwashing is the most important way to prevent spread of pneumonia from one patient to another via the hands of hospital personnel.
3. Reducing the likelihood of gram-negative colonization of patients is a primary consideration. For this reason, many hospitals have instituted tighter control policies on the use of antibiotics except in situations where a review panel of physicians approves their use. A reduction in use of antibiotics also reduces the incidence of antibiotic-resistant hospital flora, which are the source of many nosocomial infections (see Chapter 15).

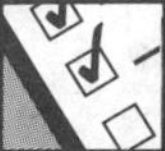

**Guidelines for Care of the Person With Pneumonia**

1. Limit the impact of infection.
2. Maintain effective airway clearance.
3. Maintain adequate gas exchange.
4. Promote comfort.
5. Promote adequate hydration and nutrition.
6. Teach patient how to lower the risk of recurrence.

### Facilitating Learning

The major teaching emphasis is on prevention.

1. Assess patient's understanding of pneumonia with questions concerning such information as how transmitted and risk factors.
2. Teach proper handling of secretions. Cover nose and mouth with tissue when coughing or sneezing. Expectorate into container provided.
3. Stress importance of handwashing after coughing, sneezing, and expectorating.
4. Reinforce importance of follow-up care.
5. Reinforce need for immunization.
   a. Two vaccines are now available to prevent respiratory infections: influenza vaccine and pneumococcal vaccine
   b. Persons at high risk for developing complication of influenza (pneumonia) should be immunized unless they are allergic to eggs or egg products or have had a previous reaction to vaccine.
      (1) Influenza vaccine is given yearly.
      (2) *Pneumonia polysaccharide* vaccine is given only every 3 to 5 years.

■ ■ ■

The Guidelines box above summarizes general care of the person with pneumonia.

## ✸ SPECIAL CONSIDERATIONS FOR CARE OF THE GERONTOLOGIC PATIENT

Nurses working with elderly patients need to be aware of their vulnerability to pneumonia. Interventions are directed toward preventing pneumonia by teaching them to receive a vaccination for influenza yearly and for pneumonia every 3 to 5 years. Also, nurses should

## GERONTOLOGIC PATIENT CONSIDERATIONS

### ASSESSMENT

Assess lung sounds; diminished lung sounds are common in elderly persons because of thickened alveoli and decreased rib cage expansion (thorax stiffening).

Assess respiratory status with activity; dyspnea with exertion may occur from decreased pulmonary oxygen diffusion.

Monitor effects of drugs that may interfere with breathing, such as narcotics and hypnotics. Elderly persons may have decreased drug clearance from decreased glomerular filtration rate (GFR) and nephron activity or from decreased hepatic function.

Monitor for signs of pneumonia, to which elderly persons are highly susceptible. Elderly patients may have symptoms of mental confusion, tachycardia, or dyspnea rather than the customary signs of cough, fever, and rales (crackles).

### INTERVENTIONS

Encourage as much activity as the person can tolerate to promote ventilation, such as paced walking.

Suggest patient sit upright for meals and for 20 to 30 minutes after meals to prevent pulmonary aspiration during eating.

Encourage pneumococcal and influenza vaccine prophylaxis.

Teach patient the importance of oral care to help prevent pneumonia.

For elderly patient with pneumonia, maintain good hydration (with close monitoring to prevent fluid imbalances), and assist with respiratory therapy and position changes.

### COMMON DISORDERS IN ELDERS

Pneumonia
Lung cancer
COPD

emphasize how elderly persons can care for themselves by maintaining activity and good health practices (see Gerontologic Patient Considerations box).

## ♦ EVALUATION

To evaluate the effectiveness of nursing interventions, compare patient behaviors with those stated in the expected patient outcomes. Successful achievement of patient outcomes for the person with pneumonia is indicated by the following:

1. Cough and sputum are reduced, and lung sounds are clear.
2. $PaO_2$, $PaCO_2$, and pH are within normal limits.
3. Is free of chest pain.
4. Does not develop superinfection.
5. States the need to receive an influenza shot yearly in September and a pneumonia shot every 3 to 5 years.
6. Verbalizes the need for medical attention if cough persists, a fever lasts for more than 48 hours, fatigue is overwhelming, or generalized achiness is present.
7. Verbalizes that failure to seek medical attention after a prolonged bout of influenza was the factor that lead to pneumonia.
8. Has improved appetite, and weight is only 2 pounds less than it was before admission.

## ❦ HOME CARE CONSIDERATIONS

Persons discharged from the hospital after being admitted with community-acquired pneumonia (CAP) who are otherwise in fairly good health still require 4 to 6 weeks before they feel completely well. Attention to their recuperation includes obtaining extra rest and gradually assuming activities such as returning to work. Many find it easier to start back to work part-time until they have more energy. An adequate balanced diet is essential, as are rest periods and adequate sleep at night.

As a general rule, the older the person, the longer is the period of recovery, although many young people recovering from pneumonia remark, "I can't believe how tired I am."

Persons with hospital-acquired pneumonia have an even more protracted period of recovery because their pneumonia was superimposed on a chronic condition such as COPD. They are likely to be even more restricted in their activities because of chronic shortness of breath and resultant fatigue.[33]

Persons living alone should have someone in the home at least part of each day to assist with ADL such as bathing, dressing, and meal preparation. The nurse caring for the patient or a social worker should make a referral to a home health agency before the patient is discharged, unless the patient has a significant other who can assist them with these activities. They also need to be monitored closely by their health care provider and often need assistance in going to follow-up appointments. For some persons, Meals on Wheels can provide them with a hot meal daily until they are well enough to prepare their own meals. Some persons, however, receive Meals on Wheels for several months.

### Complications

With the advent of antibiotics and better diagnostic measures such as x-ray procedures, complications during or after pneumonia are rare in otherwise healthy persons. Atelectasis, delayed resolution, lung abscess, pleural effusion, empyema, pericarditis, meningitis, and relapse are complications that were common in the past. Because pneumonia and influenza rank fifth as a cause of death in the United States, this is an impressive reason for strict adherence to the prescribed medical treatment. Careful and accurate observation and sufficient time for convalescence also help to ensure that the average patient has a smooth recovery. Elderly persons and those with a chronic illness are likely to have a relatively long course of convalescence from pneumonia, and a greater possibility of developing complications exists. There has been an increase in the incidence of *staphylococcal pneumonia* subsequent to influenza. *Consolidation of lung tissue, pleural effusion,* and *empyema* frequently occur soon after onset of this type of pneumonia and may cause death.

## Tuberculosis

In 1900, tuberculosis (TB) was the leading cause of death in the United States. It remained a major cause of death until the introduction of antituberculosis drug therapy in the late 1940s and early 1950s. The most effective of these agents is isoniazid, which first became available clinically in 1952. The use of isoniazid in combination with two agents introduced earlier, streptomycin and paraaminosalicylic acid, resulted in a striking decrease in TB mortality rates. It also made it possible for patients with TB to be treated on an outpatient basis. However, some patients still have to be hospitalized during their illness, and most nurses will care for a patient with TB at some time in their careers.

### Etiology

TB is an infectious disease caused by the bacillus *Mycobacterium tuberculosis* or the tubercle bacillus, an acid-fast organism.

### Epidemiology

Although TB is considered a preventable and curable disease, it is a disease that demands constant public health surveillance. The case rates for TB in the United States declined steadily from 1953, when there were 84,304 reported cases, to 1984, when there were 22,225 reported cases. Beginning in 1986, when the number of cases increased by 3%, the rates continued to increase yearly. From 1985 to 1992, new cases of TB increased by 20%. In 1992 the CDC reported 26,673 new cases. The figures for 1993 show a small decrease to 25,313 cases. This decrease is believed to be the result of increased funding at federal and state levels and more aggressive outreach programs to find and treat persons with active TB. Public health officials caution that the battle is far from over and that continued efforts and financial support will be necessary.

The case rates per 100,000 population for states in the United States and Puerto Rico and the U.S. Virgin Islands are shown in Figure 37-5. Fifteen states and the District of Columbia reported increases in TB cases in 1993: Alabama, Delaware, District of Columbia, Indiana, Iowa, Kansas, Kentucky, Maine, Missouri, Montana, New Hampshire, Oregon, Rhode Island, South Carolina, Tennesee, and Virginia.

As one can see in Figure 37-6, the case rate differs by race and ethnicity, with the largest portion of cases in non-Hispanic blacks and non-Hispanic whites. When figures for 1990 and 1993 are compared, there was a small decrease in cases in non-Hispanic blacks (−1.5%) and non-Hispanic whites (−2.0%), whereas there was a

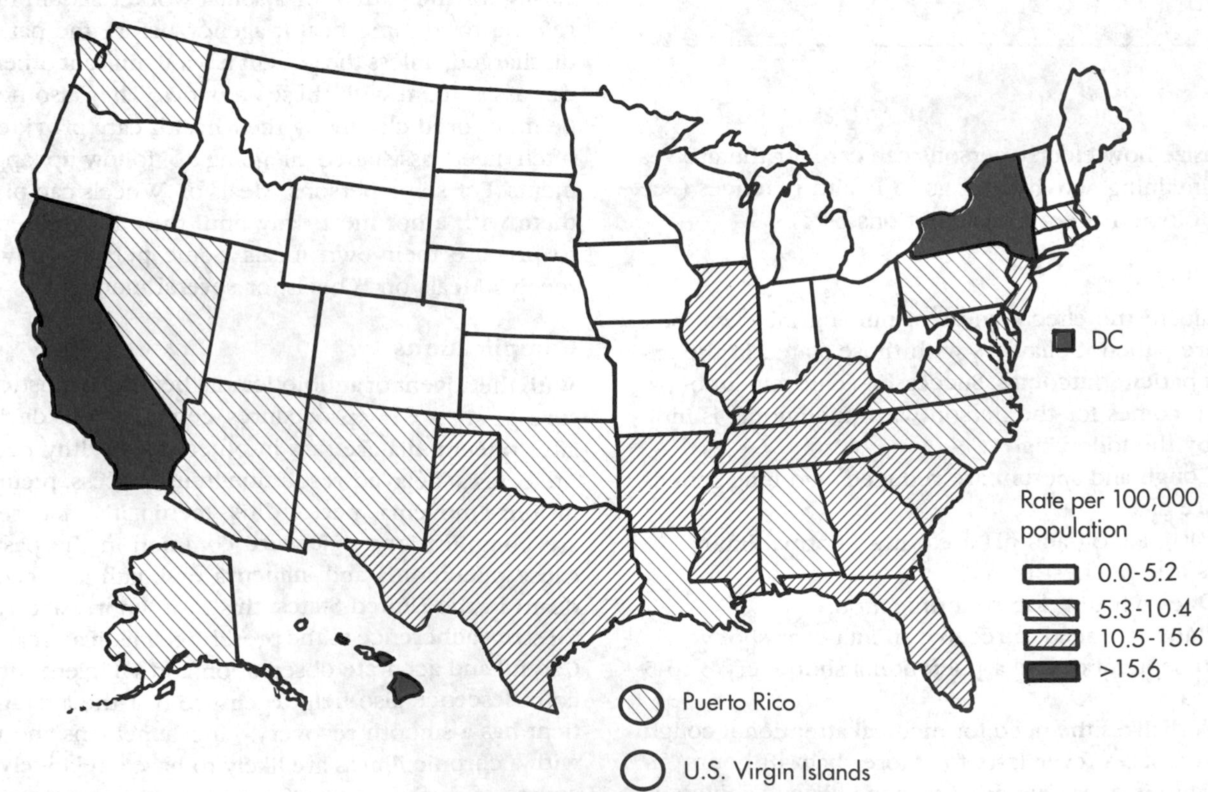


**FIGURE 37-5** Tuberculosis rates by state, United States, 1992. (From Centers for Disease Control: *MMWR* 41[55]:13-64, 1993.)

2.1% increase in Asian/Pacific Islanders and a 1.7% increase in Hispanics. The Native American/Native Alaskan group had a 0.3% decrease in their case rate.

The new cases were not evenly distributed throughout the population, however, and some differences bear mentioning. The highest number of cases were in the 25- to 44-year-old age-group. This is a change from the 1970s and early 1980s, when the highest case rates were in white males aged 65 years and older.

In addition, the highest case rates between 1985 and 1990 were found in Miami, Atlanta, San Francisco, Newark, Tampa, and New York City.[16] These cities have the highest number of persons positive for the human immunodeficiency virus (HIV), especially among drug abusers. These cities also have many immigrants, many of whom come from countries in which TB is endemic. Of particular concern has been an increase in TB cases among children under age 15. It is assumed that most of these children were infected by persons in the 25- to 44-year-old age-group, in whom the incidence of TB is highest. Also of concern is that many persons with HIV infection have organisms resistant to most chemotherapeutic agents used to treat TB. When this is true, infected persons pass their resistant organisms to those they infect, making treatment of newly infected persons particularly difficult.

Because HIV infection is an important risk factor for developing clinically apparent TB among persons already infected with the tubercle bacillus, the CDC recommends that all HIV-infected persons be screened for TB and latent infection and, if infected, receive appropriate therapy. Also, persons with TB and known tuberculin-positive persons should be evaluated for HIV infection so that appropriate counseling and treatment can be given.

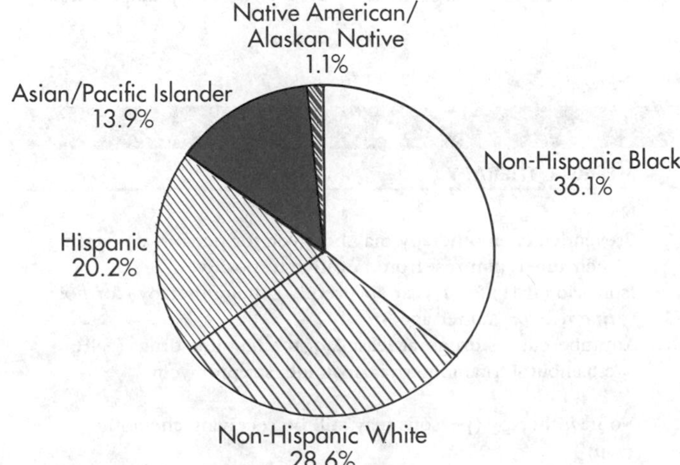


**FIGURE 37-6** Tuberculosis case rates by race and ethnicity, United States, 1992. (From Centers for Disease Control: *MMWR* 41[55]:13-64, 1993.)

**Pathophysiology**

When an individual with no previous exposure to TB (negative tuberculin reactor) inhales a sufficient number of tubercle bacilli into the alveoli, **tuberculosis infection** occurs. The body's reaction to the tubercle bacilli depends on the susceptibility of the individual, the size of the dose, and the virulence of the organisms. Inflammation occurs within the alveoli (parenchyma) of the lungs, and natural body defenses attempt to counteract the infection.

Macrophages ingest the organisms and present the mycobacterial antigens to the T cells. CD4 cells secrete lymphokines that enhance the capacity of the macrophages to ingest and kill bacteria. Lymph nodes in the hilar region of the lung become enlarged as they filter drainage from the infected site. The inflammatory process and cellular reaction produce a small, firm, white nodule called the *primary tubercle.* The center of the nodule contains tubercle bacilli. Cells gather around the center, and usually the outer portion becomes fibrosed. Thus, blood vessels are compressed, nutrition of the tubercle is interfered with, and *necrosis* occurs at the center. The area becomes walled off by fibrotic tissue around the outside, and the center gradually becomes soft and cheesy in consistency. This latter process is known as **caseation necrosis.** This material may become calcified (calcium deposits), or it may liquefy and is known as **liquefaction necrosis.** The liquefied material may be coughed up, leaving a *cavity* or hole in the parenchyma of the lung. The cavity or cavities are visible on chest x-ray films and result in the diagnosis of *cavitary disease.* Most individuals who are exposed to TB and develop a TB infection (confirmed by a positive tuberculin test) do not develop an active case of TB. The only x-ray evidence of their TB infection is a calcified nodule known as the *Ghon tubercle.* The evidence on x-ray film of enlarged hilar lymph nodes and a Ghon tubercle is referred to as the **primary complex.**

Persons who have the primary complex have become sensitized to the tubercle bacillus, and an antigen-antibody reaction results. When the person receives the antigen in the form of a purified protein derivative (PPD) or old tuberculin (OT) in a tuberculin test, the reaction results in a positive tuberculin test. This sensitization, once developed, usually remains throughout life unless something interferes with the immune response. Evidence suggests that most persons who have a tuberculin reaction and take isoniazid prophylactically for 6 months convert back to negative test results. This protection is believed to last for life. ***A positive tuberculin test does not mean that one has TB, however, and nurses should explain this to persons undergoing the test.***

TB infection is unlike other infections. Usually, other infections disappear completely when overcome by the body's defenses and leave no living organisms and generally no signs of infection. However, persons who have been infected with tubercle bacilli harbor the organism for the remainder of their lives unless they have received prophylactic isoniazid. Tubercle bacilli remain in the lungs in a dormant, walled-off, or so-called resting state. When a person is under physical or emotional stress, these bacilli may become active and begin to multiply. If body defenses are low, active TB may develop. Most persons who have active TB developed it in this manner. However, it is generally accepted that only 1 out of 10 persons with a positive tuberculin test will ever develop active TB, and the incidence is expected to be much lower among those who receive preventive therapy with isoniazid.

When tuberculosis occurs several years after the primary infection, it is known as **reactivation tuberculosis.** The development of active TB is believed to be caused by defects in T-cell or macrophage functions or both.[5]

Tuberculosis is more likely to occur in persons with HIV infection because in HIV infection, progressive depletion and dysfunction of CD4 cells occur, along with defects in macrophage and monocyte function. Epidemiologic evidence suggests that because of these changes, persons with HIV infection and a positive tuberculin test (primary infection) are at risk for reactivation tuberculosis. At the same time, persons with HIV infection who have negative tuberculin tests are at risk of progressing directly from a primary infection to active TB when exposed to someone with TB. Also, extrapulmonary TB is more common in persons with HIV infection, and when diagnosed in them, it becomes an AIDS-defining condition. This means that tuberculosis is a more opportunistic infection than is *P. carinii* and other infections that indicate that a person has progressed from HIV infection to AIDS.[5]

Two mycobacterial organisms are found in persons diagnosed as having AIDS. In developed countries the *Mycobacterium avium* intracellular complex (MAC) is the organism found in middle-class AIDS patients who have no history of intravenous drug use. Pulmonary tuberculosis caused by *M. tuberculosis* is more common in AIDS patients from developing countries and in persons from inner-city minority populations who have a history of intravenous drug use.[22]

### Classification

The classification used by states and territories of the United States when reporting TB cases to the CDC of the Public Health Service is outlined in Table 37-9. The six basic classifications cover the total child and adult population, those unexposed to TB, those uninfected even though exposed, those with evidence of infection without disease, those with disease, those with evidence of TB without current disease, and those in whom TB is suspected (diagnosis pending).

### Extrapulmonary tuberculosis

TB may affect other parts of the body besides the lungs, such as the larynx, GI tract, lymph nodes, skin, skeletal system, nervous system, urinary system, and reproductive system. TB is spread to other parts of the body hematogenously or lymphogenously.

Extrapulmonary TB has taken on increased importance because of its extremely high frequency, usually with concomitant pulmonary tuberculosis in persons with HIV infection. The most frequent site of extrapulmonary TB in persons with HIV infection are the lymph nodes; miliary disease, in which the chest x-ray film looks like millet seeds spread throughout both lungs, is also common. Involvement also occurs in bone marrow, genitourinary tract, and the CNS.

Because persons with HIV infection and TB infection usually have bacteremia, blood cultures are recommended when the diagnosis is suspected.

### Mycobacteria other than tuberculosis (MOTT)

These bacteria, formerly referred to as atypical acid-fast bacilli, were first classified by Runyon. They are *M. kan-*

**TABLE 37-9 Classification of Tuberculosis**

| CLASS | DESCRIPTION | MEDICAL THERAPY |
|---|---|---|
| 0 | No TB exposure, not infected | None |
| 1 | TB exposure, no evidence of infection | Preventive chemotherapy may be given for persons converting their tuberculin test from negative to positive |
| 2 | TB infection, no disease | Isoniazid (INH) for 1 year (preventive chemotherapy) for *positive reactors* under age 35 |
| 3 | TB: clinically active (persons with completed diagnostic evidence of TB: both a significant reaction to tuberculin skin test and clinical and/or x-ray evidence of TB) | Antituberculosis drugs: at least 2 of the first-line drugs (INH, ethambutol, rifampin, pyrazinamide, streptomycin) |
| 4 | TB: not clinically active (persons with previous history of TB or with abnormal x-ray films but no significant tuberculin skin test reaction or clinical evidence) | No new therapy (persons may still be receiving chemotherapy) |
| 5 | TB: suspect (diagnosis pending); used during diagnostic testing of suspect persons, for no longer than a 3-month period | Preventive chemotherapy with INH may be instituted |

*sasii, M. avium* complex, *M. xenopi, M. marinum, M. fortuitum,* and *M. chelonei.* The last two are classified as rapid growers, These organisms are strongly acid-fast but differ from *M. tuberculosis* on culture. They are being isolated with increasing frequency from immunocompromised patients (persons with HIV [AIDS], transplant patients, patients undergoing antineoplastic chemotherapy).[19] MOTT have been found in soil and water and less frequently in foodstuffs and are considered to be opportunistic organisms.

When they are identified in sputum specimens, it may mean that the person is *colonized* and does not have invasive disease. (See Chapter 15 for more information on colonization.) MOTT are often isolated from the sputum of patients with pneumoconiosis, chronic bronchitis, COPD, past history of TB, bronchiectasis, and chronic aspiration from esophageal disease.[19] Table 37-10 summarizes these nontuberculosis organisms.

MAC is the most common bacterial infection in patients with AIDS. It occurs in 30% to 50% of AIDS patients. Patients with MAC have fever, night sweats, weight loss, diarrhea, lymphadenopathy, and anemia. The diagnosis is usually made from isolator blood cultures, bone marrow, lymph node, or liver biopsy. It is also diagnosed by acid-fast smear of stool in patients with disseminated infection.[19]

**TABLE 37-10 MOTT Associated With Human Disease**

| ORGANISM | SITES TYPICALLY INVOLVED | SUGGESTED THERAPY |
|---|---|---|
| *M. kansasii* | Lung | INH, RIF, and EMB and sulfonamides, clarithromycin (Bioxin) for 12-18 months |
| *M. avium* complex | Lung, disseminated (AIDS) | Amikacin, clofazimine, (Lamprene), RIF and EMB and clarithromycin |
| *M. xenopi* | Lung | Amikacin, clofazimine, RIF and EMB (perhaps clarithromycin and quinolone) |
| *M. marinum* | Soft tissue | RIF and EMB for 4-6 weeks or tetracycline or trimethoprim-sulfamethoxazole as single agents |
| *M. fortuitum* | Soft tissue | Cefoxitin, cefmetazole (Zefazone), or imipenem with amikacin (perhaps clarithromycin or ciprofloxacin [Ciprol]) |
| *M. chelonae* | Soft tissue | Amikacin (tobramycin for subspecies) and/or clarithromycin |

Modified from Cynamon MH, Klemens S: Tuberculosis and other mycobacterial diseases. In Rakel RE, editor: *Conn's current therapy,* Philadelphia, 1993, Saunders.

**Multidrug-resistant TB (MDR-TB)**

MDR-TB has become a major problem in the United States. By 1993, nearly 10% of TB patients were resistant to isoniazid and/or rifampin (two of the most effective drugs for treating TB). Overall resistance to both isoniazid and rifampin was found in 35 counties in 13 states. The greatest problem was in New York City, where the MDR-TB incidence was 52.4 times that of the rest of the United States. In New York City the relative risk of MDR-TB in non-Hispanic whites was 39 compared with 229.3 in Hispanics, 420.9 in Asian/Pacific Islanders, and 701.0 in non-Hispanic blacks.[7]

The emergence of MDR-TB means that increased efforts are required to find every TB patient and to ensure that they are treated with four-drug therapy (see p. 1078) initially in an effort to prevent further drug resistance. It is also important to protect other patients and health care workers from becoming infected by patients with MDR-TB.[7] The problem is especially great in institutions caring for large numbers of patients with HIV, many of whom also have MDR-TB. Protection methods are discussed under Medical Management and Nursing Management later in this chapter.

**Prevention**

*Healthy People 2000*

The goal set in *Healthy People 2000* was to reduce the incidence of TB to no more than 3.5 cases per 100,000 from a baseline of 9.1 per 100,000 in 1988 (Figure 37-7). Since 1988, the case rate increased to 9.8 in 1993. Because minorities now account for nearly two thirds of reported cases, special target figures were set for these groups. (Table 37-11 shows these figures.)

The year 2000 target will not be easy to achieve, but it gives direction to preventive efforts, including those at the state level. In this regard, the Advisory Council for the Elimination of Tuberculosis (ACET) issued

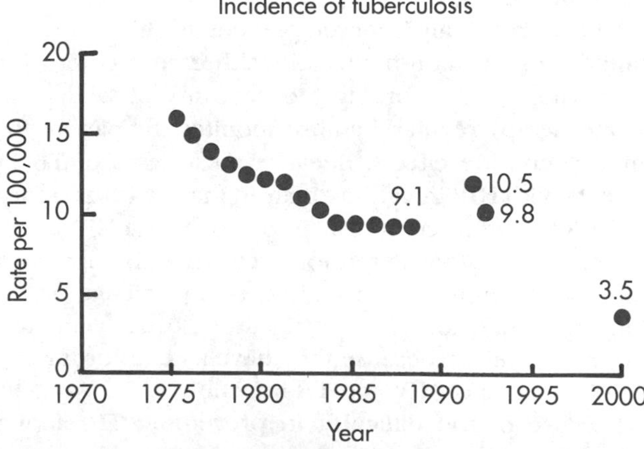


**FIGURE 37-7** Actual incidence of tuberculosis (1975 through 1993) and goal for the year 2000. (From Department of Health and Human Services: *Healthy people 2000: national health promotion and disease prevention objectives,* Washington, DC, 1990, US Government Printing Office.)

**TABLE 37-11 Special Population Targets for Decrease in the Tuberculosis Case Rate per 100,000 Persons**

| GROUP | 1988 BASELINE | 2000 TARGET |
|---|---|---|
| Asians/Pacific Islanders | 36.3 | 15 |
| Blacks | 28.3 | 10 |
| Hispanics | 18.3 | 5 |
| Native Americans/ Native Alaskans | 18.1 | 5 |

From US Department of Health and Human Services: *Healthy people 2000: national health promotion and disease prevention objectives,* Washington, DC, 1990, US Government Printing Office.

**BOX 37-8 Goals for State Tuberculosis Control Programs**

States should have systems that incorporate the following guidelines:

- Ensure the mandatory reporting of each confirmed and suspected case of TB, and observe local laws and regulations protecting patient confidentiality.
- Examine persons at high risk for TB infection and disease, prescribe the appropriate preventive or curative treatment for these persons, and monitor their treatment.
- Monitor the treatment of patients, and require that a treatment plan be devised for all hospitalized patients before they are discharged.
- Ensure the rapid laboratory examination of specimens and reporting of results to the appropriate health department and the requesting clinician.
- Ensure that TB-infected patients receive treatment until they are cured.
- Protect the health of the public by isolating and treating persons who have infectious TB and detaining persons who, although not infectious, are unwilling or unable to complete their treatment and are at risk for becoming infectious and for acquiring drug-resistant TB.
- Finance the treatment of indigent patients.

From Centers for Disease Control: *MMWR* 41(RR-5):1-23, 1992.

guidelines for state tuberculosis control programs. These goals are listed in Box 37-8.

**Primary and secondary prevention.** To eliminate TB, the organism must be prevented from being transmitted from one person to another. Preventive measures are directed toward the latest recommendations from the ACET (Box 37-9).

Persons over 35 years of age without the risk factors listed here are not given preventive chemotherapy because of the risk of isoniazid-associated hepatitis. Although the risk is small, it is age related and increases from less than 0.2% in those under age 20 to up to 2.3% in those 50 to 64 years of age.

If isoniazid-associated hepatitis occurs, the symptoms are mild, nonspecific, and resemble those of any viral illness. (See Chapter 42 for a discussion of viral hepatitis.)

Contraindications to the use of isoniazid preventive therapy are (1) previous isoniazid-associated liver disease; (2) severe adverse reactions to isoniazid, including fever, chills, rash, and arthritis; and (3) *acute* liver disease of any cause.

Persons receiving isoniazid preventive chemotherapy should be seen monthly by a health care provider for the purpose of reinforcing the necessity of taking the chemotherapy regularly and to monitor the patient for any serious side effects. Because most cases of TB in patients with HIV infection occur in those with a history of a positive tuberculin test, all persons with HIV infection should be considered for preventive therapy with isoniazid. Groups that should receive particular attention are intravenous (IV) drug users, prison inmates, and the homeless, because they have an extraordinarily high incidence of HIV and TB infection.[5]

Because of the difficulty in preventing TB among homeless persons, special recommendations have been made for this group.[16]

1. The highest priority should be given to (1) detection, evaluation, and reporting of current symptoms of active TB in homeless persons and (2) completion of an appropriate course of treatment by those diagnosed with active TB.
2. The second priority should be screening and preventive therapy for homeless persons who have, or are suspected of having, HIV infection.
3. The third priority should be the examination and appropriate treatment of persons with recent TB that has been inadequately treated.
4. The fourth priority should be screening and appropriate treatment of persons exposed to an infectious (sputum-positive) case of TB. Because contacts are difficult to define in a shelter population, it is usually necessary to screen all residents of a shelter when an infectious case is identified.
5. The fifth priority should be screening and preventive therapy for homeless persons with known medical conditions that increase the risk of TB, for example, diabetes mellitus and other conditions listed in Box 37-9.

Preventive chemotherapy in the United States is isoniazid daily for 6 months. The usual adult dose is 300 mg in a single dose daily. If the person has antibodies to HIV, isoniazid is given daily for 1 year.

In 1989 the CDC's ACET published *A Strategic Plan for Elimination of Tuberculosis in the United States.* The committee recommended that a goal be established to eliminate TB by the year 2010. To achieve the goal, a case rate of 0.1 per 100,000 persons was set for the year 2010, with an interim goal of a case rate of 3.5 per 100,000 population by the year 2000. This goal may not

**BOX 37-9 Priorities for Preventive Therapy With Isoniazid Among TB-Infected Persons**

1. Persons with HIV infection
2. Recent contacts of persons with infectious TB
3. Persons with recent skin test conversions
4. Persons with recent TB disease who have been inadequately treated
5. Persons with negative sputum cultures and stable fibrotic lesions on chest radiographs consistent with inactive TB
6. Persons with medical conditions that increase the risk of TB
   - Leukemia or lymphoma
   - Silicosis
   - Diabetes mellitus
   - Gastrectomy
   - End-stage renal disease
   - Antibodies to HIV

be easy to accomplish, in view of the 1992 case rate of 10.5 per 100,000.[16]

**Vaccination.** Efforts continue in search of a more satisfactory TB vaccine. Presently, bacillus Calmette-Guérin (BCG) vaccine is used worldwide except in the United States and the Netherlands. The vaccine contains attenuated tubercle bacilli that have lost their ability to produce disease. It is administered only to persons who have a negative reaction to the tuberculin test. It is not widely used in the United States because of disagreements among physicians as to its safety and effectiveness.

Currently, BCG vaccination is recommended only for tuberculin-negative infants and children who have continuing exposure to persons who have isoniazid-resistant and rifampin-resistant active TB, persons who cannot take isoniazid themselves and have ongoing exposure to a person with a case of infectious TB, or persons who belong to groups where the new *M. tuberculosis* infection rates exceed 1% per year.[18]

The results of a metaanalysis of the published literature on the efficacy of BCG vaccine were published early in 1994. The conclusions from this report were that:

1. BCG significantly reduces the risk of active TB cases and deaths.
2. The overall protective effect was 50% against TB infections.
3. The vaccine protected against both pulmonary TB and disseminated TB (78% protective effect), tuberculosis meningitis (64% protective effect), and death (71% protective effect).

Institutional outbreaks and the emergence of MDR-TB are prompting reconsideration of the broader use of BCG vaccine in the United States.[18]

Most persons who have received BCG will have a skin test reaction of less than 10 mm. If a larger reaction occurs to purified protein derivative (PPD), it can be assumed that the person has a TB infection.

The vaccine should be given only by persons who have had careful instruction in the proper technique. A multiple-puncture disk is used to give the vaccine. When there is a positive reaction to skin testing with tuberculin, when acute infectious disease is present, or when there is any skin disease, BCG vaccine is not given. Possible complications following vaccination are local ulcers, which occur in a relatively high percentage of persons vaccinated, and abscesses or suppuration of lymph nodes, which occur in a small percentage.

In countries where living conditions are such that transmission of TB is to be expected, BCG vaccine is given at birth and then repeated after 12 to 15 years. The intradermal method is used to administer the vaccine so that a uniform controlled dose can be given. BCG vaccine, as mentioned earlier, is not widely used in the United States, although some highly susceptible groups such as migrant workers may be vaccinated.

### Medical management

**Diagnostic tests.** Each of the tests used to diagnose tuberculosis is described in Chapter 35. These tests are (1) tuberculin skin testing, (2) chest x-ray films, and (3) sputum smear and culture. If microscopic study of a slide prepared from the sputum of an individual reveals tubercle bacilli, the individual is said to have positive sputum, and this confirms the diagnosis of TB. However, most persons with tuberculosis will not have positive sputum on smear, and a *positive sputum culture* will be necessary to confirm the diagnosis. Patients who have a positive culture and negative smear are less infectious than are those with both a positive smear and a positive culture.

***Establishing the diagnosis of tuberculosis.*** Results of chest x-ray films and sputum examinations will either rule out the possibility or confirm a diagnosis of TB. Bacteriologic confirmation of the presence of *M. tuberculosis* is necessary to establish the diagnosis of TB. Because it is impossible to differentiate between typical bacilli and MOTT by a sputum smear, cultures are obtained on all persons. Cultures are also used for antimicrobial susceptibility (sensitivity) studies. *Despite the introduction of improved culture media, the tubercle bacillus grows slowly on artificial media, and culture reports are not available for 3 to 6 weeks.*

Blood-streaked sputum in the absence of pronounced coughing may be the first indication to the person that something is wrong. Pathologic changes may have occurred in the lungs, but sputum examination may not show tubercle bacilli. However, if the nodules produced in the parenchyma of the lung become soft in the center and then caseated and liquefied, the liquefied material may break through and empty into the bronchi and be raised as sputum. Cavities in the lung may appear on x-ray film and may be present in more than one lobe of the lung.

**Medications.** To avoid the emergence of drug-resistant organisms, the ACET recommends the following beginning therapy for TB.

1. Susceptibility testing
   a. All persons with TB from whom *M. tuberculosis* is isolated should have drug-susceptibility testing performed on the first isolate.
   b. Drug-susceptibility testing also should be performed on additional isolates from patients whose cultures fail to convert to negative within 3 months of beginning therapy.
2. Initial regimen[12]
   a. Initial treatment should be with four drugs (Table 37-12). During the first 2 months, the patient should receive INH, RIF, PZA, and EMB or SM. When drug susceptibility results are available, the regimen should be altered as appropriate.
   b. Health care and correctional facilities that are experiencing outbreaks of TB resistant to INH and RIF or are resuming treatment of a patient who has been treated for TB in the past may need to begin patient treatment with five or six drugs as initial therapy.
   c. Patients whose organisms are susceptible to INH and RIF should receive these two drugs for a full 6 months, supplemented with PZA for the first 2 months.
3. Immunosuppressed patients. HIV infection and other factors that compromise a patient's immune system make them *more susceptible to the development of resistant organisms.* For this reason, it is recommended that patients with HIV and TB be treated for a total of 9 months and for at least 6 months after their sputum converts to negative. If drug susceptibility results are not available, EMB or SM should be considered for the entire course of therapy because of the rapid progression of TB while the patient is receiving inadequate therapy.
4. Treatment of extrapulmonary TB. The regimen that is used for treating pulmonary disease is also used to treat extrapulmonary disease. Some experts believe that therapy should be for 9 months instead of 6 months for patients with disseminated TB, miliary disease, TB of bone and joints, and TB of the lymph glands.
5. Treatment of TB during pregnancy. Therapy is essential for pregnant women who have TB. SM is not used because it may cause congenital deafness. Routine use of PZA is not recommended because the risk of birth defects in the fetus has not been determined.

**TABLE 37-12 Drugs Used To Treat Tuberculosis**

| DRUG | CLASSIFICATION | COMMON SIDE EFFECTS | TESTS | REMARKS |
|---|---|---|---|---|
| Isoniazid (INH) | Bactericidal; penetrates all body tissues and fluids, including cerebrospinal fluid (CSF) | Peripheral neuritis, hepatitis, rash, fever | AST (formerly SGOT), ALT (formerly SGPT) (not as routine) | Daily alcohol intake interferes with metabolism of isoniazid and increases risk of hepatitis; antacids containing aluminum interfere with absorption of INH. |
| Rifampin (RIF) | Bactericidal; penetrates all body tissues, including CSF | Hepatitis, febrile reactions, thrombocytopenia (rare), hepatotoxicity increases when given with INH | AST, ALT, platelet count (not as routine) | Urine, sweat, tears may turn orange temporarily; decrease effectiveness of oral contraceptives, anticoagulants, corticosteroids, barbiturates, hypoglycemics, and digitalis. |
| Ethambutol (EMB) | Bacteriostatic; does not penetrate CSF; penetrates other body fluids | Optic neuritis (reversible with discontinuation of drug; very rare at 15 mg/kg skin rash) | Visual acuity; red-green color discrimination; GI irritation | No significant reaction with other drugs. Check vision monthly; give with food. |
| Pyrazinamide (PZA) | Bacteriostatic or bactericidal depending on susceptibility of mycobacterium | Hyperuricemia, hepatitis, arthralgia, GI irritation | Uric acid, AST, ALT | Obtain baseline liver function tests and repeat regularly. Give with food; drink 2 L of fluid daily. |
| Streptomycin (SM) | Bactericidal, aminoglycoside; disrupts protein synthesis; poor penetration into body tissues and CSF | Eighth cranial nerve damage (vestibular or ocular); damage often irreversible; nephrotoxicity | Vestibular function; audiograms; creatinine level determined before therapy started | Monitor kidney function monthly, monitor vestibular function with caloric stimulation test monthly. Monitor hearing with audiograms monthly. Meningitis is treated with intrathecal or subarachnoid instillation of SM. |

Nine months of therapy with INH, RIF, and EMB is recommended. Women may breast-feed while receiving TB therapy because the concentration of the drugs in breast milk is so low that drug toxicity does not develop in the newborn.

6. **Directly observed therapy (DOT)**[12]
   a. A major cause of drug-resistant TB and treatment failure is patient nonadherence to prescribed treatment. Treatment failure and drug-resistant TB can be life-threatening and pose other serious public health problems because they lead to prolonged infectiousness of the patient and increased transmission of TB in the community. For this reason, direct observation of the patient taking the drugs is recommended.
   b. Effective use of DOT requires a setting where the patient goes to receive drugs either daily, 2 times a week, or 3 times a week depending on the regimen ordered. The setting can be a TB clinic, community health center, homeless shelter, prison or jail, nursing home, school, drug treatment center, or other settings that agree to serve as treatment centers.
   c. In some situations, a responsible person other than a health care worker may administer DOT. These include correctional facility personnel, staff of community-based organizations, clergy, or other community leaders.
   d. The use of incentives and enablers may promote patient adherence to a DOT program.
      (1) Providing transportation or car/bus fare to the DOT site
      (2) Use of combined preparations of INH and RIF, which reduce the number of pills the patient has to take
   e. Outreach workers who go into the community to talk with patients are often helpful in stressing to patients the urgency of taking the drugs as prescribed.

## NURSING MANAGEMENT

### ♦ ASSESSMENT

#### Subjective Data

It is important to determine whether the patient was exposed to a person with TB. Often the *source* of the infection is unknown and may never be determined. At the same time, close contacts of the patient need to be identified so that they may undergo follow-up to determine if they are infected and have active disease or a positive tuberculin test.

The most common patient complaints are productive cough and night sweats.

#### Objective Data

Data to be collected to assess the patient with TB include the following:

Productive cough
Afternoon temperature elevation
Tuberculin skin test reaction of 10 mm induration or more (see Chapter 35)
X-ray film showing a pulmonary infiltrate (see Chapter 35)

### ♦ NURSING DIAGNOSES

Nursing diagnoses are determined from analysis of patient data. Nursing diagnoses for the person with tuberculosis may include but are not limited to the following:

| Diagnostic Title | Possible Etiologic Factors |
|---|---|
| Airway clearance, ineffective | Increased sputum, decreased energy/fatigue |
| Fear | Long-term illness requiring long-term chemotherapy, life-style changes until no longer infectious |
| Knowledge deficit about tuberculosis: spread and treatment | Lack of exposure to information |

### ♦ EXPECTED PATIENT OUTCOMES

Expected patient outcomes for the person with tuberculosis may include but are not limited to the following:

1. Explains how TB is spread and those measures necessary to prevent spread of TB (remain on chemotherapy, cover mouth and nose when coughing or sneezing).
2. Explains basic food groups and how a nutritionally adequate diet will be achieved.
3. States name, dose, actions, and side effects of prescribed medications.
4. States why two, three, or four chemotherapy agents must be taken together.
   a. Explains drug-resistant organisms and relates this to the need to take chemotherapy as directed.
   b. Explains why the health care provider should be notified immediately if for any reason (e.g., side effects) chemotherapy cannot be taken.
5. States where to receive new supply of chemotherapy and date it is to be obtained.
6. States plans for follow-up care.
   a. Lists signs and symptoms that indicate need for immediate medical care (increased cough, hemoptysis, unexplained weight loss, fever, night sweats).
   b. States when next sputum test or x-ray film is to be taken and where.
   c. States plans for ongoing follow-up care.

### ♦ INTERVENTIONS

The major nursing responsibility is to teach the patient about TB and how it is transmitted. Preventing contamination of air with tubercle bacilli is accomplished by the following: (1) treating the patient with antituberculosis drugs and (2) preventing contamination of air

**Guidelines for Preventing the Transmission of Tuberculosis**

Patient must take antituberculosis drugs as prescribed.
- Drugs are always taken as combination of at least four drugs initially.
- Drugs must be taken uninterruptedly.
- Both of the above are necessary to prevent development of resistant strains of *M. tuberculosis.*

Preventing contamination of air with *M. tuberculosis.*
- Cover nose and mouth with disposable tissues when coughing, sneezing, or laughing.
- Place used tissues in paper bag, which should be burned.

with the tubercle bacilli. The most effective way to achieve both of the above is by patient teaching (see the Guidelines box above).

The most important factor in the transmission of TB is overcrowded living conditions. This is why outbreaks of TB occur in schools, homeless shelters, jails, prisons, and other settings where people are crowded together. To prevent the transmission of TB from person to person it is necessary to prevent contamination of the air with *M. tuberculosis.* This is achieved in two ways:

1. Teach the patient to cover nose and mouth when coughing, sneezing, and laughing so that droplet nuclei are not discharged into the air.
2. Adequate treatment of the patient with antituberculosis drugs. Most persons who adhere to the prescribed therapy and do not have other mitigating factors such as immunosuppression convert their sputum from positive to negative in a relatively short time (2 to 3 weeks). See the Guidelines box (above) for a summary of patient teaching about the transmission of tuberculosis.

## PROTECTION OF HEALTH CARE WORKERS

Nurses and other health care workers need to know the protective measures they can use when caring for patients who have a positive TB smear or culture. The following measures are indicated.[10]

1. As mentioned earlier, the first emphasis should be on preventing *M. tuberculosis* from being expelled into room air by the patient. Most patients will cooperate and cover their nose and mouth when coughing and sneezing. Those who are too ill to do so or who are confused can have a surgical mask put over their nose and mouth.
2. The patient is placed in a private room, and the door to the hallway is kept closed.
3. If the patient must leave the room for tests or procedures in another part of the hospital, he or she should wear a particulate respirator with a one-way valve.
4. The air pressure in the room should be negative, which allows air to flow into the room when the door is opened and prevents room air from moving out into the hallway.
5. The air in the room should be exchanged at least six times every hour, with two of the exchanges being with fresh air from the outside. Air from the patient's room should be directly vented to the outside and not recirculated within the hospital.
6. High-energy particulate air (HEPA) filters can be installed in ventilation ducts.
7. Some institutions use ultraviolet lights high on walls or ceilings in patient rooms to disinfect room air. They are placed so that they do not cause a risk to the patients or health care workers.
8. Personnel caring for the patients should wear a disposable particulate respirator. The respirator should fit snugly over the nose and mouth to prevent as much room air as possible from getting in around the edges. The particulate respirator filters out organisms as small as 1 μ. *M. tuberculosis* organisms are 3 to 5 μ.
9. All health care workers should know their tuberculin status. Most younger workers will be tuberculin negative, and the goal is to keep them that way. All workers should be tested yearly with PPD. Those who have not had a recent test should receive a baseline tuberculin test on employment and then yearly. Workers who have inadvertently been exposed to a patient with TB (often before the diagnosis of TB is made) should have a tuberculin test 8 to 12 weeks after exposure. It takes this period for a test to convert from negative to positive. The CDC recommends that health care workers involved in the care of patients receiving cough-inducing procedures such as bronchoscopy and tracheal suctioning should be tuberculin tested at least every 6 months.
10. Health care workers who convert from a negative to a positive tuberculin test should have an examination to rule out active TB. Isoniazid prevention therapy is offered to those who do not have active TB.
11. Once patients have three negative smears for TB, they are considered noninfectious, and health care workers do not need to wear a mask when caring for them.

## Lung Abscess

### Etiology

A lung abscess is an area of localized suppuration within the lung. It usually is caused by bacteria that reach the lung through *aspiration.* Some experts suggest that it might better be called *aspiration lung abscess* because aspiration is the common factor.

### Pathophysiology

The infected material lodges in the small bronchi and produces inflammation. Partial obstruction of the bronchus results in retention of secretions beyond the obstruction and the eventual *necrosis of tissue.* The ne-

**BOX 37-10 Clinical Manifestations of Acute Lung Abscess**

High fever: 39° C (102° F)
Chills and prostration
Cough and sputum production common
Night sweats, pleuritic chest pain, anemia, and occasionally hemoptysis
Putrid sputum in about 50% of patients—foul odor evident in patient's room
Weight loss in about 40% of patients (foul-smelling and foul-tasting sputum often causes anorexia)
Mortality rate of primary abscess is 5%.
Up to one third of patients 45 years of age and older have a lung abscess associated with carcinoma.
A diagnostic bronchoscopy should be considered for all high-risk patients, even if they respond well to therapy.

From Baier H: Primary lung abscess. In Rakel RE, editor: *Conn's current therapy,* Philadelphia, 1993, Saunders.

crotic lung tissue is coughed up, and an air-filled cavity is left in the lung.

Food particles and perigingival debris, which contain both aerobic and anaerobic organisms, are the most frequently aspirated substances. Laboratory cultures of sputum or transtracheal aspirates are necessary to identify the causative organism. When only normal oropharyngeal flora is found, aerobic cultures may demonstrate the presence of fusospirochetal organisms, peptostreptococci, and *Bacteroides* species. All these organisms are typically found in gingival infections. The most common aerobic bacteria causing lung abscess are *Staphylococcus aureus* and *Klebsiella pneumoniae.* Aerobic gram-negative organisms are found most frequently in persons with nosocomial infections (see Chapter 15) or in persons who are immunosuppressed. Sputum should also be examined for tumor cells and for tuberculosis and fungal organisms. Before the advent of antibiotics and specific chemotherapy, lung abscess was a fairly frequent complication after pneumonia.

Lung abscess may follow bronchial obstruction caused by a tumor, foreign body, or stenosis of the bronchus. Children particularly may aspirate foreign materials such as a peanut, and a lung abscess results. Metastatic spread of cancer cells to the lung parenchyma may also cause an abscess, and occasionally the infection appears to have been borne by the bloodstream. In recent years the incidence of lung abscess caused by infection has decreased, and secondary lung abscess after bronchogenic carcinoma has increased.[4] Bronchoscopy may be used to identify the infected segment and to obtain specimens for culture. Box 37-10 lists clinical manifestations of lung abscess.

### Medical management

The course of lung abscess is influenced by the cause of the abscess and by the type of drainage that can be established. If the purulent material drains easily, the patient may respond well to segmental postural drainage, antibiotic therapy, and good general supportive care. When obstruction interferes with drainage into the bronchi, bronchoscopic procedures should be used not only to improve drainage but also to rule out obstructing foreign bodies or neoplasms. Today, surgical treatment to establish drainage has become increasingly less necessary; but, if after several weeks of medical treatment a cavity persists, a segmentectomy or lobectomy may be performed[4] (see p. 1095).

Penicillin G is the drug of choice, and 2 to 3 million units is given intravenously every 4 hours until the fever is relieved and the patient's condition shows marked improvement. Penicillin VK in doses of 500 mg four times daily is then given orally. When the patient has a sensitivity to penicillin, clindamycin (Cleocin), 600 mg every 8 hours, is prescribed. For staphylococcal infections, oxacillin or nafcillin, 6 to 8 g intravenously in divided doses, is often prescribed. Lung abscesses caused by gram-negative organisms are treated with appropriate antibiotics, as determined by in vitro sensitivity tests.

Antibiotic therapy is continued until all signs of the illness have subsided and the chest x-ray films show that the cavity has completely disappeared or has reduced significantly in size. Most cavities close within 6 weeks, but occasionally a cavity may persist for months. Foul-smelling sputum usually disappears within a few days, whereas cough and nonfoul sputum may continue for a longer period. Usually the patient begins to feel better during the first week of therapy, but it may take up to 2 months for the temperature to return to normal.

If the patient does not improve with the therapy just discussed, bronchoscopy is performed to search for a possible obstruction to drainage, such as carcinoma or a foreign body.

Medical treatment cannot cause a walled-off abscess to disappear, and surgery may be necessary. If surgery is necessary, the portion of lung containing the abscess is removed. If the abscess is caused by carcinoma, the surgery may be much more extensive.

### Nursing management

The person with a lung abscess is very ill and will be admitted to the hospital. Other persons already in the hospital are at risk of aspiration and lung abscess. These include persons with suppressed levels of consciousness such as found in head injury, after anesthesia, CVA, alcoholism, seizure disorders, drug overdoses, persons with compromised immunologic defenses, and elderly persons, especially if immobile.

Nursing responsibilities include the following:

1. Prevention of aspiration in hospitalized patients
   a. Monitoring patients who are at risk of aspiration
   b. Frequent mouth care to persons with diminished levels of consciousness
   c. Close monitoring of persons receiving tube feedings to ensure that tube is in stomach

### Guidelines for Care of the Person With Lung Abscess

Monitor vital signs at least every 4 hours because temperature may spike in afternoon and may persist for as long as 2 weeks.
Place patient in comfortable position. If patient is conscious, usually can make more comfortable with head rest at 45 to 90 degrees.
Help patient cough up sputum. This helps drain abscess.
Collect sputum for culture and sensitivity tests to determine organism and antibiotic therapy. This monitors effectiveness of therapy and whether resistant organisms are developing.
Do postural drainage. This facilitates drainage from the abscess.

d. If patient is vomiting, place on side in postanesthesia position to reduce aspiration.
e. If patient is unable to expectorate secretions from mouth and oropharynx, oral suctioning may be necessary.

2. Care of patient with a lung abscess is outlined in the Guidelines box above.

## Bronchiectasis

### Etiology

Bronchiectasis is irreversible dilation of the bronchial tree. It has declined greatly since the advent of antibiotics.[28]

### Pathophysiology

When infection attacks the bronchial lining, inflammation occurs, and an exudate forms. The progressive accumulation of secretions obstructs the bronchioles. The obstructed bronchioles then break down, and ciliated columnar epithelium is replaced by nonciliated cuboidal epithelium and sometimes fibrotic tissue, resulting in localized areas of dilation or saccules. The expulsive force of the bronchioles is diminished, and they may remain filled with exudate. Only forceful coughing and postural drainage will empty them. Bronchiectasis may involve any part of the lung parenchyma, but it usually occurs in the dependent portions or lobes except in TB, when it is usually in the upper lobes. Before the widespread use of antibiotics in treating persons with respiratory tract infections, this disease began to develop in young people, with many showing symptoms in childhood or by age 20. Although the incidence of childhood bronchiectasis is decreasing, it is increasing in individuals with cystic fibrosis, immunodeficiency diseases, or atopic asthma, in which repeated respiratory infections have been successfully treated with antibiotics. These persons now survive the acute episodes of bacterial infection that complicate their underlying disease but sometimes develop bronchiectasis as a sequela.

A contributing factor in bronchiectasis may be a congenital weakness in the structure of the bronchi that results in impairment of elasticity. Bronchiectasis may occur without previous pulmonary disease, but it usually follows such diseases as bronchopneumonia, lung abscesses, TB, cystic fibrosis, or asthma. A computed tomography (CT) scan is used for diagnosis. Box 37-11 lists clinical manifestations.

### BOX 37-11 Clinical Manifestations of Bronchiectasis

Signs and symptoms of bronchiectasis vary with the severity of the condition and may include the following:

**SIGNS**

Cyanosis
Clubbing of fingers
Fine rales and coarse rhonchi
Dull or flat sounds over areas of mucous plugs
Increased vocal and tactile fremitus over middle and lower lobes
Decreased diaphragmatic excursion
Paroxysms of coughing on arising in morning and when lying down

**SYMPTOMS**

Severe coughing productive of copious amounts of purulent sputum
Hemoptysis
Dyspnea
Fatigue and weakness
Loss of appetite and weight loss

The condition may develop so gradually that the person is frequently unable to tell when the symptoms first began.

### Medical management

Treatment of bronchiectasis includes the following:

1. Antibiotics
2. Postural drainage to assist in removing secretions and prevent coughing (see p. 1146)
3. Bronchoscopy to remove thicker secretions

### Surgical management

Surgery is used only for patients who continue to have signs and symptoms of bronchiectasis despite medical therapy. The goal in surgery is to preserve as much functional lung as possible. Therefore a segmentectomy or lobectomy is given priority. (See p. 1095 for discussion of these procedures.) Some patients have bilateral disease. In this situation, the most involved lung is operated on first to see how much improvement occurs before treating the other side.[28]

### Nursing management

Nursing care should stress good general hygiene, which may contribute to relief of symptoms. Adequate diet, rest, exercise, and diversional activity are important; avoiding superimposed infections such as colds should be emphasized. Frequent mouth care is essential, and cleansing the mouth with an aromatic solution before meals often makes food more acceptable.

**BOX 37-12 Clinical Manifestations of Empyema**

The patient with a lung infection or chest injury may develop empyema and should be observed closely for the following signs and symptoms of empyema:

- Cough (usually nonproductive)
- Dyspnea
- Tachypnea
- Tachycardia
- Elevation of temperature
- Unilateral chest expansion
- Malaise
- Decreased appetite

The diagnosis can usually be made from the signs and symptoms and the medical history, but it is confirmed by a chest x-ray film that demonstrates the presence of a pleural exudate. A thoracentesis is performed to obtain a sample of the pus for culture and sensitivity studies and to relieve the patient's respiratory symptoms.

## Empyema

### Etiology

Empyema is pus within a body cavity, usually the pleural cavity.

### Epidemiology

Empyema occurs as a result of or in association with other respiratory diseases such as pneumonia, lung abscess, TB, and fungal infections of the lung and also after thoracic surgery or chest trauma. It now occurs fairly often as a complication of staphylococcal pneumonia.

Box 37-12 lists clinical manifestations of empyema.

### Medical management

The aim of treatment of empyema is to drain the empyema cavity completely and thus obliterate the pleural space. The cavity can be drained in the following ways:

1. Initial treatment is often daily thoracentesis with aspiration of the cavity and instillation of antibiotics into the pleural space. Oral or IV antibiotics may also be given. If the cavity cannot be evacuated within a few days or if the lung fails to reexpand to obliterate the space, surgery is necessary.
2. The type of surgery depends on the situation and may include the following:
   a. *Closed-chest drainage,* in which a trochar is inserted between the ribs at the base of the cavity. A chest catheter is inserted through the trochar, the trochar is removed, and the tube is connected to water-seal drainage (see p. 1095). Pus then drains from the cavity into the collection chamber. For closed drainage to be successful, the pus must be thin enough to drain out of the pleural space, and the lung must be able to reexpand to fill the pleural space.
   b. Rib resection with *open-chest drainage* is necessary when empyema is chronic and the lung is incapable of reexpanding to obliterate the pleural space. A portion of one or two ribs is removed, and a large drainage tube is inserted into the empyema cavity. This allows pus to drain into a heavy chest dressing, which will need to be changed once or twice daily. The tube is changed weekly. If the treatment is effective, granulation tissue will form in the space from the inside out, thus obliterating the pleural space.
   c. *Decortication* is necessary in instances of chronic empyema where a fibronous peel has formed on the visceral pleura, preventing the lung from reexpanding and filling the space left after the empyema cavity was drained. In decortication, the fibrinous peel is removed from the visceral pleura by blunt dissection, freeing the lung so that it can reexpand and fill the pleural space. Two chest tubes are inserted into the pleural space and connected to water-seal drainage with additional suction. See p. 1095 for a discussion of chest drainage.
   d. *Thoracoplasty* (the removal of one or more ribs) may be necessary if none of the preceding procedures are successful in obliterating the pleural space. The removal of ribs alters the shape of the thorax, and the chest wall is brought inward to obliterate the pleural space (see p. 1104).

### Nursing management

Nursing care depends on the type and effectiveness of the procedure. In some cases the patient will go through several treatments before the empyema space is closed. This can be frustrating, and the patient can become very discouraged. A major nursing role is to support the patient and family during the various procedures.

# FUNGAL INFECTIONS

There are three major fungal infections of the lungs: **histoplasmosis, coccidioidomycosis,** and **blastomycosis.** They are classified as deep mycoses because there is involvement by the parasite of deeper tissues and internal organs. The etiology, epidemiology, and prevention of these fungal (mycotic) infections are discussed in Table 37-13.

## Histoplasmosis

### Etiology

Inhalation of spores of *Histoplasma capsulatum* causes histoplasmosis.

### Epidemiology

See Table 37-13.

### Pathophysiology

The spores are inhaled and phagocytized by alveolar macrophages within which they germinate. They form yeast cells and multiply by budding. In persons previ-

**TABLE 37-13 Etiology, Epidemiology, and Prevention of Fungal Lung Infections**

| DISEASE | ETIOLOGY | EPIDEMIOLOGY | PREVENTION |
|---|---|---|---|
| Histoplasmosis | Inhalation of spores of *Histoplasma capsulatum*<br>Soil contaminated with fowl excreta; possibly bats infected and areas they inhabit (caves, attics, hollow trees); can be extremely infectious | Most common systemic mycotic disease in United States; endemic areas in Missouri, Kentucky, Tennessee, Southern Illinois, Indiana, and Ohio; more than 40 million in these areas infected | Locate areas where soil is infected with fowl excreta. Teach public to avoid inhalation of dust from infected soil. Infants and elderly persons are especially susceptible. |
| Coccidioidomycosis (Valley fever, San Joaquin Valley fever) | Inhalation of spores of *Coccidioides immitis*<br>Soil contaminated with spores; growth of fungus enhanced by heavy rainfall in desert; inhibited by sunlight; anthrospores which are inhaled, dispersed by liberation of dust in spring | Endemic to well-defined areas in southwestern United States, Mexico, and South America. In United States, endemic in San Joaquin Valley, Southern Arizona, New Mexico, and Southwestern Texas | Encourage wearing of masks by persons working in desert dust, archeologists, construction workers. |
| Blastomycosis | Believed to be inhalation of *Blastomyces dermatitidis*<br>Soil contaminated with spores that are carried on air currents and inhaled by humans and animals; dogs can acquire the disease; not believed to be spread from animals to man; believed that both humans and animals infected by inhaling spores | Most prevalent in the United States and Canadian valley areas surrounding the Mississippi, Missouri, Ohio, and St. Lawrence rivers; also present in Africa, South America, Mexico, and Asia | Avoid inhalation of spores in soil in areas where cases have been identified. |

ously uninfected, there is a primary or initial infection that resembles the infection in primary TB with involvement of regional lymphatics and early dissemination via lymphatic and blood to other organs. Yeast cells spread hematogenously and are phagocytized by reticuloendothelial cells in the liver, spleen, and bone marrow. *The process in the lung is similar to that seen in TB with necrosis and healing by fibrotic encapsulation.* Eventually, the original parenchymal foci in the lung and in the hilar lymph nodes show calcification. Usually the initial infection is self-limiting, and does not require antifungal chemotherapy. However, some persons such as infants and adults with immunologic incompetence (lymphoma) may develop a rapidly progressive primary infection that will be fatal without antifungal therapy.

*Reinfection histoplasmosis* and *progressive histoplasmosis* can also occur. Reinfection with *Histoplasma* causes an illness resembling the initial infection. Since some degree of immunity to histoplasmosis is conferred by the initial infection, the extent of disease will be modified by the degree of fungal immunity. Heavy inoculation may cause pneumonitis, which is usually self-limiting over days to weeks. The onset is acute with nonproductive cough, fever, malaise, and dyspnea. Some persons who are fully immune may develop a hypersensitivity-like pneumonitis with small, discrete granulomatous foci that may give a miliary appearance on x-ray examination. This means that the infection is spread throughout the lung, giving the appearance of the presence of small millet seeds throughout the lung.

Progressive histoplasmosis is usually chronic; chronic pulmonary histoplasmosis is the most frequently encountered symptomatic form of the disease. It develops almost exclusively in middle-aged white men who have COPD. There are recurrent episodes of necrotizing segmental or lobar granulomatous pneumonitis, which have a tendency to cavity formation, contraction, fibrosis, and compensatory emphysema.

*Progressive disseminated histoplasmosis* usually occurs as a consequence of the initial infection in persons with very low resistance to the infection (infants, persons with immunologic incompetence). Rarely, it can occur in adults of both genders and all ages with no known immune disorder. These persons have fever, weakness, weight loss, hepatosplenomegaly, leukopenia, and mucous membrane ulceration involving the oropharynx, tongue, or larynx. Adrenal insufficiency occurs in about 50% of these persons. See Table 37-14 for signs and symptoms and medical therapy.

## Coccidioidomycosis

### Etiology

Inhalation of spores of *Coccidioides* causes coccidioidomycosis.

**TABLE 37-14 Signs and Symptoms and Medical Therapy for Fungal Lung Infections**

| TYPE OF INFECTION | SIGNS AND SYMPTOMS | MEDICAL THERAPY |
|---|---|---|
| Histoplasmosis | Severe infections; acute onset with fever, chest pain, dyspnea, prostration, weight loss, widespread pulmonary infiltrates, hepatomegaly, and splenomegaly; no symptoms in some persons, benign acute pneumonitis in others | Drug(s) of choice: amphotericin B (Fungizone IV); 75% of patients are cured.<br>Ketoconazole (Nizoral), 400 mg orally daily at bedtime or with meals; without treatment, patient with disseminated disease will die. |
| Coccidioidomycosis (Valley fever, San Joaquin Valley fever) | Asymptomatic upper respiratory tract infection in about 60% of those who inhaled spores: 40% have symptoms ranging from flulike illness to frank pneumonia | Amphotericin B IV<br>Therapy required for only 10% of those with symptoms; remainder have spontaneous remission.<br>Ketoconazole orally. |
| Blastomycosis | Skin lesions that appear as small papular or pustular lesions on exposed parts of the body such as hands and face<br>Peripheral development of lesions, may become raised but do not itch | Amphotericin B IV; mandatory in immunocompromised patients<br>Ketoconazole orally<br>Miconazole (only for patients who cannot tolerate amphotericin or ketoconazole) |

**Epidemiology**

See Table 37-13.

**Pathophysiology**

The process following inhalation of spores is believed to be very similar to that described under histoplasmosis. The arthrospores reach the alveoli, where they are phagocytized. If the disease becomes disseminated, there is marked hilar adenopathy, and fungi can be isolated from lymph nodes. A pneumonic disease with necrosis and cavitation may occur after development of delayed hypersensitivity. The disease process is controlled and resolved in most persons as the result of cell immunity to infection. Thus, progressive disseminated coccidioidomycosis or progressive pulmonary disease is found only in those persons whose ability to resist infection or develop immunity has been compromised in some way. Susceptibility to infection is in part genetically determined. Coccidioidomycosis is 50 times more common in Filipino men and 10 times more common in black men than it is in white men. This increased susceptibility to progressive disease in these groups of men parallels their susceptibility to tuberculosis. The increased susceptibility of some races to diseases such as coccidioidomycosis and tuberculosis is believed to be the result of a genetically determined impairment of their capacity to develop cellular immunity to infection.

Skin testing with coccidioidin, 1:10 or 1:100, is available to test for the disease. The test is read in 48 hours. It takes 3 to 6 weeks after exposure for the test to become positive. In severe disseminated disease the test may be negative, indicating that the patient's immune system is no longer able to respond.

X-ray films of the chest may show pneumonic infiltrate, hilar adenopathy, pleural effusion, or a cavitary lesion. About 5% of persons with primary pulmonary involvement will have residual lung lesions such as cavities or nodules. Only about 0.5% of infected individuals go on to develop a severe, progressive mycosis.

Extrapulmonary dissemination of coccidioidomycosis can occur. One of the sites of dissemination is the meningeal surfaces of the brain. If there is any indication of involvement of the CNS, a lumbar puncture is performed. A positive complement fixation titer in the spinal fluid is diagnostic of meningitis.

Dissemination can also occur to skin, soft tissue, liver, and bones; the patient is monitored by physical examination of the skin, gallium scanning of soft tissue, and bone scans. A bone scan should be performed before starting amphotericin B therapy. See Table 37-14 for information about signs, symptoms, and medical therapy.

Surgical intervention for lesions that are localized may involve either excision or drainage to facilitate healing.

## Blastomycosis

**Etiology**

Blastomycosis is caused by inhalation of *Blastomyces dermatitidis.*

**Epidemiology**

See Table 37-13.

**Pathophysiology**

Although skin lesions are the first evidence of blastomycosis, it is believed that the initial site of infection is in the lung. It is assumed that spores are inhaled and phagocytized in the alveoli as part of the primary infection. Thus the pathogenesis of blastomycosis is similar to that of TB, histoplasmosis, and coccidioidomycosis. The infection is spread throughout the body by the lymphatics. The skin lesions represent metastatic infection from the primary pulmonary disease.

*Acute pulmonary blastomycosis* in the form of a self-limiting pneumonia can occur. Otherwise, blastomycosis is a chronic progressive disease with a mortality of about 90% when untreated. For this reason, treatment is recommended for every person in whom the diagnosis is established.

### Primary Prevention

The only way to prevent these mycotic infections is to avoid inhaling spores of the organisms. See Table 37-13 for specific details.

### Medical Management

The signs and symptoms and the medical therapy for the three fungal diseases are presented in Table 37-14.

Diagnostic tests include the following:

1. Direct demonstration of intracellular yeasts in smears of bone marrow and biopsy of lymph nodes, liver, and spleen; cultures of bone marrow, blood, or sputum
2. Serologic tests. (Aggulutination, precipitation and complement-fixation tests are used to help establish diagnosis of histoplasmosis and coccidioidomycosis. Serology tests become positive about 1 month after the primary infection. Titers of serial tests are used to determine activity of the infection.)
3. Skin testing. (Skin test for histoplasmosis is only used for screening purposes. In endemic areas, 90% to 95% of young adults have positive test results. The person should be tested with histoplasmin, tuberculin, blastomycin, and coccidiodin because of the likelihood of cross-reaction. The strongest reaction indicates the likely cause of the infection.)
4. In histoplasmosis and coccidioidomycosis, chest films demonstrate a nodular infiltrate similar in appearance to TB. In blastomycosis, chest films may be nonspecific.
5. WBC count is usually normal. In acute cases it may increase to 13,000/mm$^2$.
6. Leukopenia and anemia may be present in persons with disseminated disease.

### Nursing Management

#### Promoting comfort

Promoting comfort includes the following:

1. Place patient in position to facilitate breathing.
2. Take measures to reduce fever (if present), such as use of cool sponge baths.
3. Maintain room temperature desired by patient.

#### Administering and monitoring medications

The role of the nurse is as follows:

1. Administer medications as prescribed and monitor patient for side effects.
   a. Amphotericin B (Fungizone IV) is the standard therapy for mycotic infection. The dose and length of therapy are determined by the difficulty in eradicating the infection and the likelihood of relapse. The therapy may last 2 to 3 weeks or 2 to 3 months.
   b. Amphotericin B must be given intravenously and has many toxic properties, including local phlebitis, systemic reactions, renal toxicity, hypokalemia, and anemia. In rare instances, anaphylaxis, bone marrow suppression, and cardiovascular and hepatic toxicity develop.
   c. Systemic toxicity (chills, fever, aching, nausea, and vomiting) can be lessened by premedication with 600 mg of aspirin or acetaminophen along with 25 to 50 mg of diphenhydramine (Benadryl) or promethazine (Phenergan) or 10 mg of prochlorperazine (Compazine) orally. Heparin and hydrocortisone succinate (Solu-Cortef) are sometimes added to the infusions to minimize phlebitis.
   d. A reversible azotemia occurs regularly when amphotericin B is administered. The level of azotemia is monitored by biweekly BUN or serum creatinine determinations. A BUN of greater than 40 or a creatinine nearing 3 indicates a need to reduce the drug or temporarily stop it. Therapy is not continued until the azotemia is improved. Serum potassium levels are checked biweekly, and hypokalemia is treated with oral potassium. Anemia is common, and the hematocrit usually stabilizes at 25% to 35%.
   e. Ketoconazole (Nizoral) is administered orally and is effective in the treatment of systemic mycotic infections. It is given daily for a minimum of 6 months. Toxicity appears to be minimal; pruritus, minor GI intolerance, and liver function abnormalities have been reported.
2. Teach patient about medications and follow-up therapy.

#### Providing emotional support

Patients with mycotic infections can be quite ill and may require long-term therapy (as long as 2 to 3 months) with IV antibiotics. Because these diseases are not well understood by the public, the patient needs to feel free to discuss concerns with the nurse. The nurse needs to provide factual information, clarify misconceptions, and help the patient understand the disease and therapy.

## OCCUPATIONAL LUNG DISEASES

### ETIOLOGY

Many pulmonary diseases are believed to be caused by substances inhaled in the workplace. They are more common (1) in blue-collar workers than in white-collar workers, (2) in industrialized areas than in rural areas, and (3) in small and medium-sized businesses than in larger industrial plants.

In some instances it is debatable whether a person's lung disease is clearly occupation specific. This is especially true in cases of bronchitis, asthma, emphysema, or cancer, since all these conditions can be caused or aggravated by several factors found in many different occupations and by nonoccupational factors such as smoking and pollution of the atmosphere.

**TABLE 37-15 Major Occupational Lung Diseases**

| TYPE | ETIOLOGY AND EPIDEMIOLOGY | PATHOPHYSIOLOGY | CLINICAL MANIFESTATIONS AND PREVENTION |
|---|---|---|---|
| **PNEUMOCONIOSES*** | | | |
| Chronic silicosis | 1 million people in United States run risk of developing silicosis<br>Inhaled silica dust; most frequent form seen in miners, foundry workers, and others who inhaled relatively low concentrations of dust for 10-20 years | Dust accumulated in tissue → tissue reaction with whorl-shaped nodules throughout lungs | Breathlessness with exercise |
| Complicated silicosis | 20%-30% of persons with chronic silicosis develop this | Progressive massive fibrosis (PMF) throughout lungs → ↓ lung function and cor pulmonale | Breathlessness, weakness, chest pain, productive cough with sputum, respiratory cripple, dies of heart failure |
| Acute silicosis | Rapidly progressive disease, leading to severe disability and death within 5 years of diagnosis | Inflammatory reaction within alveoli, diffuse fibrosis | Early symptoms, difficulty in breathing, weight loss, fever, cough<br>Prevention: dust control, wetting down of mines, and improved ventilation can reduce dust levels; sandblasters in enclosed spaces can use special suits and breathing apparatuses; some experts believe such protective measures are still inadequate |
| Coal worker's pneumoconiosis (CWP; "black lung disease") | 150,000 coal miners in the United States at risk; amount, size, and nature of dust in air vary according to type of coal, machinery, and technique used, efficiency of ventilation, and other dust control measures; 10%-30% of all coal miners develop simple form of the disease, more prevalent in miners of anthracite or hard coal; other minerals found in miner's lung (silica, kaolin, mica, beryllium, copper, cobalt, others); unknown whether these minerals contribute to development or progression of CWP | Simple CWP; dust accumulation in lungs visible on x-ray film; over years dust piles up, and respiratory bronchioles are dilated (called focal emphysema) | Simple CWP, no symptoms, no respiratory difficulty |
| Complicated CWP or progressive massive fibrosis (PMF) | 3% of persons with simple CWP develop complicated form; more often occurs in miners with heavy deposits of coal dust in lungs; may appear suddenly years after miner has left the mines; can stop suddenly for no discernible reason; smoking seems to have no effect on development of CWP, but smoking has adverse effect on miners' health; miners who smoke have 5 to 6 times more lung obstruction than nonsmoking miners; cigarette smoking causes chronic bronchitis and emphysema as in nonminers | Fibrosis develops in some of dust-laden areas; fibrosis spreads and fibrotic areas coalesce; eventually most of lung is stiffened and useless; silica plays some role in fibrosis but despite international research, role of silica in CWP is not understood | PMF shortens life span; may die from respiratory failure, cor pulmonale, or superimposed infection<br>Prevention: dust control; reduced levels of coal dust can lower simple CWP and reduce number of miners who develop complicated CWP |

From American Lung Association: *Occupational lung diseases: an introduction,* New York, 1979, The Association. *Continued.*

*Also known as "dust in the lungs."

| TABLE 37-15 Major Occupational Lung Diseases—cont'd | | | |
|---|---|---|---|
| **TYPE** | **ETIOLOGY AND EPIDEMIOLOGY** | **PATHOPHYSIOLOGY** | **CLINICAL MANIFESTATIONS AND PREVENTION** |
| **ASBESTOS-RELATED LUNG DISEASE*** | One of the most dangerous occupational hazards; can cause both fibrosis and cancer in asbestos workers; also a general environmental hazard because of its extensive use before health hazards were recognized; most dangerous to those who mine the ores and process the crude material into pure form; no asbestos mines in United States, but processed and used in United States; federal agencies and state governments have tightened controls on use of asbestos; lung cancer associated with all types of asbestos; 20%-25% of deaths of workers with heavy exposure are from lung cancer; cancer related to degree of asbestos and to *cigarette smoking, which enhances carcinogenic properties of asbestos,* asbestos worker who smokes is 90 times as likely to develop lung cancer as smoker who never worked with asbestos | Asbestos occurs in several different forms or ores; commercially important ores are chrysolite, crocidolite, and amosite; most hazardous medically are crocidolite and amosite, fibrosis caused by asbestos called *asbestosis;* asbestos fibers accumulate around terminal bronchioles; body surrounds fibers with iron-rich tissue → asbestos body with characteristic picture on x-ray film; more asbestos bodies as more fibers are inhaled; after 20-30 years of exposure, fibrosis begins in lungs, if heavy exposure, fibrosis appears in 4-5 years | After fibrosis begins, cough, sputum, weight loss, increasing breathlessness; most die within 1-5 years of first symptoms |
| | Mesothelioma (cancer of the pleura) accounts for 7%-10% of deaths of asbestos workers; inoperable and always fatal; can occur after very little exposure to crocidolite; has been reported in wives of asbestos workers and in persons living near asbestos plants; cigarette smoking not a contributing factor; only a few fine, straight crocidolite fibers are necessary; asbestos workers have higher incidence of other cancers (esophagus, stomach, intestines); swallowing of asbestos-contaminated sputum responsible for these cancers | Occurs in persons exposed to crocidolite fibers of a certain size; a few cases involve amosite fibers; needlelike shape of crocidolite fibers enables them to pass through lung tissue to pleura | Radical pleurectomy and pneumonectomy; survival only 1-2 years<br>Prevention: number of asbestos-related diseases has been increasing despite recognition of hazards and dust-control measures; much tighter controls are needed; some countries have taken such steps; there is need for massive efforts to educate general public of dangers of asbestos |
| **SOME OTHER PNEUMOCONIOSES** | | | |
| Aluminum | Inhaled particles of a certain size induce disease | | |
| Beryllium | Greatest risk of exposure in plants that extract beryllium from crude ore; beryllium is metal used in metallurgy, certain machine tools, making of ceramics, and nuclear power industry | Affects most body systems; in lung produces a severe chemical pneumonia after acute exposure; chronic form called *berylliosis* | |
| Chronic berylliosis | Disease of hypersensitivity; unrelated to level of exposure; beryllium exposure also associated with ↑ rates of cancer of lung, liver, and gallbladder | Diffuse fibrosis over 15-20 years → cor pulmonale | Difficulty in breathing |

*Asbestos is a fire-proofing and insulating agent.

**TABLE 37-15 Major Occupational Lung Diseases—cont'd**

| TYPE | ETIOLOGY AND EPIDEMIOLOGY | PATHOPHYSIOLOGY | CLINICAL MANIFESTATIONS AND PREVENTION |
|---|---|---|---|
| Talc | Inhaled by miners and millers of crude ore and soapstone and by workers in cosmetic, paint, pottery, asphalt, and rubber industries; high incidence of lung cancer; not known whether high incidence is caused by asbestos in talc or whether increased incidence in those who smoke | *Pure* talc produces a characteristic pneumoconiosis; less fibrosis than with silica inhalation; evaluation of fibrosis is difficult because most talc contains traces of asbestos and silica | |
| **MIXED-DUST PNEUMOCONIOSES** | Many workers exposed to a mixture of dusts; foundry, steel, and iron workers inhale dust from a variety of ores and may also inhale fumes; miners exposed to mixed dusts; some workers are exposed to one dust, then change jobs and are exposed to another dust | Individual dusts usually deposit in patterns that can be recognized on x-ray film; mixed dusts result in different patterns; patient's work history important in diagnosing occupational lung diseases | |
| | Not known whether mixed dusts in lungs are additive (1 + 1 = 2) or potentiating (1 + 1 = 5) | Amount of fibrosis present depends on amount of silica inhaled | |
| **HYPERSENSITIVITY DISEASES** | Hypersensitivity diseases fall into occupational category when antigen is found primarily in workplace; lung hypersensitivity can occur in bronchi, bronchioles, or alveoli; coarse dust causes bronchial reactions; fine dust provokes small airway and alveolar reactions | | |
| Occupational asthma | More common in 10% of population who are atopic (genetic tendency to develop an allergy); nonatopic persons can also become sensitized; substances with antigenic properties include detergent enzymes, platinum salts, cereals and grains, certain wood dusts, isocyanate chemicals used in polyurethane paints and other products, agents used in printing, and some pesticides | Hypersensitivity reaction mediated by histamine → bronchoconstriction and ↑ mucus production; repeated attacks if cause unrecognized and asthma is untreated; may lead to permanent obstructive lung disease; asthmatic response that is well established can be provoked by other factors (house dust, cigarette smoke) and by fatigue, breathing cold air, and coughing | Wheezing is major symptom<br>Prevention: total elimination of antigen; desensitization not successful |
| Allergic alveolitis (farmer's lung) | Hypersensitivity disease caused by fine organic dust inhaled into smallest airways; cause of farmer's lung is moldy hay; other dusts can cause allergic alveolitis: these include moldy sugar cane and barley, maple bark, cork, animal hair, bird feathers and droppings, mushroom compost, coffee beans, and paprika; often disease is named for cause (mushroom worker's lung, etc.); fungus spores growing in the apparent antigen are thought in many cases to be real cause of disease | Alveoli are inflamed, inundated by WBCs, sometimes filled with fluid; if exposure infrequent or level of dust low, symptoms are mild, and treatment not sought, chronic form develops over time; eventually, fibrosis occurs, and fibrosis may be so well established that it cannot be arrested | Symptoms begin some hours after exposure to offending dust and include fatigue, shortness of breath, dry cough, fever, and chills; symptoms may be severe enough to require emergency treatment and hospitalization; acute attacks treated with steroids; recovery may take 6 weeks, and patient may have residual lung damage; real cure is permanent separation of patient and antigen<br>Prevention: properly dried and stored farm products (hay, straw, sugar cane) do not cause allergic alveolitis; presumably fungi only grow in moist conditions |

*Continued*

**TABLE 37-15 Major Occupational Lung Diseases—cont'd**

| TYPE | ETIOLOGY AND EPIDEMIOLOGY | PATHOPHYSIOLOGY | CLINICAL MANIFESTATIONS AND PREVENTION |
|---|---|---|---|
| Byssinosis (brown lung) | Occupational disease occurs in textile workers; mainly in cotton workers but also afflicts workers in flax and hemp industries; cause is found in bales of raw cotton that contain not only cotton fibers but fragments of cotton plant; something in plant matter, rather than pure cotton, is cause | Chronic bronchitis and emphysema develop in time; constriction of bronchioles in response to something in crude cotton; symptoms of asthma and allergy persist as long as there is exposure to cotton antigen | Tightness in chest on returning to work after a weekend away (Monday fever); strong relationship between amount of dust inhaled and symptoms; persistent productive tight chest with chronic bronchitis and emphysema; person leaves industry as respiratory cripple<br>Prevention: dust control measures; pretreating bales of cotton by washing with steam and other agents may inactivate causative agent; try to detect persons who are likely to become sensitized to cotton dust and keep them out of high-risk areas |

## EPIDEMIOLOGY

Millions of Americans are believed to have job-related diseases. Because these diseases are not reportable, exact statistics do not exist. The U.S. Department of Health and Human Services (HHS) has estimated that 400,000 persons develop job-related diseases each year. They also estimate that there are 100,000 deaths each year from occupational diseases. The National Heart, Lung, and Blood Institute reports that lung diseases cause more than half of these deaths. More than $5 billion a year is paid out in workers' compensation for job-related illnesses and injuries.

## PREVENTION

### *Healthy People 2000*

The year 2000 national health goal for occupational lung disease is to establish in the 50 states exposure standards to prevent the major occupational lung diseases to which their worker populations are exposed (byssinosis, asbestosis, coal worker's pneumoconiosis, silicosis). Because these diseases are not reportable, no baseline data were available. The reader is urged to contact his or her state's department of health to see what progress has been made in establishing exposure standards for these diseases.

### Primary Prevention

*Occupational lung diseases are preventable.* However, there must be a concerted effort by the public, governmental agencies, and industry if these diseases are to be prevented.

Governmental action has been slow and has only occurred, in some instances, in response to public interest groups that have lobbied for stricter regulation of harmful substances. However, countervailing political pressures have sometimes prevented laws from being passed or have resulted in less strict laws being passed because of the costs involved in meeting the strict standards required to control certain hazards.

The ALA recommends several measures to reduce the incidence of occupational-related lung diseases: (1) public education about the relationship between polluted air in the workplace and lung diseases; (2) general commitment to reduce, eliminate, or avoid air pollution in the workplace; and (3) elimination of the most prevalent and notorious lung hazard: cigarette smoke.

Education of the public includes not only employers and employees but also engineers and planners who design operations; buyers and purchasers who select ingredients, cleaning agents, and equipment; and physicians who see persons with occupation-related diseases. Many times, workers who are instructed about the hazards involved in certain occupations and workplaces are helpful in deciding what preventive measures need to be taken to combat or minimize the effects of hazards. The commitment to reduce, eliminate, or avoid pollution of workplace air requires full consideration of possible health effects whenever operations are planned and improvement of conditions whenever possible.

It is well documented that smokers develop occupational lung disease more often than nonsmokers and that smokers' lungs are more vulnerable to the effects of these diseases than are nonsmokers' lungs. The combined effects of cigarette smoke and industrial pollutants are very great. The risk of developing chronic bronchitis, emphysema, lung cancer, and heart disease is much increased when the worker smokes. Some of these risks, such as lung cancer in asbestos workers who also smoke, are becoming more widely known.

Occupational lung diseases can be divided into several categories. The major ones are (1) the pneumoconioses, including silicosis and coal worker's pneumoconiosis (black lung disease); (2) asbestos-related lung disease; (3) other pneumoconioses such as chronic berylliosis; (4) mixed-dust pneumoconioses; and (5) hypersensitivity diseases, including occupational asthma, allergic alveolitis (farmer's lung), and byssinosis (brown lung disease). The etiology, epidemiology, pathophysiology, clinical manifestations, and prevention of the major occupational lung diseases are presented in Table 37-15.

### MEDICAL MANAGEMENT

Medical therapy of these patients depends on the patient's signs, symptoms, and complications. The reader is referred to other sections of this chapter for discussion of these topics.

### NURSING MANAGEMENT

The major role of nurses is to be knowledgeable about the cause and prevention of occupational lung diseases so that appropriate information and teaching can be presented to the public.

## OTHER RESTRICTIVE DISEASES: SARCOIDOSIS

### ETIOLOGY

Sarcoidosis is a systemic granulomatous disease of unknown cause.

### EPIDEMIOLOGY

Although sarcoidosis is worldwide in distribution, it is most likely to be diagnosed where the medical community is alert to the disease and diagnostic facilities are available. It is most common in adults between 20 and 40 years of age. The incidence is almost equal in men and women, but it is twice as common in women in childbearing years. In the United States, it is 10 times more common in blacks than in whites. Some evidence suggests that the incidence is higher in blacks than whites in other parts of the world, especially if the disease is sought out.

### PATHOPHYSIOLOGY

There is evidence of an antigen-antibody reaction manifested by reticuloendothelial response in which both thymus-derived (T) cells and plasma (B) cells participate (see Chapter 70 for more information). It is believed that the antigen is airborne, because bilateral hilar lymphadenopathy is frequently present at the onset and bronchopulmonary macrophages are increased.

The central pathologic event involves the growth of granulomas and proliferation of lymph tissue. Pulmonary sarcoidosis typically is seen on chest x-ray films as enlarged lymph nodes in the hilar area. The patient with sarcoidosis may initially complain only of vague symptoms of malaise, fever, aching in the joints, or weakness. In addition to mediastinal lymph node enlargement, ocular manifestations, such as uveitis and conjunctivitis, and dermatologic changes, such as erythema nodosum, are often found.

Diagnosis of sarcoidosis is based on x-ray film findings, transbronchial lung biopsy, and positive skin test. The Kveim-Siltzback test involves the injection of sarcoid tissue; if the reaction is positive, a visible, palpable nodule develops at the site 3 to 6 weeks after the antigen is injected. A biopsy of the nodule is then performed to confirm the presence of granulomatous tissue. The Kveim-Siltzback test is not always used as part of the diagnostic process, however, because it is difficult to obtain the active antigen and because the test is associated with frequent false-negative results. Organ biopsy yields the most conclusive evidence of sarcoidosis and is most helpful in differentiating it from Hodgkin's disease and TB.

Newer diagnostic methods in pulmonary sarcoidosis include gallium scan and bronchoalveolar lavage (BAL) with flexible fiberoptic bronchoscopy. The fluid obtained from BAL is examined to determine the degree of active inflammation in the lung and need for therapy. The patient's symptoms and pulmonary function tests (especially lung volume) are still widely used, however, in deciding whether treatment is required.

### MEDICAL MANAGEMENT

In many patients, sarcoidosis is a benign, self-limiting process that resolves with no residual damage within 2 years of diagnosis. Other patients will have an acute or chronic form of the disease.

Treatment of acute disease is with systemic steroids. Patients are treated with prednisone, 60 mg daily for 2 months, followed by 40 mg of prednisone daily for 2 months. The steroids are then slowly tapered off to a maintenance dose of 15 mg daily. Most patients are treated for 18 to 24 months. The patient is then followed medically for several years for signs of relapse. Relapse usually occurs within 3 to 6 months after the steroids are discontinued.

In chronic forms of sarcoidosis, patients are treated with small doses of steroids (5 to 10 mg every other day) for years.[30] About 10% of patients develop the chronic form of sarcoidosis. In this form the disease proceeds to nodular granulomatous depositions in lung tissue and eventual pulmonary fibrosis. In severe cases, pulmonary hypertension and cor pulmonale develop.

### NURSING MANAGEMENT

Nursing care depends on severity of patient's signs and symptoms and medical therapy. Teaching the patient about the precautions and side effects of steroid therapy is a major nursing function.

# CANCER OF THE LUNG

## ETIOLOGY

Cancer of the lung may be either metastatic or primary. Metastatic tumors may follow malignancy anywhere in the body. Metastasis from the colon and kidney is common. Metastasis to the lung may be discovered before the primary lesion is known, and sometimes the location of the primary lesion is not determined during the person's life.

## EPIDEMIOLOGY

During the past 50 years there has been a startling increase in the incidence of cancer of the lung.

The ACS estimates 172,000 new cases in 1994 and 153,000 deaths. Since 1986, cancer of the lung has surpassed breast cancer to become the number-one cancer killer of women. Thus lung cancer is now the leading cause of death from cancer in both men and women.[2]

The increase in death rates for both men and women is directly related to cigarette smoking. A history of smoking, especially for 20 years or more, is considered to be a prime risk factor. Other risk factors include exposure to certain industrial substances such as arsenic, certain organic chemicals, and asbestos, particularly in those who smoke.

It is estimated that asbestos workers who smoke have six to ten times more cancer of the lung than the general population. Some evidence also suggests a genetic predisposition to lung cancer.[40]

In the United States the age-adjusted death rate from cancer has been steadily increasing. Most of the increase is directly related to rise in lung cancer death rates. Age-adjusted rates for other cancer sites have been leveling off and in some cases declining. There has been a decline in cancer death rates for all age–groups, for males and females, and for blacks and whites, except in people 55 years old and older, in whom the cancer death rate has been increasing.[40]

The cause of cancer of the lung is closely related to cigarette smoking. Box 37-13 shows the extreme increase in mortality from lung cancer in those persons who smoke. Prevention is the best protection against cancer of the lung because early detection of the disease is difficult. The cancer death rate for male cigarette smokers is more than double that for nonsmokers, and the rate for female smokers is 67% higher than that for nonsmokers.[40]

**BOX 37-13 Effects of Smoking on Lung Cancer Risk**

- Smokers are 10 times more likely to develop lung cancer than those who never smoked.
- Heavy smokers more likely to die of lung cancer than light smokers, suggesting dose-response effect.
- Risk associated with smoking increases with number of years person smokes.
- Risk decreases steadily after person stops smoking.
- Cigarette smokers have higher death rate than pipe smokers.
- Nonsmoking wives of smokers have significantly higher risk of lung cancer than nonsmoking wives married to nonsmokers.

From Harvey JC, Beattic EJ: *Clin Symp* 45(3):2, 1993.

Because no effective treatment exists for lung cancer, emphasis is placed on prevention. *Nearly 90% of persons with lung cancer die within 5 years of diagnosis.* This percentage could be reduced with early diagnosis and treatment. Unfortunately, about one third of the persons with lung cancer are inoperable when first seen by a physician. Another one third are found to be inoperable when an exploratory thoracotomy or thoracoscopy is performed.

## PATHOPHYSIOLOGY

Because most new growths in the lungs can arise from the bronchi, the term *bronchogenic carcinoma* is widely used. The signs and symptoms that a patient has depend on several factors including the location of the lesion.

Signs and symptoms of lesion in the bronchus and lung include the following:

1. Ten percent of patients are asymptomatic and are identified on routine chest x-ray film.
2. Seventy-five percent have a cough.
3. Fifty percent have hemoptysis.
4. Shortness of breath and a unilateral wheeze are common.

If *peripheral pulmonary lesions* perforate into the pleural space, there will be extrapulmonary intrathoracic signs and symptoms. These include:

1. Pain on inspiration
2. Friction rub
3. Pleural effusion
4. If the superior vena cava is involved, edema of face and neck
5. Fatigue
6. Clubbing of fingers

In the later stage of the disease, weight loss and debility usually indicate metastases, especially to the liver. Cancer of the lung may metastasize to nearby structures such as the prescalene lymph nodes, the walls of the esophagus, and the pericardium of the heart or to distant areas such as the brain, liver, or skeleton.

## PREVENTION

### Healthy People 2000

The goal set for year 2000 in *Healthy People 2000* is to *slow the rise* in lung cancer deaths to no more than 42 per 100,000 people as compared with an age-adjusted baseline of 37.9 per 100,000 in 1987. Thus the only hope is to slow the number of deaths because *decreasing* the number of deaths appears to be impossible at this time.

## MEDICAL MANAGEMENT

The treatment of lung cancer depends on the type and stage of the disease. Histologically, lung cancer is divided into four major subgroups: small cell carcinoma, squamous cell carcinoma, adenocarcinoma, and large cell carcinoma. Table 37-16 shows the types, percentage of cases in the subtypes, and recommended therapy. As with other types of cancer, lung cancer is staged (see Chapter 16 for more details about staging). The International Tumor, Node, Metastasis (TNM) Staging for Lung Cancer is presented in Box 37-14.

Because patients with early lung cancer have no symptoms they are often inoperable by the time they are seen. Some patients with cancers of the lung are first diagnosed after a chest x-ray film as part of a routine physical examination. Other patients are not diagnosed until they seek medical treatment for symptoms related to metastases.

Survival rates of patients with non–small cell lung cancer (NSCLC) depend on the size of the tumor, nodal status, and degree of metastases. Table 37-17 gives the 5-year survival rates for patients with NSCLC.

Some patients who undergo surgical resection (pneumonectomy or lobectomy) may also receive radiation

**TABLE 37-16 Histologic Subtypes of Cancer of the Lung and Therapy for Each Type**

| TYPE | CLASSIFICATION AND PERCENTAGE OF CASES | THERAPY |
|---|---|---|
| Small cell carcinoma | Small cell lung cancer (SCLC): 15%-25% of cases | Combination chemotherapy such as (1) cyclophosphamide, doxorubicin, and vincristine, or (2) cyclophosphamide, doxorubicin, and etoposide, or (3) cisplatin plus etoposide |
| Adenocarcinoma; most common type: 35%-45% of cases<br>Squamous cell carcinoma: 30%-40% of cases<br>Large cell carcinoma: about 10% of cases | All three classified as non–small cell lung cancer (NSCLC): 75%-85% of cases | Pulmonary resection—only one third are operable; one third inoperable because of advanced lung cancer; one third inoperable because of distant metastases |

**BOX 37-14 International TNM Staging System for Lung Cancer**

**TUMOR (T)**

| | |
|---|---|
| TX | Occult carcinoma (malignant cells in sputum or bronchial washings, but tumor not visualized by imaging studies or bronchoscopy) |
| $T_1$ | Tumor ≤3 cm in diameter, surrounded by lung or visceral pleura but not proximal to lobar bronchus on bronchoscopy |
| $T_2$ | Tumor ≥3 cm in diameter, or with involvement of main bronchus at least 2 cm distal to carina, or with visceral pleural invasion, or with associated atelectasis or obstructive pneumonitis extending to the hilar region but not involving the entire lung |
| $T_3$ | Tumor invading chest wall, diaphragm, mediastinal pleura, or parietal pericardium; or tumor in main bronchus within 2 cm of carina but not invading it; or atelectasis or obstructive pneumonitis of entire lung |
| $T_4$ | Tumor invading mediastinum, heart, great vessels, trachea, esophagus, vertebral body, or carina; or ipsilateral malignant pleural effusion |

**NODES (N)**

| | |
|---|---|
| $N_0$ | No regional lymph node metastases |
| $N_1$ | Metastases to ipsilateral peribronchial or hilar nodes |
| $N_2$ | Metastases to ipsilateral mediastinal or subcarinal nodes |
| $N_3$ | Metastases to contralateral mediastinal or hilar nodes or to any scalene or supraclavicular nodes |

**DISTANT METASTASES (M)**

| | |
|---|---|
| $M_0$ | No distant metastases |
| $M_1$ | Distant metastases |

**STAGE GROUPINGS**

| | | | |
|---|---|---|---|
| **Occult** | TX | $N_0$ | $M_0$ |
| **Stage I** | $T_{1-2}$ | $N_0$ | $M_0$ |
| **Stage II** | $T_{1-2}$ | $N_1$ | $M_0$ |
| **Stage IIIA** | $T_3$ | $N_{0-1}$ | $M_0$ |
| | $T_{1-3}$ | $N_2$ | $M_0$ |
| **Stage IIIB** | $T_4$ | $N_{0-2}$ | $M_0$ |
| | $T_{1-4}$ | $N_3$ | $M_0$ |
| **Stage IV** | Any T | Any N | $M_1$ |

Modified from American Joint Committee on Cancer.

**TABLE 37-17 Five-Year Disease-Free Survival Rates for Surgical Resection in Patients With Non–Small Cell Lung Cancer**

| | STAGE | 5-YEAR DISEASE-FREE (%) |
|---|---|---|
| I | $T_1, N_0, M_0$ | 70-85 |
| | $T_2, N_0, M_0$ | 55-65 |
| II | $T_1, N_1, M_0$ | 30-50 |
| | $T_1, N_2, M_0$ | 25-30 |
| IIIA | $T_3, N_0, M_0$ | 25-35 |
| | $T_3, N_1, M_0$ | 15-20 |
| | $T_{1\text{-}2}, N_2, M_0$ | 9-24 |
| | $T_3, N_2$ | 0-5 |

From Bonomi P: Primary lung cancer. In Rakel RE, editor: *Conn's current therapy*, Philadelphia, 1993, Saunders.

therapy or chemotherapy. These adjuvants are given mainly to treat metastases and in an attempt to relieve some of the patient's symptoms.

## SURGICAL MANAGEMENT

### Diagnostic Tests

1. Histologic examination of tumor necessary to confirm diagnosis of lung cancer. Four methods used to collection tissue samples:
   a. Sputum collection: a 3-day pooled sample provides more reliable evidence than a single sample. Sputum is examined for bacteria and cancer cells.
   b. Fiberoptic bronchoscopy can be used to remove tissue samples from visible tumors or to perform brushing and washing of peripheral lesions. When hilar or mediastinal lymph nodes are involved, transbronchial needle biopsy (with a bronchoscope) is used to obtain node tissue for examination.
   c. Percutaneous transthoracic needle biopsy used to biopsy lesions visible on fluoroscopy, especially when they are close to the surface of lung. Analysis of tissue samples can provide a specific diagnosis and sometimes cell type. A small number of patients develop a pneumothorax requiring chest tube drainage (see p. 1095).
   d. Excision of lesion. A lesion is removed through a small incision. Video-assisted thoracoscopy or thoracotomy is useful for performing small diagnostic wedge excisions; mechanical staplers or lasers are used with these procedures.
2. Staging techniques
   a. Imaging techniques: chest x-ray films, CT scans, and magnetic resonance imaging (MRI) all used for clinical staging of lung cancer.
      (1) Lateral chest x-ray film is able to depict tumors, especially those on periphery.
      (2) CT (contrast enhanced) or MRI can differentiate an underlying mass from atelectasis or inflammation.
      (3) Chest wall invasion: MRI can be used to differentiate involvement of visceral pleura from involvement of parietal pleura.
      (4) CT also used to reveal malignant pleural effusions, which usually mean inoperability. Malignant cells should be identified in pleural fluid before a decision is made about inoperability.
   b. Thoracentesis is routinely performed if there is evidence of pleural effusion clinically or on CT. Up to 1000 ml of fluid may be removed.
   c. Thoracoscopy and mediastinoscopy: thoracoscopy is useful for evaluating pleural seeding and for examining mediastinal nodes. Mediastinoscopy is better than CT or MRI for assessing mediastinal metastases and effectiveness of preoperative radiation therapy or chemotherapy.

Assessment of surgical risk for pulmonary resection is based on age, pulmonary reserve, cardiovascular disease, and disease so extensive it would require a pneumonectomy. Each is discussed briefly next.

*Age.* Mortality and morbidity related to pulmonary resection increase significantly in persons older than 70 years. Some studies suggest higher mortality and morbidity in those 60 to 65 years of age.

*Pulmonary reserve.* ABGs and pulmonary function tests (PFTs) are used to measure pulmonary reserve. A $Pco_2$ greater than 45 mm Hg indicates inoperability, whereas a $Po_2$ less than 60 mm Hg suggests pulmonary resection would be very risky, unless the low $Po_2$ is caused by complete airway obstruction that results from desaturated blood entering the pulmonary veins from perfused but nonventilated lung (V/Q mismatch). PFTs are used to evaluate risk of pulmonary resection. A predicted postoperative forced expiratory volume ($FEV_1$) of more than 800 ml is required in most adults. Most patients with a predicted $FEV_1$ less than 30% are usually unable to tolerate pneumonectomy.

*Cardiovascular disease.* Coronary artery disease is present in about 80 of every 1000 patients older than age 65. Previous myocardial infarction, especially when surgey would be necessary less than 6 months after infarction, increases the risk. *Left ventricular dysfunction,* including signs of congestive heart failure, indicates high risk of death after pulmonary resection. *Unstable angina* must be controlled before resection. Hypertension has to be under control. Frequent premature ventricular contractions (PVCs) are signs of severe heart disease and are associated with increased perioperative complications and death.

*Pneumonectomy.* Particularly for patients age 70 and over and especially with surgery of right lung (which normally does 60% to 70% of breathing), pneumonectomy is associated with higher risk than lesser procedures.

## Thoracic Surgery

Intelligent nursing care of patients undergoing thoracic surgery depends on knowledge of the anatomy and physiology of the chest, of the surgery performed, and of procedures and practices that assist the patient to recover from the procedure. When endotracheal anesthesia became possible, surgery of the chest was given a great impetus.

### Principles of resectional surgery

Principles of resectional surgery are as follows:

1. Endotracheal anesthesia is used for surgery involving the lung in which the pleural space is entered.
2. With endotracheal anesthesia it is possible to keep the uninvolved ("good") lung expanded and functioning when the chest is opened and atmospheric pressure enters the pleural space.
3. To understand resectional surgery and the purpose of chest tubes and closed drainage system, an understanding of the following is necessary.
   a. *Physiology of breathing*
      (1) The pressure in the pleural space (the space between the visceral and parietal pleura) is subatmospheric (less than 760 mm Hg) and is referred to as *negative.*
      (2) The pressure in the pleural space is usually 756 mm Hg and goes down to 751 mm Hg before inspiration. This change in pressure allows air (atmospheric pressure) to enter the lungs.
      (3) When the pleura is entered surgically or with trauma to the chest wall, atmospheric pressure enters the pleural space, and the lung on that side collapses.
   b. *Purpose of chest tubes and closed drainage system*
      (1) After resectional surgery of the lung (except pneumonectomy), one or two drainage tubes are inserted into the pleural space. Each tube is connected to a negative-pressure closed drainage system (Figure 37-8, *A* and *B*).
      (2) This system allows air and fluid to drain from the pleural space and prevents air or fluid from entering the pleural space.
      (3) In all resectional surgery (except pneumonectomy), the remaining portions of the lung must overexpand and fill the space left by the resected portion.
      (4) The removal of air and fluid from the pleural space accomplishes two basic purposes: (1) to aid in the expansion of the remaining portion of the lung as air *(positive pressure)* and fluid escapes through the drainage tubes, and (2) to reestablish negative pressure in the pleural space.
      (5) Nursing actions necessary to maintain the integrity of the chest tubes and closed drainage system are discussed under postoperative care.
      (6) Older closed-chest drainage systems such as water-sealed bottles may be used (Figure 37-8, *B*).

### Types of resectional surgery

Box 37-15 presents the types of resectional surgery and the indications for the use of each type. A brief discussion of each type of resectional surgery follows.

**Exploratory thoracotomy.** An exploratory thoracotomy is performed to confirm a suspected diagnosis of lung or chest disease. The usual approach is by a posterolateral parascapular incision through the fourth, fifth, sixth, or seventh intercostal space. Occasionally, an anterior approach is used. The ribs are spread to give the

**BOX 37-15 Types of Thoracic Surgery and Indications for Their Use**

**EXPLORATORY THORACOTOMY**

To confirm suspected diagnosis of lung or chest disease, especially carcinoma; to obtain a biopsy

**PNEUMONECTOMY**

Removal of a lung; bronchogenic carcinoma when lobectomy will not remove all of lesion; tuberculosis when other surgery will not remove all of diseased lung

**LOBECTOMY**

Removal of one lobe of lung; bronchogenic carcinoma confined to a lobe, bronchiectasis, emphysematous blebs or bullae; lung abscess, fungal infections, benign tumors; tuberculosis

**BILOBECTOMY**

Removal of two lobes from right lung; bronchogenic carcinoma when lobectomy will not remove all of disease

**SLEEVE LOBECTOMY**

Resection of main bronchus or distal trachea with reanastomosis to a distal uninvolved bronchus; bronchogenic carcinoma to preserve functional parenchyma

**SEGMENTAL RESECTION**

Segmentectomy; removal of one or more lung segments; bronchiectasis; lung abscess or cyst; metastatic carcinoma

**WEDGE RESECTION**

Removal of pie-shaped section from surface of lung; well-circumscribed benign tumors, metastatic tumors, or localized inflammatory disease, including TB

**DECORTICATION**

Removal of a fibrinous peel from visceral pleura; chronic empyema

**THORACOPLASTY**

Removal of ribs; residual air space after surgery; chronic empyema space

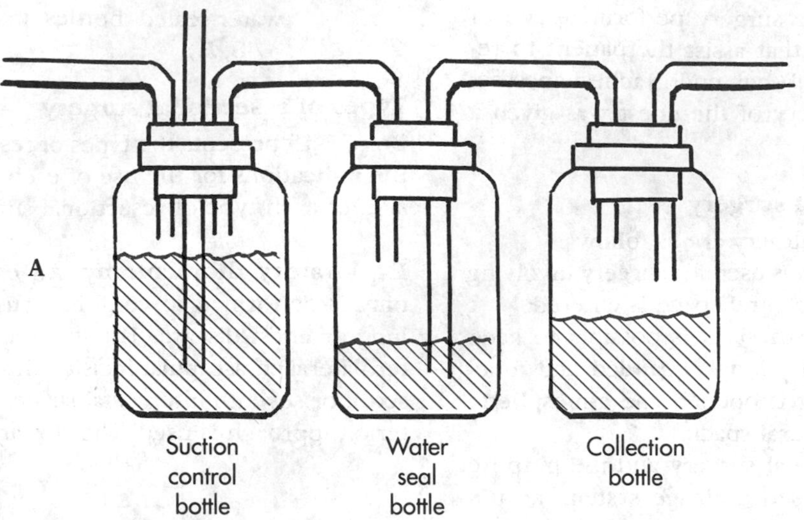


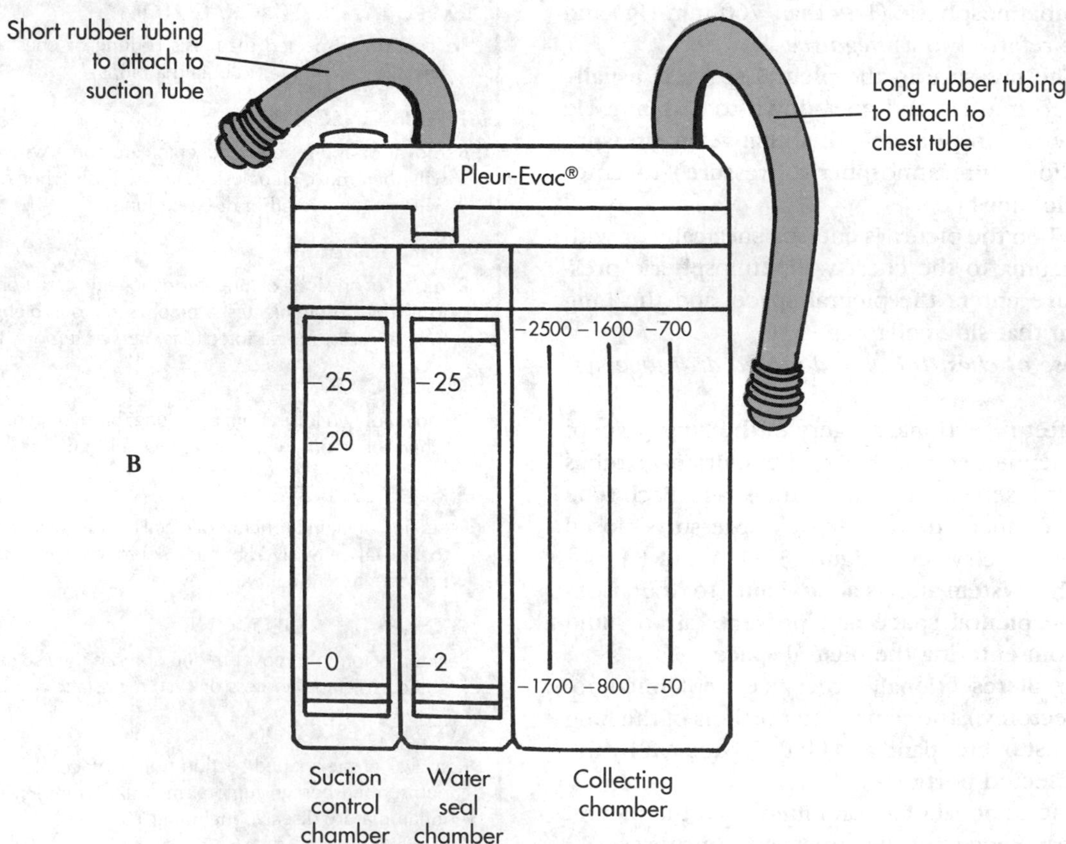


**FIGURE 37-8** **A,** Water-sealed closed-chest drainage system (original three-bottle design). **B,** Pleur-Evac, one of several available brands of disposable chest drainage systems based on the three-bottle design. The unit collects drainage, maintains a seal to prevent air from entering the pleural cavity, and prevents excessive build-up of negative pressure.

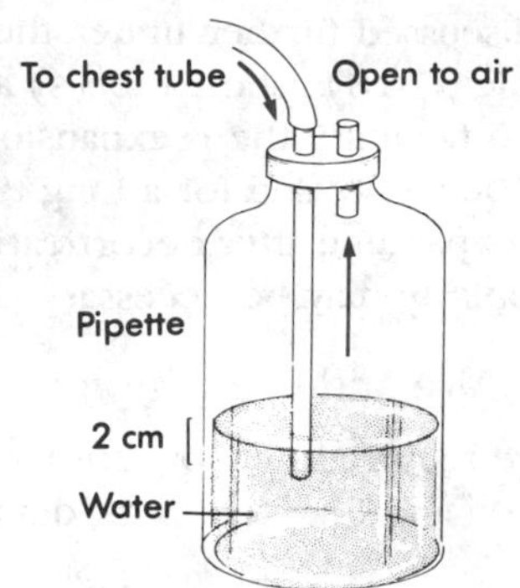


**FIGURE 37-9** Water-sealed closed-chest drainage showing type of tube under water. (From Abel LF: *Mosby's manual of critical care,* St Louis, 1979, Mosby.)

best possible exposure of the lung and hemithorax. The pleura is entered and the lung examined; a biopsy usually is taken; and the chest is closed. This procedure may also be used to detect bleeding in the chest or other injury after trauma to the chest. Because the pleural space was entered, a chest tube and closed drainage system are necessary (Figure 37-9).

**Pneumonectomy.** A pneumonectomy, the removal of an entire lung, is most often performed to treat bronchogenic carcinoma (Figure 37-10, *B*). It may also be used to treat TB. However, a pneumonectomy is only performed in those instances when a lobectomy or segmental resection will not remove all the diseased tissue. A thoracotomy is made in either the posterior or anterior chest using the method described under exploratory thoracotomy. Before the lung can be removed, the pulmonary artery and vein are ligated and then cut. The main-stem bronchus leading to the lung is clamped, divided, and sutured or stapled. To ensure an airtight closure of the bronchus, a pleural flap may be placed over it and sutured into place. This is not necessary if staples are used. The phrenic nerve on the operative side is crushed, causing the diaphragm on that side to rise and reduce the size of the remaining space. Because there is no lung left to reexpand, drainage tubes are not used. Ideally, the pressure in the closed chest is slightly negative. The fluid left in the space will consolidate in time, preventing the remaining lung and heart from shifting toward the operative side (mediastinal shift).

**Lobectomy.** In a lobectomy, one lobe of the lung is removed (Figure 37-10, *C*). It is used to treat bronchiectasis, bronchogenic carcinoma, emphysematous blebs or bullae, lung abscess, benign tumors, fungal infections, and TB. For a lobectomy to be successful, the disease must be confined to one lobe, and the remaining lung tissue must be capable of overexpanding to fill the

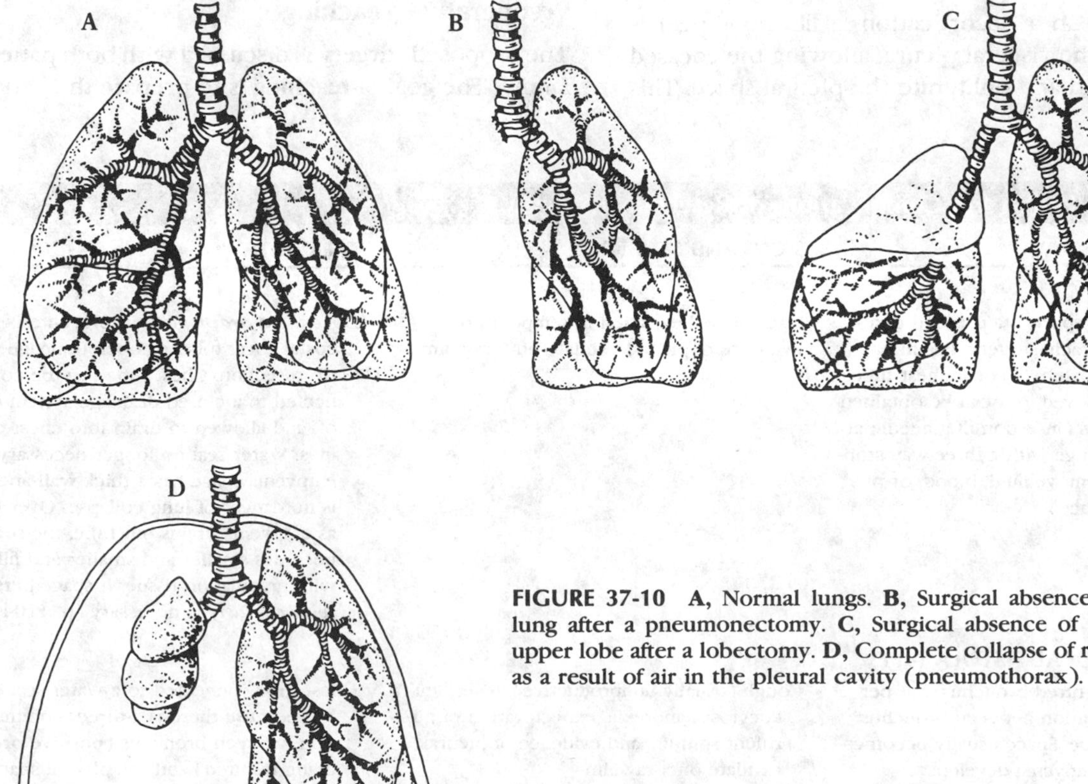


**FIGURE 37-10** **A,** Normal lungs. **B,** Surgical absence of right lung after a pneumonectomy. **C,** Surgical absence of the right upper lobe after a lobectomy. **D,** Complete collapse of right lung as a result of air in the pleural cavity (pneumothorax).

space of the resected lobe. One or two chest tubes are connected to a closed drainage system for postoperative drainage.

**Segmental resection (segmentectomy).** In a segmental resection, one or more segments of the lung are removed. This procedure is used in an attempt to preserve as much functioning lung tissue as possible. It is a very taxing procedure for the surgeon, because the dissection between segments must be performed very carefully and slowly, and the identification of the segmental pulmonary artery and vein and bronchus is more difficult than when a lobe is involved. Because there are 10 segments in the right lung and eight segments in the left lung, only a portion of a lobe or lobes may need to be removed. The most common indication for segmentectomy is bronchiectasis. It is also used to treat the other conditions listed in Box 37-15. Chest tube(s) and a closed drainage system are necessary postoperatively. Because of air leaks from the segmental surface, the remaining lung tissue may take longer to reexpand.

**Wedge resection.** In a wedge resection, a well-circumscribed diseased portion is removed without regard to the segmental planes. The area to be removed is clamped, dissected, and sutured or stapled. Chest tube(s) and a closed drainage system are used postoperatively.

**Decortication.** In a decortication, a fibrinous peel is removed from the visceral pleura, allowing the encased lung to reexpand and obliterate the pleural space. This procedure is discussed further under the treatment of empyema (Table 37-18). Chest tube(s) and chest suction are used to facilitate the reexpansion of the lung. If the lung has been encased for a long time, it may be incapable of reexpanding after decortication. In this situation, thoracoplasty may be necessary.

## Preoperative Care and Evaluation

Special tests are required by a patient having chest surgery (see p. 1094 and Chapter 35 for details about each test).

### Bronchoscopy

As mentioned earlier, bronchoscopy is performed as part of the diagnostic workup (see p. 1094). For the patient being considered for pneumonectomy, the evaluation is even more precise, because it must be determined if the uninvolved lung will be able to maintain the patient's respiration after the diseased lung is removed.

### Pulmonary function tests

PFTs are used to determine the patient's ability to withstand pneumonectomy and are discussed earlier (see p. 1094). The nurse should be sure that the patient understands what tests are to be performed and the preparation for them. The person's significant others also are kept informed. PFTs are described in Chapter 35.

# NURSING MANAGEMENT

## Preoperative Teaching

The proposed surgery is discussed with both patient and family. The goal of teaching is to prepare the patient for

**TABLE 37-18 Long-Term Complications of Resectional Surgery**

| COMPLICATIONS | SIGNS AND SYMPTOMS | TREATMENT |
|---|---|---|
| **EMPYEMA** | | |
| Pus in the pleural space is a dreaded complication of thoracic surgery. Pus may drain from chest tube(s) or if chest tubes are already removed, pus can be obtained on thoracentesis (insertion of a needle attached to a syringe with a three-way stopcock used to remove fluid, blood, or pus from pleural space). | Unexplained elevation in temperature<br>Evidence of pleural exudate on x-ray film | *Dependent drainage* by thoracentesis, intercostal chest tube, or open drainage with rib resection. Chest tube may be connected to a closed drainage system or cut off and allowed to drain into chest dressings. Water seal no longer necessary if empyema space has a thick wall and there is no danger of lung collapse. Over time as empyema drains out tube, the space becomes smaller and smaller and fills in with granulation tissue. If space persists, a *thoracoplasty* is necessary (p. 1104). |
| **BRONCHOPLEURAL FISTULA (BPF)** | | |
| Opening in the sutured bronchus that permits communication between bronchus and pleural space. Space usually becomes infected, and empyema develops.<br>Use of an automatic stapling machine to close the bronchus has reduced the incidence of BPF. | Cough (usually nonproductive), fever, leukocytosis, anorexia, expectoration of purulent sputum, and evidence of pleural exudate on x-ray film | Chest tube connected to a water-seal chamber because there is a direct communication between bronchus (positive pressure being inspired) and the pleural space. A persistent bronchopleural fistula is treated by thoracoplasty and a muscle implant to seal off the bronchus. |

what he or she is expected to do postoperatively. In some hospitals, nurses from the operating room, recovery room, or ICU do the preoperative teaching. Even when this is so, the nurse caring for the patient is responsible for determining what the patient understands about the impending surgery and to be sure that preoperative teaching is completed.

Points to be discussed in teaching include:

1. Patient's knowledge of procedure
2. Explanation of procedure as necessary, including intubation for anesthesia, site of incision, and chest tube(s) and drainage system
3. Where patient will go immediately following surgery
   a. To recovery room—for how long
   b. To ICU—for how long
4. Oxygen
5. IV and/or blood administration
6. Pain medication, including patient-controlled analgesia (PCA) if used
7. What patient will be asked to do
   a. Coughing and deep breathing
   b. Arm exercises
   c. Ambulation

## Postoperative Care

The care of the patient after thoracic surgery centers on promoting ventilation and reexpansion of the lung by maintaining a clear airway, promoting comfort by proper maintenance of the closed drainage system, promoting arm exercises to maintain full use of the patient's arm on the operated side, promoting nutrition, and monitoring the incision for bleeding and subcutaneous emphysema.

In most hospitals the patient will go from the recovery room to the ICU. The immediate postoperative nursing care is outlined here.

### Oxygen therapy

Oxygen is attached to the endotracheal tube. After extubation, oxygen is given by cannula usually at 6 L/min. An oxygen mask is not used because of a need to have the patient cough and raise secretions frequently.

### Hemodynamic monitoring

The patient is usually attached to a cardiac monitor, and a Swan-Ganz catheter and central venous pressure line are used for hemodynamic monitoring.

### Position of patient in bed

The patient is kept flat in bed or with head elevated slightly (20 degrees) until blood pressure is stabilized to preoperative levels. Once blood pressure is stabilized, the patient can usually breathe best in semi-Fowler's position with a pillow under the head and neck but not under the shoulder and back because of the subscapular incision.

### Monitoring vital signs

Vital signs are taken every 15 minutes until the patient is well recovered from anesthesia, every hour until condition has stabilized, and then every 2 to 4 hours. It is not unusual for blood pressure to fluctuate during the first 24 to 36 hours, and close monitoring of the patient is essential. A persistently low blood pressure is reported to the surgeon.

### Initiating coughing and deep-breathing exercises

The patient should be assisted to cough as soon as conscious and extubated. If the blood pressure is stable, the patient is assisted to a sitting position, and the incision is supported anteriorly and posteriorly by the nurse's hands. Firm, even pressure over the incision with the open palm of the hands is a most effective method. The nurse's head should be behind the patient when the patient is coughing (Figure 37-11). The patient is encouraged to breathe deeply, exhale, and then cough. Sips of fluids, especially warm ones such as tea or coffee, often facilitate coughing. Mist therapy may be used to loosen secretions. *Coughing keeps the airway patent, prevents atelectasis, and facilitates reexpansion of the lung.* The patient should be assisted to cough every hour for the first 24 hours, and then every 2 to 4 hours. The patient should cough until the chest sounds clear. Otherwise, secretions will accumulate in the tracheobronchial tree.

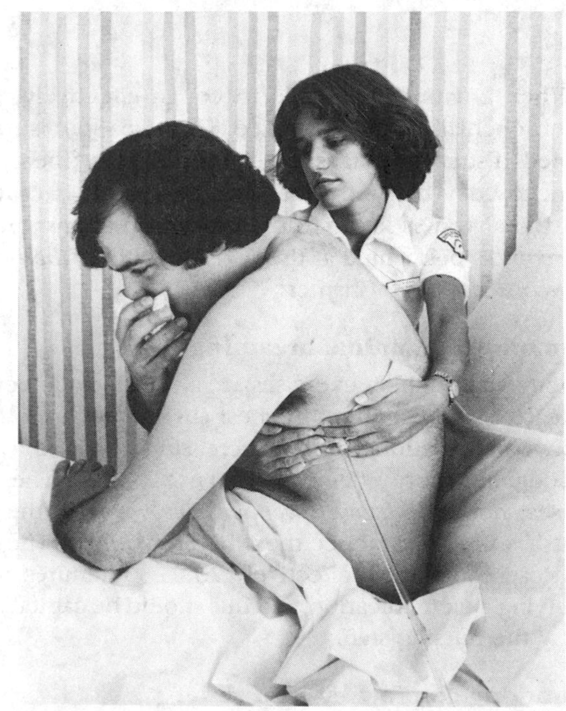

**FIGURE 37-11** Nurse helps patient cough by splinting incision with firm support from hands. This lessens muscle pull and pain as patient coughs. Note that nurse keeps her head behind patient while he coughs, and patient uses tissue to cover mouth.

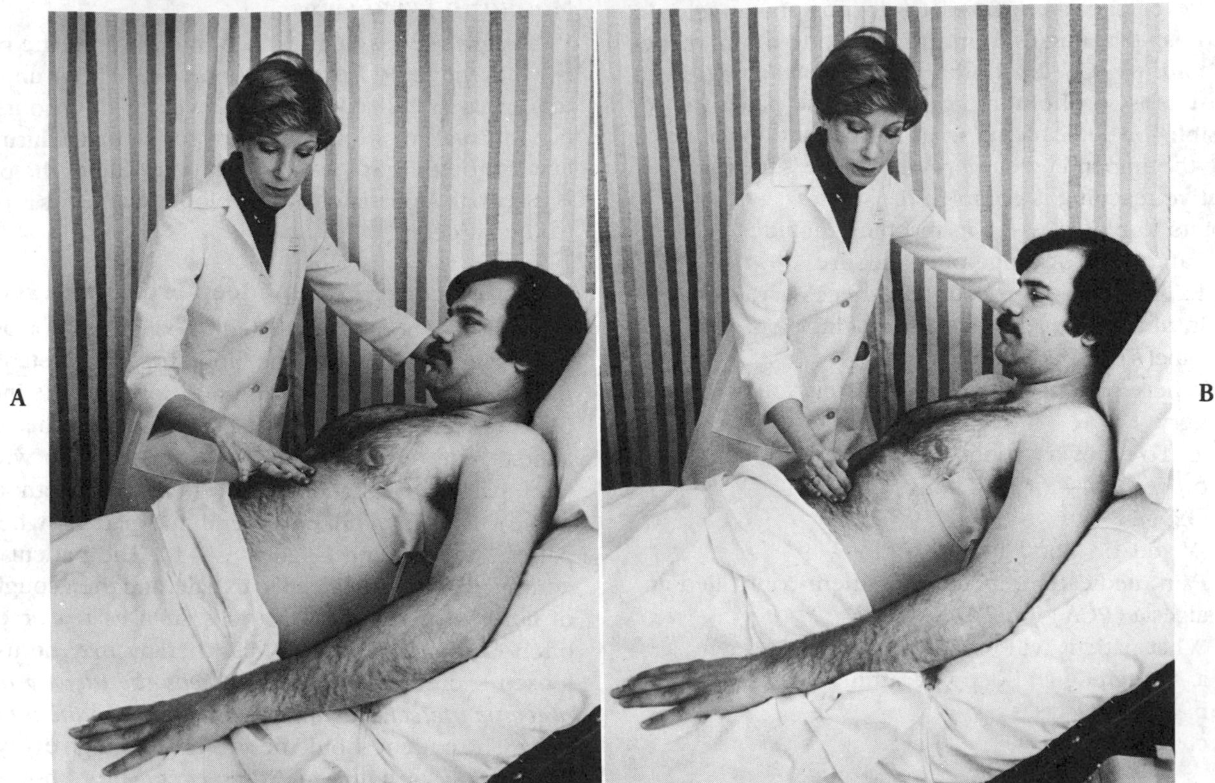


**FIGURE 37-12** **A,** Physical therapist assists patient in learning augmented abdominal breathing. Patient is instructed to inhale through nose, using abdominal muscles and concentrate on moving lower ribs under therapist's hand. This exercise improves ventilation of bases of lungs. **B,** Physical therapist places hand on upper abdomen in assisting patient to exhale fully.

When a patient is unable to cough effectively, tracheobronchial suctioning (see Chapter 36) is performed. If suctioning fails to clear the airway, fiberoptic bronchoscopy may be necessary, because it is crucial that the airway is kept clear. In these situations, *bronchoscopy* is performed at the bedside with a *fiberoptic bronchoscope* (see Chapter 35).

### Promoting abdominal breathing

Abdominal breathing exercises are a valuable adjunct to the care of the patient with chest surgery because they improve ventilation without increasing pain and assist in coughing more effectively (Figure 37-12). The exercises should be *taught preoperatively* so that the patient has time to practice them before surgery. The patient can cough most effectively 20 to 30 minutes after receiving pain medication, and this should be capitalized on by the nursing staff.

### Promoting comfort by pain relief

Morphine or meperidine hydrochloride is usually ordered for pain. Medication for pain should be given as needed and may be required as often as every 3 to 4 hours during the first 48 to 72 hours. The patient is extremely uncomfortable and will not be able to cough or turn unless there is relief from pain. In some instances the dose of the narcotic is decreased so that it may be given more frequently and yet not depress respirations. The tubes in the chest cause pain, and the patient may attempt rapid, shallow breathing to splint the lower chest and avoid motion of the catheters. This impairs ventilation, makes coughing ineffective, and causes secretions to be retained. Thus it is a nursing responsibility to make the patient comfortable, because this facilitates deep breathing and coughing. *Pain medication should never be withheld without first consulting with the surgeon because undermedication is counterproductive.* If, despite all efforts, patient's discomfort is interfering with adequate chest excursion, an intercostal nerve block may be performed.

### Promoting arm exercises

Passive arm exercises are usually started the evening of surgery. The purpose in putting the patient's arm through ROM is to prevent restriction of function. Most patients are reluctant to move the arm on the operative side, but with proper preoperative instruction and postoperative follow-through, they do so readily. It is important for both the patient and the nurse to understand that the longer the arm is unexercised, the stiffer it will become. The patient should put both arms through active ROM two or three times a day within a few days. The recommended exercises are similar to those done after mastectomy (see Chapter 54). The exercises are best performed when the patient is upright or lying on the abdomen. Exercises such as elevating the scapula and clavicle, "hunching the shoulders," bringing the scapulae as close together as possible, and hyperextending the arm can only be performed in these positions. Since lying on the abdomen may not be possible at first, these exercises are performed with the patient sitting on the edge of the bed or standing.

### Promoting nutrition

The patient is encouraged to take fluids postoperatively and to progress to a general diet as soon as it is tolerated. Forcing fluids helps to liquefy secretions and makes them easier to expectorate. A diet adequate in protein and vitamins (especially vitamin C) facilitates wound healing.

### Monitoring the incision for bleeding or subcutaneous emphysema

The dressing is checked periodically for evidence of bleeding. *Blood on the dressing is unusual and should be reported to the surgeon at once.* The time and amount of blood are recorded in the patient's record. The surgeon may reinforce the dressing, and in the rare instance when bleeding persists, the patient may be taken back to surgery. The chest wall will be reopened and the source of bleeding located and ligated.

**Subcutaneous emphysema** is not unusual after chest surgery. In subcutaneous emphysema, air leaks from the pleural space through the thoracotomy incision or around the chest tubes into the soft tissues. When palpating the chest, the presence of air under the skin is readily detected and has been described as feeling like "tissue paper" or "Rice Krispies" under the skin. Subcutaneous emphysema is most notable in the neck and chest, and if considerable air is leaking, the patient's face and neck will become considerably enlarged. Small amounts of air will reabsorb over time and cause no problem; but if subcutaneous emphysema is worsening, the chest tube may be changed by the surgeon and a larger one inserted, because air is leaking into the tissues faster than it is being removed by the tube. Additional suction (usually wall suction) may also be applied to the chest tube(s) in an attempt to remove air more rapidly. Rarely a patient will need to return to surgery for closure of air leaks.

The patient with a pneumonectomy should have only a small amount of (if any) subcutaneous emphysema. *Progressive subcutaneous emphysema after pneumonectomy is very serious and should be reported to the surgeon immediately because it could indicate a major leak in the bronchial stump.* This is a rare occurrence, requiring immediate return to surgery for reclosure of the bronchial stump.

### Maintaining chest tube(s) and drainage

All patients who have resectional surgery of the lung, except those having a pneumonectomy, will require

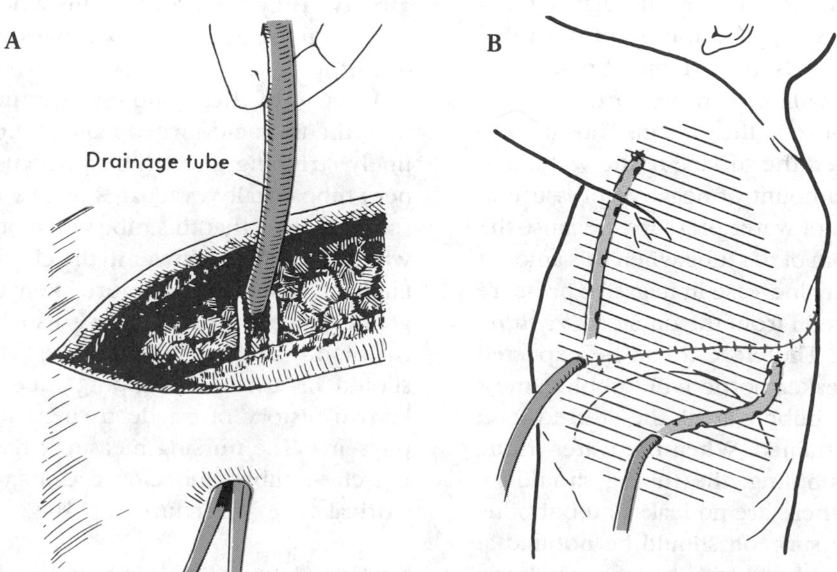


**FIGURE 37-13** **A,** Drainage tube being inserted into pleural space. **B,** Note that upper and lower tubes are placed well into pleural space. (From Johnson J, MacVaugh H III, Waldhausen JA: *Surgery of the chest, a handbook of operative surgery,* ed 4, St. Louis, 1970, Mosby.)

drainage of the pleural space by one or two chest tubes connected to closed drainage. Usually two tubes are used, although some surgeons may prefer only one tube. At the completion of the surgical resection, each tube is inserted into the pleural space through a stab wound in the chest wall. When two tubes are used, one catheter is inserted in the anterior chest wall above the resected area. This is referred to as the *anterior* or *upper tube.* It is used to remove air from the pleural space. The second tube is inserted in the posterior chest and is referred to as the *posterior* or *lower tube.* It is primarily for the drainage of serosanguineous fluid that accumulates as the result of the procedure. The lower tube may be of a larger diameter than the upper tube to prevent it from becoming plugged with clots. Figure 37-13 shows the placement of tubes within the pleural space. When only one chest tube is used, it is usually placed anteriorly above the resected area of the lung.

To initiate chest tube drainage, the chest tubes are connected to a closed-chest drainage system. The systems currently used are plastic disposable units; one of the most frequently used is the Pleur-Evac. In looking at Figure 37-8, *A* and *B,* it can be seen that the Pleur-Evac functions as a three-bottle water-seal drainage system. Bottle one to the right is connected to the patient's chest tube and allows blood from the pleural space to drain out. The middle bottle is water-sealed; that is, the tip of the tube is underwater, allowing fluid and air to drain from the pleural space and preventing air from entering the pleural space. The third bottle is a suction control bottle, sometimes called a "breaker bottle." The stopper in the control bottle has three openings. One is connected to the water-seal bottle, one is connected to the suction source, and the third contains a glass rod that is underwater and open to the outside. The amount of suction produced is determined by the distance between the surface of the water and the tip of this tube. When the suction source is turned on, the level of water in the open tube will sink in proportion to the amount of negative pressure in the system. Thus if there is 15 cm of water between the surface of the water and the tip of the tube, the amount of negative pressure in the system will be 15 cm of water pressure. Because the water will be at the bottom of the tube when this amount of pressure is reached, any increase in negative pressure will cause air to be drawn in from the outside, *breaking* the suction at this level. Therefore it can be expected that the water in the breaker bottle will bubble almost continuously. If it fails to bubble at all, the desired level of suction is not being attained. When the water in the breaker bottle is not bubbling, the tubing should be checked for air leaks. If there are no leaks and bubbling still does not occur, the surgeon should be notified at once, since the air leak in the pleural surface may be so great that the amount of negative pressure is not sufficient to overcome it. In this instance, water may be added to the breaker bottle to increase the distance between the surface of the water and the tip of the tube, thereby increasing the amount of negative pressure being exerted on the pleural space. The distance the tube is placed underwater in the breaker bottle is ordered by the surgeon.

Some thoracic surgeons want to have the chest tubes "milked" or "stripped" every hour to prevent formation of clots that could plug the tubes; the practice of routinely stripping chest tube(s) is becoming less common, however, because it increases the negative pressure exerted on the pleural space. A study by two clinical nurse specialists revealed the following: (1) the pressure generated by stripping was considerably higher than the suction pressures of −15 to −20 cm of water typically applied to chest drainage system; (2) the amount of pressure was directly related to the length of the tubing stripped; and (3) even stripping only a few centimeters produced pressures near −100 cm of water, and stripping the entire tube produced pressures exceeding −400 cm of water. They also found that higher negative pressures resulted when a roller was used to strip the tubes rather than the hands.

Undesirable side effects of increased levels of negative pressure reported in the literature include (1) lung entrapment in the thoracic tube eyelets and focal tissue infarction and (2) persistent pneumothorax. The persistent pneumothorax occurs when the pleural surface of lung, which normally has air leaks at the close of the procedure, does not "seal off." It is usually the case that fibrin will seal the air leaks; however, the presence of an increased amount of negative pressure may prevent the air leaks from sealing off and may even increase the size of the air leaks. This is why some thoracic surgeons do not attach additional suction to the closed drainage system for the first 24 hours or more after surgery. They believe that this amount of time is sufficient in most instances to allow the pleural surface to seal off.

In view of these findings, the nurse should consult with the thoracic surgeon about the desirability of routinely stripping chest tubes. Because the anterior (upper) tube usually evacuates mainly air, there is less reason to believe that this tube will clot off. Posterior tubes, which are inserted lower in the chest, usually drain more fluid and blood and are more likely to clot off. However, gentle squeezing of the tube is usually sufficient to move the bloody drainage along in the tubing. Special caution should be used in stripping tubes of patients with a known history of fragile tissue, such as occurs in emphysema. The nursing measures necessary in maintaining chest tubes and closed drainage are listed in the Critical Care Procedure, p. 1103.

**Suction.** Suction is usually used to speed reexpansion of the lung after surgery, using either wall suction or a portable suction machine (e.g., an Emerson [Figure 37-14, *B*]).

PROCEDURE FOR CRITICAL CARE

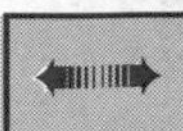

## MAINTAINING CHEST TUBES AND CLOSED CHEST DRAINAGE

1. Consult directions attached to the Pleur-Evac chest drainage unit.
2. Fill the water-seal chamber through the short suction tube to the "Fill to here" line on the water-seal pressure scale. Approximately 70 ml of sterile water or saline is needed. This is the 2 cm water level.
3. A funnel is provided to facilitate filling. To fill, attach the funnel to the connector on the suction tubing. Hold the funnel so that it is below the level of the top of the Pleur-Evac with the suction tubing crimped. Fill with sterile saline or water to the fill line. Then raise the funnel above the Pleur-Evac and release the crimp in the tubing. Water will enter the water-seal chamber to the level of the dotted line.
4. Connect the long tube from the collection chamber to the patient's chest tube.
5. Connect the short tubing to the suction source.
6. A dial to set the suction control is located on the upper left side of the unit behind the face. No water is needed in this chamber.
7. To set the suction control, turn the dial until the orange stripe appears in the semicircular window at the prescribed suction level line. Suction can be set at −10 to −40 cm water. The amount of suction is ordered by the surgeon.
8. Turn on the suction source and increase it until the orange float appears in the suction control indicator window. The setting of the suction control dial determines the approximate amount of suction regardless of the amount of source suction as long as the orange float appears in the indicator window.
9. If a suction setting is changed from a *higher level* to a *lower level,* the pressure being exerted on the patient's pleural space may remain at the higher level unless the amount of pressure in the closed system is relieved. Use the high-negativity relief valve on top of the unit to reduce negativity to the desired level.
10. Maintain fluid level at the fill line. Additional sterile water or saline may need to be added to the system periodically.
11. Samples of drainage fluid may be withdrawn from the self-sealing sampling port in the connector tubing. Use an 18-gauge or larger needle attached to a syringe for withdrawing samples.
12. Record the amount of drainage on the front of the unit.
13. To dispose of the Pleur-Evac chest drainage system, tie off drainage tubes and wrap the unit tightly in a plastic bag to prevent any leakage. Dispose of according to hospital policy for contaminated materials.

### PRECAUTIONS TO BE OBSERVED WITH ANY TYPE OF CLOSED DRAINAGE SYSTEM

1. Fasten tubing to the bed so that there are no dependent loops between the drainage system and the bed (Figure 37-14). Dependent loops allow fluid to collect in the tubing and prevent removal of air and fluid from the pleural space.
2. If the fluid is not fluctuating in the water-seal chamber:
   a. Be sure patient is not lying on tubes.
   b. Check connections to be sure chest tube system is intact.
   c. Ask patient to cough or change position to see if fluctuation is restored.
   d. Fluctuation will stop when lung is reexpanded. Call the surgeon if the tubes are not patent (column of fluid not fluctuating).
3. Keep two hemostats at the bedside so that the chest tube can be clamped if the system becomes disconnected or broken. When this occurs, the chest catheter should be clamped and then reconnected to a sterile setup as soon as possible. Sterile water should be used in the chamber. As soon as the system is reconnected, the clamp should be removed. *Except in an emergency, most thoracic surgeons prefer that tubes not be clamped, and a specific order is written if clamping is desired.*
4. When chest tubes are clamped, air (positive pressure) may be trapped in the pleural space and further collapse the lung. If a patient is being transported from one place to another, such as the radiology department, tubes should not be clamped unless it is necessary for only a few minutes.
5. An alternative method with no clamping of tubes is to keep a liter bottle of sterile water at the bedside at all times. If the patient's chest drainage unit breaks or cracks:
   a. Insert the end of the patient's chest tube into the bottle of sterile water.
   b. Remove any of the cracked or broken system.
   c. Obtain new system and reconnect it to the patient's tube as soon as possible.
6. Never lift the closed drainage system (Pleur-Evac above the level of the patient's chest) because this would allow fluid to be pulled into the pleural space.
7. If chest tube is accidentally pulled out of chest (a rare occurence):
   a. Apply gloves in accordance with body substance isolation (BSI) policy.
   b. Pinch skin opening together with fingers.
   c. Apply petroleum jelly gauze and sterile 4 × 4 dressing.
   d. Cover dressing with adhesive tape. Call surgeon immediately.

**Ambulation.** There is no contraindication to ambulating with a chest tube in place. As long as the closed drainage system remains below the level of the chest, the patient may assume any position of comfort in bed or may be out of bed in a chair. The patient is urged to be up at least twice daily.

**Removal of chest tubes.** Chest tubes are removed when there is no fluctuation of fluid in the water-seal chamber and when x-ray films confirm the full reexpansion of the lung. Most patients have their chest tube(s) removed in 48 to 72 hours postoperatively. If there is a persistent air space in the apex of the lung, the upper tube may be left in longer. *Surgeons are concerned about leaving tubes in very long because of the risk of an ascending tube track infection.* The patient should receive medication for pain 30 minutes before removal of the tube. Physicians vary in the exact procedure used

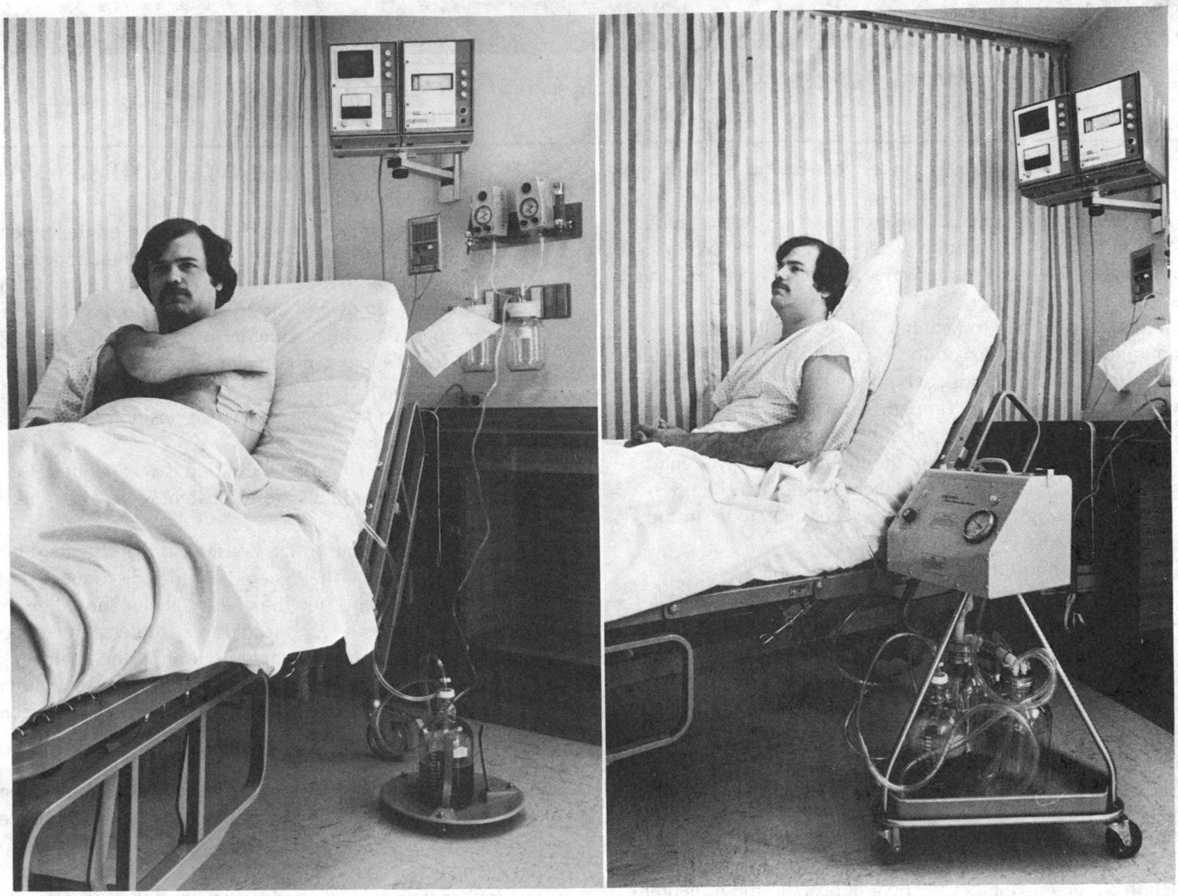

A

B

**FIGURE 37-14** Chest tube with water-seal suction. **A,** Wall outlet provides source of suction. Note holder used to secure bottle in upright position. **B,** Emerson suction machine as source of vacuum.

to remove the tube, but generally a sterile scissors, 4 × 4-inch gauze squares, and adhesive tape are required. The suture holding the tube in place is cut, the patient is asked to exhale deeply, and the tube is removed. If a pursestring suture was used, it is retied, and a dry sterile dressing is placed over the site. Some physicians cover the site with a Telfa dressing instead of gauze squares to ensure an airtight dressing. The dressing is covered securely by three overlapping strips of 2-inch adhesive tape.

An accepted practice has been to give the patient pain medication 30 minutes before removal of chest tube(s). However, a recent study of sensations experienced by patients during chest tube removal raises questions about this practice. In this study, burning was the most frequently reported sensation, followed by pain, pulling, and pressure (see Research box, p. 1105). Nurses should review this study with their surgeon colleagues to see if modifications might be made in the practice in their institutions.

### Care after pneumonectomy

The postoperative care discussed in the Critical Care Procedure applies to all patients with resectional surgery except those having a pneumonectomy. The special care required after pneumonectomy is outlined in the Guidelines box, p. 1105.

### Thoracoplasty

A **thoracoplasty** is an extrapleural procedure involving the removal of ribs to reduce the size of the chest cavity. Before the widespread use of resectional surgery, thoracoplasty was the basic surgical treatment for TB. Today, thoracoplasty is used infrequently and then only to prevent or treat the complications of resectional surgery. When it is thought that a patient's lung may not be able to expand sufficiently after a resection to fill the space, a thoracoplasty is performed 2 to 3 weeks before the resection. It also may be performed before pneumonectomy because this will reduce the chance of mediastinal shift after surgery. This type of thoracoplasty is

## RESEARCH

Gift AG, Bolgiano CS, Cunningham J: Sensations during chest tube removal, *Heart Lung* 20:131-137, 1991.

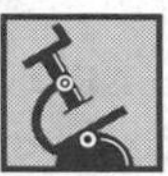

Despite information in nursing literature that persons experience pain during chest tube removal, no empiric studies supported this contention. This study examined the actual sensations experienced by 36 postoperative patients. The sample consisted of 24 men and 12 women between the ages of 32 and 83 years. Twenty of the subjects had mediastinal tubes, and the other 16 had pleural tubes. Chest tubes were removed after a standard procedure, and within 15 minutes of removal, subjects were asked to describe the sensations experienced. The intensity of each sensation mentioned was measured using a visual analog scale (VAS) with values ranging from 0 (low) to 100 (high). The most frequently reported sensation was burning (33% of reported sensations) followed by pain or hurting (29%) and pulling or yanking (20%). Some subjects reported more than one sensation. Burning was also the most intensely experienced sensation, with a mean value of 64; however, the values ranged from 34 to 100. The location of the tube did not influence the report of sensations. Age and gender of the subjects did not influence the type of sensation reported, but younger patients reported more intense sensations than did older patients. There was no difference between patients who received analgesia before chest tube removal and those who did not. The researchers suggested that further research is needed to explain variation in sensations reported and that frequently used analgesic medications may not be effective in the prevention of burning sensations.

often called a *preresection* or *tailoring* thoracoplasty; that is, the chest wall is tailored to reduce its size.

If the remaining portions of the lung fail to reexpand sufficiently postoperatively or if another complication such as empyema occurs, a thoracoplasty is performed. In general, it is used when there is a space in the chest that cannot be obliterated by other means. Usually, no more than three ribs are removed; therefore paradoxical motion after thoracoplasty is seldom seen anymore. Paradoxical motion is discussed under chest injuries (see p. 1114).

### Complications of chest surgery

In the immediate postoperative period (24 to 48 hours), hypotension, cardiac dysrhythmia, pulmonary edema, and subcutaneous emphysema (see p. 1101) may occur. Long-term complications include a residual air space, which results from failure of the remaining portions of the lung to reexpand and fill the space. If this space is small, no treatment is indicated. Two major complica-

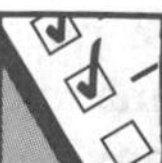

## Guidelines for Care of the Person After Pneumonectomy

1. Chest tubes are not necessary because there is no lung left to reexpand on the operative side.
2. Patient may lie on back or *operated side only*. Patient is not allowed to lie with operative side uppermost because of fear that the sutured bronchial stump may open, allowing fluid to drain into the unoperated side and drown the patient.
3. Pressure in the operative side will be checked in the operating room after the chest is closed. A pneumothorax apparatus (which can instill or remove air) will be used to check the pressure in the operative space, and air will be removed or instilled as necessary to bring the pressure to slightly negative (slightly less than 760 mm Hg).
4. The surgeon will palpate the patient's trachea at least daily to determine if it is in midline. Deviation of the trachea toward either the operated or unoperated side is a sign of *mediastinal shift*. If pressure builds up in the operated side, the trachea will deviate toward the unoperated side. The treatment is to remove air (positive pressure) with a pneumothorax apparatus. Mediastinal shift toward the "good" lung can seriously compromise ventilation and needs to be treated promptly. Deviation of the trachea toward the operated side indicates that more pressure (air) needs to be instilled into the empty space.
5. The patient with a mediastinal shift resembles the patient in congestive heart failure. Neck veins are distended, the trachea is displaced to one side, pulse and respirations are increased, and dyspnea is present.
6. Serous drainage will collect in the operated space and over time will congeal to the consistency of axle grease. This is often sufficient to keep the mediastinum from shifting toward the operative side. Persistent mediastinal shift toward the operative side may have to be treated with *thoracoplasty* (removal of ribs) to reduce the size of the remaining space and assist in maintaining the mediastinum in midline. Thoracoplasty is described on p. 1104.
7. It usually takes 2 to 4 days for the remaining lung to adjust to the increase in blood flow. For this reason the amount of fluids and blood given intravenously is monitored closely to prevent fluid overload. Central venous pressure monitoring is usually done. Rales are often heard over the base of the remaining lung, and vascular markings will be more prominent on x-ray films. Any increase in rales, in pulse or blood pressure, and in dyspnea may indicate circulatory overload and should be reported immediately. Treatment may include diuretics and/or digitalization along with discontinuing IV fluids.
8. Deep-breathing, coughing, and arm exercises are the same as described earlier (pp. 1099 and 1100).
9. Patients who have had a lung removed may have a lowered vital capacity, and exercise and activity should be limited to that which can be performed without dyspnea. Because the body must be given time to adjust to having only one lung, the patient's return to work may be delayed.
10. If the diagnosis is cancer, radiation therapy is usually given, and it may be started before the patient leaves the hospital. (See Chapter 16 for further discussion of nursing care for patients receiving radiation therapy.)
11. The patient who has had a pneumonectomy for cancer is urged to report to the physician at once if hoarseness, dyspnea, pain on swallowing, or localized chest pain develops because these symptoms may be signs of complications.

tions of chest surgery tend to occur later in the postoperative period and require treatment: empyema and bronchopleural fistula. The patient may have empyema alone or empyema and a bronchopleural fistula. The signs and symptoms and treatment of these two complications are outlined in Table 37-18.

# ADULT RESPIRATORY DISTRESS SYNDROME

## ETIOLOGY

**Adult respiratory distress syndrome (ARDS)** is the name given to a syndrome of acute hypoxemic respiratory failure without hypercapnia. The syndrome was first described by T.J. Petty in 1967.

## EPIDEMIOLOGY

ARDS is often fatal and is characterized by severe dyspnea, hypoxemia, and diffuse bilateral pulmonary infiltrations after lung injury in previously healthy persons. Recently, the term ***hyperpermeability pulmonary edema*** (HPPE) has been used to describe the condition that affects 150,000 to 200,000 critical care patients yearly. Causes of ARDS are presented in Box 37-16.

**BOX 37-16 Clinical Conditions Associated With ARDS/HPPE**

1. Shock
   a. Septic
   b. Hemorrhagic
   c. Cardiogenic
   d. Anaphylactic
2. Trauma
   a. Pulmonary contusion
   b. Nonpulmonary, multisystem
3. Infection
   a. Pneumonia
      (1) Viral
      (2) Bacterial (staphylococcal or streptococcal)
      (3) Legionellosis
   b. Miliary tuberculosis
4. Disseminated intravascular coagulation (DIC)
5. Fat emboli
6. Near-drowning
7. Aspiration: highly acid gastric contents (pH <2.5)
8. Inhaled toxic agents
   a. Smoke
   b. Phosgene
   c. Oxides of nitrogen
9. Pancreatitis
10. Oxygen toxicity
11. Narcotic drug abuse
    a. Heroin
    b. Methadone
    c. Propoxyphene (Darvon)
12. Radiation pneumonitis
13. Drugs
    a. Ethchlorvynol
    b. Salicylates

Adapted from Petty TL: Adult respiratory distress syndrome. In Kryger M: *Pathophysiology of respiration,* New York, 1981, John Wiley & Sons.

## PATHOPHYSIOLOGY

The pathophysiologic alterations that result in ARDS are typically initiated by a major trauma to the body, often a physical insult to a body system other than the pulmonary system (Figure 37-15). The following physiologic alterations result in the clinical syndrome identified as ARDS:

1. As a consequence of the precipitating insult, the complement cascade is activated, which in turn increases capillary wall permeability.
2. Fluid, granular leukocytes, red blood cells (RBCs), macrophages, cell debris, and protein leak into the interstitial spaces between the capillaries and alveoli and ultimately into the alveolar spaces.
3. Because of the fluid and debris in the interstitium and alveoli, surface area for oxygen and carbon dioxide exchange is decreased, resulting in low ventilation/perfusion (V/Q) ratios and hypoxemia.
4. Compensatory hyperventilation of functional alveoli occurs, resulting in hypocapnia and respiratory alkalosis.
5. Cells that normally line the alveoli are destroyed and replaced by cells that do not produce surfactant, thus increasing alveolar surface tension and resulting in atelectasis and increased alveolar opening pressures.

The normal function, pathophysiology, and clinical picture of a person with ARDS/HPPE are presented in Table 37-19.

ARDS usually occurs in a person who has had a recent physical trauma, although it can appear in persons who appeared to be healthy immediately before onset (e.g., someone with sudden onset of an acute infection). There is usually a latent period of 18 to 24 hours from the time of lung injury to the development of symptoms. The syndrome runs a variable course from a few days to several weeks' duration. Patients who appear to be recovering from ARDS may suddenly relapse into acute pulmonary disease from secondary insult such as pneumothorax or overwhelming infection. Box 37-17 lists clinical manifestations of ARDS.

## PREVENTION

Prompt treatment of the underlying cause of ARDS is the major focus of preventive care. Additionally, judicious use of the mechanical ventilator and oxygen therapy is required to avoid inducing ARDS as an untoward complication of these treatment modalities.

## MEDICAL MANAGEMENT

Patients with ARDS are critically ill and are best managed in an ICU. Medical management focuses on the following aspects of care:

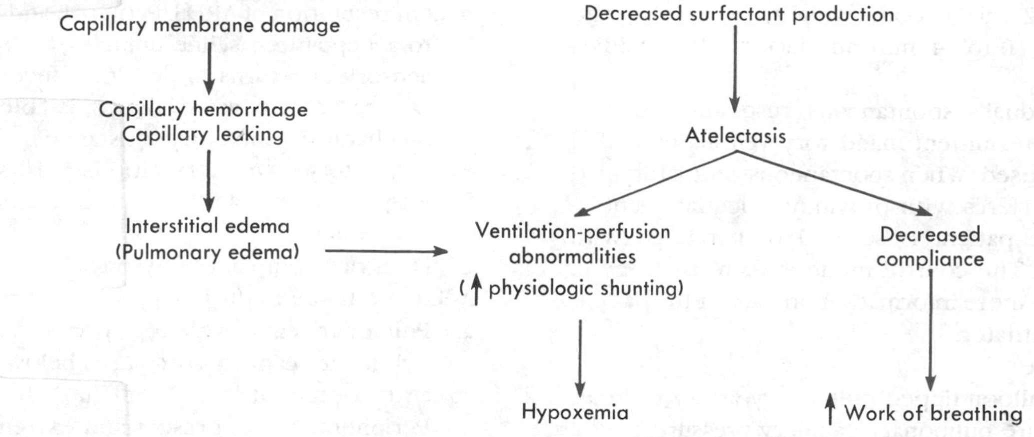


**FIGURE 37-15** Pathophysiologic events in adult respiratory distress syndrome.

**TABLE 37-19 Normal Function, Pathophysiology, and Clinical Manifestations of a Person With ARDS/HPPE**

| NORMAL FUNCTION | PATHOPHYSIOLOGY | CLINICAL MANIFESTATIONS |
|---|---|---|
| **ALVEOLOCAPILLARY MEMBRANE** | | |
| Oxygen and carbon dioxide exchange between alveolar air and pulmonary capillaries | Increased capillary wall permeability; blood plasma contents infiltrate interstitial and alveolar spaces, resulting in hypoxemia, alveolar hyperventilation, and respiratory alkalosis. | $Pa_{O_2}$ ↓<br>$Pa_{CO_2}$ ↓<br>pH ↑<br>Fine crackles auscultated throughout lungs |
| **LUNG PARENCHYMA** | | |
| Lung tissue that makes up the alveoli | Destruction of normal lung tissue, in particular, alveolar septal walls, normal cells replaced by nonsurfactant producing cells, and presence of edema and debris results in decreased lung compliance (stiff lung). Fibrosis may also develop. | Functional residual capacity and need to use high pressures to ventilate patient<br>Dyspnea at rest |

1. Oxygenation
   a. Initially may need to administer highest concentration of oxygen available (100%—using nonrebreathing face mask). However, oxygen delivered at levels greater than 50% is associated with oxygen toxicity that worsens already existing ARDS pathology. Oxygen concentrations can usually be lowered below 50%, by using **positive end-expiratory pressure (PEEP)** to open closed alveoli for increased ventilation.
   b. Goal is $Pa_{O_2}$ of 50 to 60 mm Hg.
   c. Gradually reduce $Fi_{O_2}$ while maintaining adequate arterial oxygen levels.
2. Ventilatory support: if oxygen therapy alone is unsuccessful in providing adequate arterial oxygenation, the patient is intubated and placed on a mechanical ventilator.
   a. A volume-limited ventilator is preferred.
   b. Ventilator is set to provide tidal volume equal to

**BOX 37-17 Clinical Manifestations of ARDS**

Signs and symptoms of ARDS include the following:
1. Acute respiratory distress: tachypnea, dyspnea, accessory muscle breathing, and central cyanosis
2. Dry cough and fever that develop over a few hours or days
3. Fine crackles throughout both lung fields
4. Altered sensorium ranging from confusion and agitation to coma

Radiologic and laboratory findings include the following:
1. Chest x-ray films: reveal diffuse, bilateral, and usually symmetric interstitial and alveolar infiltrations
2. ABGs
   Hypoxemia, $Pa_{O_2}$ less than 50 mm Hg
   Hypocapnia
   Respiratory alkalosis
   End stage: hypercapnia and respiratory acidosis, death

10 to 12 ml/kg body weight, respiratory rate equal to 10 to 14/min, and $FiO_2$ of 50%; PEEP is used.
   c. If individual's spontaneous respiration is adequate, intermittent mandatory ventilation (IMV) mode is used. When spontaneous ventilatory pattern interferes with providing adequate ventilation, the patient is sedated or paralyzed with Pavulon. The control mode is then used. See p. 1161 for more information on care of the patient on a ventilator.
3. Fluid volume
   a. Insert balloon-tipped pulmonary artery catheter to measure pulmonary capillary pressure.
   b. Diuretics, fluid volume expanders, and hypotensive medications are administered as indicated to maintain optimal fluid volume.
4. Treat underlying cause of ARDS.

## NURSING MANAGEMENT

### ♦ ASSESSMENT

Nursing assessment of the patient with ARDS must be tailored to maximize information obtained without increasing respiratory distress.

#### Subjective Data

Background information and history of present illness can be obtained from family members because the patient is usually too ill to give details.

#### Objective Data

The process of gathering objective data is the same as that described for respiratory failure (see p. 1159).

### ♦ NURSING DIAGNOSES

Nursing diagnoses are determined from analysis of patient data. Nursing diagnoses for the person with ARDS may include but are not limited to the following:

| Diagnostic Title | Possible Etiologic Factors |
|---|---|
| Gas exchange impaired | V/Q inequality |
| Tissue perfusion, altered (cardiopulmonary) | Fluid mobilization to (and from) third space (interstitium and alveolar space) |
| Anxiety | Threat of death |
| | Physiologic factors (ABG derangements) |
| Nutrition, altered: less than body requirements | Unable to take in adequate nutrition to meet increased metabolic workload from increased work of breathing |

### ♦ EXPECTED PATIENT OUTCOMES

Expected patient outcomes for the person with ARDS/HPPE may include but are not limited to the following:

1. Improved ventilation and oxygenation.
   a. $PaO_2$ is maintained at 50 to 60 mm Hg during acute phase of illness.
   b. On resolution of ARDS, $PaO_2$, pH, and $PCO_2$ return to acceptable baseline limits.
   c. Sensorium returns to preillness level.
   d. During acute phase of illness, is able to tolerate mechanical ventilatory assistance.
   e. Inspiratory/expiratory ratio is 5:10 seconds.
   f. Respiratory rate and tidal volume are within normal limits.
   g. Does not complain of dyspnea.
2. Adequate tissue perfusion.
   a. Pulmonary capillary wedge pressure (measure of pulmonary capillary pressure) below 18 mm Hg.
   b. Urine output at least 30 ml/hr.
   c. Peripheral pulses present and extremities warm to touch.
3. Increased physiologic and psychologic comfort and decreased anxiety.
   a. Tolerates ventilator and artificial airway.
   b. Acknowledges and expresses fears.
   c. Communicates personal needs effectively with staff and family.
   d. Cooperates and assists with care.
4. Stable body weight within 5 pounds of preillness weight.

### ♦ INTERVENTIONS

#### ➠ Managing Critical Care

Patients with ARDS are critically ill and are best cared for in an ICU (see also Nursing Care Plan for a Patient on Ventilator Support Receiving PEEP, p. 1164). Their care centers around the following measures.

#### Maintaining Adequate Gas Exchange

**Oxygenation**

1. Maintain oxygen therapy as ordered.
2. Monitor for signs of hypoxemia (see p. 1158).

**Ventilatory support**

1. Maintain a patent airway.
2. If artificial airway present (endotracheal tube or tracheostomy), provide necessary care (see Chapter 36).
   a. Secure tube to avoid movement either in or out of established position.
   b. Position patient for optimal oxygenation; usually head of bed elevated 45 to 90 degrees.
   c. Auscultate lungs hourly to assess placement of endotracheal tube (may slip into right mainstem bronchus).
3. Suction endotracheal tube as needed.
4. Administer bronchodilators as ordered.
5. Check ventilator settings frequently.

#### Maintaining Adequate Tissue Perfusion

The maintenance of adequate tissue perfusion is a nursing responsibility.

1. Monitor pulmonary capillary wedge pressure.
   a. Notify physician if pressure is above or below established range.
   b. If pressure is below established range, administer plasma volume expanders or hypotensive medications as ordered.
   c. If pressure is high, administer diuretics or vasodilators as ordered.
2. Assess urine output, vital signs, and extremities hourly.

### Decreasing Patient and Family Anxiety

1. Ensure proper ventilator function to deliver adequate tidal volume and oxygen concentration. If patient appears in respiratory distress although ventilator is functioning properly, assess ABG gas levels.
2. Identify a way for patient to be able to communicate concerns and express feelings (if unable to verbalize because of intubation, try alternative ways of communication).
3. Provide simple explanations about procedures; orient patient to surroundings, and repeat explanations regularly.
4. Offer explanations of care routines and environment to family. Encourage family to approach, talk to, and touch patient, as they desire.

### Maintaining Adequate Nutrition

Nutritional interventions for patients are the same as those for the patient with COPD (see p. 1139 and Nursing Care Plan for Person on Mechanical Ventilation Receiving PEEP on p. 1163).

## ♦ EVALUATION

To evaluate the effectiveness of nursing interventions, compare patient behaviors with those stated in the expected patient outcomes. Successful achievement of patient outcomes for the patient with ARDS is indicated by the following:

1. Is able to maintain own ventilation without mechanical assistance.
   a. $Pao_2$ is 75 mm Hg.
   b. $Paco_2$ is 45 mm Hg.
   c. Inspiratory/expiratory ratio is 5:10 seconds.
   d. Respiratory rate and tidal volume are within normal limits.
2. Is able to maintain adequate tissue perfusion.
   a. Pulmonary capillary wedge pressure is 17 mm Hg.
   b. Urine output is 150 to 200 ml at each voiding.
   c. Peripheral pulses present and extremities are warm to touch.
3. Appears calm and relaxed.
   a. Able to sleep at night.
   b. Expresses any concerns freely.
   c. Appears calm in interactions with family.
4. Body weight is below preillness level, but appetite is improving and patient is gaining weight daily.

# PULMONARY VASCULAR DISEASE

## PULMONARY EMBOLI AND PULMONARY INFARCTION

### Etiology

**Pulmonary embolism (PE)** is the lodging of a clot, usually from a deep vein thrombosis (DVT), or other foreign matter in a pulmonary arterial vessel. Pulmonary infarction is the extravasation of blood and, rarely, the necrosis of lung parenchyma resulting from the occlusion of a medium-sized pulmonary artery.

### Epidemiology

Emboli formation rarely occurs without the presence of certain risk factors (Box 37-18).

PEs result from damage to blood vessel walls (surgery), blood stasis (varicosities), or blood hypercoagulability (estrogen therapy).

### Pathophysiology

Emboli travel from their site of origin through the right side of the heart and lodge in the pulmonary vasculature. The size of the pulmonary artery and the number of emboli determine the severity of symptoms.

Blood flow is obstructed, causing localized tissue hypoxia and ultimately a decrease in the pulmonary vascular bed. Pulmonary vessels vasoconstrict in response to the hypoxia. The resultant V/Q inequality (ventilation greater than perfusion) causes arterial hypoxemia. The normal function, primary pathophysiology, and the clinical picture of a patient with PE are presented in Table 37-20.

If the embolus blocks a larger vessel, the person may complain of sudden, sharp upper abdominal or thoracic pain, become dyspneic, cough violently, and have hemoptysis; shock may develop rapidly. If the area of infarction is small, the symptoms are much milder. The patient may have cough, tachypnea, pleuritic chest pain, slight hemoptysis, elevation of temperature, and an increased leukocyte count. An area of dullness or crackles may be detected when checking breath sounds.

**BOX 37-18 Predisposing Factors in the Occurrence of Pulmonary Emboli**

- Thrombophlebitis—deep vein thrombus (DVT)
- Immobility
- Recent surgery
- Obesity
- Congestive heart failure/myocardial infarction
- Recent fracture
- Estrogen therapy

**TABLE 37-20 Normal Function, Primary Pathophysiology, and Clinical Manifestations of Pulmonary Embolism**

| NORMAL FUNCTION | PATHOPHYSIOLOGY | CLINICAL MANIFESTATIONS |
|---|---|---|
| **PULMONARY VASCULATURE** | | |
| To carry venous blood received from right side of heart to alveolocapillary membrane in lung for oxygen/carbon dioxide exchange | Occlusion of pulmonary vessels because of increased vascular resistance, decreased cardiac output (usually occurs only in massive emboli), decreased lung perfusion | Elevated pulmonary artery pressure<br>Dyspnea<br>Hypotension<br>Tachycardia<br>High V/Q ratio as shown on lung scan<br>Hypocapnia and elevated arterial blood pH |
| **AIRWAYS** | | |
| Carry oxygenated air to alveolocapillary membrane for exchange and deoxygenated air out of lung | Airway constriction from lowered alveolar carbon dioxide levels | Underventilated lung areas as shown on lung scan<br>Hypoxemia<br>Tachypnea<br>Cough |
| **ALVEOLI** | | |
| Lung site where gas exchange takes place (alveolocapillary membrane) | Infarction of alveolar tissues caused by complete obstruction, resulting in extravasation of blood cells into alveoli (NOTE: occurs only in more severe cases) | Hemoptysis<br>Radiologic opacity |
| **PLEURA** | | |
| Maintain close approximation of lungs and chest wall<br>Minimize friction during lung expansion and contraction | Transudate from damaged vascular structures | Pleural friction rub<br>Chest pain during inhalation/exhalation |

The diagnosis of PE is not easy to make. Clinical history, changes in blood chemistries, and plain chest x-ray films often are not definitive in establishing the diagnosis. The ultimate standard for the diagnosis of PE is pulmonary arteriography.[38]

## Prevention

The best treatment for PE is prevention. Preventive measures for hospitalized patients are presented under nursing interventions. The person at high risk of PE should be counseled to:

1. Avoid prolonged sitting or standing.
2. Avoid restrictive clothing.
3. Smokers should stop smoking.

## Medical Management

A major component of medical treatment or PE is anticoagulant therapy. Anticoagulant therapy may be either prophylactic for high-risk persons or curative for the actual pathologic event (Box 37-19).

When the patient is not responsive to heparin therapy or when anticoagulant therapy is contraindicated, surgical intervention may be required. Two procedures may be used to treat pulmonary emboli:

1. *Thrombolytic therapy.* This is a new therapy still undergoing trials. It can promote immediate dissolution of the embolus with prompt return of pulmonary function. In this procedure, one of the thrombolytic agents, urokinase, streptokinase, or *recombinant* tissue-type plasminogen activator (rt-PA), is used. Therapy can be delivered either systemically or directly into the pulmonary artery via selective catheterization, although systemic therapy appears to be superior. The most popular regimen involves the administration of 100 mg rt-PA as a continuous peripheral infusion over 2 hours. Thus far, the reported results indicate that this strategy is effective in achieving clot dissolution in more than 80% of patients, with bleeding complications occurring in less

**BOX 37-19 Anticoagulant Therapy for Pulmonary Emboli**

1. Prophylactic: often used for high-risk persons
   a. Low-dose heparin: 5000 U subcutaneously every 12 hours preoperatively and every 8 to 12 hours postoperatively until patient is ambulatory
   b. Oral anticoagulants: warfarin, 5-10 mg daily for 3 days, then maintenance on the basis of prothrombin time
2. Curative treatment
   a. Heparin, approximately 5000 to 15,000 U IV bolus, then continuous infusion approximately 1000 U every hour or 2500-5000 U IV every 4 hours
   b. Long-term treatment with warfarin, 5-10 mg daily

than 5%. This form of therapy is often not applicable to many postsurgical patients because of the increased risk of bleeding complications at their surgical site. A small group of patients with PE fail to respond to immediate aggressive medical support, and pulmonary embolectomy should be considered.[38]

2. *Pulmonary embolectomy.* PEs are extracted from the pulmonary vasculature. This procedure is usually performed with the patient under general anesthesia, although it may be performed with a special IV suction catheter under local anesthesia. The survival rate for this procedure is about 60%.[38]

## NURSING MANAGEMENT

### ♦ ASSESSMENT

#### Subjective Data

Data to be collected to assess the patient with PE include the following:

1. Determine the presence of risk factors (see Prevention section).
2. Assess for the recent onset of any of the following symptoms:
   Dyspnea
   Substernal chest pain
   Hemoptysis
   Chest palpitations
   Pleuritic pain
   Cough
   Apprehension
   Diaphoresis

#### Objective Data

Data to be collected to assess the patient with PE include the following:

1. Assess general appearance: patient often appears apprehensive.
2. Assess vital signs for the following:
   - Tachypnea
   - Tachycardia
   - Elevated temperature
3. Perform pulmonary examination
   - Inspection, palpation, and percussion usually normal unless there is an underlying pulmonary disease
   
   Auscultation, listening for:
   - Pleural friction rub
   - Localized, decreased breath sounds and crackles
4. Assess laboratory findings for the following:
   
   ABGs
   - Hypoxemia
   - Respiratory alkalosis
   
   Chest x-ray film: often normal
   
   Lung scan
   - Perfusion scan positive
   - Ventilation scan may indicate underventilated areas
   
   Pulmonary angiography
   - If positive, is definitive for PE
   - Positive findings indicate vessel filling defect and cut-off (abrupt ending of vessel)

### ♦ NURSING DIAGNOSES

Nursing diagnoses are determined from analysis of patient data. Nursing diagnoses for the person with PE may include but are not limited to the following:

| Diagnostic Title | Possible Etiologic Factors |
|---|---|
| Tissue perfusion, altered in pulmonary vascular and lung | Vascular obstruction from emboli resulting in decreased or absent blood flow to region |
| Gas exchange, impaired | High V/Q ratio |
| Pain | Pleural effusion |
| Knowledge deficit: condition and its treatment | Lack of exposure or unfamiliarity with information sources |

### ♦ EXPECTED PATIENT OUTCOMES

Expected patient outcomes for the person with PE may include but are not limited to the following:

1. Demonstrates adequate tissue perfusion.
   a. Extremities are warm and dry to touch, and pulses are present.
   b. Coagulation studies: prothrombin (PT) time and partial prothrombin time (PPT) are within normal limits.
   c. IV sites are intact and nonreddened.
2. Demonstrates adequate ventilation.
   a. $Pa_{O_2}$ is 80 to 100 mm Hg.
   b. $Pa_{CO_2}$ is 40 mm Hg.
   c. pH is 7.35 to 7.45.
3. States that pain is relieved.
4. Patient or significant others are able to:
   a. List behaviors that would increase the risk of pulmonary emboli.
   b. Identify the signs and symptoms of pulmonary emboli.
   c. State the reason for anticoagulant therapy, the prescribed dose and time of administration of medications, any adverse side effects, and need to take medications as prescribed.
   d. State plans for follow-up care, including periodic blood coagulation tests.

### ♦ INTERVENTIONS

#### Promoting Tissue Perfusion

1. Provide antiembolism stockings.
2. Perform hourly active foot dorsiflexion.
3. Elevate lower extremities (do not use Gatch bed).
4. Perform ROM exercises.
5. Assess legs for adequate pulses and leg size (do not massage legs).
6. Inspect IV sites regularly.
7. Administer anticoagulants as ordered.
8. Monitor PT and PPT; withhold anticoagulant and

notify physician if PT or PPT falls below accepted levels.

### Promoting Gas Exchange

1. Assist patient to deep-breathe hourly and to cough unless coughing is contraindicated.
2. Administer oxygen therapy as ordered.
3. Maintain prescribed activity while avoiding overexertion.

### Promoting Comfort

1. Elevate the head of the bed 30 to 40 degrees.
2. Maintain a quiet, calm environment.
3. Administer pain medications as ordered.

### Facilitating Learning

Teach patient about risk factors associated with PE and how to avoid them.

1. Do not wear constrictive clothing such as rolled garters.
2. Avoid standing or sitting for prolonged periods. Be sure to move about at least every 2 hours. Do active dorsiflexion of feet while sitting.
3. Stop smoking. Refer to resource that assists patients to stop smoking.

The patient needs to understand the common signs and symptoms of PE so immediate assistance can be sought if they occur. These include:

1. Dyspnea
2. Substernal chest pain
3. Hemoptysis
4. Chest palpitations
5. Cough
6. Diaphoresis
7. Apprehension

## ♦ EVALUATION

To evaluate the effectiveness of nursing interventions, compare patient behaviors with those stated in the expected patient outcomes. Successful achievement of patient outcomes for the patient with PE is indicated by the following:

1. Demonstrates adequate tissue perfusion.
   a. Extremities are warm and dry, and pulses are present.
   b. Coagulation studies: PT and PPT are within normal limits.
   c. IV sites are intact and give no indication of bleeding from them.
2. Demonstrates adequate ventilation.
   a. $Pao_2$ is 85 to 100.
   b. $Paco_2$ is 40 mm Hg.
   c. pH is 7.35 to 7.45.
3. Lists behaviors that would increase the risk of PE.
   a. Does not sit in one position for a long time without getting up and moving about.
   b. Verbalizes signs and symptoms of PE: dyspnea; sharp pain in chest, especially when taking a deep breath and when exhaling; cough; rapid heartbeat.
4. States that he or she is taking a "blood thinner" to prevent future thrombi and emboli. Knows the dose and time of medications he or she will take after discharge and side effects such as bruising easily and bleeding gums.
5. Shows card indicating next appointment for blood test. Verbalizes the importance of having blood drawn as scheduled. Also verbalizes that if for any reason appointment cannot be kept, physician should be called for assistance with alternative plan (sending someone to patient's home to draw blood, assisting patient with transportation, etc.).
6. Carries card stating is on "blood thinner."

# CHEST TRAUMA

## ETIOLOGY

Trauma to the chest is a major problem most often seen first in the emergency department. Injury to the chest may affect the bony chest cage, pleurae and lungs, diaphragm, or mediastinal contents.

Injuries to the chest are broadly classified into two groups: blunt and penetrating (Box 37-20). **Blunt injuries** or nonpenetrating injuries damage the structures within the chest cavity without disrupting chest wall integrity. **Penetrating injuries** disrupt chest wall integrity and result in alteration in intrathoracic pressures.

## EPIDEMIOLOGY

The leading cause of blunt chest injuries in the United States is motor vehicle steering wheel impaction in the person not wearing a seat belt. Blows to the chest with blunt objects or as a result of a fall also cause nonpenetrating chest injury. Penetrating wounds usually result from gunshot or stabbing injuries.

## RIB FRACTURES

### Pathophysiology

Rib fractures are the most common blunt injury. Ribs 3 through 10 are most often fractured because they are less protected by the chest muscles. The ribs usually fracture at the point of maximal impact, but they may fracture at a distant site from impact. Rib fractures are caused by blows, crushing injuries, or strain caused by severe coughing or sneezing spells. If the rib is splintered or the fracture displaced, sharp fragments may penetrate the pleura and lung, resulting in a **hemothorax** or **pneumothorax,** which are penetrating injuries.

Common signs and symptoms of rib fracture include the following:

1. Pain at the site of injury, increasing on inspiration
2. Localized tenderness and crepitus on palpation
3. Splinting of chest and shallow breathing

Fractures are confirmed by chest x-ray findings.

**BOX 37-20 Penetrating and Nonpenetrating (Blunt) Chest Injuries**

**PENETRATING**

Open pneumothorax (sucking chest wound)
Hemothorax
Tracheobronchial injury
Pulmonary contusion
Diaphragm rupture
Mediastinal injury

**BLUNT (NONPENETRATING)**

Closed pneumothorax
Tension pneumothorax
Tracheobronchial injury
Flail chest
Diaphragm rupture
Mediastinal injury
Fractured ribs

### Prevention

Nurses can promote prevention of chest trauma through public education programs focused on safe practices in vehicle use and in the workplace. The major preventable focus is promoting the use of seat belts when operating a motor vehicle.

### Medical Management

Treatment is individualized on the basis of the patient's age, whether there is preexisting chronic pulmonary disease history, and the number and location of ribs fractured. Medical treatment includes the following:

1. Analgesics as needed for pain
2. If pain is severe, a regional nerve block (intercostal) or epidural anesthesia

## NURSING MANAGEMENT

## ♦ ASSESSMENT

### Subjective Data

Data include the nature of the injury and when it occurred. If patient is unable to answer questions, data are obtained from those with the patient.

### Objective Data

Data to be collected to assess the patient with rib fracture include the following:

Pain at site of injury that increases on inspiration
Area tender to the touch
Patient splints chest and takes shallow breaths

## ♦ NURSING DIAGNOSES

Nursing diagnoses are determined from analysis of patient data. Nursing diagnoses for the person with rib fracture may include but are not limited to the following:

| Diagnostic Title | Possible Etiologic Factors |
|---|---|
| Airway clearance, ineffective | Pain/trauma to rib cage |
| Breathing pattern, ineffective | Pain, musculoskeletal impairment |
| Pain | Trauma to rib cage |
| Anxiety | Threat to change in health status |
| Knowledge deficit: condition and its treatment | Lack of exposure to information |

## ♦ EXPECTED PATIENT OUTCOMES

Expected patient outcomes for the person with fractured ribs may include but are not limited to the following:

1. Maintains a patent airway.
2. Is breathing effectively.
3. States that pain is improved.
4. Is less anxious.
5. Understands follow-up therapy.
6. Understands that physician is to be notified if shortness of breath, hemoptysis, chest pain, or temperature elevation occurs after discharge.

## ♦ INTERVENTIONS

### Initial Care for Fractured Ribs

If ribs are fractured and the rib has not penetrated the pleura, give analgesics as needed for pain and to slow respiratory rate in the patient who is anxious and may be hyperventilating.

### Maintaining the Airway

Persons with rib fractures may develop atelectasis secondary to their shallow breathing and their reluctance to expand their lungs fully. They should be assisted to periodically expand their lungs fully:

1. Administer analgesics to reduce pain.
2. Coordinate lung-expanding maneuvers such as deep breathing, coughing, sighing, or yawning to coincide with the analgesics' peak effect time.
3. Splint the fracture site with your hands to assist lung-expanding exercises.
4. Reposition patient every 2 hours.

### Assisting with Comfort and ADL

1. Place patient in position of comfort; may be able to breathe best in Fowler's or semi-Fowler's position.
2. Give prescribed analgesics.
3. If pain persists despite analgesics, notify the physician, who may infiltrate the intercostal spaces above and below the fractured rib(s) with 1% procaine.

## ♦ EVALUATION

To evaluate the effectiveness of nursing interventions, compare patient behaviors with those stated in the expected patient outcomes. Successful achievement of patient outcomes for the patient with fractured ribs is indicated by the following:

1. Is able to manage own secretions.
2. Respirations are 16 and regular.
3. States that he or she is free of pain.
4. Appears calm.
5. Has appointment for a chest x-ray in 2 weeks.
6. States he or she should notify physician if signs of complications occur.

## FLAIL CHEST

### Pathophysiology

When multiple ribs or the sternum is fractured in more than one place, a portion of the chest wall becomes separated from the chest cage, resulting in a **flail chest.** Thus the chest wall no longer provides the rigid bony support that is necessary to maintain the bellows function required for normal ventilation. This causes **paradoxical breathing,** or paradoxical respiratory movement. On inspiration the dislocated segment is pulled inward by the subatmospheric intrapleural pressure. During expiration the dislocated segment bulges outward as intrapleural pressure becomes less negative (Figure 37-16, *A* to *D*).

Flail chest usually causes localized atelectasis secondary to decreased ventilation, resulting in hypoxemia. Because of the increased work of breathing, the individual may also develop hypercapnia and respiratory acidosis. Pulmonary contusion is a common occurrence in persons with a flail chest.[24] Box 37-21 lists clinical manifestations of a flail chest.

### Medical Management

Treatment for flail chest includes the following:

1. Stabilize the flail segment. After initial stabilization the individual is usually intubated and placed on a **volume-cycled ventilator.** Mechanical ventilation provides internal stabilization of the chest, decreases the work of breathing, and initiates the bellows function normally provided by the intact

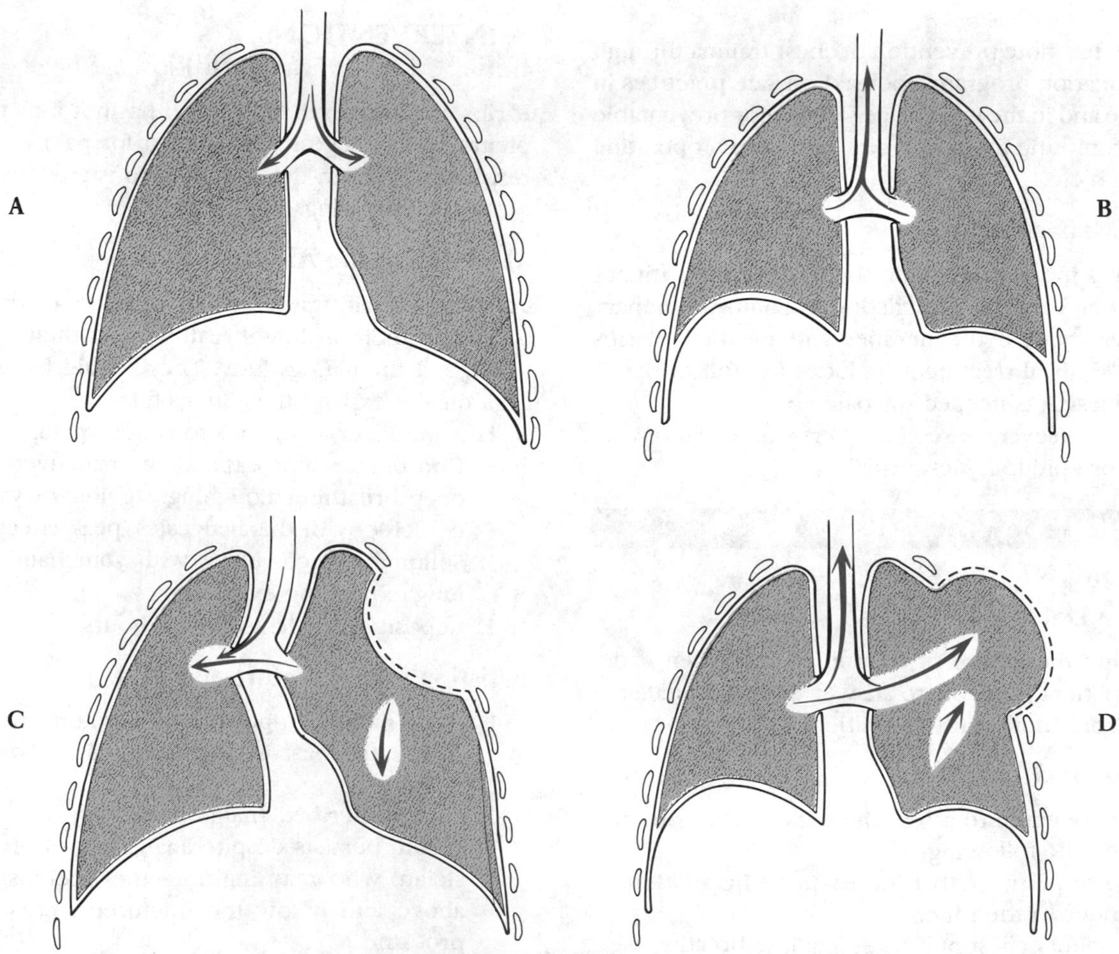


**FIGURE 37-16** Normal respiration: **A,** inspiration; **B,** expiration. Paradoxical motion: **C,** inspiration, area of lung underlying unstable chest wall sucks in on inspiration; **D,** same area balloons out on expiration. Note movement of mediastinum toward opposite lung on inspiration.

**BOX 37-21 Clinical Manifestations of a Flail Chest**

Severe chest pain
Paradoxical breathing or chest movement with movement toward unaffected side with inspiration and returning toward midline on expiration
Oscillation of mediastinum, increasing dyspnea
Tachypnea with shallow respirations
Accessory muscle breathing
Decreased breath sounds on auscultation
Anxiety related to above signs and symptoms

bony chest cage. If prolonged ventilatory support is required, a tracheostomy is performed.

2. Provide supplemental oxygen.
3. Correct acid-base imbalance. Mechanical ventilation is used to correct *respiratory* acid-base imbalance.
4. Provide analgesics for pain control.
5. For severe pain, epidural anesthesia may be used.
6. Avoid fluid overload.

## NURSING MANAGEMENT

### ♦ ASSESSMENT

#### Subjective Data

Data to be collected include nature of the injury and when it occurred. Often the patient is too badly injured to answer questions, and data are obtained from those accompanying the patient.

#### Objective Data

Data to be collected to assess the patient with flail chest include the following:

Pain is severe and increases with each respiratory movement.
Mediastinum oscillates, or "flutters," with each respiration.
Decreased breath sounds on auscultation.
If there is severe interference with cardiac function, neck veins will be distended.
Vital signs: increased pulse and respiratory rate. Blood pressure will fall if paradoxical motion is not relieved.

#### Diagnostic Tests

Chest x-ray examination to determine extent of trauma
ABGs to determine $PaO_2$ and $PaCO_2$

### ♦ NURSING DIAGNOSES

Nursing diagnoses are determined from analysis of patient data. Nursing diagnoses for the person with a flail chest may include but are not limited to the following:

| Diagnostic Title | Possible Etiologic Factors |
|---|---|
| Airway clearance, ineffective | Trauma to chest wall |
| Gas exchange, impaired | V/Q abnormality |
| Pain | Trauma to chest wall |

### ♦ EXPECTED PATIENT OUTCOMES

1. Airway is improved.
2. $PaO_2$ and $PaCO_2$ are improved.
3. Has normal respiration.
4. Is more comfortable.

### ♦ INTERVENTIONS

#### ➠ Managing Critical Care

#### Improving Airway Clearance

Nursing interventions focused on effective airway clearance are a critical component of care for the person with flail chest who is intubated and cannot clear own airway. Shallow breathing and retained secretions can result in a fatal pulmonary infection.

The following nursing actions are indicated:

1. Suction airway as needed to maintain patency.
2. Liquefy pulmonary secretions by providing adequate fluid intake and humidification of the respiratory tract.
3. After extubation, time coughing maneuvers to coincide with peak effect of analgesics.

#### Improving Gas Exchange

Nursing interventions to promote adequate oxygen and carbon dioxide exchange are aimed at stabilizing the flail segment and include the following:

1. Initially, provide direct support to the flail segment with the hands or sandbags.
2. After spinal injury is ruled out, turn the patient on to the affected side. This provides stabilization of the flail segment and also encourages lung expansion on the unaffected side until the patient can be intubated and attached to a volume-cycled ventilator.

#### Promoting Comfort

Interventions to promote comfort include the following:

1. Administer analgesics liberally as needed.
2. Splint the flail segment with hands during coughing and movement (see Figure 37-11).

### ♦ EVALUATION

To evaluate the effectiveness of nursing interventions, compare patient behaviors with those stated in the expected patient outcomes. Successful achievement of patient outcomes for the person with flail chest is indicated by the following:

1. Has been weaned from the ventilator and is extubated.

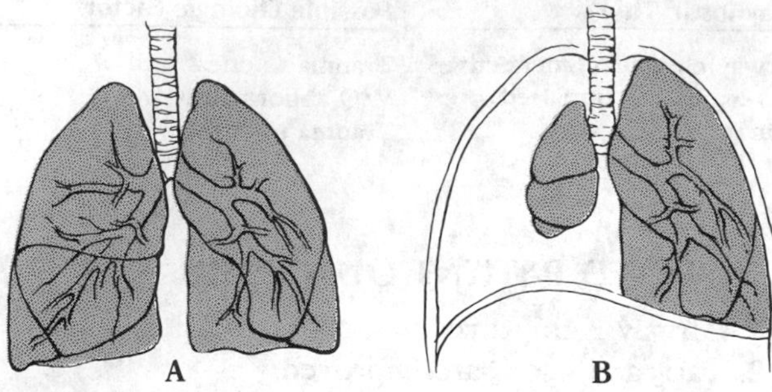


**FIGURE 37-17** **A,** Normal expanded lungs. **B,** Complete collapse of right lung caused by air in pleural cavity (pneumothorax).

2. $PaO_2$ is 90 mm Hg; $PaCO_2$ is 40 mm Hg; and pH is 7.35.
3. Respirations are 18 and regular.
4. Moves about freely without pain.

## PNEUMOTHORAX

### Etiology

Pneumothorax is a condition in which there is air in the pleural space between the lung and the chest wall. It can occur as a result of penetrating or nonpenetrating chest injuries or can occur spontaneously.

### Pathophysiology

A **closed pneumothorax** is caused by a blunt injury resulting in fractured ribs piercing the pleural membranes or by a sudden compression of the rib cage. Air enters the pleural space, increasing intrapleural pressure and collapsing the lung (Figure 37-17, *B*). A variant of a closed pneumothorax is a **spontaneous pneumothorax** that can result from the rupture of an emphysematous bleb on the lung surface, but it may also follow severe bouts of coughing in persons with a chronic pulmonary disease such as asthma. Rather frequently it occurs as a single or recurrent episode in an otherwise healthy young male. If large enough and left untreated, a closed pneumothorax can become a tension pneumothorax.

A **tension pneumothorax** occurs when air enters the pleural space on inspiration but cannot leave it on expiration. Although usually a result of a closed pneumothorax, a tension pneumothorax can be caused by a penetrating chest injury. The accumulating air builds up positive pressure in the chest cavity, resulting in:

1. Lung collapse on the affected side
2. Mediastinal shift toward the unaffected side
3. Compression of mediastinal contents (heart, great vessels) resulting in decreased cardiac output and decreased venous return

An **open pneumothorax** occurs when a penetrating chest wound opens the intrapleural space to atmospheric pressure. Each time the person inspires, air is sucked into the intrapleural space, increasing intrapleural pressure. An open pneumothorax is also called a sucking chest wound because the wound makes a sucking sound on inspiration and expiration. Blood also may leak into the pleural cavity creating a **hemothorax.**

### Clinical Manifestations and Medical Management

The clinical manifestations and medical management of the various types of pneumothorax are presented in Table 37-21.

### Nursing Management

Nursing diagnoses and interventions associated with the specific types of pneumothorax are presented in Table 37-22.

**BOX 37-22 Clinical Manifestations of Pulmonary Contusion**

Pulmonary contusion may vary from total absence of symptoms to the full spectrum of symptoms associated with noncardiogenic pulmonary edema. The onset of signs and symptoms (some of which may be delayed) include the following:

- Increasing dyspnea
- Tachypnea
- Increasing restlessness
- Crackles noted on auscultation
- Hemoptysis

## PULMONARY CONTUSION

### Etiology

Contusion of the pleurae or lung parenchyma is a penetrating injury. It usually results from sudden compression, followed by rapid decompression of the thoracic cavity, causing blood to extravasate into the pulmonary tissue.

### Pathophysiology

The contusion is usually self-limiting because pulmonary vasculature is a low-pressure system. However, extensive contusion can precipitate pulmonary edema, with resultant hypoxemia, hypercapnia, and respiratory acidosis. Box 37-22 lists the clinical manifestations.

### Medical Management

Medical treatment of pulmonary contusion depends on the severity of the injury. Treatment may vary from outpatient monitoring to intubation and mechanical ventilatory support when pulmonary edema is present.

### Nursing Management

1. Administer analgesia as ordered every 3 hours.
2. Monitor for fluid overload.
   a. Keep accurate record of all intake and output.
   b. Monitor vital signs every 30 minutes. Pulse and

**TABLE 37-21 Clinical Manifestations and Medical Management of Pneumothorax**

| PNEUMOTHORAX | CLINICAL MANIFESTATIONS | MEDICAL MANAGEMENT |
|---|---|---|
| Closed (spontaneous) | Small or slowly developing pneumothorax may produce no symptoms.<br>Larger or rapidly developing pneumothorax results in the following:<br>1. Sharp pain on inspiration<br>2. Increasing dyspnea<br>3. Increasing restlessness<br>4. Diaphoresis<br>5. Hypotension<br>6. Tachycardia<br>7. Absence of chest movement on affected side<br>8. Breath sounds absent on affected side<br>9. Hyperresonance on affected side | Observation on outpatient basis<br>Supplemental oxygen<br>Needle aspiration of air from pleural space, if present; insertion of chest catheter connected to a flutter valve or closed drainage system<br>If frequent recurrences, tetracycline or talc instilled into pleural space to cause adhesions between pleurae; if this procedure fails, lung portion with defect resected and parietal pleura abraded |
| Tension | 1. Severe dyspnea<br>2. Agitation<br>3. Trachea deviated from midline toward unaffected side—mediastinal shift<br>4. Jugular venous distention<br>5. Absence of chest movement on affected side<br>6. Hypotension, tachycardia<br>7. Breath sounds absent on affected side<br>8. Hyperresonance on affected side<br>9. Diminished heart sounds<br>10. Shock<br>11. Subcutaneous emphysema<br>12. Ineffective ventilation | True emergency<br>Defect in chest wall covered with a sterile dressing<br>Insertion of chest tube connected to a flutter valve or closed drainage system |
| Open | 1. Sucking sounds at wound site with respiration<br>2. Tracheal deviation (trachea moves toward unaffected side during inspiration and returns toward midline with expiration) | Occlusion of open wound<br>Same as for closed pneumothorax |

**TABLE 37-22 Nursing Diagnoses and Interventions for Pneumothorax**

| PNEUMOTHORAX | NURSING DIAGNOSES | NURSING INTERVENTIONS |
|---|---|---|
| Closed (spontaneous) | Knowledge deficit: condition and treatment | For outpatient or for patient after chest tube removal, instruct to:<br>1. Report any increased dyspnea to physician.<br>2. Avoid strenuous exercise or activity that increases rate and depth of breathing.<br>3. Avoid holding breath.<br>4. Follow physician's instructions about resuming normal activity. |
| | Impaired gas exchange | Perform the following:<br>1. Place in semi-Fowler's position.<br>2. Administer oxygen.<br>3. Obtain thoracentesis tray and closed drainage equipment (see p. 1101 for care of the patient with chest tubes). |
| Tension | Knowledge deficit<br>Impaired gas exchange | Same discharge instruction as for patient with closed pneumothorax<br>Life-threatening event; imperative that interventions be carried out immediately to relieve increased intrapleural pressure; interventions same as those listed for closed pneumothorax |
| | Decreased cardiac output | Perform the following:<br>1. Monitor vital signs frequently.<br>2. Observe for cardiac dysrhythmias.<br>3. Palpate for subcutaneous emphysema in upper chest and neck. |
| Open | Knowledge deficit<br>Impaired gas exchange | Same discharge instruction as for closed pneumothorax<br>Perform the following:<br>1. Occlude wound with nonporous covering.<br>2. Same interventions as for closed pneumothorax.<br>3. Same discharge instructions as for closed pneumothorax. |

respirations can be expected to increase with fluid overload.
   c. Monitor breath sounds every 30 minutes.
3. Monitor ventilatory status every 30 minutes.
   a. Check for signs of respiratory distress:
      (1) Dyspnea
      (2) Increase in respirations
      (3) Change in breath sounds
   b. Check ABG results.
4. Monitor for signs and symptoms of a flail chest, which frequently accompanies pulmonary contusion.
5. Support patient to stay in bed until physical status is stabilized.
   a. Stay with patient and listen to concerns and explain what is planned.
   b. Assist with ADL so patient can conserve energy and demands made on the cardiopulmonary system.

# CHRONIC AIRFLOW LIMITATION—OBSTRUCTIVE PULMONARY DISEASE

## CHRONIC OBSTRUCTIVE LUNG DISEASE

### Etiology

As indicated at the beginning of this chapter, although chronic airflow limitation has been recommended as the most appropriate terminology, COPD and OAD continue to be used interchangeably with chronic airflow limitation. Chronic airflow limitation uses pathophysiologic criteria to specify which disease entities should be included within this category (Box 37-23). Based on criteria for chronic airflow limitation, more disease entities are included within this category than has traditionally been the case under the classifications of COPD and OAD. Table 37-23 compares the diseases that fall under chronic airflow limitation to those that are traditionally identified with COPD or OAD.

The disease entities identified as the components of COPD are the major airflow limitation diseases. Because COPD is the term most often used by clinicians, it is used in this book to refer to a pathophysiologic state characterized by limitation to airflow on expiration. The major disease entities identified under the rubric of COPD include a variable combination of asthma, chronic bronchitis, and pulmonary emphysema (Table 37-24).

The processes that result in the pathophysiologic changes associated with COPD are neither static nor necessarily progressive. Thus all stages are possible, from reversible abnormalities to relentlessly progressive cardiopulmonary insufficiency.

### Epidemiology

In 1988, nearly 13 million persons in the United States reported that they had chronic bronchitis or emphysema. When persons with asthma are included in this statistic, the total number of persons affected by COPD totals 17 million. Persons with chronic bronchitis or emphysema had 169 million days of restricted activity per year, or nearly 2 months of restricted activity yearly

**BOX 37-23 Major Physiologic Components of Chronic Airflow Limitation**

Chronic mucus hypersecretion (a clinical diagnosis based on history)
Pulmonary emphysema (destruction of parenchyma)
Airway hyperreactivity (asthma, reversible airflow limitation)
Changes in small airways (including respiratory bronchiolitis)

Bates DV: *Respiratory function in disease,* ed 3, Philadelphia, 1989, Saunders.

**TABLE 37-23 Comparison of Disease Entities Included Under the Classification of Chronic Airflow Limitation and COPD**

| CHRONIC AIRFLOW LIMITATION* | COPD |
|---|---|
| Chronic bronchitis | Chronic bronchitis |
| Asthma | Asthma |
| Emphysema | Emphysema |
| Bronchiolitis | |
| Cystic fibrosis | |
| Parenchymal fibrosis or granulomatosis | |
| Pulmonary lymphangiomyomatosis | |
| Tracheal stenosis | |

*Disease entities included under chronic airflow limitation are from Bates DV: *Respiratory function in disease,* ed 3, Philadelphia, 1989, Saunders.

**TABLE 37-24 Possible Variants of COPD***

| PREDOMINANT DISEASE ENTITY | ASSOCIATED OBSTRUCTIVE DISEASE | | |
|---|---|---|---|
| | ASTHMA | CHRONIC BRONCHITIS | EMPHYSEMA |
| Asthma | Pure asthma | Asthma with bronchitis | Asthma with emphysema |
| Chronic bronchitis | Chronic bronchitis with asthma | Pure chronic bronchitis | Chronic bronchitis with emphysema |
| Emphysema | Emphysema with asthma | Emphysema with chronic bronchitis | Pure emphysema |

*In addition to these nine variants, the individual can have a combination of asthma, bronchitis, and emphysema.

for each person. For employed persons with these diseases, frequent absences from work are likely to threaten their jobs.[40]

Both the prevalence of COPD and the death rates attributed to it have reached epidemic proportions. COPD is the fifth cause of death in the United States, following heart disease, cancer, CVAs, and accidents. According to the CDC, the death rate increased 32.9% from 1979 to 1989. For this reason, there is little hope of reducing the death rate by the year 2000. The goal set for that year is to slow the rise in deaths from COPD to no more than 25 per 100,000 people. The age-adjusted baseline was 18.7 deaths per 100,000 in 1987. If this trend continues, the CDC estimates that the death rate for COPD will reach 26 to 28 deaths per 100,000 in the year 2000. Given the difference between 18.7 deaths per 100,000 and 26 deaths per 100,000, considerable change will have to occur if the year 2000 goal is to be achieved.

The increase in the death rate from COPD is believed to be related to (1) the growing tendency of physicians to list it as a primary cause of death, (2) the greater use of PFTs, and (3) more emphasis in medical literature on the importance of this syndrome. Despite these facts, it is believed that the mortality is even higher than reported because many persons who were reported to have died from pneumonia, asthma, or congestive heart failure probably had COPD. The major factor in this increase in mortality, in addition to improved reporting and the increased aging of the population, is a history of cigarette smoking.

Various causes are related to the onset of COPD. Table 37-25 identifies these causative factors on the basis of predominant obstructive disease with which they are associated.

Although asthma, chronic bronchitis, and emphysema are classified under the common category, it is clinically important to identify the predominant type of pulmonary disease that is the basis for the individual's COPD. Therefore, in the following presentation, COPD is divided into three major obstructive diseases: chronic bronchitis, emphysema, and asthma. Because the clinical management of chronic bronchitis and emphysema is similar, the care for patients with either of these diseases is presented together. (See Nursing Care Plan and Critical Pathway for person with COPD on pp. 1120-1123.)

**RESEARCH**

Cosette S, Levesque L: Caregiving tasks as predictors of mental health of wife caregivers of men with chronic obstructive pulmonary disease, *Res Nurs Health* 16:251-263, 1993.

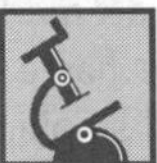

The relationships between caregiving tasks and selected mental health outcomes of 89 wives of COPD patients were examined in this cross-sectional study. All the husbands lived at home and were moderately to severely impaired by their condition. Data were collected by interview. As a group, the wives had high scores on measures of depression, obsession-compulsion, and somatization. Forty percent of the wives used psychotropic drugs. The total number of caregiving tasks performed and the number of tasks that involved supervising the husbands (e.g., preventing them from doing dangerous activities or those that could result in breathing problems) were predictors of many mental health outcomes. In addition, tasks involving provision of emotional support to the husbands were especially disturbing to the wife caregivers. Few wives received formal social support, and most thought that informal support received from family members was more helpful than that received from friends.

Appropriate interventions can minimize the progression of COPD. A comprehensive management program will benefit all patients, even those with severe disease (see Research box above). Management programs should be designed to do the following: educate patients, retard the progression of airflow limitation, minimize airflow limitation, correct secondary physiologic problems, and optimize functional capabilities.[23]

## CHRONIC BRONCHITIS

Chronic bronchitis is defined ***clinically*** by hypersecretion of mucus and recurrent or chronic productive cough for a minimum of 3 months per year for at least 2 consecutive years in patients in whom other causes have been excluded. It is characterized ***physiologically***

**TABLE 37-25 Factors in Development of COPD**

| ASTHMA | CHRONIC BRONCHITIS | EMPHYSEMA |
|---|---|---|
| Allergy | Cigarette smoking | Cigarette smoking |
| Hypersensitivity | Atmospheric contaminants | Atmospheric contaminants |
| Infection | Infection | Antienzyme and enzyme deficiencies ($\alpha$, $\alpha_1$, $\alpha_2$) |
| Environment | Chronic irritation | Advanced pulmonary fibrosis |
| Drugs | Gastroesophageal dysfunction (mainly gastric reflux) | Destruction of lung parenchyma (necrosis, ischemia) |
| Emotions | | |
| Social conditions | | |
| Exercise | | |

# NURSING CARE PLAN

## PERSON WITH CHRONIC OBSTRUCTIVE PULMONARY DISEASE (COPD)

**DATA:** Mrs. D. is a 54-year-old housewife with a past medical history of severe COPD with cor pulmonale. She has a 75-pack-year history of cigarette smoking and stopped smoking 2 years ago (husband still smokes). Patient states: "I am unable to walk back from the bathroom to the living room without 30 to 60 minutes of rest." Lung sounds are diminished throughout. Chest x-ray film indicates overinflation of the lungs. PFTs show severe obstructive ventilatory dysfunction with hyperinflation. ABGs are pH = 7.34, $Paco_2$ = 48, $Po_2$ = 69, oxygen saturation = 94%. Current medications include metaproterenol inhaler, Theo-Dur, terbutaline, hydrochlorothiazide, K-Lyte, and nitroglycerin sublingual tablets as needed for chest pain. She is seeking outpatient rehabilitation, including muscle reconditioning and education.

The nursing history identified the following:

- Mrs. D. continues to be exposed to cigarette smoke because of her husband's continued cigarette smoking. Patient stated, "He's never without a cigarette in the house."
- Mrs. D. indicated that her husband's smoking makes it hard for her not to smoke. Patient indicated that she occasionally had a cigarette.
- Mrs. D. is fearful of becoming a "bedridden invalid like my mother." Patient's mother had COPD and in her last years had a CVA, which left her totally dependent on her daughter for care until her death 5 years ago.

Collaborative nursing activities include those to (1) assess Mrs. D.'s current pulmonary function status, (2) establish individualized rehabilitation, and (3) evaluate current theophylline levels. Nursing actions include the following:

- Prepare patient for PFTs. Review her role in the testing procedure and determine what she felt during previous testing.
- Participate in rehabilitation team meetings for planning Mrs. D.'s program. Encourage Mrs. D. to actively participate in the planning process to establish realistic individualized program goals. Elicit feedback to assess Mrs. D.'s understanding of the program activities and goals.
- Assess theophylline blood levels and presence of any medication side effects.

### ■ NURSING DIAGNOSIS

Activity intolerance related to tissue hypoxia associated with impaired gas exchange/fatigue

| Expected Patient Outcome | Nursing Interventions | Rationale |
|---|---|---|
| Demonstrates increased tolerance for activity. | Provide frequent rest periods.<br>Instruct patient in energy-saving techniques.<br>Reinforce use of pursed-lip breathing.<br>Gradually increase activity. | Improve activity tolerance. |

### ■ NURSING DIAGNOSIS

Impaired gas exchange related to decrease in effective lung surface

| Expected Patient Outcome | Nursing Interventions | Rationale |
|---|---|---|
| Dyspnea is decreased. | Assess respiratory status. | Obtain baseline information. |
| | Provide prescribed low-flow oxygen. | Many persons with COPD depend on hypoxemia as stimulus to breathe. |
| | Provide breathing retraining. | Decrease work of breathing. |
| | Provide rest periods. | Improve tolerance. |

### ■ NURSING DIAGNOSIS

High risk for infection related to increased secretions/decreased motility in lungs

| Expected Patient Outcome | Nursing Interventions | Rationale |
|---|---|---|
| Infections are minimized. | Restrict persons with upper respiratory infections.<br>Teach patient measures to prevent infections.<br>Encourage patient to obtain annual influenza immunization. | Decrease exposure to infection. |

## NURSING CARE PLAN

### PERSON WITH CHRONIC OBSTRUCTIVE PULMONARY DISEASE (COPD)—cont'd

**■ NURSING DIAGNOSIS**

Self-esteem disturbance related to changes in life-style/dependence on others

| Expected Patient Outcome | Nursing Interventions | Rationale |
|---|---|---|
| Participates in necessary activities. | Give patient opportunities to express concerns about limitations. | Allow for communication. |
| | Provide rationale for necessary activities. | Maintain sense of control. |
| | Discuss with family and friends the need for patient to maintain role relationships. | |
| | Assist patient to identify personal strengths. | Increase self-esteem. |
| | Provide rationale for necessary community resources. | |

**■ NURSING DIAGNOSIS**

Knowledge deficit related to lack of exposure/lack of recall

| Expected Patient Outcome | Nursing Interventions | Rationale |
|---|---|---|
| Describes therapeutic regimen and health maintenance. | Teach patient:<br>1. Nature of COPD and need to follow prescribed therapy and activities<br>2. Home medication and treatment plans<br>3. Home exercise plan<br>4. Avoidance of respiratory irritants and infections<br>5. Signs requiring medical attention<br>6. Professional and community resources | Increase self-care abilities and self-esteem. |

by hypertrophy and hypersecretion of the bronchial mucus glands and structural alterations of the bronchi and bronchioles.

### Etiology

As indicated in Table 37-25, chronic bronchitis is caused by the inhalation of physical or chemical irritants or by viral or bacterial infections. The most common inhaled irritant is cigarette smoke, and heavy cigarette smoking is believed to be the major cause of the disease.

### Epidemiology

Occupations in which dust or other irritants are inhaled may cause bronchitis, but the evidence for this is not conclusive. However, in Great Britain it has been recognized for years that the highest incidence of bronchitis occurs in large industrial cities with high levels of air pollution.

### Pathophysiology

The two pathologic changes that typify chronic bronchitis are hypertrophy of mucus-secreting glands and chronic inflammatory changes in the small airways. First, there is glandular hypertrophy. *Mucous gland hypertrophy* and *hyperplasia* from chronic irritation cause excessive mucus production. The excessive mucus and impaired ciliary movement associated with chronic bronchitis increase susceptibility to infection. Bacteria proliferate in the mucous secretions in the lumen of the bronchi. The most common infectious agents are *Streptococcus pneumoniae* and *Haemophilus influenzae.* As bacteria multiply, they exert a neutrophilic chemotaxis, and pus cells migrate from between bronchial epithelial cells to produce a mucopurulent exudate in the lumen, or the disease may progress to ulceration and destruction of the bronchial wall. The presence of granulation tissue and peribronchial fibrosis results in stenosis and

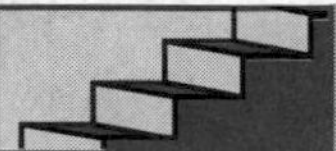

## CRITICAL PATHWAY Chronic Obstructive Pulmonary Disease Without Intubation

**DRG #: 088; expected LOS: 6**

| | Day of Admission Day 1 | Day 2 | Day 3 |
|---|---|---|---|
| **Diagnostic Tests** | CBC, UA, SMA/18,* ABGs, sputum C & S, ECG, PFTs, chest x-ray film | SMA/6,† ABGs | Chest x-ray |
| **Medications** | IV @ TKO, digitalis, antibiotic, diuretic, bronchodilator, aerosol Tx, medication for rest | IV @ TKO, digitalis, antibiotic, diuretic, bronchodilator, aerosol Tx, stool softener, medication for rest | IV to saline lock, digitalis, antibiotic, diuretic, bronchodilator, stool softener, medication for rest |
| **Treatments** | I & O q8hr, weight, $O_2$, VS q4hr, cardiac monitor, assess cardiopulmonary systems and level of consciousness (LOC) q4hr, elastic leg stockings | I & O q8hr, weight, $O_2$, VS q4hr, cardiac monitor, assess cardiopulmonary systems and LOC q4hr, elastic leg stockings | I & O q6hr, weight, $O_2$, VS q6hr, cardiac monitor, assess cardiopulmonary systems and LOC q6hr, elastic leg stockings |
| **Diet** | Full liquids, low sodium | Advance diet to soft diet, provide 6 small meals/day, high protein and calorie, low sodium | Soft diet, provide 6 small meals/day, high protein and calorie, low sodium |
| **Activity** | Bedrest, head of bed (HOB) elevated 30 degrees | Bedrest, HOB elevated 30 degrees, up to bathroom with assistance | HOB elevated 30 degrees while in bed, up in chair 4 times with help |
| **Referral/ Consultation** | Resp ther, pulmonary medicine | Home health, dietary, resp rehab | Resp rehab team |

*Serum calcium, phosphorus, triglycerides, uric acid, creatinine, BUN, total bilirubin, alkaline phosphate, aspartate aminotransferase (AST, formerly serum glutamic oxaloacetic transaminase [SGOT]), alanine aminotransferase (ALT, formerly serum glutamic oxaloacetic transaminase [SGPT]), lactic dehydrogenase (LDH), total protein, albumin, sodium, potassium, chloride, total $CO_2$, glucose.
†Serum sodium, potassium, chloride, total $CO_2$, glucose, BUN.

airway obstruction. Small airways may be completely obliterated, and others may become dilated. This chain of events further traps secretions and promotes multiplication of bacteria. There is some evidence that the pathologic changes occur initially in small airways and move to larger bronchi.

Second, persons with chronic bronchitis develop increased airway resistance as a result of bronchial wall tissue changes, mucosal edema, and excessive mucus production. Excess mucus in the airways not only obstructs airflow but also often causes bronchospasm, which further increases airway resistance.

Third, there is altered oxygen/carbon dioxide exchange. Airway obstruction resulting from all the pathophysiologic changes that increase airway resistance may impair the ability of the lungs to exchange oxygen and carbon dioxide. Obstructed airways cause V/Q mismatching at the alveolocapillary membrane by decreasing the amount of oxygenated air that reaches the alveoli. Additionally, the obstructed airways may lead to atelectasis, which further diminishes the surface area available for respiration. The result of these pathophysiologic alterations is hypercapnia, hypoxemia, and respiratory acidosis (see discussion of ABGs; see Chapter 35).

Fourth, right ventricular decompensation (cor pulmonale) may result. The hypercapnia and hypoxemia typically associated with chronic bronchitis cause pulmonary vascular vasoconstriction. The increased pulmonary vascular resistance results in pulmonary vessel hypertension that in turn increases vascular pressure in the right ventricle of the heart.

Signs and symptoms of chronic bronchitis are manifestations of the underlying physiologic abnormalities that have occurred. Table 37-26 relates normal function, primary pathophysiology, and the clinical picture observed in chronic bronchitis.

The earliest symptom of chronic bronchitis is a productive cough, especially on awakening. This symptom is often ignored by cigarette smokers, who become so accustomed to an early-morning cough that they take it for granted; some of them even refer to it as their "cigarette cough."

Persons with chronic bronchitis often unconsciously reduce their activity level to accommodate their respiratory symptoms in their daily lives. Thus they do not seek medical help until they experience a severe exacerbation of their symptoms, usually precipitated by a respiration infection.

PFTs reveal a limitation to airflow on expiration, as evidenced by a diminished forced expiratory volume. Vital capacity is also reduced, indicating diminished air movement both in and out of the lungs. Lung volumes are usually within normal limits until later in the course of the disease, when the lung volumes may be increased. There usually is no loss of diffusing capacity.

Early in the course of chronic bronchitis, the symp-

| Day 4 | Day 5 | Day of Discharge Day 6 |
|---|---|---|
| SMA/6,† ABGs | Chest x-ray, ECG | |
| IV saline lock, adjust drugs for home use, stool softener, medication for rest | IV saline lock, adjust drugs for home use, stool softener, medication for rest | Discontinue IV saline lock, adjust drugs for home use |
| I & O q8hr, weight, $O_2$, VS q8hr, discontinue cardiac monitor, assess cardiopulmonary systems and LOC q8hr, elastic leg stockings | I & O q8hr, weight, discontinue $O_2$ unless chronic use, VS q8hr, assess cardiopulmonary systems and LOC q8hr, elastic leg stockings | Weight, discontinue I & O, VS q8hr, Assess cardiopulmonary systems and LOC q8hr, elastic leg stockings |
| Soft diet, provide 6 small meals/day, high protein and calorie, low sodium | Soft diet, provide 6 small meals/day, high protein and calorie, low sodium | Soft, low sodium, provide 6 small meals/day, high protein and calorie |
| HOB elevated 30 degrees, up in hallway 4 times with help and in chair 4 times<br>Resp rehab | Up in hallway 6 times with help and chair as desired<br>Resp rehab | Up walking in hallway as desired |

toms tend to be episodic in nature. As the disease progresses in severity, the patient's symptoms are constantly present to some degree. The patient appears increasingly dyspneic, using accessory muscles to breathe. Chronic hypoxemia resulting in polycythemia causes the patient to appear to be cyanotic. Increased pulmonary vascular resistance caused by respiratory acidosis and hypoxemia increases pressure on the right side of the heart, ultimately resulting in right-sided heart failure (cor pulmonale). The person with late-stage chronic bronchitis and cor pulmonale appears stout or overweight from edema, and the skin appears dusky.

Patients with chronic bronchitis complicated by cor pulmonale often have chronic respiratory failure (gradual onset of $Pa{O_2} < 50$ mm Hg and a $Pa{CO_2} > 50$). They are also prone to develop acute respiratory failure (sudden onset of a $Pa{O_2} < 50$ and a $Pa{CO_2} > 50$) as a complication of a respiratory infection superimposed on their already diseased lung.

## Prevention

The overall focus for prevention of chronic bronchitis is to alleviate whatever irritant appears to be causing the associated symptoms in the individual. Of all the known risk factors, the most clearly implicated is smoking. The continued inhalation of tobacco smoke leads to worsening of bronchial inflammation and hypersecretion. Thus smoking cessation is an essential step for the prevention of chronic bronchitis. Additionally, such preventive measures as avoidance of repeated infections and prompt treatment of upper and lower respiratory infections are important steps to avoid disease progression. National standards for air quality and governmental actions related to improving the quality of the air we breathe should be of concern to everyone.

Progress in the prevention of chronic bronchitis has been impeded by the slow and insidious onset of the disease. Advances in PFTs have allowed identification of abnormalities in the small airways of the lungs. It is believed that peripheral airway changes occur early in the development of COPD. Research has indicated that some of the abnormalities associated with small airway changes may be reversible. Thus, if high risk populations could be identified and a feasible screening test developed, preventive measures could be insitituted before permanent lung damage and chronic disease occur.

## Medical Management

The process of medical diagnosis of chronic bronchitis may include any of the following investigative modalities.

1. Patient history
2. Physical examination
3. Diagnostic studies
   a. Chest x-ray film: typical findings with chronic bronchitis are increased bronchovascular markings.

**TABLE 37-26 Normal Function, Primary Pathophysiology, and Clinical Manifestations in Chronic Bronchitis, Emphysema, and Asthma**

| NORMAL FUNCTION/ PATHOPHYSIOLOGY | CLINICAL MANIFESTATIONS | | |
|---|---|---|---|
| | CHRONIC BRONCHITIS | EMPHYSEMA | ASTHMA |
| Bronchial mucus-secreting glands produce mucus to trap foreign particles and transport them out of lungs | Productive chronic cough, grayish white sputum; when infected sputum is yellow, inspiratory; crackles (rales) | | Inflammation, hypersecretion; eosinophils in sputum |
| **BRONCHI AND BRONCHIOLES** | | | |
| Carry oxygenated air to alveoli and carry deoxygenated air out of lungs | Inspiratory, expiratory rhonchi; dyspnea: episodic or continual; ↓ FEV, ↓ VC with small response to bronchodilators | Early onset dyspnea on exertion, which progresses to continuous dyspnea; rhonchi, crackles, accessory muscle breathing; ↓ FEV, ↓ VC with no response to bronchodilators | Episodic dyspnea, accessory muscle breathing; inspiratory/expiratory wheezing; ↓ FEV, ↓ VC with good response to bronchodilators; ↑ work of breathing, pulsus paradoxus |
| **ALVEOLOCAPILLARY MEMBRANE** | | | |
| Semipermeable membrane where oxygen diffuses from alveoli to blood and carbon dioxide diffuses from blood to alevoli | Respiratory acidosis, hypoxemia, polycythemia, tachycardia, cyanosis | Early stage: normal or mild hypoxemia, respiratory alkalosis; late stage: hypoxemia respiratory acidosis, ↓ diffusing capacity | Respiratory alkalosis with mild hypoxemia; status asthmaticus: respiratory acidosis with hypoxemia |
| **RIGHT SIDE OF HEART** | | | |
| Carries deoxygenated blood to pulmonary vasculature for oxygen/carbon dioxide exchange | Jugular vein distention, hepatomegaly, peripheral edema | Right ventricular decompensation | |
| **LUNG AND CHEST WALL COMPLIANCE** | | | |
| Relationship between lung and chest wall ability to expand and contract curing inhalation and exhalation | | ↑ Anteroposterior diameter, ↓ lateral expansion, ↓ diaphragmatic excursion, ↓ breath, heart, and voice sounds, ↑ RV, ↑ FRC, ↑ TLC, hyperresonance, complaint of episgastric fullness | ↓ Fremitus, ↓ lateral expansion, hyperresonance, ↓ breath sounds, ↓ diaphragmatic excursion |

FEV, Forced expiratory volume; VC, vital capacity; RV, residual volume; FRC, functional reserve capacity; TLC, total lung capacity.

b. Sputum studies for culture and sensitivity: neutrophils and bronchial epithelial cells usually present in chronic bronchitis.
c. ABG studies: see discussion in Chapter 35.
d. Hematology studies: complete blood count.
e. PFTs: see discussion in Chapter 35.

Effective health care management programs for persons who have chronic bronchitis or any of the variant combinations of pulmonary diseases that make up COPD require a multidisciplinary approach. The multidisciplinary approach to the management of COPD is included in the discussion of implementation of care for patients with COPD later in this chapter.

Medical management of chronic bronchitis is included in Table 37-27, which summarizes a typical multidisciplinary program for a person with COPD.

## Medication

Two categories of bronchodilators, sympathomimetic (adrenergic) agents and xanthine compounds, are used to improve efficiency of breathing patterns. These bronchodilators act at different sites and appear to work synergistically when used together. Table 37-28 lists the frequently used sympathomimetics and their doses. Adrenergic agents that work at beta-2 ($\beta_2$-) sites located in smooth muscles of the airways have fewer cardiac side effects than do $\beta_1$-agents with receptor sites in the myocardium. For this reason, albuterol, bitolterol, pirbuterol, metaproterenol, and terbutaline may be prescribed for COPD patients who have hypertension or who have excessive palpitations or tachycardia from $\beta_1$-agents. All the drugs in Table 37-28 have $\beta_2$-agonist activity with little $\beta_1$-agonist activity.

**TABLE 37-27 Etiology, Signs and Symptoms, and Medical Therapy for Chronic Bronchitis and Pulmonary Emphysema**

| BRONCHITIS | PULMONARY EMPHYSEMA |
|---|---|
| **ETIOLOGY** | |
| Inhalation of physical or chemical irritants or viral or bacterial infections<br>Most common inhaled irritant—cigarette smoke | Not known; believed that some change in the enzyme-inhibitor balance occurs, allowing proteolytic enzymes to attack lung tissue<br>Not known why some smokers develop bronchitis and others develop emphysema; α-antitrypsin deficiency in some persons who develop severe, disabling emphysema early in life; familial tendency for this type of emphysema |
| **SIGNS AND SYMPTOMS** | |
| **Early Symptoms** | |
| Productive cough on awakening; often ignored by cigarette smokers, who refer to it as their "cigarette cough" | Dyspnea on exertion, may be in acute respiratory distress<br>Using accessory muscles to breathe; ruddy color<br>Thin with a "barrel chest"<br>Usually able to maintain resting $Po_2$<br>Cyanosis uncommon |
| **Later Symptoms** | |
| Significant physical incapacity; breathlessness even when walking on a flat surface, noticeable shortness of breath and use of accessory muscles to breathe; cyanosis common; ankle edema, bloated appearance, distended neck veins | |
| **Late in Disease** | |
| Frequent complications: cor pulmonale (right ventricular hypertrophy), right-sided heart failure, and respiratory failure | ↑ $Pco_2$<br>Cor pulmonale and respiratory failure possible complications |
| **PULMONARY FUNCTION TEST FINDINGS** | |
| ↓ Expiratory flow rates<br>↓ Vital capacity (VC)<br>↑ Residual volume (RV)<br>Total lung capacity (TLC) usually within normal limits | ↓ Expiratory flows rates, especially forced expiratory volume, and maximal midexpiratory flow<br>↑ TLC<br>↑ RV<br>VC normal or slightly reduced until late stages of disease, $FEV_1$/VC ratio changed |
| **ARTERIAL BLOOD GAS FINDINGS** | |
| Low resting $Po_2$<br>Elevated $Pco_2$ (if obstruction severe)<br>During exercise $Pco_2$ ↑ and $Po_2$ may also ↑ | $Po_2$ normal or slightly reduced at *rest* but falls during exercise<br>Normal $Pco_2$<br>Late in disease ↑ $Pco_2$ |

**MEDICAL THERAPY**

Medical therapy for chronic bronchitis and pulmonary emphysema is similar and depends on symptoms, PFT results, and ABG findings. Therapy may include all or some of the modalities outlined here.

**SUPPORTIVE MEASURES**

Education of patient and family about the following:
- Avoidance of cigarette smoke
- Avoidance of other inhaled irritants
- Avoidance of persons with upper respiratory infections
- Control of environmental temperature and humidity
- Proper nutrition
- Adequate hydration

**SPECIFIC THERAPY**

Medications

Bronchodilators (see Table 37-28)

$\alpha_1$-Antitrypsin replacement for those with ↓ levels

Antimicrobials
- Ampicillin or amoxicillin usually prescribed to treat respiratory tract infections

Corticosteroids
- May be prescribed to alleviate acute symptoms; prednisone most often used

Digitalis
- May be prescribed to treat left ventricular failure if present

*Continued*

**TABLE 37-27 Etiology, Signs and Symptoms, and Medical Therapy for Chronic Bronchitis and Pulmonary Emphysema—cont'd**

| BRONCHITIS | PULMONARY EMPHYSEMA |
|---|---|

**RESPIRATORY THERAPY**

**Aerosol Therapy**

Used to deliver bronchodilators through metered cartridge devices or hand-bulb nebulizers

**Oxygen Therapy**

Required for patients who are unable to maintain a $Pa_{O_2}$ of 50 mm Hg or more at rest or who cannot carry out ADL without becoming short of breath; 1 to 2 L of $O_2$ given by nasal prongs

**PHYSICAL CONDITIONING**

**Relaxation Exercises**

Progressive relaxation exercises encouraged; best practiced before meals or 2 hours or more after eating because digestion seems to interfere with ability to relax

**MEDITATION**

Meditation becoming more widely used to assist patients to relax

**Breathing Retraining**

Pursed-lip breathing
Leaning forward position for exhalation
Abdominal breathing
Inhalation-exhalation exercises
Exhalation with exertion

**Rehabilitation**

Muscle reconditioning programs specific for patient

**TABLE 37-28 Sympathomimetic Drugs and Their Dosages for Metered-Dose Inhalers and Nebulized Solutions**

| DRUG | DOSE | mg/PUFF | NEBULIZATION |
|---|---|---|---|
| Albuterol (Proventil) | 2-3 puffs q 4-6 hr | 0.09 | 0.3-0.5 ml 0.5% solution in 3 ml saline q 4-6 hr |
| Bitolterol (Tornalate) | 2-3 puffs q 6-8 hr | 0.37 | |
| Metaproterenol (Alupent, Metaprel) | 2-3 puffs q 4-6 hr | 0.65 | 0.3 ml 5% solution in 2.5 ml saline q 4-6 hr |
| Pirbuterol (Maxair) | 2-3 puffs q 4-6 hr | 0.20 | |
| Terbutaline (Brethaire) | 2-3 puffs q 4-6 hr | 0.20 | |

Modified from Alex CG, Tobin MJ: Chronic obstructive pulmonary disease. In Rakel RE, editor: *Conn's current therapy,* Philadelphia, 1993, Saunders.

**Theophylline.** The role of theophylline (a methylxanthine) in the treatment of COPD is controversial.[23] Theophylline preparations may have little bronchodilator effect beyond that of inhaled agents. However, administering long-acting theophylline, 300 to 900 mg/day in the evening, has been shown to reduce overnight decline in forced expiratory volume and morning respiratory symptoms. Theophylline may also increase collateral ventilation, respiratory muscle function, mucociliary clearance, and central respiratory drive and may reduce airway inflammation[23] (see Guidelines box).

**Corticosteroids.** The use of corticosteroids in the treatment of COPD is also controversial.[23] Some patients benefit from both short-term and long-term administration of steroids, but it is not possible to predict which patients will benefit. A closely monitored trial of steroids for patients who have continuing symptoms or severe airflow limitation is warranted despite maximal therapy with other agents. Long-term treatment with oral corticosteroids should be prescribed only for patients who have documented improvement in airflow or exercise performance. The lowest possible dose is used. There is no evidence that administering steroids on alternate days or giving them by inhalation is beneficial to patients with COPD.[23]

Steroid preparations used to treat COPD include methylprednisolone (Solu-Medrol), 0.5 mg/kg for 3 days (burst therapy). In *burst therapy,* large doses of steroids are given for a short time. This avoids the long-term side effects of the steroids.[11] Probably the most frequently ordered corticosteroid is prednisone. A typically or-

### Guidelines for Care of the Person Receiving Methylxanthine Medications

1. Monitor theophylline plasma level results. Therapeutic levels = 10 to 20 μg/ml, although individual response to theophylline levels varies. Notify physician if these levels are exceeded before administering the next dose of medication.
2. Certain types of theophylline formulations must be specifically taken with or without food. Food present in the stomach can either slow or speed up absorption of certain types of theophylline.
3. Cigarette or marijuana smoking significantly increases plasma clearance of theophylline. Patients who quit smoking may experience onset of side effects of higher levels of these medications. Counsel patients to notify their physician if they quit smoking.
4. Various medications interact with theophylline, altering plasma absorption rates. Counsel patients to inform their physician when they begin any new medication.
5. Liver cirrhosis, hepatitis, cardiac decompensation, cor pulmonale, and viral respiratory infections decrease plasma clearance of theophylline.

dered dose is 40 mg/day for 14 days and then tapered off over several days.

Persons should have a tuberculin test before initiation of long-term steroid therapy. Those with a tuberculin reaction of 10 mm or more are candidates for isoniazid therapy (see Table 37-13).

**Anticholinergic agents.** Recently, ipratropium (Atrovent) was reported in the literature to produce greater bronchodilation than conventional doses of β-agonists, although maximal doses of β-agonists probably produce the same degree of bronchodilation.[23] The recommended dose of ipratropium, a synthetic quaternary ammonium, when administered as an aerosol inhalant, is two puffs every 4 to 6 hours.[1] It is well tolerated. Some patients will have a cough and dry mouth, which are side effects of anticholinergic agents.

**Antibiotics.** During acute exacerbations of COPD, antibiotics may be ordered. Although viruses are the usual organisms contributing to a flare-up of COPD, colonizing organisms such as *S. pneumoniae, H. influenzae,* and *Moraxella catarrhalis* also play a pathologic role.[1] The airways of the patient with chronic bronchitis provide a rich culture medium for these organisms.

Recommended antibiotics are ampicillin, 500 mg every 6 hours; amoxicillin, 500 mg every 8 hours; tetracycline, 500 mg every 6 hours; trimethoprim-sulfamethoxazole, 160 to 1800 mg every 12 hours; or ciprofloxacin, 500 mg every 6 hours for 7 to 10 days.[1]

If the person has frequent flare-ups, some experts recommend that a different antibiotic than the one usually prescribed be used. Prophylactic administration of antibiotics in persons with COPD is not recommended.[1]

### Guidelines for Teaching the Person To Use an Inhaler With a Spacer

1. Exhale fully.
2. Position nebulizer in mouth *without* sealing lips around it.
3. Take a deep breath while releasing a puff of medication into spacer.
4. Hold breath for 3 to 4 seconds at full inspiration.
5. Exhale slowly through pursed lips.
6. Usually one or two puffs is prescribed.
7. Several breaths may be necessary to receive the entire dose from the spacer.
8. The mouth should be rinsed after completing treatment.
9. The inhaler and spacer are washed with warm soapy water, rinsed, and dried thoroughly after each use.

**Mucolytics and expectorants.** Patients with chronic bronchitis usually have thick, tenacious sputum. Recent literature suggests that the overall efficacy of mucolytics and expectorants remains unproven.[1] For this reason, they are not ordered as often as they once were. Patients who have been using these agents for years and found them to be helpful may want to continue to use them while hospitalized. The patient or the nurse may convey this information to the physician.

**Alpha$_1$-antitrypsin replacement therapy.** In patients with API deficiency, pulmonary function declines more rapidly than in patients with COPD who have normal levels of API. A normal API level ranges from 180 to 280 mg/dl. Although it is expensive, 60 mg/kg of active API may be given intravenously as a weekly dose. Other experts suggest that taking it every 2 to 4 weeks may be equally effective.[23] The long-term effects of replacement therapy in the API-deficient population with emphysema is unknown.[1] However, a national registry has been formed to monitor the effectiveness of API therapy.[23]

#### Treatment

**Aerosol therapy.** Aerosol therapy is one of the most effective ways to deliver bronchodilators, corticosteroids, and cromolyn. The most frequently used ways to deliver an aerosol include a freon-propelled metered-dose cartridge inhaler (MDI), hand-held nebulizer, or intermittent positive-pressure breathing (IPPB) machine. IPPB is used less frequently and is reserved for persons who cannot inhale repetitively enough to near total lung capacity or who are unable to use a hand-held nebulizer or MDI because of lack of coordination or fatigue. Directions for teaching patients to use an inhaler with a spacer are given in the Guidelines box above, and directions for teaching patients to use a hand-held nebulizer are found in the Guidelines box on p. 1128. When bronchodilators are administered, the solution should be diluted with either water or saline. Some ex-

**Guidelines for Teaching the Person To Use a Hand-Held Nebulizer**

1. Exhale fully.
2. Position nebulizer in mouth *without* sealing lips around it.
3. Take a deep breath through mouth while squeezing the bulb of the nebulizer *once*.
4. Hold breath for 3 to 4 seconds at full inspiration.
5. Exhale slowly through pursed lips.
6. Usually one inhalation is sufficient. Several inhalations of a bronchodilator may cause medication overdosage and result in side effects (e.g., tachycardia, palpitation, nervousness).

perts recommend that the diluent be water because saline solutions already contain a solute (NaCl) in water. All bronchodilator solutions are high-molecular-weight concentrated solutions and have a high solute content. When they are diluted with water, there is a maximal decrease in solute concentration; thus smaller particle size and deeper deposition of the aerosol in the smaller airways result.

Aerosol devices are excellent sites for bacterial growth, and patients using such equipment at home should be advised on how to clean them appropriately.

When a spacer (Figure 37-18), a molded plastic chamber, is fitted on an inhaler, medication can be delivered more safely and effectively for the following reasons: (1) large droplets of the aerosol, which would tend to settle in the mouth and on the vocal cords, land on the walls of the spacer instead; (2) the finer droplets in the aerosol disperse more fully within the spacer and can be carried farther into the airways; (3) it is not necessary to coordinate breathing as carefully as it is with the standard inhaler, and thus patients are medicated more effectively; and (4) spacers can reduce the number and volume of puffs required, thereby reducing the cost of medication because each dose is used more efficiently.

After the medication is in the spacer, the patient can take several breaths, inhaling each time from the spacer, to receive the entire dose. Inhalers with spacers can be used to deliver steroids, $\beta_2$-agents, and cromolyn.

A newer device, a breath-activated MDI, is becoming available. As its name indicates, inhaling triggers the inhaler to release a premeasured dose of bronchodilator. This device offers another way to ensure that patients receive the prescribed bronchodilator in the correct dosage.

**Diet**

See discussion on p. 1139.

**Activity**

Patients should be up and about as much as possible. Some will have to use portable oxygen while walking or doing other tasks (see p. 1134 for further information).

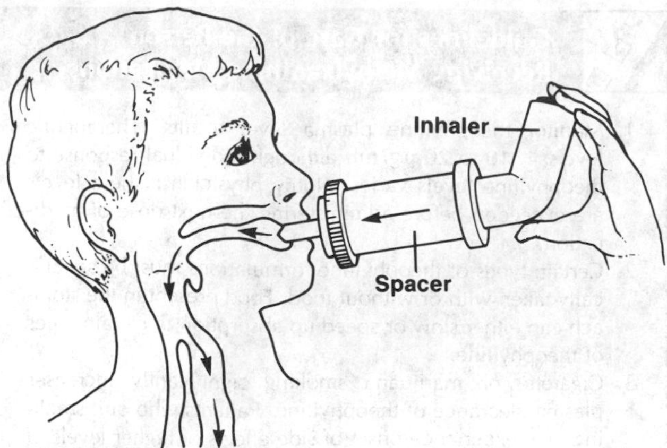


**FIGURE 37-18** Patient using inhaler with spacer attached to allow for better dispersal of medication.

**Referral/Consultation**

In some settings the nurse assumes responsibility for making referrals to other services. Common referrals for the patient with chronic bronchitis include respiratory therapy, physical therapy, dietary therapy, and social work.

## NURSING MANAGEMENT

### ♦ ASSESSMENT

#### Subjective Data

Data to be collected to assess the patient with chronic bronchitis include the following:

1. History of character of onset and duration of:
   a. Cough
   b. Sputum production (amount, color, consistency)
   c. Dyspnea
   d. Pain in right upper quadrant (hepatomegaly)
2. Smoking history
3. Disease history
   a. Influenza
   b. Pneumonia
   c. Repeated respiratory tract infections
   d. Chronic sinusitis
4. Past or present exposure to environmental irritants at home or at work
5. Self-care used to treat symptoms
6. Medications taken and their effectiveness in relieving symptoms

#### Objective Data

Data to be collected to assess the patient with chronic bronchitis include the following:

1. Assess general appearance.
   a. Patient may appear overweight or bloated, and skin is dusky.
   b. Check for dependent edema and jugular vein distention.

   c. Abdominal assessment may indicate hepatomegaly.
2. Assess vital signs.
   a. Elevated temperature
   b. Tachycardia
   c. Tachypnea
3. Pulmonary examination
   a. Inspection
      (1) Accessory muscle breathing
      (2) Forward leaning posture
      (3) Central cyanosis
      (4) Clubbing of fingers
      (5) Altered sensorium (restlessness or lethargy)
   b. Palpation: increased tactile fremitus
   c. Percussion: normal
   d. Auscultation
      (1) Inspiratory crackles (rales)
      (2) Inspiratory and expiratory rhonchi
4. Assess laboratory findings.
   a. ABGs
      (1) Respiratory acidosis
      (2) Hypoxemia
   b. Hematology
      (1) Elevated hemoglobin and hematocrit
      (2) Elevated WBC
   c. PFTs
      (1) Decreased $FEV_1$
      (2) Normal diffusing capacity
      (3) Normal lung volumes (in end-stage chronic bronchitis, lung volumes may appear similar to those found with emphysema)

## ♦ NURSING DIAGNOSES

Nursing diagnoses are determined from assessment of patient data. Nursing diagnoses for the person with chronic bronchitis may include but are not limited to the following:

| Diagnostic Title | Possible Etiologic Factors |
|---|---|
| Gas exchange, impaired | Low V/Q ratio |
| Airway clearance, ineffective | Hypersecretion, tracheobronchial infection, decreased energy/fatigue |
| Breathing pattern, ineffective | Decreased energy/fatigue, airway changes |
| Activity intolerance | Imbalance between oxygen demand and requirement |
| Fluid volume excess | Pulmonary hypertension with resultant increased cardiac workload |
| Nutrition, altered: less than body requirements | Dyspnea, anorexia, sputum production, medication side effects, fatigue |
| Infection, high risk for | Decreased lung defenses |
| Fear | Long-term illness and disability, change in role functioning |
| Knowledge deficit: condition and its treatment | Lack of exposure/recall, cognitive limitation, unfamiliarity with information source |

## ♦ EXPECTED PATIENT OUTCOMES

Expected outcomes for patients with COPD are similar, regardless of the underlying obstructive airway disease. Thus outcomes for patients with chronic bronchitis are included later in this chapter under the outcomes for patients with COPD (see p. 1132).

## EMPHYSEMA

Emphysema is defined *pathologically* by destructive changes in alveolar walls and enlargement of air spaces distal to the terminal nonrespiratory bronchioles. It is characterized *physiologically* by increased lung compliance, decreased diffusing capacity, and increased airway resistance.

### Etiology

The cause of emphysema is not known; however, evidence suggests that proteases released by polymorphonuclear leukocytes or alveolar macrophages are involved in the destruction of the connective tissue of the lungs. Connective tissue in the lungs is primarily composed of elastin, collagen, and proteoglycan, which can be damaged and destroyed by enzymes such as proteases and elastase. It has been demonstrated that protease/antiprotease imbalances and cigarette smoke are involved. Cigarette smoke directly blocks the inhibitory capacity of API and promotes an excess of neutrophils through the attractant effects of alveolar macrophages. The neutrophils release elastases, which are capable of destroying the elastin structure of the lung. Cigarette smoking is also associated with goblet cell metaplasia and bronchiolitis, which contribute to airway obstruction.[1]

It has been known since 1965 that some persons have a deficiency of $\alpha_1$-antitrypsin (AAT) and that these persons develop severe, disabling emphysema early in life, usually of the bullous type.

### Epidemiology

Although it is not known when emphysema actually begins, there appear to be many years between the initial pathophysiologic changes and the onset of overt symptoms. Symptoms associated with emphysema usually appear in the fourth decade, and disability from disease usually occurs in the fifth or sixth decade of life. The typical individual with emphysema is a male of about 55 years of age with a history of tobacco smoking.

It is not known, however, why some smokers develop bronchitis and others develop emphysema. Differences in susceptibility and the predominant type of disease are believed to be influenced by hereditary or environmental factors or those related to the patient's history. It is established, however, that there is familial tendency to AAT deficiency and that relatives of persons with this type of emphysema should be screened and provided with counseling, as discussed later.

It is estimated that 1% of persons with COPD have a AAT deficiency. The mean age for onset of dyspnea related to COPD is 40 to 45 years in persons with AAT deficiency. Their mean life expectancy is 50 to 65 years of age with smokers dying about 10 years earlier than nonsmokers.

Patients with AAT deficiency can be treated with human $\alpha_1$-proteinase inhibitor (Prolastin), which has been approved by the U.S. Food and Drug Administration (FDA). The cost of Prolastin, which is given intravenously once a week, is estimated to be about $30,000 a year. Evidence indicates that treating patients with AAT deficiency would be cost-effective because it would decrease complications in those with AAT deficiency and increase their life span. Because AAT deficiency cannot be prevented, it is important that persons who have it not smoke.

## Pathophysiology

The type of emphysema can be determined only by descriptive morphology. There are two principal types of emphysema morphologically: *centrilobular* emphysema (CLE) and *panlobular* emphysema (PLE). In CLE, there is distention and damage of the respiratory bronchioles selectively. Openings develop in the walls of the bronchioles; they become enlarged and confluent and tend to form a single space as the walls enlarge. The disease tends to be unevenly distributed throughout the lung but usually is more severe in the upper portions.

In PLE, there is a more uniform enlargement and destruction of the alveoli in the pulmonary acinus. PLE is usually more diffuse and is more severe in the lower lung. It is found in elderly persons who have no evidence of chronic bronchitis or impairment of lung function. It occurs just as often in women as in men, but PLE is less common than CLE. PLE is a characteristic finding in persons with homozygous AAT deficiency.[3]

The clinical diagnosis of emphysema is inferred from the presence of signs and symptoms that are manifestations of known pathophysiologic changes associated with the disease. Physiologic abnormalities characteristic of emphysema include the following alterations:

1. *Increased lung compliance.* Loss of elastic recoil resulting from destruction of elastin in lung parenchyma causes the lungs to become permanently overdistended. Thus, compared with normal lungs, emphysematous lungs have a larger increase in volume relative to the pressure change that occurs during inhalation.
2. *Increased airway resistance.* Destruction of elastic lung tissue causes the small airway to either collapse or narrow, particularly during expiration. Thus air becomes trapped in the distal air spaces, contributing to the lungs' overdistended state. The overdistended lungs press down against the diaphragm, diminishing its ventilatory effectiveness. Accessory muscle breathing, which is a compensatory attempt to force the trapped air out of the lungs, causes an increase in intrapleural pressure, which further accentuates airway collapse.
3. *Altered oxygen/carbon dioxide exchange.* Destruction of alveolar and respiratory bronchiole walls decreases alveolocapillary membrane surface area, which in turn may diminish gaseous diffusion. Persons with emphysema are able to compensate for these destructive changes by increasing their respiratory rate. Thus ABGs remain relatively normal, although mild hypoxemia may be present. Late in the course of the disease, extensive surface area loss coupled with V/Q inequalities usually cause respiratory acidosis and hypoxemia.

Normal function, pathophysiology, and clinical manifestations of emphysema are presented in Table 37-26.

Typically, the first symptoms heralding the onset of emphysema is dyspnea on exertion (DOE), which progresses to continual dyspnea. Sputum production tends to be scant or absent. Persons with emphysema usually appear thin and manifest a "barrel chest" with an increased anteroposterior (AP) diameter from hyperinflation. The characteristic breathing pattern of the emphysematous individual includes accessory muscle breathing, an increased respiratory rate, and a prolonged expiratory phase resulting from airway narrowing or collapse on expiration. These individuals will spontaneously exhibit pursed-lip breathing (Figure 37-19), which facilitates effective air exhalation. (Pursed-lip breathing elevates end-expiratory pressures, which inhibits airway collapse during expiration.)

Pulmonary function studies demonstrate an increased residual volume (RV), functional residual capacity (FRC), and total lung capacity (TLC). Diffusing capacity is significantly reduced because of lung tissue destruction. Diminished respiratory air flow is demonstrated by a decreased forced expiratory volume (FEV) and maximal midexpiratory flow rate (MMFR). The vital capacity (VC) may be normal or only slightly reduced until late in the disease progression; thus the $FEV_1/VC$ ratio is decreased. The degree of respiratory impairment may be estimated on the basis of the ratio of FEV to forced vital capacity (FVC) (Box 37-24). A significant finding that differentiates emphysema from the other obstructive airway pathologies is the failure to demonstrate improvement in PFT results in response to the administration of bronchodilators.

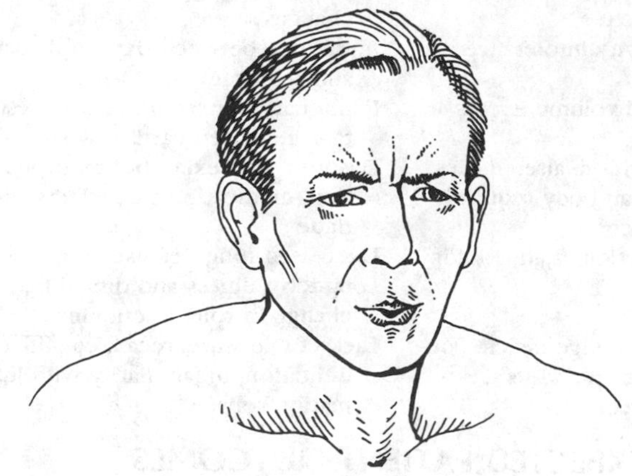

**FIGURE 37-19** Pursed-lip breathing.

**BOX 37-24 Estimate of Pulmonary Dysfunction Based on FEV/VC Ratio**

Normal lung function: greater than 80% predicted values
Mild impairment: 65% to 85% of predicted values
Moderate impairment: 50% to 64% of predicted values
Severe impairment: 49% or less of predicted values

ABGs are often near normal because of the individual's ability to compensate through increased respiratory rate and tidal volume. Indeed, many people with emphysema overcompensate and develop a mild respiratory alkalosis from hyperventilation. Because resting hypoxemia is absent and ventilation is high, these individuals maintain a normal $PaCO_2$ despite abnormal gas exchange. A person exhibiting these symptoms of pure emphysema is classified as having type A COPD. Late in the course of the disease, the $PaCO_2$ is elevated, which promotes the development of cor pulmonale and respiratory failure.

The terms "blue bloater" and "pink puffer" represent the two extremes seen in persons with chronic airway obstruction. Recently, it has been suggested that the underlying disease alone does not determine whether the person is "blue" or "pink," but rather the interaction between the lung disease and the person's drive to breathe. For example, the pink puffer may just fight harder to maintain a normal $PaCO_2$, whereas the blue bloater settles for less work and allows the $PaCO_2$ to rise.

## Primary Prevention

The cornerstone of prevention of emphysema is education. Public education must focus on the pulmonary health risks associated with inhaled irritants, regardless of their source. Increased public awareness of the vital role clean air plays in pulmonary health is essential for the success of any legislative actions promoting air quality standards. Individuals must also be educated to understand the importance of personal responsibility to decrease their own health risk through smoking cessation.

Persons with a family history of emphysema should be screened for AAT deficiency. It is imperative that persons with this enzyme deficiency take active measures to prevent additive lung damage from smoking, air pollution, and infection. Persons identified as being at high risk for emphysema may require vocational counseling if their current work environment is known to have inhaled irritants. These individuals also should be counseled to receive the influenza vaccine yearly and the pneumococcal vaccine every 3 to 5 years.

## Medical Management

The process of medical diagnosis of emphysema may include any of the following investigative modalities:

1. Patient history
2. Diagnostic studies
   a. Chest x-ray film: positive finding indicates increased radiolucency of lungs with diaphragm in a low flat position.
   b. ABG studies
   c. PFTs
   d. Hematology
      (1) AAT assay
      (2) CBC; usually normal
   e. Sputum for culture and sensitivity

Table 37-27 summarizes the components of medical therapy used in the treatment of both chronic bronchitis and emphysema.

### Medication

See p. 1124.

### Treatment

See p. 1127.

### Diet

See p. 1139.

### Activity

Patients should be up and about as much as possible. They will often have to use portable oxygen when walking and doing other activities.

### Referral/Consultation

Critical pathways (also referred to as "collaborative care paths" or "care maps") have been developed in some inpatient and outpatient settings to guide both medical and nursing management. These critical pathways are collaboratively developed along time lines and include the information described previously for specific hours, days, or visits. Pertinent information about discharge planning and patient teaching to be implemented at specified times also is included. Because the nurse has a major role in these two aspects of care, these are discussed under Nursing Management. Common referrals for the person with emphysema include respiratory therapy, physical therapy, dietary therapy, and social work.

# NURSING MANAGEMENT

## ♦ ASSESSMENT

### Subjective Data

Data to be collected to assess the patient with emphysema include the following:

1. History of and onset of the following:
   a. Dyspnea: important to investigate if patient correlates the occurrence of dyspnea with any specific illness or other life event; establish how the patient's dyspnea affects ADL.

b. Cough: usually mild or may be absent
c. Sputum production: usually scant white sputum
2. Smoking history
3. Family history of emphysema
4. Past or present exposure to environmental irritants at home or at work
5. Self-care modalities
6. Medications or other prescribed therapies and their effectiveness in relieving symptoms

## Objective Data

Data to be collected to assess the patient with emphysema include the following:

1. Assess general appearance: patient usually appears thin with a large chest. (NOTE: this is a normal variant in the elderly; thus it does not always signify pulmonary disease.)
2. Assess vital signs for:
   a. Tachycardia
   b. Tachypnea
3. Pulmonary examination
   a. Inspection
      (1) Accessory muscle breathing
      (2) Forward-leaning posture
      (3) Pursed-lip breathing
      (4) Prolonged expiration
      (5) Barrel chest, increased AP diameter
   b. Palpation
      (1) Decreased lateral expansion
      (2) Decreased fremitus
   c. Percussion
      (1) Hyperresonance
      (2) Low diaphragm
      (3) Decreased diaphragmatic excursion
   d. Auscultation
      (1) Decreased breath and heart sounds
      (2) Late inspiratory crackles
      (3) Rhonchi (NOTE: adventitious sounds are often not present with emphysema.)
4. Assess laboratory findings.
   a. ABGs
      (1) Early-stage emphysema–respiratory alkalosis with mild hypoxemia
      (2) Late-stage emphysema–respiratory acidosis with hypoxemia
   b. Hematology: positive AAT assay
   c. Pulmonary function
      (1) Decreased $FEV_1$, VC, and diffusing capacity
      (2) Increased TLC, FRC, and RV

## ♦ NURSING DIAGNOSES

Nursing diagnoses for patients with COPD are similar regardless of the underlying obstructive airway disease.

Nursing diagnoses are determined from analysis of patient data. Nursing diagnoses for the person with COPD may include but are not limited to the following:

| Diagnostic Title | Possible Etiologic Factors |
|---|---|
| Gas exchange, impaired | Low V/Q ratio |
| Breathing pattern, ineffective | Decreased energy/fatigue, airway changes |
| Airway clearance, ineffective | Hypersecretion, tracheobronchial infection, decreased energy/fatigue |
| Nutrition, altered: less than body requirements | Dyspnea, anorexia, sputum production, medication side effects, fatigue |
| Infection, high risk for | Decreased lung defenses |
| Fluid volume excess* | Pulmonary hypertension with resultant increased cardiac workload |
| Activity intolerance, high risk for | Imbalance between oxygen demand and requirement |
| Sleep pattern disturbance | Dyspnea |
| Fear | Long-term illness and disability, change in role functioning |
| Knowledge deficit: condition and its treatment | Lack of exposure/recall, cognitive limitation, unfamiliarity with information source |

*More common with bronchitis.

## ♦ EXPECTED PATIENT OUTCOMES

The following expected patient outcomes and intervention sections apply to patients with chronic bronchitis, emphysema, or any combination of these two obstructive airway diseases.

1. Demonstrates improved ventilation and oxygenation.
   a. Arterial blood pH and $P_{CO_2}$ returns or stays within acceptable baseline limits.
   b. $Pa_{CO_2}$ is at optimal level for individual.
   c. Explains how and when to use oxygen therapy.
2. Demonstrates an effective breathing pattern.
   a. Inspiratory to expiratory ratio is 5:10 seconds.
   b. Uses pursed-lip breathing (see Figure 37-19).
   c. Appropriately uses leaning-forward postures.
   d. Uses diaphragmatic breathing (abdominal muscle breathing).
   e. Exhales with activity.
   f. Respiratory rate is within near-normal limits, with moderate tidal volume.
3. Demonstrates adequate airway clearance.
   a. Uses effective methods of coughing.
   b. Appropriately uses nebulizers, humidifiers, mistometers, IPPB machine, and medications.
4. Explains dietary changes required after discharge.
   a. Maintains optimal weight for height, age, and gender.
   b. Explains food and fluid requirements and daily plan for achieving them.
   c. Lists specific foods to be avoided.
   d. Explains plan for frequent, small feedings that are soft and that do not require much chewing and the need for increased time required for eating if indicated.

5. Remains infection free.
   a. Temperature remains normal.
   b. Sputum does not change in color, amount, or consistency.
   c. If the above occur, health care provider should be informed.
6. Achieves a normal fluid balance.
   a. Daily weight remains stable.
   b. Electrolyte levels remain within expected levels.
   c. Takes diuretics and digitalis, if prescribed, as ordered.
   d. If signs of edema (weight gain, increase in dyspnea) occur, health care provider is notified.
7. Maintains or works toward an optimal activity level.
   a. Paces activities.
   b. Plans for simplification of activities.
   c. Participates in planned muscle-conditioning program.
8. Demonstrates activities to control stress response to symptoms.
   a. Uses muscle relaxation.
   b. Uses meditation.
   c. Participates in support group.
9. Uses effective measures to promote sleep
   a. Determines best position in bed (number of pillows) to minimize dyspnea.
   b. Practices methods that promote sleep (relaxation exercises, meditation, guided imagery, soft music).
10. Lists common signs and symptoms that require reporting to the health care provider:
    a. Change in sputum color, amount, and consistency
    b. Increased coughing
    c. Change in behavior (argumentative, combative)
    d. Increased fatigue
    e. Increased dyspnea
    f. Weight gain or loss
    g. Peripheral edema
    h. Elevated temperatures
11. Demonstrates how to carry out the specific exercise program to be followed at home, including:
    a. Specific exercises to be completed
    b. Frequency of each exercise
    c. Criteria for monitoring physical response to exercises, such as heart rate increase or perceived fatigue
12. Demonstrates comprehension of self-care activities.
    a. Explains health maintenance or therapeutic follow-up program.
    b. Describes any home medication or treatment program.
    c. Explains exercise program to be followed at home.
    d. Describes how to obtain professional and community resources necessary to structure a satisfactory environment at home.
    e. States plans for ongoing follow-up care.
13. Explains the following aspects of home medication or treatment regimens:
    a. Name, dose, action, and side effects of each medication to be used at home
    b. How and when to use medications ordered on an as-needed basis (e.g., bronchodilators, antibiotics, steroids, antacids)
    c. Techniques necessary for follow-up care (e.g., segmental postural drainage, clapping and vibrating, inhalation therapy treatments)
    d. How to obtain and maintain any needed equipment or supplies (e.g., oxygen, nebulizers, humidifiers, mistometers, IPPB machine, syringes, medications)
14. Lists names and telephone numbers of appropriate community support services such as the Visiting Nurse Association and a home medical equipment supplier.

## ♦ INTERVENTIONS

COPD and all of its actual or potential impact on the individual's life are most effectively managed by a multidisciplinary team. Pulmonary health care teams consisting of physicians, nurses, respiratory therapists, occupational therapists, physical therapists, dietitians, social workers, and psychologists or psychiatrists provide a comprehensive approach to assist patients to attain or maintain their optimal level of function within the constraints of their pulmonary disability.

Although it is difficult to measure the physiologic effects of these programs, hospitalization of patients who have participated in them is less frequent, and most people state that they feel better.

The complex multidisciplinary rehabilitation team is the ideal, but the nurse functioning in a small community hospital or community health agency can provide effective rehabilitation activities for the person with COPD.

Nursing interventions for persons with chronic bronchitis and pulmonary emphysema are the same, and discussion of specific medications and aerosol therapy are discussed under chronic bronchitis (see p. 1124). Other medications less often used are discussed next.

### Administering Medications

#### Digitalis and diuretics

Digitalis may be prescribed for patients with COPD and left ventricular failure. The patient receiving a digitalis preparation should be carefully monitored for side effects (see Chapter 31).

Patients with increased dyspnea secondary to pulmonary edema or with right ventricular failure or corticosteroid-induced fluid retention may benefit from diuretics. When diuretics are given, the patient should be carefully monitored for side effects. Those taking thiazide diuretics need to be told to eat foods high in potassium, such as bananas, oranges, prunes, and raisins.

#### Psychopharmacologic agents

Psychopharmacologic agents may need to be prescribed for some patients with severe emotional disturbances. The type of agent and size of dose are individually determined, but in general, the older the patient, the smaller the dose. When these agents are prescribed, a pharmacology book should be referred to for information about the side effects and precautions to be used in administering these agents.

### Improving Gas Exchange

ABGs are monitored for indications of hypoxemia, respiratory acidosis, and respiratory alkalosis.

Hypoxemia and hypercapnia often occur simultaneously, and the signs and symptoms of each are similar. These include headache, irritability, confusion, increasing somnolence, asterixis (flapping tremors of extremities), cardiac arrhythmias, and tachycardia.

If hypocapnia is developing, tachypnea, vertigo, tingling of the extremities, muscular weakness, and spasm are often present. It is important to remember that the presence of signs and symptoms associated with altered levels of $Pa{O_2}$ and $Pa{CO_2}$ depend more on the *rate of change* than on the *degree of change* in the levels. ***Rapidly changing signs usually indicate a rapid worsening of the patient's condition.*** At the same time, patients with long-standing hypoxemia and hypercapnia may be relatively asymptomatic because they have physiologically accommodated to increased levels of $Pa{CO_2}$ and decreased levels of $Pa{O_2}$.

#### Oxygen therapy

Oxygen therapy is required for patients with COPD who are unable to maintain a $Pa{O_2}$ greater than 55 mm Hg or an oxygen saturation greater than 85% or more at rest and for those who cannot carry out ADL (breathing, eating, dressing, toileting) without becoming very short of breath. In these patients, 1 to 2 L oxygen is usually given via nasal prongs to relieve hypoxemia and decrease pulmonary hypertension, which in turn decreases the load on the right side of the heart. It has been demonstrated that patients receive the best benefits from oxygen therapy if the oxygen is used continuously. A common misunderstanding expressed by patients requiring ongoing oxygen therapy is that they should only use their oxygen when they are symptomatic (i.e., short of breath) to avoid becoming habituated to the oxygen and thus requiring higher levels of oxygen. It is imperative that the nurse clarify the importance of continual oxygen use in order to receive maximal benefits of the therapy.

Because many patients with COPD have chronic carbon dioxide retention, their stimulus to breathe is their low $Pa{O_2}$ level. It is of critical importance that patients understand that high flow rates of oxygen (greater than 6 L/min) and high concentrations (greater than 40%) may elevate their $Pa{O_2}$ to a level that removes the stimulus by which they breathe, resulting in respiratory failure (see section on respiratory failure later in this chapter).

Pursed-lip breathing is also helpful in improving gas exchange in people with COPD. It has been shown to decrease $Pa{CO_2}$ levels and improve $Pa{O_2}$.

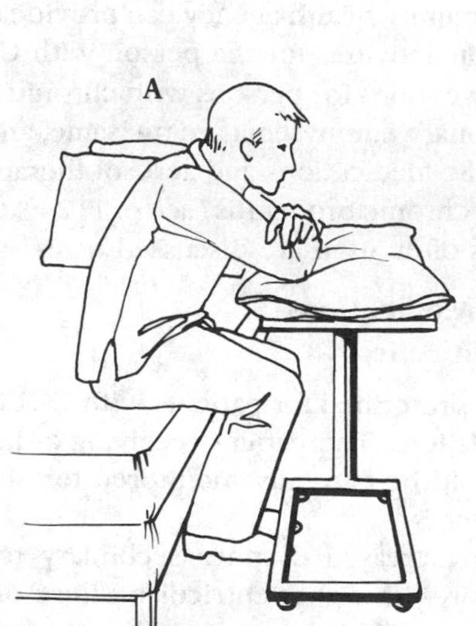


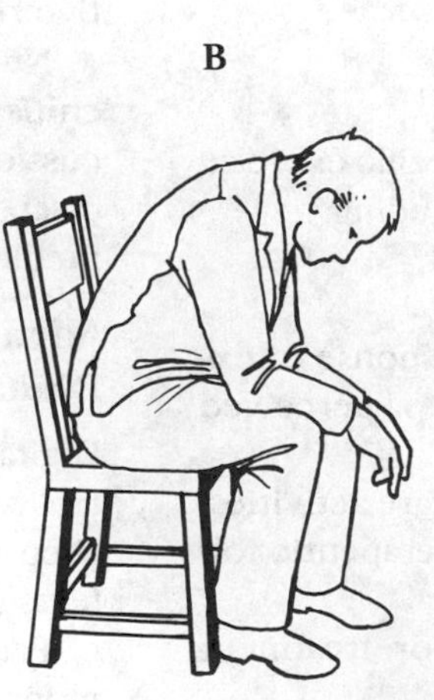


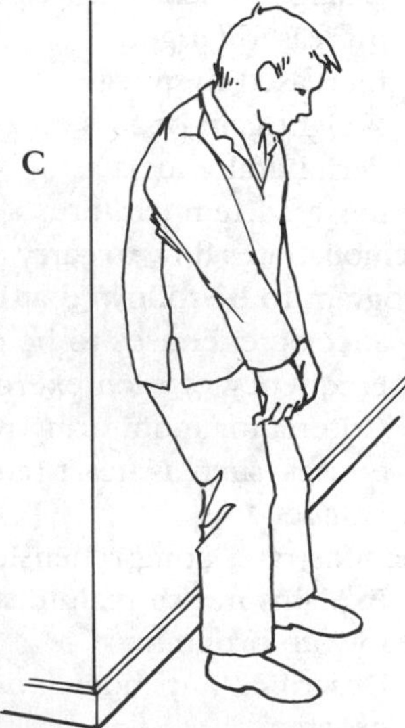


**FIGURE 37-20** Forward-leaning position. **A,** Patient sits on edge of the bed with arms folded on pillow placed on elevated bedside table. **B,** Patient in three-point position. Patient sits in chair with feet approximately 1 foot apart and leans forward with elbows on knees. **C,** Patient leans against wall with feet spread apart, allowing shoulders to sag forward with arms relaxed.

## Improving Efficiency of Breathing Pattern

1. Teach patient to slow respiratory frequency and to breathe slowly and rhythmically.
2. Discourage patient from taking large gulps of air.
3. Teach patient to increase inspiratory/expiratory ratio so that expiration takes twice as long as inhalation.
   a. Teach patient to count in seconds and to concentrate on increasing time taken to exhale.
   b. Count to 5 on inhalation and to 10 on exhalation.

Teach pursed-lip breathing if the patient is not already using it (see Figure 37-19). Teach the forward-leaning position for exhalation. Using a forward-leaning position of 30 to 40 degrees with the head tilted at a 16- to 18-degree angle is a very effective way to improve exhalation (Figure 37-20). As mentioned earlier, patients with emphysema have increased TLC and RV with the diaphragm in a fixed flattened position. For this reason, the diaphragm cannot assist in exhalation as it does normally. Leaning forward allows more air to be removed from the lungs on exhalation. The leaning-forward position can be achieved in either a sitting or standing position. For example, (1) the patient can sit on the edge of the bed or a chair and lean forward on two or three pillows placed on a table or overbed stand; (2) the patient can sit in a chair with the legs spread apart shoulder width (or wider, if obese) with the elbows on the knees and the arms and hands relaxed; or (3) the patient can stand with the back and hips against the wall with the feet spread apart and about 12 inches (30 cm) from the wall. The patient then relaxes and leans forward. In these positions the patient cannot use the accessory muscles of respiration, and the upward action of the diaphragm is improved.

### Abdominal breathing and exercises

Teach abdominal breathing, leg-raising exercises, inhalation-exhalation exercises, and muscle-reconditioning exercises.

*Abdominal breathing* improves the breathing efficiency of persons with COPD because it assists the patient to elevate the diaphragm. Abdominal breathing can be taught in the sitting or lying position. In the sitting

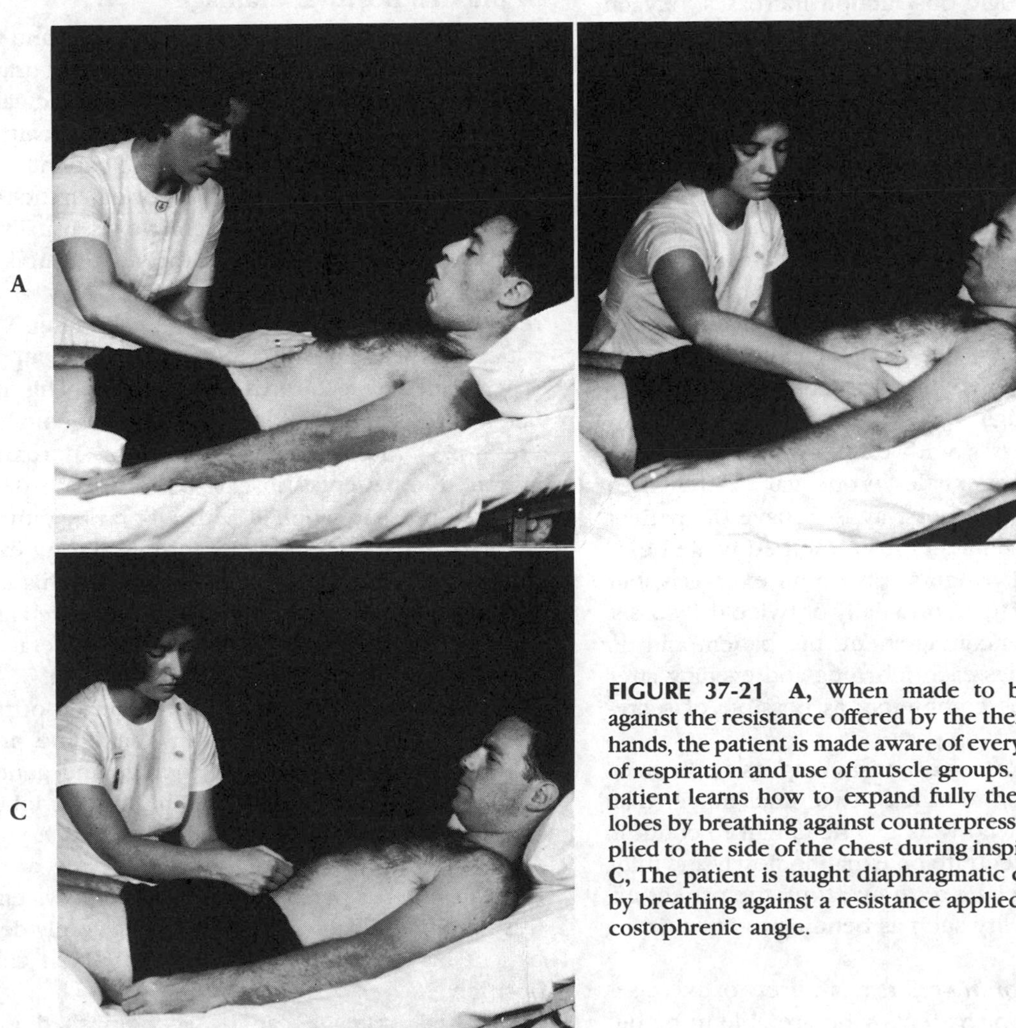


**FIGURE 37-21** **A,** When made to breathe against the resistance offered by the therapist's hands, the patient is made aware of every phase of respiration and use of muscle groups. **B,** The patient learns how to expand fully the lower lobes by breathing against counterpressure applied to the side of the chest during inspiration. **C,** The patient is taught diaphragmatic control by breathing against a resistance applied in the costophrenic angle.

position, the patient sits on the side of the bed or in a chair and holds a small pillow or a book against the abdomen. The patient then exhales slowly while leaning forward and pressing the pillow or book against the abdomen. In the lying position, a small pillow or a book is placed on the abdomen and the patient is asked to "puff out" the abdomen and raise the pillow or book as high as possible. The patient then exhales slowly through pursed lips while pulling in on the abdominal muscles. Manual pressure on the upper abdomen during expiration facilitates this maneuver (Figure 37-21). In addition to abdominal breathing, exercises to strengthen the abdominal muscles assist patients to use their abdominal muscles more effectively in emptying their lungs.

This "controlled" breathing pattern is to be used while performing various ADL: from sitting, standing, walking, and climbing stairs to more complex activities. As this pattern becomes natural, it will be used automatically during periods of increased shortness of breath. Persons who do not know how to use controlled breathing tend to increase their respiratory rate and their work of breathing when they are short of breath. As a result, physiologic obstruction increases, oxygen requirements increase, and effective ventilation decreases. Changing a person's respiratory pattern requires much effort by both the individual and those providing care.

This same method of teaching augmented abdominal (diaphragmatic) breathing can be used to teach the patient to cough. The difference is that expiration is forced down to RV. This maneuver often stimulates the cough reflex. If it does not, the person is taught to cough actively at the end of full expiration. Physiologically, forced expiration simulates the effects of a cough and is therefore more effective than telling the patient to take a deep breath and then cough.

*Leg-raising exercises,* with each leg being raised alternately as the patient exhales, is one way to strengthen abdominal muscles. Another way is to have the patient raise the head and shoulders from the bed while he or she exhales. Not all patients can do all exercises, but most can do some of them on a daily or twice-daily basis. With practice and encouragement, the patient can do the exercises 10 times each morning and evening after clearing the lungs as completely as possible of secretions.

*Inhalation-exhalation exercises* emphasize the need to prolong exhalation to at least two times longer than inhalation. Patients who walk can be taught to count in seconds and to concentrate on exhaling slowly and fully. While learning to *exhale with exertion,* the patient exhales during an activity such as bending over or sitting down.

*Muscle reconditioning* refers to a variety of exercises that tone muscles. For patients who are able to be out of bed, walking, using a treadmill, or riding a stationary bicycle is helpful. The exercise period is started slowly with 10 minutes twice daily three times a week, increasing to 20 minutes twice daily three times a week. The patient needs to be assessed for his or her ability to carry out such an exercise program, and a staff member should be present during the exercise period.

### Pulmonary physiotherapy

The person who has difficulty breathing may be taught how to increase the efficiency of his or her breathing pattern. Breathing exercises are usually a part of pulmonary physiotherapy, which may also include **segmental postural drainage, clapping,** and **vibrating.** Although pulmonary physiotherapy activities may be performed by a physical therapist, they are often part of a nurse's responsibility. Regardless of where the primary responsibility lies, nurses must be familiar with the techniques so that they can demonstrate and reinforce them and ensure that the individual is doing them correctly. Also, the need for pulmonary physiotherapy may occur at a time when the physical therapist is not available to the patient.

### Segmental postural drainage

Segmental postural drainage with clapping and vibration is a technique used to combine the force of gravity with the natural ciliary activity of the small bronchial airways to move secretions upward toward the main bronchi and the trachea. From this point the patient can cough secretions up, or they can be suctioned. In the treatment of COPD, drainage of all segments is usually accomplished by placing patients in various postural drainage positions (Figure 37-22). Treatment may also be directed at draining specific areas of the lung. While the patient is in each position, *clapping* with a cupped hand is performed over the area being drained. This maneuver helps to loosen secretions and stimulate coughing (Figure 37-23). After clapping the area for approximately 1 minute, the patient is instructed to breathe deeply. *Vibrating* (pressure applied with a vibrating movement of the hand on the chest) is performed during expiratory phase of the deep breath (Figure 37-24). This assists the patient to exhale more fully. The procedure is repeated as necessary. When the patient cannot tolerate a head-down position, a modified position is used.

Positions that provide gravity drainage of the lungs can be achieved in several ways, and the procedure selected usually depends on the age and general condition of the person as well as the lobe or lobes of the lungs where secretions have accumulated. A young person usually can tolerate greater lowering of the head than an elderly person whose vascular system adapts less rapidly to change of position. A severely debilitated patient may only be able to tolerate slight changes in position.

Postural drainage can be accomplished in several ways. Electric hospital beds can be tilted into a head-

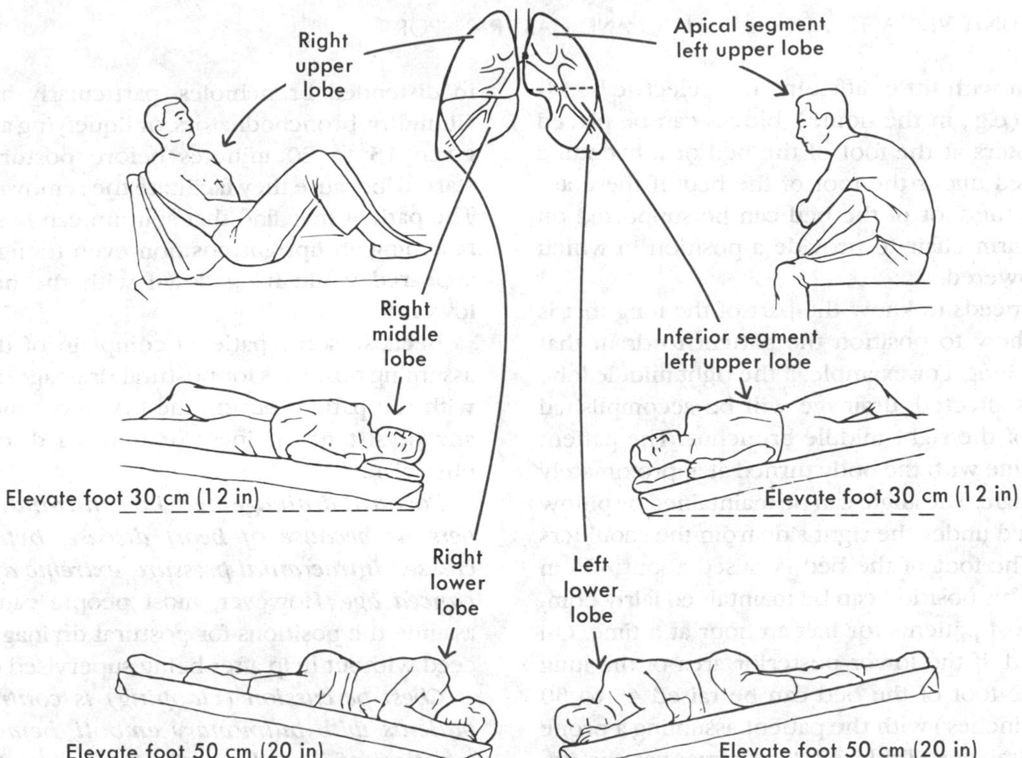


**FIGURE 37-22** Postural drainage requires that the patient assume various positions to facilitate the flow of secretions from various portions of the lung into the bronchi, trachea, and throat so that they can be raised and expectorated more easily. Drawing shows the correct position to drain various portions of the lung.

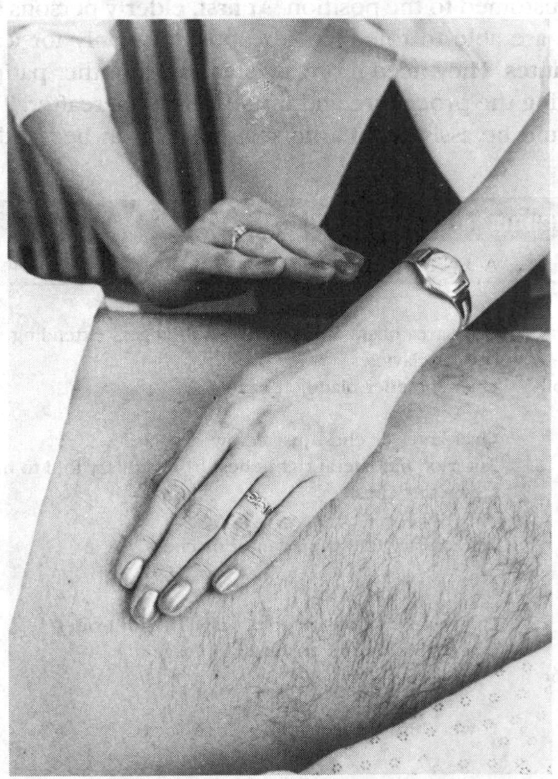

**FIGURE 37-23** Position of the hands for clapping the chest to loosen secretions. Upper hand is cupped in preparation for clapping. Lower hand at end of clapping motion.

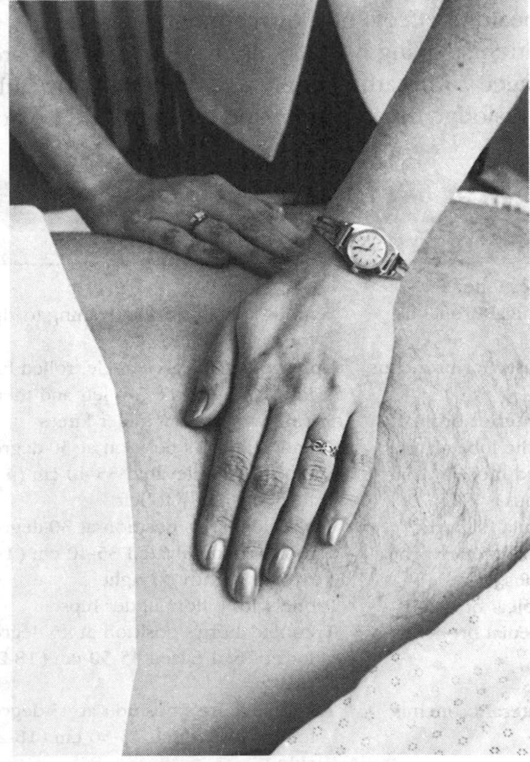

**FIGURE 37-24** Position of the hands for vibrating the chest at the end of prolonged expiration.

down position with little difficulty. If an electric bed is not available (e.g., in the home), blocks can be placed under the casters at the foot of the bed or a hydraulic lift can be used under the foot of the bed. If these are not available, the foot of the bed can be supported on the seat of a firm chair to provide a position in which the head is lowered.

The nurse needs to know the part of the lung that is affected and how to position the patient to drain that portion of the lung. For example, if the right middle lobe of the lung is affected, drainage will be accomplished best by way of the right middle bronchus. The patient should lie supine with the body turned at approximately a 45-degree angle. The angle can be maintained by pillow supports placed under the right side from the shoulders to the hips. The foot of the bed is raised about 30 cm (12 inches). This position can be maintained fairly comfortably by most patients for half an hour at a time. On the other hand, if the lower posterior area of the lung is affected, the foot of the bed can be raised 45 to 50 cm (18 to 20 inches) with the patient assuming a prone position for drainage. Table 37-29 summarizes the positions for segmental postural drainage.

Postural drainage and clapping should be planned so as to achieve maximal benefit. The best time is generally in the morning soon after arising and at night before retiring. Frequency of treatments depends on each person's needs, but care should be taken to avoid exhaustion, which results in shallow ventilation and negates the positive effects of the treatment.

Patients having postural drainage of any kind are encouraged to breathe deeply and to cough forcefully to help dislodge thick sputum and exudate that are pooled in distended bronchioles, particularly after inactivity. Humidity, bronchodilators, or liquefying agents often are given 15 to 20 minutes before postural drainage is started, because they facilitate the removal of secretions. The patient may find that sputum can best be raised on resuming an upright position even though no drainage appeared while lying down with the head and chest lowered.

Because some patients complain of dizziness when assuming positions for postural drainage, the nurse stays with the patient during the first few times and reports any persistent dizziness or unusual discomfort to the physician.

*Postural drainage may be contraindicated in some persons because of heart disease, hypertension, increased intracranial pressure, extreme dyspnea,* or *advanced age.* However, most people can be taught to assume the positions for postural drainage and can proceed without help after being supervised once or twice.

*Chest percussion (clapping) is contraindicated in patients with pulmonary emboli, hemorrhage, exacerbation of bronchospasms,* or *severe pain* and *over areas of resectable carcinoma.* Often, patients with a chronic pulmonary problem need to be taught to perform postural drainage independently so that they can continue it at home. The position usually is maintained for 10 minutes at first, and the period of time is gradually lengthened to 15 to 30 minutes as the patient becomes accustomed to the position. At first, elderly persons usually are able to tolerate these positions only for a few minutes. They need more assistance than other patients during the procedure and immediately thereafter. They should be assisted to a normal position in bed and re-

**TABLE 37-29 Positions for Segmental Postural Drainage, Clapping, and Vibrating**

| AREA OF LUNG | POSITION OF PATIENT | AREA TO BE CLAPPED OR VIBRATED |
|---|---|---|
| Upper lobe | | |
| Apical bronchus | Semi-Fowler's position, leaning to right, then left, then forward | Over area of shoulder blades with fingers extending over clavicles |
| Posterior bronchus | Upright at 45-degree angle, rolled forward against a pillow at 45 degrees on left and then right side | Over shoulder blade on each side |
| Anterior bronchus | Supine with pillow under knees | Over anterior chest just below clavicles |
| Middle lobe (lateral and medial bronchus) | Trendelenburg's position at 30-degree angle or with foot of bed elevated 35-40 cm (14-16 inches), turned slightly to left | Anterior and lateral right chest from axillary fold to midanterior chest |
| Lingula (superior and inferior bronchus) | Trendelenburg's position at 30-degree angle or with foot of bed elevated 35-40 cm (14-16 inches), turned slightly to right | Left axillary fold to midanterior chest |
| Apical bronchus | Prone with pillow under hips | Lower third of posterior rib cage on both sides |
| Medial bronchus | Trendelenburg's position at 45-degree angle or with foot of bed raised 45-50 cm (18-20 inches) on right side | Lower third of left posterior rib cage |
| Lateral bronchus | Trendelenburg's position at 45-degree angle or with foot of bed raised 45-50 cm (18-20 inches) on left side | Lower third of right posterior rib cage |
| Posterior bronchus | Prone Trendelenburg's position at 45-degree angle with pillow under hips | Lower third of posterior rib cage on both sides |

quired to lie flat for a few minutes before sitting up or getting out of bed. This helps to prevent dizziness and reduces the danger of accidents from orthostatic hypotension.

The patient may feel nauseated because of the odor and taste of sputum. Therefore the procedure should be timed so that it comes at least 1 hour before meals. A short rest period following the treatment often improves postural drainage. Aromatic mouthwashes should be available for frequent use by any patient who is expectorating sputum freely.

## Improving Airway Clearance

Patients can be taught the following measures to improve airway clearance:

1. Teach effective coughing maneuvers. Have patient sit upright and instruct patient to:
   a. Inhale slowly through the nose.
   b. Lean forward and exhale slowly through pursed lips to promote open airways.
   c. Repeat these steps several times to mobilize secretions and move them upward in the airway.
   d. Take a slow maximal inhalation through the nose when secretions reach the oropharynx. During exhalation, use short repeated coughs to minimize bronchospasm.
   e. Inhale maximally after coughing to reinflate alveoli.
2. To thin secretions, a fluid intake of 3 to 4 L has traditionally been encouraged unless contraindicated. However, evidence suggests that this quantity of fluids may not be needed to keep secretions mobile.
3. Teach postural drainage, clapping, and vibrating as discussed in Table 37-29.
4. Research indicates that airway clearance maneuvers may be enhanced by strengthening respiratory muscles.

Although expectorants are sometimes prescribed, some experts believe they do more harm than good. Water is still considered to be the best expectorant, and adequate hydration without fluid overload should be encouraged.

## Improving Nutritional Intake

Persons with COPD often demonstrate excessive weight loss. Some of the factors that may contribute to weight loss are:

1. A feeling of satiety with small amounts of food because of compression of abdominal contents by the flattened diaphragm
2. Dyspnea interfering with eating
3. Increased dyspnea when eating caused by stomach pushing up against the diaphragm
4. Decreased appetite secondary to chronic sputum production
5. Gastric irritation associated with bronchodilators and steroids
6. Increased work of breathing requiring increased caloric intake to maintain weight; makes it imperative that the patient with COPD maintain adequate nutritional levels because:
   a. Diminished total weight is correlated with a dramatic decrease in respiratory muscle (especially the diaphragm) size and strength.
   b. Inadequate nutritional status and in particular deficiencies in vitamins A and C decrease resistance to infection.
   c. Protein insufficiency decreases colloid osmotic pressure, which increases the risk of pulmonary edema.

Nursing acuons focused on assisting the patient with COPD to maintain adequate nutrition include the following:

1. Explore usual dietary habits (collect a 24-hour diet history).
2. Counsel patient to select foods that provide a high-protein, high-caloric diet (Box 37-25).
3. Encourage vitamin supplementation. It is important to counsel the patient to select foods that provide higher calorie levels through higher fat content rather than by high carbohydrate levels. Persons with advanced chronic bronchitis or emphysema are unable to breathe off the excess carbon dioxide that is a natural end product of carbohydrate metabolism. Therefore calories obtained from high-carbohydrate foods may elevate $Paco_2$ levels in persons with COPD.
4. Prepackaged food supplements such as milk shakes or snack bars taken between meals provide an excellent source of protein and calories.
5. Smaller, more frequent meals are often tolerated better than three larger meals.

**BOX 37-25 Foods To Increase Protein and Caloric Intake***

Offer frequent small feedings of foods high in protein and calories such as the following:
- Milk shakes
- Flavored gelatin or pudding with whipped cream
- Cream soups made with half-and-half
- Peanut butter spread on crackers, bananas, pears, or apples
- Crackers and cheese, nuts, dried fruits, and ice creams readily available for snacks

*Excellent sources for suggestions to increase protein and calorie intake are McCauley K, Weaver R: Cardiac and pulmonary diseases—nutritional implications, *Nurs Clin North Am* 18:81-95, 1983; Spector N: Nutritional support of the ventilator-dependent patient, *Nurs Clin North Am* 24:407-414, 1989; and Cerrato PL: The special nutritional needs of a COPD patient, *RN* 11:75-76, 1987.

6. Consider financial and ethnic background when planning for meals.

## Preventing Infection

The ***most common complication of COPD,*** and cause of most hospital readmissions, is ***respiratory infection.*** Pulmonary system response to the infectious process includes increased respiratory rate, mucosal irritation, and increased mucus production. Because of these localized responses, patients may have bronchospasm and a change in their pattern of sputum production. If the infection remains untreated, the result is an overall increased work of breathing with eventual respiratory failure. Thus, for the person with COPD, it is imperative that respiratory infections be avoided. The patient should be counseled to take the following steps to ***decrease*** the chance of contracting a pulmonary infection.

1. Avoid large crowds, especially during known influenza seasons.
   a. Avoid contact with people who have an upper respiratory infection.
   b. Receive influenza and pneumonia immunizations.
2. Contact health care provider if the following common signs and symptoms occur:
   a. Change in sputum color, amount, and consistency
   b. Increased cough
   c. Change in behavior (e.g., more argumentive than usual) that indicates an increase in $Paco_2$
   d. Increased fatigue
   e. Increased dyspnea
   f. Weight gain
   g. Peripheral edema
   h. Elevated temperature

Antimicrobial agents prescribed to treat respiratory tract infections in persons with COPD are discussed on p. 1127.

## Preventing Fluid Volume Excess

Low $Pao_2$ is a potent pulmonary vasoconstrictor. Pulmonary vasoconstriction increases pulmonary arterial pressure. If pulmonary hypertension exists for a prolonged time, the increased workload on the heart's right ventricle will ultimately result in ***right ventricular failure*** and what is known as pulmonary heart disease or ***cor pulmonale.*** Depending on its severity and duration, cor pulmonale may be characterized by neck vein distention, hepatomegaly, dependent peripheral edema, and, as oncotic pressure is exceeded, ascites and pleural effusions. Nursing interventions for fluid volume excess resulting from cor pulmonale are based on the understanding that the disease is treated by intervening with the underlying cause of the pulmonary hypertension. Therefore, nursing interventions focus on promoting adequate ventilation for optimal oxygen/carbon dioxide exhange and relieving symptoms that result from the fluid volume excess. Thus a nursing plan of care for the person with COPD that promotes optimal ventilation also intervenes with fluid volume excess resulting from cor pulmonale. Additionally, interventions focused on the symptoms of fluid volume excess include:

1. Weigh daily in the same amount of clothing and at the same time of day on the same scale.
2. Monitor intake and output accurately. (NOTE: although it is unknown if fluid restriction is effective in the actual treatment of cor pulmonale, excess fluid intake may overwhelm an already compromised cardiac system.)
3. Encourage moderate exercise or change patient's position frequently to promote adequate perfusion in lung.
4. Measure abdominal girth at regular intervals to assess the possible presence of or progression of ascites.
5. Administer diuretics as ordered. When diuretics are given, the patient should be carefully monitored for side effects. Those taking thiazide diuretics will need to be taught about eating foods high in potassium, such as bananas, oranges, prunes, and raisins.
6. Administer digitalis as ordered. (NOTE: digitalis is of questionable usefulness in pure right-sided heart failure.) Persons receiving digitalis should be carefully monitored for side effects.

### Guidelines for Teaching the Person Progressive Relaxation Exercises

1. Contract each muscle to a count of 10 and then relax it.
2. Do exercises in quiet room while sitting or lying in a comfortable position.
3. Do exercises to relaxing music, if desired.
4. Have another person serve as a "coach" by giving command to contract specific muscle, count to 10, and relax muscle.
5. The following are examples of exercises helpful to some persons with COPD.
   a. Raise shoulders, shrug them, and relax for 5 seconds; then relax them completely.
   b. Make a fist of both hands, squeeze them tightly for 5 seconds, and then relax them completely.

## Assisting with Breathing and Rest

1. Place patient in position of comfort, usually Fowler's or high Fowler's.
2. Assist patient with progressive relaxation exercises and meditation (see Guidelines boxes above).

## Assisting with Control of Environment

Abrupt changes in weather or hot or cold environments can increase sputum production and bronchial obstruction.

### Guidelines for Teaching the Person Meditation Exercises

1. Sit or lie quietly with eyes closed and attempt to relax all muscles, beginning with feet and moving upward.
2. Breathe in through the nose slowly (may help to count slowly to 4 on inhalation) and exhale slowly through pursed lips (mentally count to 6) with a natural rhythm, relaxed and peaceful (this can be coached or done privately).
3. Survey the body for points of tension. Consciously relax the tense areas. The body is peaceful and relaxed.
4. Continue breathing as above, aware of the feeling of well-being throughout your body. This can be continued for 10 to 20 minutes, or after 5 minutes go to Step 5.
5. Listen for (or visualize) a special relaxing sound (or image). Listen to it closely (or visualize) all the while breathing as above.
6. At this point, positive suggestion can be used; for example, "I am in control of my body. When I find myself getting tense, I can take a moment to stop and breathe in all the air that I need and let the tension flow away."
7. After mental suggestion, continue breathing easily and slowly come back to normal alert mental state.
8. Meditation can be used at any time to induce a relaxed state of mind (e.g., to promote sleep).

**Temperature and humidity**

1. Humidity of 30% to 50% is ideal. This can be achieved by a humidifier as necessary.
2. An air conditioner may reduce dyspnea by controlling temperature and preventing pollutants from outside air from entering. The cost of an air conditioner is a medically deductible expense for persons with COPD.
3. Wearing a scarf over the nose and mouth in cold weather helps to warm the air and prevent bronchospasm. Masks for this purpose are also available.
4. Moving to another climate is usually not advised unless there is some other medical indication for doing so. Persons living at high altitudes may be advised to move to a lower altitude or use supplemental oxygen continuously.
5. Travel by airplane is possible. The airline needs to be informed in advance of the need for supplemental oxygen during the flight.

**Avoiding inhaled irritants**

Air pollution is a common problem in modern civilization and is a real threat to persons with COPD, who should observe the following:

1. Heed announcements on radio and television regarding pollution alerts, and avoid being outdoors when an alert is in effect.
2. Use an air conditioner or high-efficiency particulate air filter (HEPA) or electrostatic filter to remove particulate matter from air.
    a. Keep filters clean.
    b. Follow manufacturer's directions for use.
3. Use an activated charcoal filter if offending odors or gas pollutants are a problem.
4. Avoid second-hand smoke.

### Improving Activity Tolerance

1. Allow ample time for activities; do not rush patient.
2. Provide oxygen as needed before and during activities.
3. Encourage gradual increase in activities such as walking.
4. Provide positive feedback on progress and encourage new endeavors when patient is ready.

### Assisting With Sleep Pattern

Persons with COPD usually only sleep for short periods. Most are most comfortable sleeping in an upright position in bed or in a lounge chair with footrest.

1. Assist with relaxation exercises at bedtime.
2. Give backrub at bedtime and encourage family member to do so at home.
3. Provide relaxing music at bedtime and encourage same at home.
4. Ascertain preferred position for sleep, usually high Fowler's.
5. Establish regular bedtime to meet patient's usual schedule.
6. Give bedtime snack, if desired.

### Assisting With Fear Reduction

Persons who are short of breath are very anxious and frightened.

1. Encourage patient to talk about anxiety and fears with nurse and family members.
2. Take measures already discussed to improve airway clearance and breathing.
3. Do not leave patient alone during periods of breathlessness.
4. Explain to family reason for not leaving patient at home alone for long periods; assist them with securing community resources to assist as necessary (e.g., Homemakers, Visiting Nurses' Association).

### Facilitating Learning

Persons with COPD play a major role in monitoring their own condition and in maintaining their physical and psychologic functioning at the maximal possible level.

For these reasons, it is imperative that the nurse thoroughly assess the patient's knowledge about COPD, including its cause and treatment. Individualized teaching plans based on the patient's knowledge level can then be developed. The Guidelines box (p. 1142) lists areas that may be included in the teaching program.

According to the CDC, only 30% of persons at high risk for influenza-related complications, such as persons with COPD, are vaccinated. A year 2000 national health objective is to achieve influenza vaccination levels of at

## Guidelines for Teaching the Person With COPD

The following areas should be addressed in a typical teaching program for persons with chronic bronchitis or emphysema:

I. Patients should be able to explain, in lay terms, the basic function and pathology of their lungs. The ALA offers several excellent booklets for the lay population. (Your local branch of the ALA can provide you with a complete listing of their various publications.)

II. The avoidance of respiratory irritants and maintenance of a proper environment should be emphasized to people with COPD. As discussed earlier, inhaled irritants (especially cigarette smoke) pose a serious threat to these persons. Steps the patient can take to reduce or avoid exposure to these irritants are listed below.
   A. Stop smoking. There are many community agencies, including the ALA, AHA, and ACS that offer programs for persons who want to stop smoking. The nurse should be familiar with community programs and give a list of them to the patient.
   B. Ask other persons not to smoke in the immediate environment. Inhalation of secondary smoke can exacerbate symptoms.
   C. Pay heed to announcements on radio and television warning of pollution alerts. Do not go outside during an alert.
   D. Use an air conditioner or HEPA filter or electrostatic filter to remove particulate matter from air.
      1. Keep filters clean.
      2. Follow manufacturer's directions for use.
   E. Use an activated charcoal filter if offending odors or gas pollutants are a problem.
   F. Avoid abrupt environmental temperature or humidity changes because they can increase sputum production and cause bronchospasm.
      1. Use an air conditioner in hot weather.
      2. Use a face mask when going out in cold weather.
      3. Use a dehumidifier or humidifier as appropriate to maintain a humidity of 30% to 50%.
   G. If air travel is required, check with physician about the need for supplemental oxygen.
   H. Avoid large crowds, especially during known influenza seasons.
      1. Avoid contact with people who have an upper respiratory infection.
      2. Receive influenza and pneumonia immunizations.

III. The patient should be able to explain the following aspects of the home medication or treatment regimen.
   A. State name, dose, action, and side effects of each medication.
   B. Explain how and when to use medications ordered on an as needed basis (e.g., bronchodilators, antibiotics, steroids, antacids).
   C. Demonstrate techniques necessary for follow-up care (e.g., postural drainage, clapping and vibrating, aerosol therapy).
   D. Describe how to obtain and maintain any needed equipment or supplies (e.g., oxygen, nebulizers, humidifiers, aerosols, IPPB machines, syringes, medications).

IV. The patient should demonstrate how to carry out the specific home exercise program:
   A. Specific exercises to be completed
   B. Frequency of each exercise
   C. Criteria for monitoring physical response to exercises, such as heart rate increase or perceived fatigue

V. The patient should be able to list the names and telephone numbers of appropriate community support services, such as the Visiting Nurses' Association and a home medical equipment supplier.

least 60% in noninstitutionalized high-risk persons. Unless more persons who are at high risk can be convinced to receive influenza vaccine, it is obvious that this goal will not be reached by the year 2000.[40]

## ♦ EVALUATION

To evaluate the effectiveness of nursing interventions, compare patient behaviors with those stated in the expected patient outcomes. Successful achievement of patient outcomes for the person with COPD is indicated by the following:

1. Ventilation and oxygenation are improved.
   a. $PaO_2$, $PaCO_2$, and pH are at acceptable levels.
   b. Verbalizes need to use oxygen therapy almost continuously. If not using continuously, use while sleeping and exercising.
2. Breathing pattern is effective.
   a. Takes twice as long to exhale as to inhale: 5:10 seconds.
   b. Uses pursed-lip breathing when exhaling.
   c. Leans forward on an overstuffed chair to increase ability to exhale.
   d. Concentrates on abdominal breathing when lying in bed and when up and about.
   e. Inhales before beginning an activity and exhales while doing activity.
   f. Has respiratory rate of 24 to 28/minute and moderate tidal volume.
3. Airway clearance is improving.
   a. Uses inhaler with bronchodilator as necessary to clear secretions.
   b. Is well hydrated.
   c. Inhales deeply and exhales down to RV to initiate cough reflex.
4. Verbalizes dietary changes after discharge.
   a. Prefers to eat several small feedings daily because it causes less shortness of breath.
   b. Verbalizes that "gas-producing" foods such as cabbage, baked beans, and raw green pepper and radishes are to be avoided because they cause discomfort and "bloating."
5. Remains infection free.
   a. Temperature is normal.
   b. Sputum is clear.

   c. Knows to call health care provider if sputum color changes to yellow, green, or rusty or if streaked with bright-red blood.
6. Fluid balance is normal.
   a. Weight remains stable.
   b. Electrolyte levels are within normal range.
   c. Is taking hydrochlorothiazide, 50 mg daily.
   d. Verbalizes need to call health care provider if has weight gain, dyspnea, or dependent edema.
7. Maintains or works toward improving activity level.
   a. Does muscle-reconditioning activities daily at home and participates in group reconditioning sessions twice weekly at support group sponsored by local branch of ALA.
   b. Paces activities, using oxygen most of the time.
8. Is able to control stress response.
   a. Demonstrates muscle relaxation.
   b. Verbalizes how to meditate using taped music to improve relaxation.
   c. Participates in support group at local ALA office.
9. Verbalizes measures used to support sleep.
   a. Uses five pillows to achieve upright position with each arm supported on a pillow.
   b. Practices relaxation exercises and meditates to soft music.
10. Verbalizes signs and symptoms that should be reported to health care provider:
   a. Change in sputum color, amount, and consistency
   b. Increase in cough
   c. Irritability, inability to control temper (both signs of increased $PaCO_2$)
   d. Fatigue, especially when unusual for activity being undertaken
   e. Increase in dyspnea
   f. Weight gain or weight loss of more than 5 pounds
   g. Swollen feet and legs
   h. Elevated temperature
11. Demonstrates exercises being done at least 3 times/week.
12. Demonstrates how to carry out activities with the least expenditure of energy.
   a. Has repositioned several pieces of furniture at home to meet needs to have things used frequently nearby.
   b. Knows community resources to call for oxygen equipment and other assistance.
   c. Family member has been taught how to assist with postural drainage. Nurse or physical therapist from home health agency comes in weekly to check progress with activities and exercise.
13. Knows names, dose, action, and side effects of all medications.
14. Has developed own phone directory of community resources.

## ASTHMA

Asthma is discussed separately from bronchitis and emphysema because it results in intermittent rather than continuous, irreversible airway obstruction. Its onset is sudden as opposed to the slow insidious progression of symptoms seen in bronchitis and emphysema.

### Etiology

Asthma is characterized by increased responsiveness of the trachea and bronchi to various stimuli that cause narrowing of the airways and difficulty in breathing.

### Epidemiology

Asthma is known to affect nearly 10 million persons in the United States, two thirds of whom are adults. Both hospitalizations for treatment of asthma and deaths from it have been increasing. In 1978, there were just under 2000 deaths from asthma. This number more than doubled in the 1980s and was 4800 in 1988. Although no firm figures are available as yet for the 1990s, both morbidity and mortality are believed to be increasing. The reasons for these increases are not well understood. The figures available show that the death rate for blacks is higher than that for whites. Some experts have suggested that the reason is that more blacks are among the medically underserved. Women have higher death rates than men, but the highest death rates are among elderly persons (age 65 and over). Deaths in elderly persons show increases during December through February, suggesting that a concomitant respiratory infection (influenza, pneumonia) contributed to the severity of asthma, the need for hospitalization, and the number of deaths.

### Pathophysiology

An asthmatic attack results from several physiologic alterations, including altered immunologic response, increased airway resistance, increased lung compliance, impaired mucociliary function, and altered oxygen/carbon dioxide exchange. Each of these alterations is discussed here.

#### Altered immunologic response

No matter what the precipitating factors, the basis of asthma appears to be genetic or immunologic factors. The basis of nonimmunologic asthma is less well understood than is immunologic asthma.

Immunologic asthma is the result of an antigen-antibody reaction in which chemical mediators are released. The chemical mediators, which include histamine, slow-releasing substance of anaphylaxis (SRS-A), eosinophilic chemotactic factor of anaphylaxis (ECF-A), and perhaps others, cause three main reactions: (1) constriction of smooth muscles of both the large and the small airways, resulting in bronchospasm; (2) increased capillary permeability that results in mucosal edema and further narrows the ariways; and (3) increased mucous gland secretion and increased mucus production. As a result, the person with an asthmatic attack struggles to breathe through a narrowed airway that is in spasm. Because breathing is labored, the person breathes through the mouth, which dries the mucus and further occludes the airway.

Box 37-26 lists common factors triggering an asthmatic attack. Although allergic mechanisms are important in the pathogenesis of asthma, the many nonimmunologic precipitating factors indicate that other pathophysiologic processes, such as parasympathetic and sympathetic nervous system reactivity, are active in the onset of asthma. *Hypoxemia, hypercapnia, and overuse of bronchodilators may lead to an acute asthma attack.*

### Increased airway resistance

Increased airway resistance results from bronchial smooth muscle spasm, mucosal inflammation, and hypersecretion of mucus. These airway changes cause obstruction to airflow both in and out of the lungs.

### Increased lung compliance

The lungs become hyperinflated during an acute asthmatic attack as a result of air that becomes trapped in the distal air spaces. During the acute attack, the person with asthma demonstrates the same symptoms of increased lung compliance that are observed in the patient with emphysema.

### Impaired mucociliary function

Hypertrophy of mucus-secreting glands, thickened mucus, and slowed ciliary movement are common findings in persons with asthma. During an asthma attack, increased mucus production combined with slowed clearance of mucus caused by decreased ciliary movement results in *increased water loss from mucus.* Thus the *mucus becomes increasingly viscous and can ultimately result in the development of mucous plugs, which may block airways.*

### Altered oxygen/carbon dioxide exchange

Increased airway resistance and hyperinflation cause the respiratory muscles to work harder, resulting in muscle fatigue and ultimately exhaustion. In mild or short-term asthmatic attacks, the individual compensates with an increased respiratory rate, which results in respiratory alkalosis. Mild hypoxemia from altered V/Q ratios usually accompanies the alkalosis.

In a severe or prolonged attack, if the increased work of breathing cannot be relieved, respiratory muscle exhaustion will result in hypoventilation, which in turn causes respiratory acidosis and severe hypoxemia. If the process cannot be reversed, the person may die.

The signs and symptoms associated with asthma are correlated with normal lung functions and underlying pathophysiologic origins (see Tables 37-26 and 37-30). The character of asthmatic attacks can vary on a continuum from chronic or acute mild intermittent attacks to life-threatening status asthmaticus.

With chronic mild asthma, symptoms are not noticeable when the person is at rest. However, after exertion such as laughing, singing, vigorous exercise, or emotional excitement, dyspnea and wheezing develop rapidly. These attacks are controlled with medications, and patients usually can continue their mode of living with a few modifications and no serious lung changes. They are not hospitalized, but they sometimes come to outpatient clinics for medical supervision.

**BOX 37-26 Common Factors Triggering an Asthmatic Attack**

- Environmental factors
  - Change in temperature, especially cold air
  - Change in humidity: dry air
- Atmospheric pollutants
  - Cigarette and industrial smoke, ozone, sulfur dioxide, formaldehyde
- Strong odors: perfume
- Allergens
  - Feathers, animal dander, dust mites, molds, allergens; foods treated with sulfites (beer, wine, fruit juices, snack foods, salads, potatoes, shellfish, fresh and dried fruits)
- Exercise
- Stress or emotional upset
- Medications
  - Aspirin and nonsteroidal antiinflammatory drugs (NSAIDs), β-blockers (including eye drops), cholinergic drugs (to promote bladder contraction and as eye drops for glaucoma)
  - Enzymes, including those in laundry detergents
  - Chemicals: toluene and others used in solvents, paints, rubber, and plastics

**TABLE 37-30 Asthma Syndromes Classified by Precipitating Factor and Response Pattern**

| ASTHMA SYNDROMES | CHARACTERISTICS |
|---|---|
| Atopic asthma | Childhood onset, allergic rhinitis, allergic dermopathy, identifiable environmental precipitating events |
| Exercise-induced asthma | Airway contriction after exercise |
| Aspirin-hypersensitivity triad | Presence of nasal polyps, urticaria, and asthma after aspirin ingestion |
| Bronchospasm associated with nonbacterial upper respiratory tract infections | As described by patient |
| Industrial asthma | Bronchoconstriction associated with certain industrial precipitating factors |

Acute asthmatic attacks often occur at night. The person awakens with a sensation of choking caused by the mucosal inflammation and hypersecretion of mucus. Bronchospasm, with resultant increased airway resistance, causes audible *expiratory* and *inspiratory wheezing. During the acute attack, patients appear to be in acute respiratory distress and typically demonstrate tachypnea, accessory muscle breathing, and nasal flaring. They appear to be apprehensive and diaphoretic, and their attention is totally focused on their breathing.* If the treatment is successful, the attack usually ends with the coughing up of large quantities of thick, tenacious sputum. Most attacks subside in 30 minutes to 1 hour, although repeated asthmatic attacks associated with infection may continue for days or weeks. The person is usually exhausted and should rest quietly after the attack.

Persons who are severely affected by asthma and who have attacks that are difficult to control with the usual medications may develop *status asthmaticus.* In this case, the symptoms of an acute attack continue despite measures to relieve them. *Air trapping in the distal air spaces ultimately leads to respiratory muscle exhaustion and severe V/Q abnormalities with resultant respiratory failure and hypoxemia.*

Patients with status asthmaticus often demonstrate respiratory distress so severe that they are unable to talk. They may be moving minimal air in and out of the lungs; thus, audible wheezing and adventitious lung sounds may *not* be present. *During this phase of the attack, the patient will appear cyanotic and may demonstrate both pulsus paradoxus and sensorium changes.* This is a medical emergency, and the patient requires immediate therapy. Most patients arrive in the emergency room, where treatment is begun. Patients remain in the emergency room until their condition is stablized. Most patients are then admitted to the hospital for ongoing therapy and observation.

Repeated attacks of status asthmaticus may cause irreversible emphysema, resulting in a permanent decrease in total breathing capacity.

PFTs characteristic of asthma show reduction in $FEV_1$ to less than 25% of the predicted value. The FEV is usually greatly reduced in proportion to the FVC, although the FVC may also be decreased. Improved flow rates after administration of bronchodilators indicating reversible bronchospasm is a characteristic finding with asthma.

The results of ABG studies can vary from respiratory alkalosis with mild hypoxemia to severe respiratory acidosis with profound hypoxemia, depending on the severity and duration of the asthmatic attack.

## Prevention

### *Healthy People 2000*

The goal set by *Healthy People 2000* is to reduce to no more than 10% the proportion of people with asthma who experience activity limitation, from a baseline of 19.4% during 1986-1988.[40]

Prevention of immunologic (atopic) asthma is focused on identification of the allergens to which the person is sensitive. In nonimmunologic or mixed asthma, factors precipitating the exacerbation of symptoms may be obscure. However, identification of causative or aggravating factors is still imperative in order to avoid or decrease the incidence of asthma attacks.

There is perhaps no disease in which knowing the patient well is more important than in asthma. Because sensitivity tests can be performed with only a very small fraction of the substances with which the patient is in contact, the physician usually makes the diagnosis on the basis of a careful history. Knowing about the person's life-style, such as the type of work, leisure-time activities, and even food preferences, may give useful clues as to what precipitates the asthmatic attack. Box 37-27 lists nursing strategies for identifying causes.

*It is imperative to understand that even though psychologic factors may precipitate an attack, the response to the attack is physiologic and requires the same treatment as that prescribed for an attack precipitated by an allergen or any other factor.*

## Medical Management

The objectives of medical management of asthma are to promote normal functioning of the individual, prevent recurrent symptoms, prevent severe attacks, and prevent side effects from medication. The chief aim of various medications is to afford the patient immediate, progressive, ongoing bronchial relaxation. One approach is presented in Table 37-31.

### Maintenance therapy

Concern has been raised recently that many patients may be undertreated and that this may have contributed to the increase in death rates.

**BOX 37-27 Identifying Factors Precipitating Asthma**

1. Be alert for casual comments about daily activities the patient might consider insignificant.
2. Encourage patient to keep a symptom diary. Ask patient to perform the following tasks:
   a. Use a small notebook that can be carried at all times.
   b. Record everything that occurred and was present during 24 hours before and during the onset of the attack. When the attack began: What were you doing? Where were you? Who or what else was present? What was the weather like?
   c. Note the time and date that the attack occurred.
3. Write down what you think caused the symptoms to occur, even if it is a guess.
4. Observe patient's interaction with others and reaction to stressors that might aggravate and/or precipitate an attack.

**TABLE 37-31 Treatment of an Acute Asthmatic Attack**

| THERAPY | EFFECTS AND PRECAUTIONS |
|---|---|
| Inhaled β-agonist such as albuterol sulfate (Proventil, Ventalin) or metaproterenol sulfate (Alupent, Metaprel) in normal saline | Stimulates $\beta_2$-receptors in bronchial smooth muscle resulting in relaxation.<br>Starts to act in 10 minutes; effects last 4-6 hours.<br>Monitor vital signs, lung sounds, and peak expiration flow rate (PEFR) before and after each treatment. |
| *If above is not successful:* | |
| Methlyprednisolone (Solu-Medrol) IV: q loading dose, 2 mg/kg or about 125 mg q 6 hr then 60-125 mg q 6 hr for 48 hours total or until patient stable. | Reduces inflammation and edema of airway and decreases hyperactivity of airway.<br>Benefit seen within 6 hours, full effect in 6-8 hours. |
| When patient is *stabilized,* change IV to 60 mg prednisone daily or every other day. | Oral prednisone should be tapered off by 7-10 days. Taper 60 mg over 2 days, 40 mg over 2 days, 30 mg over 2 days, and 10 mg over 2 days. |
| Nebulized atropine sulfate may be tried, or aminophylline may be given IV; a pump is used for better control of infusion. | Relax bronchial smooth muscle. |
| Loading dose of aminophylline: 4 to 6 mg/kg over 15 to 30 minutes and then continuous infusion of 0.45 to 0.70 mg/kg/hr. Patients who have been taking aminophylline at home will be placed on continuous IV therapy. Rate of infusion is determined by theophylline blood level. Desired level is 10 to 20 μg/ml. | *Too rapid an infusion may cause severe hypotension, premature ventricular contractions, and cardiac arrest.*<br>Monitor heart rate and rhythm closely, and report any changes immediately.<br>Theophylline metabolized by the liver. For persons with liver disease, smaller doses are used. Patients taking cimetidine, erythromycin, or ciprofloxacin require smaller doses. Smokers and those taking phenytoin require larger doses to maintain blood levels. |

As a result, more consideration is being given to the role of inflammation as the fundamental process in asthma. Thus inhaled steroids along with inhaled $\beta_2$-adrenergic agents are being ordered more frequently. The use of inhaled steroids ensures that the drugs reach deeper into the lung and do not cause the side effects associated with oral steroids.

It is recommended that the inhaled $\beta_2$-agonist be given first to open the airway, and then the inhaled steroid will be more beneficial.

In one study, patients were given peak-flow meters and taught how to use them. If their peak expiratory flow rate (PEFR) was below 70% of normal, inhaled medication was increased; if below 50%, oral steroids were added; below 30%, emergency measures were called for, and the patient called the physician and went to the emergency room for treatment with oxygen and additional drug therapy.

In Great Britain the use of peak-flow meter regimen was compared with a program based on symptoms alone. Patients were taught what to do if their breathing felt tighter, if they awoke at night with wheezing, if the inhaled bronchodilator lasted less than 2 hours or if relief lasted only 30 minutes, or they had difficulty talking. The study found that the daily use of peak-flow meters made no significant contribution. The important factor was that patients had a systematic way to evaluate their symptoms and knew what to do when they occurred.

The National Heart, Lung, and Blood Institute, which is part of the U.S. Department of Health and Human Services, convened an expert panel of physicians to address the rise in asthma morbidity and mortality. This group, the National Asthma Education Program (NAEP), published guidelines to help in the diagnosis and management of asthma. Box 37-28 presents one of these guidelines, which is addressed to patients.

# NURSING MANAGEMENT

## ♦ ASSESSMENT

### Subjective Data

Data to be collected to assess the patient with asthma include the following:

- History of asthma onset and duration
- Precipitating factors
- Current medications
- Medications used to relieve asthma symptoms
- Any recent changes in medication regimen
- Self-care methods used to relieve symptoms

### Objective Data

Data to be collected to assess the patient with asthma include the following:

1. Assess general appearance.
   a. Does patient appear apprehensive?
   b. Is there any evidence of altered sensorium?
2. Assess vital signs.
   a. Tachycardia
   b. Pulsus paradoxus (diminished pulse with inspiration, confirmed by a 6 to 8 mm Hg drop in systolic blood pressure during inspiration)
   c. Tachypnea
3. Perform pulmonary examination
   a. Inspection

**BOX 37-28 Sample Action Plan for Asthma Episodes: Adults**

Assess severity of the episode by rating the severity of symptoms and/or measuring peak flow.

**MILD EPISODE**

Symptoms: Mild wheeze, cough, chest tightness, shortness of breath occurring with activity but not at rest
Peak flow: 70%-90% of baseline (personal best or predicted, as determined by the clinician)
Actions: Take inhaled bronchodilator. If improved, continue medication on regular basis for 24-48 hours. If not improved, take action as indicated for moderate episode.

**MODERATE EPISODE**

Symptoms: Wheeze, cough, chest tightness, and shortness of breath while at rest; symptoms may interfere with daily activity.
Peak flow: 50%-70% of baseline
Actions: Repeat inhaled bronchodilator every 20 minutes for 1 hour. If improved, continue medication every 3-4 hours for 24-48 hours. If not improved in 2-6 hours after initial treatment, begin or increase prednisone. Contact your clinician.

**SEVERE EPISODE**

Symptoms: Severe shortness of breath, wheeze (wheeze may disappear with very severe episode), cough, and chest tightness at rest; difficulty walking and talking; perhaps retraction of muscles in chest or neck
Peak flow: Less than 50% of baseline and little response to bronchodilator
Actions: Repeat inhaled bronchodilator, 4-6 puffs, every 10 minutes up to 3 times. Begin or increase prednisone. Contact your clinician if available. **If there is no significant improvement after 20-30 minutes, seek emergency care immediately.**

**Be prepared:**

Have a plan for receiving emergency care quickly in the event of a sudden episode. Keep emergency phone numbers handy. Always carry an inhaler of bronchodilator medication with you.

From US Department of Health and Human Services: *National Asthma Education Program Guidelines for the Diagnosis and Management of Asthma,* Washington, DC, 1991, US Government Printing Office.

(1) Accessory muscle breathing
(2) Forward-leaning posture
(3) Dyspnea
(4) Prolonged expiration
(5) Cyanosis

b. Palpation
(1) Decreased lateral expansion
(2) Decreased fremitus

c. Percussion
(1) Hyperresonance
(2) Decreased diaphragmatic excursion

d. Auscultation (NOTE: *as patient approaches exhaustion from increased work of breathing, breath sounds and adventitious sounds may be absent or faint.*)
(1) Inspiratory and expiratory wheezing
(2) Rhonchi

4. Assess laboratory findings.
a. ABGs
(1) Short-term or moderate attack: respiratory alkalosis with mild hypoxemia
(2) Prolonged or severe attack: respiratory acidosis with severe hypoxemia
b. Sputum: for eosinophilia
c. PFT: decreased FEV and VC

## ♦ NURSING DIAGNOSES

Nursing diagnoses are determined from analysis of patient data. Nursing diagnoses for the person with asthma may include but are not limited to the following:

| Diagnostic Title | Possible Etiologic Factors |
|---|---|
| Airway clearance, ineffective | Ineffective technique, decreased energy/fatigue, impaired mucociliary clearance mechanism, inadequate fluid intake |
| Anxiety | Threat of unknown or death |
| Breathing pattern, ineffective | Bronchoconstriction, underuse of bronchodilator medications |
| Gas exchange, impaired | Mucous plugs, V/Q imbalance |
| Knowledge deficit: predisposing factors, prevention, treatment | Lack of exposure to information, unreceptiveness to information, unfamiliarity with information sources |

## ♦ EXPECTED PATIENT OUTCOMES

Expected outcomes for the person with asthma may include but are not limited to the following:

1. Demonstrates effective airway clearance.
   a. Effective methods of coughing
   b. Appropriate use of medication and equipment
2. Demonstrates activities to control anxiety response to symptoms.
   a. Muscle relaxation
   b. Meditation
   c. Appropriate use of medications
3. Demonstrates effective breathing patterns.
   a. Inspiratory/expiratory ratio of 5:10 seconds
   b. Respiratory rate within near-normal limits
4. Demonstrates improved ventilation and oxygenation.

   a. Arterial blood pH and $Paco_2$ that return to or stay within acceptable limits
   b. $Pao_2$ at optimal level for individual
5. Patient or significant other states the factors most likely to precipitate an asthmatic attack (e.g., stress, allergens, infections).
6. Patient or significant other states the importance of keeping a diary of symptoms and medications (time and dose) during an asthmatic attack.
7. If the cause is allergic, states how to prepare an environmentally controlled bedroom.
8. Patient or significant other explains any home medication program.
   a. Gives name, dose, action, and side effects of each medication.
   b. States conditions under which medications might be increased (e.g., infection: start or increase antibiotics; increased stress or worsening of symptoms: increase corticosteroids).
9. Patient or significant other demonstrates how to take inhaled medications (see p. 1127).
10. Patient or significant other describes what to do when an acute attack occurs (e.g., take medication and be quiet).
11. Patient or significant other states signs and symptoms that indicate need for immediate medical attention (e.g., asthmatic attack unrelieved by usual treatment).
12. If receiving corticosteroid therapy, shows card to be carried at all times giving data about the drug, dose, and name of physician; alternative is to wear Medic-Alert bracelet.
13. States plans for ongoing follow-up care, including plans for desensitization if appropriate.

## ♦ INTERVENTIONS

### Administering Medications

1. Give medications as ordered. Monitor IV rates closely.
2. Monitor patient closely for side effects of medications (Table 37-32).

### Improving Airway Clearance

During an asthmatic attack, secretions tend to become viscous and can plug airways, causing increased airway obstruction. By mobilizing secretions, the need for intubation and artificial ventilation can often be prevented.

1. Ensure adequate systemic fluid intake. (NOTE: research findings suggest that overhydration may not increase secretion clearance above levels obtained by normal hydration levels.)
2. Provide adequate nutritional levels.
3. Provide extra humidity.
4. Medicate with bronchodilators.
5. Teach effective cough maneuver (see p. 1136).

**TABLE 37-32 Medications Used in Treatment of Asthma**

| MEDICATIONS | DOSAGE | ACTION | SIDE EFFECTS |
|---|---|---|---|
| Epinephrine 1:1000 | 0.3-0.5 ml subcutaneously, may need to repeat 2 or 3 times at 20 to 30-minute intervals | Short-acting bronchodilator | Tachycardia<br>Palpitations<br>Elevated blood pressure |
| Ephedrine | 25-50 mg PO q 4-6 hr | Long-acting bronchodilator | Cerebral agitation (often given with phenobarbital) |
| Terbutaline | 2.5 mg PO | Bronchodilator | Tachycardia<br>Tremors<br>Headache<br>Spasms in extremities |
| Isoproterenol 0.25% (Isuprel) | 1 or 2 inhalations, q 3 hr (maximum, 8/day) | Bronchodilator | Headache<br>Tremors |
| Metaproterenol (Alupent, Metaprel) | 20 mg PO tid or 1 or 2 inhalations | Bronchodilator | Tachycardia<br>Tremors<br>Nausea |
| Cromolyn sodium (Intal) | 20 mg qid inhaled | Antiasthmatic mast cell stabilizer used as prophylactic against asthma attacks | Nasal congestion<br>Nausea<br>Bronchospasm |
| Corticosteroids | | | |
| Hydrocortisone | 200-400 mg IV (up to 1 g first 24 hours) PO ov IV | Antiflammatory | Corticosteroid withdrawal syndrome, sodium retention, GI disturbance |
| Dexamethasone | Varies with individual response and disease severity | | |
| Beclomethasone | Inhaled: 100 μg 3-4 times/day | | |
| Theophylline | Dosage to maintain serum concentrations of 10-20 μg/ml | Bronchodilator | Nausea and vomiting<br>CNS irritability<br>Tachycardia<br>Hypotension |

6. If cough ineffective to produce sputum, administer chest physiotherapy (see p. 1136).

## Providing Emotional Support and Preventing Anxiety

1. Never leave patient alone during an asthmatic attack.
2. Encourage relaxation techniques.
3. Guide/assist patient with respiratory maneuvers.
4. Assess for possible medication overuse.

## Improving Breathing Patterns

The nursing role in improving breathing patterns and gas exchange is as follows:

1. Place in high Fowler's position.
2. Encourage slow, rhythmic breathing.
3. Encourage patient to breathe through nose and exhale through pursed lips.
4. Administer bronchodilator and antiinflammatory medication as ordered. Monitor patient for both therapeutic response and side effects to medications. Table 37-32 lists medications, dosage, action, and side effects of medications typically used to treat asthma.

## Improving Gas Exchange

Blood gas results should be monitored as follows:

1. If respiratory alkalosis is present, encourage slower breathing.
2. If respiratory acidosis and hypoxemia are present:
   a. Administer oxygen as prescribed.
   b. If oxygen does not relieve the attack, intubation and ventilatory assistance may be required.

## Facilitating Learning

After the patient has recovered from an acute attack, the patient's knowledge about asthma is assessed, and the following points are stressed:

1. Keep a symptom diary (see Box 37-27) to help identify:
   a. Possible precipitating factors
   b. Symptom patterns
   c. Efficacy of self-treatment modalities (include time and dose of any medications self-administered)
2. Signs and symptoms
   a. Tightness in chest
   b. Restlessness or vague feeling of uneasiness
   c. Dyspnea
   d. Increased wheezing
   e. Productive cough
3. Self-treatment of signs and symptoms
   a. Take bronchodilator as ordered.
   b. Take epinephrine if prescribed by physician.
   c. State conditions under which medication might be increased (e.g., infection: start or increase antibiotics, increased stress or worsening of symptoms: increase inhaled corticosteroid).
   d. If another person is not present, call someone so patient will not be alone.
   e. Try to remain calm and breathe slowly; use relaxation techniques at first sign of attack.
   f. If symptoms are not relieved, call physician or go to nearest emergency facility.
4. Know how to use special equipment: MDI (see Guidelines box below, left), inhaler with spacer (see Guidelines box, p. 1127), nebulizer (see Guidelines

### Guidelines for Teaching the Person How To Use a Metered-Dose Inhaler

1. Inhale through nose, then slowly breathe out completely.
2. Place mouthpiece in mouth.
3. Press down on inhaler while simultaneously inhaling one puff deeply. Breathe in air from around the mouthpiece while inhaling.
4. Hold breath for a few seconds, then exhale.
5. Repeat second puff if one is ordered.

*Caution:* Some persons with asthma may experience bronchoconstriction after using a MDI. Patients who complain of chest tightness after using a MDI may be reacting to the propellant gases used to deliver metaproterenol.

### RESEARCH

Janson-Bjerklie S, Shnell S: Effect of peak flow information on patterns of self-care in adult asthma, *Heart Lung* 17:543-549, 1988.

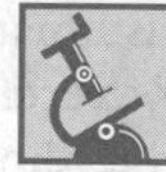

The purpose of this study was to identify self-care strategies used to control asthma symptoms and to determine the effect of peak-flow meter information on selection of self-care strategies. Twenty-eight adults with physician-diagnosed asthma were randomly assigned to a control group ($N = 15$). They were interviewed and instructed to keep an asthma care log. An experimental group ($N = 13$) was interviewed, instructed to keep an asthma care log, and instructed to use and record peak-flow meter rate three times at the beginning and end of each asthma attack. Results indicated that subjects with access to peak-flow meter information used self-treatment strategies less frequently and believed their strategies were less effective than those subjects who depended solely on bodily or emotional sensations to assess their asthma status. The researchers speculated that the physiologic feedback about degree of airway obstruction provided by the peak-flow meter might have promoted more appropriate use of self-treatment modalities or may have limited subjects' use of additional information about their respiratory status that bodily sensations may have provided. The findings suggest that patients can use objective airway obstruction information to guide self-treatment. Patient teaching for people who use peak-flow meters to monitor asthma status needs to include instruction to pay close attention to body sensations and to correlate them with individual peak-flow measurements.

box, p. 1128), and peak-flow meter (see Research box, p. 1149) if one is prescribed.

## ♦ EVALUATION

To evaluate the effectiveness of nursing interventions, compare patient behaviors with those stated in the expected patient outcomes. Successful achievement of patient outcomes for the patient with asthma is indicated by the following:

1. Airway clearance is effective.
   a. Taking a deep breath and blowing it out through pursed lips help to initiate cough reflex.
   b. Inhaled medication is effective in dilating bronchioles, as evidenced by a decrease in wheezing.
2. Patient's anxiety is improved.
   a. Demonstrates muscle relaxation while concentrating on breathing pattern.
   b. Practices meditation after acute symptoms subside.
   c. Listens to soft music.
3. Breathing pattern is effective.
   a. Is concentrating on increasing time of exhalation to twice that of inhalation by counting to 5 seconds for inhalation and 10 seconds for exhalation.
   b. Respirations are quieter and slower at 28/minute.
4. Ventilation and perfusion are improving; $PaO_2$, $PaCO_2$, and pH are returning to patient's baseline levels.
5. States factors most likely to precipitate an asthmatic attack; for example, attacks are frequently exercise induced and are more likely to occur during times of increased stress.
6. Has kept a symptom diary for years, and the cues from a review of it have assisted in reducing the frequency of attacks.
7. Knows name, dose, and side effects of prescribed medications.
8. Has had asthma since childhood. Sleeps in an environmentally controlled room with approved bedding, washable throw rug on hardwood floor, sealed closet doors, and daily damp dusting of furniture and floors. Does not have a dog or cat.
9. Demonstrates correct use of inhaler.
10. Verbalizes steps to take when an acute attack is beginning. Has peak-flow meter and uses it to determine how much bronchodilator to take and how often.
11. Verbalizes when physician needs to be called or when a trip to nearest emergency room is indicated.
12. Wears a Medic-Alert bracelet indicating that he or she takes steroids.
13. Knows importance of ongoing medical follow-up and has appointment for a complete evaluation in 2 weeks.

## CYSTIC FIBROSIS*

### Etiology

Cystic fibrosis (CF) continues to be the most common lethal genetic disease among whites. It is an autosomal recessive disease, and one of every 22 individuals carries the CF gene. When both parents are carriers (heterozygotes), there is a one in four chance with each pregnancy that their child will have CF (Figure 37-25).

### Epidemiology

Approximately 25,000 individuals with CF live in the United States. Of that population, 6500 individuals are adults according to the Cystic Fibrosis Foundation Patient Care Registry. More important, the number of adults with CF continues to increase steadily because of increased life expectancy and diagnostic advances (Figure 37-26).

Two groups make up this adult CF population: (1) those diagnosed when infants and children and (2) adolescents and adults. Statistics indicate that approximately 20% of the adult CF population is diagnosed after age 15.[21]

Reaching adulthood is now a realistic expectation for infants and children with CF. The average life expectancy is 29.4 years with a maximum survival of 30 to 40 years. The major contributing factors to this increased life expectancy include diagnostic advances and therapeutic interventions.

### Pathophysiology

CF is an exocrine gland disease involving various systems (pulmonary, pancreatic/hepatic, GI reproductive). Obstruction of the exocrine gland ducts or passageways occurs in nearly all adult patients with CF. Exocrine gland secretions are known to have a decreased water content, altered electrolyte concentration, and abnormal organic constituents (especially mucous glycoproteins); however, the specific biochemical or physiologic defect that leads to obstruction is not known.

The following physiologic alterations are found in adults with CF.

1. *Pulmonary damage.* Mucus obstruction, inflammation, edema, and smooth muscle restriction of airways are found in this COPD. Changes in the airways predispose the person to respiratory infection, which can be life-threatening. Frequent, recurrent pulmonary infections erode blood vessels, such as brachial arteries, which branch from the aorta and the lung at high pressures and are most at risk for bleeding *(hemoptysis).*

Other complications of damage to the airways include *pneumothorax, respiratory insufficiency,* and *cor pulmonale.* These complications account for 95% of the deaths in adults with CF. The normal function, primary pathophysiology, and clinical manifestations in CF are outlined in Table 37-33.

*The section on cystic fibrosis has been revised by Denise Kresevic and Mary Naccaroto.

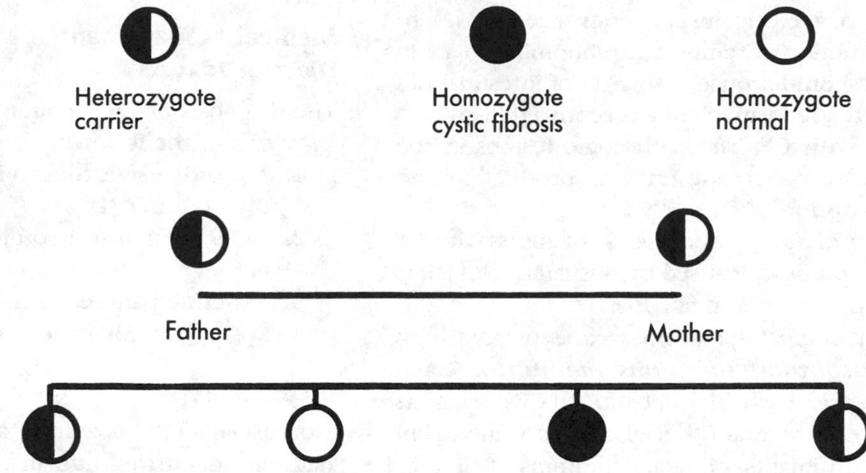


**FIGURE 37-25** Inheritance of cystic fibrosis (CF) when both mother and father are carriers of CF gene. (Modified from *CF Foundation Fact Sheet,* Bethesda, Md, 1980, CF Foundation.)

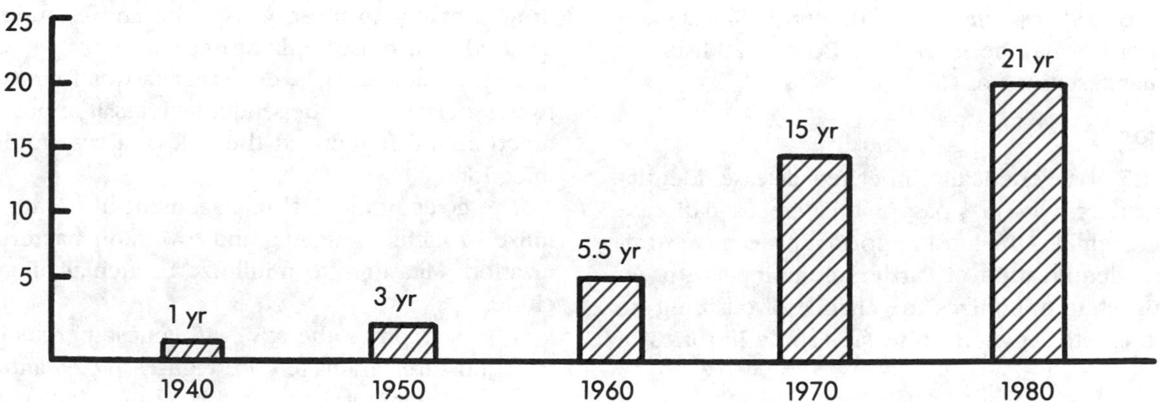


**FIGURE 37-26** Life expectancy of children born with CF. The number of children surviving to adulthood continues to increase. (Modified from *CF Foundation Fact Sheet,* Bethesda, Md, 1980, CF Foundation.)

**TABLE 37-33 Normal Function, Primary Pathophysiology, and Clinical Manifestations in Cystic Fibrosis**

| NORMAL FUNCTION | PATHOPHYSIOLOGY | CLINICAL MANIFESTATIONS |
|---|---|---|
| Mucus production by goblet cells lubricates airways and entraps foreign particles. | 1. Excessive amounts of mucus production | 1. Increased cough and mucus production |
| | 2. Inflammation of small airways, causing hyperinflation of alveoli | 2. Fatigue, shortness of breath |
| | 3. Chronic bacterial infections | 3. Fever, fatigue, shortness of breath |
| | 4. Eroding of a major blood vessel secondary to infection | 4. Hemoptysis |

2. *Gastrointestinal and pancreatic involvement.* Intestinal obstruction occurs in 20% of adult patients with CF. Generally, pancreatic insufficiency predisposes to intestinal obstruction. Cramps and abdominal pain in adults with CF should arouse suspicion of intestinal obstruction. Pancreatic insufficiency is reported in 80% to 90% of adults with CF. The pathologic lesions in the pancreas decrease pancreatic enzyme production and lead to malabsorption of fat.

3. *Glucose intolerance.* About 40% of adults with CF have glucose intolerance caused by obstruction of islets of Langerhans by pancreatic fibrosis.

Three major clinical symptoms are associated with CF: *recurrent respiratory infections, malnutrition,* and *excessive salt losses.* Early identification of CF often rests on the presence of several otherwise unexplained clinical symptoms. In infants, clinical symptoms of CF may include meconium ileus and failure to thrive. Excessive salt losses in infants may first be detected by the infant's mother who reports that the child tastes salty when kissed. Older children should be suspected of having CF when recurrent respiratory infections and failure to thrive despite large appetites cannot otherwise be explained. Excessive salt losses in older children and young adults with CF may be manifested by *heat exhaustion* after exercise or exposure to hot weather, or *dehydration* after fevers. In young adults, the *only* clinical manifestation of CF may be *infertility.* Box 37-29 lists the clinical manifestations of CF.

## Prevention

Because CF is a genetically inherited disease, identification of carriers who may pass on the defect and disease to offspring remains the most important preventive strategy. Early identification of carriers combined with genetic counseling minimizes the chance of offspring inheriting this lethal genetic disease. Family histories of possible incidences of CF should be followed up by genetic testing.

**BOX 37-29 Clinical Manifestations of Cystic Fibrosis**

Specific clinical manifestations by system are listed below. Pulmonary signs and symptoms of CF include:

1. Chronic productive cough and/or recurrent bronchitis or pneumonia
2. Crackles and rhonchi, decreased pulmonary compliance, digital clubbing (Figure 37-27)
3. Shortness of breath and dyspnea on exertion, wheezing, and weight loss occur with respiratory complications and usually indicate need for vigorous therapy.

GI signs and symptoms include:

1. Frequent, bulky, greasy stools
2. Weight loss
3. Cramps and abdominal pain—should arouse suspicion of obstructional obstruction

Glucose intolerance signs and symptoms include:

1. Polyuria, polydipsia, polyphagia
2. Absence of ketoacidosis even with above signs

## Medical Management

### Diagnostic tests

The diagnosis of CF is confirmed by the presence of *at least two* of the following:

1. A positive sweat test with a chloride level greater than 60 mEq/L
2. COPD demonstrated clinically and on chest x-ray film
3. Exocrine pancreatic insufficiency
4. Positive family history of CF

### Medication

Dornase-alfa (Pulmozyme), a recombinant form of the naturally occurring human enzyme deoxyribonuclease I (DNase I), which is responsible for the breakdown of extracellular deoxyribonucleic acid (DNA), was subjected to extensive clinical trials with 968 CF patients before it was approved by the FDA late in 1993.

Dornase-alfa is administered by inserting an ampule in an aerosol mist, compressed air–driven nebulizer. The dose is 2.5 mg in a single-dose ampul daily. The dose may need to be increased in patients over 21 years of age, who may need a second dose daily. Because the drug contains no preservative, the entire ampule must be used or it must be discarded.

In the clinical trials, dornase-alfa was found to have two associated but independent effects: it improved lung function and it reduced the risk of a respiratory tract infection.

The goals of medical management of CF are to minimize bronchial plugging and to inhibit bacterial colonization. Measures to minimize bronchial plugging include:

1. Chest physiotherapy with chest percussion and postural drainage (see Figures 37-23 and 37-24) for 20 minutes two to three times daily and sometimes much more frequently
2. Administration of dornase-alfa, 2.5 mg ampule in compressed air–driven nebulizer
3. Mucolytic agents may be ordered to thin secretions, although ensuring that the patient is well hydrated may be sufficient to thin secretions.

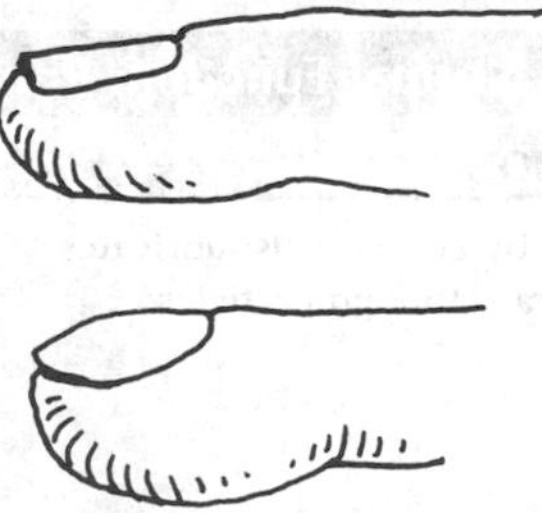

**FIGURE 37-27** Comparison of normal nail *(top)* and digital clubbing *(bottom).*

4. Humidification of air is controversial because it has been associated with bronchospasm and bacterial colonization. It may be helpful for some patients, however, and some physicians may prescribe it.

To minimize bacterial colonization during acute phases of the disease, sputum should be cultured and tested for sensitivity. Antibiotics are prescribed based on the results of these tests. Combination therapy with two or three antibiotics is recommended to prevent bacterial resistance and is usually prescribed for 14 days. Shorter courses of antibiotic therapy are associated with reexacerbation of symptoms. Oral antibiotics may be prescribed for long-term therapy to inhibit bacterial colonization, although there is little scientific basis for this practice. Inhaled antibiotics are given in very high doses because only about 10% of the inhaled drug is absorbed.

### Pulmonary infections

Pulmonary infections compromise respiratory status and usually result in the patient being hospitalized for routine pulmonary physiotherapy or "clean out." This includes:

1. Vigorous postural drainage and clapping. Some patients will spend up to 8 hours a day consumed by clapping, vibrating, and postural drainage (see p. 1146). Mechanical vibrators may be purchased by the patient with CF when physical therapists, nurses, respiratory therapists, or family members are not able to provide the necessary therapy. Most patients must have postural drainage with clapping every 4 hours. Respiratory personnel and nurses share the treatments.
2. Room humidification if ordered.
3. Aerosols with a bronchodilator such as Brokosol R or antibiotics may be administered before postural drainage and clapping.

### Hemoptysis

Hemoptysis occurs when a blood vessel is eroded as a result of pulmonary disease. The patient may expectorate as much as 300 to 500 ml of blood in 24 hours. When a patient with a pulmonary disease such as CF has an uncontrollable urge to cough, this usually indicates blood in the airways from hemoptysis. The patient will be very anxious and should not be left alone.

Nursing and medical care during hemoptysis includes the following:

1. Elevate head of bed 45 to 90 degrees.
2. Turn patient's head to left side to facilitate expectoration of blood.
3. Have emesis basin and tissues ready for expectoration of blood.
4. Provide clean basin frequently so that patient is not made more anxious by amount of blood.
5. Measure amount of hemoptysis and record time and amount.
6. Postural drainage and clapping are contraindicated when hemoptysis is present. Treatment is withheld during acute episodes of bleeding, usually for at least 24 hours.
7. Vitamin $K_1$ (Mephyton) is sometimes ordered by mouth or subcutaneously to control bleeding.
8. Stay with patient until bleeding has subsided and patient is made comfortable and is feeling less fearful.
9. Hemoptysis usually subsides without surgical intervention. If hemoptysis becomes life-threatening, surgical intervention, such as removal of the bronchiectatic lobe, may be necessary. Unfortunately, in most patients, the pulmonary disease is too extensive to permit surgery.[17]
10. Bronchoscopy with endobronchial tamponade may be successful in stopping bleeding in patients with minimal bleeding.

### Pneumothorax

Pneumothorax occurs when apical cysts rupture, allowing air from the lung to enter the pleural space. Sudden sharp chest pain in adults with CF should suggest spontaneous pneumothorax. Pneumothorax occurs in 20% of adult CF patients and has a recurrence rate of 50%. Symptomatic pneumothoraces (increasing shortness of breath, mediastinal shift) are treated with intercostal drainage as follows:

1. Stab wound is made between ribs, and chest tube is inserted.
2. Chest tube is connected to closed drainage system (see p. 1103).
3. After the lung is reexpanded, pleural sclerosis with tetracycline or guinacrine may be used. This procedure causes the visceral pleura to adhere to parietal pleura, obliterating the pleural space.
4. If there is a persistent air leak or pleural sclerosis fails, a partial pleurectomy may be performed. In a partial pleurectomy, the portion of pleura overlying the cysts that ruptured is removed.

### Cor pulmonale

As the airways become progressively plugged, *atelectasis* and *air trapping* occur. The result is a progressive V/Q mismatch, resulting in progressive ***hypoxemia***. Cor pulmonale (right-sided heart failure secondary to pulmonary hypertension) can be expected to develop in patients with cystic fibrosis and advanced lung disease. A resting $PaO_2$ less than 50 mm Hg and a $PaCO_2$ greater than 45 mm Hg usually indicate cor pulmonale. Treatment of cor pulmonale includes the following:

1. Supplemental oxygen to help reverse pulmonary vasoconstriction caused by the hypoxemia and to improve myocardial performance. Oxygen therapy via cannula during sleep is usually prescribed for patients with a daytime resting $PaO_2$ less than 60 mm Hg. Continuous oxygen is prescribed for

patients with daytime resting $PaO_2$ less than 50 mm Hg.

2. Long-term diuretic therapy and fluid restriction may be effective therapy. The patient is monitored closely for electrolyte imbalances.
3. Digoxin is of questionable value in patients with right ventricular failure. However, many patients with CF have biventricular failure, and digoxin may be of therapeutic value. Patients are monitored closely for hypoxemia and hypokalemia, which would increase the risk of digitalis toxicity.

#### Gastrointestinal problems

GI problems are common and are treated as follows:

1. Supplemental fat-soluble vitamins are used to aid digestion and improve weight.
2. Most patients take multivitamins and vitamin E.
3. Pancreatic enzyme supplement doses are individualized and titrated by patients to control fatty stools to less than three per day.
4. When a patient can take nothing by mouth, minimal doses of pancreatic supplements are necessary.
5. If adequate intake cannot be maintained orally, IV feedings or gastrostomy may be necessary.

## NURSING MANAGEMENT

### ♦ ASSESSMENT

Assessment data need to be collected to assess the patient with CF in three areas: pulmonary, nutritional/GI, and psychosocial. Data to be collected in each of these areas include the following:

#### Pulmonary

**Subjective data**

Onset and description of symptoms such as shortness of breath, dyspnea on exertion, fatigue, and wheezing
Patient's understanding of CF pathophysiology and treatment regimens, including postural drainage and clapping; antibiotics; aerosol therapy with dornase-alfa, bronchodilators, and antibiotics; and nutritional supplements such as pancreatic enzymes and vitamins

**Objective data**

Auscultation for adventitious breath sounds
Chest pain on inspiration
Cyanotic mucous membrane
Digital clubbing (Figure 37-27)
Productive cough and color of sputum
Presence of fever, tachypnea
Review ABGs for indications of falling $PaO_2$ or rising $PaCO_2$; review results of pulmonary function tests (decrease in tidal volume, $FEV_1$)
Signs and symptoms of antibiotic toxicity that may cause renal toxicity
Side effects of aerosols (bronchodilators) that may cause tachycardia

#### Nutritional/Gastrointestinal

**Subjective data**

Patient's description of color, consistency, and frequency of stools
Patient's description of color, smell, and frequency of urination
Patient's description of appetite and ability to swallow food
Patient's description of daily eating pattern
Medications taken at home and their effectiveness in decreasing stool frequency
Onset and duration of abdominal discomfort
Signs or symptoms of gastric reflux
Weight loss; when began

**Objective data**

Color, consistency, and frequency of stools
Appears thin
Presence of polyuria, polydipsia, or polyphagia
Dietary intake
Intensity, frequency, and location of abdominal pain
Absence of bowel sounds

#### Psychosocial

**Subjective data**

Description of daily routines as it relates to work or school, pulmonary regimen, medications, and leisure activities
Description of current coping strategies and support network
Concerns about sexuality or fertility
Method of financial support (job, family, other forms of assistance)
Patient and family's understanding of CF

**Objective data**

Identify stage of grieving; symptoms that would infer that patient is grieving: anxiety, sleeplessness, hallucinations.
Identify patient and family strengths.
Identify patient support structure.
Identify normal adult developmental needs (see Chapter 3).
Identify need for genetic counseling, career counseling, social services.

### ♦ NURSING DIAGNOSES

Nursing diagnoses are determined from analysis of patient data. Nursing diagnoses for the adult with CF may include but are not limited to the following:

| Diagnostic Title | Possible Etiologic Factors |
|---|---|
| Airway clearance, ineffective | Obstruction/thick secretions, tracheobronchial infection, hemoptysis |
| Fatigue | Decreased oxygenation, inadequate nutrition, inadequate rest |
| Gas exchange, impaired | V/Q imbalance |
| Grieving, dysfunctional | Loss of fertility/loss of independence/loss of job or role/loss of control of one's life; unhealthy grief work/withdrawal, preoccupation, sleeplessness |
| Infection, high risk for | Increased mucus in airway, decreased nutrition |
| Nutrition, altered: less than body requirements | Pancreatic insufficiency resulting in malabsorption, glucose intolerance/weight loss; shortness of breath makes eating difficult |

## ♦ EXPECTED PATIENT OUTCOMES

Expected patient outcomes for the person with CF may include but are not limited to the following:

1. Has improved airway clearance.
   a. Decreased mucus production
   b. Clear breath sounds
   c. Decreased fatigue and shortness of breath
   d. Absence of fever
   e. Absence of hemoptysis
2. Fatigue is improved.
   a. Oxygenation improved and has less shortness of breath.
   b. Is able to sleep better.
3. Gas exchange is improved.
   a. $PaO_2$ 50 mm Hg or above
   b. $PaCO_2$ less than 45 mm Hg
4. Improves grieving skills.
   a. Verbalizes actual and potential losses.
   b. Identifies own strengths and personal goals.
   c. Identifies support person to assist with coping and achievement of goals.
5. Decreased potential for infection.
   a. Decreased mucus in airway
   b. Environment free of pathogenic bacteria
   c. Nutrition improved
6. Demonstrates improved nutrition.
   a. Maintains weight within 20% of ideal weight.
   b. Maintains normal blood glucose.
   c. Is able to eat small frequent feedings that permit eating when less fatigued and short of breath.

## ♦ INTERVENTIONS

Because the adult with CF is most often admitted to the hospital when the airway is compromised, considerable nursing care is necessary. The care of the adult with CF centers around the following measures.

### Improving Airway Clearance

The nurse's role is as follows:

1. Provide with postural drainage with clapping every 2 to 4 hours, depending on the severity of the infection (see p. 1146).
2. Assist to cough effectively.
3. Assess breath sounds before and after each treatment.
4. Encourage patient to increase fluid intake to 3 to 4 L every 24 hours unless contraindicated.
5. Monitor food intake; provide frequent snacks when energy level is improved.
6. Provide quiet environment with frequent monitoring and reassurance.
7. Maintain cool room with temperature below 70° F (21.1° C).

### Monitoring Fatigue

The nurse is responsible for monitoring the patient's fatigue and instituting methods to improve it.

1. Assess fatigue frequently.
2. Provide rest periods between activities.
3. Provide frequent small feedings, which will increase energy stores.

### Improving Gas Exchange

The nursing role is as follows:

1. Place in high Fowler's position.
2. Encourage slow, rhythmic breathing.
3. Encourage patient to breathe through nose and exhale through pursed lips.
4. Monitor ABG findings.

### Helping the Patient Cope With Grief

The nurse can play a major role in helping the patient work through the grieving process.

1. Identify stage of grieving.
2. Allow time for patient to verbalize feelings, hopes, and fears.
3. Support expressions of hope but avoid false reassurance.
4. Support patient and family through grief work. Recommend CF support group as indicated.
5. Refer as appropriate for genetic counseling, career counseling, or social service.
6. Intervene for pathologic symptoms of grief such as anxiety, sleeplessness, and hallucinations.
7. Be aware of your own feelings of grief and share these with peers or a support group for nurses and other health care providers.

### Monitoring for Infection

Because the adult with CF is very vulnerable to infection or superinfection, the nurse needs to be aware of providing an environment that is as free of pathogens as possible.

1. Monitor patient's temperature frequently.
2. Monitor color, volume, and consistency of sputum.
3. Collect sputum specimens correctly and send for culture and sensitivity as indicated.
4. Give antibiotics as prescribed and on time to maintain adequate blood level.
5. Keep all persons with upper respiratory infections away from patient.
6. Wash own hands frequently and encourage visitors to wash hands before touching the patient.
7. Provide frequent mouth care, especially after postural drainage.
8. Assist patient to wash hands after coughing.

### Promoting Adequate Nutrition

Because the patient with CF often has difficulty in maintaining nutrition, the nurse may need to be ingenious in promoting nutrition.

1. Perform baseline and periodic assessment of nutrition, including food history, recording of daily intake/output and daily weight.
2. Monitor blood glucose levels so that insulin can be given as prescribed according to blood glucose findings.
3. Provide small, frequent feedings.
4. Work with dietitian and patient to provide feedings that will appeal to patient.
5. Administer pancreatic enzymes and vitamins as ordered.

### Facilitating Learning

Because the adult patient has had CF for several years, teaching is more in the form of review and reinforcement. In addition to the teaching guidelines for patients with COPD (see p. 1142), the following areas should be addressed with the patient with CF:

1. Review daily nutrition requirements, vitamins, and the need to check weight daily.
2. Review daily pulmonary exercises and treatments.
   a. Postural drainage and clapping
   b. Aerosol medication before postural drainage
3. Review medications in terms of usual dose, expected effects, and side effects. In some sections of the United States, medications can be obtained at substantial discount through the local Cystic Fibrosis Foundation.
4. Review clinical symptoms that indicate that the health care provider should be notified.
   a. Signs of an acute respiratory infection such as fever, increased fatigue, shortness of breath, increased production of sputum, or change in color of sputum
   b. Hemoptysis
   c. Sudden sharp chest pain
5. Assess patient's knowledge and understanding of fertility, genetic testing, and contraceptive methods.
6. Assess patient and family knowledge of community and social resources for assistance with health care reimbursement programs, disability insurance, and finding an appropriate support group.

## ♦ EVALUATION

To evaluate the effectiveness of nursing interventions, compare patient behaviors with those listed in expected patient outcomes. Successful achievement of patient outcomes for the adult with CF admitted for treatment of a respiratory infection is indicated by the following:

1. Is able to mobilize secretions and clear own airway.
2. Plans daily schedule to allow ample time for activities so that fatigue is avoided.
3. Has $PaO_2$ of 75 mm Hg and $PaCO_2$ of 40 mm Hg.
4. Verbalizes feelings about this latest hospitalization.
5. Has no signs of infection.
6. Is ½ pound below admission weight.

### Complications

#### Respiratory failure

Patients with CF eventually succumb to progressive respiratory and cardiac failure.[17] Because these patients have a fatal disease, they usually have do not resuscitate (DNR) orders and are not intubated or placed on mechanical ventilation. The patient and family have to be involved in the DNR decision, and nurses play an important role in supporting the patient and family in their decision. The median age of death of adults with CF is approximately 22 for women and 28 for men.

### Research

There is considerable ongoing research in CF. Table 37-34 summarizes research projects, findings, and future goals. The identification of the CF gene in 1989 was a major breakthrough and has raised hope for future progress in preventing and treating CF.

## RESPIRATORY INSUFFICIENCY AND RESPIRATORY FAILURE

The terms respiratory insufficiency and respiratory failure describe two states of altered lung function that differ primarily in their degree of severity. **Respiratory insufficiency** exists when the oxygen and carbon dioxide exchange is inadequate to meet the body's needs during normal activities and is usually accompanied by symptoms such as dyspnea. **Respiratory failure** exists when hypoxemia, hypercapnia, and respiratory acidosis exceed predetermined values.

**TABLE 37-34 Research in the Prevention and Treatment of Cystic Fibrosis**

| SUBJECT | TOPIC | FINDINGS | FUTURE GOALS |
|---|---|---|---|
| Prevention | CF gene | Gene identified in 1989: location, size mutations, and defective protein | To define protein structure and function<br>To treat or alter defective protein<br>To identify and change sodium and chloride ion movement in CF cell<br>To identify causes of CF |
| | Vaccinations | | To develop vaccines to prevent lung infections |
| | Genetic counseling | Phosphatase and pancreatic trypsin for neonatal diagnosis | To identify CF carriers—prenatal and neonatal diagnosis |
| Treatment | Antibiotics | Prophylactic use, early use, aerosolized antibiotics, oral route effectiveness | To treat lung infections effectively<br>To decrease side effects of frequent treatment<br>To decrease hospitalizations |
| | Dornase-alfa | Improve lung function, reduce risk of respiratory infections | Same as for antibiotics |
| | Lung transplantation | | To replace damaged lungs |

## ETIOLOGY

Many disorders can lead to or are associated with both respiratory insufficiency and failure (Table 37-35).

## PATHOPHYSIOLOGY

The respiratory system is made up of two basic parts: the gas exchange organ (the lungs) and the pump (the respiratory muscles and the respiratory control mechanisms). Any alteration in the function of the gas exchange unit or the pump mechanism can result in respiratory insufficiency or failure.

Regardless of the underlying condition, the resultant events or processes that occur in respiratory failure are the same. With inadequate ventilation, the arterial oxygen falls, and tissue cells become hypoxic. Carbon dioxide accumulates, leading to a fall in pH and **respiratory acidosis.**

Lung or gas exchange unit respiratory failure is usually seen in persons with underlying primary pulmonary disease such as COPD. In this situation, respiratory failure is a result of pathology directly affecting the respiratory unit.

Pump failure is associated with the extrapulmonary disorders that may precipitate respiratory failure. In this situation the underlying disorder decreases the ability of the lungs to move oxygen and carbon dioxide in and out of the lungs by altering either the central ventilatory control mechanism (e.g., drug overdose), neuromuscular function (e.g., Guillian-Barré syndrome), or chest wall movement (e.g., flail chest).

As indicated earlier, respiratory failure is defined by predetermined physiologic criteria. Box 37-30 lists physiologic parameters that define acute respiratory failure.

Hypercapnia and hypoxemia are present in chronic respiratory failure and respiratory insufficiency. In these disorders the pH usually stays within the range of 7.35 to 7.40 because of compensation. Patients with chronic respiratory failure or respiratory insufficiency develop ***acute respiratory failure*** as a result of a secondary insult to their already compromised pulmonary system, usually

**TABLE 37-35 Disorders Associated With Respiratory Insufficiency and Failure**

| PULMONARY DISORDERS | NONPULMONARY DISORDERS |
|---|---|
| Severe infection<br>Pulmonary edema<br>Pulmonary embolus<br>COPD<br>CF<br>ARDS<br>Cancer<br>Chest trauma<br>Severe atelectasis<br>Airway compromise secondary to trauma, infection, or surgery | CNS disturbance secondary to drug overdose, anesthesia, head injury<br>Neuromuscular disorders (e.g., Guillain-Barré syndrome, myasthenia gravis, multiple sclerosis, poliomyelitis, muscular dystrophy, spinal cord injury)<br>Postoperative reduction in ventilation following thoracic and abdominal surgery<br>Prolonged mechanical ventilation |

**BOX 37-30 Physiologic Criteria for Acute Respiratory Failure**

Sudden onset of:
- $Pa_{O_2}$ 60 mm Hg or less (measured on room air)
- $Pa_{CO_2}$ 50 mm Hg or more
- pH 7.35

in the form of a respiratory infection. The individual can no longer compensate for the altered lung function, and a dramatic decrease in pH (below 7.35), accompanied by severe hypoxemia, occurs. Because carbon dioxide retention (hypercapnia) preexists in these individuals, the $Paco_2$ is less relevant than pH and $Pao_2$ in determining respiratory status. In fact, these patients often display few clinical signs or symptoms, even though they may have major blood gas derangements.

Underlying blood gas alterations are the basis for the clinical signs and symptoms associated with respiratory failure. Box 37-31 lists the common signs associated with hypoxemia, hypercapnia, and respiratory acidosis. The signs and symptoms are presented together because the blood gas derangements causing them usually occur simultaneously.

In acute respiratory failure, there is a marked decrease in vital capacity (VC). However, PFTs are only useful if the patient is alert and able to cooperate. VC can be measured at the bedside with a Wright respirometer. It is important for the nurse to recognize that the signs and symptoms associated with hypoxemia and hypercapnia depend more on the rate of change in value than on absolute value. The patient with COPD may show few signs until severe acute respiratory failure occurs. The normal function, pathophysiology, and clinical manifestations of a person with acute respiratory failure are presented in Table 37-36.

**BOX 37-31 Signs and Symptoms Associated With Hypercapnia, Hypoxemia, and Respiratory Acidosis**

| | |
|---|---|
| Headache | Cardiac dysrhythmias |
| Irritability | Tachycardia |
| Confusion | Hypotension |
| Increasing somnolence, coma | Cyanosis |
| Asterixis (flapping tremor) | |

## PREVENTION

Prevention of both respiratory insufficiency and failure is focused on early identification of persons at high risk of developing either of these disorders. In the inpatient setting, a preventive plan of care should be developed for every person with an increased risk of developing either respiratory insufficiency or failure. A preventive plan of care should include but is not limited to the following:

1. Keeping airway clear
   a. Instituting regularly performed deep-breathing and coughing maneuvers
   b. Nasotracheal suctioning if necessary
2. Optimal activity level
3. Judicious use of sedatives or analgesics
4. Assessing regularly for signs and symptoms indicating deterioration of respiratory status

Persons with COPD have an increased risk of developing respiratory insufficiency or failure as a complication of their chronic disease. They should be counseled to contact their physician if they experience any change in the following:

**TABLE 37-36 Normal Function, Primary Pathology, and Clinical Manifestations in Acute Respiratory Failure**

| NORMAL FUNCTION | PATHOLOGY | CLINICAL MANIFESTATIONS |
|---|---|---|
| **ALVEOLOCAPILLARY MEMBRANE** | | |
| Site of oxygen and carbon dioxide exchange | Interstitial and alveolar edema, airway obstruction from mucus and bronchoconstriction causing inadequate $O_2$ and $CO_2$ transport and exchange, with resultant hypoxemia, hypercapnia, and acidosis | Headache, cardiac arrhythmias, ↑ $Paco_2$, ↓ $Pao_2$, ↓ pH, irritability, cyanosis confusion, tachycardia, hypotension, asterixis (flapping tremor), increasing somnolence with eventual coma |
| **RESPIRATORY MUSCLES** | | |
| Expand and contract chest and lungs | Respiratory muscle strength and endurance unable to counterbalance mechanical load placed on muscles | Increased work of breathing, dyspnea, exhaustion, and ↓ vital capacity |
| **CENTRAL AND PERIPHERAL CHEMORECEPTORS** | | |
| Controls rate and depth of ventilation in response to pH and $CO_2$ in CSF (central) or low levels of $Po_2$ (peripheral) | Decreased or absent response to $CO_2$, pH, or $PO_2$ levels | Increasing somnolence progressing to coma if untreated, worsening hypoxemia, hypercapnia, and acidosis |
| **RIGHT-SIDED CARDIAC OUTPUT** | | |
| Right side: receive unoxygenated blood from systemic circulation and carry deoxygenated blood to lungs for reoxygenation | Increased pulmonary vascular resistance from hypoxemia or lung pathology increases pressure on right side of heart, causing increased venous pressure | Peripheral edema, neck vein distention, hepatomegaly |

**BOX 37-32 Medical Management of Respiratory Failure**

1. Medical therapy is based on degree of severity
   a. Severe acute respiratory failure: focus on immediate oxygenation and ventilation
   b. Less severe acute respiratory failure: underlying cause determined and treated concurrently while treating hypoxemia and hypercapnia
2. Clinical evaluation
   a. Diagnostic studies
      (1) ABGs
      (2) Chest x-ray film
      (3) Bedside pulmonary spirometry
      (4) Sputum for culture and sensitivity (C & S)
   b. Treatment
      (1) Oxygen therapy
      (2) Ventilation: may require intubation and mechanical ventilatory support
      (3) Treatment of complications
      (4) Treatment of underlying cause

1. Sputum production
2. Degree of dyspnea
3. Activity tolerance
4. Changes in ability to think clearly, unexplained irritability, and so on
5. Any change in medications

## MEDICAL MANAGEMENT

Medical management of respiratory failure is presented in Box 37-32.

## NURSING MANAGEMENT

### ♦ ASSESSMENT

#### Subjective Data

Data to be collected to assess the patient with respiratory insufficiency or failure include the following:

1. History of past or present associated disorders (see Table 37-35)
2. Recent onset of change in respiratory status
   a. Change in sputum (color, viscosity, smell)
   b. Increased dyspnea
   c. Change in mental status
   d. Complaints of chest tightness or pain
3. Current medications: any recent changes in medication regimen
4. Self-care modalities

If available, a family member or friend may be able to provide objective information about changes in the patient.

#### Objective Data

Objective data include the following:

1. Assess general appearance.
2. Assess mental status: may vary from agitation to somnolence.
3. Assess vital signs.
   a. Tachycardia
   b. Tachypnea, bradypnea, or apnea
   c. Hypotension
4. Perform pulmonary examination.
   a. Select components of pulmonary examination that patient can tolerate. Findings will depend on underlying cause of respiratory failure.
   b. Assess laboratory findings.
      (1) ABGs for blood gas derangements associated with acute respiratory failure
      (2) Sputum C&S: frequently positive
      (3) Bedside spirometry: VC is less than 15 ml/kg ideal body weight

### ♦ NURSING DIAGNOSES

Nursing diagnoses are determined from analysis of patient data. Nursing diagnoses for the person with respiratory failure may include but are not limited to the following:

| Diagnostic Title | Possible Etiologic Factors |
|---|---|
| Gas exchange, impaired | V/Q imbalance |
| Airway clearance, ineffective | Fatigue, tracheobronchial infection, airway obstruction |
| Cardiac output, decreased | Increased pulmonary vascular resistance |
| Nutrition, altered: less than body requirements | Unable to maintain intake large enough to balance increased metabolic needs from increased work of breathing |
| Knowledge deficit: prevention and treatment | Lack of exposure or recall, cognitive impairment |

### ♦ EXPECTED PATIENT OUTCOMES

Expected patient outcomes for the person with respiratory failure may include but are not limited to the following:

1. Demonstrates improved ventilation and oxygenation.
   a. ABG, pH, and $Paco_2$ return to or stay within acceptable baseline limits.
   b. $Pao_2$ is at optimal level for individual.
   c. Explains how and when to use oxygen therapy.
   d. Sensorium returns to or is maintained at pre–respiratory failure level.
   e. Respiratory rate is within or near to normal levels, with moderate tidal volume.
   f. Absence of dyspnea or dyspnea returns to preacute illness level.
2. Demonstrates effective airway clearance.
   a. Effective coughing maneuvers
   b. Appropriate use of nebulizers, humidifiers
3. Demonstrates adequate cardiac output.
   a. Absence of pulsus paradoxus
   b. Blood pressure within acceptable limits
   c. Heart rate and rhythm within acceptable limits
   d. Pulses equal and present in all extremities
   e. Urine output greater than 30 ml/hr

4. Demonstrates adequate nutritional intake to balance metabolic needs.
   a. Weight stabilizes at pre–acute illness weight.
   b. If preillness weight outside acceptable limits for size and age, weight progresses toward an established goal weight.
5. Describes signs and symptoms that should be reported to the physician.

Patients with underlying COPD also meet the outcome criteria for persons with COPD (see p. 1132).

## ♦ INTERVENTIONS

The level of nursing interventions for acute respiratory failure will depend on the patient's immediate status. The patient's condition may vary from critically ill, requiring immediate life support measures (cardiopulmonary resuscitation), to less urgent, in which aggressive nursing interventions can prevent further deterioration of physical status. Nursing interventions for acute respiratory failure include the following.

### Improving Gas Exchange

#### Oxygenation

Severe hypoxemia is incompatible with life. Thus it is imperative to initiate oxygen therapy rapidly if severe hypoxemia is present. General oxygen therapy is discussed on p. 1134.

The effectiveness of oxygen therapy is evaluated with ABG measurements. Supplemental oxygen should be provided to maintain a $PaO_2$ of 60 to 90 mm Hg. Persons without underlying pulmonary disease can receive oxygen by either high-flow or low-flow systems. However, hazards are associated with prolonged exposure to high concentrations of oxygen.

**BOX 37-33 Oxygen Therapy for the Person With Elevated $PaCO_2$**

Oxygen therapy resulting in elevated $PaO_2$ levels may decrease the ventilatory drive in patients who retain carbon dioxide and are chronically hypoxemic. Decreased ventilatory drive causes hypoventilation, which causes elevated $PaCO_2$ levels, respiratory acidosis, and, ultimately, carbon dioxide narcosis.

*Oxygen toxicity* is the term used to describe the damage to lung tissue that results from prolonged exposure to high oxygen concentrations. Although the exact effects of oxygen in any one individual may depend on the person's underlying pathologic condition, it is believed that exposure to greater than 60% oxygen for more than 36 hours or exposure to 100% oxygen for more than 6 hours will result in atelectasis and alveolar collapse. Breathing very high concentrations of oxygen (80% to 100%) for prolonged periods (24 hours or more) is often associated with the development of ARDS. Thus it is a firm general principle that the lowest amount of oxygen that will achieve an acceptable $PaO_2$ is the amount that should be used.

Special precautions must be taken when administering oxygen to patients with COPD who are carbon dioxide retainers to avoid further elevation of their $PaCO_2$ levels, resulting in carbon dioxide narcosis or coma (Box 37-33).

Patients with COPD (who are carbon dioxide retainers) must receive supplemental oxygen via a low-flow controlled oxygen therapy system. The Venturi mask provides oxygen at controlled ranges of 24% to 40% (Figure 37-28). Low-flow oxygen can also be provided

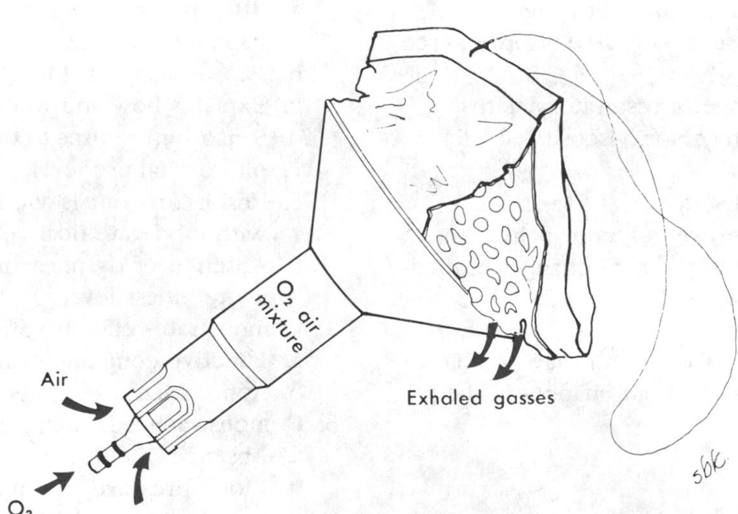


**FIGURE 37-28** Venturi mask allows air to be mixed with oxygen to provide diluted oxygen to patient. (From Wade JF: *Comprehensive respiratory care,* ed 3, St Louis, 1982, Mosby.)

by nasal cannula. However, the actual concentration of oxygen delivered to the lungs by cannula depends on the patient's ventilatory pattern. Regardless of the oxygen delivery system used, the patient's response to oxygen therapy can only be accurately assessed by ABG measurements.

It must be remembered that adequate oxygenation is essential for life. Therefore, if adequate oxygenation cannot be maintained without a concurrent rise in $PaCO_2$ (hypercapnia), oxygen therapy must still be continued. In this situation, mechanical ventilation is instituted to combat the hypercapnia.

Although it is important to realize that carbon dioxide narcosis might be precipitated if a chronically hypoxemic person receives high concentrations of oxygen, research has failed to support this standard clinical practice. Medical research on the effect of administering high oxygen concentrations to patients with COPD who were in respiratory failure showed little change in their respiratory drive. These findings can be balanced in care of the chronically hypoxemic patient in acute respiratory failure by basing practice on the principle that the first priority for survival in a person experiencing acute respiratory failure is to receive adequate oxygen. However, these patients may also be at risk of developing carbon dioxide narcosis; therefore they must be monitored continuously during oxygen therapy in order to intervene if a loss of ventilatory drive should occur.

### Ventilatory support

Ventilatory support is focused on reversing hypercapnia caused by hypoventilation. Aggressive nursing interventions to improve ventilation can often be effective in preventing the need for intubation and artificial ventilatory support (see interventions to improve airway clearance following the discussion on mechanical ventilation).

### Mechanical ventilation

If, despite all the measures discussed, the person is unable to maintain ventilation (as indicated by a rising arterial $PaCO_2$), mechanical ventilation is necessary.

The goal of mechanical ventilation is to deliver a minute ventilation (respiratory rate × tidal volume) with an enriched concentration of oxygen sufficient for adequate tissue oxygenation. The usual tidal volume delivered by a ventilator is in the range of 10 to 15 ml/kg, compared with a spontaneous tidal volume of 5 ml/kg.

Because of the complexity of mechanical ventilation, the ideal place for these patients is in the intensive care unit where experienced nursing staff can care for them. Additionally, ventilators are constantly being improved, and new models are introduced periodically. For this reason, an ongoing staff development program is mandatory. The general principles for care of patients on ventilators follow. However, it must be stressed that a nurse can only become proficient in working with the patient after repeated experience under the preceptorship of more experienced nurses.

Many different kinds of ventilators are available. In general, there are two types: pressure cycled and volume limited. The Bird and Bennett (PR series) are pressure-limited ventilators. They are mainly used for IPPB treatments. Volume-cycled ventilators include the Air Shields, Bennett MA series, Puritan-Bennett 7200 (Figures 37-29 and 37-30), BEAR 2 (Figure 37-31), Emerson, Engstrom, Ohio 560, and Siemens-Servo. Table 37-37 lists the types of ventilators and their mode of function.

**Volume-cycled ventilators** are currently the most often used. They provide a wide range of flexibility to meet individual requirements for adequate oxygen and carbon dioxide exchange. Box 37-34 lists the functions that can be adjusted on the volume-cycled ventilator.

With a volume-cycled machine a *constant volume* of air is delivered with each breath. The volume is preset and is delivered to the patient at whatever pressure is necessary to attain that volume. A volume-cycled machine should have a pressure cutoff valve. Such a mechanism allows a pressure limit to be set. If the pressure required to deliver the set volume exceeds the pressure limit, the machine will turn off before the entire volume is delivered. The pressure limit on a volume-cycled ma-

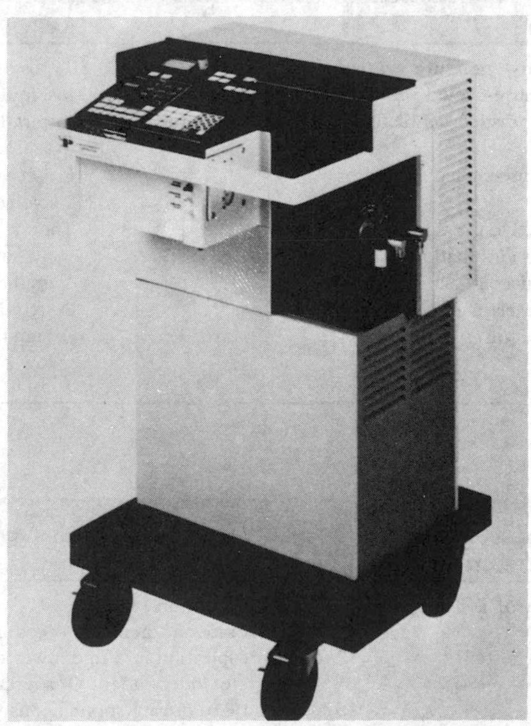

FIGURE 37-29 Puritan-Bennett 7200 ventilator shown with optional pedestal and compressor. (Courtesy Puritan-Bennett Corp, Kansas City, Mo.)

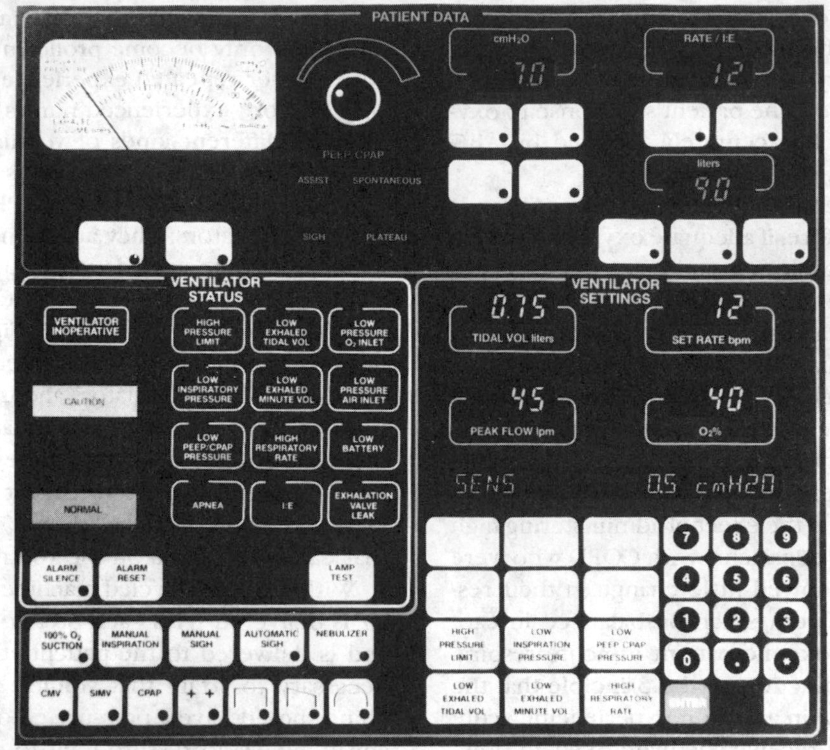


**FIGURE 37-30** Control panel of Puritan-Bennett 7200 microprocessor ventilator. (Courtesy Puritan-Bennett Corp, Kansas City, Mo.)

## TABLE 37-37 Types of Mechanical Ventilators

| TYPES | | BASIC FUNCTION MODE |
|---|---|---|
| Positive-pressure ventilator | Require intubation | Types of positive-pressure ventilators are based on how inspiratory phase is ended. |
| Pressure-cycled ventilator | | Inspiration ends at a preset pressure limit; time and volume are variable. |
| Time-cycled ventilator | | Inspiration is preset for a given time interval; volume and pressure are variable. |
| Volume-cycled ventilator | | Preset volume of air is delivered. Time and pressure are variable. However, volume-cycled ventilators often have pressure- and time-cycled capacities. |
| Negative-pressure ventilator (intubation not required) | | Thorax, at least, is encapsulated. When ventilator expands, it creates negative pressure by pulling the thorax outward. Air rushes into the airways because of the pressure gradient created. |
| High-frequency ventilation (requires intubation) | | System is still under clinical investigation. There are several variants of this system. All high-frequency ventilators use high respiratory rates to deliver small tidal volumes at low pressures. |

## TABLE 37-38 Control Modes of Volume-Cycled Ventilators

| VENTILATORY MODE | FUNCTION | RESPIRATORY STATUS |
|---|---|---|
| Control/assist | Cycles inspiration<br>Controls rate and depth of breathing | Apnea<br>Used for person requiring PEEP |
| Intermittent | Cycles inspiration at a rate lower than patient's respiratory rate; independent $O_2$ source maintains predetermined $FiO_2$ during spontaneous ventilation | Patients who have spontaneous but inadequate ventilatory drive; also used to wean patient from ventilator |
| PEEP | Increases volume of air in lungs at FRC, thus alveoli that would collapse are kept open to increase gas exchange; used either with control/assist or IMV mode | Used for patients who are hypoxemic; increases $PaO_2$ at lower $FiO_2$; effective with decreased lung compliance; can cause dangerous decrease in cardiac output in presence of increased lung compliance |

$FiO_2$, Fraction of impaired $O_2$; FRC, functional residual capacity; IMV, intermittent mandatory ventilation (see Chapter 35).

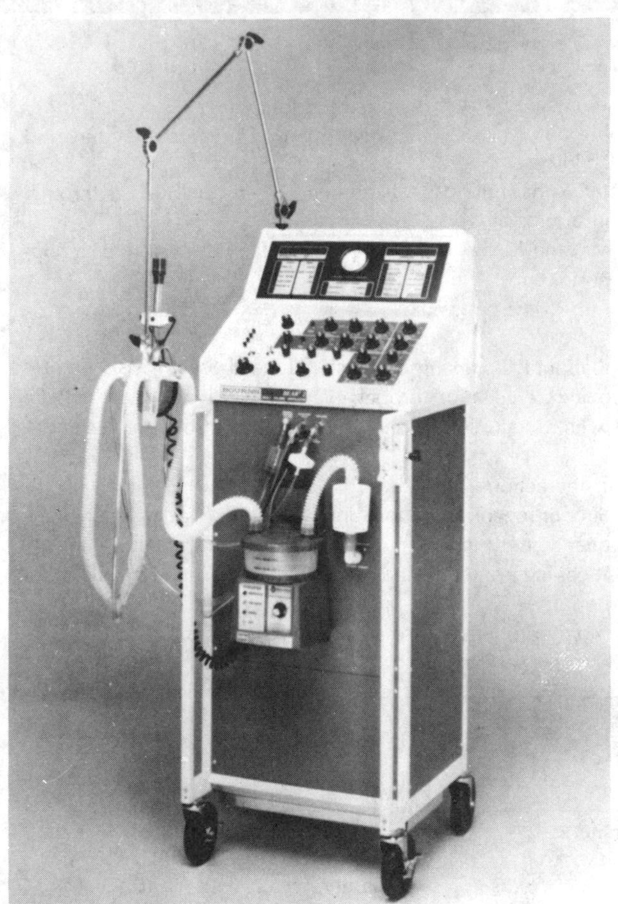

**FIGURE 37-31** BEAR 2 adult volume-cycled ventilator. (Courtesy BEAR Medical Systems, Inc, Riverside, Calif.)

chine usually has an audible alarm. The nurse can set the limit slightly above (approximately 5 cm of water) the pressure required to ventilate the patient. The alarm will then go off if the patient coughs, accumulates secretions, or starts to resist the machine.

Regardless of which type of ventilator is used, mechanisms for various regulations are necessary if the machine is to be adjusted to each patient. It is preferable to have a ventilator that can be used to assist or control the patient's breathing. *Assist* means that the *patient's own inspiratory effort triggers* (turns on) *the machine.* Most respirators have a *sensitivity control knob* that can be adjusted to respond to weak inspiratory efforts. *Control* implies the use of *automatic cycling.* The patient may be apneic and the machine set at the desired rate; the patient's own respiratory rate may be too slow, and the automatic cycling can be used to force an increase in the rate; or the patient's own respiratory efforts can be ignored and an automatic rate used to ventilate the patient. (Some machines with automatic cycling do not allow for the latter adjustment.) It is also helpful to be able to regulate the flow rates at which the gas is delivered to the patient. For example, patients breathing

**BOX 37-34 Functions That Can be Adjusted With Volume-Cycled Ventilators**

Tidal volume—volume of air in a normal breath

$FiO_2$—oxygenation concentration delivered through the ventilator

Alarm systems—vary from machine to machine; basic alarms usually present are:

1. High-pressure alarm—increased resistance somewhere in system from lungs to machine
2. Low-pressure alarm—system not reaching minimal pressure required for ventilation
3. Low-volume alarm—when volume of ventilation does not equal the amount set

Control modes—degree of ventilation that is controlled by the ventilator; can vary from complete ventilator control to almost total patient control (Table 37-38)

at rapid rates and high volumes need faster flow rates than those breathing slowly and at moderate volumes. A final necessity is the ability to regulate the inspired concentration of oxygen from 20% (room air) to 100%.

**Positive-end expiratory pressure.** Positive end-expiratory pressure (PEEP) is a ventilator mode that has been shown to increase the effectiveness of mechanical ventilation in certain patients. PEEP involves the maintenance of positive pressure at the end of expiration, rather than allowing airway pressure to return to normal (atmospheric) as usually occurs (Figure 37-32, *A*). By maintaining positive pressure, alveoli that would otherwise collapse on expiration are held open, thus increasing the opportunity for gas exchange across the alveolocapillary membrane. This is accomplished by the increase in FRC. The result is a decrease in physiologic shunting and the ability to achieve a higher level of $PaO_2$ with lower concentrations of delivered oxygen ($FiO_2$). PEEP has its greatest use in the treatment of ARDS but is also used in treating any patient who would otherwise require unacceptably high concentrations of oxygen.

PEEP can be hazardous because of the increase in intrathoracic pressure. Most serious of the dangers related to PEEP is the increased incidence of pneumothorax, particularly in those with friable lung tissue, as seen in persons with emphysema or lung cancer. The sudden disappearance of breath sounds on one side, in conjunction with signs of respiratory distress, in the patient being ventilated with PEEP *must be taken as an indication of a pneumothorax.* This can develop into a life-threatening episode if the pneumothorax is large, and the physician must be called immediately. Another less serious consequence of PEEP may be a reduction in venous return, caused by the increased intrathoracic pressure, and a subsequent fall in cardiac output. This effect seems to be particularly common in patients who are relatively dehydrated and can sometimes be avoided by careful fluid administration. (See accompanying Nursing Care Plan.)

# NURSING CARE PLAN

## PERSON ON MECHANICAL VENTILATION WITH PEEP

**DATA:** Mr. R. is a 28-year-old married male admitted to the surgical intensive care unit after a motor vehicle accident. Injuries sustained include a ruptured spleen and liver laceration resulting in hypovolemic shock. Mr. R. was taken to the operating room, where his injuries were repaired and blood losses replaced. His early postoperative course was unremarkable. On Mr. R.'s third postoperative day, he began to experience some respiratory difficulties with a deterioration in his ABGs. Because of severe hypoxemia, Mr. R. was intubated. His chest x-ray film revealed diffuse interstitial and alveolar infiltrates. He had developed ARDS and eventually required PEEP.

Mr. R.'s wife visited her husband daily and often attempted to communicate with him. She would reassure and calm him when he became anxious and resisted the ventilator. Mrs. R. would ask the nurse many questions about her husband's status.

The nursing history identified the following:

- Mr. and Mrs. R. have been married 5 years; they have no children.
- Mr. R. has full hospitalization and medical coverage through insurance at work.
- Mr. and Mrs. R. come from large families that appear supportive.
- Mr. R. is a nonsmoker.

Collaborative nursing actions include those to assist in improving oxygenation through evaluating $FIO_2$ and levels of PEEP as well as techniques used to wean Mr. R. from the ventilator.

Nursing actions include:

- Supporting oxygenation and ventilation to maintain $PaO_2$ over 60 mm Hg and to maximize functional residual capacity
- Weaning from $FIO_2$ and levels of PEEP gradually while monitoring ABGs
- Monitoring patient for signs of hypoxia

### ■ NURSING DIAGNOSIS

Impaired gas exchange related to ARDS

| Expected Patient Outcome | Nursing Interventions | Rationale |
|---|---|---|
| Remains adequately oxygenated, as evidence by:<br>1. $PaO_2$ on ABG >75 mm Hg<br>2. Adequate color<br>3. Adequate peripheral circulation | Monitor ABGs to determine $PaO_2$.<br>Suction only when necessary to prevent loss of PEEP secondary to disconnection from ventilator.<br>Monitor required levels of PEEP and $FIO_2$.<br>Assess peripheral circulation for pulses, color of extremities and warmth.<br>Monitor mixed venous blood oxygen levels. | ARDS is an acute lung injury that results in increased capillary permeability, which permits proteins and fluids to leak out into alveoli and interstitial spaces, thus preventing normal gas exchange to occur. |

### ■ NURSING DIAGNOSIS

Decreased cardiac output related to decreased venous return

| Expected Patient Outcome | Nursing Interventions | Rationale |
|---|---|---|
| Does not experience hemodynamic compromise related to PEEP. | Monitor vital signs q h and as needed.<br>Monitor hemodynamic parameters for signs of decreased cardiac output, hypotension, elevated CVP, and oliguria.<br>Monitor intake and output.<br>Check peripheral circulation every 2 to 4 hr and as needed.<br>Elevate foot of bed 10 to 20 degrees to encourage venous return.<br>Perform passive range of motion exercises q 4 to 6 hr to encourage venous return.<br>Administer adrenergic agents as ordered to improve cardiac output.<br>Notify physician of hemodynamic complications. | PEEP may cause decreased cardiac output by increasing intraalveolar pressures, thereby decreasing venous return to the heart. |

# NURSING CARE PLAN

## PERSON ON MECHANICAL VENTILATION WITH PEEP—cont'd

### ■ NURSING DIAGNOSIS

Ineffective breathing pattern related to altered lung/thoracic pressure relationship

| Expected Patient Outcome | Nursing Interventions | Rationale |
|---|---|---|
| Does not experience pulmonary complications secondary to PEEP:<br>1. Atelectasis<br>2. Pneumothorax<br>3. Pneumomediastinum<br>4. Subcutaneous emphysema | Monitor respirations q-h and as needed.<br>Assess breath sounds for adventitious findings.<br>Administer pulmonary toilet q 2 hr and as needed:<br>1. Frequent turning<br>2. Chest physiotherapy<br>Monitor for signs of pulmonary complications and respiratory distress:<br>1. Asymmetric chest excursion<br>2. Sudden sharp pain<br>3. Cyanosis<br>4. Anxiety<br>Assess for subcutaneous emphysema.<br>Keep chest tube set up at bedside.<br>Monitor ABGs as needed.<br>Notify physician of respiratory complications. | When walls of alveoli cannot withstand the positive pressure from PEEP, perforation may occur.<br>As a result, air leaks into the pleural space, mediastinum, and/or its subcutaneous space.<br>The result is a pneumothorax, pneumomediastinum, or subcutaneous emphysema, respectively. |

### ■ NURSING DIAGNOSIS

Altered nutrition less than body requirements related to intubation

| Expected Patient Outcome | Nursing Interventions | Rationale |
|---|---|---|
| Receives adequate nutritional intake while intubated. | Administer hyperalimentation or arterial feedings as prescribed.<br>Monitor intake and output.<br>Weigh daily.<br>Administer albumin or volume expanders as prescribed.<br>Monitor serum albumin level. | Nutritional status must be maintained to assist in weaning process; proteins and volume expanders will increase serum colloidal osmotic pressure, thus maintaining fluid in the intravascular compartment. |

### ■ NURSING DIAGNOSIS

Anxiety related to ARDS, intubation, and discomfort from PEEP

| Expected Patient Outcome | Nursing Interventions | Rationale |
|---|---|---|
| Mr. and Mrs. R. exhibit behavioral signs of decreased stress and anxiety. | Assess for signs of anxiety.<br>Explain ARDS to family, including rationale for mechanical ventilation and PEEP.<br>Allow Mr. and Mrs. R. to express concern and fears.<br>Explain procedures before performing them.<br>Provide comfort measures.<br>Provide for a means of communication between Mr. R. and his wife.<br>Attempt to anticipate their needs.<br>Administer light sedation/antianxiety medications if necessary, as ordered. | Intensive care unit, mechanical ventilation, the inability to communicate, and fear of the unknown all contribute to feelings of stress and anxiety for the patient in the ICU as well as significant others. |
| | Attempt to calm and reassure Mr. R. if he begins to "buck" or resist the ventilator.<br>Provide Mr. R. and his wife distraction from the ICU environment:<br>■ Soft music, TV<br>■ Breaks from the ICU for Mrs. R. | Positive-pressure exhalation is often uncomfortable for the patient, who often responds by resisting ventilator. |

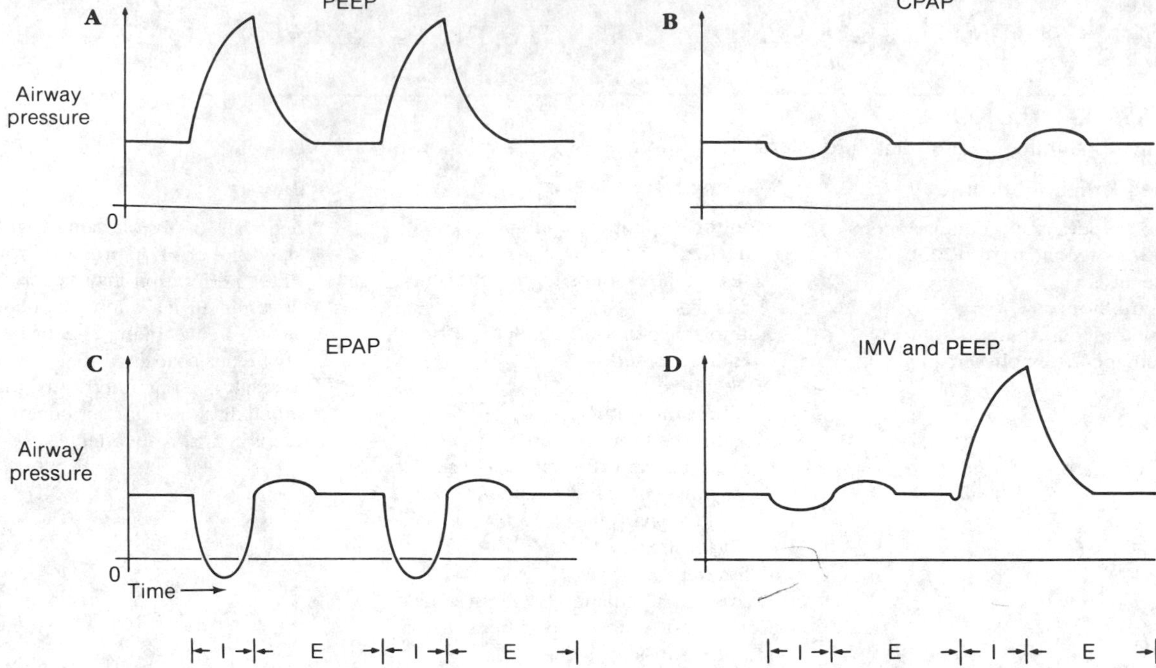


**FIGURE 37-32** Four forms of positive expiratory pressure. End positive airway pressure (EPAP) is not used in clinical practice. (From Dupuis YG: *Ventilators: theory and clinical applications,* ed 2, St Louis, 1992, Mosby.)

**Continuous positive airway pressure.** Continuous positive airway pressure (CPAP) is a technique that maintains positive pressure in the lung during spontaneous ventilation (Figure 37-32, *B*).[36]

CPAP is used most often with spontaneously breathing patients, although it also can be delivered through the tubing circuits of a volume-controlled ventilator. CPAP maintains positive pressure at the end of expiration. In this way it is similar to PEEP, which is used only for patients being mechanically ventilated. With CPAP, expiration is controlled by a valve in the expiratory circuit that measures airway pressure and stops expiration before airway pressure returns to zero.

One disadvantage of CPAP is that the work of breathing may be increased because of resistance in initiating gas flow. The level of CPAP chosen should be as low as possible to obtain a $Pao_2$ greater than 60 mm Hg with a relatively safe $Fio_2$ of less than 0.6. With CPAP there is lack of backup mandatory ventilation, and careful monitoring of oxygen saturation with oximeters is very important. Respiratory rates, level of agitation, and ABGs must be monitored to prevent unrecognized hypercapnia.

**Pressure support ventilation.** Pressure support ventilation (PSV) is another mode of ventilation. It relies on patient effort to determine tidal volume and frequency. This mode differs from CPAP in that the patient's inspiratory efforts trigger ventilator airflow until a preset airway pressure is reached. Airflow continues as long as the patient is making sufficient inspiratory effort to keep airway pressure below the preset limit. The advantages of pressure support ventilation may include overcoming the circuit-resistance breathing associated with spontaneous breathing through a ventilator. By decreasing the level of "pressure support" over time, this mode of ventilation can be an effective weaning technique.

**Biphasic airway pressure.** A recent addition to the ventilator mode is biphasic airway pressure (BiPAP), which delivers pressure support ventilation (PSV) for inspiration and CPAP on expiration. It is used primarily to assist breathing during sleep for patients with neuromuscular disorders such as muscular dystrophy and central sleep apnea. To deliver BiPAP, a small mask is fitted over the nose. The use of BiPAP during sleep allows the patient to obtain a restful night's sleep and to awake feeling more refreshed.

**Suctioning the patient.** When the patient on a ventilator needs suctioning, a closed system is preferred. In closed-system endotracheal suctioning, an adaptor is inserted at the endotracheal tube–ventilatory circuitry interface. This allows patients to be suctioned without disconnecting them from the ventilator. The potential benefits of this form of suctioning are (1) continuation of oxygen supply and (2) the stability of PEEP.

**General care of the person on a ventilator.** When care is planned for the patient on a mechanical ventilator, it is imperative to know the patient's ability to breathe spontaneously in the event of accidental disconnection from the ventilator. In most facilities, respiratory therapists regularly monitor ventilator function and settings, but the nurse is also responsible for ensuring that the ventilator settings are maintained. Usually a checklist is used to verify the ventilator settings on an hourly basis.

The patient should be assessed on a regular basis and any time a ventilator alarm sounds. The cause of an alarm sounding can be a dysfunction anywhere from the person's lungs to the machine. Trouble-shooting should be carried out in a systematic manner, starting with the patient and moving toward the machine. Assessment should include the following:

1. Patient assessment
   a. Inspection
      (1) Does the person appear to be in respiratory distress?
      (2) Is the person's chest moving with machine-cycled inspiration?
      (3) Is the chest moving bilaterally?
   b. Auscultation
      (1) Are breath sounds present?
      (2) Are adventitious sounds present?
      (3) Are breath sounds coordinated with ventilator inspiration?
2. Tubing to machine assessment: inspection
   a. Is there an air leak around the endotracheal cuff?
   b. Is there excess condensation in the tubing? (Always remove water from tubing system. Do not empty back into humidifier reservoir). NOTE: Not all ventilators have humidifiers.
   c. Check all ventilator settings and readouts.

If the alarm continues to sound and the cause cannot be determined or the patient is in respiratory distress, the patient is disconnected from the machine and manually ventilated with an AMBU bag (or anesthesia bag) with oxygenated air until the problem can be resolved.

**Weaning from the ventilator.** The decision to wean a person from the ventilator is based on clinical evidence of improved physical status. Weaning is most successful when performed by a nurse who has developed a trust relationship with the patient. Underlying pathology that compromised the patient's respiratory status must be stabilized. Weaning is initiated when the patient meets certain physiologic criteria such as:

1. Acceptable ABGs
2. Tidal volume greater than 10 ml/kg
3. VC greater than 15 ml/kg
4. $FiO_2$ less than 0.5
5. Maximal inspiratory pressure greater than −20 (usually prefer −30 to −40)
6. Normal hematocrit. Most patients on long-term ventilator support have hematocrits below 30. They are usually not transfused unless their hematocrit falls to about 25. There is general agreement that weaning is more successful if the patient's hematocrit is 30 or higher.

The weaning process should be individualized to meet the patient's needs. The three major methods of weaning are as follows:

1. T-piece weaning
   a. Place patient in upright sitting position.
   b. Deflate endotracheal or tracheostomy cuff.
   c. Disconnect patient from ventilator.
   d. Connect a T piece (Figure 37-8) to endotracheal tube cuff to provide oxygenated humidified air.
2. Intermittent mandatory ventilation (IMV) weaning (particularly useful for the person who is difficult to wean from the ventilator). Figure 37-32, *D,* illustrates IMV and PEEP. In comparing *A* and *B* of Figure 37-32, it can be seen that IMV and PEEP are a combination of PEEP and CPAP.
   a. Patient remains connected to the ventilator. The number of mandatory breaths delivered by the machine is gradually reduced, allowing the patient to take an increasing number of breaths independently.
   b. Patient is disconnected from the ventilator when predetermined physiologic criteria are maintained.
3. PSV as previously described. It is a newer method and less widely used than IMV or T-piece weaning. This mode can be used alone or with IMV.

A recent article on weaning divides the process into three phases: *preweaning, weaning,* and *extubation.*

During the *preweaning* stage, special attention is given to ensuring that the patient will have normal electrolytes, including phosphate, calcium, and magnesium. Malnutrition is to be avoided, but the patient should not be overfed. Overfeeding with carbohydrates and extra calories may result in increased carbon dioxide production and increased ventilatory demand. The recommended 24-hour caloric intake is 1500 to 2500 calories, which should ensure adequate calories for energy expenditure. Protein intake is important and 1 to 1.5 mg/kg has been suggested. Tube feedings containing these requirements are given to prepare the patient for weaning. Nursing interventions during the weaning process include the following:

1. Before initiating weaning, prepare the patient. Teach effective breathing techniques. Inform the patient that weaning may take several attempts.
2. Obtain baseline vital signs, tidal volume, and vital capacity.
3. Stay with the patient during the initial weaning process.
4. Coach the patient as needed to breath slower and deeper with emphasis on increasing the time of exhalation.

5. Suction as needed.
6. Monitor for the clinical signs of hypoxemia and hypercapnia (tachycardia, dysrhythmias, increased blood pressure, agitation, diaphoresis, or increased somnolence).
7. If patient cannot breathe on own, reconnect to ventilator.
8. Weaning may require several attempts for longer periods of time before the ventilator can be disconnected.

Several authors have suggested that success in weaning is determined more by the ability of the respiratory muscle to cope with an increased respiratory workload than any other factor.[39]

**Failure to wean successfully.** There are several reasons why some patients cannot be weaned from a ventilator. These include congestive heart failure, prolonged muscle weakness, diaphragmatic paralysis (occurs when the phrenic nerve is severed unintentionally during cardiac surgery), and COPD, which is discussed previously in this chapter.

**Care of the patient who cannot be weaned.** For those patients who are unable to be weaned from the ventilator, there are three options available to them. In a conference with the patient and his or her significant others, there needs to be a clear discussion of each of the options. These options are (1) being discharged home on the ventilator, (2) being discharged to a nursing home on the ventilator, or (3) being taken off the ventilator and allowed to die (terminal weaning).

Very few patients find it possible to go home on a ventilator because of the lack of suitable space and the lack of a significant other who can assume responsibility for the ventilator 24 hours a day for 7 days a week. If the patient is economically well off, he or she may be able to employ a nurse to provide 24-hour care at home. If the patient and significant others decide on the patient being discharged home, careful planning is required to ensure that the home can accommodate the patient and the necessary equipment. The assessment of the home is best made by a nurse from a health care agency that will be following the patient and monitoring care at home. (See Chapter 27 for more information on home health nursing care.)

The option of being discharged to a nursing home does not appeal to many patients. Also, not all nursing homes can accommodate patients on ventilators, and those who can usually have a limited number of beds for these patients.

The option of being taken off the ventilator and being allowed to die is being chosen by an increasing number of patients. Once the patient indicates that this is his or her choice, the care team meets to discuss how the patient's wishes can best be accommodated. Most patients elect to have a significant other(s) with them when the ventilator is removed. A morphine drip is usually started before the ventilator is disconnected to ease the patient's anxiety. A recent article by the daughter of a man who chose terminal weaning gives a moving account of the experience.[6] In the article she describes her own struggle with her father's decision and points out:

> Finally, Dad confronted the truth: his lungs could never sustain him without the ventilator. He had struggled long and he fought hard, but in the end he knew that if he could not live independently, he did not want to live at all. He made his decision to be disconnected from the ventilator and, as difficult as it was, we all supported him.

## Improving Airway Clearance

Airways clogged with excess mucus are one of the most reversible components precipitating acute respiratory failure. Nursing interventions that promote a patent airway and can prevent deterioration of respiratory status include:

1. Effective cough maneuvers
   a. Have patient sit upright.
   b. Inhale slowly through the nose.
   c. Lean forward and exhale slowly through pursed lips to promote open airways.
   d. Repeat these steps several times to mobilize secretions and move them upward in the airway.
   e. Take a slow maximal inhalation through the nose when secretions reach the oropharynx. During exhalation, use short repeated coughs to minimize bronchospasm.
   f. Inhale maximally after coughing to reinflate alveoli.
2. A sufficient fluid intake to mobilize secretions (From 3 to 4 L, unless contraindicated, has traditionally been encouraged, but some evidence suggests that this quantity may not be needed.)
3. Frequent deep-breathing exercises
4. Position changes every 2 hours
5. Elevation of head and chest
6. Nasotracheal suctioning if patient is unable to cough effectively (see Chapter 36).

## Improving Breathing Pattern

Nursing interventions for patients in acute respiratory failure must be implemented in a firm, assured, but empathetic manner. The patient may be agitated or nearly exhausted from hypoxemia, hypercapnia, and the increased work of breathing. It is imperative that the patient be gently guided in respiratory maneuvers to improve breathing. The nurse must be alert for signs and symptoms indicating that the patient's condition has changed from acutely ill but adequately ventilating to critically ill with insufficient ventilation to maintain body functions. Nursing interventions include the following:

1. Encourage forward-leaning postures (see Figure 37-20).
2. "Coach" patient to a slow, rapid respiratory rate and to avoid gulping large quantities of air.
3. If ordered, assist with IPPB treatments. Although the therapeutic effect of IPPB has been questioned, the treatment, at least for the short term, helps to slow respiratory rate and decreases the work of breathing.

### Improving Cardiac Output

Decreased cardiac output may be a complication of acute respiratory failure or may be a precipitating factor related to underlying *cor pulmonale*. Diminished cardiac output causes tissue hypoxia, which creates a metabolic acidosis in addition to the respiratory acidosis caused by the respiratory failure. Specific aspects of care include the following:

1. Limiting fluid intake as ordered
2. Monitoring for signs of inadequate tissue perfusion (urine output less than 30 ml/hour, cool extremities with decreased peripheral pulses)
3. Administering medications as ordered

See Chapter 31 for detailed care of the patient with decreased cardiac output.

### Maintaining Adequate Nutrition

Individuals with acute respiratory failure are at increased risk for nutritional deficits because of the increased work of breathing. Nursing interventions are the same as those for the patient with COPD (see p. 1133). Additional aspects of care must be considered for patients who require mechanical ventilatory support. The overall focus of nutritional interventions is to prevent or correct malnutrition. Nutritional intake affects ventilatory drive, respiratory muscle function, and the amount of oxygen consumed and carbon dioxide produced from metabolic processes. Persons who have fasted for a few days or have been maintained on 5% dextrose intravenously may have severely depleted glycogen stores necessary for adequate respiratory function. Thus nutritional status can have a major impact on the individual's ability to be successfully weaned from the ventilator. Actions must focus on providing appropriate nutrition to meet their specific metabolic needs while on the ventilator and during and after weaning from it. Nutritional support by either enteral supplementation or parenteral hyperalimentation may be necessary. Whenever feasible, the GI route should be used rather than parenteral therapy because it poses fewer risks and is more economical.

### Facilitating Learning

Patients with respiratory failure who have underlying COPD require the same interventions as those listed in Box 37-32.

If respiratory failure is a complication of a disease other than COPD, the patient's knowledge needs to be assessed as to causative and contributing factors. Appropriate teaching is then instituted. All patients need to be able to explain home-going medications and treatments and plans for follow-up care.

## ♦ EVALUATION

To evaluate the effectiveness of nursing interventions, compare patient behaviors with those listed in expected patient outcomes. Successful achievement of patient outcomes for the patient with respiratory insufficiency or respiratory failure is indicated by the following:

1. Demonstrates improved ventilation and oxygenation.
   a. $Pa{O_2}$, $Pa{CO_2}$, and pH have returned to patient's baseline level.
   b. Is able to maintain $Pa{O_2}$ at optimal level.
   c. Verbalizes how and when to use oxygen therapy (when exercising, when feeling very fatigued).
   d. Is able to think and speak clearly.
   e. Respiratory rate is 20.
   f. Dyspnea is greatly improved.
2. Demonstrates effective airway clearance.
   a. Coughs effectively and does not tire self with ineffective coughing.
   b. Uses inhaler correctly.
3. Demonstrates adequate cardiac output.
   a. Pulsus paradoxus is absent.
   b. Blood pressure is stable.
   c. Heart rate and rhythm are within acceptable limits.
   d. Pulses are equal and present in all extremities.
   e. Urine output is 40 to 50 ml/hour.
4. Demonstrates adequate nutritional intake to balance metabolic needs; weight is returning to pre–acute illness level.
5. Describes signs and symptoms to be reported to physician.

## QUESTIONS TO CONSIDER

- What is the quality of air in the community in which you reside? If air pollution is a problem, what are the major contributing factors (industries, automobile exhaust, etc.)? Are there community groups working to improve the problem? If so, what activities are they involved in, and how might a nurse be helpful to their efforts?
- Where is the branch of the American Cancer Society and the American Lung Association nearest your community? What services do they provide for health professionals and for patients?
- What is the tuberculosis case rate in the area in which you live? Is this higher or lower than the national rate of 9.8 per 100,000 population? List the factors that contribute to a higher or lower case rate in your community.

## QUESTIONS TO CONSIDER—cont'd

- List the services available in your community to assist persons who wish to stop smoking and to which you could refer patients or friends.
- Design a teaching plan or project that you believe would help convince teenagers they should not smoke. Would you use a different approach for females than for males?
- Plan a 3000-calorie, high-protein diet for a 60-year-old man with pulmonary emphysema who is very short of breath and finds eating to be a chore.
- Mrs. Jones has just been admitted to your unit. She has a long-standing history of COPD with chronic respiratory failure. She recently developed a viral bronchitis. She arrives on your unit with ABGs of $Pao_2$ = 55, $Paco_2$ = 80, pH = 7.30. She appears extremely short of breath and is very restless. What information do you need to obtain to assess this patient's current status? What is your immediate plan of care?
- Describe the unique developmental needs of young adults with CF.
- Considering the trend of increasing life expectancy for patients with CF, what moral and ethical developments may the nurse encounter when caring for them?
- Discuss the clinical manifestations of CF in adults.
- Explain current therapy used to treat adults with CF.
- Describe the nature of respiratory failure and the care of the patient with an artificial airway and mechanical ventilation.

## CRITICAL THINKING ACTIVITIES

- What aspects of nursing care can be generalized to individuals with infectious diseases of the respiratory tract (e.g., acute bronchitis, pneumonia, bronchiectasis, histoplasmosis)?
- How would nursing management of a 42-year-old with emphysema differ from the care of a 58-year-old with chronic bronchitis? How would care be similar?
- Integrate teaching principles related to hospitalized patients requiring oxygen therapy into a teaching plan for the client receiving oxygen in the home. What aspects of the teaching plan would be different?

## CHAPTER SUMMARY

### CLASSIFICATION OF PULMONARY DISORDERS

- Pulmonary disorders can be classified by the way ventilation is altered. The three major categories of pulmonary disorders are restrictive, obstructive, and vascular.
- In restrictive diseases, lung volume and lung compliance are reduced.
- Restrictive lung diseases include acute bronchitis, pneumonia, tuberculosis, fungal infections, occupational lung diseases, ARDS/HPPE, and cancer of the lung.

### INFECTIOUS DISEASES OF THE RESPIRATORY TRACT

- Acute bronchitis may be caused by viruses; bacteria such as *S. pneumoniae, H. influenzae, M. catarrhalis,* and *B. pertussis;* and other organisms (*Mycoplasma pneumoniae, Chlamydia pneumoniae* [Twar strain]). The better term to describe bronchitis would be tracheobronchitis because bronchitis without tracheitis is never seen.
- A newer way to classify bacterial pneumonia is community-acquired (CAP) and hospital-acquired (nosocomial) pneumonia.
- *Streptococcus pneumoniae* causes 50% to 80% of cases of CAP in young adults and 20% to 50% in elderly and debilitated persons. Several of the organisms causing CAP are resistant to penicillin and require other antibiotics. Staphylococci *(S. aureus, S. epidermidis)* infections develop in residents of nursing homes or chronic-care facilities, patients with Hickman catheters, IV drug abusers, and persons with diabetes or renal failure. *Mycoplasma pneumoniae* is the cause of 20% to 30% of CAP in adults under age 35 and 3% to 10% of those over age 60.
- Gram-negative bacteria are responsible for the greatest number of cases of hospital-acquired pneumonia. The largest number of cases are caused by Enterobacteriaceae and *Pseudomonas aeruginosa.*
- Risk factors for the development of nosocomial pneumonia include the following: being a patient in an ICU, being on mechanical ventilation, having an endotracheal or tracheostomy tube, having recent surgery, being debilitated or malnourished, having invasive devices, neuromuscular disease, or depressed levels of alertness, aspiration, antacid use, age 60 or older, prolonged hospital stay, or any prolonged underlying disease.
- The major nursing responsibility is in preventing aspiration by patients who have diminished levels of consciousness, who are reacting from anesthesia, who are receiving tube feedings, or who are having difficulty expectorating sputum.
- Prevention of pneumonia includes pneumonia vaccine for those aged 65 years or older.
- Regardless of the causative agent, pneumonia results in acute inflammation of lung tissue. Inflamed tissue often involves both the conducting airways and the alveolar tissue; thus, both airway clearance and gas exchange may be impaired.
- The number of cases of tuberculosis had been on the decline until 1986, when they began increasing. Some of the reasons for the increase in the number of TB cases is an increase in the number of persons with HIV and AIDS who are particularly susceptible to any

infection. Other causes are homelessness and IV drug abuse.

- The mycobacterium responsible for TB in middle-class AIDS patients is the *Mycobacterium avium* intracellular complex (MAC). *M. tuberculosis* is more common in AIDS patients from developing countries and inner-city minority populations who have a history of IV drug abuse.
- Mycobacteria other than TB (MOTT) are strongly acid-fast bacteria that are being isolated more frequently from immunocompromised patients.
- Multidrug-resistant TB (MDR-TB) has become a major problem in the United States, especially in New York City and other areas with many patients with HIV.
- Primary prevention of respiratory infections such as tuberculosis includes prevention of the spread of infection by teaching the infected person to cover nose and mouth when coughing or sneezing so that droplet nuclei are not released into the air.
- Histoplasmosis, coccidioidomycosis, and blastomycosis are three major fungal infections of the lungs. Amphotericin B is the standard therapy for mycotic infection.
- Lung abscess is usually caused by bacteria that reach the lung from aspiration. It can also follow bronchial obstruction caused by a tumor, foreign body, or stenosis. Up to one third of these patients 45 years and older have lung abscess associated with carcinoma.
- Although bronchiectasis is not as common as it once was, it occurs in persons with cystic fibrosis, immunodeficiency diseases, or asthma who have had repeated respiratory infections.

## OCCUPATIONAL LUNG DISEASES

- Occupational lung diseases are caused by microscopic substances inhaled in the workplace. They can cause severe lung damage especially to persons who inhale these substances for years. Examples are "black lung disease" found in coal miners and mesothelioma, cancer of the pleura, which occurs in asbestos workers.
- Occupational lung diseases are more common among smokers than nonsmokers, and smokers often have a more severe form of the disease.

## OTHER RESTRICTIVE DISEASES: SARCOIDOSIS

- Sarcoidosis is a systemic granulomatous disease of unknown cause. In the United States it is 10 times more common in blacks than whites. It is treated with steroids.

## CANCER OF THE LUNG

- Cancer of the lung is the leading cause of death from cancer in both men and women. Because there is no cure from cancer of the lung, the goal set for the year 2000 in *Healthy People 2000* is to slow the rise in lung cancer deaths because it is impossible to decrease the number of deaths.
- The treatment of choice for lung cancer is surgical removal of the tumor. Unfortunately, one third of persons are inoperable when they first see a surgeon. Another one third are found to be inoperable on exploratory examination, and 90% of the persons who do survive are dead within 5 years.
- Because there is no cure for cancer of the lung, the emphasis is on prevention, which focuses on keeping persons from starting to smoke and convincing those who smoke to quit because smokers are 10 times more likely to develop lung cancer than nonsmokers.

## PULMONARY VASCULAR DISEASE

- A newer therapy still undergoing trials in the care of patients with pulmonary embolism is thrombolytic therapy with urokinase, streptokinase, or recombinant tissue-type plasminogen activator (rt-PA). If this treatment is not successful, a pulmonary embolectomy may be used to extract emboli from the pulmonary vasculature.

## CHEST TRAUMA

- Chest trauma is divided into blunt and penetrating injuries. The most common blunt injury is fractured ribs.
- The major cause of chest trauma is automobile accidents in which the chest hits the steering wheel.
- Chest trauma is managed by stabilization of the fracture site and analgesics to reduce pain.
- When several ribs or the sternum is fractured in more than one place, the patient may develop a flail chest with paradoxical breathing.
- Nursing management of the person with a flail chest includes improving gas exchange and airway clearance and promoting comfort.
- A pneumothorax occurs when air enters the pleural space between the lung and chest wall. There are three main types of pneumothoraces: closed or spontaneous, open, and tension.
- If an open sucking wound of the chest has been sustained, the wound should be covered immediately to prevent air from entering the pleural cavity and causing a pneumothorax.
- After resectional surgery of the lung (except for pneumonectomy), one or two chest tubes are inserted into the pleural space and connected to a closed drainage system.
- Postoperative nursing care of the patient after thoracic surgery centers on promoting ventilation and reexpansion of the lung by maintaining a clear airway, promoting comfort by pain relief, promoting reexpansion of the lung by proper maintenance of the closed drainage system, promoting nutrition, and monitoring the incision for bleeding and subcutaneous emphysema.

- Bronchopleural fistula and empyema are long-term complications of resectional surgery of the lung.
- Effective breathing patterns can be facilitated by proper positioning, and the use of respiratory assistive devices such as incentive spirometery, and possibly IPPB.

### CHRONIC AIRFLOW LIMITATION—OBSTRUCTIVE PULMONARY DISEASE

- Obstructive lung diseases result in an obstruction to airflow, predominantly on expiration.
- COPD is an umbrella label for a variety of pulmonary disorders that cause a chronic limitation of airflow. The most common chronic airflow disorders are emphysema, chronic bronchitis, and asthma.
- Hypoventilation results in elevation of arterial carbon dioxide. Hyperventilation results in lowered arterial carbon dioxide.
- To facilitate breathing, the nurse teaches the person with COPD abdominal breathing, leaning-forward postures, inhalation-exhalation exercises, muscle-reconditioning exercises, and pursed-lip breathing.
- Respiratory failure is defined by the physiologic criteria of $Pao_2$ = 60 mm Hg or less, $Paco_2$ = 50 mm Hg or greater, and a pH = 7.35 or less.
- Persons with COPD who have chronically elevated carbon dioxide and low oxygen levels are considered to have chronic respiratory failure. These chronically ill people are at high risk of developing acute respiratory failure, in addition to their chronic failure.
- Cystic fibrosis is an inherited disease that causes airway obstruction. It usually develops in childhood.
- Because of better treatment, more patients with CF are living into their 20s.

### RESPIRATORY INSUFFICIENCY AND RESPIRATORY FAILURE

- When a patient is unable to maintain ventilation, the $Paco_2$ will increase and mechanical ventilation will be necessary.
- There are two major types of ventilators, pressure cycled and volume cycled. Currently, volume-cycled ventilators are more commonly used. Before attaching the ventilator, the patient will be intubated with either an endotracheal or a tracheostomy tube.
- A volume-cycled ventilator delivers a constant volume of air at a preset pressure with each breath. These ventilators have a cutoff valve, which will stop the cycle if the pressure required to deliver the desired volume exceeds a preset level.
- The patient on a ventilator requires constant attendance and is best managed in an intensive care unit.
- After the patient's underlying pulmonary problem is improved, the patient will be weaned from the ventilator. Weaning is best carried out by a nurse who has developed a trust relationship with the patient.
- There are three major methods of weaning: T piece, intermittent mandatory ventilation (IMV), and pressure support ventilation (PSV). Several attempts for increasing periods of time may be necessary before the ventilator can be discontinued.
- Nursing management to facilitate aeration of alveoli requires interventions that promote optimal airway function, promote effective breathing patterns, and manage pulmonary secretions. Measures to achieve these include hydration, humidification of the airways, nebulizer therapy, segmental postural drainage, and breathing exercises.
- When the patient cannot manage secretions, tracheobronchial suctioning may be necessary. If this is not successful in clearing the airway, fiberoptic bronchoscopy may be used to remove impacted secretions.
- Maintaining transportation of oxygen to body tissues requires several interactive physiologic processes. These include ventilation, perfusion, and diffusion. Also required are sufficient hemoglobin and an adequate cardiac output.
- Several modes are used to deliver oxygen to the patient. These include nasal cannulae and several types of face masks that can deliver various concentrations of oxygen.
- ARDS results in severe hypoxemia without hypercapnia. Patients with ARDS/HPPE usually require mechanical ventilation with PEEP in order to provide adequate oxygen safely.

## REFERENCES


1. Alex CG, Tobin MJ: Chronic obstructive pulmonary disease. In Rakel RE, editor: *Conn's current therapy,* Philadelphia, 1993, Saunders.
2. American Cancer Society: *Cancer facts and figures—1994,* Atlanta, 1994, The Association.
3. American Lung Association: *Chronic obstructive pulmonary disease,* New York, 1981, The Association.
4. Baler H: Primary lung abscess. In Rakel RE, editor: *Conn's current therapy,* Philadelphia, 1993, Saunders.
5. Barnes P et al: Tuberculosis in patients with human immunodeficiency virus infection, *N Engl J Med* 324:1644-1649, 1991.
6. Benner KL: Terminal weaning: a loved one's vigil, *Am J Nurs* 93(5):22-25, 1993.
7. Bloch AB et al: Nationwide survey of drug-resistant tuberculosis in the United States, *JAMA* 271(9):665-671, 1994.
8. Brown WD, Campbell GD: Histoplasmosis. In Rakel RE, editor: *Conn's current therapy,* Philadelphia, 1993, Saunders.
9. Centers for Disease Control: Cigarette smoking among adults—United States, 1992, and changes in the definition of current cigarette smoking, *MMWR* 43(19):342-346, 1994.
10. Centers for Disease Control: Guidelines for preventing the transmission of tuberculosis in health-care settings, with special focus on HIV-related issues, *MMWR* 39(RR-17):1-29, 1990.
11. Centers for Disease Control: Guidelines for school health programs to prevent tobacco use and addiction, *MMWR* 43(RR-2):1-15, 1994.
12. Centers for Disease Control: Initial therapy for tuberculosis in the era of multidrug resistance: recommendations of the Advisory Council for the Elimination of Tuberculosis, *MMWR* 42(RR-7):1-8, 1993.

13. Centers for Disease Control: Prevention and control of influenza. Part I. Vaccines, *MMWR* 43(RR-9):1-13, 1994.
14. Centers for Disease Control: Preventing tobacco use among young people: a report of the surgeon general, *MMWR* 43(RR-4):1-10, 1994.
15. Centers for Disease Control: Prevention and control of tuberculosis among homeless persons: recommendations of the Advisory Council for the Elimination of Tuberculosis, *MMWR* 41(RR-5):1-23, 1992.
16. Centers for Disease Control: Update—tuberculosis elimination—United States, *MMWR* 39(10):153-156, 1990.
17. Cherniak R: *Current therapy of respiratory disease,* ed 2, Toronto, 1986, Decker.
18. Colditz GA et al: Efficacy of BCG vaccine in the prevention of tuberculosis, *JAMA* 271:698-702, 1994.
19. Cynaman MH, Klemens S: Tuberculosis and other mycobacterial diseases. In Rakel RE, editor: *Conn's current therapy,* Philadelphia, 1993, Saunders.
20. D'Amico TA, Sabiston DC Jr: Carcinoma of the lung. In Sabiston DC Jr, Lyerly HK, editors: *Sabiston essentials of surgery,* ed 2, Philadelphia, 1994, Saunders.
21. Davis PB: Pathophysiology of pulmonary disease in cystic fibrosis, *Semin Respir Med* 6(4):261-269, 1985.
22. Dowling PT: Return of tuberculosis: screening and preventive therapy, *AFP* 43(2):457-467, 1991.
23. Ferguson GT, Cherniack RM: Management of chronic obstructive pulmonary disease, *N Engl J Med* 328:1017-1022, 1993.
24. Fink MP: Trauma. In Sabiston DC Jr, Lyerly LK, editors: *Sabiston essentials of surgery,* ed 2, Philadelphia, 1994, Saunders.
25. George RB: Blastomycosis. In Rakel RE, editor: *Conn's current therapy,* Philadelphia, 1993, Saunders.
26. Gift AG, Bolgiano CS, Cunningham J: Sensations during chest tube removal, *Heart Lung* 20(2):131-137, 1991.
27. Harvey JC, Beattie EJ: Lung cancer, *Clin Symp* 45(3):1-32, 1993.
28. Hill RC: Bronchiectasis. In Sabiston DC Jr, Lyerly HK, editors: *Sabiston essentials of surgery,* ed 2, Philadelphia, 1994, Saunders.
29. Hill RC: The pleura and empyema. In Sabiston DC Jr, Lyerly HK, editors: *Sabiston's essentials of surgery,* ed 2, Philadelphia, 1994, Saunders.
30. Kataria YP, Halter JF: Sarcoidosis. In Rakel RE, editor: *Conn's current therapy,* Philadelphia, 1993, Saunders.
31. Larsen RA: Coccidioidomycosis. In Rakel RE, editor: *Conn's current therapy,* Philadelphia, 1993, Saunders.
32. Lederberg J, Shape RE, Oaks SC Jr: *Emerging infections: microbial threats to health in the United States,* Washington, DC, 1992, National Academy Press.
33. Lynch JP: Bacterial pneumonia. In Rakel RE, editor: *Conn's current therapy,* Philadelphia, 1993, Saunders.
34. Moran JF: Surgical treatment of tuberculosis. In Sabiston DC Jr, Lyerly LK, editors: *Sabiston essentials of surgery,* ed 2, Philadelphia, 1994, Saunders.
35. O'Brien LM, Bartlett KA: TB plus HIV spells trouble, *Am J Nurs* 92(5):28-34, 1992.
36. Ramsey BW, Smith AL: Reduced incidence of respiratory tract infections in cystic fibrosis patients using aerosolized dornase alfa, *Dornase Alfa Clin Series* 1(1):1-5, 1994.
37. Rich EA, Eliner JJ: Acute bronchitis. In Rakel RE, editor: *Conn's current therapy,* Philadelphia, 1993, Saunders.
38. Schwartz LB, Sabiston DC Jr: Pulmonary embolism. In Sabiston DC Jr, Lyerly HK, editors: *Sabiston essentials of surgery,* ed 2, Philadelphia, 1994, Saunders.
39. Tobin MJ: Mechanical ventilation, *N Engl J Med* 330:1056-1061, 1994.
40. US Department of Health and Human Services: *Healthy people 2000: national health promotion and disease prevention objectives,* Washington, DC, 1990, US Government Printing Office.
41. US Department of Health and Human Services: *National Asthma Education Program Guidelines for the Diagnosis and Management of Asthma,* Washington, DC, 1991.
42. US Department of Health and Human Services, Public Health Service, National Heart, Lung, and Blood Institute: *Teach your patients about asthma: a clinician's guide,* Bethesda, Md, 1992.

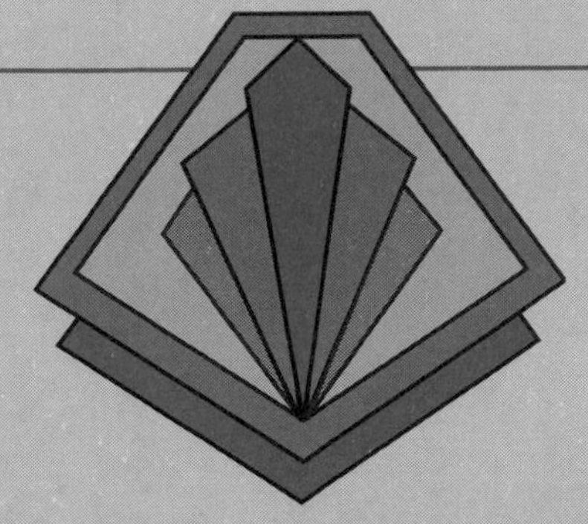

U N I T V I I

# *Alterations in Metabolism*

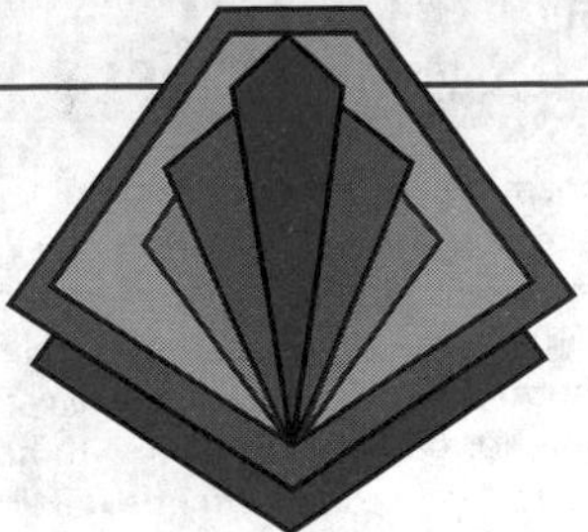

CHAPTER 38

# Assessment of the Endocrine System

*Dorothy R. Blevins*
*Virginia L. Cassmeyer*

## CHAPTER OBJECTIVES

***After studying this chapter, the learner should be able to do the following:***

1 Describe the locations of various endocrine glands in the body and the mechanisms that control hormone synthesis and release from these glands.
2 Describe the functions of the hormones secreted by the pituitary, thyroid, parathyroid, adrenal cortex, and adrenal medulla glands and the pancreas.
3 Compare biologic effects that occur when there is a deficit or an excess of endocrine hormones.
4 Identify the physiologic changes that occur within the endocrine system with aging.
5 Identify subjective and objective data that should be collected on persons with actual or potential health problems of the endocrine system.
6 Describe the common diagnostic tests used to identify endocrine dysfunction and explain the meaning of the results.

## KEY TERMS

androgens
carrier proteins
catecholamines
Chvostek's sign
counterregulatory hormone
diabetes insipidus
feedback control
glucagon
glucocorticoids
glycosylated proteins
hormone
insulin
intrinsic rhythmicity
mineralocorticoids
paracrine
pheochromocytoma
receptors
target cell
Trousseau's sign

The complexity of the human body and the specialization of cells and tissues require an internal communication system that integrates processes so that several body parts can function as a unit to meet selected needs. Two systems, the endocrine and nervous systems, function together to coordinate body processes so that an appropriate response can be made to changes in the environment.

The endocrine system consists of the anterior and posterior pituitary, thyroid, parathyroid, adrenal cortex, adrenal medulla, pancreas, gonads, pineal body, and thymus. There are also specialized endocrine cells located in various parts of the gastrointestinal (GI) tract. The hormones from these endocrine glands are vital to the important life transactions of the organism, including differentiation, reproduction, growth and development, adaptation, and senescence.[11] This is the first of three chapters that focus on the role in these processes of the anterior and posterior pituitary, thyroid, parathyroid, adrenal cortex, and adrenal medulla glands, and endocrine pancreas. The neuroendocrine response to stressors, which involves the nervous system, the adrenal medulla and other endocrine glands, is discussed in Chapter 7; the GI hormones are discussed in Chapter 43; and the gonads are discussed in Chapter 51. The thymus, which is critical to development of immunocompetent T lymphocytes, is discussed in Chapters 13 and 69.

## ANATOMY AND PHYSIOLOGY

### GENERAL ENDOCRINE PROCESSES

The endocrine system integrates body functions by the synthesis and release of hormones. **Hormones** are

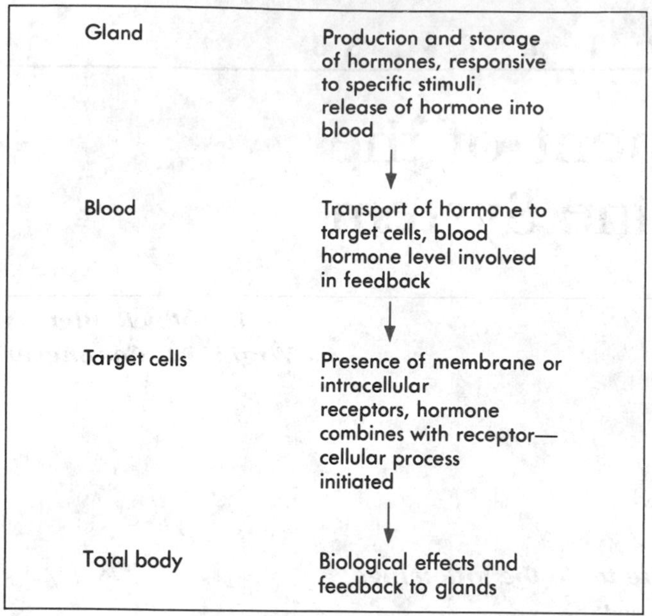


**FIGURE 38-1** Summary of processes involved in activity of endocrine glands and hormones.

**BOX 38-1 Major Chemical Classes of Hormones and Specific Hormones in Each Class**

| Class | Hormones |
|---|---|
| Biogenic amines | Dopamine, epinephrine, norepinephrine |
| Amino acids | Thyroxine ($T_4$), triiodothyronine ($T_3$) |
| Peptides | Antidiuretic hormone (ADH, vasopressin), oxytocin, corticotropin-releasing hormone (CRH), gonadotropin-releasing hormone (GnRH), growth hormone–releasing hormone (GHRH), growth hormone–inhibiting hormone (somatostatin, GHIH), thyrotropin-releasing hormone (TRH) |
| Proteins | Adrenocorticotropin (ACTH), calcitonin, glucagon, growth hormone (GH), insulin, prolactin (PRL), parathyroid hormone (PTH) |
| Glycoproteins | Follicle-stimulating hormone (FSH), luteinizing hormone (LH), thyroid-stimulating hormone (TSH) |
| Steroids | Adrenal androgens, aldosterone, estrogens ($E_2$, $E_3$), glucocorticoids, progesterone ($P_4$), testosterone (T), vitamin D (cholecalciferol) |

chemical substances that are secreted into body fluids, usually blood, by a group of specialized cells, so that they may exert a physiologic effect at another site. Hormones can travel moderate to long distances, such as from the pituitary to the ovaries, or very short distances, such as from one cell group in the pancreas to another. When hormones influence cells close to the site of origin, this is referred to as **paracrine** functioning.

A hormone acts only on cells or tissues that have **receptors** for the specific hormone. The cell or tissue that responds to a particular hormone is called the **target cell** or target tissue. Hormones, when stimulating cells, set in motion various intracellular processes so that metabolic responses, growth and development changes, and response to stressors occur as needed by the body. Hormones themselves do not produce these responses; rather, hormones set in motion a chain of events necessary to produce the desired and needed response. A summary of the processes involved in the activity of endocrine glands and their hormones is shown in Figure 38-1. Hormones can be classified by chemical structure into six groups, as shown in Box 38-1.

## Control of Hormone Levels

The level of hormones must be kept within very definite limits, because the amount of hormone available to a tissue is critical for its health. One factor responsible for controlling levels is **feedback control.** A simple closed-loop, negative-feedback system is illustrated in Figure 38-2. This diagram reveals a basic type of feedback. Gland A is stimulated to produce hormone X. Hormone X stimulates organ B to change (increase or decrease) substance Y. The change in substance Y inhibits the production and secretion of hormone X. This simple system illustrates the negative-feedback regulation of, for example, parathyroid hormone, antidiuretic hormone, and insulin (Table 38-1).

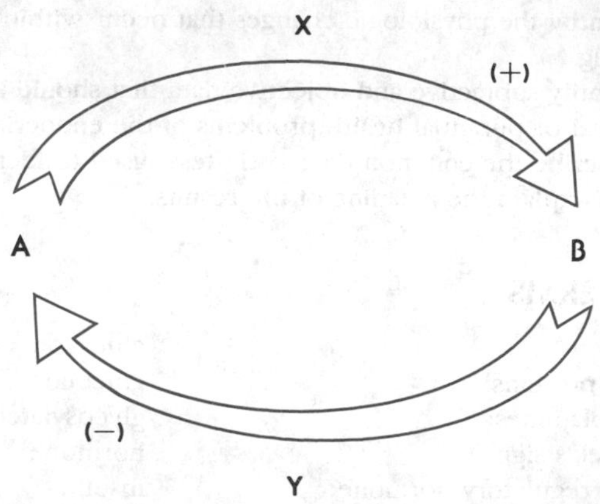


**FIGURE 38-2** Closed-loop, negative-feedback system. This principle of control applies to all endocrine glands.

A more complex feedback mechanism controls the levels of other hormones. The most elaborate feedback mechanism is demonstrated by the interaction of the hypothalamus and the anterior pituitary with the thyroid gland, the adrenal cortex, and the gonads. The basic parts of this feedback loop are illustrated in Figure 38-3. When the level of hormone produced by the thyroid gland, the adrenal cortex, or the gonads is adequate, the release of trophic hormones by the pituitary gland and/or of releasing hormone by the hypothalamus is inhibited by negative feedback. The level of trophic hormone and/

**TABLE 38-1 Examples of Negative-Feedback Regulation of Parathyroid Hormone, Antidiuretic Hormone, and Insulin**

| STIMULUS | | GLAND A | | HORMONE X | | ORGAN B | | SUBSTANCE Y |
|---|---|---|---|---|---|---|---|---|
| Decreased serum calcium | → + | Parathyroid gland ↑⊖ | → | Parathyroid hormone | → | Kidney, bone, gastrointestinal tract | → | Increased serum calcium |
| Increased serum osmolality | → + | Posterior pituitary ↑⊖ | → | Antidiuretic hormone | → | Kidney | → | Reabsorption of water leads to decreased serum osmolality |
| Increased serum glucose | → + | Beta cells of pancreas ↑⊖ | → | Insulin | → | Fat cells, liver muscle cells | → | Increased uptake of glucose leads to decreased serum glucose |

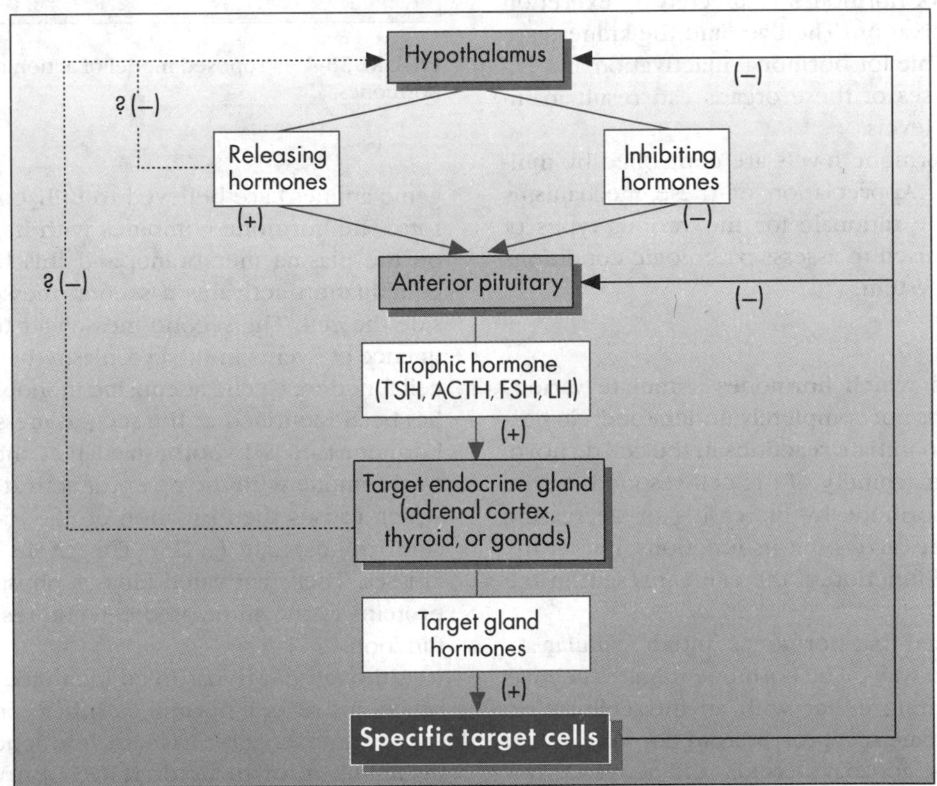


**FIGURE 38-3** Complex feedback system between hypothalamus, anterior pituitary gland, target endocrine glands, and specific target cells.

or releasing hormone may, in turn, exert a negative feedback on the hypothalamus. Also, to control the level of selected hormones, the hypothalamus synthesizes and releases inhibiting hormones (Figure 38-3). The amounts of prolactin and growth hormone released by the anterior pituitary are in part controlled by a prolactin-inhibiting hormone (dopamine) and a growth hormone–inhibiting hormone (somatostatin, GHIH).

Although negative-feeback control is a distinguishing feature of the endocrine system, not all hormones are controlled by it. For example, estrogen in males, testosterone in females, placental hormones, and hormones produced by ectopic tumors are not under feedback control.[12]

A second factor regulating hormone levels is **intrinsic rhythmicity.** The intrinsic rhythms can vary over minutes, days, or weeks. For example, adrenocorticotropic hormone (ACTH), cortisol, glucocorticoids, and growth hormone demonstrate daily circadian rhythms (24-hour patterns), whereas the reproductive hormones in females demonstrate a pattern that varies over several weeks.

These intrinsic rhythms are controlled by various factors. The environmental factor of sleep-wake patterns influences in some unknown way the circadian rhythms of growth hormone, ACTH, and cortisol. Age, growth, and development influence the intrinsic rhythmicity of gonadotropins and gonadal steroids. Neurogenic factors influence the intrinsic rhythm of other hormones such as prolactin.

Extrinsic factors such as pain, trauma, infection, and other stressors are a third factor influencing levels of selected hormones. These extrinsic factors can override the normal feedback mechanisms or intrinsic rhythmicity and increase secretion of hormones above normal levels.

Last, the level of hormones is affected by excretion or metabolic inactivation. The liver and the kidneys are primarily responsible for hormonal inactivation and excretion, and diseases of these organs can result in increased hormone levels.

In summary, hormone levels are controlled by multiple mechanisms. Appreciation of these mechanisms helps to clarify the rationale for the various types of diagnostic testing used to assesss pathologic conditions of the endocrine system.

## Receptors

The exact way in which hormones stimulate various cellular responses is not completely understood. No hormone is believed to initiate reactions in the cell de novo. The biochemical machinery of the cell responds to the presence of the hormone by increasing or decreasing the rate at which it carries out its functions, but all the equipment for the function of the cell is present in the cell.

It is hypothesized that hormones initiate cellular activity in one of two ways. The hormone initiates cellular activity by combining either with an intracellular receptor or a membrane receptor. Steroid hormones such as adrenal steroids, gonadal steroids, and active derivatives of vitamin D and thyroid hormone, which are lipid soluble, are believed to use intracellular receptors. These hormones freely cross the plasma membrane and combine with their specific intracellular receptor. The steroid-receptor complex is changed in size and conformation and is translocated to the nucleus, where it combines with acceptor sites located in the nucleus near the deoxyribonucleic acid (DNA) sequences. The binding of the hormone-receptor complex initiates transcription of DNA, translation of ribonucleic acid (RNA), and synthesis of protein. A summary of this model of hormone activation is shown in Figure 38-4.

Water-soluble hormones (hypothalamic-releasing hormones, anterior and posterior pituitary hormones, parathyroid hormone, calcitonin, insulin, glucagon, biogenic amines) are believed to utilize membrane receptors. The hormone combines with its specific receptor on the plasma membrane, and this hormone-receptor combination activates a second messenger located inside the cell. The second messenger then initiates a sequence of events in the cytoplasm that results in altered cell function. Cyclic adenosine monophosphate (cAMP) has been identified as the second messenger for several hormones. It is hypothesized that the combination of the hormone with the receptor activates adenyl cyclase, which causes the formation of 3′,5′-cAMP from adenosine triphosphate (ATP). The cAMP activates protein kinases. These activated kinases phosphorylate specific proteins in the stimulated cell and result in altered cell function.

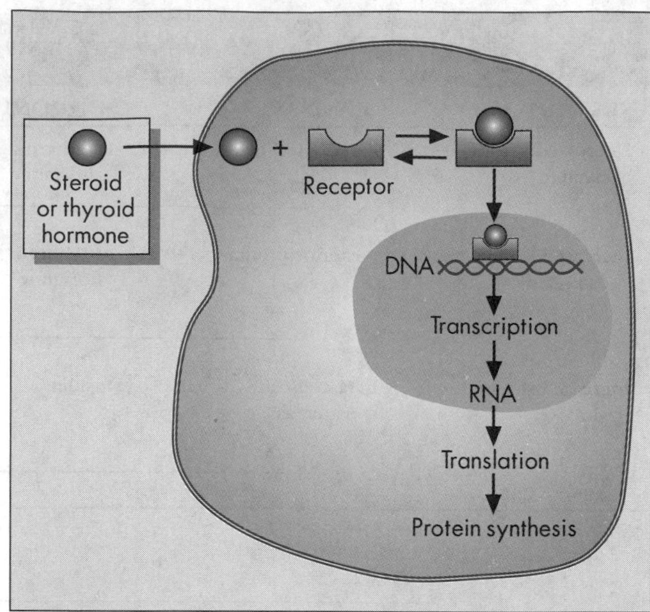


**FIGURE 38-4** Proposed model of action of steroid or thyroid hormones.

Although cAMP has been identified as a second messenger for several hormones, other compounds serve as second messengers. Growth hormone is mediated by insulin-like growth factor 1(IGF-1), or somatomedin, its second messenger.[5] Calcium ions, calmodulin, adenosine, and prostaglandins are some of the other potential second messengers. A summary of this model hormone activation is presented in Figure 38-5.

In summary, hormones initiate cellular activity by combining with specific receptors. Although hormone-receptor interaction has been hypothesized to fall into one of two major models, there may be hormones that use both models of hormone action.[6] Research on receptors is ongoing.

# LOCATION OF GLANDS AND FUNCTION OF HORMONES

The various endocrine glands are located throughout the body (Figure 38-6). In addition to the glands de-

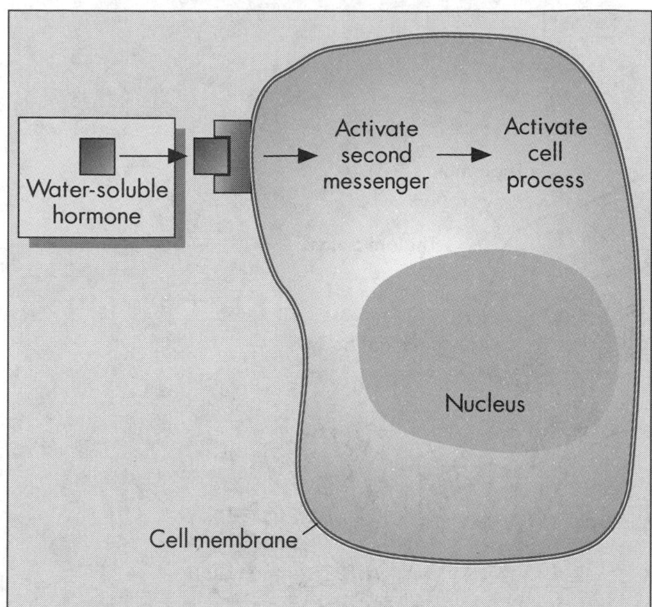


**FIGURE 38-5** Proposed model of action of water-soluble hormones.

picted, there are endocrine cells throughout various parts of the GI tract.

## Hypothalamus and Pituitary Gland

The hypothalamus, a part of the diencephalon, consists of numerous poorly defined nuclei. The hypothalamus forms the lower portion of the lateral walls and the floor of the third ventricle. It is bordered anteriorly by the optic chiasma. The hypothalamic sulcus and thalamus lie on the dorsal border; the internal capsule, subthalamic nuclei, and basis pedunculi form the lateral boundaries. On its inferior surface the hypothalamus is continuous with the pituitary stalk. Figure 38-7 shows a sagittal section through the brain. The anterior, dorsal, and inferior boundaries are depicted. Although the hypothalamus is a very small area of the brain, it receives input directly or indirectly from almost every other part of the brain and is a major controller of the anterior and posterior pituitary gland.

The pituitary gland, which is approximately 1 cm in size and weighs 500 mg, lies in the sella turcica of the sphenoid bone. This gland is composed of two functionally distinguishable components: the adenohypophysis (anterior pituitary) and the neurohypophysis (posterior pituitary). The posterior pituitary is a continuation of the pituitary stalk. The anterior pituitary, which makes up 75% of the total gland, arises embryonically from an outpouching of ectoderm and fuses with the posterior pituitary.

### Hypothalamic-pituitary relationship

The hypothalamus serves as a critical link between the rest of the nervous system and the endocrine system. It controls both the posterior and the anterior pituitary glands. By its control of the anterior pituitary gland, the hypothalamus exerts global control over the entire endocrine system. Figure 38-8 depicts the connections between the hypothalamus and the pituitary gland. The hypothalamus is connected to the posterior pituitary gland by nerve tracts that originate in the paraventricular and supraoptic nucleus of the hypothalamus. Posterior pituitary hormones are actually synthesized in the hypothalamus and transported along nerve axons to the posterior pituitary gland, where they are stored.

The hypothalamus and anterior pituitary gland are

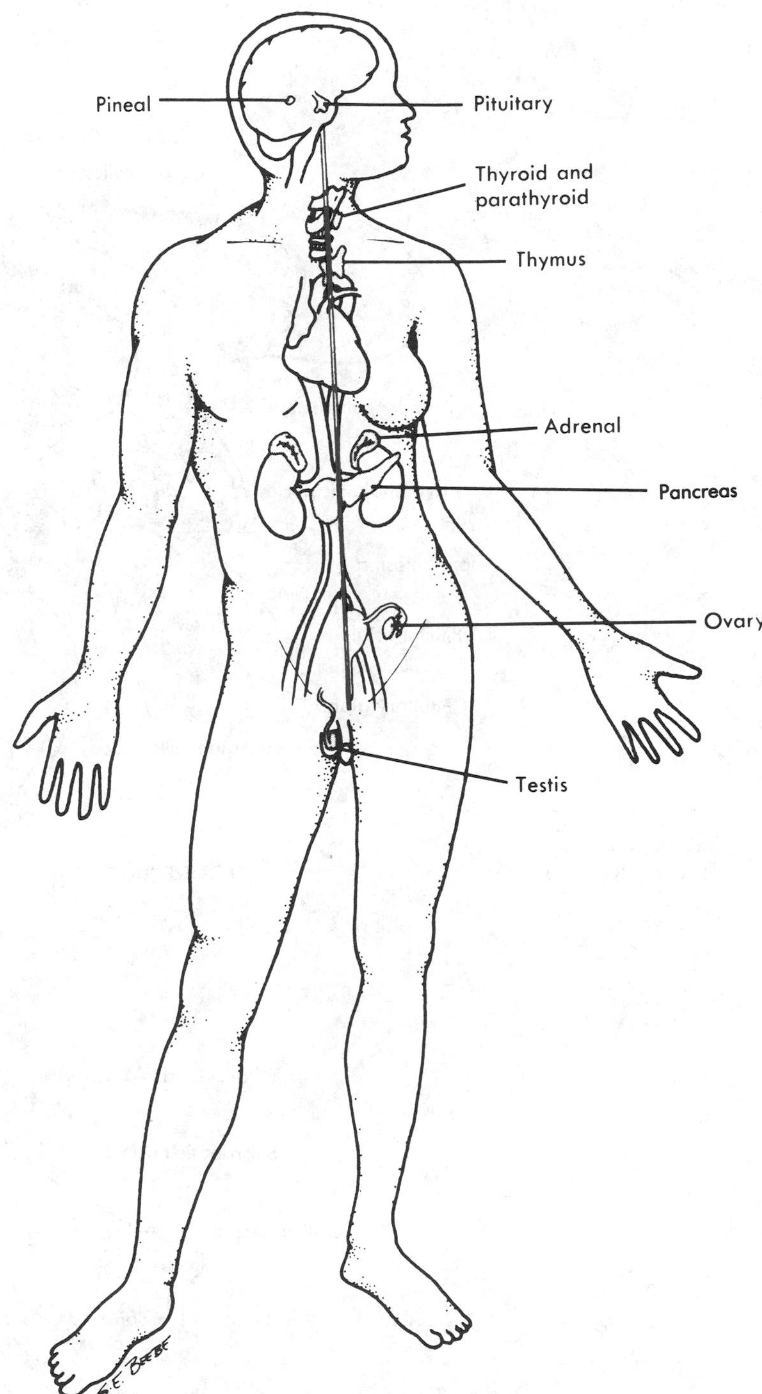


**FIGURE 38-6** Endocrine system. (From Tucker SM et al: *Patient care standards,* ed 5, St Louis, 1992, Mosby.)

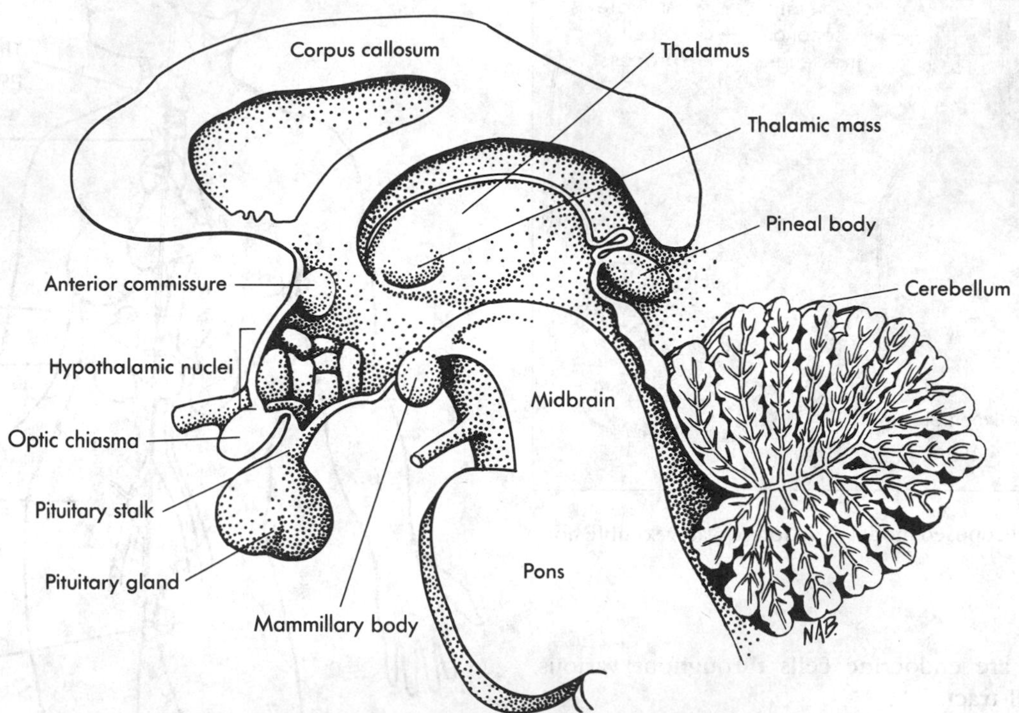


**FIGURE 38-7** Sagittal section through the brain.

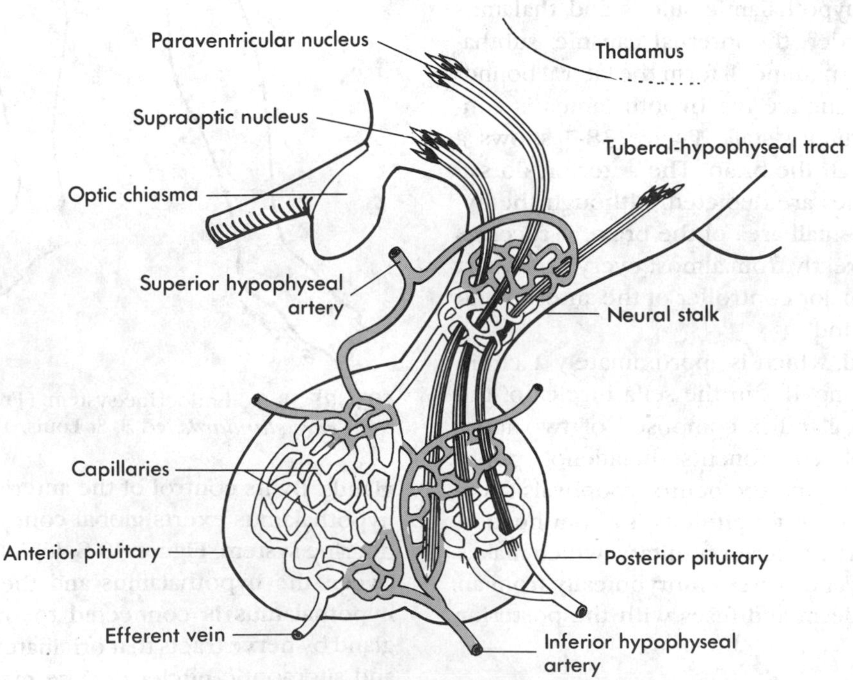


**FIGURE 38-8** Hypothalamic pituitary connections. Hypothalamus connects to posterior pituitary gland by nerve tracts. Connection between hypothalamus and anterior pituitary gland is vascular.

connected by the hypothalamic-hypophyseal portal blood supply. Blood entering the anterior pituitary gland has first passed through the hypothalamus. The hypothalamus regulates anterior pituitary function by the synthesis and secretion of releasing or inhibiting hormones into the hypothalamic-hypophyseal portal blood supply. These hormones are released in the anterior pituitary gland and stimulate the release of or inhibit the release of appropriate hormones.

The exact number and types of releasing and inhibiting hormones are unknown. Research has been extensive in this area. At present six releasing/inhibiting hormones have been identified: growth hormone–releasing hormone (GHRH), growth hormone–inhibiting hormone (GHIH, somatostatin), thyrotropin-releasing hormone (TRH), corticotropin-releasing hormone (CRH), gonadotropin-releasing hormone (GnRH), and dopamine (prolactin-inhibiting hormone [PIH]).

Some researchers believe there is another PIH, as yet not chemically identified. Data also support the presence of a prolactin-releasing hormone (PRH), but this substance has not been identified. GnRH stimulates the release of both gonadotropins from the anterior pituitary gland.

### Pituitary hormones

The posterior pituitary gland stores and releases two hormones: antidiuretic hormone (ADH), or vasopressin, and oxytocin. Both these hormones are synthesized in the paraventricular and supraoptic nucleus of the hypothalamus. The blood level of these two hormones is controlled by multiple factors that act either as stimu-

**TABLE 38-2 Posterior Pituitary Hormones: Their Regulation and Function**

| HORMONE/REGULATION | FUNCTION |
|---|---|
| **ANTIDIURETIC HORMONE (ADH, VASOPRESSIN)** | |
| **Stimulators** | Target organ: kidneys |
| ***Primary*** | Major regulator of osmolality and body water volume |
| Increased serum osmolality (as little as 1% increase) via hypothalamic osmoreceptors | Increases permeability of collecting ducts in kidney to water, resulting in increased water reabsorption |
| ***Others*** | May stimulate water intake by stimulating perception of thirst |
| Modest volume depletion via atrial volume receptors | |
| Modest hypotension via baroreceptors | |
| Stressors | |
| Psychologic | |
| Pain | |
| Nausea and vomiting | |
| Chemicals | |
| Cholinergic agonist | |
| Beta-adrenergic agonist | |
| Barbiturates | |
| Morphine | |
| Nicotine | |
| **Inhibitors** | |
| ***Primary*** | |
| Decreased serum osmolality (as little as 1%) via osmoreceptors | |
| Modest increased volume and blood pressure via atrial volume receptors and baroreceptors | |
| Chemicals | |
| Alcohol | |
| Alpha-adrenergic agonist | |
| **OXYTOCIN** | |
| **Stimulators** | Target organ: breast tissue and uterus |
| ***Primary*** | Results in milk "let-down" in lactating breast |
| Suckling via neurogenic reflex conducted from afferent fibers in nipple to hypothalamus | Causes increased uterine contraction after labor has begun; role in initiating labor unclear |
| ***Others*** | |
| Uterine contraction via neurogenic reflex from afferent fibers in uterus | |
| **Inhibitors** | |
| Stressors | |
| Psychologic | |
| Physical | |
| Alpha-adrenergic stimulation | |

**TABLE 38-3 Anterior Pituitary Hormones: Their Regulation and Function**

| HORMONE/REGULATION | FUNCTION |
|---|---|
| **GROWTH HORMONE (GH)** | |
| Controlled by GHRH/GHIH<br>GH shows episodic secretion with increases after eating (particularly a high-protein diet) and after onset of deep sleep (usually within 1-2 hours after sleep)<br>Other stimuli that increase GH<br>Exercise (strenuous)<br>Hypoglycemia<br>Stressors<br>Chemicals<br>Arginine infusion<br>L-dopa<br>Clonidine<br>TRH in acromegaly<br>Adrenergic agonists<br>Beta-adrenergic antagonists<br>Hyperglycemia decreases GH | Target organ: whole body<br>Possibly works on most tissue through action of somatomedin(s)<br>Concerned with growth of cells, bones, and soft tissues<br>Increases mitosis<br>Affects carbohydrate, protein, and fat metabolism<br>Increases blood glucose by decreasing glucose utilization; insulin antagonist<br>Increases protein synthesis<br>Increases lipolysis, free fatty acid levels, and ketone formation<br>Increases electrolyte retention and extracellular fluid volume |
| **PROLACTIN (PRL)** | |
| Controlled by PRH and PIH; PRL chronically inhibited by hypothalamus<br>PRL shows episodic secretions occurring during later hours of sleep<br>Other stimulants<br>Stressors<br>Suckling<br>Chemicals<br>Estrogen<br>TRH<br>Dopamine antagonist<br>Chlorpromazine<br>Chemicals that are dopamine agonists (L-dopa, bromocriptine) inhibit PRL | Target organ: breast, gonads<br>Necessary for breast development and lactation<br>Regulator of reproductive function in males and females |
| **THYROID-STIMULATING HORMONE (TSH)** | |
| Controlled by TRH and negative feedback from plasma $T_4$ levels<br>Increase $T_4 \rightarrow$ decrease TSH<br>Decrease $T_4 \rightarrow$ increase TSH | Target organ: thyroid gland<br>Necessary for growth and function of thyroid; controls all functions of thyroid |
| **ADRENOCORTICOTROPIN (ACTH)** | |
| Controlled by CRH and negative feedback by cortisol levels<br>ACTH shows episodic secretion with rhythm that peaks between 6 and 8 AM<br>Circadian pattern (24-hour pattern) related to sleep-wake pattern and caused by increased CRH<br>Physiologic and psychologic stressors (e.g., hypoglycemia, infections, pain, anxiety) increase ACTH caused by increased CRH (override negative feedback); changes in cortisol influence ACTH<br>Increase cortisol → decrease ACTH<br>Decrease cortisol → increase ACTH | Target organ: adrenal cortex gland<br>Necessary for growth and maintenance of size of adrenal cortex<br>Controls release of glucocorticoids (cortisol) and adrenal androgens<br>Minor role in release of mineralocorticoids (aldosterone) |
| **GONADOTROPINS**<br>**Follicle-Stimulating Hormone (FSH)**<br>**Luteinizing Hormone (LH) (Also Previously Called Interstitial Cell–Stimulating Hormone [ICSH] in Males)** | |
| Secretion controlled by GnRH<br>Amount of FSH secreted is decreased by inhibin in males<br>Amount of LH secreted is decreased by testosterone in males<br>Sex steroids in females exert positive feedback on FSH and LH at certain times in normal menstrual cycle and negative feedback at other times | Target organs: gonads<br>Stimulates gametogenesis and sex steroid production in males and females |

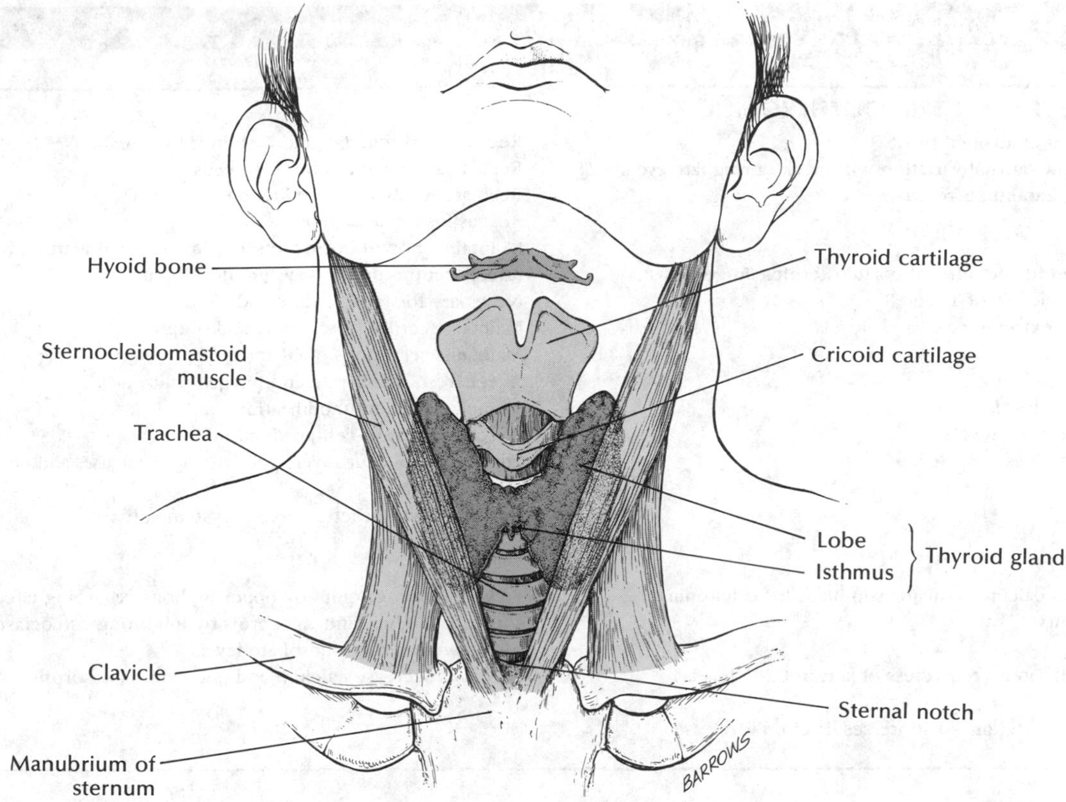


**FIGURE 38-9** Midline neck structures; note thyroid gland in anterior aspect of neck. (From Barkauskas VH et al: *Health and physical assessment,* St Louis, 1994, Mosby.)

lators or inhibitors. Table 38-2 outlines the regulation and function of ADH and oxytocin.

The anterior pituitary gland produces six hormones. These hormones are produced in specific cells located throughout the anterior pituitary gland. Table 38-3 outlines the hormones and their regulation and functions.

## Thyroid Gland

The thyroid gland (Figure 38-9) is located in the anterior aspect of the neck just below the cricoid cartilage. It consists of two lobes connected by the isthmus that lies on the upper part of the trachea. The gland weighs approximately 20 g and is composed of two distinct cell types: follicular cells and parafollicular cells. The follicular cells are responsible for thyroxine ($T_4$) and triiodothyronine ($T_3$) hormone production. These processes are carried out under the control of thyroid-stimulating hormone (TSH) and TRH. Multiple steps are involved in the production of thyroid hormone (Box 38-2). Most important, iodine is necessary to produce thyroid hormone.

The parafollicular cells (C cells) synthesize and secrete the hormone calcitonin, which is involved in calcium metabolism. Table 38-4 outlines the thyroid hormones and their regulation and functions.

**BOX 38-2 Production of Thyroid Hormone**

*Steps in production of thyroid hormones by follicular cells*

1. Uptake of iodide and oxidation of iodine
2. Production of thyroglobulin
3. Organification of thyroglobulin (iodine binds to tyrosine residues in thyroglobulin) to form 3-monoiodotyrosine and 3,5-diiodotyrosine
4. Coupling of monoiodo and diiodo compounds to form thyroxine ($T_4$) or triiodothyronine ($T_3$)
5. Hormone stored in follicle attached to thyroglobulin
6. With appropriate stimulation, proteolysis cleaves $T_4$ and $T_3$ off thyroglobulin
7. $T_3$ and $T_4$ released and thyroglobulin recycled

## Parathyroid Gland

The parathyroid gland consists of four minute glands, one located on the posterior aspect of the upper and lower poles of each lobe of the thyroid. Occasionally, normal extra parathyroid glands are found. These may be on the thyroid gland, in the mediastinum, or behind the esophagus.

The parathyroid gland produces one hormone: para-

**TABLE 38-4 Thyroid Gland Hormones: Their Regulation and Function**

| REGULATION | FUNCTIONS |
|---|---|
| **THYROXINE ($T_4$) AND TRIIODOTHYRONINE ($T_3$)** | |
| $T_4$ and $T_3$ levels controlled by TSH | Regulates protein, fat, and carbohydrate catabolism in all cells |
| Hormones show diurnal variation with peak during late evening | Regulates metabolic rate of all cells |
| Influences on amount secreted | Regulates body heat production |
| Gender | Acts as insulin antagonist |
| Pregnancy | Maintains growth hormone secretion, skeletal maturation |
| Gonadal steroid and adrenal corticosteroids; increased steroids = ↑ levels of $T_4$ and $T_3$ | Affects central nervous system development |
| Exposure to extreme cold = ↑ levels | Necessary for muscle tone and vigor |
| Nutritional state | Maintains cardiac rate, force, and output |
| Chemicals | Maintains secretions of GI tract |
| GHIH = ↓ levels | Affects respiratory rate and oxygen utilization |
| Dopamine = ↓ levels | Maintains calcium mobilization |
| Catecholamines = ↑ levels | Affects red blood cell production |
| | Stimulates lipid turnover, free fatty acid release, and cholesterol synthesis |
| | Regulates sympathetic nervous system activity |
| **CALCITONIN** | |
| Elevated serum calcium—major stimulant for calcitonin | Lowers serum calcium by opposing bone-resorbing effects of PTH, prostaglandins, and calciferols by inhibiting osteoclastic activity |
| Other stimulants | Also lowers serum phosphate levels |
| Gastrin | May also decrease calcium and phosphorus absorption in GI tract |
| Calcium-rich foods (regardless of serum $Ca^{++}$ levels) | |
| Pregnancy | |
| Lowered serum calcium—suppresses calcitonin release | |

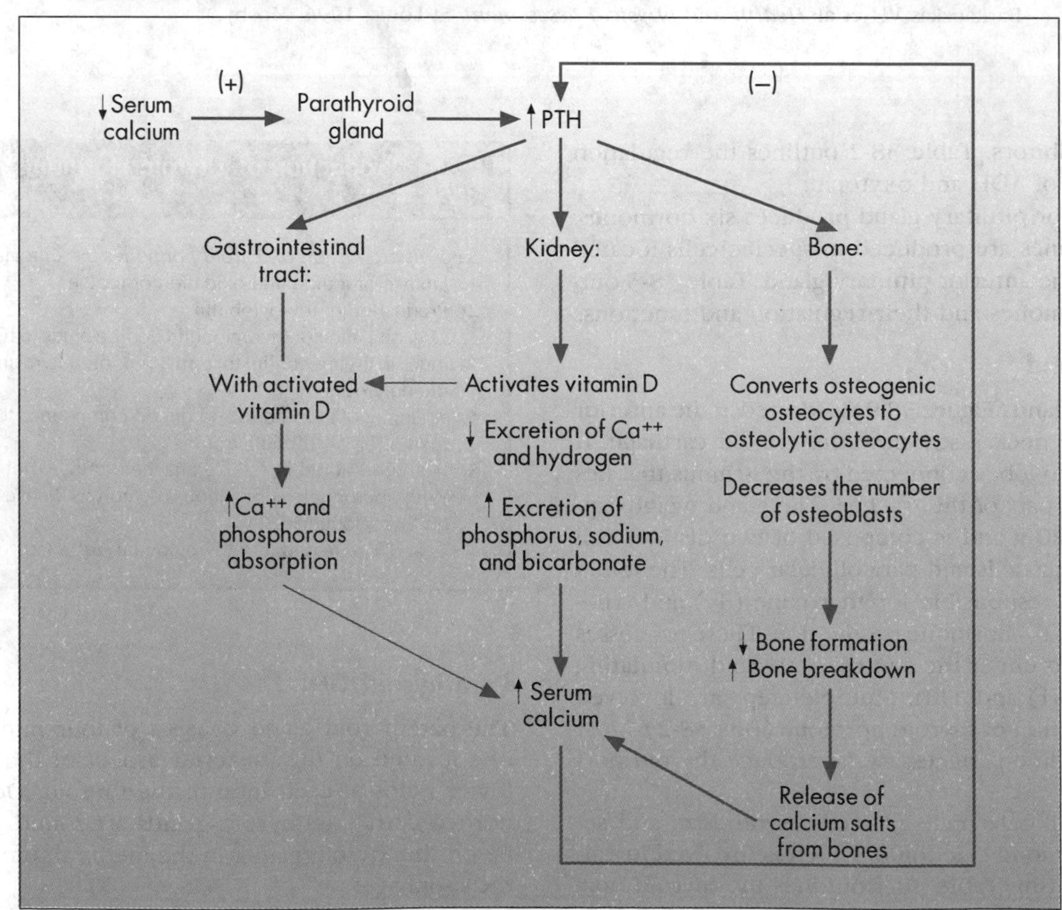


**FIGURE 38-10** Regulation and function of PTH.

**TABLE 38-5 Adrenal Cortex Hormones: Their Regulation and Functions**

| REGULATION | FUNCTIONS |
|---|---|
| **GLUCOCORTICOIDS (CORTISOL)** | |
| Level of cortisol is controlled by CRH/ACTH.<br>Cortisol shows episodic secretion with a circadian rhythm that peaks between 6 and 8 AM; this circadian pattern follows the circadian pattern of CRH/ACTH.<br>Physiologic and psychologic stressors (e.g., hypoglycemia, hypoxia, pain, infection, trauma, anxiety) result in increased cortisol via increased CRH and ACTH. This stress response overrides negative feedback cortisol normally exerts on ACTH. | Overall effect: maintain blood glucose level by increasing gluconeogenesis and decreasing rate of glucose utilization by cells<br>Increases protein catabolism<br>Promotes lipolysis<br>Antiinflammatory<br>Degrades collagen<br>Decreases T-lymphocyte participation in cellular-mediated immunity by decreasing circulating level of T lymphocytes<br>Increases neutrophils by increasing release and decreasing destruction<br>Decreases new antibody release<br>Decreases eosinophils, basophils, and monocytes<br>Decreases scar tissue formation<br>Increases red blood cell formation and possibly increases platelet formation<br>Increases gastric acid and pepsin production<br>Promotes sodium and water retention<br>Maintains emotional stability |
| **MINERALOCORTICOIDS (ALDOSTERONE)** | |
| Major regulator is renin-angiotensin system. When vascular volume or sodium is decreased, the renin-angiotensin system is activated (see Chapters 7, 20, and 48), and angiotensin II stimulates release of mineralocorticoids.<br>Other regulators<br>Increased serum potassium ($K^+$) directly stimulates adrenal cortex to release mineralocorticoids.<br>CRH/ACTH system is a weak regulator. | Maintains sodium and volume status<br>Increases sodium reabsorption in distal tubules<br>Increases potassium and hydrogen excretion in distal tubules |
| **ADRENAL ANDROGENS** | |
| Major regulator is CRH/ACTH system. | Responsible for some secondary sex characteristics in females; in males, work like gonadal steroids |

thyroid hormone (PTH). This hormone is continually synthesized. Figure 38-10 depicts the primary regulator of PTH and its function.

There are two factors related to parathyroid gland function that should be remembered. First, other factors like calcitonin levels and serum phosphate levels influence PTH secretion, probably by decreasing serum calcium. Second, the biologic regulators probably never totally depress PTH secretion.

## Adrenal Gland

The adrenal glands are retroperitoneal abdominal organs that cap the upper pole of each kidney. Each gland consists of two glands: the outer gland is the *adrenal cortex,* and the inner core is the *adrenal medulla.* The cortex consists of the three zones: the zona glomerulosa, zona fasciculata, and the zona reticularis.

### Adrenal cortex hormones

The adrenal cortex produces three hormones: **mineralocorticoids** (aldosterone), produced in the zona glomerulosa; **glucocorticoids** (cortisol) and **androgens,** produced in the zona fasciculata and zona reticularis. The glucocorticoids and mineralocorticoids are not only secreted and used daily but are two major hormones that are secreted as part of the physiologic stress response to stressors, which is discussed in Chapter 7. The mineralocorticoids and glucocorticoids are necessary for life. Table 38-5 outlines the regulation and functions of the adrenocortical hormones.

### Adrenal medulla secretions

The adrenal medulla makes up approximately 10% of the total adrenal gland and produces two secretions: *epinephrine* and *norepinephrine.* The adrenal medulla arises embryonically from the neural crest and is really a modified sympathetic ganglion. The adrenal medulla is innervated by preganglionic splanchnic nerves. With stimulation to the sympathetic nervous system via the hypothalamus and medulla oblongata, the adrenal medulla is stimulated, and two **catecholamines** (epinephrine and norepinephrine) are released. The catecholamines travel by blood to parts of the body and stimulate target cells. The catecholamine norepinephrine is also released from the terminal of postganglionic sympathetic fibers.

The healthy adrenal medulla secretes approximately 85% epinephrine and 15% norepinephrine. These catecholamines have different effects in the body because of the different receptors on body organs. These receptors are classified as alpha-($\alpha$-) adrenergic and beta-($\beta$)-adrenergic. $\beta$-Receptors are subdivided into $\beta_1$ and $\beta_2$. $\beta_1$-Receptors are located primarily in the heart, and $\beta_2$-receptors occur elsewhere in the body. $\alpha$-Receptors also can be subdivided in two types: $\alpha_1$, which occur on target organs and are excitatory; and $\alpha_2$, which occur at presynaptic sites and, when stimulated, inhibit release of the catecholamines. Much of what is known about adrenergic receptors is based on the effects of various pharmacologic agents.

Norepinephrine is a more potent stimulator of $\alpha$-receptors, whereas epinephrine stimulates $\alpha$- and $\beta$-receptors. The final effect on an organ of stimulation of the sympathetic nervous system and adrenal medulla depends on the type of receptors in a particular organ. Table 38-6 lists the effects of adrenal-medullary-sympathetic stimulation on body organs.

A small quantity of catecholamines is released at all times, and this helps to maintain homeostasis. In the presence of a major stressor, either physiologic or psychologic, increased amounts of catecholamines are released in an attempt to overcome the stressor and all the effects listed in Table 38-6 may be seen. This increased adrenal-medullary-sympathetic stimulation is part of the *physiologic stress response,* which is discussed in more detail in Chapter 7.

**TABLE 38-6 Effects of Adrenal-Medullary-Sympathetic Stimulation on Body Organs**

| ORGAN | EFFECT* |
|---|---|
| Heart | Increased conduction velocity, automaticity, contractility, rate, and stroke volume caused by $\beta_1$-stimulation |
| Blood vessels | |
| Coronary vessels, brain, lungs | Dilation caused by $\beta_2$-stimulation and autoregulatory phenomena |
| Skin, mucosa, abdominal viscera, renal and salivary gland vessels | Constriction caused by $\alpha_1$-receptor stimulation; renal vessels have dopaminergic receptors also |
| Veins | Constriction caused by $\alpha_1$-stimulation |
| Bronchial muscles | Relaxation caused by $\beta_2$-stimulation |
| Gastrointestinal tract | Inhibition of production of gastrointestinal secretions; decreased motility and contraction of sphincters |
| Gallbladder | Relaxation |
| Kidney | Increased renin secretion caused by $\beta_2$-stimulation |
| Urinary bladder | Relaxation of detrusor muscle and contraction of sphincter |
| Skin | Pilomotor muscle contraction and localized sweating |
| Liver | Glycogenolysis and gluconeogenesis caused by $\beta_2$-stimulation |
| Pancreas | Decreased secretion of exocrine cells; $\beta_2$-stimulation causes increased secretion of islet $\beta$-cells, but $\alpha$-stimulation causes decreased secretion of islet cells; $\alpha$-effect predominates |
| Fat cells | Lipolysis |
| Brain | Increased alertness, restlessness |
| Eyes | Dilation of pupils and relaxation of ciliary bodies |

*These total effects would be seen in the physiologic response to stressors, as discussed in Chapter 7.

## Pancreatic Endocrine Functions

The pancreas is both an exocrine and an endocrine gland. It lies retroperitoneally behind the stomach, with its head and neck in the curve of the duodenum, its body extending horizontally across the posterior abdominal wall, and its tail touching the spleen. The cells of the pancreas that serve the endocrine function are the *islets of Langerhans.* There are over 1 million islet cells spread throughout the total pancreas; these cells make up 1% to 2% of the pancreatic mass. The islets of Langerhans consist of four cell types: (1) $\alpha$-cells, which make up 20% of the cells and secrete glucagon; (2) $\beta$-cells, which make up 70% of the cells and secrete insulin; (3) delta cells, which make up 10% of the cells and secrete somatostatin; and (4) F-cells, which secrete pancreatic polypeptide. The purposes of somatostatin and pancreatic polypeptide are unclear. The secretions of the $\alpha$- and $\beta$-cells are discussed next.

### Insulin

Insulin is a protein hormone that is secreted as a prohormone. The removal of a connecting peptide (C-peptide) fragment results in the active hormone. Both insulin and C-peptide are secreted into the blood in equal amounts. Insulin has an unstimulated basal secretion that controls metabolism between meals. Insulin also shows meal-related increases. The major stimulus is glucose, but insulin secretion is also stimulated by the intake of amino acids. Acetylcholine increases insulin secretion, whereas catecholamines acting on $\alpha$-adrenergic receptors inhibit insulin secretion.

Overall, **insulin** is an anabolic hormone; it promotes the utilization of ingested food and the storage of nutrients in excess of body needs. Although it can affect every cell in the body, its major effects are seen in liver cells, adipose tissue, and muscles (Table 38-7).

### Glucagon

Glucagon, along with epinephrine, growth hormone, and glucocorticoids, functions as a **counterregulatory hormone** to insulin. **Glucagon**'s overall function is to increase blood glucose. It is stimulated by a decreased

TABLE 38-7 Action of Insulin

| LIVER CELLS | ADIPOSE TISSUE | MUSCLE |
|---|---|---|
| Increases glycogenesis | Increases fatty acid synthesis | Increases glycogenesis |
| Increases fatty acid synthesis | Increases glycerol synthesis and formation of triglycerides | Increases amino acid uptake and protein synthesis |
| Decreases glycogenolysis, gluconeogenesis, and ketogenesis | Decreases lipolysis | Decreases protein catabolism |

blood glucose level and increased amino acid levels. The primary target of glucagon is the liver, where it stimulates *glycogenolysis* (breakdown of glycogen to glucose). When the need for glucose is greater than can be provided by glycogenolysis, glucagon promotes amino acid transport from the muscle and stimulates *gluconeogenesis* (formation of glycogen from fatty acids and proteins rather than carbohydrates). Glucagon also promotes lipolysis and ketone formation. Glucagon works with epinephrine, glucocorticoids, and growth hormone in carrying out the metabolic function designed to maintain blood glucose in times of fasting, starvation, or stress.

## PHYSIOLOGIC CHANGES WITH AGING

Changes in the endocrine system are associated with normal aging. Endocrine dysfunction may result from cellular damage caused by aging, wear and tear on the endocrine tissue from long-term use, or genetically programmed cellular changes.[8] Endocrine changes may result in altered synthesis and secretion of hormones, altered metabolism of hormones, altered circulatory levels of hormones, altered biologic activity, and altered target cell and target tissue responsiveness, or altered intrinsic rhythms.[3] Although findings are not consistent, the following is a summary of the major alterations in endocrine function that are most frequently reported:

1. The most frequently seen change is decreased ovarian functioning, resulting in increased gonadotropins and changes in reproductive and sexual functioning. No similar change in males has been reported.
2. Impaired secretion of hypothalamic hormones or impaired response to feedback may influence endocrine system responsiveness to alterations in the internal environment and thus to stressors. Decreased secretion of GHRH has been reported.[5]
3. The anterior pituitary gland shows morphologic changes with increased fibrosis and microadenoma formation, a decrease in basal levels of prolactin in females, and a decrease in growth hormone and somatomedins.
4. Antidiuretic hormone secretion in response to changes in serum osmolality is increased, resulting in increased levels of ADH. However, elderly persons have alterations in renal function that decrease the ability to concentrate urine and can result in hyponatremia. Nocturia is typically present.
5. Various changes in thyroid gland structure, including glandular atrophy, fibrosis, nodularity, and infiltrates, have been found. The following changes in thyroid hormone levels have been reported:
   a. Decreased $T_4$ secretion and metabolism
   b. Decreased plasma $T_3$ levels
   c. Increased basal plasma TSH levels
   d. Decreased responsiveness in TSH secretion to TRH

   Hypothyroidism occurs often in elderly persons. Whether all these changes in thyroid structure, function, or disease can be attributed to the aging process is unclear. Some of the early clinical manifestations of hypothyroidism, such as skin and hair changes, neurologic changes, or GI changes, can be seen in elderly persons for other reasons, leading health care professionals to ignore or potentially misdiagnose the changes.
6. Calcium homeostasis is altered in the older adult. Changes found include decreased intake of calcium, negative calcium balance, bone loss, decreased intestinal adaptation to varied calcium intake, hypercalciuria, and decreased vitamin D levels. Age-related alterations in PTH may explain some of the changes in calcium homeostasis, but more research is needed.
7. The adrenal cortex gland, which is small and contains fibrous tissue, responds to feedback mechanisms and maintains circadian patterns of cortisol secretion in response to circadian patterns of ACTH. However, the amount of cortisol secreted is decreased because of decreased metabolic clearance and decreased usage. Thus increased blood cortisol levels result in decreased secretion. The amount of androgens secreted by the adrenal cortex is decreased, and the renin-aldosterone response to postural changes and volume depletion is depressed.
8. Impaired glucose tolerance in elderly persons is multifactorial. Delayed glucose-induced insulin secretion, altered hepatic handling of glucose, and impaired insulin-mediated glucose uptake are all part of the problem and result in elevated blood glucose levels after glucose loads, such as eating. These changes may result in blood glucose values that are higher than what are usually considered normal but are not diagnostic for diabetes mellitus.
9. Non–insulin-dependent diabetes mellitus is one of the more common chronic diseases of elderly persons.[13]

If the changes described in the preceding section are ignored, elderly persons may be misdiagnosed. Particularly, they may be diagnosed as having diabetes mellitus when further assessment reveals this to be untrue, although diabetes mellitus does occur more frequently in elderly individuals. Changes in serum sodium and potassium must be carefully evaluated to differentiate changes related to aging from those that might be caused by drugs such as diuretics, other diseases such as congestive heart failure, or diet. The potential role of changes in PTH in development of metabolic bone disease needs more exploration. It is important to remember that the hypothalamic-pituitary-adrenal axis and the hypothalamic-pituitary-thyroid axis, which are important in daily living and response to stressors, are intact but may be slower to respond.

Beside the changes just listed, changes in response to actual endocrine pathologic conditions have been reported. Some elderly persons with hyperthyroidism have subtle signs and symptoms that make diagnosis difficult. Elderly persons tolerate hypothyroidism better, and there may be a great insufficiency of thyroid hormone when they are first diagnosed. Also, early signs of hypothyroidism may be overlooked because they can occur in normal aging in the absence of a thyroid pathologic condition.

## SUBJECTIVE DATA

A review of the normal functions of all hormones as described on the preceding pages reveals that they influence four broad domains: maintenance of a normal internal environment; energy production, storage, and utilization; growth and development; and reproductive and sexual function. Alterations in endocrine function lead to varied manifestations because of disruption in maintenance of a normal internal environment; inadequate energy production, stores, and utilization; abnormal growth and development; and abnormal reproductive and sexual function. Systemic assessment of multiple parameters is necessary to define the healthiness of a person's endocrine system or needs. The anatomic location of endocrine glands precludes their direct assessment. A thorough history from the patient or significant others is absolutely necessary. Special attention should be paid to the patient's history regarding fluid and nutritional intake, elimination pattern, energy level, perception of changes in body characteristics, reproductive and sexual function, and tolerance to stressors.

### FLUID/NUTRITIONAL INTAKE

Endocrine abnormalities can lead to alteration in fluid and food intake (increased or decreased) that may or may not be associated with weight loss or weight gain. Many of the endocrine problems are chronic and require long-term special diets and, at times, fluid restrictions. Qualitative and quantitative assessment of food intake is necessary to determine the cause of weight loss or gain, adequacy of intake for normal metabolic needs, and adherence to any special diet. Having the patient list food and fluid taken on the previous day is an excellent way to assess fluid and nutritional intake. The history must include alcohol and snacks. The preferences of the patient with regard to types of food, as well as times of eating, are important in providing a diet that meets nutritional needs. Elements such as a pleasant environment, mouth care before meals, and small meals to decrease anorexia and nausea may be necessary. Assessment of how the patient is tolerating foods and fluids must be ongoing.

### ELIMINATION PATTERN

The endocrine system is involved in maintenance of water and electrolyte balance. The history should include information on the frequency, approximate amount, and color of urinary elimination. The presence of *nocturia* or *dysuria* is also noted. In endocrine disease, depending on the cause, there may be a history of increased output and increased thirst, or decreased output and increased weight. Some patients may be on diuretics, and their adherence to the therapy should be assessed. The frequency and color of bowel movements also are determined. Information concerning constipation or other changes in bowel habits that may be caused by changes in water balance, dietary intake, or sluggishness of the bowel may be elicited. Treatment of pathologic conditions may include changes in diet and fluid intake that will influence elimination. The patient's previous pattern of elimination will help the nurse teach about needed changes such as decreasing fluid intake after dinner to decrease nocturia.

### ENERGY LEVEL

Because the endocrine system is directly involved in the metabolism (storage and utilization) of nutrients for engery, pathologic conditions will usually decrease the person's energy level. Many patients will complain of "not being able to do their normal things." It is important to assess the person's energy level and to use this as a guide for helping plan activities of daily living. Some persons need help in adjusting their activities to allow for rest periods; they may need assistance in eliminating activities or in changing the ways they do activities to conserve energy.

Most endocrine problems can be well controlled so that permanent changes in life-style will not be necessary. Recovery may be slow, however; and the patient's physical status may be so damaged that, although the energy level may be normal, additional time will be required for complete recovery.

### PERCEPTIONS OF CHANGES IN BODY CHARACTERISTICS

Changes in hair distribution, body proportions, voice, skin pigmentation, and facial appearance may accompany problems of the endocrine system. A description of changes by patients or their significant others is very important, because characteristics of persons vary so greatly and changes may not be so extensive or rapid that observation alone will pick them up.

The collection of information regarding changes in body characteristics is important not only in helping to define the physiologic problem but also in identifying potential or present emotional or psychologic problems. Some of the changes that occur with endocrine problems are irreversible even when problems are controlled. Body characteristics are part of the identity of the person, and the person may have problems dealing with the changes. (See Chapter 9 for a detailed discussion of body image.)

### REPRODUCTIVE AND SEXUAL FUNCTION

The endocrine system is very involved with reproductive functions. A thorough reproductive and sexual history must be obtained. Data regarding the menstrual cycle (onset, frequency of menses, duration, amount of flow), presence of problems with the cycle (e.g., menorrhagia), presence of impotence, and any perceived problems with fertility should be obtained. The history should also include information about satisfaction with sexual relationships for two reasons. First, sometimes the first changes in reproductive functioning will manifest themselves as changes in sexual satisfaction. Second, reproductive changes may not be a problem for the patient if sexual satisfaction is maintained. For example, infertility may not be a concern if childbearing is not a desired outcome (see Chapters 11 and 51).

### TOLERANCE TO STRESSORS

The endocrine system helps the body respond to all types of physical and psychologic stressors. The patient or significant others should be questioned in relation to the person's ability (or change in ability) to tolerate stressors. Such things as intolerance to heat and cold, increased frequency of infections, increased irritation, euphoria, depression, increased crying, or increased anger may be elicited. Depending on the person's ability to handle stressors, special environmental controls to decrease the chance of infection and to maintain a consistent physical and emotional environment may be necessary.

### OTHER SUBJECTIVE INFORMATION

Each endocrine problem has unique clinical manifestations, which are described in Chapters 39 and 40. As part of the history for a patient with a known diagnosis, the patient should be asked if continued signs and symptoms associated with the specific uncontrolled pathologic condition are still present. In addition, information regarding whether the patient is experiencing any signs and symptoms of any uncontrolled endocrine pathologic condition is elicited. The last area to be assessed concerns the patient's teaching-learning needs. The person's learning style, adherence to the prescribed therapeutic regimen, difficulty in carrying out the regimen, and other self-management skills are determined.

## OBJECTIVE DATA

The collection of objective data about the endocrine system may require a complete physical examination. The major areas in which abnormalities may be found are discussed next. Collection of this data requires a thorough inspection and use of the techniques of palpation and auscultation. (See Box 38-3 for outline of areas to be examined with a head-to-toe approach.)

Inspection should be used to assess the patient's growth and developmental status. Such things as height, weight, body proportions, amount and distribution of muscle mass, fat distribution, skin pigmentation, and hair distribution should be assessed. A great variation in these parameters exists in the general population, and often the changes are not obvious. Inspection of family members for like characteristics provides information as to whether the characteristics seen in the patient are caused by hereditary or pathophysiologic alterations. The patient's alertness, responsiveness, and speech patterns can be assessed when the history is being collected.

**BOX 38-3 Summary of Objective Data Using a Head-to-Toe Approach**

**GENERAL**

General appearance, body proportions (normal for age), height, weight, general body characteristics, any skin abrasions, sores, wounds, temperature, respiratory rate, type of respiration

**SKIN**

Pigmentation, turgor, presence of edema, sweating, flushing

**FACE/SCALP**

Hair distribution, change in amount of facial/scalp hair, presence of exophthalmos

**ORAL CAVITY**

Mucous membrane moisture

**NECK**

Jugular veins, thyroid gland

**CARDIOVASCULAR**

Blood pressure and pulse, check for orthostatic changes; temperature; more extensive evaluation indicated if problem identified

**ABDOMEN**

Abdominal striae, central obesity

**MUSCULOSKELETAL**

Muscle mass, strength, joint enlargement or deformity

**NERVOUS SYSTEM**

Alertness, responsiveness, mood, tremors; possible necessity of a more extensive evaluation if problem is evident

The endocrine system plays a major role in growth and development, metabolism of food products, and regulation of sex hormones. All of these functions, if affected, cause changes in body characteristics. Some examples of specific changes are (1) *dwarfism* caused by thyroid and pituitary problems; (2) changes in fat distribution, producing *buffalo hump* and *thickened girdle* from adrenocortical excess; (3) presence of *purplish striae* instead of white striae because of adrenocortical excess; (4) *muscle wasting* with a wide variety of endocrine problems; and (5) *change in sexual characteristics* because of abnormalities of hormonal levels. All these changes can be identified during inspection.

Inspection and palpation are used to check skin turgor, mucous membrane moisture, and jugular vein distension (JVD) and to check for the presence of edema. All these data will give information about the fluid and electrolyte status of the person, which can be changed with almost any endocrine problem.

Following are changes that may be found:

1. The finger should slide over the mucous membrane easily. In states of fluid depletion as would be seen in uncontrolled diabetes mellitus, adrenocortical insufficiency, and possibly diabetes insipidus, the mucous membranes are sticky.
2. Edema as might be seen in adrenocortical excess can be graded from 1+ to 4+ (see Chapter 20).
3. Skin turgor can be checked on the forearm, on the forehead, or over the sternum.
4. Abnormal JVD may be present with fluid overload.

Assessment of cardiovascular status is imperative. A minimal assessment includes checking orthostatic blood pressure and pulse. If fluid volume or electrolyte problems are present, a more extensive evaluation of such things as rhythm and heart sounds will be necessary.

Of all the endocrine organs discussed, only the thyroid is routinely examined. In disease states, sometimes the pancreas and parathyroid gland can be palpated. The thyroid gland is usually examined along with examination of the head and neck. Palpation of the thyroid provides information about the size, shape, and symmetry of the gland and the presence of nodules or tenderness. Auscultation may be used to assess for bruits.

## DIAGNOSTIC TESTS

Endocrine dysfunction in most instances can be classified as resulting from hypersecretion or hyposecretion. The excess or deficient secretion can result from (1) *primary* dysfunction of any of the endocrine glands; (2) abnormal function of the pituitary gland, resulting in *secondary* thyroid, adrenal, or gonadal dysfunction; (3) abnormal endocrine gland functioning caused by a nonendocrine disease; (4) *ectopic* secretion of hormones by nonendocrine tissue; or (5) *iatrogenic* causes. Although most diseases can be classified into one of these categories, endocrine dysfunction also can result from abnormal receptor functioning or intracellular responses.

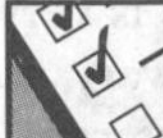

**Guidelines for Preparing the Person for Diagnostic Tests**

- Physical preparation as ordered
- Explain purpose of test
- Explain what to expect before and during the test
- Explain any special care after the test

Diagnostic tests are used to evaluate (1) the level of hormone in the blood (both basal and cyclic changes); (2) the adequacy of endocrine tissue in secreting hormone in response to exogenous stimulants; (3) the interrelationships among the hypothalamus, anterior pituitary gland, and other endocrine glands controlled by the anterior pituitary hormones; and (4) the various substrates controlled by the endocrine system.

Usually several tests are necessary in the evaluation of an endocrine gland and its functioning. Most of the tests of the endocrine system require taking samples of blood; some cause discomfort, and some require fasting. The nurse is responsible for preparing the patient appropriately. The routine physical preparation for any test will vary from institution to institution. Besides carrying out the physical preparation, the nurse teaches the patient as appropriate (see Guidelines box above).

Because the endocrine system affects fluid and electrolytes, patients with suspected pathologic conditions or those being evaluated to establish total health status will have serum electrolytes evaluated. In this section specific diagnostic tests for evaluation of particular glands will be described. The diagnostic tests for each gland are discussed separately.

### PITUITARY FUNCTION TESTING

Pituitary gland malfunction can lead to a variety of symptoms, depending on which hormone is in excess or in deficit. The pituitary gland, as described previously, is interrelated with functions of the thyroid, the adrenal glands, and the gonads. The tests for the function of the pituitary with regard to TSH, ACTH, and gonadotropins are discussed when the diagnostic tests of these glands are outlined.

#### Radiologic Tests

Pituitary malfunction may be associated with pituitary tumors, and skull x-ray films to assess the size of the pituitary gland are carried out. Computed tomography (CT) scanning or magnetic resonance imaging (MRI) may be used to demonstrate the presence of sella turcica masses. In some instances, pneumoencephalograms may be necessary to define the size of the mass or to exclude empty sella syndrome.

## Growth Hormone

The absence or deficit of growth hormone (somatotropin GH) leads to dramatic changes in appearance.

### Laboratory tests

Assay of GH is possible. GH release follows a diurnal pattern; basal levels can best be determined in the morning, but they are usually less than 3 μg/ml. Levels at other times are less than 10 ng/ml. GH secretion can be stimulated by L-dopa, bromocriptine, and hypoglycemia. The provocative tests are done as follows: (1) basal levels of GH are determined; (2) L-dopa (500 mg orally), bromocriptine (5 mg orally), or insulin (0.1 U/kg IV) is given; and (3) blood is drawn at intervals up to 120 minutes after stimulation. GH usually peaks at approximately 60 minutes after provocative stimulation.

### Radiologic tests

Diagnostic tests for abnormalities related to somatotropin include skeletal x-ray films to assess changes in bone structure.

## Prolactin

Prolactin excess is seen in the presence of some pituitary tumors, or it may be idiopathic. Prolactin deficiency may result in failure of postpartum lactation.

### Laboratory tests

Levels of prolactin can be measured by radioassay; the normal level is 2 to 15 ng/ml. Provocative tests for prolactin with the use of chlorpromazine or thyroid-releasing hormone (TRH) are available. The tests are done as follows: (1) basal levels of prolactin are measured; (2) chlorpromazine (0.7 mg/kg IM) or TRH (400 μg IV) is given; and then (3) serum levels of prolactin are drawn at timed intervals up to 240 minutes.

## Antidiuretic Hormone (ADH)

Absence of ADH leads to a disease called **diabetes insipidus.** The major symptom of this problem is an output of large quantities of dilute urine (greater than 7 to 11 L/day). Before diabetes insipidus can be conclusively diagnosed, the patient must be shown to have a deficiency in ADH, and the patient's kidney must be able to respond to ADH. Exogenous sources of ADH have no effect if the patient's kidney cannot respond. Exogenous ADH will increase the osmolality of the urine, whether the dilute urine is caused by excess intake of water or by diabetes insipidus. The differentiation is made between these two conditions by demonstrating response or lack of response to osmolality changes in the serum.

### Laboratory tests

A *water deprivation test* is used if problems with ADH are suspected. Water is withheld for 4 to 18 hours, and the person's response to this deprivation is documented. A person without diabetes insipidus will respond with a rapid decrease in urine volume and an increase in urine osmolality. A patient with diabetes insipidus will have no decrease in volume and no increase in urine osmolality, but the serum osmolality will increase to more than 300 mOsm/kg. The person who cannot produce ADH is susceptible to vascular collapse, because the massive output of urine will continue unabated. Close monitoring for impending collapse during the test is required. Monitoring should include hourly vital signs, urine output, and specific gravity. If a weight loss greater than 3% of body weight occurs or if tachycardia or significant hypotension develops, the test should be terminated. The patient with *psychogenic polydipsia* may have extreme behavioral problems associated with the deprivation of water and will need emotional support during this period.

**TABLE 38-8 Provocative Tests of Thyroid Function**

| FUNCTION TEST/PROCEDURE AND PREPARATION | INTERPRETATION |
|---|---|
| **TRH STIMULATION TEST** | |
| TRH is given IV and then serum thyroid-stimulating hormone (TSH) levels are repeatedly measured. Patient may feel facial flushing, the urge to urinate, or nausea for 5 minutes after injection. These are self-limiting but not complications. | Normal serum TSH begins to rise at 10 minutes and peaks at 45 minutes; subnormal tests reflect diminished TSH reserve; supranormal response occurs in patients with hypothyroidism of thyroid origin; no response occurs in most patients with thyrotoxicosis except when it is caused by excess TSH. |
| **TSH STIMULATION TEST** | |
| Baseline levels of radioactive iodine uptake (RAIU) and protein-bound iodine (PBI) are taken, TSH injection is given, and repeat RAIU and PBI levels are taken. | Test assists in differentiating between primary and secondary hypothyroidism; in primary hypothyroidism repeat level of RAIU and PBI stays the same; if they become normal, this indicates hypothyroidism caused by too little TSH (secondary). |
| **THYROID SUPPRESSION TEST** | |
| RAIU test and serum $T_4$ levels are done. Patient is given thyroid hormone for 7-10 days, and RAIU and serum $T_4$ tests are repeated. | If euthyroid (normal), repeat RAIU and serum $T_4$ levels will be low; failure of hormone therapy to suppress RAIU and serum $T_4$ indicates hyperthyroidism. |

**TABLE 38-9 Radiographic Tests of Thyroid Gland**

| FUNCTION TEST/PROCEDURE AND PREPARATION | INTERPRETATION |
|---|---|
| **RADIOACTIVE IODINE UPTAKE (RAIU)** | |
| Tracer dose of radioactive iodine is given orally. At 2, 6, and 24 hours after administration, scintillation detector is placed over neck and amount of accumulated iodine is measured. Urine is collected for 24 hours; decreased amounts in urine indicate hyperthyroid state. No precautions necessary. | Normal thyroid will take up 5% to 35% of tracer dose. Increased uptake occurs in hyperthyroidism. Excess iodine in foods, cough medicine, x-ray media, other medications, and enriched iodine foods affect test by giving low readings. Diarrhea gives low readings from absorption of tracer dose. Decreased excretion with renal failure gives elevated readings. |
| **THYROID SCAN** | |
| Dose of radioactive iodine or labeled pertechnitate is given, and scintillation scan is done. Scanner is moved over thyroid, and a picture of distribution of radioactivity is recorded. No radiation precautions necessary. | Size, shape, and anatomic function of gland are assessed; areas of increased uptake are noted. |
| **THYROID ULTRASOUND** | |
| Thyroid is assessed by ultrasound. | Test is helpful in defining "cold" areas as cystic or solid. |

The water deprivation test may be followed by a *vasopressin test* to determine whether the kidney can respond to vasopressin (exogenous ADH). After 5 units of aqueous pitressin is given subcutaneously, urine osmolality should increase. Failure to show an increase in osmolality confirms the diagnosis of nephrogenic diabetes insipidus.[2]

## THYROID FUNCTION TESTING

Testing for thyroid function can be made at the hypothalamic, pituitary, thyroid, or serum levels. The major tests and their procedures, preparations, and interpretations are presented in Tables 38-8 and 38-9.

### Laboratory Tests

The most frequently used tests are *serum thyroxine ($T_4$), serum triiodothryronine ($T_3$), serum thyroid-stimulating hormone (TSH),* and *free thyroxine index ($FT_4I$)* (Table 38-10). Serum levels of $T_4$ and $T_3$ reflect total thyroid hormone concentration in the blood, both the metabolically active (free) portion and the inactive (bound) portion. It is difficult and expensive to measure free $T_4$ and free $T_3$; other tests are used to estimate these levels indirectly: the *thyroid resin uptake test ($T_3U$)* and the *$FT_4I$ test.*

The largest part (99%) of $T_4$ and $T_3$ is bound to **carrier proteins:** thyroid-binding proteins (TBG [thyroid-binding globulins] and TBA [thyroid-binding albumin]). The carrier proteins have a greater affinity for $T_4$ than for $T_3$, allowing free $T_3$ to enter cells more rapidly.[10] The $T_3U$ ($T_3RU$, $RT_3U$) test indirectly measures whether unusual levels of thyroid-binding proteins are influencing the serum levels of $T_3$. The $FT_4I$ is calculated as the product of the result of the $T_3U$ and the $T_4$ level.[4] Usually, the order for an $FT_4I$ is written as an *$F_7$* or *$F_{12}$ test,* which is really a $T_4$ test and $T_3U$ test with a calculated $FT_4I$. Because the $FT_4I$ is not affected by the TBG, it reflects hormonal status more accurately than does the total $T_4$.

Further laboratory studies may be done to determine functioning of the hypothalamic-pituitary-thyroid (HPT) axis and the level at which dysfunction exists. (See Table 38-8 for several provocative tests that may be used to stimulate or depress the HPT axis.)

### Radiologic Tests

The most frequently used tests are thyroid ultrasound and thyroid scan (see Table 38-9 for details).

## PARATHYROID FUNCTION TESTING

Because the maintenance of normal calcium and phosphorus metabolism involves multiple systems beside the parathyroid (skeletal, GI, urinary), when parathyroid function is being assessed, the patient will also have diagnostic tests of these other systems. This is necessary to determine whether the problem with calcium and phosphorus metabolism is caused by altered parathyroid metabolism or by other disease states. In addition, because calcium has a very important role in the maintenance of normal neuromuscular irritability and because hypocalcemia can be lethal, the patient will be assessed and continually monitored for the presence of Trousseau's and Chvostek's signs when hypoparathyroidism is suspected (see Chapter 20). Increased neuromuscular irritability can result in carpopedal spasm, hypertonic flexion, or rigidity of the fingers and/or toes. This sign is seen in the fingers when a blood pressure cuff is inflated on the arm **(Trousseau's sign).** Tapping of the finger over the facial nerve can evoke a muscular tic on that side of the face **(Chvostek's sign).**

### Laboratory Tests

The specific tests of parathyroid function consist of serial laboratory determinations of serum calcium and phosphorus, urinary calcium, and serum alkaline phosphatase. Calcium and phosphorus are evenly proportional, so both must be measured. Normally, serum calcium

**TABLE 38-10 Tests of Thyroid Function**

| FUNCTION TEST/PROCEDURE AND PREPARATION | INTERPRETATION |
|---|---|
| **SERUM $T_4$ CONCENTRATION** | |
| Radioassay of blood is done; no special preparation is needed. | Test measures circulating thyroxine that is bound to TBG and free $T_4$; normal values are 4.7-11 μg/dl. Hyperthyroidism and increased TBG such as occurs in pregnancy and estrogen therapy cause increased $T_4$ values. Hypothyroidism and decreased TBG, as seen with glucocorticoid therapy and hypoproteinemia, cause decreased $T_4$ values. |
| **FREE $T_4$ INDEX ($FT_4I$)** | |
| Serum $T_4$ and $T_3U$ are measured. | $FT_4I$ is product of serum $T_4$ and $T_3U$; changes in TBG cause reciprocal alterations in serum $T_4$ and $T_3U$ so that $FT_4I$ stays normal. |
| **SERUM $T_3$ CONCENTRATIONS** | |
| Radioassay of blood sample is done; no special preparation is needed | Test measures circulating $T_3$ that is bound to TBG and free $T_3$; normal values are 110-230 ng/dl and are elevated in $T_3$ thyrotoxicosis; variations in TBG can influence test results as they do for serum $T_4$. |
| **SERUM TSH CONCENTRATION** | |
| Radioassay of blood is done; no special preparation is needed. | Test measures circulating TSH; normal values are 5 to 10 ng/dl. Elevated levels reflect pituitary hypersecretion of TSH. |
| **TRIIODOTHYRONINE RESIN UPTAKE ($T_3U$)** | |
| Blood sample is drawn; in laboratory, resin and radioactive $T_3$ are added to sample of blood. Radioactive $T_3$ will bind to unoccupied sites of TBG. Excessive radioactive $T_3$ will bind to resin. Radioactive counts are done on blood and resins to determine amount of $T_3$ (radioactive) bound to resin. | Normally 25% to 30% of radioactive $T_3$ will bind to resin; in hyperthyroidism, where there are increased amounts of endogenous thyroid hormone, value of amount binding to resin will be increased; in hypothyroidism, $T_3$ resin uptake will be low. This test is not a measure of the patient's endogenous $T_3$ level. Test is affected by total amount of TBG. In wasting diseases where amount of TBG may be decreased, reading may be falsely elevated. In conditions such as pregnancy and estrogen therapy, abnormal amounts of TBG may be available, and a false-low resin uptake may be obtained; phenytoin (Dilantin) and salicylates compete with thyroxine for TBG sites and may give false-negative $T_3$ resin uptake. |

levels are 9.0 to 10.5 mg/dl, serum phosphorus levels are 2.5 to 4.5 mg/dl, urinary calcium excretion in 24 hours is 1 to 300 mg (depending on diet and need) and serum alkaline phosphatase measures 30 to 85 IU/L.

## ADRENAL FUNCTION TESTING

The adrenal function tests can be divided into those designed to test *cortical* function and those designed to test *medullary* function.

### Adrenocortical Function Tests

Because the adrenal cortex affects so many physiologic functions, tests that are diagnostic for many disorders may be ordered.

**Laboratory tests**

Analysis of blood to ascertain electrolyte balance, a glucose tolerance test to determine the ability of the patient to use carbohydrates, and a test of the ability of the renal tubules to concentrate and dilute urine will probably be done. In addition, x-ray films of the kidney area may be taken to ascertain the presence of adrenal tumors.

Diagnostic tests of adrenocortical function include tests of all three types of hormonal secretions. Plasma cortisol and ACTH follow a diurnal pattern. Each can be measured at 8 AM and 4 PM (or later) to ascertain whether the normal diurnal pattern is present. A high serum value of cortisol and/or ACTH and loss of the diurnal pattern are associated with hypercortisolism (Table 38-11). A below-normal serum level of cortisol or a normal level of cortisol in a stressed patient indicates adrenal insufficiency. Confirmation of adrenal insufficiency is by a blunted or absent response to ACTH.[7] The rapid ACTH stimulation test is particularly useful in

**TABLE 38-11 Diurnal Pattern of Serum Cortisol and Adrenocorticotropic Hormone (ACTH) Levels**

| SERUM VALUES | 6 AM | 4 PM (OR LATER) |
|---|---|---|
| Cortisol | 6-28 ng/dl | 2-12 ng/dl |
| ACTH | 15-100 pg/ml | 50 pg/ml |

**TABLE 38-12 Tests of Adrenocortical Function**

| FUNCTION TEST/PROCEDURE AND PREPARATION | INTERPRETATION |
|---|---|
| **ACTH STIMULATION TEST (VARIOUS TESTS AVAILABLE)** | |
| Synthetic adrenocorticotropic hormone (ACTH) is given in 500-1000 ml of normal saline at 2 U/24 hr; then 17-OHCS and plasma cortisol levels are measured; alternative ways is to infuse 25 units of ACTH over 8 hours on 2-3 days and measure 17-OHCS and plasma cortisol levels on these days. | Normally, 17-OHCS excretion increases to 25 mg/24 hr, and plasma cortisol increases to 40 μg/dl or greater; in patients with secondary adrenal insufficiency, the 17-OHCS rate is 3-20 mg/24 hr, and the cortisol level is 10-40 μg/dl. |
| **SCREENING ACTH STIMULATION TEST; COSYNTROPIN TEST** | |
| Cosyntropin, 250 ng, is given IV and plasma cortisol level is measured before and 30-60 minutes after this dose. | Normally, plasma cortisol increases >18 μg/dl; this increase confirms a functional HPA axis and rules out adrenal insufficiency. |
| **CORTISONE SUPPRESSION TEST** | |
| Twenty-four–hour urine specimen for 17-OHCS is collected for baseline; dexamethasone, 0.5 mg, is given every 6 hours for 2 days; 24-hour urine is collected for these 2 days. | Dexamethasone suppresses pituitary secretion of ACTH and thus steroid levels; normally by second day of dexamethasone, 24-hour urinary level of OHCS should drop more than 50% below baseline. Patients with adrenocortical excess (primary) will not show decrease in 24-hour urine levels; patients with secondary adrenocortical excess will have drop, but less than 50%. |
| **SCREENING SUPPRESSION TEST; MINERALOCORTICOID SUPPRESSION TEST (VARIOUS TESTS ARE AVAILABLE)** | |
| Dexamethasone, 1 mg, is given at 12 PM. At 8 AM cortisol level is drawn. | Normally, cortisol should be less than 5 μg/dl. |
| Saline, 500 ml/hr for 4 hours, is infused IV. | Normally, saline infusion depresses plasma aldosterone to <8 μg/dl if patient has been on a sodium-restricted diet and to <5 μg/dl if patient has been on a normal sodium diet. |
| An alternative is that patient is placed on normal sodium diet (100 mEq) or high sodium diet (200 mEq). After patient is in sodium balance, deoxycorticosterone acetate (DOCA) (10 mg q 12 hr) is administered IM for 3-5 days. | Normal persons in sodium balance from diet will have a 70% decrease in aldosterone. |

the critically ill patient. Plasma aldosterone, angiotensin II, and renin are measured to evaluate the renin-angiotensin-aldosterone system. Plasma levels of aldosterone are increased by dietary potassium loading, sodium restriction, and assumption of an upright position. Aldosterone levels may be measured before and after manipulating these factors. Plasma levels of androgens are also measured to evaluate the adrenal androgen system.

Twenty-four–hour urine collections may also be analyzed for 17-ketosteroids (17-KS), 17-ketogenic steroids (17-KGS), and 17-hydroxycorticosteroids (17-OHCS). These compounds are metabolites of the hormones produced by the adrenal gland. These 24-hour urine collections require special preservatives, and the nurse should know the institution's requirements and make sure the appropriate container is available.

In addition to the above studies, other definitive tests are available to determine whether hypofunction or hyperfunction of the adrenal cortex is present and to establish whether the malfunction is caused by a primary adrenocortical problem or whether the malfunction is secondary to pituitary malfunction. These studies are described in Table 38-12.

## Adrenomedullary Function Tests

### Laboratory tests

The function of the adrenal medulla can be assessed by the assay of catecholamines in plasma or in urine. Most often, the initial screening test is of a metabolite in the urine, vanillylmandelic acid (VMA). Table 38-13 gives the normal values of 24-hour urine measurements. In **pheochromocytoma,** a catecholamine-secreting tumor, basal levels of plasma and urinary catecholamines are elevated; and, further, they are not suppressed by the oral administration of 300 mg of clonidine. Clonidine normally suppresses the secretion of catecholamines; hypotension, bradycardia, and somnolence may occur as side effects.

The *clonidine suppression test* is now more frequently used than are pressor tests that manipulate the blood pressure.[9] It yields fewer false-positive and false-negative results and is less risky. In the *histamine test,* 0.01 to 0.25 mg of histamine is administered intravenously; this can provoke a hypertensive crisis. In pheochromocytoma, a dramatic rise in blood pressure is seen. In the *Regitine test,* phentolamine (Regitine), 5 mg, is administered intravenously; this agent can provoke a hypotensive crisis. In pheochromocytoma the blood

**TABLE 38-13 Urinary Tests of Adrenomedullary Secretions**

| SPECIFIC TESTS | NORMAL VALUES |
|---|---|
| Epinephrine | 5-40 ng/24 hr |
| Norepinephrine | 10-80 ng/24 hr |
| Metanephrine | 24-96 ng/24 hr |
| Dopamine | 65-400 ng/24 hr |
| Vanillylmandelic acid (VMA) | 1-9 mg/24 hr |

pressure drop is diagnostic when there is a decrease of 35 mm Hg systolic and 25 mm Hg diastolic. In either test, close monitoring is necessary and preparations should be made to treat a crisis if it develops.

### Radiographic tests

Because 10% of catecholamine-secreting tumors are extraadrenal, radiographic tests are not limited to the adrenal gland and kidney. The $^{131}$I- or $^{123}$I-labeled metaiodobenzylguanidine *(MIBG)* scintigraphy may be the initial study done to locate a pheochromocytoma.[9] Other techniques to locate tumors and to plan surgical treatment may include CT, MRI, ultrasonography, arteriography, and retroperitoneal air sufflation.

## PANCREATIC ENDOCRINE FUNCTION TESTING

The major endocrine disorder of the pancreas is caused by disturbance in production, action, or metabolic rate of utilization of insulin. The relative lack of insulin leads to elevated blood glucose levels and the presence of glucose in the urine.

### Laboratory Tests

Tests to assess blood glucose levels are described in Table 38-14, and a more detailed explanation of them is given in Chapter 40.

The *fasting blood glucose (FBG)* and *glucose tolerance (GTT)* tests are used to diagnose diabetes mellitus, which has insulin deficit as a key feature of the disease. Plasma assays of insulin and glycogen are available but are infrequently used in clinical practice. The C-peptide test can be helpful in determining whether a patient is secreting insulin; this is particularly useful in a patient receiving exogenous insulin because exogenous insulin does not contain the C-peptide fragment.

**TABLE 38-14 Diagnostic Blood Tests for Pancreatic Endocrine Function**

| FUNCTION TEST/PROCEDURE AND PREPARATION | INTERPRETATION |
|---|---|
| **FASTING BLOOD GLUCOSE (FBG)**<br>NPO after midnight | Normal level should be at 60-120 mg/dl; elevated level indicates a need for further study to rule out diabetes mellitus. |
| **TWO-HOUR POSTPRANDIAL BLOOD GLUCOSE**<br>Blood glucose measured 2 hours after heavy meal or 2 hours after receiving loading dose of 100 g of sugar | Blood glucose should be within normal limits; levels above 120 mg/dl should be investigated further. |
| **GLUCOSE TOLERANCE TEST (GTT)**<br>NPO after midnight; samples of blood and urine collected at beginning of test; patient given mixture of glucose to drink or a meal containing 150-300 g of carbohydrate; blood and urine collected at intervals of ½, 1, and 2 hr (2-hr GTT); samples may be collected at 3-, 4-, and 5-hour intervals (5-hour GTT); presence of GI disorder that interferes with oral glucose absorption requires administration of IV glucose; test done in same manner as for oral GTT | Interpretation of results differs according to source of blood, method of analysis, and critical levels established by various authorities; levels established by the National Diabetes Data Group (1979) as diagnostic for diabetes mellitus in nonpregnant adults are as follows:<br>Source / Fasting (mg/dl) / 2 hr after glucose load (mg/dl)<br>Venous plasma / >140 / >200<br>Venous whole blood / >120 / >180<br>Capillary whole blood / >120 / >200 |
| **CORTISONE-GLUCOSE TOLERANCE TEST**<br>Performed similar to GTT except that cortisone is administered at start of test | Used when GTT results are inconclusive. Cortisone causes an abnormal increase in blood glucose, and decreased peripheral utilization of glucose in persons predisposed to diabetes; blood glucose level of 140 mg/dl at end of 2 hours is considered positive test. |
| **C-PEPTIDE TEST**<br>10- to 12-hour fasting blood sample drawn before ingestion of glucose and after 1 hour | Normal values: fasting, 2-20 μg/ml; after glucose, up to 120 μg/ml. Levels of C-peptide fragment correlate with level of virologically active insulin molecule endogenously secreted. |

**Glycosylated proteins** (proteins bonded with glucose) can be measured; the amount of glycosylation correlates with average blood glucose levels over the life span of the protein. For the glycosylated hemoglobin ($HbA_{1C}$) test, the life span is 9 to 12 weeks; the time is shorter for albumin and fructosamide. Glycosylated protein tests (usually $HbA_{1C}$) can be helpful in evaluating whether the current blood glucose level is a marked change from those in the past. (See Table 38-14 for details of the test.)

Laboratory tests of venous blood to measure FBG, postprandial blood glucose, premeal blood glucose, and $HbA_{1C}$ are used periodically to evaluate the effectiveness of blood glucose control in treated persons with diabetes. Therapeutic goals are established for each patient individually; the goals may be set at normal blood glucose levels or higher. For example, goals might include a fasting blood sugar of 140 mg/dl or lower; blood glucose at other times of 180 mg/dl or lower, and $HbA_{1C}$ at every 3 months to be 7 or less.[1]

In addition to laboratory tests of blood glucose, nurses use blood glucose monitors to measure capillary blood for frequent testing each day of patients in hospitals or nursing homes (bedside glucose monitoring). Patients use capillary blood for self–blood glucose monitoring as an important part of daily self-management. The most common times for blood glucose monitoring are fasting, before meals (ac), and at bedtime (hs). (See Chapter 40 for information about teaching patients about the use of self–blood glucose monitoring.)

Testing of *urine* for glucose yields inaccurate findings, and urine tests have been supplanted by blood glucose monitoring in most instances. Testing for glycosuria is part of a urinalysis. Several products are available, including reagents incorporated into tablets (Clinitest), test strips (Chemstrip UG and UGK, Diastix, Clinistix), and tapes (Test-Tape). It is most important to follow directions on the product label to ensure accuracy. The products vary in their sensitivity to glucose and in the ranges of glycosuria levels that they detect.

Acetest tablets may be used to test for acetone. Urine is dropped on the tablet. If acetone is present, varying shades of lavender will appear and can be compared with a color chart. Ketostix is a strip product that can also be used to detect the presence of ketones. Testing of urine for *ketones* to detect accelerated fat metabolism is used when blood glucose levels are 200 mg/dl or higher.

## CRITICAL THINKING ACTIVITIES

- What is the relationship of the hypothalamus, anterior pituitary gland, and thyroid gland in terms of thyroid hormone secretion?
- Compare and contrast the functions and systems effects of glucocorticoids and mineralocorticoids.
- Summarize the age-related alterations that occur in each of the endocrine glands and describe the consequences or results of these hormonal changes (i.e., increased ADH from the posterior pituitary = hyponatremia, SIADH).

## CHAPTER SUMMARY

### ANATOMY AND PHYSIOLOGY

- Normal differentiation of tissue, reproduction, growth and development, adaptation, aging, and senescence depend on a healthy endocrine system.
- The endocrine system integrates body functions so that appropriate body parts will respond as a unit to meet selected needs.
- Hormone levels are finely regulated by various types of feedback mechanisms.
- Many hormones display intrinsic rhythms that vary minute to minute, daily, or over longer periods.
- A hormone acts only on tissue that has an appropriate receptor for the hormone.
- Steroid hormones and thyroid hormones are lipid soluble and enter cells to combine with intracellular receptors.
- Other types of hormones (biogenic amines, small peptides, protein hormones, glycoproteins) are water soluble and combine with membrane receptors; the combination of hormone and membrane receptor stimulates a second messenger such as cyclic AMP.
- The hypothalamus serves as a major link between the rest of the nervous system and the endocrine system by its control of the pituitary gland, as well as its communication with other parts of the brain and the autonomic nervous system.
- Posterior pituitary hormones, antidiuretic hormone (ADH), and oxytocin are synthesized in the hypothalamus and stored in the pituitary.
- ADH controls serum osmolality, and oxytocin is involved in lactation and uterine contraction.
- The hypothalamus controls anterior pituitary gland function by synthesis of releasing or inhibiting hormones. The hypothalamus secretes prolactin-inhibiting and prolactin-releasing hormones, growth-hormone–releasing and growth-hormone–inhibiting hormone, corticotropin-releasing hormone, gonadotropin-releasing hormone, and thyrotropin-releasing hormone.
- The anterior pituitary secretes six hormones: growth hormone, prolactin, follicle-stimulating hormone, lu-

teinizing hormone, thyroid-stimulating hormone, and adrenocorticotropin.

- Control of anterior pituitary secretion is regulated by the hypothalamus and by negative feedback.
- The thyroid gland consists of two cell types: follicle cells, which synthesize thyroid hormone; and C-cells, which synthesize calcitonin.
- Control of thyroid function is from the hypothalamus, the anterior pituitary gland, and external factors.
- Thyroid hormone alters protein, carbohydrate, and fat metabolism; calorigenesis; growth and development; cardiac, respiratory, musculoskeletal, neurologic, and reproductive function; and function of the sympathetic nervous system.
- Calcitonin is involved in calcium homeostasis.
- The parathyroid glands are four small glands lying on the posterior aspect of the thyroid; parathyroid hormone is responsible for maintaining serum calcium levels.
- The adrenal cortex gland secretes the adrenal androgens, aldosterone, and glucocorticoids. Androgens are involved in development of secondary sex characteristics. Aldosterone is a major controller of sodium balance and volume status. Glucocorticoids are involved in gluconeogenesis, protein catabolism, and lipolysis, are antiinflammatory and suppress immune responsiveness, alter mood, and maintain emotional stability.
- Glucocorticoid production is controlled by the hypothalamus, the anterior pituitary gland, and external factors such as glucose level and physiologic and psychologic stressors. Aldosterone levels are controlled by the renin-angiotensin system, which responds to changes in sodium and volume, and by the serum potassium level.
- The adrenal medulla produces and secretes epinephrine and norepinephrine and works with the sympathetic nervous system in a coordinated response to stressors; all body systems are affected.
- The adrenomedullary sympathetic response is designed to stimulate organ systems that are necessary for life, such as the cardiovascular, respiratory, and neurologic systems, and to inhibit systems such as the gastrointestinal, hepatic, and pancreatic.
- The endocrine functions of the pancreas are carried out by the islet cells.
- The β-cells secrete insulin, which works on muscle, hepatic, and fat cells to lower blood glucose, store carbohydrates and fat, and synthesize protein.
- The α-cells secrete glucagon, which elevates blood glucose and mobilizes fat. Glucagon works with cortisol, growth hormone, and epinephrine to counterbalance the effects of insulin.
- Aging alters endocrine functioning, specifically pituitary, adrenal, pancreatic, thyroid, and parathyroid functioning.
- Aging is associated with altered bone and calcium metabolism, hypothyroidism, and diabetes mellitus.
- Most disorders of the endocrine system result in hypersecretion or hyposecretion of hormones.

### SUBJECTIVE DATA

- Endocrine dysfunction affects fluid intake, nutritional intake, elimination, energy level, body characteristics, reproductive and sexual functioning, tolerance to stressors, and almost every physiologic system.

### OBJECTIVE DATA

- An entire endocrine system history must be completed, along with a thorough head-to-toe physical examination.
- Because many endocrine problems are chronic, the history must also focus on learning styles and needs and home care skills.

### DIAGNOSTIC TESTS

- Diagnostic tests of the endocrine system focus on hormone levels; the interrelationships among the hypothalamus, the anterior pituitary gland, and other endocrine glands; or the substrates controlled by the hormone.

## REFERENCES


1. American Diabetes Association: Office guide to diagnosis and classification of diabetes mellitus and other categories of glucose intolerance (Position Statement), *Diabetes Care* 16 (suppl 2):4, 1993.
2. Batcheller J: Disorders of antidiuretic hormone secretion, *Crit Care Nurs* 3(2):370-378, 1992.
3. DeGroot L et al: *Endocrinology,* ed 2, Philadelphia, 1989, WB Saunders.
4. Isley WL: Thyroid disorders, *Crit Care Nurs Q* 13(3):39-49, 1990.
5. Kaplan S: The newer uses of growth hormone in adults, *1993 Adv Intern Med* 38:2287-3001, 1993.
6. King RJB: Enlightenment and confusion over steroid hormone receptors, *Nature* 312:20, 1984.
7. Lee L, Gumowski J: Adrenocortical insufficiency: a medical emergency, *AACN Clin Issues Crit Care Nurs* 3(2):319-330, 1992.
8. McCance KL, Huether SE: *Pathophysiology: the biological basis for disease in adults and children,* St Louis, 1990, Mosby.
9. Shapiro B, Gross MD: Pheochromocytoma, *Crit Care Clin* 7(1):1-2, 1991.
10. Spittle L: Diagnoses in opposition: thyroid storm and myxedema coma, *AACN Clin Issues Crit Care Nurs* 3(2):300-308, 1992.
11. Tepperman J: *Metabolic and endocrine physiology: an introductory text,* ed 5, Chicago, 1987, Year Book.
12. Wilson J, Foster D: *Williams' textbook of endocrinology,* ed 7, Philadelphia, 1992, Saunders.
13. Wingard DL et al: Community-based study of prevalence of NIDDM in older adults, *Diabetes Care* 13(2):3-8, 1990.

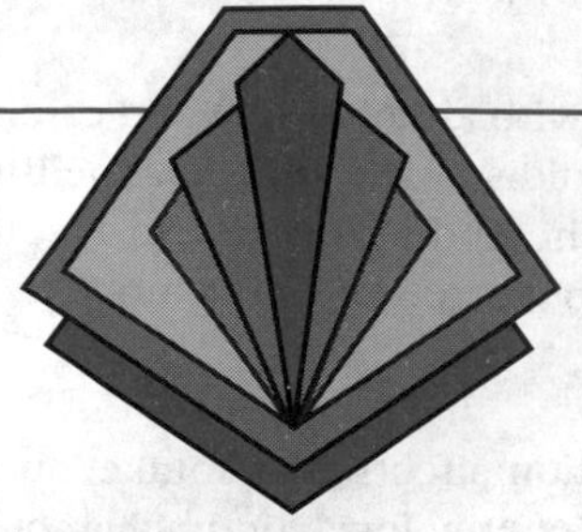

C H A P T E R 39

# Management of Persons With Problems of the Pituitary, Thyroid, Parathyroid, and Adrenal Glands

*Dorothy R. Blevins*
*Virginia L. Cassmeyer*

## CHAPTER OBJECTIVES

***After studying this chapter, the learner should be able to do the following:***

1 Describe the pathophysiology of hypersecretion and hyposecretion of the anterior and posterior pituitary, thyroid, parathyroid, and adrenal glands.
2 Describe the clinical manifestations, including history, physical examination, and diagnostic test findings, associated with hypersecretion and hyposecretion of the anterior and posterior pituitary, thyroid, parathyroid, and adrenal glands.
3 Develop a nursing plan of care, including identification of appropriate nursing diagnosis, patient outcomes, and interventions, for a patient with hypersecretion or hyposecretion of the anterior or posterior pituitary, thyroid, parathyroid, or adrenal gland.
4 Identify reasons for surgery of the pituitary, thyroid, parathyroid, or adrenal gland.
5 Develop a nursing plan of care for an individual having surgery on the pituitary, thyroid, parathyroid, or adrenal gland.
6 Identify self-care skills needed by a patient receiving long-term hormonal replacement therapy for pituitary, thyroid, parathyroid, or adrenocortical insufficiency.
7 Develop a teaching plan for a patient receiving long-term hormonal replacement therapy for pituitary, thyroid, parathyroid, or adrenocortical insufficiency.

## KEY TERMS

ablation
acromegaly
adenectomy
adrenal crisis
adrenocortical insufficiency
aldosteronism
bilateral hemianopsia
cretinism
Cushing's disease
Cushing's syndrome
diabetes insipidus
galactorrhea
gigantism
goiter
Graves' disease
halo ring
Hashimoto's thyroiditis
hyperparathyroidism
hyperpituitarism
hypoparathyroidism
hypophysectomy
hypopituitarism
myxedema
ophthalmopathy
pheochromocytoma
panhypopituitarism
pituitary apoplexy
primary glandular disorder
secondary glandular disorder
tetany
thyroid crisis (storm)
thyrotoxicosis
toxic multinodular goiter

Alterations in function of the endocrine system result in a variety of physiologic changes. Dysfunction of the endocrine system is serious and can be fatal because of the vital functions regulated by the hormones from the pituitary, thyroid, parathyroid, and adrenal glands. The result of most pathologic processes affecting the endocrine glands is depression or elevation of blood levels of hormones.

Many types of pathologic processes can result in destruction of endocrine tissue and decreased blood levels of hormones. Selected types of problems that result in decreased blood hormone levels include:

1. Destruction of glands by infiltrative processes, infarction, infection, autoimmune and immunologic processes, and tumor
2. Abnormal embryonic development, resulting in structural problems or inadequate capacity for synthesis
3. Destruction of glands by surgical removal, radiation therapy, or trauma

The target cells for the selected hormones can become nonresponsive to the hormones. Although in this type of problem the blood hormone levels may be normal or even high, the condition mimics those seen with depression of blood hormones.

Selected types of problems that result in increased blood levels of hormones include:

1. Hyperplasia or hypertrophy of endocrine glands
2. Benign or malignant tumor growth with capacity to secrete hormone
3. Stimulation of glands by trophic factors liberated from ectopic nonendocrine sites
4. Secretion of hormones by ectopic nonendocrine tissues
5. Exogenous administration of hormones
6. Decreased metabolism of hormones, resulting in prolonged activity of hormones

For those endocrine glands controlled by the hypothalamus and pituitary gland, which include the thyroid and adrenocortical glands and the gonads, **glandular disorders** resulting in hypersecretion or hyposecretion can be classified as **primary** or **secondary.** Primary problems occur when the thyroid gland, adrenocortical gland, or gonads are diseased. Secondary dysfunction occurs when the problem results from hypothalamic or anterior pituitary dysfunction.

Benign and malignant cell growth of endocrine glands can occur. Although hormonal levels are often not immediately affected by the tumor growth, progressive growth can either destroy normal tissue, resulting in hyposecretion of hormones, or the tumor can be made up of secreting tissue, resulting in hypersecretion. Also, the treatment of the tumor by surgery, radiation, or drug therapy often results in *iatrogenic-induced* depressed blood levels of hormones.

# PITUITARY GLAND

## ANTERIOR PITUITARY GLAND: HYPERPITUITARISM

### Etiology

**Hyperpituitarism** of the anterior portion of the pituitary gland may involve only a single hormone or two or more hormones. The cause may be a primary problem in the pituitary gland or secondary to hypothalamic dysfunction. Pituitary adenomas are a common cause of hyperpituitarism. Pituitary adenomas of the anterior pituitary gland account for 6% to 18% of all intracranial tumors.[42]

### Epidemiology

In most patients the cause of adenomas of the anterior pituitary gland is unknown, and no family history exists. Pituitary adenomas are almost always *secreting* or *functioning* tumors. These tumors are usually benign, but some can grow very aggressively. A nonfunctional tumor is nonsecreting. Previously, adenomas were classified as chromophilic, eosinophilic, or basophilic based on the staining characteristics of the tumor cells, but this method has proved to be inadequate. Classification usually is now based on the specific hormone secreted, for example, prolactinoma, somatotroph tumors, corticotroph tumors, or gonadotroph adenomas. Tumors are also classified by size and invasiveness of the sella turcica (Box 39-1).

Prolactin-secreting tumors *(prolactinomas)* account for 30% of all pituitary tumors.[34] The next most frequently occurring tumor secretes growth hormone (GH) (somatotroph tumor). Tumors that secrete adrenocorticotropic hormone (ACTH) (corticotroph tumors) are the third most frequently occurring tumors. Gonadotroph adenomas, reported in the past to be rare, may be more common than initially thought. It is possible that adenomas once classified as nonsecreting actually secrete gonadotropins or their subunits.[35] Thyroid-stimulating hormone–(TSH-)secreting tumors are still considered to be rare. Pituitary adenomas can occur as part of multiple endocrine neoplasia, type 1 (MEN I).[24] MEN I is a hereditary disorder that consists of primary hyperparathyroidism, pancreatic islet cell tumor, and pi-

**BOX 39-1 Classification of Pituitary Adenomas**

| | |
|---|---|
| Enclosed | No invasion into the floor of the sella turcica |
| Invasive | Destruction of part or all of the sella turcica |
| Microadenoma | Enclosed tumors <10 mm in diameter |
| Macroadenoma | Enclosed tumors >10 mm in diameter; these tumors may show suprasellar extension |

tuitary adenoma. The pituitary adenoma in MEN I is secreting and usually secretes GH, but some have been found to secrete prolactin or ACTH.

Pituitary hyperfunctioning also can result from hyperplasia of pituitary tissue. The cause of hyperplasia is not always known, but one hypothesis is that altered feedback signals can cause the hypersecretion.[40] Diminished feedback from target organ secretions can result in hyperplasia and hypersecretion.

## Pathophysiology

Two alterations in physiologic functioning that occur with pituitary tumors result from the presence of a space-occupying mass in the cranium and from the effects of the excessive secretion of hormones by functional neoplasms. In contrast, another alteration may result from the compression of glandular tissue by the tumor mass; this can cause hyposecretion of one or more anterior pituitary hormones and is caused by a *nonfunctional adenoma*[34] (see p. 1212).

### Neurologic alterations

Neurologic alterations occur because the growing tumor presses on the dura, diaphragm sellae, or adjacent structures. The optic chiasm lies anteriorly and superiorly, and tumors that extend upward press on it. In some patients, cranial nerves III, IV, and VI also may be involved with lateral extension of tumors. The most common sign of compression is a **bilateral hemianopsia** (blindness in half the visual field), often identified during visual field testing in a routine eye examination. The tumor may involve the neighboring bony structures or the temporal or frontal lobe, and very large tumors may compress or infiltrate the hypothalamus.

Hemorrhage into the tumor can result in a sudden increase in size, with rapid onset of various neurologic signs and symptoms.

### Endocrine alterations

Depending on which hormone is being secreted by the tumor, a variety of effects may be seen. This section focuses on hypersecretion of prolactin, GH, and gonadotropins. The pathophysiologic factors associated with increased secretion of ACTH or TSH are the same as those seen with adrenocortical hormone or thyroid hormone excess and are discussed in later sections.

**Prolactin hypersecretion.** Prolactin excess usually results from pituitary tumors but can also result from pharmacologic agents such as psychotropics, antihypertensives, estrogens, and opiates or from central nervous system (CNS) disease that interferes with dopamine secretion. It also may be idiopathic. Prolactin hypersecretion interferes with the hypothalamic-pituitary-gonadal axis. It inhibits the normal release of gonadotropins and gonadal steroids in both females and males. Excessive secretion of prolactin stimulates breast development and milk production in persons with near-normal levels of ovarian steroids. **Galactorrhea** (inappropriate milk production) is a common symptom of hypersecretion.

**Growth hormone hypersecretion.** In conditions of GH excess, secretion remains episodic, but the number, duration, and amplitude of pulses are increased and occur randomly throughout the day. The excessive secretion of GH produces excessive amounts of somatomedins and the characteristic proliferation of bone, connective tissue, cartilage, and soft tissue resulting in gigantism or acromegaly. GH excess that occurs in childhood and adolescence before closure of the epiphyseal plate produces proportional growth of the skeleton and **gigantism. Acromegaly** results when GH excess occurs in adult life.[23] It involves overgrowth of soft tissue and terminal skeletal structures such as the nose, jaw, forehead, hands, and feet.

Excessive GH exaggerates the normal depression of carbohydrate metabolism, increasing insulin resistance and depressing glucose uptake. Changes in GH can alter fat metabolism and renal excretion of phosphorus and calcium.

**Gonadotropin hypersecretion.** Gonadotropin tumors occur most often in middle-aged persons and are found in males more frequently than in females. Hypersecretion of follicle-stimulating hormone (FSH) is most common, although the tumors can secrete luteinizing hormone (LH) or both hormones.[35] The hypersecretion occurs both basally and in response to stimulation. The hypersecretion of gonadotropins frequently causes no clinical changes, although hypersecretion of FSH without LH can result in secondary hypogonadism.[29] Impor-

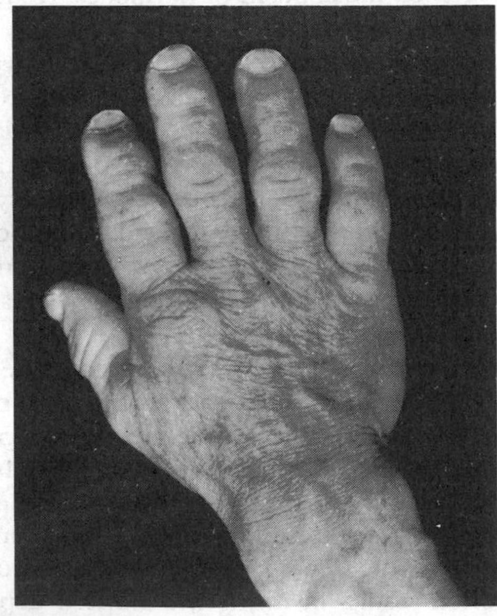

**FIGURE 39-1** Hand showing characteristics of acromegaly. (From Schottelius B, Schottelius D: *Textbook of physiology*, ed 18, St Louis, 1978, Mosby.)

**BOX 39-2 Clinical Manifestations of Pituitary Hormone–Secreting Tumors**

**NEUROLOGIC**

1. Visual defects often first seen as losses in superior temporal quadrants with progression to hemianopia or scotomas and finally to total blindness
2. Headache
3. Somnolence
4. Occasional signs of increased intracranial pressure (hydrocephalus, papilledema)
5. With very large tumors, disturbance in appetite, sleep, temperature regulation, and emotional balance because of hypothalamic involvement
6. Behavioral changes and seizures with expansion causing compression of the temporal or frontal lobe

**ENDOCRINE**

**Prolactin Hypersecretion**

1. Females
   a. Menstrual disturbances, such as irregular menses, anovulatory periods, oligomenorrhea, or amenorrhea
   b. Infertility
   c. Galactorrhea
   d. Manifestations of ovarian steroid deficit, such as dyspareunia, vaginal mucosal atrophy, decreased vaginal lubrication, decreased libido
2. Males
   a. Decreased libido and possible impotence
   b. Reduced sperm count and infertility
   c. Gynecomastia
3. Both males and females: depressed levels of gonadal steroids

**Growth Hormone (GH) Hypersecretion (Acromegaly)**

1. Macroadenomas with resultant headache and visual changes
2. Changes in facial features (coarsening of features; increased size of nose, lips, and skin folds; prominence of supraorbital ridges; growth of mandible resulting in prognathism and widely spaced teeth; soft tissue growth resulting in facial puffiness)
3. Increased size of hands and feet (Figure 39-1), weight gain
4. Deepening of voice from thickening of vocal cords
5. Increases in vertebral bodies resulting in thoracic kyphosis
6. Enlarged tongue, salivary glands, spleen, liver, heart, kidney, and other organs; cardiomegaly may result in increased blood pressure and signs and symptoms of congestive heart failure.
7. Elevated blood pressure even without cardiac failure
8. Snoring, sleep apnea, and respiratory failure
9. Dermatologic changes: acne, increased sweating, oiliness, development of skin tags
10. Hypertrophy progressing to atrophy of skeletal muscles
11. Backache, arthralgia, or arthritis from joint damage and bony overgrowth
12. Peripheral nerve damage, such as carpal tunnel syndrome or neuropathies, from bony overgrowth and changes in nerve size
13. Impaired glucose tolerance progressing to diabetes mellitus with its manifestations
14. Changes in fat metabolism resulting in hyperlipidemia
15. General changes in mobility: presence of lethargy and fatigue
16. Radiographic findings indicative of bony proliferation in hands, feet, skull, ribs, vertebrae
17. Electrolyte changes: increased urinary excretion of calcium; elevated blood phosphate level

**Gonadotropin Hypersecretion**

1. Usually no clinical manifestations
2. If signs and symptoms present: secondary hypogonadism, such as changes in secondary sexual characteristics or atrophy of external genitalia, with history of normal pubertal development and fertility

tantly, the patient gives a history of normal pubertal development and fertility even if hypogonadism is currently present.

Clinical manifestations vary depending on the type of tumor and are summarized in Box 39-2.

## Prevention

### Primary prevention

No known primary prevention exists for pituitary tumors or pituitary hyperplasia. There is concern about nonmedical use and increased availability of GH, now produced by ribonucleic acid (RNA) recombinant gene technology. Current research is studying the effects of GH excess and long-term consequences of its use in healthy persons to increase height in short-statured persons, to increase athletic ability, and to combat aging.[20]

### Secondary prevention

Screening examinations also can detect early visual field deficits from compression by tumors.

### Tertiary prevention

Once patients have been diagnosed and early treatment started, monitoring for side effects of the treatment and for recurrences of tumors is necessary to limit complications.

## Medical Management

The goal for discharge of patients with pituitary adenoma as determined by diagnosis-related groups (DRGs) is 5.1 days for medical management and 10.1 days for surgical management. The nurse works collaboratively with the physician for implementation of prescribed medical therapy.[34] Because the nurse has a major role in discharge planning and patient teaching, these are discussed under nursing management.

Untreated GH-secreting tumors can result in major neurologic alterations and continual systemic changes if the hormone level does not return to normal and if tumor growth is not inhibited. Treatment consists of surgery, radiation, or pharmacologic agents.

For prolactin-secreting tumors, some authorities[40] have recommended no treatment for persons with a microadenoma who have no annoying symptoms and do not want to become pregnant. Studies have shown that the incidence of microadenomas progressing to macroadenomas is very low.[25] However, the ovarian dysfunction and the low estrogen state that can be associated with elevated prolactin levels may result in premature osteoporosis; thus other experts recommend that all prolactin-secreting tumors be treated.

**Diagnostic tests**

The specific tests used in pituitary disorders are explained in Chapter 38. One or more radiographic examinations, including one of the head; computed tomography (CT); magnetic resonance imaging (MRI); and digital subtraction angiography may be used to identify presence, size, and features of a pituitary tumor. Of special interest is the integrity of the sella turcica and the surrounding tissues.

Endocrine studies of hormonal secretions of the pituitary and target glands are performed to confirm hypersecretory states and to determine pretreatment serum levels and responses to provocative testing.

A complete eye examination is performed. If surgery is planned, the usual preoperative evaluations of cardiovascular, renal, hematologic, respiratory, neurologic, and fluid and electrolyte status are done.

**Medication**

When treatment is recommended for prolactinoma, the dopamine agonist bromocriptine (Parlodel) is used for enclosed tumors. A dosage of 2.5 to 15 mg daily usually returns hormone levels to normal, restores fertility, and decreases tumor size in most patients. Bromocriptine is a dopamine agonist and is effective in lowering GH levels but not always to the level needed; therefore it is used mainly if surgery and radiation have not been effective. Higher doses may be necessary for GH-secreting tumors. The major side effects are mild nausea, vomiting, and headache. Gastric irritation can be decreased by teaching the patient to take the medicine with food.[34] Continual hormonal analysis is carried out to monitor the effectiveness of therapy.

Because the use of bromocriptine during gestation is very limited, patients who become pregnant after successful bromocriptine therapy are treated in various ways. In persons with microadenomas, the drug may be stopped during pregnancy and the patient monitored for signs and symptoms of tumor enlargement. The patient needs clear understanding of the use of bromocriptine and its relationship to the inducing of regular menstrual cycles, the use and timing of contraceptives in relation to bromocriptine therapy, and whether the drug is to be withheld if a menstrual period is late.[34] Visual testing is used to monitor for enlargement, and if enlargement is suspected, a CT scan or MRI is done. After delivery and if surgery was not done, bromocriptine is restarted. If necessary, the drug may be reinstituted during pregnancy. For larger tumors, prepregnancy surgery may be done. In some instances, bromocriptine may be continued throughout pregnancy.

A long-acting somatostatin analog (octreotide [Sandostatin], SMS 201-995) is available and has been approved by the U.S. Food and Drug Administration (FDA) for use in treating carcinoid.[1] In experimental studies with persons with acromegaly, it has been found to be effective in reducing plasma GH levels and in relieving some clinical manifestations of GH excess, such as headache, arthropathy, swelling of soft tissue, excess perspiration, sleep apnea, and neuropathy. If discontinued, hypersecretion recurs. Sandostatin must be given by subcutaneous injection three or four times daily. It also can be given by continuous subcutaneous infusion. Side effects include pain at injection site, diarrhea, steatorrhea, abdominal cramps, and flatulence. This drug has also been used preoperatively and appears to improve the success of surgery. The routine use of somatostatin analogs for persons with acromegaly will depend on future research.[39]

If patients are placed on the somatostatin analog, they may need to be taught how to self-administer the drug by subcutaneous injection, how to prepare the injection site, how to prepare the subcutaneous injection, how to store the drug, how to care for syringes and needles, and so forth. The information is similar to that taught to persons with diabetes mellitus about subcutaneous injections (see Chapter 40).

**Treatment**

Radiation therapy may be used as an adjunct to surgery or as an alternative. It is frequently used when tumors have extended beyond the sella turcica and surgery has resulted in incomplete removal of the tumor. Skin changes, alopecia, or oral complications may occur. Concerns surround the use of postsurgical radiation because of the rate of recurrences of tumor in these patients and the development of brain tumors in some patients.[34] Radiation therapy is done on an outpatient basis. Radiation treatments are usually given over 4 to 6 weeks. The response to radiation is slow, and hypopituitarism develops in many patients. Deficiencies of ACTH and gonadotropins typically occur, although a deficiency in TSH may occur also.[40]

Patient education should focus on how the procedure is done. A visit to the radiation therapy department should be planned. Patients need to know the number of visits required and when they will begin to see or experience effects. They also should be told of possible hormonal deficits as a side effect. The nurse should emphasize that these do not occur until many years after the therapy. Radiation therapy can cause damage to surrounding tissue and swelling of the tumors[34] and worsen neurologic signs and symptoms. The patient must know

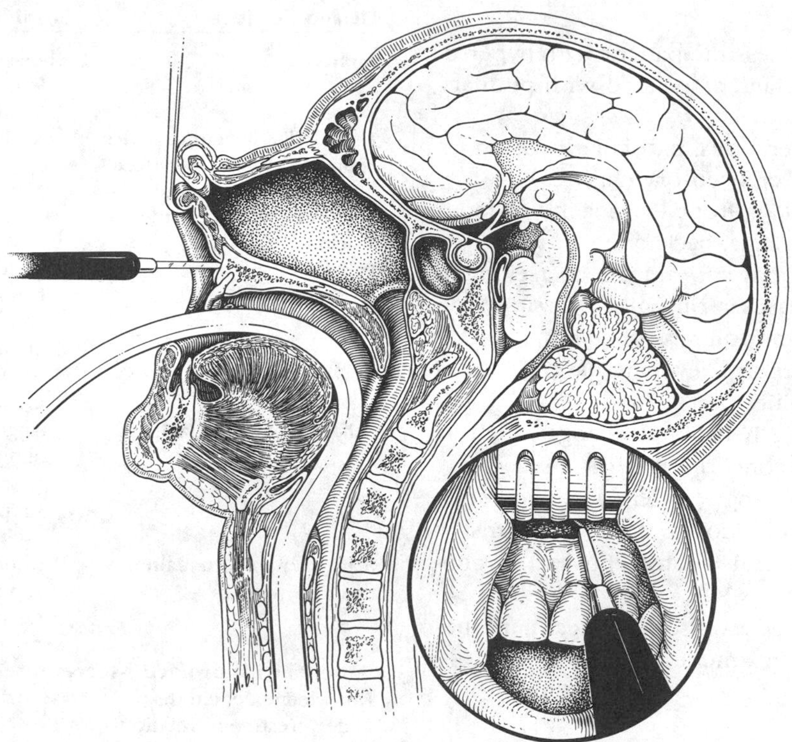

**FIGURE 39-2** Diagram of transsphenoidal approach in anterior pituitary surgery with incision in the gingival mucosa. (From Tindall GT, Barrow DL: *Disorders of the pituitary,* St Louis, 1986, Mosby.)

to report any worsening of signs and symptoms and to keep follow-up appointments indefinitely.

### Diet

Dietary changes may be necessary if hypersecretory states of acromegaly or Cushing's syndrome are present. Carbohydrate intolerance or frank diabetes mellitus may be associated with both these disorders. (See Chapter 40 for interventions related to dietary management of diabetes mellitus.) Congestive heart failure may occur in patients with acromegaly, and sodium and lipid restrictions may be necessary (see Chapter 31).

### Activity

No specific activity is prescribed for persons with pituitary tumors. Efforts should be made to maintain or improve mobility status of patients with acromegaly who have bone, muscle, or joint problems.

### Referral/Consultation

In some settings the nurse assumes responsibility for making referrals to other services. The patient with acromegaly may benefit from referral to physical therapy or occupational therapy. The patient with visual loss may benefit from occupational therapy and visual rehabilitative services. Social work services can be helpful when an acute crisis or the burdens of chronic illness stress financial, personal, and family resources.

## Surgical Management

The surgical removal of a pituitary tumor may be an **adenectomy** if tumors are small or a **hypophysectomy** if complete removal of anterior pituitary tissue is required for large, invasive tumors. An adenectomy preserves anterior pituitary function in most patients, whereas a hypophysectomy results in hypopituitarism.

Hypopituitarism is discussed in the next section. Usually, microsurgery and a transsphenoidal approach are used for microadenomas and some macroadenomas. Figure 39-2 illustrates the surgical incision made through the upper gingival mucosa, along one side of the nasal septum, and through the sphenoid sinus to the sella turcica. For large, invasive tumors, a transfrontal craniotomy may be the procedure of choice. (See Chapter 57 for nursing care related to a craniotomy.) The nursing care of patients undergoing transsphenoidal surgery of the pituitary is discussed in the section on surgical management.

## NURSING MANAGEMENT

### ♦ ASSESSMENT

Assessment of the patient with potential hyperpituitarism of the anterior pituitary gland focuses on identification of manifestations of these problems, particularly as they relate to the patient's total health.

## Subjective Data

Data to be collected to assess the patient with hypersecretion of the pituitary gland associated with pituitary tumor include the following:

- History of sensory alterations, particularly vision, as well as other peripheral sensory changes
- Discomforts: temporal or frontal headache of moderate intensity, arthralgia, backache
- History of changes in body appearance: coarsening of facial features; increases in ring, glove, or shoe size; increase in sweating or oiliness of skin
- History of change in energy level (lethargy, fatigue) or decrease in mobility
- Psychosocial concerns: behavioral changes such as anxiety, irritability, concerns about self-image
- History of menstrual changes in females, impotency in males, changes in libido; infertility concerns
- Drug history: taking oral contraceptives, psychotropic drugs
- Knowledge level related to disorder, treatment, potential outcome of treatment

## Objective Data

Data about neurologic and endocrine effects include the following:

- Functioning of cranial nerves II, III, IV, and VI (see Chapter 56)
- Retinal changes indicative of papilledema or elevated blood pressure
- Mental status: alertness, emotional status
- Peripheral nerve functioning (see Chapter 56)
- Body appearance, description
- Mobility and joint functioning (see Chapter 63)
- Vital signs: blood pressure, pulse, respirations, temperature
- Body weight and height
- Presence of organomegaly, particularly cardiac and hepatic, and signs associated with these changes

## Diagnostic Test Findings

Confirmation of pituitary tumor and/or a hypersecretory state may include the following:

1. Radiographic evidence of tumor
2. Elevated levels of serum prolactin, GH, TSH, FSH, and LH or subunits of gonadotropic hormones; ACTH and cortisol; or TSH and triiodothyronine ($T_3$) and thyroxine ($T_4$)
3. Elevated levels of urinary hormones and/or their metabolites

## ◆ NURSING DIAGNOSES

Nursing diagnoses are determined from analysis of patient data. Nursing diagnoses for the patient with hypersecretion of the anterior pituitary gland associated with pituitary tumor may include but are not limited to the following:

| Diagnostic Title | Possible Etiologic Factors |
|---|---|
| Anxiety | Uncertainty about cause of problem and outcomes of treatment |
| Knowledge deficit: disorder and treatment, expected outcomes, expected complications or side effects | New diagnoses and treatment |
| Pain | Headache from intracranial mass: from pressure on nerve roots and on nerves associated with changes in joints and vertebrae related to abnormal bone growth |
| Self-esteem disturbance | Changes in body characteristics and functions associated with hormonal excess, visual loss, sexual dysfunction, impaired mobility |
| Sensory/perceptual alterations: visual | Pressure on optic chiasma disrupting functioning of cranial nerve II or pressure on cranial nerves III, IV, and VI |
| **Patients with prolactin-secreting tumors—pretreatment** | |
| Knowledge deficit: disorder, treatment, relationship of disorder to sexual functioning | New diagnoses and treatment |
| Sexual dysfunction | Alteration in menstrual cycle, decreased libido, or impotence associated with increased secretion of prolactin |
| **Patients with GH-secreting tumors—pretreatment** | |
| Knowledge deficit: disorder, treatment, effect of treatment on signs and symptoms | Newly diagnosed disorder and new treatment |
| Mobility, impaired physical | Pain from pressure on nerve roots |
| Pain | Pressure on nerves associated with changes in joints and vertebrae related to growth |
| **Patients with any type of tumor treated with surgery** | |
| Fluid volume deficit, high risk for | Disruption in normal antidiuretic hormone (ADH) secretion or adrenocortical functioning associated with surgical trauma |
| Gas exchange, impaired | Inadequate deep breathing; instructions not to cough and presence of nasal packing |
| Infection, high risk for | Loss of barriers to organisms associated with disruption of external incision in mucous membrane from improper care; disruption of internal incision through dura associated with increased intracranial pressure (ICP) resulting in cerebrospinal fluid (CSF) leak |
| Knowledge deficit: procedure, expected outcomes, expected complications | New treatment so no previous exposure to information |

| Diagnostic Title | Possible Etiologic Factors |
|---|---|
| **Patients with any type of tumor treated with radiation** | |
| Injury, high risk for | Inability to maintain homeostasis, cardiac output, respiratory functioning, and fluid and electrolyte balance associated with ACTH and/or TSH deficiency |
| Knowledge deficit: procedure, expected outcomes, potential complications | Newly prescribed treatment so no previous exposure to information |
| Sexual dysfunction | Impotency, decreased libido, change in menstrual cycles associated with long-term loss of adequate synthesis and secretion of gonadotopins |
| **Patients with any type of tumor treated with drug therapy** | |
| Knowledge deficit: drugs, self-administration techniques, expected results, potential side effects | Newly prescribed treatment so no previous exposure to information |

## ♦ EXPECTED PATIENT OUTCOMES

Expected patient outcomes for the person with hypersecretion of the anterior pituitary gland associated with pituitary tumor may include but are not limited to the following:

**All patients—pretreatment**

1. Describes anxiety level as tolerable, amount of sleep as adequate, and identifies one or more anxiety-reducing strategies.
2. Explains nature of the disorder, how signs and symptoms relate to the disease, and how the disease will alter activities of daily living (ADL).
3. Describes the purpose of each diagnostic test and special pretest and posttest requirements.
4. Explains (a) dietary regimen and plans to implement the regimen; (b) medications: knowledge about the drug and administration, expected results, and potential side effects; (c) measures to relieve signs and symptoms, as appropriate; and (d) plans for follow-up care.
5. States headache is controlled by prescribed interventions and environmental modifications.
6. Talks positively about self when discussing body characteristics and functions that are reversible and those that will not change.
7. Is able to function independently in the hospital or at home.

**Patients with prolactin-secreting tumors—pretreatment**

1. Attains adequate knowledge, as evidenced by patient's and significant others' ability to describe how the sexual dysfunction relates to prolactin excess and what effects treatment has on sexual functioning.
2. Sexual dysfunction will cause no long-term problems, as evidenced by statements and explanation that treatment should resolve the problem.

**Patient with GH-secreting tumors—pretreatment**

1. Has adequate knowledge, as evidenced by patient's and significant others' ability to describe the effects of treatment on signs and symptoms.
2. Is independent in ADL and states ability to participate in all activities enjoyed.
3. States that interventions prescribed control back and joint discomfort and that discomfort does not limit activity.

**Patients with any type of tumor treated with surgery**

1. Does not develop fluid volume deficit, as evidenced by decreased blood pressure, poor skin turgor, unrelieved thirst, or hemoconcentration.
2. Maintains adequate gas exchange, as evidenced by clear breath sounds, $PaO_2$, $PaCO_2$, and $O_2$ saturation within normal limits, no tachycardia, and appropriate response to interactions.
3. Remains free of infection and has no CSF leak.
4. Describes procedure, outcomes, and complications correctly.

**Patients with any type of tumor treated with radiation**

1. No injuries occur because of patient's and significant others' ability to state signs and symptoms they should monitor for and report immediately.
2. Has adequate knowledge, as evidenced by patient's and significant other's ability to explain radiation procedure, expected outcomes, and potential complications.

**Patients with any type of tumor treated with drug therapy**

Has adequate knowledge, as evidenced by patient's and significant others' ability to name drugs, state how to administer, and describe the expected results and potential side effects.

## ♦ INTERVENTIONS

The patient with a hormonal excess caused by a secreting pituitary tumor will seek care for various reasons.[34] These reasons include symptoms and signs such as frequent or persistent headache, visual changes, or changes in body characteristics or function; anxiety may be high.

### Reducing Anxiety

1. Assess anxiety level, particular stressors, and patient's use of stress-reducing strategies.
2. Provide clear instructions for and explanations of diagnostic tests and treatment measures.

3. Provide opportunity for patient to express concerns and to use resources perceived as helpful.
4. Provide support as necessary to maintain optimal level of independence in ADL, decision making, and planning for discharge.

The level of anxiety of the patient with pituitary hypersecretion related to a tumor varies with the individual responses to the particular body changes induced by neurologic or endocrine alterations, uncertainty about diagnosis, treatment method, and effects of treatment. Particular stressors may include visual loss, infertility, sexual dysfunction, or immobility. Although some patients who are diagnosed with neurologic symptoms require immediate surgical treatment, most patients have a diagnostic work-up in the outpatient setting and time to learn about their illness and its implications. The nurse can help the patient reduce stress by attending to the emotional impact of the illness. The major nursing need at this stage of the illness is patient education. The patient and significant others need to know:

1. How the patient's symptoms relate to a pituitary tumor and hormone excess.
2. What is meant by the term *tumor*; some people automatically assume that tumor means cancer. These tumors usually are not malignant.
3. What diagnostic tests are planned, including blood tests; skull roentgenogram, CT scan, or MRI; and visual assessment.
4. What treatment is available for the tumor. Based on the signs and symptoms, the physician has a high index of suspicion for the type of tumor and potential treatment. This is the information that the physician shares at this time and the nurse reinforces.
5. What outcomes are expected from the treatment, including reversibility or irreversibility of signs and symptoms.

This knowledge assists the patient in dealing with the physiologic changes and should help to relieve uncertainty and decrease anxiety. Usually this teaching is done in an outpatient setting. The nurse can have a model of a brain available, which may be used to help the patient understand better what is happening, as well as written material for the patient to read. The nurse should also provide the name and telephone number of someone (nurse, physician) who can be contacted if the patient thinks of more questions.

### Facilitating Learning

1. Assess knowledge of disease, diagnostic tests, therapeutic measures, barriers to learning, and information patient desires.
2. Provide dietary instruction about prescribed changes as needed, and help patient/family plan ways of meeting dietary requirements.
3. Teach patient about medication therapy: hormonal agents used as *replacement therapy* (in diabetes insipidus; hypopituitarism; insufficiency of cortisol, $T_4$, and/or sex hormones) and *hormonal suppressant drugs:* bromocriptine and Sandostatin.
4. Assess ability to perform subcutaneous injection if Sandostatin is prescribed; provide teaching and multiple opportunities for practice and return demonstration.
5. Refer to visual rehabilitation services as needed, or provide patient/family with necessary information.
6. Clarify understanding about need and plans for follow-up care.

### Promoting Comfort

1. Monitor pain using pain scales and flow sheets (see Chapter 17) every 4 hours; assess for nonverbal signs of pain. Ask patient to be specific about location and type of pain.
2. Assess for factors that increase or decrease pain.
3. Implement measures to reduce pain:
   a. Assist with nonpharmacologic measures for pain relief (e.g., music, massage, distraction, relaxation, imagery, heat or cold, exercise).
   b. Identify optimal pain schedule and administer prescribed analgesics; assess for response; anticipate and prevent common side effects.
4. Consult physician if pain-reducing measures fail to provide adequate pain relief.
5. Ensure adequate rest and sleep.

The patient may need immediate treatment for headache, such as mild nonnarcotic analgesics. Other helpful measures include sitting and lying with the head elevated. Relaxing in a dark room, listening to quiet music, meditation, and other types of relaxation may also help. The nurse needs to identify, in cooperation with the patient, measures that help relieve the headache. The patient with a GH-secreting tumor requires comfort measures to manage joint and back pain and impaired mobility. These measures may include nonnarcotic analgesics, warm baths, range of motion (ROM) exercises, and moist or dry heat.

Nursing care related to visual disturbances, self-esteem disturbances, and sexual dysfunction is primarily educational at this stage of care; low self-esteem may hinder learning.

### Minimizing Low Self-Esteem

1. Assess for factors posing a threat to self-esteem and for statements of negative self-appraisal.
2. Provide support for patient in asking questions, in seeking information, in obtaining needed resources, and in decision making about care.
3. Reassure patient about normalcy of individual responses to stressors.
4. Enable patient to maintain optimal level of independence in ADL and personal control.
5. Clarify patient knowledge about disease, its treat-

ment, and anticipated effects on body appearance and functions.

The patient who has just learned of a tumor in the pituitary gland, enclosed within the skull, and who must make choices about type of treatment may be overwhelmed and feel helpless. Threats to self-esteem might be increased by visual disturbances, infertility, immobility, or changes in body appearance. Chronic or stable low self-esteem may be a usual attribute of the patient; however, stressors may induce temporary low self-esteem in any person (situational low self-esteem).[3] Self-esteem is protected through the cognitive processes of (1) searching for meaning in the experience, (2) regaining mastery over the event or exerting personal control, and (3) self-enhancement.[37]

## ♦ EVALUATION

To evaluate the effectiveness of nursing interventions, compare patient behaviors with those stated in the expected patient outcomes. Successful achievement of patient outcomes for the person with hypersection of the anterior pituitary gland associated with pituitary tumor is indicated by the following:

1. Reports that anxiety is at a tolerable level, uses anxiety-reducing strategies, and perceives ability to manage stressors.
2. Explains diagnostic and treatment effects and implications for self-management.
3. Reports that comfort is at an acceptable level.
4. Comments positively about self-attributes, abilities, and participation in activities to regain optimal functioning.

The patient and significant others need to know that changes in body characteristics and vision are not always reversible, but that progressive changes will be stopped and they will be helped to cope with irreversible changes. Sexual dysfunction associated with prolactin excess is usually reversible. The patient must be assessed for the ability to maintain a safe environment if visual disturbances are present. Although severe visual disturbances rarely occur, interventions such as those discussed in Chapter 60 for the person with blindness may be necessary.

## NURSING MANAGEMENT OF THE PATIENT UNDERGOING PITUITARY SURGERY

After a transsphenoidal adenectomy, the patient's care has three additional focuses: prevention of fluid volume deficit, prevention of respiratory complications, and prevention of infection.[2] Patient education continues to be important.

### Assessment

Refer to previous Nursing Management section for assessment specific to patients with pituitary adenoma and hormonal imbalance and to Chapter 25 for usual assessment of any postoperative patient.

### Nursing Diagnoses

Refer to previous Nursing Management section for nursing diagnoses and possible etiologic factors related to patient education. Diagnoses related to surgical intervention include but are not limited to those listed previously under Patients with any type of tumor treated with surgery.

### Expected Patient Outcomes

Expected patient outcomes for the patient with transsphenoidal adenectomy or hypophysectomy may include but are not limited to the following:

1. Exhibits physical signs of fluid balance:
   a. Weight returns to patient's baseline weight.
   b. Has good skin turgor and moist mucous membranes.
   c. Blood pressure and pulse are within patient's normal range.
   d. Serum electrolytes and hematocrit are within normal limits.
   e. Urine specific gravity is 1.010 to 1.025.
2. Has a fluid intake of 2500 to 3000 ml/day, orally or parenterally (unless restrictions are prescribed).
3. Explains measures to prevent fluid deficit.
4. Has adequate gas exchange, as evidenced by:
   a. Normal arterial blood gases (ABGs): pH 7.35 to 7.45, $P_{CO_2}$ 35 to 45 mm Hg, $P_{O_2}$ 90 to 100 mm Hg, $O_2$ saturation 90% to 100% (if available)
   b. Usual mental status and skin color
   c. Usual respiratory depth, rate, and effort
   d. Tolerance to activity
5. Remains free of infection, as evidenced by absence of persistent headache, of CSF leak, and of nuchal (nape of neck) rigidity.
6. See p. 1207 related to knowledge deficit.

### Interventions

#### Preventing fluid volume deficit

1. Assess risk factors for fluid deficit and correct when possible.
2. Weigh daily before breakfast with patient wearing same clothing, with empty bladder, and on same scale.
3. Monitor every 8 hours for signs of fluid deficit: decreased skin turgor, dryness of mucous membranes, postural hypotension, tachycardia, extremes of specific gravity of urine. Monitor available laboratory reports: serum osmolality and sodium levels, hematocrit.
4. Encourage fluid intake to 2500 to 3000 ml/day unless contraindicated, collaborating with patient preferences.
5. Maintain prescribed parenteral therapy.
6. Teach patient/family about diet and fluid needs and measures to prevent fluid deficit, as appropriate.

Fluid volume deficit is a potential problem in any patient during the postoperative period. However, the patient who has had a transsphenoidal adenectomy or hypophysectomy is at higher risk because *diabetes insipidus* may be caused by inadequate release of ADH. Diabetes insipidus, if it does occur, is usually temporary because ADH is produced in the hypothalamus and adequate amounts can be released from it even if damage occurs to the posterior pituitary gland. It usually develops within the first 24 hours. In a few patients, remission occurs for 1 to 14 days, then a recurrence of diabetes insipidus ensues.[32]

Polyuria (urine output greater than 200 ml/hour) and continuously dilute urine (specific gravity of 1.000 to 1.005) are signs of diabetes insipidus. Intake and output measurements every 4 to 8 hours, specific gravity checks of each urine specimen, daily patient weighing, and assessment for complaints of thirst help to identify the presence of diabetes insipidus early. If a deficit in ADH does occur, treatment depends on the severity. If the deficit is mild and the patient can take in enough fluids to maintain fluid volume and still receive adequate rest during the night, replacement of fluids guided by the patient's thirst is the only treatment. The patient should have easy access to cold water. If the deficit of ADH is more severe, requiring frequent awakenings for urination and water intake and thus inadequate sleep, or if the patient is unable to take in adequate fluids, vasopressin is given. In the immediate postoperative period, aqueous vasopressin, given subcutaneously or intramuscularly, is the drug of choice if replacement therapy is necessary. Parenteral use of desmopressin is also reported as effective.[4]

Although rare following adenectomy, ACTH deficiency resulting in glucocorticoid deficiency is a potential problem and can result in severe fluid volume deficit, as well as other complaints and needs.

After a hypophysectomy, cortisol replacement is necessary to maintain life. In fact, intravenous (IV) administration of a cortisol drug is started preoperatively. All patients should be monitored for potential glucocorticoid deficiency. The monitoring should identify early signs and symptoms of adrenal insufficiency, as described on p. 1267. It includes the monitoring just described to assess for the adequacy of ADH, as well as vital signs every 4 hours and observation of energy level, alertness, patient's stated feelings of well-being, and appetite. If abnormalities in these data are found, serum sodium, potassium, and glucose levels may be obtained. Increased urine output, hypotension while lying or orthostatic hypotension, persistent nausea, vomiting, fatigue and tiredness, low sodium level, increased potassium level, hypoglycemia, and acidosis indicate inadequate ACTH and glucocorticoid secretion. Hydrocortisone (Cortef) or other high-potency corticoids and fluid replacement are provided. If the deficit in ACTH is permanent, the patient will have to be treated as discussed later in this chapter for persons with chronic adrenal insufficiency.

**Promoting gas exchange**

1. Monitor gas exchange status every 4 hours, including ABG values (if available), vital signs, mentation, and skin color, and report signs of decreased gas exchange.
2. Place patient in semi-Fowler's position (or as ordered) to facilitate breathing by diaphragm expansion. Turn patient every 2 hours.
3. Administer oxygen therapy as ordered.
4. Teach deep breathing, sighing, and mouth breathing and how to avoid coughing.
5. Initiate activities within limits of dyspnea and ABGs, increasing gradually as tolerated.

Because of the caution against coughing and the nasal packing necessitating mouth breathing, patients are at some risk for ineffective gas exchange. Patients should be instructed about mouth breathing and deep breathing exercises before surgery, have an opportunity to do a return demonstration, and then be monitored for compliance with deep breathing exercises at least every 2 hours for the first 1 to 3 postoperative days. Assessment of vital signs and breath sounds every 4 to 8 hours helps to identify any impairment of air exchange. Maintenance of adequate fluid intake helps to prevent drying of mucous secretions and the formation of mucous plugs.

**Preventing infection**

1. Use proper handwashing technique before and after contact with patient.
2. Assess for signs of infection every shift, including elevated temperature, rhinorrhea, nuchal rigidity, and persistent headache.
3. Assess for halo ring on each change of nasal sling dressing; send drainage to laboratory for glucose analysis if halo ring is present.
4. Provide frequent, gentle mouth rinsing with prescribed mouthwash or normal saline; use mouth care sponges for cleansing teeth. Avoid brushing teeth.
5. Teach patient the importance and methods of mouth care.

With transsphenoidal adenectomy, the sella turcica is entered from below through the sphenoid sinus, and the tumor is removed. An external incision is made between the upper gum and lip, and an internal incision is made through the sella turcica and dura. Care to prevent disruption of both these incisions and to prevent infection are nursing concerns. Care of the incision in the mouth consists of rinsing the mouth with saline or mouthwash and cleansing the teeth with a Toothette or cotton swab. Brushing the teeth is forbidden until the suture line heals.

Oral fluids and a clear-liquid diet are given as soon

as the patient is alert and no longer nauseated from the anesthetic. The diet can progress to solid foods as soon as tolerated, which is usually by the second or third meal after surgery. Because of the mouth incision, rough foods that could irritate the mucous membrane and disrupt the suture line must be avoided. The discomfort associated with eating rough food usually serves as a limiting guideline.

The major occurrence that can disrupt the incision made through the sella turcica and dura is increased cerebrospinal fluid (CSF) pressure. After the tumor is resected, the sella turcica is packed with muscle or fat from the abdomen or thigh. (NOTE: it is important that the patient be prepared for this additional incision.) The floor of the sella turcica is reconstructed with bone or cartilage. This patching, although strong, can be disrupted by increased intracranial pressure (ICP), which in turn increases pressure on the incisional site. Activities such as bending over, straining, coughing, sneezing, and blowing the nose are forbidden. The head of the patient's bed should be elevated at least 30 degrees when the patient is reclining. In most cases, these interventions will prevent disruption of the patch and incision.

CSF leakage will occur if the patching and incision in the sella turcica are disrupted. The nurse monitors for signs and symptoms of such leakage. After surgery the patient's nose is packed for 24 to 48 hours, and a gauze sling is worn under the nose to absorb drainage (see Chapter 36). A CSF leak may be identified by:

1. Complaints of postnasal drip, even with packing in place
2. Observation that the patient is constantly swallowing or stating that he or she needs to swallow constantly
3. Appearance of a **halo ring** on the gauze sling (CSF is clear and, when mixed with serous fluid on gauze, will form a halo surrounding the serous drainage.)

Nasal drainage can be differentiated from CSF based on glucose content. Although the nurse can assess the glucose content of nasal drainage with Tes-Tape, this is unreliable, and fluid should be sent to a laboratory for accurate assessment. If a CSF leakage occurs or is suspected, bedrest with the patient's head elevated is reinstituted and maintained until the leakage is ruled out or clears. Occasionally, patients will have to return to surgery for repair of the site in the sella turcica.

If a CSF leak occurs and has been established as such, the patient is at high risk for infection, including meningitis. Besides instituting restriction of activities to prevent or control a CSF leak, the nurse should begin careful monitoring to identify early signs of an infection. Monitoring includes temperature checks at least every 4 hours and evaluation for presence of nuchal rigidity (see Chapter 56) or headaches at the same time. Antibiotics should be administered as prescribed.

#### Facilitating learning

The first focus of patient education is similar to that for any patient during the postoperative period and includes preparing the patient for day-to-day care (see Chapter 25). The second focus of patient education in the postoperative period is to prepare the patient for resuming self-care and discharge and assuming responsibility for any special follow-up care. The patient should know when to return to see the physician (usually within 1 to 2 weeks), again in 1 month, and then every 6 to 12 months. The first follow-up visit allows for the assessment of the patient's general recovery from surgery and hormonal status. The other visits allow for assessment for recurrence of the tumor.

The third focus of patient education is to prepare the patient to manage any hormonal deficiencies that have occurred. If antidiuretic hormone (ADH) or ACTH and glucocorticoid deficiency occurred postoperatively, diagnostic tests are done before the patient leaves the hospital to identify whether the deficiencies are permanent. If permanent, the patient needs the same education required by any patient with diabetes insipidus or adrenocortical insufficiency (see later discussions in this chapter).

If a deficiency of ACTH and glucocorticoid occurs, secretion of other hormones from the anterior pituitary gland, such as TSH or gonadotropins, may also be deficient. These deficiencies do not cause immediate postoperative concerns and may not even be evident in the immediate postoperative period. However, the adequacy of anterior pituitary secretion of these hormones is assessed before discharge or at the return visits. If the patient develops no deficiency during the postoperative period, approximately 4 to 6 weeks after surgery, diagnostic tests to evaluate the hormonal response to surgery and the adequacy of other hormone synthesis and secretions are completed.

The last focus of patient education is to reinforce care needs for irreversible changes in body appearance, joint and back pain, and visual problems. Information shared may include ways to minimize body changes with makeup and clothes, frequent showers to help control increased sweating and oily skin, pain management techniques (see Chapter 17), modification of activities to decrease stress and strain on the joints and back (see Chapter 65), and referral to the Society for the Visually Impaired.

#### Promoting comfort

Incisional discomfort and headache may occur after surgery and are treated with nonnarcotic analgesics or codeine. Persistent headaches may indicate meningitis and should be reported to the physician immediately. A firm mattress, ROM exercises, back massage, ambulation frequently throughout the day, and heat may be used to help decrease back and joint discomfort in persons with

GH-secreting tumors. Ambulation as soon as possible helps to prevent deterioration in mobility and joint movement. Visual problems should be managed as they were preoperatively, and the patient's vision should be monitored for deterioration postoperatively. Rearranging the room so that needed articles are placed in line with intact vision or other interventions (see Chapter 60) may be necessary. Although visual complications following transsphenoidal resection are rare, the visual pathway can be damaged during surgery or as a result of hemorrhage.[1]

## Complications

Common complications of pituitary tumors and their management have been discussed previously; these are summarized in Box 39-3. In addition, **pituitary apoplexy** can occur. This syndrome is the result of a sudden enlargement of the tumor by hemorrhagic necrosis occurring from damage to the tumor's fragile vascular supply. Other causes of pituitary hemorrhage include head injury, pregnancy and delivery, long-term ventilatory support, meningoencephalitis, estrogen drug therapy, anticoagulation, and radiation therapy.

There is sudden onset of severe headache, vomiting, visual impairment, and altered mental and autonomic functioning (hypotension, hyperthermia). Laboratory abnormalities include leukocytosis, xanthochromic or bloody CSF, and increased CSF pressure. Radiographic examination may show an enlarged sella turcica.

The treatment of these patients is still controversial. Most authorities agree that corticosteroids should be given to correct any adrenal insufficiency and decrease cerebral edema.[40] Most patients with visual or mental changes are treated with decompression surgery using a transsphenoidal approach. Many patients recover with normal endocrine function, but if deficiencies occur later, care is similar to that described next.

### BOX 39-3 Complications of Pituitary Tumors

**NEUROLOGIC**

Increased ICP
Compression of optic chiasma and/or other brain tissue: visual loss
After surgery: CSF leak, meningitis, increased ICP, neurologic deficit, worsening of vision
Pituitary apoplexy

**ENDOCRINE**

Syndromes of excess hormone: acromegaly, Cushing's syndrome; suppression of gonadotropic hormones; infertility and/or sexual dysfunction
Iatrogenic syndromes of hormonal deficit: diabetes insipidus, adrenal insufficiency, hypopituitarism (deficit in one or more anterior pituitary hormones: ACTH, TSH, GH, gonadotropin)
Recurrence of pituitary tumor

# ANTERIOR PITUITARY GLAND: HYPOPITUITARISM

## Etiology

Several disorders can interfere with the function of the anterior pituitary gland and cause hyposecretion of one or more hormones, or **hypopituitarism** (Box 39-4). **Panhypopituitarism** (deficiency of all anterior pituitary hormones and of ADH from the posterior pituitary gland) may be present, or there may be isolated deficiency of one anterior pituitary hormone. If panhypopituitarism occurs, unless it results from surgical removal of the pituitary gland, the deficiencies of the anterior pituitary hormones usually do not appear simultaneously. Deficits of GH and gonadotropins usually occur first, followed by deficits of TSH and then ACTH.

## Epidemiology

Incidence of hypopituitarism is unknown; more is known about the incidence of specific disease states, and these are discussed under the appropriate sections. Because prolactinomas are the most common pituitary tumors, one can assume that related gonadotropic insufficiency is the most common pituitary deficiency in adults. The course of illness in treated children with GH deficiency is expected to change, since replacement of GH is now more accessible and may involve larger doses than in the past.

## Pathophysiology

In hypopituitarism the symptoms vary widely depending on the cause and the endocrine dysfunction present. If a tumor is the cause, the patient may have some of the symptoms previously described for secreting pituitary tumors. These include symptoms resulting from growth of a space-occupying lesion in the cranium, effects resulting from pressure on the optic chiasm, and potential disturbances of cranial nerves III, IV, and VI. If the tumor arises from regions surrounding the pituitary, such as Ratke's pouch (craniopharyngiomas), the hypothalamus, or the third ventricle, the neurologic signs and symp-

### BOX 39-4 Causes of Hypopituitarism

Tumors: craniopharyngioma, primary CNS tumors, nonsecreting pituitary tumors
Ischemic changes: Sheehan's syndrome (ischemic changes following postpartum hemorrhage or infection resulting in shock)
Developmental abnormalities
Infections: viral encephalitis, bacteremia, tuberculosis
Autoimmune disorders
Radiation damage, particularly after treatment of secreting adenomas of pituitary gland
Trauma, including surgery

toms will be more severe and include manifestations of increased ICP.

The endocrine dysfunction may be the result of hypothalamic damage or primary pituitary disease. The most frequent pathophysiologic alteration results from lack of synthesis and secretion of gonadotropins. The second most frequently encountered problem is deficiency of GH synthesis and secretion. The symptoms associated with deficiency of individual anterior pituitary hormones are summarized in Figure 39-3. The patient with hypopituitarism exhibits all or only selected aspects of these deficiencies. Usually the pathologic alteration progresses slowly.

The exact manifestations vary depending on the cause of the anterior pituitary problem and the type of hormonal deficiency. The major manifestations are listed in Box 39-5.

## Medical Management

Medical management is directed toward identifying patients with deficiency syndromes, treating the underlying problem, and supplying the appropriate hormonal replacement. The target gland hormone (thyroid, cortisol, or gonadal steroids) is replaced as necessary. If a childbearing female desires fertility, gonadotropins must be replaced. However, prolactin does not need to be replaced.

Replacement therapy of GH in adults with GH deficiency is a recent development. Clinical trials have demonstrated that GH (insulin-like growth factor 1 [IGF-1]) administration for 4 to 12 months improves metabolic status, energy level, muscle strength, cognitive function, and mental attitude. Side effects have included fluid retention and arthralgia.[20] Replacement therapy of GH is used for all short children with GH deficiency. The source of GH in the past had been human cadaver pituitaries, but the occurrence of lethal infection in persons receiving this form of GH caused great concern and limited use. Biosynthetic human GH is now available as somatrem (Protropin) and somatropin (Humatrope). Each can be given intramuscularly at individually prescribed doses three times a week. In the first year of treatment, there is a rapid catch-up pattern of growth, but the growth pattern then returns to normal. GH replacement also has been effective in some children with short stature who have normal GH levels.[11]

# NURSING MANAGEMENT

## ♦ ASSESSMENT

Assessment focuses on identifying signs and symptoms of the hormonal deficiencies and etiologic factors. In addition, data are collected on how well the patient is dealing with the disorder. In this section, only data rel-

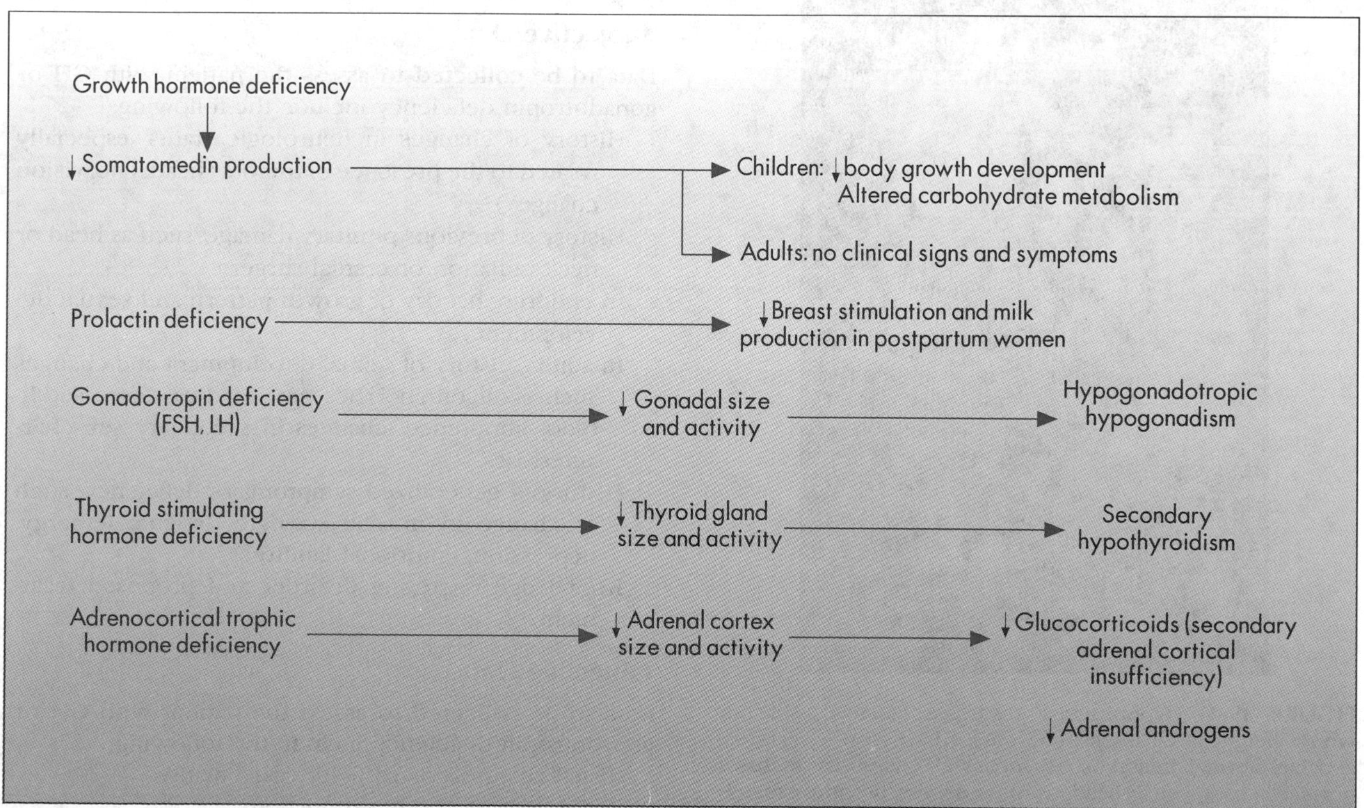


**FIGURE 39-3** Pathophysiologic findings associated with individual anterior pituitary hormone deficiency.

**BOX 39-5 Clinical Manifestations of Hypopituitarism**

1. Manifestations based on cause, such as bacteremia, viral hepatitis, autoimmune disorders, and trauma
2. Manifestations such as vision changes, papilledema, or hydrocephalus if cause is tumor
3. Manifestations of gonadotropin deficiency
   a. Decreased serum levels of FSH, LH, and gonadal steroids
   b. Children—delayed puberty
   c. Adults
      (1) Females—oligomenorrhea or amenorrhea, uterine and vaginal atrophy, potential atrophy of breast tissue, loss of libido, decrease in body hair
      (2) Males—loss of libido, decreased sperm count, possible impotence, decreased testicular size, decreased total body hair
4. Manifestations of GH deficiency
   a. Children
      (1) Stunted growth (below third percentile) with normal body proportions (Figure 39-4), excessive subcutaneous fat, poor muscle development
      (2) Immature facial features, immature voice
      (3) Slow growth of nails and thin hair
      (4) Delayed puberty but eventual normal sexual development
      (5) Decreased levels of GH
   b. Adults
      (1) Severe, short stature
      (2) Immature facies
      (3) Moderate obesity
      (4) Decreased muscle mass and weakness
      (5) Lassitude
      (6) Emotional lability
      (7) Decreased basal levels of GH or decreased response to provocative testing
      (8) Some persons may have normal GH levels with low level of somatomedins (IGF-I)
5. Manifestations of prolactin deficiency
   a. Failure to lactate in the postpartum female
   b. Decreased serum levels of prolactin
6. Manifestations of TSH deficiency
   a. Signs and symptoms of secondary hypothyroidism
   b. Decreased serum level of TSH and thyroid hormone
7. Manifestations of ACTH deficiency
   a. Signs and symptoms of secondary ACTH insufficiency; *no hyperpigmentation*
   b. Decreased serum levels of ACTH, glucocorticoids, and adrenal androgens (aldosterone levels may be normal)

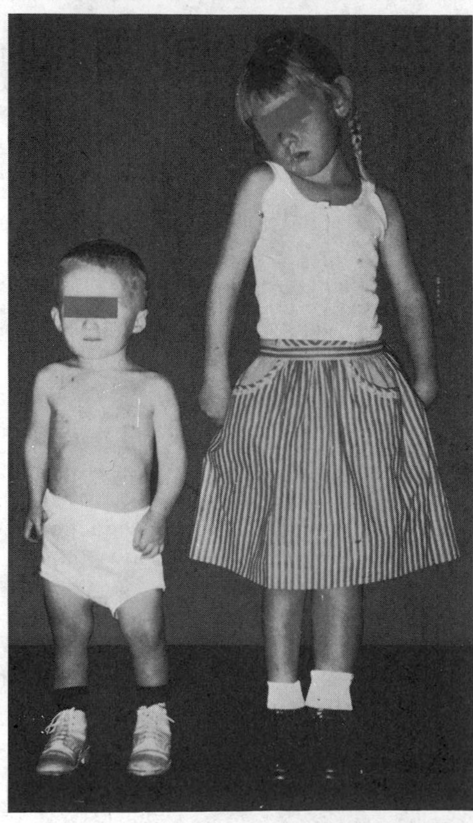

**FIGURE 39-4** Hypopituitary dwarfism in 4-year-old boy whose height is 25 inches (62 cm). Girl is also 4 years old and has normal height of 39 inches (97 cm). Dwarf has a normal face, as well as head, trunk, and limbs of approximately normal proportions. (From Brashear HR, Raney RB: *Shand's handbook of orthopaedic surgery,* ed 9, St Louis, 1978, Mosby.)

evant to GH and gonadotropin deficiencies are described. (TSH and ACTH deficiencies are described later in the chapter.)

## Subjective Data

Data to be collected to assess the patient with GH or gonadotropin deficiency include the following:

History of changes in neurologic status, especially related to the presence of tumors (headache, vision changes)

History of previous pituitary damage, such as head or neck radiation or cranial surgery

In children, history of growth pattern and sexual development

In adults, history of sexual development and changes such as oligomenorrhea, amenorrhea, decreased libido, impotence, changes in secondary sex characteristics

History of generalized symptoms of deficiency, such as change in muscle strength, fatigue, lethargy, depression, emotional lability

Knowledge regarding disorder and proposed treatment

## Objective Data

Data to be collected to assess the patient with GH or gonadotropin deficiency include the following:

Visual changes: visual field, visual acuity

Facial features, body proportions

Distribution of fatty tissue and hair

Presence or absence of secondary sex characteristics

### Diagnostic Test Findings

Confirmation of a hyposecretory state may include the following:

1. Decreased serum levels and levels of urinary metabolites of pituitary and target gland hormones
2. Decreased serum levels and levels of urinary metabolites in response to provocative testing

## ♦ NURSING DIAGNOSES

Nursing diagnoses are determined from analysis of patient data. Nursing diagnoses for the person with GH or gonadotropin deficiency may include but are not limited to the following:

| Diagnostic Title | Possible Etiologic Factors |
|---|---|
| Body image disturbance | Lack of normal sexual development (child), lack of normal growth (child), change in sexual characteristics (adult) |
| Coping, ineffective (individual) | Lack of learned coping strategies, uncertainty about cause of problem |
| Knowledge deficit: disease procedures, treatment, nursing care needs | New disease, never exposed to information |
| Sensory/perceptual alterations: visual | Growth of mass in cranium causing pressure on optic chiasm or cranial nerves III, IV, or VI |
| Sexual dysfunction | Alteration in desire or functioning associated with alterations in gonadotropin levels |

## ♦ EXPECTED PATIENT OUTCOMES

Expected patient outcomes for the person with a deficiency of GH or gonadotropin may include but are not limited to the following:

1. Body image improves, as evidenced by describing self in positive terms and describing ways to minimize body image changes.
2. Coping improves as evidenced by listing coping strategies helpful in dealing with the stressors related to hormonal deficiencies.
3. Describes the hormonal deficiency causing the problem, how it relates to the signs and symptoms, any tests planned, and the treatment planned.
4. Does not have any injuries related to the vision loss, and maintains independence in ADL.
5. Describes how therapy can reverse sexual dysfunction.

## ♦ INTERVENTIONS

### Promoting Positive Body Image

One focus of care is helping the patient manage disturbances or alterations in body image. The patient should know what changes are reversible. Treatment with sex steroids helps to initiate the development of sexual characteristics in the adolescent entering puberty. Treatment with sex steroids restores secondary sexual characteristics in adults, and treatment with gonadotropins restores fertility in the female with normal menstrual cycles. Replacement of GH increases growth in the child with short stature. The parents and child should know what growth outcome is expected so that unrealistic goals are not set. (Refer to Chapter 9 for additional information on how to assist persons with alterations in body images.)

### Promoting Coping

Another focus of care is to help patients cope with signs and symptoms that are not reversible or that take a long time to reverse. Helping them see their positive attributes is one alternative. Another alternative is helping them develop positive coping strategies, such as relaxation techniques and new hobbies. Patients with GH deficiency report high rates of unemployment and social isolation.[20] Improved sense of well-being and increased energy level (resulting from GH therapy) may make patients more interested in exploring coping strategies. (See Chapter 7 for additional information on coping.)

### Facilitating Learning

Patient education is another focus of care. The patient must be prepared for various diagnostic tests, including blood tests and roentgenograms, CT scans, or MRI of the head. If a tumor is the cause of the deficiency, the tumor is removed. A transsphenoidal approach is usually used, or the tumor is treated by radiation. Hormonal replacement of GH in children and therapy with gonadal steroids and gonadotropins in adolescents and adults are individualized. The patient needs to be taught how to take the hormones. GHs are given subcutaneously. Gonadal steroids are given orally to restore sexual characteristics, and gonadotropin or clomiphene citrate is used in females to induce ovulation if pregnancy is desired. An important focus of teaching is for patients to realize the need for adequate steroids to prevent premature bone demineralization. Patients who decline hormonal therapy, particularly women, need to be monitored periodically for accelerated bone loss and must take adequate calcium.[2]

If visual changes are present, care as described in Chapter 60 is necessary. In relation to the sexual dysfunction, patient education about the cause of the problem and the replacement therapy described previously are the major interventions.

## ♦ EVALUATION

To determine the effectiveness of nursing interventions, compare patient behaviors with those stated in the expected patient outcomes. Successful achievement of patient outcomes for the person with a deficiency of GH or gonadotropin is indicated by the following:

1. Describes self positively.
2. Shows improved coping strategies to deal with related stressors, and identifies at least three techniques that help reduce the stress response.

3. Accurately describes how the hormonal deficiency relates to signs and symptoms.
4. Has no visual injuries, and reports increased initiation and completion of ADL.
5. Accurately describes how therapy can reverse sexual dysfunction.

## POSTERIOR PITUITARY GLAND: HYPERFUNCTION

### Syndrome of Inappropriate Antidiuretic Hormone

#### Etiology/Epidemiology

Many factors cause the syndrome of inappropriate antidiuretic hormone (SIADH) (Box 39-6). This disorder is associated with various pathologic processes, as well as with drug therapy.

#### Pathophysiology

In SIADH, total body water increases because of water retention and a hypoosmolar state results from hyponatremia (low serum sodium concentration). In SIADH the ADH release follows one of four patterns[30,42]:

1. ADH release is erratic and unrelated to plasma osmolality.
2. ADH release varies with the plasma osmolality, but the osmostat has been reset, and ADH release occurs at a lower plasma osmolality.
3. ADH release is normal in response to a normal or elevated plasma osmolality, but ADH is not reduced as the plasma osmolality is lowered.
4. ADH release is normal, but the patient is more sensitive to the released ADH, or some "unmeasured factor" that increases water retention is released.

The abnormally released ADH or the increased sensitivity of cells to ADH increases the permeability of the distal renal tubules and collecting ducts to water, and water resorption by the kidney increases. Intravascular volume increases, but edema is not present, as would be seen in congestive heart failure (see Chapter 31) or cirrhosis (see Chapter 42). Edema does not occur because the volume expansion in SIADH results in *natriuresis* (urinary sodium excretion). The natriuresis results because of enhanced glomerular filtration and decreased proximal tubular sodium reabsorption, even with hyponatremia.

It is important to note that a reduction in plasma sodium level to 119 mEq/L from 139 mEq/L within 2 hours can result in death, whereas a reduction to as low as 99 mEq/L in 16 days results only in lethargy.[30] The following are some guidelines for understanding the potential changes that may occur in patients and for planning the monitoring that needs to be done[30]:

1. As serum sodium levels falls below 125 mEq/L, the patient complains of nausea and malaise.
2. At serum sodium levels between 115 and 120 mEq/L headache, lethargy, and obtundation may appear.
3. Seizures and coma are not usually seen until the plasma sodium concentration falls below 110 to 115 mEq/L.

The hyponatremia results in hypoosmolality and creates an osmolar gradient across the blood-brain barrier and other cellular membranes. This osmolar gradient results in water movement into the brain and other cells and cellular overhydration.

Box 39-7 summarizes clinical manifestations of SIADH.

#### Medical management

Medical management in acute SIADH focuses on treatment of the etiologic factor (e.g., carcinoma, infection) and correcting, or at least restoring toward normal, the plasma sodium level and plasma osmolality. Water restriction is the first priority of management. Water may be restricted to as little as 500 ml/day. Oral salt intake is increased if the patient is able to take in oral nutrients.

**BOX 39-6 Etiologic Factors Associated With SIADH**

- Pulmonary disorders: malignant neoplasms (e.g., oat cell adenocarcinoma of lung), tuberculosis, ventilator patients receiving positive pressure
- Other malignancies: duodenum, pancreas, prostate lymphoma, sarcoma, leukemia
- CNS disorders: tumors, infection, trauma, surgery[26]
- Endocrine disorders that result in hypovolemia and impaired free water excretion, particularly if associated with fluid replacement (adrenal insufficiency, anterior pituitary insufficiency)
- Drugs such as clofibrate, chlorpropamide, thiazides, vincristine, cyclophosphamide, morphine
- Stressors: fear, acute infections, pain, anxiety, trauma, surgery

**BOX 39-7 Clinical Manifestations of SIADH**

**FLUID AND ELECTROLYTE CHANGES**

- Decreased plasma sodium and plasma osmolality
- Increased urinary sodium and urinary osmolality
- Decreased urinary volume
- Increased weight
- Absence of edema

**NEUROLOGIC CHANGES***

- Lethargy, headache, mild disorientation that progresses to seizures
- Emotional/behavioral changes, such as anxiety, irritability, uncooperativeness, hostility
- Gastrointestinal (GI) changes: anorexia, nausea, vomiting

*Depending on severity of serum sodium depression and rapidity of the reduction in plasma sodium concentration.

If the patient's plasma sodium level is less than 120 mEq/L and the patient is exhibiting CNS manifestations such as nausea, vomiting, lethargy, and headaches, more rapid correction of the low plasma sodium is necessary. This severe *hyponatremia* is treated with hypertonic saline (3% sodium chloride) and a loop diuretic such as furosemide (Lasix) or ethacrynic acid.[20a,38] The goal of this later therapy is not to return the plasma sodium level to normal, but to increase it to 125 to 130 mEq/L or to administer enough sodium chloride to relieve symptoms or increase the plasma sodium by 25 mEq/L. This correction needs to be done cautiously because of potential complications from either too rapid or too slow correction. Verbalis[38] recommends that the plasma sodium should be increased as necessary but that the rate of increase should be no faster than 0.5 to 2 mEq/L/hour. Too fast a correction of plasma sodium can worsen the neurologic manifestations.

Too rapid of an increase in the plasma sodium can produce a plasma solution that is relatively hypertonic compared with the intracellular compartment and a shifting of fluids from the intracellular to the extracellular compartment. A rapid shift of fluids can result in central pontine myelinolysis, which is demyelination of the pons. This demyelination results in dysfunction of the nerve tracts that travel through or originate in the pons, causing bulbar palsies, quadriplegia, coma, and death.[38] During treatment with hypertonic saline or loop diuretics, plasma osmolality and serum sodium are monitored every 2 to 4 hours. Note that 3% sodium chloride is used for sodium replacement, not for volume replacement.

Chronic SIADH and hyponatremia are treated at first with water restriction. If water restriction alone cannot prevent hypoosmolality, pharmacologic treatment is added. Demeclocycline, a tetracycline derivative, blocks the action of ADH on the renal tubule and collecting duct cells and decreases urine osmolality. Diuretics may be used on a long-term basis, and a high-sodium diet may be continued.

#### Nursing management

Nursing interventions are as follows:

1. Perform assessment.
   a. Identify patients at high risk.
   b. For high-risk patients,[19] monitor daily weights, daily intake and output, daily serum and urinary sodium levels and osmolality, and vital signs and neurologic status every 4 hours. Report any decrease below normal in serum sodium (if the level is below 125 mEq/L, report laboratory results immediately), any signs of fluid retention (increased weight, decreased output), and any neurologic changes (complaints of headaches or nausea, decreased responsiveness).
   c. For patients with diagnosed SIADH being treated aggressively with hypertonic sodium or loop diuretics, frequency of monitoring is increased to every 1 to 2 hours. Any deterioration in neurologic status is reported immediately.
   d. For patients with chronic SIADH, monitor weights daily to weekly and report any increases not attributed to dietary changes or any complaints of nausea, headache, or lethargy. Monitoring by the nurse in the outpatient department is the same as that described for high-risk patients.
2. Provide supportive care.
   a. Restrict fluids as prescribed.
   b. Control discomfort from thirst.
      (1) Space fluids throughout 24-hour period.
      (2) Use ice chips, which allow more frequent relief of thirst with less fluid intake.
      (3) Provide frequent mouth care.
   c. Administer drugs or fluids as ordered.
3. Provide care appropriate to specific etiologic factor (varies).
4. Initiate patient teaching.
   a. Review purpose of fluid restriction and how to manage it.
   b. Review self-monitoring required on a long-term basis (intake and output measurement, weight change).
   c. Discuss drug therapy as appropriate.

Box 39-8 lists the drugs that have been used in treatment of SIADH. Diuretics may be used on a long-term basis, and a high-sodium diet may be continued. In some patients, salt tablets are used with diuretics to replace urinary sodium losses and prevent volume depletion.

## Diabetes Insipidus

### Etiology/Epidemiology

Pituitary **diabetes insipidus** (DI) results from lack of sufficient ADH. The cause may be a *central* brain or pituitary tumor, head trauma, encephalitis, meningitis, hypophysectomy, or cranial surgery. The cause is often *idiopathic. Nephrogenic* DI is a second form of the disorder and results from failure of the renal tubules to respond to ADH. A rare hereditary form of nephrogenic DI occurs.[16] Diabetes insipidus may be transient or permanent. Postsurgical DI is discussed earlier in this chapter. Transient DI associated with pregnancy is caused by an excessive amount of placental secreted vasopressinase that neutralizes ADH activity.[21]

**BOX 39-8 Drugs Used in SIADH**

Demeclocycline
Furosemide
Lithium carbonate
Phenytoin

**BOX 39-9 Clinical Manifestations of Diabetes Insipidus**

1. Polyuria: as much as 20 L urine/day may be excreted; urine is dilute, with a specific gravity of 1.005 or less or an osmolality of 200 or less
2. Polydipsia secondary to increased thirst
3. Only slightly elevated serum osmolality because water intake is usually maintained
4. Abnormal results on tests for urine concentration
   a. Water deprivation test (see Chapter 38): no increase in urine concentration with either pituitary or nephrogenic DI
   b. ADH replacement: increase in urine osmolality with pituitary DI but no response with nephrogenic DI
5. Sleep disturbance from polyuria
6. Inadequate *water replacement* results in:
   a. Hyperosmolality: irritability, mental dullness, coma, hyperthermia
   b. Hypovolemia: hypotension, tachycardia, dry mucous membranes, poor skin turgor

**TABLE 39-1 Drugs Used for Treatment of Diabetes Insipidus**

| DRUG | DOSAGE | ROUTE |
|---|---|---|
| Arginine vasopressin* (vasopressins for injection) Aqueous solution | 0.25-0.5 mg | SC, IM |
| Lysine vasopressin* (Lypressin, Diapid) Aqueous solution | 3-8 doses/24 hr | Nasal spray |
| Pitressin tannate in oil* | 10-40 ng 1-3 doses/wk | IM |
| Desmopressin (DDAVP)† | 5-10 ng dose; 1 or 2 doses/24 hr | Nasal instillation[4] |
| Parenteral solution | 1-2 ng dose; 1 or 2 doses/24 hr | IM |

*These preparations interact with $V_1$ and $V_2$ receptors; thus, pressor side effects can occur (abdominal cramping, hypertension, angina).
†DDAVP interacts with $V_2$ receptors only; thus, pressor side effects do not occur.

### Pathophysiology

The lack of adequate ADH or ineffective kidney response to ADH results in insufficient water reabsorption by the kidney. The loss of excessive water from the body (polyuria) stimulates the perception of thirst (polydipsia). If the problem is long-standing, the kidney, pelvis, and urinary bladder may show changes caused by the large urine volume. When inadequate water replacement occurs, CNS and vascular changes from hyperosmolality and volume depletion can occur. Box 39-9 lists clinical manifestations of DI.

### Medical management

The person with pituitary DI is treated with vasopressin replacement; four preparations of ADH are available (Table 39-1).

Vasopressin, or its synthetic analogs, binds with $V_2$ receptors in the renal tubule; vasopressin also binds with $V_1$ receptors found in smooth muscle of arterioles and other tissues. The action of ADH on $V_1$ receptors is responsible for *pressor* side effects of exogenous ADH (abdominal cramping, hypertension, angina). These pressor effects occur because of vasoconstriction and are seen in all preparations except *desmopressin* (DDAVP), which acts only on $V_2$ receptors.[32] DDAVP is also much more potent in its antidiuretic effect and has a longer duration of action; for these three reasons, it is the drug of choice for chronic DI. For persons who have some residual pituitary function, chlorpropamide and clofibrate, which stimulate release of endogenous ADH, may be prescribed.

Temporary DI associated with head trauma or surgery is treated with aqueous vasopressin, 5 to 10 IU subcutaneously, until nasal administration of lysine or DDVP becomes appropriate. After transsphenoidal surgery, nasal packing and edema of the mucosa are present. In addition, the physician may choose the shorter-acting aqueous vasopressin until the hormonal status stabilizes. Administration of DDAVP by intramuscular (IM) injection in the immediate postoperative period has been reported to be an alternative.[4]

The most common treatment for persons with nephrogenic DI is a low-sodium, low-protein diet and thiazide diuretics. The low-sodium diet and thiazide diuretics induce a mild volume depletion. This volume depletion enhances sodium chloride and water reabsorption in the proximal part of the kidney tubule, resulting in less water being delivered to the collecting tubules where ADH should be; therefore, less water is excreted. The diuretic also increases the osmolality of the medullary interstitial space and thus promotes more water resorption in collecting tubules that are less permeable because of inadequate ADH. The protein restriction helps control water loss by decreasing solute excretion. A last therapy in nephrogenic DI is administration of nonsteroidal antiinflammatory agents, which impair prostaglandin production in the kidney and increase urinary concentrating ability.[30]

If the patient is showing *hypernatremia* and clinical signs and symptoms such as mental changes and hyperthermia are present, replacement of water must be instituted. Water replacement must be done carefully over 48 hours[30] to avoid cerebral edema, seizures, or even death. Too rapid a correction of hypernatremia by fluid administration may result in the establishment of an osmotic gradient, with the plasma osmolality being less than the intracellular osmolality and the entry of water into the brain. The water deficit for a patient with hypernatremia is estimated, and this deficit, along with continual insensible water loss or dilute urinary loss, is replaced over 48 hours. The exact fluid administered will vary depending on the patient's needs. If pure water loss is present, free water is given orally or in the form of dextrose in water. If the patient is hypotensive as well as hypernatremic, isotonic saline is given until *vascular volume* is adequate, and then free water is given. If the patient has a slight deficit in sodium along with free water deficit, one-quarter strength sodium chloride is used. During fluid replacement, serial measurement of plasma sodium level and assessment of mental and circulatory status are required every 1 to 2 hours.

### Nursing management

Nursing interventions for the person with DI focus on maintenance of fluid and electrolyte balance, provision of rest, and teaching.

1. Maintain fluid and electrolyte balance.
   a. Monitor intake and output, daily weights, urine specific gravity, vital signs (orthostatic), skin turgor, and neurologic status every 1 to 2 hours during the acute phase, then every 4 to 8 hours until discharge, and then on return to physician or outpatient clinic.
   b. Provide fluids; be sure that they are within reach of patient.
2. Provide daily rest periods during time when nocturia interferes with sleep.
3. Provide patient teaching.
   a. Diagnostic tests: purposes, procedures, and required monitoring (see Chapter 38)
   b. Self-management: drug therapy
      1. Administration: method and frequency
      2. Effectiveness: if nasal congestion occurs, drug effectiveness may decrease and polyuria and thirst occur
      3. Side effects: particularly signs of volume excess (weight gain, edema)

# THYROID GLAND

Disorders of the thyroid gland are relatively common endocrine problems. They are second to diabetes mellitus in occurrence. Alterations in the thyroid gland may be associated with hypersecretion, hyposecretion, or normal secretion of thyroid hormone.

A goiter is a typical finding in many patients with thyroid problems. **Goiter** is an enlargement of the thyroid gland that causes the gland to form a protuberance on the anterior aspect of the neck. Goiters occur because of hypertrophy of the gland when it is being stimulated by increased amounts of TSH or any substances that act as TSH. Goiter can be associated with hyperthyroidism, hypothyroidism, or euthyroidism.

## HYPERSECRETION OF THYROID HORMONE: HYPERTHYROIDISM

### Etiology

Hyperthyroidism, also called **thyrotoxicosis,** is a condition that results when tissues are stimulated by excessive thyroid hormone. The numerous causes of hyperthyroidism are summarized in Table 39-2. The two

**TABLE 39-2 Causes and Definitions of Types of Hyperthyroidism**

| CAUSE | DEFINITION |
|---|---|
| Toxic diffuse goiter (Graves' disease) | See discussion in text. |
| Toxic multinodular goiter | See discussion in text. |
| Toxic adenoma | Single or occasionally multiple adenomas of follicular cells that secrete and function independent of TSH |
| Thyroiditis | Increased amount of thyroxine ($T_4$) and triiodothyronine ($T_3$) released during acute inflammatory process; transient hyperthyroid state followed by return to euthyroid state, and eventually to hypothyroid state as gland is destroyed by the recurring inflammatory exacerbations; hyperthyroid state usually requires no treatment. |
| $T_3$ thyrotoxicosis | $T_3$ level elevated but cause unknown; $T_4$ normal or low; should be suspected in patients who have normal $T_4$ but have signs and symptoms of thyrotoxicosis |
| Hyperthyroidism caused by metastatic thyroid cancer | Rare because thyroid cancer cells do not usually concentrate iodine efficiently; may occur with large follicular carcinomas |
| Pituitary hyperthyroidism | Rare; pituitary adenomas may secrete excess TSH; treatment involves removal of pituitary tumor. |
| Chorionic hyperthyroidism | Chorionic gonadotropin has weak thyrotropin activity; tumors such as choriocarcinoma, embryonal cell carcinoma, and hydatiform mole have high concentrations of chorionic gonadotropins that can stimulate $T_4$ and $T_3$ secretion; hyperthyroidism disappears with treatment of tumor. |
| Struma ovarii | Ovarian dermoid tumor made up of thyroid tissue that secretes thyroid hormone. |
| Factitious hyperthyroidism | Results from ingestion of exogenous thyroid extracts |
| Iodine-induced hyperthyroidism (Jod-Basedow) | Overproduction of thyroid hormone resulting from administration of supplemental iodine to a person with endemic goiter |

most common causes are Graves' disease and toxic multinodular goiter.

### Graves' disease

**Graves' disease** is a disorder characterized by one or more of the following: *diffuse goiter, hyperthyroidism,* and *infiltrative ophthalmopathy.*[8] Occasionally, *infiltrative dermopathy* is seen. It is important to note that ophthalmopathy or dermopathy can occur without hyperthyroidism.

### Toxic multinodular goiter

**Toxic multinodular goiter** is a disorder characterized by the presence of many thyroid nodules and a milder form of hyperthyroidism than that seen with Graves' disease. The multinodular goiter is probably caused by mild iodide deficiency.[18] Unlike Graves' disease, it does not have an autoimmune basis.

## Epidemiology

Incidence rates of hyperthyroidism in all adults have been estimated at 0.02% to 0.06% in different surveys.[40] Community screening programs have shown prevalence rates of subclinical hyperthyroidism of about 1% and have shown limited identification of unsuspected cases of overt hyperthyroidism. Because subclinical disease is usually not treated, screening in the wide community is not recommended. Certain disorders have been associated with hyperthyroidism and are sometimes considered risk factors (see p. 1212).

The most common cause of hyperthyroidism is Graves' disease, which occurs seven to nine times more often in women than in men and most often in persons under age 40. The disease often occurs after severe emotional stress. A hereditary influence is manifested by the higher frequency of Graves' disease in persons with specific haplotypes and the higher rate in monozygotic twins. The exact incidence of Graves' disease is uncertain.[40]

The second most common cause, *toxic multinodular goiter,* usually occurs after age 50 in persons who have had multinodular goiter for many years.

## Pathophysiology

### Hypermetabolism

In hyperthyroidism from any cause, the normal regulatory control of thyroid function is lost, resulting in an increased concentration of thyroid hormone and increased peripheral manifestations of thyroid hormone excess. Thyroid hormone increases metabolic rate and calorigenesis; alters protein, fat, and carbohydrate metabolism; directly stimulates some body systems, such

**TABLE 39-3 Hyperthyroidism: Normal Function, Pathologic Alterations, and Clinical Manifestations**

| NORMAL FUNCTION | ALTERATIONS | CLINICAL MANIFESTATIONS |
|---|---|---|
| Regulates metabolic rate, calorigenesis, and oxygen consumption | Increased metabolic rate, heat production, and oxygen consumption: peripheral vasodilation, increased nutrient requirements | General: increased body temperature and intolerance to heat<br>Skin: warm, moist<br>Hair: fine, friable<br>Increased appetite |
| Regulates protein, fat, and carbohydrate (CHO) metabolism | Altered CHO, protein, and fat metabolism:<br>1. Increased protein synthesis, glycogenolysis, and lipolysis | Metabolic fatigue, increased appetite, weight loss, muscle weakness |
| | 2. Increased glucose absorption and degradation of insulin | Blood glucose levels may increase in patients with diabetes mellitus |
| | 3. Decreased lipid metabolism, especially lipid degradation | Decreased serum triglycerides and cholesterol |
| | 4. Hepatic dysfunction in severe cases | Signs of hepatic dysfunction |
| | 5. Increased intestinal motility | Increased frequency of stools |
| Sensitizes cells to catecholamines | Altered cardiovascular functioning<br>Hypermetabolic and adrenergic state: increased myocardial oxygen consumption, shortened systolic time intervals, increased cardiac output | Tachycardia, palpitations, increased blood pressure, dyspnea, angina, atrial fibrillation, congestive heart failure |
| Regulates rate of cellular functions; interacts with other hormones and systems | Increased and altered CNS function | Nervousness, restlessness, decreased attention span; insomnia; emotional lability; hyperkinesis; fine, rhythmic tremors of hands, tongue, and eyelids |
| Regulates bone resorption of calcium and phosphorylation of creatine | Increased excretion of calcium and phosphorus; sometimes associated with demineralization of bones | Hypercalcemia, mild osteoporosis, fractures; muscle weakness and wasting, most prominent in proximal muscles |
| Regulates reproductive system | Altered reproductive function, altered secretion and metabolism of gonadotropins and gonadal steroids | Prepubertal: delayed sexual development<br>Postpubertal: increased libido, altered menses, decreased fertility; failure to conceive |

as bone and bone marrow; and increases sympathetic (adrenergic) activity.

The pathophysiologic factors just described are related to specific clinical manifestations, as noted in Table 39-3. One must remember that the underlying pathophysiology of all manifestations of hyperthyroidism is not known. However, the effects of hyperthyroidism on body systems are well known and occur in large part because of the interaction of the hypermetabolic state, increased circulation, and adrenergic stimulation.

Tachycardia is present, and more severe illness can lead to atrial fibrillation, other dysrhythmias, angina, and congestive heart failure. In addition, thyroid storm can develop; this life-threatening crisis is discussed on p. 1226.

The typical patient with hyperthyroidism from any cause is nervous and has tremors, muscle weakness, fatigue, weight loss, and intolerance to heat. The patient usually demonstrates emotional lability and may give a history of insomnia, and in females, amenorrhea.

### Ophthalmopathy

In Graves' disease, **ophthalmopathy** may precede, occur at the same time, or follow hyperthyroidism. In ophthalmopathy the retrobulbar connective tissue and extraocular muscle volume are expanded. This volume expansion occurs because of fluid retention resulting from the accumulation of glycosaminoglycans. The increase in tissue mass forces the eye forward (proptosis) up to the limits of the restraining action of the extraocular muscles (exophthalmos). The pressure in retrobulbar space increases because of an increase in retrobulbar tissue and limited forward movement and causes periorbital and lid edema and pressure on the optic nerve.[10] The stretched enlarged extraocular muscles do not function well.

**BOX 39-10 Ophthalmopathy in Graves' Disease**

**SIGNS**

Bright-eyed stare: results from retraction of upper eyelid
Lid lag: on downward gaze, upper lid lags behind globe movement, and sclera seen between lid and limbus
Globe lag: globe lags behind lid with upward gaze
Lid movement: jerky and spasmodic
Eyes partly open when sleeping
Periorbital edema

**SYMPTOMS**

Sense of irritation and excessive tearing
Feeling of pressure behind eyes
Complaints of blurred, double vision, easy tiring of eyes

**COMPLICATIONS**

Corneal ulceration
Optic nerve involvement (optic neuropathy)
Myopathy of extraocular muscles

Glycosaminoglycans and fluid accumulation also occur in the connective tissue in other parts of the body. This accumulation is particularly seen in the pretibial area. Box 39-10 lists other signs and symptoms of ophthalmopathy, and Figure 39-5 illustrates the eye's appearance.

Research supports the contention that Graves' disease is caused by stimulation of the gland by immunoglobulins of the IgG class. It is believed that the thyroid-related immunoglobulins are a heterogenous group of antibodies directed at varying sites within the thyroid cell membrane. These immunoglobulins are called *thyroid-stimulating immunoglobulins* (TSIs). The cause of the abnormal development of immunoglobulins is unknown. Heredity, gender, and perhaps emotions have a role.[40]

### Goiter

A goiter results from increased stimulation of the thyroid gland by TSH or TSH-like substances. Goiters are seen in toxic diffuse goiter (Graves' disease), toxic multinodular goiter, pituitary hyperthyroidism (secondary hyperthyroidism), thyroiditis, $T_3$ thyrotoxicosis, and iodine-induced hyperthyroidism. Chorionic hyperthyroidism may or may not be associated with a goiter. In toxic adenomas, small well-defined nodules occur, whereas with cancer there are poorly defined nodules. Persons with hyperthyroidism resulting from struma ovarii and persons with factitious hyperthyroidism do not have goiters.

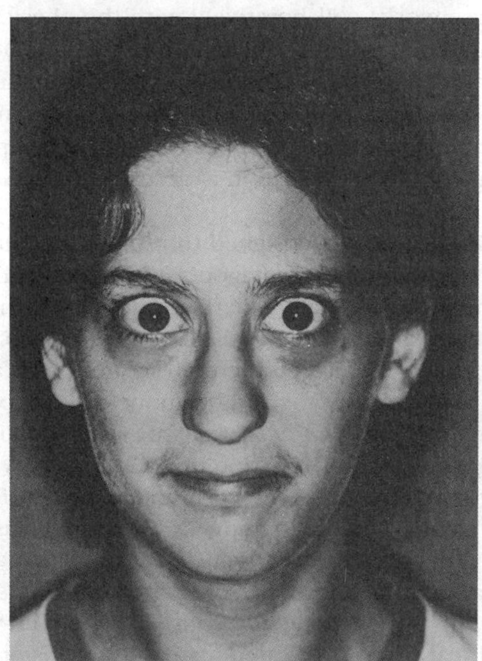

**FIGURE 39-5** Ophthalmopathy of Graves' disease. Patient has typical noninfiltrative changes (stare with severe upper and lower lid retraction). (From Rose L, Kaye D: *Fundamentals of internal medicine,* St Louis, 1983, Mosby.)

**BOX 39-11 Risk Factors for Hyperthyroidism**

Family history of thyroid disease
Autoimmune disorders
Women over age 40
People over age 65

## Prevention

Only two of the causes of hyperthyroidism are preventable: factitious (artificial) hyperthyroidism and iodine-induced hyperthyroidism. *Primary prevention* of factitious hyperthyroidism is possible through appropriate health teaching regarding safe measures for weight reduction and weight control. To prevent iodine-induced hyperthyroidism, persons with endemic goiter who are treated with supplemental iodine must be monitored very closely. *Secondary prevention* for persons with hyperthyroidism includes early detection of signs and symptoms and early prompt treatment to prevent disease progression. Screening is recommended in clinic patients with risk factors shown in Box 39-11. The "sensitive" TSH assay of blood is used most often.[15] Prompt treatment and adequate follow-up can reduce the incidence and severity of complications of hyperthyroidism (*tertiary prevention*).

## Medical Management

The goal for discharge of patients with hyperthyroidism with atrial fibrillation as determined by DRGs is 7 days. The nurse works collaboratively with the physician for implementation of prescribed medical therapy. Because the nurse has a major role in discharge planning and patient teaching, these are discussed under nursing management. A sample Critical Pathway for hyperthyroidism with atrial fibrillation is described at the end of the chapter.

Medical therapy is designed to reduce the output of thyroid hormone and to antagonize the effects of thyroid hormone on peripheral tissue. Two approaches that may be used to achieve these goals are (1) the use of drugs to antagonize the effects of thyroid hormone and to reduce the output of thyroid hormone or (2) **ablation** (therapy to remove or destroy tissue) of thyroid tissue by surgery or radioactive iodine (RAI) therapy. Drug therapy is often used first to promote a euthyroid state before using ablation therapy in Graves' disease and multinodular goiter. However, RAI therapy is usually the first treatment in elderly persons with Graves' disease.[31] RAI therapy is now generally considered safe in women of childbearing age, although many physicians prefer to try medications first.[12] Women of childbearing age might also prefer antithyroid medications (exception: iodides) or surgery instead of RAI therapy. The choice of therapeutic measures is individualized based on age, size of goiter, severity of hyperthyroidism, duration of illness, reproductive status, and cause of hyperthyroidism.[12]

### Diagnostic tests

When hyperthyroidism is suspected, various diagnostic tests are necessary to confirm the diagnosis. (See Chapter 38 for a complete description of tests used.) The first tests done are measurement of serum $T_4$ and free $T_4$ or free $T_4$ index. In most cases of hyperthyroidism, these levels are elevated. If these tests are not conclusive, a serum $T_3$ level and free $T_3$ are done. In $T_3$ thyrotoxicosis, these levels are elevated with normal $T_4$ and free $T_4$ index.

TSH levels are ordered and are low in most patients with hyperthyroidism if "sensitive" TSH assays of blood are used. (TSH levels would be high if there were a pituitary hypersecretory state.) The "sensitive" TSH assay is able to differentiate low serum levels from normal levels of TSH: previous TSH assays were unable to do this.[6] Radioactive iodine uptake (RAIU) is elevated in all types of hyperthyroidism except thyroiditis, factitious thyrotoxicosis, and struma ovarii. RAIU findings are inaccurate if there has been iodine ingested or administered in the past few weeks. Other tests, such as thyroid-binding globulin (TBG), may be used to calculate the $T_4$ index in such cases.[6] Further clarification of the hormonal status can be done with provocative testing; however, the "sensitive" TSH test has reduced the use of the TRH stimulation test or thyroid suppression tests. Patients with hyperthyroidism usually show blunted TSH response to thyrotropin-releasing hormone (TRH) and no suppression of RAIU with exogenous thyroid therapy. (See Chapter 38 for a description of radiographic tests that might be used in the diagnosis of hyperthyroidism.)

### Medication

Three classes of medications are used in the treatment of hyperthyroidism: the antithyroids, or *thioamides,* which inhibit the synthesis of thyroid hormones; the *iodides,* which primarily inhibit the release of thyroid hormones; and beta *($\beta$)-adrenergic blockers* (propranolol) and *calcium antagonists,* which antagonize the effects of thyroid hormone on body cells. The severity of the hyperthyroidism is a major factor in whether drugs from one, two, or three of these classes may be used in any given patient. Table 39-4 provides details of these drugs and of others that may be used as alternate choices.

**Thioamides.** *Propylthiouracil* (PTU) and *methimazole* (Tapazole) are the most frequently used *antithyroid* drugs. The action of these drugs is slow, and it usually takes 2 to 4 weeks before improvement is noticeable. This is because these drugs block thyroid hormone synthesis and not the secretion of the hormone itself. The supply of hormone stored in the gland must be reduced before improvement is seen, and this takes from 2 to 4 weeks. The patient usually is started on a

**TABLE 39-4 Drugs Used in Treatment of Hyperthyroidism**

| CLASS | MAJOR ACTIONS | MAJOR SIDE EFFECTS OR PROBLEMS |
|---|---|---|
| **ANTITHYROIDS/THIOAMIDES** | | |
| Propylthiouracil (PTU)<br>Methimazole (Tapazole) | Inhibit biosynthesis of thyroid hormone<br>Stops production step of iodination<br>PTU inhibits conversion of $T_4$ to more active $T_3$ | Agranulocytosis, hypersensitivity reactions |
| **IODIDES** | | |
| Lugol's solution<br>Saturated solution of potassium iodide | Inhibit release of thyroid hormone<br>Preoperative use: see text | Iodine-induced thyrotoxicosis in some patients; limits use of RAIU and RAI for several weeks |
| **ALTERNATIVES TO IODIDES** | | |
| Lithium | Blocks hormone release | Toxicity |
| Corticosteroids (dexamethasone [Decadron]) | Dexamethasone also blocks conversion of $T_4$ to $T_3$ | Wide range of doses, multiple side effects |
| **THYROID BLOCKERS OR ANTAGONISTS** | | |
| Propranolol | β-adrenergic blocking agent | Negative inotropic effects, hypotension, worsening of cardiac or airway disease |
| Reserpine, guanethidine, clonidine | Catecholamine-depleting agents | Hypotension |
| Verapamil, diltiazem | Calcium antagonists | Negative inotropic effects, hypotension, worsening of cardiac or airway disease |

relatively large dose of the antithyroid drug (PTU, 300 to 450 mg/day in three divided doses; methimazole, 30 to 45 mg/day in three divided doses). Then the dosage is gradually reduced to a level sufficient to maintain the euthyroid state (PTU, 100 to 150 mg/day, or methimazole, 10 to 15 mg/day, both given in divided doses). When antithyroid drugs are used as the primary therapy, they usually are continued for 6 to 18 months or longer. Approximately one-half the persons with Graves' disease will develop a spontaneous remission of their hyperthyroidism. Although it is impossible to predict which persons will go into remission, persons whose goiters decrease in size and who remain euthyroid as drug dosage is decreased are the most likely candidates. No guarantee exists that patients will remain in remission. In one study the remission rate 1 year after discontinuance of medications was only 38%.[12] The patient should see the physician regularly after drugs are discontinued so that early signs of recurrence can be detected. Patients who redevelop hyperthyroidism require drug therapy, RAI therapy, or surgery.

Antithyroid drugs must be taken several times a day to maintain an adequate blood level and drug effect. This administration schedule is a disadvantage to using drugs as a primary therapy.

Patients are instructed to look for toxic signs of the drugs, such as fever, sore throat, and skin eruptions or any signs of infection and to call their physician immediately if these signs appear. The signs of infection need to be reported immediately because they may indicate *agranulocytosis* (lack of production of granulocytes). If this occurs, the drugs are stopped immediately. Almost all patients recover from agranulocytosis; however, the patient's hyperthyroidism must be treated with some alternative therapeutic measure, as discussed next.

**Iodides.** Iodides reduce the metabolic rate rapidly because they block the release and synthesis of thyroid hormone, reduce glandular vascularity, and increase colloid formation. These actions help to prevent hemorrhage and make the thyroid firmer, an advantage in manipulation of the gland during surgery.

*Lugol's solution* is more palatable given in milk or fruit juice. It should be taken through a straw because it may stain the teeth. A brassy taste in the mouth and sore teeth and gums are signs of toxicity, but these complications rarely occur.

There are limitations to iodide treatment.[41] First, iodides can be used only for a short time, about 10 days, because of an escape mechanism called the *Wolff-Chaikoff effect.*[41] Autoregulation of thyroid hormone secretion limits the time iodides can affect the gland in most persons. However, a defective or absent escape mechanism is present in some patients who develop *iodide-induced thyrotoxicosis* when given iodide-containing medication or when exposed to iodide loading in radiographic examinations. Second, once iodide is administered, RAI must be delayed until the iodide-uptake capacity of the thyroid gland has been restored.

The treatment of *iodine-induced hyperthyroidism* is the withdrawal of all sources of iodide and the administration of potassium perchlorate and often, methimazole.[41] If the source of iodide cannot be withdrawn, thyroidectomy may be the choice of therapy. (One example: amiodarone, an antidysrhythmic drug, has high iodine content; sometimes its use must be continued because no alternative drug is appropriate for the patient.)

**Alternatives to iodides.** *Lithium* has been found to block hormone release. However, it is used less often than other drugs and is saved for times when patients develop toxicity to other drugs or as an adjunct to other therapy during thyrotoxic crisis. Because lithium has the ability to block the release of thyroid hormone, hypothyroidism can occur as a side effect of lithium therapy.

*Dexamethasone,* the most potent glucocorticoid, is effective in blocking hormone release in patients with Graves' disease. It also inhibits the conversion of $T_4$ to $T_3$ in the periphery. These two actions make it most useful in acute crises.

**Thyroid blockers or antagonists.** The *β-adrenergic blockers,* such as propranolol (Inderal), are used to treat symptoms from increased sympathetic nervous system stimulation, such as tachycardia, dysrhythmias, and angina. These blockers reduce the signs and symptoms rapidly because they block beta receptors. Thus the catecholamines, even if present, cannot stimulate the receptors. These agents block beta receptors on all organs in the body, producing widespread effects. The blocking of the actions of catecholamines helps to prevent critical complications of thyroid hormone excess.

β-Adrenergic blockers also improve tremors, restlessness, anxiety, and sometimes myopathy. Propranolol, 20 to 40 mg every 4 to 6 hours, may be given for symptom control except in persons with congestive heart failure or bronchial asthma. Worsening of these conditions can occur from the negative inotropic side effects of β-adrenergic blockers. Alternative drugs used to treat adrenergic symptoms include calcium antagonists or drugs that deplete catecholamines. These drugs have fewer negative inotropic side effects than do the β-blockers.[28]

### Treatment

**Radioactive iodine therapy.** RAI therapy with $^{131}$I is increasingly being used because it (1) can be given on an outpatient basis; (2) is safer for a wider range of patients, including elderly persons, who are poorer surgical risks; (3) can result in faster improvement in thyroid function than antithyroid drug therapy; and (4) although still controversial, can be used in women of childbearing age. RAI is given orally in one dose. The dosage is individualized, but on the average, it is 80 to 90 μCi/g of thyroid tissue or equivalent to 6000 to 7000 rad. Although symptoms of hyperthyroidism will decrease in approximately 3 weeks, *a euthyroid state will not be achieved for 6 months.* The treatment must be repeated in about 20% of patients.

The RAI is eliminated in a very short time after treatment, approximately 2 days. Because of this short excretion time, no tests are used to monitor RAI elimination from the body. RAI is excreted in urine, saliva, sweat, and feces. The major precaution to protect others is care with body secretions, particularly urine.

**Guidelines for Instructing the Person Receiving Radiation Therapy of the Thyroid Gland**

- Flush the toilet two or three times after each use.
- Increase intake of fluids to aid in the RAI's excretion.
- Use separate eating utensils and separate towels and washcloths; wash these and underclothes and bed linens separately.
- Rinse bathroom sinks and tubs thoroughly after use, and wash hands carefully after using the bathroom.
- Sleep alone for a few days, and avoid kissing and intercourse (although the amount of radiation in the patient's body is minimal).
- Avoid prolonged physical contact with anyone, including holding a baby.
- Do not breast-feed.
- Delay pregnancy for 6 months after therapy.

Breast-feeding is not allowed. The length of time these restrictions are required varies, but it is usually only for a few days, sometimes only 2 days.

Radiation precautions are dose dependent; instructions are individualized for each patient (see the Guidelines box above). RAI is not used in pregnant women because of the potential teratogenic effects on the fetus; the placenta transports iodine easily. If RAI is used in women of childbearing years, pregnancy should be delayed for 6 months after therapy.

The major side effect of RAI therapy is hypothyroidism. Although different authorities[12,42] report different figures for the percentage of persons developing hypothyroidism each year after $^{131}$I therapy, eventually almost 100% of all persons become hypothyroid. Persons must be told about this complication before treatment; they are monitored for hypothyroidism, should know the signs and symptoms (see p. 1235), and must report their onset to the physician.

### Diet

Increased food intake and loss of weight are characteristic of untreated hyperthyroidism. Increased nutrient and calorie intake are necessary to meet the increased food requirements. Weight gain in the treated patient can signal the return of the euthyroid state in elderly patients.[31] While hyperthyroidism is present, caloric intake needs to be increased, with attention to appropriate distribution of calories from macronutrients. Supplemental vitamins and trace minerals may be prescribed.

### Activity

Activity may be self-limited because of the fatigue the patient experiences. Often, no activity restrictions are related to work unless the patient has symptoms of tachycardia, atrial fibrillation, or other cardiovascular problems. (See Chapter 31 for activity interventions for these problems.) Thyroid storm mandates complete bedrest and admission to an intensive care unit.

The patient is advised to rest. Symptoms of fatigue and insomnia may help patients accept and plan for rest periods during the day; however, hyperkinetic activity may make trying to rest at any one time very frustrating. Work requiring concentration for long periods may be difficult to perform. Financial and work-related barriers to compliance with rest prescriptions should be explored carefully.

**Referral/Consultation**

In some settings the nurse assumes responsibility for making referrals to other services. Concerns about personal, family, or financial resources may be identified. Decreased emotional stability and energy level may decrease ability to cope or solve problems. Barriers to compliance with treatment recommendations are explored carefully to maximize compliance and thereby prevent recurrence of symptoms or onset of thyroid storm. Appropriate patient-specific referrals are made.

### Surgical Management

Surgery is the treatment of choice for patients with Graves' disease who have large goiters and whose thyroid glands have low RAUI. Surgery is frequently still used as primary therapy for children. Surgery and/or treatment with antithyroid drugs is used in treating the pregnant woman with hyperthyroidism. RAI therapy is not used during pregnancy because iodine is a teratogenic agent[40] and the placenta transports iodine easily.

Surgical techniques include the removal of one lobe, 75% to 80% of the gland *(subtotal thyroidectomy),* or removal of 100% of the gland *(total thyroidectomy).* Subtotal thyroidectomy has the advantage over RAI therapy in that the incidence of hypothyroidism is much less. However, hyperthyroidism may occur from hypertrophy of the remaining tissue over time. The risks associated with thyroid surgery are very minimal in patients treated by experienced surgeons. Nursing management of the patient undergoing thyroid surgery is discussed on p. 1243.

## NURSING MANAGEMENT

## ♦ ASSESSMENT

As described, hyperthyroidism can affect almost every system of the body and cause major physiologic and psychosocial problems.

### Subjective Data

Data to be collected to assess the patient with hyperthyroidism include the following:

- History of emotional and mental status changes
- Complaints of palpitations or chest pain
- Complaints of dyspnea, with or without exercise
- History of changes in hair, skin, nails, or amount of sweating
- Complaints of visual disturbances and irritations; reports of eyes tiring easily
- Appetite, history of nutritional intake and weight changes
- History of increased stool frequency and stool bulk
- History of intolerance to heat
- Complaints of weakness, fatigue, decreased ability to complete ADL
- History of changes in menses or change in libido
- Knowledge: disease, treatment, care needs

### Objective Data

Data to be collected to assess the patient with hyperthyroidism include the following:

- Mental status changes: shortened attention span, emotional lability, hyperkinesia, tremor
- Cardiovascular status changes: increased systolic blood pressure, decreased diastolic pressure, tachycardia at rest, dysrhythmias, murmurs
- Skin and hair changes: warm, flushed, moist skin; dermopathy; fine, thinning hair
- Eye changes: lid lag, globe lag, diplopia, injection of conjunctiva, decreased acuity
- Nutritional/metabolic changes: decreased weight, increased appetite and intake, decreased serum triglycerides and cholesterol
- Musculoskeletal changes: muscle weakness, decreased muscle tone, difficulty rising from sitting position

### Diagnostic Test Findings

1. Elevations of serum $T_3$, $T_4$, and $T_4$ index
2. Decreased serum levels of TSH measured by "sensitive" assay

Other tests may be used to interpret accurately the results of the above tests, as discussed in Chapter 38. Among the factors that can make $T_3$, $T_4$, and serum TSH levels poorly reflect true hormonal status is total binding proteins (TBG). Other factors are elevation of $T_3$ or $T_4$ and the suppression of TSH by acute or severe illness and the effects of drugs such as iodides.[15]

## ♦ NURSING DIAGNOSES

Nursing diagnoses are determined from analysis of patient data. Nursing diagnoses for the person with hyperthyroidism may include but are not limited to the following:

| Diagnostic Title | Possible Etiologic Factors |
|---|---|
| Activity intolerance, high risk for | Muscle weakness and wasting associated with altered metabolism |
| Cardiac output, decreased | Dysrhythmias associated with increased sympathetic activity |
| Coping, ineffective (individual) | Altered processing of sensory input, decreased attention span, emotional lability |

| Diagnostic Title | Possible Etiologic Factors |
|---|---|
| Home maintenance management, impaired | Delay between initiation of therapy and return of euthyroid state |
| Hyperthermia | Increased heat production greater than dissipation |
| Knowledge deficit: disease, treatment, outcomes, self-monitoring needs | Never presented with new information |
| Nutrition, altered: less than body requirements | Increased metabolic needs |
| Sensory/perceptual alterations: visual | Disruption of function of optic nerves or extraocular muscles of eyes associated with infiltrative changes |
| Sleep pattern disturbance | Increased metabolic rate, restlessness |

## ♦ EXPECTED PATIENT OUTCOMES

Expected patient outcomes for the person with hyperthyroidism may include but are not limited to the following:

1. Demonstrates no further decrease in activity tolerance, and shows a gradual increase in activity over 2 to 3 months.
2. Shows evidence of adequate tissue perfusion and cardiac output: no change in mental status, breath sounds clear, no edema formation, heart rate within 20 beats of baseline, and gradual decrease in resting heart rate.
3. Shows effective coping:
    a. Rates self as less anxious or less stressed on a scale of 1 to 10, with 1 meaning no stress and 10 the worst stress.
    b. Lists three ways to cope with feelings.
4. Identifies home maintenance difficulties, and states how these can be taken care of until health is stable.
5. Has normal body temperature.
6. Describes how hyperthyroidism causes the signs and symptoms present, lists treatment options available, lists expected outcomes of treatment with realistic time frames, lists signs and symptoms requiring self-monitoring (signs/symptoms of hypothyroidism, hyperthyroidism, agranulocytosis), and lists precautions to be observed if RAI therapy is used.
7. Does not lose more weight; weight will return to within 0.5 kg of preillness weight.
8. Does not complain of eye pain, diplopia, or a decrease in visual acuity.

## ♦ INTERVENTIONS

A nursing care plan for a specific patient is presented at the end of the chapter and illustrates some of the care needs of persons with hyperthyroidism. Many patients with hyperthyroidism are managed outside the hospital setting.

### Managing Critical Care

**Thyroid crisis** or **storm** is a medical emergency in which patients develop severe manifestations of the signs and symptoms of hyperthyroidism, including an elevated temperature; increased tachycardia or onset of dysrhythmias; worsening tremors and restlessness; worsening mental status, including a delirious or psychotic state or coma; and sometimes complaints of abdominal pain. Blood pressure and respiratory rate increase above baseline. This state is usually seen in persons with Graves' disease, and symptoms result from a severe increase in metabolism and are usually precipitated by a major stressor such as infection, trauma, or surgery. The use of medications to suppress thyroid activity before surgery decreases the risk of thyroid storm, since less hormone is released into the blood with manipulation of the gland. Thyroid crisis also may occur in a person who has been inadequately treated or who stops taking prescribed therapy.

Patients with thyroid storm must be hospitalized. The immediate focus of care is to lower the metabolic rate as fast as possible, remove the precipitating cause, and support physiologic functioning. The typical therapeutic regimen is outlined in the Guidelines box below. Note that the doses of medicines in the box are higher than those used in less critically ill patients. Doses of drugs are adjusted according to patient response. Patients may require continual monitoring during rapid treatment.

### Guidelines for Care of the Person With Thyroid Crisis or Storm

Monitor the patient's temperature, intake and output, neurologic status, and cardiovascular status every hour.

Initiate an IV line for medications and fluids.

Administer increasing doses of oral propylthiouracil as ordered (200 to 300 mg every 6 hours may be given) after a loading dose of 800 to 1200 mg orally.[28,36]

Administer iodide preparations as ordered. Sodium iodide given IV twice daily or an oral preparation may be ordered.

Administer dexamethasone, 2 mg IV every 6 hours. Glucocorticoids help to inhibit the release of thyroid hormone.

Administer propranolol, 20 to 80 mg PO or 2 to 10 mg IV, as ordered. Propranolol (β-adrenergic blocker) can worsen asthma or congestive heart failure because it constricts bronchial smooth muscles and causes a decrease in cardiac output.

Initiate measures to lower body temperature, including external cooling devices, cold baths, and acetaminophen. Salicylates are contraindicated because they inhibit thyroid hormone binding to protein carriers and thus increase free thyroid hormone levels.

Initiate other support therapy as ordered, including oxygen, cardiac glycosides, and treatment measures for the precipitating event.

Maintain a quiet, calm, cool, private environment until crisis is over.

Maintain continuity of care.

Decrease stressors by use of patient education, comfort measures, or family support.

Priority interventions are directed toward the management of the fever and the cardiovascular responses seen in thyroid storm.[36] Atrial fibrillation is often the first cardiac alteration noted; other dysrhythmias are possible. Angina and congestive heart failure may occur in hyperthyroid patients in intensive care units; often these patients have underlying heart disease. Interventions include the following:

1. Maintain cardiac output.
   a. Monitor cardiovascular status every hour.
   b. Report any changes to the physician, such as increased tachycardia, dysrhythmias, or signs of congestive heart failure (see Chapter 31).
   c. Decrease cardiac workload by decreasing physical and emotional stressors.
2. Maintain normal body temperature.
   a. Monitor temperature every hour: report any elevations.
   b. Use external cooling devices as ordered.
   c. Maintain room temperature in cool range.

As the acute crisis subsides, there should be continued attention to maintaining cardiac output and normal temperature.

## Providing Recuperative Care

As recovery ensues, the nurse must continue to provide interventions that address the outcomes related to hyperthyroidism. These include but are not limited to the following:

1. Promote adequate rest.
   a. Provide quiet, comfortable environment.
   b. Provide back rubs.
   c. Use home remedies such as hot milk to assist in promoting sleep.
   d. Encourage quiet periods even if the patient does not sleep.
2. Maintain and increase activity tolerance.
   a. Encourage short walks if cardiac output is stable.
   b. Space activity between rest periods.
3. Maintain adequate nutrition intake.
   a. Monitor intake and output every 8 hours.
   b. Weigh daily.
   c. Monitor nutritional intake.
   d. Provide frequent high-protein, high-calorie meals.
4. Promote good eye care.
   a. Monitor cornea for damage, visual acuity, and patient complaints every shift.
   b. Initiate appropriate measures such as dark glasses, elevating head of bed, use of artificial tears, and taping eyelids closed at various intervals.
   c. Report any new complaints immediately.
5. Facilitate improved coping; offer patients interventions to help them relax, such as music; back rubs, and distraction. (See Research box on right for a description of research supporting the effectiveness of different relaxation measures.)
6. Enhance patient knowledge.
   a. Describe the disease and how it causes signs and symptoms.
   b. Clarify treatment options.
   c. List the expected outcomes, such as relief of symptoms in 4 weeks if receiving drug therapy, need for drug therapy for extended periods, and the potential complications of therapy.
   d. List signs and symptoms the patient must self-monitor.
   e. List precautions if the patient received RAI, such as how long he or she should sleep alone, refrain from intimate contact, limit physical contact with children, and handle own clothes and eating utensils separately.
   f. List planned follow-up care.

## Preparing for Discharge

The nurse can assist the patient in learning how to incorporate the therapeutic regimen into ADL. In addition,

### RESEARCH

Hyman RB et al: The effects of relaxation training on clinical symptoms: a meta-analysis, *Nurs Res* 38:216-220, 1989.

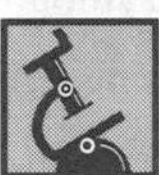

Many clinical problems are associated with anxiety and tension. These states elicit a stress response. Several relaxation techniques have been proposed as useful treatments for these problems. This study was a meta-analysis to determine (1) the overall effectiveness of relaxation techniques in relieving clinical symptoms and (2) the effectiveness of some techniques over others in relation to specific symptoms.

Relaxation training was defined as nonpharmacologic, nonmechanical-assisted techniques to facilitate a relaxed state and included Benson's relaxation technique, Jacobson's progressive muscle relaxation, rhythmic breathing, imagery, Lamaze, meditation, autogenic training, hypnosis, transcendental meditation (TM), yoga, and zen. Biofeedback-assisted relaxation was not included. Studies were used from 1970 that investigated relaxation training on adult subjects not hospitalized for psychiatric reasons. The literature search resulted in 100 studies, 48 of which fit the criteria.

The most common problems for which relaxation was prescribed included insomnia, acute pain, anxiety, and hypertension. Relaxation treatments often included more than one treatment. The analysis revealed that relaxation techniques do affect some clinical symptoms. The treatment worked better for nonsurgical subjects than for surgical subjects. All treatments, except Benson's relaxation, showed evidence of effectiveness. The problems most consistently improved were hypertension, headache, and insomnia. Effectiveness of techniques for pain and anxiety were low to moderate. The results for acute pain were very low. Research is still needed to study whether the effectiveness of relaxation techniques varies depending on symptoms as well as the acuteness or chronicity of the problem.

# NURSING CARE PLAN

## PERSON WITH HYPERTHYROIDISM

**DATA:** Mrs. T., a 28-year-old housewife, is admitted for diagnostic evaluation before a thyroidectomy, which is scheduled to be performed in 2 weeks. Graves' disease was diagnosed 2 days ago; hospitalization was delayed until child-care arrangements were made for her 6-year-old stepson. (The marriage occurred 3 months ago.) Initial therapy, started 2 days ago, is Tapazole and Lugol's solution. The ECG report is sinus tachycardia (rate 132).

The nursing history identified the following about the patient:

- She feels overwhelmed, cries frequently, and fears losing control of temper.
- She has lost 15 pounds in 2 months and is always hungry, although she is eating large amounts of food.
- She is bothered by heat, others' noisiness, and her own clumsiness.
- She expects medicine to make her feel better and dreads surgery.

The physical examination revealed the following:

- Blood pressure: 140/60; pulse: 132, respiration: 24
- Staring gaze of eyes with proptosis (equal bilaterally); lid lag and globe lag present; right eye slightly reddened
- Skin warm and perspiration present
- Increased muscle tone with weakness of lower extremities; quick muscle response to sudden noise; fine tremor of both hands
- Diffuse visible enlargement of thyroid
- *Bruit* present over thyroid

Collaborative nursing actions include those to prevent further environmental stressors that could make the patient more uncomfortable and increase her signs and symptoms.

Nursing actions include monitoring the following: temperature, pulse, respiration, blood pressure, weight, excessive hunger, and tremulousness.

### ■ NURSING DIAGNOSIS

Decreased cardiac output related to increased sympathetic stimulation

| Expected Patient Outcomes | Nursing Interventions | Rationale |
|---|---|---|
| Pulse rate is less than 20 above baseline during first 72 hours.<br>Pulse rate decreases gradually after 72 hours.<br>Undetected cardiac dysrhythmias do not occur. | Assess vital signs, especially heart rate and rhythm, at least 4 hr; if worsens, assess q hr.<br>Instruct patient to report palpitations, chest pain, and dizziness.<br>Assess daily weight, daily intake and output; assess for signs of edema, jugular vein distention, and pulmonary congestion q 8 hr.<br>Decrease known stressors; explain all interventions, and listen to patient.<br>Balance periods of activity with rest.<br>Administer prescribed drugs and monitor therapeutic response.<br>Report any changes to physician. | Early detection of atrial fibrillation or thyroid storm allows prompt treatment and prevents cardiovascular crisis. |

### ■ NURSING DIAGNOSIS

Ineffective individual coping related to personal vulnerability to environmental stimuli

| Expected Patient Outcomes | Nursing Interventions | Rationale |
|---|---|---|
| Explains reason for change in behavior.<br>Decreases emotional lability.<br>Identifies at least one coping mechanism that will help during periods of nervousness. | Discuss reasons for emotional lability.<br>Maintain calm, relaxed environment.<br>Encourage visitors who are calm and will not upset Mrs. T.<br>Provide privacy (e.g., a single room).<br>Suggest that others avoid sharing distressing news with Mrs. T.<br>Explain all interventions.<br>Avoid stimulants such as coffee, caffeine, and alcohol.<br>Help Mrs. T. identify previous coping mechanisms or explore new ones.<br>Offer measures to help Mrs. T. relax.<br>Include family in discussions. | A supportive environment can reduce environmental stimuli and stressors and assist patient in coping. |

# NURSING CARE PLAN

## PERSON WITH HYPERTHYROIDISM—cont'd

### ■ NURSING DIAGNOSIS

Altered nutrition: less than body requirements related to increased metabolic needs

| Expected Patient Outcomes | Nursing Interventions | Rationale |
|---|---|---|
| Maintains normal weight.<br>Gains at least 0.5 kg/wk if weight below normal. | Monitor weight qod to weekly.<br>Monitor serum albumin, hemoglobin, and lymphocyte levels.<br>Help her plan for high-calorie, high-protein, high-carbohydrate diet with selection from all food groups.<br>Suggest six small meals per day or between-meal snacks. | Increased nutrient intake meets increased metabolic demand. |

### ■ NURSING DIAGNOSIS

Sensory/perceptual alterations (potential visual) related to infiltrative changes associated with Graves' disease

| Expected Patient Outcomes | Nursing Interventions | Rationale |
|---|---|---|
| Vision does not worsen.<br>Explains measures to protect eyes. | Assess visual acuity, ability to close eyes, and photophobia.<br>Protect eyes from irritants:<br>1. Use patches or glasses when in high wind.<br>2. Use artificial tears, if prescribed.<br>3. Elevate head of bed at night.<br>Instruct patient not to lie prone.<br>If eyes do not close completely, check about using shields at night. | These measures can prevent corneal injury and minimize risk of loss of vision. |

### ■ NURSING DIAGNOSIS

Hyperthermia related to increased heat production greater than dissipation

| Expected Patient Outcomes | Nursing Interventions | Rationale |
|---|---|---|
| States that she feels more comfortable.<br>Has normal body temperature. | Control environmental temperature for comfort (fans may be helpful).<br>Suggest that she take frequent showers.<br>Encourage adequate fluid intake and monitor fluid losses.<br>Monitor temperature q 4 hr. | These measures keep her comfortable by increasing heat loss. |

### ■ NURSING DIAGNOSIS

Activity intolerance related to generalized muscle weakness

| Expected Patient Outcomes | Nursing Interventions | Rationale |
|---|---|---|
| States fatigue is decreased.<br>Maintains current activity level. | Assess activity schedule.<br>Suggest ways to modify fatiguing activities.<br>Identify activities that can be done by others until condition is controlled.<br>Schedule rest periods between activities.<br>Encourage activities that promote sleep at night.<br>At present, keep activities at current level. | Reduction of energy expenditure is necessary to reduce fatigue in persons with increased metabolism until treatment decreases metabolism. |

*Continued.*

## NURSING CARE PLAN

### PERSON WITH HYPERTHYROIDISM—cont'd

#### ■ NURSING DIAGNOSIS

Impaired home maintenance management related to delay in initiation of therapy and stabilization of patient

| Expected Patient Outcome | Nursing Interventions | Rationale |
|---|---|---|
| States plan for home maintenance management. | Assist her to identify home maintenance difficulties.<br>Assist her to identify persons who can provide temporary help.<br>Make referrals as needed, such as to social services.<br>Identify persons who can help monitor her compliance with medical regimen.<br>Help Mrs. T. plan own schedule to allow for rest. | These measures increase resources available to Mrs. T. and reduce stress from inability to meet expectations of role. |

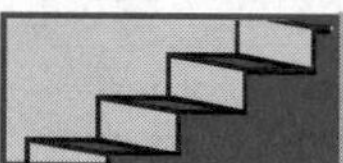

## CRITICAL PATHWAY Hyperthyroidism with Atrial Fibrillation

**DRG #: 300; Expected LOS: 7**

| | Day of Admission Day 1 | Day 2 | Day 3 |
|---|---|---|---|
| **Diagnostic Tests** | CBC; UA; SMA/18*; serum TSH and free $T_4$ index or free $T_4$ concentration; total $T_4$ or $T_3$ concentrations as necessary; ECG; C & S blood/UA/ sputum if necessary; $O_2$ saturation on room air, ABGs if necessary | CBC; $O_2$ saturation on room air, ABGs if necessary | SMA/18,* ECG |
| **Medications** | IV @ TKO; propylthiouracil; antiatrial fibrillation medication (possibly including digitalis, coumadin, propranolol, or calcium channel blockers); medication for congestive heart failure (CHF) as necessary; eye drops OU q2hr PRN for dryness; multivitamins; medication for rest/sleep if necessary; stool softener | IV @ TKO; propylthiouracil; antiatrial fibrillation medication; medication for CHF as necessary; eye drops OU q2hr PRN for dryness; multivitamins; medication for rest/sleep if necessary; stool softener | IV @ TKO; propylthiouracil; antiatrial fibrillation medication; medication for CHF as necessary; eye drops OU q2hr PRN for dryness; multivitamins; medication for rest/sleep if necessary; stool softener |
| **Treatments** | I & O q4hr; VS q hr 4 times then q2hr; $O_2$ PRN; cardiac monitor; weight; record food intake; assess moisture to eyes q2hr; assess neuro-cardio-pul-circ systems q2hr 4 times then q4hr | I & O q8hr; VS q4hr; $O_2$ PRN; cardiac monitor; weight; record food intake; assess moisture to eyes q2hr; assess neuro-cardio-pul-circ systems q4hr | I & O q8hr; VS q4hr; $O_2$ PRN; cardiac monitor; weight; record food intake; assess moisture to eyes q2hr; assess neuro-cardio-pul-circ systems q4hr |
| **Diet** | Soft diet with high calories, protein, and CHO; serve 6 meals; NO STIMULANTS | Soft diet with high calories, protein, and CHO; serves 6 meals; NO STIMULANTS | Soft diet with high calories, protein, and CHO; serve 6 meals; NO STIMULANTS |
| **Activity** | Bedrest with BRP; minimize environmental stressors (keep room cool, calm, quiet; provide rest periods) | Bedrest with BRP; minimize environmental stressors | Up in room 4 times; minimize environmental stressors |
| **Referral/ Consultation** | Social services | Dietary, home health if necessary | |

*Serum calcium, phosphorus, triglycerides, uric acid, creatinine, blood urea nitrogen (BUN), total bilirubin, alkaline phosphate, aspartate aminotransferase (AST) (formerly serum glutamic oxaloacetic transaminase [SGOT]), alanine aminotransferase (ALT) (formerly serum glutamic oxaloacetic transaminase [SGPT]), lactic dehydrogenase (LDH), total protein, albumin, sodium, potassium, chloride, total $CO_2$, glucose.

## NURSING CARE PLAN

### PERSON WITH HYPERTHYROIDISM—cont'd

**■ NURSING DIAGNOSIS**

Knowledge deficit (disease, treatment, expected outcomes) related to new information and no previous exposure to information

| Expected Patient Outcome | Nursing Interventions | Rationale |
|---|---|---|
| Explains medical regimen and care needs. | Explain how and when to take prescribed medications.<br>Describe symptoms of infection to be reported to physician, such as sore throat or fever.<br>Describe ways to plan prescribed dietary intake.<br>Provide required teaching about care needs (comfort, sleep, rest).<br>Explain the reason for the delay before surgery. | These measures increase likelihood of compliance with therapy used to achieve euthyroid state and optimal physical status before surgery. |

| Day 4 | Day 5 | Day 6 | Day of Discharge Day 7 |
|---|---|---|---|
| | CBC, SMA/18* | | |
| IV saline lock; adjust propylthiouracil, antiatrial fibrillation medication, and other medications for home use; eye drops OU q2hr PRN for dryness; multivitamins; medication for rest/sleep PRN; stool softener | IV saline lock; adjust propylthiouracil, antiatrial fibrillation medication, and other medications for home use; eye drops OU q4hr PRN for dryness; multivitamins; medication for rest/sleep PRN; stool softener | IV saline lock; adjust propylthiouracil, antiatrial fibrillation medication, and other medications for home use; eye drops OU q4hr PRN for dryness; multivitamins; medication for rest/sleep PRN; stool softener | Discontinue saline lock; continue propylthiouracil, antiatrial fibrillation medication, and other medications for home use; eye drops OU q4hr PRN for dryness; multivitamins; medication for rest/sleep PRN; stool softener; provide info for $^{131}I$ radioactive isotope as outpatient in 6 wk |
| I & O q8hr; VS q6hr; discontinue $O_2$; cardiac monitor; weight; record food intake; assess moisture to eyes q4hr; assess neuro-cardio-pul-circ systems q6hr | Discontinue I & O; VS q8hr; weight; discontinue cardiac monitor; assess moisture to eyes q8hr; assess neuro-cardio-pul-circ systems q8hr | VS q8hr; weight; assess moisture to eyes q8hr; assess neuro-cardio-pul-circ systems q8hr | VS q8hr; weight; assess moisture to eyes q8hr; assess neuro-cardio-pul-circ systems q8hr |
| Regular diet with high calories, protein, and CHO; serve 6 meals; NO STIMULANTS | Regular diet with high calories, protein, and CHO; serve 6 meals; NO STIMULANTS | Regular diet with high calories, protein, and CHO; serve 6 meals; NO STIMULANTS | Regular diet with high calories, protein, and CHO; serve 6 meals; NO STIMULANTS |
| Up in room ad lib; minimize environmental stressors | Up in room ad lib | Up ad lib | Up ad lib |

the patient needs to plan how to achieve rest, adequate nutrition, and energy conservation at home and at work.

During this time, the patient may be exploring with the physician the options of definitive treatment that are appropriate and recommended. The nurse can support information seeking about risks, benefits, consequences of the treatment, and the requirements for follow-up care. The patient's beliefs and desires need to be valued, and the patient should be supported in expressing any concerns to the physician. A common concern is the effect of environmental radiation if RAI therapy is an option.

The teaching plan should include interventions to help the patient:

1. Describe the disease and how it causes signs and symptoms.
2. Clarify treatment options.
3. List the expected outcomes, such as relief of symptoms in 4 weeks if receiving drug therapy, need for drug therapy for extended periods, and the potential complications of therapy.
4. Explain each medication, purpose, dose and schedule, and side effects to report.
5. List precautions if the patient received RAI (see Guidelines box, p. 1224).
6. List signs and symptoms patient must self-monitor.

## ♦ EVALUATION

To evaluate the effectiveness of nursing interventions, compare patient behaviors with those stated in the expected patient outcomes. Successful achievement of patient outcomes for the person with hyperthyroidism is indicated by the following:

1. Reports increased energy level, activity endurance, and activity completion.
2. Has pulse rate less than 80 at rest.
3. Rates anxiety as reduced and tolerable.
4. States plans for home maintenance that address rest and required resources.
5. Has temperature of 37.2° C (99° F) or below.
6. Describes dosage schedule, rationale, and importance of drug therapy.
7. Maintains weight or increases weekly by at least 0.5 kg.
8. Reports no visual problems or loss of visual acuity.

## ✸ SPECIAL CONSIDERATIONS FOR CARE OF THE GERONTOLOGIC PATIENT

1. Elderly patients have less clear-cut clinical findings of hyperthyroidism. There may be weight loss, fatigue, and irritability, but goiter, tachycardia, eye changes, or tremor may be absent. In fact, subclinical hyperthyroidism, or "apathetic" or "masked" hyperthyroidism, is typical in elderly persons.
2. Hyperthyroidism may be the cause of new onset of atrial fibrillation.
3. Nonthyroid disease may or may not raise the serum $T_3$ and/or $T_4$ in elderly persons and may suppress serum TSH. Elderly persons typically have more than one chronic illness.
4. RAI therapy is the treatment of choice in elderly patients.
5. Common drug interactions with hyperthyroidism include increased metabolism of drugs typically taken by elderly persons: digoxin, theophylline, and warfarin.

## ❦ HOME CARE CONSIDERATIONS

The nurse focuses on assessment of the patient's and family's ability to manage the therapeutic regimen and to adapt resources to meet patient needs. The patient and family need to understand the therapy and expected results and to plan how to incorporate therapeutic requirements into daily life. The nurse can help the patient and family:

1. Increase resources for home maintenance while fatigue is present.
2. Increase food supplies and monitor weight weekly.
3. Plan for increased rest periods during the day.
4. Plan strategies for insomnia, hyperkinesis, increased stool frequency, and heat intolerance.
5. Understand importance of adherence to therapy and follow-up monitoring.

## COMPLICATIONS

Various ocular changes occur in Graves' disease. Patients usually have some degree of ophthalmopathy (see earlier discussion). In addition, more serious ocular conditions resulting from infiltrative changes may be present.

None of the therapy previously described directly attacks the basic pathophysiologic process, that is, the infiltrative changes. The therapy does not inhibit the production of glycosaminoglycan in the retrobulbar tissue. Better understanding of this pathophysiologic process will lead to new treatment measures. (For a detailed discussion of the surgical eye procedures, the reader should refer to Chapter 60.)

## HYPOSECRETION OF THYROID HORMONE: HYPOTHYROIDISM

### Etiology

Hypothyroidism is a metabolic state resulting from a deficiency of thyroid hormone that may occur at any age. Congenital hypothyroidism results in a condition called cretinism. Hypothyroidism may result from the following:

1. Loss or atrophy of thyroid tissue: autoimmune thyroiditis, ablative therapy for hyperthyroidism, thyrotoxic drugs, congenital agenesis, maldevelopment, radiation for head and neck malignancies
2. Loss of trophic stimulation: pituitary dysfunction

**BOX 39-12 Goitrogenic Factors**

Iodine deficiency
Foods with goitrogenic factors: cabbage, turnips, soybeans
Drugs: lithium, thiocarbamides, sulfonylureas
Intrinsic abnormality in thyroid hormone syntheses

(pituitary or secondary hypothyroidism), hypothalamic dysfunction

3. Miscellaneous alterations: deficit in hormone biosynthesis, peripheral resistance to thyroid hormone, idiopathic factors, environmental factors (iodine deficiency)

In the United States, the most frequent causes of hypothyroidism are autoimmune thyroiditis and ablative therapy, whereas in the world, iodine deficiency is the leading cause. Goiter formation occurs as the pituitary gland secretes more TSH in response to lower levels of thyroid hormone in the blood. Over time, the resultant enlargement of the gland (goiter) is unable to maintain sufficient hormonal output, and hypothyroidism develops.

### Goiter

Any enlargement of the thyroid gland is called a goiter. If this enlargement is not associated with hyperthyroidism or hypothyroidism, cancer, or inflammation, it is referred to as *simple goiter. Endemic goiters* refer to those that occur in a particular geographic region and from a common cause, such as iodine deficiency. *Sporadic goiter* describes those that occur sporadically in regions that are not the locus of endemic goiters. (See Box 39-12 for goitrogenic factors.) In most cases of simple goiter in the United States, no extrinsic factors can be identified. Simple goiter is seen most frequently in females (3:1 ratio with males)[42] and occurs most often during pregnancy or adolescence. Goiter also occurs more frequently in particular families.[40]

#### Autoimmune disorders

Hashimoto's disease is the leading cause of hypothyroidism in the United States. Autoimmune changes in the thyroid gland occur often in persons over age 60. In this chronic disease, immunologic changes lead to goiter and may lead to hypothyroidism. Early in the disease, there may be hormonal imbalance or episodic hyperthyroidism because of inappropriate release of hormones from the thyroid gland. When atrophy occurs later, the condition is called *atrophic thyroiditis* and is more frequently found in elderly persons.[31] Other forms of thyroiditis, acute and chronic, are described in Table 39-5.

#### Ablation therapy

Total thyroidectomy, hypophysectomy, and radiation therapy of the pituitary or thyroid gland cause *iatrogenic hypothyroidism.* Patients undergoing these treatments must take thyroid hormone replacement for life.

## Epidemiology

Hypothyroidism is estimated to affect 1% of the population and to be particularly underdiagnosed in elderly

**TABLE 39-5 Thyroiditis: Types and Characteristics**

| TYPE | CHARACTERISTICS |
|---|---|
| **ACUTE THYROIDITIS** | |
| Acute pyogenic thyroiditis | Rare form of thyroiditis; results from infection of thyroid by pyogenic organism; symptoms include pain and tenderness in thyroid, dysphagia, fever, malaise; treated symptomatically. |
| **SUBACUTE NONSUPPURATIVE THYROIDITIS** | |
| De Quervain's thyroiditis<br>Granulomatous thyroiditis | Rare form of thyroiditis; results from viral infection of thyroid gland; may follow an upper respiratory infection; most often seen in 4th and 5th decades of life; symptoms include pain in thyroid, fever, hoarseness, dysphagia, feelings of palpitation, nervousness, lassitude, thyroid moderately enlarged; subsides in a few months; treatment usually symptomatic; aspirin for mild cases; glucocorticoids when disease unresponsive to other measures. |
| **SUBACUTE LYMPHOCYTIC THYROIDITIS** | |
| Painless thyroiditis<br>Lymphocytic thyroiditis | Form of thyroiditis increasing in frequency; etiologic factor unknown but possible autoimmune factor; symptoms include self-limiting form of hyperthyroidism and nontender enlarged thyroid gland, which may be followed by hypothyroidism; treatment symptomatic during hyperthyroidism phase and may include β-adrenergic blockers but not propylthiouracil (not effective); monitor annually for hypothyroidism. |
| **CHRONIC THYROIDITIS** | |
| Hashimoto's thyroiditis | See text. |
| Riedel's thyroiditis | Rare form of thyroiditis; cause unknown; extensive fibrosis of gland occurs; symptoms include insidious onset; symptoms from compression of trachea, esophagus, and recurrent laryngeal nerve; gland enlarged, hard; hypothyroidism can occur; treatment is symptomatic with surgery for symptoms of compression; thyroid replacement for hypothyroidism. |

persons. Prevalence rates are greater in elderly women (10%) than in elderly men (2.3%).[31] Hypothyroidism is detected in 1 of every 4000 to 5000 newborns.[40]

## Pathophysiology

### Goiter

The patient with hypothyroidism may or may not have a goiter. An enlarged thyroid gland is seen when the disease results from thyroiditis, defective hormone biosynthesis, peripheral resistance to thyroid hormone, and environmental factors. All these conditions reduce thyroid hormone production, and as a result, TSH secretion is increased because of lack of negative feedback. Increased thyroid mass then results from the increased stimulation. In contrast, if hypothyroidism results from a lack of TSH (secondary hypothyroidism), growth of the thyroid gland is not stimulated.

### Thyroiditis

There are three types of thyroiditis (inflammation of the thyroid): acute, subacute, and chronic. **Hashimoto's thyroiditis,** a form of chronic thyroiditis, is the most common form of thyroiditis and is described here.

In Hashimoto's thyroiditis the thyroid is infiltrated with lymphocytes and antithyroid antibodies. These findings support the belief that Hashimoto's thyroiditis is an autoimmune disease, and it is generally believed that it is one of the triad of autoimmune thyroid disorders that include Graves' disease and primary thyroid atrophy. The mechanisms for the autoimmunity are not understood, although significant association exists between Hashimoto's thyroiditis and specific haplotypes, as well as other autoimmune diseases.

The lymphocytic infiltration in Hashimoto's thyroiditis results in obliteration of thyroid follicles and fibrosis. The destruction of the gland decreases the serum levels of $T_4$ and $T_3$ and thus increases TSH. The increase in thyroid tissue is not usually associated with overproduction of thyroid hormone, although transient hyperthyroidism can occur early in the disease. The increase in thyroid tissue and hyperfunction help to maintain an euthyroid state for some time, but eventually hypothyroidism and atrophy will develop.

The major clinical finding in Hashimoto's thyroiditis is *diffuse thyroid enlargement,* found as a goiter on examination. The thyroid gland is firm and smooth, moves freely, and is usually painless. Both lobes are enlarged, but one lobe may be larger than the other. Some persons may experience dysphagia or choking.

### Hypometabolism

Regardless of the cause, a lack of thyroid hormone results in a general depression of basal metabolic rate and slows the development or functioning of almost every system of the body. Alterations in the integumentary, cardiovascular, nervous, musculoskeletal, alimentary, and reproductive systems are often seen. One major change is an accumulation of hyaluronic acids and alteration of ground substances producing mucinous edema **(myxedema)** and third-space fluid effusions. Figure 39-6 illustrates the puffiness characteristic of *myxedema facies.* In the periphery the edematous tissues feel thickened or "doughy." Table 39-6 lists the pathophysiologic alterations seen in hypothyroidism and relates the clinical manifestations seen with each.

The manifestations of hypothyroidism in infants are not usually seen until several months after birth, when signs such as retardation of mental and physical development occur and are usually irreversible. Figure 39-7 clearly shows the effect of severe, untreated infantile hypothyroidism, **cretinism.**

In adults, early signs and symptoms are vague and may go unrecognized. A typical clinical picture is as follows. Early complaints may consist of tiredness, lethargy, and weakness resulting in the inability to carry out a normal day's activities. Intolerance to cold and constipation develop. There may be alterations in menstrual cycles, menorrhagia, and inability to conceive. Loss of interest in sexual activity may be noted by men or women. As the disease progresses, mental dysfunction occurs, appetite decreases, changes in physical characteristics are noted, muscle and joint discomforts are present, and chest pain occurs. If not treated, myxedema coma will develop.

### Myxedema coma

Myxedema coma represents the most severe form of hypothyroidism and ultimately can occur in any patient with untreated prolonged hypothyroidism. Precipitating factors include sedative drugs and narcotics, exposure to cold, surgery, infections, and trauma. The patient has all the classic symptoms of hypothyroidism and also is comatose and has severe hypothermia. (See Table 39-6 for further discussion.)

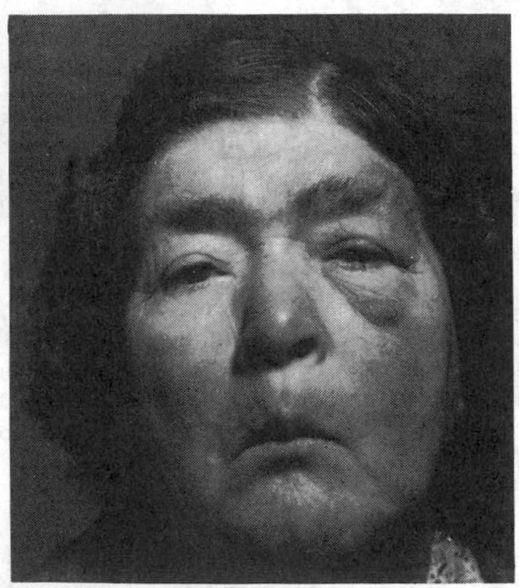

**FIGURE 39-6** Adult with severe hypothyroidism showing typical puffiness around eyes. (From Schottelius B, Schottelius D: *Textbook of physiology,* ed 18, St Louis, 1978, Mosby.)

**TABLE 39-6 Hypothyroidism: Normal Function, Pathologic Alterations, and Clinical Manifestations**

| NORMAL FUNCTION | PATHOPHYSIOLOGIC ALTERATIONS | CLINICAL MANIFESTATIONS |
|---|---|---|
| Regulates metabolic rate, calorigenesis, and oxygen consumption | Decreased metabolic rate, heat production, and oxygen consumption<br>May be vasoconstriction in periphery<br>Decreased nutrient requirements<br>Decreased sweat gland and sebaceous gland activity<br>Myxedema | General: decreased body temperature; intolerance to cold; skin: cool, pale; hair: thin, dry; deepened voice; decreased appetite; dry, thickened, scaly skin<br>Myxedema facies: large tongue, peripheral edema, deepened voice |
| Regulates protein, fat, and carbohydrate metabolism | Altered carbohydrate, protein, and fat metabolism<br>Decreased protein synthesis, gluconeogenesis, and glycogen storage<br>Increased interstitial fluid with polysaccharide deposits and increased albumin content<br>Decreased glucose absorption and cellular uptake; decreased degradation of insulin<br>Decreased lipid metabolism, especially degradation of lipid<br>Decreased erythropoietin production<br>Hypercarotenemia | Metabolic: decreased appetite, weight gain, (edema), slow wound healing<br>Myxedematous tissues: peripheral organs, tongue, vocal cords<br>Hypoalbuminemia<br>Decrease in blood glucose possible in patients with diabetes mellitus<br>Increased serum triglycerides and serum cholesterol<br>Anemia; yellow cast to skin and nails |
| Sensitizes cells to catecholamines | Altered cardiovascular functioning<br>Hypometabolic state, decreased inotropic and chronotropic effects on heart, polysaccharide infiltrate of myocardium<br>Decreased cardiac output, decreased contractility and rate<br>Increased interstitial fluid and third-space fluids | Cardiovascular: bradycardia, enlargement of heart, pericardial effusion, pleural effusion, decreased excretion of water load, hyponatremia, possible increased blood pressure |
| Regulates rate of cellular functions: multiple interactions of thyroid hormone with other hormones and systems | Altered CNS function<br>Altered reproductive function | CNS: apathy, slow slurred speech, lethargy, somnolence, coma, paresthesia, slow deep tendon reflexes<br>Reproductive: decreased libido, failure to conceive, changes in menses, anovulation in women, oligospermia and impotence in men |

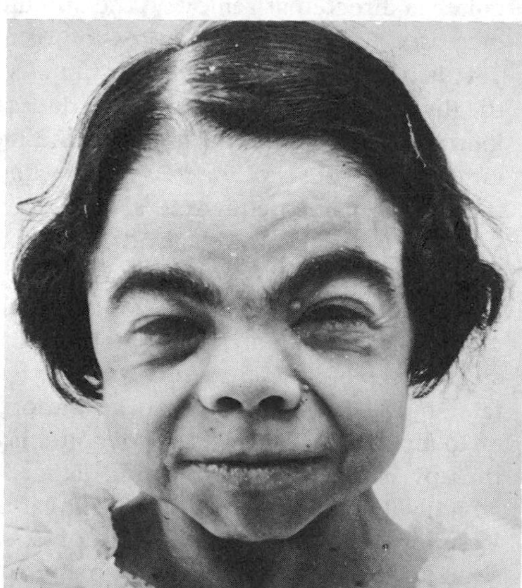

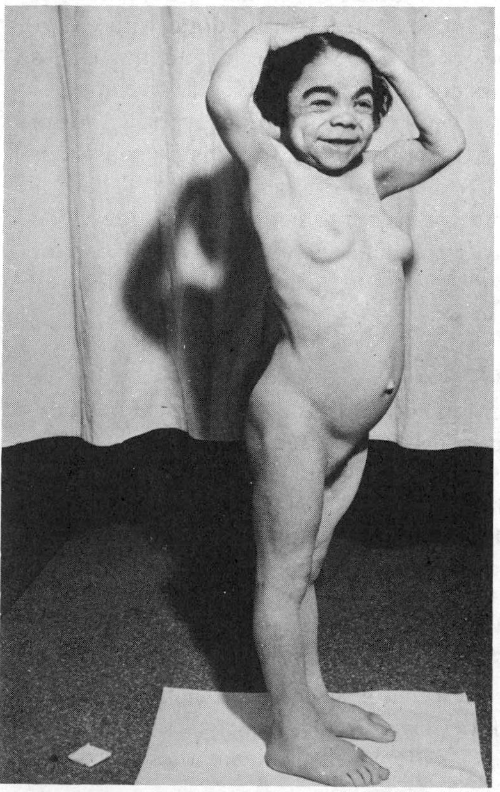

**FIGURE 39-7** Adult cretin (33 years old, untreated). Note cretinoid features, dwarfism (height 44 inches [104 cm]), absent axillary and scant pubic hair, poorly developed breasts, truncal obesity, and small umbilical hernia. Patient has primary amenorrhea. (From Schneeburg NG: *Essentials of clinical endocrinology,* St Louis, 1970, Mosby.)

## Prevention

### Primary prevention

Primary prevention of hypothyroidism is concerned with the prevention of iodine deficiency and its consequences. Iodine is necessary for proper growth and development of the brain of the fetus, infant, and child. Hypothyroidism from iodine deficiency is a global health problem and is recognized as the most important preventable cause of mental defects in the world. The World Health Organization (WHO) estimates that more than 200 million people have goiter and 20 million have some degree of brain damage from the effects of iodine deficiency during pregnancy.[40]

People at risk for iodine deficiency live in geographic areas lacking iodine in soil and in the water supplies. In the United States the Great Lakes region is lacking in sufficient iodine. Foods grown in these areas also lack iodine. Public health measures can be used to increase iodine intake in diet through additives to salt, water, sauces, or oil. In the United States, iodized salt has been an effective means for reducing the incidence of goiter. Programs to educate the public about iodine intake and the use of iodized salt date from the 1920s.

**BOX 39-13 Risk Factors for Hypothyroidism**

- Past history of thyroid disease
- Past history of radiation to neck
- Autoimmune disorders
- Family history of thyroid disease
- History of treatment with lithium, amiodarone, or iodine
- Increased serum cholesterol

### Secondary prevention

Target populations for secondary prevention of hypothyroidism are newborn infants and persons over age 60, especially women, and those persons with risk factors as listed in Box 39-13. Screening of all newborns is done in the United States by the use of $T_4$ tests.[6] Prompt treatment of newborns with congenital deficiencies of thyroid hormone is necessary to prevent irreversible brain damage and dwarfism (cretinism). Screening of adults in clinics and hospitals can be done with either the serum assays of $T_4$ or TSH. The former test is less sensitive and less costly. Community-wide screening of older adults is rarely done because most hypothyroidism in older adults is subclinical, and there is no consensus about when to treat asymptomatic patients.[31] There is consensus that those asymptomatic persons identified to have laboratory test findings for higher TSH and for lower $T_4$ serum levels should be followed and monitored at certain intervals.

### Tertiary prevention

Tertiary prevention includes the appropriate replacement of iodide in patients with iodine-deficient states and the administration of thyroid hormone to treat those with thyroid hormone deficiency. Efforts to increase compliance with thyroid hormone replacement drugs are important measures to prevent complications.

## Medical Management

### Diagnostic tests

Studies of thyroid function useful for diagnosing hypothyroidism include serum free $T_4$ index and a "sensitive" serum TSH assay. As in hyperthyroidism, these tests may need repeating. Other tests may be needed to determine the true hormonal status (see Chapter 38).

Decreased levels of $T_4$ and $T_3$ and an elevated TSH level can confirm the diagnosis of a patient who has primary thyroid hyposecretion and no other disease.[15] Two factors may alter $T_3$, $T_4$, and TSH results: acuity of illness and presence of nonthyroid disease. In nonthyroid disease, there is a decreased conversion of $T_4$ to $T_3$. As a result, 70% of all patients in intensive care units have low serum levels of $T_3$ and normal TSH levels. As patients recover, levels of $T_3$ increase (low $T_3$ state). $T_4$ and TSH levels may also be affected by illness.

When Hashimoto's disease is suspected, the physician will order antithyroid antibody tests and perhaps a fine-needle biopsy to confirm the presence of chronic thyroiditis or to identify other pathologic factors.

### Medication

**Goiter suppression.** Medical management of simple goiter is directed at removing the stimulus causing the increased thyroid mass. Suppression of the increase in TSH is necessary to correct the stimulus for growth of the thyroid gland. Correction also reduces the associated increase in turnover of iodine and the increased $T_4/T_3$ ratio in thyroid secretion.[42] With elevated TSH, the patient has remained euthyroid at the expense of the elevated TSH and an enlarged gland. If extrinsic factors such as goitrogenic drugs or foods are the cause, they are eliminated. Iodine deficiency, although very rare, is ruled out and replacement instituted if appropriate.[13] Only small doses of iodide, such as saturated solution of potassium iodide (SSKI) or Lugol's solution, are needed.

In most instances the cause of goiter is unknown, and therapy is directed at supplying exogenous hormone, which will inhibit TSH secretion. Similar therapy is used to suppress TSH secretion in goiter associated with Hashimoto's disease. Sodium L-thyroxine in doses of 150 to 200 μg is usually necessary. The adequacy of the dosage in suppressing TSH secretion is verified by an RAIU test that should have a value of less than 5%. Surgery is sometimes necessary if obstruction is not relieved with other therapy. Surgery will result in hypothyroidism requiring lifelong replacement of thyroid hormone.

**TABLE 39-7 Replacement Therapy in Hypothyroidism***

| DRUG | COMMENTS |
|---|---|
| Sodium L-thyroxine: levothyroxine (Synthroid, Levoid) | Synthetic $T_4$ only; $T_3$ levels increased by peripheral conversion of $T_4$ to $T_3$; parenteral and oral forms available; most frequently used drug; normal dosage, 1.8 μg/kg body weight |
| Sodium L-triiodothyronine (Cytomel, Trionine) | Synthetic $T_3$; therapeutic effects more difficult to monitor; may experience peaks in serum $T_3$ levels |
| Synthetic combinations of $T_3$ and $T_4$ liotrix (Euthroid, Thyrolar) | Synthetic $T_4$ and $T_3$; therapeutic effects more difficult to monitor; may experience peaks in $T_3$ levels |
| Natural combination of $T_3$ and $T_4$: thyroid extract | Natural preparation of $T_3$ and $T_4$ from animal thyroid; potency may vary |

*Therapeutic equivalence: L-thyroxine 100 μg = L-triiodothyronine 25 μg = liotrix 1 unit = thyroid extract 60 mg.

**Replacement therapy.** Hypothyroidism is treated with replacement of thyroid hormone. Various preparations are available (Table 39-7); most often, L-thyroxine is used. The major precaution is to initiate drug therapy slowly, particularly if the patient has heart dysfunction or is elderly. The initial daily dose usually should not exceed 12.5 to 25 μg of L-thyroxine. This dose is increased by increments of 25 to 50 μg every 2 to 4 weeks until a normal metabolic rate is attained.[40,42]

The optimal maintenance dose of replacement therapy varies and is determined by the clinical state. The earliest clinical response is diuresis, resulting in weight loss and regression of puffiness. The pulse rate then increases, appetite improves, constipation is relieved, and mental and motor activity increase.[40]

The major side effects of thyroid replacement therapy are (1) inadequate treatment, with the patient continuing to show signs and symptoms of hypothyroidism; (2) excessive treatment, resulting in signs and symptoms of hyperthyroidism; (3) increases in drug dose at too fast a rate, resulting in cardiac problems such as angina, palpitations, tachycardia, or cardiac failure; and (4) bone loss and decreased bone density.[27] During the initiation of therapy, the patient is seen every 2 to 4 weeks. After the patient's condition is stable, thyroid hormone replacement should be monitored annually by such tests as serum free $T_4$ index, TSH level, and serum $T_3$ level.

### Treatment

Treatment of hypothyroidism consists of pharmacologic therapy, as previously described. Surgery may be performed for large goiters (see following discussion).

### Diet

Adequate nutrition (well-balanced meals) is promoted for patients with hypothyroidism. They are advised to follow prescribed caloric intake and therapeutic goals regarding weight loss as therapy proceeds. If iodine deficiency or excessive intake of goitrogenic foods has been identified, remedial instruction is given. In severe hypothyroidism, apathy, anorexia, and self-care deficit may combine to limit food intake, and attention must be given to achieve adequate intake. Fluid restriction and occasionally sodium modifications are necessary if hyponatremia is severe.

### Activity

Fatigue may limit activity initiation or endurance in any patient with hypothyroidism. Usually, these patients need to be encouraged to maintain and increase activity tolerance until treatment has been underway for some time. Fatigue may become more severe, and angina and dyspnea on exertion can occur.

### Referral/Consultation

In some settings the nurse assumes responsibility for making referrals to other services. Appropriate referrals might include home care nursing, physical therapy, and social services if family or personal resources are limited.

### Surgical Management

Thyroidectomy may be used to treat large goiters, particularly those causing compression of adjacent tissues. If the goiter is very large, it may displace or compress the esophagus or trachea and cause dysphagia, a choking sensation, or inspiratory stridor. Compression of the recurrent laryngeal nerve may lead to hoarseness, although this sign is more suggestive of cancer. Narrowing of the thoracic inlet decreases venous return from the head, neck, and upper limbs and results in venous engorgement. This obstruction is accentuated with elevation of the person's arms and results in dizziness and syncope (Pemberton's sign).

## NURSING MANAGEMENT

### ♦ ASSESSMENT

### Subjective Data

Hypothyroidism affects every system of the body. The early manifestations will most likely be identified by a thorough history. The history should focus on assessing the following areas for changes:

- Changes in physical energy level and activity or mental/neurologic status
- Changes in skin, hair (head, body), nails
- Presence of chest pain, occurrence of syncope
- Changes in appetite and weight with a typical nutrition intake
- Changes in bowel elimination
- Presence of discomfort: headache, muscle or joint pain, intolerance to cold

Changes in sexual function:
(a) Women: changes in menses, libido, difficulty conceiving
(b) Men: changes in libido
Knowledge level: dysfunction, diagnostic tests, treatment

### Objective Data

Data are collected using a head-to-toe approach, with particular emphasis on the following systems. The nurse is assessing to see if the typical signs of hypothyroidism are present.

Mental status: intellectual functioning; memory; speech pattern; presence of somnolence, lethargy, or confusion
Body weight and temperature
Skin: pigmentation, temperature, presence of nonpitting edema
Neck/hair: quality and quantity of head and body hair, thyroid examination
Cardiovascular: pulse rate, blood pressure at rest and with exercise, heart size
Respiratory: rate, breath sounds
Abdomen: bowel sounds
Motor: muscle strength, tone, and mass; ROM; deep tendon reflexes; joint movement

### Diagnostic Test Findings

The first studies ordered are $T_4$ level, free $T_4$ index, and TSH assay. If hypothyroidism is confirmed, findings would include the following:

1. Increased serum levels of TSH
2. Decreased $T_4$, $T_3$, free $T_4$, and free $T_4$ index

These tests may need to be repeated if findings are inconclusive, as discussed earlier.

To confirm Hashimoto's disease, test findings would include the following:

1. Presence of antithyroid antibodies
2. Chronic thyroiditis findings on pathology report of biopsy

## ♦ NURSING DIAGNOSES

Nursing diagnoses are determined from analysis of patient data. Nursing diagnoses for the person with hypothyroidism may include but are not limited to the following:

| Diagnostic Title | Possible Etiologic Factors |
|---|---|
| Activity intolerance | Poor work capacity associated with poor cardiac function, decreased breathing capacity, and muscle stiffness |
| Body image disturbance | Change in appearance (weight gain, hair and skin changes), change in functioning (decreased mental and physical function) |
| Constipation | Decreased peristaltic action, decreased physical activity |
| Hypothermia | Decreased heat production associated with decreased metabolic rate |
| Knowledge deficit: disease, treatment, expected outcomes, self-monitoring, follow-up care | New interventions with no previous exposure to information |
| Nutrition, altered: more than body requirements | Decreased metabolic rate |
| Pain | Headache and joint pain associated with chronic thyroid problems |
| Self-care deficit, total (varies): bathing-hygiene, dressing-grooming, feeding, toileting | Inability to perform care associated with altered thought process and mental functioning |
| Sexual dysfunction | Alterations in menstrual cycle, ovulation, sperm production, and libido |
| Skin integrity, impaired | Mucinous deposits in skin, decreased circulation, immobility |
| Thought processes, impaired | Slowing of intellectual functions associated with chronic deficit of thyroid hormone |

## ♦ EXPECTED PATIENT OUTCOMES

Expected patient outcomes for the person with hypothyroidism may include but are not limited to the following:

1. Shows a gradual increase in activity tolerance over 2 to 3 months.
2. Relates body image changes to hypothyroidism and verbalizes that most changes are reversible.
3. Maintains a bowel pattern that was typical before onset of illness.
4. Maintains a body temperature of 36° to 37° C (96.8° to 98.6° F).
5. Patient and significant others are able to:
   a. Explain the disease in simple terms.
   b. Explain that treatment is lifelong drug therapy.
   c. Explain that treatment should reverse most signs and symptoms.
   d. Describe self-monitoring needs and planned follow-up.
6. Nutritional status will improve, as evidenced by a gradual decrease in body weight.
7. States pain is controlled.
8. Self-care needs are met.
9. Understands that sexual function will increase as thyroid status returns to normal.
10. Skin remains intact.
11. Alteration in thought processes does not lead to injuries or loss of dignity, as evidenced by no injuries and participation in decisions as much as possible.

## ♦ INTERVENTIONS

The nursing interventions required by the patient with hypothyroidism vary greatly depending on the severity of disease. Not every patient has all the nursing diagnoses previously listed. Many persons are treated as out-patients.

## Managing Critical Care

Hypothyroid patients requiring intensive care are the rare patients with myxedema coma and those with respiratory failure and heart failure secondary to hypothyroidism.[18] The most frequent cause of death in this population is ventilatory failure. Mortality rate of patients with myxedema coma is 25%.[8] Assessment and management priorities are directed toward support of respiratory and cardiac function.[36]

Isley[18] discusses several factors in severe hypothyroidism that are significant in intensive care units.

1. Respiratory function may be compromised by a large tongue and sleep apnea; it may be decreased by hypoxic and hypercapneic ventilatory drives and respiratory muscle weakness.
2. Cardiac output is low as a result of bradycardia and a decrease in stroke volume; frank congestive heart failure usually occurs in patients with an underlying cardiac disorder.
3. Metabolism of digoxin is slowed, so cardiac glycosides must be used cautiously.
4. Long-standing hypothyroidism can cause secondary adrenal insufficiency; stress doses of corticosteroids are recommended.
5. Early treatment of myxedema coma improves patient outcome.

It is important to understand that myxedema coma is often a clinical diagnosis; treatment often must start before laboratory test findings are conclusive.

Therapy for patients with *myxedema coma* includes supportive care (cardiovascular, respiratory, fluid balance support), treatment of the underlying precipitating factor, and administration of thyroid hormone. Thyroid hormone is given intravenously. Usually, L-thyroxine, 2 μg/kg, is given as the initial dose, with an additional 100 μg every 24 hours. Hydrocortisone (100 mg daily) is recommended by some authorities because adrenocortical insufficiency is frequently present.[42] The patient is kept warm enough to avoid additional heat loss without overwarming to avoid vascular collapse. Tracheal intubation and mechanical ventilation may be necessary. Improvement is seen in 3 to 24 hours.

Nursing interventions include care of the comatose patient; surveillance of respiratory, cardiovascular, and fluid status; care of the patient with respiratory insufficiency; preventive care for problems of immobility; and assistance with the institution of the medical regimen.

## Providing Recuperative Care

The hypothyroid state is reversed slowly, so the patient will not return to the premorbid health state for 2 to 3 months. Potential nursing interventions include:

1. Promote activity to the level of patient tolerance.
   a. At first the patient will have a very limited tolerance and may only be able to move around in the room. Activities should be increased gradually.
   b. Monitor the cardiovascular response to new activities. If the patient complains of chest pain or develops an unacceptable heart rate above baseline, stop the activity and then restart at a slower rate.
   c. Monitor blood pressure, pulse, and respirations before, during, and after each new activity.
2. Promote positive body image.
   a. Provide information that helps the patient and significant others understand how body changes relate to the hypothyroidism.
   b. Educate about reversible body changes.
   c. Help the patient see the positive changes that have occurred.
3. Promote normal bowel elimination.
   a. Monitor bowel elimination.
   b. Maintain adequate fluid intake.
   c. Increase bulk in the diet.
4. Treat hypothermia.
   a. Monitor temperature every 2 to 4 hours.
   b. Maintain an environmental temperature that is comfortable for the patient.
   c. Use blankets to increase body temperature if necessary.
5. Facilitate intake of nutritional diet that is low in calories and includes food from all food groups.
6. Promote comfort.
   a. Use nonmedicinal comfort measures such as massage, cool or warm heat, and distraction to promote pain control.
   b. If medications are used, monitor patient carefully. Patient will have a lower tolerance for sedative and depressant medications.
7. Provide for self-care needs. At first the patient may require complete care for hygiene, toileting, and dietary needs.
8. Facilitate patient's understanding of the relationship between the sexual problems and the hypothyroidism.
9. Maintain skin integrity.
   a. Monitor skin condition each shift.
   b. Institute preventive care measures such as sheepskin pads and soft sheets.
   c. If patient is unable to or does not turn by self, assist in turning every 2 hours.
10. Facilitate a safe environment and orientation to environment.
    a. Monitor neurologic status every shift.
    b. Incorporate into contacts with the patient information about date, place, time, current events, and current activities to facilitate orientation.
    c. Maintain a safe environment: remove any clutter, keep bed low, and keep bed rails up.

**TABLE 39-8 Characteristics of the Five Types of Thyroid Cancer**

| | CANCERS OF FOLLICULAR EPITHELIUM | | | | CANCER OF PARAFOLLICULAR TISSUE |
|---|---|---|---|---|---|
| CHARACTERISTICS | PAPILLARY | FOLLICULAR | ANAPLASTIC | THYROID LYMPHOMA | MEDULLARY |
| Incidence of all thyroid cancers | 65% | 20% | 5% | 5% | 5% |
| Age | Young persons | After 40 | After 60 | After 40 | After 50 |
| Female/male ratio | 2-3:1 | 2-3:1 | F > M | F > M | F = M |
| Metastasis | By intraglandular lymphatics; slow-growing tumor | By blood vessels to distant sites (bone, lung, liver); occurs early | By direct invasion to adjacent structures; highly malignant | By lymphatic system; gland fixed to other structures | By intraglandular lymphatics and blood vessels |
| Prognosis | Good; rarely causes death in young persons if occult or intrathyroidal | Good if minimally invasive lesion | Prognosis varies with cell type; for giant cell, very poor (<6 months from diagnoses); for small cell, better (5-year survival rate of 20% to 50%) | Good | Moderate; 10-year survival is estimated as 2 of 3 persons |
| Symptoms | Asymptomatic | Goiter may have been present for years | Hoarseness, inspiratory stridor, dysphagia (signs of invasion of adjacent areas) | May have long history of previous goiter; rapid enlargement of goiter, hoarseness, dysphagia, pressure sensation, dyspnea, some pain | Because tumor produces hormones, possible paraendocrine manifestations such as carcinoid syndrome, watery diarrhea, Cushing's syndrome |
| Tumor | Occult (<1.5 cm in diameter), intrathyroidal (>1.5 cm in diameter but does not extend through thyroid surface), and extrathyroidal (extends through thyroid surface); well differentiated; psammoma body found in 40% of tumors and virtually diagnostic of malignant nature; tumors appear as "cold" spots on thyroid scan | Well differentiated to poorly differentiated; cyst formation and calcification possible; tumors may appear as "hot" areas on thyroid scan | Two cell forms: giant cell and small cell | Usually of nodular histocytic form | Tumor of C cells of thyroid; not encapsulated; some appear as "cold" spots on thyroid scan; may produce ACTH, prostaglandin, or carcinoembryonic antigen |

d. Use frequent stimulation; at dusk, as well as at night, use nightlights to prevent confusion.
e. Inform significant others of relationship between mental status and hypothyroidism.
f. Involve patient, as possible, in decisions about care.

## Preparing for Discharge

The nurse helps the patient and family caregivers learn how to continue the plan of care after discharge. The importance of compliance with medications and follow-up care should be stressed. The teaching plan should include the following:

1. Nature of the disorder, diagnostic tests, treatment; need for lifelong replacement therapy
2. Medications: dosage, method of administration, side effects
3. Self-monitoring of vital signs, body weight, any signs of skin breakdown, and any signs of constipation

**TABLE 39-8 Characteristics of the Five Types of Thyroid Cancer—cont'd**

| | CANCERS OF FOLLICULAR EPITHELIUM | | | | CANCER OF PARAFOLLICULAR TISSUE |
|---|---|---|---|---|---|
| CHARACTERISTICS | PAPILLARY | FOLLICULAR | ANAPLASTIC | THYROID LYMPHOMA | MEDULLARY |
| Other | Growth partially dependent on TSH; thyroid hormone can cause regression of metastatic lesions; $^{131}$I may be used for nonresectable lesions; may have history of radiation therapy to head and neck | Suppressive thyroid therapy can cause regression of metastatic lesions; radiation therapy with $^{131}$I may be used when vascular invasion or metastasis present | — | Strong association with Hashimoto's thyroiditis; may have lymphoma at other sites | Occurs as a familial form as part of multiple endocrine neoplasia (MEN) type IIa or MEN IIb; in MEN IIa, there is medullary carcinoma, adrenomedullary hyperplasia, or bilateral pheochromocytomas and hyperparathyroidism; in MEN IIb, there is medullary carcinoma, bilateral pheochromocytomas, and an unusual phenotype with ganglioneuromas of eyelids, oral mucosa, tongue, and labia, marfanoid habitus; skeletal abnormalities; and prominent corneal nerves; also occurs as a non-MEN familial form |

4. Methods to prevent skin breakdown and constipation
5. Need for periods of rest alternating with activity
6. Need for continued follow-up care

The patient with a large goiter may need help with altered body image related to disfigurement. An open and trusting relationship is necessary so that the patient can share feelings and concerns. The goiter may be concealed by the use of scarves, high collars, and make-up.

## ♦ EVALUATION

To evaluate the effectiveness of nursing interventions, compare patient behaviors with those stated in the expected patient outcomes. Successful achievement of patient outcomes for the person with hypothyroidism is indicated by the following:

1. Demonstrates increasing ability to ambulate and participate in ADL.
2. Attributes body changes to disease and its treatment.
3. Reports resumption of usual elimination patterns.
4. Temperature remains between 36° and 37° C (96.8° to 98.6° F).
5. Patient and significant others accurately explain disease and need for lifelong intake of a thyroid drug even though symptoms will be alleviated.
6. After diuresis has occurred, weight will decrease no more than 2 kg/week (or by prescribed amount).
7. Reports absence of severe headache or joint pain.
8. Reports initiation and completion of increased number of self-care activities.
9. Explains how therapy should increase sexual function.
10. Skin remains intact.
11. Experiences and reports no injuries.

## ✸ SPECIAL CONSIDERATIONS FOR CARE OF THE GERONTOLOGIC PATIENT

1. Assess for signs and symptoms of decreased alertness, decreased mobility, or increased susceptibility to cold, which may be signs and symptoms more typically noted with hypothyroidism in elderly persons.
2. Assess for signs of myxedema, as seen with untreated hypothyroidism.

3. Assess for signs of drug toxicity because of decreased metabolic activity from diminished endocrine function.
4. Assess for signs of infection because thymic activity is decreased.
5. Assist elderly patient to plan a way for remembering to take replacement therapy; without a plan, the apathetic patient may forget to take the thyroid hormone replacement.
6. Teach patient and significant others the following:
   a. Monitor for drug side effects.
   b. Report signs of angina or congestive heart failure, which may result from initial doses of thyroid hormone replacement.
   c. Take precautions to avoid infections.
   d. Take measures to prevent constipation, which often occurs with hypothyroidism, especially in elderly persons.

## ❦ HOME CARE CONSIDERATIONS

Family involvement is usually necessary to ensure appropriate care and compliance with the therapeutic regimen in the elderly myxedematous patient.

## CANCER OF THE THYROID

### Etiology/Epidemiology

Cancer of the thyroid is less prevalent than other forms of cancer and only a very small percentage of thyroid neoplasms are malignant (1% of invasive neoplasms). Two general types of malignant neoplasms are found: those arising from follicular epithelium (papillary, follicular, anaplastic) and those arising from parafollicular tissue. Non-Hodgkin's lymphomas can also develop in thyroid tissue. Table 39-8 presents characteristics for the five forms of primary thyroid malignant neoplasms. Papillary carcinoma is the most common (65% of thyroid malignancies).[40]

Thyroid nodules occur in 4% of the population. One of 1000 nodules is maligant.[31] The incidence of malignancy in nodules is much higher in children (50%) and in very elderly persons. The female/male ratio of malignancy is 4:1. A history of radiation to the thyroid in amounts of 6.5 to 2000 rad is linked with a 7% incidence of thyroid cancer.[9]

### Pathophysiology

Diagnosis of thyroid cancer has been simplified by the acceptance of fine-needle biopsy in obtaining tissue samples from solid tumors or fluid from cysts. It is most reliable in detecting papillary cancers. It is less reliable in detecting follicular cancers and other types; therefore follow-up open biopsy is done if pathologic analysis is inconclusive. This procedure can be done in the office setting and allows earlier detection of malignancy. Many factors are now being studied to develop more fully a consensus on the staging classification of thyroid malignancy. (See Chapter 16 for principles related to diagnosis, staging, and treatment of all malignancies.)

Three tests help differentiate benign and malignant nodules. Briefly, radionuclide imaging is based on the concept that cancer cells do not concentrate iodine and thus are labeled as "cold" on scans. Only 20% of "cold" nodules seen on thyroid scans are malignant. Ultrasound aids in differentiating cystic nodules (usually benign) from solid nodules. Thyroid suppression tests discover whether the nodule decreases in size; if so, it is likely to be benign. Serum calcitonin and carcinoembryonic antigens (CEAs) may be measured and may be high in some patients with medullary carcinoma. Serum TSH levels are used as the first test to determine thyroid function. Most patients with thyroid cancer are euthyroid.

### Medical Management

Medical management of persons with thyroid cancer includes use of all modalities of cancer treatment: surgery,[33] radiation, hormonal suppression, and chemotherapy. For occult papillary cancer, treatment consists of lobectomy and isthmectomy followed by thyroid hormone suppression therapy (administration of thyroid hormone preparation to suppress TSH). For extrathyroidal papillary carcinoma and invasive follicular carcinoma, a total thyroidectomy followed by $^{131}$I therapy is frequently done. Removal of the entire thyroid gland in follicular carcinoma increases the effectiveness of treatment of distant metastasis with $^{131}$I. Follicular cancer does trap iodine but not nearly as well as normal thyroid tissue. A total thyroidectomy allows for the metastatic tissue to trap the iodine without competition.

Treatment of intrathyroidal papillary carcinoma and noninvasive follicular carcinoma is more controversial. Some authorities recommend the conservative approach used for occult papillary carcinoma, and others recommend the approach used for extrathyroidal papillary and invasive follicular carcinoma.[31,42] For both papillary and follicular cancer, involved lymph nodes are resected during surgery. Also, these patients may be seen every 2 to 3 months, and any recurrence is treated with $^{131}$I therapy. Suppressive thyroid hormone therapy and $^{131}$I therapy are frequently used after surgery.

Anaplastic thyroid cancer may be treated aggressively with surgery, radiation therapy, and chemotherapy,[9] but frequently the cancer is too far advanced and only palliative surgery is done.[42]

Thyroid lymphoma usually is treated using radiation and chemotherapy; however, very small lymphomas may be treated surgically. Medullary carcinoma is treated with total thyroidectomy. These tumors do not respond to $^{131}$I therapy or thyroid hormone suppression. Recurrence and metastatic lesions have been treated with surgery and sometimes radiation therapy. Calcitonin levels can be used to monitor for recurrence.

For some patients with certain tumors and lymph

node involvement, a modified neck dissection is recommended by some authorities.[9] (See Chapter 36 for a discussion of neck dissection.)

## Nursing Management

Care of the patient with a thyroid nodule first focuses on helping the patient through the diagnostic process. Thyroid nodules occur frequently, and most are not cancerous. No one diagnostic test is completely reliable. Depending on patient characteristics and physician philosophy, various tests may be performed. The nurse prepares the patient for each test, particularly focusing on education.

### Preoperative care

The patient having surgery of the thyroid needs care directed toward producing and maintaining a euthyroid state (see earlier sections on hyperthyroidism or hypothyroidism), if this is not already present. Patients with both hyperthyroidism and hypothyroidism have been treated medically for varying lengths of time to induce the euthyroid state, and this care must be continued. Because patients who have recently experienced alteration in thyroid hormone levels may have an altered nutritional status, extra attention should be paid to promoting and maintaining positive nitrogen balance.

The patient with previous abnormal thyroid hormone levels may still be having difficulty coping effectively. The patient with a diagnosis of cancer may be experiencing major disruption in coping because of that diagnosis. Therefore the patient who is to have surgery of the thyroid requires a nonstressful environment (quiet room and calm, relaxed approach by staff). General measures to induce relaxation, such as back rubs, a consistent nurse, and a consistent schedule, should be included in patient care.

Patient teaching regarding general preoperative and postoperative care (see Chapter 23) is given. The patient also needs to learn how to cough and to move the head and neck postoperatively without placing strain on the suture line. Thus the patient is taught preoperatively to support the neck by placing both hands behind the neck when moving the head or when coughing.

### Postoperative care

Immediate interventions for postoperative care are listed in the Guidelines box above. In addition to routine monitoring, the patient is monitored for major complications that can occur following thyroid surgery: recurrent laryngeal nerve injury, hemorrhage, tetany, and respiratory obstruction. Signs of these complications are reported immediately to the surgeon. Although the signs of laryngeal nerve damage may be related to intubation during surgery, such hoarseness should clear gradually. If hoarseness persists or worsens, it is reported immediately to the surgeon. Hoarseness may be a first sign of laryngeal nerve damage, which can result in vocal cord spasm and respiratory obstruction. An emergency tracheostomy may be necessary, and equipment for this should be available on the nursing unit.

The patient is monitored for presence of hemorrhage for the first 12 to 24 hours postoperatively. Hemorrhage can result in incisional bleeding or in compression of the trachea or surrounding tissue. If hemorrhage causes compression, the patient will complain of signs of compression. If these signs should occur and if loosening of the dressing does not relieve respiratory distress and medical assistance is not immediately available, the

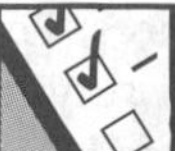

### Guidelines for Care of the Person After Thyroid Surgery

1. Monitor for and report signs of complications.
   a. Laryngeal nerve damage; hoarseness, weak voice
   b. Hemorrhage or tissue swelling
      (1) Bleeding on dressing: check back of dressing by slipping hand gently under neck and shoulders
      (2) Choking sensation
      (3) Difficulty in coughing or swallowing
      (4) Sensation of dressing being too tight even after it is loosened
   c. Calcium deficiency (tetany)
      (1) Early signs: tingling around mouth or of toes and fingers, decreasing serum calcium levels
      (2) Later signs: positive Chvostek's and Trousseau's signs (Chapter 38), grand mal seizures
   d. Respiratory distress associated with any of signs just listed
2. Provide emergency care.
   a. Keep emergency supplies readily available:
      (1) Tracheostomy set (for laryngeal nerve damage), oxygen and suction equipment, suture removal set (for respiratory obstruction from hemorrhage)
      (2) IV calcium gluconate or calcium chloride (for tetany)
   b. For acute respiratory distress:
      (1) Call for immediate medical help.
      (2) Raise head of bed.
      (3) Loosen dressing over incision.
      (4) Give calcium as ordered, if signs and symptoms of tetany are present.
      (5) If loosening the dressing does not relieve symptoms of respiratory distress and if medical help is not readily available, remove clips or sutures as instructed.
3. Provide comfort.
   a. Avoid tension on suture lines; encourage patient to support head when turning by placing both hands behind neck.
   b. Give prescribed analgesics as necessary.
4. Maintain nutritional status.
   a. Start soft foods as soon as tolerated (only fluids may be tolerated initially).
   b. Encourage a high-carbohydrate, high-protein diet.
5. Teach patient:
   a. ROM exercises to neck when suture line is healed, to prevent permanent limitations
   b. Need for lifelong thyroid hormone replacement therapy after a total thyroidectomy
   c. Any special care measures related to the underlying disease
   d. Need for follow-up care

nurse may be instructed to remove clips or sutures. The patient may need to be taken back to surgery for retying of the blood vessels and resuturing of the wound.

Although the occurrence of tetany is minimal, the parathyroid glands can be injured during surgery, or inflammation may block the normal release of parathyroid hormone. If the level of parathyroid hormone drops, symptoms of calcium deficiency can occur. If not treated promptly, calcium deficiency can result in contraction of the glottis, respiratory obstruction, and death. Tetany may appear from 1 to 7 days postoperatively. Treatment for calcium deficiency is calcium chloride or calcium gluconate given intravenously. Oral calcium is then necessary until normal parathyroid function returns.

The nurse must know that respiratory obstruction can occur from (1) recurrent laryngeal nerve damage causing vocal cord spasms that close off the larynx, (2) tracheal compression from hemorrhage, (3) tissue swelling, or (4) tetany. The nurse should be prepared to manage all these problems.

A patient who had surgery for hyperthyroidism, although treated to promote a euthyroid state before surgery, requires extra monitoring of cardiovascular and respiratory status after surgery to assist in identifying early any problems caused by the hyperthyroid state. During surgery with manipulation of the gland, extra hormone can be released, and this may precipitate a thyroid storm or crisis. If a total thyroidectomy was done, the patient needs to be monitored for signs of hypothyroidism (see p. 1235) and started on replacement therapy.

# PARATHYROID GLAND

## HYPERSECRETION OF PARATHYROID HORMONE: PRIMARY HYPERPARATHYROIDISM

### Etiology

Primary **hyperparathyroidism** (PHPT) is being diagnosed with increased frequency because of the more frequent routine measurements of serum calcium levels.[14] An elevated serum calcium level is the key clinical feature of PHPT.

The most frequent cause of PHPT is benign adenomas, although hyperplasia and malignant tumors may also be causes. The cause of adenomas, hyperplasia, or malignant tumors is not known, but a history of earlier radiation of the neck has been reported in some patients.[14,40] There is no evidence that postmenopausal estrogen causes tumors of the parathyroid gland; however, it may unmask effects of preexisting tumors.[14]

Another theory is that the "set point" at which ionized calcium inhibits parathyroid gland tissue may be increased so that the normal negative feedback control between calcium and parathyroid gland function is lost. A genetic component is present in some patients who have PHPT as part of the syndrome of multiple endocrine neoplasia, type I (MEN I) (PHPT is associated with islet cell tumors and pituitary adenoma)[24] or part of MEN IIa (PHPT is associated with medullary thyroid carcinoma and pheochromocytoma).

### Epidemiology

PHPT is seen most frequently in women over age 40 and is found in 2% of white women over age 60.[14] Most patients are asymptomatic or have mild symptoms of malaise, muscle weakness, and mental depression; they may have hypertension and mild osteoporosis. This "typical picture" is very different from that found 20 years ago; the change is attributed to the development of technology that allows more accurate serum calcium measurements and parathyroid hormone (PTH) assays.[14] More widespread screening and earlier detection have followed. In the past the typical picture was that of a patient with severe hypercalcemia, bone pain, and renal stones.

### Pathophysiology

The alteration in physiologic functioning associated with PHPT is the result of one or two major problems:

1. The exaggeration of the normal effects of PTH on the skeletal, renal, and gastrointestinal (GI) systems
2. The associated hypercalcemia

The primary function of PTH is the maintenance of a normal serum level of calcium. Hypersecretion of PTH results in continual stimulation of target organs and elevates serum calcium. The normal negative feedback of serum calcium on PTH secretion is lost or ineffective. Increased PTH (1) increases bone resorption, (2) enhances the reabsorption of calcium from the glomerular filtrate, and (3) increases calcium absorption through the GI tract.

In the skeletal system, increased PTH increases bone resorption, resulting in osteopenia and, in very severe cases, cysts and fractures from *osteitis fibrosa cystica.* Joint changes also occur. In the renal system, increased PTH enhances the reabsorption of calcium from the glomerular filtrate, reabsorption of phosphate, and alteration in the excretion of bicarbonate. Production of activated vitamin D increases. Elevated PTH effects on the GI tract are indirect and occur through the action of vitamin D. The activated vitamin D results in increased calcium absorption through the GI tract.

The processes just described result in elevated serum calcium, which in itself leads to neurologic, musculoskeletal, cardiac, GI, and renal alterations. The alterations in the various systems caused by hypercalcemia result in most of the clinical manifestations. The relationship between the pathophysiology of hyperparathyroidism and the clinical manifestations is presented in Table 39-9.

Because calcitonin from the C cells of the thyroid opposes the effect of PTH, it would be logical to assume

**TABLE 39-9 Hypersecretion of Parathyroid Hormone: Normal Function, Primary Pathophysiologic Factors, and Clinical Manifestations**

| NORMAL FUNCTION | PATHOPHYSIOLOGIC FACTORS | CLINICAL MANIFESTATIONS |
|---|---|---|
| Maintenace of normal serum calcium | Hypersecretion, continual stimulation of target organs | Increased serum calcium |
| Regulates bone resorption of calcium | Increase bone resorption resulting in osteopenia, cysts, and fractures *(osteitis fibrosa cystica)*; bone formation increased but less than resorption | Bone pain, arthralgia, osteopenia |
| Regulates reabsorption of calcium from glomerular filtrate | Early in disease, hypocalciuria in response to increase blood calcium level; later, hypercalciuria as reabsorptive capacity is overwhelmed | Early, hypocalciuria; later, hypercalciuria and polyuria, polydipsia, thirst, urinary calculi, renal failure |
| Regulates phosphate and bicarbonate excretion in kidney tubule | Ineffective bicarbonate reabsorption and phosphate clearance | Hyperchloremic acidosis: anorexia, nausea, vomiting |
| Regulates calcium absorption in intestines; influenced by estrogen in women and activated vitamin D (1,25-dihydroxy cholecalciferol, calcitriol) | Increased calcium absorption from intestines adds to hypercalcemia; increased gastrin secretion, increased calcitriol production | Hypercalcemia: possible peptic ulcer and pancreatitis |
| Calcium regulates pores of cell membranes, movement of sodium, and thus depolarization and resultant action potential in nerves and muscles | Hypercalcemia blocks cell membrane permeability and depresses nerve and muscle activity | *Neuromuscular*<br>Impaired mentation, apathy, lethargy, somnolence, coma, hypoactive reflexes, fasciculation of tongue, muscle weakness/aches (lower limbs more than upper) |
| | Depresses activity of cardiac muscle | *Cardiovascular*<br>Electrocardiographic (ECG) changes: shortened QT intervals, dysrhythmias, hypertension |
| | Slows intestinal motility | *Gastrointestinal*<br>Anorexia, nausea and vomiting, constipation |

that in response to the increased serum calcium, calcitonin secretion would increase. This is not seen in PHPT.

## Prevention

### Primary prevention

No known primary prevention exists for PHPT.

### Secondary prevention

Target populations for secondary prevention are persons over age 60, those who have a history of radiation to the neck, and those who are found to be hypercalcemic. PHPT is only one of the causes of hypercalcemia.

### Tertiary prevention

In most patients, tertiary prevention includes surgery as the therapy of choice to prevent bone and renal complications of PHPT. In other patients, it includes regular monitoring of calcium levels and treatment when symptoms appear.

## Medical Management

The goal for discharge of patients with PHPT as determined by DRGs is 5 days. The nurse works collaboratively with the physician for implementation of prescribed medical therapy. Because the nurse has a major role in discharge planning and patient teaching, these are discussed under nursing management.

### Diagnostic tests

An increased serum PTH level and persistent hypercalcemia are criteria for establishing the diagnosis of PHPT; other causes of hypercalcemia (Box 39-14) and increased serum PTH must be ruled out. Another disorder (e.g., malignancy) may coexist with PHPT. Table 39-10 gives details of tests typically used in parathyroid diseases. In addition to these tests, the physician studies the renal and skeletal systems for radiographic evidence of PHPT complications: urine stones, changes in bone density, and cysts or signs of demineralization in bone. If the patient is severely hypercalcemic, treatment is started before findings of most tests are received.

**BOX 39-14 Causes of Hypercalcemia (Other Than Hyperparathyroidism)**

Malignancy
Leukemia, lymphoma, multiple myeloma
Vitamin D intoxication
Hypervitaminosis A
Granulomatous diseases
Other endocrine disorders: thyrotoxicosis, adrenal insufficiency
Milk-alkali syndrome
Immobilization

**TABLE 39-10 Diagnostic Tests for Parathyroid Function**

| TEST | PROCEDURE | INTERPRETATION |
|---|---|---|
| **SERUM** | | |
| Total calcium 9.6-10.4 mg/dl | Blood sample | Measures both bound and ionized calcium; increased in PHPT; decreased in hypoparathyroidism or with low albumin |
| Phosphorus 2.8-4.5 mg/dl | Blood sample | Decreased with hypercalcemia and elevated in hypocalcemia and renal failure |
| Alkaline phosphatase 2-5 Bodansky units | Blood sample | Increased in bone demineralization, liver disease, and by certain drugs |
| Parathyroid hormone (PTH) by radioimmunoassay | Blood sample | Elevated in hyperparathyroidism and decreased in hypoparathyroidism |
| **URINE** | | |
| Calcium | Collect single specimen | Decreased in hypoparathyroidism |
| Quantitative | 24 hour collection | Elevated in hyperparathyroidism |
| Phosphorus | 24 hour collection | Elevated in hypocalcemic states and PTH excess; decreased with PTH lack and renal failure |
| **FUNCTION TESTS** | | |
| Ellsworth-Howard excretion test (PTH infusion test) | Fasting required; 200 units of PTH extract administered IV; hourly urine collections | Normal response is 5-6 times increased urinary phosphate excretion; an increase of 10 times is found in hypoparathyroidism |
| Urinary cyclic adenosine monophosphate (cAMP) | Urine sample | High levels of AMP found in hyperparathyroidism |

The control of elevated calcium levels is the first priority of treatment. While the upper limits of blood calcium levels are 10.1 to 10.4 mg/dl (or those established by a laboratory), aggressive treatment may not be instituted until the patient becomes symptomatic or the calcium levels are 13 mg/dl or higher. The immediate treatment is with *normal saline infusion* to ensure a well-hydrated state in order to have less concentration of blood calcium and to promote calcium clearance in the kidney tubule. In addition, the excretion of sodium enhances excretion of calcium. Patients often have a history of anorexia, nausea, and vomiting and thus are hypovolemic and require fluid replacement as well.

### Medication

Once hydration has been ensured, the next therapeutic agent is a *loop diuretic* (furosemide or ethacrynic acid), given intravenously or orally. Drugs that increase serum calcium (e.g., thiazides) are avoided. In a severe crisis, more potent *anticalcemic drugs* sometimes are used. These increase urinary excretion of calcium, as do the loop diuretics; and they also inhibit bone resorption and/or intestinal absorption of calcium. Anticalcemic agents are toxic drugs, and their use is limited to one or two doses, if possible.

*Mithramycin,* sometimes used as a cytotoxic neoplastic agent, is a very potent anticalcemic. *Edetate disodium* is a chelating agent, binding calcium in the blood so that the resultant complexes can be excreted in the urine. Nephrotoxicity has limited its use. *Calcitonin (salmon)* and *dexamethasone* are other choices of treatment, but their effectiveness is limited in PHPT. Dexamethasone is particularly effective in hypercalcemia related to bone malignancy.

In PHPT, serum phosphate levels are usually low. In this type of hypercalcemia, *phosphates* may be used as anticalcemic agents; however, caution is necessary. Phosphates lower serum calcium levels by inhibiting bone resorption, and if an acute elevation of serum phosphate occurs, calcium phosphate salts precipitate out. Extensive precipitation of calcium phosphate salts can result in hypocalcemia, renal stones, and renal failure. Cautious use of phosphates includes oral administration rather than IV; careful monitoring of blood urea nitrogen (BUN), serum calcium, and phosphate levels; and monitoring for signs of hypocalcemia and renal stones. If medications are not effective or not appropriate for a particular patient, severe hypercalcemia can be treated by dialysis.

While the anticalcemic drug therapy is underway, it is important to maintain the high infusion rate of sodium chloride. It is necessary to replace electrolytes as needed, and serum calcium, potassium, magnesium, and phosphate levels are monitored.

### Treatment

Once the diagnosis has been made and hypercalcemia treated, options for treatment of PHPT are considered. Although surgical removal of the parathyroid glands is the therapy of choice, some controversy surrounds the selection of patients for surgery.[7,14] The issues involve whether to offer surgery to the asymptomatic patient or to the one who has mild symptoms and slight elevations of serum calcium.

Medical management, as an alternative to surgery, consists of continuing hydration, use of one of the loop diuretics, replacement of electrolytes, and sodium chloride, 300 to 400 mEq/24 hours. Repeat monitoring and follow-up of the patient is necessary to detect worsening of the hypercalcemia and the onset of renal or bony lesions. Use of an anticalcemic agent sometimes is necessary. Medical management may be the only treatment used in patients who are not suitable candidates for surgery.

#### Diet

In the past, a calcium-restricted diet was ordered for patients with PHPT who were treated medically. At present, not all physicians prescribe low-calcium diets; some believe these diets reduce urinary excretion of calcium and should not be used.[7]

#### Activity

There are no restrictions of activity unless the patient has severe hypercalcemia and/or pathologic bone conditions. In fact, maintaining activity is advised because stress on long bones helps reduce calcium resorption.

#### Referral/Consultation

In some settings the nurse assumes responsibility for making referrals to other services. Careful assessment should be made of the patient's and/or family caregivers' ability to manage the therapeutic regimen at home and to continue with required follow-up care. Appropriate referrals might include home nursing, physical therapy, and social services.

## NURSING MANAGEMENT

### ♦ ASSESSMENT

#### Subjective Data

Nursing assessment includes identifying the presence of signs and symptoms of hyperparathyroidism and the resultant hypercalcemia. Data to be collected to assess the patient with PHPT include the following:

- Mental status: history of change in mentation, personality, or alertness
- Skeletal system: presence of bone or joint pain
- Renal system
  - Changes in urine output, particularly polyuria or nocturia
  - Symptoms of renal colic or pyelonephritis
- GI system
  - Normal 24-hour intake
  - Symptoms of anorexia, nausea, vomiting
  - Changes in bowel elimination
- Neuromuscular system
  - Symptoms of fatigue or weakness
  - Changes in ability to carry out ADL
  - Presence of pruritus
  - Presence or absence of flank pain

#### Objective Data

Data to be collected to assess the patient with PHPT include the following:

- Mental status: short-term memory, affect, alertness, orientation
- Skeletal system: ROM, presence of excessive immobility
- Renal system: urine output, characteristics of urine
- GI system: fluid/food intake, bowel movements, bowel sounds, weight
- Neuromuscular system: muscle strength, peripheral sensory function, reflexes
- Cardiovascular system: blood pressure, pulse (rhythm, rate), electrocardiogram (ECG)

#### Diagnostic Test Findings

Results of tests indicative of PHPT include the following:

1. Laboratory tests
   a. Blood: elevated serum calcium, decreased serum phosphate, elevated PTH levels
   b. Urinary: elevated urinary cyclic adenosine monophosphate (cAMP)
2. Radiographic: abnormalities particularly noticeable in the phalanges: cysts, demineralization
3. Radiographic: renal abnormalities such as calculi

### ♦ NURSING DIAGNOSES

Nursing diagnoses are determined from analysis of patient data. Nursing diagnoses for the person with PHPT may include but are not limited to the following:

| Diagnostic Title | Possible Etiologic Factors |
|---|---|
| **For patients treated medically on long-term basis and acutely before surgery** | |
| Injury (trauma), high risk for | Muscular weakness, altered mental status, bone demineralization |
| Cardiac output, decreased | Dysrhythmias associated with altered electrical conduction |
| Pain | Bone changes, joint changes, potential renal colic and pruritus |
| Urinary elimination pattern, altered | Polyuria |
| Activity intolerance | Muscular weakness, decreased cardiac output associated with changes in electrical activity of heart |
| Nutrition, altered: less than body requirements | Anorexia, nausea, vomiting |
| Constipation | Decrease in GI motility |
| Knowledge deficit: immediate treatment, diagnostic tests, surgery, follow-up, long-term treatment | New problem and treatment with no previous exposure to information |
| **For patients after surgery** | |
| Breathing pattern, ineffective | Tracheal obstruction associated with spasm of vocal cords or hemorrhage, laryngeal stridor associated with low serum calcium level |

| Diagnostic Title | Possible Etiologic Factors |
|---|---|
| Injury (trauma), high risk for | Hemorrhage, increased neuromuscular excitability associated with low serum calcium level |
| Knowledge deficit: follow-up care after surgery | No previous exposure to information |

## ♦ EXPECTED PATIENT OUTCOMES

Expected patient outcomes for the patient with PHPT include but are not limited to the following:

1. Reports no injuries; falls or dislodged arterial lines do not occur.
2. Maintains cardiac output, as evidenced by stable blood pressure; dysrhythmias or ECG changes are detected.
3. States that pain reduction measures are effective; activities or self-care is not limited because of pain; signs of renal colic (bloody urine, pain, nausea) do not occur.
4. Activity level does not decrease any further; gradually increases activity, as evidenced by more ambulation.
5. Maintains normal nutritional status, as evidenced by maintenance of weight or, if necessary, a return to normal weight, with a gain of 1 to 2 lb/week; the patient eats 75% to 100% of every meal.
6. Maintains normal patterns of bowel elimination (as established by assessment).
7. Output equals intake and is at least 2000 ml/day.
8. Patient and significant others:
   a. Describe the disease accurately, how signs and symptoms relate to the disease, and how the disease will alter ADL.
   b. Describe the purpose of each diagnostic test and special pretest and posttest requirements.
   c. Explain the following:
      (1) Dietary regimen and plans to implement the regimen
      (2) Medications: knowledge about the drug and administration
      (3) Measures to relieve signs and symptoms, as appropriate
      (4) Plans for follow-up care

## ♦ INTERVENTIONS

Care of the patient varies depending on the treatment. This section describes the care during the acute preoperative period for patients treated medically. Nursing management of the postoperative patient is discussed at the end of this section.

### Promoting Safety

PHPT may increase the likelihood of the patient being injured in a fall because of weakness or because of changes in mental status. If altered mental functioning is present, patients are placed in an environment where they can be observed closely, measures to increase orientation are used, and side rails are kept up. Soft restraints may be necessary but should be the last alternative.

If weakness is a factor, the patient must be assisted when up, have nonskid slippers for ambulation, and be provided with a room that is free of unnecessary equipment. A gradual increase in activity or the incorporation of isometric exercise may increase endurance. A physical therapist may be helpful in planning an exercise strengthening program.

### Maintaining Cardiac Function

Hypercalcemia associated with PHPT presents a risk for decreased cardiac functioning. The patient is monitored frequently (every 2 to 4 hours) to detect early signs and is instructed to report any episodes of palpitations or vertigo. If dysfunction occurs, the patient may need to be placed on continuous cardiac monitoring. The patient receiving digitalis therapy is monitored closely for digitalis toxicity because the myocardium is unusually sensitive to digitalis in the presence of hypercalcemia. The dose may be decreased.

### Promoting Comfort

The exact cause of patient discomfort must be identified. If bone or joint pain is present, proper positioning, support of joints and body parts, and gentleness in moving the patient are required. If renal colic is the cause of pain, the pain is severe and narcotics are necessary for relief; their effectiveness must be documented. Measures are taken to relieve pruritis as necessary (see Chapter 67); antihistamines or mild tranquilizers may be required.

### Promoting Urinary Elimination

The first intervention for alteration in urinary elimination is to increase the patient's fluid intake, which will decrease the urinary mineral concentration and thus decrease urinary stone formation. A fluid intake of at least 3 L/day should be the goal unless other physiologic alterations such as cardiac or renal problems are present. Fluids are given throughout the 24 hours. The urine is strained through a gauze mesh to collect any small stones that pass, and the patient is monitored continually for recurrence of stone formation. Monitoring includes assessing intake and output and observing for presence of flank pain from renal colic, hematuria, and nausea and vomiting.

### Promoting Activity

The patient with PHPT may have activity intolerance and needs to be involved in some weight-bearing activities that provide bone stress. This helps lower serum calcium levels. Thus a schedule of progressive activities is planned with the patient. Activities are spaced so fatigue is lessened. Goals should be identified with the

**BOX 39-15 Foods High in Calcium**

| | |
|---|---|
| Almonds | 332 mg/1 cup |
| Blackstrap molasses | 137 mg/1 tbsp |
| Brazil nuts | 260 mg/1 cup |
| Broccoli spears | 132 mg/1 cup |
| Cabbage (cooked) | 220 mg/1 cup |
| Canned mackerel | 221 mg/3 oz |
| Cheese (blue cheese, cheddar, American) | About 100 to 150 mg/1 oz |
| Collards (cooked) | 289 mg/1 cup |
| Custard | 280 mg/1 cup |
| Dandelion greens (cooked) | 252 mg/1 cup |
| Egg | 27 mg/1 egg |
| Green beans | 80 mg/1 cup |
| Ice cream | 175 mg/1 cup |
| Ice milk | 292 mg/1 cup |
| Kale (cooked) | 147 mg/1 cup |
| Lima beans | 75 mg/1 cup |
| Macaroni (enriched) and cheese, baked | 398 mg/1 cup |
| Milk (whole, 2%, skim, buttermilk) | 290 mg/1 cup |
| Mustard greens (cooked) | 193 mg/1 cup |
| Oranges | 50 mg/1 orange |
| Oysters | 226 mg/1 cup |
| Peanut halves | 107 mg/1 cup |
| Pizza (cheese) | 107 mg/1 slice |
| Raisins | 124 mg/1 cup |
| Rhubarb (cooked) | 212 mg/1 cup |
| Salmon, pink, canned | 167 mg/3 oz |
| Sardines | 372 mg/3 oz |
| Spinach (drained solids) | 212 mg/1 cup |
| Turnip greens (cooked) | 250 mg/1 cup |
| White sauce, medium | 305 mg/1 cup |
| Yogurt | 295 mg/1 cup |

patient to provide motivation and encourage increased activity. Activities such as bathing may require assistance to conserve energy for ambulation.

### Promoting Nutrition

If a low-calcium diet is prescribed, a dietary consultation should be requested. A low-calcium diet is not ordered as frequently now as in the past (see p. 1247). The diet is monitored for foods high in calcium (Box 39-15), and those foods are avoided. This may help decrease the hypercalcemia. The nurse should note that very few groups of food are high in calcium. Anorexia is often present, and measures such as environmental control of noxious stimuli, providing rest, and giving oral hygiene are taken to encourage the person to eat.

### Promoting Bowel Elimination

The patient's bowel movements are monitored because constipation is a major problem. Fluids, dietary fiber, and ambulation are increased for prevention of constipation (see Chapter 47). If preventive measures are ineffective, stool softeners or laxatives may be prescribed by the physician.

### Facilitating Learning

1. Assess knowledge of disease, diagnostic tests, therapeutic measures, barriers to learning, and information patient wants.
2. Provide dietary instruction about calcium, as needed, and help patient/family plan ways of meeting dietary requirements.
3. Teach patient about medication therapy (specify): name, purpose, dosage, side effects, signs and symptoms to report immediately, and special administration requirements. Provide written instructions as needed.
4. Assess ability to perform skills of prescribed regimen (specify); provide teaching and multiple opportunities for practice and return demonstration.
5. Refer to community agencies (specify type) as needed, or provide patient/family with necessary information.
6. Clarify patient/family understanding about need and plans for follow-up care.

Teaching can help the patient cope more effectively with changes that are occurring. Frequent reexplanations may be required for the person with altered mental functioning.

The family is included in the teaching. Because the patient's condition can be critical and may change rapidly, it may be helpful to plan with the family for daily formalized updates. Patients receiving medical therapy need instructions regarding comfort measures, safety, diet, activities, increased fluid intake, prevention of constipation, medications, and planned follow-up. Much of the care the patient required as an inpatient must be provided at home. Written and verbal instructions are helpful.

Patients who have undergone surgery need the general teaching described in Chapter 23.

### Providing Postoperative Care

Most patients with PHPT are treated surgically. Postoperatively, the care requirements are very similar to those required after thyroidectomy (see p. 1243). Potential physiologic complications include hemorrhage, hypocalcemia, and airway obstruction. The patient's fluid volume, neurologic, respiratory, and cardiovascular states are monitored routinely. The serum calcium level will decrease within 24 hours, and the patient is monitored for tetany. Parathyroid function usually returns to normal within 5 to 7 days after a partial parathyroidectomy because the remaining tissue resumes normal functioning.

If mild hypocalcemia occurs, calcium is replaced orally. Severe hypocalcemia can occur if there has been extensive bone demineralization. With the removal of the elevated PTH, the calcium-deficient bones extract larger-than-normal quantities of calcium from the extracellular fluids. For patients with severe hypocalcemia, calcium chloride or calcium gluconate is given intravenously. These calcium preparations should be readily available for immediate administration if necessary. If permanent hypoparathyroidism results because the remaining tissue does not resume normal secretion or because a total parathyroidectomy is done, the patient will need continued treatment.

The Guidelines box below outlines postoperative care after surgery of the parathyroid gland.

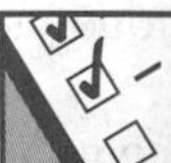

**Guidelines for Care of the Person After Parathyroidectomy**

**ASSESSMENT**

1. Monitor vital signs q 2-4 hr.
2. Monitor quality of voice and presence or absence of stridor, complaints of dyspnea, and choking sensation q 1 hr for 8 hours, then q 2 hr for 4 to 8 hours, and then q 4 hr.
3. Monitor serum calcium levels, presence of signs of tetany and paresthesias.

**NURSING DIAGNOSES**

1. Breathing pattern, ineffective: tracheal obstruction associated with spasm of vocal cords or hemorrhage, laryngeal stridor associated with low serum calcium
2. Injury (trauma), high risk for: hemorrhage, increased neuromuscular excitability associated with low serum calcium level
3. Knowledge deficit (follow-up care after surgery): no previous exposure to information

**EXPECTED PATIENT OUTCOMES**

1. Maintains adequate air exchange, as evidenced by adequate breath sounds throughout lung field, ABGs within normal range, and absence of signs of respiratory distress.
2. No injuries occur; shows no undetected changes in vital signs or neuromuscular excitability.
3. Patient and significant others can:
   a. Describe reason for frequent vital signs and neurologic assessments.
   b. Describe symptoms they should report immediately.
   c. Describe plans for follow-up care.

**INTERVENTIONS**

1. Have a tracheostomy set and IV calcium preparations readily available.
2. Report any sign of hemorrhage, hypocalcemia, or airway obstruction.
3. Provide a safe environment appropriate to assess mental status and weakness.
4. Encourage deep breathing, coughing, and turning q 2-4 hr.
5. Increase ambulation at patient's tolerance; take into account mental status and weakness.
6. Maintain fluid intake at prescribed level or enough to achieve 1000 ml or more if serum calcium levels are normal, 2000 ml or more if they are higher.
7. Teach patient and significant others about:
   a. Prescribed drugs
   b. Prescribed diet, if any
   c. Electrolyte replacement, if any
   d. Fluid intake requirements
   e. Wound care
   f. Symptoms to report: those indicating infection, hypocalcemia, or hypercalcemia
   g. Follow-up care requirements

## ♦ EVALUATION

To evaluate the effectiveness of nursing interventions, compare patient behaviors with those stated in the expected patient outcomes. Successful achievement of patient outcomes for the patient with PHTH is indicated by the following:

1. Reports no injuries.
2. Maintains stable blood pressure within acceptable parameters.
3. Reports no episodes of flank pain, bloody urine, or bone pain.
4. Maintains activity level at baseline or increases.
5. Maintains weight at desired or prescribed level.
6. Reports bowel pattern restored to preillness level and no rectal or abdominal discomfort.
7. Output equals intake and is at least 2000 ml/24 hours.
8. Patient and significant others describe disease and effects on ADL and explain medication and dietary regimens.

For patients after surgery:

1. Breath sounds are clear; if available, ABGs are within normal range.
2. Blood pressure, pulse, and respiratory rate remain within specific parameters that are normal for patient.
3. Explanations of symptoms, treatment, and needed follow-up care are accurate.

## SECONDARY AND TERTIARY HYPERPARATHYROIDISM

### Etiology/Epidemiology

*Secondary hyperparathyroidism* is a disease characterized by excessive production of PTH resulting from chronic hypocalcemia. *Malabsorption* and *chronic renal failure* are two common causes of secondary hyperparathyroidism. *Tertiary hyperparathyroidism* is the result of long-standing secondary hyperparathyroidism. It is characterized by the development of autonomous parathyroid gland functioning that is not under normal homeostatic control mechanisms. When tertiary hyperparathyroidism occurs, the patient with chronic renal failure or malabsorption syndrome will develop *hypercalcemia*. In many instances, with removal of the chronic stimulus of hypocalcemia to the parathyroid gland, the hyperplasia will regress.

### Pathophysiology

In these conditions the calcium level is chronically low. In chronic renal failure the low calcium results from *hyperphosphatemia*, a decrease in production of activated vitamin D, and a decrease in calcium absorption. There also may be a decreased sensitivity of the bones to the action of PTH.[40] The low calcium level is a chronic stimulus to the parathyroid glands and results in their hyperplasia. The hyperplasia and excessive production of PTH are usually able to keep the calcium level close to normal, but at the expense of bone destruction. The bone lesions are characterized by osteomalacia, osteosclerosis, and osteitis fibrosa cystica.

## Medical Management

Treatment for secondary hyperparathyroidism is directed at decreasing the chronic stimulation of the parathyroid gland by improving the calcium level. In patients with malabsorption, calcium supplements and vitamin D are used. In patients with chronic renal failure, the treatment is first directed toward (1) lowering the phosphorus level with a phosphorus-depleting agent such as aluminum hydroxide or calcium carbonate and (2) increasing the calcium level with calcium and vitamin D supplementation. There is concern about using aluminum hydroxide over a long time because of toxicity in the bone.[42] If medical therapy does not lower the phosphorus level and thus elevate the calcium level and halt the chronic stimulation of the parathyroid gland and the bone destruction, a subtotal parathyroidectomy may be done.

If a single adenoma is the problem, it is removed. With hyperplasia, usually three complete glands and part of the fourth are removed. In hyperplasia a total parathyroidectomy sometimes is performed, with transplantation of some parathyroid tissue into the muscle of the forearm to avoid loss of function of the residual tissue in the neck resulting from vascular failure, which is a complication of surgery.

If no abnormal glands are found during the exploration of the neck, the search may be extended into the retroesophageal and retropharyngeal spaces to search for ectopic glandular tissue. Later surgical exploration may be necessary if no abnormal tissue is found during the initial surgery. This latter surgery is only carried out after instituting localizing procedures. Subsequent surgery may require mediastinal exploration.

Serum calcium levels decline within 24 hours after successful surgery, and subnormal levels may be present for 4 to 5 days. Severe postoperative hypocalcemia may occur. The hypocalcemia may result from "hungry bone syndrome," which causes an increase in new bone formation. This syndrome is treated with calcium replacement. Most patients develop hypocalcemia because of temporary hypoparathyroidism. This is also treated with calcium replacement and usually resolves in 1 week. If permanent hypoparathyroidism occurs, the patient is treated as described on p. 1252.

The usual treatment for tertiary hyperparathyroidism is to prevent complications of hypercalcemia by hydration, diuretics, and restriction of calcium intake, until the gland returns to normal. In some patients the glandular hyperplasia does not regress, and a partial parathyroidectomy is necessary.

## Nursing Management

The care for patients who undergo partial parathyroidectomies for secondary or tertiary hyperparathyroidism is the same as for patients who have partial parathyroidectomies for primary hyperparathyroidism. Nurses have a major role in helping patients with malabsorption syndrome or chronic renal failure to follow prescribed regimens so that secondary or tertiary hyperparathyroidism is prevented. Nursing management of the patient undergoing surgery of the parathyroid gland is discussed in the previous section.

# HYPOSECRETION OF PARATHYROID HORMONE: HYPOPARATHYROIDISM

## Etiology/Epidemiology

The causative factors of true **hypoparathyroidism** may be classified into three major categories: surgically induced, idiopathic, and functional.[42] Hypoparathyroidism occurs mainly from trauma of the anterior neck during surgery, particularly thyroid surgery, parathyroid surgery, or radical neck surgery. In rare instances, hypoparathyroidism may result from radioactive iodine therapy for hyperthyroidism of thyroid cancer. *Idiopathic* hypoparathyroidism is deficient hormone production from unknown causes. It may be seen at an early age and is probably the result of a genetic defect. There may be an autoimmune basis for early-age idiopathic hypoparathyroidism because many of these persons have abnormal antibodies directed against the parathyroid gland.[42] Late-onset idiopathic hypoparathyroidism has no known cause. *Functional* hypoparathyroidism is the result of chronic hypomagnesemia, which may be seen in malabsorption or alcoholism and appears to impair PTH release.

In *pseudohypoparathyroidism* the secretion and release of PTH are normal, but there is target tissue resistance to PTH. The cause of the resistance is unknown.

## Pathophysiology

A deficiency of or tissue resistance to PTH results in decreased bone resorption, decreased activation of vitamin D (and thus decreased intestinal absorption of calcium), increased renal excretion of calcium, and decreased renal excretion of phosphorus. The result is hypocalcemia and hyperphosphatemia. The major physiologic alterations result from the effects of low calcium levels on neuromuscular irritability. Nerves show decreased thresholds of excitation, repeated responses to a single stimuli, and, in severe cases, continuous activity or muscular spasms **(tetany).** Cardiac activity is altered. Calcification of basal ganglia and the lens of the eye may occur.

The severity of the hypocalcemia and the chronicity of the problem dictate the signs and symptoms seen with *true hypoparathyroidism.* In mild cases, which result in only mildy decreased serum calcium levels, the patient may be asymptomatic. In more severe cases, any or all of the clinical manifestations listed in Box 39-16 may be seen.

The patient with pseudohypoparathyroidism may have the same signs and symptoms as seen with true hypoparathyroidism. In addition, such patients may have

**BOX 39-16 True Hypoparathyroidism: Clinical Manifestations**

1. Neuromuscular manifestations: changes in nerve activity affect peripheral motor and sensory nerves
   a. Numbness and tingling (paresthesia) around mouth, tips of fingers, and sometimes in the feet
   b. Tetany with positive Chvostek's and Trousseau's signs (see Chapter 38), spasms of wrists, fingers, and forearms or feet and toes
   c. Convulsions that may consist of tonic spasms of the total body or the more typical tonic-clonic activity
   d. Laryngeal stridor and dyspnea
   e. Other neurologic signs: headache, papilledema, elevated cerebrospinal fluid (CSF) pressure, local signs that mimic a cerebral tumor; extrapyramidal neurologic signs and symptoms, including gait changes, tremors, rigidity, and spasms; possible signs and symptoms of parkinsonism (see Chapter 57)
2. Emotional-mental manifestations: irritability, depression, anxiety, emotional lability, memory impairment, confusion, frank psychosis
3. Cardiovascular manifestations (effect of hypocalcemia)
   a. Prolonged QT and ST intervals and occasional dysrhythmias
   b. Resistance to effects of digitalis preparations
   c. Decreased cardiac output from congestive heart failure
4. Eye manifestations (calcification of lens)
   a. Cataract formation
   b. Eventual loss of all sight
5. Dental manifestations (depending on age of onset)
   a. Enamel defects seen on the tooth crown
   b. Delayed or absent tooth eruption
   c. Defective dental root formation
6. Integumentary manifestations: fragile nails, thin patchy hair, dry scaly skin, skin infections (usually candidiasis), vitiligo
7. GI manifestations: malabsorption, steatorrhea

skeletal and developmental abnormalities, including short stature, round face, short neck, stocky body, and discrete bone lesions. The most common bone lesion is unilateral or bilateral shortening of the fourth and fifth metacarpal and metatarsal bones. Mental retardation may also be present. The patient has low serum calcium and high serum phosphorus with normal to high PTH level on radioimmunoassay.

### Medical Management

The first priority of treatment is correction of calcium levels to prevent tetany. This is achieved by giving IV calcium gluconate or calcium chloride. Airway patency must be maintained. Maintenance of a calcium level of about 7 mg/dl usually prevents signs and symptoms such as laryngeal stridor and convulsions.

The cause of hypoparathyroidism is then identified, and long-term therapy is started as soon as possible. Normal serum calcium levels are maintained by supplemental dietary and elemental calcium, by dietary phosphate restriction and phosphate-binding agents such as aluminum hydroxide, and by vitamin D therapy to increase GI absorption of calcium. Vitamin D preparations include ergocalciferol (Drisdol, Geltabs), dihydrotachysterol (Hytakerol), or the cholecalciferol metabolites calcifediol (Calderol) or calcitriol (Rocaltrol).

It takes several weeks before the full effect of vitamin D therapy is seen. Major complications of therapy are vitamin D toxicity and renal calculi formation. Renal calculi can occur in the hypoparathyroid patient even in the presence of normal serum calcium because the lack of PTH results in excessive urinary calcium excretion. The patient is monitored at 6- to 12-month intervals to evaluate the effectiveness of treatment and to assess for side effects.

## NURSING MANAGEMENT

### ♦ ASSESSMENT

Assessment focuses on identifying signs and symptoms of hypocalcemia and on identifying the patient's and significant others' knowledge level regarding the altered health state.

#### Subjective Data

Data to be collected to assess the patient with hypoparathyroidism include the following:

Neuromuscular/emotional-mental status: history of paresthesia, episodes of spasms in extremities, convulsions, and changes in behavior, mood, memory, or orientation

Cardiovascular status: complaints of palpitations, syncope, edema

Eyes: history of visual changes

Integumentary status: changes in pigmentation, reports of skin dryness or hair loss

Knowledge level: disease process, relationship of signs and symptoms and functional changes to disease, medical therapy

#### Objective Data

Data to be collected to assess the patient with hypoparathyroidism include the following:

Neuromuscular/emotional-mental status: Chvostek's and Trousseau's signs, affect, memory, orientation

Cardiovascular status: blood pressure, pulse rate and rhythms, heart sounds, presence of edema, weight

Eyes: visual acuity

Teeth: abnormal dentation (lack of eruption, enamel defects)

Integumentary status: pigmentation, presence of infection, hair loss

Musculoskeletal status: height, body proportions, hand defects (shortened fourth and fifth fingers)

#### Diagnostic Test Findings

Laboratory tests for the patient with hypoparathyroidism may show the following findings (see Chapter 38 and p. 1246):

1. Decreased serum calcium and increased serum phosphate levels
2. Low to undetectable levels of PTH by radioimmunoassay
3. Low basal levels of urinary cAMP and increased levels after exogenous PTH administration.

## ♦ NURSING DIAGNOSES

Nursing diagnoses are determined from analysis of patient data. Nursing diagnoses for the person with hypoparathyroidism may include but are not limited to the following:

| Diagnostic Title | Possible Etiologic Factors |
|---|---|
| Anxiety | Uncontrollability or alarming quality of signs and symptoms |
| Breathing patterns, ineffective | Obstruction to air exchange associated with laryngeal spasm, hyperventilation caused by anxiety |
| Cardiac output, decreased | Impaired electrical activity and contractility associated with low serum calcium level |
| Injury (trauma), high risk for | Altered mental status associated with tetany |
| Knowledge deficit: disease, diagnostic tests, treatment, side effects, follow-up | New diagnoses and no previous exposure to information |
| Sensory/perceptual alterations: visual | Calcification of lens |

## ♦ EXPECTED PATIENT OUTCOMES

Expected patient outcomes for the person with hypoparathyroidism may include but are not limited to the following:

1. Shows no signs of anxiety, such as restlessness, constant motion, or jitteriness.
2. Maintains adequate air exchange, as confirmed by adequate ABGs; stridor and dyspnea are absent.
3. Maintains blood pressure; undetected dysrhythmias do not occur.
4. Reports no injuries from convulsions or undetected tetany.
5. Patient and significant others can explain planned diagnostic tests and treatments, long-term therapy and follow-up, and self-monitoring for signs of tetany or hypercalcemia.
6. Maintains independent activities.

## ♦ INTERVENTIONS

Nursing care includes dealing with anxiety; monitoring and intervening to prevent respiratory distress, cardiac dysfunction, or injury; and patient education.

### Controlling Anxiety

The alarming quality of the signs and symptoms of hypoparathyroidism and hypocalcemia can provoke great anxiety and alter breathing patterns. A major intervention is to establish confidence in the patient that the nurse understands the patient's physical status, understands the symptoms, and is available. The patient should be placed in a room so the nurses' station is visible. The patient's call light should be answered promptly. The nurse needs to follow up on any patient complaint. *Hyperventilation,* which can accompany anxiety, worsens the hypocalcemia because hyperventilation causes respiratory alkalosis, which in turn causes more of the ionized calcium to bind to serum protein. The decrease in ionized calcium exacerbates symptoms of hypocalcemia. Thus the patient should be supported to prevent hyperventilation. Keeping patients informed of their serum calcium levels will also help them feel in control and may lessen anxiety.

### Monitoring/Supporting/Preventing Injury

A routine schedule for monitoring is developed, and monitoring may need to be done as frequently as every hour. Parameters to monitor include the following:

1. Chvostek's and Trousseau's signs (see Chapter 38)
2. Airway patency
3. Mental status: orientation
4. Emotional status: anxiety, irritability
5. Vital signs, particularly pulse rate and rhythm

Any abnormal changes that are detected are reported immediately so that treatment can be instituted and convulsions prevented. The initiation of maintenance therapy does not immediately correct the physiology problem, and therapy is adjusted to maintain a normal serum calcium level without complications. Monitoring is continued during this period of adjustment or with any future changes.

A high priority for care is the maintenance of a safe environment. Seizure precautions such as padded bed rails, suctioning equipment, a tracheostomy tray, and IV calcium must be readily available. The patient should be in a room that facilitates easy and frequent observation.

If visual changes are present, the environment is structured to allow the patient to function as independently as possible. If confusion or memory deficits are present, the patient is reoriented frequently. The room should be free of clutter. A chest restraint may be necessary.

### Preparing for Discharge

The potential convulsions and spasms and the necessity for diagnostic tests and frequent monitoring need to be explained to the patient and significant others. The nurse must explain the relationships among the signs and symptoms, tests, monitoring, the disease, and each new intervention. Patient teaching includes the following:

1. Nature of the disease and need for long-term therapy
2. Medication administration
   a. Prescribed calcium, phosphate-binding agents, and vitamin D to be taken daily
   b. Monitor for signs of:

(1) Ineffective treatment: recurrence of tetany
(2) Signs of hypercalcemia: thirst, polyuria, lethargy, decreased muscle tone, constipation
(3) Complications: renal stones (flank pain or pain radiating down into groin)

3. Need for continual follow-up care every 6 to 12 months
4. Dietary changes: increased calcium and decreased phosphorus

## ♦ EVALUATION

To evaluate the effectiveness of nursing interventions, compare patient behaviors with those stated in the expected patient outcomes. Successful achievement of patient outcomes for the person with hypoparathyroidism is indicated by the following:

1. Reports no episode of restlessness or constant motion or jitteriness and has no complaints of paresthesias.
2. Demonstrates no respiratory stridor and has no complaint of dyspnea.
3. Maintains blood pressure within established parameters for patient.
4. Reports no convulsive activity.
5. Patient and significant others explain how treatment controls disorders and symptoms.
6. Initiates increasing number of ADL.

# ADRENAL GLAND

The *adrenal cortex* is essential to life. Without the hormones cortisol and aldosterone, the body's metabolic processes respond inadequately to even minimal physical and emotional stressors such as changes in temperature, exercise, or excitement. More severe stressors such as serious infections, surgery, or extreme anxiety may result in shock and death.

The *adrenal medulla* is not essential to life because the sympathetic nervous system produces similar although slower responses. Dysfunction of the adrenal gland can be manifested as an increased or decreased function of the cortex or increased function of the medulla (Figure 39-8).

## HYPERFUNCTION OF THE ADRENAL CORTEX: CORTISOL EXCESS

### Etiology

Excessive levels of glucocorticoids, whatever the cause, result in a constellation of symptoms known as **Cushing's syndrome.** The causes of Cushing's syndrome may be divided into three major groups.

1. Primary Cushing's syndrome: excessive cortisol production resulting from adrenal adenomas or carcinomas; also called *adrenal Cushing's syndrome*
2. Secondary Cushing's syndrome: excessive cortisol production resulting from adrenal hyperplasia because of excessive ACTH production. The excessive ACTH production may result from either:
   a. Increased release of ACTH from the pituitary gland because of pituitary or hypothalamic problems; also called **Cushing's disease** or *pituitary Cushing's syndrome*
   b. Increased release of ACTH from ectopic nonpituitary sites such as bronchogenic carcinoma, pancreatic carcinoma, and bronchial adenoma; also called *ectopic Cushing's syndrome*
3. *Iatrogenic Cushing's syndrome:* excessive cortisol levels resulting from chronic glucocorticoid therapy

### Epidemiology

Ten million Americans receive glucocorticoid therapy each year. Although estimates of iatrogenic Cushing's syndrome are imprecise, it is the most common cause of cortical excess. The second highest incidence of cortisol excess occurs with *ectopic ACTH syndrome,* estimated at 660 cases per 1 million persons per year. This

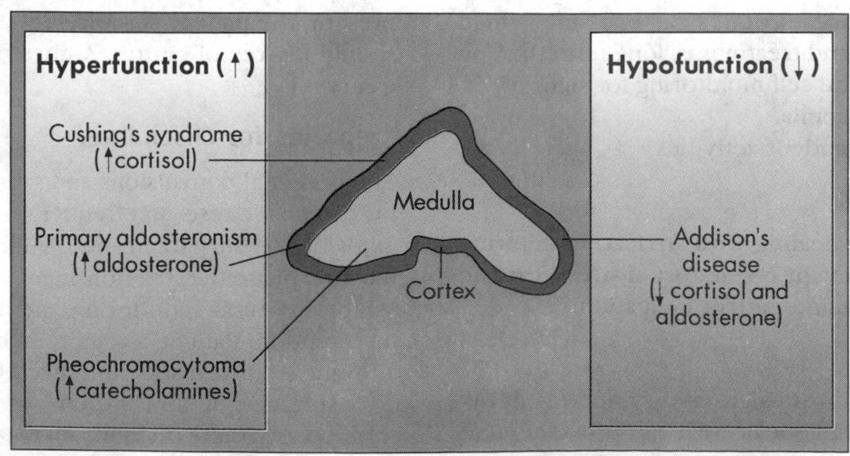


**FIGURE 39-8** Adrenal gland dysfunctions.

high incidence is attributed to patients with small cell lung cancer. One percent of patients with lung cancer have ectopic ACTH syndrome.[40] In the past, ectopic ACTH syndrome was found more often in men than women; this pattern is changing as women smokers increase. The incidence of Cushing's disease (ACTH-dependent cortisol excess) is estimated at 5 to 25 cases per 1 million persons per year. Women have a higher incidence than men of Cushing's disease, which occurs most frequently in women 25 to 45 years of age. The incidence of adrenal tumors is also higher in women than men (four to five times). There is no known explanation for the gender differences.

## Pathophysiology

The major result of Cushing's syndrome is excessive production of cortisol. Early in the noniatrogenic disorders, the most prominent alteration is loss of the normal diurnal secretory pattern. With loss of the diurnal pattern, the morning level of cortisol production may not be abnormally elevated, but levels during the day do not show the normal decrease below the morning peak. At later stages, cortisol is elevated at all times.

The pathophysiologic factors associated with cortisol excess primarily result from exaggeration in all the known actions of glucocorticoids and include alterations in the following:

**TABLE 39-11 Hypersecretion of Glucocorticoids, Aldosterone, and Androgens (Cushing's Syndrome, CS): Normal Function, Pathophysiologic Alterations, and Clinical Manifestations**

| NORMAL FUNCTION | PATHOPHYSIOLOGIC ALTERATIONS | CLINICAL MANIFESTATIONS |
|---|---|---|
| **GLUCOCORTICOIDS** | | |
| Organic metabolism<br>Protein catabolism<br>Gluconeogenesis<br>Changes peripheral tissue sensitivity to insulin<br>Role in maintenance of blood glucose | Increased catabolism of protein (including bone matrix) and of fats: in particular, lipolysis and mobilization of fats<br>Increased blood glucose from glycogenolysis and gluconeogenesis | Hyperglycemia, onset of worsening of diabetes: osteoporosis, muscle wasting, purple striae, poor wound healing, easily bruised<br>Appearance: moon face, buffalo hump, central obesity, thin musculature |
| Negative feedback on secretion of ACTH | Variable effects on hypothalamic-pituitary-adrenal (HPA) axis: primary disease—suppression of ACTH; secondary (ACTH-dependent) and ectopic CS—increased ACTH and melanocyte-stimulating hormone (MSH) | Hyperpigmentation seen in ACTH-dependent CS |
| Potentiate response to catecholamines | Increased catecholamine sensitivity; vasoconstriction increases peripheral resistance<br>In combination with alterations of aldosterone excess (see below), increases workload of heart | Hypertension and manifestations of altered aldosterone excess (see below) |
| Antiinflammation and immunosuppression | Increased susceptibility to infection, impaired localization (fibrin deposition) of infection | Increased incidence of infections, suppression of local signs of infection: redness, heat, edema, pain |
| Maintain emotional stability | Emotional instability | Mood swings, anxiety, depression, low tolerance for frustration; possible psychoses |
| Maintain fluid and electrolyte balance: effects similar to aldosterone (see below) | In ACTH-dependent CS, increased aldosterone secretion (see below); in primary CS, possibly minimal effects | Manifestations similar to those of aldosterone excess (see below) |
| Some androgenic effects | In ACTH-dependent CS with adrenal hyperplasia, excess of androgens present (see below) | Effects: clinical manifestations of androgen excess (see below) |
| **ALDOSTERONE** | | |
| Renin-angiotensin system is major controller of production.<br>Aldosterone acts at kidney tubules, particularly distal nephrons, to increase sodium reabsorption with consequent expansion of intravascular and extracellular fluid volume.<br>Potassium excretion is increased. | Abnormal increase in sodium and water retention; increased potassium excretion, hypervolemia, and increased cardiac output; cardiovascular effects heightened when combined with catecholamine effects (see above) | Hypertension, hypokalemia, edema; potential for dysrhythmias and congestive heart failure |
| **ANDROGENS** | | |
| Some role in establishment and maintenance of secondary sexual characteristics | Androgen excess; in ACTH-dependent CS with adrenal hyperplasia, excess androgen secretion present | Effects: clinical manifestations of androgens; in females, hirsutism and virilization |

1. Protein, fat, and carbohydrate metabolism
2. Inflammatory and immune response
3. Water and mineral metabolism
4. Emotional stability
5. Red blood cell (RBC) and platelet levels

Excessive cortisol may also disturb secretion of other anterior pituitary hormones (prolactin, thyrotropin, LH, GH) and alterations in sleep patterns. Some of these alterations may contribute to the clinical picture.[40]

In many instances, cortisol excess is also associated with excessive production of androgen; this results in virilization in females. Adrenal tumors may secrete cortisol, androgens, and mineralocorticoids in various proportions. Depending on which hormone is produced in excess, the patient will have (1) the clinical picture associated with Cushing's syndrome, (2) only the effects of androgen excess, (3) a clinical picture similar to that for hyperaldosteronism, or (4) any combination of these three.

Table 39-11 lists the normal function, pathophysiologic alterations in function, and clinical manifestations of excess corticosteroids. Box 39-17 presents the clin-

**BOX 39-17 Pathophysiologic Alterations in Corticosteroid Excess**

### ALTERATION IN PROTEIN, FAT, AND CARBOHYDRATE METABOLISM

#### Altered Protein Metabolism

Excessive catabolism of proteins results in loss of muscle mass, causing following symptoms:

1. Muscle wasting, particularly of extremities, resulting in thin arms and legs, difficulty getting up from low chairs, difficulty climbing stairs, or generalized weakness and fatigue
2. Depletion of protein matrix of bone, resulting in osteoporosis, compression fractures of spine, backache, bone pain, and pathologic fractures
3. Loss of collagen support of skin, resulting in thin, fragile skin that bruises easily, ecchymosis at trauma sites, and pink to purple cutaneous striae
4. Poor wound healing

#### Altered Fat Metabolism

Changes in fat metabolism cause obesity, with abnormal deposition of fat in face producing *moon face* (Figure 39-9), in intrascapular area producing the *buffalo hump,* and in mesenteric bed producing *truncal obesity*. Redistribution of fat with these characteristic features may be seen in patients without obesity. Body weight usually is increased.

#### Altered Carbohydrate Metabolism

Increased hepatic gluconeogenesis and impaired insulin use result in postprandial hyperglycemia and occasionally frank diabetes mellitus with all its signs and symptoms (see Chapter 40). Patients with concurrent diabetes mellitus may have worsening of signs and symptoms of their diabetes.

### ALTERATION IN INFLAMMATORY AND IMMUNE RESPONSE

Cortisol excess results in decreased lymphocytes, particularly T lymphocytes; decreased cell-mediated immunity; increased neutrophils; and altered antibody activity. These changes make persons particularly vunerable to viral and fungal infections. Depression in inflammatory and immune responsiveness results in opportunistic infections such as *Pneumocystis carinii* or other fungal infections. Early signs of infection, such as fever, may not be seen. Poor wound healing may also be related to infections.

### ALTERATIONS IN WATER AND MINERAL METABOLISM

Cortisol itself possesses mineralocorticoid activity; therefore, cortisol excess results in characteristic signs and symptoms of increased mineralocorticoid activity even though level of aldosterone is normal. These include the following:

1. Sodium and water retention, which may accentuate body weight increase and may cause edema; serum sodium usually normal.
2. Hypertension, which is found in almost every patient with excessive cortisol and may be caused by increased volume or by increased sensitivity of arterioles to circulating catecholamines
3. Hypokalemia, hypochloremia, and metabolic alkalosis if cortisol excess is severe because of increased excretion of potassium and chloride (most often seen with ectopic Cushing's syndrome)
4. Increased calcium resorption from the bones and renal calculi from hypercalciuria (resulting in renal colic)

### ALTERATION IN EMOTIONAL STABILITY

Various emotional changes may occur: from irritability and anxiety, to mild depression and poor concentration and memory, to severe depression and psychosis. Euphoria and sleep disorders are frequently noted.

### HEMATOLOGIC ALTERATIONS

Various changes in blood components, which occur as the result of excessive cortisol:

1. High to normal RBC count, hemoglobin, and hematocrit (may account in part for facial plethora [appearance of increased facial circulation])
2. Leukocytosis, lymphopenia, eosinopenia
3. Increases in various clotting factors and platelets, resulting in thromboembolic phenomena

### EXCESSIVE ANDROGEN ACTIVITY

If excessive androgens are present, female patient exhibits virilization, which includes following signs:

1. Hirsutism, manifested as fine, downy coat of hair on face and total body
2. Loss of scalp hair
3. Acne
4. Changes in menstrual cycle, varying from irregularities to oligomenorrhea to amenorrhea
5. Changes in libido

### OTHER FINDINGS

Hyperpigmentation may be present and indicates elevation of ACTH, usually from ectopic site. ACTH has melanotrophic activity. Hyperpigmentation is seen on skin and mucous membranes.

ical manifestations according to the ways in which they alter the patient's normal adrenocortical physiologic status.

## Prevention

### Primary prevention

Most causes of excessive cortisol production are not preventable except for the ectopic secretion of ACTH from bronchogenic carcinoma. Elimination of smoking would decrease the occurrence of bronchogenic carcinoma.

### Secondary prevention

No screening tests are available for secondary prevention. Evaluation of adrenal function depends on the clinical suspicion of the primary health care provider.

### Tertiary prevention

Tertiary preventive activities should be a major focus of nursing care. Nurses should help patients deal with their chronic health problems, carry out self-monitoring practices to identify exacerbations early, and maintain their therapeutic regimens. These practices help prevent progression of problems. One patient group of particular importance because of their large number is those receiving long-term glucocorticoid therapy. Through their patient educator roles, nurses can help patients maintain their therapy in the safest manner possible.

## Medical Management

The goal for discharge of patients with ectopic ACTH and bilateral adrenalectomy as determined by DRGs is 10.1 days. The nurse works collaboratively with the physician for implementation of prescribed medical therapy. Because the nurse has a major role in discharge planning and patient teaching, those are discussed under nursing management.

Medical management is directed toward identifying the cause of the problem and removing the cause of cortisol excess, if possible. In iatrogenic Cushing's syndrome, care is directed toward control of signs and symptoms if the chronic therapy cannot be terminated.

For patients with pituitary Cushing's syndrome resulting in adrenal hyperplasia, six therapeutic options are available (Table 39-12), although transsphenoidal removal of the pituitary tumor is the first line of therapy. When pituitary tumor removal is not possible or successful, other methods are used as adjunctive therapy.

For patients with the ectopic syndrome, the first line of therapy is to remove the source of the ectopic ACTH secretion. If this is not possible, drugs that inhibit cortisol production (Table 39-12) may be used. In some instances, when the site of ectopic ACTH cannot be found and the signs and symptoms cannot be controlled, bilateral adrenalectomy may be done.

For adrenal tumors, the treatment of choice is tumor removal. If the tumor is localized to one gland, a unilateral adrenalectomy is done. When there has been excessive cortisol production by one gland, the negative feedback has caused a decrease in ACTH and subsequent atrophy of the unaffected gland. Thus the patient needs glucocorticoid replacement therapy for some time until normal function of the other adrenal gland returns. If the adrenocortical tumors are bilateral, bilateral adrenalectomy is done, and the patient will receive lifetime hormone replacement therapy.

A

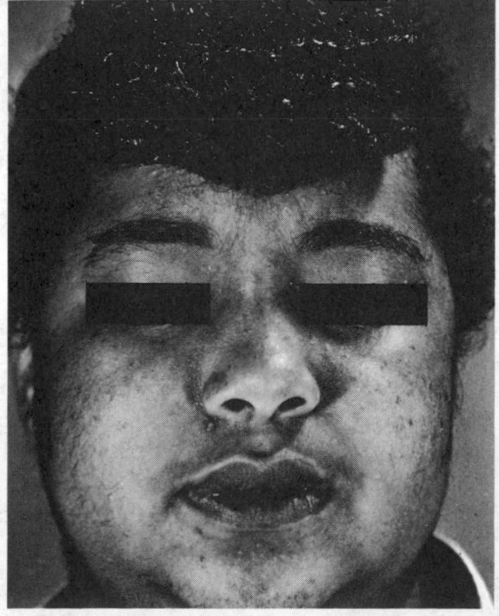

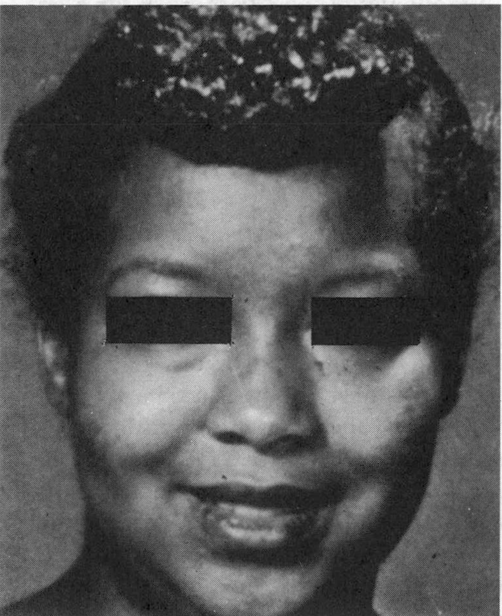

B

**FIGURE 39-9** Facial changes characteristic of increased cortisol hormone. **A,** Before treatment. **B,** Six months after treatment. (From Thibodeau GA, Anthony CP: *Structure and function of the body,* ed 8, St Louis, 1988, Mosby.)

**TABLE 39-12 Medical Management of Patients With Pituitary Cushing's Syndrome**

| TREATMENT | COMMENTS | COMPLICATIONS |
|---|---|---|
| Transsphenoidal adenectomy | First approach for pituitary tumors; preserves normal pituitary function; very successful for microadenomas; less successful for macroadenomas or invasive tumors | Complete recovery of gland requires a year or so; patients may require glucocorticoids for some time. |
| Transsphenoidal hypophysectomy | Gives 100% cure but removes total pituitary; may be used for invasive tumors or macroadenomas | Patient requires replacement therapy of glucocorticoids, thyroid hormone, gonadal steroids, and possibly ADH for life. |
| Radiation therapy by conventional methods, heavy particles of implants | Implants successful if no evidence of exact tumor found; conventional and heavy particle therapy used as adjunct to surgery | Complete remission not always possible; patient may develop hypopituitarism or damage to visual system. |
| Bilateral total adrenalectomy | Produces complete cure of signs and symptoms of cortisol excess; does not decrease ACTH | Replacement therapy of glucocorticoids and mineralocorticoids required for life; hyperpigmentation occurs because ACTH still elevated; visual problems result from a continually growing tumor (Nelson's syndrome). |
| Drug therapy (work at level of adrenal gland)<br>Aminoglutethimide (inhibits cholesterol synthesis)<br>Mitotane (inhibits cortisol production; can destroy gland)<br>Metyrapone (partially inhibits adrenal cortex steroid synthesis) | Used as adjunct to surgery of pituitary or radiation when complete remission not achieved; used for unresectable malignant tumors producing ACTH or unresectable adrenal carcinoma | All drugs have toxic effects; control symptoms but do not cure; can result in permanent adrenal insufficiency (mitotane); all patients require adrenal steroid replacement during therapy; patient can develop Nelson's syndrome because pituitary tumor remains. |
| Drug therapy (work at level of pituitary gland)<br>Cyproheptadine (serotonin antagonist that inhibits ACTH release) | Thus far used only in a few patients who have had recurrence after pituitary adenectomy | Effective only as long as drug is given; some patients show no response. |

### Diagnostic tests

Various diagnostic procedures are performed to confirm the diagnosis and differentiate among the various causes of cortisol excess. Positive test results, regardless of the cause, include the following (see Chapter 38 for a detailed discussion of these tests):

1. Elevated serum cortisol level or elevated excretion of urine-free cortisol
2. Elevated urinary levels of 17-ketogenic steroids (17-KGS) and 17-hydroxycorticosteroids (17-OHCS)
3. Loss of diurnal rhythms of cortisol production
4. Loss of suppression of endogenous cortisol with the normal and screening cortisone suppression tests
5. Abnormalities in serum electrolytes, chemistry, and hematology, as described earlier

Secondary Cushing's syndrome from either pituitary disease or diseases that cause ectopic ACTH secretion results in elevated plasma ACTH, whereas persons with primary Cushing's syndrome have ACTH levels too low to measure. Pituitary and ectopic Cushing's syndromes are differentiated by response to the high-level dexamethasone suppression test (2 mg dexamethasone given every 6 hours). Pituitary production of ACTH and thus of cortisol is suppressed with this high level of drug, whereas no suppression occurs in ectopic Cushing's syndrome. The presence of pituitary, ectopic, or adrenal tumors may be demonstrated by CT scans, ultrasound, and angiographic studies.

To analyze the results of the diagnostic tests accurately, various factors that cause false-positive results *must* be eliminated (Box 39-18).

### Medication

The previous discussion identified two classes of drugs used in treatment of cortisol excess: inhibitors of cortisol production and serotonin antagonists that may inhibit the release of ACTH (see Table 39-12).

### Treatment

Surgical intervention is a treatment option in some patients with cortisol excess. Surgical procedures include pituitary adenectomy or hypophysectomy, adrenal adenectomy, and unilateral or bilateral adrenalectomy. In addition, any of various surgeries might be involved in removing an ectopic source of ACTH or cortisol. Radiation therapy can be ablative to the pituitary or used as adjunctive therapy.

### Diet

Modifications of diet are prescribed according to individual patient needs. Common restrictions include calories, sodium, lipids, and cholesterol. Depending on

**BOX 39-18 Factors Causing False-Positive Tests for Cortisol Excess**

**Persons with acute or chronic illnesses:** acute stressors may result in high cortisol levels and abnormal dexamethasone tests; these tests must be repeated after patient's condition is stable.

**Obesity:** results in high levels of urinary 17-OHCS and 17-KGS and abnormal screening suppression tests, but urine-free cortisol, serum cortisol, and response to normal suppression test are normal.

**Pregnancy, estrogen therapy, and oral contraceptives:** elevated estrogen associated with these states can increase serum cortisol and give abnormal results on a screening cortisol suppression test, but urine-free cortisol and response to normal suppression test are normal.

**Alcoholism:** alcoholics may have both clinical and diagnostic characteristics of Cushing's syndrome, but abstinence from alcohol reverses signs, symptoms, and abnormal test results.

**Depression:** endogenous depression results in increased cortisol levels, loss of diurnal rhythm, increased urine-free cortisol, increased urine 17-OHCS and 17-KGS, and abnormal suppression tests; however, patients with depression have increased cortisol in response to insulin-induced hypoglycemia, whereas patients with true Cushing's syndrome do not.

blood glucose patterns and the development of diabetes mellitus, dietary management of blood glucose levels may be appropriate.

### Activity

The patient with untreated Cushing's syndrome has persistent fatigue and obesity and may have muscle weakness and/or pathologic bone conditions. Maintenance of optimal activity is encouraged; restrictions of activity are related to particular complications.

### Referral/Consultation

Only through individual assessment of patient and family can the nurse learn their perceptions of issues related to the patient's health and the ease or difficulty they have in incorporating the medical regimen in daily living. Problems in home maintenance and role performance in the family and workplace may reveal a need to strengthen the resources available to the patient and/or family. Referral or consultation with social services, home nursing, or other services may be helpful.

## NURSING MANAGEMENT

## ♦ ASSESSMENT

### Subjective Data

Data to be collected to assess the patient with cortisol excess include the following:

- General data
  - Changes noted in body proportions, weight, hair distribution, pigmentation, bruising, delayed wound healing
  - History of discomfort, particularly back pain
  - History of frequent infections: skin respiratory
- Neurologic data: changes noted in behavior, concentration, memory
- Nutritional data
  - Usual 24-hour food/fluid intake
  - History of increase in thirst
- Musculoskeletal data: complaints of weakness, fatigue, or difficulty doing normal activities
- Elimination data: changes in urine output
- Sexuality data
  - Females: changes in menstrual history, secondary sexual characteristics, libido, or feelings about self
  - Males: changes in libido, secondary sexual characteristics, or feelings about self
- Knowledge level: condition, treatment, diagnostic tests

### Objective Data

Data to be collected to assess the patient with cortisol excess include the following:

- General: body appearance (presence of moon facies, buffalo hump, truncal obesity, thin arms and legs, hyperpigmentation, striae, bruises, ecchymoses, fragile skin, facial plethora, unhealed wounds)
- Neurologic: affect and its appropriateness to situation, short-term memory, concentration
- Cardiovascular: blood pressure, pulse, weight, presence of edema, jugular vein distention
- Nutrition: intake of food and fluids
- Musculoskeletal: muscle mass, strength, ability to stand up from a sitting position or do knee bends
- Elimination: urine output, presence of glycosuria
- Sexuality: female secondary sexual characteristics, body hair distribution, scalp hair changes, presence of acne

### Diagnostic Test Findings

Typical test results in cortisol excess include the following:

1. Elevated serum cortisol level or elevated excretion of urine-free cortisol
2. Elevated urinary levels of 17-KGS and 17-OHCS
3. Loss of diurnal rhythms of cortisol production
4. Loss of suppression of endogenous cortisol with the normal and screening cortisone suppression tests
5. Abnormalities in serum electrolytes, chemistry, and hematology, as described earlier

## ♦ NURSING DIAGNOSES

Nursing diagnoses are determined from analysis of patient data. Nursing diagnoses for the person with cortisol excess may include but are not limited to the following:

| Diagnostic Title | Possible Etiologic Factors |
|---|---|
| **For patients during acute period before definitive treatment or if definitive treatment not possible** | |
| Activity intolerance | Muscle weakness, abnormal carbohydrate metabolism, abnormal electrolyte balance |
| Body image disturbance | Changes in body characteristics, change in functioning |
| Coping, ineffective (individual) | Inability to mount a normal physiologic response to stressors, possible lack of learned coping strategies, emotional lability |
| Fluid volume excess | Abnormal retention of sodium and water |
| Infection, high risk for | Inability to fight organisms because of depression of immune and inflammatory responsiveness |
| Injury (trauma), high risk for | Falls associated with muscle weakness and bone changes |
| Knowledge deficit: disease, diagnostic tests, treatment, side effects, expected outcomes | New disease, new tests, never exposed to information previously |
| Nutrition, altered: more than body requirements | Increase in appetite with increased cortisol, alteration in metabolism |
| Pain | Demineralization of bone resulting in compression fractures |

## ♦ EXPECTED PATIENT OUTCOMES

Expected patient outcomes for the patient with cortisol excess may include but are not limited to the following:

### For patients during acute period before definitive treatment or if definitive treatment is not possible

1. Improves activity tolerance as evidenced by maintenance of current activity level and a weekly increase in activity
2. Has improved body image, as evidenced by speaking about self in positive terms.
3. Shows adequate coping, as evidenced by absence of signs of uncontrolled stress (restlessness, lack of attention, increased heart rate or blood pressure).
4. Fluid volume returns to normal, as evidenced by elimination of signs of hemodilution or edema.
5. Detects early signs and symptoms of infections.
6. Does not fall or injure self.
7. Patient and significant others can:
   a. Explain the rationale and procedure for diagnostic tests.
   b. Explain the cause of the disease and how signs and symptoms relate to the disease.
   c. Describe the treatment and the expected effects.
   d. Describe replacement or other medication therapy (drug, dosage, frequency, side effects).
   e. Describe plans for follow-up care.
   f. State need for bracelet, necklace, or identification card if receiving replacement therapy.
8. Maintains adequate nutritional status, as evidenced by a gradual decrease in weight and a decrease in caloric intake.
9. States pain is controlled; activities are not limited because of pain.

## ♦ INTERVENTIONS

The patient with excessive cortisol secretion needs skilled nursing care. The patient can be critically ill. During the acute period, the primary focus of care is on the high-priority needs of supporting coping, restoring fluid balance, and preventing infections and injuries. In the more stable patient, these needs are still a focus of care, but the focus will expand to the other needs described by the additional nursing diagnoses listed earlier.

### Providing Physical Care

1. Decrease controllable stressors.
   a. Provide continuity of care.
   b. Explain all procedures slowly and carefully.
   c. Spend time with patient and listen carefully.
   d. Avoid sudden noises, temperature changes, drafts, and unnecessary invasion of privacy.
   e. Promote relaxation.
2. Monitor physiologic coping ability.
   a. Ensure blood pressure and pulse remain stable.
   b. Take vital signs at least every 2 to 4 hours.
3. Control fluid volume excess.
   a. Restrict fluids as prescribed; distribute fluids throughout the 24 hours; use ice chips to prevent thirst.
   b. Provide a diet low in sodium as necessary.
   c. Provide potassium replacement as ordered, and increase intake of foods high in potassium.
   d. Monitor daily weight, intake and output every 4 to 8 hours, and laboratory values of sodium, potassium chloride, bicarbonate, and pH.
4. Prevent infection and falls.
   a. Monitor temperature every 4 hours.
   b. Assess mouth, lungs, and skin every shift for early signs of infection; report signs immediately.
   c. Limit staff and visitors with signs and symptoms of upper respiratory infections.
   d. Institute preventive care: sterile technique for invasive procedures; routine turning, coughing, and deep breathing every 2 hours; oral hygiene before breakfast, after meals, and at bedtime.

### Maintaining and Increasing Activity

As the patient begins to recover from the acute episode, the goal is to maintain the patient's current activity level. This requires assisting with some activities that require energy, such as bathing. In addition, the nurse should space out activities and provide rest periods between them. When electrolyte and fluid balance and glucose metabolism have been stabilized, the patient's energy level will increase and more activities can be added gradually on a week-by-week basis.

### Promoting Nutritional Balance

Patients with cortisol excess are usually overweight. The nurse should provide a diet that restricts calories but is high in protein and that meets special needs based on glucose metabolism. Because cortisol excess can increase appetite, patients need assistance in controlling calories; the approach to this is individualized (see Chapter 6) for a discussion of techniques that can be used). The patient's nutritional status should be monitored by checking weight, actual food intake, and blood glucose level. Blood glucose levels should be monitored every 4 to 8 hours until the patient is stable.

### Promoting Comfort

Pain occurs because of demineralization of bones and compression fractures. Measures that can be used to promote comfort include (1) providing a mattress with good support, (2) instituting back rubs to promote relaxation, and (3) using pain medications as appropriate. If these measures are unsuccessful, the nurse should consult the physician and physical therapist about other alternatives, including braces. It is important to remember that pain must be controlled so that ambulation and activity can be maintained.

### Promoting Positive Body Image

Another major focus of care is helping the patient deal with changes in body image, sexuality, and self-concept. Patients should know that some body changes are reversible with treatment, and they are helped to accentuate positive attributes. To help increase their self-concept as they recover, they are assisted in setting realistic goals within their physiologic tolerance. Clear explanations about changes in sexual characteristics and changes that will occur with treatment help patients to cope better.

### Facilitating Learning

Education of patients and significant others is ongoing. At first the patient needs basic information regarding the care being given and any restrictions such as diet and limitation of some visitors. Many diagnostic tests may be necessary, and careful explanations are given. Over time the patient needs information about the disease process and planned treatment, long-term care needs related to the disease process, and specific care for complications such as adrenal insufficiency, which can occur with some treatments.

## ♦ EVALUATION

To evaluate the effectiveness of nursing interventions, compare patient behaviors with those stated in the expected patient outcomes. Successful achievement of patient outcomes for the person with cortisol excess is indicated by the following:

1. Reports that activity level is increased from baseline.
2. Comments positively about self.
3. Shows no excessive restlessness.
4. Reports decreasing weight and a decrease in peripheral edema, if present.
5. Maintains body temperature within specified parameters.
6. Reports no injuries.
7. Patient and significant others accurately explain disease and symptoms, diagnostic test requirements, expected effects of treatment, and dietary and medication requirements.
8. Discusses future plans, including ways to decrease food intake.
9. States pain is controlled and does not restrict activity.

## IATROGENIC CUSHING'S SYNDROME

### Etiology/Epidemiology

Iatrogenic Cushing's syndrome occurs when large doses of exogenous glucocorticoids are taken for their therapeutic antiinflammatory effects. As described in Chapter 38, the glucocorticoids have profound antiinflammatory and immunosuppressive effects. Because of these effects, glucocorticoids are frequently prescribed in therapeutic doses to suppress undesirable inflammatory reactions and immune responses. Box 39-19 presents examples of clinical situations in which glucocorticoids might be used for their antiinflammatory and immunosuppressive effects. See p. 1254 for epidemiologic information about this most common cause of cortisol excess.

**BOX 39-19 Therapeutic Use of Glucocorticoids: Clinical Situations**

1. Eye surgery or trauma: usually given as drops, ointment, or intraorbital, so systemic effects are minimal
2. Dermatologic disorders: used as ointments; can have systemic effects if used over large part of body or used daily
3. Autoimmune diseases: rheumatoid arthritis, lupus erythematosus, scleroderma
4. Hematologic disorders: hemolytic anemia, thrombocytopenia, lymphomas, leukemias
5. Allergic reactions: anaphylaxis, contact dermatitis, transfusion reactions
6. GI disorders: ulcerative colitis, Crohn's disease, hepatitis
7. Nephrologic disorders: nephrotic syndrome
8. Neurologic disorders: head trauma and surgery to prevent cerebral edema and increased intracranial pressure
9. Cardiopulmonary disorders: asthma, chronic obstructive pulmonary disease, myocarditis
10. Transplantations: renal, liver, heart, and β-cell transplantation
11. Other: glucocorticoids are part of many protocols for various malignancies

Regardless of the purposes, when glucocorticoids are given for any reason other than replacement therapy, the person receives dosages that will elevate the serum glucocorticoid level above normal. Adrenocorticosteroids used in this manner can cause problems when they are prescribed for long-term, continuous use and when they are withdrawn after long-term use. The total dosage and the duration of therapy determine the side effects. The larger the dose and the longer the time during which glucocorticoids are used, the greater are the side effects.

## Pathophysiology

Long-term therapeutic doses of glucocorticoids can result in the full clinical picture of Cushing's syndrome. However, at other times the clinical picture seen with iatrogenic Cushing's syndrome can be different. Suppression of growth in children can be more severe than in endogenous Cushing's syndrome, and it is irreversible. Bone changes may be greater in iatrogenic Cushing's syndrome, and patients often develop vascular necrosis. Fluid and electrolyte disturbances may not be as severe because synthetic glucocorticoids possess less mineralocorticoid activity than natural glucocorticoids. Severe *myopathy* can occur. *Peptic ulcers* occur more often in patients who receive glucocorticoid therapy for more than 30 days.[40] Patients receiving glucocorticoid therapy are very susceptible to *cataract formation,* which is not seen in endogenous Cushing's syndrome. It is important to remember that patients receiving long-term glucocorticoid therapy are very susceptible to all types of infection.

## Medical Management

A different type of problem, *cortisol deficit,* can occur when glucocorticoids are given for a prolonged period. They must be withdrawn slowly to prevent adrenal insufficiency. The reason is that the high blood levels of exogenous glucocorticoids cause negative feedback to the hypothalamus and anterior pituitary gland, and the production of corticotropin-releasing factor (CRF) and ACTH is suppressed. The lack of ACTH results in depression of the hypothalamic-pituitary-adrenal (HPA) axis and adrenal atrophy. Thus, if glucocorticoids are stopped suddenly, the patient develops signs and symptoms of *adrenal insufficiency* because of an inability to produce the glucocorticoids internally. It has been found that it may take as long as 9 months for return of normal HPA function.[40]

To prevent depression of the HPA axis, some physicians prescribe every-other-day glucocorticoid therapy. In these instances, *double the patient's daily dose is given at 8 AM every other day.* The benefit of this schedule is that it allows the serum glucocorticoid level to drop low enough every other day to prevent the negative inhibition of the hypothalamus and the anterior pituitary gland. Thus, every other day the person has a normal secretion of endogenous CRF and ACTH and normal stimulation of the adrenal cortex, and atrophy of the adrenal cortex glands does not occur. Even though the glucocorticoid level drops low enough to prevent negative feedback, the antiinflammatory effect is not reduced. Even though every-other-day therapy should prevent HPA axis depression, the dose of glucocorticoids is still tapered when they are withdrawn. In some instances after withdrawal, the patient may be able to produce enough glucocorticoids to meet body needs in nonstressful times but may need additional glucocorticoids during increased stress.

## Nursing Management

### Promoting self-care

Patients receiving prolonged therapeutic glucocorticoid therapy need considerable *teaching* to be able to manage therapy and to identify signs and symptoms of complications (see Guidelines box below). In addition, *counseling* is usually needed to help the patient cope with changes in appearance and behavior.

The disturbances associated with long-term therapeutic doses of glucocorticoids cannot be completely avoided, but they often can be minimized and complications avoided. The changes in body structure may not be avoidable. Patients should be aware of these side effects and be supported in dealing with these changes. Instructions on use of clothes, makeup, and so on may be incorporated into care.

**Guidelines for Teaching the Person Receiving Long-Term Therapeutic Doses of Glucocorticoids**

1. Take drugs as prescribed.
   a. Do not miss a dose or stop medication suddenly.
   b. Drug must be withdrawn slowly under a physician's supervision.
   c. If nausea and vomiting occur and drug cannot be taken, notify physician immediately.
   d. Keep sufficient tablets on hand to avoid missing a dose.
   e. Take drug with food or antacids.
   f. With every-other-day therapy, take twice the normal dose every other day at 8 AM.
   g. If traveling, *carry* medications (do not ship them).
2. Monitor self for and report side effects of weight gain, edema, behavior changes, GI bleeding, increased urination or thirst, or signs of infection.
3. Check blood glucose level if directed.
4. Prevent infections.
   a. Avoid persons with infections, especially children.
   b. Avoid crowded, poorly ventilated places.
   c. Care for wounds carefully.
   d. Report signs of infection, which may include feelings of increased weakness, feeling poorly, and having less energy.
5. Maintain a nutritious diet, including foods from all food groups (see Chapter 6); follow directions for any prescribed diet (low calorie, high potassium, low sodium).
6. Carry out a regular exercise program; walking will help to strengthen muscles and decrease bone problems.
7. Have yearly eye examinations.
8. Consult physicians regularly as instructed.

**RESEARCH**

Streiff LD: Can clients understand our instructions?, *Image* 18:48-52, 1986.

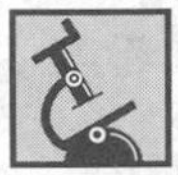

Written instructions are an important tool for patient education. Twenty percent of people in the United States are functionally illiterate in that they are not able to read at a fourth- to fifth-grade level. This study was designed to determine whether clients in an ambulatory care setting read at a level that allowed them to comprehend the written materials. Interviews and assessment of reading level, using the Wide Range Achievement Test (WRAT), was performed on 106 adults. The last grade completed in school, and thus the reported level of reading skills, for the subjects ranged from 3 to 18 grades with a mean of 9.9. The actual reading skills ranged from 1.7 to 13.5 grades with a mean of 6.8.

The readability level of 28 different patient education materials was assessed by three methods. The mean readability level calculated from the averages of the three tests for each pamphlet was 11.2 grades.

In conclusion, most of the study participants read at a level that does not allow comprehension of this material. Several recommendations were made by the researcher:

1. Clients should be tested by use of the WRAT or some other method for their reading levels.
2. Written material should be assessed for readability level, and this should be published with the material.
3. Materials developed by nurses should be written at lower readability levels.

The patient and significant others must be aware of potential changes in behavior that may occur. Usually, patients adjust to the therapy, but if behavior changes occur, the physician should be notified immediately. Written and verbal instructions should be given (see Research box above).

**Promoting nutrition and fluid balance**

Blood glucose levels may be monitored frequently, particularly if there is a family history of diabetes mellitus. If hyperglycemia develops, dietary control is necessary to control blood glucose levels. Some patients may develop insulin-dependent diabetes mellitus (see Chapter 40).

Most persons experience an increase in appetite. If weight gain is a problem, a calorie-restricted diet may be necessary. To prevent GI problems, steroids should be taken with food or antacids. Stools should be guaiac-tested regularly to monitor for early signs of GI irritations.

If fluid retention becomes a problem, the patient is placed on a sodium-restricted diet. The patient is weighed frequently, and the extremities are observed for signs of edema; changes are reported as soon as possible because diuretic therapy may be necessary. To prevent hypokalemia, the person should be on a diet high in potassium, and a potassium replacement may be prescribed unless some underlying condition results in potassium retention.

**Promoting activity**

The effects of glucocorticoids on muscle wasting and bone demineralization can best be minimized by promoting a regular exercise regimen incorporating weight bearing, adequate dietary protein, and ambulation.

**Preventing infection**

The person receiving prolonged glucocorticoid therapy must avoid anyone with an infection. Because young children frequently have upper respiratory infections, close contact with them may have to be limited. Crowded, poorly ventilated environments should also be avoided. The patient is monitored constantly for signs of infection, and the primary caregiver should be notified immediately if any signs of infection occur.

**Preventing complications**

To prevent adrenal insufficiency secondary to sudden withdrawal, patients taking glucocorticoids for a prolonged time must have the steroids withdrawn gradually to allow the HPA axis to recover. During the time the drug is being withdrawn, these patients should be monitored for signs and symptoms of adrenal insufficiency. If symptoms occur, withdrawal is slowed. To prevent sudden withdrawal in emergency situations, the patient should wear an identification bracelet or carry an identification card that states the name and dosage of the prescribed glucocorticoid. If the patient is ill or injured and requires emergency care, those treating the patient will be able to determine if more glucocorticoids are needed because of the increase in stressors; additional glucocorticoids can be given intravenously if they cannot be tolerated by mouth.

It may take some time for the adrenal cortex to recover sufficiently to respond to additional stressors after withdrawal of therapeutic doses of glucocorticoids. Therefore, patients with a recent history of glucocorticoid therapy are monitored for manifestations of adrenal insufficiency, particularly at times of stress.

Although most of the emphasis in this section has been on care of patients receiving oral therapy, the information applies equally to those receiving prolonged steroids intravenously or topically.

## HYPERFUNCTION OF ADRENAL CORTEX: ALDOSTERONE EXCESS

### Etiology/Epidemiology

Aldosterone excess, **aldosteronism**, can be either primary (Conn's syndrome) or secondary. *Primary aldosteronism* results from bilateral nodular hyperplasia or from a single aldosterone-producing adenoma. *Secondary aldosteronism* occurs frequently and results from

**BOX 39-20 Exogenous Causes of Secondary Aldosteronism**

- Cardiac failure
- Liver disease
- Nephrosis
- Renal artery stenosis
- Bartter's syndrome (hypertrophy and hyperplasia of the juxtaglomerular cells)
- Idiopathic cyclic edema
- Pregnancy
- Hypovolemic states
- Estrogen therapy

**BOX 39-21 Laboratory Test Results With Primary Aldosteronism**

**BLOOD TESTS**

- Lower serum potassium level (hypokalemia)
- High serum sodium level (hypernatremia)
- Elevated serum bicarbonate level and pH (alkalosis)
- Low serum magnesium level (hypomagnesemia)
- Elevated plasma aldosterone with low plasma renin levels

**URINE TESTS**

- Low specific gravity (dilute urine)
- Increased urinary protein
- Increased urinary aldosterone

the presence of exogenous conditions that stimulate the renin-angiotensin-aldosterone system (Box 39-20).

Primary aldosteronism is a rare disorder affecting approximately 2% of the hypertensive population. It is twice as common in women as in men and occurs most frequently in the third to fifth decades of life.

## Pathophysiology

In primary aldosteronism, excessive aldosterone is secreted and stimulates the reabsorption of sodium in the kidney in exchange for potassium and hydrogen. The increased sodium retention is accompanied by water retention and results in volume expansion and hypertension. The hypertension may result in ECG and radiologic changes of left ventricular enlargement and in retinopathy. Although the extracellular volume is expanded, edema is not usually present. Headache is a typical clinical finding.

The loss of intracellular and extracellular potassium changes the excitability of muscle membrane, resulting in muscular weakness, intermittent paresthesia, and sometimes diminished deep tendon reflexes. Paralysis can also occur. Low potassium can result in ECG changes, dysrhythmias, and hypersensitivity to digitalis preparations. Severely low levels of potassium result in loss of the concentrating ability by the kidney tubules, leading to increased water loss, polyuria, nocturia, and polydipsia. The increased loss of water by the kidney can result in hypernatremia. Excessive loss of hydrogen ions results in hypokalemic alkalosis, producing signs and symptoms of tetany.

Aldosterone secretion is high with low plasma renin activity. The aldosterone level does not decrease in response to sodium loading and does not increase in response to volume and sodium depletion or assuming the upright position. Laboratory test results are listed in Box 39-21.

Secondary aldosteronism results when increased renin secretion is stimulated by the various pathologic factors. Usually the increased renin activity results from decreased perfusion pressure or decreased effective plasma volume to the kidney. The increased aldosteronism leads to hypokalemia and alkalosis. Hypertension may or may not be present, and some of the patients have edema. Sodium concentration is normal or low.

## Medical Management

The major treatment for primary aldosteronism from an adenoma is surgical resection. The electrolyte imbalance and volume excess are corrected with sodium restriction, potassium replacement, and spironolactone or amiloride before surgery. Spironolactone is prescribed in doses as high as 200 to 400 mg/day and amiloride in doses of 20 to 40 mg/day. Spironolactone is a mineralocorticoid antagonist. It blocks the effect of aldosterone on the kidney tubule, and thus blocks the abnormal reabsorption of sodium and potassium excretion. Potassium is conserved with spironolactone. Amiloride also is a potassium-sparing diuretic.

For bilateral hyperplasia, medical treatment with sodium restriction, potassium replacement, and spironolactone is the treatment of choice. If the hypertension is not controlled by this treatment, traditional antihypertensive therapy is used. Some patients respond to suppression of aldosterone secretion by glucocorticoids.[42]

In secondary aldosteronism, medical treatment for the abnormal sodium and water retention is sodium restriction, potassium replacement, and diuretics. In addition, treatment is directed toward the underlying pathologic factors.

## NURSING MANAGEMENT

Nursing care is directed toward assisting with implementation of medical therapy, monitoring for effectiveness of therapy, monitoring for side effects of therapy (e.g., fluid overload), and preventing or detecting complications that may result from the patient's changed mental status (particularly respiratory depression). Monitoring for fluid status may include vital signs taken as often as every 15 minutes, hourly intake and output, and daily weights. Temperature is monitored hourly because hyperpyrexia is often present.

## ♦ ASSESSMENT

### Subjective Data

Data to be collected to assess the patient with aldosterone excess include the following:

- History of weakness, paresthesias, palpitations
- History of visual changes, headaches
- History of polyuria, nocturia, increased thirst, kidney infections
- Nutritional intake
- History of edema, weight change
- Knowledge of the disease, planned tests, therapy

### Objective Data

Data to be collected to assess the patient with aldosterone excess include the following:

- Vital signs, especially blood pressure
- Heart sounds, point of maximal impulse (PMI)
- Weight
- 24-hour fluid intake and output
- Visual acuity
- Muscle strength, deep tendon reflexes, sensory perception
- Edema

## ♦ NURSING DIAGNOSES

Nursing diagnoses are determined from analysis of patient data. Nursing diagnoses for the person with aldosterone excess (before surgery or while being treated medically only) may include but are not limited to the following:

| Diagnostic Title | Possible Etiologic Factors |
|---|---|
| Activity intolerance | Muscle weakness and fatigue associated with electrolyte imbalance, especially hypokalemia |
| Fluid volume excess | Abnormal retention of sodium and water associated with increased aldosterone |
| Knowledge deficit: disease, diagnostic tests, treatment, side effects, expected outcomes | New disease, new treatment, never given information previously |
| Pain | Headache associated with hypertension |

## ♦ EXPECTED PATIENT OUTCOMES

Expected patient outcomes for the person with aldosterone excess (before surgery or while being treated medically only) may include but are not limited to the following:

1. Shows improvement in tolerance to activity as potassium level improves.
2. Maintains fluid balance, as evidenced by normal serum sodium levels.
3. Patient and significant others can:
   a. Describe the disease and its relationship to patient problems.
   b. Explain the purpose and procedures of diagnostic tests.
   c. Describe planned treatments and expected effects.
   d. Explain the need for long-term care.
   e. Explain when the physician or nurse should be contacted.
4. Controls headaches.

## ♦ INTERVENTIONS

Nursing interventions are directed toward managing critical care, increasing activity tolerance, maintaining fluid balance, promoting comfort, and preparing for discharge.

### ➠ Managing Critical Care

Potential complications include hypertension, hypokalemia, tetany, and alkalosis. Until the patient's condition is stabilized, vital signs are monitored at least every 4 hours. If hypertension is present, hourly vital signs may be necessary. Any increases are reported immediately and managed as directed. Cerebral dysfunction may indicate uncontrolled hypertension. Care is designed to prevent activities that increase blood pressure, such as Valsalva maneuver, straining at stool, or heavy exertion. If antihypertensive drugs are ordered, monitoring for side effects must be included.

Assessment of serum electrolytes (especially potassium) and the presence of weakness, cardiac dysrhythmias, and Chvostek's and Trousseau's signs should be ongoing.

Complications are present preoperatively, and hypertension remains a potential complication for some time after surgery. It may take as long as 1 month for the blood pressure to return to normal. In addition, hypoaldosteronism may occur postoperatively and result in sodium loss and potassium retention. A high sodium intake prevents sodium deficit in the postoperative period.[40]

### Increasing Activity Tolerance

Care is spaced to allow for rest periods. Activity is increased gradually, and as potassium is returned and maintained at a normal level, strength should increase. A high-potassium diet, potassium replacement, and spironolactone are given as prescribed.

### Maintaining Fluid Balance

The patient's fluid volume status is monitored by checking daily weights, intake and output, and serum electrolytes. A sodium-restricted diet may be necessary preoperatively, and a high-sodium diet may be necessary when surgery is performed. If the patient is treated medically, a long-term sodium-restricted diet is maintained.

### Promoting Comfort

Headache may be eased by use of cold packs, relaxation therapy, and analgesics. Polydipsia may be controlled by making sure the patient has ready access to ice water and receives good oral hygiene.

### Preparing for Discharge

Ongoing teaching is necessary and includes the following:

1. Preoperative
   a. Information about diagnostic tests and proposed surgery
   b. Need for long-term care
2. Postoperative
   a. Prescribed diet: may include a high-sodium diet to be followed for several weeks or longer
   b. Monitoring for unstable blood pressure and fluid volume deficit
3. Patient treated medically
   a. Medication (diuretics): dosage, frequency, side effects
   b. Signs and symptoms of uncontrolled disease to be reported to physician
   c. Need for continued medical follow-up care

## ♦ EVALUATION

To determine the effectiveness of nursing interventions, compare patient behaviors with those stated in the expected patient outcomes. Successful achievement of patient outcomes for the person with aldosterone excess is indicated by the following:

1. Reports increased initiation and completion of ADL.
2. Maintains serum sodium levels within normal limits, and has no edema.
3. Patient and significant others accurately describe disease and symptomatology, diagnostic tests and their purpose, planned treatments and long-term replacement therapy, and symptoms to report.
4. Reports infrequent and mild headache.

## HYPOFUNCTION OF THE ADRENAL CORTEX: CORTISOL INSUFFICIENCY

### Etiology/Epidemiology

Inadequate secretion of cortisol may occur as a result of (1) insufficient secretion of ACTH resulting from hypothalamic-pituitary disease *(secondary adrenocortical insufficiency)*, (2) insufficient secretion of ACTH and adrenal atrophy resulting from suppression of hypothalamic-pituitary function by long-term exogenous glucocorticoids given in therapeutic doses (iatrogenic), or (3) destruction of the adrenal cortex itself (primary). Primary insufficiency, also called *Addison's disease*, can result from several causes (Box 39-22).

**BOX 39-22 Causes of Addison's Disease**

Idiopathic atrophy, probably caused by an autoimmune abnormality
Infection of adrenal glands
Infiltration of adrenal glands with cancer
Impairment of blood flow from vasculitis or thrombosis
Hemorrhage and infarction secondary to septicemia (Waterhouse-Friderichsen syndrome)
Destruction of adrenal glands by chemicals such as mitotane
Congenital hypoplasia
Surgical removal of adrenal glands

*Iatrogenic adrenal insufficiency*, resulting from glucocorticoid therapy, is the most frequent cause of adrenal insufficiency. In *primary adrenocortical insufficiency*, clinical signs of **adrenocortical insufficiency** develop when 90% of both glands is destroyed. Under stress, clinical signs may develop when a smaller amount of integral tissue is present.[5] The most common causes of primary adrenocortical insufficiency are autoimmune destruction (70%) and tuberculosis (20%).[22,40]

Autoimmune destruction is termed *idiopathic atrophy* of the adrenal gland; the disorder probably has a genetic component because it often occurs in families and is associated with specific haplotypes. It can be part of multiple endocrine defects caused by autoimmune processes, such as those associated with thyroid and parathyroid gland dysfunction.

Metastasis from malignancy is a frequent cause of adrenal insufficiency in oncology patients.[40] In critical care settings the most frequent acute adrenal insufficiency is caused by hemorrhage of the adrenal glands. Adrenal hemorrhage is associated with conditions of overwhelming sepsis, concurrent infections of human immunodeficiency virus (HIV), and other disorders.[5,40]

### Pathophysiology

Adrenocortical insufficiency, whether primary or secondary, is a rare problem. When it occurs, however, it is life-threatening because the adrenocortical hormones are necessary for existence. The disorder can occur abruptly, as with hemorrhage and infarction, or slowly, as with idiopathic insufficiency. With slow progressive destruction, the adrenal cortex initially may be able to meet the hormonal needs of daily living, but when a stressor occurs, insufficiency becomes evident because the gland cannot meet the extra needs associated with the stress response.

#### Biologic effects

Primary adrenocortical insufficiency deprives the body of both mineralocorticoids and glucocorticoids. These hormonal losses decrease the body's ability to retain sodium and secrete potassium. The loss of sodium decreases extracellular electrolytes and fluid volume. The decreased volume, along with decreased vascular tone, diminishes cardiac output and decreases renal perfusion. Excretion of waste products is inhibited.

**TABLE 39-13 Hyposecretion of Glucocorticoids, Aldosterone, and Androgens (Addison's Disease): Normal Function, Primary Pathophysiologic Alterations, and Clinical Manifestations**

| NORMAL FUNCTION | PATHOPHYSIOLOGIC ALTERATIONS | CLINICAL MANIFESTATIONS |
|---|---|---|
| **GLUCOCORTICOIDS** | | |
| Organic metabolism<br>Protein catabolism<br>Fat metabolism<br>Gluconeogenesis<br>Changes peripheral tissue sensitivity to insulin<br>Role in maintenance of blood glucose | Inadequate metabolism of protein, carbohydrates, and fats; in particular, inadequate gluconeogenesis and glycogen stores<br>Increased insulin sensitivity in periphery | Potential low fasting blood glucose; inability to tolerate prolonged fasts; experiences hunger, weakness, lightheadedness; fatigue and weakness possibly extreme; nausea and vomiting leading to emaciation |
| Negative feedback on secretion of ACTH | Diminished negative feedback on secretion of ACTH; ACTH stimulates MSH | Hyperpigmentation particularly in areas exposed to light, pressure areas, hand creases, and buccal mucosa |
| Potentiate response to catecholamines | Diminished catecholamine activity; poor response to stressors | Hypovolemic shock, as seen by hypovolemia, hypotension, and tachycardia |
| Antiinflammation and immunosuppression | Poor response to any trauma, infection, or stress | May give history of many infections, frequent sick days, not ever really feeling well |
| Maintain emotional stability | Emotional lability | Mood changes: often depressed, lack of interest, sad, mild neuroses |
| Maintain fluid and electrolyte balance: effects similar to aldosterone (see below) | Effects similar to those seen with aldosterone deficiency, but if client produces aldosterone without glucocorticoids, pathophysiologic effects not as severe (see below) | Effects similar but milder than those seen with aldosterone deficiency (see below) |
| Some androgenic effects | Androgen deficiency similar to that seen with decreased adrenal androgens (see below) | Clinical picture similar to that seen with decreased adrenal androgens (see below) |
| **ALDOSTERONE** | | |
| Renin-angiotensin system is major controller of production.<br>Aldosterone acts at kidney tubules, particularly distal nephrons, to increase sodium reabsorption with consequent expansion of intravascular and extracellular fluid volume.<br>Potassium excretion is increased. | Abnormal increase in water and sodium loss; abnormal potassium conservation; inadequate maintenance of blood volume, decreased cardiac output, and decreased blood pressure | Dehydration and hypovolemia (decreased weight, increased BUN, increased hematocrit, poor skin turgor); hyponatremia; hyperkalemia; decreased bicarbonate; acidosis; postural hypotension to shock; muscle weakness and fatigue |
| **ANDROGENS** | | |
| Some role in establishment and maintenance of secondary sexual characteristics | Androgen deficiency in females | In females, loss of hair in axillae, pubis, and over lower extremity; may give history of menstrual irregularities |

The loss of glucocorticoids in primary adrenocortical insufficiency decreases hepatic gluconeogenesis and increases tissue glucose uptake. Muscle strength is lost. Various GI disorders occur, and mental and emotional functioning and stability are impaired. The loss of negative feedback of glucocorticoids with pituitary secretion of ACTH results in uncontrolled ACTH release along with β-lipotropin. The β-lipotropin is hydrolyzed to β-melanocyte-stimulating hormone (β-MSH). Thus excessive amounts of ACTH and β-MSH are present in the serum. Various changes in sexual characteristics may result from a decrease in adrenal androgen or from the general debility associated with the insufficiency (Table 39-13).

Secondary adrenal insufficiency results in similar pathophysiologic disturbances, except that the fluid and electrolyte imbalances are not usually as severe because the adrenal cortex can still produce mineralocorticoids (aldosterone) in response to the renin-angiotensin system. In addition, because ACTH secretion is diminished, no increase occurs in serum levels of β-MSH.

In chronic insufficiency the earliest symptoms are vague, and the clinical picture is not easy to recognize. Clinical signs of acute and chronic insufficiency include those listed in Box 39-23.

### Adrenal crisis (addisonian crisis)

**Adrenal crisis** (addisonian crisis) is a severe exacerbation of adrenal insufficiency. It may occur in any person with chronic insufficiency regardless of the cause.

**BOX 39-23 Clinical Manifestations of Adrenal Insufficiency**

1. *Mental and emotional changes* are some of earliest symptoms and may include lethargy, loss of vigor, depression, irritability, and loss of ability to concentrate. Patient can become increasingly apathetic and not be able to participate in any ADL.
2. *Hypoglycemia* is seen in about 50% of patients with adrenocortical insufficiency. Periods of fasting may exacerbate problem.
3. *Weakness* and *fatigue* are some of most common findings in adrenocortical insufficiency. At first, this may be episodic but can progress to general prostration. Muscle changes may be associated with muscle pain.
4. *Anorexia, nausea,* and *vomiting* are very common manifestations. Diarrhea or constipation may be present. Abdominal pain occurs frequently, and all patients experience weight loss.
5. *Electrolyte changes* include low serum sodium and high serum potassium levels. However, total body potassium is low because potassium moves out of cells in response to extracellular hypoosmolality. Some potassium is lost through GI tract and kidney, and less potassium is taken in. Low serum sodium level can result in dizziness, confusion, and neuromuscular irritability; some patients give history of salt craving. High serum potassium level can result in ECG changes (peaked T wave and broadened QRS complex) (see Chapter 20) and, if very severe, cardiac standstill. Muscles become weaker, and flaccid paralysis can occur.[40] Occasionally, high serum calcium levels may be present because of increased protein concentration associated with volume deficit.

   Along with the sodium deficit, a *fluid volume deficit* also occurs. Signs of dehydration, such as poor turgor, sunken eyeballs, and dry mucous membranes, are present. Hypotension is seen initially with postural changes but eventually is always present. Complete vascular collapse (shock) may occur.
6. *Hyperpigmentation* is seen only in primary adrenocortical insufficiency when ACTH and possibly β-MSH are elevated. It appears as a bronzing seen with a normal suntan in light-skinned persons or generalized darkening in dark-skinned persons. The hyperpigmentation affects both exposed and unexposed skin areas, as well as mucous membranes. It is often exaggerated over pressure areas such as knuckles, knees, elbow, and ischial tuberosities. Palmar creases, thumbnails, and dorsum of tongue may also show the unusual pigmentation.
7. Most females experience loss of body and axillary hair and menstrual changes. *Menstrual changes* may be related more to weight loss than to changes in adrenal androgens. Males experience *impotence,* probably related to generalized debility associated with adrenocortical insufficiency.

It is usually seen in an undiagnosed person who undergoes a major stressor, in a person who has abrupt withdrawal of therapeutic glucocorticoids, or in a person with a poorly controlled condition who enters a stressful situation. It may also be precipitated in a previously well person by adrenal hemorrhage.

Severe hypovolemia (up to 20% of circulating volume can be lost) can lead quickly to hypovolemic shock, hypoperfusion, and lactic acidosis. Patients may experience mental status changes and coma, dysrhythmias, azotemia, and vascular collapse. Hyperkalemia and hyponatremia are present. Acute adrenal insufficiency is a life-threatening crisis and must be treated rapidly.

## Medical Management

This section first discusses the treatment of adrenal crisis, then management of chronic adrenal insufficiency.

### Adrenal crisis

For patients having a known history of adrenal insufficiency or clinical symptoms of the disorder, treatment is begun with a minimum of testing. The short ACTH test is very helpful in confirming or ruling out adrenal insufficiency. Serum cortisol levels are drawn at 0, 30, and 60 minutes after administration of ACTH (cosyntropin, 250 ng) intravenously. When a patient is severely stressed, baseline levels of serum cortisol less than 5 ng/dl are diagnostic, and levels less than 10 ng/dl are suggestive of adrenal insufficiency.[22] A blunted or absent elevation of serum cortisol at 30 and 60 minutes in response to the ACTH is diagnostic for adrenal insufficiency. (See Chapter 38 for details of this test and others used in evaluating ACTH and cortisol secretion.) The rapid or short ACTH test does not differentiate between primary and secondary adrenal insufficiency.

Treatment of adrenal crisis includes the following:

1. *Administration of glucocorticoids and mineralocorticoids.* Hydrocortisone, 100 to 200 mg, is given intravenously, first as a bolus and then for repeated doses every 8 hours in the patient with known adrenal insufficiency. In the undiagnosed patient, dexamethasone (Decadron), 4 to 10 mg, may be chosen instead of hydrocortisone because dexamethasone does not cross-react with cortisol, which can influence tests of cortisol function. Hydrocortisone has some mineralocorticoid activity, whereas dexamethasone does not; fludrocortisone (Florinef) is more likely needed when dexamethasone is prescribed.

2. *Initiation of volume replacement.* Volume replacement with IV normal saline is started immediately at a rapid rate (e.g., 500 to 1000 ml the first hour and 2000 to 3000 ml the next 2 to 3 hours[5]). Typically, glucose is added to the first liter as 5% dextrose in normal saline.

3. *Administration of glucose.* The results of blood glucose testing can quickly determine whether additional IV glucose needs to be given. Patients are often nauseated and vomiting and may complain of abdominal pain, so food ingestion is not an appropriate source of glucose.

4. *Administration of vasopressors.* If glucocorticoid and fluid therapy do not improve vascular status, vasopressors may be started.

5. *Treatment of cause.* Identification and the initiation

**TABLE 39-14 Comparison of Antiinflammatory and Mineralocorticoid Potency of Derivatives of Adrenocorticosteroids**

| DRUG | ANTIINFLAMMATORY POTENCY* | MINERALOCORTICOID POTENCY† |
|---|---|---|
| Hydrocortisone (cortisol) | Potency = 1 | Potency 0.03 times that of Doca |
| Cortisone acetate | Potency 0.8 times that of hydrocortisone | Potency 0.03 times that of Doca |
| Prednisone | Potencyy 4 times that of hydrocortisone | Potency 0.04 times that of Doca |
| Methylprednisolone | Potency 6 times that of hydrocortisone | Potency 0.02 times that of Doca |
| Triamcinolone | Potency 5 times that of hydrocortisone | No mineralocorticoid activity |
| Dexamethasone | Potency 30 times that of hydrocortisone | Only mild natriuretic effect |
| Desoxycorticosterone (DOC) | Zero antiinflammatory effect | Potency = 1 |
| Fludrocortisone | Potency 10 times that of hydrocortisone | Potency 4.2 times that of Doca |

*Potency relative to hydrocortisone, whose potency = 1.
†Potency relative to Doca (desoxycorticosterone acetate), whose potency = 1.

of treatment of the precipitating factor is carried out as rapidly as possible.

### Chronic adrenal insufficiency

Chronic adrenal insufficiency is treated by hormone replacement. In primary insufficiency a glucocorticoid, usually cortisone, 37.5 mg daily (25 mg on awakening and 12.5 mg before 4 PM; or hydrocortisone, 20 mg in the morning and 5 mg before 4 PM), and a mineralocorticoid, usually fludrocortisone (0.1 to 0.2 mg daily), are prescribed. Other forms of these drugs may be prescribed. If a different adrenocortical derivative with glucocorticoid properties (e.g., prednisone) is prescribed, the dosage is equivalent to the antiinflammatory potency of hydrocortisone. For example, the dosage of prednisone is approximately 10 mg/day. Table 39-14 presents a comparison of the antiinflammatory potency of the adrenocortical steroids relative to the glucocorticoid potency of hydrocortisone and the mineralocorticoid potency of desoxycorticosterone acetate (Doca). In secondary insufficiency, only glucocorticoid replacement is necessary.

The dose of glucocorticoids or mineralocorticoids is adjusted until the patient has no symptoms. The dosage of glucocorticoids is temporarily tripled or doubled in situations such as psychologic stressors, vacations, infections, trauma, or dental work. When the stressors have dissipated, the dosage is returned to normal.

Some physicians have the patient keep a parenteral form of cortisol at home and instruct significant others in its administration for emergency purposes. Patients may also carry a vial of hydrocortisone with a syringe for use when away from home.

## NURSING MANAGEMENT

### ♦ ASSESSMENT

Because the clinical manifestations in chronic adrenal insufficiency are subtle and affect a variety of systems, a thorough assessment is necessary.

### Subjective Data

Data to be collected to assess the patient with cortisol insufficiency include the following:

- General: history of weakness, fatigue, muscle pain, dizziness, changes in behavior, lethargy, depression; attention or ability to do work and activities
- Appearance: history of changes in pigmentation
- Nutrition: history of anorexia, nausea, vomiting, salt craving, weight loss, and abdominal pain; usual 24-hour food/fluid intake
- Elimination: history of changes in bowel habits; urine output
- Sexual
  - Females: menstrual history, history of changes in body/axillary hair
  - Males: history of impotence
- Knowledge: disease, treatment, expectations

### Objective Data

Data to be collected to assess the patient with cortisol insufficiency include the following:

- Emotional-mental status: affect, attention, activity level
- Integumentary status: hyperpigmentation, axillary/body hair distribution, skin turgor, eyeball softness
- Cardiovascular status: blood pressure and pulse, especially with postural changes; heart rhythm
- Gastrointestinal status: weight, 24-hour intake and output, abdominal tenderness
- Musculoskeletal status: muscle strength; presence of wasting; ability to do ADL, rise up from sitting position, or walking

### Diagnostic Test Results

Findings from diagnostic tests include the following:

1. Low serum sodium and glucose, high serum potassium levels
2. Increased serum BUN from hemoconcentration and decreased renal perfusion
3. Normal basal levels of cortisol may be noted; low

to normal levels during acute illness indicate adrenocortical insufficiency.

4. Response to ACTH stimulation
   a. Low or no plasma cortisol with primary insufficiency
   b. Normal response to repeated stimulation with secondary insufficiency
5. Elevated ACTH serum levels with primary insufficiency
6. Abnormal ACTH response to metyrapone or hypoglycemia with secondary insufficiency

## ♦ NURSING DIAGNOSES

Nursing diagnoses are determined from analysis of patient data. Possible nursing diagnoses for the patient with cortisol insufficiency include but are not limited to the following:

| Diagnostic Title | Possible Etiologic Factors |
|---|---|
| Activity intolerance | Muscle weakness, postural hypotension, electrolyte imbalance |
| Coping, ineffective (individual) | Inability to mount normal response to stressors, insufficient learned coping mechanisms |
| Fluid volume deficit | Sodium and water loss associated with deficiency of adrenal cortex hormones |
| Injury (trauma), high risk for | Instability associated with weakness, electrolyte imbalance |
| Knowledge deficit: disease, diagnostic tests, treatment, side effects, expected outcomes | New disease, new treatment, no previous exposure to information |
| Nutrition, altered: less than body requirements | Decreased intake associated wih anorexia, nausea, vomiting |
| Pain | Abdominal discomfort |
| Self-esteem disturbance | Change in functional ability, change in body characteristics |

## ♦ EXPECTED PATIENT OUTCOMES

Expected patient outcomes for the person with cortisol insufficiency may include but are not limited to the following:

1. Improves activity tolerance, as evidenced by increased activity level.
2. Improves coping, as evidenced by no signs and symptoms of stress; avoids stressors when possible.
3. Maintains fluid intake of approximately 3000 ml/day, and signs of fluid deficit decrease.
4. Experiences no injuries.
5. Patient and significant others can describe:
   a. Effect of stressors on the disease and measures to be taken to reduce them
   b. Home medication program, need for continued treatment if replacement is necessary, and situations that require an increase in medication dosage
   c. Medical follow-up plan
      (1) Symptoms indicating adrenal crisis and need for medical attention
      (2) Need for continual medical follow-up
      (3) Need to carry identification card with information concerning physician and current medication
6. Has improved nutritional status, as evidenced by increase in weight; eats and retains 100% of prescribed diet.
7. States pain is controlled.

## ♦ INTERVENTIONS

### ➠ Managing Critical Care

Management priorities in adrenal crisis are restoration of fluid volume and electrolyte balance, administration of glucose, and support to patient and family.[22] Frequent monitoring of the patient is necessary to detect changes, to evaluate effectiveness of therapy, to detect side effects of therapy (e.g., fluid overload), and to prevent or detect complications. Of particular concern are the changes in mental status and respiratory depression. Monitoring for fluid status may include vital signs taken as often as every 15 minutes, hourly intake and output, and daily weights. Temperature is monitored hourly because hyperpyrexia is often present. Hemodynamic monitoring may be used to help determine the exact amount of fluids needed. The fluid deficit is usually corrected in 4 to 6 hours.

Until the patient's condition is stabilized, serum values are monitored daily or more frequently as necessary. During the early phase of illness, a neurologic assessment is made at least every 4 hours for signs of *hyponatremia* (dizziness, confusion, neuromuscular irritability); this assessment can be done while taking vital signs.

If serum potassium levels are elevated, the patient should be placed on a cardiac monitor to check for changes in T wave or QRS complexes or for changes in rhythm. The *hyperkalemia* usually disappears with cortisol and fluid therapy, and the patient may actually need potassium after the acute period. Until serum potassium level returns to normal, the nurse should make sure the patient does not inadvertently receive potassium in IV fluids or medications. Measures to prevent infections and trauma, which can increase cell death and the liberation of potassium into the extracellular space, are incorporated into the nursing care.

Monitoring for signs and symptoms of *hypoglycemia* and monitoring of blood glucose levels are done on a routine basis, such as every 4 hours. Glucose is given in IV fluids as prescribed and, when food is allowed, snacks may be incorporated between meals to avoid long periods of fasting. If symptoms of hypoglycemia occur, the blood glucose is checked, if possible, and treatment initiated for the hypoglycemia (see Chapter 40).

A focus of care is avoiding additional stressors. These patients should do absolutely nothing for themselves and should be protected from all stimuli and from exposure to infection. To decrease stressors, the same nurse should provide care for the first several hours, during which time the patient's condition stabilizes. One-to-one care may be necessary. To prevent aspiration, the patient is given nothing by mouth until nausea and vomiting are relieved and until mental status is normal. After several hours, oral liquids may be given, and oral glucocorticoids may be started within 48 hours. The patient may experience a severe headache that may be relieved by an ice bag.

After the patient's condition is stabilized, attention is directed toward achieving an improved state of well-being and preparing for discharge; the plan of care is modified as the patient recovers from crisis to a state of chronic adrenal insufficiency. A sample nursing care plan is presented at the end of this chapter. *Acute adrenal insufficiency* or *addisonian crisis* is a potential complication for any patient with adrenal insufficiency. The management for this condition is described on p. 1268.

## Providing Restorative Care

Nursing care that relates to identified nursing diagnoses includes the following:

1. Promote activity tolerance.
   a. Limit activities until vascular volume is stable and blood pressure is normal.
   b. Gradually increase activity and monitor for fatigue and weakness.
   c. Schedule rest periods throughout the day.
2. Facilitate coping.
   a. Provide stressor-reduced environment: quiet private room, controlled temperature; limit visitors but promote visits by persons who have a calming effect.
   b. Avoid surprises; explain everything carefully before proceeding with care.
   c. Use preventive measures for infection or trauma, such as sterile technique, coughing and deep breathing, and good skin care.
   d. Provide continuity of care.
   e. Help patient identify daily stressors and ways to avoid and cope with these stressors.
3. Promote fluid balance.
   a. Monitor for fluid deficit:
      (1) Weight every day
      (2) Intake and output every 1 to 8 hours
      (3) Laboratory values for signs of hemoconcentration every day
      (4) Skin turgor every 4 hours
      (5) Vital signs every 1 to 4 hours
   b. Report signs of increasing fluid deficit immediately.
   c. Maintain fluid intake at several liters a day.
   d. Provide diet with "normal" sodium (approximately 4 g sodium chloride) level.
4. Prevent injury from falls.
   a. Remove unnecessary equipment from room.
   b. Assist patient with ambulation.
   c. Use side rails as necessary and keep bed low to floor.
5. Promote good nutrition.
   a. After patient is stable, provide high-calorie diet incorporating foods from all food groups.
   b. Provide good oral hygiene before meals.
   c. Provide an environment conducive to eating.
6. Promote comfort: back rubs and relaxation techniques; promote stress reduction.
7. Improve self-esteem.
   a. Help patient and significant others understand relationship between changes in self and the disease process; explain that physical changes are reversible.
   b. Help patient set short-term realistic goals.
   c. Compliment patient on accomplishments.
   d. Involve patient in decision making, even if patient is unable to perform physical activities.

## Preparing For Discharge

The initial teaching during the acute phase relates to proposed diagnostic tests and immediate interventions. After the patient's condition is stable, information is given about the disease and long-term needs. Instructions about replacement therapy are similar to those given to patients taking therapeutic doses of glucocorticoids, but some important differences exist (see Guidelines box, p. 1272).

Surgery results in complete remission of symptoms in most patients; therefore discharge teaching for most patients is directed toward helping the patient plan for resumption of normal activities, maintenance of an adequate diet, and follow-up care.

## ♦ EVALUATION

To determine the effectiveness of nursing interventions, compare patient behaviors with those stated in the expected patient outcomes. Successful achievement of patient outcomes for the person with cortisol insufficiency is indicated by the following:

1. Reports more activity tolerance.
2. Identifies at least three techniques that help in reducing stress responses.
3. Describes strategies to monitor fluid intake and to drink 3000 ml/24 hours.
4. Reports no injuries.
5. Patient and significant others accurately describe symptomatology in relation to disease, daily schedule of medication times, names/purpose of drugs, and particular situations in which crisis or symptoms must be followed up by physician; carries identification card.
6. Eats 100% of planned caloric intake every 24 hours.
7. Reports no severe pain.

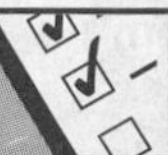

**Guidelines for Instructing the Person on Replacement Doses of Glucocorticoids and Mineralocorticoids**

1. Follow medication regimen.
   a. Take drugs with meals or snacks.
   b. Glucocorticoids: take ⅔ of dose at approximately 8 AM and ⅓ of dose at approximately 4 PM.
   c. Mineralocorticoids: take medication in the morning.
   d. Do not omit a drug dose.
   e. Keep sufficient medication on hand.
   f. If unable to retain oral form of drug, take parenteral form as instructed.
   g. Carry drugs when traveling; do not ship drugs with luggage; make sure traveling companion knows how to give the injectable form of glucocorticoid.
2. Wear a Medic Alert bracelet or necklace that lists condition, drugs and dosage, and name and phone number of physician.
3. Monitor self for presence of increased stressors (fever, infections, dental work, accidents, family or personal crises) and increase dose of glucocorticoids as instructed or consult physician (normal dose covers only daily needs; it does not provide for additional stressors).
4. Monitor self daily for signs and symptoms of insufficient drug therapy (anorexia, nausea, vomiting, weakness, depression, dizziness, polyuria, weight loss) and report immediately (larger drug dose may be necessary).
5. Monitor self daily for signs and symptoms of excessive drug therapy (rapid weight gain, round face, edema, hypertension) and report immediately (smaller drug dose may be necessary).
6. Eat a well-balanced diet, choosing foods from all food groups.
7. Maintain a regular schedule with adequate sleep, regular meals, and regular exercise (irregular health habits increase glucocorticoid needs).
8. Eliminate as many work and home confrontations as possible to decrease stress response that increases glucocorticoid needs.
9. See physician as instructed; consult as necessary if questions arise concerning therapy.

## HYPERSECRETION OF THE ADRENAL MEDULLA: PHEOCHROMOCYTOMA

### Etiology/Epidemiology

**Pheochromocytoma** is a catecholamine-producing tumor of the sympatheticoadrenal medullary system that causes hypertension. Although pheochromocytomas account for less than 1% of the cases of hypertension, it is important that they be diagnosed because these persons can be cured.

A single benign adrenomedullary tumor is the most common pathologic finding. They occur most frequently between the fourth and fifth decades of life and are slightly more common in females. The tumors are most frequently found in the abdomen around or in the adrenal medulla, but they can be found anywhere along the sympathetic nervous system trunk. The tendency to develop pheochromocytomas may be inherited and may be part of the MEN syndromes. Pheochromocytomas may be found in MEN IIa in association with hyperparathyroidism and medullary thyroid carcinoma or in MEN IIb in association with medullary thyroid carcinoma and multiple mucosal neuromas.

### Pathophysiology

Pheochromocytomas of the adrenal medulla release excessive amounts of catecholamines, both epinephrine and norepinephrine. A tumor of the sympathetic nervous system trunk releases excessive amounts of norepinephrine. The hormone release may be constant or episodic, producing constant or episodic clinical manifestations.

A paroxysm or crisis may be precipitated by any lifting, straining, bending, or exercise that increases intraabdominal pressure or moves abdominal contents. Palpation of the abdomen may also precipitate a paroxysm. Anxiety or stress does not usually precipitate an attack.[40] In some patients, no precipitating factors can be identified. The frequency of paroxysms varies but usually increases as the disease progresses.

Release of norepinephrine causes an exaggeration of its effects on alpha ($\alpha$-)receptors, producing massive vasoconstriction. Release of epinephrine causes an exaggeration of its effects on beta ($\beta$-)receptors, producing cardiac stimulating effects and alterations in metabolism.

The most common manifestation of pheochromocytoma is hypertension that is usually sustained. Blood pressure is usually very labile with superimposed paroxysms.[40] Occasionally, patients show true paroxysms, with elevation of blood pressure only present intermittently. The hypertension is resistant to treatment by traditional antihypertensive drugs. Along with the hypertension, orthostatic hypotension is frequently present, resulting from a decrease in plasma volume and loss of tone of postural reflexes.[42]

Other manifestations frequently present include the following:

1. Signs of cardiac stimulation: tachycardia, palpitation, chest pain, ECG changes, angina
2. Headaches that are throbbing, abrupt, and severe
3. Increased metabolic rate manifested by heat intolerance, sweating, fever, wasting of fat stores, and weight loss
4. Elevated blood glucose level
5. Nausea, vomiting, and epigastric pain
6. Tremors, weakness, and nervousness or anxiety
7. Flushing
8. Tachypnea

The diagnosis is confirmed by assays of catecholamines and their metabolites in urine (see Chapter 38). Pharmacologic tests are used infrequently; these tests either demonstrate the dependence of the hypertension on catecholamines by evaluating response to an α-receptor antagonist or provide a paroxysm. Both types of tests are very hazardous. Results of CT scans, arteriography, and venography, used to localize the tumor, are abnormal.

## Medical Management

Before surgery, treatment consists in controlling hypertension and symptoms of cardiac stimulation. An α-adrenergic blocker such as phenoxybenzamine (usual dose, 10 to 20 mg every 6 to 8 hours) or prazosin (usual dose, 2 to 5 mg twice a day) is given to help control blood pressure and paroxysms and to increase blood volume. This therapy is started 1 to 2 weeks before surgery. Phentolamine may also be given if hypertensive crisis occurs. A liberal salt diet is prescribed to restore blood volume. If necessary, saline and blood products are given 12 to 24 hours before surgery.

Tachycardia, dysrhythmias, sweating, and angina are controlled with a β-blocker such as propranolol. This is started only after α-adrenergic blockade is established.

Surgical resection of the tumor is the treatment of choice. Postoperative management is directed toward maintaining a normal blood pressure. Immediately after surgery the patient may be hypertensive; this hypertension is first managed with diuretics and then with phentolamine if necessary. Later the patient may need fluid replacement for hypotension.

Some tumors are not resectable because of disseminated malignancy or other illnesses. Pheochromocytomas do not respond to radiotherapy or chemotherapy. The tumors are slow growing, and morbidity results from excessive catecholamine secretion. The disease is controlled with α- and β-adrenergic blocking agents and α-methyl-para-tyrosine, which reduces the production of catecholamines.

## Nursing Management

### Preoperative care

Preoperatively, nursing care is directed toward instituting measures to help stabilize the patient's hemodynamic status, monitoring the clinical state, preparing the patient for tests and surgery, and preventing paroxysms. Patients experiencing hypertensive crisis should be in an intensive care unit because cardiac, blood pressure, and neurologic monitoring is required as frequently as every 15 to 60 minutes. If phentolamine infusion is necessary, the blood pressure is checked every 15 minutes, and the drug is given by controlled infusion at a rate to keep the blood pressure at a prescribed level. During this time the patient must be informed about planned diagnostic tests and planned treatment and is prepared for surgery. Activities that precipitate paroxysms, such as bending, Valsalva maneuver, and lifting, should be limited.

### Postoperative care

The patient continues to need close monitoring of blood pressure, pulse, cardiac rhythm, neurologic status, and the effectiveness of treatment. After the hypertensive period, hypotension may occur; thus, nursing care is directed toward continual monitoring and administration of fluids or plasma expanders as prescribed.

Surgery results in complete remission of symptoms in most patients; therefore, discharge teaching for most patients is directed toward helping the patient plan for resumption of normal activities, maintenance of an adequate diet, and follow-up care. For those who did not have complete remission, discharge teaching is directed toward helping the patient arrange antihypertensive therapy.

### Care of the nonsurgical patient

For patients treated medically, nursing care is directed toward helping the patient attain skills necessary for self-care. Patient teaching includes the following:

1. Knowledge about the disease and its relationship to the signs and symptoms
2. Medication regimen: purpose, dosage, expected effects, side effects
3. Blood pressure self-measurement
4. Methods to prevent paroxysms: preventing constipation, avoiding Valsalva maneuver, avoiding bending or flexion of the body
5. Importance of follow-up care

# SURGERY OF THE ADRENAL GLAND

Adrenalectomy, either unilateral or bilateral, may be done for a variety of reasons (Box 39-24).

## Preoperative Care

The patient who has dysfunction of the adrenal glands is very fragile before surgery. Medical treatment is used to stabilize the patient's condition hormonally before

**BOX 39-24 Disorders That Respond to Adrenalectomy**

**UNILATERAL**

Single adrenocortical adenomas or carcinomas
Single adrenomedullary tumors

**BILATERAL**

Bilateral adrenal hyperplasia if other forms of therapy are ineffective
Bilateral adrenocortical adenomas or carcinomas
Bilateral adrenomedullary tumors
Removal of source of excessive cortisol secretion in response to ectopic ACTH secretions if ectopic site not controllable and Cushing's syndrome severe

# NURSING CARE PLAN

## PERSON WITH ADRENAL INSUFFICIENCY

**DATA:** Mr. J. is admitted from the emergency room with complaints of feeling so tired that he is unable to get out of bed. He also complains of nausea, vomiting, and diarrhea and having no appetite. He gives a history of feeling poorly for the last 2 months with increasing fatigue. Mr. J. thought he just could not recover from the flu that had been prevalent in the winter. He is an accountant and had been working every day; he also believed that his work partly caused his fatigue.

Physical examination reveals the following:

- 52-year-old white male with "good tan" (NOTE: Mr. J. denies sun exposure)
- Looks ill
- Skin cool, sweaty
- Complains of lightheadedness when head of bed (HOB) elevated
- Lungs clear
- Heart rate—sinus tachycardia; jugular vein distention—flat when HOB elevated 15 degrees
- Skin turgor poor; mucous membranes dry
- Blood pressure: lying, 90/60; sitting, 70/50
- Pulse, 110
- Respirations, 20
- Temperature, 36.5° C
- Weight, 70 kg (lost 3 kg in last month)

Laboratory results were:

- White blood cells, 16,000
- Blood glucose, 60 mg/dl
- Sodium, 130 mEq/L
- Chloride, 86 mEq/L
- Hematocrit, 46%
- Hemoglobin, 15 g/dl
- BUN, 39 mg/dl
- Creatinine, 0.8 mg/dl
- Potassium 5.4 mEq/L

### ■ NURSING DIAGNOSIS

Activity intolerance related to postural hypotension

| Expected Patient Outcome | Nursing Interventions | Rationale |
|---|---|---|
| Increases activity level gradually. | Provide bedrest for first 24 hours.<br>Avoid any unnecessary activities, such as bathing, for first 12 hours.<br>Explain that when hormone level returns to normal, Mr. J. will feel stronger. | Activities should only be increased when serum glucocorticoid levels return to normal. |

### ■ NURSING DIAGNOSIS

Ineffective individual coping related to inability to mount normal response to stressors

| Expected Patient Outcome | Nursing Interventions | Rationale |
|---|---|---|
| Stressors and signs of stress decrease. | Decrease stressors from noise, lights, and temperature changes.<br>Explain everything to Mr. J.<br>Maintain consistent persons caring for patient for first 24 hours.<br>Pad door to prevent slamming.<br>Set temperature to comfortable level.<br>Keep stressful news from reaching Mr. J.<br>If family members are comforting, have one stay with Mr. J.<br>Make sure family members are calm. | Because of lack of glucocorticoids, patient can not respond physiologically to any stressor; nurse should limit stressors. |

### ■ NURSING DIAGNOSIS

Fluid volume deficit related to inability to conserve fluid

| Expected Patient Outcomes | Nursing Interventions | Rationale |
|---|---|---|
| Fluid intake is approximately 3000 ml/day.<br>Signs of fluid deficit decrease. | Monitor intake and output hourly.<br>Monitor blood pressure and pulse hourly until normal.<br>Weigh daily. | Surveillance will identify any problems with replacement therapy early so that solutions can be changed. |

## NURSING CARE PLAN

### PERSON WITH ADRENAL INSUFFICIENCY—cont'd

| Expected Patient Outcomes | Nursing Interventions | Rationale |
|---|---|---|
| | Monitor hematocrit, hemoglobin, and BUN daily.<br>Administer IV fluids (usually 5% dextrose in normal saline) as ordered.<br>Administer cortisol as ordered. | Fluid volume deficit results from excessive loss of sodium and water and lack of glucocorticoids. |

■ **NURSING DIAGNOSIS**

High risk for injury (trauma) related to weakness and hypoglycemia

| Expected Patient Outcome | Nursing Interventions | Rationale |
|---|---|---|
| Experiences no injury. | Keep bed low.<br>Keep bed rails up.<br>Maintain quiet environment and consistent nurse for 24 hours.<br>Monitor blood glucose q 4 hr.<br>Instruct Mr. J. to stay in bed. | Hypoglycemia and weakness can lead to injury; nurse should provide safe environment. |

■ **NURSING DIAGNOSIS**

Knowledge deficit related to new problem with no previous exposure to information

| Expected Patient Outcome | Nursing Interventions | Rationale |
|---|---|---|
| Mr. J. and significant others can explain what will happen over next 24 hours. | Explain all care to patient and family so that no unexpected event occurs.<br>Focus only on care to be given for next 24 hours.<br>Help Mr. J. and family know that he will be much more stable in 24 hours. | Mr. J. can only handle minimal knowledge, so limit to what must be provided in first 24 hours; knowledge helps to decrease stress. |

surgery. The patient's nutritional status should be stabilized by a high-protein, high-calorie diet with adequate minerals and vitamins. Electrolyte imbalances (sodium, potassium, acid-base) are corrected. On the night before surgery, the morning of surgery, and during surgery, the patient is given a soluble preparation of cortisol. If hypotension occurs during surgery, additional cortisol and fluids are given as needed. Care is the same regardless of whether a unilateral or bilateral procedure is performed.

## Postoperative Care

The patient having an adrenalectomy is usually sent to the intensive care unit postoperatively because of the high risk of adrenal crisis and the careful monitoring needed to maintain fluid and electrolyte balance. Immediately after bilateral adrenalectomy, the patient is depleted of both glucocorticoids and mineralocorticoids, and the patient who is not managed correctly will develop adrenal crisis (see p. 1268). Hemodynamic monitoring (central venous pressure, blood pressure, pulse, at times pulmonary wedge pressure) is done continuously. In addition, daily serum electrolytes and blood glucose levels every 4 hours, daily weights, and hourly intake and output are monitored.

Intravenous cortisol replacement is continued for at least the first 24 hours postoperatively and usually for 48 hours. Fluids are given based on the clinical data and usually include saline/dextrose solutions. On the second day postoperatively, mineralocorticoids may be started. By the third day, the patient is usually able to tolerate oral glucocorticoids and a normal diet. If unusual weakness or anorexia, nausea, or vomiting occurs, glucocorticoids are increased. If unusual hypotension occurs, mineralocorticoids and fluids are adjusted appropriately.

A major complication of surgery is poor wound healing and infection. Strict aseptic technique is used with wound care. Splinting the incision during coughing o turning prevents stress on the suture line and promo comfort. Other postoperative needs are similar to th described for the patient with adrenal insufficiency Nursing Care Plan). Replacement therapy is nec throughout life.

For the patient who has had a unilateral ad

## Guidelines for Care of the Person Undergoing Adrenal Surgery

### PREOPERATIVE

1. Provide supportive care.
2. Assist patient with usual preoperative care.
3. Maintain nutritional status with a high-protein, prescribed-calorie diet with adequate minerals and vitamins.
4. Assist with correction of fluid and electrolyte imbalance.
5. Assist with hormonal therapy as prescribed.
6. Assist with measures used to prevent or treat crisis of adrenal hormonal excess or deficit.
7. Administer prescribed IV fluids and glucocorticoids before surgery.

### POSTOPERATIVE

1. Establish monitoring schedule to detect complications of surgery and:
   a. Adrenal crisis
   b. Blood pressure alterations
   c. Blood glucose alterations
   d. Fluid and electrolyte imbalances
2. Because the patient may have unusual activity intolerance, pace postoperative activities with alternate periods of rest and a gradual increase in self-care.
3. Provide measures to minimize effects of postural hypotension:
   a. Supply Ace bandages or elastic stockings.
   b. Assess effects of posture on blood pressure.
   c. Assist or accompany the patient during ambulation while blood pressure remains labile.
4. Provide measures to decrease risk of infection in the immunosuppressed patient (e.g., strict surgical asepsis, deep breathing, avoiding contact with persons with upper respiratory infections).
5. Administer cortisol replacement as typically prescribed:
   a. IV route for the first 24 to 48 hours
   b. Oral route when patient is able to tolerate food by mouth
6. Administer mineralocorticosteroid (fludrocortisone) replacement, if prescribed; typically prescribed when cortisol replacement is less than 40 to 50 mg/24 hours in the patient with bilateral adrenalectomy.
7. Assist patient and family in learning about required hormonal replacement:
   a. Bilateral adrenalectomy—maintenance dose of cortisol and mineralocorticoids
   b. Unilateral adrenalectomy—doses of cortisol depend on degree of suppression of HPA axis.

tomy, monitoring, hormonal support, fluid therapy, and other care needs are the same during the immediate postoperative period as for the patient with a bilateral adrenalectomy. After the patient is stabilized and has successfully passed any physiologic and psychologic crises, the glucocorticoid support is slowly withdrawn because eventually a single gland can maintain enough hormonal secretion for both daily living and additional stressors. When glucocorticoids are withdrawn, monitoring for signs and symptoms of adrenal insufficiency and crisis must be continued because the remaining gland may have atrophied and may not have fully recovered. If signs and symptoms occur, glucocorticoids are restarted and then again slowly withdrawn.

It is important to remember that a patient who has chronic adrenal insufficiency and who requires surgery for an unrelated adrenal problem requires the preoperative and postoperative care just described.

The Guidelines box above summarizes preoperative and postoperative care.

## QUESTIONS TO CONSIDER

- Which endocrine gland dysfunction causes each of the following?
  1. Major problems in a fluid status
  2. Major alterations in energy production and use
  3. Major alterations in mineral/electrolyte balance
- What are some techniques that can be used to help patients in complying with dietary restrictions that are a common part of the therapeutic regimen for many endocrine problems?
- What instructions should be given to a person taking long-term glucocorticoids for their antiinflammatory effect?
- What are several techniques that can be used to help patients remember to take drugs on a regular schedule?
- What are 10 self-care activities that persons with immunosuppression resulting from elevated glucocorticoid levels should learn and implement? Give a rationale for each activity.
- Differentiate the effects of elevated and depressed calcium levels on the neurologic system, cardiac system, and renal system.
- Contrast the abnormalities in the cardiac system caused by hypothyroidism and hyperthyroidism.
- What are the ethical issues in administering growth hormone to healthy children of short stature? To healthy elderly persons as a possible way to retard aging?

## CRITICAL THINKING ACTIVITIES

- Janine, 57, has known thyroid dysfunction and is exhibiting signs and symptoms of shock, hyperthermia, and heart failure. Joseph, 62, also has known thyroid dysfunction present with hypothermia and hypotension. Analyze these data, draw conclusions about each patient's thyroid status, and form an opinion about appropriate emergency medical management for which the nurse must be prepared to facilitate.
- Toni, 38, is diagnosed with adrenal dysfunction, rule out adrenal insufficiency. What questions or methods of inquiry would you use to facilitate differential diagnosis?
- Think about the implications of an endocrine disorder on body image and self-esteem. Plan strategies for improving a patient's adjustment/adaptation to a disorder such as Cushing's syndrome.

## CHAPTER SUMMARY

- Various pathologic processes, including tumor growth, hyperplasia, atrophy, autoimmune processes, infections, and ischemic changes, can affect the endocrine glands. The pathophysiologic alteration that occurs in the endocrine glands can be classified as hypoactivity and hyposecretion or hyperactivity and hypersecretion.
- Endocrine dysfunction can also result from resistance to the action of a hormone at the level of the target cell; this type of problem mimics those seen with hyposecretion of hormone.
- Cancer tumors of the endocrine glands can be made up of (1) secreting cells that result in hypersecretion or (2) nonsecreting cells that do not change hormone level or cause hyposecretion by depressing the function of normal tissue.

### ANTERIOR PITUITARY GLAND: HYPERPITUITARISM

- Hypersecretion of the anterior pituitary gland is usually of one hormone: prolactin resulting in amemorrhea and galactorrhea or GH resulting in gigantism in children and acromegaly in adults.
- Hypersecretion of the anterior pituitary gland is usually caused by an adenoma; these adenomas can cause neurologic problems, vision changes, headache, and changes in mentation by their compressions on normal neural tissue.
- Prolactin-secreting tumors are controlled by drug therapy; GH-secreting tumors are resected.
- Surgical removal of the pituitary tumor does not usually disrupt normal pituitary action.
- Nursing care for the patient with a pituitary adenoma consists of (1) helping the patient deal with the irreversible changes (growth changes, bone changes in acromegaly, possible visual changes); (2) helping the patient achieve a stable metabolic status before surgery; (3) preparing the patient for surgery; (4) caring for the patient after surgery, with a particular focus on monitoring fluid and electrolytes status, monitoring for signs of hormonal deficit (ADH, adrenocortical hormones), preventing increases in intracranial pressure and stress on suture line, and preventing infection; and (5) preparing for home care.

### ANTERIOR PITUITARY GLAND: HYPOPITUITARISM

- Hyposecretion of the anterior pituitary gland can be of one hormone or all anterior pituitary hormones and ADH (panhypopituitarism).
- Hyposecretion of gonadotropins results in reproductive problems; hyposecretion of prolactin results in problems in lactation in postpartum patients; hyposecretion of TSH results in hypothyroidism; and hyposecretion of ACTH results in adrenocortical insufficiency.

### POSTERIOR PITUITARY GLAND: HYPERFUNCTION

- Syndrome of inappropriate antidiuretic hormone (SIADH) results from hypersecretion of the posterior pituitary gland.
- SIADH causes abnormal water reabsorption, as well as hyponatremia and hypoosmolality, which cause fluid movement from the extracellular to the intracellular compartment and change electrical activity of nerves, potentially resulting in seizures.
- Nursing care in SIADH is focused on increasing osmolality and sodium by water restriction, monitoring for and reporting critical changes (sodium $<$120 mEq/L, neurologic changes), maintaining a safe environment, and patient education.
- Diabetes insipidus, a deficiency of ADH, results from posterior pituitary gland insufficiency.
- Although diabetes insipidus can cause volume deficit and hypernatremia, it usually does not because the thirst precipitated will cause increased fluid intake.
- Vasopressin in a nasal spray is used to treat permanent diabetes insipidus.

### HYPERSECRETION OF THYROID HORMONE: HYPERTHYROIDISM

- Hypersecretion of thyroid hormone most frequently results from Graves' disease, which is caused by an autoimmune process.
- Graves' disease can include hyperthyroidism, goite pretibial myxedema, and ophthalmopathy.
- Hyperthyroidism results in increased activity of neurologic system, increased GI motility, incr metabolism, heat production and calorigenes

creased cardiac activity, increased respiratory activity, and muscle wasting. Many of these changes result from hyperactivity of the sympathetic nervous system.

- Thyroid crisis results from worsening hyperthyroidism when critical increases occur in metabolism, calorigenesis, and sympathetic stimulation.
- Hyperthyroidism is treated with antithyroid drugs, radiation therapy, or surgical resection. Use of radioactive iodine after stabilizing the patient is the treatment of choice.
- The major nursing needs of the patient with hyperthyroidism include potential decrease in cardiac output, hyperthermia, activity intolerance, ineffective coping, home maintenance problems, nutritional problems, sleep pattern disturbances, and visual deficits.
- Except for surgery, treatment of hyperthyroidism does not result in immediate improvement; that is, the return to a euthyroid state may not be observed for 6 to 8 weeks.

## HYPOSECRETION OF THYROID GLAND: HYPOTHYROIDISM

- Hypothyroidism is seen most frequently in elderly women; has a slow, insidious onset; and causes neurologic, respiratory, cardiovascular, GI, and metabolic dysfunction.
- Untreated hypothyroidism in neonates can result in severe mental and physical retardation.
- Hypothyroidism requires lifelong hormonal replacement.
- Nursing interventions for patients with hypothyroidism need to address activity intolerance, body image disturbances, constipation, hypothermia, pain, self-care deficits, sexual dysfunction, impaired skin integrity, altered mental status, and knowledge deficits.
- The problems of patients with hypothyroidism vary from minimal dysfunction to severe dysfunction, in which the patient requires complete care, is unresponsive, and may have respiratory failure and diminished cardiac reserve.
- Myxedema coma is the diagnostic title given the condition in which the patient has critically depressed physiologic function resulting from hypothyroidism.

Various processes, including infection and an autoim-
...une process, can result in an inflammatory process
...e thyroid; this process can be acute, subacute, or

...'s thyroiditis is the most frequently occur-
...thyroiditis. It is an autoimmune disease
...ations and remissions.
...hyroiditis the thyroid is enlarged,
With disease progression, the
...stroyed and hypothyroidism
...rbations, before the gland
can experience episodes of

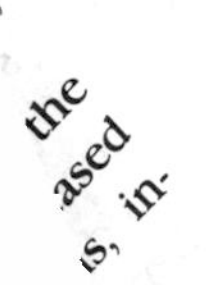

- A goiter is an enlargement of the thyroid gland. It can result from iodine deficiency, exposure to goitrogens, hypothyroidism, or hyperthyroidism.

## CANCER OF THE THYROID

- Cancer of the thyroid is more rare than other forms of cancer. It can be classified into one of five types: papillary, follicular, anaplastic, medullary, or thyroid lymphoma.
- The prognosis in thyroid cancer varies from very good for patients with papillary and follicular cancer to very poor (less than 6-month survival from diagnosis) for those with anaplastic tumors.
- Most cancers of the thyroid are treated with total thyroidectomy. Thus, after surgery, the patient requires hormonal replacement therapy.
- Nursing interventions for patients with thyroid cancer focus on preparing them for diagnostic tests, preparing them for surgery, helping them to cope with the diagnosis, and caring for them postoperatively.
- The major nursing needs after thyroid surgery relate to monitoring for respiratory distress or any of its etiologic factors: internal hemorrhage, which can cause compression on the trachea; laryngeal damage to the vocal cords and obstruction of the airway; or tetany, which can cause laryngeal spasms. Any signs of respiratory distress or its causes need to be reported immediately.
- The tetany results from damage to the parathyroid glands during thyroid surgery. The nurse should have an intravenous preparation of calcium available as well as a tracheostomy tray.

## HYPERSECRETION OF PARATHYROID HORMONE: HYPERPARATHYROIDISM

- Hyperparathyroidism can be primary, secondary, or tertiary. Primary hyperparathyroidism results from adenomas and hyperplasia; secondary from chronic hypocalcemia, which causes chronic stimulation of the parathyroid gland; and tertiary from the development of an autonomous parathyroid gland chronically stimulated by a hypocalcemic state.
- In primary hyperparathyroidism, continual bone resorption and changes in renal and GI processing of calcium occur. The results are hypercalcemia and changes in neurologic, GI, and cardiac functioning. Renal stones can occur; bone density decreases.
- Secondary hyperparathyroidism is a compensatory process that maintains the plasma level of calcium at the expense of bones; chronic renal failure is a major cause.
- Hypercalcemia is treated before parathyroid surgery by hydration with normal saline, and diuretics such as furosemide or ethacrynic acid; thiazide diuretics are not used because they inhibit calcium excretion.

- Primary hyperparathyroidism is treated by surgery; three to three and one-half glands are removed.
- The major complications following parathyroid surgery are hypocalcemia and laryngeal spasms from tetany and respiratory obstruction for compression of the trachea by hemorrhage or from laryngeal nerve damage.
- The calcium level declines within 24 hours after parathyroid surgery, and hypocalcemia may occur.

### HYPOSECRETION OF PARATHYROID HORMONE: HYPOPARATHYROIDISM

- Hypoparathyroidism can result from trauma or surgery or be idiopathic.
- Hypoparathyroidism results in hypocalcemia, which leads to cardiac and neurologic problems; the latter result from increased excitability of neurons.
- The treatment for hypoparathyroidism is vitamin D and calcium replacement.

### HYPERFUNCTION OF THE ADRENAL CORTEX: CORTISOL EXCESS

- The adrenal cortex secretes glucocorticoids and mineralocorticoids that are essential for life and adrenal androgens.
- Glucocorticoid excess (Cushing's syndrome) can result from excessive production of ACTH by the pituitary gland, excessive production of ACTH by ectopic tumors, excessive production of glucocorticoids by the adrenal glands, or intake of large doses of exogenous steroids.
- Glucocorticoid excess results in increased protein breakdown and muscle wasting, abnormal metabolism of fats with changes in fat stores and increased serum lipid levels, and increased glucose production. Abnormal retention of sodium and water with increased excretion of potassium and hydrogen ions also occurs. Bone demineralization results. Suppression of the immune system and the inflammatory response is a major result of glucocorticoid excess.
- Patients with glucocorticoid excess have fluid volume excess, hypernatremia, hypocalcemia, alkalosis, infections, muscle wasting, osteoporosis, hyperglycemia, peptic ulcers, mental changes, body changes (thin extremities, truncal obesity, moon face, kyphosis), poor wound healing, and bruising.
- Nursing care for patients with Cushing's syndrome focuses on the nursing diagnoses of activity intolerance, disturbances in body image, ineffective coping, fluid volume excess, high risk for infection and injury, nutrient excess, pain, and knowledge deficit.
- The most frequent cause of Cushing's syndrome is iatrogenic, and the treatment focuses on dealing with the signs and symptoms of glucocorticoid excess.
- When patients have been taking long-term steroids, drug therapy must be tapered as it is discontinued.

### HYPERFUNCTION OF THE ADRENAL CORTEX GLAND: ALDOSTERONE EXCESS

- Aldosterone excess results in sodium and water excess, volume expansion, hypokalemia, and hypertension.
- Treatment for aldosterone excess is designed to lower blood pressure using sodium restriction and spironolactone or amiloride diuretics or surgery.

### HYPOFUNCTION OF ADRENAL CORTEX

- Adrenocortical insufficiency is a medical emergency because the person is not able to mount a compensatory response to a major stressor. When glucocorticoids are deficient and a stressor is present, the person is unable to retain needed water and sodium, maintain blood pressure, and produce energy substrates (glucose, fatty acids).
- Untreated glucocorticoid deficiency results in shock.
- Patients deficient in glucocorticoids require lifetime replacement therapy. They must know what to monitor to identify signs of a deficit or an excess, must know when to take additional hormones, and must wear or carry appropriate identification.
- Hyperpigmentation occurs in patients with Cushing's syndrome resulting from increased ACTH and primary adrenocortical insufficiency, which is associated with increased ACTH.

### HYPERSECRETION OF ADRENAL MEDULLA

- Tumors of the adrenal medulla cause excessive production of catecholamines and are called pheochromocytomas.
- Hypertension, constant or paroxysmal, is the major sign of pheochromocytoma.
- Activities such as increased abdominal pressure, Valsalva maneuver, straining, and bending over can increase release of catecholamines and worsen hypertension in pheochromocytoma.
- Before surgery for pheochromocytoma, blood pressure is lowered using alpha-adrenergic blockers.
- Surgery is the treatment of choice for patients with pheochromocytoma. If bilateral tumors are present, after surgery the patient will be deficient in glucocorticoids and will need lifelong replacement therapy.

## REFERENCES

1. Barkan A et al: Preoperative treatment of acromegaly with long-acting somatostatin analog SMS 201-995: shrinkage of invasive pituitary macroadenomas and improved surgical cure rate, *J Clin Endocrinol Metab* 67:1040-1048, 1988.
2. Black P, Zervas NT, Candia GL: Incidence and managem of complications of transsphenoidal operation for pitui adenomas, *Neurosurgery* 20(6):920-924, 1987.
3. Carpenito LJ: *Nursing diagnosis: application to clinical tice,* ed 5, Philadelphia, 1993, Lippincott.
4. Chanson P, Jedynak CP, Czernichow L: Management

postoperative diabetes insipidus with parenteral desmopressin, *Acta Endocrinol* 117:513-514, 1988.
5. Chin R: Adrenal crisis, *Crit Care Clin* 7:23-41, 1991.
6. Crapo LM: Thyroid function testing. In the Endocrine Society: 45th Post Graduate Annual Assembly syllabus, Bethesda, Md, 1993, The Society.
7. Davies M: Primary hyperparathyroidism: aggressive or conservative treatment? *Clin Endocrinol* 36:326-332, 1992.
8. DeGroot LJ: Complications of Graves' disease. In the Endocrine Society: 41st Post Graduate Annual Assembly syllabus, Bethesda, Md, 1989, The Society.
9. Greenspan FS: Medical management of thyroid nodules and thyroid cancer. In the Endocrine Society: 45th Post Graduate Annual Assembly syllabus, Bethesda, Md, 1993, The Society.
10. Gorman CA: Thyroid orbitopathy: the gravest problem in Graves' disease. In the Endocrine Society: 41st Post Graduate Annual Assembly syllabus, Bethesda, Md, 1989, The Society.
11. Grumbach MM: Evaluation or treatment of the child with short stature. In the Endocrine Society: 41st Post Graduate Annual Assembly syllabus, Bethesda, Md, 1989, The Society.
12. Harada T et al: Current treatment of Graves' disease, *Surg Clin North Am* 67:299-314, 1987.
13. Hetzel BS: The control of iodine deficiency, *Am J Pediatr* 83:494-495, 1993.
14. Heath H: Primary hyperparathyroidism: recent advances in pathogenesis, diagnosis, and management, *Adv Intern Med* 37:275-293, 1992.
15. Hershman JM: Effect of nonthyroid illness on thyroid function. In the Endocrine Society: 45th Post Graduate Annual Assembly syllabus, Bethesda, Md, 1993, The Society.
16. Holzman EJ et al: Brief report: a molecular defect in the vasopressin V2-receptor gene causing nephrogenic diabetes insipidus, *N Engl J Med* 328:24, 1993.
17. Hyman RB et al: The effects of relaxation training on clinical symptoms: a meta-analysis, *Nurs Res* 38:216-220, 1989.
18. Isley WL: Thyroid disorders, *Crit Care Nurs Q* 13:(3):39-49, 1990.
19. Illowsky BP, Kirch DG: Polydipsia and hyponatremia in psychiatric patients, *Am J Psychiatry* 145:675-683, 1988.
20. Kaplan S: The newer uses of growth hormone in adults, *Adv Intern Med* 38:287-301, 1993.
20a. Kinzier BJ: Management of the syndrome of inappropriate secretion of antidiuretic hormone, *Clin Pharm* 6:833, 1987.
21. Krege J, Kagtz VL, Bowes WA: Transient diabetes insipidus of pregnancy, *Obstet Gynecol Surv* 44:789-795, 1989.
22. Lee LM, Gumowski J: Adrenocortical insufficiency: a medical emergency, *AACN Clin Issues Crit Care Nurs* 3:319-330, 1992.
23. Melmed S: Acromegaly, *N Engl J Med* 322:966-975, 1990.
24. Miyagawa K et al: Multiple endocrine neoplasia type I with Cushing's disease, primary hyperparathyroidism, and insulin—glucagonoma, *Cancer* 61:1232-1236, 1988.
25. Molitch M: Lactation and prolactinomas. In the Endocrine Society: 41st Post Graduate Annual Assembly syllabus, Bethesda, Md, 1989, The Society.
26. Murty GE, Lamballe MB, Welch AR: Early inappropriate secretion of antidiuretic hormone after transsphenoidal pituitary adenomectomy, *J Laryngol Otol* 104:894-895, 1990.
27. Paul T et al: Long-term L-thyronine therapy is associated with decreased hipbone density in premenopausal women, *JAMA* 295:3137-3141, 1988.
28. Reasner CA II, Isley WL: Thyrotoxicosis in the critically ill, *Crit Care Clin* 7:57-73, 1991.
29. Rebar R: Amenorrhea. In the Endocrine Society: 41st Post Graduate Annual Assembly syllabus, Bethesda, Md, 1989, The Society.
30. Rose DB: *Clinical physiology of acid-base and electrolyte disorders,* ed 3, New York, 1989, McGraw-Hill.
31. Sawin CT: Thyroid dysfunction in older persons, *Adv Intern Med* 37:223-247, 1992.
32. Seck JR, Dunger DB: Diabetes insipidus: current treatment recommendations, *Drugs* 44:216-224, 1992.
33. Siperstein AE, Clark CH: Surgical management of thyroid nodules and thyroid cancer. In the Endocrine Society, 45th Post Graduate Annual Assembly syllabus, Bethesda, Md, 1993, The Society.
34. Smith-Rooker JL, Garrett A, Hodges LC: Case management of the patient with pituitary tumor, *Med Surg Nurs* 2:265-274, 1993.
35. Snyder PJ: The myth of the nonsecreting pituitary adenoma. In the Endocrine Society: 41st Post Graduate Annual Assembly syllabus, Bethesda, Md, 1989, The Society.
36. Spittle L: Diagnoses in opposition: thyroid storm and myxedema coma, *AACN Clin Issues Crit Care Nurs* 3(2):300-308, 1992.
36a. Streiff LD: Can clients understand our instructions? *Image* 18:48-52, 1986.
37. Taylor S: *Positive illusions,* New York, 1989, Basic Books.
38. Verbalis JG: SIADH and other hyponatremic states. In the Endocrine Society: 41st Post Graduate Annual Assembly syllabus, Bethesda, Md, 1989, The Society.
39. Wass JSH, Popovic V, Chayvialle JA: Proceedings of the discussion, "Tolerability and Safety of Sandostatin," *Metabolism* 41(9)(suppl 2):80-82, 1992.
40. Wilson JD, Foster DW, editors: *Williams' textbook of endocrinology,* ed 8, Philadelphia, 1992, Saunders.
41. Woeber KA: Iodine and thyroid disease. In the Endocrine Society: 45th Post Graduate Annual Assembly syllabus, Bethesda, Md, 1993, The Society.
42. Wyngaarden JB, Smith LH, editors: *Cecil's textbook of medicine,* ed 19, Philadelphia, 1992, Saunders.

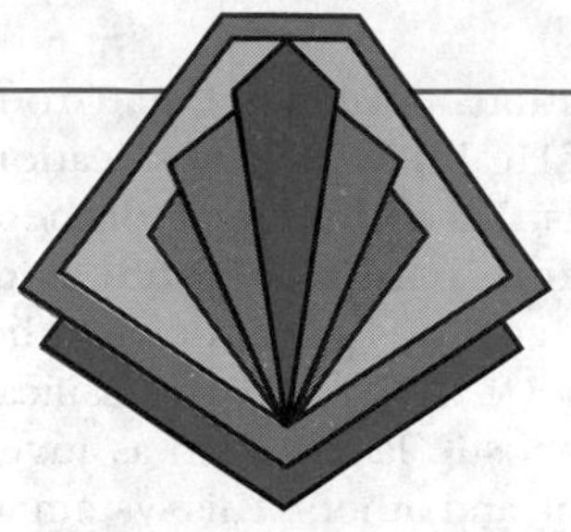

C H A P T E R 40

# Management of Persons With Diabetes Mellitus and Hypoglycemia

**George Ann Eaks**
**Virginia L. Cassmeyer**

## CHAPTER OBJECTIVES

***After studying this chapter, the learner should be able to do the following:***

1 Differentiate between insulin-dependent diabetes mellitus (IDDM), non-insulin-dependent diabetes mellitus (NIDDM), gestational diabetes mellitus (GDM), malnutrition-related diabetes mellitus, and other types of diabetes mellitus.
2 Describe the epidemiologic and etiologic factors of IDDM and NIDDM.
3 Describe primary, secondary, and tertiary preventive interventions for persons with diabetes mellitus or impaired glucose tolerance.
4 Explain the pathophysiologic basis for IDDM, NIDDM, diabetic ketoacidosis (DKA), and hyperosmolar, hyperglycemic, nonketotic coma (HHNC).
5 Describe the common manifestations of IDDM, NIDDM, DKA, and HHNC.
6 Describe the medical management of IDDM, NIDDM, DKA, and HHNC.
7 Describe the major focus of dietary management for persons with diabetes.
8 Explain the role of exercise in management of IDDM and NIDDM.
9 Describe types of insulin, insulin regimens, and complications of the regimens.
10 Describe oral hypoglycemic agents: how they work, normal dosages, and side effects.
11 Describe chronic complications of diabetes mellitus, the relationship between the complications and metabolic control of the disease, and the management of the complications.
12 Develop a nursing care plan, including nursing diagnoses, patient outcomes, and interventions, for persons with stable diabetes.
13 Describe precautions to be taken after an acute illness.
14 Explain special needs of the person who has diabetes mellitus and is undergoing surgery.
15 Define hypoglycemia.
16 Describe the various causes of fasting and reactive hypoglycemia.
17 Describe the medical and nursing management of hypoglycemia.

## KEY TERMS

diabetes mellitus
diabetic ketoacidosis (DKA)
diabetic nephropathy
diabetic foot
diabetic retinopathy
dietetic
gestational diabetes mellitus (GDM)
glycemic index
glycogenesis
glycosuria
hyperglycemia
hyperglycemic, hyperosmolar, nonketotic coma (HHNC)
hypoglycemia
impaired glucose tolerance (IGT)
incidence
insulin
insulin resistance
insulin-dependent diabetes mellitus (IDDM)
ketones
non-insulin-dependent diabetes mellitus (NIDDM)
polydipsia
polyphagia
polyuria
postprandial
preprandial
prevalence
self-monitoring of blood glucose (SMBG)
Somogyi phenomenon
type I
type II

**Diabetes mellitus** is a multifactorial, systemic disease characterized by hyperglycemia and frequently hyperlipidemia. The symptoms are caused by a decrease in the secretion of **insulin** or a decrease in the effectiveness of the insulin. Diabetes mellitus is frequently associated with problems of the microvascular and macrovascular systems, neuropathic disorders, and dermopathic lesions.

By its very nature, diabetes mellitus can be significantly influenced by the treatment components. These treatment components can be delivered only by self-care. No other disease demands so much of the patient's own self-knowledge and skills. Thus the professional nurse has the challenge and responsibility to help patients gain the knowledge, skills, and attitudes necessary for self-management.

## CLASSIFICATION

Part of the early frustration in diabetes care was the need for a uniform classification of glucose abnormalities. Before 1980, there was no uniform method of classifying diabetes. Then a classification system (Table 40-1) was developed by an international work group, sponsored by the National Diabetes Data Group of the National Institutes of Health.[60] This classification system clearly separated **insulin-dependent diabetes mellitus (IDDM)** and **non-insulin-dependent diabetes mellitus (NIDDM)** and was accepted by the World Health Organization (WHO).[77] This classification replaced previous diagnostic labels such as juvenile diabetes, ketosis-resistant, and others. This system was modified by the WHO in 1985, and malnutrition-related diabetes mellitus was added as a separate category.

Because most cases of diabetes mellitus are either IDDM or NIDDM, this chapter focuses on these two classifications. Most of the information, however, applies to the other classifications. Table 40-2 compares the characteristics of the two major types of diabetes mellitus. Both the classifications and their characteristics are significant information for the nurse in understanding the remainder of this chapter.

## ETIOLOGY

In a recent *Diabetes Forecast,* the following words began an article on research: Will diabetes ever yield its dark secrets to the light of reason? Researchers say, 'Yes, in

**TABLE 40-1 Classification System for Diabetes Mellitus and Other Categories of Glucose Intolerance**

| CLASS | DEFINING CHARACTERISTICS |
|---|---|
| Insulin-dependent diabetes mellitus (IDDM): **Type I** | Persons are deficit in insulin (insulinopenic) and depend on exogenous insulin to prevent ketoacidosis and to sustain life.<br>Abrupt onset of symptoms, usually as a youth and almost always before age 30.<br>Certain HLA types, an autoimmune mechanism, and precipitation by an environmental factor, such as a viral infection, have been associated with susceptibility and onset. |
| Non-insulin-dependent diabetes mellitus (NIDDM): **Type II** | Persons do not depend on insulin to sustain life but may be treated with insulin; they are resistant to ketoacidosis except during periods of excessive stress.<br>Onset is usually after age 40, without classic symptoms.<br>Associated with endogenous insulin levels that may be mildly depressed, normal, or high, and with insulin resistance.<br>Obesity and heredity have been associated with susceptibility and onset. |
| Gestational diabetes mellitus (GDM) | Persons have onset of glucose abnormality during pregnancy.<br>Women with known diabetes mellitus who become pregnant are not classified in this group.<br>After delivery, the woman is reclassified on the basis of blood or plasma glucose testing. |
| Malnutrition-related diabetes mellitus | Persons require insulin.<br>Diabetes mellitus found in tropical areas.<br>It occurs in young adults with histories of nutritional deficiencies.<br>Ketosis is not usually present. |
| Other types of diabetes mellitus | Diabetes mellitus associated with other disorders such as pancreatic disease, other endocrine diseases, drugs, and genetic syndromes.<br>Persons usually require insulin. |
| Impaired glucose tolerance (IGT)<br>a. Obese<br>b. Nonobese<br>c. Associated with other conditions | Persons have glucose levels higher than normal but lower than those considered diagnostic for diabetes mellitus.<br>Persons may be subclassified as obese or nonobese, or be included with persons with other conditions such as pancreatic disease, other endocrinopathies, or drug history. |
| d. Previous abnormality of glucose intolerance (PreAGT) | Persons have history of glucose intolerance but now have normal glucose levels.<br>It is designed for epidemiologic and research purposes. |
| e. Potential abnormality of glucose (PotAGT) | Persons have no history of glucose intolerance but have a potentially higher risk because of historical factors such as delivering large babies, obesity, or relatives with diabetes mellitus. |

time.'[14,49] In regard to the causation and treatment, this statement sums up the frustration of both health care giver and patients. On the hopeful side, there is currently in existence an array of hard data on the etiology of diabetes. Throughout the world, researchers continue to make great strides in diabetes research. Table 40-3 identifies the role of genetics, heredity, autoimmunity, and environmental factors in the cause of IDDM and NIDDM.

The cause of each type of diabetes mellitus is still unfolding. In relation to IDDM, it seems that genetics have a permissive role that allow environmental factors to trigger onset of diabetes by stimulating an autoimmune process. The increased understanding of the role of genetics, heredity, autoimmunity, and environmental factors in the cause of IDDM has allowed for research, which is in progress, directed at halting the onset of IDDM in susceptible persons. Clinically significant information from Table 40-3 that is used in patient care is measurement of islet cell antibodies (ICAs). This test is often positive before the onset of symptoms and the diagnosis is made.[63] In addition, the presence of a positive ICA in a previously diagnosed, poorly controlled patient gives impetus toward initiating insulin.

The etiologic factors for NIDDM involve the same factors as for IDDM. Overweight adults, especially those

**TABLE 40-2 Characteristics of Type I and Type II Diabetes Mellitus**

| CHARACTERISTICS | INSULIN DEPENDENT (IDDM) TYPE I | NON-INSULIN-DEPENDENT (NIDDM) TYPE II |
|---|---|---|
| Insulin status | Insulin secretion ↓ | Insulin secretion ↑, ↓, or normal |
| Age | Usually in young but may occur at any age | Usually over 40 but may occur at any age |
| Onset | Rapid | Slow |
| Body build | Lean | 80%-90% overweight |
| Family history | Questionable | Strong |
| Islet cell antibodies | Present at onset | Absent |
| HLA association | Positive | Negative |
| Incidence | 10% of total | 90% of total |
| Symptoms | Polyuria, polydipsia, polyphagia, weight loss | None, or the same as type I, especially if stressed |
| Ketones | Prone | Resistant except during infection or with stressors |
| Complications—vascular/neurologic | After 5 or more years | Frequent (may be present at diagnosis) |
| Treatment | Insulin, diet, exercise | Diet, exercise, oral agents, insulin |
| Racial distribution | More common in whites | More common in African-Americans and Hispanics; highest in Native Americans |

**TABLE 40-3 Etiologic Factors in IDDM and NIDDM**

| FACTORS | IDDM | NIDDM |
|---|---|---|
| Genetic | Associated with HLA antigens located on chromosome 6 (particularly DR3 and DR4) | Not associated with HLA antigens except in three specific populations (Pimas, Xhosas, Fijians)[69]<br>A2 allele of human glycogen synthase gene on chromosome 19 identifies a subgroup of patients with NIDDM who have a strong family history of NIDDM and in whom hypertension and insulin resistance are prevalent. This may be a marker.[41,53] |
| Heredity | Unknown: familial aggregates rare; less than 50% concordance in monozygotic twins | Unknown except for subclass of NIDDM in the young (also called *maturity onset DM of the young [MODY]*, which is dominant[69])<br>Probably multifactorial because familial aggregates are common, shows 55%-100% concordance in monozygotic twins |
| Autoimmune basis | Strong autoimmune basis as seen by:<br>Occurrence of IDDM in patients with other autoimmune disease<br>Insulinitis (inflammation of the islet of Langerhans, with lymphocytic infiltration)<br>Presence of islet cell antibodies (ICAs)<br>Presence of insulin autoantibodies (IAAs) | Possible autoantibodies to islet amyloid seen in 20% of patients with NIDDM[16] |
| Environmental factors | Frequent coincidence between IDDM and viral infections | Modern life-style of poor eating habits (resulting in obesity) and inactivity provides stimulus for those who are genetically predisposed. |

with a family history of diabetes, are at high risk for NIDDM. A prior history of **impaired glucose tolerance (IGT)** or **gestational diabetes mellitus (GDM),** particularly in obese persons, are risk factors for NIDDM. Approximately 25% of persons with IGT and 30% of women with GDM develop NIDDM. Other contributing factors to the cause of diabetes include deposits of amylin in the beta (β-) cells. Amyloid deposits eventually result in destruction of all cells of the islets.[16] Glucose toxicity may be another causal factor in NIDDM. Several studies have indicated hyperglycemia to be toxic to β-cells.[16] Insulin resistance has a role in the cause of NIDDM and in the pathogenesis of NIDDM. This is a term often confusing to patients. Insulin resistance acts like a block in the uptake of glucose in the muscle and fat cells, increasing the glucose in the bloodstream, which increases the resistance to insulin and worsens hyperglycemia.[59] Insulin resistance increases with obesity. However, weight loss is not the simple solution. There appear to be two separate defects or blocks in glucose uptake by the muscle and fat cells. One defect is inherited, and then if obesity occurs, resistance to insulin is acquired.[65]

When skeletal and fat muscle start to develop resistance to insulin, a vicious cycle begins. Compensation for this resistance begins, with the pancreas secreting more and more insulin to keep blood glucose levels within a normal range. Finally, the pancreas becomes exhausted and slows down or stops production of insulin. Other factors that increase insulin resistance include natural aging (there is a loss of muscle mass and increased fat), counterregulatory hormones (glucagon, epinephrine, cortisol, growth hormone), and certain medications such as glucocorticoids.[65]

## EPIDEMIOLOGY

"If diabetes is a disease you can live with, why do 150,000 people die from it each year?" These words come from a poster developed by the American Diabetes Association.[6] The poster gives the definite message that diabetes is a major health problem. Today in the United States, more than 14 million people have diabetes. More than half are unaware that they have the disease. It is the fourth leading cause of death by disease in the United States. It is a chronic disease that has no cure. Prevalence (Box 40-1) increases with age, with about half the cases in people older than 55. Prevalence also increases by race and gender and is highest in African-American women.[6] Race prevalence is shown in Figure 40-1. Regional variations in prevalence have been reported, and the highest rates of diabetes are in the Southeast and North Central states.[75] Incidence indicates the new cases of diabetes. About 750,000 new cases are diagnosed each year, with the majority being diagnosed as having NIDDM.[4]

**BOX 40-1 Definitions of Prevalence and Incidence**

- **Prevalence**—total number of people known to have the disease at a particular time
- **Incidence**—number of people diagnosed with a disease for the first time in the previous year (new cases)

Epidemiologic studies not only define the prevalence and incidence of diabetes, but also the incidence of complications and who is at risk for development of complications.[76] Figure 40-2 depicts the risks of major complications of diabetes when persons with diabetes are compared with nondiabetic persons. In addition to the complications depicted in Figure 40-2, as many as 50% of men with diabetes and 35% of women with diabetes have sexual problems from neuropathy. As demonstrated in Figure 40-2, diabetes mellitus is a costly disease not only in terms of dollars (diabetes accounts for 5% of the total health cost, and treatment costs $20 million annually), but also in terms of morbidity.

## PATHOPHYSIOLOGY

Although there are many unanswered questions about IDDM and NIDDM, one question has a definite answer: "When is diabetes present?" When a deficiency exists in amount or activity of insulin, hyperglycemia results and

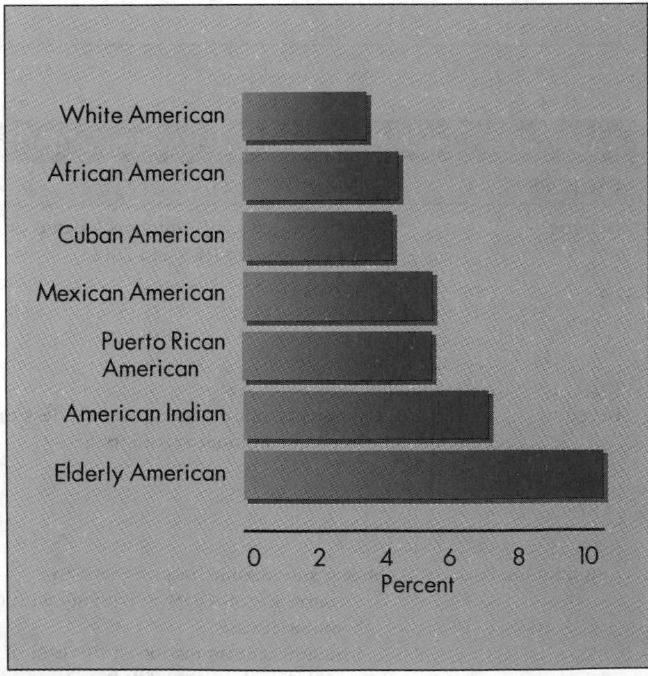


**FIGURE 40-1** Americans with diagnosed diabetes. (From US Department of Health and Human Services, Public Health Service: *Diabetes in the United States: a strategy for prevention* (map reference), National Center for Chronic Disease Control and Prevention, Division of Diabetes Translation, Washington, DC, 1992, US Government Printing Office).

**hyperglycemia** (elevated serum/blood glucose) is diabetes. This lack of insulin can be *absolute,* when the pancreas does not produce enough insulin or produces none at all, as is seen in IDDM. Alternately, the lack can be *relative,* when the body produces normal amounts of insulin, but for some reason that amount is not enough or the insulin is ineffective. That is, insulin resistance is present, as is seen in NIDDM (Figure 40-3). This absolute or relative insulin deficiency results in significant abnormalities in the metabolism of the body fuels. The body needs fuel for all its functions, for building new tissue, and for repairing tissue. The fuel comes from the food that is ingested, which is composed of carbohydrates, proteins, and fats. It is important to understand and emphasize to patients that diabetes is not a disease of "sugar" alone, although the diagnostic criteria that have been devised use the serum glucose level as the marker for the diagnosis and control of the disease. Because the most common word used in the diabetes vocabulary is "sugar," it is understandable how patients with long-standing or new diabetes can believe that if sugar is eliminated from the diet, the battle is won. It is important that nurses help patients understand that diabetes is a disease that affects how the body utilizes all foods (carbohydrates, fats, proteins).

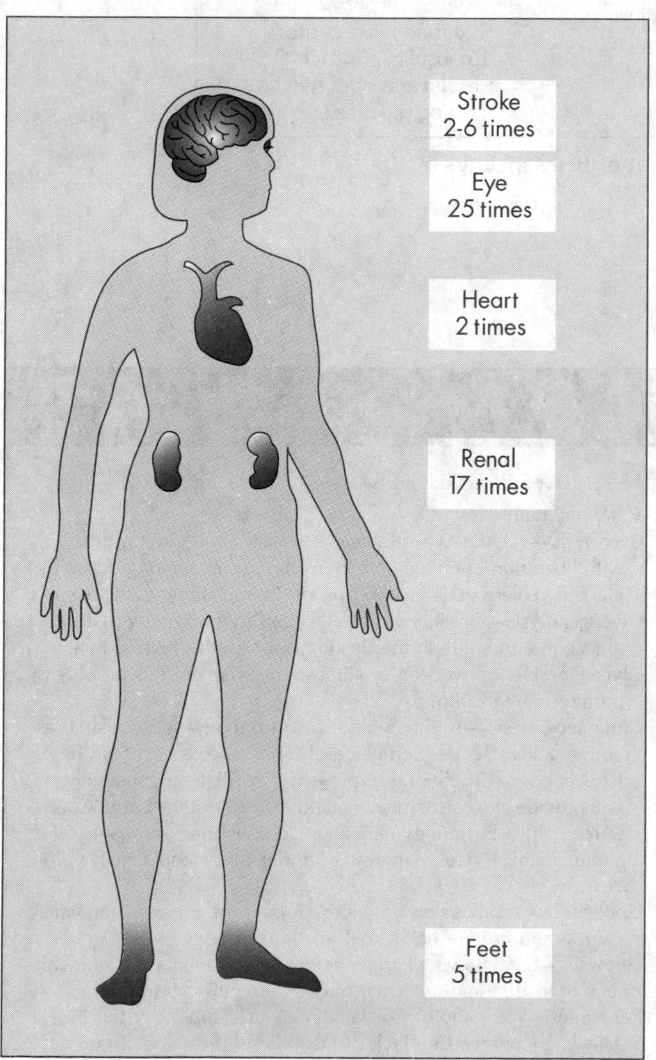


**FIGURE 40-2** Diabetes complications.

## HORMONES

Diabetes is one of the most difficult diseases to understand for both caregivers and patients. Understanding of this disease is enhanced by studying the "star players" in diabetes mellitus[52] (Box 40-2).

The hormones (Table 40-4) act like a "board of directors" in relation to metabolism; that is, their role is directing and controlling activity. The board has representation from the pancreas (insulin and glucagon), pituitary gland (growth hormone [GH] and adrenocorticotropic hormone [ACTH]), adrenal cortex (cortisol), and autonomic nervous system (ANS) (norepinephrine) and adrenal medulla (epinephrine).[36]

Insulin is the first member of the board of directors to be discussed. Of all the hormones involved in glucose metabolism (Table 40-4), insulin is the only one that lowers the blood glucose. (The other members of the board of directors are called *counterregulatory hormones* and elevate blood glucose.) Insulin is the hormone that is either absolutely or relatively deficient in diabetes mellitus. Insulin is synthesized by the β-cells located in the islets of Langerhans within the pancreas. It is insulin's role to see that the body can use fuel to work. Insulin acts like a key that unlocks and opens the doors to let fuel into cells. Insulin fits into little locks (receptors) on the surface of the cells. This unlocking triggers a series of reactions on the cell membrane and inside the cell (postreceptor) that allow for the entry of glucose and amino acids. Without insulin, glucose and other metabolic products build up in the bloodstream and cannot get into the cells to be used for energy.

The best way to understand all of the players in normal metabolism is to use Figure 40-4. This figure incorporates some hospital analogies to which patients can relate. As Figure 40-4 depicts, raw food is digested in the gastrointestinal (GI) tract to the basic forms of glucose, fats, and amino acids. These simple compounds can be absorbed from the GI tract into the bloodstream (hospital hallway). First, for these food particles to get out of the bloodstream (hallway), insulin (member of the board of directors) is required. Insulin allows the liver (patient admitting) to take up and process glucose, amino acids, and fats. The liver stores some products (glucose in the form of glycogen) in the presence of insulin. Many products are sent from the liver (patient admitting) to muscle cells and fat cells (patient rooms). At these cells (patient rooms), if insulin is available, these products are taken up and processed into storage forms of fuel.

In fasting states (between meals and during sleep), insulin levels are decreased and the other hormones

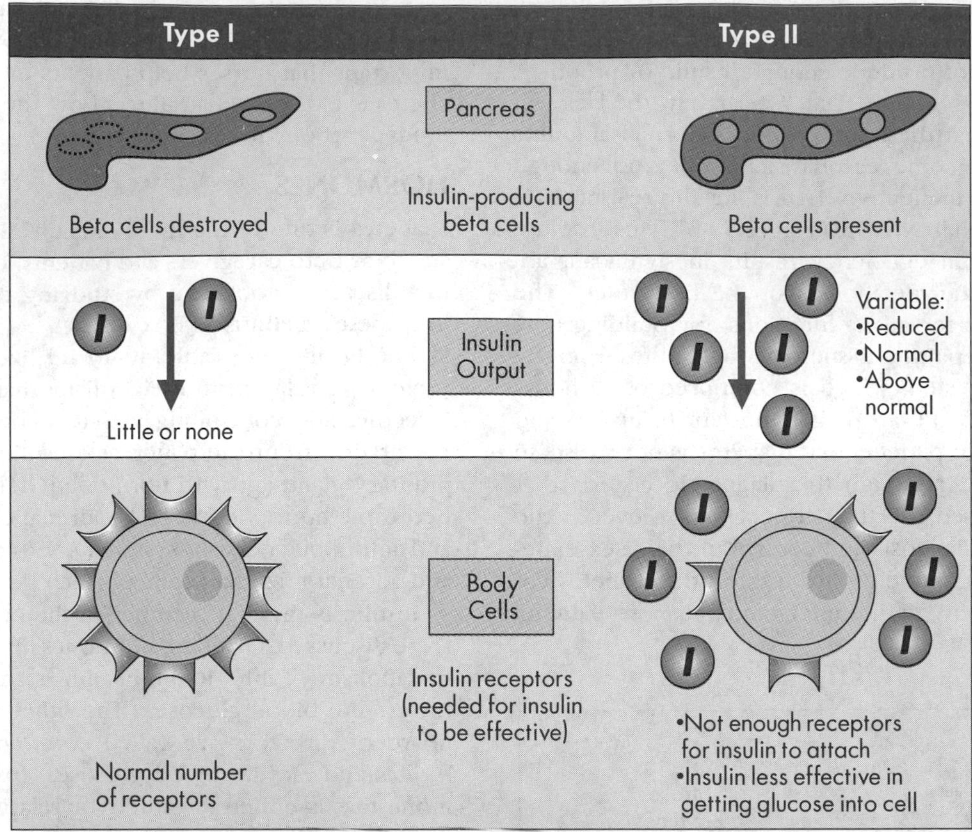


**FIGURE 40-3** Insulin defects in type I and type II diabetes mellitus.

## BOX 40-2 "Star Players" in the Pathophysiology of Diabetes

### BOARD OF DIRECTORS

Hormones: insulin, glucagon, growth hormone (GH), adrenocorticotropic hormone (ACTH), cortisol, norepinephrine, epinephrine

### STARS

Body substrates: carbohydrates, fats, proteins

### SUPPORTING STARS

Cells: liver, adipose cells, muscle

### PRODUCERS

Metabolism: breaking down (catabolism) without insulin or building up (anabolism) with insulin of substrates. Glycogen, triglycerides, and proteins are the anabolic products made from glucose, fatty acids, and amino acids. These anabolic products are reconverted to basic forms of glucose, amino acids, and fatty acids and broken down further during catabolism; anabolism and catabolism depend on all hormones.

### ASSOCIATE PRODUCERS

Metabolic pathways:

**Glycolysis**—breakdown of glucose to water and carbon dioxide, with liberation of energy. Need insulin for uptake of glucose by all cells. Liver needs insulin to start the metabolic pathways.

**Glycogenolysis**—breakdown of glycogen to glucose by action of glucagon and epinephrine. Insulin opposes this breakdown.

**Glycogenesis**—conversion of glucose to glycogen; this process is promoted by insulin.

**Gluconeogenesis**—building of glucose from new sources such as amino acids, lactate, and glycerol. This process occurs in liver. If not enough carbohydrate is present in the diet, gluconeogenesis will provide glucose to meet metabolic needs for the brain. Counterregulatory hormones (glucagon, epinephrine, cortisol, GH) stimulate this process. Thyroid hormone also stimulates this process.

**Lipogenesis**—conversion of excess food substances to fat; after calorie and protein needs met, insulin supports.

**Lipolysis**—breakdown of triglycerides. This is encouraged with lack of insulin and presence of counterregulatory hormones.

**Ketogenesis**—metabolism of fatty acids to ketones (by the liver). This is encouraged by lack of insulin and presence of counterregulatory hormones.

**TABLE 40-4 Hormones (Also Called the "Board of Directors") and Their Roles in Glucose, Protein, and Fat Metabolism**

| PANCREAS | | PITUITARY | | ADRENAL CORTEX | ANS AND ADRENAL MEDULLA |
|---|---|---|---|---|---|
| **INSULIN** | **GLUCAGON** | **ACTH** | **GH** | **CORTISOL** | **CATECHOLAMINES** |
| Promotes glucose storage | Breaks down glycogen | Controls secretion of cortisol | Decreases cellular use and uptake of glucose | Increases gluconeogenesis by liver 6- to 10-fold | Promotes glycogenolysis |
| Prevents fat breakdown | Stimulates gluconeogenesis | | Reinforces function of epinephrine and cortisol | Increases lipolysis | Increases breakdown of fats<br>Inhibits insulin release |
| Increases fat synthesis | Increases lipolysis | | | | Maintains blood glucose in presence of stressors |
| Increases protein synthesis | Increases protein breakdown | | | | Very important in hypoglycemia |
| Lowers blood sugar | Very important in hypoglycemia | | | | |

**TABLE 40-5 Metabolic Alterations Seen in Deficiency of Insulin and its Action**

| CELL TYPE | CARBOHYDRATE | PROTEIN | FAT |
|---|---|---|---|
| Liver cell | ↑ Glycogenolysis<br>↑ Gluconeogenesis | ↑ Protein catabolism | ↑ Ketogenesis |
| Muscle cell | ↑ Glycogenolysis liberating lactate and pyruvate<br>↓ Glucose uptake | ↑ Protein catabolism<br>↑ Liberation of amino acids<br>↓ Amino acid uptake | |
| Fat cell | ↓ Glucose uptake | | ↑ Lipolysis<br>↓ Lipogenesis |

(other members of the board of directors) take over. These counterregulatory hormones and the lack of insulin allow glycogen in the liver and muscles to be used as fuel. Lipids also can be released from the fat cells and transported to the liver, where they are metabolized for energy. Every day, all these hormones are involved in the metabolism of nutrients so that cellular processes are maintained.

## EFFECTS OF DEFICIENCY OF INSULIN SECRETION OR ACTION

A relative or an absolute lack of insulin results in hyperglycemia and impaired fat metabolism. Table 40-5 and Figure 40-5 present the alterations in metabolism associated with diabetes mellitus. In Figure 40-5, the hospital analogies are used. After a meal, because of the deficiency in the action or amount of insulin (insulin member of the board of directors not working), glucose is not taken up from the portal vein (hallway) by the liver (patient admitting). Thus, glucose remains in the general circulation, and **glycogenesis** (formation of glycogen from glucose) is inhibited. In addition, because of cellular starvation, the liver (patient admitting) continues to produce glucose (via glycogenolysis or gluconeogenesis) and to release this glucose into the bloodstream. These processes worsen the hyperglycemia. Insulin-dependent peripheral tissues, such as resting skeletal muscle and adipose tissue (patient rooms), do not extract glucose from the blood as they normally would; muscle cells metabolize their own glycogen supply and then break down protein.

Amino acid transport into muscle cells also requires insulin; thus amino acid uptake and protein synthesis in muscles are impaired. In fact, proteins are actually catabolized (broken down), and amino acids are used to provide the substrate necessary for gluconeogenesis. Amino acids go from the muscle (their storage site) to the liver and are used in the process of gluconeogenesis.

The metabolism of triglycerides, fatty acids, and glycerol is altered. Instead of lipogenesis (formation of tri-

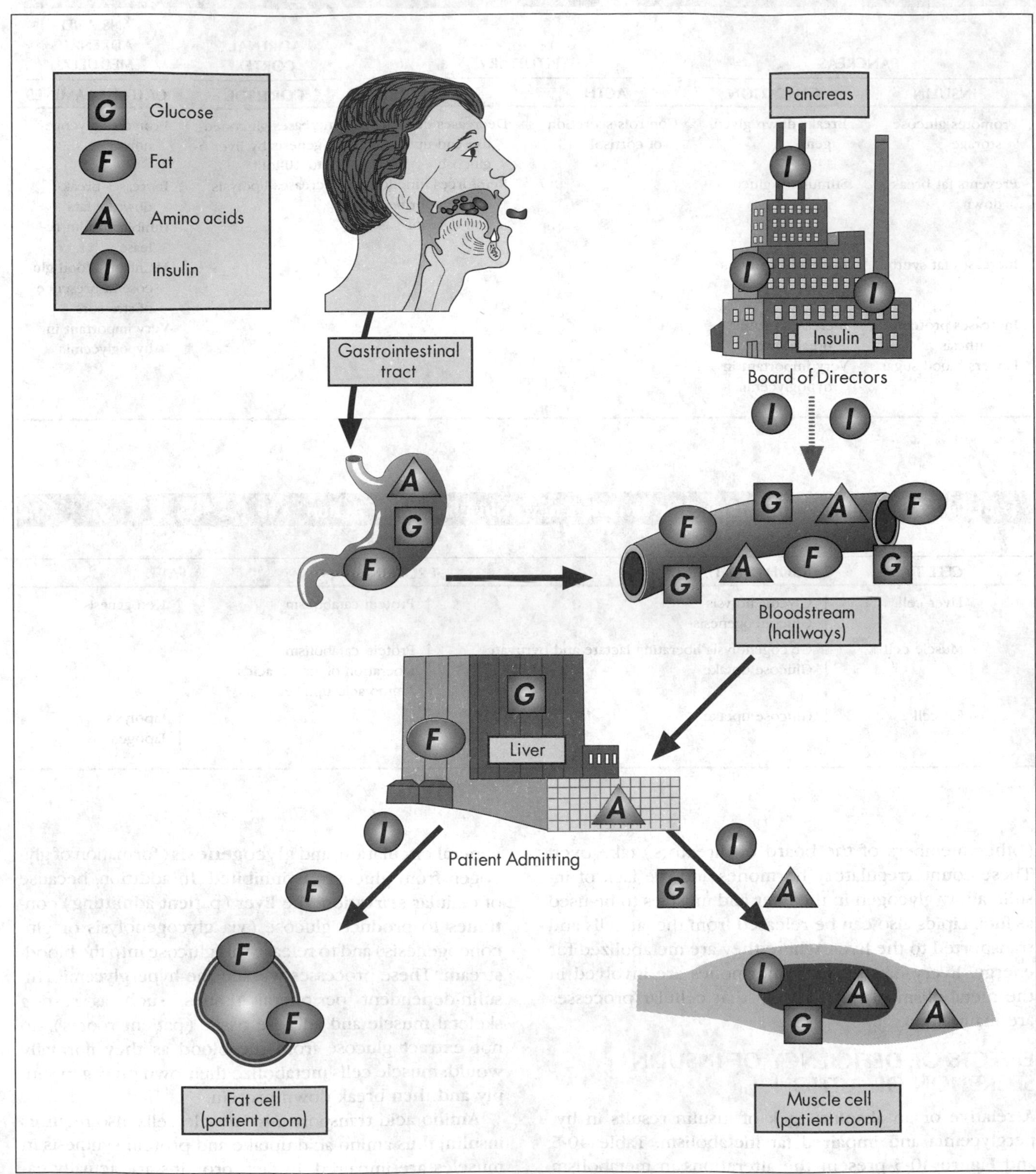


**FIGURE 40-4** Depiction of normal metabolism in terms of insulin's role: analogy to the hospital.

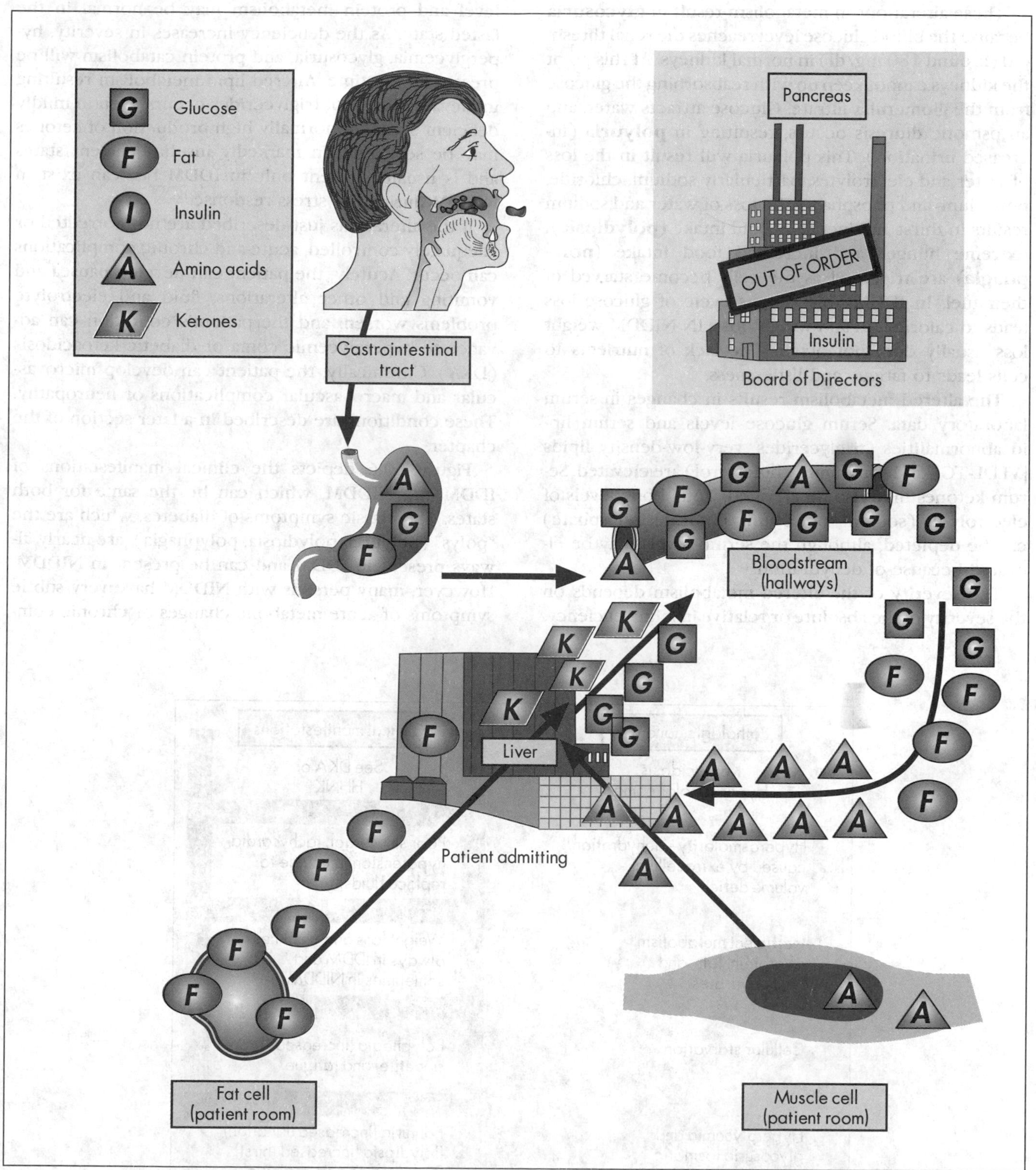


**FIGURE 40-5** Abnormal metabolism in diabetes mellitus: analogy to the hospital.

glycerides), lipolysis (breakdown of triglycerides) occurs. The liver will continue the formation of or increase the formation of ketone bodies from fatty acids.

These alterations in metabolism result in **glycosuria** because the blood glucose level reaches the renal threshold (around 180 mg/dl) in normal kidneys. At this point the kidneys cannot keep up with reabsorbing the glucose from the glomerular filtrate. Glucose attracts water, and an osmotic diuresis occurs, resulting in **polyuria** (increased urination). This polyuria will result in the loss of water and electrolytes, particularly sodium, chloride, potassium, and phosphate. The loss of water and sodium results in thirst and increases fluid intake **(polydipsia).** Extreme hunger and increased food intake **(polyphagia)** are triggered as the cells become starved of their fuel. In IDDM, this vicious cycle of glucose loss leads to calorie loss and weight loss. IN NIDDM weight loss usually does not occur. The lack of nutrients to cells leads to fatigue and listlessness.

The altered metabolism results in changes in serum laboratory data. Serum glucose levels and serum lipid abnormalities (triglycerides, very-low-density lipids [VLDL-TG], and sometimes cholesterol) are elevated. Serum ketones may also be elevated. Total body levels of electrolytes (sodium, potassium, chloride, phosphate) can be depleted, although the serum levels may be elevated because of dehydration.

The severity of the altered metabolism depends on the severity of the absolute or relative insulin deficiency. In mildly deficient conditions, altered glucose metabolism with hyperglycemia and glycosuria may occur only after meals. In these mildly deficient conditions, glucose level and protein metabolism may be normal in the fasted state. As the deficiency increases in severity, hyperglycemia, glycosuria, and protein catabolism will be present all the time. Altered lipid metabolism resulting in elevated levels of triglycerides occurs even in mildly deficient states. Abnormally high production of ketones may be seen only in markedly insulin-deficient states and is usually present only in IDDM but can exist in NIDDM during the stress response.

If the alterations just described are not corrected or adequately controlled, acute and chronic complications can occur. Acutely, the patient can develop nausea and vomiting and other alterations, fluid and electrolyte problems worsen, and the patient's condition can advance to hyperglycemic coma or diabetic ketoacidosis (DKA). Chronically, the patient can develop microvascular and macrovascular complications or neuropathy. These conditions are described in a later section of the chapter.

Figure 40-6 depicts the clinical manifestations of IDDM and NIDDM, which can be the same for both states. The classic symptoms of diabetes, which are the "polys" (polyuria, polydipsia, polyphagia), are nearly always present in IDDM and can be present in NIDDM. However, many persons with NIDDM have very subtle symptoms of acute metabolic changes or chronic com-

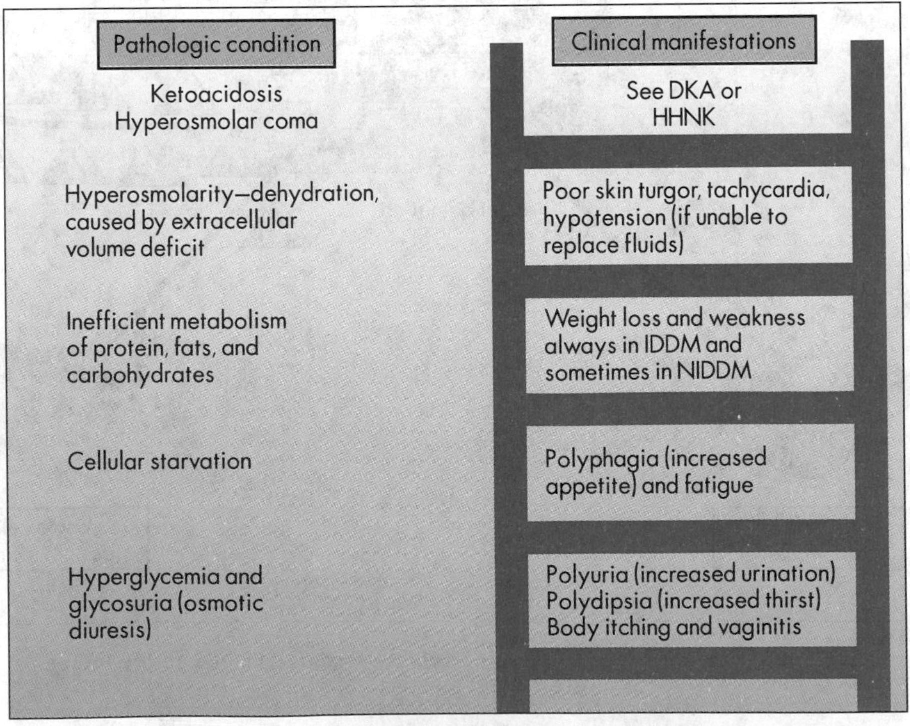


**FIGURE 40-6** Clinical manifestations of diabetes mellitus. Like a ladder, the beginning clinical manifestations start on the bottom rung.

plications, such as extreme fatigue, blurred vision, and falling asleep in the chair. As with a ladder, the beginning clinical manifestations start on the bottom rung.

## PREVENTION

Preventive health care for diabetes mellitus may be primary (prevention of the primary disease), secondary (early detection and control of the disease), or tertiary (control of complications).

*Healthy People 2000*[74] is a report of the U.S. Public Health Services that identifies goals for health care for the year 2000. These goals as related to diabetes are listed in the following preventive stages.

### PRIMARY PREVENTION

Patients frequently ask, "How can diabetes be prevented?" Although there is no definite answer, a responsibility exists to discuss the following: (1) risk factors that either directly cause diabetes or are statistically associated with it and (2) research and experimental approaches to preventing diabetes. Prevention of both IDDM and NIDDM involves knowledge of risk factors (Box 40-3). How to use these risk factors is not completely clear. Experimental treatment for preventing diabetes mellitus is being used in IDDM. Currently, by using antibody tests, the risk for IDDM can be identified. At this time, experimental therapy such as immunosuppressive agents, nicotinamide, β-cell rest, and reprogramming of the immune system is being used.[23]

Primary prevention of NIDDM may involve identifying metabolic abnormalities such as hyperglycemia and hyperinsulinemia, which may predict risk of IGT and NIDDM. Data show that persons who are lean or obese and have these two metabolic markers are at much higher risk for developing glucose intolerance than obese subjects who have normal glucose and insulin levels.[80] This is not a clear package of information that the nurse can give to patients, but it does clearly reveal there may be other factors that should give risk factor counseling more impetus. To simply encourage diet and exercise will not ensure prevention. Background information that comes from evolving studies helps the caregiver put preventive education into focus. For example, it is clear that exercise, moderate or strenuous, is clearly associated with improved insulin sensitivity, modification of cardiovascular risk factors, and lower prevalence of NIDDM.[80]

Obesity has long been discussed in association with NIDDM; however, a newer culprit in this area is the distribution of the weight, upper-body weight (apple shape), and lower-body weight (pear shaped). NIDDM often occurs in association with upper-body obesity, and studies have shown that regular exercise can result in greater loss of abdominal compared with midthigh fat tissue in certain subjects.[22] Therefore primary prevention should be directed toward life-style changes that include exercise, weight control or weight loss, and knowledge of risk factors. Genetic counseling is still not recommended because of the unknown nature of the pattern of transmission. It is important that persons with diabetes are made aware of the familial tendencies and risks for siblings of the individual with either type of diabetes and that they be discussed[16,74,75] (Table 40-6).

The surgeon general's report *Healthy People 2000*[74] established several goals that give the previously discussed primary prevention recommendations more momentum. One goal is to reduce overweight prevalence to not more than 20% among people aged 20 or older (baseline: 26% for people age 20 through 74 in 1976-1980, 24% for men and 27% for women). For people ages 20 years and older, overweight is defined as body mass index (BMI) equal to or greater than 27.8 for men and 27.3 for women. BMI is calculated by dividing weight in kilograms by the square of height in meters. Another goal from *Healthy People 2000* that has relevance for prevention of NIDDM pertains to exercise. The goal is to increase to at least 30% the proportion of people ages 6 years and older who engage regularly, preferably daily, in light to moderate physical activity for at least 30 minutes per day (baseline: 22% of people ages 18 and older were active for at least 30 minutes five or more times per week, and 12% were active seven

**BOX 40-3 Risk Factors for Diabetes Mellitus**

- Family history of diabetes
- Obesity
- Race (Native American, Hispanic, or African-American)
- Age
- Previously identified IGT
- Hypertension or hyperlipidemia
- Women (history of GDM or delivery of babies >9 pounds)
- Presence of islet cell antibodies

**TABLE 40-6 Estimated Risk of Developing Diabetes Mellitus**

| RELATIONSHIP TO PERSON WITH DIABETES | APPROXIMATE RATE OF DEVELOPING DIABETES |
|---|---|
| No diabetes in family | Type I: 0.3% |
| Identical twin with type I | Type I: 36% |
| One parent with type I | Type I: 3% |
| Sibling with type I | Type I: 3% |
| No diabetes in family | Type II: 14% |
| Identical twin with type II | Type II: almost 100% |
| One parent with type II | Type II: 20%-30% |
| Both parents with type II | Type II: 35%-55% |

Data from Bode BW et al: *DiabetesDek—how to control and manage diabetes mellitus*, Atlanta, 1992, Lifescan Infodek.

or more times per week in 1985). Light to moderate physical activity requires sustained, rhythmic muscular movements; is at least equivalent to sustained walking; and is performed at less than 60% of maximal heart rate for age. Maximal heart rate equals about 220 beats per minute minus age. Examples of light to moderate physical activity include walking, swimming, cycling, dancing, gardening and yard work, various domestic and occupational activities, and games and other childhood pursuits.

The urgency of primary prevention is blatant when looking at the objective from *Healthy People 2000* to reduce diabetes-related deaths to no more than 34 per 100,000 people (age-adjusted baseline: 38 per 100,000 in 1986). Cardiovascular disease is the leading cause of death among people with diabetes, accounting for more than half of all deaths. Health behaviors aimed at modifying the risk of cardiovascular disease by reducing cardiovascular disease risk factors (Box 30-6, p. 814) could have a major effect on morbidity and mortality from diabetes mellitus.

## SECONDARY PREVENTION

Much of the primary prevention discussed is in the research stage, and until this information becomes certain, secondary prevention is necessary. Surveys conducted by the National Institutes of Health have emphasized the importance of screening for NIDDM. Two surveys conducted by the National Center for Health Statistics used 75 g, 2-hour oral glucose tolerance tests, interviews, and examinations of several thousand persons to estimate the prevalence of diagnosed and undiagnosed diabetes in the general population and in the Hispanic population. In the U.S. population, the prevalence of diabetes was 20% at ages 65 to 74. Undiagnosed diabetes represented about half the group. About 10% of the adult population over age 50 had undiagnosed diabetes. These results suggest that about 4.5 million non-Hispanic whites have undiagnosed diabetes. There is a 50% greater prevalence of undiagnosed diabetes in blacks and a 60% greater prevalence of undiagnosed diabetes in Hispanics. This comes to about 6.3 million individuals with undiagnosed diabetes in the United States. According to the surveys, many of the undiagnosed individuals had substantial elevations in blood glucose, with 40% having 2-hour blood glucose levels greater than 250 mg/dl and 25% with levels greater than 300 mg/dl.[74] Screening criteria can be obtained from the American Diabetes Association and can be carried out successfully in most settings.[7]

Because of the number of persons with undiagnosed diabetes and the strong association between diabetes and hypertension, atherosclerotic heart disease, and pe-

**TABLE 40-7 Prevention of Long-Term Complications of Diabetes Mellitus**

| COMPLICATIONS | EARLY DETECTION | EARLY INTERVENTION |
|---|---|---|
| Eye problems | Ophthalmoscopic examination | Care by an ophthalmologist or retinal specialist<br>Control of hyperglycemia<br>Control of hypertension<br>Laser photocoagulation<br>Referral for low vision evaluation, optical aids, and rehabilitation |
| Kidney problems | Examination of urine for albumin and/or protein excretion<br>Measurement of serum creatinine and creatinine clearance | Control of hyperglycemia<br>Control of hypertension and other cardiovascular risk factors<br>Consultation with a nephrologist<br>Limiting protein intake<br>Avoiding nephrotoxic agents<br>Early treatment of urinary tract infections |
| Atherosclerosis | History of risk factors and symptoms<br>Examination: electrocardiogram and serum lipids measurements, peripheral pulses | Control of hyperglycemia<br>Control of hypertension<br>Weight control<br>Exercise<br>Consultation with specialist: cardiologist, neurologist, vascular surgeon |
| Neuropathy | History of symptoms of pain, numbness, etc.<br>Examination: orthostatic blood pressures, muscle strength, reflexes, and sensory function | Control of hyperglycemia<br>Avoidance of neurotoxic agents<br>Education about the importance of routine evaluation, foot care, and specific treatment of neuropathy |
| Foot problems | History of symptoms of numbness, infection, and peripheral vascular insufficiency<br>Complete foot examination | Control of hyperglycemia<br>Control of atherogenic risk<br>Education about the importance and methods of foot care<br>Referral to a podiatrist and vascular surgeon<br>Referral for special shoes, shoe inlays, assistive mobility devices, and rehabilitation services |

Data from Herman W: *The prevention and treatment of complications of diabetes: a guide for primary care practitioners,* Atlanta, 1990, 6-1 to 6-4, US Department of Health and Human Services, Centers for Disease Control.

ripheral vascular disease, health promotion behaviors that diminish the risk for the latter will help diminish complications in persons with both known and undiagnosed diabetes. Health-teaching programs should involve persons of all ages in schools, industry, or senior citizen groups.

Persons with known diabetes must have access to education, dietary support, social support systems, medical care, and nursing care so that prevention and early detection of complications are possible. Services need to include programs for hypertension detection and control, smoking cessation, eye care, and foot care.

## TERTIARY PREVENTION

Both chronic and acute complications occur often, and nurses who work with persons who have diabetes must be involved in tertiary prevention if complications are to be lessened. Another national goal for the year 2000 is to reduce the most severe complications of diabetes, as shown in Table 40-7.[45] Major emphasis on tertiary preventive education will be on the ability of nurses to counsel the patient about the early detection and interventions listed in Table 40-7.

The importance of patient education is clear, and the need for its availability was outlined in one of the goals of *Healthy People 2000.*[74] The goal is to increase to at least 40% the proportion of people with chronic and disabling conditions who receive formal patient education including information about community and self-help resources as an integral part of the management of their condition. (The specific target for the year 2000 for patient education of people with diabetes is 75%; the 1983-1984 baseline was 32% [classes] and 68% [counseling].)

# MEDICAL MANAGEMENT

The expected length of stay of patients with diabetes mellitus as determined by diagnosis-related groups (DRGs) is 5 to 6 days. In the past, patients with diabetes were often hospitalized to initiate management. This is done now only if the patient is experiencing severely worsening acute or chronic complications. Currently, no cure exists for diabetes, so patients need to establish goals with their health care team members for management of their diabetes. The focuses of medical therapy are:

1. Implementing diagnostic tests for presence of diabetes mellitus or complications
2. Establishing goals related to level of daily control
3. Using medications, treatments, diet, and activities to manage diabetes on a day-to-day basis
4. Using medications, treatments, and diet to manage acute and chronic complications of diabetes

The way to achieve the goals of metabolic control is through the use of medications, diet, activity, monitoring, and education. By its very nature, diabetes can be significantly influenced by each of these management components (Figure 40-7). Common medical therapy for management is discussed next.

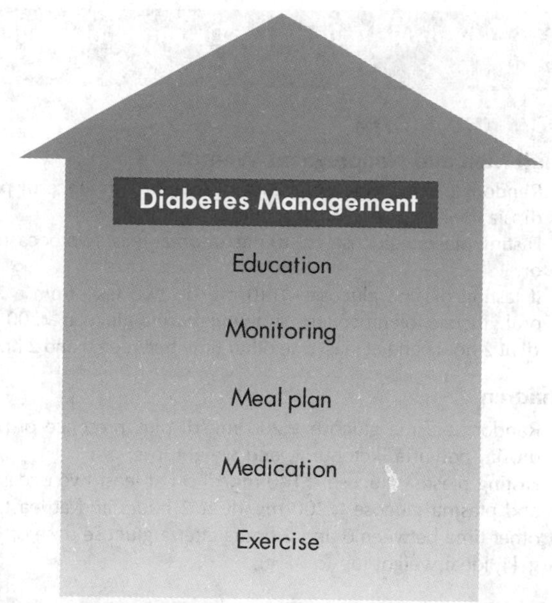


**FIGURE 40-7** Diabetes management.

## DIAGNOSTIC TESTS

The diagnosis of diabetes is not always easy, and controversy has existed especially with the elderly population. Where does that leave the nurse? A general consensus would be the "criteria for diagnosis" stated in the position statement by the American Diabetes Association (ADA).[7] These criteria are listed in Box 40-4.

## ESTABLISHING GOALS RELATED TO LEVEL OF CONTROL

Criteria for levels of metabolic control vary depending on (1) the philosophy of the health team about the benefits of meticulous control in avoiding the long-term manifestations of deficiency of insulin or its action and (2) what the health team believes is realistic for an individual patient based on the patient's age, ability, other health problems, support, and desires. It is important to remember that data[8] support that long-term complications can be prevented or arrested by normalizing the metabolic environment; therefore the goal frequently is to achieve good-to-excellent metabolic control. However, the achievement of excellent or ideal control increases the risk of hypoglycemia and can place a tremendous burden and risk on the patient. The patient must participate in establishing the goals of therapy, and everyone involved must know what those goals are.

The level of control is evaluated in several ways. The indexes used to evaluate level of control and indications of good-to-excellent control in adults with IDDM or NIDDM can be found in Table 40-8. In addition to meet-

**BOX 40-4 Metabolic Criteria for Diagnosis of Diabetes Mellitus**

**IDDM AND NIDDM**

**Adult Men and Nonpregnant Women**

1. Random plasma glucose ≥200 mg/dl plus presence of polydipsia, polyuria, polyphagia, and weight loss, or
2. Fasting plasma glucose ≥140 mg/dl on at least two occasions, or
3. If fasting plasma glucose <140 mg/dl, two tests from a 75-g oral glucose tolerance test; showing plasma glucose ≥200 mg/dl at 2 hours and at least one other time between 0 and 2 hours.

**Children**

1. Random plasma glucose ≥200 mg/dl plus presence of polydipsia, polyuria, ketonuria, and weight loss, or
2. Fasting plasma glucose ≥140 mg/dl on at least two occasions and plasma glucose ≥200 mg/dl at 2 hours and at least one other time between 0 and 2 hours after a glucose dose of 1.75 g/kg ideal weight (up to 75 g).

**GDM: Pregnant Women**

Two plasma glucose values ≥ the following fasting or after 100 g of oral glucose:
Fasting ≥ 105 mg/dl
1 hour ≥ 190 mg/dl
2 hour ≥ 165 mg/dl
3 hour ≥ 145 mg/dl.

**IMPAIRED GLUCOSE TOLERANCE**

**Adult Men and Nonpregnant Women**

1. Fasting plasma glucose concentration <140 mg/dl, *and*
2. 1-2 hour oral glucose tolerance test plasma glucose ≥140 mg/dl but <200 mg/dl, *and*
3. An intervening oral glucose tolerance test plasma glucose ≥200 mg/dl.

**Children**

1. Fasting plasma glucose concentration <140 mg/dl, *and*
2. A 2-hour oral glucose tolerance test plasma ≥140 mg/dl.

ing the criteria of these indexes, the patient should be attaining or maintaining a normal weight. Level of control must not be a blanket number. Each person's situation must be considered in setting control goals.

## MEDICATION

Although medication is the first management component listed, it is not first in clinical application and cannot stand alone without the most significant part of the treatment regimen: diet. Insulin is necessary for every person with IDDM; insulin or oral hypoglycemic agents may be necessary for some patients with NIDDM.

### Properties of Insulin

Four properties of insulin preparation may be identified in the prescription: source, purity, strength, and type of action.[24,28,38]

#### Insulin species source and purity

Insulin sources that are currently available are beef, pork, and human. The different insulin types are either beef, pork, beef/pork combination, biosynthetic recombinant human derived from bacteria (Lilly brand),[28] and biosynthetic recombinant human derived from yeast (Novolin). Pork and beef differ from human insulin by one amino acid (pork) and three amino acids (beef). Insulin antigenicity can decrease insulin receptor effectiveness. In the past, most insulin was prepared from a combination of beef and pork pancreata. Pork most closely resembles human insulin and is considered the least antigenic animal insulin.

Now, human insulin is often used and recommended by most endocrinologists. It has less antigenicity than animal insulin, and it greatly expands the insulin resources of the world. Human insulin is available as regular, lente, NPH, ultralente, 70/30, and 50/50. The latter two are mixtures of 70% NPH/30% regular and 50% NPH/50% regular. Generally, when changing a person from animal source to human source, no change in dosage is required; however, patients should be directed to check blood sugar more frequently as the human insulin is more like their own and may work better to lower the blood glucose.

Purity of insulin preparations is reflected by the amount of proinsulin (noninsulin pancreatic proteins) in the preparation. Today, insulins are defined as *purified* when they contain less than 10 parts per million (ppm) of proinsulin. Standard insulins (beef/pork, beef, pork) contain less than 10 ppm. Insulins labeled as purified or human contain less than 1 ppm. Most insulin products contain less than 1 ppm. Purified insulins are associated with reduced incidence of allergic responses.

### TABLE 40-8 Laboratory Indexes for Evaluating Level of Control in Adults with IDDM or NIDDM

**TARGET BLOOD GLUCOSE FOR HEALTHY YOUNG INDIVIDUALS WITH DIABETES**

| TIME | mg/dl | mM |
|---|---|---|
| Fasting | 70-130 | 3.9-7.2 |
| 1-hour postprandial | 100-180 | 5.6-10.0 |
| 2-hour postprandial | 80-150 | 4.4-8.3 |
| 0200-0400 postprandial | 70-120 | 3.9-6.7 |

**TARGET BLOOD GLUCOSE FOR TYPE II DIABETES**

| | |
|---|---|
| Normalize fasting plasma glucose: | Ideally <115 mg/dl (<6.4 mM) |
| | Minimally <140 mg/dl (<7.8 mM) |
| Postprandial plasma glucose: | Ideally <140 mg/dl (<7.8 mM) |
| | Minimally <200 mg/dl (<11.1 mM) |

The American Diabetes Association's response to the Diabetes Control and Complications Trial (June 1993)

Level of glucose control for persons with IDDM who are intellectually, emotionally, physically, and financially able to attempt target control: mean blood glucose of 155 mg/dl and $HbA_{1c}$ of 7.29%; normal 4% to 6.5%

Target Blood Glucose is not "cut and dry," and the following should be considered:

- Age of patient
- Status of health
- Pregnancy
- Ability to recognize insulin reaction

**LIPID LEVELS FOR ADULTS**

| RISK FOR ADULT DIABETIC PATIENTS | CHOLESTEROL (mg/dl) | HDL CHOLESTEROL (mg/dl) | LDL CHOLESTEROL (mg/dl) | TRIGLYCERIDES (mg/dl) |
|---|---|---|---|---|
| Acceptable | <200 | ≥60 | <130 | <200 |
| Borderline | 200-239 | — | 130-159 | 200-399 |
| High | ≥240 | ≤35 | ≥160 | ≥400 |

Data from American Diabetes Association: *Diabetes Care* 16(suppl 2):1-66, 1993; American Diabetes Association: ***Report on diabetes control and complications trial,*** National Meeting, Las Vegas, June 1993; and Lebovitz HE, editor: ***Therapy for diabetes mellitus and related disorders,*** Alexandria, Va, 1991, American Diabetes Association.

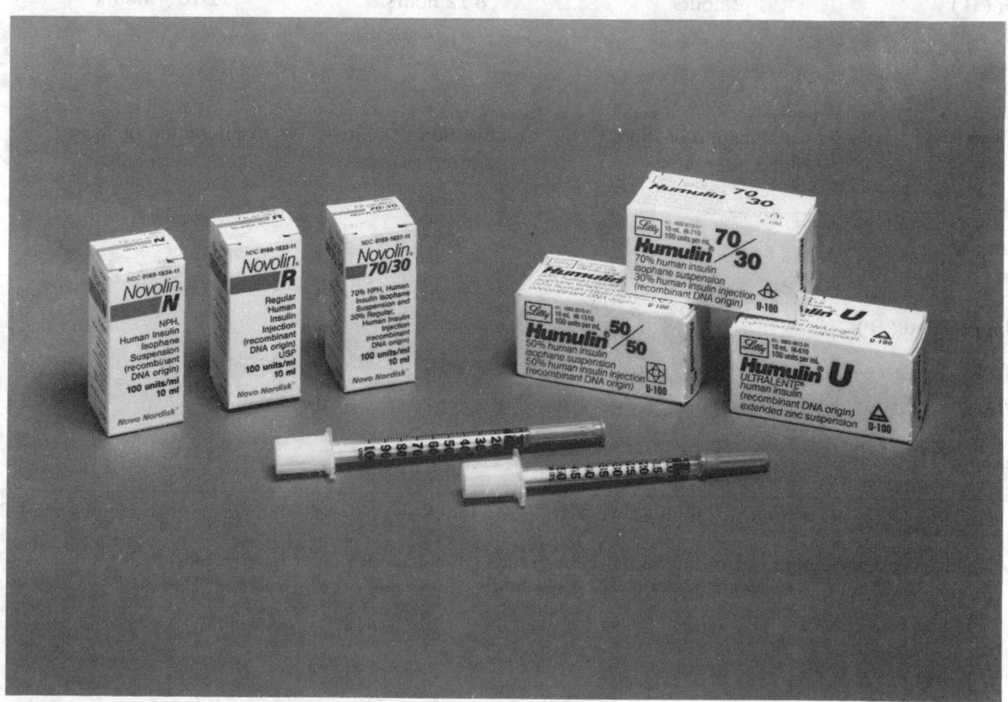


**FIGURE 40-8** Containers of various types of insulin, including U-100 Novolin N, U-100 Novolin R, Novolin 70/30, Humulin 50/50, Humulin 70/30, U-100 Humulin Ultralente, and U-100 Becton-Dickinson insulin syringe.

**TABLE 40-9 Onset, Peak, Duration, and Appearance of Different Brands and Types of Insulin**

| TYPE OF INSULIN* | ONSET | PEAK | DURATION | APPEARANCE |
|---|---|---|---|---|
| **SHORT ACTING** | | | | |
| **Lilly** | | | | |
| Regular Iletin (B/P) | ½-1 hour | 2-4 hours | 6-8 hours | Clear |
| Regular Iletin II (P) | " | " | " | " |
| (R) Regular Humulin (H) | " | " | " | " |
| **Novo Nordisk** | | | | |
| Regular (P) | " | " | " | " |
| Velosulin (H) | " | " | " | " |
| (R) Regular Novolin (H) | " | " | " | " |
| (R) Regular Pen-fill (H) | " | " | " | " |
| **INTERMEDIATE ACTING** | | | | |
| **Lilly** | | | | |
| (R) NPH Humulin (H) | 1-2 hours | 4-12 hours | 10-14+ hours | Cloudy |
| NPH Iletin I (B/P) | " | " | " | " |
| NPH Iletin II (P) | " | " | " | " |
| (R) Lente Humulin (H) | 2 hours | 8-12 hours | 12-16+ hours | " |
| Lente Iletin I (B/P) | " | " | " | " |
| Lente Iletin II (P) | " | " | " | " |
| **Novo Nordisk** | | | | |
| (R) NPH Novolin (H) | 1-2 hours | 4-12 hours | 10-14+ hours | Cloudy |
| (R) NPH Novolin Pen-fill (H) | " | " | " | " |
| NPH Purified (P) | " | " | " | " |
| NPH Standard (B) | " | " | " | " |
| (R) Lente Novolin (H) | 2 hours | 8-12 hours | 12-16+ hours | " |
| Lente Purified (P) | " | " | " | " |
| **MIXTURE OF NPH/REGULAR** | | | | |
| **Lilly** | | | | |
| (R) 70/30 Humulin (H) | Combination of short and intermediate | Combination of short and intermediate | Combination of short and intermediate | Cloudy |
| (R) 50/50 Humulin (H) | | | | " |
| **Novo Nordisk** | | | | |
| (R) 70/30 Novolin (H) | " | " | " | " |
| (R) 70/30 Novolin Pen-fill (H) | " | " | " | " |
| 70/30 Mixtard (P) | " | " | " | " |
| (R) 70/30 Novolin prefilled (H) (disposable) | " | " | " | " |
| **LONG ACTING** | | | | |
| **Lilly** | | | | |
| (R) Ultralente Humulin (H) | 8 hours | 18 hours | 24-36 hours | Cloudy |

*P,* Pork; *B/P,* beef and pork; *B,* beef; *H,* human (both Eli Lilly [human] and Novo Nordisk [human] are of recombinant DNA origin); *(R),* recombinant DNA.

*Onset and duration differ across time range according to different brands. They can also differ from person to person.

### Strength

The strength of insulin correlates to the number of units of insulin per milliliter. In the very recent past, four strengths were available in the United States (U-40, U-80, U-100, U-500). Today, two strengths are available: U-100 and U-500 (U-500 can be obtained only by special request from Eli Lilly and Co.). Persons who are resistant to insulin and require more than 100 units may need to be treated with U-500 insulin. Insulin syringes are calibrated in units per milliliter. Elimination of U-40 and U-80 strengths of insulin has decreased errors of use of either wrong strength or wrong syringe (Figure 40-8).

### Type of action

All insulins are hypoglycemic, but they differ in speed of effect (onset), time of greatest action (peak), and how long they act (duration). Insulins are classified as short, intermediate, and long acting (Table 40-9). Food and activity must be coordinated with insulin action so that (1) insulin is available for optimal metabolism when the food that was eaten is absorbed, and (2) food is available while insulin is acting to prevent hypoglycemic reactions.

Three principles are useful in coordinating food and hypoglycemic medications:

1. Food must be taken after insulin within the time of onset of insulin action; for example, with regular insulin, food must be taken within 1 hour after injection, but regular insulin should be given 30 minutes before meals so it is available with the food.
2. Intermediate- or long-acting insulin requires that a supplemental feeding (snack) be given to match the peak action of the insulin; for example, a 3 PM snack after a 7 AM injection of NPH insulin.
3. Intermediate- or long-acting insulin requires a bedtime snack.

Because of the many changes being made in insulin preparations, the nurse must clarify the insulin prescription if the type, strength, purity, or species is unclear. A change in any one of the properties may lead to differences in action. When the insulin prescription is changed, careful patient monitoring is necessary to identify the extent of clinical effect.

## Insulin Regimens

Insulin therapy may include various regimens.[1,61] In persons with IDDM, the goal usually is to mimic, as closely as possible, normal endogenous insulin secretion patterns. In persons without diabetes, there is a meal-related increase in insulin secretion, with basal secretion between meals. There is also a tendency for glucose to reach its lowest peak at 3 to 4 AM and for basal insulin secretion to rise between 5 and 8 AM, before breakfast (dawn phenomenon). Descriptions of various regimens are presented in Box 40-5; regimens 3 to 6 are designed to mimic the normal endogenous secretion pattern. Regimens 5 and 6 are often described as intensive therapy.

Each regimen has advantages and disadvantages. Regimen 3 requires only two injections, but because intermediate-acting insulin peaks 8 to 12 hours after administration, it may peak during the night. This peak, along with the normal 3 to 4 AM drop in blood glucose, may cause nocturnal hypoglycemia. Regimen 4 should lessen the chance of nocturnal hypoglycemia and provide better coverage for the normal prebreakfast rise (dawn phe-

**BOX 40-5 Insulin Therapy Regimens**

1. One injection of intermediate-acting insulin per day
   a. Most frequently used in persons with NIDDM who are not controlled with diet and/or oral hypoglycemic agents
   b. Does not mimic the normal endogenous pattern
2. Two injections of intermediate-acting insulin per day
   a. Also used mostly in persons with NIDDM
   b. Does not mimic the normal endogenous pattern
3. Split and mixed insulin regimen: injection of rapid-acting insulin and intermediate-acting insulin at breakfast and supper
   a. Used in many persons with IDDM and some with NIDDM
   b. Theoretically, the morning rapid-acting insulin covers breakfast and early morning, the morning intermediate-acting insulin covers lunch and afternoon, the evening rapid-acting insulin covers the evening meal, and the evening intermediate-acting insulin covers the bedtime snack, the basal level needed during the night, and the normal prebreakfast rise (dawn phenomenon) in glucose
4. Split and mixed insulin regimens similar to regimen 3, except that the evening intermediate-acting insulin is given at bedtime instead of at the evening meal
   a. Used in persons with IDDM and some with NIDDM
   b. Theoretically provides better basal nighttime coverage and provides coverage for the natural prebreakfast glucose elevation (dawn phenomenon)
5. Multidosage regimen: three injections of rapid-acting insulin, one before each meal; one injection of intermediate insulin at bedtime
   a. The rapid-acting insulin provides coverage for each meal
   b. The bedtime intermediate-acting insulin provides the nighttime basal level and coverage for the natural prebreakfast glucose elevation (dawn phenomenon)
6. Multidose regimen: three injections of rapid-acting insulin, one before each meal; one injection of long-acting insulin at breakfast or at supper, or split between breakfast and supper (provides the same coverage as regimen 5)

Data from: American Diabetes Association: Physicians' guide to insulin-dependent (type I) diabetes: diagnoses and treatment, Alexandra, Va, 1988, The Association.
Novo Nordisk: Product reference guide, chart, Princeton, NJ, 1992, Novo Nordisk Pharmaceuticals.

nomenon) of blood glucose, but it requires three injections. Neither of these regimens allows flexibility in meal size or time; the person must eat on time or hypoglycemia can occur. For example, the morning intermediate-acting insulin will begin working in 1 to 4 hours and will peak in 8 to 14 hours, so if food is not provided at lunchtime, a hypoglycemic reaction can occur.

Regimen 5 requires four injections per day, but allows flexibility in meal size because the dose of rapid-acting insulin can be increased or decreased on the basis of the planned meal. Meals should still be on a relatively consistent basis so that insulin is taken on a consistent basis because there is no basal insulin coverage during the day. The **preprandial** (before meal) insulin must be taken in adequate time (usually 30 minutes) before meals to prevent **postprandial** (after meal) hyperglycemia. Regimen 6 allows the same flexibility in meal size as regimen 5. It also allows flexibility in meal time, because basal insulin coverage is provided between meals by the long-acting insulin. The preprandial insulin must still be taken in adequate time before meals to prevent postprandial hyperglycemia. With regimen 6, there is a large subcutaneous depot of long-acting insulin available all the time; if something occurs that increases absorption or if a meal is missed completely, hypoglycemia can occur.

Regimens 3 through 6 (particularly 5 and 6) require frequent blood glucose self-monitoring, before and after meals, to determine how much insulin is needed. An algorithm is usually developed for the patient using regimen 5 or 6, and although adherence to this algorithm will increase metabolic control, it requires a large investment of the patient's time and interest every day. Regimens 5 and 6, because they provide tighter control, also predispose the patient to hypoglycemia. Algorithms also may be developed for patients on regimens 3 and 4.

### Insulin pumps

Use of a portable infusion pump (Figure 40-9) to deliver insulin continuously can mimic a physiologic state. The pump is programmed to deliver a basal level of rapid-acting insulin continuously, with the basal level varied so that it is lower from 12 midnight to 4 AM, when glucose is naturally dropping, and higher from 5 to 8 AM, when glucose is normally increasing. It is manually activated to deliver a bolus of rapid-acting insulin in the preprandial period (the bolus must be taken an adequate time before a meal).

The use of an insulin pump prevents multiple injections (injection site is changed every 24 to 36 hours) and prevents the subcutaneous deposit of insulin that provides 24-hour basal coverage with regimen 6.

The pump allows flexibility in meal size and time. It requires intensive self-monitoring of blood glucose, adherence to an algorithm that requires an intense investment of the patient's time and interest, and wearing of the pump at all times. Interest, time, and repeated practice are required to learn how to program the pump. The pump has an alarm that informs the person if the battery is low, if insulin is infusing too rapidly, or if there is an occlusion in the line. Pumps are expensive; however, some insurance companies reimburse the expense.

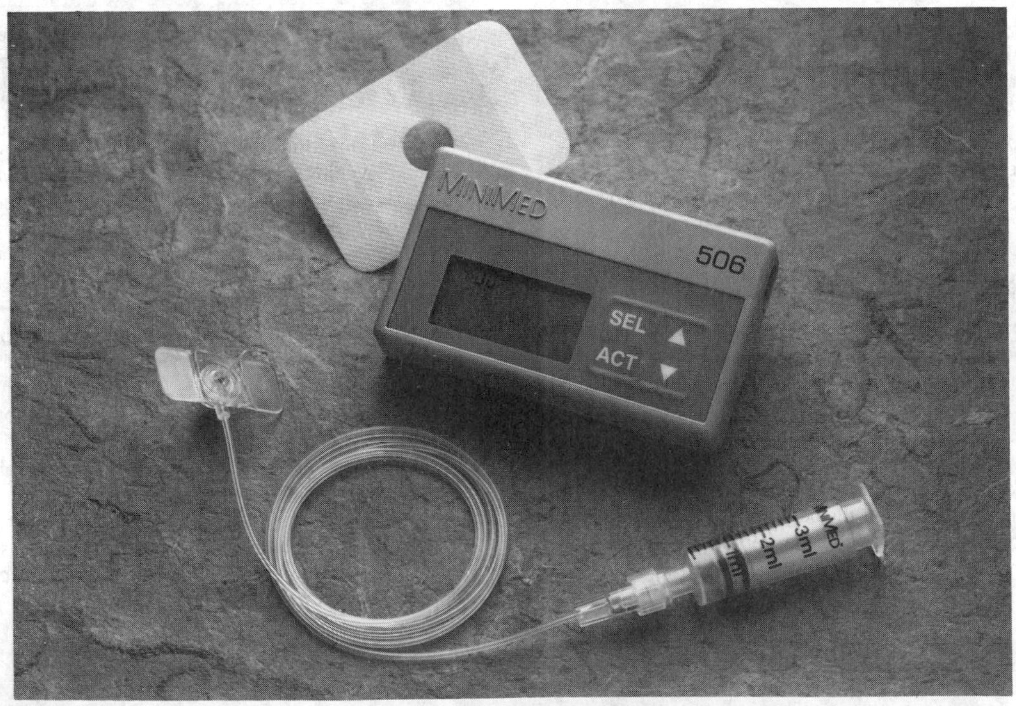


**FIGURE 40-9** Insulin infusion pump. (Courtesy MiniMed Technologies, Sylmar, Calif.)

## Oral Hypoglycemic Agents

Oral hypoglycemic agents are used in treating persons with NIDDM who are not controlled by diet and exercise alone. These agents are not insulin; to refer to them as oral insulin is a misnomer.

Six oral hypoglycemic agents are currently used in the United States[24] (Table 40-10). These agents are all sulfonylureas, which are thought to help control hyperglycemia by (1) increasing the ability of the islet cells of the pancreas to secrete insulin, (2) increasing the insulin sensitivity of extrapancreatic tissues, and (3) decreasing the rate of glucose production by the liver. Persons taking oral hypoglycemic agents need to adhere to the prescribed doses and the prescribed diet, maintain the usual amount of exercise, carry out prescribed self-monitoring, and take general health precautions.[2] Metformin, a biguanide, should be available in the United States in 1995.

Because of a study conducted in the 1970s by the University Group Diabetes Program (UGDP), much controversy has surrounded the use of these agents. The researchers in this study reported that the death rate from cardiovascular disease was two and one-half times higher in persons receiving tolbutamide than in those receiving a placebo. The results of the UGDP study have been challenged by numerous groups, but the Food and Drug Administration (FDA) recommends that oral hypoglycemic agents be limited to persons with symptomatic NIDDM who cannot be adequately controlled by diet or weight loss alone and in whom the addition of insulin to the therapeutic regimen is impractical or unacceptable. Oral hypoglycemic agents are not to be used in treating persons with IDDM or GDM. The sulfonylureas are metabolized by the kidneys and liver; thus the person with liver or kidney dysfunction may be at higher risk for development of side effects, particularly hypoglycemia.

Complications of oral hypoglycemic agents, besides hypoglycemia, include allergic skin reactions, gastrointestinal distress, and hematologic disorders. Chlorpropamide causes water retention and dilutional hyponatremia. Complications are rare, but hypoglycemic reactions that result from oral hypoglycemic agents may take several days to resolve because of the long duration of action of these drugs and the blood levels that will be present for some time. Many drugs interact with oral hypoglycemic agents and can potentiate, prolong, or shorten the action of the agents. Consult a pharmacist or physician if drug interactions are suspected. Patients should take most oral agents ½ hour before eating and be reminded to eat three meals a day. Some patients with NIDDM may be treated with a combination of insulin and oral agents. Theoretically, the oral agents should increase the patient's tissue sensitivity to both endogenous and exogenous insulin. The exogenous insulin replaces insulin that might be inadequate. This therapy is used only after other therapies are tried.

## Complications of Medication

### Insulin hypersensitivity and resistance

Insulin hypersensitivity occurs in some patients. Most reactions are local, consisting of wheals at injection sites, but systemic symptoms and anaphylactic reactions can

**TABLE 40-10 Onset, Peak, Duration, and Dosage of Oral Hypoglycemic Agents**

| BRAND NAME | GENERIC NAME | WHEN IT STARTS TO WORK | WHEN IT WORKS THE HARDEST | HOW LONG IT WORKS | TABLET SIZE | DOSE RANGE | DOSE/DAY | EXCRETION |
|---|---|---|---|---|---|---|---|---|
| **FIRST GENERATION** | | | | | | | | |
| Orinase | Tolbutamide | 1 hour | 4-6 hours | 6-12 hours | 250/500 | 500-3000 | 2-3 | Kidney |
| Tolinase | Tolazamide | 1 hour | 4-8 hours | Approx. 24 hours | 100/250/500 | 100-1000 | Once a day | Kidney |
| Dymelor | Acetohexamide | 1-2 hours | 8-12 hours | Approx. 18 hours | 250/500 | 250-1.5 g | 1-2 | Kidney |
| Diabinase | Chlorpropamide | 1 hour | 3-6 hours, up to 36 hours | Up to 60 hours | 100/250 | 100-500 | Once a day | Kidney |
| **SECOND GENERATION** | | | | | | | | |
| Micronase | Glyburide (non-micronized) | 1 hour | 4-8 hours | 12-24 hours | 1.25/2.5/5 | 1.25-20 | 1-2 | 50% kidney 50% bile |
| Diabeta | Glyburide (non-micronized) | 1 hour | 4-8 hours | 12-24 hours | 1.25/2.5/5 | 1.25-20 | 1-2 | 50% kidney 50% bile |
| Glynase | Glyburide (micronized) | 1 hour | 2-6 hours | 12-24 hours | 3 mg Pres-tabs | 1.5-12 | 1-2 | 50% kidney 50% bile |
| Glucotrol* | Glipizide | 10-30 minutes | 1-3 hours | 12-24 hours | 5/10 | 2.5-40 | 1-2 | 80% kidney 20% bile |
| Glucotrol XL | Glipizide Extended Release | | Up to 24 hours | 24 hours | 5/10 | 5-20 | Once a day | Feces |

*For best results must be taken 30 minutes before eating.
All other oral agents may be taken at any time, but work best if taken before eating. For all medications listed, action may vary from person to person.

occur. The hypersensitivity may be the result of several factors, including improper injection technique, sensitivity to the alcohol used to prepare the skin, sensitivity to the modifying proteins in the insulin, or sensitivity to the species source.

Treatment for hypersensitivity varies depending on the cause. Improper technique or hypersensitivity to the alcohol is ruled out first, proper injection technique is ensured, then a more purified form of alcohol or a different antiseptic agent is used to prepare the skin. If the modifying protein in the insulin is thought to be the causative factor, the patient may be switched from NPH to lente insulin. If the species source is thought to be the cause, the patient is switched to another species source. If the hypersensitivity is severe, an antihistamine may be given to treat the symptoms until the allergic response disappears. Corticosteroids may be used for severe reactions. If the patient is found to be allergic to all types of insulin, desensitization may be necessary.

**Insulin resistance,** defined as an insulin requirement greater than 200 U/day for longer than 2 days in the absence of infection or other factors that would increase insulin need, can also occur. The cause of insulin resistance is unknown but is thought to be the result of the development of antibodies that render insulin inactive. All patients who have been on insulin for 6 weeks to 3 months develop some antibodies to insulin. Usually, these antibodies are not sufficient to interfere with the response to insulin and the control of diabetes.

Insulin resistance may be treated by a different species of insulin. In some instances, adrenocorticotropic hormone (ACTH) or adrenal glucocorticoids may be used for short-term treatment. In most instances, insulin resistance is self-limiting. For this reason, some physicians do not use adjunctive therapy such as glucocorticoids; instead, they treat the patient with a higher dose of insulin during the period of resistance. When high doses of insulin are used to treat resistance, the patient must be monitored carefully for signs and symptoms of hypoglycemia; the dose will need to be decreased when the resistance period passes.

### Hypoglycemia

**Hypoglycemia** (frequently defined as plasma glucose level less than 50 mg/dl) is a major complication of insulin therapy or oral hypoglycemic agents. Note that less than 50 is too low for many patients and 70 would be more appropriate for persons who are not healthy or are elderly. Hypoglycemia is caused by an excess of insulin or oral hypoglycemic agent in relation to food intake or energy expenditure (Box 40-6). The signs and symptoms of hypoglycemia can be related to two factors (these signs and symptoms are discussed on p. 1330): increased sympathetic nervous system activity and the deprivation of the central nervous system (CNS) of glucose. The exact signs and symptoms seen in a particular individual vary with the rapidity of the drop in blood glucose level and the duration of hypoglycemia. A rapid drop in plasma glucose results primarily in manifestations from increased sympathetic nervous system activity. In slow-developing hypoglycemia, as might be seen with long-acting insulin or with oral hypoglycemic agents, the CNS signs and symptoms predominate. If a rapid drop occurs and is allowed to persist, all signs and symptoms usually occur.

**BOX 40-6 Causes of Hypoglycemia From Exogenous Insulin or Oral Hypoglycemic Agents**

1. Excessive dose of insulin or oral hypoglycemic agents or prolonged action of these drugs
2. Too little food intake (meal delayed or skipped), delayed gastric emptying, vomiting, or diarrhea
3. Excessive exercise in relation to food intake and insulin or oral hypoglycemic agent doses
4. Unknown causes
5. Kidney disease
6. Liver disease
7. Ingestion of other hypoglycemic agents or alcohol

Hypoglycemia may occur during sleep, particularly in persons on multidose insulin regimens, and the only symptoms may be nightmares, sweating, and headache on arising. Nighttime hypoglycemia may be part of the *Somogyi phenomenon.*

Patients with diabetes mellitus who are treated with β-adrenergic antagonists may be at special risk for hypoglycemia. The β-adrenergic agents block or inhibit the appearance of early signs and symptoms of hypoglycemia by blocking the sympathetic nervous system. In addition, these drugs prevent or block gluconeogenesis and glycogenolysis, thus inhibiting the normal endogenous response to hypoglycemia, making it more difficult to reverse the problem.

Signs and symptoms similar to those of hypoglycemia may occur when the blood glucose level is elevated and drops rapidly to a level that is still in an elevated range. The sudden rapid drop in blood sugar, regardless of the final level reached or the levels at which this occurred, is a stimulus for the physiologic neuroendocrine response to stressors to come into play. Thus a patient whose glucose level drops from 500 mg/dl to 300 mg/dl very rapidly may demonstrate the same signs and symptoms as a patient whose glucose drops to 30 mg/dl. Patients with uncontrolled diabetes may complain of feeling hypoglycemic, even though their plasma glucose levels are high. The patient is often labeled as a "malingerer" or "uncooperative" because health team members may believe that the patient is trying to obtain more food. The nurse who is aware of this phenomenon may be able to help others understand the patient's complaints and help avoid such labeling.

The treatment for hypoglycemia is fast-acting carbohydrates. If a question exists about the validity of the diabetic person's feelings about an impending hypoglycemic reaction, blood should be drawn immediately for a blood glucose test and sugar given at once. The nurse should understand that, when in doubt, it is always safer to give sugar than to risk nervous system damage from hypoglycemia. Usually 10 to 15 g of carbohydrate is sufficient to overcome hypoglycemia. If the individual is already unconscious, 50% glucose usually is given intravenously. When the person's symptoms have cleared, a snack consisting of complex carbohydrates and proteins such as cheese or peanut butter and crackers should be given. If the next meal is due soon, it can be eaten instead of the snack.

Glucagon, a pancreatic hormone that acts primarily by mobilizing hepatic glycogen, may be given to treat insulin reaction. The effects of this glycogen conversion last about 1½ hours; therefore treatment with sugar, complex carbohydrates, and proteins will also be required to prevent a recurrence of the hypoglycemia. Glucagon is given subcutaneously or intramuscularly, and some physicians instruct their patients to take it when an insulin reaction occurs. If the patient is unconscious, the family administers the drug and then seeks medical assistance.

The patient who develops hypoglycemia while taking oral hypoglycemic agents may need treatment for several days, and hospitalization may be mandatory. These patients may need dextrose infusion and glucocorticoids to promote gluconeogenesis along with the other therapy. The reason any hypoglycemic episode is serious is that it interferes with the oxygen consumption of nervous tissue. Repeated or prolonged attacks can cause irreparable brain damage.

The following are *pertinent nursing implications of the medication component:*

1. Being knowledgeable of the time/action of insulin and oral agents and how this relates to meal planning, activity, and potential time for hypoglycemia
2. Being knowledgeable of the names of the insulin that fit into the categories of rapid acting, intermediate acting, and long acting
3. Being knowledgeable that there are multiple insulin regimens and oral agent/insulin regimens and therefore more options for patients
4. Being knowledgeable about the complications of insulin and oral agents and how to manage these

## TREATMENT

No specific treatments exist for persons with diabetes mellitus.

## DIET

A true and frequently used statement is, "Nutritional management is the cornerstone of therapy in all types of diabetes mellitus." Since diet is a part of medical management and should be the first component of management, patients need to be referred early to a registered dietitian (RD) for nutritional education and the development of meal plans that are flexible and fitting for their life-styles. Food issues are never simple to patients, and a good understanding from the beginning can often determine the success of their management. Patients are often fearful about what to put into their mouths. If this fear is not addressed through education, at first eating will be curtailed but later all caution goes to the wind and it is difficult to make a new beginning. Here lies the rationale for an early referral to an RD. If no dietitian is

### BOX 40-7 Target Nutritional Goals for Persons with Diabetes

**CALORIES**

Sufficient to achieve and maintain reasonable body weight

**CARBOHYDRATE**

Varies in relation to assessment and protein and fat intake; usually 45% to 60% calories

Liberalized individualized emphasis on unrefined carbohydrate with fiber

Modest amounts of sucrose and other refined sugars may be acceptable contingent on metabolic control and body weight

**PROTEIN**

Usual dietary intake of protein is double the amount needed.

Exact ideal percentage of total calories is unknown; however, usual intake is 12%-20% of total calories.

RDA is 0.8 g/kg body weight for adults; it is modified for children, pregnant and lactating women, elderly persons, and those with special medical conditions.

**FAT**

Usually ≤30% of total calories, but may be as high as 40%.

Polyunsaturated fats, 6%-8%

Saturated fats, 10%

Monounsaturated fats, remaining percentage

Cholesterol <300 mg/day

**FIBER**

Up to 40 g/day

25 g/1000 kcal for low-calorie intakes

**ALTERNATIVE SWEETENERS**

Use of various nutritive and nonnutritive sweeteners is acceptable

**SODIUM**

≤3000 mg/day

Modified for special medical conditions

**ALCOHOL**

≤1-2 equivalents 1-2 times per week

1 equivalent = 1.5 oz distilled liquor, 4-oz glass of wine, 12-oz glass of beer

**VITAMINS/MINERALS**

No evidence that diabetes mellitus influences need

**TABLE 40-11 Guidelines for Estimating Calorie Requirements**

| LEVEL | ACTIVITIES | CALORIE REQUIREMENTS |
|---|---|---|
| Light, >55 years, obese, and/or inactive | Less than for "light" below | 10 calories/lb (22 kcal/kg) Desired body weight (DBW) |
| Light | Ambulating in hospital, washing clothes, walking 2.5 to 3 miles/hour, carpentry, electrical work, golfing, sailing | 10-12 calories/lb (22-26 kcal/kg) DBW |
| Moderate | Weeding and hoeing, bicycling, dancing, tennis, walking 3.5 to 4 miles/hr, scrubbing floors, work involving loading and stocking | 12-14 calories/lb (26-32 kcal/kg) DBW |
| Heavy | Climbing, walking uphill with a full load, basketball, football, swimming | 14-16 calories/lb (31-35 kcal/kg) DBW |
| Weight reduction | | Subtract 500 calories from total calories for the day |

available, the nurse should be able to give basic nutritional information to suffice until the patient can see a dietitian.

The current nutritional management for diabetes is to maintain reasonable weight and control blood glucose and lipid levels without compromising health. Current nutritional recommendations for people with diabetes are similar to those for healthy individuals without diabetes, as developed by the National Research Council, the American Heart Association, and the American Cancer Society. Box 40-7 can assist the nurse with current recommendations for people with diabetes. Controversy has developed over the amount of fat and starch to be utilized in the diabetes diet. The current recommendations in the table are supported by the American Diabetes Association policy statement and the Diabetes Care and Education Dietetic Practice Group.[7,8a,21,57]

Most persons need 25 kilocalories (kcal)/kg of desired body weight (DBW) to maintain their weight and meet basic metabolic needs. With this as the basis, kilocalories are added or subtracted, based on activity level, age, and need to lose weight (Table 40-11).

Another dietary component that is manipulated is fiber. A high-fiber, high-carbohydrate diet has been shown to decrease insulin requirements and cholesterol, both fasting and postprandial glucose serum levels. Fiber can increase satiety, which might help with weight reduction. Fiber delays gastric emptying and decreases peak blood glucose, so when it is introduced in the diet, blood

**TABLE 40-12 Fiber Content of Selected Foods**

| FOOD | SERVING SIZE | FIBER (g) |
|---|---|---|
| **BREADS/CEREALS** | | |
| 100% bran cereal | ½ cup | 10 |
| Kidney beans | ½ cup | 4.5 |
| Peas | ½ cup | 5.2 |
| Potatoes, white | 1 small | 3.8 |
| Rice, brown | ½ cup | 1.3 |
| Bread, whole-grain wheat | 1 slice | 2.7 |
| **FRUITS** | | |
| Apple, uncooked | 1 small | 3.9 |
| Orange | 1 small | 2.1 |
| Strawberries | ¾ cup | 2.4 |
| Peach | 1 medium | 1.0 |
| **COOKED VEGETABLES** | | |
| Beets | ½ cup | 1.7 |
| Broccoli | ½ cup | 2.6 |
| Carrots | ½ cup | 2.2 |
| Lettuce, uncooked | ½ cup | 0.5 |

glucose should be monitored and insulin or any oral agents may need to be adjusted.

This dietary manipulation requires that 25 to 40 g of plant fiber be added to the diet each day.[11,12] The fiber source should be a natural one, not a commercial fiber supplement. Some high-fiber foods are listed in Table 40-12. A review of this table reveals that increasing fiber content to the 40 g range takes careful planning and may not be warranted in a low-calorie diet.[11]

Research to define fully the benefits of a high-fiber diet and its side effects is ongoing. Fiber should be added gradually to avoid abdominal discomfort, and water intake should be increased. For additional information about this diet, consult the listed references.[11,12]

Future recommendations for nutritional management may be influenced by the knowledge that foods do not all cause the same rise in blood glucose levels. The term **glycemic index** is used to describe the change in blood glucose levels from ingestion of specific foods. With glucose given a glycemic index of 100%, potatoes, white rice, honey, and carrots have an index of 70%; peanuts, lentils, and kidney beans have an index less than 30%.[31] The physical form of the food and the combination of nutrients are important factors in the glycemic index. At this time, information about the glycemic index of foods is applied on an individual basis only and has not been incorporated into general recommendations for diabetic diets.

## Principles of Dietary Management

If the person with diabetes mellitus has a nutritional history that incorporates the dietary recommendations described in the preceding section, few dietary changes will be needed. The diabetic diet is one that all persons

**TABLE 40-13 Examples of Food Exchanges***

| EXCHANGES | FOOD SERVING SAMPLE | |
|---|---|---|
| **STARCH/BREAD EXCHANGE** | | |
| (Includes starchy vegetables) | 1 slice bread | ½ bagel, 1 tortilla |
| Calories—80 | ½ hamburger bun | ½ small baked potato |
| CHO (g)—15 | ⅓ C corn, ½ C peas | ½ C oatmeal |
| Protein (g)—3 | ½ C cooked pasta | ⅓ C rice |
| Fat (g)—trace | 6 saltines | |
| **MEAT EXCHANGE** | | |
| **Lean** | **Lean** | |
| Calories—55 | 1 oz lean beef, pork, veal, or poultry without skin | |
| CHO (g)—0 | 2 oz fish | |
| Protein (g)—7 | ¼ C dry cottage cheese | |
| Fat (g)—3 | ¼ C tuna, mackerel | |
| | 1 oz diet cheese (<55 calories/oz) | |
| **Medium** | **Medium-Fat** | |
| Calories—75 | 1 oz 15%-fat beef, boiled ham, or liver | |
| CHO (g)—0 | 1 egg | |
| Protein (g)—7 | | |
| Fat (g)—5 | | |
| **High** | **High-Fat** | |
| Calories—100 | 1 oz 20%-fat beef, ground pork, duck, or regular cheeses | |
| CHO (g)—0 | 1 frankfurter | |
| Protein (g)—7 | 1 oz lunch meat | |
| Fat (g)—8 | 1 T peanut butter (contains unsaturated fats) | |
| **VEGETABLE** | | |
| Calories—25 | ½ C cooked, 1 C raw—beets, carrots, brussel sprouts, onions, sauerkraut, eggplant, asparagus, cabbage, green or wax beans, or mustard greens | |
| CHO (g)—5 | 1 medium tomato | |
| Protein (g)—2 | | |
| Fat (g)—0 | | |
| **FRUIT EXCHANGE** | | |
| Calories—60 | 1 small apple, orange, peach, tangerine, or pear | |
| CHO (g)—15 | ½ C applesauce | |
| Protein (g)—0 | ½ banana or grapefruit | |
| Fat (g)—0 | ⅓ cantaloupe | |
| | ⅛ honeydew melon | |
| **MILK EXCHANGE** | | |
| Calories—80 | 1 C skim or nonfat milk | **Calories—120, Fat (g)—5:** |
| CHO (g)—12 | 1 C plain nonfat yogurt | 1 C lowfat (2%) milk |
| Protein (g)—8 | 1 C skim buttermilk | 1 C lowfat (2%) yogurt |
| Fat (g)—trace if skim | | |
| **FAT EXCHANGE** | | |
| Calories—45 | 1 t margarine | ⅛ avocado |
| CHO (g)—0 | 1 t oil | 1 strip crisp bacon |
| Protein (g)—0 | 1 t regular mayonnaise | 1 T reduced-calorie mayonnaise |
| Fat (g)—5 | 1 T cream cheese | |
| **FREE EXCHANGE** | | |
| Calories—0 | Unsweetened gelatin | |
| CHO (g)—0 | Calorie-free beverages | |
| Protein (g)—0 | Coffee, tea, spices, bouillon | |
| Fat (g)—0 | | |

From American Diabetes Association and American Dietetic Association: *Exchange lists for meal planning,* Alexandria, Va, 1986, The Association.
*This table shows a sample of the type and size of food servings from each food group (exchange). For complete exchange list, see reference 9.
*C,* Cup; *CHO,* carbohydrate; *T,* tablespoon; *t,* teaspoon.

should follow; however, given the dietary habits of most Americans, some dietary changes are usually necessary. Recommendations need to be made with the awareness that eating habits are difficult to change.

To increase success, dietary planning should include consideration of the following:

1. Religious, cultural, and personal preferences of the patient
2. Life-style components: family eating patterns, finances, and hour-work schedule
3. Activity/rest patterns: amount, timing, and level of exercise, work, and sleep
4. Actions of prescribed hypoglycemic agents: onset, duration, and peak
5. Self-perception of DBW

Calories, carbohydrates, fats, and proteins must be distributed on a consistent basis so that the blood level of nutrients matches the blood level of insulin or any oral hypoglycemic agent. Consistency in timing of meals is also important for the person who needs to lose weight. Distribution of calories over 24 hours with frequent meals helps to prevent large increases in postprandial blood glucose and allows the blood glucose to return to the preprandial level before the next meal regardless of whether the patient is receiving a hypoglycemic agent.

## Systems for Learning and Maintaining Dietary Plans

Once the goals of nutritional therapy are established, patients are taught one of several methods for manipulating calories and food.

### Exchange system

The exchange system (Table 40-13) is the most frequently used method. The American Dietetic Association and the American Diabetes Association have divided foods into six groups called exchange lists (or choices). Each list is based on the amount of carbohydrate, protein, and fat contained in foods. There are six exchange lists: starch/bread, meat and meat substitutes, vegetables, fruit, milk, and fat. Each exchange list contains foods in specific serving sizes that contain approximately equal amounts of carbohdyrates, proteins, and fats, and calories. Because of this, these foods can be substituted or "exchanged" for one another. For example, in the fruit list, 1 apple = 12 cherries = ½ cup orange juice. What is important is using suggested serving size. Foods can be measured by tablespoons and measuring cups and meats by ounces. The exchange system offers an infinite number of foods and combinations of foods that can be eaten. It is simply a matter of knowing the calorie, carbohydrate, protein, and fat content of different foods. Labels on food products, convenience foods, and special

**TABLE 40-14 Selection of Diets With Exchange List**

| CALORIES | CHO (g)* | PROTEIN (g) | FAT (g) | BREAD LIST 1† | MEAT LIST 2‡ | VEGETABLE LIST 3 | FRUIT LIST 4 | MILK LIST 5† | FAT LIST 6 |
|---|---|---|---|---|---|---|---|---|---|
| 1000 | 139 | 53 | 26 | 4 | 3 | 2 | 3 | 2 sk | 1 |
| 1100 | 154 | 56 | 32 | 5 | 3 | 2 | 3 | 2 sk | 2 |
| 1200 | 154 | 63 | 37 | 5 | 4 | 2 | 3 | 2 sk | 2 |
| 1300 | 179 | 70 | 38 | 6 | 4 | 4 | 3 | 2 sk | 2 |
| 1400 | 179 | 70 | 44 | 6 | 4 | 4 | 3 | 2 sk | 3 |
| 1500 | 194 | 70 | 48 | 6 | 4 | 4 | 4 | 2 sk | 4 |
| 1600 | 209 | 73 | 54 | 7 | 5 | 4 | 4 | 2 sk | 4 |
| 1700 | 224 | 75 | 55 | 8 | 5 | 4 | 4 | 2 sk | 4 |
| 1800 | 239 | 77 | 61 | 9 | 5 | 4 | 4 | 2 sk | 5 |
| 1900 | 244 | 79 | 66 | 9 | 5 | 5 | 4 | 2 sk | 6 |
| 2000 | 274 | 81 | 67 | 10 | 5 | 5 | 5 | 2 sk | 6 |
| 2100 | 274 | 88 | 72 | 10 | 6 | 5 | 5 | 2 sk | 6 |
| 2200 | 289 | 90 | 73 | 11 | 6 | 5 | 5 | 2 sk | 6 |
| 2300 | 304 | 92 | 79 | 12 | 6 | 5 | 5 | 2 sk | 7 |
| 2400 | 319 | 94 | 80 | 13 | 6 | 5 | 5 | 2 sk | 7 |
| 2500 | 334 | 94 | 85 | 13 | 6 | 5 | 6 | 2 sk | 8 |
| 2600 | 349 | 103 | 91 | 14 | 7 | 5 | 6 | 2 sk | 8 |
| 2700 | 364 | 105 | 92 | 15 | 7 | 5 | 6 | 2 sk | 8 |
| 2800 | 379 | 107 | 93 | 16 | 7 | 5 | 6 | 2 sk | 8 |
| 2900 | 394 | 109 | 99 | 17 | 7 | 5 | 6 | 2 sk | 9 |
| 3000 | 409 | 111 | 100 | 18 | 7 | 5 | 6 | 2 sk | 9 |

From Amick BL, Lopes GL: *Kansas diet manual*, ed 6, Topeka/Kansas City, 1992, Kansas Dietetic Association.
*Carbohydrate grams are approximately 60%-65% of calories for all diets shown.
†In the exchange lists for meal planning, trace of fat is listed for bread and skim milk (sk) exchanges. For calculation purposes, 1 g of fat was added to each serving.
‡Based on medium-fat meat values.
NOTE: Grams of carbohydrate, protein, and fat should be adjusted to meet individual needs.

foods and recipe books list carbohydrate, protein, and fat content. The total number of exchanges for each day is determined from the total calorie, carbohydrate, fat, and protein prescription. A convenient reference that puts this in perspective is the chart entitled *Selection of Diets with Exchange Lists* from the *Kansas Diet Manual,* 1992, which is shown in Table 40-14. To the extreme left of the chart is the caloric level, and to the right of the page are the exchange lists. Therefore, if a person were given a 1600-calorie meal plan, to identify the number of choices from the bread list, follow the line from 1600 to the bread. The answer is seven. Those seven exchanges from the bread and starch list are used throughout the day using choices the person wants (e.g., potato, cereal, pasta, peas).

Using Table 40-11 to calculate calories, Table 40-14 to identify types and number exchanges per day, and Table 40-13 to identify specific foods, a nurse could help make a tentative meal plan—tentative in that it is always best to have counseling by a dietitian if one is available. Once the dietary prescription has been made and the caloric amount decided on, a meal plan such as in Figure 40-10 can be made. There are resources other than the one depicted in the figure. Some are simple and have pictures of foods and a place to write in the number of exchanges from each group to be used. Examples of other plans can be obtained from the American Diabetes Association, Novolin *How to Choose What I Can Eat, Personal Guidelines* from Kentucky Diabetes Foundation, and *Diabetes—An Owner's Manual* from Cray Diabetes Education Center.[18,26,50,61]

Other questions the nurse must be able to help patients with include these: How can a McDonald's hamburger be worked into the meal plan? What about my

**MY MEAL PLAN**

Meal Plan for: JOHN DOE Date: 8/16/93

Dietitian: JANE SMITH Phone:

| | Grams | Percent |
|---|---|---|
| Carbohydrate | 199 | 55 |
| Protein | 79 | 20 |
| Fat | 44 | 25 |

Calories 1580

| Time | Meal Plan | Menu Ideas | Menu Ideas |
|---|---|---|---|
| BREAKFAST | 2 Starch | 1/2 CUP OATMEAL, 1 SLICE WHOLE GRAIN TOAST | |
| | Meat | | |
| | Vegetable | | |
| | 1 Fruit | 1/2 BANANA | |
| | 1 Milk | 1 CUP SKIM MILK | |
| | 1 Fat | 1 TSP MARGARINE | |
| | | | |
| LUNCH | 2 Starch | 2 SLICES WHOLE GRAIN BREAD | |
| | 2 Meat | 2 SLICES TURKEY BREAST (2OZ) LETTUCE LEAF, TOMATO SLICE (FREE) | |
| | 1 Vegetable | 1/2 CUP BROCCOLI/CAULIFLOWER MARINATED IN 1 TBSP LOW-CALORIE ITALIAN DRESSING (FREE FOOD) | |
| | 1 Fruit | APPLE | |
| | Milk | | |
| | 1 Fat | 1 TSP MAYONNAISE | |
| AFTERNOON SNACK | 1 STARCH | 3 GRAHAM CRACKERS | |
| | 1 MEAT | 1 TBSP PEANUT BUTTER | |
| DINNER | 2 Starch | 1 LARGE POTATO | |
| | 2 Meat | MEATLOAF (2OZ) TOSSED SALAD WITH 1 TBSP LOW-CALORIE ITALIAN DRESSING (FREE FOOD) | |
| | 1 Vegetable | 1/2 CUP GREEN BEANS | |
| | 1 Fruit | 1 1/4 CUPS FRESH STRAWBERRIES | |
| | Milk | | |
| | 1 Fat | 1 TSP MARGARINE | |
| BEDTIME SNACK | 1 STARCH | 1/2 BAGEL | |
| | 1 FAT | 1 TBSP LITE CREAM CHEESE | |
| | 1 MILK | 1 CUP SKIM MILK | |

FIGURE 40-10 Sample meal plan.

**BOX 40-8 Nutrition Information per Serving**

Serving size........................... 1 ounce (1¼ cup)
Serving per package ................. 20 (1-ounce servings)
Calories ........................................... 110
Protein, grams ........................................ 4
Carbohydrate, grams ................................ 20
Sodium, milligrams ................................. 320
Percentage of vitamins and minerals listed next
Ingredients: Whole oat flour, wheat starch, salt, sugar, calcium carbonate, etc.

favorite cereal? Patients need to read the values listed on fast food exchange handouts (provided by the fast food business) and labels on cereal boxes.[33] A McDonald's Big Mac has 560 calories, 43 g carbohydrate, 25 g protein, and 32 g fat. The McLean hamburger has 320 calories, 35 g carbohydrate, 22 g protein, and 10 g fat.[58] The nutrition information in Box 40-8 is an example of what can be found on cereal boxes. In comparing the amounts of carbohydrate, protein, and fat to the exchange list (see Table 40-13), one serving, 1¼ cup of this cereal, would be equal to about 1⅓ bread exchanges.

### Other systems

Another system that can be used to help patients with meal plans could include the Food Guide Pyramid (provided by the Kansas LEAN Food Professionals Task Force and the Wheat Food Council) (Figure 40-11).[73] This guide recommends less meat and poultry than the exchange list does.

**Points system.** Another system is point counting. With this system, foods are assigned points for calorie and carbohydrate, protein, and fat content. The total daily food allowance is written as number of calorie and carbohydrate points, and the person is instructed to select foods according to a point distribution. This system is similar to the exchange list but less well known.

**Total available carbohydrate.** This system counts the amount of carbohydrate available in the total meal. Only carbohydrates are tracked. Some persons prefer this plan because they are directed to give insulin according to total available carbohydrates.[62] This system is also less well known.

Some individuals who have difficulty with the systems described are given a rigid menu plan that states the amount and type of food to eat or drink at each meal and snack. For example, the breakfast plan could be this: ½ grapefruit, 1 cup oatmeal, 1 slice toast with 1 teaspoon margarine, 1 cup 2% milk, and coffee. This system is used until the person is ready for more independence.

Many tools are available to meet the needs of a variety of patients. Exchanges teach good nutrition and are very flexible. A paperback book entitled *Meal Planning Approaches in the Nutrition Management of the*

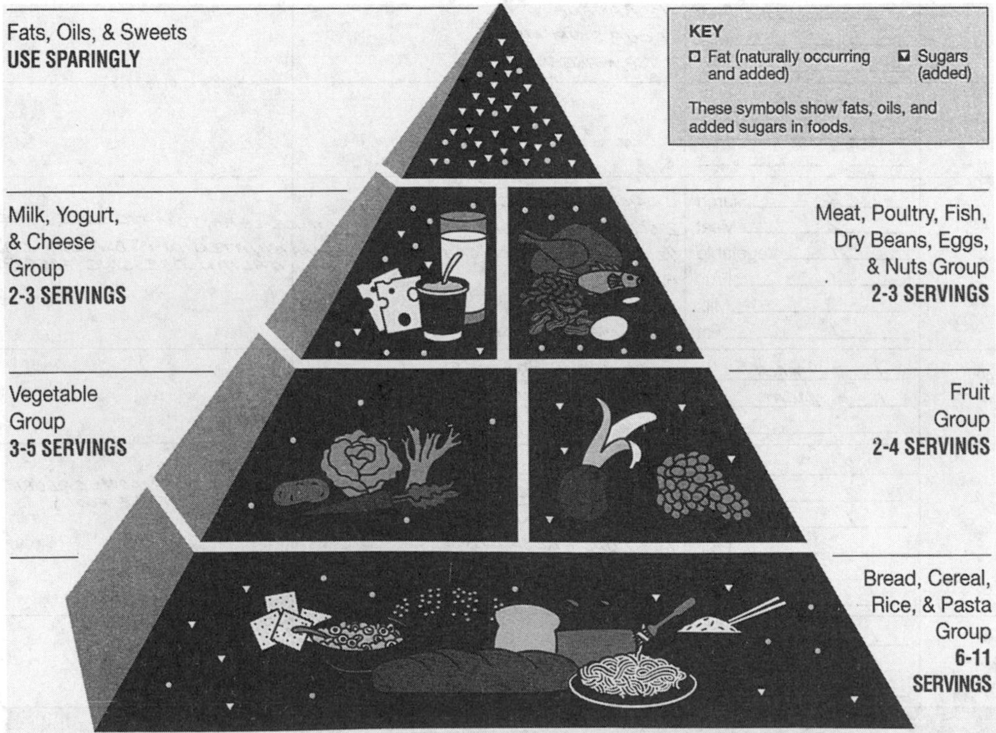


**FIGURE 40-11** Food guide pyramid.

*Persons with Diabetes* is an economical source that outlines many of the existing plans for nutrition. With any of the educational tools for nutrition, patients will more then likely need to learn in small steps; therefore, select the meal plan that is best suited for the patient at the point at which he/she is.

## Dietetic Foods, Sweeteners, and Alcohol

The diabetic diet does not require the use of special or **dietetic** foods. Dietetic, diet, and dietary mean the same thing when used on labels. If used, these foods must be counted into the meal plan, since they are products that have had a substitution made and the substitution does not necessarily mean the product is low in calories or useful for people with diabetes.

Various sweeteners other than sugar are available in the United States, including saccharin, aspartame (Equal), acesulfame-K (Sunette), and sucralose (the first sugar substitute made from sugar). All these products are called low- or no-calorie sweeteners. Patients frequently ask how much of the sweeteners can be consumed safely. The *accepted daily intake* (ADI) is quite generous and is usually reported as an amount per kilogram of body weight (2.2 pounds equals 1 kg). For example, 50 mg/kg is the ADI for aspartame. What this means is for a 110-pound person, this represents twelve 12-ounce cans of 100% aspartame-sweetened soda pop or 71 packets of Equal per day for a lifetime. Other sweeteners that contain calories include fructose, sorbitol, and mannitol.[35] Fructose is a natural sugar found in many fruits. Because it is absorbed slowly and because part of its metabolism does not depend on insulin, it has been proposed as a sweetener for persons with diabetes mellitus. However, because part of its metabolism requires insulin and because it yields 4 kcal/g when metabolized, fructose must be calculated into the dietary prescription. Sorbitol may be found in certain prepared foods. It is metabolized to fructose in the liver; therefore the precautions decribed for fructose apply. Excessive sorbitol can lead to diarrhea from slow gastrointestinal absorption.

Alcohol does not furnish carbohydrate, protein, or fat, but it yields 7 kcal/g when metabolized and must be included in caloric calculations if weight loss is necessary. Some alcohol may be permitted, but the patient must be instructed about the caloric value of pure alcohol; the high carbohydrate content of beer, cordials, wine, and mixed drinks; the inhibiting effect of alcohol on gluconeogenesis with the possible precipitation of hypoglycemia; and the alcohol-induced increase in triglyceride levels.[2] Hypoglycemia is especially common if alcohol is consumed while fasting, particularly in the person with diabetes who may have insulin available from a prior injection.[1]

# ACTIVITY

In all persons with diabetes, activity is an important part of the medical management and deserves careful and thorough explanation before implementation. Physical activity has important physiologic and psychologic implications. Table 40-15 gives a succinct overview of the physiologic hormonal responses to exercise.[67] Again, the "board of directors" (see Table 40-4) raise their boastful heads in an attempt to make the reader understand the gravity of their existence in diabetes care. Exercise increases the uptake of glucose by active muscle cells without the need for insulin and can increase tissue sensitivity to insulin. Overall activity has a hypoglycemic effect. In obese persons, exercise can decrease insulin resistance and help in weight loss. Exercise by persons with diabetes, particularly if they receive insulin or an oral hypoglycemic agent, must consider the dietary plan and medications. Fair to good control should be achieved before starting an exercise program.[34]

Just as IDDM and NIDDM differ in other aspects, they do so in regard to the activity programs. Exercise programs have not been exclusively shown to improve glycemic control in people with IDDM, and because of

**TABLE 40-15 Hormonal Response to Exercise**

| HORMONE | EFFECT | RESULT |
|---|---|---|
| Insulin | Decreased | Increases glucose output from liver<br>Stimulates glucose utilization by exercising muscle cells<br>Increases adipose tissue lipolysis<br>Restrains glucose utilization by nonexercising muscle cells |
| Counterregulatory hormones | | |
| Epinephrine | Increased | Stimulates rapid breakdown of muscle glycogen stores at start of exercise<br>In response to high-intensity exercise and declining blood glucose, stimulates hepatic glycogenolysis and adipose tissue lipolysis |
| Growth hormone and cortisol | Increased | Less important in short-term exercise; increases lipolysis and decreases glucose uptake in peripheral tissues<br>Over longer periods of exercise; increases gluconeogenesis |
| Glucagon | Increased | Stimulates glucose production by the liver |

Data from Pollock ML, Wilmore JH: *Exercise in health and disease—evaluation and prescription for prevention and rehabilitation,* ed 2, Philadelphia, 1990, Saunders.

**BOX 40-9 Benefits of Exercise for the Person with Diabetes**

Improves insulin sensitivity
Lowers blood glucose during and after exercise
Improves lipid profile
May improve some hypertension
Increases energy expenditure
- Assists with weight loss
- Preserves lean body mass

Promotes cardiovascular fitness
Increases strength and flexibility
Improves sense of well-being

From Horton ES: In Lebovitz HE, editor: *Therapy for diabetes mellitus and related disorders,* Alexandria, Va, 1991, American Diabetes Association.

**BOX 40-10 Risks of Exercise for the Person with Diabetes**

Precipitation or exacerbation of cardiovascular disease, angina, arrhythmias, sudden death
Hypoglycemia, if taking insulin or oral agents
- Exercise-related hypoglycemia
- Late-onset postexercise hypoglycemia

Hyperglycemia after very strenuous exercise
Worsening of long-term complications
- Proliferative retinopathy
- Peripheral neuropathy
- Autonomic neuropathy

From Horton ES: In Lebovitz HE, editor: *Therapy for diabetes mellitus and related disorders,* Alexandria, Va, 1991, American Diabetes Association.

increased risk of exercise, experts still debate whether exercise should be recommended for all persons with IDDM.[46] Insulin resistance and excess weight are present in many persons with NIDDM. Any type of therapy that lessens resistance and helps in weight loss has potential benefit. Exercise helps in both cases. Both clinical experience and various studies have shown exercise to be of value in both insulin resistance and weight loss. For maximal benefit, the exercise program should be done on a regular basis. Even then, the effect on glucose may be short-lived.

Exercise plans for persons with diabetes cannot be discussed without exploring the risks and benefits of such a program.[46] Box 40-9 lists some of the benefits of exercise for persons with diabetes. Entering into an exercise plan can pose certain risks for patients with diabetes (Box 40-10). Both benefits and risks must be carefully investigated before launching an exercise prescription. The exercise prescription may look something like Figure 40-12 and consists of the following parts: type of exercise, intensity, duration, and frequency. The center part of the prescription is called a perceived exertion scale. A *perceived exertion scale,* developed by Borg, determines how hard the person is working by having a person rate how he or she feels.[67] Such a prescription is not always used; however, its structure gives better direction to patients.

Before entering into any type of exercise program, all patients should have a complete history and physical examination with particular attention to the cardiovascular system and any existing long-term complications. An exercise stress electrocardiogram (ECG) is recommended for all patients over 35 years of age.[46] By doing this test, silent ischemic heart disease and exaggerated hypertensive responses to exercise can be identified. Once the patient has been cleared for an exercise program, special precautions may be indicated. General guidelines for exercise are listed in the Guidelines box, p. 1310.

## MONITORING FOR GLUCOSE AND URINE KETONES

**Self-monitoring of blood glucose (SMBG)** has been widely accepted as an important tool in the management of diabetes. The American Diabetes Association[78] has identified four functions of SMBG:

1. To guide physicians in long-term treatment planning
2. To guide patients in short-term adjustments in insulin and diet
3. To signal possible emergency situations
4. To enhance patient education

SMBG is now the preferred way to monitor glycemic control.[7] Urine testing for ketones remains an important but frequently forgotten part of monitoring diabetic control. Urinary ketones may be an indication of impending ketoacidosis. Urine should be tested for ketones when blood glucose is over 250 mg/dl (in either IDDM or NIDDM as sometimes under stress the person with NIDDM will show ketones) and when illness or stressors occur regardless of the blood glucose. In some situations, when food intake is compromised, blood glucose can drop and ketones are positive because of starvation ketosis. This situation warrants a visit to the emergency room for fluids. Nursing implications related to SMBG are discussed in detail under nursing management.

## PATIENT EDUCATION

Medical management has been discussed. However, a person with diabetes cannot succeed without education. In no other disease is there so great a need for patient education. It has been said that most of the management of diabetes is up to the patient. Frequently referrals, consultations, and physician orders will state, "Do patient education or diabetes teaching."

In the last few years, because of the American Diabetes Association recognition program, much more emphasis is being placed on diabetes programs and the quality of those programs. The recognition program is

Name: ______________________ Date: ______________

Mode: (type of exercise)*

( ) Cycling ( ) Jumping Rope
( ) Walking
( ) Swimming ( ) Other ______________
*Can change/rotate

Intensity: (how hard)

Perceived exertion scale

6
7 Very, very light
8
9 Very light
10
11 Fairly light
12
13 Somewhat hard
14
15 Hard
16
17 Very hard
18
19 Very, very hard
20

Duration: (how long)*

Slow (stretch–warm up) __________
Faster (training) __________
Slow (cooling down) __________
*Start slow and build up

| Frequency: (how often) | Type of exercise | How often |
|---|---|---|
| Aerobic: | __________ | __________ |
| Other: | __________ | __________ |

Physician: ______________

**FIGURE 40-12** Sample exercise prescription.

similar to an accreditation program such as the joint commission, but for diabetes programs only. Programs offering diabetes education must qualify and meet criteria or standards (in 1984 the National Diabetes Advisory established a set of standards to be used for ensuring the quality of diabetes patient education programs) to become formally recognized. This process affects all persons, including the consumer. It is believed that meeting the national standards and obtaining recognition will result in improvements in the overall quality of diabetes patient education programs. In addition, recognition is seen as a prerequisite to obtaining third-party reimbursement for diabetes patient education services. In order to become recognized, the program must offer materials in the 15 areas listed in Box 40-11.[3,5,71a] This list is included because it gives the novice or the expert guidelines for patient education. It can be given to patients for them to identify areas for which they would like more information. The "how to teach" this content is addressed in the nursing management section.

## REFERRAL/CONSULTATION

In some settings the nurse assumes responsibility for making referrals and consultations to other services. This depends on the area in which the nurse is working. From the hospital setting, frequent needs exist for referrals to

**Guidelines for Exercise Program for the Person With Diabetes**

**EXERCISE TYPE**

Aerobic (low impact for NIDDM)
Start with **light level.**

**EXERCISE SESSION**

Each session should eventually include:
1. 5-10 minutes of warm-up stretching and limbering exercises
2. 20-30 minutes of aerobic exercise and heart rate in target zone (as defined by physician) or perceived exertion rating
3. 15-20 minutes of light exercise and stretching to cool down

**EXERCISE FREQUENCY**

3 to 5 times per week

**SPECIAL PRECAUTIONS**

1. Consider the insulin/oral agent regimen (may need to ↓ insulin).
2. Consider the plan for food intake:
   Eat meal 1-3 hours before exercise.
   Take extra carbohydrate during exercise if over 30 minutes and vigorous.
3. Check blood glucose before, during, and afterward (for baseline):
   If <100 mg/dl, eat a preexercise snack.
   If 100-250 mg/dl, it is probably okay to exercise.
   If 250 mg/dl, check urine ketones.
4. Check urine ketones (if glucose over 250 mg/dl):
   If negative, okay to exercise.
   If positive, take insulin; do not exercise until ketones are negative.
5. Exercise should not cause shortness of breath and should be stopped with any onset of chest pain.
6. Carry diabetes ID card or bracelet.
7. Carry a source of easily absorbed carbohydrate.
8. Avoid exercise in extreme heat or cold.
9. Inspect feet daily and after exercise.

**PRECAUTIONS FOR SELECTED PERSONS**

1. Persons with insensitive feet should avoid running and jogging and choose good shoes for walking. Swimming and cycling may also be included.
2. Persons with proliferative retinopathy should avoid exercises associated with Valsalva maneuvers or that cause jarring and jolting of head or exercises with head in low position.
3. Persons with hypertension should avoid exercises associated with Valsalva maneuvers and exercises involving intense exercises of torso and arms. (Exercises involving the lower extremities are preferred.)

social service, dietary, diabetes nurse educator, and home health. In the outpatient setting, referrals may differ and include referrals and consultations to ophthalmology clinic, vocational rehabilitation, and various clinical nurse specialists. A system that can be used to identify potential referrals and resources is to match particular areas of patient education to potential resources (Table 40-16).

Critical pathways (also referred to as "collaborative care paths" or "care maps") have been developed in some inpatient and outpatient settings to guide both medical and nursing management. These critical pathways are collaboratively developed along time lines and include the information previously described for specific hours, days, or visits. Pertinent information about discharge planning and patient teaching to be implemented at specified times also is included. Because the nurse has a major role in these two aspects of care, these are discussed under Nursing Management. A sample of a critical pathway for the areas of diagnostic tests, medications, treatments, diet, activity, and consultants for a patient with NIDDM and hyperosmolar, hyperglycemic, nonketotic coma (HHNC) is presented at the end of the chapter. A nursing care plan for a patient with NIDDM is also included.

## SURGICAL MANAGEMENT

Surgery is not part of the usual management for persons with diabetes mellitus to treat the metabolic abnormalities. However, most persons with diabetes mellitus will have surgery at some point in their life. Nursing management of the person with diabetes having surgery is discussed at the end of the chapter.

## NURSING MANAGEMENT

### ♦ ASSESSMENT

Assessment of the patient with IDDM or NIDDM has several focuses, depending on the stage of illness and the reason the patient is seeking health care. The following assessment data pertain to the stabilized patient (meaning the patient is not in an acute situation such as DKA). Most information is the same whether the patient is newly diagnosed or previously diagnosed.

#### Subjective Data

Data to be collected to assess the patient with diabetes include the following:

- Psychosocial/emotional
  - Perception of meaning of diagnosis and how it will affect person's life
  - Loss of identity (temporarily have a loss of who he or she is)
  - Fear of what lies ahead
  - Uncertainty about day-to-day activities (work, social activities, family role, meals, etc.)
  - Identification of life stressors
  - Coping strategies currently used
  - Support system
- Knowledge level: concept of diabetes, effect of uncontrolled metabolic state, potential treatment
- Family patterns: food buying, cooking, history of diabetes
- Cardiovascular: drugs, history of blood pressure problems, chest pain or leg pain with exercise
- Respiratory: smoking history

## BOX 40-11 Fifteen Content Areas of Diabetes Education

1. *Overview of diabetes mellitus*
   - Definition of diabetes mellitus
   - Effects of alterations in metabolism of carbohydrates, proteins, and fats
   - Classification of diabetes (type I, type II, gestational, etc.)
2. *Stress and psychological adjustment*
   - Grieving and adaptation to living with a chronic disease
   - Expressing feelings openly
   - Unrealistic expectations
   - Effect of stress on metabolic control
   - Recognizing the need for professional help
   - Stress management
3. *Family involvement and social support*
   - Diabetes as a family challenge
   - Learning to recognize and work with adverse family dynamics
   - Need for support
4. *Nutrition*
   - Individualized meal plan to control weight, glucose, and lipids
   - Composition of the diet
   - Achieving and maintaining desired body weight and glucose control
   - Advice on alcohol use
   - Eating on special occasions
   - Reading and interpreting nutrition labels
5. *Exercise and activity*
   - Benefits/risks
   - Effects of exercise on therapeutic plan
   - Preparing for exercise (food and medication; companion)
   - Heart rate monitoring
   - Monitoring necessary before starting exercise
   - Monitoring necessary when establishing an exercise program
6. *Medications*
   - Goals of treatment
   - Oral agents
     - Action on blood glucose
     - Side effects
     - Drug interactions
   - Insulin
     - Action on blood glucose
     - Cautions (especially Somogyi effect)
     - Strengths/purities
     - Injection techniques
     - Complications of treatment: hypoglycemia, antibodies, lipodystrophy
   - Glucagon
     - How to buy, store, and use
7. *Monitoring and use of results*
   - Goals
   - Types of blood glucose monitoring available
   - Quality control of monitors
   - How to use blood glucose monitoring to achieve and maintain good glucose control: performing tests accurately, interpreting test results, frequency of testing, taking action appropriate to test results
   - Urine ketone testing
   - Glycosylated hemoglobin test: how to relate to average blood glucose level
8. *Relationships among nutrition, exercise, medication, and blood glucose levels*
   - Balancing nutrition, exercise, and medications
   - Adjusting each factor in relation to the others
   - Adjusting times of monitoring
   - Identify times for snacks
   - Effects of exercise on blood glucose
9. *Acute complications: hyperglycemia and hypoglycemia*
   - Definition of hyperglycemia and hypoglycemia
   - Prevention of each
   - Early recognition/treatment/record-keeping
   - Hypoglycemia unawareness
   - Dawn and Somogyi phenomena
   - What to do for diabetic ketoacidoses/hyperosmolar coma
   - Effects of illness on diabetes
   - Monitoring glucose/ketones
   - Sick day guidelines (including diet)
10. *Chronic complications: prevention, detection, and treatment*
    - Kinds of complications—microvascular and macrovascular; neuropathy
    - Examples of each kind of complication (especially those likely to occur in your population)
    - Possible causes of complication
    - Self-care for prevention or delay of complications
    - Coping strategies (support groups, counseling, stress management)
11. *Foot, skin, and dental care*
    - Daily self-care measures
    - Relationship of problems to diabetes care
    - The need for regular evaluation of feet and teeth
12. *Behavioral change strategies, goal setting, risk factor reduction, and problem solving*
    - Changing behaviors through goal setting
    - Rights of patient
    - Responsibility of patient
    - Patient-professional partnership in planning care
    - Taking care of self when sick
13. *Benefits, risks, and management options for improving glucose control*
    - DCCT results
    - Therapeutic care plans—maps to good health and quality of life
14. *Preconception care, pregnancy, and gestational diabetes*
    - See maternity texts and Ref. 3 for detailed statement of goals and care for this content area
15. *Use of health care systems and community resources*
    - Planned follow-up (times and tests that are part of 1000 mile check-up)
    - Patient's responsibility
    - Names and telephone numbers of health care team members
    - Emergency care
    - Community resources
    - Planning for travel
    - Educational resources and need for continuing education
    - Insurance and employment regulations and reimbursement

---

**With permission from American Diabetes Association, Goals for Diabetes Education, Clinical Education Program, 2nd edition, Alexandria, VA (in press); Task force to revise the national standards: National standards for diabetes self-management education programs, *Diabetes Care* 18(1):141-148, 1995.**

**TABLE 40-16 Potential Community Resources for the Person With Diabetes**

| CATEGORY | RESOURCES |
|---|---|
| 1. Overview of diabetes mellitus | American Diabetes Association (ADA), Juvenile Diabetes Foundation (JDF), diabetes team, public library |
| 2. Stress/psychological adjustment | ADA and other community support groups, hospital department of social services, community mental health program |
| 3. Family involvement/ social support | ADA, local diabetes group classes, your health care team, department of social services, family and children's service, home health care agencies |
| 4. Nutrition | ADA, Dial-A-Dietitian, diabetes classes, American Heart Association, Meals on Wheels, health department, food kitchens, nutrition sites, Weight Watchers, hospital nutrition programs, public library |
| 5. Exercise and activity | ADA, diabetes classes, health care team, fitness centers, YMCA, YWCA, senior citizens' programs, walk clubs, Outdoor Club of KC, hospital physical therapy programs, TV programs, exercise videos, public library |
| 6. Medications | Financial assistance programs such as Medicaid, ADA for information and sometimes insulin on emergency basis, information from classes, printed materials—*Diabetes Forecast,* local pharmacy |
| 7. Monitoring and use of results | Financial assistance programs, local representatives from monitoring companies, insurance company, health care team, other persons with diabetes |
| 8. Relationships among nutrition, exercise, medication, and blood glucose levels | Classes, printed materials, ADA, Learning Library at local diabetes center, public library |
| 9. Acute complications: hyperglycemia and hypoglycemia | Diabetes supply stores, drug stores (for glucose tablets, ID bracelets), ADA meetings |
| 10. Prevention, detection, and treatment of chronic complications | There is an agency for almost every disease or health-related problem: eye, kidney, heart; Impotence Anonymous; ADA; Centers for Disease Control; state department of health; local health department; hospital; Rehabilitation Centers for Visual Impairment; Program for the Deaf; etc. |
| 11. Foot, skin, and dental care | Podiatrist, skin specialist, dental schools, classes |
| 12. Behavioral change strategies, goal setting, risk factor reduction, and problem solving | Materials on helping persons establish goals and use of contracts; classes on change |
| 13. Benefits, risk, and management options for improving glucose control | ADA, classes, health care team, materials on patient-health team partnerships, results of DCCT study |
| 14. Preconception care, pregnancy, and gestational diabetes | Prenatal classes, dairy council, WIC, physician specialist in high-risk pregnancy |
| 15. Use of health care system/community resources | Know about Vocational Rehabilitation Act of 1973 and the Americans with Disabilities Act of 1990—its implications for you/your rights as an employee with diabetes (physical handicap); know about insurance—can you get it; know about patient rights and responsibilities<br>Look in yellow pages for physician specialty; look in the blue pages of the telephone book for self-help agencies |

- Neuromuscular: history of changes in vision or speech, dizziness, confusion, headache, or symptoms of neuropathy (tingling, numbness, pain at rest that disappears with activity)
- Gastrointestinal: weight changes, history of GI problems (indigestion, diarrhea, constipation)
- Urinary: history of changes in urinary frequency or incontinence
- Sexual function:
  - Females: menstrual history, history of changes noted with intercourse (if sexually active)
  - Males: problems with impotence or amount of ejaculate (if sexually active)
- Vision: history of blurring, decreased acuity
- Financial security, insurance

## Objective Data

Data to be collected to assess the patient with diabetes include the following:

- Emotional/mental: emotional state, responsiveness, attention, alertness, comprehension, appropriateness of response
- Neuromuscular:
  - Eyes: visual acuity (with and without glasses)
  - Motor: range of motion, muscle strength (both upper and lower extremities)
  - Sensory: touch, temperature, pain, vibratory sense (especially lower extremities), position sense
- Cardiovascular: blood pressure (both lying and standing), peripheral pulses

- Gastrointestinal: weight and height
- Urinary: output and fluid intake
- Vagina: discharge, irritation
- Skin: intactness, temperature, presence of lesions, moisture, hair distribution, texture (especially in lower extremities), turgor

### Diagnostic Test Findings

1. Increased fasting blood/plasma glucose levels; increased postprandial blood/plasma glucose levels
2. Glycosylated hemoglobin level twice normal
3. Serum lipids abnormal (triglycerides >200 mg/dl, VLDL-TG greater than normal, decreased HDL-C)
4. Urine acetone positive

## ♦ NURSING DIAGNOSES

Nursing diagnoses are determined from analysis of patient data. Possible nursing diagnoses for the person with diabetes mellitus may include but are not limited to the following:

| Diagnostic Title | Possible Etiologic Factors |
|---|---|
| Fluid volume deficit, high risk for | Excess urination, limited access to fluids, inadequate knowledge |
| Fatigue | Inadequate nutrition (from glycemic state), muscle weakness |
| Infection, high risk for | Elevated blood glucose |
| Nutrition, altered: less or more than body requirements | Alteration in metabolism, decreased nutrition, lack of knowledge |
| Fear | Long-term illness, taking insulin, life-style changes (loss of job) |
| Knowledge deficit: disease, drugs, self-care skills (insulin injection, SMBG), diet needs, activity needs | New information and skills; never been exposed before |

## ♦ EXPECTED PATIENT OUTCOMES

Expected patient outcomes for the patient with diabetes may include but are not limited to the following:

1. Exhibits physical signs of fluid balance:
   a. Weight returns to patient's baseline weight.
   b. Skin turgor and mucous membranes are normal.
   c. Blood pressure and pulse are within patient's normal range and do not vary by more than 10 mm Hg or 10 beats/minute with activity.
   d. Serum electrolytes and hematocrit are within normal limits.
2. The patient:
   a. Has an oral fluid intake of 2500 to 3000 ml/day.
   b. Explains how to prevent deficits.
3. Exhibits signs of nutritional adequacy:
   a. Maintains weight, or loses or gains as appropriate.
   b. Glycosylated hemoglobin and lipid measurements moving toward normal.
   c. Food is distributed throughout the day.
4. Fatigue is improved:
   a. States fatigue level is decreased by a lower rating on a scale of 1-10 (1 = no fatigue, 10 = most fatigue).
   b. Verbalizes need to do regular glucose monitoring in order to take action with high blood glucoses.
5. Risk for infection is decreased:
   a. Verbalizes need to do blood glucose monitoring at least three times a week.
   b. Identifies factors that increase blood glucose.
   c. Lists signs and symptoms of infection.
6. Patient's fear is decreased:
   a. Expresses feelings about having diabetes.
   b. Verbalizes a plan to be retrained for different work; acknowledges losses.
7. An adequate level of knowledge is attained:
   a. Verbalizes that diabetes is a disease in which the body is unable to use all foods properly because of lack of insulin or inability to use insulin.
   b. Demonstrates correctly how to give insulin and rotate injection sites.
   c. Demonstrates correctly how to monitor for blood glucose and urine ketones (knows when and who to call for help).
   d. Verbalizes the definitions of hypoglycemia and hyperglycemia.
   e. Verbalizes symptoms and treatment of hypoglycemia.
   f. Verbalizes how to take oral agents and side effects to report.
   g. Verbalizes dietary plan and ways to achieve.
   h. Verbalizes exercise plan, safety precautions, and what to report.

## ♦ INTERVENTIONS

### Improving Fluid Status

To improve fluid status, the patient's metabolic status needs to be improved, and the patient needs to take in an adequate amount of fluids. Explore with the patient, using patient terminology, possible causes for loss of fluid (dehydration). Relate the fluid loss to the high blood sugar. Use terminology such as sugar attracts water, and when blood sugar is high, sugar goes out the urine, pulling water with it, thus increasing urination. Relate increased thirst to nature's way of telling the person to drink more. If the person is not drinking, fluid losses will not be controlled. Relate symptoms of high blood glucose from Figure 40-6 to the fluid loss. This illustration can help the patient visualize how to manage the diabetes using tools such as SMBG and testing for urine ketones. Teach the patient and family about diet, medications, and fluid needs. Teach SMBG and urine tesing for ketones. If there are any questions about follow-through in the home, initiate a home care referral.

## Promoting Adequate Nutrition

The registered dietitian who is part of the health team is usually responsible for the nutrition component of the educational program for the person with diabetes, but the nurse is also involved. A dietary history should be part of the nurse's initial assessment. Any pertinent data are shared with other health team members, particularly the dietitian.

Because of the difficulty in changing food habits, the patient should be involved in setting goals for dietary changes. Some of the compromises that may be necessary are:

1. Identifying an acceptable weight loss schedule for the obese person
2. Incorporating an alcoholic beverage into the daily plan
3. Distributing food in a different pattern (e.g., a large noon meal and a small evening meal)
4. Adding desserts to some meals
5. Adding dietetic candies and cookies

Information about cultural or social food habits that are identified in the dietary history need to be incorporated into the dietary plan. For example, make accommodations for a vegetarian diet or for a large amount of fast foods in the diet.

The system for maintaining the dietary plan will usually be identified by the patient and the registered dietitian. The selected system is documented in the nursing care plan so that everyone involved uses the same terminology and food groupings. The mutually established goals, including compromises and sociocultural practices, are also documented so the patient is not given conflicting information. Significant others should be included in the teaching.

After dietary goals are established, help the patient to apply dietary knowledge through:

1. Simulations in which the person chooses foods from the hospital menu, food models, or other learning tools
2. Patient participation in documenting food intake, blood and urine results, activity, and medications and in discussing how these interrelate

Evaluate the patient's and significant other's satisfaction with the plan. Additional needs may be identified over time and communicated to the dietitian, to be incorporated into the plan.

Skills that the patient should possess after the initial management period are: (1) ability to manage the diet for stable condition over 1 week; (2) knowing who to contact if unusual events requiring adjustments occur; and (3) knowing how to handle sick days.

As persons gain ability, they will be able to:

1. Manage their diets on a daily basis, making adjustment for normal life changes
2. Select appropriate foods from restaurant menus or at social occasions
3. Handle dietary needs while traveling or for shift work
4. Handle dietary needs at unplanned social events (e.g., "happy hour" after work, unexpected business dinner, unexpected company)
5. Evaluate their success in dietary management through evaluating weight changes and hemoglobin $A_{1c}$ levels or through blood glucose self-monitoring
6. Make a conscious effort to include adequate vitamins and minerals, eliminate excess salt, decrease saturated fat intake, decrease caffeine intake
7. Keep up-to-date on new findings about dietary management and consult health team members about the new recommendations
8. Avoid "quack" recommendations
9. Manipulate diet, exercise, and medications together to cover a vast number of daily situations
10. Work with others in the household to help them incorporate principles of healthy eating into the diet

## Decreasing Fatigue

Measures to improve metabolic control will improve fatigue. However, because the patient may have loss of muscle mass and be deconditioned, metabolic control will usually improve before the fatigue. Therefore the patient will need help in developing a schedule to promote graded increase in activity and adequate rest and sleep. The patient and the family need to understand the basis of the fatigue. Teach that diabetes is a disease in which the body is unable to use foods properly because of lack of insulin. The metabolic abnormalities result in loss of fluids and other body chemicals such as potassium and sodium. The food eaten cannot be used for energy when there is a lack of insulin. These abnormalities result in the body breaking down its own stores of muscle and fat, resulting in fatigue. Teach that fatigue is reversible but will take time to improve.

## Preventing Infection

Again, improvement in metabolic control is the primary way to prevent infections. This is achieved by patient education about the relationship of poor blood glucose control to infection. The patient and family must understand the effects of infection on diabetic control; that is, infection can worsen blood glucose. They must know the signs and symptoms of infection and how to manage sick days (Box 40-12).

## Decreasing Fear

Before the patient is ready to take on self-care, fears must be controlled. The nurse should anticipate the presence of fears by asking straightforward questions about fear of loss of job, giving self-injections, or relationships with others. Possible conflicting factors such as life-style changes should be identified. The nurse needs to eliminate misconceptions that can increase fear. Patients must have permission to feel grief for losses

**BOX 40-12 Short-Term Sick Day Checklist**

*When to call your physician/nurse about being sick or "out of sorts"* (just go through the checklist and check what you have):

_____ If you are sick longer than 1-2 days
_____ If you are unable to eat regular foods for more than 1 day
_____ Signs of infection: redness, warmth, swelling, pus, tenderness any place
_____ Symptoms of dehydration: dry mouth, fever, thirst, dry flushed skin, vomiting, abdominal pain, severe nausea, diarrhea, rapid breathing
_____ Vomiting and diarrhea lasting longer than 6 hours
_____ Increased urination and increased thirst
_____ Have cough and bring up yellow or green material
_____ Have fever and questions about what to eat or drink
_____ Any symptoms getting worse
_____ SMBG consistently elevated beyond specified levels
_____ Fever present
_____ Ketones present
_____ Have any questions about how to take care of yourself and control your diabetes
_____ Have questions about adjusting insulin/oral agents

*Information to have ready for physician/nurse when you call:*

_____ Length of time you have been sick
_____ Your temperature
_____ What's bothering you (a list of symptoms)
_____ Test results: urine ketones and blood glucose
_____ Diabetes medication: type, time you take, and amount and what you have taken
_____ Other medications you take: any medication allergies and what you have taken
_____ Pharmacy phone number

*Remember:*

1. Always take your insulin or oral agent unless your blood glucose is extremely low for you.
2. Drink plenty of fluids.
3. Test urine ketones and do blood glucose every 4-6 hours; write down results.
4. Eat 50 g of carbohydrates or food equal to 200 calories every 3-4 hours. Use frequent small feedings.
5. If you are sick for more than 1 day and cannot eat carbohydrates or take in any food, call your physician or nurse or the emergency room.
6. Know all your caregivers' numbers and names.

(When you get better, return to your normal eating plan and medication dosage. This information applies to *short-term* illness [1-2 days]. If you are unable to eat, or have vomiting or diarrhea, call immediately.)

being experienced, must know that everyone feels like they are "falling apart," and that with time they will get better and feel better. Referrals to social workers, counselors, or ministers for emotional support will be necessary.

## Facilitating Learning

A major responsibility of the professional nurse is helping persons gain self-management skills for any chronic health problem through teaching and counseling. Self-management skills are probably the major determinant of how well the health problem is controlled and the quality of life maintained.[42] This is particularly true for persons with diabetes. Research supports the idea that patient education has a positive effect on patient outcomes (see Research box at right).

The major problem confronting the nurse when dealing with the problem of knowledge deficit in the person with diabetes mellitus is, "What do I teach and how much do I teach?" Remember, the medical management covered seven areas, six nursing diagnoses have been discussed, and there are 15 content areas of education the patient needs to be offered. Even though there is overlap in the topics from these three focuses, it can be an awesome task. Diabetes learning and diabetes teaching have been compared to "taking a drink from a fire hydrant—there's just too much to take in." So where does one start?

The bottom line is patients have to survive in the real world. This requires ability to perform survival day-to-day skills. Wherever you find yourself, *always* validate that your patients can perform survival/initial skills. Regardless of whether a patient has had diabetes 10 days or 10 years, survival/initial skills must be validated.

**RESEARCH**

Brown, SA: Effects of educational interventions in diabetes care: a meta-analysis of findings, *Nurs Res* 37:223-230, 1988.

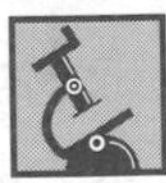

Meta-analysis techniques were used to analyze data from 47 studies about the effects of patient teaching on knowledge, self-care behavior, and metabolic control. The analysis was designed to answer the following research question: What is the magnitude of the effect of patient teaching in diabetic adults? In this analysis, patient teaching appeared to enhance patient outcomes and have a positive effect on knowledge, self-care behavior, and metabolic control.

The American Diabetes Association has suggested that diabetes education take place in three stages and is continuous:

1. Survival/initial stage
2. In-depth stage
3. Continuous stage

Stages two and three place emphasis on knowledge and skills needed to be completely self-sufficient in daily management and knowledge and skills needed to gain flexibility in management, insight, and self-determination.[3,32] A tool such as the Professional Prompter Worksheet (Box 40-13) can help in facilitating learning.

This tool provides the survival/initial knowledge that must be mastered by the person with type I or type II diabetes mellitus. The survival/initial information is identified on the tool. Other areas, such as dealing with complications and in-depth knowledge about hyperglycemia and ketoacidosis, are left for stages 2 and 3 teaching. The Professional Prompter Worksheet provides information on what to teach and on teaching strategies and available tools.

### Obtaining teaching tools

Many teaching tools are available from drug vendors such as Eli Lilly, Boehringer Mannheim, Novolin, Upjohn, Roerig, and so forth. Nurses can gain access to this information by contacting the drug or medical equipment representative for the institution or region in which they work. Teaching materials also are available from the American Diabetes Association.[3] The book *Learning to Live with Diabetes* from the International Diabetes Center, DCI Publishing, Minneapolis, is also valuable. Other resources can be obtained from the Cray Diabetes Center, University of Kansas Medical Center, Kansas City, Kans. Almost every institution with a diabetes center will have materials similar to those listed on the Professional Prompter Worksheet that can be purchased or borrowed. The diabetes clinical nurse specialist is also a source of information and assistance.

The rest of this section provides more detail on medication management, nutrition management, exercise knowledge, self-monitoring, managing hypoglycemia, psychologic adjustment, hygiene and foot care, and economic issues related to diabetes.

## Managing Medications

### Insulin knowledge

Patients taking insulin should be able to name their prescribed type and species source of insulin, their dose and the peak effects, and how the exercise regimen and diet are coordinated with the insulin. They should know insulin measurement (units) and the need for similarly calibrated syringes. In addition, they must know how to handle insulin needs on sick days.

### Insulin self-administration

For safe insulin administration, patients must know how to draw insulin into the syringe, mix two insulins (if pertinent), select and prepare the injection site, rotate sites, and inject insulin. The essential teaching points are summarized on the Professional Prompter Worksheet (Box 40-13). Most persons will have some fears related to self-injection and will want to delay learning this skill. Repeated practice may be necessary, so patients should be started on self-injections as soon as insulin treatment is deemed necessary.

**Preparing insulin dose.** The patient is taught to rotate or roll the insulin bottle to return any precipitated particles to solution and to draw the required dose of insulin into the syringe using correct technique. The procedure can be practiced using saline solution and a syringe or by using expired insulin and injecting into foam. For the first injection, the nurse may elect to delay teaching about the preparation and focus first on self-injection. Adults may be better able to focus on preparing the syringe after experiencing self-injection.

#### Guidelines for Mixing Two Insulins in One Syringe

1. Gather equipment.
2. Wash hands.
3. Roll bottle of modified insulin.
4. Cleanse tops of bottles.
5. Draw up air equivalent to dose of modified insulin, and inject the air into modified insulin vial. (Do not draw up this insulin.) Remove needle from vial.
6. Draw up air equivalent to dose of regular insulin, inject the air into the bottle, and withdraw the regular insulin to the correct dose. Remove all air, and readjust to correct dose.
7. Return to bottle of modified insulin, and draw up correct dose.
8. Discard insulin in syringe and start over if an error is made.

**Mixing two insulins.** If the patient is using two insulins, they may be mixed in one syringe so only one injection is necessary (see Guidelines box above). Regular insulin can be mixed with any other insulin. Lente insulins can be mixed with each other, but not with other insulins (except regular). Mixing two insulins in the same syringe is one of the more complex psychomotor skills the patient has to learn; therefore it needs to be started early.

A major complication with mixing two insulins in one syringe is that each of the two vials of insulin can be contaminated with the insulin from the other vial. This first concern is controlled by always withdrawing from the regular insulin vial first because injecting minute amounts of regular insulin into a vial of intermediate is less problematic than when the regular insulin is contaminated with the intermediate. Another concern is the dead space of the needle. The first insulin drawn up fills the dead space and is actually included in the measurement of the second insulin. New syringes with little or no dead space eliminate this last concern for the most part, and if the two insulins are always drawn up in the same sequence, the amount will always be the same.

If the patient has difficulty mastering the skill of mixing two insulins, several alternatives are available:

1. Take two separate injections each time.
2. Have a family member, friend, or community health nurse prefill the syringes; a week's supply can be drawn up at one time.
3. Premix a 4-week supply in one mixing bottle. For example, if the prescription is 16 U NPH and 8 U

*Text continued on p. 1324.*

## BOX 40-13 Professional Prompter Worksheet for Diabetes Education

SI = Survival information/skills for type I
SII = Survival information/skills for type II

**SURVIVAL/INITIAL TEACHING**

| Survival/Initial Skills | Type I Survival/Initial Skills | Type II Survival/Initial Skills |
|---|---|---|
| 1. Concentrate on survival. These are the skills every patient must know before discharge. It is necessary, and patient cannot go further without this foundation.<br>2. Start with survival skills regardless how long person has had diabetes. | 1. Psychologic and family.<br>2. Can patient give insulin correctly; i.e., see the increments, inject correctly, use proper sites, reuse syringe, know time action.<br>3. Monitor sugar and ketones.<br>4. Recognize and treat an insulin reaction. | 1. Psychologic and family.<br>2. Explanation of what diabetes is.<br>3. Treatment with diet, oral agent, and insulin if necessary.<br>4. Monitor sugar and ketones.<br>5. Recognize and treat an insulin reaction if on oral agent or insulin. |

**Tools To Use for Survival/Initial Teaching**

- Barrier check
- Initial assessment
- Take home Instruction Sheet
- American Diabetes Association (ADA) Curriculum Guidelines
- Refer to group class in local hospital

| ASSESSMENT | SI & SII |
|---|---|
| Complete assessment, including diabetes knowledge | |

**BARRIERS** SI & SII

| Define Barrier | Teaching Tools |
|---|---|
| 1. Fatigue/pain | 1. Do instructions another time. |
| 2. High anxiety | 2. Identify why and work on anxiety before proceeding. |
| 3. Blindness | 3. Audio material and devices. |

Developed by George Ann Eaks, RN, MN, CDE. From Cray Diabetes Center, University of Kansas Medical Center, Kansas City, Kans.

*Continued.*

**BOX 40-13 Professional Prompter Worksheet for Diabetes Education—cont'd**

**OVERVIEW OF DIABETES** SII

| Patient Can Verbalize/Demonstrate | Teaching Tools |
|---|---|
| 1. Diabetes is a disease in which the body is unable to utilize *all* foods properly due to lack of insulin or inability to use insulin. | ▶ Videotapes<br>■ Boehringer Mannheim: *Understanding Your Diabetes*<br>■ Lilly: *Managing Your Diabetes*<br>■ *Understanding Diabetes and Living a Healthy Life* |
| 2. Define high blood sugar in terms of blood glucose. Normal versus diabetes. List symptoms. | |
| 3. Define which of the types of diabetes patient has. | ▶ Refer to module<br>■ *Diabetes: What You Need To Know* |
| 4. Describe essential parts of diabetes management: Knowledge, self-care, meal planning, exercise, and medication. Know the effect each of these has on the blood glucose. | ▶ Refer to audiotape notebooks<br>■ Type I—*Diabetes: What You Need to Know*<br>■ Type II—*What IS Type II Diabetes?* |
| 5. Know effect of activity on blood glucose. | ▶ Refer to the International Diabetes Center's book, *Learning to Live Well with Diabetes* |
| 6. Know effect of illness/stress on blood glucose. | ▶ Chalkboard review |

**STRESS AND PSYCHOLOGICAL ADJUSTMENT** SI & SII

| Patient Can Verbalize/Demonstrate | Teaching Tools |
|---|---|
| 1. That patient has adapted to having diabetes. | ▶ Refer to two sources on emotions<br>■ The chapter on emotions from the International Diabetes Center's book, *Managing Type II Diabetes*<br>■ *Diabetes: Caring For Your Emotions as Well as Your Health* |
| 2. That patient expresses feelings about having diabetes. | ▶ Diabetes Center handouts on the grieving process<br>■ *Emotional/Grief Responses to Chronic Disease*<br>■ *Stages of Adaptation to a Chronic Disease* (2 parts) |
| 3. Acknowledges losses—grief process (fear, anxiety, denial, anger, bargaining, depression, acceptance).<br><br>Discussion with nurse or social worker. | ▶ Videotapes<br>■ *Type I Diabetes: One Man's Story*<br>■ Tom Parks in: *Diabetes—A Positive Approach* |

**BOX 40-13 Professional Prompter Worksheet for Diabetes Education—cont'd**

**FAMILY INVOLVEMENT AND SOCIAL SUPPORT** SI & SII

| Patient Can Verbalize/Demonstrate | Teaching Tools |
|---|---|
| 1. Family can identify one feeling a person with diabetes may experience.<br>2. Ways diabetes has affected the family.<br>3. A support person. | ▶ Refer to chapter on family involvement from the book, *Learning to Live Well With Diabetes*<br>▶ Refer to book, *Diabetes: Caring For Your Emotions as Well as Your Health*<br>▶ Specific articles from the journal, *Diabetes Forecast*<br>■ The Family Affair, Jan-Feb '84<br>■ Strategies for Living: Diabetes Is a Family Affair, May '89<br>▶ Frank discussion with nurse or social worker |

**NUTRITION** SI & SII

| Patient Can Verbalize/Demonstrate | Teaching Tools |
|---|---|
| 1. Individualized meal plan.<br>2. Reason for maintaining consistency (if appropriate of: meal spacing, proper meal times, and snacks to avoid hypo/hyperglycemia).<br>3. Relationship of insulin or oral agent, activity, and calorie intake.<br>4. Diet changes for sick day management, exercise, use of alcohol, change in meal schedule, and restaurant dining.<br>5. The importance of attaining and maintaining ideal body weight.<br>6. Effects of slow-burning foods (logs) and fast-burning foods (paper). | ▶ ADA Meal Plan<br>▶ ADA Sheets<br>▶ Novolin "Picture" Sheets<br>▶ Kentucky Guidelines[50]<br>▶ Vendor literature<br>■ Novolin<br>■ Lilly<br>▶ Refer to module<br>■ Sick Day Guidelines<br>▶ Videos<br>■ Novo Care's *Eat Well, Feel Good*<br>■ *Diabetes & Food: The Challenge of Choices*<br>▶ Pyramid Food Poster<br>▶ Logs and Paper Sheet<br>▶ If Dietitian unavailable, instruct patient to:<br>■ Eat three meals.<br>■ Two snacks (3 PM and hs); hs snack needs to be a log.<br>■ Assist patient in making an appointment to see dietitian if cannot be done before discharge. Diet is the foundation of diabetes care. |

**EXERCISE AND ACTIVITY**

| Patient Can Verbalize/Demonstrate | Teaching Tools |
|---|---|
| 1. How exercise affects diabetes control.<br>2. Cautions and risks of exercise.<br>3. When one should not exercise.<br>4. What is patient's personal exercise program? | ▶ ADA guidelines<br>▶ ADA books<br>▶ Exercise prescription handout sheet<br>▶ Refer to the International Diabetes Center's book, *Learning to Live Well with Diabetes*<br>▶ Vendor literature |

*Continued.*

**BOX 40-13 Professional Prompter Worksheet for Diabetes Education—cont'd**

| MEDICATIONS | SI & SII |
|---|---|
| **Patient Can Verbalize/Demonstrate** | **Teaching Tools** |
| *Insulin:*<br>1. What is function of insulin?<br>▶ Species/source.<br>▶ Intermediate, quick or long acting. | ▶ Have a bottle of expired insulin sample(s) to demonstrate how cloudy and clear appear.<br>▶ Use casting foam for patient to inject real expired insulin into. |
| 2. Differentiation of types of insulin. | |
| 3. Medication schedule—amounts and times taken. | ▶ If patient's extremely anxious, draw up a syringe of normal saline and let them quickly inject the needle into their skin to get over the anxiousness; otherwise, can first draw up insulin from insulin bottle(s) and inject into foam, then do self-injection. |
| 4. Correct technique for insulin preparation:<br>▶ Rotates bottle to mix (cloudy insulin).<br>▶ Injects air.<br>▶ Withdraws proper amount of insulin.<br>▶ Rids syringe of air bubbles. | ▶ Demonstrate injection sites on their own body (use injection site form). |
| 5. Correct technique for insulin preparation, two types:<br>▶ Rotates bottle to mix (cloudy) insulin.<br>▶ Injects air into both bottles.<br>▶ Withdraws clear (regular) insulin first.<br>▶ Adds proper amount of second insulin. | ▶ View videotape on insulin injection.<br>▶ Give handout on insulin injection.<br>▶ Chalkboard review of how insulin works; i.e., time of onset and peak action. Correlate this with food and blood testing. (Best done when discussing hypoglycemia.) |
| 6. Correct technique for insulin administration:<br>▶ Cleans site with alcohol.<br>▶ Pinches skin and inserts needle all the way.<br>▶ Injects insulin, holding needle steady (needle should go in straight unless person is very thin).<br>▶ Rotates injection site: abdomen, arm, leg. | ▶ Tie in hypoglycemia and monitoring.<br>▶ Use food models. |
| 7. Storage of insulin:<br>▶ Best to store in refrigerator.<br>▶ For travel okay at room temperature up to 1 month (57°-85° F). | ▶ Encourage patient to give insulin early while in hospital. If you do injection, teach as you go.<br>▶ Have patients begin injection from the time they enter the hospital so it is not so frightening when they go home. |
| 8. Discard syringes in sealable can (old coffee can). | |
| 9. Can cause hypoglycemia. | ▶ Use posters of insulin. |
| *Oral Agents:*<br>1. Action of oral agent. | ▶ Show time of action of medication, and demonstrate on chalkboard so patient understands importance of eating three meals a day.<br>▶ Refer to videos<br>■ Boehringer Mannheim: *In Balance In Control: Diabetes Medication as Directed*<br>■ Medcom: *Diabetes—Diet, Exercise and Self Care*<br>■ Upjohn: *Diabetes—What you Need to Know*<br>■ Roerig: *You're In Control—Managing Your Diabetes* |
| 2. Medication schedule—amount and *time* to be taken. | |
| 3. Need to eat 3 meals a day, spread throughout the day. | ▶ Refer to module<br>■ *Diabetes: What you Need to Know*<br>▶ Refer to audiotape notebook<br>■ *What is Type II Diabetes* |
| 4. Can cause hypoglycemia. | ▶ Show handout<br>■ *Oral Hypoglycemic Agents* |

**BOX 40-13 Professional Prompter Worksheet for Diabetes Education—cont'd**

| RELATIONSHIPS AMONG NUTRITION, EXERCISE, MEDICATION, AND BLOOD GLUCOSE LEVELS SI & SII | |
|---|---|
| **Patient Can Verbalize/Demonstrate** | **Teaching Tools** |
| 1. Effect of food on blood sugar.<br>2. Effect of insulin oral agents on blood sugar.<br>3. Effect of physical activity on blood sugar.<br>4. Effect of illness on blood sugar. | ▶ Diagram on board<br>▶ Chalkboard review |

| MONITORING AND USE OF RESULTS SI & SII | |
|---|---|
| **Patient Can Verbalize/Demonstrate** | **Teaching Tools** |
| 1. Explain need for monitoring glucose.<br>2. Normal range of blood glucose for self.<br>3. Capillary blood glucose monitoring:<br>▶ Loads and operates lancing device.<br>▶ Holds arm down to the side to get better drop of blood.<br>▶ Obtains large hanging drop of blood.<br>▶ Places blood on strip properly.<br>▶ Waits appropriate amount of time according to directions.<br>▶ Reads visual and records results.<br>▶ Uses meter (knows name of meter, strips to use, how to calibrate, use control solutions, how to clean, insert battery, and understand readout).<br>4. Checking urine ketones:<br>▶ Knows how to do.<br>▶ Knows when to do.<br>5. Knows when to call for help. | ▶ Show-and-tell<br>■ Demonstration<br>■ Have patients do return demonstration.<br>▶ Videotapes on SBGM<br>▶ Monitoring module<br>▶ Have patients begin all this from the time they enter the hospital so it's not so frightening when they go home.<br>▶ Realize there are many monitoring machines. Mention these to patients. Ask your diabetes nurse if not familiar. Help fit diabetes into patients' life-style by giving them a choice.<br>▶ Give patients monitoring journal and show how to use.<br>▶ Chalkboard review (demonstrate when to check blood sugar and how to look for patterns).<br>▶ Scorecard<br>▶ Monitor checklist |

*Continued.*

**BOX 40-13 Professional Prompter Worksheet for Diabetes Education—cont'd**

**ACUTE COMPLICATIONS: HYPERGLYCEMIA**

| Patient Can Verbalize/Demonstrate | Teaching Tools |
|---|---|
| 1. Definition and cause of hyperglycemia. | ▶ Visual aid of hyperglycemic effects<br>▶ Videotapes<br>■ *Hyperglycemia and Ketoacidosis*<br>▶ Refer to modules<br>■ *Insulin Reaction*<br>■ *Sick Day Guidelines*<br>■ *Hyperglycemia and Ketoacidosis* |
| 2. Symptoms of hyperglycemia. | ▶ Review what should be in a sick day kit<br>■ Nutrition handouts<br>■ Sick day foods<br>■ Food models<br>■ Log and paper<br>■ *Short-Term Sick Day Checklist*<br>■ *Sick Day Guidelines module*<br>■ Audiotape notebook: *Sick Day*<br>■ *Guidelines* |
| 3. Illness and sick day rules:<br>▶ What to do about insulin/oral agents when ill.<br>▶ How often to check sugar and ketones.<br>▶ When to call physician.<br>▶ Sick day eating. | ▶ Vendor literature<br>■ Becton Dickinson<br>■ Novolin<br>■ Lilly<br>▶ Novo Care posters |

**ACUTE COMPLICATIONS: HYPOGLYCEMIA** **SI & SII**

| Patient Can Verbalize/Demonstrate | Teaching Tools |
|---|---|
| 1. Definition and cause of hypoglycemia. | ▶ Videotape<br>■ Hypoglycemia<br>▶ Vendor literature<br>■ Becton Dickinson<br>■ Novolin<br>■ Lilly |
| 2. Symptoms of hypoglycemia. | ▶ Refer to module<br>■ *Insulin Reaction*<br>▶ Actual food models to be used for treatment (show and tell) |
| 3. Treatment of hypoglycemia (wears diabetes ID). | ▶ Logs and paper<br>▶ Chalkboard review of a simulated day (use time of action of insulin, when to eat—refer to diagram in audiotape notebook on *Insulin Reaction*) |
| 4. When to call physician. | ▶ Novo Care posters<br>▶ Give ID card. |

**BOX 40-13 Professional Prompter Worksheet for Diabetes Education—cont'd**

**CHRONIC COMPLICATIONS**

| Patient Can Verbalize/Demonstrate | Teaching Tools |
|---|---|
| 1. Possibility of long-term complications. | ▶ Chalkboard review<br>▶ Boehringer Mannheim: *Body Link Tool* |
| 2. Importance of prevention. | ▶ Cray Diabetes Center: *Owner's Manual*[26]<br>▶ Videotapes<br>■ *Diabetic Complications: Reducing the Odds*<br>■ Others |
| 3. The trouble spots at risk for diabetes.<br>▶ Eyes<br>▶ Blood vessels<br>▶ Sexual dysfunction<br>▶ Blood pressure<br>▶ Feet<br>▶ Kidneys<br>▶ Nerves | ▶ Visual aid<br>▶ Refer to module<br>■ *Why the Fuss about Feet* |
| 4. Reasons for good foot care:<br>▶ Daily cleansing and inspection. | ▶ Vendor literature<br>■ Foot care<br>■ Novo Care posters |
| 5. Reason for yearly eye examination (and last date). | ▶ Resource books/journals<br>■ International Diabetes Center books<br>■ Others<br>■ *Diabetes Forecast* |
| 6. Need for blood pressure control.<br>▶ Knows blood pressure. | ▶ *Foot Inspector's Guide* |

**FOOT, SKIN, AND DENTAL CARE**

| Patient Can Verbalize/Demonstrate | Teaching Tools |
|---|---|
| 1. Importance of good health habits.<br>▶ Dental<br>▶ Skin<br>▶ Feet<br>▶ Signs of infection<br>▶ Effect of smoking, alcohol, and drug abuse | ▶ *Diabetes Forecast*<br>▶ Resource books<br>▶ Videotapes<br>▶ Vendor literature |

**BEHAVIOR CHANGE STRATEGIES, GOAL SETTING, AND PROBLEM SOLVING**

| Patient Can Verbalize/Demonstrate | Teaching Tools |
|---|---|
| 1. The need for a planned system of medical care.<br>▶ Follow-up and education | ▶ Local diabetes center's materials<br>▶ Local diabetes center's newsletter |
| 2. The benefits and responsibilities of goal setting for self-help care. | ▶ Resource books/journals |
| 3. The importance of being well-informed, equal partners to make choices. | ▶ Selected handouts |

**USE OF HEALTH CARE SYSTEM AND COMMUNITY RESOURCES**

| Patient Can Verbalize/Demonstrate | Teaching Tools |
|---|---|
| 1. The need to identify one or two resources that can help them.<br>▶ Home Health<br>▶ American Diabetes Association<br>▶ Self-management classes<br>▶ Services for the blind | ▶ Where to Turn<br>▶ ADA handouts<br>▶ Local diabetes center's class schedule of Self-Management Series Class for Persons with Diabetes |

*Continued.*

**BOX 40-13 Professional Prompter Worksheet for Diabetes Education—cont'd**

| NECESSARY TAKE-HOME | SI & SII |
|---|---|
| **Patient Can Verbalize/Demonstrate** | **Teaching Tools** |
| 1. Feel comfortable doing all skills under survival. | ▶ Seek information from diabetes nurse. |
| 2. Know the skills and be able to simulate them in a normal day; i.e., take you through a day and list all diabetes-related activities as they would do them. | ▶ Fill out and complete forms.<br>▪ *Choices To Better Daily Living*<br>▪ *Take Home Instruction* |
| 3. Know whom to call, the telephone number, and when to call. | |
| 4. Have a return appointment card with physician name and phone number listed. | ▶ Give schedule of classes |
| 5. Have instructions written on:<br>▶ *Take Home Instruction* form<br>▶ *Choice to Better Daily Living* form | ▶ Make sure patient has supplies<br>▪ Syringes<br>▪ Medication (insulin or oral agent)<br>▪ Blood glucose test strips<br>▪ Ketone test strips<br>▪ Pricking device<br>▪ Lancets<br>▪ Cotton balls<br>▪ Alcohol wipes<br>▪ Monitor (if necessary)<br>▪ ID card |
| 6. Have a schedule of the diabetes classes if they choose to attend them. | |
| 7. Have a meal plan—have patient seen by dietitian. If dietitian unavailable and you must instruct on meal plan, refer to section on Nutrition. | |

regular insulin, the ratio is 2:1; 10 ml of NPH could be mixed with 5 ml of regular insulin, and a dose of 24 U is then measured from the mixing bottle. This alternative works only if the patient is on a relatively fixed insulin regimen. The diaphragm on the mixing vial lasts for about 3 months.

4. Use commercially premixed insulin (Novolin 70/30 and Mixtard Human 70/30 are two such preparations) if appropriate for treatment. (NOTE: These ratios frequently do not reflect the patient's needs. People do not fit one "recipe.")

**Selection and preparation of injection sites.** Any area of subcutaneous tissue can be used for injection. The recommended sites are illustrated in Figure 40-13. When selecting a site, the patient's ability to use it must be considered. Some patients have difficulty using the arms and buttocks because of dexterity, and some the abdomen, because patients pattern the procedure used in the hospital, where the abdomen is rarely used. The best site for the first injection is the abdomen. It is easy to work with and has the most rapid absorption, and absorption is not affected by physical activity.

Be aware that it is known that insulin absorption from the different body areas varies (abdomen > arm > thigh). That is why all sites on one area are used before moving to another site. Some recommend that arms and legs be avoided if the person will be using the extremities in physical activities, because it may cause faster absorption. (Some researchers do not agree with this.) If the patient exercises infrequently and has only one injection a day, it may be possible to avoid using the arms and legs. However, with daily exercise and a multiple injection regimen, avoiding the arms and legs is impractical; teaching should focus on the principles related to rotating the site. In preparing the site, all that is needed is to cleanse the area with alcohol.

**Rotation of sites.** Injection sites must be rotated to achieve proper absorption. Lipodystrophy can occur with repeated injections at the same site, causing poor absorption of the medications. Two forms of lipodystrophy can occur: hypertrophy and atrophy. *Hypertrophy* is thickening of an injection site due to development of fibrous scar tissue from repeated injections. A hypertrophic area is usually devoid of nerve endings, and the patient likes to reuse it because injections are painless, but absorption is erratic. *Atrophy* is loss of subcutaneous fat from unknown causes; however, an immunologic process is implicated. Lipodystrophies may be partially caused by impurities in insulin; development of purified insulins has decreased this problem, but rotation of sites is still important (Figure 40-14). The principles governing site rotation follow.

1. Do not use a site more than once every 4 to 6 weeks.
2. Sites should be 1 to 1½ inches apart.
3. Use all sites in one geographic area, then move to the next area.
4. Document site use.

Each injection area has multiple sites, as indicated by the X's in Figure 40-13.

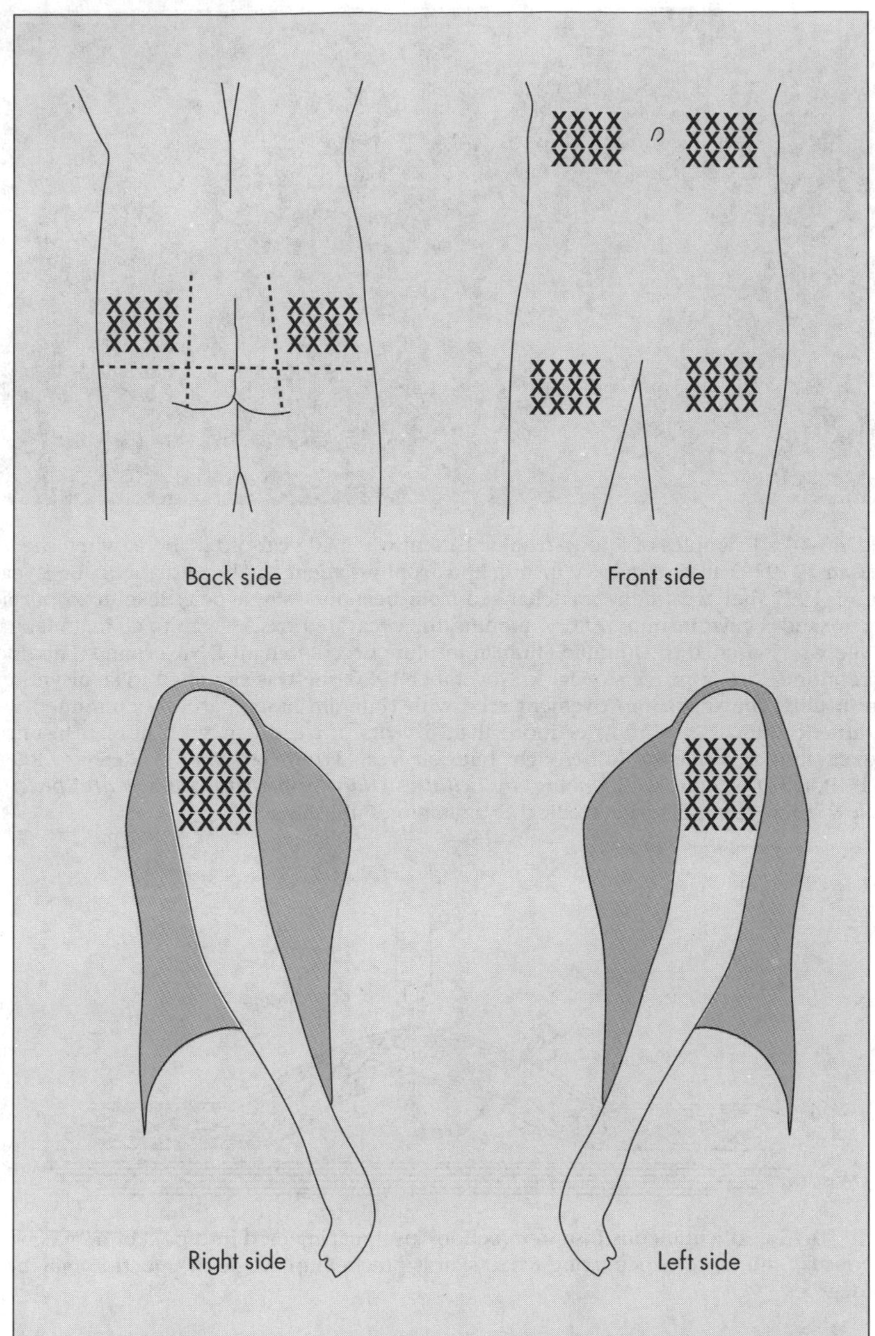


**FIGURE 40-13** Recommended injection rotation sites.

**Injection of insulin.** Insulin should be administered directly under the subcutaneous tissue (Figure 40-15). This can be achieved by pinching up the skin and injecting at a 45- to 90-degree angle. If the person has considerable fatty tissue (> 1 inch) a 90-degree angle is safe. Use a 45-degree angle when the fatty tissue is less than 1 inch. The needle length is usually ½ inch. (Consult a principles of nursing text if necessary for principles of correct subcutaneous injection.) Jet spray injectors are available for insulin injection. They are expensive but may be helpful to persons coping with multiple daily injections (Figure 40-16).

**Storage of insulin and other supplies and care of syringe.** Patients need to develop a home storage system for equipment (syringes, alcohol, cotton balls) and the currently used bottle of insulin and extra insulin. Insulin is stable for 30 days at room temperature; however, it is a good idea to have patients keep extra insulin in a refrigerator because what temperature room tem-

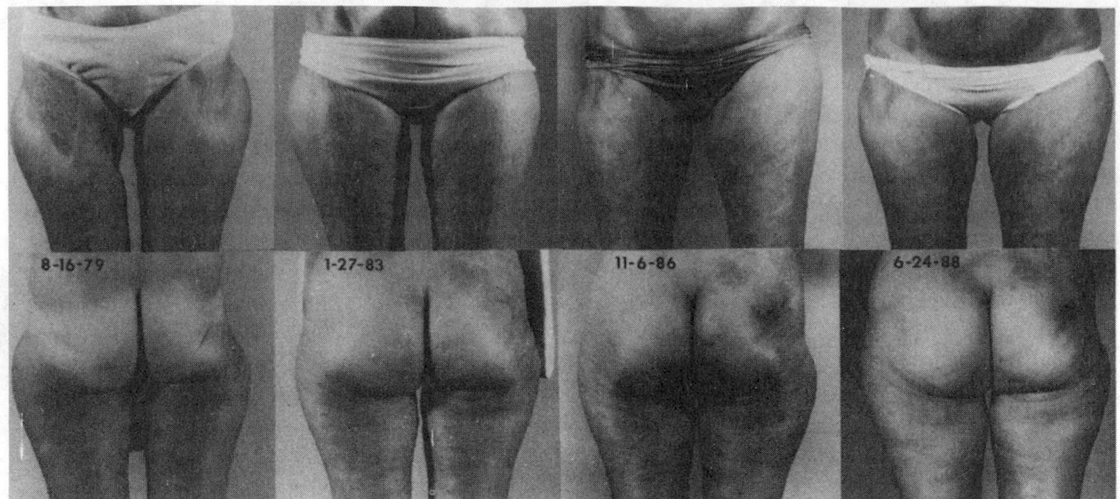


**FIGURE 40-14** Examples of lipodystrophy. Patient was a 50-year-old diabetic when she was referred in 1979 because of marked insulin lipoatrophy. Patient had been diabetic for 3 years. In August 1979, her treatment was changed from beef-pork single-peak insulin to purified pork Lente and regular insulins. After 4 months, the excavated areas began to fill in. In January 1983, she was switched to Humulin (human insulin of recombinant DNA origin). The lipoatrophy continued to improve slowly. In November 1986, she was switched to semisynthetic human insulin. The slight improvement seen with Humulin has apparently continued with semisynthetic human insulin. After more than 5 years of treatment with human insulin, a large excavated area persists in her right buttock area. (From Galloway JA, deShazo RD: In Rifkin H, Porte D Jr, editors: *Ellenberg and Rifkin's Diabetes mellitus: theory and practice,* ed 4, New York, 1990, Elsevier Medical Examination Publishing.)

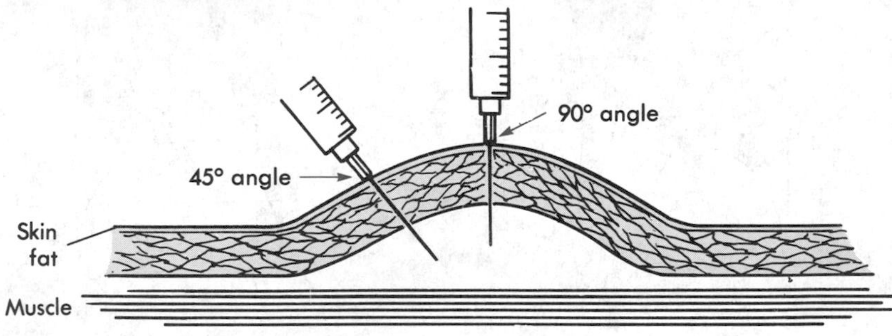


**FIGURE 40-15** Subcutaneous insulin injection. Insulin is injected into pocket between subcutaneous fat and muscle, occurring when skin is pinched up. Angle of injection may be 45 or 90 degrees.

perature is differs from individual to individual. *The current recommendation is to keep the currently used insulin bottle and the other supplies together at room temperature and to store extra bottles of insulin in the refrigerator. Store prefilled syringes in the refrigerator with the needles facing upward.*

Patients should always have an extra bottle of each type of insulin they use. Insulin has an expiration date, which should be checked at purchase; purchase only the amount that can be used before the expiration date. When traveling, insulin and supplies should be hand-carried to prevent loss.

Almost all patients use disposable syringes, and many patients reuse them. Although research has shown no infections on reuse of disposable syringes, normal flora was cultured from some reused syringes.[68] The American Diabetes Association position statement of 1992[7] suggests that reuse of syringes can be considered unless patients have poor hygiene, acute concurrent illness, open wounds on hands, or decreased resistance to infection.

A few persons still use glass reusable syringes, which are less expensive than others. These patients must learn one of two sterilization techniques: (1) immerse syringe and needle in 70% alcohol between injections and boil weekly for 10 minutes, or (2) boil syringe and needles daily for 10 minutes. A strainer placed in a saucepan simplifies draining and handling the boiled equipment.

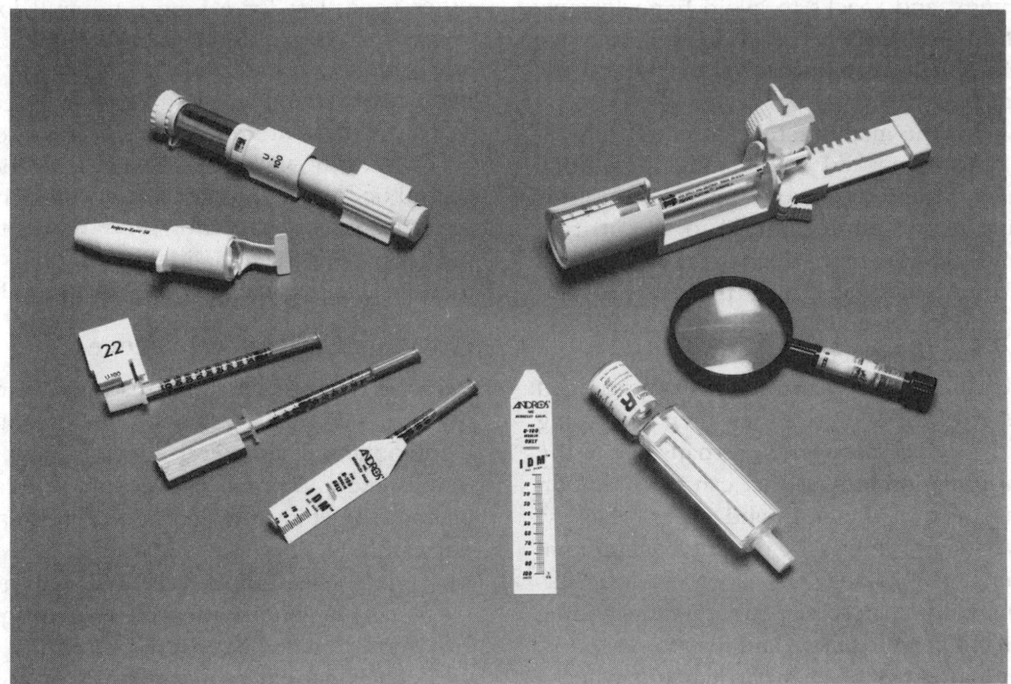

**FIGURE 40-16** Insulin injection devices. These are particularly well suited for visually impaired persons, but the jet injector and Inject-Ease can be used by persons who have trouble injecting themselves. *Left to right:* Jet Injector, Inject-Ease, BD chip, generic syringe chip, Andros IDM on syringe, Andros IDM, BD Magnifier, generic magnifier, Insul-ease device.

Because patient and family must learn many details, disposable syringes may be used until the patient feels more comfortable with other skills before learning the sterilization methods.

**Measures to assist the sensory-impaired person.** Adaptation of equipment may be necessary for the sensory-impaired person. A number of aids available for the visually handicapped are advertised in diabetic publications or are available from the American Foundation for the Blind (15 West 16th St., New York, NY 10011). Special syringes with plunger locks, attachable devices for locking the plunger, and attachable needle and insulin bottle guides to facilitate entry of the needle into the bottle can be purchased. Persons who have failing vision may also use a small magnifying adapter that can be clipped to a syringe (see Figure 40-16).

Persons with poor vision may draw air instead of insulin into the syringe. They must be cautioned to invert the bottle completely and insert the needle only a short distance. They are often advised to use only about two thirds of a bottle of insulin. Some persons have a community health nurse or a friend draw the last doses from a bottle of insulin. Another option is to know how long to use a vial before the level gets so low the needle is not covered (e.g., 1000 units in vial—if person is taking 40 units a day, he or she should stop using vial on the 22nd day unless assisted by sighted person).

Some individuals who are not able to prepare an insulin dose accurately because of motor or sensory problems are still capable of giving their own injections. Prefilled syringes may be used. Automatic injectors may be used for some persons with physical handicaps (see Figure 40-16).

### Oral hypoglycemic agents

Although care is less complex, patients receiving oral hypoglycemic agents must be equally prepared to handle their medication. Each patient must know the name of the drug, dose, and peak effects, and how the diet and exercise regimens are coordinated with the drug therapy. It is important to encourage patients to eat three meals a day. Give patients a specific time to take medications. They must be taught about hypoglycemia symptoms and treatment. Patients must know how to handle their drug on sick days. Oral hypoglycemic agents should be kept out of reach of children and in a place that is dark and cool. The medication should be hand carried when traveling to prevent loss.

## Managing Nutrition

Since diet is the cornerstone of treatment for the person with diabetes, it is important to be able to teach the patient information on the Professional Prompter Worksheet under nutrition (see Box 40-13). Nurses can help reinforce the individualized meal plan and must be aware of maintaining consistency of meal spacing, proper meal times, and snacks to avoid hypoglycemia (if on medication). All diabetes teaching will interface with the relationship of insulin or oral agent, activity, and calorie intake.

Weight is one of the major factors in monitoring diabetes control. Attaining and maintaining ideal body weight are major criteria in diabetes management; this needs the whole team's effort. Central to all nutrition management information that will help the patient is stressing the importance of eating three meals and snacks. When patients are taking insulin, snacks also become a part of the treatment plan. Meals should be spaced throughout the day. This should be encouraged for all persons regardless of whether they are taking insulin or oral hypoglycemic agents. Perhaps one of the most important nutrition lessons that can be passed on to patients is the use of the "logs and paper" analogy. Information overload prohibits the patient from remembering everything. The analogy of "paper and logs" has been helpful clinically to increase patient understanding of types of foods to use for snacks and insulin reactions. In practice, the patient is asked what happens when a piece of *paper* is put into a fire in a fireplace. The answer is usually, "It burns fast and it's gone." This is what fruits, juices, real soda pop, and candy do. They raise the blood sugar quickly, and it goes down quickly. *Logs,* on the other hand, last for a long time and do not cause an immediate rise in blood glucose. Some examples of log and paper foods are listed in Figure 40-17. When written instructions are given and "log" is listed for bedtime snack, the patient knows exactly what to eat and why. When asked how to treat an insulin reaction, the answer should be "paper" followed by a "log." This has been an effective nutritional analogy and frequently puts a smile on the patient's face. Using food models or pictures of food makes this analogy more memorable.

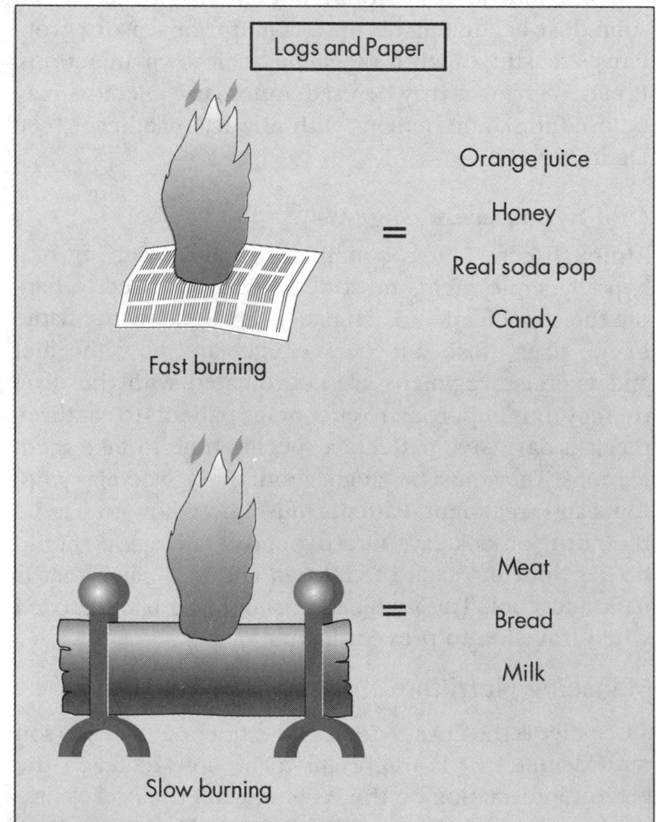


**FIGURE 40-17** "Logs" and "paper." (From Cray Diabetes Center, University of Kansas Medical Center, Kansas City, Kan.)

## Providing Exercise Knowledge

Exercise is another major area of patient education for persons with diabetes mellitus. Nursing activities include obtaining an exercise history, helping the person understand and obtain a preexercise examination, and planning an enjoyable and safe exercise program.[15] The nurse should:

1. Help select an exercise that will not cause problems if conditions such as neuropathy or proliferative retinopathy are present.
2. Refer patient to a podiatrist for correct footwear for the chosen exercise.
3. Help establish a regular exercise routine to reduce the risk of hypoglycemia.
4. Explain the components of a safe exercise program and special needs of the person with diabetes.
5. Teach how to monitor cardiovascular tolerance (e.g, by pulse rate or level of exertion).
6. Identify the parameters to monitor before daily exercise (blood glucose level, ketone level, environmental temperature).
   a. Patient should not exercise if blood glucose is greater than 300 mg/dl or if there are ketones in the urine.
   b. If weather is hot, suggest exercising in an air-conditioned area, such as a shopping mall or gymnasium, or using an exercise bicycle to avoid dehydration.

See Boxes 40-9 and 40-10 for the risks and benefits of exercise.

## Self-monitoring of Metabolic Status

All patients need to do some self-monitoring.

### Self-monitoring of blood glucose

Various types of home tests for SMBG correlate well with laboratory measurement of blood glucose level. A reflectance meter adds to the cost of monitoring, but it gives a precise numeric value. Newer meters are small; some are the size of fountain pens and credit cards and thus are more convenient. Some test strips (Chemstrip bG) do not require a meter, but instead indicate the range of blood glucose; for some patients, knowing the range is sufficient and thus a meter is not required. (Good vision and color vision are necessary for visual readings.)

SMBG has been found to facilitate attainment of glycemic control in IDDM and pregnant women. It is always used by those with multiple-injection regimens or infusion pumps and by many on diet only, oral agent, or less frequent insulin injection regimens. SMBG can be used to validate subjective symptoms of hypoglycemia or hyperglycemia, and it provides more immediate feedback about the effects of nonadherence with the prescribed regimen. There is great variability in physicians' recommendations for frequency of blood glucose testing. Many patients are advised to test before and after meals and at bedtime for a short period, then after meals and at bedtime for a short period, and once they are stable, four times a day on only 1 day each week and whenever they feel sick. Persons who manipulate their insulin may need to test four or more times daily at all times. To do the test, the person sticks a finger and applies a drop of blood to a commercially prepared glucose oxidase stick or a sensor strip. Timing of the reading and preparation of the specimen are very important in obtaining accurate results. Research has shown that, although most patients experience difficulty at first, especially sore fingers, and inconvenience, these disappear for most persons. Research also shows that most patients decrease their frequency of monitoring below that prescribed.[30] This may be appropriate for most, but if not, the nurse must reinforce the need for continual monitoring. SMBG is expensive. Most insurance companies will reimburse for the reflectance meter, but not always for the test strips. Figure 40-18 shows sticking devices and different glucose meters.

### Urine testing

Urine testing for **ketones** should be encouraged for *any* person with diabetes who is ill or if blood glucose is greater than 240 mg/dl. Urine ketones are rarely positive in persons with NIDDM even when the blood glucose is 240 or greater. Urine tests are described in Chapter 38.

### Other types of patient self-monitoring

Although health professionals emphasize use of physiologic parameters to monitor glucose status, patients continue to use symptoms as guides for self-regulation.[43] In the presence of some chronic illnesses, even when patients are told the disease may be asymptomatic, they report that symptoms guide them. One research study has shown that not only do patients use symptoms for self-regulation, but they also take action on the basis of these symptoms (see Research box, p. 1330). Further studies are investigating the accuracy of the symptoms in relation to actual blood glucose levels.[43] Results of this type of study have important implications for future patient education of the person with diabetes mellitus.

### Patient teaching regarding self-monitoring

Techniques for appropriate monitoring must be part of the teaching plan. Teaching should include knowledge

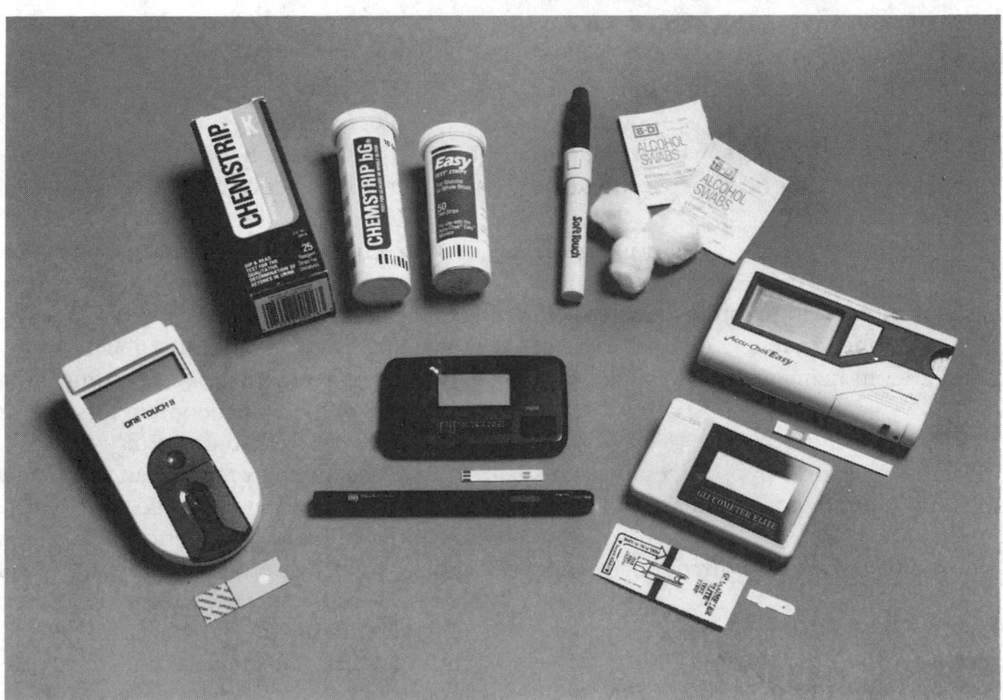


**FIGURE 40-18** Self-monitoring devices for blood glucose. *Left to right, top row:* Chemstrip K, Chemstrip bG, Accu-Chek Easy Strips, Soft-Touch pricker device, Accu-Chek Easy Meter. *Bottom row:* One Touch II Meter, Medisense Companion and Pen sensor, Glucometer Elite Meter and strips.

## RESEARCH

Hamera E et al: Self-regulation in individuals with type II diabetes, *Nurs Res* 37(6):363-367, 1988.

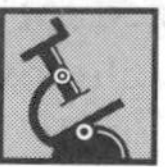

In this study, a model for self-regulation of diabetes was tested. The model proposed that individuals monitor their disease status by comparing their current status with an internal standard of well-being. When a discrepancy was noted and associated with a change in blood glucose, action was taken to relieve the symptom and thereby regulate blood glucose. Data from interviews with 173 persons with NIDDM were used to test the variables symptom associating and action taking from the model. Most subjects did associate symptoms, and of those, most took action. Symptom associating and action taking were not related to metabolic control. Women and persons who were currently taking insulin were more likely to associate symptoms with high or low blood glucose, but insulin taking was not related to action taking. Actions taken included eating or drinking caloric foods, taking fluids, and resting. Not all actions were logical for the associated blood glucose level (e.g., exercise for symptoms associated with low blood glucose or eating for symptoms associated with high blood glucose) but were logical for the symptoms. The authors suggest that potential use of this type of self-regulation must be considered in the care plans of persons with diabetes.

about testing procedures, demonstrations, return demonstrations by patients, and information about what to do with the collected data. All patients should use a diary or log to record date, time, and monitoring results. Other diary notations may include medications, food intake, activity level, and illnesses so the persons can begin to see the relationship between blood glucose or urine ketone levels and their regimens.

As patients gain flexibility and self-determination, they may manipulate insulin/diet/exercise independently on the basis of monitoring results. Patients will progress toward more independence on the basis of ability, interest, and encouragement by caregivers.

### Managing Hypoglycemia

Patients receiving insulin or oral hypoglycemic agents must have information about hypoglycemia, also known as *insulin shock,* including:

1. Signs and symptoms associated with hypoglycemic reaction
2. Assistance with recall of symptoms of a hypoglycemic reaction
3. Knowledge of appropriate treatment of hypoglycemia
4. How to obtain an identification card or Medic-Alert bracelet or necklace and the importance of carrying or wearing it at all times
5. The importance of carrying a quickly absorbed glucose source
6. The importance of identifying why the hypoglycemic reaction occurred so it can be avoided in the future (see p. 1300)

**BOX 40-14 Signs and Symptoms of Hypoglycemia**

**SYMPATHETIC NERVOUS SYSTEM ACTIVITY**

| | | |
|---|---|---|
| Pallor | Palpitation | Weakness* |
| Perspiration* | Nervousness* | Trembling |
| Piloerection | Irritability | Hunger |
| Tachycardia | | |

**CENTRAL NERVOUS SYSTEM ACTIVITY**

| | |
|---|---|
| Headache | Fatigue |
| Blurred vision | Numbness of lips, tongue |
| Diplopia | Mental confusion |
| Incoherent speech | Convulsion* |
| Emotional changes | Coma |

Data from Paulk LH: *Hypoglycemic reactions from the diabetic's perspective,* unpublished master's thesis, Kent, Ohio, 1983, Kent State University.
*Signs most often reported by patients.

**BOX 40-15 Carbohydrates (10 to 15 g) for Relief of Hypoglycemia**

½ cup pure fruit juice
½ cup carbonated soda drink with sugar
½ cup regular gelatin dessert
4 cubes or 2 packets of sugar
2 squares of graham crackers
2 to 3 pieces of hard candy

The common signs and symptoms of hypoglycemia are caused by activation of the sympathetic nervous system or depression of CNS activity. These signs and symptoms are listed in Box 40-14. The treatment for hypoglycemia is 10 to 15 g of fast-acting carbohydrate. Some examples of foods that contain this amount of fast-acting carbohydrate are listed in Box 40-15.

Because hypoglycemia can occur suddenly, family members and friends should also learn the symptoms and how to handle a reaction. If a patient is awake but groggy, another person can be taught to place a teaspoon of corn syrup, honey, or cake icing in the patient's mouth between the gum and cheek. This will be absorbed through the oral mucosa, and the patient will usually arouse sufficiently to take a glass of juice, milk, or sugar-sweetened coffee or tea. If glucagon is prescribed for hypoglycemic reactions, a family member is taught how to give the injection.

All information about hypoglycemia should be taught

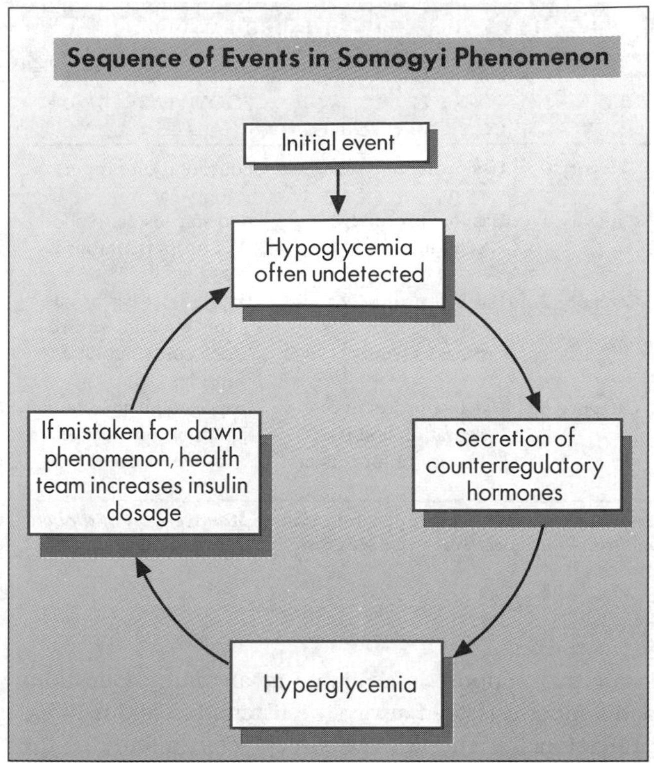


**FIGURE 40-19** Somogyi phenomenon.

as part of the survival skills during the initial management phase. A good time to teach about hypoglycemia is after teaching about insulin injection and self-monitoring has been completed. It is helpful to illustrate survival teaching using simulation and going through a typical day with patients, letting them guide you through all the diabetes-related activities in sequence. At this time, information about insulin reaction can be taught in relationship to time/action of insulin.

### Somogyi phenomenon

The **Somogyi phenomenon** is a reaction characterized by alternating hypoglycemic reactions and periods of hyperglycemia. This phenomenon is most frequently seen during initial periods of blood glucose regulation. The person being treated with intermediate- or long-acting insulin may experience hypoglycemia at peak times of insulin activity. As is true with healthy persons without diabetes, the hypoglycemia in persons with diabetes stimulates the production of counterregulatory hormones (glucagon, glucocorticoids, growth hormone, epinephrine). These hormones promote glycogenolysis and gluconeogenesis. In normal persons the blood glucose level is brought only to the normal range because, as it is elevated, insulin secretion is stimulated and the blood glucose level is again lowered. In persons with diabetes, the blood glucose goes to abnormally high levels because insulin secretion does not respond in the normal way. In some instances, the signs and symptoms of hypoglycemia are not obvious enough to be detected. In some instances, the *hyperglycemia* following the *hypoglycemia* is recognized in the early morning and may be mistaken for the *dawn phenomenon*. The assumption is made that the patient needs higher doses of insulin, but this treatment worsens the problem. Figure 40-19 illustrates this cycle.

The signs and symptoms of the Somogyi phenomenon can be any of those normally associated with hypoglycemia, but frequently they consist only of nighttime sweats, nightmares, and a headache on arising (however, this can happen anytime). There may be weight gain in the presence of glycosuria, relatively normal blood glucose with positive ketones (remember that counterregulatory hormones stimulate lipolysis and β-oxidation of fats), and wide fluctuations in blood glucose unrelated to meals.

Treatment consists of identifying the phenomenon and then decreasing insulin dose. A primary nursing role is to document complaints of hypoglycemia, glucose intake, and laboratory results and to look for complaints of night sweats, nightmares, and early-morning headaches. The nurse should also correlate these complaints and laboratory results with the times of meals. Such data help to identify the phenomenon.

## Providing Hygiene and Foot Care

### Hygiene

Persons with diabetes are susceptible to infection. The effectiveness of the skin as a first line of defense is diminished. Uncontrolled diabetes leads to loss of fat deposits under the skin, loss of glycogen, and catabolism of body proteins. Protein loss can hamper inflammatory response and wound healing and impair leukocyte function, migration of leukocytes to site of infection, phagocytosis, and bacterial killing, all of which are involved in combating infection. Decreased circulation to selected body parts can also delay healing. The skin must be kept supple and as free of pathogenic organisms as possible. This is especially true in warm, moist areas that encourage growth of organisms (between the toes, under the breasts, and in the axillae and groin). It is very important that persons with diabetes carry out hygienic measures for prevention of infection daily, with special emphasis on foot care. They should also avoid persons with upper respiratory tract infections and must seek medical attention immediately if an infection occurs.

### Foot care

The need for foot care cannot be overemphasized. The patient's feet should be visually assessed at every follow-up visit (Box 40-16). This action by caregivers may reinforce the need for the person to practice preventive self-care at home. Semmes-Weinstein monofilaments are currently the most common form of quantifiable testing today. The mylar filaments are similar to a stiff fishing line. The test is performed by applying a force to one

**BOX 40-16 Assessment of Feet of the Person With Diabetes**

**Color:** Compare one foot with the other.
**Temperature:** Compare both feet with upper legs; assess for line of demarcations.
**Sensory function:** Test for pinprick and vibratory sense (Semmes-Weinstein monofilament).
**Reflexes:** Test Achilles tendon reflex.
**Pulses:** Check dorsalis pedis and posterior tibialis.
**Lesions:** Examine for calluses, cuts, bruises, cracks, or infection.
**Self-care:** Discuss self-care regimen being used.

**TABLE 40-17 Risk Categories and Associated Footwear Guidelines**

| | CLINICAL FINDINGS | FOOTWEAR CHANGES |
|---|---|---|
| Category 0 | Has protective sensation | Education on proper footwear |
| Category 1 | Has lost protective sensation | Add soft insole to shoe of proper contour and fit |
| Category 2 | Has lost protective sensation and has foot deformity | Depth footwear or custom shoe for severe deformity, molded insoles |
| Category 3 | Has lost protective sensation and has history of foot ulcer | Inspect type and condition of footwear and insoles at every visit |

From Coleman W: In Haire-Joshu D, editor: *Management of diabetes mellitus—perspectives of care across the life span,* St Louis, 1992, Mosby.

end of the filament and pressing against the patient's skin. Persons who do not feel the filament are at high risk for foot problems.

Now that protective sensory loss can be assessed, the risk of the patient's foot being injured can be categorized. A program using the risk categories has been used for some years at the Hansen's Disease Center in Carville, La. The risk categories used by the team at Carville are listed in Table 40-17.

The patient must practice preventive care on a daily basis. If neuropathy or other changes occur, a podiatric consultation is necessary. The podiatrist can help the patient by treating calluses and corns and by relieving pressure areas through custom-made shoes. The Guidelines box (p. 1333) outlines teaching about foot care.

## Managing Concurrent Illnesses

All illnesses influence the status of diabetes control. In most instances, the person with diabetes needs increased insulin during a concurrent illness (especially infection), but many mistakenly believe that if they cannot eat, they do not need to take the prescribed insulin or oral hypoglycemic agent. Patients with IDDM who fail to take insulin when they are sick frequently develop ketoacidosis. These persons must take carbohydrate in some form. Box 40-12 presents data that patients must be taught related to managing concurrent illnesses.

## Assisting With Psychologic Adjustment

Adjustment to a chronic illness such as diabetes is ongoing. The degree to which persons with diabetes mellitus adjust, as evidenced by taking control of the disease management, often depends on how well they adapt emotionally to their diagnosis.[55]

Helping the person begin to cope with chronic illness must be one of the first nursing care priorities. Patients must have a chance to work through their feelings of loss, shock, disbelief, identity change, or anger in response to the crisis. They need to feel accepted, regardless of their behavior.

Teaching and management are instituted in a manner to avoid overwhelming the patient. The patient must know that support is available at all times. Questions and concerns should always be listened to and handled professionally. The concerns may seem minute to the health team members, but they are great for the patient.

Giving the patient a chance to master a skill and take control is often very helpful because it increases the person's confidence and self-esteem. Patients master skills at different rates, and the grief process interferes with learning. Thus the nurse must always approach each patient as an individual and move at the patient's pace. Because patients are not hospitalized as long as they used to be, the community health nurse is often involved and must be informed before discharge regarding how well the patient is coping.

Family members and friends are included, as appropriate, to give them a better perspective of what the patient is dealing with. Local chapters of the American Diabetes Association and the Juvenile Diabetes Association sponsor support groups in some communities. Patients and families may find these groups helpful, both initially and over time.

As patients deal with chronic illness, they may deviate from parts of their regimens as a means of testing importance, either because of the effect on their life-style or because they do not know if the regimen is really necessary. If this behavior occurs, the nurse must show understanding and then help the patient get back on target with the therapeutic regimen. Health care team members should never be judgmental.

The behavior must be accepted without value judgment, and the cause of the deviation identified. The nurse must not assume that knowledge deficit is the cause of nonadherence; adherence to the diabetic regimen requires a large investment of the patient's energy and time, which may be difficult to do every day. The patient needs support to return to the regimen.

## Guidelines for Foot Care for the Person With Diabetes

1. Inspect feet daily for color changes, temperature changes, swelling, cuts, cracks, redness, blisters, or other signs of trauma; report changes immediately. (A mirror can be used to see bottom of feet.)
2. Wear well-fitting shoes and clean stockings when walking; never walk barefoot.
   a. Inspect shoes, before putting them on, for foreign objects, nail points, or wrinkles.
   b. There should be enough room in shoes to allow the toes to wiggle easily.
   c. Break in new shoes gradually.
3. Bathe feet daily and dry them well, paying particular attention to area between the toes.
4. Immediately after bathing, when toenails are soft, cut (or have someone else cut) nails straight across; smooth cut nails with an emery board.
5. If feet are dry, apply bland cream or petroleum jelly to heels and feet (but not toes).
6. Do not self-treat calluses, corns, or ingrown toenails; consult a podiatrist if these are present.
7. Bath water should be 30° to 32° C (84° to 90° F) and should be tested with a bath thermometer or elbow before immersing the feet.
8. Heating pads and hot-water bottles should not be used; wear socks if feet are cold.
9. Measures that increase circulation to the lower extremities should be instituted, including:
   a. Avoid smoking.
   b. Avoid crossing legs when sitting.
   c. Protect extremities when exposed to cold.
   d. Avoid immersing feet in cold water.
   e. Use socks or stockings that do not apply pressure to the legs at specific sites.
   f. Institute an exercise regimen.
10. Do not walk or jog in the dark; have a light source.
11. Obtain proper shoes before jogging.

Ultimately, patients are the final decision makers about self-care. The health team provides the teaching, the support, the guidance, and the counseling, but the patient makes the final decisions. Time for psychologic counseling should be available in every follow-up visit.

## Follow-up

Follow-up of patient teaching may be accomplished in a clinic, physician's or nurse's office, home, hospital, or ambulatory education program. It must be continuous and meet the identified patient needs. It is often incorporated into routine return visits for assessment of disease control and thus can be forgotten or missed when time is limited. The nurse responsible for this follow-up should identify the goals for each visit ahead of time so time is used effectively and teaching needs are met. Because of shortened hospital stays and because of the complexity of skills the patient with diabetes mellitus must master, a home health nurse may provide some of the follow-up nursing care.

## Teaching Materials for Patient Education

The teaching needs described in the preceding sections are summarized in Box 40-13. In addition to planning and implementing an individualized teaching plan, the professional nurse is responsible for developing materials that can be used to complement or supplement any verbal exchanges. Written instructions should be provided for all parts of the diabetic education program so that the patient has a resource to consult at home. Culture-sensitive literature augments teaching.

The teaching materials available from drug companies, private clinics, various diabetes education programs, and local chapters of the American Diabetes Association were designed for the "typical" person; they must be evaluated for usefulness for a particular person. Streiff[71] found, from an evaluation of various printed materials for diabetic education, that a high-school reading level was required; an evaluation of 106 adults revealed an average reading level of less than seventh grade (6.8). The patient's reading abilities must therefore be part of the initial assessment. Information about reading level and targeted population should be included when developing new materials.

## Economic Issues Related to Diabetes

Diabetes mellitus is an expensive disease for the patient and for society. Even the well-controlled person with stable diabetes and no complications will be affected by economics. The cost of the medications, syringes, and self-monitoring equipment alone may be prohibitive. Nurses need to be aware of this and economize wherever possible. For example, limit SMBG to what is necessary, continue to evaluate the possibility of reusing syringes, and so on.

Another economic issue that nurses must be aware of is health insurance coverage. Many persons with diabetes do not have adequate coverage, because (1) the cost of private insurance may be prohibitive and (2) some companies will not insure people with diabetes. Also, many large companies are self-insured; they use their own funds to pay claims. Self-insurance is exempt from many of the laws regulating insurance companies, which could have a severe effect on the person with diabetes.[70] Prepaid capitation plans also have rules that may not adequately support the needs of persons with chronic illnesses. Therefore, even if a person is part of a group plan, the plan may be inadequate.

Nurses should either refer patients with diabetes to social workers or help them obtain information needed to evaluate insurance plans that may be available to them. Questions that patients need to ask include:

1. Are routine visits to diabetes specialist, podiatrist, dietitian, and ophthalmologist covered?
2. Does the insurance cover reflectance meters or external infusion pumps?
3. Will the cost of blood glucose test strips be covered?

4. Are syringes, alcohol pads, insulin, or oral hypoglycemic agents covered?
5. Would special footwear be covered?
6. Would procedures/medications for complications be covered?
7. Is diabetes education covered?

Nurses will indirectly help patients with the economic issues related to insurance through patient education. However, nurses should also work on a societal level to promote adequate reimbursement (particularly for diabetes education) and to promote formation of "pooled risk plans" as insurance alternatives.

The patient with diabetes also may have trouble obtaining other types of insurance, such as disability and life. Often the premiums can be prohibitive.

A third economic issue affected by diabetes is employment. Persons with diabetes may not qualify for some jobs because of poor vision or presence of peripheral vascular disease, which would interfere with walking, but they may also face discrimination. Problem areas include (1) the armed forces (diabetes makes the person ineligible; if onset occurs after acceptance, it may result in termination) and (2) law enforcement agencies, including the FBI. In regard to employment, both health care members and patients need to be familiar with the American Disability Act.

Employment may also be limited because of inability to obtain necessary licenses. Individual drivers' licenses are not automatically withheld because of diabetes, but most states require a physician's statement to confirm the person's ability to drive safely, and the state can place restrictions on driving despite the physician's recommendation. The few studies that have been conducted do not support a major increase in motor vehicle accidents among people with diabetes.[70]

Persons who have IDDM or NIDDM and are receiving insulin are prohibited from driving a commercial motor vehicle in interstate or foreign commerce.[70] Also, people who are being treated with medications for diabetes are, at present, prohibited from obtaining licenses to fly noncommercial airplanes. These restrictions may prevent persons from reporting their medications or cause them to avoid insulin, regardless of their clinical state. Saudek and Segal-Polin[70] reported no knowledge of restrictions on obtaining retail or professional licenses. The terms *prediabetes* and *chemical diabetes* should not be used; they are not diagnoses but can cause problems for patients.

## ♦ EVALUATION

To evaluate the effectiveness of nursing interventions, compare patient behaviors with those stated in the expected patient outcomes. Successful achievement of patient outcomes for the patient with diabetes is indicated by the following:

1. Fluid balance is improved:
   a. Weight has increased or decreased at about 2 pounds per week toward normal.
   b. Urination has returned to normal, and skin turgor shows no tenting.
   c. Blood pressure and pulse are normal and show no orthostatic changes.
   d. Sodium and chloride levels are normal, as well as hematocrit.
2. The patient:
   a. Has an intake of fluid of about 2½ liters.
   b. Describes correctly how to prevent dehydration.
3. Signs of nutritional adequacy are present:
   a. Maintains weight changes as listed above.
   b. Has a glycosylated hemoglobin measurement that has decreased and serum lipid levels that have decreased.
   c. Appropriately describes food type, amount, and distribution.
4. Fatigue is improved:
   a. States that no fatigue is present.
   b. Demonstrates how to perform glucose monitoring correctly.
5. Risk for infection is decreased:
   a. States importance of checking glucose on regular basis.
   b. Correctly describes how infections affect blood glucose.
   c. Correctly lists signs and symptoms of infection.
6. Fear is decreased:
   a. States that fear is lessened.
   b. Explains way to obtain vocational rehabilitation.
7. An adequate level of knowledge is evidenced:
   a. Correctly describes the disease process of diabetes.
   b. Correctly demonstrates how to inject insulin and rotate sites.
   c. Correctly defines hypoglycemia.
   d. Correctly describes signs, symptoms, and treatment of hypoglycemia.
   e. Correctly describes dosage, time, and side effects of oral hypoglycemic agents.
   f. Correctly describes exercise plan and safety precautions.

## NURSING MANAGEMENT OF THE PATIENT WITH DIABETES HAVING SURGERY

Most nurses working in acute care centers at some time will work with persons with diabetes who are undergoing surgery. The perioperative management of the diabetic patient is complicated by the metabolic abnormalities of the disease and by the presence of atherosclerotic disease, diabetic nephropathy, and autonomic neuropathy.[13] There is also an increased risk of postoperative wound infection in patients with diabetes mellitus. Additionally, the counterregulatory hormones of the "board of directors" (Table 40-4) make an appearance during anesthesia and surgery when there is change in food and fluid intake and exposure to various stressors.

### Effects of Surgery on Metabolic Control of Diabetes

The person with diabetes mellitus faces the risk of developing hypoglycemia or hyperglycemia during the perioperative period. To explain this, a brief review of factors that change insulin needs follows. During the perioperative period, persons are not usually given anything by mouth and are given intravenous (IV) fluids. This decreases total calorie intake and may also decrease insulin needs; however, the effects of surgery on counterregulatory hormones usually increase the need for insulin. The stressors of surgery cause the release of glucocorticoids and catecholamines, which elevate blood glucose.

There are many ways to manage the person with diabetes during periods of fasting. To minimize the disruption in metabolic control, the person should be thoroughly regulated before surgery, and the surgery should be scheduled for early morning to minimize variations from normal control measures. Persons with diabetes are kept on their usual food, fluid, and medication routines until the night before surgery if possible.

### Management of Glucose Control During Surgery in Persons Treated with Insulin

Various protocols may be used to maintain glucose control in the person receiving insulin. Neither hyperglycemia nor hypoglycemia should be allowed to occur. One of the most frequently used perioperative protocols is starting an IV infusion of glucose the morning of surgery and giving one-half the usual insulin dose subcutaneously. The IV glucose will usually cover this insulin during the intraoperative period and prevent hypoglycemia, and the insulin will cover, in part, the glucose needs. If the surgery is long, blood glucose levels may be checked during surgery; insulin or extra glucose can be given as needed.

During the postoperative period, the person is maintained by IV glucose infusion until food can be taken. Insulin is given either by dividing the normal daily dose equally over a 24-hour period and giving it subcutaneously or by adding regular insulin directly to the IV fluids. If the person is receiving a standard dose of insulin, extra insulin may be administered based on blood glucose checks. These checks must be performed every 4 to 6 hours. Some patients may receive no daily insulin dose and instead will be given insulin based on the amount of blood glucose. This latter method does not provide the best control.

### Management of Glucose Control During Surgery in Persons Not Normally Receiving Insulin

Persons with diabetes who are not normally managed with insulin will receive an IV infusion of glucose on the morning of surgery, after fasting during the night. Such patients may be able to meet their usual insulin needs with their endogenous insulin supply, but in times of stress they may require exogenous insulin. After surgery, blood glucose and urine acetone levels are checked every 4 to 6 hours; if hyperglycemia is present, exogenous insulin may need to be given.

### Management During Surgery of Persons Unable to Eat Prescribed Diet

All persons with diabetes, whether or not they are treated with insulin, should receive 125 to 250 g of carbohydrates per day until their normal diet is resumed. Fewer carbohydrates than this may result in starvation ketosis. The patient's normal diabetic regimen should be reinstituted as soon as possible. Blood glucose and urine ketone levels should be monitored frequently, even after the patient's usual diet and medication are resumed. The increase in catabolism because of the surgery will remain for some time, and additional insulin may still be needed. By the time patients are discharged, they should be back on their normal regimens. Other postoperative care measures are similar to those for all surgery patients. Initiation of these measures should prevent complications.

## ✷ SPECIAL CONSIDERATIONS FOR CARE OF THE GERONTOLOGIC PATIENT

Diabetes in elderly persons is a special consideration for nurses because America is growing old. By the year 2000, it is expected that more than 22% of the population will be over 65. By then, there will be more than 50 million people over age 65. Diabetes mellitus poses an important health problem in elderly persons. Hyperglycemia is not a benign condition in elderly persons, and it needs to be considered seriously.

Elderly does not mean "ill," but certainly the complications of diabetes and some of the natural aging changes carry an extra burden for the aging person (i.e., skin, eye, teeth, renal impairment, macroangiopathy, neuropathy, change in the senses). Factors that predispose elderly people to development of diabetes mellitus include genetics, drugs, decreased physical activity, more fat-to-muscle ratio, age-related insulin resistance, age-related decreased insulin secretion, and coexisting illness.

As with anyone else, elderly persons need to be considered as individuals rather than a "blanket label" and be assessed for their individual needs. Target blood glucose levels should be more liberal in elderly persons who have any type of cardiovascular problems or a cognitive disorder. Hypoglycemia should be avoided; thus, early identification of risk factors for hypoglycemia is necessary. The risk factors for hypoglycemia in the elderly include impaired autonomic nervous system function, impaired counterregulatory responses, poor or irregular nutrition, possible cognitive disorder, use of alcohol or other sedating medications, and kidney or liver failure.

Nurses working with elderly persons need to know that there are special strategies for educating this age population just as there are for children and adults. Healthy elderly persons want to be participants and have a need for psychologic growth and fulfillment.[25] Teaching strategies for elderly patients include self-instructional, self-paced, short learning sessions and control over the session; use of low voice tones, large black print on nonglare paper, with ample white space between letters; conversational style; and terminology that best fits the generation and ability to learn in the home.[25]

## HOME CARE CONSIDERATIONS

With the day of short hospitalization or no hospitalization coupled with the overwhelming amount of information to be learned, home care is a high priority for persons with diabetes mellitus. Frequently, ability to be mobile is hindered, and changes in vision may hamper the drawing up of insulin or other care. Often there is a missing piece as to why control cannot be obtained. Often that missing link can be found during a home visit. The onset of complications often necessitates home care. Diabetes caregivers and home care agencies often team up to provide good care for elderly persons. For those living alone, the initiation of a referral provides a lifeline and method to stay in the home. Home care personnel network with other community resources to help increase the elderly person's quality of life or help deal with economic issues.

# COMPLICATIONS

The complications of diabetes fall into two categories, acute and long term (or chronic). Acute complications include (1) hypoglycemia, (2) diabetic ketoacidosis, and (3) hyperglycemic, hyperosmolar, nonketotic coma. Hypoglycemia in persons with diabetes mellitus is discussed on pp. 1300-1301.

## DIABETIC KETOACIDOSIS

**Diabetic ketoacidosis (DKA)** is one of the most serious outcomes of "out of control" diabetes; primarily seen in IDDM, it can be seen in NIDDM. Before insulin therapy was available, DKA was the predominant cause of death from diabetes. Although DKA can easily be prevented or treated, it is responsible for more than 160,000 hospital admissions each year.[29] DKA is identified in approximately 40% of patients with newly diagnosed IDDM.[54] DKA occurs with severe insulin deficiency. It can occur in the undiagnosed person with diabetes; in the diagnosed person whose insulin needs become greater than the prescribed therapy because of infection, trauma, emotional upsets, or other stressors; or in the person who stops treatment. As previously stated, it is usually seen in persons with IDDM but can occur in those with NIDDM.

The pathophysiology of DKA (Figure 40-20) is a continuation of that described for the effects of a deficiency of insulin and its actions. However, an increase in the counterregulatory hormones (glucagon, growth hormone, cortisol, catecholamines) is important in the pathogenesis of DKA. These four hormones accentuate the hyperglycemic state resulting from insulin deficiency and the lipolysis and ketogenesis. In DKA, there is a constant state of hyperglycemia with its resultant osmotic diuresis, a constant state of protein breakdown with the liberation of potassium and increased urea nitrogen formation leading to more diuresis, and massive ketone formation.

The ketones are an acid source and use the body's alkali reserve for buffering, resulting in acidosis. Ketones are also excreted in the urine, increasing diuresis. The diuresis resulting from the excretion of glucose, urea, and ketones results in the loss of sodium, water, potassium, and phosphate. The sodium loss prevents the formation of bicarbonate, and the alkali reserve of the body cannot be replaced. When the alkali reserve is depleted, the pH of the blood decreases, and compensatory mechanisms to control the metabolic acidosis are stimulated. These responses cause the kidney to try to excrete even more acids, which worsens the fluid and electrolyte imbalance even more. The lungs try to compensate by excreting hydrogen ions as carbon dioxide with Kussmaul's breathing, but because acid is continually formed, complete compensation cannot occur and the pH remains low, altering cellular functioning.

The diuresis from all the processes just described results in hyperosmolality, dehydration, hemoconcentration, and shock. The hyperosmolality causes fluids to move from the intracellular to the extracellular compartment, which also causes altered cellular functioning. Poor tissue perfusion from shock contributes to the altered cellular functioning. With shock and tissue hypoxia, lactic acidosis can occur and worsen the acidotic state. If this process is not interrupted, the patient will lapse into coma.

Signs and symptoms resulting from the pathogenesis of DKA may be the initial manifestations for some persons with IDDM, although DKA is most frequently seen in persons who have been previously diagnosed and experience additional stressors, such as an infection, or who stop taking their insulin[72] or greatly increase their food intake. It has been reported that 20% of the episodes of DKA occur in undiagnosed persons with diabetes and that 80% occur in previously diagnosed persons with diabetes.[69] Table 40-18 summarizes the clinical manifestations of DKA and compares these with HHNC. The onset can be gradual or relatively sudden.

## HYPERGLYCEMIC, HYPEROSMOLAR, NONKETOTIC COMA

**Hyperglycemic, hyperosmolar, nonketotic coma (HHNC)** can occur when the action of insulin is severely inhibited. HHNC is seen in patients with NIDDM. It can occur in a person with undiagnosed NIDDM or in a

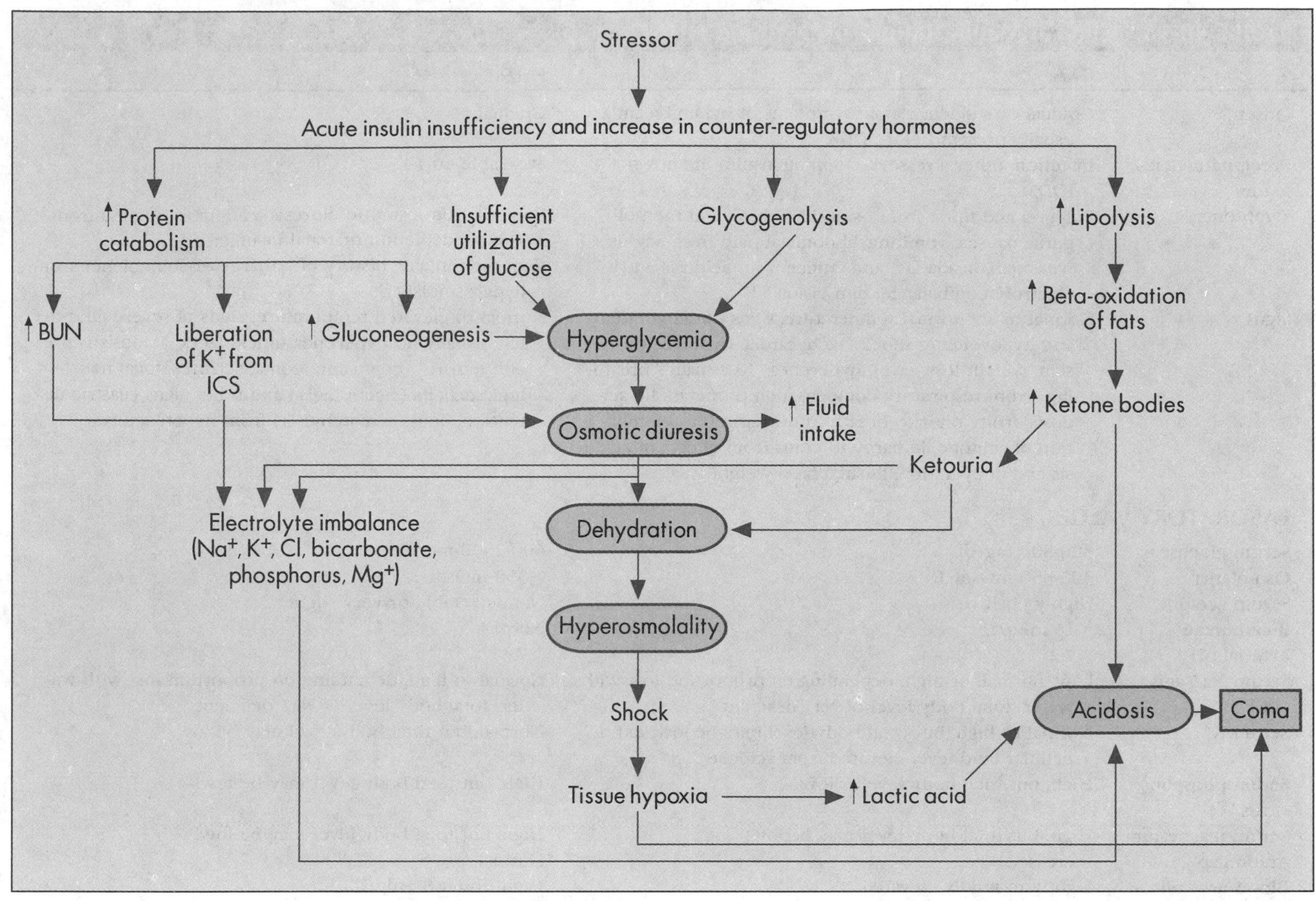


**FIGURE 40-20** Summary of pathogenesis of diabetic ketoacidosis (DKA) coma.

poorly treated patient and is almost always precipitated by a specific factor (Table 40-19). HHNC is primarily seen in elderly persons with NIDDM.

The pathophysiology of HHNC is, in part, a continuing condition of that described previously for the effects of a deficiency of insulin and its action, but the serum glucose level becomes extremely high (≥600 mg/dl).[69] The reason for the high glucose level is that, although early in the pathogenesis of HHNC the patient has an osmotic diuresis from the hyperglycemia, which helps eliminate some of the excessive glucose, this diuresis is not maintained. The diuresis is inhibited, primarily because of a contraction of the extracellular fluid volume resulting from lack of adequate fluid intake. The lack of fluid intake may result from failure to respond to the stimulus of thirst or inadequate administration of fluids. The patient may also be losing excess fluids from other processes such as vomiting or inability to concentrate urine. The contraction of extracellular fluid volume decreases the glomerular filtration rate and therefore the excretion of glucose.

Thus glucose is not being lost from the vascular space through diuresis or by uptake into the cell, but it is continually added because of the ineffective insulin metabolism. Glucose may actually be added in greater quantities because of the effects of glucagon, cortisol, growth hormone (GH), and epinephrine. These hormones also inhibit cellular uptake of glucose, which results in severe hyperglycemia and hyperosmolality.

The hyperosmolality initiates a major shift of fluids from the intracellular to the extracellular space, which may initially lead to additional diuresis. Eventually, both intracellular and extracellular dehydration occur. Intracellular fluid loss results in dysfunction. The extracellular fluid loss may be so severe that it results in shock and hypoxia. Cellular dysfunction and coma then occur.

A major difference between DKA and HHNC is that HHNC is not associated with ketosis and acidosis. Acidosis, if present, is usually very mild and occurs as a result of lactic acidosis from shock or other illnesses. The reason for the lack of ketosis is not fully understood. It is known that free fatty acid levels are usually lower in HHNC than in DKA; this decreases the availability of substrate for ketogenesis.[69] It was previously believed that higher insulin levels in NIDDM prevented lipolysis and thus inhibited ketogenesis, but peripheral insulin levels have not been found to be higher in HHNC than in DKA. It is possible that the person with HHNC has

**TABLE 40-18 Clinical Manifestations of DKA and HHNC**

| | DKA | HHNC |
|---|---|---|
| Onset | Gradual or sudden; classic symptoms of hyperglycemia usually present before DKA | Gradual |
| Precipitating factors | Infection, other stressors, stopping insulin in known IDDM | See Table 40-19 |
| Symptoms | Polyuria and thirst from osmotic diuresis and then oliguria; nausea, vomiting, abdominal pain from acidosis; weakness, headache, and fatigue from acidosis and electrolyte imbalance; dim vision | Polyuria from osmotic diuresis leading to oliguria from volume depletion or renal insufficiency<br>Poor fluid intake; history of lethargy or somnolence from hyperosmolality |
| Signs | Normal or subnormal temperature; signs of dehydration and hypovolemic shock (tachycardia, hypotension, dry skin, weight loss, etc.); hyperpnea (Kussmaul's breathing) from respiratory compensation of metabolic acidosis; fruity odor to breath from respiratory elimination of acetone; lethargy to coma from effects of acidosis and dehydration; flushed face; weight loss | Normal to elevated temperature; signs of severe fluid deficit; usually no hyperpnea unless lactic acidosis is present; lethargy, confusion, coma, seizures, focal neurologic deficits (hemiplegia) and other signs (gastric distention, ileus, hematemesis) from hyperosmolality |
| **LABORATORY VALUES** | | |
| Serum glucose | 300-800 mg/dl | 600-2000 mg/dl |
| Osmolarity | 300-350 mOsm/L | >350 mOsm/L |
| Serum acetone | Highly positive | Nondetectable or very slight |
| Bicarbonate | <15 mEq/L | Normal |
| Arterial pH | <7.2 | >7.3 |
| Serum $Na^+$ and $Cl^-$ | Low, normal, or high, depending on proportion lost with water; total body level of $Na^+$ deficient | Normal to high, depending on proportion lost with water; total body level of $Na^+$ deficient |
| Serum $K^+$ | Normal to high, but total body level may be low; extracellular fluid level elevated from acidosis | Normal, but total body level may be low. |
| Serum phosphorus | High, but total body level is low | High, but total body level may be low. |
| Serum magnesium | High, but total body level may be low, | High, but total body level may be low. |
| Anion gap | Increased | Normal |
| Blood urea nitrogen (BUN) | Lightly to mildly elevated | High, about 87 mg/dl |
| Others | Elevated white blood cells (WBCs) | Elevated WBCs, triglycerides, and cholesterol |

**TABLE 40-19 Factors That Precipitate HHNC**

| FACTOR | EXAMPLES |
|---|---|
| Associated illness | Infections (pneumonia, acute pyelonephritis, septicemia)<br>Renal failure<br>Lactic acidosis<br>Myocardial infarction<br>Cerebrovascular accidents (CVAs)<br>Gastrointestinal (GI) hemorrhage<br>Subdural hematoma<br>Pancreatitis<br>Arterial thrombosis<br>Congestive heart failure<br>Cognitive dysfunction resulting in lack of thirst perception |
| Therapeutic procedures | Dialysis: peritoneal<br>Total parenteral nutrition<br>Hyperosmolar tube feedings<br>Surgery, stress |
| Drugs | Glucocorticoids, diuretics, diphenylhydantoin, β-adrenergic blocking agents, immunosuppressive agents, diazoxide |

higher hepatic insulin levels, even though peripheral insulin levels are low, and this would inhibit ketogenesis. It is also possible that extremely high hyperglycemia and hyperosmolality block the formation of ketones by inhibiting lipolysis.[69] Figure 40-21 summarizes the pathogenesis of HHNC.

Signs and symptoms resulting from the pathogenesis of HHNC may be the initial manifestation for some persons with NIDDM. These manifestations are usually precipitated by one of the factors listed in Table 40-19. HHNC is seen slightly more frequently in persons who have been previously diagnosed and experience a precipitating factor, although it occurs very frequently in persons with undiagnosed NIDDM. Table 40-18 summarizes the clinical manifestations of HHNC and compares these with DKA. Onset is very gradual, and a precipitating factor is almost always present.

## MEDICAL MANAGEMENT OF DKA AND HHNC

The management of DKA and HHNC, when present, becomes a medical priority, whether these are part of the initial manifestations of diabetes mellitus or occur after

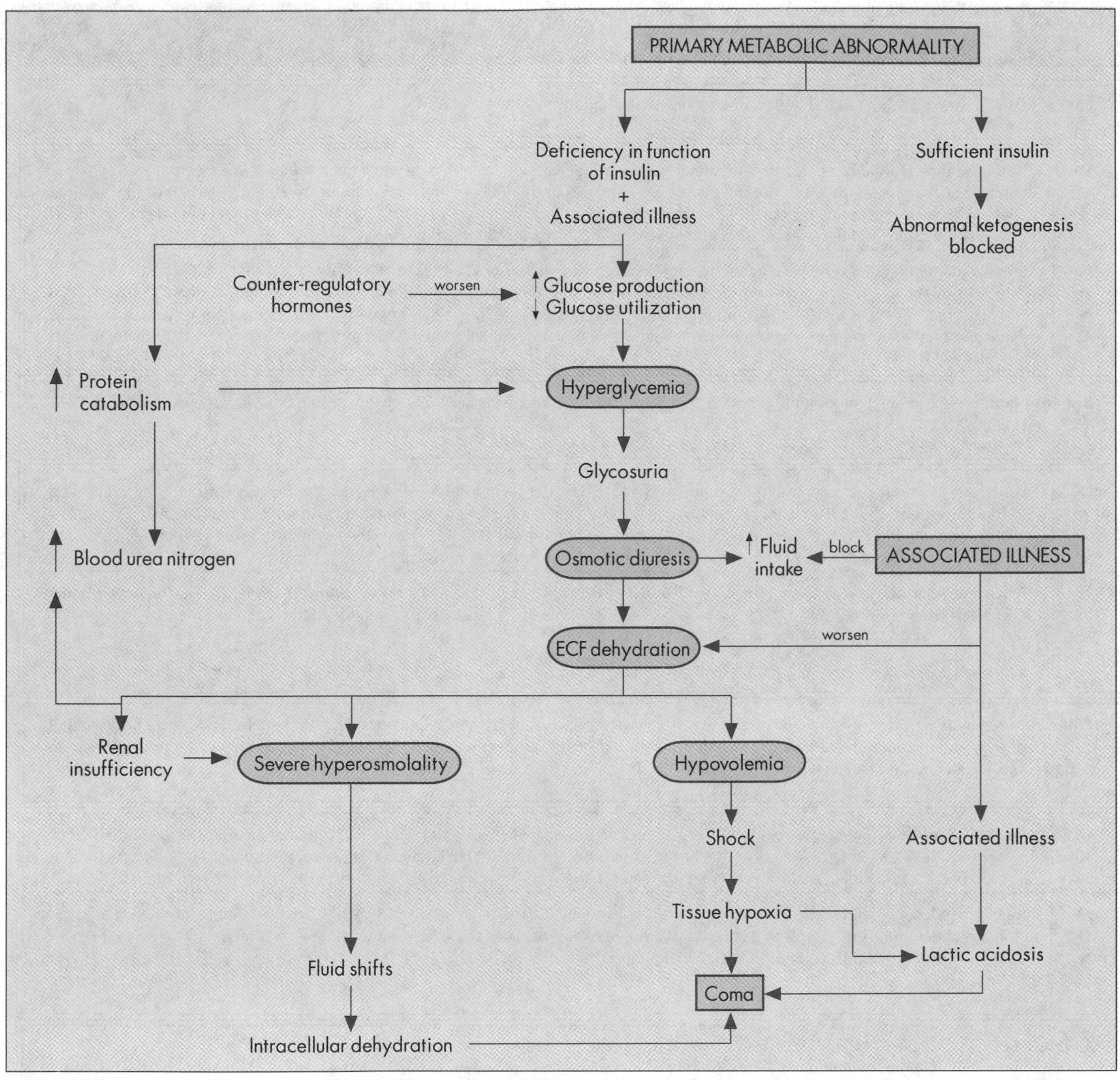


**FIGURE 40-21** Summary of pathogenesis of HHNC.

the onset of diabetes. Management involves fluid and electrolyte replacement, insulin therapy, and other measures based on the severity of the problem and continual assessment. Treatment also involves measures for the precipitating factors. The management of DKA and HHNC are similar; generalized management guidelines for adults are present in Box 40-17 (also Critical Pathway).

## NURSING MANAGEMENT OF DKA AND HHNC

Since DKA and HHNC are acute situations that demand emergency treatment, nurses in this situation usually find themselves in the emergency room or the critical care unit. Monitoring is the major nursing management at this time. The sicker the patient, the more frequently he or she should be monitored. The information in Box 40-18 outlines the monitoring parameters in DKA (HHNC is very similar).

The most valuable messages in nursing management of DKA and HHNC are monitoring the parameters on the flow sheet, prevention, and referral. Prevention can be initiated by immediate screening of blood sugar of any patient presenting with coma, shock, dehydration, stroke-like symptoms, and respiratory distress. If this rule is followed, new-onset cases of diabetes that present

### BOX 40-17 Medical Management Guidelines for Adults With DKA or HHNC

**Fluids:** Major priority; adequate fluid replacement alone will decrease hyperglycemia.

| | |
|---|---|
| DKA | Isotonic saline is fluid of choice unless patient has history of hypertension or congestive heart failure; give fluids at rate of 1 to 2 L for first hour, slow to 1 L/hr for next 2 to 3 hours, then slow to 500 ml/hr; total amount, type, and rate based on continual assessment of intake and output, weight, hemodynamic status, mental status, and laboratory determinations; dextrose added as 5% glucose in saline when plasma glucose reaches 250 mg to 300 mg/dl. |
| HHNC | Usually start with 0.5 saline because of hyperosmolality; give at rate of 1.5 L/hr for first hour, 1 L/hr for next 2 hours, then 500 to 750 ml/hr for next hour; when serum osmolarity is $<320$ mOsm/L switch to normal saline; add dextrose (5% in saline) when glucose is 250 to 300 mg/dl; monitor central venous pressure or pulmonary capillary wedge pressure (see Chapter 22), weight, intake and output, blood pressure, pulse and respiration, mental status; laboratory determinations will guide treatment. |

**Insulin:** Plasma glucose level should fall about 75 to 100 mg/dl/hr if adequate insulin is given. (Insulin needs are very similar in DKA and HHNC.)

| | |
|---|---|
| DKA | Low-dose protocol most common; IV bolus of 5 to 10 U of regular insulin followed by continuous infusion, by controlled administration, of 5 to 10 U/hr (0.1 U/kg body weight) until plasma glucose level reaches about 250 mg/100 ml (which takes 4 to 6 hours) and pH = 7.30 and $HCO_3 \geq 18$ mEq/L (which takes 8 to 12 hours), then switch to usual insulin regimen.<br>Hourly IM injections of 5 to 10 U regular insulin may be used instead of IV route. |
| HHNC | Low-dose regimen similar to that for DKA; give 5 to 10 U regular insulin as IV bolus followed by 5 to 10 U/hr until plasma glucose level is 250 to 300 mg/dl; then decrease to 2 to 3 U/hr; when stable switch to usual insulin regimen.<br>Hourly IM insulin injections may be used. |

**Potassium:** Replacement is individualized, the major electrolyte needed is potassium. (Potassium is started after an adequate urine output is established, after obtaining serum for potassium level and an electrocardiogram (ECG); ECG can be used to monitor the serum potassium level (T-wave changes).

| | |
|---|---|
| DKA | Potassium replaced based on plasma $K^+$ levels; guidelines for adults[69]: if serum $K^+$ is $< 3$ mEq/L, give $K^+$ 40 to 60 mEq/hr; if serum $K^+$ is 3 to 4 mEq/L, give $K^+$ 30 mEq/hr; if serum $K^+$ is 4 to 5 mEq/L, give $K^+$ at 20 mEq/hr; if serum $K^+$ is 5 to 6 mEq/L, infuse $K^+$ at 10 mEq/hour; if serum $K^+$ is greater than 6 mEq/l, withhold $K^+$ until serum $K^+$ is less than 6 mEq/L. |
| HHNC | Recommended guidelines for potassium replacement in HHNC[69]: if serum $K^+$ is $<3$ mEq/L, give one dose of $K^+$ (60 mEq/hr) and recheck; if serum $K^+$ is 3 to 4 mEq/L, give 40 mEq/hr twice and recheck; if serum $K^+$ is 4 to 5 mEq/L, give $K^+$ at 20 mEq/hr; if serum $K^+$ is greater than 5 mEq/L do not give $K^+$. |

**OTHER ELECTROLYTES INCLUDE:**

| | |
|---|---|
| DKA | Bicarbonate: most experts do not recommend bicarbonate for routine use in DKA; if used, give only if arterial pH is $<7.0$ and patient has other problems such as hypotension, shock, or arrhythmia; give as an infusion of 1 to 2 mEq/kg over 2 hours.<br>Phosphate: hypophosphatemia may occur during treatment; modest reduction in phosphate could result in changes in myocardial, diaphragmatic, and skeletal muscle function; outcome of care has not been shown to be affected by replacement, so not all authorities recommend replacement; if administered, give at rate of 1.5 mEq/kg/24 hr as potassium phosphate; hyperphosphatemia can cause hypocalcemia.<br>Magnesium: sample to be drawn, not usually given. |
| HHNC | Phosphate: phosphate replacement guidelines are the same as those listed for DKA.<br>Magnesium: no recommendation for routine replacement in HHNC; give if serum level is low or signs of tetany are present; deliver 500 ml of 2% $MgSo_4$. |

Compiled from American Diabetes Association: ***Physician's guide to insulin-dependent (type I) diabetes, diagnosis and treatment,*** ed 2, Alexandria, Va, 1994, The Association; American Diabetes Association: ***Physician's guide to non-insulin-dependent (type II) diabetes, diagnosis and treatment,*** ed 3, Alexandria, Va, 1994, The Association; Genuth S: In Lebovitz H, editor: ***Therapy for diabetes mellitus and related disorders,*** Alexandria, Va, 1991, American Diabetes Association; and Rifkin H, Porte D, editors: ***Ellenberg and Rifkin's diabetes mellitus, theory and practice,*** ed 4, New York, 1990, Elsevier.

**BOX 40-17 Medical Management Guidelines for Adults With DKA or HHNC—cont'd**

**OTHER MEASURES MAY INCLUDE:**

Nasogastric intubation to prevent vomiting and aspiration if bowel sounds decreased and patient is obtunded; maintain airway and oxygenation if patient is obtunded.

Monitor cardiovascular function with ECG to assess effects of $K^+$ on cardiac rhythm and adequacy of replacement and to assess for complications, such as myocardial infarction (MI) or cardiac ischemia, that may have been the precipitating event; monitor fluid status: central venous pressure, Swan-Ganz catheter, indwelling urinary catheter.

**BOX 40-18 Parameters, Frequency, and Other Information in DKA**

| | |
|---|---|
| 1. Glucose | Every 1-2 hours by fingerstick and confirmed by laboratory when indicated |
| 2. Fluid intake and output (I & O) | Every 1-2 hours (catheter) |
| 3. Insulin | Should be charted hourly; route of administration |
| 4. Vital signs | Every 1-2 hours |
| Mental state | Every 1-2 hours |
| Temperature | Every 4 hours |
| 5. Potassium | At onset, 1 hour, and 2 hours: when normal at 2- to 4-hour intervals |
| 6. Arterial blood gas (ABG) | Hourly until the pH is greater than 7.2; after that, only needed if patient not doing well |
| 7. Plasma sodium, chloride, bicarbonate, serum ketones | Every 4 hours (urine ketones if voiding) |
| 8. ECG | Admission; repeat if follow-up plasma potassium abnormal or unavailable |
| 9. Complete blood count, blood urea nitrogen (BUN), creatinine, UA, appropriate cultures, chest x-ray film | Admission |
| 10. Plasma phosphate, magnesium, calcium | Admission; if low, repeat every 4 hours |

with DKA should never be missed. The mnemonic for changes in mental status (AEIOU, TIPS) is useful in evaluating patients with such changes and suspected DKA. The mnemonic stands for **a**lcohol, **e**ncephalopathy (metabolic or neurologic), **i**nsulin, (i.e., DKA, HHNC, or hypoglycemic coma), **o**verdose, **u**remia, **t**rauma, **i**nfections, **p**sychosis, and **s**yncope.[44]

Referral in this situation applies to the astute observation of repeated DKA admissions, which should alert health care personnel to the need for referral and consultation for possible psychosocial treatment of recurrent DKA.[44,55,56]

## LONG-TERM PROBLEMS (CHRONIC COMPLICATIONS)

Long-term changes associated with insulin deficiency or its action lead to a number of pathologic changes that involve alterations in structure and function of vessels and nerves and occur in all types of diabetes. These changes involve small and large blood vessels, cranial and peripheral nerves, the skin, and the lens of the eye. These lesions lead to hypertension, renal failure, blindness, autonomic and peripheral neuropathy, amputations of the lower extremities, myocardial infarction, and cerebrovascular accidents (see Figure 40-2). Research continues in an effort to identify whether the altered metabolism associated with a deficiency of insulin or its action causes these problems or whether some pathologic process causes both the deficiency in insulin or its action and the vascular and nerve changes. These changes occur at variable times during the disease, although they rarely occur within the first 5 to 10 years after diagnosis of IDDM; many persons with NIDDM may first be diagnosed as having diabetes when they enter the health care system with complaints related to these long-term complications. To reiterate, the resulting alterations are classified as macrovascular changes, microvascular changes, and neuropathy. Major problems include cardiovascular disease, renal disease, blindess, autonomic neuropathy, and diabetic foot problems.

### Macrovascular Changes

Persons with diabetes mellitus develop macrovascular changes from atherosclerosis that are the same as those seen in persons with diabetes. However, it is well known that persons with diabetes are prone to develop atherosclerosis at an earlier age and that the disease progresses faster and is more severe and extensive. Persons with NIDDM develop macrovascular changes more frequently than persons with IDDM. The exact mechanism underlying the formation of atheromatous lesions is unknown but probably involves the interaction of many factors. It has been hypothesized that the initial event involves endothelial injury, which is followed by the proliferation of smooth muscle cells with an accumulation of intracellular matrix. Endothelial lesions can result from mechanical and chemical factors, such as hypertensive lipid disorders, tissue hypoxia, and possibly hyperglycemia. The smooth muscle cell proliferation, lipid accumulation, and extracellular matrix formation that result are accelerated by various factors, such as presence of abnormal lipids, tissue hypoxia, platelet changes, and hormonal changes. Diabetes is associated with several of these atherogenic factors.

Insulin has a major role in the metabolism of lipids. Lipid disorders are frequently found in persons with diabetes mellitus. The hyperlipoproteinemia seen in diabetes is usually identified as Type IV or Type V, and it is often the result of an excess of triglycerides, VLDL-TG, and low-density-lipoprotein-cholesterol (LDL-C). Diabetes is also considered to be a contributing factor in the development of hypertension.

Macrovascular changes result in decreased lumen size, compromised blood flow, and decreased delivery of oxygen to tissues, resulting in tissue ischemia. The result is usually cerebrovascular disease, coronary artery disease, renal artery stenosis, or peripheral vascular disease. Cardiovascular complications cause the deaths of many persons with IDDM or NIDDM. Diabetes mellitus is an independent risk factor for arteriosclerotic cardiovascular disease, and 25% to 75% of all persons with diabetes have some lipid abnormality.[1]

## Microvascular Changes

Microvascular changes seen in persons with diabetes do not occur in persons without diabetes. These changes are characterized by thickening of the capillaries and damage to the basement membrane and result in diabetic nephropathy and retinopathy. The causes of the changes are unknown but believed to be related to uncontrolled diabetes. Various factors, such as the role of protein fractions, glycoproteins, lipids, and lipoproteins, have been studied; however, no conclusive evidence is yet available about the relationship between these factors and the microvascular changes seen in persons with diabetes.

### Diabetic nephropathy

One of the major results of microvascular changes is alteration in renal structure and function. Renal failure frequently results from the changes, and **diabetic nephropathy** may account for 30% of the persons receiving long-term renal dialysis.[69] Four types of kidney lesions can occur: (1) glomerular lesions, (2) arteriosclerosis of the renal arteries, (3) tubular lesions, and (4) pyelonephritis.

Three types of glomerular lesions can occur. Diffuse glomerulosclerosis, resulting in severe proteinuria and renal failure, is one type of glomerular lesion. A second type is nodular glomerulosclerosis (Kimmelstiel-Wilson syndrome), which involves nodular masses of laminated hyaline material that occur randomly throughout the kidney and result in a nephrotic syndrome with proteinuria, edema, and hypertension. This lesion is found only in persons with diabetes and occurs in 10% to 35% of all persons with diabetes. A third type of glomerular lesion is an exudative one in which eosinophilic fibrinoid deposits are found in the Bowman's capsule or over the outer surface of glomerular capillary loops. These glomerular lesions, along with arteriosclerosis, obliterate vascular channels and glomeruli and lead to renal failure. Tubular lesions result from deposits of glycogen, fat, and mucopolysaccharide, within the epithelial cells of the distal tubules and the descending limb of Henle's loop.

Although renal abnormalities can be identified through renal biopsy early in the onset of diabetes, clinical problems are often not seen until 10 or more years after onset. One of the earliest visible signs is microalbuminuria, which is reversible with meticulous treatment. The level of proteinuria has been thought to relate to protein intake by some authorities but not all.[47] Eventually, intermittent and constant proteinuria occurs, followed by renal insufficiency, progressing to renal failure.

Hypertension is the factor that most often accelerates nephropathy associated with diabetes mellitus.[79] Aggressive treatment of hypertension is necessary, and the blood pressure should be normalized. Obstructive nephropathy, repeated infections, and nephrotoxic drugs, such as contrast media used for x-ray films, can also accelerate the progression of diabetic nephropathy to renal failure.

### Diabetic retinopathy

**Diabetic retinopathy** is a leading cause of blindness in the United States. Retinopathy will affect 50% to 80% of all persons with diabetes 10 to 15 years after diagnosis.[1]

The primary lesion is the formation of microaneurysm in the retinal vessels, followed by hemorrhage and exudate formation. These early retinal changes, called ***background*** or ***simple retinopathy,*** may progress to a more serious state, ***proliferative retinopathy,*** in which new blood vessels form on the retina. These new vessels bleed, causing vitreous hemorrhage and retinal detachment. The bleeding is usually repetitive and leads to permanent loss of vision.

There are no symptoms of early retinal change, and persons with diabetes are encouraged to have yearly eye examinations by an ophthalmologist. Hypertension, which can worsen the retinopathy, should be screened for and adequately controlled.[4,79]

Cataracts also occur in persons with diabetes. Cataracts may be caused by prolonged hyperglycemia, resulting in polyol-increased metabolism via the polyol pathway, with increased sorbitol formation. Intra-lens hyperosmolality, swelling, and opacity formation result in cataracts and glaucoma.

## Neuropathy

Persons with IDDM or NIDDM usually have one or more alterations that affect peripheral nerves, the autonomic nervous system (ANS), the spinal cord, or the CNS. Symmetric peripheral neuropathy and autonomic neuropathy are by far the most common disorders and are the focus of this discussion.

Neuropathies unique to diabetes may occur from increased metabolism via the polyol pathway that results from hyperglycemia. Metabolism via this pathway causes accumulation of sorbitol in nerve cells. Sorbitol accumulation can result in hyperosmolality, fluid shifts with swelling, and subsequent nerve dysfunction. Sorbitol accumulation can also lower nerve myo-inositol content, and this change disrupts sodium/potassium adenosine triphosphatase (ATPase) activity, decreases energy metabolism, and can result in nerve dysfunction and structural damage. The result of the nerve changes is altered nerve conduction.

#### Symmetric peripheral polyneuropathy

The most common type of neuropathy is symmetric peripheral polyneuropathy. Sensory changes and then sensory loss in the distal lower extremities are the most common nerve involvement. Eventually, motor loss in the lower extremities and sensory and motor loss in the upper extremities can occur. The impairments occur slowly and are progressive.

#### Autonomic neuropathy

Autonomic neuropathy is also common. Alteration of the ANS's control of the bladder, sexual function, GI tract, sweating mechanisms, and cardiovascular reflexes can occur (Box 40-19). The impairments occur slowly and are progressive. A patient may experience some or all of the dysfunctions.

### The Diabetic Foot (Insensitive Foot)

The macrovascular and microvascular changes and the neuropathy all contribute to changes in the lower extremity called the **diabetic foot.** One major factor is sensory neuropathy, which may lead to painless trauma, ulceration, and infection. Sensory and motor neuropathy contribute to bone changes and deformed feet that change gait and pressure distribution and contribute to infection. Autonomic neuropathy can result in anhidroses and resultant cracking of the skin, which also contributes to infection. Macrovascular and microvascular changes produce tissue ischemia and skin changes that can cause ulcerations and infections and prevent healing. The interrelationship of all these factors, as they contribute to lesions that result in gangrene and ultimately amputation, is illustrated in Figure 40-22. It is important to note that the vascular changes (angiopathy) may actually worsen neuropathy, and vice versa. Either may contribute to the occurrence of foot lesions.

Gangrene can be either dry or wet. Dry gangrene occurs when tissue death is not associated with inflammatory changes. Autoamputation of affected toes is the treatment of choice. The area must be kept dry, or wet gangrene can occur. Wet gangrene is gangrene coupled with inflammation; septicemia and septic shock may occur.

Prevention is the key to care of the insensitive diabetic foot. It is estimated that prevention could result in a 50% to 75% reduction in the need for amputation.[51]

Prevention is the major focus of care for long-term manifestations associated with changes in the vascular bed and neuropathy. It is important to remember that for some patients with NIDDM, signs and symptoms of these changes may be the initial manifestations of diabetes mellitus. Table 40-20 summarizes some general medical treatment modalities used for various problems resulting from the vascular changes of neuropathies.

**BOX 40-19 Autonomic Neuropathic Changes With Diabetes Mellitus**

Bladder: Becomes hypotonic or atonic and empties poorly; neurogenic bladder
Sexual function: Inability to have an erection (male), change in lubrication (female)
GI system: Delayed gastric emptying, impaired gastric acid secretion, constipation or diarrhea
Sweating: May be inhibited or excessive; ANS response to changes in environmental temperature is lost or decreased
Cardiovascular reflexes: Impaired maintenance of blood pressure and cerebral blood flow during position changes or in response to other stimuli; heart rate may be high at rest because of loss of parasympathetic function but remains fixed with activity

## NURSING MANAGEMENT OF COMPLICATIONS

From *When Diabetes Complicates Your Life*,[48] a paperback book for patients written by a physician who is blind, the following paragraph warrants quoting:

> You'll note I constantly stress the positive, even when I must delve into the negatives of long-term complications. Please, always keep in mind that *knowledge is strength*. The more you know about and understand diabetes, the more powerful your control. Your determination to strive for knowledge and understanding is a key factor to your overall health.

This paragraph was quoted because, in a nutshell, it is the answer to nursing management of complications. Knowledge is the strength . . . for patients. This means that nursing has the charge to educate patients about the complications of diabetes, the causes, and the prevention of long-term problems. Next, our challenge is to join the Centers for Disease Control and Prevention (CDC) in their effort to lessen the complications of diabetes by the year 2000. By learning ourselves and teaching patients early recognition of signs and symptoms of complications, this is possible. Early recognition requires regularly scheduled examinations. The "1000-Mile Check-up Chart" in Boxes 40-20 and 40-21 de-

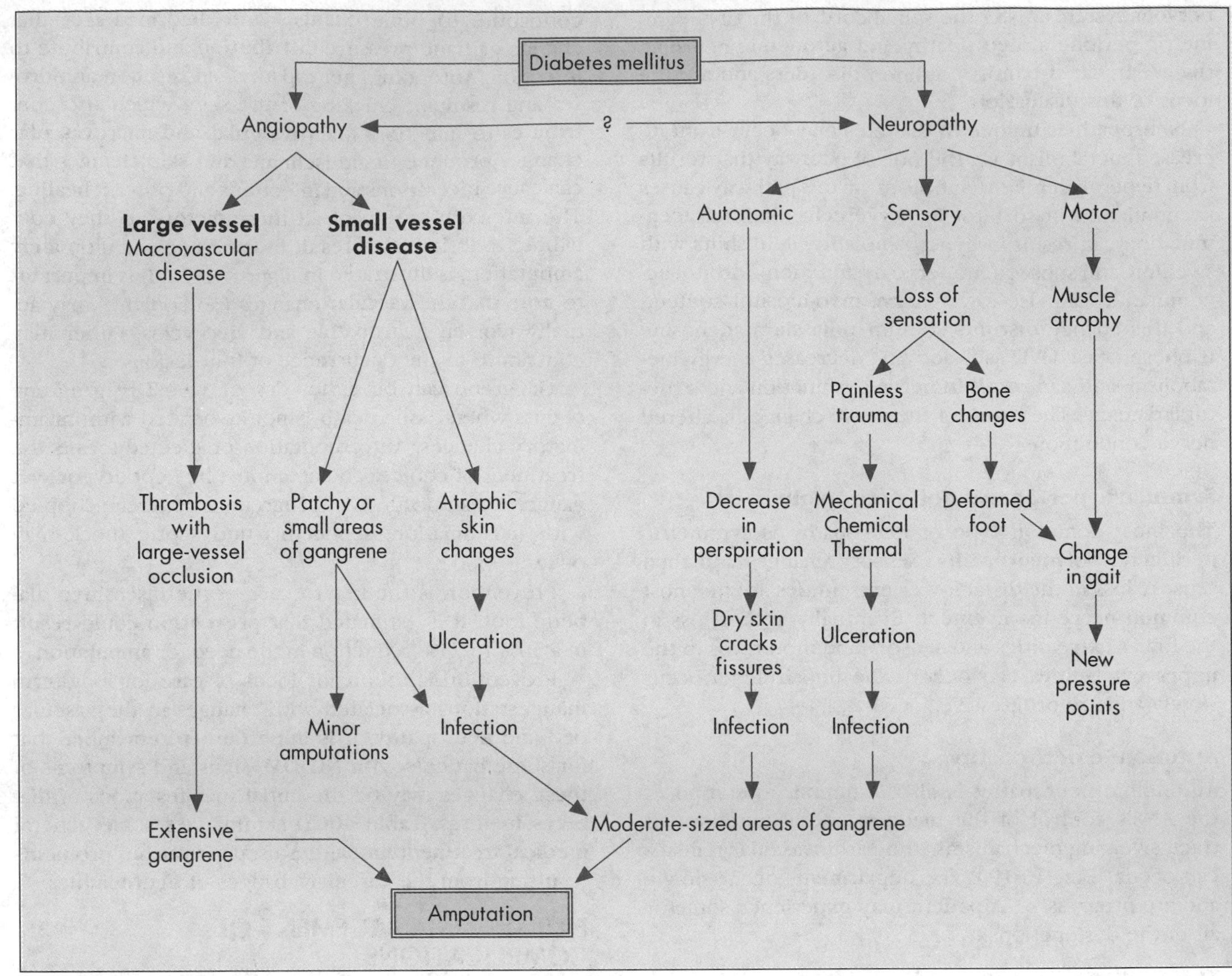


**FIGURE 40-22** Pathogenesis of diabetic foot lesions. (From Levin ME, O'Neal LW, editors: *The diabetic foot,* St Louis, 1988, Mosby.)

scribes what this entails. Education, early recognition, and regular follow-up with certain expectations are what we must do to limit long-term complications. The CDC has granted monies to many states for studying ways to help decrease these complications. One method is to help educate caregivers who are on the front line with persons with diabetes. *The Prevention and Treatment of Complications of Diabetes* is a paperback guide for primary care practitioners. It outlines background information, clinical manifestations, prevention, detection, treatment, referral, and patient education principles.[45] Another way to achieve the goal for 2000 is to teach simultaneously the patients the same information that is in this book. One of the states that received a CDC grant developed a small book for patients entitled *Diabetes—An Owner's Manual.*[26] A major theme to this book is prevention. It is a teaching tool to help the patient obtain knowledge and know what to ask for and expect in a visit for diabetes care. It also lists the preventive maintenance tests that patients should know about. In the Preventive Maintenance (Trouble Spots) chapter, the body map in Figure 40-23 is included to heighten the patient's awareness of the possible "trouble spots" associated with diabetes mellitus and provide some explanation. This body map can be a good teaching tool, if presented positively with preventive care. Also important are the "1000 Mile Check-Up" charts, which give the nurse a tool to help patients prevent the possible complications/trouble spots on the body map. Box 40-20 depicts what a patient should expect to discuss at a routine diabetic visit (according to *Standards of Care for Patients with Diabetes Mellitus* by the American Diabetes Association).[7] Box 40-21 is the second part of the "1000 Mile Check-Up" chart. It describes the necessary tests to be done to provide early detection about areas on the body map. It also lists the frequency, description, and purpose of the test.

You will encounter patients with painful neuropathy

**TABLE 40-20 Summary of Medical Treatment for Problems Related to Vascular Changes and Neuropathies**

| PROBLEMS | TREATMENT |
|---|---|
| **Cerebrovascular and cardiovascular dysfunction** secondary to macrovascular changes (CVA, MI, hypertension) | Same treatment as that prescribed for persons without diabetes; metabolic control of diabetes must be attained for the most effective treatment of problems; after CVA or CV problems, diabetic control may be decreased in tightness. |
| **Renal insufficiency or failure** secondary to diabetic nephropathy | Rigorous control of hypertension to help prevent renal damage; same treatment as prescribed for person without diabetes; persons with diabetes placed on peritoneal dialysis may have difficulty with glucose regulation because of glucose in the dialysate. Insulin may be added to dialysate.<br>Less insulin is usually needed in the presence of renal insufficiency because insulin is excreted more slowly. |
| **Pyelonephritis** | Same treatment as that prescribed for persons without diabetes. |
| **Retinopathy** secondary to microvascular changes | Photocoagulation and vitrectomy are prescribed; hypertension must be controlled. |
| **Cataracts** secondary to increased polyol pathways | Same treatment is prescribed for persons without diabetes. |
| **Symmetric peripheral polyneuropathy** | Treatment is primarily symptomatic, cold compressses at night or capsaicin 0.076% (Zostrix), a topical analgesic cream, has been used[19]; nonnarcotic analgesics including phenytoin, carbamazepine, and amitriptyline also have been used.<br>Aldose-reductase inhibitors (sorbinol), which inhibit formation of sorbitol from glucose, are being tested.[1,2,69]<br>Myo-inositol supplements and B vitamins also have been used to prevent or reverse neuropathy, but data are inconclusive.[69] |
| **Autonomic neuropathies:** | |
| Pseudomotor dysfunction with resultant heat intolerance | Prevention of heatstroke and hyperthermia is necessary. |
| Bladder dysfunction | Bladder is to be emptied regularly (every 3 to 4 hours while awake).<br>Cholinergic stimulation with drug such as bethanechol chloride is advisable.<br>Resection of internal bladder sphincter to decrease resistance to emptying has been used. |
| **Sexual dysfunction** | **Females:** For lack of lubrication, over-the-counter lubricants; to thicken vaginal walls and decrease dyspareunia, estrogen creams.<br>**Males:** For erection problems, injection of papaverine and phentolamine, which are injected directly into corpus and cause luminescence for ½ to 2 hours if a rubber band is placed at base of penis after injection; yohimbine, an $\alpha_2$-adrenergic blocker, increases blood flow into the corpus and is effective when the problem is vascular in nature; suction (to draw blood into the corpus); penile prosthesis (simple or complex) that requires surgery is available. |
| **Gastroparesis** | For delayed gastric emptying: small, low-fiber diets, metoclopramide (Reglan), or bethanechol chloride.<br>For constipation (the most frequent GI symptom): stool softeners, laxatives, cathartics, or metoclopramide.<br>For diarrhea (from decreased sympathetic inhibition, bacterial overgrowth, pancreatic insufficiency or bile salt malabsorption): antibiotics, bile salt sequestrants, or diphenoxylate hydrochloride and atropine (Lomotil). |
| **Orthostatic hypotension** | After identifying cause, therapy may include volume repletion, high-salt diet, mineralocorticoid therapy, or waist-high Jobst stockings. |
| **Hypoglycemic unawareness** | Rigorous control of blood glucose (not allowed to go too low) if possible; frequent blood glucose checks; avoid hypoglycemia-inducing activities. |
| **Diabetic foot** | Prevention is the key.<br>For **dry gangrene:** Keep area dry; monitor for infection and extension of gangrene.<br>For **wet gangrene:** Bedrest; antibiotic therapy; cleansing and debridement; application of platelet drive growth factors is being tested on many types of ulcers[51]; amputation (see Chapter 64) may be necessary if wet gangrene spreads. |
| **Skin** | |
| Infections | Treat infections. |
| Other lesions specific to diabetes | No specific treatment. |

and other problems, and today, no cure for diabetes or even a good treatment for some complications (e.g., neuropathy) exists. This should not stop you. As the quotation from the book *When Diabetes Complicates Your Life* alluded to, each of us has the option to reach for an answer to help solve some problem such as painful neuropathy. *The Diabetes Educator* and other magazines for persons with diabetes often have good suggestions, such as use of audio tapes, visualization, and transcutaneous electrical nerve stimulation (TENS) units to help decrease pain. In the 1990s, none of us can go it alone. In other words, the patient is the expert on his or her life, and the health care team has knowledge of diabetes. It will only be through a partnership that the goals for

## BOX 40-20 1000-Mile Checkup, Part One

Make sure you and your health care providers discuss the following items on each clinic visit.

| Check and date per visit: | | | | | | |
|---|---|---|---|---|---|---|
| Blood sugar (for control) | | | | | | |
| Weight (for food intake) | | | | | | |
| Blood pressure (for pressure changes and blood vessels) | | | | | | |
| Eye examination (for retinopathy) | | | | | | |
| Feelings: emotional, spiritual, physical (checks your ability to function) | | | | | | |
| Meal plan | | | | | | |
| Activity | | | | | | |
| Maintenance record (blood sugar, ketones) | | | | | | |
| Medications | | | | | | |
| Tobacco use | | | | | | |
| Pregnancy plans | | | | | | |
| Foot examination | | | | | | |

## BOX 40-21 1000-Mile Checkup, Part Two

These items should be checked as follows: *every 3 to 6 months; †random and yearly visits.

| Check and date per visit: | | | | | | |
|---|---|---|---|---|---|---|
| *Glycosylated hemoglobin—$HgA_{1c}$ (checks overall blood sugars for past 6-8 weeks) | | | | | | |
| *Pulses and nervous system (checks circulation and neuropathy) | | | | | | |
| †24-hour urine and serum creatinine clearance (checks kidney functioning) | | | | | | |
| †Routine urinalysis | | | | | | |
| †Microalbumin | | | | | | |
| †24-hour urine for protein | | | | | | |
| †Cholesterol—fasting test (checks fat level in blood) | | | | | | |
| †HDL (good cholesterol greater than 35) | | | | | | |
| †LDL (bad cholesterol less than 130) | | | | | | |
| †Thyroid (palpate gland and do blood test) | | | | | | |

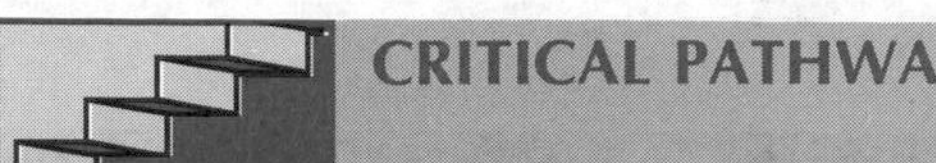

## CRITICAL PATHWAY Hyperglycemic, Hyperosmolar, Nonketotic Coma (HHNC)

**DRG #: 294; expected LOS: 5**

| | Admission to ICU Day of Admission Day 1 | Day 2 | Transfer out of ICU Day 3 | Day 4 | Day of Discharge Day 5 |
|---|---|---|---|---|---|
| **Diagnostic Tests** | CBC; SMA/18*; UA; ECG; ABGs; urine, blood, and sputum C & S; chest x-ray film; ? CT scan | FBS and 2-hour postprandial with SMA/6† | FBS and 2-hour postprandial | FBS and 2-hour postprandial with SMA/6† | FBS |
| **Medications** | IVs (0.5 NS at rate 1.5 L first hour, 1 L over next hour, then 500 ml for 1 hour; when serum osmolarity is <320 mOsm/L, switch to NS); IV insulin bolus and drip; add dextrose (5% saline) when glucose is 250 to 300 mg/dl; $K^+$ replacement to maintain serum levels of 4-5 mEq/L; IV antibiotics; evaluate home medications. | Continue with appropriate IV solutions and medications; IV antibiotics; continue with appropriate home medications. | IV to saline lock; return to prehospital treatment for DM and insulin on sliding scale; IV antibiotics. | IV saline lock; return to prehospital treatment for DM; antibiotics; evaluate medications for home use. | Disc saline lock; adjust medications for home use. |
| **Treatments** | VS q hr until neuro status stable, then q2hr for 12 hours; I & O including Foley q hr for 4 hours, then q2h for 12 hours; weight; capillary blood glucose (CBG) q hr while range <60 and/or >200, then q4hr; monitor hemodynamic parameters q hr; assess cardiovascular, pulmonary, and neurologic systems q hr; assess skin and feet and give special care q2hr. | VS q2hr; I & O q4hr; weight; CBG q4hr and PRN; assess cardiovascular, pulmonary, and neurologic systems q2hr; assess skin and feet and give special care q2hr. | VS q6hr; I & O q8hr; disc Foley and central lines; weight; CBG AC and HS and PRN; assess cardiovascular, pulmonary, and neurologic systems q4hr; assess skin and feet and give special care q4hr. | VS q8hr; disc I & O; weight; CBG AC and HS and PRN; assess cardiovascular, pulmonary, and neurologic systems q8hr; assess skin and feet and give special care q8hr. | VS q8hr; weight; CBG AC and HS and PRN; assess cardiovascular, pulmonary, and neurologic systems q8hr; assess skin and feet and give special care q8hr. |
| **Diet** | NPO, clear liquids when fully awake | Full liquid American Diabetes Association (ADA) diet with appropriate calorie restriction. | ADA diet with appropriate calorie restriction; add between meal snacks as appropriate. | ADA diet with appropriate calorie restriction; add between-meal snacks as appropriate. | ADA diet with appropriate calorie restriction; add between-meal snacks as appropriate. |
| **Activities** | Bedrest, T & DB q2hr; patient safety considerations (bed in lowest position, suction ready, etc.) until neurologic status stable | Up in chair with help, T & DB q2hr; continue with patient safety considerations. | Up in room and walk in hallway with help. | Up in room ad lib and walk in hallway with help. | Up ad lib |
| **Referral/ Consultation** | Endocrinologist | | Dietary, social service, home health, diabetes education | | |

*Serum calcium, phosphorus, triglycerides, uric acid, creatinine, BUN, total bilirubin, alkaline phosphate, aspartate aminotransferase (AST) (formerly serum glutamic oxaloacetic transaminase [SGOT]), alanine aminotransferase (ALT) (formerly serum glutamic oxaloacetic transaminase [SGPT]), lactic dehydrogenase (LDH), total protein, albumin, sodium, potassium, chloride, total $CO_2$, glucose.
†Serum sodium, potassium, chloride, total $CO_2$, glucose, BUN.

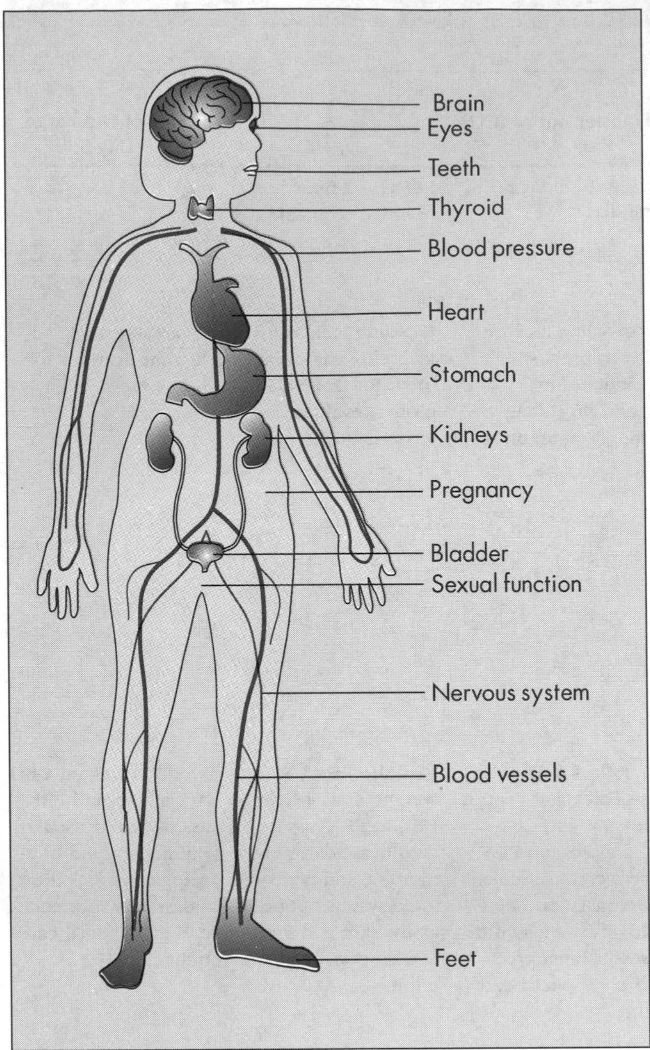


**FIGURE 40-23** The body map. (From *Diabetes—an owner's manual,* Cray Diabetes Education Center, University of Kansas Medical Center.)

year 2000 will be reached and persons with diabetes will have preventive peace.[37]

## HYPOGLYCEMIC STATES

**Hypoglycemia** is the condition in which the plasma or blood glucose concentration falls below normal. It may be clinically serious because a sudden drop in blood glucose deprives the nervous system of its energy supply.

### ETIOLOGY/EPIDEMIOLOGY

Hypoglycemia is classified as either fasting or reactive. The former is seen after periods of fasting that range from a few to several hours; the latter occurs only after the intake of a meal.

*Fasting* hypoglycemia is most often seen as a side effect of insulin therapy or of oral hypoglycemic agents and in persons with diabetes mellitus who take or accumulate too much insulin or oral hypoglycemic agent, who have decreased intake or decreased absorption of carbohydrate, or who exercise more than usual. Fasting hypoglycemia also occurs from underproduction of glucose or overproduction of insulin (see Box 40-22). With autoimmune disease, antibodies against insulin bind up insulin, allowing a large inactive supply to be present in the blood. Antibodies then suddenly release insulin, resulting in relative overproduction or the antibodies mimic insulin at the insulin receptor.[40]

**BOX 40-22 Causes of Fasting Hypoglycemia**

**BOTH AN INCREASE IN INSULIN AND A DECREASE IN GLUCOSE**

Improper treatment of diabetes mellitus

**UNDERPRODUCTION OF GLUCOSE**

Hormonal deficiencies: ACTH, cortisol, glucagon, and catecholamines
Acquired liver disease
Drugs: alcohol, propranolol, salicylates

**OVERPRODUCTION OF INSULIN OR INSULIN-LIKE MATERIAL**

Insulinoma
Extrapancreatic tumors
Autoimmune disease

*Reactive* hypoglycemia (also called *functional*) is the second most frequently diagnosed cause of hypoglycemia. True reactive hypoglycemia is seen in persons after surgery of the stomach or duodenum, such as gastrectomy or gastrojejunostomy, which results in rapid gastric emptying. Reactive hypoglycemia is idiopathic in most instances.

Reactive hypoglycemia may be overdiagnosed. Frequently, no abnormal decrease in blood glucose can be found except after a prolonged (5 hours) glucose tolerance test; this decrease does not correspond to the occurrence of symptoms. The term *idiopathic postprandial syndrome* has been used to differentiate this condition from true reactive hypoglycemia, where there is documented decrease in blood glucose at the time of symptom occurrence.

### PATHOPHYSIOLOGY

Regardless of the cause of fasting hypoglycemia or reactive hypoglycemia, the result is an imbalance between the body's need for glucose and the blood glucose concentration. Normally the blood glucose level is kept within fine limits by counterregulatory hormones. During fasting states, insulin is decreased, and counterregulatory hormones promote hepatic glucose production and decreased glucose use by tissues other than the nervous system.

# NURSING CARE PLAN

## PERSON WITH DIABETES MELLITUS

**DATA:** Mrs. F. is an obese, 72-year-old married woman with NIDDM diagnosed 8 years ago. She was referred to a short-term ambulatory diabetes education program by her physician for instruction on insulin administration because blood glucose control had not been achieved with dietary measures alone or in conjunction with oral hypoglycemic agents.

The nursing history identified the following:

- She saw referral as necessary but perceived the need for insulin and her inability to control weight as personal failures.
- She maintained inconsistent sleep/activity schedule.
- She had accurate knowledge about dietary modifications and had participated successfully in several weight reduction programs with 20- to 40-pound weight loss each time.
- She did regular checks of feet and wore proper shoes.
- She did not exercise consistently.
- She has performed blood glucose monitoring on others and once or twice on self.
- She stated that church activities were important to her; satisfactions were derived from church group socialization and it "keeps me busy."
- She feared that her husband would die suddenly at home. Two years ago, CPR had to be performed when he had a cardiac arrest at home.

Objective data included the following:

- Blood glucose (fasting), 220 mg/dl
- Weight, 200 pounds
- Height, 5'4"
- Blood pressure, 134/84
- Urine negative for ketones
- Urine negative for microalbuminuria
- Peripheral pulses present
- Legs warm and dry, color even with rest of body
- Patellar and Achilles tendon reflexes 3+ (on 1 to 4 scale)
- Identified touch in lower extremities
- Discriminated between sharp and dull in lower extremities
- Felt vibration in lower extremities
- Vision 20/20 on Snellen chart eye examination.

Collaborative nursing actions included teaching Mrs. F. those measures that would help her achieve control of blood glucose (diet, insulin, exercise) and teaching her to detect, prevent, and treat hypoglycemic reactions.

### ■ NURSING DIAGNOSIS

Knowledge deficit: self-injections, care of equipment, and self-monitoring of blood glucose (SMBG) related to lack of exposure to information

| Expected Patient Outcomes | Nursing Interventions | Rationale |
|---|---|---|
| Independently adminsters injection to self. | Support patient as necessary to self-inject insulin. | Adults who perform this task have minimal discomfort and realize they are capable of giving own insulin. |
| Performs self-monitoring of blood glucose (SMBG) accurately. | Observe patient's skill in SMBG; correct as necessary. | Evaluation of patient technique is necessary to ensure accuracy. |
| Uses measurements obtained by SMBG to achieve fasting blood glucose below 140 mg/dl. | Review, with patient, effect of activity, dietary intake, and insulin on blood glucose. Instruct patient on frequency and timing of SMBG. | SMBG gives almost immediate feedback about previous behaviors and reinforces value of therapeutic measures. |
| Describes symptoms of hypoglycemia and knows how to treat. | Review, with patient, signs and symptoms and treatment measures for hypoglycemia. | This knowledge ensures that patient can safely give own insulin and decreases fear of reaction. |
| Describes how to care for insulin and supplies. | Review with patient information about care of insulin and supplies. | This knowledge ensures that insulin and equipment will be stable. |
| Describes how diet will be changed because of insulin. | Refer to dietitian for modification of diet necessary with insulin and verification of diet knowledge. | The dietitian is appropriate person to teach about diet. |

*Continued.*

## NURSING CARE PLAN

### PERSON WITH DIABETES MELLITUS—cont'd

#### ■ NURSING DIAGNOSIS

Altered health maintenance related to ineffective coping skill

| Expected Patient Outcome | Nursing Interventions | Rationale |
|---|---|---|
| States at least one change that will improve blood glucose control. | Counsel patient about effects of stress, lack of exercise, and activity pattern on blood glucose. | Patient's understanding of how stress impairs health is necessary before change. |
| | Explore with Mrs. F. willingness and ability to change behaviors: sleep/activity, coping, and exercise. | Goals are more likely to be achieved if patient makes realistic choices after considering cost and benefits. |
| | Engage Mrs. F. in mutual problem solving; refrain from prescribing. | Increasing patients' sense of control can help with self-esteem and enhance attitudes toward change. |
| | Explore sources for long-term support in learning more effective coping skills. Suggest support groups:<br>1. For spouses of patients with MI<br>2. For weight loss *and maintenance* of weight loss<br>3. For exercise | Changing life-style, eating behaviors, and coping skills is very difficult; support over long periods is usually required. |

This fine regulation is not maintained in either type of hypoglycemia because there is either more insulin than normal or glucose production is inhibited. The result is low blood glucose; counterregulatory hormones (glucagon, epinephrine, cortisol, growth hormone) are secreted to the extent possible but are not effective in bringing the glucose to normal. The epinephrine that is secreted produces symptoms by increasing the activity of the epinephrine-sensitive organs or tissues (e.g., heart, sweat glands). The CNS is deprived of its source of energy, and dysfunction results. Remember the nervous system has no stores of glucose; it is dependent on the blood level.

The signs and symptoms seen in fasting hypoglycemia and reactive hypoglycemia are the same as those described for hypoglycemia associated with diabetes mellitus. The diagnosis of fasting hypoglycemia is based on history, plasma insulin and plasma glucose levels, and identification of one of the listed etiologic factors. The patient may be admitted for fasting for up to 72 hours to see if hypoglycemia develops.

The diagnosis of reactive hypoglycemia should be based on a mixed-meal tolerance test. In this test, a standardized meal is ingested, and plasma glucose and symptoms are checked every 30 minutes for 5 hours. If the blood glucose level drops and the patient has symptoms, reactive hypoglycemia is diagnosed.[40] An oral glucose tolerance test should not be used to diagnose this problem.[40]

## MEDICAL MANAGEMENT

Medical therapy consists of treating symptoms of hypoglycemia with glucose replacement (50% glucose solution, by infusion or orally). Oral therapy is the preferred method. After the cause is identified, treatment may include the following:

1. Surgery for insulinomas or extrapancreatic tumor
2. Diazoxide therapy for inoperable insulinomas to suppress insulin secretion
3. Discontinuance of drugs that induce hypoglycemia (alcohol, propranolol, salicylates)
4. Correction of hormonal deficiency
5. Correction of hepatic disease

The dietary control usually recommended is a low-carbohydrate, high-protein diet, but its efficacy has not been established by research. The major medical therapy is avoidance of simple sugars and of fasting so hypoglycemia does not occur.

## NURSING MANAGEMENT

Nursing care of the person with hypoglycemia is directed toward the following nursing diagnoses:

1. Anxiety related to sympathetic symptoms
2. Injury (trauma), high risk for, related to CNS dysfunction
3. Knowledge deficit: disease; tests and treatments related to new diagnosis

During the early phase of illness, the patient is monitored for the presence of changes in CNS function that might indicate hypoglycemia. A protocol for treatment of symptoms should be established and instituted; symptoms, such as sweating, trembling, and shakiness, which result with increased sympathetic stimulation, may cause considerable discomfort. Cool baths and a cool environment may relieve some discomfort. Relaxation therapy that includes backrubs, relaxation exercises, music, or distraction may also be helpful.

Patient teaching includes:

1. Diagnostic tests: purpose, procedures
2. Cause and treatment
3. Dietary management: avoidance of simple sugars and fasting
4. Preparation for surgery (see Chapter 23)

## QUESTIONS TO CONSIDER

- How can you use the Professional Prompter Worksheet, and what does "survival" teaching entail?
- How would you determine whether poor control by a patient diagnosed with diabetes mellitus is caused by knowledge deficit, noncompliance, ineffective coping, or lack of resources? Be specific.
- How would you determine whether a person with diabetes is developing problems associated with autonomic neuropathy? Be specific.
- How is hypoglycemia treated? What is the rationale for each part of treatment?
- What physiologic parameters are monitored in a person with DKA? Make a flow chart indicating frequency. Are the parameters different for a person with HHNC?

## CRITICAL THINKING ACTIVITIES

- You are assigned to care for two patients. Jim has non-insulin-dependent diabetes mellitus (NIDDM), and Tim has insulin-dependent diabetes mellitus (IDDM). Without any additional information, how may you anticipate that your care of these two men will differ? How will their care be the same?
- After discussing your patient's diet with her, she states that she cannot afford to buy expensive diabetic foods. How should you respond?
- While teaching Molly, a new diabetic patient, how to give her own insulin dose, you note that she tends to use the same site for each injection. When requested to use another site, Molly states that she prefers to use her right thigh because it feels more comfortable to her. How should you intervene?

## CHAPTER SUMMARY

### CLASSIFICATION

- Diabetes mellitus is a complex metabolic disorder, which may be clinically categorized in one of five different classifications. The two major classifications are non-insulin-dependent diabetes mellitus (NIDDM) and insulin-dependent diabetes mellitus (IDDM).

### ETIOLOGY

- Genetics, heredity, autoimmunity, and environmental factors have a role in the causes of both IDDM and NIDDM.

### EPIDEMIOLOGY

- Diabetes occurs more often in Native Americans, Hispanics, African-Americans, and elderly people.

### PATHOPHYSIOLOGY

- Insulin deficit is a central feature of the disease; insulin deficit may be absolute, when β-cells do not secrete insulin, or relative, when β-cell defect and peripheral resistance to insulin is present.
- Insulin deficit and hyperglycemia lead to many immediate alterations in metabolism, including hyperosmolarity and osmotic diuresis, glycosuria, cellular starvation, calorie loss, and increased fat metabolism and catabolism.
- The classic signs and symptoms of IDDM are polyuria, polydipsia, polyphagia, weight loss, weakness, and fatigue. Patients with IDDM may have these symptoms or signs and symptoms of diabetic ketoacidosis; patients with NIDDM may have the same symptoms, except that they usually have weight gain instead of weight loss, or they may have signs and symptoms of hyperglycemic, hyperosmolar, nonketotic coma or vascular changes and neuropathy.

### PREVENTION

- Taking measures to prevent and treat obesity is the focus of primary prevention of NIDDM; screening to detect undiagnosed cases (50%) is the focus of secondary prevention; detecting and preventing progression of complications is the focus of tertiary prevention.
- The five primary modalities of treatment for diabetes mellitus are diet, exercise, hypoglycemic agents, monitoring, and education.
- Dietary recommendations include calorie distribution of carbohydrate (CHO) (40% to 60%); fat (usually ≤30% but may be as high as 40%) with restriction in saturated fat to 10%; protein (20%); limitation of cholesterol, sodium, and refined simple CHO; and increased use of complex, unrefined CHO.
- Exercise has a hypoglycemic action in most instances; it can increase hyperglycemia if blood glucose levels are above 300 mg/dl or if exercise is intense. Exercise

does aid in cardiovascular fitness and weight reduction and maintenance, and it decreases peripheral resistance to insulin.

## MEDICAL MANAGEMENT

- Insulin is used in all persons with IDDM and many with NIDDM; nurses and patients must be careful to use prescribed insulin: strength, species, length of action, purity.
- Oral hypoglycemic agents are used in NIDDM; they stimulate the pancreas and decrease peripheral resistance. They may induce hypoglycemia.
- Self-monitoring of blood glucose (SMBG) is always used by patients using insulin pump therapy or multiple injections. *Patients treated in other ways use SMBG.* This technology has made it possible to achieve normoglycemia in well-educated patients.
- Hemoglobin $A_{1c}$ measures the amount of glycosylation of normal hemoglobin A; it correlates with the average blood glucose levels over the past 3 months.

## NURSING MANAGEMENT

- Assessment of the patient includes collecting objective data about metabolic status and assessing cardiovascular-renal status, vision, and nerve function. The lower extremities should be examined carefully.
- Because patients must be responsible for diabetes management, nurses must assess the knowledge and coping skills of patients early in hospitalization so that appropriate education and counseling can proceed.
- A well-educated person will be assertive in describing special needs relating to patterns of food intake, exercise, monitoring, medication, and foot care.
- An educational program for persons with diabetes mellitus has 15 components: these components include knowledge, skills, and attitudes for effective diabetes management.
- Diabetes education must be individualized and planned over time. Initial instruction should be restricted to "survival/initial skills" with plans for continued education.
- The impact of diagnosis of diabetes mellitus and living with this chronic illness may be expressed by patients emotionally, in concerns about the future, in family conflicts, and in noncompliance.
- The treatment of hypoglycemia must be prompt; 10 to 15 g of simple CHO is given as soon as symptoms are detected. The first signs present are those of epinephrine excess; later signs are those of cerebral dysfunction. The signs and symptoms may be prolonged if the patient is taking oral hypoglycemic agents.
- Insulin or oral hypoglycemic agents should not be omitted when short illness occurs; about 50% of normal daily CHO intake should be distributed over 24 hours. Monitoring should dictate the need for more or less medication.
- Foot care includes daily inspection, measures to maintain integrity of skin, and prevention of injury. Referral to podiatric services is highly recommended. Patient should verbalize knowledge of feet at risk.
- Evaluation of nursing interventions includes assessment of whether the metabolic balance is improved, whether the patient has the requisite knowledge and coping skills for self-management, and whether appropriate referrals were made. The Professional Prompter Worksheet is a guide for nurses that outlines what to teach and how to teach.
- Diabetes treatment is expensive. Persons with diabetes may have difficulty getting health insurance and certain jobs.

## NURSING MANAGEMENT OF THE PATIENT WITH DIABETES HAVING SURGERY

- Patients fasting or undergoing surgery require modifications of insulin and food intake and increased monitoring of metabolic status.

## COMPLICATIONS

- Diabetic ketoacidosis (DKA) and hyperglycemic, hyperosmolar, nonketotic coma (HHNC) are two life-threatening situations that occur in uncontrolled diabetes mellitus; they are usually precipitated by infection, stressors, or failure to follow regimen.
- Medical management of DKA and HHNC includes intensive fluid replacement, low-dose insulin infusion, and potassium replacement. The patient may also need phosphate and magnesium replacement.
- Hyperglycemia, from poorly controlled diabetes mellitus, seems to be a major predictor of the development of microvascular lesions (nephropathy, retinopathy), macrovascular lesions (atherosclerotic disease), and neuropathy (autonomic and peripheral).
- Amputation of a limb may be necessary because of alterations in blood vessels and nerve trauma, tissue trauma, or infections occurring in persons with inadequate skin integrity and insensitivity to pain and pressure. Proper foot care, which helps to prevent an infection, can reduce the chance of amputation.
- The major nursing focuses in patients with DKA or HHNC are (1) monitoring intake and output, weight, vital signs, mental status, ECG, blood glucose, urine ketones, serum electrolytes, and osmolality; (2) implementing the medical plan; (3) reporting unexpected changes immediately; and (4) providing a safe environment.

## HYPOGLYCEMIC STATES

- Hypoglycemia can occur separately from diabetes mellitus.
- Hypoglycemia can be classified as fasting (includes excessive insulin production from insulinomas) or reactive (hypoglycemia after a meal).
- The signs and symptoms of fasting or reactive hypoglycemia are caused by the release of epinephrine and inadequate glucose levels for normal neurologic function.

- Reactive hypoglycemia can be inappropriately diagnosed if oral glucose tolerance testing is used; the diagnostic test of choice is a mixed-meal tolerance test.
- Insulinomas, which cause fasting hypoglycemia, are treated surgically; reactive hypoglycemia is treated with dietary manipulation.

## REFERENCES


1. American Diabetes Association: *Physician's guide to insulin-dependent (type I) diabetes, diagnosis and treatment,* ed 2, Alexandria, Va, 1994, The Association.
2. American Diabetes Association: *Physician's guide to non-insulin-dependent (type II) diabetes, diagnosis and treatment,* ed 3, Alexandria, Va, 1994, The Association.
3. American Diabetes Association: *Goals for Diabetes Education,* Clinical Education Program, ed 2, Alexandria, Va, The Association. (In press.)
4. American Diabetes Association: *Diabetes—1991 vital statistics,* Alexandria, Va, 1991, The Association.
5. American Diabetes Association: *Meeting the standards—a manual for completing the American Diabetes Association application for recognition,* ed 3, Chicago, 1991, The Association.
6. American Diabetes Association, Diabetes Facts, 1-page handouts, Alexandria, Va, 1992, The Association.
   The Dangerous Toll of Diabetes
   Diabetes: Facts You Need To Know
   Diabetes Among Hispanics
   Diabetes Among Seniors
   Diabetes Among Youth
   Diabetes Among American Indians
   Diabetes Among Black Americans
   Direct and Indirect Costs of Diabetes in the United States
7. American Diabetes Association: Clinical practice recommendations 1992-1993, *Diabetes Care* 16(suppl 2):1-66, 1993.
8. American Diabetes Association: *Report on diabetes control and complications trial,* Las Vegas, National Meeting, June 1993.

8a. American Diabetes Association: Position statement—Nutrition recommendations and principles for people with diabetes mellitus, *Diabetes Care* 17:519-522, 1994.

9. American Diabetes Association and American Dietetic Association: *Exchange lists for meal planning,* Alexandria, Va, 1986, The Association.
10. Amick BL, Lopes GL: *Kansas diet manual,* ed 6, Topeka/Kansas City, 1992, Kansas Dietetic Association.
11. Anderson JW et al: Dietary fiber and diabetes, a comprehensive review and practical application, *J Am Diet Assoc* 87:1189-1197, 1987.
12. Anderson J, Clark JT: The promise of fiber, *Diabetes Forecast* 40(12):47-48, 50, 52, 1987.
13. Ashley D: Surgery and the diabetic patient, *Post Anesth Nurs* 1:205-207, 1986.
14. Atkinson MA, MaClaren NK: What causes diabetes? *Sci Am* 263:62-67, 1990.
15. Blevins D, Cassmeyer, VL: The patient with diabetes mellitus. In Long B, Phipps WJ, Cassmeyer VL, editors: *Medical-surgical nursing—a nursing process approach,* ed 3, 1993, St Louis, Mosby.
16. Bloomgarden ZT: Epidemiology, diagnosis, and treatment of type II diabetes—a meeting report, *Pract Diabetol* 12(2): 4-9, 1993.
17. Bode BW et al: *DiabetesDek—how to control and manage diabetes mellitus,* Atlanta, Ga, 1992, Lifescan Infodek.
18. Breckenridge BP: *Diabetes guide sheet—please tell me about what I can eat,* Princeton, NJ, 1992, Novo Nordisk Pharmaceuticals.

18a. Brown SA: Effect of educational interventions in diabetes care: a meta-analysis of findings, *Nurs Res* 37:223-230, 1988.

19. Capsaicin Study Group: Effect of treatment with capsaicin on daily activities of patients with painful diabetic neuropathy, *Diabetes Care* 15(2):159-165, 1992.
20. Coleman W: Foot care and diabetes mellitus. In Haire-Joshu D, editor: *Management of diabetes mellitus—perspectives of care across the life span,* St Louis, 1992, Mosby.
21. Daly A, Arky RA: Nutritional management. In Lebovitz HA, editor: *Therapy for diabetes mellitus and related disorders,* Alexandria, Va, 1991 American Diabetes Association.
22. Depres JP et al: Loss of abdominal fat and metabolic response to exercise training in obese women, *Am J Physiol* 261:E, 159-167, 1991.
23. Dinsmoor RS: Better prediction spurs new approaches to prevention, *JDF Countdown* 14(1):6-13, 1993.
24. *Drug facts and comparisons, 1993,* St Louis, 1993, Wolters Kluwer Co.
25. Eaks GA: *An evaluation of a self-instructional teaching package for the elderly with diabetes mellitus,* unpublished master's thesis, Kansas City, 1976, University of Kansas School of Nursing.
26. Eaks GA: *Diabetes—an owner's manual,* Kansas Diabetes Control Project Cray Diabetes Education Center, Kansas City, 1990, University of Kansas Medical Center.
27. Eaks GA: *Professional Prompter Worksheet,* Cray Diabetes Education Center, Kansas City, 1993, University of Kansas Medical Center.
28. Eli Lilly: *Characteristics of Lilly insulins,* Indianapolis, 1993, Eli Lilly.
29. Fleckman AM: Diabetic ketoacidosis, *Pract Diabet* 10(3):1-8, 1991.
30. Fox MA et al: Blood glucose self-monitoring usage and its influence on patients' perceptions of diabetes, *Diabetes Educator* 10:27-31, 1984.
31. Franz MJ: Evaluating the glycemic response to carbohydrates, *Clin Diabetes* 11:127-130, 1986.
32. Franz MJ: *Goals for diabetes education,* American Diabetes Association Task Group on Goals for Diabetes Education, American Diabetes Association, Clinical Education Program, Alexandria, Va, 1989, The Association.
33. Franz MJ: Fast food facts—nutritive and exchange values for fast-food restaurants, Minneapolis, 1990, International Diabetes Center, DCI Publishing.
34. Franz MJ: Exercise and diabetes. In Haire-Joshu D, editor: *Management of diabetes mellitus,* St Louis, 1992, Mosby.
35. Franz MJ, Cooper N: Meal planning—adding flexibility. In Weiler C, editor: *Learning to live well with diabetes,* Minneapolis, 1991, International Diabetes Center, DCI Publishing.
36. Feldman JM: Pathophysiology of diabetes mellitus. In Galloway JA, editor: *Diabetes mellitus,* ed 9, Indianapolis, 1988, Eli Lilly.
37. Funnell MM: Empowerment, *Pract Diabetol* 10(3):15-18, 1991.
38. Galloway JA, deShazo RD: Insulin chemistry and pharmacology: insulin allergy, resistance, and lipodystrophy. In Rifkin H, Porte D Jr, editors: *Ellenberg and Rifkin's diabetes mellitus, theory and practice,* ed 4, New York, 1990, Elsevier.
39. Genuth S: Diabetic ketoacidosis and hyperglycemic hyperosmolar coma in adults. In Lebovitz H, editor: *Therapy for diabetes mellitus and related disorders,* Alexandria, Va, 1991, American Diabetes Association.
40. Gorden P: *The clinical spectrum of hypoglycemia.* In Endocrine Society: 41st Post Graduate Annual Assembly syllabus, Bethesda, Md, 1990, The Endocrine Society.

41. Groop LC et al: Association between polymorphism of the glycogen synthase gene and non-insulin dependent diabetes mellitus, *N Engl J Med*, 328(10):568-570, 1993.
42. Guthrie DW, Guthrie RA: *Nursing management of diabetes mellitus*, ed 3, New York, 1991, Springer.
43. Hamera E et al: Self-regulation in individuals with type II diabetes, *Nurs Res* 37:363-367, 1988.
44. Henderson G: The psychosocial treatment of recurrent diabetic ketoacidosis: an interdisciplinary team approach, *Diabetes Educator* 17(2):119-123, 1991.
45. Herman W: *The prevention and treatment of complications of diabetes mellitus—a guide for primary care practitioners*, US Department of Health and Human Services, Public Health Service, Centers for Disease Control, National Center for Chronic Disease Prevention and Health Promotion, Division of Diabetes Translation, Washington, DC, 1992, US Government Printing Office.
46. Horton ES: Exercise. In Lebovitz HE, editor: *Therapy for diabetes mellitus and related disorders*, Alexandria, Va, 1991, American Diabetes Association.
47. Jameel N et al: Dietary protein intake is not correlated with clinical proteinuria in NIDDM, *Diabetes Care* 15(2):178-183, 1992.
48. Juliano J: *When diabetes complicates your life*, Minneapolis, Mn, 1993, Chronimed.
49. Keegan A et al: Bringing research to light, *Diabetes Forecast* 45(9):34-43, 1992.
50. Kentucky Diabetes Foundation: *Personal guidelines—a guide to servings*, Lexington, Ky, 1984, Kentucky Diabetes Foundation.
51. Knighton DR: Treating diabetic foot ulcers, *Diabetes Spectrum* 3(1):51-56, 1990.
52. Krall L, Beaser R: *Joslin diabetes manual*, ed 12, Philadelphia, 1989, Lea & Febiger.
53. Leahy JL, Boyd AE: Diabetes genes in non-insulin dependent diabetes mellitus, *N Engl J Med* 328(1):56-57, 1993.
54. Lebovitz H, editor: *Therapy for diabetes mellitus and related disorders*, Alexandria, Va, 1991, American Diabetes Association.
54a. Levin ME, O'Neal LW, editors: *The diabetic foot*, St Louis, 1988, Mosby.
55. Lloyd CE et al: Psychosocial factors and complications of IDDM, *Diabetes Care* 15(2):166-172, 1992.
56. Lorber DL: Important considerations: acute glycemic complications, *Pract Diabetol* 11(2):33-35, 1992.
57. Lyon R, Vinci DM: Nutrition management of insulin-dependent diabetes mellitus in adults, *Am Dietetic Assoc* 93(3):309-317, 1993.
58. McDonald's: *Food exchanges for McDonald's menu items*, Oak Brook, Ill, 1992, McDonald's.
59. Moller DE, Flier JS: Insulin resistance—mechanisms, syndromes, and implications, *N Engl J Med* 324(13):938-948, 1991.
60. National Diabetes Data Group: Classification and diagnoses of diabetes mellitus and other categories of glucose intolerance, *Diabetes* 28:1039-1057, 1979.
61. Novo Nordisk: *Product reference guide*, chart, Princeton, NJ, Novo Nordisk Pharmaceuticals, 1992.
62. Oexmann MJ: *Total available glucose—a diabetic food system*, New York, 1989, William Morrow.
63. Palmer JP: Predicting IDDM—use of humoral immune markers, *Diabetes Rev* 1(1):104-112, 1993.
64. Parillo M et al: Prevention of early-morning hyperglycemia in IDDM patients with long-acting zinc insulin, *Diabetes Care* 15(2):173-177, 1992.
65. Pasmantier R: Muscle cells' resistance to insulin may start decades before diagnosis of type II, *Diabetes News* 12(2):14-16, 1993.
66. Paulk LH: *Hypoglycemic reactions from the diabetic's perspective*, unpublished master's theisis, Kent, Ohio, 1983, Kent State University.
67. Pollock ML, Wilmore JH: *Exercise in health and disease—evaluation and prescription for prevention and rehabilitation*, ed 2, Philadelphia, 1990, Saunders.
68. Poteet GW et al: Outcome of multiple usage of disposable syringes in the insulin-requiring diabetic, *Nurs Res* 36:350-352, 1987.
69. Rifkin H, Porte D, editors: *Ellenberg and Rifkin's diabetes mellitus, theory and practice*, ed 4, New York, 1990, Elsevier.
70. Saudek CD, Segal-Polin S: Economic aspects: insurance, employment, and licensing. In Rifkin H, Porte D, editors: *Ellenberg and Rifkin's diabetes mellitus, theory and practice*, ed 4, New York, 1990, Elsevier.
71. Streiff LD: Can clients understand our instructions? *Image* 18:48-52, 1986.
71a. Task Force to Revise the National Standards: National Standards for Diabetes Self-Management Education Programs, *Diabetes Care* 18(1):141-148, 1995.
72. Ulchaker MM, Sheehan JP: Iatrogenic brittle diabetes: the hold-the-insulin decision, *Diabetes Educator* 17(2):111-113, 1991.
73. US Department of Agriculture/HNIS: *Food guide pyramid—a guide to daily food choices*, Washington, DC, 1992, USDA/HNIS.
74. US Department of Health and Human Services, US Public Health Service: *Healthy people 2000: national health promotion and disease prevention*, Pub 91-50213, Washington, DC, 1991, US Government Printing Office.
75. US Department of Health and Human Services, US Public Health Service: *Diabetes in the United States: a strategy for prevention* (map reference), National Center for Chronic Disease Control and Prevention, Division of Diabetes Translation, Washington, DC, 1992, US Government Printing Office.
76. Vinicor FA: Epidemiology of diabetes complications—defining risk factors and frequency of complications, *Diabetes Spectrum* 5(2):86-121, 1992.
77. World Health Organization: WHO expert committee on diabetes mellitus, second report, *WHO Tech Rep Series* 646:1-80, 1980.
78. Wysocki T: SMBG—Has the promise been fulfilled? *Diabetes Spectrum* 1(2):83-87, 1988.
79. Zehrer J, Rode S: Hypertension and diabetes, *Drugs* 35(suppl 6):135-141, 1988.
80. Zimmet PZ: Challenges in diabetes epidemiology—from West to the rest, *Diabetes Care* 15(2):232-252, 1992.

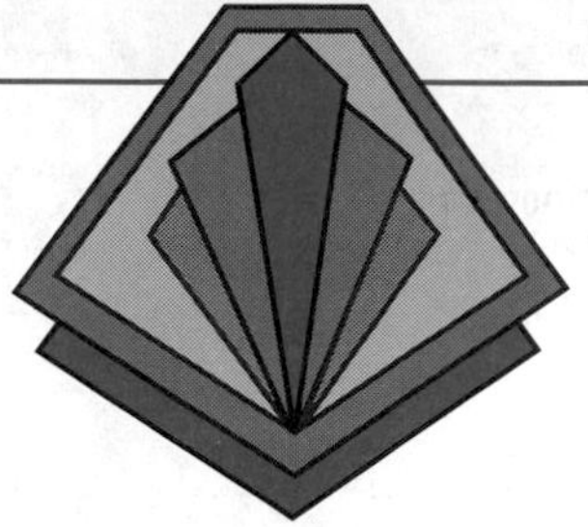

CHAPTER 41

# Assessment of the Hepatic System

*Debera Jane Thomas*

## CHAPTER OBJECTIVES

***After studying this chapter, the learner should be able to do the following:***

1 Describe the normal anatomy of the liver.
2 Describe the role of the liver in metabolism and maintenance of energy balance.
3 Explain the basis for subjective and objective data that must be collected to identify problems of the hepatic system.
4 Describe the various laboratory and diagnostic tests used in identifying the pathophysiologic states of the liver.
5 Develop a plan of care for patients undergoing the radiologic and special tests used in diagnosing hepatic dysfunction.

## KEY TERMS

ascites
bile
bile salts
bilirubin
chylomicrons
clotting factors
colloid osmotic pressure
common bile duct
cystic duct
detoxification
endoscopic retrograde cholangiopancreatography (ERCP)
fatty acids
gluconeogenesis
glycogenesis
glycogenolysis
hepatic duct
hypoalbuminemia
jaudice
lipogenesis
liver biopsy
liver lobule
paracentesis
pruritus
transamination
urobilinogen

The liver is of prime importance in metabolism and in the maintenance of normal energy stores. Because the liver has multiple functions (more than 400), pathologic conditions of the liver can cause a variety of problems that impact the entire body.

## ANATOMY AND PHYSIOLOGY

### ANATOMIC CONCEPTS

The liver is one of the largest organs in the body and weighs 1.3 to 1.8 kg. It consists of two lobes, which are divided by the falciform ligament and attaches the liver to the diaphragm. Anatomically, it extends up under the ribs and is 4 to 8 cm in height in the midsternal line and 6 to 12 cm in height in the midclavicular line. The liver normally extends from the fifth intercostal space to just below the right costal margin (Figure 41-1).

The liver receives 25% of the cardiac output from two sources, the portal vein and the hepatic artery. Most of blood flow (75%) is derived from the portal vein; thus the liver receives mostly unoxygenated blood (Figure 41-2). The liver is innervated by the sympathetic and parasympathetic nervous systems. Sympathetic fibers innervate the hepatic artery branches and the bile ducts. Parasympathetic innervation is supplied to the intrahepatic and extrahepatic biliary tract system. Stimulation of the sympathetic and parasympathetic nervous systems affects blood flow and the flow of bile within the biliary tract, but the function of the hepatic cells or parenchymal cells is not influenced.

The functional unit of the liver is the **liver lobule** (Figure 41-3). Each lobule is composed of multiple

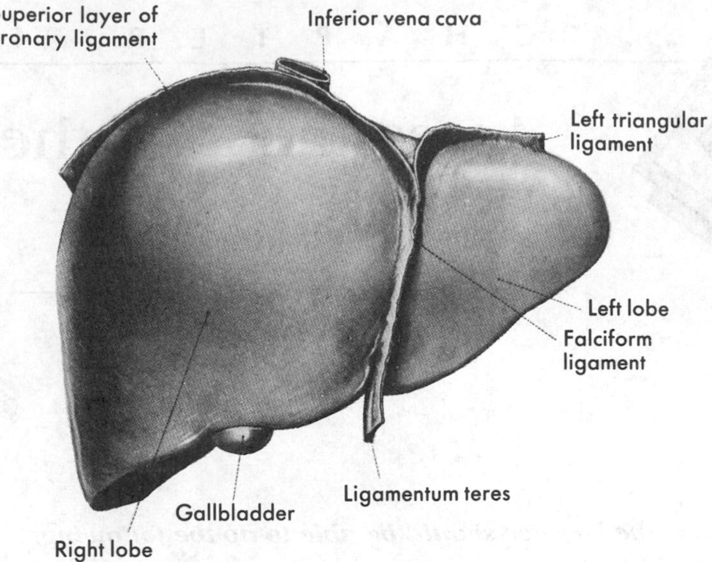


**FIGURE 41-1** Anterior view of liver. (From Hamilton WJ, editor: *Textbook of human anatomy,* ed 2, St Louis, 1976, Mosby. By permission of Macmillan, London & Basingstoke.)

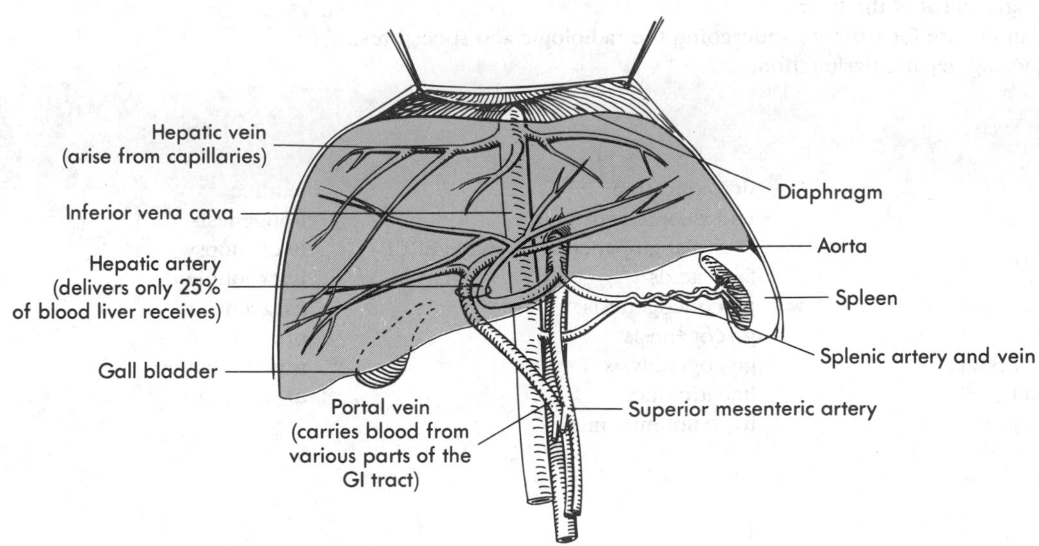


**FIGURE 41-2** Diagram demonstrating circulation of liver. (Modified from Porth C: *Pathophysiology: concepts of altered health status,* Philadelphia, 1982, Lippincott.)

plates of hepatic cells. Between the individual cells of the cellular plate are biliary canaliculi, which empty into the bile ducts. The terminal bile ducts join to form the **hepatic duct,** which merges with the **cystic duct** of the gallbladder to form the **common bile duct.** On each side of the cellular plate is a venous sinusoid, which receives blood from branches of the portal vein and hepatic artery. As blood flows through the sinusoids, substances can be exchanged between the hepatic cells and the blood.

The sinusoids are lined with phagocytic cells of the reticuloendothelial system (Kupffer cells). These cells remove bacteria and other foreign substances from the blood. Because the portal blood originates in the gastrointestinal (GI) tract, some bacteria or other foreign substances always need to be removed.

The blood from the venous sinusoids empties into the central vein and then into the hepatic vein. The hepatic vein empties into the inferior vena cava.

## PHYSIOLOGIC CONCEPTS

The liver can be thought of as a metabolic factory and a waste disposal plant. As should be evident from the anatomic description of the blood and bile flow, the liver

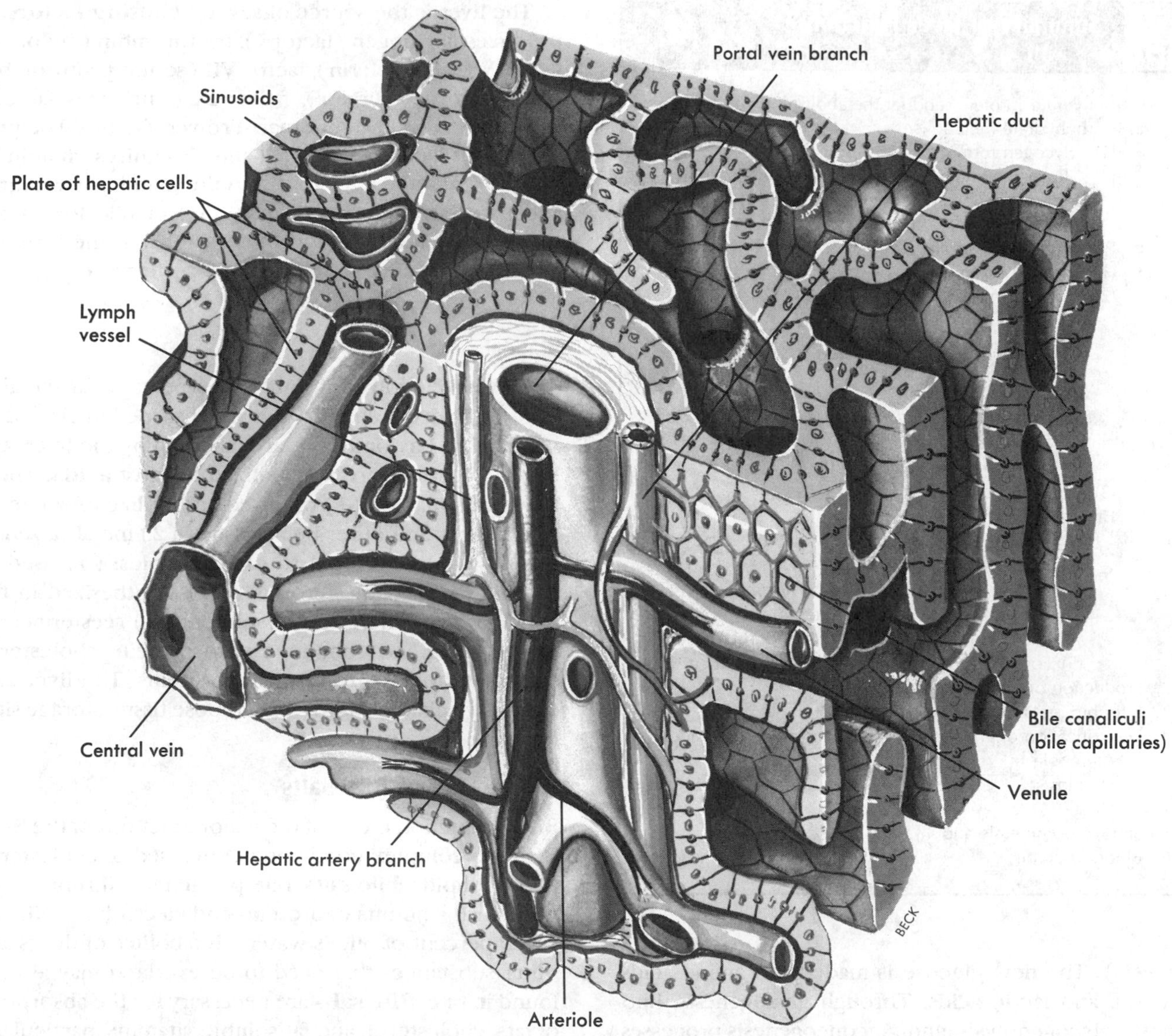


**FIGURE 41-3** Liver lobule. Blood from branches of the portal vein and hepatic artery passes through sinusoids between plates of hepatic cells. Sinusoidal blood empties into central vein, which leads to the hepatic veins. Bile canaliculi empty bile into bile ducts. (From Anthony CP, Thibodeau GA: *Textbook of anatomy and physiology,* ed 11, St Louis, 1983, Mosby.)

is ideally structured to carry out its multiple metabolic and waste disposal functions. The major functions of the liver are summarized in Box 41-1. Each of these functions is presented in more detail in the following sections.

## Carbohydrate, Protein, and Fat Metabolism

The liver has a significant role in the metabolism of each of the three major food nutrients. The liver either oxidizes these components for energy, uses the nutrients to synthesize storage forms of substances for future use, or uses the nutrients to synthesize other essential compounds.

### Carbohydrate

Immediately after meals, the liver extracts glucose, fructose, and galactose from the blood. These simple sugars are metabolized into glycogen **(glycogenesis)** to replenish liver stores. If the diet ingested is low in carbohydrates, the liver converts protein to glucose to replenish glycogen stores. If more carbohydrate is ingested than is needed to replenish glycogen stores or to supply energy, the excess carbohydrate is converted to fat **(lipogenesis).** Between meals and during other fasting states, the liver assists in maintaining the blood glucose concentration. It does this by breaking down glycogen **(glycogenolysis)** or forming new glucose **(gluconeo-**

**BOX 41-1 Summary of Liver Functions**

1. Carbohydrate, protein, and fat metabolism
   a. Carbohydrate metabolism
      (1) Glycogen formation and storage
      (2) Glucose formation from glycogen (glycogenolysis) and from amino acids, lactic acids, and glycerol (gluconeogenesis)
   b. Protein metabolism
      (1) Protein catabolism
      (2) Protein synthesis
         (a) Albumin
         (b) alpha-(α) and beta-(β)Globulins
         (c) Clotting factors
         (d) C-reactive protein
         (e) Transferrin
         (f) Enzymes
         (g) Ceruloplasmin, and so on
      (3) Formation of needed amino acids
   c. Fat metabolism
      (1) Oxidation of fatty acids for energy
      (2) Ketone formation
      (3) Synthesis of cholesterol and phospholipids
      (4) Formation of triglycerides from dietary lipids and excessive dietary carbohydrates and proteins
      (5) Formation of lipoproteins
2. Production of bile salts
3. Bilirubin metabolism
4. Detoxification of endogenous and exogenous substances
   a. Ammonia
   b. Steroids
   c. Drugs
5. Storage of minerals and vitamins
6. Blood reservoir

**genesis).** The new glucose is made from amino acids, glycerol, and lactic acids. Through glycogenesis, lipogenesis, glycogenolysis, and gluconeogenesis processes, which are under hormonal control, the liver helps to maintain a normal blood glucose level, preventing high levels immediately after eating (postprandial) and hypoglycemia between meals or during other periods of fasting.

### Proteins

The liver is vital to normal protein metabolism. It provides needed amino acids through transamination. **Transamination** is the process of nitrogen metabolism in which the liver transfers an amino group ($NH_2$) to form nonessential amino acids. The liver also is the only source of some of the major plasma proteins. One of these major proteins is albumin, which is necessary for the maintenance of a normal internal environment and for fluid and electrolyte balance. *Albumin,* produced only in the liver, is responsible for maintaining **colloid osmotic pressure** and thus the proper distribution of fluids between the vascular and interstitial compartments.

The liver is the source of several **clotting factors.** It produces fibrinogen (factor I), prothrombin (factor II), factor V (proaccelerin), factor VII (serum prothrombin conversion accelerator), factor IX (Christmas factor), and factor X (Stuart, or Stuart-Prower, factor). The production of factors II, VII, IX, and X requires vitamin K. Because vitamin K is a fat-soluble vitamin, it requires adequate production and excretion of bile for its absorption. In addition to protein synthesis, the liver catabolizes proteins as necessary for energy or glucose production.

### Fats

The liver is involved in multiple aspects of fat metabolism. Triglycerides in the diet are absorbed in **chylomicrons.** The chylomicrons are taken up by the liver, and the triglycerides are metabolized to **fatty acids.** These fatty acids may be (1) oxidized and utilized for energy by the liver and other body tissues; (2) metabolized to ketones; (3) converted to phospholipids; (4) used to combine with cholesterol, which is synthesized in the liver, to form cholesterol esters; or (5) reesterified to triglycerides and combined with protein, cholesterol, and phospholipids to form lipoproteins. The liver also uses fatty acids released from adipose tissue storage sites for these same processes.

## Production of Bile Salts

Bile production is one of the major functions of the liver. **Bile** is a complex compound composed of cholesterol, phospholipids, bile salts, bile pigments (bilirubin), and very small amounts of proteins and electrolytes. Ninety-seven percent of bile is water. Metabolites of drugs and other substances that need to be excreted may also be found in bile. **Bile salts** are necessary for the absorption of fats, cholesterol, and fat-soluble vitamins, particularly vitamin K. Bile is released from the liver and concentrated and stored in the gallbladder. The liver secretes approximately 700 ml of bile daily. The bile salts released during each meal are reabsorbed into the enterohepatic circulation and recycled two or three times during a meal. Bile is reabsorbed along the total intestinal tract, but the terminal ileum has a major role in its active reabsorption. If the terminal ileum is diseased or resected, reabsorption of bile does not occur and abnormal fat absorption results.

## Bilirubin Metabolism

**Bilirubin** is a byproduct of the *heme* portion of red blood cells and is released when these cells are destroyed. The released bilirubin is not water soluble (unconjugated). Unconjugated bilirubin is carried in the blood bound to albumin and other proteins. The liver extracts the unconjugated bilirubin from the blood and combines it with glucoronide into a water-soluble form (conjugated). The conjugated bilirubin is secreted into the bile and then enters the duodenum. In the GI tract, bilirubin is metabolized to urobilinogen. **Urobilinogen** is excreted in feces as stercobilin, giving feces its brown color, or it is reabsorbed. Most of the reabsorbed urobilinogen is extracted from the blood by the liver and recycled; some is excreted in the urine.

### Detoxification

The liver has a prime role in **detoxification** of endogenous and exogenous substances. Ammonia ($NH_3$) is a major toxic product handled by the liver. Ammonia is produced in the gut and the liver from the deamination of amino acids, that is, the removal of the amino group ($NH_2$) from amino acids. Bacteria in the GI tract are responsible for the ammonia formation in the gut. Peripheral blood ammonia levels are kept very low because the ammonia from the gut is extracted from the enterohepatic circulation by the liver and it, along with the ammonia produced in the liver, is detoxified by conversion into urea, which is then excreted by the kidneys.

Steroid hormones (estrogen, progesterone, testosterone, corticosterone, aldosterone) are inactivated by the liver. Liver diseases may depress this inactivation, resulting in pathologic levels of these hormones.

The liver detoxifies many drugs; all barbiturates (except phenobarbital and barbital) and many sedatives are inactivated by the liver. The status of the liver has an important role in the effectiveness or toxicity of these and other drugs.

### Storage of Minerals and Vitamins

The liver stores reserves of various minerals and vitamins. This storage prevents abnormal internal levels from occurring, although the oral intake may be very irregular. Vitamins A, D, and $B_{12}$ are stored in sufficient quantities to prevent deficiencies for months. Vitamins E and K are also stored. Iron in the form of *ferritin* is stored and can be used to resupply iron for hemoglobin formation as needed; copper is stored as well.

### Blood Reservoir

The liver, because of its tremendous vascular supply and sinusoidal system, can act as a reservoir for blood. When the venous vascular volume becomes greater than can be handled by the right side of the heart, the excess blood can accumulate in the liver.

## PHYSIOLOGIC CHANGES WITH AGING

As the body ages, a decrease occurs in the number and size of hepatic cells, which results in an overall decrease in the size and weight of the liver. In addition, an increase occurs in the formation of fibrous tissue within the liver, resulting in decreased protein synthesis and possible changes in the production of enzymes that assist in the metabolism of drugs, particularly anticonvulsants, psychotropics, and oral anticoagulants. The nurse should be alert to the signs and symptoms of drug toxicity even when the drugs are administered in normal doses because the decreased metabolism in the liver can cause an accumulation of the drug. The common liver function tests are usually normal in elderly persons unless pathology exists.

# SUBJECTIVE DATA

A thorough history is necessary to assess adequately the health status of people with potential dysfunction of the hepatic system. These data assist in identifying immediate nursing needs and providing information necessary for helping patients to live with chronic problems of the hepatic system. The assessment focuses on comfort status; nutritional status; fluid and electrolyte status; elimination patterns; energy level; perception, motion, and cognition; and potential exposure to toxins, as well as general living conditions and life-style.

## COMFORT STATUS

Discomfort resulting from abdominal pain or **pruritus** (itching) may be one of the major problems of people with hepatic dysfunction. The person may complain of continuous upper abdominal discomfort or a dull ache in the upper right quadrant. The discomfort does not usually alter normal functioning, although it can cause ineffective breathing secondary to the abdominal pain. The discomfort is most significant in that it provides verification for the underlying pathologic process. Comfort status may be altered because of the general body aching associated with acute viral infections of the hepatic system. Most distressing to the patient is the pruritus usually associated with **jaundice,** which may cause significant discomfort. The elevated serum bilirubin that occurs with jaundice causes capillary dilation in the skin, which is the source of the pruritus; in addition, bilirubin is an irritating substance to the chemosensitive area of the skin. The history should include an assessment of factors that worsen itching and of measures that help to relieve it.

## NUTRITIONAL STATUS

Persons with hepatic dysfunction often experience alterations in nutritional status. Some hepatic problems result in anorexia, nausea, and vomiting, and the patient should be questioned about the occurrence of such episodes. Assessment should include onset, precipitating factors, association with food or alcohol intake, and measures that provide relief.

Poor nutritional habits and malnutrition resulting from life-style patterns or food intolerances may be present. A useful tool to assess the patient's nutritional status is to ask the patient what he or she has eaten in the past 24 hours and ascertain whether this is the typical eating pattern.

Alcohol use should also be assessed. Weight loss may have been noticed by the patient but can be hidden by water retention. The patient may have noticed changes in muscle mass, even though overall weight may have stayed the same. Also, alcohol, which provides calories but has no nutrient value, may hide the weight loss normally associated with malnutrition.

Persons with chronic problems of the hepatic system often require treatment with special diets, such as low sodium, altered protein intake, water restriction, and so forth. In anticipation of these needs, the history should include information about food intolerances and food preferences.

### FLUID AND ELECTROLYTE STATUS

Hepatic dysfunction can be associated with volume deficit from nausea and vomiting or even from acute bleeding with cirrhosis. Fluid volume excess typically occurs in people with hepatic dysfunction as a result of renal retention of sodium and water that is initiated by peripheral vasodilation. This expansion of the vascular space effectively decreases the circulating blood volume, which results in the release of renin, angiotensin, and aldosterone. These hormones increase sodium and water retention. Another factor causing fluid volume excess is the **hypoalbuminemia** that is associated with liver disease. The hypoalbuminemia decreases the osmotic pressure in the vasculature, causing fluid to leave the vascular space and enter the interstitial space, resulting in edema. Levels of electrolytes, particularly sodium, potassium, hydrogen, and bicarbonate, can be elevated or decreased.

To establish the patient's needs, the history collected should include information about:

1. Normal fluid and food intake and output
2. Abnormal fluid and electrolyte losses, such as vomiting, diarrhea, or bleeding
3. Changes in weight, both losses and gains
4. Occurrence of signs and symptoms of fluid or electrolyte deficit, such as weakness, dizziness, syncope, and weight loss
5. Occurrence of signs and symptoms of fluid or electrolyte excess, such as edema in hands, feet, and legs; an increase in abdominal girth; and weight gain

### ELIMINATION PATTERNS

Intestinal and urinary elimination may be altered in people with liver problems. If there is an obstruction of bile flow, the person may give a history of grayish white stools (sometimes called clay colored) and have dark amber, brown, or mahogany-colored urine. Blood in the urine or stools may also be reported by people with cirrhosis. The nurse can test for occult blood in the urine by using a reagent strip, often referred to as a "dipstick," and test the stool by performing a Hematest or guaiac test. A reported decrease in urine output or the occurrence of nocturia may result from sodium and water retention.

### ENERGY LEVEL

Because of altered nutrient intake, abnormal fluid and electrolyte status, and increased metabolic needs, people with hepatic problems often report an activity intolerance to normal daily activities or simply fatigue. Weakness may be reported, and nursing care should be adjusted to provide for the patient's safety. As the underlying liver condition resolves, the fatigue and weakness may resolve, although the patient and family must understand that the energy level may take a long time to return to normal.

### PERCEPTION, MOTION, AND COGNITION

Chronic health problems of the hepatic system can cause changes in neurologic functioning, particularly in relation to the peripheral nervous system and higher cognitive functions. The patient should be asked about alterations in sensation in extremities, any noticeable changes in memory, episodes of forgetfulness or blackouts, and alterations in coordination or in ability to do fine motor tasks. The *onset* of any alterations, *pattern* of changes (continuous or intermittent), and *duration* of any changes should be determined.

### EXPOSURE TO TOXINS

Hepatic dysfunction can be caused by various agents, such as alcohol, drugs, industrial chemicals, and viruses. A history of exposure to any toxins must be elicited. A *drug and alcohol history* is necessary to determine whether the patient has been exposed to these two toxins. The drug history should focus on prescription, over-the-counter, and street drugs. For example, acetaminophen is a drug often used by adolescents to commit suicide and can cause severe liver damage in doses just 10 times greater than the recommended dose. The liver damage is intensified by the combination of acetaminophen and alcohol. The alcohol history should focus on normal amount of intake and time since last intake. An *occupational history* helps to identify potential toxins in the work environment. An *environmental/social history* might identify potential sources of viruses. (See Box 41-2 for significant sources of contact with the hepatitis viruses.) The environmental/social history also can help identify particular persons, factors, or places associated with substance abuse, if a problem exists. Data about persons, factors, or places associated with substance abuse are needed for long-term management of drug and alcohol abuse (see Chapter 19).

## OBJECTIVE DATA

To assess the functioning of the hepatic system completely, a thorough assessment of the total body is required. First, examination of the overall appearance of patients is necessary. Do they appear chronically or acutely ill? Are they attentive, restless, or lethargic? Do they appear nourished, or malnourished? Is their skin jaundiced? Do they have yellow sclera? In darker-

**BOX 41-2 Health History Necessary to Identify Exposure to Hepatitis Viruses**

Contact with persons with jaundice
Travel or visits to environments with poor sanitation (camping trips, travel to less well-developed countries, and so on)
Ingestion of shellfish or raw fish
History of recent ear piercing or tattooing
History of recent blood transfusions
Intravenous drug abuse (sharing of contaminated needles)
Occupational exposure (health service personnel with frequent blood contact, personnel in day-care centers, personnel in centers of custodial care, and so forth)
History of hemodialysis
History of multiple sex partners; male bisexual or male homosexual life-style

skinned people, are the palms of the hands or soles of the feet jaundiced? Are their oral mucous membranes yellow? Are there any other signs of hepatic dysfunction, such as enlarged abdomen, palmar erythema, change in secondary sexual characteristics, bruises, muscle wasting, or edema?

After the general inspection, the assessment should focus on fluid status. Vital signs, including orthostatic changes, weight, temperature, skin turgor, mucous membrane moisture, presence of edema, and behavior, should be assessed. To assess energy level and nutritional status, the patient's total muscle mass and muscle strength should be examined.

While performing the assessment mentioned previously, the patient's mental status, affect, and alertness should be noted. Note changes in facial expression, responsiveness, level of consciousness, and affect. Are there periods of confusion or disorientation? Is the affect appropriate for this situation? Because handwriting or the ability to draw a box, triangle, or square deteriorates with worsening of liver function, a sample of handwriting or a drawing of a geometric figure may be obtained from the patient.

After a general impression of the total patient is obtained, the assessment should focus on the abdomen. The abdomen is inspected for enlargement, presence of distended or dilated periumbilical veins (caput medusae), and ascites. **Ascites** is characterized by distention of the abdomen with tight, glistening skin, protruding umbilicus, and bulging flanks. Palpation or percussion of the abdomen to ascertain the presence of a fluid wave and shifting dullness, which are indicative of ascites, should be performed. Palpation and percussion are also used to assess for hepatic tenderness, size, and consistency and the presence of hepatic masses. The spleen often is enlarged in the patient with chronic hepatic dysfunction and should be percussed to determine the size and location, but palpation should be deferred because of the fragility of the enlarged spleen. Last, abdominal girth should be measured.

# DIAGNOSTIC TESTS

Various tests help in assessing the status of the hepatic system. Many of the tests require taking samples of blood; other tests are more extensive and may cause discomfort; still others may require fasting. The nurse is responsible for preparing the patient for the tests. The physical preparation of the patient will vary from institution to institution, and the nurse needs to learn the routine preparation. In addition to the physical preparation, the nurse carries out appropriate teaching and monitoring of the patient before, during, and after the diagnostic tests.

## LABORATORY TESTS

Multiple tests may be necessary to determine the extent and seriousness of hepatic disease. Many tests require serial readings to be of benefit. The procedure, special preparation, and interpretation of frequently used blood, stool, and urine studies for evaluation of liver function are summarized in Table 41-1.

## RADIOLOGIC TESTS

Radiographic tests are used to assist in identifying the cause of hepatic dysfunction. Besides the examinations described in the following section, abdominal films, barium swallow, barium enema, and gastroscopy may be ordered. These tests help to identify the presence of pathologic GI conditions that may cause similar signs and symptoms as found in hepatic dysfunction or that may result from complications of hepatic dysfunction.

### Ultrasonography

Ultrasonography of the liver may be done to differentiate between causes of jaundice associated with increased serum bilirubin levels and to identify hepatic metastases, hematomas, and abscesses.

The preparation of the patient for ultrasonography is relatively simple. Usually the patient is not allowed to eat for 8 to 12 hours before the procedure, because bowel gas in the GI tract will interfere with the test. Any residual barium needs to be eliminated from the GI tract before the test. The patient must be well hydrated, because dehydration can decrease the ability of ultrasonography to distinguish between the liver and surrounding tissues. Ultrasound is used intraoperatively to identify hepatic tumors.[1]

### Computed Tomography (CT Scan)

Computed tomography can also be used to assess patients with potential hepatic problems. It is helpful in identifying problems similar to those described for ultrasonography. Contrast medium can be used with the CT scan to intensify the appearance of vascular structures and hepatic parenchyma. The patient should eat nothing for 8 to 12 hours before the test; if contrast medium is to be used, the patient should be assessed for allergies to iodine or contrast media. Adequate hy-

## TABLE 41-1 Laboratory Tests of Liver Function

| FUNCTION AND TEST | PROCEDURE AND PREPARATION | INTERPRETATION |
|---|---|---|
| **Fat metabolism** | | |
| Serum total cholesterol and cholesterol esters | Venipuncture; fasting may be required | Normal level is 140-220 mg/dl of blood; approximately 70% is cholesterol ester; in hepatocellular disease, amount of total serum cholesterol and cholesterol ester may be decreased; in obstructive biliary tract disease, total serum cholesterol is increased, but amount of esterified cholesterol is decreased; normal cholesterol levels rise with age. |
| Serum phospholipids | Venipuncture; no special preparation | Normal level is 150-250 mg/dl; serum phospholipids tend to be low in severe hepatocellular disease and high in obstructive biliary tract disease. |
| **Protein metabolism** | | |
| Total serum protein | Venipuncture; no special preparation | Normal level is 6-8 g/dl; measures all serum protein; may be normal in hepatocellular disease because increased serum globulin will replace decreased serum albumin; increased serum globulin is seen in chronic inflammatory disease, neoplastic diseases, and biliary obstruction. |
| Albumin | Venipuncture; no special preparation | Normal level is 3.4-5.0 g/dl; albumin made only in liver; in hepatocellular disease there may be a decrease in serum albumin level. |
| Protein electrophoresis | Venipuncture; no special preparation; protein fraction of blood will migrate in characteristic directions in electrical field; after separation of fractions, specimen stained, and densitometer used to measure amounts of various serum protein | Normal fractions in relation to total serum protein (100%) are albumin, 52%-68%; α-globulins, 12%-17%; β-globulins, 7%-15%; and immune serum globulins (γ-globulins), 9%-19%; in severe hepatocellular damage, amount of albumin may be decreased; inflammatory processes of the liver may produce increased amounts of $\alpha_1$-globulins, neoplastic disease is associated with increased levels of $\alpha_2$-globulins, and some patients with obstructive biliary tract disease may have high levels of β-globulins. |
| Immunoglobulins | Venipuncture; no special preparation | Five classes of antibodies; IgA, IgG, IgM, IgE, and IgD; IgA and IgG are often increased in the presence of cirrhosis; IgG is elevated in the presence of chronic active hepatitis; biliary cirrhosis and hepatitis A cause an increase in the IgM component. |
| Blood urea nitrogen (BUN) | Venipuncture; no special preparation | Normal is 10-20 mg/dl; in severe hepatocellular disease if portal venous flow is obstructed, level may decrease; varies with dietary protein intake and fluid volume. |
| Serum prothrombin time (PT) | Venipuncture; no special preparation; reflects activity of extrinsic and common coagulation pathways, including prothrombin, fibrinogen, and factors V, VII, IX, and X | Normal PT is 12-15 sec; it is compared with a control level; the normal PT is calculated based on the institution's control and therefore may differ between institutions; PT reflects activity of extrinsic and common coagulation pathways, including prothrombin, fibrinogen, and factors V, VII, IX, and X; PT may be increased in hepatocellular disease because of the inability of liver to produce clotting factors or in obstructive hepatic or biliary tract disease because of the malabsorption of vitamin K; persistence of abnormal PT after parenteral administration of vitamin K indicates hepatocellular damage. May be expressed as International Normalized Ration (INR). |
| Serum partial thromboplastin time (PTT) and activated partial thromboplastin time (APTT) | Venipuncture; no special preparation; reflects activity of intrinsic and common coagulation pathways | Normal PTT is 68-82 sec with standard technique, APTT is 32-46 sec; as with the PT, the normal value may differ between institutions depending on the control used; PTT reflects activity of intrinsic and common coagulation pathways; PTT and APTT will be increased in hepatocellular disease because of the inability of liver to produce clotting factors. |
| Blood ammonia levels | Venipuncture; may require fasting | Normal level is less than 75 μg/dl; may be elevated in severe hepatocellular disease because of obstruction of portal blood flow and rarely because of decreased urea synthesis. |

**TABLE 41-1 Laboratory Tests of Liver Function—cont'd**

| FUNCTION AND TEST | PROCEDURE AND PREPARATION | INTERPRETATION |
|---|---|---|
| Bilirubin metabolism | | |
| Total bilirubin<br>Conjugated (direct)<br>Unconjugated (indirect) | Venipuncture; no special preparation | Total serum bilirubin measures both conjugated and unconjugated bilirubin; normal total serum bilirubin values range from 0.1-1 mg/dl; conjugated bilirubin acts directly with diazo reagents; unconjugated bilirubin requires addition of methyl alcohol; thus the terms *direct* and *indirect;* conjugated bilirubin increases in the presence of hepatocellular or obstructive biliary tract disease; unconjugated bilirubin is elevated in the presence of increased hemolysis of red blood cells or hepatocellular disease. |
| Urine bilirubin | Spot urine specimen; no special preparation | Normally no bilirubin is excreted in urine; urine with abnormal bilirubin is mahogany colored and has a yellow foam when shaken *(foam test);* unconjugated bilirubin even in excess is not excreted in urine because it is not water soluble; conjugated serum bilirubin levels greater than 0.4 mg/dl will lead to conjugated bilirubin being excreted in urine because it is water soluble and indicates hepatocellular or obstructive biliary tract disease; bilirubinuria may be present before jaundice. |
| Urine urobilinogen | 24-hr urine collection or 2-hr afternoon collection | Normally 0.2-1.2 units found in specimen; fresh urine urobilinogen is colorless; decreased amounts of urine urobilinogen found in obstructive biliary tract disease; increased amounts found in hepatocellular disease; alterations in intestinal flora by broad-spectrum antibiotics may change test. |
| Fecal urobilinogen | Stool specimen; no special preparation | Normally 90-280 mg/day; presence of fecal urobilinogen (stercobilin) gives stool brown color; absence of stercobilin causes stools to become clay (grayish white) to white colored; increased amounts of stercobilin found with increased hemolysis of red blood cells; absence of fecal stercobilin indicates obstructive biliary tract disease. |
| Serum enzymes | | |
| Asparate aminotransferase (AST), formerly called serum glutamic-oxaloacetic transaminase (SGOT)<br>Alanine aminotransferase (ALT), formerly called serum glutamic pyruvic transaminase (SGPT)<br>Lactic dehydrogenase (LDH)<br>Gamma-glutamyl transpeptidase (GGT) (γ-glutamyltransferase) | Venipuncture; no special preparation | Normal values vary depending on measurement used; these enzymes are present in hepatic cells; and with necrosis of hepatic cells, enzymes are released and elevated serum levels will be found; GGT is found in high levels in liver cells as well as kidneys; ALT is primarily present in liver cells; AST is also present in high levels in skeletal and heart muscle; LDH is also present in heart cells, kidney cells, skeletal muscle cells, and erythrocytes, but in each tissue the LDH enzyme has a characteristic composition: thus the tissue source of elevated serum LDH levels can be determined by isoenzyme tests; with the other three enzyme tests, necrosis of other organs must be ruled out; GGT is elevated early in liver disease, and elevation persists as long as cellular damage continues; GGT is routinely elevated in alcohol-induced liver disease, and increased levels are often seen before other abnormal test results occur. |
| Alkaline phosphatase | Venipuncture; no special preparation | Normal values vary depending on measurement used; this enzyme originates in liver, bone, intestine, and placenta; alkaline phosphatase is slightly to moderately elevated in hepatocellular disease but extremely elevated in obstructive biliary tract and bone disease. |

*Continued*

**TABLE 41-1 Laboratory Tests of Liver Function—cont'd**

| FUNCTION AND TEST | PROCEDURE AND PREPARATION | INTERPRETATION |
|---|---|---|
| Antigens and antibodies of viral hepatitis | Venipuncture; no special preparation | Normally, no hepatitis antigens are found in the serum or other body fluids; ***hepatitis A virus (HAV)*** can be found in the stool during the last part of the incubation period and early prodromal phase; ***IgM-class anti-HAV*** appears in the acute and early convalescent period and is used to diagnose hepatitis A; ***IgG-class anti-HAV*** becomes detectable during the convalescent period and confers enduring protection; hepatitis B has many associated serum particles; complete ***hepatitis B virus (HBV)*** is also called Dane particle; a ***core antigen*** ($HB_cAg$) can be found in the liver, an ***antibody*** (anti-$HB_c$) can be found in the blood, and the presence of anti-$HB_c$ indicates past infection with HBV at some undefined time; a ***surface antigen*** ($HB_sAg$) and several subtypes and ***antibody*** (anti-$HB_s$) are also measurable; $HB_sAg$, previously called Australia antigen, is one of the antigens measured to diagnose hepatitis B, and its presence indicates infectivity; presence of anti-$HB_s$ indicates past infection and immunity to HBV, presence of passive antibodies from HBIG, or immune response from HBV vaccine; ***hepatitis*** $B_e$ ***antigen*** ($HB_eAg$) indicates high infectivity and its ***antibody*** (anti-$HB_e$) chronic infectivity; enzyme-linked immunosorbent assay (ELISA) has detected antibodies to hepatitis C ***(anti-HCV)*** in people who have been exposed to hepatitis C; however, the antibodies do not appear in most people until at least 5 months after exposure to the virus; an enterically transmitted virus that was previously related to hepatitis non-A non-B has been identified and labeled ***hepatitis E (HEV); anti-HEV*** has been detected using ELISA but is not available in the United States at this time.[2,3] |

dration is necessary when a contrast medium is used. Barium studies should be done at least 4 days before the CT scan or after the scan because the barium can interfere with test results.

## Radionuclide Imaging

The liver may be outlined by radionuclide imaging techniques. Selected radioisotopes are given intravenously. After the injection of the radioisotope, the patient is placed supine, and a scintillation detector is passed over the abdomen in the area of the liver. The radiation coming from the isotopes immediately beneath the probe of the scanner is detected, amplified, and recorded. Scanning helps to differentiate nonfunctioning areas from normal tissue and helps to identify hepatic tumors, cysts, and abscesses. Usually a nonfunctioning area will appear as an area of decreased activity. However, gallium-67 ($^{67}$Ga) is preferentially taken up by hepatocellular carcinomas and abscesses, and these areas will appear as areas of very heavy radioactivity. Adverse reactions to the radioisotopes used for radionuclide imaging are unusual, and the procedure is relatively safe. Discomfort is minimal and is related to the intravenous injection and the position on the x-ray table. Only small amounts of radioactive material are given, and radiation precautions are *not* necessary. Except for $^{67}$Ga scanning, no special preparation is required. Gallium-67 is excreted by the GI tract. To avoid absorption of the radioisotope by the GI contents, cleansing of the bowel with laxatives and enemas is prescribed. The exact preparation will vary from institution to institution. The toilet should be flushed twice for bowel movements after the $^{67}$Ga scanning to ensure the safety of the patient and others. Radionuclide imaging is being used less than other tests such as CT scan or ultrasonography in patients with potential hepatic dysfunction.[1]

## Angiography and Portal Pressure Measurements

Catheterization of the hepatic artery, portal venous system (by various routes), and the hepatic vein allows the injection of a contrast medium and the visualization of the vascular supply of the hepatic system. The patency of the system and the presence of tumors, abscesses, collateral circulation, varices, and bleeding may be determined by use of angiography.

Portal and hepatic vein pressure (wedged hepatic vein pressure [WHVP]) can be measured. These readings may be done in conjunction with angiography or as a separate study. These measurements help in determining the degree of portal hypertension.

The presence of allergy to contrast media must be ascertained before angiography is done. After both angiography and pressure readings, the site of insertion is observed for bleeding, and the patient's vital signs are checked frequently (such as every 15 minutes for 1 hour, every 30 minutes for 1 hour, every hour for 4 hours, and then if the patient is stable, every 4 hours). The patient is kept on bedrest for 24 to 48 hours.

### Magnetic Resonance Imaging

Magnetic resonance imaging (MRI) is sometimes used to detect liver tumors. Because magnetic fields are used instead of radioactive isotopes to produce the image, no special preparation of the patient is necessary. It is important to inform the patient that this test is painless. The patient should be instructed to remove any jewelry, dentures and partial dentures if they contain metal, or any other item that contains metal, such as hairpins or limb prostheses.

## SPECIAL TESTS

### Biopsy of the Liver

A biopsy of the liver may be used to aid in establishing the cause of liver disease. In this procedure a specially designed needle is inserted through the chest or abdominal wall into the liver, and a small piece of tissue is removed for study. This procedure is contraindicated in a patient who has an infection of the right lower lobe of the lung, ascites, a blood dyscrasia, or a problem with blood clotting, as well as in any patient unable to cooperate by holding his or her breath. To avoid hemorrhage, vitamin K may be given parenterally for several days before and after the biopsy is taken. A biopsy usually is not done if the prothrombin time is below 40%. The physician should explain the procedure to the patient; for example, the importance of being able to hold one's breath and remain absolutely still when the needle is introduced. Movement of the chest may cause the needle to slip and to tear the liver covering. Most hospitals require that the patient sign a written permission form for the procedure to be done. Food and fluids may be withheld for several hours preceding the test, and a sedative usually is given about 30 minutes before the biopsy.

A **liver biopsy** is performed as follows. The patient lies supine; the skin over the area selected (usually the eighth or ninth intercostal space) is cleansed and anesthetized with procaine hydrochloride. A nick is made in the skin with a sharp scalpel blade. Then the patient is instructed to take several deep breaths and then to hold his or her breath while the needle is introduced through the intercostal or subcostal tissues into the liver. The special needle assembly is rotated to separate a fragment of tissue and then is withdrawn. The specimen is placed into an appropriate container, which is labeled and sent to the pathology laboratory. A simple dressing is placed over the wound.

The dangers of liver biopsy, which is done relatively "blind," are accidental penetration of blood vessels, causing hemorrhage, or accidental penetration of a biliary canniculi, causing a chemical peritonitis from leakage of bile into the abdominal cavity. After the procedure the nurse should assess the patient for signs of hypovolemia and shock. The patient's pulse and blood pressure should be monitored every 30 minutes for the first few hours after the procedure and then hourly for 24 hours. The patient's temperature should be taken at least every 4 hours to determine a baseline and detect peritonitis. The physician may order pressure applied to the biopsy site to help stop any bleeding. An effective way to apply pressure is to have the patient lie on the right side with a small pillow or folded bath blanket placed under the costal margin for several hours after the biopsy. Bedrest is maintained for 24 hours after the test.

### Paracentesis

A **paracentesis,** or peritoneal tap, can be done to remove peritoneal fluid (ascitic fluid) for cytology or other laboratory studies or to drain large volumes of ascitic fluid. When such conditions as respiratory distress, severe abdominal discomfort, or cardiac dysfunction, are present because of the ascites, a paracentesis may be necessary. It is important to note that repeated paracenteses are not the treatment of choice for controlling chronic, recurring ascites because of complications.

When paracentesis is performed, the skin is cleansed and the abdominal wall anesthetized. A long, aspiration needle is inserted, and fluid is aspirated for diagnostic tests or drained as necessary. In preparation for the procedure, the patient is given a complete explanation, a consent form is signed, and the patient should void immediately before the procedure to diminish the risk of puncturing the bladder. Sterile technique must be maintained during the procedure.

The complications of paracentesis include peritonitis, if sterility is not maintained, and peritoneal bleeding resulting from trauma to blood vessels. The patient's vital signs, including temperature, urine output, and skin temperature and moisture, should be monitored for signs of peritonitis or bleeding. The patient's abdomen should be assessed for rigidity and his or her sensorium for confusion.

Removal of large amounts of fluid from the peritoneal space can result in hypovolemia and shock because additional fluid can shift from the intravascular compartment into the peritoneal cavity, although this risk is minimal in the patient with cirrhosis and edema. Other substances that are lost with removal of large amounts of ascitic fluid are protein and potassium. Postprocedural monitoring of vital signs, mental status, urine output, skin temperature and moisture, mucous membrane moisture, and so forth should be instituted to monitor for hypovolemia. Laboratory studies should be monitored to determine whether protein and potassium levels are normal.

### Peritoneal Lavage

Peritoneal lavage may be used to assess damage to the liver from abdominal trauma in persons with altered states of consciousness who cannot give a satisfactory history. It may also be used in patients with abdominal trauma when unexplained hypotension is present, when unreliable physical examination results are present, or when the patient requires general anesthesia for other injuries.

Peritoneal lavage can be done by either the closed or open method. In the *closed method,* a peritoneal dialysis catheter is inserted, and the peritoneal space is aspirated for gross blood. If no gross blood is found, lavage is carried out with normal saline. In the *open method* the peritoneum is exposed completely and then opened enough to allow entry of a dialysis catheter. Again, gross blood is aspirated first, and if no blood is found, lavage is carried out.

Peritoneal lavage requires a complete explanation to the patient and significant others and informed consent. A nasogastric tube and Foley catheter are inserted before the procedure to prevent penetration of the intestines or bladder. In the closed method a local anesthetic is used, whereas in the open method general anesthesia is necessary. Postprocedural care involves monitoring for peritonitis and bleeding in patients who have closed peritoneal lavage. Patients who have open peritoneal lavage require general postanesthetic care (see Chapter 25).

## ENDOSCOPY

The hepatic system and gallbladder can be examined by several types of endoscopic procedures. The endoscope can be inserted directly through the peritoneum (peritoneoscopy), thus affording direct visualization of the abdominal organs and the taking of biopsies. An esophagoscopy or gastroscopy may be done to visualize esophageal varices or injection sclerotherapy. An **endoscopic retrograde cholangiopancreatography (ERCP)** can be done to visualize and provide radiographic examination of the liver, gallbladder, and the pancreas. All these procedures require that the patient be fasting at least 12 hours before the test. Before ERCP the patient should be asked about allergies or sensitivities to x-ray dye.

After the procedure, the nurse should assess the patient's ability to swallow. The patient's gag reflex may not return for 1 to 2 hours. After ERCP, the patient should be monitored for signs of complications, which include perforation, sepsis, and pancreatitis. Vital signs are usually taken every 30 minutes for several hours and then hourly for 4 hours. Preprocedural and postprocedural sedation may be given.[4,5]

## CRITICAL THINKING ACTIVITIES

- Explain what kinds of data or methods of inquiry you would use in the process of distinguishing between hemolytic jaundice, hepatocellular jaundice, and obstructive jaundice.
- Outline social, personal, and lifestyle factors that are significant to assessment of the individual with suspected liver dysfunction.
- A 72-year-old male patient who is scheduled for a liver scan is fearful of radiation exposure. How would you alleviate his fears?

## CHAPTER SUMMARY

### ANATOMY AND PHYSIOLOGY

- The liver is important for adequate energy production and waste disposal.

### SUBJECTIVE DATA

- Pathophysiologic conditions of the liver result in discomfort, inadequate nutrition, fluid and electrolyte deficit or excess, bleeding, altered elimination, fatigue, and altered perception, cognitive, and motor functioning.

### OBJECTIVE DATA

- Pathophysiologic conditions of the liver can result from exposure to various toxins, including drugs, alcohol, chemicals, and viruses.

### DIAGNOSTIC TESTS

- Liver dysfunction results in multiple abnormalities in blood studies, which are used to help identify the pathophysiologic state or other nursing needs.
- Radiologic, endoscopic, and other invasive tests are used to help in identifying the exact pathophysiologic condition. These tests all require special preparation and postprocedural care.

## REFERENCES


1. Clouse ME: Current diagnostic imaging modalities of the liver, *Surg Clin North Am* 69(2):193-234, 1989.
2. Gurevich I: Enterically transmitted viral hepatitis: etiology, epidemiology, and prevention, *Heart Lung* 22(4):370-372, 1993.
3. McMillan-Jackson M, Rymer TE: Viral hepatitis: anatomy of a diagnosis, *Am J Nurs* 94(1):43-48, 1994.
4. Renkes J: GI endoscopy: managing the full scope of care, *Nursing '93,* 23(6):50-55, 1993.
5. Wilkinson M: Nursing implications after endoscopic retrograde cholangiopancreatography, *Gastroenterol Nurs* 13(2):105-109, 1990.

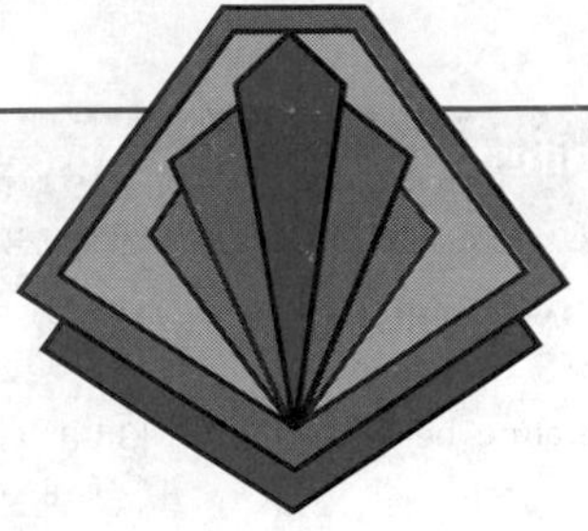

C H A P T E R 42

# Management of Persons With Problems of the Hepatic System

***Debera Jane Thomas***
***Virginia L. Cassmeyer***

## CHAPTER OBJECTIVES

***After studying this chapter, the learner should be able to do the following:***

1. Describe the medical and nursing care needs of patients with liver abscesses, tumors, and trauma.
2. Contrast the differences between pathophysiology and signs and symptoms of focal liver disease and diffuse hepatocellular liver disorders.
3. Differentiate between toxic and viral hepatitis.
4. Differentiate between hepatitis A, B, C, D, and E.
5. Describe the pathophysiologic basis of the clinical manifestations in cirrhosis and the complications of cirrhosis.
6. Develop a plan of care for patients with viral or toxic hepatitis or cirrhosis.
7. Describe the common medical and nursing needs of a patient with ascites, esophageal varices, portal-systemic encephalopathy, or hepatorenal syndrome.

## KEY TERMS

amebic abscess
ascites
cirrhosis
diffuse hepatocellular disorder
esophageal varices
esophagoscopy
extrahepatic obstruction
focal hepatocellular disorders
hepatic arterial infusion
hepatic resection
hepatitis
hepatitis A
hepatitis B
hepatitis C
hepatitis D
hepatitis E
hepatoma
hepatorenal syndrome
hepatotoxin
injection sclerotherapy
intrahepatic cholestasis
jaundice
Laënnec's cirrhosis
liver abscess
peritoneal venous shunt
peritonitis
portal hypertension
portal-systemic encephalopathy (PSE)
postnecrotic cirrhosis
pyogenic abscess
toxic hepatitis
transjugular intrahepatic portosystemic shunt (TIPS)
viral hepatitis

The liver, or hepatic system, is affected by a variety of disorders that produce many physiologic and psychosocial needs for patients, as well as many nursing care challenges. Some patients with liver problems are critically ill and will require intensive care nursing; some problems of the liver are chronic in nature and require nursing care that helps the patient make the changes necessary to control the problem and prevent its progression. Patients with chronic problems often have acute exacerbations, so there will be periods in which intensive, total care is required; as stabilization of the alteration occurs, emphasis on regaining self-management skills is required.

Severe liver problems can result from a variety of causes such as infective organisms, neoplastic growths, toxic agents, and trauma. The pathologic states that result can be classified in several ways. In this chapter, disorders are classified as **focal hepatocellular dis-**

**BOX 42-1 Common Liver Disorders**

FOCAL HEPATOCELLULAR DISORDERS

1. Abscess of the liver
2. Trauma to the liver
3. Tumors of the liver

DIFFUSE HEPATOCELLULAR DISORDERS

1. Hepatitis
2. Cirrhosis
3. Sequelae of chronic diffuse hepatocellular disorders
   a. Portal hypertension
   b. Ascites
   c. Esophageal varices
   d. Portal-systemic encephalopathy
   e. Hepatorenal syndrome

**BOX 42-2 Clinical Manifestations of Liver Abscess**

SIGNS AND SYMPTOMS RESULTING FROM INFECTIOUS PROCESS

Fever and chills (temperature between 102° F [38.8° C] and 106° F [41.1° C])
Cough
Diaphoresis
Difficulty breathing
Abnormal breath sounds from pleural involvement
Right upper quadrant abdominal pain and tenderness
Anorexia
Nausea and vomiting
Signs and symptoms of peritonitis (see Box 42-3)

SIGNS AND SYMPTOMS RESULTING FROM HEPATIC DYSFUNCTION

Hepatomegaly
Jaundice and pruritus
Splenomegaly
Abdominal distention and ascites

**orders** (localized to one portion of the liver) and **diffuse hepatocellular disorders** (spread through a major portion of the liver) (Box 42-1).

## FOCAL HEPATOCELLULAR DISORDERS

Three of the more common focal hepatocellular disorders are discussed next.

### LIVER ABSCESS

#### Etiology

**Liver abscesses** may result from a variety of organisms, including *Escherichia coli, Staphylococcus, Streptococcus, Pseudomonas, Proteus,* and *Klebsiella.* In patients with depressed immune functioning, such as those with neutropenia or leukemia, systemic candidiases with multiple hepatic abscesses have been found. Many people with abscesses have multiple bacteria involved.[18] *Entamoeba histolytica* is an important worldwide cause of amebic liver abscess and dysentery.

#### Epidemiology

Liver abscess is an uncommon disorder in the United States but is associated with a high mortality. Amebic liver abscess is relatively common worldwide, particularly in countries in tropical and subtropical climates, although it is found in temperate regions of the United States and in people who have traveled in tropical climates.

#### Pathophysiology

**Pyogenic abscesses** can occur as either a singular large abscess or multiple small and/or microscopic abscesses. Amebic liver abscesses are typically large and singular.

Liver abscesses are usually a secondary site of infection. Pyogenic organisms originating in various areas of the body reach the liver through the biliary, vascular, or lymphatic systems. In addition, pyogenic organisms may be introduced by penetrating injuries to the liver or by direct continuous extension. In amebic abscesses, the vegetative form of the organism moves from the gut to the small portal vessels and into the hepatic tissue, where it becomes activated. The organisms cause necrosis of the liver tissue and abscess formation.

The abscess formation may disrupt hepatic function, but most of the altered physiologic function is caused by the presence of an acute infective process. If liver abscesses are not identified, they continue to increase in size and can perforate into the pleural cavity, the peritoneal cavity, or the pericardial cavity. The major manifestations of liver abscess are caused by the infection rather than by changes in hepatic functioning. The person usually has history of not feeling well for several weeks. Common clinical manifestations are listed in Box 42-2.

The patient with *pyogenic abscesses,* particularly multiple small or microscopic abscesses, may have clinical manifestations of sepsis and septic shock. The patient with **amebic abscesses** may have signs and symptoms of intestinal amebiasis or give a history of previous intestinal signs and symptoms such as bloody, mucoid diarrhea; generalized abdominal pain; rectal tenesmus; dehydration; and hypotension. However, many patients with amebic abscess report no previous history of intestinal signs and symptoms.

**Diagnostic test results**

Diagnostic tests usually reveal leukocytosis and elevated erythrocyte sedimentation rate due to the infection and moderate elevation of serum alkaline phosphatase and minimal elevation of serum transaminases (AST, ALT) from liver cell damage. Hyperbilirubinemia and hypoalbuminemia result from impaired liver function. In amebic liver abscesses, serologic laboratory tests such as immunoglobulins against antigens, indirect hemagglutination (IHA) titers, complement fixation tests, and latex agglutination tests are highly diagnostic for amebic infection. Hepatic radioisotope scans, ultrasonic scanning, and computed tomography (CT) scans also are used in diagnosis and follow-up evaluation and reveal the presence of abscesses.

### Medical Management

The medical management for the patient with liver abscesses includes the following:

1. Supportive measures—fluid and electrolyte replacement and control of temperature elevation.
2. Surgical drainage of the abscess and antimicrobial therapy for pyogenic abscesses.
3. Metronidazole (Flagyl), chloroquine, and dehydroemetine, or emetine for amebic abscesses. Needle aspiration or surgical drainage of amebic abscesses is only indicated in select patients because these abscesses respond very well to medication alone.

## NURSING MANAGEMENT

### ♦ NURSING DIAGNOSES

Nursing diagnoses are determined from assessment of patient data. Nursing diagnoses for the person with liver abscess may include but are not limited to the following:

| Diagnostic Title | Possible Etiologic Factors |
|---|---|
| Fluid volume deficit | Fever, nausea and vomiting, diaphoresis, decreased intake |
| Pain | Stretching of liver capsule, muscle aches with febrile illness, pruritus associated with jaundice |
| Nutrition, altered: less than body requirements | Anorexia and increased metabolic needs |
| Knowledge deficit: immediate needs and long-term needs | New disease and no previous exposure to information |

### ♦ INTERVENTIONS

Nursing management is directed toward assisting with (1) fluid and nutritional deficits, (2) the control of discomfort including dealing with pruritus if jaundice is present (see p. 1376), (3) the medical regimen (diagnostic tests and therapeutic measure), and (4) helping the patient attain appropriate knowledge for self-management. In the very acute situation, nursing management may incorporate the care needs described for a patient with sepsis and septic shock (see Chapter 22) or severe intestinal colitis, appendicitis, and megacolon (see Chapter 47). The first priority of care is to help with treatment of fluid volume deficit or shock, if present. The next priority is to provide comfort measures. The high temperature, episodes of chills and diaphoresis, pruritus, anorexia, and abdominal pain all cause discomfort. During periods of chills, adequate blankets to provide comfort without increasing temperature will be necessary. Cool sponge baths may help lower the temperature. The gown and bed linens should be changed if the patient is diaphoretic. Pruritus can be controlled with cool sponge baths, use of soft linens, prevention of dry skin, and cool environmental temperatures.

Another aspect of care is to provide adequate fluids and nutrition. At first the patient may only tolerate intravenous (IV) fluids or at least need IV fluids to replace deficits. The effectiveness of these measures is evaluated by monitoring the patient's daily weight and skin turgor and assessing laboratory values for hemoconcentration or dilution. Food should be given in small amounts, and the patient's preference should be incorporated to help overcome anorexia. Frequent oral hygiene (at least once every 8 hours) is necessary because fever and fluid loss cause drying of the mucous membranes and may worsen anorexia. The environment should be clean, free of odors, and relaxed.

In assisting with the medical regimen, the nurse is primarily involved with preparing patients physically for tests (instituting nothing by mouth status or other preparations as necessary, as described in Chapter 41 for specific test). The patient also needs appropriate education about the various tests (what will be done, purpose of test, and special care necessary as described in Chapter 41). The nurse is involved in preparing those patients having surgical drainage of abscesses for surgery and providing appropriate postoperative care similar to that needed by any patient (see Chapter 25). The nurse also is involved in administering the prescribed antimicrobials and amebicidal agents. This involves not only appropriate administration, but also monitoring for side effects.

Patient education for long-term care is also a major nursing responsibility. For some patients with liver abscesses, the medication may need to be taken for some time (several weeks to several months). The patient must be instructed about the importance of continual adherence to the medication regimen. In addition, the patient should be instructed to report immediately any signs and symptoms of recurrence of infection (recurring chills, fever, diaphoresis), of spread of infection (worsening abdominal pain, increased difficulty breathing), or of deteriorating liver function (e.g., jaundice, ascites), as well as any side effects of the medication. Instructions about the need for continual follow-up should be emphasized.

### Discharge Teaching

For the person with amebic abscesses, prevention of recurrence is important. The nurse should help the patient identify potentially contaminated sources of food and water and help to identify ways to decontaminate or avoid these sources, such as using iodine-releasing tablets in water and scalding of vegetables or not eating peelings of fresh fruits.

## LIVER TRAUMA

### Etiology/Epidemiology

Because of its location and size, the liver is frequently subjected to trauma, which may be either penetrating (gunshot wounds, stab wounds) or blunt (collision with steering wheel during automobile accidents, falls). If the injury is severe, rupture of the liver may occur, with severe internal hemorrhage.

### Pathophysiology

The pathophysiology seen varies with the types of injury. Liver injuries are graded on a scale of one to five.[14] In grade one, there is laceration and capsular tear with minimal damage to the parenchyma. In grades two through five, there is increasing parenchymal damage with fractures of the liver. In grade five, the damage extends into the retrohepatic vasculature. The liver is a highly vascular organ, receiving 25% of the cardiac output, and severe hemorrhage that results in hypovolemic shock may occur. Stab wounds often make a relatively superficial incision and may do no more damage than a needle biopsy of the liver. Gunshot wounds and blunt trauma often result in significant hemorrhage that results in hypotension or shock and leakage of bile from the biliary canniculi. Hypovolemic shock may occur. If the peritoneal cavity has been contaminated by blood or bile, **peritonitis** occurs (Box 42-3). Less severe blunt trauma may result in subcapsular hematoma only.

Late complications of liver trauma may include the following:

1. Severe hemorrhage, resulting from disseminated intravascular coagulation that often accompanies shock during the total course of treatment
2. Degeneration and sloughing of segments of the liver that have had disruption in circulation with resultant hemorrhage
3. Intrahepatic abscess formation
4. Traumatic hepatic cyst formation
5. Infections of other areas of body following hepatic trauma
6. Subphrenic abscess formation
7. Biliary fistulas

The mortality for liver trauma has decreased over the years. The mortality depends on the type of injury (highest for blunt trauma because of the larger portion of liver damaged and because of other associated injuries), the severity of the injury (highest for those requiring resection of a large amount of liver), and the presence of associated injuries (increasing mortality with each additional injury to another organ).

The manifestations of liver trauma vary with type of injury (Box 42-4). If peritoneal contamination from hemorrhage or bile has occurred, signs and symptoms of peritonitis may be present (see Box 42-3).

#### Diagnostic test results

In some instances, the only sign of hepatic trauma is the presence of blood in peritoneal lavage (see Chapter 28) for a description of this test). Laboratory studies may reveal a decreasing hematocrit and hemoglobin from blood loss and leukocytoses from peritoneal infection and inflammation.

### Medical Management

The immediate medical management for patients with suspected liver trauma is the same as that for any patient with intraabdominal trauma and includes the following:

1. Maintenance of airway
2. IV therapy
3. Type and crossmatch for blood replacement
4. Venipuncture for laboratory tests
5. Urine output monitoring
6. Mean arterial pressure monitoring
7. Treatment of shock with fluids, dextran, and blood components (see Chapter 22)
8. Immediate surgical exploration of the abdomen to detect the presence of abdominal hemorrhage, trauma to liver or other organs, presence of necrotic tissue, or presence of bile drainage
9. Treatment of peritonitis

### Nursing Management

The *first* major nursing focus for the patient with suspected liver trauma is to establish and implement a sys-

**BOX 42-3 Signs and Symptoms of Peritonitis**

Abdominal tenderness
Rebound tenderness
Muscle rigidity or spasms
Decreased or absent bowel signs
Sometimes a fluid wave is present

**BOX 42-4 Clinical Manifestations of Liver Trauma**

SIGNS OF SHOCK
Pale, cool, clammy skin
Diaphoresis
Hypotension
Tachycardia
Mental confusion

PENETRATING TRAUMA
Entry and sometimes exit wounds

BLUNT TRAUMA
Abdominal pain exaggerated by breathing
Shoulder pain indicating diaphragmatic irritation

tem of assessment that focuses on cardiovascular and volume status, neurologic status, and signs and symptoms of peritonitis (see the Guidelines box below). This assessment is required from the moment the patient is first seen through the postoperative period.

The *second* major focus for the nurse is to assist with the initiation of monitoring devices such as the Foley catheter and Dynamap (mean arterial pressure monitor), administration of fluids and blood, and collection of specimens for laboratory tests. The nurse should anticipate the possibility of surgery and prepare the patient for this procedure.

The *third* major nursing focus is to help the patient and family control their fear and anxiety by using simple explanations of all activities and maintaining a calm environment. Continuity of care is essential to minimizing fear and anxiety.

The *fourth* major nursing focus is to provide information and support for the patient's family or significant others. A specific time should be set aside for the family and significant others to ask questions and verbalize their fears. Spiritual support is extremely important to many patients and their families and should be considered when planning care.

After the acute/critical period, which includes the postoperative period for some patients, continual monitoring as already described plus provision of emotional support for the patient and family are still needed. The patient will also need help with self-care, gradual increase in activity, and comfort measures. Over the long term, the patient needs to be able to do self-monitoring for signs and symptoms of residual liver damage that result from a decrease in the normal function of the liver and to be aware of the importance of continual follow-up for several months.

## LIVER TUMORS

Liver neoplasms or tumors may be either benign or malignant. Benign lesions include hemangioma, cysts, and, rarely, adenoma. Most benign tumors are asymptomatic, but occasionally they enlarge enough to become symptomatic. If they become symptomatic, surgical intervention may be required. The care would be the same as that described later for the patient having surgical resection for malignant neoplasms. The focus of this section is malignant neoplasms.

**Guidelines for Assessing the Person With Suspected Liver Trauma**

- Vital signs every 15 minutes (blood pressure, pulse)
- Mean arterial pressure every hour
- Other hemodynamic monitoring, such as intraarterial pressure monitoring and cardiac output measurements, as ordered
- Urine output and other fluid losses documented hourly
- Intake documented hourly
- Serum and urinary electrolytes and osmolality at least daily
- Hematocrit and hemoglobin daily
- Neurologic checks for responsiveness and motion every hour
- Consciousness monitored every hour using Glasgow Coma Scale
- Respiratory status (rate, breath sounds, blood gases)
- Skin temperature, color, and moisture every hour
- Bowel sounds, pain, abdominal tenderness

### Etiology

Malignant tumors are either primary or metastatic. Because the liver is a highly vascular organ, it is a common site for metastatic cancer spread from the gastrointestinal (GI) tract, the lungs, the breasts, the kidneys, and malignant melanomas. Primary liver tumors arise in the liver cell (hepatocellular) or the bile duct cell (cholangiocellular), or they can be of mixed origin. The incidence of primary liver cancer is increased in people with chronic liver disease.

### Epidemiology

Hepatocellular tumors **(hepatomas)** are the most common type of primary liver cancer but account for only 1% to 2% of malignant tumors found at death in the United States. Primary liver cancer is one of the most common malignancies in other parts of the world, particularly in Africa. This geographic difference in incidence probably results from the prevalence of chronic liver disease from hepatitis B and nutritional deficiencies in other countries. Metastatic liver tumors occur 20 times more frequently than primary tumors and rank second only to cirrhosis as a cause of fatal liver disease in the United States.

### Pathophysiology

Primary tumors arise from liver cells or bile ducts or from both. The lesions are multiple or singular, diffuse or nodular, and may spread to only a lobe or to the entire liver. The cancerous cells compress the surrounding normal liver cells and spread by invading the portal vein branches. Some cells infiltrate the gallbladder, mesentery, peritoneum, and diaphragm by direct extension. Primary cancers also tend to cause hemorrhage by extension into the vascular tissue of the liver and necrosis by depriving normal hepatic tissue of adequate circulation. The most common site for metastasis of the primary liver lesion is the lung, but it can also metastasize to the adrenal glands, spleen, vertebrae, kidney, ovary, or pancreas. Primary lesions grow rapidly, sometimes without signs or symptoms, and often the patient lives only a short time after the diagnosis.

Metastatic carcinoma of the liver varies from a few small nodules to large nodules. Adjacent nodules may eventually go together and compress the surrounding liver tissue. Usually different parts of the liver are uniformly involved; thus liver biopsy may be a useful diagnostic aid.

The signs and symptoms of liver cancer depend on

**BOX 42-5 Clinical Manifestations of Liver Cancer**

**EARLY SIGNS**
Right upper quadrant mass
Epigastric fullness
Pain
Fatigue
Weight loss
Changes in liver function tests

**LATER SIGNS**
Fatigue
Ascites
Liver failure
Fever
Hepatic bruits
Jaundice
Variceal bleeding
Portal-systemic encephalopathy (PSE)

**METASTATIC LIVER TUMORS**
Fatigue
Anorexia
Weakness
Weight loss followed by weight gain resulting from ascites
Hepatomegaly
Hepatic bruits
Jaundice
PSE

the size and extent of the tumor, the amount of hepatocellular damage, and the presence of liver failure. Box 42-5 lists clinical manifestations of liver cancer.

#### Diagnostic tests

Diagnostic tests include blood studies, radioisotope scans, MRI, liver biopsy, ultrasonography, and CT scans. The blood studies may show increased erythrocyte sedimentation rate associated with generalized inflammation of the liver, anemia resulting from increased metabolism and decreased food intake, hyperbilirubinemia, elevated alkaline phosphatase, aspartate aminotransferase (AST), and alanine aminotransferase (ALT), decreased blood glucose, and hypoalbuminemia. The number of abnormalities depends on the severity of hepatocellular damage. A special test that is used to help diagnose primary liver carcinoma is serum concentrations of alpha-fetoprotein (AFP). AFP in concentrations of 500 ng/ml to 5 mg/ml is found in up to 70% of patients with hepatocellular cancer. It is also found in a small percentage of patients with metastatic carcinoma or viral hepatitis, but rarely at the same high levels. High levels that occur in any adult without obvious GI tract tumors strongly suggest primary liver cancer. Radioisotope and CT scans and ultrasonography may reveal lesions in the liver. A liver biopsy is necessary for definitive diagnosis of cancer.

### Medical Management

The goal for discharge of patients with hepatic cancer as determined by diagnosis-related groups (DRGs) is 6 days (medical treatment) or 15 days (surgical treatment). The nurse works collaboratively with the physician for implementation of prescribed medical therapy. Because the nurse has a major role in discharge planning and patient teaching, these are discussed under nursing management.

For many primary or metastatic tumors, no medical and surgical treatment exists, because the lesion is too far advanced at the time of diagnosis. Treatment is supportive and similar to that used in cirrhosis.

#### Medication

Chemotherapy has been used to induce regression of primary and metastatic tumor growth. Chemotherapeutic agents have been given systemically or by infusion into the hepatic artery. Theoretically, arterial infusion allows more drug to be delivered directly to the tumor and decreases systemic side effects. Regional chemotherapy results have been promising. 5-Fluorouracil (5-FU), 5-fluorodeoxyuridine (FUDR), and doxorubicin are agents that have been used in combination with radiation. Doxorubicin, 5-FU, methyl CCNU, carmustine, streptozotocin, and mitomycin have been given systemically alone or in combination. 5-FU and FUDR are the drugs most frequently given by hepatic artery infusion.

#### Treatment

Radiation therapy may be used to control pain. It does not prolong survival. Immunoradiotherapy, which combines specific immunoglobulins directed toward an antigen of a primary hepatic tumor with an isotope for therapeutic radiation, is being tested experimentally and clinically. The primary hepatic tumor has two antigens, ferritin and alpha-fetoprotein, for immunoradiotherapy targeting.[16] Hepatic dearterialization, which decreases the oxygen delivered to the tumor, can decrease tumor mass and may help control pain.[6]

#### Diet

There is no special diet unless signs and symptoms of cirrhosis occur.

#### Activity

Activity as tolerated is encouraged.

#### Referral/Consultation

In some settings the nurse assumes responsibility for making referrals to other services. Common referrals for patients with hepatic tumors include social services, cancer support groups, and cancer specialists.

### Surgical Management

For solitary primary tumors and some metastatic solitary tumors, surgery may be performed. The remarkable regenerative capacity of the liver permits resection of as much as 90% of it. Nursing management of the patient with a hepatic resection is discussed next. Orthotopic transplantation (removal of recipient's liver and replacement with a graft liver) have been performed for patients with primary liver tumors with varying success. Liver transplantation is discussed in Chapter 72.

## NURSING MANAGEMENT

The nursing management of the patient with hepatic tumors is guided by nursing diagnoses.

### ♦ NURSING DIAGNOSES

Nursing diagnoses are determined from assessment of patient data. Nursing diagnoses for the person with hepatic tumors may include but are not limited to the following:

| Diagnostic Title | Possible Etiologic Factors |
|---|---|
| Pain | Stretching of liver capsule by growth of tumor, metastasis to other body areas |
| Fear | Diagnosis of cancer |
| Anxiety | Uncertain outcome of tests, prognosis |
| Injury, high risk for | Altered hepatic function |
| Coping, ineffective (individual) | Situational crisis |
| Fluid volume excess | Compromised regulatory mechanisms from ascites |
| Nutrition, altered: less than body requirements | Increased metabolic needs with decreased intake |
| Home maintenance management, impaired | Fatigue and weakness associated with cancer and treatment or progression of disease |
| Greiving, anticipatory | Poor prognosis |
| Self-esteem disturbance | Change in role and appearance, the illness |
| Knowledge deficit: diagnostic tests, treatment, expected outcomes | New information with no previous exposure to information |

### ♦ INTERVENTIONS

The nursing management of patients with hepatic tumors varies, depending on the stage of the illness and the treatment modalities being used. All patients need help coping with the anxiety and fear associated with the diagnosis of cancer and require education regarding diagnostic tests and treatment. In addition, the patient and significant others may need assistance in dealing with the psychosocial and physiologic alterations associated with cancer, such as grieving, changes in home maintenance management, changes in self-esteem, pain, and alteration in nutrition (see Chapter 16).

When no surgical or medical treatment is possible, the care is directed toward the needs arising from the diagnosis of cancer, as listed previously. Other interventions are needed to manage physiologic changes that occur as liver failure progresses, such as fluid volume excess, alteration in thought processes, and pain associated with pruritus. Interventions for these needs associated with liver failure are discussed in detail on pp. 1388-1411.

### Care of the Patient Having Hepatic Resection

#### Preoperative care

For the patient having surgical resection of a hepatic tumor **(hepatic resection)**, skilled preoperative and postoperative care is necessary. Preoperative teaching about the preoperative preparation, the procedure itself, and postoperative care is needed. The patient may need vitamin K for defects in clotting factors, as well as other vitamins if deficits are present. Preparation of the bowel is the same as for intestinal surgery (see Chapter 47). If blood volume deficit is present, blood will be given. The goal is to make the patient as physically stable as possible before surgery.

#### Postoperative care

Postoperatively the patient will be in a critical care unit because close monitoring is necessary. Hypovolemia from blood loss is a complication. Sepsis is the most common complication. Vital signs should be monitored every 15 minutes until stable and then every hour. Dressings should be checked for oozing or bleeding. Intake and output, serum electrolytes, and hematocrit or hemoglobin levels are carefully monitored. Weights should be recorded daily. Assessment of the cardiorespiratory system (cardiac rhythm, breath sounds, blood gases) is also necessary. Temperature should also be monitored at least every 4 hours.

Assessment not only focuses on the potential for sepsis, hypovolemic shock, and cardiorespiratory complications, but should also include decreased liver function (blood glucose, coagulation status, serum albumin levels, neurologic status). The nurse should anticipate the possibility of administering glucose, albumin, and blood. Restriction of protein is necessary if the patient is not able to metabolize adequately the ammonium released during the breakdown of proteins.

The patient may have a chest tube attached to water-seal drainage if the surgery is performed through a thoracoabdominal incision. The care of patients with water-seal chest drainage is discussed in Chapter 37. To promote turning and deep breathing, the nurse must ensure adequate pain control by giving the patient medications as ordered, splinting the incision, and positioning the patient properly (upright). Because most analgesics, narcotic and nonnarcotic, are metabolized in the liver, no "safe" analgesic exists for the patient with liver dysfunction, and the nurse should monitor closely for signs of toxicity.

The patient has nothing by mouth for several days and has a nasogastric tube attached to suction. Frequent mouth care every 4 hours and monitoring of the nasogastric suction are indicated. Food is started on approx-

## Guidelines for Care of the Person Undergoing Liver Resection

### PREOPERATIVE CARE

Teaching
- Explain special postoperative procedures (e.g., chest tube drainage, nasogastric intubation, parenteral fluids for several days).
- Teach deep breathing exercises and leg exercises.
- Teach use of side rails to facilitate turning in bed without exerting pull on the abdominal muscles.

Preventing hemorrhage
- Give prescribed vitamin K.

Bowel preparation
- See Chapter 47.

### POSTOPERATIVE CARE

Promoting oxygenation
- Encourage turning and deep breathing exercises.
- Encourage activity/ambulation as ordered.

Maintaining fluid and electrolyte balance
- Check dressings for oozing or bleeding.
- Maintain patency of GI tube.
- Maintain prescribed flow of parenteral fluids.
- Monitor for signs of fluid imbalance (daily weight changes, hematocrit, lung congestion, dry skin and mucous membranes).

Promoting comfort
- Give analgesics on a regular basis during the first 48 hours to minimize severe pain.
- Give frequent oral hygiene until oral fluids are resumed.

Teaching
- Explain menu choices for a low-protein diet.
- Reinforce information about a low-sodium diet.

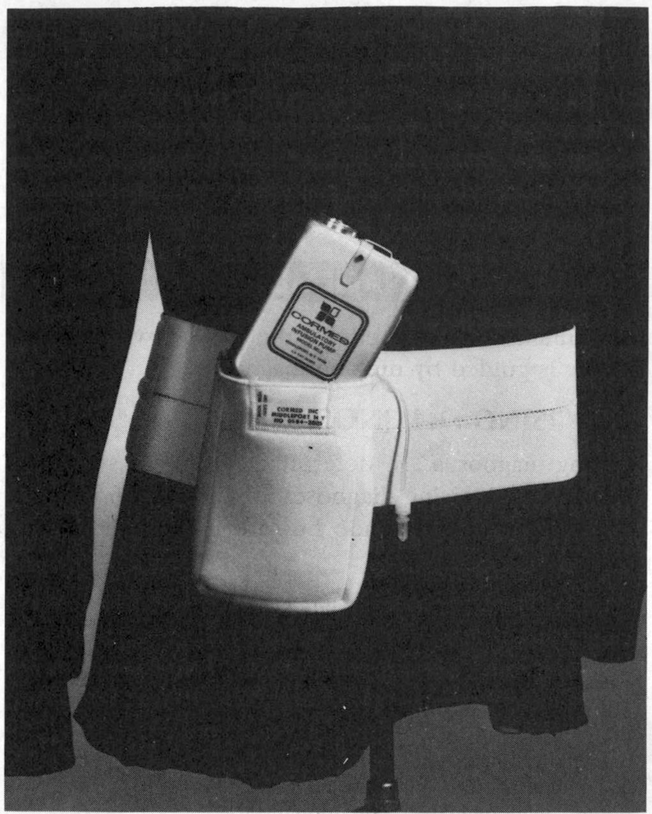

**FIGURE 42-1** External infusion pump. Lightweight, battery-operated infusion pump for ambulatory patient. Flow rate is adjustable; power pack operates for 7 days before needing recharging. (Courtesy CORMED, Middleport, NY.)

imately the fifth postoperative day. At first, liquids are given, and then the diet is advanced as tolerated based on appetite and bowel function. The patient needs adequate calories, protein, vitamins, and minerals. The nurse must monitor the patient for adequacy of intake by monitoring caloric intake. The patient's tolerance to protein nitrogenous waste products must be monitored. If the patient cannot metabolize protein adequately because of loss of liver tissue, a low-protein diet (as used for portal-systemic encephalopathy, see p. 1408) is necessary. If the patient can adequately detoxify ammonium, a high-protein diet is given.

After surgery, the patient may sit on the side of the bed and be out of bed by the second or third postoperative day. Close monitoring of vital signs, tolerance for activity, and respiratory status are required. The care of the patient undergoing hepatic resection is summarized in the Guidelines box above.

### Discharge care

In preparation for discharge, the patient should receive instructions concerning any dietary restrictions. The patient's liver function will be limited for up to 6 months after surgery, and dietary protein and sodium are restricted. Corticosteroids are given to enhance regeneration and prevent fibrosis, and if they are to be continued after discharge, the patient needs to receive written and verbal instructions regarding dosage, purpose, how to take, and side effects that need to be reported to the physician. The patient's activity tolerance will gradually increase. The patient will need instruction on activities that are permitted and activities to avoid, such as heavy lifting. The patient needs to know how to monitor himself or herself in relation to activity tolerance. Usually the patient uses his or her feeling of fatigue and tiredness as indicators of what can or cannot be done. The patient will not be able to assume all activities of daily living (ADL) immediately because of fatigue, and the nurse must assess whether self-care and home care needs can be met by the family or if outside help is necessary. Appropriate referrals should be made if necessary for home health care.

## Care of the Patient Having Chemotherapy

Chemotherapy is increasingly being used to treat primary and metastatic tumors of the liver. It may be given systematically or by perfusion into the hepatic artery. All chemotherapeutic agents have major side effects, and one of the major focuses of nursing is to help the patient and family deal with these side effects (see Chapter 16).

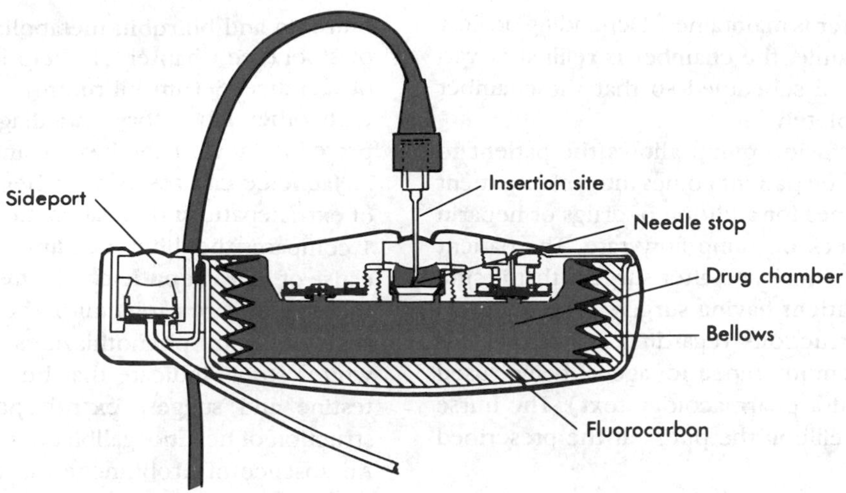


**FIGURE 42-2** Implantable infusion pump. Infusaid pump.

**BOX 42-6 Characteristics of Infusaid Pump**

1. The pump has two chambers: one for the drug solution and one that contains a fluorocarbon fluid.
2. The two chambers are separated by a flexible metal bellows.
3. The drug reservoir has a capacity of approximately 50 ml (model 400) and is refilled every 2 weeks by percutaneous injection into the insertion site with the use of a special needle.
4. The fluorocarbon is temperature sensitive and converts from a liquid to vapor at body temperature.
5. The vapor exerts pressure on the bellows, forcing the drug solution from its reservoir into the catheter. This occurs at a constant preset rate, and typically 2 to 3 ml/day of solution is delivered.
6. *Drug dosage* is controlled by manipulating the concentration of the chemotherapeutic agent.
7. The fluorocarbon vapor is reliquefied as the drug chamber is refilled; vaporization again occurs, and the next dosage is delivered.

**INSTRUCTIONS REGARDING SELF-CARE FOR PATIENTS WITH IMPLANTED PUMPS**

1. Avoid deep-sea diving, mountain climbing, or long-distance airplane trips. These activities change atmospheric pressure and can change vaporization of the fluorocarbon and thus the delivery rate.
2. Monitor body temperature daily, and report elevations immediately.
3. Avoid long hot baths, saunas, and spas. These activities can change the flow rate.
4. Avoid contact sports because they can damage the pump.
5. Wear a Medic-Alert bracelet or necklace that indicates the presence of an implantable pump and gives information such as the physician's name.
6. Return for follow-up care as prescribed, usually every 2 weeks.
7. Contact the nurse/physician/outpatient department any time questions arise.
8. Individualized instructions are given about side effects of the specific chemotherapeutic agents that need to be monitored for and reported.

From Gullate MM, Foltz AT: *Am J Nurs* 83:1674-1678, 1983.

In addition, patients may need to learn to care for an external infusion pump, as shown in Figure 42-1, or an internal pump, as shown in Figure 42-2.

### Hepatic arterial infusion

Patients receiving chemotherapy through the hepatic artery have additional needs. **Hepatic arterial infusion** can be accomplished by one of two methods. In the first method, a percutaneous catheter is inserted into the hepatic artery using fluoroscopy. The catheter is attached to an external infusion pump that is filled with the appropriate chemotherapeutic agent and programmed to deliver the agent over a desired period. The catheter is removed after each drug treatment cycle. In the second method, a catheter is surgically inserted into the hepatic artery and connected to an implanted infusion pump (Figure 42-2). Characteristics of the Infusaid pump (an internal pump) are described in Box 42-6.

The implanted pump can be filled with the correct amount of drug and programmed to deliver the chemotherapeutic agent over a desired time and at a desired dosage. In chemotherapy-free intervals, the pump is filled with a heparin solution so that patency of the hepatic artery catheter is maintained. Depending on flow rates and drug schedule, the chamber is refilled at various intervals that are scheduled so that the chamber never empties completely.

The implanted infusion pump allows the patient to be treated at home. The patient comes into an outpatient site at prescribed times for addition of drugs or heparin solution and a recheck of pump flow rate. The patient needs physical care before and after surgery that is similar to that of any patient having surgery (see Chapters 23 to 25), and instructions regarding self-care needs related to the chemotherapeutic agent being used (see Chapter 16 and a pharmacology text). The nurse also is involved in refilling the pump at the prescribed intervals.

## DIFFUSE HEPATOCELLULAR DISORDERS

**Jaundice** is a major problem in patients with diffuse hepatocellular disorders. It is caused by a disturbance in bilirubin metabolism (see Chapter 41 for an explanation of bilirubin metabolism). With jaundice, an excess of bilirubin in the blood is distributed to the skin, mucous membranes, sclera of the eye, and other body fluids and tissues. This high total serum bilirubin (usually greater than 2.5 mg/dl; normal: 0.5 to 1.0 mg/dl) is responsible for the characteristic yellow discoloration of these tissues. If the bilirubin has been processed by the liver (extracted, conjugated, and secreted), it is water soluble and can be excreted in urine, which is darker than usual. The presence of bilirubin in the skin causes pruritus (itching) in about 20% to 25% of the patients who have jaundice. The changes in concentration of bilirubin and bilirubin metabolites in the serum, urine, or stool (see Chapter 41) help in determining the type of jaundice. Serum bilirubin levels must be combined with other laboratory and diagnostic tests and interpreted in view of the history and clinical findings.

Jaundice can result from hemolysis and obstruction of extrahepatic and intrahepatic biliary ducts. Table 42-1 compares the different causes of jaundice. A common cause of **intrahepatic cholestasis** (stasis of bile within the small biliary canniculi of the liver) is drug reactions such as from phenothiazines. Clay-colored (grayish white) stools indicate that bile is not reaching the intestine and suggest **extrahepatic obstruction** (obstruction of hepatic, gallbladder, or common bile duct). An absence of urobilinogen in the urine supports this inference because bile and bilirubin must reach the intestines for the normal formation of urobilinogen, some of which is usually excreted in the urine. Frequent causes of extrahepatic obstruction are gallstones lodged in the common bile duct, pancreatitis, and carcinoma of the head of the pancreas, all of which are discussed in Chapter 46.

In hepatocellular damage, there is interference with uptake, conjugation, and excretion of bilirubin into bile. Excretion is the most profoundly affected process, and a predominantly conjugated hyperbilirubinemia is seen. The level of jaundice does not correlate with the severity in hepatitis; but in cirrhosis, jaundice suggests a poorer prognosis.

### HEPATITIS

Hepatitis is defined as any acute inflammatory disease of the liver. Although the term **hepatitis** is most often used in conjunction with viral hepatitis, the disease can be caused by viruses, bacteria, or toxic injury to the liver.

**TABLE 42-1 Types of Jaundice**

| CATEGORY | PATHOLOGY | POSSIBLE FINDINGS |
|---|---|---|
| **OBSTRUCTIVE** | | |
| Intrahepatic | Suppression of bile flow in canaliculi or small biliary ductiles (cholestasis) | Direct* bilirubin elevated; alkaline phosphatase elevated; no enlargement of bile ducts seen on scan or ultrasound |
| Extrahepatic (bile duct obstruction) | Obstruction of bile flow in large bile ducts, as in gallbladder disease | Direct* bilirubin elevated; alkaline phosphatase elevated; enlargement of bile ducts documented by scan, ultrasound; absence of urobilinogen in urine |
| **HEPATOCELLULAR** | Hepatocyte injury from toxins (toxic hepatitis), from viruses (viral hepatitis), or as part of syndrome of cirrhosis (all types) | Transaminases (ALT, AST) elevated 10- to 15-fold; both direct* and indirect† bilirubin may be elevated (direct more than indirect); prolonged prothrombin time |
| **HEMOLYTIC** | Excessive amounts of bilirubin are released from red blood cells (RBCs) as would be seen in sickle-cell anemia or other hemolytic anemias; liver is unable to excrete bilirubin as rapidly as it forms | Usually mild elevation of total bilirubin (indirect more than direct) |

*"Direct" measures conjugated bilirubin.
†"Indirect" measures unconjugated bilirubin.

Although some differences exist in the pathologic and clinical phenomena of viral, bacterial, and toxic hepatitis, the clinical management of the person with any of these types of hepatitis is quite similar. The particular aspects of care for toxic and viral hepatitis are discussed next. It should be pointed out that almost any form of hepatitis can result in **postnecrotic cirrhosis** (p. 1388), unless the hepatitis responds to treatment.

## Toxic Hepatitis

### Etiology

Because the liver has a primary role in the metabolism of foreign substances, many agents, including drugs and alcohol, industrial toxins, and plant poisons, can cause **toxic hepatitis** (Table 42-2). Many health care workers are concerned about hepatic injury caused by adverse drug reactions from the drugs they handle (especially those needing to be mixed from powder).

**TABLE 42-2 Selected Hepatoxins and Class of Hepatotoxins**

| AGENTS | TYPE OF HEPATOTOXIN |
|---|---|
| **INDUSTRIAL TOXINS** | |
| Carbon tetrachloride and other chlorinated hydrocarbons | Predictable; direct |
| Yellow phosphorus | Predictable; direct |
| **PLANT POISONS** | |
| Mushroom poisoning (*Amanita phalloides* and related poisons) | Predictable; direct |
| **DRUGS** | |
| Ethanol | Predictable; indirect |
| Tetracycline | Predictable; indirect |
| Methotrexate | Predictable; indirect |
| L-Asparaginase | Predictable; indirect |
| Puromycin | Predictable; indirect |
| 6-Mercaptopurine | Predictable; indirect |
| Acetaminophen | Predictable; indirect |
| Mithramycin | Predictable; indirect |
| Urethane | Predictable; indirect |
| Cholecystographic dyes | Predictable; indirect |
| Rifamycin B | Predictable; indirect |
| Phenytoin | Nonpredictable |
| Para-aminosalicylic acid (PAS) | Nonpredictable |
| Isoniazid (INH) | Nonpredictable |
| Chlorpromazine | Nonpredictable |
| Androgens and anabolic steroids | Nonpredictable |
| Chlorpropamide | Nonpredictable |
| Imipramine | Nonpredictable |
| Methyldopa | Nonpredictable |
| Monoamine oxidase inhibitors | Nonpredictable |
| Oral contraceptives | Nonpredictable |
| Sulfonamides | Nonpredictable |
| Allopurinol | Nonpredictable |
| Clindamycin | Nonpredictable |
| Erythromycin esters | Nonpredictable |
| Nitrofurantoin | Nonpredictable |
| Oxacillin | Nonpredictable |

### Epidemiology

Only a minor number of the cases of acute hepatic disease in health care workers are the result of adverse drug reactions. However, up to 25% of all cases of fulminant hepatic failure are the result of adverse drug reactions.[12,15]

### Classification of the hepatotoxins

The agents that produce hepatic injury are categorized into two major groups: *predictable (intrinsic)* hepatotoxins and *nonpredictable (idiosyncratic)* hepatotoxins. The predictable hepatotoxins are further divided into two subgroups: *direct* and *indirect* (Box 42-7). The selected agents listed in Table 42-2 have been classified according to type of **hepatotoxin.** As should be noted, most drugs are nonpredictable (idiosyncratic) hepatotoxins. Acetaminophen, which is a predictable hepatotoxin, produces injury at high doses and has been increasingly used in suicide attempts.

### Pathophysiology

The morphologic changes produced in the liver by the toxins vary, depending on the specific hepatotoxin. For example, carbon tetrachloride, tetracycline, and ethanol cause fatty infiltration and/or necrosis. Oral contraceptives, cholecystographic dyes, and chlorpromazine produce cholestasis and portal inflammation. Regardless of the morphologic changes, some alteration in liver function occurs. The alteration may result in only minimal manifestations of altered liver function such as slightly elevated serum enzymes or major manifestations associated with terminal liver failure (see pp. 1388-1411). Box 42-8 lists clinical manifestations of toxic hepatitis.

**BOX 42-7 Classification of Hepatotoxins**

**PREDICTABLE HEPATOTOXINS**

Agents cause toxic hepatitis with predictable regularity and produce injury in a high percentage of persons exposed to them; occurrence of toxic hepatitis is dose dependent.

**NONPREDICTABLE HEPATOTOXINS**

Agents produce hepatic injury only in unusually susceptible persons and in only a small percentage of persons exposed to them; occurrence is not dose dependent.

**DIRECT PREDICTABLE HEPATOTOXINS**

Agents have direct effect on hepatic cells and organelles, producing structural changes that lead to metabolic defects.

**INDIRECT PREDICTABLE HEPATOTOXINS**

Agents first interfere with normal metabolic function, and this alteration in metabolic function produces structural changes.

**BOX 42-8 Clinical Manifestations of Toxic Hepatitis**

**EARLY MANIFESTATIONS**
Anorexia
Nausea and vomiting
Lethargy
Elevated ALT and AST

**LATER MANIFESTATIONS**
Icterus
Hepatomegaly
Hepatic tenderness
Dark urine
Elevated serum bilirubin
Elevated urine bilirubin

### Prevention

**Primary prevention.** The nurse can assist in the prevention of toxic hepatitis by teaching the danger of injudicious use of materials that are known to be injurious to the liver and by emphasizing the need for a diet (well-balanced diet with recommended dietary requirements of nutrients and with minimal or no alcohol) that is protective to the liver.

Because cleaning agents, solvents, and related substances sometimes contain products that are harmful to the liver, the public should read instructions on labels and should follow them explicitly. Dry-cleaning fluids may contain carbon tetrachloride, which can cause liver injury if warnings to avoid inhalation of the fumes and to keep windows open are not heeded. If people must use these agents inside the home, a good practice is to open the windows wide; use the cleaning materials as quickly as possible; and then vacate the room, the apartment, or the house for several hours, leaving the windows open.

Many solvents used to remove paint and plastic material and to stain and finish woodwork contain injurious substances and should be used outdoors and not in the basement, since dangerous fumes may spread throughout the house. Cleaning agents and finishes for cars should be applied outdoors or in the garage with the door open. Nurses in industry have a responsibility to teach the importance of observing regulations to avoid industrial hazards. Nitrobenzene, tetrachloroethane, carbon disulfide, and dinitrotoluoyl are examples of injurious compounds used in industry.

**Secondary prevention.** Some drugs that are known to cause mild damage to the liver must be used therapeutically. However, the nurse should warn the public about the use of preparations that are available without prescription that can cause liver injury. Many drugs, prescription and nonprescription, reach the market before dangers resulting from their extensive use have been conclusively ruled out; for example, the prescription drug chlorpromazine, which was being widely used as a tranquilizer, has been found to cause stasis of bile in the canaliculi of the liver, which can lead to serious hepatic damage. A safe rule to follow is to avoid taking any medication except that specifically prescribed by a physician for a specific ailment.

### Medical management

Attention is directed toward identifying the toxic agent and removing or eliminating it. Gastric lavage and cleansing of the bowel may be indicated to remove the hepatotoxin(s) from the intestinal tract. In some instances, there is a specific treatment for a particular hepatotoxin. For example, acetylcysteine, a mucolytic agent, can be given within 16 hours (immediately is preferred) of ingestion of an acetaminophen overdose. Acetylcysteine prevents hepatotoxicity by possibly maintaining or restoring glutathione levels or acting as an alternate substrate for the toxic metabolite of acetaminophen. The drug may be given orally or intravenously, although only the oral form has been approved for use in the United States at this time. However, in most instances of toxic hepatitis, medical treatment is supportive and directed toward particular manifestations, such as treatment of cirrhosis, portal-systemic encephalopathy, or accompanying renal failure.

### Nursing management

The major focus for nursing management occurs in the community or other outpatient setting and is directed toward the nursing diagnosis, potential for injury related to improper use of chemicals at home, exposure to chemicals in the work environment, or injudicious use of drugs or other materials. The nursing care involves patient education, as discussed in the section on prevention (see p. 1378).

For the patient with acute toxic hepatitis, the nursing management in the acute care setting is directed toward promoting comfort, maintaining normal fluid and electrolyte balance, promoting a well-balanced diet when food and fluid are allowed, and promoting rest as discussed in the section on viral hepatitis (see pp. 1385-1386). The nurse also assists with the implementation of any medical regimen. If cirrhosis develops or portal-systemic encephalopathy occurs, the patient may require all the interventions described for the patient with cirrhosis (see pp. 1388-1411).

## Viral Hepatitis

Viral hepatitis is by far the most important infection that affects the liver. It is a major health problem in the United States and in many other countries. The term **viral hepatitis** is used to refer to several clinically similar but etiologically and epidemiologically distinct infections.

### Etiology

Five major categories of viruses have been identified as causing viral hepatitis: **hepatitis A** (HAV), **hepatitis B**

**TABLE 42-3 Etiologic/Epidemiologic/Transmission Characteristics of Hepatitis**

| HEPATITIS A | HEPATITIS B | HEPATITIS C | HEPATITIS D | HEPATITIS E |
|---|---|---|---|---|
| **AGE-GROUP** | | | | |
| Older children and young adults | Young adults because of life-style | All age-groups but highest in adults because of more frequent blood transfusions | Same as for hepatitis B | All age-groups |
| **TRANSMISSION** | | | | |
| Primarily person to person through fecal contamination; common source epidemics from contaminated food and water; rare transmission by blood; *not* transmitted by shared utensils and kissing | Percutaneous or permucosal routes through infected blood or body fluids introduced by contaminated needles and sexual contact; spread by personal contact in households and among children; rare transmission by blood transfusion, since screening of blood for presence of HBV surface antigen ($HB_sAg$) | Parenterally transmitted form is spread percutaneously through infected blood transfusion and parenteral drug abuse; a large percentage of persons have no known risk factors | Routes same as those for hepatitis B | Oral—fecal contaminated water |
| **INCUBATION PERIOD** | | | | |
| 15-50 days; average 28-30 days | 45-160 days, average 60-120 days | Variable—14-150 days; average 50 days | Same as for HBV | 2-9 weeks |
| **SECRETIONS THAT HAVE BEEN FOUND TO CONTAIN INFECTIVE AGENT** | | | | |
| Stools: 2 weeks before jaundice<br>Blood: incubation and acute phase | Highest in blood and serous fluids; also found in saliva, semen, urine, nasopharyngeal washings, feces, and pleural fluid | Blood | Blood | Feces possible |
| **GREATEST INFECTIVITY** | | | | |
| 2 weeks before onset of jaundice | — | — | Infections occur as either coinfection with HBV or superinfection in HBV carrier | — |
| **CLINICAL ONSET** | | | | |
| Abrupt | Insidious | Insidious | Insidious | Resembles hepatitis A |
| **DIAGNOSTIC SEROLOGIC TESTS** | | | | |
| Confirmed by presence of immunoglobin against HAV (IgM-class anti-HAV) in serum (found during acute and early convalescent period) | Confirmed by $HB_sAg$, hepatitis $B_e$ antigen ($HB_eAg$), antibody against $HB_eAg$ (anti-$HB_e$), antibody against core antigen (anti-$HB_c$) (see Chapter 41 for discussion) | Antibody to HCV (anti-HCV) has been identified | Antibody to HDV (anti-HDV), HDAg (HDV antigen) | Antibody to HEV (anti-HEV) |
| **INDICATION OF PROTECTIVE IMMUNITY** | | | | |
| IgG-class anti-HAV appears during convalescent period and indicates immunity | Antibody against hepatitis$_s$ antigen (anti-$HB_s$) indicates immunity | No tests available; people have had repeated infections | No test available but can only occur if HBV is present | No test available |

Modified from Advisory Committee on Immunization Practices (ACIP): *MMWR* 39(52):1-26, 1990.

*Continued*

**TABLE 42-3 Etiologic/Epidemiologic/Transmission Characteristics of Hepatitis—cont'd**

| HEPATITIS A | HEPATITIS B | HEPATITIS C | HEPATITIS D | HEPATITIS E |
|---|---|---|---|---|
| **CHRONIC CARRIERS** | | | | |
| None demonstrated | Frequent—6% to 10% of adult persons with HBV become carriers; 90% of infected infants and 25% to 50% of infected children become carriers | 8% of persons with HCV become carriers | 80% of those persons who have superinfection with HDV become carriers with superinfection | Unknown |
| **MORTALITY** | | | | |
| Infrequent (<0.6%) | 1%-2% | Unknown | Increased | Unknown |
| **SUBSEQUENT CHRONIC DISEASE** | | | | |
| Absent | About 10% develop chronic disease | High—20% to 70% develop chronic disease | Frequent in persons who contact a superinfection of HDV | No |
| **HIGH-RISK GROUPS** | | | | |
| Staff and children at day-care centers where children in diapers are cared for; staff and persons in institutions for custodial care (prisons, institutions for developmentally disabled); international travelers to developing countries | Immigrants/refugees from areas of high HBV endemic areas; clients and staff in institutions for developmentally disabled; users of illicit parenteral drugs; fetuses of infected mothers; homosexually active men; household and sexual partners of HBV carriers; patients on hemodialysis; male prisoners; health care workers with frequent contact with blood | Persons receiving frequent transfusions; international travelers to endemic area | Same as for HBV | Immigrants/travelers from HEV-epidemic areas and developing countries |

(HBV), **hepatitis C** (HCV), **hepatitis D** (HDV or delta virus), and **hepatitis E** (HEV). Two other forms of hepatitis, hepatitis F and G, have been identified but occur rarely. Table 42-3 provides a summary of the modes of transmission for each viral type.

## Epidemiology

Viral hepatitis is a reportable disease in all states in the United States. Statistics from the Centers for Disease Control and Prevention (CDC) indicate that viral hepatitis is one of the most frequently reported infectious diseases in the United States. The most common type of hepatitis worldwide is HAV, with 40% of the reported cases of hepatitis being caused by HAV.[9,17]

The incidence of HBV infection is reported to be about 5% of the world's population. Fifty-nine percent of the reported cases of HBV infection in the United States occur in heterosexuals with multiple sex partners, homosexual men, and IV drug users. The incidence of HBV in health care workers is about 3% of all reported cases.[17]

Twenty percent of all cases of viral hepatitis reported to the CDC are caused by HCV infection, and 50% of these persons will develop chronic hepatitis. HDV is endemic among persons with HBV in areas around the Mediterranean and Middle East. HEV is extremely rare in the United States but occurs in epidemic proportions in areas of India. It has also been reported in Mexico, Asia, and Africa.[9]

The vast majority of cases of hepatitis that are seen clinically are caused by HAV or HBV. Most cases of all types of hepatitis occur in young adults. Factors such as the viral agent, transmission, and high-risk groups vary for the five types of hepatitis. Table 42-3 summarizes the difference between the five types of hepatitis.

## Pathophysiology

Viral hepatitis causes diffuse inflammatory infiltration of hepatic tissue with mononuclear cells and local, spotty, or single cell necrosis. The liver cells may be very swollen. With typical viral hepatitis, there is no collapse of lobules, no loss of lobular architecture, and minimal or

**BOX 42-9 Atypical Life-Threatening Variants of Hepatitis**

| | |
|---|---|
| Fulminant viral hepatitis | Sudden, severe degeneration and atrophy of liver, resulting in hepatic failure |
| Subacute fatal viral hepatitis | Severe but slower degeneration of liver |
| Confluent hepatic necrosis—submassive or massive | Destruction of substantial groups of adjacent cells with necrosis of portions of a lobule (submassive) or entire lobule (massive); can result in chronic active disease or cirrhosis, but most patients will recover |

no fibrosis. Inflammation, degeneration, and regeneration occur simultaneously, distorting the normal lobular pattern and creating pressure within and around the portal vein areas and obstructing the bile channels. These changes are associated with elevated serum transaminase levels, prolonged prothrombin time, slightly elevated serum alkaline phosphatase level, and elevated bilirubin.

The outcome of viral hepatitis is affected by such factors as the following:

1. Virulence of the virus
2. Amount of hepatic damaged sustained
3. Natural individual barriers to damage and disease of the liver, such as immune status, nutritional status, and overall health of individuals
4. Supportive individual care the patient receives

Most patients recover normal liver function, but the disease can progress to atypical life-threatening variants (Box 42-9). Chronic sequelae can occur with all types of hepatitis but are virtually absent with HAV and HEV. Because of the continual destruction of the liver in *chronic active hepatitis,* there are continual signs and symptoms of liver impairment and histopathologic changes on a liver biopsy. Chronic active hepatitis is usually indicative of a poor prognosis but can revert to an inactive form. *Chronic relapsing hepatitis* is characterized by the reappearance of symptoms and signs after recovery from an acute episode is believed to have occurred (usually within 6 months). *Chronic persistent hepatitis* refers to cases of hepatitis with a benign course where all the signs and symptoms do not resolve in the usual time frame. The patient may be asymptomatic, except for minimal abnormalities in serum transaminase levels. There is no indication of progression to severe hepatic dysfunction, and eventually full recovery occurs.

Manifestations of the various forms of hepatitis are not clinically distinct from each other, except that, with HAV, the manifestations may be more abrupt in onset. The signs and symptoms and abnormal diagnostic tests

**BOX 42-10 Pathophysiology and Clinical Manifestations of Viral Hepatitis**

| PATHOPHYSIOLOGY | CLINICAL MANIFESTATIONS |
|---|---|
| | **Preicteric and Icteric Phase** |
| Necrosis and inflammation of hepatic cells with decreased liver function | Elevated temperature, chills, nausea, vomiting, dyspepsia, anorexia; right upper quadrant tenderness and enlarged liver; fatigue, weakness, and malaise; enlarged lymph nodes; elevated serum transaminases (ALT, AST) and alkaline phosphatase |
| | **Preicteric Phase** |
| Circulating immune complexes and complement system activation | Arthralgia, headache, urticaria |
| | **Icteric Phase** |
| Impaired bilirubin metabolism and obstruction to bile flow | Jaundice with elevated total, conjugated, and unconjugated serum bilirubin; dark-amber urine with bilirubinuria and increased urobilinogen; light-brown to grayish white stools (depending on the amount of bile obstruction); pruritus |
| | **Preicteric, Icteric, and Posticteric Phases** |
| Viral infection | Presence of viral antibodies, antigens, or virus particles |

can be grouped into three phases: preicteric, icteric, and posticteric phases. Box 42-10 lists pathophysiology and related clinical manifestations.

## Prevention

### Healthy People 2000

The goal of *Healthy People 2000* is to decrease the incidence of HAV from a 1987 occurrence of 31 per 100,000 to a target of 23 per 100,000 by the year 2000.[17] HAV vaccines are undergoing clinical trials and may be available before the target date. High-risk groups that are identified are Native Americans and IV drug users.

Since the identification of HCV, screening of blood transfusions has reduced the incidence of posttransfusion hepatitis from HCV to about 5%. The goal by the year 2000 is to decrease the rate of HCV to 13.7 per 100,000 from 18.3 per 100,000 in 1987.[17]

HBV vaccine has the potential for decreasing the incidence of HBV infection dramatically. *Healthy People 2000* has set a target goal of a 37% reduction in HBV occurrence by the year 2000. This will be achieved through education and vaccination of high-risk groups.[17]

Health care workers are at a higher risk for becoming infected with HBV. The CDC estimates that 12,000 health care workers become infected each year. The goal of *Healthy People 2000* is to reduce HBV infections among occupationally exposed workers to an incidence of no more than 1250 cases.[17]

**Primary prevention.** Prophylaxis can be instituted either before exposure for persons at high risk and/or after exposure. The recommendations for prophylaxis vary for the different types of hepatitis and are reevaluated continually by the CDC.

***Hepatitis A.*** For HAV, the following recommendations have been made by the CDC.[1]

*Preexposure prophylaxis* is recommended for travelers to developing countries who will be eating in settings of poor or uncertain sanitation or visiting extensively with local people. The recommended therapy is immune globulin, 0.02 ml/kg, for people traveling for less than 3 months and 0.06 ml/kg every 5 months for those traveling for prolonged periods.

Postexposure prophylaxis is recommended for selected people who have had contact with a person known to be positive for HAV, if the prophylaxis is given *within* 2 weeks of exposure. Postexposure prophylaxis for the following people is recommended:

1. Close household and sexual contacts of people with HAV
2. Staff and attendees of day-care centers, if HAV cases are recognized among attendees or employees, or two or more households of center attendees have recognized cases; household members of families with children in diapers, if three or more families of attendees report cases
3. Residents and staff in institutions for custodial care who have close contact with people with HAV
4. Hospital staff who have close contacts with patients with HAV (only if outbreaks occur)
5. People exposed to a common source of infection (infected food or water), if identified within 2 weeks of exposure
6. Food handlers working with a handler diagnosed as having HAV; patrons of food establishments only treated in rare instances

***Hepatitis B.*** HBV is a vaccine-preventable disease. As the cost of the vaccine decreases, worldwide use will become more realistic. The vaccine provides active immunity (HBV vaccine) and an immune globulin with high amounts of anti-$HB_s$ (HBIG). The HBV vaccine is used in both preexposure and postexposure prophylaxis.

HBV vaccine is given as a series of three intramuscular injections (deltoid in adults and children; anterolateral thigh muscles in infants and neonates), with the second and third doses given 1 and 6 months after the first dose. The vaccine has shown an efficacy of 85% to 95%.[4] The effect of the vaccine on the developing fetus is not known. Because HBV infection in pregnant women results in a severe infection in the mother and chronic infection in the infant and because the vaccine contains only noninfectious $HB_sAg$ particles, pregnancy should not be considered a contraindication for its use if necessary. Soreness at injection site is the most common side effect.[1]

HBV vaccine causes *no adverse effects or benefits* in HBV carriers. Because HBV vaccine has no benefits for HBV carriers and because of the cost of the vaccination (approximately $110/person), prevaccination serologic screening for anti-$HB_c$ and anti-$HB_s$ may be done to identify both carriers and previously infected noncarriers who have adequate immunity. The cost of screening is weighed against the cost of unnecessary but harmless vaccination to identify whether screening before vaccinating should be performed.

Preexposure vaccination is recommended for everyone with highest priority for the following[1,4]:

1. Health care workers at high risk for exposure (medical technologists or staff, phlebotomists, most nurses in acute and critical care settings, surgeons, pathologists, oncology and dialysis unit staff, dentists, oral surgeons, dental hygienists, laboratory and blood bank technicians, emergency medical technicians, morticians)
2. Clients and staff of institutions for developmentally disabled
3. Hemodialysis patients
4. Sexually active persons with multiple partners
5. IV drug users sharing needles
6. Recipients of frequent blood products, particularly patients with clotting disorders who receive frequent transfusions of clotting factors
7. Household and sexual contacts of HBV carriers
8. Some American populations, including infants, such as Alaskan Inuits, native Pacific islanders, and immigrants and refugees and their infants from areas where HBV is endemic, such as Eastern Asia; adoptees from countries of high HBV endemicity; and families of adoptees with positive $HB_sAg$ tests
9. Long-term correctional facility inmates
10. International travelers who plan to reside in areas with a high endemic incidence of HBV for 6 months or longer

Postexposure prophylaxis for HBV should be considered for the following[1]:

1. Infants born to $HB_sAg$-positive mothers
2. Persons who have percutaneous or permucosal exposure to $HB_sAg$-positive blood
3. Persons who have sexual contact with $HB_sAg$-positive persons
4. Infants less than 12 months old exposed to primary caregiver who has acute HBV

Infants exposed perinatally are given HBIG at birth, and the HBV vaccination series is started at the same time, if possible. Persons who have percutaneous or permucosal exposure and are unvaccinated are also treated with HBIG, and the HBV vaccination series is started. If the exposed person has been vaccinated, he or she is checked for anti-$HB_s$ and given HBIG immediately plus a booster dose of HBV vaccination. The CDC also makes recommendations about prophylaxis after percutaneous or permucosal exposure from a source with unknown hepatitis B virus status.[1]

Booster immunization doses, described previously, are recommended for previously vaccinated persons who experience percutaneous or needle exposure to $HB_sAg$-positive blood. In addition, it is recommended that patients on hemodialysis be assessed semiannually by antibody testing, and if their antibody level declines below 10 U/ml, they should be given a booster dose. For persons with normal immune status, booster doses and routine serologic testing to assess antibody level are not necessary.[1]

Although the HBV vaccine has been available since 1981, the incidence of the disease has not decreased.[4,9] This lack of decrease may be caused by health care workers who are uninformed about who should be vaccinated, the inability of health care workers to reach high-risk groups, unfounded patient concerns about the safety of the vaccine, and incomplete identification of high-risk persons. With regard to this last factor, it has been shown that 30% of the people with acute HBV infection do not indicate any source of contact or definable risk even when questioned thoroughly.[1]

***Hepatitis C and E.*** Prophylaxis for HCV and HEV is not as effective as that for HBV. For travelers to countries where HEV occurs in endemic proportions, preventive health teaching is the best prophylactic measure. The value of immunoglobulin in this situation is unknown. For postexposure prophylaxis in persons exposed through breaks in the skin to blood from a patient with HCV, immunoglobulin may be given, but its value is uncertain.[1]

***Hepatitis D.*** HDV requires the presence of HBV; thus the preexposure and postexposure prophylaxes that are recommended for HBV should suffice to prevent delta hepatitis.[1] Currently, no prophylaxis exists for preventing HDV infection in HBV carriers except health teaching.

**Secondary prevention.** The major activity that can assist in the general prevention of the spread of hepatitis is thorough universal precautions for all body fluids for all people. All feces, urine, blood and other body fluids should be considered potentially infectious for a wide variety of organisms and disposed of properly. Nurses should be involved in the promotion of the development of adequate sewage disposal systems to prevent contamination of food and water supplies that may result in endemic forms of HAV.

Because HBV, HCV, HDV, and possibly HAV, as well as carrier states of some types of hepatitis, can be spread by contaminated needles and other equipment that comes in contact with infected blood and body fluids, disposable and nondisposable needles, syringes, and other equipment used in patient care must be handled with great care. *All equipment should be treated as if it had been used on an infected person and handled using universal precautions no matter who the patient.*

Needles should *not be recapped.* They should be discarded in puncture-resistant containers designated for this purpose. Other disposable equipment should also be discarded in appropriate containers; the containers are marked contaminated to alert persons handling the rubbish.

Nondisposable equipment should be rinsed, packaged so sharp objects do not accidentally puncture someone, and sterilized by dry heat and steam under pressure (autoclaving) or by gas sterilization. If invasive reusable equipment is used in an environment in which autoclave sterilization is not available and boiling is the only available way to sterilize, the nurse should see that everything placed in the water sterilizer is covered completely and boiled for at least 30 minutes. The nurse should realize that the boiling time needed to destroy hepatitis viruses is unknown and that water sterilization of invasive equipment, such as catheters, to be used for another patient is *not* an acceptable method for preventing the transmission of hepatitis.

**Preventive measures used with persons with known hepatitis.** Patients with known HAV should be placed on *enteric precautions* which is part of universal precautions, during the time of infectivity. Children should be in private rooms, but responsible adults do not require one. Good handwashing after fecal and urine elimination is essential. Anyone handling feces or potentially contaminated articles (bedpan, diapers, rectal thermometer) must wear gloves and gowns and wash hands thoroughly after completing care (see Research box, p. 1384). Separate toilet facilities are sometimes used, but this is not necessary if fecal contamination, which might occur in a person who is confused, is not a problem. The toilet should be cleansed thoroughly daily. All disposable and nondisposable equipment and linens should be bagged properly and labeled correctly before being removed from the patient's room.

For patients with HBV, HCV, or HDV, good handwashing and blood/body fluid precautions (also part of universal precautions) are used. Any time blood or body fluids are handled, gown and gloves must be worn. The benefit of double-gloving is unknown. If splattering of contaminated blood and body fluids is likely, goggles and a mask are worn. Care must be taken to avoid contact

## RESEARCH

Korniewicz DM et al: Integrity of vinyl and latex procedure gloves, *Nurs Res* 38:144-146, 1989.

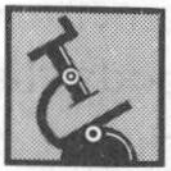

The use of protective gloves in the delivery of nursing care is a critical component in preventing the spread of HBV and human immunodeficiency virus (HIV). The risk of transmission of HBV exceeds that for HIV. The effectiveness of gloves in preventing transmission of HBV or HIV depends on the integrity of the gloves during use. This study was designed to determine the integrity of vinyl and latex procedure gloves under in-use conditions that are present in clinical practice.

In this study, 645 latex and vinyl gloves from 28 lot numbers and five manufacturers were first tested for presence of visible defects when filled with water and allowed to hang vertically for 2 minutes. Next, 90 vinyl and 90 latex gloves with no visible defects were checked for permeability to dye after being worn by one of 28 subjects during one of three levels of hand manipulation, some of which mimicked activities performed during routine patient care. The permeability of the gloves to *Serratia marcescens* was also tested using 50 of each type of glove.

Visible defects were present in 4.1% of the vinyl gloves and 2.7% of the latex gloves. Fifty-three percent of vinyl and 3% of the latex gloves showed dye penetration, and 20% of latex gloves and 34% of vinyl gloves that were watertight allowed for penetration of *S. marcescens*.

Glove standards set by the American Society for Testing and Materials (ASTM) allow for a failure rate of 1.5% for sterile surgical latex gloves and 2.5 for nonsterile latex gloves by the watertight method. When the watertight test was used in this study, the latex glove failure rate was equal to the standards established by ASTM, whereas the vinyl glove failure rate was much higher. When more sensitive tests were used to examine the gloves, both the latex and the vinyl gloves showed failure rates higher than the standard.

Latex gloves maintained better integrity when tested after in-use conditions than did vinyl gloves in all tests. Because all gloves showed leakage, this finding reemphasizes the need for excellent handwashing before and after all patient care activities, the importance of not reusing gloves, and the importance of not just washing the gloved hands between patient contacts. Additionally, in situations where high stress is placed on the gloves during patient care, gloves may need to be changed.

between the blood and body fluids of an infected person and open cuts, the mucous membranes, or eyes of another person. All invasive equipment such as needles, lancets, and dental drills should be disposed of properly or sterilized properly. All contaminated items should be bagged and labeled correctly. A history of viral hepatitis precludes blood donation because of the possibility of being a carrier. Intimate sexual contact should be avoided during the period of infection. Protection of household and sexual contacts of persons who become HBV carriers is discussed later in this chapter.

### Medical management

The goal for discharge of patients with viral hepatitis as determined by DRGs is 6 days. The nurse works collaboratively with the physician for implementation of the prescribed medical therapy. Common medical therapy includes the following.

**Diagnostic tests.** Blood tests are done for viral antibodies and antigens and for actual viral particles (see Table 42-3).

**Medication.** Vitamin K is given if the prothrombin time is prolonged. Antihistamines are given for pruritus associated with jaundice, and antiemetics are given for nausea. Essentially, all analgesics are metabolized in the liver and therefore are given only sparingly in people with liver dysfunction. Fulminant viral hepatitis may be treated with corticosteroids, but this is controversial.

**Diet.** If liver function is not impaired, a well-balanced diet is adequate. Protein and sodium are restricted if liver function is compromised. Abstinence from alcohol is essential.

**Activity.** Rest is the foundation of treatment for viral hepatitis. Activity can be increased as tolerated by the patient.

## NURSING MANAGEMENT

### ♦ ASSESSMENT

Nursing assessment focuses on identifying the changes related to viral hepatitis and sources of transmission that are controllable.

### Subjective Data

Data to be included to assess the patient with viral hepatitis include the following:

- Presence of discomfort: headache, right upper abdominal quadrant tenderness, arthralgia, itching
- Presence of GI alterations: history of anorexia, nausea, vomiting, dyspepsia
- Changes in nutritional intake of food and fluids
- History of changes in weight
- History of episodes of fever, chills, or adenopathy
- Reports of weakness/malaise not relieved by rest
- History of potential exposure to hepatitis virus: work environment, child-care facilities, recent international travel, injections of illegal drugs, recent blood transfusions, contaminated food and water, recent sexual contact with infected person, homosexual or bisexual life-style
- Knowledge about the disease
- Length of time since onset of symptoms

### Objective Data

Data to be included to assess the patient with viral hepatitis include the following:

Skin/sclera: adequacy of skin turgor, presence of jaundice or lesions from scratching; if jaundice is present, the nurse should assess the patient for the presence of petechiae or bruises
Lymph nodes: enlargement
Abdomen: liver enlargement, guarding in right upper quadrant
Documented nutritional and fluid intake and output
Temperature
Weight/height
Musculoskeletal: strength, ability to do activities

## ♦ NURSING DIAGNOSES

Nursing diagnoses are determined from analysis of patient data. Nursing diagnoses for the patient with viral hepatitis may include but are not limited to the following:

| Diagnostic Title | Possible Etiologic Factors |
|---|---|
| Fatigue | Imbalance between energy level and demand, decreased rest, feeling of malaise |
| Activity intolerance | Fatigue, weakness |
| Fluid volume deficit, high risk for | Vomiting, sweating, decreased intake, elevated temperature |
| Infection, high risk for | Length of infectivity and transmission to others through blood and/or body fluids |
| Knowledge deficit: diagnostic tests, manifestations, isolation, prophylaxis for others, treatment, prevention of future cases | Anxiety, new diagnosis, multiple tests |
| Nutrition, altered: less than body requirements | Anorexia, inadequate intake, increased metabolic needs |
| Pain | Arthralgia, itching, headaches, abdominal tenderness |
| Health maintenance, altered | Lack of knowledge or indifference to "safe sex" practices, needle sharing |
| Skin integrity, high risk for impaired | Jaundice, itching, scratching |
| Social isolation | Physical isolation, fear of others catching disease |
| Injury (trauma), high risk for | Altered clotting or prothrombin time |

## ♦ EXPECTED PATIENT OUTCOMES

Expected patient outcomes for the person with viral hepatitis may include but are not limited to the following:

1. Is able to explain why fatigue occurs and indicates a decrease in fatigue, as evidenced by giving it a lower rating on a scale of 1 to 5, with 1 indicating no fatigue.
2. Slowly increases activity until former activity level is achieved.
3. Maintains good skin tone, stable weight, and adequate and balanced intake and output and demonstrates no significant orthostatic postural changes in blood pressure (decrease in systolic between lying and standing of ≤10 mm Hg) or pulse (increase in pulse between lying and standing of ≤10 beats/min).
4. Is able to demonstrate adequate isolation precautions while hospitalized and describes appropriate precautions for use at home.
5. Is able to list the diagnostic tests prescribed, explain why isolation precautions are necessary, list significant others who require prophylaxis, describe the purpose of all treatments, and describe care necessary for prevention of future infections.
6. Increases food intake until adequate in amount and content for body size.
7. Verbalizes that pain is controlled and/or rates pain on a scale from 1 (no pain) to 10 (severe pain).
8. Is able to explain safe sex practices and use and describe the risk of needle sharing (see Chapter 19).
9. Skin remains intact and free of lesions.
10. Expresses the feeling that isolation is not distressing and shares information that reveals he or she is being kept up to date about family affairs.
11. Does not experience undetected bleeding.

## ♦ INTERVENTIONS

The patient with hepatitis needs general supportive care that promotes rest, fluid balance, prevention of injury, prevention of spread of disease, adequate knowledge, adequate nutrition, comfort, prevention of impairment of skin integrity, and prevention of social isolation. If the patient with HBV or HDV has a history of multiple sex partners, counseling and patient education about safe sex practices, as described in Chapters 55 and 71, are necessary. If a history of illegal drug use is elicited, the patient needs the care described in Chapter 19. The spread of the human immunodeficiency virus (HIV) and the hepatitis virus can be stopped in users of IV drugs if the practice of sharing equipment ceases. Some persons have suggested that sterile needles/syringes should be distributed to persons who are addicted to IV drugs, and some communities are doing so.

### Monitoring Fatigue

The patient with hepatitis will need considerable rest during the acute phase of the illness. The level of physical activity allowed will be individually determined on the basis of the amount of fatigue and severity of the disease. Rest periods should be interspersed throughout the day, and patient care should be scheduled to allow for uninterrupted periods for napping and relaxation. If hepatic enzyme levels increase with resumption of near-normal activities, limitations on activity will be reimposed.

## Reducing Activity Intolerance

The patient should be instructed to increase activity slowly as tolerated. An adequate diet will provide needed energy for increasing activity.

## Maintaining Fluid Intake and Nutritional Status

During the acute phase of the illness, the patient needs 3000 ml/day of fluids because of the increased fluid needs associated with febrile illness and vomiting. The fluid can usually be given orally if nausea and vomiting are not severe. When nausea and vomiting are severe, IV infusions are given. Intake, output, and weight should be monitored to assess the patient for adequacy of intake. Fluids such as fruit juices and carbonated beverages that provide both volume and nutrients are encouraged. Because patients with impaired liver function may not produce adequate levels of albumin and may not metabolize aldosterone, abnormal fluid retention can occur. Although abnormal retention of fluids is rare in acute viral hepatitis, the patient should be monitored for abnormal fluid retention.

No special dietary restrictions are required in most patients. The diet should be well balanced and provide adequate nutrients and calories based on the patient's size and age. The diet should be planned with the patient so that it is appealing. Frequent, small meals are usually better tolerated than larger meals. Fats may need to be restricted if poorly tolerated. Intolerance to fatty foods can occur if bile obstruction is severe. Good oral hygiene and the maintenance of a clean, pleasant environment may enhance appetite. Antiemetics may be used and should be given ½ hour before meals. Alcoholic beverages should be avoided, since they are metabolized in the liver and can damage it.

## Preventing Spread of Infection

All patients with hepatitis require precautions to prevent spread of the virus. For patients with HAV, the following *enteric precautions* or universal precautions are necessary:

1. Good handwashing by patient and staff
2. Wearing gloves when handling feces/urine
3. Wearing a gown when soiling of uniform is likely
4. Cleansing of toilet daily and use of private toilet
5. Private room necessary only if patient cannot take care of self regarding proper disposal of feces and urine
6. Proper cleansing, bagging, and labeling of contaminated items such as bed linens and bedpans
7. Discarding contaminated items such as rectal thermometers

For the patient with HBV, universal precautions are used and include the following:

1. Good handwashing by patient and staff
2. Wearing gloves when handling blood or body fluids
3. Wearing a gown, goggles, and/or mask when splattering of blood or body fluids is likely
4. Proper cleansing, bagging, and labeling of contaminated equipment and linens
5. Proper disposal of needles or any items exposed to the patient's blood or body fluids
6. Careful labeling of blood specimens to protect personnel working with them
7. Avoidance of contamination of open cuts and mucous membranes with patient's blood or body fluid
8. Teaching patients to avoid intimate sexual contact until liver function tests have returned to normal

The nurse in the hospital at times and particularly the nurse in the community are also involved in identifying patient contacts who will require prophylaxis. Prophylactic therapy should be administered to contacts as described on p. 1382.

## Facilitating Learning

A major focus of care is patient education. Most patients are treated at home for the duration of their illness. The nurse must prepare these persons for adequate home care by teaching them about the measures previously described for the provision of adequate rest, provision of adequate fluid and nutritional intake, relief of discomfort, identification of signs and symptoms of bleeding, and maintenance of adequate isolation. The patient must be able to detect changes indicating a worsening of his or her condition (e.g., increasing fatigue, uncontrolled nausea and vomiting, onset of bleeding, worsening of upper quadrant discomfort, water retention) and be instructed to report these changes immediately.

All patients, whether treated in the hospital or at home, should understand that it may take several months or longer for complete recovery and that they must be evaluated frequently for repeated assessment of blood studies to monitor their progress. Blood studies may be performed weekly for several weeks and then monthly until they return to normal. If blood studies do not show the expected improvement from the care being given, more invasive procedures, such as a liver biopsy, will be necessary to identify why. The patient will be followed for at least 1 year after liver function tests have returned to normal to ensure that relapse does not occur.

## Providing Comfort Measures and Promoting Skin Integrity

During the early phase of the illness, the patient may have headaches and arthralgia, resulting in discomfort. The use of general comfort measures, relaxing baths, backrubs, fresh linen on the bed, and a quiet, dark environment may help make the patient more comfortable. During the icteric phase of the illness, the presence of bile pigments in the skin may cause severe pruritus. The cause of pruritus is unknown, but it is aggravated by the presence of bile pigments in the skin and by tissue anoxia and dilation of capillaries. Pruritus can be exhausting and demoralizing to the patient.

Measures to control pruritus include the following:

1. Use of cool, light, nonrestrictive clothing and avoidance of clothes or blankets made of wool
2. Use of soft, dry, clean bedding; use of warm, not hot, tub baths
3. Application of emollient creams and lotions to skin
4. Avoidance of activities that promote sweating and increase body temperature
5. Maintenance of a cool environment
6. Administration of antihistamines as ordered
7. Use of diversional activities such as reading, television, and radio to reduce the patient's perception of pruritus

The major aim of care is to prevent scratching with resultant injury to the skin. It is impossible for people with pruritus not to scratch. Sometimes the person may be given a soft cloth with which to rub the skin. The patient's fingernails should be kept short, and the patient's hands should be kept clean to decrease the likelihood of excoriation or infection, if scratching occurs.

### Supporting Health Maintenance

The nurse must provide an open and honest environment where frank discussions about dangerous sexual practices and drug use can be undertaken. The risk of contracting viral hepatitis through multiple sex partners should be addressed. Sharing of IV drug equipment should be discouraged, and alternatives, such as drug treatment, should be suggested.

### Avoiding Social Isolation

The nurse must work with the patient and significant others so that they understand that the needed isolation does not prohibit social interaction and visiting. Fear of spread of the infection can lead others to avoid the patient. Proper teaching can ensure that both isolation and the patient's need for support from significant others are maintained.

### Preventing Injury

In a patient with a prolonged prothrombin time, bleeding may be a major problem. The patient should be assessed carefully for signs of bleeding. This includes monitoring the urine and stools for fresh or old blood, monitoring any incisions for recurrent bleeding, monitoring the skin for petechiae, monitoring vital signs, and monitoring prothrombin time, hematocrit, and hemoglobin. Minor procedures such as drawing of blood can result in hematoma formation, if precautions are not instituted. Care to prevent *hematoma formation* includes the following:

1. Planning so that all blood samples are collected at one time to avoid several punctures
2. Avoiding intramuscular and subcutaneous injections, if possible
3. Applying pressure to injection sites and venipuncture site for 5 minutes after the procedure

Other precautions to prevent bleeding include:

1. Using soft toothbrushes or swabs to avoid injury to gums and resultant bleeding
2. Testing stools for occult blood

If prothrombin time is prolonged, vitamin K may be administered.

## ♦ EVALUATION

To evaluate the effectiveness of nursing interventions, compare patient behaviors with those stated in the expected patient outcomes. Successful achievement of patient outcomes for the patient with viral hepatitis is indicated by the following:

1. States why fatigue is present and that fatigue remains at a rating of 2 or less if rest periods are interspersed throughout the day.
2. Increases activity level without an increase in fatigue.
3. Has good skin tone and an intake that equals output and is adequate for age and body size; no orthostatic blood pressure changes are present; and weight has returned to normal and is stable.
4. Correctly describes isolation precautions for home, including using separate bathroom from family; flushing stool twice after using; handling own body secretions; not sharing razors, toothbrushes, and food or drinks; abstaining from intimate relationships until infection has subsided; and washing hands as appropriate.
5. Correctly describes blood tests; explains why isolation is necessary; identifies persons in household who may have been exposed to same source of infection from contaminated foods and fluids, hygiene practices, sharing of needles, or sexual relationships; explains need for high-protein, high-calorie, well-balanced diet, adequate rest, and avoidance of alcohol; explains hygiene practices, safe sex practices, and avoidance of sharing of needles to avoid future infections; and states plans for obtaining vaccinations for self and others as appropriate.
6. Calorie intake and food selections are appropriate for body size and metabolic need.
7. States that itching and arthralgia are controlled and that no scratching, restlessness, or grimacing is present.
8. Correctly explains safe sex practices and dangers of sharing needles.
9. Skin is intact.
10. States that he or she is aware of family affairs.
11. Hematocrit and hemoglobin levels remain within normal limits, prothrombin time is within normal limits, and no undetected bleeding episodes occur.

### Complications

Complications of viral hepatitis include the possibility of developing chronic active hepatitis with subsequent

**TABLE 42-4 Types of Cirrhosis**

| TYPE | ETIOLOGY | DESCRIPTION |
|---|---|---|
| Laënnec's cirrhosis (nutritional, portal, or alcoholic cirrhosis) | Alcoholism, malnutrition | Massive collagen formation; liver in fatty and hepatitis stages is large and firm; in late state, it is small and nodular. |
| Postnecrotic cirrhosis | Massive necrosis from hepatotoxins, usually viral hepatitis | Liver is decreased in size with nodules and fibrous tissue. |
| Biliary cirrhosis | Biliary obstruction in liver and common bile duct | Chronic impairment of bile drainage; liver is first large, then becomes firm and nodular; jaundice is major symptom. |
| Cardiac cirrhosis | Right-sided congestive heart failure (CHF) | Liver is swollen, and changes are reversible if CHF is treated effectively; some fibrosis occurs with long-standing CHF. |
| Nonspecific, metabolic cirrhosis | Metabolic problems, infectious diseases, infiltrative diseases, GI diseases | Portal and liver fibrosis may develop; liver is enlarged and firm. |

cirrhosis and liver failure. These complications are discussed on pp. 1388-1411.

## CIRRHOSIS OF THE LIVER

**Cirrhosis** of the liver is the term applied to chronic disease of the liver characterized by diffuse inflammation and fibrosis of the liver resulting in drastic structural changes and significant loss of liver function. The basic changes in cirrhosis are liver cell death and replacement of normal tissue by regeneration of cell mass and scar tissue that results in nodules of normal liver parenchyma surrounded by fibrous tissue. These changes result in loss of function and distortion of the structure with a resultant obstruction of hepatic blood flow.

Cirrhosis of the liver can be classified in various ways. Table 42-4 lists the major types of cirrhosis based on a pathologic classification.

### Etiology

As can be seen from Table 42-4, cirrhosis can result from liver disease secondary to intrahepatic and extrahepatic cholestasis, viral hepatitis, and other hepatotoxins (drugs, chemicals). Alcoholism and malnutrition are two major predisposing factors for development of Laënnec's cirrhosis. Less common causes of cirrhosis are right-sided congestive heart failure, hemochromatosis, Wilson's disease, glycogen storage disease, cystic fibrosis, and small bowel bypass. In some patients the cause is not identifiable.

### Epidemiology

**Postnecrotic cirrhosis** from hepatotoxins is the most common type of cirrhosis worldwide. **Laënnec's cirrhosis** is the most common type in North America and accounts for 75% of all cases of cirrhosis.

The role of alcohol in the development of cirrhosis is still under study. It is known, however, that approximately 15% of all alcoholics will develop cirrhosis and that the volume of alcohol rather than the type of alcohol is the important factor. Most persons with Laënnec's cirrhosis have a history of consumption of the equivalent of a pint of whiskey a day for 15 years.

Cirrhosis as a cause of death in the United States now ranks fourth in middle-aged men and women, accounting for 350,000 deaths each year. Cirrhosis can occur in any age-group, but in the United States it is more common in 45- to 64-year-old white men and in nonwhites of both sexes.

### Pathophysiology

In Laënnec's cirrhosis caused by alcoholism and in other types of cirrhosis, fatty infiltration of the liver is the first alteration seen. This fatty infiltration is usually reversible if the causative factor (alcohol, malnutrition, or biliary obstruction) is halted or reversed. If the degenerative process continues, acute inflammation (alcoholic hepatitis) and cirrhosis result.

The result of any type of cirrhosis is loss of liver function and obstruction of hepatic portal blood flow. Alterations in physiology are usually seen late in the progression of the disease because of the large reserve capacity of the liver. As much as three fourths of the liver can be destroyed before physiologic function is altered.

In the United States the pathophysiology seen most often is a result of both cirrhosis and long-term alcohol abuse. The relationships between normal functions of the liver and alterations seen in cirrhosis are presented in Table 42-5.

The fibrotic changes in the liver that result from continual destruction distort the hepatic structures and result in obstruction of splanchnic veins and portal blood flow. This obstruction can result in additional problems with fluid retention, including increasing edema, ascites, and hydrothorax. Increased portal pressure and splanchnic venous congestion result in splenomegaly and altered spleen function, which can cause leukopenia, thrombocytopenia, and anemia. Portal hypertension causes increased venous pressure, vascular hemostasis, varicose veins, hemorrhoids, and esophageal varices.

**TABLE 42-5 Relationship Between Normal Liver Functions and Altered Functions Associated With Cirrhosis**

| NORMAL LIVER FUNCTIONS | ALTERED PHYSIOLOGIC FUNCTIONS |
|---|---|
| Maintenance of normal size and drainage of blood from GI tract | Liver inflammation<br>↓<br>Venous congestion of GI tract → Altered GI function<br>↓<br>GI symptoms |
| Metabolism of carbohydrates | Increased glycogenesis and decreased glycogenolysis and gluconeogenesis<br>↓<br>Altered glucose metabolism<br>↓<br>Decreased energy |
| Metabolism of fats | Increased fatty acid and triglyceride synthesis and decreased fatty acid oxidation and triglyceride release<br>↓ Fatty liver ↓ Hepatomegaly<br>↓ Decreased energy production; weight loss |
| Protein metabolism | Decreased production of albumin → decreased colloidal osmotic pressure → edema and ascites<br><br>Decreased production of clotting factors<br>↓<br>Altered clotting studies<br>↓<br>Bleeding tendencies<br>↓<br>Blood loss → anemia<br><br>Decreased protein synthesis in general<br>↓<br>Alteration in immune function and alteration in healing |
| Detoxification of endogenous substances | Decreased metabolism of sex steroids (estrogen, progesterone, testosterone)<br>↓ Male ↓ Loss of masculine characteristics and development of some feminine characteristics from excessive estrogen<br>↓ Female ↓ Loss of feminine characteristics and development of some masculine characteristics from excessive testosterone<br><br>Decreased metabolism of aldosterone<br>↓ Sodium and water retention ↓ Edema, ascites<br>↓ Increased potassium and hydrogen excretion ↓ Hypokalemia and alkalosis<br><br>Decreased metabolism of ammonia (usually resulting from blood bypassing liver rather than loss of parenchymal cell function) → increased ammonia levels<br>↓<br>Hepatic encephalopathy<br>↓<br>Changes in coordination, memory, orientation, etc. |

*Continued*

**TABLE 42-5 Relationship Between Normal Liver Functions and Altered Functions Associated With Cirrhosis—cont'd**

| NORMAL LIVER FUNCTIONS | ALTERED PHYSIOLOGIC FUNCTIONS |
|---|---|
| Detoxification of exogenous substances | Decreased metabolism of drugs → Altered drug effects and potential increase in toxicities and side effects |
| Metabolism and storage of vitamins and minerals | Decreased stores of vitamins and minerals → Decreased red blood cell production → Anemia; Decreased stores of vitamins and minerals → Decreased energy production |
| Bile production and excretion | Obstruction to bile flow → Decreased fat absorption → Decreased vitamin K absorption → Decreased clotting factors → Bleeding/blood loss |
| Bilirubin metabolism | Decreased uptake of bilirubin from circulation → increased unconjugated bilirubin → jaundice, pruritus, scratching, and skin lesions<br>Decreased conjugation and release of bilirubin → increased conjugated bilirubin and increased urine bilirubin → jaundice, pruritus, scratching, and skin lesions<br>Decreased excretion of bilirubin to bowel → light-colored stools (clay or grayish white)<br>Decreased reuptake of urobilinogen → ↑ urine urobilinogen → dark urine |

**BOX 42-11 Clinical Manifestations and Sequelae of Cirrhosis**

- History of failing health
  - Nausea
  - Vomiting
  - Anorexia
  - Indigestion
  - Flatulence
  - Constipation
- Weight loss masked by water retention
- Malnutrition
- Abdominal pain (usually right upper quadrant)
  - Dull
  - Mild
  - Steady or wavelike
- Late signs occurring gradually
  - Ascites
  - Jaundice
  - Edema
  - Anemia
  - Bleeding

(Figure 42-3, *A*, depicts the venous drainage of splanchnic organs, and Figure 42-3, *B*, depicts the massive ascites and dilated vasculature that can be seen in cirrhosis.)

A variety of signs and symptoms can be seen in persons with cirrhosis. The patient may exhibit any or all of the signs and symptoms. Most manifestations can be directly related to the pathophysiology (Table 42-5 and Figure 42-4). Box 42-11 lists clinical manifestations of cirrhosis.

## Prevention

### *Healthy People 2000*

The goal of ***Healthy People 2000*** is to reduce the number of deaths from cirrhosis to no more than 6 per 100,000 people, with African-American men, Native Americans, and Alaskan Inuits being targeted populations.[17] Even though cirrhosis among African-American and Native-American men has decreased in the last decade, the death rate for nonwhite men is 70% higher than for white men.[17]

#### Primary prevention

In the United States, programs aimed at the prevention of cirrhosis are designed primarily to control the ingestion of alcohol. The loss of time from work related to alcoholism is estimated to cost billions of dollars annually. Many large corporations have or are organizing programs to help employees control their alcohol intake (see Chapter 19).

#### Secondary prevention

Early detection of cirrhosis is difficult because three fourths of the liver can be destroyed before signs of cirrhosis become evident. For this reason, cessation of alcohol intake is the focus of prevention.

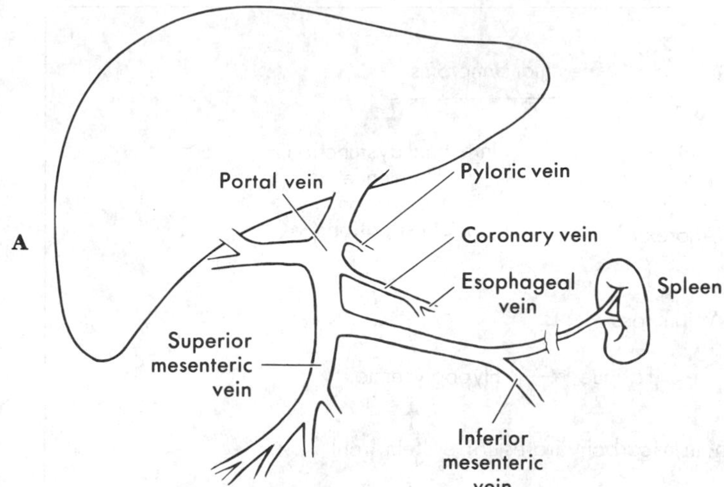


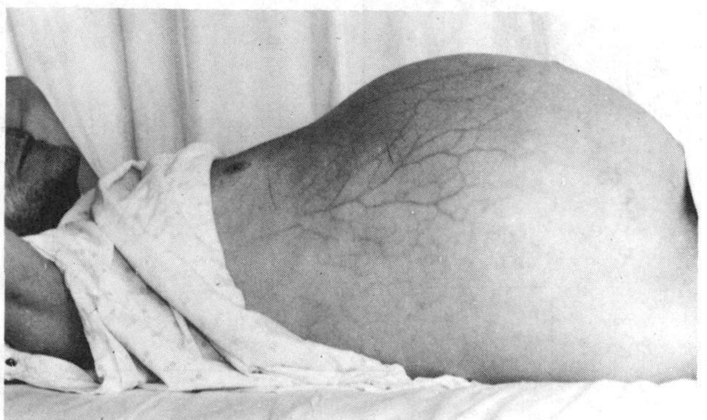


**FIGURE 42-3** **A,** Splanchnic veins. Venous drainage of splanchnic organs. When portal hypertension develops, other vessels can become engorged, leading to stasis and hypoxia of respective organs. **B,** Massive ascites. Note bulging flanks, dilated upper abdominal veins, and everted umbilicus. (**A** from Groer ME, Shekleton ME: ***Basic pathophysiology: a conceptual approach,*** ed 2, St Louis, 1983, Mosby; **B** from Prior JA, Silberstein JS, Stang JM: ***Physical diagnosis: the history and examination of the patient,*** ed 6, St Louis, 1981, Mosby.)

## Medical Management

The goal for discharge of patients with cirrhosis as determined by DRGs is 7 days. The nurse works collaboratively with the physician for implementation of prescribed medical therapy. Because the nurse has a major role in discharge planning and patient teaching, these are discussed under nursing management. A sample Critical Pathway is described at the end of the chapter.

No specific medical management exists for the treatment of cirrhosis. Management is directed toward removal or treatment of causative factors such as alcoholism, biliary obstruction, infections, and cardiac problems and toward preventing additional liver damage.

### Diagnostic tests

The patient with cirrhosis will have various abnormalities in blood and urine laboratory data as depicted in Figure 42-4; such as increased levels of total, unconjugated, and conjugated bilirubin; increased urine bilirubin; increased urine urobilinogen; increased prothrombin time; decreased platelets, white blood cells, and red blood cells; decreased serum albumin and serum glucose; hypokalemia; hyponatremia; and elevated levels of serum enzymes (ALT, AST, lactic dehydrogenase, alkaline phosphatase). Other studies, such as liver biopsy, CT scan, endoscopy, barium contrast, and angiography, may be done if the clinical manifestations are vague or inconsistent. The results of these later diagnostic tests depend on what complications the patient has developed.

### Medication

Drug therapy depends on the signs and symptoms the patient exhibits and includes the following medications: antihistamines for pruritus; potassium for hypokalemia; diuretics (particularly aldosterone antagonists for edema because the patient with cirrhosis does not catabolize aldosterone appropriately and has hyperaldosteronism); and folic acid, thiamine, and other vitamins and minerals for vitamin deficiency and anemia. Persons with alcoholism are particularly deficient in thiamine and folic acid because these water-soluble vitamins have been depleted and thus deficits occur rapidly with lack of intake of nutrients. Sodium and fluids are also usually restricted. Occasionally, albumin may be given for hypoalbuminemia; however, its effects last only a short time. If ascites causes severe distress, paracentesis may be done. Additional therapy is used to treat complications of chronic liver disease and is described later.

### Diet

Because alcoholism and malnutrition are major factors in the development of cirrhosis, supplying an adequate diet (well-balanced, normal nutrients) and helping the patient control alcohol intake are important.

### Activity

The patient is usually fatigued and does not tolerate activity well. The patient is encouraged to limit activity to what is comfortable for him or her.

### Referral/Consultation

In some settings the nurse assumes responsibility for making referrals to other services. Common referrals for persons with cirrhosis include gastroenterology and alcohol treatment and Alcoholics Anonymous (AA). Social service, dietary, and home health also may be consulted.

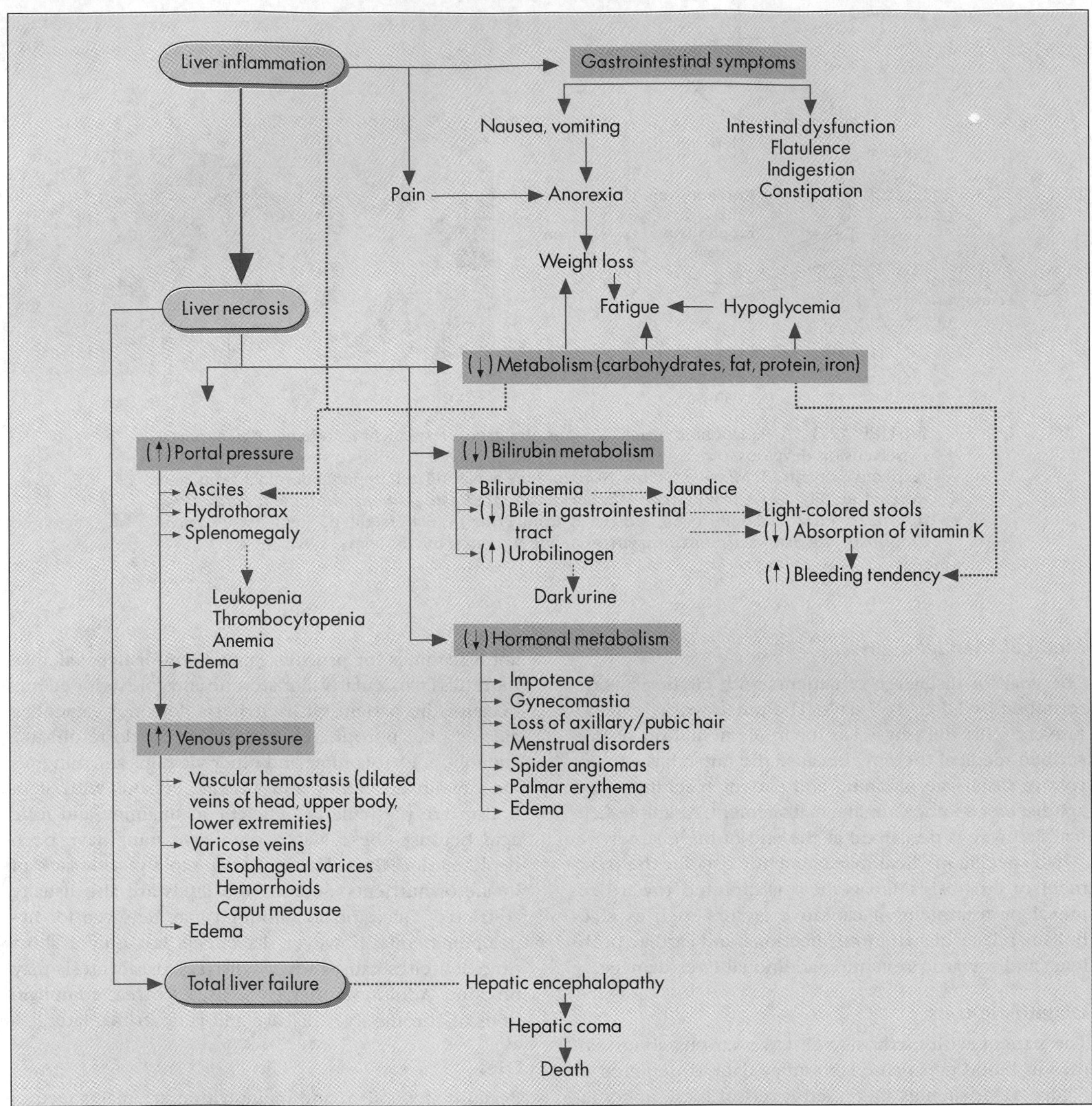


**FIGURE 42-4** Progression of liver cell failure. Pathophysiology of signs and symptoms that occur in cirrhosis. NOTE: Process can be arrested if adequate liver regeneration occurs. Regeneration is rarely complete, and there is always some liver cell deficiency.

## NURSING MANAGEMENT

### ♦ ASSESSMENT

A thorough nursing assessment is necessary to define adequately the multiple nursing diagnosis that can occur.

#### Subjective Data

Data to be included to assess the patient with cirrhosis include the following:

Overview of patient's complaints, including length of time patient has had them; a history of temperature elevations; history of frequent infections

General body characteristics: history of changes in color of skin or sclera or history of skin marks such as bruising and hematomas; history of changes in secondary sex characteristics (external genitalia, body hair distribution, breast tissue); history of increase in abdominal size (belt size); history of edema; any complaints of itching

Social habits: drug and alcohol use, amount, factors that precipitate use, any attempts to quit, limitations on success, reasons for failure; last time patient had a drink; work environment

Nutritional history: daily 24-hour intake for past 1 to 3 days, history of recent change in appetite

GI system: complaints of nausea, vomiting, anorexia, indigestion, flatulence, or abdominal tenderness

Elimination: history of any changes in amount or color of urine, changes in bowel movements, or changes in color of feces

Neuromuscular: any complaints of weakness, fatigue, history of decreased ability to do work; history of any changes in memory or coordination; any history of tremors

Sexuality: history of impotence (males), decreased libido (males and females), or change in menstrual patterns (females)

## Objective Data

Data to be included to assess the patient with cirrhosis include the following:

Vital signs, including orthostatic blood pressure and pulse, temperature, weight

Skin and sclera: presence of jaundice, bruises, hematomas, petechiae, spider angiomas, palmar erythema, dilated vessels on upper body or lower extremities, loss of chest hair (males), gynecomastia (males), edema of lower extremities, lesions from scratching

Abdomen: bowel sounds, presence of abdominal distention or guarding, presence of ascites (fluid wave or shifting dullness), increased abdominal girth, increased liver size, presence of hepatic bruits, enlarged spleen, presence of dilated veins on abdomen *(caput medusae)*

Neuromuscular: muscle wasting, decreased muscle strength, presence of deficits in memory or coordination, presence of tremors, asterixis, exaggerated deep tendon reflexes, changes in orientation, behavior or emotional changes, presence of apraxia

GI/elimination: volume of urine output, color of urine and stools, presence of testicular atrophy

Respiratory: breath sounds, presence of dullness in right lower lobe (RLL)

# ♦ NURSING DIAGNOSES

Nursing diagnoses are determined from analysis of patient data. Nursing diagnoses for the person with cirrhosis may include but are not limited to the following:

| Diagnostic Title | Possible Etiologic Factors |
|---|---|
| Breathing pattern, ineffective | Increased restriction of chest movement from ascites or hydrothorax; decreased depth of breathing from limited mobility |
| Fatigue | Energy needs greater than energy production associated with anemia, altered metabolism, and poor food intake; electrolyte imbalance |
| Fluid volume, excess | Abnormal fluid retention associated with increased circulating aldosterone, decreased colloidal osmotic pressure or hepatorenal syndrome |
| Health maintenance, altered | Inability to make appropriate judgments because of alcoholism |
| Infection, high risk for | Decreased immune competence associated with altered protein metabolism and alcoholism; loss of normal phagocytic function of liver or decreased leukocytes secondary to splenomegaly; alterations in external immune barriers (skin and GI mucosal integrity) |
| Injury (trauma), high risk for | Alteration in clotting mechanism, enhancing bleeding; alteration in neurologic function and strength that could lead to falls |
| Knowledge deficit: diagnostic tests, treatment, home care, follow-up care | Lack of exposure to information; potential cognitive limitations |
| Nutrition, altered: less than body requirements | Impaired metabolism, nausea, decreased intake |
| Pain: itching | Enlarged liver and pruritus associated with jaundice |
| Self-esteem disturbances | Inability to accept physical changes of abdominal girth, jaundice, and change in secondary sexual characteristics; changes in roles and relationships |
| Skin integrity, high risk for impaired | Scratching, edema, impaired mobility |

Many other nursing diagnoses that might be identified result from the complications associated with cirrhosis. These vary from patient to patient.

# ♦ EXPECTED PATIENT OUTCOMES

Expected patient outcomes for the person with cirrhosis may include but are not limited to the following:

1. Shows no increase in dullness on percussion of thorax and has normal breath sounds and normal chest x-ray films.
2. Demonstrates a gradual increase in activities, is able to meet self-care needs, and ambulates an increased amount each day.
3. Has an output of urine that is greater than fluid intake until excess fluids are excreted, has a daily decrease in weight, has resolution of edema, has a decrease of abdominal girth, and has a return of electrolytes to normal.
4. Verbalizes that alcohol is a problem, states that alcohol has caused his or her problem, lists resources available for assisting with alcohol problem, and contacts one resource (alcohol counselor, AA, inpatient center).
5. Develops no new infection(s) and has a return to normal temperature.

6. Does not develop any undetected bleeding, maintains normal vital signs, and has no falls or injuries.
7. Patient or significant other can perform the following:
   a. List prescribed diagnostic tests.
   b. Describe the planned treatment regimen and patient's long-term role in treatment.
   c. Explain the dietary plan to be followed at home.
   d. Explain prescribed fluid restrictions.
   e. Explain prescribed medications, such as diuretics and vitamins (dosage, expected effects, and side effects to report).
   f. Explain ways to prevent bleeding, infections, and progression of disease.
   g. Explain plans for follow-up care and signs and symptoms (weight gain, increased temperature, bleeding, change in behavior) that should be reported to physician.
8. Eats food from all food groups (unless restricted) in adequate amounts to meet caloric needs and experiences a decrease in signs of muscle wasting.
9. Reports that itching is controlled and is not observed scratching.
10. Describes self in positive terms, discusses accomplishments, and sets realistic goals.
11. Maintains intact skin and shows healing of any lesions.

## ♦ INTERVENTIONS

The patient with cirrhosis may be acutely ill and may require critical nursing care or may be relatively free of acute problems and require teaching, counseling, and support. The nurse must set priorities for care on the basis of the patient's needs. Care for the various patient outcomes is described next and in the nursing care plan on pp. 1396-1399.

### Supporting Respiration

The patient with cirrhosis has decreased resistance to infection and may be particularly prone to respiratory infection because of the presence of a hydrothorax and/or shallow breathing. The patient may experience dyspnea because of pressure on the diaphragm from ascites.

A high Fowler's position may assist respiratory exchange. The patient for whom bedrest is prescribed should be encouraged to turn frequently and to take deep breaths to prevent stasis of secretions. Hydrothorax is sometimes treated with thoracentesis (see Chapter 37). The nurse should prepare the patient for this procedure, assist with the procedure, and monitor the patient's response during the procedure and afterward.

### Controlling Fatigue

Patients with cirrhosis have various levels of fatigue. The amount and type of activity encouraged depend on the individual's energy level, level of consciousness and coordination, and whether any complications of cirrhosis are present. If the patient has severe fluid excess and ascites or signs and symptoms of other complications, bedrest is usually required. When bedrest is required, special attention to skin care is necessary, particularly if the patient also has severe peripheral edema. Alternating pressure mattresses or flotation pads may be helpful. If bedrest is not required, the patient should be ambulated within the room or hall as tolerated. Level of tolerance is based on the patient's statement about the level of fatigue and/or pulse changes (pulse should not increase by more than 10 beats above baseline with activity).

### Maintaining Fluid and Electrolyte Balance

Most patients with cirrhosis have sodium retention and hypokalemia. A great majority of patients have ascites, and some also have peripheral edema. The exact management of these varies depending on the patient's needs.

Potassium replacement will be given for ***hypokalemia.*** It is usually given orally, and the nurse should monitor the patient's serum $K^+$ values to verify that the patient is not developing hyperkalemia. Some patients with cirrhosis develop hepatorenal syndrome and have decreased renal function, which impairs the excretion of potassium and can develop hyperkalemia quite rapidly.

Sodium imbalance and ascites are treated in several ways. Restriction of sodium aids greatly in limiting the formation of ascitic fluid. The basis for determining the amount of dietary restriction necessary to reduce sodium and water retention may initially be a collection of urine for 24 hours to determine sodium loss. Sodium is generally restricted to 1 g daily. The sodium restriction along with bedrest may be enough to relieve the ascites and edema.

If bedrest and sodium restriction do not improve ascites, diuretics may be used. Spironolactone A (aldactone A), which inhibits the reabsorption of sodium in the distal tubules and promotes potassium retention by inhibiting the synthesis and renal effects of aldosterone, is frequently used. The therapy is adjusted on an individual basis. Sometimes furosemide (Lasix) or another diuretic is used with spironolactone. Because furosemide causes potassium excretion and can worsen hypokalemia, the patient's serum potassium level is monitored frequently, and the patient is observed for signs and symptoms of hypokalemia such as abdominal distention, nausea, vomiting, anorexia, decreased bowel sounds, weakness, or irregular pulse.

Removal of fluid through the kidneys has the advantage of not removing essential body protein, such as occurs when fluid is removed from the abdominal cavity by paracentesis. However, diuretic therapy may cause serious side effects for the patient with cirrhosis. An extremely rapid diuresis can precipitate ***oliguria*** and ***uremia*** caused by the rapidly diminished blood volume.

According to one expert, ascites cannot be mobilized at rates greater than 500 ml/day or approximately 1 lb/day.[3] If the patient has a fluid loss that is greater than 400 to 500 ml greater than intake, unless the patient has peripheral edema, which could contribute to a fluid loss greater than 400 to 500 ml/day, nonascitic extracellular fluid is being lost.[3] Infusions of albumin in 25 g units to promote retention of an adequate vascular volume may be given to prevent *azotemia* and *encephalopathy* by maintaining adequate perfusion to the kidneys and the brain and to promote diuresis. The administration of salt-poor albumin may expand the blood volume rapidly, and the patient should be monitored carefully for signs of congestive heart failure and *pulmonary edema* during and after administration.

Fluid restriction is used if hyponatremia is caused by fluid retention. Fluid restriction is monitored closely because it may lead to decreased output and the hepatorenal syndrome (see p. 1410). When fluids are restricted, the nurse must work with the patient to provide fluids that are tolerated best and to spread the allotted fluids throughout the total 24 hours. Fluids will have to be distributed to provide some at each meal and some for required medicine. Some fluids should be given on all three shifts while the patient is hospitalized. At home the patient should distribute fluids over the waking hours.

To evaluate further the effectiveness of therapy, daily weights are required. Measurements of abdominal girth assist in determining the gross amount of abdominal swelling. Patients need to be taught the importance of monitoring and reporting weight gain or rapid increase in abdominal girth after discharge. When ascites is intractable to the therapies mentioned, other procedures such as a peritoneal venous shunt may be used. Peritoneal venous shunts are described in the section on complications (see p. 1403).

## Helping Patient Avoid Alcohol

A major nursing focus for many patients is helping them to deal with alcoholism. Helping patients cope with alcohol requires that they trust the health team is interested in their well-being. The patient must admit that he or she has a drinking problem. Confrontation may sometimes be used to help the patient recognize the problem. (See Chapter 19 for a discussion of various techniques and support systems to assist persons with alcohol problems.)

## Preventing Infection

The loss of the normal phagocytic function of the liver and the leukopenia and malnutrition associated with cirrhosis require that precautions be taken to avoid infection. These precautions involve proper handwashing, observing sterile technique with all invasive procedures, respiratory preventive care, and avoidance of contact with people with infections. The patient must be monitored carefully for presence of infection, and any increase in temperature should be reported immediately so that appropriate measures can be taken.

## Preventing Bleeding and Falls

The patient with cirrhosis is at great risk for bleeding because of poor vitamin K absorption, impaired production of clotting factors, and thrombocytopenia. In addition, the patient may have gastritis, esophageal varices, and hemorrhoids that are easily injured by any substance that comes in direct contact with these dilated vessels. Nursing care should focus on monitoring for the presence of bleeding (see Guidelines box below) and instituting measures that decrease the risk of bleeding from trauma or injury to varices (see Guidelines box below). The information to be shared about diagnostic tests is described in Chapter 41. Treatment measures that will need to be explained include the dietary restrictions (sodium, protein), the fluid restrictions, the diuretics, potassium supplements, and vitamin and mineral supplements. If bedrest is prescribed, the reason this is necessary must also be explained.

*Text continued on p. 1400.*

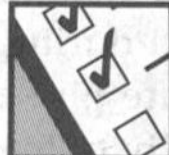

### Guidelines for Monitoring to Detect Bleeding in the Person With Cirrhosis

1. Monitor urine and stool for blood.
2. Check the patient's body daily for purpura, hematomas, and petechiae.
3. Check mouth, especially gums, carefully for signs of bleeding.
4. Check vital signs at least every 4 hours.
5. Monitor prothrombin time, partial thromboplastin time, and thrombocyte count frequently.

### Guidelines for Decreasing Risk of Bleeding in the Person With Cirrhosis

1. Avoid all intramuscular and subcutaneous injections, if possible.
2. Use the smallest-gauge needle possible when giving an injection.
3. Apply pressure to injection sites and venous puncture sites for at least 5 minutes and to arterial puncture sites for at least 10 minutes.
4. Give vitamin K as ordered.
5. Use or instruct patient to use a soft-bristled toothbrush or cotton swabs for oral hygiene.
6. Instruct patient not to strain at stool and to avoid vigorous blowing of nose or coughing.
7. Instruct patient to avoid foods (e.g., spicy, hot, raw) that can traumatize esophageal varices.
8. Provide assistance to avoid falls.
9. Make sure that room is free of clutter, that floors are dry, and that shoes or slippers are worn to avoid injuries.

# NURSING CARE PLAN

## PERSON WITH CIRRHOSIS

**DATA:** Mr. S. is a 55-year-old salesman with portal hypertension who is admitted to the hospital with upper GI bleeding. Endoscopy revealed enlarged esophageal and upper gastric veins and a bleeding ulcer. Gastric lavage with iced saline controlled bleeding; 1 U of packed red blood cells was given. Treatment orders included protein (20 g/day) and sodium (1000 mg/day) restrictions, fluid (1000 ml/day) restriction, neomycin (1 g every 4 hours), thiamine (1 ml intramuscularly), vitamin K subcutaneously once a day, and spironolactone (25 mg twice a day). A physical examination revealed slight jaundice of sclera and skin; ascites and peripheral edema; thin legs and arms and poor musculature; signs of increased estrogen; orientation to person, place, and time; and coherence; blood pressure of 116/60 mm Hg; pulse of 90 beats/min; and respiration rate of 32.

The nursing history identified the following:

- Mr. S. has participated in AA for 1 year; he has not been drinking since then.
- Mr. S. has had influenza-like symptoms the past 2 weeks but continued with his busy schedule. He complains of fatigue, anorexia, and itching.

Collaborative nursing actions include interventions to prevent further impairment of physical status from hemorrhage and ammonia toxicity and to assist in treatment of the gastric ulcer and fluid excess. Nursing actions include monitoring for the following:

- Signs of hemorrhage: hematemesis, decreased blood pressure, tachycardia, restlessness, stools testing positive for guaiac, and cool, moist skin
- Signs of hepatic encephalopathy: change in mental status, asterixis, and change in handwriting, tremors

### ■ NURSING DIAGNOSIS

Fatigue related to muscle wasting, blood loss, and potential anemia

| Expected Patient Outcome | Nursing Interventions | Rationale |
|---|---|---|
| Indicates on a weekly basis that he is less fatigued; shows improved rating of fatigue on a scale of 1 (no fatigue) to 10 (severe fatigue); shows a gradual increase in activities on a weekly basis. | Ensure or maintain bedrest as prescribed during the acute phase.<br>After acute phase, encourage increasing activity interspersed with rest periods as tolerated.<br>Intervene if patient shows fatigue after or during visits by family or friends.<br>Make sure diet is well balanced nutritionally and that patient takes calories, protein, and sodium within proper restrictions. | Graduated increase of activity is important so as not to overtax patient who has poor nutritional status and activity intolerance. |

### ■ NURSING DIAGNOSIS

Altered nutrition less than body requirements related to anorexia and flu-like symptoms

| Expected Patient Outcome | Nursing Interventions | Rationale |
|---|---|---|
| Ingests required nutrients and adequate calories on a daily basis; signs of muscle wasting lessen. | Assess knowledge of nutrient needs.<br>On a daily basis, plan and implement well-balanced, high-carbohydrate, low-protein diet with adequate vitamins.<br>Decrease roughage in diet.<br>Encourage use of salt substitute or alternative seasonings (e.g., Mrs. Dash).<br>Give antiemetics as prescribed and mouth care if nausea is present.<br>Suggest six small, frequent meals daily.<br>Use measures that encourage eating, such as a clean environment and making sure patient is rested and comfortable.<br>Support continuation of AA activities while patient hospitalized. | Food intake within prescribed limitation can influence liver regeneration; nursing measures can influence amount of intake in anorectic patient. Low-roughage diet is necessary because of esophageal varices.<br>It is important that patient continue AA participation as he has for past year. AA representatives should be allowed to see patient as condition permits. |

# NURSING CARE PLAN

## PERSON WITH CIRRHOSIS—cont'd

### ■ NURSING DIAGNOSIS

Fluid volume excess related to impaired metabolism of aldosterone and hypoalbuminemia

| Expected Patient Outcomes | Nursing Interventions | Rationale |
|---|---|---|
| Weight and abdominal girth decrease daily.<br>Edema resolves.<br>Serum sodium and potassium levels remain within normal limits. | Monitor weight daily, blood pressure q 4 hr; assess edema every shift; and measure abdominal girth daily.<br>Monitor intake and output on every shift until excess fluid is excreted.<br>Teach patient rationale for sodium restriction when he shows interest.<br>Provide bedrest for ascites.<br>Give the patient prescribed diuretics.<br>Restrict fluids; provide those that are best tolerated, and space the fluids throughout 24 hours. | Diuresis in cirrhosis is undertaken slowly using very conservative measures because of the contracted intravascular fluid volume. Diuresis in excess can jeopardize renal perfusion and precipitate portal-systemic encephalopathy, so careful monitoring is necessary. |

### ■ NURSING DIAGNOSIS

Ineffective breathing pattern related to ascites and immobility and potential status of secretions

| Expected Patient Outcomes | Nursing Interventions | Rationale |
|---|---|---|
| Dyspnea is decreased or does not worsen, as indicated on a scale of 1 (no dyspnea) to 5 (severe dyspnea).<br>Breath sounds are clear. | Monitor respirations and breath sounds q 4 hr.<br>Place in high Fowler's position.<br>Encourage patient on bedrest to turn frequently, q 2 hr.<br>Encourage deep breathing q 2 hr. | Nursing measures to encourage deep chest excursions are important when ascites and immobility are present. High Fowler's position can relieve pressure on diaphragm, which can decrease chance of stasis of secretions. |

### ■ NURSING DIAGNOSIS

High risk for impaired skin integrity related to immobility, poor nutrition, edema, and jaundice

| Expected Patient Outcome | Nursing Interventions | Rationale |
|---|---|---|
| Skin remains intact. | Assess patient's skin daily for signs of possible breakdown.<br>Use measures such as flotation mattress and routine turning schedule to prevent skin breakdown.<br>Keep skin clean and moisturized. Clean and apply lotion every shift.<br>Keep nails short and clean.<br>Provide soft cloth to rub skin. | Patient has poor nutrition, edema, immobility; all these are risk factors for pressure ulcers requiring preventive care. Jaundice could lead to scratching and requires preventive care. |

*Continued.*

# NURSING CARE PLAN

## PERSON WITH CIRRHOSIS—cont'd

### ■ NURSING DIAGNOSIS

Pain: itching related to jaundice and environmental stimuli

| Expected Patient Outcome | Nursing Interventions | Rationale |
|---|---|---|
| States that he feels more comfortable and that itching is decreased. Patient not observed scratching. | Avoid heat and heavy clothing; provide a cool environment.<br>Apply antipruritic lotion as prescribed to skin as needed at least every shift.<br>Give patient prescribed antihistamines.<br>Use diversional activities such as music.<br>Keep patient's fingernails short and clean.<br>If patient must scratch, provide soft cloth to prevent excoriations.<br>Use tepid water for bathing. | Nursing measures relieve or lessen the effects of environmental stimuli, reduce itching, and promote comfort. |

### ■ NURSING DIAGNOSIS

High risk for infection related to immunosuppression

| Expected Patient Outcome | Nursing Interventions | Rationale |
|---|---|---|
| Develops no infections; temperature remains normal. | Monitor patient for signs of infection every shift.<br>Use sterile technique for all invasive procedures.<br>Encourage pulmonary hygiene, such as turning and deep breathing q1-2 hr.<br>Restrict exposure to persons with infections. | Infection in patient with cirrhosis can be life-threatening because they can cause sepsis and can precipitate failure, which may result in hepatic encephalopathy and septicemia.<br>Measures to prevent infection are essential in persons whose immune systems are suppressed.<br>Early detection is important for early treatment. |

### ■ NURSING DIAGNOSIS

Ineffective individual coping related to health crisis

| Expected Patient Outcome | Nursing Interventions | Rationale |
|---|---|---|
| Describes at least one coping mechanism to deal with health crisis. | Assess patient's perception of health and present illness.<br>Identify and support patient's coping strategies, such as prayer, music, and conversation.<br>Listen actively if patient expresses feeling of powerlessness, fears, or spiritual distress. Plan time daily for listening.<br>Assess and facilitate family support. Meet with family or significant other on a scheduled basis. | Support of patient undergoing a health crisis can facilitate use of intrapersonal family resources. One can expect this patient to be discouraged and fearful. |

# NURSING CARE PLAN

## PERSON WITH CIRRHOSIS—cont'd

### ■ NURSING DIAGNOSIS

High risk for injury (bleeding, falls) related to decreased metabolic function of liver

| Expected Patient Outcomes | Nursing Interventions | Rationale |
|---|---|---|
| No undetected bleeding occurs. | Monitor the following for bleeding: urine, stool, skin, and mucous membranes. | Patient's esophageal varices and cirrhosis make him a candidate for bleeding and falls; surveillance is the major nursing focus, as well as decreasing precipitating factors. |
| Vital signs return to normal. | Check patient's vital signs q 4 hr and prothrombin and partial thromboplastin levels and thrombocytes daily.<br>Avoid injections if possible; apply pressure at all puncture sites for 5 minutes.<br>Give prescribed vitamin K.<br>Teach patient to use soft toothbrush and to avoid straining or coughing. | |
| No falls occur. | Provide support when patient is ambulating to prevent falls.<br>Maintain safe environment. | |

### ■ NURSING DIAGNOSIS

Self-esteem disturbance related to inability to accept physical changes of increased abdominal girth, jaundice, and change in secondary characteristics and potential changes in role

| Expected Patient Outcome | Nursing Interventions | Rationale |
|---|---|---|
| Describes self in realistic terms, which include positive characteristics. | Encourage patient to participate in goal setting and decision making.<br>Help patient identify personal strengths and give positive feedback.<br>Assist family to understand patient's need for a positive self-concept and how they can help.<br>Assist patient to explore ways to diminish overt signs of jaundice and ascites and thus help body image. | Poor self-esteem can lead to poor coping, causing the patient to resume alcohol consumption. |

### ■ NURSING DIAGNOSIS

Knowledge deficit: follow-up care and home care related to change in health status and previous inability to cope with information

| Expected Patient Outcome | Nursing Interventions | Rationale |
|---|---|---|
| Describes nature of cirrhosis and therapeutic regimen. | Assess patient's knowledge and clarify the following, as necessary: basis of signs and symptoms and therapeutic regimen, dietary and fluid restrictions, medication therapy, avoidance of infection and bleeding, and signs (increased temperature, bleeding, worsening jaundice, change in mental status, etc.) requiring immediate medical follow-up. | Patient has had the problem for some time, so first assess his knowledge, he may not need teaching. |

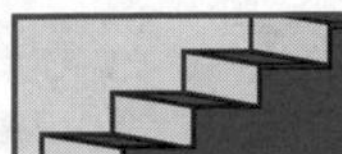

## CRITICAL PATHWAY Cirrhosis of Liver with Gastrointestinal Bleeding

**DRG #: 202; expected LOS: 7**

| | Admit to ICU<br>Day of Admission<br>Day 1 | Day 2 | Day 3 |
|---|---|---|---|
| **Diagnostic Tests** | CBC, UA, SMA/18,* type and cross-match, PT/PTT, ABG | H & H, ABG, gastroscopy, hema-test stools | H & H, SMA/18,* hema-test stools |
| **Medications** | IVs, blood transfusions as indicated, IV cimetidine, antacids via NG tube after gavage | IVs, blood transfusions as indicated, IV cimetidine, Tylenol PRN for fever and discomfort after sclerotherapy, antacids via NG tube | IVs, IV/PO cimetidine, Tylenol PRN for fever and discomfort, antacids, (?diuretics, $K^+$ replacement), multivitamins, folic acid, ferrous sulfate |
| **Treatments** | I & O q hr (including Foley and NG); VS q hr until stable, then q2hr; weight; measure abdominal girth; assess cardio-pul-neuro-circ systems q2hr; assess skin and mouth, give special care q2hr; NG gavage with NaCl for acute bleeding. | I & O q hr (including Foley and NG); VS q2hr; weight; measure abdominal girth; assess cardio-pul-neuro-circ systems q2hr; assess skin and mouth, give special care q2hr; injection sclerotherapy as necessary. | I & O q4hr (discontinue Foley and NG); VS q2hr; weight; measure abdominal girth; assess cardio-pul-neuro-circ systems q4hr; assess skin and mouth, give special care q2hr. |
| **Diet** | NPO | NPO | Clear liquids and, as necessary, low sodium/protein and fluid restriction |
| **Activities** | Bedrest, T & DB q2hr | Bedrest, T & DB q2hr | Bedrest, up to bathroom with help, T & DB q2hr |
| **Referral/Consultation** | Gastroenterologist, other specialist as needed for other medical problems | | Social services, home health, dietary |

*Serum, calcium, phosphorus, triglycerides, uric acid, creatinine, BUN, total bilirubin, alkaline phosphate, aspartate aminotransferase (AST) (formerly serum glutamic oxaloacetic transaminase [SGOT]), alanine aminotransferase (ALT) (formerly serum glutamic oxaloacetic transaminase [SGPT]), lactic dehydrogenase (LDH), total protein, albumin, sodium, potassium, chloride, total $CO_2$, glucose.

### Guidelines for Teaching the Person With Cirrhosis

1. Avoidance of further hepatic damage: abstain from alcohol; abstain from any drugs not prescribed by physician, including over-the-counter drugs, such as analgesics or cold remedies; work environment hazards; home hazards
2. Dietary regimen (may include sodium and/or protein restrictions) but usually should be well balanced and include sources high in protein such as milk, eggs, fish, and poultry
3. Fluid restriction if required; how to incorporate restrictions throughout the day
4. Signs and symptoms requiring immediate follow-up: weight gain, increased abdominal girth, recurrence of edema, fever, bleeding (blood in urine, stool, or vomitus; epistaxis; cuts that continue to bleed), change in mental function or behavior
5. Measures that lessen chance of bleeding
6. Drug therapy (diuretics, potassium, antihistamines)
7. Activity plan that promotes adequate rest
8. Care measures that help to control pruritus

## Facilitating Learning

All patients need to be prepared for diagnostic tests, to understand their treatment, and to learn to meet long-term care needs. Information should be given verbally and supplemented with written information, depending on the patient's physical status; the information may need to be repeated several times and given in small amounts. Family members or significant others should be included so that they can help reinforce the information or participate in the patient's care. Long-term care usually requires major changes in life-style (diet, fluid intake, alcohol intake), and thus continual support is necessary. Specific information that the nurse may want to include in the teaching plan is highlighted in the Guidelines box at left.

## Promoting Nutrition

Most patients with cirrhosis will require a well-balanced high-protein, high-carbohydrate diet with adequate vitamins to provide nutrients for repair of the liver. When nausea is a problem, antiemetics should be given 30 minutes before meals to help increase food tolerance.

| Transfer out of ICU Day 4 | Day 5 | Day 6 | Day of Discharge Day 7 |
|---|---|---|---|
| Hema-test stools | H & H, hema-test stools | SMA/18* | CBC |
| IV to saline lock, PO cimetidine, Tylenol PRN for fever and discomfort, antacids, (?diuretics, $K^+$ replacement), multivitamins, folic acid, ferrous sulfate | IV saline lock, PO cimetidine, Tylenol PRN for fever and discomfort, antacids, (?diuretics, $K^+$ replacement), multivitamins, folic acid, ferrous sulfate | IV saline lock, PO cimetidine, discontinue Tylenol, antacids, (? diuretics, $K^+$ replacement), multivitamins, folic acid, ferrous sulfate; adjust medications for home use. | Discontinue saline lock, continue cimetidine, antacids, vitamins, and other medications for home use |
| I & O q8hr; VS q6hr; weight; measure abdominal girth; assess cardio-pul-neuro-circ systems q8hr; assess skin and mouth, give special care q4hr. | I & O q8hr; VS q6hr; weight; measure abdominal girth; assess cardio-pul-neuro-circ systems q8hr; assess skin and mouth, give special care q4hr. | Discontinue I & O; VS q8hr; weight; measure abdominal girth; assess cardio-pul-neuro-circ systems q8hr; assess skin and mouth, give special care q6hr. | VS q8hr; weight; measure abdominal girth; assess cardio-pul-neuro-circ systems q8hr; assess skin and mouth, give special care q8hr. |
| Soft diet, high carbohydrate (CHO) and, as necessary, low sodium/protein and fluid restriction | Soft diet, high CHO and, as necessary, low sodium/protein and fluid restriction | Regular diet, high CHO and, as necessary, low sodium/protein and fluid restriction | Regular diet, high CHO and, as necessary, low sodium/protein and fluid restriction |
| Bedrest, up in chair twice with help | Up in chair 4 times with help, up walking in hall with help twice | Up ad lib, up walking in hallway with help 4 times | Up ad lib |
| | Chemical dependency counseling if appropriate | | |

Sodium restriction is frequently necessary, and this restriction can make finding a palatable diet more difficult. Salt substitutes and information on alternative seasonings may help. The liver dysfunction and the presence of portal hypertension, which results in portal vessel blood being shunted around the liver, result in an impairment in the metabolism of ammonia. Ammonia, which originates from deamination of protein, is very toxic to the body. Protein restriction is necessary for the patient with cirrhosis who cannot metabolize ammonia, which would be evident by the onset of signs and symptoms of portal systemic encephalopathy (see p. 1408).

Frequent oral hygiene and a pleasant environment should be provided to help increase food intake. The patient's food preferences should be incorporated into the diet. Food should be served in small, frequent amounts. Because persons with cirrhosis need increased calories but often have poor appetites, measures to increase calories without increasing the volume of food should be used. These measures include use of butter as a seasoning, adding dry milk to appropriate foods, and using gravies and sauces. The patient with cirrhosis has the same nutritional needs after discharge, and the person who shops and cooks for the patient must be included in the teaching. The patient's economic situation should be assessed to determine his or her ability to purchase the food required for the prescribed diet. A social service referral may be necessary to help the patient obtain financial assistance. For the person who eats out frequently, instruction on how to select appropriate meals from a restaurant menu is necessary. If the patient's meals are obtained through a service such as Meals on Wheels, arrangements can be made for some special dietary requirements.

### Controlling Pruritus

The management of pruritus is similar to that discussed earlier under care of patients with hepatitis (p. 1387).

### Promoting Positive Self-Esteem

The patient with cirrhosis may experience changes in body appearance and in roles and relationships. If the patient is not helped to establish or maintain positive self-esteem, this can add to the problem of alcoholism. The nurse is in a prime position to help promote positive self-esteem by giving the patient as much control as possible. Positive self-esteem can be facilitated by:

1. Involving the patient in goal setting
2. Allowing the patient to make as many decisions as possible
3. Giving positive feedback for accomplishments
4. Supporting the patient in times of failure, whatever the failure might be, including conflicts with family or friends or participation in drinking
5. Helping the patient recall past accomplishments
6. Helping significant others provide positive feedback
7. Helping the patient learn ways to disguise jaundice or ascites

### Providing Skin Care

Because of pruritus, malnutrition, and the edema often associated with cirrhosis, the patient is prone to skin lesions and pressure ulcer formation. Preventive nursing care to avoid skin breakdown, such as air mattresses, frequent turning, backrubs, and massage of bony prominences, should be instituted. Measures to prevent pruritus assist in preventing damage to the skin resulting from the patient's scratching.

## ♦ EVALUATION

To evaluate the effectiveness of nursing interventions, compare patient behaviors with those stated in the expected patient outcomes. Successful achievement of patient outcomes for the patient with cirrhosis is indicated by the following:

1. Has clear breath sounds throughout lung fields and normal percussion results from thoracic cavity.
2. Increases involvement in daily self-care activities and ambulation in hospital hallways.
3. Loses 1 to 2 lb/day until dry weight is reached; has decreasing edema, decreasing abdominal girth, and urine output of 500 to 1000 ml greater than intake until dry weight is reached.
4. States that alcohol is the cause of problem and is not controllable without some outside support, and attends one counseling session or one AA meeting.
5. Has normal body temperature and no indications of infections of any body organs or sites.
6. Shows normal prothrombin time and hematocrit; hemoglobin levels that are increasing; no orthostatic vital sign changes; and no falls, cuts, or other injuries.
7. Patient or significant other correctly performs the following:
   a. Describes diagnostic tests.
   b. Describes treatment regimen and long-term role.
   c. Explains diet plan.
   d. Explains sodium and fluid restrictions and avoidance of hepatotoxins, including alcohol.
   e. Describes any medications, including dosage, expected effects, and side effects to report.
   f. Explains what to do if signs of bleeding or infections occur or if other signs of disease progression occur.
   g. Explains planned follow-up and any times that immediate help should be sought.
8. Maintains adequate food intake to regain or keep weight as appropriate with incorporation of foods from all food groups and restriction of sodium and protein as necessary.
9. Shows no evidence of scratching, and states that itching is decreased and controlled.
10. Makes positive statements about self and realistic statements about future goals.
11. Maintains intact skin and appropriate healing of any lesions.

### Complications

Persons with cirrhosis very frequently develop portal hypertension that can result in ascites, esophageal varices, and/or portal-systemic encephalopathy. Each of these major complications is discussed next.

#### Portal hypertension

As structural damage occurs, the portal vascular system may become obstructed. This obstruction to blood flow causes a rise in portal venous pressure and results in **portal hypertension.** The obstruction to portal blood flow can cause splenomegaly because of increased vascular pressure and venous congestion in the spleen, contribute to ascites by causing leakage of albumin and fluid from the vascular compartment of the liver into the peritoneal cavity, and cause the development of collateral channels of circulation that bypass the obstruction. Collateral channels are most likely to occur in the paraumbilical and the hemorrhoidal veins and at the cardia of the stomach extending into the esophagus.

**Management.** The nursing and medical management of portal hypertension is directed first to treatment of the consequences of portal hypertension: ascites and esophageal varices. The only way to achieve permanent lowering of portal pressure is surgical treatment to reduce blood flow through the obstructed portion of the portal system (see p. 1407). Because of the risks of the surgery and the frequent fatalities from hepatic failure after surgical treatment with a portacaval shunt, the shunt procedure is used only in persons who have esophageal varices (see p. 1403), have bled from the varices, and do not respond to other therapy. Surgical care is discussed later in this chapter.

#### Ascites

As mentioned earlier, **ascites** is one of the most frequent complications of cirrhosis of the liver and results in part from the portal hypertension. Other contributing factors are decreased hepatic synthesis of albumin, increased levels of aldosterone, and obstruction of hepatic lymph flow. Ascites may occur with or without peripheral edema. Because ascites is so frequently seen, the required therapy and nursing care are discussed earlier in the section related to general care needs of patients with cirrhosis. This section describes care related to use of a peritoneal venous shunt.

**Peritoneal venous shunt (PV shunt).** In chronic and resistant ascites caused by cirrhosis, a LeVeen or Denver **peritoneal venous shunt** may be used (Figure 42-5). The shunt allows for the continuous reinfusion of ascitic fluid back into the venous system through a silicone catheter with a one-way pressure-sensitive valve. One end of the catheter is implanted in the peritoneal cavity, and the tube is channeled through subcutaneous tissue to the superior vena cava, where the other end is implanted. The valve opens when there is a pressure differential greater than 3 mm of water between the peritoneal cavity and the vein in the thoracic cavity, allowing fluid to move from the peritoneal cavity into the superior vena cava.

Persons treated with a shunt may also receive furosemide therapy, and the two together have been successful in relieving ascites in some patients. Persons who have a shunt may still have severe problems, including disseminated intravascular coagulation (DIC), bleeding esophageal varices, and congestive heart failure.[3]

A modification of the original LeVeen peritoneal venous shunt, the Denver shunt, is sometimes used when ascites is severe and is the result of malignancy. Malignant ascites may contain particulate matter that can stop the flow of ascitic fluid through the tubing. The Denver shunt has a subcutaneous pump that can be compressed manually to irrigate the tubing. Increased comfort and improvement of renal and respiratory function have been reported when the Denver shunt is used.

When shunts are first implanted and functioning, there can be dramatic changes, such as hemodilution of intravascular fluid, decrease in abdominal girth, and increase in renal output. As peritoneal fluid is removed, less of a pressure gradient exists between the peritoneal cavity and the superior vena cava, and thus less fluid is removed. To force the valve open, deep breathing is encouraged at regular intervals (every 1 to 2 hours) with the patient in the supine position.

### Esophageal varices

**Pathophysiology.** Bleeding **esophageal varices** are the most dangerous complication of portal hypertension.

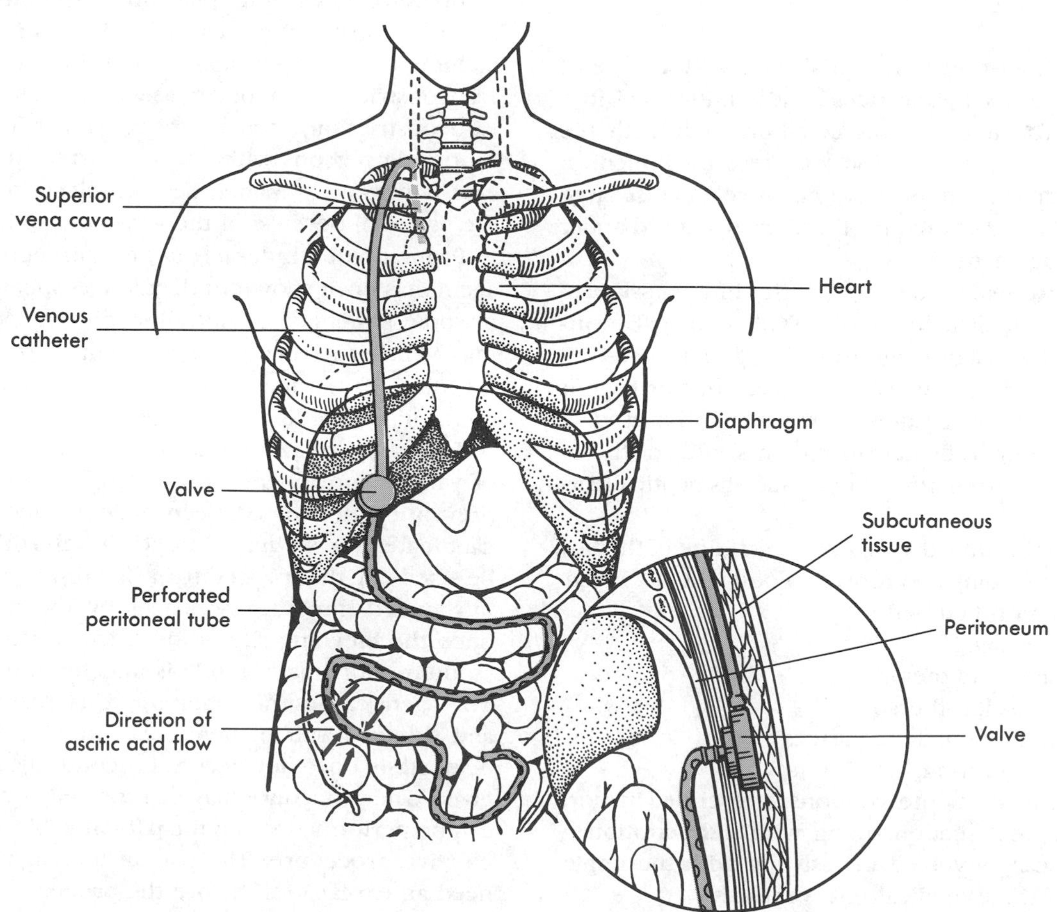


**FIGURE 42-5** LeVeen shunt, showing placement of catheter.

The mortality associated with variceal hemorrhage is 50%.[3] In portal hypertension, the azygos and vena cava veins become distended where they join the smaller vessels of the esophagus. This distention occurs because of the greater volume of blood flowing through these vessels as a result of higher pressure within the portal system. Normal portal pressure is about 9 mm Hg. The higher portal venous pressure causes the blood, which would normally flow through the liver, to be forced into these other vessels (see Figure 42-3, *A*, for a diagram of the relationship between these various blood vessels). These small vessels were not designed to carry much blood and become tortuous and fragile. The changes in the structure of these vessels make them prone to injury by mechanical trauma from ingestion of coarse foods and acid pepsin erosion, which may result in bleeding. Bleeding may also occur as a result of coughing, vomiting, sneezing, straining at stool (Valsalva maneuver), or any physical exertion that increases abdominal venous pressure. The major clinical manifestation is upper GI bleeding. Bleeding is frequently abrupt and painless. If bleeding is slow, melena and decreasing hemoglobin and hematocrit may be the only signs. Severe hematemesis and resultant shock may follow, requiring emergency treatment. The patient exhibits signs and symptoms of hypovolemic shock (see Chapter 22) or may exhibit signs and symptoms of portal-systemic encephalopathy (see p. 1408).

**Medical management.** The goal for the discharge of patients with esophageal varices as determined by DRGs is 12 days. The nurse works collaboratively with the physician for implementation of prescribed medical therapy. Because the nurse has a major role in discharge planning and patient teaching, these are discussed under nursing management.

***Diagnostic tests.*** The first priority in medical management is to establish the source of GI bleeding. **Esophagoscopy** is the major diagnostic tool, and, if this is not possible, *angiography* is used. If severe hemorrhage is not present, barium studies or scans may be used. It must be remembered that, in patients with cirrhosis, bleeding may be from other causes such as peptic ulcers and gastritis.

***Treatments.*** After diagnosis, the first line of therapy is to control bleeding and replace blood volume. Bleeding may be controlled with:

1. Gastric lavage
2. Pharmacologic therapy
3. Injection sclerotherapy
4. Balloon tamponade of varices
5. Surgery—ligation and shunts

Each of these medical interventions is described in more detail in the next section, along with a description of the nursing care involved in assisting with the implementation of these medical interventions.

**Nursing management.** The first priority of nursing care in the management of patients with esophageal varices is to establish monitoring parameters of cardiac output; adequacy of vascular volume; effectiveness of tissue perfusion; adequacy of hemostasis treatment; and adequacy of fluid and electrolyte, respiratory, renal, and neurologic status. Surveillance must be instituted immediately on admission of the patient and continued on a frequent basis (every 15 to 60 minutes), because the patient can lose several units of blood within 1 hour if hemorrhage is severe. The nurse, in collaboration with the physician, decides what physiologic parameters to measure and what minimal and maximal values are acceptable.

If the hemorrhage is considered to be minor, introduction of a nasogastric (NG) tube by the nurse or physician and administration of an antacid through the tube may be sufficient to control the hemorrhage. The NG tube removes gastric secretions, and the antacids neutralize gastric acids that may irritate esophageal varices. If hemorrhage is more severe, pharmacologic therapy will be started. Pharmacologic therapy includes vasopressin administration and sometimes use of propranolol (Inderal).

***Pharmacologic therapy.*** Vasopressin is given intravenously mixed in 120 to 200 ml of dextrose either intermittently or as a continuous infusion. It lowers portal pressure by causing splanchnic vasoconstriction and can thus stop or control esophageal bleeding. Side effects include abdominal cramping and pallor. Coronary artery vasoconstriction can occur, as well as mesenteric artery vasoconstriction; thus vasopressin must be used with caution in persons with coronary artery disease and in elderly persons.[3,5] Sometimes nitroglycerine is added to the protocol because of the vasoconstriction.[5]

Propranolol (Inderal), a beta-adrenergic blocking agent, has been shown to decrease esophageal bleeding in some patients, but not all studies support this finding.[3,5] Thus it is still used experimentally to treat variceal bleeding. If pharmacologic therapy is not effective in controlling bleeding, sclerotherapy is used.

***Injection sclerotherapy.*** For emergency treatment of varices and longer-term control or for control and prevention of rebleeding in patients who may not be candidates for surgery, **injection sclerotherapy** may be used. In this procedure a fiberoptic endoscope is introduced into the esophagus by the physician, and once the bleeding site is identified, a sclerosing agent (sodium morrhuate, 5 ml) is injected into the varices. This agent causes thromboses and sclerosis of the vessel and should result in hemostasis in 3 to 5 minutes. If hemostasis does not occur, a second injection may be given. The procedure may be repeated as necessary and can be performed while the patient is bleeding or as an elective procedure. The patient and significant others need an explanation before the procedure, and the pa-

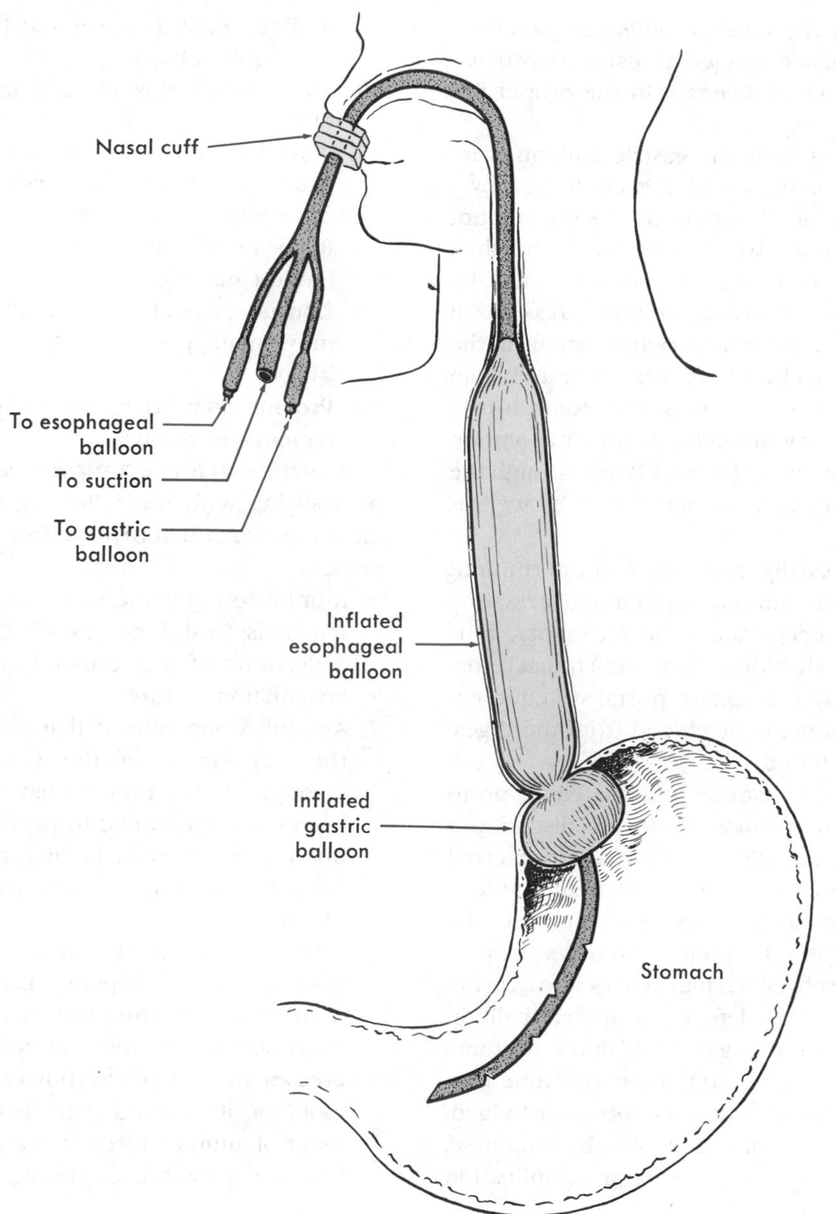


**FIGURE 42-6** Sengstaken-Blakemore tube with esophageal and gastric balloons inflated. (Redrawn from *Rubber appliances in surgery and therapeutics,* Providence, RI, Davol.)

tient should receive nothing by mouth for at least 6 hours. A mild sedative and a local anesthetic are given. After the procedure, the nurse monitors the patient for complications (perforated esophagus, aspiration pneumonia, pleural effusion, worsening of ascites). Respiratory support to ensure adequate air exchange must be provided. *Retrosternal pain* is often present and is treated with analgesics; fever is common for several days. The procedure has shown very favorable results in some patients.

***Esophageal tamponade.*** If bleeding is not controlled by the preceding methods, balloon tamponade of varices may be instituted. The esophagogastric tubes (Sengstaken-Blakemore or Minnesota) are three-lumen or four-lumen tubes with two balloon attachments. One lumen serves as an NG suction tube, the second is used to inflate the gastric balloon, and the third is used to inflate the esophageal balloon (Figure 42-6). The Minnesota esophagogastric tamponade tube has a fourth lumen used for esophageal aspiration. The tube is passed by the physician through the nose into the stomach with the balloons deflated. When the tube is in the stomach, the gastric balloon is inflated and the lumen clamped; the tube is then pulled out slowly so that the balloon is held tightly against the *cardioesophageal junction.* A football helmet–shaped device is used to provide traction on the tube, which keeps it in the proper position.

If bleeding continues after the gastric balloon is inflated, the esophageal balloon, which is connected by a Y tube to a manometer, is inflated to the desired amount of pressure, as determined by the physician, and then clamped. To stop the bleeding, the pressure must be greater than the patient's portal venous pressure. If bleeding is from esophageal varices rather than from the gastric mucosa, blood will no longer be aspirated from the stomach. If blood is still present, the stomach may be lavaged with a small amount of ice water, or a solution of iced alcohol and water may be circulated through the gastric balloon to provide vasoconstriction as well as pressure.

The NG lumen is usually connected to intermittent gastric suction, which permits easy appraisal of cessation of bleeding and also keeps the stomach empty. It is important to remove all blood from the stomach, because its presence may precipitate portal-systemic encephalopathy from ammonia produced from the digestion of protein in the blood.

The esophageal balloon can be left inflated for up to 48 hours without tissue damage or severe discomfort. The fully inflated gastric balloon with traction exerted on it, however, compresses the stomach wall between the balloon and the diaphragm, causing ulceration of the gastric mucosa and severe discomfort. To offset the possibility of necrosis, the physician may release the traction on the gastric balloon and deflate the gastric balloon pressure periodically. If the gastric balloon ruptures (and the patient is not intubated), the entire tube may move up and obstruct the airway; if the tube is dislodged, the esophageal balloon is deflated at once by the nurse, and the entire tube is removed. The major complication of the tube is ulceration.

Nursing care of the patient with esophageal tamponade includes the following:

1. Explain procedure and provide continued support to patient during the procedure.
2. Monitor vital signs every 15 minutes until blood pressure is stable, and then monitor hourly or every 2 hours.
3. Measure and record pressures in the esophageal balloon every hour; maintain pressure at prescribed level.
4. Ensure that patient does not pull on the tube.
5. Provide care to mouth and nares every 1 to 2 hours.
   a. Provide patient with tissues, and encourage spitting of saliva into tissues.
   b. Have patient rinse mouth well to remove any old blood; a Water Pik under low pressure may be helpful.
   c. *Gently* suction mouth and throat if patient is too weak to expectorate secretions on own.
   d. Keep nostrils clean and lubricated with water-soluble jelly.
6. Maintain transfusions and infusions at prescribed rates.
7. If iced solutions are used in the balloons, report patient chilling to the physician, who may then order a warming blanket.
8. Record intake and output; test GI output for occult blood (guaiac).
9. Consult physician concerning permissible patient movement; passive range of motion is usually allowed.
10. Provide comfort measures (e.g., rub back, change patient's position).

***Additional therapeutic measures.*** The nurse will be assisting with the following additional therapeutic measures when hemorrhage from esophageal varices is present:

1. Administering prescribed fresh whole blood and IV infusions; fresh blood avoids the increased ammonia and citrate of stored blood and has relatively more coagulation factors
2. Administering saline cathartics as prescribed through the NG lumen of the esophagogastric tube or through an NG tube to hasten expulsion of blood from the GI tract and to prevent an increase in production of ammonia. Enemas may also be ordered to decrease gut content and bacterial action on the blood
3. Administering lactulose or neomycin prevents portal-systemic encephalopathy. Lactulose is given either orally or by retention enema. Lactulose promotes the excretion of ammonia in the stool because it decreases the pH of the bowel, thereby keeping ammonia in its ionized state. This facilitates the movement of ammonia from the blood to the stool. Also, bacterial growth is discouraged by the acid environment.

Neomycin is a broad-spectrum antibiotic that destroys the normal flora of the bowel. Bacteria in the bowel normally break down protein, including blood protein in the GI tract, producing ammonia. Therefore neomycin is given to decrease the protein breakdown by bacteria in the bowel.

***Shunt procedures.*** Shunt procedures are one of the last measures used to treat bleeding esophageal varices. Portal decompression can be obtained by several shunt procedures, most of them requiring surgery. The mortality rate for shunt surgery is 5% to 15%, and if emergency shunt surgery is necessary, the mortality rate increases to 50%.

***Nonsurgical shunt procedure.*** A new alternative to the surgical shunt procedure that has been developed is the **transjugular intrahepatic portosystemic shunt (TIPS).** This shunt placement is performed in the radiology suite and uses the normal vasculature of the liver to create a shunt between the portal and systemic venous circulation. The right internal jugular vein is used to cannulate the portal and hepatic veins. After the portal and hepatic veins are located, a connection between the two vessels is made to form a new path of blood flow. This path is enlarged by balloon dilation and then a stent(s) is (are) placed. The goal is to decrease the pressure gradient in the liver to 10 mm Hg, which is effective in decreasing esophageal bleeding.[2,7]

The benefit of the TIPS procedure is that it is less invasive and is successful in 92% to 96% of patients. It has been shown to decrease ascites in 80% to 90% of patients. Liver transplantation remains a possibility because there is no surgical invasion of the abdominal cavity with resultant scar tissue and adhesions, as occurs with traditional shunting procedures.[2,7]

The TIPS procedure is not without complications. Because it is performed through the jugular vein and without direct visualization, bile duct trauma and vascular trauma of the liver are possible. Other complications are stent thrombosis and stent migration, although migration is unlikely because the stent is endothelialized in 7 to 10 days. Nursing management of patients after a TIPS procedure is similar to the care following traditional shunt procedures and is discussed next.

***Surgical shunt procedures.*** Depending on the location of the obstruction, various operative procedures

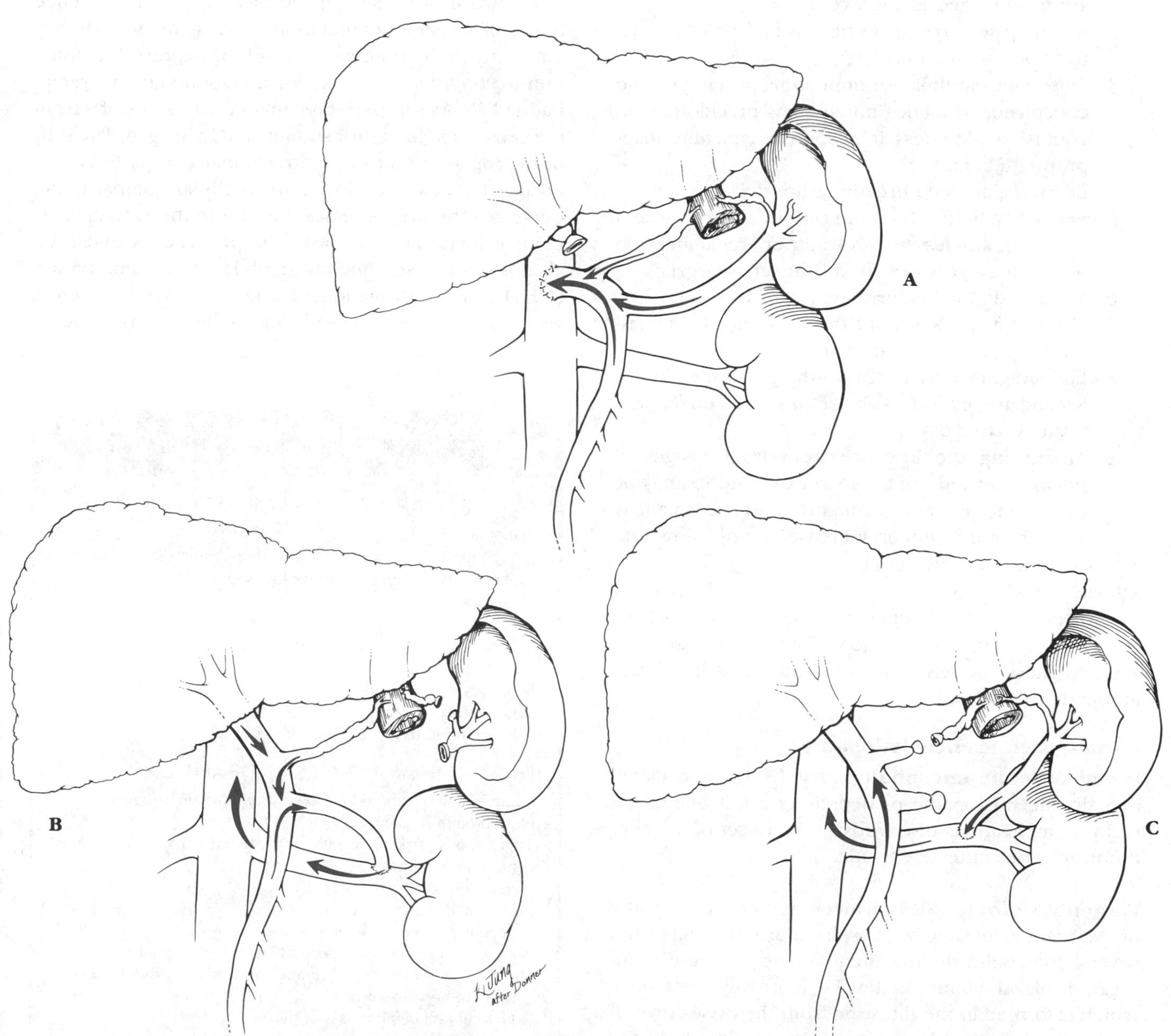


**FIGURE 42-7** Decompression procedures for portal hypertension. **A,** End-to-side portacaval shunt. **B,** Splenorenal shunt. **C,** Distal splenorenal shunt.

may be used (Figure 42-7). The purpose of all procedures is to decrease the blood flow through the portal vascular system and thus decrease portal hypertension. Portal hypertension is lowered by shunting blood around the liver. The lowering of portal hypertension decreases the pressure in the esophageal vessels and the bleeding from the varices. Preoperatively, the patient's vascular volume is stabilized with fluids and blood as necessary. Vitamin K may be given to correct coagulation problems, antibiotics may be given prophylactically, and nutritional status is improved as much as possible.

Postoperatively, the patient needs intensive care and constant attention regarding the following:

1. Administering narcotics for pain (the amount given is usually guarded because most narcotics are metabolized in the liver)
2. Avoiding sedative drugs because of their toxic effects on the diseased liver
3. Observing carefully for impending portal-systemic encephalopathy (beginning signs include mental confusion, slowness in response, generally inappropriate behavior)
4. Encouraging deep breathing hourly
5. Recording fluid intake and output accurately, and reporting any lessening of output (renal function sometimes decreases for a time after surgery)
6. Monitoring for hemorrhage (signs of shock)
7. Monitoring for signs of thrombosis at site of anastomosis (pain, distention, fever, nausea)
8. Encouraging activity within the prescribed limits; leg and arm exercises are often started on the first postoperative day
9. Monitoring the lower extremities for signs of edema; elevation of the lower extremities may be ordered to prevent edema formation (edema may form from the sudden increase of blood flow into the inferior vena cava)

All patients who have had a portal-systemic shunt are at risk for portal-systemic encephalopathy. Some patients will require lifelong restriction of protein because the shunted blood bypasses the liver and thus limits ammonia detoxification.

### Portal-systemic encephalopathy

**Portal-systemic encephalopathy (PSE),** also called hepatic encephalopathy or hepatic coma, is one of the major complications of cirrhosis. The onset of the condition may be acute or chronic.

**Pathophysiology.** PSE is a metabolic encephalopathy of the brain associated with liver failure. It results from several metabolic derangements; a major cause is increased blood ammonia levels. Normally, ammonia, which is formed in the intestine from the breakdown of protein by intestinal bacteria, is carried directly to the liver and converted to urea through the *Krebs-Henseleit cycle* in the liver. In liver failure, ammonia levels may be increased at the same time that the liver's detoxification ability is decreased or when blood is shunted past the liver. Many factors can increase ammonia levels.

A second hypothesis related to the onset of PSE has been called the false-neurotransmitter hypothesis. It has been shown that patients with PSE have increased levels of aromatic or short-chain amino acids (SCAAs) and a decrease in branched-chain amino acids (BCAAs). Normally, SCAAs are cleared by the liver. With liver failure, they are not cleared, and the levels are increased. These SCAAs cross the blood-brain barrier. The SCAAs such as phenylalanine, trytophan, and tyrosine act as weak neurotransmitters and compete with regular neurotransmitters, resulting in an impairment of normal neurologic function.

A third major cause in the onset of PSE is presence of any of a number of metabolic derangements that may indirectly increase ammonia levels or depress liver function. ***Hypokalemia*** is a major metabolic factor precipitating PSE. As serum potassium decreases, it shifts from the cells in exchange for sodium and hydrogen. The shift of hydrogen ion into the intracellular compartment increases the acid level in the intracellular compartment, decreases the pH, increases the base in the extracellular compartment, and increases the pH. The extracellular alkalosis increases liberation of $H^+$ from ammonium ($NH_4$) and the formation of ammonia ($NH_3$), which is gaseous and crosses readily into cells, where it accu-

**BOX 42-12 Common Factors Associated With Portal-Systemic Encephalopathy**

**FACTORS DEPRESSING CNS OR LIVER FUNCTION**

Hypoxia
- Secondary to hemorrhage and hypovolemic shock
- Secondary to morphine and other sedatives

Infections

Exercise
- In patients with chronic liver disease who are in impending coma

Sedatives

Abdominal paracentesis
- Resulting in reduction of plasma volume

**FACTORS INCREASING LEVEL OF AMMONIA**

GI ammonia (old blood in bowel from GI hemorrhage)

High-protein intake

Transfusions, especially with stored blood because it contains more ammonia

Hypokalemia
- Secondary to thiazide diuretics
- Secondary to potassium loss from the bowel

Alkalosis secondary to hyperventilation or hypokalemia

Shunting of blood into systemic circulation without passing through hepatic sinusoids
- Natural collateral bypass of liver
- Surgical bypass of liver

Constipation

mulates and exerts toxic effects. Increased accumulation of base in the extracellular compartment from other causes can precipitate the same type of response.

Constipation may also increase formation and absorption of ammonia from the gut, or it may induce straining and thus precipitate bleeding from esophageal varices or hemorrhoids. Other metabolic factors such as exercise and infection may precipitate PSE by causing increased ammonia formation or decreased liver function.

A fourth major causative event in the onset of PSE is increased cerebral nervous system sensitivity to depressants. Any hypoxic insult or sedative, which can increase the sensitivity of the central nervous system (CNS) to any substance, can precipitate PSE.

Common factors that can precipitate PSE are summarized in Box 42-12.

The manifestations of PSE vary and may occur quickly or gradually over the course of a few days. PSE results in alterations in the state of consciousness, in intellectual function, in behavior and personality, and in neuromuscular function. These changes have been graded in four stages (Table 42-6).

**Medical management.** Medical management of PSE includes identifying the precipitating factors and treating them (hypokalemia, hemorrhage, hypoxia), reducing serum ammonia levels, and providing supportive care.

***Diagnostic tests.*** Patients with PSE have the abnormal liver function as described earlier for patients with cirrhosis. An elevated serum ammonia level provides the definitive diagnosis, but not all patients show an increase in ammonia. Therefore treatment is determined by the signs and symptoms and not the serum ammonia level.

***Medication.*** Lactulose and neomycin are given to decrease the serum ammonia levels. Lactulose also causes diarrhea, which helps eliminate blood from the GI tract in those patients with bleeding esophageal varices.

***Diet.*** A low-protein diet may be prescribed, but this practice is being questioned. Some researchers have found that increasing the calories and protein in patients with alcoholic liver disease did not make the encephalopathy worse and did make them stronger nutritionally.[10]

**Nursing management.** Nursing management is directed toward the following four goals:

1. Providing continual, regular monitoring of patients at high risk of PSE
2. Assisting with the therapeutic regimen
3. Providing supportive care
4. Providing long-term care

***Providing continual monitoring.*** As can be seen from a review of Table 42-6, the early indications of PSE are very subtle and can easily be missed if regular, objective assessments are not made. The nurse must (1) be as descriptive as possible, (2) assess skills such as handwriting or the ability to draw a circle, box, or square, and (3) maintain continuity of care so that the staff becomes familiar with the patient's behavior. Early detection of symptoms allows for more rapid treatment and consequently improves the patient's chance of recovery.

The continual monitoring should also focus on the patient's vital signs (particularly pulse, respiration, and temperature) and on the patient's total cirrhotic status to identify worsening of the patient's basic condition, which could be seen by the onset of fever or worsening of laboratory studies (e.g., serum enzymes [ALT, AST], prothrombin time, bilirubin, albumin) and can increase the risk of PSE.

***Assisting with therapeutic regimens.*** If encephalopathy is present, a major focus of nursing is to implement the prescribed regimen. The first treatment may be directed toward eliminating the causes of PSE, such as GI bleeding or hypokalemia, if known.

The second approach is directed toward decreasing ammonia levels. Interventions include the following:

1. Eliminating protein intake or severely restricting it
2. Increasing carbohydrate intake to decrease metabolism of endogenous proteins
3. Administering oral cathartics or enemas to empty the bowel and decrease ammonia formation

**TABLE 42-6 Stages of Portal-Systemic Encephalopathy**

| STAGE 1 (PRODROMAL) | STAGE 2 (IMPENDING) | STAGE 3 (STUPOROUS) | STAGE 4 (COMA) |
|---|---|---|---|
| Change in sleep pattern | Lethargy | Confused, somnolent | Unconscious |
| Slow response | Disorientation to time | Stupor, but arousable | No intellectual functioning |
| Shortened attention span | Impaired computation | Disorientation to place | Loss of deep tendon reflexes |
| Depressed or euphoric | Decreased inhibition | Anger, rage, paranoia | If responsive, only to deep pain |
| Irritable | Anxiety or apathy | Increased reflexes | Hyperventilation |
| Tremors | Inappropriate behavior | Clonus | Fetor hepaticus (musty, sweet breath odor) |
| Some incoordination | Speech slurred | Babinski reflex | Increased temperature and pulse rate |
| Writing impaired | Decreased reflexes | Asterixis | |
| | Ataxic | | |
| | Asterixis | | |

4. Administering intestinal antibiotics such as neomycin to kill bacteria in the GI tract
5. Administering lactulose
   a. Lactulose is a synthetic disaccharide that is degraded by bacteria in the lower intestines, causing acidification of the intestinal lumen and increased formation and GI elimination of $NH_4$.
   b. Lactulose also acts as an inhibitor of coliform growth and stimulates fecal excretion.
   c. Lactulose can be given orally or as an enema and is often one of the first agents used.

***Providing supportive care.*** The patient with PSE is very ill and requires excellent care directed toward prevention of respiratory problems. This includes turning and deep breathing and may include administration of oxygen, suctioning, or even ventilatory support. Coughing is prohibited if the patient has esophageal varices. The patient also needs care to prevent skin breakdown that may be worsened by malnutrition, ascites, and frequent or incontinent stools. Infections must also be prevented.

Many patients with PSE die of renal failure secondary to an inadequate circulating blood volume (hypovolemia). In some patients, renal function progressively deteriorates without any apparent cause. The treatment of PSE requires a careful balancing of fluid administration to maintain adequate perfusion of the kidney without creating an excessive load on the cardiovascular system. Therefore, when IV solutions are being administered, the desired flow rate is monitored very closely, and the patient is observed for signs of cardiovascular overload. To monitor renal function adequately, an indwelling catheter is often inserted, especially if the patient is being maintained on IV. Central venous pressure (CVP) monitoring is also frequently used. The nurse is alert to changes in the CVP readings suggestive of either hypervolemia or hypovolemia. The supportive nursing care required by any patient with hepatic disease, as well as by any unconscious patient, should be given.

Because most narcotics and sedatives must be detoxified by the liver, they are contraindicated in patients with impaired liver function. If a sedative must be used, drugs such as chlordiazepoxide (Librium), barbital, or phenobarbital, which are excreted by the kidney, are prescribed. If any sedatives, analgesics, or hypnotics are used, they should be given in smaller than normal doses, and the patient's response in terms of development of signs and symptoms of PSE, such as behavioral or mental changes and asterixis, should be evaluated carefully.

Maintenance of adequate nutrition is a major nursing focus. A low-protein diet is often less palatable. Providing good oral hygiene, maintaining a pleasant clean environment, and serving small attractive meals may help increase appetite. If proteins need to be severely restricted for some time, the use of a dietary or IV supplement that provides selected BCAAs and is lower in SCAAs may be used. Commercial oral preparations and IV preparations are available. These supplements also provide carbohydrates. Vitamins and minerals are added as necessary.[10]

***Providing long-term care.*** Some patients may always be under the threat of developing PSE and may be kept on a low-protein diet (20 to 40 g/day) indefinitely. Lactulose and neomycin may also be used indefinitely. The patient and family will need instructions regarding the dietary restrictions and how to take medications. They also must be taught to be alert for subtle changes in the patient's behavior that indicate worsening or onset of PSE and to seek medical attention immediately if the patient shows any behaviors indicative of worsening PSE. In addition to these needs, the patient and family have all the other needs as other patients with cirrhosis (see earlier).

### Hepatorenal syndrome

**Hepatorenal syndrome** is a poorly understood complication of cirrhosis. It is characterized by sudden renal failure for no known cause in a patient with progressively worsening liver failure.

The pathogenesis of hepatorenal failure is uncertain but includes a marked decrease in renal cortex blood flow because of intrarenal vasoconstriction. The intrarenal vasoconstriction can possibly result from the following[15,18]:

1. An increase in renin
2. A decrease in prostaglandin production by the kidney
3. The release of endotoxin in the body because of liver failure
4. A change in sympathetic activity, causing vasoconstriction
5. The production of a vasoconstrictor by the diseased liver

The patient with hepatorenal failure has oliguria and azotemia. Blood pressure may be elevated or decreased. The patient complains of anorexia, fatigue, and weakness. Fluid retention leads to hyponatremia and a decrease in urine osmolality. The continual accumulation of waste products and alterations in fluid and electrolytes cause neurologic changes that can resemble those of PSE. Blood pressure continues to drop. Hepatorenal failure carries a very poor prognosis.

The first focus of medical management is to identify whether the oliguria is caused by decreased cardiac output, hepatorenal syndrome, or acute tubular necrosis. Any of these processes can occur in the person with cirrhosis. Once the diagnosis of hepatorenal syndrome is made, the management is designed to improve hepatic function and support renal function. Fluid and electrolytes are given to maintain hemodynamic status. Potentially nephrotoxic drugs such as neomycin are stopped. Some patients have shown improvement after a portacaval shunt has been implemented for other reasons, and others have shown improvement with a decrease in ascites. Liver transplantation is the major intervention for most patients.[13] Hemodialysis has been successful in treating hyperkalemia. Continuous arteriovenous hemodialysis or ultrafiltration may be used to treat fluid overload and pulmonary edema. Note that these last treatments only improve symptoms and not the hepatorenal syndrome itself, because the basic problem is in the liver and not in the kidney.

## HEPATIC TRANSPLANTATION

Hepatic transplantation is performed for various reasons, including biliary atresia, chronic active hepatitis, fulminant hepatitis, end-stage cirrhosis with complications, metabolic diseases of the liver, and hepatic malignancy. Liver transplantation and the related nursing care are discussed in Chapter 72.

## QUESTIONS TO CONSIDER

- How do patients who have developed a chronic carrier state for hepatitis B need to change their lifestyles to prevent the spread of hepatitis B?
- What questions should you incorporate in your assessment that would identify persons at high risk for exposure to hepatitis B?
- How do neomycin, lactulose, a low-protein diet, and prevention of constipation and gastrointestinal bleeding prevent hepatic encephalopathy?
- What factors play a role in increasing the chance of bleeding or infections in a person with cirrhosis?
- Explain the significance of the presence of anti-$Hb_s$ in a patient's serum.

## CRITICAL THINKING ACTIVITIES

- Examine the scientific principles underlying the nursing management of individuals with cirrhosis of the liver, and determine those that could be applied or broadened to nursing care related to all types of liver disorders.
- Differentiate the characteristics of hepatitis A from hepatitis B. Identify principles of prevention with regard to transmission that are universal to all types of hepatitis.

## CHAPTER SUMMARY

### FOCAL HEPATIC DISORDERS

- Liver abscesses may be pyogenic and treated with broad-spectrum antibiotics and surgery, or they may be amebic and treated with amebicidal drugs.
- Metastatic tumors of the liver are 20 times more prevalent than primary tumors of the liver. Symptoms occur late; jaundice, ascites, and weakness are common.
- Malignant lesions of the liver are treated with resection, palliative use of radiation, and chemotherapy by systemic routes or hepatic arterial infusion.
- New forms of treatment such as immunoradiotherapy and hepatic dearterialization for malignant lesions of the liver are being experimentally tested.
- Injury to the liver, which frequently results from trauma, can lead to major hemodynamic changes.

### DIFFUSE HEPATOCELLULAR DISORDERS

- The incidence of toxic hepatitis may be reduced by decreased use or proper use of toxins such as petroleum distillates.
- There are five types of viral hepatitis. Measures to control hepatitis A and E are directed toward handwashing, thus interrupting the fecal-oral route of transmission. The other three types are spread through blood and body fluid routes.
- Many tests use serologic markers (antigens, antibodies) for differentiating the type of hepatitis; $HB_sAg$ is one test for hepatitis B (HBV). Hepatitis A (HAV) is detected by the presence of IgM class anti-HAV. Hepatitis C (HCV) is detected by the presence of anti-HCV.
- The Centers for Disease Control and Prevention considers HBV to be the greatest occupational hazard for health care workers. Measures to decrease risk include HBV vaccination, handwashing, and universal precautions.
- Preexposure and postexposure prophylaxis for HAV and HBV include immune globulin (passive immunity for HAV) and HBIG (passive immunity for HBV) and HBV vaccine (active immunity for HBV). A vaccine for HAV is being tested.
- Anorexia and influenza-like symptoms are often more acute in HBV, but these symptoms occur in all types of hepatitis. They occur before icterus (jaundice) appears.
- Most persons with viral hepatitis recover within 6 months and have no residual liver damage. HBV and HCV may lead to a carrier state, atypical course of illness, chronic hepatitis, or cirrhosis.
- All types of jaundice involve increased serum levels of bilirubin. Hemolytic jaundice is a problem of excessive red blood cell breakdown; obstructive jaundice is associated with an elevation of conjugated bilirubin (direct) and an absence of urinary urobilinogen, and hepatocellular jaundice is often associated with elevated serum transaminases.
- In the United States, cirrhosis is most often a result of chronic alcoholism and is characterized by multiple abnormal hepatic function tests. Portal hypertension and bleeding esophageal varices are two life-threatening problems.
- Patients with cirrhosis can have a long history of vague gastrointestinal complaints and failing health.
- Cirrhosis eventually leads to fatigue, hypoglycemia,

fluid and electrolyte disturbances, bleeding, immune incompetence, poor wound healing, ascites, edema, muscle wasting, jaundice, and changes in secondary sexual characteristics if the process is not stopped. The major focus of nursing care is on supporting the patient by dealing with problems related to altered liver function and helping patients deal with the alcoholism that is frequently the cause.

- The major complications of cirrhosis are portal hypertension, varices, ascites, portal-systemic encephalopathy, and hepatorenal syndrome.
- Varices are treated pharmacologically, with sclerotherapy, with balloon tamponade, and in some instances, with shunting procedures.
- Ascitic fluid must be decreased slowly at a rate of no greater than 500 ml/day to prevent hypokalemia, elevated blood urea nitrogen, oliguria, and hepatic encephalopathy.
- Resistant ascites may be treated with use of peritoneal venous shunt or transjugular intrahepatic portosystemic shunt.
- Hepatic encephalopathy causes subtle neurologic changes that can be missed unless assessment focuses on collecting objective neurologic data.
- Hepatic encephalopathy can be precipitated by increased ammonia from gastrointestinal bleeding or increased protein in the diet, by electrolyte imbalances such as hypokalemia and alkalosis, and by depressed central nervous system states such as hypoxia and sedation.
- Hepatic encephalopathy is treated with neomycin, lactulose, and a low-protein diet.
- Hepatorenal syndrome is renal failure from no known cause in persons with hepatic failure; it has a very poor prognosis.
- Liver transplantation is increasingly being performed for a variety of liver problems.
- Patient education is a major nursing intervention for most patients with diffuse liver disease because of the chronicity of the liver problems.

## REFERENCES


1. Advisory Committee Immunization Practices (ACIP): Recommendation for protection against viral hepatitis, *MMWR* 39(S-2):1-26, 1990.
2. Adams L, Soulen MC: TIPS: a new alternative for variceal bleeder, *Am J Crit Care* 2(3):196-201, 1993.
3. Arora S, Kaplan MM: Cirrhosis. In Rakel RE, editor: *Conn's current therapy,* ed 28, Philadelphia, 1989, Saunders.
4. Bloom BS et al: A reappraisal of hepatitis B virus vaccination strategies using cost-effectiveness analysis, *Ann Intern Med* 118(4):298-306, 1993.
5. Burns SM et al: Evaluation and revision of a vasopressin/nitroglycerin protocol for use in variceal bleeding, *Am J Crit Care* 2(3):202-207, 1993.
6. Clouse ME: Hepatic artery embolization for bleeding and tumors, *Surg Clin North Am* 69:419-432, 1989.
7. Doherty MM, Carver DK: Transjugular intrahepatic portosystemic shunt: new relief for esophageal varices, *Am J Nurs* 93(4):58-63, 1993.
8. Gullate MM, Foltz AT: Hepatic chemotherapy via implantable pump, *Am J Nurs* 83:1674-1678, 1983.
9. Gurevich I: Hepatitis. Part I. Enterically transmitted viral hepatitis: etiology, epidemiology, and prevention, *Heart Lung* 22:370-372, 1993.
10. Kearns PJ et al: Accelerated improvement of alcoholic liver disease with enteral nutrition, *Gastroenterology* 102:200-205, 1992.
11. Korniewicz DM et al: Integrity of vinyl and latex procedure gloves, *Nurs Res* 38:144-146, 1989.
12. Kucharski SA: Fulminant hepatic failure, *Crit Care Nurs Clin North Am* 5(1):141-151, 1993.
13. Mudge C, Carlson L: Hepatorenal syndrome, *AACN Clin Issues Crit Care Nurs* 3(3):614-632, 1992.
14. Semonin-Holleran R: Critical nursing care for abdominal trauma, *Crit Care Nurse* 8(3):48-58, 1988.
15. Sherlock S: Fulminant hepatic failure, *Adv Intern Med* 38:245-267, 1993.
16. Sitzman J, Order SE: Immunoradiotherapy for primary nonresectable hepatocellular carcinoma, *Surg Clin North Am* 89:393-400, 1989.
17. US Dept of Health and Human Services, Public Health Service: *Healthy people 2000: national health promotion and disease prevention objectives,* Washington, DC, 1990, US Government Printing Office.
18. Wungaarden JB, Smith LH, Bennett JC, editors: *Cecil textbook of medicine,* ed 19, Philadelphia, 1992, Saunders.

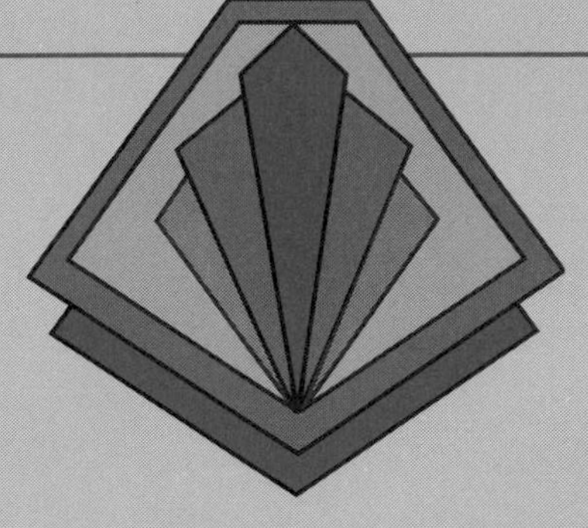

UNIT VIII

# Alterations in Digestion and Elimination

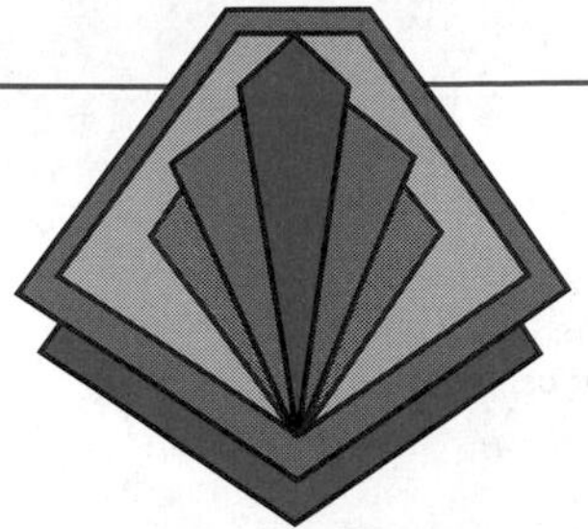

CHAPTER 43

# Assessment of the Gastrointestinal, Biliary, and Exocrine Pancreatic Systems

*Judith K. Sands*

## CHAPTER OBJECTIVES

***After studying this chapter, the learner should be able to do the following:***

1 Describe the functions of the mouth, esophagus, stomach, gallbladder, biliary ductal system, exocrine pancreas, and intestines.
2 Discuss the physiologic changes that occur in the gastrointestinal system in response to aging.
3 Identify the subjective and objective data components of the nursing assessment of the gastrointestinal system.
4 Identify the data that may be obtained from the diagnostic tests used for problems of the gastrointestinal tract.
5 Describe the nursing responsibilities associated with common diagnostic tests used for problems of the gastrointestinal tract.

## KEY TERMS

barium enema
Bernstein test
borborygmi
cecum
cholangiography
cholecystography
chyme
colonscopy
common bile duct
Diagnex blue test
duodenum
ERCP
esophagogastroduodenoscopy
gastric analysis
hepatic duct
ileum
intestinal villus
jejunum
melena
pancreas
rugae
Schilling test
steatorrhea
villus

The gastrointestinal (GI) system, also termed the *digestive system* and *alimentary canal,* consists of the GI tract and its accessory organs. Its primary function is to convert ingested nutrients and fluids into a form that can be used by the cells of the body. This goal is accomplished through the processes of ingestion, digestion, and absorption. The second major function of the GI system is the storage and final excretion of the solid waste products of digestion. Proper functioning of the GI system is essential to the maintenance of proper nutrition and health.

## ANATOMY AND PHYSIOLOGY

The upper portion of the GI tract consists of those structures that aid in the ingestion and digestion of food. They include the mouth, esophagus, stomach, and duodenum, plus the related organs of the biliary system and exocrine pancreas. The lower GI tract consists of the small and large intestines. The structures of the GI system are illustrated in Figure 43-1. The GI system is primarily composed of a hollow, muscular tube approximately 9 m in length that stretches from the mouth to the anus.

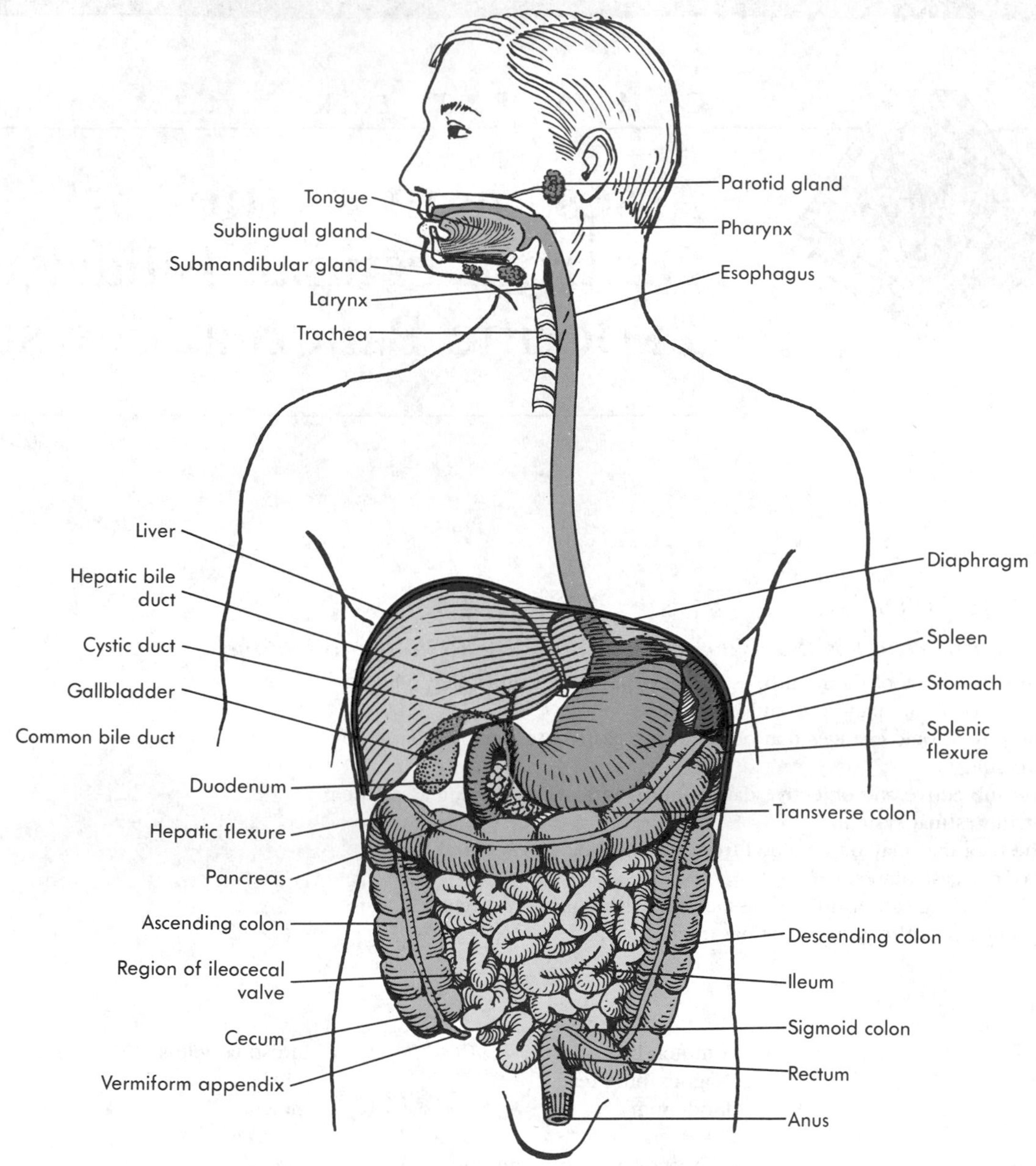


**FIGURE 43-1** The organs of the GI system and related structures.

Although the tube is located within the body, it is really an extension of the external environment. The walls of the GI tract successfully prevent most harmful agents from entering the body. The walls also prevent the escape of essential body fluids and materials. It is composed predominantly of smooth muscle, although some voluntary muscle is found at each end of the tract.

## MOUTH

The mouth is made up of the lips, cheeks, tongue, hard and soft palates, teeth, and salivary glands (Figure 43-2). These structures begin the digestive process by mechanically breaking down and lubricating the food. Because digestive enzymes can function only on the exposed surfaces of food particles, the teeth begin the breakdown of food. No other portion of the GI system can perform the function of the teeth in their absence. This cutting and grinding action also influences the overall rate of digestion.

The lubrication of food is accomplished by mixing it with the watery and mucous secretions of the salivary, parotid, sublingual, and submandibular glands of the mouth. Saliva also contains ptyalin (amylase), which hydrolyzes starch to maltose. Small amounts of saliva are produced continually to keep the tissues of the mouth moist and clean. IgA antibodies to many normal environmental microorganisms are found in saliva. After chewing and moistening are completed, the muscular

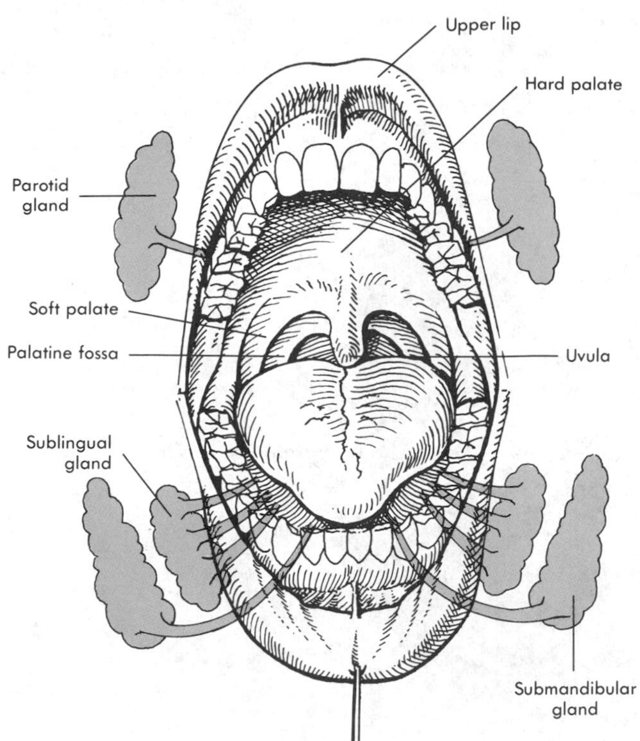


**FIGURE 43-2** The structures of the mouth.

tongue pushes the food bolus back to the pharynx to initiate swallowing (deglutition).

## ESOPHAGUS

The esophagus begins at the lower end of the pharynx. It is a hollow, muscular tube 10 inches (25 cm) in length that lies behind the trachea, passes through the thorax, and connects the mouth and stomach. The upper third is composed of skeletal muscle, and the lower two thirds are smooth muscle. Both ends of the esophagus are protected by sphincters that help to prevent the reflux of gastric contents. Both sphincters are normally closed, except during the act of swallowing.

The primary function of the esophagus is to move the food bolus by peristalsis from the pharynx to the stomach. No enzymes are secreted by the esophagus, and only mechanical digestion takes place. The secretion of mucus assists in the movement of the food bolus and protects the walls of the esophagus from abrasion by partially digested food.

Swallowing is a complex physiologic mechanism that must be accomplished without compromising respiration. It consists of three phases: a voluntary phase in which the tongue forces the bolus of food into the pharynx, an involuntary pharyngeal phase in which the food moves into the upper esophagus, and an esophageal phase during which food moves from the pharynx down into the stomach. The esophageal muscles are activated by the glossopharyngeal and vagal nerves, which create rhythmic peristaltic waves that propel the food toward the stomach. Food is prevented from passing into the trachea by closing of the epiglottis and the opening of the esophagus.

## STOMACH

The stomach is roughly J-shaped and lies in the upper abdomen to the left of midline. It is positioned to the left of the liver, to the right of the spleen, and posterior to both organs. It is a muscular pouch whose shape changes with its contents. Its three major regions are the fundus, body, and antrum. The cardiac sphincter protects the opening from the esophagus, and the pyloric sphincter protects the exit to the duodenum. The **rugae,** or longitudinal folds, of the stomach enable it to quadruple in size and increase from a resting volume of 50 ml to a capacity of approximately 1500 ml for food digestion without major changes in pressure. The stomach has an outer serous layer and three layers of smooth muscle. The outermost layer of smooth muscle is longitudinal, the middle layer is circular, and the inner layer is oblique (Figure 43-3). The rugae are found on the inner mucosal layer.

The stomach primarily serves as a reservoir but also has digestive and secretory functions. Food is stored in the stomach until partially digested. The fundus contains chief cells, which secrete digestive enzymes, and parietal cells, which secrete water, hydrochloric acid (HCl), and the intrinsic factor that is essential for the absorption of vitamin $B_{12}$. The HCl is responsible for the highly acidic medium of the stomach (pH of 0.9 to 1.5), which is needed to activate the enzymes that begin protein digestion. This highly acidic pH also serves as a protective barrier, destroying most ingested microorganisms. Gastric acid secretion is under the control of parasympathetic stimulation via the vagus, as is the secretion of gastrin and histamine. Gastrin is a hormone secreted from endocrine cells in the gastric glands of the stomach in response to vagal stimulation and mechanical distention of the stomach. The secretion of histamine 2 ($H_2$) also increases gastric acid secretion. Approximately 2 to 2.5 L of gastric secretions is produced each day.

The gastric mucosa is covered by a thick mucous gel layer produced by the densely packed epithelial cells of the mucosa. The mucous layer is almost completely impermeable to hydrogen ions. The mucosal epithelial cells also secrete bicarbonate, which acts as a buffer and helps to neutralize the acidic secretions. The combined actions of these two mechanisms are so effective that, while the gastric secretions have a pH of less than 2, the intraluminal pH of the mucosa is maintained at about 7.[16]

Gastric emptying is controlled by both hormonal and autonomic nervous system activity. Parasympathetic stimulation by the vagus nerve increases both peristalsis and secretion. Sympathetic stimulation inhibits them. The peristaltic contractions of the stomach propel the chyme toward the antrum and occur at a frequency of

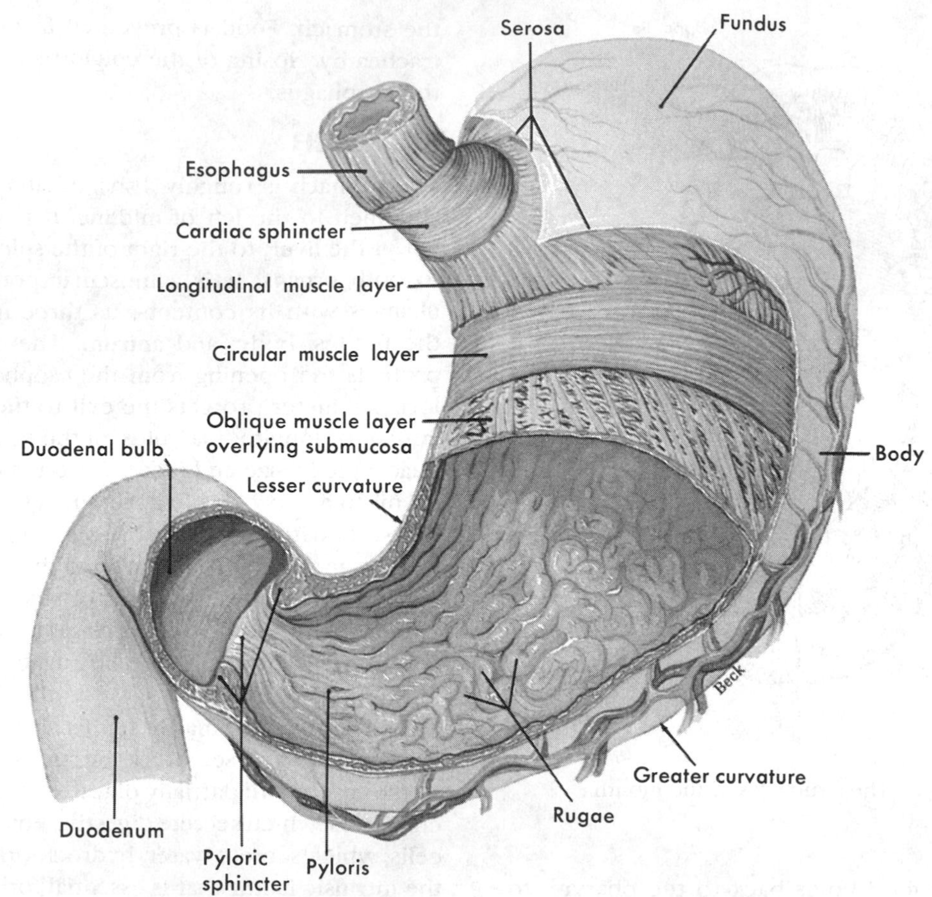


**FIGURE 43-3** The stomach. (From Thibodeau GA: *Anthony's textbook of anatomy and physiology,* ed 13, St Louis, 1990, Mosby.)

about three to five contractions per minute. The pylorus closes during antral contraction, and larger food particles are propelled back toward the body of the stomach for further mixing. Gastric contents are emptied into the duodenum *between* peristaltic contractions. Although the pylorus is not a true anatomic sphincter, it does help to prevent the backflow of duodenal contents and bile salts into the stomach.[12]

## GALLBLADDER AND BILIARY DUCTAL SYSTEM

The gallbladder is a pear-shaped organ that lies on the inferior surface of the liver. It is composed of serous, muscular, and mucous coats and has a usual capacity of 50 ml, although it can increase in size under normal conditions. Innervation of the gallbladder is from the parasympathetic and sympathetic nervous system. The cystic duct connects the gallbladder with the remaining structures of the ductal system—the hepatic ducts and common bile duct.

The major function of the gallbladder is to store and concentrate bile. Bile, which is formed in the liver, is excreted into the **hepatic ducts,** which unite to form the **common bile duct.** It passes behind the pancreas, is joined by the pancreatic duct, and empties into the duodenum. The sphincter of Oddi regulates the flow of bile into the duodenum (Figure 43-4). A second sphincter (sphincter of Boyden) is located above the junction with the pancreatic duct and controls the flow of bile in the common bile duct. When this sphincter is closed, bile moves back into the gallbladder, where it is concentrated fivefold to tenfold. Because bile can be released directly into the duodenum, the gallbladder is not essential to life. Bile salts facilitate fat digestion by emulsifying fats for action by intestinal lipases and facilitate the absorption of fats, fat-soluble vitamins, and cholesterol.

The release of bile from the gallbladder or liver is controlled by cholecystokinin (CCK). Approximately 600 to 800 ml of bile is produced daily. CCK is released from the walls of the duodenal intestinal mucosa when lipids, amino acids, and hydrogen ions enter the duodenum from the stomach. It travels by the blood to the gallbladder and causes contraction of the gallbladder's smooth musculature and relaxation of the sphincter at the end of the common bile duct (the sphincter of Oddi), so that bile can be emptied into the duodenum.

Most of the bile salts are reabsorbed from the intestine

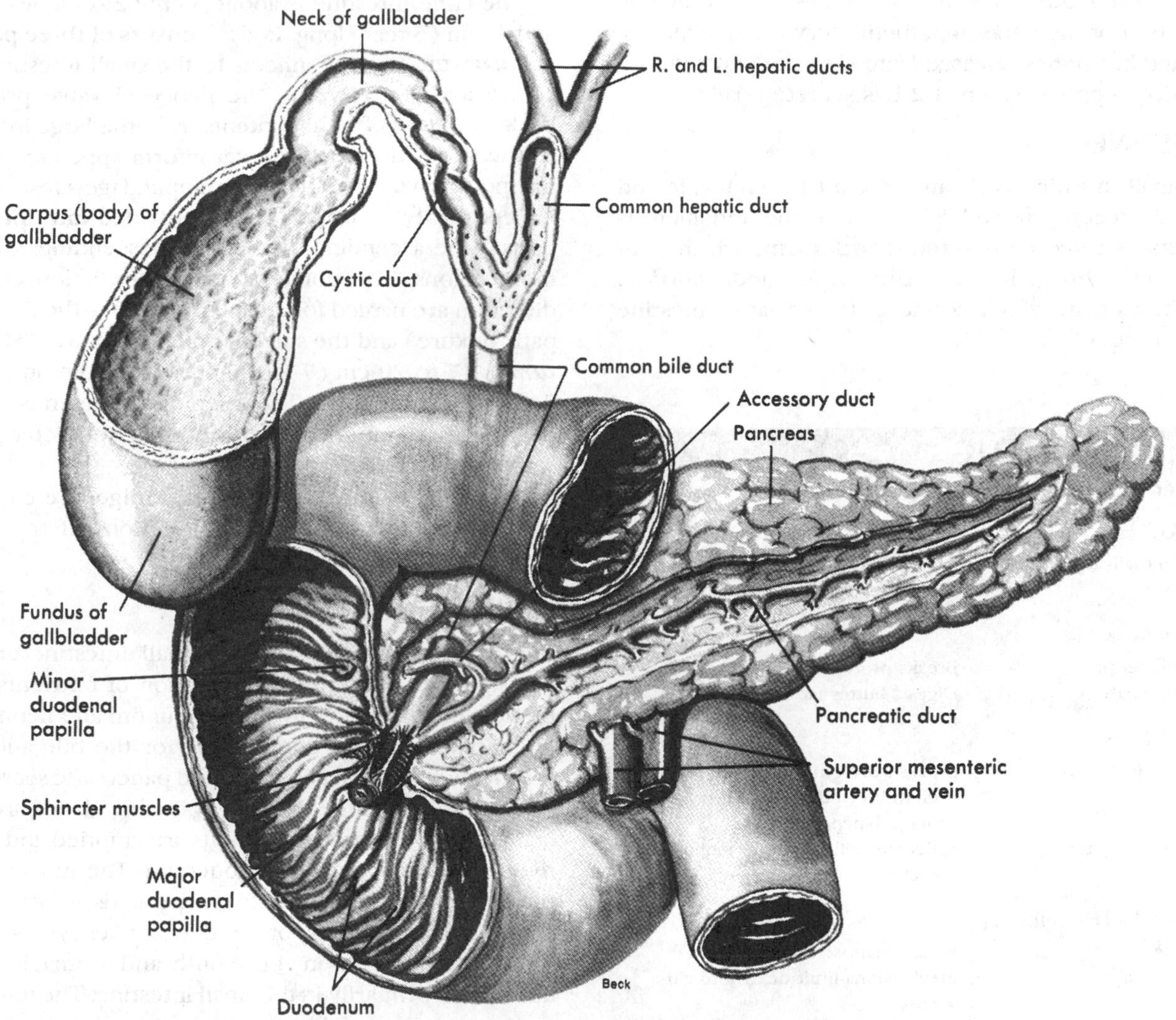


**FIGURE 43-4** The biliary and pancreatic ductal systems. Note that the head of the pancreas completely surrounds the common bile duct. (From Thibodeau GA: *Anthony's textbook of anatomy and physiology,* ed 13, St Louis, 1990, Mosby.)

into the enterohepatic circulation and returned to the liver, where they can be recirculated. The system is so efficient that only 15% to 25% of the bile salt pool needs to be replaced each day.

## PANCREAS

The **pancreas** is an elongated, flattened organ located in the posterior abdomen, with its head lying within the curve of the duodenum and its tail resting against the spleen. The pancreas has both exocrine and endocrine functions. The exocrine functions are carried out by the acinar cells and duct system, and the endocrine functions are carried out by islets of Langerhans cells. The endocrine function of the pancreas is discussed in Chapter 39.

The pancreas is divided into three parts, which are composed of lobules. The lobules are formed from groups of secretory cells called *acini,* which drain into a ductal system that ultimately reaches the main pancreatic duct of Wirsung. This major duct extends the entire length of the gland. At the head of the pancreas the ductal secretions enter the duodenum through the ampulla of Vater. The sphincter of Oddi controls its opening (see Figure 43-4).

Approximately 2 L of pancreatic secretions is produced daily. The ductal epithelium secretes a balanced electrolyte secretion, and the acinar cells secrete digestive enzymes in an inactive precursor state. The pancreatic secretions contain proteolytic enzymes, which break down protein; pancreatic amylase, which breaks down starch; and lipase, which hydrolyzes fat into glycerol and fatty acids. The pancreatic acinar cells also produce an enzyme inhibitor that prevents the activation of the secretions until they reach the duodenum. The production of the pancreatic secretions is controlled by the action of the parasympathetic nervous system, gastrin, and hormones released from the duodenum during digestion. Approximately 1.2 L is secreted daily.

## INTESTINES

The small intestine is about 2.5 cm (1 inch) wide and 6 m (20 feet) long and fills most of the abdomen. It consists of three parts—the **duodenum,** which connects to the stomach; the **jejunum,** or middle portion; and the **ileum,** which connects to the large intestine (see Figure 43-1).

The large intestine is about 6 cm (2½ inches) wide and 1.5 m (5 feet) long. It also consists of three parts—the **cecum,** which connects to the small intestine; the *colon;* and the *rectum.* The ileocecal valve prevents backward flow of fecal contents from the large intestine to the small intestine. The vermiform appendix, which has no known function, is an appendage close to the ileocecal valve. The colon is subdivided into four sections—the ascending, transverse, descending, and sigmoid colons. The points at which the colon changes direction are named for adjacent organs—the liver (hepatic flexure) and the spleen (splenic flexure). The *rectum* is 17 to 20 cm (7 to 8 inches) long, ending in the 2- to 3-cm anal canal. The opening of the anus is controlled by a smooth muscle internal sphincter and a striated muscle external sphincter.

Table 43-1 summarizes the major digestive enzymes, and Table 43-2 summarizes the actions of the major gastrointestinal hormones.

**TABLE 43-1 Digestive Enzymes**

| SOURCE | ACTION |
|---|---|
| **MOUTH** | |
| Pytalin (salivary amylase) | Breaks starch into maltose (polysaccharides to disaccharides) |
| **STOMACH** | |
| Gastric pepsin | Breaks protein into polypeptides |
| Gastric lipase | Digests butter fat |
| **PANCREAS** | |
| Pancreatic amylase | Breaks starch into maltose (polysaccharides to disaccharides) |
| Trypsin | Splits polypeptide chains |
| Pancreatic lipase | Splits emulsified fat into monoglycerides |
| **SMALL INTESTINE** | |
| Maltase | Breaks maltose into glucose |
| Dextrinase | Breaks alpha-limit dextrin to glucose |
| Lactase | Breaks lactose into galactose and glucose |
| Sucrase | Breaks sucrose into glucose and fructose |
| Enterokinase | Activates trypsin |
| Peptidases | Splits polypeptides into amino acids |
| Intestinal lipase | Splits neutral fats into glycerol and fatty acids |

### Small Intestine

The primary functions of the small intestine are the digestion of food and the absorption of nutrients. This process occurs primarily in the jejunum and ileum. The duodenum contains the opening for the bile and pancreatic ducts, which allow bile and pancreatic secretions to enter the intestine. Mucus-producing glands are concentrated where gastric contents are emptied and digestive secretions enter the duodenum. The mucus helps to protect the duodenum from the acids in the gastric chyme and the actions of the digestive enzymes.

Digestion begins in the mouth and stomach, but it takes place primarily in the small intestine. The intestinal mucosa is impermeable to most large molecules, so proteins, fats, and complex carbohydrates must be broken down into small particles before they can be absorbed. The intestinal mucosa also secretes surface enzymes that aid in digestion and about 2 L per day of serous fluid that acts as a diluting agent to facilitate absorption.

Carbohydrate digestion, which began in the mouth, is completed in the small intestine as disaccharides are

**TABLE 43-2 Major Gastrointestinal Hormones**

| HORMONE | ACTION | STIMULUS FOR SECRETION |
|---|---|---|
| Gastrin | Stimulates secretion of gastric acid and pepsinogen; increases gastric blood flow; stimulates gastric smooth muscle contraction and motility | Secreted from antrum of stomach and duodenum in response to vagal stimulation, epinephrine, solutions of calcium salts, and alcohol; inhibited by an antral stomach pH of less than 2.5 |
| Secretin | Stimulates secretion of bicarbonate-containing solution by the pancreas and liver; inhibits gastric acid secretion and motility | Secreted by duodenum in response to low pH chyme (less than 3.0) entering the duodenum |
| Cholecystokinin | Stimulates the contraction of the gallbladder and the secretion of pancreatic enzymes; slows gastric emptying | Secreted in duodenum and jejunum in response to the presence of fatty and amino acids |
| Enterogastrone | Inhibits gastric secretion and motility; relaxes sphincter of Oddi | Secreted in duodenum in response to the presence of partially digested proteins and fats |

broken down into monosaccharides (glucose, fructose, and galactose) by the action of intestinal enzymes and pancreatic amylase. Protein digestion, which began in the stomach, is completed as polypeptides are broken down into peptides and amino acids by the action of pancreatic trypsin. Fat digestion is accomplished by emulsification into small droplets by the action of bile and pancreatic lipase. The droplets are then further broken down into glycerol and fatty acids. The release of digestive secretions is stimulated by the hormones *secretin* and *cystokinin-pancreozymin* (CCK-PZ), as well as by the action of the parasympathetic nervous system.

The inner mucosal surface of the small intestine is covered with millions of villi, which are the functional units for absorption. Each **villus** is equipped with a blind-end lymph vessel (lacteal) in its center, which is surrounded by capillaries, venules, and arterioles (Figure 43-5). These structures bring blood to the surface of the intestine and provide a network for absorption into the portal blood or lymphatic system.[12] Ninety percent of absorption occurs within the small intestine by either active transport or diffusion. Active transport requires a metabolic energy expenditure and is used to absorb amino acids, monosaccharides, sodium, and calcium. Fatty acids and water diffuse passively, primarily into the lymphatics.

The contents of the small intestine **(chyme)** are propelled toward the anus by regular peristaltic movements. Both segmental and propulsive movements occur. The segmental movements involve primarily the circular muscles of the intestine. Slow contractions move the chyme back and forth in small segments of the intestine (1 to 4 cm). This movement mixes the chyme and facilitates digestion and absorption. Segmental peristaltic movements increase after meals. The propulsive peristaltic movements involve intestinal segments of 10 to 20 cm in length.[16] Contraction occurs in the proximal segment, with relaxation in the distal segment. Chyme

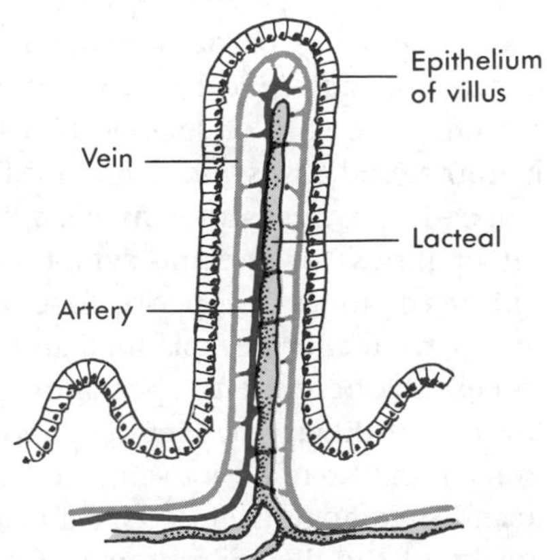


**FIGURE 43-5** The intestinal villus. Note the circulatory vessels surrounding the lacteal, which drains into the lymphatic system.

moves slowly and normally takes 3 to 10 hours to move from the stomach to the colon. Parasympathetic stimulation, primarily through branches of the vagus nerve, increases peristaltic activity. Sympathetic stimulation is primarily inhibitory.

### Large Intestine

Very little chemical digestion takes place in the large intestine. It functions primarily to absorb water and electrolytes from the chyme and store the food waste (feces) until defecation. Reabsorption occurs predominantly in the right or ascending colon. The colon can absorb 6 to 8 times more fluid than is delivered to it daily, and only approximately 100 ml of fluid is left in the colon to be mixed with the fecal residue.

The large number of microorganisms found in the large intestine further break down the residual proteins that were not digested or absorbed in the small intestine. The breakdown of amino acids produces ammonia, which is converted to urea by the liver. These intestinal bacteria also play a vital role in the synthesis of vitamin K and some of the B vitamins. The only significant secretion of the colon is mucus, which protects the walls and helps the fecal matter adhere into a mass.

Approximately 450 ml of chyme reaches the cecum each day. The transit time in the large bowel is slow, taking about 12 hours to reach the rectum. The fecal contents in the colon are pushed forward by mass movements that occur only a few times each day. These mass movements are stimulated by gastrocolic reflexes initiated when food enters the duodenum from the stomach, especially after the first meal of the day.

The rectum is well innervated with sensory fibers. Parasympathetic fibers are responsible for the contraction of the rectum and relaxation of the internal sphincter of the anus. The defecation reflex occurs when feces enter the rectum. Afferent impulses are transmitted to the sacral segments of the spinal cord, and reflex impulses are transmitted back to the sigmoid and rectum, initiating relaxation of the internal anal sphincter.

## PHYSIOLOGIC CHANGES WITH AGING

Gastrointestinal complaints are extremely common in elderly persons, and it is clear that distinct changes occur in the GI system with aging, although these changes are incompletely understood. Most of the aging-related changes do not interfere with normal functioning, however, unless the elderly person also experiences problems associated with other chronic illnesses, such as diabetes. The effects of co-morbidity are usually much more important than are the effects of aging itself.[1] Documented changes in GI function are summarized in Box 43-1.

In the mouth, teeth darken and may loosen or fracture and gums recede. Salivary gland output decreases, which causes mouth dryness and increased susceptibility to infection and breakdown. Aging causes decreased mo-

**BOX 43-1 Physiologic Changes in GI Tract Functioning with Aging**

**MOUTH AND TEETH**
Teeth darken and may loosen or fracture
Decreased saliva

**ESOPHAGUS**
Decreased peristalsis
Weakening of lower esophageal sphincter

**STOMACH**
Decreased gastric motility and emptying
Decreased secretion of gastric acid

**BILIARY SYSTEM**
Increased cholesterol content of bile, gallstones

**PANCREAS**
Decreased secretion of pancreatic enzymes

**SMALL INTESTINE**
Impaired nutrient absorption, particularly carbohydrates
Defective vitamin D absorption
Impairment of calcium active transport
Decreased production of secretory IgA

**LARGE INTESTINE**
Increased incidence of polyps and diverticula

**RECTUM**
Decreased elasticity and volume

NOTE: Although GI complaints are common, most GI problems are related to the effects of chronic illnesses rather than aging.

tility and strength of peristalsis in the esophagus, but these changes appear to have minimal significance in healthy persons. Some deterioration in the lower esophageal sphincter may increase the frequency of esophageal reflux.[1]

Gastric motility and emptying diminish slightly but progressively with age, and gastric acid secretion also decreases steadily after age 50. Achlorhydria is relatively common. These changes can produce minor problems in digestion but are usually asymptomatic. Chronic gastritis is common in elderly persons, but the condition is a result of bacterial colonization by *Helicobacter pylori* and not aging.

No significant changes in biliary system morphology are associated with aging. However, the composition of the bile becomes increasingly lithogenic, possibly related to an increase in biliary cholesterol. The incidence of gallstones increases with each decade.[4]

The pancreas exhibits ductal hyperplasia and fibrosis with aging, but these changes are not necessarily associated with altered functioning. The output of pancreatic secretions steadily declines after age 40, but related problems with absorption cannot be documented.

Aging-related changes in small intestinal function are important and can lead to poor nutrition even with adequate intake. Nutrient absorption is clearly impaired, particularly the absorption of carbohydrates. Absorption of water-soluble vitamins remains intact, but the absorption of vitamin D is defective in many elderly persons, and the active transport of calcium is also impaired. Decreased production of secretory IgA can lead to an increase in the frequency and severity of infections.[3]

Although chronic constipation is one of the most common complaints in elderly persons, the segmental mass movements and contractions of the large intestine have been found to be unchanged as long as the individual remains physically active. The incidence of both diverticula and polyps in the colon rises with age. There is a decrease in elasticity in the rectum and a steady decrease in the rectal volume, which can result in sphincter failure. However, the sensation of rectal fullness remains intact, and most problems with bowel incontinence in elderly persons are not attributable to the effects of aging.[2]

# SUBJECTIVE DATA

A thorough health history is necessary to adequately assess the health status of persons with potential dysfunction of the GI system.

## PATIENT/FAMILY HISTORY

The nurse asks the patient about previous GI problems, hospitalizations, and surgeries. This includes past and current medication use, both over-the-counter and prescribed. The use of antacids and laxatives is particularly important. The nurse inquires about the presence of GI problems in the nuclear or extended family, including cancer and such disorders as inflammatory bowel disease, which have a documented hereditary link.

## DIET AND NUTRITION

The adequacy of the diet, in terms of both quality and quantity, can be quickly estimated through comparison of the diet with recommended food intake patterns. The nutritional assessment has particular significance in GI disorders, because it may reveal changes in eating patterns that are characteristic of specific illnesses or disorders. The nutritional assessment includes an exploration of usual eating patterns and any changes that may be the result of illness or specific symptoms. The assessment explores changes in appetite, food preferences and intolerances, food allergies, planned and unplanned changes in weight, adherence to special or therapeutic diets, and the use of dietary or vitamin supplements. A 24-hour dietary recall may be a useful tool to approximate caloric and specific nutrient intake and analyze the overall adequacy of the diet. Symptoms related to food intake should also be carefully assessed. Changes in appetite and the presence of such symptoms as dysphagia, nausea, and discomfort are carefully explored.

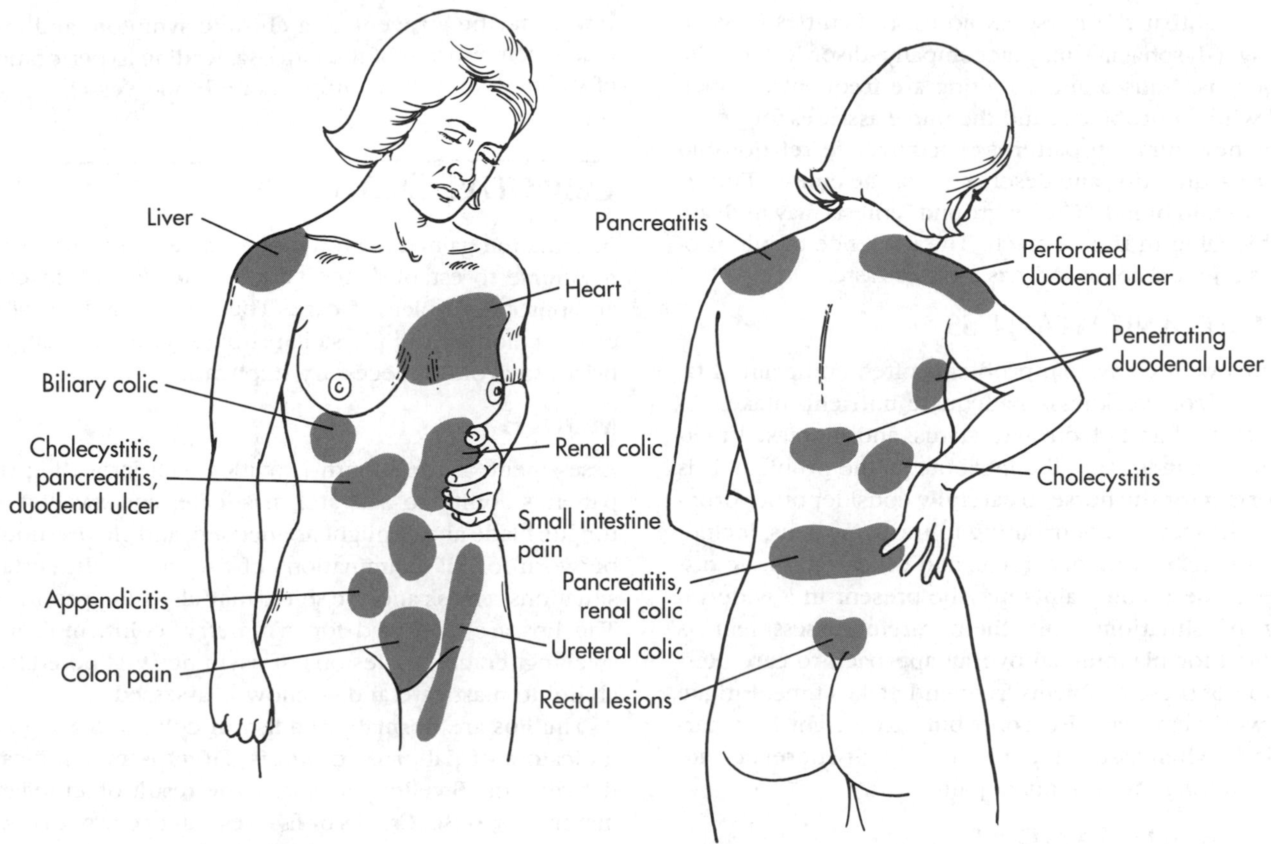


**FIGURE 43-6** Common sites of referred abdominal pain. Note that the pain's location may not be directly over or even near the site of the organ.

Life-style, economic, and cultural factors affecting nutrition are also assessed. Food has multiple social and emotional values for individuals that are quite distinct from its role in nutrition. Financial resources, access to food preparation and storage facilities, and religious or social beliefs may all influence both the quality and quantity of the diet. Life-style factors can have a direct or indirect effect on GI function. GI symptoms frequently develop in response to life stressors or worsen in response to those stressors. Open-ended questions are most effective for exploring beliefs and feelings about food.

Complete nutritional assessment includes an evaluation of the patient's use of sugar and salt substitutes, coffee, alcohol, and tobacco (both chewing and smoking). The presence of dentures is an essential consideration, because dentures may significantly influence food selection and chewing.

## ABDOMINAL PAIN

Although pain is neither an early nor common manifestation of GI disease, it is frequently the reason individuals seek medical attention. The nurse assesses its onset, duration, character, location, and relationship to meals, stressful events, or activity. Pain may be experienced anywhere along the length of the GI tract in a specific localized pattern, a general nonspecific pattern, or referred to another somatic or skeletal region that shares the same nerve innervation[7] (Figure 43-6). Abdominal pain may be continuous, episodic, or associated with eating. The pain sensation is thought to arise from the distention or sudden contraction of a hollow viscus; therefore local stretching or traction on pain-sensitive structures will elicit the pain stimulus. The painful area may demonstrate local muscle guarding, which serves as a protective mechanism as the overlying muscles contract. The pain associated with pancreatic or biliary dysfunction is frequently very severe.

Abdominal pain or discomfort may be reported as heartburn, indigestion, or stomachache and requires further clarification,. The pain may interfere with chewing or swallowing food. Specific foods, such as those that are spicy, very hot, or very cold; alcohol; or smoking may initiate or aggravate the pain. Abdominal pain may have been self-treated with a variety of over-the-counter preparations.

The term *indigestion* is frequently used by patients to describe heartburn (usually the result of reflux), uncomfortable fullness or distention after meals, or the excessive production of gas. The nurse clarifies the patient's use of the term and the nature of the symptom.

Abdominal pain is frequently associated with other

symptoms that the nurse explores. Difficulties in swallowing (dysphagia) may accompany disorders of the esophagus. Nausea and vomiting are frequently associated with GI problems, and the nurse assesses for onset, frequency, duration, patterns of occurrence, relationship to meals, quantity, and description of the emesis. Emesis may contain blood. "Coffee-ground" emesis may indicate old bleeding in the stomach. The presence of bile produces a green color and has a bitter taste.

### FATIGUE AND WEAKNESS

Persons with GI system problems often complain of fatigue and/or weakness. Inadequate nutrient intake, abnormal fluid and electrolyte status, and increased metabolic demands may all contribute to the problem. It is important for the nurse to carefully consider other problems that may be contributing to the symptoms, including cardiac, respiratory, renal, and other metabolic disorders. These complaints may be present in a wide variety of situations, but their careful assessment is essential for planning an overall approach to care. Resolution of these problems frequently takes time. Fatigue and weakness may also contribute to weight loss, particularly when associated with persistent anorexia, nausea, vomiting, or abdominal pain.

### ELIMINATION PATTERNS

Patterns of bowel elimination vary significantly among healthy individuals, and these patterns are frequently altered by GI system disorders. The nurse assesses the individual's usual elimination pattern and explores any changes that have occurred. The use of laxatives, suppositories, or other products to support bowel elimination is carefully assessed.

Changes in the normal pattern of bowel elimination may represent a physiologic alteration, a pathologic condition, or simply a change in normal diet and activity patterns. Constipation—defined as the presence of small, hard stools that are passed with difficulty at infrequent intervals—is a classic example. It may be a temporary response to inactivity and a diet change or a sign of bowel obstruction. Diarrhea and stools containing mucus, pus, and possibly undigested food may indicate enteritis or invasion by a parasite. Partial obstruction of the descending colon may produce small, ribbon-shaped stools, whereas no stool is passed if obstruction is complete. Diarrhea and constipation may also result from medical therapy or surgical intervention.

When fat absorption is abnormal, **steatorrhea** (bulky, foul, fatty stools) may occur. If biliary obstruction is present, the patient may give a history of clay-colored (grayish) stools. Bright red blood in the stool indicates lower GI bleeding. Blood from the upper GI tract is changed by digestive secretions, and the stool appears black and sticky (tarry), although the presence of blood in the GI tract acts as a powerful cathartic and may produce abrupt, severe diarrhea. Blood in the stool **(melena)** may be a recent or a chronic symptom and may result from erosion of the mucosa, leading to perforation of the muscle wall or rupture of a blood vessel.

## OBJECTIVE DATA

Information gained from the physical assessment assists the nurse to establish the patient's needs and develop an appropriate plan of care. The history and physical examination by the physician should be used as appropriate to avoid unnecessary duplication.

### MOUTH

Assessment of the mouth provides data indicating the patient's ability to salivate, masticate, and swallow. A tongue blade and penlight are needed, and gloves should be worn for all examinations of the mouth. In certain situations, a mask and eye shield may also be appropriate. The lips are observed for symmetry, color, moisture, swelling, cracks, or lesions. If asymmetry is noted, the ability to masticate and swallow is assessed.

The lips are normally reddish in color and are good indicators of pallor or cyanosis. Dryness may indicate dehydration. Swelling is usually the result of an inflammatory response. Cracks or fissures can occur with overdryness or exposure to cold or, if in the corners of the mouth *(angular stomatitis),* from lack of dentures, poorly fitting dentures, or a riboflavin deficiency.

Lesions on the lips may be benign or malignant. A frequently encountered benign lesion is *herpes simplex* (cold sore, fever blister), which is caused by a virus and can create enough discomfort to limit mastication. The enamel surface of the teeth should be white but will darken with surface stains (tea, coffee, tobacco). Commonly found abnormalities include caries, loose or broken teeth, and absence of some or all teeth. The gums—or *gingivae*—are normally pink in color, attach to the teeth, and fill the interdental surfaces. If the person is partially or completely edentulous, the gingivae are examined for areas of redness caused by improperly fitting dentures, partial plates, or implants. The person is then asked to insert the dentures to assess correct fit and comfort for adequate mastication. Recession of the gum line is not uncommon in older individuals.

The buccal mucosa is light pink, although patchy pigmentation is seen in dark-skinned individuals. The mucosa is examined for moisture, white spots or patches, debris, areas of bleeding, or ulcers resulting from ill-fitting dentures or braces. Dryness and debris may indicate dehydration. White, curdy patches—which are removable with some effort—may be caused by *candidiasis* (thrush). White, nonremovable patches *(leukoplakia);* white plaques within red patches; or red, granular patches may be premalignant lesions and should be reported to the physician. A round or oval white ulcer surrounded by an area of redness is indicative of an *aphthous ulcer* (canker sore). (See Chapter 44.)

When the tongue is depressed with a tongue blade and the person says "Ah," the soft palate is observed for symmetry and the effective functioning of cranial nerve X (necessary for effective swallowing). The uvula, soft palate, tonsils, and posterior pharynx are observed for signs of inflammation. Tongue mobility and function are essential to mastication, taste, and swallowing. Normally, there is no limitation to movement in any direction, but the tongue will deviate to the paralyzed side with paralysis of the twelfth cranial nerve (hypoglossal). A thin, white coating and presence of large papillae on the dorsum of the tongue are normal findings. A thick coating indicates poor oral hygiene, and a smooth, red surface suggests a nutritional deficiency. The ventral surface is examined for leukoplakia, ulceration, or nodules, any of which may indicate malignancy.

Any distinctive odor of the breath is noted. A foul odor may occur after the ingestion of certain foods, with poor hygiene or oral infections, and with some metabolic dysfunctions, such as diabetic ketoacidosis, liver disease, and bowel obstruction. Normally the mandible will slide forward and down with ease. A normal "cracking" sound may be heard when the mouth is opened widely. The interior of the mouth should also be carefully examined with a gloved finger to check for areas of tenderness, ulcers, and lumps.

## ABDOMEN

Examination of the abdomen determines the presence or absence of (1) tenderness, (2) organ enlargement, (3) masses, (4) spasm or ridigity of the abdominal muscles, and (5) fluid or air in the abdominal cavity. Physical examination of the abdomen is performed in the following order: inspection, auscultation, percussion, and palpation. Auscultation is performed before percussion and palpation, because the latter two may alter the frequency and intensity of bowel sounds.

The surface of the abdomen may be described anatomically in either four quadrants or nine regions (Figure 43-7). The patient should be in a supine position and as relaxed as possible. Bending the patient's knees slightly and placing a small pillow under the head can help the patient to relax the abdominal muscles and make palpation easier. Good lighting should be available.

### Inspection

The skin of the abdomen is inspected for color, texture, scars, rashes, lesions, symmetry, contour, and visible peristalsis. The abdomen is normally flat but will be rounded in an obese person and may appear scaphoid in the thin or emaciated person. The integrity and turgor of the skin are reliable indicators of total body hydration.

Abdominal distention may be caused by air or fluid in the GI tract or fluid in the peritoneal space (ascites). Air may collect from swallowing or from gas produced by bacterial action in the bowel. Decreased peristalsis prevents the accumulated air from moving through the GI tract. Fluid may also accumulate from decreased peristalsis and be a symptom of partial or complete bowel obstruction. Ascites usually results from increased portal hypertension secondary to liver or heart disease.

Measurement of abdominal girth provides a baseline

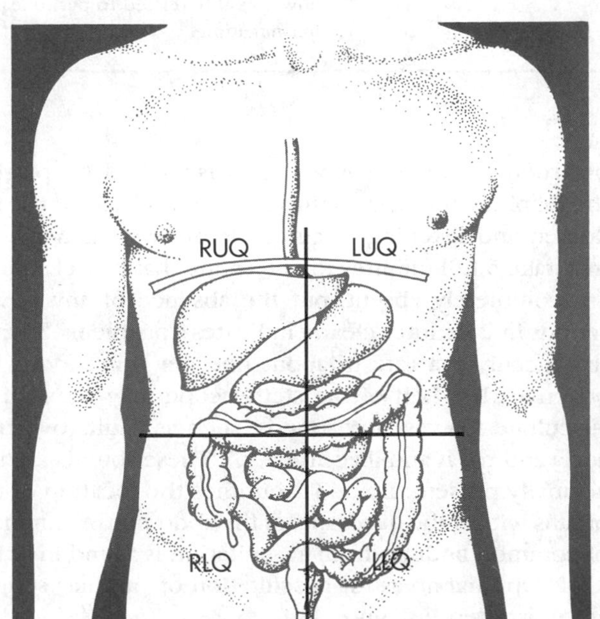


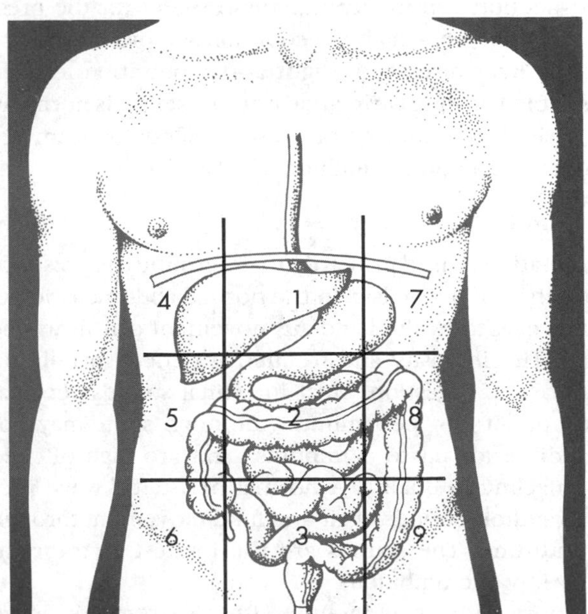


**FIGURE 43-7** Regions of the abdomen. *Left:* The abdomen divided into four quadrants. *Right:* The abdomen divided into nine topographic regions: *1,* epigastrium; *2,* umbilical; *3,* suprapubic; *4,* right hypochondrium; *5,* left hypochondrium; *6,* right lumbar or flank; *7,* left lumbar or flank; *8,* right inguinal or iliac, and *9,* left inguinal or iliac.

**TABLE 43-3 Common Findings from Abdominal Inspection**

| FINDING | INTERPRETATION |
|---|---|
| Scars or striae | May be result of pregnancy, obesity, ascites, tumors, edema, surgical procedures, or healed burned areas |
| Engorged veins | May be caused by obstruction of vena cava or portal vein and circulation from abdomen |
| Skin color | Observe for evidence of jaundice or inflammation (redness) |
| Visible peristalsis | May be caused by pyloric or intestinal obstruction; normally peristalsis not visible except for slow waves in thin persons |
| Visible pulsations | Normally slight pulsation of aorta, visible in epigastric region |
| Visible masses and altered contour | Observe for hernias, distention of ascites, and obesity; instructing patient to cough may bring out hernia "bulge" or elicit pain or discomfort in the abdomen; marked concavity may be caused by malnutrition |
| Spider angioma | Appear on upper portion of body and blanch with pressure; commonly result from liver disease |

for the evaluation of increase or decrease in size because of distention. A measuring tape is placed around the abdomen at the level of the umbilicus or 2.5 cm below, and the reading is taken. It is important to lightly mark the site for measurement on the patient's skin, so that all subsequent measurements are taken at the same level for accurate evaluation.

Inspection will incorporate assessment for the presence of jaundice, which is a common symptom in biliary tract or liver disease. A slight aortic pulsation may be present in the epigastric area, but peristalsis is normally not visible. A summary of common findings from abdominal inspection is included in Table 43-3.

## Auscultation

Auscultation is used primarily to determine the presence or absence of peristalsis. In the normal abdomen, bowel sounds caused by fluid and air movement can always be heard. The intensity and frequency depend mainly on the phase of digestion. Most intestinal sounds occur at a rate of 5 to 34 per minute (although some may not be audible for up to 5 minutes) and are high pitched and gurgling in quality. A normal peristaltic wave produces audible sounds of air and fluid movement through the intestine. The sounds are the loudest to the right and below the umbilicus.

Abnormalities may include either extreme. A virtual absence of normal sounds occurs when bowel motility is inhibited by inflammation or paralytic ileus. Exaggerated peristalsis produces waves of loud, gurgling sounds called **borborygmi** and may result from infection or obstruction. Bowel sounds are auscultated by placing the diaphragm of the stethoscope lightly against the abdomen and listening to all quadrants systematically. It may take 5 full minutes to determine that bowel sounds are completely absent, but the absence of any bowel sounds in 2 minutes clearly indicates a problem.[9] Sounds that occur at a rate of about one per minute are hypoactive. The bell of the stethoscope may be used to auscultate for vascular sounds, such as bruits over the aorta and renal and iliac arteries.[10] These sounds are not normally present. Box 43-2 outlines the location of the organs within the quadrants of the abdomen. A summary of common findings from auscultation is found in Table 43-4. Optimal areas for auscultation of vascular sounds are illustrated in Figure 43-8.

**BOX 43-2 Anatomic Location of Organs within Each Abdominal Quadrant**

| RIGHT UPPER QUADRANT (RUQ) | LEFT UPPER QUADRANT (LUQ) |
|---|---|
| Liver<br>Gallbladder<br>Duodenum<br>Right kidney<br>Hepatic flexure of colon | Stomach<br>Spleen<br>Left kidney<br>Pancreas<br>Splenic flexure of colon |
| **RIGHT LOWER QUADRANT (RLQ)** | **LEFT LOWER QUADRANT (LLQ)** |
| Cecum<br>Appendix<br>Right ovary and tube | Sigmoid colon<br>Left ovary and tube |

**TABLE 43-4 Common Findings from Abdominal Auscultation**

| FINDING | INTERPRETATION |
|---|---|
| Absence of sounds in 5 minutes | Peritonitis, paralytic ileus, pneumonia, and hypokalemia |
| Repeated, high-pitched sounds occurring at frequent intervals | Increased peristalsis heard in gastroenteritis, early pyloric obstruction, early intestinal obstruction, and diarrhea |
| Bruit | Presence of abnormal sounds (turbulence of blood flow through partially occluded or diseased aorta or renal artery) |
| Hum and friction rub | Heard over liver and splenic areas, indicating an increased venous blood flow, possibly related to peritoneal inflammation |

## Percussion

Percussion of the abdomen has relatively limited value. It is used primarily to confirm the size of various organs

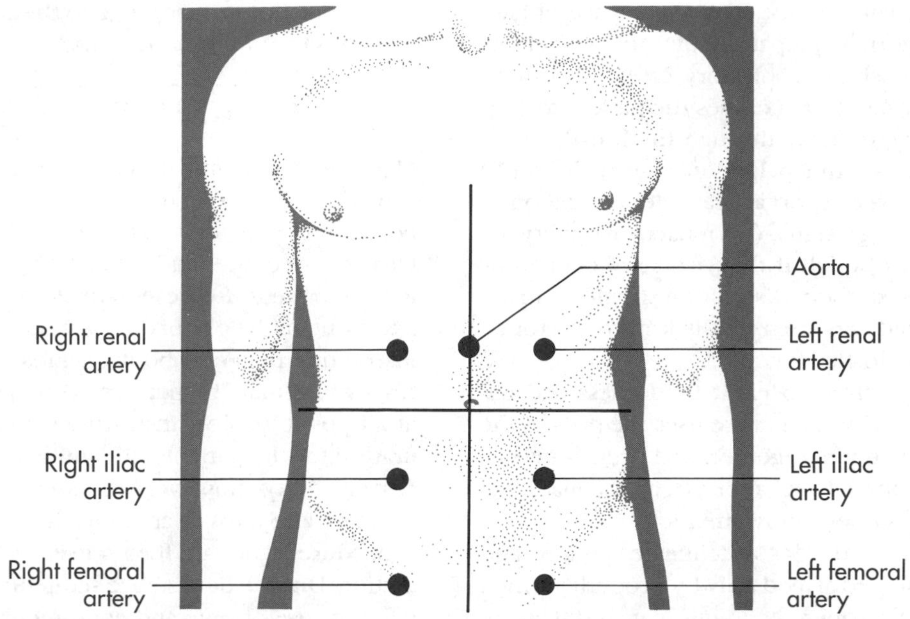


**FIGURE 43-8** Sites for auscultation of vascular sounds in the abdomen.

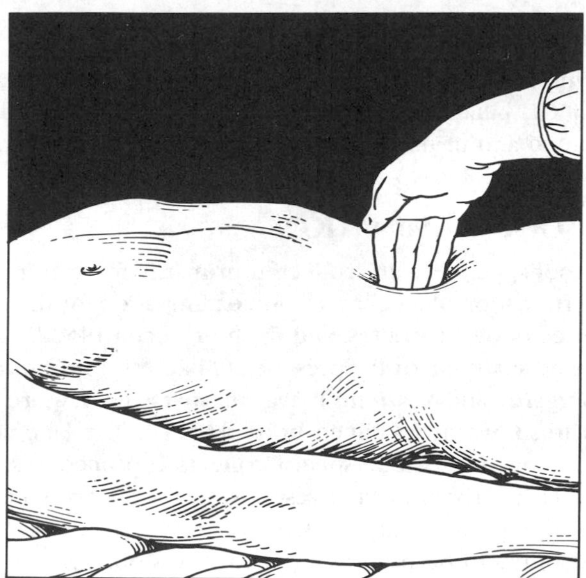

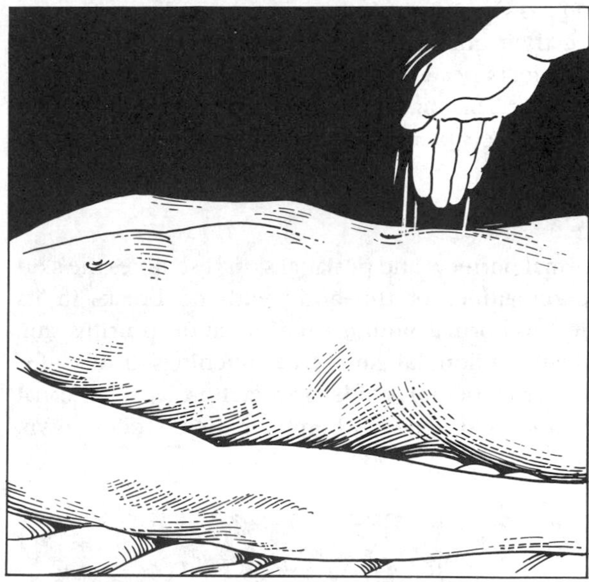

**FIGURE 43-9** Palpating for rebound tenderness.

and to determine the presence of excessive amounts of fluid or air. Normally, percussion over the abdomen is tympanic because of the presence of a small amount of swallowed air within the GI tract. A dull or flat percussion note is found over a solid structure. Dull sounds normally occur over the liver and spleen or a bladder filled with urine. Abnormal percussion findings occur because of the presence of ascites or abnormal masses. Ascites classically produces a shifting dullness, which is caused by fluid movement to dependent areas. Interpreting the sounds of abdominal percussion may be difficult in obese individuals.

The four quadrants are percussed beginning with the thorax area and moving downward systematically. The degree of tympany, from soft to pronounced, is recorded. Tympanic sounds should be heard beginning at the ninth interspace in the left upper quadrant of the abdomen.

## Palpation

Palpation is of value in determining the outlines of the abdominal organs, determining the presence and characteristics of any abdominal masses, and identifying the presence of direct tenderness, guarding, rebound tenderness, and muscular rigidity. In the presence of gallbladder disease, normal palpation of the liver elicits sharp pain and a positive inspiratory arrest (Murphy's sign). The acute onset of pain causes the patient to stop inspiration abruptly, midway through the breath.

Abnormal findings from palpation may include (1) direct tenderness over an organ capsule, (2) rebound tenderness (Blumberg's sign), (3) muscular rigidity, or (4) masses that may be felt if they are large enough or close enough to the surface. Distinction should be made between a distended abdomen that is firm to the touch and one that is soft to the touch.

Light palpation is used to elicit tenderness and cutaneous hypersensitivity. The nurse uses the pads of the fingertips, with the fingers together, and presses gently, depressing the abdominal wall about 1 cm. All quadrants are palpated using smooth movements.[5]

Deep palpation is used to delineate organs and masses. It should be performed only by properly trained persons, because improper technique can result in injury. The nurse again uses the palmar surface of the fingers but presses more deeply using a single- or two-handed technique. Rebound tenderness is tested by pressing slowly but firmly over the painful site. The fingers are then quickly withdrawn. Acute pain on withdrawal reflects peritoneal inflammation (positive Blumberg's sign).[8] This maneuver (illustrated in Figure 43-9) can be extremely painful and should never be performed unnecessarily.

### RECTUM

The normal perineal and perianal skin resembles the skin on the remainder of the body with no breaks in its integrity. Abnormal findings may include pruritus ani, coccygeal or pilonidal sinus tract openings, fistulas, fissures, external hemorrhoids, or rectal prolapse. Internal hemorrhoids may appear when the patient strains down.

### GERONTOLOGIC PATIENT CONSIDERATIONS

**SUBJECTIVE DATA**

- History of GI problems or surgery
- Use of medications, particularly antacids and laxatives
- Usual diet—food intolerances, anorexia
- Nutritional adequacy
- Heartburn, reflux, indigestion—frequency, severity, treatment
- Financial resources
- Facilities for shopping and cooking
- Fatigue and weakness
- Elimination patterns—problems with constipation or incontinence; frequency, severity, treatment

**OBJECTIVE DATA**

- Condition of mouth and teeth—dentures, adequacy of fit; dry mouth
- Body weight and comparisons with norms

Modifications appropriate to the assessment of elderly persons are summarized in the box below.

## DIAGNOSTIC TESTS

Many of the examinations and tests performed for diagnosis of problems of the GI system are both time-consuming and unpleasant. Several of the tests are intrusive procedures and as such may present added stress for the patient. Representatives from the radiology department or laboratory may assume responsibility for instructing patients about diagnostic tests, because the tests will usually be performed on an outpatient basis if at all possible. Most institutions also have prepared literature for the patient and family. It remains the nurse's responsibility, however, to assess the patient's understanding and answer any questions concerning the test procedure, rationale for its use, and specific test preparation. Diagnostic tests are sequenced to make the most effective use of time and equipment. The nurse ensures that the patient is prepared physically and mentally to avoid the preventable repetition of time-consuming and expensive tests.

### LABORATORY TESTS

Numerous tests may be used as part of the evaluation of GI, biliary, and exocrine pancreas function. Major blood and urine tests that may be ordered are summarized in Table 43-5.

### STOOL EXAMINATION

Stool specimens are collected primarily for culture, determination of fat content, and examination for the presence of ova, parasites, and fresh or occult blood. Stools to be analyzed for the presence of bacteria (*Salmonella, Shigella,* and *S. aureus*), ova, and parasites require that a fresh, warm specimen be received in the laboratory and may necessitate special collection procedures.

Fecal urobilinogen is responsible for the brown color of the stool. Biliary obstruction may cause decreased amounts to be present and turn the stool light or clay colored. These specimens should also be sent promptly to the laboratory, because urobilinogen breaks down rapidly. Table 43-6 identifies other fecal color changes that may occur.

Detection of *occult blood* in the stool is useful in identifying bleeding in the GI tract. Occult blood may be identified by one of three tests—guaiac (Hemoccult), benzidine, or orthotoluidine (Occultest). The guaiac test is the least sensitive and does not require special preparation. Meat, poultry, or fish can cause a false-positive test, and vitamin C in quantities of greater than 500 mg/day may cause a false-negative test; therefore these substances must be omitted from the diet for 3 days before testing with benzidine or orthotoluidine. Determination of fecal fat may be done as part of a workshop for malabsorption. Elevations in fecal fat will be present with

## TABLE 43-5 Major GI, Biliary, and Exocrine Pancreas Blood and Urine Tests

| BLOOD TEST | RANGE OF NORMAL VALUES | DESCRIPTION AND PURPOSE |
|---|---|---|
| Stomach gastrin | <200 pg/ml (200 ng/L) | Gastrin is a gastric hormone that is a powerful stimulus for gastric acid secretion. Elevated levels are found in those with pernicious anemia and Zollinger-Ellison syndrome. |
| **BILIARY SYSTEM** | | |
| Total bilirubin | 0.1 to 1.0 mg/dl | Bilirubin is excreted in the bile. Obstruction in the biliary tract contributes primarily to a rise in conjugated (direct) values. |
| Conjugated (direct) | 0.1-0.3 mg/dl | |
| Unconjugated (indirect) | 0.1-0.8 mg/dl | |
| Alkaline phosphatase | 30-85 ImU/ml | Alkaline phosphatase is found in many tissues with high concentrations in bone, liver, and biliary tract epithelium. Obstructive biliary tract disease and carcinoma may cause significant elevations. |
| **PANCREAS** | | |
| Amylase | 80-150 Somogyi units | Amylase is secreted normally by the acinar cells of the pancreas. Damage to these cells or obstruction of the pancreatic duct causes the enzyme to be absorbed into the blood in significant quantities. It is a sensitive yet nonspecific test for pancreatic disease. |
| Lipase | 0-110 units/L | Lipase is a pancreatic enzyme normally secreted into the duodenum. It appears in the blood when damage occurs to the acinar cells. It is a specific test for pancreatic disease. |
| Calcium | 9.0-11.5 mg/dl | Calcium levels may be low in cases of severe pancreatitis or steatorrhea, because calcium soaps are formed from the sequestration of calcium by fat necrosis. |
| **INTESTINE** | | |
| Total protein (albumin/globulin) | Total protein: 6-8 g/dl<br>Albumin: 3.2-4.5 g/dl<br>Globulin: 2.3-3.4 g/dl | Although primarily a reflection of liver function, serum protein level is also a measure of nutrition. Malnourished patients have greatly decreased levels of blood protein. |
| D-xylose absorption test | Blood levels of 25-40 mg/dl 2 hr after ingestion | D-xylose is a monosaccharide that is easily absorbed by the normal intestine but not metabolized by the body. It does not require biliary or pancreatic function. D-xylose is administered orally and assists in the diagnosis of malabsorption. |
| Lactose tolerance test | Rise in blood glucose level of >20 mg/dl | An oral dose of lactose is administered. In the absence of intestinal lactase, the lactose is neither broken down nor absorbed and plasma glucose levels do not rise. The test assists in the diagnosis of lactose intolerance. |
| Carcinoembryonic antigen (CEA) | <5 ng/ml | CEA is a protein normally present in fetal gut tissue. It is typically elevated in persons with colorectal tumors. Although not useful as a screening tool, it is useful in determining prognosis and response to therapy. |
| **URINE** | | |
| 5-hydroxyindoleacetic acid (5-HIAA) | 2-9 mg/2 hr | Carcinoid tumors are serotonin secreting and are derived from neuroectoderm tissue—e.g., the appendix and intestine. These neurohormones are metabolized to 5-HIAA by the liver and excreted in the urine. |
| Urine bilirubin | None | Bilirubin is not normally excreted in the urine. Biliary stricture, inflammation, or stones may cause its presence. |
| Urobilinogen | 24-hr collection: 0.2-1.2 units<br>24-hr collection: 0.05-2.5 mg | A sensitive test for hepatic or biliary disease. Decreased levels are seen in those with biliary obstruction and pancreatic cancer. |
| Urine amylase | 10-80 amylase units/hr | A rise in level usually mimics the rise in serum amylase. The level remains elevated for 7-10 days, however, which allows for retrospective diagnosis. |

**TABLE 43-6 Interpretation of Feces Color**

| COLOR | INTERPRETATION |
|---|---|
| White | Barium |
| Gray, tan (clay) | Lack of bile, biliary obstruction |
| Red | Lower gastrointestinal bleeding, food intake (e.g., beets) |
| Black | |
| Tarry | Upper GI bleeding |
| Dry | Rapid peristalsis with bile present |
| Green | Rapid peristalsis with bile present |

NOTE: Stool color may also vary in response to food intake and artificial colors in foods.

biliary or pancreatic obstructions and many intestinal malabsorption disorders.

## RADIOLOGIC TESTS

Visualization of the GI tract may be performed by barium swallow, upper GI series, or barium enema. Barium is a radiopaque substance that, when ingested or given by enema in solution, outlines the passageways of the GI tract for viewing by fluoroscopy or x-ray films. Nursing responsibilities frequently involve cleansing of the GI tract with enemas and laxatives. It is important for the nurse to monitor the patient's fluid and electrolyte status, because the severe bowel cleansing may cause significant fluid losses, particularly in elderly persons.

### Upper GI Series

An upper GI series involves visualization of the esophagus, stomach, duodenum, and upper jejunum through the use of a contrast medium. It is a fluoroscopic and x-ray test that permits the examination of the structure, position, peristaltic activity, and motility of the organs. It can assist in the detection of tumors, ulceration, inflammation, abnormal anatomy, or malposition.

The procedure involves swallowing the contrast medium (usually barium), which is prepared in a milk shake form. The barium outlines the structures as it flows by gravity through the esophagus and stomach into the intestinal loops. Films are taken at intervals during the test, and the entire test takes about 45 minutes. The procedure may also be termed a *barium swallow* if just the function of the esophagus is to be evaluated. This shortened procedure takes about 15 minutes. If the small bowel is the primary focus of the test, it may be termed a *small bowel series.* The procedure is essentially the same, although it may take a little longer.

No special preparation is necesasry before a GI series, although the patient maintains NPO status for at least 6 hours before the test. After an upper GI series, the patient is prescribed a laxative to hasten elimination of the barium; barium that remains in the colon may become hard and difficult to expel, leading to fecal impaction. The stool should return to the normal color (barium is white) after the barium is expelled.

### Barium Enema

A **barium enema** clearly outlines most of the large intestine through the use of a contrast medium. It is used to detect colon polyps, tumors, and chronic inflammatory bowel disease. If both an upper GI series and a barium enema are to be performed, the barium enema is done first, before barium from the upper GI series reaches the colon.

The procedure involves the instillation of barium through a rectal tube with an inflatable balloon to hold the barium in the colon. The patient is then placed in various positions while the radiologist observes on a monitor as the barium flows through the colon. The procedure takes about 30 minutes, and the instillation and retention of the barium cause the patient considerable discomfort.

Preparation for a barium enema involves thorough cleansing of the bowel by laxatives and/or enemas. Thorough preparation is essential, because retained fecal material obscures the normal bowel anatomy. The patient may be asked to restrict dairy products and follow a liquid diet for 24 hours before the test. The patient typically maintains NPO status for at least 8 hours before the test. Laxatives are again administered *after* the test to facilitate the removal of the barium. The stools may be white-tinged for several days. Inpatients are closely monitored for complications after the test, such as perforation of the bowel. Outpatients are instructed to report the development of abdominal pain and to monitor carefully for constipation.

### Ultrasonography

Ultrasonography involves the use of high-frequency sound waves that are transmitted into the abdomen and create echoes that vary with tissue density. The echoes bounce back to a transducer and are electronically converted into pictorial images of the organs. It can reveal organ size, shape, and position and is extremely useful in diagnosing cysts, tumors, and stones. It has gradually become the procedure of choice for diagnosing gallbladder disease, because it does not expose the patient to radiation. The procedure is both painless and safe.

Patient preparation is straightforward. The patient maintains NPO status for 8 to 12 hours before the test, because gas in the bowel may interfere with the results. If the gallbladder is the focus of the test, the patient is instructed to eat a low-fat meal the evening before the test, so that bile will accumulate in the gallbladder, thereby enhancing visualization. The patient resumes a normal diet and activity after the test.

### Computed Tomography

Computed tomography (CT scan) can also be used to assess patients with gallbladder, biliary ductal system, or pancreatic problems. It is helpful in identifying problems similar to those described for ultrasonography. Multiple x-rays are passed through the abdomen. A computer reconstructs the data into two-dimensional images on a television screen. Still photographs can also be taken of the images. Contrast medium can be used with the CT scan to better visualize the biliary tract or to accentuate differences in tissue density of the pancreas. The test is about equal to ultrasonography in effectiveness. It is used less often because of its significantly higher cost and moderate radiation exposure for the patient. It is extremely useful with obese individuals, however, because increased tissue density limits the effectiveness of ultrasound transmission.[11]

The patient should maintain NPO status for 8 to 12 hours before the test. If contrast medium is to be used, the patient should be assessed for allergies to iodine or contrast medium. Barium studies, if necessary, should be done at least 4 days before CT scan or after the scan, because the barium can interfere with test results. There are no special aftercare considerations. The patient may resume pretest diet and activity.

### Radionuclide Imaging (GI Bleeding Scan, GI Scintigraphy)

GI scintigraphy may be used to localize the site of GI bleeding. Endoscopy provides excellent visualization of gastric or esophageal bleeding, but other areas of the GI tract are much more difficult to visualize and pinpoint. An intravenous injection of $^{99m}$TC sulfur colloid is administered. Pooling of the radionuclide will occur at the bleeding site.[6] No pretest preparation is required, and no discomfort is experienced. Patients in unstable condition may not be able to travel safely to the nuclear medicine department for the 30 minutes required for the test.

### Cholecystography

Oral **cholecystography** involves the radiographic examination of the gallbladder after the administration of a contrast medium. A normal liver will remove radiopaque drugs—such as iodoalphionic acid (Priodax), iopanoic acid (Telepaque), and iodipamide methylglucamine (Cholografin Meglumine)—from the bloodstream and store and concentrate them in the gallbladder. The dye-filled gallbladder shows on x-ray examination as a dense shadow. If no shadow is seen, this indicates a nonfunctioning gallbladder. Stones, which are not radiopaque, show as dark patches on the film. Visualization of the gallbladder depends on absorption of the dye through the intestinal tract, isolation of it by the liver, and a free passageway from the liver to the gallbladder.

Ultrasonography has gradually replaced this once commonly used test in the diagnosis of gallbladder disease. Cholecystography is primarily used today when the ultrasound picture is inconclusive.

Patient preparation involves instruction to eat a fat-free meal the evening before the test and to avoid all additional intake except water until the test is completed. The patient is carefully assessed for allergies to contrast dyes, seafood, or iodine. The radiopaque substance (usually iopanoic acid) is administered orally 2 to 3 hours after the evening meal. The dose is based on body weight, and the tablets are administered one at a time at 5- to 10-minute intervals with several swallows of water after each pill. Side effects of the iodine-based tablets may include abdominal cramping, vomiting, or diarrhea. The patient then maintains NPO status until the test. A high-fat food or drink may be administered during the procedure to stimulate emptying of the gallbladder. No specific care is indicated after the test.

### Cholangiography

**Cholangiography** involves the x-ray examination of bile ducts to demonstrate the presence of stones, strictures, or tumors. The radiopaque substance may be administered intravenously or injected directly into the common bile duct with a needle or catheter at the time of surgery. After surgery on the common bile duct, the radiopaque drug—usually iodipamide methylglucamine—may be instilled through a drainage tube—such as the T-tube—to determine the patency of the duct before the tube is removed (T-tube cholangiography). This dye also may be injected through the skin and abdominal wall directly into a bile duct within the main substance of the liver *(percutaneous transhepatic cholangiography)*. The technique is useful in visualizing the location and extent of a pathologic process, such as obstructive jaundice. It permits decompression of the liver for improved function. The procedure helps the surgeon identify the location of pathologic processes before surgery, or it may indicate that surgery is not necessary. The hazards of the examination occasionally may include bile leakage leading to bile peritonitis or bleeding caused by accidental rupture of a blood vessel. The patient maintains NPO status for about 8 hours before the test. The injection of the contrast medium may cause temporary pain or a feeling of pressure or epigastric fullness. The patient is carefully monitored for bleeding or adverse reactions to the dye. Vital signs are monitored, and the patient typically rests in bed for about 6 hours after the test, lying on the right side as much as possible. The needle insertion site is carefully monitored for signs of bleeding or infection.

## SPECIAL TESTS

### Esophageal Function Tests

Several diagnostic tests may be used to evaluate the functioning of the esophagus and aid in the diagnosis of esophageal reflux or motility problems.

#### Manometry

This test is used to measure the pressure in the lower esophageal sphincter and record the duration and sequence of peristaltic movements within the esophagus. Readings are taken at various levels in the esophagus with the patient at rest and during swallowing. Baseline sphincter pressure is normally about 20 mm Hg. The test is used primarily to diagnose esophageal reflux, but the graphic record of muscular activity during swallowing may also help document the presence of achalasia or esophageal spasm.[11]

### pH test

Despite its proximity to the highly acidic medium of the stomach, the esophagus normally maintains a pH of more than 6.0. This test evaluates the competency of the lower esophageal sphincter by measuring the esophageal pH via an electrode attached to a manometry catheter.

### Esophageal clearance test

This test is usually performed in conjunction with pH or manometry testing for reflux. Normal esophageal function allows for the complete clearance of acid material from the esophagus in less than 10 swallows. When reflux is demonstrated through manometry and pH testing, the rate and efficiency of acid clearance is assessed.

### Acid perfusion test (Bernstein test)

When there is confusion about the origin of heartburn symptoms, the **Bernstein test** may be used to attempt to reproduce the pain. Small quantities of HCl are instilled into the distal esophagus by NG tube. The test is positive if the acid produces pain. Saline is instilled to rinse out the acid, and an antacid may be administered to relieve the pain.

All of these tests can be performed by having the patient swallow two or three tiny tubes that are attached to an external transducer. Once the tubes are in the stomach, they are slowly pulled back into the distal esophagus at varying levels. They can measure lower esophageal sphincter pressure, graph swallowing activity, measure pH, and assess the effectiveness of clearance.

The entire series can be completed in about 30 to 45 minutes, although 24-hour pH monitoring is now considered to be the gold standard for the accurate diagnosis of reflux. No special preparation is required, but the individual maintains NPO status for about 8 hours before the test. Sedation is not required but may be used if the individual experiences persistent choking or gagging. Antacids, $H_2$-receptor antagonists, cholinergics, and anticholinergics should not be administered before the test, if possible. The individual is instructed to avoid alcohol and smoking the day before the test. A mild sore throat after the removal of the tubes is quite common.

## Tests of Gastric Function

### Gastric analysis (basal gastric secretion and gastric acid stimulation tests)

Examination of the fasting contents of the stomach may be used in establishing a diagnosis of gastric disease. The purpose is to quantify gastric acidity in the fasting and stimulated states. Abnormal secretion may be related to ulcers, malignancy, pernicious anemia, or Zollinger-Ellison syndrome. A nasogastric tube is inserted, and gastric contents are aspirated. Gastric contents may then be aspirated every 15 minutes for 1½ hours. The patient is instructed to restrict food, fluid, and smoking for 8 to 12 hours before the test. The flow of gastric acid is then stimulated by betazole hydrochloride, histamine phosphate, or pentagastrin given subcutaneously. The person may experience side effects of the medication, including flushing, feeling of warmth, slight headache, or itching. Epinephrine is given to counteract the effects of histamine if sensitivity occurs.

### Tubeless gastric analysis (Diagnex blue test)

Tubeless gastric analysis may be used for detection of gastric achlorhydria. The test will indicate the presence or absence of free hydrochloric acid but cannot be used to determine the *amount* of free hydrochloric acid, if any is present. For a tubeless gastric analysis, a gastric stimulant—such as caffeine—is given. One hour later, a cation exchange resin containing azure A is given orally with water on an empty stomach. If there is free hydrochloric acid in the stomach on the introduction of this resin, a substance will be released in the stomach that will be absorbed from the small intestine and excreted by the kidneys within 2 hours. Absence of detectable amounts of blue dye in the urine indicates that free hydrochloric acid probably was not secreted.

### Schilling test

The **Schilling test** evaluates vitamin $B_{12}$ absorption. In the normal GI tract, vitamin $B_{12}$ combines with the instrinsic factor that is produced by the parietal cells in the gastric mucosa, and is absorbed in the distal portion of the ileum. Pernicious anemia will develop if instrinsic factor is lacking or malabsorption exists. The test can identify problems of absorption.

The patient is administered an oral preparation of radioactive vitamin $B_{12}$, followed by an intramuscular injection of nonradioactive vitamin $B_{12}$ to saturate the tissue-binding sites. Urinary $B_{12}$ levels are measured after urine collection for 24 to 48 hours. With normal absorption of vitamin $B_{12}$, the ileum absorbs more vitamin $B_{12}$ than the body needs and excretes the excess into the urine. With impaired absorption of vitamin $B_{12}$, little or no vitamin $B_{12}$ is excreted into the urine. Intrinsic factor preparations may also be administered to differentiate intestinal problems from pernicious anemia. The person is instructed to maintain NPO status for 8 to 12 hours before the test, except for water. Laxatives should not be used during the duration of the test, but no specific aftercare is indicated.

## Biopsy

### Upper gastrointestinal biopsy

A biopsy of the oral cavity or tongue may be done on any lesion or ulcerated area that requires a differential diagnosis. This procedure is usually performed with a local anesthetic. After the biopsy, the biopsy site is assessed for bleeding. Biopsy of the stomach is typically performed during fiberoptic endoscopy.

**Intestinal biopsy**

Biopsy of the small or large bowel may also be performed during the course of endoscopic examination to allow tissue analysis of lesions, polyps, or masses. A knife blade or snare is typically used to obtain the tissue sample. The procedure is not generally painful, although a feeling of pressure may be experienced. Bleeding from the site of the biopsy is uncommon. The patient is instructed to report any signs of rectal bleeding and to curtail physical activity until examined by a physician.

## ENDOSCOPY

Endoscopy allows for direct visualization of portions of the GI tract by means of a long, flexible, fiberoptic lighted scope. Images are provided through an eyepiece or onto a video screen. The remote control tip moves in four directions. Endoscopy may be used for direct inspection, biopsy, and removal of polyps and stones and to control bleeding through laser or photocoagulation or the injection of sclerosing agents. Most endoscopic examinations are performed in special procedures laboratories, but in emergency situations they can be done at the bedside. The patient typically is conscious but sedated.[13] The upper GI tract may be visualized as far as the duodenum by insertion of a fiberscope through the mouth. A fiberscope inserted through the rectum is used for visualization of the rectum (proctoscopy), sigmoid colon (sigmoidoscopy) or the entire colon (colonoscopy).

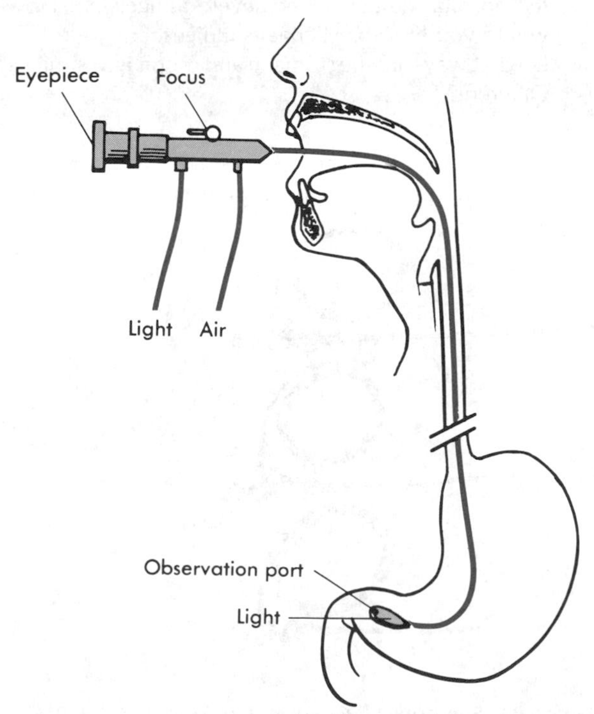


**FIGURE 43-10** Fiberoptic endoscopy of the stomach.

### Esophagogastroduodenoscopy

Upper GI endoscopy may be limited to the esophagus (esophagoscopy), stomach (gastroscopy), or duodenum (duodenoscopy), or it may involve examination of the entire region **(esophagogastroduodenoscopy)** (Figure 43-10). It is particularly useful for identifying upper GI bleeding and for differentiating gastric malignancies from benign ulcers, and gastric ulcers from duodenal ulcers. Other uses include visualization of esophageal strictures, varices and tumors, achalasia, and hiatal hernias and surgical removal of gastric polyps. Preparation simply involves instructing the patient to maintain NPO status for 8 hours before the test.

The insertion of the endoscope is uncomfortable and may cause choking or gagging, despite the use of a topical anesthetic spray or gargle. Discomfort is minimized by premedication with an IV sedative, such as midazolam (Versed) or diazepam (Valium), or an analgesic, such as meperidine (Demerol). The patient is conscious but sedated and frequently experiences amnesia for the experience when higher doses are administered. Air is typically introduced as the endoscope is advanced to improve visibility, and this may produce a feeling of pressure or fullness. The entire test lasts about 15 to 30 minutes, unless additional treatments are planned.

After the procedure the patient is monitored carefully for signs of dyspnea, pain, bleeding, or acute dysphagia. Vital signs are taken every 30 minutes for 3 to 4 hours, and no oral food or fluids are administered until the nurse determines that the gag reflex is intact. Throat lozenges or gargles may be used to relieve sore throat after the test. Complications are rare but could include aspiration, perforation, or bleeding.

### Endoscopic Retrograde Cholangiopancreatography (ERCP)

**ERCP** also involves the oral insertion of an endoscope, but this device has a side-viewing tip and a cannula that can be maneuvered into the ampulla of Vater (Figure 43-11). Dye may be injected to outline the pancreatic and biliary ducts. The procedure may be combined with papillotomy to enlarge the sphincter and release gallstones.[15] Glucagon may be administered to minimize spasm in the duodenum and sphincter. Care after the procedure is similar to that just described. The patient is monitored carefully for signs of abdominal pain, nausea, and vomiting, which might indicate the development of pancreatitis.

### Colonoscopy

Fiberoptic **colonoscopy** allows the examination of the entire colon in most patients. It may be used to evaluate benign and malignant growths, remove polyps, take biopsy specimens, and localize sites of bleeding. The colonoscope is 105 to 185 cm (42 to 72 inches) in length (Figure 43-12).

Thorough bowel preparation is essential before the

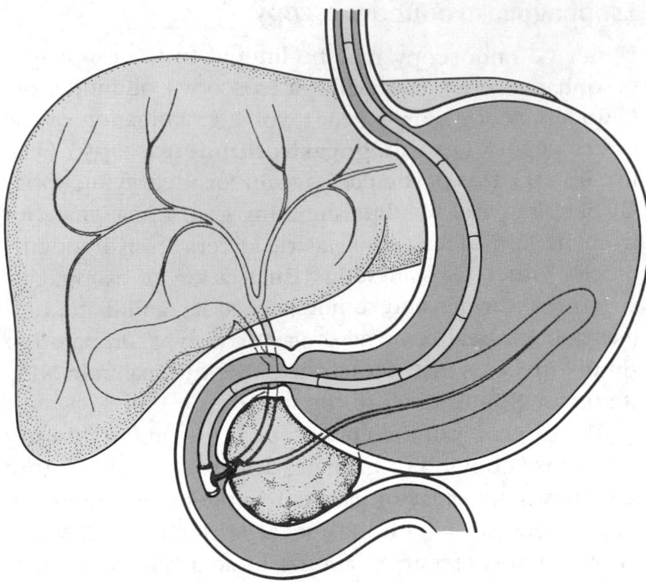

**FIGURE 43-11** Endoscopic retrograde cholangiopancreatography (ERCP). (From Pagana KD, Pagana TJ: *Diagnostic and laboratory test reference,* St Louis, 1992, Mosby.)

test. The patient may receive a 2- to 3-day preparation involving a clear liquid diet, strong laxatives, and an enema the day of the test. A 1-day preparation with an oral osmotic solution has become fairly standard, because it reduces overall electrolyte loss. A gallon of polyethylene glycol (Colyte) solution is administered rapidly (8 oz every 15 minutes) and induces a profuse watery diarrhea within 30 to 60 minutes, which lasts about 4 hours.[13] The patient is then NPO for about 8 hours before the test. Midazolam (Versed), diazepam (Valium), or meperidine (Demerol) is administered before the test and augmented as needed during the test.

The procedure lasts from 20 to 60 minutes. Air is introduced as the colonoscope is inserted to increase visualization of the mucosa. The air frequently causes abdominal cramping. After the test the patient is carefully monitored for changes in vital signs and the development of severe abdominal pain, rectal bleeding, or fever. The nurse ensures that someone is available to provide the patient with transportation home.

Sigmoidoscopy may be performed rather than colonoscopy. This procedure allows for visualization of the anus, rectum, and distal sigmoid colon. Approximately 75% of all polyps and tumors of the large intestine can be visualized in this way. The test may be performed with either a rigid or flexible sigmoidoscope. Pretest preparation instructions vary widely. The patient may be instructed to prepare with a 2-day clear liquid diet and pretest fasting. Fleet's enemas may be ordered, or a cleansing enema may be preferred. The knee-chest position and a strong urge to defecate that is produced by the larger diameter sigmoidoscope make this both an uncomfortable and unpopular procedure for patients. Sedation is not usually employed.[6] Aftercare involves monitoring for distention, increased tenderness, or bleeding. The patient may initially pass large amounts of flatus from the instillation of air during the procedure. Slight rectal bleeding may occur if biopsies have been taken.

## CRITICAL THINKING ACTIVITIES

- On his return to work after lunch, Michael was involved in a car accident. Although he was not seriously injured, he was very frightened. Upon leaving the hospital he developed severe indigestion. How would you explain Michael's indigestion?
- In what ways are the stomach and esophagus similar? Different?

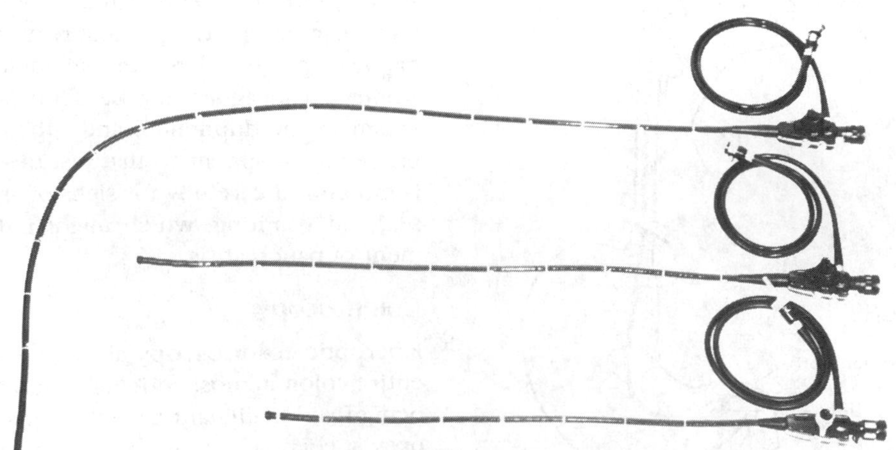

**FIGURE 43-12** Flexible colon fiberscopes. (From Given BA, Simmons SJ: *Gastroenterology in clinical nursing,* ed 4, St Louis, 1984, Mosby.)

## Chapter Summary

### ANATOMY AND PHYSIOLOGY

- Functions of the GI tract include the following: salivation and mastication in the mouth, swallowing in the esophagus, digestion in the stomach and small intestines, and absorption in the large intestine.
- Carbohydrate digestion begins in the mouth and continues in the small intestine with the action of pancreatic and intestinal enzymes.
- Protein digestion begins in the stomach and continues in the small intestine with the action of pancreatic and intestinal enzymes.
- Fat digestion takes place primarily in the small intestine with the action of the pancreatic enzymes and bile salts.

### ASSESSMENT

- Changes in the GI system that occur with aging usually do not interfere with normal functioning, unless chronic illnesses are present. Common changes include the following: mouth—tooth loss and a decrease in saliva; esophagus—decreased motility; stomach—decreased secretion of gastric acids; biliary system—increased cholesterol content in bile; pancreas—gradual decline in pancreatic secretions; small intestine—impaired absorption of nutrients, particularly carbohydrates; and large intestine—decreased rectal elasticity.
- Subjective data for GI assessment include patient/family history; diet and nutrition; presence of abdominal pain, anorexia, or vomiting; fatigue and weakness; and elimination patterns.
- Objective data include assessment of the mouth, abdomen, and rectum.
- The abdomen is divided into either four quadrants or nine regions for assessment. Auscultation precedes percussion and palpation, because the activities may alter the frequency and intensity of bowel sounds.

### DIAGNOSTIC TESTS

- Laboratory tests include analysis of stool and urine and a variety of blood tests, including those for pancreatic enzymes, protein, bilirubin, and alkaline phosphatase.
- Major radiologic tests include barium contrast studies of the entire GI tract, endoscopic examinations of the upper and lower GI tract, ultrasonography, and cholecystography. Special tests include esophageal studies and gastric analyses.
- Endoscopy and ultrasonography are the mainstays of diagnosis in GI system disease. Ultrasound is safe and painless for the patient, and endoscopy allows for direct visualization.

## REFERENCES


1. Altman DF: Changes in gastrointestinal, pancreatic, biliary and hepatic function with aging, *Gastroenterol Clin North Am* 19(2):227-233, 1990.
2. Bell JE, Dixon L, Sehy YA: Physical assessment: the breast and the pulmonary, cardiovascular, gastrointestinal, and genitourinary systems. In Chenitz WC, Stone JT, Salisbury SA, eds: *Clinical gerontological nursing,* Philadelphia, 1991, WB Saunders.
3. Esberger KK: Guide to gastrointestinal problems of elders, *Geriatr Nurs* 12(2):74-75, 1991.
4. Hogstel MO: Gastrointestinal system. In *Clinical manual of gerontological nursing,* St Louis, 1992, Mosby.
5. Holmgren C: Abdominal assessment, *RN* 55(3):28-33, 1992.
6. *Illustrated guide to diagnostic tests,* Springhouse, Pa, 1994, Springhouse.
7. Jarvis C: *Physical examination & health assessment,* Philadelphia, 1992, WB Saunders.
8. Lindsey M: Abdominal assessment, *Orthop Nurs* 8(4):34-38, 1989.
9. McConnell E: Auscultating bowel sounds, *Nurs 90,* 20(6):76-79, 1990.
10. O'Toole M: Advanced assessment of the abdomen and gastrointestinal problems, *Nurs Clin North Am* 25(4):771-76, 1990.
11. Pagana KD, Pagana TJ: *Mosby's diagnostic and laboratory test reference,* St Louis, 1992, Mosby.
12. Porth CM: *Pathophysiology: concepts of altered health states,* ed 3, Philadelphia, 1990, JB Lippincott.
13. Renkes J: GI endoscopy—managing the full scope of care, *Nurs 93,* 23(6):50-55, 1993.
14. Sleisenger MH, Fordtran JS: *Gastrointestinal disease,* ed 4, Philadelphia, 1989, WB Saunders.
15. Wilkinson M: Nursing implications after endoscopic cholangiopancreatography, *Gastroenterol Nurs* 13(2):105-109, 1990.
16. Yamada T et al: *Textbook of gastroenterology,* Philadelphia, 1992, JB Lippincott.

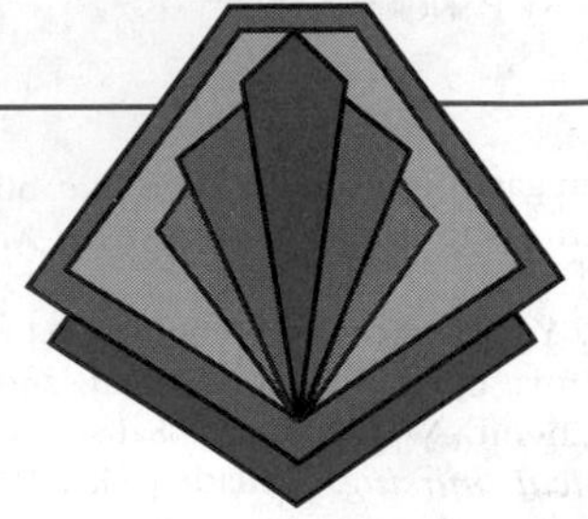

C H A P T E R 44

# Management of Persons With Problems of the Mouth and Esophagus

***Judith K. Sands***

## CHAPTER OBJECTIVES

***After studying this chapter, the learner should be able to do the following:***

1. Describe life-style modifications for the prevention of common oral and esophageal disorders.
2. Discuss the pathophysiology underlying common problems of the mouth and esophagus.
3. List the major clinical manifestations of common oral and esophageal disorders.
4. Discuss the medical and surgical options for management of common problems of the mouth and esophagus.
5. Use the nursing process to describe nursing care of patients with common oral and esophageal disorders.

## KEY TERMS

achalasia
aphthous stomatitis
barium swallow
candidiasis
diverticula
dysphagia
erythroplakia
erythroplasia
gastrostomy
GERD
gingivitis
glossectomy
halitosis
herpes simplex
hiatal hernia
leukoplakia
nicotine stomatitis
Nissen fundoplication
odynophagia
parotitis
Valsalva maneuver
Vincent's angina
water brash
xerostomia

Problems involving the mouth and esophagus include a number of common disorders that affect millions of individuals throughout the adult life span. The majority of the disorders are managed by the individual in the home and rarely involve the acute care setting. The nurse's role includes teaching individuals strategies for prevention and health promotion.

## PROBLEMS OF THE MOUTH

## DENTAL DISORDERS

Progressive tooth loss used to be considered a virtually inevitable consequence of aging. Advances in our understanding of dental health and new approaches to tooth maintenance have changed these perspectives substantially, and today major efforts are expended toward preserving natural teeth into advanced age.

### DENTAL CARIES

Tooth decay is by far the most common problem affecting the teeth. It is the result of a pathologic process that causes the gradual destruction of the enamel and dentin of the teeth. Plaque formation is the most important aspect of the decay process. Dental plaque is a soft mass composed of proliferating bacteria in a matrix of polysaccharides and salivary glycoproteins. It adheres to the teeth and is both transparent and colorless. Acids produced by the bacteria slowly decalcify the inorganic tooth enamel. Food, particularly carbohydrates, stimulates bacterial acid production. Simple sugars have the greatest effect. The plaque begins to collect on the teeth within 2 hours of eating, and the longer or more frequently carbohydrates are ingested, the longer it takes for the pH of the mouth to return to normal. Cavity formation is the visible clinical evidence of the progression of the decay process.

Plaque is clearly the most important aspect of tooth decay, but familial tendency, poor oral hygiene, and poor health are also factors. A diet high in simple or refined sugars may also play a role.

Several approaches are available for preventing or minimizing plaque formation and tooth decay, and these practices should be instituted in childhood. Good oral hygiene, with frequent brushing and daily flossing, is a mainstay, and widespread fluoridation of water supplies has had significant positive effects. Fluoride makes tooth enamel more resistant to acids. It is commonly added to drinking water in many localities and is widely available in toothpastes, dental rinses, and mouthwashes. It may also be applied in concentrated forms by a dentist. Sealants and bonding preparations may be applied in childhood to increase tooth resistance to decay. Restricting the amount of simple sugars in the diet is a standard recommendation. Adequate or supplemental vitamin C is also believed to reduce plaque. Regular dental examinations for thorough cleaning and evaluation are the final component of prevention. Treatment routinely includes the removal of decayed tooth structures and their replacement with restorative barriers.

### PERIODONTAL DISEASE

The periodontium is the tissue that surrounds and supports the teeth. Disease affecting this structure is the most common cause of tooth loss in adults after age 50. It is estimated that, at any time, from 25% to 75% of the adult population with natural teeth has some evidence of the disease.[5] Bacterial plaque is again the most important contributor to the problem, but dental malocclusion, caries, dietary deficiencies, and systemic diseases such as diabetes may also play a role.

**Gingivitis** is the earliest form of periodontal disease. It is characterized by color alterations in the gums, swelling, and easy bleeding. Inflammation causes the gingivae to separate from the tooth surface. Pockets form in the gingivae that can collect bacteria, food particles, and pus. As the process gradually worsens over time, the gums recede, the alveolar bone is resorbed, and the teeth loosen (Figure 44-1).

Bleeding of the gums with normal toothbrushing is a common early sign. There is usually no pain. Prevention is the best strategy, with emphasis on regular and frequent brushing, flossing, and professional cleaning. Regular checkups allow for correction of local factors if needed, or intervention with aggressive measures such as scaling or root planing for advancing disease.

If control of the disease is not possible, the individual may need to face tooth extraction and the fitting of dentures. Proper sizing and fitting by a skilled professional are key elements. Even with a correct fit, however, adjusting to dentures requires patience because the action and feel of routine chewing are altered. Careful regular cleansing remains important, as well as daily inspection for evidence of local irritation or gingivitis, which can be warning signs of more serious oral problems.

## MOUTH INFECTIONS

Any of the structures of the mouth may develop infections. They may be primary mouth infections or may occur as the result of other systemic diseases, treatments, or vitamin deficiencies. Their presence can seriously affect the ability of the patient to adequately ingest food and fluids by mouth.

### APHTHOUS STOMATITIS

**Aphthous stomatitis** (canker sore) produces ulcers on the soft tissues of the mouth, including the lips, tongue, insides of the cheeks, pharynx, and soft palate. The lesions are noncontagious and are of uncertain, although perhaps autoimmune, cause. They are possibly associated with emotional stress, vitamin deficiency, or local reactions to food. The ulcers are typically well circumscribed with an erythematous border and are acutely painful, particularly if multiple lesions are present. Treatment is basically palliative and may involve mouth-

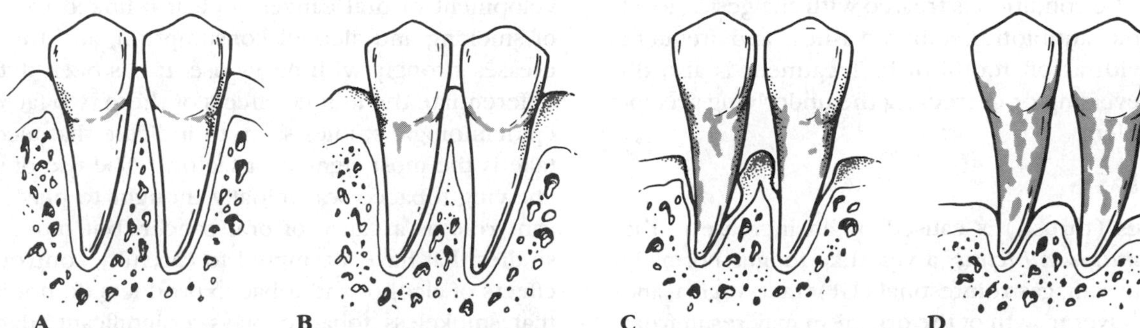


**FIGURE 44-1** The progression of periodontal disease. **A,** Calculus deposited on teeth at gum line. **B,** Gingivae become swollen and tender. **C,** Inflammation spreads, pockets develop between gums and gingivae, and gums recede. **D,** Alveolar bone is destroyed and teeth loosen. (From Lewis MN, Collier IC: *Medical surgical nursing,* ed 3, St Louis, 1992, Mosby.)

washes, oral steroid solutions or ointments, and topical analgesics or antibiotics if secondary infection is suspected. Healing is usually achieved within 1 to 3 weeks.

### HERPES SIMPLEX VIRUS

**Herpes simplex** is an extremely common viral infection that produces characteristic blisters that are commonly called *cold sores* or *fever blisters.* The individual usually acquires the virus in early childhood. It is variously estimated that as many as 80% of the adult population have been infected. The virus is harbored by cells in the sensory nerve ganglia in a dormant state. Reactivation of the virus can occur with emotional stress, fever, or exposure to cold or ultraviolet light.

The lesions appear most commonly on the mucocutaneous border junction of the lips in the form of small vesicles, which then erupt and form sore shallow ulcers. Some individuals experience itching and burning in the prodromal period. Although uncomfortable, the lesions usually require no treatment. Severe herpetic lesions are treated with acyclovir (Zovirax) administered topically or systemically. A lysine-rich diet or supplements of lysine may be prescribed for patients prone to recurrent attacks. Patients are also encouraged to limit their intake of arginine-rich foods such as nuts and chocolate. The lesions typically heal in 7 to 10 days and are contagious while present. Good hand washing is essential to limit transmission during the infectious period.

### VINCENT'S ANGINA

**Vincent's angina** (called *necrotizing ulcerative gingivitis or trench mouth)* is an acute inflammatory gum disease caused by a tremendous proliferation of normal mouth flora, such as spirochetes and fusiform bacilli. It is commonly triggered by poor oral hygiene, nutritional deficiencies, alcoholism, infection, or immunocompromise. Individuals develop ulcerative lesions that are covered by a grayish pseudomembrane and surrounded by erythematous areas.

The disorder is accompanied by pain, bleeding gums, tonsilitis, fever, foul mouth odor, and lymphadenopathy. The lesions do not recur, but they will not heal spontaneously. The condition is treated with analgesics, local and systemic antibiotics, mouthwashes, and frequent brushing with a soft toothbrush. Treatment is also directed at reversing or correcting the underlying precipitating problem.

### CANDIDIASIS

**Candidiasis** (thrush) is caused by an increase in the level of *Candida albicans,* a yeastlike fungus normally found in the skin, gastrointestinal (GI) tract, vagina, and oral cavity. Overgrowth of the organism may result from antibiotic depletion of normal flora or immunosuppression from steroid therapy, chemotherapy, or HIV infection.

The classic feature of candidiasis is the presence of creamy white patches of exudate that can be rubbed off with gauze, leaving a reddened base that bleeds easily. The condition is painful and, if widespread, may interfere with oral nutrition.

Treatment is aimed at reducing the quantity of the fungus and restoring the balance of the normal flora. The most effective agent is clotrimazole (Mycelex) given by lozenge to dissolve in the mouth.[1] The traditional nystatin (Mycostatin, Nilstat) in tablet or oral suspension may also be used. Ketoconazole (Nizoral) provides another treatment alternative, and amphotericin B may be needed to treat patients with HIV-related infections. Efforts may be made to repopulate the GI tract through the ingestion of buttermilk or yogurt with active cultures, or the administration of lactobacillus tablets.

### PAROTITIS

**Parotitis** is an inflammation of the salivary or parotid glands. The viral inflammation known as *mumps* occurs primarily in the pediatric population, although it can occur in adults. Nonviral parotitis, sometimes referred to as *surgical mumps,* typically occurs in debilitated patients in whom dehydration, minimal oral intake, or medications have resulted in chronic dry mouth. As the natural secretions diminish, bacteria invade the gland. Poor oral hygiene also is usually present, and elderly persons are particularly susceptible. The causative organism is often *Staphylococcus.*

Symptoms appear abruptly and include fever, swelling, and pain in the glands. Treatment involves the administration of antibiotics, local heat or cold application, frequent oral hygiene, adequate hydration, and stimulation of salivary secretion with lozenges or hard candies. Complications may include stone formation in the gland, with the need for incision and drainage. Table 44-1 summarizes common mouth infections and their treatment.

## CANCER OF THE MOUTH

### ETIOLOGY

Cancer may develop on the lips, tongue, palate, floor of the mouth, or other portion of the oral cavity. The development of oral cancer is clearly linked to a history of smoking and alcohol consumption, and the risk increases strongly with heavy use. It has been difficult to differentiate the unique effects of these two factors, but epidemiologic studies seem to indicate that alcohol intake is the most significant factor.[14] The use of snuff or chewing tobacco was initially thought to play a significant role as a cause of oral cancer, but more precise studies that have attempted to carefully control for the effects of alcohol and tobacco products do not indicate that smokeless tobacco plays a significant identifiable role.[3] The issue of smokeless tobacco use by adolescents remains unclear, however, and adolescents seem to show a different and more virulent response pattern.[14]

The combination of alcohol and smoking is theorized

**TABLE 44-1 Mouth Infections**

| TYPE | ETIOLOGIC FACTORS | CLINICAL SIGNS | MANAGEMENT |
|---|---|---|---|
| Aphthous stomatitis (canker sore) | Autoimmune disorder | Painful, small ulceration on oral mucosa; heals in 1 to 3 weeks; is recurrent | Palliative: mouthwashes, hydrocortisone-antibiotic ointment; fluocinonide (Lidex) ointment in Orabase |
| Herpetic stomatitis (cold sore, fever blister) | Herpesvirus type I | Painful vesicles and ulcerations of mouth, lips, or edge of nose; fever, malaise, lymphadenopathy may occur | Palliative: mouthwashes, fluids, soft diet, topical or systemic acyclovir (Zovirax) in severe cases |
| Vincent's angina (trench mouth) | May be caused by overgrowth of normal oral spirochetes or fusiform bacilli | Painful hemorrhagic gums with ulceration, fever, lymphadenopathy | Oral antibiotics, analgesics, topical hydrogen peroxide, good oral hygiene, referral to dentist for removal of plaque or tartar |
| Candidiasis (thrush) | *Candida albicans* | Creamy white, curdlike patches closely adherent to mucosa; mucosa bleeds and ulcerates when patches scraped off | Oral nystatin, ketoconazole, clotrimazole; amphotericin B for the immunocompromised person |
| Parotitis | Viral and nonviral forms (surgical mumps) | Fever, swelling, and pain in the glands with an abrupt onset | Local heat and cold, frequent oral hygiene, adequate hydration. Broad-spectrum antibiotics occasionally needed |

to cause a breakdown in the body's defense mechanisms, as evidenced by a decrease in the levels of immunoglobulin A (IgA) in the saliva. The role of viruses, particularly oncogenic viruses acquired through sexual contact, is also being thoroughly researched.

## EPIDEMIOLOGY

Oral cancers account for approximately 4% of cancers in men, 2% of cancers in women, and 3.5% of cancers overall.[14] More than 90% of these cancers occur in persons over 45 years of age, and the incidence increases with age. Oral cancers have shown a steady increase in women over the past 50 years as major changes in female life-styles have caused generational exposure to alcohol and tobacco that now approximates that of men. Speculation exists that the incidence of oral cancer in women has not yet peaked, because smoking cessation efforts in general have been less successful with women than with men.

## PATHOPHYSIOLOGY

The vast majority of oral cancers arise from the squamous cells, which line the surface oral epithelium; epidermoid, basal cell, and other carcinomas also may arise. Tumors frequently develop at the base of the tongue or floor of the mouth and may go unnoticed by the patient. The tongue has an abundant vascular supply and lymphatic drainage channels, and spread of the cancer to adjacent structures may be rapid. Metastasis to the neck has already occurred in 60% of patients at the time the diagnosis is made. The mortality rate is high. The cure rate for cancer involving the lips, on the other hand, is high, because the lesion is so readily apparent. Early metastasis is rare, although rapid extension to the mandible or floor of the mouth is possible. Tumors that involve the parotid gland are usually benign, although those arising in the submaxillary glands have a high rate of malignancy and tend to grow rapidly.

Malignant lesions of the mouth are usually asymptomatic and difficult to detect in early stages. Masses in the neck require careful evaluation and frequently are accompanied by ear pain. Biopsy is usually recommended if new growths do not resolve in 1 to 2 weeks, although biopsy of the parotid gland is not usually recommended because of the risk of tumor seeding.

### Premalignant Lesions

Premalignant lesions of the mouth include **leukoplakia** (white patches), **erythroplasia** (red granular patches), and **erythroplakia** (white patches within red patches). They may or may not progress toward malignancy. Leukoplakia lesions are the result of hyperkeratinization of the oral mucosa with sclerosis of the underlying tissue. The cause is usually a chronic irritant, and the site of the lesion is usually the best clue to its cause. Leukoplakia represents a diagnosis of exclusion in the presence of white plaque in the mouth that cannot be wiped off. Biopsy is important, particularly in the patient over 50 years of age.

**Nicotine stomatitis** is a leukoplakia unique to pipe smokers. It appears on the hard palate and is theorized to be related to the heat of the pipe smoke. It disappears rapidly with smoking cessation and is rarely malignant. Snuff dipper's lesion is a second classic form of leukoplakia. It appears wherever the snuff or smokeless tobacco is typically pouched and also disappears rapidly with chewing cessation. It appears to require prolonged exposure to represent any kind of cancer risk, except

**RESEARCH**

Sterling TD, Rosenbaum WL, Weinkam JJ: Analysis of the relationship between smokeless tobacco and cancer based on data from the National Mortality Followback Survey, *J Clin Epidemiol* 45(3):223-231, 1992.

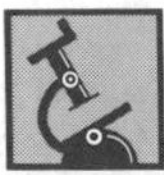

The study investigated the potential link between the use of smokeless tobacco and oral cancer or cancer of the digestive organs. Two major data sources were used from the National Mortality Followback Survey (NMFS). These surveys are based on stratified national samples. Statistical analysis of the data revealed that risks of oral cancer were significantly related to increasing age, drinking, and smoking. The risks associated with smoking and drinking increase with consumption levels, and the effects of the combination are particularly high. Of the two factors, the highest risk is associated with alcohol consumption. The use of smokeless tobacco *alone* was not found to be associated with an increased risk of oral or digestive system cancer.

perhaps in adolescents. Researchers express concern that direct local application and prolonged contact of known carcinogens with immature oral mucous membranes in adolescence may decrease the period of latency and significantly accelerate the onset of neoplastic transition. This is particularly important in situations in which alcohol is also used.[3] Further study is ongoing. Leukoplakia is also a common manifestation of HIV-related infection. See Research box above.

## PREVENTION

### *Healthy People 2000*

The *Healthy People 2000* report includes multiple objectives related to improved oral health for persons of all ages. Pertinent objectives include the following[16]:

1. Increase to at least 45% the proportion of people ages 35 through 44 who have never lost a permanent tooth because of dental caries or periodontal diseases. (Baseline: 31% of employed adults had never lost a permanent tooth for any reason by 1985-86.)
2. Reduce to no more than 20% the proportion of people ages 65 and older who have lost all of their natural teeth. (Baseline: 36% in 1986.)
3. Reduce the prevalence of gingivitis among people ages 35 through 44 to no more than 30%. (Baseline: 42% in 1985-86.)
4. Reduce destructive periodontal diseases to a prevalence of no more than 15% among people ages 35 through 44. (Baseline: 24% in 1985-86.)
5. Reduce deaths related to cancer of the oral cavity and pharynx to no more than 10.5 per 100,000 men ages 45 through 74 and 4.1 per 100,000 women ages 45 through 74. (Baseline: 12.1 per 100,000 men and 4.1 per 100,000 women in 1987.)
6. Increase to at least 75% the proportion of people served by community water systems providing optimal levels of fluoride. (Baseline: 62% in 1989.)
7. Increase use of professionally administered or self-administered topical or systemic (dietary) fluorides to at least 85% of people not receiving optimally fluoridated public water. (Baseline: an estimated 50% in 1989.)
8. Extend to all long-term institutional facilities the requirement that oral examinations and services be provided no later than 90 days after entry into these facilities. (Baseline: nursing facilities receiving Medicaid or Medicare reimbursement will be required to provide for oral examinations within 90 days of patient entry beginning in 1990; baseline data unavailable for other institutions.)
9. Increase to at least 70% the proportion of people ages 35 and older using the oral health care system during each year. (Baseline: 54% in 1986.)
10. Extend requirement of the use of effective head, face, eye, and mouth protection to all organizations, agencies, and institutions sponsoring sporting and recreation events that pose risks of injury. (Baseline: only National Collegiate Athletic Association football, hockey, and lacrosse; high school football; amateur boxing; and amateur ice hockey in 1988.)

### Primary Prevention

**Primary prevention** is clearly directed toward significantly limiting or eliminating the use of tobacco and alcohol. The two present the greatest risk when used in combination. Alone, tobacco appears to be less significant, except perhaps in adolescents. The new links with oncogenic viruses reinforce the importance of safe sex techniques for the sexually active, again particularly teenagers. Good oral hygiene and care of the teeth and gums are also important.

### Secondary Prevention

**Secondary prevention** focuses on early identification. Early detection of oral cancer can help increase the patient's chance of survival. Any person with a mouth lesion or swelling that does not heal within 2 weeks is urged to seek immediate medical evaluation. Regular dental care and assessment are important, particularly for the evaluation of any premalignant lesions. Treating decayed or broken teeth removes a common source of chronic irritation in the mouth. Proper fitting of dentures is essential for the older population.

## MEDICAL MANAGEMENT

The expected length of stay of patients with oral cancer as determined by DRG is 9.1 days. Common medical therapy for management of oral cancer includes the following.

## Diagnostic Tests

Biopsy is the primary diagnostic test used in cases of suspected oral cancer. It may be used to evaluate leukoplakias, ulcers, lesions, or neck masses that do not resolve spontaneously within 1 to 2 weeks. Ultrasonography is an excellent adjunct to evaluate masses that are close to the surface. CT scans may be used to evaluate deeper, less defined masses, and MRI is most useful in the effort to evaluate deep masses of inconclusive structure.

## Medication

Pharmacotherapy does not play a role in the treatment of oral cancer except to increase patient comfort and correct any concurrent or underlying infection.

## Treatment

Treatment of oral cancer depends on the location and staging of the tumor. Early stage cancer is usually treated by either radiation or surgery, depending on the size and accessibility of the tumor. More invasive cancers may require both modalities, and advanced oral cancers are treated palliatively. Radiation may be delivered by external beam or through the insertion of needles or seeds. If both radiation and surgery are planned, the radiation therapy is usually administered *after* the surgery, since irradiated tissue is more susceptible to infection and breakdown. The method and effects of the radiotherapy need to be fully explained to the patient before the start of treatment. Care of the patient with implanted radioactive needles in oral tissue is summarized in the Guidelines box at right. For a more complete discussion of radiotherapy and associated nursing care, see Chapter 16.

Secondary effects of radiation therapy to the mouth and neck include mucositis, **xerostomia** (dryness in mouth), and dental decay. Some of these changes may be permanent. Tissue may also slough and create a foul mouth odor.

*Dryness of the mouth* begins 1 to 2 weeks after radiation is started and may persist throughout life. The dryness makes the mouth feel uncomfortable and gives an unpleasant taste. Frequent drinks of water, mouthwashes, and increased humidification of the air contribute to added moisture and comfort.

*Dental decay,* especially at the gingival margins, results from decreased salivary secretion and altered pH of the saliva. An active control program is started before radiation therapy is initiated and includes a conscientious tooth-care regimen using fluoride toothpaste, a soft toothbrush, and dental floss. Fluroide treatments for the teeth may also be given.

## Diet

No specific diet modifications are associated with the treatment of oral cancer. The treatment approach selected, however, may necessitate modifications in food selection and feeding methods to maintain adequate nutrition. As previously discussed, high-dose radiation therapy commonly causes stomatitis and/or xerostomia, as well as changes in taste, which may be long-term. Extensive oral surgery may radically alter the patient's ability to ingest, chew, or swallow food and fluid. Specific strategies are discussed under Nursing Management.

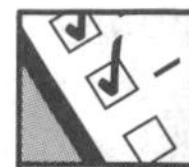

### Guidelines for Care of the Person with Radioactive Needle Implants in Oral Tissue

**IMPLANT CARE**

1. Do not pull on the strings. Any movement could alter the placement or direction of the radiation or cause the needles to loosen.
2. Check needle patency several times each day.
3. Monitor linens, bed areas, and emesis basin for needles that may dislodge.
4. Ensure that a protective container is present in the room to contain any needles that might dislodge.

**PATIENT CARE**

1. Assist with gentle oral hygiene q 2 hr while awake.
2. Encourage the patient to avoid hot and cold foods and beverages, as well as smoking.
3. If the patient has dentures, encourage their removal at night for comfort. Assess gums for irritation and bleeding whenever dentures are removed.
4. Provide viscous lidocaine (Xylocaine) solutions or lozenges as needed when oral discomfort interferes with nutrition.
5. Provide the patient with an alternate means of communication; talking around implanted needles is frequently difficult or impossible.
6. Assist the patient to implement the mouth care regimen prescribed by the physician.

## Activity

Patients with oral cancer are encouraged to remain as active as possible. The only restrictions will be the fatigue associated with radiotherapy and surgery, and the patient's willingness to resume daily activities.

## Referral/Consultation

In some settings the nurse assumes responsibility for making referrals to other services. Common referrals for persons with oral cancer include speech and occupational therapy. Most forms of treatment at least temporarily interfere with the patient's oral communication. The dietitian and occupational therapist may also be involved in devising strategies to improve oral nutrition and assisting the patient to relearn chewing and swallowing after treatment.

# SURGICAL MANAGEMENT

Surgery is the preferred mode of treatment for most early- and middle-stage oral cancers. Although confined local excision may be possible in some situations, many of the operations are radical procedures involving extensive resection. Examples include partial mandibulectomy, partial (hemiglossectomy) or total **glossectomy** (removal of the tongue), and resections of the floor of the mouth or buccal mucosa. Because oral cancers frequently metastasize early to the cervical lymph nodes, the surgical procedure usually also includes functional or radical neck dissection, with removal of the regional and deep cervical lymph nodes and their channels. In a functional dissection the lymph nodes and channels are removed but the other structures are preserved. In advanced cases the surgery may also include removal of the sternocleidomastoid muscle or other neck muscles, the internal jugular vein, thyroid gland, submaxillary gland, and spinal accessory nerve (Figure 44-2). The surgery can create significant functional and cosmetic problems for the patient. A temporary or permanent tracheostomy may be performed. Reconstructive surgery may be planned for a future time. Discussion of nursing management of the patient undergoing surgery for oral cancer follows.

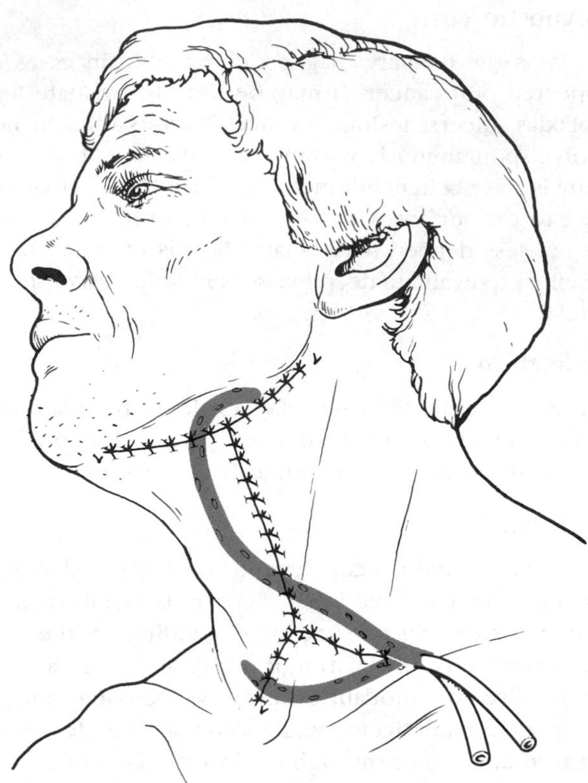

**FIGURE 44-2** Radical neck incision with drainage tubing in place. (From Lewis MN, Collier IC: *Medical surgical nursing,* ed 3, St Louis, 1992, Mosby.)

## NURSING MANAGEMENT: The Patient Undergoing Surgery for Oral Cancer

### ♦ ASSESSMENT

#### Subjective Data

Data to be collected to assess the patient undergoing surgery for oral cancer include the following:

- History of alcohol and/or tobacco use—amount and duration
- History of exposure to or treatment for sexually transmitted diseases
- Oral and dental hygiene habits
- Presence of mouth soreness, pain, or irritation—nature, duration, and self-treatment strategies used
- Presence of ear pain
- Knowledge and understanding of planned surgery and its expected outcomes—functional and cosmetic

#### Objective Data

Data to be collected to assess the patient undergoing surgery for oral cancer include the following:

- Condition of mouth and teeth
- Presence of leukoplakia, erythroplakia, or ulcers
- Presence of lesions—location, appearance, severity
- Mouth odor

#### Diagnostic Test Findings

1. Tissue biopsy—diagnosis and staging
2. CT scan or sonogram—evaluates deeper structure tumors

### ♦ NURSING DIAGNOSES

Nursing diagnoses are determined from analysis of patient data. Nursing diagnoses for the patient undergoing surgery for oral cancer may include but are not limited to the following:

| Diagnostic Title | Possible Etiologic Factors |
|---|---|
| Communication, impaired verbal | Tissue resection, tracheostomy |
| Nutrition altered: less than body requirements | Chewing and swallowing difficulties, discomfort, or foul taste |
| Mucous membranes, altered oral | Excessive or inadequate secretions, discomfort |
| Airway clearance, ineffective | Excessive secretions, loss of protective reflexes, swallowing difficulties |
| Body image disturbance | Disfiguring surgery, functional changes, or loss of oral communication |

### ♦ EXPECTED PATIENT OUTCOMES

Expected patient outcomes for the patient undergoing surgery for oral cancer may include but are not limited to the following:

1. Successfully uses alternative methods to communicate needs.
2. Follows suggested diet and life-style changes.
   a. Adapts feeding method to functional limitations.
   b. Ingests a nutritionally balanced diet.
   c. Maintains a stable body weight.

3a. Oral and neck incisions heal without infection.
   b. Adapts mouth care regimen to functional changes.
   c. Controls drooling, or uses strategies to keep mouth moist and odor free.

4a. Learns techniques to successfully remove secretions from the mouth.
 b. Maintains an intact airway.
5a. Accepts altered body image, and speaks positively of self.
 b. Interacts with others, and gradually resumes social activities.

## ♦ INTERVENTIONS

### Preoperative Care

The mouth is thoroughly cleansed before surgery to reduce the number of bacteria present. Antibiotics may also be started at this time. Impressions of the palate and jaw will be made before radical surgery if use of prostheses is planned to replace resected tissue. The actual prosthesis is fitted when surgical healing is completed. The nurse provides the patient with careful explanations of all planned activities and treatments, with special attention to the feeding and communication adaptations that may be necessary in the immediate postoperative period. Emotional support in the preoperative period is an essential intervention; the changes the patient faces may be extensive. The remainder of the preparation is similar to that required before any major surgery (see Chapter 23).

### Postoperative Care

Postoperative care of the patient focuses on promoting an adequate airway, mouth drainage, oral hygiene, comfort, nutrition, and speech. Specific interventions related to the primary nursing diagnoses follow. Care of the patient after surgery for oral cancer is summarized in the Guidelines box below.

#### Facilitating verbal communication

The ability to speak is commonly lost for short or long periods after surgery, but if the vocal cords are intact, speech will eventually be restored. Phrasing questions

**Guidelines for Care of the Person After Surgery for Oral Cancer**

**PREOPERATIVE CARE**

1. Clarify the patient's knowledge of changes expected after surgery
2. Explain expected postoperative measures (including suctioning, nasogastric tube)
3. Provide opportunities for the patient to begin to express feelings about changes in body image

**POSTOPERATIVE CARE**

1. Monitoring
   a. Assess facial movement for facial nerve damage (if parotid gland excised): ask the patient to raise the eyebrows, frown, smile, show the teeth, pucker the lips
   b. Assess the degree and character of drainage
      (1) Amount of drainage and presence of blood should be minimal
      (2) Hemorrhage may occur with wide resection of the tongue
2. Maintaining an adequate airway
   a. Place the patient in side-lying position initially
   b. Place the patient in Fowler's position when fully alert
   c. Suction the mouth (except for lip surgery)
   d. Gauze wick may be used to direct saliva into an emesis basin
   e. Maintain patency of drainage tubes, if used
3. Promoting oral hygiene and comfort
   a. Clean involved areas of the mouth with a cotton applicator moistened with hydrogen peroxide and saline
   b. Mouth irrigations
      (1) Use sterile equipment
      (2) Use a solution of sterile water, diluted hydrogen peroxide, normal saline, or sodium bicarbonate (avoid commercial mouthwashes)
      (3) Protect any dressings from getting wet
      (4) A catheter may be inserted along the side of the cheek and the solution injected with gentle pressure; a spray may also be used
      (5) Give analgesics as indicated (pain is *not* usually severe)
4. Promoting nutrition
   a. Tube feedings will be used initially with hemiglossectomy
   b. Oral fluids: place in back of throat with aseptic syringe or feeding cup with attached tubing
   c. Eating soft foods
      (1) Encourage the patient to feed self when possible
      (2) Teach the patient to drink clear water after all meals to cleanse the mouth
      (3) Avoid using a fork, which may traumatize new tissue
   d. Foods
      (1) Avoid long-term use of commercial preparations such as instant breakfast drinks (may cause diarrhea or constipation)
      (2) Give fruit-flavored yogurt preparations, which are less irritating than gelatin preparations and are easier to swallow
      (3) Avoid very hot or cold foods (hot foods irritate new tissue; cold foods may cause facial pain or paralyze oral functions)
5. Promoting speech
   a. Limit patient responses initially to *yes* or *no*, which can be answered by gestures
   b. When speech returns, encourage the patient to speak slowly
   c. Listen carefully and validate communication before acting on requests
   d. Speak in a soft, clear voice
   e. Refer the patient to a speech therapist if necessary
6. Promoting a positive body image
   a. Prepare all visitors for visible outcomes of surgery
   b. Include the family in all teaching
   c. Encourage the patient to ventilate feelings about changes
   d. Encourage socialization with others

initially in a *yes* or *no* format enables the patient to respond effectively with gestures, head nods, or simple sounds. The nurse validates all communication by repeating answers or questions before acting on perceived requests. Loud noises may be disturbing to the patient because the loss of oral tissue may create a channel that amplifies sound; the person should therefore be addressed in a soft, clear voice. As speech begins to return, the patient is encouraged to speak slowly and to use the throat rather than the lips to achieve clarity. Speech retraining may be necessary, and referrals for speech therapy are usually initiated. A tape recorder may be useful so that the person can hear his or her own voice and work on improvements.

**Promoting adequate oral nutrition**

The problems that the patient faces related to oral nutrition after oral surgery depend entirely on the nature and extent of the surgical procedure.

Chewing is difficult without an intact tongue, and the person often has a problem getting the food to the posterior pharynx. Sensation in the mouth is decreased, and the patient has difficulty locating the position of the food in the oral cavity. One method of eating is for the person to use the forefinger to push the food to the posterior pharynx.

A syringe or tube is commonly used to assist the patient to successfully direct fluids toward the back of the mouth. The tube may be placed and anchored by the surgeon at the time of surgery. Tube feeding is used while tissue healing takes place, and it may be a permanent approach to nutrition when extensive tissue removal is necessary.

Most patients can suction and feed themselves a few days after mouth surgery and are happier doing so. With practice, the patient develops confidence in self-care and is often more adept than the nurse in placing the catheter or tube in a position where fluids can be received into the mouth and swallowed without difficulty. A mirror often helps. Privacy is essential during the initial period. The patient should not be hurried and is observed very carefully to determine how much assistance is needed. Forks are *not* used, since they may traumatize healing tissues. Both very hot and very cold foods are avoided because they may irritate healing tissue or produce facial pain.

Patients are instructed to carefully rinse the mouth with clear water or with the prescribed solution after finishing each meal. Some patients experience persistent problems with choking or nasal regurgitation, which can significantly interfere with the social nature of meals.

**Promoting oral hygiene**

Good mouth care after surgery is essential for comfort, prevention of infection, and promotion of healing. Tooth brushing is usually contraindicated because of discomfort and potential trauma. Sterile equipment is used to prevent introduction of exogenous organisms. Patients are encouraged to assist in their oral hygiene as soon as possible.

Mouth irrigations are standard postoperative interventions and are performed every few hours and after feedings. Commercial mouthwashes are avoided in preference for sterile water, dilute peroxide and saline, or bicarbonate solutions. The solution is typically introduced into the mouth via a catheter, which is gently inserted along the cheek line, or with a spray. A cotton tipped applicator moistened with peroxide and saline may be used to reach difficult or painful areas. The nurse encourages self-care and teaches the patient to use mirrors to increase visualization.

**Maintaining a patent airway**

Removal of secretions is the primary concern immediately after surgery. Tissue and nerve trauma may impair the natural protective reflexes and leave the airway vulnerable. A side-lying position is used until the patient is fully alert, followed by a head-elevated Fowler's position. Oral suction is kept available at the bedside, and the nurse instructs the patient in its proper use. An emesis basin or gauze wicks may also be used to collect saliva. The nurse carefully monitors the airway, auscultates the lungs, and maintains the patency of any drainage tubes in use.

**Facilitating adaptation of body image**

Treatment for cancer of the mouth interferes with major oral functions such as eating and speaking and thus creates major changes in the person's life. Changes in the patient's ability to speak will vary from some limitation to complete inability to speak, depending on the amount of tissue resected or destroyed. Eating patterns will be changed in terms of the consistency of foods, as well as methods of ingestion. Persistent drooling is a common problem. The person's facial appearance will also change, depending on the extent of tissue removed or destroyed, and even with reconstructive surgery, noticeable changes will be present.

Therefore one of the major problems that the person will have to cope with and adapt to is the change in body image. Patients need to know in advance the changes that will occur and the measures that will be taken to assist them during the adjustment period. The impact of the loss may be slightly minimized when the grieving process begins early. The full emotional impact of the loss, however, occurs after surgery.

Problems with speaking and eating may cause the patient to avoid interactions with family, friends, or strangers. Family is included, if possible, in all teaching, and the nurse encourages them to include the patient in mealtimes and social occasions as soon as possible. Visiting is encouraged, but all visitors need to be prepared in advance concerning the visible changes and functional problems created by the surgery. Body image changes are discussed in depth in Chapter 9.

## ♦ EVALUATION

To evaluate the effectiveness of nursing interventions, compare patient behaviors with those stated in the expected patient outcomes. Successful achievement of patient outcomes for the patient undergoing surgery for oral cancer is indicated by the following:

1. Communicates needs effectively.
2a. Can feed self.
 b. Ingests a balanced, nutritional diet.
 c. Has a stable body weight.
3a. Has clean, healed neck incisions.
 b. Performs adequate mouth care.
 c. Controls drooling, dry mouth, and mouth odor.
4a. Controls and eliminates oral secretions.
 b. Has an intact airway.
5a. Has positive attitudes and expressions about physical self.
 b. Interacts socially with family and friends.

## ✵ SPECIAL CONSIDERATIONS FOR CARE OF THE GERONTOLOGIC PATIENT

The incidence of oral cancer is increased in the elderly population. Oral cancer appears to be primarily a reaction to long-term exposure to alcohol and tobacco, and the cumulative effects are typically seen in the aging population. The importance of seeking prompt evaluation of any mouth lesion is stressed with elderly individuals.

Surgical intervention for oral cancer is typically radical, and it may be a significant stressor for an elderly person with less adaptive reserve. The need to learn new approaches to secretion removal, oral feeding, and communication may pose significant challenges to an older adult, particularly if psychomotor abilities are compromised by arthritis. Discharge planning needs to be carefully undertaken, because social isolation may become a reality for elders who live alone. The nurse is an essential link in the process of identifying persons who will need home care assistance.

## ❦ HOME CARE CONSIDERATIONS

Home care considerations are primarily related to the extent of the surgery and its impact on speech and oral nutrition. When wound healing is prolonged, the patient may need ongoing assistance or supervision in performing oral care or feedings. If nutritional needs are not being met, home administration of tube feedings or gastrostomy feedings may be initiated. Ongoing work with a speech therapist is frequently necessary.

### COMPLICATIONS

Complications are primarily related to the progression of the original disease process or treatment-related problems.

Tissue necrosis and severe pain can occur in advanced cancer of the mouth, either from failure of treatment or from death of tissue as a result of radiation. The patient usually experiences difficulty in swallowing, fear of choking, and the constant accumulation of foul-smelling secretions. The danger of severe and even fatal hemorrhage must always be considered. It is very difficult to assist these patients to take sufficient nourishing fluids. A gastrostomy may be done to permit direct introduction of food into the stomach. Family members caring for the person at home need considerable support from hospice or other community health nurses.

# TRAUMA OF THE MOUTH AND JAW

### ETIOLOGY/EPIDEMIOLOGY

Injuries to the mouth and jaw usually result from blows, motor vehicle accidents, or foreign objects. Soft tissue injuries are extremely common outcomes of contact sports and domestic violence. Trauma to the jaw bone results most commonly from high speed and force contact. Soft tissues of the mouth may be bruised or lacerated, and the jaw may be fractured.

### PATHOPHYSIOLOGY

Soft tissue injuries usually involve bleeding, bruising, and extensive edema. Unless suturing is required, most injuries, although temporarily disfiguring, resolve with rest and conservative care. Fractures create a greater challenge. The mandible, although a bone of significant size and strength, is frequently vulnerable to fracture injury where it articulates with the temporal bones. Restoring mandibular continuity is essential for the normal occlusal relationship of the teeth, and mandibular fixation may be necessary for healing.

### MEDICAL MANAGEMENT

Lacerations and bruises of the mouth and jaw are cleansed and sutured, if their severity warrants it, and then are treated with analgesics and the local application of ice to reduce swelling. Antibiotics may be prescribed for major lacerations because of the large amounts of bacteria that are found in the mouth.

Fractures of the jaw are treated by closed or open reduction and intermaxillary fixation. The teeth are wired, and the upper and lower teeth are connected by rubber bands or tie wires to immobilize the jaw. Because of the excellent blood supply to the jaw, fractures usually heal in 5 to 8 weeks.

### NURSING MANAGEMENT

Edema may be pronounced after trauma to the mouth and may interfere with respiration. Usually the head of the bed is elevated to a semi-Fowler's position to aid venous drainage from the area and thereby lessen edema. Tight dressings about the face must be checked carefully because they may contribute to development of edema and may cause headache.

Immediately following wiring of the teeth, the nurse observes the patient for nausea and vomiting resulting from the presence of blood or other swallowed material, anesthetic, or emotional trauma. Care must be taken to prevent aspiration of vomitus. Vomitus and secretions must be removed by suction because the patient cannot expectorate them through the mouth. A catheter may be inserted through the nasopharynx or into the mouth through a gap created by missing teeth or in the space behind the third molar, but this approach may not be feasible if there are multiple loosened teeth and dental stability is a priority. Scissors or a wire cutter should be at the bedside so that the wires can be cut or the elastic bands released if necessary. Specific orders should state the circumstances under which wires or rubber bands should be released.

Persons who have fixation by wiring often must subsist on liquids and may be taught to take a high-calorie liquid diet through a catheter or straw. In other settings patients may be instructed in a "sip" technique, sucking small amounts of liquid placed between the lips. The method is very tiring, and adequate time must be allowed for meals. The patient also often experiences considerable pain from muscle spasms in the immobilized jaw. The spasms can be severe enough to necessitate muscle relaxants, which are typically administered in an elixir form. Teaching will also include methods for mouth hygiene and the importance of promptly reporting the sudden development of swelling or new pain after discharge.

# PROBLEMS OF THE ESOPHAGUS

## GASTROESOPHAGEAL REFLUX DISEASE

### ETIOLOGY

*Gastroesophageal reflux disease* **(GERD)** is a term that refers to a heterogenous syndrome resulting from esophageal reflux. Most cases are attributed to the inappropriate relaxation of the lower esophageal sphincter (LES) in response to an unknown stimulus. Reflux allows gastric and duodenal contents to move back into the distal esophagus. The presence of a hiatal hernia, which displaces the LES into the thorax, was formerly commonly assumed to be the primary cause of GERD. However, hiatal hernia has subsequently been found to be a common condition in the adult population and, although most persons with hiatal hernias do experience reflux, the reverse has not been found to be true.[13] The two conditions are better considered as related but separate. A number of environmental and physical factors have been identified that appear to influence the tone and contractility of the LES, and these may play an etiologic role in some cases of GERD. LES pressure is lowered by dietary factors such as fatty foods, chocolate and xanthine; nicotine; pharmacologic agents such as ganglionic stimulants and beta adrenergic drugs; elevated levels of estrogen and progesterone; delayed gastric emptying; and the elevated intraabdominal pressure that is commonly associated with pregnancy, obesity, or heavy lifting.

### EPIDEMIOLOGY

GERD can occur in any age-group from infancy to old age. It is estimated to produce daily symptoms in as much as 10% of the general population, and monthly symptoms in as much as 40%.[2] It is theorized that the actual incidence of mild disease may be even higher, because many individuals simply accept reflux as a normal periodic problem and attribute its occurrence to periods of stress or overindulgence in food. There are no documented gender or cultural patterns associated with the disease.

### PATHOPHYSIOLOGY

Two zones of high pressure, one at each end of the esophagus, normally prevent reflux of gastric contents. The zones are constricted except during the act of swallowing. Although they are termed the *upper* and *lower esophageal sphincters,* they are not really distinct anatomic structures. Esophageal reflux occurs when gastric volume or intraabdominal pressure is elevated or when LES sphincter tone is decreased. Periodic reflux occurs normally in most persons and is usually asymptomatic. However, the esophagus has only a limited ability to withstand the damaging effects of acid reflux, and GERD will develop when an inflammatory response occurs and the mucosal barrier breaks down.

The degree of esophageal inflammation is related to the number, duration, and acidity or alkalinity of the reflux episodes. The effectiveness and efficiency of esophageal clearance also are important. Refluxed material is returned to the stomach by rapid peristaltic waves, increased saliva, and gravity. These factors are particularly important at night when the swallowing rate decreases by two thirds and a recumbent position interferes with clearance. An inflamed esophagus gradually loses its ability to clear refluxed material quickly and efficiently, and the duration of each episode gradually increases.

Hyperemia and erosion occur in the face of chronic inflammation. Minor capillary bleeding is common, although frank bleeding is rare. Repeated episodes of inflammation and healing can gradually produce a change in the epithelial tissue, which makes it more resistant to acid. However, the presence of this new tissue, termed *Barrett's epithelium,* is also associated with a higher risk of adenocarcinoma. Over time, fibrotic tissue changes can also result in esophageal stricture, which can progressively impair normal swallowing.

The clinical manifestations of GERD are very consistent in their nature, but they vary substantially in severity. The irritation of chronic reflux produces the primary symptom, which is heartburn (pyrosis). The pain is described as a substernal or retrosternal burning sensation that tends to radiate upward and may involve the neck, jaw, or back. The pain typically occurs 20 minutes to 2 hours after eating. An atypical pain pattern that closely mimics angina may also occur and needs to be carefully differentiated from true cardiac disease. The second major symptom of GERD is regurgitation, which is not associated with either belching or nausea. The individual experiences a feeling of warm fluid moving up the throat. If it reaches the pharynx, a sour or bitter taste is perceived. **Water brash** occurs less commonly. This is a reflex salivary hypersecretion that does not have a bitter taste.

In severe cases GERD can produce dysphagia or **odynophagia** (painful swallowing). Belching and a feeling of flatulence are other fairly common complaints. The frequency, severity, and duration of the reflux episodes usually determine the severity of the symptoms. The clinical manifestations of GERD are summarized in Box 44-1.

**BOX 44-1 Clinical Manifestations of GERD**

**Heartburn**—substernal or retosternal burning sensation that may radiate to the back or jaw
NOTE: In some cases the pain may mimic angina
**Regurgitation** (not associated with nausea or belching)—a sour or bitter taste is perceived in the pharynx
**Water brash**—a reflex hypersecretion that does not have a bitter taste
**Frequent belching**
**Flatulence**
**Dysphagia** or **odynophagia** (difficult or painful swallowing)—usually occurs only in severe cases

## PREVENTION

**Primary prevention** does not play a major role in GERD because the condition does not have readily identifiable preventable etiologic factors. Standard preventive measures might include maintaining an optimal body weight and avoiding episodes of overeating, particularly at night. The most significant factor in **secondary prevention** is for health care professionals to directly inquire about a patient's experience with heartburn. Studies have shown that patients rarely report heartburn to their health care provider unless directly asked, or until the symptoms have become severe.[2] If identified and recognized early, the disease may be more responsive to diet and life-style modification measures. Situations occur in which reflux is severe and persistent and will worsen and necessitate more aggressive management, but complications can be prevented and symptoms significantly reduced in most cases of uncomplicated GERD.

## MEDICAL MANAGEMENT

Patients with GERD are rarely admitted to the acute care setting unless they require surgery or experience serious complications. The problem is usually managed in the outpatient setting. Common medical therapy for GERD includes the following.

### Diagnostic Tests

Mild cases of GERD are diagnosed from the classic symptoms. More involved cases may require other screening tools. The "gold standard" for diagnosis is 24-hour pH monitoring, which accurately records the number, duration, and severity of reflux episodes and is considered to be 85% sensitive. The esophageal motility and Bernstein tests are usually performed in conjunction with pH monitoring to evaluate LES competence, quantify reflux episodes, and evaluate the response of the esophagus to acid infusion. These tests are described in more detail in Chapter 43. The barium swallow with fluoroscopy is widely used to document the presence of hiatal hernia, but it can demonstrate only gross disease. Endoscopy is rarely necessary to establish the diagnosis, but it is routinely performed to rule out malignancy. The classic signs of esophageal erosion and inflammation are readily apparent on endoscopy.

### Medication

Drug therapy is an important aspect of GERD management, and it is usually initiated by the patient with antacid use as needed. Antacids are effective in dealing with occasional heartburn because of their acid neutralizing effect. They usually produce prompt relief of symptoms. Either aluminum or magnesium products may be used, but combination mixtures such as Maalox and Mylanta are usually best tolerated since they control the incidence of common side effects such as diarrhea or constipation. The nurse instructs the patient to take 30 ml of antacid 1 hour before and 2 to 3 hours after each meal, or as needed for control of heartburn. Gaviscon, a combination of alginic acid and antacid, may be used as an alternative. It creates a viscous foam that floats on the gastric contents and theoretically reduces the incidence of reflux. It is also the first substance to enter the esophagus when reflux occurs and thus limits acid contact with the mucosa.

Antacids are usually inadequate for the control of frequent reflux symptoms because their duration of action is too short. Histamine ($H_2$) receptor antagonists such as cimetidine (Tagamet), ranitidine (Zantac), famotidine (Pepcid), or nizatidine (Axid) may be used for more severe GERD. Although they do not influence reflux directly, they reduce gastric acid secretion and provide symptomatic improvement. They also support tissue healing. These drugs may be prescribed for use at intervals, or in a single large dose at bedtime to significantly reduce the effects of nightime reflux. Gastric secretion is reduced by 60% to 70% over the 24-hour

**TABLE 44-2 Drug Therapy For GERD**

| DRUG | ACTION | USUAL DOSAGE | NURSING INTERVENTION |
|---|---|---|---|
| Antacids:<br>Aluminum or magnesium-based product | Neutralize gastric acids | 30 ml PO 1 hr before meals, 2-3 hr after meals, at bedtime, and PRN for heartburn | Evaluate effectiveness<br>Monitor frequency of use<br>Monitor for constipation or diarrhea, and assist patient to adjust product use as needed |
| Antacid plus alginic acid:<br>Gaviscon | Neutralizes gastric acid; forms viscous foam that prevents reflux or buffers its effects | 1 tablet, or 10-20 ml PO using same dosage pattern as for antacids | Same as for antacids |
| Histamine ($H_2$) receptor antagonists: | Reduce gastric acid secretion and support tissue healing | | |
| Cimetidine (Tagamet) | | 300 mg PO qid or 900-1200 mg at bedtime | Instruct patient to take drugs with meals if ordered at intervals |
| Ranitidine (Zantac) | | 150 mg PO bid | Monitor for common side effects: fatigue, headache, diarrhea |
| Famotidine (Pepcid) | | 20 mg PO bid or 40 mg at bedtime | |
| Nizatadine (Axid) | | 300-600 mg PO at bedtime | |
| Bethanecol (Urecholine) | Increases LES pressure; increases esophageal clearance | 25 PO qid | Monitor for common cholinergic side effects: abdominal cramping, diarrhea, urinary urgency; instruct patient to continue antacid or $H_2$ receptor antagonist drugs since bethanecol increases gastric secretions |
| Metoclopramide (Reglan) | Increases the rate of gastric emptying; may increase LES pressure | 10 mg PO tid or qid | Instruct patient to take drug before meals<br>Monitor for common side effects of long-term use: anxiety, ataxia, restlessness, or hallucinations (occur in up to ⅓ of users) |
| Proton pump inhibitors:<br>Omeprazole (Prilosec) | Inhibits enzyme system of gastric parietal cells and suppresses gastric acid secretion by more than 90% | 20 mg PO daily for 4-8 weeks | Instruct patient to take the drug before meals; monitor for side effects: abdominal cramping, headache, diarrhea |

period, and the drugs are considered safe for long-term use.

Bethanecol (Urecholine) or metoclopramide (Reglan) may be added to the regimen in severe cases. Bethanecol increases LES pressure and the rate of esophageal clearance, but its cholinergic action also increases gastric acid secretion and necessitates the simultaneous use of a histamine ($H_2$) receptor antagonist. Metoclopramide directly increases the rate of gastric emptying, but it does not reduce acid secretion or assist in healing, and its multiple side effects make it inappropriate for long-term use. The nurse instructs the patient to take these drugs before meals and discusses their multiple potential side effects.

A new category of drugs, the proton pump inhibitors, is being researched for the treatment of GERD. These potent drugs reduce acid secretion by 90% over 24 hours and promote rapid healing; they may be given in a single daily dose. Relapses are common, however, after the drug is discontinued, and safety for long-term use has not been clearly established.

The nurse also explores the patient's use of other medications. Anticholinergics, calcium channel blockers, xanthine derivatives, and diazepam all appear to lower the LES pressure, and their use should be avoided if possible. Drug therapy for GERD is summarized in Table 44-2.

## Treatment

GERD is typically managed using a combination of drug therapy, life-style modification, and surgical intervention if necessary. There are no specific treatments included in the standard medical plan of care.

## Diet

The modification of diet and eating patterns may significantly relieve symptoms in mild GERD. Certain foods have been clearly demonstrated to affect LES pressure.

Fatty foods, cola, coffee, tea, chocolate, and alcohol all clearly decrease LES pressure and should be avoided. Adequate dietary protein stimulates the release of gastrin and cholecystokinin, which increase LES pressure. Spicy and acidic foods are usually restricted until healing occurs and then may be resumed if they do not produce pain. Weight loss and avoiding overeating may also reduce the frequency of reflux episodes.

### Activity

Activities that increase intraabdominal pressure and the likelihood of reflux are restricted. Lifting heavy objects, straining, constrictive clothing, and working in a stooped or bent-over position are all contraindicated.

### Referral/Consultation

Referrals are rarely necessary for persons with uncomplicated GERD, but the nurse may encourage the patient to seek assistance for weight loss or smoking cessation as indicated.

## SURGICAL MANAGEMENT

Antireflux surgery is usually performed in patients with severe GERD who do not respond to aggressive medical management. The procedures are the same as those used to correct hiatal hernia and are discussed on p. 1452. They involve fundoplication, the wrapping and suturing of the gastric fundus around the esophagus, which reinforces the LES area and anchors it below the diaphragm.

The placement of the synthetic Angelchik prosthesis (Figure 44-3) is occasionally used as an alternative to antireflux surgery. It entails a relatively minor surgical procedure, including a laparotomy to tie a C-shaped silicone prosthesis around the distal esophagus. The prosthesis anchors the sphincter in the abdomen and reinforces the LES. Success rates vary by study, and complications are associated with dysphagia and the presence of a foreign body. European surgeons tend to view the procedure more favorably than do American surgeons.[1]

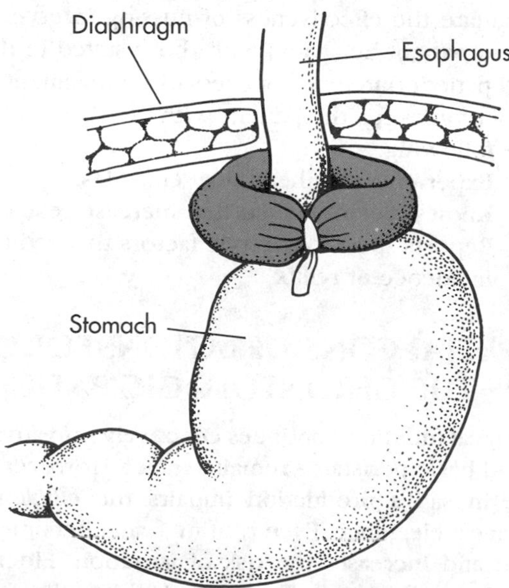


**FIGURE 44-3** The Angelchik antireflux prosthesis in place around the distal esophagus.

## NURSING MANAGEMENT

### ♦ ASSESSMENT

### Subjective Data

Data to be collected to assess the patient with gastroesophageal reflux disease include the following:

- Heartburn—severity and duration
- Regurgitation or water brash—presence and severity
- Relationship of symptoms to food, meal pattern, and activity
- Dysphagia and odynophagia—presence and severity
- Belching or flatulence
- Diet and meal pattern
- Use of over-the-counter medications, particularly antacids

### Objective Data

Data to be collected to assess the patient with gastroesophageal reflux disease include the following:

- Body weight
- Auscultation for signs of reflux aspiration
- Hoarseness or wheezing—day or night

### Diagnostic Test Findings

1. 24-hour pH monitoring and esophageal studies—abnormal results support the presence of reflux
2. Endoscopy—evidence of esophageal inflammation or ulceration

### ♦ NURSING DIAGNOSES

Nursing diagnoses are determined from analysis of patient data. Nursing diagnoses for the person with GERD may include but are not limited to the following:

| Diagnostic Title | Possible Etiologic Factors |
|---|---|
| Pain | Acid reflux in the esophagus |
| Knowledge deficit | Diet and life-style modifications needed to control reflux |

### ♦ EXPECTED PATIENT OUTCOMES

Expected patient outcomes for the patient with GERD may include but are not limited to the following:

1. Reports minimal or no episodes of heartburn.
2. Can list diet and life-style changes that will control reflux and incorporates these changes into daily living.

## ♦ INTERVENTIONS

### Promoting Comfort

The nurse discusses the medication regimen with the patient and ensures that written information about the safe use and expected side effects of all medications is provided. The nurse encourages the patient to use antacids as ordered 1 hour before and 2 to 3 hours after meals, and at bedtime, during the healing phase of management. Antacids should not be restricted to an as needed status for actual heartburn episodes. The nurse informs the patient about the common bowel problems that accompany extensive antacid therapy and suggests strategies such as alternating mixtures or using combination products to maintain a normal pattern of bowel elimination.

### Modifying the Diet

The patient is encouraged to eliminate or significantly reduce consumption of foods that have been shown to lower LES sphincter pressure. A low-fat diet with limited use of caffeine-containing beverages, such as tea, alcohol, and chocolate, is ideal. Adequate protein intake is encouraged for its LES sphincter enhancing ability. The nurse explores barriers to adherence in the patient's usual diet pattern and involves the family if possible to support needed changes.

Patients are also encouraged to modify their basic meal pattern. Eating four to six small meals daily is recommended. Large meals both increase gastric pressure and volume and delay gastric emptying. These factors increase the frequency and severity of reflux episodes. Avoiding evening snacking is particularly important. The individual should not eat for at least 3 hours before bedtime. Nighttime reflux, when both recumbency and inactivity dramatically decrease the effectiveness of esophageal clearance, is a serious problem in GERD that is significantly worsened by evening snacking.

Reducing body weight helps to lower intraabdominal pressure and may be very helpful for obese patients. Simple strategies such as eating slowly and chewing thoroughly facilitate digestion and reduce belching. The nurse works with the patient to carefully evaluate which strategies most effectively reduce the incidence and severity of symptoms.

### Promoting Life-style Changes

Teaching the patient to elevate the head of the bed from 6 to 12 inches for sleep is the highest priority life-style change. Nighttime reflux is the most difficult to manage. Wooden blocks have traditionally been recommended, but recent research indicates that the use of foam wedges can also achieve satisfactory results.[10] The nurse must introduce this crucial intervention with tact and care, since a change affects both the patient and his or her sleeping partner. See Research box above.

The nurse will recommend other life-style changes, including avoiding increases in intraabdominal pressure caused by constrictive clothing, straining, lifting heavy weights, or working in a bent-over or stooped position. Smoking cessation is another critical and sensitive area. Smoking causes a rapid and significant drop in LES pressure and should be reduced or eliminated if at all possible. Evening smoking, particularly while resting in bed, is of particular concern. The combination of evening snacking and smoking receives the highest priority. Diet and life-style changes recommended for GERD are summarized in the Guidelines box, p. 1451.

> **RESEARCH**
>
> Hamilton JW, Boisen RJ, Yamamoto DT, Wagner JL, Reichelderfer M: Sleeping on a wedge diminishes exposure of the esophagus to refluxed acid, *Dig Dis Sci* 33(5):518-522, 1988.
>
> 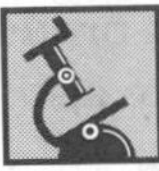
>
> The purpose of the study was to compare the effect of three sleeping positions on the incidence of gastroesophageal reflux. A group of 15 patients with severe GERD was consecutively studied in the flat position, elevated on 8-inch high bed blocks, and elevated on a 10-inch high foam bed wedge. Reflux was monitored via continuous intraesophageal pH monitoring. Reflux frequency was the same in each position. Both methods of elevation decreased the esophageal clearance time, and the wedge caused a significant decline in the duration of the episodes. Elevation on bed blocks has been the conventional recommendation, but this study indicates that the use of a foam wedge can achieve comparable results without significant impact on the furniture or sleeping habits of the partner.

## ♦ EVALUATION

To evaluate the effectiveness of nursing interventions, compare patient behaviors with those stated in the expected patient outcomes. Successful achievement of patient outcomes for the patient with GERD is indicated by the following:

1. Experiences no heartburn episodes.
2a. Knows dietary factors that increase reflux.
b. Reports specific life-style factors that reduce the incidence of reflux.

## ✷ SPECIAL CONSIDERATIONS FOR CARE OF THE GERONTOLOGIC PATIENT

Esophageal function continues effectively into advanced age, and basic peristalsis remains intact. However, a decrease in saliva production impairs the efficiency of esophageal clearance. Even routine reflux becomes protracted and increases the risk of irritation. Elderly individuals need to be clearly assessed for heartburn, since they are found to routinely underreport their symptoms. They also appear to be particularly vulnerable to alkaline

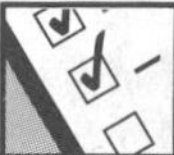

**Guidelines for Diet and Life-style Modifications for GERD**

**DIET**

Eat 4-6 small meals daily.
Follow a low-fat, adequate protein diet.
Reduce intake of chocolate, tea, and all foods and beverages that contain caffeine.
Limit or eliminate alcohol intake.
Eat slowly, and chew food thoroughly.
Avoid evening snacking, and do not eat for 2-3 hr before bedtime.
Remain upright for 1-2 hr after meals when possible, and never eat in bed.
Avoid any food that directly produces heartburn.
Reduce overall body weight if indicated.

**LIFE-STYLE**

Eliminate or drastically reduce smoking.
Avoid evening smoking, and never smoke in bed.
Avoid constrictive clothing.
Avoid activities that involve straining, heavy lifting, or working in a bent-over position.
Elevate the head of the bed 6-8 in for sleep, using wooden blocks or a thick foam wedge.
Never sleep flat in bed.

reflux from the duodenum. It typically occurs at night and causes respiratory symptoms such as choking, paroxysmal coughing, and wheezing. Patients with frequent nighttime awakenings from coughing should be evaluated for GERD. The risk of aspiration is high. Treatment approaches are the same as those outlined for other forms of GERD.

## HOME CARE CONSIDERATIONS

The plan of care that has been outlined takes place almost exclusively in the home setting, with the patient in charge of the self-care regimen. Written instructions are provided about all aspects of the plan to reinforce verbal teaching. The nurse involves the spouse or partner and family where possible, as changes in diet and meal patterns affect the entire family. Major life-style changes are not necessary, but even relatively minor regimen restrictions require planning and support if they are to be successful.

### COMPLICATIONS

If GERD is not successfully controlled, it can progress to serious and even life-threatening problems. Esophageal ulceration and hemorrhage may result from severe erosion, and chronic nighttime reflux is accompanied by a significant risk of aspiration. Adenocarcinoma can develop from the premalignant tissue termed Barrett's epithelium. Gradual or repeated scarring can permanently damage esophageal tissue and produce stricture and dysphagia.

## HIATAL HERNIA

### ETIOLOGY

The opening in the diaphragm that allows the esophagus to pass from the thorax to the abdomen is called the *esophageal hiatus.* **Hiatal hernias** (also called *diaphragmatic hernias*) develop when the distal esophagus, and possibly a portion of the stomach, move into the thorax through the hiatu. There are two major types. One type is the sliding hernias, which accounts for 90% of the total.[6] In these hernias the distal esophagus, gastric junction, and possibly a portion of the stomach are simply displaced upward into the thorax (Figure 44-4, *A*). The hernia is usually freely movable and slides back and forth in response to changes in position or abdominal pressure. Sliding hernias are believed to develop from muscle weakness in the esophageal hiatus, which undermines the supports. The defect is consistent with the aging process, although congenital weakness, trauma, surgery, or prolonged increases in intraabdominal pressure may also play a role.

The second and relatively unusual form of hiatal hernia is the paraesophageal, or rolling, hernia. In this situation the gastric junction remains anchored below the diaphragm, but the fundus of the stomach, and possibly portions or even all of the greater curvature, rolls into the thorax next to the esophagus (Figure 44-4, *B*). Muscle weakening does not appear to play a major role. It is theorized that an anatomic defect causes the stomach to not be firmly anchored below the diaphragm.

### EPIDEMIOLOGY

Hiatal hernias are quite common in the adult population. Their incidence is roughly estimated at as high as 30% in the general population to as high as 60% in the over-60 age-group.[6] Hiatal hernias affect women much more commonly than men, although their incidence increases in both sexes with aging.

### PATHOPHYSIOLOGY

Although hiatal hernias may be present from birth, individuals rarely develop symptoms until middle age. It is estimated that as many as 80% of persons with hiatal hernias are completely unaware of the problem and experience only rare or occasional symptoms.[6]

The major pathophysiologic concern with sliding hernias is the development of gastroesophageal reflux and its complications. Reflux occurs from the chronic exposure of the LES to the low-pressure environment of the thorax, where its function is significantly impaired. Although the classic hernia-related problems of volvulus (twisting) or obstruction do exist, they rarely occur and the structural hernia itself causes few, if any, problems.

Reflux is rarely a concern with paraesophageal hernias, since the LES remains anchored below the diaphragm. The anatomic risks of volvulus, strangulation, and obstruction are quite high. In addition, venous ob-

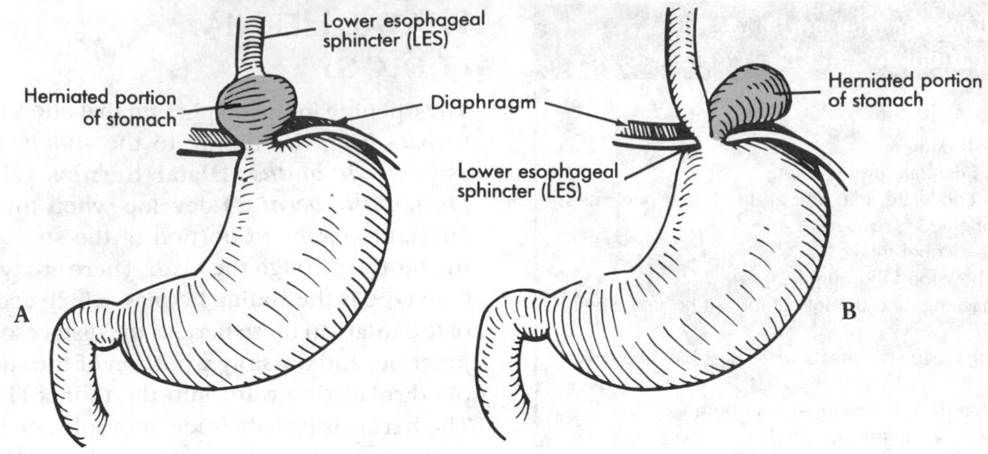


**FIGURE 44-4** Hiatal hernia. **A,** Sliding hernia. **B,** Paraesophageal hernia.

struction in the herniated portion of the stomach causes the mucosa to become engorged and to ooze. Slow bleeding leads to the development of iron deficiency anemia, but significant bleeding or hemorrhage is quite rare.

Unless acute complications develop, most hiatal hernias are diagnosed as part of a workup for GERD and both the clinical manifestations (see Box 44-3) and diagnostic tests are quite similar.

## PREVENTION

**Primary prevention** does not play a major role in the management of hiatal hernia, since the disorder is primarily related to heredity and the effects of aging. Once the hernia is diagnosed, **secondary prevention** strategies include the diet and life-style modifications designed to reduce the incidence and severity of reflux such as changing diet, managing weight, avoiding straining and heavy lifting, and eliminating smoking.

## MEDICAL MANAGEMENT

Patients with hiatal hernia are rarely admitted to the acute care setting except for planned surgical repair or to manage complications. The expected length of stay of patients undergoing surgical repair of hiatal hernia as determined by DRG is 8 days. Common medical therapy for management of hiatal hernia includes the following.

### Diagnostic Tests

The **barium swallow** with fluoroscopy is the most useful test for diagnosing hiatal hernia. Paraesophageal hernias are usually clearly visible, and sliding hernias can be easily demonstrated when the individual is moved into positions that increase intraabdominal pressure. Any or all of the tests used as part of a reflux workup may be used to evaluate the degree of esophageal damage (see Chapter 43). Findings in individuals with paraesophageal hernias may include low hemoglobin and hematocrit levels from chronic low grade bleeding, which will be evident on routine blood tests.

### Medication

Antacids, histamine receptor antagonists, and other antireflux agents are used as needed to manage the reflux that may accompany hiatal hernia. See the discussion on p. 1447 under Gastroesophageal Reflux Disease.

### Treatment

There are no specific treatments utilized in the management of hiatal hernia. Management approaches include drug therapy, life-style modifications, and surgery.

### Diet

The recommended diet modifications for hiatal hernia follow the general guidelines outlined under antireflux therapy. The diet also focuses on reducing obesity if possible. Obesity can significantly increase intraabdominal pressure and worsen the severity of both the hernia and the symptoms of reflux.

### Activity

Activities that increase intraabdominal pressure and reflux are restricted as discussed under Gastroesophageal Reflux Disease (see p. 1449).

### Referral/Consultation

Referrals are rarely necessary for the management of hiatal hernia, except possibly to assist the individual with weight loss and smoking cessation, which are critical components in managing reflux.

## SURGICAL MANAGEMENT

Surgery is performed for paraesophageal hernias when they are diagnosed because the risk of serious complications is significant. The surgery involves straight anatomic repair; there is no need to alter or modify LES function.

The repair of sliding hernias is more complex, because simple repair of the defect in the diaphragm rarely corrects the reflux problem. Restoring LES competence becomes a second major consideration. Several different

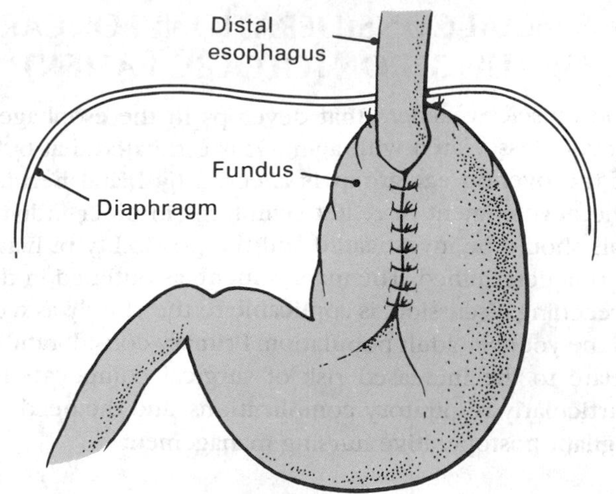


FIGURE 44-5 Nissen fundoplication for repair of hiatal hernia. (From Lewis MN, Collier IC: *Medical surgical nursing,* ed 3, St Louis, 1992, Mosby.)

surgical procedures exist, but each involves LES reinforcement through fundoplication, or wrapping of the stomach fundus around the LES zone.

The **Nissen fundoplication** is the most common (Figure 44-5); it involves wrapping the fundus a full 360 degrees around the lower esophagus, using an abdominal approach. The Hill repair wraps 180 degrees but also restructures the angle of His to make it more acute. The Belsey repair wraps 270 degrees and usually utilizes a thoracic approach. There are advantages and disadvantages to each procedure, and there are no clear indications for the use of one approach over another.

Discussion of nursing management of the patient undergoing surgery for hiatal hernia repair follows.

## NURSING MANAGEMENT: The Patient Undergoing Hiatal Hernia Surgery

### ♦ ASSESSMENT

#### Subjective Data

Data to be collected to assess the patient undergoing hiatal hernia surgery include the following:

- Symptoms of reflux: heartburn, regurgitation, and water brash—presence and severity
- Response of symptoms to position changes—recumbency, bending, stooping
- Belching and flatulence
- History of smoking and/or alcohol use
- Chest pain or odynophagia (rare)
- Episodes of breathlessness (paraesophageal hernias)
- Use of over-the-counter medications, particularly antacids
- Diet and meal pattern
- Knowledge and understanding of planned surgery

#### Objective Data

Data to be collected to assess the patient undergoing hiatal hernia surgery include the following:

- Body weight
- Lung auscultation, particularly if patient has a history of smoking

#### Diagnostic Test Findings

1. Barium swallow with fluoroscopy—demonstrates presence of hernia
2. Abnormal esophageal and pH studies—demonstrate presence of reflux
3. Anemia—results from chronic low level bleeding

### ♦ NURSING DIAGNOSES

Nursing diagnoses are determined from analysis of patient data. Nursing diagnoses for the patient undergoing hiatal hernia repair may include but are not limited to the following:

| Diagnostic Title | Possible Etiologic Factors |
|---|---|
| Airway clearance, ineffective | Incisional pain |
| Swallowing, impaired | Functional changes of fundoplication surgery |

### ♦ EXPECTED PATIENT OUTCOMES

Expected patient outcomes for the patient undergoing hiatal hernia repair may include but are not limited to the following:

1. Maintains clear breath sounds without evidence of congestion or atelectasis.
2. Ingests a normal oral diet without aspiration or discomfort.
3. Maintains a stable body weight.
4. Adjusts eating style to avoid gas bloat and discomfort.

### ♦ INTERVENTIONS

#### Preoperative Care and Teaching

Preoperative teaching focuses on instructing the patient in deep breathing, correctly using incentive spirometry, and splinting the incision effectively for coughing. The surgical approaches all involve the diaphragm, and these exercises are essential to the prevention of respiratory complications. The high incision makes pulmonary hygiene painful, and it is essential to discuss the plan and approach to pain management with the patient. If a thoracic approach is used, teaching will also include the management of chest tubes. Individuals who are overweight are encouraged to lose weight if possible before surgery, and smokers are encouraged to significantly reduce or eliminate their use of tobacco. The nurse also teaches the patient about the nasogastric (NG) tube that will be inserted during surgery and will remain in place for several days, even when oral intake is restarted.

#### Facilitating Airway Clearance

Prevention of respiratory complications is the primary postoperative consideration. The head of the bed is elevated 30 degrees to facilitate lung expansion. The nurse assists the patient out of bed as soon as possible and supports the incision for coughing. Regular lung auscultation, incentive spirometry, and chest physiotherapy are routinely employed. Adequate analgesia is essential to the success of the respiratory protocol. It should be provided via patient-controlled analgesia, or through aggressive nursing management, particularly before ambulation or chest physiotherapy. Patients with a smoking or pulmonary disease history need to be managed even more aggressively.

### Facilitating Swallowing

A large-diameter NG tube is usually inserted during surgery to prevent the fundoplication from being made too tightly. The nurse monitors the tube postoperatively for secure anchoring and patency and regularly assesses the drainage, which should return to normal yellowish green gastric secretions within the first 8 hours after surgery. It should not contain fresh blood. It is essential that the stomach remain decompressed to prevent vomiting, which could disrupt the fundoplication sutures. Frequent oral and nasal hygiene is important for comfort, because the large tube is very irritating.

The patient is offered oral fluids after peristalsis has been reestablished. Some surgeons prefer to use **gastrostomy** feedings to facilitate healing, but most patients progress to a near-normal diet within 6 weeks. Temporary dysphagia is fairly universally present. The food storage area of the stomach is decreased after surgery. The nurse encourages the patient to eat multiple small meals throughout the day, gradually exploring tolerance to different foods and consistencies. Few foods ever need to be completely restricted. An upright position is also helpful. Support and encouragement during early feeding attempts are essential.

Many patients also experience temporary or persistent gas bloat from a compromised ability to belch as needed. The nurse teaches the patient to avoid carbonated beverages and gas-producing foods, and to remember to drink through a straw. Patients who swallow a lot of air need to eat and drink slowly and chew food thoroughly. Excess air in the stomach that cannot be relieved by belching produces significant abdominal discomfort. Frequent position changes and ambulation are often effective strategies for clearing air from the GI tract.

## ♦ EVALUATION

To evaluate the effectiveness of nursing interventions, compare patient behaviors with those stated in the expected patient outcomes. Successful achievement of patient outcomes for the patient with hiatal hernia repair is indicated by the following:

1. Has clear breath sounds and no evidence of atelectasis.
2. Ingests a normal oral diet.
3. Maintains stable body weight.
4. Report no gas bloat.

## ✸ SPECIAL CONSIDERATIONS FOR CARE OF THE GERONTOLOGIC PATIENT

The muscle weakness that develops in the esophageal hiatus is associated with aging. It is estimated that 60% of the over-60 age-group is affected by hiatal hernia.[6] The development of reflux symptoms in older individuals should be investigated and the possibility of hiatal hernia determined. The management, as outlined in the preceding discussion, is applicable to the elderly as well as the younger adult population. Primary considerations relate to the increased risk of surgical complications, particularly respiratory complications, and the need for vigilant postoperative nursing management.

## HOME CARE CONSIDERATIONS

Minimal ongoing care is required after hiatal hernia surgery, but lifting and stair climbing will be restricted until healing is complete. Relatively few dietary restrictions are in place at discharge, but the patient should continue to incorporate measures designed to facilitate swallowing and prevent air accumulation. Even with successful surgery, reflux may continue to some degree, and antireflux diet and life-style modifications may need to continue indefinitely. This can be discouraging to the individual who anticipated a complete cure from the procedure.

## COMPLICATIONS

Routine complications of hiatal hernia surgery include persistent dysphagia and gas bloat. In some cases dilation may be necessary to support effective swallowing. The surgery is not uniformly effective, and the individual may still face chronic and debilitating problems with gastroesophageal reflux.

**BOX 44-2 Causes of Dysphagia**

**INCOORDINATION OF SWALLOWING**

Upper motor neuron lesions such as CVA

**PHARYNGEAL WEAKNESS**

Disease or trauma of cranial nerves V, IX, and X
Brainstem disorders causing bulbar palsy (poliomyelitis, amyotrophic lateral sclerosis, multiple sclerosis)
Diseases affecting neuromuscular transmission (myasthenia gravis, botulism)
Diseases affecting striated muscle (muscular dystrophy, polymyositis)

**ESOPHAGEAL DISORDERS**

Obstructive disorders
- External compression by enlarged thyroid
- Internal narrowing by tumors or strictures

Motor esophageal disorders
- Achalasia, esophageal spasm

# ACHALASIA

## ETIOLOGY/EPIDEMIOLOGY

**Achalasia** is an uncommon disorder in which the lower esophageal muscles and sphincter fail to relax appropriately in response to swallowing. Its characteristic feature is chronic and progressively worsening **dysphagia.** Other conditions that can result in dysphagia are summarized in Box 44-2. The cause of true achalasia is unknown, although a familial factor is possible. Symptoms may be worsened by stress or overeating. Achalasia usually occurs in early or middle adulthood, although approximately one third of cases begin after age 60.[4] Both sexes are affected about equally, and there are no apparent cultural differences.

## PATHOPHYSIOLOGY

Although the exact pathophysiologic factors remain unclear, achalasia is theorized to result from a neuromuscular defect that is localized in the inner circular muscle layer of the esophagus. Degeneration of ganglion cells causes a loss of the nerves that innervate the smooth muscle. This causes both a failure of peristalsis and severe muscle spasm. Although no gross lesion is observable in the early stages, as the disease progresses, the portion of the esophagus around the constriction becomes dilated and the muscle walls hypertrophy (Figure 44-6). Although the severity of achalasia varies widely, the spasm may be extremely painful and so severe that little or no food can enter the stomach. In extreme cases the esophagus may hold a liter or more of food and fluid above the constricted area and slight or massive regurgitation may occur. **Halitosis** (foul mouth odor) and weight loss may be present. The classic "bird's beak" narrowing plus dilation are readily observable with barium studies. Esophageal manometry reveals an elevated resting LES pressure, combined with diminished or absent peristaltic waves. Clinical manifestations include:

1. Gradual onset dysphagia (usually includes both solids and liquids)
2. Pain—sometimes substernal
3. Regurgitation—slight or massive
4. Weight loss
5. Halitosis—from regurgitated or retained food

Other factors that should be considered in any workup of dysphagia are summarized in Box 44-3.

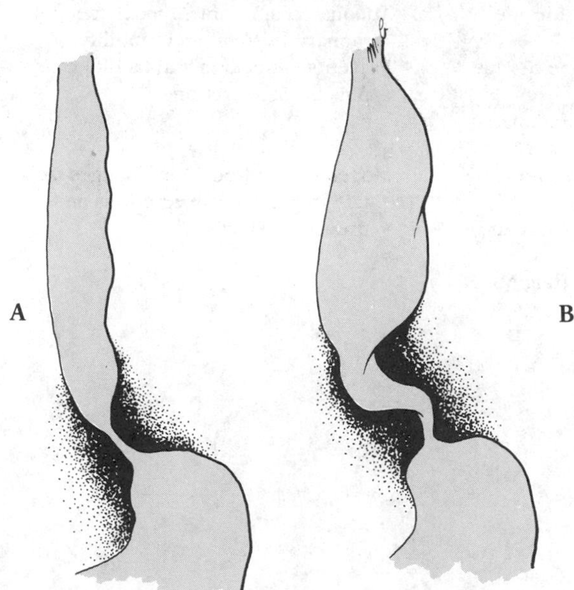


**FIGURE 44-6** Esophageal achalasia **A,** Early stage showing narrowing of lower esophagus. **B,** Advanced stage showing dilated middle esophagus. (From Price S, Wilson L: *Pathophysiology: clinical concepts of disease processes,* ed 4, St Louis, 1992, Mosby.)

## MEDICAL MANAGEMENT

Various categories of medications have been investigated in the attempt to lower esophageal pressures and relax the LES. Anticholinergics, nitrates, and calcium channel blockers have all been used, but none has proven to be of consistent value or effectiveness. Analgesics may be needed when pain is severe.

Forceful dilation of the esophagus has been a mainstay of treatment for achalasia, literally for centuries. The procedure, which is performed on an outpatient basis, involves passing polyurethane balloons on a catheter across the esophageal junction with the aid of fluoroscopy. The balloon is inflated to a predetermined level for 30 to 60 seconds. Some rupture of the esophageal sphincter muscle is expected. The procedure is repeated as needed. Motility is rarely improved, but 70% of patients report improvement in swallowing, and the procedure may be repeated in 2 to 3 months if needed.[8]

The surgical approach to achalasia involves esophagomyotomy, which uses longitudinal incisions to release the sphincter and facilitate passage of food. A success rate of 90% is reported with the surgery, which may use either a thoracic or abdominal approach. Antireflux fundoplication may be included, based on surgeon pref-

**BOX 44-3 Assessment of Dysphagia**

**SUBJECTIVE DATA**

Is there greater dysphagia with liquids or with solids?
Is dysphagia intermittent, or does it occur each time swallowing is attempted?
Are there other associated symptoms, such as pain with swallowing (odynophagia)?
What approaches to eating has the person found to be more effective?

**PHYSICAL ASSESSMENT**

Assessment of the gag reflex
Presence of drooling or facial droop
Movement of the larynx during swallowing

# NURSING CARE PLAN

## PERSON WITH HIATAL HERNIA

**DATA:** Mr. K. is a 56-year-old businessman with a 5-year history of progressively worsening heartburn. The pain is most severe at night. Recently he has noted the occurrence of regurgitation—sometimes of just "water" and other times of sour, acidic fluid. He has self-treated his problem with liquid antacid, but recently his wife has been urging him to seek medical help since he "always seems to be taking that stuff." He otherwise has an unremarkable medical history and considers himself to be in good health.

Mr. K.'s physician sent him for esophageal studies, which documented severe reflux. A barium swallow under fluoroscopy revealed a large sliding hiatal hernia, which shifted into the thorax with minimal position changes. An esophagoscopy revealed inflamed and minimally ulcerated tissue but no signs of cancer. The size of the hernia and rapid progression of his symptoms caused the physician to recommend surgical repair.

Mr. K. is admitted for hiatal hernia repair via Nissen fundoplication. In addition to the above data, the nursing history identified the following:

- Mr. K. has always been overweight but now carries about 40 extra pounds, concentrated in his abdomen.
- He has an almost 40-year history of cigarette smoking. He has made sincere efforts to cut down but still smokes about one half pack per day.
- Mr. K. considers his job to be quite stressful. He gets frequent headaches for which he takes aspirin or ibuprofen, usually several days each week.
- He is a moderate social drinker, stating, "Food is my real vice. There is nothing I enjoy more than a big meal." He snacks at night frequently while reading or when relaxing in bed and watching TV.
- He is extremely anxious about the surgery because he has never been hospitalized before.

Collaborative nursing actions before surgery include preparing Mr. K. for his imminent surgery, including:

- Clarifying knowledge and expectations concerning surgery.
- Preparing Mr. K. for the expected postoperative care, particularly the importance of respiratory hygiene.
- Implementing preoperative orders and providing Mr. K. with support and reassurance.

Mr. K. is returned to the unit directly after surgery. The surgery was successful and uneventful. He has an NG tube connected to low suction and IVs with boluses of Cimetidine and antibiotics. His incision is intact, with a Jackson Pratt drain. The planned abdominal approach was successful, and no chest tubes were utilized. He is groggy but alert when addressed by name and appears to be in significant pain.

### ■ NURSING DIAGNOSIS

Ineffective airway clearance related to incisional pain and limited mobility

| Expected Patient Outcome | Nursing Interventions | Rationale |
|---|---|---|
| Maintains clear breath sounds and effectively coughs up secretions. | Maintain head of bed in a semi-Fowler's position (at least 30 degrees). | Drops diaphragm and lungs to facilitate ventilation. |
| | Perform lung assessment q 2-4 hr. | Assesses for atelectasis and retained secretions. |
| | Monitor PCA pump or provide adequate narcotic analgesia. | Adequate pain control facilitates pulmonary hygiene and mobility. |
| | Supervise pulmonary hygiene q 4 hr.<br>Incentive spirometry.<br>Chest percussion and vibration.<br>Deep breathing q 1-2 hr. | Prevents atelectasis and facilitates expulsion of secretions. |
| | Assist with position changes and ambulation.<br>Splint incisions for movement and position changes.<br>Medicate ½ hr before getting Mr. K. out of bed. | Movement and position changes facilitate expulsion of secretions and prevent atelectasis. |

# NURSING CARE PLAN

## ■ NURSING DIAGNOSIS

Impaired swallowing related to the functional changes of fundoplication surgery

| Expected Patient Outcome | Nursing Interventions | Rationale |
|---|---|---|
| Successfully progresses from clear liquids to a normal diet without aspiration or discomfort. | Maintain initial NPO status and monitor patency of NG tube.<br>Do not irrigate or reposition the tube.<br>Report the incidence of any fresh blood in the drainage after 8 hr postop.<br>Offer frequent oral and nasal hygiene. | NG tube used is very large to preserve esophageal lumen.<br>Stomach must remain decompressed to prevent vomiting.<br>Tube movement or vomiting could disrupt the sutures.<br>Fresh bleeding indicates incisional complications. |
| | Initiate feedings with 30 ml of clear liquids once peristalsis is reestablished.<br>Evaluate presence and severity of dysphagia.<br>Advance to multiple small feedings.<br>Progress from liquids to solids as patient tolerates.<br>Encourage thorough chewing of small food boluses. | The food storage area of the stomach is significantly reduced, and the fundoplication induces a feeling of dysphagia.<br>Ability to swallow should improve slowly and steadily. |
| | Teach Mr. K. to avoid air swallowing and gas bloat.<br>Avoid carbonated beverages, use of straws, and gas producing foods.<br>Eat slowly and chew thoroughly.<br>Always eat sitting up.<br>Avoid excessive talking while eating.<br>Ambulate after meals. | The fundoplication usually makes belching difficult if not impossible.<br>Retained air and gas produce significant abdominal discomfort. |

## ■ NURSING DIAGNOSIS

Altered health maintenance related to lack of knowledge concerning measures to prevent reflux

| Expected Patient Outcome | Nursing Interventions | Rationale |
|---|---|---|
| Correctly identifies dietary and life-style changes to reduce the incidence of reflux. | Provide Mr. K. with instructions about diet modifications.<br>Eat small frequent meals.<br>Follow a low-fat diet and avoid excess tea, coffee, chocolate, and other caffeine-containing foods.<br>Strictly limit or eliminate alcohol.<br>Eat 4-6 small meals daily.<br>Eat slowly and chew food thoroughly.<br>Remain upright 1-2 hr after meals.<br>Never eat in bed.<br>Avoid evening snacking.<br>Reduce overall body weight.<br>Avoid any food that induces heartburn. | Fundoplication reduces the severity of reflux but does not eliminate it.<br>Foods that lower the LES pressure should be avoided. |
| | Discuss life-style modifications that can reduce the incidence of reflux.<br>Enroll in a smoking cessation program.<br>Avoid activities such as straining, lifting, and stooping.<br>Avoid constrictive clothing.<br>Never sleep flat in bed.<br>Elevate the head on a foam wedge for sleep.<br>Use antacids for occasional heartburn. Report frequent or severe episodes. | Smoking decreases the LES pressure significantly and can induce reflux.<br>Heavy lifting and straining increase abdominal pressure and can induce reflux. Reflux is more common and severe at night in the recumbent position. |

erence. The major drawbacks are related to the necessity for major abdominal or thoracic surgery.

## NURSING MANAGEMENT

Diet and life-style modifications play a role in the management of achalasia. The nurse encourages the individual to experiment with various types and consistencies of foods and meal sizes to evaluate their influence on swallowing. Small, frequent, semisoft meals are usually best tolerated. Warm liquids are recommended, and extremes of temperature should be avoided because they usually worsen the spasm. The nurse also advises the patient to experiment with changing positions during eating. Some individuals can swallow more effectively if they arch their back. The use of the **Valsalva maneuver** (bearing down with a closed glottis) while swallowing may help to propel food beyond the LES. Nocturnal reflux of retained food and fluid presents a significant risk for aspiration. The nurse instructs the patient to sleep on a foam wedge or with the head of the bed elevated.

Patients who undergo esophageal dilation are monitored after treatment for signs of perforation such as chest or shoulder pain, fever, subcutaneous emphysema, dyspnea, or shock. The nurse also assesses for hemoptysis and instructs the patient to expectorate rather than swallow secretions. The diet is restricted to liquids for about 24 hours. Care after myotomy is similar to that required for fundoplication (see p. 1449), with additional monitoring for complications such as perforation. Care after thoracotomy is discussed in Chapter 31.

# ESOPHAGEAL CARCINOMA

## ETIOLOGY

Both benign and malignant tumors occur in the esophagus. Benign tumors, usually leiomyomas, are extremely rare and frequently asymptomatic; they require no care unless symptoms necessitate local excision.

Malignant tumors of the esophagus are not common, but they assume increased importance because of their virulence. Cancer of the esophagus is almost always fatal, with 5-year survival rates at less than 8%.[12] The tumor is almost never diagnosed early enough to allow for effective treatment.

Both geographic and environmental factors play a role in the development of esophageal cancer. The long-term heavy use of alcohol and tobacco appear to be the most significant etiologic factors in the Western world. In other parts of the world, however, where esophageal cancer is quite common, development of the tumor is clearly linked to high levels of nitrosamines and other contaminants in the soil and foods. Diets that are chronically inadequate in fresh fruits, vegetables, vitamins, and certain proteins are also implicated. The long-term effects of other esophageal problems, such as stricture, achalasia, and particularly GERD, also are linked, but only in a relatively minor way.

## EPIDEMIOLOGY

Although there have been statistically significant annual increases in the incidence of cancer of the esophagus over the past several decades, particularly among the African-American population, the tumor still accounts for less than 2% of all newly diagnosed cancers and 7% of gastrointestinal tract cancers in the United States.[9]

The disease typically affects men between the ages of 50 and 80 years. It occurs in men four times as often as in women and in African-Americans four times as often as in whites. The racial differences are even more dramatic in the mortality statistics. Death from cancer of the esophagus now ranks second in cancer deaths behind death from lung cancer for the African-American male population.[9] Asian males also have a significantly higher incidence of and mortality from esophageal cancer.

Low incidence statistics for esophageal cancer are unique to the United States and the Western world. Localized areas of China, the former Soviet Union, Iran, and southern Africa have such high incidence that 30% to 40% of the local population are at risk of dying from cancer of the esophagus.[12] The environmental factors involved in such extreme variations are under close investigation.

## PATHOPHYSIOLOGY

Tumors may develop at any point along the length of the esophagus, but the majority occur in the middle and lower two thirds. Squamous cell tumors have typically predominated. They tend to develop in the middle third and are clearly related to the risk factors of smoking and alcohol use. Adenocarcinomas represent the remaining minority of tumors. These tend to develop in the lower third of the esophagus and may evolve from the Barrett's epithelium, which develops in response to the irritation of chronic reflux. An alarming trend has recently been noted in the incidence statistics. Adenocarcinomas have increased dramatically, particularly in middle-aged white men, but reasons for the shift are unknown.

Esophageal tumors of all types appear to emerge as part of an initially slow process that begins with benign tissue changes. Local growth of the tumor is rapid, and early spread is common because of the rich lymphatic supply found in the esophagus. Tumors are characteristically intraluminal and ulcerating, with a tendency to encircle the esophageal wall, as well as extend up or down the length.

Spread of the carcinoma is by local invasion or through the bloodstream or lymphatics. Neoplasms of the upper and middle esophagus may extend into the pulmonary system and those of the lower esophagus into the diaphragm, vertebrae, or heart. Metastasis is present in about 80% of esophageal cancers at the time of diagnosis.

Early diagnosis is rare, and tumors of less than 10 cm are considered small. Persons typically complain of symptoms related to obstruction, dysphagia, or reflux.

**BOX 44-4 Clinical Manifestations of Esophageal Cancer**

- Early disease is largely asymptomatic
- Gradually progressive dysphagia
  - Usually not present until 60% of diameter is obstructed
  - Progresses typically from solids to liquids
  - Continuous, not intermittent
- Odynophagia—typically a steady, dull substernal pain
- Regurgitation—foul breath from retained food in esophagus
- Heartburn
- Vomiting
- Anorexia
- Weight loss—up to 40 lb in 2-3 mo is common

Pulmonary complications such as fistula formation or aspiration are common, and complete obstruction is inevitable without successful therapy. Box 44-4 summarizes the common clinical manifestations of esophageal cancer.

## PREVENTION

The incidence of cancer of the esophagus in the United States is clearly linked to the heavy and long-term use of tobacco and alcohol. **Primary prevention** strategies focus on moderation or elimination of consumption, particularly in the African-American male population. Ensuring adequate intake of fresh fruits and vegetables to maintain appropriate levels of vitamins A and C is recommended. **Secondary prevention** focuses on early diagnosis, which represents the only hope for successful treatment. Any individual who has difficulty swallowing, no matter how trivial, is urged to seek medical advice promptly. Adequate control and treatment of other esophageal disorders, such as reflux or achalasia, are also recommended.

## MEDICAL MANAGEMENT

The expected length of stay of patients with cancer of the esophagus as determined by DRG is 14 days. Common medical therapy for management of cancer of the esophagus includes the following.

### Diagnostic Tests

The barium swallow with fluoroscopy is the primary diagnostic tool. Large masses will be clearly outlined. Endoscopy allows for direct visual inspection and the obtaining of cytologic samples and biopsy specimens. CT scans may be employed to evaluate the extent of the tumor.

### Medication

Primary treatment of esophageal cancer increasingly includes combinations of various antineoplastic agents. Chemotherapy is most effective when combined with radiation and/or surgery. Cisplatin is frequently included in the protocol. Antacids and analgesics may also be included for symptom management.

### Treatment

Treatment decisions are based on the location and size of the tumor, degree of metastasis, and the individual's health status. Nonsurgical options are usually selected when the individual is unable or unwilling to undergo radical surgery. They focus on palliation of symptoms. Options include radiation therapy, dilation of strictures, and prosthesis insertion, as well as chemotherapy.

#### Radiation therapy

Radiation therapy is the treatment of choice for palliation. It reduces tumor size and gives consistent long-term symptom relief, but it may lead to debilitating stricture or stenosis, since esophageal tissue is extremely sensitive to radiation. The treatment is spread over 6 to 8 weeks to minimize the edema and epithelial desquamation, which often lead to acute esophagitis and odynophagia. Anorexia, nausea, and vomiting may also occur.

The nurse assesses the individual frequently. Regular, gentle mouth care is essential because the patient is at risk for monilial esophagitis. The nurse encourages the use of oral lidocaine before meals. The diet is modified to increase comfort while still supporting nutritional needs. Small, frequent meals and soft or semiliquid foods are recommended. Sweet, light foods may be best tolerated, and protein powder drink supplements are a useful strategy. Additional interventions for radiation therapy are discussed in Chapter 16. Palliative relief may also be obtained through the YAG laser, which "vaporizes" a part of the tumor to open the esophagus.

#### Dilation

Esophageal dilation is performed as needed throughout therapy to relieve dysphagia resulting from either tumor obstruction or radiation stricture. The malignant esophageal tumor may be dilated safely by skilled physicians, and the treatment is employed as needed to preserve swallowing (see discussion under Achalasia, p. 1455).

#### Prosthesis insertion

A semirigid prosthesis may be inserted into the esophagus to bypass an obstruction or fistula. The procedure preserves swallowing and a patent esophagus, but it carries the significant risk of aspiration, dislodgement, or esophageal perforation. The prosthesis disrupts the function of the LES and permits free reflux of gastric contents. The nurse encourages the patient to eat small, frequent meals, eat only in an upright sitting position, and carefully follow all guidelines for positioning and activity to prevent reflux. Lying flat in bed could be life-threatening with the risk of reflux aspiration.

### Diet

Maintaining adequate nutrition as the disease progresses is the primary consideration. The diet is modified as

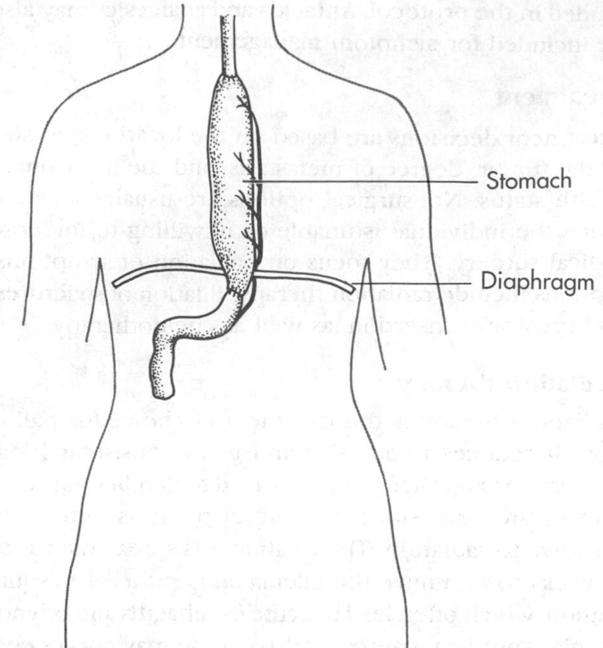

FIGURE 44-7 Esophagogastrostomy for esophageal cancer.

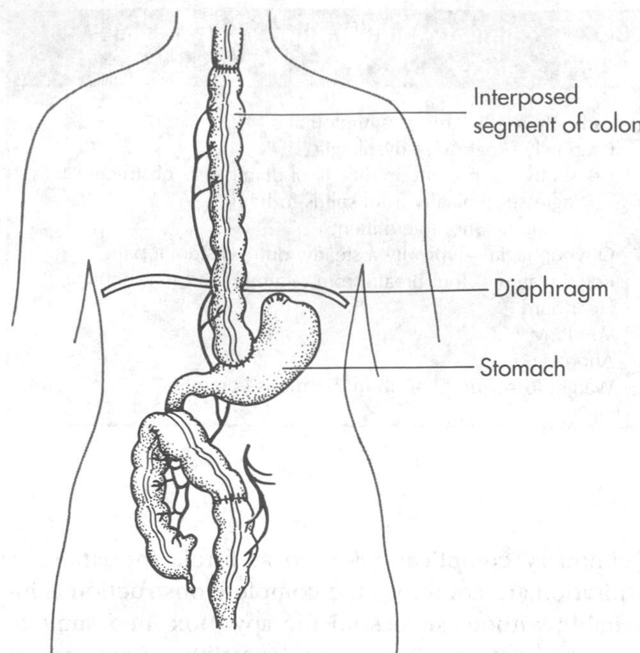

FIGURE 44-8 Esophagectomy with colon interposition.

needed as dysphagia worsens. Tube or gastrostomy feedings and short-course hyperalimentation may all be needed at some point in the disease process.

## Activity

The individual is encouraged to remain as active as the condition and treatment allow. Positioning and activity restrictions are important for individuals experiencing frequent reflux or regurgitation. The nurse teaches the patient to remain upright for several hours after meals, to avoid all bending, stooping, or lifting, and to never lie down in a flat position. The head should always be elevated at least 30 to 45 degrees.

## Referral/Consultation

In some settings the nurse assumes responsibility for making referrals to other services. Nutritional support services are frequently needed to plan feeding approaches for the patient and to ensure adequate nutrients. Patients also frequently need significant assistance at home, particularly after radical surgery, and the nurse coordinates these referrals as part of the discharge planning.

# SURGICAL MANAGEMENT

Radical surgery is the only definitive treatment for esophageal cancer, and it is the treatment of choice for otherwise healthy individuals. The surgeries are extensive, with a high mortality rate, especially for patients with concurrent health problems. Disease survival rates are extremely low, even with radical procedures. Subtotal or total esophagectomy is usually required. Although several procedural options exist, the preferred surgery is the esophagogastrostomy in which the diseased portion of the esophagus is removed. The cervical stump is anastomosed to the stomach, which is drawn up into the thorax through the esophageal hiatus (Figure 44-7). The procedure is the simplest, but it still involves both laparotomy and thoracotomy incisions. If the tumor also involves the stomach, the surgeon may perform a colon interposition by substituting a portion of the right or left colon for the esophagus (Figure 44-8).

In addition to the usual complex surgical risks of shock, hemorrhage, and infection, these procedures also create a serious risk of leakage at the anastomosis site, particularly with colon interpositions. Even when surgical healing is successful, the patient remains at serious risk for aspiration from the elimination of the sphincter protection of the LES. Discussion of nursing management of the patient undergoing surgery for cancer of the esophagus follows.

# NURSING MANAGEMENT: The Patient Undergoing Surgery for Cancer of the Esophagus

## ♦ ASSESSMENT

### Subjective Data

Data to be collected to assess the patient undergoing surgery for cancer of the esophagus include the following:

Early symptoms are quite rare

Dysphagia (appears once the esophagus is 60% obstructed)[11]
- Duration, severity, and extent
- Progressive from solids to liquids
- Continuous rather than intermittent

Diet patterns and modifications made in response to dysphagia
Presence of anorexia or nausea
Presence of odynophagia—steady, dull, substernal pain
Regurgitation and vomiting—frequency and severity
History of alcohol and/or tobacco use
Knowledge and understanding of planned surgery and its functional outcomes

## Objective Data

Data to be collected to assess the patient undergoing surgery for cancer of the esophagus include the following:

Current weight and recent weight loss—up to 40 pounds in 2 to 3 months is common
Height/weight balance
Nutritional status
Presence of foul breath odor—retained food in the esophagus

## Diagnostic Test Findings

1. Barium swallow—outlines tumor obstruction
2. Positive biopsy and/or cytology findings

# ♦ NURSING DIAGNOSES

Nursing diagnoses are determined from analysis of patient data. Nursing diagnoses for the patient undergoing surgery for esophageal cancer may include but are not limited to the following:

| Diagnostic Title | Possible Etiologic Factors |
|---|---|
| Aspiration, high risk for | Loss of LES sphincter function |
| Nutrition, altered: less than body requirements | Acute dysphagia |
| Grieving, anticipatory | Shortened life expectancy |

# ♦ EXPECTED PATIENT OUTCOMES

Expected outcomes for the patient undergoing surgery for esophageal cancer may include but are not limited to the following:

1a. Maintains a patent airway.
b. Lungs are clear to auscultation.
2a. Does not lose additional weight.
b. Consumes sufficient nutrients and calories to meet daily needs.
3. Adapts to the physical changes and prognosis as evidenced by:
a. Seeking support from family and friends.
b. Discussing losses.
c. Making realistic plans for the future.

# ♦ INTERVENTIONS

## Preoperative Preparation

The duration of preoperative preparation is largely determined by the patient's nutritional status. Nutritional support is provided as needed via tube feedings or hyperalimentation. Intake and output, total daily calories, and body weight are all carefully monitored. The nurse encourages the patient to perform frequent mouth care to reduce the risk of postoperative infection, since the patient may be regurgitating retained food particles, blood, or pus from the tumor. Mouthwashes can help to control foul mouth odors and make oral intake more palatable. Dental problems will also usually be corrected before surgery, particularly if radiation treatment is planned.

The nurse ensures that the patient and family are knowledgeable about the planned surgery and its expected outcomes. Specific teaching will include the purpose, number, and location of all incisions, lines, and tubes; wound drainage, chest, and NG tubes; and intravenous (IV) lines. Pulmonary hygiene is a major focus of postoperative care, and the nurse instructs the patient about the importance of turning and deep breathing regimens and other aspects of chest physiotherapy. Practice time is provided. The possibility of temporary ventilator support is also introduced. If a colon interposition procedure is planned, a complete bowel preparation will also be necessary in the preoperative period.

The nurse encourages the patient to verbalize feelings and concerns related to this extensive surgery. It is natural for the patient to be both extremely anxious and ambivalent about the surgery. Family members are encouraged to be involved in all teaching sessions, and all caregivers should be familiar with the patient's wishes as expressed through advance directives.

## Protecting the Airway

The patient receives routine but meticulous postoperative care, since the extensive nature of the surgery increases the risk of serious complications. Respiratory care is the highest priority. The patient typically remains intubated for the first 24 hours. Respiratory assessment is documented every 1 to 2 hours, and vigorous turning, deep breathing, coughing, suctioning, and chest physiotherapy routines are utilized. Adequate analgesia is essential to the achievement of respiratory goals. The nurse assists the patient to adequately splint major incisions for turning and coughing, and ensures that appropriate narcotic analgesia is being provided.

The patient is placed in a semi-Fowler's or high Fowler's position to support ventilation and prevent regurgitation and reflux. Supplemental oxygen is administered routinely, and blood gases or $O_2$ saturation is monitored. The nurse ensures the patency of the chest tubes and water seal drainage system.

The multiple incisions and drains significantly increase the potential for problems with wound healing.

Anastomosis leakage is a serious complication that can compromise the airway or pulmonary gas exchange. The risk is highest 5 to 9 days after surgery. Prompt identification of leakage is essential. The nurse monitors for signs of inflammation, fever, or fluid accumulation. Early symptoms of shock such as tachycardia, tachypnea, or restlessness may be the first warnings.

## Promoting Adequate Nutrition

The patient is usually allowed nothing by mouth for 4 to 5 days until GI motility is well reestablished. The NG tube is carefully secured and monitored frequently to prevent movement or dislodgement, which might disrupt the sutures at the anastomosis sites. The tube is *not* irrigated or repositioned. The initial NG drainage is bloody, but it should gradually resume a normal greenish-yellow color by the end of the first postoperative day. The continued presence of blood might indicate oozing at the suture line. Frequent oral hygiene is provided.

After an initial period of stabilization, the patient is given 3 to 5 ml of water every 15 to 30 minutes throughout the day. The quantity is gradually increased if it is tolerated. The nurse supervises the patient during all initial swallowing efforts, and ensures that an upright position is maintained. The NG tube remains in place while oral fluids are introduced because esophageal tissue is very friable and bleeds easily. The surgical area needs to remain decompressed to protect the anastomoses.

The patient is slowly progressed to a pureed or semisolid diet if problems do not develop. The nurse assists the patient to carefully determine the amount and type of foods and fluids that can be safely and comfortably swallowed. Small meals are essential because the food storage area of the stomach is radically decreased. Initially patients may experience a feeling of fullness in the chest, or shortness of breath with meals. Adjusting meal size and progressing slowly usually alleviates these problems. The process of gradually resuming oral nutrition will continue into the postdischarge period and requires patience. Calorie counts and daily weights assist in the ongoing evaluation of the patient's nutritional status.

## Promoting Grief Resolution and Coping

Despite the radical surgery, the patient with esophageal cancer still has a terminal illness and dramatically shortened life expectancy. Considerable psychologic support is provided to the individual patient and family in their efforts to cope with the diagnosis, prognosis, and physical limitations of the disease. The nurse places emphasis on the improved quality of life that treatment affords. Realistic planning is important, since the patient's condition will inevitably worsen. The nurse encourages the patient and family to talk about the situation together, make realistic plans, and seek out supports available in the community.

### Guidelines for Care of the Person Experiencing Esophageal Surgery

**PREOPERATIVE CARE**

1. Encourage improved nutritional status
   a. High-protein, high-calorie diet if oral diet is possible
   b. Total parenteral nutrition may be necessary for severe dysphagia or obstruction
2. Give good mouth care; breath may be foul
3. Give preoperative preparation appropriate for thoracic surgery
4. Give prescribed antibiotics before esophageal resection or bypass

**POSTOPERATIVE CARE**

1. Promote good pulmonary ventilation
2. Maintain chest drainage system as prescribed
3. Maintain gastric drainage system
   a. Small amounts of blood may drain from nasogastric tube for 6 to 12 hr after surgery
   b. Do not disturb nasogastric tube (to prevent traction on suture line)
4. Maintain nutrition
   a. Start clear fluids at frequent intervals when oral intake is permitted
   b. Introduce soft foods gradually, and slowly progress to several small meals of bland foods
5. Prevent aspiration if LES is removed or disrupted
   a. Always raise the head of the bed for swallowing food or liquid
   b. Head of the bed must be elevated for sleeping
   c. Bending or stooping must be avoided
   d. Keep suction apparatus available at the bedside

## ♦ EVALUATION

To evaluate the effectiveness of nursing interventions, compare patient behaviors with those stated in the expected patient outcomes. Successful achievement of patient outcomes for the patient undergoing surgery for cancer of the esophagus is indicated by the following:

1a. Has a patent airway.
 b. Has clear lung fields on auscultation.
2a. Has a stable weight.
 b. Ingests adequate daily calories and nutrients.
3a. Utilizes family and friendship supports.
 b. Verbalizes loss and grief.
 c. Has established realistic plans for the future.

The Guidelines box above summarizes major nursing care considerations following esophageal surgery.

# ✷ SPECIAL CONSIDERATIONS FOR CARE OF THE GERONTOLOGIC PATIENT

Cancer of the esophagus is usually identified in late middle age or in the elderly population. These patients have a high incidence of chronic health problems, which makes the risks of radical surgery more extensive. Postoperative complications are both more common and more severe. These patients are also less likely to have family and support networks to help them manage their care after discharge. The nurse must be vigilant in assessing the need for postdischarge assistance and initiating needed referrals.

## ❦ HOME CARE CONSIDERATIONS

Most patients with cancer of the esophagus require a significant amount of assistance after discharge. Even without major postoperative complications, the patient will need to deal with ongoing respiratory care, wound healing concerns, and nutrition support. The care initiated in the hospital continues after discharge, and both the patient and family need to be well informed about its components. Essential concerns include pulmonary hygiene, which may include chest physiotherapy. Any surgery that removes or disrupts the LES necessitates constant care with positioning to protect the airway and prevent reflux or regurgitation. No anatomic protection remains, and the risk of aspiration is constant. Wound healing also remains a concern, and the incisions need to be inspected regularly for signs of infection. Nutritional recovery is ongoing. The patient and family will slowly explore the range of food tolerance to meet nutrient needs. Home preparations of egg nogs or milkshakes may be used to supplement calories and nutrients. The family may also need to learn to manage tube feedings or hyperalimentation. The nurse encourages the family to seek out and utilize supports such as those available from the American Cancer Society. Hospice referrals may be appropriate for later stage disease.

### COMPLICATIONS

Esophageal cancer is a terminal illness, and complications are expected. Tumor regrowth may cause recurrent dysphagia and obstruction. Weight loss may persist. The very high risk of aspiration from regurgitation makes pulmonary complications common. Tumor regrowth, invasion, and metastasis create problems with chronic pain, bleeding, and fistula development.

## ESOPHAGEAL DIVERTICULA

### ETIOLOGY/EPIDEMIOLOGY

An esophageal diverticulum is an outpouching of the esophageal mucosa and submucosa that creates a blind pouch in which foods and liquids are trapped. After a sufficient quantity of food material accumulates in the pouch, it overflows back into the esophagus and is frequently regurgitated. Although **diverticula** may develop at any point along the esophagus, they are most commonly found at the pharyngoesophageal junction (Zenker's diverticulum). Diverticula may develop from congenital weaknesses of the esophageal wall, esophageal trauma, or the development of fibrotic scar tissue in response to chronic inflammation or erosion. The incidence of all types is rare.

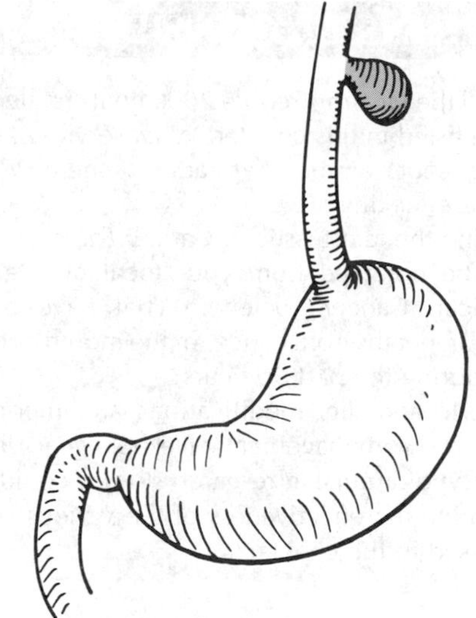

**FIGURE 44-9** Esophageal diverticulum.

### PATHOPHYSIOLOGY

Diverticula result when a portion of the muscular layer of the esophagus becomes weakened (Figure 44-9). Since the herniated portion of the esophageal mucosa is without the protection of the muscle layer, the diverticulum creates a significant risk of perforation. There is also always a danger that some of the regurgitated material may be aspirated into the trachea and lungs, especially during sleep.

Patients often complain of symptoms similar to those of achalasia. Typical symptoms include dysphagia, regurgitation, halitosis, feelings of pressure or fullness in the throat, and nocturnal cough.

### MEDICAL MANAGEMENT

Diverticula can be readily diagnosed on barium swallow. Endoscopy is performed with care to reduce the risk of accidental perforation. Conservative management includes positioning and diet modifications. Surgical management involves excision of the herniated sac and reapproximation of the mucosa.

### NURSING MANAGEMENT

The nurse assists the patient to explore variations in food texture, consistency, and quantity. Small meals composed of semisoft foods are usually best tolerated and may reduce or eliminate the problems of pressure and reflux. Frequent oral hygiene along with mouthwashes is encouraged to control odor. The nurse encourages the patient to sleep with the head elevated to reduce the risk of nighttime reflux and aspiration. Nursing care of the patient undergoing esophageal surgery is summarized in the Guidelines box, p. 1462.

## QUESTIONS TO CONSIDER

- Reread the *Healthy People 2000* goals related to oral health listed in this chapter. What services are available in your community to address them? What services are lacking?
- Examine the latest issue of *Cancer Facts and Figures* (may be obtained from your local chapter of the American Cancer Society). What have been the trends in deaths from cancer of the mouth and esophagus during the past 30 years?
- Life-style and diet modifications are important aspects in the management of esophageal disorders. What type of nursing research studies could help to determine the effectiveness of the various strategies discussed in the chapter?

## CRITICAL THINKING ACTIVITIES

- You are reviewing the history and physical assessment of Mrs. Frost, 79, a newly admitted patient to the medical unit. You note that she has a history of polymyositis, asthma, and diverticulitis. Her primary complaint is that she has had difficulty swallowing over the past 3 to 4 months, and she states that she has lost 10 pounds recently. All other data are within normal limits. Is additional data required to plan care for this patient? If so, what other information should be gathered?
- From the case just mentioned, what data in Mrs. Frost's history would lead the nurse to think that Mrs. Frost may be suffering from achalasia?

## CHAPTER SUMMARY

### DENTAL DISORDERS

- Oral health can be promoted by good nutrition, good oral hygiene, fluoridation of water supplies, regular dental examinations and care, and avoidance of alcohol and tobacco use.

### MOUTH INFECTIONS

- Common infections of the mouth include aphthous stomatitis (canker sore), herpetic stomatitis (cold sore, fever blister), Vincent's angina, thrush, and parotitis.
- Mouth care for mouth infections includes frequent rinsing with alkaline mouthwash or diluted hydrogen peroxide and cleaning gums and teeth with a toothette or a gauze-wrapped tongue blade if a toothbrush causes pain. Hot, spicy, or irritating foods should be avoided.

### CANCER OF THE MOUTH

- Contributing factors to cancer of the mouth and esophagus include alcohol and heavy smoking.
- Carcinoma of the mouth can occur on the lips, the anterior tongue and floor of the mouth, and in the salivary glands. Treatment is by surgery and/or radiation.
- After surgery of the mouth for cancer, the patient may have problems with body image, verbal communication, eating, and mouth discomfort.

### PROBLEMS OF THE ESOPHAGUS

- Common esophageal disorders include gastroesophageal reflux, hiatal hernia, cancer, achalasia, and diverticuli. Dysphagia is a common symptom of esophageal disorders.
- Gastroesophageal reflux may result from an incompetent lower esophageal sphincter (LES), pregnancy, obesity, ascites, or hiatal hernia, or after resection of the lower esophagus. Heartburn is a major symptom. Management includes medications (antacids, histamine [$H_2$] receptor antagonists); surgery for hiatal hernia; high-protein, low-fat diet; avoidance of smoking and alcohol, as well as foods and beverages containing caffeine or xanthines; avoidance of activities that increase abdominal pressure; and sleeping with the head elevated to prevent reflux.
- Achalasia results from aperistalsis and a failure of the LES to relax in response to swallowing. Treatment consists of dilation with pneumatic dilators or cardiomyotomy.
- Esophageal diverticula are outpouches of the esophagus where food collects, causing regurgitation and possible obstruction. Treatment is by surgical excision or myotomy.
- There are two types of hiatal hernias: sliding and paraesophageal. They are usually asymptomatic but may cause problems with reflux.
- Hiatal hernias may be treated surgically if symptoms are severe. There is a variety of procedures, but all of them involve some form of fundoplication (wrapping the stomach fundus around the distal esophagus to reinforce the LES).
- Risk factors for cancer of the esophagus include smoking, alcohol, and achalasia. Any person with dysphagia should be urged to consult a physician.
- Cancer of the esophagus has a poor prognosis, because metastasis is usually present when the diagnosis is made. Treatment is by surgery, radiation, and chemotherapy.
- Postoperative care for esophageal cancer includes promotion of pulmonary ventilation, maintenance of gastric drainage systems, encouragement of good nutrition when eating is permitted, and good mouth care.

## REFERENCES


1. Bhaskar SN, Lilly GE, Pratt LW: A practical, high yield mouth exam, *Patient Care* 24(2):53-74, 1990.
2. Castell DO, Holtz A: Gastroesophageal reflux—don't forget to ask about heartburn, *Postgrad Med* 86(5):141-148, 1989.
3. Chen J, et al: Changing trends in oral cancer in the United States, 1935 to 1985: a Connecticut study, *J Oral Maxillofac Surg* 49(11):1152-1158, 1991.
4. Clouse RE, Abramson BD, and Todorczvk JR: Achalasia in the elderly, *Dig Dis Sci* 36(2):225-228, 1991.
5. Coleman GC, Nelson JF: *Principles of oral diagnosis,* St Louis, 1993, Mosby.
6. Ellis FH: Diaphragmatic hiatal hernias, *Postgrad Med* 88(1):113-124, 1990.
7. Evans DF et al: An objective evaluation of the Angelchik antireflux prosthesis, *Ann Royal Coll Surg* 73(6):355-360, 1991.
8. Ferguson MK: Achalasia: current evaluation and therapy, *Ann Thorac Surg* 52(2):336-342, 1991.
9. Foltz AT: Nutritional factors in the prevention of gastrointestinal cancer, *Semin Oncol Nurs* 4(4):239-245, 1988.
10. Hamilton JW, et al: Sleeping on a wedge diminishes exposure of the esophagus to refluxed acid, *Dig Dis Sci* 33(5):518-522, 1988.
11. Kelsen D, et al: Alarming trends in esophageal cancer, *Patient Care* 26(16):72-122, 1992.
12. Mayer R: Gastrointestinal cancer. In Rubenstein E, Federman D, editors: *Scientific American medicine,* New York, 1988, Scientific American.
13. Medvec BR: Esophageal cancer: treatment and nursing interventions. *Semin Oncol Nurs* 4(4):246-256, 1988.
14. Richter JE: Gastroesophageal reflux: diagnosis and management, *Hosp Pract* 27(1):59-66, 1992.
15. Sterling TD, Rosenbaum WL, Weinkam JJ: Analysis of the relationship between smokeless tobacco and cancer based on data from the National Mortality Followback Survey, *J Clin Epidemiol* 45(3):223-231, 1992.
16. U.S. Department of Health and Human Services, Public Health Service: *Healthy People 2000: summary report,* Boston, 1992, Jones & Bartlett.

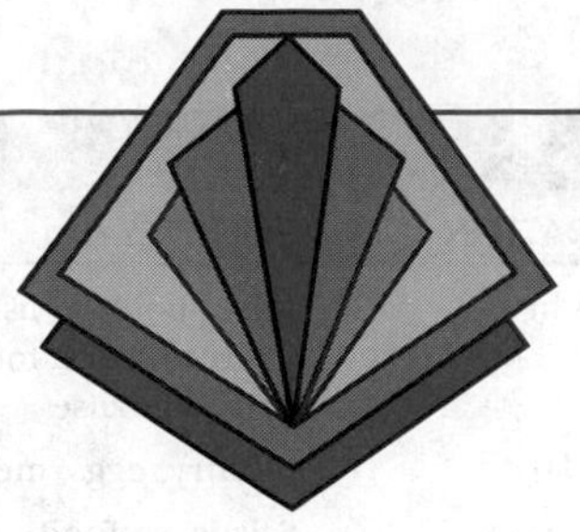

C H A P T E R 45

# Management of Persons With Problems of the Stomach and Duodenum

*Judith K. Sands*

## CHAPTER OBJECTIVES

***After studying this chapter, the learner should be able to do the following:***

1. Discuss the etiology and epidemiology of common problems affecting the stomach and duodenum.
2. Describe the roles of acid oversecretion, impaired mucosal defenses, and *Helicobacter pylori* infection in the development of gastritis and peptic ulcer disease.
3. Discuss the medical and surgical management of peptic ulcer disease and its complications.
4. Describe appropriate nursing interventions for the management of peptic ulcer disease and its complications.
5. Explain the role of surgery in the management of morbid obesity.
6. Discuss the medical and nursing management of gastric cancer.
7. Outline essential nursing care associated with gastric surgery.

## KEY TERMS

| | | |
|---|---|---|
| antrectomy | gastritis | Roux-en-Y gastric bypass |
| dumping syndrome | gastroplasty | stress ulcer |
| duodenal ulcer | *H. pylori* | truncal vagotomy |
| gastrectomy | peptic ulcer | vagotomy |
| gastric ulcer | peritonitis | Zollinger-Ellison syndrome |
| gastrinoma | pyloroplasty | |

# GASTRITIS

## ETIOLOGY/EPIDEMIOLOGY

**Gastritis,** which is a diffuse or localized inflammation of the gastric mucosa, is the most common pathologic condition of the stomach. It may be acute or chronic and can be triggered by a variety of factors.

*Acute gastritis* is a short-term inflammatory process that may be related to the ingestion of chemical agents or food products that irritate and erode the gastric mucosa. Examples include food seasonings and spices, alcohol, drugs (nonsteroidal antiinflammatory drugs [NSAIDs], aspirin, iron salts), and corrosive agents such as cleaning fluids or kerosene. Acute gastritis is a common problem after radiation treatment or cancer chemotherapy. Bacteria such as salmonella or staphylococci also can produce acute gastritis if they contaminate food. Agents involved in bacterial food poisoning are summarized in Table 45-1.

*Chronic gastritis* is a separate entity from acute gastritis rather than a chronic form of it. It can be subdivided into types A and B. Type A is believed to be basically autoimmune in nature and involves all of the acid-secreting gastric tissue, particularly the tissue in the fundus. Circulating antibodies are produced that attack the gastric parietal cells and eventually may cause pernicious anemia from loss of the intrinsic factor. Type B is more common and is almost always associated with infection by ***Helicobacter pylori,*** which is currently believed to be a direct cause of the gastritis rather than a secondary invader.[6] It involves primarily the fundus and the antrum of the stomach. The infection damages the

**TABLE 45-1 Bacterial Food Poisoning**

| ORGANISM | VOMITING | DIARRHEA | FEVER | ONSET | DURATION | SOURCES |
|---|---|---|---|---|---|---|
| *Staphylococcus aureus* | Severe | Occasionally | — | 1-8 hr | 8-24 hr | Meat, poultry, fish, cream-filled foods, mayonnaise |
| *Salmonella* | Occasionally | + | + | 8-48 hr | 2-5 days | Poultry, eggs, meat |
| *Shigella* | Occasionally | + | + | 24-72 hr | 3-7 days | Salads, seafood |
| *Escherichia coli* | Rare | + | — | 24-72 hr | 1-3 days | Uncooked foods, contaminated water |
| *Campylobacter jejuni* | — | Severe | + | 1-10 days | 2-7 days | Meat, poultry, fish, mushrooms, contaminated water |
| *Clostridium perfringens* | Occasionally | Severe | — | 8-16 hr | 1-4 days | Rewarmed foods |
| *Clostridium botulinum* | Occasionally (diplopia, dysphagia, respiratory failure may occur) | Rare | — | 24-96 hr | High mortality | Improperly canned foods |

mucosal protective mechanisms and leaves the mucosa vulnerable to the effects of alcohol, smoking, gastric acid, and alkaline reflux from the duodenum (see discussion of peptic ulcer disease beginning on p. 1469 for a more complete discussion of the role of *H. pylori* infection).

## PATHOPHYSIOLOGY

Acute gastritis develops when the protective mechanisms of the mucosa are overwhelmed by the presence of bacteria or irritating substances. Mucus is a poor protector against chemical injury. Regeneration of the gastric mucosa after injury is both prompt and efficient, however, and the disorder usually is self-limiting once the irritating agent is removed. Common symptoms include anorexia, nausea and vomiting, abdominal cramping or diarrhea, epigastric pain, and fever. Painless gastrointestinal (GI) bleeding may occur and is more likely if the person uses aspirin or NSAIDs regularly.

Type A chronic gastritis is associated with atrophy of the gastric glands and thinning or deterioration of the mucosa. There is an eventual decrease in gastric secretions. The antibody attack on the parietal cells is believed to be autoimmune in nature. Atrophic gastritis may be a precursor to gastric cancer. The condition is frequently asymptomatic until problems related to pernicious anemia develop.

Type B chronic gastritis is characterized by the presence of *H. pylori* bacteria. The bacteria can survive in the strongly acidic environment of the stomach and impair the normal mucosal protections. The presence of *H. pylori* bacteria creates an environment that is conducive to ulceration. Again the condition may be asymptomatic, or the patient may have mild dyspepsia or classic ulcer symptoms.

## MEDICAL MANAGEMENT

Mild acute gastritis is treated symptomatically. The patient is encouraged to follow a bland or liquid diet until discomfort resolves. Antacids are used for symptomatic relief. Severe cases may necessitate hospitalization for fluid and electrolyte replacement or the treatment of bleeding or complications.

Treatment of type A chronic gastritis focuses on the management of the underlying systemic disease. Vitamin $B_{12}$ is administered if pernicious anemia occurs. Type B is treated symptomatically with standard ulcer medications such as antacids, sucralfate, or histamine$_2$ ($H_2$) receptor antagonists. Definitive treatment also includes medications to eradicate the presence of *H. pylori* (see discussion of peptic ulcer disease).

## NURSING MANAGEMENT

The role of the nurse while caring for patients with acute gastritis primarily involves preventive health teaching, monitoring, and offering supportive care. The nurse teaches the patient about the cause-and-effect relationship between alcohol, smoking, and mucosal irritation. Bacterial food poisoning represents a serious public health concern, and that concern is reflected in the *Healthy People 2000* goals (Box 45-1).[25] General measures to prevent food poisoning are outlined in Box 45-2.

Care of the patient with chronic gastritis is mainly supportive. The nurse emphasizes the cause-and-effect relationship between alcohol, smoking, and mucosal irritation and encourages the patient to avoid food substances that cause discomfort. The nurse also encourages the patient to avoid overeating, which can distend the atrophied and irritated mucosa. Careful and faithful ad-

**BOX 45-1 *Healthy People 2000* Goals Related to Food Safety**

Reduce infections caused by key food-borne pathogens to incidences of no more than:

| *Disease (per 100,000)* | *1987 Baseline* | *2000 Target* |
|---|---|---|
| *Salmonella* species | 18 | 16 |
| *Campylobacter jejuni* | 50 | 25 |
| *Escherichia coli* 0157:H7 | 8 | 4 |
| *Listeria monocytogenes* | 0.7 | 0.5 |

Reduce outbreaks of infections due to *Salmonella enteritidis* to fewer than 25 outbreaks yearly. (Baseline: 77 outbreaks in 1989)

Increase to at least 75% the proportion of households in which principal food preparers routinely refrain from leaving perishable food out of the refrigerator for over 2 hours and wash cutting boards and utensils with soap after contact with raw meat and poultry. (Baseline: For refrigeration of perishable foods, 70%; for washing cutting boards with soap, 66%; and for washing utensils with soap, 55%, in 1988)

Extend to at least 70% the proportion of states and territories that have implemented model food codes for institutional food operations and to at least 70% the proportion that have adopted the new uniform food protection code ("Unicode") that sets recommended standards for regulation of all food operations. (Baseline: For institutional food operations currently using FDA's recommended model codes, 20%; for the new Unicode to be released in 1991, 0%, in 1990)

From US Department of Health and Human Services, Public Health Service: *Healthy people 2000: summary report*, Boston, 1992, Jones & Barlett.

**BOX 45-2 Prevention of Food Poisoning**

1. Wash hands before handling food.
2. Do not thaw foods on the kitchen counter.
3. Keep meats, fish, poultry, mayonnaise, and cream-filled foods refrigerated.
4. Wash hands and utensils after contact with raw meat or poultry.
5. Never leave perishable foods unrefrigerated for more than 2 hours—less in hot weather.
6. Use a meat thermometer when cooking large pieces of meat, especially pork.
7. Stuff poultry immediately before roasting (warm stuffing is a good medium for bacterial growth).
8. Avoid slow cooling of meat and poultry.
9. Freeze or refrigerate leftovers promptly.
10. Can low-acid foods (foods other than tomatoes or fruits) under pressure to prevent botulism.
11. Discard any can that bulges.

herence to the prescribed medication regimen is critical, and the nurse explains the action and rationale of all drugs, as well as the management of any anticipated side effects. Ongoing medical follow-up is emphasized.

# PEPTIC ULCER DISEASE

**Peptic ulcers** are ulcerations that involve the mucosa and often the deeper structures of the upper gastrointestinal tract. They may occur anywhere in the esophagus, stomach, duodenum, or jejunum, but the term *peptic ulcer* usually refers to gastric and duodenal ulcers. Peptic ulcers, one of the most common GI disorders, are a chronic problem characterized by a pattern of exacerbations and remissions. There are several types of ulcers and multiple causes, and they consistently share only one common feature—the presence of a mucosal crater. Peptic ulcers frequently are considered to be a symptom rather than a distinct disease entity,[12] and controversy exists as to whether all ulcers need to be either prevented or treated, particularly when they are asymptomatic and discovered incidentally during endoscopy.[24]

## ETIOLOGY

The etiology of peptic ulcer disease remains elusive despite extensive research. Ulcers once were believed to be the direct result of acid oversecretion in response to stressful, hard-driving life-styles. It is clear today, however, that no such simple explanation can accurately describe the disease process. Genetic predisposition, environmental factors, and infection have been shown to alter the ongoing processes of mucosal breakdown and repair, and they all are considered to be major factors involved in ulcer development.

### Genetic Factors

There appear to be certain intrinsic elements in the development of ulcers that cannot be related to external environmental factors. Both gastric and duodenal ulcers occur 2 to 3 times more often when there is a family history of ulcers. The nature of the familial link is not clear, but it may be related to an increase in parietal cell mass, with a corresponding increase in acid secretion. Unexplained links also have been noted between ulcer incidence and particular blood groups. Numerous studies have explored various racial and cultural factors without uncovering any clear trends.

### Environmental Factors

Numerous environmental factors have been targeted in research studies, with very few clear and unequivocal results. Although social and emotional factors are intuitively believed to be involved in ulcer etiology, numerous studies have uncovered no clear links.

The role of smoking as a causative factor has been extensively studied. Smoking has been shown to adversely affect the mechanisms of gastric mucosal protection and ulcer healing,[12] but its role in initial ulcer development is less apparent. Although heavy smokers appear to have a higher incidence of peptic ulcer, quitting smoking does not *clearly* affect the long-term course of the disease in a positive manner.[6] The role of alcohol is similarly contradictory. Alcohol can cause direct and severe mucosal damage and local bleeding, but again, the reduction or elimination of alcohol shows questionable benefit for ulcer healing and long-term management. Although beer causes a significant increase in acid secretion, the effect is not produced by its alcohol content.[12] The causative effects of combined smoking and alcohol use on ulcer development and healing have been difficult to separate and track.

The role of caffeine also is controversial. Coffee appears to act as a strong acid secretagogue, but it is unclear whether caffeine is the primary cause.[15] No agreement has been reached at present over the role or influence of caffeine-containing colas and other beverages such as tea. No direct evidence links other dietary factors with the development of peptic ulcers.

The role of life stress in the development of peptic ulcers is also unclear. Acute stress ulcers, which occur in response to overwhelming physical stimuli, represent a unique situation, which is discussed on pp. 1483-1484. The role of stress in peptic ulcer disease has been researched since Beaumont first observed direct mucosal responses to stress in a patient with a fistula in the early nineteenth century.[19] Persons with ulcers have not been found to have more life stress than persons without ulcers, but they tend to react to stress more negatively. Chronic stressors appear to be more important than acute ones, as does a poor ability to cope with life events.[21] Stress also may play a role in the perceived link between peptic ulcers and chronic illnesses such as chronic obstructive pulmonary disease, cirrhosis, and arthritis, but the complicating variables of smoking and alcohol use have proved difficult to control.

### Drug Effects

The NSAIDs are believed to play a causative role in the development of gastric ulcers and some duodenal ulcers, particularly in elderly persons. These drugs significantly impair mucosal defenses by suppressing prostaglandins, which are the endogenous mediators of bicarbonate secretion. The effects are systemic and far more significant than simple local irritation. Aspirin damages the surface mucosa directly, and corticosteroids typically contribute to mucosal injury through stimulation of increased gastric secretion. These ulcerogenic drugs may contribute directly to the development of a peptic ulcer, exacerbate an existing ulcer, or cause a recurrence.

### Infection

Although the etiology of peptic ulcers is clearly heterogeneous, it is increasingly accepted that *H. pylori* bacteria must be present for ulcers to develop, except in cases that can be clearly attributed to the effects of NSAIDs.[12] A final understanding of the role of the bacteria in ulcer etiology depends on a more complete knowledge of its prevalence in the normal population. These data are not available at present. The relationship is, therefore, largely inferential. Researchers agree, however, that *H. pylori* infection definitely plays a permissive role in ulcer development, making the mucosa more vulnerable to damage from other factors. The presence of these bacteria may simply be innocuous in some ulcer patients, but they significantly impair defenses in specific populations.[16] *H. pylori* is strongly associated with chronic gastritis, and the incidence of chronic gastritis increases with age. However, there is no clear explanation at present as to why active ulcers actually develop in so few persons in whom the bacteria have colonized. The presence of the bacteria is now considered to be *the* major determinant of ulcer relapse, but its direct role in initial ulcer development remains controversial.

### Zollinger-Ellison Syndrome

**Zollinger-Ellison syndrome** is an ulceration syndrome of the duodenum or jejunum caused by a **gastrinoma** (gastrin-producing tumor). The tumor is commonly found in the noninsulin-producing islet cells of the pancreas. Most patients have a single tumor that eventually becomes malignant. This rare syndrome occurs more commonly in men, usually in early or middle adulthood.

The tumors produce an enormous quantity of gastrin, which massively overstimulates gastric acid secretion. The resulting ulcers frequently do not respond to conventional therapy, and complications are common. Diarrhea is another common symptom. It is caused by a relative lack of the pancreatic lipase needed for fat digestion. The diagnosis of Zollinger-Ellison syndrome is differentiated from standard duodenal ulcers by radioimmunoassay measurements of high serum gastrin levels. A CT scan may be used to localize the pancreatic tumor, and the tumor is removed if possible. The ulcers are treated as outlined for peptic ulcer disease.

## EPIDEMIOLOGY

Peptic ulcer disease currently is estimated to affect 1% of the total adult population.[24] This figure reflects dramatic changes over the past 100 years. The problem was rare in the nineteenth century but became common in the early twentieth century. In the 1940s, peptic ulcer disease was roughly estimated to affect as many as 10% to 15% of the adult male population. No satisfactory explanation for this dramatic rise has ever been found. The rate has been steadily declining since that peak.[12] The incidence statistics increase sharply with age, particularly in persons who use NSAIDs. No identifiable racial, ethnic, or cultural patterns have been found.

**Duodenal ulcers** have traditionally been reported as occurring 4 times more frequently than **gastric ulcers** and 4 times more frequently in men than in women. Peak ages were identified as 40 to 50 years. Today, however, both of these classic patterns are steadily shifting. All ulcer patients are older, and women represent an ever-increasing percentage.[12] The general aging of the population and the routine use of NSAIDs in arthritis management are steadily increasing the representation of both women and gastric ulcers in the overall incidence statistics. A bimodal incidence pattern is still apparent, however, with duodenal ulcers predominantly affecting younger adults and gastric ulcers predominantly affecting older adults. In the most vulnerable age-groups, peptic ulcers are estimated to still affect up to 10% of the general population. Although the incidence of duodenal ulcers continues to exceed that of gastric, the mortality rate of gastric ulcers equals or exceeds that of duodenal.[24]

## PATHOPHYSIOLOGY

Acid secretion is controlled by endocrine, neural, and paracrine factors, as outlined in Figure 45-1. Gastric acid is secreted by the parietal cells of the fundus of the stomach in response to gastrin (secreted by cells in the pyloric region), acetylcholine (cholinergic action of the vagus nerve), and histamine (found in cells throughout the gastric mucosa). There are two types of cellular receptors to histamine in the body. $H_1$ receptors are found in the cells of smooth muscle and capillaries, and they mediate smooth muscle contraction and capillary dilation. $H_2$ receptors are found in cells of the stomach and mediate secretion of hydrochloric acid (HCl). The basic paradigm of peptic ulcer development is an imbalance between gastric acid and pepsin secretion and the protective mechanisms of the mucosa.

The protection of the gastric and duodenal mucosa is a biologic imperative. Two primary mechanisms are involved. Primary protection is provided by the constant presence of a thick mucus layer that coats the mucosa. The network of mucus-producing cells is so tight that the mucus layer is almost completely impermeable to the effects of HCl. The second mechanism involves the secretion of bicarbonate from the surface epithelial cells in both the stomach and duodenum. This maintains a protective pH gradient for the mucosa. Sufficient bicarbonate is secreted to neutralize 50% of gastric secretions in the duodenum. The secretion of pancreatic bicarbonate also assists in neutralizing acid. The combined effects of the mucus and bicarbonate secretion are so powerful that mucosal pH is maintained at a level greater than 6, even when the gastric luminal pH is as low as 1.5.

### Acid Oversecretion

A variety of heterogeneous pathologic factors appear to result in ulceration. Duodenal and gastric ulcers share overlapping features but also have some distinct features. Acid oversecretion is one pathologic element. Only one third of ulcer patients have documented increases in acid secretion,[16] and these are almost exclusively associated with **duodenal ulcers**. The acid oversecretion theoretically is traced to a 1.5 to 2 times increase in parietal cell mass, which causes a moderate increase in both gastric and peptic acid activity. This increase in cell mass is believed to be genetically predetermined. Patients with duodenal ulcers also may

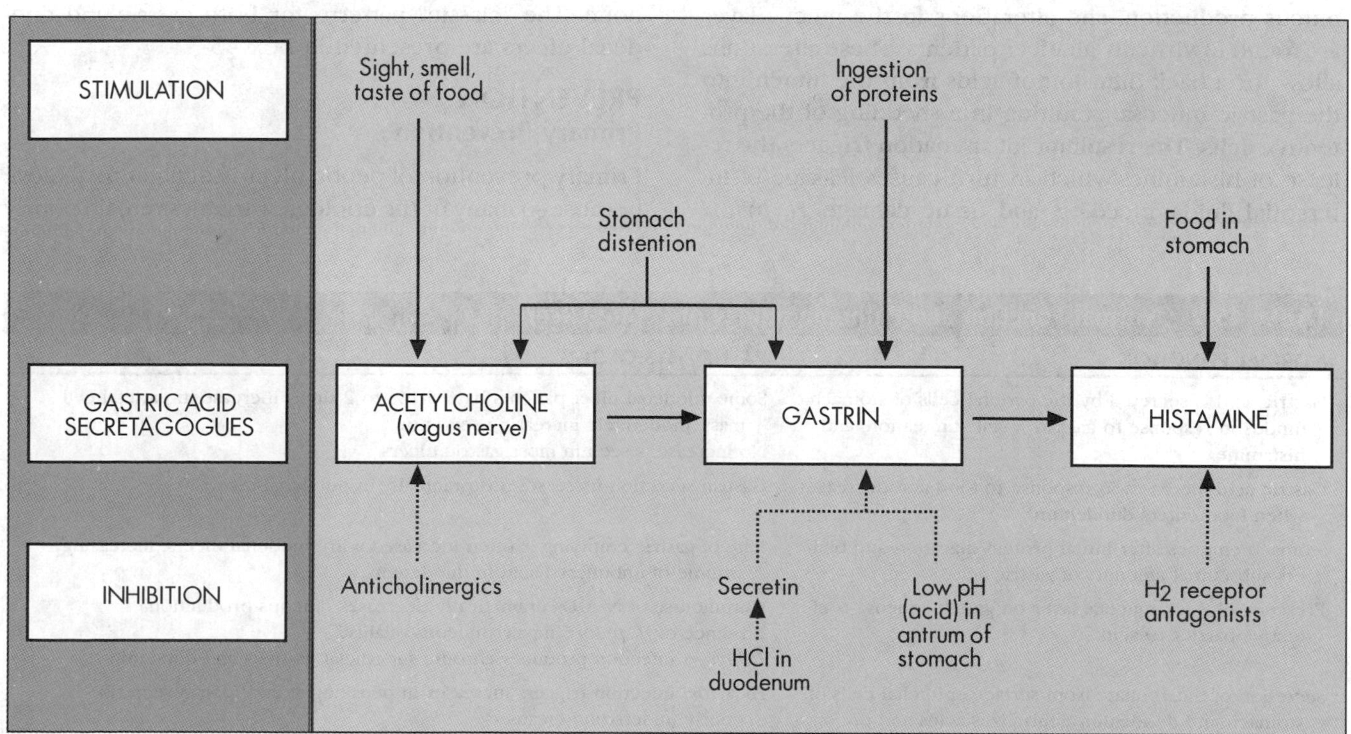


**FIGURE 45-1** Stimulation and inhibition of gastric acid.

show elevated levels of gastrin secretion postprandially. The gastrin levels typically are normal when the stomach is empty. Some patients also exhibit an increased rate of gastric emptying. The ability of protein to buffer gastric acid is therefore impaired, and more unbuffered acid moves into the duodenum. If secretion is typically at normal or even low levels, acid oversecretion rarely occurs in the presence of gastric ulcers.

### Impaired Defenses

The second major pathologic element of ulcer development is impairment of mucosal defenses. These defenses may be breached in several ways, but the presence of *H. pylori* infection and the chronic use of NSAIDs are by far the most significant.

The prostaglandins are endogenous mediators of mucus production, and the chronic use of NSAIDs can dramatically block their function. This causes the mucosa to become extremely vulnerable to acid injury. The effect of NSAIDs is *systemic* and not attributable simply to ulcerogenic local irritation. These agents also appear to mildly impair bicarbonate secretion.

When ulceration cannot be directly connected with chronic NSAID use, it is frequently associated with gastritis. *H. pylori* infection is the primary cause of chronic active gastritis. *H. pylori* can be found in the stomachs of 95% to 100% of persons with duodenal ulcers and in 60% to 80% of persons with gastric ulcers.[16] Superficial gastritis is associated with increased secretion of pepsinogen and increased levels of serum gastrin in response to meals, although both the how and why are unclear. Infection with *H. pylori* also causes abnormal mucus production, and alterations in the mucus layer are found in virtually all ulcer patients. These alterations allow for a back diffusion of acids from the lumen into the gastric mucosa, resulting in a shedding of the protective cells. The resultant inflammation triggers the release of histamine, which in turn causes leakage of interstitial fluids, bleeding, and tissue damage. *H. pylori* infection also appears to impair bicarbonate secretion in a manner as yet not understood. Asymptomatic *H. pylori* infection increases dramatically with age. It is extremely rare in persons younger than 20 years of age and is present in 50% of persons aged 55 to 64 years and in 75% of those older than 65 years.[5] No satisfactory explanation exists as to why ulcers actually develop in so few of these affected individuals. Current research focuses on the possibility that certain strains of the bacteria secrete a toxin that directly affects mucosal defenses. Table 45-2 summarizes the differences between normal function and peptic ulcer pathophysiology, which also are illustrated in Figure 45-2.

The symptoms of peptic ulcer disease, when they are present, appear to correlate well with the pathophysiologic changes and location of the ulcer. The problem is that a large number of persons never have any symptoms at all. This is particularly true with older persons and those whose ulcers are related to NSAID use.

Pain is the classic feature of peptic ulcers. The pain traditionally has been attributed to the irritation of gastric acid over the eroded mucosa. During endoscopy, however, rubbing, cutting, and burning the mucosa produce little or no perceived pain. Even the direct instillation of HCl onto an active ulcer produces pain in only 40% of patients.[12] Further, both antacids and placebos can produce the same symptomatic relief of pain. Duodenal and gastric ulcers frequently manifest different profiles, and when "classic" features are present, a diagnosis is easily established. The problem is the considerable overlap in the symptoms associated with both types of ulcers, and many patients experience few or none. The "classic" patterns for both gastric and duodenal ulcers are presented in Box 45-3.

## PREVENTION

### Primary Prevention

Primary prevention of peptic ulcer is difficult to achieve because so many of the etiologic variables remain poorly

**TABLE 45-2 Normal Function and Pathophysiology of Peptic Ulcers**

| NORMAL FUNCTION | PATHOPHYSIOLOGY |
|---|---|
| Gastric acid is secreted by the parietal cells of stomach fundus in response to gastrin, vagal stimulation, and histamine. | Some duodenal ulcer patients have a 1½ to 2 times increase in parietal cell mass, moderately increasing secretion.<br>No increase is seen in most gastric ulcers. |
| Gastric acid increases in response to food and decreases when food enters duodenum. | Gastrin secretion increases postprandially in duodenal ulcers. |
| Stomach empties after initial protein digestion and buffers substantial amounts of gastric acid. | Rate of gastric emptying is often increased with duodenal ulcers, increasing volume of unbuffered acid in duodenum. |
| Presence of thick mucous layer on gastric mucosa is effective barrier to acid. | Chronic use of NSAIDs dramatically decreases mucous production.<br>Presence of *H. pylori* impairs mucous quality.<br>*H. pylori* infection produces chronic superficial gastritis and duodenitis. |
| Secretion of bicarbonate from surface epithelial cells of stomach and duodenum neutralizes acids and prevents back diffusion. | *H. pylori* infection triggers increases in pepsinogen and gastrin secretion by poorly understood means.<br>*H. pylori* impairs bicarbonate secretion by unclear mechanisms. |

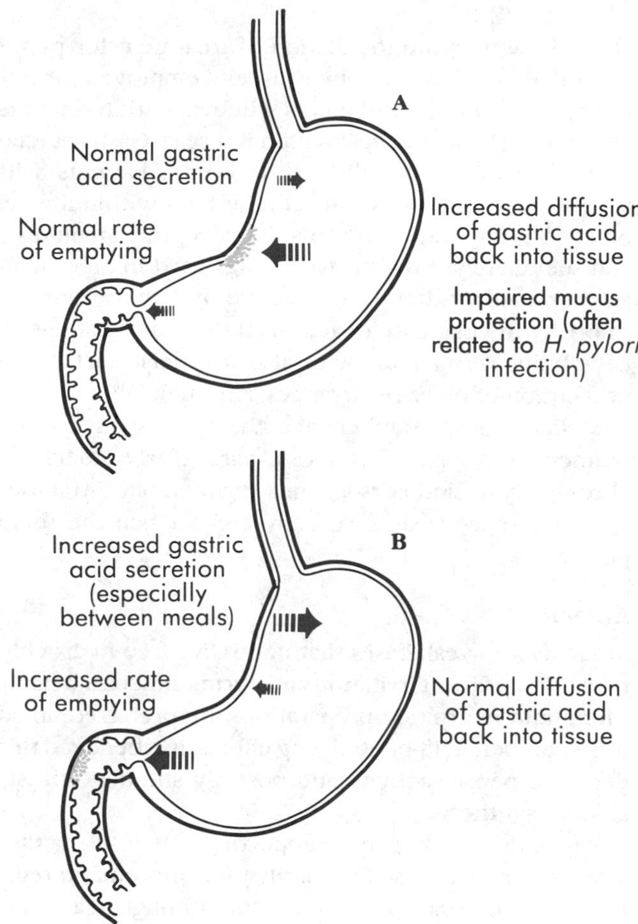


**FIGURE 45-2** Pathophysiology of peptic ulcer. **A,** Gastric ulcer. **B,** Duodenal ulcer. Note that the major alteration in gastric ulcer is increased back diffusion, whereas with duodenal ulcer, acid secretion and gastric emptying are increased.

understood. Some early evidence exists that a diet high in fiber and complex carbohydrates and low in saturated fats may support the normal protective mechanisms of the mucosa, but the links are not clear.[15] Eliminating smoking and limiting the use of alcohol also are potentially beneficial. The same kind of general recommendation includes following a healthy life-style that balances work and play and incorporates active stress-management techniques.

The most specific preventive recommendation involves the use of NSAIDs and other known ulcerogenic medications. The link between chronic NSAID use and gastric ulceration is clear, and yet these drugs are essential components of basic arthritis management for millions of elders. Patients should be taught to always buffer ulcerogenic drugs with food or antacid, but this strategy will not prevent the systemic effects of NSAID use. Until such time as synthetic prostaglandins are readily available and of proved effectiveness, the long-term use of NSAIDs remains a medical judgment.

**BOX 45-3 "Classic" Clinical Manifestations of Duodenal and Gastric Ulcers**

**DUODENAL ULCER**

May be completely asymptomatic

Pain

- Epigastric location near midline; may radiate around costal border to back
- Described as gnawing, burning, aching
- Occurs 2-4 hr after meals and at night
- Usually relieved by food or antacid

**GASTRIC ULCER**

Frequently completely asymptomatic

Pain

- Epigastric location near midline; may radiate around costal border to back
- Described as gnawing, burning, aching
- Occurs 1-2 hr after meals
- May be relieved *or* worsened by food or antacid

**BOTH**

Dyspepsia syndrome: fullness, epigastric discomfort, vague nausea, distention, and bloating

Weight gain or loss

### Secondary Prevention

Secondary prevention largely revolves around the role of *H. pylori* in peptic ulcer disease. The identification and effective treatment of *H. pylori* infection are now recognized as the most essential components of long-term ulcer relapse prevention. Patients who experience ulcers, particularly the relapse of an ulcer, should always be evaluated for treatment of *H. pylori* infection.

## MEDICAL MANAGEMENT

Patients with peptic ulcer disease rarely are hospitalized except for the treatment of complications. Common medical therapy for the management of peptic ulcer disease includes the following measures.

### Diagnostic Tests

A presumptive diagnosis of peptic ulcer can be made on the basis of a classic symptom pattern (see Box 45-3). An upper GI series can be used to identify the presence of an ulcer, but endoscopic examination is considered to be the definitive diagnostic test.[14] The ability to obtain a biopsy specimen is the primary diagnostic advantage of endoscopy. Gastric cancer is extremely rare in young adults, but its incidence increases rapidly after the fifth decade. Ulceration is usually one of the first signs of gastric cancer, and only multiple biopsy specimens can accurately differentiate between benign and malignant ulcers. *H. pylori* sampling also can be performed during endoscopy. In addition, gastric analysis can be used to document or rule out the presence of acid oversecretion.

**TABLE 45-3 Commonly Used Antacids**

| GENERIC NAME | TRADE NAME | COMMENTS |
|---|---|---|
| Aluminum hydroxide | Amphojel<br>ALternaGEL<br>Alu-Cap<br><br>Dialume | Slow buffering effect<br>Constipating<br>Decreased absorption of phosphates<br>Contains sodium<br>Edema of feet and legs with large doses |
| Aluminum carbonate | Basaljel | Same as for aluminum hydroxide |
| Aluminum and magnesium hydroxide | Maalox | A preferred antacid<br>Good buffering effect<br>Good taste<br>Nonconstipating<br>Low sodium content |
| Aluminum hydroxide and magnesium trisilicate | Gaviscon | Slower buffering effect<br>Coats and protects ulcer<br>Nonconstipating |
| Magaldrate | Riopan | A chemical combination of magnesium and aluminum hydroxide<br>Intermediate buffering action<br>Nonconstipating<br>Low sodium content<br>No acid rebound |
| Calcium carbonate | Alka-2<br>Tums<br><br>Rolaids | Rapid buffering effect<br>Constipation may be severe<br>Calcium may cause acid rebound<br>May cause hypercalcemia<br>Not suitable for long-term therapy |
| Magnesium and calcium carbonate | Marblen | Slow buffering effect<br>Neutralizes more acid than do other antacids<br>Nonconstipating<br>Low sodium content |
| **ANTACIDS WITH SIMETHICONE** | | |
| Aluminum and magnesium hydroxide, with simethicone | Mylanta<br>Maalox Plus<br>Gelusil | Same actions as aluminum and magnesium hydroxide alone<br>Simethicone is non–gas-forming: lowers the surface tension of gas bubbles |

## Medication

Drug therapy is the foundation of treatment for peptic ulcer disease. Drug therapy is usually employed for 6 to 8 weeks; with it 75% of ulcers will heal within 4 weeks, and 85% to 90% will heal within 8 weeks. Gastric ulcers typically heal at a slightly slower rate. Patients with symptoms will experience relief of pain within a week or even a few days. Antacids, $H_2$ receptor antagonists, and sucralfate are the primary drugs used in ulcer management. All of them are effective, but they vary substantially in cost, ease of administration, and patient acceptability. Drug therapy is also a crucial part of the prevention of ulcer recurrences, although few definitive guidelines exist. Maintenance therapy usually is recommended for patients at risk, particularly elders, the chronically ill, and persons on a regimen of NSAID therapy. Maintenance doses usually are one-half the therapeutic dose.

### Antacids

Antacids are weak bases that neutralize free hydrochloric acid to prevent irritation and permit mucosal healing. Aluminum hydroxide preparations are preferred; in addition to their acid-neutralizing effects, it is believed they decrease pepsin activity and possibly stimulate prostaglandin synthesis.

Antacids usually play a supporting role in ulcer therapy today and are used primarily for symptomatic relief. However, they can also *heal* ulcers, although at a slower rate than other products. The main disadvantage to antacid therapy is the frequency with which the antacids must be administered. Their effect is transitory, and for maximum effectiveness the nurse instructs the patient to take the antacid 1 and 3 hours after meals and at bedtime. Even with this frequent administration, however, antacids are ineffective for buffering nighttime acid secretion because they are rapidly cleared from the empty stomach. Administration in tablet rather than liquid form prolongs the buffering effect slightly and is recommended. Antacids should never be given concurrently with other ulcer drugs such as $H_2$ blockers inasmuch as they will interfere with drug absorption. Because aluminum hydroxide products used alone frequently cause constipation, they typically are combined with magnesium hydroxide for its laxative effect. Table 45-3 summarizes the commonly used antacids.

### Histamine ($H_2$) receptor antagonists

Several different generations of $H_2$ receptor antagonists have been developed. They vary in potency and cost but are equally effective in healing peptic ulcers after an average of 4 weeks of therapy. $H_2$ receptor antagonists inhibit HCl secretion by binding to the histamine $H_2$ receptors on stomach cells and blocking the release of histamine, which is a secretagogue for HCl. Gastric emptying is unaffected by their use.

Recommended dosage schedules for the $H_2$ receptor

antagonists have varied over the years. The doses can be spread throughout the day and given with meals, but a single bedtime dose has been shown to be extremely effective in suppressing the 60% of daily acid that is secreted at night when the stomach is empty. Overall drug side effects are quite low, and these drugs have an excellent record of safety. Potential side effects may include diarrhea and abdominal cramps, as well as confusion, dizziness, and weakness, which are more common in elderly patients. The drugs in current use include the following:

Cimetidine (Tagamet) 800 mg—oldest and least expensive

Ranitidine (Zantac) 300 mg—more potent and usually side-effect–free

Famotidine (Pepcid) 40 mg—drug of choice when the possibility of adverse reactions with other prescribed medications is a concern

Nizatidine (Axid) 300 mg—newest and most costly

Cimetidine has been shown to have antiandrogenic effects that may cause gynecomastia, decreased libido, or impotence in some men. It also has the potential to interfere with the metabolism of drugs such as phenytoin, theophylline, benzodiazepine, and tricyclic antidepressants. It is not recommended for use in situations in which drug interactions are of concern. Famotidine usually is substituted when carefully titrated drug protocols must be continued. Cimetidine, ranitidine, and famotidine are all available in intravenous forms to address acute and emergency situations.

### Sucralfate (Carafate)

Sucralfate originally was believed to coat an ulcer and provide a sealant protection against acid irritation. Additional research has indicated that it also acts as a cytoprotective agent and increases prostaglandin synthesis. It neither inhibits acid secretion nor neutralizes gastric acid, but it has an excellent record of ulcer healing. Its only common side effect is constipation. One gram of sucralfate is taken four times daily on an empty stomach 30 to 60 minutes before meals and at bedtime. The tablet is large and may be dissolved in water if it is difficult to swallow.

### Misoprostol (Cytotec)

Misoprostol is a synthetic prostaglandin analogue that offers a new dimension to ulcer management. It enhances mucosal defenses by replacing gastric prostaglandins, and it also appears to have some antisecretory properties. It is the only drug of its type approved for routine use. Its use at present is recommended in conjunction with prescribed NSAIDs to prevent the development of gastric ulceration. The effectiveness of NSAIDs does not appear to be diminished by the action of misoprostol. The drug is used for prevention and does not play a role in ulcer healing at present. The dosage is 100 to 200 μg four times daily and may cause crampy abdominal pain or diarrhea. The drug is contraindicated for use in pregnancy and should be used with caution in women of childbearing age. See Research box above.

#### RESEARCH

Walt RP: Misoprostol for the treatment of peptic ulcer and antiinflammatory–drug-induced gastroduodenal ulceration, *N Engl J Med* 327(22):1575-1580, 1992.

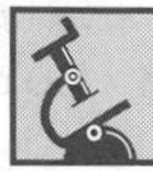

Misoprostol was the first analogue of prostaglandin $E_1$ to be made commercially available. This article reviews the pool of research accumulated on the drug's uses and effectiveness. Misoprostol has been shown to be an effective healing agent for both gastric and duodenal ulcers. It prevents much of the early ulceration associated with NSAID use, but its long-term efficacy is not yet clear. The drug has more side effects than traditional histamine ($H_2$) receptor antagonists and cannot be used in pregnant women because it increases uterine contractility. It cannot be recommended as a first-line peptic ulcer drug at this time, and routine prophylaxis is not recommended, although ongoing research is indicated. Its use for high-risk patients is clearly recommended.

### Omeprazole (Prilosec)

Omeprazole is the only proton pump inhibitor approved for clinical use in the United States at present. It virtually eliminates acid secretion and significantly improves the rate of healing for an ulcer, but the clinical benefit for long-term management is not proved. Its use is currently limited to 8 weeks of therapy, and the healing effects have not been shown to be sustained after that time frame. It cannot be used for maintenance. The present use of omeprazole is restricted to patients at extremely high risk for whom prompt healing is a priority concern.

### *H. pylori* drug treatment

The most controversial decision in current peptic ulcer drug therapy concerns when and whom to treat for *H. pylori* infection. Although its role in ulcer development remains under investigation, it is generally agreed that *H. pylori* infection is the major determinant of ulcer relapse. Triple therapy usually is recommended because of concern over the development of resistant organisms. A typical regimen includes the following:

Bismuth compounds (e.g., Pepto-Bismol)—exert a direct antibacterial effect on the organism's attachment to the mucosa; 1 to 2 tablets with meals and at bedtime

Amoxicillin or tetracycline—250 to 500 mg four times daily

Metronidazole (Flagyl, Protostat)—250 mg four times daily

Treatment should continue for a minimum of 3 weeks. GI side effects are quite common and may be severe, which makes adherence to effective therapy a problem.

### Treatment

Most peptic ulcers are responsive to the aggressive pharmacologic approach already discussed. There are no routinely ordered treatments. If an ulcer should bleed, obstruct, or perforate, however, the management will shift dramatically. Treatments for these problems are discussed under Complications (see pp. 1481-1483).

### Diet

The role of diet in peptic ulcer disease management has changed dramatically over the past 40 years. The Sippy and Hurst milk-based therapy was used for years in the belief that constantly diluting and neutralizing acid would facilitate ulcer healing.[14] Although milk-based diets provide symptomatic relief, they do not influence healing. In fact, research has shown that the amino acids and calcium in milk actually increase acid secretion regardless of its fat content. Current management reflects the understanding that no special diet is required for ulcer healing, that bland diets are not helpful in facilitating healing, and that patients should be encouraged to simply eliminate or restrict foods that cause discomfort.

### Activity

Patients with ulcers do not need to restrict their activity in any particular way to support the healing of the ulcer. Most care is managed at home, and patients are able to continue with their usual activities while undergoing treatment. Adequate rest is encouraged because it appears to promote ulcer healing.

### Referral/Consultation

Consultation usually is not needed for management of uncomplicated ulcers. The nurse may encourage patients to seek community support for reducing alcohol intake and smoking. Surgical consultation may be indicated if ulcer complications develop.

## SURGICAL MANAGEMENT

The emergence of effective drug therapy for peptic ulcer disease has caused a massive change in the role of surgery in disease management. Surgery is used today primarily for the management of acute complications and the treatment of intractable ulcers that are resistant to standard therapy or that continue to recur despite aggressive treatment.[20] Patients who require surgery often are older and usually have significant comorbid conditions. Surgery is required in men more often than in women. Various surgical procedures may be performed. The choice of procedure is tailored to the individual patient's risk profile. The physiologic basis for the various surgical procedures is summarized in Box 45-4.

**BOX 45-4 Physiologic Basis for Various Ulcer Surgeries**

**VAGOTOMY**

Removes cholinergic drive; requires a drainage procedure
Reduces parietal cell sensitivity to gastrin
Reduces basal and maximal acid output by 85% and 50%, respectively

**SELECTIVE VAGOTOMY**

Removes cholinergic drive to parietal cells
Denervates antropyloric motor complex; requires a drainage procedure
Preserves extragastric vagal function

**HIGHLY SELECTIVE VAGOTOMY**

Removes cholinergic drive to parietal cells
Preserves innervation of antrum and pylorus; does not require a drainage procedure
Preserves extragastric vagal function

**VAGOTOMY PLUS ANTRECTOMY**

Removes cholinergic drive
Removes gastrin drive
Reduces acid secretion profoundly

**GASTRECTOMY**

Removes antrum, source of gastrin
Reduces parietal cell mass

### Truncal Vagotomy and Drainage

**Vagotomy** reduces acid production by decreasing cholinergic stimulation of the parietal cells and limiting the response to gastrin. **Truncal vagotomy** severs the vagus on the distal esophagus where the nerve enters the stomach. It reduces basal acid secretion by 70% and stimulated acid secretion by 50% (Figure 45-3). Because truncal vagotomy creates gastric stasis and poor gastric emptying, it usually is combined with a **pyloroplasty,** which widens the gastric outlet to ensure adequate drainage (Figure 45-4). The Heineke-Mikulicz procedure, which is technically easy and safe, is used most frequently. Mild diarrhea and dumping syndrome are common problems after surgery, and ulcer recurrence is still a problem in some cases.

### Proximal Gastric Vagotomy

The proximal gastric vagotomy is more selective than the truncal vagotomy. It divides and severs the vagus nerve branches that supply the parietal cells while preserving those that innervate the antrum and pylorus of the stomach. Vagal stimulation to other abdominal organs is preserved, and there are fewer side effects. This surgery ensures more normal gastric function, but it is a much more technically difficult procedure, and ulcer recurrence rates, typically about 10% to 15%, can be as high as 30%.

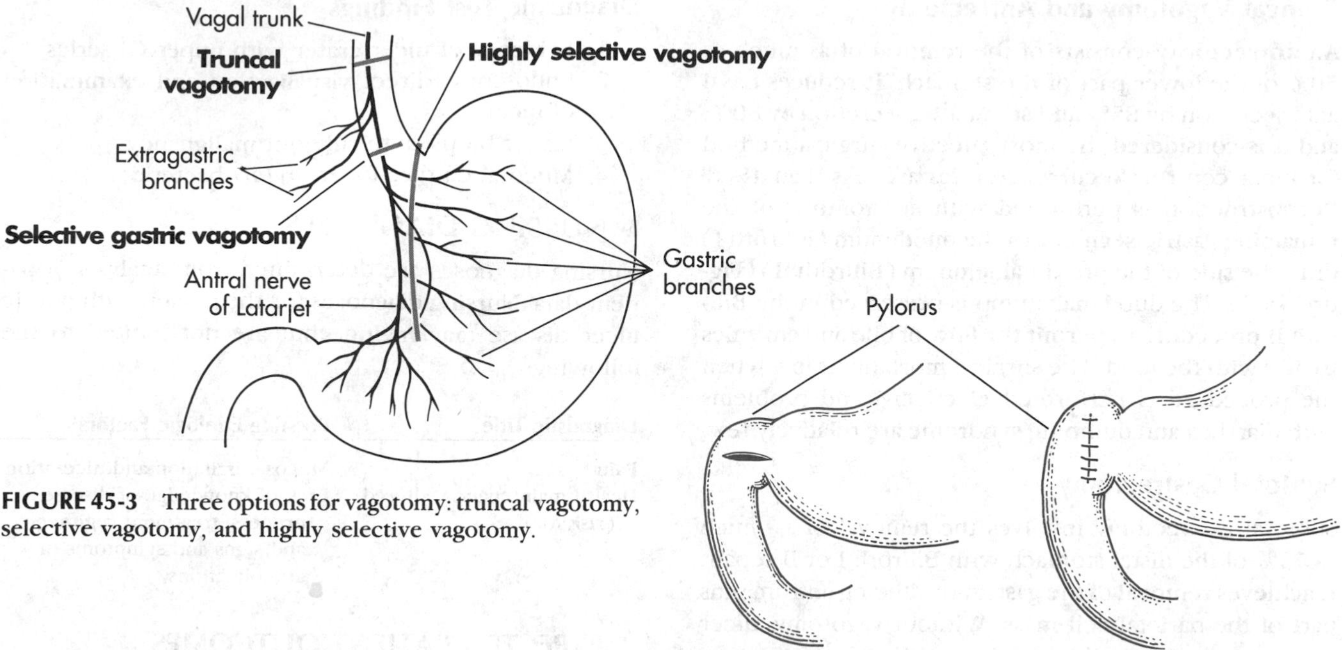


**FIGURE 45-3** Three options for vagotomy: truncal vagotomy, selective vagotomy, and highly selective vagotomy.

**FIGURE 45-4** Heineke-Mikulicz pyloroplasty. Longitudinal incision across pylorus is pulled apart and closed in transverse position to widen pyloric outlet.

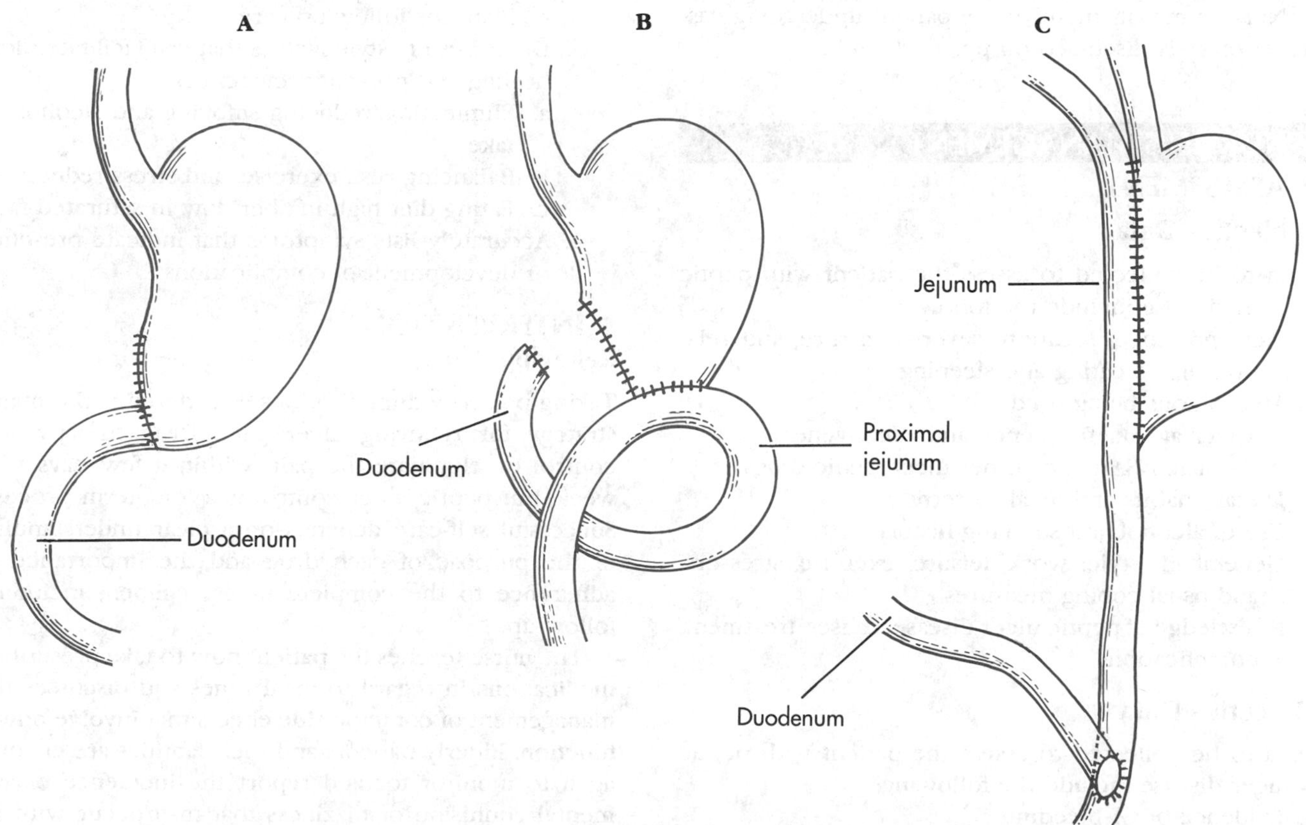


**FIGURE 45-5** Types of gastric resections with anastomoses. **A,** Billroth I anastomosis of gastric segment to duodenum. **B,** Billroth II, anastomosis of gastric segment to the proximal jejunum. **C,** Roux-en-Y anastomosis of small gastric segment to middle of jejunum with patching of duodenum to lower segment.

### Truncal Vagotomy and Antrectomy

An **antrectomy** consists of the removal of as much as 50% of the lower part of the stomach. It reduces basal acid secretion by 85% and stimulated secretion by 80%, and it is considered the most effective surgical method for ulcer control. Recurrence rates are less than 1%.[20] Reconstruction is performed with anastomosis of the remaining gastric segment to the duodenum (Billroth I) or to the side of the proximal jejunum (Billroth II) (Figure 45-5). The duodenal stump is preserved in the Billroth II procedure to permit the flow of bile and enzymes to mix with the food. The surgical mortality is low when the procedure is performed electively, and problems with diarrhea and dumping syndrome are relatively few.

### Subtotal Gastrectomy

Subtotal gastrectomy involves the removal of as much as 75% of the distal stomach with Billroth I or II repair. It achieves removal of the gastrin-producing antrum plus part of the parietal cell mass. Without vagotomy, ulcer recurrence rates are higher than with antrectomy, and dumping syndrome is more severe and common. Alkaline reflux can be a problem after any Billroth I or II repair but is more common after subtotal gastrectomy. If alkaline gastritis persists, the Roux-en-Y procedure, which patches the duodenum lower on the jejunum, may be necessary (see Figure 45-5).

Nursing management of the patient undergoing gastric surgery is discussed on pp. 1490-1494.

## NURSING MANAGEMENT

## ♦ ASSESSMENT

### Subjective Data

Data to be collected to assess the patient with peptic ulcer disease include the following:

- Pain: presence, location, severity, nature, and relationship to eating and sleeping
- Medications being used
  - Ulcer agents: frequency and effectiveness
  - Aspirin, NSAIDs, or other ulcerogenic drugs
- Dietary habits and meal patterns
- Use of alcohol and smoking history
- General life-style: work, leisure, exercise, stressors, and usual coping measures
- Knowledge of peptic ulcer disease: causes, treatment, complications

### Objective Data

Data to be collected to assess the patient with peptic ulcer disease include the following:

- Evidence of GI bleeding
  - Occult blood in stool
  - Decreased Hgb/Hct and RBC counts
- Weight loss or gain from baseline

### Diagnostic Test Findings

1. Evidence of ulcer crater with upper GI series
2. Endoscopy: direct visualization and examination of ulcer
3. Crater biopsies to rule out malignancy
4. Mucosal culture for *H. pylori* bacteria

## ♦ NURSING DIAGNOSES

Nursing diagnoses are determined from analysis of patient data. Nursing diagnoses for the person with peptic ulcer disease may include but are not limited to the following:

| Diagnostic Title | Possible Etiologic Factors |
|---|---|
| Pain | Mucosal irritation and ulceration |
| Health maintenance, altered (risk for) | Lack of knowledge of disease process, treatment regimen, and signs and symptoms of complications |

## ♦ EXPECTED PATIENT OUTCOMES

Expected patient outcomes for the patient with peptic ulcer disease may include but are not limited to the following:

1. Describes pain as decreased, minimal, or absent.
2. Describes components of disease management:
   a. Medication schedule and control of side effects
   b. Plans for follow-up care
3. Describes life-style factors that can facilitate ulcer healing and prevent recurrence:
   a. Eliminating/reducing smoking and alcohol intake
   b. Balancing rest, exercise, and stress reduction
   c. Eating diet high in fiber, low in saturated fat
4. Accurately lists symptoms that indicate presence or development of complications.

## ♦ INTERVENTIONS

### Relieving Pain

Taking prescribed medications as ordered is the major strategy for relieving ulcer pain. Drug therapy will control or eliminate the pain within a few days to a week, but peptic ulcer control is a long-term process. Successful self-care depends on a clear understanding of the purpose of each drug and the importance of adherence to the complete ulcer regimen, including follow-up.

The nurse teaches the patient how to take prescribed medications in regard to meal times and discusses the management of common side effects that involve bowel function. Elderly patients and their families are encouraged to monitor for and report the incidence of any mental confusion or dizziness that may occur with cimetidine use. Patients are taught never to abruptly discontinue their use of antiulcer medications because of the danger of severe acid rebound.

## Promoting a Healthy Life-Style

There is no conclusive, research-based evidence that modifying the diet in any way promotes ulcer healing, and no special diet is required. The nurse encourages the patient to avoid any food that causes discomfort and to avoid overdistention of the stomach and binge eating. There is no research evidence that a pattern of small, frequent feedings is any more effective in ulcer management than a standard three-meal-a-day pattern, but overeating should be avoided.[15] Eating slowly and chewing thoroughly prevent overdistention and reflux. Bedtime snacking may promote nighttime acid secretion and should be avoided.

The nurse may encourage the patient to limit the use of foods that have been shown to have a strong acid-stimulating effect. These include coffee, tea, cola drinks, and chocolate. Direct irritants such as spices and red and black pepper also should be limited. Milk products may be used, but large quantities should be avoided. Early research findings indicate that a diet high in fiber and low in saturated fats may support the natural mucosal defenses, and the nurse can recommend this dietary pattern that is beneficial to the heart and colon as well.

The nurse encourages the patient to eliminate the use of alcohol during the period of ulcer healing. Alcohol, although not directly ulcerogenic, is irritating to the mucosa and should not be consumed on an empty stomach. Beer has been shown to be a strong stimulator of acid secretion separate from its alcohol content and should be used only in moderation. The nurse encourages smokers to quit if possible because of the link between smoking and ulcer relapse.

## Coping

The role of stress in peptic ulcer disease remains unclear. The physiologic effects of stress may be traced to vagal stimulation of acid secretion. The nurse encourages the patient to establish a pattern of regular aerobic exercise and to explore appropriate approaches to stress reduction at home and work. Specific stress management and relaxation techniques can be learned (see Chapter 7). The Guidelines box on right summarizes the major points involved in teaching self-care management to the patient with peptic ulcer diseases. A nursing care plan for the patient with peptic ulcer disease is found on pp. 1480-1481.

### Guidelines for Teaching the Person With a Peptic Ulcer

**MEDICATIONS**

1. Know dosage, administration, action, and side effects.
2. Continue drug for prescribed time, even when symptoms abate.
3. Keep antacids available at all times.
4. Anticipate increased need for antacids during periods of stress.
5. Avoid self-medication with systemic antacids (such as bicarbonate of soda) that alter acid-base balance.
6. Avoid ulcerogenic drugs such as salicylates, ibuprofen, and corticosteroids.
7. Use acetaminophen (Tylenol) or buffered aspirin (if tolerated) for relief of pain.

**EATING**

1. Eat three balanced meals a day.
2. Eat between-meal snacks if this helps to relieve pain.
3. Avoid any foods that increase discomfort.
4. If alcohol is taken, drink minimally and not on an empty stomach.
5. Avoid stress at mealtimes and plan for a quiet time after eating.

**SMOKING**

1. Stop smoking if possible.
2. If complete abstinence causes increased discomfort from stress, try to decrease number of cigarettes smoked.

**RELAXATION AND REDUCTION OF STRESS**

1. Participate in recreation and hobbies that promote relaxation.
2. Participate in a reasonable exercise program for promotion of well-being.
3. Structure home and work environment to keep stressors at a reasonable level.

## ♦ EVALUATION

To evaluate the effectiveness of nursing interventions, compare patient behaviors with those stated in the expected patient outcomes. Successful achievement of patient outcomes for the patient with peptic ulcer disease is indicated by the following:

1. States that ulcer pain is no longer present.
2. Correctly describes medication schedule and management of side effects.
3. Makes appointments for medical follow-up.
4. Correctly describes diet and life-style changes to be made to prevent ulcer recurrence.

# ✷ SPECIAL CONSIDERATIONS FOR CARE OF THE GERONTOLOGIC PATIENT

Although the incidence of peptic ulcer disease in the general population has been steadily declining, a significant rise in incidence has been noted in elderly persons. Hospitalization rates for elders with peptic ulcer disease also have risen steadily in the face of a continuing overall decline in hospitalization for the disease.[10] Most of the complications and mortality associated with ulcers occur in elderly patients with more than 80% of ulcer-related deaths in the over-65 age-group.

Peptic ulcer disease is clearly a more serious problem in elderly persons, and elderly persons are also more prone to complications. It is ironic that susceptibility to ulceration should increase at the exact time when nor-

# NURSING CARE PLAN

## PERSON WITH PEPTIC ULCER

**DATA:** Mr. J. is a single, 42-year-old computer operator with a history of duodenal ulcer 4 years ago. He has had periods of epigastric distress for the past month with partial relief from Maalox. He was admitted 2 days ago with hematemesis, tarry stools, faintness, and a blood pressure of 96/54 (usual 124/84). IV fluids were initiated, and an NG tube was inserted for tap-water lavage. When the bleeding persisted, an endoscopic examination was performed for local treatment of the recurrent duodenal ulcer. Antacids were administered hourly through the NG tube after the endoscopy. Cimetidine was administered by IV push.

Mr. J's BP is now stable, and the NG tube was removed early today. He is taking oral fluids and has been started on a soft diet. The cimetidine has been changed to 300 mg with meals and at bedtime. Maalox 30 ml is ordered 1 hour and 3 hours after meals and as needed.

The nursing history also identified the following:

- Mr. J. is vague about the nature of peptic ulcer disease, its treatment, or potential complications.
- He takes aspirin fairly regularly for headaches caused by "computer eyestrain."
- He smokes 1½ packs/day; he has tried several times unsuccessfully to quit.
- He spends two to three evenings a week at a local bar and "puts down quite a few beers."

Collaborative nursing actions include monitoring for the following:

- Signs of further hemorrhage: hematemesis; decreased blood pressure; restlessness; cool, moist skin; stools that show positive reaction to guaiac test
- Signs of perforation: severe, sudden, sharp abdominal pain

### ■ NURSING DIAGNOSIS

Epigastric pain related to mucosal irritation and ulceration

| Expected Patient Outcome | Nursing Interventions | Rationale |
|---|---|---|
| States epigastric pain is decreased or absent | Administer prescribed cimetidine with meals and at bedtime (8 AM, 12 noon, 5 PM, and 10 PM). | Cimetidine facilitates ulcer healing by decreasing gastric acid secretion; it is given with meals to inhibit food-stimulated HCl secretion |
| | Give prescribed antacid 1 and 3 hr after meals (9 AM, 11 AM, 1 PM, 3PM, 6 PM, and 8 PM) and as needed. | Antacids neutralize HCl and quickly reduce pain; they interfere with absorption of cimetidine if given concurrently. They must be given frequently as they are cleared rapidly from the stomach. |

### ■ NURSING DIAGNOSIS

Risk for altered health maintenance related to lack of knowledge of disease process, treatment regimen, and signs and symptoms of complications

| Expected Patient Outcome | Nursing Interventions | Rationale |
|---|---|---|
| Accurately describes: | Encourage patient to avoid: | |
| ▪ Components of disease process | ▪ Any food that causes pain | Diet modifications will not heal peptic ulcers. |
| ▪ Life-style modifications to facilitate ulcer healing<br>▪ Symptoms of complications | ▪ Foods that have a strong acid-stimulating effect, e.g., tea, coffee, chocolate, cola, and milk products | Diet changes are directed primarily at relieving discomfort. |
| | Encourage patient to eat a high-fiber, low saturated–fat diet. | This diet is believed to support the natural defenses of the GI mucosa. |
| | Teach patient the links between aspirin use, smoking, and alcohol consumption on ulcer relapse.<br>▪ Encourage reduction of intake or use. | Aspirin and ibuprofen contribute to mucosal breakdown; alcohol is a direct irritant to the mucosa; beer is a strong gastric acid secretagogue, and smoking appears to be related to an increased rate of ulcer relapse. |
| | ▪ Refer to community smoking cessation programs.<br>▪ Suggest substituting acetaminophen for aspirin or ibuprofen. | |

## NURSING CARE PLAN

### PERSON WITH PEPTIC ULCER—cont'd

| Expected Patient Outcome | Nursing Interventions | Rationale |
|---|---|---|
| | ▪ Suggest eye examination or environmental modification to reduce eye strain. | |
| | Explore new patterns of recreation and stress-reduction techniques. | Ulcer recurrence is more common in patients with chronic anxiety and poor coping skills; stress reduction may aid in changing nonhealthful recreation patterns. |
| | Explain side effects of prescribed medications and relationship to bowel elimination. | Antacids may have either a cathartic or constipating effect depending on their constituents; bowel elimination may need to be supported through diet changes. |
| | Instruct Mr. J. to monitor for and report the following:<br>▪ Persistent epigastric pain<br>▪ Sudden severe abdominal pain<br>▪ Tarry stools<br>▪ Persistent vomiting<br>▪ Bloody or brown vomitus | These symptoms may indicate ulcer complications, e.g., GI bleeding, perforation, or obstruction. |

mal basal acid secretion is in decline and moving toward achlorhydria. Increasing use of NSAIDs is considered to be a crucial element, but it alone cannot explain all of the problems. Changes in structure and blood flow also may play a role, especially in women, in whom postmenopausal changes result in the loss of some hormonally mediated mucosal protections.

Peptic ulcer disease often manifests in an atypical manner in elders. Symptoms tend to be more poorly defined and variable, and the standard pain characteristics frequently are not present. The discomfort, if present at all, often is poorly localized and vague, radiating in ways that cause confusion and overlap with angina, gallbladder disease, and dysphagia. Because early accurate diagnosis is rare, the ulcers tend to be larger at diagnosis or are already exhibiting complications. The analgesic effect of NSAIDs may play a role in masking symptoms and also may increase the tendency of the ulcers to bleed. Elderly women are at particular risk, and the use of NSAIDs is estimated to increase the risk of peptic ulcer complications and death by a factor of 2 to 4.[10]

Diagnosis and treatment of peptic ulcer disease in elders follow the same general guidelines outlined in the remainder of the discussion. Elderly persons are at greater risk for recurrence and usually require full-dose maintenance therapy. Therapeutic dilemmas arise when complications develop, inasmuch as the mortality rates for both conservative and aggressive therapies are high in this population.

## ❦ HOME CARE CONSIDERATIONS

Standard management of peptic ulcer disease is achieved by the individual patient and family in a home-based self-care regimen. Adherence issues are important as they relate to medication administration, the restriction of alcohol, and the cessation of smoking. The severity of symptoms provides an initial impetus for regimen compliance, but this effect is difficult to sustain once symptom control has been achieved. The nurse's teaching concerning the regimen and its rationale is essential to long-term success in management.

## COMPLICATIONS

The major complications of peptic ulcer disease are hemorrhage, perforation, and obstruction of the pyloric outlet.

### Hemorrhage

Peptic ulcers account for approximately 80% of all episodes of GI bleeding and result in emergency hospitalization for more than 300,000 persons annually.[26] Although the overall incidence of peptic ulcer is steadily declining, the incidence of complications has remained fairly steady and primarily affects elderly persons. Bleeding is by far the most common complication, occurring in 15% to 20% of patients with ulcers. It occurs at least 2 to 3 times more often than does perforation or obstruction.[8] Bleeding occurs more commonly from gastric ulcers, and the associated mortality is also higher and increases with the patient's age.

The severity of ulcer bleeding ranges from slight oozing to frank profuse hemorrhage. The presence of occult blood in the stool, or tarry stools, indicates that enzymes in the GI tract have had time to oxidize the blood and to break down the blood proteins. Emesis that is dark or of coffee-ground appearance indicates that the blood has been in the stomach long enough for HCl to alter it. Bright-red bleeding, which indicates a very recent onset, usually is associated with higher mortality. Significant bleeding is almost always arterial in nature and originates from a single eroded vessel in the base of the ulcer. Small arteries typically are involved, but deep erosion (greater than 1 mm) may affect the larger arterial trunks. Clinical manifestations vary with the extent of the bleeding. The most common sign is hematemesis, although patients with duodenal ulcers may experience only rectal bleeding. The rapid movement of large amounts of blood through the GI tract may produce significant abdominal cramping and discomfort. Severe bleeding also will be accompanied by early signs of shock (tachycardia, tachypnea, restlessness, and orthostatic hypotension).

### Medical management

It is estimated that bleeding from an ulcer will stop spontaneously in as many as 85% of patients.[14] Standard interventions include placement of a nasogastric (NG) tube for gastric lavage. A large-bore NG tube helps to clear the stomach of excess blood and clots and prepares it for diagnostic endoscopy. Room-temperature tap water is recommended for lavage.[8,9,26] Iced saline no longer is advised because it can significantly lower the patient's core body temperature, particularly in elderly persons, and it does not result in vasoconstriction or a reduction in bleeding. The chilling also may trigger cardiac dysrhythmias. The addition of epinephrine to lavage solutions has not been shown to reduce bleeding.

If the bleeding is profuse, fluid replacement and blood transfusions are administered as necessary. Fluid replacement typically begins with normal saline or a crystalloid solution such as Ringer's lactate. Blood products typically are used when the patient's hemoglobin drops below 10 g/dl.[9] Providing supplemental oxygen by nasal cannula is standard, particularly if the patient is elderly. (See Chapter 22 for a more complete discussion of shock management.)

Drug therapy during a bleeding episode usually involves the intravenous administration of cimetidine, rantidine, or famotidine. The effectiveness of the $H_2$ receptor antagonists in bleeding episodes is not proved, but these agents will begin immediately to reduce gastric secretion and promote healing of the ulcer. Early studies of the use of omeprazole, the potent proton pump inhibitor, during episodes of bleeding appear promising, but it is too early to determine if it will replace the standard use of $H_2$ receptor antagonists. Despite their proved ability to support ulcer healing, neither antacids nor sucralfate is used in initial management of bleeding because these agents interfere with endoscopic visualization and add no therapeutic benefit.[8]

Endoscopic examination is essential to enable the physician to isolate and evaluate the bleeding site. Lavage is employed primarily to prepare the stomach for endoscopic evaluation. Therapeutic endoscopy also may be employed. Both thermal coagulation and injection therapy have been studied extensively as means of controlling bleeding. Thermal coagulation, which seals the bleeding vessel, may be achieved by electrocautery, heater probe, and laser. Although controversy exists, the heater probe appears to produce the most consistent results.[9] It is easy to use, portable, and relatively inexpensive. Lasers produce excellent results, but they require extremely expensive equipment, which often is not portable, and a highly trained operator. Injection therapy—with epinephrine, absolute alcohol, or other sclerosing agent—is an alternative primary or adjunct therapy. It is also the easiest and least expensive approach.

Surgery has long been a mainstay of treatment for bleeding. Associated mortality rates can be quite high, but it is an essential option for patients with persistent, recurrent, uncontrollable bleeding. Endoscopic treatment usually is attempted first, but it is essential that surgery be performed before the onset of severe comorbid complications that would significantly increase the surgical risk, particularly in elderly persons.

### Nursing management

The nursing role in the management of GI hemorrhage revolves around careful ongoing assessment, prevention of complications, and support of the patient. A patient at risk for hemodynamic instability usually will be placed in an intensive care unit. Large-bore IV access is established, and the nurse monitors fluid infusions and all vital signs. The nurse may be responsible for the gastric lavage, which often involves instilling about 250 ml of water and then aspirating it after it has been in the stomach for 2 minutes. The procedure is repeated until the returns are light red and free of clots. A piston type of syringe usually is easiest to use.

Hematemesis presents a serious risk for aspiration, particularly when large clots are present. Maintaining a patent airway is critical. The nurse turns the patient to the side and keeps the head of the bed elevated about 45 degrees unless the vital signs become unstable. Suction should be present at the bedside and used as needed to help clear the mouth. Mouth care after vomiting episodes is important for comfort.

Acute bleeding can be terrifying for the patient. The nurse maintains a calm and confident approach and remains at the bedside to provide reassurance to the patient. All interventions should be carefully explained. Ensuring warmth also is important. Gastric lavage, IV solutions, and chilled blood products can induce chilling and shivering. This will significantly increase the body's need for oxygen. Management

### Guidelines for Management of Gastrointestinal Bleeding

Insert NG tube and institute gastric lavage:
- Instill 250 ml room-temperature tap water
- Allow a 2-min dwell time
- Aspirate and evaluate the returns using a piston type of syringe
- Repeat as needed until returns are light-colored and free of clots

Monitor vital signs frequently for signs of shock.
Measure and record all output.
Establish at least one large-bore IV access:
- Instill normal saline or Ringer's lactate as ordered

Draw blood for CBC, type, and crossmatch.
Administer IV $H_2$ receptor antagonist as ordered.
Start oxygen by nasal cannula as ordered:
- Extremely important in elderly persons

Turn vomiting patient on side to protect the airway.
Raise head of bed 45 degrees if vital signs remain stable.
Provide oral suction at bedside to help clear blood.
Provide mouth care after vomiting episodes.
Reassure patient and maintain a calm manner.
Administer blood products as ordered.
Prepare patient for therapeutic endoscopy.
Maintain the patient NPO.

of the patient with GI bleeding is summarized in the Guidelines box above.

## Perforation

Perforation involves the erosion of a peptic ulcer through the muscular wall of the stomach or duodenum, with spillage of gastric secretions into the abdominal cavity. It occurs more commonly with duodenal ulcers. A chemical **peritonitis** quickly develops from contact with the GI contents, and a bacterial peritonitis follows within 12 hours. The clinical presentation of perforation usually is dramatic in younger adults, but it may be subdued in elderly persons. This fact typically causes delays in seeking treatment and contributes to the high mortality associated with perforation in older patients.[9] Perforations, which frequently seal spontaneously in younger adults, are less likely to do so in elderly persons.

The classic clinical picture of ulcer perforation includes (1) severe, sharp abdominal pain, (2) an abdomen that becomes rigid, with rebound tenderness, and (3) tachycardia, tachypnea, and diaphoresis.

A perforation usually is diagnosed by the symptom pattern and supported by the finding of subdiaphragmatic free air on abdominal x-ray film.

### Management

Emergency surgery is the definitive treatment for perforation. Controversy exists over whether the surgery should simply repair the defect with an omental patch or include definitive ulcer correction.[20] If surgery is delayed for 24 hours or more, which frequently is the case in elderly persons, the operative mortality is about 10% overall and 30% to 50% in elders.

Immediate care consists of establishing IV access to replace fluids and inserting an NG tube for drainage of the GI tract. High-dose antibiotics usually are administered in anticipation of sepsis. The patient is kept in low Fowler's position in the attempt to contain the escaped secretions in a limited area of the abdomen. The nurse provides the patient with emotional support and reassurance, offers comfort measures, and attempts to prepare the patient for surgery.

## Obstruction

The incidence of gastric outlet obstruction has declined dramatically with increasingly effective ulcer therapy. Obstruction is usually the result of long-standing, symptomatic duodenal ulcer disease. Repeated cycles of ulceration and healing can lead to scarring, chronic edema, and fibrotic tissue changes, which may obstruct the gastroduodenal junction (pylorus). It usually develops insidiously over a period of days or weeks and proceeds to complete obstruction.

Initially the patient may experience dyspepsia symptoms, including anorexia and nausea, as the stomach fails to empty completely. Weight loss and malnutrition will develop if the diagnosis is delayed, and this is the common occurrence in elderly persons. Vomiting occurs when the chyme is completely unable to pass into the duodenum. The diagnosis usually can be established by abdominal x-ray films that show gastric distention and large fluid levels. Endoscopy usually is performed to rule out the presence of an obstructing tumor and may be used to relieve uncomplicated obstructions.

The initial management of obstruction involves fluid and electrolyte replacement and gastric decompression with an NG tube. $H_2$ receptor antagonists may be used, but medical management is rarely of definitive benefit. Improvement usually occurs within 72 hours, although a longer preoperative period may be needed if significant fluid and electrolyte imbalances exist. Truncal vagotomy plus antrectomy with a Billroth II reconstruction usually is recommended for patients at low risk. Even high-risk elders generally can tolerate surgery fairly well if attention has been paid to careful preoperative stabilization and preparation. Truncal vagotomy and pyloroplasty may be used if the patient is not a candidate for more definitive surgery.

## STRESS ULCERS

### Etiology/Epidemiology

Inflammation, erosion, and bleeding of the gastroduodenal mucosa can develop rapidly after major physical trauma or illness. The development of acute duodenal ulceration was first described by Curling in 1842 in a group of extensively burned patients. Acute gastric ulceration was similarly described by Cushing in patients with extensive central nervous system trauma or surgery.[17] The development and widespread use of intensive care units in the past two decades have resulted in a tremendously increased recognition of **stress ulcers** in critically ill patients.

Lesions can occur within hours of injury. The classic presentation is the development of painless upper GI bleeding, usually within 3 to 7 days of a precipitating major physiologic stress. It is generally agreed that, without treatment, stress ulceration will occur in most critically ill patients. Overt bleeding will occur in at least 15% of them and carries an associated mortality rate of 50% to 75%.[9] Curling's ulcers, which typically involve multiple sites in the superficial mucosa of the duodenum, are associated with burns, trauma, hemorrhage, sepsis, and respiratory and renal failure. Cushing's ulcers typically manifest as single, deep lesions and are associated with central nervous system injury or surgery. The likelihood of severe stress ulceration increases dramatically in a patient with multiple risk factors. Hemorrhage is the most common complication, but perforation also occurs frequently.

### Pathophysiology

The major factor that causes stress ulceration is a loss of the ability to maintain the integrity of the mucosa. The maintenance of mucosal homeostasis is a complex process involving mucus production, mucosal blood flow, prostaglandin secretion, bicarbonate production, and maintenance of the needed pH gradient. The stress state decreases gastric mucosal blood flow, and this event triggers a series of changes that ultimately result in mucosal breakdown. The epithelial cells of the mucosa are extremely sensitive to hypoxia, and the process of cellular necrosis can begin within minutes. Stress ulceration cannot occur without the presence of acid and pepsin, but overproduction of acid has not been found to be the cause of stress ulcers in most situations. In fact, acid secretion frequently is temporarily diminished in the acute stress state. Mucosal resistance therefore is believed to be the key.[16] The exceptions are central nervous system trauma and sepsis, which are commonly associated with massive increases in acid secretion, often exceeding 3 to 4 L/day. Stress ulcer lesions tend to be more shallow than standard peptic ulcers and resemble acute bleeding gastritis. There are usually numerous ulcerated areas rather than a single well-defined lesion.

Painless GI bleeding in a critically ill patient is the hallmark of stress ulceration. It may begin as bloody NG aspirate, melena, or a massive hematemesis accompanied by clinical signs of volume depletion. The lesions develop most frequently in the fundus or midbody of the stomach: within 24 to 48 hours of admission to an ICU, 75% to 100% of patients show evidence of gastric injury on endoscopic examination.

### Medical Management

The key to stress ulcer management lies in aggressive prevention. The major emphasis is on reduction of gastric acidity through continuous IV infusion of $H_2$ receptor antagonists to keep the pH above 3.5. Although antacids can be used for this purpose, they require such frequent administration that the incidence of side effects is quite high. Concern has arisen that the prophylactic neutralization of gastric secretions may be leaving ICU patients vulnerable to nosocomial infection, particularly in the form of gram-negative pneumonias. These organisms can colonize the stomach within 2 to 5 days.[5] Research is ongoing concerning the effectiveness of sucralfate for prophylaxis, inasmuch as it does not affect the gastric pH. Early results are promising although the necessity for oral administration remains a drawback.

If bleeding does occur, the associated mortality is very high. Management efforts may include therapeutic endoscopy with cauterization, laser photocoagulation, vasopressin administration, or emergency surgery.

### Nursing Management

The nursing role in the management of stress ulceration traditionally has involved continuous bedside monitoring of the patient and administration of medications. The NG tube is used to aspirate gastric secretions, measure gastric pH, and check for the presence of active or occult bleeding. Assessment of gastric pH typically is performed every 2 to 4 hours. NG tubes are now available that have pH electrodes at their tip to allow for continuous monitoring of the patient's gastric pH. A new approach involves the GI tonometer and sump tube.[18] See Research box, p. 1485. This special NG tube has a saline-inflated semipermeable balloon near its tip that is permeable to gas. It measures the changes in carbon dioxide and hydrogen ion concentration that occur in response to ischemia. This device allows for a measurement of the pH of the gastric *mucosa* rather than just the gastric *secretions.* It is thought that, in addition to increased accuracy in predicting stress ulceration, this device also allows for earlier and more accurate data concerning hypovolemia, sepsis, and other conditions that may result in GI ischemia.

# CANCER OF THE STOMACH

## ETIOLOGY

The cause of cancer of the stomach remains unknown, and yet its highly erratic worldwide incidence pattern clearly suggests the involvement of multiple environmental, genetic, and possibly cultural factors. The steady decline in incidence of gastric cancer in the United States from the 1950s to the 1980s has been attributed primarily to changes in dietary and food-handling practices. These include reduced intake of smoked, highly salted and preserved foods, increased intake of fresh fruits and vegetables, and improved refrigeration and shipping practices. Specifically, researchers attribute the decline in incidence to reduced consumption of nitrates and nitrites, which are converted in the body to carcinogenic nitrosamines. Increased consumption of vitamin C also appears to prevent nitrosamine formation.[22]

## RESEARCH

Neill KM, Rice KT, Ahern HL: Comparison of two methods of measuring gastric pH, *Heart Lung*, 22(4):349-355, 1993.

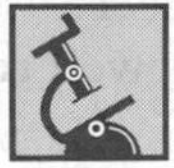

This study compared the degree of agreement between two methods of measuring pH—the NG tube with a pH sensor in the tip and testing actual gastric aspirate with litmus paper. The study took place with 39 ICU patients who had undergone surgery. The pH measurements were taken every 2 hours for 48 hours. Although there was substantial agreement in values, the pH sensor provided more consistent and accurate data with a significantly smaller standard deviation in values. It also was viewed as safer, faster, and more satisfactory by the ICU nurses.

Gastric cancer is related to the presence of chronic achlorhydria, pernicious anemia, and villous adenoma. Some studies indicate a higher risk after gastric resection surgery.[1] The risk of benign ulcers becoming malignant is extremely small, and at present the role of *H. pylori* bacteria, if any, is unclear.

Patterns of familial clustering occasionally occur in gastric cancer, and a family history in a first-degree relative is considered a risk. The most famous historic example is the incidence of gastric cancer in Napoleon Bonaparte's family, in which his father, grandfather, brother, and three sisters died of the disease. Worldwide, an inverse relationship is seen between incidence and socioeconomic status. Cigarette smoking has now been conclusively tied to gastric cancer. The risk for smokers in general is 2½ times greater than for nonsmokers, and it is 5 times greater in heavy smokers (more than 30 cigarettes per day).[13]

## EPIDEMIOLOGY

The incidence of gastric cancer in the United States has declined steadily over the past 40 years, but recent statistics indicate that this encouraging trend may be reversing. From 1950 to the mid-1980s the incidence dropped sharply from 22.8 to 9.0 cases per 100,000 population for men, and from 12.3 to 4.3 cases per 100,000 for women.[3] Both incidence and mortality figures appear to have bottomed out, however, and approximately 24,400 new cases are now being diagnosed annually. The 13,000 annual deaths from gastric cancer represent 3% of all cancer deaths. This cancer traditionally has been found in the distal portion of the stomach. The recent increase in cases of gastric cancer has been located primarily in the gastric cardia. These increases parallel the new site statistics reported for the increased incidence of esophageal cancer. These proximal tumors are showing a 4:1 preference for men, particularly white males.[1] Distal gastric cancers are more common in African-American males.

Gastric cancer traditionally has followed a highly varied pattern internationally. Japan, Chile, and Costa Rica have the greatest incidence of the disease. Gastric cancer accounts for more than half of all cancer deaths in Japan.[11] The United States has the lowest worldwide incidence rate. The link to environmental and dietary factors appears clear, inasmuch as the risk of immigrants drops sharply by the second generation. The cancer is rare before the age of 40 years and occurs most frequently in persons between 50 and 70 years of age.

## PATHOPHYSIOLOGY

Gastric cancers are virtually all primary adenocarcinomas that are derived from the epithelium. They have been found traditionally in the pyloric and antral regions, particularly along the lesser curvature. The recently noted upswing in incidence has been for tumors of the gastric cardia. Adenocarcinomas occur in polypoid, ulcerative, or infiltrating forms. Growth of the tumors is either by expansion, forming discrete tumor nodules, or by individual cell infiltration. Gastric cancer may spread directly through the stomach wall into adjacent tissues; to the lymphatics; to the regional lymph nodes of the stomach; to the esophagus, spleen, pancreas, and liver; or through the bloodstream to the lungs or bones. Involvement of regional lymph nodes occurs early. There is a tendency toward intraperitoneal seeding, particularly to the peritoneal cul-de-sac. Prognosis depends on the depth of invasion and extent of metastasis. Three fourths of patients with gastric carcinoma have metastases at the time of diagnosis.

Gastric cancer is typically incurable by the time it is diagnosed because symptoms rarely develop until the growth spreads to adjacent organs. Vague and persistent symptoms of gastric distress, flatulence, loss of appetite, nausea, gradual weight loss, and loss of strength may be the only patient complaints. These vague symptoms should never be ignored, and the person is encouraged to seek immediate medical advice. However, these symptoms are not necessarily symptoms of cancer. Pain does not usually appear until late in the disease, and the absence of this symptom is often the reason for the delay in seeking medical help. If the disease progresses untreated, marked cachexia develops and eventually a palpable mass may be felt in the region of the stomach. Frequently there are no early gastric symptoms. Typical clinical manifestations are summarized in Box 45-5.

## PREVENTION

Most of the etiologic factors identified for gastric cancer do not translate well into *primary prevention* strategies. The clear exception appears to be cigarette smoking, which is now believed to play a causative role. Dietary avoidance of heavily processed or cured foods that contain nitrates is recommended, and a diet with adequate quantities of fresh vegetables and of fruits with vitamin C is advised. *Secondary prevention* focuses on early detection in patients at high risk. Mass fluoroscopic and endoscopic screening is used in Japan for early detec-

**BOX 45-5 Clinical Manifestations of Gastric Cancer***

Dyspepsia: early satiety, bloating, anorexia
Epigastric pain or burning (usually mild and relieved by antacids)
Mild nausea
Weight loss (may be rapid and severe)
Fatigue and weakness
Changes in bowel habits: constipation or diarrhea

*Gastric cancer typically is asymptomatic in early stages.

tion, but it is not believed to be cost effective in the United States. Aggressive screening is warranted, however, in patients older than 40 years of age who experience persistent vague abdominal complaints or have been losing weight for no apparent cause. All patients with documented or suspected gastric ulcers should be screened for cancer of the stomach.

## MEDICAL MANAGEMENT

The only potentially curative intervention for gastric cancer is surgical. The expected length of stay of patients with gastric cancer as determined by DRG is 6.3 days. Common medical therapy for management of gastric cancer includes the following approaches.

### Diagnostic Tests

Biopsy is considered to be the diagnostic procedure of choice when gastric cancer is suspected. Multiple specimens are obtained through endoscopy. Many gastric cancers can be located by barium contast upper GI x-ray films, but only biopsy can confirm the diagnosis. The decision to use endoscopy in cases where complaints are vague and inconclusive is a difficult one because of the invasive nature and expense of the test. Again, the cost benefits of mass screening by endoscopy are questionable given the low incidence of gastric cancer in the United States. CT scanning and endoscopic ultrasonography also may be used to define the tumor and to search for distant metastasis.

### Medication

Medications do not play a role in the management of gastric cancer except when chemotherapy is used. Adjuvant therapy guidelines for gastric cancer are not well developed, and the use of chemotherapy has not proved to be of clear benefit. Chemotherapy is, however, the mainstay of treatment for nonresectable tumors. Several new drug and combination chemotherapy/radiotherapy protocols are under investigation today at major cancer research centers.

If the cancer has an ulcerative component, the patient may receive peptic ulcer drug therapy for symptomatic relief as outlined on pp. 1474-1475.

### Treatment

Radiotherapy is being researched as a treatment option for gastric cancer. At present it shows little proved effectiveness. It usually is used in combination with chemotherapy for nonresectable or recurrent cancer cases, and its role in palliation of bone metastases is well recognized.

### Diet

There are no specific dietary considerations for the treatment of gastric cancer. Patients may experience severe weight loss and cachexia and eventually require nutritional support. If a patient experiences ulcer-related pain, the standard recommendations for avoiding spicy and irritating foods will be made. The patient is encouraged to work within the scope of individual preferences to maintain adequate nutrition. Patients who undergo gastric resection may develop significant problems with dumping syndrome and malabsorption. Management of these disorders is discussed on pp. 1492-1493.

### Activity

The patient with gastric cancer does not need to restrict activity in any way. Patients are encouraged to remain as active in their usual life-styles as their activity tolerance permits. Treatment for gastric cancer is rigorous and may take a significant toll on the patient's energy level and stamina. The nurse encourages patients to make any necessary modifications in their daily activities to accommodate the demands of the treatment protocol.

### Referral/Consultation

The treatment of resectable gastric cancer is primarily surgical. Referral to consultants usually is not necessary in the early period. The primary ongoing concerns are maintenance of desired weight and nutritional status. If digestion and absorption problems become severe, the patient may be referred to a nutritional support team for guidance and management.

## SURGICAL MANAGEMENT

The only potentially curative treatment for gastric cancer is surgical resection. The procedure of choice depends on the location and extent of the tumor. The major stages of gastric cancer are outlined in Box 45-6. Most surgeons perform subtotal gastrectomies and attempt to remove all the tumor. Total **gastrectomy** is not recommended because of the serious digestive difficulties that may result. It also appears to have no positive effects on disease mortality. The extensive experience of Japanese surgeons with gastric cancer emphasizes the importance of performing more extensive lymph node dissections than have been standard in the United States.[23] The trend is to attempt to remove as much of the stomach's lymphatic drainage network as possible. Antrectomy plus vagotomy is performed if pos-

**BOX 45-6 Stages of Gastric Cancer**

| | |
|---|---|
| Stage I | Tumor limited to mucosa (Ia) or submucosa (Ib); no lymph node or distant metastases |
| Stage II | Tumor involves gastric wall but not serosa; no metastases |
| Stage III | Tumor similar to stage II; positive lymph nodes but no distant metastases |
| Stage IV | Tumor may extend beyond gastric walls; positive lymph nodes and distant metastases |

sible. Tumors that are high in the cardia, however, present more technical challenges to resection and anastomosis. Removal of other abdominal organs appears to have no positive impact at all on survival. Despite aggressive intervention, 5-year survival remains at 5% to 15%.

## NURSING MANAGEMENT

Nursing management of the patient undergoing gastric surgery is discussed at the end of the chapter on pp. 1490-1494.

## ✷ SPECIAL CONSIDERATIONS FOR CARE OF THE GERONTOLOGIC PATIENT

Gastric cancer is rare before the age of 40 years and typically occurs in persons between 50 and 70 years of age. Therefore the entire discussion related to the medical and nursing management of gastric cancer is targeted primarily toward elderly persons who are most likely to be affected by this deadly disease process.

## ❦ HOME CARE CONSIDERATIONS

The dumping syndrome is the most common complication of the surgical treatment of gastric cancer, and the patient will need to make multiple dietary adjustments to control its symptoms. Chronic diarrhea and malabsorption also may become daily struggles. Management of these problems is discussed on pp. 1492-1493. Nutritional support may become necessary in certain situations and will be essential if further active treatment is planned.

Pain control is a frequent home care issue for patients with advanced disease. The appropriate use of long-acting oral narcotics, epidural catheters, and infusion pumps can make it possible for patients to remain in their home environments with home health or hospice support.

# SURGICAL TREATMENT FOR OBESITY

## ETIOLOGY/EPIDEMIOLOGY

Surgery for obesity is reserved for persons with massive or morbid obesity who have diligently tried other methods of weight control and failed. Opinions vary as to its appropriateness and effectiveness, but there is general consensus that it can be lifesaving if used by a skillful surgeon and under the right circumstances. Criteria for the surgery generally include (1) age between 18 and 55 years, (2) at least 100 pounds over ideal body weight, (3) morbid obesity for at least 5 years, (4) evidence of serious dieting efforts, and (5) absence of major illnesses.

## PATHOPHYSIOLOGY

Morbid obesity has multiple effects on the body that often manifest as comorbid conditions. Obesity is listed as an independent risk factor for coronary artery disease. It also is implicated in hypertension, reflux esophagitis, arthritis, stress incontinence, non–insulin-dependent diabetes mellitus, and sleep apnea. The psychosocial toll that is extracted from an obese individual by a society fixated on thinness and physical perfection is difficult to overestimate.

## MEDICAL MANAGEMENT

Several procedures have been used to facilitate permanent weight loss, but only two currently have widespread approval. Jaw wiring is effective in achieving rapid weight loss but accomplishes little or nothing in the way of long-term benefits. Patients typically regain the lost weight very rapidly after the wires are removed. The use of intragastric balloons also has been discontinued. The gastric balloon is a polyurethane balloon with a hollow central channel that is inserted into the stomach by endoscopy. The balloon is inflated with approximately 200 ml of air through a catheter attached to a self-sealing valve. The balloon occupies about 25% of the total volume of the stomach and produces early satiety that theoretically reduces food intake. The stomach can enlarge, however, to accommodate extra intake. The presence of the balloon created many problems for patients, including nausea, pain, and a sensation of hunger. Gastritis and ulceration developed in some patients, and the risk of deflation that required surgery for removal was high. The balloons are no longer used in the United States.[2]

The two procedures in current use are the **gastroplasty** (gastric stapling, tucking, partitioning) and the **Roux-en-Y gastric bypass.** Gastroplasty appears to be the most successful and safest procedure. The stomach is made smaller by the placement of horizontal or vertical sutures through the stomach wall, which create a small pouch and significantly limit the amount of food that can be consumed without pain or vomiting (Figure 45-6). A small outlet to the duodenum is created, approximately 10 mm, that also limits the rate at which food exits the stomach, prolonging satiety. The partition staple line must be reinforced to reduce the risk of dehiscence. The procedure has a solid safety record and has been shown to be effective in fairly large samples.[4]

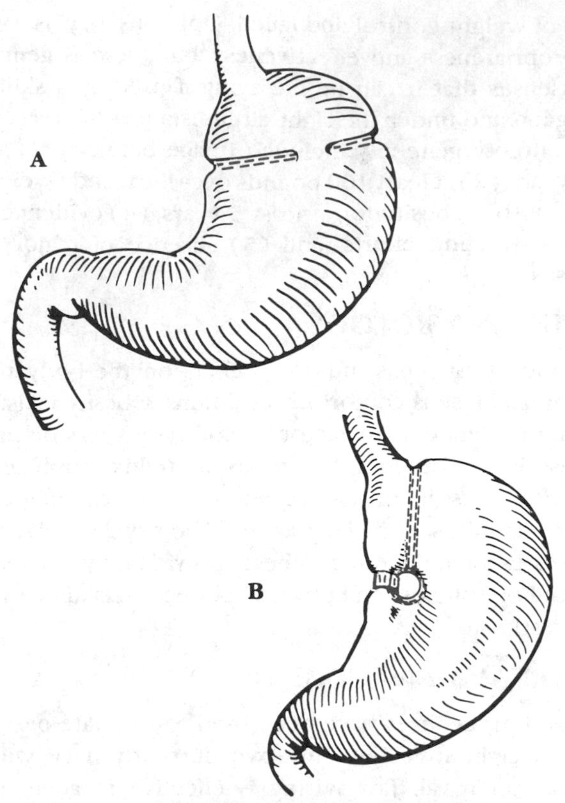


FIGURE 45-6 Gastric partitioning. **A,** Horizontal stapling. **B,** Vertical stapling.

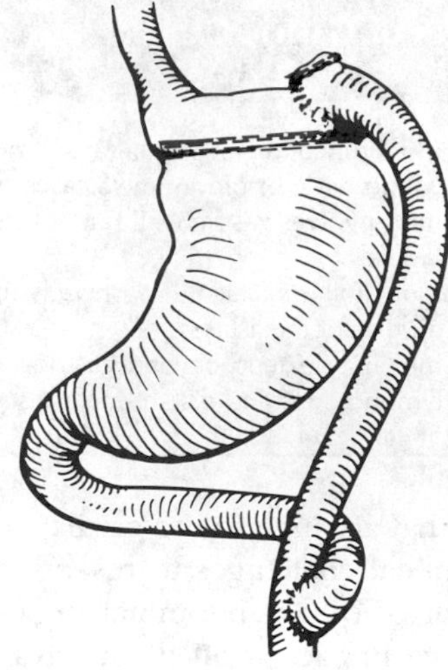

FIGURE 45-7 Roux-en-Y retrocolic gastric bypass. The stomach is completely stapled horizontally, jejunum is resected from duodenum and connected to stomach entrance, and distal duodenal stump is connected to jejunum to permit drainage of intestinal secretions.

A Roux-en-Y gastric bypass consists of a gastrojejunostomy with the jejunum attached to a closed-off pouch of the upper stomach (Figure 45-7). Food then bypasses most of the stomach and duodenum. Intestinal bypass, in which more than a foot of jejunum also was bypassed before the anastomosis, rarely is performed today because of its extensive complications. Weight loss from bypass is significant but seems to result primarily from malabsorption of food. Patients experience significant problems with the dumping syndrome regardless of eating habits. Complications can be severe and may include persistent diarrhea, electrolyte imbalance, and vitamin deficiency. Weight loss is substantial but appears to stabilize after about 2 years.

## NURSING MANAGEMENT

Preoperative preparation for gastric partitioning or Roux-en-Y bypass is similar to that required for any abdominal surgery, but morbidly obese patients are at particular risk. Concerns focus on the respiratory system, and smoking cessation before surgery is essential. The nurse teaches the patient about incisional splinting, deep breathing, coughing, and other pulmonary hygiene interventions that will be used in the postoperative period. Emotional support is critical because these patients typically are extremely anxious and even ambivalent about the need for the planned surgery.

Postoperative care is similar to that of any patient after abdominal surgery, with particular attention to pulmonary hygiene and wound healing. The head of the bed is elevated 30 to 45 degrees to support respirations. Patient-controlled analgesia is useful because appropriate narcotic doses are more difficult to calculate in the obese person. The nurse carefully monitors wound healing and is alert to the increased risk of wound infection or dehiscence, or both.

An oral diet of clear liquids is resumed 2 to 3 days after surgery. The nurse teaches the patient about the dietary restrictions in food type and amount that need to be followed to prevent discomfort or the dumping syndrome. Small feedings are essential, and the patient is encouraged to avoid the consumption of soft, high-calorie foods that can be easily digested but that will block the planned weight loss of the surgery. Vitamin supplements may be needed.

The nurse encourages the patient to use peer support groups in the community to support continued weight loss. The surgical procedures are not miracles or panaceas. To achieve maximum benefit from the surgery, the patient needs to explore and resolve food-related issues in daily life. As weight drops, aerobic exercise will become an essential component of continued weight loss and improved health and well-being. See Research box, p. 1489.

# NAUSEA AND VOMITING

## ETIOLOGY/EPIDEMIOLOGY

Nausea and vomiting, which often occur together but may occur independently, are common and important

## RESEARCH

Bufalino J et al: Surgery for morbid obesity: the patient's experience, *Appl Nurs Res* 2(1):16-22, 1989.

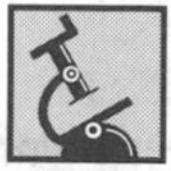

This study explored the physical and psychosocial outcomes of surgery for morbid obesity from the perspective of 137 respondents who underwent treatment between 1971-1985. Overall the respondents perceived improvements in energy level, exercise tolerance, and general mobility. Food tolerances showed wide variation ranging from virtually unlimited to broadly intolerant of most foods. Most of the study participants expressed general satisfaction with the decision to have the surgery and an improved self-perception after surgery. They also readily acknowledged the physical discomfort of the surgery itself and the strong need for follow-up counseling and support as important aspects of healing.

GI symptoms. They are part of the body's protective mechanisms and are usually a response to chemical or bacterial/viral insults to the body's integrity. They are present in a wide array of disorders and, if persistent, can lead to serious consequences. Chronic problems with nausea and vomiting may develop during pregnancy, in severe metabolic imbalances associated with uremia or alcoholism, and during cancer chemotherapy.

## PATHOPHYSIOLOGY

The vomiting center, which is located in the medulla, may be stimulated directly by the vagus nerve and the sympathetic nervous system. Visceral receptors in the GI tract and other organs can be stimulated by spasms or inflammation and can produce vomiting directly. Increased intracranial pressure also can trigger the vomiting center directly. Indirect stimulation comes from the chemoreceptor trigger zone (CTZ), which is located on the floor of the fourth ventricle. The chemical effects of a wide variety of medications can activate the CTZ. The labyrinthine stimulation associated with motion sickness also can activate the CTZ. In addition, it appears that the cerebral cortex can trigger nausea and vomiting in response to pain, stress, or intense sensation from any of the five senses. The exact mechanism of this cerebrocortical influence is not understood, but it is believed to be extremely important. A strong conditioned response to certain specific sensations or situations develops in most persons with chronic problems related to nausea and vomiting. Intense nausea and vomiting therefore can be triggered by association with events or settings. In certain persons it may occur in *anticipation* of events or situations.

Short-term episodic nausea and vomiting is distressing to almost everyone, but prolonged vomiting can have serious physiologic effects. Prolonged and severe vomiting interferes with nutrition and causes fluid and electrolyte imbalance—specifically dehydration, metabolic alkalosis, and loss of potassium, chloride, and hydrogen ions. The act of vomiting strains the abdominal muscles, and in postoperative patients it may cause wound separation or bleeding. Vomiting is especially dangerous for anesthetized patients or persons in coma because they are likely to aspirate the vomitus into the lungs. Aspiration may cause atelectasis, pneumonitis, or asphyxia, especially in the elderly person whose protective reflexes work less efficiently.

Nausea is difficult to describe because it is a subjective experience. It frequently is accompanied by weakness, hypersalivation, and diaphoresis. Gastric tone and peristalsis are typically slowed or absent. Vomiting is a complex phenomenon that begins with rhythmic contractions of the respiratory and abdominal muscles and culminates in the forceful expulsion of gastric contents from the mouth. It may be accompanied by "retching" or "dry heaves" and should be distinguished from the classic regurgitation that may accompany gastroesophageal reflux.

The color of the vomitus may be greenish-yellow, red, or brownish. A greenish-yellow color is caused by gastric juice mixing with bile that has been forced back into the stomach. Bright-red vomitus indicates overt bleeding of recent origin. Blood that has been in the stomach for a period of time becomes partly digested by the gastric juices and has a dark brown, "coffee-grounds" appearance. This blood may have originated in the stomach, or it may have been swallowed from the nose, mouth, or throat. Vomitus with a fecal odor indicates lower gastrointestinal obstruction.

## MEDICAL MANAGEMENT

The treatment of nausea and vomiting depends on the cause. Medications or other substances known to cause nausea and vomiting are discontinued if possible, and fluid and electrolyte imbalances are corrected. Fluids may be given intravenously if vomiting persists.

Antiemetic medications may be necessary. Drugs that are classified as antiemetics are theorized to function as a form of pharmacologic blockade to stimuli that may trigger nausea and vomiting (Table 45-4). Most of the drugs also are believed to have some direct sedative action on the CTZ. Antiemetics are prescribed orally if the patient is able to retain the tablets, but they often need to be given by rectal, IM, or IV route. Any of the antihistamine and phenothiazine drugs may cause dizziness and sedation, and patients are cautioned about these effects for work and driving. None of the traditional antiemetic agents have been highly effective against the nausea and vomiting induced by chemotherapy. Metoclopramide (Reglan) has been shown to be effective in blocking the effects of highly emetic chemotherapy protocols such as cisplatin (Platinol), but it is completely effective in only about 40% to 50% of patients. Meto-

**TABLE 45-4 Common Antiemetic Medications**

| DRUG | ACTION | ROUTE | CLINICAL USE |
|---|---|---|---|
| **ANTIHISTAMINES** | | | |
| Buclizine hydrochloride (Bucladin) | May depress neural pathways from labyrinth | PO | Motion sickness, vertigo |
| Cyclizine hydrochloride (Marezine) | Exact action unknown<br>As above | PO | Motion sickness, vertigo, postoperative nausea and vomiting |
| Meclizine hydrochloride (Antivert) | As above | PO | Motion sickness, vertigo |
| Dimenhydrinate (Dramamine, Dimetabs) | As above | PO | Motion sickness, vertigo |
| Hydroxyzine hydrochloride, hydroxyzine pamoate (Atarax, Vistaril) | Depression of CNS at limbic and subcortical levels | PO, IM | Postoperative nausea and vomiting |
| **PHENOTHIAZINES** | | | |
| Prochlorperazine (Compazine) | Depressant effect on CTZ<br>Suppresses vomiting center in large doses | PO, IM, suppository | Nausea and vomiting; postoperative and other conditions |
| Thiethylperazine (Torecan) | Depressant effect on CTZ | PO, IM, suppository | Nausea and vomiting; postoperative and other conditions |
| **OTHER** | | | |
| Trimethobenzamide hydrochloride (Tigan) | Depressant effect on CTZ | PO, IM, suppository | Limited value in controlling nausea and vomiting from various causes |
| Benzquinamide hydrochloride (Emete-Con) | Inhibits the CTZ | IM, IV | Postoperative nausea and vomiting |
| Diphenidol hydrochloride (Vontrol) | Inhibits the CTZ | PO | Vertigo, postoperative nausea and vomiting |
| Dronabinol (Marinol) | Derivative of marijuana; mode of action is unknown | PO | Nausea and vomiting from chemotherapy |
| Metoclopramide hydrochloride (Reglan) | Increases GI motility and lower esophageal sphincter tone; blocks dopamine receptors in CTZ | PO, IV | Nausea and vomiting from chemotherapy |
| Ondansetron hydrochloride (Zofran) | Prevents serotonin binding in GI tract and CTZ by blocking receptor sites | PO, IV | Nausea and vomiting from chemotherapy; under investigation for postoperative use |

clopramide facilitates gastric emptying and prevents bloating. It also blocks dopamine receptors in the CTZ. A new drug, ondansetron (Zofran), is extremely effective in preventing acute chemotherapy-related nausea and vomiting.[7] It is believed to work by binding serotonin receptors in the GI tract and brainstem. Chemotherapeutic agents are theorized to release serotonin from specialized cells in the GI tract. With the use of ondansetron, the receptor sites are blocked and the emetic impulse aborts. The drug is given intravenously for patients undergoing highly emetic protocols, and it may be used in oral form for mild or moderately emetic regimens. Ondansetron is not useful in the treatment of delayed emesis. It is now being tested for its effectiveness against postoperative nausea and vomiting.

## NURSING MANAGEMENT

The nursing management of nausea and vomiting is tailored to the specific needs and symptoms of the individual patient. It necessitates a careful search for both causes and successful interventions. Most persons will experience less vomiting if the emotional components of its cause are addressed, and measures to reduce anxiety should be instituted. Possible nursing interventions for the patient with nausea and vomiting are summarized in the Guidelines box, p. 1491.

# NURSING MANAGEMENT OF THE PATIENT WITH GASTRIC SURGERY

Gastric surgery may be indicated for patients with peptic ulcer disease who do not respond to traditional therapy or for those who experience potentially life-threatening complications such as hemorrhage, perforation, or obstruction. It also is performed to treat gastric cancer or to control morbid obesity. Most procedures involve some degree of partial gastrectomy with anastomosis to either the duodenum or jejunum.

## Guidelines for Management of Nausea and Vomiting

**ASSESSMENT**

Pattern of nausea/vomiting
- Time of day and duration
- Relationship to meals

Color, odor, quantity of vomitus

**SAFETY AND COMFORT**

Keep head of bed elevated and emesis basin handy.
Protect airway with suction and positioning if patient is not alert.
Provide frequent mouth care.
Control sights and odors in room.
Reduce anxiety if possible.
Provide quiet or distraction on the basis of patient response.
Modify environmental stimuli (cool cloth, dim light), and evaluate response.

**DIET MODIFICATIONS**

Maintain NPO if vomiting is severe.
Explore use of clear liquids:
- Serve liquids cool or room temperature
- Try effervescent drinks and evaluate effect
- Avoid fatty foods
- Keep meals small, avoid overdistention

**DRUGS**

Administer medications before vomiting occurs, if possible.
Evaluate patient response to medications.
Maintain patient safety and assess for sedation or confusion.

## PREOPERATIVE CARE

It is not uncommon for gastric surgery to be performed on an emergent basis in the attempt to control a life-threatening complication. When circumstances permit, however, every effort is made to ensure that the patient is in optimal nutritional status to undergo the rigors of major surgery. Correction of nutritional deficits may involve preoperative enteral feedings or short-term parenteral nutrition.

### Patient Teaching

A high abdominal incision is standard practice with gastric surgery. This incision limits respiration and places the person having gastric surgery at high risk for postoperative respiratory complications. The nurse focuses preoperative teaching on pulmonary hygiene and the importance of deep breathing, effective coughing, splinting the incision, frequent position changes, incentive spirometry, and chest physiotherapy if indicated. These teaching interventions are even more critical if the patient has a history of smoking.

Most patients undergoing gastric surgery have an NG tube in place for several days after surgery, because of decreased peristalsis from manipulation of the GI tract organs during surgery and for prevention of trauma or pressure on suture lines. The nurse teaches the patient about the NG tube and its purpose, the necessity for an initial NPO status, and the planned use of any other wound-drainage device.

Relieving anxiety if possible is the final area addressed by the nurse in the preoperative period. Gastric surgery frequently is necessitated by serious and even life-threatening conditions. The nurse provides the patient with accurate information and encourages the patient to verbalize concerns.

## POSTOPERATIVE CARE

### Maintaining a Patent Airway and Ventilation

The patient who has had gastric surgery tends to lie still and breathe shallowly to limit incisional pain. Pain medications are provided frequently, or patient-controlled analgesia is used and monitored. Adequate pain management is essential to achieving respiratory goals. Turning, deep breathing, incentive spirometry, and ambulation are stressed during the 30- to 90-minute period when the pain medication is at its peak effectiveness. A semi-Fowler's position assists with natural chest expansion. The nurse routinely auscultates the lungs to monitor pulmonary status and consistently encourages the patient in all pulmonary hygiene routines.

### Supporting Adequate Nutrition

The patient is given nothing by mouth until peristalsis resumes and initial surgical healing occurs. Drainage from the NG tube usually contains some blood for the first 6 to 12 hours, but bright-red blood, large amounts of blood, or excessive bloody drainage is reported to the surgeon at once. If the NG tube stops draining, the surgeon also is notified immediately because a buildup of gas or fluid can cause pressure on the suture line, resulting in rupture or dislodgment of the sutures.

To protect the healing suture line, the nurse does not routinely irrigate or reposition the NG tube. Fluids are given parenterally until the tube is removed and the patient is able to drink enough fluids orally. The nurse offers or provides the patient with frequent mouth care. It is important for gastric drainage and urinary output to be accurately measured and recorded.

Fluids by mouth may be restricted for 12 to 24 hours after the NG tube is removed. Small amounts of fluid are then given frequently, and the patient is observed for signs of leakage, such as difficulty in breathing, pain, or rise in temperature. Foods are added as tolerated by the patient. The dietary regimen must be adapted to the individual, because some persons tolerate increasing amounts of food and fluids better than others.

When the cardia of the stomach has been removed, the patient may complain of nausea and vomiting. This difficulty usually is caused by irritation of the esophageal mucosa by the gastric juices that reflux into the esophagus when the patient lies flat. The patient should never lie flat in bed and should avoid bending and stooping.

Early satiety is a common problem after gastric surgery. Regurgitation after meals also occurs and may be caused by eating too fast, eating too much, or postoperative edema around the suture line that prevents the food from passing into the intestines. If regurgitation occurs, the patient is encouraged to eat more slowly and to temporarily decrease the size of each meal.

Anorexia and weight loss are common problems after gastric surgery, particularly if the dumping syndrome and early satiety occur. The ongoing involvement of a dietitian or nutritionist may be necessary.

## Managing Complications

A variety of major and minor complications may occur after gastric surgery. Early complications include bleeding and duodenal stump leakage. Later complications include dumping syndrome, anemia, and fat malabsorption.

### Early postoperative complications

Bleeding at the anastomosis site is a fairly common problem. Sometimes it stops spontaneously. Major risk periods include the first 24 hours after surgery and again between the fourth and seventh days when nonhealing becomes apparent. The nurse carefully monitors the NG tube drainage for blood and avoids unnecessary irrigation or repositioning of the tube.

Any of the anastomosis sites are at risk for leakage in the early postoperative period. The blind-end duodenal stump that is created with a Billroth II or Roux-en-Y procedure appears to be particularly vulnerable. The nurse monitors for classic peritonitis symptoms such as severe abdominal pain, rigidity, and fever. Surgical drainage and closure often are necessary.

### Dumping syndrome

**Dumping syndrome** is the term used for a group of unpleasant vasomotor and gastrointestinal symptoms that occur after gastric surgery in as many as 50% of patients. The pathophysiology of dumping syndrome is not well understood. It is a complex process with several contributing causative factors. One major element is believed to be the rapid entry of hypertonic food directly into the jejunum without undergoing usual changes and dilution in the stomach. The chyme—more hyperosmolar than the jejunal secretions—causes fluid to be drawn from the bloodstream into the jejunum, decreasing blood volume and leading to hypotension. Another factor involved in the dumping syndrome appears to be related to the ingestion of sugar, the most osmotically active food. There is a sudden rise in blood sugar (hyperglycemia) with the entrance of glucose into the bloodstream, followed by an increased secretion of insulin and a subsequent fall in blood sugar to subnormal levels (hypoglycemia). The rapid gastric emptying and the propulsion of chyme into the small intestine are also thought to initiate an intensive gastrocolic reflex and to cause diarrhea and a feeling of fullness and discomfort.

The nurse instructs the patient about the nature of the problem and assesses for its presence once oral feedings are resumed. Patients typically experience weakness, faintness, palpitations of the heart, and diaphoresis. Feelings of fullness, discomfort, and nausea often occur, and diarrhea may develop. The onset of symptoms may occur during the meal or from 5 to 30 minutes after the meal. The attack may last 20 to 60 minutes.

Prevention is the most effective means of controlling dumping syndrome. The nurse instructs the patient to follow a moderate-fat, high-protein diet with limited carbohydrates. Simple sugars should be avoided completely. Fluids with meals are discouraged because they increase total volume. Lying down on the left side for 20 to 30 minutes to delay gastric emptying is helpful in some patients. Anticholinergic or antispasmodic drugs may be helpful. Surgical correction occasionally is needed through narrowing of the gastric outlet. Management of the dumping syndrome is summarized in Box 45-7.

### Malabsorption

After gastric surgery, malabsorption of fat may occur from decreased acid secretion, decreased availability of pancreatic enzymes, and increased upper gastrointestinal motility, which prevents adequate mixing of the chyme with biliary and pancreatic secretions. It is particularly troublesome after Billroth II repairs. The pa-

**BOX 45-7 Management of Dumping Syndrome**

**PATHOPHYSIOLOGY**

Multifactorial, poorly understood
Rapid entry of food into jejunum
- Chyme is hypersmolar
- Fluids shift from bloodstream into jejunum for osmotic dilution

Simple sugars trigger rise in blood sugar
Rebound secretion of insulin triggers hypoglycemia
Rapid gastric emptying triggers gastrocolic reflexes

**CLINICAL MANIFESTATIONS**

Weakness
Dizziness
Diaphoresis
Feeling of fullness or discomfort
Nausea
Diarrhea
Onset of symptoms is usually 5-30 min after eating and may last for 20-60 min

**MANAGEMENT**

Prevention is the key:
- Small frequent meals
- Moderate-fat, high-protein diet
- Limited carbohydrates, no simple sugars
- Minimal liquids with meals
- Avoid very hot and very cold foods and beverages
- Rest on left side for 20-30 min after eating
- Anticholinergic or antispasmodic medications

tient experiences steatorrhea, diarrhea, and weight loss. Deficiencies in fat-soluble vitamins may occur. Diet adjustments are made to test the patient's responsiveness to various amounts of dietary fat. Pancreatic enzymes or antispasmodic agents may be helpful.

The combined effects of dumping syndrome and steatorrhea can result in fairly significant weight loss over a relatively short time. The patient is encouraged to monitor body weight at least weekly and to experiment with food supplements as tolerated to meet nutritional needs.

### Vitamin $B_{12}$ deficiency

Gastrectomy procedures result in a partial or total loss of the intrinsic factor that is secreted by the parietal cells of the stomach. Intrinsic factor is essential to the

**TABLE 45-5 Nursing Care of the Patient After Gastric Surgery**

| INTERVENTION | RATIONALE |
|---|---|
| **PREOPERATIVE CARE** | |
| 1. Teach breathing exercises. | Exercises learned preoperatively have a greater probability of being performed postoperatively. |
| 2. Explain special postoperative measures: nasogastric tube and parenteral fluids until peristalsis returns. | Knowing what to expect may decrease anxiety. |
| **POSTOPERATIVE CARE** | |
| 1. Promote pulmonary ventilation. | |
| a. Encourage patient to turn, breathe deeply, and cough at least q 2 hr (or less until ambulating well); splint or support incision during coughing. | The high abdominal incision will cause patient to splint chest and breathe shallowly; supporting incision will help patient cough more deeply. |
| b. Give pain medication before activities. | Patient will be more active if feeling comfortable; activity will increase ventilation. |
| c. Position patient in mid- or high-Fowler's position. | Position promotes chest expansion. |
| 2. Provide comfort. | |
| a. Provide good mouth care until oral fluids can be resumed. | Oral dryness and debris result from NPO status. |
| b. Provide adequate analgesics during first few days; patient-controlled anesthesia (PCA) is effective. | Pain is expected; giving analgesics before pain becomes severe will increase effectiveness of analgesic. |
| c. Splint incision with hands or towel before patient coughs. | A pulling sensation on incision will make patient hesitant to cough; splinting supports the incision. |
| d. Encourage ambulation. | Encourages ventilation, comfort, and improved morale (see Chapter 25). |
| 3. Promote nutrition. | |
| a. Measure NG drainage accurately; monitor for blood in drainage. Do not irrigate or reposition tube unless ordered. | Drainage is measured for maintenance of fluid and electrolyte balance; the amount of fluid lost by gastric drainage will be replaced by IV fluids. Movement can weaken sutures. |
| b. Monitor for signs of leakage of anastomosis (dyspnea, pain, fever) when oral fluids are initiated. | Anastomotic leakage will be most evident when fluids first pass anastomosis site. |
| c. Add food in small amounts at frequent intervals until well tolerated. | Edema from surgery will further decrease stomach reservoir. |
| d. Monitor for early satiety and regurgitation. | Contents from a very full stomach may be regurgitated into esophagus, causing discomfort and esophagitis. |
| e. If regurgitation occurs, tell patient to eat less food at a slower pace. | This gives stomach time to adapt and prevents early satiety and distention. |
| f. Report signs of dumping syndrome (weakness, faintness, palpitations, diaphoresis, nausea, diarrhea). | Diet will need to be changed to low-carbohydrate, high-fat, high-protein foods. |
| g. Monitor weight. | Slow weight loss can be expected from decreased intake; weight gain indicates fluid retention. |
| 4. Provide patient teaching. | |
| a. Gradually increase amount of food each meal until able to eat 3 to 6 meals/day, if possible. | The stomach will expand and adapt slowly. |
| b. If discomfort occurs after eating, decrease size of meals and amount of fluids with meals; eat more slowly. | Ingestion of fluids leads to early satiety; eating too fast promotes air swallowing and gaseous feeling. |
| c. Avoid stress during and immediately after meals; plan a rest period after eating. | Stress stimulates blood flow to vital organs and away from stomach (decreases digestion); activity redirects blood flow to muscles. |
| d. Elevate head when lying down (if cardia of stomach removed). | This prevents gastroesophageal reflux (heartburn) by gravity flow. |
| e. Monitor weight regularly. | Weight loss >10% should be reported to physician; this may indicate partial obstruction. |
| f. Report signs of complications: vomiting after meals, increasing feelings of abdominal fullness or weakness, hematemesis, tarry stools, persistent diarrhea. | Facilitates early treatment of complications. |

absorption of vitamin $B_{12}$ in the intestine. Without its presence, the patient will gradually develop the symptoms of pernicious anemia, which can be fatal if not treated. The nurse teaches the patient about the vitamin deficiency and explains why oral vitamin replacement is not possible. A 100- to 200-μg monthly injection of vitamin $B_{12}$ will prevent the deficiency. Replacement therapy will be lifelong. The digestive changes associated with gastrectomy also increase the risk of iron deficiency anemia, and ferrous sulfate may be prescribed.

Care of the patient who has had gastric surgery is summarized in Table 45-5.

## QUESTIONS TO CONSIDER

- Review the *Healthy People 2000* goals related to food safety (p. 1469). What type of program(s) or approaches would you recommend to help your community address these goals?
- What recommendations would you make to a friend or family member who was considering gastric partitioning or gastric bypass surgery?
- Consider your current life-style and meal pattern. What changes would you have to make to prevent or treat dumping syndrome?
- Design a research project to test the effectiveness of antacids versus $H_2$ receptor antagonists in preventing stress ulcers in ICU patients.

## CRITICAL THINKING ACTIVITIES

- Your neighbor confides in you that he is afraid to go to the doctor because he fears he has stomach cancer. Upon further questioning you learn that he has had frequent episodes of indigestion and increased flatulence. He also comments that he has been under a lot of pressure at work, which has caused him to become nauseated on a few occasions. He does not have a family history of stomach cancer. What is the best approach to take in this situation?
- Ruth has had a gastrostomy and is going home in the morning. You are teaching her about home care. After your discussion Ruth comments, "I'm glad I'm going to lose weight without exercising. I really don't enjoy aerobics." Does Ruth require any further teaching, or is she ready for discharge?

## CHAPTER SUMMARY

### GASTRITIS

- Gastritis may be acute or chronic. Acute gastritis results from severe irritation by chemicals, foodstuffs, drugs, or bacteria. Chronic gastritis either is caused by an autoimmune process that results in atrophic problems or is related to chronic infection with *H. pylori* bacteria.

### PEPTIC ULCER DISEASE

- The exact causes of peptic ulcer disease remain unclear. It occurs from a combination of acid oversecretion and breakdown of the protective mechanisms of the gastric mucosa. Genetic, environmental, and infectious processes are all important aspects.
- The overall incidence of peptic ulcer disease has declined, and it is now typically a disease of older adults. Duodenal ulcers still occur more frequently than gastric and are more common in men.
- The chronic use of NSAIDs is a primary cause of gastric ulcers in elderly persons, particularly women.
- Actual oversecretion of acid is relatively rare in peptic ulcers. In duodenal ulcers acid may be secreted excessively postprandially, and an increase in parietal cell mass often is noted. Oversecretion is extremely rare in gastric ulcers.
- The role of *H. pylori* infection in peptic ulcers continues to be researched. It produces chronic gastritis and interferes with mucous and bicarbonate production by the mucosa, impairing mucosal defenses.
- Pain is a common symptom in peptic ulcers, but it may not be present. Classic duodenal ulcer pain is located in the epigastrium, is relieved by food or antacid, and is worse at night. Pain from gastric ulcers has a similar quality but occurs more rapidly after meals and is often poorly relieved by food or antacid.
- Drug therapy is the core of peptic ulcer management. Antacids, sucralfate, and $H_2$ receptor antagonists all are effective in ulcer healing, which usually is accomplished in 6 to 8 weeks.
- Misoprostol may be given to patients taking NSAIDs. It is a synthetic prostaglandin that supports the integrity of the gastric mucosal defenses.
- Recurrence is a major problem of peptic ulcer management. When relapse occurs, patients may be given triple therapy with bismuth products and antibiotics to eradicate the *H. pylori* infection, which is theorized to cause most recurrences.

### NURSING MANAGEMENT

- Nursing care of patients with peptic ulcers involves teaching about the medication regimen, fostering adherence, and exploring life-style changes to reduce recurrence risk, e.g., eliminating smoking and alcohol.
- No special diet is required for ulcer healing. Patients are encouraged to avoid any foods that cause pain and

to follow a "heart healthy" high-fiber, low–saturated fat diet.

- The most common complication of peptic ulcer is hemorrhage; treatment consists of stabilization of shock, gastric lavage, drugs for peptic ulcer therapy, and endoscopic treatment of the bleeding site. Surgery may be needed if bleeding persists.
- Perforation of an ulcer through the stomach wall is treated with parenteral fluids, nasogastric suction, antibiotic therapy, and surgery.
- Surgical treatment for peptic ulcers may consist of severing the vagus nerve in one of three places, where it innervates the stomach and widening the pyloric outlet (vagotomy and drainage), or removing the lower half of the stomach and severing the vagus nerve where it enters the stomach (antrectomy with vagotomy).

### STRESS ULCERS

- Stress ulcers can develop very rapidly after major trauma, surgery, or other critical illness. Mucosal ischemia triggers the ulcerative cycle. Aggressive prevention with $H_2$ receptor antagonists or other drugs is essential because mortality is very high.

### CANCER OF THE STOMACH

- The incidence of gastric cancer has declined significantly. Its cause is unknown but related to achlorhydria, heavy cigarette smoking, and genetic vulnerability. Virtually all gastric tumors are malignant.
- Most gastric tumors are incurable by the time symptoms appear. Mortality is extremely high. Surgical resection (partial gastrectomy) is the preferred treatment.

### SURGICAL TREATMENT FOR OBESITY

- Surgery for morbid obesity usually consists of gastroplasty (most effective) and gastric bypass.

### NAUSEA AND VOMITING

- Nausea and vomiting is a complex problem that has physiologic, cognitive, and emotional components. The vomiting center is located in the medulla and may be stimulated by the sympathetic nervous system or the chemoreceptor trigger zone or indirectly by the cortex.
- Antiemetics are usually only partially effective in controlling nausea and vomiting. Nursing interventions focus on reducing anxiety, manipulating the environment, and experimenting with diet modifications.

### NURSING OF THE PATIENT WITH GASTRIC SURGERY

- Postoperative care after gastric surgery focuses on promoting pulmonary ventilation, promoting nutrition, providing comfort, and teaching about self-care.
- Dumping syndrome is a postoperative complication that results from rapid entry of hypertonic chyme directly into the jejunum, causing fluid from the bloodstream to be drawn into the jejunum. There is a sudden rise in blood glucose (from absorbed glucose) followed by hypoglycemia. Therapy consists of a low-carbohydrate, moderate-fat, and high-protein diet with fluids restricted between meals.

## REFERENCES


1. Barkin JS et al: What's new in stomach cancer? *Patient Care* 26(8):22-59, 1992.
2. Black J, Mangan M: Body contouring and weight loss surgery for obesity. *Nurs Clin North Am* 26(3):777-789, 1991.
3. Cady B, Rossi RL, Silverman ML: Gastric adenocarcinoma: a disease in transition, *Arch Surg* 124(3):303-308, 1989.
4. Calloway CW et al: Obesity: a quartet of approaches, *Patient Care* 26(14):157-199, 1992.
5. Clearfield HR: *Helicobacter pylori:* aggressor or innocent bystander? *Med Clin North Am* 75(4):815-827, 1991.
6. Clearfield HR, Wright RA: Update on peptic ulcer disease, *Patient Care* 24(3):28-40, 1990.
7. Distasio S: Zofran makes chemo bearable, *RN* 13(5):56-59, 1993.
8. Dudnick R, Martin P, Friedman LS: Management of bleeding ulcers, *Med Clin North Am* 75(4):947-963, 1991.
9. Gervin AS, Gostout CJ, Zinner MJ: Upper GI bleeding: treatment options, *Patient Care* 25(2):59-77, 1991.
10. Gilinsky NH: Peptic ulcer disease in the elderly, *Gastroenterol Clin North Am* 19(2):255-268, 1990.
11. Hisamichi S: Screening for gastric cancer, *World J Surg* 13(1):31-37, 1989.
12. Katz J: The course of peptic ulcer disease, *Med Clin North Am* 75(4):831-840, 1991.
13. Kneller RW, McLaughlin J, Bjelke E: A cohort study of stomach cancer in a high risk American population, *Cancer* 68(3):672-678, 1991.
14. Mamel JJ: Use of endoscopy in peptic ulcer disease, *Med Clin North Am* 75(4):841-850, 1991.
15. Marotta RB, Floch MH: Diet and nutrition in ulcer disease, *Med Clin North Am* 75(4):967-978, 1991.
16. Mertz HR, Walsh JH: Peptic ulcer pathophysiology, *Med Clin North Am* 75(4):799-812, 1991.
17. Pilchman J, Lefton HB, Barden GL: Cytoprotection and stress ulceration, *Med Clin North Am* 75(4):853-863, 1991.
18. Prevost SS, Oberle A: Stress ulceration in the critically ill patient, *Crit Care Nurs Clin North Am* 5(1);163-169, 1993.
19. Rubin W: Medical treatment of peptic ulcer disease, *Med Clin North Am* 75(4):981-998, 1991.
20. Sachdeva AK, Zaren HA, Sigel B: Surgical treatment of peptic ulcer disease, *Med Clin North Am* 75(4):999-1012, 1991.
21. Schindler BA, Ramchandani D: Psychologic factors associated with peptic ulcer disease, *Med Clin North Am* 75(4):865-874, 1991.
22. Schorah CJ, Sobala GM, Sanderson M: Gastric juice ascorbic acid: effects of disease and implications for gastric carcinogenesis, *Am J Clin Nutr* 53(1) Supplement, 1991.
23. Smith JW, Shiu MH, Kelsey L: Morbidity of radical lymphadenectomy in the curative resection of gastric carcinoma, *Arch Surg* 126(12):1469-1473, 1991.
24. Spiro HM: Some perspectives on peptic ulcer, *Med Clin North Am* 75(4):941-946, 1991.
25. US Department of Health and Human Services, Public Health Service: *Healthy people 2000: summary report,* Boston, 1992, Jones & Bartlett.
26. Wardell TL: Assessing and managing a gastric ulcer, *Nursing '91* 21(3):34-41, 1991.

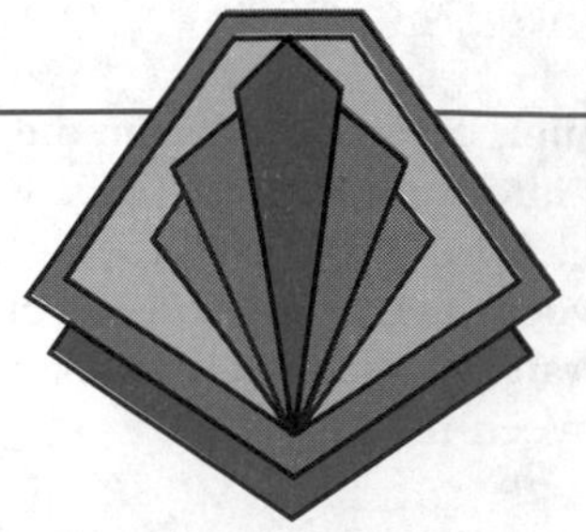

CHAPTER 46

# Management of Persons With Problems of the Gallbladder and Exocrine Pancreas

*Virginia L. Cassmeyer*

## CHAPTER OBJECTIVES

***After studying this chapter, the learner should be able to do the following:***

1. Describe the etiology, epidemiology, and pathophysiology of cholelithiasis and cholecystitis and cancer of the biliary tract.
2. Describe primary and secondary preventive techniques for gallbladder disease.
3. Describe the nursing care needs of patients with disorders of the biliary system.
4. Develop nursing diagnoses, patient outcomes, and plans of interventions for patients with cholelithiasis, cholecystitis, and cancer of the biliary tract.
5. List the causes of acute and chronic pancreatitis.
6. Describe primary and secondary preventive techniques for pancreatic disease.
7. Explain the pathophysiologic basis for signs and symptoms of acute and chronic pancreatitis and pancreatic tumors.
8. Develop nursing diagnoses, patient outcomes, and plans of interventions for patients with acute or chronic pancreatitis, cancer of the pancreas, or pancreatic surgery.

## KEY TERMS

acalculous cholecystitis
autodigestion
biliary colic
bilirubinuria
cholecystectomy
cholecystitis
cholecystostomy
choledocholithiasis
choledochostomy
cholelithiasis
cholestasis
conjugated hyperbilirubinemia
extracorporeal shock wave lithotripsy (ESWL)
extrahepatic
gallstone colic
hepatocellular
hyperbilirubinemia
icterus
intrahepatic
jaundice
laparoscopic cholecystectomy (LC)
pancreatectomy
pancreatic pseudocyst
pancreatitis
unconjugated hyperbilirubinemia

The major focuses of this chapter are diseases of the biliary system and exocrine pancreas. Because jaundice is a major finding in biliary disease and, at times, in pancreatic disease, it will be discussed first.

## JAUNDICE

### DEFINITION

**Jaundice** (also called **icterus**) is yellowish discoloration of the mucous membranes, sclera, and skin caused by the retention of bilirubin. Carotene can cause yellowing of the skin but does not affect the sclera.[14] Jaundice occurs when the total serum bilirubin is three to four times normal.[14]

### TYPES OF JAUNDICE

Jaundice and the associated **hyperbilirubinemia** (increased bilirubin in the blood) can be classified as *unconjugated* or *conjugated,* based on the predominate form of bilirubin in the blood. **Unconjugated hyper-**

**bilirubinemia** (increased non-water-soluble form of bilirubin in the blood) results from disorders of red blood cells, circulatory disturbances involving the liver, and functional problems with the uptake or conjugation of bilirubin.[14] **Cholestasis** (stasis or obstruction of any part of the biliary duct system from the biliary canaliculi to the sphincter of Oddi) and liver disease that is **hepatocellular** (affecting the parenchymal cells of the liver) in origin cause conjugated hyperbilirubinemia. **Conjugated hyperbilirubinemia** (increased water-soluble bilirubin in the blood) results from (1) blockage of secretion of conjugated bilirubin into canaliculi and (2) blockage of conjugated bile flow through the biliary tract—both the intrahepatic and extrahepatic ducts.

## Differentiating Types of Jaundice

When jaundice occurs or when an elevation in total serum bilirubin is discovered, the challenge is to diagnose the cause. Serum and urine bilirubin tests can be used to differentiate the two types of jaundice.

### Conjugated versus unconjugated jaundice

The simplest test for conjugated hyperbilirubinemia is to test the urine for **bilirubinuria** (bilirubin in the urine). It should be remembered that normally no bilirubin is found in the urine because the blood level is less than the renal threshold. Elevation of unconjugated bilirubin does not lead to bilirubinuria because it is not water soluble. Conjugated bilirubin, being water soluble, can be found in the urine even before jaundice is present clinically because the renal threshold is less than 1.0 mg/dl.

### Hepatocellular versus cholestatic jaundice

Once conjugated hyperbilirubinemia is identified, the next challenge facing the clinician is to separate hepatocellular jaundice from cholestatic jaundice. One major difference is that itching of the palms and soles occurs in 75% of persons with cholestatic jaundice.[14] Other laboratory differences between the major causes of jaundice are presented in Table 46-1. It should be noted that persons with hepatocellular disease can have intrahepatic cholestasis. This is found in alcoholic liver disease and viral hepatitis. Also, prolonged cholestasis of any type can cause hepatocellular disease. Last, uncontrolled cholestasis and hepatocellular disease both lead to cirrhosis. In these last three situations the differentiation of hepatocellular disease from cholestasis will require other tests.

### Intrahepatic versus extrahepatic jaundice

The next challenge is to localize the site of blockage. That is **intrahepatic** (within the liver) versus **extrahepatic** (in the biliary tract outside of the liver). This differentiation is made based primarily on the history and physical examination. Factors supportive of an extrahepatic site of obstruction include the following[14]:

**TABLE 46-1 Tests to Differentiate Cholestatic Jaundice From Hepatocellular Jaundice**

| TESTS | CHOLESTATIC JAUNDICE | HEPATOCELLULAR JAUNDICE |
|---|---|---|
| Serum bile acids | Very high | Moderately high |
| Steatorrhea | Common | Uncommon |
| Serum alkaline phosphatase | > three times normal | < three times normal |
| Serum cholesterol | Increased | Decreased |
| Serum transaminases (AST [SGOT] and ALT (SGPT]) | Seldom >300 IU | Can be >1000 IU |
| Effectiveness of vitamin K on prothrombin time | Good effect | No effect |

Adapted from Ostrow, JD: Jaundice and disorders of bilirubin metabolism. In Stein JH, editor: *Internal medicine,* ed 4, St Louis, 1994, Mosby.

1. Palpable gallbladder
2. Severe jaundice without other systemic symptoms of liver disease (see Chapter 42)
3. *Clay-colored* (grayish-white) stools for more than 2 weeks
4. Right upper quadrant pain that is colicky and associated with chills
5. Older age

Intrahepatic jaundice is seen in younger persons with a history of etiologic factors supportive of liver disease and an enlarged liver.[14]

## PERTINENT NURSING CARE RELATED TO JAUNDICE

The care for the patient with jaundice has four focuses:

1. Patient education and care related to the diagnostic tests—explanations about the purposes of tests, preparation for the tests, and care after the tests.
2. Control of itching by:
   a. Avoiding wool clothes and linens and restrictive clothing.
   b. Using soft, dry linens (not new).
   c. Using warm water for bathing instead of hot water.
   d. Maintaining a cool environment.
   e. Avoiding activities that increase body temperature or cause sweating.
   f. Applying emollient creams and lotions to dry skin.
   g. Administering antipruritic medicines as ordered.
3. Care directed toward the underlying problem (hemolytic, hepatic, gallbladder).
4. Care to prevent bleeding if prothrombin time is prolonged (see Guidelines box, p. 1498).

**Guidelines for Decreasing the Risk of Bleeding in the Person With Jaundice and Prolonged Prothrombin Times (PT time)**

1. Avoid all intramuscular or subcutaneous injections if possible.
2. Use the smallest gauge needle possible when giving an injection.
3. Apply pressure to injection sites and venous puncture sites for at least 5 minutes and to arterial puncture sites for at least 10 minutes.
4. Give vitamin K as ordered.
5. Use a soft-bristled toothbrush or cotton swabs for oral hygiene.
6. Instruct patient not to strain at stool and to avoid vigorous blowing of nose or coughing.
7. Provide assistance when patient is up to avoid falls.
8. Make sure that room is free of clutter, that floors are dry, and that patient wears shoes or slippers to avoid injuries.

# BILIARY SYSTEM

The biliary system is affected by stones and obstruction, inflammation and infection, and cancer. Each of these pathologic conditions is discussed.

## CHOLELITHIASIS/CHOLECYSTITIS/ CHOLEDOCHOLITHIASIS

**Cholelithiasis** is stone formation in the gallbladder. This is the most common problem of the biliary system. **Cholecystitis** is an inflammation of the gallbladder that can be acute or chronic and is usually precipitated by gallstones. **Choledocholithiasis** is stone formation in the common bile duct and can occur alone but usually occurs with the other two problems. Gallstones can occur anywhere in the biliary tree (Figure 46-1).

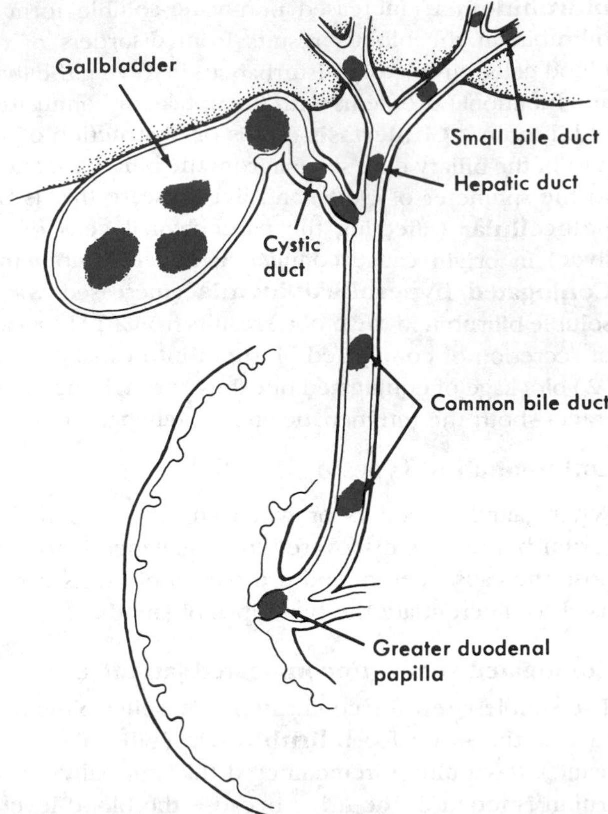


**FIGURE 46-1** Common sites of gallstones.

### ETIOLOGY

The two primary types of gallstones are *cholesterol stones* and *pigmented stones.* The pigmented stones are classified as black or brown. The etiology of gallstones is unknown but consists of any factors that increase the level of the components of stones—cholesterol, bile salts, calcium, bilirubin, and proteins. Various conditions associated with changes in cholesterol formation and excretion are associated with cholesterol stone. These risk factors include the following[5]:

1. Clinical states such as obesity, pregnancy, rapid weight loss (greater than 5 lbs/wk), and high plasma triglycerides with or without low levels of HDL-cholesterol.
2. Diseases and injuries such as primary biliary cirrhosis, hypothyroidism, and spinal cord injury.
3. Hypolipidemic drugs, such as clofibrate and gemfibrozil, and estrogen therapy.

Diabetes mellitus, long thought to be a risk factor for cholesterol stones, is not an independent factor when obesity, hypertriglyceridemia, and ethnic origin are considered.[3] Diet also is not an independent risk factor.[3] Gender (women), ethnic origin (American Indians), and advancing age also are risk factors for cholesterol stones.

Pigmented stones also have associated risk factors. These include chronic hemolysis, alcoholic cirrhosis, advancing age, ileal disease or resection, long-term treatment with total parenteral nutrition (TPN), and advanced AIDS.[5]

### EPIDEMIOLOGY

Cholelithiasis is a common health problem in the Western World. It affects 15% of the U.S. population, with an estimated 1 million new cases per year.[3] Cholelithiasis is one of the most common reasons for surgery.[22]

Cholelithiasis is two times more common in women, occurs most frequently in middle-aged and older persons, and affects American Indians, Mexican-Americans, and whites more frequently than African-Americans and Asians, although the incidence in Asians is increasing.[3]

### PATHOPHYSIOLOGY

Most of the gallstones in the body, although classified into two categories, are not pure stones. Most cholesterol stones contain only 70% cholesterol. The rest of the stone is made up of pigments, calcium, and other components. Most pigmented stones contain some cholesterol, along with calcium and other components.

Gallstone formation involves three major processes. First, the bile must become supersaturated with one of the insoluble substances—cholesterol or bilirubin pigments. The insoluble substance must form a nucleus or kernel and then precipitate. Last, the precipitate grows.

In persons who form cholesterol stones there is a relative increase in cholesterol compared with the bile salts. Cholesterol gallstone formation is also enhanced by production of a mucin glycoprotein, which traps cholesterol particles. Another factor in the pathogenesis of cholesterol stones is a decrease in the motility of the gallbladder resulting in stasis of gallbladder secretions.

Cholesterol stones usually contain some calcium, can be large (up to 4 cm), are hard and white or yellow-brown in color, and are radiolucent. The stones most frequently occur in multiples but can be solitary and are usually in the gallbladder.[3] Cholesterol stones, pure or mixed, account for 70% to 80% of all stones.

Pigmented stones are of two types—black and brown.[3] Black pigmented stones are the result of an increase in unconjugated bilirubin and calcium with a decrease in bile salts. Gallbladder motility may be impaired. These stones are primarily in the gallbladder, small (2 to 5 mm), multiple, and radiopaque. Brown pigmented stones occur mostly in the intrahepatic and extrahepatic ducts and are preceded by bacterial invasion of the duct system.[3] These stones are radiolucent and occur in multiples.

Cholecystitis may be acute and results from a blockage of the cystic duct caused by stones (95%) or blockage of the duct caused by edema and spasm initiated by the passage of the gallstone. The cystic duct can be blocked by sludge, particularly if associated with trauma, major stress, or dehydration. This type of cholecystitis is called **acalculous cholecystitis.** The blockage results in distention of a gallbladder with edema of its walls. This leads to inflammation and ischemia; the inflamed wall allows absorption of bile salts from the lumen, further increasing the inflammation. A *secondary infection* with one of several organisms that can reach the gallbladder through blood, lymph, or the biliary duct occurs within several days. In acute cholecystitis the gallbladder is enlarged and tense. The walls may become friable and necrotic, and perforation may occur, resulting in peritonitis. The gallbladder may adhere to surrounding structures. The bacterial infection is the cause of most serious consequences of cholecystitis.

*Cholecystitis may be chronic* and follow several acute attacks. But most frequently chronic cholecystitis is the result of mechanical and chemical injuries precipitated by stones that result in scarring, thickening, and ulceration of the gallbladder wall. A secondary bacterial infection also may be present in chronic cholecystitis. The gallbladder is pearly white and contains turbid bile and debris.

The patient with cholelithiasis and/or cholecystitis may have various manifestations. Cholelithiasis may cause no signs and symptoms. In some studies, 80% of study populations have been found to have asymptomatic gallstones, and most of these remain silent.[20] Asymptomatic patients have only a 1% to 2% chance of becoming symptomatic. If a stone becomes lodged in a biliary duct or inflammation occurs, symptoms can occur. However, a history of indigestion after consuming high caloric, fatty foods, occasional discomfort in the right upper quadrant of the abdomen, and more trouble than the normal person has with gaseous eructation after eating are common complaints.

If a stone lodges in the duct system, **gallstone colic** or **biliary colic** can occur. The pain comes on suddenly and may start in the midepigastrium, spread to the right upper quadrant of the abdomen, and radiate through to the back under the scapula and to the right shoulder. The pain may be extremely severe and is usually associated with tachycardia, diaphoresis, and nausea and vomiting. Frequently the patient paces or moves and turns constantly when laying in bed. Occasionally complete prostration occurs.

If cholecystitis is present, the patient may have chills and fever. Anorexia, nausea, and vomiting can occur. Jaundice can occur with or without choledocholithiasis. Bowel sounds may be absent. Palpation of the right upper quadrant (RUQ) causes a severe increase in pain and temporary inspiratory arrest *(Murphy's sign).*[2] The episode of cholecystitis usually subsides in 1 to 4 days.[3]

If the obstruction occurs in the common bile duct (choledocholithiasis), bile will be inhibited from reaching the GI tract, total and conjugated serum bilirubin will increase, and jaundice will occur. The excessive conjugated bilirubin will be excreted in the urine. Because no (or less) bile reaches the GI tract, urine urobilinogen will be decreased and clay-colored (grayish white) stools will result. The absorption of fat and fat-soluble vitamins will also be impaired. If vitamin K absorption is disrupted, a prolonged prothrombin time will occur.

Persons having an acute attack of cholecystitis may be very ill. If perforation and peritonitis occur, the patient may have signs and symptoms of peritonitis, which include sudden, severe abdominal pain, distention, and rigidity; extreme tenderness; decreased or absent bowel sounds; tachypnea; tachycardia; and leukocytosis. Bacteremia and septic shock may occur.

The patient with chronic cholecystitis usually has a history of several previous attacks of acute cholecystitis or a history indicative of cholelithiasis. There is usually a history of intolerance to fatty foods. Pain may be severe and usually is limited to the right upper quadrant. Nausea and vomiting may be present. Very frequently patients with chronic cholecystitis do not seek help until jaun-

**TABLE 46-2 Relationship of Normal Function of the Gallbladder to Pathophysiology and Clinical Manifestations of Gallbladder Disease**

| NORMAL FUNCTION | PATHOPHYSIOLOGY | CLINICAL MANIFESTATIONS |
|---|---|---|
| Concentration and storage of bile | Stasis of bile → stone formation → obstruction of bile flow | ↑ total conjugated serum bilirubin, ↑ urinary bilirubin and ↓ urine urobilinogen; jaundice; pruritus; clay-colored (grayish white) stools; impaired vitamin K absorption → prolonged prothrombin time |
| | Smooth muscle contractions | Biliary colic and generalized symptoms from severe pain |
| | Impairment of fat absorption | Intolerance of fatty foods, indigestion, eructation, nausea, and vomiting → hypovolemia → ↓ blood pressure, tachycardia, tachypnea, and diaphoresis; hypokalemia |
| | Acute or chronic inflammation or infection of gallbladder | Chills, fever, and elevated white blood cell count; bacteremia and septic shock |
| | Perforation | Peritonitis |

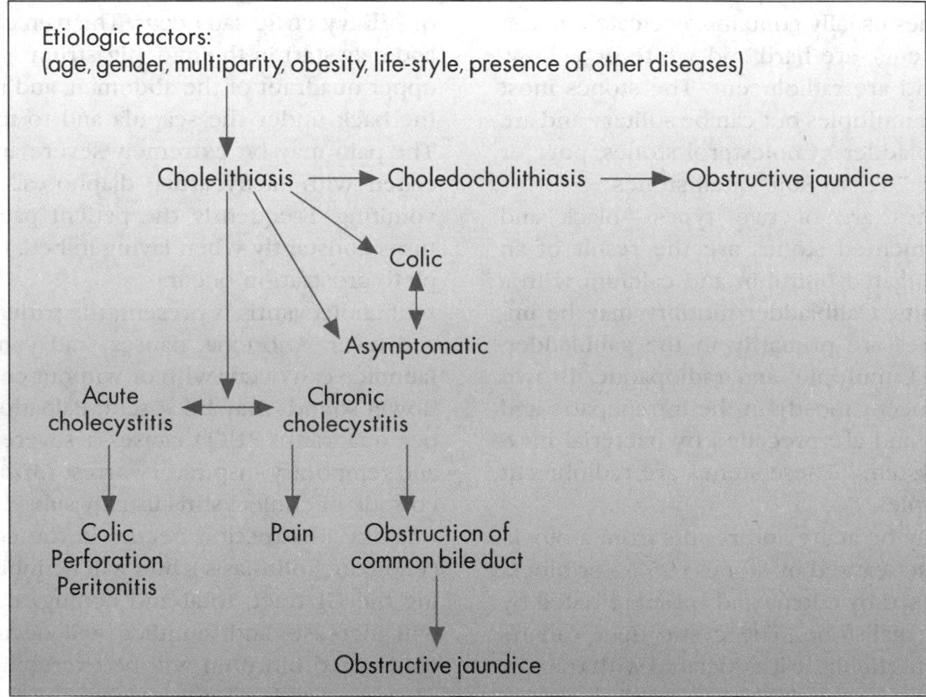


**FIGURE 46-2** Relationship between cholelithiasis and cholecystitis and other complications of biliary system disease.

dice or an acute obstruction occurs. Table 46-2 depicts the relationship between pathophysiology and clinical manifestations of cholelithiasis and cholecystitis. Figure 46-2 depicts the relationship between cholelithiasis and cholecystitis and other complications.

# PREVENTION

## Primary Prevention

The risk factors for gallbladder disease are described in the etiology section. There are two groups of patients in whom therapy is recommended to prevent gallstone formation.[3] These are patients receiving total parenteral nutrition (TPN) for 3 months or longer and persons undergoing rapid weight loss. Daily intravenous cholecystokinin-octapeptide (CCK-OP) is recommended for TPN patients; ursodiol 8 to 10 mg/kg/day is recommended for periods of rapid weight loss.[3] Control of obesity and chronic illnesses such as hemolytic anemia, hyperlipidemia, and hypothyroidism also will help to prevent gallstone formation.

## Secondary Prevention

Secondary prevention is directed at prevention of cholecystitis in selected persons with asymptomatic gallstones. **Cholecystectomy** is recommended for the following groups of persons with asymptomatic disease:

1. Persons who need to live in areas without adequate medical facilities
2. Persons with diabetes with nonfunctioning gallbladders, but not all persons with diabetes mellitus

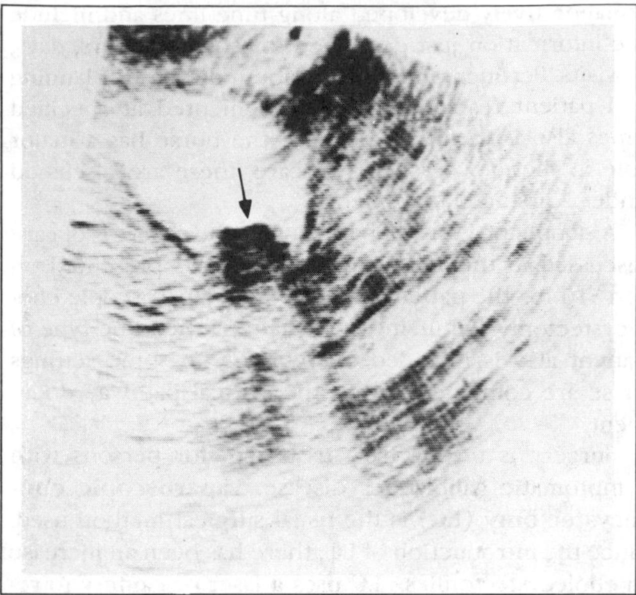

**FIGURE 46-3** Ultrasonogram demonstrating a large gallstone *(arrow)* in a dilated gallbladder. Note acoustic shadowing. (From Apstein MD, Carey MC: Biliary tract stones and associated diseases. In Stein JH, editor: *Internal medicine,* ed 4, St Louis, 1994, Mosby.)

3. American Indian women to prevent cancer
4. Persons with solitary stones that are >3.0 cm in diameter

## MEDICAL MANAGEMENT

The expected length of stay of patients with cholelithiasis and cholecystitis as determined by DRG is 2 to 6 days based on type of treatment. Common medical therapy for management of cholelithiasis and cholecystitis includes the following.

### Diagnostic Tests

Ultrasonography is the major test used in acute situations (Figure 46-3). If it is inadequate, oral cholecystography is done (Figure 46-4). Additional tests are those necessary to rule out other causes of abdominal pain. Serum laboratory tests including white blood cell count and serum transaminase, alkaline phosphatase, serum amylase, and serum bilirubin levels are conducted to identify the presence of cholecystitis and choledocholithiasis. Serum electrolyte level is done to assess fluid and electrolyte status.

### Medication

If biliary colic is present, pain is controlled by use of meperidine hydrochloride (Demerol). If nausea, vomiting, and dehydration are present, intravenous fluids are necessary. Broad-spectrum antibiotics are necessary if cholecystitis is present. If jaundice is present and the prothrombin time is prolonged, vitamin K is given.

In persons with mild, symptomatic cholelithiasis

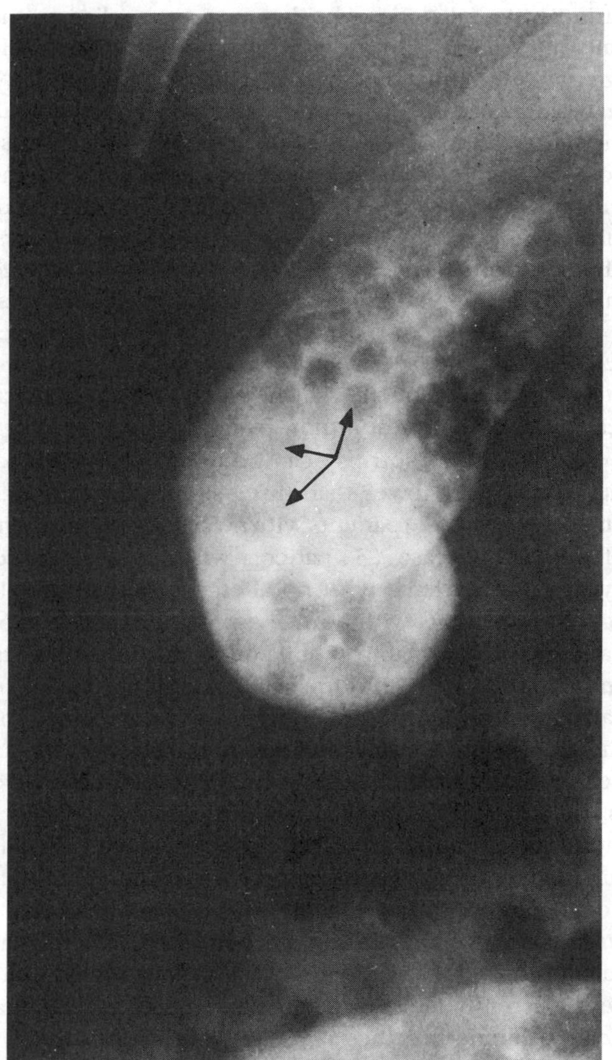

**FIGURE 46-4** Oral cholecystogram. Opacified gallbladder with multiple radiolucencies *(arrows)* caused by gallstones. (From Apstein MD, Carey MC: Biliary tract stones and associated diseases. In Stein JH, editor: *Internal medicine,* ed 4, St Louis, 1994, Mosby.)

when stones are small, in patients who refuse surgery, or in patients who are poor risk for surgery, dissolution therapy is used. Ursodiol (Actigall) dissolves stones by decreasing biliary cholesterol secretion and desaturating bile.[3] This therapy takes a long time and is expensive.[5] In addition, recurrence of stones is high.[13]

Direct dissolution therapy where methyl tert butyl ether (MTBE) is instilled through a percutaneous transhepatic catheter is experimental therapy that is used only for persons with lucent stones who are very-high-risk surgical patients.[21]

### Treatment

**Extracorporeal shock wave lithotripsy (ESWL)** is an experimental treatment available to treat selected patients. Lithotripsy involves the use of shock waves to disintegrate gallstones. Shock waves are applied to the gallstones in the gallbladder or common and hepatic bile ducts, which are located by use of ultrasound. The shock waves are usually passed through a water medium, although some machines are "dry" lithotripters and use liquid couplers contained by membranes between the shock wave source and the patient's skin.[1] Approximately 1500 shocks are delivered over 1 to 2 hours. The fragments of the disintegrated stones are excreted through the common bile duct into the small intestines.

Use of lithotripsy for patients with bile duct stones requires that the patient have an endoscopic sphincterotomy or percutaneous transhepatic catheterization at least 5 days before the lithotripsy.

At this time lithotripsy can be used only in (1) patients who have fewer than three stones that are <3.0 cm in diameter, (2) patients with no acute complications of gallstone disease, (3) patients with no acute cholecystitis, (4) patients with no allergy to iodine or bile acids, (5) patients with normal coagulation profiles, (6) patients with normal liver and pancreatic function tests, and (7) patients with no pacemakers or artificial heart valves.[1,10] The gallstones must be located so that the shock waves, which disintegrate the gallstones, do not penetrate the lung or head of the pancreas. Lithotripsy is usually used in combination with dissolution agents. Modifications in the lithotripters have altered the body surface area over which the shock wave enters the patient. Some lithotripters allow the waves to penetrate a larger skin area, decreasing the pain.[1] Also, lithotripters vary in the actual pressure delivered to the second focus.[1] Currently, most lithotripters can be applied to patients using no anesthesia or only light IV sedation.[1]

### Diet

There is no special diet for persons with gallstones to prevent stone formation. Low-fat, small meals may decrease symptoms before definitive therapy. After definitive treatment the patient is allowed to eat what is tolerated.

### Activity

There are no special activity restrictions for persons with cholelithiasis, cholecystitis, or choledocholithiasis.

### Referral/Consultation

In some settings the nurse assumes responsibility for making referrals to other services. Common referrals for persons with cholelithiasis and cholecystitis include (1) surgeon if surgery is anticipated and (2) other specialist as needed for pregnancy or hypothyroidism.

## SURGICAL MANAGEMENT

Critical pathways (also referred to as "collaborative care paths" or "care maps") have been developed in some inpatient and outpatient settings to guide both medical and nursing management. These critical pathways are collaboratively developed along time lines and include the information just described for specific hours, days, or visits. Pertinent information about discharge planning and patient teaching to be implemented at specified times also is included. Because the nurse has a major role in these two aspects of care, these are discussed under Nursing Management.

A sample of a critical pathway for the six areas of care discussed in this management section is presented on p. 1510 for the patient undergoing a laparoscopic cholecystectomy. A nursing care plan for the same type of patient also is included on p. 1510. In some settings these are combined within the critical pathway document.

Surgery is the primary treatment for persons with symptomatic gallbladder disease. **Laparoscopic cholecystectomy (LC)** is the usual surgical method used. Since the introduction of LC, there has been an increase in cholecystectomies.[4] LC uses a laser or cautery to remove the gallbladder. The first LC was performed in the United States in 1988. LC offers several advantages over the common abdominal cholecystectomy including: (1) less invasive and thus less chance of wound infection or respiratory impairment, shorter healing time, and shorter recuperative time; (2) no unsightly scar; and (3) less pain and thus much more rapid return to normal activities. The mortality and morbidity associated with LC are no greater than those associated with the traditional cholecystectomy, which are very low.[18] Most patients are discharged on the day of surgery or on the first postoperative day.

LC involves preprocedure preparation of the patient similar to that of any patient having abdominal surgery, including NPO after midnight, an enema to reduce the mass of the colon, and an antibiotic given with any premedications for anesthesia. In the operating room the patient receives a general anesthetic, has a nasogastric tube and Foley catheter inserted, and has intravenous fluids started.

The surgery is carried out using video monitors and instrumentation through four cannulas introduced by trocars into the peritoneal cavity via four small (5 mm to 10 mm) incisions. These incisions are made at the umbilicus, midline in the epigastric region and in the right upper quadrant at the midclavicular line and at the anterior axillary line. After the first incision is made at the umbilicus, carbon dioxide is introduced to insufflate the abdominal cavity, which allows for the insertion of the instruments. The carbon dioxide is removed at the end of the surgery.

An LC is not the surgery of choice for everyone. Persons who have had extensive abdominal surgery may have too many adhesions to allow for this procedure. Gallstones within the common bile duct cannot be removed with this procedure. Of course, persons who cannot tolerate general anesthesia cannot be treated with this procedure. Potential complications of the pro-

**BOX 46-1 Surgeries of the Biliary Tract**

**CHOLECYSTECTOMY**
Removal of gallbladder

**CHOLECYSTOSTOMY**
Creation of an opening into gallbladder for drainage

**CHOLEDOCHOSTOMY**
Incision into common bile duct

**CHOLEDOCHOLITHOTOMY**
Incision into common bile duct to remove a stone

**CHOLEDOCHODUODENOSTOMY**
Anastomosis of common bile duct with duodenum

**CHOLEDOCHOJEJUNOSTOMY**
Anastomosis of common bile duct with jejunum

**CHOLECYSTOGASTROSTOMY**
Anastomosis of gallbladder with stomach

cedure include injury to the hepatic or common bile duct, injury to the bowel, wound infection, abdominal abscess formation, and retained stones in the common bile duct.

The alternative surgical approach to LC is removal of the gallbladder through an abdominal incision. An abdominal incision may be used for other types of surgery on the gallbladder or duct system. Other types of surgical procedures that may be carried out are defined in Box 46-1. The terminology used to indicate specific biliary tract surgery is self-explanatory once common terms are understood. *Cholecyst* refers to the gallbladder, *choledocho* refers to the common bile duct, and *lith* refers to a stone. Biliary tract anastomoses are palliative operations to provide biliary drainage to the intestine by bypassing an obstructed area.

External biliary drainage is used in empyema, for fistulas, when chronic decompression of the biliary tract is required, and often after abdominal cholecystectomy when the common bile duct has been explored. Drainage is provided by a catheter inserted into the gallbladder **(cholecystostomy)** or by a T-tube inserted into the common bile duct **(choledochostomy)** (Figure 46-5). Usually stab wounds are used to bring these tubes through the skin.

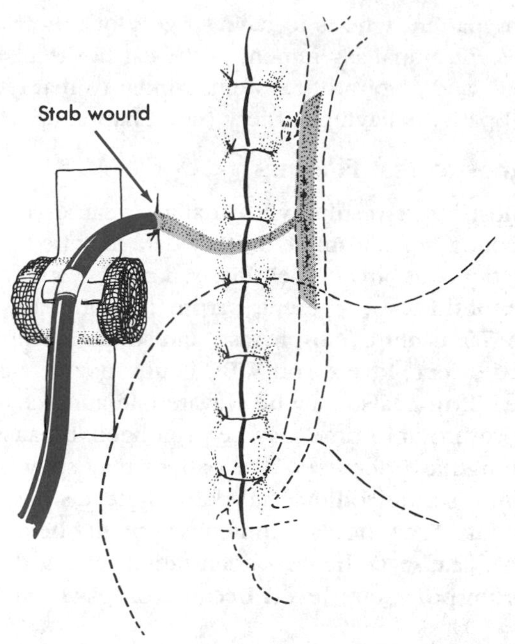


**FIGURE 46-5** Section of T-tube emerging from stab wound may be placed over roll of gauze anchored to skin with adhesive tape to prevent its lumen from being occluded by pressure.

## NURSING MANAGEMENT

### ♦ ASSESSMENT

Although some patients are admitted in a relatively stable state for surgery or lithotripsy, other patients are acutely ill. Nursing assessment will provide direction for nursing care.

#### Subjective Data

Data to be collected to assess the patient with gallbladder disease include the following:

Presence of pain: RUQ or epigastric pain with referral to scapular area or the posterior chest wall; pain intense for 1 to 4 hours; pain onset with large or rich meals

GI symptoms: nausea, vomiting, anorexia, eructation, fat intolerance, bloating, heartburn, regurgitation, change in stool color

History of fever and chills, previous attacks, jaundice

History of change in urine color

Knowledge of problem, treatment, and expectations of treatment

#### Objective Data

Data to be collected to assess the patient with gallbladder disease include the following:

1. Vital signs: blood pressure, pulse, respiration, temperature may be normal unless cholecystitis—then pulse and temperature will be mildly elevated
2. Fluid status: weight, skin turgor, mucous membrane moisture, intake and output may be normal, but signs of deficit may be present
3. Presence of jaundice
4. Abdomen: distention, tenderness, and guarding in right upper quadrant; Murphy's sign
5. Dark-colored urine, clay-colored (grayish-white) stools

The patient who is to have surgery or lithotripsy requires additional assessment of the cardiovascular, neurologic, and respiratory systems similar to that required by all patients having surgery (see Chapter 23).

## Diagnostic Test Findings

Diagnostic test results will usually reveal an abnormal ultrasonogram. Serum laboratory data may be normal if the patient has only cholelithiasis. If cholecystitis or choledocholithiasis is present, serum transaminases (ALT and AST), alkaline phosphatase, and serum bilirubin (total and direct) levels, and WBC count may be elevated. Urine bilirubin also may be elevated. If jaundice is present, prothrombin time may be prolonged. If nausea and vomiting have occurred, the patient may show an elevation in serum sodium and chloride levels because of dehydration, an increase in hematocrit and hemoglobin levels because of hemoconcentration, and a decrease in serum potassium levels because of loss from the GI tract.

# ♦ NURSING DIAGNOSES

Nursing diagnoses are determined from analysis of patient data. Nursing diagnoses for the person with biliary tract disease before definitive medical treatment may include but are not limited to the following:

| Diagnostic Title | Possible Etiologic Factors |
|---|---|
| Pain | Biliary colic and jaundice |
| Knowledge deficit: diagnostic and therapeutic measures | Lack of exposure to information |
| Nutrition, altered: more than body requirements | Excessive intake in relation to metabolic needs, lack of knowledge |

Nursing diagnoses after laparoscopic cholecystectomy may include but are not limited to the following:

| Diagnostic Title | Possible Etiologic Factors |
|---|---|
| Pain | Incisions, carbon dixoide insertion |
| Knowledge deficit: needs immediately after treatment and at discharge | Lack of exposure to information |

Nursing diagnoses after abdominal cholecystectomy or shock-wave lithotripsy treatment may include but are not limited to the following:

| Diagnostic Title | Possible Etiologic Factors |
|---|---|
| Breathing pattern, ineffective | High surgical incision, abdominal distention |
| Fatigue | Surgical or lithotripsy procedure, malnourishment before surgery or lithotripsy |
| Fluid volume deficit, high risk for | Nausea and vomiting after surgery, bleeding, loss of fluids through external drainage tubes |
| Injury, high risk for | Obstruction of T-tube after surgery or obstruction of bile duct by fragment of stone after lithotripsy |
| Knowledge deficit: needs immediately after treatment and at discharge | Lack of exposure to information |
| Nutrition, altered: high risk for less than body requirement | Nausea and vomiting after treatment |
| Pain | Incisional, spasms of ductal system associated with obstruction of T-tube or of cystic or common bile ducts from stone fragments |
| Skin integrity, impaired | Incision, potential long-term drainage tubes, potential bile drainage irritating the skin |

# ♦ EXPECTED PATIENT OUTCOMES

Expected patient outcomes for the patient with biliary tract disease before definitive medical treatment may include but are not limited to the following:

1. States pain is controlled and does not demonstrate behaviors associated with discomfort.
2. Describes the purpose of diagnostic and therapeutic measures.
3. Describes ways to reduce caloric and fat content in the diet.

Expected patient outcomes for the patient after laparoscopic cholecystectomy may include but are not limited to the following:

1. States pain is controlled and does not demonstrate behaviors associated with pain.
2. Describes care needs after discharge, signs and symptoms to report immediately, and follow-up care.

Expected patient outcomes for the patient after abdominal cholecystectomy or shock-wave lithotripsy treatment may include but are not limited to the following:

1. Breath sounds are clear and present in all lobes.
2. States fatigue is gradually improved and rates fatigue as lessened on a 1 to 5 scale (1 = no fatigue; 5 = severe fatigue).
3. Maintains normal fluid volume as evidenced by stable weight, moist mucous membranes, adequate skin turgor, and balanced intake and output with adequate amounts for age and size of person.
4. Has no undetected obstruction of T- tube drainage; reports immediately recurrence of colicky pain, jaundice, nausea and vomiting, or fever.
5. States immediate care needs, pain relief methods, activity allowed, dietary requirements, signs and symptoms to report immediately, and follow-up care.
6. Consumes a balanced diet with food from all food groups and restricted in fat if the patient had lithotripsy.

7. States pain is controlled; activity not inhibited because of pain.
8. Incision heals without complications.

## ♦ INTERVENTIONS

### Promoting Comfort

Pain control is a need of all persons with biliary tract disease before definitive treatment. Analgesics such as meperidine will be needed to control the pain from biliary colic adequately and should be freely administered. Measures to decrease nausea and vomiting, such as maintenance of an NPO status or dietary fat restriction, will be necessary.

Pain control remains a need in the posttreatment period regardless of the treatment, although pain is much less after laparoscopic cholecystectomy. For the patient who has an abdominal cholecystectomy, pain remains a problem for up to 6 weeks. Immediately after either LC or abdominal surgery, injectable analgesics are necesary. After the person is ambulating well and eating well, oral analgesics are usually satisfactory. For patients who had lithotropsy treatment, pain may continue for some time until the disintegrated stones are passed into the duodenum. Pain control is necessary to allow for adequate ambulation, deep breathing, and nutritional intake after definitive treatment.

Dressings, such as those present after abdominal surgical treatment of biliary tract disease, are monitored for moisture, which is uncomfortable and increases the risk of infection. Moist dressings are changed immediately. In addition, care is taken to avoid tension on biliary drainage tubes—another source of discomfort.

### Promoting Learning

The time available for preoperative or prelithotripsy teaching is often limited because patients may be acutely ill and undergoing diagnostic procedures and treatments to prepare them for surgery or lithotripsy within a short time. Conversely, the patient scheduled for elective surgery or lithotripsy may come to the hospital the morning of treatment 1 to 2 hours before the treatment. The nurse must be prepared to give essential information in the brief period that is available, as well as to address the patient's expressed concerns.

After treatment, carefully assessing the patient's understanding of treatment care measures is important.

Patients who have had an LC will be discharged on the day of surgery or the first day after surgery. Before discharge, patients should be eating without difficulty, be walking, and have no abdominal distention, evidence of bleeding, or bile leakage. They are instructed to report immediately any severe pain, any tenderness in the right upper quadrant, any increase in abdominal girth, any leakage of bile-colored drainage from the puncture sites, any increase in pulse, or any symptoms of low blood pressure. Patients are instructed that they usually can return to work in 3 days and can resume full activity after 1 week. Patients should know that oral analgesics control incisional pain and a heating pad usually relieves shoulder pain, which results from insertion of carbon dioxide into the abdomen during surgery.

Patients who have an abdominal cholecystectomy are discharged 5 to 6 days after surgery. They need to know that recovery at home takes 3 to 6 weeks. The patient is instructed to increase activities gradually as tolerated but to limit heavy lifting (nothing greater than 10 pounds) until full recovery is achieved at about 6 weeks. The patient also is taught how to monitor for signs and symptoms of infection, jaundice, or bile leakage and to report any signs or symptoms immediately. The nurse teaches the patient that oral analgesics should control any pain.

Patients who have had lithotripsy treatment need to know how to control pain with analgesics and low-fat diets and the importance of maintaining an adequate fluid intake to assist with the passage of the disintegrated stones. Patients should know that nausea, vomiting, and hematuria may be present for 24 hours and are treated symptomatically. The patient is instructed to report reoccurrence of fever, jaundice, prolonged nausea and vomiting, or pain, all of which indicate obstruction of the biliary tract. Patients who have had lithotripsy treatment are monitored by ultrasound and laboratory tests for passage of stones 6 weeks, 3 months, and 6 months after the procedure.

Persons with prolonged illness, as with biliary tract

**Guidelines for Teaching the Person With a Chronic Biliary System Disorder**

**DIETARY RESTRICTIONS**

Low-fat diet if fat is poorly tolerated
Low-calorie diet if weight reduction is necessary

**DRUG THERAPY, IF APPROPRIATE**

Medication: importance in preventing recurrence of symptoms
Medications: when and how to use

**DRESSINGS OR DRAINAGE TUBE**

Biliary drainage: expected amount
Dressing change or emptying of drainage bag: how to do and frequency
Dressings: need to keep dry and skin clean (soap and water is sufficient by time of discharge); a daily shower may be permitted
Dressing change: technique and availability of supplies
Signs to report to physician: excessive drainage, leakage, obstruction (jaundice, grayish-white stools)

**FOLLOW-UP CARE**

Signs and symptoms to report to health care provider (pain, fever, jaundice, dark urine, grayish-white stools, pruritus, tube dislodgement)
Planned return appointments

fistulas or metastatic carcinomas, need supportive care and instructions related to specific symptoms including fatigue and activity intolerance. They may need instructions on dealing with chronic biliary drainage and dietary restrictions. They also need to know signs and symptoms to report. Important teaching points for patients with chronic biliary system disorders are summarized in the Guidelines box, p. 1505).

## Promoting Adequate Nutrition

Many persons with gallbladder disease are obese. Also, hyperlipidemia is associated with increased risk of gallstone formation. Last, some persons will have food intolerance. Patients will need beginning assistance to match caloric intake to need. The major way nursing assists in this is to help the patient identify the problem, establish goals, and find resources to help meet the goal.

After surgery or lithotripsy, nausea and vomiting may decrease intake over a short period. The patient needs assistance in finding foods that can be tolerated. A balanced diet needs to be encouraged. Once the patient is recovered from surgery or lithotripsy treatment, the patient may need help to refocus on a diet that promotes weight loss.

## Promoting Physiologic Stability

Postoperative and postlithotripsy care are focused on the nursing diagnoses. In the immediate postoperative period care focuses on comfort measures, maintenance of fluid status, and prevention or detection of complications such as respiratory problems or obstruction of T-tube or bile duct. Other care needs relate to reducing fatigue and promoting normal activity, providing a palatable diet, promoting skin integrity, and preparing the patient for home.

On recovery from anesthesia the patient is usually placed in a low-Fowler's position. Because breathing is painful, the patient may take shallow breaths to splint the incision and lessen pain. Based on ongoing pain assessment, medications for pain should be given fairly liberally during the first 48 to 72 hours, and the patient must be urged to breathe deeply at regular intervals (every 1 to 2 hours) to avoid atelectasis. The patient must also be helped and encouraged to change position and to move about in bed frequently. If a nasogastric tube is in use, it is attached to suction. Because essential electrolytes and abdominal gas are removed by this procedure, it is discontinued as soon as possible, usually within 24 hours if bowel sounds are normal and abdomen is soft and not distended. An infusion of 5% glucose in distilled water or in some concentration of saline is usually administered. When the nasogastric tube is removed, the patient is given clear fluids by mouth. Sweet, effervescent drinks such as ginger ale usually are tolerated best at first. Within a few days the patient usually is able to eat a soft diet. Appetite will probably remain poor if bile is not flowing into the duodenum. The patient should be assessed for tolerance of oral fluids and foods. Tolerance is indicated by absence of nausea and vomiting, maintainence of soft abdomen, and lack of abdominal distention.

Dressings are checked frequently for the first few hours after surgery because, although hemorrhage from the wound is rare, it can occur. Occasionally, internal hemorrhage follows surgery of the gallbladder and bile ducts, particularly if the inflamed gallbladder was adherent to the liver. A decrease in blood pressure, increase in pulse rate, tachypnea, decreased urine output, restlessness, complaints of thirst, poor skin turgor, and so forth potentially indicate internal hemorrhage and are reported to the surgeon at once.

## Promoting Activity

Patients are usually permitted out of bed the evening of or the day after surgery. If a T-tube or a cholecystostomy tube is present, it may be attached to a small drainage bottle or plastic bag to permit greater freedom of movement. It may be placed in a pocket of the patient's bathrobe or attached to the robe below the level of the common duct. Patients may need help and encouragement because dressings are uncomfortable and they fear spilling the drainage when moving about. Patients benefit from a regular schedule of getting up and walking with assistance. This activity helps the patient to cope with fatigue. In preparation for discharge the patient should be given a schedule that incorporates a gradual increase in activity with rest periods. Heavy lifting (>10 pounds) must be avoided for some time (up to 6 weeks) after discharge, and plans must be made with family members so that they perform activities requiring heavy lifting.

## Maintaining T-tube Drainage

If the gallbladder is removed, the cystic duct is ligated and a drain usually is inserted near its stump and brought out through a stab wound on the abdomen. This drain allows drainage of bile and small amounts of blood and other serous fluid or exudates onto the dressings. It is usually removed within 5 days when drainage has almost subsided.

If a *cholecystostomy* has been performed, a self-retaining catheter is inserted through an opening in the gallbladder and is attached to straight drainage. Bile will drain out through this catheter until it is removed, usually between 6 weeks and 6 months.

After exploration of the common duct, a T-tube with the short end placed into the common duct will probably be used. The long end of the soft rubber tube is brought out through a stab wound and sutured to the skin. The section of the T-tube emerging from the stab wound may be placed over a roll of gauze anchored to the skin with adhesive tape to prevent it from occluding (see Figure 46-5). The T-tube is inserted to preserve patency of the common duct and to ensure drainage of bile out of the body until edema in the common duct has subsided enough for bile to drain into the duodenum normally. If the T-tube was clamped while the patient was being transported from the recovery room, it must be released *immediately* on arrival in the patient's room. The nurse should check the operative sheet carefully and seek clarification if the physician's written directions are not clear. The tube is usually connected to closed-gravity drainage similar to that used to drain the urinary bladder. Sufficient tubing should be attached so that the patient can move without restriction. The purpose of the tube should be explained, and the patient should be told why it must not be kinked, clamped, or pulled. The drainage should be checked for color and amount at least every 2 hours on the operative day. Some blood and blood-stained fluid may have drained from the tube during the first several hours, but drainage of more than a small amount of blood should be reported to the surgeon at once. The amount of drainage is measured and recorded daily. At first the entire amount of bile produced (normally 500 to 100 ml/day) may flow through the tube, but within 10 days most of the bile should be flowing into the duodenum.

Before the T-tube is removed, the patency of the common bile duct must be assessed. The tube is clamped for variable intervals, and the patient is monitored for signs of distress. If distress occurs, the tube is unclamped immediately and the surgeon is informed. A cholangiogram (Chapter 43) is usually performed to confirm the patency of the duct before the tube is removed. After the removal of the T-tube, the patient may have chills and fever that usually subside within 24 hours. They are caused by edema and a local reaction to the bile. Occasionally, flow of bile into the abdominal cavity causes *peritonitis,* and therefore any abdominal pain should be reported at once. The T-tube removal occurs at no specific time. Removal follows an x-ray examination that reveals no stones and the free flow of injected dye and a 5- to 7-day asymptomatic period in which the T-tube is clamped. Also, the patient should be reporting an improved feeling of well-being and having stools that have returned to a brown color.

After surgery the bile should either drain out through the drainage tube or flow into the intestine. If it does not do so, it can be assumed that the flow of bile is obstructed and that bile is being forced back into the liver and into the bloodstream. The nurse should observe the patient closely for jaundice, particularly in the sclerae. Urine should be examined for the brown color that is indicative of bilirubin: specimen should be saved for the surgeon's inspection when bilirubin is observed in the urine. The nurse may observe the patient's progress by noting the appearance of the stools. A light grayish-white color is usual if all the bile is flowing out through the drainage tubes (unless bile salts are being given by mouth). The normal brown color of the stool should gradually reappear as bile drainage diminishes and finally disappears.

## Guidelines for Discharge Teaching Regarding Care of the T-Tube

1. The patient must have instructions about whether the tube should be connected to continuous drainage, clamped continuously, or drained intermittently.
   a. If the T-tube is drained continuously, the patient must know how to empty the bag, the importance of keeping the bag below the level of the T-tube insertion site, and ways to maintain mobility with a continuous drainage system.
   b. If the T-tube is drained intermittently, the patient must know how to unclamp the tube and attach it to a drainage bag, how long to drain the tube, how to reclamp the tube, and how to measure drainage.
   c. If the T-tube is kept clamped, the tube and insertion site can be covered with a dry, sterile dressing.
2. The patient must have instructions about cleansing the insertion site. Usually a daily shower is all the cleansing that is necessary. A dry sterile dressing is reapplied every day.
3. The patient should be instructed on techniques that can be used to protect the skin, such as zinc oxide or karaya gel.
4. The patient must be instructed about the self-monitoring that will be necessary.
   a. Assessment for infection (redness, warmth, and swelling at insertion site, temperature elevation, or purulent drainage from T-tube site)
   b. Assessment for obstruction (recurrence of pain in right upper quadrant, bile drainage *around* T-tube, recurrence of nausea and vomiting, clay-colored (grayish-white) stools, brown urine, or jaundice)
   c. Assessment for tube dislodgement (sudden decrease in drainage or evidence that tube has shifted)
5. The patient should be instructed to report signs and symptoms of complications immediately.

Patients should be told about any drainage tubes, and they should know if much bile is expected on the dressings so that they will not become alarmed by soiling of dressings, gowns, or bedclothes. Outer dressings usually should be changed frequently when there is excessive drainage, since the drainage is irritating to the skin and wet dressings interfere with the patient's comfort and rest. Soap and water will remove bile from the skin. Montgomery straps make the changing of dressings much easier. Occasionally patients will be discharged with a T-tube in place. They must be taught how to care for it and how to monitor for complications that need to be reported to the surgeon (see the Guidelines box above).

### Maintaining Skin Integrity

The surgical incision of the T-tube is treated the same as most incisions (see Chapter 25). The nurse should remove any soiled dressing and cleanse the skin around the drains or tubes to remove any bile. If the T-tube is left in place for a prolonged period, the patient must institute care as described in the Guidelines box above. The nursing care for persons having abdominal surgery on the gallbladder is described in the Guidelines box, p. 1508.

## Guidelines for Care of the Person Undergoing Abdominal Surgery to Treat Biliary Tract Disease

**PREOPERATIVE**

Carry out actions used in preparing any patient with abdominal surgery (see Chapter 23).

Pay particular attention to improving respiratory function, because the high incision and right upper quadrant (RUQ) pain predispose the patient to *atelectasis* and *right lower lobe pneumonia*.

Explain the types of biliary drainage tubes that are anticipated.

Provide care required because of severity of acute symptoms or the presence of jaundice.

Administer intravenous fluids and antibiotics as prescribed.

Administer analgesics (usually meperidine) as prescribed and required.

Provide comfort measures for pruritus, nausea and vomiting, and pain.

Administer vitamin K as prescribed.

**POSTOPERATIVE**

Place patient in low-Fowler's position; assist to change position frequently.

Urge patient to deep breathe at regular intervals (every 1 to 2 hours) and to cough if secretions are present until ambulating well.

Monitor frequently for signs of hemorrhage (shock) the first few hours postoperatively (hemorrhage is rare but may occur when the inflamed gallbladder was adherent to the liver and difficult to remove).

Give analgesics fairly liberally the first 2 to 3 days.

Maintain a dry, intact dressing; usually a drain is inserted near the stump of the cystic duct; some serous fluid drainage is normal initially.

Encourage progressive ambulation when permitted.

Increase diet gradually to regular with fat content as tolerated when appropriate (appetite and fat tolerance may be diminished if there is external biliary drainage).

**BILIARY DRAINAGE**

Connect any biliary drainage tubes to closed gravity drainage.

Attach sufficient tubing so the patient can move without restriction.

Explain to patient the importance of avoiding kinks, clamping, or pulling of the tube.

Monitor the amount and color of drainage frequently; measure and record drainage at least every shift.

Report any signs of peritonitis (abdominal pain, rigidity, or fever) to the physician immediately.

Monitor color of urine and stools; stools will be grayish-white if bile is flowing out a drainage tube, but the normal color should gradually reappear as external drainage diminishes and disappears.

## ♦ EVALUATION

To evaluate the effectiveness of nursing interventions, compare patient behaviors with those stated in the expected patient outcomes. Successful achievement of patient outcomes for the patient with cholelithiasis and cholecystitis is indicated by the following:

*Before definitive medical treatment:*

1a. States that no pain is present.
 b. Does not demonstrate splinting, grimacing, shallow breathing, or other behaviors indicative of pain.
2a. Correctly describes diagnostic tests.
 b. Correctly explains planned treatment.
3. Appropriately describes and selects a low-calorie, low-fat diet.

*After laparoscopic cholecystectomy:*

1a. States that no pain is present.
 b. Does not demonstrate splinting, grimacing, shallow breathing, or other behaviors indicative of pain.
 c. Ambulates well.
2. Correctly describes self-care after discharge including the following:
   a. Oral analgesic as necessary for pain.
   b. That diet allowed is well balanced with no restrictions.
   c. Activities as tolerated.
   d. Return to work can occur in 3 days and full activities in 7 days.
   e. Shower as desired.
   f. Return for follow-up in 2 weeks.

*After abdominal cholecystectomy and lithotripsy:*

1. Has breath sounds that are clear and present in all lobes; does not splint.
2. States that fatigue is controlled and improving.
3. Has stable weight, moist mucous membranes, and normal serum electrolytes.
4. Has decreasing jaundice, normal temperature, and no return of biliary colic, nausea, and vomiting.
5. Shows no evidence of splinting, grimacing, or decreased ambulation.
6. Has adequate diet intake that contains food from all food groups; if post lithotripsy, eats decreased fat diet.
7. States pain is controlled and does not demonstrate behaviors associated with discomfort.
8. Edges of incision are approximated; no drainage present.

## ✸ SPECIAL CONSIDERATIONS FOR CARE OF THE GERONTOLOGIC PATIENT

Gallbladder disease is seen more frequently with advancing age but is treated in the same manner. Elderly persons may present with more subtle symptoms and signs in the presence of cholecystitis. Thus they can develop bacteremia before they seek help. Because of the normal decrease in immune function with aging, they are at greater risk for septic shock.

Elderly patients have more risks with surgery just because of their age. They are at more risk for any complications so they need very close monitoring.

Elderly persons may need more assistance at home when they have "same day" surgery or are discharged the day after surgery because of decreased indepen-

## NURSING CARE PLAN

### PERSON EXPERIENCING LAPAROSCOPIC CHOLECYSTECTOMY

**DATA:** Mrs. C. is a 50-year-old woman admitted for elective surgery. She gives a history of 3 months of episodes of food intolerance with vomiting at times. No recent (within past week) vomiting. All preoperative laboratory tests are normal. She is a smoker. The following is a proposed plan of care for the postsurgical period.

#### ■ NURSING DIAGNOSIS
Ineffective breathing pattern related to anesthesia

| Expected Patient Outcomes | Nursing Interventions | Rationale |
|---|---|---|
| Breath sounds are clear.<br>Respirations are within baseline range. | 1. Monitor respirations and breath sounds (especially RLL) q2hr to q4hr until patient is ambulating well.<br>2. Place patient in low-Fowler's position and encourage patient to change position frequently.<br>3. Encourage deep breathing exercises at least q1hr to q2hr until patient is ambulating. Encourage coughing if secretions present.<br>4. Splint incisions to encourage deep breathing.<br>5. Encourage use of incentive spirometer q1hr to q2hr until ambulating well.<br>6. Encourage ambulation.<br>7. Give analgesics before ambulation based on assessment. | This monitoring will help the nurse identify early any respiratory problems; deep breathing and ambulation will prevent atelectasis, a major respiratory complication. Incentive spirometer helps the patient increase deep breathing efforts. |

#### ■ NURSING DIAGNOSIS
Fatigue related to surgical procedure

| Expected Patient Outcome | Nursing Interventions | Rationale |
|---|---|---|
| States fatigue is lessening. | 1. Space activities between rest periods, and evaluate tolerance before increasing activity.<br>2. Assist patient with activities like bathing to conserve energy for ambulation.<br>3. Teach patient about need to continue to get adequate rest after discharge. | Fatigue is a common problem and is self-limiting. This care will prevent fatigue from becoming so severe that the patient does not participate in ambulation. |

#### ■ NURSING DIAGNOSIS
High risk for fluid volume deficit related to nausea and vomiting

| Expected Patient Outcomes | Nursing Interventions | Rationale |
|---|---|---|
| Maintains normal fluid volume as evidenced by stable weight, moist mucous membranes, adequate skin turgor, and balanced intake and output. | 1. Monitor intake and output and NG drainage every shift, and blood pressure and pulse q4hr.<br>2. Administer fluids and electrolytes as ordered.<br>3. Provide oral fluids as tolerated after establishing presence of normal bowel sounds. | The monitoring will allow for detection of early signs of volume deficit and to assure that adequate fluid volume is maintained. |

*Continued.*

## NURSING CARE PLAN

### PERSON EXPERIENCING LAPAROSCOPIC CHOLECYSTECTOMY—cont'd

| Expected Patient Outcomes—cont'd | Nursing Interventions—cont'd | Rationale—cont'd |
|---|---|---|
| Describes self-care needs. | 1. Teach patient:<br>a. Techniques of dressing change if drainage is still occurring at time of discharge.<br>b. Any prescribed dietary changes such as low fat or low calories.<br>c. Signs to report to physician (fever, unusual drainage).<br>d. Return to work in 3 days and full activities in 7 days. | Adequate knowledge will help the patient to take care of self. |

## CRITICAL PATHWAY Laparoscopic Cholecystectomy Without Complications

**DRG #: 195 Expected LOS: 2**

| | Day of Surgery<br>Day of Admission<br>Day 1 | Day of Discharge<br>Day 2 |
|---|---|---|
| **Diagnostic Tests** | Preoperative: CBC, UA<br>Postoperative: Hgb and HCT | |
| **Medications** | POST-PAR: IVs decreased to saline lock after nausea subsides; IV analgesic, then PO | Disc saline lock; PO analgesic |
| **Treatments** | POST-PAR: I & O q shift; VS q4hr × 4, then q8hr; assess bowel sounds q4hr; check drainage on bandages q2hr | Disc I & O; VS q8hr; assess bowel sounds q8hr; remove bandages and reapply bandages after shower if necessary |
| **Diet** | NPO until nausea subsides, then clear liquids; advance to full liquids, low fat | Regular diet, low fat |
| **Activity** | Up in room with assistance about 6 to 10 hr after surgery; T & DB q2hr | Up ad lib, OK to shower |
| **Consultations** | | |

dence. Services such as Meals-On-Wheels and transportation systems for the elderly may be helpful.

## ❦ HOME CARE CONSIDERATIONS

There are no special home care needs for most persons with cholelithiasis and cholecystitis unless patients are sent home with T-tubes. A home health referral might be necessary to ensure that a patient can manage all the care described in the Guidelines box, p. 1508.

## CARCINOMA OF THE BILIARY SYSTEM

### ETIOLOGY/EPIDEMIOLOGY

The cause of carcinoma of the biliary system is unknown, although the role of gallstones is being investigated. As noted earlier, cholecystectomy is indicated in selected asymptomatic cholelithiasis patients because of the increased risk of cancer. Cancer of the biliary system is the fifth most common cancer of the alimentary tract and accounts for 6500 deaths per year. It is more common in women and occurs in the sixth decade of life.

### PATHOPHYSIOLOGY

Carcinoma can occur anywhere in the biliary system. It has a very insidious onset and can metastasize by direct extension, through the lymphatics, and through the blood system. Many patients have no symptoms that are referable to the gallbladder. Other patients have symptoms similar to those seen with cholelithiasis and cholecystitis because of obstruction and inflammation. Pain that is intermittent and in the upper abdomen is the most common symptom. Anorexia, nausea, vomiting, weight loss, and jaundice may also be present. The patient may have a palpable abdominal mass. Signs and symptoms indicative of metastasis to the liver or pancreas may also be present.

Various tests used to diagnose other diseases of the gallbladder (Chapter 43) may be used but are often not definitive.

### MEDICAL MANAGEMENT

The major treatment for carcinoma of the biliary system is surgical, and surgery is performed as soon as the condition is recognized if possible, in the hope that complete surgical removal of the lesion is possible. Radiation therapy is used for palliation in some cases of bile duct cancer, but it is not effective in gallbladder cancer. Chemotherapy has no current role. Surgery may involve resection of part of the liver. Patients often benefit from surgery even when cure of the carcinoma is impossible, because surgical procedures can help to restore the flow of bile into the gastrointestinal tract. These surgeries can bring about remarkable relief of symptoms, and patients may feel relatively well for a time. Percutaneous insertion of tubes or catheters to bypass obstructions will also be used. Other medical treatment is directed toward generalized support.

### NURSING MANAGEMENT

One focus of care will be preoperative and postoperative management similar to that described for the patient with cholecystitis and cholelithiasis having an abdominal cystectomy (pp. 1504-1508). If resection to the liver also is done, the patient will need care as described in Chapter 42. Another focus of care will be that required for any patient with the diagnosis of cancer (see Chapter 16).

In addition, the patient often will need teaching with regard to dealing with an external or internal-external bile drainage system. For an external drainage system, teaching will be the same as that for a patient who is discharged with T-tube (see the Guidelines box, p. 1508). For an internal-external drainage system, a multiperforated catheter is passed through the liver past the obstruction and into the duodenum. The catheter is attached at first to continuous drainage and then plugged if no complications such as fever, chills, or leakage are present. The patient must learn how to care for the skin around the tube, how to monitor for signs and symptoms of obstruction, and how to irrigate the tube. The tube must be irrigated daily to keep the perforations open.

**BOX 46-2 Causes of Acute Pancreatitis**

- Alcoholism
- Biliary tract disease
- Postoperative—abdominal or nonabdominal surgery
- Postendoscopic retrograde cholangiopancreatography
- Blunt abdominal trauma
- Metabolic problems (increased serum calcium [hyperparathyroidism and postrenal transplant patients], hypertriglyceridemia)
- Idiopathic
- Infections (especially viral)
- Connective tissue disease with vasculitis such as systemic lupus erythematosus
- Drugs (antihypertensives, diuretics, antimicrobials, immunosuppressives, and oral contraceptives)
- Intestinal diseases such as regional enteritis and penetrating duodenal ulcers

# PANCREATIC DISORDERS

## PANCREATITIS

**Pancreatitis** is a serious inflammatory disorder of the pancreas that can be *acute* or *chronic*. Because patient needs are different in acute and chronic pancreatitis, the disorders are discussed separately.

## ACUTE PANCREATITIS

Acute pancreatitis can occur as a single episode or as recurrent attacks (recurrent acute pancreatitis). It can be classified by pathologic changes (edematous, hemorrhagic). The unique morphologic feature of acute or recurrent acute pancreatitis is that, except in cases of alcohol-induced pancreatitis, the pancreas returns to normal after successful treatment and there are no irreversible sequelae. The illness episode of a patient with acute pancreatitis can range from a mild illness to a critical illness.

### ETIOLOGY

Numerous factors have been identified as causative agents of acute pancreatitis (Box 46-2). In the United States the most common factor is alcoholism. The second most common cause is cholelithiasis and cholecystitis.

### EPIDEMIOLOGY

The epidemiology of acute pancreatitis is unknown. However, it is a common problem.[16]

### PATHOPHYSIOLOGY

Although there are many known causes of pancreatitis, the manner in which they result in acute inflammation is unknown. The currently favored pathologic factor leading to the acute inflammation is **autodigestion.** This theory proposes that proteolytic enzymes, particularly trypsinogen, are activated within the pancreas itself. Once it is activated to trypsin, trypsinogen can activate itself and other proteolytic enzymes. The activated proteolytic enzymes digest pancreatic and surrounding tissues and cellular membranes. This autodigestion results

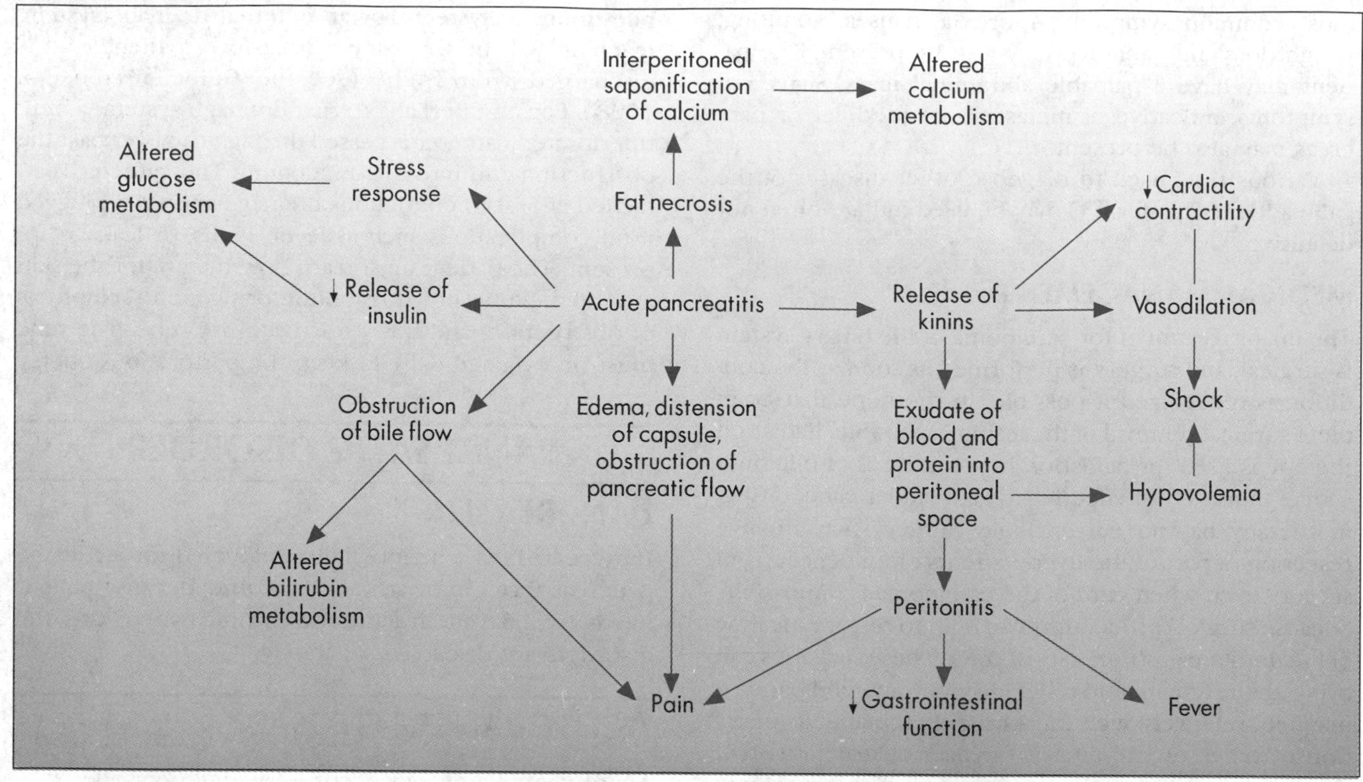


**FIGURE 46-6** Summary of major pathologic events that occur in acute pancreatitis.

in edema, interstitial hemorrhage, vascular damage, coagulation necrosis, fat necrosis, and parenchymal cell necrosis. The injured tissue releases histamine and bradykinin, which increase vascular permeability and vasodilation and cause more edema. The initiation of activation of the proteolytic enzymes is thought to result from reflux of bile, obstruction of the pancreatic duct or ampulla of Vater, ischemia, direct toxic effects, trauma, endotoxins, and exotoxins.

Regardless of the cause, the acute inflammatory process and autodigestion result in a spectrum of physiologic alterations that can occur as a mild to a very critical event. Figure 46-6 depicts some of the major pathophysiologic events seen in acute pancreatitis.

The majority of patients (80% to 90%) with acute pancreatitis recover without any residual dysfunction. The mortality is 5% to 10%.[16] Table 46-3 lists two scoring systems used to estimate the severity and prognosis of acute pancreatitis. Multiple complications can occur as a result of acute pancreatitis.[8,17] These complications can affect all systems (Box 46-3). The major symptom of acute pancreatitis is *pain.* The pain varies from *mild* to *severe,* is *constant,* and is *incapacitating.* The pain may be experienced in the epigastrium and other parts of the abdomen, and it may radiate to the back, flanks, and substernal area. It is usually more intense when the person is lying supine. Other common symptoms are nausea, vomiting, and abdominal distention.

The patient with acute pancreatitis normally has a low-grade fever and signs and symptoms of fluid deficit (poor skin turgor, dry mucous membranes, postural hypotension, tachycardia, and weight loss). Sometimes all the signs and symptoms of shock will be present. Abdominal tenderness and rigidity and diminished bowel sounds are present. Ten to twenty percent of patients develop respiratory problems, and decreased breath sounds or rales may be auscultated. Other signs that might be present are jaundice from obstruction of the common bile duct, purplish discoloration of the flanks (Grey Turner's sign) or the periumbilical area (Cullen's sign) from hemorrhagic necrosis of the pancreas, or tetany from low calcium.

## PREVENTION

### Primary Prevention

Because the major etiologic factors for acute pancreatitis are alcoholism and gallbladder obstruction, primary prevention of these two problems would help to prevent acute pancreatitis. Primary prevention of alcoholism is described in Chapter 19. Primary prevention of gallbladder disease is described in an earlier section of this chapter.

### Secondary Prevention

Secondary prevention measures focus on early detection of signs and symptoms indicative of complications. Early detection allows for early initiation of interventions to prevent complications.

**TABLE 46-3 Representative Prognostic Scoring Systems in Acute Pancreatitis***

| RANSON | GLASGOW |
|---|---|
| **ADMISSION** | |
| Age >55 years | Age >50 years |
| WBC >20,000 cell/mm$^3$ | WBC >15,000 |
| LDH >350 IU/L | Glucose >180 mg/dl |
| AST >250 IU/L | BUN >45 mg/dl |
| **INITIAL 48 HRS** | |
| Hematocrit decrease >10% | $Po_2$ <60 mm Hg |
| BUN increase >5 mg/dl | Albumin <3.2 g/dl |
| Calcium <8 mg/dl | Calcium <8 mg/dl |
| $Po_2$ <60 mm Hg | LDH >600 IU/L |
| Base deficit >4 | |
| Estimated fluid sequestration >6 liters | |

Data from Ranson JAC et al: *Surg Gynecol Obstet* 143:209, 1976 and Neoptolemos VP et al: *Lancet* 2:979, 1988. From Regan PT, Go VLW: Pancreatic diseases. In Steen JH, editor: *Internal medicine,* ed 4, St Louis, 1994, Mosby.
*Presence of 3 or more factors indicates poor prognosis.

## MEDICAL MANAGEMENT

The expected length of stay of patients with acute pancreatitis as determined by DRG is 14 days. A discussion of common therapy for management of acute pancreatitis follows.

### Diagnostic Tests

Diagnostic tests of the greatest value in establishing a diagnosis are serum enzyme levels. A *serum amylase* level of greater than 300 Somogyi units in the presence of the symptoms just outlined usually establishes the diagnosis of acute pancreatitis. *Serum amylase* levels usually become elevated within 24 to 48 hours of the onset of acute pancreatitis and may range from 300 to 800 U. There is no apparent relationship between the severity of the disease and the height of the enzyme levels. Isoenzymes of amylase can be measured and provide even more specificity in diagnosing pancreatitis. Assays for isoenzymes are not yet widely available so they are not routinely measured. *Serum lipase* also increases in pancreatitis and reaches its peak in 72 to 96 hours after the onset of the acute pancreatitis. In the absence of kidney failure, *urinary amylase* levels may also be used to diagnose acute pancreatitis.

Other laboratory findings include leukocytosis, anemia, increased serum bilirubin, altered laboratory values consistent with dehydration, and hyperglycemia. In severe cases hypocalcemia may be present. Elevation of ALT, AST, or alkaline phosphatase may be present and suggest gallstones as a cause of the pancreatitis if no history of excessive alcohol consumption or other etiologic factors responsible for elevation of these enzymes are present.

Other diagnostic tests that may be used are: (1) abdominal x-ray examination to reveal GI changes, such as distention associated with pancreatitis; (2) chest x-ray to identify respiratory changes, such as atelectasis, plural effusion, or pulmonary infiltrates; (3) ultrasonography to rule out an edematous pancreas and pseudocyst; and (4) endoscopic retrograde cholangiopancreatography (ERCP) to identify obstructions.

**BOX 46-3 Major Complications of Acute Pancreatitis**

**CARDIOVASCULAR**
Hypotension/shock from hypovolemia or hypoalbuminemia

**HEMATOLOGIC**
Leukocytosis from generalized inflammation or secondary infections, anemia from blood loss, disseminated intravascular coagulation (DIC) from unknown causes

**RESPIRATORY**
Atelectasis, pneumonitis, pleural effusion, adult respiratory distress syndrome (ARDS)

**GASTROINTESTINAL**
Hemorrhage from peptic ulcers, gastritis

**PANCREATIC/LIVER**
Hemorrhage from varices; pancreatic pseudocysts, abscesses, or pancreatic ascites

**RENAL**
Oliguria and increased blood urea nitrogen (BUN) from hypovolemia

**METABOLIC**
Increased blood glucose from decreased insulin release associated with the stress response or destruction of beta cells of pancreas; increased triglycerides from the stress response and changes in insulin release or secretion; decreased calcium associated with low albumin, precipitation of calcium with free fatty acids to form calcium soaps, and unknown causes

**NEUROLOGIC**
Encephalopathy

### Medication

Usually meperidine (Demerol) is used for pain management. In addition, intravenous fluids and colloids are used to return the vascular volume to normal. If hypocalcemia is present, intravenous calcium will be necessary. Insulin might be necessary if hyperglycemia is present. Drug therapy to decrease pancreatic secretions including glucagon, cimetidine, somatostatin, and the enzyme inhibitor aprotinin has been tried but has not been found to be effective.

### Treatment

Nasogastric suctioning is usually used to reduce pain, rest the pancreas, and relieve ileus. Peritoneal lavage to remove peritoneal toxic chemicals has provided some improvement in symptoms but not in survival or prevention of complications.[9,16]

### Diet

During the acute period the patient will be placed on NPO status. TPN is recommended for the acute period.[9,11] After symptoms decrease and the patient is stabilized, food will be restarted. The patient is started on liquids in small amounts and then increased as tolerated. There are no long-term restrictions on food substances except for alcohol.

### Activity

Patients with acute pancreatitis are acutely or critically ill. Bed rest is required until the patient is hemodynamically stable. Then activity is restarted gradually within the patient's tolerance.

### Referral/Consultation

In some settings the nurse assumes responsibility for making referrals to other services. Common referrals for persons with acute pancreatitis include respiratory therapy for respiratory complications, nutritional support team, dietitian, and potentially any medical specialist, depending on how the patient progresses. Surgery to remove necrotic tissue, place drains, or treat associated gallbladder disease may be necessary, and thus surgical consultations will be necessary.

Critical pathways (also referred to as "collaborative care paths" or "care maps") have been developed in some inpatient and outpatient settings to guide both medical and nursing management. These critical pathways are collaboratively developed along time lines and include the information just described for specific hours, days, or visits. Pertinent information about discharge planning and patient teaching to be implemented at specified times also is included. Because the nurse has a major role in these two aspects of care, these are discussed under Nursing Management.

## SURGICAL MANAGEMENT

Surgery is not a routine part of the management of acute pancreatitis, but some procedures may be necessary to control related gallbladder problems, pseudocyst, or abscess. Also, necrotic tissue may be resected. Patients with acute pancreatitis requiring surgery are very ill. Nursing management of the patient with surgery of the pancreas is discussed on pp. 1520-1521.

## NURSING MANAGEMENT

### ♦ ASSESSMENT

The patient with acute pancreatitis requires a thorough nursing assessment.

### Subjective Data

Data to be collected to assess the patient with acute pancreatitis include the following:

Presence of pain: sharp, constant pain in epigastric region associated with abdominal tenderness and nausea and vomiting; food and alcohol intake precipitate pain

GI complaints: nausea, vomiting, recent food and liquid intake

History of causes: alcoholism, gallbladder disease, recent trauma, recent surgery

Respiratory complaints: any dyspnea, shortness of breath, pain with breathing

Miscellaneous: any episodes of temperature elevation

### Objective Data

Data to be collected to assess the patient with acute pancreatitis include the following:

General: affect—patient looks distressed; posture—sits with knees pulled toward abdomen; temperature—usually has fever

Fluid status: weight, intake and output, skin turgor, and mucous membrane moisture may be normal, but may show signs of severe fluid deficit

Cardiovascular status: blood pressure, including orthostatic changes, and pulse possibly normal, but may show signs of hypovolemic shock

Respiratory status: tachypnea and dyspnea are common, breath sounds may be diminished, or crackles may be present

Abdomen: presence of tenderness, palpable, mass, or rigidity, presence of bowel sounds, presence of cyanotic or greenish yellow-brown discoloration on abdomen around the umbilicus and flank area (Grey Turner's sign and Cullen's sign)

Others: jaundice and positive Chvostek's and Trousseau's signs caused by hypocalcemia

### Diagnostic Test Findings

The major finding is an elevated serum amylase, which is detectable shortly after the onset of symptoms and returns to normal in 1 to 4 days if the pancreatitis resolves. Urinary amylase also will be elevated. Serum lipase levels, although not frequently measured, are elevated. The patient may show an elevated white blood cell count, slightly elevated serum glucose level, elevated triglyceride level, and hypocalcemia (a very serious finding). Most patients will have mildly to severely elevated levels of serum electrolytes and low potassium levels because of fluid deficit. Computed tomography (CT) will reveal an enlarged pancreas. Plain abdominal films may reveal the presence of ileus.

### ♦ NURSING DIAGNOSES

Nursing diagnoses are determined from analyses of paient data. Nursing diagnoses for the person with acute pancreatitis may include but are not limited to the following:

| Diagnostic Title | Possible Etiologic Factors |
|---|---|
| Pain | Inflammation of pancreas or peritoneum |

| Diagnostic Title | Possible Etiologic Factors |
|---|---|
| Fluid volume deficit | Vomiting; lack of intake; pancreatic hemorrhage |
| Self-care deficit: variable | Weakness; pain |
| Nutrition, altered: less than body requirements | Nausea and vomiting; pain; life-style patterns |
| Knowledge deficit: disease management | New diagnosis; no previous exposure to information |
| Health maintenance, altered | Unhealthy life-style patterns, including alcoholism, poor nutrition, and obesity |

Potential complications that might occur and should be a focus of nursing are respiratory failure, shock, hypocalcemia, and hyperglycemia.

## ♦ EXPECTED PATIENT OUTCOMES

Expected patient outcomes for the person with acute pancreatitis may include but are not limited to the following:

1. States that pain is controlled and does not appear to be in pain (does not display distressed appearance, limited body movement, or limited activity).
2. Will have adequate fluid volume as demonstrated by normal blood pressure, absence of orthostatic changes, normal skin turgor, and moist mucous membranes.
3. Will have self-care needs met
4. Will consume a well-balanced diet and show an increase in weight when able to eat
5. The patient and significant others will be able to do the following:
   a. Describe the disease, the need for specific tests, and the purpose of various interventions.
   b. Explain the relationship between the etiologic factor (e.g., alcoholism, biliary disease) and pancreatitis.
   c. Describe dietary needs.
   d. Explain plans for follow-up care.
6. Will assume safe and adequate health practices (e.g., improve diet, control obesity, or control alcoholism if present as an etiologic condition of acute pancreatitis

## ♦ INTERVENTIONS

The patient with acute pancreatitis may be acutely ill and require critical care. Interventions for the priorities of care are presented first, followed by a discussion of interventions for other needs.

### ➠ Managing Critical Care

Many patients with acute pancreatitis will require critical care. The focus in critical care is pain relief, improving fluid and electrolyte status, and monitoring for complications. Each of these is discussed next.

#### Controlling pain

Control of pain is a major priority. Meperidine hydrochloride, 75 to 100 mg every 3 to 4 hours, may be necessary to reduce pain. Morphine and codeine are not used because of their spasmogenic effects. Some patients find that the pain is decreased if they assume a sitting position with the trunk flexed or with their knees drawn up to the abdomen in a side-lying, knee-chest position. Sympathetic nerve blocks and epidural anesthesia can be used if pain is persistent and not relieved by meperidine.

The measures used to rest the pancreas (NPO status and nasogastric suctioning) will also assist with pain control by decreasing the continual autodigestive process and associated edema and inflammation. In addition, the nurse should help the patient initiate relaxation techniques, such as deep breathing and imagery, and distraction techniques such as music, TV, and sewing, to help with pain control (see Chapter 17). These measures should be introduced after the patient has adequate pain control from analgesic drugs. If the patient is highly distressed, these techniques are not easily used. It is important to implement comfort measures such as backrubs and purposeful touch.

#### Maintaining fluid and electrolyte balance

As soon as the patient is admitted, the nurse should institute monitoring related to fluid and electrolyte status, cardiac output, and renal status. It is a critical need. Monitoring includes intake and output; vital signs; daily weights; daily electrolytes; and as necessary, blood urea nitrogen (BUN), creatinine, and hemodynamic measurements. An indwelling catheter may be necessary, since decreased renal function can occur in association with hypotension and shock. Monitoring parameters and frequency of monitoring will depend on the stability of the patient's condition. Fluids, electrolytes, colloids, or blood will be given as necessary. The nurse is responsible for administering these and for monitoring the patient's response to them. Frequent adjustments in therapy may be necessary in relation to the patient's response to fluid therapy. If the patient develops shock, all the care described in Chapter 22 will be necessary.

#### Monitoring for potential complications

In addition to monitoring fluid and electrolyte, cardiovascular, and renal status as mentioned earlier, the patient must be monitored for the onset of respiratory problems, hypocalcemia, and hyperglycemia. Breath sounds should be monitored at least every shift. If any signs of respiratory distress are present, blood gases and a chest x-ray examination will be necessary. Preventive respiratory care, including routine turning and deep breathing are essential. The serum calcium level is checked frequently, and the patient is monitored for signs of hypocalcemia (tetany, positive Trousseau's and Chvostek's signs, muscle twitching, jerking, and irritability). If any of these occur, they must be reported immediately because calcium replacement will be necessary. The patient also is monitored for hyperglycemia, and frequent checks of blood glucose should be carried out. If hyperglycemia occurs, it may be treated with insulin.

### Providing Self-Care

During the acute phase of the illness the patient will need assistance with all care. Dehydration and potential malnutrition make the patient particularly prone to skin breakdown. Because of the amount of monitoring and the total care that is necessary, a schedule must be established that provides for the necessary monitoring, meeting care needs, and rest periods.

### Promoting Adequate Nutrition

The patient will be placed on NPO status and often has a nasogastric tube in place. Institution and maintenance of the NPO status are major interventions. Good oral hygiene will be necessary to decrease discomfort from NPO status and from the nasogastric tube. TPN is recommended to be used during the critical phase of the illness. When the acute symptoms decrease (3 to 5 days), oral fluids and food are restarted. The patient is started on clear liquids and then advanced to a low-fat, bland diet, distributed over five to six small feedings daily. When refeeding starts, the patient must be observed carefully for pain, nausea, and vomiting, all of which indicate continuing inflammation. If these occur, the physician should be notified and the methods described previously for inhibition of pancreatic activity will be reinstituted. After discharge from the hospital, patients are advised to avoid alcohol.

### Patient Teaching

Teaching the patient and significant others will be ongoing. At the beginning of hospitalization, the patient and significant others need basic instructions about the disease, the diagnostic tests, and the treatment. Because of the pain and the distress it causes and because of potential fluid status and cardiovascular instability, the patient and family may be experiencing tremendous stress and anxiety. Therefore explanations and instructions should be brief and as simple as possible and may need to be repeated. Support and continuity of care also need to be instituted to help decrease anxiety. Long-term education will be directed toward prevention of future attacks by avoiding alcohol, maintaining a nutritious diet, and continuing medications as prescribed. The patient must know that any recurrence of signs and symptoms should be reported immediately. Follow-up care must be explained in detail.

### Promoting Healthy Life-Style Patterns

If unhealthy life-style patterns such as diet, obesity, or alcoholism are indicated as a cause of acute pancreatitis, the nurse must work with the patient on these problems. This care will not be instituted until the patient is stabilized, but it must be introduced before the patient leaves the hospital. See Chapter 19 for further information on coping with alcoholism.

## ♦ EVALUATION

To evaluate the effectiveness of nursing interventions, compare patient behaviors with those stated in the expected patient outcomes. Successful achievement of patient outcomes for the patient with acute pancreatitis is indicated by the following:

1a. States no pain.
 b. Does not splint, grimace, and breathe shallowly.
2. Hemodynamic measures are within normal limits, weight returns to normal, and intake equals output.
3. Hygiene, mouth care, nutrition, and rest needs are met.
4a. NPO status is maintained as appropriate.
 b. By discharge is consuming a well-balanced diet without nausea, vomiting, or pain.
 c. Weight returns to normal.
5a. Appropriately describes the disease, tests, and planned interventions.
 b. Appropriately describes the relationship between etiologic factors and the disease.
 c. Appropriately describes and selects well-balanced diet.
 d. Lists appropriately the planned follow-up.

## ✸ SPECIAL CONSIDERATIONS FOR CARE OF THE GERONTOLOGIC PATIENT

Pancreatic secretions do decrease with age so elderly persons may have some complaints of food intolerance even without disease. Acute pancreatitis after abdominal surgery is a common complication for the elderly. Therefore every elderly patient recovering from abdominal surgery should be monitored carefully for pancreatic problems. The elderly, because of co-morbid problems, may become more critically ill faster with acute pancreatitis.

## ❦ HOME CARE CONSIDERATIONS

Most patients with acute pancreatitis will have no sequel of the illness and no major changes in daily activities except the need to avoid alcohol. Thus the only home care needs relate to any assistance the patient needs to return to the preillness level of functioning. The elderly patient recovering from acute pancreatitis may need home care to help regain physical strength and return to full functioning.

# CHRONIC PANCREATITIS

In chronic pancreatitis there is permanent and progressive destruction of the pancreas, with normal tissue being replaced by fibrous tissue. Chronic pancreatitis can eventually lead to chronic insufficiency of pancreatic hormones.

## ETIOLOGY/EPIDEMIOLOGY

The major cause of chronic pancreatitis in adults in the United States is alcoholism. A major cause in children is cystic fibrosis; approximately 85% of patients with cystic fibrosis have impaired pancreatic exocrine function. Other causes include the following: trauma; gastric or pancreatic surgery; neoplasms of the pancreas, islet cells, or duodenum; and severe protein and calorie malnutrition. The epidemiology of chronic pancreatitis is unknown.

## PATHOPHYSIOLOGY

The organ destruction that occurs in chronic pancreatitis occurs in the same manner as that described for acute pancreatitis (p. 1511); that is, autodigestion.

In chronic pancreatitis caused by alcohol abuse the pancreatic juices secreted contain decreased bicarbonate, increased protein, and a decreased amount of substances that inhibit trypsin activation.[19] In addition, the pancreatic juices of persons with chronic pancreatitis may be altered in other ways that allow for calcium precipitation. These changes would allow for formation of protein plugs that block the pancreatic ducts and initiate inflammation, fibrosis, and stenosis with loss of normal cell function.

The loss of normal cellular mass results in a deficiency of pancreatic exocrine secretion. Ductal obstruction and dilation have been thought to be the cause of the pain associated with chronic pancreatitis, but they cannot always be identified as a cause.

The patient with chronic pancreatitis may initially have signs and symptoms identical to those described for the patient with acute pancreatitis, with *pain* being the *major manifestation.* The pain occurs in the right or left upper quadrant, in the back, or throughout the total abdomen. It is severe and constant and does not respond to normal food ingestion or antacids. It may be worsened by alcohol or high fat intake. Nausea, vomiting, and abdominal distention may be present, but they are usually secondary to the pain and its treatment. The patient also has a history of weight loss, diarrhea, steatorrhea, and malnutrition. Mild fever may be present, and jaundice is common. Ascites and an abdominal mass may be seen. Signs and symptoms of diabetes mellitus may also be present.

Laboratory tests reveal leukocytosis. Bilirubin and alkaline phosphatase levels may be elevated if obstruction of the common bile duct is present. Serum lipase and amylase are usually not helpful in diagnosing chronic pancreatitis because of acinar cell atrophy and replacement of cells by fibrous tissue. Other specialized diagnostic tests that may be abnormal in chronic pancreatitis are tests of pancreatic secretion of bicarbonate-rich fluid or enzymes in response to the administration of secretin or cholecystokinin (CCK). Patients with chronic pancreatitis will show decreased amounts of bicarbonate-rich fluids or enzymes in response to these tests. The Bentiromide test is an indirect test of pancreatic secretory capacity. This compound requires chymotrypsin for its digestion before absorption. The amount of metabolic product excreted in urine after a 500 mg dose will be decreased in chronic pancreatitis. A D-xylose test will be used to rule out small bowel disease as the cause of

**TABLE 46-4 Relationship Between Normal Physiology of the Pancreas and Pathophysiology and Clinical Manifestations of Chronic Pancreatitis**

| NORMAL FUNCTION | PATHOPHYSIOLOGY | CLINICAL MANIFESTATIONS |
|---|---|---|
| Production and secretion of digestive enzymes | Alteration in pancreatic secretions ↓ | |
| Production and secretion of bicarbonate-rich isoosmolar solution | Plugging of pancreatic ducts ↓ | Pain → nausea, vomiting, and abdominal distention; fever |
| | Inflammation ↓ | |
| | Stenosis and fibrosis ↓ | |
| | Acinar cell mass diminished ↓ | Steatorrhea, diarrhea, weight loss, and malnutrition; dehydration and electrolyte imbalance |
| | Decreased enzyme and isoosmotic secretions to duodenum | |
| | Obstruction of biliary drainage | Increased bilirubin, jaundice, increased alkaline phosphatase |
| | Islet cells destroyed → Decreased insulin | Hyperglycemia and all other symptoms of diabetes mellitus |

malabsorption. Other abnormal findings include increased amounts of undigested meat fibers and split and neutral fat in the stool and elevated stool fat. Plain films of the abdomen, ultrasound examination of the abdomen, or CT scan of the abdomen may reveal pancreatic calcification. Endoscopic retrograde cholangiopancreatography (ERCP) of the pancreas may also show calcification and distortion of the pancreatic duct system. The relationship between normal pancreatic function and the pathophysiology and the clinical manifestations of chronic pancreatitis is depicted in Table 46-4.

## MEDICAL MANAGEMENT

The initial focus of treatment during an acute exacerbation of chronic pancreatitis may be the same as that for acute pancreatitis: analgesics for pain, nothing by mouth and nasogastric intubation to rest the pancreas, fluid and electrolyte replacement for fluid deficit, and supportive care for complications such as respiratory problems.

Once the patient is stabilized or for the less critically ill patient, a major focus of medical care is to confirm the diagnosis if it is not clear. Then the focus is to control pain, diarrhea, steatorrhea, weight loss, and diabetes mellitus.

For severe pain, narcotic analgesics will be used at first. Chronic control of pain and control of exocrine insufficiency are achieved with pancreatic extract replacement. In patients in whom this therapy is ineffective in controlling pain, an ERCP (see Chapter 43) will be used to identify the presence of duct obstruction or pseudocysts that may require surgery. Sometimes antacids and cimetidine may be used to decrease gastric acid secretion and thus pancreatic stimulation. Dietary manipulation, including avoiding high-protein foods, caffeine, and alcohol (which increase gastric secretions and pancreatic stimulation), will often be tried to help control pain. As stated previously, diarrhea, steatorrhea, and malabsorption will be treated with pancreatic enzyme replacement. If it is present, diabetes mellitus is treated as described in Chapter 40.

## NURSING MANAGEMENT

For patients with chronic pancreatitis, the nursing assessment is the same as that described for acute pancreatitis. In some instances the nursing diagnoses, outcomes, and interventions are the same. Other diagnoses include the following.

| Diagnostic Title | Possible Etiologic Factors |
|---|---|
| Pain | Chronic inflammation of pancreas |
| Nutrition, altered: less than body requirements | Malabsorption |
| Health maintenance, altered | Alcohol abuse or unhealthy life-style pattern |
| Knowledge deficit: disease and treatment | New diagnosis, lack of previous exposure to information, inability to accept information at early exposure |

The nurse must focus first on the patient's priority, which usually is the pain. This requires that the pain be adequately controlled, possibly with analgesics at first so that the patient is open to alternative therapeutic measures such as relaxation or massage. The patient must believe that dietary manipulations—pancreatic extract and abstinence from alcohol—will be effective to help control pain. In some instances the patient has had negative experiences with pain management during previous hospitalizations for exacerbations and thus believes that analgesics are not being given because the health team does not care about him or her. Thus it is important that a trusting relationship be established between the patient and the nurse.

The patient must take large quantities of pancreatic extract with each meal. The patient must also learn to manipulate necessary dietary changes (avoiding any foods that increase symptoms). And of course the patient must be helped with the alcoholism problem, if present, as described in Chapter 19.

If the therapy is effective, the patient should have adequate pain control, regain weight, and have less or no diarrhea. The patient needs to understand that it may take some time to achieve complete control of symptoms. Signs and symptoms that require immediate follow-up (recurrence of pain, occurrence of nausea and vomiting, occurrence of abdominal distention, recurrence or worsening of steatorrhea and diarrhea, and occurrence of signs and symptoms of diabetes mellitus) must be understood by the patient. If surgery is required, the nursing needs will be similar to those described on pp. 1520-1521.

# PANCREATIC PSEUDOCYSTS

A **pancreatic pseudocyst** is a potential complication of acute and chronic pancreatitis, pancreatic trauma, or carcinoma. A pseudocyst is a collection of tissue, fluid, debris, and blood that fills a cavity contiguous with or surrounding the pancreas. The pseudocyst frequently disrupts the duct system of the pancreas. The signs and symptoms of pseudocysts are similar to those seen in acute pancreatitis, with pain being the most common symptom. An epigastric mass may be palpable.

Pseudocysts are serious for the following reasons: they worsen pain; they may rupture with or without bleeding; they may result in gastrointestinal bleeding because of erosive gastritis, peptic ulcer, or esophageal varices; they may result in pancreatic abscess formation; and they may cause ascites. Pancreatic pseudocysts may resolve spontaneously over 6 weeks. If no signs of complications are present, they are usually monitored by serial ultrasound examinations. If resolution does not occur, if the cyst increases in size, or if complications are present, surgery to drain the pseudocyst will be necessary. The care needs of the patient having surgery of the pancreas are described on pp. 1520-1521.

# CANCER OF THE PANCREAS

## ETIOLOGY/EPIDEMIOLOGY

The cause of cancer of the pancreas is unknown, but it is diagnosed more often in smokers. Cancer of the pancreas also is associated with diets high in meat and fat, high coffee consumption, high alcohol consumption, and exposure to chemicals.[6] Cancer of the pancreas is the fourth leading cause of death from cancer. Pancreatic cancer affects men more than women. It usually occurs in the elderly.[7]

## PATHOPHYSIOLOGY

Most malignant tumors of the pancreas appear to begin in the ductal areas, causing eventual blockage and resulting in chronic pancreatitis. Direct extension of the lesion may cause its spread to the posterior wall of the stomach, the duodenal wall, the colon, and the common bile duct. The tumor may be diffusely spread over the entire gland, or it may be a well-defined growth. It commonly grows in a rapid manner and is highly invasive. Vascular, lymphatic, and perineural metastases frequently occur. The 5-year survival is less than 5%.[16]

Symptoms of pancreatic malignancies are not usually detectable until late in the course of the disease. Pain occurs in about 85% of the patients. This may be preceded by vague anorexia, nausea, and weight loss over a period of months. Jaundice frequently occurs because of common duct obstruction but is seldom a primary sign. Changes in stools may occur if the pancreatic ducts are obstructed. Pain may be colicky or intermittent and often radiates to the back, abdomen, and chest. About half of the patients develop diabetes mellitus.

Definitive diagnosis before surgery is difficult. Diagnostic studies include CT scan, ERCP, duodenal cytology, pancreatic scans, and arteriography.

## MEDICAL MANAGEMENT

The primary treatment of the patient with pancreatic cancer is surgery, although the prognosis is usually poor. Surgery may be used for its curative effect in only a small percentage of cases. One procedure used for tumors of the head of the pancreas is pancreatoduodenal resection (Whipple's procedure) (Figure 46-7). Another procedure is total pancreatectomy with resection of parts of the gastrointestinal tract. Other procedures to help restore normal bile flow and the maximum pancreatic flow possible may be used.

Nonsurgical treatment with radiation and chemotherapy may be used. Other medical care focuses on general supportive measures such as nutritional support, comfort measures, and maintenance of physical functioning.

## NURSING MANAGEMENT

The nursing care for patients with cancer of the pancreas varies. In some patients, the focus will be related to care needs related to the surgery (see next section). In many patients the cancer is not resectable; thus care will be related to the needs induced by chemotherapy, radiation

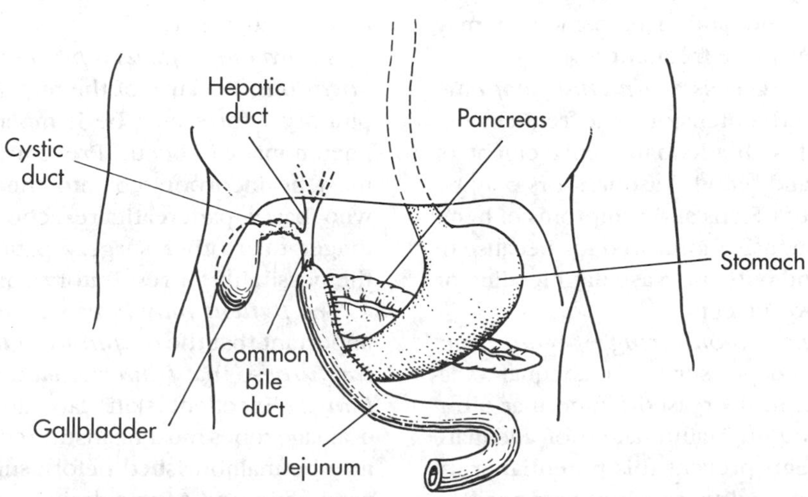


**FIGURE 46-7** Pancreatoduodenectomy (Whipple's procedure) with anastomosis.

therapy, and the diagnosis itself as described in Chapter 16. This care includes the following: pain relief measures; nutritional, fluid, and electrolyte support; other comfort measures; promotion of maximum functioning and activity; and dealing with the grief, fear, and anxiety of the patient and the family.

## NURSING MANAGEMENT OF THE PATIENT WITH SURGERY OF THE PANCREAS

Surgery of the pancreas may be used to treat pseudocysts, cancer, intractable pain, and calcification associated with chronic pancreatitis, traumatic injuries, and acute fulminant pancreatitis. The various surgical procedures are described in Table 46-5. The preoperative and the postoperative care described below applies to patients undergoing partial or total **pancreatectomy** or the Whipple's procedure.

**TABLE 46-5 Selected Surgical Procedures of the Pancreas**

| PROCEDURES | USES |
|---|---|
| Drainage procedures: drainage systems possibly established to drain fluid and debris from pancreas into adjacent structures such as stomach (cystogastrostomy) or jejunum) (cystojejunostomy); also may involve placement of tube for external drainage | For pseudocysts |
| Resection of tail of pancreas and adjacent organ (spleen) | Cancer of tail of pancreas, chronic pancreatitis |
| Pancreatoduodenectomy (Whipple's procedure): removal of head of pancreas, ampulla of Vater, lower end of common bile duct, duodenum, and distal portion of stomach with anastomoses of stomach, pancreas and common bile duct to jejunum (Figure 46-7) | Carcinoma of the head of the pancreas, ampulla of Vater, duodenum, or common bile duct |
| Total pancreatectomy | Resectable cancers, trauma, intractable pain of chronic pancreatitis |
| Pancreatojejunostomy | Decompression of main pancreatic duct (palliative therapy for cancer of pancreas) |
| Cholecystoenterostomy | Decompression of biliary tract obstructed by pancreatic cancer |
| Partial pancreatectomy | For removal of portions of pancreas severely diseased with chronic pancreatitis; for liver donor tissue for transplantation for diabetes mellitus |

### Preoperative Care

Before surgery the patient should be as stable and as physically strong as possible. Fluid and vascular status should be normal. Nutritional status may be improved before surgery with hyperalimentation. If jaundice is present, the prothrombin time may be prolonged. This problem, if present, must be corrected with vitamin K or clotting factors. Before surgery the patient also needs the routine care described in Chapter 23. This includes collection of adequate baseline data, patient and family education, physical preparation, and emotional support of patient and family.

### Postoperative Care

After surgery the patient will be in an intensive care unit. The nurse must immediately establish the parameters that should be monitored continuously. Vital signs, output (e.g., urinary and drainage tubes), intake, and hemodynamic parameters (CVP and arterial blood pressure) need to be monitored at least hourly. Laboratory measurements of hematocrit, blood gases, albumin, glucose, electrolytes, and serum and urine osmolality may be made at least daily or more frequently.

A *major focus* after surgery is *maintenance of adequate tissue perfusion.* Hypotension is a frequent occurrence and is treated with adequate replacement of fluids and electrolytes and blood. Vasopressors may be needed for 24 to 48 hours. Signs and symptoms of hemorrhage must be continuously monitored for because of the massive resection and potential vascular bleeding or because of clotting factor defects.

A *second major focus* is *monitoring of renal function.* A decrease in blood pressure or inadequate vascular volume can result in decreased glomerular filtration rate (GFR) and output. Maintenance of adequate vascular volume also helps prevent this potential problem. The fluid needs and/or drug needs are assessed on the basis of the continual monitoring carried out by the nurse. The importance of this surveillance cannot be overstated. An output of 20 to 50 ml/hr of urine is considered normal.

A *third major focus* is *prevention of respiratory complications.* Because of the high abdominal incision, respiratory efforts may be hampered and atelectasis and pneumonia can occur. Preventive respiratory measures must be incorporated into the care plan. The patient who has a pancreatic resection may be on bed rest longer than other surgery patients, and this increases the possibility of respiratory complications.

The *patient may have various drainage tubes.* It is important that the *output from these tubes be measured carefully* so that *fluid* and *electrolyte balance* is *maintained.* Excellent skin care around T-tubes or other drainage tubes must be instituted. Because these patients may be malnourished before surgery and because bile, pancreatic, and gastric drainage are extremely irritating to the skin, breakdown can easily occur.

The nurse must *monitor* the patient for *wound in-*

*fection* and *infection* at *insertion sites* of *invasive* lines. The tubing and dressing for IV lines and wound dressings must be managed with aseptic technique. Temperature should be monitored carefully. Any signs of infection should be reported immediately.

*Pain control* is *another major focus of care*. Adequate pain control is necessary so that the patient is able to turn, cough, and deep breathe.

*Maintenance* of *nutritional status* is a *focus of care during* both the *preoperative and postoperative periods*. The poorly nourished patient will often start on hyperalimentation before surgery, and this will be continued after surgery. When oral food and fluids are allowed, clear fluids will be started first and advanced as tolerated. If a total pancreatectomy was performed, the patient will require pancreatic exocrine enzyme replacement. This may also be necessary if a large amount of the pancreas is removed during a partial resection. The patient's stools should be monitored for the presence of steatorrhea, which is used to assess the adequacy of exocrine replacement or the need for replacement. Weight changes will also help identify nutritional status. Also, if a portion of the stomach was removed, the *dumping syndrome* may occur and is managed as described on p. 1492. Management of the patient's nutritional status is an ongoing need.

Glucose metabolism must also be assessed. With a partial pancreatectomy in association with chronic pancreatitis, the islet cell mass will be decreased and may be insufficient to maintain normal glucose metabolism. If a total pancreatectomy is performed, insulin replacement will be necessary. After partial or total pancreatectomy, all patients should have blood glucose monitored routinely and insulin replacement should be given as needed. If insulin deficiency is present, it is treated as type I diabetes mellitus is treated (see Chapter 40).

Psychologic support will also be a major need because of the diagnosis, the acuity of the problem, the need for long-term dietary and drug management, and the physical debility that might have been present preoperatively and will be present after surgery. Support and encouragement must be provided during patient care. The patient needs help in recognizing progress and also must be helped to set realistic goals. The patient and family must be kept informed about all care measures.

An additional problem for the patient who is having pancreatic resection for intractable pain from chronic pancreatitis is potential narcotic addiction. The narcotic addiction may have occurred as a result of the previous management of the pain associated with chronic pancreatitis and must be dealt with. Immediately after surgery, the patient will continue to need narcotics for pain control, but once physical recovery is established, the patient and health team should work at decreasing and eliminating narcotic use. Some patients may need the assitance or support and counseling available in specialized hospital units or hospitals that treat the chemically dependent person (see Chapter 19). It is crucial to remember that adequate pain control with narcotic analgesics will be necessary during the immediate postoperative period and that the patient's addiction will not be addressed until he or she is physiologically stable and physical sources of pain are thought to be controlled.

## QUESTIONS TO CONSIDER

- Contrast the priority nursing needs of a patient with acute pancreatitis with those of a patient with chronic pancreatitis.
- Contrast the care needs of a patient with cholelithiasis with those of a patient with cholecystitis.
- What are some pain control measures besides narcotics that can be employed in chronic pancreatitis, cancer of the pancreas, or cancer of the biliary system?

## CRITICAL THINKING ACTIVITIES

- Mrs. Blue has a T-tube present after an abdominal cholecystectomy. What may normally occur after the removal of her T-tube? What complication should the nurse be alert for? Why? How should she respond?
- In what ways would your assessment findings on a person with chronic pancreatitis differ from those of a person with acute pancreatitis?
- Mr. Ryan, 57, is being treated for acute pancreatitis related to drug therapy for hypertension. What aspect of this type of pancreatitis differs from acute alcohol-induced pancreatitis?

## CHAPTER SUMMARY

### JAUNDICE

- Jaundice is yellowish discoloration of the mucous membranes, skin, and sclera, resulting from increased bilirubin. Jaundice occurs in hemolytic, hepatic, and gallbladder diseases.
- Jaundice is associated with itching and potential bleeding.

### CHOLELITHIASIS/CHOLECYSTITIS/ CHOLEDOCHOLITHIASIS

- Cholelithiasis and cholecysitis are common health problems that could be decreased in incidence by decreasing obesity and controlling health problems such as hypertriglyceridemia.
- Biliary tract surgery by laparoscopic cholecystectomy (LC) is the treatment of choice for gallbladder disease, even though lithotripsy and dissolving agents are available and used for some persons.
- Nursing needs before medical or surgical treatment of gallbladder disease focus on pain and knowledge deficits.

- If cholecystitis occurs, fluid and electrolyte problems, jaundice, and bleeding may be of concern.
- Patient problems of concern after LC include pain and knowledge deficit.
- Patient problems requiring nursing attention after abdominal surgical treatment or lithotripsy of gallbladder disease include ineffective breathing pattern, fatigue, fluid volume deficits, obstruction of T-tube or bile duct, knowledge deficit, and pain.

### CARCINOMA OF THE BILIARY SYSTEM

- Carcinoma of the biliary system is insidious and can be asymptomatic until late in the disease.
- Care needs of the patient with biliary carcinoma may vary and may be focused on care after surgery, care to provide comfort, and care for a person with a terminal illness.

### PANCREATIC DISORDERS

- Pancreatitis may be acute or chronic.
- Acute pancreatitis can result in critical fluid and electrolyte problems, metabolic disturbances, and pain. It is reversible but has a high mortality.
- Chronic pancreatitis is progressive and usually results from alcoholism. It is not reversible.
- The patient with chronic pancreatitis will have acute exacerbations.
- Chronic pancreatitis results in pain, malnutrition, possibly diabetes mellitus, and variable fluid and electrolyte problems.
- Pain control measures and measures to prevent malabsorption are the major focus of nursing care for all persons with chronic pancreatitis; many patients with chronic pancreatitis will also need measures to assist them in dealing with alcoholism.
- Cancer of the pancreas is insidious and has a very poor prognosis.
- Pancreatic cancer may result in chronic pancreatitis, jaundice, and pain.
- In rare instances of pancreatic cancer, a pancreatoduodenectomy may be performed.
- Postoperative care for the patient who has a pancreatoduodenectomy should focus on maintaining tissue perfusion, renal function, vascular volume, respiratory function, and skin integrity; preventing infections; controlling pain; and maintaining glucose metabolism and nutritional status.

## REFERENCES


1. Adwers JR: Clinical trials of gallstone lithotripsy, *Hosp Prac* 24(7):83-90, 1989.
2. Anderson KN, Anderson LE, Glanze WD, editors: *Mosby's medical nursing, and allied health dictionary,* ed 4, St Louis, 1994, Mosby.
3. Apstein MD, Carey MC: Biliary tract stones and associated diseases. In Stein JH, editor: *Internal medicine,* ed 4, St Louis, 1994, Mosby.
4. Diehl AK: Laparoscopic cholecystectomy: too much of a good thing? *JAMA* 270(12):1469-1470, 1993.
5. Farha GJ, Beamer RL: New options for treating gallstone disease, *AFP* 44(4):1295-1304, 1991.
6. Fontham E, Correa P: Epidemiology of pancreatic cancer, *Surg Clin North Am* 69:551-567, 1989.
7. Greifzu S, Dest V: When the diagnosis is pancreatic cancer, *RN* 22(9):38-44, 1991.
8. Jeffres C: Complications of acute pancreatitis, *Crit Care Nurs* 9(4):38-48, 1989.
9. Krumberger JM: Acute pancreatitis, *Crit Care Nurs Clin North Am* 5(1):185-202, 1993.
10. Lancaster S, Biaro-Marshall D: Gallstone lithotripsy, *Am J Nurs* 88:1629-1630, 1988.
11. Latifi R, McIntosh K, Dudrick S: Nutritional management of acute and chronic pancreatitis, *Surg Clin North Am* 71:579-595, 1991.
12. Neoptolemos VP et al: Controlled trial of urgent endoscopic sphincterotomy versus conservative treatment for acute pancreatitis due to gallstones, *Lancet* 2:979-983, 1988.
13. O'Donnell LD, Heaton KW: Recurrence and re-recurrence of gallstones after medical dissolution: a longterm follow-up, *Gut* 29:655-658,1988.
14. Ostrow JD: Jaundice and disorders of bilirubin metabolism. In Stein JH, editor: *Internal medicine,* ed 4, St Louis, 1994, Mosby.
15. Ranson JHC et al: Prognostic signs and nonoperative peritoneal lavage in acute pancreatitis, *Surg Gynecol Obstet* 143:209-215, 1976.
16. Regan PT, Go VLW: Pancreatic disease. In Stein JH, editor: *Internal medicine,* ed 4, St Louis, 1994, Mosby.
17. Smith A: When the pancreas self-destructs, *Am J Nurs* 91(9):38-48, 1991.
18. Southern Surgeons Club: A prospective analysis of 1518 laporoscopic cholecystectomies, *N Engl J Med* 324(16):1073-1078, 1991.
19. Steer ML: Classification and pathogenesis of pancreatitis, *Surg Clin North Am* 69:467-480, 1989.
20. Thistle JL et al: The natural history of cholelithiasis: the national cooperative gallstone study, *Ann Intern Med* 101:171-175, 1984.
21. Thistle JL et al: Dissolution of cholesterol gallbladder stones by methyl tert butyl ether administered by percutaneous transhepatic catheter, *N Engl J Med* 320:633-639, 1989.
22. Way LW, Sleisenger MH: Cholelithiasis: chronic and acute cholecystitis. In Sleisenger MH, Fordtran JS, editors: *Gastrointestinal disease,* ed 4, Philadelphia, 1989, WB Saunders.

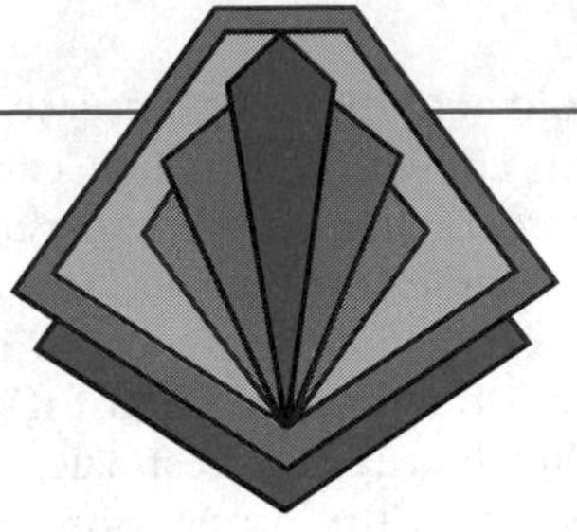

# CHAPTER 47

# Management of Persons With Problems of the Intestines

*Judith K. Sands*

## CHAPTER OBJECTIVES

***After studying this chapter, the learner should be able to do the following:***

1. Discuss life-style modifications for the management of constipation, diarrhea, and flatulence.
2. Compare the common forms of intestinal infections and their management.
3. Describe current pharmacologic and nursing management of inflammatory bowel disease.
4. Discuss the use of enteral and parenteral feedings in the management of malabsorption and malnutrition.
5. Compare the pathophysiology of hernias, cancer, and volvulus as causes of bowel obstruction.
6. Discuss the nursing management of the patient with an ostomy.
7. Compare the various surgical approaches to the management of common anorectal disorders.
8. Discuss preoperative and postoperative care of the patient undergoing bowel surgery.

## KEY TERMS

amebiasis
anal abscess
anal fissure
anal fistula
appendicitis
barium enema
colonoscopy
colostomy
constipation
Crohn's disease
diarrhea
diverticula
diverticulitis
diverticulosis
enteral nutrition
flatulence
gastrostomy
giardiasis
hemorrhoids
hernia
home total parenteral nutrition (HTPN)
ileostomy
intussusception
irritable bowel syndrome
malabsorption syndrome
occult blood
paralytic ileus
peristalsis
peritonitis
polyps
protein-calorie malnutrition
sigmoidoscopy
steatorrhea
stoma
strictureplasty
total parenteral nutrition (TPN)
trichinosis
ulcerative colitis
volvulus

Disease and disorders that affect the intestines constitute major health problems in the United States. Digestion, absorption, and elimination may be affected. The scope of problems range from mild to life-threatening. The categories of intestinal disorders discussed in this chapter include common bowel dysfunctions, infections, inflammatory bowel disease, malabsorption and malnutrition, bowel obstructions, and anorectal disorders.

## COMMON BOWEL DYSFUNCTIONS

### FLATULENCE

#### Etiology/Epidemiology

**Flatulence** is one of the most common gastrointestinal (GI) discomforts. The complaint usually refers to a sensation of bloating and abdominal distention that is accompanied by excess flatus (gas) or belching, or both.

A person normally passes between 400 and 1500 ml of flatus each day. The exact volume varies widely, depending on diet, amount of air swallowed, the action of the intestinal bacteria, and the amount of carbon dioxide formed by the action of bicarbonate with hydrochloric or fatty acids.

Bacterial flora produce hydrogen through the action of the bacteria on ingested fermentable matter. Some vegetables (e.g., legumes), fruits (e.g., raw apples or melons), and whole grains contain some polysaccharides that cannot be digested; thus they serve as a substrate for bacterial action with the production of hydrogen.

### Pathophysiology

Swallowed air that is not belched passes into the intestines and diffuses passively between the intestinal lumen and the bloodstream, depending on the partial pressure difference of the gas. Different quantities of gas are present in the intestinal lumen at different times. In addition to the standard gases, methane gas is produced by bacteria in about one third of the adult population. This appears to be a familial trait resulting from early-childhood environmental factors.

Persons who complain of excess flatus usually are not excreting larger amounts of gas than symptom-free persons. The symptoms probably are related to a disorder of intestinal motility and not the quantity of gas itself. Persons experiencing abdominal distention or discomfort from gas may have problems with altered GI motility or malabsorption syndromes. These conditions need to be ruled out if the person experiences marked discomfort.

### Medical Management

It usually is not necessary for the physician to intervene in situations involving occasional flatulence. Successful management usually can be achieved with diet and life-style modifications. Flatulence may become a more significant problem, however, when it accompanies the decreased peristalsis or ileus that commonly follows abdominal surgery. The intermittent use of nasogastric (NG) or rectal tubes may be ordered to attempt to relieve distention. Simethicone (Mylicon, Gas-X) also may be ordered. This drug has a defoaming action and helps to break up mucus-surrounded gas pockets in the intestines.

### Nursing Management

Simple modification in diet and life-style may provide the affected person greater comfort. An increase in exercise, particularly walking, can stimulate intestinal peristalsis and help with the passage of gas. Because gas bubbles rise, an erect position after eating assists the escape of gas. If the patient is confined to bed, positioning on the right side will move stomach contents toward the pylorus and allow gas to move freely to the cardia for expulsion through belching. The nurse also encourages the patient to avoid activities that increase air swallowing such as gum chewing, drinking carbonated beverages, using a straw, or talking while eating.

Dietary measures include avoiding gas-forming carbohydrates that increase discomfort, such as legumes, onions, cucumbers, radishes, and foods in the cabbage family. A high-fiber diet increases intestinal peristalsis, and a low-fat diet decreases the production of carbon dioxide. The nurse explores the patient's usual dietary pattern and makes suggestions concerning changes that may be beneficial.

## CONSTIPATION

### Etiology/Epidemiology

The term **constipation** refers to an abnormal infrequency of defecation or the passage of abnormally hard stools, or both. The term lacks precise definition because it has different meanings to different people. Almost everyone experiences occasional constipation, and it is a common complaint among elderly persons. Lack of physical activity, stress, diet changes, and lack of fluids can contribute to occasional episodes of constipation. A great number of persons in the United States spend vast amounts of money annually on over-the-counter laxatives and other aids to intestinal elimination. Lack of dietary fiber and inadequate fluid intake can lead to infrequent, dry stools. Dietary fiber increases the amount of water content of the stool, and bacterial degradation of the fiber enhances colonic motility. If the body lacks fluid (dehydration), the colon will reabsorb an increased amount of water from the stool, leading to a hardened stool.

Defecation, which is initiated when the feces enter the rectum, can be voluntarily controlled by contraction of the external anal sphincter. If the defecation urge is not heeded, it soon disappears and the feces remain in the rectum. The defecation urge occurs most frequently after meals, particularly breakfast, as a result of stimulation of the gastrocolic reflex from food entering the stomach. Most people defecate on a regular pattern, but this pattern varies widely among persons, from three times a day to once every 2 or 3 days. True constipation is defined as a stool frequency of less than three per week.

### Pathophysiology

Constipation may be associated with disorders of the bowel, hypometabolism, and neurogenic or psychogenic disorders. Physiologically, constipation may result from decreased motility of the colon or from retention of feces in the lower portion of the colon, or rectum. In either case the longer the feces remain in the colon, the greater is the amount of water that is reabsorbed and the drier the stool becomes. The stool is then more difficult to expel. Occasional constipation is not detrimental to health, but habitual constipation leads to decreased intestinal muscle tone, increased use of Valsal-

**BOX 47-1 Factors That Place Patients at High Risk for Constipation and Fecal Impaction**

- Nutritional depletion
- Dehydration
- Constipating medications:
  - Aluminum- and calcium-based antacids
  - Narcotics
  - Anticholinergics
  - Antidepressants/antipsychotics
  - Iron, calcium, and bismuth salts
  - Antihistamines
- Barium studies
- Abdominal surgery
- Prolonged bed rest
- Confusion, disorientation
- Spinal cord injury
- Interruption of usual bowel routine

va's maneuver as the person bears down in the attempt to pass the hardened stool, and an increased incidence of hemorrhoids. Chronic laxative use can lead to hypokalemia, sodium depletion, and dehydration.

## Medical Management

The treatment of constipation is related to its underlying cause and may include the use of stool softeners, suppositories, laxatives, or occasionally enemas. These drugs are used for the shortest possible time period, and every effort is made to return the person to a drug-free pattern of elimination. Factors that place patients at high risk for constipation and impaction are listed in Box 47-1. Common examples of drugs used in the treatment of constipation are summarized in Table 47-1.

If the stool is permitted to remain in the colon until it becomes exceedingly hard, a fecal impaction can occur. The impaction blocks the rectum and must be removed. If it cannot be softened and removed by oil retention and cleansing enemas, digital removal with a gloved finger may be necessary. This is an uncomfortable experience for the patient, and gentleness is required. The stimulation of vagal nerve endings in the rectum may cause slowing of the heart during digital removal. Impaction can be prevented by regular assessment of bowel elimination and early intervention for patients at high risk, such as those placed on bed rest, elders, and patients receiving frequent or high-dose narcotics.

## Nursing Management

Nursing management of constipation focuses on careful assessment of all patients at risk and teaching about lifestyle factors that can facilitate a normal pattern of elimination. Diet modification is important. The nurse teaches patients to eat a high-fiber diet and to avoid highly refined foods. Bran may be used as a supplement in a limited way. Patients should attempt to drink at least 2500 to 3000 ml of fluid daily, unless their medical condition contraindicates a liberal fluid intake. Regular exercise and a planned daily time for defecation are important measures. Any patient who is placed on bed rest or receives regular doses of narcotics should be started on a plan to prevent problems with constipation. Hospitalization inevitably interferes with a person's normal patterns of exercise and eating. The nurse monitors all hospitalized patients for constipation and records all bowel elimination. For greatest success, bowel programs need to be initiated *before* problems with constipation

**TABLE 47-1 Commonly Used Drugs in the Management of Constipation**

| CLASSIFICATION AND EXAMPLES | ACTION | PATIENT TEACHING |
|---|---|---|
| **STOOL SOFTENERS (EMOLLIENTS)** | | |
| Dioctyl sodium Sulfosuccinate (Colace)<br>Docusate calcium (Surfak) | Docusate salts act as detergents in the intestine, reducing surface tension, which facilitates the incorporation of liquid and fat, softening the stool. | Preparations lose effectiveness with long-term use; patient should not rely on this measure alone.<br>Discontinue if abdominal cramping occurs. |
| **BULK FORMERS** | | |
| Psyllium (Metamucil)<br>Methylcellulose (Citrucil)<br>Bran | Polysaccharides and cellulose derivatives mix with intestinal fluids, swell, and stimulate peristalsis. | Ensure adequate fluid intake to prevent impaction or obstruction; take separately from prescribed drugs to avoid problems with absorption. |
| **LUBRICANTS** | | |
| Mineral oil | Soften fecal matter by lubricating the intestinal mucosa, facilitating easy stool passage. | Do not take with meals or drugs because oil can impair absorption; swallow carefully to prevent lipid aspiration. |
| **STIMULANTS/IRRITANTS** | | |
| Cascara sagrada<br>Senna (Senokot)<br>Bisacodyl (Dulcolax)<br>Castor oil | Directly stimulate and irritate the intestine, promoting peristalsis. | Cramps and diarrhea can occur; monitor for fluid and electrolyte imbalance if reaction is severe. |
| **SALINE/OSMOTICS** | | |
| Milk of Magnesia<br>Magnesium citrate<br>Lactulose (Cephulac) | Alter stool consistency by drawing water into the intestines by osmosis, thus stimulating peristalsis. | Monitor for fluid and electrolyte imbalance or dehydration if reaction is severe; liquid preparations are more effective than tablets. |

**Guidelines for Patient Teaching to Prevent or Correct Constipation**

**DIET**

Eat a high-fiber diet:
- Whole grain cereals and breads
- Fresh fruits and vegetables
- Use supplemental bran only in moderation (can cause flatulence, diarrhea, or obstruction): begin with a low dose (6-10 tsp/day) and increase gradually if needed.

Drink 2500-3000 ml of liquid daily distributed throughout the day unless contraindicated by a fluid restriction.

**ACTIVITY**

Participate in daily active exercise (walking is ideal exercise).

Set aside a regular time each day for defecation (do not suppress the normal defecation stimulus).

**LAXATIVES**

Avoid laxative use if possible; use only when other measures fail.

Use a stool softener or bulk laxative if possible for occasional constipation.

arise. Teaching measures to correct constipation are outlined in the Guidelines box above.

## DIARRHEA

### Etiology/Epidemiology

The definition of **diarrhea** is based on the consistency of the stool (watery), not necessarily the number of stools expelled per day. Diarrhea occurs primarily as a result of infections and diseases of the GI tract, hypermetabolism, food allergies, as a reflex triggered from adjoining pelvic organs, or after vagotomy surgery. Diarrhea also can occur in hospitalized and institutionalized patients who experience severe constipation and impaction. Diarrhea occurs as pressure builds around the impaction. Because of its diverse causes, it is often more difficult to prevent diarrhea than constipation.

Diarrhea may be caused by changes in the fecal contents (solutes exerting an osmotic effect or a fluid content increase) or by a decrease in intestinal transit time so that less fluid can be reabsorbed. The final result is passage of feces high in water content.

Acute diarrhea usually is self-limiting and of short duration. Chronic diarrhea usually is related to changes in the GI tract that alter the transport of fluid, electrolytes, and solids. Infectious diarrhea may be severe and typically is related to a recurring cycle of oral ingestion and anal excretion of the organism.

### Pathophysiology

Large-volume diarrhea is caused by a hypersecretion of water and electrolytes by the intestinal mucosa. This secretion occurs in response to the osmotic pressure exerted by nonabsorbed food particles in the chyme or from direct irritation of the mucosa. **Peristalsis** is increased, and the transit time through the intestine is significantly decreased. Increased peristalsis also may result from inflammation as mucosal cells hypersecrete water in the presence of infectious organisms such as *Shigella, Escherichia coli, Staphylococcus,* and *Campylobacter jejuni.* Diarrhea may be accompanied by severe abdominal cramping, tenesmus (persistent spasm) of the anal area, abdominal distention, and borborygmus (loud bowel sounds). It also may be painless, particularly if it is a result of stress. Defecation may be precipitated by the intake of food or may occur irrespective of time or situation.

Fluid and electrolyte imbalances can result from diarrhea, depending on its severity. Mild diarrhea in adults can lead to losses of sodium and potassium (causing metabolic alkalosis). Severe diarrhea causes dehydration, hyponatremia, hypokalemia, and metabolic acidosis (from the loss of large amounts of bicarbonate). Malnourished or elderly persons tolerate severe diarrhea less well than do younger or well-nourished persons. Persistent diarrhea readily leads to skin breakdown in the perianal region.

### Medical Management

Inasmuch as diarrhea usually is caused by a pathologic condition or as a side effect of medications, medical treatment consists primarily of correcting the underlying cause. Other measures include providing electrolyte replacement, allowing the bowel to rest, and administering antidiarrheal medications.

Severe diarrhea may necessitate hospitalization for fluid replacement and control. Total parenteral nutrition (TPN) may be required if a prolonged period of bowel rest is necessary. Common drugs used in the treatment of diarrhea are summarized in Table 47-2.

### Nursing Management

If patients are hospitalized with acute diarrhea, the nurse maintains an accurate record of diarrhea incidence and severity, estimates fluid losses, assesses for fluid and electrolyte disturbances, and promotes patient comfort. Sitz baths can be extremely comforting when perianal skin becomes irritated; they usually are contraindicated, however, if actual skin breakdown has occurred. The prevention of perianal skin breakdown is an important nursing intervention. The nurse may need to assist a weakened patient in keeping the area clean and dry. Skin ointments and barriers (e.g., zinc oxide) are reapplied as needed after each episode of diarrhea. A fecal incontinence pouch may be applied if the frequency or severity of the diarrhea overwhelms the anal sphincters. General measures to be employed in the management of diarrhea are summarized in the Guidelines box, p. 1527.

**TABLE 47-2 Commonly Used Drugs in the Management of Diarrhea**

| CLASSIFICATION/ EXAMPLES | ACTION | PATIENT TEACHING |
|---|---|---|
| **LOCAL ACTING** | | |
| Kaolin and pectin (Kaopectate) | Soothes the intestinal mucosa and increase absorption of water, nutrients, and electrolytes | Shake liquids well before using. |
| Bismuth subsalicylate (Pepto-Bismol) | Bismuth preparations bind bacterial toxins | Bismuth products may turn the stool black. |
| **SYSTEMIC ACTING** | | |
| Loperamide (Imodium)<br>Tincture of opium (paregoric)<br>Diphenoxylate hydrochloride with atropine (Lomotil) | Acts systemically to reduce peristalsis and GI motility | Drugs are part of the narcotic family.<br>Loperamide is a narcotic analog with no associated physical dependence.<br>Lomotil has a lower potential for dependency than most narcotics and paregoric acts as a traditional narcotic. |
| **ANTIBIOTICS** | | |
| Doxycycline (a tetracycline)<br>Trimethoprim<br>Sulfamethoxazole (a sulfa drug) | May be prescribed in situations in which infectious diarrhea is present | Follow prescription carefully as to dose and frequency; keep fluid intake high. |

**Guidelines for Management of Diarrhea**

**FOOD AND FLUID**

Withhold food for 24 hours if diarrhea is severe.
Continue oral fluids as tolerated.
- Gatorade, which contains 23 mEq of sodium, 17 mEq of chloride, 3 mEq of potassium, and 7 mEq of phosphate in a 5% glucose solution, is recommended.
- A home preparation of 1 tsp of salt, 1 tsp of bicarbonate of soda, and 4 tsp of sugar added to 1 L of drinking water is also effective (this solution lacks potassium).
- Avoid beverages that contain caffeine or alcohol.

Restart diet with small feedings of a low-fiber, low-fat, bland diet.
Limit use of milk products because a transient lactase deficiency is fairly common after an episode of diarrhea.
Avoid very hot and iced foods and beverages.

**ACTIVITY**

Rest in bed when diarrhea is severe.
Rest after meals to avoid stimulating peristalsis.

**COMFORT MEASURES**

Perform perianal hygiene after *each* stool, and avoid excessive abrasion with toilet paper.
Keep perianal area clean and dry to prevent skin breakdown.
Provide sitz baths three times a day if skin is intact.
Use a protective ointment (such as zinc oxide) on perianal area.
Keep environment odor-free with deodorizers as necessary.

## FECAL INCONTINENCE

### Etiology/Epidemiology

Problems with bowel incontinence may be associated with aging, disability, and loss of self-care potential. There are a variety of causes of fecal incontinence. The external anal sphincter may be relaxed, the voluntary control of defecation may be interrupted in the central nervous system or messages may not be transmitted to the brain because of a lesion within or external pressure on the spinal cord. The disorders that cause breakdown of conscious control of defecation include cortical clouding or lesions, spinal cord lesions or trauma, and trauma to the anal sphincter (e.g., from fistula, abscess, or surgery). Perineal relaxation and actual damage of the anal sphincter often are caused by injury from perineal surgery, childbirth, or anal intercourse. Relaxation of the sphincter usually increases with the general loss of muscle tone in aging. The normal changes that occur with aging are not of sufficient significance to cause incontinence, however, unless concurrent health problems predispose the patient to the disorder.

### Pathophysiology

Normally the contents of the bowel are moved by mass movements toward the rectum. The rectum then stores the stool until defecation occurs. Distention of the rectum initiates nerve signals that are transmitted to the spinal cord and then back to the descending colon, initiating peristaltic waves that force more feces into the rectum. The internal anal sphincter relaxes, and if the external sphincter also is relaxed, defecation results. Defecation occurs as a reflex response to the distention of the rectal musculature, but this reflex can be voluntarily inhibited. Voluntary inhibition of defecation is learned in early childhood, and control typically lasts throughout life. Voluntary regulation is under cortical control. Emptying of the rectum occurs when the external anal sphincter (under cortical control) relaxes and the abdominal and pelvic muscles contract.

Reflex defecation continues to occur even in the presence of most upper or lower motor neuron lesions, because the musculature of the bowel contains its own nerve centers that respond to distention through peristalsis. Reflex defecation therefore often persists or can be stimulated even when motor paralysis is present. Defecation occurs primarily in response to mass peristaltic

**Guidelines for a Bowel Training Program**

Include person and the family or a friend in the planning.
Determine when bowel evacuation usually occurs; the most common times are after breakfast or dinner.
Determine whether a morning or evening program is more suitable for the person.
Insert a glycerine or bisacodyl (Dulcolax) suppository 30 minutes before expected time of defecation; give suppository at same time every day.
If possible, have the person sit on the toilet for defecation.
If necessary, massage the abdomen toward the sigmoid (left lower quadrant) to encourage defecation; digital rectal stimulation also may stimulate defecation.
Keep a daily record to determine whether program is producing desired results.

movements that follow meals or whenever the rectum becomes distended.

### Medical Management

Bowel training is the major approach to managing fecal incontinence. If a person can sit on a toilet or commode and actively concentrate on defecation, it is often possible to teach *automatic* defecation. A specific routine of activities such as familiar surroundings, consistent time of day, and timing with meals allows many persons to defecate predictably and remain continent for the remainder of the day. Consistency in the approach is the most crucial aspect of a bowel training program. Principles are summarized in the Guidelines box above.

### Nursing Management

The nurse helps the patient implement the bowel training program. The nurse initially collects data about the nature and frequency of the incontinence problem, particularly its relationship to meals or other regular activity. Another important component involves assessment of the ability and motivation of the patient and family to participate in the program. An effective program demands consistency from the staff, but it also requires cooperation and commitment from the patient and family members. It is a team effort and involves a significant amount of time *and* effort.

To plan the most effective approach the nurse gathers specific information concerning the person's general physical and cognitive condition, ability to contract the abdominal and perineal muscles on command, and awareness of the need or urge to defecate. The nurse provides a high-fiber diet and ensures that the patient consumes at least 2500 to 3000 ml of fluid daily. The need for a regular stool softener or bulk former is evaluated. The nurse offers ongoing psychosocial support and encouragement to the patient because it may take time before positive gains are achieved.

Despite significant honest efforts on the part of nursing staff members and patient, the fecal incontinence may remain uncontrolled. The nurse then shifts efforts toward maintaining the person's psychologic integrity and preventing problems with the skin.

Loss of control over intestinal elimination may be associated with feelings of regression, inadequacy, guilt, and uncleanliness. The person needs to feel accepted as an adult and to have the condition accepted by others as a situational physical condition and not as a personal inadequacy. Incontinence is a major issue in home care and frequently is cited as the most common cause for elderly persons to be admitted to nursing homes.

Protective disposable pants are available and provide the person with a sense of security and dignity. Cleansing of the anal and perineal areas as soon as possible after fecal incontinence helps to maintain skin integrity and removes a source of discomfort and odor. Adequate intake of fiber-rich foods and fluids, when possible, assists in defecation of a normal stool at less frequent intervals.

# ACUTE INFECTION/INFLAMMATION OF THE INTESTINES

## APPENDICITIS

### Etiology/Epidemiology

The vermiform appendix is a small, fingerlike projection that is attached to the cecum usually just below the ileocecal valve (Figure 47-1). The appendix is approximately 10 cm (4 inches) long and has no clearly identified function. It is an integral part of the cecum and fills with chyme and empties by peristalsis along with the rest of the bowel.

**Appendicitis** is an acute inflammation of the appendix, which is one of the most common surgical emergencies. The cause rarely is clear-cut, but the lumen of the appendix is quite small, making it vulnerable to incomplete emptying or obstruction, which can lead to infection. Kinking of the appendix or obstruction by fecaliths (hardened feces) or foreign bodies also may trigger the acute inflammatory response.

Appendicitis occurs most commonly in teen-agers and young adults between the ages of 10 and 30 years. Appendicitis can occur at any age, however, and is an extremely serious condition in elders. Males are affected more commonly than females during the teen-age and young adult years. Approximately 7% of the population is affected by the disorder at some point. Appendicitis appears to occur more commonly in societies in which the diet is low in fiber and high in refined carbohydrates. The higher incidence of constipation associated with this diet pattern is theorized to increase the chance of developing obstructive fecaliths.

### Pathophysiology

The inflammatory process of appendicitis can involve all or part of the appendix. Intraluminal pressure increases,

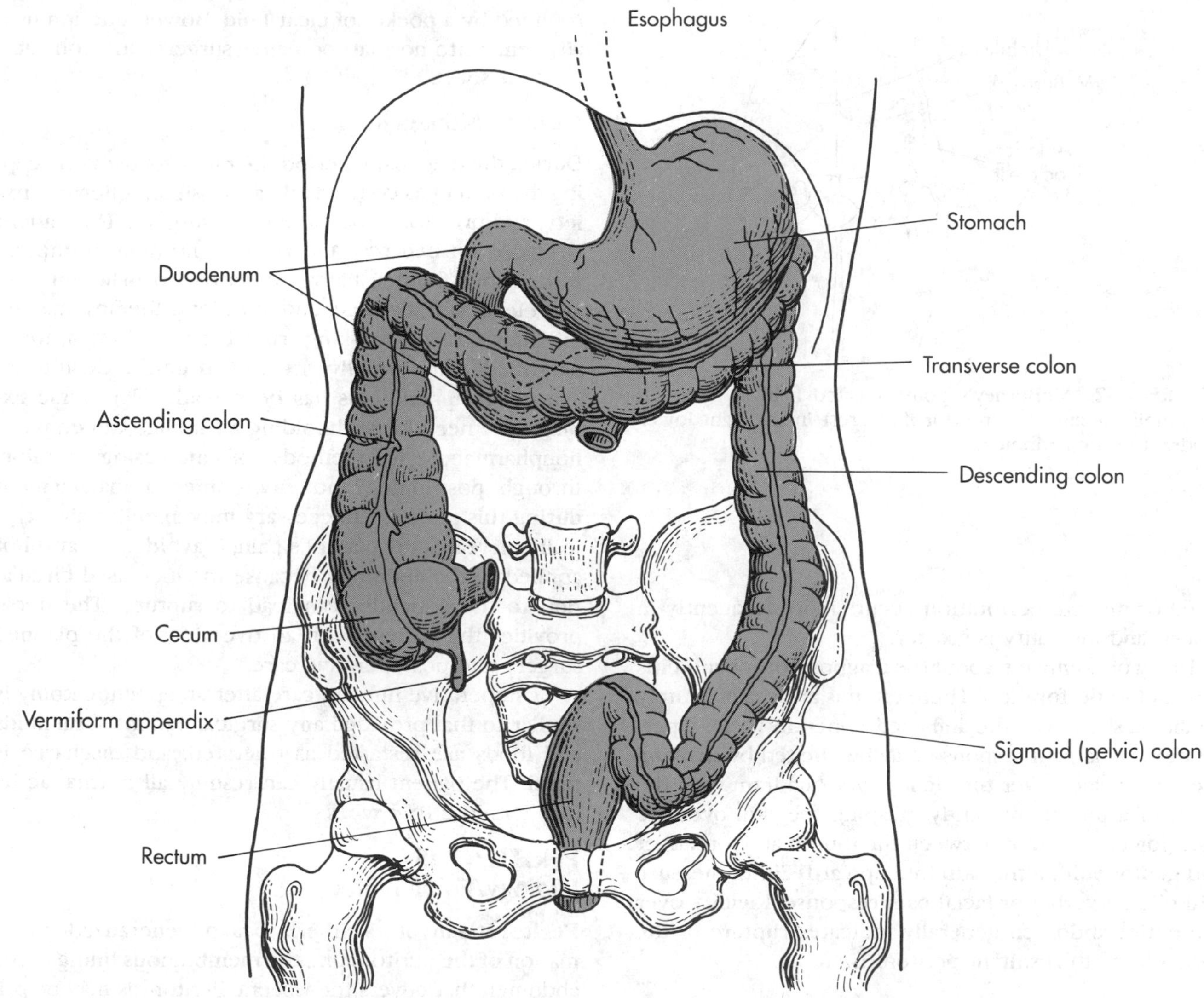


**FIGURE 47-1** The appendix at the beginning of the ascending colon.

leading to lymphoid swelling, decreased venous drainage, thrombosis, and bacterial invasion. An abscess may develop in the appendiceal wall or surrounding tissue and, unless treated, can progress to gangrene and perforation within 24 to 36 hours. If the inflammatory process develops fairly slowly, the infection may be successfully walled off in a local abscess. In more rapidly developing cases, the risk of rupture and acute peritonitis is quite high.

The classic clinical manifestation of appendicitis typically begins with acute abdominal pain that comes in waves. The pain typically starts in the epigastric or umbilical region but gradually becomes localized in the right lower quadrant of the abdomen. Localization at McBurney's point, halfway between the umbilicus and the anterior spine of the ileum (Figure 47-2), is considered classic. The pain is intermittent at first but typically becomes steady and severe over a short period. Pain frequently is accompanied by nausea, anorexia, and vomiting. Light palpation of the abdomen elicits pain in the right lower quadrant. Rebound tenderness is a common finding (see Chapter 43). The abdominal muscles overlying the area of inflammation in the right lower quadrant may feel tense as a result of voluntary rigidity. The person with appendicitis often is noted to be lying on the side or back with knees flexed in an attempt to decrease muscle strain on the abdominal wall. Other symptoms may include temperature elevations in the range of 38° to 38.5° C (100.5° to 101.5° F) accompanied by an elevation in WBC count above 10,000/mm$^3$ and a neutrophil count above 75%.

Some patients with appendicitis may have less well-defined local symptoms because of small variations in the location of the appendix. Elderly patients are less likely to experience classic acute symptoms. Their response to pain is decreased, and their symptoms frequently are mild or vague. Because appendicitis is relatively rare in this age-group, the diagnosis may be de-

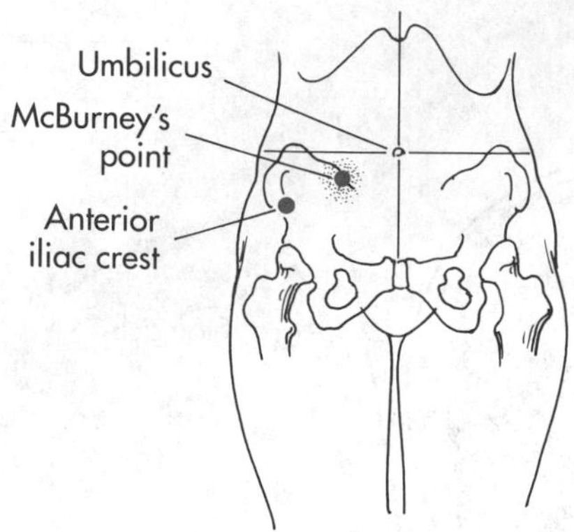


**FIGURE 47-2** McBurney's point, located halfway between the umbilicus and the anterior iliac crest in the right lower quadrant of the abdomen.

layed or missed. Perforation occurs more frequently in elders, and mortality is greater.

Delay or confusion about the diagnosis of appendicitis can lead to perforation. There often is an area of acutely sensitive skin over the inflamed appendix before perforation. This pain response may be elicited by stroking the skin surface over the right lower quadrant with the point of a pin or by lightly grasping the skin over the right lower quadrant between the thumb and forefinger and gently pulling the skin fold upward. Either measure will elicit a verbal or facial pain response. Rigidity over the entire abdomen generally indicates rupture of the appendix with resultant peritonitis.

### Medical Management

The diagnosis of appendicitis is made from the classic physical and laboratory indicators if they are present. When the clinical picture is unclear, however, urinalysis and an intravenous pyelogram may be employed to rule out acute pyelitis or a ureteral stone. Many other diseases can produce symptoms similar to appendicitis, and these problems may need to be ruled out before a positive diagnosis of appendicitis can be made. Some of the related disorders include acute salpingitis, regional ileitis, mesenteric lymphadenitis, ovarian cyst, mittelschmerz, and biliary colic.

The appendix is removed surgically (appendectomy) as soon as possible to prevent rupture with subsequent peritonitis. When the surgery is performed promptly, mortality is less than 0.5%. If the diagnosis is not promptly established, the incidence of complications rises dramatically. The appendix is removed through a small incision over McBurney's point or through a right paramedial incision. The incision usually heals with no need for external drainage. Drains are inserted when an abscess is discovered, when the appendix has ruptured, or when the appendix is severely edematous and surrounded by a pocket of clear fluid. Bowel function usually returns to normal soon after surgery, and convalescence is short.

### Nursing Management

During the diagnostic period the nurse focuses on keeping the patient as comfortable as possible, relieving anxiety, and preparing the patient for surgery. The patient is placed on bed rest and is given nothing by mouth. Intravenous fluids usually are started to maintain fluid and electrolyte balance, and antibiotic therapy may be initiated. To avoid masking critical changes in symptoms, pain medication usually is withheld until a definite diagnosis of appendicitis has been made. The nurse explains the need for withholding analgesics and employs nonpharmacologic methods of increasing comfort through positioning and environmental management during this period. Unnecessary movement, which typically increases the patient's pain, is avoided. Heat is not applied to the abdomen because the increased circulation to the appendix can lead to rupture. The nurse provides the patient with an overview of the planned surgery and postoperative care.

Postoperative nursing care after an appendectomy is similar to that provided any surgical patient. Oral fluids and foods are restarted as tolerated, and discharge is rapid. The patient usually can resume all normal activities within 2 to 4 weeks.

## PERITONITIS

### Etiology/Epidemiology

**Peritonitis** involves either a local or generalized inflammation of the peritoneum, the membranous lining of the abdomen that covers the viscera. Peritonitis may be primary or secondary, aseptic or septic, and acute or chronic. Primary peritonitis usually is caused by bacterial infection whereas secondary peritonitis often results from trauma, surgical injury, or chemical irritation.

A ruptured appendix, perforated peptic ulcer, diverticulitis, pelvic inflammatory disease, urinary tract infection or trauma, bowel obstruction, and surgical complications are possible causes of primary peritonitis. Secondary bacterial invasion occurs within hours of the initiating event and is an important component of all forms of peritonitis. Common organisms for bacterial invasion include *E. coli,* streptococci, staphylococci, pneumococci, gonococci, *Klebsiella,* and *Pseudomonas.*

### Pathophysiology

The body uses natural barriers to attempt to control the inflammation associated with peritonitis. Adhesions form rapidly and may be successful in limiting involvement to only a portion of the abdominal cavity. The end result may be abscess development. Adhesions are more likely to develop in the lower portion of the abdomen. As healing progresses, the adhesions may shrink and virtually disappear, or they may persist as constrictions that bind the involved structures together, possibly creating intestinal obstruction.

The peritoneal lining serves as a semipermeable membrane lining that allows the flow of water and electrolytes between the bloodstream and peritoneal cavity. When peritonitis occurs, fluid can shift into the abdominal cavity at a rate of 300 to 500 ml/hr in response to the acute inflammation. The inflammatory process also shunts extra blood to the inflamed areas of the bowel to combat the secondary bacterial infection, and peristalsis typically ceases. The bowel increasingly becomes distended with gas and fluid. The circulatory, fluid, and electrolyte changes can rapidly become critical. Local reactions of the peritoneum include redness, inflammation, and the production of large amounts of fluid that contains electrolytes and proteins. Hypovolemia, electrolyte imbalance, dehydration, and finally shock can develop. The loss of circulatory volume is proportional to the severity of peritoneal involvement. The fluid usually becomes purulent as the condition progresses and as the bacteria become more numerous. The bacteria also may enter the blood and cause septicemia.

The clinical manifestations of peritonitis are both local and systemic. They depend to some degree on the site and extent of the inflammation. Abdominal findings include pain and tenderness that may be local or diffuse and often includes rebound tenderness. Guarding and rigidity are classic signs. Distention and paralytic ileus develop as the inflammation progresses. Systemic signs may include fever and elevated white blood cells (WBCs), nausea and vomiting, and symptoms of early shock such as tachycardia, tachypnea, oliguria, restlessness, weakness, pallor, and diaphoresis. The symptoms initially are much less severe in elderly persons, and the diagnosis may be overlooked until the condition is extremely serious. Patients receiving high levels of corticosteroids also may exhibit mild or ambiguous symptoms, and thus early diagnosis is difficult.

### Medical Management

The diagnosis of peritonitis is made primarily on the basis of the symptom pattern, laboratory findings, and x-ray studies that may show abnormalities in gas and air patterns in the abdomen. Free air or fluid in the abdominal cavity is indicative of perforation. Specimens of blood and peritoneal fluid are obtained for culture before the initiation of antibiotic therapy. WBC counts frequently are elevated to 20,000/mm$^3$ or higher. Electrolyte values are carefully monitored.

The primary curative intervention for peritonitis is surgery to correct the underlying cause and remove infected material. Surgical healing is impaired if sepsis or ischemia occurs, and complications associated with wound healing are common. Peritoneal lavage with warm saline may be performed during surgery, followed by the insertion of drainage tubes to facilitate healing. Surgery may need to be delayed until the patient's condition can be medically stabilized.

Fluid, electrolyte, and colloid replacement is the major focus of medical care. The fluid shifts that cause massive hypovolemia and shock need aggressive management. Broad-spectrum antibiotics are administered against suspected organisms and then adjusted as needed in response to culture and sensitivity reports. Nutritional management with TPN solutions may be necessary when sepsis is severe and recovery is expected to be prolonged. The overall mortality of patients with severe peritonitis is about 40%.

### Nursing Management

The patient with peritonitis is critically ill and requires careful monitoring of all vital parameters. Placement in a critical care environment frequently is indicated. The nurse monitors vital signs and intake and output frequently and adjusts IV lines and medications as ordered. A nasogastric tube is inserted to help relieve abdominal distention. Bed rest in a semi-Fowler's position is maintained to support ventilation and increase patient comfort. The nurse encourages the patient to deep breathe frequently because pain and distention can significantly impair ventilation. The nurse also provides comfort measures whenever possible, including frequent mouth care, basic hygiene, and measures to reduce anxiety. (More thorough discussion of the nursing management of the patient in shock is presented in Chapter 22.) The patient receives standard postoperative care after surgery (see p. 1584 and Chapter 25), with particular attention to respiratory care and wound healing. If the abdominal contamination is extensive, there may be multiple incisions and drains. Complications are common, and recovery frequently is prolonged.

## DIVERTICULAR DISEASE/DIVERTICULITIS

### Etiology/Epidemiology

**Diverticula** are small outpouchings or herniations of the mucosal lining of the gastrointestinal tract. Diverticula, commonly found in the colon, become inflamed when food, fecal matter, or bacteria are trapped within the pouches. The presence of asymptomatic multiple diverticula is termed **diverticulosis** (Figure 47-3). It is a progressive disorder, and the number of diverticula tends to increase with age. **Diverticulitis** occurs when trapped fecal material and bacteria combine to produce acute inflammation and infection. The inflammation can progress to microperforation and possibly abscess.

Diverticulosis rarely occurs before age 35; the probability then increases progressively with age and may be as high as 60% in older persons. The number of persons who have diverticulosis is merely estimated, however, because most persons with diverticulosis are symptom-free. The incidence of diverticulitis is approximately 10% of the general population and also increases sharply with age. About 20% of persons with diverticular

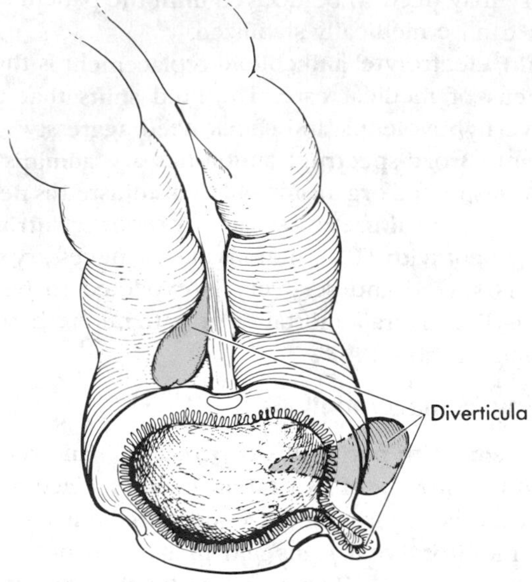


**FIGURE 47-3** Diverticuli in the colon.

disease will experience diverticulitis at some point. Diverticula can form virtually anywhere in the GI tract, but more than 90% occur in the descending and sigmoid colon.[20]

Diverticulosis has been described as a disease of Western civilization because of its high incidence in developed countries and the low incidence in nonindustrialized countries and Japan. The cause is thought to be the relatively low intake of fiber-rich foods by persons in most developed countries. Vegetarians have been shown to have a markedly lower incidence of diverticular disease.

## Pathophysiology

The development of intestinal diverticula is theorized to be related to low fecal volume in the colon, increased intraluminal pressure, and decreased muscle strength in the colon wall. Diverticula tend to form in the colon wall at points where blood vessels penetrate the mucosal and muscular layers, creating points of relative weakness. It is theorized that increased muscular contractions in the sigmoid colon that are generated to push stool into the rectum increase both the thickness of the muscle and the intraluminal pressure. The weaker connective tissue then herniates between the circular muscle bands and forms the diverticula.

Diverticulitis frequently develops in a single diverticulum in response to irritation initiated by trapped fecal material. Blood supply to the area decreases, and bacteria invade the diverticulum. The inflammation tends to spread to surrounding bowel walls, causing spasticity and instability of the bowel. Partial obstruction of the diverticulum can cause thickening of the bowel wall and scarring from chronic inflammation. The inflammation may wall itself off or proceed to local abscess formation, bleeding, or perforation. Generalized peritonitis may occur.

The clinical manifestations of diverticulitis reflect the inflammation of the diverticula or the development of complications. Crampy lower left quadrant abdominal pain accompanied by low-grade fever is classic. The pain is triggered by muscle spasms of the sigmoid colon and usually is acute and persistent in nature. The pain worsens with movement, coughing, or straining. Nausea and vomiting occur frequently. The abdomen is tender and may be distended. Occult bleeding occurs frequently and hemorrhage is possible, although unusual. The development of an abscess or perforation triggers the symptoms of localized peritonitis (see p. 1531). The traditional symptoms tend to be less pronounced or underreported by elders.

Although diverticulosis itself is symptomless, the person may experience occasional left lower quadrant crampy pain, chronic constipation, bowel irregularity, and episodes of diarrhea. The problem usually is identified during radiographic testing for other illnesses.

### Meckel's diverticulum

Meckel's diverticulum is a congenital abnormality in which a blind tube, similar in structure to the appendix, is present, which usually opens into the distal ileum near the ileocecal valve. The tube may be attached to the umbilicus by a fibrous band. It occurs in about 2% of the population and is more common in men. Although it usually is symptomless throughout life, its mucosal lining may become inflamed and lead to intestinal obstruction or perforation, causing peritonitis. The symptoms resemble appendicitis, but the pain localizes around the umbilicus. The treatment involves surgical excision of the diverticulum.

## Medical Management

The preliminary diagnosis of diverticulitis may be made from the history and presenting symptoms. A computed tomography (CT) scan or abdominal ultrasound examination reveals the presence of an abscess. A barium enema can show the thickened muscle layers and narrowed colon, but it is not performed until after the acute inflammation subsides. Direct visualization is possible by means of sigmoidoscopy or colonscopy but increases the risk of perforation.

Diverticulosis is managed by the prevention of constipation through the use of a high-fiber diet. Bulk-forming laxatives also may be used to increase the mass and water content of the stool. An episode of diverticulitis is managed by resting the bowel. Mild cases of diverticulitis can be managed successfully in the home environment. The patient is instructed to rest and limit oral intake to clear liquids. Hospitalization may be required in acute situations. The patient is given nothing by mouth and placed on a regimen of intravenous fluids, antibiotics, analgesics, and anticholinergics (propantheline bromide [Pro-Banthine]) to reduce bowel spasm. Nasogastric intubation also may be used if vomiting or distention is severe. An oral diet gradually is resumed as the acute inflammation subsides. The patient usually is prescribed bulk-forming laxatives and stool softeners to ensure that the fecal mass passes easily through the inflamed area. These interventions also reduce the bacterial load of the colon by increasing the movement of intestinal contents.

Acute diverticulitis usually subsides with conservative medical management. About 25% of cases, however, may need surgical intervention to deal with complications. Surgical resection of the involved portion of the bowel with an end-to-end anastomosis is performed if possible. In complex cases it may be necessary to construct a temporary colostomy to divert the fecal flow from the diseased portion of bowel. Reanastomosis at a future point usually is possible.

### Nursing Management

The management of patients with symptomless diverticula focuses on prevention. The nurse encourages the patient to maintain a liberal fluid intake of 2500 to 3000 ml/day and to ingest a diet that contains soft foods high in fiber, such as peas and prunes. Fruits, vegetables, and whole grains are added as tolerated. The person is advised to avoid eating items such as nuts and seeds, which can become trapped in the diverticula and trigger inflammation. Small amounts of bran may be added to regular foods, or bulk-forming agents may be used daily to increase stool mass and softness, increase the diameter of the colon, and reduce intraluminal pressure associated with straining at hard stool. Diet suggestions for the patient with diverticular disease are summarized in Box 47-2. High-fiber foods are not to be used when symptoms of inflammation are present because they can be highly irritating to the mucosa. The patient also is encouraged to avoid activities that increase intraabdominal pressure. Weight loss may be recommended in the attempt to lower the baseline levels of intraabdominal pressure.

Nursing care during an acute episode is largely supportive and focused on patient comfort. The nurse teaches the patient the rationale for bed rest and bowel rest and the role these interventions play in bowel healing. The nurse monitors fluid and electrolyte balance and the status of the patient's pain. The abdomen is regularly assessed for signs of complications.

**BOX 47-2 Diet Suggestions for the Person With Diverticular Disease**

**FOODS TO INCLUDE**

Foods high in fiber with emphasis on cellulose and hemicellulose types:

| | |
|---|---|
| Wheat bran | Lettuce |
| Whole grain breads and cereals | Peaches |
| | Prunes |
| Peas | Seedless grapes |
| Carrots | |

**FOODS TO AVOID**

Foods high in indigestible fibers or containing nuts and seeds:

| | |
|---|---|
| Cucumbers | Strawberries |
| Celery | Raspberries |
| Tomatoes | Figs |
| Corn/popcorn | Nuts and seeds (sesame, caraway) |

## PARASITIC INFECTIONS

Parasites can easily enter the GI tract and cause infections. The usual mode of infection is through the oral-fecal route, often from contaminated food or water. The resulting infections may be mild or produce serious gastroenteritis. Parasitic infections often are endemic in developing countries, and they may be acquired during international travel. A few of the more common infections are briefly described here.

### Amebiasis

#### Etiology/Epidemiology

Amebae are protozoa that move by ameboid action. Only a few infect human beings, the most significant being *Entamoeba histolytica*, which causes amebic dysentery. **Amebiasis**, which primarily affects the large intestine, can be found worldwide. It is estimated that as much as 10% of the world's population is infected. Although it is a problem primarily in tropical countries, where infection rates can run as high as 30%, the disease can occur anywhere that sanitation is poor. The parasite is transmitted by direct contact from person to person, by insects, and through contaminated water, milk, and other foods. Sexual transmission accounts for a high incidence rate of amebiasis among homosexual men in some urban communities.

#### Pathophysiology

The active, motile form of the protozoa, the trophozoite, is not infectious. If it is ingested, it can be easily destroyed by the digestive enzymes. The inactive form (cyst) of the protozoa, however, is highly resistant to extremes in temperature, most chemicals, and the digestive juices. When the cyst is swallowed in contaminated food or water, it easily passes into the intestines, where the active trophozoite is released and enters the intestinal wall. It feeds on the mucosal cells, causing ulceration of the intestinal mucosa.

The cyst can survive for long periods outside the body. Most infected persons are symptom-free. Symptoms usually begin from 1 week to several months after infection and depend on the extent of tissue invasion. Mild disease is accompanied by abdominal cramping, intermittent diarrhea, and flatulence. Severe infections cause copious diarrhea that may contain blood and mucus, colicky abdominal pain, rectal spasms (tenesmus), and fever.

Two significant aspects of amebiasis are its chronicity and ability to trigger liver abscesses. Attacks of dysentery may occur at intervals of several months. Constipation is a common complaint during the interim period. Migration of the parasite to the liver via the portal vein makes liver abscess the most common complication. Abscesses gradually increase in size and number, progressively damaging liver function.

#### Medical management

The definitive diagnosis of amebiasis is made by identification of trophozoites or cysts in a fresh stool specimen. Fecal material for analysis also may be obtained by means of proctoscopy, colonoscopy, or biopsy. In addition, serologic ELISA tests can be used to detect the parasite.

The goals of treatment are to provide symptomatic relief, eradicate the parasite, and prevent spread of the amebae. Optimal treatment has not been determined, and most patients require serial treatment with more than one drug. Amebicides may be effective against the parasite within the intestinal lumen (luminal amebicide) or only on the trophozoites within the intestinal wall. The drug of choice for mild or moderate amebiasis is metronidazole (Flagyl). The usual dosage is 750 mg orally three times daily for 5 to 10 days. Drinking alcohol while taking metronidazole may make the patient very ill. The drug also interacts with disulfiram (Antabuse) and with oral anticoagulants. For severe infection, additional luminal amebecides must be given and may include diiodohydroxyquin (iodoquinol), paromomycin (Humatin), chloroquine (Aralen), dehydroemetine (emetine), or tetracycline.

During acute exacerbations the person may require hospitalization because of dehydration, exhaustion, or severe anemia. Fluid and electrolyte replacement and blood transfusions may be necessary. Opiates may be required to reduce bowel motility. A bland, low-residue, high-protein diet is commonly prescribed after the acute period has subsided.

#### Nursing management

Nursing management is primarily directed at monitoring the patient during the acute phase, promoting comfort, and preventing transmission of the parasite. If the diarrhea is severe, the patient is placed on bed rest and given intravenously administered fluids. The nurse records strict intake and output by all routes and monitors for signs of fluid and electrolyte imbalances. Oral fluids are encouraged. Gentle cleansing of the anal area after each episode of diarrhea helps prevent skin breakdown. Sitz baths may be comforting. Scrupulous enteric precautions need to be followed during care (see p. 1526 for discussion of the management of diarrhea).

Teaching is another emphasis of care. The nurse instructs the patient to take the medication after meals to limit side effects and to avoid alcohol during the course of the treatment. The ingestion of alcohol during the course of metronidazole may cause an acute reaction, including severe headache, nausea, and vomiting. The nurse reinforces the importance of completing the full course of treatment and returning for repeat stool examinations as needed to verify the effectiveness of treatment. Persons who travel to countries where the incidence of amebiasis is high should be encouraged to avoid eating fresh uncooked foods or drinking local milk and unbottled water. Boiling water for 10 minutes is required to kill both cysts and trophozoites. Freezing does not destroy the cysts.

### Giardiasis

#### Etiology/Epidemiology

**Giardiasis** is a protozoan infection of the small intestine caused by the flagellate *Giardia lamblia.* Giardiasis is a common cause of traveler's diarrhea and occurs worldwide in both developing and industrialized countries. It is transmitted by person-to-person contact and through drinking contaminated water.

#### Pathophysiology

The *Giardia* parasite is waterborne and can exist in both trophozoite and cyst form. Transmission usually occurs in the highly resistant cyst form. It affects *only* the intestinal system. The typical clinical manifestations include persistent watery diarrhea accompanied by abdominal cramping and weight loss. In mild cases the disease may be symptomless or cause a constant bloated feeling with abdominal discomfort. Malabsorption of fats and vitamins may occur in severe cases. The disease usually is self-limiting within 2 to 6 weeks but can, in severe cases, recur persistently until effective treatment is instituted.

#### Medical management

Giardiasis can be diagnosed by identifying the parasite in samples of fresh stool. A mucosal biopsy specimen also shows the trophozoites. The treatment of choice is a full course of quinacrine (Atabrine) or metronidazole (Flagyl). The stool is reexamined 2 weeks after the start of treatment to evaluate the effectiveness of the drug therapy.

#### Nursing management

Teaching focuses on prevention strategies for traveling. Bottled water is recommended, and raw fruits and vegetables should be avoided in areas where giardiasis is endemic. Scrupulous personal hygiene, particularly frequent handwashing, is a standard recommendation. The organism can be found in canine stools, and special care should be taken if a person comes into direct contact with stool from household pets or strays.

## Trichinosis

### Etiology/Epidemiology

**Trichinosis** (trichinellosis, trichiniasis) is caused by the larvae of a species of roundworm, *Trichinella spiralis,* which lives in the intestines of human beings, pigs, and rats. The larvae become encysted in the striated muscles and usually are transmitted by ingestion of undercooked pork or pork products. Trichinosis has a worldwide distribution with the highest incidence occurring in Europe and the United States. It occurs more often in hogs that have been fed garbage than in those fed grain. The larvae become encysted only in humans and therefore are not visible to the naked eye and cannot be seen by food inspectors.

### Pathophysiology

When infected food is eaten, the larvae mature within the intestine of the host. They mate and produce eggs that hatch in the uterus of the female worm. Larvae are then discharged in huge numbers (approximately 1500 per worm) into the lymphatic and lacteal vessels of the host's small intestine, usually over a 6-week period. They pass into the muscles of the host, where they become encysted by the reaction of the host's body and may remain for many years.

Persons with trichinosis may be symptom-free, but the clinical manifestations typically include GI symptoms in the early phase. Nausea, anorexia, abdominal cramping, and diarrhea are common. Muscle pain, especially with movement, develops in weeks 2 to 8 and often is accompanied by fever, weakness, and periorbital edema.

The more commonly involved muscles are in the back, eyes, jaw, throat, and diaphragm. Chewing and breathing may be painful. The infection may spread to the meninges, cardiac muscle, lungs, and kidneys in severe cases. Recovery usually begins during the second month, but it may be prolonged after severe illness. Vague muscle pains and malaise may persist for many months.

### Medical management

The diagnosis of trichinosis is confirmed by the finding of larvae in a biopsy specimen taken from the deltoid or gastrocnemius muscle in the fourth week of infection. Treatment focuses primarily on symptomatic relief. The person is instructed to rest and eat a high-calorie, high-protein diet. Analgesics are given as needed for muscle pain, and antiinflammatory steroids such as prednisone or dexamethasone may be prescribed to relieve fever, edema, and muscle pain. Mebendazole (Vermox) or thiabendazole (Mintezol) is administered during both the intestinal and muscular phases of the disease.

### Nursing management

The most essential aspect of intervention for trichinosis is education for prevention. Trichinae can be killed by cooking meat at the recommended temperature of 77° C (170° F) or by freezing meat at −15° C (5° F) for 20 days. The trichinae are not killed by smoking, pickling, or other methods of processing and may not be completely destroyed by microwave cooking. Sausage and other infected pork products carelessly prepared are a common source of infection in human beings. The nurse also reinforces the importance of scrupulous hygiene and frequent handwashing during food preparation.

# Inflammatory Bowel Disease

## IRRITABLE BOWEL SYNDROME

### Etiology/Epidemiology

The term **irritable bowel syndrome,** also known as spastic colon or mucous colitis, refers to symptoms of abdominal pain and altered bowel habits, usually diarrhea, in the absence of demonstrable organic disease. Irritable bowel syndrome is the diagnosis in as much as 30% to 50% of patients cared for in gastroenterology practice.[3] It is the most frequent GI condition encountered by physicians, and it is estimated that many thousands of other persons self-manage mild forms of the disorder without medical assistance. At least half of those with the diagnosed problem have an onset of symptoms before 35 years of age, and many can trace their problems to adolescence. A North Carolina study identified the symptom pattern in 10% to 15% of college students.[3] Two thirds of those seeking medical help are women although in other cultures the incidence is higher in men. Willingness to seek medical help is a primary consideration in many mild cases and may clearly skew the incidence statistics. The etiology remains largely unknown.

### Pathophysiology

Multiple minor pathophysiologic abnormalities in bowel motility occur in patients with irritable bowel syndrome. It is estimated that up to 85% of patients exhibit some of these changes, but the relative importance of any of the individual factors remains unknown. Motility in the proximal small bowel is increased, as well as the frequency and amplitude of muscular contractions in the colon. There are no demonstrable changes in the bowel mucosa, and inflammation is not present. The disorder creates multiple life-style problems for the patient but does not appear to create any serious health problems.

The symptoms of irritable bowel syndrome occur intermittently and vary among persons, although each person has a characteristic pattern. There appear to be two major symptom patterns: (1) spastic colon type, characterized by (a) colicky abdominal pain relieved by passing gas or stool and (b) periodic constipation and diarrhea, and (2) painless diarrhea type, characterized by urgent diarrhea during or after meals. The stool of either type may contain excess mucus, but all other physical findings are normal. The symptoms may be precipitated by stress, anxiety, or dietary factors.

## Medical Management

Spasticity of the colon can be visualized on radiographs and endoscopy, and it often is worsened by the stimulus of the diagnostic examinations themselves. Changes in myoelectric activity in the bowel can be elicited after eating, and exaggerated sigmoid contractions can be traced in response to meals, especially fatty foods. The irritable bowel syndrome diagnosis is made by the physician after ruling out other pathologic conditions, and the person needs to know that the condition is benign and is related to bowel irritability. Treatment involves life-style modifications and symptomatic care.

## Nursing Management

Most persons learn to control the symptoms of irritable bowel syndrome by modifying their diet and life-style. Symptoms usually are worsened by the ingestion of rich, fatty foods. The nurse provides instruction about the elements of a low-fat diet and encourages the patient to limit the quantity of gas-producing foods and carbonated beverages. The person is encouraged to eat a well-balanced diet and to follow a regular schedule for meals. Some patients respond well to the use of a high-fiber diet, but no direct benefits have been found from adding bran to the diet. Alcohol, smoking, and other gastric stimulants should be reduced or eliminated from the daily routine.

Bulk-forming laxatives such as psyllium (Metamucil) may be helpful in adding soft bulk to the stools. Heat may be applied to the abdomen for comfort, but analgesics are not commonly used. Narcotics have been shown to induce a hyperactive response in the sigmoid, worsening the pain. Antidiarrheal agents such as loperamide (Imodium) and diphenoxylate hydrochloride with atropine (Lomotil) may be used to control diarrhea during exacerbations (see Table 47-2). Because these drugs have a narcotic base, they are not prescribed for long-term use.

Persons with irritable bowel syndrome need support in coping with life stress. Health-promoting routines such as regular physical exercise and relaxation sessions are recommended. Support groups or counseling may be encouraged in certain situations. Efforts at problem solving may be successful in lessening the frequency or severity of irritable bowel syndrome symptoms.

# CROHN'S DISEASE/ULCERATIVE COLITIS

## Etiology

**Crohn's disease** and **ulcerative colitis,** the two classic forms of inflammatory bowel disease (IBD), are two distinctly different disease processes that share many overlapping features. Their hallmark characteristic is bowel inflammation. Despite extensive research, the etiology of IBD remains unknown. A clear familial link has been demonstrated through sibling and twin studies, but no genetic markers have been isolated. In first-degree relatives, Crohn's disease occurs from 12 to 30 times the expected rate, and the genetic link is unquestioned.[10] A clear familial link also can be seen in ulcerative colitis, but the incidence rates in relatives are much lower.

Environmental factors have been extensively explored. No clear answers have emerged. The erratic incidence patterns that occur worldwide appear to point clearly to specific environmental influences, but what these factors are remains elusive. The effect of smoking is a typical example. Smoking appears to have some kind of masking effect on the development of ulcerative colitis. Former smokers show a higher incidence of the disease than do nonsmokers. The opposite appears to be true with Crohn's disease. Smokers have a two- to four-times greater risk of developing the disease, and the effect is not dose-dependent.[30] An apparent increased incidence of Crohn's disease in women who use birth control pills is under investigation.

A similar frustrating pattern of inconclusive trends is seen in research regarding a possible infectious origin, either bacterial or viral. Persons with ulcerative colitis frequently have a high antibody titer to strains of *E. coli* that are not pathologic in nonaffected persons. The usefulness of this finding is not clear at present, and no definitive research support exists at this time for a transmissible cause of any form of IBD. The same types of patterns occur in dietary research as well. Altered immune status may play a role, but exactly how is not known. Stress and emotional factors once were believed to play an important etiologic role in IBD, but research has shown *no* indications of support for a psychogenic cause. The diseases are clearly multifactorial in origin, and the interplay of environmental factors is believed to occur at an early age for genetically susceptible persons.[30]

## Epidemiology

Inflammatory bowel disease occurs worldwide with an annual incidence rate of approximately 3 to 20 new cases per 100,000 population.[30] The incidence is significantly higher in the United States, northern Europe, and the United Kingdom, and approximately 1 million Americans deal with the problem on a daily basis.[16] The worldwide ratio of ulcerative colitis to Crohn's disease varies widely, but ulcerative colitis usually is more prevalent. Although the incidence statistics for ulcerative colitis have remained fairly stable in recent years, Crohn's disease has shown a distinct increase in incidence.[30] IBD, which is prevalent in white persons, is rare in African-Americans and Native Americans. No gender pattern is evident in racially mixed groups, but white women appear to be at particular risk. A link with the use of birth control pills in this population is under investigation.[30] One of the most unusual aspects of the incidence statistics is a higher incidence among American and Eu-

**TABLE 47-3 Comparison of Ulcerative Colitis and Crohn's Disease**

| ULCERATIVE COLITIS | CROHN'S DISEASE |
|---|---|
| **USUAL AREA AFFECTED** | |
| Left colon, rectum | Distal ileum, right colon<br>Can occur anywhere in GI tract |
| **EXTENT OF INVOLVEMENT** | |
| Diffuse areas, contiguous | Segmental areas, noncontiguous |
| **INFLAMMATION** | |
| Mostly mucosal | Transmural |
| **MUCOSAL APPEARANCE** | |
| Shallow mucosal ulcerations, edematous, superficial bleeding | Cobblestone effect, granulomas<br>Thickened walls, narrowed lumen |
| **COMPLICATIONS** | |
| Loss of absorption and elasticity<br>Replacement of mucosa by scar tissue<br>Development of pseudopolyps that may become malignant<br>Toxic megacolon<br>Hemorrhoids<br>Hemorrhage | Fistulas<br>Perianal disease<br>Strictures<br>Abscesses<br>Perforation<br>Anemia<br>Malabsorption of fat and fat-soluble vitamins |

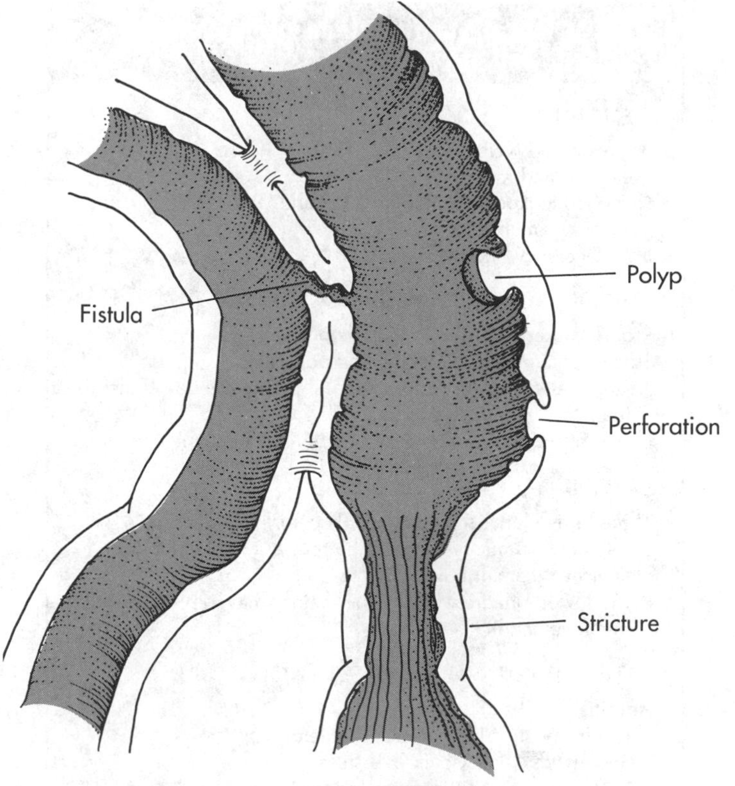


**FIGURE 47-4** Common complications of inflammatory bowel disease.

ropean Jews. This higher incidence does not occur among native-born Israelis and appears to point to some as yet unidentified genetic and environmental interaction. Although IBD can occur at any age, its peak period of onset is in young adulthood between the ages of 15 and 25 years. There is another smaller peak between 55 and 60 years in some countries.

## Pathophysiology

Although inflammation is the hallmark of both Crohn's disease *and* ulcerative colitis, the two disorders are markedly different in their effect on the intestinal tract. The diseases are distinguished largely by the nature of the inflammation, the location in the GI tract, the pattern of distribution, and the degree of mucosal penetration. See Table 47-3 for comparison of the major pathophysiologic features of each disease process.

Ulcerative colitis creates a diffuse continuous process of inflammation characterized by edema and shallow mucosal ulceration. It primarily affects the distal colorectal area, and if the disease is confined to this region, it usually is milder and responsive to topical therapy. More extensive disease is termed *left-sided* and involves the colon up to the splenic flexure. In severe disease the inflammatory process extends all the way to the hepatic flexure or ileocecal junction. The mucosa develops many superficial bleeding points and becomes increasingly thickened and edematous. The bleeding points gradually enlarge and become ulcerated. The continuous healing process and the formation of scar tissue that accompany it may cause the colon to lose its normal elasticity and absorptive capability. Normal mucosa gradually is replaced by scar tissue, and the colon becomes thickened, rigid, and pipelike. The mucosa also may undergo structural changes over time, forming pseudopolyps that can become malignant.

Crohn's disease can occur anywhere in the GI tract, but it is found most often in the proximal colon and ileocecal junction, making it a right-sided disease. The inflammation of Crohn's disease is transmural, affecting all layers of the intestinal wall. It follows a "skip" or "cobblestone" pattern in which affected areas are separated by normal tissue. Mucosal granulomas, luminal narrowing, thickening of the intestinal wall, mucosal nodularity, and ulceration are characteristic features. The lesions may perforate and form fistulas that connect with the colon, bladder, or vagina. Scar tissue may form as the lesions heal, preventing the normal absorption of nutrients, and strictures may form, causing intestinal obstruction. Mesenteric lymph nodes are enlarged and firm. Figure 47-4 illustrates several of the common complications of IBD.

IBD is characterized by a pattern of exacerbation and

**BOX 47-3 Clinical Manifestations of Inflammatory Bowel Disease**

**GENERAL**

Anorexia and weight loss
Weakness and malaise
Fever and leukocytosis (a high fever and WBC > 15,000/$mm^3$ suggests an abscess)
Iron deficiency anemia

**SPECIFIC TO ULCERATIVE COLITIS**

Profuse watery diarrhea (15-20 stools per day)
Stools contain blood, mucus, and possibly pus
Abdominal cramping can be present before the bowel movement
Losses of sodium, potassium, bicarbonate, and calcium

**SPECIFIC TO CROHN'S DISEASE**

Three to five large semisolid stools per day
Stool contains mucus and possibly pus but rarely blood
Steatorrhea if small bowel affected
Right lower quadrant cramping pain—may be severe and mimic appendicitis

**EXTRAINTESTINAL MANIFESTATIONS**

Arthritis (4%-23%)
- Involvement of large joints, nondeforming
- Spondylitis—back pain and stiffness
- Hypertrophic clubbing and periostitis

Ocular (4%-10%)
- Uveitis, episcleritis
- Serous retinopathy

**SKIN**

Erythema nodosum: raised red tender nodules on anterior tibial surfaces
Pyoderma gangrenosum: painful necrotizing ulcerations most common on legs
Stomatitis (6%-20%): aphthous ulcers often precede an exacerbation; linear ulcerations and fissures

**HEPATOBILIARY DISEASE**

Cholelithiasis
Fatty liver, cirrhosis
Cholangitis

**RENAL (4%-23%)**

Kidney stones
Ureteral obstruction
Vesical fistulas

remission. Although there is a great deal of potential overlap in the symptoms, ulcerative colitis and Crohn's disease have different characteristic features. Diarrhea is a classic symptom of ulcerative colitis. The diarrhea usually is profuse, as much as 15 to 20 liquid stools a day, and contains blood, mucus, and pus. Abdominal cramps sometimes occur before the bowel movement. As the scarring within the bowel progresses, the feeling of the urge to defecate is lost, leading to involuntary leakage of stool. With severe diarrhea there may be losses of sodium, potassium, bicarbonate, and calcium.

Diarrhea also is a feature of Crohn's disease, but it is more likely to consist of three to five large semisolid stools daily that contain mucus and pus but no blood. Steatorrhea may be present if the ulceration extends high in the small intestine. The abdominal colicky pain is relieved with a bowel movement. Fat-soluble vitamins—that is, A, D, E, and K—may be poorly absorbed with marked steatorrhea.

Right lower quadrant *abdominal pain* also is characteristic of Crohn's disease and may be accompanied in the same area by a tender mass of thickened intestines. During an acute episode the symptoms may closely resemble those of appendicitis.

In addition to these classic symptoms IBD frequently causes anorexia, weakness, and malaise from the chronic inflammation. Weight loss is common and may become a problem if the absorption capability of the bowel is significantly impaired. Intermittent fever and leukocytosis frequently accompany an exacerbation, and iron deficiency anemia may develop from both chronic mucosal bleeding and poor iron absorption. The clinical manifestations of IBD are summarized in Box 47-3.

### Extraintestinal symptoms of inflammatory bowel disease

Extraintestinal and systemic manifestations occur commonly in patients with IBD and often complicate their disease management. Involvement of virtually every organ system is possible. Although it generally is accepted that extraintestinal symptoms are systemic disorders, their etiology is not understood. They appear to reflect some type of generalized tissue vulnerability and usually are considered to be immunologic phenomena.[22] They may precede or accompany the underlying bowel disorder. A patient with one extraintestinal manifestation has an increased risk of developing others.

Arthritis is the most common manifestation and occurs in 4% to 23% of patients with IBD. A wide range of ocular problems may occur, for example, uveitis, corneal ulceration, and retinopathy. The incidence is about 4% to 10%. Skin lesions also are common. A grouping of small bowel–related problems appears to be associated with Crohn's disease. Cholelithiasis, for example, has an incidence of 13% to 34% in Crohn's disease versus 10% to 15% in the general population.[22] Extraintestinal manifestations are summarized in Box 47-3. Table 47-4 compares normal function and the pathophysiology of IBD.

## Prevention

There is no *primary prevention* for IBD because causative factors remain largely unknown. No known dietary or life-style factors can prevent its development. Environmental factors are believed to be extremely important, but research findings at present do not support any particular recommendations or factors.

*Secondary prevention* takes the form of early diagnosis. Either Crohn's disease or ulcerative colitis initially may be mistaken for irritable bowel syndrome, espe-

**TABLE 47-4 Normal Function, Pathophysiology, and Clinical Presentation of Chronic Inflammatory Bowel Disease**

| NORMAL FUNCTION | PATHOPHYSIOLOGY | CLINICAL PRESENTATION |
|---|---|---|
| Chyme is liquid on entering colon; water is absorbed in colon; blood is not normally present | UC: Hemorrhagic ulcerations in lower colon walls interfere with reabsorption of water from the chyme; stool remains liquid | UC: frequent liquid stools; bloody with severe disease |
| | CD: Lesions are in ileum or ascending colon; some water is reabsorbed in the nonaffected colon; no bleeding | CD: 3-5 or more semisoft stools per day |
| Nutrients are absorbed in the small intestines | UC: Loss of fluid and blood by diarrhea | UC: anorexia, weight loss, anemia |
| | CD: Inflamed and scarred walls interfere with absorption of nutrients; fat is excreted in the stools | CD: same as for UC; steatorrhea |
| Chyme flows freely through intestinal lumen | CD: Edema and inflammation of intestinal wall cause narrowing of intestinal lumen leading to partial obstruction | UC: occasional mild abdominal discomfort<br>CD: Cramping abdominal pain; may be severe |

*UC,* Ulcerative colitis; *CD,* Crohn's disease.

cially in early stages or with mild disease. The person may put off seeking help and attempt self-management of symptoms at home, which could result in unnecessary delay in initiating efforts to establish a full remission. All persons with IBD symptoms should be encouraged to seek a work-up by a skilled physician to establish an accurate diagnosis and treatment plan.

## Medical Management

The goal for discharge of patients with IBD as determined by DRGs is 7 days. The nurse works collaboratively with the physician for implementation of prescribed medical therapy. Because the nurse has a major role in discharge planning and patient teaching, these are discussed under nursing management.

### Diagnostic tests

The diagnosis of IBD begins with a careful history that includes the symptom pattern and its severity and duration. A stool examination for leukocytes, parasites, blood, and culture also is performed to rule out an infectious origin for the symptoms. Laboratory tests may include CBC, erythrocyte sedimentation rate (ESR), and serum albumin value.

A barium enema usually is ordered to evaluate the physical changes in the bowel; it provides accurate data about the structure of the colon, can be performed rapidly, and provides a permanent record for future disease comparison. An upper GI series also may be prescribed to evaluate small bowel involvement if Crohn's disease is suspected. Endoscopy procedures such as sigmoidoscopy or colonoscopy also may be ordered to evaluate any premalignant lesions, to establish the spread of the disease, and to complete a differential diagnosis in cases of unclear diagnosis. Colonoscopy is not routinely included in the work-up for IBD because of the need for both vigorous bowel preparation and sedation.[29]

### Medication

Medications are used in the treatment of IBD in an effort to relieve symptoms, induce remission, postpone the need for surgery, and improve the quality of life.[9] Inasmuch as the cause of IBD remains basically unknown, the components of drug therapy are empirically based on a combination of clinical trials and practical experience.

*Sulfasalazine* (Azulfidine) was developed in the 1930s specifically for use in treating arthritis. Arthritis was then believed to have an infectious origin, and sulfasalazine combined the proved effectiveness of aspirin with a sulfonamide antibiotic.[23] Its application was quickly broadened to include IBD, and it has been a mainstay of treatment ever since. It remains the foundation of treatment for mild and moderate forms of ulcerative colitis and plays a role in symptom management of Crohn's disease. The exact mechanism of action of sulfasalazine is unknown, but it combines bacterial suppression with the antiinflammatory effects of aspirin. It successfully induces and sustains remission in most patients. Sulfasalazine is split by bacteria in the colon into its two components. 5-ASA is poorly absorbed and thus maintains prolonged contact with the inflamed mucosa. Sulfapyridine, its second component, has no proved effectiveness against the disease. Therefore efforts have focused on developing 5-ASA products that can be delivered intact to the colon. Two drugs of this type are being tested—olsalazine (Dipentum) and resin-coated mesalamine (Asacol). These drugs are well tolerated if started in graduating doses and taken buffered with food. Toxicity appears minimal.[23] The most common side effects are GI and include nausea, vomiting, and diarrhea. Photosensitivity may develop.

Sulfasalazine-derivative drugs also can be used topically for the 25% or more of patients with ulcerative colitis whose disease is confined to the rectal and sigmoid area. These drugs can be administered by enema, which provides for homogeneous delivery to the inflamed lower colon. Enemas provide high local concentrations of the drug, with minimal systemic absorption, and have been shown to be more effective than steroids

**TABLE 47-5 Drug Therapy for Inflammatory Bowel Disease**

| DRUG | TYPICAL DOSAGE | COMMON SIDE EFFECTS | PATIENT TEACHING |
|---|---|---|---|
| **SULFONAMIDE/ASPIRIN** | | | |
| Sulfasalazine (Azulfidine) | 2-4 g/day PO | Anorexia, nausea and vomiting, headache | Question for allergy to sulfonamides or aspirin.<br>Take in divided doses.<br>Take with full glass of fluid or with food.<br>Maintain a liberal fluid intake (2500-3000 ml daily).<br>Report incidence of skin rash or other adverse effects.<br>Photosensitivity may occur. |
| Olsalazine (Dipentum) | 250 mg/day PO initially—increased gradually to 1-3 g/day | As above; also may cause mild to moderate diarrhea | Take in divided doses.<br>Take with full glass of fluid or with food.<br>Maintain a liberal fluid intake (2500-3000 ml daily).<br>Monitor presence and severity of diarrhea. |
| Mesalamine (Asacol)<br>Mesalamine in suspension for retention enema<br>Mesalamine suppository | 800-4800 mg/day PO<br>4 g/day (60 ml)<br>500-mg suppository bid | Generally well tolerated; occasional abdominal discomfort | Take in divided doses.<br>Maintain a liberal fluid intake (2500-3000 ml daily).<br>Swallow tablets whole; do not chew or break outer coating.<br>Administer enema while positioned on left side—retain as long as possible. |
| **CORTICOSTEROIDS** | | | |
| Hydrocortisone<br>Intrarectal foam (Cortifoam)<br>Retention enema (Cortenema)<br>Intravenous (Solu-Cortef) | <br>90 mg daily or bid<br>100 mg/day (60 ml)<br>100-500 mg at intervals | Adrenal suppression (osteoporosis, infection, mood disorders, fluid retention, etc.) | Give with food or fluid.<br>Monitor weight gain; assess for edema.<br>Have blood pressure checked regularly.<br>Be alert to signs of infection and report promptly.<br>Be aware that mood swings occur commonly.<br>Do not change dose or schedule or abruptly discontinue drug.<br>Maintain good personal hygiene; keep perianal area clean and dry. |
| Adrenocorticotropic hormone (ACTH) | 120 U/day IV by infusion | Adverse effects are related to increased secretion of glucocorticoids as above | As above. |
| Prednisone | 40-60 mg/day PO | As above | As above. |
| **IMMUNOSUPPRESSIVES** | | | |
| Mercaptopurine (Purinethol) | 50-100 mg/day up to 2 mg/kg/day PO | Bone marrow suppression, rashes, occasional nausea and vomiting, hepatotoxicity | Report any signs of infection.<br>Be alert to easy bruising.<br>Return for laboratory work as scheduled.<br>Maintain liberal daily fluid intake (2500-3000 ml daily). |
| Azathioprine (Imuran) | 50-100 mg/day up to 2 mg/kg/day PO | Same as above | Give with food or after meals.<br>As above. |
| Cyclosporine (Sandimmune) | Effective dosage not established | Renal dysfunction, hypertension, hirsutism, paresthesias, tremor | Oral solution may be mixed in glass and given with milk or orange juice at room temperature—avoid refrigeration.<br>Monitor blood pressure.<br>Report hematuria or any change in urinary function. |

in many situations.[26] Suppository forms of the drugs also have been developed in the attempt to increase patient acceptability. Patients frequently find daily enemas to be unacceptable for long-term therapy. Drug therapy for IBD is summarized in Table 47-5.

*Corticosteroids* also have played an important role in IBD management for many years. The potent antiinflammatory effects of steroids have proved effective in inducing remission. Although both local and systemic steroids are used, their widespread and severe side effects limit their long-term use. Steroids can be administered rectally, but most forms absorb readily from the rectal mucosa and produce systemic effects. Newer, less absorbable steroids such as budesonide and beclomethasone dipropionate (BDP) are being extensively researched.[9] Corticosteroids have a major role in the management of Crohn's disease, which is less responsive to sulfasalazine derivatives unless the disease is confined to the colon, but they have not been shown to maintain remission.

Other potent antiinflammatory *immunosuppressive* agents also are being studied for use in the treatment of IBD. Study results are mixed, and controversy continues over both their safety and effectiveness. These agents typically are associated with fairly severe side effects. However, because IBD is presumed to involve a disorder in immune regulation, this category of drugs will continue to be researched. Azathioprine (Imuran), mercaptopurine (Purinethol), and cyclosporine (Sandimmune) are being studied.

*Antibiotics,* although not a primary treatment, may play an important role in the management of both ulcerative colitis and Crohn's disease. Some studies have shown metronidazole (Flagyl) to be as effective as sulfasalazine in the management of disease confined to the colon.[9] Antibiotics also are appropriate for severely ill patients at risk for infection and in situations in which bowel stricture causes stasis and bacterial overgrowth in the bowel.

Drug therapy for IBD also may include the use of antidiarrheal medications when disease activity is high (see Table 47-2). These drugs are administered for symptomatic relief, and an accurate record needs to be maintained of their administration and effectiveness in controlling symptoms. Vitamin supplements frequently are necessary, particularly when anorexia and nausea are present. Replacement of vitamin $B_{12}$ is provided when large amounts of the ileum are lost and absorption is compromised. When severe anemia is present, an iron-dextran complex (Imferon) may be administered, inasmuch as oral iron cannot be effectively absorbed from the ulcerated bowel.

### Treatment

No specific treatment comprises IBD management. Patients with primarily rectal involvement may follow a regimen of daily enema administration. Other prescribed treatments may be related to the management of skin breakdown or excoriation that may accompany severe diarrhea.

### Diet

Diet does not cause IBD and cannot influence the course of the disease, but diet is an important consideration in patient comfort. Nutritional concerns also become extremely important during exacerbations of the disease when diarrhea may be severe and the patient is unable to meet nutritional needs through an oral diet.

Diet recommendations are tailored to the needs of the individual patient, but as a general rule patients with diarrhea or abdominal pain are encouraged to restrict their intake of raw fruits and vegetables, as well as fatty and spicy foods. Constipation may be a problem in distal colon or rectal disease and usually is controlled with the use of bulk hydrophilic laxatives such as psyllium (Metamucil). The general guideline for ulcerative colitis is that when patients feel well, they can eat almost anything, but when they feel sick, they should limit what they eat.[9]

Nutrition is considered to be more significant in Crohn's disease, and specific foods may trigger disease flare-ups. Constipation can be a problem when strictures develop in the bowel, and it may not be possible to safely increase bulk in the diet. Bowel rest can play a role in Crohn's disease management, and elemental diets or supplements may be used. These preparations are completely digested and absorbed in the duodenum and ileum and place no demands on the large bowel. Recent attention has been focused on the possible suppressive effect of fish oil on the inflammatory process. Lactose intolerance also is a common problem in persons with IBD, and patients may be encouraged to evaluate the effectiveness of restricting dairy products in their diet.

Acute exacerbations of IBD present a challenge to the maintenance of adequate nutrition. Total parenteral nutrition may be necessary to ensure minimal essential nutrients and prevent complications. This can be particularly important if the patient requires surgery.

### Activity

Activity levels may be restricted during acute exacerbations of IBD in response to fever, fatigue, and malaise. Reduced activity also may be useful in slowing peristalsis and decreasing the frequency of diarrhea episodes. When remission is established, patients are encouraged to resume all aspects of their normal life-styles and no activity restrictions are required.

### Referral/Consultation

In some settings the nurse assumes responsibility for making referrals to other services. Common referrals for persons with inflammatory bowel disease include nutrition support and counseling.

**Nutrition support.** The assessment of nutritional status and determination of the most appropriate approach to improving or maintaining nutrition may involve a skilled nutritionist. Diet modification, supplement selection, and management of total parenteral nutrition may be coordinated through this service.

**Counseling.** Although it has been clearly established that neither stress nor personality is part of the etiology of inflammatory bowel disease, it also is clear that coping with the effects of IBD can put a tremendous strain on a person's adaptive abilities. Times of disease exacerbation may leave the patient particularly vulnerable to depression and even despair. Support services in this area can be extremely important.

Critical pathways (also referred to as *collaborative care paths* or *care maps*) have been developed in some inpatient and outpatient settings to guide both medical and nursing management. These critical pathways are collaboratively developed along time lines and include the information previously described for specific hours, days, or visits. Pertinent information about discharge planning and patient teaching to be implemented at specified times also is included. Because the nurse has a major role in these two aspects of care, these are discussed under nursing management.

## Surgical Management

Surgical intervention may be a valid alternative to medical therapy in certain IBD situations. Newer procedures are offering the opportunity for definitive disease management earlier in the overall disease process. Even in Crohn's disease, in which surgical management is not curative, patients can experience a significantly improved quality of life as a result of surgery.

The primary indications for surgery in IBD include perforation, toxic megacolon, hemorrhage requiring transfusion, high-grade cellular dysplasia or cancer, acute exacerbations that do not respond to aggressive therapy within 10 to 14 days, and failure of medical therapy for long-term control. In addition, the development of bowel obstruction, fistula, abscess, or serious infection in Crohn's disease may necessitate surgery.

### Surgery for ulcerative colitis

Surgical approaches to ulcerative colitis involve the removal of the entire colon and are therefore curative. Their effectiveness has been well documented over the years, but the profound lifelong challenges of living with an ileostomy have spurred the development of several new approaches in recent years.

**Proctocolectomy with ileostomy.** This is the oldest and best established colectomy procedure; its effectiveness is widely acknowledged. The proctocolectomy involves removal of the colon, rectum, and anus with permanent closure of the anus. The **ileostomy** is created

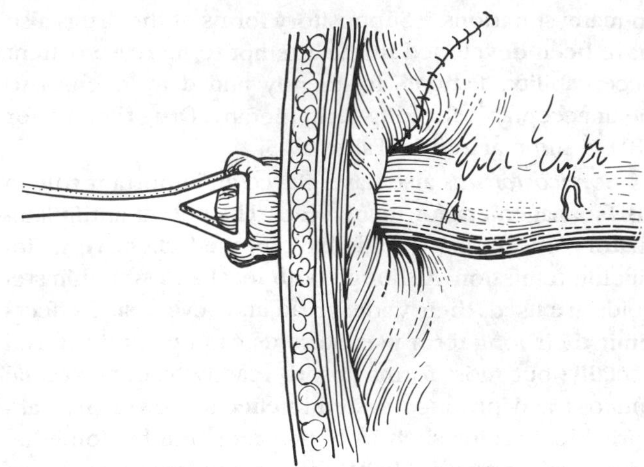

FIGURE 47-5 Construction of an ileostomy.

when the end of the terminal ileum is brought out through the abdominal wall to form a **stoma.** Ileostomy drainage initially is profuse and watery. The stoma drains continuously as long as peristalsis is intact. The volume of stool decreases over time as the terminal ileum dilates and begins to function somewhat like the cecum. The consistency of the drainage eventually is thickened and pastelike.

After ileostomy surgery, the ulcerative colitis is cured and the risk of cancer is virtually eliminated. When patients are in good nutritional status and care is exerted to create a well-placed stoma, healing is prompt and physical problems are fairly mild. The permanent ileostomy (Figure 47-5) can create profound adjustment problems for patients, however, related to fears of leakage, embarrassment from noise and odor, and negative impact on self-concept, body image, and sexuality. Male impotence is a frequently expressed concern but is not a problem if the surgeon dissects carefully past the autonomic nerves in the pelvis.

**Continent ileostomy.** In the late 1960s Dr. Nils Kock developed a surgical procedure to spare patients some of the challenges of traditional ileostomy. The procedure (the Kock pouch) involves the creation of an abdominal reservoir to store the feces by use of a piece of terminal ileum. A portion of the ileum is intussuscepted to form a nipple valve that is flush with the abdomen (Figure 47-6). A catheter is used to empty the pouch, and a small dressing or adhesive bandage is worn over the stoma between emptyings. The pouch eventually can expand to hold about 500 ml.[11] Nipple slippage occurs in up to 15% of situations, which has limited the acceptance and use of the procedure. A laparotomy is required to repair the nipple. The procedure no longer is recommended as a primary intervention.

**Colectomy and ileoanal anastomosis.** This was the first procedure developed to avoid the need for any type of ileostomy. It is a simpler procedure than traditional

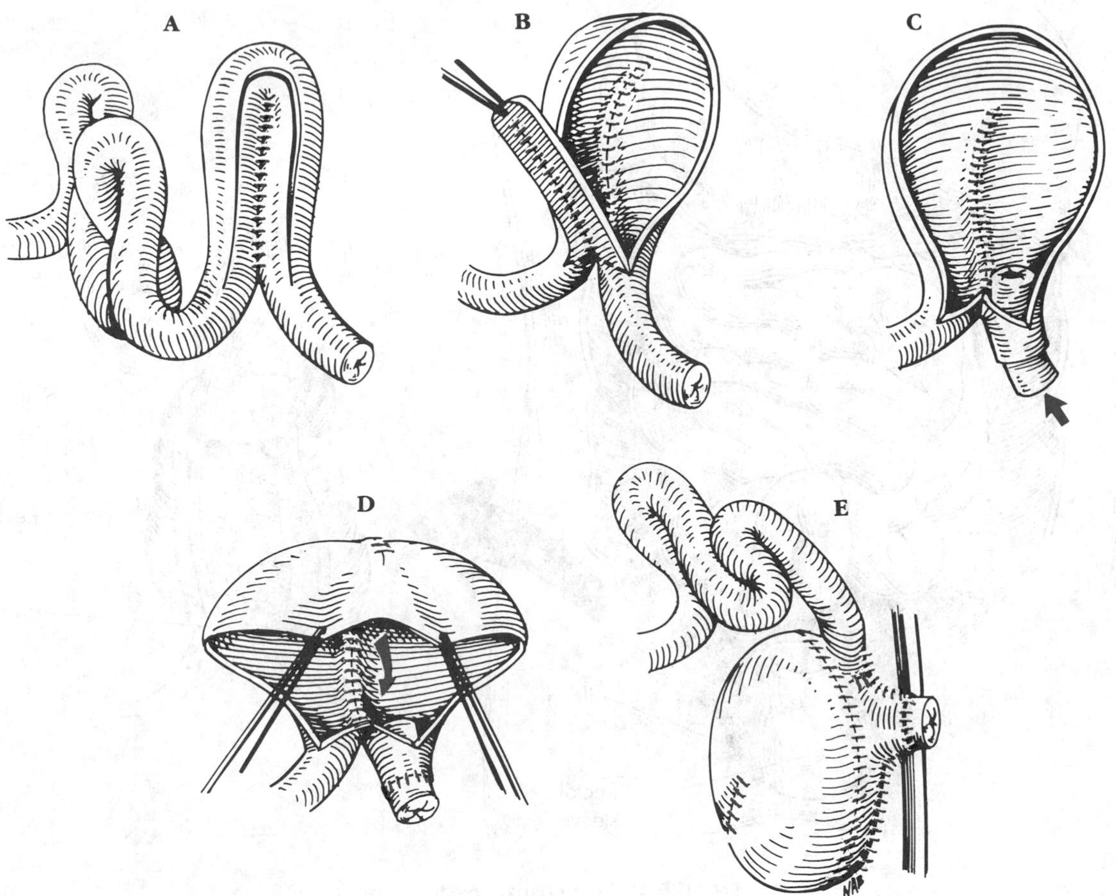


**FIGURE 47-6** Continent ileostomy (Kock pouch). **A,** Loop of bowel sewn together. **B,** Removal of anterior portion. **C,** Nipple valve made by pushing bowel back on itself. **D,** Pouch formation. **E,** End brought through stoma.

ileostomy and results in lower surgical morbidity. It leaves a rectal stump, 12 to 15 cm, after the colon is removed, and the small bowel is placed inside this rectal sleeve for anastomosis (Figure 47-7). The major concern is associated with the remnant of the rectum, which is virtually always affected by the ulcerative colitis disease process and may become a management problem. The risk of rectal cancer also is present although the risk is not as great as was originally theorized.[11] This procedure has had greater acceptance in Europe than in the United States despite success rates in excess of 90%.

**Ileoanal reservoir.** The current procedure of choice for colectomy involves the creation of a pouch from the terminal ileum that is sutured directly to the anus. The anal sphincter is preserved for continence plus approximately 1 inch of rectum that is stripped of its mucosa to remove the last vestige of ulcerative colitis. A temporary loop colostomy is formed until healing of all anastomosis incisions is complete, making this a two-stage surgery. The loop ileostomy usually can be closed within 3 to 4 months. Several different approaches to reservoir construction have been developed. A J-shaped anastomosis is shown in Figure 47-8. W- and S-shaped pouches also are being used. Functional results continue to improve for up to 12 months after surgery, and most patients have three to eight bowel movements per day. Slight fecal incontinence is a problem—sometimes a persistent one, especially at night—but the normal function and relative continence make this a popular procedure. It usually is not used in persons older than 55 years who may experience sphincter deterioration related to aging.

### Surgery for Crohn's disease

The major management challenge of Crohn's disease is the fact that it is stubbornly incurable even in the face of aggressive medical or surgical intervention. Because recurrence of the disease process is virtually inevitable, surgical approaches to Crohn's disease focus on sparing and conserving as much of the bowel as possible, particularly when the small bowel is involved. A wide margin exists, but the loss of more than 100 cm of bowel almost inevitably results in short bowel syndrome and persistent problems with malabsorption.[7] *Segmental resection* with reanastomosis has been the primary sur-

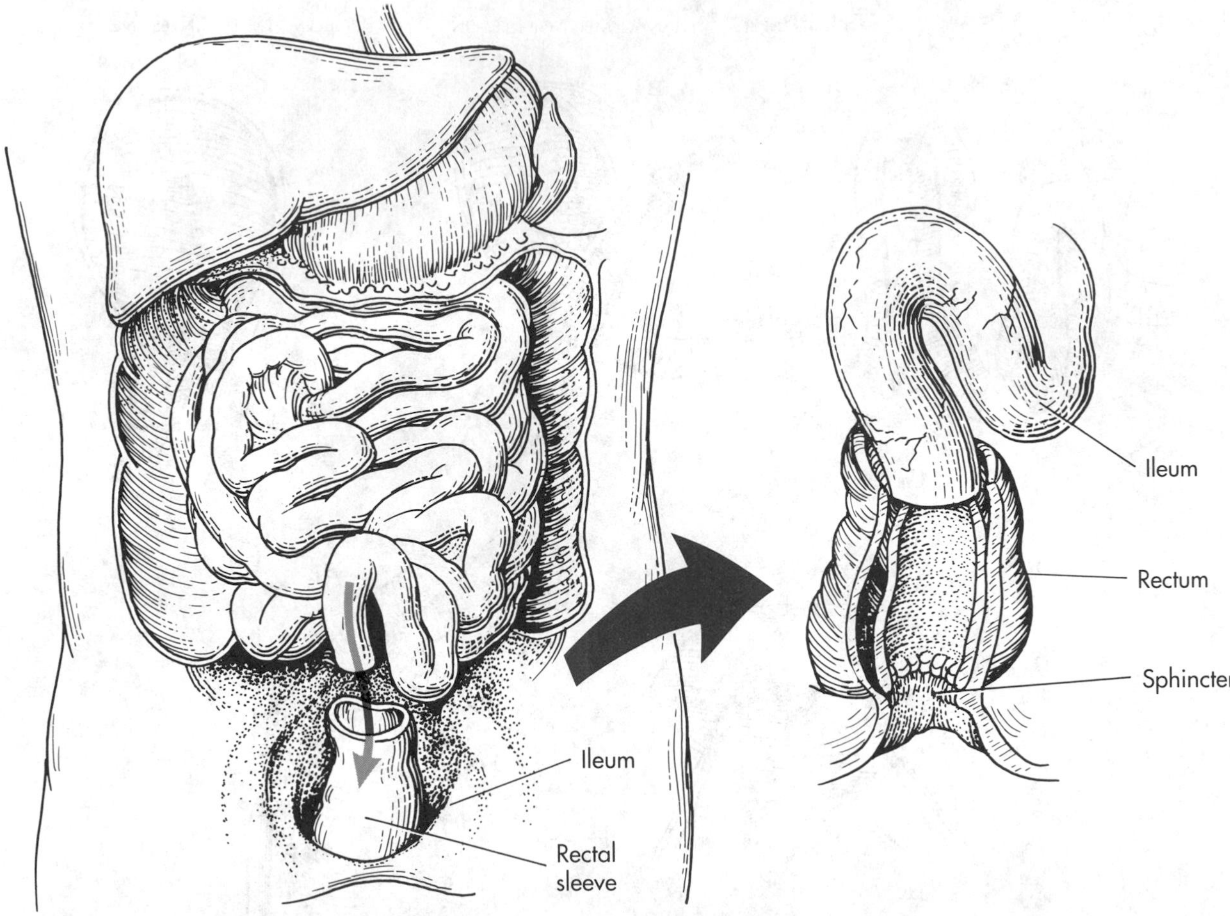

Ileum
Rectum
Sphincter
Ileum
Rectal
sleeve

**FIGURE 47-7** Ileoanal anastomosis.

A
S-shaped reservoir
B
Blind end of
distal ileum
J-pouch
reservoir
Rectum
Anus

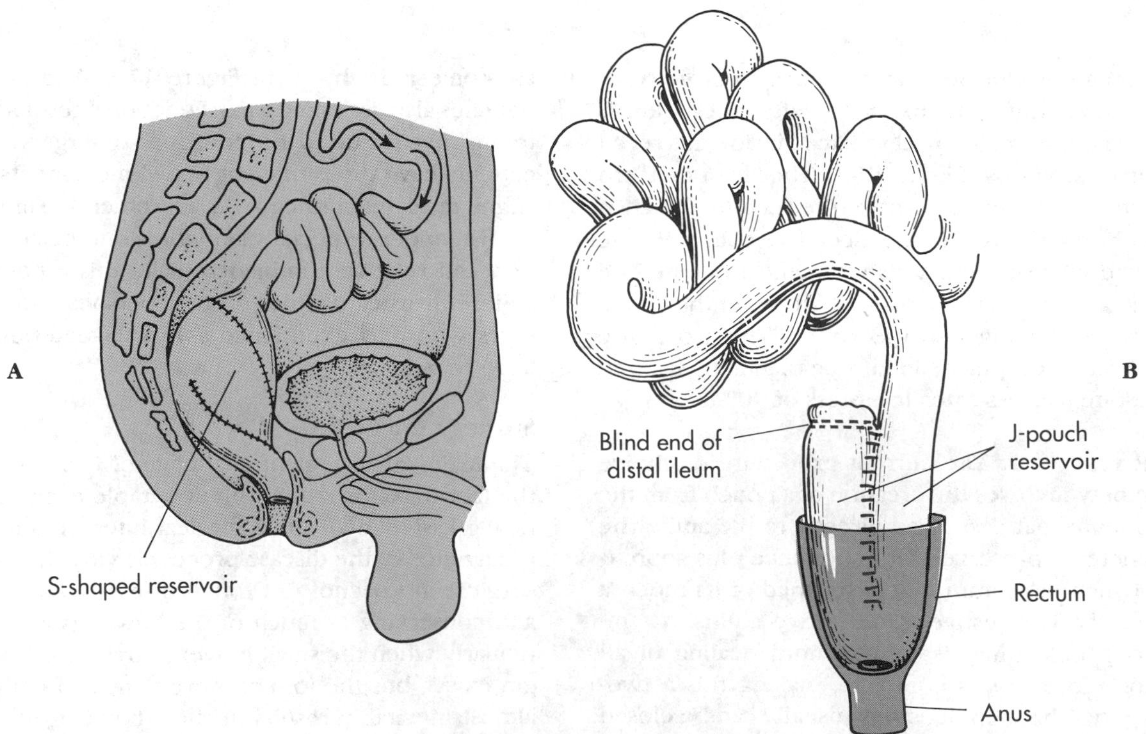

**FIGURE 47-8** Ileoanal reservoir. **A,** S-shaped reservoir. **B,** J-shaped reservoir.

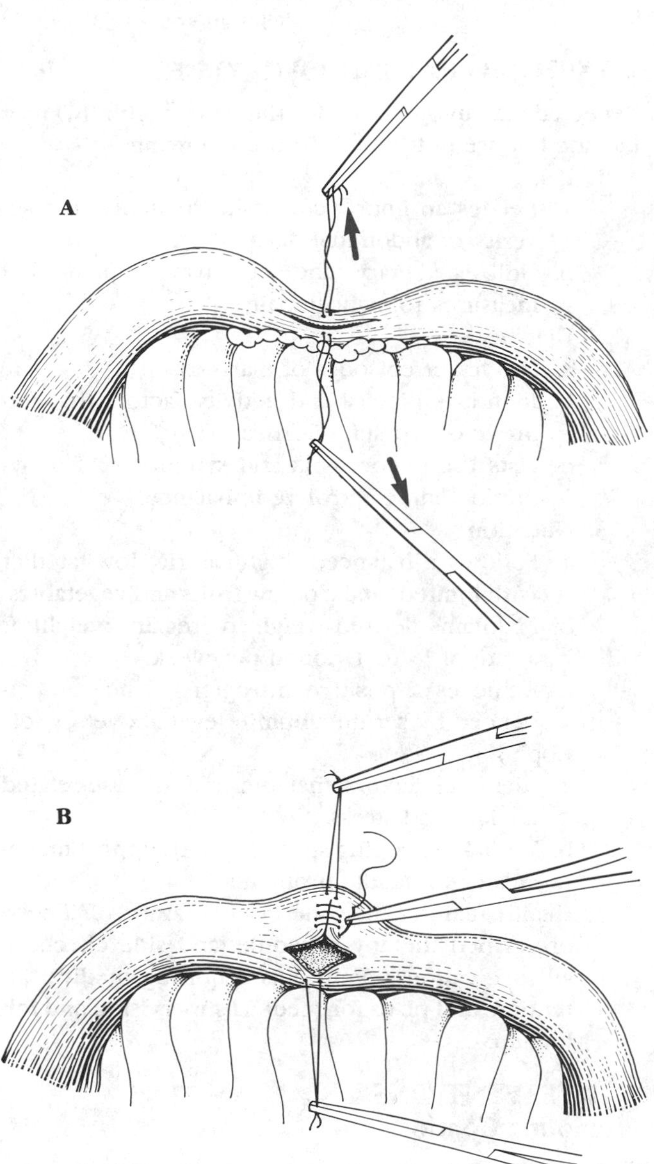


FIGURE 47-9 Strictureplasty. **A,** A linear incision is made at and beyond the stricture site. The site is spread open. **B,** The widened site is sutured closed.

## Guidelines for Teaching the Person With Inflammatory Bowel Disease

### DIET AND FLUIDS

Eat a high-calorie, high-protein diet.
Modify diet to bland, low-residue during disease exacerbations.
Avoid any foods that increase symptoms (e.g., fresh fruits and vegetables, fatty foods, spicy foods, alcohol).
Limit the use of dairy products, and assess the effect of this restriction on symptoms.
Take a multivitamin/mineral supplement daily.
Ensure a liberal fluid intake—2500-3000 ml daily:
  Drink Gatorade or other commercial products, if tolerated during flare-ups, to replace lost electrolytes.

### ELIMINATION

Take medication as prescribed.
Keep rectal area clean and dry; use analgesic rectal ointment or sitz baths for rectal discomfort.
Consult with physician about the appropriateness of bulk laxatives if constipation develops.

### REST AND COPING

Maintain a regular sleep schedule.
Schedule daily activities to avoid fatigue; take rest periods as necessary.
Use relaxation measures such as breathing exercises when emotional tension is present.
Discuss concerns with family or support person.
Attend local IBD support group if available.

### HEALTH MAINTENANCE

Report signs requiring medical attention:
  Change in pattern or severity of abdominal pain or diarrhea
  Development of constipation
  Change in stool character
  Unusual discharge from rectum
  Fever
Plan for regular follow-up care.

gical approach. Surgeons typically resect the bowel 5 to 10 cm above and below the macroscopically visible disease. The disease consistently reappears at or near the site of anastomosis. Recurrence symptoms appear at a rate of approximately 10% per year,[24] but they do not always necessitate repeat surgery. Although at least 70% of patients with Crohn's disease require surgery at some point, only 45% require a second procedure and 25% require three or more.

Although bowel resection is necessary to repair the effects of acute inflammation and perforation, a newer procedure may be appropriate for dealing with obstruction related to Crohn's strictures. **Strictureplasty** (Figure 47-9), which is analogous to pyloroplasty, permits the release of strictures that may form around multiple skin lesions in the bowel. It also corrects obstruction without the physical loss of bowel segments. Strictured segments tend to be fibrous rather than acutely inflamed and initially show a restricture rate of less than 2%.[7] It is theorized that the obstruction itself triggers the infection and inflammation in response to trapped bowel contents. The inflammation resolves with relief of the stricture. Nursing management of the patient undergoing surgery for inflammatory bowel disease is discussed beginning on p. 1548 and summarized in the Guidelines box, p. 1550.

# NURSING MANAGEMENT

## ♦ ASSESSMENT

### Subjective Data

Subjective data to be collected to assess the patient with IBD include the following:

Patient's knowledge base and understanding of the disorder
Pain: location, nature, severity, frequency; relationship to eating; measures used to self-treat
Bowel elimination pattern: constipation or diarrhea, frequency and character of stools; presence of blood, fat, mucus, or pus
Nutritional status: usual meal pattern and intake; recent weight changes, food intolerances and allergies, appetite, fatigue or weakness, nausea
Social relationships: support network; impact of illness on family, employment, life-style, and sexuality
Perceived life stress and usual coping patterns
Medications in current use—prescribed and over the counter; dosage and side effects; perceived effectiveness in managing disease and symptoms

### Objective Data

Objective data to be collected to assess the patient with IBD include the following:

Body weight
Skin turgor and condition of mucous membranes
Presence of fever
Bowel sounds: presence, character
Condition of perianal skin

### Diagnostic Test Findings

1. Stool specimen: positive findings for blood and leukocytes
2. Decreased hemoglobin and albumin levels; elevated ESR; decreased serum potassium
3. Barium enema showing structural abnormalities, for example, dilated loops of bowel, strictures, fistulas
4. Endoscopy findings of characteristic superficial ulceration and bleeding (ulcerative colitis) or cobblestone (skip pattern) regions (Crohn's disease)

## ♦ NURSING DIAGNOSES

Nursing diagnoses are determined from analysis of patient data. Nursing diagnoses for the patient with IBD may include but are not limited to the following:

| Diagnostic Title | Possible Etiologic Factors |
|---|---|
| Pain, chronic | Inflammatory process in intestine |
| Diarrhea | Chronic inflammation in intestine |
| Nutrition, altered: less than body requirements | Anorexia and nausea, abdominal cramping with meals, malabsorption of food |
| Coping, ineffective (individual) | Persistent symptoms and lack of curative treatment |
| Health maintenance, altered | Lack of knowledge of condition, treatment, or recognition of complications |

## ♦ EXPECTED PATIENT OUTCOMES

Expected patient outcomes for the patient with IBD may include but are not limited to the following:

1. Pain
   a. Relates an improvement in frequency and severity of abdominal discomfort.
   b. Utilizes dietary and noninvasive pain-relief measures to manage pain.
2. Diarrhea
   a. Has fewer episodes of diarrhea.
   b. Identifies dietary and activity factors that improve or worsen diarrhea.
   c. Lists the major signs and symptoms of dehydration and electrolyte imbalance.
3. Nutrition
   a. Follows a balanced, high-calorie, low-fat diet with limited intake of raw fruits and vegetables.
   b. Maintains desired weight or regains weight at a rate of ½ to 1 pound per week.
   c. Achieves a positive nitrogen balance as evidenced by serum albumin level above 4 g/dl.
4. Coping
   a. Identifies factors that increase disease-related anxiety and stress.
   b. Verbalizes coping strategies and support mechanisms to handle problems.
5. Health maintenance: describes nature of illness, prescribed therapy schedule, and side effects of all medications; symptoms requiring medical attention; and plans for medical supervision and follow-up.

## ♦ INTERVENTIONS

### Promoting Comfort

The nurse encourages the patient to accurately document the character and severity of the pain and to determine its relationship to eating, drinking, and the passage of stool or flatus. Anticholinergic or antispasmodic medications such as propantheline bromide (Pro-Banthine) may be prescribed to reduce the cramping, but narcotics are not used because of their negative effect on peristalsis. A warm heating pad to the abdomen often is comforting but should *not* be used during acute exacerbations. The nurse assists the patient with position changes and encourages the practice of relaxation strategies and diversional activities. The nurse documents the patient's pain pattern and response to interventions.

### Controlling Diarrhea

Chronic diarrhea often becomes a focus of care during exacerbations of the disease process. Patients may feel trapped by the frequency and urgency of their need to defecate. The nurse encourages the person to keep accurate records of the frequency, severity, and character of each diarrhea episode, particularly if blood or pus is present.

The medication regimen is designed to control the inflammation and eventually the diarrhea, but this process may take days or weeks. The patient is encouraged to limit activity when diarrhea is severe and to lie down for 20 minutes after meals to limit peristalsis. Patients are encouraged to use the toilet or commode whenever possible, but a weak, acutely ill person usually wants the bedpan accessible at all times. The bedpan should be emptied as often as it is used, which may be frequently for ulcerative colitis. Room deodorizers may be necessary. Patients who brace themselves on the bedpan by leaning on their elbows may develop pressure areas; these areas will need to be protected and massaged frequently.

The anal region often becomes excoriated from the frequent stools. Painful anal fissures and fistulas may develop. The anal area needs to be kept clean and dry. Medicated wipes (such as Tucks) can provide greater comfort than toilet tissue. Sitz baths three times a day also promote comfort and cleanliness. Ointments such as Desitin or zinc oxide may be used to protect the perianal skin.

Profuse diarrhea can lead to severe losses of fluids and electrolytes. If the patient is taking an oral diet, the nurse encourages a liberal fluid intake (at least 2500 to 3000 ml daily) and explores the patient's tolerance to solutions such as Gatorade, which can help replace lost electrolytes. The nurse records accurate intake and output and monitors the patient's weight daily.

## Promoting Nutrition

During acute exacerbations of IBD, the patient usually is malnourished from anorexia, inflammation of the bowel, and malabsorption. The method of feeding depends on the type and extent of the disorder. With severe or extensive disease, especially in Crohn's disease in which absorption is decreased or when complications are present, the patient is given nothing by mouth, and TPN may be necessary. Bowel rest is important in Crohn's disease but has no proved therapeutic benefit in ulcerative colitis.

Elemental feedings similar to that given in tube feedings are started as soon as possible; these feedings are absorbed rapidly in the upper GI tract, causing minimal demand on the colon. Palatability is a problem with the oral intake of elemental diets. Serving the fluids chilled and offering a variety of flavors increase patient acceptance. A low-residue, high-protein, high-calorie diet is then gradually introduced.

During periods of remission, patients are advised to continue to eat a well-balanced, high-protein, high-caloric diet. Only those foods that are known to cause problems are restricted. The person with ulcerative colitis often needs to avoid intestinal stimulants such as alcohol, caffeinated beverages, high-fat foods, and very high–fiber foods such as *raw* fruits and vegetables (cooked fruits and vegetables usually are better tolerated). Milk often is poorly tolerated, and the nurse encourages the patient to evaluate the effect of milk product restriction on the severity of symptoms. Multivitamin and mineral supplements are regularly used.

## Promoting Effective Coping

Inflammatory bowel disease is characterized by periods of exacerbation and remission throughout the patient's adult life. It can significantly disrupt the patient's preferred life-style. Although emotions and stress do *not* play a role in disease etiology, they are believed to influence the severity and frequency of disease exacerbations. Frustration, depression, and a sense of powerlessness are common responses to the disease, and they may precipitate hostile or dependent behaviors. Patients frequently become preoccupied with their physical symptoms.

The nurse encourages the patient to become an active participant in all decisions related to disease management and to assume control of the basic components of daily life. The nurse encourages the patient to verbalize concerns and feelings related to the disease and treatment, as well as explores potential diversional, relaxation, and coping strategies. The nurse provides the patient with information about local support groups and encourages involvement with the National Foundation for Ileitis and Colitis.

Fatigue is a common problem in IBD and can worsen the patient's psychologic response to the disease. Fatigue is common because of increased energy demands as a result of the inflammatory process and decreased energy supply from inadequate nutrition and anemia. Planned rest periods should be included in the daily activities. The patient's complaints of fatigue and an evaluation of pulse stabilization after activity are criteria used to determine the amount of rest necessary. When the acute episode begins to subside, progressive activity is encouraged. During periods of remission the person is encouraged to participate in social activities but should not overexert to the point of fatigue. Sexual response also may be affected by IBD, which can interfere with sexual relationships. Malnutrition and frequent diarrhea often lead to decreased libido, and the presence of an ileostomy may be associated with a sense of diminished sexual attractiveness. The nurse encourages the patient to express sex-related concerns and explore them openly with the spouse or partner. IBD support groups can be excellent resources for strategies to manage concerns over odor and leakage during sexual activity, particularly after colectomy surgery.

## Promoting Effective Self-Care

Accurate knowledge about the disease process and therapeutic modalities can be extremely influential in helping the patient achieve a sense of control. The nurse explores the patient's existing knowledge base about the cause, course, prognosis of the disease, treatment options, and the identification and management of complications. Prepared written materials should be provided to the patient from the National Foundation for Ileitis and Colitis. The nurse ensures that the patient understands the importance of careful adherence to the medication regimen and has a plan for scheduled medical follow-up. Major points to be included in teaching the patient with IBD are summarized in the Guidelines box, p. 1545.

## ♦ EVALUATION

To evaluate the effectiveness of nursing interventions, compare patient behaviors with those stated in the expected patient outcomes. Successful achievement of patient outcomes for the patient with IBD is indicated by the following:

1. Pain
   a. States that abdominal pain is less frequent and severe.
   b. Successfully uses noninvasive pain-relief strategies to manage abdominal pain.
2. Diet
   a. Reports fewer or no episodes of diarrhea.
   b. Successfully modifies diet to reduce diarrhea.
   c. Correctly identifies major warning signs of fluid and electrolyte imbalance (see Chapter 20).
3. Nutrition
   a. Adheres to a high-calorie, high-protein, low-fat diet.
   b. Maintains optimal body weight.
   c. Achieves serum albumin levels within normal range.
4. Coping
   a. Identifies personal life-style factors that increase stress.
   b. Uses community support mechanisms to enhance coping strategies.
5. Health maintenance: accurately describes nature of illness and prescribed therapy, schedule and side effects of medications, symptoms needing medical attention, and appointments scheduled for follow-up care.

## NURSING MANAGEMENT OF THE PATIENT UNDERGOING ILEOSTOMY SURGERY

The general care of the patient undergoing bowel surgery for any reason is discussed beginning on p. 1584. This discussion focuses on the unique needs of the patient undergoing ileostomy. The patient with IBD also may undergo surgery for bowel resection, temporary colostomy, or continent colectomy.

### Preoperative Care

An ileostomy may be created as a permanent cure for ulcerative colitis or as a temporary measure while the multiple anastomoses of ileoanal reservoir surgery heal and strengthen. Although the surgery usually is performed on an elective basis, it can be abruptly required by an acute exacerbation of the disease or the development of complications.

During the preoperative period the nurse assesses the patient's knowledge and understanding of the proposed surgery and its outcomes. It is essential that an enterostomal therapist (a nurse specially educated and certified in ostomy care) be involved in both the initial teaching and the selection and marking of the optimal stoma site. Many common stoma complications can be avoided by appropriate site selection in which the shape and contour of the skinfolds of the abdomen in both a sitting and upright position are considered.

Emotional preparation for ileostomy surgery is extremely important. The nurse encourages the patient to verbalize feelings related to this radical change in body image and function. Validating the appropriateness of these concerns lays the foundation for an effective working relationship with the patient. The patient may need to progress through the grieving process, and if the person is in the shock state, specific factual teaching may be ineffective. The nurse offers acceptance of all feelings and reinforces the importance of open communication.

The preparation phase may include nutritional support, possibly TPN, if the patient's nutritional state is inadequate for surgery. The nurse discusses the management of postoperative pain, the nature and appearance of all incisions and drains, and the purpose of the NG tube, perineal packing, and IV lines. The patient should know what to expect in the postoperative period. Bowel cleansing also is performed and may include the use of enemas, laxatives, and antibiotics to reduce intestinal bacterial flora.

### Postoperative Care

The nurse provides general abdominal surgery care. Nasogastric suction is maintained for 4 to 5 days after surgery, and the patient is given nothing by mouth to prevent distention or pressure on the suture lines. The rectal packing typically is removed by the end of the first week. The general care for an ostomy is discussed in detail on p. 1575. Unique considerations for a patient undergoing an ileostomy are discussed next.

#### Maintaining fluid and electrolyte balance

Attention to fluid and electrolyte balance is crucial for the person with an ileostomy. After surgery the fecal drainage from the ileostomy is liquid and may be constant. The patient will have fecal outputs ranging from 1000 to 1500 ml every 24 hours. This amount should begin to decrease slightly within 10 to 15 days as the terminal ileum begins to absorb more water and the stool becomes thicker. The losses still are significant, however, and careful intake and output records are essential. The ileostomy patient becomes dehydrated easily. The stool may not thicken if the patient has had previous small bowel resections or resections of the ileum for Crohn's disease. The more intestine that has been resected, the greater the chance for a high-volume output of very liquid stool. Some patients require medications to help decrease the output and control the loss of fluid.

The output from the ileostomy will still be watery as the patient begins to learn self-care for discharge. The pouch may need to be emptied every 1 to 2 hours. Volumes greater than 1500 ml in 24 hours are considered to be excessive. The nurse instructs the patient that diarrhea accompanied by nausea and vomiting can rapidly progress to dehydration. The nurse provides the patient with a list of signs of dehydration and electrolyte imbalance. The patient needs to know how to safely replace lost fluids and when to seek medical attention. Persons with ileostomies also may become dehydrated if they are given laxatives or routine preparations for diagnostic procedures. The ileostomy stoma is not irrigated.

Enteric-coated, time-released medications or hard tablets may not be absorbed in a patient with an ileostomy. Liquid or chewable forms of medications are preferred. Because the remaining ileum develops a bacterial flora, antibiotic therapy also can cause diarrhea. Vitamin supplementation is a standard measure inasmuch as colon absorption and synthesis are eliminated.

#### Maintaining skin integrity

An ostomy pouch is placed over the new stoma at the conclusion of the surgery. The ileostomy drainage is both continuous and erosive, and it is essential that the pouch be tight and properly fitted. Ileostomy drainage contains residual digestive enzymes that will quickly break down the peristomal skin if they are allowed to make contact with it. The use of a skin barrier with the pouch is an important means of protecting the peristomal skin (see Figure 47-22). The nurse teaches the patient to change the pouch or skin barrier immediately if leakage occurs and implements this approach during the hospitalization. The goal is for the patient to establish a routine of pouch changes before stool leakage occurs. The usual wearing time for an ileostomy pouch is 5 to 7 days, with the pouch emptied every 4 to 6 hours. The nurse instructs the patient to empty the pouch when it is one-third to one-half full. The pouch is changed during inactive times and before meals so there is less chance of the stoma functioning during the change. The skin is carefully inspected at each pouch change for any signs of redness or irritation.

The drainage from an ileostomy is not strongly foul-smelling. A foul odor may indicate a problem such as infection or obstruction. Odor-proof pouches are available that can be emptied without removal. If the pouch seal is intact, no odor will be present except during emptying. Diet modification also can be recommended if the patient is concerned about potential odor. Foods such as eggs, fish, onions, cabbage, and greens increase odor, and foods such as spinach, parsley, and yogurt decrease it. Deodorizing solutions and tablets also may be placed in the pouch. The nurse reminds the patient never to prick the bag for release of gas because the odor of the drainage also will be released.

#### Maintaining nutrition

General guidelines for nutrition after ileostomy surgery include eating slowly and chewing food thoroughly. Overeating of any kind should be avoided. Persons with an ileostomy need to avoid high-fiber or high-residue foods for 4 to 6 weeks after surgery. These foods may then be added one at a time in small amounts. If cramping or a problem passing the food occurs, the person should wait a few weeks and try again. If unable to tolerate the food after two or three trials, the person should eliminate it from the diet. Most persons can tolerate a nearly normal diet after healing is complete.

Ileostomy patients should be aware of the potential for obstruction. Obstruction usually is caused by a large mass of undigested food that becomes lodged at a narrow point in the bowel and blocks the intestinal lumen. After ileostomy surgery some persons discover they can eat foods such as coconut, corn, or celery only in limited amounts.

If the ileostomy becomes obstructed, the person should get into a knee-chest position and gently massage the area below the stoma. Stomal edema will develop with a food blockage; the pouch should be changed and the flange opening enlarged to accommodate the swelling. Diarrhea usually follows the passage of the obstruction, and fluids must be replaced. Abdominal pain in the peristomal area generally is present for 3 to 5 days after the obstruction is relieved. If the obstruction is not relieved within a few hours, the physician should be notified. It may be necessary for the person to be admitted for an ileostomy lavage, which is the gentle insertion of normal saline, 30 to 50 ml, through the stoma with a small 14F or 16F catheter and a bulb syringe. Careful measurement of the fluid inserted and returned is required. This procedure may be repeated until the obstruction is released.

Specific principles related to ileostomy care are summarized in the Guidelines box, p. 1550.

## ✱ SPECIAL CONSIDERATIONS FOR CARE OF THE GERONTOLOGIC PATIENT

Although both forms of inflammatory bowel disease typically begin in young adulthood, the onset can occur after age 60 years. The presentation, clinical course, and response to treatment generally are similar in both age-groups. Ulcerative colitis typically manifests as a severe initial attack, but if this first episode can be brought under control, the overall outlook is good. The disease usually takes the form of proctitis, and local treatment

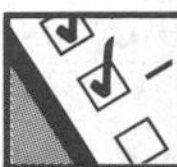

## Guidelines for Care of the Person Undergoing Ileostomy Surgery*

### PREOPERATIVE CARE

Assess knowledge base concerning procedure and outcomes.
Consult with enterostomal therapist for:
- Initial teaching concerning ileostomy management
- Introduction to pouching products to be used
- Site selection and marking

Encourage patient to verbalize feelings and concerns:
- Determine grieving stage and adjust teaching appropriately.

Assist with nutritional preparation:
- TPN may be used to improve nutritional status.

Implement components of the bowel preparation as ordered:
- Laxatives, enemas, and antibiotics (neomycin)

Explain the need for and function of all tubes and drains:
- NG, IV, wound drains

### POSTOPERATIVE CARE

Provide routine care for extensive abdominal surgery.*
Implement standard stoma monitoring and teaching.*

#### Fluids and Electrolytes

Monitor and record all output (NG, stoma, urinary).
Ensure adequate IV replacement.
Assess for imbalances.
Weigh daily.

### TEACHING

#### Fluid Balance

Maintain a liberal fluid intake (2500-3000 ml daily).
Be alert to dehydration in hot weather or during viral illness.
Drainage will thicken over time but always has a high water content.
Do not take laxatives or irrigate stoma.

#### Skin Care

Prevention and a properly fitted pouch are the keys; monitor for signs of skin irritation.
Ileostomy drainage is erosive.
Use a skin barrier at all times to protect the skin from the ileostomy drainage.
Pouch is changed every 5 to 7 days.
Establish schedule for changing pouch before leakage.
Empty pouch when it is one-third to one-half full.
Change the pouch during a time when the stoma is inactive.

#### Nutrition

Eat slowly and chew thoroughly; food transit time is greatly reduced.
Avoid high-fiber or high-residue foods for 4 to 6 weeks, and then add new foods carefully, assessing the response of the bowel.
Take a multivitamin supplement daily.
Avoid enteric-coated or time-released medications that will not be absorbed before excretion.
Adjust diet as needed for odor control.

*See pp. 1575 and 1584 for a complete discussion of general nursing care related to bowel surgery and general measures for ostomy management.

is effective. Complications usually are related to comorbidity problems rather than the primary IBD, but toxic megacolon occurs frequently. Once the disease is controlled, the person with ulcerative colitis is less likely to have a relapse, and the risk of disease-related cancer is minimal. Crohn's disease in elders tends to be localized in the distal colon and rectum, and generalized involvement is unusual.[8] When surgery is necessary, the risk of disease recurrence is small. Because both forms of IBD tend to concentrate in the distal colon and rectum, the differential diagnosis may be unclear in elderly patients. This is particularly true if the disease does not have an acute onset.

## HOME CARE CONSIDERATIONS

The patient with inflammatory bowel disease has a chronic lifelong condition that will be primarily managed in the home with family support. Two particular situations may necessitate the involvement of home care supports. Patients may need short- or long-term home administration of TPN for nutrition support. The monitoring of this therapy will involve home health nurses. In addition, patients who undergo ileostomy procedures will be referred to community enterostomal therapy services for ongoing teaching and follow-up. The patient will need to know where ostomy supplies can be purchased in the local community and is encouraged to contact a local ostomy support group for peer assistance.

## COMPLICATIONS

The primary complications of inflammatory bowel disease are hemorrhage, obstruction, perforation, toxic megacolon, and cellular dysplasia that can lead to cancer. The management of the first three is similar to that discussed elsewhere in this chapter. Toxic megacolon involves an extreme dilation of a segment of the diseased colon (frequently the transverse colon) that typically results in complete obstruction. The patient is at risk for toxic megacolon during acute exacerbations. The problem may develop after distention from a barium enema or bowel preparation or from the negative effects of narcotics and anticholinergics on peristalsis. Bacteria rapidly invade the inflamed tissue, creating the acute state. The condition may respond to conservative management or may require surgical correction.

The development of cellular dysplasia and eventually carcinoma from the chronic irritation of ulcerative colitis has been a concern for many years. Patients who have had the disease for 7 to 10 or more years need routine surveillance inasmuch as dysplasia develops frequently. The risk of cancer increases exponentially after this duration of exposure, and is estimated to be 30 times that of the average 40- to 60-year-old person.[13] The risk is also greater with widespread than with localized disease. Colectomy, of course, eliminates this risk. Dysplasia is estimated to be present in 50% to 80% of patients before the development of the cancer.[13] Sigmoidoscopy and colonoscopy are the primary tools for detecting dysplasia. Colonoscopy allows for improved visualization and greater accuracy of diagnosis. Because dysplasia, if present, is an unstable condition, specific monitoring guidelines are ineffective. In general it is recommended that colectomy be performed if mass lesions or high-grade dysplasias are found. If lower-grade dysplasia is found, conservative management consists of repeat colonoscopy at 3-month intervals or less.

It was formerly believed that patients with Crohn's disease did not have an increased risk of cancer. This premise is no longer accepted, and a cancer incidence six times that of normal populations has been found in research samples.[13] Recommendations for routine cancer surveillance do not exist at present. The tendency of cancer to develop at sites grossly involved with Crohn's disease means that these sites frequently are resected surgically before the slowly evolving cancer has a chance to develop. Standards for the early detection of cancer in patients with Crohn's disease are still under study.

**BOX 47-4 Causes of Intestinal Malabsorption**

**ALTERED DIGESTION**

Subtotal gastrectomy
Pancreatic insufficiency: pancreatitis, cancer of pancreas, cystic fibrosis, Zollinger-Ellison syndrome
Liver disease, biliary tract obstruction, enteric fistulas
Drugs that precipitate bile salts (neomycin, cholestyramine)
Intestinal bacterial overgrowth

**ALTERED MUCOSAL CELL TRANSPORT**

Lactase deficiency
Crohn's disease, celiac disease, tropical sprue, Whipple's disease, infectious or allergic enteritis, parasitic infections, small bowel ischemia
Intestinal resection or bypass
Paraaminosalicylic acid, colchicine, irritant laxatives, neomycin
Radiation enteritis

**ALTERED LYMPH/BLOOD TRANSPORT**

Lymphoma
Superior mesenteric thrombosis

# MALABSORPTION AND MALNUTRITION

## MALABSORPTION

### Etiology/Epidemiology

To maintain adequate nutrition the GI tract must be able to both break down foodstuffs into an appropriate nutrient form and transport these nutrients across the mucosa of the intestine to gain access to the bloodstream. A large volume of ingested and secreted fluids and food components pass through the GI tract each day. Approximately 7 to 10 L of liquid chyme moves through on an average day. Reabsorption in the small intestine is so efficient, however, that all but 600 to 800 ml of this volume is reabsorbed before it reaches the ileocecal valve. If this complex process is interrupted in any way, the body may be unable to adequately absorb one or more of the major nutrients. This can result in the syndrome of malabsorption.

Malabsorption results when there are (1) alterations of digestion so that nutrients are not broken down into a form that can be transported across the cell membranes—for example, deficiencies of pancreatic enzymes, bile salts, or bacteria, (2) alterations in the transport of nutrients across the cell membranes of the villi—for example, disruption of the mucosal lining, and (3) alterations in the transport of nutrients into the lymphatic or circulatory systems. Severe inflammatory bowel disease affecting the small intestine significantly impairs the mucosal lining of the intestine and is a common cause of malabsorption. Gastrointestinal surgery is a common secondary cause of malabsorption. Removal of short segments of the jejunum or ileum do not cause malabsorption, but if more than 50% of the small intestine is resected or bypassed, nutrient absorption will be severely compromised. Box 47-4 summarizes the major conditions that can result in malabsorption.

### Pathophysiology

**Malabsorption syndrome** is a group of signs and symptoms resulting from inadequate absorption of fat, protein, or carbohydrates in the small intestine. Because fat-soluble vitamins (A, D, E, and K) require fat for absorption, decreased absorption of fat also typically results in a deficiency of these vitamins. Fat malabsorption is the most common problem, but it also may be accompanied by a decreased absorption of protein, carbohydrate, and minerals. Different signs and symptoms specific to various nutrient deficiencies result from malabsorption of nutrients other than fat.

The characteristic sign of malabsorption syndrome is **steatorrhea**, or excess loss of fat in the stool. The fat gives the stool a light, greasy, bulky, mushy appearance and a foul odor. The stools float because of their low specific gravity and because of gas produced by action of intestinal bacteria on the undigested fat. Stools may be limited to one bulky stool a day or may occur frequently. Steatorrhea causes flatulence with borborygmi (loud bowel sounds) and abdominal distention. The decreased fat absorption leads to weight loss, weakness, fatigue, and anorexia.

Signs and symptoms of vitamin deficiencies can include bleeding (ecchymoses, hematuria), bone pain, fractures, hypocalcemia, anemia, glossitis, cheilosis, muscle tenderness, peripheral neuritis, and dermatitis. Protein deficiency results in edema, hypoalbuminemia, and loss of muscle mass. The person with malabsorption syndrome appears pale and emaciated and has dry, scaly

**TABLE 47-6 Three Primary Malabsorption Diseases of Adulthood**

| DISORDER | PATHOPHYSIOLOGY | TREATMENT |
|---|---|---|
| **CELIAC SPRUE** | | |
| Nontropical sprue, gluten enteropathy<br>Familial; high incidence of childhood celiac disease in relatives | Hypersensitivity response to the gluten fraction of grains (wheat, rye, barley, oats), which causes destruction of the absorbing surface of the intestine; proximal jejunum affected most seriously | Anatomic and clinical problems can be reversed with a well-balanced, gluten-free diet; vitamin and mineral replacement needed |
| **TROPICAL SPRUE** | | |
| Endemic to the Caribbean, India, and Southeast Asia; may have both a nutritional and an infectious basis | Unknown toxic factors result in mucosal inflammation plus partial atrophy of the intestinal villi | Remission of symptoms can be achieved with antibiotics (tetracycline), folic acid therapy, and a balanced diet high in protein and normal in fat; folic acid supplement is ongoing |
| **ADULT LACTASE DEFICIENCY** | | |
| Affects up to 80% of African-American and other nonwhite races; usually a congenital problem but may develop after gastric surgery or secondary to IBD | Deficiency of the intestinal enzyme lactase needed to hydrolyze lactose<br>Undigested lactose acts as an osmotic agent, creating diarrhea and interfering with absorption of other nutrients | Restriction of lactose-containing foods until tolerance level reached; includes milk and other dairy products, commercially prepared foods processed with lactose, instant coffee, chocolate, cold cuts, hot dogs |

skin that may be hyperpigmented. The three primary diseases that cause adult malabsorption are summarized in Table 47-6. They have many overlapping manifestations but wide variations in incidence and causes.

### Medical Management

Medical treatment for malabsorption is based on the underlying cause. Diagnostic studies may be necessary to determine the specific disorder responsible. Nutrition is the major problem associated with malabsorption syndromes, and dietary intervention is the primary approach to management. Diet modifications may be successful in compensating for the malabsorption on a daily basis, but more aggressive management may be necessary during disease exacerbations. Either enteral or parenteral (TPN) feedings may be necessary.

### Nursing Management

The nurse assists the patient to incorporate needed dietary changes into the daily life-style and works with the family on strategies to promote adherence. Major diet changes can have profound psychosocial ramifications that are rarely related to the actual food restriction. The nurse ensures that the patient understands the rationale for all prescribed dietary and drug interventions. The severely malnourished person also may require good mouth care to increase comfort and prevent oral inflammations, as well as good skin care to prevent skin breakdown.

## PROTEIN-CALORIE MALNUTRITION

### Etiology/Epidemiology

Many disease conditions can result in negative nitrogen balance, particularly those that affect the GI tract. A poor nutritional state is a common problem in both acute and long-term care settings, and the problem of **protein-calorie malnutrition** has been receiving increasing attention as the importance of nutrition to such factors as wound healing, immunocompetence, and ventilator weaning is acknowledged. The actual incidence of protein-calorie malnutrition is unknown, but some authorities estimate that it may occur in up to 20% to 50% of hospitalized adults.[6] Elders are particularly vulnerable. Box 47-5 identifies some of the typical causes of malnutrition in hospitalized patients. Intake may be deficient in all elements or just in needed protein.

### Pathophysiology

If a diet provides adequate carbohydrates and fats, the body uses these nutrients to meet its energy needs. When intake of these nutrients is inadequate, however, the body meets its energy needs by utilizing body proteins. Most severely ill hospitalized adults experience a deficiency of all dietary elements. The process of protein synthesis in the body is constant. The body can synthesize certain amino acids from its stored pools, but it depends on ingested protein sources for others. Amino acids that are not used are excreted. Negative nitrogen balance occurs when more nitrogen (which is an end product of amino acid breakdown) is excreted than is ingested via dietary proteins.

Ongoing severe protein loss leads to decreases in both muscle and visceral mass. Cardiac output decreases, respiratory muscles weaken, and malabsorption occurs in the GI tract. Immunocompetence is impaired, and the risk of infection increases. The greatest impairment is noted in cell-mediated immunity. The number of T cells declines. Weight loss, decreased muscle mass, and weakness are common, but the affected person may have few overt signs.

**BOX 47-5 Causes of Malnutrition in Hospitalized Patients**

**DECREASED INTAKE**

| | |
|---|---|
| Anorexia and nausea | Self-care deficits |
| NPO status | Dysphagia |
| Pain | Depression |
| Medication effects | |

**INCREASED LOSSES**

| | |
|---|---|
| Vomiting | Open wounds |
| Diarrhea | GI suctioning |

**INCREASED NEEDS**

| | |
|---|---|
| Fever | Trauma |
| Infection | Surgery |

## Medical Management

The primary approach to malnutrition management is recognizing patients at risk, monitoring physical and laboratory parameters, and intervening with oral supplements, tube feedings, or TPN as indicated. The evidence of weight loss is an important basic component. Serial measurements of serum albumin and transferrin levels are obtained. Albumin levels below 3.5 g/dl indicate early malnutrition. Prealbumin levels are followed during treatment inasmuch as they provide an analysis of protein changes during the previous 48 hours. Total lymphocyte counts also are followed as a basic measure of immunity. A nutrition-support team, if available, will guide decision making concerning dietary supplements or replacements (see discussion of tube feedings and total parenteral nutrition, below).

## Nursing Management

The nursing role in malnutrition varies on the basis of the patient's ability to take oral nutrients. Fatigue is common, and the nurse provides the patient with frequent rest periods and spaces needed treatments and activities throughout the day. A high-calorie, high-protein diet is encouraged if the patient can eat. The nurse ensures that the environment is conducive to eating, arranges for small frequent feedings rather than large meals, and encourages the patient to avoid empty calories. It is essential to involve the patient and family in all nutritional planning. Assisting the patient with meals and reinforcing self-care skills are important. The nurse keeps an accurate record of the patient's weight and records calorie counts if ordered. Care for the patient receiving tube feedings or total parenteral nutrition is discussed on pp. 1556 and 1578.

# ENTERAL AND PARENTERAL NUTRITION

## Enteral Nutrition

**Enteral nutrition** refers to the delivery of nutrients directly into the GI tract. It may be used as a nutritional supplement or as a method of meeting the total nutritional needs of patients who cannot meet their needs orally because of an underlying illness or condition. Enteral nutrition is used only with patients who have normal GI motility and absorption. It is not administered to persons with malabsorption, trauma to the lower portion of the abdomen, or insufficient lengths of bowel to absorb nutrients. It is considered to be a safer nutritional alternative in many situations than TPN because of the serious infectious and metabolic risks associated with central venous catheter use. Other advantages to the use of enteral feedings include the following[12]:

- Preservation of normal GI integrity
- Preservation of normal sequence of intestinal and hepatic metabolism
- Maintenance of normal insulin-glucagon ratios
- Maintenance of lipoprotein synthesis by the intestinal mucosa and liver

Tube feedings may be delivered to the stomach (nasogastric) or to the distal duodenum or proximal jejunum (nasointestinal). Long-term enteral nutrition is preferably delivered via a permanent access, which usually is a gastrostomy, but the jejunum may be used (jejunostomy).

### Enteral feeding tubes

Enteral tubes generally are described in terms of their external diameter, composition, length, and the presence or absence of a weighted tip. A wide variety of containers, tubes, catheters, and delivery systems are available for use in enteral feedings. The most common types of feeding tubes are constructed of polyurethane or silicone. The polyurethane tubes have a larger inside diameter and have been shown to facilitate greater fluid flow. Enteral feeding tubes come in different sizes: 8F to 10F (small bore), 12F to 14F (medium bore), and 16F to 18F (large bore). Some tubes have a monofilament or stainless steel stylet for easy insertion. A tube with a weighted end may be used to help pass the tube through the pylorus into the duodenum or jejunum. A typical small bore feeding tube is shown in Figure 47-10.

Nasogastric tubes are appropriately used with patients who have intact gag-and-swallow reflexes and a competent lower esophageal sphincter. The nasointestinal route is used for persons who are at risk for aspiration or have dysfunction of the gastric outlet. These tubes are smaller in diameter and usually have a weighted tip. A stylet usually is needed to guide their insertion. Small-bore tubes are more easily tolerated, but certain types of feedings may congeal and block their lumen. Small-bore tubes also collapse with suction; therefore aspiration of stomach contents for checking residual volumes often cannot be performed. (See Research box, p. 1554.)

### Gastrostomy

Insertion of a gastrostomy tube is an alternative approach to enteral nutrition for patients who are unable to take oral nutrients for long periods. The procedure

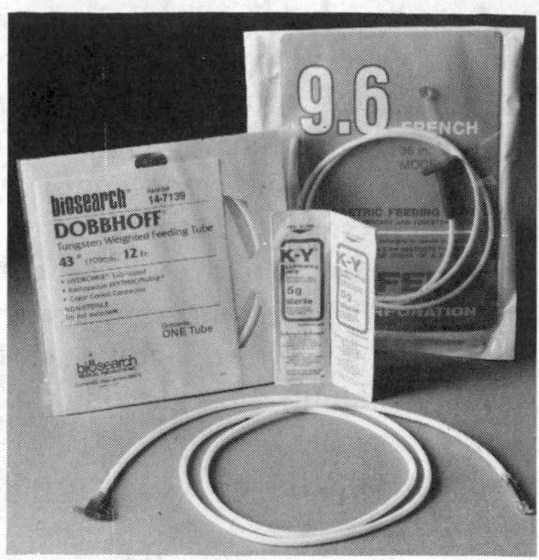

**FIGURE 47-10** Typical small-bore feeding tube. (From Perry AG, Potter PA: *Clinical nursing skills and techniques,* ed 3, St Louis, 1994, Mosby.)

## RESEARCH

Eisenberg P, Metheny N, McSweeney M: Nasoenteral feeding tube properties and the ability to withdraw fluid via syringe, *Appl Nurs Res* 2(4):168-172, 1989.

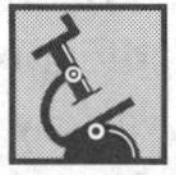

Most enteral feeding tubes in use today are of the soft small-bore variety. These are more comfortable for patients but make it difficult to aspirate fluid to assess pH or measure residual. This study sought to determine if the diameter or material of the feeding tube significantly affected the ability to aspirate fluid from the tube.

The sample consisted of 108 feeding tubes of various diameters and from various manufacturers. Half of the sample tubes were made of silicone and half of polyurethane. Both tube material and diameter were found to be significant. Mean volumes that could be aspirated were greater for size 10F than for either size 8F or size 12F. Products vary widely in internal diameter because of the presence of double lumens or thick walls. The internal diameter was found to be the key variable, but polyurethane was consistently superior to silicone.

involves the creation of an opening into the abdominal cavity and insertion of a catheter through the stomach wall either surgically or via endoscopy and local anesthesia.

The *percutaneous endoscopic gastrostomy* (PEG) does not require incision into the abdominal cavity and is a safe and rapid method of creating a **gastrostomy.** It is performed via endoscopy and local anesthesia; the patient is mildly sedated. A small incision is made on the skin of the abdomen, and a cannula is pushed through the adjacent abdominal and gastric walls while the site is observed through a gastroscope. A long silk suture is threaded through the cannula, grasped through the endoscope, and pulled up through the endoscope, which

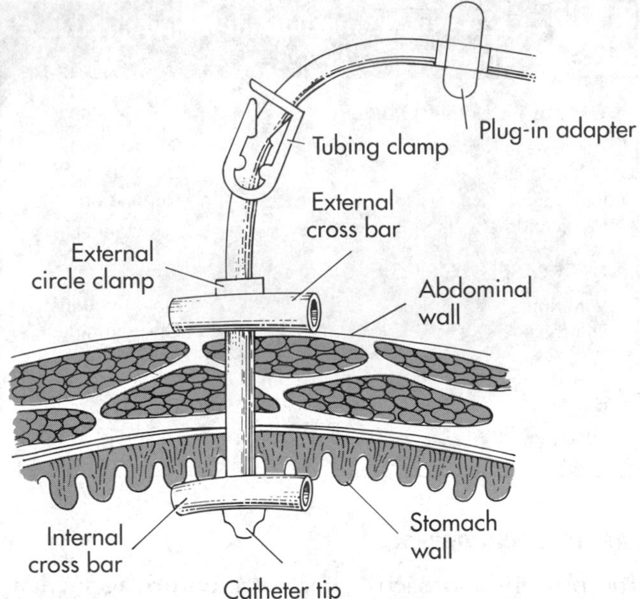


**FIGURE 47-11** A percutaneous endoscopic gastrostomy (PEG) tube in place in the stomach.

is then removed. The exit end of a specially prepared mushroom catheter is attached to the thread, and the catheter is then pulled in retrograde fashion through the esophagus and stomach and out the abdominal wall. Internal and external dams hold the catheter in place. A jejunostomy tube may be inserted by a similar method (Figure 47-11).

The catheter inserted into a gastrostomy usually is large (18F to 24F). Traditionally a Foley catheter has been used, which allows the balloon to serve as an anchor against the stomach wall. PEG tubes are smaller (12F to 16F) and usually are anchored by a 1 to 2-inch cross-linked latex tube placed inside the stomach. Principles of administration are the same as for other types of tube feedings. A dressing is not generally used. Keeping the site open helps to prevent skin maceration, breakdown, and infection. The skin around the gastrostomy may be cleaned with hydrogen peroxide solution to remove crusts and rinsed with normal saline or water.

An alternate type of gastrostomy that does not require a tube and therefore lessens the chance of complications from tube irritation or obstruction may be used in certain situations. This "button" gastrostomy is constructed by making a small tube from the wall of the stomach and then pushing it in to form an intussusception valve. The "valve" is brought out flush with the skin surface to create a flat stoma. The valve prevents leakage of stomach contents; therefore no skin care or dressings are needed. A feeding tube is inserted through the valve for feedings. The stoma can be closed at a later date.

### Enteral feeding solutions

Many types of feeding solutions are available to meet the multiple and diverse needs of patient populations.

All formulas contain some balance of the essential nutrients. They differ in the balance of the constituents, as well as the amount of digestion and absorption that is required to utilize them.

*Protein* usually is considered to be the most critical component of the formula. The solution may contain intact nutrients and resemble a puréed diet. These products require normal levels of pancreatic enzymes to break down the protein into small polypeptides and free amino acids for absorption. Most of these solutions are lactose-free and derived from soybean protein or hydrolyzed lactalbumins. Formulas also may contain hydrolyzed proteins, among others, derived from meat, soy, and lactalbumin. These proteins have been predigested to dipeptides and free amino acids and do not require further digestion. GI absorption must be adequate, however. Crystalline amino acid formulas are composed of amino acids that require no digestion and readily transport across the intestinal mucosa for easy absorption. Incomplete formulas are available for patients with renal or liver failure. They provide essential amino acids but a low overall protein content.

The major issues in the *carbohydrate* content of feeding solutions have related to lactose content and total calorie needs. Increasing awareness of the pervasiveness of partial lactose intolerance has stimulated the development of formulas without a milk base. Carbohydrates in standard formulas usually are easily utilized as long as intestinal absorption remains intact. Components include starch and polysaccharides, disaccharides, and monosaccharides. Effective carbohydrate use also depends on the person having adequate amounts of insulin, glucagon, norepinephrine, and vitamins, among other elements. Any imbalance or deficiency in these elements can produce watery diarrhea.

*Fats* in the formula provide a source for concentrated calories and essential fatty acids and serve as a carrier for fat-soluble vitamins. Fat digestion depends on pancreatic enzymes, bile salts, and normal intestinal flora. Short-, medium-, and long-chain fatty acids may be included in both saturated and polyunsaturated forms. Various vegetable oils and coconut oil may be used as sources.

*Caloric density* (the number of calories per unit volume) is an extremely important consideration. High-density formulas tend to be more hypertonic and may contribute to diarrhea. Lower-density formulas require a larger volume of solution to provide needed levels, which may be an issue if fluids must be restricted.

*Osmolality* is another essential consideration for enteral solutions. Isotonic formulas approximate the osmolality of plasma (280 to 300 mOsm/kg) and can be administered at full strength with the rate adjusted to patient tolerance. Even isotonic solutions cause the extracellular fluids to become hyperosmolar unless adequate hypotonic fluids also are administered to the patient. The osmolality is primarily a reflection of the concentration of proteins and carbohydrates in the solution. Hypertonic formulas typically have osmolalities ranging from 400 to 1100 mOsm/kg and usually need to be diluted initially or administered at an extremely slow rate until patient tolerance increases. Formulas with simple (predigested) proteins often have a higher osmolality, and patients receiving them need careful monitoring. Table 47-7 compares the various components of a few sample formulas. All formulas are supplemented with substantial quantities of essential vitamins and minerals.

**TABLE 47-7 Sample Tube Feeding Composition**

| FORMULA | CARBOHYDRATE | PROTEINS | OSMOLALITY (mOsm) |
|---|---|---|---|
| **LIQUID WHOLE FOOD** | | | |
| Ensure, Isocal, Sustacal, Osmolite | Complex carbohydrates | Intact proteins | 300-600 |
| **SUPPLEMENTAL** | | | |
| Precision, Vital | Complex carbohydrates | Peptides | 450-600 |
| **PREDIGESTED/ELEMENTAL** | | | |
| Vivonex, Flexical, Pregestimil | Simple carbohydrates | Amino acids | 500-800 |

### Enteral feeding techniques

Feeding schedules may be planned on an intermittent, bolus, or continuous basis. Because normal eating patterns are intermittent, an intermittent schedule is clearly preferable when nasogastric feedings are being used. An intermittent schedule also allows the patient to be free of the feeding equipment for intervals of time. The intestinal mucosa, however, receives nutrients from the stomach in slow peristaltic waves over several hours in an almost continuous rather than a bolus pattern. If a nasointestinal route is being used for enteral feeding, the formulas ideally should be delivered by constant infusion, preferably with use of a mechanical pump to maintain a constant rate. Intermittent scheduling would increase the potential for "dumping syndrome" and diarrhea.[6]

Residual gastric volume is checked before each intermittent feeding and then returned to the patient. If more than 100 to 150 ml can be withdrawn, the feeding usually is postponed and the residual checked again before the next scheduled feeding. The physician is notified if the excess residual occurs again. Intermittent feedings are delivered by gravity and regulated to infuse over 30 to 60 minutes.[6] The tube is irrigated with 30 to 50 ml of tap water before and after the feeding to prevent clogging. The delivery set bag and tubing are washed

## RESEARCH

Metheny N et al: Effectiveness of pH measurements in predicting feeding tube placement, *Nurs Res* 38(5):280-285, 1989.

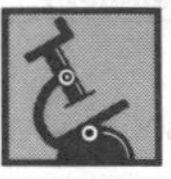

This study was designed to test the effectiveness of the pH method of predicting the placement of feeding tubes in the stomach, intestine, or respiratory system. The sample consisted of 181 patients—94 with small-bore nasogastric tubes and 87 with nasointestinal tubes. None of the patients received antacid therapy. Color-coded pH paper was used for the measurements and compared with pH meter readings for the same specimen in about half the cases. The two readings correlated well. Timing of the testing was adjusted to make it as close to scheduled x-ray position determinations as possible.

The pH readings were successful in predicting gastric versus intestinal placement in most situations. Failures included patients with severe metabolic disarray and those receiving $H_2$ receptor antagonist therapy and other medications. Only one testing involved tube migration to the lung. The aspirate had an alkaline pH but no coloring from bile as would be expected in the duodenum.

## RESEARCH

Metheny N et al: Effectiveness of the auscultatory method in predicting feeding tube location, *Nurs Res* 39(5):262-266, 1990.

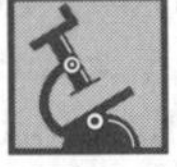

The auscultatory method of confirming the placement of nasogastric tubes has been routinely recommended. This study attempted to determine the accuracy of this method for determining the location of the tube in the GI tract or lungs. Auscultation data were obtained from 85 acutely ill adult patients. In the procedure 30 ml of air were injected into each tube five times, and the abdominal sounds produced were recorded at five separate locations—right and left upper and lower quadrants and the epigastrium. The study resulted in 115 usable tapes that were analyzed by a team of five skilled clinicians.

The auscultatory method was ineffective in specifying feeding tube location. The air sounds were audible at all testing sites. Sounds are freely dispersed throughout the abdomen, and the correct classification was only 34%, slightly above chance. Interrater reliability also was extremely low. Even with three patients whose tubes were inadvertently placed in the bronchi, the sounds were readily heard in the abdomen.

with warm water with vigorous agitation after each feeding and allowed to dry. The set is discarded after 24 to 48 hours depending on institutional policy. Medical asepsis should be ensured in all aspects of tube feeding administration.

Similar principles of cleanliness and scheduling guide continuous infusion feedings. The volume delivered usually is about 50 to 125 ml/hr. Long-term tube patency is promoted by irrigation with 30 to 50 ml of tap water every 4 hours. Care of the patient receiving an enteral tube feeding is summarized in the Guidelines box at right.

### Managing complications

**Tube obstruction.** Feeding tube obstructions are relatively common problems that can cause a patient considerable expense and discomfort if replacement is necessary. Pill fragments, formula residue adhering to the tube lumen, and formula/medication incompatibilities are common causes. Acidic medications, slow formula delivery rates, and use of silicone tubes appear to increase the risk of clogging. The Guidelines box, p. 1557, left, summarizes strategies to prevent tube clogging.

**Regurgitation/aspiration.** Pulmonary complications are the most dangerous problems associated with enteral feedings. A tube of any size may enter the tracheobronchial tree on insertion or migrate there with vigorous coughing or suctioning. Patients who are obtunded and have impaired cough or gag reflexes are at particular risk.

## Guidelines for Care of the Person Receiving an Enteral Tube Feeding

Check the placement of the feeding tube:
- Aspirate gastric secretions if possible.
- Measure gastric residual–return residual to stomach.
- Inject 10-30 ml of air into feeding tubes, and auscultate over left upper quadrant of abdomen.

Place patient in high Fowler's position if permitted.

Attach syringe to feeding tube (for intermittent feedings):
- Elevate syringe 18 inches above the patient's head.
- Fill syringe with formula.
- Allow feeding to empty by gravity.
- Keep syringe filled to avoid infusion of air.

Hang tube feeding bag about 18 inches above patient's head (for continuous feedings), and set prescribed rate for flow.

Flush tube with 30-50 ml of water at the end of the feeding or q 4 hr for continuous feedings; always flush tube before and after medication administration.

Record all administered volumes and residuals on intake and output record.

Traditional methods for checking tube position frequently are inadequate with the use of flexible small-lumen tubes. The injection of air with simultaneous auscultation of the abdomen can be misleading inasmuch as sounds are readily transmitted throughout the abdomen. Small-bore tubes collapse easily when attempts are made to aspirate gastric contents, even when tube positioning is accurate. See Research boxes above.

### Guidelines for Preventing Enteral Feeding Tube Obstruction

Use a polyurethane feeding tube if possible.
Flush the tube with at least 30 ml of water q 4 hr; do this before and after administering medications and before and after checking gastric residuals.
Use a controller pump for slow rates.
Administer medications in elixir form if possible. If pills are given, crush thoroughly and dissolve in an appropriate solvent.
If the tube obstructs, attempt to irrigate it with water or cola. Avoid using meat tenderizer.

Modified from Kohn CL, Keithley JK: *Nurs Clin North Am* 24(2):339-351, 1989.

Tube position after insertion should be confirmed by x-ray film, and repeat radiographs may be needed if tube patency or position is questioned. In addition, the head of the bed should be kept elevated 30 to 40 degrees at all times if possible. Enteral feedings usually are temporarily discontinued if the patient needs to be transported off the unit for x-ray examination or other treatments or tests. The use of transpyloric tubes with weighted tips for patients at high risk diminishes the incidence of reflux.

Routine care includes monitoring tube position by any and all means every 4 hours. This includes pulmonary auscultation, checking residuals, and monitoring for active bowel sounds.

**Diarrhea.** Diarrhea is the most commonly encountered complication of enteral feedings, and it may be caused by a variety of factors. The diarrhea may be related to prescribed medications, such as antibiotics, $H_2$ receptor antagonists, and elixirs containing sorbitol, rather than to the tube feeding itself. Hypertonic solutions frequently are diluted, and patients receiving antibiotics may be given a *Lactobacillus acidophilus* preparation to help restore normal GI flora.

Malnutrition, particularly hypoalbuminemia, is associated with a decrease in intestinal absorption and also can contribute to diarrhea. This problem is corrected as the patient's nutritional status is improved, but it may require formula readjustment or direct replenishment of the serum albumin.

Diarrhea also may be directly related to the formula in use. Formulas with lactose, high-fat content, or low-fiber content have been implicated in the development of diarrhea.[12] High osmolality also appears to be important, particularly with severely malnourished patients. Strategies may include the use of bulking agents, slow delivery rates, and formula dilution if the malabsorption is severe.

Bacterial contamination is a significant cause of diarrhea. Formula can become contaminated at any point in the preparation and delivery process. Formulas with higher osmolalities appear to be *less* likely to support bacterial growth. The length of time the formula hangs at room temperature also is a factor. Hospital-prepared formulas that contain milk are the most vulnerable. The Guidelines box, above, summarizes measures to help reduce the risk of bacterial contamination of formula.

### Guidelines for Preventing Bacterial Contamination of Tube Feeding Formulas

Use prefilled, ready-to-use sets if available.
Follow strict aseptic technique in handling all components; good handwashing is essential.
Use full-strength ready-to-use formula; dilution and reconstitution increase the chances of contamination.
Rinse the delivery set with water before adding new formula.
Hang commercially prepared formulas for no more than 8 to 12 hours (hospital-prepared formulas for no more than 6 hours).

**Hyperglycemia.** Hyperglycemia may become a problem for patients who are receiving high–caloric density formulas or corticosteroids or who have diabetes. Elderly persons are at increased risk. The urine may be monitored for glucose and ketones, or blood glucose monitoring may be utilized. Sliding-scale insulin may be necessary to control the hyperglycemia. It is essential that dehydration be prevented through adequate amounts of free water. The greater the formula's osmolality the more water that is needed. High-carbohydrate contents in formulas also may increase carbon dioxide production to the point at which it places a strain on the respiratory system. This factor can be extremely important in weaning patients from ventilators and with patients who are at risk for respiratory failure. Frequent monitoring of respiratory effort status is important.

## Parenteral Nutrition

Parenteral nutrition is a method of giving highly concentrated solutions (1800 to 2200 mOsm/L) intravenously to maintain a patient's nutritional balance when oral or enteral nutrition is not possible. Indications for this therapy include (1) major GI diseases, fistulas, or inflammatory diseases, (2) severe trauma or burns, (3) severe GI side effects from radiation or chemotherapy, (4) congenital malformations of the GI tract, and (5) severe malnutrition.

Parenteral nutrition is commonly administered through the central venous route, but it can be administered by peripheral vein as well. Peripheral administration typically is used as maintenance nutrition for patients who will be without oral intake for at least 1 week and have some nutritional compromise. Its main disadvantage is the fact that solutions that contain glu-

**TABLE 47-8 Commonly Used Central Venous Catheter Options**

| CATHETER TYPE | CHARACTERISTICS |
|---|---|
| **SUBCLAVIAN CATHETERS** | |
| Single and multilumen | Short-term use (usually less than 60 days)<br>Sutured in place (Figure 47-12, *A*)<br>Sterile occlusive dressing required for duration of catheter use<br>Regular heparinization of lumen required |
| **TUNNELED CATHETERS** | |
| Single and multilumen<br>Hickman-Broviac | Long-term use (1-2 yr)<br>Subcutaneously tunneled in place (Figure 47-12, *B*)<br>Sterile cover dressing required only until exit site heals<br>Scheduled heparin flushes required when not in use |
| **GROSHONG CATHETER** | |
| Central venous catheter with valve and closed distal tip | Same characteristics as tunneled catheter<br>Requires vigorous scheduled flushing when not in use |
| **IMPLANTABLE PORTS** | |
| Single and dual lumen | Long-term use (1-2 yr)<br>Metal or plastic portal chamber is connected to the venous catheter and implanted beneath the skin (Figure 47-13, *A*)<br>Requires Huber needle for port access; port septum is self-sealing for approximately 2000 punctures<br>Monthly heparinization of port required<br>No dressing needed when not in use |
| **PERIPHERALLY INSERTED CENTRAL CATHETERS** | |
| PICC lines<br>Single or dual lumen | May be inserted by nurses with special training in IV devices<br>Catheter-tip location is verified by radiograph<br>Pressure dressing is placed over insertion site for 24 hr<br>Sterile occlusive dressing is required for duration of catheter use<br>Regular heparinization of lumen required |

Modified from LaRocca JC, Otto SE: *Pocket guide to intravenous therapy,* ed 2, St Louis, 1993, Mosby.

cose as the primary calorie source and are high in osmolality may be extremely irritating to peripheral veins. Therefore a large-fluid volume is required to deliver acceptable osmolalities. The peripheral solutions rely on lipid emulsions that are isotonic as the main nonprotein calorie source. **Total parenteral nutrition (TPN)** usually is selected when a patient is expected to need extensive nutritional support over an extended period. Hypertonic concentrations of dextrose and amino acids may be given to maintain or increase the patient's lean body mass.

### Central venous catheters

A variety of options exist for the delivery of TPN solutions. Whenever hypertonic solutions are used, a central venous catheter is inserted to allow for rapid mixing and dilution of the solution. Subclavian, tunneled, and implantable port catheters are available in single-lumen and multilumen forms. Table 47-8 summarizes the features of some of the most commonly used options. Infection is the primary concern related to the administration of TPN. It is believed that catheter contamination at the point of entry into the skin and migration of bacteria along the catheter are the major sources of TPN sepsis. Rigorous dressing care is essential, but there are wide variations in institutional protocols. Further research is needed to determine the optimal interval for dressing changes and the effectiveness of the various dressing materials.

### Total parenteral nutrition

TPN solutions are complex formulas that provide all the known essential nutrients in quantities that will support wound healing, anabolism, weight gain or maintenance, and growth in children. All TPN solutions contain water, protein, carbohydrates, fat, vitamins, and trace elements. The various proportions of each element are individualized to the patient's unique clinical situation and needs.

TPN solutions usually consist of 25% to 35% dextrose, 3% to 5% amino acids, electrolytes, minerals, and vitamins. Intravenous fat emulsions in 10% to 20% concentrations also may be added. Dextrose and fat are given for their caloric value. The body uses them to meet its energy needs. This permits the administered amino acids to be utilized for anabolism. Fat provides twice the caloric value of dextrose, exerts minimal osmotic pressure, and prevents fatty acid deficiency. Regular insulin may be added to the solution or given to support glucose utilization.

TPN solutions provide good culture media for bacteria. They are therefore prepared under strict aseptic conditions in the pharmacy under a laminar airflow hood. The solutions are kept refrigerated until ready for use and are left at room temperature for 30 minutes before administration. Prepared formulas ideally should be used within 24 hours to prevent contamination, but institutional protocols may vary slightly.

TPN solutions are started slowly and advanced as patient tolerance permits. Blood glucose levels are checked frequently at the beginning of treatment while endogenous insulin production adjusts to the increased

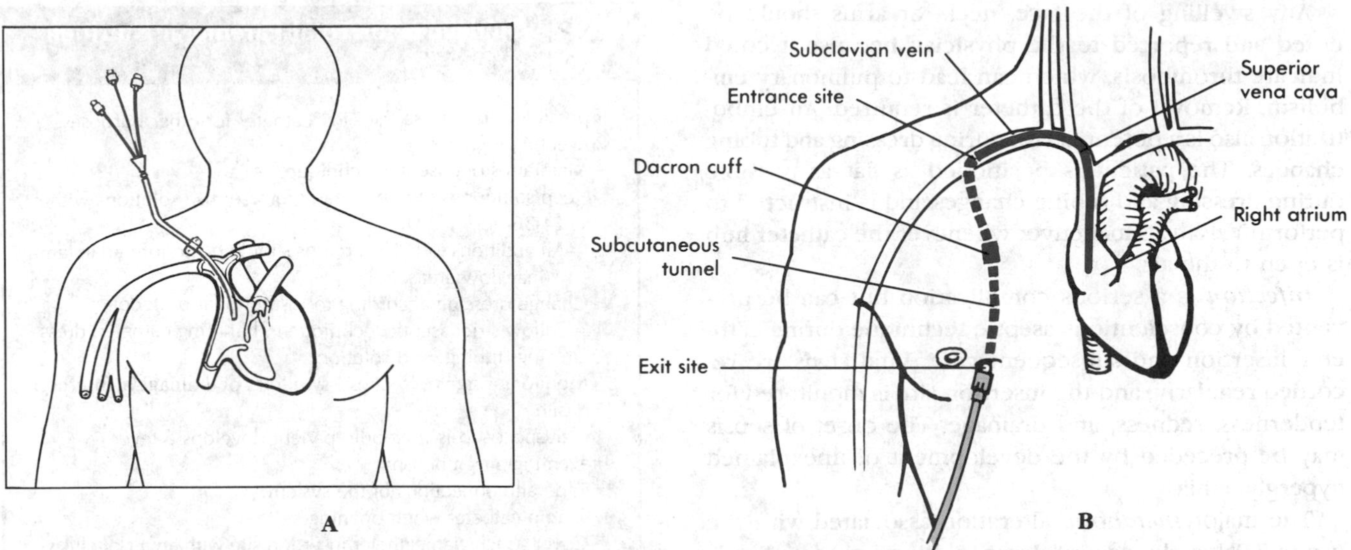


**FIGURE 47-12** **A,** Multilumen central venous (subclavian) catheter. **B,** Hickman tunneled catheter. (**A** from LaRocca JC, Otto SE: *Pocket guide to intravenous therapy,* ed 2, St Louis, 1993, Mosby.)

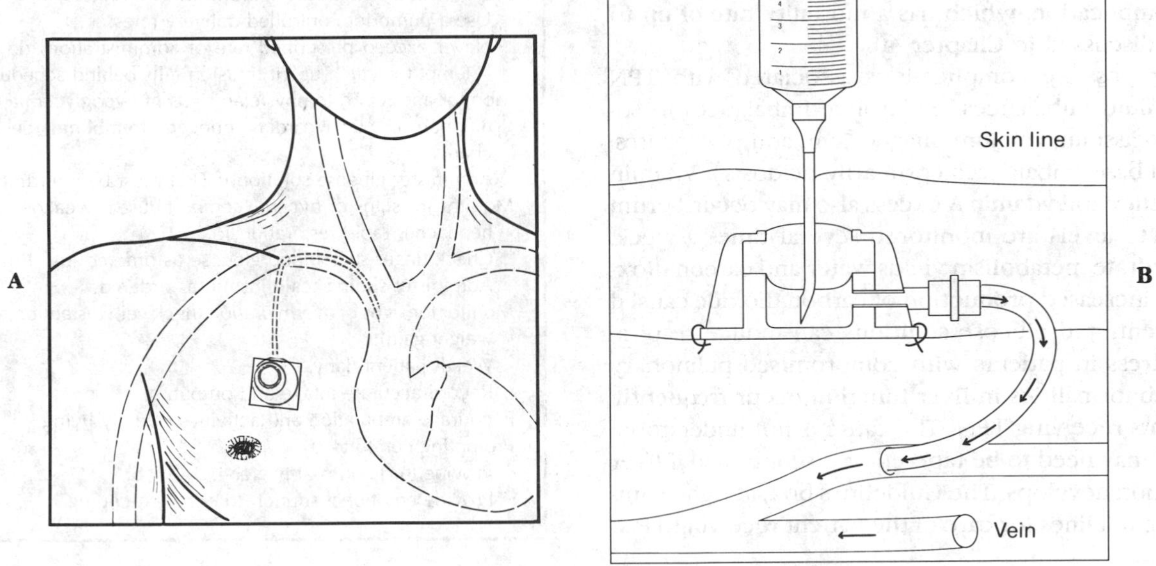


**FIGURE 47-13** **A,** Implantable port. **B,** Cross section of port with needle access. (From LaRocca JC, Otto SE: *Pocket guide to intravenous therapy,* ed 2, St Louis, 1993, Mosby.)

glucose load. A steady infusion rate is ensured through the use of a pump controller. If TPN administration needs to be interrupted for any reason, infusions of at least 5% dextrose should be administered to prevent rebound hypoglycemia. TPN administration should be tapered and not abruptly discontinued. Lipid emulsions may be mixed with the TPN solution, given through a separate peripheral IV line or a Y connector in the main IV line close to the catheter hub. The large size of the fat molecules necessitates the use of unfiltered tubing. The use of filters with TPN solutions remains controversial. The purpose of filters is to reduce bacterial contamination, but concern exists that these filters also may absorb drugs. Institutional protocols vary.

### Preventing complications

Complications of TPN may be mechanical, infectious, or metabolic. *Mechanical* problems may include pneumothorax, hemothorax, air embolism, catheter misplacement, brachial plexus injury, and thromboembolism. These complications are rare with correct catheter insertion and maintenance.

Any swelling of the face, neck, or arms should be noted and reported to the physician because it could indicate thrombosis, which can lead to pulmonary embolism. Removal of the catheter is required. Air embolization also is a potential risk during dressing and tubing changes. The patient is positioned as flat as possible during dressing and tubing changes and is instructed to perform Valsalva's maneuver whenever the catheter hub is open to the air.

*Infection* is a serious complication but can be prevented by conscientious aseptic technique during catheter insertion and subsequent care. Vital signs are recorded regularly, and the insertion site is monitored for tenderness, redness, and drainage. The onset of sepsis may be preceded by the development of unexplained hyperglycemia.

The major *metabolic* alteration associated with the use of TPN is glucose intolerance. Blood glucose levels must be carefully monitored through finger sticks every 6 hours. Insulin may be added to the TPN solution or administered on a sliding scale if needed. Severe osmotic diuresis can result from uncontrolled hyperglycemia and may lead to hyperglycemic, hyperosmolar, nonketotic coma (HHNC), particularly in elderly persons. This serious complication, which has a mortality rate of up to 50%, is discussed in Chapter 40.

Other possible complications associated with TPN include fluid imbalances; electrolyte imbalances in sodium, potassium, calcium, magnesium, and phosphates; and acid-base imbalances (primarily acidosis). Vitamin D deficiency and vitamin A excess also may occur. Serum electrolyte levels are monitored several times a week. Carbohydrate metabolism yields water and carbon dioxide. The increased production of carbon dioxide caused by concentrated glucose solutions can induce respiratory distress in patients with compromised pulmonary status. Abnormalities in liver function occur frequently in patients receiving TPN. The cause is not understood, but TPN may need to be tapered or discontinued if liver dysfunction develops. The Guidelines box, at right, summarizes guidelines for care of the patient receiving TPN.

### Guidelines for Total Parenteral Nutrition

If possible, do not use the TPN catheter for other purposes.

Preventing infection:
- Maintain strict aseptic technique.
- Keep solutions cold until ready for use; use solutions within 24-36 hr.
  - —All additions to TPN solutions should be performed in laminar flow areas.
- Change dressing according to institutional protocol.
  - —Follow strict aseptic technique in handling catheter, dressing, tubing, and solution.
- Monitor for signs of redness, swelling, or drainage at insertion site.
  - —Suspect sepsis if afebrile patient develops a fever.

Preventing air embolism:
- Tape all connections of the system.
- Clamp catheter when opening system.
- Cover subclavian catheter insertion site with an air-occlusive dressing (covered with adhesive tape) or transparent polyurethane (Op-site) dressing.
- Position patient as flat as possible for dressing and tubing changes.
- Instruct patient to perform Valsalva's maneuver whenever catheter hub is open to the air.

Maintaining fluid and electrolyte balance:
- Maintain a continuous uniform infusion rate.
- Use a pump for controlled delivery rates.
- Never exceed prescribed rate of administration; do not attempt to "catch up" if infusion falls behind schedule.

Monitor and report to physician signs of *hypoglycemia* (pallor, diaphoresis, tachycardia, hunger, trembling, behavioral changes):
- Administer glucose solution if TPN must be interrupted.

Monitor for signs of *hyperglycemia* (nausea, weakness, thirst, headache, rapid respirations):
- Check finger-stick blood glucose as ordered (q 6 hr).
- Administer sliding scale insulin as ordered.

Monitor for signs of *overhydration* (neck vein distention, cough, weight gain):
- Weigh patient daily.
- Record accurate intake and output.

Encourage ambulation and activities of daily living.

Promoting comfort:
- Provide for good oral hygiene.
- Provide emotional support to enhance coping.

### Home parenteral nutrition

The administration of total parenteral nutrition in the home setting—**home total parenteral nutrition (HTPN)**—has allowed thousands of patients to avoid dependence on the acute care hospital and resume their lives in the community. More than $170 million is expended annually to achieve this goal. The largest percentage of patients receiving HTPN have inflammatory bowel disease (about 38%). Most of these patients require lifelong nutritional support. Advanced cancer, AIDS, and swallowing disorders are other common problems that require long-term parenteral nutrition. Most patients with chronic bowel problems can return to productive employment when their disease is controlled, but insurance stipulations frequently require that recipients be unemployed to receive disability benefits. Because HTPN costs $40,000 to $80,000 a year, this reimbursement is absolutely essential for most families.

Families often experience anxiety related to learning about the complicated technologic care required for HTPN. However, the tremendous improvement in the patient's condition as a result of TPN is a great motivator. Nevertheless, over time, as the procedure becomes an accepted part of daily activities, it is not uncommon for patients to have problems with depression related to loss of control, cost factors, and lifelong dependence. Food and eating are associated with many social and emotional rewards in our society. Disruption of these patterns removes a major source of pleasure for the patient. Relationship and role changes within the family are almost inevitable. Caregivers and patients fre-

## RESEARCH

Heaphey L: Survey results provide insight into psychosocial issues, *Lifeline Lett Oley Foundation* 9(6):1-2, 1988.

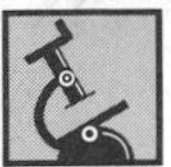

A survey by the Oley Foundation of 172 HTPN families indicates that family members' and patients' perspectives differ on the problems experienced and the resources most helpful in adapting to HTPN. Spouses reported guilt about their ability to eat, distress at social gatherings with food, and concern about eating out. However, patients indicated that a spouse's ability to eat and eating out were not problems. Body image distortions and sexual difficulties were problems patients ranked as continuing and significant, although spouses did not report these as important issues. The third-ranked problem listed by both patient and spouse was "relationships with spouse," especially communication. Yet patients ranked their spouse as their number-one resource for helping with psychosocial problems. The nurse from the physician's office or home care service was ranked second, gastroenterologist third, hospital nurse fourth, and another family member fifth. Very few patients listed another HTPN patient or someone outside the family as a helpful resource.

## BOX 47-6 Sample Teaching Plan for Home Total Parenteral Nutrition

Review purpose and procedures for the HTPN regimen.
Validate presence of detailed written instructions for each procedure and piece of equipment.
Validate understanding of all home equipment:
  Provide additional instruction as needed inasmuch as equipment and supplies used in the hospital frequently differ from those available through home health care.
Validate aseptic technique and skills.
Evaluate adequacy of home refrigeration and supply storage.
Teach patient/family about ordering replacement supplies.
Establish record keeping system for body weights, temperatures, finger sticks, and sliding scale insulin if ordered.
Reinforce importance of aseptic technique and safe disposal of equipment.
Discuss trouble shooting of common equipment problems.
Review symptoms related to infection, air embolism, and other complications; provide written instructions of actions to be taken in the event of a complication.
Provide listing of appropriate emergency telephone numbers.

## TABLE 47-9 Potential Problems of Home Total Parenteral Nutrition

General Guidelines to Prevent HTPN Problems:
- Wash hands thoroughly before any procedures.
- Wear gloves for all procedures, particularly if cuts, scrapes, or rashes are present on the hands.
- Keep all supplies dry and sterile during storage.
- Use aseptic technique for any procedures.

| PROBLEM | SYMPTOMS | PATIENT INSTRUCTIONS |
|---|---|---|
| Possible leak in internal catheter | Swelling of skin over catheter insertion site; sensations of pain, heat, burning near site | Call home health nurse or physician.<br>Do not use catheter to give fluids.<br>Tape the catheter securely to the skin so that it does not dangle.<br>Avoid rough contact or sports that could dislodge catheter. |
| Possible loose cap or leak in external catheter | Leak of blood from injection cap or catheter | Clamp catheter.<br>Change cap and heparin lock.<br>Call physician or go to emergency room for catheter repair. |
| Water intoxication | Puffy eyes, neck vein distention, increased urination, and confusion | Contact physician and go to emergency room for laboratory tests. |
| Possible air embolism—air may be drawn into the vein if catheter is not clamped during cap change | Cough, shortness of breath, chest pain | If giving fluids, stop and place heparin lock on catheter.<br>Lie on left side.<br>Call physician or go to emergency room. |
| Skin infection or irritation | Redness, swelling, drainage, tenderness at exit site | Call home health care nurse or physician.<br>Change bandage and clean daily. |
| Possible infection within the bloodstream | Chills, fever, fatigue, aches, weakness, hyperglycemia | Change the bandage and clean around the catheter if bandage gets wet or soiled.<br>Go to emergency room for tests. |

quently see the issue very differently (see Research box, p. 1561).

**Nursing management of home total parenteral nutrition.** Acute care medical centers and commercial home care agencies have developed skilled teams to assist patients and families with learning to administer and manage HTPN. A nutrition-support team, if available, usually initiates the educational process before the patient's discharge. The nurse typically coordinates the home care team, which may include the physician, dietitian, social worker, pharmacist, and counselor or psychiatrist. Successful management demands a team approach. Patient teaching includes basic information about HTPN; discussion about symptoms, problems, and complications; and practical planning concerning the acquisition of equipment, location and storage of supplies, and special telephone service to cover emergencies. A sample teaching plan for HTPN is outlined in Box 47-6.

Once initial mastery of the technique has been achieved by the patient and/or caregiver, the nurse primarily monitors ongoing management of HTPN and assesses for complications. The nurse assesses the patient's ongoing physical status and determines whether improvement or deterioration is occurring. Factors include the patient's weight, condition of the catheter and insertion site, presence of fever or systemic signs of infection, blood glucose variations, and coping problems related to the therapy. A sample of common HTPN complications is summarized in Table 47-9. The ongoing adequacy of home resources is another concern. The nurse may need to solve problems relating to equipment availability and cost issues or arrange respite care for overwhelmed family members. The nurse also needs to offer support and encouragement to the patient and family caretaker. HTPN is a demanding therapy that requires a major time commitment. It is easy for caretakers to feel isolated and alone with the demands of the task.

Documentation is always a major and crucial issue in home care. Standard Medicare reimbursement is limited to 2 to 3 weeks of intermittent visits. Ongoing professional involvement by the nurse depends on clear documentation of exceptional circumstances that support that need. Documentation also is a crucial component of quality assurance determinations. The data may be used to project trends, identify personnel needs, test treatment protocols, establish the cost effectiveness of nursing interventions, and plan for future services.

# INTESTINAL OBSTRUCTION

## ETIOLOGY

Normal functioning of the small and large intestines depends on the presence of an open lumen or passageway for the movement of intestinal contents, as well as adequate circulation and nervous innervation to sustain rhythmic peristalsis. Any factor or condition that either narrows that intestinal passageway or interferes with peristalsis can result in bowel obstruction. Obstructions commonly are classified as either mechanical (affecting the intestinal lumen) or nonmechanical (related to peristalsis) and can be either partial or complete.

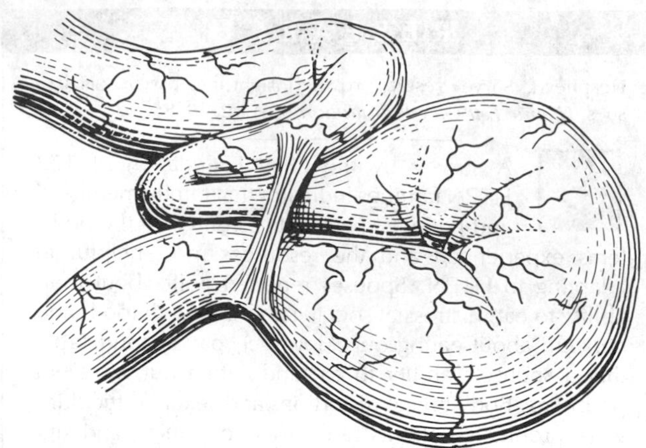

**FIGURE 47-14** A band of adhesions causing intestinal obstruction in the small bowel.

### Causes of Mechanical Obstruction

**Adhesions.** Adhesions may form after abdominal surgery for unknown reasons, perhaps related to inflammatory responses in the healing bowel. Adhesions are the most common cause of small bowel obstruction, accounting for about 60%.[5] In some persons the adhesions may become massive. The fibrous bands of scar tissue can loop over bowel segments, either causing the bowel to kink or compressing the loop with external pressure (Figure 47-14).

**Hernias.** A hernia can result in bowel obstruction if the abdominal wall defect through which the hernia protrudes becomes so tight that the bowel segment becomes strangulated. (See p. 1568 for a discussion of abdominal hernias.)

**Tumor.** A tumor mass gradually will restrict the internal lumen of the bowel as it enlarges. Eventually a fecal mass may be unable to pass through the constriction, leading to partial or complete obstruction. Bowel cancer accounts for approximately 80% of obstructions of the large intestine, with most occurring in the sigmoid colon.[5] (See p. 1569 for a discussion of bowel cancer.)

**Volvulus.** A twisting of the bowel upon itself, usually at least a full 180 degrees, obstructing the intestinal lumen both proximally and distally, is called a **volvulus,** (Figure 47-15). The acute obstruction can quickly result in bowel infarction and can be life-threatening as a result of necrosis, perforation, and peritonitis.

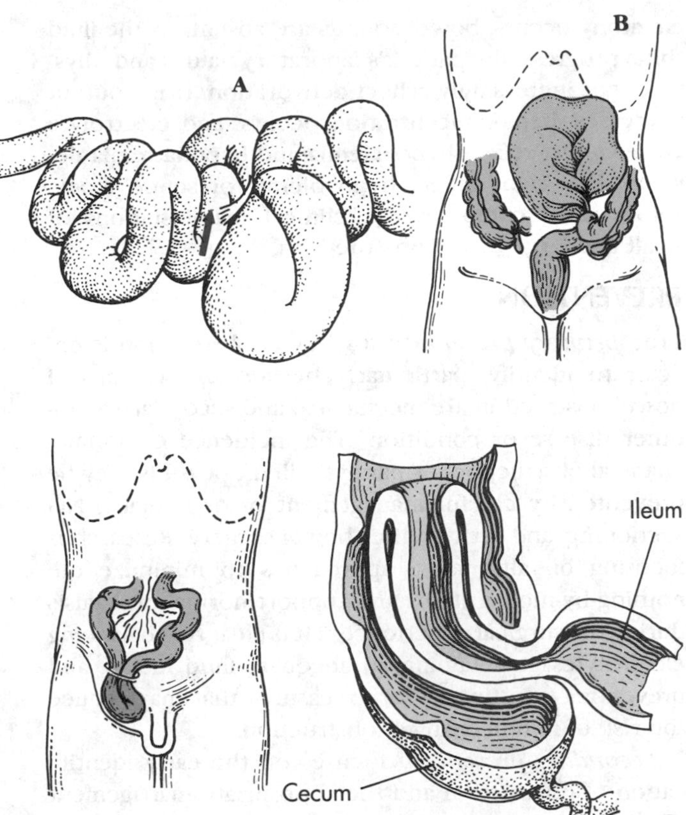


FIGURE 47-15 Common causes of intestinal obstruction. **A,** Constriction by adhesions. **B,** Volvulus of the sigmoid colon. **C,** Strangulated inguinal hernia. **D,** Ileocecal intussusception.

**Intussusception. Intussusception** involves a telescoping of the bowel on itself (see Figure 47-15). The invagination occurs with peristalsis and, in the adult, often is triggered by the presence of a tumor mass. The bowel segment containing the mass is propelled by peristalsis into the adjacent bowel segment. Constriction is immediate, and strangulation of the trapped segment can develop.

Other possible causes of mechanical obstruction include fecal impaction, gallstones, strictures resulting from diverticulitis, and IBD.

### Causes of Nonmechanical Obstruction

**Paralytic ileus.** Adynamic or **paralytic ileus** results from a lack of peristaltic activity, usually as a result of neurogenic impairment. It is a common temporary problem after abdominal surgery, particularly if the bowel has been extensively handled. In addition to direct irritation, paralytic ileus also can occur as a response to major trauma, sepsis, and electrolyte imbalances (particularly hypokalemia).

**Mesenteric vascular occlusion infarction.** Any occlusion of the vascular supply to the bowel can interfere with bowel function. It may result from extensive atherosclerosis of the mesenteric arteries or mesenteric thrombosis. It is a possible complication of heart disease, particularly in elderly persons. The nature and extent of the problem are determined by the size of the occluded vessel and the length of the bowel segment affected. It may be symptomless, or it can cause reversible symptoms related to periodic ischemia or create an acute surgical emergency. The superior mesenteric arteries are the most common sites, affecting circulation to the distal jejunum and ileum.

## EPIDEMIOLOGY

Bowel obstruction can occur at any point in the life span. It occurs in both genders and all races. It is estimated that bowel obstruction is the cause of about 20% of all cases of acute abdominal pain.[5] Because bowel obstruction usually is a secondary effect of a primary problem, incidence statistics are unreliable. The close relationship of large bowel obstruction to cancer of the colon and small bowel obstruction to abdominal surgery and adhesions creates a few clear patterns. Obstruction is more common in elderly persons, who are more vulnerable to colon cancer. The occurrence of volvulus obstruction also has been tied to chronic constipation in elders.

## PATHOPHYSIOLOGY

Intestinal obstruction triggers a series of events in the GI tract whose clinical manifestations depend largely on the location of the obstruction and the degree of circulatory compromise. Approximately 7 to 10 L of electrolyte-rich fluid is secreted into the small intestine each day. In the normal bowel all but approximately 600 to 800 ml is reabsorbed before the chyme enters the cecum. About 200 ml is lost daily in the stool. Even when the forward movement of chyme is obstructed, GI secretion continues, at least initially. Fluid and air accumulate proximal to the site of the obstruction and create distention. There is an initial increase in peristaltic waves, increasing intraluminal pressure. This increase in peristalsis is an attempt to move the intestinal contents past the obstructed area. The increased peristaltic efforts usually are accompanied by colicky pain.

If these compensatory measures fail, the proximal intestine dilates, the smooth muscle becomes atonic, and peristalsis ceases. Elevated intraluminal pressure causes the bowel wall to become edematous, and increased capillary permeability allows massive amounts of isotonic fluid to move from the plasma and interstitial spaces into the distended bowel. Normal reabsorption processes in the bowel are blocked by the tissue edema and decreased mucosal blood flow. Gas accumulates in the bowel from both air swallowing and the action of intestinal bacteria on stagnant bowel contents. This worsens the abdominal distention. The stagnant and distended bowel also becomes increasingly permeable to bacteria. Organisms can enter the peritoneal cavity and lead to peritonitis. The loss of extracellular fluid can range from 2 to 6 L within 2 to 3 days of a mechanical bowel obstruction. The resulting hypovolemia may be mild or severe enough to compromise renal perfusion and induce dehydration, electrolyte imbalance, and shock. The release of bacterial endotoxins can lead to sepsis. The concentration of the blood can result in vascular thrombosis and intestinal gangrene. Mortality as a result of small bowel obstruction is 10% and 30% for large bowel obstruction. If the bowel is strangulated, these percentages rise to 20% in the small bowel and 60% in the large.[5]

Although the exact clinical manifestations vary depending on the site of the obstruction, abdominal pain is a relatively consistent symptom. Pain typically decreases as the obstruction worsens. Approximately 80% of all bowel obstructions are located in the small intestine where the bowel lumen is the smallest, and these obstructions usually are accompanied by vomiting, which may be profuse. During the early phases of obstruction, auscultation of bowel sounds typically reveals loud, frequent, high-pitched sounds. Once smooth muscle atony occurs, bowel sounds are absent. As the fluid shifts progress, the patient's laboratory values and physical signs increasingly reflect dehydration. Urine output decreases, hemoconcentration occurs, and electrolyte changes that reflect hypokalemia and hyponatremia develop. Late signs reflect hypovolemic or septic shock. Table 47-10 compares the clinical manifestations of small and large bowel obstructions.

**TABLE 47-10 Clinical Manifestations of Mechanical Small and Large Bowel Obstructions**

| | SMALL BOWEL | LARGE BOWEL |
|---|---|---|
| Etiology (major) | Adhesions, hernia | Tumor, stricture, etc. |
| Onset | Rapid | Gradual |
| Pain | Midportion to upper portion of abdomen, episodic, crampy; may become severe and continuous | Suprapubic, lower abdominal, colicky |
| Vomiting | Usually present; may be severe if higher portion of bowel involved; fecal odor if lower in small bowel | Late symptom; may be fecal if ileocecal valve fails |
| Abdominal distention | Present, usually nontender | Present in late stages |
| Bowel sounds | Early: high-pitched, tinkling, intermittent<br>Late: decreased or absent | Early: increased, high-pitched, crescendo or borborygmus sounds<br>Late: decreased or absent |
| Laboratory values | Rapid hyponatremia, hypokalemia, hemoconcentration | Late developing changes |

## PREVENTION

True *primary prevention* for bowel obstruction is difficult to identify, particularly because most types of bowel obstruction are mechanical and secondary to another disease or condition. The incidence of nonmechanical obstruction, or paralytic ileus, possibly may be prevented by careful management of oral intake, NG suctioning, and activity after bowel surgery. Research is focusing on alternative approaches to minimize the nothing-by-mouth status and support normal peristalsis during the surgical experience.[18] It is clear that balancing electrolytes, maintaining an adequate fluid intake, and preventing constipation are measures that may reduce the risk of nonmechanical obstruction.

*Secondary prevention* focuses on the early identification of obstruction and the appropriate management of associated primary disorders and conditions. The most significant of these is clearly the early identification of colorectal cancer (see p. 1571). Patients at risk for obstruction—for example, persons with IBD, extensive abdominal surgery, or bowel atony—should be informed of the symptoms associated with obstruction so that they can know when to seek medical evaluation.

## MEDICAL MANAGEMENT

Intestinal obstruction is diagnosed primarily from its clinical manifestations. In addition, abdominal radiographs generally show clear patterns of air and fluid entrapment in the obstructed area. Obstruction cannot be ruled out, however, by the presence of apparently normal x-ray findings. A barium enema may be used to localize the site of the obstruction if the risk of perforation is not great, but ingested barium will not be used because it cannot be excreted from the GI tract.

The goal for discharge of patients with bowel obstruction as determined by DRGs is 5 days. The nurse works collaboratively with the physician for implementation of prescribed medical therapy. Because the nurse has a major role in discharge planning and patient teaching, these are discussed under nursing management.

### Diagnostic Tests

There are no laboratory tests that can confirm or rule out a diagnosis of bowel obstruction. WBC counts may be elevated in the presence of strangulation but otherwise are normal. Once hypovolemia becomes severe, hemoconcentration elevates hemoglobin and hematocrit values and serum potassium levels typically fall.

### Medication

Pharmacologic treatment plays no real role in the management of bowel obstruction. Analgesics rarely are used, even in the presence of moderate to severe abdominal pain. Their negative effects on peristalsis mitigate against their use, and the pattern and severity of the pain may be important in establishing a correct diagnosis. Antibiotics may be administered to counter the effects of the significant overgrowth of bacteria in the bowel.

### Treatment

The treatment of bowel obstruction is directed toward relieving the obstruction, if possible, and correcting the fluid and electrolyte imbalances. Intervention usually begins with nasogastric or intestinal intubation to decompress the abdomen. This procedure usually is successful in removing gas and fluid. Decompression also typically relieves any associated vomiting and prevents aspiration. In cases of partial obstruction, decompression alone may relieve the problem.

Intestinal tubes may be used if the obstruction is located in the small intestine. Intestinal tubes are longer (180 to 300 cm) to permit passage into the intestinal tract. They are constructed with a small balloon at the tip that, when filled with water or mercury, acts like a bolus of food and stimulates peristalsis. The tube advances in this way along the intestinal tract. Even in the absence of peristalsis, the weighted tip usually is able to pull the tube along. Intestinal tubes are avoided by some physicians because their insertion is more difficult and uncomfortable for the patient. Common examples of intestinal tubes (Figure 47-16) include the following:

*Cantor tube.* A single-lumen 300-cm tube with just one opening used for drainage; its balloon is injected with 4 to 5 ml of mercury before insertion of the tube.

*Harris tube.* A single-lumen 180-cm tube with a metal tip; its single lumen is used for drainage or irrigation and is weighted with a prefilled mercury balloon.

*Miller-Abbott tube.* A double-lumen 300-cm tube with markings to indicate how far it has passed. One lumen leads to the balloon, which is filled with mercury after it has been inserted; the second lumen has openings along its course to allow for drainage and irrigation.

*Dennis tube.* A three-lumen 300-cm tube with one lumen for suction, one for irrigation or venting, and one for insertion of mercury into a distal balloon.

### Diet

No particular dietary management is associated with bowel obstruction. The patient is given nothing by mouth during the acute period. Ice chips may be permitted to relieve the thirst and dry mouth associated with hypovolemia and nasogastric or intestinal intubation. The patient is restarted gradually on a regular diet, with an emphasis on the prevention of constipation.

### Activity

No specific activity restrictions are necessary for the treatment of bowel obstruction. Initially the patient rests in bed in response to abdominal pain, distention, and possible vomiting. Once the acute period is past, the patient is encouraged to be up and ambulating to support the return of effective peristalsis and the expulsion of gas.

### Referral/Consultation

Referral to consultants usually is not necessary in the management of bowel obstruction. Surgical correction of the obstruction frequently is required if the underlying cause is mechanical. Then referral to a general surgeon is the standard practice.

## SURGICAL MANAGEMENT

Surgical correction of mechanical bowel obstruction frequently is necessary after bowel decompression. Specific surgical procedures depend on the nature and location of the obstruction. Release of adhesions, bowel resection with reanastamosis or temporary colostomy, or embolectomy may be the appropriate procedure. The existence or development of bowel strangulation or vascular compromise necessitates that corrective surgery be performed on an emergent basis. Discussion of care of the patient undergoing bowel surgery begins on p. 1584.

## NURSING MANAGEMENT

### ♦ ASSESSMENT

### Subjective Data

Subjective data to be collected to assess the patient with an intestinal obstruction include the following:

- Abdominal pain, initially colicky in nature
  - Gradually decreasing severity
- Bloating and distention
- Nausea
- Knowledge of diagnosis and planned treatment

### Objective Data

Objective data to be collected to assess the patient with an intestinal obstruction include the following:

- Visible peristaltic waves (early)
- Unequal bowel sounds in different abdominal quadrants
- Borborygmi (early)
- Absence of bowel sounds (late)

Abdominal distention
- Taut shiny skin over abdomen
- Increasing abdominal girth

Vomiting
- Early and profuse if obstruction above ileum
- Foul odor, possible fecal contamination

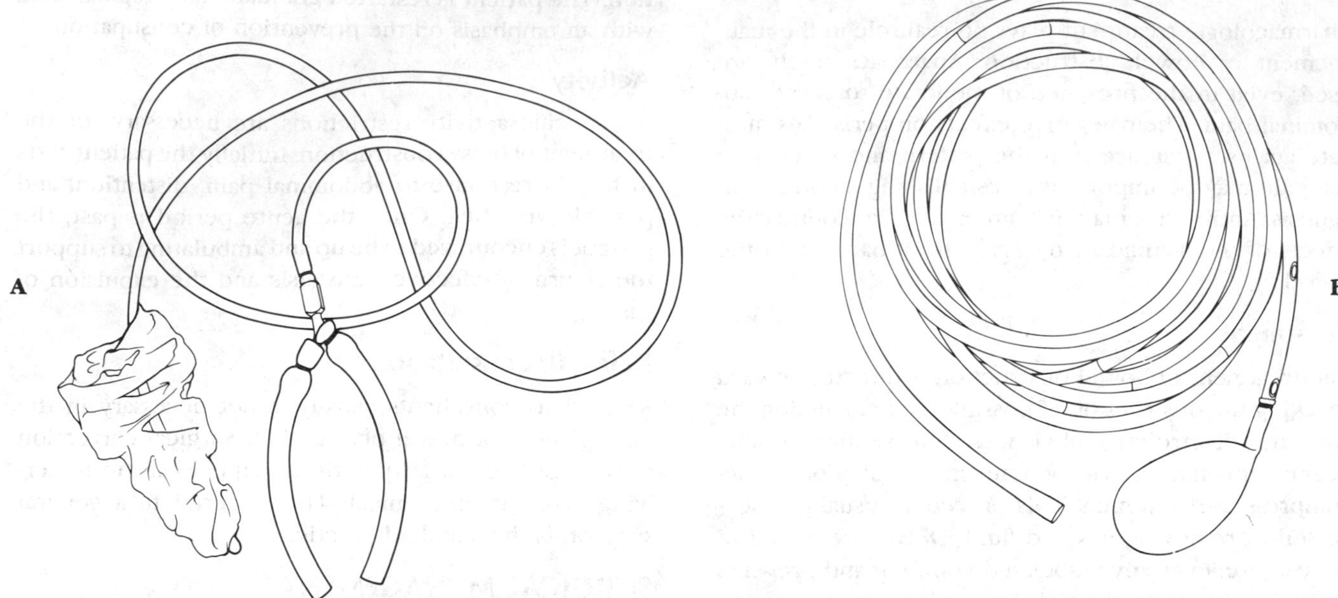


**FIGURE 47-16** Intestinal tubes. **A,** Miller-Abbott tube. **B,** Cantor tube.

Fecal breath odor
Obstipation (passage of neither stool nor gas)
Singultus (hiccups)

## Diagnostic Test Findings

1. Diagnosis established primarily from symptoms
2. Abdominal radiographs showing air and fluid in obstructed area
3. Laboratory tests indicating hypovolemia: elevated hemoglobin and hematocrit values, hypokalemia

## ♦ NURSING DIAGNOSES

Nursing diagnoses are determined from analysis of patient data. Nursing diagnoses for the patient with an intestinal obstruction may include but are not limited to the following:

| Diagnostic Title | Possible Etiologic Factors |
|---|---|
| Fluid volume deficit | Loss of reabsorption in the bowel; fluid shifts |
| Pain | Abdominal distention, hyperperistalsis |

## ♦ EXPECTED PATIENT OUTCOMES

Expected patient outcomes for the patient with an intestinal obstruction may include but are not limited to the following:

1. Exhibits physical signs of fluid balance: body weight returns to baseline; good skin turgor and moist mucous membranes; vital signs in normal range for patient; serum electrolytes and hematocrit values within normal limits; and urine specific gravity of 1.010 to 1.025.
2. Verbalizes that pain is decreased or absent.

## ♦ INTERVENTIONS

### Promoting Fluid and Electrolyte Balance

Nursing management focuses on careful monitoring of all physical parameters. The nurse monitors the patient's vital signs, urine output, and NG output frequently. Changes are compared with the symptoms of early shock (see Chapter 22). The nurse administers IV fluids as ordered and monitors for symptoms of electrolyte imbalance. Fluid replacement is provided for all patients with intestinal obstruction because fluid losses usually are significant. Supplemental potassium usually is added to IV lines to compensate for losses through vomiting and fluid shifts.

Third spacing of fluids is typical with intestinal obstruction. The nurse assesses for edema and measures abdominal girth every 2 to 4 hours. Fluid losses and shifts trigger nagging thirst, and small amounts of ice chips may be comforting. Frequent oral hygiene is offered or provided by the nurse.

### Relieving Pain and Discomfort

General comfort measures include positioning the patient with the head of the bed elevated to relieve abdominal pressure and providing frequent position changes. A side-lying position often is the most comfortable. Oral and nasal care is offered every 2 to 4 hours to counter the drying and irritating effects of the NG tube and nothing-by-mouth status.

The nurse regularly assesses the patient's pain and records the response that is obtained to all interventions. Analgesics rarely are given to patients with bowel obstruction; thus it is critical for the nurse to explore non-

### Guidelines for Care of the Person With an Intestinal Tube

**FACILITATING MOVEMENT OF THE TUBE**

Position patient:
- Two hours on right side
- Two hours on back with head elevated
- Two hours on left side

Encourage ambulation once tube has passed the pylorus (assessed by radiograph).

Gently advance the tube 2-10 cm (1-4 inches) as prescribed to provide slack for movement.

Do not tape tube until desired location has been reached; pin extra tubing to clothing.

**FACILITATING DRAINAGE**

Use intermittent low suction with single-lumen tubes to prevent mucosal injury.

Constant suction may be used with sump action tubes.

Use normal saline to irrigate tube if there is no drainage or patient becomes nauseated.
- It is rarely possible to aspirate returns back through a long intestinal tube.

**PROMOTING COMFORT**

Tape tube securely to nostril once the desired location has been reached.

Pin tube to clothing to support its weight.

Apply water-soluble lubricant to nares for comfort and to prevent secretion crusting.

Provide frequent mouth care:
- Offer hard candy and occasional ice chips.
- Provide throat lozenges or saline rinses for sore throat.

Assess mucous membranes for signs of irritation or infection.

pharmacologic measures to increase comfort. If the patient's pain increases significantly or shifts from a cramping to a constant character, it should be reported promptly. It may indicate strangulation or perforation of the bowel.

The patient may be extremely anxious during the initial treatment period. It is important for the nurse to explain all tests, procedures, and planned care thoroughly. Support and reassurance are important, especially if corrective bowel surgery is planned.

The nasogastric or intestinal tube that is inserted to decompress the abdomen also increases the patient's comfort as excess gas and fluid are eliminated. These tubes are connected to intermittent or continuous suction depending on the location and structure. Output from the tube is carefully measured and recorded. Nursing care associated with the use of an intestinal tube is summarized in the Guidelines box above.

## ♦ EVALUATION

To evaluate the effectiveness of nursing interventions, compare patient behaviors with those stated in the expected patient outcomes. Successful achievement of patient outcomes for the patient with an intestinal obstruction is indicated by the following:

1. Shows physical indicators of appropriate fluid balance: stable body weight; good skin turgor and moist mucous membranes; stable vital signs in normal range for patient; serum hematocrit and electrolytes values within normal limits; and urine specific gravity of 1.010 to 1.025.
2. Has no abdominal pain.

## SPECIAL CONSIDERATIONS FOR CARE OF THE GERONTOLOGIC PATIENT

Of mechanical obstructions of the large bowel, 80% are caused by the presence of a tumor. Because bowel cancer affects primarily older adults, the elderly population is at particular risk for obstruction at this site. Large bowel obstructions tend to be less acute than do those of the small bowel, however, so that the risks to elders are not significant. The challenge primarily comes from dealing with the actual diagnosis of cancer and facing the possibility of needing ostomy surgery. The relatively brief period involved in the management of the bowel obstruction thus becomes less significant unless an acute strangulation or infarction has occurred. The necessary care and concerns are the same as for any other patient. Nursing care associated with bowel cancer is discussed beginning on p. 1574.

## HOME CARE CONSIDERATIONS

Discharge planning is tailored to the unique needs of the patient. Recovery from intestinal obstruction may be prolonged or swift based on the location and severity of the obstruction. Many patients will have undergone surgery to relieve the obstruction. Home care needs revolve around issues related to wound healing, reestablishing a normal diet, and regular bowel habits. Teaching is provided concerning the prevention of constipation through a fiber-rich diet, adequate fluids, and exercise.

Patients who undergo colostomy surgery because of cancer or bowel complications need ongoing support and supervision as they adjust to new self-care patterns. Referral to a home health care agency is initiated.

## COMPLICATIONS

The development of complications from bowel obstruction is related to the nature and severity of the obstructive process. Prompt diagnosis and intervention are crucial components. Early in the obstructive process patients may be vulnerable to hypovolemic shock. If the obstructed loop of bowel is strangulated or incarcerated (compromised blood flow plus necrosis), the risk of perforation, peritonitis, and septic shock is extremely high. Strangulation in the small bowel is associated with a 20% to 75% mortality. Strangulation in the large bowel causes a 60% mortality.[5] Age and comorbidity are clearly associated with poorer outcomes.

# ABDOMINAL HERNIAS

## ETIOLOGY/EPIDEMIOLOGY

A **hernia** is a protrusion of an organ or structure from its normal cavity through a congenital or acquired defect, usually in the muscle of the abdominal wall. Depending on its location, the hernia may contain peritoneum, omentum, a loop of bowel, or a section of bladder. Hernias can develop in the abdominal wall through a weakness or opening in the muscle wall at the umbilicus, at the site of a previous incision, or adjacent to a colostomy or ileostomy stoma. Inguinal and umbilical hernias usually result from congenital weakness of the muscle, whereas incisional hernias typically develop as a complication of surgery.

The most important factors in the development of a hernia are congenital or acquired muscle weakness and intraabdominal pressure increases related to heavy lifting, obesity, and pregnancy. Hernias can occur at any age and are more common in men and elders.

Hernias of the groin are by far the most common type and are the result of primary muscular defects. They account for approximately 80% of all hernias. *Indirect inguinal* hernias develop from weakness of the abdominal wall at the point through which the spermatic cord emerges in the male during fetal development. A parallel weakness is found in the female from the emergence of the round ligament. Indirect hernias are much more common in men than in women. The higher incidence probably is explained by the need for the testes to pass through the inguinal ring in fetal development. Indirect inguinal hernias account for more than 50% of the total hernia incidence. Figure 47-17 illustrates the indirect inguinal hernia. The protruded bowel may rest in the inguinal canal or move down into the scrotum in males and, on rare occasions, into the labia in females.

*Direct inguinal hernias* pass through the posterior inguinal wall at a point of muscle weakness. They typically are caused by increased intraabdominal pressure. These hernias also occur more frequently in men. They are the most technically difficult to repair and are likely to recur after surgery. They occur most often in elderly persons.

*Femoral hernias* develop when a loop of intestine passes through the femoral ring and down the femoral canal. They appear as a round bulge below the inguinal ligament and are thought to be caused by changes related to pregnancy in women. Femoral hernias are rare in men.

Several other terms are used to describe abdominal hernias and reflect the severity of the problem. A *sliding* hernia moves freely in and out of the hernia sac. If the protruding structure requires manipulation to return it to its proper position, the hernia is termed *reducible.* If the protruding structure cannot be returned to its proper position, the hernia is called *irreducible* or *incarcerated.* The term *incarcerated* usually is reserved for an irreducible hernia in which bowel obstruction occurs. The size of the defect largely determines whether the hernia can be reduced. When the blood flow to the trapped segment is compromised by pressure from the surrounding muscle ring, the hernia is said to be *strangulated.* Intestinal obstruction occurs, and gangrene of the viscera can develop rapidly.

## PATHOPHYSIOLOGY

The muscular portion of the abdominal wall consists of four overlapping muscle layers. The major pathologic concern associated with hernias is the constant risk of strangulation and bowel obstruction. Once present, hernias tend to extend and the risk of major complications increases.

The person with a hernia typically has a lump in the groin, around the umbilicus, or protruding from an old surgical incision. The lump or swelling may always have been present, or it may have appeared suddenly after coughing, straining, lifting, or other vigorous exertion. Hernias frequently cause no other symptoms. The pro-

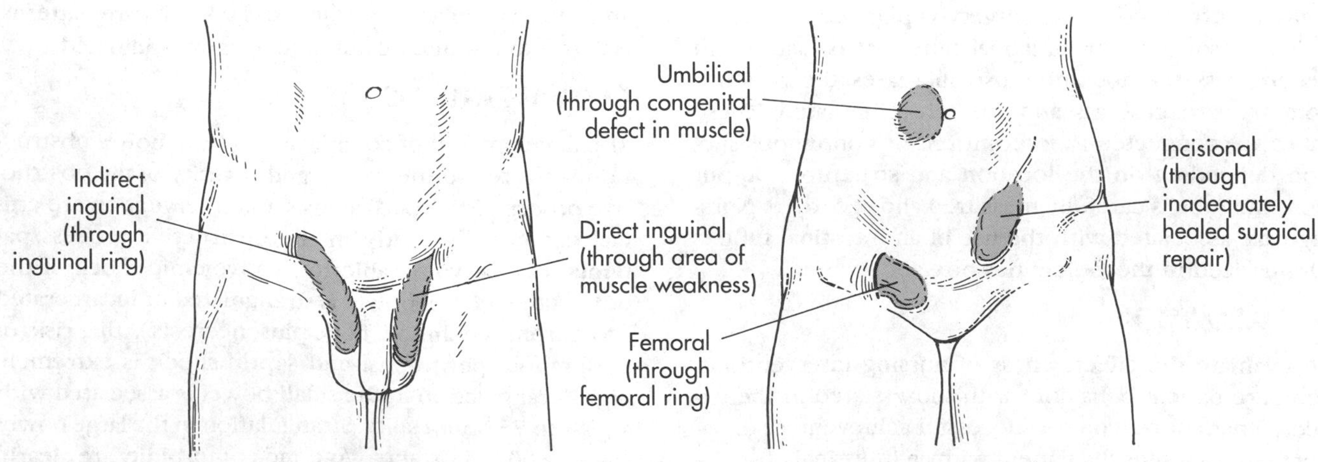


**FIGURE 47-17** Common sites of abdominal herniation.

trusion usually disappears when the person lies down and reappears with standing, coughing, or lifting.

The person may perceive a vague discomfort as the hernia contents slide in and out of the abdominal defect, but little actual pain is experienced as long as the hernia is freely reducible. A "dragging" sensation or feeling of heaviness is common, especially with groin hernias. If pain is present, it may be caused by local irritation of the parietal peritoneum or by traction on the omentum. An irreducible hernia may become strangulated, causing severe pain and symptoms of intestinal obstruction such as nausea, vomiting, and distention. These complications require emergency surgery, and a portion of bowel may have to be resected if gangrene develops from compromised circulation.

### MEDICAL MANAGEMENT

A diagnosis of hernia is readily established by reviewing the patient's history and results of the physical examination. Palpation of the herniated area reveals the contents of the sac as soft and nodular (omentum) or smooth and fluctuant (bowel). Fingertip palpation is used to feel the edges of the hernial ring and its contents by inserting the examining fingertip into the ring and feeling for the impulse as the person coughs. Attempts generally are not made to reduce strangulated hernias because of the high risk of rupture of the strangulated contents.

A femoral hernia may be palpated by placing the index finger of the right hand over the femoral artery in the patient's right leg. The middle finger will then lie over the femoral vein, and the ring finger will lie over the femoral canal. As the person coughs, the examiner's fingertips will feel the movement if the herniated sac is in the canal area.

Hernias should always be repaired by elective surgery if at all possible. Strangulation is an everpresent risk, and if it should occur, the surgical repair would need to be performed on an emergent basis. This emergency surgery is accompanied by a high incidence of postoperative complications. Hernia surgery often is performed in ambulatory surgical centers with the patient under local or spinal anesthesia.

The patient is discharged directly home after the repair. Before surgery the patient should be free of upper respiratory symptoms such as sneezing or coughing that could weaken the repair. The herniated tissues are returned to the abdominal cavity, and the defect in the fascia or muscle is closed with sutures (herniorrhaphy). To prevent recurrence of the hernia and to facilitate closure of the defect, a *hernioplasty* may be performed. This procedure uses fascia or a variety of synthetic materials to strengthen the muscle wall.

### NURSING MANAGEMENT

Recovery from hernia repair usually is rapid and without incident. Standard postoperative interventions are employed, but the nurse encourages the patient to deep breathe rather than cough. Fluid and food are resumed as tolerated. Ice bags are applied after inguinal hernia repair to minimize edema, particularly in the scrotum. A scrotal support may make initial ambulation easier and less painful. Fluids are encouraged, and IV infusions are continued until the patient is able to successfully empty the bladder.

Discharge teaching includes the avoidance of any heavy lifting, pushing, or pulling for about 6 weeks. Driving and stair climbing initially are restricted. The nurse instructs the patient to monitor the incision for signs of infection. Postoperative ecchymosis should disappear in a few days. Stool softeners or bulk laxatives usually are prescribed to prevent straining at defecation. The nurse also reassures the patient that sexual functioning is not affected by the surgery and may be resumed once healing is complete and comfort assured.

## COLORECTAL CANCER

### ETIOLOGY

The cause of bowel cancer remains elusive despite extensive research. Environmental factors are clearly implicated inasmuch as the incidence rates vary substantially worldwide. Diet has received the most attention in recent years. Because the cancer is significantly more common in industrialized societies, research has focused on the detrimental role of a diet that is low in fiber and high in fat, protein, and refined carbohydrates. The results are inconclusive and a direct causative relationship has not been proved, but the trends are strongly suggestive. It is theorized that by unclear mechanisms harmless foodstuffs are transformed in the bowel into metabolic and bacterial end products that act as carcinogens. Low-fiber diets increase colon transit time and increase the overall contact time of the mucosa with these carcinogenic agents.

A genetic link in colorectal cancer has been recognized for many years. New research indicates that approximately one in seven cases of colon cancer can be traced to a mutant gene that creates a predisposition to cancer by promoting mutations in other genes. It is estimated that some form of cancer will develop in 95% of persons carrying the defect, with colorectal cancer developing in 60%.[27] Future testing will focus on persons with a strong family history of colon cancer (three or more relatives with the disease, at least one younger than 50 years of age), and it is hoped that simplified screening techniques will be available within 5 to 10 years.

The risk of colon cancer also is strongly associated with long-standing ulcerative colitis, granulomas, adenomas, and familial polyposis. The presence of an adenoma in the colon is considered to be a primary risk factor. However, even though virtually all colon cancers appear to develop from adenomas, only about 5% of

**BOX 47-7 Risk Factors for Colorectal Cancer**

- Age > 40 years
- Diet low in fiber, and high in fat, protein, and refined carbohydrates
- Obesity (nature of the link is unclear at present)
- History of chronic constipation
- History of inflammatory bowel disease, polyposis, or colon polyps
- Family history of colon cancer
- Presence of a genetic defect that causes repeated gene mutations toward malignant growth

colon adenomas ever become malignant. Villous adenomas appear to have the highest potential for malignant growth. Familial polyposis is an autosomal dominant hereditary disorder that causes the early development of multiple adenomatous polyps in the colon and rectum. The risk of cancer reaches nearly 100% by midlife.[25] Risk factors are summarized in Box 47-7.

## EPIDEMIOLOGY

Cancer of the colon and rectum is the third most common type of cancer in men and second most common type in women. The mortality is second only to that of lung cancer. Approximately 147,000 new cases are diagnosed annually, with 60,000 deaths and an average 5-year survival rate of approximately 52%.[2] The mean age at onset is 63 to 67 years. The disease shows significant variations worldwide, but there have been only minor changes in the incidence and death rates in the United States in recent years. The incidence rates are significantly higher in the industrialized Western world than in Asia and Africa. The rates in immigrant families rapidly increase to match those of the larger society, however, again supporting a strong environmental and possibly dietary link. Approximately 50% of the tumors develop in the distal colon and rectum (Figure 47-18), and most of these develop from adenomatous polyps. The incidence of right colon cancer has been increasing steadily in recent years, however, and occurs more frequently in women. The development of cancer in the small intestine is extremely rare and accounts for less than 1% of all GI tract malignant tumors.

## PATHOPHYSIOLOGY

Colorectal cancers are almost all adenocarcinomas that arise from the epithelial lining of the intestine. The cancer typically develops from adenomatous **polyps.** In the cecum and ascending colon the lesions grow as cauliflower-like masses that project into the lumen of the colon (Figure 47-19). These lesions may ulcerate, but obstruction is rare because of the semiliquid nature of the stool in this region. Over time the lesions penetrate the colon wall and extend into surrounding tissue. In

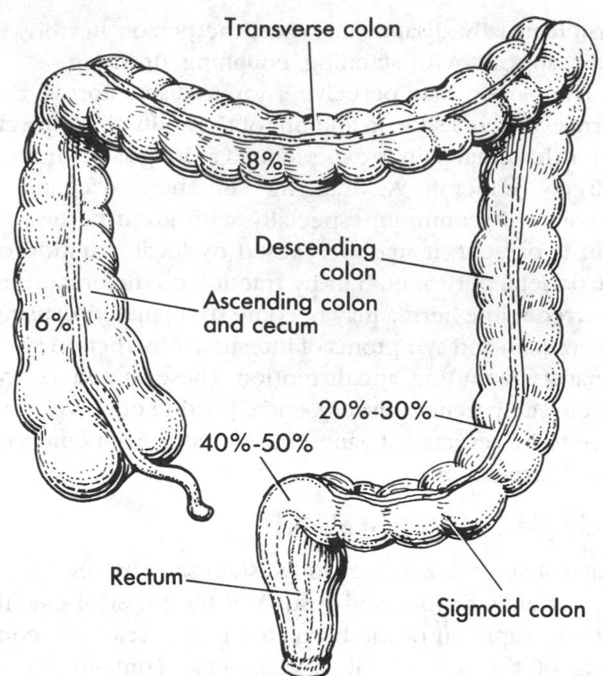


**FIGURE 47-18** Incidence of cancer in various segments of the colon and rectum.

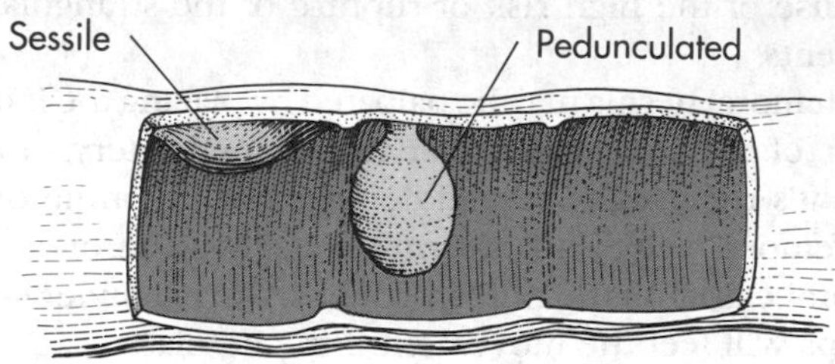


**FIGURE 47-19** Colon polyps.

the distal colon the lesions are more likely to be annular and placquelike. They grow circumferentially, encircling the colon wall. The lumen becomes narrow and constricted. Obstruction occurs when formed stool is unable to pass through the narrowed lumen.

Cancer of the colon may spread by direct extension or through the lymphatic or circulatory systems. It may seed at distant points in the peritoneum or at distant points in the colon. The liver and lungs are the major organs of metastasis. Box 47-8 summarizes the Dukes' classification system used for colorectal cancer. Note that the stage of bowel cancer is determined by the degree of invasion of the tumor and not its size. Staging is used to establish the appropriate level of intervention and treatment. Persons with stage A disease have an 80% to 90% 5-year survival rate; those with stage D have less than a 5% 5-year survival rate.

The clinical manifestations of colon cancer vary with the location of the tumor. There are often *no* early symp-

**BOX 47-8 Dukes' Classification of Colorectal Cancer**

Stage A: confined to bowel mucosa
Stage B: invading muscle wall
Stage C: lymph node involvement
Stage D: metastases or locally unresectable tumor

**BOX 47-9 Clinical Manifestations of Bowel Cancer**

| ASCENDING (RIGHT) COLON | DISTAL COLON/RECTUM |
|---|---|
| Occult blood in stool | Rectal bleeding |
| Anemia | Changed bowel habits |
| Anorexia and weight loss | Constipation or diarrhea |
| Abdominal pain (above umbilicus) | Pencil or ribbon-shaped stool |
| Palpable mass | Tenesmus |
| | Sensation of incomplete bowel emptying |

toms, particularly with cancer in the right ascending colon. Cancer in the distal colon and rectum typically produces symptoms related to partial obstruction. The patient may experience a change in bowel habits and rectal bleeding. The bleeding may be overt or occult.

Weakness, malaise, anorexia, anemia, and weight loss are nonspecific symptoms that occur frequently in patients with colorectal cancer. The tumor occasionally may perforate into the peritoneal cavity, and acute peritonitis occurs before the person notices any other signs of illness. The clinical manifestations of bowel cancer are summarized in Box 47-9.

## PREVENTION

### Primary Prevention

No specific primary prevention measures have proved effective against bowel cancer. All persons generally are encouraged to follow a high-fiber, low-fat diet, maintain an appropriate body weight, and avoid constipation. However, a research-based cause and effect relationship has not yet been established.

### Secondary Prevention

Secondary prevention primarily involves early detection. The American Cancer Society has developed recommended guidelines for screening persons older than 40 years of age (Box 47-10), but these suggestions are being carefully scrutinized in the light of rigorous new research studies. The importance of early detection is unquestioned, however. It is estimated that 75% of patients with colorectal cancer could be cured if the cancer were detected and treated early.[25]

**BOX 47-10 American Cancer Society's Recommended Guidelines for Early Detection of Colorectal Cancer**

Digital rectal examination yearly after age 40
Occult blood stool test yearly after age 50
Proctosigmoidoscopy every 5 years after age 50, following two negative results of yearly examinations

The value of digital rectal examination is unquestioned. Approximately 50% of colorectal cancers are found in the rectosigmoid area, and fully one third can be felt on a digital examination. **Sigmoidoscopy** with a flexible fiberoptic sigmoidoscope easily identifies more than 60% of colorectal cancers, with an accompanying 60% to 70% decrease in mortality.[25] The major drawbacks to routine screening are its unacceptability to patients and its potentially enormous cost if applied to the entire population over age 50. Study results are contradictory concerning the frequency of screening required. It appears, however, that 3- to 5-year intervals are clearly sufficient, and 10-year intervals eventually may be adequate for persons at low risk.[21] The issue of cost has no easy answer.

The routine use of fecal **occult blood** screening is being seriously reexamined. It has a high degree of patient acceptability and a relatively low cost, but its validity as a screening tool is questioned. In a major series of studies, fecal blood screening failed to detect more than 70% of colorectal cancers and 90% of polyps.[1] Both Hemo Quant and Hemoccult were shown to be similarly insensitive in symptom-free patients. Strong advocates for fecal blood screening exist as well, and the issue is unresolved. Most reported success is found in persons with symptoms. The symptomless population remains a challenge. At present it seems that without the development of sensitive new approaches, the routine use of fecal blood screening is questionable from a diagnostic and economic perspective.

Similar limitations exist with the carcinorembryonic antigen (CEA) screen. CEA is a tumor marker, a substance secreted in association with colon and breast cancer. It has not been found to be useful for diagnosis because it is not specific only to cancer. The cancer also tends to be advanced by the time the level is measurable. It is a useful tool for evaluating response to treatment and monitoring for recurrences.

## MEDICAL MANAGEMENT

The goal for discharge of patients with colorectal cancer as determined by DRGs is 10 days. The nurse works collaboratively with the physician for implementation of prescribed medical therapy. Because the nurse has a major role in discharge planning and patient teaching, these are discussed under nursing management.

### Diagnostic Tests

The diagnosis of bowel cancer is made from the history, physical examination, barium enema, sigmoidoscopy or colonoscopy, and biopsy (see Chapter 43). **Colonoscopy** and **barium enema** have been found to be approximately equal in their ability to detect lesions of 7 to 10 mm or greater, but colonoscopy offers in addition the ability to remove or to obtain a biopsy specimen of colonic polyps.[15] *Early* detection is the primary diagnostic challenge. More sophisticated imaging tests such as CT or MRI scans and the use of ultrasonography may play a role, but they are primarily useful in staging the cancer. CT and MRI scans provide data about lymph node involvement and spread beyond the colorectal region. Results of ultrasound examination yield data about the depth of bowel wall penetration by the tumor.

### Medication

Surgery is the primary treatment for bowel cancer. Chemotherapy has no role in the primary treatment, but it can play a significant role in adjuvant treatment (interventions provided in addition to primary therapy). Chemotherapy commonly is combined with radiation therapy. Adjuvant chemotherapy is used routinely in conjunction with the newer sphincter-preserving surgeries. Fluorouracil (Adrucil) is the drug with the best established effectiveness record. Combination drug protocols have offered no substantial benefit to date.

### Treatment

Radiotherapy is an important component of the management of rectal cancer, but it has minimal value in the management of colon cancer.[17] External beam radiation or endocavitary irradiation, in which the radiation source is placed directly on the tumor, may be used. Radiation may be used to shrink a tumor preoperatively, and it appears to be essential in preventing recurrence of rectal cancer after conservative sphincter-sparing surgeries. Radiation enteritis is a common complication during treatment, but the incidence of serious complications is only 5% to 6% at major centers.

### Diet

No special diet restrictions are ordered for patients with colorectal cancer. Anorexia and weight loss are common early symptoms, and concern may develop over the adequacy of the patient's nutritional status. The standard treatment approaches also may compromise the patient's nutritional status. Bowel surgery frequently necessitates as much as a week of nothing-by-mouth status or limited oral intake. Aggressive chemotherapy may be accompanied by nausea and/or vomiting, and both external beam and endocavitary irradiation can trigger radiation enteritis.

Low levels of serum albumin are associated with a higher incidence of postoperative complications, especially in elders.[27] It is essential to improve and sustain the patient's nutritional status during all planned treatments.

### Activity

The diagnosis of bowel cancer may affect the patient's activity level in several ways. Anemia and fatigue are common early signs of colon cancer. Severe anemia and fatigue frequently accompany aggressive chemotherapy and radiotherapy. Bowel surgery is initially very painful and significantly restricts the patient's activity. The patient is encouraged to modify and space activities throughout the day to remain involved in the usual activities of daily living. The patient is encouraged to remain as active as possible throughout all phases of treatment.

### Referral/Consultation

In some settings the nurse assumes responsibility for making referrals to other services. Common referrals for persons with bowel cancer include the following:

1. Enterostomal therapy. Because most patients are still treated with surgical procedures that result in permanent ostomies, it is essential that an enterostomal therapy specialist be involved in the patient's care from the point of admission.
2. Nutrition support. The involvement of a nutrition-support team may be appropriate at any point in the treatment plan. The team may perform a detailed nutritional assessment and plan for the appropriate use of scheduled meals and supplements to meet the varying needs of the patient. Ensuring adequate protein and calories for healing is essential.

Critical pathways (also referred to as *collaborative care paths* or *care maps*) have been developed in some inpatient and outpatient settings to guide both medical and nursing management. These critical pathways are collaboratively developed along time lines and include the information already described for specific hours, days, or visits. Pertinent information about discharge planning and patient teaching to be implemented at specified times also is included. Because the nurse has a major role in these two aspects of care, these are discussed under nursing management.

A sample of a critical pathway for the six areas of care discussed in the medical management section is presented at the end of the chapter. A nursing care plan for the patient with bowel cancer also is included. In some settings these are included within the critical pathway document.

## SURGICAL MANAGEMENT

Surgery is the definitive treatment for colorectal cancer. It typically involves removal of the tumor, surrounding colon, and lymph nodes. When the tumor is located in the ascending, transverse, or descending colon, it usually is possible for the surgeon to perform a resection with end-to-end anastomosis that preserves the natural pro-

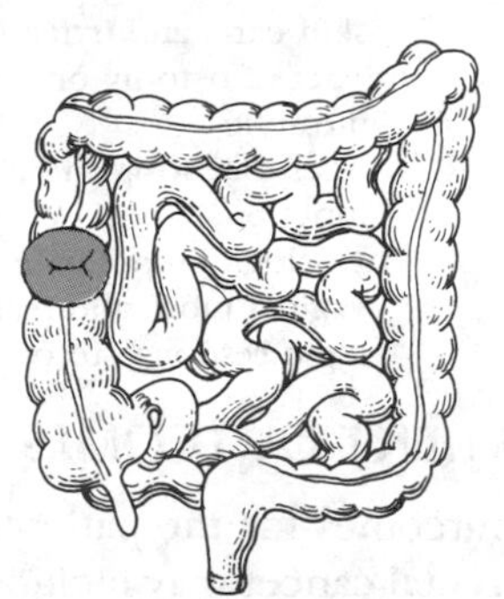
The **ascending colostomy** is done for right-sided tumors.

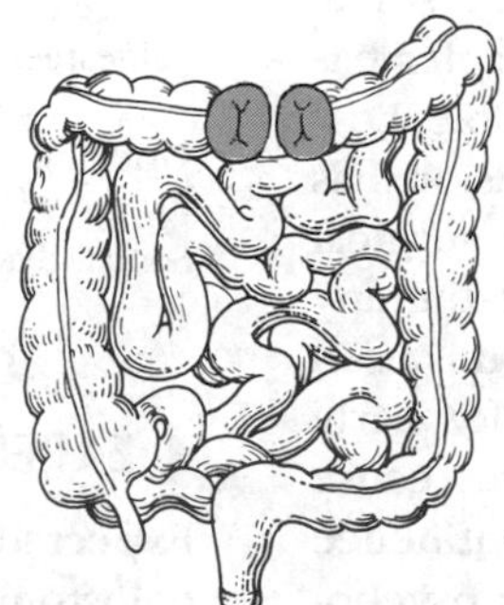
The **transverse (double-barreled) colostomy** is often used in such emergencies as intestinal obstruction or perforation because it can be created quickly. There are two stomas. The proximal one, closest to the small intestine, drains feces. The distal stoma drains mucus.

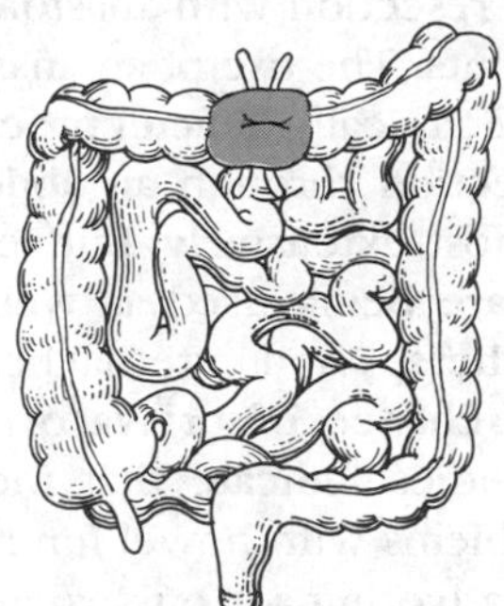
The **transverse loop colostomy** has two openings in the transverse colon, but one stoma.

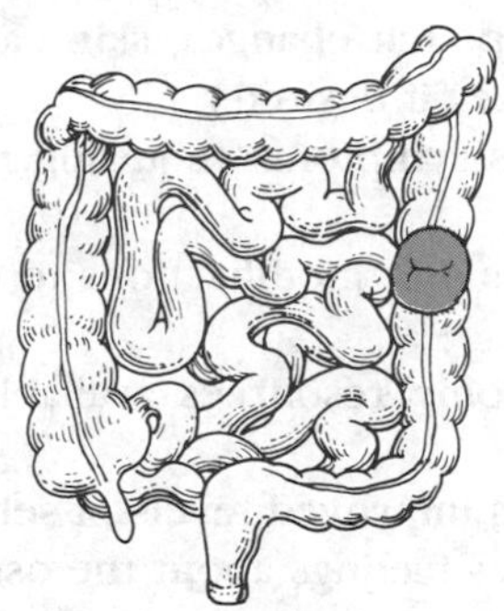
**Descending colostomy**

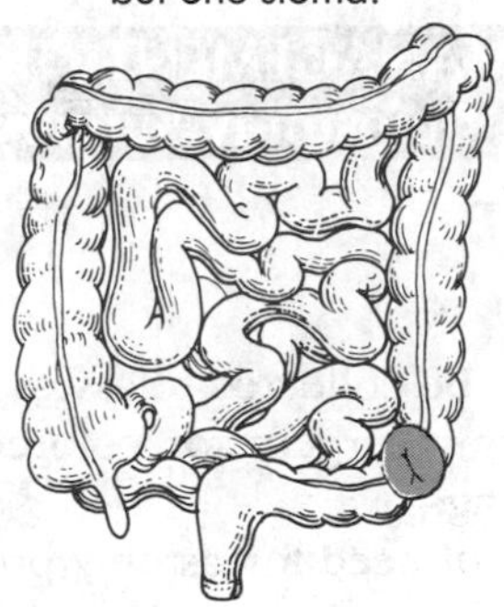
**Sigmoid colostomy**

**FIGURE 47-20** Types of colostomies.

cess of defecation. The specific type of surgery performed depends on the exact location and size of the tumor and the overall condition of the patient. Tumors in the rectum traditionally have been treated by removing the entire rectum and anus through a dual incision procedure called an *abdominoperineal resection.* The procedure necessitates permanent **colostomy** and leaves a significant perineal wound that heals slowly around active drains. The anus is sutured closed. Other types of colon cancers also may necessitate the creation of an ostomy. Tumors frequently cause bowel obstruction with inflammation. Creation of a temporary colostomy allows for bowel rest and healing. A temporary colostomy usually is required to treat perforation and fistulas as well. Closure of the colostomy is scheduled in about 6 months. Examples of various colostomy procedures are illustrated in Figure 47-20 and described in Box 47-11. General nursing management of the patient undergoing colostomy surgery for colorectal cancer is discussed in the next section. The unique care required by patients undergoing ileostomy was discussed beginning on p. 1548.

Persons with stage I rectal cancers that are believed

**BOX 47-11 Types of Colostomies**

**END STOMA**

The proximal bowel is brought out through an incision, folded over to form a cuff, and sutured to the skin. The remaining distal bowel is removed or oversewn.

**LOOP STOMA**

The bowel is brought through the incision, a support is placed under it, and an opening is made into the upper wall of the bowel. The posterior wall remains intact. There is one stoma with two openings, and the procedure usually is temporary.

**LOOP-END STOMA**

As with an end stoma the proximal bowel is brought out through an incision. The end is oversewn and the stoma created from an intestinal loop just proximal to the oversewn end. The loop is supported on the skin surface by a supporting rod and opened during or after surgery.

**MUCOUS FISTULA**

The distal bowel from an end stoma may be preserved and brought to the skin surface to form another stoma. It secretes mucus and requires dressings rather than a pouch.

to be localized are clear candidates for the newer sphincter-sparing treatments. These procedures involve regional rectal resection with anastomosis of the residual bowel segments. The use of an anastomotic stapler has made these technically difficult procedures feasible. Low anterior resection through an abdominal incision has been used most extensively, but several other surgical approaches are being used as well. Adjuvant therapy with chemotherapy and external beam radiation is used to reduce the chances of survival of residual tumor. Early outcomes studies indicate that the procedures cause minimal problems with bowel function and continence and less negative impact on sexuality.[19] Their psychosocial advantages are obvious. Mild and infrequent diarrhea is the most common complaint.

## NURSING MANAGEMENT: The Patient Undergoing Colostomy Surgery

### ♦ ASSESSMENT

#### Subjective Data

Subjective data to be collected to assess the patient undergoing colostomy surgery for colorectal cancer include the following:

Understanding of need for ostomy procedure
Knowledge of planned surgical procedure and stoma location
Previous exposure to ostomy or ostomy care
Emotional response to need for surgery and usual coping strategies
Available support mechanisms

#### Objective Data

Objective data to be collected to assess the patient undergoing colostomy surgery for colorectal cancer include the following:

Nutritional status
Manual dexterity
Cognitive ability, memory, vision
Ostomy site planning and marking (with enterostomal therapist)

#### Diagnostic Test Findings

1. Barium enema, sigmoidoscopy, or colonoscopy outlining presence of tumor
2. Positive findings on tissue biopsy
3. CT/MRI evidence of lymph node involvement if present
4. Ultrasound data concerning depth of tumor penetration

### ♦ NURSING DIAGNOSES

Nursing diagnoses are determined from analysis of patient data. Nursing diagnoses for the patient undergoing colostomy surgery for colorectal cancer may include but are not limited to the following:

| Diagnostic Title | Possible Etiologic Factors |
|---|---|
| Health maintenance, altered | Lack of knowledge concerning stoma, skin care, and irrigation |
| Self-esteem disturbance | Impact of ostomy on body image and life-style |
| Grieving | Cancer diagnosis and altered body function |
| Sexual dysfunction | Physiologic impotence, decreased vaginal lubrication, and psychologic response to ostomy |

### ♦ EXPECTED PATIENT OUTCOMES

Expected patient outcomes for the patient undergoing colostomy for colorectal cancer may include but are not limited to the following:

1. Participates in self-care activities:
   a. Demonstrates components of ostomy care, including pouch changes, skin care, and irrigation technique (if desired).
   b. Identifies symptoms requiring medical intervention.
   c. Discusses diet modifications to control odor and flatus.
   d. Lists ostomy resources available in home community.
2. Experiences improved levels of self-esteem
   a. Verbalizes feelings about the ostomy.
   b. Actively participates in stoma care.
3. Expresses grief and discusses personal meaning of the loss.
4. Verbalizes concerns with spouse or partner and identifies alternatives to deal with physical problems.

### ♦ INTERVENTIONS

#### Preoperative Care

The immediate reaction to the need for a colostomy is typically shock and disbelief. Whether it is to be temporary or permanent, it usually is difficult for the patient to accept. The nurse supplements and reinforces all teaching provided by the physician and adjusts the content in response to the patient's anxiety level and readiness. Written materials and booklets may be helpful. Minimally the patient should be informed about the nature of the ostomy and the management it will require. Content for initial teaching is summarized in the Guidelines box, p. 1575. Referral to an enterostomal therapist for assistance in developing a teaching plan for colostomy self-care is desirable. Family or other support persons should be included in all teaching sessions, with the patient's approval.

Sexual dysfunction is a potential problem after rectal surgery, particularly if widespread lymph node dissection is performed. The surgeon will inform the patient about this risk. The nurse will clarify any misconceptions, answer the patient's questions, and encourage the patient to verbalize feelings with the spouse or sexual partner.

The nurse prepares the patient for abdominal surgery

**Guidelines for Preoperative Teaching for an Ostomy**

- Provide brief overview of GI tract structure and function.
- Mark on drawing sections of bowel to be removed and location of stoma.
- Describe stoma appearance, sensation, and function.
- Provide brief overview of care regimen.
- Develop outline of postoperative teaching plan.
- Arrange for United Ostomy Association visitor if acceptable to patient.
- Provide written materials from United Ostomy Association and American Cancer Society.

and general anesthesia as outlined in Chapter 23. A thorough bowel cleansing is required. This is accomplished by diet modification, mechanical cleansing, and pharmacologic suppression of colon bacteria. The patient begins with a low-residue diet and moves toward clear liquids as surgery approaches. Laxatives and enemas are administered to thoroughly empty the bowel. Oral antibiotics such as neomycin are administered to reduce bacterial flora. If the patient is in good physical condition, much of this preparation will be performed at home before admission.

#### Site selection

The potential stoma site is selected and marked by the surgeon or the enterostomal therapy nurse. It should be visible to the patient when sitting or standing, lie within the rectus muscle, and be away from scars, bony prominences, and skinfolds. The patient's belt line also should be avoided. The stoma site frequently is the most significant factor influencing the patient's ability to maintain a good pouch seal and manage the colostomy independently after surgery.

### Postoperative Care

The nurse provides routine postoperative care after surgery as outlined in Chapter 25 and discussed on p. 1584. The extensive nature of the surgical procedure necessitates careful attention being paid to fluid and electrolyte balance, pulmonary hygiene, and pain management.

#### Managing the perineal wound

The abdominal perineal resection has been the gold standard for the treatment of rectal cancer for many years. It is still the treatment of choice for managing highly invasive disease. Postoperative care is more complex because of the presence of a major perineal wound that may require up to 6 months to completely heal. The patient's convalescence is prolonged.

The perineal wound is created by the removal of the entire rectum and anus plus muscle and fatty tissue. The large gap that is created gradually fills in with granulation tissue. The remaining pelvic organs shift slightly to fill the remaining space. The wound may be left open and loosely filled with packing. Wound irrigations and absorbent dressings are used until the wound closes. The perineal wound may instead be partially closed with drains inserted, or it may be sutured closed with stab wounds formed for drainage and irrigation. The drainage initially is copious and serosanguineous. It must be effectively drained away to prevent infection and abscess formation. The drainage tubes may work passively by gravity or be attached to a suction apparatus. Wound irrigations, usually with normal saline, are initially performed by catheter, but the patient gradually may progress to a hand-held shower massage or water pik. The dressings are changed as needed. A T binder may be useful in holding the dressings in place in the perineum. The top of the T binder is wrapped around the waist, and the strap is brought up between the patient's legs. Sitz baths may be substituted for irrigations once the patient is ambulatory, but a free flow of water on the perineal wound is preferred.

The perineal wound makes it difficult for the patient to sit or find a comfortable position. Foam pads or soft pillows may increase comfort while the patient is sitting. The nurse instructs the patient to avoid the use of air or rubber rings that separate the buttocks and stress the healing wound. The side-lying position usually is preferred. Phantom rectal sensations and itching may occur after healing. The origin of these sensations is unknown.

#### Stoma monitoring

The patient who has undergone colostomy surgery typically returns from surgery with an ostomy pouch system in place. The nurse observes the stoma regularly for redness and edema. Color reflects perfusion, and a dark, dusky, or brown-black stoma indicates ischemia and necrosis. Color changes should be reported immediately. Initial stoma edema is expected in response to surgical manipulation. The pouch opening will need to be adjusted to accommodate the changing stoma size. Edema typically resolves in 5 to 7 days. A small amount of bleeding from the stoma is expected, but any significant bleeding is reported to the surgeon immediately.

The abdominal incision and sutures anchoring the stoma are inspected for intactness. Some of the stoma mucosa may pull away from the abdominal skin before healing is complete. Superficial separations heal by granulation, but deeper problems may require packing or resuturing.

The stoma drainage consists initially of mucus and serosanguineous secretion. As peristalsis returns, flatus is produced. Flatus and fecal drainage usually begin in 4 to 7 days. The drainage initially is liquid and becomes thicker as the diet progresses. The pouch should be emptied when it is one-third to one-half full of stool or more frequently if excess gas is present.

A loop colostomy may be opened during surgery or in the patient's room 48 to 72 hours later. A cautery is used to open the bowel and creates two openings, one proximal and one distal, in the one stoma (see Figure 47-20). The nurse reassures the patient that the procedure causes no pain inasmuch as the stoma has no sensory nerves endings for pain sensation. It creates a distinct burning smell, however, and the procedure can be quite frightening. The nurse offers support and reassurance during the loop opening. The supporting rod for the loop is removed after 7 to 10 days when adhesions prevent the stoma from retracting into the incision.

## Teaching for Self-Care

It is essential that the patient acquire basic colostomy self-care skills during the postoperative period. Successful self-care provides the foundation for both independence and a reintegration of body image that includes the ostomy. The nurse teaches the patient the principles of colostomy care, but providing information is only one tool. The patient needs to acquire the psychomotor skills involved in self-care. The nurse provides the patient with the opportunity to handle, assemble, and use all equipment. Time for practice is essential. The process rarely can be completed during the hospitalization, particularly with elderly persons, and the nurse initiates referral to appropriate home health care and community ostomy services. Involvement of a family member or supportive friend can be helpful if acceptable to the patient.

### Stoma care

Teaching begins with the first pouch change. The patient may or may not be ready to view the stoma, but the nurse gently encourages the patient to look at and touch it. The nurse briefly explains each step of the procedure in a factual manner. The nurse reminds the patient that the stoma has no touch sensation, but the rest of the abdomen will still be tender and sore from the surgery. Surgical pain should be thoroughly controlled before any teaching session.

A systematic plan should have been developed before surgery to guide teaching the colostomy regimen. Teaching sessions should be spaced throughout the hospitalization to allow for repetition and assimilation. Pouches are changed more frequently than needed to allow for adequate practice time. Written instructions and resource materials are invaluable supplements to instruction. A basic colostomy teaching plan is summarized in Box 47-12.

**Pouch selection.** An effective pouch system protects the skin, contains stool and odor, molds to the body's contours, allows for movement, and is inconspicuous under clothing. It is the most important aspect of ostomy management. The basic issues involve ostomy type, size and contour of the abdomen, peristomal skin condition, financial considerations, and personal preferences.

Products for ostomy care are available in a variety of styles, shapes, and sizes. Disposable pouches are available in one- and two-piece systems, with skin barriers attached, and in a variety of materials (Figure 47-21). Reusable pouches are worn, cleansed, and worn again. Drainable pouches are easier to keep clean and are more economical than closed nondrainable pouches. Drainable pouches usually are changed every 3 to 7 days if there are no problems with leakage. They are available in one- and two-piece systems in a variety of materials.

A properly applied pouch system is odor-free except during changes. If odor persists, it is usually the result of inadequate cleansing of the drainage spout or a poor pouch seal. Pin holes in a pouch destroy its odor-proof quality and should not be used to release gas. The skin wafer is gently removed by peeling it carefully down from the top. The nurse instructs the patient to use this opportunity to carefully assess the stoma and peristomal skin.

**BOX 47-12 Components of a Colostomy Teaching Plan**

**CHARACTERISTICS OF A HEALTHY STOMA**

Normal color varies from pink to deep pink–red. Purple or black color indicates compromised circulation and should be reported immediately. The surface is moist.
Stoma has no touch or pain sensation.
Shape changes slightly throughout the day in response to peristalsis.

**STOMA CARE SYSTEMS**

One-piece versus two-piece systems
Drainable versus nondrainable disposable pouches
- Drainable are more economical

**POUCH CHANGE PROCEDURES**

Nondrainable pouches are changed when one-half full
Drainable pouches changed every 3 to 7 days
Manufacturer's guidelines should be followed
Measuring the stoma and reapplying the pouch

**PERISTOMAL SKIN CARE AND PROTECTION**

Peristomal skin is cleansed with warm water during each pouch change
Skin barriers
Managing skin irritation or erosion

**MANAGEMENT OF PROBLEMS**

Odor: diet modifications, medications, equipment management
Gas: diet and activity modifications

**SUPPLIES AND SUPPORT**

Supplies and price lists for equipment
Services available through
- American Cancer Society
- United Ostomy Association
- Community enterostomal therapy agencies

Insurance coverage for costs

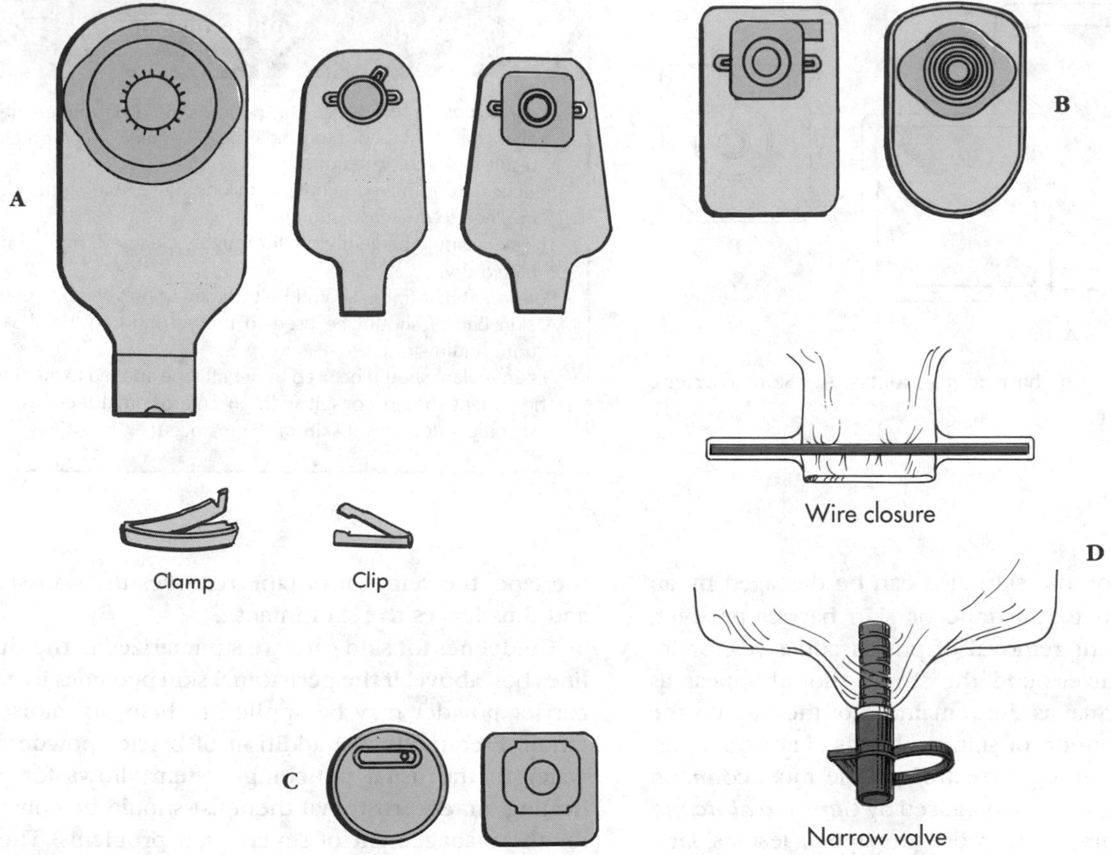

FIGURE 47-21 Common ostomy pouch products, closures, and patches. **A,** Drainable pouches. **B,** Nondrainable pouches. **C,** Patches for regulated colostomies. **D,** Pouch closures.

It is essential that the patient learn to properly measure the stoma to ensure a proper fit. The stoma may shrink dramatically during the first week after surgery and will continue to change size slightly during the first year. Thus it is important for the patient to measure the stoma accurately during each pouch change in the first weeks and then every few months.

To ensure a proper fit the pouch should closely surround the stoma but not press or rub against it. Cutouts of various diameters are included in the box of pouches. The skin barriers are cut slightly larger than the stoma (approximately one-eighth inch) to accommodate stomal swelling with peristalsis. The pouch change procedure is outlined in more detail in the Guidelines box, at right.

The nurse ensures that the patient has an adequate temporary supply of equipment before discharge, a complete list of supplies that will be needed for home management, and information about where supplies can be obtained in the local community. A prescription may be needed for Medicare or insurance reimbursement.

**Skin care.** Skin exposure to stool can be a major problem for a person with a colostomy. In addition to irri-

## Guidelines for Changing a Pouch

### STOMA MEASUREMENT

Use the measuring guide and sample diameters, and cut the colostomy appliance to fit—pattern should be one-eighth to one-quarter inch larger than the stoma.

Use the same procedure to prepare the skin barrier. NOTE: The pouch opening is cut slightly larger than the skin barrier to prevent the paper from cutting the stoma.

### REMOVING OLD POUCH

Empty drainable pouch to prevent spills.

Disconnect pouch from skin wafer if two-piece system is used.

Gently peel the wafer away from the skin beginning at the top.

### SKIN CARE

Cleanse the skin with warm water and dry thoroughly; use soap only if stool adheres to skin. Rinse thoroughly with water.

Assess peristomal skin and stoma carefully for signs of irritation or infection.

Pat peristomal skin dry thoroughly.

### APPLYING NEW POUCH

Center the pouch opening over the stoma. Ask patient to tense abdominal muscles to make easier application.

Gently press into place and hold for at least 30 seconds to seal.

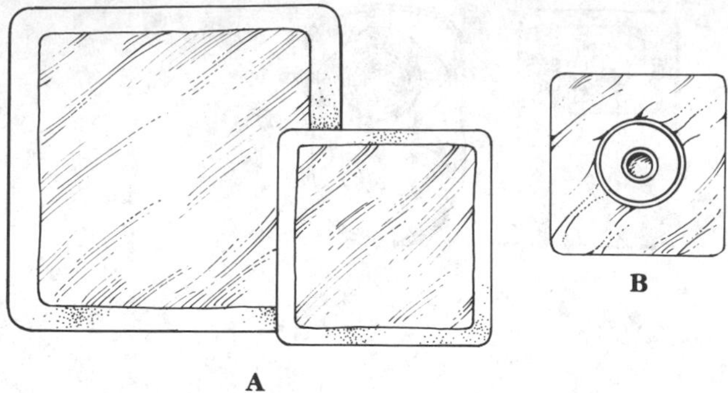


FIGURE 47-22 Skin barrier products. **A,** Skin barriers. **B,** Wafer.

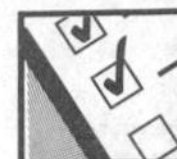

## Guidelines for Colostomy Skin Care

When a pouch seal leaks, the pouch should be immediately changed, not taped. Stool held against the skin can quickly result in severe irritation.
Pouches are removed gently, with one hand holding the skin in place to decrease pulling.
The skin should be gently but thoroughly cleansed, rinsed, and patted dry.
Peristomal hair (men) should be trimmed to prevent folliculitis.
A skin barrier should be used to protect the peristomal skin from liquid stool.
A skin sealant should be used under all tape applied to the skin.
The patient should consult with an enterostomal therapist for specific guidelines if skin problems occur.

tation from stool, the skin also can be damaged by an allergic reaction to the tape or skin barrier product, rough or frequent removal of pouch adhesives, or infection. The skin around the stoma should appear as healthy and normal as the remainder of the skin on the abdomen. Prevention of skin problems is always easier and less expensive than treatment. The most common peristomal skin infection is caused by *Candida albicans.* The skin becomes bright red with papular lesions. Dryness and scaling develop if the condition persists. It is treated with nystatin (Mycostatin) powder.

The use of a skin barrier is an important means of protecting the peristomal skin. Skin barriers come in several basic forms: powder, paste, washer, or wafer (Figure 47-22). Skin barriers include such products as karaya, Stomahesive (Convatec), Hollihesive (Hollister), ReliaSeal (Bard), Skin Barrier (Coloplast), and Mason Colly-Seal Disc. Skin barriers attached to the pouches are available as one- or two-piece systems, as well as single-use items that can be used with any pouch.

***Powder.*** A pouch will not adhere to powder, cream, or ointment. If powder is applied to the skin, it must be sealed in before applying the pouch. Karaya powder releases an acid that may sting irritated skin, but stomadhesive powder works well.

***Paste.*** Paste is available for use around the stoma, to fill in creases or folds, and to supplement skin barriers for a longer seal. The use of paste has made it easier to keep a pouch seal intact in poor locations.

***Skin barrier wafers.*** These may be used with a variety of pouches and protect the skin from stool. The opening in the wafer is carefully measured so that it fits at the base of the stoma without rubbing into or onto the stoma.

***Skin sealants.*** These come in sprays, liquids, gels, and wipes. These products coat the skin with a clear film and are useful under pouch adhesives. When tape is removed from the skin, it removes the stratum corneum layer of the skin. When a skin sealant is used under the tape, the removal of tape removes the skin sealant and thus leaves the skin intact.

Guidelines for skin care are summarized in the Guidelines box above. If the peristomal skin becomes irritated, barrier powder may be applied to help dry moist irritation. Frequently the addition of barrier powder or a wafer to the usual pouching system allows for rapid healing. An enterostomal therapist should be consulted for the management of severe skin problems. The use of antacids or products that contain alcohol on the skin should be avoided inasmuch as they dry the skin and alter the pH, leaving it vulnerable to infection.

**Colostomy irrigation.** A colostomy irrigation is an enema given through the stoma to stimulate bowel emptying at a regular and convenient time. The procedure is no longer routinely recommended and is used only with sigmoid colostomies where the stool is formed. A patient who uses irrigations successfully may be able to dispense with a standard pouch and wear a stoma cap—a small adhesive pouch with an absorbent dressing. Because the ostomy continues to secrete mucus and release flatus, a gas filter is desirable.

If irrigations are planned, they typically are initiated about 5 to 7 days after surgery. The procedure is described in the Guidelines box, p. 1579, and common equipment is illustrated in Figure 47-23. A variety of equipment is commercially available, and most sets include irrigating sleeves, a cone tip for insertion into the stoma, a bag to hold the solution, and clips to close the sleeve. The procedure is ideally taught in the bathroom. Cramping during an irrigation may be caused by instilling the water too rapidly or solutions that are too cold or too hot. The flow should be halted until cramping subsides.

**Managing odor.** Colostomy pouches are made of odorproof plastic, but a leaking seal or improperly cleaned pouch end can emit an unpleasant odor. The inside of

### Guidelines for Colostomy Irrigation

Assemble all equipment:
- Water container, irrigating sleeve, and belt
- Skin care items
- New pouch system, ready for use

Remove old pouch and dispose.
Clean the stoma and peristomal skin with water and assess.
Apply the irrigating sleeve and belt.
- Place open end of sleeve in toilet.

Fill irrigating container with 500 to 1000 ml of lukewarm water, and suspend container at shoulder height.
Run water through the tubing to remove air.
Gently insert the irrigating cone into stoma, and slowly start the flow of water. Catheters are inserted no more than 2 to 4 inches into the stoma. Do not force. If cramping occurs, stop the irrigation and wait.
Allow approximately 15 to 20 minutes for stool to empty.
Rinse sleeve, dry the bottom, roll it up, and close off the end. Patient should go about regular activities for 30 to 45 minutes.
Remove sleeve, clean stoma, and apply new pouch.
Clean and store the irrigating equipment.

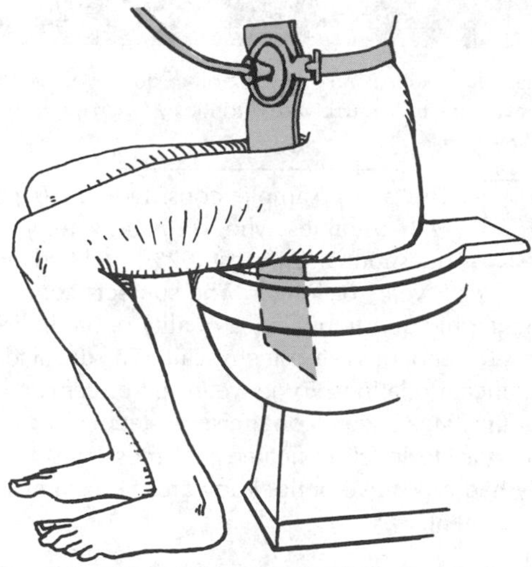

**FIGURE 47-23** Colostomy irrigation with person sitting on the toilet; irrigating sleeve drains into the toilet.

the pouch should be rinsed with tepid water after emptying and the pouch outlet wiped with toilet paper. If the patient desires, a pouch deodorizer may be used or a small amount of mouthwash can be applied with a squeeze bottle.

The nurse encourages the patient to eat a balanced diet at regular intervals and to chew foods slowly and thoroughly. No special diet is required; however, patients need to be informed about foods that increase gas and odor. Dairy products, highly seasoned foods, fish, and a variety of vegetables are known to increase the odor of the stool. Individual responses to gas-producing foods tend to be variable, with known exceptions such as beans, cabbage, and brussel sprouts. The patient will need to experiment with diet modifications that reflect individual food tolerances. Closed pouches usually have a charcoal filter at the top that releases and deodorizes gas. Pouches should be opened to release accumulated gas but never pricked. A puncture in the pouch would create a constant odor problem.

**Supporting a positive self-concept**

The formation of a stoma frequently is viewed as mutilating surgery, and most patients need time and the support of others to work through their feelings. The nurse encourages the patient to view the stoma and cares for it in a matter-of-fact manner. Emotional support is incorporated into all self-care sessions, and the nurse encourages the patient to verbalize concerns and feelings about the stoma and its anticipated effects on daily life. The nurse provides positive support and reinforcement for all self-care efforts. The nurse encourages the patient to meet with a visitor from the United Ostomy Association and to incorporate family members into the teaching-learning process.

Patients are encouraged to gradually resume all their usual activities. No clothing restrictions are necessitated by the stoma except the avoidance of tight belts or waistbands directly over it. Pouches hold well in baths and showers, and normal hygiene patterns may be resumed as soon as the incision is healed. There are no specific restrictions on exercise or recreational activities.

The nurse reminds the patient always to carry ostomy supplies when traveling and not to place them in checked luggage. Extra care with food choices is helpful. The quality of water is of particular concern inasmuch as traveler's diarrhea could create serious problems.

**Resolving grief**

Removal of any part of the body involves a sense of loss and grief. The stoma causes the patient to experience a change in body image and may trigger feelings of guilt or shame. The nurse encourages the patient to express these feelings of loss and makes no attempt to suppress them or minimize their validity. The nurse acknowledges the work involved in grief resolution and explores the patient's usual coping strategies for handling grief. Counseling and referral to community support groups may be helpful. The Research box, p. 1580, discusses a study of quality of life issues among persons with ostomies.

**Preventing sexual dysfunction**

Many patients will not directly verbalize their concerns about sexuality after ostomy surgery; thus it is usually necessary for the nurse to address the topic deliberately. The nurse provides the patient with specific suggestions for dealing with sexual concerns such as the following:

**RESEARCH**

Kelman G, Minkler P: An investigation of quality of life and self-esteem among individuals with ostomies, *J Enterostom Ther* 16:4-11, 1989.

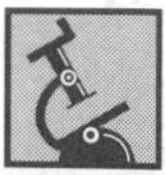

The study sample consisted of 50 persons with ostomies who voluntarily returned the questionnaires. Most (62%) had had their ostomies for 5 years or longer. The subjects completed a demographic questionnaire, a quality of life index, and Morris Rosenberg's self-esteem scale. The data indicated a significant relationship between self-esteem and quality of life. Mean scores on the self-esteem scale and the quality of life index indicated that most persons in the study had a positive outlook toward the ostomy and its management.

Exploring positions that minimize stress and pressure on the pouch

Emptying and cleaning the pouch before sexual activity

Using a smaller-sized pouch or pouch cover during sexual activity

Use of a binder or special underwear to hold the pouch secure

The nurse's primary role is encouraging and facilitating partner discussions about sexual matters. It is not uncommon for patients to move into their own rooms or twin beds after surgery. The emotional distancing may be difficult to repair. Role playing or visualizing worst-case scenarios helps some patients to acknowledge their fears. The use of a community support group can be particularly helpful for getting practical advice about sexual matters. The use of a protective covering on the bed may add a sense of security for persons concerned about pouch leakage. About 15% of male ostomates have decreased sexual activity that may be related either to nerve injury or to psychologic responses. Counseling may be helpful if nerve injury is not present and yet sexual difficulties are being experienced. A penile prosthesis may be an option for the man with nerve damage (see Chapter 53). Ostomy surgery does not interfere with contraception, pregnancy, or delivery; and pregnancy seldom produces complications with stoma care. A pamphlet entitled *Sex and the Osteomate* is available from the United Ostomy Association.

## ♦ EVALUATION

To evaluate the effectiveness of nursing interventions, compare patient behaviors with those stated in the expected patient outcomes. Successful achievement of patient outcomes for the patient with ostomy surgery is indicated by the following:

1. Participates in self-care activities
   a. Accurately performs pouch changes and irrigations, using appropriate skin barriers.
   b. Lists symptoms that indicate stoma problems.
   c. Identifies foods to limit in daily meals.
   d. Identifies ostomy resources in home community.
2. Demonstrates positive self-esteem
   a. Expresses beginning acceptance of ostomy.
   b. Cares for ostomy with minimal coaching.
3. Acknowledges loss and change in body functions and selects support mechanisms for resolving loss.
4. Discusses sexual concerns with partner and identifies strategies to compensate for physical limitations.

## SPECIAL CONSIDERATIONS FOR CARE OF THE GERONTOLOGIC PATIENT

The incidence of cancer of the bowel is strongly skewed toward the elderly population, and the entire discussion of the disease is really aimed at that population. The issues of comorbidity and general health, therefore, become extremely important. Healthy elders can withstand the rigors of treatment well, but the concurrent existence of other chronic health problems increases the risk for postoperative complications.

Early diagnosis frequently is difficult in the older population. Symptoms tend to be underreported and attributed to the effects of aging. This is particularly true concerning symptoms related to digestion and elimination. Chronic constipation is a frequent complaint in this population, and changes in bowel habits may not be reported until the disease is well established.

The challenges of learning an ostomy self-care regimen also may be more significant for older persons who are acknowledged to have some difficulty in processing new information and tasks. The presence of arthritis or failing vision may make it difficult for elders to acquire the psychomoter skills necessary for self-care. The teaching plan will need to be structured to address these concerns and probably will need to move at a slower pace.

## HOME CARE CONSIDERATIONS

As the acute care hospitalization phase of treatment continues to get shorter and shorter, home care considerations for patients with colorectal cancer become increasingly important. It is extremely unlikely that sufficient in-hospital time will be available for the nurse to ensure that the patient can be safely independent in self-care, especially if the patient is elderly and has a colostomy.

Discharge planning must begin at admission. The nurse assesses the patient's home environment and the supports that are available to meet physical and emotional needs. For elderly patients, particularly those who live alone, this assessment includes extended family and friendship networks. The involvement of a social worker may be helpful to determine insurance and financial qualifications for home care assistance.

Referral for postdischarge assistance is likely to be necessary. The patient may need direct assistance in caring for a perineal wound or may need further teaching and supervision to become independent with the colostomy self-care regimen. Plans for adjuvant treatment with radiation or chemotherapy will further deplete the patient's physical and emotional resources. The American Cancer Society and United Ostomy Association can provide much-needed services and support, and direct referral should be made to these groups. Peer counselors also can be extremely helpful in making the transition to home care.

## COMPLICATIONS

Immediate complications related to bowel cancer are primarily surgical. The surgeries that have been described are extensive and wound complications are a real risk, particularly for elderly patients and those with diabetes. Complications include infection, bleeding, anastomosis leakage, and fistula development. Close monitoring is required in the initial days and weeks.

Longer-term complications are primarily related to stoma complications and disease recurrence and metastasis. The 5-year survival after the diagnosis of colorectal cancer is only 52%; thus ongoing medical surveillance for disease recurrence is essential. Stoma-related problems are also possible, including peristomal skin breakdown or infection, obstruction, and inversion of the stoma. Early recognition of these problems is important and frequently depends on the quality and success of the original self-care teaching plan.

# Anorectal Disorders

A variety of common disorders can affect the perianal area. Persons who experience anorectal disorders typically seek medical care for symptoms such as pain, tenderness, itching, or the development of rectal bleeding. Many of the disorders can be treated on an outpatient basis.

## HEMORRHOIDS

### Etiology/Epidemiology

**Hemorrhoids** are masses of dilated blood vessels that lie beneath the lining of the skin in the anal canal. They are extremely common and estimated to be present in up to 50% of the population by age 50.[14] They affect persons of all ages, but they typically cause more problems with increasing age. Pregnancy is clearly recognized as an initiating or aggravating condition for hemorrhoids. Other conditions associated with the development or aggravation of hemorrhoids include obesity, congestive heart failure, and chronic liver disease, which results in portal hypertension. These conditions are all associated with chronic elevations in intraabdominal

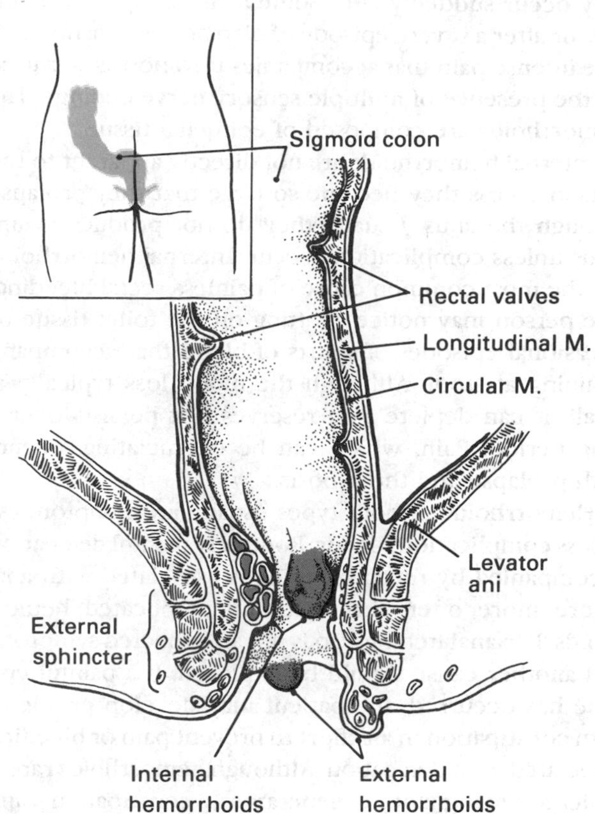


**FIGURE 47-24** Internal and external hemorrhoids.

pressure. Sedentary occupations that involve long periods of sitting or standing also are implicated, although the exact mechanism is not known.

Hemorrhoids usually are classified into two types. Those that occur above the anal sphincter are termed *internal* hemorrhoids and those that occur below the anal sphincter are termed *external* hemorrhoids (Figure 47-24). A person can have both forms at the same time. Although hemorrhoids usually are a chronic health problem, they may cause acute episodes.

### Pathophysiology

Hemorrhoids traditionally have been viewed as varicose veins of the rectum. The superior hemorrhoidal veins contain no valves and are vulnerable to overdistention when the person is in an upright position. Additional studies have documented that hemorrhoids actually are composed of spongy vascular tissue with multiple direct arteriovenous connections.[14]

External hemorrhoids can be detected by the affected persons. The classic "skin tag" consists of small lumps of fibrous tissue and folds of anal skin that have been stretched by bulging of the hemorrhoids. They rarely bleed and seldom cause pain exept when they become inflamed and edematous as a result of thrombosis or subcutaneous rupture of an external vein with hematoma formation. A thrombosed external hemorrhoid may occur suddenly after some form of vigorous exercise or after a severe episode of diarrhea or constipation. The intense pain that accompanies thrombosis is caused by the presence of multiple sensory nerve endings. The hemorrhoids are composed of epithelial tissue.

Internal hemorrhoids are not directly apparent to the person unless they become so large that they prolapse through the anus. Usually they do not produce symptoms unless complications occur. Internal hemorrhoids are the most common cause of painless rectal bleeding. The person may notice spotting on the toilet tissue or occasional episodes of spurts of blood that accompany straining at stool. Although the blood loss typically is small, it can deplete iron reserves if it persists over a long period. Pain, which can be excruciating, occurs with prolapse and thrombosis.

Hemorrhoids of both types usually are symptomless unless complications occur. Routinely painful defecation accompanied by rectal bleeding is associated with anal fissure more often than with uncomplicated hemorrhoids. Perianal itching also is not an expected symptom, and another cause should be explored. If a painful episode has occurred, the patient may develop problems with constipation in an effort to prevent pain or bleeding associated with defecation. Although hemorrhoids rarely undergo malignant degeneration, constipation and bleeding also are symptoms of cancer of the rectum. For this reason all persons with these symptoms should have a medical examination to rule out cancer.

## Medical Management

The diagnosis of hemorrhoids is fairly straightforward. The person's presenting symptoms establish the initial diagnosis, which usually can be confirmed by inspection and digital palpation. Proctoscopy or colonoscopy to confirm the diagnosis also may be scheduled for patients who are middle-aged and experiencing rectal bleeding.

Both forms of hemorrhoids can be managed conservatively if their symptoms are not severe. Conservative management includes a high-fiber diet, bulk laxatives, warm sitz baths, and gentle cleansing. If severe pain, bleeding, or thrombosis are present, however, more definitive management may be indicated. Treatment options for internal hemorrhoids include sclerotherapy, cryosurgery, and rubber-band ligation, as well as traditional surgical hemorrhoidectomy. Infrared photocoagulation and bipolar diathermy are newer adaptations that can be used to affix the mucosa to the muscle. External hemorrhoids may be managed by evacuating the hematoma or surgical hemorrhoidectomy.

### Sclerotherapy

The injection method can be effective for small, bleeding internal hemorrhoids. It is not effective for external hemorrhoids. A sclerosing solution such as 5% phenol in oil is injected into the submucous areolar tissue in which the hemorrhoidal veins lie, producing an inflammatory reaction. Fibrous induration, which surrounds and constricts the veins, occurs at the site of the injection in 2 or 3 weeks. The hemorrhoid shrinks and has less tendency to prolapse. Bleeding from the hemorrhoids usually stops within 24 to 48 hours. The procedure is palliative and not curative, and repeat injection may be required in the future. However, it is extremely economical and rarely associated with complications, making it an appropriate choice for selected patients.

### Cryosurgery and photocoagulation

Cryosurgical hemorrhoidectomy involves freezing hemorrhoidal tissue through a probe that carries liquid nitrogen or another agent for a sufficient time to cause tissue necrosis. The procedure usually is performed with the patient under local anesthesia and requires expensive equipment. The patient will have a foul-smelling discharge for several weeks while the decayed tissue is being sloughed from the body. This has decreased the popularity of the approach. Also, the incidence of residual hemorrhoids is high.[14]

During photocoagulation the physician inserts an infrared photocoagulator probe through an anoscope and applies radiation to each involved area for 1.5 seconds. The hemorrhoidal tissue then becomes necrotic and sloughs off. The procedure is repeated in three or four adjacent areas to completely destroy the hemorrhoid. A second treatment, if needed, may follow in 7 to 10 days. Although the treatment is successful, at present it is also extremely expensive.

### Ligation

Internal hemorrhoids may be treated by ligation with latex bands. The hemorrhoid is grasped with forceps and pulled down into a special instrument that, when

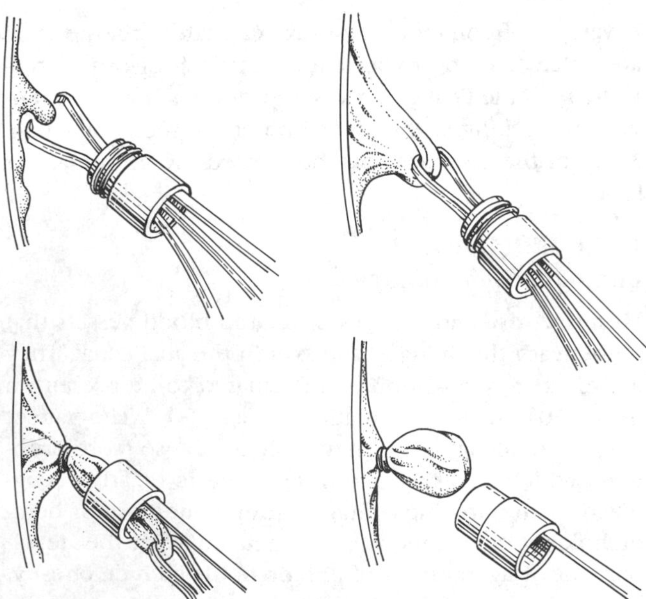

FIGURE 47-25 Rubber-band ligation of an internal hemorrhoid.

the trigger handle is pressed, slips a latex band over it (Figure 47-25). The band constricts the circulation and causes necrosis; the destroyed tissue usually sloughs off within a week. An enema is given before the treatment to prevent a bowel movement for 24 hours and thus prevent straining that would cause the band to break or slip off. No anesthesia is required. Local discomfort is minimal and usually is successfully relieved by aspirin or acetaminophen.

### Hemorrhoidectomy

Surgical excision (hemorrhoidectomy) is the treatment used for external or internal hemorrhoids that do not respond well to more conservative treatment or that must be treated on an emergent basis because of acute strangulation.

## Nursing Management

Limited problems with hemorrhoids often can be successfully managed through a combination of strict personal hygiene and prevention of constipation and straining. The nurse encourages the patient to follow a high-residue diet rich in fruit and vegetable fiber. Bran may be added to ease stool passage. Liberal fluids and regular exercise also are encouraged to promote normal bowel function. If necessary, a bulk-forming hydrophilic laxative may be added to the daily routine.

Local treatment promotes comfort during symptom flare-ups. The local application of ice, warm compresses, or analgesic ointments such as dibucaine (Nupercaine) provides temporary relief from pain and reduces the edema around external or prolapsed internal hemorrhoids. Sitz baths also are extremely helpful in relieving pain.

Acutely thrombosed or prolapsed hemorrhoids may require surgical hemorrhoidectomy. The patient often is in extreme pain and may not be able to focus on the elements of preoperative teaching. Treatment consists of excision of the entire mass. Care of the patient after anorectal surgery is summarized in the Guidelines box below.

### Guidelines for Care of the Person Undergoing Anorectal Surgery

**PREOPERATIVE CARE**

An enema may not be prescribed if rectal pain is acute.
Stool softeners may be given to promote a soft stool before surgery.

**POSTOPERATIVE CARE**

**Promotion of Comfort**

Administer analgesics as prescribed (considerable rectal discomfort may be present).
Suggest side-lying position.
Provide sitz baths as ordered (monitor for hypotension secondary to dilation of pelvic blood vessels in early postoperative period).

**Promotion of Elimination**

Administer prescribed stool softeners.
Encourage patient to defecate as soon as the inclination occurs (prevents strictures and preserves the normal anal lumen). Considerable anxiety is usually present.
Administer an analgesic a short time before initial defecation.
Monitor for hypotension (dizziness, faintness, rapid pulse) during first defecation.
If an enema must be given, use a small-bore rectal tube.

**Patient Teaching**

Clean rectal area after each defecation until healing is complete (sitz bath is recommended).
Avoid constipation with a high-fiber diet, high-fluid intake, regular exercise, and regular time for defecation.
Use stool softeners until healing is complete.
Seek medical consultation for rectal bleeding, suppurative drainage, continued pain on defecation, or continued constipation despite preventive measures.

## ANAL FISSURE, ABSCESS, AND FISTULA

### Etiology/Epidemiology

Anal fissures, fistulas, and abscesses are relatively common problems that develop from trauma or infection in the anorectal area. An **anal fissure** is an elongated laceration between the anal canal and the perianal skin. Fissures may be primary or secondary. Most primary fissures are idiopathic. Secondary fissures are associated with chronic constipation and the passage of hard stool, trauma, or the presence of chronic ulceration from inflammatory bowel disease. An **anal abscess** results most often from the obstruction of gland ducts in the anorectal region by feces, but they also may complicate the presence of a fissure. Stasis of duct contents results in infection that can spread to adjacent tissue. An **anal fistula** involves the development of an abnormal communication between the anal canal and skin outside the anus. The rupture and drainage of an abscess frequently cause an anal fistula.

### Pathophysiology

Most acute anal fissures are superficial and heal spontaneously or in response to conservative therapy. If healing does not occur, however, the fissure may cause significant bleeding or develop local infection. The infection of an abscess may be relatively minor and confined to a single rectal crypt or become widespread. Widespread infection or sepsis may develop in patients with immunodeficiencies. The development of a fistula may necessitate extensive surgical repair.

Pain is the primary problem associated with anal fissure and abscess. It can be severe and prolonged from pressure on the somatic nerves in the perianal area. Any position can be painful inasmuch as the pain often is reflected. Constipation is inevitable because the patient attempts to avoid pain by preventing defecation. Local swelling, erythema, and acute tenderness accompany abscess development. Pruritus in the anal region fre-

**TABLE 47-11 Treatment Options for Anal Fissure, Abscess, and Fistula**

| LESION | DESCRIPTION | CLINICAL MANIFESTATIONS | MEDICAL MANAGEMENT |
|---|---|---|---|
| Fissure | Slitlike ulceration in epithelium of anal canal | Pain with defecation; bleeding; pruritus; constipation | Stool softeners; analgesic ointments; sitz bath; sphincterotomy or fissurectomy if medical therapy ineffective |
| Abscess | Abscess in tissue around anus | Persistent throbbing; anal pain with walking, sitting, defecation; systemic signs of infection | Incision and drainage of abscess |
| Fistula | Hollow track leading through anal tissue from anorectal canal through skin near anus | Purulent discharge near anus; pain; pruritus | Fistulotomy or fistulectomy |

quently accompanies both fissure and fistula. When a fistula is present, the patient notices periodic purulent drainage, which stains undergarments.

### Medical Management

The degree of medical intervention necessary depends on the exact nature and severity of the problem. Medical treatment options are outlined in Table 47-11.

### Nursing Management

Initial nursing interventions for anal disorders focuses on improving the patient's comfort level. This may include analgesics, sitz baths, and the local application of heat, cold, or preparations such as witch hazel. These interventions also are initially important if the patient is undergoing surgical excision or repair.

Preventing recurrences focuses on the importance of careful perianal hygiene and avoiding constipation. All standard measures are presented, including a diet rich in fiber, the selective addition of bran to the diet, adequate fluids and exercise, and the use of stool softeners or bulk laxatives to prevent straining. The repair of fistulas is technically more involved, and nursing interventions focus on restoring and maintaining skin integrity and ensuring adequate nutrition for healing.

# NURSING CARE OF THE PATIENT UNDERGOING BOWEL SURGERY

## PREOPERATIVE CARE

Preparation for bowel surgery may be completed over several days depending on the patient's overall physical condition, need for nutritional support, and the urgency of the surgery. Preparation may begin at home with the use of a low-residue diet to diminish the amount of fecal material in the bowel. Clear liquids typically are given the day before surgery, with supplemental intravenous fluids. Boluses of vitamins K and C may be given to support clotting and wound healing in the postoperative period. The synthesis and absorption of these vitamins are impaired by the vigorous bowel preparation.

Preparation of the bowel for surgery may involve the use of either laxatives or enemas, or both. Bowel preparation is performed to cleanse the colon and suppress bacterial growth that might lead to infection in the postoperative period. A solution such a Golytely (sodium sulfate and polyethylene glycol) provides for an osmotic cleansing of the entire bowel. Up to 4 L are administered orally in divided doses 10 to 15 minutes apart. The cleansing usually is complete in about 4 hours. Systemic or oral antibiotics also may be administered to reduce colonic bacteria. Oral neomycin is a standard preparation. Depending on the urgency of the need for surgery, complete bowel preparation may not be possible.

Teaching is another focus of preoperative nursing care. The nurse teaches the patient about the planned surgery and its expected outcomes including incisions, nasogastric and wound drainage, and the need for an ostomy if applicable. Most patients are extremely concerned about the severity of postoperative pain, and the nurse discusses the plan for postoperative pain management, including the use of patient-controlled analgesia (PCA) (see Chapter 17) if indicated. Pulmonary hygiene is extremely important in the early postoperative period, and the nurse reviews the correct technique for deep breathing, splinting for effective coughing, and use of incentive spirometers. The nurse also stresses the importance of early ambulation in preventing respiratory complications.

## POSTOPERATIVE CARE

### Maintaining Fluid and Electrolyte Balance

The patient usually receives nothing by mouth for brief or extended periods after surgery, and nasogastric suctioning may be in use. Output from the tube is carefully assessed and recorded, and the tube is irrigated as needed to maintain patency. The nurse evaluates intake and output balance, maintains IV fluids as ordered, records daily weight, and monitors for electrolyte imbalance. Monitoring continues as the patient is gradually advanced to a normal diet. An adequate nutrient intake is essential for wound healing, and the nurse carefully assesses the adequacy of the patient's oral intake.

# NURSING CARE PLAN

## PERSON UNDERGOING BOWEL RESECTION WITHOUT COLOSTOMY

**DATA:** Mrs. P. is a 63-year old retired schoolteacher. She is married and the mother of three children and six grandchildren. During the last several months she had noticed several episodes of blood in her stool and a change in bowel habits, with the development of chronic constipation. She underwent colonoscopy 2 weeks ago, which revealed a tumor in her transverse colon. She is admitted on an elective basis for surgery. A colon resection with anastomosis is planned.

The nursing history identified the following:

- Mrs. P. has been in good health her entire life. Her only hospitalizations have been for childbirth. The cancer diagnosis is very frightening to her.
- She is about 20 pounds overweight, which she reports "has been a problem for years."
- She takes a beta blocker for mild hypertension.
- She has osteoarthritis in her right hip and lower back but is active and walks several times a week.
- Mr. P. is attentive and concerned. He is also in good health. Her children are arriving to lend support to their parents.

Mrs. P. completes her bowel preparation and is prepared for surgery. The nurse reinforces teaching about deep breathing, position changes, leg exercises, and use of patient-controlled analgesia (PCA) after surgery. Mrs. P. is very nervous but in control.

Mrs. P. returns from successful surgery very groggy but arousable. She has an IV infusion in place, a second IV line with a PCA pump, an NG tube to low intermittent suction, a midline abdominal dressing, and a Jackson-Pratt wound drain. Collaborative nursing actions include the following:

- Frequent monitoring of vital signs
- Monitoring all intake and output
- Assessing level of consciousness
- Monitoring for complications such as shock, hemorrhage, dehiscence

### ■ NURSING DIAGNOSIS

Acute pain related to surgical procedure

| Expected Patient Outcome | Nursing Interventions | Rationale |
|---|---|---|
| States pain is relieved by medication and other pain-relief measures. | Encourage Mrs. P. to use the PCA pump:<br>Review technique as needed.<br>Reinforce understanding of safeguards to prevent overdosage. | Surgical pain is severe after abdominal surgery. Narcotic doses administered by PCA are small and should be used before pain becomes extreme to maintain effectiveness. Drowsiness occurs after surgery, and patient needs to be reminded to self-medicate. |
| | Assess effectiveness of pain relief obtained by PCA use.<br>If inadequate, encourage more frequent use. | Prescribed doses for PCA use are based on averages. They will be effective only if used promptly to control pain. |
| | If still inadequate, contact physician to seek medication change. | The dose may need to be increased if it remains ineffective in controlling pain. |
| | Assess vital sign changes in response to narcotic. | Narcotics can depress the respiratory center. |
| | Provide nonpharmacologic pain-relief measures to augment PCA, for example:<br>Position changes<br>Distraction<br>Ice chips and mouth care<br>Back rub or massage | Not all discomfort related to surgery is incisional. These measures help restore a sense of control and can be utilized by family as well. |

### ■ NURSING DIAGNOSIS

Ineffective airway clearance related to pain, immobility, and postanesthesia effects

| Expected Patient Outcome | Nursing Interventions | Rationale |
|---|---|---|
| Lungs will be clear to auscultation. | Reinforce preoperative teaching concerning the importance of deep breathing, coughing, and changing positions. | Delayed effects of anesthesia and the immediate pain of surgery decrease adherence. Verbal reminders may increase use of measures. |

*Continued.*

# NURSING CARE PLAN

## PERSON UNDERGOING BOWEL RESECTION WITHOUT COLOSTOMY—cont'd

| Expected Patient Outcome | Nursing Interventions | Rationale |
|---|---|---|
| | Promote and assist patient to<br>▪ Take 10 maximal deep breaths each hour<br>▪ Change positions q 1-2 hr<br>▪ Splint the incision to cough effectively and clear the airway<br>▪ Use incentive spirometer if ordered | Breathing exercises and position changes promote maximal lung expansion and the clearance of secretions, preventing atelectasis. |
| | Auscultate lungs q 4 hr. | Diminished breath sounds may indicate atelectasis. Retained secretions will create rales. |
| | Monitor I&O, and ensure adequate pain relief. | IV fluids must be adequate to keep patient hydrated and secretions thin.<br>Pain inhibits deep breathing and promotes atelectasis. |

### ▪ NURSING DIAGNOSIS

Colonic constipation related to decreased peristalsis secondary to surgical manipulation of intestines, effects of narcotics, and decreased mobility

| Expected Patient Outcome | Nursing Interventions | Rationale |
|---|---|---|
| Will resume preoperative bowel elimination pattern. | Auscultate abdomen for return and character of bowel sounds. | Return of bowel sounds is an indication of restored peristalsis. |
| | Encourage patient to be out of bed and ambulating.<br>Ensure adequate pain relief before activity. | Activity stimulates peristalsis through improved abdominal muscle tone.<br>The presence of pain will decrease activity. |
| | Introduce liquids and diet as ordered once peristalsis is restored.<br>Instruct patient about fiber-rich food before discharge.<br>Encourage daily fluid intake of ≥2000 ml or more. | Food and fluid are needed to restore a normal bowel pattern after surgery.<br>Adequate fiber promotes regular elimination. |

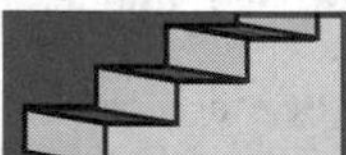

## CRITICAL PATHWAY Colon Resection Without Colostomy

**DRG #: 152 Expected LOS: 8**

| | Day of Admission<br>Day 1 | Day of Surgery<br>Day 2 | Day 3 | Day 4 |
|---|---|---|---|---|
| **Diagnostic Tests** | CBC, UA, SMA/18,* chest x-ray films, ECG, T & X | CBC, electrolytes | | CBC, electrolytes |
| **Medications** | IV saline lock; IV antibiotics; colon cleansing, e.g., oral laxatives, enemas | IVs, IV antibiotics, IV analgesic | IVs, IV antibiotics, IV analgesic | IVs, IV antibiotics, IV analgesic |
| **Treatments** | Wt, VS q8hr | I & O q8hr, including NG and Foley; check drainage on dressing q2hr; elastic leg stockings; mouth and nares care q2hr | I & O q8hr, including NG and Foley; check dressing for drainage q4hr, VS q4hr; wt; elastic leg stockings; mouth and nares care q2hr; assess bowel sounds q4hr | I & O q8hr, including NG and Foley; check dressing for drainage q4hr, VS q6hr; elastic leg stockings; mouth and nares care q2hr; assess bowel sounds q4hr |
| **Diet** | Clear liquids; NPO p̄ MN | NPO | NPO | NPO |
| **Activity** | Up ad lib | Bed rest; up in chair with assistance × 1; T, C & DB q2hr | Bed rest; up in room with assistance × 4; T, C & DB q2hr | Bed rest; up in chair with assistance × 6; T, C & DB q2hr |
| **Consultations** | Anesthesiologist; other specialist as needed for other medical problems | | | SNU care/or home health |

*CBC,* Complete blood cell count; *Disc,* discontinue; *I & O,* intake and output; *LOS,* length of stay; *p MN,* after midnight; *SMA,* sequential multiple analysis; *SNU,* skilled nursing unit; *T, C & DB,* turn, cough, and deep breathe; *T & X,* type and crossmatch; *UA,* urinalysis; *VS,* vital signs; *Wt,* weight.

## NURSING CARE PLAN

### PERSON UNDERGOING BOWEL RESECTION WITHOUT COLOSTOMY—cont'd

**■ NURSING DIAGNOSIS**

Altered health maintenance related to insufficient knowledge of incision care and signs and symptoms of complications

| Expected Patient Outcomes | Nursing Interventions | Rationale |
|---|---|---|
| Can describe:<br>Wound care<br>Factors that influence wound healing<br>Signs and symptoms to be reported to physician | Explain and demonstrate care of healing abdominal incision:<br>■ Washing gently with soap and water<br>■ Using dry sterile dressing to cover if preferred<br>Teach factors to promote continued wound healing:<br>■ Avoiding frequent bending or lifting<br>■ Eating a balanced diet with adequate protein, vitamins, and fluid | Operative incisions are sealed within 24 hr and do not require special sterile care. However, a dry sterile dressing may be used to prevent pulling on retained sutures or staples. Healing wounds need increased levels of protein, carbohydrate, and vitamin intake to support scar formation. Excessive activity suppresses skin regeneration and increases risk of dehiscence. |
| | Teach signs and symptoms of complications to be reported:<br>■ Wound separation, redness, swelling or discharge<br>■ Fever; change in sputum quantity or color<br>■ Urinary frequency, burning, or foul-smelling urine<br>■ Pain, swelling, and warmth in calf or leg | Early detection minimizes severity of complications: signs of wound infection, dehiscence, pneumonia, urinary tract infection, and deep venous thrombosis (DVT). |
| | Provide written instructions to go home with patient. | Written instructions provide a resource for home use. |

| Day 5 | Day 6 | Day 7 | Day of Discharge Day 8 |
|---|---|---|---|
| | | | |
| IV rate decreased as PO fluid increased; IV antibiotics; IM to PO analgesic | IV to saline lock; IV antibiotics; PO analgesic, stool softener | Disc antibiotic; PO analgesic, stool softener | Disc saline lock |
| I & O q8hr (?Disc NG and Foley); check dressing for drainage q6hr, VS q6hr; elastic leg stockings; mouth and nares care q2hr; assess bowel sounds q4hr | I & O q8hr, VS q8hr; wt; assess bowel sounds q8hr; elastic leg stockings | Disc I & O; VS q8hr; assess bowel sounds/q8hr; elastic leg stockings | VS q8hr; elastic leg stockings |
| Begin clear liquids | Clear liquids; advance to soft diet | Soft | Soft |
| Up walking in hallway with assistance × 3; up in chair × 6 | Up walking in hallway with assistance × 4; up in chair ad lib | Up ad lib; walking in hallway | Up ad lib; walking in hallway |

*Serum calcium, phosphorus, triglycerides, uric acid, creatinine, BUN, total bilirubin, alkaline phosphate, aspartate aminotransferase (AST) (formerly serum glutamic-oxaloacetic transaminase [SGOT]), alanine aminotransferase (ALT) (formerly serum glutamate pyruvate transaminase [SGPT]), lactic dehydrogenase (LDH), total protein, albumin, sodium, potassium, chloride, total $CO_2$, glucose.

## RESEARCH

Tittle MB, Long MC, McMillan SC: Measurement of pain in postoperative abdominal surgery patients, *Appl Nurs Res* 5(1):26-31, 1992.

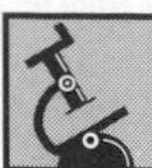

This study was designed to determine whether pain decreased between the first and third days after abdominal surgery. It involved 100 patients from two different institutions. The mean scores on the pain scales used indicated that pain decreased significantly from the first to third day for most patients but was still present. For 18% to 20% of the study participants at each hospital, however, pain intensity *increased* over the 3 postoperative days. A wide range of terms was used by study participants to describe their pain. The findings confirm the importance of assessing and planning interventions for pain on an individual basis.

### Promoting Ventilation

Incisional pain typically is severe with abdominal surgery, and pain can interfere with lung excursion (see Research box above). The nurse monitors the effectiveness of the patient-controlled analgesia system or ensures that adequate narcotic analgesia is provided to allow for early ambulation and regular deep breathing. The nurse auscultates regularly for signs of atelectasis and encourages the use of incentive spirometry to open the alveoli. Deep breathing must be performed hourly in the early postoperative days to prevent pulmonary complications.

### Supporting Peristalsis

Temporary paralytic ileus is an expected complication of bowel surgery in which manipulation of the intestines takes place. Prolonged ileus may indicate an abdominal abscess or obstruction. The passage of gas rectally indicates the beginning return of peristalsis. The nurse auscultates the patient's abdomen for bowel sounds every 4 hours and assesses for the movement of gas or presence of distention. Ambulation facilitates the return of peristalsis, and the nurse encourages the patient to be as active as possible. The diet and activity changes plus loss of bowel tissue that accompany resection may make it difficult initially for the patient to resume a normal elimination pattern. Diarrhea may occur initially, but it usually is temporary and self-limiting. The nurse teaches the patient to avoid constipation through regular exercise, adequate fluids, and adjusting the fiber content of the diet. Laxatives should be avoided if possible.

Some surgeons are investigating the theory that preserving GI function after abdominal surgery can drastically reduce the incidence of postoperative complications. This "accelerated recovery" approach utilizes a triple-lumen Moss tube that is inserted during surgery. It provides for simultaneous gastric decompression and intestinal feeding. Elemental tube feedings are initiated in the recovery room. Theoretically this intervention supports normal functioning of the small intestine and prevents the gastric distention that is theorized to contribute to paralytic ileus. Metoclopromide (Reglan) also is administered to promote GI motility. The tube is removed after about 18 hours, and the average hospital stay is significantly reduced. See Nursing Care Plan (pp. 1584-1587) and corresponding Critical Pathway (pp. 1586-1587) for the patient undergoing bowel resection without colostomy.

## QUESTIONS TO CONSIDER

- Compare and contrast ulcerative colitis, Crohn's disease, and diverticular disease.
- Suppose you have recently been diagnosed as having ulcerative colitis. Your weight is 110 pounds, down from your normal 130 pounds. You have diarrhea about once every hour with occasional leakage. You feel tired and listless and have lost your appetite. What changes would you have to make in your life? What particular concerns do you think you might have? What kind of help would you seek?
- Compare and contrast small and large bowel obstruction.
- Obtain a copy of the most recent issue of *Cancer Facts and Figures* from your local chapter of the American Cancer Society. How does the incidence of colorectal cancer compare with other cancers among men and women? What are the recent trends?
- What resources are available in your community for persons with a colostomy? Where can supplies be purchased? What would be the average monthly cost? Discuss with an enterostomal therapist common problems experienced by persons with ostomies.

## CRITICAL THINKING ACTIVITIES

- Ms. Butler has been in the hospital for over 3 weeks. Her initial diagnosis was that of diverticulitis. However, she developed a perforation, which led to the development of peritonitis. While you were giving her a bath, she asks why she became so sick, and what will be done for her now. How could you best explain the complication of peritonitis, and its treatment, to her?
- You are Mr. Freeman's home health nurse, and Mrs. Freeman calls you in a panic state. She tells you that Mr. Freeman's Groshong site is red and swollen. He has been running a fever of 101° F. What problem do you suspect, and what plan of action would you take to reduce their anxiety and address the problem?

## Chapter Summary

### COMMON BOWEL DYSFUNCTIONS

- Flatulence is one of the most common GI complaints. Increasing exercise and reducing gas-producing foods in the diet can improve a patient's comfort.
- Constipation refers to the passage of abnormally infrequent or hard stools. Although a wide variety of drug therapies exist, it is best managed by increasing dietary fibers, fluids, and exercise.
- Diarrhea refers to abnormally watery stools and may be caused by food allergies, GI infections, hypermetabolism, or malabsorption disorders. Medical treatment is aimed at correcting the underlying cause and may involve drug treatment with local or systemic-acting agents.
- Fecal incontinence may result from CNS lesions or injury or trauma to the anal sphincter. Management involves bowel training programs that combine the use of suppositories and conditioned responses.

### ACUTE INFECTION/INFLAMMATION OF THE INTESTINES

- Appendicitis involves acute inflammation of the appendix and is a common surgical emergency. Classic features include acute right lower quadrant abdominal pain, localization and rebound tenderness at McBurney's point, anorexia, and nausea.
- Peritonitis is an inflammation of the peritoneum from trauma or rupture of an organ. Loss of fluids into the peritoneal cavity leads to dehydration and shock; peristalsis may cease. Treatment consists of fluid replacement and antibiotic therapy; surgery may be necessary.
- Diverticular disease involves small outpouchings, usually of the colon wall; diverticulitis is the associated inflammatory condition. It is related to chronic constipation and managed with a high-fiber diet and bulk laxatives. Surgical resection may be necessary to treat acute episodes or perforation.
- Parasitic infections of the intestine include amebiasis and giardiasis, which are caused by protozoa, and trichinosis caused by roundworm infestation. Treatment involves appropriate antibiotics and teaching to prevent reinfestation.

### INFLAMMATORY BOWEL DISEASE

- Ulcerative colitis primarily affects the rectum and left colon. Mucosal involvement is continuous and causes profuse diarrhea, which contains blood but rarely fat.
- Crohn's disease affects primarily the distal ileum but may occur anywhere in the GI tract. It involves all layers of the bowel and appears in scattered segmental sections. Fistulas and strictures are common. The frequent semisoft stools contain fat but rarely blood.
- Care of the patient with inflammatory bowel disease involves a low-residue, high-protein, and high-calorie diet; drug therapy with sulfasalazine and other antiinflammatory agents; comfort measures; and facilitation of coping.
- Total colectomy is curative for ulcerative colitis. Continent procedures that preserve the anal sphincter are used more commonly today than the traditional ileostomy.
- Surgery in Crohn's disease is used to treat strictures, fistulas, or perforation. Although the disease frequently recurs after surgery, quality of life usually is significantly improved.

### MALABSORPTION AND MALNUTRITION

- Malabsorption syndrome results from inadequate absorption of fat in the small intestine; it often is accompanied by decreased absorption of protein, carbohydrates, and minerals. It can result from IBD, extensive gastric surgery, pancreatic insufficiency, and extensive liver disease. Long-term nutritional support often is necessary.
- Tropical sprue is a malabsorption disorder that appears to have both nutritional and infectious bases; treatment is with tetracycline, folic acid, and a diet high in protein but normal in fat.
- Celiac sprue results from an intolerance to gluten found in grains, causing atrophy of intestinal villi in the proximal jejunum; treatment consists of a gluten-free diet.
- Adult lactase deficiency causes an accumulation of lactose in the GI tract, which acts as an osmotic agent in the intestinal lumen, causing diarrhea. Treatment involves a lactose-free diet.
- Protein-calorie malnutrition occurs in hospitalized patients who have difficulty or disinterest in eating, who have nutrient losses through the GI tract, or who have cancer, prolonged infection, or fever.
- Persons with protein-calorie malnutrition may be fed orally, enterally (tube feedings, gastrostomy), or by total parenteral nutrition (TPN).
- Tube feeding solutions differ in terms of carbohydrate or protein content, osmolality, consistency, palatability, flavor, and expense.
- Gastrostomy may be performed surgically through the abdomen or by percutaneous endoscopy.
- TPN solutions are deposited into the superior vena cava to provide greater dilution of the highly concentrated solutions.
- Complications of TPN include infection, air embolism, electrolyte imbalances, overhydration, hyperglycemia, hypoglycemia, vitamin D deficiency, and vitamin A excess.
- Long-term TPN may be administered successfully in the home setting with careful teaching and supervision of the patient and caretaker. IBD is one of the most common causes of need for long-term administration of TPN.

## INTESTINAL OBSTRUCTION

- Intestinal obstruction may result from inhibition of peristalsis (paralytic ileus) or from mechanical obstruction caused by such factors as adhesions, volvulus, intussusception, hernias, or cancer. Large amounts of fluid and electrolytes are lost from the circulation into the intestinal lumen, resulting in fluid and electrolyte imbalances and finally shock. Therapy consists of inserting an NG tube, restricting oral intake, and removing the source of obstruction, if possible.
- Bowel infarction may result from interruption of blood flow in the mesenteric blood vessels, leading to interruption of bowel function. Surgery to remove the gangrenous bowel usually is indicated.
- Paralytic ileus is cessation of peristalsis from neurogenic impairment, usually as a result of irritation of the GI tract during surgery. Gastrointestinal intubation with suction provides removal of excess fluid and gas until peristalsis returns; surgery to decompress the bowel is sometimes necessary.

## ABDOMINAL HERNIAS

- Hernias may occur in the inguinal, femoral, or umbilical areas from mural defects or in weakened scars from previous abdominal surgeries. Of concern is the possible entrapment (incarceration) of a loop of bowel. The treatment is surgical repair.

## COLORECTAL CANCER

- Risk factors for bowel cancer (the second most common form of cancer) are age—40 years or older; history of colon polyps, colon cancer, cancer of the reproductive organs, or ulcerative colitis; or a family history of colorectal cancer or polyposis disorder.
- Recommendations for early detection of colorectal cancer include a digital rectal examination yearly after 40 years of age; occult blood stool test yearly after age 50; and proctosigmoidoscopy every 3 to 5 years after age 50, following two negative results of yearly examinations.
- Current research does not support the effectiveness of currently available occult stool tests as a mass screening tool for colorectal cancer.
- More than half of all colorectal cancers occur in the distal sigmoid colon or rectum. Most are detectable by digital rectal examination.
- Surgery for cancer of the colon and upper rectum usually consists of resection with anastomosis; surgery for cancer involving the lower rectum has traditionally involved abdominoperineal resection plus colostomy. Sphincter-sparing surgeries that avoid colostomy are being increasingly used for distal cancers.
- Types of stomas include end stoma (end of bowel brought out abdominal wall to form a single stoma), loop stoma (loop of bowel brought out abdominal wall and opened to create one stoma with two openings), and loop-end stoma (end of bowel oversewn and stoma made from intestinal loop close to end).
- Care of a person with a colostomy or ileostomy includes preparing the person for the surgery, monitoring the stoma, assessing readiness of the person to view the stoma, promoting acceptance of body changes, teaching the person stoma care, and informing the person of community support services.
- Teaching the person with a colostomy includes promoting nutrition and elimination, promoting return to normal activities and sexuality, and preventing complications.
- Stoma care includes cleaning of the skin to prevent skin breakdown, early treatment of excoriated skin, application of pouches to prevent leakage, and irrigation techniques to control timing of stool elimination.

## ANORECTAL DISORDERS

- Inflammatory anorectal lesions include anal fissures, anal abscesses, and anal fistulas; hemorrhoids are varicose veins of the rectum. Relief of discomfort from anal lesions may include measures to prevent constipation (which irritates the lesions) and sitz baths.
- Care after anorectal surgery includes giving prescribed analgesics and sitz baths for comfort, stool softeners to promote early defecation with less trauma, and teaching the patient measures to prevent constipation.
- Care of the patient after bowel surgery includes breathing exercises to promote oxygenation, ensuring adequate fluid intake, monitoring for return of peristalsis, giving analgesics for pain, and teaching to avoid constipation and laxative use.

# REFERENCES


1. Ahlquist DA et al: Accuracy of fecal occult blood screening for colorectal neoplasia, *JAMA* 269(10):1262-1267, 1993.
2. American Cancer Society: *Cancer facts and figures,* New York, 1992, The Society.
3. Bayless TM, Harris ML: Inflammatory bowel disease and irritable bowel syndrome, *Med Clin North Am* 74(1):21-28, 1990.
4. Brostrom O: Prognosis in ulcerative colitis, *Med Clin North Am* 74(1):201-218, 1990.
5. Bryant G: When the bowel is blocked, *RN* 55(2):58-66, 1992.
6. Eisenberg P: Enteral nutrition: indications, formulas and delivery techniques, *Nurs Clin North Am* 24(2):315-338, 1989.
7. Fazio VW: Conservative surgery for Crohn's disease of the small bowel: the role of strictureplasty, *Med Clin North Am* 74(1):169-181, 1990.
8. Grimm IS, Friedman LS: Inflammatory bowel disease in the elderly, *Gastroenterol Clin North Am* 19(2):361-385, 1990.
9. Hanauer SB, Peppercorn MA, Present DH: Current concepts, new therapies in IBD, *Patient Care* 26:79-102, 1992.
10. Hellers G, Bernell O: Genetic aspects of inflammatory bowel disease, *Med Clin North Am* 74(1):13-19, 1990.
11. Jagelman DG: Surgical alternatives for ulcerative colitis, *Med Clin North Am* 74(1):155-167, 1990.

12. Kohn CL, Keithley JK: Enteral nutrition: potential complications and patient monitoring, *Nurs Clin North Am* 24(2):339-351, 1989.
13. Korelitz BI: Considerations of surveillance, dysplasia and carcinoma of the colon in the management of ulcerative colitis and Crohn's disease, *Med Clin North Am* 74(1):189-198, 1990.
14. Leibach JR, Cerda JJ: Hemorrhoids: modern treatment methods, *Hosp Med* 27(8):53-68, 1991.
15. MacCarty RL: The case for barium enema, *Mayo Clin Proc* 67(3):253-257, 1992.
16. Meize-Grochowski AR: When the DX is Crohn's disease, *RN* 54(2):52-55, 1991.
17. NIH Consensus Group: Adjuvant therapy for patients with colon and rectum cancer, *JAMA* 264:1444-1450, 1990.
18. Novak LT: Accelerated recovery technique: a new approach to abdominal surgery, *RN* 56(3):19-23, 1993.
19. O'Connell MJ, Rich TA, Steele GD: Low rectal Ca: sphincter-sparing strategies, *Patient Care* 25:32-48, 1991.
20. Palmer RC: Diverticular disease: dietary and other measures that help control the lesions, *Consultant* 28(5):75-82, 1988.
21. Ranashoff DF, Lang CA: Sigmoidoscopic screening in the 1990's, *JAMA* 269(10):1278-1281, 1993.
22. Rankin GB: Extraintestinal and systemic manifestations of inflammatory bowel disease, *Med Clin North Am* 74(1):39-50, 1990.
23. Ruderman WB: Newer pharmacologic agents for the therapy of inflammatory bowel disease, *Med Clin North Am* 74(1):133-150, 1990.
24. Sachar DB: The problem of postoperative recurrence of Crohn's disease, *Med Clin North Am* 74(1):183-188, 1990.
25. Selby JV: How should we screen for colorectal cancer, *JAMA* 269(10):1294-1296, 1993.
26. Sutherland LR: Topical treatment of ulcerative colitis, *Med Clin North Am* 74(1):119-130, 1990.
27. Vandel JS et al: Reducing mortality from colorectal cancer by screening for fecal occult blood, *N Engl J Med* 328(19):1365-1371, 1993.
28. Wallach CB, Kurtz RC: Gastrointestinal cancer in the elderly, *Gastroenterol Clin North Am* 19(2):419-432, 1990.
29. Waye JD: Endoscopy in inflammatory bowel disease, *Med Clin North Am* 74(1):51-64, 1990.
30. Whelan G: Epidemiology of inflammatory bowel disease, *Med Clin North Am* 74(1):1-12, 1990.

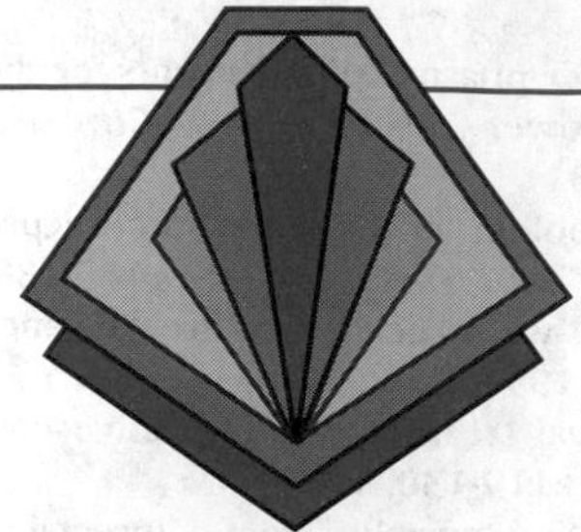

CHAPTER 48

# Assessment of the Renal System

*Marilyn Rossman Bartucci*

## CHAPTER OBJECTIVES

***After studying this chapter, the learner should be able to do the following:***

1 List seven major functions of the kidneys.
2 Apply subjective, objective, and laboratory data to assess renal and urinary function.
3 Analyze the relationships among glomerular filtration rate, creatinine clearance, blood urea nitrogen, and serum creatinine as indicators of renal function.
4 List seven symptoms related to urination and the possible urinary problems they may indicate.
5 Describe the nursing implications of eight common radiologic examinations of the urinary tract.

## KEY TERMS

anuria
clean-catch specimen
collecting duct
composite specimen
creatinine clearance test
cystometric examination
cystoscopy
distal convoluted tubule
dysuria
erythropoiesis
frequency
glomerular filtration rate (GFR)
hematuria
hesitancy
intravenous pyelogram (IVP)
kidney, ureter, bladder (KUB) x-ray film
loop of Henle
micturition
midstream void
nephron
nocturia
oliguria
open renal biopsy
percutaneous renal biopsy
polyuria
proximal convoluted tubule
renal angiography
renal cortex
renal medulla
renal sinus
residual urine
retrograde pyelogram
sodium excretion test
trigone
ultrafiltrate
ultrafiltration
urgency
urinary incontinence

An essential process for living tissue is *metabolism,* the process by which an organism is able to convert raw materials into energy. During metabolism, toxic waste products are formed. Maintaining *homeostasis,* or the state of equilibrium of the internal cellular environment, becomes essential for the continuation of life. There must be a means by which metabolic wastes are removed from living cells. Furthermore, the body must regulate fluid volume, electrolyte composition, and acid-base balance. The kidneys and other structures of the urinary system (Figure 48-1) play major roles in the regulation of the internal environment. In addition to the role the kidneys play in maintaining the composition of body fluids and electrolytes within critical limits—providing a vehicle by which metabolic wastes are excreted from the body and regulating the acid-base balance—these organs serve several other functions (Box 48-1).

## ANATOMY AND PHYSIOLOGY

### ANATOMY

#### Upper Urinary Tract

The kidneys are two reddish-brown, lima bean-shaped organs that lie behind the parietal peritoneum, against

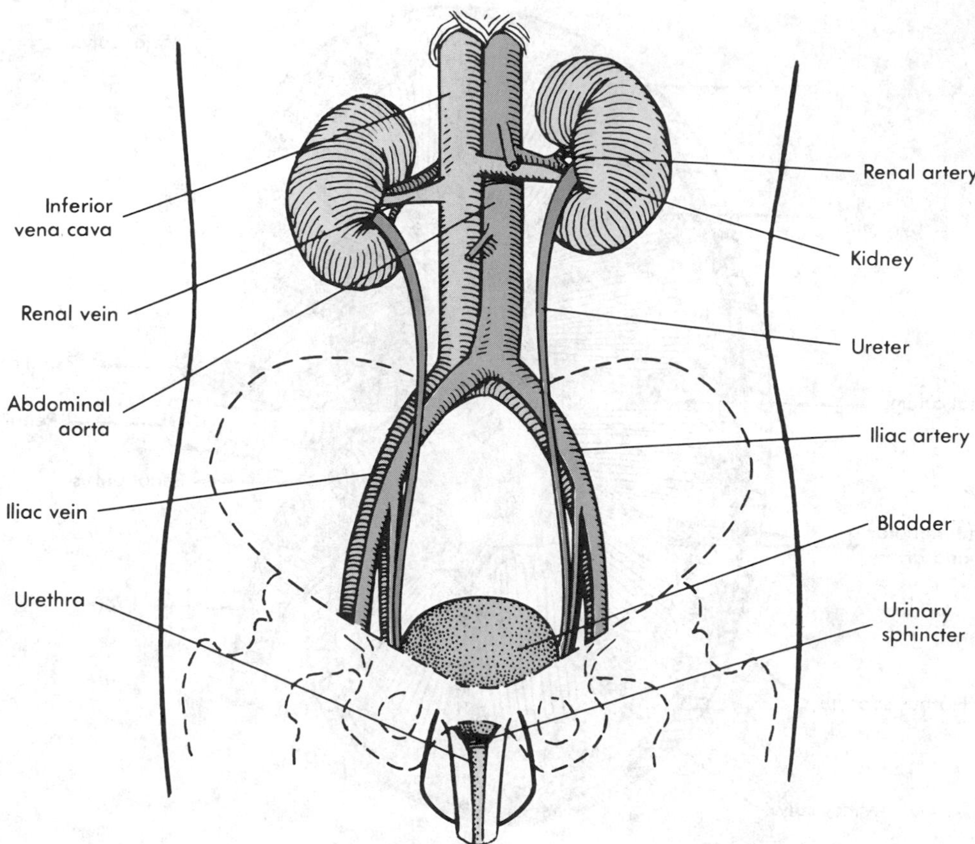


**FIGURE 48-1** Organs and structures of urinary system.

the posterior abdominal wall at the costovertebral angle. The kidneys lie on either side of the abdominal aorta, inferior vena cava (see Figure 48-1), and lumbar spine between the twelfth thoracic and third lumbar vertebrae. The liver pushes the right kidney down to a level slightly lower than the left.

The kidneys are encased in a tough white fibrous coat known as the *renal capsule.* In addition, each kidney is surrounded by a mass of perinephric fat that provides protection against injury. An adrenal gland lies above each kidney within the perinephric fat. The renal fascia and surrounding organs help to hold the kidneys in place. On the medial aspect of each kidney is a concave notch known as the *hilum.* The renal arteries and nerves enter and the renal veins, lymphatics, and ureters exit the kidney at the hilum (Figure 48-2).

When the kidney is cut longitudinally and opened, three distinct areas of the kidney can be seen: the cortex, the medulla, and the renal sinus (Figure 48-2). The **renal cortex** is pale and has a granular appearance. Most parts of the nephron, the functional unit of the kidney, lie in this area.

The middle section, the **renal medulla,** has a striated appearance. In the medulla there are 8 to 10 triangular wedges or pyramids. The bases of the pyramids face the cortex, and their apexes or renal papillae face the center of the kidney. The pyramids have a striated appearance because of the segment of the nephrons and collecting ducts located here.

The third section of the kidney is the **renal sinus.** It is a cavity almost completely filled with blood vessels and structures formed by the expanded upper end of the ureter. Before entering the kidney, the ureter dilates to form the renal pelvis. The renal pelvis branches into two or three calyces. Each major calyx branches into several minor calyces. The minor calyces collect the urine that drains from the collecting ducts.

### BOX 48-1 Major Functions of the Kidneys

**HOMEOSTASIS OF INTERNAL ENVIRONMENT**

Fluid-volume control
Electrolyte regulation
Acid-base balance
Excretion of metabolic wastes, toxins, and drugs

**REGULATION OF BODY PROCESSES**

Regulation of blood pressure
Stimulation of red blood cell production
Regulation of calcium-phosphate metabolism

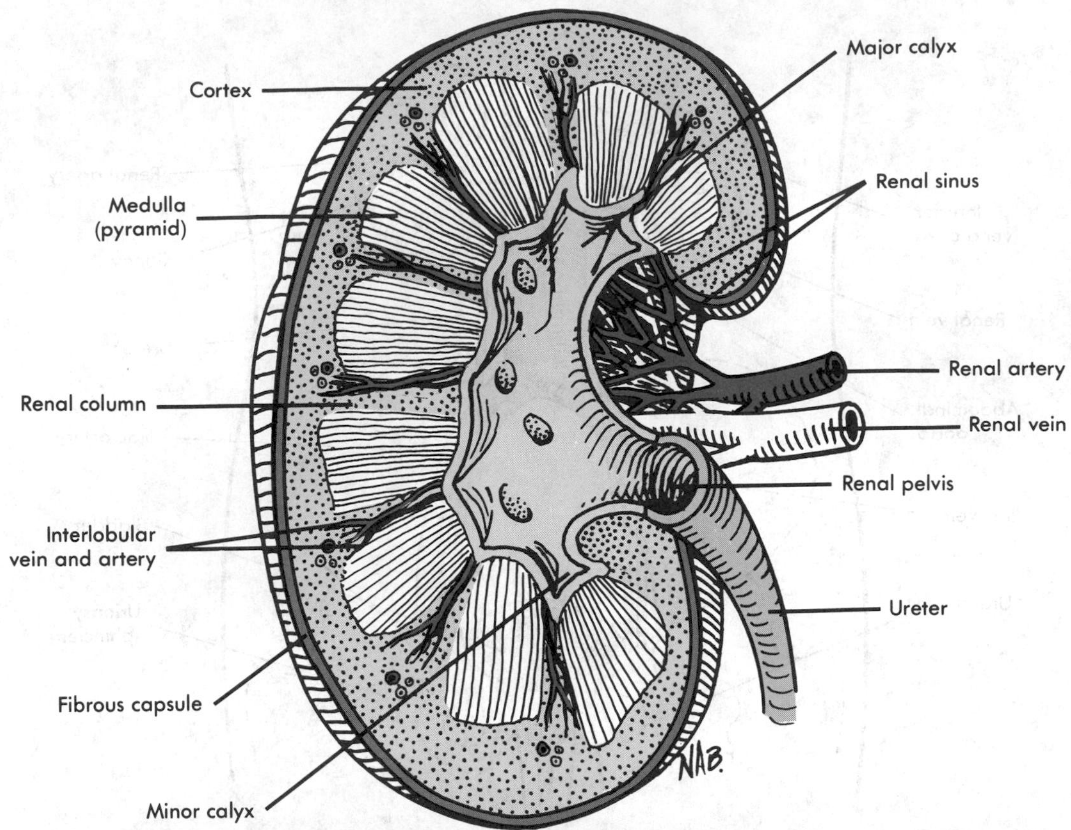


**FIGURE 48-2** Frontal section of kidney.

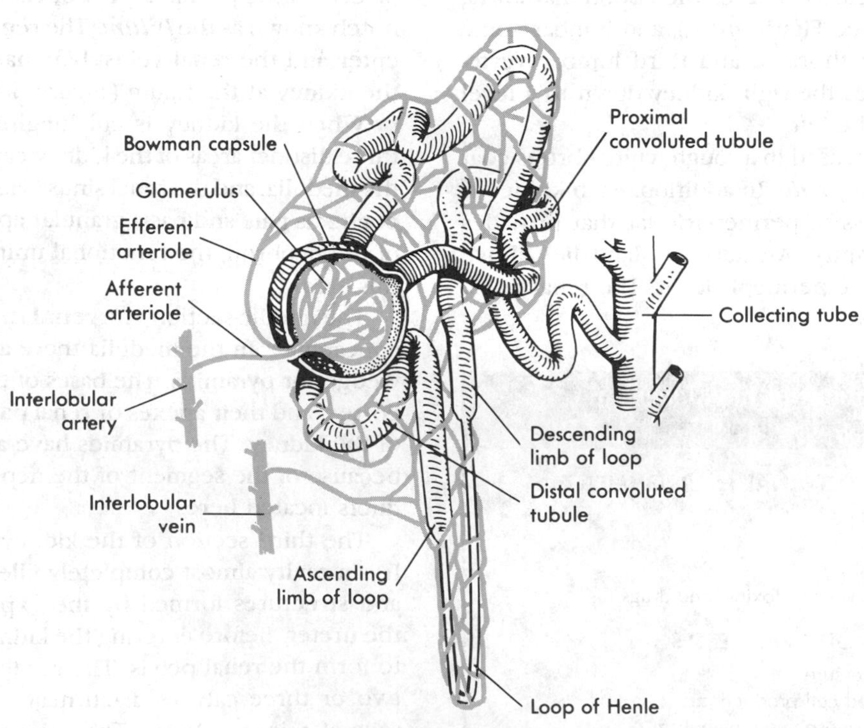


**FIGURE 48-3** Nephron.

The **nephron** is the functional unit of the kidney. Each kidney contains approximately 1 million nephrons. There are two types of nephrons, cortical and juxtamedullary, named according to the location of their glomeruli within the renal parenchyma. The cortical nephrons comprise 85% of the total nephrons and perform excretory and regulatory functions. The juxtamedullary nephrons make up the remaining 15% and play an important role in the concentration and dilution of urine by generating a steep interstitial fluid osmotic gradient between the cortex and deep medulla.[3] The structures of the nephron involved in the process of urine formation include the renal corpuscle, the renal tubules, and the collecting duct (Figure 48-3). The *renal corpuscle* consists of the glomerulus and Bowman's capsule and is responsible for the formation of ultrafiltrate from the blood. The *renal tubules* consist of the **proximal convoluted tubule,** the **loop of Henle,** and the **distal convoluted tubule** and are responsible for the reabsorption and secretion that alter the volume and composition of the ultrafiltrate to form the final urine product. The **collecting duct** receives tubular fluid from many nephrons and transports the fluid from the cortex to the minor calyx.

The kidneys are highly vascular organs, receiving about 20% of the cardiac output in the resting state.[3] Arterial blood is supplied by the renal arteries, which branch directly off the abdominal aorta (see Figure 48-1). Although 70% of human beings have one renal artery supplying each kidney, about 30% have one or more accessory renal arteries that also branch off the aorta and supply a portion of the kidney.

The renal artery branches into approximately five segmental arteries, dividing the kidney into vascular segments. The segmental arteries branch to form the lobar arteries, one of which supplies each pyramid. The lobar arteries divide into two or three interlobar arteries, which ascend toward the cortex on either side of the pyramid in the renal columns. The interlobar arteries turn at right angles to form the arcuate arteries where the cortex and medulla meet. The arcuate arteries have multiple branches known as the *interlobular* arteries, which ascend at right angles into the cortex.

The vascular structure of the kidney is unique. It has two capillary beds separated from each other by the efferent arteriole. The afferent arteriole branches off the interlobular artery to supply blood to the glomerular capillaries. Blood leaving the glomerulus does not enter a vein but instead enters a second arteriole, the efferent arteriole (Figure 48-3).[6]

Blood drains from the peritubular capillaries into the interlobular veins, beginning the venous system in the kidneys. The veins of the kidney follow the same pattern as the renal arteries. Blood flows from the interlobular veins into the arcuate veins and then to the interlobar veins, ultimately forming the renal vein, which empties into the inferior vena cava. Most persons have one renal vein, but some may have one or more accessory veins.

The *ureters* (see Figure 48-1) arise as extensions of the pelvis and empty into the bladder in an area known

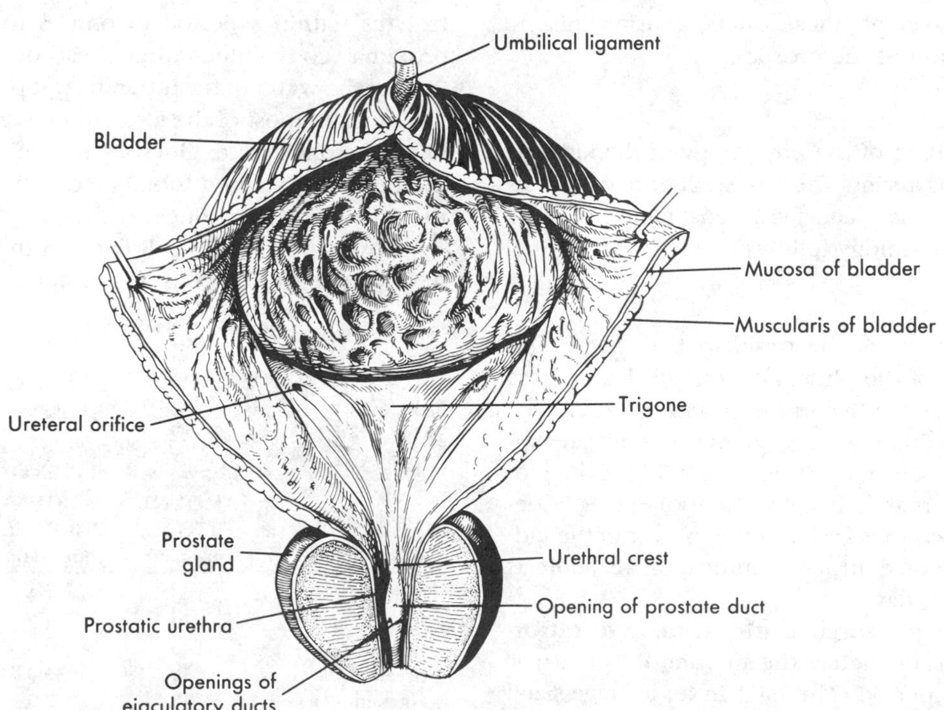


**FIGURE 48-4** Interior of urinary bladder and some associated structures. (From McClintic JR: *Human anatomy,* St Louis, 1983, Mosby.)

as the **trigone** (Figure 48-4). The trigone is a fold of mucous membrane that serves as a valve preventing the backflow or reflux of urine into the ureter when the bladder contracts. The ureters are composed of smooth muscle and are innervated by the sympathetic nervous system. The function of the ureters is to propel urine from the renal pelves to the bladder.

### Lower Urinary Tract

The *bladder,* located behind the symphysis pubis in the pelvic region (see Figure 48-1), serves as a collecting bag for the urine. The mucous membrane is arranged in folds called *rugae* that, together with the elasticity of the muscular walls, can distend the bladder considerably to hold large amounts of urine. A layer of skeletal muscle encircles the base of the bladder, forming the *external urinary sphincter.* The bladder is innervated by both the sympathetic and parasympathetic nervous systems. The urethral sphincter, operating under voluntary control, allows the urine to pass into the urethra.

The *urethra* serves as the outlet for urine from the bladder. The male urethra is about 20 cm (8 in) in length, whereas the female urethra is about 4 cm (1.5 in) long. The urinary meatus is the opening through which urine is excreted from the body.

The *prostate gland* is a male reproductive gland about the size of a walnut that encircles the upper portion of the male urethra (see Figure 48-4). It is doughnut-shaped with the urethra passing through the "hole." When the prostate is enlarged, the urethra is squeezed, causing obstruction of urinary flow. Numerous prostatic ducts empty into the urethra. Bacteria from urinary tract infections may travel up these ducts, causing inflammation and infection of the prostate.

## PHYSIOLOGY

A clear understanding of the physiology of the kidneys is essential to mastering the constellation of physiochemical changes that occur with renal failure. A short review of renal physiology follows.

### Ultrafiltration

As blood passes through the capillary bed of the glomerulus, filtration of the plasma occurs. In this process of **ultrafiltration,** primitive urine *(glomerular filtrate)* is formed. The volume of the glomerular filtrate approximates 180 L/day. Of this volume, 99% of the glomerular filtrate is reabsorbed by the kidneys. It is because of this tremendous reabsorptive power of the kidneys that the average urinary output of an adult is between 1 and 2 L/day.

Ultrafiltration is measured as **glomerular filtration rate (GFR).** GFR is defined as the amount of glomerular filtrate in a given period. The GFR in an average-sized adult is approximately 125 ml/min (7.5 L/hr). At this rate a volume of approximately 60 times the plasma volume is filtered each day. The average GFR of a woman is about 10% less than that of a man. The same forces that affect fluid transport between vascular and interstitial spaces in other tissues of the body also affect filtration in the nephron. These factors include hydrostatic pressure and oncotic pressure (see Chapter 20).

The kidneys receive approximately 20% of the cardiac output, resulting in renal blood flow rates of about 1200 ml/min. This rapid blood flow rate exceeds the metabolic and oxygen needs of the kidneys but facilitates efficient clearance of metabolic waste products.[5] Severe or prolonged interruptions in cardiac output or renal perfusion as a result of vascular obstruction have profound effects on the formation of urine, as well as on the viability of the cells responsible for maintaining the consistency of the body's internal environment.

After passing through a series of progressively smaller arteries, blood enters the afferent arteriole that branches into the glomerular capillaries. The glomerulus, located in Bowman's capsule, is the first functional portion of the nephron. When blood enters the glomerular capillaries at a pressure greater than 60 to 70 mm Hg, an **ultrafiltrate** (primitive urine) is formed.[4] The ultrafiltrate contains approximately the same concentration of elements as plasma. It is important to note that in a normal person there should not be any plasma in the ultrafiltrate. As the ultrafiltrate passes through the remainder of the nephron, reabsorption and secretion occur to produce the actual urine that is excreted from the body. Table 48-1 summarizes the average filtration rates and reabsorption rates of several substances.

Were it not for the conserving mechanisms in the kidneys, a person would be depleted of fluid and electrolytes within a period of only 3 to 4 minutes. The proximal convoluted tubule reabsorbs up to 85% to 90% of the water in the ultrafiltrate; up to 80% of filtered sodium; and most of the filtered potassium, bicarbonate, chloride, phosphate, glucose, and amino acids. It is in the distal convoluted tubule and collecting tubule that the final urine is produced.

Dehydration would still occur if the kidneys did not have the ability to conserve water in the ultrafiltrate.

**TABLE 48-1 Average Filtration and Reabsorption Values for Several Common Substances**

| SUBSTANCE | AMOUNT FILTERED (per day) | AMOUNT EXCRETED (per day) | PERCENT REABSORBED |
|---|---|---|---|
| Water (L) | 180 | 1.8 | 99.0 |
| Sodium (g) | 630 | 3.2 | 99.5 |
| Glucose (g) | 180 | 0.0 | 100.0 |
| Urea (g) | 54 | 30.0 | 44.0 |
| Potassium (g) | 35 | 2.0 | 94.0 |
| Calcium (g) | 5 | 0.2 | 96.0 |
| Amino acids (g) | 10 | 0.3 | 97.0 |

This mechanism depends on hormonal control. Antidiuretic hormone (ADH), a hormone produced by the pituitary gland, concentrates urine to 1% of the daily filtered volume. Through reabsorption, the kidneys vary the amount of fluid excreted so that intake over the required fluid balance is excreted. Reabsorption, leading to further concentration of urine, occurs when fluid intake falls short of that required for normal fluid balance. The kidney can vary the amount of fluid excreted so precisely that intake over that required for normal fluid balance is excreted and intake under that required for normal fluid balance leads to further concentration of the urine. The mechanisms responsible for this increased urine-concentrating ability and precision in excreting appropriate urine volume are found in the *loop of Henle* and the distal convoluted and collecting tubules. The loop of Henle reaches into the medullary portion of the kidney, which is highly hypertonic in comparison to the filtrate. In the descending portion of the loop, sodium diffuses into the filtrate as the tubule passes deeper into the medullary area, and water moves out of the primitive urine in response to the high sodium concentrations. The results are a reduction in volume of the glomerular filtrate and a dramatic increase in its osmolality. In the ascending limb of the loop of Henle, sodium is reabsorbed into the interstitial tissues, but the loop is impermeable to the movement of water either into or out of the tubule. The primitive urine now presented to the distal convoluted and collecting tubules is greatly reduced in volume but is hypotonic because of the reabsorption of sodium. The influence of ADH on these last two segments of the tubules allows water to be reabsorbed into the interstitial tissue in an amount compatible with maintenance of proper fluid balance. The reabsorption of water from the ultrafiltrate increases osmolality and results in the excretion of hypertonic urine.[7]

## Electrolyte Balance

Electrolyte balance is achieved mainly in the distal and collecting tubule portions of the nephron. As with fluid, the major conservation site for electrolytes is the proximal convoluted tubule where most of all filtered electrolytes are reabsorbed, thus preventing the depletion of these substances. The precise regulation of body electrolyte composition occurs in the distal tubular segments. Depending on the concentrations of electrolytes presented to the tubule cells in the primitive urine and the concentrations of these substances in the interstitium, tubular cells further reabsorb or secrete electrolytes into the urine. This regulation is by both *passive* and *active* mechanisms. Passive movement of electrolytes occurs across a concentration gradient; that is, electrolytes move from an area of higher concentration to an area of lower concentration. Active movement of electrolytes occurs by ion transport mechanisms and, therefore, can move electrolytes without respect to concentration gradients. Active transport requires the expenditure of energy. Table 48-2 summarizes reabsorption and secretion by the nephron.

**TABLE 48-2 Major Sites of Reabsorption and Secretion Within the Nephron**

| REABSORPTION | SECRETION | LOCATION |
|---|---|---|
| Glucose | Creatinine | Proximal tubule |
| Amino acids | Hydrogen ions | |
| Uric acid | Penicillin | |
| Sodium | | |
| Potassium | | |
| Calcium | | |
| Magnesium | | |
| Bicarbonate | | |
| Phosphate | | |
| Chloride | | |
| Water | | |
| Urea | | |
| Sodium chloride | | Loop of Henle |
| Chloride | Ammonium | Distal tubule |
| Water | Hydrogen ions | |
| Bicarbonate | Potassium | |
| Water | | Collecting duct |
| Urea | | |

## Acid-Base Balance

The metabolic processes of the body generally produce excess acid. The body uses two major mechanisms for the maintenance of acid-base balance within a narrow range: respiratory and renal. Acid-base balance is maintained partially through the reabsorption of bicarbonate in the proximal tubule. More precise control of acid-base status is achieved through the reabsorption of bicarbonate and secretion of hydrogen ions into the urine. Hydrogen ions are passively secreted in the proximal tubule and actively secreted in the distal tubule in exchange for sodium ions.

## Excretion

***Metabolic wastes*** are excreted in the glomerular filtrate. Creatinine contained in the glomerular filtrate is excreted unchanged in the urine. Other wastes, such as urea, are excreted unchanged in the glomerular filtrate but undergo reabsorption during passage through the nephron. The amount of waste material excreted in urine is only a portion of that which was originally contained in the glomerular filtrate. As electrolytes are reabsorbed by the nephron, so are most waste materials. It is important to remember that most drugs are either excreted directly by the kidneys or metabolized by the liver to inactive forms, then excreted by the kidneys. Because of this role of the kidneys, some drugs are contraindicated and the dose of others must be adjusted when renal function is impaired. Examples of drugs that are affected by renal failure include many classes of antibiotics, digitalis, salicylates, and long-acting barbiturates.

### Blood Pressure Regulation

The kidneys play an active role in the regulation of blood pressure. Four mechanisms have been identified by which the kidneys regulate blood pressure: regulation of plasma volume, aldosterone, renin-angiotensin-aldosterone system, and prostaglandins.

The kidneys play a role in the regulation of plasma volume in two ways. The first of these is through the direct reabsorption of water to maintain plasma volume. The kidneys also regulate plasma volume by controlling the composition of extracellular fluids. Aldosterone, an adrenal cortical hormone, conserves body sodium by stimulating renal tubular reabsorption. This results in the conservation of water.

Renal regulation of blood pressure also is controlled by the renin-angiotensin-aldosterone system. *Renin* is a hormone released by the juxtaglomerular apparatus of the nephron in response to sodium depletion, renal artery hypoperfusion, or stimulation of the renal nerves through the sympathetic pathway. *Angiotensinogen,* which is produced in the liver, is activated to *angiotensin I* in the presence of renin. An enzyme in the lungs converts *angiotensin I* to the active form, *angiotensin II.* Angiotensin II is a powerful vasoconstrictor and also stimulates the release of aldosterone. The combined effects of these two mechanisms is an elevation in blood pressure. The systemic hypertension associated with renal disease (i.e., renal artery occlusion, chronic renal failure, and acute renal rejection) results from the inappropriate activation of the renin-angiotensin-aldosterone system. In these conditions, the circulating blood volume is adequate, but renal perfusion is diminished, resulting in activation of the renin-angiotensin-aldosterone system.

In addition, prostaglandin and bradykinin are two hormones produced by the kidney and other tissues. They are considered local hormones because they are synthesized in the same location in which they exert their effect and they are rapidly inactivated. Prostaglandin production is promoted by the presence of angiotensin II, bradykinin, ADH, sympathetic stimulation, and renal ischemia.[2]

### Erythropoiesis

Red blood cell (RBC) production is controlled by the kidneys. *Erythropoietin* stimulates bone marrow to produce RBCs and prolongs the life of existing RBCs. Erythropoietin is produced in response to decreased oxygen delivery to the cells of the kidney. Persons with chronic renal failure often have serum hematocrit values of 18% to 30% (normal values are 37% to 49%). This decrease in hematocrit is the result of decreased secretion of erythropoietin from the diseased kidneys compounded by bone marrow toxicity, decreased life span of RBCs, and increased bleeding, all of which are associated with the altered metabolic state present in chronic renal failure.

### Regulation of Phosphate and Calcium

The kidneys also control calcium and phosphate metabolism. Vitamin D prohormone is converted to its active form by the kidneys. Active vitamin D regulates not only gastrointestinal (GI) absorption of calcium but also its deposition within the bone matrix, as well as the metabolism of calcium and phosphorus. Parathyroid hormone (PTH) stimulates the tubular reabsorption of calcium and excretion of phosphate.

## MICTURITION

Urine flows from the kidney pelvis and is propelled through the ureters by peristaltic action. About 200 to 300 ml of urine can collect in the bladder before the person feels the urge to void. As the bladder wall is stretched, baroreceptors cause reflex stimulation of parasympathetic nerves to the bladder, resulting in bladder contractions. When the motor nerves to the external urinary sphincter are inhibited, the muscle relaxes, opening the sphincter and permitting urine to be expelled. Stimulation of the sphincter muscles can keep the sphincter contracted against strong bladder contractions. Voluntary control over micturition can be exerted by a stimulus transmitted over descending spinal pathways from the brainstem.

Use of a large balloon (30 ml) indwelling catheter (such as after a transurethral resection of the prostate) can stimulate the parasympathetic nerves, causing uncomfortable bladder contractions. Pressure on the sphincter by the balloon also can create an urge to void, although the bladder has been emptied by the catheter.

## PHYSIOLOGIC CHANGES WITH AGING

A direct relationship exists between blood supply to the kidneys and renal function. The rate of blood flow to the kidneys is about five to ten times greater than that to the heart, liver, and brain. Glomerular capillary pressure, which is the force that promotes ultrafiltration, is controlled by blood flow to the kidneys. Therefore physiologic alterations in the vascular bed can lead to changes in renal function.

Arteriosclerotic changes in renal arteries are the most common form of renovascular pathologic conditions. Arteriosclerotic changes occur to some extent in the normal aging process. The degree of morphologic change depends on the specific arteries affected and the extent of involvement within those arteries.

Aging also is known to cause predictable increases in both systolic and diastolic blood pressure. This slow increase in blood pressure begins early in life and continues through adulthood. This relationship between aging and increasing blood pressure is so well accepted that normal systolic blood pressure commonly is described as 100 mm Hg plus the person's age. Although this definition is not entirely accurate, it does emphasize the effect of aging on blood pressure. Untreated hypertension further accelerates the development of atherosclerosis, which can lead to renal failure.

Prostatic hypertrophy is a common physiologic change associated with aging discussed in detail in Chapter 53. Prostatic hypertrophy that goes untreated will result in urinary obstruction that can lead to renal failure.

## SUBJECTIVE DATA

### URINATION

Obtaining baseline data concerning the person's usual voiding patterns, such as the frequency and amount of urine with each void, is helpful when changes are anticipated. Persons who are admitted to a hospital or other nursing facility are questioned about their ability to carry out toileting independently. All persons should be questioned about any changes noted in voiding patterns. If changes have occurred, more detailed information must be obtained pertaining to onset, duration, and any measures that the person has taken to deal with these problems.

**TABLE 48-3 Exploring Causes of Urinary Symptoms**

| SYMPTOM | CAUSE | RELEVANT QUESTION |
|---|---|---|
| Dysuria | Urinary tract infection | "Do you experience pain or burning on urination?" |
| Frequency of urination | Urinary tract infection<br>Retention with overflow<br>Excess fluid intake | "How frequently do you void?" |
| Urgency | Bladder irritation as result of inflammation<br>Trauma<br>Tumor | "Do you experience urgency or the need to void immediately?" |
| Nocturia | Increased fluid intake<br>Diuretics<br>Enlarged prostate<br>Early renal failure | "Are you awakened at night with the need to void?" |
| Hesitancy | Partial urethral obstruction | "Do you have difficulty starting or maintaining your stream of urine?" |
| Decreased force and flow of urinary stream | Partial urethral obstruction | "Has the force of your stream of urine changed?" |
| Urinary incontinence | Stress<br>Spinal cord injury<br>"Do you dribble urine?"<br>CNS disease<br>Urinary tract infection<br>Partial urethral obstruction<br>Trauma<br>Prostatectomy | "Do you have difficulty controlling voiding?" |

When asking questions about urination, it is important to recognize that some persons may be somewhat reluctant to answer, either because of embarrassment or misunderstanding. A calm, matter-of-fact approach by the interviewer will assist in putting the person at ease. Many persons are not familiar with terms such as "voiding" or "urination," and more colloquial words may need to be used in certain situations. The interviewer should be sure to confirm that the person understands the questions, thus ensuring the validity of responses to these questions.

Specific questions are directed at eliciting the presence of abnormal conditions (Table 48-3). **Dysuria** (painful urination) usually is described as "burning with urination" and usually is associated with frequency and urgency when urinary tract infection is present. **Frequency** of urination is voiding at frequent intervals, either in small or large amounts; therefore the approximate amount must be ascertained when this symptom is present. Voiding in small amounts may be caused by infection. Voiding in large amounts may be the result of an increased fluid intake or the effect of diuretics. If frequency is associated with suprapubic discomfort and the sense of fullness of the bladder but not with dysuria, the cause may be retention of urine in the bladder with frequent overflow of the excess amounts. **Urgency** refers to the need to void immediately. It commonly accompanies frequency in persons with urinary tract infections. A person with **nocturia** awakens at night with the need to urinate. Additional data that are collected when a person complains of nocturia include the number of times this occurs at night, the amount of fluid intake in a 24-hour period, and whether this is a change in the usual voiding pattern.

**Hesitancy** refers to difficulty in initiating voiding. This often is accompanied by a decrease in the force and flow of the urinary stream. Persons with difficulties initiating voiding are asked if they have to strain to start or maintain the urinary flow. In men the most common partial obstruction is an enlarged prostate, whereas in women there may be weakened perineal muscles or meatal stenosis.

**Urinary incontinence** is the lack of control over voiding. Incontinence is assessed by determining the specific nature of the problem: occurrence continually or only with stress (such as exercise or coughing), the presence or absence of a sensation of fullness before voiding, health conditions associated with the incontinence, and the person's feelings about incontinence.

Many persons are unwilling to admit that they have this problem, and assessment can be difficult. Any methods the person or family members use to control the incontinence also must be identified.

### PAIN

Pain resulting from urinary disorders is located in different areas of the body, depending on the organ involved. Referred pain also is fairly common with some urinary disorders. Pain from the kidney usually is experienced over the kidney site in the back between the twelfth rib and the iliac crest (costovertebral angle). Pain from the ureters may begin over the kidney area but radiate to the front along the course of the ureter and down the groin. Pain from the bladder usually is perceived in the suprapubic area. Any discomfort from prostatic disease usually is felt in the perineum. Data are collected regarding characteristics of the pain (see Chapter 17).

### RENAL DISEASE

Whenever a urinary tract disorder is suspected, a complete assessment of renal history and functioning must be made. The following subjective data are useful guidelines for making a nursing assessment of a person with renal disease:

1. Person's perception of illness
   a. Factors leading person to seek health care
   b. Expectations about current health care
2. Previous or concurrent illness
   a. Other chronic health problems
   b. Medication currently taken
3. Social needs
   a. Availability of supporting others
   b. Current occupation; capacity to continue present work
4. Fluid balance: dyspnea, visual changes, headaches
5. Electrolyte balance: lethargy, memory function, muscle weakness
6. Nutrition: anorexia, nausea and vomiting, history of special diets, knowledge of dietary restrictions, usual eating pattern
7. Elimination: bowel pattern, laxative use, urinary pattern
8. Comfort: pruritus (extent, relief measures), sleep pattern, pain (nature, extent), mouth discomfort (odors, debris)
9. Mobility: fatigue, weakness, numbness, tingling, usual activity pattern
10. Sexuality: menses pattern (if appropriate), concerns about reproduction or sexuality

## OBJECTIVE DATA

### URINARY OUTPUT

Most persons have a urinary output approximately equal to their fluid intake. **Polyuria** (urinary output greater than 2500 ml/day) may occur with an intake greater than 2500 ml/day, uncontrolled diabetes mellitus, or renal disease. **Oliguria** (urinary output less than 400 ml/day) may be the result of suppression of urine formation by the kidneys or retention of urine in the bladder. When urinary retention is present, the person experiences suprapubic discomfort and the enlarged bladder may be palpated above the symphysis pubis. Percussion usually reveals a dull sound. The frequent voiding of small amounts of urine is often a sign of retention with overflow. **Anuria** (urinary output less than 100 ml/day or the cessation of urinary output) is associated with renal failure.

Obtaining an accurate assessment of urinary output is often difficult in a hospital setting. Urine may be inadvertently discarded, or the patient may void into the toilet. The nurse should explain the importance of accurate urine collection. A communication system should be implemented to alert all staff members to patients whose output is being measured. In some cases, such as with shock or acute renal failure, when it is essential to accurately assess urinary output, an indwelling urinary catheter may be inserted. The risks and benefits of inserting an indwelling urinary catheter always should be assessed before placement.

### URINE CHARACTERISTICS

The urine is inspected for gross variations from normal. Normal urine varies in color from pale to deep yellow, depending on specific gravity. A very dark shade suggests that urine may be concentrated (high specific gravity) or that there may be an increased excretion of bilirubin. Certain medications and foods also can change the color of urine.

**Hematuria** (blood in the urine) may be detected overtly or may be present microscopically. In gross hematuria the urine may be pink-tinged to cherry red. If blood is observed in the urine of a woman having her menstrual period, the vaginal orifice can be blocked with cotton balls and another specimen obtained to ascertain the source of the blood. Hematuria with pain may be the result of calculi, a clot from renal bleeding, or bladder infection.

Cloudy urine may result from precipitation of phosphate salts in an alkaline urine or from bacterial growth. A urinary or vaginal discharge also may give the urine a cloudy appearance. Urine collection methods are discussed in the section on diagnostic tests.

### RENAL DISEASE

Objective data pertinent to specific renal diseases and to renal failure are discussed in Chapters 49 and 50, respectively. The following factors provide some general data parameters:

1. Behavior: behavioral changes, level of alertness and orientation, apprehension, scratching, sleeping during day, grimacing, or showing other signs of pain

2. Vital signs
   a. Respirations: rate, depth
   b. Pulse: irregularities
   c. Blood pressure: postural
   d. Temperature (fever)
3. Weight: direction and rate of change
4. Skin and mucous membranes: lesions, moisture
5. Mouth: odor, presence of debris, condition of teeth
6. Chest: breath sounds (wheezing, rhonchi), pericardial friction rub
7. Extremities: peripheral edema, decreased muscle tone, decreased sensation, decreased balance
8. Urinary output: amount/hour, amount/day in relation to intake
9. Laboratory values
   a. Urine: urinalysis, specific gravity, culture
   b. Blood: electrolytes, pH, creatinine, BUN

## PHYSIOLOGIC CHANGES WITH AGING

It is particularly important to recognize the physiologic changes that occur with aging so that normal variations can be distinguished from those caused by aging. Of all age-groups, elders show the greatest diversity.[1] Important changes occurring with aging that affect the assessment of urinary function include nocturia, frequency, and urgency, which result from decreased bladder and pelvic muscle tone. Sphincter muscles become also weakened; however, urinary incontinence is not a normal part of aging and its presence always should be thoroughly evaluated.

Glomerular filtration rate also is affected. Glomeruli become scarred with age and become nonfunctional. In addition, decreased reabsorption results in less efficient urine concentration. As a result of these physiologic changes, serum creatinine and BUN levels are slightly elevated. Glucose reabsorption also may be decreased, resulting in normal serum values (for elderly persons) of 52 to 135 mg/dl (compared with standard values of 70 to 110 mg/dl). Care of elderly persons with urinary problems is summarized in the Gerontologic Patient Considerations box at right.

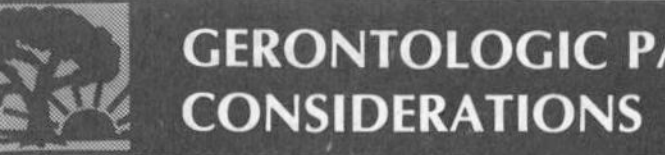

### GERONTOLOGIC PATIENT CONSIDERATIONS

**ASSESSMENT**

Determine urinary habits, especially if patient has any difficulty with urinary control.

Assess for mobility problems, diuretics, or mental changes that may contribute to functional (environmental) incontinence.

Assess for signs of urinary tract infections commonly experienced by elderly persons. Usual signs of fever and pain or burning with urination may be minimal or absent; confusion and anorexia may be the only symptoms.

Monitor kidney function when elders undergo extensive testing that may lead to dehydration, which can compromise marginal kidney function in some elderly persons.

**INTERVENTION**

Refer person with incontinence to a physician for further work-up; this condition is *not* a normal concomitant of aging.

Give diuretics early in day so patient will not need to use toilet frequently after bedtime.

Arrange environment to facilitate toileting, such as moving furniture, using bedside commode, ensuring grab bars by the toilet (or raised seat), and keeping call light within reach.

Schedule fluid intake to match toileting time, about every 2 hours while awake.

Maintain patient's usual routines as much as possible.

Limit stimulants such as coffee and tea.

Plan for increased need for toileting if patient is receiving intravenous therapy.

Try to avoid use of urinary catheters; if catheter is necessary, use good aseptic technique to prevent urinary tract infection.

Teach patient to report to health care provider any change in the urine or presence of blood; be aware that the patient may not be able to monitor own urine if vision is diminished.

**COMMON DISORDERS IN ELDERS**

Urinary incontinence
Urinary tract infections
Benign prostatic hyperplasia
Cancer of kidney, bladder, or prostate
Renal failure

# DIAGNOSTIC TESTS

Special examinations of the urinary system are performed to identify the location and nature of existing disease. The accuracy of findings in many of the following tests depends on the assistance of the person in restricting or augmenting intake of fluids or in collecting specimens at designated time intervals. The person should be given clear, precise directions; written instructions are a valuable supplement to verbal directions.

Many of the diagnostic tests used to assess renal function are performed on an ambulatory basis. Therefore it is important to assess the understanding of the patient about all instructions in preparation for the test. Some examinations must be performed with the patient under sedation; if so, the patient is instructed to make prior arrangements for someone to provide transportation after the procedure.

## EXAMINATION OF THE URINE

### Urinalysis

In identifying disease of the urinary tract, one of the first tests performed is urinalysis. This test yields information about probable locations and causes of urinary disease and some information as to the extent of the illness. Urinalysis is a test that assists in establishing tentative diagnoses, as well as the need for additional tests and observations required to make precise diagnoses. Urinalysis also indicates abnormalities of nonrenal and nonurologic origin (e.g., diabetes mellitus). Table 48-4 indicates possible normal and abnormal findings.

### Clean-Catch Specimens

Ideally the urine specimen is collected from the first voiding of the day. This sample is preferred because it

**TABLE 48-4 Urinalysis Findings**

| TEST | NORMAL | ABNORMAL |
|---|---|---|
| Color | Amber-yellow | Red indicates hematuria (possibly urinary obstruction, renal calculi, tumor, renal failure, cystitis) |
| Clarity | Clear | Cloudy: debris, bacterial sediment (urinary infection) |
| pH | 4.6-8.0 (average 6.0) | Alkaline on standing or with urinary tract infection<br>Increased acidity with renal tubular acidosis |
| Specific gravity | 1.010-1.026 | Usually reflects fluid intake; the less the fluid intake, the higher the specific gravity<br>If specific gravity remains low (1.010-1.014), renal disease or pituitary disease (deficit of ADH) is suspected |
| Protein | 0-8 mg/dl | Proteinuria may occur with high-protein diet and exercise (particularly prolonged)<br>Seen in renal disease |
| Sugar | 0 | Glycosuria occurs after a high intake of sugar or with diabetes mellitus |
| Ketones | 0 | Ketonuria occurs with starvation and diabetic ketoacidosis |
| RBCs | 0-4 | Injury to kidney tissue (see color, above) |
| WBCs | 0-5 | Urinary tract infection (UTI) |
| Casts | 0 | UTI, renal disease |

is concentrated and abnormal constituents are more likely to be present. The person is given a clean container in which to catch urine. Cleansing the meatus before collecting the specimen decreases the likelihood of external contamination; mild soap followed by water or a special antiseptic solution may be used. The patient uses a midstream technique to obtain a **clean-catch specimen.** At least 50 to 100 ml of urine is collected for the test to ensure a sufficient amount to measure specific gravity and to perform microscopic analysis. If analysis of the urine cannot be performed immediately, the specimen must be refrigerated to retard bacterial growth.

## Composite Specimens

A **composite specimen,** a specimen of all the urine excreted over a specific period of time, often is required for urologic diagnosis. The duration of urine collections may vary from 2 to 24 hours. Specimens are examined for sugar, protein, sediment (blood cells and casts), 17-ketosteroids, electrolytes, catecholamines, and breakdown products of protein metabolism. These tests provide information on (1) the ability of the kidneys to excrete and conserve various solutes, (2) the production in the body of excessive hormones that are excreted in the urine, (3) changes in the body's regulation of glucose metabolism, (4) identification of organisms difficult to recognize through routine urine cultures, and (5) presence of abnormal cells and debris in the urine.

The accuracy of findings in this type of test depends on proper collection of the specimen. Whether the specimen is to be obtained in the hospital or in the home, the person needs to be told exactly how to collect it. Instructions for a composite urine specimen are found in the Guidelines box at right.

Composite urine tests also may involve collecting urine from multiple sources from the body. For instance, the person may pass urine from the urethra and also have a nephrostomy tube from which urine drains. In addition, ureteral catheters may be in place, with urine being collected from each kidney separately. Depending on the function of the test—whether the purpose is to measure the identified element in the urine as a whole or to measure separately the excretion of this element from each kidney—the urine collected from each source may be combined into one specimen container or collected into separate, appropriately labeled containers.

## Urine Culture

Urine cultures are used to confirm suspected infections, to identify causative organisms, and to determine ap-

### Guidelines for Collecting a Composite Urine Specimen

1. The bladder is emptied and the urine *discarded* at the appointed time to start the test.
2. Urine from *all* subsequent voidings is saved.
3. Specific directions for storing the urine should be given. Some specimens need to be kept cold during the collection period; some need preservatives added, and some need no special care.
4. The person should void into a separate receptacle before defecation to prevent contamination of the specimen.
5. The bladder is emptied and the urine *added* to the collection at the appointed time to end the test.
6. The designated amount (properly labeled) is sent to the laboratory.
7. If an aliquot (5-10 ml sample of the total specimen) is the designated amount, the total amount collected is (a) measured and recorded on the specimen requisition and (b) mixed well before the aliquot is removed.

propriate antimicrobial therapy. Cultures also are obtained for periodic screening of urine when the threat of urinary tract infection (UTI) exists.

Urine in a properly collected and stored sample is considered to be normal if it contains 10,000 or fewer organisms per milliliter. Organisms of this magnitude are the result of normal urethral flora and do not signify UTI. A UTI is diagnosed when bacterial counts in a properly collected and stored sample reach 100,000 or more organisms per milliliter and the organisms are of one or very largely one bacterial type. It is most likely that contamination of the urine specimen during collection has occurred when bacterial counts include predominant colonies of *Staphylococcus, Streptococcus,* and diphtheroids; when two or more organisms contribute significantly to the total bacterial count; or when repeated cultures yield differing results. Each of these results indicates a need to repeat the culture, paying particular attention to the collection of the specimen and to its handling.

Specimens for urine culture may be obtained either by catheterization or by **midstream void** (see the Guidelines box below). It should be made clear, however, that *urethral catheterization never should be used routinely in collecting urine for culture because of the risk of introducing additional bacteria into the bladder.* Catheterization may be necessary to obtain a sterile urine specimen when the person is unable to void after adequate hydration or if the person is incontinent of urine. When a catheter is passed, meticulous attention is given to nontraumatic aseptic technique. After urine flow from the catheter is established, 5 to 10 ml of urine should be collected directly into a sterile specimen container. Care must be taken to ensure that the rim and the inside of the container are not touched by the catheter or by the hands. If a culture tube with a cotton plug is used as a specimen container, care must be taken to keep the tube upright to prevent moistening the cotton and thereby contaminating the specimen. Cultures also may be ordered on the urine taken from the renal pelvis during ureteral catheterization or when ureterostomy or nephrostomy tubes are in place.

In collecting a voided specimen for culture, the nurse must decide if the patient is capable of independently obtaining the specimen or if nursing or medical personnel will need to collect a midstream specimen. Most persons who are ambulatory and are given precise and unhurried directions are able to collect their own midstream urine specimen.

The first voided specimen of the day should be used, whenever possible, because bacteria will be more numerous. If the specimen is not cultured immediately, refrigeration is mandatory to prevent growth of organisms in the specimen.

### Guidelines for Collecting a Midstream Urine Specimen

**EQUIPMENT NEEDED**

Sterile container for the urine

Three sponges (cotton or gauze) saturated with cleansing solution

**GENERAL DIRECTIONS**

Only outside of collecting container is touched

Urine is collected in container well after urinary stream is started

**SPECIAL DIRECTIONS**

**Female**

Labia are kept separated throughout procedure

Meatus is cleansed with one front-to-back motion with each of the three cleansing sponges

**Male**

Foreskin is retracted if man is uncircumcised

Glans is cleansed with each of the three cleansing sponges

## EVALUATION OF BLADDER FUNCTION

### Measurement of Residual Urine

Normally the bladder contains little or no urine after voiding; however, certain disease states inhibit the bladder from emptying completely. Some common conditions in which incomplete emptying of the bladder occurs are benign prostatic hypertrophy, urethral strictures, and interruptions in bladder innervation. Urine left in the bladder after voiding is called **residual urine.**

One way to determine the amount of residual urine is to *catheterize* the person immediately after voiding. This may be ordered by the physician on a one-time or on a repeated basis. Before catheterizing the person, the physician is consulted about the plan for establishing urinary drainage. If a large amount of residual urine is suspected, the physician may wish the catheter to be left in place in the bladder. *Residual urine volumes of 50 ml or less indicate near-normal or returning bladder function.*

To avoid passing a catheter to measure residual urine volumes, x-ray film examination of retained urine may be performed. In this procedure a radiopaque substance excreted by the kidneys is injected intravenously. As the dye is excreted in the urine, it passes into the bladder. A sufficient amount of urine containing the radiopaque material is allowed to accumulate in the bladder before the person is instructed to void. Immediately after voiding, an x-ray film is taken. Any urine retained in the bladder will be visualized on the x-ray film. This means of determining residual urine is used in conjunction with other studies requiring visualization of the urinary tract.

### Cystometrography

**Cystometric examination** is performed to evaluate bladder tone. In general, the examination is indicated in the presence of incontinence or evidence of neurologic dysfunction of the bladder. A Foley catheter is

## TABLE 48-5 Selected Renal Function Tests

| NORMAL RESULTS | PURPOSE OR SIGNIFICANCE | NURSING IMPLICATIONS |
|---|---|---|
| **SPECIFIC GRAVITY OF URINE** | | |
| 1.010-1.026 | Test measures ability of kidneys to concentrate urine. | First morning void usually is in the high normal range in healthy person.<br>False high is caused by presence of radiographic dyes. |
| **OSMOLALITY OF URINE** | | |
| 500-800 mOsm/L | Test is excellent indication of renal function.<br>Osmolality is total concentration of particles in solution. | No special preparation needed. |
| **FISHBERG CONCENTRATION TEST** | | |
| Urine volume 300/ml/12 hr<br>Specific gravity of 1.024 or greater<br>Urine osmolality of 850 mOsm or greater | Test is used to determine ability of kidney to conserve fluid and to establish differential diagnosis for diabetes insipidus and psychogenic polydipsia. | No fluid can be taken during test period.<br>Test period is 8 to 12 hr, usually during night.<br>First morning void ensures maximal concentration.<br>Three hourly urine specimens are collected for volume, specific gravity, and osmolality after test period.<br>Patient should be observed for signs of vascular collapse. |
| **URINE CHEMISTRY** | | |
| Sodium: 100-260 mEq/24 hr<br>Potassium: 39-90 mg/24 hr<br>Calcium: 100-300 mg/24 hr | Urine electrolytes reflect ability of kidney to excrete and reabsorb electrolytes. | Abnormal results may be caused by disease processes other than renal disorders; for example, elevated urine calcium in hyperparathyroidism or prolonged immobilization. |
| **CREATININE CLEARANCE** | | |
| Men: 90-140 ml/min<br>Women: 85-125 ml/min | Results provide rate at which kidneys remove creatinine from the plasma.<br>Because diet and metabolic state have little influence on it, creatinine clearance provides a rough estimate of glomerular filtration rate (GFR). | *Procedure*<br>1. Patient empties bladder and time is noted.<br>2. *All* urine is saved for 24 hr.<br>3. Exactly 24 hr after start of procedure the patient voids, and specimen is saved.<br>4. Total urine volume and urine creatinine are measured.<br>5. Serum creatinine is determined at end of 24-hr period.<br>6. Creatinine clearance is then calculated by formula:<br>$\text{Clearance} = \frac{UV}{P}$<br>U = Urine creatinine concentration<br>V = Urine volume<br>P = Plasma creatinine concentration |
| **SERUM CREATININE** | | |
| Men: .85-1.5 mg/100 ml<br>Women: .7-1.25 mg/100 ml | Test indicates ability of kidneys to excrete creatinine.<br>Serum creatinine gives a rough estimate of GFR. | No specific preparation is needed for test.<br>Diet and metabolic rate have little effect on serum creatinine value. |
| **BLOOD UREA NITROGEN (BUN)** | | |
| 5-20 mg/100 ml | Test indicates ability of kidneys to excrete nitrogenous wastes. | BUN can be affected by high-protein diet, blood in GI tract, and catabolic state (injury, infection, fever, poor nutrition). |
| **PHENOSULFONPHTHALEIN (PSP) EXCRETION TEST** | | |
| 30%-50% of PSP dye excreted in 15 min | Test measures tubular secretion rates. | *Procedure*<br>1. Patient drinks 8-10 glasses of water.<br>2. 1 ml PSP dye is given intravenously.<br>3. Urine specimens are collected at 15-, 30- and 60-min intervals.<br>4. The exact time the urine specimen is collected must be recorded to calculate excretion rates. |

inserted before the examination. After the person assumes a supine position, a liter bag of normal saline or sterile distilled water and a cystometer are connected to the catheter. Fluid is instilled at a constant and specified rate; measurements of the pressure exerted on the fluid by the bladder musculature are recorded after the instillation of every 50 ml of fluid. The person is asked to report feelings of fullness, the need to void, and any urgency or discomfort. Fluid is instilled until urgency occurs or it is determined that the sensation is absent. During cystometric examination, bethanechol chloride (Urecholine) may be administered to determine its effect on enhancing the tone of a flaccid bladder, or an anticholingeric medication may be given to assess relaxation in a hyperactive bladder. There is no specific care required after cystometric examination.

*Electromyography* may be used to evaluate sphincter tone and to determine whether nerve pathways are intact.

**BOX 48-2 Normal Values of Selected Serum Electrolytes**

**SODIUM**
135-145 mEq/L

**POTASSIUM**
3.5-5.0 mEq/L

**CHLORIDE**
90-110 mEq/L

**BICARBONATE**
23-27 mEq/L

**CALCIUM**
9.0-10.5 mg/dl (total)

**PHOSPHORUS**
2.5-4.5 mg/dl

## EVALUATION OF RENAL FUNCTION

When findings of the general physical examination or urinalysis suggest renal disease, tests of renal function are conducted. A summary of selected renal function tests is presented in Table 48-5. It should be remembered that the best overview of the patient's clinical condition is obtained by comparing the results of a number of tests. Therefore it is common for a series of renal function tests to be ordered.

Serum electrolyte values do not provide conclusive results in terms of renal function. Many factors influence serum electrolyte levels. In renal failure the serum electrolyte value may be normal, elevated, decreased, or any combination of these. Serum electrolyte levels are monitored closely in patients with renal failure so that their levels can be adequately regulated. The normal ranges for the most commonly measured electrolytes are shown in Box 48-2.

### Clearance Tests

When renal disease is suspected, the physician will want to determine the amount of damage, if any, that has already occurred. Clearance tests are the most practical and efficient way to identify losses in renal function. These tests measure the amount of blood that a person's kidneys can "clear" of a substance in a given amount of time. When the results are compared with normal values, changes in renal function become apparent. Clearance tests also are used to monitor the direction of change and the rate of change in renal function over time.

The **creatinine clearance test** is the most practical and widely used of all clearance tests. Creatinine is a substance that results from the breakdown of muscle tissue. It is produced at a relatively fixed and uniform rate throughout the day, it can be measured readily in the blood, and it is not influenced by dietary intake. Creatinine is excreted through the kidneys; it is filtered in the glomerulus and passes practically unchanged through the renal tubules. It is an ideal naturally occurring substance that, when blood and urine values are compared, allows one to estimate changes in glomerular filtration rates and overall kidney function. A person's creatinine clearance value is expressed in terms of milliliters per minute and is determined according to the following formula:

$$\text{Creatinine clearance (ml/min)} = \frac{\text{Urine volume (ml/min)} \times \text{Urine creatinine concentration (mg/ml)}}{\text{Plasma creatinine concentration (mg/ml)}}$$

For this test, a morning-to-morning 24-hour urine collection is obtained. (Refer to collection of composite urine specimens on p. 1602.) Immediately after the final urine specimen is collected, a blood specimen is drawn to determine the serum creatinine level. Both blood and urine specimens are sent together for analysis. Analysis of the total urine volume for the test period is essential for accurate determination of renal function. If one void is accidentally discarded, the test must be repeated. The nurse must ensure accurate collection of all urine in the prescribed time. A shorter time may be used in instances in which it is not possible to obtain an accurate 24-hour urine collection.

The **sodium excretion test** measures tubular function. Specifically, this test provides information about the kidney's ability to appropriately excrete or conserve this electrolyte; in chronic renal failure either inappropriate retention or excretion of sodium can occur. Knowledge of urinary excretion of this electrolyte is helpful in calculating the patient's sodium intake requirements. To determine change in direction and degree of tubular functions, comparison of current and past sodium excretion studies is made. The test is performed

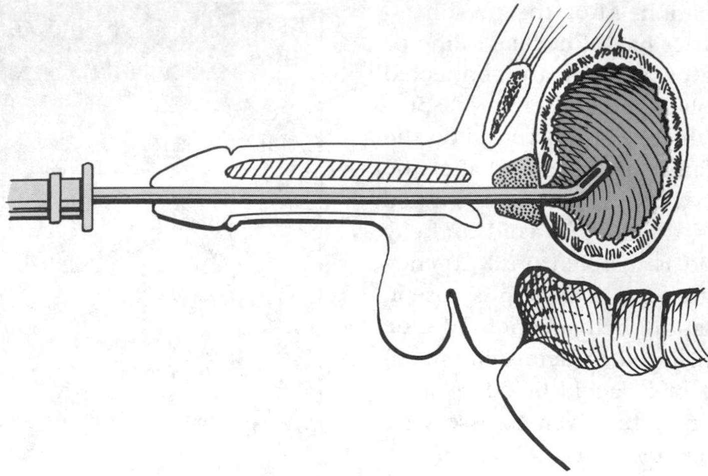

**FIGURE 48-5** Cystoscope inserted for examination of bladder.

by analyzing the sodium content of a 24-hour urine collection.

## VISUALIZATION OF THE URINARY TRACT

Technologic advances in the last several years have made it possible to visualize the urinary tract by both direct and indirect means. These tests allow for assessment of both structure and function of the organs and tissues of the urinary tract. Visualization of the urinary tract is used not only for diagnosis but also for evaluation of the patient's response to therapy over time.

### Cystoscopy

**Cystoscopy** is the direct examination of the bladder by use of an instrument called a *cystoscope* (Figure 48-5). The cystoscope relies on a flexible optic fiber to provide illumination into the urinary tract. The instrument is attached to the illuminating source and then slowly passed through the urinary tract, thus enabling direct visualization of the urethra, ureteral orifices, and bladder.

Most hospitals require a signed permit before cystoscopy is performed after the person is given an explanation of the procedure, along with the risks and benefits. Fluids usually are forced for several hours before the procedure. This ensures a continuous flow of urine in the event specimens need to be collected and aids in preventing multiplication of bacteria that may be introduced during the procedure. If general anesthesia is to be used, fluids may be administered intravenously. If x-ray films are to be taken during the procedure, bowel preparation may be ordered.

The cystoscopic examination may be performed with or without anesthesia. General anesthesia is required for cystoscopic examination when the person is apprehensive or when painful manipulation is anticipated. In these instances, anesthesia reduces the possibility of trauma to the urethra or perforation of the bladder caused by sudden vigorous movement of the patient during the examination. Children usually are given a general anesthetic for this procedure.

Much of the discomfort felt during this procedure is the result of contraction or spasm of the bladder sphincters; this can be decreased through deep-breathing exercises and general relaxation. A sedative such as diazepam (Valium) or midazolam (Versed) and a narcotic such as morphine or meperidine hydrochloride (Demerol) usually are given an hour before the examination.

If the patient is relatively comfortable, the cystoscope should be passed with little pain, provided there is no obstruction in the urethra. A local anesthetic such as procaine (usually 4%) may be instilled into the urethra before insertion of the cystoscope.

When the patient is awake, passing the instrument will be followed immediately by a strong desire to void. This occurs as a result of the pressure the instrument exerts against the internal sphincter. During the examination, the bladder is distended with normal saline for visualization. As the bladder becomes increasingly distended, the urge to void increases.

During cystoscopic examination a number of tests may be performed on the urinary system. *Cystography* involves the injection of a radiopaque dye such as methiodal (Skiodan) or air as a contrast medium to visualize the bladder and determine its size, shape, and any irregularities. Bladder capacity can be measured through instillation of distilled water. A ***voiding cystourethrogram*** can reveal reflux of urine into the ureters on voiding, a bladder malfunction that can lead to pyelonephritis.

*Ureteral catheterization* (with a nylon, radiopaque, size 4F to 6F catheter) can be performed through the cystoscope. The catheter is inserted into the ureteral

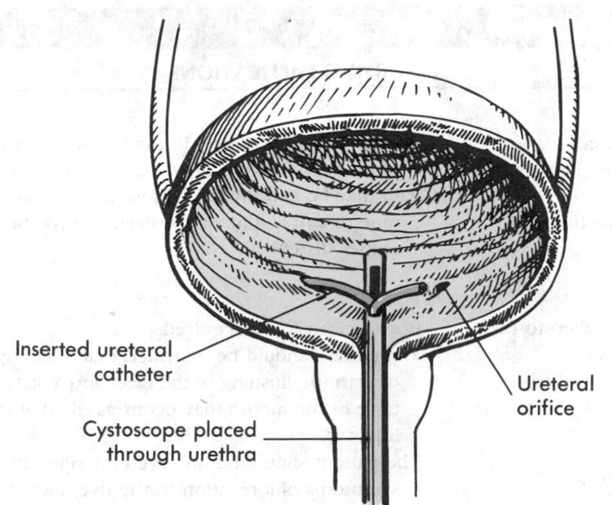


**FIGURE 48-6** Ureteral catheterization through cystoscope. Note ureteral catheter inserted into left orifice. Right ureteral catheter is ready to be inserted.

opening in the bladder, carefully advanced up the ureter, and into the renal pelvis (Figure 48-6). This procedure may involve one or both ureters. It is performed (1) when culture and analysis of urine from individual kidneys are required, (2) when tests of renal function are to be performed on the kidneys separately, and (3) when visualization of the urinary tract is desired and intravenous pyelogram visualization has been inadequate, obstruction is present, or sensitivity to intravenous radiopaque material is noted.

The nurse validates the person's understanding of the procedure as part of the preoperative teaching. If local anesthesia is to be used, the nurse must be certain to describe what the patient can expect during the procedure. The patient should not stand or walk alone immediately after cystoscopic examination because blood that has drained from the leg while in the lithotomy position will flow back into the vessels of the feet and legs as standing is assumed. Accidents caused by dizziness and fainting can occur from the sudden change in distribution of blood.

The patient needs to be observed for three complications of cystoscopic examination: bleeding, perforation of the bladder, and spread of infection throughout the urinary tract or into the bloodstream (sepsis). Observation for frank bleeding (pink-tinged urine is normal) is necessary. Urinary output and voiding pattern are monitored to detect obstruction, and fluid intake is increased to prevent stasis. Mild analgesics are given for discomfort, and warmth is provided if the patient complains of being chilled. Vital signs are monitored as necessary. The patient should be instructed that the first void after cystoscopic examination can be uncomfortable. Warm tub baths may provide comfort. (See Nursing Care Plan on p. 1609.)

### Radiologic Examination

A number of radiologic examinations are used to visualize the urinary tract (Table 48-6). Because the kidneys lie retroperitoneally, any accumulation of flatus or feces in the intestine can obstruct the view on the x-ray film. To ensure adequate visualization, bowel evacuation is necessary before the x-ray films are taken.

X-ray films of the urinary tract may be ordered in conjunction with other abdominal studies. Problems may arise in visualizing the urinary system if the patient has recently undergone barium studies. This problem can be prevented by scheduling tests so that examination of the urinary tract precedes barium contrast x-ray films of the GI tract.

## RENAL BIOPSY

Renal biopsy is potentially the most accurate diagnostic tool for determining the type and stage of progression of a pathologic condition of the renal system. Specifically, this test aids in differentiating diagnoses, following the progression of disease processes, assisting in selection of therapy most beneficial to the patient, and determining prognosis of the illness. The biopsy can be performed either through a skin puncture (percutaneous) or through an incision **(open renal biopsy)** over the kidney.

Because the kidney is such a vascular organ, hemorrhage after a biopsy is a potential threat. Throughout the procedure, care is given to prevent and detect early loss of blood. Before biopsy is performed, a thorough medical evaluation with particular attention to detection of any abnormality in bleeding or coagulation time is completed. The patient's blood usually is typed and crossmatched with two units of blood; the blood is held for the patient until any threat of bleeding has passed. The largest risk of bleeding is in the first 12 hours after biopsy.

An open biopsy carries less risk of hemorrhage and provides better visualization of the kidney, but it is a more invasive procedure with risks of anesthesia, wound infection, and longer recovery time.

Preparation before biopsy includes discussing the procedure with the patient. Topics covered should include the necessity for the examination, the procedure itself, and the care to be anticipated after the procedure. The patient is encouraged to ask any questions regarding the procedure. The preparation of the patient is shared by the physician and the nurse. In most institutions it is necessary to have the patient sign a special permit before having the biopsy performed. The biopsy may be performed in the patient's room, the operating room, or in the radiology department.

The procedure for **percutaneous** (closed) **renal biopsy** is as follows: Before the biopsy, the patient is taken to the radiology department for localization of the kidney. This is accomplished with a plain film, a dye contrast film, or fluoroscopic location. The lower pole of the

**TABLE 48-6 Common Radiologic Examinations of the Urinary Tract**

| PURPOSE | PROCEDURE | NURSING IMPLICATIONS |
|---|---|---|
| **RETROGRADE PYELOGRAPHY** | | |
| Visualization of urinary tract | 1. Ureteral catheterization required<br>2. Radiopaque material (Hypaque, Renografin) gently injected<br>3. X-ray films taken of renal collecting structures | Patient may experience discomfort in region of kidneys as dye is injected.<br>Pain may be experienced if too large a volume of dye is injected and renal pelvis becomes distended. |
| **INTRAVENOUS PYELOGRAPHY (IVP)** | | |
| Determination of size and location of kidneys<br>Demonstration of presence of cysts or tumors<br>Outline of filling of renal pelvis<br>Outline of ureters and bladder | 1. X-ray film of abdomen (KUB) taken to identify size and position of kidneys<br>2. Radiopaque dye given intravenously<br>3. X-ray films of kidneys taken at 3-, 5-, 10-, and 20-min intervals | Bowel cleansing is required.<br>The patient should be informed that a feeling of warmth, flushing of the face, and a salty taste in the mouth may occur as the dye is injected.<br>The patient should be observed for signs and symptoms of a reaction to the dye, including respiratory distress, diaphoresis, urticaria, instability of vital signs, or unusual sensations.<br>CPR equipment and emergency medications should always be available for immediate use. |
| **KIDNEY, URETER, AND BLADDER (KUB) X-RAY FILMS** | | |
| Gross visualization of KUB<br>Location of calcifications and stones possible | X-ray film of abdominal region obtained | Bowel cleansing sometimes is ordered. |
| **URETHROGRAPHY** | | |
| Visualization of urethral size and shape | X-ray films of urethra taken after instilling 20 ml of radiopaque water-soluble lubricant | No special preparation is needed. |
| **COMPUTED TOMOGRAPHY (CT)** | | |
| Visualization of kidneys and renal circulation | Whole body CT scanner segments kidneys<br>Can be performed with IV contrast dye | If dye is used, the same implications apply as listed for IVP. |
| **RENAL ANGIOGRAPHY** | | |
| Visualization of renal circulation<br>Particularly useful in evaluating renal artery stenosis | Similar to IVP; however, contrast dye often injected directly into femoral artery by passing a catheter through artery to level of renal arteries | Nursing implications are the same as in IVP.<br>Patient must be observed for dye-induced acute renal failure and bleeding at arterial puncture site, especially within first 4 hr. The pressure dressing should be checked for fresh bleeding. The puncture site should be checked for tenderness or swelling. Vital signs and distal pulses must be assessed frequently (q 15 min × 4 hr). Bed rest should be maintained for 8 hr after the procedure. |
| **RENOGRAPHY** | | |
| Visualization of urinary tract<br>Measurement of renal blood flow<br>Measurement of renal tubular and excretory function | Involves scintillation scanning or photography<br>Radioactive isotope such as iodohippurate sodium tagged with iodine-125 or iodine-131 injected intravenously<br>Scintillating probes placed over kidneys to record photographs | Because only trace doses of bound isotopes are used, no special precautions are necessary. |
| **ULTRASOUND** | | |
| Used to distinguish between abnormal fluid collections and solid masses; used to identify obstructions and detect abscesses; often used to diagnose abscesses, ureteral leaks, and obstructions in renal transplant recipients | Sound waves used to outline internal body structures; procedure accomplished by computer interpretation of tissue densities | Procedure is painless and noninvasive. A full bladder assists in outlining structures. |

## NURSING CARE PLAN

### PERSON AFTER CYSTOSCOPY

**DATA:** Mr. K. is a 64-year-old retired accountant. He reports that up until last month he was in good health. He has no significant medical history and has never been hospitalized. He is currently taking no prescription medications. Mr. K. visited his family physician 2 weeks ago and complained of urinary dribbling, which has increased significantly in the past several days. On further questioning, he states he has experienced nocturia for the last several months. He also has experienced increasing difficulty in initiating urination. On physical examination the physician noted a grossly enlarged prostate. Mr. K. was admitted for cystoscopic examination.

#### ■ NURSING DIAGNOSIS

Altered urinary elimination pattern: nocturia related to anatomic obstruction

| Expected Patient Outcome | Nursing Interventions | Rationale |
|---|---|---|
| Will not experience nocturia. | Limit fluid intake in evening hours; have Mr. K. empty bladder before going to bed. | Reduce urine production at time of sleep; empty bladder will reduce need to wake during night. |

#### ■ NURSING DIAGNOSIS

Knowledge deficit (cystoscopy) related to lack of exposure to information

| Expected Patient Outcome | Nursing Interventions | Rationale |
|---|---|---|
| Can describe what to expect during and after cystoscopy. | Teach about procedure and stress sensations he may experience. Describe postprocedure routine. Instruct patient about postprocedure limitations. | Understanding procedure will reduce anxiety and facilitate compliance and relaxation.<br>Providing information on restrictions may prevent postprocedure injury. |

kidney is located and marked on the skin in ink. The lower pole is the site for obtaining the biopsy specimen because it contains the fewest number of blood vessels. The patient is then transported to the area where the biopsy will be performed. The procedure may be accomplished with computed tomography (CT) used as the guide for placing the biopsy needle. Sedation usually is not required except for patients who are restless and unable to relax sufficiently to follow necessary instructions during the procedure. The patient is placed in a prone position over a sandbag or firm pillow and an additional soft pillow. The physician identifies the location for biopsy, and a local anesthetic agent is injected. As the biopsy needle is inserted, the patient is instructed to take a breath and hold it because the kidneys move up and down with respiration. Pressure pain may be felt in the kidney region as the needle punctures the tough renal capsule and the tissue sample is taken. The needle is withdrawn immediately, and direct pressure is applied to the site for 20 minutes. A pressure dressing is then applied, and the patient is turned supine and kept flat for at least 4 hours. A small sandbag may be placed over the biopsy site to prevent bleeding. The nursing care requirements are summarized in the Guidelines box at right.

The procedure for an *open* biopsy is similar to that used in kidney surgery. The nursing care for this type of surgery is discussed in Chapter 49. Most biopsies are performed by the percutaneous method.

#### Guidelines for Care of the Person After Percutaneous Renal Biopsy

1. Patient must remain on bed rest, flat, in a supine position, and motionless for 4 hours after the biopsy.
2. Coughing must be avoided for first 4 hours after the biopsy.
3. Blood pressure and pulse should be taken on the following schedule:
   a. Every 15 minutes for 1 hour
   b. Every 30 minutes for 1 hour
   c. Every hour for additional 2 hours or until stable
   
   The responsible physician should be notified of increases in pulse of more than 10 to 20 beats/min above the baseline or decreases in blood pressure of more than 10 mm Hg, unless the physician instructs otherwise.
4. Patient should remain on bed rest for 24 hours.
5. Urine is observed for hematuria for first 24 hours after the biopsy.
6. Patient should avoid heavy lifting for 10 days after the biopsy.

## CRITICAL THINKING ACTIVITIES

- ► Ron is a 23-year-old man and Tim is an 80-year-old man. How may their renal status differ based on normal renal physiology?
- ► At 4 PM when assessing your patient who had a renal biopsy at 9 AM, you note that she is lying flat on her back with a sandbag to her right side. She states that she is experiencing no pain at the site but is beginning to experience a backache from lying on her back. How should you respond to this patient?

## CHAPTER SUMMARY

### ANATOMY AND PHYSIOLOGY

- The kidneys play an essential role not only in maintaining hemostasis but also in the excretion of drugs.
- The major functions of the kidneys include fluid and electrolyte regulation; acid-base balance; excretion of metabolic wastes, toxins, and drugs; regulation of blood pressure; RBC production; and regulation of calcium and phosphate.

### SUBJECTIVE DATA

- In gathering data about urinary function, it is important to validate the person's understanding of all the questions asked, because many euphemisms exist about body elimination.

### DIAGNOSTIC TESTS

- The nurse must have a clear understanding of diagnostic tests to appropriately prepare and support the patient.
- The nurse must validate that the person understands all instructions related to diagnostic testing and provide written information whenever possible.

## REFERENCES


1. Andreesen G: A fresh look at assessing the elderly, *RN* 52(6):28-40, 1989.
2. Carretero O, Scicli A: Kallikrein-kinin system. In Massry S, Glassock R, editors: *Textbook of nephrology,* ed 2, Baltimore, 1989, Williams & Wilkins.
3. Chmielewski C: Renal anatomy and overview of nephron function, *ANNA J* 19(1):34-40, 1992.
4. Guyton A: *Textbook of medical physiology,* ed 8, Philadelphia, 1991, WB Saunders.
5. Holechek MJ: Glomerular filtration rate and renal hemodynamics, *ANNA J* 19(3):237-248, 1992.
6. Peschman P: Renal physiology. In Clochesy L et al, editors: *Critical care nursing,* Philadelphia, 1993, WB Saunders.
7. Preisig P: Urinary concentration and dilution, *ANNA J* 19(4):351-355, 1992.

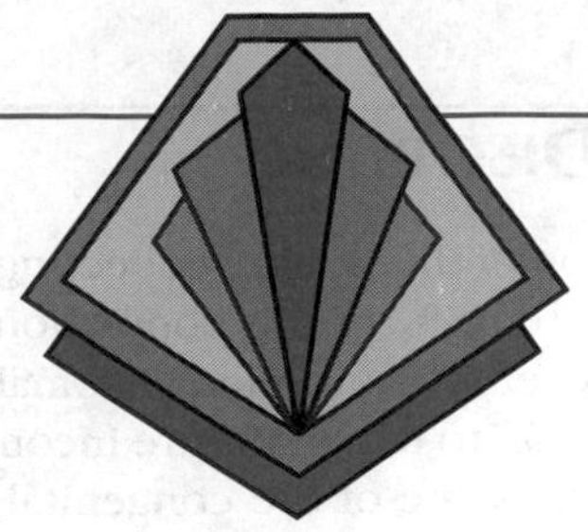

CHAPTER 49

# Management of Persons With Problems of the Kidney and Urinary Tract


***Marilyn Rossman Bartucci***

***Rebecca Anne Roberts***


## CHAPTER OBJECTIVES

***After studying this chapter, the learner should be able to do the following:***

1 Identify six major health problems of the urinary system.

2 Describe the pathophysiology and management of polycystic kidney disease.

3 Describe etiology, pathophysiology, and management of lower urinary tract infections and pyelonephritis, including the importance of public awareness and patient teaching.

4 Compare glomerulonephritis and the nephrotic syndrome in relation to pathophysiology, clinical manifestations, and management.

5 Describe management of persons requiring assisted drainage.

6 Describe the pathophysiology and interventions for renal calculi.

7 Compare different approaches to prostatectomy and the related nursing interventions.

8 Differentiate types of urinary incontinence and their management.

9 Develop a plan of care for patients undergoing urologic surgery.

10 Compare and contrast the four types of urinary diversion procedures and management of urinary stomas.

## KEY TERMS

bladder retraining
calculi
colon conduit
continent ileal reservoir
continent urostomy
cutaneous ureterostomy
cystectomy
cystitis
cystostomy
cystotomy
diabetic nephropathy
diverticuli of bladder
epispadias
extracorporal shock wave lithotripsy
glomerulonephritis
hydronephrosis
hydroureter
hypospadias
ileal conduit
ileal loop
ileocecal pouch
intermittent catheterization
litholapaxy
nephrectomy
nephritis
nephrolithotomy
nephropexy
nephroptosis
nephrosclerosis
nephrostomy
nephrotic syndrome
neurogenic bladder
overflow incontinence
percutaneous lithotripsy
polycystic kidney disease
pyelolithotomy
pyelonephritis
pyeloplasty
pyelostomy
renal artery stenosis
renal colic
residual urine
retention with overflow
segmental resection
stoma
stress incontinence
ureterolithotomy
urethral stricture
urethritis
urge incontinence
urinary incontinence
urinary retention
vesicourethropexy

A major cause of morbidity and a significant cause of mortality in the United States is disease of the urinary system. Mortality from disease of the urinary system is generally associated with damage to the interstitial kidney tissue. When a disease process involves the kidney, renal function is directly threatened. If disease is present in the urinary drainage system, it not only affects tissues at the site of the disease but also can threaten renal function by two mechanisms: spread of the disease process or destruction of the kidney from obstruction of urine flow. The primary objective for treatment of disease in any part of the urinary tract should be early detection and adequate therapy directed toward preserving or improving renal function; without renal function, life can be maintained for only a few days.

During the last 2 decades, some of the most striking developments in the treatment of urinary system diseases have evolved in both diagnosis and treatment. Advances in computed tomography (CT) and ultrasound have made major contributions to diagnosis. New technologies in membrane development have provided improved dialysis while surgical and immunologic advances have greatly improved the success of transplantation.

Nurses can provide valuable assistance in significantly reducing morbidity related to the urinary system. This can be achieved by (1) increasing public awareness of preventive measures, (2) assisting in early detection of signs and symptoms of renal disease, (3) providing ongoing health teaching for persons with renal disease, and (4) providing long-term care to the growing population of chronically ill individuals with urinary tract disease. This chapter describes common disorders of the urinary system and their management.

Major health problems of the urinary system can be divided into six categories as follows:

1. Congenital disorders
   a. Structural malformations of the urinary system
   b. Renal cystic disorders
2. Inflammatory disorders
   a. Urinary tract infection
   b. Pyelonephritis
   c. Chemical-induced nephritis
   d. Glomerulonephritis
   e. Nephrotic syndrome
3. Vascular disorders
   a. Nephrosclerosis
   b. Renal artery stenosis
   c. Diabetic nephropathy
4. Obstructive disorders
   a. Calculi
   b. Neoplasms
   c. Prostatic hypertrophy
   d. Urethral strictures
5. Urinary incontinence
6. Trauma

# CONGENITAL DISORDERS

Structural malformation of the urinary collecting system occurs in about 10% to 15% of the population. These deviations range in severity from minor anomalies that do not require correction to those that are incompatible with life. Box 49-1 lists some of the congenital malformations that can potentially influence urinary function in adult life.

Details about the management of congenital disorders can be found in most pediatric nursing texts. However, renal cystic disorders contribute to significant adult morbidity and are discussed in this chapter.

## RENAL CYSTIC DISORDERS

Renal cystic disorders encompass a relatively large group of diseases typified by the formation of one or more fluid-filled cavities within the kidneys. Cysts can arise in all parts of the kidney. Renal cysts may develop in utero, may be acquired after birth, and may be congenital or hereditary. Cysts may be slightly larger than

**BOX 49-1 Congenital Malformations of Urinary Tract**

**Duplication of ureters** (Partial or complete)
**Hydroureters** Dilation of ureters
**Exstrophy of urinary bladder** Eversion of bladder on outer abdominal wall
**Epispadias** Opening of urethra on dorsum of penis (Figure 49-1, *B*)
**Hypospadias** Opening of urethra on underside of penis (Figure 49-1, *A*)

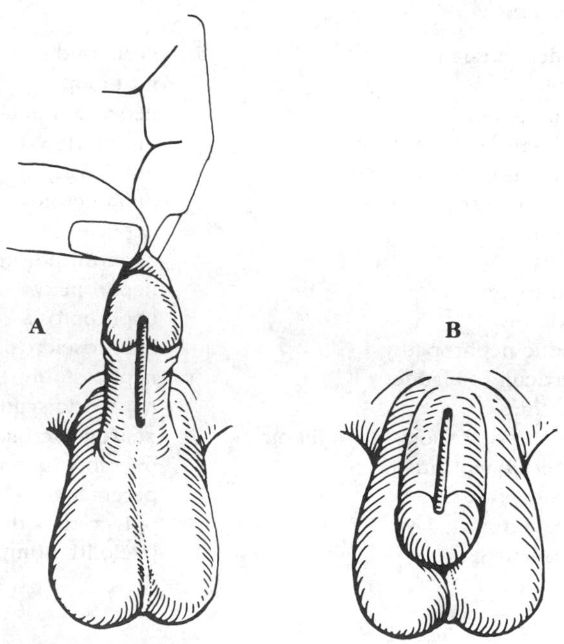


**FIGURE 49-1** **A,** Hypospadias. **B,** Epispadias.

a single nephron in their formative stage, or they may be so large as to compress the abdominal viscera. Renal cysts may be benign occupants or may compromise function, causing renal failure. Cysts may be the primary renal disorder or may appear in association with non-renal disorders.

## Polycystic Kidney Disease

### Etiology/Epidemiology

**Polycystic kidney disease** is the most common renal cystic disorder. The adult form of polycystic kidney disease (APKD) may be recognized in utero, shortly after birth (Figure 49-2, *A*), or after several decades of "normal" life. There is an autosomal dominant pattern of inheritance, although the gene for this disorder has a high degree of penetrance. In the United States, it has been estimated that 1:500 to 1:1000 persons have APKD (200,000 to 400,000 people).[10]

### Pathophysiology

APKD is usually a bilateral disorder; that is, it affects both kidneys in 95% of patients.[16] Cysts are diffusely scattered through the renal parenchyma, with islands of normal tissue between the cysts (Figure 49-2, *B*). The cysts arise from all segments of the nephron and collecting system. The kidneys are larger than normal (as much as five times normal size) and are studded with cysts of various sizes. As the cysts enlarge, they compress adjacent parenchyma, destroy it by ischemia, and occlude normal tubules. One of the most devastating features is that APKD undergoes relentless progression to end-stage renal failure in a high percentage of patients, usually in the fourth or fifth decade of life. Abnormalities may affect other organs: liver cysts occur in 20% to 40% of patients; a few have pancreatic cysts; and 10% to 20% have aneurysms of the cerebral artery or the abdominal aorta.

Pain in one or both kidneys is the most common initial complaint in patients with APKD. The pain may be a dull aching, a vague sense of heaviness, or knifelike and stabbing. Medium-size blood vessels rupture occasionally and cause extravasation of blood either into cysts or into perinephric tissue. Hemorrhage may cause the cyst to rupture into the kidney pelvis and be associated with moderate to severe hematuria. These patients are prone to infections of the cysts and serious infections of the kidney parenchyma manifested by pain, fever, leukocytosis, pyuria, and positive blood and urine cultures. Hypertension develops in 60% to 70% of patients at some time in the course of the disease. Hypertension often antedates measurable functional renal impairment by several years. If uncontrolled, it accelerates renal destruction. Serum and urine electrolytes, as well as creatinine clearance tests, provide data about renal function.

### Prevention

Prevention is the key to decreasing the incidence of APKD. Prevention can be realized only by prospectively identifying those with the disorder so that they may have

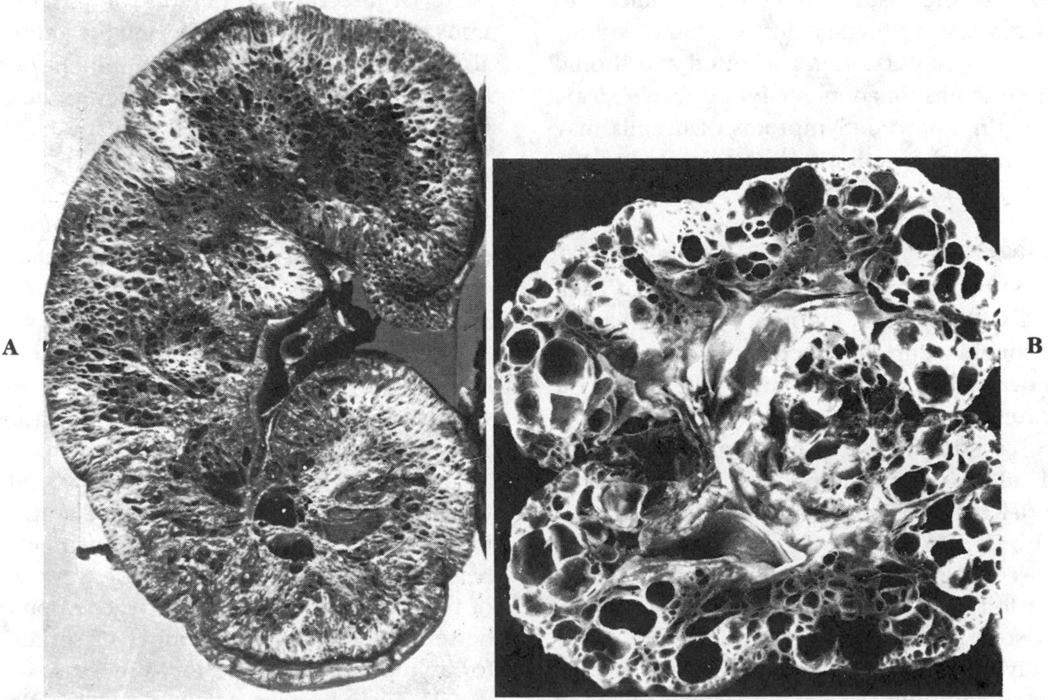


**FIGURE 49-2** Polycystic kidney disease. **A,** Newborn. **B,** Adult. (From Anderson WAD, Kissane JM: *Pathology,* ed 7, St Louis, 1977, Mosby.)

the opportunity of determining whether to bear children. Because APKD is an autosomal disorder, patients with the gene may expect that each child will have a 50/50 chance of having the gene.

The family history is a crucial part of the counseling process; however, many family members are unwilling to reveal that they or other family members have had this disease. Guilt and denial are prominent coping patterns in these families. Often, persons do not learn they have the APKD gene until beyond the childbearing period. Some believe it is advisable to evaluate all persons at risk for APKD. Recent studies using combined sonography and CT scanning indicate that the presence of the disease in young persons can probably be established with a 95% degree of certainty. For the individual found not to have renal disease, the future is clear: there is little chance the disease will be passed on. However, for the young person found to have early APKD, several socioeconomic problems have been identified. The most difficult problem is that nothing can be done to prevent the disease's progression. Second, the early discovery in the young person of a potentially disabling or life-threatening disease may affect future employability and insurability. These factors must be carefully discussed with the individual before screening for APKD.

#### Medical management

The goals of medical management are to alleviate symptoms and slow the onset of renal dysfunction. Hypertension is closely monitored and controlled. Infections are treated vigorously because the scarring leads to further progression of the disease. Infection is difficult to eradicate and can lead to further destruction of kidney tissue. Antibiotic therapy is often instituted and should be given on time to ensure adequate blood levels. Urine output is closely monitored. Symptoms of uremia may be present when renal function has deteriorated to the point of end-stage renal disease.

#### Nursing management

Analgesic drugs may be necessary for control of flank pain associated with enlarged kidneys. Tepid baths will also provide comfort during infections. When urinary bleeding from ruptured cysts becomes severe, bedrest is often instituted.

Because polycystic disease is bilateral and leads to chronic renal failure, ongoing support and health teaching are essential nursing interventions. The patient is instructed to be alert to signs and symptoms of infection and bleeding. The emotional overtones of this illness can be severe for both the individual and the family. Challenges exist in helping the person deal with an illness on an individual basis when relatives have died of the same disease and children have not yet developed symptoms. Counseling may be required about family health care and the individual's role in passing on a potentially fatal disease to children. Patients are instructed to monitor urine output and report changes to their physician.

Most patients require no modification in physical activity or life-style until they approach the end stage of their illness. Some patients are unusually susceptible to physical trauma to the abdomen. Cyst rupture has been caused by seat-belt constraints in automobiles and airplanes. This does not mean that patients are exempt from wearing seat belts, but they should be cautioned against strapping the lap belt too tightly across the abdomen. In male patients with massive kidneys, the use of suspenders for pants rather than constrictive belts is recommended. Patients with APKD should not participate in strenuous athletic events such as wrestling, boxing, football, and horseback riding. Although no evidence suggests that cyst rupture adversely affects renal function, the constant bouts of pain caused by cyst rupture can be avoided to some extent by tailoring the physical activity.

# INFLAMMATORY DISORDERS

The kidneys are susceptible to inflammation caused by bacterial infection, altered immune response, drugs and other chemicals, toxins, and radiation. Inflammation may be acute or chronic. This section addresses the most common inflammatory disorders of the urinary system.

## LOWER URINARY TRACT INFECTIONS

Urinary tract infections (UTIs) are a significant source of morbidity in the United States and the most common bacterial infections in persons of all ages. These infections contribute to illness during the acute infection and also are significant in the development of chronic renal failure. Infection occurs in both acute and chronic stages in all portions of the urinary tract.

### Etiology/Epidemiology

Table 49-1 summarizes factors contributing to infection of the urinary tract. Although the great majority of uncomplicated UTIs are asymptomatic and clear spontaneously, a significant enough number warrant consideration as a health problem. Because untreated UTIs can lead to more serious problems, they must be taken seriously. No controversy exists among those practicing preventive health care about the need for screening for asymptomatic infections; however, it is difficult to identify the specific groups at risk in whom detection and treatment yield significant improvement in health. As health care becomes more oriented toward prevention of health problems, specific target populations will be better defined, and the number of screening programs for asymptomatic UTIs should increase.

UTI occurs more frequently in females than males. Contributing factors include a shorter urethra with proximity to the vagina and rectum and the lack of prostatic fluid that provides protection from UTI for males. In-

**TABLE 49-1 Risk Factors Associated With Development of Urinary Tract Infections**

| RISK FACTORS | COMMON EXAMPLES |
|---|---|
| Female | Short urethra |
| Structural abnormality | Strictures<br>Incompetent ureterovesical junction anomalies |
| Obstruction | Tumors<br>Prostatic hypertrophy<br>Calculi<br>Iatrogenic causes |
| Impaired bladder innervation | Congenital spinal cord malformation<br>Spinal cord injury<br>Multiple sclerosis |
| Chronic disease | Gout<br>Diabetes mellitus<br>Hypertension<br>Sickle cell disease<br>Polycystic kidney disease<br>Multiple myeloma<br>Glomerulonephritis |
| Instrumentation | Catheterization<br>Diagnostic procedures |

fection rates for females are approximately 1% in school-aged girls. This rate increases to approximately 2.5% for women in the childbearing years and 20% in women aged 65 to 70. For the elderly (over 80 years) living at home or in a chronic care facility, the incidence increases to 30%.[11] Risk of infection also increases with increased sexual activity. Pregnancy does not seem to increase UTI rates, although spontaneous clearing of infections is decreased during pregnancy. Infection of the lower urinary tract also increases the incidence of acute kidney infections as a result of ascending microorganisms.

Structural and functional abnormalities of the urinary tract, obstruction to the flow of urine, and impaired bladder innervation promote UTI. Mechanisms that result in infection include stasis of urine that promotes a culture medium for bacterial growth, reflux of infected urine higher into the urinary tract, and increasing hydrostatic pressure.

Several chronic health problems (Table 49-1) predispose an individual to UTI by changing the metabolism of tissues, creating extrarenal obstruction, and altering the function and structure of kidney tissue.

Instrumentation of the urinary tract is also associated with high rates of UTI. Catheterization, even when performed without break in aseptic technique, results in a significant rate of infection of the bladder. Nosocomial infections account for a sizable percentage of all UTIs and should be closely monitored. Drug-resistant strains of *Staphylococcus* and *Pseudomonas,* along with various other organisms typically found in hospitals, are frequently those involved in nosocomial UTI. Prevention and control of all UTIs can be most significantly influenced through a lowering of the rate of nosocomial infection.

Lower UTIs involve the urinary bladder **(cystitis)** and the urethra **(urethritis).** Upper UTIs may involve the kidney **(pyelonephritis).**

The mode of entry of bacteria into the genitourinary tract cannot always be traced with certainty. Four major pathways exist:

1. *Ascending* infection from the urethra is the most common cause of genitourinary tract infection in men and UTI in females. Because the female urethra is short and rectal bacteria tend to colonize the perineum and vaginal vestibule, females are especially susceptible to ascending UTI. Sexual intercourse has been shown to be a major precipitating factor of UTI in women.
2. *Hematogenous* spread occurs infrequently, with the exception of tuberculosis, renal abscesses, and perinephric abscesses. Bacteremia is more likely to complicate UTI when structural and functional abnormalities exist than when the urinary tract is normal.
3. *Lymphatogenous* spread is rare. Some researchers speculate that bacterial pathogens travel through the rectal and colonic lymphatics to the prostate and bladder and through the periuterine lymphatics to the female genitourinary tract.
4. *Direct extension from another organ* occurs with intraperitoneal abscesses, especially those associated with inflammatory bowel disease, fulminant pelvic inflammatory disease in women, paravesical abscesses, and genitourinary tract fistulas.

The etiologic factors and general preventive and management principles for UTI are the same for infection elsewhere in the urinary tract. Pyelonephritis is discussed in greater detail on pp. 1617-1618.

## Pathophysiology

Most UTIs result from gram-negative organisms, such as *Escherichia coli, Klebsiella, Proteus,* or *Pseudomonas,* that originate in the person's own intestinal tract and ascend through the urethra to the bladder. During micturition, urine may flow back up the ureters (vesicoureteral reflux) and carry bacteria from the bladder up through the ureters to the kidney pelvis (Table 49-2). Whenever stasis of urine occurs, such as with incomplete emptying of the bladder, renal calculi, or genitourinary obstructions, the bacteria have a greater opportunity to grow. Urinary stasis also promotes a more alkaline urine, which facilitates bacterial growth.

UTIs occur primarily when host resistance is impaired. The major factors preventing UTI are tissue integrity and blood supply. A break in the surface of the mucous membrane lining of the urinary tract permits the bacteria to invade tissue and cause infection. Breaks

**TABLE 49-2 Normal Function, Pathophysiology, and Clinical Manifestations in Lower Urinary Tract Infection**

| NORMAL FUNCTION | PATHOPHYSIOLOGY | CLINICAL MANIFESTATIONS |
|---|---|---|
| Urine produced in kidneys flows unobstructed through urinary tract. Urine is sterile until it reaches urethra. | Urine stasis promotes bacterial growth. Bacteria may ascend urethra into bladder and ureters, leading to infection. Inflamed tissues may bleed. | Frequency, urgency, dysuria<br>Fever and chills<br>Hematuria<br>Bacteriuria |

in tissue integrity result from erosions caused by tips from indwelling catheters, trauma, or rough-edged renal stones; from neoplasms; or from invasion of the tissue by parasites such as *Schistosoma.* In the bladder, blood supply to tissues can be compromised when the pressure within the bladder is greatly increased, as may occur with overdistention of the bladder, contracture of the bladder neck, or obstruction of the urethra by an enlarged prostate, metastatic growth, or urethral stricture.

*Symptoms* that bring the person with UTI to seek medical attention typically include frequency, urgency, burning on urination (dysuria), cloudy or foul-smelling urine, and hematuria. Most persons, however, are asymptomatic or minimally symptomatic. In these cases the UTI is identified only on routine examination of the urine. Bacteriuria and positive urine cultures serve as the basis for diagnosing lower UTIs. Infection is indicated by growth of a single pathogen in excess of $1 \times 10^5$ organisms/ml of urine in a properly obtained and stored midstream specimen (Chapter 48).

## Prevention

The most important defenses against UTI are large urine volume, free urine flow, and complete emptying of the bladder to prevent urinary stasis. Three considerations are important in preventing lower UTI: (1) preventing or minimizing morbidity that can accompany these infections, (2) preventing recurrence of the infection, and (3) preventing renal damage from untreated or inadequately treated ascending infections. Persons with lower UTIs seek medical attention as a result of symptoms or are identified through routine urinalysis or screening. Education of the public (Box 49-2) and efforts of the health care community assist in decreasing UTI and its complications.

## Medical Management

### Diagnostic tests

It is crucial that urine cultures be obtained before initiating drug therapy to confirm the organism's sensitivity to antimicrobial medications and to decrease the development of resistant organisms. The urine should be recultured every few months during the following year to reconfirm urine sterility.

A more extensive urologic work-up, including intravenous pyelogram (IVP) and voiding cystogram, may be performed for men and young children after a repeated, or even first, UTI or when infection does not abate. This work-up is performed on women when infection occurs repeatedly or cannot be cleared with treatment. The rationale for this extensive work-up is that UTIs are not common in men and children. A significant portion of infection in these populations and in women with persistent infection involves a urinary tract abnormality.

### Medication

Medications typically used in the treatment of UTI include urinary tract antiseptics such as sulfisoxazole (Gantrisin) or nitrofurantoin (Furadantin). Systemic antibiotics are also frequently prescribed. Sulfonamides are widely used and are usually effective against the organisms causing a large percentage of UTIs. Sulfonamides are relatively safe and are less likely than most systemic antibiotics to contribute to growth of resistant organisms.

For persons with chronic bacteriuria, urine-acidifying agents may be prescribed. The effect of these medications is to provide a less suitable environment for bacterial growth and to enhance the effectiveness of antibiotic and urinary antiseptics. When bacteriuria becomes constant, prophylaxis may be undertaken with antimicrobial drugs.

### Treatment

Additional treatment includes increasing fluid intake to 3 to 4 L/day unless contraindicated. Increased fluid helps to dilute the urine, lessen irritation and burning, and provide a continual flow of urine to minimize stasis and multiplication of bacteria in the urinary tract. Sitz baths may provide comfort for individuals with urethritis.

No special dietary or activity requirements are prescribed.

# NURSING MANAGEMENT

## ♦ ASSESSMENT

### Subjective Data

The subjective data should include assessment of symptoms of frequency, urgency, and burning on urination (dysuria). Chills and fever may be present. Data should be collected on predisposing factors, such as use of bubble baths or contraceptive jellies and a history of previous infections.

### Objective Data

A urine culture is obtained because bacteriuria serves as the basis for diagnosis of lower UTI. The urine should also be tested for occult blood.

**BOX 49-2 Information To Be Included in Public Education Programs About Urinary Tract Infection**

- Symptoms of UTI
- Need for prompt medical attention when symptoms of UTI occur
- Need to continue drug therapy even though symptoms abate
- Importance of follow-up care and repeat urine cultures
- Maintenance of fluid intake of 3 to 4 L/day if the person's health permits

## ♦ NURSING DIAGNOSES

Nursing diagnoses are determined from analysis of patient data. Nursing diagnoses for the person with UTI may include but are not limited to the following:

| Diagnostic Title | Possible Etiologic Factors |
|---|---|
| Urinary elimination patterns, altered | Urinary infection |
| Pain | Inflammation |
| Knowledge deficit | Lack of exposure/recall |

## ♦ EXPECTED PATIENT OUTCOMES

Expected patient outcomes for the person with UTI may include but are not limited to the following:

1. Kidney function is stabilized or improved.
2. Sterile urine or urine bacteria count is less than $1 \times 10^5$ organisms/ml of urine.
3. States that symptoms of UTI are relieved.
4. Describes the following:
   a. Signs and symptoms of UTI.
   b. Rationale and means of increasing fluid intake to 3 to 4 L/day.
   c. Risk factors for UTI.
   d. When and how to take prescribed medications.
   e. Plan for follow-up care, including urine cultures.

## ♦ INTERVENTIONS

### Facilitating Healing and Comfort

Antibiotic therapy must be given on time on a regular schedule to ensure adequate blood levels. If the patient is to undergo instrumentation, the nurse reinforces instructions about the specific procedure. Knowledge about potential sensations during instrumentation and deep breathing exercises during the procedure may assist in relaxing the patient.

Individuals with urethritis may experience pain or itching in the perineum. Sitz baths may provide relief of symptoms.

### Facilitating Learning

Patient education concerning the specific problem, the requirements for drug therapy, and follow-up care should facilitate completion of drug regimens for eradication of bacteria and early identification of recurrence of infection. Success in both these areas depends directly on patient understanding and compliance and allows the patient to assist in overcoming this health problem. Female patients should be instructed in good perineal hygiene and to void after intercourse.

## ♦ EVALUATION

To evaluate the effectiveness of nursing interventions, compare patient behaviors with those stated in the expected patient outcomes. Successful achievement of patient outcomes for the person with a UTI are indicated by the following:

1. Kidney function does not deteriorate further, as demonstrated by follow-up tests.
2. Infection not present, as demonstrated by urine bacteria count less than $1 \times 10^5$ organisms/ml of urine.
3. States that no pain, frequency, or urgency are present.
4. Correctly describes the following:
   a. Signs and symptoms of UTI and need for prompt medical attention when they occur.
   b. Rationale for increasing fluids to 3 to 4 L/day.
   c. Risk factors for UTI.
   d. Routine for taking prescribed medication with regard to dose, frequency, and length of therapy.
   e. Follow-up care, including return visit to health care professional and repeat urine culture.

## PYELONEPHRITIS

### Etiology/Epidemiology

Pyelonephritis is an infectious inflammatory disease that involves both the parenchyma and the kidney pelvis. This infection usually begins in the lower urinary tract and ascends into the kidneys. Lower UTI may be asymptomatic, and kidney involvement may be the first indication of lower urinary tract disease. Diagnostic workup of a person with pyelonephritis often reveals previously unknown urinary tract obstruction or the presence of another chronic kidney disease. *Escherichia coli* is the most common organism identified in pyelonephritis, and resistance to antibiotic therapy is rare. Pyelonephritis is most frequently associated with (1) cystitis, (2) pregnancy, or (3) obstruction, instrumentation, or trauma of the urinary tract. Other risk factors include septicemia and chronic health problems, including diabetes, analgesic abuse, polycystic kidney disease, and hypertensive kidney disease.

### Pathophysiology

Infection of the kidney occurs in both acute and chronic forms. Although *acute* pyelonephritis may temporarily affect renal function, this rarely progresses to renal failure. *Chronic* pyelonephritis destroys renal tissue permanently through repeated inflammation and scarring (Table 49-3). The process of developing chronic renal

**TABLE 49-3 Normal Function, Pathophysiology, and Clinical Manifestations in Pyelonephritis**

| NORMAL FUNCTION | PATHOPHYSIOLOGY | CLINICAL MANIFESTATIONS |
|---|---|---|
| Fluid regulation<br>Electrolyte regulation<br>Blood pressure regulation<br>Excretion of metabolic wastes | Acute inflammation results in hyperemia and suppuration of tissues (inflammatory response). | *Acute:* flank pain, fever, chills, malaise, leukocytosis, WBCs and bacteria in urine |
| | Chronic inflammation results in scarring and atrophy, leading to chronic renal failure. | *Chronic:* persistent bacteriuria; hypertension, ↑ BUN, ↓ creatinine clearance in late stages |

failure from repeated kidney infections occurs over a number of years or after several extensive and fulminant infections. It is estimated that pyelonephritis represents the original diagnosis in one third of all persons with chronic renal failure.

*Signs and symptoms* of acute pyelonephritis may include those of lower UTI in addition to the following typical signs of inflammation: chills and fever, malaise, flank pain, costovertebral angle tenderness, and leukocytosis. Urinalysis demonstrates presence of white blood cells (WBCs), casts, and bacteria. In chronic pyelonephritis the only symptoms may be persistent bacteriuria until extensive scarring and atrophy result in renal insufficiency, as manifested by hypertension, increased blood urea nitrogen (BUN), and decreased creatinine clearance.

## Prevention

The most significant efforts in preventing pyelonephritis are through early detection and adequate treatment of lower UTIs.

## Medical Management

Optimal treatment of pyelonephritis includes early detection of the bacterial infection through urine culture, antibacterial therapy based on identified sensitivities, and detection and treatment of any underlying systemic disease or urinary abnormality. The course of antibiotic therapy may extend over weeks. The urine is recultured 2 weeks after drug therapy has been discontinued and monthly for several months thereafter. If infection becomes chronic, maintenance drug therapy may continue indefinitely; the goal is to reduce and control the bacterial population of the urinary tract to prevent renal damage.

## Nursing Management

It is important to maintain sufficient urinary flow to remove byproducts of the inflammation and to prevent urinary stasis with further bacterial growth. Fluid intake of 3 L/day is encouraged in persons with normal excretory function.

During the acute phase the patient is encouraged to rest. Prescribed analgesics may be given for flank pain. Back massage often provides short-term relief of discomfort. Pain eases as the inflammation resolves.

### Facilitating learning

Persons with pyelonephritis may be treated at home; therefore patient teaching is important. Instruct the patient to do the following:

1. Continue antibiotic therapy even after symptoms resolve.
2. Drink 3 L/day of fluids unless otherwise instructed.
3. Monitor urinary output; report to physician an output considerably less than fluid intake.
4. Weigh self daily; report a sudden weight gain to physician.
5. Take measures to prevent infection; report signs of urinary infection (increased flank pain, fever, chills, frequency, urgency) to physician.
6. Continue with medical follow-up and have follow-up urine cultures as instructed.

# TUBERCULOSIS OF THE KIDNEY

## Etiology/Epidemiology

Renal tuberculosis is caused by *Mycobacterium tuberculosis.* Renal tuberculosis is an example of a kidney infection that is secondary to an infection in a different site (pulmonary tuberculosis). Tuberculosis of the kidney is acquired by hematogenous spread of the mycobacterium and is most common in men 20 to 40 years of age.

## Pathophysiology

Signs and symptoms of renal tuberculosis are mild and usually include loss of appetite, unexplained weight loss, and intermittent fever. Hematuria may also be present. Diagnostic tests usually include screening for pulmonary tuberculosis. Urine samples are also obtained and screened for the presence of *M. tuberculosis.*

## Prevention

Prevention is primarily through the control of pulmonary tuberculosis by early detection and treatment.

## Medical Management

Treatment is usually through the institution of antituberculosis medication, alone or in combination (see Chapter 37). Medications typically used include isoniazid, rifampin, and ethambutol. Drug therapy is usually given for 9 to 18 months.

**TABLE 49-4 Substances Associated With Chemical-Induced Nephritis**

| CATEGORY | SUBSTANCE |
|---|---|
| Solvents | Carbon tetrachloride<br>Methanol<br>Ethylene glycol |
| Heavy metals | Lead<br>Arsenic<br>Mercury |
| Antibiotics | Kanamycin<br>Gentamicin<br>Amphotericin B<br>Calistin<br>Neomycin<br>Phenazopyridine |
| Pesticides | |
| Poisonous mushrooms | |

### Nursing Management

Nursing interventions are the same as those for pyelonephritis (increased fluid intake, medications, rest).

## CHEMICAL-INDUCED NEPHRITIS

### Etiology/Epidemiology

Chemical-induced **nephritis** is an idiosyncratic reaction that results in damage to the kidney tubules and interstitium. This disease process was first noted in patients who were sensitive to the sulfonamide drugs. Many other substances are now associated with chemical-induced nephritis, including those listed in Table 49-4.

### Pathophysiology

Chemical-induced nephritis usually begins within 15 days of exposure to the chemical. The inflammatory process disrupts the ability of the glomeruli to filter. Furthermore, the capillary membrane is altered to the extent that it becomes permeable to plasma proteins and red blood cells (RBCs) resulting in proteinuria and hematuria.

*Signs and symptoms* of nephritis include fever, eosinophilia, hematuria, mild proteinuria, and rash. Oliguria or urine output of 400 ml or less in a 24-hour period occurs in approximately 50% of all patients. Urinalysis is used to demonstrate protein or RBCs in the urine. Serum toxicology screening may identify the source of the nephritis.

### Prevention

Prevention of chemical-induced nephritis is best managed by identifying causative agents and removing them from the environment. Many people are exposed to these agents as a result of their medical regimen. The health care professional must be aware of these agents and the signs and symptoms associated with chemical-induced nephritis. With early detection and removal of the causative agent as soon as possible, the prognosis is improved.

A major risk factor is industrial exposure to chemicals. Occupational health professionals should be aware of potential risks and should educate employees regarding appropriate preventive measures.

### Medical Management

Medical management usually includes immediate withdrawal of the suspected chemical. Hemodialysis may be required to remove the nephrotoxins from the blood. Steroids are often administered because of their antiinflammatory effect. If renal function is severely compromised, dietary sodium and protein restrictions may be instituted.

### Nursing Management

The patient is assessed for fluid and electrolyte imbalance, including the presence of edema, blood pressure changes, and adventitious breath sounds. The person needs to know the rationale for maintenance of fluid balance and any sodium restrictions. Care is similar to that for the patient with acute renal failure (see Chapter 50).

## ACUTE GLOMERULONEPHRITIS

### Etiology/Epidemiology

**Glomerulonephritis** is a disease that affects the glomeruli of both kidneys. Etiologic factors are many and varied; they include immunologic reactions (lupus erythematosus, streptococcal infection), vascular injury (hypertension), metabolic disease (diabetes mellitus), and disseminated intravascular coagulation (DIC). Glomerulonephritis exists in acute, latent, and chronic forms.

The most common form of *acute* glomerulonephritis occurs 2 to 3 weeks after a streptococcal infection. Common sites of the primary infection include the pharynx or tonsils and the skin (impetigo). Preschool-age and grade-school-age children are most likely to develop the illness. Of all individuals developing acute poststreptococcal glomerulonephritis, approximately 1% to 2% will develop end-stage renal failure requiring renal replacement therapy (dialysis or transplantation). Approximately 90% of children and 50% of adults with acute glomerulonephritis attain full recovery from illness, although recovery may require as long as 2 years.[17] Little can be inferred from the severity of the acute episode regarding prognosis. Persons with mild illness may develop chronic disease, and those with severe illness may completely recover and have no recurrence of the illness.

### Pathophysiology

Acute poststreptococcal glomerulonephritis is a result of an *antigen-antibody reaction* with glomerular tissue that produces swelling and death of capillary cells. The antigen-antibody reaction activates the complement pathway (see Chapter 13), resulting in chemotaxis of polymorphonuclear (PMN) leukocytes with release of lysosomal enzymes that attack the glomerular basement membrane (GBM). The response in the membrane is an increase in all three types of glomerular cells (endothelial, mesangial, epithelial), causing an *increase in membrane porosity* with resultant proteinuria and hematuria. Renal function is depressed by scarring and obstruction of the circulation through the glomerulus.

Typical patient complaints include shortness of breath, mild headache, weakness, anorexia, and flank pain. The usual *signs* associated with acute glomerulonephritis are the following:

1. Proteinuria
2. Hematuria
3. Increased urine specific gravity
4. Mild generalized edema
5. Elevated antistreptolysin O titer
6. Hypertension
7. Decreased urinary output
8. Elevated serum urea nitrogen
9. Elevated serum creatinine levels
10. Elevated sedimentation rate

Signs and symptoms reflect damage to the glomeruli, with leaking of protein and RBCs into the urine, and varying degrees of decreased glomerular filtration, with retention of metabolic waste products, sodium, and water.

## Prevention

Prevention of acute poststreptococcal glomerulonephritis involves prompt medical treatment of sore throats and upper respiratory infections. Cultures should be obtained and antibiotics prescribed when indicated.

## Medical Management

### Diagnostic tests

Urinalysis provides important data, such as the presence of proteinuria, hematuria, and cell debris. Serum BUN and urine creatinine clearance tests indicate renal function status.

### Medication

Persistent infection is treated promptly to help prevent increase in antigen-antibody complex formation. Patients with poststreptococcal glomerulonephritis are given a course of prophylactic antibiotics; the drug of choice is penicillin. Prophylactic therapy may be continued for months after the acute phase of illness. Diuretic therapy is implemented when severe fluid overload develops. Elevated blood pressure is controlled by antihypertensive drugs only after fluid control has proved to be unsuccessful.

### Treatment

No specific treatment exists for acute glomerulonephritis. General management is directed toward preventing overhydration and hypertension. Exposure to any infection must be avoided because even mild infection may reactivate nephritis.

### Diet

Fluid retention is often a problem and is managed by dietary sodium restrictions. Dietary protein is reduced when BUN and creatinine levels are elevated. It is important that the diet contain sufficient carbohydrates to prevent protein being used for energy, resulting in muscle wasting and nitrogen imbalance.

### Activity

Bedrest is usually instituted until clinical signs of nephritis have resolved.

## NURSING MANAGEMENT

### ♦ ASSESSMENT

#### Subjective Data

General questions to ask the patient include: Have you experienced shortness of breath, headaches, weakness, or anorexia? Have you noticed a change in your pattern of urination, either frequency or volume? Do you recall a recent infection or symptoms of a virus?

#### Objective Data

Data to be collected to assess the patient with acute glomerulonephritis include the following:

Frequent assessment of vital signs
Daily assessment for edema
Intake and output
Daily weights

### ♦ NURSING DIAGNOSES

Nursing diagnoses are determined from analysis of patient data. Nursing diagnoses for the person with acute glomerulonephritis may include but are not limited to the following:

| Diagnostic Title | Possible Etiologic Factors |
|---|---|
| Fluid volume excess | Compromised regulatory mechanism, renal impairment |
| Infection, high risk for | Decreased immune response |
| Coping, ineffective (individual) | Activity restrictions |
| Knowledge deficit | Lack of information |

### ♦ EXPECTED PATIENT OUTCOMES

Expected patient outcomes for the person with acute glomerulonephritis may include but are not limited to the following:

1. Fluid balance is achieved; edema is decreased; weight is stable.
2. Infection does not occur.
3. Expresses concerns and feelings about restricted activity; does not express boredom with prolonged bedrest.

4. Describes the rationale for therapy, dietary restrictions, medication program, measures to prevent infection, and signs and symptoms requiring medical attention.

## ♦ INTERVENTIONS

### Maintaining Fluid Balance

Edema and fluid overloading are anticipated and treated initially with dietary sodium restrictions. The amount of sodium restriction depends on the severity of fluid retention and is maintained until dependent edema and circulatory overload are no longer present. Keep strict records of fluid intake and output. Calculate the difference between fluid intake and loss, and determine the net fluid change. Fluid restrictions must be maintained.

Be constantly alert for signs and symptoms of fluid overload. Weigh the patient daily using correct procedure. Use a metric scale, if possible, because it is easier to calculate fluid changes. Take vital signs at least daily, including apical pulse. Listen for presence of a dysrhythmia. Assess for neck vein distention indicating fluid overload and congestive heart failure. Assess for periorbital, pretibial, pedal, and sacral edema. Measure edematous legs to assess changes in size. Administer antihypertensive and diuretic therapy as prescribed. Monitor serum potassium levels closely, especially for those diuretics that eliminate potassium (see Chapter 31).

### Preventing Infection

Mild infections may reactivate nephritis; therefore minimize patient exposure to any infection. The patient must avoid contact with any persons with upper respiratory infections (URIs). If a URI is suspected, cultures are usually obtained, and when indicated, appropriate antibiotics should be prescribed. When possible, avoid any procedures that may lead to nosocomial infection.

### Facilitating Coping

Bedrest is instituted until clinical signs disappear; this may involve a period of several months. Ambulation is allowed when blood sedimentation rates and blood pressure are normal and edema abates. If ambulation causes an increase in proteinuria or hematuria, bedrest is reinstituted. Since the period of bedrest may be extensive, the nurse may need to continue to reinforce the importance of bedrest as the patient starts to feel better. The importance of diversional activities should not be ignored. When bedrest is reinstituted after a period of ambulation, the person may become depressed as a result of the perceived setback in recovery. Helping the patient express concerns can serve as the impetus for making realistic plans about the illness and its sequelae.

### Facilitating Learning

The recovery period for acute glomerulonephritis may take as long as 2 years; therefore patient teaching is important. Proteinuria, hematuria, and cellular debris may exist microscopically, even when other symptoms subside. Although fatigue may be present, these persons usually feel well; thus they often need to be convinced of the importance of follow-up care. Teaching includes the following:

1. Nature of the illness and effect of diet and fluids on fluid balance and sodium retention.
2. Diet teaching regarding prescribed sodium and fluid restrictions (provide written information regarding sodium content of foods, as necessary)
3. Medication regimen: dose frequency, side effects, need to continue regimen as instructed by physician
4. Need to pace activities with rest if fatigue is present
5. Avoidance of infection, which may exacerbate the illness
6. Signs and symptoms indicating need for medical attention (hematuria, headache, edema, hypertension)
7. Importance of follow-up care

## ♦ EVALUATION

To evaluate the effectiveness of nursing interventions, compare patient behaviors with those stated in the expected patient outcomes. Successful achievement of patient outcomes for the patient with acute glomerulonephritis are indicated by:

1. Edema is decreased or absent and weight is stable.
2. Infection does not occur.
3. Carries out activity restrictions, participates in diversional activities, and does not express boredom.
4. Makes correct descriptions of the nature of the illness, dietary and fluid restrictions, importance of preventing URIs, signs and symptoms to be reported to physician, and importance of follow-up care.

## CHRONIC GLOMERULONEPHRITIS

### Etiology/Epidemiology

Although chronic glomerulonephritis (CGN) may follow the acute disease, most persons give no history of the disease. Usually no evidence of predisposing infection can be found. The course of CGN is extremely variable. Some persons with minimal impairment in renal function continue to feel well and show little progression of disease. With other individuals, the progression of renal deterioration may be slow but steady, resulting in end-stage renal disease. In still other individuals, the progression to end-stage disease is rapid.

### Pathophysiology

CGN is characterized by *slow progressive destruction* (sclerosis) of glomeruli and gradual loss of renal function. The glomeruli have varying degrees of hypercellularity and become sclerosed (hardened). The kidney decreases in size. Eventually there is tubular atrophy,

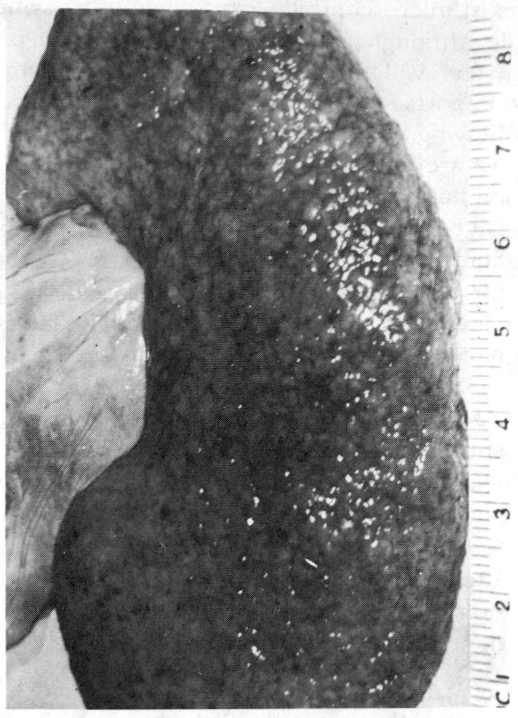

**FIGURE 49-3** End-stage chronic glomerulonephritis. Note pebbly surface corresponding to surviving hypertrophied nephrons and atrophy. (From Anderson WAD, Kissane JM: *Pathology,* ed 7, St Louis, 1977, Mosby.)

chronic interstitial inflammation, and arteriosclerosis (Figure 49-3).

Various symptoms of renal dysfunction may lead the person to seek health care. These include headache, especially in the morning; dyspnea on exertion; blurring of vision; lassitude; and weakness or fatigue. Signs of CGN may also include edema, nocturia, and weight loss.

Early in the disease process, urinalysis may show albumin, casts, and blood, despite normal renal function tests. The ability of the kidneys to regulate the internal environment will begin to decrease as more glomeruli become scarred, resulting in fewer functional nephrons. When few nephrons remain intact, hematuria and proteinuria decrease, the specific gravity of the urine becomes fixed at 1.010 (same as plasma), and the nonprotein nitrogen level in the blood increases.

## Prevention

Because predisposing factors have not been identified for CGN, no preventive measures can be instituted. Known infections should be treated promptly, as discussed under acute glomerulonephritis, to reduce the possibility of the acute disease progressing to CGN. Chronic diseases should be treated and controlled.

## Medical Management

No specific therapy exists to arrest or reverse this disease process. Treatment of renal failure begins when the illness progresses to end stage (see Chapter 50).

**TABLE 49-5 Normal Function, Pathophysiology and Clinical Manifestations in Nephrotic Syndrome**

| NORMAL FUNCTION | PATHOPHYSIOLOGY | CLINICAL MANIFESTATIONS |
|---|---|---|
| Glomerular capillaries are impermeable to serum proteins. Plasma proteins create colloid osmotic pressure to retain intravascular fluid. | Glomerular capillaries become permeable to serum proteins, resulting in proteinuria and decreased serum osmotic pressure. Glomerular filtration rate decreases. | Severe generalized edema; pronounced proteinuria; hypoalbuminemia; hyperlipidemia |

With any exacerbation of hematuria, hypertension, and edema, the client is returned to bedrest, and treatment similar to that for acute glomerulonephritis is instituted. Signs of pulmonary edema and congestive heart failure are closely monitored.

Women with CGN who become pregnant appear to be susceptible to toxemia and to spontaneous abortion. The woman who has had nephritis of any nature should be urged to see a physician if she plans on pregnancy. When pregnancy does occur, she should be followed closely by an obstetrician who specializes in high-risk pregnancies.

## Nursing Management

Care involves teaching the client to live healthfully, to avoid infections, to eat a balanced diet within prescribed limits, to take prescribed medications appropriately, to maintain follow-up health care, and to report (to the physician) any exacerbation in signs or symptoms. In the event of complications, specific treatment is symptomatic and supportive.

# NEPHROTIC SYNDROME

**Nephrotic syndrome** (nephrosis) is not a single disease entity but a constellation of symptoms. In nephrotic syndrome, damage to the glomeruli occurs, and large quantities of protein are lost in the urine.

## Etiology/Epidemiology

Nephrotic syndrome has been associated with allergic reactions (insect bites, pollen, acute glomerulonephritis), infections (herpes zoster), systemic disease (diabetes mellitus, sickle cell disease), circulatory problems (severe congestive heart failure, chronic constrictive pericarditis), and pregnancy. Known glomerular disease is the most common precipitating event in adults. In 50% to 75% of adults who develop nephrosis, the disease progresses to renal failure within 5 years.[17] Many

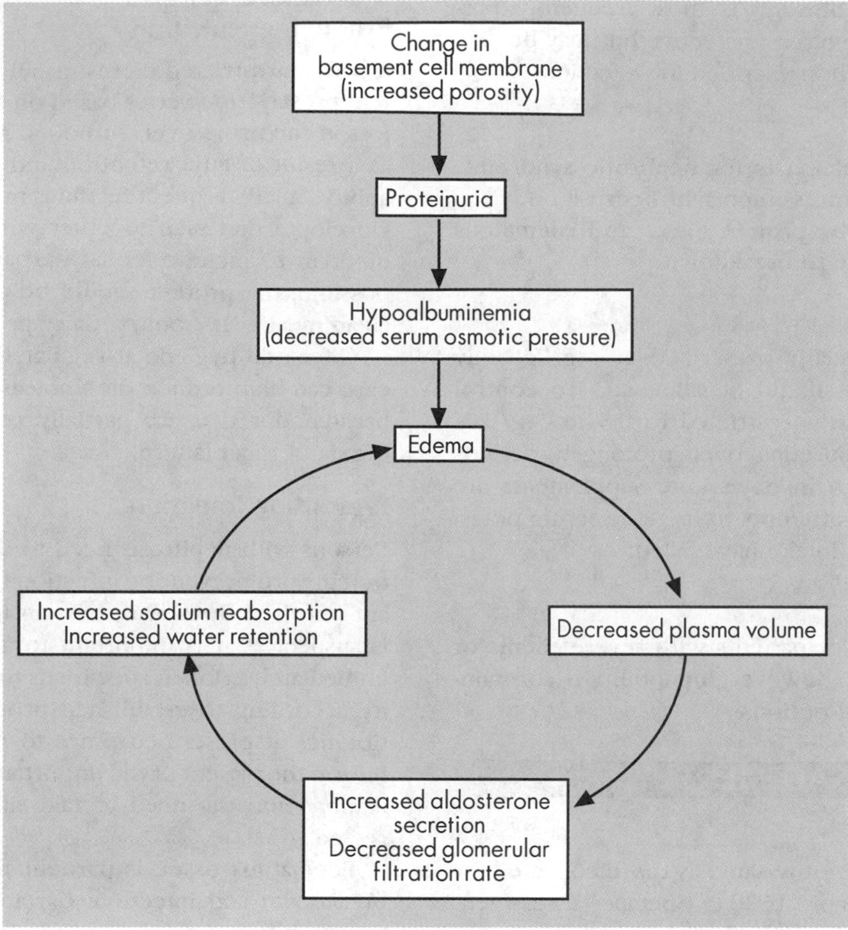


**FIGURE 49-4** Pathophysiologic changes in nephrotic syndrome.

individuals will have periods of remission and exacerbation. Nephrosis may also exist in chronic forms.

## Pathophysiology

The initial physiologic change in nephrotic syndrome is a derangement of cells in the glomerular basement membrane, resulting in increased membrane porosity with loss of large amounts of protein in the urine (proteinuria). As protein continues to be excreted, serum albumin is decreased (hypoalbuminemia), thus decreasing the serum osmotic pressure (Table 49-5). The capillary hydrostatic fluid (push) pressure in all body tissues becomes greater than the capillary osmotic (pull) pressure, and generalized edema results (Figure 49-4). As fluid is lost into the tissues, the plasma volume decreases, stimulating secretion of aldosterone to retain more sodium and water, thereby decreasing the glomerular filtration rate to retain water. This additional fluid also passes out of the capillaries into the tissue, leading to even greater edema.

Clinical manifestations of nephrotic syndrome include severe generalized edema, pronounced proteinuria, hypoalbuminemia, and hyperlipidemia. Urine volumes and renal function may be either normal or greatly altered. Altered renal function and development of symptoms of renal failure occur as a result of progressing glomerulonephritis. Loss of appetite and fatigue are common. Women usually experience amenorrhea and other disturbances in the reproductive cycle.

## Prevention

Other than treating the underlying illness, little can be done to prevent occurrence or recurrence of nephrosis.

## Medical Management

Treatment of nephrotic syndrome is directed toward reducing albuminuria, controlling edema, and promoting general health.

### Diagnostic tests

Laboratory tests include urinalysis for protein, casts, and erythrocytes and serum tests for protein and lipid analysis. Periodic determinations of proteinuria and measures of renal function are performed to monitor response to treatment and level of kidney function. Renal biopsy is sometimes used to obtain a definitive diagnosis.

### Medication

Corticosteroids may be useful in controlling the illness, but the response will vary from remission of nephrosis to no response. Prednisone is most frequently prescribed. Diuretics are often ineffective but may be prescribed. Antibiotics are prescribed for infections.

### Treatment

No specific treatment exists for nephrotic syndrome. Prevention of infection is important because body defenses are impaired by protein losses and edematous tissues are susceptible to breakdown.

### Diet

Dietary protein is usually prescribed at 1 g/kg body weight/day. Calories should be adequate. To control edema, sodium intake is restricted to 0.5 to 1 g/day. Patients receiving diuretics over prolonged periods should eat foods high in potassium. Supplements are prescribed only after attempts to increase serum potassium through dietary intake have failed.

### Activity

Bedrest is indicated for patients with severe edema or those with infections; however, immobility is contraindicated for prolonged periods.

## NURSING MANAGEMENT

### ♦ ASSESSMENT

The subjective data are the same as those collected for glomerulonephritis (p. 1620). Specific assessment should include the following objective data:

- Edema: amount, location, and degree of pitting
- Intake and output
- Daily weight
- Abdominal girth
- Condition of skin (severe edema may lead to skin breakdown)
- Respiratory status: signs of pulmonary edema
- Signs and symptoms of infection

### ♦ NURSING DIAGNOSES

Nursing diagnoses are determined from analysis of patient data. Nursing diagnoses for the person with nephrosis may include but are not limited to the following:

| Diagnostic Title | Possible Etiologic Factors |
|---|---|
| Nutrition, altered: less than body requirements | Anorexia, edema |
| Infection, high risk for | Decreased nutrition, immobility, edema |
| Knowledge deficit | Lack of exposure/recall |

### ♦ EXPECTED PATIENT OUTCOMES

1. Eats a diet high in protein and calories and low in sodium.
2. Maintains stable weight.
3. Maintains intact skin.
4. Describes dietary and drug therapy, measures to prevent infection, and symptoms requiring medical attention.

### ♦ INTERVENTIONS

#### Promoting Nutrition

A sodium-restricted diet is usually prescribed. The protein prescription varies based on the amount of protein lost in the urine over 24 hours. Appetite is diminished as a result of fluid retention and decreased food palatability. Small, frequent feedings may be better tolerated. Develop a diet plan together with patient, family, and dietitian to include foods the patient likes. Whenever possible, the protein should be of high biologic value (lean meat, fish, poultry, dairy products).

Offer oral hygiene at regular intervals. Good mouth care can help reduce the unpleasant metallic taste and breath odor that are partially responsible for the anorexia of renal failure.

#### Preventing Infection

Persons with nephrosis need to direct particular attention toward preventing infection because body defenses are impaired by urinary protein losses. When infection is suspected, it is important to attend to the problem immediately. Obtain specimens for culture and sensitivity according to established protocols. Administer antibiotics at prescribed times to maintain blood levels. Inform the patient of the importance of prescribed medications and the need to take all the antibiotic as directed.

Edematous tissue is particularly susceptible to skin breakdown and infection. Careful positioning and frequent changes in position may increase comfort while also protecting the skin. Air or water mattresses may increase comfort and relieve skin pressure. Males may develop edema of the scrotum; a sling to support the scrotum not only provides comfort but also aids in reducing swelling.

#### Facilitating Learning

Although nephrosis is often progressive, health teaching can help the patient maintain as much comfort as possible. Teaching includes the following:

1. Medication regimen: name, dose, actions, side effects, need to finish antibiotic prescription (as appropriate).
2. Nutrition: increased calories, adequate protein, decreased sodium.
3. Self-assessment of fluid status, including signs and symptoms of hypovolemia and hypervolemia.
4. Signs and symptoms requiring medical attention: increased edema, dyspnea, fatigue, headache, infection.
5. Need for follow-up care.

### ♦ EVALUATION

To evaluate the effectiveness of nursing interventions, compare patient behaviors with those stated in the expected outcomes. Successful achievement of patient outcomes for the patient with nephrotic syndrome are indicated by:

1. Eats meals high in calories, low in sodium, and following the protein prescription.
2. Maintains stable weight.
3. Shows no evidence of redness or breaks in skin integrity.
4. Describes medication regimen, nutrition prescription, measures to assess fluid status, signs and symptoms requiring medical attention, and need for follow-up care.

# VASCULAR DISORDERS

Vascular renal disease results from one of two processes: (1) disease of the main renal arteries or renal artery stenosis and (2) sclerosis of renal arterioles or nephrosclerosis.

## RENAL ARTERY STENOSIS

### Etiology/Epidemiology

**Renal artery stenosis** is the cause of approximately 5% of all cases of hypertension. Stenosis of the renal artery is usually classified as either arteriosclerosis or fibromuscular dysplasia. In either case, the end result is a narrowing of the lumen of the arteries supplying the kidneys. Obstruction of the renal arteries can be caused by aneurysm, thrombosis, and emboli.

### Pathophysiology

Renal artery stenosis results in a major reduction in blood flow to the kidneys. This change in renal perfusion causes increased secretion of renin and activation of the renin-angiotensin-aldosterone system.[6] The end result is acceleration of hypertension, which, if untreated, leads to further pathologic changes in the kidneys. Box 49-3 lists the signs of renal artery stenosis.

### Prevention

Prevention centers around the underlying disease entities that may lead to thrombosis and emboli. Measures may also be taken to reduce risk of arteriosclerosis (see Chapter 30).

**BOX 49-3 Clinical Manifestations of Renal Artery Stenosis**

- Hypertension
- Disparity in kidney size
- Delayed appearance of contrast medium in renal arteriogram
- Hyperconcentration of contrast media in kidney's calyceal system on intravenous pyelogram
- Lesion evidenced on renal arteriogram
- Increased serum creatinine with captopril challenge
- Changes in blood flow on duplex Doppler ultrasonography
- Detection of change in blood flow within vessels on magnetic resonance imaging

### Medical Management

Medical treatment includes vigorous antihypertensive therapy to control blood pressure. When a well-defined lesion exists in the renal artery, angioplasty or surgical bypass of the stenotic area may be performed to improve circulation.[6]

## NEPHROSCLEROSIS

### Etiology/Epidemiology

Whereas renal artery stenosis results in hypertension, hypertension can cause **nephrosclerosis.** Hypertension is the second major cause of end-stage renal disease. It is estimated that approximately 10% of individuals with essential hypertension will develop severe renal damage and that approximately 1% will develop end-stage renal disease and die unless supportive care is provided.[13]

### Pathophysiology

The renal vasculature is affected in ***benign*** nephrosclerosis. The renal arterial vessels show thickening and narrowing of their lumina, and some glomerular capillaries are sclerosed and collapsed. Renal blood flow can be reduced as a result of these vascular changes. The renal tubules can also be affected, resulting in tubular atrophy. Signs and symptoms are usually mild and include mild proteinuria from glomerular damage. Nocturia may occur from moderate loss of tubular concentrating ability. Casts may be present in the urine from tubular injury. Although the renal insufficiency is relatively mild, these patients are at risk for acute failure.

In ***malignant*** nephrosclerosis, the major changes are necrosis and thickening of the arterioles and glomerular capillaries and diffuse tubular loss and atrophy. Gross hematuria occurs with RBC casts, heavy proteinuria, and elevated plasma creatinine. Malignant nephrosclerosis is a medical emergency, and high blood pressure must be lowered to prevent permanent renal damage as well as damage to other vital organs.

*Signs and symptoms* of nephrosclerosis are the same as those for chronic renal failure (see Chapter 50). By the time the signs and symptoms develop, the disease has progressed to an extreme point. Deterioration in renal function progresses gradually. However, if an acute or malignant phase of hypertension occurs, the process may accelerate.

### Prevention

Prevention is best accomplished by routine screening to detect hypertension and to provide adequate treatment and follow-up care. Regular blood pressure screening of persons with elevated blood pressure is a minimal preventive measure.

### Medical Management

Treatment of nephrosclerosis is directed toward early detection and treatment of hypertension. Causative factors are sought, and treatment to lower blood pressure is initiated (see Chapter 34). When significant renal damage exists, stabilizing the person's current level of function or slowing deterioration of the kidney tissue is the goal. Control of hypertension is continued.

For hypertensive emergencies, potent vasodilators such as diazoxide and sodium nitroprusside are used. These intravenous (IV) medications usually act rapidly. Diazoxide is given as an IV bolus by a physician.

### Nursing Management

Management of end-stage renal disease and uremic symptoms provides for comfort and increased independence in daily living, although renal function may not improve.

Monitor the patient closely for tachycardia, hypotension, hyperglycemia, and marked sodium and water retention. Sodium nitroprusside is given as a continuous IV drip. Monitor the patient continuously for headache, hypotension, muscle twitching, tachycardia, restlessness, and retrosternal or abdominal pain.

Nursing management of patients with nephrosclerosis is the same as outlined for chronic renal failure (see Chapter 50).

## DIABETIC NEPHROPATHY

### Etiology/Epidemiology

Persons with diabetes mellitus develop vascular changes at a more accelerated rate than do nondiabetic persons. The end result of these vascular changes can be **diabetic nephropathy,** which is the leading cause of end-stage renal disease (ESRD). Approximately 30% of patients who begin treatment for ESRD are diabetic, and 50% with type I diabetes develop renal failure within 15 to 18 years of disease onset.[10]

### Pathophysiology

Vascular changes have been identified as a normal component of the aging process. A process of accelerated vascular change is most evident in the patient with type I diabetes, which often develops in childhood. In controlling the carbohydrate intake of the person with diabetes, abnormal metabolism of fat occurs, resulting in elevated serum cholesterol levels. Immunofluorescent and electron microscopic studies of the renal vasculature suggest that large quantities of lipids leak into these blood vessels and precipitate in the vessel walls. The vasculature changes caused by diabetes result in two distinct processes: glomerulosclerosis and nephrosclerosis. As described earlier, nephrosclerosis develops from sclerosing of the renal arterioles. Glomerulosclerosis is the scarring of the capillary loops in the glomerulus. Pathologic changes also occur in the the basement membrane. The first indication of renal involvement in the person with diabetes is usually proteinuria.

*Signs and symptoms* of diabetic nephropathy are the same as those for chronic renal failure (see Chapter 50).

### Prevention

The most effective preventive measure for diabetic nephropathy is adequate control of blood glucose. Routine monitoring of renal function is necessary to detect early renal dysfunction.

### Medical Management

The medical management of the patient with diabetic nephropathy is the same as that listed for nephrosclerosis. Adequate control of the diabetes is essential.

### Nursing Management

The nursing assessment and implementation for persons with diabetic nephropathy are the same as those outlined for chronic renal failure (see Chapter 50).

## OBSTRUCTIVE DISORDERS

Urinary tract obstruction can occur in any portion of the urinary tract from the urinary calyces to the meatus. Patients with obstructions have characteristic signs and symptoms, depending on the location and extent of the obstruction. If urinary obstruction is not corrected, renal failure may result. This section describes the major concepts related to obstruction of the urinary system and the care of patients with obstructive disorders. Subsequent sections discuss specific obstructive disorders (renal calculi, urinary strictures, tumors). Benign prostatic hypertrophy is discussed in Chapter 53.

## HYDRONEPHROSIS

### Etiology/Epidemiology

**Hydronephrosis** is the dilation of the renal pelvis and calyces with urine. Hydronephrosis may occur either unilaterally or bilaterally. Table 49-6 summarizes causes of obstruction of the urinary tract.

**TABLE 49-6 Causes of Urinary Tract Obstruction**

| LOCATION | MAJOR CAUSES |
|---|---|
| Lower urinary tract | Bladder neoplasms |
| | Urethral strictures |
| | Calculi |
| | Tumors |
| | Benign prostatic hypertrophy (BPH) |
| Ureteral obstruction | Calculi |
| | Trauma |
| | Nephroptosis ("floating" or "dropped" kidney) |
| | Enlarged lymph nodes |
| | Lymphosarcoma |
| | Reticulum cell sarcoma |
| | Hodgkin's disease |
| | Congenital anomaly |
| Kidney | Calculi |
| | Ptosis |
| | Polycystic kidney disease |

## Pathophysiology

Obstruction of any part of the urinary system from the kidney to the urethra will generate pressure that may cause functional and anatomic damage to the renal parenchyma. When any part of the urinary tract is obstructed, urine collects behind the obstruction, producing a dilation of the urinary collecting structures. Muscles of the affected area contract in an effort to push the urine around the obstruction. Partial obstruction may produce slow dilation of structures above the obstruction without functional impairment. As the obstruction increases, however, pressure builds up in the tubular system behind the obstruction, causing a backflow of urine and dilation of the ureter **(hydroureter)** (Figure 49-5). The urine backup eventually reaches the kidney, causing dilation of the kidney pelvis (hydronephrosis). Pressure build-up in the renal pelvis leads to destruction of kidney tissue and eventually renal failure.

With obstruction, urine flow is decreased even to the point of stagnation. This stagnant urine provides a culture medium for bacterial growth, and rarely is obstruction seen without some infection. The specific effects that occur with obstruction depend on the location of the obstruction, the extent of obstruction (partial or complete), and the duration. Obstruction in the lower urinary tract causes bladder distention. If this is prolonged, muscle fibers become hypertrophied, and **diverticuli** (herniated sacs of bladder mucosa) develop between the hypertrophied muscle bands. Since the diverticulum holds stagnant urine, infection often occurs and bladder stones may form.

Obstruction of the upper urinary tract leads even more quickly to hydronephrosis because of the small size of the ureters and kidney pelvis. Increased pressure causes partial ischemia between the renal cortex and medulla and the dilation of the renal tubules leading to tubular damage. Stasis of urine in the dilated pelvis leads to infection and calculi, which add to the renal damage. Some urine can flow back up the renal tubules into the veins and lymphatics as a compensatory mechanism. The unaffected kidney then takes on increased elimination of waste products. With prolonged obstruction, the unaffected kidney hypertrophies and may function almost (80%) as effectively alone as both kidneys did before

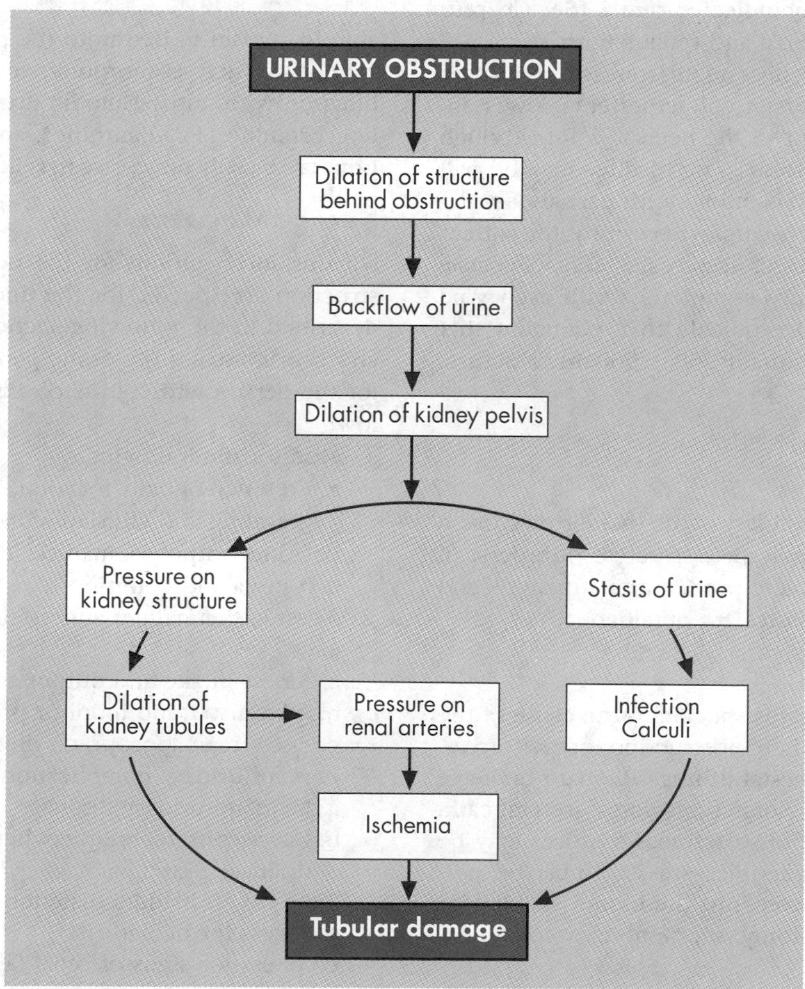


**FIGURE 49-5** Pathophysiology of uncorrected urinary obstruction.

the obstruction. Obstruction of both kidneys leads to renal failure.

Hydronephrosis can occur without any symptoms as long as kidney function is adequate and urine can drain. An *acute* upper urinary tract obstruction will cause pain, nausea, vomiting, local tenderness, spasm of the abdominal muscles, and a mass in the kidney region. The pain is caused by stretching of the tissues and by hyperperistalsis. Since the amount of pain is proportional to the rate of stretching, a slowly developing hydronephrosis may cause only a dull flank pain; whereas a *sudden blockage of the ureter,* such as may occur from a stone, causes a severe stabbing *(colicky)* pain in the flank or abdomen. The pain may radiate to the genitalia and thigh and is caused by the increased peristaltic action of the smooth muscles of the ureter in an effort to dislodge the obstruction and force urine past it.

The nausea and vomiting frequently associated with acute obstruction are caused by a reflex reaction to the pain and will usually be relieved as soon as the pain is relieved. An extremely dilated kidney, however, may press on the stomach, causing continued gastrointestinal symptoms. If renal function has been seriously impaired, nausea and vomiting may indicate uremia. (See Chapter 50 for discussion of uremia and renal failure.)

When the bladder is distended from lower urinary tract obstruction, the person will experience lower abdominal discomfort and feel the need to void although voiding may not be possible. The bladder may be palpated above the symphysis pubis. With partial obstruction, as seen in benign prostatic hypertrophy, the patient first complains of increasing urinary frequency because the bladder fails to empty completely with each void and therefore refills more quickly to the amount that causes the urge to void (usually 250 to 500 ml). Nocturia may also be present.

**TABLE 49-7 Summary of Tests Used for Diagnosis of Obstructive Disorders**

| | RENAL CALCULI | RENAL NEOPLASMS | PROSTATIC HYPERTROPHY | URETHRAL STRICTURES |
|---|---|---|---|---|
| Cystoscopy | X | X | X | X* |
| Retrograde pyelography | X | X | | |
| Intravenous pyelography | X | X | X | X* |
| Kidney, ureters, and bladder | X | X | | |
| Urethrography | | | X | X |
| Computed tomography | | X | | |
| Renal angiography | | X | | |
| Renography | | | | |
| Ultrasound | | X | | |
| Renal biopsy | | X | | |

*Not always completed.

## Medical Management

### Diagnostic tests

Table 49-7 provides a summary of the specific diagnostic tests used in the diagnosis of obstructive disorders. In addition to these diagnostic procedures, urinalysis and serum renal function studies are obtained.

### Treatment

The medical management is specific to the cause of the urinary obstruction. When obstruction occurs, treatment centers around reestablishing adequate drainage from the urinary system, such as placing a ureteral catheter above the point of obstruction. Strictures may be successfully dilated. Sometimes surgery must be performed to insert a catheter into the kidney or bladder (nephrostomy, ureterostomy, suprapubic cystostomy).

### Medication

The person with a sudden obstruction is frequently acutely ill and may have severe colic but will not be able to remain in bed until the pain has been relieved. Narcotics, such as morphine and meperidine, in combination with antispasmodic drugs, such as propantheline bromide (Pro-Banthine), and belladonna preparations are usually necessary to relieve severe colicky pain.

## Nursing Management

Nursing interventions for the person with urinary obstruction are specific for the underlying cause and are described in the following sections on calculi, tumors, and urinary strictures. Some general principles of care for the person with a urinary obstruction are listed below:

1. Monitor the following:
   a. Presence of pain: location, intensity, character, aggravating and alleviating factors
   b. Urine: output, hematuria, dysuria
   c. Nausea and vomiting
2. Assist in the maintenance of fluid and electrolyte balance.
   a. Assess intake and output at least every 8 hours.
   b. Administer and monitor prescribed IV fluids.
   c. Encourage appropriate diet.
3. Prevent urinary complications.
   a. Maintain urinary drainage systems.
   b. Use aseptic technique when working with urinary drainage systems.
   c. Assess for bladder distention at least every 8 hours.
   d. Assess for hematuria.
   e. Assess for signs of renal failure (oliguria, proteinuria, anorexia, lethargy).
   f. Encourage activity, as tolerated, to prevent urinary stasis.

4. Promote comfort.
   a. Maintain a calm environment to decrease anxiety.
   b. Administer analgesic or antispasmodic as necessary.
   c. Assist with activities of daily living (ADL) as necessary.
   d. Encourage self-care and independence as tolerated.
5. Patient teaching
   a. Prescribed diet and fluid restrictions
   b. Necessary care if patient is discharged with an indwelling catheter
   c. Desired action, side effects, dosage, and frequency of prescribed medications
   d. Need for following the prescribed medical regimen to prevent further problems

## URINARY RETENTION

**Urinary retention** is the inability to empty the bladder. The kidney is producing sufficient urine, but the person is unable to expel the urine from the bladder.

### Etiology/Epidemiology

Causes of urinary retention are either mechanical or functional. Mechanical causes may be congenital or acquired and include anatomic blockage of urine flow in the lower urinary tract. Functional causes include impairment of urine flow in the absence of mechanical obstruction. Box 49-4 summarizes causes of urinary retention.

**BOX 49-4 Causes of Urinary Retention**

**MECHANICAL CAUSES**

**Congenital**

Urethral stricture
Urinary tract malformation
Spinal cord malformation

**Acquired**

Calculus
Inflammation
Trauma
Tumor
Hyperplasia
Pregnancy

**FUNCTIONAL CAUSES**

Neurogenic bladder dysfunction
Ureterovesical reflux
Decreased peristaltic activity of the ureter
Detrusor muscle atrophy
Anxiety, i.e., fear of pain after surgery
Medications, i.e., anesthetics, narcotics, sedatives, and antihistamines

### Pathophysiology

Inability to void results from blockage of the urethra so that urine cannot be expelled from the bladder. A key symptom of urinary retention is inability to void. The bladder becomes distended with urine and is sometimes displaced to either side of the midline. Percussion over a full bladder produces a "kettle drum" sound. Discomfort occurs from pressure of the bladder on other organs, and the person has an urge to urinate. Restlessness and diaphoresis also may occur with a full bladder.

Voiding 25 to 50 ml of urine at frequent intervals often indicates **retention with overflow.** The intravesicular pressure increases as the bladder continues to fill with urine and overcomes the sphincter's restraining capability. A small amount of urine flows out of the bladder to reduce the intravesicular pressure to the level where the sphincter can control the flow of urine once again. The patient may state that the bladder continues to feel full. The bladder fills again, and the cycle is repeated. The urine specific gravity is normal or high in the presence of retention with overflow because the kidney's ability to produce urine is not impaired.

### Medical Management

Urinary retention is a urologic emergency and, if untreated, can lead to kidney damage. Interventions for urinary retention are aimed at reestablishing urine flow. Some mechanical obstructions must be corrected by surgical intervention; others, such as that caused by an enlarged prostate, may require temporary urethral catheter drainage. Bethanechol chloride (Urecholine) may be prescribed to initiate voiding by stimulation of the detrusor muscle of the bladder. Intermittent catheterization may be used for long-term problems rather than maintaining an indwelling catheter.

## NURSING MANAGEMENT

### ♦ ASSESSMENT

Persons experiencing urinary retention may be unable to void any urine (retention) or may void small amounts of overflow urine but be unable to empty the bladder completely (retention with overflow). Urine remaining in the bladder is a good medium for bacterial growth, leading to urinary tract infection (UTI).

### Subjective Data

Data to be collected to assess the person with urinary retention include the following:

Voiding pattern
Pain or burning on urination (probable UTI)
Sense of need to void or bladder fullness immediately after voiding (retention with overflow)

### Objective Data

Data to be collected to assess the person with urinary retention include the following:

Frequency of voiding and volume of each void
Characteristics of urine (color, clarity, odor)
Palpation of bladder above symphysis pubis after voiding
Comparison of fluid intake versus output

## ♦ NURSING DIAGNOSES

Nursing diagnoses are determined from analysis of patient data. Nursing diagnoses for the person with urinary retention may include but are not limited to the following:

| Diagnostic Title | Possible Etiologic Factors |
|---|---|
| Urinary retention | Obstruction, position for voiding, immobility, inability to initiate stream |
| Infection, high risk for | Indwelling catheter |
| Knowledge deficit | Lack of exposure/recall |

## ♦ EXPECTED PATIENT OUTCOMES

Expected patient outcomes for the person with urinary retention may include but are not limited to the following:

1. Voids several times a day.
2. Bladder is not palpable after voiding.
3. Describes signs of retention or UTI (for indwelling catheter).
4. If catheter in place, no signs of UTI are present.
5. Describes need to maintain fluid intake.

## ♦ INTERVENTIONS

### Promoting Micturition

If the patient is having difficulty eliminating urine from the bladder in the absence of mechanical obstruction, measures that encourage voiding are attempted before catheterization is instituted. These measures may include ensuring a position that facilitates voiding (positional stimuli: male standing upright, female sitting upright), running water (auditory stimuli), or pouring water over the perineum or placing the patient's hands in water (tactile stimuli). Sitting in lukewarm water may help relax the urinary sphincters. Providing privacy and encouraging use of the bathroom whenever possible also help to promote voiding.

### Facilitating Assisted Urinary Drainage

Assisted urinary drainage is used in a variety of clinical situations in both acute and chronic care. Major reasons for catheter drainage are to:

1. Relieve temporary anatomic or physiologic obstruction.
2. Permit healing of the urinary system postoperatively.
3. Permit accurate measurement of urine output in severely ill patients.
4. Relieve inability to void.
5. Achieve continence.
6. Prevent retention of urine in persons with neurogenic bladder.
7. Permit irrigation to prevent obstruction or urine flow.

**TABLE 49-8 Types of Catheters**

| TYPE OF CATHETER | DESCRIPTION | USE |
|---|---|---|
| Whistle-tip | Open slant end | Hematuria or blood clots in urine |
| Robinson | Close end, many "eyes" | Intermittent catheterization |
| Foley | Balloon (5 or 30 ml) to secure catheter in bladder | Constant drainage |
| Coudé | Tapered curved end | Suspected prostatic hypertrophy |
| Ureteral | 4 to 6 Fr size (urethral catheters are usually 14 to 16 Fr) | Drain ureters |
| Malecot | "Batwing"-shaped tip | Drain renal pelvis, nephrostomy drainage |
| Pezzar | Mushroom-shaped tip | Drain renal pelvis, nephrostomy drainage |

Reestablishing urine flow is an immediate treatment goal. The type of catheter used to provide drainage in the presence of obstruction will depend on the location of the blockage. Table 49-8 summarizes the use of specific types of catheters.

#### Urethral drainage

Urethral catheterization is the most common means of draining the bladder, and insertion of this type of catheter is often the nurse's responsibility. The Foley catheter is most frequently used for this purpose. *Catheterization is the major cause of UTIs,* and strict asepsis must be practiced during insertion and in assembling the drainage equipment. The need for urethral catheterization must be carefully evaluated and should never be undertaken for nursing convenience.

If the nurse finds it difficult to insert the catheter, the procedure is discontinued and the physician notified. Traumatic catheterization predisposes the patient to UTIs, formation of urethral strictures, and bleeding. In patients who have urethral disorders, resistance may be encountered with a standard catheter; special equipment, such as catheter directors or filiform catheters, may be needed. Neither the use of such equipment nor the catheterization of a patient in the immediate postoperative period after urethral or bladder surgery is a nursing procedure.

The urethral catheter is changed when it is in danger of becoming obstructed by sediment within its lumen.

The person who will have an indwelling urethral catheter at home needs to learn to change the catheter or have a family member demonstrate the ability to insert a catheter before discharge.

### Direct bladder drainage: cystostomy tube

When obstruction occurs below the bladder, constant drainage must be provided to prevent damage to the kidney, which may occur because of inadequate emptying of the lower urinary system. One means of providing drainage is by the use of a *cystostomy* tube (usually a Foley, Malecot, or Pezzar catheter), which is placed directly into the bladder through a suprapubic incision. This method is usually used when the urethra is completely obstructed or when the prolonged use of a urethral catheter is to be avoided in a male patient. During some operative procedures, both a cystostomy tube and a small urethral catheter will be inserted to drain the bladder. Both catheters must be monitored for patency. If patency is assured, it is not necessary to record the output from each catheter separately, since both tubes drain the bladder. The catheters will not necessarily drain equal amounts of urine. As is true with nephrostomy tubes and ureteral catheters, securely anchoring these catheters is also necessary.

### Drainage of kidney, pelvis and ureters

If a ureter becomes obstructed, a catheter must be placed directly into the renal pelvis. This prevents kidney damage that otherwise would occur as pressure increases because of continued urine formation. When a ureter is completely obstructed, a **nephrostomy** or **pyelostomy** tube may be inserted surgically or under guidance of a radiologist into the renal pelvis (Figure 49-6). The surgical incision is located laterally and posteriorly in the kidney region. Catheters used as nephrostomy or pyelostomy tubes are usually of the Pezzar (mushroom) or Malecot (batwing) types. An alternate form of drainage for a ureteral obstruction is the surgical placement of a ureterostomy tube (a whistle-tip or many-eyed Robinson catheter, size 6 or 8 Fr) that is passed through an incision in the upper outer quadrant of the abdomen into the ureter above the obstruction. The catheter is then passed through the ureter to the renal pelvis.

If the ureter is unobstructed or partially obstructed, the renal pelvis may be drained by a ureteral catheter, which is passed up the ureter to the renal pelvis through a cystoscope (see Figure 48-6). Ureteral catheterization is performed before gynecologic and lower abdominal surgery when there is danger of not recognizing and accidentally injuring the ureter during the operation. Ureteral catherization is also used after surgery involving the ureters to prevent stricture as the ureter heals. When used for this purpose, the catheter is referred to as a *stent* (see Figure 49-6). Whether it is expected to drain urine will depend on its relation to other catheters used.

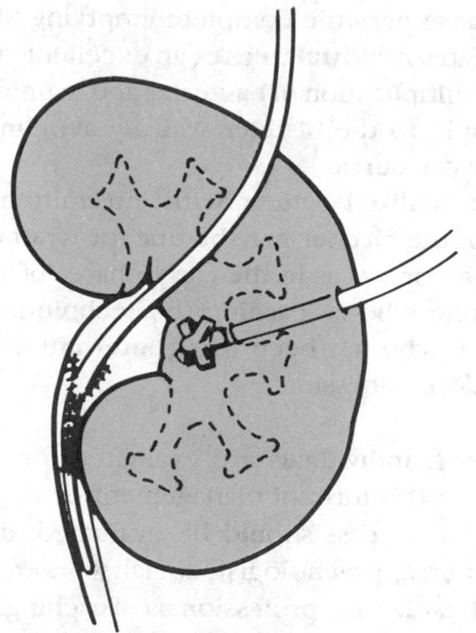

**FIGURE 49-6** Placement of stent after repair of ureteropelvic stricture. Note use of nephrostomy tube for urinary drainage during healing of anastomosis.

The *nephrostomy* and *ureteral* catheters must be firmly anchored to prevent accidental dislodging and trauma to the tissues. The openings made for these tubes are essentially fistulas that rapidly decrease in size on removal of the catheter. Even 30 minutes after removal of this type of catheter, it is often impossible to reinsert a similar-sized tube. When a catheter is inserted during surgery, it is usually sutured in place and affixed to the skin. When not sutured in place, the tube should be anchored to the skin at *two points* using adhesive, with some slack in the tubing between the anchor points.

Free drainage of catheters leading to the renal pelvis is of the utmost importance. Since the normal renal pelvis has only a 5 to 8 ml capacity, great pressure can be exerted on renal structures even when these catheters are obstructed for only a few minutes. Care must be taken to prevent kinking of the tubes while the patient is in the side-lying position in bed.

In some cases, nephrostomy tubes may be left in place for several months, with the patient returning to the hospital later for their removal. Occasionally, the nephrostomy tube serves as a form of urinary diversion for long-term use. The person at home with a catheter draining the kidney pelvis must know how to obtain medical assistance quickly should the catheter become obstructed or dislodged.

### Intermittent catheter drainage

**Use. Intermittent catheterization** of the urinary bladder is used in the treatment of neurogenic bladder dysfunction secondary to spinal cord trauma, birth defects, urinary retention, and some chronic diseases. Infections are often decreased, even when a clean technique is used, because periodic complete emptying of the bladder eliminates **residual urine** (an excellent culture medium for multiplication of bacteria) and maintains a good blood supply to the bladder wall by avoiding high intrabladder pressures.

The hospitalized patient with intermittent catheter drainage of the bladder may be one for whom the treatment is temporary (as in the early phases of spinal cord trauma), one who is learning the technique for home use, or one who has been using intermittent catheterization before admission.

**Assessment.** Individuals are evaluated for the appropriateness of this form of management by the urologist. Potential for success should be evaluated, using input from the nurse, psychologist, social worker, and other involved health care professionals. Teaching, however, is generally a nursing responsibility. An individual catheterization regimen is planned using either clean or sterile technique, as appropriate. The goals of intermittent catheterization are generally to prevent urinary retention and its sequelae (UTI, kidney damage) and to achieve continence. The patient needs to know the expectations of the treatment plan to promote cooperation.

**Method.** Even though the clean technique is suitable for home use, sterile technique is necessary during hospitalization to decrease the possibility of hospital-acquired infection when the catheterization is performed by hospital personnel. When hospitalized, the patient who customarily performs self-catheterization may continue to use clean technique if this method is used at home, but preferably a sterile catheter will be used each time or special precautions are taken to store the reusable catheter in a closed container. Specimens for culture must be obtained by the usual sterile catheterization technique to avoid contamination of the specimen. The patient is informed about the reason why sterile precautions are necessary in the hospital setting.

In the hospital, the size 14 Fr Robinson catheter is generally used for an adult. A special silicone catheter is used for intermittent catheterization. The volume of urine obtained with each catheterization is recorded so schedule adjustments can be made when necessary. The adult bladder should not be permitted to hold more than 300 ml at any time, since greater amounts lead to overdistention of the bladder and increased susceptibility to infection. The frequency of catheterization is determined by the amount of residual urine.

The person voids and then performs self-catheterization to determine the amount of urine remaining in the bladder. A large amount of residual urine (>100 ml) means that more frequent catheterization is necessary, usually every 4 to 6 hours. If there is only a small amount of residual urine (<100 ml) after voiding, self-catheterization may only be necessary every 8 to 12 hours. Some persons eventually will be able to manage with once-a-day catheterization. Catheterization is rarely required during the night unless a large urine output occurs at night, particularly if the patient is receiving IV fluids. Frequency of catheterization is usually a nursing judgment, although the physician may make the decision in some instances. A prescribed schedule may need to be altered if excess urine volumes are being obtained.

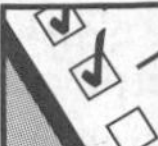

### Guidelines for Teaching the Person With Intermittent Catheterization

The patient or significant others can:

1. Explain the reason for the intermittent catheter drainage.
2. State the need for regular, periodic, complete emptying of the bladder.
3. Demonstrate self-catheterization using clean technique unless sterile technique is prescribed.
4. Describe how to adapt the catheterization routine to the individual life-style.
5. State how to obtain needed supplies.
6. Describe symptoms of UTI requiring medical care.
7. State plans for ongoing urologic care.

**Patient teaching.** The person needs to understand the rationale for intermittent catheter drainage and for regularity of bladder emptying (see Guidelines box above). Basic anatomy of the genitalia and urinary tract is illustrated to alleviate fears of causing damage by misplacement of the catheter.

Most persons require much support during the actual teaching but usually become comfortable with the procedure. Initially, a mirror is used to teach women where to place the catheter. The woman should learn to catheterize while sitting on the commode, using palpation to locate the urethral meatus. Men may sit or stand for self-catherization. It is important that men use generous amounts of lubricant to avoid urethral irritation; women generally do not require lubrication. Family members may be taught catheterization if the patient is unable to perform self-catheterization.

## Following Catheter Removal

It is normal to note some dribbling of urine for a few hours after a urethral catheter has been removed because of dilation of the sphincter muscles by the catheter. Dribbling of urine that persists longer than a few hours should be reported to the physician; this symptom may indicate damage to the sphincters. In determining the type of intervention necessary to reestablish bladder control, information about the nature of the incontinence is gathered. Incontinence is described as complete (constant dribbling) or occurring only on urgency or stress. Assessment should include whether incontinence is present in all positions (lying, sitting, standing). If muscular weakness of the sphincters is the major problem, incontinence is least likely to occur when the person is in a prone position and most likely to be a problem when standing or walking. Perineal exercises (p. 1645) may help to regain control of voiding.

Another problem that may arise after removal of a catheter is inability to void. The patient is encouraged to drink fluids and then attempt to void. The nurse carefully assesses the patient's bladder for distention. Efforts are made to provide comfortable positioning and privacy to facilitate voiding. No patient with an adequate intake should go longer than 8 hours without voiding. A patient with edema of the bladder neck may require temporary reinsertion of a catheter to facilitate urinary drainage.

Color and clarity of the urine are noted. *Cystitis* (inflammation of the bladder) may develop after cathether removal because of incomplete emptying of the bladder as muscle tone is being reestablished. Any abnormalities in color, odor, or sediment in the urine are reported.

Educating the patient about signs and symptoms of urinary retention, changes in the color and clarity of the urine, and incontinence and dysuria is undertaken when bladder drainage is discontinued. Often the first indicators of dysfunction are subjective comments from the patient. This information enhances detection of early recurrence of urinary drainage problems.

## ♦ EVALUATION

To evaluate the effectiveness of nursing interventions, compare patient behaviors with those stated in the expected patient outcomes. Successful achievement of patient outcomes for the patient with urinary retention is indicated by the following:

1. Voids several times a day in amounts of 150 to 400 ml/void.
2. Bladder is not palpable after voiding.
3. Describes signs of urinary retention or UTI (for indwelling catheter) to be reported to physician.
4. If catheter is in place, catheter drains freely and signs of UTI are not present (fever, back pain, increased serum WBC).
5. Describes need to maintain fluid intake of 2000 to 2500 ml/day.

## HOME CARE CONSIDERATIONS

Clean (not sterile) catheterization technique usually is prescribed for home use. Handwashing is required before each catheterization, and the meatal area is cleansed with soap and water. After the catheter is inserted and the bladder is drained, the catheter is removed, washed with soap and water, and dried on a clean surface. Once dry, the catheter is stored in a closed container for the next use. The catheter is reused until it becomes either too soft or too hard to be directed properly.

If sterile catheterization technique is needed for home use, careful explanation of sterile technique and sterilization of equipment must be given. More time is needed for the person to learn good sterile technique.

If the hospital or outpatient teaching time is short, follow-up may be required by a home health care nurse to help the person adapt the catheterization routine to life routines and to assist with any difficulties the patient may be having. Ongoing urologic care is essential, with periodic urine cultures.

### Preventing Urinary Tract Infection

An indwelling catheter provides a potential source for microorganisms to enter the urinary system; therefore good sterile technique is essential for catheter care during hospitalization. Fluid intake of at least 2000 to 2500 ml is essential to prevent urinary stasis leading to bacterial growth.

For home care, the person or care provider must be helped to understand the importance of cleanliness of the catheter and genitalia. Instructions should include the following:

- Good handwashing before and after working with the catheter
- Twice-daily cleansing of the meatal-catheter junction with soap and water
- Minimizing disconnection of the catheter and drainage tubing

The tubing is disconnected at night to change from a leg bag to the overnight drainage bag and again in the morning to resume leg-bag drainage. To lessen contamination, the caregiver is taught to wash the hands and then wipe the catheter and tubing with 70% alcohol before disconnection and reconnection. The disconnected ends of the drainage bags are protected with sterile gauze secured in place with a rubber band or protected with a connector cap. The drainage system, such as collection bags and tubing, should be kept as clean as possible by daily washing with soap and water. Teaching also includes the need to keep the drainage collection bag at a level lower than the cavity being drained to prevent urine reflux.

### Facilitating Learning

Persons requiring catheter drainage at home on a temporary or permanent basis must be able to maintain safely the urinary drainage system or have a family member instructed in all necessary care. Written instructions are provided. Teaching includes care of the catheter and drainage system as previously described. A written list of needed specific supplies and where they can be obtained is helpful to avoid confusion because so many products are available.

The person needs to be well informed about adaptations that can be made with the urinary drainage system to allow a return to an optimal level of activity. A *shower* or *tub bath* with a catheter in place is generally permitted unless there is an unhealed surgical incision. The adhesive tape holding the catheter in place needs to be replaced after bathing. *Leg bags* are available in a variety of sizes and are concealed by clothing. Men or women do not need to remove an indwelling catheter before *intercourse.* This information should be included in all teaching because patients may hesitate to ask. The male can fold the indwelling catheter over the penis to facilitate insertion during intercourse.

The person with a urinary catheter of any type needs continued urologic surveillance. Instructions include the need to contact the physician if back pain, fever, or other urinary tract symptoms are present.

## RENAL CALCULI

Urinary stones *(urolithiasis)* may develop at any level in the urinary system but are most frequently found within the kidney *(nephrolithiasis).* Figure 49-7 illustrates the most common locations of **calculi** formation.

### Etiology/Epidemiology

It is estimated that at least 1% of all people in the United States will develop urolithiasis. About one third of the individuals that have recurrent upper urinary tract calculi will eventually have the affected kidney removed.

Renal calculi (stones) are crystallizations of minerals around an organic matrix such as pus, blood, or devitalized tissue. The mineral composition of renal calculi varies. Most stones consist of calcium salts (oxalates, phosphates) or magnesium-ammonium phosphate; the remainder are cystine or uric acid stones.

No demonstrable cause can be found for more than half the renal stones that occur *(idiopathic).* A major predisposing factor is the presence of UTI. Infection increases the presence of organic matter around which the minerals can precipitate and increases the alkalinity of the urine (by the production of ammonia). This results in precipitation of calcium phosphate and magnesium-ammonium phosphate. Stasis of urine also permits precipitation of organic matter and minerals.

### Pathophysiology

Because most stones are calcium oxalates, anything that leads to hypercalciuria is a predisposing factor to renal stones (Table 49-9). In persons for whom no underlying pathology can be identified, hypercalciuria may result from increased calcium absorption from the intestine or from decreased reabsorption of calcium by the kidney tubules. These persons do not have hypercalcemia because the calcium is eliminated in the urine. Hypercalcemia leading to hypercalciuria may be present with an increased calcium intake (milk, alkali); prolonged immobilization (loss of bone calcium); hypervitaminosis D (increased calcium absorption from the intestines); hyperparathyroidism, multiple myeloma, Paget disease, or cancer (loss of bone calcium); Cushing's syndrome or prolonged intake of corticosteroids (loss of bone calcium); and renal tubular acidosis (increased calcium secondary to defective ammonia formation). Increased uric acid in the urine leading to uric acid stones may

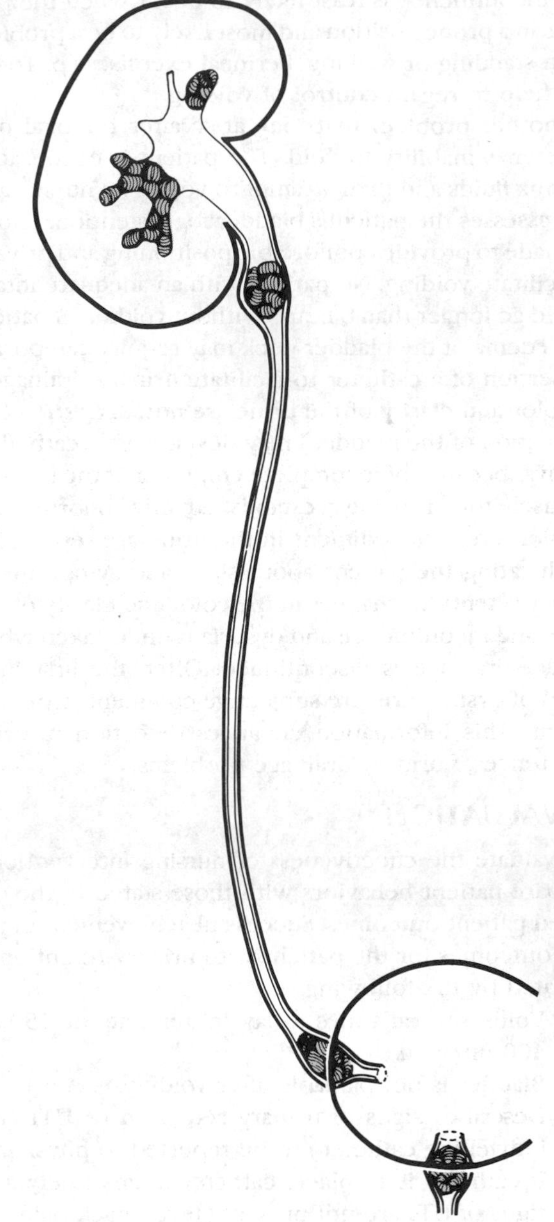

**FIGURE 49-7** Most common locations of renal calculus formation.

**TABLE 49-9 Renal Calculus Composition and Contributing Factors**

| COMPOSITION OF STONE | FACTORS CONTRIBUTING TO STONE FORMATION |
|---|---|
| Calcium (oxalate and phosphate) | Hypercalcemia and/or hypercalciuria resulting from hyperparathyroidism, vitamin D intoxication, multiple myeloma, immobilization, severe bone disease, renal tubular acidosis, and prolonged intake of steroids |
| Uric acid | High purine diet, gout |
| Cystine | Cystinuria resulting from genetic disorder of amino acid metabolism |

be seen with gout, with some leukemias, or in patients treated with cancer chemotherapeutic agents. Cystine stones usually result from a genetic defect. Both uric acid and cystine precipitate in acid urine.

Pain **(renal colic)** is the primary symptom in an acute episode of renal calculi. The location of the pain depends on the location of the renal stone. If the stone is in the kidney pelvis, the pain is caused by hydronephrosis and is more dull and constant in character, occurring primarily in the costovertebral angle. As the stone moves along the ureter, the pain can be excruciating and is intermittent in character. It is caused by spasm of the ureter and anoxia of the ureter wall from the pressure of the stone. The pain follows the anterior course of the ureter down to the suprapubic area and radiates to the external genitalia. Nausea and vomiting often accompany renal colic.

Patients frequently have two or three attacks of acute renal colic before the stone passes. This is probably because the stone becomes lodged at a narrow point in the ureter, causing temporary obstruction. The ureters are normally narrower at the ureteropelvic and ureterovesical junctions and at the point where they pass over the iliac crest into the pelvis. If the stone is to pass along the ureter by peristaltic action, the patient will have some pain.

Gross hematuria may occur if the stone has rough edges. Microhematuria is almost always present. Signs and symptoms of UTI (p. 1616) may also be present. Often a stone is "silent," causing no symptoms for years. This is especially true of very large stones that develop over a long period before resulting in symptoms. Extremely small smooth stones may be passed asymptomatically.

## Prevention

Measures can be taken to decrease the potential for renal stones in persons at high risk. Adequate hydration (intake of 2500 ml/day or more unless contraindicated) will help to prevent urinary stasis that can lead not only to stone formation but also to UTI. Persons confined to bed should be encouraged to turn and move frequently, exercising arms and legs whenever possible. Urinary stasis can be prevented by sitting up in a chair or by changing the body position of an immobile bedridden patient. Even with exercises and the use of sitting in a chair, paraplegics and quadriplegics often develop renal calculi. Persons with indwelling catheters need scrupulous aseptic technique in catheter care to prevent infection and require adequate hydration and good catheter drainage to wash away minerals that can deposit at the catheter tip.

Renal stone formation can often be controlled by regulating urinary pH. Table 49-10 provides a summary of diet principles applied to renal calculi. Persons at risk for developing calcium oxalate, calcium phosphate, or magnesium-ammonium phosphate stones may be placed on an acid-ash diet (Table 49-11) to promote excretion of an acid urine. Catheter irrigations using acetic acid solution or hemiacidrin (Renacidin) help provide an acid environment and thus decrease precipitation of calcium and phosphate. Persons at risk for developing uric acid or cystine stones may be placed on an alkaline-ash diet because uric acid and cystine are soluble in an alkaline urine.

## Medical Management

### Diagnostic tests

The diagnostic tests performed to determine the presence of renal stones include kidney, ureters, and bladder (KUB); IV or retrograde pyelography; ultrasound; computed tomography (CT); cystoscopy; and urinalysis.

Because recurrence of renal calculi is common, additional studies are carried out after the acute episode has subsided. Successive determination of serum calcium, phosphorus, protein, electrolytes, and uric acid are performed to identify the underlying disease that can influence stone formation. The urine pH is measured with a dipstick each time the patient voids to determine the urine acidity or alkalinity. A ***nitroprusside urine test***

**TABLE 49-10 Summary of Diet Principles in Renal Stone Disease**

| STONE CHEMISTRY | NUTRITION MODIFICATION | DIET ASH URINARY pH |
|---|---|---|
| Calcium | Low calcium (400 mg) | Acid ash |
| Phosphate | Low phosphorus (1-1.2 g) | |
| Oxalate | Low oxalate | |
| Struvite ($MgNH_4PO_4$) | Low phosphorus (1-1.2 g) (associated with UTI) | Acid ash |
| Uric acid | Low purine | Alkaline ash |
| Cystine | Low methionine | Alkaline ash |

From Coe FL, Parks JH, Asplin JR: *N Engl J Med* 327(16):1141-1152, 1992.

**TABLE 49-11 Acid-Ash and Alkaline-Ash Food Groups Used To Control pH of Urine**

| ACID ASH | ALKALINE ASH | NEUTRAL |
|---|---|---|
| Meat | Milk | Sugars |
| Whole grains | Vegetables | Fats |
| Eggs | Fruit (except cranberries, prunes, plums) | Beverages |
| Cheese | | Coffee |
| Cranberries | | Tea |
| Prunes | | |
| Plums | | |

From Williams, SR: *Nutrition and diet therapy,* ed 7, St Louis, 1993, Mosby.

may be performed to check the presence of cystine. An accurate 24-hour urine is collected to measure calcium, oxalate, phosphorus, and uric acid levels. The 24-hour urine may be collected with the patient eating a normal diet or following a 3-day low-calcium, low-phosphorus diet.

### Treatment

**Acute care.** About 90% of urinary calculi are passed spontaneously. A person who is up and moving is more likely to pass a stone than one who is in bed. The urine is strained and observed closely for stones. The person is permitted to carry out usual activities. If there is no infection or obstruction, the stone may be left in the ureter for several months. Fluids are prescribed at 2500 ml/day or more to promote passage of the stone and to prevent infection.

If some obstruction is present and the stone fails to pass, one or two ureteral catheters may be passed through a cystoscope up the ureter and left in place for 24 hours. The catheters dilate the ureter, and when they are removed, the stone may pass into the bladder. If signs of infection exist, an attempt is made to pass a ureteral catheter past the stone into the renal pelvis. The catheter is left as a drain, since pyelonephritis will quickly follow if adequate urinary drainage is not reestablished. Patients with ureteral catheters are usually confined to bed to prevent catheter dislodgement.

Stones in the lower ureter may be removed by cystoscopic manipulation. General anesthesia may be required, and care is similar to that after cystoscopy (see Chapter 48).

**Percutaneous lithotripsy. Percutaneous lithotripsy** is a technique that requires a percutaneous nephrostomy tract created through an incision of ¼ to ½ inch over the kidney region. An endoscope is then passed through the tract, and a snare basket is used to retrieve the calculi. If the calculi cannot be removed, ultrasonic lithotripsy is used to disintegrate the stone. Complications of the surgery are rare; however, hemorrhage, urinoma, sepsis, and abscess may develop. Postoperatively, the patient usually experiences pain similar to renal colic caused by the presence of calculi. Pain is controlled by administering meperidine hydrochloride. The patient may also have large amounts of drainage from the nephrostomy tract. Dressings should be changed frequently to prevent infection. Urinary drainage from the incision may be experienced for 3 to 4 days after the procedure. Patients usually receive a 2-week course of antibiotic therapy after surgery.

**Extracorporeal shock wave lithotripsy.** With **extracorporeal shock wave lithotripsy,** the patient is submerged in a large tank of distilled water, at the bottom of which is placed the shock wave electrode. The shock waves produced by the electrode fragment the renal stone. The shock waves are focused and directed at the stone by an alpha-dimensional radiographic scanning system and are keyed to follow the R wave of the patient's electrocardiogram (ECG).[14] The water bath is necessary to allow for the passage of the shock waves into the body. It may require 1000 to 1500 or more shock wave pulses to break up a large stone. The patient may be sedated with diazepam (Valium) during the procedure. Pain of moderate intensity may be experienced during the passage of each sound wave; therefore an epidural (preferred) or general anesthesia also may be used.

Newer lithotriptors have eliminated the need for a water bath and can be used without anesthesia. They use ultrasound to localize the stone and generate shock waves by a variety of mechanisms.

After lithotripsy, small particles are passed in the urine over the next several days. The patient is observed for signs of bleeding. Blood pressure is monitored frequently for the first several hours after the procedure. Urine output is also closely monitored for both quantity and quality. Blood initially may turn the urine cherry red to pink for the first several hours. The urine should then clear. Immediately after the procedure, the patient may experience redness or bruising on the skin at the lithotripsy site. Pain may also be experienced in this region from the force of the ultrasonic shock waves. Pain is usually localized to the skin as a result of the shock waves entering the body. The patient can be discharged within a few days after the procedure if there are no complications.

The patient may also experience pain similar to renal colic after lithotripsy. This is usually a result of the passage of fragments of the pulverized renal stone through the lower urinary tract. Renal colic is usually controlled by use of narcotic analgesics. Since renal colic often occurs 3 or more days after lithotripsy, the patient should be made aware of this potential complication and informed about the use of pain medications and signs requiring physician notification.

Occasionally, urinary obstruction may occur as a result of stone fragments blocking the flow of urine. The patient is instructed to observe the volume of urine output for several days after discharge. Daily weight should be obtained to detect urinary retention. Flank pain may also indicate urinary obstruction. When these symptoms are present, the patient should contact the physician immediately.

**Candela laser therapy.** The Candela laser is a pulsed-dye laser system designed to break up calculi that have migrated to the lower ureters. The laser probe is inserted through a ureteroscope. A new 2.4 mm flexible probe is expected to decrease the minor ureteral injury often caused by a wider probe and ureteroscope. An advantage of the Candela laser system is that it spares the patient the discomfort and cost of lithotripsy or surgery.

### Diet

Persons who have recurrent renal calculi benefit from ongoing prophylactic therapy determined by the type of stone being produced. For *calcium* stones, foods high in calcium are sometimes restricted, but a very low-calcium diet is not very appealing.

### Medication

Sodium or potassium phosphate may be prescribed to decrease urinary calcium; these drugs are contraindicated if the kidney is infected. Thiazide diuretics, particularly hydrochlorthiazide (HCTZ), decrease the calcium content in the urine by increasing reabsorption of calcium in the renal tubules.

*Phosphate* calculi develop in alkaline urine; therefore, their prevention depends on keeping the urine acidic and preventing UTIs. Cranberry juice can be taken (200 ml four times daily) to keep the urine acidic. Ascorbic acid may also be prescribed to acidify the urine.

Prophylaxis for *uric acid* stones consists of alkalinizing the urine by the administration of sodium bicarbonate or citrate solution. Allopurinol (Zyloprim) is usually prescribed to inhibit synthesis of uric acid.

## Surgical Management

Surgical intervention is indicated when a large stone (greater than 1 cm) is producing pain, obstruction, or infection. The procedure for removal of a stone from the ureter is a **ureterolithotomy** (Figure 48-6, *C*). A radiograph is taken immediately preceding surgery, since the stone may have moved, so that the incision into the ureter is made directly over the stone. If the stone is in the lower third of the ureter, a rectus incision is made. If it is in the upper two thirds, a flank approach is used. If the patient has a ureteral stricture that causes stones to form, a plastic surgery procedure to relieve the stricture may be carried out as part of the procedure.

Removal of a stone through or from the renal pelvis is known as **pyelolithotomy** (Figure 49-8, *A*). Removal of a stone through the parenchyma is a **nephrolithotomy** (Figure 49-8, *B*). Occasionally, the kidney may have to be split from end to end (a kidney split) to remove the stone. Patients in whom such a split is performed are at risk for hemorrhage after surgery.

*Bladder stones* may be removed through a suprapubic incision, or they may be crushed with a lithotrite (stone crusher) that is passed transurethrally. This procedure is known as **litholapaxy.** After bladder stone removal, the bladder may be irrigated (intermittently or constantly) with an acid solution such as magnesium and sodium citrate (G solution) or Renacidin to counteract the alkalinity caused by the infection and to help wash out the remaining particles of stone. If a suprapubic incision has been made, the care of the incision is similar to that after a suprapubic prostatectomy. (See p. 1648 for care of the patient requiring urologic surgery.)

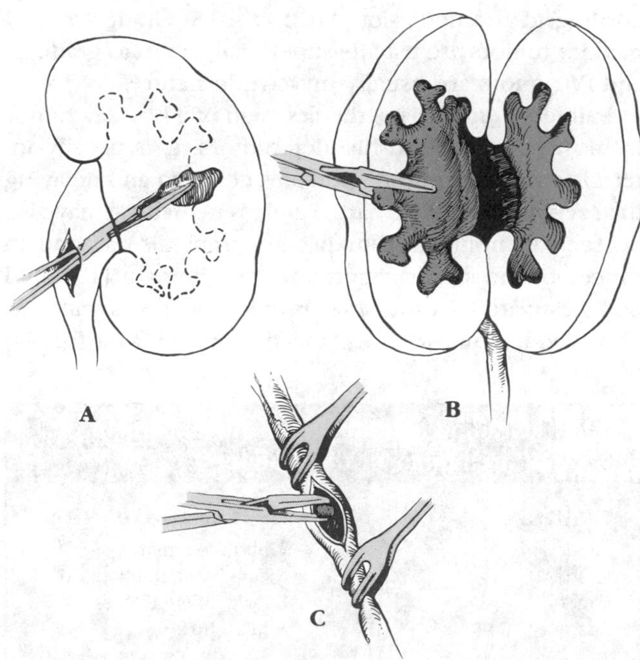


**FIGURE 49-8** Location and methods of removing renal calculi from upper urinary tract. **A,** Pyelolithotomy, removal of stone through renal pelvis. **B,** Nephrolithotomy, removal of staghorn calculus from renal parenchyma (kidney split). **C,** Ureterolithotomy, removal of stone from ureter.

## Nursing Management

The urine of all persons with relatively small stones should be strained. Urine can be strained easily by placing two opened 4 × 8 inch gauze sponges over a funnel. Stones vary in size and may be no larger than the head of a pin. The stones are saved for inspection by the physician and sent to the laboratory for analysis.

Renal colic is an excruciating type of pain. The patient usually determines when medication is needed. Morphine or other opiates are given in doses to control the pain. Antispasmodics, such as atropine or methantheline bromide (Banthine), may also be prescribed to depress the smooth muscles of the ureter and lessen pain from spasm.

Monitor intake and output and encourage fluids to 2500 ml/day or more to promote passage of the stone and prevent infection.

### Facilitating learning

The person who has had urinary calculi needs to know how to prevent development of further stones. Patient teaching includes the following:

1. Prevent UTIs.
    a. Drink at least 2500 ml fluids/day.
    b. Avoid situations that lead to urinary stasis, if possible (e.g., long periods of inactivity).
2. Follow any dietary prescriptions.
3. Know name, dosage, and side effects of medications prescribed to acidify or alkalinize the urine.

4. Report to physician signs of recurrence of calculi (costovertebral pain or pain radiating to external genitalia).
5. Report to physician signs of UTI (burning on urination, frequency, urgency, fever).

# TUMORS OF THE KIDNEY

## Etiology/Epidemiology

Malignant renal tumors, primarily adenocarcinomas, account for 3% of all cancers. Small benign tumors (adenomas) may occur without causing significant damage or symptoms. Renal cell carcinomas rarely occur before the age of 30 years, are more often seen in the 50- to 70-year age range, and occur twice as often in men as in women.

## Pathophysiology

Renal carcinomas usually develop unilaterally but may occur bilaterally. In stage I the tumor margins are well defined (encapsulated) and compress the kidney parenchyma during growth rather than infiltrating the tissue. The upper pole of the kidney is usually involved, and the tumor is usually large at the time of diagnosis. In stage II the tumor invades the fat surrounding the kidney. Stage III consists of local metastasis either through direct extension or through the renal vein or lymphatics (lymph node involvement). Distant metastases during stage IV are primarily in the lungs or bone, but other areas, such as the liver, spleen, or brain, may also be involved.

*Hematuria* is the most frequent sign of renal cell carcinoma. Unfortunately, the hematuria is often intermittent, lessening the person's concern and causing procrastination in seeking medical care. Any person with hematuria should have a complete urologic examination, since it is only by immediate investigation of the first signs of hematuria that any hope of cure exists. Other signs and symptoms include dull flank pain, flank mass, unexplained weight loss, fever, and polycythemia. Hypertension may also be present as a result of stimulation of the renin-angiotensin system.

An IV pyelogram may show a distortion of renal outline suggesting a kidney tumor. Small tumors in the parenchyma may not be apparent on a routine pyelogram but may be identified by a computed tomography (CT) scan (see Chapter 48) or by magnetic resonance imaging (MRI). CT is also useful in differentiating between renal cell carcinoma and a renal cyst. Angiography may also be performed to differentiate a cyst from a tumor.

## Medical Management

Unless the person is a poor surgical risk or has extensive metastases, the diseased kidney is removed **(nephrectomy)** through a transabdominal, thoracoabdominal, or retroperitoneal approach. The first two approaches are preferred to secure the renal artery and vein and to prevent any spread of malignant cells. (See p. 1647) for care of the person requiring urologic surgery.)

Radiation has not proved to be beneficial, except for symptomatic bone metastases, and chemotherapy is also of limited value. Therapy with interferon-α appears to be promising. Five-year survival rates after treatment of stages I, II and IIIA are 70%.[4]

# TUMORS OF THE BLADDER

## Etiology/Epidemiology

The bladder is the most common site of cancer in the urinary tract. Cancer of the bladder occurs three times more often in males than in females, and multiple tumors are common. About 25% of patients have more than one lesion at the time of diagnosis. This figure increases to about 50% in persons with papilloma grade I carcinoma over a 5-year period. Approximately 40% of all tumors involve the trigone, and an additional 45% involve the posterior and lateral walls of the bladder.

## Pathophysiology

Tumors of the bladder range from small benign papilloma to large invasive carcinomas. Most neoplasms are of the transitional cell type because the urinary tract is covered with transitional epithelium. These neoplasms begin as papillomas; therefore, all papillomas of the bladder are considered premalignant and are removed when identified. Squamous cell carcinoma occurs less frequently and has a poorer prognosis. Other neoplasias include adenocarcinoma (which is often inoperable) and rhabdomyosarcoma (seen most frequently in infants).

Carcinomas of the bladder are graded and staged according to the definitions in Box 49-5. Grade I and II bladder tumors are usually superficial, whereas grade III and IV tumors are usually invasive in nature.

Painless hematuria is the first sign of a bladder tumor in most patients with bladder tumors. It is usually intermittent, lessening the person's concern and delaying the seeking of medical care. Painless hematuria may also be seen in nonmalignant urinary tract disease and in cancer of the kidney; therefore, any hematuria should be investigated. Cystitis may provide the first symptoms of a bladder tumor, since the tumor acts as a foreign

**BOX 49-5 Grading and Staging of Advancement of Carcinomas of the Bladder**

| GRADES | DIFFERENTIATION |
|---|---|
| Grade I | Well differentiated |
| Grade II | Medially differentiated |
| Grade III | Poorly differentiated |
| Grade IV | Anaplastic |

| STAGES | TISSUE INVOLVEMENT |
|---|---|
| Stage O | Mucosa |
| Stage A | Submucosa |
| Stage B | Muscle |
| Stage C | Perivesical fat |
| Stage D | Lymph nodes |

body in the bladder, causing inflammation. Symptoms of renal failure resulting from obstruction of the ureters is sometimes the reason for seeking medical care. Vesicovaginal fistulas may occur before symptoms develop. The presence of renal failure or vesicovaginal fistulas indicates a poor prognosis because they usually occur after the tumor has infiltrated widely.

Cytologic examination of the urine may reveal malignant cells before the lesion can be visualized by cystoscopy. The diagnosis is established by cystoscopic visualization and biopsy of the bladder. Clinical determination of the invasiveness of the tumor is important in establishing a therapeutic regimen and in predicting the prognosis. Any person who has had a papilloma removed should have a cystoscopic examination every 3 months for 2 years and then at less frequent intervals if there is no evidence of new lesions. Repeated cystoscopies may seem unacceptable to persons who dread them; the necessity for frequent examination should be fully explained by the urologist and the explanation reinforced by the nurse. Emphasis is placed on the necessity for repeated cystoscopies, since papillomas tend to recur without symptoms until they are far-advanced tumors.

## Prevention

Known factors predisposing to bladder cancer are exposure to the chemicals β-naphthylamine and xenylamine, infestation with *Schistosoma haematobium,* and cigarette smoking. Therefore, exposure to these substances should be avoided.

## Medical Management

The treatment of bladder tumors depends on the size of the lesion and the depth of the tissue involvement.

### Surgery

Small tumors with minimal tissue layer involvement may be adequately treated with *transurethral fulguration* or *excision.* A Foley catheter may or may not be inserted after surgery. The urine may be pink tinged, but gross bleeding is unusual. Burning on urination may occur and is relieved by drinking increased fluids to dilute the urine. Heat applied over the bladder and sitz baths may provide relief. The patient is usually discharged within 1 to 2 days after surgery.

If the tumor involves the dome of the bladder, a segmental resection of the bladder may be performed. More than half the bladder may be resected. A **cystectomy** (complete removal of the bladder) usually is performed only when the disease appears curable. Complete removal of the bladder requires permanent urinary diversion. Urinary tract surgery is discussed on p. 1647.

### Radiation

*External cobalt radiation* of large invasive tumors may be recommended before surgery to retard tumor growth. Supervoltage irradiation can be given when the patient physically cannot tolerate surgery. Radiation is not curative and has little value in patient management if the tumor is deemed inoperable. Internal radiation (radioisotopes or radon seeds) is rarely used because of the availability of external radiation.

### Chemotherapy

Chemotherapy is primarily palliative. CMV (cisplatin, methotrexate, vinblastine) with or without doxorubicin hydrochloride (Adriamycin) are the most frequently used agents. Thiotepa may be instilled into the bladder as a topical treatment. The patient is dehydrated 8 to 12 hours before thiotepa treatment, and the drug remains in the bladder for 2 hours.

# URETHRAL STRICTURES

## Etiology/Epidemiology

A **urethral stricture** is a narrowing or constriction of the lumen of the urethra. Urethral strictures can be congenital or acquired. Congenital urethral strictures can occur in isolation or in combination with other urinary tract anomalies. Acquired urethral stricture can result from trauma secondary to accident or instrumentation; infection (especially gonorrhea); muscle spasm; or pressure from the outside, by adjacent structures, or by growing tumors. Urethral strictures occur more often in men than women, primarily because of the length of the urethra.

## Pathophysiology

Narrowing of the urethra can result from chronic infection that leads to inflammation of the lining. The inflammation causes a hyperplasia of the lining, and the stricture develops. Trauma may completely sever the urethra. When the urethra is anastomosed, stricture frequently occurs at the surgical site. The third leading cause of urethral stricture is the growth of a tumor that puts pressure against the exterior of the urethra, resulting in a stricture of the lumen.

The first *symptom* of urethral stricture is usually a decrease in the urinary stream and difficulty initiating the stream. Other symptoms are those of UTI and urinary retention. Severe urethral strictures result in complete urinary obstruction, leading to the signs and symptoms of hydronephrosis (p. 1628).

## Prevention

Primary prevention of urethral strictures is accomplished by prompt treatment of any underlying infection. Care should also be taken whenever the patient is to undergo urethral instrumentation.

## Medical Management

Urethral strictures are often repaired with urethroplasty (p. 1648). Strictures may also be corrected by dilation of the urethra. Dilation is accomplished by inserting splinting catheters into the urethra past the area of the stricture. The size of the splinting catheters can be increased to dilate the urethra.

**TABLE 49-12 Major Causes of Urinary Incontinence**

| CAUSE OF URINARY INCONTINENCE | FACTORS INVOLVED: AWARENESS OF NEED TO VOID | CORTICAL ABILITY TO INHIBIT VOIDING | REFLEX ARC | BLADDER RESPONSE TO FILLING | RESULT |
|---|---|---|---|---|---|
| Cerebral clouding | Impaired | Impaired | Intact | Normal | Uncontrolled voiding because of reflex response |
| Infection | Intact | Intact, but overcome by strong reflex response | Abnormally stimulated | Heightened | Voiding because of strong reflex response (urgency) |
| Disturbance of central nervous system pathways (cortical lesions) | Diminished | Impaired | Intact | Heightened | Voiding because of reflex response |
| Disturbance of urethrobladder reflex | | | | | |
| Upper motor neuron lesion | Destroyed | Destroyed | Intact but deranged | Heightened | Voiding because of reflex response |
| Lower motor neuron lesion | Destroyed | Destroyed | Destroyed or impaired | Diminished to absent | Distention or incomplete emptying |
| Tissue damage | Intact | Intact, but not functional because of poor muscle response | Intact | Normal | Loss of control of voiding because of muscular impairment |

# URINARY INCONTINENCE

## ETIOLOGY/EPIDEMIOLOGY

**Urinary incontinence** is the involuntary expulsion of urine from the urinary tract. Urinary incontinence is encountered in several temporary and permanent conditions (Table 49-12). It can be caused by pathologic, anatomic, or physiologic factors affecting the urinary tract, as well as by factors outside of it. Many of these factors can be reversed, such as infection, atrophic vaginitis, acute confusional states, restrictions in mobility, fecal impaction, medical conditions that cause polyuria or nocturia, and drug side effects. Inability to control urination is a problem that frequently leads to emotional distress and can seriously impair a person's social activities. Incontinence must be managed in a way that makes the person feel both physically and emotionally comfortable and socially acceptable.

More than 10 million Americans have urinary incontinence. It is estimated that more than $10 billion a year is spent in managing patients with incontinence. As the U.S. population continues to age, the incidence of incontinence will increase. For noninstitutionalized persons older than 60 years, the incidence ranges from 15% to 30%, with women having twice the incidence of men. Among the more than 1.5 million nursing facility residents, the incidence is greater than 50%. Because of underdiagnosis and underreporting, the problem of urinary incontinence may be even more widespread.

Changes that occur with aging lead to decreased sensation and bladder muscle control, resulting in urinary incontinence. Because persons are often embarrassed about the loss of bladder control, they do not seek assistance and often become isolated from social interactions.

## TYPES OF INCONTINENCE

Three distinct types of urinary incontinence are described in the literature. The exact pattern of incontinence may vary among patients; however, incontinence can be categorized into one of these three types: stress, urge, or overflow.

**Stress incontinence** occurs as a result of incompetence of the bladder outlet or urethral closure. Because of this incompetence, any activity leading to an increase in intraabdominal pressure on the bladder can result in urinary incontinence. Activities leading to stress incontinence include lifting, exercising, coughing, sneezing, or laughing.

**Urge incontinence** is the involuntary loss of urine associated with an abrupt and strong desire to void (urgency). It occurs as a result of uninhibited detrusor contractions. When active detrusor contractions overcome urethral resistance, urine leakage occurs. This type of incontinence is seen in patients with multiple sclerosis or after a cerebrovascular accident (stroke).

Involuntary loss of urine associated with overdistention of the bladder is called **overflow incontinence.** It may have a variety of presentations, including frequent or constant dribbling, or have urge or stress incontinence symptoms. Overflow incontinence can result from spinal cord injury, stroke, or diabetic neuropathy or after radical pelvic surgery.

# PATHOPHYSIOLOGY

## Physiology of Urinary Continence

Bladder sphincter control is necessary to have urinary continence. Such control requires normal voluntary and involuntary muscle action coordinated by a normal urethrobladder reflex. As the bladder fills, the pressure within the bladder gradually increases. The detrusor muscle within the bladder wall responds by relaxing to accommodate the greater volume. When the bladder has filled to capacity, usually between 400 and 500 ml of urine, the parasympathetic stretch receptors located within the bladder wall are stimulated. The stimuli are transmitted through afferent fibers of the reflex arc for micturition. Impulses are then carried through the efferent fibers of the reflex arc to the bladder, causing contraction of the detrusor muscle. The internal sphincter, which is normally closed, reciprocally opens, and urine enters the posterior urethra. Relaxation of the external sphincter and perineal muscles follows, and urine is released. Completion of this reflex arc can be interrupted and voiding postponed through release of inhibitory impulses from the cortical center, which results in voluntary contraction of the external sphincter. If any part of this complex control system is interrupted, urinary incontinence will result.

## Disturbances of Cerebral Control

*Cerebral clouding* is most common in elderly persons. In many instances the person is incontinent because of a lack of awareness of a full bladder. This type of incontinence is often not associated with any definite pathologic problem at the cerebral level. Cerebral clouding also occurs in acutely ill persons—a result of dulled cerebration as a function of the illness. These patients may not have the energy to exercise voluntary control of bladder function. Likewise, a comatose patient is incontinent because of loss of ability to control voluntary use of the external sphincter. As soon as urine is released into the posterior urethra on bladder filling, the bladder contracts and empties. This is why voiding sometimes occurs when a patient is under anesthesia.

*Disturbance of the central nervous system pathways* may occur in diseases such as cerebral embolus, cerebral hemorrhage, brain tumor, meningitis, or traumatic injury of the brain. Adequate voluntary (cortical or cerebral) control of bladder function is prevented in these situations. Urgency incontinence may be present as a result of the inability to inhibit completion of the urethrobladder reflex by the higher centers.

## Disturbances of Urethrobladder Reflex

Disturbance of the urethrobladder reflex may result from lesions of the spinal cord or damage to peripheral nerves of the bladder. This form of incontinence may be seen in persons with spinal cord malformations, injuries, or tumors and in those with compression of the spinal cord caused by fractures of the vertebrae, herniated disk, metastatic tumor, or postoperative edema of the spinal cord. This type of difficulty can result in two types of responses known as **neurogenic bladder:** *automatic* and *flaccid.* The person with a neurogenic bladder has no control over bladder function.

Lesions above the S2 level of the spinal cord or impairment of the cerebrocortical centers do not destroy the reflex arc for voiding, although they may affect control. Such lesions destroy the potential for cortical control to inhibit the reflex. The result is an "upper motor neuron" or "automatic" bladder. The bladder is hypertonic and has a small capacity of usually less than 150 ml. The increased detrusor tone and increased sensitivity to small amounts of urine present in the bladder result in precipitous voiding and the potential for vesicoureteral reflex.

Damage to nerves in the cauda equina or sacral segments of the spinal cord may cause destruction of the reflex arc by interruption of the afferent, efferent, or central components. The result is a "lower motor neuron" or "flaccid" bladder. The bladder is hypotonic with large capacities, sometimes of 750 ml or more. Overflow incontinence, retention of residual urine, and the potential for vesicoureteral reflux are problems imposed by a hypotonic bladder.

## Bladder Disturbances

Overflow incontinence is caused by overdistention of the bladder. This type of incontinence may result from an underactive or a contractile detrusor or from bladder outlet or urethral obstruction, leading to overdistention and overflow.

*Infection* anywhere in the urinary tract may lead to incontinence, since bacteria in the urine causes irritation of the bladder mucosa. The resulting inflammation stimulates the urethrobladder reflex abnormally.

*Tissue damage* to the sphincters of the bladder from instrumentation, surgery, trauma, scarring from urethral infection, lesions involving the sphincter, or relaxation of the perineal structures may cause urinary incontinence. The latter cause of incontinence is seen occasionally after childbirth. The problem is local in nature and does not involve the nervous system.

## Relaxed Musculature

Stress incontinence is seen primarily in women who have relaxed pelvic musculature, but it may also occur in men after prostatectomy. When bladder pressure is suddenly increased, urine enters the proximal third of the urethra, then returns to the bladder when pressure is decreased after exertion. Some of the urine escapes through the urethra.

# MEDICAL MANAGEMENT

Medical management of incontinence includes treatment of any underlying disorders.

## Sphincter Dysfunction

Repair of a sphincter that has been cut is almost impossible. When the *external sphincter* has been damaged, the person will be incontinent on urgency. A voiding schedule can be planned so that voiding occurs before the bladder is full enough to exert sufficient pressure to open the internal sphincter involuntarily. When the *internal sphincter* is damaged, the person may have no acute feeling of the need to void. Here the problem is not one of incontinence but of retention. To ensure routine emptying of the bladder, a regular voiding schedule is necessary. *If both sphincters are damaged, total incontinence will occur.*

## Stress Incontinence

Surgery may be indicated for severe stress incontinence. A **vesicourethropexy** (Marshal-Marchetti procedure) consists of fixation of the urethra to the fascia of the rectus muscle of the abdomen with support given to the neck of the bladder. A suprapubic incision is usually made, but a transvaginal approach may be used if scar tissue is around the urethra from vaginal surgery. A urethral catheter is inserted postoperatively and maintained for 5 to 6 days. The urine may be pink, but the urethral catheter is not irrigated as a rule. The person may have difficulty voiding immediately after the indwelling catheter is removed. The woman is observed for signs of vaginal bleeding. Straining and use of Valsalva's maneuver should be avoided until healing has occurred, and mild laxatives may be given to prevent straining from constipation. Surgeons differ in the amount of activity permitted in the early postoperative period.

Less invasive is the *Stamey* procedure, a suspension of the bladder neck by sutures passed adjacent to the ureterovesical junction. A small incision is made above and lateral to the symphysis pubis. The needles are introduced suprapubically by endoscopy, and the positions are checked by cystoscopy before suturing. The procedure is then repeated on the opposite side. A percutaneous suprapubic catheter is inserted after the suturing; the catheter is removed when spontaneous voiding occurs, which may take several days. There is minimal postoperative discomfort. Antibiotics are given for 2 weeks postoperatively. The patient should refrain from sexual activity for about 1 to 2 months.

## Urgency

Incontinence caused by urinary tract infection (UTI) is generally temporary, responding to treatment of the UTI by systemic antibiotics. Specific causes of infection such as obstruction must be identified and corrected when possible. Provision must be made for adequate fluid intake of 3000 ml or more per day unless contraindicated by the person's medical condition.

The person who has a brain tumor, meningitis, or traumatic injury to the brain that prevents adequate voluntary control of bladder function and causes urgency incontinence by inhibiting cortical control over the urethrobladder reflex may respond to a bladder retraining program. If the person's condition or response prohibits such a program, an internal or external drainage device should be used.

## Neurogenic Bladder Dysfunction

Persons with injuries of the spinal cord experience a transitory period of "spinal shock" in which urinary retention occurs (see Chapter 58). This is treated with continuous or intermittent catheter drainage that aims to prevent UTI and overdistention of the bladder. After this acute stage, further management depends on the exact nature of any residual neurogenic bladder dysfunction. Persons with a lesion *above the sacral segments* and who have an intact urethrobladder reflex may initiate voiding by pinching or stroking trigger areas of the thighs or suprapubic area. In persons with a *lower motor neuron lesion,* the use of the *Credé method,* which consists of exerting manual pressure over the bladder, may provide more complete bladder emptying. The appropriateness of this technique must be determined by the physician based on the person's complete urologic status. An increasing number of persons with neurogenic bladder dysfunction are being taught intermittent self-catheterization using clean technique to prevent infection and manage incontinence. Maintenance of a regular schedule is stressed, and the frequency of catheterization is determined on an individual basis.

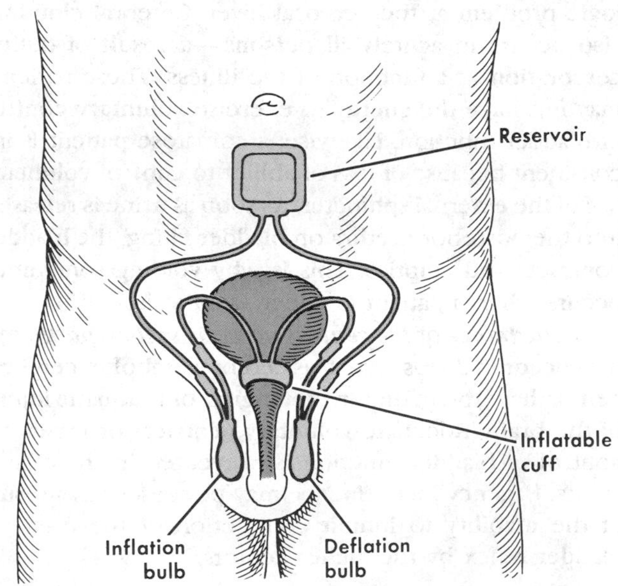


**FIGURE 49-9** Artificial bladder sphincter. Compression and release of inflation pump bulb inflates cuff surrounding urethra, stopping urine flow. Compression and release of deflation pump bulb deflates inflatable cuff, returning fluid to storage reservoir. This releases urethral constriction, permitting urine to flow.

Certain medications are given alone or in conjunction with an intermittent catheterization program in the management of incontinence related to neurogenic bladder dysfunction. α-Adrenergic drugs such as ephedrine sulfate are used to increase urethal resistance. Anticholinergic drugs such as propantheline (Pro-Banthine) are prescribed to control the reflex bladder activity.[15]

### Artificial Sphincter

Implantation of an artificial urinary sphincter may be used to achieve continence when other methods have failed. In this procedure, a hydraulically activated sphincter mechanism is placed around the urethra or bladder neck. The sphincter is made to open and close at will by squeezing one of two bulbs implanted under the skin of the labia or scrotum (Figure 49-9). Postoperative nursing care of the person with such an implant includes observation for and reporting of fever or pain on inflation of the device, swelling of the genitalia, and recurrence of incontinence. Complications of the procedure include erosion of the urethra, abscess, cellulitis, and mechanical malfunctions in the system. Men have had more success with the artificial sphincter than women.

## NURSING MANAGEMENT

## ♦ ASSESSMENT

### Subjective Data

Questions to ask the patient when assessing for urinary incontinence include: What is the frequency of incontinence? Can anything be associated with precipitating incontinence (stress, fear, coughing, sneezing, laughing, exercise)? Is pain or burning present with incontinence? Is there a state of awareness to void before incontinence?

### Objective Data

Data to be collected to assess the person with urinary incontinence include the following:

Volume of output
Characteristics of urine
Patient's ability to follow directions
Physiologic reason for incontinence (e.g., spinal cord injury)

## ♦ NURSING DIAGNOSES

Nursing diagnoses are determined from analysis of patient data. Several nursing diagnoses could be made for the incontinent patient for which the interventions are not specific for urinary incontinence and thus are not discussed in this section. Some of these nursing diagnoses include skin integrity, impaired; self–bathing-hygiene deficit; mobility, impaired physical; and coping, ineffective individual. Nursing diagnoses specific for the incontinent patient may include but are not limited to the following:

| Diagnostic Title | Possible Etiologic Factors |
|---|---|
| Incontinence (specify type) | Relaxed pelvic muscles, altered environment, sensory deficit, neurologic impairment, overdistention, decreased bladder capacity |
| Self-esteem, situational low | Loss of urinary control |
| Knowledge deficit | Lack of exposure/recall |

## ♦ EXPECTED PATIENT OUTCOMES

Expected patient outcomes for the person with urinary incontinence may include but are not limited to the following:

1. Achieves optimal urinary control.
2. Verbalizes feelings and concerns without self-deprecating statements.
3. Socializes with others.
4. Demonstrates perineal exercises (if appropriate).
5. Describes actions to control voiding (as appropriate), measures to maintain skin integrity, and plans for follow-up care.

## ♦ INTERVENTIONS

### Assisting With Urinary Control

#### Bladder retraining

When incontinence is caused by dulled cerebration in elderly persons, by confusion, or by acute illness, control can usually be established if a persistent **bladder retraining** schedule is carried out. A voiding schedule is developed and strictly adhered to until the person gradually relearns to recognize and react appropriately to the urge to void. A successful program of this type (Box 49-6), leading to complete rehabilitation, or continence, requires mental competence of the individual. Otherwise, someone else must always remind the person to follow the schedule.

People ordinarily void on awakening, before retiring, and before or after meals. If a diuretic such as coffee has been taken, it is usually necessary to void about 30 minutes later. Using this knowledge, the nurse can begin to set up a schedule for placing the person on a bedpan or

**BOX 49-6 Bladder Retraining**

- Establish patient's usual voiding patterns.
- Plan toileting based on the patient's usual pattern; assist patient as necessary.
- If no voiding pattern can be determined, plan toileting for every 1 to 2 hours.
- Encourage patient to use normal toilet position.
- Encourage patient to empty bladder completely.
- Provide for a fluid intake of 3000 ml/day for adequate urine volume.
- Schedule most fluids to be taken before 4 PM.

taking the person to the toilet. Then, if a record is kept for a few days of the times the person voids involuntarily, it is usually possible to determine the normal voiding pattern. If the schedule based on the pattern of incontinence is not successful, toileting every 1 to 2 hours should be carried out on a 24-hour basis.

During the retraining program, *mobilization* of the individual, attention to the *position* assumed for voiding, and adequate *fluid intake* contribute to reduction of the possibility of infection. Complete emptying of the bladder eliminates the possibility of residual urine acting as a medium for bacterial growth, whereas a high fluid intake provides for internal bladder irrigation.

When it is possible, *toileting* should be carried out in surroundings that will remind the person of the voiding function; that is, the person should be taken to the bathroom where the toilet can be used. If this is not possible, a bedside commode can be an adequate substitute. Many men can void into a urinal more easily if allowed to stand at the bedside. The use of a bedpan is unfamiliar and distasteful to most persons, but in instances where women must remain in bed, voiding into a bedpan can be facilitated if the head of the bed is rolled up as high as allowed. This form of positioning is more consistent with the position normally assumed for voiding and facilitates complete emptying of the bladder. Few persons can void adequately in the supine position.

Providing adequate amounts of *fluids,* a minimum of 3000 ml per day, is necessary to ensure that adequate amounts of urine are produced and present in the bladder to stimulate the voiding reflex at the proper times. Fluids may be given at scheduled times, the largest portion being given during the day *before 4 PM* to decrease the frequency of voiding through the night. Persons on fluid restriction because of medical problems should receive no more fluids than the amount prescribed.

### External urinary drainage

Occasionally, justifications exist for the use of an indwelling catheter for the incontinent patient. Such reasons include the need to protect a surgical incision or to permit healing of a decubitus ulcer in the area. Indwelling catheterization, however, presents many potential dangers, such as UTI, urethritis, epididymitis, and urethral fistulas. All other means to manage the incontinence should be tried before resorting to catheterization.

For the man, external drainage can be accomplished by applying a watertight apparatus to the penis. Several commercial products are available for external urinary drainage and should be used whenever possible. The following is an alternative method. Select a condom of the correct size. Puncture a hole in the closed end of the condom with an applicator stick. Attach the punctured end of the condom to a firm rubber or plastic drainage tube with either a 3 mm (⅛ inch) piece of rubber tubing or a strip of adhesive tape (Figure 49-10).

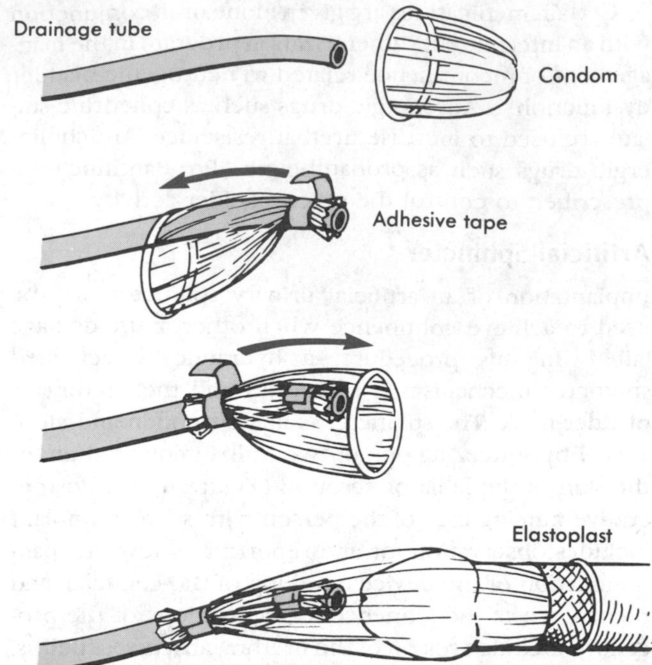


**FIGURE 49-10** One method of making an external drainage apparatus.

Before applying the condom, clean and dry the penis thoroughly and check it for edema, skin breaks, or discoloration. Invert the condom and roll it onto the penis. There should be no roll at the top that could cause constriction. At least 2.5 cm (1 inch) of the condom should remain between the meatus and drainage tube to allow for penile erection. There should not be so much slack as to cause twisting and subsequent interference with drainage. Elastoplast is then applied over the condom and around the penis (never touching the skin). *Under no circumstances should adhesive tape be used.* The Elastoplast must not be constricting.

The external catheter should be removed daily and the skin washed and checked. Frequent checking is necessary to determine whether edema or irritation is present and to ensure proper drainage. This is especially important in men with loss of sensation. The external device is attached to straight drainage or to a leg bag.

For persons who need external catheter drainage indefinitely, a rubber urinary appliance (sometimes called an *incontinence urinal*) may be used (Figure 49-11). Several models are available, and the one best suited to the person's needs is selected. Two appliances are recommended to allow for cleaning and drying. They should be washed in mild soap, turned inside out, and thoroughly dried before application.

Most persons prefer to manage their own incontinence if they are at all able to do so. The nurse supports and encourages this, offering assistance as necessary and instruction in basic principles of skin care, equipment

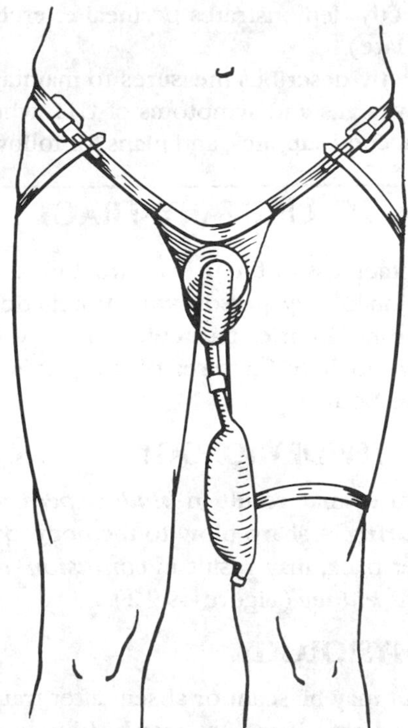

**FIGURE 49-11** Rubber urinary appliance. Bag is emptied by drain valve at bottom bag.

selection, and maintenance. The choice of management method should take into account the person's ability to manage as independently as possible.[12]

## Facilitating Coping

If none of the previous measures is appropriate or successful, nursing goals of assisting the person to remain clean, free of odor, and free of decubiti may require external urinary protection. The type varies with the person's gender, functional status, and physical status.

Those who are incapacitated by critical illness or unconscious depend on the nursing staff to manage their incontinence by protective pants or external catheter drainage. Others may be capable of some or all of their own management. Men and women may wear protective waterproof pants lined by disposable or washable absorbent pads. A resourceful person may be able to improvise equipment that is as comfortable and is less costly than commercially available pants. Zippers, Velcro, elastic, and a variety of waterproof materials may be used. Bedding and furniture can be protected with waterproof materials such as commercially available squares of absorbent cellucotton backed with light plastic.

Whatever the type of padding, liners, or pants used, frequent changing is required for skin protection and comfort. The perineal and genital areas are thoroughly washed with soap and water and dried well at each changing. If possible, the person is bathed in a tub of

### Guidelines for Teaching Perineal Exercises

1. Tighten the perineal muscles as if to prevent voiding; hold for 3 seconds, then relax.
2. Inhale through pursed lips while tightening perineal muscles.
3. Bear down as if to have a bowel movement. Relax then tighten perineal muscles.
4. Hold a pencil in the fold between the buttock and thigh.
5. Sit on the toilet with knees held wide apart. Start and stop the urinary stream.

warm water at least once a day. Periodic exposure of the perineal area to air is beneficial. A moisture barrier product (e.g., A&D ointment) helps protect the skin. Zinc oxide powder can be applied to lessen irritation. Excess amounts of powder are avoided, since this will cake on the skin and cause irritation. Deodorant sprays for use on dressings and liners are valuable, but they may cause skin irritation in persons who develop a hypersensitivity to them. Deodorant room fresheners may be helpful if the odor is strong.

If the person can be up, a favorite chair can be equipped with a commode seat. Special commode wheelchairs are also available, making it possible for the person to be more comfortable and to mingle socially with others.

## Promoting Self-Esteem

Elderly persons isolated from their families and familiar surroundings, confused by institutionalization, or with feelings of loss of self-esteem frequently respond well to mobilization in bladder retraining programs. Their circulation is enhanced by the imposed mobility, their awareness is increased, and they respond to the attention given them. When nurses believe that it is easier to change bed linen than to establish an appropriate bladder retraining program, a disservice is done to the individual and more work is actually created for the nurse. The person becomes subject to UTI and skin breakdown, and feelings of worthlessness are increased. For those who can be continent, incontinence is an indignity.

## Facilitating Learning

Teaching is an important aspect of care for the incontinent person because the patient, often with family assistance, is usually involved in control of urinary continence. Explanation of the rationale for activities, such as the toileting schedule, mobility, and fluid requirements, increases the probability of the person following through with the activities.

*Perineal exercises* are helpful in controlling mild stress incontinence or strengthening muscles after withdrawal of an indwelling catheter. The exercises consist of tightening and relaxing perineal and gluteal muscles and can be performed in several ways (see Guidelines box, p. 1645). Much of the incontinence problem caused by a relaxed perineum in women can be prevented if perineal exercises are taught before and after childbirth. These exercises also may be included as part of the health teaching of any woman.

Additional teaching includes care of any drainage system, measures to maintain skin integrity, signs and symptoms of UTI (frequency, dysuria) that should be reported to the physician, and how to obtain and maintain any needed supplies and equipment (commode, protective padding, drainage system).

## ♦ EVALUATION

To evaluate the effectiveness of nursing interventions, compare patient behaviors with those stated in the expected outcomes. Successful achievement of patient outcomes for the patient with urinary incontinence is indicated by the following:

1. Achieves urinary continence through bladder retraining (if appropriate) or uses a drainage system or padding.
2. Describes self in positive terms.
3. Socializes with others.
4. Correctly demonstrates perineal exercises (if appropriate).
5. Correctly describes measures to maintain skin integrity, signs and symptoms of UTI, where to obtain needed supplies, and plans for follow-up care.

# TRAUMA TO URINARY TRACT

Assessing intactness of the urinary tract must be part of the evaluation of any person with traumatic injury to the lower trunk. Injuries particularly related to urinary tract damage include fractures of the pelvis and sharp blows to the body.

## ETIOLOGY/EPIDEMIOLOGY

Pelvic fractures may result in *bladder perforation* and *urethral tearing*. A sharp blow to the body, particularly to the lower back, may result in *contusion, tearing,* or *rupture of a kidney* (Figure 49-12).

## PATHOPHYSIOLOGY

Urine output may be scant or absent after trauma to the urinary tract. Urine, if present, may be bloody, and symptoms of peritonitis may appear. The first *symptoms* of

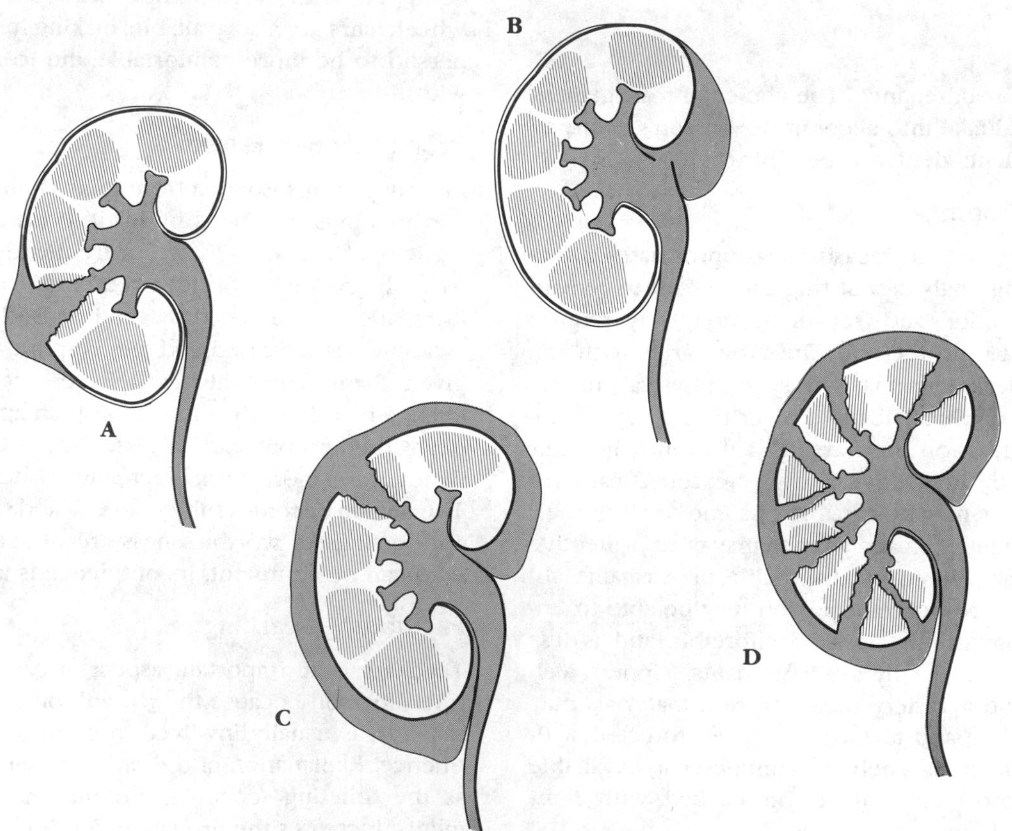


**FIGURE 49-12** Four degrees of renal trauma. **A,** Urine is extravasating from split in renal parenchyma but confined under renal capsule. **B,** Urine is extravasating through tear in renal pelvis. **C,** Urine is extravasating through rent in kidney and capsule and surrounds kidney and renal pelvis. **D,** Kidney is shattered, and urine is extravasating in all areas. (From Winter CC, Morel A: *Nursing care of patients with urologic diseases,* ed 4, St Louis, 1977, Mosby.)

trauma to the kidney usually are hematuria and pain or tenderness of the upper abdominal quadrant and flank on the involved side. Signs of shock may be present if hemorrhage is extensive.

Diagnostic tests used to facilitate diagnosis of trauma to the urinary tract include KUB, cystogram, IV pyelography, renal angiography, and CT scan. Laboratory tests include serial urinalysis, hemoglobin, BUN, and creatinine levels.

## MEDICAL MANAGEMENT

Treatment of injuries is directed toward stabilizing the patient and surgically repairing any perforations or lacerations of the urinary tract. Initial treatment includes control of bleeding, prevention of shock, and promoting drainage of urine. While stabilizing the patient, a cystotomy may be performed to provide urinary drainage when injuries involve the bladder or urethra. Vital signs, fluid balance records, and hematocrit levels are monitored to assess bleeding. Complaints of pain may indicate ureteral colic, signifying obstruction of the ureter by a clot. Surgical intervention is required to control severe hemorrhage; spontaneous healing of the kidney is otherwise permitted. Bedrest is maintained until gross hematuria clears; thereafter, activity is progressed according to tolerance and absence of hematuria.

When urethral injuries are suspected, great care must be taken when inserting urinary catheters to prevent further injury to the urethra. It may be necessary for a urologist to insert the catheter during a retrograde urethrogram or cystogram (see Chapter 48).

A kidney may become loosened and "float" or become displaced **(nephroptosis).** If symptoms of obstruction occur, the kidney may be sutured to its anatomic site **(nephropexy).** Postoperatively, the patient is positioned with the hips elevated to prevent tension on the suture line.

# UROLOGIC SURGERY

## GENERAL INTERVENTIONS

Before the detailed discussion of particular types of surgery of the urinary tract, general principles of care of the patient requiring urologic surgery are described.

### Preoperative Nursing Care

The focus of preoperative care is preparation of the patient for the impending surgery and implementation of the medical regimen. Much of the patient's concern depends on the type of surgery and diagnosis. Since the surgery will temporarily or permanently alter urinary elimination, the person will be concerned about the degree of change that will occur.

Preoperative instructions may include a discussion of the type and length of surgery; type of anesthesia; and the need for an IV line, catheter, or other drains. Instructions in coughing and deep breathing and using the incentive spirometer are crucial because inadequate ventilation is a frequent problem postoperatively. The patient is informed of the pain medication routine: whether or not it will be offered or if it must be requested. A description of methods of decreasing pain, such as by splinting the incision, should be offered. Persons having a urinary diversion require bowel preparation (p. 1651).

### Postoperative Nursing Care

The basic needs of the patient requiring urologic surgery are the same as those of any other surgical patient. Special emphasis must be placed on promotion of ventilation and adequate urine output, prevention of distention and hemorrhage, and attention to drainage tubes and dressings (see Guidelines box below).

#### Promoting ventilation

Surgery of the kidney or upper ureters usually involves a flank incision that can influence respiratory status. Because the incision is directly below the diaphragm, deep breathing is painful, and the patient is reluctant to take deep breaths or move about. Splinting of the chest is common; therefore, atelectasis or other respiratory complications must be prevented. In addition, because of the location of the incision, greater incisional pull occurs every time the person moves. The patient is often reluctant to turn in bed or to get up to ambulate. Most patients will be more comfortable turning themselves if they are given time, side rails to hold onto, and encouragement. Incisional pain usually requires a narcotic every 3 to 4 hours for 24 to 48 hours after surgery. Turning, ambulation, and deep breathing exercises should be planned so that these activities occur at the time the analgesic has the greatest effect. Patients may lie on the affected side unless a nephrostomy tube is in place. Even then, patients can be tilted to the affected side with pillows placed at the back for support. The nephrostomy tube must not be kinked and must be free of traction.

**Guidelines for Care After Urologic Surgery**

1. Promote ventilation.
   a. Encourage breathing exercises.
   b. Encourage self-turning in bed frequently.
   c. Encourage ambulation.
2. Monitor patency and output of urinary catheters.
3. Prevent complications.
   a. Change wet dressings to protect skin.
   b. Restrict food and oral fluids if paralytic ileus is present.
   c. Encourage fluids to 3000 ml/day when permitted.
   d. Monitor for bright-red blood on dressings or in urine.
4. Administer analgesics to control pain.

### Monitoring urine output

Urine output is monitored carefully for several days postoperatively. The output should be at least 50 ml/hr, preferably greater to prevent urinary stasis and subsequent infection. Urine output of 20 to 30 ml/hr in a patient with satisfactory fluid intake (at least 1200 ml/day) and in the absence of signs of urinary retention is reported immediately to the physician. Urine output includes drainage from nephrostomy or cystostomy tubes, urethral or ureteral catheters, and an estimate from urine-soaked dressings. Daily weights are compared with the preoperative weight and with previous days to identify shifts in fluid status.

### Preventing distention

After kidney surgery, most patients have some abdominal distention that may result in part from pressure on the stomach and intestinal tract during surgery. Patients who have had renal colic before surgery frequently develop paralytic ileus postoperatively. This condition may be related to the reflex gastrointestinal tract symptoms caused by postoperative pain. Because of the problem of abdominal distention after kidney surgery, food and fluids by mouth are often restricted for 24 to 48 hours postoperatively. By the fourth postoperative day, most patients tolerate a regular diet. Fluids are usually encouraged to 3000 ml/day.

### Preventing hemorrhage

Hemorrhage may follow such operative procedures as prostatectomy, nephrolithotomy, or partial nephrectomy. It occurs most often when the highly vascular parenchyma of the kidney has been incised. The bleeding may occur on the day of surgery, or it may occur 8 to 12 days postoperatively, during the period when tissue sloughing normally occurs with healing. The presence of bright-red blood on the dressing or in the urine is reported immediately to the physician. The patient is observed for signs of shock. Since many patients with urologic disease have hypertension, the blood pressure may be relatively high but still demonstrate a marked drop for the individual. Therefore, comparisons should be made with baseline data.

If hemorrhage occurs, a pressure dressing is applied over the incision while awaiting the physician's arrival. Measures to prevent shock are instituted (see Chapter 22).

### Care of dressings

Large amounts of urinary drainage may follow urologic surgery, except after nephrectomy. The drainage may be pink or dark red but should not be bright red. If the surgery involves a flank incision, drainage is usually the heaviest on the posterior edge of the dressing because of gravity. It is important, therefore, to turn the patient on the side opposite the surgery to examine the posterior edge of the dressing. When a suprapubic incision is present, drainage is heaviest on the side and in the inguinal region.

The dressings are usually held in place by Montgomery straps and must be changed frequently. Urinary drainage irritates the skin, has an unpleasant odor, and leads to discomfort. If a drain is present, the end of the drain should be placed over dressings, then covered with additional dressings to absorb the drainage. The presence of large amounts of drainage on the dressing with little drainage coming from the tube indicates blockage of the tube. If a large amount of drainage is present, a disposable drainage bag used for urinary stomas (p. 1654) may be applied over the drain site.

### Care of drain tubes

A catheter is usually inserted during surgery to drain urine from the operative area and permit healing to occur. Different types of drain tubes may be inserted, and each tube is connected to a separate drainage system. It is important to know the purpose of the catheter and the area to be drained.

## SPECIFIC TYPES OF UROLOGIC SURGERY

### Surgery of the Kidney

Removal of a kidney *(nephrectomy)* may be indicated for some congenital anomalies or for irreparable damage to kidney tissue from trauma or diseases such as renal hypertension, tumor, multiple cysts, or kidney stones. Adequate waste removal can be maintained by the remaining kidney or by even less than half of one functional kidney. In some instances, only a portion of a diseased kidney is removed *(partial nephrectomy)*. If an entire kidney is removed, a drain may be placed to remove serous fluid from the space previously occupied by the kidney. In this situation, no urinary drainage occurs. Urinary drainage occurs with partial nephrectomy.

The kidney may also be incised for removal of calculi, either through the pelvis of the kidney *(pyelolithotomy)* or through the parenchyma *(nephrolithotomy)*. A large amount of urinary drainage usually occurs after these surgeries.

A kidney may become loosened and "float" or become displaced *(nephroptosis)*. If symptoms of obstruction occur, the kidney may be sutured to its anatomic site *(nephropexy)*. Postoperatively, the patient is positioned with the hips elevated to prevent tension on the sutures.

### Surgery of the Ureters and Bladder

Removal of stones *(calculi)* blocking a ureter is termed *ureterolithotomy*. The root word "lith" refers to stones. Obstruction at the ureteropelvic junction is corrected by means of a **pyeloplasty** (plastic repair of the renal pelvis).

The bladder may be incised **(cystotomy)** for removal of calculi or as part of one method of prostate removal (suprapubic prostatectomy) (see Chapter 53). A **cystostomy** (note the "s" in the middle of the word) is an opening made into the bladder for drainage, usually by means of a tube.

Partial removal of the bladder **(segmental resection)** is usually performed for tumors of the bladder. Bladder capacity will be small initially with a capacity of no more than 60 ml immediately after surgery. However, the elastic tissue of the bladder will regenerate, so bladder capacity will increase to 200 to 400 ml within several months.

The decreased bladder size, however, is of major importance in the postoperative period. The patient will return from surgery with catheters draining the bladder both from a cystostomy and from the urethra to avoid obstruction of drainage. The bladder would become distended in only a very short time if obstruction occurred, resulting in disruption of the bladder suture line. Because bladder capacity is limited, the catheters usually cause severe bladder spasm. The urethral catheter is usually removed 3 weeks after surgery, but it may be left in place longer if the cystotomy wound is not healed.

As soon as the urethral catheter is removed, the patient becomes acutely aware of the small bladder capacity. Most patients will need to void at least every 20 minutes and be reassured that the bladder capacity will gradually increase. Total fluid intake should be 3000 ml throughout the day. Large quantities of fluid should not be ingested at one time, and fluids should be limited for several hours before going out.

If the entire bladder is removed **(cystectomy),** diversion of the urinary tract is necessary. Large amounts of surrounding tissue will also be removed if the tumor is malignant. A long, vertical abdominal incision is present, along with one or more pelvic drains. A nasogastric tube is inserted in the operating room, and the patient is given nothing by mouth until gastrointestinal function returns. The nursing care is similar to that provided for any patient after major abdominal surgery, plus the care and monitoring of the diverted urinary tract.

## URINARY DIVERSION PROCEDURES

### Purpose and Types

Urinary diversion procedures are required to treat malignancies of the urinary tract, birth defects, neurogenic bladder, chronic progressive pyelonephritis, and irreparable trauma to the urinary tract. The most common urinary diversion procedure that results in an external stoma and the need for an ostomy pouch is the ileal or colon conduit. A surgical alternative that has an external stoma, the **continent urostomy,** has an internal reservoir made from intestine that holds urine. The stoma must be catheterized at regular intervals to drain the reservoir. The Kock **continent ileal reservoir** (Figure 49-13) is formed from loops of the small intestine. The **ileocecal** (or Indiana **pouch**) consists of portions of large intestine and ileum (Figure 49-14). New surgical advances being studied consist of internal reservoirs anastomosed to the urethra.

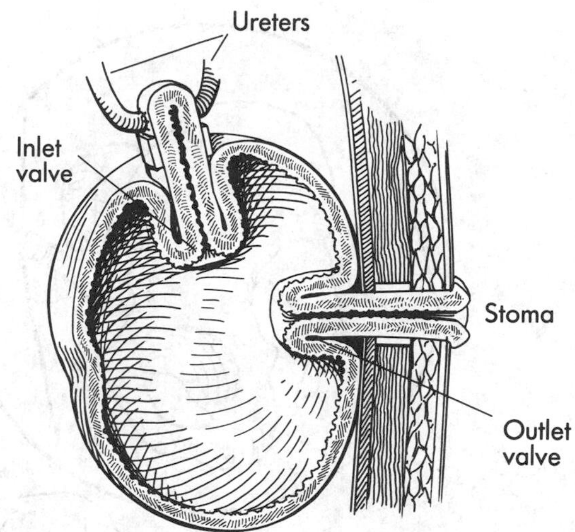


**FIGURE 49-13** Kock continent ileal urinary reservoir.

**Cutaneous ureterostomy** is used when the physical condition prohibits more extensive surgical procedures. One or both ureters are excised from the bladder and brought out through the skin, either on the flank or the anterior abdominal wall to create a small stoma. When both ureters are involved, each may be brought out to the skin surface separately, resulting in two stomas, or the ureters may be joined at some point and brought out through the abdominal wall to form only one stoma. Initially after surgery, ureterostomy stomas are pink, but they will turn very pale in several weeks. This surgery works best when the ureters are dilated from chronic reflux. Otherwise, the ureterostomy opening will be very small and may tend to become stenosed. The complications associated with ureterostomy stoma stenosis are inadequate drainage of the kidney resulting in hydronephrosis, infection, and progressive kidney damage. Urinary tract infection in persons with ureterostomy is common because of the ease of reflux of urine from the stoma to the kidney.

During the **ileal conduit, ileal loop,** or Bricker procedure, the ureters are excised from the bladder and transplanted into one end of a 15 to 20 cm (6 or 8 inch) segment of ileum that has been resected from the intestinal tract with its mesentery, which contains the blood supply. The remaining intestinal segments are anastomosed, and gastrointestinal function is expected to return to its normal preoperative state after healing. The end of the resected ileum into which the ureters are connected is sutured closed, and the other end is brought through the abdominal wall to the skin surface to create a **stoma** (Figure 49-15). The urinary bladder may be resected or left intact, depending on the reason for the diversion. The ileal segment is intended to serve as a passageway for urine flow rather than as a reservoir.

The **colon conduit** (colonic loop) is basically performed like an ileal conduit except that a segment of

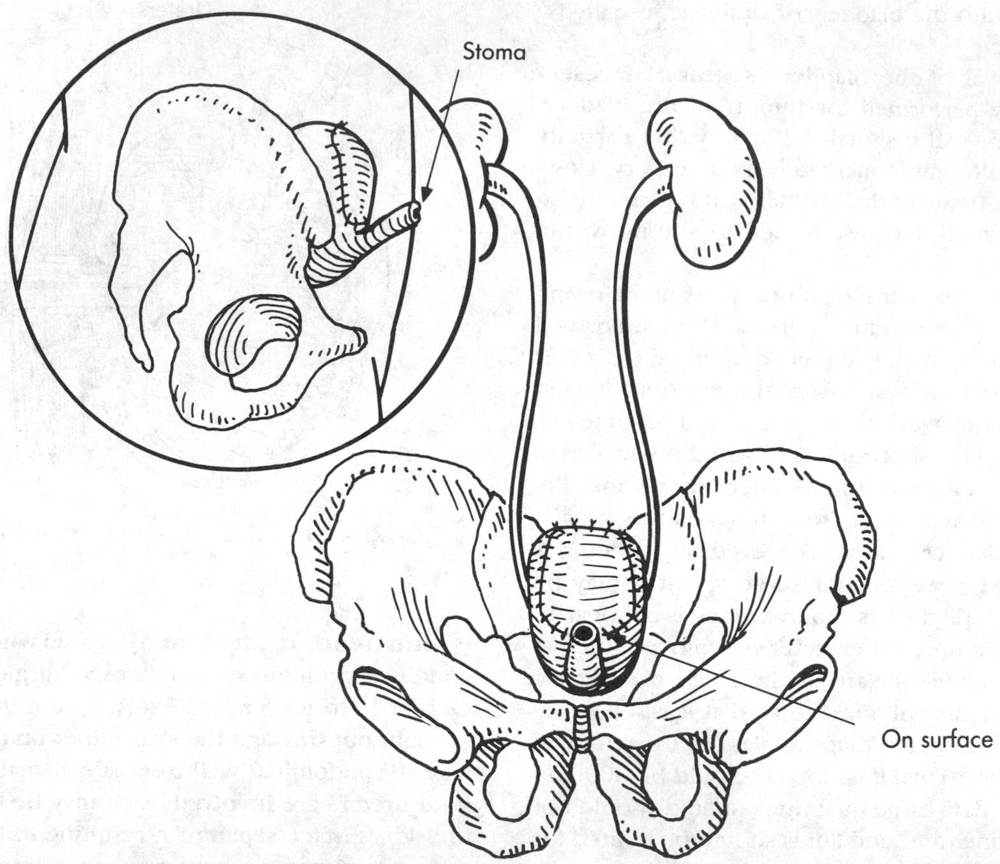


**FIGURE 49-14** Ileocecal continent urinary reservior (Indiana pouch).

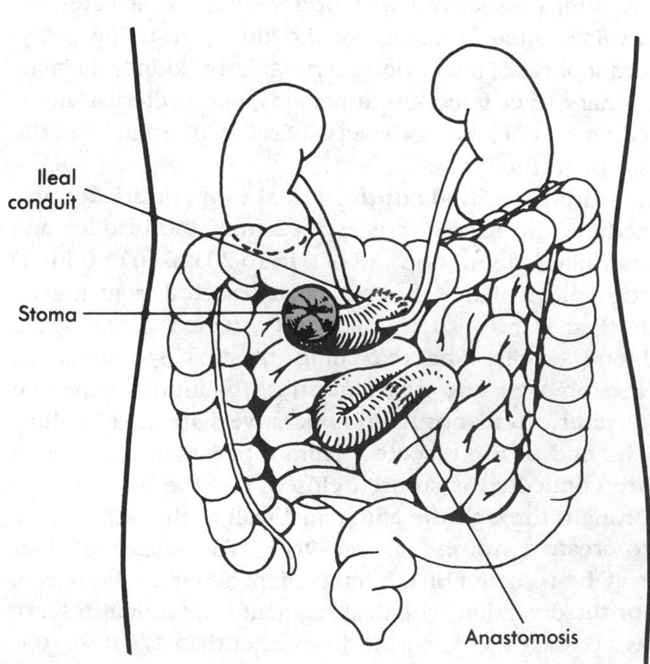


**FIGURE 49-15** Ileal conduit or ileal loop.

colon (ascending, descending, transverse, or sigmoid) instead of ileum acts as the conduit for the urine. The colon conduit has reduced the incidence of urinary reflux for some persons. Preoperative and postoperative nursing care and ongoing management are the same as those for ileal conduit surgery.

The continent urostomy *(Kock pouch, Indiana pouch)* consists of loops of intestine anastomosed together, separated from the rest of the intestine so that the gastrointestinal function occurs normally and then connected to the abdomen via the stomal segment. For the Kock pouch, ureters from the kidney are connected to the pouch above a valve. This valve prevents urine from refluxing to the kidney. The urine stays in the reservoir because a second valve is placed in the intestinal segment leading to the stoma. This valve prevents the leakage of urine, thus maintaining continence.[7] For the ileocecal or Indiana pouch, the ureters are anastomosed to the colon portion of the reservoir in a manner to prevent reflux. The ileocecal valve is used to provide continence, and the section of ileum that extends from the intestinal reservoir to the skin is made narrower (plicated) to prevent urine leakage.[8] The end of the intestinal segment is brought out onto the skin to form the stoma. The stoma for the continent urostomy is usu-

**RESEARCH**

Smith DB, Babaian RJ: *J Enterostom Ther* 16:244-246, 1989.

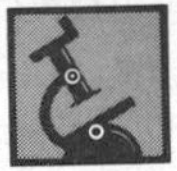

Over a 20-month period, 128 consecutive patients undergoing radical cystectomy with ileal conduit urinary diversion for treatment of bladder cancer were surveyed, comparing adjustment to the conduit by education, finances, age, occupation, activity, gender, presence of physical limitations, response of friends, response of sexual partner, change in self-image, and postoperative chemotherapy. Adjustment was significantly influenced by the patient's gender, with women scoring higher than men on the adjustment scale ($p = 0.03$); how the sexual partner responded to the patient ($p = 0.001$); whether or not the patient perceived a change in self-image ($p < 0.001$); level of preoperative activity ($p = 0.04$); response of friends ($p = 0.001$); who changes the appliance ($p = 0.001$); and whether or not postoperative chemotherapy was administered ($p = 0.03$). Factors that did not significantly affect adjustment were educational level, occupation, financial status, age, and physical handicaps. The authors concluded that adjustment is important to a patient and influences the postoperative quality of life. Support in adjusting to an ileal conduit should be incorporated into preoperative and postoperative care by the health care team. Of particular concern should be reinforcing the patient's positive self-image, encouraging self-reliance, and encouraging a supportive response from the patient's spouse or significant other.

ally flush to the skin and placed lower on the abdomen than the ileal conduit stoma.

The ileal conduit, colon conduit, and continent urostomy stomas should be a bright-red color. Early complications after surgery include breakdown of the anastomosis in the gastrointestinal tract, leakage from the ureteroileal or ureterosigmoid anastomosis, paralytic ileus, obstruction of the ureters, wound infection, mucocutaneous separation, and stomal necrosis. Complications that may occur after hospitalization include stomal problems (retraction, stenosis, hernia) and urinary infections.

Any procedure for diversion of urine that results in an external stoma leads to a significant change in body image. Reactions may vary depending on the reason for the procedure, but virtually every person will require time and much nursing support while adapting to the altered means of urine elimination (see Research box above).

## Preoperative Nursing Care

### Counseling and teaching

When the physician tells the person of the probable need for a urinary diversion, the first reaction is likely to be disbelief and disappointment. The reason for the surgery will influence the reaction. Time to grieve is essential, and the nurse can be a source of support during this time. Persons who have been well informed about the surgical procedure as well as the postoperative period and long-term management goals are generally better able to adjust to the entire experience than those who do not receive such preparation. As soon as a person learns that a urinary diversion is contemplated, many questions arise, and accurate answers must be given at this time.

The enterostomal therapy nurse specializes in the care and instruction to persons who have or will have an ostomy. If possible, a preoperative meeting with the patient and enterostomal therapy nurse should be arranged. In addition to providing information, the enterostomal therapy nurse can select and mark the site for the placement of the stoma. If time permits, a meeting with the patient and a visitor from the United Ostomy Association can be arranged. The visitor is a trained volunteer who has an ostomy and has adjusted well to it. A postoperative or home visit can be arranged.

The nurse's goals for preoperative teaching must reflect the patient's needs. However, certain basic information must be included. The patient should understand the surgical procedure and should know whether a pouch will have to be worn postoperatively.

Preoperative instruction also involves preparing the person for the appearance of the stoma. The patient should be told that the stoma will be red, that the tissue is similar to the mucosal lining of the mouth, and that it will not be painful. An anastomy chart or simple drawing supplements and clarifies explanations of the surgical procedure. The patient should be given the definition of terms such as stoma, urostomy, and pouch.

Booklets designed for the person having a urinary diversion may be given to the patient preoperatively.[2,3] Some persons need this additional information to assist them in accepting the surgery. Others may be unable to review written materials until after surgery.

Finally, a brief description of the management of the urostomy is given. The person who will be having an ileal or colon conduit is informed of the need to wear the pouch, the frequency of changing and emptying the pouch, and the function of the urinary stoma. The person having a continent urostomy procedure is informed of the need to catheterize the stoma at regular intervals and to irrigate the internal reservoir to remove mucus. Assurance is given that the nurse will provide stoma care immediately after surgery and that the patient will be assisted to master self-care before discharge.

### Physical preparation

Before an ileal or colon conduit diversion or a continent urostomy diversion, a complete cleansing of the bowel is required; this reduces the possibility of fecal contamination when the bowel is resected and used to form the conduit or internal reservoir. The cleansing routine generally consists of a clear-liquid diet for 24 hours before surgery and nothing by mouth after midnight the night before surgery. Large-volume oral bowel cleansing solutions (GoLYTELY or Colyte) or a special laxative and fluid program may be prescribed the day before surgery. Cleansing enemas may be ordered to supplement the cleanout procedure. Intestinal antibiotics such as neomycin may also be administered orally.

Determination of the exact placement for the stoma should be made by the surgeon and/or the enterostomal therapy nurse. The stoma for the ileal conduit is usually constructed on the right side of the abdomen, below the waist, and within the rectus muscle. The continent urostomy stoma is placed lower on the right or left side of the abdomen because a flat surface for a pouch is not needed. Selection of the site is ideally made before surgery and should include evaluation of the person's body when in the lying, sitting, and standing positions. Since a smooth, even skin surrounding the stoma is important for optimal adherence of the pouch, it is important that the site selected is free of scars, skin folds, and bony prominences.

## Postoperative Nursing Care

After an ileal or colon conduit procedure, stents are usually in place in the stoma for 1 week to 10 days. The stents promote urinary drainage. The person with a continent urostomy will usually have a catheter and/or stents in the stoma sutured in place to allow drainage from the reservoir. Another drain tube is placed into the pelvic area. The newly created internal reservoir must be protected from overdistention to prevent leakage at the anastomoses.

A nasogastric tube with gastric suction will be used until effective intestinal peristalsis has returned. Adequate drainage through the nasogastric tube is maintained to prevent pressure on the intestinal anastomosis. Nothing by mouth is permitted until peristalsis has returned; then a normal diet is gradually resumed, beginning with small amounts of water. IV fluids are continued until an adequate diet is tolerated.

### Maintaining skin integrity

In any type of urinary diversion, care must be taken to prevent urine leakage onto the surrounding skin and abdominal incision. For the ileal or colon conduit, a

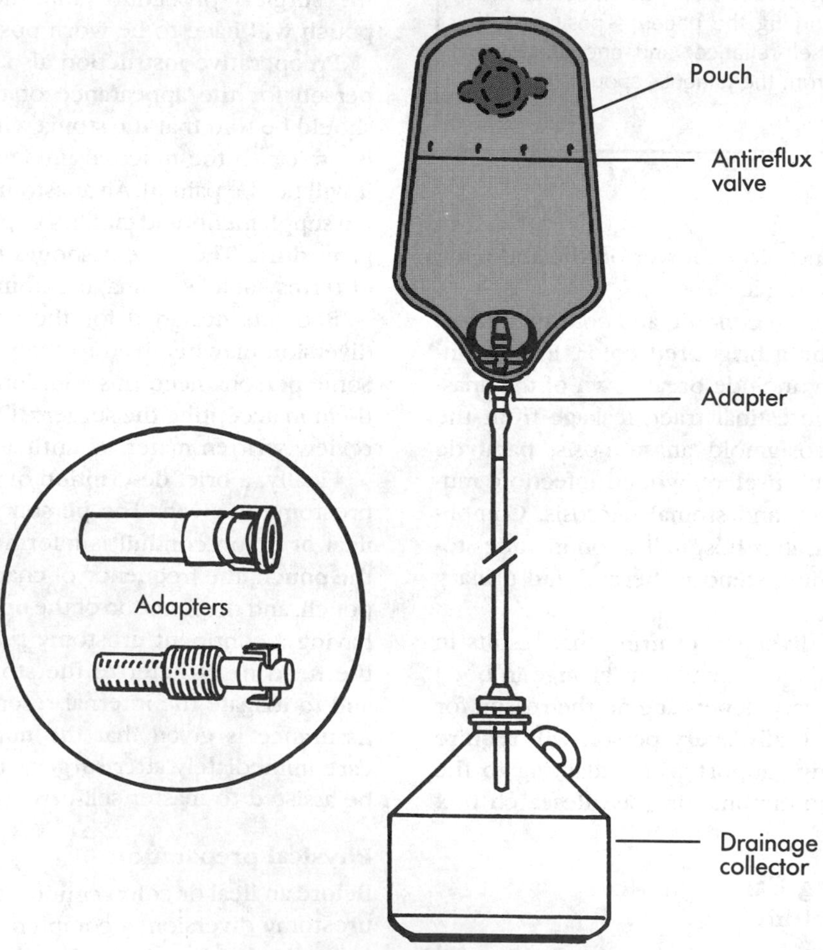


**FIGURE 49-16** Urostomy pouch connected to continuous drainage.

transparent pouch is placed around the stoma in the operating room. This allows visualization of the stoma, catheter or stents, and stoma sutures. The stoma should be bright pink or red. Any evidence of gray or black discoloration is reported to the surgeon, since this may indicate necrosis of the stoma. Careful checking of the stoma that is in contact with a catheter is imperative because improper positioning of a catheter may exert pressure on the stoma mucosa, leading to necrosis. The pouch is changed within 24 to 48 hours after surgery to allow for better visualization and assessment of the stoma and the peristomal skin.

In the early postoperative period, the pouch is positioned so that it drains to the side of the bed, facilitating drainage and emptying of the pouch. The urostomy pouch has a valve at the bottom that permits emptying. Drain tubing and a collection bag can be attached to the valve of the pouch to allow continuous drainage in the postoperative period (Figure 49-16). The procedure for changing the pouch is outlined in the Guidelines box below.

### Monitoring urine output

After any type of urinary diversion, urine output must be carefully monitored in the postoperative phase. Edema of the stoma or of the ureteral anastomosis site may cause failure of adequate urine drainage that may lead to hydronephrosis or to a break in the anastomosis. Other complications that may first be detected by decreased urine output include dehydration, obstruction of the ureters, or compromised renal function.[9]

**Guidelines for Changing a Urinary Pouch**

1. Assemble all supplies.
2. Empty the pouch and gently remove the pouch from the skin.
3. Cleanse the skin surrounding the stoma with mild soap and water. Rinse and pat dry. Mucus secretions should be washed off the stoma gently.
4. Place a rolled piece of gauze or cotton balls over the stomal opening to absorb draining urine while the skin is being cared for.
5. Measure the diameter of the stoma, and cut a corresponding opening in the skin barrier and the pouch or select the corresponding size of precut pouch.
6. Apply skin sealant around the stoma if desired. Allow the area to dry completely.
7. Attach the pouch to the skin barrier. The pouch and skin barrier may be applied to the skin separately or together. In the early postoperative period, it is easier to attach the pouch to the skin barrier and then to apply the system in one piece to the skin.
8. Apply the pouch and skin barrier around the stoma, keeping the adhesive area free of wrinkles or creases. Press gently but firmly into place. The valve at the bottom of the pouch must be closed or attached to drain tubing and a collection bag.

Decreased urine output associated with symptoms of peritonitis (fever, abdominal distention, pain) should alert the nurse to the possibility of intraperitoneal leakage caused by a leak at either the intestinal or the ureterointestinal anastomosis. If this occurs, emergency surgery is required to repair the leak.

The color and nature of the urine are also noted. Blood in the urine is expected in the immediate postoperative period with gradual clearing. Mucus, a normal discharge from the intestinal segment, is normally secreted from an ileal or colon conduit or continent urostomy.

The abdominal incision is observed *at least daily* for healing of the suture line.

### Promoting body image

A person with a urinary diversion will need time to adjust to the change in body appearance, to the loss of the usual pattern of elimination, to the presence of an external pouch or an internal reservoir, and to the presence of a stoma. An opportunity should be provided for the patient to explore feelings and to begin to cope with all the changes (see Chapter 9). Postoperative instruction in the care of the stoma is started early; mastering stomal care enhances the person's self-confidence and acceptance of the stoma.

### Facilitating learning the use and care of pouches

Postoperative instruction is started as soon as the patient feels able to participate in urostomy care. During the active phases of teaching, the pouch is removed more often than is recommended after discharge. The patient (or caregiver) must learn how to manage the assembly, application, and emptying of the selected pouch.

Postoperatively, the edema of the stoma begins to subside within 7 days, but the stoma continues to decrease gradually in size for the next 6 to 8 weeks. Therefore, before discharge, the patient is taught how to measure the stoma and how to adjust the pouch size to accommodate the smaller stoma. Too large an opening can lead to skin problems for persons with an ileal or colon conduit. Too small an opening may restrict circulation or cause trauma to the stoma. The opening should be no more than 2 to 3 mm larger than the stoma.

Several types of pouches are available (Figures 49-17 and 49-18). All have two things in common: a pouch to collect the urine and an outlet or valve at the bottom for easy emptying every 3 to 4 hours. The basic types of pouches are (1) semidisposable pouches that fit onto a permanent disk or faceplate and (2) one-piece or two-piece disposable pouches that are discarded after use. The pouches adhere to the body with a skin barrier to form a watertight seal. The type of pouch selected depends on the patient's preference, body build, and special needs, such as physical or visual impairment. The enterostomal therapy nurse can assist the patient in the assessment and selection of the appropriate pouch.

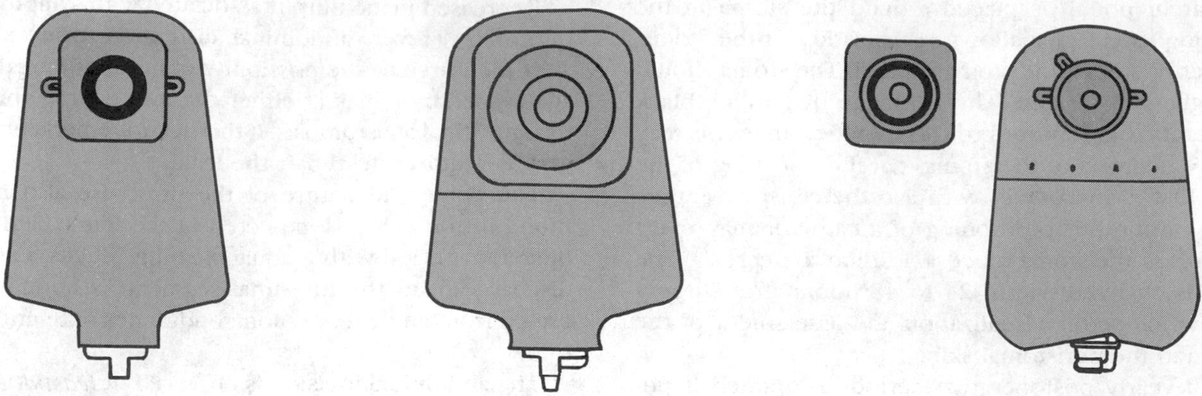

FIGURE 49-17 Disposable one- and two-piece pouches.

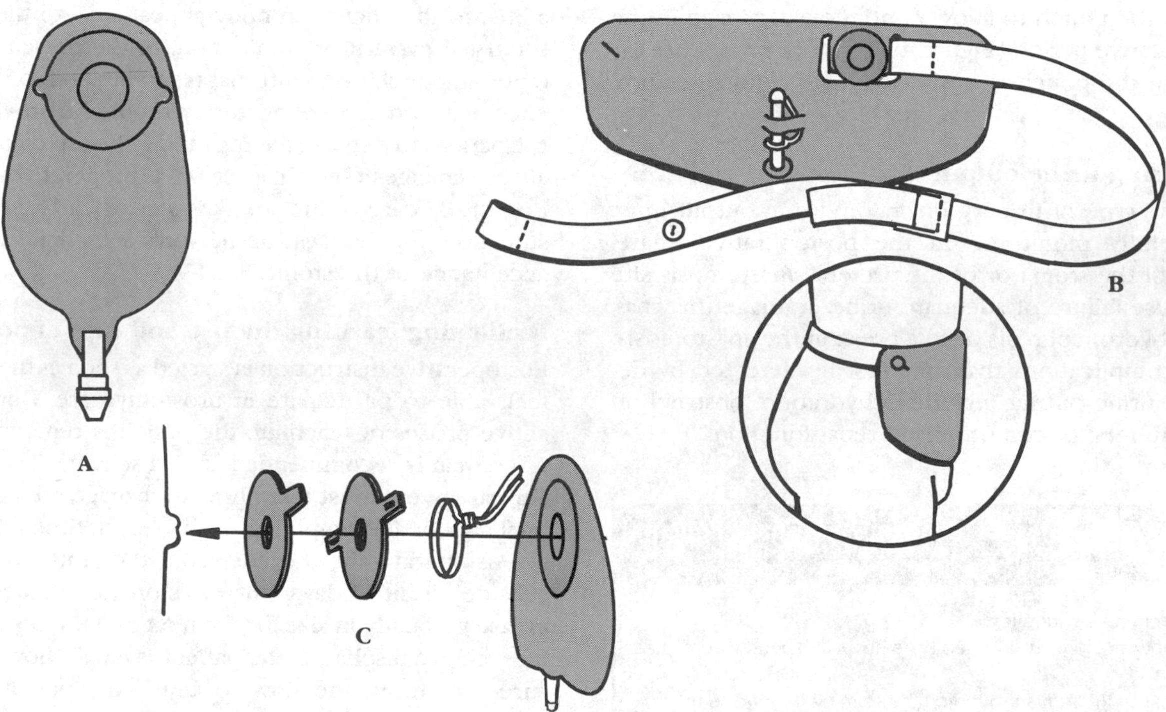


FIGURE 49-18 Reusable pouches. A, One-piece pouch. B, One-piece nonadhesive pouch. C, Two-piece reusable faceplate and reusable or disposable pouch.

Most persons can wear a pouch for 3 to 5 days between changes. An interval longer than 7 days should be discouraged because of the risk of infection. An appropriate schedule that eliminates leakage and provides the best skin protection needs to be determined. For example, if the pouch tends to show signs of impending leakage or skin redness on the fifth day, it should be changed every 3 to 4 days—before leakage and skin problems occur. This individualized schedule provides security and prevents skin problems.

## Potential Problems of Urinary Diversions

The person with a urinary diversion is at greater risk for *urinary tract infection* (UTI) because of the shorter distance from the urinary diversion to the kidneys. The patient must be taught the signs and symptoms of UTI (cloudy urine, blood in urine, strong odor to urine, flank pain, fever, malaise). Urine cultures are correctly obtained by catheter from the ileal or colon conduit stoma. A specimen taken from the pouch is likely to be contaminated. A pouch with an antireflux valve is recommended to reduce infection from bacteria found in the pouch.

Problems with the *peristomal skin* include erythema and irritation from contact with urine, candidal infections, allergic dermatitis, and pseudoverrucous lesions. Table 49-13 lists measures to relieve these problems.

*Problems with the stoma* include bleeding, stenosis,

**TABLE 49-13 Peristomal Skin Problems**

| PROBLEM | DESCRIPTION | THERAPY |
|---|---|---|
| Erythema | Redness from contact with urine | Correct pouch opening for better fit around stoma.<br>Change pouch system if leakage occurs. |
| Candidal infection | Red rash surrounding stoma | Administer antifungal powder. |
| Allergic skin reaction | Redness, weeping | Change pouch system.<br>Eliminate offending products.<br>If severe, refer patient to dermatologist. |
| Pseudoverrucous lesions | Raised, painful, wartlike areas next to stoma | Cover exposed skin by recalibrating stomal opening.<br>Protect affected skin area. |

Modified from Hampton BG, Bryant RA: *Ostomies and continent diversions,* St Louis, 1992, Mosby.

or hernia. A small amount of bleeding from the stomal mucosa may occur when the stoma is cleansed. This generally stops within a few seconds. If bleeding persists or is unusually severe, the physician is notified. Blood that originates from the urinary tract rather than the stoma may be related to complications such as infection or calculi. Patients also need to be forewarned about medicines that will discolor the urine; for example, doxorubicin (Adriamycin) will produce red urine. Peristomal hernia is treated by surgery; however, some patients may elect not to have the hernia repaired. The pouch opening may need to be adjusted or enlarged to accommodate the stoma.

Electrolyte imbalance may develop if the urine is retained in the conduit because of stomal or loop stenosis. The conduit mucosa reabsorbs chloride from the urine, and the patient may develop a ***metabolic hyperchloremic acidosis.*** A person with optimal renal function has no difficulty excreting the reabsorbed chloride. When renal function is compromised, the patient is more likely to develop electrolyte problems. This reabsorption can also occur in those with internal reservoirs because the urine is retained within the internal pouch until the stoma is catheterized and the urine drained.[1] Follow-up urologic visits and electrolyte studies are imperative.

## Discharge Planning

Before the patient is discharged from the hospital, the nurse must be certain that the individual can manage the urinary drainage and can detect any deviations from normal. A return visit or an opportunity for telephone consultation with the primary nurse involved in the teaching or the enterostomal therapy nurse is extremely helpful so that questions that arise after discharge can be addressed. Home health care nurse assistance may be required for a period of time, as well as ongoing urologic care.

In summary, at the time of discharge the person should be able to explain the nature of the urinary diversion, expected appearance of the stoma, care of the stoma and pouch, and signs and symptoms to be reported to the physician.

## QUESTIONS TO CONSIDER

- What are the differences between upper and lower urinary tract infections in terms of causative organisms, clinical manifestations, and treatment? Why is it important to stress prevention of UTIs to patients who are at risk for infection?
- What are the differences and similarities among acute and chronic glomerulonephritis and nephrotic syndrome?
- What are the effects of obstruction of urinary flow? How do symptoms differ depending on the site of obstruction? What is the most important difference between care given to persons with drainage from the renal pelvis and those with drainage from the bladder?
- Mrs. G., age 45, married with two children, had a urinary diversion 3 days ago. She is refusing to look at the stoma and feigns sleep during pouch changes. What factors may be influencing her behavior? What approaches would be helpful to move her toward self-care?

## CRITICAL THINKING ACTIVITIES

- Mary's older sister recently developed chronic renal failure as a result of polycystic kidney disease. Mary is very concerned because she has three teenaged children. Are Mary's concerns warranted, since neither she nor her children have any symptoms of kidney disease? What interventions are appropriate on Mary's behalf?
- After outpatient surgery, Mr. Clark complains that he needs to urinate. The nurse provides privacy and gives him a urinal. He voids about 50 ml of urine. About an hour later, he again complains of needing to urinate and voids only 30 ml of urine. What is your assessment of this situation, and what should the nurse do? Why is urinary retention considered a urologic emergency?

# CHAPTER SUMMARY

- The major health problems of the urinary system include congenital, inflammatory, vascular, and obstructive disorders; urinary incontinence; and trauma to the urinary tract.

## CONGENITAL DISORDERS

- Polycystic kidney disease is an inherited disease in which cysts form in the kidneys and enlarge and rupture, causing scarring with loss of kidney function. Treatment is symptomatic with control of infection.

## INFLAMMATORY DISORDERS

- Chronic health problems predisposing to urinary tract infections (UTIs) include diabetes mellitus, gout, hypertension, polycystic kidney disease, multiple myeloma, and glomerulonephritis.
- UTIs may occur in the lower urinary tract (most common) or ascend into the kidney (pyelonephritis).
- The most important defenses against UTI are large urine volume, unobstructed flow, and complete emptying of the bladder to prevent urinary stasis.
- It is essential to teach the patient receiving antibiotic therapy for UTI to continue antibiotics for the entire prescribed course even if symptoms resolve.
- Acute glomerulonephritis usually follows a streptococcal infection and is a result of an antigen-antibody reaction; the significant effect is loss of glomerular basement membrane porosity. Proteinuria, hematuria, and fluid retention result. Management consists of bedrest, maintenance of fluid balance, and prevention of infection.
- Chronic glomerulonephritis may follow the acute disease or may develop from unknown causes; it is characterized by slow, progressive glomerular destruction terminating in renal failure. No specific therapy exists; patients are taught to live with their disease and report signs of exacerbation.
- Nephrotic syndrome is a constellation of symptoms (severe generalized edema, pronounced proteinuria, hypoalbuminemia, hyperlipidemia) resulting from kidney damage; it often progresses to kidney failure. Management consists of administering steroids and diuretics, promoting comfort (because of fatigue and massive edema), encouraging a restricted protein and sodium diet, and teaching the patient self-care.

## VASCULAR DISORDERS

- Vascular disorders include renal artery stenosis characterized by hypertension and nephrosclerosis caused by hypertension; treatment consists of control of hypertension and correction of the stenosis.

## OBSTRUCTIVE DISORDERS

- Disorders that may obstruct the urinary tract include urinary calculi, tumors of the kidney or bladder, prostatic hyertrophy, or urethral strictures. Backup of urine causes hydronephrosis, leading to kidney damage. General interventions include monitoring for signs of additional obstruction, promoting fluid balance and comfort, preventing urinary complications, and patient teaching.
- Urinary retention is the inability to empty the bladder; small amounts of urine voided frequently may result from retention with overflow; causes may be mechanical or functional. Methods of urinary drainage include urethral catheter drainage, direct bladder drainage with cystostomy tube, and catheter drainage of kidney pelvis and ureters. Intermittent catheter drainage can be taught to the patient for home care of urinary retention.
- The most common urinary stones are calcium oxalates; the stones cause renal colic from urine backup or from irritation or stretching of the ureters. If the stone does not pass spontaneously and is causing symptoms or damage, it must be removed surgically or broken up by lithotripsy or laser treatment.
- Recurrence of some renal stones can be controlled by an alkaline-ash or acid-ash diet (depending on the type of stone).
- Bladder cancer is more common than malignant renal tumors; both are removed surgically. If the entire bladder is removed, permanent urinary diversion is necessary.

## URINARY INCONTINENCE

- Urinary incontinence is not a normal part of aging; whenever urinary incontinence is present, the cause should be thoroughly investigated.
- Major types of urinary incontinence include stress, urge, and overflow incontinence; two other forms are reflex and total incontinence. Control largely depends on cause. Stress incontinence may be controlled surgically. Nursing interventions include teaching perineal exercises and bladder retraining. Keeping the person dry is of utmost importance; waterproof pants or external urinary drainage may be used when control is inadequate.

## UROLOGIC SURGERY

- Postoperative care for patients having urologic surgery includes promoting ventilation, monitoring urine output, observing for signs of distention and hemorrhage, protecting the skin from urinary drainage through the incision, and patient teaching.

- Two types of urinary diversion procedures include ileal or colon conduit and continent urostomy.
- Postoperative care after a urinary diversion procedure includes maintaining skin integrity, monitoring urine output, promoting body image, and facilitating learning the use and care of pouches.

## REFERENCES


1. Benson M, Olsson C: Urinary diversion, *Urol Clin North Am* 19(4):779-795, 1992.
2. Bristol-Myers Squibb Company: *For a better way of living with a urostomy: the Durahesive Sur-Fit way,* Princeton, NJ, 1992, Convatec.
3. Bristol-Myers Squibb Company: *Living with an urostomy the easy, Active Life Way,* Princeton, NJ, 1992, Convatec.
4. Carroll PR: Urothelial carcinoma: cancers of the bladder, ureter, and renal pelvis. In Tanagho EA, McAninch JW, editors: *Smith's general urology,* East Norwalk, Conn, 1992, Appleton & Lange.
5. Coe FL, Parks JH, Asplin JR: The pathogenesis and treatment of kidney stones, *N Engl J Med* 327(16):1141-1152, 1992.
6. Davidson RA, Wilcox CS: Newer tests for the diagnosis of renovascular disease, *JAMA* 268(23):3353-3358, 1992.
7. Hampton BG, Bryant RA: *Ostomies and continent diversions,* St Louis, 1992, Mosby.
8. Heneghan GM et al: The Indiana pouch: a continent urinary diversion, *J Enterostom Ther* 17:231-236, 1990.
9. Licklinder D, Mauffray D: Conventional urostomy vs continent urostomy, *Ostomy/Wound Management* 34:26-29, 1991.
10. McAninch JW: Disorders of the kidneys. In Tanagho EA, McAninch JW, editors: *Smith's general urology,* East Norwalk, Conn, 1992, Appleton & Lange.
11. Meares EM: Nonspecific infections of the genitourinary tract. In Tanagho EA, McAninch JW, editors: *Smith's general urology,* East Norwalk, Conn, 1992, Appleton & Lange.
12. Powers I, William D: Urinary incontinence, *Nurs '92* 22(12):46-47, 1992.
13. Smith DB, Babaian RJ: Patient adjustment to an ileal conduit after cystectomy, *J Enterostom Ther* 16:244-246, 1989.
14. Spirnak JP, Resnick MI: Urinary stones. In Tanagho EA, McAninch JW, editors: *Smith's general urology,* East Norwalk, Conn, 1992, Appleton & Lange.
15. Tanagho EA, Schmidt RA: Neuropathic bladder disorders. In Tanagho EA, McAninch JW, editors: *Smith's general urology,* East Norwalk, Conn, 1992, Appleton & Lange.
16. Vincenti FG, Amend WJC: Diagnosis of medical renal diseases. In Tahagho EA, McAninch JW, editors: *Smith's general urology,* East Norwalk, Conn, 1992, Appleton & Lange.
17. Wiseman KC: Nephrotic syndrome: pathophysiology and treatment, *ANNA J* 18(5):469-478, 1991.

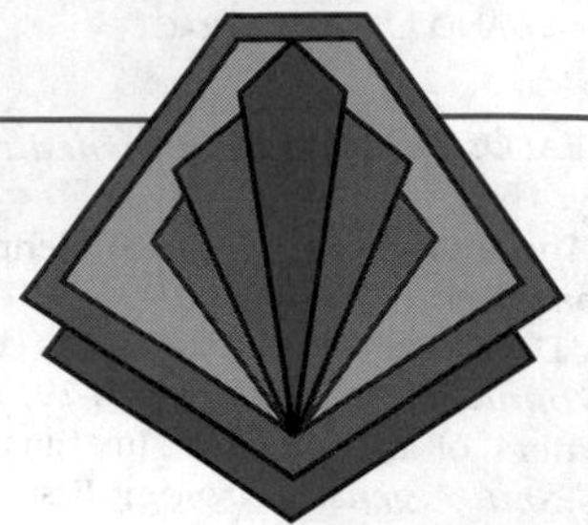

C H A P T E R 50

# Management of Persons With Renal Failure

*Marilyn Rossman Bartucci*

## CHAPTER OBJECTIVES

***After studying this chapter, the learner should be able to do the following:***

1 Explain the pathophysiologic changes and clinical manifestations of acute and chronic renal failure.
2 Compare and contrast the medical and nursing management of patients during the oliguric and diuretic phases of acute renal failure.
3 Explain the benefits of continuous renal replacement therapy for patients with acute renal failure.
4 Identify treatment goals for patients with chronic renal failure.
5 Explain the physiologic principles of dialysis.
6 Compare and contrast nursing assessment and management of patients undergoing hemodialysis, peritoneal dialysis, and kidney transplantation.

## KEY TERMS

acute renal failure (ARF)
anuria
azotemia
chronic renal failure
continuous ambulatory peritoneal dialysis (CAPD)
continuous arteriovenous hemodialysis (CAVHD)
continuous arteriovenous hemofiltration (CAVH)
continuous cyclic peritoneal dialysis (CCPD)
continuous renal replacement therapy (CRRT)
dialysate
dialysis
diffusion
disequilibrium phenomenon
diuresis
end-stage renal disease (ESRD)
epoetin alfa (EPO)
hemodialysis
kinetic modeling
oliguria
osmosis
peritoneal dialysis
renal failure
renal insufficiency
slow continuous ultrafiltration (SCUF)
ultrafiltration
uremia

**Renal failure** is the state of total or nearly total loss of kidney function. The kidneys have a tremendous ability to adapt to a decreasing number of functioning nephrons. With less than 25% of the original nephrons functioning, the kidneys are able to excrete waste products and maintain fluid and electrolyte balance.[13] As renal failure develops, laboratory tests reflect the changes in homeostasis, and the person appears clinically ill. The person in renal failure cannot independently sustain life.

Renal failure may be acute in onset or may develop slowly and progressively over a course of several years. When renal failure occurs suddenly, as within a few days, biochemical changes are often dramatic, and the person has little time to adjust to these changes. The person becomes very ill and is frequently treated in a critical care area.

When renal failure occurs as the end result of a chronic kidney illness in which kidney is destroyed progressively over the course of several months or years, control of symptoms and preservation of functional abilities are achievable goals. Dietary adjustment, medications, and attention to preventing additional illnesses must compensate for loss of renal function in the early stages of progressing renal failure. As renal function continues to deteriorate, dialysis or transplantation becomes necessary to maintain life.

**Renal insufficiency** exists when a significant loss of renal function occurs but enough functioning remains to maintain an internal environment consistent with life. When renal insufficiency exists, any additional physiologic stressor, such as illness, dietary indiscretion, or nephrotoxic drugs, can lead to renal failure. The individual experiencing renal insufficiency may appear and feel well, even though laboratory data reflect deterioration in renal function. Renal insufficiency occurs as a phase in gradually but chronically progressive renal disease.

# Acute Renal Failure

## ETIOLOGY/EPIDEMIOLOGY

**Acute renal failure (ARF)** occurs as a sudden and frequently reversible decrease or cessation of kidney function related to prerenal, renal, or postrenal factors. It generally follows an identifiable trauma of either toxicity, ischemia, infection, or obstruction.[1] The health of the individual before the insult is usually good.

Recovery from an episode of ARF depends on the underlying illness, the patient's condition, and the careful, supportive management given during the period of renal shutdown. Mortality associated with ARF approaches 40% to 50%. In postsurgical or trauma patients, mortality rates as high as 60% to 80% have been reported.[16] These statistics largely reflect the deaths of severely ill persons in whom renal failure is a sequela to extensive underlying illness. Because of the availability of dialysis, mortality from potassium intoxification, fluid overload, and acidosis has been reduced. The potential for recovery of renal function for those who survive acute tubular necrosis (ATN) is good. Although recovery statistics indicate that the kidney may regenerate more completely after toxic injury in comparison with ischemic injury, follow-up studies of persons several years after episodes of ATN show normal or near-normal renal function.

For those in whom ARF has been caused by glomerular disease or severe infection of the kidneys, the prognosis may not be as favorable. Return of renal function is determined by the extent of scarring and obliteration of functional nephrons that has occurred during the acute episode of kidney failure.

Box 50-1 lists the major causes of ischemic, toxic, and obstructive injuries to the kidney that can lead to ARF. Additionally, other conditions can precipitate ARF:

1. Acute glomerular disease
2. Acute severe kidney infection
3. Bilateral occlusion of the renal arteries
4. Intravascular hemolysis
5. Malignant hypertension

All of these conditions lead to massive and rapid destruction of kidney tissue.

**BOX 50-1 Conditions and Substances That Produce Ischemic, Nephrotoxic, or Obstructive Injury to the Kidneys**

**ISCHEMIC CAUSES* (PRERENAL)**

Hypovolemia
Blood loss (surgery, trauma)
Plasma loss (burns, surgery, acute pancreatitis)
Sodium and water loss (prolonged diarrhea or vomiting, gastrointestinal tract drainage, sustained high fever)
Cardiac failure
Myocardial infarction
Cardiac dysrhythmias
Congestive heart failure
Septic shock

**TOXIC SUBSTANCES† (RENAL)**

Solvents (carbon tetrachloride, methanol, ethylene glycol)
Heavy metals (lead, arsenic, mercury)
Antibiotics (kanamycin, gentamicin, polymyxin B, amphotericin B, colistin, neomycin, phenazopyridine)
Pesticides
Mushrooms

**OBSTRUCTION (POSTRENAL)**

Ureteral: calculi, blood clot, retroperitoneal tumor
Bladder: prostatic hypertrophy, carcinoma, tumor
Urethral: stricture, stenosis

*Inadequate perfusion of the kidney.
†Direct injury to functional components of kidney cells.

## PATHOPHYSIOLOGY

Renal ischemia occurs when blood flow to the kidneys is reduced. The response of the normal kidney is *vasoconstriction,* which compounds the problem of reduced renal blood flow and increases renal ischemia. Perfusion problems affect both kidneys. When ischemia is prolonged, renal tubular necrosis and frank renal failure develops.

Substances that are toxic to the tubules affect the kidneys bilaterally. The kidney, with its large blood flow and ability to concentrate fluid in the medullary portion (where the tubules are located), creates conditions in which exposure of tubular cells to toxins is maximized. Damage to the cells leads to decreased glomerular permeability and tubular obstruction.

The course of ARF is usually characterized by an initial oliguric phase followed in a number of days (10 to 15) to a few weeks by a diuretic period. Major problems during the *oliguric* phase include inability to excrete fluid loads, regulate electrolytes, and excrete metabolic waste products (Table 50-1). During the *diuretic* phase, large amounts of fluid (4 to 5 L/day) and electrolytes are lost.

### Oliguric Phase

#### Inability to excrete fluid loads

Because of decreased kidney function, fluids are retained in the body, resulting in fluid overload and edema (see Chapter 20). When fluid overload is excessive, congestive heart failure and pulmonary edema may occur. Hypertension accompanies ARF when the person is hypervolemic.

Inability to excrete fluid loads leads to decreased urine output. Either **oliguria** (urine output less than 400 ml/day) or **anuria** (urine output less than 100 ml/

**TABLE 50-1 Symptoms Caused by Physiologic Changes in Acute Renal Failure**

| PHYSIOLOGIC EFFECT | FINDINGS | SYMPTOMS |
|---|---|---|
| **OLIGURIC PHASE** | | |
| Inability to excrete metabolic wastes | Increased serum:<br>Urea nitrogen<br>Creatinine | Nausea, vomiting<br>Drowsiness, confusion<br>Coma<br>Gastrointestinal bleeding<br>Asterixis<br>Pericarditis |
| Inability to regulate electrolytes | Hyperkalemia<br>Hyponatremia<br>Acidosis<br>Hypocalcemia<br>Hyperphosphatemia | Nausea, vomiting<br>Cardiac dysrhythmias<br>Kussmaul's breathing<br>Drowsiness, confusion<br>Coma |
| Inability to excrete fluid loads | Fluid overload<br>Hypervolemia | Edema<br>Congestive heart failure<br>Pulmonary edema<br>Neck vein distention<br>Hypertension |
| Hematologic dysfunction | Anemia<br>Platelet dysfunction<br>Leukopenia | Fatigue<br>Bleeding<br>Infection |
| **DIURETIC PHASE** | | |
| Increased production of urine (deficit in concentrating ability of tubules and osmotic diuretic effect of high BUN). Slowly increasing excretion of metabolic wastes | Hypovolemia<br>Loss of sodium<br>Loss of potassium<br>High blood urea nitrogen (BUN) initially<br>BUN gradually returns to baseline | Urine output of up to 4-5 L/day<br>Postural hypotension<br>Tachycardia<br>Improving mental alertness and activity<br>Weight loss<br>Thirst<br>Dry mucous membranes<br>Decreased skin turgor |

day) may be present, although oliguria is more common. Classically, the patient in ARF shows a fall in urine output within 1 to 2 days to between 50 and 400 ml/day. The urine *specific gravity is low* (1.010), and the osmolality of the urine approaches that of the person's serum (280 to 320 mOsm). Specific gravity and urine osmolality remain within this fixed range because the tubules have lost the ability to excrete sodium and water.[14]

The three major electrolyte problems are retention of potassium, excretion of sodium, and metabolic acidosis.

**Potassium imbalance.** In the normal individual, the potassium ion is exchanged in the distal convoluted tubule of the nephron for either sodium or hydrogen ions; healthy persons cannot conserve the potassium ion. However, in the individual with ARF in whom many tubular cells are no longer functioning, no mechanism exists to remove potassium from the body. *Hyperkalemia* (the most sudden hazard in oliguric ARF) is said to exist when the serum concentration of this ion reaches a level of 5.5 mEq/L or higher. Serum concentrations of 7 to 10 mEq/L can be quickly reached in ARF and are incompatible with normal cardiac function and life.

In monitoring for signs of potassium toxicity, electrocardiography and laboratory determinations of serum potassium are the most reliable indicators. Occasionally, neuromuscular symptoms such as paresthesias and paralysis (distal moving to proximal) are seen.[18] Pulse changes must not be relied on to indicate the degree of rise of potassium in the patient's system.

**Sodium imbalance.** *Hyponatremia* in ARF most often develops with overhydration. The oliguric patient cannot excrete large volumes of urine; when the administration of sodium-free or low-sodium intravenous or oral fluids continues, the serum is diluted and the serum concentration of sodium falls.

In this situation, hyponatremia is accompanied or caused by hypervolemia. In the very acutely ill patient, the situation typically occurs when the person receives numerous drugs and fluids in an attempt to treat coexisting life-threatening problems. When the volume of drugs and fluids cannot be reduced to a safe level, dialysis is required to remove the excess fluid and restore sodium balance.

Signs and symptoms of hyponatremia include warm, moist, flushed skin; muscle weakness; muscle twitching; and mental status changes such as confusion, delirium, coma, and convulsions. Serum sodium concentrations are less than 130 mEq/L. The hematocrit and hemoglobin values fall suddenly in the absence of bleeding because of hemodilution.

*Increases in total body content of sodium* also occur in ARF when the patient is receiving medications high in sodium content and excess sodium in the diet. Edema and increasing blood pressure indicate retention of sodium and water, even though the serum sodium concentration is normal or below normal.

**Metabolic acidosis.** Acidosis develops when hydrogen ion secretion and bicarbonate ion production diminish in the tubules. The pH of the blood decreases, the carbon dioxide content decreases, and central nervous system symptoms of drowsiness progressing to stupor and coma may appear. Although the lungs cannot compensate totally for the increasing acid load, they help determine the rate at which acidosis develops and the frequency or need for dialysis. In compensating for increased metabolic acid loads, the lungs attempt to excrete more carbon dioxide. Kussmaul's breathing is noted.

**Inability to excrete metabolic wastes**

Decreased kidney function alters the body's ability to eliminate metabolic waste products, producing typical signs and symptoms referred to as **uremia.** Blood urea nitrogen (BUN) and serum creatinine values rise sharply. In the person who has already sustained illness and trauma, BUN values may increase at a rate of 30 mg/dl/day. Signs and symptoms include neurologic manifestations such as confusion, convulsions, coma, and asterixis. Gastrointestinal bleeding may result from uremic gastritis or colitis. Decreased cellular immunity causes an increased risk of infections to develop. Bruising and bleeding result from changes in blood coagulation factors. Pericarditis is thought to develop as a result of pericardial irritation from accumulated metabolic wastes. A pericardial friction rub may be present on auscultation.

### Diuretic Phase

After a period of oliguria or anuria that may last a few days to several weeks, patients recovering renal function pass into another distinct phase of illness, **diuresis,** which is characterized by increased urine output. Increased output indicates that the damaged nephrons are healing and are able to begin excreting urine. At first, daily urine volume increases slowly, although within 1 to 2 days, diuresis up to or exceeding 4 to 5 L/day may occur. Although fluid can be excreted, the kidneys are not yet healed. Often the person is unable to excrete proportional amounts of waste products, and BUN and creatinine may rise or remain elevated as urine volume increases. At times, excessive excretion of sodium and potassium occurs during diuresis. Complete recovery of renal function is slow and requires anywhere from days to several months. Renal function is normal or near normal when the kidney can both concentrate and dilute urine, control serum electrolytes, and excrete nitrogenous wastes.

## PREVENTION

### Primary Prevention

The incidence of ARF can be reduced by the identification and control of environmental risk factors. A significant factor in preventive care is the control of nephrotoxic drugs. Attempts to control the distribution and identification of nephrotoxic drugs and chemicals are primarily accomplished through the Food and Drug Administration (FDA). Identification of nephrotoxic drugs and chemicals, enforced labeling of these substances, and drug dispensing by prescription only are examples of the FDA's attempts to promote public health. Proper labeling and storage of potentially toxic drugs and chemicals in the home can further reduce the number of accidental ingestions of nephrotoxic substances.

### Secondary Prevention

Prevention of ARF includes increased medical supervision of persons with sore throats and upper respiratory infections and increased case finding and treatment of individuals with bacteriuria and obstructive disease of the urinary system. The greatest incidence of ARF occurs in persons with major trauma, extensive burns, surgery of the heart or large blood vessels, massive blood loss, and severe myocardial infarction. Frequent monitoring of urine output and detection of excessive losses of body fluid of these patients will help to identify instances of inadequate renal perfusion before renal failure develops.

## MEDICAL MANAGEMENT

Medical management of the patient is specific to the cause and phase of ARF. During the *oliguric* phase, the goals are to control fluids, regulate electrolytes, control and promote excretion of metabolic wastes, and reduce tissue catabolism. This is accomplished by conservative management with medications, fluid restriction, and a diet prescription that includes low-sodium, low-potassium, low-protein, and high-carbohydrate recommendations. In severe cases of ARF, when conservative management is not effective, dialysis is required. **Dialysis,** the process by which waste products in the blood are filtered through a semipermeable membrane, is indicated when the patient with ARF is fluid-overloaded and/or has rapidly progressive **azotemia** (high BUN), hyperkalemia, and metabolic acidosis. Three methods of dialysis are used: hemodialysis (see p. 1679), peritoneal dialysis (see p. 1687), and continuous renal replacement therapy.

### Continuous Renal Replacement Therapy

**Continuous renal replacement therapy (CRRT)** provides continuous (8 to 24 hours or more) ultrafiltration of extracellular fluid and clearance of uremic toxins.[15] It must be administered in a critical care setting. This therapy does not require the use of a hemodialysis machine; instead, it relies on the patient's own blood pressure to power the system. The ultrafiltration system is composed of arterial and venous tubing, the hemofilter, and an ultrafiltration collection receptacle. The success of CRRT depends on the maintenance of blood flow through the hemofilter. Both arterial and venous vascular access are required. Blood flows up to 200 ml/min can be obtained using an external arteriovenous shunt or percutaneous femoral catheter. In most patients, a mean arterial blood pressure of 60 mm Hg is required to maintain adequate blood flow.[18]

During CRRT, water, electrolytes, and other solutes are removed as the patient's blood passes over the semipermeable membrane in the hemofilter. The resulting ultrafiltrate is a protein-free fluid with a solute and electrolyte concentration similar to plasma. The plasma proteins and cellular components of the blood remain in the hemofilter circuit and return to the venous circulation. The mass transfer of water and solutes across a semipermeable membrane is a result of convection and diffusion. The convection forces applied across the hemofilter depend primarily on the patient's arterial blood pressure. The higher the blood pressure, the greater is the hydrostatic pressure within the hemofilter. Diffusion is the process by which solutes are passively transported across a semipermeable membrane (p. 1678). It depends on the presence of a concentration gradient across the membrane. In CRRT, a concentration gradient is established by infusing dialysate into the nonblood side of the hemofilter.

Removal of plasma water and electrolytes by CRRT is a gradual process that closely resembles the kidney's normal function. Because the process is gradual, rapid fluctuations in fluid and electrolyte status do not occur. Therefore CRRT is recommended for patients with ARF who are too hemodynamically unstable to tolerate hemodialysis or peritoneal dialysis. Patients who may benefit from CRRT are those with advanced cardiac disease, abdominal wounds, cerebral edema, or sepsis.

Three variations of CRRT are in use: slow continuous ultrafiltration, continuous arteriovenous hemofiltration, and continuous arteriovenous hemodialysis. Each of these is designed to meet the renal replacement needs of a specific group of patients.

**Slow continuous ultrafiltration (SCUF)** slowly removes small amounts of plasma water and solutes at a rate of 150 to 300 ml/hr. It is used to control fluid balance and is highly effective in patients with severe congestive heart failure who do not respond to diuretic therapy. Fluid removal by ultrafiltration can achieve significant preload reduction in these patients. SCUF is unsuitable for patients with ARF who are azotemic or have significant electrolyte abnormalities, because only small amounts of solutes are removed.

**Continuous arteriovenous hemofiltration (CAVH)** removes large amounts of plasma water and solutes at rates of 400 to 800 ml/hr. Control of fluid volume and electrolyte balance is achieved through large-volume fluid exchanges. Hourly ultrafiltrate loss is replaced by prescribed amounts of a sterile intravenous electrolyte solution. CAVH provides a mechanism of diluting the patient's plasma by selective replacement of solutes. It can be used as the primary dialysis therapy for patients with ARF who have mild to moderate azotemia and electrolyte disturbances.

**Continuous arteriovenous hemodialysis (CAVHD)** combines the convective transport of CAVH with diffusion dialysis. Sterile dialysate fluid is infused into the ultrafiltration compartment of the hemofilter. The dialysate flows countercurrent to the blood flow, which increases diffusion of solutes from the blood to the ultrafiltration compartment. Solute removal is much greater than in CAVH. CAVHD can be used as primary dialysis therapy in a wide variety of critically ill patients, including patients with ARF who have severe azotemia, electrolyte imbalances, and acid-base disturbances.

The goals of nursing management for patients undergoing CRRT are optimization of the patient's fluid volume and hemodynamic status, maintenance of ultrafiltration system patency, prevention of blood loss from line disconnection, and prevention of infection.

During the *diuretic* phase, medical management centers around maintaining adequate fluid balance and regulating electrolytes. Even though the patient may be excreting large volumes of urine, dialysis may still be necessary to control electrolyte balance adequately. Protein restrictions are continued until BUN and serum creatinine levels decline.

## NURSING MANAGEMENT

### ♦ ASSESSMENT

#### Subjective Data

Data to be collected from the person with ARF or significant other include the following:

- Voiding patterns, including any recent changes
- Weight gain (fluid retention)
- Nausea and vomiting
- Patient and family history of renal disease
- Medication use (prescription and over the counter)
- Recent surgery, anesthesia, or trauma
- Muscle weakness
- Mental status changes

#### Objective Data

Data to be collected from the person with ARF or significant other include the following:

- Amount of urine excreted in 24 hours
- Blood pressure, particularly postural changes
- Fluid status: presence of peripheral, periorbital, or sacral edema; lung sounds; skin turgor; daily weights
- Halitosis as a result of acidosis and/or ammonia secretion
- Changes in mental status
- Pulse rate and rhythm

### ♦ NURSING DIAGNOSES

Nursing diagnoses are determined from analysis of patient data. Nursing diagnoses for the person with ARF may include but are not limited to the following:

| Diagnostic Title | Possible Etiologic Factors |
|---|---|
| Fluid volume deficit/excess | Abnormal fluid loss, compromised regulatory mechanism |
| Nutrition, altered: less than body requirements | Anorexia, nausea, restricted diet |
| Activity intolerance | Biochemical alterations |
| Injury, high risk for | Sensorimotor deficits, mental confusion |
| Infection, high risk for | Decreased nutrition, decreased immune response |
| Coping, ineffective (individual) | Changes in health status |
| Knowledge deficit | Lack of exposure/recall |

## ♦ EXPECTED PATIENT OUTCOMES

Expected patient outcomes for the person with ARF during the *oliguric* phase may include but are not limited to the following:

1. Controls fluids, electrolytes and waste products:
   a. Absence of pulmonary edema, absence or control of peripheral edema.
   b. Control of blood pressure (range between 140/90 and 100/60 mm Hg.
   c. Control of electrolyte balance: sodium 125 to 145 mEq/L, potassium 3.0 to 6.0 mEq/L, bicarbonate greater than 14 mEq/L.
   d. Control of protein catabolism: BUN less than 100 mg/dl, creatinine less than 12 mg/dl, absence of skin breakdown.
2. Eats diet high in calories and fat and restricted in protein and potassium.
3. Does not express fatigue.
4. Does not fall; bleeding does not occur.
5. No infection occurs.
6. Describes alternative ways of coping.
7. During the *diuretic* phase, states nature of illness, diet therapy, signs and symptoms to be reported to physician, and plans for follow-up care.

## ♦ INTERVENTIONS

### Maintaining Fluid and Electrolyte Balance

Control of fluids is essential during the oliguric phase of ARF because of the decreased ability of the kidneys to excrete urine. Nursing care is directed toward three broad objectives: (1) monitoring for signs of fluid overload, (2) maintaining the patient's energy expenditure at a level compatible with the individual's state of health, and (3) controlling or helping to control fluid intake.

All observations about the patient's state of hydration need to be recorded so that hour-to-hour and day-to-day comparisons can be made. Any finding indicating retention of fluids is reported to the physician. Edema can first be noted in dependent areas such as the feet and legs, in the presacral area, and around the eyes. It is important to remember, however, that edema may not be detected until the person has gained 5 to 10 pounds (2 to 5 kg) in fluid. The person is observed carefully for signs of pulmonary edema and congestive heart failure (see Chapter 31).

Central venous lines or arterial monitoring lines will help to provide data for short-term comparison in managing the fluid balance of the critically ill person. Positioning and activity are determined daily based on assessment of the energy level and ability to breath adequately.

All fluids (parenteral and oral) must total only slightly more than daily output if severe overhydration is to be avoided. Devices that allow precise control of intravenous fluids are added safety measures when giving fluids parenterally to anuric or oliguric patients. Accuracy in fluid balance records is essential.

### Promoting Nutrition

Most patients with ARF are too ill to tolerate oral feedings, either initially or for sustained periods. Some patients who are able to tolerate fluids orally find that eating food compounds the nausea they experience as a result of the altered biochemical environment and accompanying gastrointestinal tract irritation. If the patient is able tolerate ***oral feedings, dietary protein and potassium are restricted to modest amounts,*** thus increasing protein available for tissue building and increasing the palatability of the diet without leading to metabolic waste build-up or hyperkalemia.

A ***high-carbohydrate, high-fat*** diet is encouraged. Calories in the form of carbohydrates and fats provide energy and spare body protein stores, thus decreasing nonprotein nitrogen production. The body recycles urea to synthesize amino acids for protein building so that some regeneration of tissues can occur even though protein intake is curtailed.

### Promoting Rest/Activity Balance

The patient is placed on strict bedrest in the acute phase to decrease metabolic activity. Provide assistance with activities of daily living (ADL). Provide rest periods to conserve patient energy. Encourage ambulation when permitted and provide assistance as required.

### Preventing Injury

The patient with ARF is weak, may be confused, and may have visual changes, thus increasing risk of falls. The amount of supervision required during daily care must be assessed continually and appropriate actions taken to prevent injury. The confused, agitated, or restless patient must be protected from injury; keep side rails elevated and pad them if necessary. To allay patient/family anxiety, explain the rationale for the mental status change (electrolyte imbalance, uremia). (Care of the disoriented patient is described in Chapter 12.) Use meticulous skin care to prevent skin breakdown from edema.

Bleeding may occur from changes in blood coagulation factors. Use measures to prevent bleeding (see Guidelines box, p. 1664, left). (Further information on protection from bleeding can be found in Chapter 34.)

### Preventing Infection

Infection leads to tissue breakdown with production of metabolic wastes, which the patient with ARF has difficulty eliminating. Aseptic technique must be ***rigorously*** pursued during all treatments, especially with indwelling lines and catheters. ***The patient should be isolated from anyone with an infection,*** including patients, visitors, and hospital personnel. Pruritus frequently occurs and may lead to skin lesions from scratching. Measures to relieve pruritus include bathing the patient every day (or more often if necessary) using superfat soap. Administer prescribed antipruritics.

In compensating for increased metabolic acid loads, the lungs attempt to excrete more carbon dioxide. Pul-

### Guidelines for Care of the Person With Acute Renal Failure

1. Maintaining fluid and electrolyte balance
   a. Maintain fluid restrictions.
   b. Monitor intravenous fluids carefully.
   c. Keep accurate records of intake and output.
   d. Weigh patient daily.
   e. Monitor vital signs frequently, including postural signs.
   f. Assess fluid status of patient frequently.
   g. Administer phosphate-binding medications as prescribed.
   h. Monitor serum electrolytes.
   i. During diuretic phase:
      (1) Assess for changes in mental status indicative of low serum levels.
      (2) Assess for presence of irregular apical pulse indicative of hypokalemia.
2. Maintaining nutrition
   a. Provide fluid in small amounts during oliguric phase; ginger ale and other effervescent soft drinks may be tolerated better than other fluids.
   b. Provide a diet:
      (1) Restricted in protein, as prescribed.
      (2) High in carbohydrates and fat during protein restriction.
      (3) Low in potassium during hyperkalemia and high in potassium during hypokalemia.
   c. Take measures to relieve nausea (antiemetics, comfort measures).
3. Maintaining rest/activity balance
   a. Maintain bedrest in the acute phase.
   b. Assist patient with ADL to conserve energy.
   c. Promote early ambulation when renal status permits.
   d. Provide for planned rest periods.
4. Preventing injury
   a. Assess orientation; orient confused patient.
   b. During bedrest, keep side rails raised and use padded rails as necessary.
   c. When patient is ambulatory, assess motor skills and monitor ambulation; assist patient as necessary.
   d. Assess patient for signs of bleeding.
   e. Protect patient from bleeding: instruct patient to use soft toothbrush; perform guaiac tests on stool, emesis, and nasogastric returns.
5. Preventing infection
   a. Avoid patient contact by anyone with an infection.
   b. Assess for signs and symptoms of infection.
   c. Maintain asepsis for indwelling lines or catheters.
   d. Facilitate pulmonary hygiene while patient on bedrest.
   e. Turn weak or immobile patients frequently.
   f. Provide meticulous skin care.
   g. Bathe patient at least daily with superfat soap.
   h. Administer prescribed antipruritics.
6. Facilitating coping
   a. Encourage development of nurse-patient relationship to assist patient to express feelings as desired.
   b. Promote patient independence during diuretic phase.
   c. Assist patient to explore alternative ways of coping.

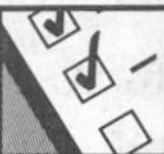

### Guidelines for Teaching the Person With Acute Renal Failure

1. Cause of renal failure and problems with recurrent failures
2. Identification of preventable environmental or health factors contributing to the illness, such as hypertension and nephrotoxic drugs
3. Prescribed medication regimen
4. Prescribed dietary regimen
5. Explanation of risk of hypokalemia and reportable symptoms (muscle weakness, anorexia, nausea and vomiting, lethargy)
6. Signs and symptoms of returning renal failure (decreased urine output without decreased fluid intake, signs of fluid retention)
7. Signs and symptoms of infection
8. Need for ongoing follow-up care

monary hygiene should be carried out to maximize this pathway for acid excretion, to maintain maximal lung expansion, and to prevent atelectasis.

## Promoting Coping

During the oliguric phase of illness, the biochemical alterations may affect not only the level of awareness but also the patient's personality. Family members and occasionally the patient will be aware of these changes, such as faltering memory or an inability to think clearly. Reassure patient and family that mental capacities will return with recovery of physical health. Structuring environment and activities may help with coping in the initial phase. During the diuretic phase, the patient can be helped to explore feelings concerning the nature of the illness and find alternative ways of coping, as necessary.

## Facilitating Learning

Most of the patient teaching takes place during the diuretic phase; the patient is usually ready to learn about kidney disease at this time. Items to include in the teaching plan are listed in the Guidelines box above.

## ♦ EVALUATION

To evaluate the effectiveness of nursing interventions, compare patient behaviors with those stated in the expected patient outcomes. Successful achievement of patient outcomes for the patient with ARF is indicated by the following:

1. Lack of respiratory distress, peripheral edema, or hypertension indicating fluid volume excess.
2. Blood pressures range between 140/90 to 100/60.
3. Serum electrolytes are controlled: sodium 125 to 145 mEq/L, potassium 3.0 to 6.0 mEq/L, bicarbonate greater than 14 mEq/L.
4. Protein catabolism is controlled: BUN less than 100 mg/dl, creatinine less than 12 mg/dl, absence of skin breakdown.

5. Eats diet high in calories and fat and restricted in protein and potassium.
6. Statements of feeling rested.
7. No falls or bleeding occurs.
8. No signs of infection are present.
9. Uses alternative ways of coping, as appropriate; manages ADL independently.
10. Correct explanation of nature of illness, diet therapy, signs and symptoms to be reported to physician, and plans for follow-up care.

# Chronic Renal Failure

## ETIOLOGY/EPIDEMIOLOGY

**Chronic renal failure** exists when the kidneys are no longer capable of maintaining an internal environment that is consistent with life and damage to the kidneys is irreversible. For most individuals, the transition from health to a state of chronic or permanent illness is a slow process that may occur over a number of years. Recurrent infections and exacerbations of nephritis, obstruction of the urinary tract, and destruction of blood vessels from diabetes and long-standing hypertension can lead to scarring in the kidney and progressive loss of renal function. Some individuals, however, develop total irreversible loss of renal function acutely. Such loss of renal function usually develops in a few hours or days and follows direct traumatic kidney insult.

Chronic renal failure remains a significant health problem in the United States. In 1991, more than 200,000 patients received renal replacement therapy. The leading causes of **end-stage renal disease (ESRD)** in order of occurrence are (1) diabetes mellitus, (2) hypertension, and (3) glomerulonephritis.[3]

## PATHOPHYSIOLOGY

Chronic renal failure differs from acute renal failure in that it is progressive and irreversible damage to the kidneys. Progression of the disorder is essentially through four stages: decreased renal reserve, renal insufficiency, renal failure, and ESRD (Box 50-2). However, in practice, no sharp division of these stages is apparent. Severe symptoms occur at the renal failure stage.

The specific pathophysiologic mechanisms depend on the underlying disease causing the destruction of the kidney. The following general pathophysiologic mechanism summarizes these changes. During chronic renal failure, some of the nephrons (including the glomeruli and tubules) are thought to remain intact while others are destroyed (intact nephron hypothesis). The intact nephrons hypertrophy and produce an increased volume of filtrate with increased tubular reabsorption despite a decreased glomerular filtration rate (GFR). This adaptive method permits the kidney to function until about three fourths of the nephrons are destroyed. The solute load then becomes greater than can be reabsorbed, producing an osmotic diuresis with *polyuria*

**BOX 50-2 Stages of Chronic Renal Failure**

**DECREASED RENAL RESERVE (RENAL IMPAIRMENT)**

GFR 40%-50% of normal
BUN and serum creatinine normal
Patient asymptomatic

**RENAL INSUFFICIENCY**

GFR 20%-40% of normal
BUN and serum creatinine begin to rise
Mild anemia; mild azotemia, which worsens with physiologic stress
Nocturia, polyuria

**RENAL FAILURE**

GFR 10%-20% of normal
BUN and serum creatinine increase
Anemia, azotemia, metabolic acidosis
Urine specific gravity low
Polyuria, nocturia
Symptoms of renal failure

**END-STAGE RENAL DISEASE (ESRD)**

GFR <10% of normal
BUN and serum creatinine at high levels
Anemia, azotemia, metabolic acidosis
Urine specific gravity fixed at 1.010
Oliguria
Symptoms of renal failure

and *thirst.* Eventually, as more nephrons are damaged, oliguria occurs with retention of waste products.

The clinical course of chronic renal failure varies greatly from individual to individual; however, some common features exist. Signs and symptoms result from disordered fluid and electrolyte balance, alterations in regulatory functions of the body, and retention of solutes. *Anemia* results from impaired red blood cell (RBC) production because of decreased secretion of erythropoietin by the kidney. In addition, the life span of RBCs is shortened because of the uremia and superimposed nutritional anemia resulting from dietary restrictions. *Azotemia* (excess nitrogenous products in the blood) and *acidosis* are always present. Potassium and hydrogen ion excretion is impaired. Fluid and sodium balance is abnormal and may involve either abnormal retention or secretion of sodium and water; thus urine volume can be increased, normal, or decreased.[20]

With ESRD, *hyperuricemia* is a common finding, although the varied serum levels of uric acid seem to have no definite relationship to the exact level of kidney function. Increased levels of serum phosphate are characteristic, and calcium levels may be low or normal. These findings result from decreased renal excretion of phosphate and simultaneous reduction in ionized serum calcium. Through increased production of parathormone, the body may reestablish a normal serum calcium level,

**TABLE 50-2 Body System Manifestations in Chronic Renal Failure**

| CAUSES | SIGNS/SYMPTOMS | ASSESSMENT PARAMETERS |
|---|---|---|
| **HEMATOPOETIC SYSTEM** | | |
| Suppression of RBC production | Anemia | Hematocrit |
| Decreased survival time of RBCs | Leukocytosis | Hemoglobin |
| Loss of blood through bleeding | Defects in platelet function | Platelet count |
| Loss of blood during dialysis | Thrombocytopenia | Observe for bruising, hematemesis, melana. |
| Mild thrombocytopenia | | |
| Decreased activity of platelets | | |
| **CARDIOVASCULAR SYSTEM** | | |
| Fluid overload | Hypervolemia | Vital signs |
| Renin-angiotensin mechanism | Hypertension | Body weight |
| Fluid overload, anemia | Tachycardia | Electrocardiogram |
| Chronic hypertension | Dysrhythmias | Heart sounds |
| Calcification of soft tissues | Congestive heart failure | Monitor electrolytes. |
| Uremic toxins in pericardial fluid | Pericarditis | Assess for pain. |
| Fibrin formation on epicardium | | |
| **GASTROINTESTINAL SYSTEM** | | |
| Change in platelet activity | Anorexia | Monitor intake and output. |
| Serum uremic toxins | Nausea and vomiting | Hematocrit |
| Electrolyte imbalances | Gastrointestinal bleeding | Hemoglobin |
| Urea converted to ammonia by saliva | Abdominal distention | Guaiac test for all stools |
| | Diarrhea | Assess quality of stools. |
| | Constipation | Assess for abdominal pain. |
| | Uremic fetor (halitosis) | |
| **NEUROLOGIC SYSTEM** | | |
| Uremic toxins | Lethargy, confusion | Level of orientation |
| Electrolyte imbalances | Convulsions | Level of consciousness |
| Cerebral swelling resulting from fluid shifting | Stupor, coma | Reflexes |
| | Sleep disturbances | Electroencephalogram |
| | Unusual behavior | Electrolyte levels |
| | Asterixis | |
| | Muscle irritability | |
| **SKELETAL SYSTEM** | | |
| Decreased calcium absorption | Osteodystrophy | Serum phosphorus |
| Decreased phosphate excretion | Renal rickets | Serum calcium |
| | Joint pain | Assess for joint pain. |
| | Retarded growth | |
| **SKIN** | | |
| Anemia | Pallor | Observe for bruising. |
| Pigment retained | Pigmentation | Assess color of skin. |
| Decreased size of sweat glands | Pruritus | Assess integrity of skin. |
| Decreased activity of oil glands | Ecchymosis | Observe for scratching. |
| Dry skin; phosphate deposits | Excoriation | |
| **GENITOURINARY SYSTEM** | | |
| Damaged nephrons | Uremic frost | Monitor intake and output. |
| | Decreased urine output | Serum creatinine |
| | Decreased urine specific gravity | BUN |
| | Proteinuria | Serum electrolytes |
| | Casts and cells in urine | Urine specific gravity |
| | Decreased urine sodium | Urine electrolytes |
| **REPRODUCTIVE SYSTEM** | | |
| Hormonal abnormalities | Infertility | Monitor intake and output. |
| Anemia | Decreased libido | Monitor vital signs. |
| Hypertension | Impotence | Hematocrit |
| Malnutrition | Amenorrhea | Hemoglobin |
| Medications | Delayed puberty | |

although this is accomplished at the expense of the bone matrix.

Hypertension may or may not be present. Often with the development of ESRD, blood pressure is elevated because of increased total body water, a renally released vasopressor, and inadequately secreted vasodepressors. Glucose intolerance may be seen, although usually not of sufficient severity to warrant treatment. The rising blood sugar level appears to be the result of an altered biochemical environment produced by the failing kidneys and does not signify the development of diabetes mellitus. As renal failure progresses, the patient develops *increased pigmentation* of the skin; the skin becomes sallow or brownish in color. With more advanced and insufficiently treated renal failure, the patient may develop muscular twitching, numbness in the feet and legs, pericarditis, and pleuritis. These signs usually resolve when the patient is treated by dietary modifications, medication, and/or dialysis.

The symptoms of uremia usually develop so slowly that the patient and family often cannot identify the time of onset. Symptoms generally noted as *uremia* (more correctly called *azotemia*) develop, including lethargy, headaches, physical and mental fatigue, weight loss, irritability, and depression. Anorexia, persistent nausea and vomiting, shortness of breath on either mild or no exertion, and pitting edema are symptomatic of severe loss of renal function. Pruritus may be absent, mild, or severe. Table 50-2 provides a summary of the body systems affected by chronic renal failure.

As ESRD develops, most women note changes in their menstrual cycle. Bleeding may occur at more widely spaced intervals, may be heavier or lighter in flow than normal, or may cease altogether. This obvious change in reproductive cycle is usually accompanied by changes in fertility. Ovulation may occur normally or may occur only a few times a year. Pregnancy in uremic women is of much lower incidence than in the normal population. ESRD, however, cannot be relied on as a method of birth control. In men, impotence may occur as chronic renal failure progresses toward ESRD. Dialysis or more vigorous treatment of uremia is indicated to return or maximize reproductive function. It should be stressed that sexual activity of some persons with chronic renal failure may remain quite normal even though changes occur in reproductive ability.

The point at which the patient becomes obviously symptomatic and displays signs typical of renal failure occurs when approximately 80% to 90% of renal function has been lost (Figure 50-1). At this level of renal function, creatinine clearance values will fall to 10 ml/min or less.

## PREVENTION

### *Healthy People 2000*

A risk-reduction objective listed in *Healthy People 2000* of the U.S. Public Health Service and Department of Health and Human Services that relates to ESRD is as follows:

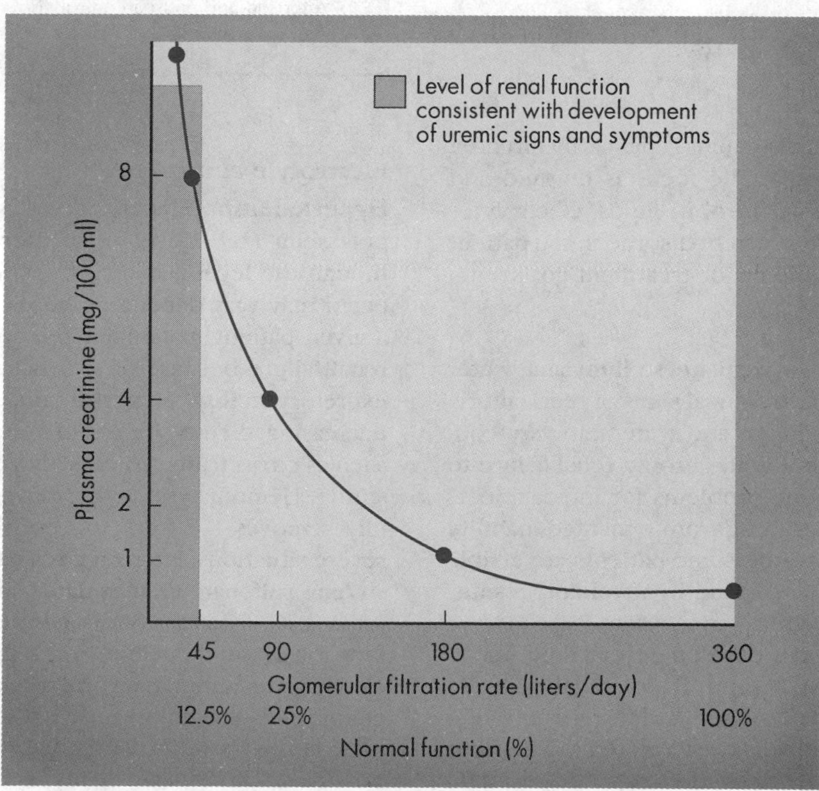


**FIGURE 50-1** Glomerular filtration and plasma creatinine levels.

Reverse the increase in end-stage renal disease (requiring maintenance dialysis or transplantation) to attain an incidence of no more than 13 per 100,000. (Baseline: 13.9 per 100,000 in 1987)

## Primary Prevention

Obstruction and infection of the urinary tract and hypertensive disease are common and often asymptomatic causes of kidney damage and renal failure. A significant reduction in the incidence of chronic renal failure can be effected through increasing attention to general health promotion. Yearly physical examinations in which blood pressure is measured, urinalysis is performed, and the person is questioned about dysuria or pain in the urinary tract assist in early detection of diseases that may lead to chronic renal failure. Meticulous blood glucose control in diabetic persons is critical to reducing renal failure.

## Secondary Prevention

General health maintenance can reduce the number of individuals who progress from renal insufficiency to frank renal failure. Care is aimed toward adequately treating medical problems and closely supervising the person's health status in times of stress (infection, pregnancy).

# MEDICAL MANAGEMENT

The medical management of patients with chronic (end-stage) renal disease can be categorized as follows:

1. Conservative management
2. Dialysis (p. 1677)
3. Renal transplantation (p. 1690)

## Conservative Management

Conservative medical management is primarily directed toward relief of symptoms. The focus is on fluid and electrolyte regulation by control of fluids, electrolytes and diet, treatment of intercurrent disorders, and patient comfort. Box 50-3 lists the major treatment goals.

### Fluid control

Changes in the ability to regulate sodium and water excretion are often the first clinical signs of renal failure. The ability to excrete sodium and water can vary considerably from one patient with chronic renal failure to the next. Although volume problems for most patients involve hypervolemia resulting from a marked inability to excrete sodium and water, some patients are unable to conserve these substances and hypovolemia results. With either marked inability to excrete or conserve body fluid, the patient can develop severe fluid imbalances in a relatively short time. Fluid imbalances are identified, and an intake of sodium and water equivalent to the amount of these substances excreted in a 24-hour period is prescribed. The desired effect is to maintain the person in a normotensive, normovolemic state.

**BOX 50-3 Treatment Goals for the Person With Chronic Renal Failure**

1. Stabilization of the internal environment as demonstrated by:
   a. Mental alertness, attention span, and appropriate interactions
   b. Absence or control of peripheral and pulmonary edema
   c. Control of electrolyte balance within the following limits:

| | |
|---|---|
| Sodium | 125 to 145 mEq/L |
| Potassium | 3 to 6 mEq/L |
| Bicarbonate | >15 mEq/L |
| Calcium | 9 to 11 mg/dl |
| Phosphate | 3 to 5 mg/dl |

   d. Serum albumin >2 g/dl
   e. Control of protein catabolism and protein metabolic wastes as indicated by the following parameters:

| | |
|---|---|
| Urea nitrogen | <100 mg/dl |
| Creatinine | <10 mg/dl |
| Uric acid | <12 mg/dl |

   f. Absence of joint inflammation and pain
   g. Control of anemia

| | |
|---|---|
| Hematocrit | ≥33% |
| Ferritin | >50-100 ng/ml |
| Iron saturation | >20% |

2. Absence of infection
3. Absence of bleeding
4. Blood pressure controlled at <140/90 mm Hg sitting, <10 mm Hg postural change on standing
5. Any intercurrent illness controlled or resolved, including:
   a. Heart failure
   b. Anemia
   c. Dehydration
6. Absence of toxicity from inadequately excreted medications
7. Nutrient intake sufficient to maintain positive nitrogen balance
8. Anorexia and nausea controlled
9. Pruritus controlled

### Electrolyte control

**Hyperkalemia.** Hyperkalemia is defined as a plasma potassium ($K^+$) level of greater than 5.5 mEq/L, although the level at which hyperkalemic complications occur may vary depending on the steady-state value for a given patient. Potassium retention occurs in chronic renal failure because of a direct reduction in nephron excretory ability. Hyperkalemia can be controlled by decreasing dietary intake of foods high in potassium, such as citrus fruits, green leafy vegetables, and salt substitute. Hemodialysis with a zero $K^+$ dialysate bath rapidly removes $K^+$ from the body and may be used in severe situations. Exchange resins, such as sodium polystyrene sulfonate (Kayexalate), are also effective in removing $K^+$ from the body. The resin exchanges sodium ions for $K^+$ and calcium in the gastrointestinal tract. It can be given either as an oral preparation or by retention enema. It is usually given with sorbitol to enhance $K^+$ loss via the bowel. A 25 g dose removes approximately 12.5 to 25 mEq of $K^+$. This method of $K^+$ removal is slower and requires 1 to 2 hours before onset of action.

The additional sodium from the resin, approximately 3 mEq/1 mEq of $K^+$ exchanged, may be contraindicated in patients with serious cardiac disease.[10]

**Metabolic acidosis.** Metabolic acidosis occurs because the damaged kidneys are unable to excrete the normal load of acids generated by metabolism. There is a reduced capacity of the distal tubules to produce ammonia and impaired reabsorption of bicarbonate. Although there is continued hydrogen ion retention and bicarbonate loss, the plasma pH is maintained at a level compatible with life by other buffering mechanisms, particularly the bone salts.

**Hypocalcemia/hyperphosphatemia.** When the kidneys fail, the ability to excrete phosphorus decreases. This leads to a vicious cycle of hypocalcemia/hyperphosphatemia that results in significant bone demineralization. Several factors are responsible for these imbalances. In a state of acidosis, there is dissolution of the alkaline salts of bone to serve as buffers because the kidney is no longer able to maintain acid-base balance and calcium and phosphorus are released into the bloodstream. Reduced glomerular filtration and excretion of inorganic phosphate lead to an elevation of plasma phosphate with a concomitant decrease in serum calcium. Decreased serum calcium concentrations stimulate the secretion of parathyroid hormone (PTH), which results in resorption of calcium from the bones. Under normal circumstances, PTH inhibits tubular reabsorption of phosphates. The kidneys are also unable to complete the synthesis of vitamin D to its active form, 1,5-dihydrocholeciferol, which is necessary for absorption of calcium from the gastrointestinal tract and deposition of calcium in the bones. This acquired resistance to vitamin D decreases calcium absorption, permits retention of phosphorus, and contributes to secondary hyperparathyroidism. The result of these complex disturbances is growth arrest or retardation in children and bone pain and deformities known as *renal osteodystrophy* in adults.[12] Treatment is aimed at decreasing the serum phosphorus levels. This can be accomplished with restriction in dietary phosphorus intake (eliminating dairy products and restricting protein) and the use of phosphate binders. The reduction of serum phosphorus toward normal is often associated with a small increase in serum calcium, a fall in serum PTH, and a reduced incidence of overt secondary hyperparathyroidism.

The goal of therapy with phosphate-binding agents is to reduce serum phosphorus to normal or near normal levels. In dialysis patients, predialysis serum phosphorus levels are ideally maintained between 4.5 and 6 mg/dl, and phosphate binders should be taken with each meal. The available agents for intestinal phosphate binding include the aluminum-containing gels (ALternaGEL, Alu-Cap, Amphojel, Basaljel), calcium carbonate, and calcium acetate. The aluminum-containing gels have been most widely used. Because of the absorption of aluminum from these compounds that can accumulate in renal failure patients, they should be used as a last resort. Calcium carbonate in doses of 4 to 12 g daily with meals is an available alternative. The risks and side effects include hypercalcemia and diarrhea. If the calcium carbonate is given with meals, less calcium is absorbed and the risk of hypercalcemia is reduced.[6] It is critical that nurses adjust the medication times to coincide with meal delivery to enhance phosphate binding and minimize calcium absorption.

Some patients may benefit from the administration of the active form of vitamin D (calcitriol, 0.25 μg daily). Indications for use include adequate control of serum phosphorus, hypocalcemia, bone pain or myopathy, and rising serum alkaline phosphatase.[9]

### Dietary Control

The goals of diet therapy are to (1) reduce the quantity of metabolic waste that requires excretion by the kidney, (2) provide sufficient calories and protein for growth and repair while limiting excretory demands on the kidney, (3) minimize metabolic bone disease, and (4) minimize fluid and electrolyte disturbances. The dietary protein restriction is calculated at 1 to 1.5 g/kg of ideal body weight. Adequate protein intake is reflected by a BUN/creatinine ratio of 10:1. Excessive intake of protein results in nausea and vomiting, apathy, weakness, and neurologic symptoms. Insufficient protein intake results in lowered serum albumin, muscle wasting, edema, and weight loss. Two thirds of the total protein consumed should be protein of high biologic value, that is, containing the essential amino acids.[4]

Ample calories are obtained from carbohydrates and fats because they do not require renal excretion of their metabolic by-products. This spares protein for growth and repair. Catabolism of existing protein stores liberates nitrogenous wastes. For this reason, sources of potential infection, such as indwelling catheters, are avoided. When infection is noted, it is immediately treated.

## Treatment of Intercurrent Disorders

### Anemia

Anemia universally accompanies chronic renal disease. Hematocrit values of 16% to 22% were not uncommon in the days before **epoetin alfa (EPO).** The introduction and subsequent clinical success of EPO, the recombinant form of human erythropoietin, have confirmed this hormone's primary role in regulating the erythropoietic cascade. Patients treated with this agent have enjoyed an increase in hematocrit, a decrease in the need for blood transfusions, and amelioration of the decreased energy and easy fatigability associated with anemia that significantly limited the renal failure patient's ability to carry out normal daily activities.[11]

EPO is administered subcutaneously, three times a

week, in a calculated dose of 50 U/kg of body weight. It is usually administered during a scheduled dialysis treatment. Patients who are in a predialysis state, receiving peritoneal dialysis, or receiving other home dialysis regimens learn to self-administer the drug at home. The medication is irritating to the subcutaneous tissue and causes a transient burning discomfort on administration.

*Iron* is a necessary component of erythropoiesis, and therapy with EPO will be hindered if patients do not have adequate iron stores. Iron stores should be evaluated before and during therapy. Iron deficiency may occur with EPO because of an internal shift of iron from stores to RBCs during the acute correction of anemia and/or the external loss of RBC iron during both the acute and maintenance phases of therapy. Because iron is necessary for continued RBC production, virtually all patients receiving EPO eventually require supplemental

**HEMODIALYSIS NURSING NOTES**
**ADMISSION HISTORY**

41 (Inpatient)/Patient Notes (Outpatient)

| DATE | HOUR | | | | | |
|---|---|---|---|---|---|---|
| | | **I. Perception of Illness** | | | | |
| | | Why, initially, did you come to the hospital? | | | | |
| | | | | | | |
| | | What does the doctor plan for you while you are here? | | | | |
| | | | | | | |
| | | What do you expect to happen to you when you start dialysis? | | | | |
| | | | | | | |
| | | **II. History of Past Illness (Include dates and hospitalizations).** | | | | |
| | | | | | | |
| | | | | | | |
| | | | | | | |
| | | | | | | |
| | | | | | | |
| | | | | | | |
| | | | | | | |
| | | MEDICATIONS | DOSE | FREQUENCY | LAST DOSE TAKEN | REASON FOR TAKING |
| | | | | | | |
| | | | | | | |
| | | | | | | |
| | | | | | | |
| | | | | | | |
| | | | | | | |
| | | | | | | |
| | | | | | | |
| | | Do you receive any special treatments or exercises? | | | | |
| | | | | | | |
| | | | | | | |
| | | | | | | |
| | | **III. Activity** | | | | |
| | | Do you have difficulty walking or getting in and out of a chair? | | | | |
| | | Can you climb stairs? | | | | |
| | | Are you employed? | | | | |
| | | What are your usual daytime activities? | | | | |
| | | What are your recreational interests? | | | | |
| | | | | | | |
| | | | | | | |

**FIGURE 50-2** Hemodialysis nursing notes: admission history.

iron. Patients should be instructed that the adverse effects caused by iron on the gastrointestinal tract, nausea and constipation, can be avoided or minimized by taking iron on a full stomach and by adding a stool softener or laxative to the medication regimen. In addition, simultaneous ingestion of iron and phosphate binders should be avoided because phosphate binders impede the absorption of oral iron.

Folate and vitamin $B_{12}$ are important cofactors in the production of RBCs and play a role in the formation and development of deoxyribonucleic acid (DNA). Shortages of these vitamins will hinder the formation of DNA and thus RBCs. Folate can be taken in pill form at a dose of 1 mg/day and $B_{12}$ can be replaced with a monthly intramuscular injection of 100 to 1000 μg based on the $B_{12}$ blood level.

Blood pressure may rise during EPO therapy, especially during the early stage of treatment when the he-

| DATE | HOUR | IV. | Nutrition | |
|---|---|---|---|---|
| | | | Are you on a special diet? | |
| | | | Do you have difficutly following a diet? | |
| | | | How many meals do you eat a day? | |
| | | | | |
| | | V. | **Sleep Habits** | |
| | | | Do you sleep through the night at home? | |
| | | | What helps in getting to sleep at night? | |
| | | | What are your usual sleeping habits? | |
| | | | | |
| | | VI. | **Elimination** | |
| | | | How often do you urinate? | |
| | | | Do you have any difficulty with urination? | |
| | | | Frequency | Pain on urination |
| | | | Urgency | Other |
| | | | Have you ever had urinary tract infections? | |
| | | | | |
| | | | 24-hour urine output | cc/24 hr |
| | | | Color of urine? | |
| | | | What are your usual bowel habits? | |
| | | | Do you have difficulty with diarrhea or constipation? | |
| | | | How often do you use enemas or laxatives? | |
| | | | | |
| | | VII. | **Reproductive System** | |
| | | | When was your most recent menses? | |
| | | | Have you recently had a change in menses? | |
| | | | Have you had any changes in sexual function recently? | |
| | | | Do you have any concerns about reproductive or sexual functions? | |
| | | | | |
| | | VIII. | **Social** | |
| | | | Do you live with anyone? | |
| | | | Upon whom do you rely when you need help? | |
| | | | What type of dwelling do you live in? | |
| | | | Do you have to climb stairs? | |
| | | | Financial resources/insurance | |
| | | | | |
| | | | | |
| | | | | |
| | | | | |
| | | | | |

Admitting Nurse ______________________________

**FIGURE 50-2, cont'd** Hemodialysis nursing notes: admission history.

matocrit is rising. About 25% of patients require initiation of or an increase in antihypertensive therapy. Regulating a dialysis patient's blood pressure involves reevaluating dietary sodium intake, the dialysis prescription, and antihypertensive medications.

Therapy with EPO resulting in an increase in hematocrit and a decrease in plasma volume can affect dialysis efficiency. In such cases the patient may require increases in blood flow rates and treatment time or changes in membrane type and size. Patients may also require increases in anticoagulation during dialysis.

Stimulation of renal and extrarenal EPO production can be achieved by the administration of *androgens.* Before EPO, androgens were the mainstay in the treatment of the anemia of ESRD. Parenteral preparations, such as nandrolone decanoate (Deca-Durabolin) or testosterone propionate, are very effective. They are given in doses of 1 to 4 mg/kg of body weight once a week

**HEMODIALYSIS NURSING NOTES**
**ADMISSION ASSESSMENT**

**41** (Inpatient)/Patient Notes (Outpatient)

| DATE | HOUR | | | |
|---|---|---|---|---|
| | | **A) Vital Signs** | | |
| | | Temperature | | |
| | | Pulses | Apical | |
| | | | Radial | |
| | | | Rhythm | |
| | | Weight | | |
| | | Height | | |
| | | | | |
| | | **B) Cardiopulmonary** | | |
| | | Vascular Access | | |
| | | Peripheral Pulses: | Right | Left |
| | | Radial | | |
| | | Femoral | | |
| | | Popliteal | | |
| | | Pedal | | |
| | | Peripheral Edema? | | |
| | | Periorbital Edema? | | |
| | | Friction Rub? | | |
| | | Neck Vein Distention? | | |
| | | Cough? | Sputum? | Smoking Habits? |
| | | Adventitious Breath Sounds? | | |
| | | Shortness of Breath? | | |
| | | Orthopnea? | | |
| | | **C) Neuromuscular** | | |
| | | Orientation | | |
| | | Level of Alertness and Responsiveness? | | |
| | | | | |
| | | Muscle Tone and Strength, Symmetry? | | |
| | | | | |
| | | Weakness or Loss of Function of Extremities? | | |
| | | | | |
| | | Balance | | |
| | | Numbness, Tingling or Tremors? | | |
| | | | | |
| | | | | |

**FIGURE 50-3** Hemodialysis nursing notes: admission assessment.

and then titrated down by increasing the dose interval. The use of androgens is associated with side effects, including hirsutism, acne, and cholestasis.

### Gastrointestinal disturbances

In patients with uremia, disturbances in fluid, electrolyte, and waste composition of body fluids produce changes in osmotic gradients in all cells. When these changes occur in the cells of the gastrointestinal (GI) tract and the central nervous system (CNS), anorexia, nausea, and vomiting result. Persons with uremia are subject to *bleeding of the GI tract,* including the oral cavity. Urea is broken down to ammonia by the action of intestinal bacteria. Because ammonia is a mucosal irritant, ulceration and bleeding can occur. In addition to GI tract problems that lead to nausea and vomiting, persons with chronic renal disease have *decreased salivary flow.* An ammonia smell and taste can quickly

| DATE | HOUR | Patient Experiencing Difficulties with: |
|---|---|---|
| | | Sight |
| | | Speech |
| | | Touch |
| | | Taste/Smell |
| | | |
| | | D) Skin |
| | | Color |
| | | Turgor |
| | | Temperature |
| | | Lesions |
| | | Condition of Nails |
| | | |
| | | E) General |
| | | Presence of: |
| | | Nausea |
| | | Vomiting |
| | | Headache |
| | | Blurring of Vision |
| | | Ability to perform ADL |
| | | |
| | | |
| | | |
| | | |
| | | |
| | | |
| | | |
| | | |
| | | |
| | | |
| | | |
| | | |
| | | |
| | | |
| | | |
| | | |
| | | |
| | | |

Admitting Nurse ____________________

**FIGURE 50-3, cont'd** Hemodialysis nursing notes: admission assessment.

accumulate in the mouth and can further compound anorexia. Vinegar mouthwashes help neutralize the ammonia and promote comfort. Treatment includes administering antacids every 2 to 4 hours to decrease GI irritation. Dietary control of uremia, perhaps augmented by dialysis, helps to control disturbances in fluid, electrolyte, and water composition of body fluids and thus help to control nausea and vomiting.

### Other conditions

From 70% to 90% of patients with renal failure are hypertensive. In most patients, hypertension can be controlled by a combination of dietary sodium and fluid restriction and sodium and water removal (ultrafiltration) during dialysis. Approximately 30% of patients require antihypertensive therapy for optimal blood pressure control. Calcium channel blockers (Procardia, DynaCirc) and angiotensin-converting enzyme inhibitors (captopril, enalapril) are often used. Other conditions that are treated include ***heart failure*** and ***infection.***

## NURSING MANAGEMENT

### ♦ ASSESSMENT

The nursing assessment of the patient with chronic renal failure is extremely complex. The assessment must include physical, psychological, and social parameters. The basis of this assessment is the same as that described in Chapter 48 for the patient with suspected renal problems. The initial nursing history and physical assessment must elicit adequate information to generate the appropriate nursing diagnoses. An example of a comprehensive nursing history is found in Figure 50-2 and an example of a physical assessment in Figure 50-3.

The extent and nature of subsequent assessments are determined by the medical regimen and nursing diagnoses for the individual patient. The frequency of assessment is a function of the medical regimen and stability of the patient. For example, the patient being managed by conservative means may be able to go several months without follow-up assessments. On the other hand, the patient being treated with hemodialysis will require a thorough assessment with each treatment.

### ♦ NURSING DIAGNOSES

Nursing diagnoses are determined from analysis of patient data. Nursing diagnoses for the person with chronic renal failure may include but are not limited to the following:

| Diagnostic Title | Possible Etiologic Factors |
|---|---|
| Fluid volume excess | Compromised regulatory mechanism |
| Nutrition, altered: less than body requirements | Anorexia, nausea, decreased salivary flow, bad taste, pain |
| Infection, high risk for | Compromised immune response |
| Injury, high risk for | Sensorimotor deficits, lack of awareness of environmental hazards, decreased level of consciousness |
| Fatigue | Uremia, anemia, insomnia |
| Pain: muscle cramping, pruritus, ocular irritation | Sodium depletion, uremia |
| Coping, ineffective (individual) | Situational crisis |
| Self-esteem, situational low | Changes in body appearance, change in social involvement |
| Knowledge deficit | Lack of exposure/recall |

### ♦ EXPECTED PATIENT OUTCOMES

Expected patient outcomes for the person with chronic renal failure vary depending on the course of the disorder and the identified nursing diagnoses. Expected patient outcomes may include but are not limited to the following:

1. Has no respiratory distress, peripheral edema, hypertension, or other signs and symptoms indicating fluid and electrolyte imbalance.
2. Correctly explains dietary plan, including fluid, protein, potassium, and sodium restrictions.
3. Shows no signs of infection; skin remains intact.
4. No injury occurs.
5. States feeling more rested and less fatigued.
6. States no muscle cramping, itching, or ocular irritation present.
7. Demonstrates mental clarity and ability to perform ADL independently and safely.
8. States satisfaction with life and self.
9. Correctly describes nature of illness, treatment regimen, and plans for follow-up care.

### ♦ INTERVENTIONS

Because the condition of the person with chronic renal failure can vary, nursing care focuses on the specific identified nursing diagnoses. Most persons, however, require some help or teaching to maintain fluid and electrolyte balance; prevent infection or injury; promote comfort, rest, and sleep; and cope with the effects of renal failure (see Guidelines box, p. 1675).

#### Maintaining Fluid and Electrolyte Balance

The person with chronic renal failure must learn how to identify signs of imbalances, take fluids in the prescribed amounts, and eat within the prescribed limits.

Controlling sodium intake can be an extremely challenging problem for both the nurse and the patient. Any sudden increase in weight indicates accumulating fluid, and the source of this fluid must be discussed with the patient. Often, when the patient is not acutely ill and is responsible for diet restrictions, the problem can be traced to excess sodium ingestion, which produces thirst. In helping to avoid this cycle of sodium-driven

## Guidelines for Care of the Person With Chronic Renal Failure

1. Maintain fluid and electrolyte balance.
   a. Monitor for fluid and electrolyte excess.
      (1) Assess intake and output every 8 hours.
      (2) Weigh patient every day.
      (3) Assess presence and extent of edema.
      (4) Auscultate breath sounds.
      (5) Monitor cardiac rhythm and blood pressure every 8 hours.
      (6) Assess level of consciousness every 8 hours.
   b. Encourage patient to remain within prescribed fluid restrictions.
   c. Provide small quantities of fluid spaced over the day to stay within fluid restrictions.
   d. Encourage a diet high in carbohydrates and within the prescribed sodium, potassium, phosphorus, and protein limits.
   e. Administer phosphate binding agents with meals as prescribed.
2. Prevent infection and injury.
   a. Promote meticulous skin care.
   b. Encourage activity within prescribed limits but avoid fatigue.
   c. Protect confused person from injury.
   d. Protect person from exposure to infectious agents.
   e. Maintain good medical/surgical asepsis during treatments and procedures.
   f. Avoid aspirin products.
   g. Encourage use of soft toothbrush.
3. Promote comfort.
   a. Medicate patient as needed for pain.
   b. Medicate with prescribed antipruritics, use emollient baths, keep skin moist, and control environmental temperature to modify pruritus.
   c. Encourage use of damp cloth to keep lips moist; give good oral hygiene.
   d. Encourage rest for fatigue; however, encourage self-care as tolerated.
   e. Provide calm, supportive atmosphere.
4. Assist with coping in life-style and self-concept.
   a. Promote hope.
   b. Provide opportunity for patient to express feelings about self.
   c. Identify available community resources.

thirst leading to increased fluid ingestion and overhydration, the patient is carefully taught about the amount of sodium and fluid allowed in the diet and what restrictions are to be observed when purchasing prepared foods. The words "sodium" and "salt" should be checked on all food labels. Salt substitutes should be avoided by all patients with chronic renal failure because these substitutes contain large amounts of potassium.

At times the patient is unable to offer an explanation for increasing thirst and sodium ingestion. At this point the question of home self-medication is raised. The person may be taking over-the-counter antacids that are high in sodium. If the cause of the hypervolemia cannot be identified, the patient is asked to list all foods and fluids ingested over the previous 3 days. This list can be used to uncover dietary indiscretions as well as serve as a teaching tool to reinforce the prescribed diet.

### Facilitating Nutrition

Persons usually need help in planning diets within the prescribed sodium, potassium, phosphorus, and protein limits. Modifying the diet to the individual's preferences can help to maintain intake of food. Dietary teaching and meal planning can be approached according to an exchange system similar to that used for persons with diabetes.

Actual eating of a modified diet can be promoted through attempting to decrease emotional tension at the dinner table. Food that is attractively arranged and well flavored is also likely to encourage eating. Herbs and other flavorings can add variety to foods that are prepared without sodium. When the GI tract is ulcerated, bland foods may be tried in an attempt to increase ingestion of food.

### Preventing Infection and Injury

Tissue breakdown leads to infection and significant rises in serum potassium and must be avoided. Potassium is largely an intracellular cation, and extensive tissue damage can liberate a lethal amount of this ion into the system of the person with chronic renal failure. Edematous skin poses a high risk for skin breakdown; therefore, meticulous skin care is important. Patients with chronic renal failure should avoid others with infections; avoid fatigue, which lowers body resistance; and seek medical attention when symptoms of infections, GI bleeding, or other problems first appear.

The risk of constipation is also high in persons with chronic renal failure because of the fluid restrictions. Stool softeners or laxatives may be needed.

Other important nursing activities include helping the patient to control blood losses. A soft toothbrush is recommended for oral care. The patient is instructed to observe for melena and to report this without delay to the physician. *Aspirin should be avoided* because it is normally excreted by the kidneys and may rapidly build to toxic levels and prolong bleeding time.

The build-up of osmotically active particles and fluid in the body that occurs with azotemia produces changes in the cells of the brain that may lead to confusion and impairment in decision-making ability. Fluid accumulation and hypertension can produce visual changes. The person's environment is assessed for potential for injury. At times the person may need help in limiting activities to a level commensurate with mental processes and level of awareness. For example, blurred vision and delayed reaction time contraindicate driving an automobile.

### Promoting Comfort, Rest, and Sleep

The patient with chronic renal failure rarely has acute, sharp pain; however, these persons are subject to a wide variety of chronic discomforts, including pruritus, muscle cramping, headaches, ocular irritation, insomnia, and bone pain.

Most patients with ESRD develop *pruritus;* they describe a sensation of deep itching. Itching is largely symptomatic, and measures that are effective in controlling it vary from person to person. Reducing levels of serum phosphorus with phosphate-binding preparations decreases itching for most patients. Medications such as trimeprazine tartrate (Temaril) may be effective for some patients. Keeping the skin moist and supple through use of lotions and bath oils, controlling the room temperature during sleep to prevent excessive warmth, and bathing with emollients or a vinegar solution are measures alone or in combination that may provide some relief from itching. (See Chapter 67 for a discussion of pruritus.) Since emotional stress seems to increase the itching, helping the patient verbalize feelings may provide resolution of conflict and help decrease itching. The urge to scratch the skin is acute in some patients. Because scratching is often vigorous, injury to the skin with subsequent infection can result. Fingernails are trimmed closely. Instead of fingernails, a soft cloth should be used to scratch the skin.

*Muscle cramping in the lower extremities and hands* is common in renal failure. Often, cramping can be correlated with sodium depletion. Primary treatment for muscle cramping involves controlling the state of uremia and fluid and electrolyte balance. Temporary measures of heat and massage are effective for some persons. Quinine sulfate, 325 mg at bedtime, often prevents cramping.

*Ocular irritation* in chronic renal failure is caused by calcium deposits in the conjunctiva that cause burning and watering of the eyes. Treatment involves controlling the plasma phosphate level through administration of oral phosphate-binding preparations. "Artificial tears" (methylcellulose) placed in the conjunctival sac every few hours also help to reduce irritation.

*Insomnia* and *chronic daytime fatigue* are common complaints of persons with chronic renal failure. This reversal of normal sleep patterns has been attributed to a variety of causes. These include (1) recurring preoccupation with thoughts concerning the disease state and resultant changes in life-style, (2) pruritus, and (3) the state of uremia itself. Reduction of high serum levels of urea nitrogen and creatinine through decreasing dietary intake of protein or dialysis may bring sleep patterns back to normal. When control of uremia fails to cure insomnia, mild CNS depressants may be prescribed.

The severely anemic person complains of extreme fatigue and shortness of breath. Because of a lack of RBCs, there is an inability to transport sufficient oxygen to cells for energy production. The anemic person may be unable to work or play without extended rest periods. Rest periods should be taken early enough in the day to prevent sleeplessness at night.

General comfort at bedtime is needed to induce sleep at any time and is especially important whenever sleeping problems arise. Comfort measures can include tepid baths, pursuing quiet activities an hour or two before bedtime, controlling itching, or anything the patient finds calming and soothing.

## Facilitating Coping With Changes in Life-Style and Feelings Regarding Self

The goals of therapy for ESRD include not only the preservation of the patient's life in the presence of ESRD, but also restoration of optimal quality of life. There is broad agreement that patients' quality of life is related to their function in the physical/medical, ADL, psychologic, and social/occupational dimensions.[19]

Optimal psychosocial care of patients with chronic renal failure requires careful and sophisticated psychosocial patient assessment. This assessment is accomplished as a collaborative effort with the physician, nurse, and social worker. The common psychological problems include dysphoric moods (anxiety, depression, frustration, anger), impaired body image (with a perceived loss of physical attractiveness), impaired self-esteem, and suicidal crises.

Noncompliance with the treatment regimen is a common behavioral problem; this may include treatment participation, diet and fluid restriction, and medication noncompliance as well as noncompliance with other medical diagnostic and therapeutic procedures. Several factors contribute to noncompliance: the intrusive and demanding aspects of chronic dialysis regimen, strong feelings of frustration and depression, a strong desire to maintain control over one's life and deny the unpleasant personal reality of chronic illness, a need to indirectly express anger toward staff members, and legitimate attempts to balance health concerns with a short-term need for pleasure. Interventions that may effectively reverse significant patient noncompliance include (1) providing further information about the rationale for treatment procedures or restrictions, (2) helping the patient regain as much constructive control as possible over life's activities, (3) communicating with staff members to gather information and to design and implement a program to reward increased patient compliance, and (4) working with family members to educate them and enlist their support.

Social problems in ESRD patients include strains in intimate relationships, loss of vocational function, and restriction of social and leisure activities. The introduction of a serious life-threatening illness such as ESRD is an added stress dimension to the already enormous demands placed on the contemporary family system. Role changes are common in these families such that spouses often take on the role responsibilities of the sick partner while maintaining their own role. This leads to reduced rest and leisure for the spouse and lowers physical reserve. Major adjustments in thinking and living must be made, and at the same time, relationships must be maintained and nurtured.[7] Nursing staff must be aware that additional social support for patients may need to be provided by professional caregivers, especially when family members take little responsibility for either physical and/or emotional support. Caregiving staff may be viewed as important "significant others" for the ESRD patient.

Vocational dysfunction is a result of decreased physical capacities, the time-intensive requirements of dialysis, depression and cognitive impairment, governmental policies about reimbursement for dialysis medical care, and the reluctance of employers to hire individuals with kidney disease. The problem of vocational function are quite complex, particularly for patients with limited skills and whose work has previously involved manual labor. Implications for nursing and social work consist of identifying patients being started on dialysis who had physically taxing occupations and providing counseling about job changes and retraining.

### Facilitating Learning

The person with ESRD presents a unique opportunity for the nurse to promote optimal health through teaching and counseling. Important points to be included in patient teaching are listed in the Guidelines box below.

**Guidelines for Teaching the Person With Chronic Renal Failure**

1. Relationships between symptoms and their causes
2. Relationships among diet, fluid restriction, medication, and blood chemistries
3. Preventive health care measures: good oral hygiene, prevention of infection, avoidance of bleeding
4. Dietary regimen, including fluid restrictions
   a. Prescribed sodium, potassium, phosphorus, and protein restrictions
   b. Means of identifying contents of foods
   c. Use of small, frequent feedings to maintain nutrient intake when anorexic or nauseated
   d. Fluid prescription and sources of fluid in diet
   e. Avoidance of salt substitutes containing potassium
5. Monitoring for fluid excess
   a. Accurate measurement and recording of intake and output
   b. Monitoring for weight gain and edema
6. Medications
   a. Actions, doses, purpose, and side effects of prescribed medications
   b. Avoidance of over-the-counter drugs, especially aspirin, cold medications, and nonsteroidal antiinflammatory drugs
7. Planning for gradual increase in physical activity, including rest periods to conserve energy
8. Measures to control pruritus
9. Planning for follow-up health care
   a. Symptoms requiring immediate medical attention: changes in urine output, edema, weight gain, dyspnea, infection, increased symptoms of uremia
   b. Need for continual medical follow-up

Education about medications should include both prescribed medications and over-the-counter or folk medicines. All medications taken by the person with chronic renal failure should be prescribed by the physician. Many cold preparations contain large amounts of sodium. Remembering to take prescribed medications can be a problem for the person who may have to take more than two dozen pills each day. Thus, "noncompliance" for medications may actually be simply difficulty in memory. Correlating pill-taking times with major activities of the day and use of aids to separate out the day's pills are helpful.

## ♦ EVALUATION

To evaluate the effectiveness of nursing interventions, compare patient behaviors with those stated in the expected patient outcomes. Successful achievement of patient outcomes for the patient with chronic renal failure is indicated by the following:

1. Lacks respiratory distress, peripheral edema, hypertension, or other signs of fluid and electrolyte imbalance.
2. Correctly explains dietary plan, including fluid, protein, potassium, and sodium restrictions.
3. Shows no signs of infection; skin remains intact.
4. No injury occurs.
5. States feeling more rested and less fatigued.
6. States that no muscle cramping, itching, or ocular irritation present.
7. Demonstrates mental clarity and ability to perform ADL independently and safely.
8. States satisfaction with life and self.
9. Correctly describes nature of illness, treatment regimen, and plans for follow-up care.

# DIALYSIS

In 1960, a person with ESRD was treated for the first time with chronic intermittent hemodialysis by means of an artificial kidney. That individual was successfully treated for more than 14 years. Before that time, many patients were treated for acute renal failure with hemodialysis; however, once it was determined that the kidney disease was irreversible, the treatment was withdrawn. This practice continues today in many industrialized countries around the world.

In 1972, the U.S. Congress enacted legislation that provides for payment of health care costs for all U.S. citizens with ESRD. Under this legislation, any person with documented chronic uremia is provided benefits under Medicare. As a result of this legislation, many persons are able to live extended lives. In 1992, almost 200,000 persons were receiving some form of dialysis.[4]

Many technologic advances have been made in the treatment of persons with ESRD. Drastic changes in artificial kidneys allow for more efficient and comfortable hemodialysis treatments. Advances in the development of dialysis machines allow individuals the convenience of treatment in their own homes. Developments in peritoneal dialysis permit patients to treat themselves with continuous peritoneal and intermittent peritoneal dialysis. These advances provide persons with the opportunity to have more control over meeting their own health care needs.

Dialysis involves the movement of fluid and particles across a semipermeable membrane. It is a treatment that can help restore fluid and electrolyte balance, control acid-base balance, and remove waste and toxic material from the body. This treatment can sustain life successfully in both acute and chronic situations where substitution for or augmentation of normal renal function is needed. Specifically, dialysis is used to remove excessive amounts of drugs and toxins in poisonings of both an intentional and an accidental nature, to correct serious electrolyte and acid-base imbalances, to maintain kidney function when renal shutdown occurs as a result of transfusion reactions, to replace renal function temporarily in persons with acute renal failure of various etiologies, and to be a permanent substitute for the loss of renal function in persons with ESRD.

## PHYSIOLOGIC PRINCIPLES OF DIALYSIS

Dialysis is based on three principles: diffusion, osmosis, and ultrafiltration (Figure 50-4). **Diffusion** involves the movement of particles from an area of greater to an area of lesser concentration. In the body, this usually occurs across a semipermeable membrane. Diffusion is involved in the clearance of solute from the patient's body in both hemodialysis and peritoneal dialysis. Diffusion results in the movement of urea, creatinine, and uric acid from the patient's blood into the **dialysate** solution. This solution contains fewer particles to be removed from the bloodstream and high concentrations of particles to be added to the blood (Figure 50-5). Since the dialysate contains no protein waste products, the concentration of these substances in the blood will decrease because of random movement of the particles across the semipermeable membrane into the dialysate. The same principle applies to the movement of potassium ions. Although the concentration of RBCs and protein is high in blood, these molecules are quite large and do not diffuse through the membrane pores; thus, they are not lost from the blood.

**Osmosis** involves the movement of water across a semipermeable membrane from an area of lesser to an area of greater concentration (osmolality) of particles. Osmosis is responsible for movement of extra fluid from the patient, particularly in peritoneal dialysis. Figure 50-5 shows that glucose has been added to the dialysate to make its particle concentration greater than that of the patient's blood. Fluid will then move through the pores of the membrane from the patient's blood to the dialysate.

**Ultrafiltration** involves the movement of fluid across a semipermeable membrane as a result of an artificially created pressure gradient. Ultrafiltration is more efficient than osmosis for removal of fluid and is used in hemo-

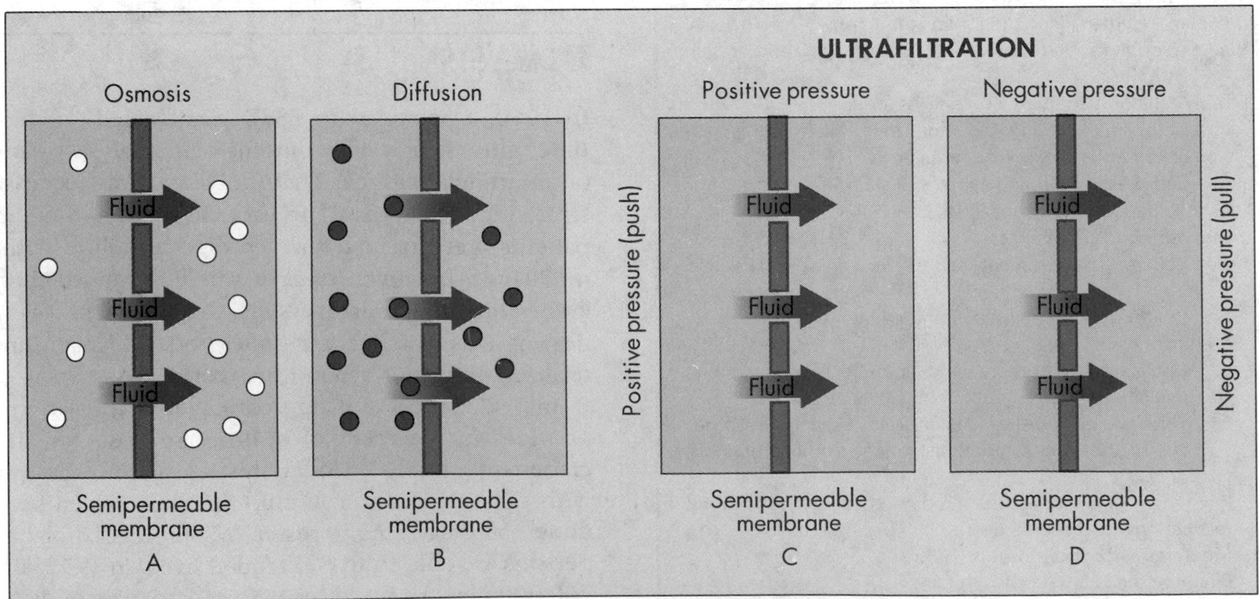


**FIGURE 50-4** Dialysis is based on principles of osmosis (**A**): diffusion (**B**) and ultrafiltration. Ultrafiltration occurs when either positive pressure (**C**) or negative pressure (**D**) is placed on system. Ultrafiltration can be maximized by exerting both positive and negative pressure on system simultaneously.

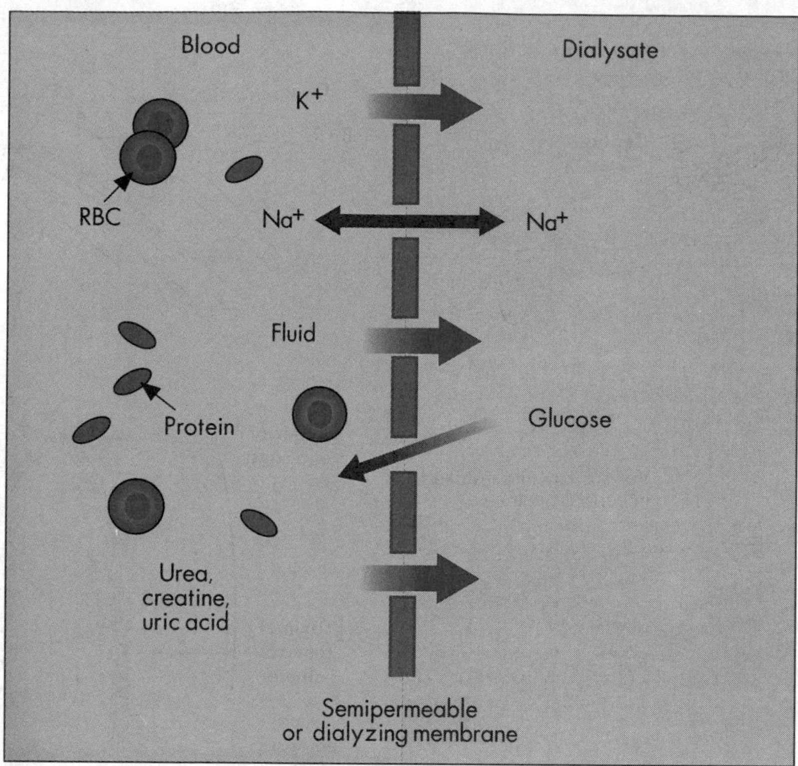


**FIGURE 50-5** Osmosis and diffusion in dialysis. Net movement of major particles and fluid is illustrated.

dialysis for this purpose. During dialysis, osmosis and diffusion or ultrafiltration and diffusion occur simultaneously.

## HEMODIALYSIS

**Hemodialysis** involves shunting the patient's blood from the body through a dialyzer in which diffusion and ultrafiltration occur and back into the patient's circulation. To accomplish hemodialysis, there must be access to the patient's blood, a mechanism to transport the blood to and from the dialyzer, and a dialyzer (area in which the exchange of fluid electrolytes and waste products occurs). Currently, five major means are available for gaining access to the patient's bloodstream. These include the following:

1. Arteriovenous fistula (Figure 50-6, *A*)
2. Arteriovenous graft (Figure 50-6, *B*)
3. External arteriovenous shunt (Figure 50-6, *C*)
4. Femoral vein catheterization (Figure 50-6, *D*)
5. Subclavian vein catheterization (Figure 50-6, *E*)

The indications and nursing implications for each access are summarized in Table 50-3.[5]

Many patients expect to leave the dialysis treatment with a feeling of well-being. Few persons feel this way; most experience some minor discomfort that diminishes within several hours after dialysis. The greatest feeling of well-being seems to occur the day after dialysis.

Immediately before dialysis, the patient is weighed, vital signs are taken, a sample of blood is drawn to determine the level of serum electrolytes and waste products, and the patient's physical status is assessed. Nursing care of the patient during hemodialysis centers around (1) monitoring physical status before and during dialysis for evidence of physiologic imbalance and change, (2) providing comfort and safety, and (3) helping the patient to understand and adjust to the care and changes in lifestyle. This latter objective involves educating the person as to the specifics of the treatment program (diet and medications in particular) and how these relate to altered kidney function. The person is encouraged to express concerns and feelings, and attempts must be made to help the individual work through these feelings. If dialysis is performed at home, the patient and dialysis partner must be able to institute all the care described. See Nursing Care Plan, p. 1682.

## NURSING MANAGEMENT

### ♦ NURSING DIAGNOSES

Nursing diagnoses are determined from analysis of patient data. Patients receiving hemodialysis are experiencing ESRD; therefore, it must be remembered that numerous nursing diagnoses are ongoing during hemodialysis that are not specific to hemodialysis. Nursing diagnoses pertinent to hemodialysis may include but are not limited to the following:

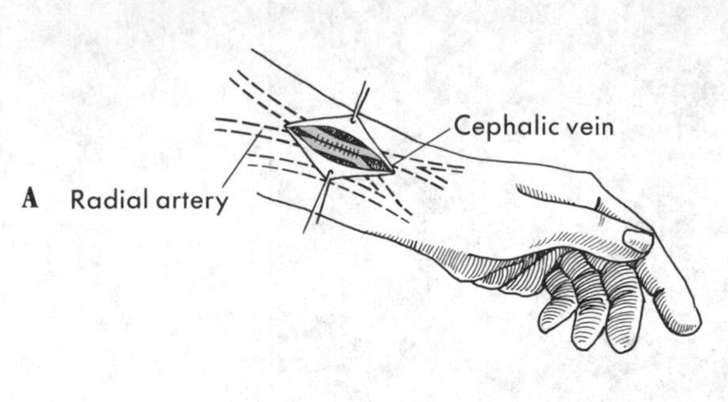


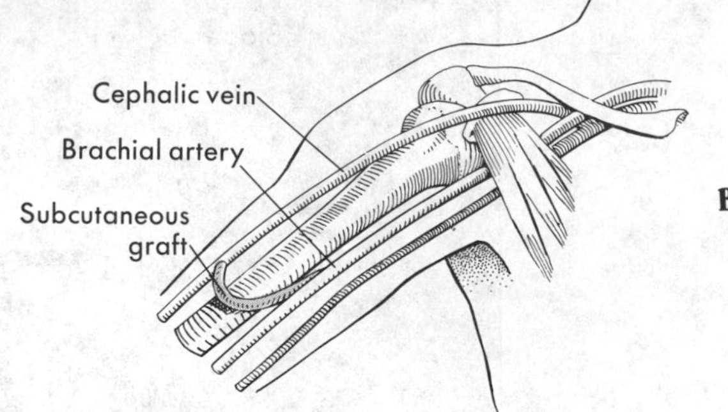


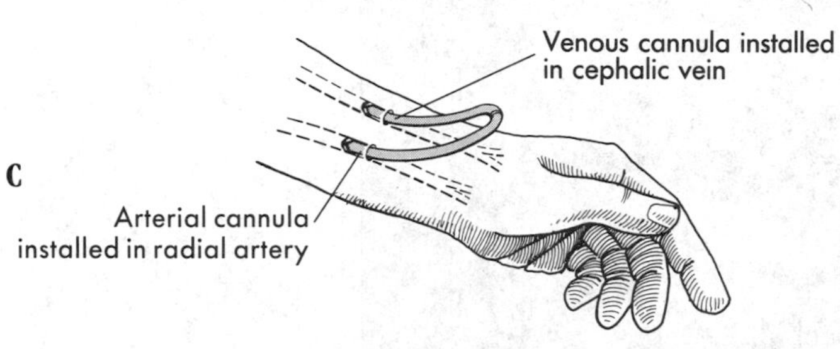


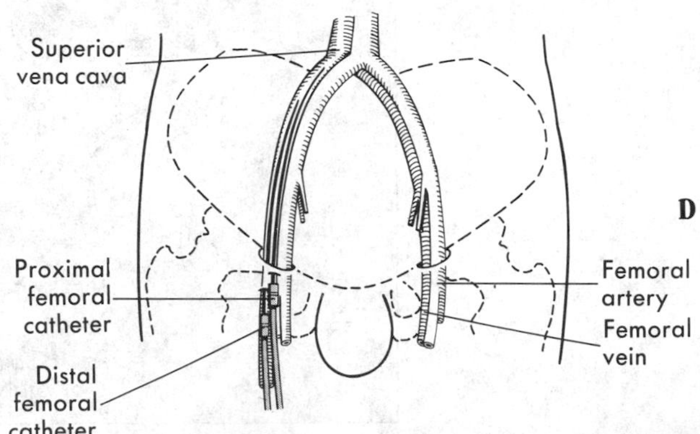


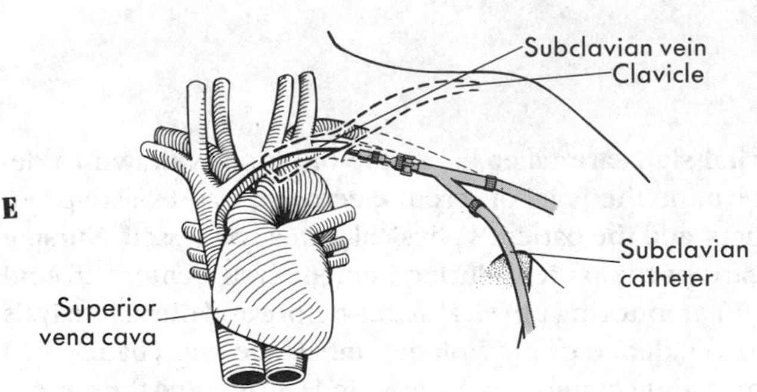


**FIGURE 50-6** Frequently used means for gaining vascular access for hemodialysis include **A,** arteriovenous fistula; **B,** arteriovenous graft; **C,** external arteriovenous shunt; **D,** femoral vein catheterization; and **E,** subclavian vein catheterization.

| Diagnostic Title | Possible Etiologic Factors |
|---|---|
| Fluid volume deficit | Overvigorous dialysis |
| Pain/discomfort | Venipuncture for dialysis, immobility, headache, nausea |
| Activity intolerance | Immobility, anemia |
| Nutrition, altered: less than body requirements | Effects of dialysis |
| Knowledge deficit | Lack of exposure/recall |

## ♦ EXPECTED PATIENT OUTCOMES

Expected patient outcomes for hemodialysis include but are not limited to the following:

1. Achieves dry weight during dialysis.
2. States that discomfort is decreased.
3. Participates in a program to maintain activity level.
4. Eats according to preference during therapy.
5. Describes nature of dialysis, care of venous access routes, side effects, and work/activity schedule.

## ♦ INTERVENTIONS

### Facilitating Fluid and Electrolyte Balance

**Preventing hypovolemia and shock**

Most physical problems that occur during dialysis are related to hypotension from removal of fluid and disequilibrium from a rapid reduction in extracellular electrolytes and wastes. *Hypovolemia* and *shock* can occur during dialysis as a result of rapid removal of fluid from the intravascular compartment. Because this can occur faster than reequilibration of intracellular and intravascular volume relationships, the person may appear edematous and yet exhibit signs of shock. Signs and symptoms that indicate that the intravascular volume is being rapidly depleted are anxiety, restlessness, dizziness, nausea and vomiting, diaphoresis, tachycardia, and hypotension.

To avoid depleting the intravascular space and pro-

**TABLE 50-3 Indications and Nursing Implications for the Major Types of Vascular Access for Hemodialysis**

| INDICATIONS | ADVANTAGES | NURSING IMPLICATIONS |
|---|---|---|
| **FEMORAL VEIN CATHETERIZATION** | | |
| Immediate access<br>Need for access seen as short duration | Ease of access<br>Can be used immediately | Assess patient frequently for bleeding from insertion sites and tubing connections.<br>This requires frequent irrigation with heparin solution to maintain patency<br>Sterile technique is essential when working with catheters. |
| **EXTERNAL SHUNT** | | |
| Long term (weeks to months) needed for vascular access<br>Access required within a few hours | Ease of access<br>Can be used immediately | Assess patient frequently for bleeding at insertion site and tubing connections.<br>Assess patency of access frequently by observing continuous flow of blood through shunt.<br>Shunt is potential source of infection. |
| **SUBCLAVIAN VEIN CATHETERIZATION** | | |
| Immediate access<br>Short or long duration of vascular access | Does not restrict patient's activity<br>Requires only one catheter | Assess patient frequently for bleeding from insertion site and infection.<br>Sterile technique is essential when working with catheter.<br>This requires irrigation with heparin solution to ensure patency. |
| **ARTERIOVENOUS FISTULA AND GRAFT** | | |
| Permanent access required | Is least likely of all the accesses to develop an infection<br>Once maintained it provides easy access | Assess patency of fistula or graft by palpating or auscultating bruit.<br>Instruct patient to avoid compression of fistula by tight clothing or carrying objects with arm bent.<br>Patient must be instructed to assess fistula for signs and symptoms of infection, including pain, redness, swelling, or excessive warmth and patency by palpating thrill.<br>Avoid blood pressure measurements and venipunctures in access arm. |

ducing shock, the blood pressure and pulse rate are checked every 30 to 60 minutes and more frequently when any of the previously mentioned signs and symptoms are present. Blood pressure readings should show only a slight gradual drop during the course of dialysis. Because the rate and pressure at which blood flows through the dialyzer are proportional to the rate and amount of fluid removed, blood flow and dialyzer pressure settings are carefully monitored. Unless the individual is severely hypertensive, rapid-acting antihypertensive medications are usually withheld the morning of dialysis until after the treatment. Additionally, sedative drugs (analgesics, tranquilizers, hypnotics) and those primarily affecting the vasculature (nitroglycerin) predispose the patient to hypotensive episodes. Self-medication with these agents before and during dialysis must be carefully reviewed with each patient.

In treating a patient who shows signs of hypovolemia, initial nursing measures include determining the blood pressure and pulse, placing the head of the bed in a flat position, and raising the patient's feet. The ultrafiltration pressure is decreased, and fluid replacement may be necessary to restore blood pressure. Throughout a hypotensive episode, vital signs, level of consciousness, and any complaints are closely monitored; vomiting frequently accompanies severe hypotension. Because an upper extremity must be fairly immobile during dialysis, the patient must be helped to a safe position to avoid aspiration if vomiting occurs.

The patient is weighed before and after dialysis to determine the amount of fluid loss during treatment. When the weight losses of several dialysis treatments are correlated with the patient's blood pressure, pulse, and other indications of hypovolemia, a pattern of tolerance to fluid removal can be determined. This trend or pattern can be used to help adjust the rate and overall effect of the dialysis in keeping with the patient's physiologic tolerance.

## NURSING CARE PLAN

### PERSON WITH CHRONIC GLOMERULONEPHRITIS AND RENAL FAILURE RECEIVING DIALYSIS

**DATA:** Mr. D. is a 52-year-old high-school teacher with a 10-year history of chronic glomerulonephritis. He worked full time until 3 months ago, when his renal disease progressed to end-stage disease requiring hemodialysis. He has been depressed and confided in the nurse that he seems to be losing control over his life.

Mr. D. is married with three active adolescent children, who were accustomed to him attending their sports activities. Mr. D. can no longer attend these activities because of fatigue and limited mobility.

Because of financial hardship, his wife started working full time as a salesclerk. She can no longer find the time to play bridge with her friends.

The nursing assessment identified the following:

- His dialysis schedule is three times weekly with 4-hour treatments each time.
- He has an arteriovenous fistula in his left arm.
- His blood pressures ranged from 190/110 to 180/100 before dialysis and 120/70 to 100/64 after the second hour of treatment.
- He often develops a headache and becomes agitated during dialysis.

#### ■ NURSING DIAGNOSIS

Fluid volume excess related to fluid accumulation since last dialysis

| Expected Patient Outcome | Nursing Interventions | Rationale |
|---|---|---|
| Maintains fluid volume status within established parameters. | Assess weight, lungs, and extremities for presence of edema.<br>Monitor intake and output and vital signs. | To determine fluid volume status as a guideline for determining treatment parameters. |
| | Monitor laboratory values: BUN; serum creatinine, sodium, potassium, calcium, magnesium, and phosphorous levels; hemoglobin and hematocrit. | Nitrogenous wastes and electrolytes accumulate between treatments; anemia is a continuing problem with chronic renal failure and blood losses associated with dialysis. |

#### ■ NURSING DIAGNOSIS

Fluid volume deficit related to rapid fluid removal during dialysis and potential blood loss

| Expected Patient Outcome | Nursing Interventions | Rationale |
|---|---|---|
| Does not exhibit signs of hypovolemia. | Monitor intake and output and vital signs during dialysis. | To recognize shifts in fluid balance. |
| | Monitor effects of anticoagulant therapy every hour during dialysis.<br>Monitor blood clotting time hourly during dialysis. | Anticoagulant therapy is necessary to prevent clotting in the dialysis tubing. The hourly checking of clotting time helps to prevent excessive bleeding in patient. |
| | Minimize blood loss by:<br>Careful drawing of blood samples for clotting times.<br>Returning all blood from hemodialysis machine to patient at end of treatment.<br>Applying pressure to fistula puncture point sites at end of dialysis. | Careful returning of all blood to patient helps prevent worsening anemia, which is a part of chronic renal failure. |
| | Monitor weight during dialysis to prevent weight loss greater than 3-4 kg during treatment. | To prevent hypovolemia. |

## NURSING CARE PLAN

### PERSON WITH CHRONIC GLOMERULONEPHRITIS AND RENAL FAILURE RECEIVING DIALYSIS—cont'd

#### ■ NURSING DIAGNOSIS

High risk for infection related to invasive procedure and possible blood transfusion requirements

| Expected Patient Outcome | Nursing Interventions | Rationale |
|---|---|---|
| Does not develop an infection. | Identify Mr. D.'s hepatitis B and C virus and human immunodeficiency virus (HIV) status; follow universal precautions for exposure to blood and body fluids. | To protect patient and nurse. |
| | Use sterile technique to start and stop procedure for shunt or fistula care.<br>Inspect shunt exit sites and fistula needle puncture sites for signs of infection. | To protect patient from potential sources of infection during procedure. |
| | Monitor temperature and white blood cell count (WBC). | To detect infection; small elevations in temperature may reflect significant infection. |
| | Follow routine testing policies; hepatitis B and C and HIV antibodies for patients and staff. | To identify change in status, patients are monitored monthly and staff yearly. |

#### ■ NURSING DIAGNOSIS

Body image disturbance related to chronic renal failure requiring machine dependency

| Expected Patient Outcome | Nursing Interventions | Rationale |
|---|---|---|
| Mr. D. and family accept the changes in body image that are part of chronic renal failure requiring dialysis. | Observe Mr. D.'s response to chronic illness, altered renal function, and other body alterations. | People vary greatly in their response to such life changes. |
| | Recognize response to dependence on a machine. | Patient may feel helpless and hopeless; deny reality; personalize the machine or accept it as a necessity. |
| | Support strengths; self-confidence, determination, and motivation to live. | Dialysis patients are not disabled in all aspects of life. |
| | Be aware of changes in social involvement; help him develop or continue interests beyond dialysis and return to as normal a life as possible. | Patient may participate in fewer social-recreational activities, experience life-style changes, and withdraw because of being different. |
| | Be alert to excessive concerns with losses, depression, self-neglect, noncompliance with medical regimen, and possibility of suicide; try to keep lines of communication open; encourage questions. | Suicide is possible, and Mr. D. has access to several methods that could be used to commit suicide. |
| | Be aware of effect that loss of libido, impotence, and decreased orgasm has on patient's marital and sexual life. | |
| | Refer for psychologic counseling as appropriate. | |
| | Try to help him develop realistic expectations of dialysis. | Hemodialysis does not reverse all signs and symptoms of chronic renal disease, and this may be difficult for Mr. D. to accept. |

*Continued.*

## NURSING CARE PLAN

### PERSON WITH CHRONIC GLOMERULONEPHRITIS AND RENAL FAILURE RECEIVING DIALYSIS—cont'd

#### ■ NURSING DIAGNOSIS

Impaired thought processes related to dialysis disequilibrium syndrome or dialysis dementia

| Expected Patient Outcome | Nursing Interventions | Rationale |
|---|---|---|
| Has no alteration in thought processes. | Monitor during and toward end of dialysis for headaches, nausea, vomiting, and agitation. | These signs indicate uneven or too rapid removal of fluid, electrolytes, and nitrogenous wastes that most often occurs toward the end of treatment. |
| | Monitor speech during dialysis; observe for myoclonus and change in behavior. | These signs appear first during hemodialysis. |

#### ■ NURSING DIAGNOSIS

Altered family processes related to need for hemodialysis

| Expected Patient Outcome | Nursing Interventions | Rationale |
|---|---|---|
| Mr. D. and family have adjusted to his lifetime need to receive hemodialysis and are prepared for his dialysis treatments to be given in the community dialysis center. | Recognize the impact that chronic renal failure and hemodialysis have on the family. | Disruption, expense, and considerable alterations in time commitments may occur. |
| | Explore with patient and family the demands that his illness has made on family. | Patient outcomes affect the family's ability to cope, and vice versa. |
| | Support coping skills of patient and family, and assist them in exploring alternatives. | |
| | Explore with patient his feelings about no longer being the family "breadwinner." | |
| | Prepare patient and family for community dialysis center by reviewing location of center and when possible introducing them to a representative from the center who will review policies and procedures with them. | Mr. D. may have separation anxiety about moving to a new environment. Preparing patient and family well in advance of the move will give them time to work through their feelings about the change. |
| | Support patient and family to express fears that they may have about leaving a familiar environment and staff for a new and unknown setting. | Meeting someone from the dialysis center can help allay fears about the unknown. |

### Preventing disequilibrium phenomenon

A **disequilibrium phenomenon** occurs for many dialysis patients. This syndrome occurs toward the end of or after dialysis. Disequilibrium results when excess solutes (urea) are cleared from the blood more rapidly than they can diffuse from the body's cells (particularly those of the CNS) into the vascular compartment. Thus, disequilibrium exists in the concentration of solute inside and outside the cells. Since particle content is greater inside the cells, water is taken in and edema results. Intracellular pH changes also occur. To some degree, this process occurs with each dialysis procedure and helps to explain why patients do not feel their best immediately after treatment. Severe disequilibrium or disequilibrium phenomenon is most likely to be seen in the person whose blood chemistry values are exceptionally high before dialysis. Signs and symptoms of disequilibrium include *headache, hypertension, restlessness, mental confusion,* and *nausea* and *vomiting.* Severe disequilibrium may result in convulsions, especially in children, when BUN levels exceed the concentration of 100 mg/ml.

Treatment includes anticipation of severe disequilibrium. For example, when a patient undergoes dialysis for the first time, the treatment is shortened and is scheduled 3 days in a row. This allows solute to be cleared from the body without producing the extremely wide swings in blood chemistry that would result in severe disequilibrium. Keeping the patient quiet, reducing environmental discomfort such as temperature extremes and bright lights, and closely supervising the patient to ensure physical safety are nursing care requirements. Mild analgesics may help to relieve headache. If disequilibrium becomes severe, the dialysis treatment may be discontinued.

#### Preventing blood loss

Care of the patient on dialysis also includes preventing blood loss. To prevent the patient's blood from clotting as it flows through the dialyzer, heparin is administered. Protamine sulfate is not generally given to the patient to counteract the effect of heparin. The patient is watched for signs of bleeding anywhere in the body. At the end of the treatment when dialysis needles are removed from the fistula, pressure dressings are applied to the puncture sites. They are observed at frequent intervals to detect hemorrhage. During and shortly after dialysis, treatments that cause tissue trauma should not be performed. These typically include venipuncture and intramuscular injections. The patient who has had recent surgery, dental extractions, or recent trauma to soft tissues will have clotting times monitored frequently during dialysis to prevent hemorrhage. These sites need to be closely observed for signs of bleeding.

### Promoting Comfort

Patients should have an opportunity to become familiar with the dialysis unit before therapy begins. They should be given an explanation of what will happen and what will be expected of them during the treatment. Patients often want to know the following:

1. What type of pain or discomfort will be experienced?
2. How long and how often will dialysis be required?
3. What will they feel like during and after the treatment?
4. What will they be allowed to do during dialysis?
5. May family members be present during therapy?

Sometimes it helps if the new dialysis patient is given the opportunity to talk with an "experienced" dialysis patient.

Pain of a moderate degree may be experienced when venipuncture is performed in an arteriovenous fistula or graft. A local anesthetic is used in most dialysis centers before insertion of the large-bore needles. Some patients find it less painful if they insert their own needles.

Patients should be told that they may experience some headache and nausea during the treatment and for a few hours afterward. *Headache* and *nausea* result from changes in fluid and acid-base balance and from nitrogenous waste removal during dialysis. The symptoms should never be extreme, and relief can be attained from rest and sleep, mild analgesics, or antiemetics. Mouth care is required if the patient is nauseated and vomiting. *Dizziness* and *faintness* may result from hypotension. Relief should be obtained within a few hours with rest. The patient is assured that all these symptoms will abate and that frequent monitoring during the procedure will help to control the degree of change that occurs during dialysis and the development of these symptoms.

### Maintaining Activity and Nutrition

A dialysis treatment lasts from 2 to 4 hours, depending on the type of dialyzer used and the time necessary to correct the fluid, electrolyte, acid-base, and nitrogenous waste imbalances. Dialysis for an *acute* problem may be carried out daily or as often as warranted. Hemodialysis for *chronic* renal failure is usually performed two or three times a week.

Lying relatively immobile for even a few hours can produce pressure over bony prominences and general restlessness. Frequent position changes can increase tolerance for restricted movement. Because the upper extremity is generally kept immobile during dialysis, the patient may need help with activities requiring the use of both hands. Activity during dialysis is largely a matter of individual preference. Some sleep throughout treatment; others read, watch TV, or socialize with other patients.

Eating during dialysis is largely a matter of individual preference. Some individuals may become quite hungry, whereas for others the smell of food causes nausea. Patients may ask that they be allowed to eat foods not generally allowed during dialysis; the best time to eat usually nonallowed foods is the night before dialysis because the food is digested and metabolized and because the waste products are already in the blood to be removed by dialysis. Practice indicates that either allowing or discouraging eating during dialysis is a matter of individual unit philosophy. Because of the frequency of nausea, vomiting, and disequilibrium experienced during hemodialysis, it may be best to discourage eating to decrease the potential of aspiration.

### Facilitating Learning

The person or significant others can state, demonstrate, or plan the following:

1. The process of hemodialysis and relate to own body needs
2. Observations required of vascular access about infection and clotting as well as means of obtaining care when these occur
3. Appropriate care of arteriovenous access
4. Common side effects of treatment, means of controlling mild symptoms, and means of obtaining medical attention for severe or persistent complications
5. Changes in medication schedule required before and after dialysis

## BOX 50-4 Example of A Teaching Plan for The Person Receiving Hemodialysis

| Date | Hour | Teaching/learning | RN signature |
|---|---|---|---|
| | | Chronic renal failure being treated by hemodialysis | |
| Start | Stop | Plan | |
| | | 1. Introduce patient to hemodialysis unit using available printed material and a visit to unit when appropriate. | |
| | | 2. Explain normal kidney function. | |
| | | 3. Explain kidney failure specific to patient's pathophysiology: | |
| | | a. Types | |
| | | b. Causes | |
| | | 4. Explain and reinforce medication regimen: | |
| | | a. Purpose of each prescribed medication | |
| | | b. Common side effects | |
| | | c. Dose and times of each medication | |
| | | d. Prescription filling procedure | |
| | | 5. Reinforce dietary instruction: | |
| | | a. Protein | |
| | | b. Potassium | |
| | | c. Sodium | |
| | | d. Fluids | |
| | | e. Calories | |
| | | 6. Instruct patient about need for and care of vascular access: | |
| | | a. Procedure for assessing presence of thrill and bruit; who to notify if thrill or bruit is absent | |
| | | b. Guarding against constriction of fistula; that is, sleeping on arm or wearing tight clothing | |
| | | c. Hygiene and removing dressing after dialysis | |
| | | d. Signs and symptoms of infection; that is, redness, swelling, or tenderness | |
| | | e. Measures to control hemorrhage should it develop while away from dialysis unit | |
| | | 7. Instruct patient about process of hemodialysis: | |
| | | a. Explain principles of dialysis in sufficient detail for learning level of patient. | |
| | | b. Describe hemodialysis in full detail to patient. | |
| | | c. Explain common sights and sounds of dialysis unit to patient. | |
| | | d. Describe common complications of hemodialysis to patient as well as usual treatments: | |
| | | (1) Hypotension | |
| | | (2) Nausea | |
| | | (3) Vomiting | |
| | | (4) Cramping | |
| | | 8. Instruct patient in interpretation of laboratory data and effects of hemodialysis, diet, and medications on these values. | |
| | | 9. Introduce patient to alternative modes of treatment of end-stage renal disease: | |
| | | a. Free-standing hemodialysis centers | |
| | | b. Self-dialysis (home) | |
| | | c. Peritoneal dialysis | |
| | | d. Transplantation | |

*Continued.*

**BOX 50-4 Example of a Teaching Plan for The Person Receiving Hemodialysis—cont'd**

| Date | | Status of problems at discharge | |
|---|---|---|---|
| | | | |
| | | | |
| | | | |
| Date | | Patient knowledge | |
| | | | |
| | | | |
| | | | |
| | | | |
| Date | | Follow-up plan | |
| | | | |
| | | | |
| | | | |
| | | | |
| | | | |
| | | | |

RN signature ______________________

6. A work and activity schedule as physical capabilities permit

An example of a teaching care plan for the person receiving hemodialysis is illustrated in the Box 50-4.

## ♦ EVALUATION

To evaluate the effectiveness of nursing interventions, compare patient behaviors with those stated in the expected patient outcomes. Successful achievement of patient outcomes for the patient receiving hemodialysis is indicated by the following:

1. Lack of excessive fluid weight gain between dialysis treatments.
2. States that no pain is present and that discomfort experienced during dialysis is decreased.
3. Participates in a program to maintain prescribed activity level.
4. Eats according to preference during therapy.
5. Correctly explains dialysis, care of venous access, common side effects, and recommended work/activity schedule.

## PERITONEAL DIALYSIS

In **peritoneal dialysis** the dialyzing fluid is instilled into the peritoneal cavity, and the peritoneum becomes the dialyzing membrane (Figure 50-7). Compared with hemodialysis treatments, which last 2 to 4 hours, peritoneal dialysis is maintained continuously for up to 36 hours. The procedure, once instituted, becomes largely a nursing responsibility. Peritoneal dialysis is used in treating acute and chronic renal failure. It can be performed in the hospital or at home (see p. 1690).

The major advantages of peritoneal dialysis include the following:

1. It provides a steady state of blood chemistries.
2. Patient can dialyze alone in any location without need for machinery.
3. Patient can readily be taught the process.
4. Patient has few dietary restrictions; because of loss of protein in dialysate, the patient is usually placed on a high-protein diet.
5. Patient has much more control over daily life.
6. Peritoneal dialysis can be used for patients that are hemodynamically unstable.

### Procedure

Access to the peritoneum is gained through introduction of a catheter into the peritoneal space. For acutely ill patients and those who are chronically ill and require sporadic dialysis, a sterile catheter is inserted for each procedure. For the chronically ill person treated on a routine basis, a special catheter can be placed into the peritoneal space; the catheter remains in place until it malfunctions or until another treatment option, such as

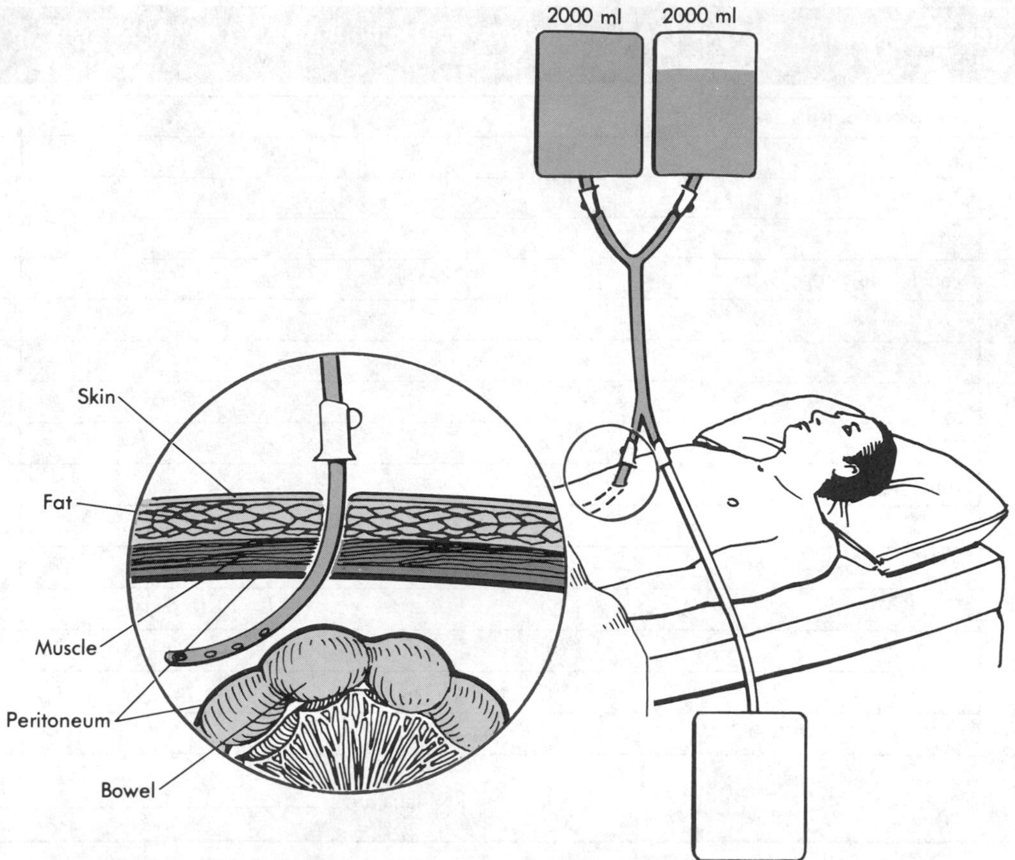


**FIGURE 50-7** Patient receiving peritoneal dialysis. Dialysis fluid is being infused into the peritoneal cavity.

transplantation, is selected. These catheters present a continued potential entrance for organisms into the peritoneum. Each patient must be thoroughly instructed in the care of the catheter and the signs and symptoms indicative of local or peritoneal infection. These must be reported to the physician.

For all patients, weight, blood pressure, and pulse are recorded before initiating the procedure. These values serve as baseline information to assess changes during treatment. For persons undergoing insertion of a peritoneal catheter before dialysis, assessment should be made of their knowledge of the procedure and their anxiety level. A mild sedative may help the severely anxious person to better tolerate the insertion of the catheter. It is important that these patients void just before catheter insertion; this decompresses the bladder and prevents accidental puncture during catheter placement.

To insert a peritoneal catheter, the physician cleanses the abdomen and anesthetizes a small area in the midline of the abdomen about 5 cm (2 inches) below the umbilicus. A small incision is made, and the many-eyed nylon catheter is inserted into the peritoneal cavity (Figure 50-7). A dressing is placed around the protruding catheter.

Approximately 2 L of sterile dialysate warmed to body temperature is attached by tubing to the catheter and allowed to run into the peritoneal cavity as rapidly as possible. This usually takes about 10 minutes. The tubing is then clamped. The maximal osmosis of fluid and diffusion of particles into the dialysate occurs in 20 to 30 minutes. At the end of the dwell time, the tubing is unclamped and the fluid is allowed to flow by gravity from the abdomen. Fluid should drain in a steady stream. Drainage time should average about 10 to 15 minutes. The first drainage may be pink tinged as a result of the trauma of catheter insertion; however, this should clear with the second or third drainage. At no time should fluid draining from the abdomen appear grossly bloody. After fluid has drained from the abdomen, another cycle is started immediately. Dialysis is initiated for the person with a permanent catheter by carefully cleansing the catheter and surrounding skin with a bactericidal agent before the catheter is connected to the dialysate line.

After the infusion of dialysate has been completed, the permanent catheter is again cleansed and a sterile cap applied to the tip.

If the procedure is temporary, the catheter is removed, and the incision is covered with a dry, sterile dressing. The small abdominal wound from the catheter should heal completely in 1 to 2 days.

## Care During Peritoneal Dialysis

Problems most often associated with peritoneal dialysis include hypotension and hypovolemia, inadequate drainage of fluid from the peritoneal space, pain, atelectasis, respiratory distress, and peritonitis.

### Regulating fluid volume and drainage

As with hemodialysis, *hypotension* is most likely a result of rapid removal of fluid from the intravascular space. In addition to checking vital signs and observing the patient's behavior, records of fluid balance are crucial in determining the amount of fluid that has been removed. The net gain or loss of fluid from the abdomen should be determined at the completion of each cycle. To decrease the amount of fluid that is being removed from the vascular space, the physician may decrease the hypertonicity of the dialysate and may increase the amount of fluid administered through an intravenous line.

*Drainage of fluid* from the abdomen can be slow or impossible to start. Generally, this problem results when the tip of the catheter has become lodged against the abdominal wall. It may also result when the catheter becomes plugged with blood or fibrin that has accumulated as a result of tissue trauma. A small amount of heparin may be added to the dialysate to decrease the chance of a clot forming in the catheter. When the dialysate does not drain freely from the abdomen, the patient should be turned from side to side in an attempt to reposition the catheter in the peritoneal cavity. In addition, firm pressure may be applied to the abdomen with both hands and the head of the bed may be raised. If the flow of the dialysate does not increase, the physician is called to irrigate the catheter or reposition it.

### Promoting comfort

Severe *pain* should not be experienced during peritoneal dialysis. Moderate levels of pressure pain are often experienced as fluid is instilled and withdrawn from the peritoneal cavity. Procaine hydrochloride may be instilled with the dialysate in an attempt to control the patient's discomfort. Mild analgesics may be ordered for administration at 3- to 4-hour intervals during the procedure.

Although the patient is generally confined to a recumbent position for the length of the dialysis, comfort and diversion can be provided. The patient may turn from side to side and move about in bed as desired as long as the catheter remains undisturbed. The patient may be provided assistance with oral care and bathing as needed. Visiting and other diversional activities should be encouraged when the patient's physical condition permits. If peritoneal dialysis is carried out at home, the patient and a dialysis partner need to be able to perform all the steps previously described.

### Preventing complications

When the patient is extremely overhydrated and shows evidence of congestive heart failure and pulmonary edema, *respiratory difficulty* may be encountered as the dialysate infuses. The quality and rate of respiration should be closely observed. The head of the bed can be raised to decrease the pressure of the dialysate on the diaphragm. The amount of dialyzing fluid used for each cycle may be decreased when respiratory distress becomes prolonged and severe. The patient, although encouraged to eat while being dialyzed, may find that this increases respiratory difficulty. To help overcome additional pressure created by a full stomach, frequent small meals may be provided.

*Peritonitis* is an ever-present threat during peritoneal dialysis. Aseptic technique must be rigidly maintained during insertion of the catheter and throughout the procedure. Care should be taken to avoid contaminating the solution or the tubing when dialysate solution is hung. Cultures of the dialysate fluid are performed routinely to ensure continued attention to asepsis and to identify organisms if peritonitis develops. The patient should be observed for signs of peritonitis. These include an elevated temperature, chills, tenderness or abdominal pain, nausea and vomiting, and cloudy outflow.

### Facilitating learning

The teaching requirements for the patient undergoing peritoneal dialysis is consistent with the teaching plan for hemodialysis. However, the patient will need to be instructed in the specifics of the process of peritoneal dialysis. If the patient will undergo continuous ambulatory dialysis, training should be accomplished in a home training center that is equipped to assist the patient in dealing with home care.

The teaching plan should include the following:

1. The process of dialysis and how the dialysis relates to the patient's own body needs
2. Signs and symptoms of infection of the peritoneal cavity or catheter site and where to obtain care if these occur
3. Appropriate care of the permanent peritoneal catheter
4. Common side effects of treatment, means of controlling mild symptoms, and means of obtaining medical attention for severe or persistent complications
5. Changes in medication schedule required before and after dialysis
6. A work and activity schedule as physical capabilities

permit, with minimal interference from scheduled dialysis time.

### Other Approaches to Peritoneal Dialysis

Several advances in the management of patients with chronic ESRD have led to two variations of peritoneal dialysis. These technologies emphasize home and self-dialysis.

**Continuous ambulatory peritoneal dialysis (CAPD)** is one method leading to safe self-dialysis that is practical, is relatively inexpensive when compared with hemodialysis, and promotes independence. Basically, CAPD involves continuous contact of dialysate with the peritoneal membrane. Approximately 2 L of dialysate is maintained in the peritoneal cavity and exchanged by the patient through a permanent peritoneal catheter 4 to 5 times each day. No special equipment is required for the exchanges, and therefore the patient can lead a fairly normal life. Exchanges can take place at home or at work by connecting an empty bag to the catheter and opening a clamp to allow drainage. A full dialysate bag is then instilled, and the patient has completed an exchange.

The second method is **continuous cyclic peritoneal dialysis (CCPD).** CCPD differs from CAPD in that a machine known as a cycler is used to instill and drain dialysate from the patient. The machine has a series of clamps that are controlled by timers. The timers open and close the clamps in sequence to allow for instillation and drainage of dialysate from the patient. The cycle times for patients with chronic renal failure generally allow for the patient to be dialyzed in 6 to 8 hours. A patient, therefore, can connect up to the cycler at bedtime, set the machine, and be dialyzed while sleeping. Several alarms are built into the cycler to protect the patient from such malfunctions as dialysate that is too hot or cold, long or short dwell times, improper return of fluid, and changes in catheter pressures. The greatest advantage of CAPD and CCPD over other forms of dialysis is that both offer the patient unprecedented freedom in managing their own care.

## EVALUATING DIALYSIS EFFECTIVENESS

**Kinetic modeling,** or prescription dialysis, is a tool developed by dialysis practitioners in the last decade for computing how much hemodialysis an individual patient needs and monitoring the effectiveness of the delivered prescription. Hemodialysis is usually prescribed by nephrologists based on the mathematical formula $Kt/V$. This formulation includes individual patient parameters of dialyzer clearance ($K$), time of dialysis ($t$), and volume of urea distribution ($V$). In addition, the normalized protein catabolic rate of the individual patient must be determined and periodically reassessed. Using serum urea levels as the kinetic factor, practitioners are able to determine an expected outcome of treatment. A $Kt/V$ equal to 1.0 represents adequate dialysis. If the $Kt/V$ is less than 1.0, a change in dialyzer and/or increase in dialysis time may be required. In a peritoneal dialysis patient, an increase in the number of dialysis exchanges may be necessary.[17]

# KIDNEY TRANSPLANTATION

The advantages of kidney transplantation are the reversal of many of the pathophysiologic changes associated with renal failure as normal kidney function is restored. It also eliminates the dependence on dialysis and the accompanying dietary restrictions, provides the opportunity to return to normal life activities, including work, and is less expensive than dialysis after the first year.

Although transplant procedures are expensive, the current success rates have made transplantation a cost-effective treatment option compared with traditional medical management. For example, a patient undergoing chronic hemodialysis in 1994 costs the federal government, through Medicare, about $40,000/yr. The cost of a kidney transplant is approximately $40,000 for the first year and $5000/yr for follow-up care. If the transplant functions for 5 years (the actual rate approaches 75%), the cost is $60,000 as opposed to $200,000 for 5-year chronic hemodialysis. Other financial factors that increase the cost-effectiveness of transplantation are the potential earning power of the transplant recipient and the discontinuation of disability benefits previously required. In short, transplantation is a therapy that can restore dignity and quality to the lives of patient and families dealing with ESRD and provide the potential for patients to become productive members of society again.[2]

(For a discussion of the methods of kidney transplantation and required care requirements, see Chapter 72.)

# INTERVENTIONS FOR THE PERSON DYING OF RENAL FAILURE

Approximately 15% to 20% of dialysis patients voluntarily choose to discontinue dialysis. Because patient autonomy in the United States is the overriding legal imperative to accepting treatment, patient wishes must be honored. If the burdens of life with impaired quality are so great that continuation of therapy offers no benefit but only prolongs a miserable existence, then discontinuing dialysis is reasonable. This is not considered suicide by the major religious groups (Protestant, Catholic, Jewish, Muslim, Buddhist). Patients are very apprehensive about the process of dying, fearing pain and discomfort. They should be counseled that death from uremia is generally quiet, peaceful, and without pain or discomfort. Hospice care is very helpful for patients who wish to remain at home.[8]

As the patient dies, it is unrealistic to continue fluid and dietary restrictions. Many patients wish to enjoy favorite foods previously denied them; this wish should be honored. As the uremia progresses, patients will restrict their own intake. The goals of nursing care are maintaining comfort and safety and providing the opportunity for patient and family to express their feelings and arrive at some degree of emotional comfort.

In providing physical comfort, frequent turning and repositioning are necessary to prevent skin excoriation and breakdown. Oral care is extremely important, because mouth sores, once developed, will not heal. Mineral oil is an acceptable protective lubricant for the alert patient; a water-soluble lubricant with a vegetable base (such as K-Y jelly) is preferable for the comatose patient. Hydrogen peroxide is helpful in removing blood from the mouth and nose. Vinegar mouthwash neutralizes the ammonia.

As death approaches and the patient's level of awareness and ability to control the environment decrease, it becomes the responsibility of the nursing staff to provide safety. (Chapter 57 describes the specific care required for the unconscious patient.)

Providing an opportunity for the patient and family to talk about their feelings is one of the more important aspects of nursing care. Thoughts concerning death and alarm over treatments can produce considerable anxiety. The wishes of the patient and family regarding spiritual counseling should be determined. Through demonstrating interest in individual needs and providing comfort measures, the nurse can do much to help the patient and family through the process of dying. (For further information on loss, grief, and dying, see Chapter 10.)

## QUESTIONS TO CONSIDER

- How does fluid and electrolyte balance differ among the oliguric and diuretic phases of acute renal failure and chronic renal failure?
- How would the nursing care plan of a patient receiving hemodialysis differ from that of a patient receiving peritoneal dialysis?
- If you were assigned a patient who is to initiate continuous cyclic peritoneal dialysis (CCPD) at home, what information would you need?
- What resources are available in your community for persons with end-stage renal disease?

## CRITICAL THINKING ACTIVITIES

- Mrs. Gray, 57, has a 10-year history of lupus erythematosus. She has been treated intermittently with prednisone to control symptoms. Her disease has been slowly progressive but has not interfered with her ability to work. Mrs. Gray is married and has two grown daughters. She is 5′4″ tall and normally weighs 132 pounds. Does Mrs. Gray have any significant risk factors for renal failure? If so, what? Explain how lupus can affect her renal status.

## CRITICAL THINKING ACTIVITIES – cont'd

- Rex, 39, makes his living as an exterminator. He is being admitted to the hospital for persistent flank pain and denies urinary frequency, urgency, or pain. He has had no recent illnesses or injuries except for a sore throat 3 weeks ago that subsided without treatment. His family history is positive for hypertension and diabetes. He is currently taking no medications. What risk factors does Rex have for the development of renal disease?

## CHAPTER SUMMARY

- Renal failure is a state of total or nearly total loss of the kidney's ability to excrete waste products and to maintain fluid and electrolyte balance.

### ACUTE RENAL FAILURE

- Signs and symptoms indicating the onset of acute renal failure (ARF) appear rapidly and are a direct result of retention of fluids, metabolic wastes, and inability to regulate electrolytes.
- The oliguric phase of ARF is characterized by inability to excrete fluid loads (oliguria), hyperkalemia, hyponatremia, metabolic acidosis, and uremia. The diuretic phase is characterized by excessive diuresis with loss of sodium and potassium; BUN remains elevated, then decreases slowly.
- Nursing care during the oliguric phase of ARF includes monitoring and controlling fluid intake, controlling protein and potassium intake, encouraging a high-carbohydrate, high-fat diet, promoting rest/activity balance, and preventing injury and infection. During the diuretic phase, monitoring of fluid and electrolyte balance continues, activity is encouraged, and learning is facilitated.

### CHRONIC RENAL FAILURE

- Chronic renal failure represents progressive and irreversible kidney damage. It is characterized by altered fluid and electrolyte balance and regulatory body functions and by retention of nitrogenous wastes (uremia).
- Chronic renal failure can be treated by conservative medical management, hemodialysis, peritoneal dialysis or its variations (CAPD, CCPD), or kidney transplantation.
- Nursing interventions for chronic renal failure include maintaining fluid and electrolyte balance, preventing infection and injury, promoting comfort, facilitating coping with life-style changes and feelings regarding self, and facilitating teaching.

## DIALYSIS

- Dialysis involves movement of fluid and particles across a semipermeable membrane by diffusion, osmosis, and ultrafiltration. *Hemodialysis* involves shunting the patient's blood through a dialyzer to exchange fluids, electrolytes, and waste materials. With *peritoneal dialysis,* the peritoneum becomes the dialyzing membrane.
- Nursing care for hemodialysis includes preventing hypovolemia, shock, disequilibrium phenomenon, and blood loss; promoting comfort; maintaining activity and nutrition; and facilitating learning.
- Nursing care for peritoneal dialysis includes regulating fluid volume and drainage, promoting comfort, preventing complications, and facilitating learning.

## KIDNEY TRANSPLANTATION

- Kidney transplantation restores normal kidney function, eliminates dependence on dialysis, and is less expensive than dialysis after the first year.

# REFERENCES


1. Baer C, Lancaster L: Acute renal failure, *Crit Care Q* 14(1):1-21, 1992.
2. Bartucci M: Organ donation. In Clochesy J et al, editors: *Critical care nursing,* Philadelphia, 1993, WB Saunders.
3. Bloembergen W, Port F: Demographics of the ESRD population. In Nissenson AR, Fine RN, editors: *Dialysis therapy,* St Louis, 1993, Mosby.
4. Butler B: Nutritional management of catabolic acute renal failure requiring renal replacement therapy, *ANNA J* 18(3):247-259, 1991.
5. Counts C: Potential complications of the internal vascular access: implications for nursing care, *Dialysis Transplant* 22(2):75-87, 105, 1993.
6. Emmett M, Hootkins R: Phosphorus binders. In Nissenson AR, Fine RN, editors: *Dialysis therapy,* St Louis, 1993, Mosby.
7. Flaherty MJ, O'Brien ME: Family styles of coping in end stage renal disease, *ANNA J* 19(4):345-349, 1992.
8. Foulks C: Ethical dilemmas in dialysis: to initiate or withdraw therapy. In Nissenson AR, Fine RN, editors: *Dialysis therapy,* St Louis, 1993, Mosby.
9. Hodsman AB: Use of vitamin D sterols in the management of renal osteodystrophy. In Nissenson AR, Fine RN, editors: *Dialysis therapy,* St Louis, 1993, Mosby.
10. Keen M: Patients with fluid and electrolyte disturbances. In Clochesy J et al, editors: *Critical care nursing,* Philadelphia, 1993, WB Saunders.
11. Latham D, Nichols E: Epoetin alfa: patient management issues and development through recombinant DNA technology, *ANNA J* 17(4):311-316, 1990.
12. Llach F: Differential diagnosis of renal osteodystrophy. In Nissenson AR, Fine RN, editors: *Dialysis therapy,* St Louis, 1993, Mosby.
13. Peschman P: Renal physiology. In Clochesy J et al, editors: *Critical care nursing,* Philadelphia, 1993, WB Saunders.
14. Preisig P: Urinary concentration and dilution, *ANNA J* 19(4):351-355, 1992.
15. Price C: Continuous renal replacement therapy: the treatment of choice for acute renal failure, *ANNA J* 18(3):239-244, 1991.
16. Shusterman N et al: Risk factors and outcome of hospital acquired acute renal failure, *Am J Med* 83:65-71, 1987.
17. Threlkeld JS: Nursing implications in kinetic modeling, *ANNA J* 19(2):178-181, 1992.
18. Whittaker A: Patients with acute renal failure. In Clochesy J et al, editors: *Critical care nursing,* Philadelphia, 1993, WB Saunders.
19. Wolcott DL: Psychosocial rehabilitation of adult dialysis patients. In Nissenson AR, Fine RN, editors: *Dialysis therapy,* St Louis, 1993, Mosby.
20. Yarian S: Patients with end-stage renal disease. In Clochesy J et al, editors: *Critical care nursing,* Philadelphia, 1993, WB Saunders.

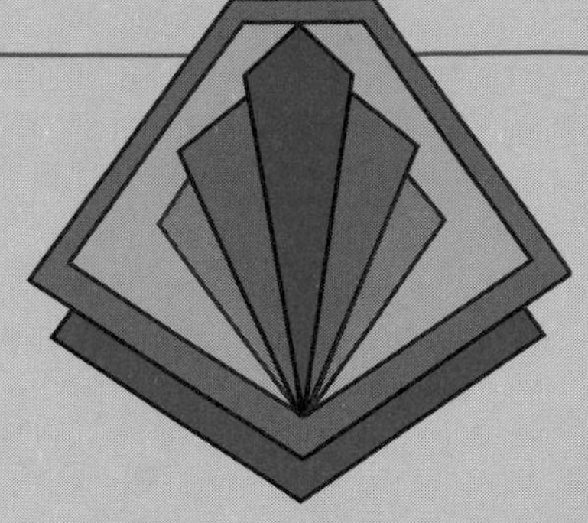

UNIT IX

# Alterations in Reproduction and Sexuality

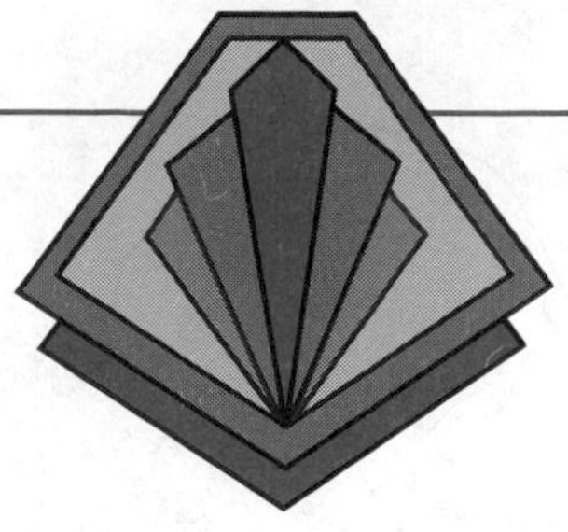

CHAPTER 51

# Assessment of Reproduction and Sexuality

*Jo Ann Lierman*
*Greer Glazer*

## CHAPTER OBJECTIVES

***After studying this chapter, the learner should be able to do the following:***

1 Describe the structures and functions of the male and female reproductive systems.
2 Explain the functions of the major hormones necessary to the structure and function of the reproductive systems.
3 Describe age-related changes in the reproductive systems.
4 Identify data related to the reproductive system and to sexual functions that should be obtained from a patient.
5 Discuss diagnostic and laboratory tests used in identifying reproductive tract problems and related nursing interventions.

## KEY TERMS

cervical intraepithelial neoplasia (CIN)
climacteric
colposcopy
culdoscopy
dilation and curettage (D & C)
estrogen
falloposcopy
hysterosalpingography
hysteroscopy
laparoscopy
luteinizing hormone (LH)
mammography
menarche
menopause
menstrual cycle
menstruation
mittelschmerz
Papanicolaou (Pap) smear
progesterone
prostate-specific antigen (PSA)
testosterone
transvaginal ultrasonography

Conditions affecting healthful functioning of the reproductive systems of men and women take a high toll in loss of life and acute and chronic physical and emotional stress. The nurse has a responsibility to assist in general health education, to refer patients to good health care, and to understand the treatment available and the nursing care needed when disease develops. A sound knowledge of the structure and functions of the reproductive system is essential to the assessment process.

## ANATOMY AND PHYSIOLOGY

### PELVIS

The bones of the pelvis are shown in Figure 51-1. The pelvis is the weight-bearing structure of the upper body and trunk. The pelvic bones consist of the innominate bones, the sacrum, and the coccyx. The two innominate bones are made up of the pubic bone, ilium, and ischium. Anteriorly, the pubic bones join at the symphysis pubis. The inferior borders of the pubic bones and symphysis form an inverted V, called the pubic arch. The sacrum and coccyx come together at the sacrococcygeal joint, which is movable.

The pelvis is divided into two parts (the true and the false pelvis) by a bony ridge called the pelvic brim. The false pelvis is the broad, expanded portion above the pelvic brim. The narrow part below the pelvic brim is the true pelvis. The true pelvis is further described as having an inlet and an outlet. The inlet is located at the pelvic brim, and the outlet is at the base of the pelvis. The iliac spines mark the midpoint between the inlet and the outlet. The distances between the bones of the true pelvis have special significance during childbirth, since it is through this bony canal that the baby must pass to be born.

As with other bones of the skeletal system, the pelvic bones undergo changes during periods of growth and development until maturity is reached. The major differences between the pelves of men and women are in the contour of the pelvis and thickness of the bones.

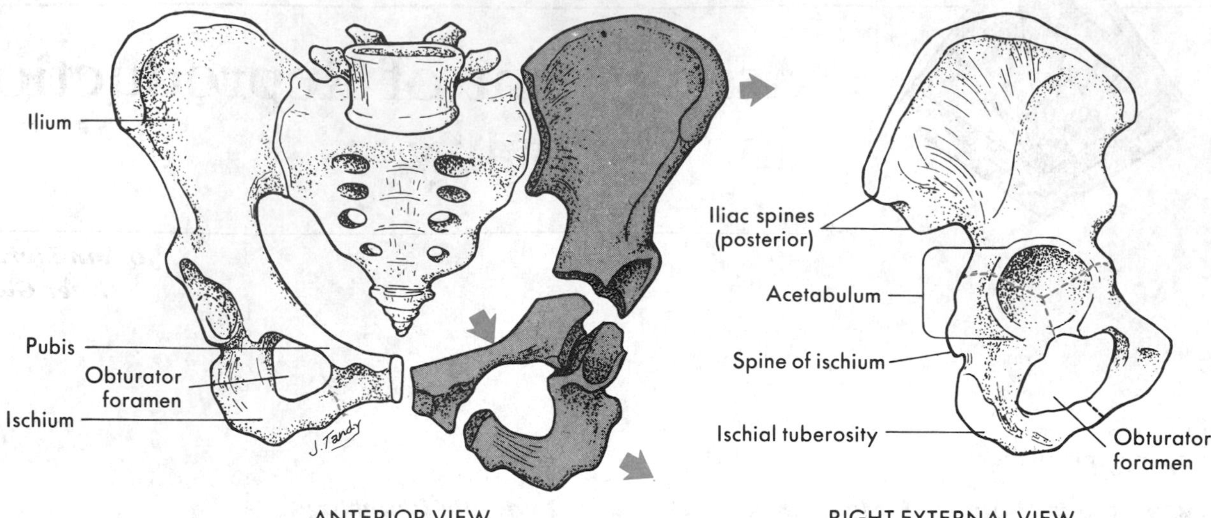


**FIGURE 51-1** Adult female pelvis, showing origin of parts from separate embryonic bones. (From Jensen MD, Benson RC, Bobak IM: *Maternity care: the nurse and the family,* ed 2, St Louis, 1981, Mosby.)

Although variations are seen in both sexes, the female pelvis is more delicate because the bones are thinner and lighter in weight. The female pelvis is wider and more shallow because of the flaring of the ilac bones; the male pelvis tends to be narrow and deep. In women, the sacrum is shorter, wider, and less curved and the coccyx is more movable. The pubic arch is wider and more rounded in women, and the ischial spines are less prominent. Pelvic dimensions vary with age and race in addition to gender. The typical architecture of the female pelvis is especially suited for childbirth.

## FEMALE GENITAL SYSTEM

### External Structures

Figure 51-2 shows the external genitalia of a female. The external genitalia consist of the mons pubis (mons veneris), labia majora, labia minora, clitoris, prepuce, frenulum, vestibule, urethral meatus, Skene's (paraurethral) glands, vaginal orifice, hymen, fossa navicularis, Bartholin's (vulvovaginal) glands, fourchet, perineum, and escutcheon. The escutcheon is the triangular pubic hair pattern from the upper portion of the pubic bone to the lateral areas of the labia majora. The *mons pubis* is the rounded area in front of the symphysis pubis. It consists of a collection of fatty tissue beneath the skin and is covered with hair after puberty.

The *labia majora* are two prominent, longitudinal folds of tissue extending back from the mons pubis. These labia are thicker in front, gradually become thinner as they extend back, and appear to flatten out as they merge with the adjacent tissues in the area of the perineum. The labia majora have two surfaces. The outer surface is covered by a thin layer of skin containing hair follicles and sebaceous and sweat glands. The inner surfaces are smooth, lack hair, and are supplied with many sebaceous follicles. The labia are homologous to the male scrotum.

The *labia minora* are two smaller folds of tissue parallel to the labia majora and sometimes concealed between the folds of the labia majora. In sexually active women and in women who have borne children, the labia minora may project beyond the labia majora. The labia minora join near the prepuce, which covers the clitoris, extend backward to enclose the urethral and vaginal openings, and merge with the labia majora in the perineum. The labia minora are made up of connective and elastic tissue and contain little fatty tissue. Sweat glands and hair follicles are absent from the labia minora, but sebaceous glands are present.

The *clitoris* is situated near the anterior folds of the labia minora. The glans of the clitoris is a small, rounded area consisting of erectile tissue enclosed in a layer of fibrous membrane. Although it is often compared with or said to be homologous to the penis in males because it consists of the glans, corpus, and crura, the clitoris is unique in that its sole physiologic functions are initiation and elevation of sexual tension levels. The clitoris serves as both receptor and transformer of sexual stimuli. Sexual stimulation initiates a process whereby the clitoris becomes enlarged, erect, and very sensitive to sexual stimuli. Female orgasm can occur from stimulation of the clitoris but also results from stimulation of other sites.

The *vestibule* is a boat-shaped fossa formed between the labia minora, clitoris, and fourchet. The *fossa navicularis* is a small depression between the fourchet and hymen. On opening the labia minora, the vaginal and urethral orifices can be seen. These surfaces are thin,

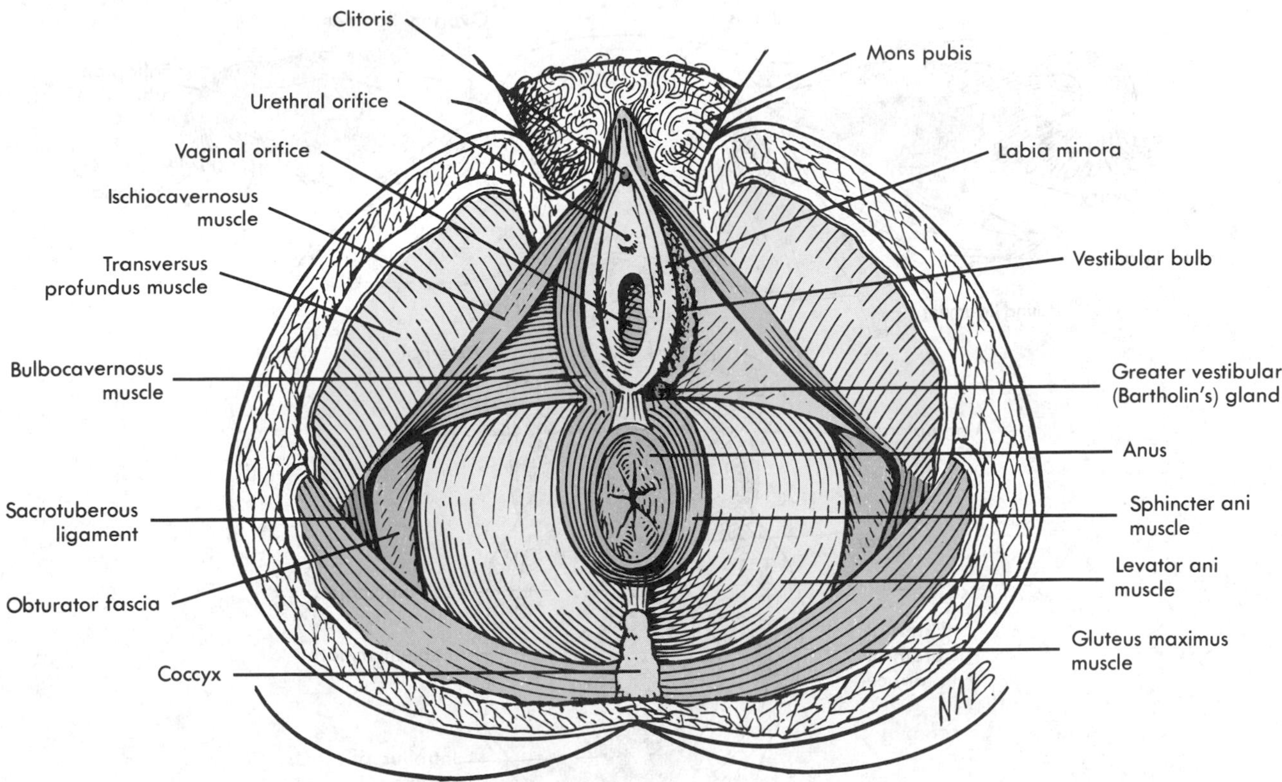


**FIGURE 51-2** Female perineum.

easily irritated, and especially subject to laceration during childbirth.

The *hymen* is an irregular membranous fold of connective tissue of varying thickness that partially covers the vaginal orifice. The hymen may be avulsed (broken) by coitus, digital examination, vigorous exercise, or surgery. Remnants of the hymen usually persist after avulsion and form an irregular border around the vaginal opening.

The location of *Skene's* (paraurethral) *glands* and *Bartholin's* (vulvovaginal) *glands* should be noted because they are common sites of infection. Skene's glands are located on each side of the urethral meatus. Bartholin's glands are situated at each side of the vaginal opening near the bases of the labia. Since both Skene's glands and Bartholin's glands are very small, their openings are just visible. They may not be palpable unless the woman is very thin or unless the glands are enlarged because of infection.

The *perineum* is the area between the vagina and anus. It is composed of muscles and subdermal and dermal tissue.

The appearance of the external structures varies with age. Before puberty, the external genitalia are characterized by absence of pubic hair, and the labia minora are more prominent than the labia majora. With deposit of body fat and hormone effects during puberty, the labia majora increase in thickness and pubic hair appears. With the onset of the menopause and gradual withdrawal of hormones, the external genitalia again become less prominent and the pubic hair begins to thin. In elderly women, the vulva may appear wrinkled, shrunken, and almost flat.

## Internal Organs

The female internal reproductive organs are shown in Figure 51-3. The internal reproductive organs are located in the true pelvis and remain there unless their size is increased by a disease process or pregnancy.

### Vagina

The vagina is a soft, tubular structure that extends upward and back from the vaginal opening connecting the vulva with the cervix and uterus. It is located between the rectum and urethra. The functions of the vagina are to receive the penis during intercourse, allow for childbirth, and permit discharge of the menstrual flow. The length of the vaginal canal varies, and the posterior wall is longer than the anterior wall. The anterior wall averages 6 to 8 cm long, whereas the posterior wall averages 8 to 9 cm.

The vagina is lined with pink mucous membrane arranged in folds called *rugae.* The rugae make it possible for the vagina to distend and to stretch during coitus and childbirth. The rugated appearance of the vaginal canal is prominent during adolescence and tends to disappear with multiparity.

The vaginal walls end in a blind pouch *around* the

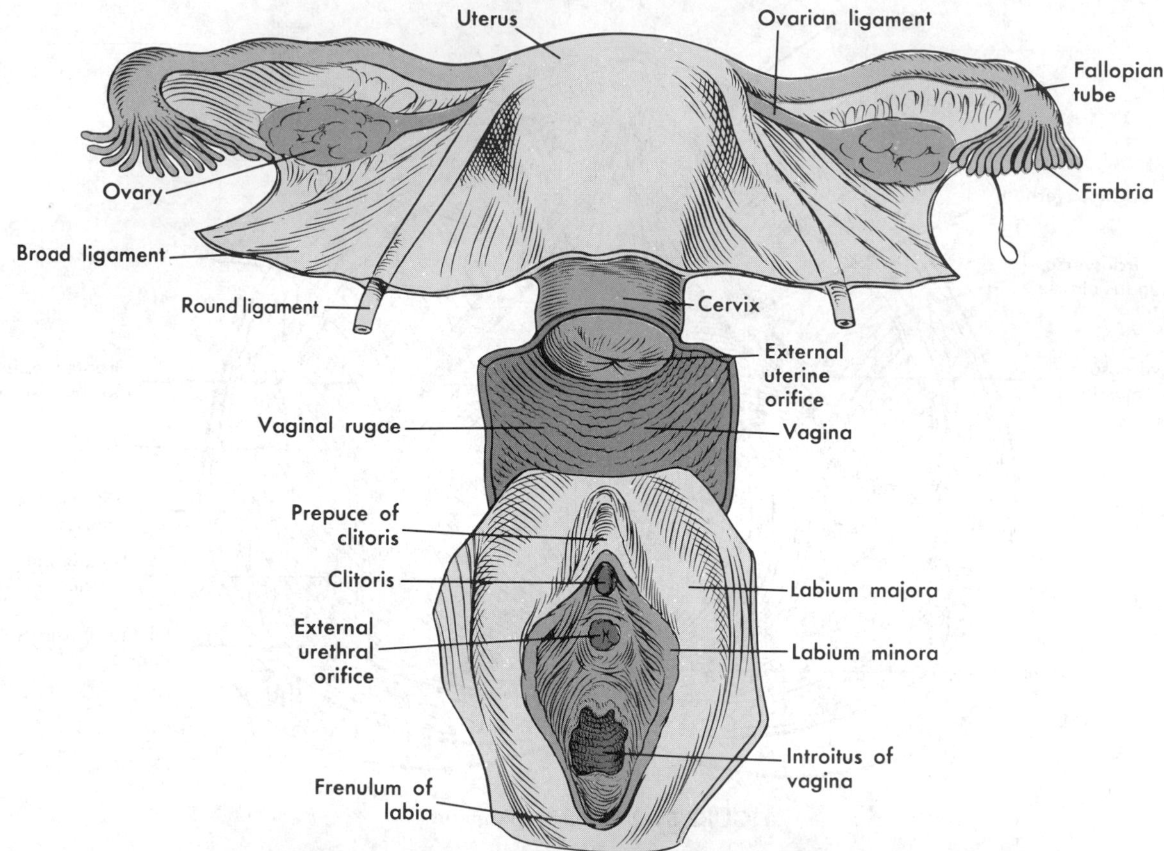


**FIGURE 51-3** Female internal organs of reproduction. Major ligaments are shown.

cervix. Note that the vaginal epithelium is continuous with the epithelium of the cervix and that the cervix projects into the upper vagina, creating a cup-shaped fornix. The groove formed by the termination of the vagina around the cervix is called the *vaginal vault.*

The vagina is lubricated by secretions from its own cells and by secretions from the cervix and Bartholin's glands. Before puberty, the vaginal pH tends to be neutral. With the onset of puberty, the pH drops to 4.0 to 5.0. The vaginal secretions remain acidic throughout the reproductive years and become even more strongly acidic during pregnancy. Neutral or alkaline values are normally found in postmenopausal women. Acidity is strongly influenced by estrogen concentration, which controls the glycogen levels of the cells. The normal vaginal flora, Döderlein's bacilli, interact with the secreted glycogen to produce lactic acid and maintain an acid pH. The importance of vaginal acidity is demonstrated by the fact that most pathogenic bacteria produce signs of vaginal infection when the pH falls below 4.0 or rises above 5.0.

Until puberty, the vaginal epithelium is thin. The epithelium thickens at the time of puberty, and this state persists through the reproductive years until the menopause, when the epithelium again becomes thin. The thickness of the vaginal epithelium is also closely related to estrogen levels.

The natural barriers to infection (thickness of the vaginal epithelium and acidity of the vagina) are minimal before puberty and after menopause, predisposing females in these age-groups to vaginal infections and trauma of the vaginal mucosa.

### Uterus

The uterus is a hollow, muscular organ located between the urinary bladder and rectum. It consists of two portions: the *corpus (body)* and the *cervix.* The body is composed of the fundus, which is the thick muscular region above insertion of the fallopian tubes; the body, which is the main portion of the uterus; and the isthmus, which is the lower region. The cervix is located between the isthmus and the vagina. The size of the uterus decreases from the fundus to the cervix, giving the contour of the uterus a triangular, pear-shaped appearance. The size of the uterus varies among women, ranging from 5.5 to 9 cm long, 3.5 to 6 cm wide, and 2 to 4 cm thick in nonparous women. All dimensions may be 2 to 3 cm larger in multiparas.

The position of the uterus is subject to considerable variation. The uterus is usually anteverted and slightly anteflexed, although it may be retroverted, retroflexed, or in midposition. The body of the uterus is normally bent forward over the bladder so that the fundus is behind the symphysis pubis. The uterus is in direct contact with the bladder and may also touch the rectum, sigmoid colon, and small intestines. The cervix curves forward. The relationship between the corpus and the cervix produces an angle of about 90 degrees. The angle is decreased as the urinary bladder fills and elevates the corpus.

During pregnancy, the uterus changes remarkably in size, shape, structure, and position and returns to its prepregnancy state within 6 to 8 weeks after delivery. During menopause, the uterus begins to atrophy and decreases in size.

The outer surfaces of the uterus are covered by peritoneum, which is reflected from the abdominal wall. The anterior and posterior reflections of the peritoneum join at the sides to enclose the fallopian tubes and ovaries. Reflection of the peritoneum over the top of the pelvic organs creates spaces between the uterus and bladder anteriorly and the uterus and rectum posteriorly. The posterior space is known as the *cul-de-sac of Douglas* and is a common entry site for culdoscopy, culpotomy, and surgical drainage of the peritoneal cavity.

The uterus has three functional layers: the parametrium, which is the peritoneal and fascial outer layer; the myometrium, which is the middle muscular layer; and the endometrium, which is the mucous membrane–type tissue. The cavity of the uterus is continuous with the cervical canal and has an average capacity of 3 to 8 ml. Near the fundus, the uterus opens into the lumen of the fallopian tubes. Thus, a direct route exists from the vagina through the cervix, uterus, and fallopian tubes to the peritoneum.

The cervix is firm, smooth, and round. It is primarily made up of elastic and fibrous connective tissue and smooth muscle. Its color is usually lighter pink than that of the vagina. The *external os* is located in the center of the vaginal portion of the cervix. Extending upward from the external os is the cervical canal, which averages 2 to 3 cm long. The cervical canal terminates as it joins the corpus, and the junction of the cervical canal and the corpus is termed the *internal cervical os.* The functions of the cervix are to secrete mucus to facilitate transport of sperm, to dilate during labor, and to provide a channel for discharge of the menstrual flow.

### Fallopian tubes

The fallopian tubes are two narrow, muscular canals ranging from 8 to 14 cm long. They extend outward from the corpus near the fundus at the cornua and are enclosed in the folds of the broad ligaments. The tubes are divided into three portions: the *isthmus* is the proximal portion of the tube nearest the cornua; the *ampulla* is the longer, middle portion where fertilization usually occurs; and the farthest, distal portion of the tube is the *infundibulum,* which terminates in fimbria (Figure 51-4).

The functions of the fallopian tubes are to serve as a site for union of the ovum and sperm and to transport the ovum to the uterus. The walls of the fallopian tubes

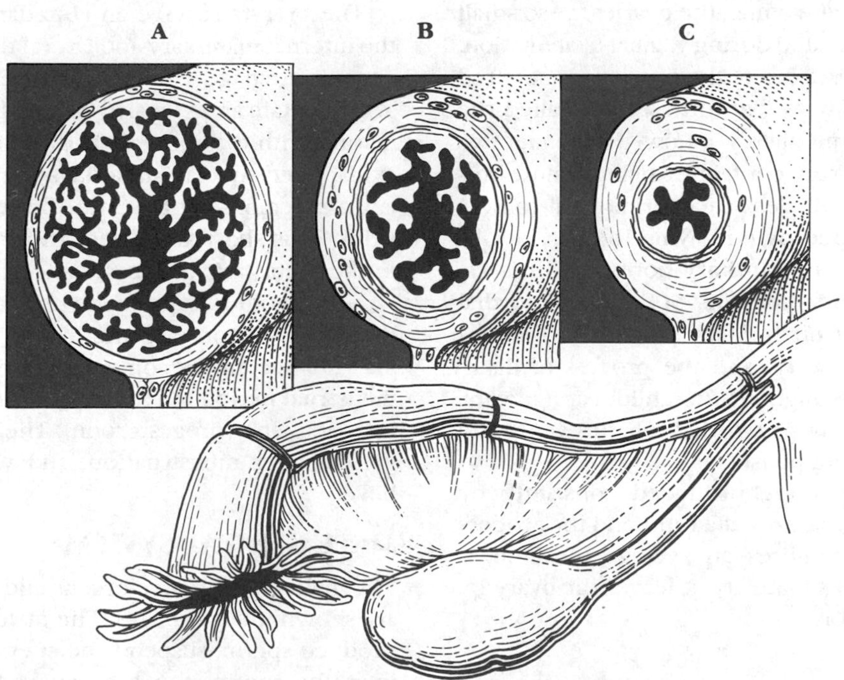


**FIGURE 51-4** Longitudinal folds of oviduct seen in cross section. **A,** Infundibulum. **B,** Ampulla. **C,** Isthmus.

contain smooth muscles that possess peristaltic properties. The fallopian tubes are lined with a mucous membrane that contains cilia. At the time of ovulation, both the peristaltic action and the ciliary action increase, and it is likely that these combined actions provide the mechanism for ovum transport.

### Ovaries

The ovaries are endocrine glands as well as reproductive organs. There are normally two almond-shaped ovaries, ranging from 3 to 4 cm long, 2 cm wide, and 1 to 2 cm thick, each lying near the fimbriae of the fallopian tubes. They are partly enclosed by the broad ligaments. Each ovary contains an outer portion (cortex) and an inner portion (medulla). The term *adnexa* refers to the ovaries, fallopian tubes, and supporting tissues. The functions of the ovaries are to store primordial follicles; to produce mature ova; and to produce and secrete estrogen, progesterone, and androgens.

The ovaries undergo physical changes in position, size, and shape during the life span. At birth, the ovaries are very small, round, smooth, and light pink and are located in the false pelvis. Between infancy and puberty, the ovaries increase in size, become more flattened, assume a grayish color, and descend into the true pelvis. During the childbearing years, the ovaries appear long and flat, have a nodular surface caused by the presence of follicles, and lie close to the pelvic walls. During pregnancy, the ovaries are lifted out of the pelvis by the enlarging uterus, but they descend into the pelvis after childbirth. After menopause, the ovaries undergo rapid regressive changes. They decrease in size, their surfaces become wrinkled, and the color fades from gray to white. In most postmenopausal women, the ovaries are so small that they cannot be palpated during vaginal examination.

After puberty, the surfaces of the ovaries are covered by connective tissue fibers that form a layer called the *tunica albuginea.* Immediately below the connective tissue is the ovarian cortex containing many minute vesicles, the primordial follicles. Each primordial follicle contains an undeveloped ovum having the capacity to respond to stimulation by pituitary hormones. It is estimated that each ovary contains 500,000 primordial follicles at the time of birth. Many primordial follicles disintegrate before puberty, and the process of disintegration continues throughout the childbearing years. Consequently, few if any primordial follicles are found in the ovaries after menopause.

Unlike sperm, which are produced constantly by males, only one ovum matures at a time, and the process of ovum maturation requires an average of 28 days. When the ovum reaches maturity, it leaves the ovary by the process of ovulation.

### Breasts

The female breasts are accessory structures of the reproductive system meant to nourish the infant after birth. They are paired mammary glands located between the second and sixth ribs, the edge of the sternum, and the midaxillary line. They develop in response to hormonal stimulation from the hypothalamus, pituitary gland, and ovaries.

The tissue of the breast has three primary components: an interconnected network of glandular and ductal tissue, fibrous tissue, and fat. The proportion of each component tissue is a reflection of the individual woman's genetic make-up, age, obstetric history, and weight. The breast is supported by Cooper's suspensory ligaments, which attach to the underlying muscles.

The external structure of the breast includes the nipple, which arises from the center of the pigmented areola near the midline. The elevations on the areola are small, round sebaceous glands termed *Montgomery's glands.* They are believed to secrete a fatty substance that offers some protection to the nipple during breastfeeding.

Internally, each mature breast is composed of 15 to 25 lobes arranged radially around the breast and separated from each other by fatty tissue. Each lobe is composed of several lobules, which in turn are composed of numerous alveoli. Each alveolus is connected by a duct to a larger duct from the lobule. These *lactiferous ducts* join to form one duct from each lobe that then converge at the nipple. Just before the nipple, the ducts expand into sinuses or ampullae, which serve as reservoirs. The epithelial linings of the alveoli synthesize and secrete the components of breast milk in response to stimulation by prolactin from the pituitary. Unless a woman is pregnant or nursing a child, there should be no milk production in the breasts or discharge of any type from the nipple.

The breasts receive an abundant blood supply from the internal mammary and lateral thoracic arteries. Their venous drainage connects to the superior vena cava. They contain an extensive lymph drainage network originating within the breast and draining radially into the axillary and subclavian nodal system. Drainage from the axillary region empties into the jugular and subclavian veins. This short and direct route assumes significance in the metastasis of breast cancer.

Many women experience noticeable changes in their breasts in response to the menstrual cycle. The breast may enlarge and become tender or nodular in the premenstrual period in response to the increasing levels of estrogen and progesterone. The cellular growth regresses after menstruation, and water retention is relieved.

## MALE GENITAL SYSTEM

The male reproductive organs and associated structures are shown in Figure 51-5. The male reproductive organs produce sperm, suspend the sperm in a liquid, and deliver the sperm into the vagina to fertilize an ovum. Another important function is secretion of male hormones, the androgens. The male genitalia include the

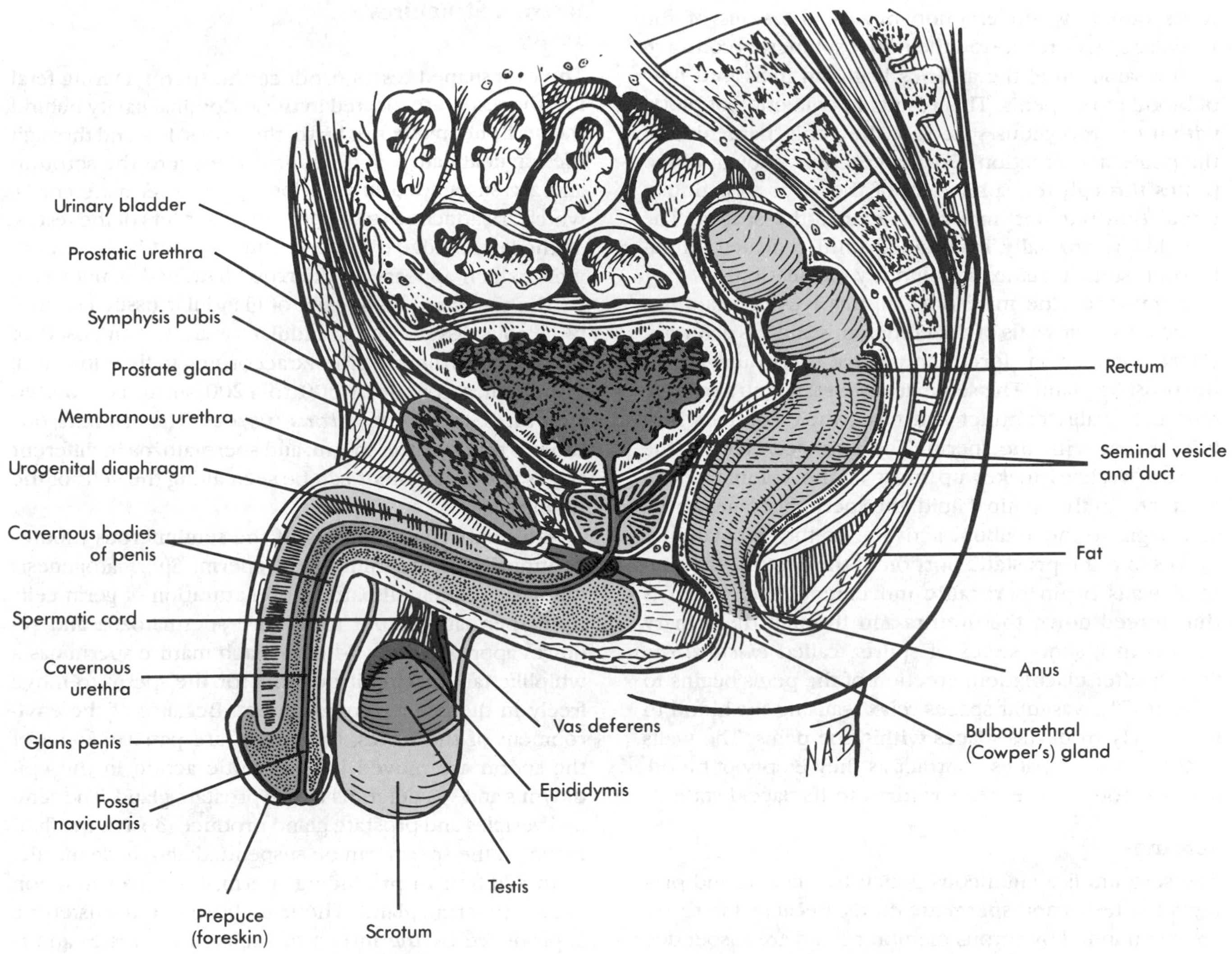


**FIGURE 51-5** Male organs of reproduction.

testes, vas deferens, seminal vesicles, ejaculatory ducts, and penis, along with the prostate and bulbourethral glands, which are accessory structures.

## External Structures

### Penis

The penis is a conduit for elimination of ejaculate and urine through the urethral opening. It is attached to the front and sides of the pubic arch. The penis consists of three masses of cavernous tissue held together by fibrous tissue. The three columns of erectile tissue are the two corpora cavernosa and the corpus spongiosum, which contains the urethra.

The skin covering the penis is dark, contains no fat, and is loosely connected to the underlying tissues. At the pubis, the skin is covered with hair in a characteristic triangular distribution. At the neck of the penis, the skin is folded on itself to form the prepuce (foreskin). The prepuce covers a variable amount of the glans at the tip of the penis. The glans is covered by a menbranous tissue that is continuous with the mucous membrane of the urethra. Small, sensitive papillae are located on the surface of the glans, the inner surface of the prepuce, and the neck of the penis. These papillae secrete a sebaceous substance and have a characteristic odor. When mixed with epithelial cells, the combined discharge is called *smegma* and is similar to the deposits found between the labial folds in women.

The penis is enclosed in a strong capsule of fascia. Numerous cords extend from the inner surface of the capsule, cross in all directions, and divide the penis into compartments. This gives the entire inner structure of the penis a spongy appearance. Within the structure of muscle fibers and fibrous and elastic tissue are the numerous blood vessels and nerves of the penis.

When the male is sexually aroused, erection of the penis occurs involuntarily. Because the penis consists largely of spaces in which blood can collect, the mechanism of erection involves the blood vessels. Each space in the penis is supplied by a vein having a small sphincter at its outlet. When erection begins, the walls of the vascular spaces relax, and the outlet sphincters contract. At the same time, the arteries bring an increased flow of blood to the penis. This results in collection of blood within the cavernous spaces of the penis, hardening of the penis, and erection. During erection, enough blood passes through the sphincters of the veins to maintain circulation but not enough to empty the spaces. The erection is normally maintained until repeated stimulation results in reflex, involuntary ejaculation.

Ejaculation, the male orgasm, involves contractions of the muscular walls of the epididymis and vas deferens. These contractions force the passive sperm upward to the prostate gland. The seminal vesicles, which also have muscular walls, contract and force their contents into the urethra with the sperm. The fluid secreted by the seminal vesicles makes up most of the volume of the ejaculate. In the seminal fluid, the sperm become motile and begin to move about actively. As the seminal fluid moves into the prostatic portion of the urethra, the urethral walls begin peristaltic movement. The semen is thus forced down the urethra and through the urinary meatus in a short series of spurts, called *ejaculation.* Shortly after ejaculation, erection of the penis begins to subside. The vascular spaces relax, causing the blood to flow freely from the spaces within the penis. The walls of the vascular spaces contract as they empty of blood, and the body of the penis returns to its flaccid state.

#### Scrotum

The scrotum is a cutaneous pouch that covers and protects the testes and spermatic cords. Because the testes are surrounded by serous membrane and are suspended in the cavity of the scrotum, the testes are capable of being moved about readily. The ease of movement of the testes within the scrotum protects them against injury.

The skin of the scrotum is thin, brownish, and very elastic because it contains rugae. Because of the rugae, the skin of the scrotum is capable of great distention, and the scrotum may become greatly enlarged when edema is present. The scrotal skin is covered by thinly scattered hair and contains sebaceous follicles. The surface of the scrotum is divided into two halves by a ridge (raphe) that extends anteriorly to the undersurface of the penis and posteriorly along the midline of the perineum to the anus. Internally, a septum divides the scrotum into two halves, each containing a testis and its epididymis and portion of spermatic cord. The left side of the scrotum normally hangs lower than the right side because the left spermatic cord is longer.

The external appearance of the scrotum varies under different conditions. In warm temperatures and in older or debilitated men, the scrotum becomes elongated and flat. In young, healthy men and in cool temperatures, the scrotum appears short, more wrinkled, and closely applied to the testes.

### Internal Structures

#### Testes

The oval-shaped testes produce the sperm. During fetal life, the testes are located in the abdominal cavity behind the peritoneum. Before birth, the testes descend through the inguinal canals and inguinal rings into the scrotum and are suspended in position by the spermatic cords, which are attached to the posterior borders of the testes. At the lateral edge of each spermatic cord is the epididymis, which appears as a narrow, flattened structure.

The testes are composed of glandular tissue covered by fibrous tissue. The glandular tissue is composed of many lobules differing in size according to their location. The lobules consist of 600 to 1200 small, convoluted structures, the *seminiferous tubules.* The seminiferous tubules produce the sperm, and spermatozoa in different stages of development can be seen along the cells of the tubules.

After puberty, the lining of the seminiferous tubules continually forms millions of sperm. Spermatogenesis follows a sequential pattern of maturation of germ cells from spermatogonium to mature spermatozoa and requires approximately 74 days. Each mature sperm has a whiplike tail, making it possible for the sperm to move freely in the proper environment. Because of the environment of the testes, the sperm are passive. Some of the sperm are moved by peristaltic action in the epididymis and vas deferens to the prostate gland. The seminal vesicles and prostate gland produce most of the fluid in which the sperm can be suspended and made motile.

In addition to producing sperm, the testes function as an endocrine gland. The male hormone testosterone is produced by the interstitial cells of the testes and is responsible for development of the genitalia during puberty and for maintaining the genitalia in a functional state during life. Androgenic hormones are also responsible for the development of secondary sex characteristics, including growth of body hair and thickening of the vocal cords.

#### Epididymis/vas deferens

The comma-shaped epididymis can be visually located at the lateral edge of the posterior segment of the testes, where it creates a bulge. It is continuous with the vas deferens. The vas deferens serves as the excretory duct of the testes, is a constituent of the spermatic cord, and separates from the spermatic cord at the inguinal ring. After taking a complex path through the pelvis, the vas deferens descends, enters the base of the prostate gland, becomes greatly narrowed, and joins the ducts of the seminal vesicles to form the ejaculatory duct.

#### Spermatic cords

The spermatic cords extend from the deep inguinal rings and consist of arteries, veins, lymphatics, nerves, and the excretory duct of the testes held together by the spermatic fascia. At the deep inguinal rings, the structures of the spermatic cords converge with the structures of the testes. The spermatic cords then pass through the inguinal canals, emerge through the superficial inguinal rings, and pass downward into the scrotum.

### Seminal vesicles

The seminal vesicles are two lobulated, membranous pouches, 5 to 10 cm long, located between the bladder and the rectum. They secrete fluid to be added to the secretions of the testes. The lower end of each seminal vesicle becomes constricted into a straight duct and joins the vas deferens to form the ejaculatory duct. The ejaculatory duct begins at the base of the prostate gland, runs posteriorly and downward, and enters the prostate gland in the midline. In the prostate gland, the ejaculatory duct opens into the prostatic portion of the urethra.

### Prostate gland

The prostate gland is located below the internal urethral orifice, behind the symphysis pubis, and close to the rectal wall, extending around the beginning of the urethra. The prostate gland grows to the size and shape of a walnut during puberty and weighs about 20 g. It is enveloped in a firm, adherent capsule. Internally, the prostate gland is partly muscular and partly glandular. The glandular substance of the prostate gland consists of numerous follicular pouches that open into long canals. These canals join to form 12 to 20 small excretory ducts. Prostatic ducts open into the prostatic portion of the urethra, thus adding the prostatic secretion to the seminal fluid.

### Cowper's glands

Cowper's (bulbourethral) glands are two small, round bodies located at the sides and to the back of the membranous portion of the urethra. They are enclosed by the transverse fibers of the sphincter muscles of the urethra. Each gland has an excretory duct that opens into the urethra. The main excretory duct of a Cowper's gland represents the joining of many ducts from the internal glandular tissue substance. Cowper's glands secrete an alkaline substance into the semen to counteract vaginal and urethral acidity.

## PELVIC LIGAMENTS AND MUSCLES

The internal and external reproductive structures are maintained in their positons by groups of ligaments and muscles. In the female, the broad ligaments (consisting of peritoneum) extend from the surfaces of the uterus to the sides of the pelvis and support the uterus in a horizontal position. The free margins of the broad ligament enclose and support the fallopian tubes and ovaries. The ovaries are suspended from the broad ligament by the ovarian ligaments (see Figure 51-3).

The round ligaments extend laterally from the anterior surface of the uterine fundus. They pass through the abdominal wall, inguinal canals, and inguinal rings and terminate by dissemination of their fibers in the labia majora and surrounding tissues, holding the corpus forward in an anteverted position over the urinary bladder. These ligaments stretch to allow enlargement and alteration of position of the uterus during pregnancy.

The uterosacral ligaments originate from the posterior surface of the uterus at the level of the internal os. They arch posteriorly and are inserted into the sacrum at the level of the second and third sacral vertebrae. Because the uterosacral ligaments exert backward tension on the cervix, they maintain the cervix and vagina at right angles to each other. The uterosacral ligaments thus prevent prolapse of the uterus by preventing the corpus from taking a position in line with the vagina. It is likely that uterosacral ligaments contain sensory nerve fibers, which may contribute to dysmenorrhea.

The cardinal ligaments arise from the base of the broad ligaments. They integrate with the pelvic fascia and fan outward around the base of the uterus. The cardinal ligaments provide the chief support for the cervix and upper vagina, preventing descent of these structures.

The pubocervical ligaments extend from the posterior surface of the pubis to the anterolateral portion of the cervix. They provide some support to the bladder and cervix.

The muscles that actively and passively support the pelvic floor in both males and females are shown in Figure 51-2. The pelvic diaphragm consists of the levator ani and coccygeus muscles together with the pelvic fascia and stretches across the bottom of the pelvic cavity. The anal cavity, the urethra, and in females the vagina pierce the pelvic diaphragm. The levator ani muscles contain striated muscle fibers that enable the vaginal and anal openings to be closed voluntarily. The pubococcygeus muscle (part of the levator ani muscle) is especially important to women in sexual functioning, in expulsion of the fetus during childbirth, and for bladder control.

In females, the perineum is wider and thicker than it is in males. The muscles of the perineum, commonly called the perineal body or perineal center, reinforce the support provided by the levator ani and coccygeus muscles. The perineal body consists of a mass of several muscles extending across the center of the pelvic outlet. It is located between the anus and vagina. Together, the pelvic diaphragm and perineum support the pelvic organs and external genitalia from below.

## BLOOD, LYMPH, AND NERVE SUPPLY

In males and females, the organs of reproduction are supplied with blood from the aorta as it branches downward and divides into the internal iliac (hypogastric) artery.

The ovarian and uterine arteries anastomose to furnish the ovaries with blood. The arteries are paired, are

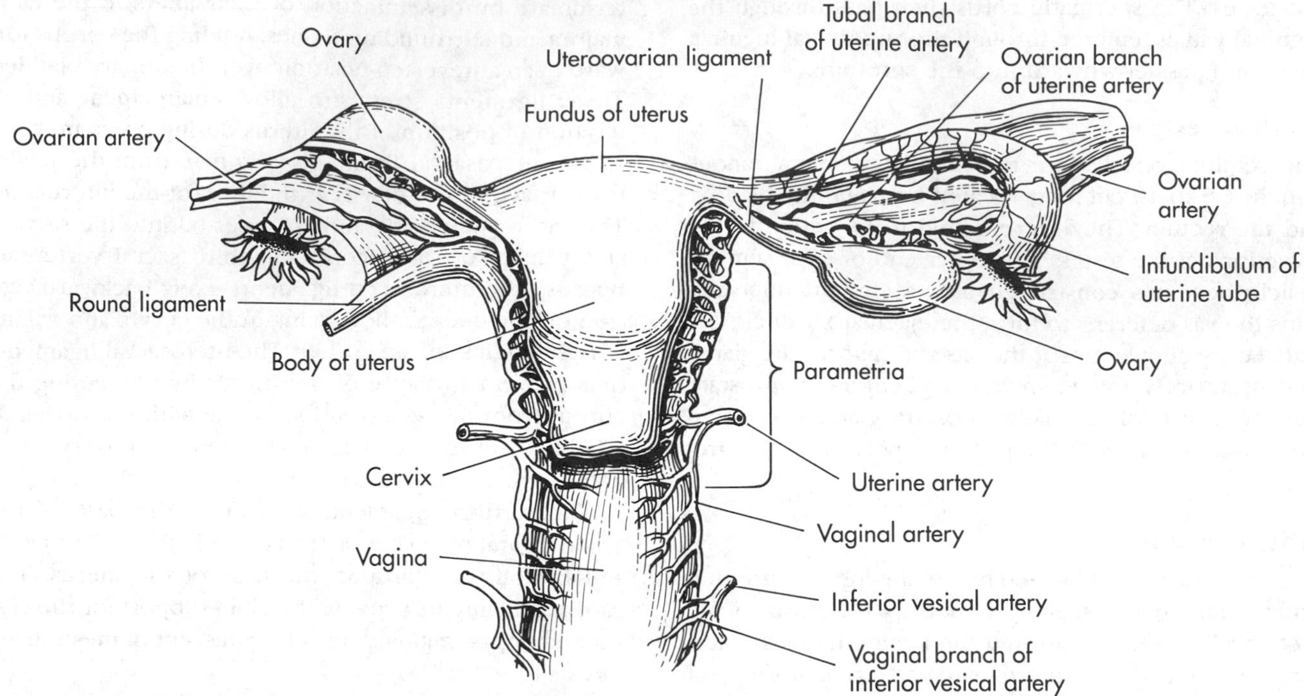


**FIGURE 51-6** Arteries of reproductive organs. Note paired arteries entering laterally and freely anastomosing with each other.

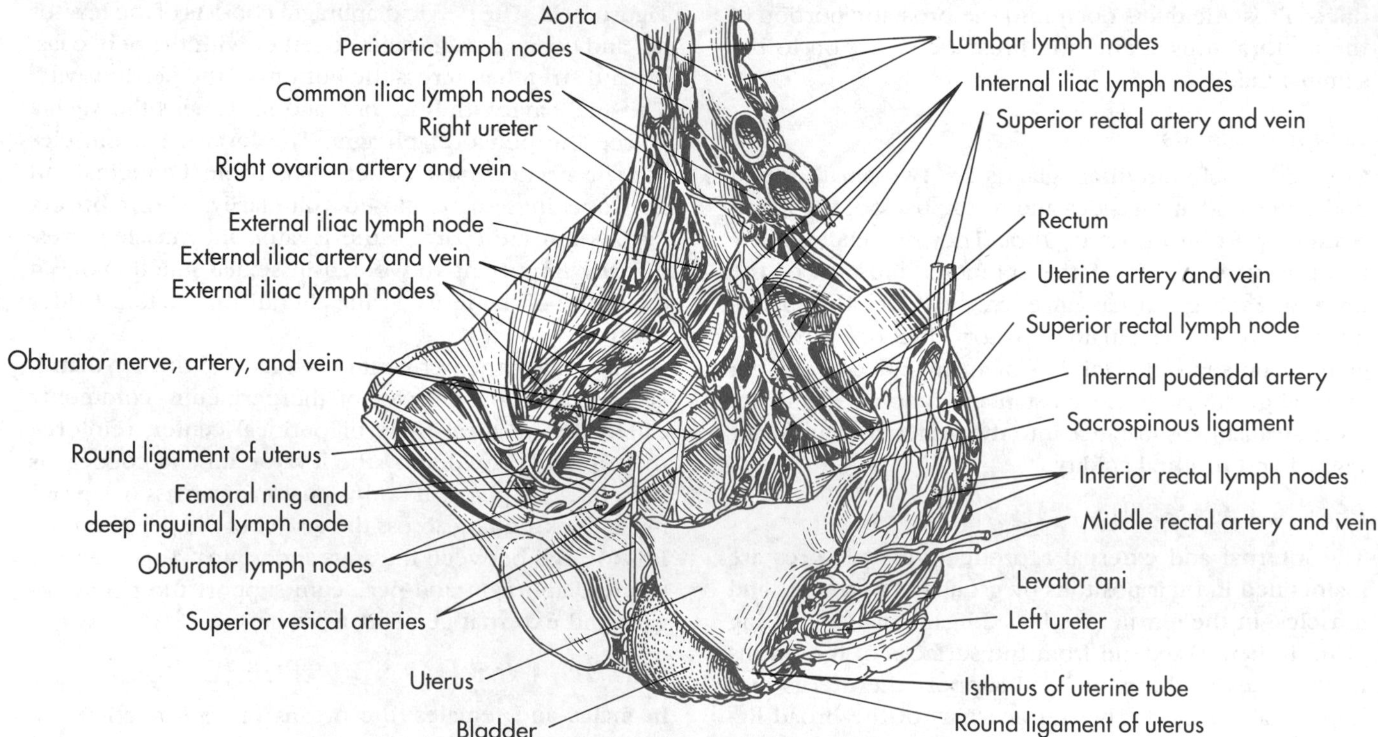


**FIGURE 51-7** Lateral view of female pelvis demonstrating extensive lymphatic network. Note that most lymphatic channels follow courses of major vessels.

bilateral, and have multiple collaterals. The pelvic reproductive viscera lie within a loosely woven basket of large veins with numerous interconnecting venous plexuses. The arteries thread their way through this interwoven mesh of veins to reach the pelvic reproductive organs, giving off numerous branching arcades to provide a rich blood supply (Figure 51-6). The venous drainage is similar to the arterial supply to the reproductive organs, with the blood vessels emptying into the vena cava.

In males, blood is similarly supplied to and drained from the reproductive organs. The pudendal branches of the aorta divide into the testicular arteries, and arteries supplying the seminal vesicles are derived from the inferior vesical and middle rectal arteries. Most blood to the penis is furnished through the internal pudendal artery. Venous return is similar to the arterial supply. Blood from the penis, testes, and prostate gland is returned to the internal iliac vein and then to the vena cava.

In both males and females, lymphatic drainage of the external and internal organs of reproduction is extensive. Both superficial and deep lymphatics empty into the external iliac, internal iliac, and preaortic lymph nodes (Figure 51-7). Nerve supply is derived from sympathetic and parasympathetic fibers of the autonomic nervous system and by spinal nerve pathways. In the female, the pudendal nerve and its branches supply the majority of both motor and sensory fibers to the muscles and skin of the vulvar region. The pudendal nerve arises from the second, third, and fourth sacral roots. In the male, the motor segment of the pudendal nerve innervates the urinary sphincter, and the sensory portion supplies the glans penis and urethra.

## ENDOCRINE FUNCTIONS

### Female Hormones

The major hormones produced by the ovaries are estrogen and progesterone. **Estrogen** is the hormone responsible for the development of secondary sex characteristics at puberty. After puberty, the primary function of estrogen is to cause development of the endometrium in preparation for implantation of a fertilized ovum. **Progesterone** enhances the preceding action of estrogen on the endometrium. The ovaries depend on stimulation from pituitary hormones to fulfill their functions.

### Male Hormones

In males, secretion of the androgenic hormones increases at puberty, resulting in appearance of secondary sex characteristics and production of mature sperm. Of the androgens, **testosterone** is most closely related to reproduction, since it specifically stimulates maturation of sperm and is responsible for maintaining the reproductive organs in a functional state. Testosterone secretion is closely related to pituitary gland function. The rate of secretion of testosterone is determined by levels of luteinizing hormone in the blood.

### Menstruation

**Menarche** is the term used to designate the onset of **menstruation,** and it reflects the time when reproduction is first possible. The onset of menarche reflects a girl's age, heredity, general health, weight, and nutritional status and cannot be accurately predicted. The average age at menarche has decreased significantly over the past 100 years and is now 12.5 to 12.8 years, with a normal range from 9.1 to 17.7 years.[7] It is believed that a critical body weight (47.8 kg, or 105 pound) and shift in body composition to a greater percentage of fat (from 16.0% to 23.5%) must be attained for the average girl to reach menarche.[3]

Normal variation exists in the intervals between menstrual periods. The greatest variance typically occurs during the perimenarchal and perimenopausal years. Most cycles occur within a normal range of 26 to 36 days. The menstrual flow usually lasts for 3 to 7 days, with an average loss of 30 to 180 ml of menstrual fluid and an average blood loss of 45 ml. Menstrual fluid does not clot unless it is retained in the uterus or vagina for a prolonged time. It is believed that the endometrium produces an anticoagulant that prevents the clotting of blood in the uterus.

Menstruation may be accompanied by a variety of symptoms, including fluid retention (up to a 5-pound weight gain); aching in the lower back, legs, or pelvis; fatigue; tenderness or fullness in the breasts; premenstrual mood swings; and lower abdominal cramping.

### Menstrual Cycle

The **menstrual cycle** is divided into phases according to uterine or ovarian changes. The uterine cycle consists of the menstrual, proliferative, and secretory phases. The follicular phase in the ovarian cycle corresponds to the menstrual and proliferative phases of the uterine cycle. The luteal phase in the ovarian cycle corresponds to the uterine secretory phase. Secretion of ovarian hormones occurs in a cyclic pattern, with each cycle requiring an average of 28 days.

The functioning of the menstrual cycle depends on the proper relationships among the central nervous system, anterior pituitary, ovaries, and uterus (Figure 51-8). In describing the ovarian-pituitary-uterine cycles, the events occurring usually are related to the phases of the menstrual cycle. The first day of the menstrual flow is the first day of the menstrual cycle.

#### Menstrual phase

During the menstrual phase of the cycle, the endometrium breaks down and is shed. Withdrawal of estrogen and progesterone before the onset of menstrual flow

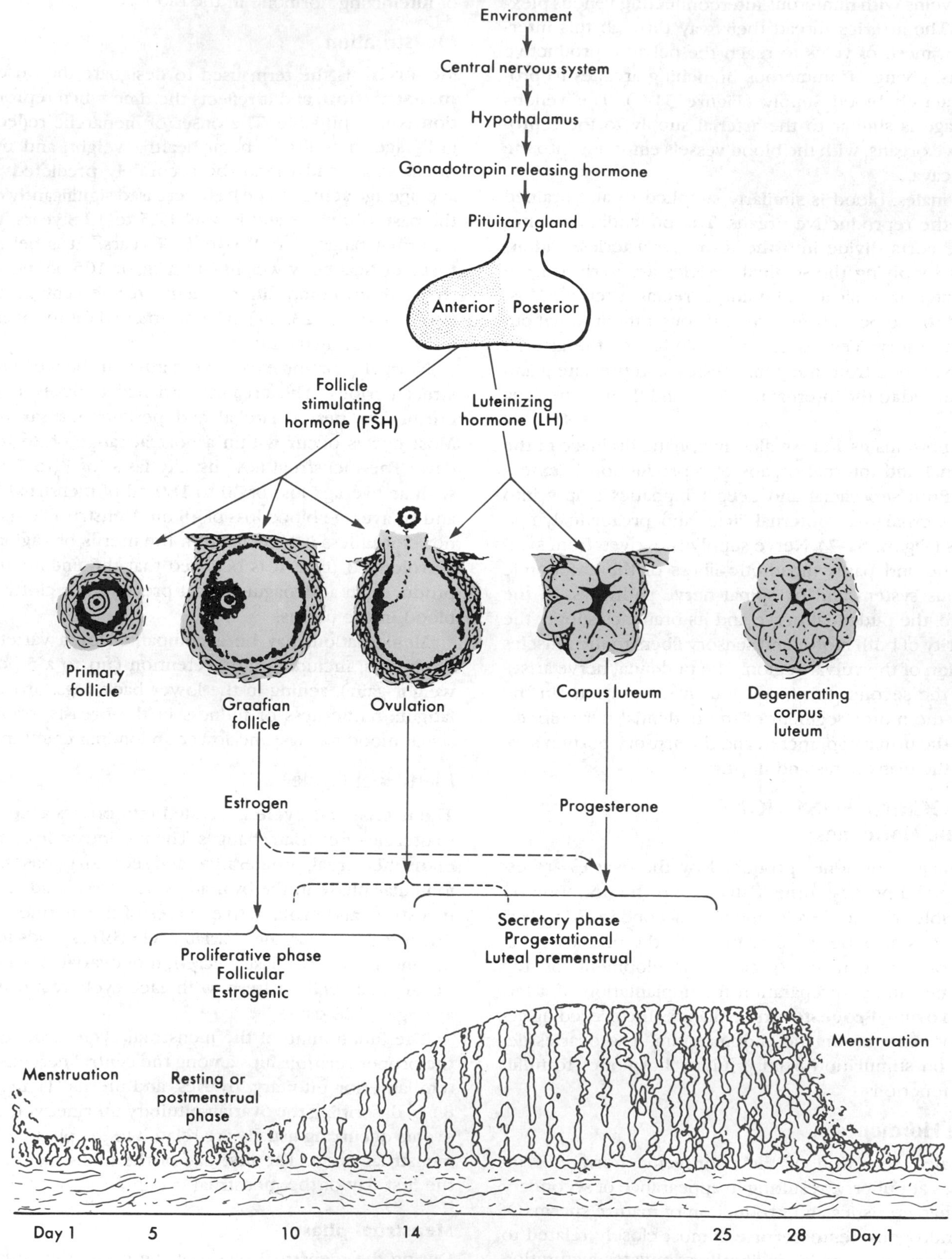


**FIGURE 51-8** Hormonal control of menstrual cycle.

results in rupture of uterine capillaries and necrosis of endometrial tissue. The menstrual phase of the cycle lasts an average of 4 days.

### Proliferative phase

When menstruation ceases, the proliferative phase begins, extends over the next 14 days, and ends with ovulation. During the proliferative (follicular) phase, the pituitary gland secretes increasing amounts of follicle-stimulating hormone (FSH), which stimulates a primordial follicle to develop into a mature graafian follicle containing a mature ovum. Because the graafian follicle produces estrogen, FSH is essential for estrogen production. While increasing in size, the graafian follicle moves toward the surface of the ovary, where it appears as a blisterlike structure. Finally, the graffian follicle ruptures (ovulation), allowing the ovum and follicular fluid to escape. The ovum enters the fallopian tube and is carried in the direction of the uterus.

As the graafian follicle matures, it secretes increasing amounts of estrogen. Estrogen causes the endometrium to become thicker and softer as it prepares for implantation of a fertilized ovum. Estrogen also causes the cervical mucus to increase in quantity and attain a clear, elastic state. This permits sperm to enter the cervix more readily. The high level of estrogen before ovulation also suppresses pituitary release of FSH and triggers release of **luteinizing hormone (LH).** A sharp rise in LH levels occurs 12 to 24 hours before ovulation, followed by a peak level about 8 hours after ovulation. This change in hormone levels is reflected in the basal body temperature, which drops just before and rises after ovulation.

On the day of ovulation, about 25% of women experience pain in the lower abdomen on the side of ovulation. This pain is referred to as **mittelschmerz** and is probably a result of peritoneal irritation from follicular fluid or blood released from the ovary with the ovum.

### Secretory phase

With ovulation, the proliferative phase ends and the secretory phase begins. The secretory phase lasts for approximately 10 to 14 days. The secretory (luteal) phase is the least variable part of the menstrual cycle. Irregular menstrual cycles are most frequently related to longer or shorter menstrual or proliferative (follicular) phases.

Under the influence of LH, the corpus luteum forms in the ovary at the site of the ruptured graafian follicle. The hormone produced by the corpus luteum is progesterone. Progesterone further alters the endometrium by stimulating growth of cells and circulation of blood to the uterus. With these additional endometrial changes, the uterine environment is prepared for implantation of a fertilized ovum.

If pregnancy occurs, the corpus luteum remains secretory by the action of human chorionic gonadotropin (HCG), which is produced within a week of conception by the placenta. By 6 to 8 weeks after conception, the placenta is developed and assumes the function of secreting progesterone to maintain the endometrium. If pregnancy does not occur, the corpus luteum degenerates in about 10 days, progesterone secretion drops greatly, and the endometrium degenerates; menstruation results, and the cycle begins again.

### Menopause

The term **menopause** refers to the cessation of menstruation. The **climacteric,** which lasts for 12 to 18 months, is the transitional phase between reproductive and nonreproductive ability. Natural menopause occurs between ages 35 and 60, with an average age of about 51 in Western societies. (See Chapter 11 for an in-depth discussion of menopause and the associated problem of osteoporosis.)

## PHYSIOLOGIC CHANGES WITH AGING

Changes in the reproductive tract in the female begin at middle age with menopause (see Chapter 11). When ovulation ceases, no progesterone is produced and estrogen diminishes. The hormonal changes lead to changes in the uterus, ovaries, and vagina (Box 51-1). The physiologic changes may lead to discomfort or complications with sexual intercourse; vaginal dryness and narrowed introitus may cause dyspareunia (painful intercourse); and vaginal infections may occur more

**BOX 51-1 Age-Related Changes in the Reproductive Tract and Sexual Function**

**FEMALE**

Mons pubis: decreased fullness because of redistribution of fat pad
Pubic hair: becomes gray to white and thinner; curly hair becomes straightened
Labia majora/minora: decrease in size; mucous membranes lining minora become dry and pale
Bartholin's glands: atrophy; produce less mucoid material
Vagina: decreased width and length; vaginal entrance (introitus) narrowed; vaginal secretions decrease and become more alkaline
Vaginal walls: become dry, smoother, thinner
Ovaries: atrophy, with decreased size; nonpalpable 3 to 5 years after menopause
Uterus: decreased size; thin lining

**MALE**

Pubic hair: becomes gray to white and thinner; curly hair becomes straightened
Testes: decreased size and firmness; change in position (lower)
Seminal fluid: decreased amount and viscosity
Prostate gland: hypertrophy (enlargement)
Penis: decreased size and sensation; easily retractable foreskin (if uncircumcised)
Ejaculation: decreased force and need
Bladder: increase in bladder neck tone
Pelvic muscles: decreased strength
Scrotum: becomes more pendulous; fewer rugae

readily in the alkaline medium. Muscle weakness may lead to cystocele, rectocele, or uterine prolapse.

In the male, the production of testosterone decreases gradually until about age 60 and then levels off. Changes can be noted in the testes, seminal fluid, prostate, and in penile erections (Box 51-1). Contrary to the inability to procreate as seen in elderly females, males may still procreate, but with less probability than when younger because of fewer, less viable sperm. Both elderly females and elderly males have the capacity for sexual response.

Changes resulting from advancing age occur at different rates and to varying degrees. Changes are usually gradual. In working with the elderly person, nurses have an important role in regard to counseling and education. For elderly persons who are concerned about their sexuality, the nurse should emphasize the normalcy of sexual activity. Education should be provided about expected physiologic changes and counseling provided about ways to accommodate these changes (see Chapter 11).

## SUBJECTIVE DATA

Men and women who present themselves for a checkup or with a complaint related to the genital tract should have a complete history taken. Some persons who at first appear to have no symptoms indicating involvement of the reproductive organs may be found to have a problem of the genital system.

Many problems that individuals bring to the attention of nurses and physicians concern subjects or body areas that they are hesitant to discuss. Careful, tactful questioning can assist them to feel more at ease, and often they are relieved that the topic has been raised by someone else. Sympathy and understanding, along with respect for personal feelings, are essential.

Chapter 11 discusses strategies for successfully assessing sexual functioning. It is critical to include sexual assessment in the overall assessment of elderly as well as younger patients.

### PERSONAL DATA

Sociocultural information is helpful to determine the patient's frame of reference and provides insight into the whole person. The data include the person's age, socioeconomic status, educational background, occupation and job history, religion, ethnic group, living arrangements, marital status, financial situation, family network and position in family structure, support systems, existence of stressors, and leisure-time activities. Many superstitions related to the reproductive system are culture specific. All these areas can influence the function of the reproductive system.

Leisure-time activities have been associated with reproductive system dysfunction. For example, women who are long-distance runners have reduced percentages of body fat and a greater risk of menstrual irregularities. Men who sit in hot tubs or saunas for extended periods may experience decreased sperm counts. Religious beliefs may influence contraceptive practices. Exposure to extremely high temperatures in the workplace may cause male infertility. Exposure to industrial agents, such as cadmium, could result in the development of carcinomas of the reproductive system. Extreme stress has been associated with reproductive dysfunction. Their perception of the quality of life, outlook for the future, general satisfaction with daily life, and available support systems directly affect decisions patients will make about treatment and how they will respond to treatment.

Information regarding self-care practices, especially in relation to personal hygiene, is important for the prevention of infections in both genders. The nurse should elicit information about the patient's usual habits as well as assess at toileting time if the patient has learning needs regarding hygiene care. For example, women may need to be taught the importance of cleansing the genital area from front to back. Men may need to be taught how to cleanse well around the meatus and the glans, especially if the man has not been circumcised.

### PAST MEDICAL HISTORY

The person's history of previous illnesses and surgery is carefully recorded and includes any previous treatment for conditions that might influence functioning of the reproductive organs.

Men should be questioned about their past history concerning pain or swelling of the scrotum or testes, sores on the penis, discharges from the urethra, urinary tract problems, ability to achieve and maintain an erection, and previous surgery or treatments for problems of the genitourinary tract. Both men and women should be questioned about a history of sexually transmitted diseases.

Men also should be questioned about the occurrence of mumps, mumps immunizations, or any indications of sterility. Mumps in young men has been associated with an increase in sterility. Women should be questioned about the occurrence of rubella, which is a concern to women of childbearing age. During the first 3 months of pregnancy, rubella can increase the possibility of congenital anomalies. If a woman has not had rubella, she should be encouraged to be immunized if not pregnant and advised not to conceive for at least 3 months after immunizations.

The nurse should assess for chronic diseases as well. Impotence in the male can result from the chemical imbalances caused by diabetes. Cardiovascular disease, hypertension, angina, thrombophlebitis, and diabetes in women can cause a higher incidence of morbidity and mortality with pregnancy or oral contraceptive use. Anemia may be present as a result of menstrual flow or may be aggravated by it.

Men who have had heart attacks frequently experience impotence because of fear of causing another attack. Genitourinary problems can impede sexual functioning and reproductive capacity. Endocrine problems such as hypothyroidism and hyperthyroidism can interfere with menstrual cycles in females and sexual performance in males.

Oral contraceptives may be contraindicated in women with some pathologic conditions. Seizures, migraine headaches, and cholecystitis are often aggravated by oral contraceptive use. Estrogen products need to be avoided in patients with liver disease because estrogen is metabolized by the liver. Oral contraceptives may be contraindicated in women with chronic obstructive pulmonary disease or asthma because progesterone causes increased viscosity of respiratory secretions.

## FAMILY HISTORY

Some chronic diseases that tend to recur in families influence functioning of the reproductive organs. A history of the mother's past pregnancies is important, especially if it involved use of diethylstilbestrol (DES), which leads to vaginal adenosis. Women exposed to this drug in utero have a higher risk for developing cervical and vaginal adenocarcinoma. Male offspring of mothers who took DES have developed congenital anomalies such as structural defects of the genitourinary tract, decreased semen levels, and cancer.

## GYNECOLOGIC-OBSTETRIC HISTORY

In securing information about the gynecologic history, as with other aspects of the history, it is important to assess the person's level of understanding and to use words that are readily understood. For example, few women can answer questions about *menarche*, but most could answer the question, "How old were you when your periods began?" Box 51-2 summarizes a typical gynecologic-obstetric history.

### BOX 51-2 Gynecologic-Obstetric History

1. Previous illness or surgery involving the reproductive organs
2. Menstrual history
   a. Age at menarche
   b. Interval and duration of menstrual periods
   c. Pain with menstruation, including days of cycle on which it occurs, duration, and factors that intensify or alleviate it
   d. Amount of flow (number of tampons or pads)
   e. Presence of clots, their size, and dates on which they appear
   f. Dates of onset of last two menstrual periods and duration of flow
3. Obstetric history
   a. Pregnancies (dates, length of gestation, type of delivery, birth weight, complications during or after pregnancy)
   b. Abortions, miscarriages (length of pregnancy, method of abortion, physical or psychologic complications)

A complete contraceptive history should be taken if the woman has been determined to be heterosexually active and of reproductive age. Information includes types of contraceptives used in the past and at present, how long each type was used, why a specific method was discontinued and another substituted, and any problems that occurred during the use of contraception.

## MEDICATIONS AND ALLERGIES

The nurse should not overlook investigating what drugs the patient may be taking besides oral contraceptives. The nurse should ask what prescribed, over-the counter, and street drugs the patient might be currently taking or has taken in the past. Many drugs prescribed for a particular purpose (e.g., hypertension, coronary artery disease) have been found to have an adverse effect on the reproductive system or sexuality. (These drug effects are discussed in more detail in Chapter 11.)

The nurse should assess if the patient has allergies to rubber or latex, which are essential ingredients in diaphragms and some condoms. Allergies can preclude the use of these agents. Sulfonamides and penicillin frequently are used to treat genitourinary symptoms, including vaginitis. It is important to obtain an allergy history and know what symptoms of sensitivity the patient experienced.

## PATIENT'S COMPLAINT

The patient's complaint is recorded in the patient's own language. The data should include the nature and location of the symptoms, duration, severity, treatment by a physician, and attempts made by the patient to relieve the problem. If pain is a complaint, the patient is asked to describe it in clear terms. The effect of coughing, changing position, having intercourse, or applying heat or cold is established.

When the patient complains of bleeding, as much specific information should be obtained as possible. For women, data about the last two menstrual periods are obtained. If the menstrual periods are irregular, the range of the cycles and duration of flow are recorded. Bleeding between menstrual periods is described in terms of number of days before or after a menstrual period and duration of bleeding at these times. In addition, characteristics of the blood lost are obtained and recorded. In men, complaints of bleeding are often related to the presence of blood in the urine, and other symptoms such as pain on voiding may be present. Frank bleeding may be present in the form of bright or dark blood on the underwear. Associated symptoms may include discharges, burning, or itching of the genitalia, sores on the genitals, and the presence of swelling or masses.

Urinary symptoms frequently are reported with reproductive problems and may be associated with a variety of disorders. Urinary symptoms such as urgency, frequency, pain, hematuria, nocturia, or incontinence should be carefully evaluated. Gastrointestinal symptoms also may occur and typically include heartburn, bloating, nausea and vomiting, or constipation.

## OBJECTIVE DATA

A complete physical examination should be performed. Men should have a rectal examination, and women should have a pelvic examination and a thorough examination of the breasts. Both men and women may delay seeking medical help concerning problems of the reproductive tract because the examination triggers an emotional response. Fear, embarrassment, and cultural mores play an important part. In our culture, people frequently fear that their anxieties concerning carcinoma, venereal disease, sterility, or the menopause will be verified (see Research box on right). Many patients are embarrassed by the required exposure of the external genitalia during examination and fear that some condition will be discovered that will require surgery resulting in sterility or impotence. The nurse who is sensitive to the many thoughts and fears that may trouble patients will be better prepared to help them accept the necessary examination. Preparation for the physical examination includes informing the patient of what is to be done, by whom and why, and when the patient will be informed of results.

### PHYSICAL EXAMINATION OF THE FEMALE

The physical examination of the reproductive system begins with an examination of the breasts in the female (see Chapter 54).

#### Abdominal Examination

Physical assessment of the reproductive organs includes a standard assessment of the lower abdomen (see Chapter 43). Any localized areas of prominence are noted, since these may indicate enlargement of the reproductive organs or adjacent structures. The skin of the abdomen and pubic area is inspected for amount, distribution, and character of hair; abnormal pigmentation; and lesions. Abdominal muscle tone is assessed by having the patient cough or raise the head. Such actions reveal muscle weakness by producing bulging around the umbilicus, inguinal region, or in the midline between the rectus muscles. Women who have been pregnant are more likely to have diastasis recti.

*Auscultation* of the abdomen does not play a significant role unless the presence and quality of peristaltic movement needs to be assessed. Since the reproductive organs are normally situated in the pelvic cavity, they are usually not palpable through the abdominal wall. Therefore abdominal *palpation* is performed to rule out or discover abnormalities. If an abdominal mass is felt, its position, size, shape, consistency, contour, tenderness, movability, and relationship to any pelvic or abdominal organ are described.

Enlargement of the uterus is detected by palpating in the midline of the lower abdomen. Palpation is started just below the umbilicus and continued in the direction of the symphysis pubis. In contrast to a full bladder, which feels soft, an enlarged uterus feels firm and may be round or asymmetric. A firm, isolated area of enlargement may be caused by the presence of a tumor of the uterus.

Enlargement of the fallopian tubes and ovaries may be detected by palpation of the right and left lower quadrants. Even when enlarged, these organs are not always palpable through the abdominal wall. However, enlargement is often associated with pain or tenderness on palpation of the lower quadrants. The round ligaments are often palpable in the lower quadrants, stretching from the iliac crests to the pubic bones, and they should not be confused with the fallopian tubes.

*Percussion* of the lower abdomen is directed chiefly to the organs or masses that are palpable. A tumor, such as an ovarian cyst or fibroid tumor of the uterus, produces a flat note (dullness), over the area.

#### Pelvic Examination

The pelvic examination is frequently a stressful event for the patient. The nurse can help the woman to overcome negative aspects such as pain, embarrassment, and anxiety by establishing a relaxed, positive atmosphere and addressing the woman's questions and concerns. Visual aids are useful when a pelvic examination is to be performed for the first time. Models of the pelvic organs and pamphlets assist with the presentation of information about the purpose of the examination, what is done, and what to expect. The nurse or examiner explains the procedure and answers questions before the patient is undressed and on the examination table.

**RESEARCH**

Lauver D, Rubin M: Women's concerns about abnormal Papanicolaou test results, *J Obstet Gynecol Neonat Nurs* 20:154-159, 1991.

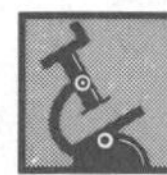

Because of the increase in and potential severity of abnormal Papanicolaou (Pap) tests, women's concerns and methods of coping with abnormal Pap results are of clinical importance. Through this study, the researchers sought to describe women's questions and identify their reactions to abnormal Pap results. The study included 118 women whose Pap tests suggested precancer. Interviews were conducted with the participants after they received the news of their Pap tests and at follow-up. On hearing the results of their Pap tests, the participants asked questions reflecting their concern about follow-up, causes, and implications. The participants' reactions at follow-up reflected their concerns about serious diseases, worry, and uncertainty about the meaning of Pap tests.

Some patients may need to see and touch the speculum before it is inserted.

Sharing information with the woman about sensory data has been found to be more important in reducing anxiety and pain than explanation of the procedure. The nurse should describe the pulling of the labia during inspection, the sensation of a finger in the vagina, the feeling of opening experienced when the speculum is inserted, and the pressure similar to having a bowel movement during the rectal examination.

The patient should have the option to use or not use drapes to cover her perineum. Some women feel that drapes prevent embarrassment and protect their modesty, whereas others feel that draping indicates something mysterious or shameful about the pelvic examination. During the examination, the examiner tells the patient what will be done next and informs her of the findings. The patient is encouraged to relax *specific* tense body parts rather than generally to relax throughout the examination.

After the pelvic examination, the nurse or examiner reviews findings and answers any patient questions. The pelvic examination is a unique opportunity to teach anatomy and physiology, as well as to discuss health practices.

Women who are scheduled ahead of time for pelvic examination should be advised to avoid douching, sexual intercourse, and applying any vaginal preparations (medicinal or deodorant) for at least 24 hours before examination. Patients should void and defecate, if needed, immediately before examination because an empty bladder and lower bowel makes palpation of the pelvic organs easier, decreases patient discomfort, eliminates possible distortion of the position of pelvic organs caused by a full bladder, and obviates the danger of incontinence during examination.

A mirror used by the examiner enables the woman to visualize her genitalia, often correcting myths about the vagina and other structures. This approach may provide many women with their first opportunity to view and identify their genitalia.

## Positioning

The most common position used for the pelvic examination is the lithotomy position (Figure 51-9, *B*). However, because the lithotomy position requires flexion of the ankles and knees and simultaneous flexion, abduction, and external rotation of the hips, it may not be suitable for elderly patients or women with arthritis or other conditions that limit mobility. Sims' position (Figure 51-9, *A*) may be used for the rectal part of the examination. The knee-chest position may be used in selected situations (Figure 51-9, *C*), but it usually carries the same drawbacks for mobility-limited persons and is both uncomfortable and highly embarrassing for women of any age or physical condition.

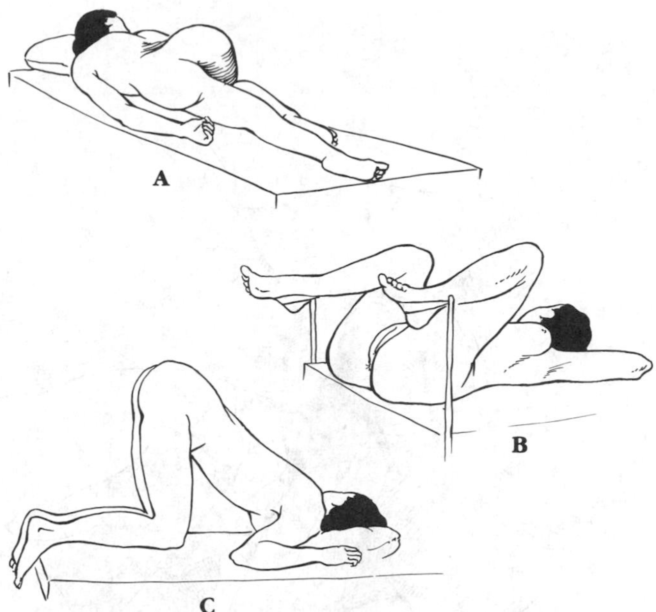


**FIGURE 51-9** Various positions that can be assumed for examination of rectum and vagina. **A,** Sims' (lateral) position. Note position of left arm and right leg. **B,** Lithotomy position. Note position of buttocks on edge of examining table and support of feet. **C,** Knee-chest (genupectoral) position. Note placement of shoulders and head.

The pelvic examination can be performed with the woman in bed if it is inadvisable for her to be moved to an examining table. The woman can be helped to assume a position across the bed, and her feet can be supported on the seats of two straight chairs. Most women are able to place their own legs in the stirrups; they should be told to raise both legs and put them in the stirrups simultaneously. The older patient may need assistance and may require additional support of her legs by attendants during the examination. Gentleness and gradual positioning are essential to prevent strain or twisting of the hip joint. Metal stirrups are the most satisfactory; however, if they are used, the patient should wear her shoes because the heels help to hold the feet in the stirrups.

Care must be taken to see that there is no pressure on the legs when sling stirrups are used, since nerve damage and impairment of circulation can occur. The buttocks need to be moved down so that they are even with the end of the table. One or more pillows may be placed under the head for comfort and to prevent dyspnea.

### Inspection of external structures

The external genitalia are examined before the internal examination. The labia are inspected for asymmetry, enlargement, exudates, altered pigmentation, varicosities, and leukoplakia. Irregularities or tissue distortions may result from healed lacerations, ulcers, or cysts of the Skene's or Bartholin's glands, which are common sites of infection, especially from the gonococcus organism.

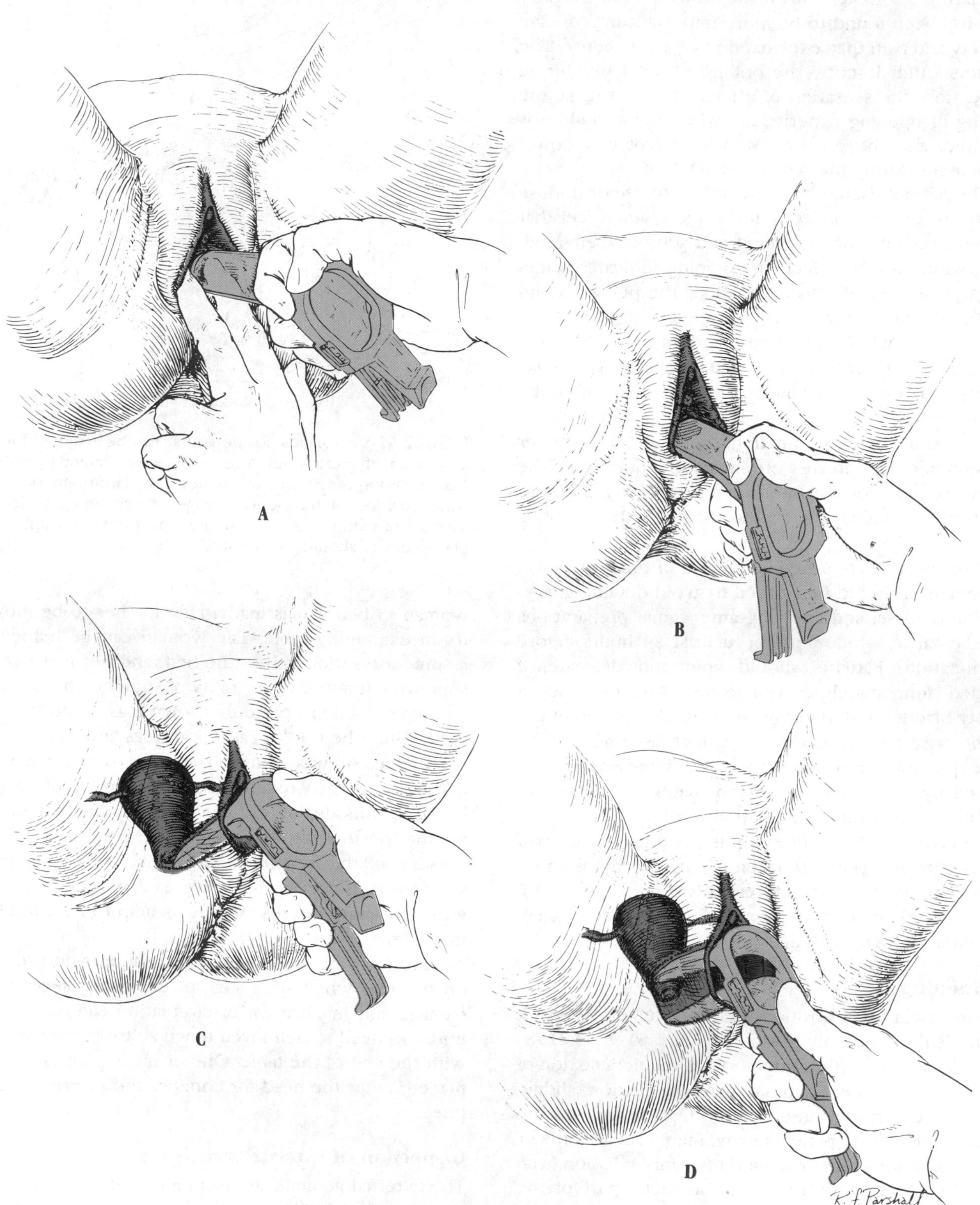

**FIGURE 51-10** Procedure for speculum examination. **A,** Opening of introitus. **B,** Oblique insertion of speculum. **C,** Final insertion of speculum. **D,** Opening of speculum blades. (From Malasanos L et al: *Health assessment,* ed 4, St Louis, 1990, Mosby.)

Clitoral enlargement or atrophy is abnormal. The clitoris is a potential site of syphilitic chancres or maligant lesions. Abnormalities of the urinary meatus may include erythema, exudates, and masses.

### Inspection of vagina and cervix

The vagina and cervix are inspected after the insertion of a vaginal speculum (Figure 51-10). The *cervix* is inspected for color, contour, position, size, symmetry, surface characteristics, discharge, and patency of the external os. In nulliparous women, the external os appears as a round, depressed area. In multiparous women, the os usually appears as a transverse slit in the center of the cervix. The color of the cervix varies but is usually pink. It becomes pale after menopause and cyanotic either during pregnancy or with any condition causing venous congestion or hypoxia.

The surface of the cervix is inspected to determine whether it is smooth, irregular, or raw and whether there is any purulent or other type of discharge from the os. A red, somewhat raw appearing area (an erosion) may be seen on the surface of the cervix. Scars may appear as white or reddened slits radiating from the cervical os and are lacerations often present in women who have borne children. Occasionally, a stalked polyp may be seen extending through the cervical os as a bright-red or dark-red mass. These polyps frequently cause bleeding and require further study.

The walls of the *vagina* are inspected as the speculum is withdrawn. The vaginal mucosa is observed for color, consistency, inflammation, ulcers, masses, presence of rugae, discharge, and color. The vaginal wall is normally pink in color but is usually pallid after menopause.

### Palpation

Palpation of the internal reproductive organs follows speculum examination. The cervix is palpated for consistency and contour. The cervix feels softer with pregnancy and harder with tumors. Areas of irregularity and abnormal tension are carefully noted in terms of site.

An attempt is made to insert a finger into the cervical os to detect masses, but excessive force should not be used. In nulliparous women, the cervix is usually closed. In multiparous women, the cervix may admit one or two fingers. Movability of the cervix in all directions is checked, and any restrictions of movement are noted. The vaginal vault is palpated for areas of tenderness and presence of masses. Feces in the rectum may be palpated and can be verified later by rectal examination.

*Bimanual palpation* follows palpation of the cervix. The purpose of the bimanual examination is palpation of the internal reproductive organs and assessment of pelvic supports. The position of the uterus is determined first. It may be anteverted, midpositioned, retroverted, anteflexed, or retroflexed (see Chapter 52). Usually, the fundus can be felt anterior to the cervix between the two hands. If not, the uterus may lie posteriorly and be palpated through the posterior vaginal vault. The size, shape, and regularity of the uterine surface are palpated. Normally, the uterus feels firm and the fundus is round. The uterus is softer during pregnancy and firmer during menopause. Localized areas of enlargement are noted, and the approximate size and shape of masses are determined. Because the uterus is normally movable and easy to displace, loss of movability is readily detected. This, too, is noted and recorded.

The areas around the fallopian tubes and ovaries require deep palpation. Normally, the fallopian tubes are not palpable; therefore, any enlargement is significant. An enlarged fallopian tube resembles an enlarged ovary to a great extent, and it may not be possible to distinguish between the two.

On bimanual examination, the ovaries are normally slightly tender to palpation and are not always palpable, especially in obese women. When palpable, the ovaries feel smooth and oval in shape if no pathologic condition exists. Any readily palpable mass in the area of the fallopian tubes and ovaries that feels irregular, round, or very firm indicates a possible deviation from normal. Because the ovaries atrophy during the menopause, any mass felt in the areas of the ovaries in postmenopausal women is usually a sign of a problem.

The *rectovaginal examination* is performed to confirm uterine position, to reassess the adnexal areas, to follow up on complaints of pain or bleeding, and to determine rectal sphincter tone. The woman is told that it may be uncomfortable and she may feel as though she has to have a bowel movement. Hemorrhoids, fistulas, and fissures can be observed.

After the pelvic examination, a woman may need assistance with removing lubricating jelly or discharge that may be on her genitalia, removing her legs from the stirrups, and getting down from the table. If a bloody discharge is present, a sanitary pad may need to be provided. Elderly women merit careful assistance after pelvic examination because unnatural positions such as the knee-chest and lithotomy positions may alter the normal circulation of blood sufficiently to cause faintness or changes in blood pressure.

## PHYSICAL EXAMINATION OF THE MALE

Examination of the male genitourinary system includes inspection and palpation of the lower abdomen, inspection and palpation of the external genitalia, and palpation of the prostate gland by rectal examination.

The *abdomen* is palpated above the symphysis pubis to determine whether the bladder is distended; if so, as evidenced by a soft, palpable mass, the patient is questioned about the time of last voiding.

The *inguinal area* is inspected for areas of bulging caused by hernias. The man is requested to hold his breath and to bear down to make presence of herniation more evident (Figure 51-11). Straining is preferable to coughing because it produces more steady sustained

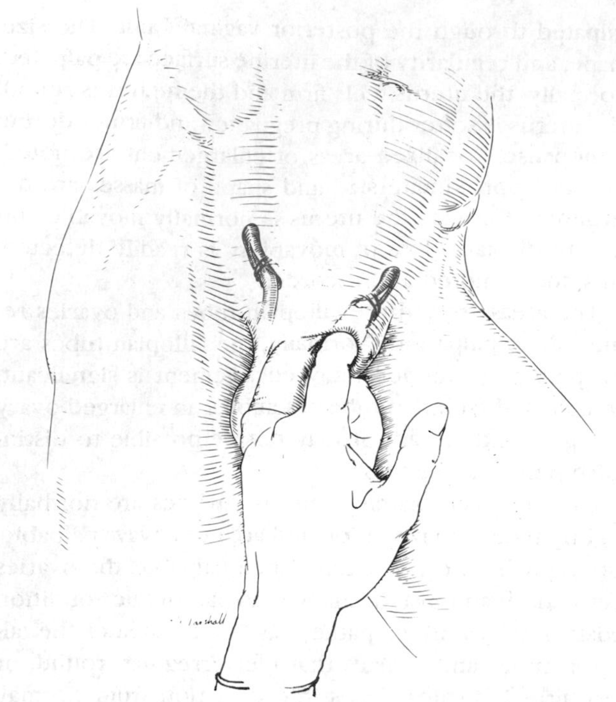

**FIGURE 51-11** Palpation of inguinal area for hernias. (From Barkauskas VH: *Health and physical assessment,* St Louis, 1994, Mosby.)

pressure. The load test is used if a hernia is not palpated despite complaints of hernia symptoms. The man lifts something heavy while the inguinal area is inspected.

The inguinal lymph nodes are palpated for enlargement, pain, or tenderness. The amount and distribution of pubic hair are noted.

The *penis* is inspected for abnormalities of prepuce, glans, and urethral meatus and for visible evidence of infection and masses. The prepuce is fully retracted to determine the presence and degree of phimosis, an abnormality of the foreskin that prevents its free retraction. It is important to note whether the urethra is centrally located or whether it opens on the upper or lower surface of the glans. The urinary meatus is inspected for lesions, periurethral abscess, and purulent or bloody discharge. If a discharge is present, a specimen is obtained by milking the penis from the base to the urethra. The skin along the shaft of the penis is checked for lesions of any type and for general color.

The *scrotum* is observed for general appearance, color of the skin, tension of the skin surfaces, symmetry, and the presence of lesions on the skin surfaces.

The left testis is lower than the right, which causes the scrotum to appear asymmetric under normal conditions. Scrotal size is determined by the tone of the dartos muscle. The scrotum may look pendulous in older age as the dartos muscle becomes atonic and when warm temperatures cause the muscle to relax. Cold temperatures cause the dartos muscle to contract, and the scrotum shrinks. The testes are inspected for shape, size, consistency, and response to pressure by simultaneous palpation between the thumb and first two fingers. The spermatic cords are palpated between the thumb and forefinger. Unilateral or bilateral enlargement usually indicates presence of a mass or edema.

Palpation of the scrotum is necessary to distinguish between enlargement caused by a mass and swelling caused by collection of fluid. The size, shape, location, tenderness, and consistency of any mass are carefully noted. Transillumination of the scrotum with a flashlight may be attempted to differentiate the cause of the scrotal mass. Serous fluid will transilluminate or produce a red glow; tissue and blood will not transilluminate.

The *prostate gland* is palpated by means of a rectal examination with the patient standing (Figure 51-12). Rectal examination on a regular basis is the most important step in the diagnosis of prostatic disease, especially carcinoma. Cancer of the prostate gland may start as a localized, hard nodule, palpable by rectal examination, before proceeding to an advanced, inoperable, or incurable stage. For this reason, it is recommended that all men, especially those over age 50 years, have a rectal examination at least once a year.

# DIAGNOSTIC TESTS

Many diagnostic tests are useful in providing data about the reproductive system. They include blood and urine tests, cytology, radiologic tests, biopsies, and endoscopic procedures.

## LABORATORY TESTS

### Blood and Urine Tests

Because the endocrine system is so closely related to reproductive function, almost any study for endocrine function may be ordered, including determination of estrogen levels and secretion in women and 24-hour urine collections for ketosteroids and pituitary gonadotropins in both sexes. Table 51-1 summarizes a sample of these tests.

Enzyme values play a role in diagnosis of cancer of the prostate gland. The enzyme tests of most value are phosphatase levels. The phosphatases are secreted in the serum of the tumor mass in the prostate gland and are reflected in changes in the blood chemistry. The phosphatases are labeled as acid or alkaline, depending on the optimal pH. Acid phosphatase usually has a pH of 4.0 to 6.0, whereas alkaline phosphatase usually ranges from 8.5 to 9.5. A rise in phosphatase value is indicative of cancer of the prostate gland but is not conclusively diagnostic. Usually, the phosphatase values are repeated for reliability because such events as rectal examination, prostate massage, or recent episodes of fever may cause either an elevation or a drop in phosphatase level. Ad-

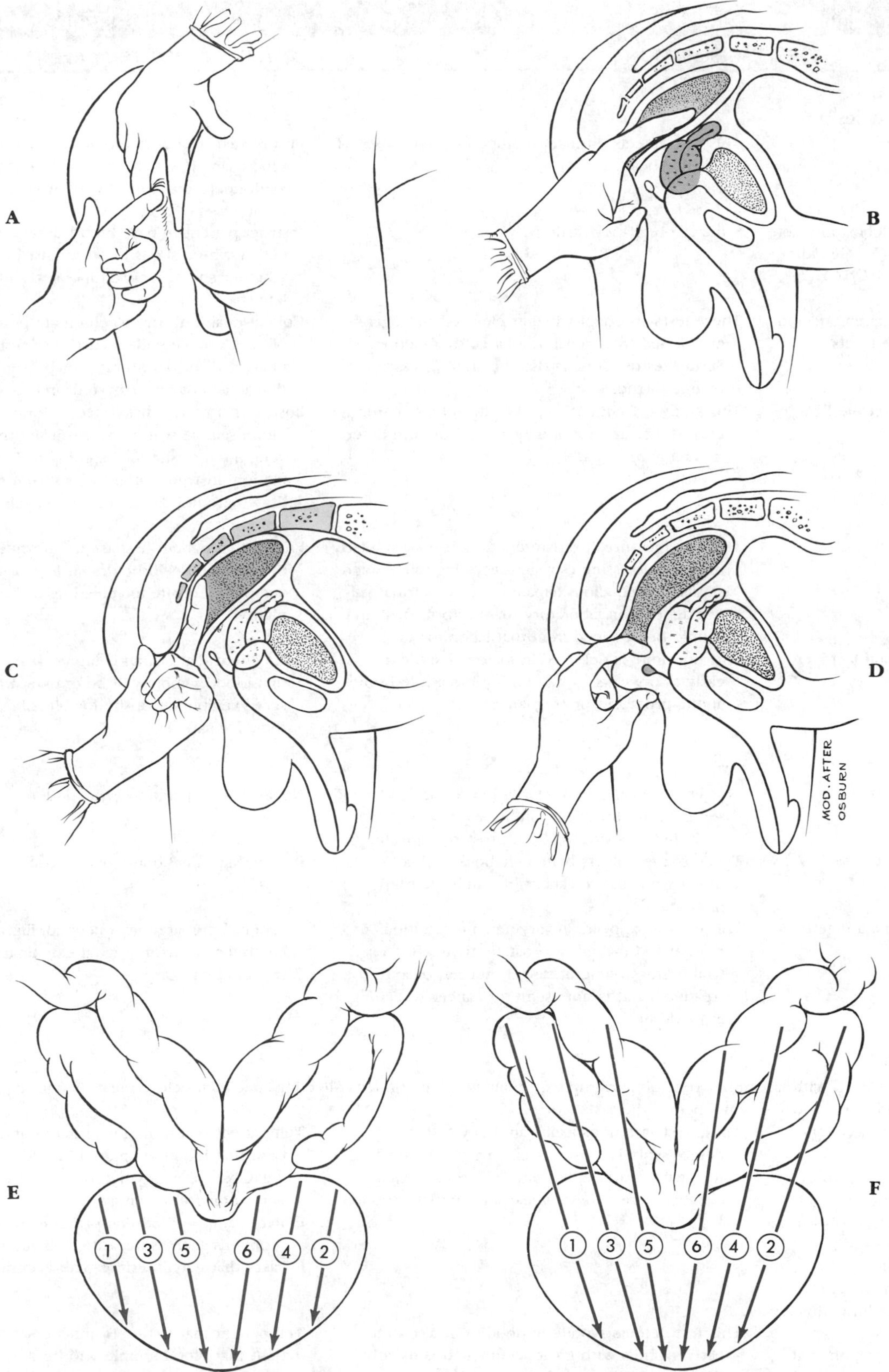


**FIGURE 51-12** Rectal examination. **A,** Introduction of protected, well-lubricated finger. **B,** Palpation of prostrate gland and seminal vesicles, lateral view. **C,** Palpation of anterior surface of sacrum and coccyx. **D,** Palpation of Cowper's glands. **E,** Massage of prostate gland for specimen collection or treatment; order of strokes is indicated by gradually working toward center (verumontanum). **F,** Massage of seminal vesicles and prostate gland. (From Campbell MF, Harrison JH: *Urology,* vol 1, ed 3, Philadelphia, 1970, Saunders.)

**TABLE 51-1 Diagnostic Studies of Male and Female Reproductive Systems—Blood and Urine Studies**

| TEST | DESCRIPTION | PRETEST AND POSTTEST CARE |
|---|---|---|
| **BLOOD** | | |
| **Endocrine Studies** | | |
| Prolactin assay | This test detects pituitary dysfunction and causes of amenorrhea. | Ensure that patient has fasted. Inform patient that blood sample will be drawn in morning. Observe venipuncture site for bleeding or hematoma formation. |
| Serum human chorionic gonadotropin (HCG) radioimmunoassay (RIA) | Same as pregnancy testing. | Instruct patient to have blood drawn in laboratory. (Elicit where she is in her menstrual cycle, whether she has missed menses, and if so, how late she is.) |
| Serum androstenedione and testosterone levels | These tests ascertain whether elevated androgens are caused by adrenal or ovarian dysfunction. Serum testosterone is also drawn to assess cause of amenorrhea. | Collect health history to eliminate potential sources of interference with accuracy of results (i.e., use of steroids or barbiturates or presence of hypothyroidism or hyperthyroidism). |
| Serum progesterone RIA | This study is frequently used to detect a functioning corpus luteum cyst. It may also be used in determining adrenal pathology. | Ensure that patient has fasted. Inform patient that blood sample will be drawn in morning. Observe venipuncture site for bleeding or hematoma formation. Instruct patient that serum must be drawn around day 24 or 25 of cycle for greatest accuracy. |
| Serum estradiol RIA | This test measures ovarian function. It is particularly useful in assessing estrogen-secreting tumors and status of precocious female puberty. Normal values depend on laboratory that performs test and should be obtained from that laboratory. | Ensure that patient has fasted. Inform her that blood sample will be drawn in morning. Observe venipuncture site for bleeding or hematoma formation. |
| Human placental lactogen (HPL) | This hormone is detected in maternal serum as early as 6 weeks' gestation. It plays a role in metabolic processes of pregnancy. | Tell patient that fasting is unnecessary. Inform her that blood sample will be drawn in morning. Observe venipuncture site for bleeding or hematoma formation. |
| **Enzyme Studies** | | |
| Acid phosphatase | This enzyme appears primarily in prostate gland and semen. High levels may indicate prostate tumor with metastasis beyond the prostatic capsule. | No special preparation is needed. |
| Alkaline phosphatase | This enzyme reflects bone metabolism. High levels in known prostate cancer may indicate bony metastasis. | Patient fasts for 8 hours before test. |
| Prostate-specific antigen | This enzyme appears in varying concentrations in normal and malignant prostatic tissue. It is used to monitor course of cancer and response to treatment but is not useful for cancer screening at this time. | No special preparation is needed. Enzyme should be collected before digital examination which triggers its release. |
| **Syphilis Studies** | | |
| *General note:* Check with laboratory regarding fasting requirements. Some prefer collecting specimen before meals. Some request that patient avoid alcohol for 24 hours before the test. | | |
| Nontreponemal serologic tests<br>Wassermann (complement fixation)<br>Venereal Disease Research Laboratories (VDRL) (flocculation)<br>Rapid plasma reagin (RPR) (agglutination) | These tests are nonspecific antibody tests used to detect syphilis. Positive readings can be made 1 to 2 weeks after appearance of primary lesion (chancre) or 4 to 15 weeks after initial infection. | Tell patient that fasting is unnecessary. Inform patient that blood sample will be drawn in morning. Observe venipuncture site for bleeding or hematoma formation.<br>Obtain data to determine presence or absence of problems such as hepatitis and autoimmune diseases that may interfere with accuracy of results. |
| Treponemal test<br>Fluorescent treponemal antibody absorption (FTA-ABS) | This test detects syphilis antibodies. It also detects early syphilis with great accuracy. It is usually performed if results of nontreponemal testing are questionable. | Tell patient that fasting is unnecessary. Inform patient that blood sample will be drawn in morning. Observe venipuncture site for bleeding or hematoma formation. |

Modified from Lewis SM, Collier IC: *Medical-surgical nursing: assessment and management of clinical problems,* ed 3, St Louis, 1992, Mosby.

**TABLE 51-1 Diagnostic Studies of Male and Female Reproductive Systems—Blood and Urine Studies—cont'd**

| TEST | DESCRIPTION | PRETEST AND POSTTEST CARE |
|---|---|---|
| **URINE** | | |
| Pregnancy testing (Pregnosticon Dri Dot [latex inhibition test], Gravindex, Pregnosticon Accuspheres [hemagglutination-inhibition]) | HCG is detected in urine to ascertain whether woman is pregnant. Hydatidiform mole and chorioepithelioma (in men and women) may also be detected. Positive result is cloudy solution. Negative result is clear solution. | Instruct patient to obtain first morning specimen. Tell her that accuracy of test is greatest 6 weeks after last menstrual period. Obtain thorough menstrual history, including birth control methods. Determine presence or absence of presumptive signs of pregnancy (e.g., breast changes, increased whitish vaginal discharge). |
| **Hormone Testing** | | |
| Total estrogen levels | Urine estrogen levels are used to detect ovarian pathology, hyperadrenalism, interstitial cell tumor of testes, liver disease, and ectopic pregnancy. A 24-hour urine collection is required. Normal levels vary, depending on menstrual cycle. | Instruct patient to save all urine for 24 hours and to keep it refrigerated. Check with laboratory to see if preservative is needed for urine collection container. Encourage patient to drink fluids during collection period. |
| Pregnanediol levels | Progesterone levels are assessed. This is most often used to detect corpus luteum cysts and sometimes threatened abortions. It may also be used to determine adrenal cortical function and causes of amenorrhea. Normal levels vary according to menstrual cycle or length of gestation. | Instruct patient to collect all urine for 24 hours and to keep it refrigerated. Check with laboratory to see if preservative is needed for urine collection container. Encourage patient to drink fluids during collection period. Assess type of drugs patient is currently taking. |
| Testosterone levels | Tumors and developmental anomalies of testes can be detected. | Instruct patient to collect 24-hour urine specimen and to keep it refrigerated. Obtain genitourinary and reproductive system history. |

ditional studies such as prostatic biopsy are done to confirm the diagnosis.

#### Prostate-specific antigen

**Prostate-specific antigen (PSA)** has received much research attention. This enzyme is secreted by normal prostate tissue and is elevated in the presence of both benign prostatic hypertrophy and prostate cancer. Since it reflects the volume and weight of the prostate, there is no accurate way to separate values that are elevated because of cancer versus values that are elevated because of benign disease. Therefore, at present, PSA levels play little role in screening for prostate cancer. However, the values are an excellent method of tracing an individual's response to treatment and monitoring for cancer recurrence.

### Syphilis Studies

Serologic testing is used for detecting syphilis. Two identifiable antibodies appear in the blood 1 to 4 months after syphilis is contracted. Two types of tests, treponemal and nontreponemal, are presently available. The tests differ in the type of antibody measured and in the antigen used to detect antibodies.

The nontreponemal tests, typically called serologic tests for syphilis (STS), measure an antibody-like substance called *reagin.* The Venereal Disease Research Laboratories (VDRL) test is the most frequently used serologic test for syphilis and is the test used most often for routine premarital and prenatal screening.

Syphilitic reagin is thought to form from tissue breakdown products resulting from the interaction of the organism and body tissues. STS are usually reported as nonreactive, weakly reactive, or reactive. If any degree of reactivity is found, a quantitative test is performed by diluting the serum progressively until an end point of reactivity is reached. Quantitative reactions are reported in ratios and reflect the ***highest dilution*** at which the serum reacts. For example, a reaction reported as 1:16 means that the person's serum was diluted 16 times and still produced reaction, but no reaction occurred when the serum was diluted more than 16 times.

Reactive STS are confirmed by alternate serologic tests. For this purpose, the fluorescent treponemal antibody-absorption test (FTA-ABS) is most often used, since it is the most sensitive and specific test for syphilis available. Reactive STS, which occur with no exposure to syphilis, frequently occurs in conjunction with a hypersensitivity reaction, acute bacterial or viral infection, recent vaccination, or chronic systemic illness such as tuberculosis, collagen disease, or malaria. Recent ingestion of alcohol can alter the test results. It is important, therefore, not to tell patients they have syphilis based on STS alone. A positive FTA-ABS must be established before the diagnosis of syphilis is made.

Because antibodies are not present in the serum of

the infected person until the organism gains entry into the circulation, STS may be negative, and the individual may still be infected. A negative syphilis test may also occur when an individual is taking antibiotics. Once antibodies are present, they do not completely disappear from the serum. Although treated and noninfected, the person may have a positive serology test indefinitely. If successful therapy is given before antibodies develop, these tests may never be positive unless the person again becomes infected and develops antibodies. Therefore, serologic tests in use today do not always indicate an active syphilitic infection and only detect the presence of antibodies. There is presently an urgent need for a specific, rapid method of detecting infection caused by syphilis, and such methods are being studied. Until new tests are developed, the patient's history, clinical symptoms (if any), and serologic testing are the means most often used to make a diagnosis of syphilis. Table 51-1 summarizes these studies.

## Cultures and Smears

Secretions may be obtained from the vagina for wet smear examination, and cultures may be obtained from any orifice and of any discharge of the male or female reproductive tract when symptoms of infection are present. Table 51-2 summarizes these diagnostic studies. Most infectious diseases of the reproductive tract produce a purulent discharge. In men, the most common site of purulent discharge is the urinary meatus. The cervix, urethra, Skene's glands, and Bartholin's glands are the most common sites of infection in women. Smears or cultures of the discharge are usually successful in identification of the organism responsible for the infection. The culture for *Neisseria gonorrhoeae* is one of the most important, since it is the only means of confirming a diagnosis of gonorrhea in an otherwise asymptomatic woman. These approaches may be used to evaluate nonspecific vaginitis, candidiasis, trichomoniasis, *Gardnerella* infection, and herpes simplex virus as well.

### Tests for chlamydial infections

Chlamydial infections are the most common cause of sexually transmitted disease (STD) and occur 10 times more often than gonorrhea. Tests for *Chlamydia* using fluorescent tagging are very specific and sensitive. For these tests, cells are obtained from the urethra or cervix rather than from exudate or cervical mucus. The material on the slide is fixed with ethyl acetate, and fluorescently tagged monocolonal antibody is added. A diagnosis can be made in 20 to 30 minutes. The enzyme-

**TABLE 51-2 Diagnostic Studies of Male and Female Reproductive Systems—Cultures and Smears**

| TEST | DESCRIPTION | PRETEST AND POSTTEST CARE |
|---|---|---|
| Dark-field microscopy | Direct examination of specimen obtained from potential syphilitic lesion (chancre) is performed to detect treponema. | Avoid direct skin contact with open lesion. |
| Wet mounts | Direct microscopic examination of specimen of vaginal discharge is performed immediately after collection. This determines presence or absence and number of *Trichomonas* organisms, bacteria, white and red blood cells, and candidal buds or hyphae. Other clues or causes of inflammation or infection may be determined. | Explain procedure and purpose to patient. Instruct patient not to douche before examination. Prepare for collection of specimens (glass slide, 10% to 20% potassium hydroxide [KOH] solution, sodium chloride [NaCl] solution, cotton-tipped applicators). |
| Cultures | Culture of specimens of vaginal, urethral, or cervical discharge is taken and used to assess presence of gonorrhea, chlamydia, or yeast. Rectal and throat cultures may also be taken, depending on data obtained from sexual history. | Obtain specific contact and sexual history, including oral and rectal intercourse. Instruct against douching before examination. Obtain urethral specimen from men before they void. Instruct women who are sexually active with multiple partners to have at least a yearly culture. Instruct sexually active men to have any discharge evaluated immediately to rule out gonorrhea strains that do not cause classic symptoms of dysuria. |
| Gram stain | This presumptive test is used for rapid detection of gonorrhea. Presence of gram-negative intracellular diplococci generally warrants initiation of treatment. | Same as for cultures. |
| **CYTOLOGIC STUDIES** | | |
| Pap smear | Microscopic study of exfoliated cells via special staining and fixation technique detects malignancy. Cells most often studied are those obtained directly from endocervix, cervix, vaginal pool, and endometrial lining of the uterine cavity. | Instruct women who are sexually active and over 18 to have yearly Pap smears. Arrange for smear at midcycle time. Instruct patients not to douche or tub-bathe for at least 24 hours before examination. Collect careful menstrual and gynecologic history. Some physicians prefer patient refrain from sexual intercourse for 24 to 48 hours before test. |

Modified from Lewis SM, Collier IC: *Medical-surgical nursing: assessment and management of clinical problems,* ed 3, St Louis, 1992, Mosby.

linked immunosorbent assay (ELISA) test (Chlamydiazyme) is another diagnostic test, but a diagnosis takes 4 hours.

Persons who should be tested for chlamydial infections are those with mucopurulent cervicitis or urethral discharge, sterile pyuria, a positive gonorrhea culture, and pelvic inflammatory disease (PID).

#### Prostatic smear

For a prostatic smear, the physician first massages the prostate gland (see Figure 51-12). The next voided urine specimen is collected, and a smear is prepared in the laboratory. Some cases of cancer and tuberculosis of the prostate gland can be detected by this method.

Most often, biopsy specimens of the prostate gland are used for diagnosis. Various methods are used to obtain tissue specimens from the prostate gland.

### Cytology

#### Papanicolaou (Pap) smear

The American Cancer Society recommends that all women who are or have been sexually active or who are at least 18 years of age have an annual **Papanicolaou (PAP) Smear** for 3 consecutive years and then every 3 years until middle age.[1] More frequent testing may be recommended at the discretion of the physician for women with a history of multiple sexual partners or STD, a family history of cervical cancer, or those whose mothers used diethylstilbestrol (DES) during pregnancy.

The PAP test makes it possible to detect abnormal cells, not all of which are malignant, as well as precancerous lesions and cervical cancer. It is 95% accurate in detecting abnormal cells. False-negative reports are most frequently the result of an inadequate sample or improperly fixed slide. The PAP test is performed by microscopic examination of cells collected from the vaginal pool, exocervix, and endocervical canal. The Guidelines box below, left, summarizes specific instructions for obtaining a PAP smear.

A woman should not douche, tub-bathe, use vaginal medications or deodorants, or have sexual intercourse for at least 24 hours before the test. Some physicians request a 48-hour delay before the test. Pap smears should be obtained preferably 5 to 6 days after menstruation termination, since menses makes interpretation difficult and may camouflage atypical cells. Infections can interfere with hormonal cytology. Pap smears should be delayed for at least 1 month after use of topical antibiotics, which produce rapid, heavy shedding of cells. Many women experience some vaginal bleeding in the form of spotting after a Pap smear has been taken. They should be advised that this is expected and normal but that any bleeding in excess of spotting is abnormal and should be reported to the health care provider.

Box 51-3 provides a classification of the cytologic findings. Over the past 10 years, there has been a movement to reclassify findings and report them in terms of **cervical intraepithelial neoplasia (CIN).** This is a simple designation of the spectrum of intraepithelial dysplasia that usually occurs before invasive cervical cancer. CIN 1 includes classes II and some of III, CIN 2 includes class III, and CIN 3 comprises classes IV and V.

When the Pap test is positive, additional tissue studies are indicated. The woman should understand that the Pap test is not necessarily conclusive and that biopsy or even surgery may be necessary to verify the diagnosis of premalignancy or malignancy. The false-positive rate is 5%.

#### Guidelines for Obtaining a Pap Smear

1. Explain the steps of the procedure to the patient.
2. Place the patient in the lithotomy position.
3. Lubricate the speculum with warm water. Using lubricating jelly on the speculum can alter the specimen.
4. Insert the vaginal speculum to expose the cervix.
5. Collect material from the cervical canal by rotating a moist, saline cotton swab or spatula within the cervical canal and in the squamocolumnar junction. Collect enough material to make a distinct blur on the slide.
6. Smear material on prelabeled glass slides.
7. Place the glass slides immediately in a wide-mouthed jar containing a fixative solution of 95% alcohol and ether (to prevent drying out and cell distortion). Place the slides in solution so that the unsmeared sides are back to back.
8. Carefully label the specimen with the patient's name, age, parity, and date of last menstrual period. The patient's medication history should be written on the laboratory request form (e.g., oral contraceptives, digitalis, and tetracycline can alter the test results by affecting the squamous epithelium).

## RADIOLOGIC TESTS

### Ultrasonography

Ultrasonography (ultrasound) has become a useful diagnostic tool for gynecologic problems. It can be used

#### BOX 51-3 Classification of Papanicolaou Smears

**TRADITIONAL CLASSIFICATION**

| | |
|---|---|
| Class I | Absence of atypical or abnormal cells (normal) |
| Class II | Atypical cells, but no evidence of malignancy (most frequently caused by inflammation of cervix) |
| Class III | Cytologic findings suggestive of but not conclusive concerning malignancy |
| Class IV | Cytologic findings strongly suggestive of malignancy |
| Class V | Cytologic findings conclusive of malignancy |

**CERVICAL INTRAEPITHELIAL NEOPLASIA (CIN) CLASSIFICATION**

| | |
|---|---|
| CIN 1 | Mild and mild-to-moderate dysplasia |
| CIN 2 | Moderate and moderate-to-severe dysplasia |
| CIN 3 | Severe dysplasia and carcinoma in situ |

**BOX 51-4 Uses of Transvaginal Sonography**

**UTERUS**
Size, position
Inspection of myometrium and endometrial lining
Detection of malformations
Identification of small fibroids
Early pregnancy determination
Early fetal heartbeats

**OVARIES**
Size, texture, location
Monitoring follicular growth
Evaluation of ovulation
Identification of corpus luteum
Identification of tumors and structural deformities
Follicular aspiration

**FALLOPIAN TUBES**
Diagnosis of tubal pathology
Detection of tuboovarian abscess
Early recognition of tubal pregnancy

**EXTRAGENITAL STRUCTURES**
Evaluation of free pelvic fluid
Detection of pelvic blood clots

to locate pelvic masses, intrauterine devices (IUDs), ectopic pregnancies, and prostatic neoplasms. **Transvaginal ultrasonography** allows for improved ultrasonic picture clarity compared with transabdominal sonography in assessing gynecologic health.[2] Transvaginal sonography is currently being used to inspect and assess the uterus, ovaries, fallopian tubes, and extragenital structures (Box 51-4). A transducer is inserted a few centimeters into the vagina while the patient is in a lithotomy position. Vaginal probes are inserted into a sterile sheath before patient use. Transvaginal probe use is increasingly common in guiding procedures involving needle puncture, such as ova retrieval for in vitro fertilization.

Transrectal ultrasonography may also be used as part of a work-up for benign prostatic enlargement or prostate cancer. It is not sensitive enough to be used alone for diagnosis of cancer, because its false-negative and false-positive results are too high, but it can be part of a more complete office work-up and be used to guide the physician in prostate biopsy. (See Table 51-3.)

## Hysterosalpingography

**Hysterosalpingography** involves radiographic visualization of the uterine cavity and fallopian tubes after the injection of contrast material through the cervix. The test is useful in the evaluation of uterine tumors, tubal obstructions, and abnormalities. The procedure is usually performed in the radiology department, and the patient is placed in a lithotomy position on a fluoroscopy table. A plastic speculum is inserted into the vagina rather than a metal one, to allow for better visualization. A cannula is filled with a water-soluble contrast material, which is injected slowly and under direct fluoroscopy. These studies are preferably performed 2 to 5 days after the end of a menstrual period to avoid interfering with ovum transport.

The ***Rubin test,*** in which carbon dioxide is forced into the uterus and fallopian tubes, is now rarely performed because of numerous false-positive and false-negative results and patient discomfort. The Rubin test has been replaced by the hysterosalpingogram.

If pregnancy is suspected, hysterosalpingography is not done. The patient should be assessed for allergy to iodine dye or shellfish. Allergic reactions are rare, however, since the contrast material is not injected intravenously. The patient may be instructed to take laxatives the night before the test. An enema or a suppository may be ordered on the morning of the test. The patient may be given a sedative or antispasmodic before the test. No food or fluid restrictions are needed. The patient should be advised that she may feel occasional transient, menstrual-type cramping and that she may have shoulder pain caused by subphrenic irritation from the dye as it leaks into the peritoneal cavity.

After the procedure, the nurse should assess the patient for nausea, faintness, and discomfort. Analgesics may be prescribed. The patient is instructed to apply a perineal pad, since vaginal drainage may be present for 1 to 2 days after the test and the radiopaque dye may stain clothing. The patient should call the physician if she notices any signs of infection such as fever, increased pulse rate, or pain. The nurse should evaluate the patient for signs of delayed reaction to the dye such as dyspnea, rash, hives, or tachycardia. (See Table 51-3.)

## Computed Tomography

Computed tomography (CT) is a leading example of advanced technology in gynecology. A CT scan image results from passing x-rays through tissue at different densities. This test is excellent in discovering extension of pelvic cancer into the fat of the retroperitoneal space. Abnormal masses are visualized, but a definitive pathologic diagnosis cannot be established until a surgical biopsy is performed, since most masses do not have distinctive enough anatomic shapes or unique density characteristics. CT scans are used extensively in gynecologic oncology. It is more useful in staging than in diagnosis. A CT scan can facilitate needle placement when a percutaneous biopsy of suspicious lymph nodes is to be performed. This type of scan is useful in diagnosing retroperitoneal metastatic disease, detecting small collections of ascites, determining ureteral obstruction, confirming diagnosis of ovarian vein thrombophlebitis, locating intraabdominal abscesses, and diagnosing partial perforations of the uterus missed by ultrasound.

A CT scan is contraindicated in very obese persons,

**TABLE 51-3 Diagnostic Studies of Male and Female Reproductive Systems—Radiographic Studies**

| TEST | DESCRIPTION | PRETEST AND POSTTEST CARE |
|---|---|---|
| Computerized tomography (CT) scan | X-ray beam is used with computer to provide three-dimensional picture. It is used to identify soft-tissue abnormalities, bony abnormalities, and various musculoskeletal trauma. CT can be done with or without contrast dye. | Explain procedure to patient. Inform patient that procedure is painless. Inform patient of importance of remaining still during procedure. If dye used, determine allergy to iodine. Determine if patient has problem with claustrophobia. Keep patient NPO 4 hours before test if dye used, and encourage fluids after test. |
| Hysterosalpingogram | This test involves instillation of radioscopic dye through cervix into uterine cavity and subsequently through and out fallopian tubes. Spot x-ray images are taken to detect abnormalities of uterus and its adnexa (ovaries, tubes) as dye progresses through them. Test may be most useful in diagnostic assessment of fertility (i.e., to detect adhesions near ovary, abnormal uterine shape, blockage of tubal pathways). | Inform patient about procedure and that it may be fairly uncomfortable. Determine possibility of dye allergy. Instruct patient to take laxative night before test. Administer enemas or suppositories morning of test if ordered. Administer sedatives or antispasmodics if ordered. Inform patient that no food or fluid restrictions are needed. Have patient void before test. Inform patient that vaginal discharge may be present for 1 to 2 days after test. |
| Magnetic resonance imaging (MRI) | Radiowaves and magnetic field are used to view soft tissue. Study is especially useful in diagnosis of avascular necrosis, dark disease, tumors, osteomyelitis, and ligament tears. Patient is placed inside scanning chamber. | Explain procedure to patient. Inform patient that it is painless. Be aware that it is contraindicated in persons with aneurysm clips, metallic implants, pacemakers, electronic devices, hearing aids, shrapnel, and extreme obesity. Ensure that patient has no metal on clothing (e.g., snaps, zippers, jewelry, credit cards). Convert intravenous to heparin lock. Inform patient of importance of remaining still throughout examination. Inform patients who are claustrophobic that they may experience symptoms during examination. Administer antianxiety agent (if indicated and ordered). Inform patient that he or she will hear loud thumping noise during test; provide earplugs if needed. Have patient void before test. |
| Mammography | Test is used to screen for breast cancer and evaluate any breast mass. Different densities in breast tissue are analyzed. | No specific preparation is required except thorough teaching. Woman should not wear deodorant, cream, or powder, which may mimic calcium deposits on x-ray film. |
| Ultrasonography (ultrasound) | This test measures and records high-frequency sound waves as they pass through tissues of variable density. It is very useful in detecting masses greater than 3 cm, such as ectopic pregnancies, IUDs, ovarian cysts, and hydatidiform moles. | Instruct patient that test is accurately performed only with full bladder. Tell patient not to empty bladder for at least 1½ to 2 hours before examination. Instruct patient to drink 200 to 350 ml water 1 hour before test. |

Modified from Lewis SM, Collier IC: *Medical-surgical nursing: assessment and management of clinical problems,* ed 3, St Louis, 1992, Mosby.

usually more than 300 pounds, and in pregnant women. Patients should be assessed for allergies to iodinated dye or shellfish. When an allergy is noted, the radiologists may prescribe a Benadryl and steroid preparation to be administered before testing. A hypoallergenic, nonionic contrast can be used during the test. If an oral contrast is to be administered, patients should not eat or drink for at least 4 hours before the test. Patients should be assessed for any problems with claustrophobia; they may be premedicated with antianxiety drugs. Visualization of structures may be obstructed by internal metallic objects such as hemostasis clips, retained barium from previous studies, or large amounts of fecal material or gas in the bowel. A tampon is often placed in the vagina because the gas within the tampon helps to delineate the vaginal cavity. Sometimes a small Foley catheter is placed in the uterine cavity to increase diagnostic landmarks. (See Table 51-3.)

## Magnetic Resonance Imaging

Magnetic resonance imaging (MRI) is a noninvasive diagnostic scanning technique that provides information about the body's biochemistry by placing the patient in a magnetic field. This test does not require exposure to ionizing radiation. MRIs have advantages over CT scans by providing better contrast between normal and pathologic tissue. Bone artifacts do not occur in MRI scanning, and blood vessels appear dark, allowing for measurement of the amount of blood flow to a specific organ. MRI is most specific in the diagnosis of conditions associated with edema, as well as evaluating vaginal anatomy, congenital defects of the müllerian system, vaginal malignancy, adenomyosis, myomas, endometrial cancer, and cervical carcinoma, both local and distant spread. It has been employed to evaluate the spread of uterine and cervical malignancy and, to a lesser degree, endometriosis and adnexal disease. No known risk exists to the patient. A major disadvantage compared with CT scans is that patients who require cardiac monitoring or have metal implants, pacemakers, or cerebral aneurysm clips cannot be exposed to MRI. Since the long-term effects of MRI are not known, patients who are pregnant should not have this test. Patients should be assessed for any problems with claustrophobia. Patients should empty their bladder before the test for comfort. They should be informed that during the procedure they will hear a loud thumping sound. Earplugs are available if the patient wishes to use them. (See Table 51-3.)

### Mammography/Xeromammography

**Mammography** is a radiologic study of the soft tissue of the breast. It is used to evaluate differences in the density of tissue, particularly small or poorly defined masses or nodules. It is capable of detecting many breast cancers that are too small to be palpated on physical examination. Mammograms are most effective in older women who have a higher percentage of fatty tissue in their breasts, which creates a greater contrast density on x-ray film. The density of benign cysts and malignant tumors may be similar, but their appearance is usually quite different. Suspicious lesions may be referred for needle aspiration or biopsy.

Recommendations for mammography screening are under constant evaluation and revision. Currently it is recommended that a woman have a single baseline mammogram taken between ages 35 and 40. Routine screening is then undertaken at the advice of the physician considering all known and suspected risk factors for breast cancer (see Chapter 54). Some sources believe that low-risk women can delay further screening until age 50. Others recommend mammography every 2 years for women in their 40s. General consensus exists concerning the appropriateness of annual screening after age 50.

No special preparation is required before a mammogram, but the woman should be instructed to avoid use of deodorant, cream, or powder, which can mimic calcium clusters on x-ray film. Pretest teaching about the test is critical, since most women are highly anxious about the examination and the possibility of breast cancer. Many institutions have created women's centers where specially trained staff conduct examinations and teaching in an environment that preserves the woman's dignity and modesty to the greatest degree possible. The woman is positioned standing next to the x-ray machine, and one breast at a time is placed between the platform and film plate. Most women experience some degree of discomfort from the breast compression. At least two views of each breast are taken.

No specific aftercare is done except for clear information concerning how and when the results of the test will be communicated to the patient. Most centers use this opportunity to reinforce skill and understanding of the purpose, technique, and timing of breast self-examination as well (see Chapter 54).

The xeromammogram provides an x-ray image with a much lower dose of radiation than that required for a traditional mammogram. The images are recorded on paper rather than film. The technique has become increasingly popular in some areas because the high contrast is easier to read and may be more accurate. (See Table 51-3.)

## SPECIAL TESTS

### Pregnancy Tests

Biologic tests for pregnancy first became available in the 1920s. They involved the injection of a urine specimen into a laboratory animal. Because of their relative lack of sensitivity and procedural difficulty, this type of test is no longer used.

Most of the frequently used pregnancy tests are based on two facts. First, human chorionic gonadotropin (HCG) is present in the serum of pregnant women within 10 to 14 days after the first missed menstrual period. Second, HCG produces antisera. Currently available methods of pregnancy testing fall into four groups: biologic, immunologic, radioreceptor assay, and immunoassay tests.

Since the early 1960s, several of commercial *immunologic tests* for pregnancy have become available (Ortho, Hyland, and Roche manufacturers). Depending on the specific test, blood or urine specimens are used. Results are obtained within 2 minutes to 2 hours. The short period for obtaining results is an advantage. However, these tests are not as sensitive in detecting pregnancy as are other tests. When used in women in whom menstruation is delayed for up to 2 weeks, they show positive results 50% of the time.

The *radioreceptor assay* test for pregnancy is rapid and reliable. The test can be performed in 1 hour and is 90% to 95% accurate by 6 to 8 days after ovulation. A blood sample from the finger is taken. This test has proved to be very reliable clinically. *Ultrasensitive immunoassay* is accurate within 7 to 14 days after conception. It can be performed in a few hours and is often used for confirmation of normal pregnancy.

Do-it-yourself pregnancy tests are available to women through department stores and drugstores. These tests are sensitive and easy to perform.

### Schiller's Test

Schiller's test is a simple test that reveals the presence of atypical cervical cells. A solution of 3.5% iodine or Lugol's solution is applied to the cervix. Atypical cells,

**TABLE 51-4 Diagnostic Studies of Male and Female Reproductive Systems—Operative and Endoscopic Procedures**

| TEST | DESCRIPTION | PRETEST AND POSTTEST CARE |
|---|---|---|
| Colposcopy | Direct visualization of cervix with binocular microscope allows study of cellular dysplasia and vascular and tissue abnormalities of cervix. This test is used as a follow-up study for abnormal Pap smears and for examination of women exposed to DES in utero. Biopsy of cervix may be taken during colposcopic examination. This test is valuable in decreasing number of false-negative cervical biopsies. | Instruct woman about this outpatient procedure. Inform her that this examination is similar to speculum examination. Explain purpose of procedure and prepare patient for it. |
| Conization | Cone-shaped sample of squamocolumnar tissue of cervix is removed for direct study. | Explain purpose and method of procedure and that it requires use of surgical facilities and anesthesia. Instruct patient to rest and avoid heavy lifting for at least 3 days after procedure. Also discuss necessity for follow-up check. |
| Culdotomy, culdoscopy, culdocentesis | Culdotomy is incision made through posterior fornix of cul-de-sac that allows visualization of peritoneal cavity (specifically, uterus, tubes, ovaries). Culdoscope can then be used to study these structures closely. This is valuable technique in fertility evaluations. Withdrawal of fluid (culdocentesis) allows examination of fluid type. | Explain purpose and method of procedure. Prepare patient for vaginal surgery with preoperative instruction and sedation. Perform assessment of bleeding and discomfort after surgery. Administer enema or vaginal douche before procedure is ordered. Tell patient to avoid douching and intercourse for 1 to 2 weeks after procedure. |
| Dilation and curettage (D & C) | This operative procedure dilates cervix and allows curetting of endometrial lining. Curetted material is studied histologically. This test is used in assessment of abnormal bleeding patterns and cytologic evaluation of lining. | Before surgery, instruct patient about procedure and sedation. Tell her that overnight hospitalization may be required. Perform postoperative assessment of degree of bleeding (frequent pad check during first 24 hours). Assess urine output. |
| Endometrial biopsy | In this outpatient procedure, small curette is used to obtain piece of endometrial lining to assess endometrial changes common to progesterone secretion after ovulation. | Tell patient that test must be performed in postovulation portion of cycle and that local anesthesia is used. Explain that procedure should cause only short period of uterine cramping. Instruct patient to rest after procedure. |
| Falloposcopy | Transcervical endoscopic examination of fallopian tubes is used to investigate infertility. | Inform patient that procedure is uncomfortable. Administer premedication as ordered. Assess vital signs, discomfort, and bleeding after procedure. |
| Hysteroscopy | This procedure is used to inspect inside of uterus and treat adhesions, retrieve lost IUDs, and evaluate uterus. Scope is inserted through cervix. | Explain purpose and method of procedure to patient. Administer preoperative medications as ordered. Prepare patient in same manner as for pelvic examination. If general anesthesia used, provide preoperative instructions; administer enema and Betadine douche if ordered. After procedure, perform assessment for bleeding and discomfort; also perform routine postanesthesia assessment. |
| Laparoscopy (peritoneoscopy) | This test allows visualization of pelvic structures via special fiberoptic scopes inserted through small abdominal incisions. Instillation of carbon dioxide into cavity improves visualization. This technique is used in diagnostic assessment of uterus, tubes, and ovaries. | Explain purpose and method of procedure. Before surgery, instruct patient about procedure, prepare abdomen, and reassure her about sedation. Keep patient NPO for 8 hours before surgery. Administer enema if ordered. Have patient void before procedure. Perform routine postoperative assessment. Assess for bleeding, perforation of viscus, and acidosis. Inform patient that she may have shoulder pain. Instruct her in wound care. Tell patient to rest for 1 to 3 days after surgery. |

Modified from Lewis SM, Collier IC: *Medical-surgical nursing: assessment and management of clinical problems,* ed 3, St Louis, 1992, Mosby.

both malignant and benign, do not contain glycogen and will fail to stain. Early cancerous lesions and benign lesions, such as cervicitis, may appear as glistening areas of a lighter color than surrounding tissue. The tissue having lighter color indicates, for example, the site from which a biopsy specimen should be taken. The test is currently used less frequently because culposcopy is a more accurate method of obtaining the same information.

## Biopsies

### Cervical biopsy

A cervical biopsy is performed to obtain a tissue specimen for pathologic examination. It is almost always performed with culposcopic direction. Although bleeding is minimal, the biopsy is ideally performed shortly after the menses when the cervix is least vascular. A punch biopsy can be safely performed as an office procedure without the use of anesthesia because the cervix has few pain receptors. Momentary discomfort may occur. The woman is instructed to leave the packing or tampon in place for 8 to 24 hours and report the incidence of excessive bleeding (in excess of a normal menses).

### Conization of cervix

Conization of the cervix may be performed as a diagnostic or therapeutic measure. It is typically performed in an outpatient setting with the woman under local anesthesia. A cone-shaped portion of the cervix containing the suspected malignant or infected tissue is removed. Bleeding from the site of conization is greater than that occurring from punch biopsy. If the bleeding is excessive or if hemorrhage seems likely, the cervix is sutured to control loss of blood. Oozing is controlled by packing, which is kept in place for 24 to 48 hours. The patient is directed to rest and to avoid heavy lifting for at least 3 days. She should be informed that her next two or three menstrual periods may be heavy and prolonged. (See Table 51-4.)

### Endometrial biopsy

Although an ideal method for screening for endometrial cancer has not been developed, a variety of methods are now in use. Less than one half of women with uterine cancer have an abnormal Pap test at diagnosis. Cells rarely exfoliate from the endometrium in the early stages of the cancer, making this an unsatisfactory method of screening and diagnosis. The best results are obtained when cervical aspiration is performed as part of the Pap test.

Endometrial cells obtained by aspiration smear show malignant changes 75% to 90% of the time when uterine cancer exists. The aspiration method is popular because of its relative simplicity; however, it is not an acceptable method for the routine screening of asymptomatic patients. In this method, a small cannula is inserted through the cervix into the uterine cavity, and suction is applied by means of a syringe attached to the cannula. The specimen obtained is prepared as for a Pap smear.

Endometrial biopsy can be used to diagnose cancer; evaluate bleeding, polyps, or inflammatory conditions; and determine whether ovulation has occurred by assessing the effects of estrogen or progesterone on the endometrium. It is performed by introducing a small curette into the uterus and obtaining several strips of endometrial tissue. The specimens are taken from several sites of the uterine cavity to increase the chances of obtaining malignant cells. For diagnosis of endometrial cancer, the biopsy method is considered to be about 90% accurate.

Complications that can occur include perforation of the uterus, uterine bleeding, interference with early pregnancy, and infection. Any temperature elevation after the biopsy should be reported to the physician because this procedure may activate PID. The patient should be advised to wear a pad after the procedure because some vaginal bleeding is to be expected. If excessive bleeding occurs (requiring more than one pad per hour), the physician should be notified. The patient should be advised that douching and intercourse are not permitted for 72 hours after the biopsy specimen removal. Instruct the patient to rest during the next 24 hours and to avoid heavy lifting to prevent uterine hemorrhage. (See Table 51-4.)

### Breast biopsy

It is widely accepted that most breast masses need to be evaluated for the possibility of cancer. Biopsy can differentiate fibrocystic lesions, fibroadenomas, and intraductal papillomas. Three major approaches are in use. An excisional biopsy removes the mass for pathologic evaluation. An incisional biopsy samples some of the tissue from the mass, and an aspiration biopsy involves the removal of fluid or tissue from the mass through a large-bore needle. The aspiration method is in widespread use. Bloody fluid aspirated from the mass indicates the possibility of cancer. If nothing can be aspirated, the mass is considered to be solid and needs to be evaluated via the incisional route. Breast biopsies are usually performed in ambulatory settings with the patient under local anesthesia. It is crucial that the woman clearly understand what procedure is planned, the anesthesia to be used, and the sensations she may experience during the procedure. This is usually an exceedingly stressful time, and the patient may not process information or teaching accurately. Aftercare is straightforward. The incision site is assessed for bleeding, edema, or infection. Mild analgesics are provided for discomfort. Numbness at the biopsy site may persist for months.

### Needle biopsy of prostate

A needle aspiration biopsy is performed to retrieve cells for histologic study. The procedure is usually performed at the same time as cystoscopy but can also be done as an office procedure with the patient under local anesthesia. Either a transrectal or a transperineal approach is used. With a transrectal approach, the needle is inserted through the rectal mucosa into the prostate gland. Aspiration may be repeated several times in different locations to sample the tissue adequately. This method is thought to be slightly more accurate than the transperineal approach, which involves insertion of the needle through the perineum into the prostate using the examiner's finger, which is placed in the rectum, as a guide.

Patient preparation for prostatic biopsy may include bowel cleansing if a rectal approach is to be used. Sepsis is a potentially life-threatening complication. Prophylactic antibiotics are usually prescribed, and any signs of infection or bleeding must be reported promptly.

### Open perineal biopsy

To obtain a specimen of tissue by open perineal biopsy, a small incision is made in the perineum between the anus and the scrotum. This technique gives the greatest accuracy because the suspect lesion can be clearly identified and multiple specimens can be taken from the prostate gland.

A dressing is required after open perineal biopsy and can be held in place for about 24 hours with a two-tailed binder. The patient is instructed not to contaminate the incision while cleansing himself after defecation by wiping from front to back. Cleansing by perineal irrigation is sometimes advised for both cleanliness and comfort. Unless the physician prescribes a solution, warm water poured from front to back over the incision can be used. After sutures are removed, sitz baths may be used and add much to the patient's general comfort. The man may be hospitalized after an open perineal biopsy until the laboratory findings are reported. If he is not hospitalized, he requires instruction in self-care, including signs to report, prevention of infection of the incision, and sitz baths.

### Testicular biopsy

Smears or biopsy specimens from the testes can be obtained by the needle method or by an incision made through the scrotum. Most often an incision is used. After a local or general anesthetic has been administered, a small incision about 2.5 cm long is made, and a small piece of the testis is removed. A dressing is applied, and postoperative management is similar to that after open perineal prostatic biopsy. Testicular biopsy specimens are sometimes used to evaluate fertility. If sperm are present in the biopsy tissue but are absent from the semen, absence of the sperm is most often the result of stricture of tubal systems beyond the testes.

## Dilation and Curettage

**Dilation and curettage (D & C)** may be performed for a variety of purposes, including evaluating infertility, treating bleeding, and inducing abortion. Diagnostically, D & C is the most prevalent and preferred method of obtaining endometrial cells for study. Because the entire uterine cavity is "scraped," a large tissue sample is obtained. This makes the likelihood of missing malignant cells minimal. Most of the procedures used for diagnosis of endometrial cancer require some dilation of the cervix to introduce instruments into the uterus. Vacuum curettage applies suction to the entire uterine cavity to obtain tissue specimens. Vacuum curettage is considered to be at least as good as conventional biopsy for diagnosing endometrial cancer.

For a D & C, metal dilators of graduated sizes are inserted into the cervical canal. Once the cervix is dilated, curettes having a sharp surface are used to remove endometrial tissue. The major complications of a D & C are hemorrhage and perforation of the uterus. Postoperative care is summarized in the Guidelines box above. Most women are discharged on the day of the procedure. Normal daily activities can be resumed, but vigorous exercise is discouraged. Sexual intercourse may be resumed when the woman feels comfortable. The menstrual cycle usually is not upset by a D & C, and all vaginal bleeding should disappear in a week to 10 days. Women are advised to report recurrence of bright-red blood or the development of a vaginal discharge with an unpleasant odor.

### Guidelines for Care of the Person After D & C

1. Place a perineal pad over perineum and anchor with a sanitary belt to ensure all blood loss will be absorbed by the pad.
2. Take vital signs every 15 minutes until stable.
3. Monitor bleeding every 15 minutes for 2 hours; if active bleeding continues, monitor every hour for about 8 hours.
4. Record each pad change and amount of blood loss in estimated milliliters (60 ml saturates a perineal pad).
5. Monitor urine output.
6. Give mild analgesics as prescribed; report immediately any abdominal pain that is continuous, sharp, and not relieved by analgesics (may indicate perforation of uterus).
7. Encourage ambulation when patient is awake and vital signs are stable.

## Infertility Tests

The purposes of an infertility evaluation are to establish the cause of infertility and determine the diagnosis, to give a prognosis for future fertility, to provide a basis for medical or surgical treatment, and to plan for assisting the couple to accept their diagnosis, treatment, and future options. The assessment and intervention can be physically painful as well as emotionally and economically stressful.

Common diagnostic tests used in infertility evaluation are listed in Table 51-5 and summarized in Table 51-6.

**TABLE 51-5 Examinations for Infertility**

| GENDER | TESTS | DATA OBTAINED |
|---|---|---|
| Male | Multiple semen examination | Determine presence, number, and motility of sperm |
| | Testicular biopsy if sperm count low or absent | Presence of sperm indicates obstruction of vas deferens |
| Female | Basal body temperature chart | Determines that ovulation is occurring |
| | Postcoital test of cervical secretions | Measure ability of sperm to penetrate cervical mucus and remain active, and measure quality of the mucus |
| | Endometrial biopsy, serum progesterone and estradiol levels, laparoscopic inspection of ovaries | Determine whether ovulation is occurring (if in question) |
| | Laparoscopy | Determine patency of fallopian tubes |
| | Hysterosalpingography (x-ray film after insertion of contrast media) | Determine patency of uterus and fallopian tubes) |
| Male/female | Hormonal tests | Determine whether the problem is hormonal |

**TABLE 51-6 Diagnostic Studies of Male and Female Reproductive Systems—Fertility Studies**

| TEST | DESCRIPTION | PRETEST AND POSTTEST CARE |
|---|---|---|
| Semen analysis | Semen is assessed for volume (2-5 ml), viscosity, sperm count (>20 million/ml), sperm motility (60% motile), and percentage of abnormal sperm (60% with normal structure). | Instruct patient to bring in fresh specimen within 2 hours after ejaculation. Protect specimen from cold. Instruct patient that specimen is to be collected after abstaining from intercourse for 2 to 5 days. |
| Basal body temperature assessment | This measurement indicates indirectly whether ovulation has occurred. (Temperature rises at ovulation and remains elevated during secretory phase of normal menstrual cycle.) | Instruct patient to take her temperature using special basal temperature thermometer (calibrated in tenths of degrees) every morning before getting out of bed. Tell her to record temperature on graph. |
| Sim-Huhner test (postcoital cervical mucus test or cervical mucus sperm penetration test) | Mucus sample from cervix is examined within 2 to 8 hours after intercourse. Total number of sperm is assessed in relation to number of live sperm. This test is performed to determine whether cervical mucus is "hostile" to passage of sperm from vagina into uterus. | Instruct couple to have intercourse at estimated time of ovulation and be present for test within 2 to 3 hours after intercourse. Instruct woman not to use vaginal lubrication, douche, or bathe until after examination. Instruct woman to remain in bed for 15 minutes after coitus. Study should be performed after 3 days of sexual abstinence. |

Modified from Lewis SM, Collier IC: *Medical-surgical nursing: assessment and management of clinical problems,* ed 3, St Louis, 1992, Mosby.

### Semen analysis

Evaluation of infertility frequently begins with the male partner because the tests are less complex, expensive, and time consuming. Multiple semen examinations are standard to determine the presence, number, maturity, and motility of the sperm. Since semen characteristics fluctuate considerably over time, two and preferably three analyses are usually recommended over a 2- to 3-month period. A single test will not diagnose infertility. Additional work-up may include postcoital tests and detailed exploration of exposure to drugs, radiation, or illness such as mumps. The vas deferens is assessed for the presence of stricture. Urology referral may be appropriate. A testicular biopsy indicates whether sperm are being produced. Recommendations can be made to compensate for a low sperm count (see Chapter 53), but if the man is aspermatic, conception is impossible.

The semen is collected after a period of abstinence, usually at least 2 to 5 days. A gross examination of the semen for its physical properties is first carried out. Semen is normally a highly viscous, opaque, grayish white fluid that spontaneously liquefies by prostatic enzymes within 10 to 45 minutes after ejaculation. After this time, the semen appears translucent, turbid, and viscous. Semen is normally slightly alkaline, with a pH of about 7.7, which protects sperm from the acid environment in the vagina. The normal volume in an ejaculation of semen is 3 to 5 ml. Five to 10 white blood cells observed by higher power field on microscopic examination may be normal. Higher amounts of white blood cells are associated with decreased fertility.

After the semen liquefies, a sperm count is taken. A count repeatedly greater than 20 million/ml is considered to be associated with normal fertility if other parameters are normal. From 20% to 25% of men who are fertile have sperm counts less than 20 million/ml at some point in their lives.

The sperm are also examined for motility and for

presence and number of abnormal forms. It is generally accepted that normal semen contains more than 70% motile sperm and fewer than 30% abnormal forms. Sperm motility less than 40% and abnormal sperm forms greater than 25% are known to lower the chance of fertilization of an ovum. Also, men who are infertile may have an increased rather than a decreased volume of semen, and the increased volume is often associated with a significantly decreased sperm count.

The measurements of motility provided by the current computer semen analysis tests are greatly improved over the previous analytic methods. However, assessment methods have not been standardized, and interpretation of these data requires specialists well versed in the testing procedures.

No single test has been devised to predict the ability of the sperm to carry out its specific physiologic functions. The *sperm penetration assay* (SPA), also known as the hamster ovum penetration assay, was controversial until recently. Research studies have led to improved predictive ability of this test in defining male infertility. The SPA can be combined with an enhanced assay of follicular fluid and is called a FF-SPA.[8]

Three tests to detect sperm-bound immunoglobulins are available:

1. Xenogenous antihuman antiserum and immunobinding: uses microsize polyacrylamide spheres covalently linked to rabbit antihuman antibodies[8]
2. Mixed agglutination reacter (MAR): Rh-positive human red blood cells previously exposed to a human anti-Rh antibody of the immunoglobulin G class are mixed with the test semen
3. Radiolabeled antiglobulin assay: use of radioiodinated xenogenous antibodies raised against human immunoglobulins to detect antibodies bound to sperm

### Ovulation studies

Infertility evaluation of the female potentially takes a heavy toll in emotion, cost, discomfort, and expectations. It is critical that a couple understand the full ramifications of what they are undertaking in the process. The presence of regular menses indicates that the ovaries are producing estrogen and progesterone, but it does not guarantee that ovulation is taking place. Beginning evaluation includes basal temperature graphing and cervical mucus analysis for pH and characteristics of the cervical mucus (spinnbarkeit) (Figure 51-13). These help to confirm the presence of ovulation. If these results are inconclusive, endometrial biopsies may be necessary to assess for ovulation. Over-the-counter ovulation kits may be used in the home, with laparoscopic confirmation that ovulation has occurred. Laparoscopy will also be used to confirm tubal patency and undertake microscopic surgery if necessary.

### Postcoital test

The postcoital test may be performed to determine if sperm are being destroyed by vaginal and cervical secretions. The test, often called the *Sims-Huhner test,* examines the cervical mucus after intercourse to assess the ability of the sperm to penetrate the mucus and remain active. For the postcoital test, mucus is aspirated from the cervical canal and examined for the presence and number of sperm. Characteristics of the cervical mucus are also studied. At the time of ovulation under normal circumstances, the amount of cervical mucus is maximal, but the viscosity is decreased. This facilitates penetration of the cervical mucus by the sperm.

## ENDOSCOPY

The pelvic organs and surrounding tissues can be visualized directly by endoscopy. The procedures by

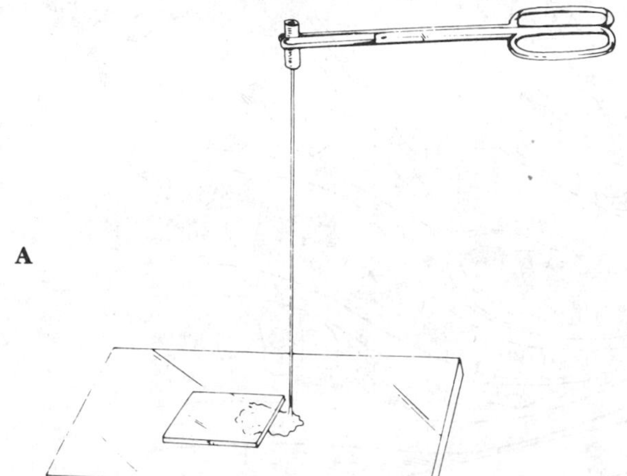


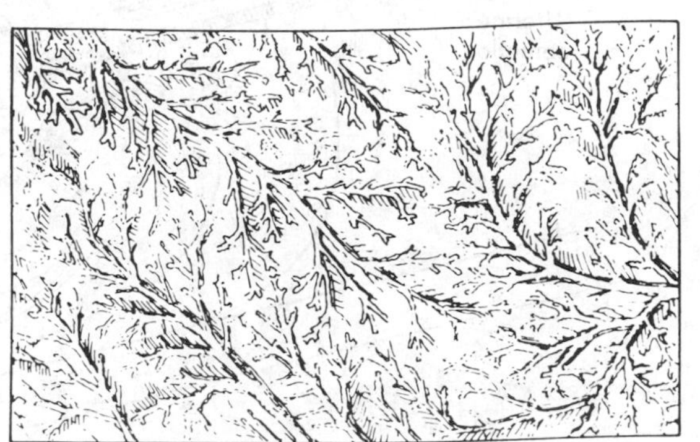


**FIGURE 51-13** **A,** Spinnbarkeit. At midcycle, mucus resembles raw egg white, being clear, stretchy, and slippery. It stretches without breaking or "spins a thread." **B,** Ferning. When allowed to dry on a slide, midcycle mucus gives fern or palm-leaf pattern. (From Fogel CI, Woods NF: *Health care of women,* St Louis, 1981, Mosby.)

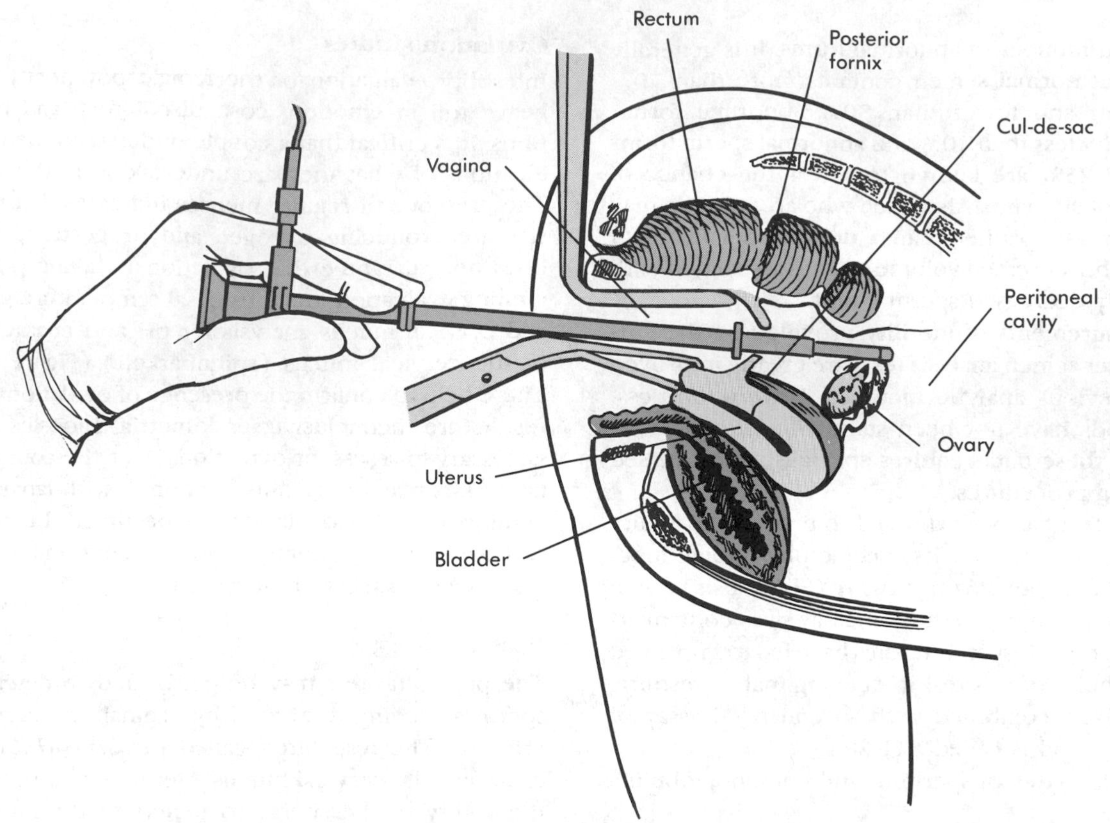


**FIGURE 51-14** With patient in knee-chest position, culdoscope is inserted through posterior fornix of vagina into cul-de-sac of Douglas. Note that ovaries can be seen.

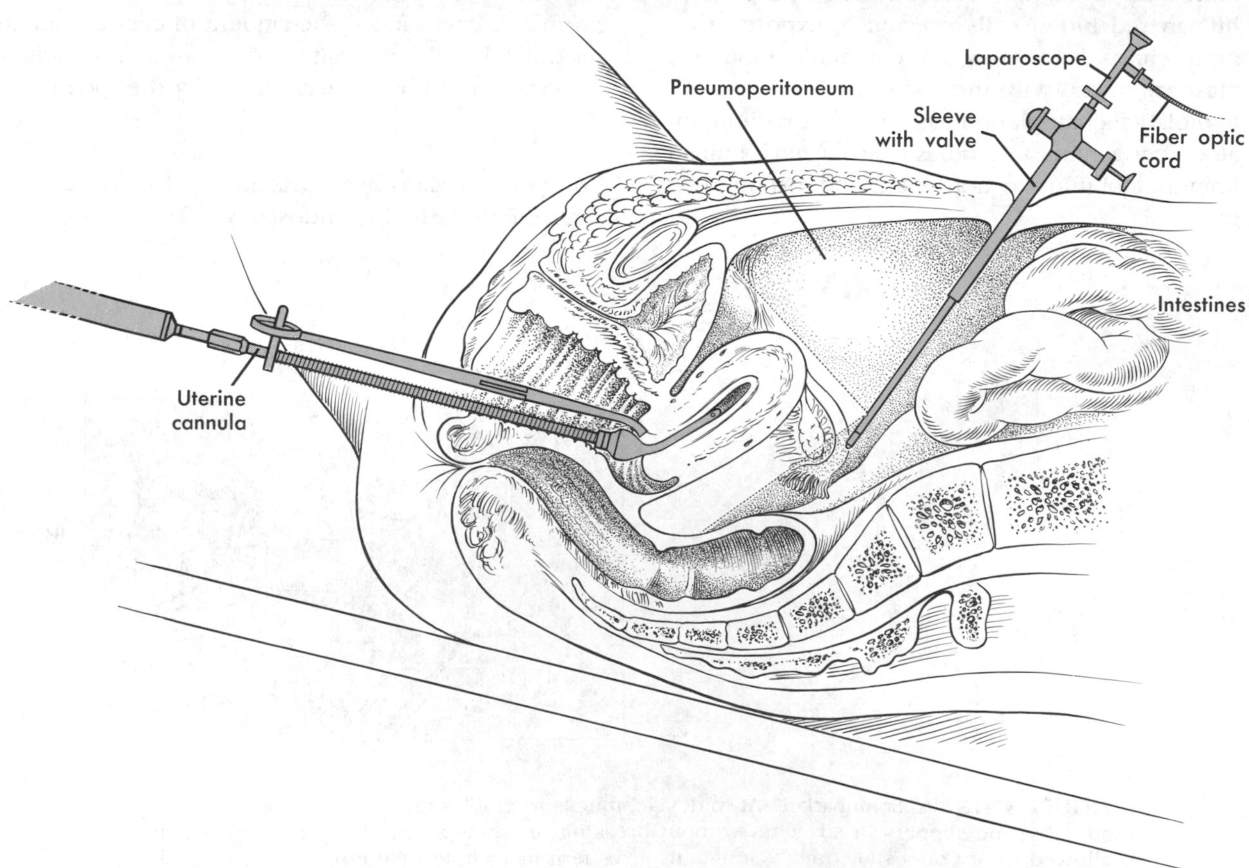


**FIGURE 51-15** Schema of gynecologic laparoscopy. (From Cohen MR: *Laparoscopy, culdoscopy, and gynecography: techniques and atlas,* vol 1, Philadelphia, 1970, Saunders.)

**BOX 51-5 Endoscopic Procedures for Visualization of Pelvic Organs**

**COLPOSCOPY**
Visualization of vagina and cervix under low-power magnification

**CULDOSCOPY**
Insertion of culdoscope through posterior vaginal vault into cul-de-sac of Douglas for visualization of fallopian tubes and ovaries (Figure 51-14)

**FALLOPOSCOPY**
Transcervical endoscopic examination of fallopian tubes[6]

**HYSTEROSCOPY**
Insertion of hysteroscope through cervix for visualization of inside of uterus

**LAPAROSCOPY**
Insertion of laparoscope (patient under local anesthesia) through small incision in abdominal wall (inferior margin of umbilicus), which is insufflated with carbon dioxide; permits visualization of all pelvic organs (Figure 51-15)

which this can be accomplished are colposcopy, culdoscopy, laparoscopy (peritoneoscopy), hysteroscopy, and **falloposcopy.** Box 51-5 defines these procedures, and Table 51-4 summarizes their associated nursing care. **Culposcopy** is used to augment a detailed examination of the vagina and cervix or to guide cervical biopsy. The associated care is the same as that for other types of cervical biopsy. The use of **culdoscopy** is declining because laparoscopy has become a standard diagnostic and treatment intervention. **Hysteroscopy** is frequently performed as part of any D & C to allow the physician to inspect directly the inside of the uterus before scraping or treatment.[5]

In the male, *cystoscopic examination* allows the physician to inspect the condition of the urethral and bladder mucosa and to detect prostatic encroachment on the urethra (see Chapter 53).

**Laparoscopy** (pelvic endoscopy or peritoneoscopy) may be used to inspect the outer surface of the uterus, fallopian tubes, and ovaries. A laparoscope is inserted through the abdominal wall through a small incision in the subumbilical area. The peritoneal cavity is filled with 3 to 4 L of carbon dioxide to separate the abdominal wall from the viscera and increase visualization. The laparoscope is then inserted to conduct the planned procedure. In addition to its role in diagnosis, laparoscopy may be used for tubal sterilization, lysis of adhesions, biopsy, and in various infertility procedures. General anesthesia is typically used. At the end of the procedure, the carbon dioxide is removed, but referred pain to the shoulder from gaseous irritation of the diaphragm and phrenic nerve often occurs. The Guidelines box above, right, summarizes nursing care.

**Guidelines for Discharge After Routine Laparoscopy**

1. Rest for the next 24 hours before resuming normal activities.
2. Avoid sexual intercourse until after postoperative visit with physician.
3. Discomfort may be experienced in shoulder and upper abdominal area. Take oral pain medications as prescribed.
4. Call the physician if abdominal pain increases, if temperature elevates, if abnormal vaginal bleeding occurs, or if there is increased redness, swelling, soreness, or foul drainage at wound sites before first postoperative visit.
5. Wound dressings may be removed in 24 hours, and you may shower.
6. Resume regular diet and drink plenty of fluids.

Most procedures used for visualizing the pelvic organs can be performed on an ambulatory basis; this allows the physician to schedule at the patient's convenience and during the appropriate time of the menstrual cycle.

Maintaining asepsis throughout any endoscopic procedure is important in preventing infection. Air may enter the abdominal cavity during the procedure and cause discomfort; a prone position with a pillow under the abdomen may increase comfort. Douching and intercourse should be avoided for about 1 week after a culdoscopy. Complications such as hemorrhage and infection are rare, but women should be cautioned to report fever or pain in the lower abdomen.

## CRITICAL THINKING ACTIVITIES

- Contrast the reproductive system of a 32-year-old woman with that of a 63-year-old woman. What assumptions can you make about hormonal levels based on the ages of these women? What reproductive problems can the 63-year-old anticipate apart from the 32-year-old and vice versa?
- Of what significance is a medical and drug history to the reproductive assessment of a 42-year-old man who is impotent?

## CHAPTER SUMMARY

### ANATOMY AND PHYSIOLOGY

- Major external structures of the female genital system include the mons pubis, labia majora, labia minora, clitoris, prepuce, frenulum, vestibule, urethral meatus, Skene's glands, vaginal orifice, hymen, fossa navicularis, Bartholin's glands, fourchet, perineum, and escutcheon.
- Major female internal reproductive organs are the vagina, uterus, fallopian tubes, and ovaries.
- The male genital system includes the testes, spermatic

cords, vas deferens, seminal vesicles, ejaculatory ducts, penis, scrotum, prostate glands, and bulbourethral glands.

- The menstrual cycle is divided into phases according to uterine or ovarian changes. The ovarian cycle consists of the follicular and luteal phase, whereas the uterine cycle consists of the menstrual, proliferative, and secretory phases.
- Menstrual cycle function depends on the interrelationship of the central nervous system, anterior pituitary, ovaries, and uterus.
- The female and male reproductive systems change with aging.

### SUBJECTIVE DATA

- An extensive history including patient's complaint in detail, medications and allergies, reproductive health history, and family and personal history is collected.

### OBJECTIVE DATA

- The physical examination of female and male reproductive systems requires use of special positioning and extensive palpation, both requiring clear explanations.
- Preparation of the woman for a pelvic examination includes use of models, films, visual aids, explanation of the procedure and answering questions, draping or nondraping per the patient's request, explanation of what is being done and findings during the examination, and sharing information about sensations she will feel.

### DIAGNOSTIC TESTS

- Laboratory tests used to assess reproductive health include tests for syphilis and chlamydia, Pap smear, endocrine studies, and smears and cultures from various sites.
- Radiologic tests used to assess reproductive health include ultrasonography, CT scan, and MRI.
- Screening tests for endometrial cancer include aspiration smear, endometrial biopsy, vacuum curettage, and D & C.
- Endoscopic procedures to assess reproductive health include colposcopy, culdoscopy, laparoscopy, hysteroscopy, and falloposcopy.
- Special tests for assessing reproductive health in males include prostatic smear, needle biopsies, open perineal biopsy, testicular smears and biopsy specimens, enzyme tests, and endoscopy.

## REFERENCES


1. American Cancer Society: 1992 cancer facts and figures, New York, 1992, ACS.
2. Fleischer AC, Kepple DM: *Transvaginal sonography,* Philadelphia, 1992, Lippincott.
3. Herbst A et al: *Comprehensive gynecology,* St Louis, 1992, Mosby.
4. Lauver D, Rubin M: Women's concerns about abnormal Papanicolaou test results, *J Obstet Gynecol Neonat Nurs* 20:154-159, 1991.
5. Lavy G: Hysteroscopy as a diagnostic aid, *Obstet Gynecol Clin North Am* 15:61-72, 1988.
6. Scudamore IW, Dunphy BC, Cooke ID: Outpatient falloposcopy: intra-luminal imaging of the fallopian tube by trans-uterine fibre-optic endoscopy as an outpatient procedure, *Br J Obstet Gynaecol* 99(10):829-835, 1992.
7. Speroff L, Glass RH, Kase N: *Clinical gynecologic endocrinology infertility,* ed 4, Baltimore, 1989, Williams & Wilkins.
8. Stenchever, MA: *Office gynecology,* St Louis, 1992, Mosby.

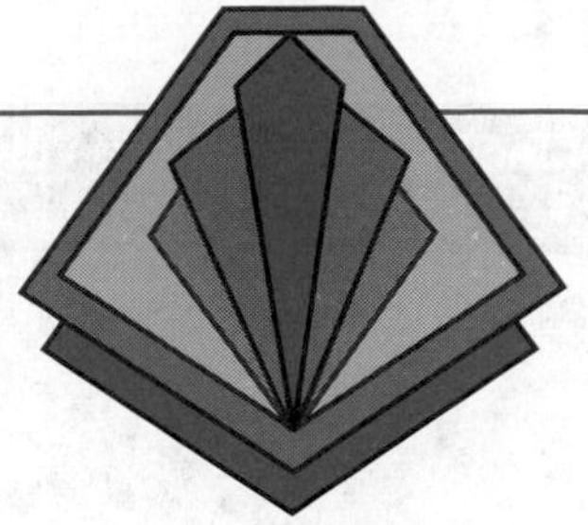

C H A P T E R 52

# Management of Women With Reproductive Problems

*Jo Ann Lierman*
*Greer Glazer*

## CHAPTER OBJECTIVES

***After studying this chapter, the learner should be able to do the following:***

1 Analyze the process of infectious diseases specific to women's reproductive health.
2 Analyze the process of development of structural problems specific to women's reproductive health.
3 Differentiate between the process of development of benign and malignant diseases specific to women's reproductive health.
4 Compare and contrast processes affecting menstruation and fertility.
5 Develop nursing diagnoses and nursing care plans related to the conditions discussed.

## KEY TERMS

amenorrhea
Bartholin's cysts
cervical intraepithelial neoplasia (CIN)
cervical polyps
cervicitis
colpotomy
culdoscopy
cystocele
dysfunctional uterine bleeding (DUB)
dysmenorrhea
endometriosis
fistula
gamete intrafallopian transfer
gestational trophoblastic neoplasia (GTN)
hysterectomy
hystero-oophorectomy
hysterosalpingectomy
in vitro fertilization
infertility
intracavitary implants
Kegel perineal exercises
laparoscopy
laparotomy
leiomyoma
leukorrhea
minilaparotomy
oophorectomy
ovum transfer
pelvic exenteration
pelvic inflammatory disease (PID)
premenstrual syndrome (PMS)
rectocele
salpingectomy
salpingo-oophorectomy
surrogate mother
toxic shock syndrome (TSS)
transcervical balloon tuboplasty (TBT)
uterine prolapse
vaginitis
vulvectomy

Despite advances in medicine, science, and technology, diseases and disorders of the reproductive system continue to threaten the lives and the physical and emotional health of millions of women, sometimes needlessly. Some of these problems are preventable; many can be treated and cured.

# INFECTIOUS PROCESSES

## VAGINITIS

### Etiology/Epidemiology

Although the vulva and vagina are considered to be relatively resistant to infection, **vaginitis** is one of the most common problems for which women seek medical care. Bacterial vaginitis accounts for 40% to 50% of the cases and includes infection by streptococci, staphylococci,

**RESEARCH**

Woolard DB, Larson J, Hudson L: Screening for *Chlamydia trachomatis* at a university health service, *J Obstet Gynecol Neonatal Nurs* 18(2):145-149, 1989.

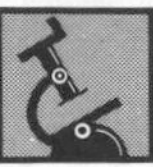

A descriptive study based on retrospective data from a nonprobability sample of 419 female students at a small midwestern university was conducted to assess the usefulness of routine screening for *Chlamydia trachomatis*. The method involved routinely screening all family-planning patients for chlamydia regardless of history of symptoms or high-risk factors such as multiple sexual partners. Results indicated that 53 students (12.6%) were positive for *C. trachomatis;* of this group, 26% had clinical signs and 74% had no clinical signs. In addition, 85% of the 53 students had no symptoms. Thus no statistical significance was found between signs and symptoms and presence of *C. trachomatis* infection. A statistically significant difference was found between those infected with *C. trachomatis* and a higher mean number of sexual partners compared with those not infected, although reliability of subject reporting of number of sexual partners was questioned. Implications for nursing include the importance of routine screening for *C. trachomatis* regardless of presence or absence of signs and symptoms and education of nurses regarding current knowledge of *C. trachomatis*.

*Escherichia coli,* chlamydiae, and *Neisseria gonorrhoeae,* among others. Candidiasis *(Candida albicans)* and trichomoniasis *(Trichomas vaginalis)* each account for 20% to 30% of all cases.[37] Viruses, parasites, chemical and mechanical irritants, and allergens are other potential causes. The Research box above discusses a study on *Chlamydia trachomatis* screening. Box 52-1 summarizes risk factors for vaginitis.

**BOX 52-1 Risk Factors for Infections of the Vulva and Vagina**

- Pregnancy
- Premenarchal age
- Low estrogen levels
- Dermatologic allergies
- Diabetes mellitus
- Oral contraceptive use
- Inadequate hygiene
- Excessive douching
- Treatment with broad-spectrum antibiotics
- Use of vaginal inserts
- Intercourse with infected partner
- Frequent intercourse with multiple partners
- Tight, nonabsorbent, and heat-retaining clothing

## Pathophysiology

The vagina is normally protected from infection by its acid pH and the presence of normal flora such as Döderlein's bacilli. If the pH is altered or the woman's resistance is decreased by aging, stress, or disease, her risk of infection is increased. The use of drugs such as steroids or antibiotics, which destroy the normal protective flora of the vagina, also increases the risk of infection. Many organisms proliferate in a less acidic medium, which becomes important for postmenopausal women, who experience a decrease in normal vaginal secretions and a rise in vaginal pH caused by a decline in estrogen secretion. Vaginitis can also be caused by insults to tissue from foreign objects such as tampons or caused by chemical irritation from strong douches, which make tissues more susceptible to invasion by organisms.

Vaginitis frequently appears as a nonspecific, superficial vaginal infection that may be caused by a variety of organisms. The organisms are typically introduced from outside sources such as clothing, hands, intercourse, or contaminated articles.[34] Reinfection can cause a prolonged problem in sexually active women. The classic symptoms of vaginitis include tissue inflammation, vaginal or urethral discharge, and pruritus. The discharge may be purulent, white, curdlike, or grayish white. Different organisms are associated with a specific type of discharge and symptom pattern, but pruritus is extremely common and frequently is severe. Table 52-1 presents a comparison of different forms of vaginitis.

## Medical Management

The diagnosis of vaginitis is made from the presence of the classic symptoms, supplemented by culture of the discharge, KOH analysis, wet smear analysis, or Gram stain. Serologic testing and urine culture may also be used. The management of vaginitis is primarily pharmacologic, and drug treatment is outlined in Table 52-1. The drugs may be administered orally or by ointment, cream, or suppository. Women should be informed that the use of metronidazole (Flagyl) causes urine to turn a dark reddish brown. It also causes numerous gastrointestinal (GI) side effects that may be reduced by taking the drug with meals. The use of alcohol can trigger an Antabuse-like reaction of severe nausea, vomiting, and abdominal distress and should be avoided during treatment.[35]

Because women have self-managed vaginitis for generations, a number of alternative treatments have arisen and are in common use; some are presented in Table 52-2. Women should receive specific instructions about the safe and appropriate use of soaks, irrigations, and douches in vaginitis treatment.

## Nursing Management

Nursing management focuses primarily on the appropriate use of prescribed therapy and measures to prevent reinfection. The woman is instructed to cleanse the genital area thoroughly with soap and water and dry well before applying any medication. The hands should be washed carefully before and after use. No supplemental

**TABLE 52-1 Common Causes, Clinical Manifestations, and Treatment of Vaginitis**

| CAUSE | CLINICAL MANIFESTATIONS | TREATMENT |
|---|---|---|
| Infections | | |
| *Candida albicans* (20%-30% of all vaginitis) | White, curdlike, cheesy discharge; characteristic patches on vaginal walls and cervix; itching; inflamed vagina and cervix | Miconazole (Monistat) cream used daily for 14 days<br>Nystatin suppositories daily or bid for 14 days |
| *Trichomonas vaginalis* (20%-30% of all vaginitis) | Yellowish to greenish, frothy, copious discharge; "strawberry spots" on cervix; foul odor; severe burning, itching, and dyspareunia | Metronidazole (Flagyl), 250 mg tid for 7 days or 2 g stat for both partners<br>Symptomatic therapy |
| Nonspecific vaginitis (bacterial vaginosis) | Grayish white, homogenous discharge; scant amount; fishy or foul odor | Oral antibiotics for both partners: ampicillin, 500 mg qid for 5 days; metronidazole (Flagyl), 250 mg tid for 7 days or 500 mg bid for 7 days |
| Foreign body | Blood-tinged, serosanguineous, or purulent discharge; usually foul odor; discharge may be thick or thin | Removal of object; antibiotics specific to secondary infection |
| Allergens or irritants | Increase in usual type and amount of secretions; itching, burning, rash | Removal of possible allergen or irritant; topical steroid ointment as needed |

Modified from Fogel CI, Woods NF: *Health care of women: a nursing perspective,* St Louis, 1981, Mosby.

**TABLE 52-2 Alternative Therapies for Vaginitis**

| INFECTION | INTERVENTION | DOSAGE | ADMINISTRATION |
|---|---|---|---|
| *Candida (Monilia)* | Gentian violet | Few drops/qt water 0.25%-2% (over-the-counter drug) | Douche or local application |
| | Vinegar (white) | 1 tbsp/1 pt water | Douche every day for 5-7 days; twice daily for 2 days |
| | Acidophilus culture | 2 tbsp/1 pt water | Douche twice daily |
| | Acidophilus yogurt<br>Plain yogurt | 1 application hourly and as needed to labia for symptom relief | |
| *Trichomonas* | 1 handful chapparel chamomile | Steep in 1 qt water for 20 min | Douche 2-3 times/wk for 2 wk |
| Nonspecific vaginitis | Vinegar douche | 5 tbsp/2 qt water | Every other day for 1 wk |
| | Salt (sea) | 1 tbsp/1 qt water | Every other day for 1 wk |
| | 1 tsp goldenseal and 1 clove minced garlic | Steep in 1 qt boiling water | Douche every day for 1 wk |
| | 1 tsp goldenseal | Steep in 1 pt water; strain with cloth | Douche every day for 1 wk |
| | Povidone-iodine (Betadine) gel | | Twice daily for 1 wk |

From Fogel CI, Woods NF: *Health care of women: a nursing perspective,* St Louis, 1981, Mosby.

over-the-counter preparations should be used without the physician's approval. The woman is advised to remain recumbent for 30 minutes after insertion of a suppository or cream to facilitate absorption and prevent loss from the vagina. If vaginal drainage is present, the woman can be encouraged to wear a minipad. Sitz baths and the local application of heat can be comforting and reduce itching. The woman should generally refrain from intercourse while the infection is being treated, and the use of a condom by the male partner is encouraged until all symptoms of inflammation have resolved.[9,21]

Prevention of reinfection is an important consideration, since vaginitis can easily become a recurrent problem. The nurse can instruct the woman concerning multiple life-style modifications that she can implement to reduce the incidence of vaginal infection. The Guidelines box on p. 1734 summarizes these measures.

## CERVICITIS

### Etiology/Epidemiology

**Cervicitis** is a vague term used to denote a number of conditions characterized by inflammation of the cervix. It can appear in an acute or chronic form. Acute cervicitis is usually associated with vaginitis or a sexually transmitted disease (STD) but may be associated with mechanical or surgical trauma. Chronic cervicitis is related to infection, instrumentation, or atrophy associated with falling estrogen levels.[3] The chronic irritation theoretically can predispose the woman to cancer.

**Guidelines for Preventing Vaginal Infection**

1. Cleanse the genital area thoroughly with mild soap and water daily.
   a. Wipe genital area from front to back after bowel movements.
   b. Avoid use of vaginal irritants (e.g., harsh deodorant and perfumed soap, deodorant sprays, perfumed douches).
   c. Avoid routine douching, which can alter the vaginal pH.
2. Use cotton rather than nylon underwear and change panties daily; avoid use of any clothing that is tight in the crotch or thighs.
3. Assess sexual partners for any sign of infection (e.g., discharge, lesions, reddened areas on genitals).
   a. Use a barrier method of contraception.
   b. Avoid any sexual practice that is painful or abrasive.
   c. Avoid anal genital intercourse.
   d. Cleanse genital area of self and partner and void before and after intercourse.
4. Change tampons or napkins frequently during menstruation.
5. Recognize the signs of infection and respond promptly.

### Pathophysiology

The gonococcus, streptococcus, staphylococcus, herpesvirus, and chlamydia organisms all can be causes of cervicitis. Cervicitis will progress from acute to chronic if it is not treated and may go unrecognized for a long period while the disease ascends into the uterus. **Leukorrhea** may be the only sign, and the amount may not be significant. On examination, the cervix is grossly erythematous and edematous, and there is usually a mucoid purulent discharge, but the amount might be so small that it is not noticed by the patient. The woman frequently has no subjective signs but may report pruritus, burning, lower abdominal pain, or dyspareunia from pelvic congestion. Cervical stenosis, salpingitis, and infertility are possible sequelae of chronic disease.[3]

### Medical Management

Vaginitis, if present, is treated first. The cervix is cultured, and appropriate pharmacologic therapy is initiated. Gonococcal cervicitis is treated with penicillin G plus tetracycline if chlamydial infection is also present.[13] Other organisms may be treated as outlined under Vaginitis. If lacerations or erosions are present, they usually are cauterized.

### Nursing Management

Care after cauterization involves leaving the packing in place as instructed, avoiding douching or intercourse until medical clearance is given, and reporting the occurrence of excess bleeding. A foul discharge may occur from sloughing of the destroyed cells about 4 to 5 days after treatment. It should not persist for more than a few days and can be controlled with warm sitz baths several times a day. Preventive measures include those outlined in the previous Guidelines box, since many cases of cervicitis develop from vaginal infection.

## BARTHOLINITIS/CYSTS

### Etiology/Epidemiology

**Bartholin's cysts** are one of the most common disorders of the vulva. They result from obstruction of a duct, which may become infected. Thickened mucus, stenosis, or mechanical trauma may initiate the process.

### Pathophysiology

The infection usually is unilateral but can be bilateral. The secretory function of the gland continues, and the duct fills up with fluid, producing severe inflammation, enlargement of the gland, and tissue edema. The area becomes tender, and even walking may become difficult. The pain is constant, and dyspareunia can be severe. The abscess may rupture, resulting in temporary symptom relief, but it usually re-forms. Occasionally, the acute inflammation resolves, leaving scar tissue that can develop into a cyst. The cyst usually is nontender but may interfere with ambulation or intercourse.

### Medical Management

Cultures are taken, and the woman is treated for any underlying infectious process. If the cysts are symptomatic, surgical treatment with incision and drainage may be performed. Because there is a tendency for recurrence, a permanent opening for drainage of the gland may be constructed. Total gland excision may be performed in older women who have suffered repeated abscess formation or when cancer is suspected.

### Nursing Management

Nursing interventions focus on comfort. Mild analgesics and sitz baths help relieve pain. Because most procedures are performed on an outpatient basis, the nurse instructs the woman on the safe use of these techniques at home and reinforces the need to report any signs of infection.

## PELVIC INFLAMMATORY DISEASE

### Etiology/Epidemiology

**Pelvic inflammatory disease (PID)** is a general term that refers to acute, subacute, recurrent, or chronic infection of the reproductive organs, pelvic peritoneum, veins, or connective tissue. The infection may be confined to just one structure or be widespread.

Between 750,000 and 1 million cases of PID are diagnosed annually in women of reproductive age in the United States, and 30,000 women undergo hysterectomy as a consequence of the disease. Sexually active young adolescents have a greatly increased risk of contracting the disease.[37] PID occurs in women using intrauterine devices (IUDs) five times more often than in women using other forms of contraception.

The risk factors for PID are the same as those for STDs

(see Chapter 55). Known risk factors include low socioeconomic status, early onset of sexual activity and multiple sex partners, and frequent douching (three or more times per month).[37] Surgery, childbearing, and abortion all lower the woman's resistance to infection and provide portals of entry for pathogens.

## Pathophysiology

The routes of pelvic infection are illustrated in Figure 52-1. Pathogenic organisms usually are introduced from outside the body and pass up the cervical canal into the uterus. Common causative organisms include gonococcus, chlamydia, *Haemophilus,* and streptococcus. They appear to cause little problem in the uterus. They invade the pelvis by way of the fallopian tubes or through uterine veins or lymphatics. Many of the pathogens lodge in the fallopian tubes and create an acute or chronic inflammatory reaction. Purulent material collects in the tubes, adhesions and strictures form, and sterility, which is one of the most serious consequences of PID, may occur. Partial obstruction of the tubes may predispose a woman to ectopic pregnancy because the fertilized ovum cannot reach the uterus. Inflammatory adhesions may become so severe that surgical removal of the uterus, tubes, and ovaries may be necessary. The infection usually remains localized in the lower abdomen and pelvis, although abscesses may form.

Clinical manifestations of acute PID include severe abdominal pain, lower abdominal cramping, intermenstrual bleeding, dyspareunia, fever and chills, malaise, nausea, and vomiting. A foul-smelling, purulent vaginal discharge may be present. Symptoms persist for a variable time. Chronic PID generally is considered to be a result of undiagnosed or inadequately treated acute infection. Dull, aching pain, backache, malaise, low-grade fever, and menstrual disturbances are typical symptoms. Abdominal palpation reveals pain and tenderness in the lower quadrants of the abdomen, which is confirmed on pelvic examination. Masses may be felt, indicating enlargement of the fallopian tubes or ovaries or the presence of an abscess.

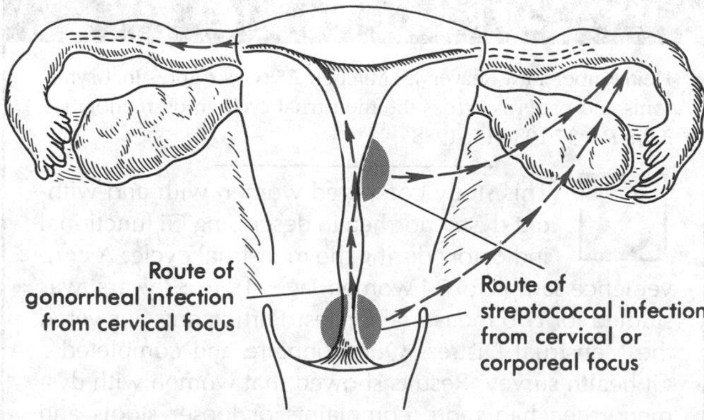


**FIGURE 52-1** Two main routes of pelvic infection. (From Novak ER, Jones GJ, Jones HW Jr: *Novak's textbook of gynecology,* ed 10, Baltimore, 1980, Williams & Wilkins.)

## Medical Management

Diagnostic studies include white cell counts and culture of any purulent secretions. A laparoscopy may be ordered to visualize pelvic structures and accomplish drainage of abscesses and lysis of obstructing adhesions. Ultrasonography may be used to evaluate masses.

Treatment is aimed at eradicating the infection and preventing complications. Hospitalization may be necessary if the woman is acutely ill. Broad-spectrum antibiotics are used until sensitivities are available. Salpingectomy may be necessary if an abscess is found, and more radical surgery is performed if all the reproductive organs have been compromised by the infection.[5] If the woman has an IUD, it is removed.

## Nursing Management

Nursing interventions are largely supportive. Bedrest in a semi-Fowler's position is recommended to assist with pelvic drainage. Heat applied to the abdomen may be comforting, but tub or sitz baths should be avoided during the period of active infection. The vaginal discharge is copious and frequently purulent and may induce pruritus and excoriation. The woman is instructed to cleanse the perineal region every 3 to 4 hours and maintain scrupulous hygiene after urination and defecation. Tampons should not be used, and drainage pads should be changed frequently. Other nursing measures include managing fever, monitoring vital signs, and balancing intake and output. A minimum of 3000 ml of fluids daily is recommended. Women treated as outpatients are reminded of the importance of seeking appropriate follow-up to monitor the progress of treatment. The woman's sexual partner may be treated with antibiotics at the same time.

# TOXIC SHOCK SYNDROME

## Etiology/Epidemiology

**Toxic shock syndrome (TSS)** is a severe disease caused by strains of staphylococci of phage group I that produce a unique epidermal toxin. TSS has occurred in infants, children, and men and has been associated with a variety of surgical procedures, including gynecologic, urologic, and orthopedic. It can occur in any situation in which staphylococcal organisms can be harbored, but it is most clearly associated with women during menstruation, particularly women who use tampons. Women at increased risk include those who use superabsorbent tampons, insert tampons with their fingers, or have chronic vaginal infections or herpes genitalis. The overall incidence is currently about 6.2 per 100,000, which is a dramatic decrease, since the link with tampon use was made in the early 1980s.[13]

## Pathophysiology

The exact mechanism by which staphylococcal toxins gain access to the circulatory system is unknown. The role of tampons remains unclear. They may cause mucosal damage, but it is theorized that superabsorbent tampons may obstruct the vagina and cause retrograde menstruation and peritoneal absorption of bacteria or toxin. Tampons may also cause an increase in aerobic bacteria from oxygen trapped in the interfibrous spaces. The longer a tampon is left in place, the greater the risk for TSS. The mortality is 3% to 6%.[13]

The onset of symptoms is usually abrupt, with high fever, vomiting, watery diarrhea, headache, and myalgia. The patient will appear acutely ill with fever of 39° C or higher, and the syndrome can progress to hypotensive shock within hours. An erythematous, sunburnlike rash will develop over the face, proximal extremities, and trunk, and both the conjunctiva and the pharynx will be erythematous. Muscle and abdominal tenderness frequently are present, but if neck rigidity, headache, or disorientation is present, a lumbar puncture usually is performed to rule out meningitis.[13] Prompt diagnosis is critical, and the key is that the woman is menstruating and using tampons.

### Medical Management

Diagnostic tests for TSS include a complete blood screen and cultures of the blood, throat, urine, vaginal secretions, and possibly cerebrospinal fluid. TSS is the operative diagnosis in any menstruating woman who develops a sudden high fever accompanied by vomiting or diarrhea. The cornerstone of medical care is beta-lactamase-resistant antibiotics such as nafcillin, cefoxitin, cefazolin, and cephalothin.[24] Penicillinase-resistant agents, antistaphylococcal agents, and corticosteroids may all be used.[13,24] Aggressive fluid and electrolyte management is indicated if the patient shows signs of shock. Mechanical ventilation may be necessary if adult respiratory distress syndrome develops. The management of shock is discussed in detail in Chapter 22.

### Nursing Management

Nursing care revolves around careful monitoring and supportive care similar to that offered any critically ill patient (see Chapter 26). If the woman is wearing a tampon, it should be removed immediately. Approximately 30% of women who develop TSS experience recurrences. The greatest risk for recurrence is during the first three menstrual periods after treatment. Recurrent episodes are usually less severe than the initial one. Women can almost entirely eliminate the risk of TSS by avoiding tampon use.[13] In addition, they should be instructed about the importance of careful perineal hygiene, avoiding douching or maintaining asepsis in cleaning douching equipment, and limiting the use of a contraceptive diaphragm to not more than 24 hours at one time.

# Disorders of Menstruation

Almost all women experience a problem with their menstrual cycle at some point in their reproductive years. Problems produce a variety of symptoms that may be directly or indirectly related to the pelvic organs. Most problems are self-managed and rarely brought to a physician's attention unless they become severe or persist.

## DYSMENORRHEA

### Etiology/Epidemiology

**Dysmenorrhea** involves uterine pain with menstruation and is commonly called "menstrual cramps." Primary dysmenorrhea is not associated with pelvic pathology and occurs in the absence of any organic disease. Its severity frequently declines after pregnancy or by age 30. Secondary dysmenorrhea occurs in response to organic disease such as PID, endometriosis, leiomyomas (uterine fibroids), and IUD use.

Although estimates vary, it is generally believed that primary dysmenorrhea affects about 75% of menstruating woman, with about 15% becoming incapacitated.[14] Studies in industry and schools have shown dysmenorrhea to be the greatest single cause of absenteeism among women. It is one of the most common health problems for which women seek treatment. Studies have indicated possible linkage between dysmenorrhea and a variety of unrelated factors, such as fatigue, lack of exercise, anemia, anxiety, immaturity, dependence, underachievement, and perfectionism.[38]

### Pathophysiology

The pain of primary dysmenorrhea is produced by a high concentration of uterine prostaglandins, which stimulate the frequency and strength of uterine contractions. The exact mechanism by which prostaglandins cause dysmenorrhea is not understood. What causes some women to have excess prostaglandins or increased sensitivity to them also remains in question, but women with dysmenorrhea have been found to have concentrations up to four times higher than in women without pain.

The pain of primary dysmenorrhea typically occurs on the first or second day of the menses. It is usually described as colicky, cramping pain in the lower ab-

**RESEARCH**

Heitkemper MN, Shaver JF, Mitchell ES: Gastrointestinal symptoms and patterns across the menstrual cycle in dysmenorrhea, *Nurs Res* 37:108-113, 1988.

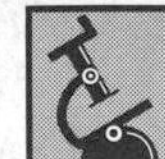

This study compared women with and without dysmenorrhea in describing GI functional indicators during the menstrual cycle. A convenience sample of 34 women, ages 19 to 37 years, was studied for two menstrual cycles. Participants answered the Menstrual Distress Questionnaire and completed a GI health survey. Results showed that women with dysmenorrhea had more complaints of looser stools and stomach pain and decreased food intake during menses. This information can be used by nurses in planning therapeutic interventions for women with dysmenorrhea.

domen that may be perceived as minor, controllable with mild analgesics, or incapacitating. Backache and other systemic symptoms, particularly involving the GI tract, may also occur (see Research box, p. 1736). The related symptoms are also thought to result from systemic prostaglandin absorption.[38]

## Medical Management

Primary dysmenorrhea is treated with prostaglandin inhibitors, which block prostaglandin synthesis and metabolism. Aspirin has been the classic drug, but ibuprofen has been found to be extremely effective for many women. Table 52-3 summarizes other options for treatment. These drugs are most effective when taken at the onset of the menses before pain becomes severe and should always be taken buffered by food or antacid. Oral contraceptives are helpful in some severe cases, although their exact mechanism of action is not known.

Treatment of secondary dysmenorrhea is aimed at correcting the underlying organic cause. Options include both pharmacologic and surgical intervention.

## Nursing Management

Women rarely seek professional help for managing mild primary dysmenorrhea. Women who are consistently unable to engage in normal activities because of menstrual pain should be encouraged to seek medical care. Related factors that the nurse can encourage a woman to consider include adequate rest, nutrition, and exercise. Constipation should be avoided. If pain occurs, the nurse can suggest that the woman (1) use local heat, which helps to dilate the blood vessels and relieve ischemia, and (2) work on strategies for systemic and psychologic relaxation.

# AMENORRHEA

## Etiology/Epidemiology

**Amenorrhea** refers to the absence of menstruation. Primary amenorrhea exists when the first menses has not occurred by age 16. It usually results from a genetic or congenital developmental defect. Gonadal dysgenesis is the single most common cause of primary amenorrhea, with uterovaginal anomalies the next most frequent. Hypothalamic/pituitary causes account for about 15% of cases.[37]

Secondary amenorrhea exists when a previously menstruating woman ceases to menstruate for more than 3 months. Skipping an occasional single period may be normal. Secondary amenorrhea is usually a response to environmental variables, such as stress or excessive exercise, or to an acquired pathology. About 55% of cases are due to hypothalamic causes, and 20% are related to ovarian dysfunction.[32] Secondary amenorrhea can be a side effect of some medications, and women who take oral contraceptives may experience amenorrhea for up to 6 months after discontinuing the pill.

## Pathophysiology

Prolonged secondary amenorrhea is common among certain groups of conditioned athletes, such as gymnasts and long-distance runners. High levels of dopamine may contribute to hypothalamic/pituitary or ovarian dysfunction. One theory is that a weight loss of 10% to 15% of total body weight can result in amenorrhea. In order for regular menstruation to be maintained after age 16, a critical percentage of fat (about 22% of body weight) must be maintained.[14]

Consequences of prolonged amenorrhea are not known, but strong evidence indicates that it is detrimental to bone density and can hasten the development of osteoporosis (see Chapter 11). Women with amenorrhea do not ovulate and cannot conceive. If estrogen is being produced, it can lead to endometrial hyperplasia and increase the risk of endometrial cancer.

## Medical Management

The diagnostic workup for amenorrhea includes a detailed history and careful examination of the reproductive system. The treatment depends on the cause. An organic problem is corrected if possible. Hormone therapy may be required.

## Nursing Management

The nursing role involves teaching about the problem, its causes, and the diagnostic studies planned. Teaching may need to include information about weight gain, stress reduction, and reducing the energy drain of strenuous exercise. Women may need extensive counseling and support to deal with the feelings of threat to their

**TABLE 52-3 Medications for Relief of Primary Dysmenorrhea**

| DRUG | DOSE | MAXIMUM DOSE/24 hr | COMMENTS |
|---|---|---|---|
| Ibuprofen (Motrin, Rufen) | 400-800 mg q 4-6 hr | 2400 mg | May be taken on an empty stomach for rapid absorption; take with milk if gastric irritation occurs |
| Mefenamic acid (Ponstel) | 500 mg initially then 250 mg q 6 hr | 1000-1250 mg | Take with meals or antacids to decrease gastric irritation; do not take for more than 7 days |
| Naproxen (Naprosyn, Anaprox) | 500 mg initially then 250 mg q 6-8 hr | 1250 mg | Same as for ibuprofen |
| Fenoprofen calcium (Nalfon) | 200-600 mg q 4 hr | 3200 mg | Same as for ibuprofen |

self-concept and fertility that may be caused by the amenorrhea.

## PREMENSTRUAL SYNDROME

### Etiology/Epidemiology

**Premenstrual syndrome (PMS)** is defined as a cluster of physical and behavioral symptoms that occur in the second half of the menstrual cycle and are followed by a symptom-free period. Anecdotal and research data report the prevalence of PMS anywhere from 5% to 95% of menstruating women. It is generally agreed that about 40% of women are significantly affected at one time or another, although severe symptoms occur consistently in only 2% to 3%.[14] The peak prevalence for PMS occurs in the 30s, with a slight decline noted in the 40s.[37]

The etiology of PMS is unknown. Researchers theorize that it is the result of a wide variety of hormonal, psychogenic, nutritional, and adrenal factors.[10,36] Research is ongoing.

### Pathophysiology

Symptoms of PMS are many and varied and may range in severity from mild to severe. The symptoms are not well defined and involve multiple body systems. The lack of a proven etiology makes it difficult to track a cause-and-effect relationship for physiologic changes and observed or reported symptoms. The symptoms appear only in the luteal phase of the menstrual cycle and disappear completely with menopause. Table 52-4 presents common symptoms grouped into a classification schema and linked with a theorized cause for each group.

### Medical Management

No objective means of diagnosing PMS exists. A woman is considered to have PMS if her symptoms interfere with activities of daily living (ADL). Identical symptoms must occur in three consecutive menstrual cycles to confirm the diagnosis. A careful clinical history is critical, and the woman is asked to keep accurate records of dates for (1) her menstrual period and (2) occurrence of symptoms and the exact nature and severity of them.

Table 52-4 outlines suggested therapies for typically occurring groups of symptoms. Numerous treatments have been suggested, including both pharmacologic and nonpharmacologic strategies, but no treatment has been clinically proved to be therapeutically effective in all

**TABLE 52-4 Common Symptoms, Possible Etiologies, and Treatment of Premenstrual Tension Symptoms***

| CATEGORY | SYMPTOMS | POSSIBLE ETIOLOGY | TRADITIONAL THERAPY |
|---|---|---|---|
| PMT-A | Anxiety:<br>Nervous tension<br>Mood swings<br>Irritability | High serum estrogen<br>Low serum progesterone<br>Elevated adrenal androgens<br>Possible disturbance of thyroid axis | Progesterone; vitamin $B_6$; limit dairy products intake; increase outdoor exercise; lorazepam |
| PMT-H | Water-related symptoms:<br>Weight gain<br>Swelling of extremities<br>Breast tenderness<br>Abdominal bloating | High serum aldosterone<br>Retention of sodium and water<br>Decreased colloid osmotic pressure in abdomen | Restrict intake of salt, coffee, tea, cola, chocolate; vitamin $B_6$; primrose oil; spironolactone; antiprostaglandins; oral contraceptives |
| PMT-C | Cravings:<br>Craving for sweets<br>Increased appetite<br>Headache<br>Heart pounding<br>Fatigue<br>Dizziness or faintness | Increased carbohydrate tolerance<br>Low red cell magnesium levels | Restrict free sugar, sodium, animal fat intake; substitute complex carbohydrate for simple sugars |
| PMT-D | Depression:<br>Forgetfulness<br>Crying<br>Confusion<br>Insomnia | Same as Category PMT-A | Increase intake of foods high in B vitamins and magnesium (green leafy vegetables, legumes, whole-grain cereals) |

| NONTRADITIONAL THERAPY FOR PMS |
|---|
| Validation |
| Education |
| Exercise |
| Family therapy |
| Peer support groups |
| Stress management |
| Assertiveness training |
| Sex and marital therapy |

Modified from Gerbie MD: In Pernoll ML: ***Current obstetric and gynecologic diagnosis and treatment,*** ed 7, East Norwalk, Conn, 1991, Appleton & Lange; Nikolai TF and others: ***J Clin Endocrinol Metab*** 70:1108, 1990; and Ryan KJ, Berkowitz R, Barbieri RL: ***Kistner's gynecology: principles and practices,*** ed 5, Chicago, 1990, Year Book.

*NOTE: The classification schema used in this table refers to PMS as premenstrual tension, or PMT.

cases.[19] The use of oral contraceptives can produce symptoms similar to PMS in some women but can also relieve symptoms in some women diagnosed with the disorder. The treatment attempts to reduce the number and severity of symptoms and restore the woman's psychologic health.

### Nursing Management

The nursing role in PMS involves helping the woman and her family to understand the possible causes of the syndrome and the rationale for any planned treatments (see Research boxes below). Simple life-style modifications can reduce symptoms and improve the woman's overall well-being. Regular aerobic exercise is strongly recommended because exercise results in a release of endorphins, which can elevate the mood. The nurse also encourages the woman to avoid fatigue, since it exaggerates the symptoms of PMS. This is particularly important in the premenstrual period. Stress management techniques are also strongly recommended. The Guidelines box below summarizes patient teaching related to PMS. The nurse can refer interested patients and families to the National Center for PMS and Menstrual Disorders, 15 Smith Rd., Bedford, NH 03102; or National PMS Society, P.O. Box 11467, Durham, NC 27703.

**RESEARCH**

Cortese J, Brown MA: Coping responses of men whose partners experience premenstrual symptomatology, *J Obstet Gynecol Neonatal Nurs* 18:405-412, 1989.

This exploratory study was designed to describe and categorize coping strategies used by partners of women with premenstrual symptoms. Eighty-six female subjects and their partners were recruited from a variety of sources for the study. Two instruments were developed for the study. Women completed the Premenstrual Symptomatology Inventory, and men were interviewed to identify coping strategies. Results indicated a variety of coping responses. Responses identified included anger and physical abuse. This study has implications for nurses in recognizing and planning care for the male partners of women with PMS.

**RESEARCH**

Rossignol AM, Bonnlander H: Caffeine-containing beverages, total fluid consumption, and premenstrual syndrome, *Am J Public Health* 80:1106, 1990.

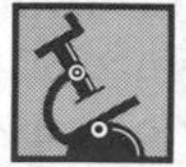

In a study of 841 college women, those with severe PMS symptoms showed a dose-dependent relationship in relation to caffeine consumption. Prevalence odds ratios for demonstrating PMS symptoms varied from 1.3 for consumers of one cup of caffeine-containing beverage to 7.0 for consumers of 8 to 10 cups per day when compared with noncaffeine users. This study has implications for nurses regarding nutritional teaching for women with PMS.

## DYSFUNCTIONAL UTERINE BLEEDING

### Etiology/Epidemiology

Abnormal, or **dysfunctional, uterine bleeding (DUB)** is defined as excessive or irregular uterine bleeding with no demonstrable cause. DUB can take many forms, including infrequent episodes, excessive flow, prolonged duration of menses, and intermenstrual bleeding.

Abnormal bleeding may be caused by a variety of factors. Table 52-5 lists and defines the various types of DUB with associated causes. Endocrine abnormalities are the most common etiologies, although the likely causes differ in women of childbearing age and postmenopausal women. Some systemic diseases can cause DUB. Liver disease may interfere with estrogen metabolism, and blood dyscrasias can produce spontaneous bleeding.[10] DUB related to the menstrual cycle is usually anovulatory and painless and generally occurs at the extremes of menstrual life, when disturbances of ovarian function are common. About 50% of DUB occurs in perimenopausal women, in whom it is a significant warning sign of uterine cancer. Cancer is diagnosed in 35% to 50% of postmenopausal women with DUB.[24]

### Pathophysiology

DUB may occur between or during the menstrual periods. When menorrhagia is present, the woman may soak a tampon or pad every few hours for a week or more. The exact cause of the anovulatory episode is not understood, but it may represent a dysfunction of the hypothalamic-pituitary-ovarian axis that results in continuing estrogen stimulation of the endometrium. The endometrium outgrows its blood supply, partially breaks down, and is sloughed in an irregular manner. Anovulation may also result from thyroid or adrenal abnormalities.[10]

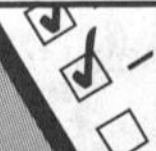

**Guidelines for Patient Teaching for Premenstrual Syndrome**

1. Teach possible causes of condition and treatments.
2. Avoid stress activities during the premenstrual period.
3. Ensure adequate rest, especially during premenstrual period. Fatigue exaggerates symptoms.
4. Encourage regular exercise program.
5. Provide diet instruction in well-balanced, high-protein diet with reduction of salt intake and refined sugars.
6. Take medications as prescribed and explain rationale.
7. Reduce or eliminate smoking and alcohol consumption.
8. Reduce or eliminate consumption of caffeine.
9. Encourage life-style changes to relieve stress.
10. Teach relaxation techniques.

**TABLE 52-5 Causes of Abnormal Gynecologic Bleeding During Childbearing and Postmenopausal Years**

| TYPE | CAUSES |
|---|---|
| **Menorrhagia**—Prolonged profuse menstrual flow during the regular period | Submucous myomas, pregnancy complications, adenomyosis, endometrial hyperplasias, malignant tumors, hypothyroidism |
| **Metrorrhagia**—Bleeding between periods | Endometrial polyps, endometrial and cervical cancer, exogenous estrogen administration |
| **Polymenorrhea**—Increased frequency of menstruation | Anovulation; shortened luteal phase |
| **Cryptomenorrhea**—Unusually light menstrual flow | Hymenal or cervical stenosis, Asherman's syndrome (uterine synechiae), oral contraceptives |
| **Menometrorrhagia**—Bleeding at irregular intervals | Any condition causing intermenstrual bleeding; sudden onset is indication of malignant tumors or complications of pregnancy |
| **Oligomenorrhea**—Menstrual periods more than 35 days apart | Anovulation from endocrine causes (pregnancy, menopause) or systemic (excessive weight loss); estrogen-secreting tumors |
| **Dysfunctional uterine bleeding**—Abnormal bleeding without known organic cause | Unknown |

## Medical Management

The diagnostic workup for DUB begins with a thorough history of the frequency, amount, and duration of bleeding. Laboratory tests may include blood counts to estimate blood loss, coagulation studies, pregnancy tests, thyroid studies, and ovulation tests. Pap smears, pelvic examinations, ultrasonography, endometrial biopsy, and hysterosalpingography may be employed to assess for structural problems and cancer (see Chapter 51).

The cause of the bleeding guides medical care. In the absence of an organic cause, the preferred treatment is usually conservative. Pharmacologic options to stop heavy bleeding or reduce future blood loss in subsequent menstrual cycles include the use of estrogens, progestins, nonsteroidal antiinflammatory drugs (NSAIDs), antifibrinolytic agents, and gonadotropin-releasing hormone agonists such as danazol.[14] Hysterectomy may be necessary for those women whose bleeding cannot be controlled with hormones, who are symptomatically anemic, and whose life-style is compromised by persistent bleeding.[10]

## Nursing Management

Because most care for DUB is provided in the outpatient setting, the nursing role is largely educational. The nurse teaches the woman how to accurately assess the amount of bleeding in terms of number of pads or tampons, type of pad or tampon, and degree of saturation. The nurse helps the woman set up and maintain an accurate record of the bleeding in the form of a diary. The nurse also encourages the woman to share her concerns and fears regarding infertility or cancer with her sexual partner.

# ENDOMETRIOSIS

## Etiology/Epidemiology

**Endometriosis** is a condition in which endometrial cells that normally line the uterus are seeded throughout the pelvis. The incidence of endometriosis appears to have been increasing over the past 25 years, but it is unclear how much of the increase is related to the increased use of laparoscopy as a diagnostic tool. Endometriosis typically affects women during their childbearing years. Although the age-specific prevalence is unknown, it is estimated that the incidence is 5% to 15%. The incidence in infertile women is 30% to 45%. Involuntarily nulliparous women in their mid-30s have the highest incidence.[14]

The etiology of endometriosis remains unknown, but there are multiple theories and lines of research. The condition may be hereditary, since it occurs more often in women whose mother had the disorder. Theories include the congenital presence of endometrial cells out of their normal location, their transfer by means of the blood or lymph system, and reflux of menstrual fluid containing endometrial cells up the fallopian tubes and into the pelvic cavity. A more recent theory associates endometriosis with the activation of polyclonal B cells, a characteristic of autoimmune disease.[1,40]

## Pathophysiology

With each menstrual period, the seeded endometrial cells are stimulated by the ovarian hormones and bleed into the surrounding tissues, causing an inflammatory response. Encased blood may lead to palpable tumor masses known as *chocolate cysts.* Occasionally, the cysts will rupture and spread endometrial cells deeper into the pelvis. Repeated inflammation and healing may create adhesions severe enough to fuse pelvic organs or cause bowel or bladder strictures.

The ovaries are the most common site of involvement, and the process is usually bilateral (Figure 52-2). The pelvic peritoneum, anterior and posterior cul-de-sac, and the uterosacral, round, and broad ligaments are other common sites.

Endometriosis progresses gradually and usually does not produce symptoms until 30 to 40 years of age. The classic feature is menstrual pain and discomfort that becomes progressively worse. Other possible symptoms include abdominal pain, dyspareunia, irregular menses,

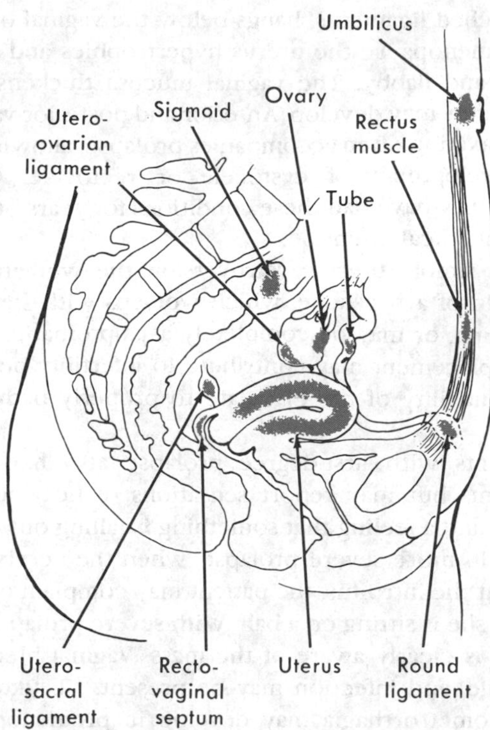


**FIGURE 52-2** Sites of endometrial implants.

bowel problems, and urinary dysfunction. Pelvic examination will reveal a fixed, retroverted uterus that is enlarged, tender, and nodular. Occasionally, the disease will be far advanced but cause no symptoms, and it may first be diagnosed as part of a workup for infertility.

## Medical Management

Laparoscopy is the only definitive method of diagnosing endometriosis. The endoscopy is used to carefully map and describe the extent of disease involvement, and biopsies of suspicious tissue may be obtained during the procedure. Ultrasound may be helpful in differentiating solid from cystic lesions, but it is otherwise of little value. Magnetic resonance imaging (MRI) is also of little value in either detecting or staging the disease. A newer approach involves the use of cancer antigen-125 (CA-125) as a chemical marker, since these levels are elevated in most patients with endometriosis and the levels continue to rise as the disease progresses.[14] The marker is not specific to endometriosis, however, and can be used only to follow the course of the disease.

Because the cause is not understood, the treatment of endometriosis is highly individualized. In rare cases, endometriosis may disappear spontaneously. Pregnancy appears to prevent the development of the condition and slow its progression because menstruation is halted during pregnancy and lactation. Some women remain asymptomatic after pregnancy. A couple may be encouraged to attempt pregnancy if children are desired, since the fertility rate is low and continues to deteriorate with time. Mild cases may be managed with mild analgesics and regular monitoring.

Oral contraceptives with minimal estrogen and high levels of progestins may be used to produce endometrial atropy. Disadvantages to this approach include irregular bleeding and symptoms such as nausea, fatigue, and depression that may be troublesome. Drugs with antigonadotropic action such as danazol may be used to suppress ovarian activity. It stops endometrial proliferation, prevents ovulation, and produces atrophy of the ectopic endometrial tissue. The treatment is expensive, costing up to $180 per month, and may cause side effects such as hot flashes, depression, and weight gain. If the condition does not respond to drug treatment, surgical intervention with total hysterectomy, oophorectomy, and salpingectomy may be necessary. The onset of menopause stops the progress of the disorder.

## Nursing Management

Because most care for endometriosis is delivered in the community, the nurse's role is largely educational and supportive. The nurse reassures the woman that endometriosis can be treated. The nurse may provide teaching concerning the prescribed drugs and the management of side effects. The importance of ongoing care and follow-up is reinforced. Referral to support groups may be beneficial. This is particularly important if infertility related to the endometriosis is diagnosed. Two excellent organizations are The Endometriosis Association, 8585 North 76th Place, Milwaukee, WI 53223; and Resolve Incorporated, 5 Water St., Arlington, MA 02174.

# STRUCTURAL PROBLEMS

## UTERINE DISPLACEMENT/PROLAPSE

### Etiology/Epidemiology

The uterus may undergo minor displacement in ways that are merely anatomic variations with little or no clinical effects (Figure 52-3). Retroversion is the most common of these variations and occurs in about 20% of women. **Uterine prolapse** represents a severe uterine problem in which the uterus protrudes through the pelvic floor aperture or genital hiatus. It is usually associated with a cystocele or rectocele. Uterine prolapse occurs most often in multiparous white women as a gradual response to childbirth injuries to the muscles and fascia of the pelvis. Systemic conditions, such as obesity and chronic pulmonary disease, and local conditions, such as ascites and uterine or ovarian tumors, can also contribute to prolapse. Prolapse is usually not seen until years after the causative event, which suggests that the effects of aging play a major role.[39] As the uterus begins to drop, the vaginal walls become relaxed and the bladder may herniate into the vagina **(cystocele),** or the rectal wall may herniate into the vagina **(rectocele).** These structural problems are illustrated in Figure

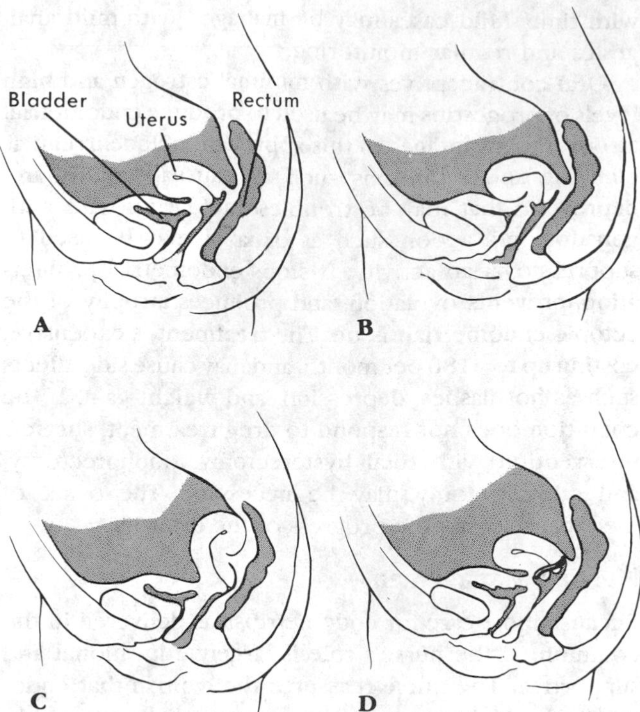


**FIGURE 52-3** Normal and abnormal positions of uterus. **A,** Normal anatomic position of uterus in relation to adjacent structures. **B,** Anterior displacement of uterus. **C,** Retroversion or backward displacement of uterus. **D,** Normal anatomic position of uterus maintained by use of rubber S-shaped pessary.

52-4. Both conditions may occur simultaneously. Cystoceles are quite common, and the woman may remain completely asymptomatic until after menopause. Estrogen helps to maintain adequate blood flow and tone of the paravaginal tissues, and its deprivation results in atrophic changes that render the tissues more subject to prolapse. The incidence of herniation is strongly associated with vaginal delivery, and one half of all parous women develop some degree of cystocele or rectocele, usually after menopause. Only 10% of these women become symptomatic.[14] Bowel habits are also related to the development of rectocele. Long-term chronic constipation with straining at stool may cause or aggravate a rectocele.

## Pathophysiology

Variations in the normal position of the uterus or prolapse can result from congenital or acquired abnormalities of the pelvic support structures. Acquired weaknesses occur after childbirth, surgery, and closely spaced pregnancies and in response to obesity and the loss of tissue elasticity with aging. The severity of the prolapse is designated by degree. In a *first-degree* prolapse, the cervix is still within the vagina. In a *second-degree* prolapse, the cervix protrudes from the vaginal orifice. In a *third-degree* prolapse, the entire uterus, suspended by its stretched ligaments, hangs below the vaginal orifice. Before menopause the uterus hypertrophies and is engorged and flabby. The vaginal mucosa thickens, and stasis ulcers may develop. Anterior and posterior vaginal wall relaxation often accompanies prolapse, allowing for the development of cystocele or rectocele. Older women may have had these conditions for years but not sought medical attention.

With simple uterine retroversion the woman may complain of a backache, which worsens with standing or walking, or may be completely asymptomatic. Anterior displacement may contribute to infertility because of the inability of the ejaculate to properly bathe the cervix.

Patients with first-degree prolapse also have few symptoms but may report sensations of heaviness or fullness and a feeling that something is falling out of the vagina. In more severe prolapse, when the cervix protrudes at the introitus, the patient may complain of feeling like she is sitting on a ball. With severe prolapse, the woman is clearly aware of the mass. Vaginal bleeding, discharge, and infection may be present.[37] Leukorrhea or menometrorrhagia may develop in premenopausal women with prolapse as a result of uterine engorgement. After menopause, discharge and bleeding with prolapse usually result from infection and ulceration.

The woman with a cystocele may complain of urinary incontinence accompanying any activity that increases intraabdominal pressure, such as coughing, laughing, or lifting. The patient with a rectocele may complain of chronic constipation and develop hemorrhoids.[39]

## Medical Management

Uterine prolapse can be readily identified on pelvic examination. If a cystocele is present, the vaginal outlet will be relaxed with a thin-walled, smooth, bulging mass present in the anterior vaginal wall below the cervix. The mass descends when the patient is asked to strain. In the presence of chronic urinary tract infection, a cystoscopy may be ordered. If a rectocele is present, palpation of the vaginal area will reveal a thin-walled rectovaginal septum projecting into the vagina. Many women are found to have both a cystocele and a rectocele.

Asymptomatic retroversion does not require medical intervention. Estrogen therapy may be used for postmenopausal women to maintain the tone and integrity of the pelvic floor muscles, and exercise therapy is suggested for all women. (Exercises for the pelvic floor are discussed under nursing management.) If pain or bleeding occurs, the uterus may be manually repositioned and supported by the insertion of a vaginal pessary (Figure 52-5). Pessaries are devices made of hard rubber or plastic that maintain the uterus in a forward position by exerting pressure on the ligaments attached to the posterior wall of the cervix.

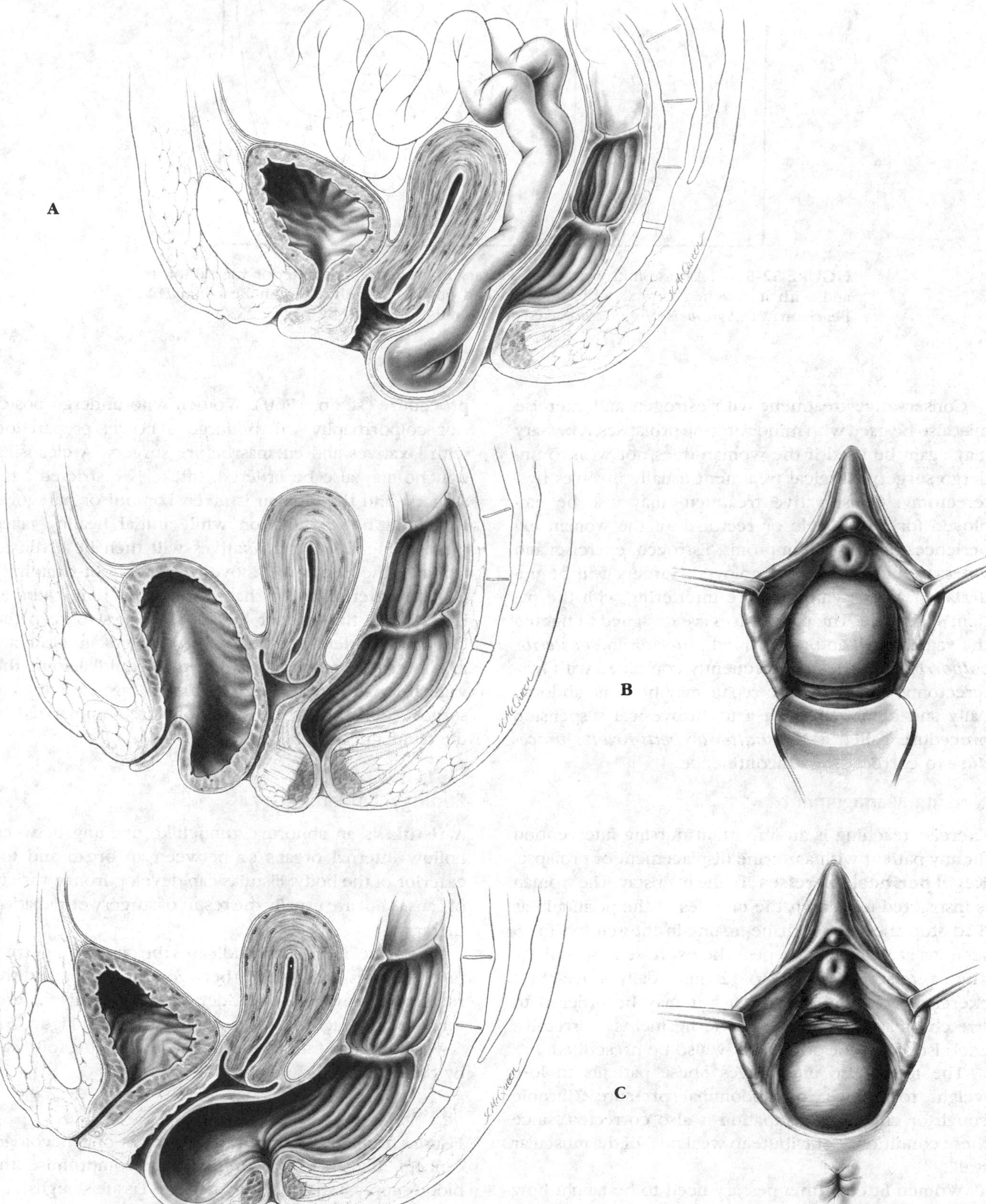


**FIGURE 52-4** **A,** Lateral view of enterocele and prolapsed uterus. **B,** Side and direct views of cystocele. **C,** Side and direct views of rectocele. (Redrawn from Symmonds RE: Relaxations of pelvic supports. In Benson RC, editor: *Current obstetric and gynecologic diagnosis and treatment,* ed 5, Los Altos, Calif., 1984, Lange Medical Publications.)

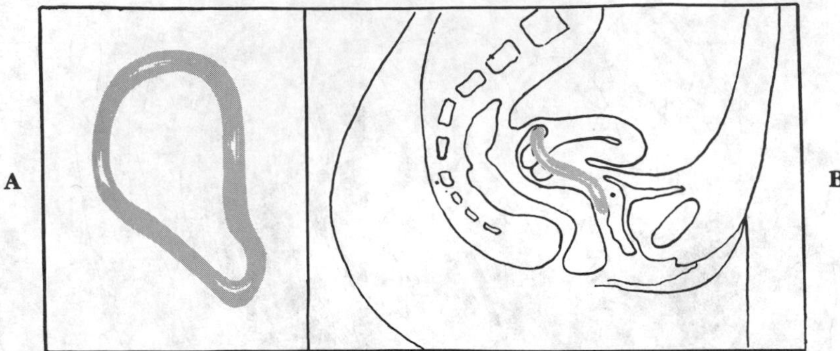


**FIGURE 52-5** **A,** Albert Smith pessary. **B,** Pessary in place to hold posterior vaginal fornix, and with it attached cervix, well backward and upward in pelvis. (From Beacham DW, Beacham WD: *Synopsis of gynecology,* ed 10, St Louis, 1982, Mosby.)

Conservative treatment with estrogen and exercise may also be used with minor uterine prolapses. A pessary may again be used if the woman does not wish to undergo surgery. Surgical treatment usually involves hysterectomy. Conservative treatment may also be employed for a cystocele or rectocele if the woman experiences only mild symptoms. Estrogen, exercise, and a pessary may again be employed. Surgery will be undertaken when symptoms are interfering with the patient's life-style. The procedures are designed to tighten the vaginal wall and are termed *anterior* and *posterior colporrhaphy.* They are frequently combined with hysterectomy. The cystocele repair may be done abdominally and combined with a urethrovesical suspension procedure called a *Marshall-Marchetti-Krantz procedure* to correct stress incontinence.

## Nursing Management

Exercise teaching is an important nursing intervention for any patient with a uterine displacement or prolapse. **Kegel perineal exercises** are the mainstay. The woman is instructed to tighten the muscles of the perineum as if to stop the flow of urine, maintain the tension for 5 seconds at a time, and repeat the exercise in sets of 10. The exercise is done 10 to 12 times daily. Knee-chest exercises are used less often but may be ordered to stretch or strengthen the pelvic ligaments. Corrective exercises for poor posture may also be prescribed.

The nurse also encourages obese patients to lose weight to reduce intraabdominal pressure. Chronic cough or chronic constipation is also corrected, since these conditions contribute to weakness of the muscular wall.

Women fitted with a pessary need to be taught how to insert it or withdraw it if the device becomes displaced or uncomfortable. Pessaries should be removed and cleaned once every few weeks or months as recommended by the physician. If the pessary is neglected, it can cause infection or fistula.

Surgical care is related primarily to the hysterectomy procedure (see p. 1760). Women who undergo posterior colporrhaphy will undergo a bowel preparation with laxatives and enemas before surgery. A cleansing douche may also be ordered. Intake is restricted after surgery, and the woman is given Lomotil or paregoric to inhibit bowel function while initial healing takes place. Mineral oil and laxatives will then be given to facilitate the first bowel movements without straining.

After anterior colporrhaphy, an indwelling catheter is placed in the bladder for about 4 days to keep the bladder completely empty. Stool softeners are again administered to reduce straining that could disrupt the vaginal repair. Guidelines for nursing care after vaginal surgery and discharge instructions are summarized in the Guidelines boxes, p. 1745.

# FISTULAS

## Etiology/Epidemiology

A **fistula** is an abnormal tunnellike opening between hollow internal organs or between an organ and the exterior of the body. Fistulas can develop from a variety of causes but are usually the result of surgery or radiation therapy.

The name of the fistula indicates the connecting structures. Fistulas can develop between the vagina and the rectum (rectovaginal), bladder (vesicovaginal), or urethra (urethrovaginal). They are illustrated in Figure 52-6. Vesicovaginal fistulas are the most common, followed by rectovaginal.[17]

## Pathophysiology

Fistulas frequently complicate treatment of gynecologic cancers. Radiation or surgery may compromise the blood supply, causing tissue damage. Tissue sloughs, and a channel gradually develops between the affected tissue and the vagina. The result is a constant drip of urine or an escape of flatus and fecal material through the vagina. This is highly distressing to the patient and creates an offensive odor. The drainage causes excoriation and irritation of the vaginal and vulvar tissue.

## Guidelines for Care of the Person After Vaginal or Perineal Surgery

1. Give perineal care after each voiding or defecation:
   a. Pour sterile normal saline over vulva and perineum.
   b. Cleanse perineum as needed with sterile cotton balls; cleanse away from vagina toward rectum.
   c. Dry perineum as needed with sterile cotton balls.
2. Encourage sitz baths after sutures are removed.
3. If douches are ordered during immediate postoperative period:
   a. Use sterile equipment and sterile solution.
   b. Insert douche nozzle very gently and rotate carefully.
4. Avoid pressure on suture line:
   a. Avoid a full bladder; keep urinary catheter patent.
   b. Use measures to prevent constipation.
   c. Teach patient to avoid Valsalva maneuver.
   d. Keep flat or in low-Fowler's position in bed.
5. Provide an ice pack for perineal discomfort (covered, sealed plastic bags or gloves make an acceptable pack).
6. Provide leg exercises.
7. Encourage deep breathing.
8. Monitor intake and output.
9. Note characteristics of urine and stool.

## Guidelines for Discharge After Vaginal or Perineal Surgery

1. Take daily douches and tub baths as prescribed.
2. Avoid straining at stool.
3. Use stool softeners and laxatives as prescribed.
4. Avoid lifting for 6 weeks.
5. Avoid sexual intercourse until physician gives permission (usually about 6 weeks).
6. Avoid jarring activities.
7. Avoid prolonged standing, walking, or sitting. Continue leg exercises for 6 weeks.
8. Reassure patient that possible loss of vaginal sensation for several months postoperatively will be temporary.
9. Instruct patient about high-fiber diet and need for 3000 ml of fluids daily.

## Medical Management

Fistulas are diagnosed primarily through pelvic examination. A *fistulogram,* which involves the injection of dye into the vagina, may be used to assess the exact location and severity of the fistula. Small fistulas may heal spontaneously if the tissue is allowed to rest. Surgery may otherwise be necessary to close the fistula tract. Tissue inflammation and edema must be treated first, and this can take months. Either anterior or posterior colporrhaphy may be used. It may be necessary to divert temporarily the urinary or fecal stream in complex situations. A Foley, ureteral, or nephrostomy catheter will be used to keep the area well drained and may

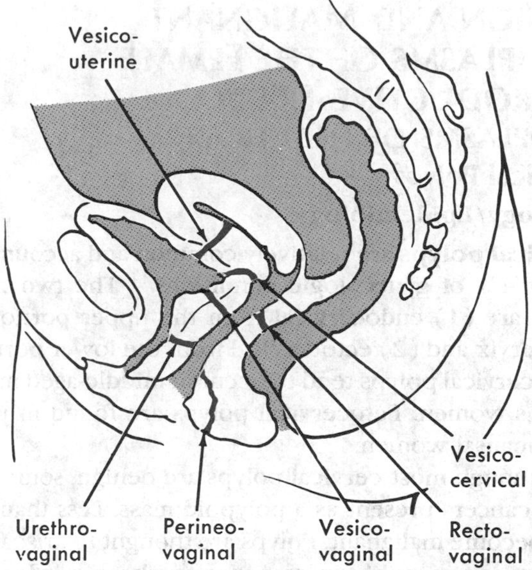


**FIGURE 52-6** Types of fistulas that may develop in vagina and uterus.

be left in place for weeks in some patients. With urine diversion, many urinary fistulas are able to heal spontaneously.[17] Bowel rest contributes to healing of rectovaginal fistulas, and the patient may be placed on total parenteral nutrition (TPN) to support spontaneous healing.[14] A diverting colostomy is performed if surgical intervention is necessary.

## Nursing Management

Nursing intervention focuses on comfort and the prevention of infection. A chlorine solution makes an effective deodorizing douche, and this solution is also excellent for perineal irrigation. A solution of 5 ml of household bleach to 1 L of water is appropriate. Douching should be performed at low pressure to prevent forcing the solution through the fistula tract. Sitz baths and careful cleansing with mild soap and water are also helpful. Although protective pads may be worn, the cleansing must be repeated at regular intervals to prevent skin breakdown and odor.

Postoperative care focuses on tissue healing. A small amount of serosanguineous drainage is expected, but the patient is carefully monitored for evidence of continued fecal or urinary drainage. Douches may be ordered, and the nurse administers them gently and at low pressure to protect healing tissue. Bedrest may be enforced for several days.

Surgical repair is not always successful, and repeat procedures frequently are needed. The risk of infection is constantly present, and the nurse anticipates that the patient may become increasingly anxious and depressed about her situation. The nurse encourages the patient to verbalize her concerns about her situation and seek support from family and friends.

# BENIGN AND MALIGNANT NEOPLASMS OF THE FEMALE REPRODUCTIVE TRACT

## NEOPLASMS OF THE CERVIX

### Cervical Polyps

#### Etiology/Epidemiology

**Cervical polyps** are relatively common and account for about 4% of gynecologic conditions.[14] The two main types are (1) endocervical from the upper portion of the cervix and (2) ectocervical from the lower portion. Endocervical polyps tend to occur in middle-aged multiparous women. Ectocervical polyps are found in postmenopausal women.

Although most cervical polyps are benign, some cervical cancers present as a polypoid mass. Less than 1% will become malignant. Polyps are thought to arise from hyperplasia, possibly in response to chronic inflammation, abnormal responses to hormonal stimulation, or localized vascular congestion. Hyperestrinism is thought to play a major role.

#### Pathophysiology

Most polyps are asymptomatic and discovered on routine pelvic examination. Endocervical polyps are usually reddish purple to cherry red, smooth, soft growths that may vary in size from a few millimeters to 2 or 3 cm in diameter and length. They are usually attached to the mucosa by a narrow pedicle and may be single or multiple in number. Ectocervical polyps are pale or flesh colored, round or elongated, and often attach with a broad pedicle. Most polypoid structures are vascular, and both types of polyps may become infected and necrotic at the tip.[15] The classic symptom is intermenstrual bleeding, particularly after intercourse or douching. A leukorrhea discharge may be present. The chronic irritation and bleeding can lead to cervicitis, endometritis, or even salpingitis.

#### Medical management

Cervical polyps are usually diagnosed by direct inspection and can be removed safely in a physician's office. Minimal bleeding is involved in most patients, but if bleeding should occur, it can be controlled by electrical or chemical cautery. All the removed tissue is sent for pathologic examination. Antibiotic therapy may be given prophylactically, particularly if there is any evidence of tissue necrosis or cervicitis.

#### Nursing management

The nurse encourages the woman to rest and avoid strenuous activity after polyp removal. A perineal pad can be provided to prevent soiling. The nurse instructs the woman to report any significant bleeding and to be alert to the development of signs of infection. The nurse instructs her to avoid tampon use, douches, and sexual intercourse for about a week while healing takes place.

### Cancer of the Cervix

#### Etiology

Although the cause of carcinoma of the cervix remains unknown, a close association exists between early and frequent sexual contact with multiple partners and cervical viral infection. Studies have shown a high incidence of the disease in prostitutes.[8,16] There is also an increased incidence in multiparous women, particularly African-Americans and Mexican-Americans. Socioeconomic factors associated with cervical cancer include poverty, early marriage, and early childbearing. Smoking, particularly long-term, high-intensity use, is now also considered a potential risk factor. Components of tobacco have been found to be secreted in the cervical mucus. Immunosuppression also increases the risk, and recent studies have indicated that women positive for the human immunodeficiency virus (HIV) are at high risk for development of cervical cancer and have a poorer disease prognosis.[20] STDs are also linked with atypical cell transformation. Dietary factors include deficiencies of vitamins A and C and derangement in folic acid metabolism.[8,20] Box 52-2 lists known and potential risk factors associated with the development of cervical cancer.

The vast majority of cervical cancers are squamous cell. Adenocarcinoma tends to have a different etiology. This cancer tends to appear in nulliparous or low-parity, diabetic women. These women also are older at the time of diagnosis. A subset of adenocarcinoma called *clear cell* develops in young women who have been exposed to diethylstilbestrol (DES) in utero.[14]

#### Epidemiology

The incidence of invasive cervical cancer has steadily decreased over the past 50 years. Cervical carcinoma in situ, a precancerous, noninvasive stage, now occurs

**BOX 52-2 Risk Factors for Cervical Cancer**

**RISK FACTORS**

- Low socioeconomic status
- Early age at first coitus
- Multiple sexual partners
- History of sexually transmitted diseases (STDs)
- Promiscuous male partner
- Early age at first pregnancy
- Race
- Prostitution

**POTENTIAL RISK FACTORS**

- Heavy use of talc
- Cigarette smoking
- Use of oral contraceptives
- Vitamins A and C deficiencies
- Derangement of folic acid metabolism
- Intrauterine exposure to diethylstilbestrol (DES)
- Diabetes
- Nulliparity
- Frequent douching

more frequently, especially in women over age 50.[2] The steady decline is attributed at least in part to improved early detection through Pap smear screening and improved surgical and radiotherapy techniques. Despite this very significant progress, cervical cancer still causes approximately 4500 deaths each year and 13,500 new cases are diagnosed annually.

**Pathophysiology**

Ninety-five percent of all cervical cancers are squamous cell, arising from the epidermal layer of the cervix. Cell dysplasia represents a precursor lesion, typically called *cervical intraepithelial neoplasia (CIN)*. It has been divided into the following three stages:

| | |
|---|---|
| CIN I | Mild to moderate |
| CIN II | Moderate to severe dysplasia |
| CIN III | Severe dysplasia to carcinoma in situ |

Women diagnosed with dysplasia may experience regression, persistence, or progression to carcinoma.[2]

Cervical adenocarcinoma arises from the mucus-producing gland cells of the cervix. It is not preceded by a well-recognized precursor state, and because of its location, it may be present for a considerable time before it can be clinically detected.[8]

Cervical cancer spreads by direct extension, blood, and lymph invasion. As the lymph nodes grow larger, venous flow is obstructed, and leg edema, ureteral obstruction, or hydronephrosis may occur. Hematogenous spread can be to the lungs, mediastinum, liver, and bone.[22]

Prognosis is based on the stage of the disease, depth of invasion, and vascular involvement of the tumor. Persistent or recurrent disease will develop in one third of the women with invasive cervical cancer. The 5-year survival rate for all cervical cancer patients is 66%. The survival rate is 88% for patients diagnosed early and virtually 100% when the disease is diagnosed in situ.[2]

Cervical cancer is asymptomatic in the early stages. As the disease progresses, the woman may experience a slight watery vaginal discharge and occasional bloody spotting, especially after intercourse. With advanced disease, a foul-smelling discharge may develop from sloughing of the epithelial tissue. Pain is usually a late sign and may involve the pelvic, flank, lower back, and abdominal area. The growing tumor may place pressure on the rectum and bladder, causing irritation and discharge. Hemorrhage is possible with advanced infiltrative tumors, which may also erode the walls of adjacent organs and create fistulas. Box 52-3 presents the clinical manifestations of cervical cancer.

**BOX 52-3 Clinical Manifestations of Cervical Cancer**

**EARLY SYMPTOMS**

Thin, watery vaginal discharge
Bloody spotting after coitus or douching
Metrorrhagia
Postmenopausal bleeding
Polymenorrhea

**LATE SYMPTOMS**

Dark, foul-smelling vaginal discharge
Pelvic, abdominal, or back pain
Flank pain
Weight loss
Anorexia
Anemia
Leg edema
Dysuria
Rectal bleeding

**Prevention**

**Primary prevention.** Primary prevention is aimed at supporting and maintaining good general health and avoiding smoking. Women should be taught the importance of condom use during sex to limit the transmission of STDs and genital viruses. Adolescent girls are encouraged to delay the onset of sexual activity and limit the number of their sexual partners. The early and effective treatment of any and all vaginal or cervical infections is stressed.

**Secondary prevention.** Early detection has played a critical role in reducing the number of deaths from cervical cancer. The American Cancer Society recommends that a Pap test should be performed annually with a pelvic examination in women who are or have been sexually active or who have reached age 18 years. After three or more consecutive annual examinations with normal findings, the Pap test may be performed less frequently at the physician's discretion. Women in high-risk groups should be examined and have a Pap test performed annually.[2] These recommendations assume even greater significance when it is recognized that many older women have not had a physical examination since their childbearing years.

**Medical management**

Common medical therapy for the management of cervical cancer includes the following.

**Diagnostic tests.** The diagnosis of cervical cancer can be confirmed only by biopsy. The Pap smear is a screening test but not a diagnostic tool. The two most common methods of obtaining a cervical biopsy are by conization or punch biopsy. Punch biopsies can easily be obtained in the physician's office. Conization is performed diagnostically when a question exists about the presence of invasive disease. It may also be used for treatment when preserving childbearing function is a priority.[14] Cone biopsy is illustrated in Figure 52-7.

Other diagnostic tests may then be performed to stage the disease. Chest x-ray films, pelvic computed tomog-

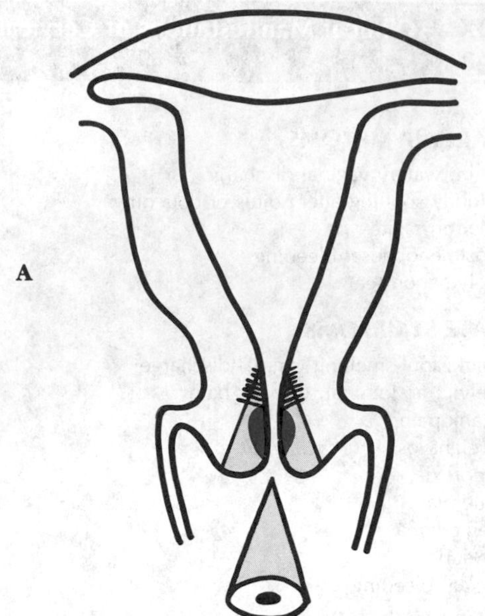


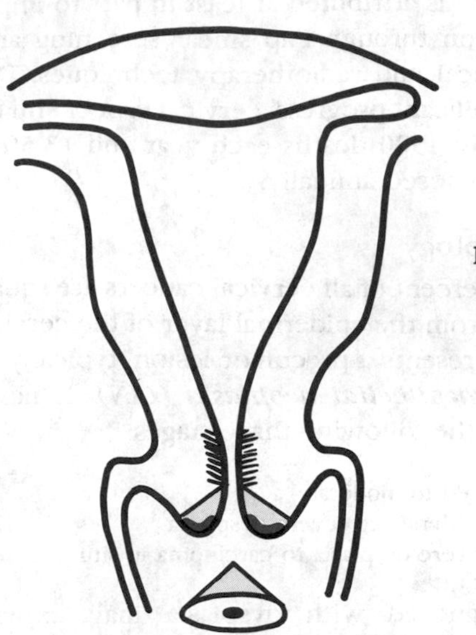


**FIGURE 52-7** **A,** Cone biopsy for endocervical disease. Limits of lesion were not seen colposcopically. **B,** Cone biopsy for cervical intraepithethial neoplasia (CIN) of exocervix. Limits of lesion were identified colposcopically. (From DiSiaia PJ, Creasman WT: *Clinical gynecologic oncology,* ed 4, St Louis, 1993, Mosby.)

raphy (CT) scans, intravenous pyelography (IVP), cystoscopy, proctosigmoidoscopy, and barium studies of the lower GI tract are all possible diagnostic adjuncts.[8] During the staging workup, the nurse ensures that the woman has all the information necessary to understand the tests and their rationale. Anxiety is typically high until the extent and invasiveness of the cancer can be established.

**Medication.** In the past chemotherapy has not played a significant role in the management of cervical cancer. Squamous cell cancers tend to be relatively unresponsive to drug treatment. Recurrent cancers tend to appear in areas previously irradiated, and the tissue is fibrotic and relatively avascular, making it difficult to obtain high tissue concentrations of the drugs. However, new research protocols have been developed that involve the administration of chemotherapy *before* other treatments when advanced disease is present. Early reports are of a drastic reduction in tumor size.[8] When used, chemotherapeutic agents are usually administered in combinations. (Nursing care related to chemotherapy is discussed in Chapter 16.)

**Treatment.** Cervical cancer is treated according to the stage of the disease (Table 52-6). Figure 52-8 illustrates the extent of anatomic involvement represented by each stage. Carcinoma in situ may be treated by excisional conization or cryosurgery, particularly if the woman is young and wants to have more children. Radiotherapy or hysterectomy may be chosen if fertility is not an issue. More invasive cancer is treated with increasingly extensive surgical procedures or radiotherapy. Table 52-7 summarizes the major treatment options for various stages of cervical cancer and their associated long-term survival projections.

***Radiotherapy.*** When radiotherapy is used in the treatment of cervical cancer, it may consist of external pelvic irradiation or intracavitary implants (Figures 52-9 to 52-11). **Intracavitary implants** are usually left in place for 24 to 72 hours. (The use of radiotherapy as a cancer treatment is discussed in detail in Chapter 16.)

During an intracavitary implant, it is important that all untreated tissues remain in their normal positions and not come in close contact with the radioactive substance. The bowel is cleansed before therapy, and the woman is maintained on a low-residue diet during treatment to prevent bowel distention and defecation. A catheter is typically inserted to keep the bladder small and decompressed. Gauze packing may be used in the vagina to support the rectum and bladder away from the treatment field. The woman is kept flat in bed during treatment to prevent dislodgement of the radioactive substance. The exact position of the implants can be verified by x-ray film.

The presence of the implants in the cervix may stimulate uterine contractions that may become severe. A foul-smelling vaginal discharge develops from the destruction and sloughing of cells. Also, the woman may develop symptoms of radiation syndrome, with nausea, vomiting, anorexia, and malaise. Local reactions may include cystitis and proctitis. After treatment, the catheter is removed and an enema may be administered to restore bowel function. The vaginal discharge will persist for

**TABLE 52-6 Clinical Stages in Carcinoma of the Cervix Uteri (FIGO System)**

| STAGE | INVOLVEMENT |
|---|---|
| Stage 0 | Carcinoma in situ, intraepithelial carcinoma |
| Stage I | Carcinoma is strictly confined to the cervix (extension to the corpus should be disregarded). |
| Stage Ia | Preclinical carcinomas of the cervix; that is, those diagnosed only by microscopy |
| Stage Ia1 | Minimal microscopically evident stromal invasion |
| Stage Ia2 | Lesions detected microscopically that can be measured. The upper limit of the measurement should not show a depth of invasion of more than 5 mm taken from the base of the epithelium, either surface or glandular, from which it originates, and a second dimension, the horizontal spread, must not exceed 7 mm. Larger lesions should be staged as Ib. |
| Stage Ib | Lesions of greater dimensions than stage Ia2, whether seen clinically or not. Preformed space involvement should not alter the staging but should be specifically recorded so as to determine whether it should affect treatment decisions in the future. |
| Stage II | Involvement of the vagina but not the lower third, or infiltration of the parametria but not out to the sidewall |
| Stage IIa | Involvement of the vagina but no evidence of parametrial involvement |
| Stage IIb | Infiltration of the parametria but not out to the sidewall |
| Stage III | Involvement of the lower third of the vagina or extension to the pelvic sidewall. All cases with a hydronephrosis or nonfunctioning kidney should be included, unless they are known to be attributable to other cause. |
| Stage IIIa | Involvement of the lower third of the vagina but not out to the pelvic sidewall if the parametria are involved |
| Stage IIIb | Extension onto the pelvic sidewall and/or hydronephrosis or nonfunctional kidney |
| Stage IV | Extension outside the reproductive tract |
| Stage IVa | Involvement of the mucosa of the bladder or rectum |
| Stage IVb | Distant metastasis or disease outside the true pelvis |

From DiSaia PJ, Creasman WT: *Clinical gynecologic oncology,* ed 4, St Louis, 1993, Mosby.

**TABLE 52-7 Summary of Treatment Options for Cervical Cancer**

| CLINICAL STAGE | TREATMENT OPTIONS | 5-YEAR SURVIVAL (%) |
|---|---|---|
| Dysplasia | Cryosurgery/conization/laser surgery | 100 |
| CIN (carcinoma in situ) | Simple hysterectomy | 100 |
| Ia<br>Ia1: Microinvasive (3 mm below basement membrane) | Simple hysterectomy or radiation (cesium implant) | 95-100 |
| Ia2: Microinvasive (3-5 mm depth) | Radical hysterectomy with nodes or radiotherapy (external and implant) | 95-98 |
| Ib and IIa | Radical hysterectomy with nodes or radiotherapy | 75-90 |
| IIb | Radiation | 50-60 |
| IIIa and IIIb | Radiation | 30-40 |
| IV | Radiation or chemotherapy | 5-14 |
| Recurrent | Pelvic exenteration, if operable, or chemotherapy | Varies according to site and extent of recurrence |

some time, and the woman may need to douche regularly at home to control odor. Slight vaginal bleeding may occur for 1 to 3 months after treatment. Discharge typically occurs within 1 day after removal of the applicators. The woman is instructed to monitor for signs of complications, such as fistula formation, cystitis, or bleeding, and report any related symptoms to her physician.

External pelvic radiation treatments are usually given over a course of 5 to 6 weeks. (General care for the patient receiving external radiotherapy is presented in Chapter 16; the nursing care of patients receiving intracavitary implants is discussed under nursing management.)

**Diet.** No special diet is required for a patient having cancer of the cervix. Any change in diet required is usually the result of radiation, chemotherapy, or surgical interventions.

**Activity.** No activity restrictions are required by the diagnosis. Sexual activity may be restricted temporarily after biopsy, radiation treatment, or surgery. General activity restrictions are also made purely in response to the short-term requirements of specific treatments.

**Referral/Consultation.** In some settings the nurse assumes responsibility for making referrals to other services. The nurse may need to refer the patient to an

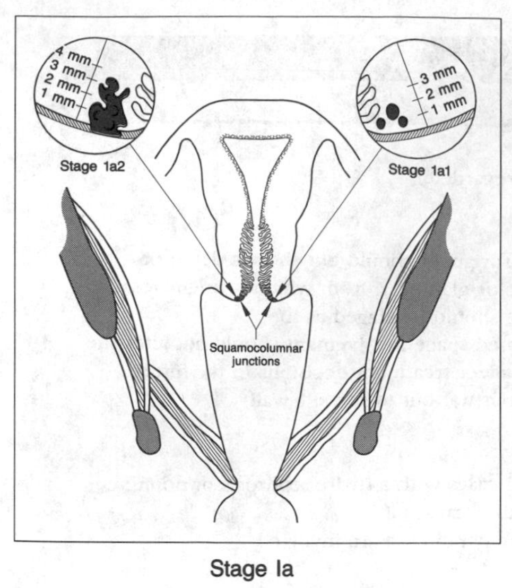


Stage Ia

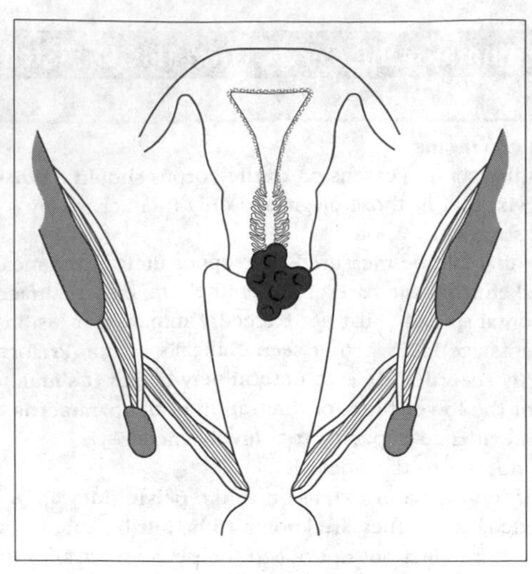

Stage Ib

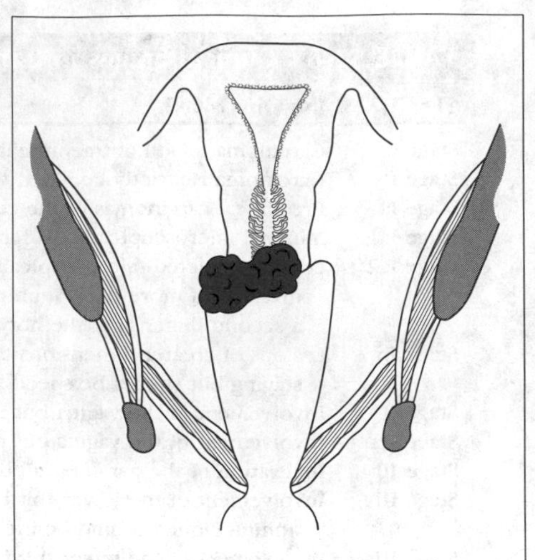

Stage IIa

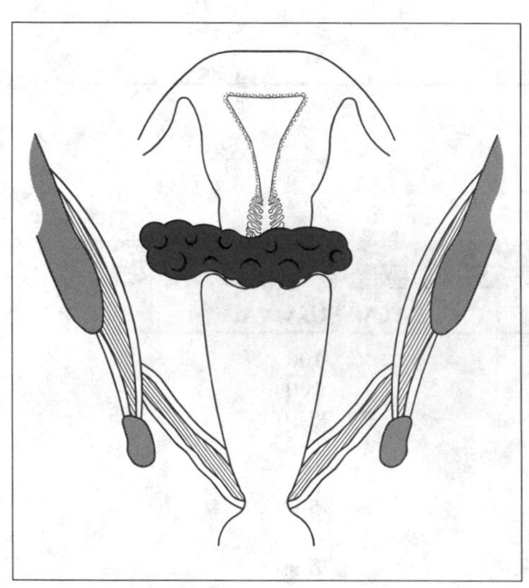

Stage IIb

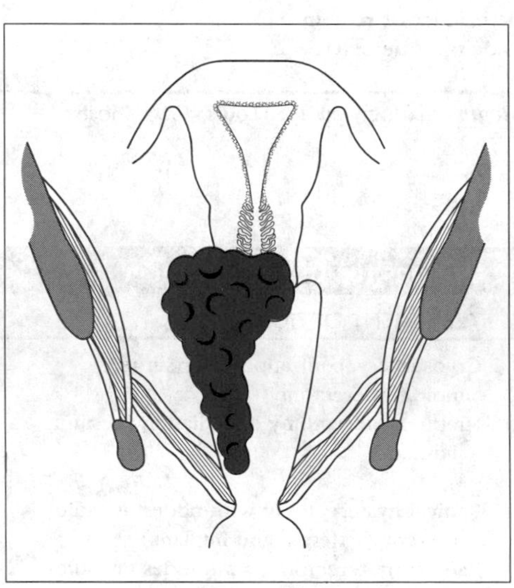

Stage IIIa

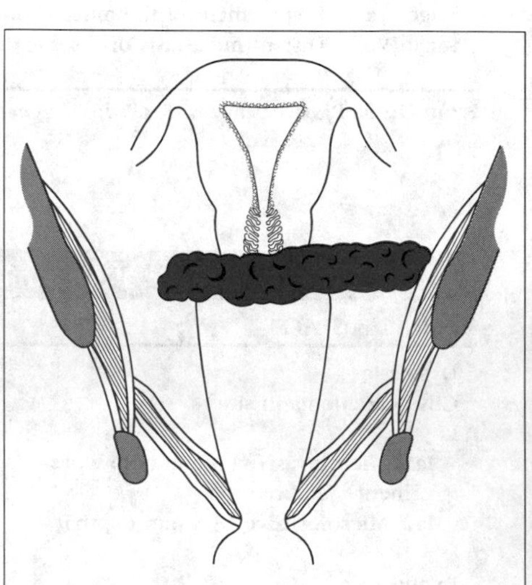

Stage IIIb

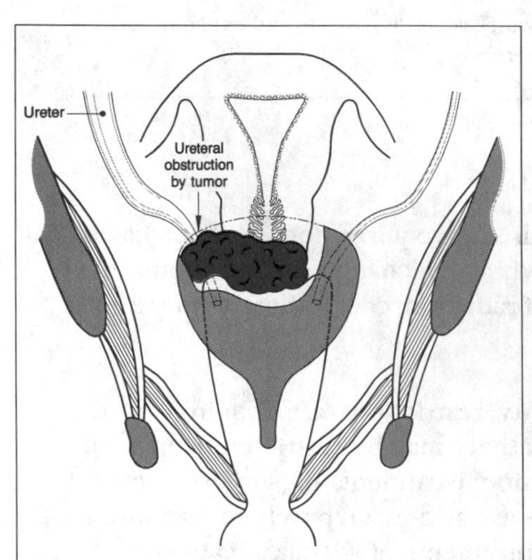


Stage IIIb (urinary)

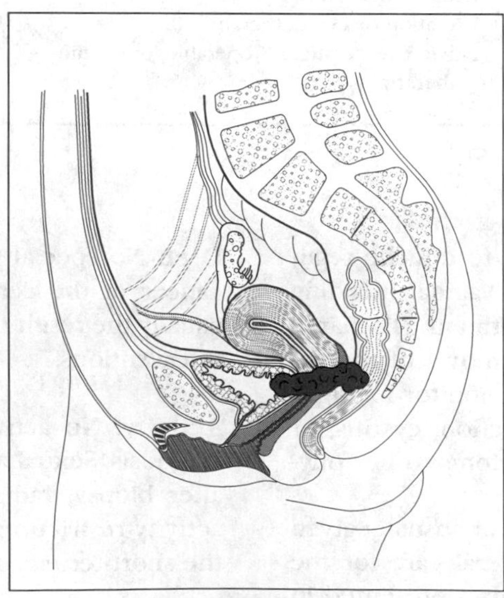

Stage IVa

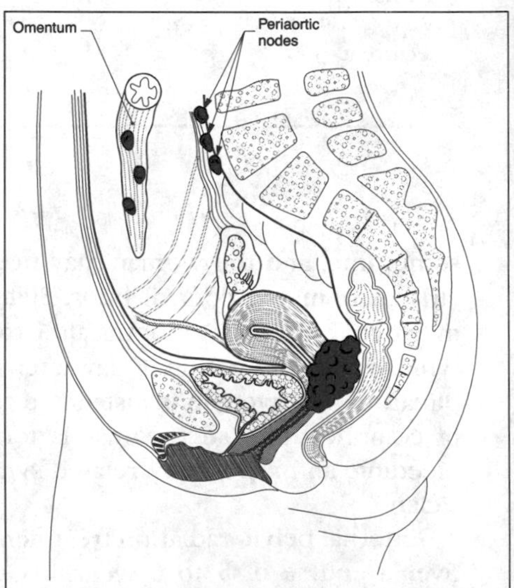


Stage IVb

**FIGURE 52-8** FIGO staging and classification of cancer of cervix. (From DiSaia PJ: *Adv Oncol* 8[2]:15, 1992.)

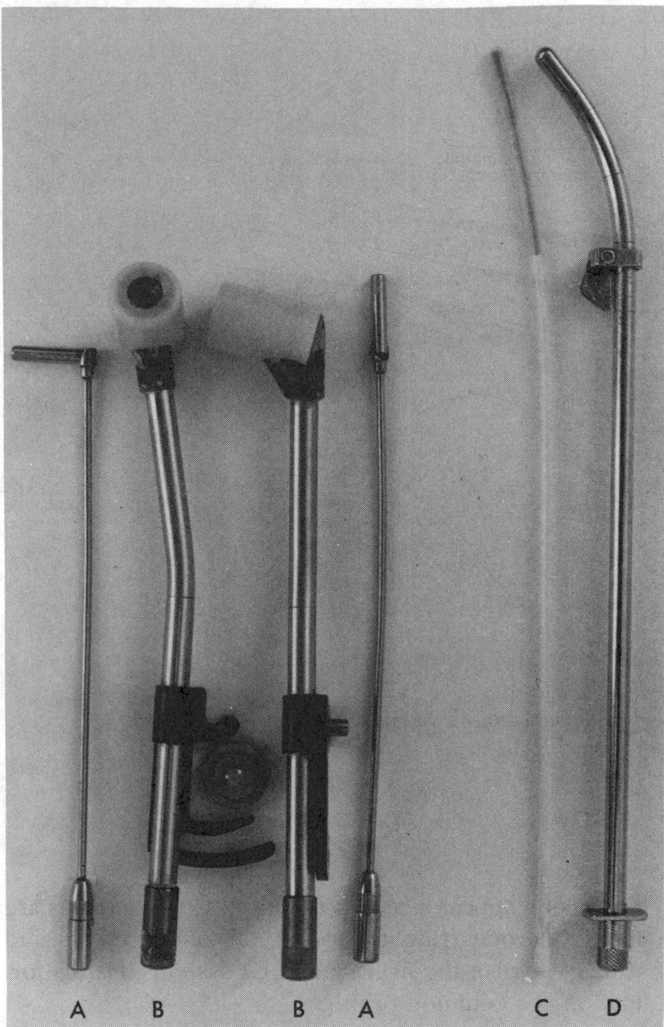


**FIGURE 52-9** Intracavitary implant for treatment of cervical cancer. **A,** Inserts for colpostats to insert radium or cesium. **B,** Colpostats. **C,** Teflon tubing to insert radium or cesium into tandem. **D,** Tandem.

enterostomal therapist for stomal care if the patient experiences a pelvic exenteration. Sexual dysfunction as a result of disease and/or treatment may necessitate a psychiatric or sexual counseling referral.

### Surgical management

Simple or radical **hysterectomy** is the most frequently recommended surgical procedure for treating stages I and II cervical cancer. A radical hysterectomy removes the uterus, supporting tissues, distal vagina, and pelvic lymph nodes (Figure 52-12). In some patients the cancer may be locally advanced but still confined to the pelvis. In these situations, a **pelvic exenteration** procedure may be considered (Figure 52-13). The surgery is still controversial, but it is lifesaving in certain malignancies, particularly advanced or recurrent cervical cancer.[8] The procedure involves removal of all the pelvic viscera, including the bladder, rectosigmoid colon, and all reproductive organs. Five-year survival rates after this radical surgery range from 20% to 62%.[8] Discovery of disease spread beyond the pelvis is an absolute contraindication to the procedure. Newer operative techniques have brought the ability to provide the patient with reconstructive surgery and the construction of a neovagina. It can be done at the time of surgery or as a second surgery later. Figures 52-14 and 52-15 illustrate approaches to vaginal reconstruction.

Nursing care of the patient undergoing hysterectomy is presented on p. 1760. Women undergoing exenteration receive this standard care but also receive care for an abdominal-perineal resection of the bowel and an ileoconduit. The extensive nature of the surgery usually necessitates at least a short stay in a critical care unit. Clear and honest teaching is a foundational component of this surgery. Women need to be fully aware of the nature and consequences of the procedures in terms of

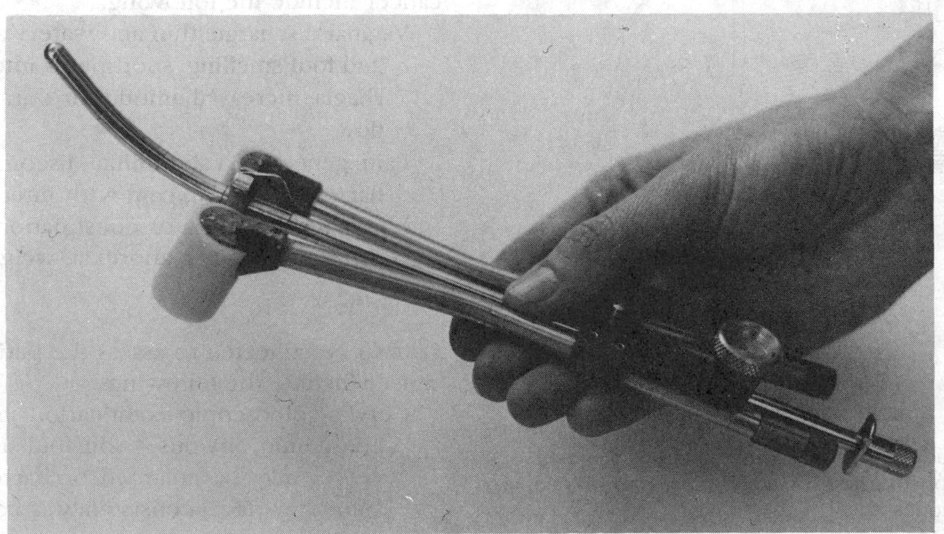

**FIGURE 52-10** Assembled configuration of tandem and colpostat before displacement.

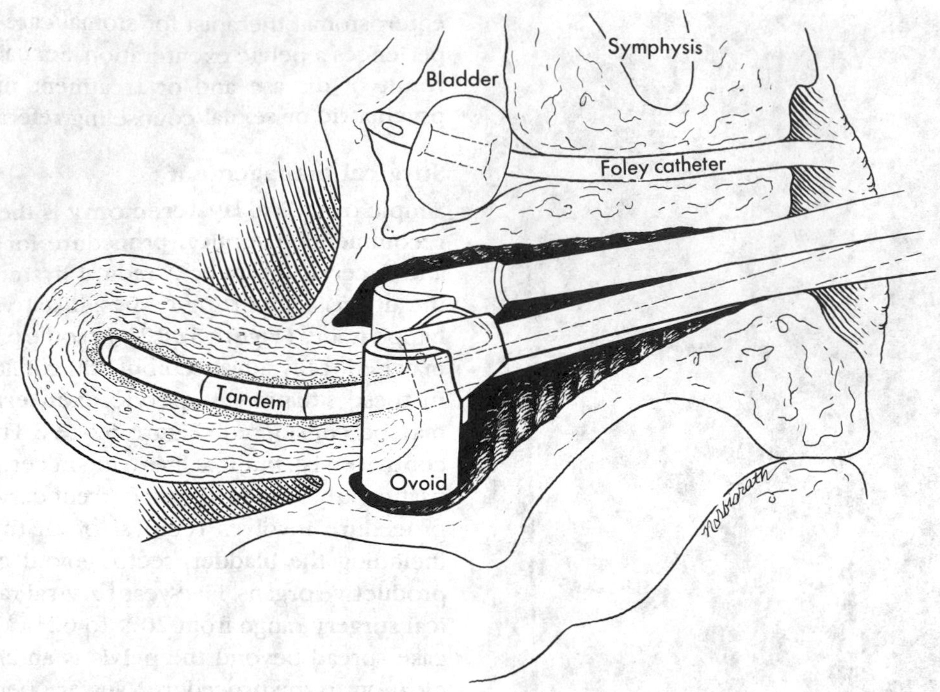


FIGURE 52-11 Placement of tandem and colpostats before vaginal packing.

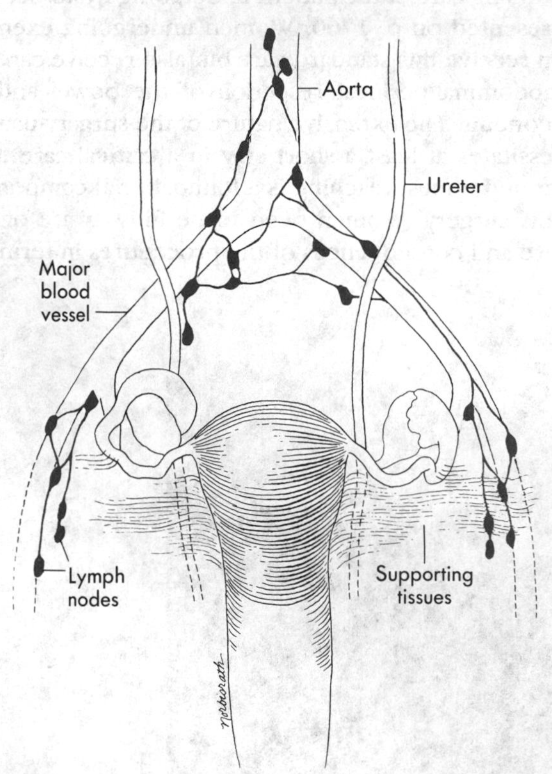


FIGURE 52-12 Radical hysterectomy includes removal of uterus, nearby supporting tissues, uppermost part of vagina, and pelvic lymph nodes.

both body appearance and function. Complications are numerous, occurring in 25% to 50% of all patients, and usually involve the urinary and GI systems. Fistula formation is a common problem.

## NURSING MANAGEMENT

### ♦ ASSESSMENT

#### Subjective Data

Data to be collected to assess the patient with cervical cancer include the following:

Vaginal discharge: thin and watery advancing to dark and foul smelling; spotting or intermittent metrorrhagia; increased amount or duration of menstrual flow

Pain: generalized abdominal discomfort; pelvic, back, flank, or leg pain; pain with intercourse

Elimination: dysuria or constipation

General complaints: anorexia, weight loss, fatigue

#### Objective Data

Data to be collected to assess the patient with cervical cancer include the following:

Cervix: colposcopic examination showing erosion of epithelium, obvious lesion; foul-smelling discharge; cervix may be enlarged or barrel shaped with a smooth surface; consistency is hard to palpation

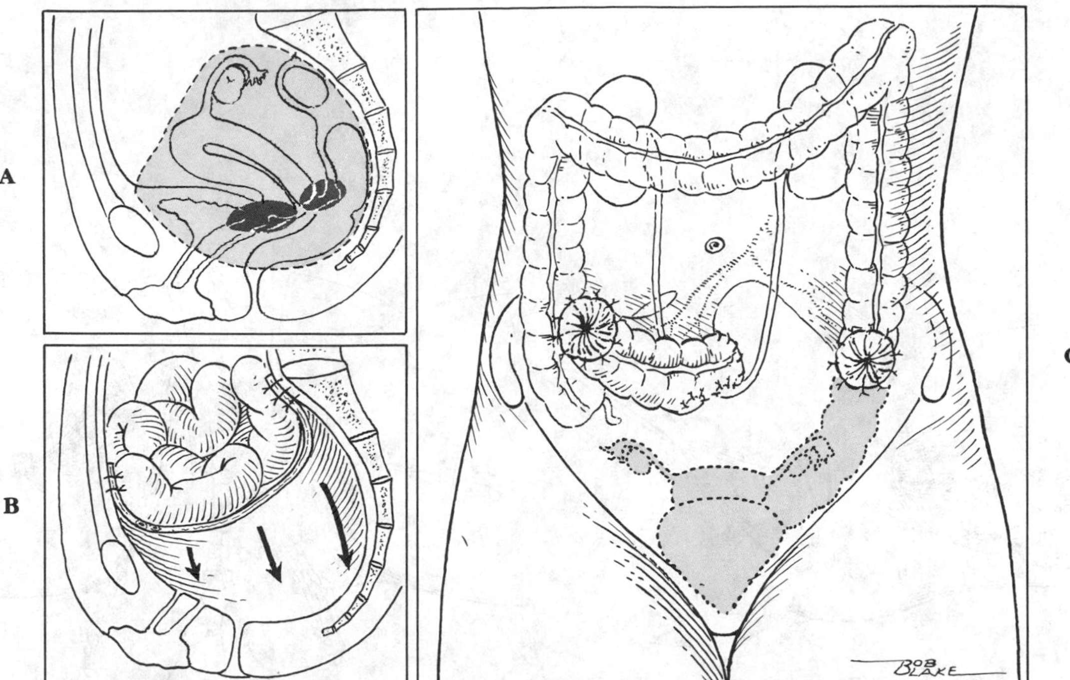


**FIGURE 52-13** **A,** Lateral view of recurrent cancer involving cervix and upper vagina with extension into bladder and rectum. Stippled area is tissue to be removed by exenteration. **B,** Lateral view after pelvic viscera have been removed. Omental "carpet" is used to keep intestines out of pelvis during immediate postoperative period. With time, omental "carpet" will descend into pelvis, and "carpet" will adhere to pelvic floor. **C,** Urinary conduit and colostomy diversion after exenteration. Dotted areas of sigmoid, bladder, and internal genitalia have been removed. (From DiSiaia PJ, Creasman WT: *Clinical gynecologic oncology,* ed 4, St Louis, 1993, Mosby.)

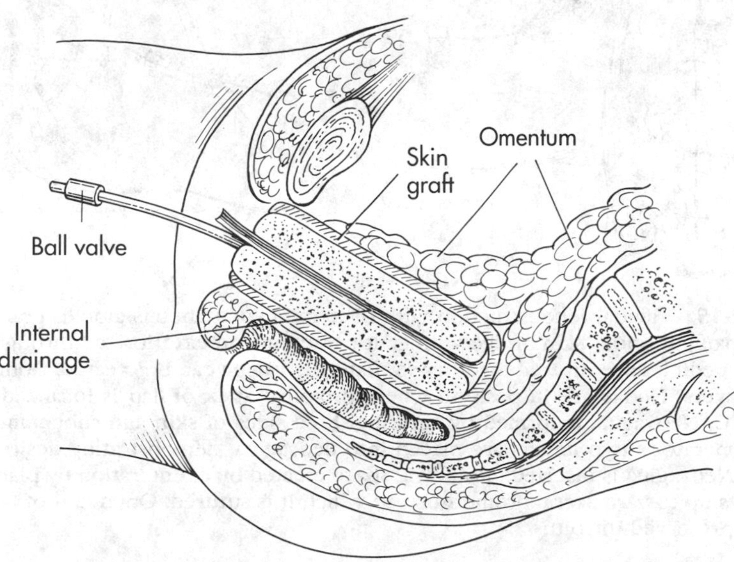


**FIGURE 52-14** Vaginal reconstruction with skin graft. Omentum is placed in pelvis and sutured to rectum posteriorly and sigmoid colon laterally to create a "pocket" for neovagina. Two split-thickness skin grafts are harvested, sutured together over a Heyer-Schulte stent, and inserted into newly created pelvic space.

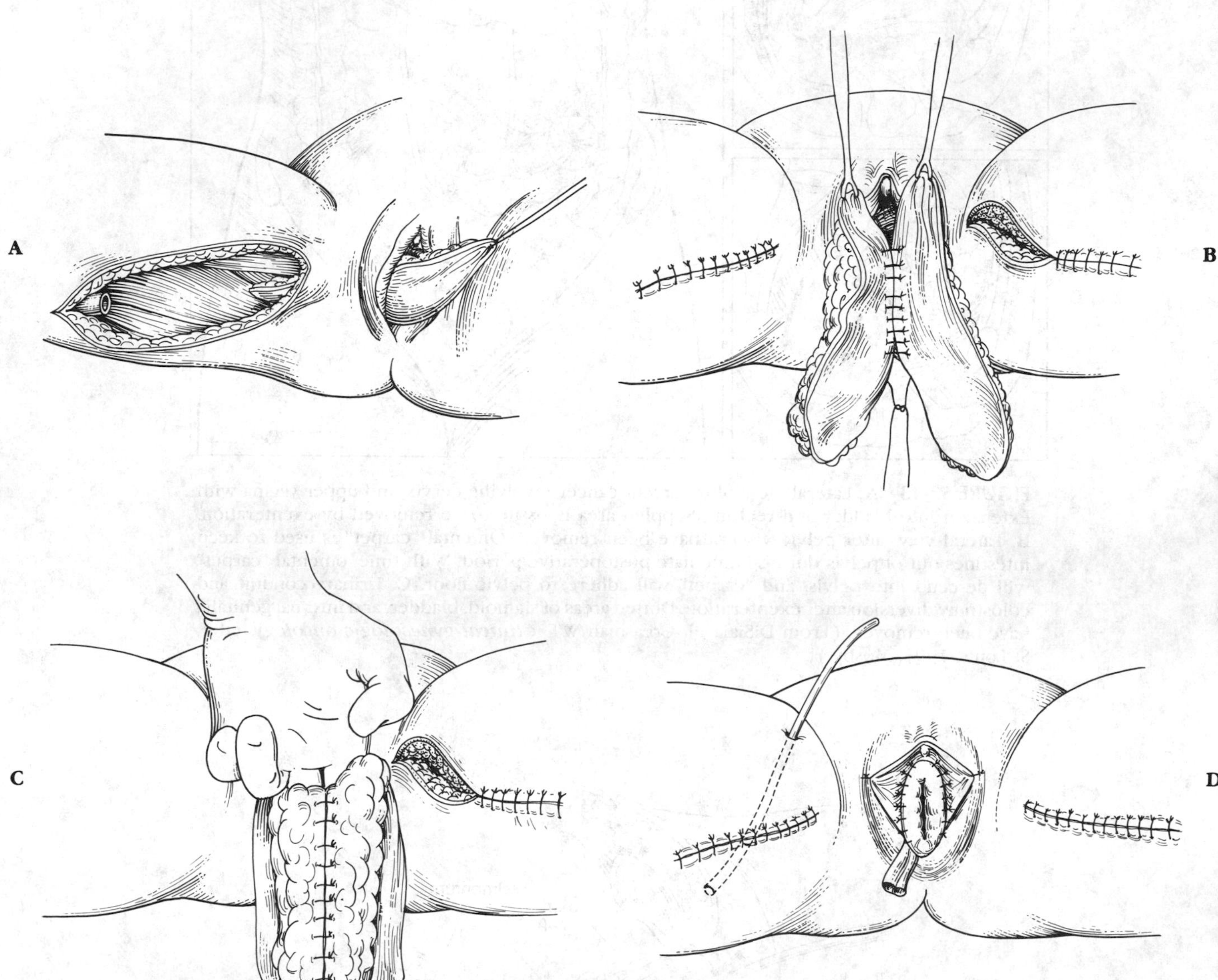


**FIGURE 52-15** Vaginal reconstruction with bilateral myocutaneous gracilis graft. **A,** Entire pedicle is brought under skin bridge with gentle traction and exteriorized through introitus. **B,** Bilateral pedicles are sutured together so that a neovagina can be created. Donor sites are closed in layers. Hooks are in position where proximal apex of flap is localized before its dissection. **C,** Neovagina is formed by suturing three sides of skin and subcutaneous tissue together. Operator's two fingers are placed into neovagina, demonstrating desired size and caliber. **D,** Neovagina is inserted into pelvic space created by exenteration by placing closed end of grafts up toward sacral promontory, to which it is sutured. Open end of neovagina is sutured to preserved introitus.

Elimination: hematuria or rectal bleeding; palpable lesion on rectal examination is late finding
Abdomen: muscle guarding or rigidity
Edema: present along entire length of leg; one leg may be larger

## Diagnostic Test Findings

1. Colposcopy showing abnormal cervical blood vessels and irregular surface contour
2. Positive Pap test and cervical biopsy
3. CT scan showing pelvic and/or paraaortic lymph node enlargement or intraabdominal masses (late finding)
4. Barium enema or proctosigmoidoscopy showing involvement of colon or rectum (late finding)
5. Cystoscopy or IVP showing involvement of urinary system—obstruction or hydronephrosis (late finding)

## ♦ NURSING DIAGNOSES

Nursing diagnoses are determined from analysis of patient data. Nursing diagnoses for the patient with cervical cancer being treated with radiotherapy may include but are not limited to the following:

| Diagnostic Title | Possible Etiologic Factors |
|---|---|
| Anxiety | Fear of radiation and its effects; diagnosis of cancer; uncertainty of outcome |
| Self-care: bathing-toileting deficit | Activity restrictions during treatment |
| Social isolation | Isolation and safety precautions necessitated by implant |
| Health maintenance, altered (risk of) | Insufficient knowledge about home care requirements |

## ♦ EXPECTED PATIENT OUTCOMES

Expected patient outcomes for the patient with cervical cancer being treated with radiotherapy may include but are not limited to the following:

1a. Verbalizes rationale for precautions followed by both staff and visitors.
b. Communicates feelings about diagnosis and treatment.
c. Expresses less anxiety about treatment and future outcomes.
2. Adapts self-care tasks to activity restrictions and accepts assistance as needed.
3a. Interacts with staff and visitors within the established safety guidelines.
b. Utilizes appropriate diversional activities.
4a. Accurately describes components of home care and need for follow-up monitoring.
b. Demonstrates competency in care skills such as vaginal dilation and perineal cleansing.
c. Correctly identifies signs and symptoms of complications.

## ♦ INTERVENTIONS

### Reducing Anxiety

A cancer diagnosis can produce a barrage of negative feelings in the patient that are frequently increased during the overwhelming diagnosis and staging period. Anxiety frequently alters how persons process information and can reduce their ability to make decisions about their own care. The nurse conveys a sense of empathetic understanding and provides reassurance with every patient encounter. The nurse encourages the woman to talk about her feelings and concerns and supports the need to ventilate emotions through anger or crying. As anxiety is controlled, effective teaching can begin concerning the condition, treatment options, and expected side effects. The nurse should assess the meaning of the diagnosis to the patient and her significant others, clarify misconceptions, and provide reliable information to enhance their understanding.

Careful teaching takes place before the insertion of the implant so the woman and her family clearly un-

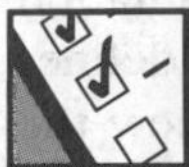

### Guidelines for Care of the Woman Undergoing Internal Radiotherapy

**PREIMPLANTATION**

Care before the insertion of the radioactive implant usually includes the following:

1. Provide cleansing enema to empty the bowel.
2. Insert Foley catheter to keep the bladder empty and small during treatment.
3. Provide Betadine douche, and shave pubic area if ordered.

**IMPLANTATION PERIOD**

Care during the 24 to 72 hours of treatment includes the following:

1. Insert gauze packing into the vagina to separate the rectum and bladder from the irradiated area. One or two stitches may be placed in the labia to support the holder in position.
2. Maintain strict bedrest.
   a. Elevate head of bed no more than 20 degrees.
   b. Tell patient turning from side to side is permitted.
3. Ensure low-residue diet and possibly antimotility agents to prevent bowel distention.
4. Administer analgesics as needed for uterine cramping, which can be severe.
5. Perform routine perineal cleansing if drainage is present; provide room deodorizer if discharge is foul smelling.
6. Ensure a minimum fluid intake of 2500 ml daily.
7. Visit patient frequently from room doorway for emotional support.
8. Provide diversional activities appropriate to activity restrictions.
9. Monitor implant for proper placement; keep long-handled forceps and a lead-lined container in the room in case of dislodgement.
10. Monitor for complications:
    a. Infection: increased vaginal redness or swelling; increasingly dark, foul-smelling drainage; cloudy urine; fever
    b. Thrombophlebitis: painful leg swelling; positive Homans' sign

**BOX 52-4 Radiation Precautions for Internal Radiotherapy**

1. Time at the bedside is limited—each contact should last no more than 30 minutes.
2. Children and pregnant women/staff should not visit during treatment.
3. Staff members should wear a dosimeter during every patient contact to monitor radiation exposure.
4. Lead shield may be installed at the side and foot of the bed.
5. Staff should use the principles of distance, time, and shielding in all contacts with the patient.
6. Implant is always handled by means of long-handled forceps, never with the hands. A lead-lined container should be present in the room for use if the implant dislodges.
7. A sign that clearly identifies the radiation hazard is posted on the room door.
8. A contact number for the radiation safety officer of the institution should be posted on the warning sign.

derstand the rationale for all restrictions and safety measures. Guidelines for care during the preimplantation and radiotherapy periods are outlined in the Guidelines box, p. 1755. It is particularly important to review the precautions related to the implant itself, which are summarized in Box 52-4. The cesium implant is a source of high-dose ionizing radiation to all who come into its range, and these risks must be minimized to the extent possible. The radiation hazard is clearly marked on the door to the room, and a radiation safety officer is available in the institution to deal with questions and concerns.

## Promoting Self-Care

The activity restrictions outlined in the Guidelines box on p. 1755 must be followed carefully during the treatment period to prevent accidental dislodgement of the device or movement of the implant that endangers normal tissue. It is critical that the woman understand the rationale for all restrictions to promote adherence with the treatment plan. The nurse supports self-care principles and ensures that all needed articles are kept within easy reach, but assistance may still be necessary because the woman must remain on flat bedrest. Hourly turning is encouraged, and back rubs may help to relieve some of the discomforts of bedrest. The foul-smelling vaginal discharge may be both physically irritating and embarrassing. The nurse assists with frequent perineal hygiene and acquires a room deodorizer.

Comfort is another concern during treatment. The uterine cramping can become severe, and narcotic analgesia may be indicated. Regular rather than as needed administration can help keep the discomfort under control. Patients may develop symptoms of radiation syndrome that make nutrition difficult. The nurse encourages the patient to maintain a fluid intake of 2500 to 3000 ml daily, even in the face of anorexia and nausea, to help relieve irritation in the urologic system. Phlebothrombosis is another concern during bedrest, and the nurse teaches the woman range-of-motion and isometric exercises that support venous return and encourages her to perform them 10 times each hour.

## Preventing Social Isolation

The woman receiving intracavitary radiation often feels alienated and depressed. The nurse can spend time talking with the patient but must remain at a safe distance and observe the time restrictions for safety. Family members are also encouraged to visit, following the same guidelines. Children or pregnant women cannot visit.

Strict bedrest rapidly creates both a boring and an uncomfortable situation for the patient. The nurse makes an effort to create a pleasant, odor-free environment. Self-care items are kept within easy reach, and diversional activities are acquired for the patient. Reading, music, telephone, and television are all easily implemented. The nursing staff maintain frequent contact with the patient, checking on her at least hourly, and ensure that the call bell is within easy reach.

## Teaching Home Care Skills

The hospitalization period for intracavitary radiotherapy is short, and the patient is discharged soon after the removal of the implant. The woman must learn several self-care skills for home management and must be aware of the signs and symptoms of potential complications. Radiotherapy induces fatigue, vaginal stenosis, loss of vaginal lubrication, and induced menopause.

The vaginal discharge will continue for some time, and the woman may need to douche for as long as discharge and odor persist. Douching is usually performed twice daily. The nurse cannot assume that the woman has either experience in or equipment for douching and should review the technique and precautions in detail. Some vaginal bleeding may also continue for a few months after treatment, and the woman should receive information from her physician about acceptable limits and quantities.

The cesium implant may lead to vaginal narrowing and fibrosis. Regular vaginal dilation is essential to minimize these effects. Regular sexual intercourse, usually at least three times per week, is one method of minimizing stenosis. The nurse needs to explore the woman's normal pattern of sexuality and ascertain whether this approach is realistic and acceptable. The woman may prefer to use a pattern of dilation with a manual obturator. The importance of this intervention is explained to women who are not sexually active as well. Even routine pelvic examination can become difficult or almost impossible if the vagina becomes severely stenosed. Dilation should be maintained at least three times a week for a year after treatment. The obturator should be lubricated before use and washed carefully in soap and water after each use. A vinegar and water douche

**RESEARCH**

Jenkins B: Patients' reports of sexual changes after treatment for gynecological cancer, *Oncol Nurs Forum* 15(3):349-354, 1988.

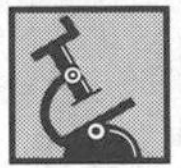

Twenty sexually active women were studied for the occurrence of sexual changes after surgical and radiation treatments for endometrial and cervical cancer. In response to a mailed questionnaire, statistically significant negative changes were reported by 95% of the women in four indicators of sexual function: frequency of intercourse and orgasm and feelings of desire and enjoyment. Regarding the amount of sexual counseling received before and after treatment, 59% reported that they received no information. Most of the information was given to patients by radiotherapists. No sexual counseling was given by nurses. Eighty-eight percent of these women wanted sexual discussions initiated by the physician or nurse.

may be ordered after treatment. The nurse informs the woman that slight bleeding may occur after dilation and that this may persist for up to a year.

Sexual intercourse may be resumed about 3 weeks after discharge, but the woman should be instructed to use a water-soluble lubricant for comfort because vaginal secretions will be decreased or absent (see Research box above). The partner should be included in all discussions about sexual activity and expected effects if the woman is comfortable with his presence.

Other self-care teaching includes gradually increasing activity, maintaining a liberal fluid intake to prevent urologic problems, and adjusting the diet to prevent bowel problems. Either constipation or diarrhea may occur in response to the radiation, and these problems may persist for several months after treatment. The woman is also informed of symptoms that may indicate the development of a complication. She should promptly report unusually heavy discharge, foul-smelling urine, low-grade fever, persistent bowel problems, or pain. Radiotherapy can result in the development of fistulas in the pelvis, either in the early posttreatment period or in the future. Written material to take home can be helpful in providing the woman with a resource for referral. The importance of follow-up care and monitoring cannot be overemphasized.

## ♦ EVALUATION

To evaluate the effectiveness of nursing interventions, compare patient behaviors with those stated in the expected patient outcomes (see Research box above right). Successful achievement of patient outcomes for the patient with cervical cancer receiving radiotherapy is indicated by the following:

1a. Correctly explains the rationale for all radiation and activity restrictions.

**RESEARCH**

Corney R et al: The care of patients undergoing surgery for gynaecological cancer: the need for information, emotional support and counseling, *J Adv Nurs* 17(6):667-671, 1992.

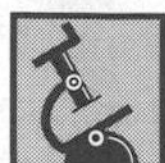

In this study, 105 patients who had undergone major gynecologic surgery for carcinoma of the cervix or vulva in the past 5 years were interviewed. A high proportion of the women were still found to be depressed and anxious when interviewed, and most reported chronic sexual problems. The women were asked if they had received enough information regarding their illness and its treatment; a high proportion would have liked to have had more information on the aftereffects of the surgery, including physical, sexual, and emotional aspects. Many of the younger women would have wanted their partner to have been included in the discussions, and 25% of the 40 partners who responded to a questionnaire stated they would have liked more information on the illness and its treatment. The women also indicated their needs for emotional support, discussion, and counseling.

b. Communicates feelings to partner, family, or staff.
c. States that anxiety is minimal or absent.

2. Performs self-care activities independently or with the use of appropriate assistance.

3a. Regularly interacts with family, friends, and staff.
b. Uses books, hobbies, music, and TV to break up the day.

4a. Correctly describes home care regimen and planned pattern for follow-up care.
b. Correctly demonstrates perineal care and use of an obturator for dilation.
c. Correctly describes signs of complications that need to be reported.

## ✸ SPECIAL CONSIDERATIONS FOR CARE OF THE GERONTOLOGIC PATIENT

Cancer of the cervix occurs in women of all ages. Early diagnosis is critical whenever the disease develops and is frequently a more complex problem in older women. After the childbearing years, many women tend to stop having routine gynecologic examinations. Symptoms are often discounted or attributed to the multiple effects of aging on the reproductive tract. Therefore it is less likely that cervical cancer will be caught in the early and curable stages. Elderly women are less able to withstand the rigors of radical surgery, are more prone to complications of treatment, and often experience exaggerated tissue responses to radiotherapy. It is critical that teaching and outreach be provided to this population of women about the ongoing importance of Pap smear screening for cancer.

## HOME CARE CONSIDERATIONS

Much of the diagnostic and conservative treatment for cervical cancer takes place in an outpatient environment. Even hospitalization for radiotherapy continues only for the duration of the implant placement. It is therefore critical that the woman be made an informed partner in her own care. Extensive teaching needs to be provided, with full understanding that the anxiety associated with the diagnosis of cancer and its treatment will make it difficult for the woman to hear and process much of the information. Repeat sessions and written reference materials are critical. Formal home care services are rarely used or needed, so the goal of knowledgeable self-care becomes even more critical. The woman's partner is included in teaching sessions if possible, since the disease and treatment have significant potential impact on the couple's patterns of sexuality, at least in the short term.

### Complications

The primary complications of cervical cancer and its treatment have been outlined in the discussion. The most significant is the risk of recurrence and metastasis. The diagnosis itself can complicate the woman's entire view concerning her body image, sexuality, and fertility. Implant therapy results in radiation menopause, which the woman must adjust to in addition to the treatments needed to keep the vagina supple enough for intercourse. Prolonged vaginal discharge does not promote an atmosphere conducive to a satisfactory sexual relationship. The woman will likely have ongoing problems with odor and drainage. Physical complications such as fistula formation, tissue fibrosis, and inflammatory bowel problems are readily addressed in discharge teaching, but the woman is frequently alone in her attempts to deal with the more subtle but overwhelming changes that result from the diagnosis of cancer.

## NEOPLASMS OF THE UTERUS

### Uterine Leiomyomas (Fibroids)

#### Etiology/Epidemiology

**Leiomyomas** (myomas) are benign tumors of muscle cell origin that contain varying amounts of fibrous tissue. They are the most common type of pelvic tumor and occur most often during the fifth decade of life. They occasionally are found in the fallopian tubes or round ligament, and approximately 5% originate from the cervix. Leiomyomas occur more frequently in African-American women, occurring in one of every two black women and one of every four white women.[14,25]

The etiology of leiomyomas is not completely understood. The stimulus for growth is unclear but is thought to be related to estrogen, since they are rare before menarche and often decrease in size after menopause. They often enlarge during pregnancy and with the use of oral contraceptives. Women who smoke tend to be relatively estrogen deficient and have been found to have a lower incidence of leiomyomas. The tumors can reach enormous proportions, weighing as much as 50 pounds. Malignant transformation is rare, estimated at less than 0.5% of myomas.[14,25]

#### Pathophysiology

Leiomyomas originate in the myometrium and are classified by the anatomic location (Figure 52-16). Submucous myomas lie just beneath the endometrium and compress it as they grow. They can develop a pedicle and protrude into the uterine cavity or even through the cervical canal. Intramural myomas lie within the uterine wall, and subserous tumors lie at the serosal surface of the uterus or may bulge outward from the myometrium. These external tumors also tend to become pedunculated.[44]

Most leiomyomas are asymptomatic even when large and may go undetected, particularly if the woman is obese. The development of symptoms depends on the location, size, and condition of the tumor. Menorrhagia is the most common symptom. Bleeding can result from distortion and congestion of surrounding vessels or ulceration of the overlying endometrium. It usually takes the form of premenstrual spotting or prolonged light bleeding after the menses. Metrorrhagia is associated with venous thrombosis or necrosis on the surface of the tumor, particularly if it extrudes through the cervix. The blood loss may be significant enough to create an iron deficiency anemia that does not respond to iron therapy.[44]

Pain is not a characteristic symptom, although it can result from tumor degeneration or with myometrial contractions that attempt to expel a subserous myoma from the uterus. If the pedicle stalk becomes twisted, pain may appear suddenly and be severe. Women often report a sensation of heaviness in the pelvis or a "bearing down" feeling, especially with large tumors. It may cause pelvic circulatory congestion and create backache, constipation, or dysmenorrhea. The woman even may notice an increase in abdominal girth.

Leiomyomas may interfere with fertility by blocking the opening of the fallopian tubes, inducing spontaneous abortion, or obstructing the cervical canal, making delivery hazardous. Sudden growth of a myoma after menopause is considered to be a classic sign of leiomyosarcoma, which necessitates hysterectomy.

Anemia is a common symptom of chronic blood loss, but women may also exhibit erythrocytosis. Although the etiology is unclear, it is speculated that compression of the ureters may increase ureteral back pressure and stimulate the production of erythropoietin by the kidneys.

#### Medical management

Myomas often can be detected by routine pelvic examination when the uterus is displaced or irregular nod-

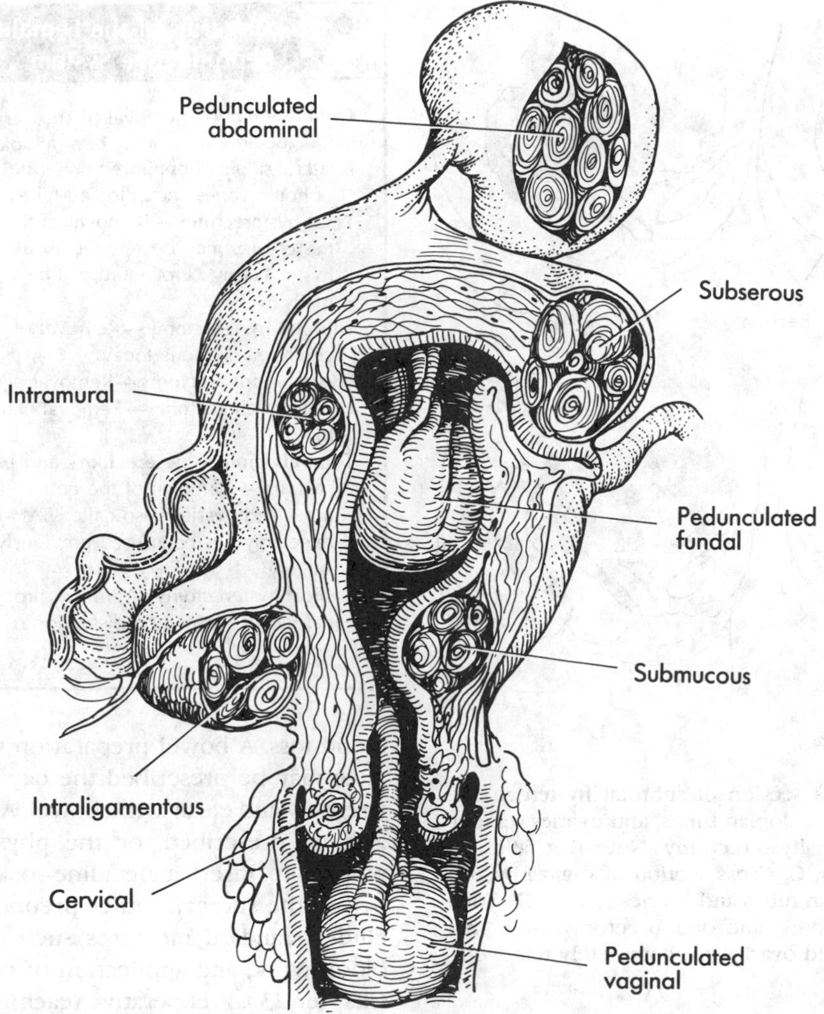


**FIGURE 52-16** Myomas of uterus.

ules are felt on the uterine surface. Diagnosis is confirmed through the use of x-ray films, pelvic sonography, IV urography, and hysterography or hysteroscopy. These tests establish the presence of the tumor(s), evaluate the degree of urologic compression, if any, and help to identify the presence of submucous myomas. Serial ultrasound may be used to monitor progression in size or evaluate response to treatment.

Small, asymptomatic myomas are simply monitored. The myomas tend to shrink as estrogen levels begin to decline. If a patient is symptomatic, a dilation and curettage (D & C) may be performed to take an endometrial biopsy to verify the diagnosis and rule out cancer. Submucous myomas may be resected via the cervical canal using the hysteroscope and laser therapy as an office procedure. Drug therapy may be used to reduce the levels of circulating estrogen. Depo-Provera, danazol, and gonadotropin-releasing hormone (GnRH) analogues have all been used in clinical trials. Results indicate that as many as 90% of patients will experience tumor reduction, but the myomas gradually return to pretreatment size with cessation of therapy. Drug treatment is successfully used in the perimenopausal period to avoid the need for hysterectomy. Some physicians prefer to use them to shrink the tumor size before surgery.[14]

Leiomyomas are one of the most common indications for hysterectomy.[14,25] The decision to undergo surgery largely depends on the woman's age, degree of symptom severity, and desire to preserve her childbearing ability. Occasionally, if the tumor is near the outer wall of the uterus, it may be removed while leaving the muscular walls of the uterus relatively intact.

### Nursing management

Most women are familiar with the term *fibroids* but have little real understanding of their development, treatment, or relationship with estrogen levels. Many women assume that hysterectomy is an inevitable necessity. Women receiving estrogen replacement therapy should understand the implications of continued estrogen stim-

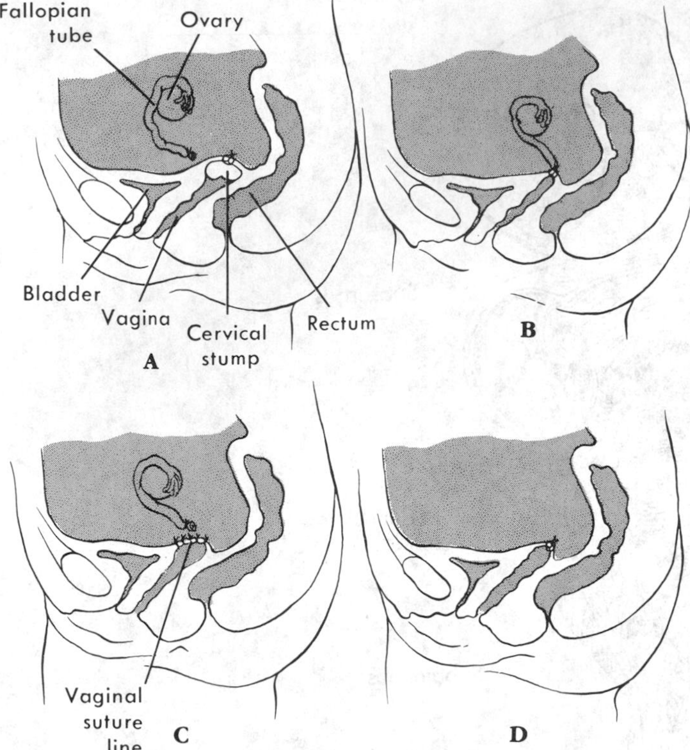


**FIGURE 52-17** **A,** Cross section of subtotal hysterectomy. Note that cervical stump, fallopian tubes, and ovaries remain. **B,** Cross section of total hysterectomy. Note that fallopian tubes and ovaries remain. **C,** Cross section of vaginal hysterectomy. Note that fallopian tubes and ovaries remain. **D,** Total hysterectomy, salpingectomy, and oophorectomy. Note that uterus, fallopian tubes, and ovaries are completely removed.

ulation on growth of the myomas. Follow-up care to monitor tumor growth is essential.

Some women experience discomfort during intercourse that may be alleviated by altering positions or using water-soluble lubricants. Local heat may be successful in relieving mild abdominal pain.

**BOX 52-5 Surgeries of the Female Reproductive System**

**Oophorectomy**—Removal of an ovary
**Salpingectomy**—Removal of a fallopian tube
**Bilateral salpingo-oophorectomy (BSO or Bil S&O)**—Removal of both ovaries and fallopian tubes
**Total hysterectomy**—Removal of the entire uterus, including the cervix; may be referred to as a TAH (total abdominal hysterectomy). Procedure can be done vaginally or abdominally.
**Subtotal hysterectomy**—Removal of the uterus except for the cervix; rarely done today
**Hystero-oophorectomy**—Removal of the uterus and an ovary
**Hysterosalpingectomy**—Removal of the uterus and a fallopian tube
**Total abdominal hysterectomy and bilateral salpingo-oophorectomy**—Removal of the entire uterus and both fallopian tubes and ovaries (also called TAH-BSO). The term *panhysterectomy* has been used previously to refer to this type of surgery.
**Radical hysterectomy** (Wertheim procedure)—TAH-BSO, partial vaginectomy, and dissection of the lymph nodes in the pelvis

## NURSING MANAGEMENT: The Patient Undergoing Hysterectomy

Hysterectomy is one of the most common surgical procedures and may be used as a treatment for a variety of reproductive tract problems, including cancer of the cervix, uterus, and ovaries; structural problems such as severe prolapse; and removal of leiomyomas, which is one of the most frequent causes. Several variations on the hysterectomy procedure differ in approach and complexity; these are illustrated in Figure 52-17. Terminology used to describe surgery of the female reproductive tract is summarized in Box 52-5. A hysterectomy may be performed vaginally or by an abdominal approach.[30]

### PREOPERATIVE CARE

Ferrous sulfate therapy may be initiated several weeks before surgery if the woman is anemic from chronic blood loss. A bowel preparation with an enema or laxative may be prescribed the day before the procedure to empty and cleanse the bowel. A Betadine douche may also be prescribed, or the physician may order the woman to insert a Betadine-soaked tampon 12 hours before the surgery. Other preoperative preparation includes standard measures such as nothing by mouth, blood work, and application of compression hose (see Chapter 23). Preoperative teaching is essential and usually is performed in the physician's office or by the preadmissions team. The nurse verifies that teaching has been provided and that the woman can accurately describe the planned surgery and associated care. Preoperative teaching is outlined in the Guidelines box, p. 1761.

### POSTOPERATIVE CARE

Much of the postoperative care provided after hysterectomy is the same as that provided after any major surgery (see Chapter 25). Unique aspects of care are addressed here.

#### Promoting Activity

Ambulation begins on the day of surgery or the first postoperative day, and the nurse encourages regular brief ambulation throughout the day. Ambulation supports oxygenation through natural deep breathing, assists in the prompt elimination of residual anesthetic, supports the return of peristalsis, and supports venous return. Venous pooling and pelvic congestion are concerns after hysterectomy because of the inflammatory response to the trauma of surgery. This is particularly important if the lithotomy position was used during surgery. The risk of thromboembolism is significant, and the physician may order subcutaneous heparin injec-

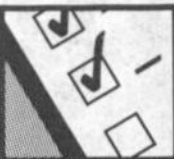

### Guidelines for Teaching the Person Undergoing Hysterectomy

Simple explanation of the anatomy of the female reproductive tract and the effects of hysterectomy on physiologic function
Explanation of events the day before and day of surgery: bowel cleansing, Betadine douche, skin scrub, preoperative medications, TED hose, length of time in surgery (depends on type of surgery being done), length of time until able to see family after surgery
Explanation of expected lines, tubes, and packing: IV lines for fluids, bladder catheter, nasogastric tube, wound drain, possible vaginal packing, compression stockings; dangling or ambulating the night of surgery or morning of the first postoperative day; leg and ankle exercises; use of incentive spirometer, deep breathing, position changes
Explanation of pain control: use of patient-controlled analgesia (PCA) or principles of PRN analgesic administration; principles of safe movement and wound splinting (if abdominal incision)
Explanation of diet: diet depends on the extent of surgery and return of bowel sounds; diet progresses from clear liquids toward a regular diet based on patient's response

tions. Routine measures include applying compression stockings, encouraging leg and foot flexion and extension exercises every 2 hours, and avoiding positioning the patient with the knees bent. Elevating the legs at intervals throughout the day may be helpful also. Routine monitoring for pain or swelling in the calf is included in the ongoing assessment.

## Supporting Urinary Elimination

Urinary problems are common after hysterectomy. The woman who undergoes vaginal hysterectomy may have a catheter left in place for 3 to 5 days to allow for a resolution of edema around the urethra. The catheter is typically removed on the first postoperative day after abdominal hysterectomy, but many women experience some difficulty in voiding spontaneously or emptying the bladder. Bladder problems may be particularly troublesome in elderly women who have weakened muscles and decreased sensitivity to the neurologic stimuli for voiding. Suppressed immune functioning also leaves them more vulnerable to infection.

A radical hysterectomy may leave the woman with some permanent bladder dysfunction. The catheter is left in place usually for 7 to 10 days and may be placed suprapubically. A self-catheterization routine may need to be taught to prevent overdistention and compensate for the overdistention of the detrusor muscle. This routine is followed until bladder sensations return and residual urine volumes are consistently less than 50 to 75 ml. An indwelling catheter is left in place for several weeks after surgery if the woman is incapable of managing self-catheterization. Bladder function rarely returns to normal, but most women are able to achieve satisfactory bladder function by the end of the first year.[42]

### Guidelines for Care of the Person Undergoing Hysterectomy

**PREOPERATIVE CARE**

Promote a stable emotional state and positive body image.
- Encourage expression of feelings and concerns.
- Provide teaching as outlined in the Guidelines box left.

Prevent infection.
- Give prescribed enemas, laxatives, and douches.
- Give or supervise prescribed skin preparation.
- Administer prescribed antibiotics.

Promote circulation and oxygenation.
- Apply antiembolic hose.
- Teach deep breathing, coughing, and use of incentive spirometer.
- Teach leg and feet exercises.

**POSTOPERATIVE CARE**

Promote comfort.
- Administer analgesics and antiemetics; assist with PCA use.
- Teach how to splint incision and change positions without putting strain on the abdomen.
- Provide frequent oral hygiene until taking oral fluids freely.

Promote circulation and oxygenation.
- Encourage turning, deep breathing, coughing, and use of incentive spirometer.
- Encourage leg and feet exercises every hour while in bed.
- Maintain use of antiembolic hose as ordered.
- Encourage frequent ambulation.
- Assess for signs of thromboembolism.
- Administer heparin as ordered.

Maintain fluid and electrolyte balance.
- Accurately record all output and drainage.
- Maintain prescribed IV fluids and encourage PO fluids when allowed.

Promote elimination.
- Maintain patency of bladder catheter.
- Teach catheter care or self-catheterization if bladder dysfunction is present.
- Monitor for signs of returning peristalsis.
- Encourage frequent ambulation.

Provide discharge teaching.
- Teach signs of urinary tract infection.
- Provide teaching regarding incision care and care of drains or catheter at home.
- Note that itching, burning, or numbness may be present around the healing incision.
- Teach diet modifications to prevent constipation.
- Encourage a daily fluid intake of 3000 ml.
- Instruct patient to avoid heavy lifting, prolonged sitting, and long car rides.
- Tell patient to refrain from coitus for about 6 weeks and not to douche unless prescribed by her physician. Vaginal bleeding or discharge may persist for up to 6 weeks.
- Help patient anticipate the occurrence of mood swings and emotional lability during healing. Emotional balance will gradually return.

A liberal fluid intake and monitoring for infection will be interventions the woman should follow permanently.

## Supporting Return of Peristalsis

Peristalsis is typically suppressed after hysterectomy, particularly if an abdominal approach with extensive handling of the GI organs has occurred. Gaseous disten-

# NURSING CARE PLAN

## WOMAN AFTER HYSTERECTOMY FOR CERVICAL CANCER

**DATA:** Mrs. Conn, age 42, saw her gynecologist 2 weeks ago because of bleeding between periods and occasional postcoital bleeding. The result of her Pap smear 5 years previously had been negative. The Pap smear this time was positive, and a cervical biopsy confirmed cancer of the cervix, Stage I. She was admitted yesterday for a total hysterectomy.

Admission notes indicate that Mrs. Conn is married and has two teenagers, a boy and a girl. Her husband accompanied her to the hospital and appeared to be supportive. Mrs. Conn is a bank teller and likes to read, knit, and watch TV. She has varicose veins but states these do not bother her. Her preoperative concerns centered mainly on the cancer: "I hope they get it all." She also stated, "Well, at least I hadn't planned any more children. My boy joked and said, 'You're going to be neutered like our cat was!' I wonder how it feels to be so-called neutered. I hope it won't affect my sex life." The nurse explored Mrs. Conn's knowledge of the surgery and explained that the surgery would not physically affect sexual relationships.

Mrs. Conn returned from the recovery room alert with an IV running and stable vital signs. The dressing was dry. She has morphine sulfate (MS) running per a patient-controlled analgesia (PCA) pump at 1 mg/hr with a bolus of 1 mg available every 8 minutes.

Nursing assessment includes monitoring the following activities:

- Vital signs
- Breath sounds
- Urine output
- Fluid intake
- Dressing checks
- Respiratory rate

### ■ NURSING DIAGNOSIS

Abdominal pain related to abdominal incision

| Expected Patient Outcome | Nursing Interventions | Rationale |
|---|---|---|
| States she is feeling more comfortable. | Maintain analgesic infusion so analgesics given on a regular basis for first 24 hours, then as necessary. | Giving the analgesic regularly will prevent severe pain and thus be more effective. |
| | Encourage frequent changes of position in bed and early ambulation. | Activity decreases pain by increasing circulation and reducing muscle tension; ambulation will also encourage peristalsis, decreasing possibility of gas pains. |

### ■ NURSING DIAGNOSIS

Potential body image disturbance related to loss of uterus and concern about personal sexuality

| Expected Patient Outcomes | Nursing Interventions | Rationale |
|---|---|---|
| Verbalizes concerns about loss of uterus. | Provide patient opportunities to express feelings and concerns about loss of uterus. Assess significant others' concerns and perceptions of body changes. | Patient may feel freer to talk about her feelings if opportunities are provided. Validates perceptions. Helps patient and significant other to ventilate doubts and resolve concerns. |
| | Provide factual information regarding anticipated bodily changes; include significant other if possible. | Provides accurate information and corrects misconceptions. |
| | Be empathetic about patient's feelings, which may include grief, guilt, shame, or remorse. | Feelings associated with grief may also be expressed when grieving over loss of a body part. |
| | Encourage her to continue activities associated with femininity, such as fixing hair, makeup, wearing own apparel. | Feelings of femininity will emphasize "feminine" rather than "neuter," and that she herself has not changed. |
| Makes plans for resuming her role. | Help her make plans for resumption of former activities. | If life pattern is not changed, her thoughts about her body changes may diminish. |

# NURSING CARE PLAN

## WOMAN AFTER HYSTERECTOMY FOR CERVICAL CANCER—cont'd

### ■ NURSING DIAGNOSIS

Potential constipation related to surgical manipulation of bowel, pain medication, and immobility

| Expected Patient Outcome | Nursing Interventions | Rationale |
|---|---|---|
| Stool is soft and formed. | Monitor stool characteristics and frequency. | Helps form basis of an effective treatment plan. |
| | Encourage ambulation q 4 hr. | Ambulation promotes peristalsis. |
| | Assess abdomen for presence of flatus. | Peristalsis may be decreased from handling of pelvic viscera; helps determine flatus buildup. |
| | Encourage oral fluids when permitted. | Hydration will promote a soft stool. |
| | Teach patient to avoid straining at stool. | Increases abdominal pain and can lead to hemorrhage. |

### ■ NURSING DIAGNOSIS

Altered patterns of urinary elimination related to loss of bladder tone; pain with muscle contraction; and discomfort from urinating position

| Expected Patient Outcome | Nursing Interventions | Rationale |
|---|---|---|
| Voids in sufficient quantities. | Monitor urine output until she voids sufficiently. | Handling of bladder during pelvic surgery may decrease bladder muscle tone, leading to urinary retention. (Mrs. Conn did not have an indwelling catheter.) Accurate I & O records detect inadequate emptying of bladder. |
| | Monitor for distention above symphysis pubis and for lower abdominal discomfort other than incisional pain, q 4 hr. | Detects bladder distention and degree of fullness. |
| | Encourage patient to void q 2 hr. | Promotes optimal bladder tone and prevents distention. |
| | Provide privacy during attempts to urinate. | Promotes elimination. |
| | Catheterize as ordered. | An overdistended bladder can cause atony, increased discomfort, and stress on internal sutures. |
| | Teach perineal care. | Helps to prevent urinary tract infections and promotes normal elimination. |

### ■ NURSING DIAGNOSIS

Altered peripheral tissue perfusion related to pelvic venous stasis from surgery

| Expected Patient Outcome | Nursing Interventions | Rationale |
|---|---|---|
| Normal circulation is present without development of thrombus, emboli, or leg or thigh pain. | Monitor for discomfort in legs/thighs or sudden dyspnea; assess for Homans' sign; check warmth, color, blanching of lower extremities q 8 hr. | Early detection will ensure early treatment of thrombophlebitis. |
| | Encourage patient to lie completely flat in bed for short periods q 4 hr for 24 hours, then q 4 hr until ambulating well. | Lying flat for periods of time will help blood return from the pelvic veins. |
| | Encourage leg exercises and frequent turning in bed until ambulating well. | Exercises promote venous return (muscle pumps). |

*Continued.*

## NURSING CARE PLAN

### WOMAN AFTER HYSTERECTOMY FOR CERVICAL CANCER—cont'd

| Expected Patient Outcome | Nursing Interventions | Rationale |
|---|---|---|
| | Avoid use of knee gatch or pillows under knees; encourage patient to keep knees flat when in bed; avoid high-Fowler's position. | Pressure on popliteal veins or sharp knee flexion may increase venous stasis. |
| | Provide antiembolic stockings and/or apply intermittent pneumatic compression stockings. | Antiembolic stockings help to prevent venous stasis. Mrs. Conn is at higher risk for thrombophlebitis because of varicose veins (sluggish circulation) and sedentary life pattern. |
| | Encourage ambulation. | Ambulation promotes venous return by contracting muscles to compress veins. |

#### ■ NURSING DIAGNOSIS

Knowledge deficit: self-care related to new needs from surgery

| Expected Patient Outcome | Nursing Interventions | Rationale |
|---|---|---|
| Describes self-care accurately. | Teach patient: | |
| | 1. When activities can be resumed (see text). | Activities are resumed gradually to permit healing; heavy activities are avoided for 6-8 weeks. |
| | 2. Signs of thrombophlebitis to be monitored and reported. | Thrombophlebitis may occur 7-10 days postoperatively, after patient goes home. |
| | 3. Signs of vaginal bleeding to be reported (excessive or persistent); possibility of slight vaginal discharge for 1-2 weeks. | Bleeding could indicate impaired healing. |
| | 4. Bathing and light activity permitted after hospital discharge. | |
| | 5. Avoid driving car for 2-4 weeks, especially with standard shift. | |
| | 6. Avoid heavy activity and active sports for 4-6 weeks. | |
| | 7. Need for medical follow-up. | To ensure that metastasis has not occurred and recovery is progressing. |
| | Include significant other if possible. | Promotes compliance with discharge teaching. |
| | Reinforce the preoperative explanations of the surgery and effect on sexual relationships; include significant other if possible. | Preoperative anxiety may have decreased her awareness; hysterectomy does not interfere with satisfactory sexual relationships. |
| | Find out what she has told her daughter about regular Pap smears. | Regular Pap smears enhance early detection of cervical cancer. |
| | Suggest she use support hose in her job as a bank teller. | Preventive measure for thrombophlebitis because of her varicose veins. |

tion is one of the most common and troublesome postoperative complaints. The woman typically receives nothing by mouth until there is some return of bowel sounds, and intravenous fluids are continued until she is taking oral fluids well. If problems do not develop, the patient moves quickly from a liquid to a regular diet. When paralytic ileus is severe, a nasogastric tube may be placed to relieve gaseous pressure. Frequent ambulation is encouraged as the most reliable means of supporting peristaltic activity. The woman's potassium level will be monitored to ensure that hypokalemia does not contribute to the ileus.

### Providing Emotional Support

Hysterectomy frequently is accompanied by some degree of emotional upset or ambivalence concerning the loss of reproductive ability, but this is not always the case. Many women are concerned about the effects of the surgery on femininity and sexuality. Postoperatively, almost all women experience some degree of depression or upset for several days and may be inexplicably tearful. Grieving for losses is both appropriate and important, and the nurse encourages the woman to deal honestly with her emotions. Family members need to be informed about these expected responses, and partners may need to be encouraged to offer the patient specific reassurance and understanding during this time. Women are instructed to avoid intercourse until the postoperative examination shows that the vaginal vault is satisfactorily healed. This usually takes about 6 weeks. Satisfactory sexual relations can then be reestablished, but many women need to adjust to changes in the nature of pelvic sensations and stimuli during sex.

The Guidelines box, p. 1761, summarizes the nursing care for the hysterectomy patient. A sample nursing care plan for the woman undergoing hysterectomy is found on pp. 1762-1764.

## Cancer of the Endometrium

### Etiology/Epidemiology

Cancer of the endometrium (uterine corpus) affects mainly older women and occurs most often in women between ages 50 and 64. Seventy-five percent of all endometrial cancers occur in postmenopausal women. The estimated annual incidence is 32,000 cases, with a mortality of 5600.[2] Multiple risk factors have been identified in addition to age. These include obesity, nulliparity, late menopause (after age 52), use of exogenous estrogens in estrogen replacement therapy (ERT), and diabetes.

### Pathophysiology

Uterine hyperplasia is somewhat analogous to dysplasia of the cervix. Some of the lesions revert to normal, some persist as hyperplasia, and a few progress to endometrial adenocarcinoma. Unfortunately, unlike cervical dysplasia, no reliable, frequently used screening method for endometrial hyperplasia exists. Most women with this condition are diagnosed because they seek medical care with symptoms of abnormal uterine bleeding. The diagnosis of endometrial hyperplasia can be made only in pathologic examination of uterine tissue.

The most common symptom associated with endometrial cancer is abnormal spotting and bleeding. Any postmenopausal woman with uterine bleeding should be evaluated for endometrial cancer. During menopause the symptoms may be mistaken for normal menopausal changes. With normal menopause, however, the periods should become lighter and farther apart. Any other pattern should be reported to the physician.[8] Other more vague symptoms include abdominal pain or pressure, nausea, and vomiting. These are late symptoms, however, and patients who have these symptoms and the subsequent diagnosis of uterine cancer usually have a history of abnormal bleeding.

### Medical management

Cancer of the endometrium is a slow-growing form of cancer and is very amenable to treatment if detected early. Women in high-risk categories may have endometrial tissue samples taken periodically. Tissue samples may be acquired in a variety of ways using outpatient facilities. Table 52-8 outlines some of the common methods and their relative effectiveness in diagnosing endometrial cancer.

Endometrial cancer is treated according to its stage. Table 52-9 outlines the staging criteria. The most common treatment is total abdominal hysterectomy with bilateral salpingo-oophorectomy (TAH/BSO). Radiation and surgery often are combined to treat early-stage disease. In high-risk stage I disease, patients often receive postoperative radiation, whereas in more advanced stages the radiation may be given preoperatively to shrink the tumor and reduce the risk of local infection.[20] Radiotherapy will be used as a primary modality if the woman is a poor risk for surgery or refuses surgery.

Hormonal therapy and chemotherapy often are added for stage III or IV disease. Progestins have been successfully used for years. They may be administered in a daily oral dose or a weekly intramuscular injection. Chemotherapy with doxorubicin, cyclophosphamide, and cisplatin, individually or in combination, has had more mixed results.

### Nursing management

The nursing care associated with hysterectomy and radiotherapy has been discussed previously. Nurses play a major role in promoting the importance of careful evaluation of all dysfunctional uterine bleeding in the postmenopausal population. This single factor is the most important route to identification of endometrial cancer in a treatable stage.

**TABLE 52-8 Methods for Detection of Endometrial Cancer**

| METHOD | EFFECTIVENESS (%) |
|---|---|
| Endometrial aspirations | 70-80 |
| Endometrial washings | 80-90 |
| Dilation and curettage (fractional) | 85-90 |
| Pap smear | 45-50 |
| Combination of above | 90 |

**TABLE 52-9 Stages of Cancer of the Endometrium**

| STAGE | INVOLVEMENT |
|---|---|
| I | Confined to corpus |
| II | Involves corpus and cervix |
| III | Extends outside corpus but not outside pelvis (vaginal wall but not bladder or rectum) |
| IV | Involves bladder, rectum, or outside pelvis |

## Gestational Trophoblastic Neoplasia

### Etiology/epidemiology

**Gestational trophoblastic neoplasia (GTN)** is the term used to describe choriocarcinoma and related diseases such as hydatidiform mole and invasive mole. GTN is extremely sensitive to chemotherapy and considered to be one of the most curable gynecologic malignancies. The etiology of GTN is not thoroughly understood. The hydatidiform mole precedes malignant disease in approximately 50% of patients. There is an antecedent normal pregnancy or abortion in the other 50%.[14]

The risk of hydatidiform mole varies significantly in different regions of the world, being 10 times more prevalent in the Far East than the United States. Both nutrition and socioeconomic factors have been correlated. Risk factors for molar pregnancy include age (under 20 and over 40) and geographic residence in Mexico or southeast Asia. Choriocarcinoma risk factors are similar.[14]

### Pathophysiology

GTN is an abnormal pregnancy characterized by a degeneration, or abnormal growth, of the trophoblastic tissue of the placenta, usually in the absence of an intact fetus. GTN produces a serum marker, human chorionic gonadotropin (HCG), whose levels are directly related to the number of tumor cells.

Early stages of GTN may be similar to normal pregnancy. As the disease progresses, most women experience uterine bleeding. Uterine growth more rapid than appropriate for gestational age occurs, often accompanied by nausea and vomiting.

### Medical management

The diagnosis of GTN usually is accomplished by ultrasonography, amniography, and analysis of HCG levels. Other diagnostic tests may be employed to rule out the presence of metastasis.

Suction curettage is the most common method used for evacuation of a molar pregnancy, although hysterectomy may be selected if the woman does not desire future pregnancies. Intravenous oxytocin may be used to assist in expulsion of tissue, which is then sent for extensive pathologic analysis. HCG titers are then monitored after treatment to assess for recurrence. The woman is advised to prevent pregnancy for at least a year, since pregnancy will cause a rise in HCG levels.[8] Chemotherapy is used in the treatment of recurrent or persistent disease. A 100% cure rate can be expected with low-risk nonmetastatic disease, and even patients with high-risk GTN are successfully treated in more than 70% of cases.

### Nursing management

Nursing care of the woman undergoing hysterectomy has been discussed previously. It is essential to address the social and emotional impact of the disease process in the overall plan of care. Patient and family teaching should include an understanding of the disease process, implications for future pregnancies, the effect of chemotherapy on future children, and the need for effective contraception during the first year after diagnosis.

# NEOPLASMS OF THE OVARIES

## Ovarian Cysts

### Etiology/Epidemiology

Many types of benign tumors affect the ovaries; 80% are classified in the epithelial group comprising serous, mucinous, endometrial, and mesonephroid lesions. These tumors are composed of supporting connective

**BOX 52-6 Characteristics of Various Types of Benign Ovarian Cysts and Tumors**

**FOLLICULAR CYSTS**

Most frequent form of cysts
Frequently multiple; range in size from a few millimeters to as large as 15 cm in diameter
Depend on gonadotropin for growth
Occur during menstrual years and usually resolve spontaneously
May cause menstrual irregularities if blood estrogen elevated

**CORPUS LUTEUM CYSTS**

Less common variety
Associated with normal ovarian function or elevated progesterone
Average diameter 4 cm
May appear purplish red from bleeding within corpus luteum
May cause delayed menstrual bleeding from progesterone secretion; menorrhagia common

**THECA LUTEIN CYSTS**

Least common variety
Usually bilateral and produce significant ovarian enlargement, up to 30 cm in diameters
Develop from prolonged or excessive stimulation by gonadotropins
Associated with hydatidiform mole 50% of the time and choriocarcinomas 10% of the time

**SEROUS TUMORS**

Found in all age-groups
Can be extremely large, filling pelvis or abdomen

**MUCINOUS TUMORS**

Occur in second to third decade of life
May be bilateral
Can reach spectacular size; largest form

**ENDOMETROID TUMORS**

Small lesions, purplish blue in color
Large tumors called "chocolate cysts" because they contain brownish fluid
Very low malignancy potential

**MESONEPHROID TUMORS**

Usually multifocal
Involve peritoneal surfaces and may cause intestinal or urinary tract complications
Characterized by papillary proliferations without mitotic activity

tissue and ovarian stroma but also have the capacity to alter the woman's hormonal status. In addition, both simple cysts and nonneoplastic cysts originating in the graafian follicle may occur. Nearly 80% of ovarian tumors are discovered during routine pelvic examination and are asymptomatic. Women between ages 45 and 60 are at greatest risk. Each of the various tumor types tends to affect a different age-group and behave in a different way.

#### Pathophysiology

Benign cysts and tumors may develop from a variety of physiologic imbalances. Elevated levels of luteinizing hormone may cause hyperstimulation of the ovaries. Follicular cysts depend on gonadotropins for growth and generally occur during the menstrual years and resolve spontaneously. Simple cysts occur frequently during menopause. Box 52-6 summarizes the characteristics of various common types of ovarian cysts and tumors.

Most ovarian tumors are asymptomatic for long periods or produce only nonspecific symptoms. Menstrual irregularities may be present when hormonal imbalance exists.[14] Dull, unilateral, lower quadrant pain may occur, especially as the cysts grow in size. Ascites and increasing abdominal girth have been reported in slender women. Complaints of fatigue or a sense of heaviness in the pelvis also may occur. Overt pain is an unusual symptom. Large tumors may cause symptoms of pelvic pressure, such as urinary frequency and constipation.

#### Medical management

Palpation of the reproductive organs during pelvic examination can usually detect any mass or enlargement of the ovary. Any mass palpated in a postmenopausal woman requires further investigation, since the ovaries normally atrophy after menopause. Ultrasonography may be employed to distinguish functional from neoplastic cysts. CT scans are capable of distinguishing solid tumors, cysts, and ascites, but laparoscopy may be performed to confirm the diagnosis.

Many ovarian cysts resolve spontaneously. If the cyst does not decrease in size, oral contraceptives may be prescribed to shrink it. Surgery is usually recommended only when the cyst is larger than 8 cm or occurs after menopause or before puberty. A cystectomy rather than oophorectomy will be performed if possible.

#### Nursing management

Because most ovarian cysts are diagnosed incidentally, minimal intervention is needed. The woman should be reminded of the importance of follow-up care to continue to monitor the tumor's size. Most women are extremely anxious concerning the effects of the tumor on fertility and should be reassured that even oophorectomy does not interrupt childbearing potential as long as the second ovary is healthy. If a laparotomy is performed, the woman will receive standard postoperative care. If both ovaries are removed, the woman will experience surgical menopause and will need to receive estrogen replacement therapy (see Chapter 11).

### Cancer of the Ovary

#### Etiology/Epidemiology

Malignant neoplasms of the ovaries occur at all ages, including infancy and childhood. It is estimated that one of every 70 women will develop ovarian cancer during her lifetime. Overall, about 21,000 new cases are diagnosed each year, and 13,000 deaths are attributed to the disease.[21] It accounts for only 4% of all cancers among women but is the most deadly form of reproductive cancer.[2] The risk of ovarian cancer increases after age 40 and peaks between 50 and 60.

The etiology of ovarian cancer is not understood, but several factors have been identified that appear to affect its incidence. Hereditary, endocrine, environmental, and dietary factors and viral agents have all been implicated. Those at highest risk appear to be middle-class and upper-class women, nulliparous women, and women who have not used oral contraceptives.[4,20] Early age at first pregnancy, early menopause, and the use of oral contraceptives appear to have a protective effect. If a woman has had breast cancer, her chances of developing ovarian cancer double.[2] The rates are high in industrialized areas, which points to environmental influences. Exposure to talc and asbestos, diets high in meat and animal fat, and high milk consumption all appear to be linked to a higher incidence. The fat content of the milk appears to be the key.[20,23] A slight familial link has been found, and unusual patterns of clusters of breast and ovarian cancers in family groups have been identified.[20]

The survival rate is 87% when the disease is diagnosed and treated early, but only about 23% of cases are detected in localized stages. Survival rates for women with regional and distant metastases are 39% and 19%, respectively.[2]

#### Pathophysiology

Ovarian cancer is a broad term that can be divided into many categories depending on the cell type of origin. The major histologic types occur in distinctive age ranges. The four main types are described in Table 52-10. Malignant germ cell tumors are most common in women under age 20, whereas epithelial cancers are primarily seen in women over 50.

**TABLE 52-10 Classification of Ovarian Neoplasms**

| SOURCE OF NEOPLASM | EXAMPLES |
|---|---|
| Epithelium | Serous, mucinous, endometroid |
| Germ cell | Teratoma (mature and immature), dysgerminoma |
| Gonadal stroma | Granulosa (theca, Sertoli's, Leydig's cells) |
| Mesenchyme | Fibroma, lymphoma, sarcoma |

The clinical manifestations of advancing disease include pelvic discomfort, low back pain, weight change, abdominal pain, nausea and vomiting, constipation, and urinary frequency. Any ovarian enlargement should be evaluated for malignancy. Palpable ovaries in premenarchal or postmenopausal women are abnormal physical findings.

#### Medical management

The early diagnosis of an ovarian neoplasm is usually by chance rather than successful screening. No useful screening test exists at present for routine use. Even ultrasonography, CT scanning, and MRI are not sufficiently specific to distinguish between benign and malignant tumors, although the use of transvaginal ultrasonography may allow for recognition of early malignancies through increased vascularity.[20] A tumor marker called CA-125 is produced by tissues derived from the coelomic epithelium. About 80% of epithelial tumors produce the marker, but since other tumors also produce the marker and false negatives are also common, the test is not specific enough to be diagnostic.[4] A variety of other tests may be employed in the search for metastasis.

**Laparotomy** is the primary tool of both diagnosis and staging. Ovarian cancer is *surgically* staged rather than clinically staged; Table 52-11 presents the staging system. Surgery is the primary therapeutic approach and usually involves total abdominal hysterectomy with bilateral salpingectomy-oophorectomy. Ascitic fluid or washings are submitted for cytology. All the tissue of the pelvis is carefully assessed, and biopsies of any suspicious tissue are sent for analysis.

Adjuvant therapy is often employed in addition to surgery. The specific approach is guided by the stage of the disease. Chemotherapy is typically used for stage I disease. Patients with stage II disease may be treated with instillation of radioactive phosphorus (32-P) into the peritoneum, external irradiation, or combined chemotherapy. Patients with stages III and IV disease undergo surgical attempts to remove as much tumor as possible. This intervention appears to be directly related to survival. Surgery is followed by aggressive combination chemotherapy. Various combinations of agents are under investigation.

**TABLE 52-11 Stages of Cancer of the Ovary**

| STAGE | INVOLVEMENT |
|---|---|
| I | Limited to ovaries |
| II | Involving one or both ovaries with pelvic extension |
| III | Involving one or both ovaries with intraperitoneal metastasis outside pelvis or positive lymph nodes |
| IV | Involving one or both ovaries with distant metastasis (e.g., liver, lungs) |

#### Nursing management

The nursing care for a patient undergoing surgical treatment for ovarian cancer is similar to that required after any major abdominal surgery. Patient teaching concerning the diagnosis, surgery, and adjuvant therapy for ovarian cancer is an integral aspect of nursing care. Support and education are offered to the patient and family throughout each aspect of diagnosis and treatment.

## NEOPLASMS OF THE VULVA

### Cancer of the Vulva

#### Etiology/Epidemiology

The incidence of carcinoma of the vulva in situ is 0.7 per 100,000 women and that of invasive carcinoma is 1.9 per 100,000. Preinvasive disease occurs primarily in women of reproductive age, whereas invasive disease is predominantly a disease of the elderly.[20] Three times as many whites are affected as blacks. Parity does not seem to play a role in the incidence.

The exact etiology of cancer of the vulva is still unknown. Etiologic factors are believed to include venereal lesions of the vulva, the use of tight-fitting apparel or nylon undergarments, perineal deodorants, and trauma. Herpes, syphilis, and other lesions have all been associated with the development of carcinoma. Immunosuppression, diabetes, and hypertension also have been linked, but the cause-and-effect relationship has not been established.[20]

#### Pathophysiology

Most cancers of the vulva are squamous in origin (90%). The initial lesion often arises from an area of intraepithelial neoplasia, which can eventually form a firm nodule that can ulcerate.[8] The diagnosis of vulvar cancer can be made only by biopsy and histologic tissue examination.

The lesion can develop anywhere on the vulva, but 70% of them arise on the labia. The lesion is usually localized and well demarcated. Common clinical manifestations include vulvar itching and burning.

#### Medical management

Treatment of carcinoma of the vulva varies significantly based on the location and extent of the disease. Preinvasive disease is usually treated surgically, although colposcopy-guided laser therapy may be used in some patients.[20,42] Carcinoma in situ may also be treated nonsurgically with topical 5-fluorouracil (1% Efudex) applied daily, but long-term results are unknown. The standard treatment for invasive carcinoma has been radical **vulvectomy,** which involves excision of the mons pubis, terminal portion of the urethra and vagina, excision of portions of the round ligaments and saphenous veins, and selected lymph node dissection (Figure 52-18). Radical surgery achieves a 70% to 80% 5-year survival rate. Radiation treatment for advanced disease is being researched. Chemotherapy has not proved useful.

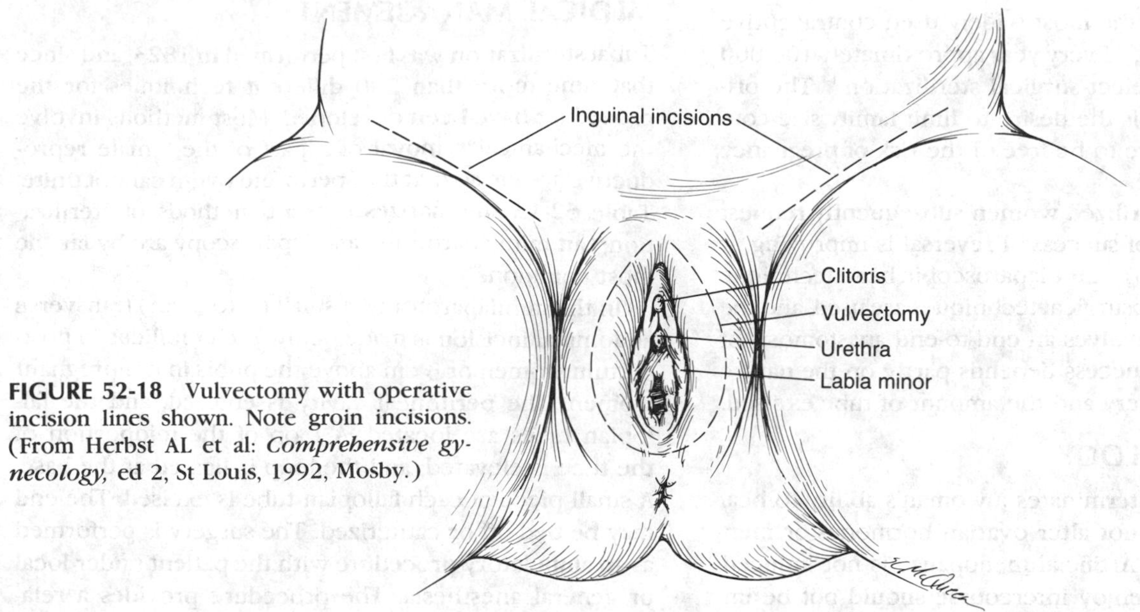

**FIGURE 52-18** Vulvectomy with operative incision lines shown. Note groin incisions. (From Herbst AL et al: *Comprehensive gynecology,* ed 2, St Louis, 1992, Mosby.)

Complications related to radical vulvectomy include wound infection and disruption because the wounds are typically left open to heal by secondary intention. Delayed complications include stenosis of the vagina from scar tissue formation, pelvic muscle relaxation leading to stress incontinence, and swelling of the legs from obstructive lymphangitis.

### Nursing management

Preoperative care focuses on careful teaching and patient support. Physical care addresses a bowel preparation and insertion of a Foley catheter.

Comfort is a major issue in the early postoperative period. Because of the widespread tissue destruction, the inguinal suture line is very tight and extremely uncomfortable. The woman will need much assistance to achieve comfortable positioning. Wound breakdown is often a problem. The vulvar wound usually is left open. Sitz baths, whirlpool therapy, and topical agents may be used to support healing. Despite meticulous care, the wounds heal very slowly. Privacy should be ensured, and the nurse encourages the woman to express her feelings concerning this disfiguring surgery. The nurse reassures the woman that sexual intercourse usually can be resumed after complete wound healing has occurred—usually 4 to 6 weeks.[7] The lymphedema of the legs is treated with compression stockings for at least 6 months after surgery. The Guidelines box, at right, summarizes nursing care for patients experiencing radical vulvectomy.

## STERILIZATION

### ETIOLOGY/EPIDEMIOLOGY

Voluntary sterilization is the most frequently used method of fertility control for married couples over 30

#### Guidelines for Care of the Person Undergoing Radical Vulvectomy

**PREOPERATIVE CARE**

Explain treatment and plan of care.
Explain about compression stockings and begin heparin therapy.
Administer enemas and douches as prescribed.
Provide emotional support.
Teach how to logroll.
Teach deep breathing exercises and feet exercises.

**POSTOPERATIVE CARE**

Maintain bedrest for 72 hours in semi-Fowler's position.
Support legs with pillows.
Avoid stress on suture lines.
Maintain patency of Foley catheter.
Provide low-residue diet.
Turn every 2 hours.
Assess discomfort level and administer analgesics.
Cleanse wound bid and after defecation.
Assess for pulmonary emboli and deep vein thrombosis.
Provide perineal hygiene and give sitz baths when ordered; keep perineum dry.
Provide diversional activities.
Encourage expression of feelings.

**DISCHARGE TEACHING**

Use support hose for 6 months; elevate legs frequently.
Can resume sexual activity in 4 to 6 weeks.
Discuss possible need for lubrication and position changes with coitus; genital numbness may be present.
Avoid straining with defecation.
Discuss signs and symptoms to report to physician.
Note the possible altered directional flow of urine.

years of age and is the most widely used contraceptive method worldwide.[12] Every year approximately 100,000 American women elect surgical sterilization.[14] The primary reason given is the desire to limit family size coupled with the desire to be free of the risk of pregnancy with advancing age.

About 1% of sterilized women subsequently request reversal. The rate of successful reversal is improving. It is approximately 75% after laparoscopic band technique procedures.[14] Microsurgical techniques are used, and the surgery typically involves an end-to-end anastomosis of the ligated tubes. Success depends partly on the nature of the original surgery and the amount of tube excised.

## PATHOPHYSIOLOGY

Tubal sterilization terminates a woman's ability to bear children but does not alter ovarian hormones or menstrual functioning. Artificial menopause is not induced, and the ability to enjoy intercourse should not be impaired. Women appear to have little regret after the surgery if they understand what to expect during and after the procedure and are able to express their feelings and have their questions answered before surgery. Occasionally, however, women who are ambivalent about the choice or have preexisting self-esteem issues develop psychologic problems after sterilization.

**TABLE 52-12 Methods of Tubal Sterilization for Women**

| DESCRIPTION | COMMENTS |
|---|---|
| **ABDOMINAL** | |
| **Minilaparotomy** | |
| Ligation or cutting of fallopian tubes under direct vision through small abdominal incision | Local or general anesthesia<br>Complications: wound infection, hematoma, bladder injury<br>Advantages: good chance for sterility reversal |
| **Laparoscopy** | |
| Electrocoagulation of segment of fallopian tubes by laparoscopy through small abdominal incision | Local or general anesthesia<br>Advantages: minimal discomfort, short procedure |
| **VAGINAL** | |
| **Culpotomy** | |
| Ligation or cutting of fallopian tube through small incision in cul-de-sac of Douglas | Local, spinal, or general anesthesia<br>Higher complication rate than laparoscopy (infection, hemorrhage) |
| **Culdoscopy** | |
| Electrocoagulation of segment of fallopian tubes by culdoscope through small incision in cul-de-sac of Douglas | Local anesthesia<br>Higher complication rate than laparoscopy |

## MEDICAL MANAGEMENT

Tubal sterilization was first performed in 1823, and since that time more than 200 different techniques for the procedure have been developed. Most methods involve the mechanical removal of a part of the female reproductive system so that the sperm and ovum cannot unite. Table 52-12 summarizes current methods of sterilization, but minilaparotomy and laparoscopy are by far the most common.[29]

In the minilaparotomy, a small (2 to 3 cm) transverse abdominal incision is made below the umbilicus in postpartum women or 3 cm above the pubis in nonpregnant women. The peritoneal cavity is entered, and the fallopian tubes are located. A loop of the midportion of the tube is elevated, and the loop is ligated at the base. A small piece of each fallopian tube is excised. The end may be tied off or cauterized. The surgery is performed as an ambulatory procedure with the patient under local or general anesthesia. The procedure provides a relatively good chance of success for reanastomosis if sterilization reversal is requested in the future.

Laparoscopic tubal sterilization is more frequently performed and requires only a small subumbilical incision for insertion of the laparoscope. A segment of each tube is grasped with the forceps, and an electric current is passed through the forceps to bring about coagulation of the tissues. Clips or rings may also be applied to the tube. The procedure is brief and safe and can be performed with the patient under local anesthesia. Sterilization is often performed in the postpartum period when the fallopian tubes have not descended back into the pelvis and are readily accessible.

The laws governing sterilization vary from state to state and have undergone many changes over the years. In general, the surgery may be performed if written, informed consent is given by a woman capable of giving

**BOX 52-7 Informed Consent Guidelines (Federal) Relating to Sterilization**

1. Choice is made by patient. No pressures are placed on choice (e.g., loss of welfare benefits, wrath of health care provider).
2. Benefits and risks of sterilization are described:
   a. Benefits: permanent, no further costs or decision making
   b. Risks: usual surgical risks, possibility of future pregnancy (i.e., not 100% effective)
3. Alternative contraceptive methods are described.
4. Patient is encouraged to ask questions.
5. Patient may withdraw from using the method without penalty.
6. Explanations are given about the entire sterilization procedure, costs, and possible side effects (effects of hormones, weight changes, menstrual changes, sexual response).
7. Written instructions and risk factors are given to patient.
8. A written consent to the procedure is signed by patient and witnessed.

permission. Patients using federal funds for payment must be at least 21 years of age, and there may be a prescribed waiting period for patients using Medicaid funds.

## NURSING MANAGEMENT

Patient teaching as the basis for true informed consent is the foundation of nursing care. The discussion of sterilization methods should be based on the federal government's informed consent guidelines (Box 52-7). The nurse confirms that the woman understands the nature and consequences of the surgical procedure. The facts concerning reversibility, including current success rate, are discussed. Lay people often equate sterilization with a loss of femininity, and even women who know the difference frequently appreciate reassurance.

Visual aids and models can be of great value in patient education. Films such as *Freedom from Pregnancy,** *Sterilization by Laparoscopy,*† and *Tubal Ligation*† and pamphlets such as *Voluntary Sterilization for Men and Women*‡ can be helpful in increasing the patient's understanding.

Postoperatively, women who have had tubal sterilization can be discharged when the effects of anesthesia have dissipated and vital signs are stable. The woman is instructed to rest for 24 to 48 hours after the procedure and avoid all heavy lifting and strenuous exercise for a week. She is instructed to abstain from sexual intercourse for 1 week if a vaginal approach was used or until the wound is completely healed if an abdominal approach was used. Women are instructed to report any signs of fever, incisional bleeding, or persistent abdominal pain to the physician. (Care of the woman after a laparoscopic procedure is discussed in Chapter 51.)

# INFERTILITY

The term **infertility** refers to the inability to achieve a pregnancy within a stipulated period of time, usually a year. The problem may be considered *primary* if the couple has never conceived or *secondary* if conception was successfully achieved in the past.

## ETIOLOGY/EPIDEMIOLOGY

It has been estimated that 10% to 15% of all couples in the United States are infertile. This represents about 10 million persons.[14] Approximately 50% of the couples who undergo assessment and treatment for infertility are likely to conceive. Infertility is most often attributed to women, but about 40% of cases result from male infertility and 20% from a combination of the partners.

The fertility of a couple is influenced by four major factors: the frequency of coitus, duration of exposure to pregnancy, and the ages of the two partners. From 80% to 90% of women will become pregnant within 1 year if they practice unprotected intercourse. Increased frequency of intercourse increases fertility by enhancing sperm motility through frequent ejaculation, unless available sperm are depleted. Fertility in women is low during the early teenage years, peaks in the mid 20s, and declines after age 30. The risk of infertility is doubled for women 35 to 44 years of age as compared with younger women, and approximately 33% of women who delay pregnancy until they are over 35 will have an infertility problem.[14] The infertility rate exceeds 60% in women over 40. Fertility reaches its peak in men in the mid 20s and subsequently declines, but the decrease is much less significant than in women. The age of men younger than 60 has little impact on conception.

There are many causes of infertility (Box 52-8). Some are treatable or preventable, and others are not. The most significant factors include failure to ovulate, tubal pathology, cervical factors, and STDs. No cause can be found in 10% to 20% of infertile women.[14]

## PATHOPHYSIOLOGY

Structural defects of the reproductive organs, previous infections, genetic abnormalities, and immunologic aberrations can all cause infertility in the female. Ovulatory

**BOX 52-8 Causes of Infertility**

**FEMALE**

1. Developmental: uterine abnormalities
2. Endocrine: pituitary, thyroid, and adrenal dysfunctions, ovarian dysfunctions (inhibit maturation and release of ova)
3. Diseases: PID (especially from gonococcus, fallopian tube obstructions, diseases of cervix and uterus that inhibit passage of active sperm)
4. Other: malnutrition, severe anemia, anxiety

**MALE**

1. Developmental: undescended testes, other congenital anomalies (inhibit development of sperm)
2. Endocrine: hormonal deficiencies (pituitary, thyroid, adrenal) (inhibit development of sperm)
3. Diseases: testicular destruction from disease, orchitis from mumps, prostatitis
4. Other: excessive smoking, fatigue, alcohol

**BOTH FEMALE AND MALE**

1. Diseases: STDs, cancer-causing obstructions (inhibit transport of ovum or sperm)
2. Other: immunologic incompatibility (inhibit sperm penetration of ovum), marital problems
3. Diethylstilbestrol exposure in utero (suggested but not proved as a cause of male infertility)

*Allend'or Productions, Inc., 3449 Cahuenga West, Hollywood, CA 90068

†Milner Fenwick, Inc., 3800 Liberty Heights Ave., Baltimore, MD 21215

‡Planned Parenthood World Population, 810 Seventh Ave., New York, NY 10019

dysfunction is a leading cause of infertility and can result from a malfunction at any point in the hormonal feedback system. Pelvic causes include a history of pelvic infections, use of IUDs, and endometriosis. Complete blockage of the fallopian tube is usually the result of salpingitis of gonorrheal origin.[41]

Infection may destroy the glands that secrete the thin, watery mucus that is beneficial to sperm survival and migration. Estrogen deficiency may decrease the volume and quality of the mucus. Malposition of the uterus may prevent the cervix from being exposed to the seminal pool when the woman is in a recumbent position. Anomalies of the uterus, including the presence of leiomyomas, may interfere with successful implantation.[43]

A number of studies have been conducted recently that suggest tobacco may be a causal factor in infertility. The pathologic action appears to be nicotine's effect on tubal transport and implantation. *Mycoplasma,* which causes cervicitis, may contribute to infertility, and the role of viruses is under investigation. Dietary deficiencies are known to adversely affect secretion of pituitary gonadotropins, and strenuous exercise such as running more than 10 miles per week has been implicated in causing infertility, either through its caloric demands or the effects of endorphins on the pituitary.[41]

Infertility can also produce profound psychologic effects. When couples find themselves unable to have children, the trauma can affect every aspect of their lives and marriage. The experience of diagnosis and treatment can be an emotional roller coaster of raised expectations and dashed hopes.

## MEDICAL MANAGEMENT

The purposes of an infertility evaluation are to establish the cause of infertility and provide a basis for determining medical or surgical treatment options. The process can be physically painful, as well as emotionally and economically stressful. The various diagnostic tests used in the diagnosis of infertility are discussed in Chapter 51 and summarized in Table 52-13.

**TABLE 52-13 Examination for Infertility**

| GENDER | TESTS | DATA OBTAINED |
|---|---|---|
| Male | Multiple semen examination | Determine presence, number, and motility of sperm |
| | Testicular biopsy if sperm count low or absent | Presence of sperm indicates obstruction of vas deferens |
| Female | Basal body temperature chart | Determine that ovulation is occurring |
| | Postcoital test of cervical secretions | Measure ability of sperm to penetrate cervical mucus and remain active; determine quality of mucus |
| | Endometrial biopsy, serum progesterone and estradiol levels, laparoscopic inspection of ovaries | Determine whether ovulation is occurring (if in question) |
| | Laparoscopy | Determine patency of fallopian tubes |
| | Hysterosalpingography (x-ray film after insertion of contrast media) | Determine patency of uterus and fallopian tubes |
| Male/female | Hormonal tests | Determine whether problem is hormonal |

The correction of structural problems is undertaken first if feasible. This may include treatment for endometriosis or uterine fibroids. **Transcervical balloon tuboplasty (TBT)** may be attempted to correct blocked or scarred fallopian tubes. A modified cardiovascular balloon is passed into the fallopian tube and inflated to clear the occlusion.

A variety of drugs may be used to induce or support ovulation. Clomiphene citrate (Clomid, Serophene) is the primary drug used for ovulation induction in women with intact pituitary function. Pergonal and Metrodin are indicated when patients have pituitary dysfunction. HCG may be used to trigger the release of mature follicles, and progesterone preparations may be used for luteal phase support.[11] The drugs may be used in various combinations. The woman is closely monitored with ultrasonograms and measurements of serum estradiol and urinary luteinizing hormone. The protocols are often confusing, time consuming, and expensive.

Multiple births can occur with ovulatory induction therapy. The onset of low abdominal pain can indicate the development of an ovarian cyst or cyst rupture. Basal body temperature is recorded to determine when ovulation has occurred. The woman is informed of the multiple drug side effects, which include hot flashes, emotional lability and depression, fatigue, nausea, and bloating.

When traditional drug therapy has failed, it may be combined with intrauterine insemination (IUI). This combined approach has achieved a success rate comparable to that of in vitro fertilization, approximately 20%.[6]

Artificial insemination is a simple, safe, inexpensive, and highly successful treatment whose major indication is male infertility. Semen may be deposited by a cervical-vaginal route, intracervically, or intrauterine. A few drops of semen are injected as close to the time of ovulation as possible. It may be homologous and use the partner's semen or heterologous when donor semen is used. Donor selection is a very important part of the procedure and is based on semen analysis, history and physical examination, and physical characteristics if that is important to the couple. The fertility of donors is carefully determined, and the sperm are screened for

**BOX 52-9 Alternative Approaches to Infertility Management**

**IN VITRO FERTILIZATION AND EMBRYO TRANSFER**

One or more ova are recovered from the ovarian follicles and fertilized with the partner's sperm in a Petri dish. Oocyte retrieval is performed by means of ultrasound-guided needle aspiration. The cleaved ova are placed in the patient's uterus through a small catheter about 48 hours after retrieval.[12] Pregnancy rates are related to the number of embryos placed and vary from 18% to 30%.[14]

**GAMETE INTRAFALLOPIAN TRANSFER**

Oocytes aspirated from follicles are mixed with washed sperm and placed in the uterine tube via laparoscopy. This approach appears to achieve a higher pregnancy rate than in vitro fertilization. The preembryo travels toward the uterus, following the natural timetable for implantation in 4 days.[28]

**SURROGATE MOTHERS**

Surrogate mothers are women who contract to conceive by artificial insemination and give the baby to the semen donor after delivery. Many social and legal implications with the process have received recent attention through some extremely public lawsuits over custody of the child.

**OVUM TRANSFER**

A donor provides the ovum and site of fertilization and carries the embryo for a short time. The ovum is fertilized with the partner's sperm. The embryo is transferred to the infertile woman's uterus after about 5 days via a small catheter. Pregnancy rates have been as high as 25% to 50%.[33]

HIV. The topic is an emotional one for some couples and may induce strong reactions. Box 52-9 summarizes other, less frequently employed approaches to infertility.

## NURSING MANAGEMENT

Infertility can produce profound psychologic effects on couples.[31] Marital bonds may be threatened and social relationships with friends and family altered (see Research box, upper right). The nurse is challenged to assess couples to be active participants in the entire infertility workup and treatment plan, carefully exploring their own feelings about the limits they wish to set on the attempt to become pregnant and the alternative options of adoption or living childless by choice. Sexual dysfunction often occurs, since this formerly pleasurable and spontaneous private activity becomes a public process to be dissected and often used as a measure of their success or failure concerning pregnancy. The nurse who works with infertile couples must be committed to encouraging their honest expression of feelings and provide time for this in their care, both together and singly.[27]

Nurses also play an important role in promoting fertility among their patients, regardless of the setting or circumstances of care. Prevention of problems is much more effective than any attempt at corrective treatment. Interventions to prevent infection of the pelvic organs, particularly with gonorrhea and chlamydia, are critical interventions in preventing infertility. Salpingitis is often the first overt sign of gonorrhea infection and can result in obstruction of the fallopian tubes. This serious consequence is preventable through early diagnosis and treatment of all vaginal and cervical infections. The prevention and treatment of STDs and PID can help prevent infertility. The nurse encourages the use of barrier contraceptives, which help reduce the risk of infection, and encourages the woman to thoughtfully limit the number of her sexual partners.

Women with ovarian and hormonal problems frequently experience symptoms such as menstrual irregularities. Many of these problems can be successfully managed with hormone therapy if identified early before problems with infertility develop. Women with irregular menstrual cycles may be advised to avoid the use of oral contraceptives, and all women using oral contraceptives are encouraged to consider a break from long-term use to reactivate normal hypothalamic controls.[18]

**RESEARCH**

Hirsch AM, Hirsch SM: The effect of infertility on marriage and self-concept, *J Obstet Gynecol Neonatal Nurs* 18:13-20, 1989.

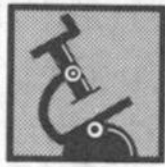

Questionnaires were completed by 92 subjects (58 seeking medical treatment for a perceived infertility problem and 34 who had not decided whether to have children) assessing the impact of infertility on their marriages and self-concept. Groups were compared as to self-esteem, marital satisfaction, sexual satisfaction, and general contentment. People experiencing infertility had greater dissatisfaction with themselves and their marriages. They experienced less sexual satisfaction and greater discontent than noninfertile persons. Infertile couples labeled noncommunicators had significantly higher levels of general discontent and marital dissatisfaction.

## QUESTIONS TO CONSIDER

- What are some of the factors that predispose a postmenopausal woman to infection of the vulva or vagina?
- What important factors must the nurse consider in caring for a patient complaining of altered patterns of sexuality related to vaginal or vulvar infection?
- What are the learning needs of patients with infections of the vagina and vulva?
- How might a nurse approach a patient who is recently diagnosed with endometriosis, complains of chronic pelvic pain, and fears future infertility?
- Explain the important areas to cover in teaching patients about prevention and treatment of pelvic inflammatory disease.
- Describe the nursing care of women who have undergone perineal surgery for structural problems of the uterus.

## QUESTIONS TO CONSIDER – cont'd

- How would the diagnosis of a genital cancer affect the sexuality of a 35-year-old woman?
- How would the diagnosis of ovarian cancer affect the life plans of a 25-year-old single woman compared with those of a 55-year-old mother of three children?
- What methods of public education may encourage the population at risk for developing vulvar cancer to seek medical attention at the time symptoms first develop?
- How would immediate pregnancy affect the follow-up of the woman recently treated for gestational trophoblastic neoplasia (GTN)?
- What nursing interventions are most effective in reducing infection after radical vulvectomy surgery?
- What self-image changes occur for the patient who undergoes radical vulvectomy?
- What are the psychologic effects of infertility on a woman?
- What approach would you consider for a couple experiencing infertility for 2 years without treatment if the woman wants to try anything available and the man wants nature to take its course?
- How would you counsel a menopausal woman who asks you, "Should I take estrogen replacement therapy for my hot flashes?"
- Outline the major teaching points that would be beneficial to the reproductive health of premenstrual girls.

## CRITICAL THINKING ACTIVITIES

- Of the following individuals, who is at the *highest* risk for developing a vaginal infection: (1) a 22-year-old nulliparous woman taking oral contraceptives; (2) a 35-year-old pregnant woman who has diabetes and is receiving ampicillin for a leg ulcer; (3) a 49-year-old premenopausal woman using vaginal creams/suppositories for birth control.
- A 38-year-old woman is admitted to the emergency room with a fever of 102° F and a sunburn-type skin reaction of the face. What should be the nurse's *first* assessment priority?

## CHAPTER SUMMARY

### INFECTIOUS PROCESSES

- Many organisms play a role in the development of infections of the vulva and vagina. In addition, women may be predisposed to developing such infections as a result of stress, malnutrition, aging, and decreased resistance.
- The clinical manifestations of such infections include inflammation of the tissues; abnormal discharge from the vagina, urethra, or Bartholin's glands; and pruritus. Each specific organism that is the causative factor of the infection produces signs and symptoms specific to that organism.
- Associated risk factors for vaginal infections include pregnancy, premenarchal age, menopausal and postmenopausal status, allergies, diabetes, oral contraceptives, inadequate hygiene, excessive douching or use of vaginal inserts, treatment with broad-spectrum antibiotics, and intercourse with an infected partner.
- The criteria for the diagnosis of bacterial vaginosis are that (1) a homogenous vaginal discharge is present; (2) the vaginal discharge has a pH of 4.7 or greater; (3) the vaginal discharge has an aminelike odor when mixed with potassium hydroxide; and (4) a wet smear of the vaginal discharge demonstrates clue cells.
- *Candida albicans* causes most cases of fungal vaginitis. It is found on most mucosal and skin surfaces and is the normal flora of approximately 25% of women, but it becomes an opportunistic pathogen when the normal ecosystem of the vagina is disturbed. *Candida* vaginitis is treated by means of topical application of one of the synthetic imidazoles or triazoles.
- The major goals of medical management of infections include cure of the infection, prevention of reinfection, prevention of complications associated with infections of the reproductive tract, and prevention of infection spread to sexual partners.
- Nursing management involves teaching regarding the prevention of infection. Such teaching includes self-care techniques, modifications of habits and activities of daily living, as well as correct adherence to therapeutic regimens.
- Nursing diagnoses associated with vaginal infections include infection, knowledge deficit, pain, altered sexual patterns, and social isolation.
- Specific conditions that require in-depth assessment, diagnosis, and management include cervicitis, pelvic inflammatory disease, toxic shock syndrome, structural problems of the uterus, ovarian tumors/cysts, fibroid tumors, endometriosis, and cervical polyps.
- Pelvic inflammatory disease (PID) is an infectious process involving the fallopian tubes, ovaries, pelvic peritoneum, pelvic veins, or pelvic connective tissue.
- To prevent PID and its serious consequences, it is important to prevent infections of the vulva, vagina, and cervix and to treat these infections promptly when they occur.
- Women need to be informed of methods of preventing infection, how to recognize infection in their sexual partners, and what to do when they suspect infection has occurred.
- Signs and symptoms of acute PID include severe abdominal pain, lower abdominal cramps, intermenstrual spotting, dyspareunia, fever and chills, malaise, nausea and vomiting, and a foul-smelling purulent vaginal discharge.

- The initial rash of toxic shock syndrome (TSS) over the first 48 hours is similar in appearance to an intense sunburn. Over the next several days, it evolves into a macular rash with fine, flake desquamation over the face and trunk and sloughing of the entire skin thickness over the palms and soles.
- Women with TSS should be treated with beta-lactamase-resistant antistaphylococcal antibiotics for 10 to 14 days.
- Women who are menstruating and develop a sudden high fever accompanied by vomiting or diarrhea should seek medical treatment and remove tampons immediately.

### DISORDERS OF MENSTRUATION

- The menstrual cycle is usually 26 to 36 days but may be altered by changes in climate, changes in working hours, emotional trauma, fatigue, exercise, illness, and surgery.
- Health teaching for menstruation includes information about the physiologic process, factors that may alter the menstrual cycle, personal hygiene, exercise, diet, and dysmenorrhea.
- PMS occurs in about 40% of all menstruating women; symptoms include behavioral changes, fatigue, signs of water and sodium retention, palpitations, headache, increased appetite, joint pain, and backache.
- Primary dysmenorrhea is caused by high levels of prostaglandin and can be treated with antiprostaglandins, some of which are now available without a prescription.
- Amenorrhea is classified as primary or secondary and results from a variety of causes.
- Abnormal types of vaginal bleeding include oligomenorrhea, menorrhagia, metrorrhagia, polymenorrhea, menometrorrhagia, cryptomenorrhea, and dysfunctional uterine bleeding.

### STRUCTURAL PROBLEMS

- Nursing diagnoses associated with women with structural problems of the reproductive system include body image disturbance, constipation, stress incontinence, knowledge deficit, pain, altered sexual patterns, and social isolation.
- Nursing care for a patient with a cystocele or rectocele includes teaching Kegel exercises; diet management to decrease weight; prevention of constipation; psychologic support; and possible instruction about use and care of a pessary.
- Preoperative preparation for surgery involving the reproductive system frequently includes a cleansing douche the morning of surgery, cathartics 24 hours before surgery, and several enemas the morning of surgery.
- Postoperative nursing care after vaginal or perineal surgery includes perineal care after elimination; use of sitz baths; prevention of constipation; maintenance of patency of Foley catheter; ice packs for perineal discomfort; and avoidance of Valsalva maneuver.

### BENIGN AND MALIGNANT NEOPLASMA OF THE FEMALE REPRODUCTIVE TRACT

- Factors placing the woman at risk for developing cancer of the cervix include first coitus at an early age, multiple sexual partners, low socioeconomic group, and exposure to herpesvirus type 2.
- The incidence of and death rate associated with invasive cervical cancer can continue to be reduced through adequate screening using the Pap smear.
- Treatment for invasive cancer of the cervix depends on the stage of the disease. Surgery and radiation therapy are the most frequently used methods. Surgical techniques include radical hysterectomy for stages IB and IIA and pelvic exenteration for locally recurrent disease. Radiation therapy includes external beam irradiation followed by two implants.
- Teaching for the woman undergoing radical hysterectomy includes information about the disease and proposed surgery; diagnostic tests; diet, exercise recommendations, and bladder function after surgery; personal impact and sexuality; and follow-up care.
- Factors placing the woman at risk for developing cancer of the endometrium include obesity, nulliparity, late menopause, diabetes mellitus, hypertension, and the use of exogenous estrogens.
- Any postmenopausal woman with vaginal bleeding should be encouraged to seek medical advice.
- Treatment for endometrial cancer is most often abdominal hysterectomy. Radiation therapy, hormonal manipulation, and chemotherapy may also be used for patients with advanced disease or those who are not good surgical candidates.
- Teaching for the woman who has endometrial, ovarian, or vulvar cancer should include information about her specific treatment plan, the disease, diagnostic tests, diet and exercise recommendations during and after therapy, personal impact and sexuality, and follow-up recommendations.
- No known risk factors are associated with ovarian cancer; nonspecific risk factors include familial history and environmental factors.
- Treatment for ovarian cancer usually includes extensive debulking surgery followed by chemotherapy.
- The usual treatment for invasive cancer of the vulva is a radical vulvectomy.
- Postoperative care for the patient experiencing a radical vulvectomy includes avoidance of stress on suture lines, maintenance of Foley catheter, avoidance of straining to defecate, low-residue diet, good perineal care, comfort measures, assessment for emboli, and emotional support.
- Gestational trophoblastic neoplasia (GTN) results from degeneration of the placental tissue; therefore, it can be considered an abnormal pregnancy. It is one

of the most curable gynecologic malignancies.

- The treatment for GTN is evacuation of the uterine contents, close follow-up of human chorionic gonadotropin (HCG) levels, and possibly short-term chemotherapy.
- Teaching for the woman being treated for GTN or monitored for its occurrence includes information about the disease and proposed treatment, the need for frequent serum evaluations of HCG level, the contraindication of pregnancy until serum HCG titers return to normal levels, personal impact and sexuality, and follow-up recommendations.

### STERILIZATION

- Sterilization is the most widely used contraceptive method worldwide. Female methods of sterilization include abdominal tubal sterilization by minilaparotomy and laparoscopy and vaginal tubal sterilization (rarely performed) by culpotomy and culdoscopy.
- Sterilization reversal is performed via microsurgical procedures.

### INFERTILITY

- Infertility affects 10% to 15% of all couples in the United States. Tests for males include multiple semen examination, hormonal tests, and testicular biopsy. Tests for females include the basal body temperature chart, postcoital test, endometrial biopsy, laparoscopy, hysterosalpingography, and hormonal tests.
- Nurses can assist couples experiencing infertility by providing emotional support, encouraging them to grieve and express their feelings, providing anticipatory guidance about testing, assisting the couple to consider their alternatives, and referring couples to support groups or other health care professionals.
- The incidence of infertility gradually increases in women after age 30.
- In the United States, approximately 10% to 15% of cases of infertility are caused by anovulation, 30% to 40% by an abnormality of semen production, 30% to 40% by pelvic disease, 10% to 15% by abnormalities of sperm transport through the cervical canal, and about 5% by uncommon causes.
- The technique of in vitro fertilization (IVF) with embryo transfer is now being widely used to treat infertile couples.

## REFERENCES


1. Adamson GD: Surgical and medical treatment of endometriosis, *Contemp Obstet Gynecol* 36(7):48-63, 1991.
2. American Cancer Society: *1992 cancer facts and figures,* New York, 1992, The Society.
3. Barclay DL: Benign disorders of the vulva and vagina. In Pernoll ML: *Current obstetric and gynecologic diagnosis and treatment,* ed 7, East Norwalk, Conn, 1991, Appleton & Lange.
4. Brucks JA: Ovarian cancer—the most lethal gynecologic malignancy, *Nurs Clin North Am* 27:835-845, 1992.
5. Centers for Disease Control: 1989 sexually transmitted disease treatment guidelines, *MMWR* 38(suppl 8):1, 1989.
6. Chaffkin LM et al: A comparative analysis of the cycle fecundity rates associated with combined human menopausal gonadotropin (hMG) and intrauterine insemination (IUI) versus either hMG or IUI alone, *Fertil Steril* 55:252-257, 1991.
7. Chamorro T: Cancer of the vulva and vagina, *Semin Oncol Nurs* 6:198-205, 1990.

7a. Corney R et al: The care of patients undergoing surgery for gynaecological cancer: the need for information, emotional support, and counseling, *J Adv Nurs* 17(6):667-671, 1992.

7b. Cortese J, Brown MA: Coping responses of men whose partners experience premenstrual symptomatology, *J Obstet Gynecol Neonatal Nurs* 18:405-412, 1989.

8. DiSaia PJ, Creasman WT: *Clinical gynecologic oncology,* ed 4, St Louis, 1993, Mosby.
9. *FDA Medical Bulletin,* 1993, Vol 23, No. 2, US Department of Health and Human Services, Rockville, Md, 1993, US Government Printing Office.
10. Gerbie MD: Complications of menstruation—abnormal uterine bleeding. In Pernoll ML: *Current obstetric and gynecologic diagnosis and treatment,* ed 7, East Norwalk, Conn, 1991, Appleton & Lange.
11. Hammond MG, Talbert LM: *Infertility: a practical guide for the physician,* ed 3, Boston, 1992, Blackwell.
12. Hatcher R: *Contraceptive technology,* ed 14, New York, 1988, Irvington.

12a. Heitkemper MN, Shaver JF, Mitchell ES: Gastrointestinal symptoms and patterns across the menstrual cycle in dysmenorrhea, *Nurs Res* 37:108-113, 1988.

13. Hemsell DL, Wendel GD, Mickal A: Sexually transmitted diseases and pelvic infections. In Pernoll ML: *Current obstetric and gynecologic diagnosis and treatment,* ed 7, East Norwalk, Conn, 1991, Appleton & Lange.
14. Herbst A et al: *Comprehensive gynecology,* St Louis, 1992, Mosby.
15. Hill EC: Benign disorders of the uterine cervix. In Pernoll ML: *Current obstetric and gynecologic diagnosis and treatment,* ed 7, East Norwalk, Conn, 1991, Appleton & Lange.

15a. Hirsch AM, Hirsch SM: The effect of infertility on marriage and self-concept, *J Obstet Gynecol Neonatal Nurs* 18:13-20, 1989.

16. Jenkins B: Patients' report of sexual changes after treatment for gynecologic cancer, *Oncol Nurs Forum* 15(3):349-354, 1988.
17. Jones, HW: Benign diseases of the vulva and vagina. In Jones HW, Wentz AC, Burnett LS, editors: *Novak's textbook of gynecology,* Baltimore, 1988, Williams & Wilkins.
18. Keating CE: The role of the expanded function nurse in fertility preservation, *NAACOGS Clin Issues Perinat Women's Health Nurs* 3:293-299, 1992.
19. Keye WR: Premenstrual symptoms: evaluation and treatment, *Compr Ther* 14:19-26, 1988.
20. Knapp RC, Berkowitz RS: *Gynecologic oncology,* ed 2, New York, 1993, McGraw-Hill.
21. Lichtman R, Papera S: *Gynecology—well-woman care,* East Norwalk, Conn, 1990, Appleton & Lange.
22. McMullin M: Holistic care on the patient with cervical cancer, *Nurs Clin North Am* 27:847-858, 1992.
23. Mettlin C, Piver MS: A case controlled study of milk drinking and ovarian cancer risk, *Am J Epidemiol* 132:871-876, 1990.
24. Mishell DR, Kirschbaum TH, Morrow CP: *Year book of obstetrics and gynecology,* St Louis, 1991, Mosby.
25. Muse KN, Wilson EA: Endometriosis. In Pernoll ML: *Current obstetric and gynecologic diagnosis and treatment,* ed 7, East Norwalk, Conn, 1991, Appleton & Lange.
26. Nikolai TF et al: Thyroid function and treatment in premenstrual syndrome, *J Clin Endocrinol Metab* 70:1108, 1990.
27. Olshansky EF: Redefining the concepts of success and failure in infertility treatment, *NAACOGS Clin Issues Perinat Women's Health Nurs* 3:343-346, 1992.

28. Pace-Owens S: Gamete intrafallopian transfer (GIFT), *J Obstet Gynecol Neonatal Nurs* 18:93-97, 1989.
29. Pernoll ML: *Current obstetric and gynecologic diagnosis and treatment,* ed 7, East Norwalk, Conn, 1991, Appleton & Lange.
30. Raz S: *Atlas of transvaginal surgery,* Philadelphia, 1992, Saunders.
31. Rosenthal M: Grappling with the emotional aspects of infertility, *Contemp Obstet Gynecol* 27:97-106, 1985.
31a. Rossignol AM, Bonnlander H: Caffeine-containing beverages, total fluid consumption, and premenstrual syndrome, *Am J Public Health* 80:1106, 1990.
32. Ryan KJ, Berkowitz R, Barbieri R: *Kistner's gynecology: principles and practices,* ed 5, Chicago, 1990, Year Book.
33. Sauer MV et al: Oocyte and pre-embryo donation to women with ovarian failure: an extended clinical trial, *Fertil Steril* 55:39-43, 1991.
34. Secor RMC: Bacterial vaginosis: a comprehensive review, *Nurs Clin North Am* 23:865-875, 1988.
35. Skidmore-Roth L: *Mosby's 1995 nursing drug reference,* St Louis, 1995, Mosby.
36. Speroff L, Glass RH, Kase N: *Clinical gynecologic, endocrinology, and infertility,* ed 4, Baltimore, 1989, Williams & Wilkins.
37. Stenchever MA: *Office gynecology,* St Louis, 1992, Mosby.
38. Sullivan N: Dysmenorrhea. In Lichtman R, Papera S: *Gynecology—well-woman care,* East Norwalk, Conn, 1990, Appleton & Lange.
39. Symmonds RE: Relaxation of pelvic supports. In Pernoll ML: *Current obstetric and gynecologic diagnosis and treatment,* ed 7, East Norwalk, Conn, 1991, Appleton & Lange.
40. Taylor PV et al: Autoreactivity in women with endometriosis, *Obstet Gynecol Surv* 42(2):127-129, 1992.
41. Taymor ML: *Infertility: a clinician's guide to diagnosis and treatment,* New York, 1990, Plenum.
42. Thompson JD, Rock JA: *Te Linde's operative gynecology,* ed 7, Philadelphia, 1992, Lippincott.
43. Toback BM: Recent advances in female infertility care, *NAACOGS Clin Issues Perinat Women's Health Nurs* 3:313-319, 1992.
44. Woodruff JD: Benign disorders of the ovaries and oviducts. In Pernoll ML: *Current obstetric and gynecologic diagnosis and treatment,* ed 7, East Norwalk, Conn, 1991, Appleton & Lange.
44a. Woolard DB, Larson J, Hudson L: Screening for *Chlamydia trachomatis* at a university health service, *J Obstet Gynecol Neonatal Nurs* 18(2):145-149, 1989.

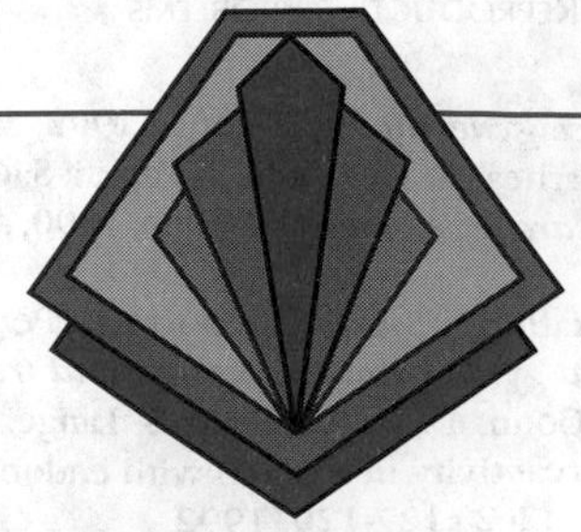

CHAPTER 53

# Management of Men With Reproductive Problems

*Carolyn W. Eddins*
*Margaret Heitkemper*
*Deborah Power*

## CHAPTER OBJECTIVES

***After studying this chapter, the learner should be able to do the following:***

1 Describe the process of infectious diseases specific to men's reproductive health.
2 Discuss the differences in nursing care associated with benign and malignant neoplasms that are specific to men's reproductive health.
3 Describe expected patient outcomes for each condition discussed.
4 Identify teaching needs of the client with impotence.
5 Discuss the common causes of impotence, both physical and psychologic.
6 Discuss nursing interventions related to the conditions described.

## KEY TERMS

| | | |
|---|---|---|
| benign prostatic hypertrophy | orchiectomy | prostatitis |
| cremasteric reflex | orchiopexy | testicular torsion |
| cryptorchidism | orchitis | transurethral prostatic resection (TURP) |
| epididymitis | paraphimosis | vasectomy |
| impotence | phimosis | |

Men's reproductive health care is one dimension of an emerging specialty area of nursing practice, men's health.[6] Currently, a gap exists between expectations of male health care consumers and the health care options available to them. As with women, men have unique biologic and social health care needs. Among these are a need for permission to have health concerns and discuss them; access to information about their bodies; instruction in self-care techniques; opportunities for physical examinations and history taking, including the sexual-reproductive system; consideration of life-styles and male role influences on physical and mental health; concern for factors such as occupation, leisure, and personal relationships related to health; a health care system sensitive to their occupational demands that compete for time; and financial support to obtain health care.

The chapter is divided into sections based on problems related to specific organ structures and functions in the male reproductive system. Included is a discussion of the most common health problems involving the reproductive system in men. Particular emphasis is placed on infectious processes, neoplasms of the reproductive tract, and the problem of impotence. Table 53-1 summarizes the problems affecting men's reproductive health discussed in this chapter. Sexually transmitted diseases and methods of contraception are discussed in Chapters 55 and 52, respectively. Figure 53-1 illustrates the male reproductive organs and associated structures.

## PROBLEMS OF THE TESTES AND RELATED STRUCTURES

The scrotal sac contains the testes, epididymis, and part of the spermatic cord; other associated structures include nerve, lymphatic, and vascular networks (Figure 53-2). These structures are responsible for sperm production and storage and provide the pathway for ejaculation. The testes are also involved in hormonal production, primarily testosterone. Any disorders related to these structures have the potential to affect male fertility adversely, as well as testosterone production.

Pathologies of these structures include problems with swelling, twisting of cords, trauma, and carcinomas. The testes are particularly sensitive to changes in scrotal

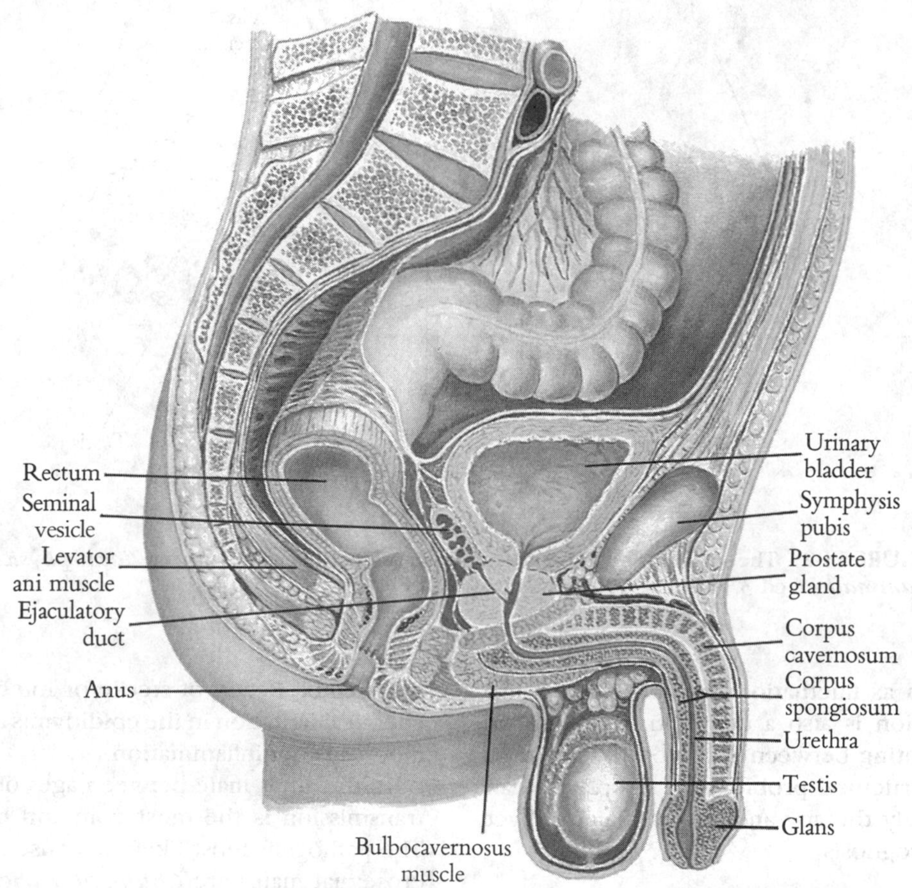


**FIGURE 53-1** Male reproductive organs and associated structures. (From Seidel HM et al: *Mosby's guide to physical examination,* ed 3, St Louis, 1995, Mosby.)

**TABLE 53-1 Major Health Problems Affecting the Male Reproductive System**

| | INFECTIONS | CANCER | IMPOTENCE | BENIGN GROWTH |
|---|---|---|---|---|
| **SCROTUM** | | | | |
| Epididymis | Epididymitis | | | |
| Hydrocele | | | | |
| Varicocele | | | | |
| Spermatocele | | | | |
| **TESTES** | | | | |
| Torsion | Orchitis | Testicular<br>Seminomatous<br>Nonseminomatous | Infertility<br>Decline in spermatogenesis | |
| **PROSTATE** | | | | |
| | Prostatitis | Prostatic | Decline in prostatic fluid or fluid loss | Benign prostatic hypertrophy |
| **PENIS** | | | | |
| | | Penile | Loss of erectile function | |

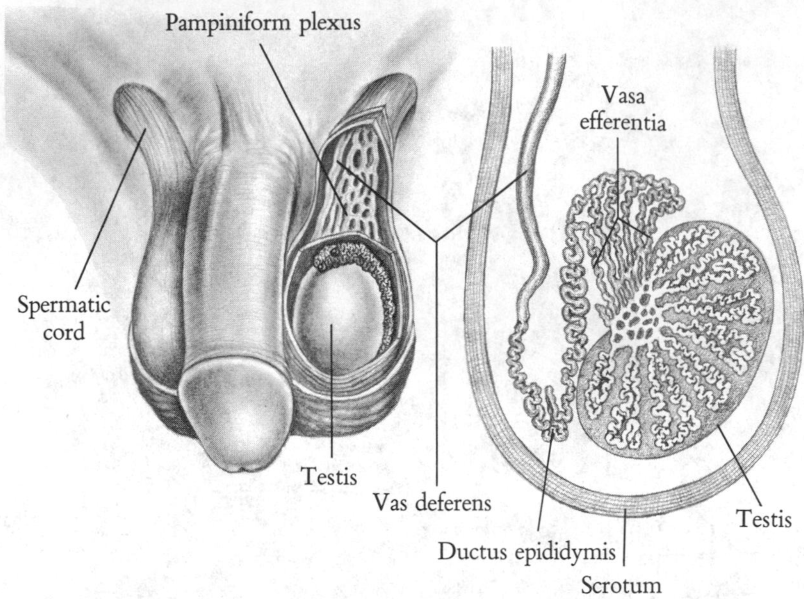


**FIGURE 53-2** The scrotum and its contents. (From Seidel HM et al: *Mosby's guide to physical examination,* ed 3, St Louis, 1995, Mosby.)

environment, such as fluctuations in temperature and blood flow. Infection is also a common problem. Accurately differentiating between pathologies related to infection versus structural problems or neoplasms can help promote timely therapy and have a major impact on the patient's prognosis.

## EPIDIDYMITIS

### Etiology/Epidemiology

The epididymis is a convoluted tubular structure within the scrotal sac that acts as a reservoir for sperm. While in this structure, sperm mature and become fertile and mobile. **Epididymitis** is an acute inflammatory process within the epididymis and is the most common intrascrotal inflammation in adult males. In the United States, epididymitis accounts for more than 600,000 visits per year to health care providers. Epididymitis is responsible for 20% of all urologic admissions in the military population. It is also the cause of more lost work days than any other disease in the military.[13] This inflammation is rarely seen in children and occurs infrequently in the elderly adult male.

Inflammation of the epididymis is most often caused by an ascending infection via the ejaculatory duct through the vas deferens into the epididymis. Infection may be introduced when surgical or diagnostic procedures are performed. This occurs more frequently among males less than 15 years old and in those over 45 years old. The most common organism for contamination in these age-groups is *Escherichia coli.*[13] In the child, structural malformations or developmental structural insufficiencies may contribute to problems of urinary reflux. Reflux of sterile or infected urine causes a chemical irritation in the epididymis and is another common cause of inflammation.

In the adult male between ages of 19 and 35, sexual transmission is the most common means of infection. The pathogens most likely to cause epididymitis in heterosexual males are *Chlamydia trichomatis* and *Neisseria gonorrhoeae.* In homosexual males, the most common pathogens are the ones that would be found in the anal canal, which are *E. coli* and *Haemophilus influenzae.* (For more information on sexually transmitted diseases and the associated pathogens, see Chapter 55.)

### Pathophysiology

Epididymitis results from inflammation of the epididymis and scrotal sac. Fluid accumulates in the scrotal sac as an inflammatory response to an infectious process occurring in the epididymis. Excess fluid loss into the interstitial space of the scrotal sac can lead to diminished blood flow, nerve damage, and resultant pain and swelling. Inflammatory fluids can also form pockets of pus called *abscesses.* Heat generated from the inflammatory process can negatively affect the testicular function of spermatogenesis. Consequently, complications of epididymitis include testicular infarction, chronic pain from nerve damage, abscess formation, and infertility.

The most common clinical manifestations are severe tenderness, pain in the scrotal area, and noticeable swelling of one or both sides of the scrotum. The onset of the pain may be insidious, gradually increasing over hours or days. The scrotal swelling can cause pain on ambulation and discomfort that is exacerbated by wearing restrictive clothing. Men with epididymitis often walk with a type of "waddle" to help spare the scrotum from rubbing up against the thighs or clothing. Elevation of the scrotum will reduce the pain (Prehn's sign). Other symptoms include an increase in temperature of the scrotum and sometimes a systemic rise in temperature. A urethral discharge may also be present, with the color and consistency varying according to the type of causative organism. Urethritis is often associated with epididymitis, and the associated symptoms include burning on urination, frequency, urgency, and general malaise.

## Medical Management

Prompt diagnosis is essential to decrease the risk of complications. Urinalysis is used to differentiate epididymitis from emergency conditions such as testicular torsion (see later discussion). If epididymitis is present, the urinalysis usually shows an increased white blood cell (WBC) count and the presence of bacteria. Urine and urethral cultures are needed to determine the specific causative organism and its sensitivity to various antibiotics, as well as provide information for needed drug therapies.

Other diagnostic tests to detect epididymitis focus on changes in blood flow to the inflamed scrotum. An initial increase in blood flow to the area would indicate inflammation and/or infection, whereas other conditions might impede blood flow initially. Scrotal ultrasound is a noninvasive diagnostic measure used when urinalysis and cultures are not conclusive. Ultrasound for this condition is usually done serially over minutes to hours. Any indication of reduced blood flow to the affected side usually indicates a more serious condition or a complication of epididymitis. Radionuclide scanning can also be performed when the diagnosis is questionable. These scans are more sensitive than ultrasound and generally show increased blood perfusion to the affected side of the scrotum if epididymitis is present.

For patients with chronic recurrent epididymitis, aspiration of fluid from the epididymis can be performed. It is a more direct method of determining the causative agent than routine cultures. This diagnostic method is rarely used, however, unless a chronic condition has been verified.

Treatment of epididymitis usually consists of medications and supportive care. Nonsteroidal antiinflammatory drugs (NSAIDs), such as aspirin, or oxyphenbutazone (Butazolidin) may be used to decrease the inflammation and relieve the discomfort and swelling. Sometimes, narcotic analgesics are prescribed if the pain is severe. Stool softeners are given to prevent constipation and reduce straining on defecation that can cause severe pain in the inflamed scrotum.

Medical treatment is also aimed at eradicating the infection, which is generally accomplished by giving oral antibiotics. Most antibiotics prescribed are broad spectrum. If sexually transmitted diseases (STDs) are present, the patient's sexual partners should also be treated at the same time.

Unless high fever and the potential for complications are present, most males with epididymitis can be treated as outpatients. Frequent return appointments to the physician's office are indicated if swelling does not resolve in a few weeks. Because this condition can be associated with other pathologies of the scrotum, an in-depth scrotal examination should be carried out after the swelling has resolved. The examination incorporates such diagnostic tests as ultrasound, magnetic resonance imaging (MRI), and aspiration of fluid from the scrotum. Also, a more comprehensive palpation of scrotal structures can be accomplished when swelling has decreased.

## Nursing Management

Assessment of the patient with symptoms of epididymitis should include a history of sexual activity. For young children, it should include questions to determine possible sexual abuse and, more often, a history of recent urinary examinations or instrumentation. In the elderly male, questions focus on history or symptoms of urinary obstruction or recent urinary examinations.

The nurse assesses whether the pain is bilateral or unilateral, and if the pain is of sudden onset or has developed over hours or days. The nurse should also note if the pain is relieved by elevating the scrotum. Any symptoms of dysuria should be documented, such as burning, frequency, urgency, fever, and general malaise. A recent history of urethral discharge or change in the discharge is important to help determine the possible type of causative organism. The color, consistency, and amount of any discharge should be documented.

The nurse observes for the classic "waddle," or a somewhat rolling gait, indicating that the patient is attempting to protect his scrotum. Swelling of the scrotum should be documented, as well as whether it is on one side or both sides. Palpation of the scrotum at this time is generally deferred to avoid causing severe pain.

Nursing interventions include comfort measures that will reduce the swelling of the scrotum. Bedrest with the scrotum elevated on a towel, application of ice packs, and the use of scrotal supports when the swelling is less severe decrease the discomfort caused by the heavy sensation resulting from the enlarged scrotum (Figure 53-3). Bedrest should be maintained until the patient is pain free, then a scrotal support should be worn for approximately 6 weeks. The patient should be instructed to avoid work that would put a strain on the lower abdomen and scrotal area.

Because STDs are the most common causes of epididymitis, it is important for the patient to be informed on means of protection. The importance of using condoms and of maintaining good hygiene should be

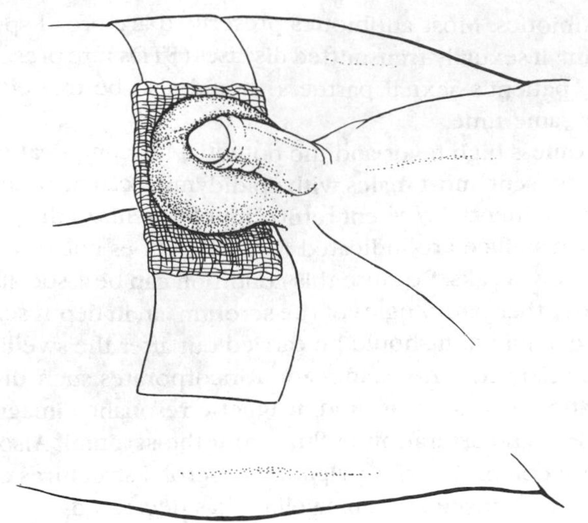

FIGURE 53-3 A simple scrotal support.

stressed in patient teaching. (Methods of preventing STDs are discussed more completely in Chapter 55.) Avoiding excessive instrumentation to the male urethra is also a means of decreasing the incidence of inflammation.

## ORCHITIS

### Etiology/Epidemiology

Inflammation or infection of the testicle is known as **orchitis.** It may be caused by pyogenic bacteria, gonococci, tubercle bacilli, or viruses (e.g., paramyxovirus, the agent responsible for mumps), or it may follow any septicemia. Orchitis occurs as a complication of mumps in approximately 20% of all cases contracted after puberty. Symptoms may develop 4 to 6 days after the onset of parotitis. If the case of mumps is mild, there may be no symptoms until the onset of orchitis.[5]

### Pathophysiology

Inflammatory fluid seeps from the testicle into the serous membrane lining the epididymis and the testicle to create unilateral or bilateral swelling. *Hydrocele* (a collection of fluid within the tunica vaginalis testis) is frequently associated with orchitis. The signs and symptoms of orchitis are the same as those of epididymitis. However, because orchitis is caused by a systemic infectious process rather than a localized infection, more systemic symptoms are present. Consequently, the patient may also have clinical manifestations of nausea, vomiting, and pain radiating to the inguinal canal.

As a result of inflammation and fibrosis, some degree of testicular atrophy occurs in 50% of patients. The atrophy of the testes may lead to sterility. Unless both testes are severely involved, however, infertility occurs infrequently.

### Medical Management

Any postpubertal boy or man who is exposed to mumps usually is given gamma globulin immediately unless he has already had the disease or been vaccinated. If there is any doubt, globulin usually is given. Although it may not prevent mumps, the disease is likely to be less severe with less likelihood of complications. Broad-spectrum antibiotics are given for common bacterial causes.

If hydrocele is present, the fluid may be aspirated to reduce pressure on the testes. If the hydrocele is surgically tapped within the first 2 days, it may decrease the atrophy; however, a tap should only be done when edema is persistent, because a chance exists that surgical decompression may exacerbate the inflammation.

### Nursing Management

Nursing management focuses on reducing discomfort from gonadal swelling and alleviating systemic symptoms. During the acute phase of gonadal swelling, the scrotum may be supported in the same methods used for the patient with epididymitis. Antibiotics are administered for bacterial causes. Rest and increasing fluid intake are encouraged for all patients. Antiinflammatory medication is given to help reduce pain and swelling.

## TESTICULAR TORSION

### Etiology/Epidemiology

**Testicular torsion** is a condition in which testicular circulation is acutely impaired by the twisting of the spermatic cord. Torsion may follow activities that put a sudden pull on the cremasteric muscle, such as jumping into cold water, blunt trauma, or bicycle riding. It may also occur at night when there is less gravitational pull from the testes on the cord, allowing more movement and consequent twisting.

Approximately 1 in 4000 males under age 25 years experiences torsion. Testicular torsion is most common between ages 12 and 18 years but can occur at any age. Forty percent of the cases reported occur spontaneously, awakening the male at night.[18]

### Pathophysiology

Torsion interrupts the blood supply to the testes, leading to ischemia and severe pain that is not relieved and may be aggravated by manual elevation of the affected side. The scrotum is swollen, tender, and red. The affected side is usually elevated because the twisting and shortening of the cord pull up the testicle. Although the scrotum appears infected because of the swelling and redness, both urinalysis and blood tests are typically normal. Fever is rarely present. Absence of pain after a time may indicate infarction and necrosis. Gangrene may be a serious sequela.

Testicular viability after torsion is directly related to the duration of the torsion episode. If torsion has occurred for less than 4 hours, there is an 80% salvage rate for the testicle. If more than 12 hours have elapsed,

**TABLE 53-2 Differentiation Between Testicular Torsion and Epididymitis**

| TORSION | EPIDIDYMITIS |
|---|---|
| **AGE** | |
| First year through adolescence; most common age, 12-18 years | Adolescence and later |
| **ONSET** | |
| Acute | May be gradual |
| **SIGNS AND SYMPTOMS** | |
| **Pain** | |
| Localized to testis and radiates to groin and lower abdomen; severe in nature; similar episodes of self-limiting pains are not unusual. | Usually localized to epididymis and testis, sometimes to groin; increasing severity of pain; similar episodes of self-limiting pains are rare. |
| **Fever** | |
| Rare | Common |
| **Vomiting** | |
| Common | Rare |
| **Dysuria** | |
| Rare | Common |
| **Physical Examination** | |
| Testis may be in elevated position with abnormal lie; testis will be swollen and tender; epididymis also may be tender. | Epididymis will be firm, tender, and swollen; testis may be normal or tender. |
| **Cremasteric Reflex** | |
| Usually negative | Usually positive |
| **Prehn's Sign** | |
| Pain constant | Pain decreased |
| **Urethral Discharge** | |
| Not found | Common with sexually acquired infections |
| **LABORATORY EXAMINATION** | |
| **Urinalysis** | |
| Usually normal | Pyuria common |

there is only a 20% salvage rate. Early recognition and treatment are imperative if the testicle is to be preserved.[18] Table 53-2 lists assessment criteria to differentiate torsion from epididymitis.

## Medical Management

The physician may perform a scrotal examination depending on the amount of swelling and tenderness. If palpation of the epididymis is possible, it may be found anteriorly instead of in the normal posterolateral position. The **cremasteric reflex,** elicited by stroking the inner aspect of the thigh to cause reflex retraction of the testicle, is usually absent on the same side that the torsion is suspected.

An orchiogram, or testicular scan, which is performed in the nuclear medicine department, can qualitatively measure the blood flow to the testis. Diminished or obstructed blood flow distinguishes torsion from an inflammatory process such as epididymitis. Doppler studies can also help to identify reduced blood flow and diagnose torsion.

Detorsion (a process of untwisting the spermatic cord) can be attempted manually. If detorsion is unsuccessful, surgical intervention is imperative within 6 to 12 hours to maintain viability of the testis. Even so, the testis may atrophy. Unless the testis is gangrenous, it is not excised, since it may still produce hormones, even if spermatogenesis is destroyed. The testis is fixed surgically to the scrotal wall **(orchiopexy)** to prevent recurrence. The contralateral testis is usually fixed prophylactically at the same time.

If the testicle is gangrenous or found to be nonviable after surgical detorsion, an **orchiectomy** (removal of the testicle) is carried out. If orchiectomy is performed, a testicular prosthesis is usually inserted.

## Nursing Management

Nursing care after orchiopexy and orchiectomy is similar. Ice bags and scrotal elevation may be ordered to reduce swelling. The nurse continues to monitor the patient for signs of testicular necrosis and fever in the case of orchiopexy. A small Penrose drain may be placed in the scrotum, which will necessitate dressing changes.

After scrotal surgery, the patient should be instructed to limit stair climbing to two flights and not to lift or carry heavy objects for 4 weeks. He is instructed to refrain from sexual activity for 6 weeks. The use of a scrotal support for at least 3 weeks is recommended to control edema. Sitz baths may help relieve any discomfort.

Body image disturbances may include fears of castration (orchiectomy), loss of masculinity, sterility, and impotence. The nurse provides specific information about how to cope with the physiologic changes resulting from testicular atrophy or surgical removal of the testicle. The patient is still able to have an erection after trauma or surgery to the testicles. Fertility may or may not be affected if there is still a remaining healthy testicle. Counseling on alternative means of having children may be suggested. The patient is reminded that the appearance of the scrotum does not change when a testicular prosthesis is inserted after orchiectomy.

# TESTICULAR CANCER

## Etiology/Epidemiology

The causes of testicular cancer are still unknown. Acquired causes being investigated include chemical carcinogens, trauma, and orchitis. Environmental factors are also being considered, since there is a greater incidence of testicular cancer in men who live in rural than in urban areas. Congenital causes implicated are familial predisposition, gonadal dysgenesis (developmental abnormality), and **cryptorchidism** (failure of the testis to descend at birth). Factors that may delay or inhibit testicular descent into the scrotum (e.g., developmental abnormalities), in utero exposure to hormone preparations (e.g., diethylstilbestrol [DES]), and oral contraceptives are also being investigated.

Because there is a 40% greater risk of cancer developing in men who have a history of cryptorchidism, orchiopexy (a surgical procedure to bring the testis into the scrotum) is being recommended for infants with cryptorchidism between ages 1 and 2 years.[15] Orchiopexy performed on male children with cryptorchidism before age 6 greatly reduces the incidence of testicular cancer in that high-risk group.

Cancer of the testis is the leading cause of death from cancer in the 15- to 35-year-old age-group.[3,12] Two to three men per 100,000 have testicular cancer, but the number is increasing. The age-groups that are most prone to testicular cancer are infants, men between 20 and 40 years, and men over age 60. Testicular cancer is more common in white than in black males. If testicular cancer is untreated, death often occurs in 2 to 3 years. If it is detected and treated early, there is a 90% to 100% chance of cure. Unfortunately, approximately half the cases are found in advanced stages, and the prognosis for these men is poor.

## Pathophysiology

Testicular neoplasms are divided into two classifications: germinal and nongerminal. Germinal cancers make up 90% to 95% of all testicular neoplasms and are further divided into two groups: seminomatous (40%) and nonseminomatous (60%) tumors. In addition, tumors with mixed cell types can occur.

The determination of cell type is crucial for treatment. The diagnostic workup includes chest x-ray films, computed tomograms (CT scans), and intravenous pyelogram, skeletal surveys if the patient's alkaline phosphatase is elevated, and lymphangiography. Lymphangiography decreases pulmonary function by 10% because of oil embolism; therefore general anesthesia is contraindicated for 48 hours after the procedure. *Biopsy of the testis is contraindicated* because of the highly metastatic character of testicular carcinoma. Manipulation and invasion of the cancer could cause it to seed to other areas. Laboratory tests include evaluation of alpha fetoprotein (AFP) and the beta subunit of human chorionic gonadotropin (beta-HCG). AFP and HCG are considered *markers* that indicate the presence of nonseminomatous disease, although a small number of men (less than 10%) with diagnosed seminoma will also have elevations in some of these marker hormones.[4] No one combination of elevated and normal markers specifically indicates testicular neoplasm. However, changes that occur in the laboratory values of these markers help to indicate the effectiveness of therapeutic interventions. These are monitored throughout the course of therapy.

Clinical manifestations of testicular cancer are often subtle and go unnoticed by the male until a feeling of heaviness or dragging is noted in the lower abdomen and the groin area. A lump or swelling may be present, which is usually nontender and painless. Other symptoms are nonspecific, such as back pain, weight loss, and fatigue. Testicular tumors are often rapidly growing. Some complex tumors have been reported to double in size in a few days.[15]

## Medical Management

In any suspected case of testicular cancer, the testis is usually removed immediately. *Orchiectomy* consists of en bloc excision of the spermatic cord, the contents of the inguinal canal, and the testis with the tunicae attached. The adjacent area is explored for metastases. The specimens are then examined to determine the cancer cell type. Staging of the disease (Box 53-1), as well as pathologic findings, determines the course of treatment.

*Seminoma* is highly responsive to radiation therapy. For stage I seminoma, irradiation is administered to the retroperitoneal nodes. In stage II, irradiation of the mediastinal and supraclavicular nodes is added. Chemotherapy is added for stage III. If tumor markers are present or elevated after irradiation, nonseminomatous involvement must be suspected. Seminoma can metastasize into a different type of cancer. It is possible to develop a second primary lesion in the remaining testis. The prognosis in that case is the same as if it were the first lesion.

*Nonseminomatous neoplasms* are radioresistant. Therefore retroperitoneal lymphadenectomy or radical node dissection is performed immediately. If the nodes are free of metastases, careful follow-up every 2 months is mandatory. Chemotherapy is given for clinical, radiologic, or tumor marker evidence of metastasis. If the lymph node dissection is positive, the patient has stage II disease. Cyclic combination chemotherapy is started for 2 years with adjuvant surgery. In stage III, intensive cyclic combination chemotherapy is instituted for 10 to 12 months, followed by surgical excision of all metastatic sites. Drugs used in combination therapy include cisplatin, vinblastine, and bleomycin.

Nongerminal testicular tumors are rare. Treatment

**BOX 53-1 Staging of Testicular Neoplasia**

| | |
|---|---|
| Stage I | No metastasis; confined to testis |
| Stage II | Metastasis to retroperitoneal lymph nodes or other subdiaphragmatic areas |
| Stage III | Metastasis to mediastinal and supraclavicular nodes or other areas above diaphragm |

consists of various combinations of the four modes of treatment (orchiectomy, radiation, lymphadenectomy, chemotherapy) used in germinal neoplasms, depending on the specific type. Table 53-3 lists treatments of testicular cancer based on tumor type.

Seminoma has the best prognosis of any of the germinal neoplasms. Five-year survival rates are as follows: for stage I, 95% to 100%; for stage II, 70% to 90%; for stage III, 50% to 70%. For those patients with advanced-stage cancer, relapse is higher and thus chemotherapy with radiation results in a higher percentage of persons with sustained remission. For nonseminomatous neoplasms, 5-year survival rates are as follows: for stage I 90%; for stage II, 60% to 85%; and for stage III, 30% to 40%.[1]

For infants with cryptorchidism, orchiopexy is being recommended between ages 1 and 2 years. Hormonal therapy may also be used to cause the testes to descend. In some cases, descent is spontaneous. The effect of early treatment on the probability of cancer is not known at this time. Although the likelihood of cancer in the testis that descends after age 5 or 6 years is comparable to the likelihood of cancer in the testis that has always been outside the scrotum, regular examination of the descended testis does increase the chance of early cancer detection: the site of the testis makes no difference in the risk of developing cancer. Patients with current cryptorchidism or a history of cryptorchidism should be observed yearly; then after the 20-year latency period when testicular cancer is prone to develop, they should be examined every 6 months. Orchiectomy instead of orchiopexy is recommended in adults with cryptorchidism as a prophylaxis against cancer.

**TABLE 53-3 Treatment of Testicular Cancer Based on Tumor Type**

| STAGE | TUMOR TYPE | TREATMENT |
|---|---|---|
| 0 | Benign | Surveillance |
| I | Seminomatous | Orchiectomy<br>Radiation therapy |
| | Nonseminomatous | Orchiectomy<br>Modified retroperitoneal lymph node dissection<br>Radiation therapy |
| II | Seminomatous | Orchiectomy<br>Radiation |
| | Nonseminomatous | Orchiectomy<br>Radiation therapy/modified or full retroperitoneal lymph node dissection |
| III | Seminomatous | Combination chemotherapy/full retroperitoneal lymph node dissection |
| | Nonseminomatous | Combination chemotherapy/full retroperitoneal lymph node dissection |

## Nursing Management

Nursing interventions for patients receiving radiation therapy and chemotherapy are discussed in Chapter 16. Although the normal testis is shielded during external radiation, it is exposed to radiation scattered from the abdomen and thighs. The nurse explains to the patient that a period of 70 days is required to determine if spermatogenesis has been affected. Spermatogenesis may be decreased for 7 months to 5 years or more. The patient is encouraged to seek genetic counseling related to questions about the effects of radiation on sperm and consequently the rare possibility of genetic defects. Sperm banking before treatment is often recommended.

The nurse explains the effects of orchiectomy on fertility to the patient. Orchiectomy alone does not result in impotence if the contralateral testis is normal. The remaining testis undergoes hyperplasia, producing sufficient testosterone to maintain sexual function, drive, and characteristics.

After a *radical node dissection*, there is danger of hemorrhage. Active movement may be contraindicated, since nodes may have been resected from around many large abdominal vessels, but gentle passive turning and leg and arm movement are essential to prevent postoperative development of pneumonia and thrombosis. After a retroperitoneal lymphadenectomy, 90% of patients experience a decreased ejaculatory ability. Decreased ejaculation results from a disruption of the sympathetic nervous system pathways. The nurse should inform the patient that ejaculation is independent of other sexual functions; orgasm is still possible.

Follow-up visits to the clinic are often done monthly for the first year after surgery to have serum tumor mark-

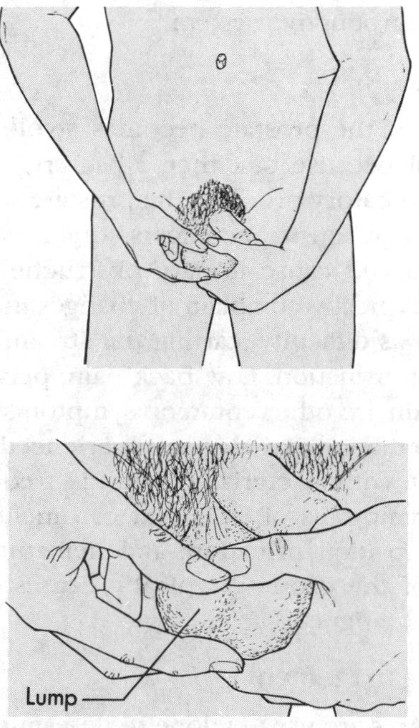


**FIGURE 53-4** Testicular self-examination.

ers drawn, chest x-ray films, and possibly a CT scan. The time between return visits often increases to 2 months for 2 more years to continue watching for signs of return of the cancer. The nurse teaches the patient how to perform regular testicular examinations. Figure 53-4 describes steps in the testicular self-examination.

## PROBLEMS OF THE PROSTATE

Infection of the prostate occurs infrequently but can result in chronic problems that are difficult to eradicate. Prostatitis can cause long-term discomfort and problems with fertility. Enlargements of the prostate are either benign or caused by cancer. These two problems are the most common of all the pathologies affecting the male reproductive system.

### PROSTATITIS

#### Etiology/Epidemiology

There are two common types of **prostatitis** (an inflammation of the prostate gland): bacterial and nonbacterial. Bacterial prostatitis can be acute or chronic. It is often caused by bacteria that also cause urinary tract infections (UTIs), such as *E. coli, and Pseudomonas.* Ascending UTIs or reflux of infected urine may be the route of bacterial contamination. Urethral instrumentation has also been cited as a means of bacterial infection. Nonbacterial prostatitis is the most common type. The organism of infection often cannot be identified. *Chlamydia trachomatis* has been suspected as the cause in many cases of nonbacterial prostatitis. Some nonbacterial inflammations may be attributed to allergic or antibody-antigen reactions.

Prostatitis is most often seen in young to middle-aged men. It is one of the more common inflammations of the male reproductive system.[17]

#### Pathophysiology

The gland of the prostate becomes swollen, inflamed, and painful because of either a bacterial infection or other inflammatory process. The prostate surrounds the urethra and, when it becomes swollen, can compress the urethra and cause urinary obstruction. Men with prostatitis typically complain of changes in voiding patterns, such as difficulty starting the stream or the need to strain on urination. Low back pain, pelvic pain, and perineal pain are other common symptoms. Pain during or after ejaculation may also be experienced. In addition, the patient with bacterial prostatitis frequently complains of symptoms of UTIs that can include urgency, frequency, painful urination, and hematuria. Bacterial infection of the prostate typically causes fever, chills, and general fatigue.

#### Medical Management

Urine cultures are usually done to determine the organisms causing bacterial prostatitis. Cultures of prostatic secretions can verify a diagnosis of bacterial infection. Nonbacterial prostatitis usually has negative urine cultures, but prostatic secretions can show increased number of leukocytes and fat containing macrophages.[17]

Treatment is usually conservative, consisting of antibiotics for 30 days to prevent chronic infection, forcing fluids, physical rest, stool softeners to decrease rectal irritation of the prostate, and local application of heat by sitz baths.

Prompt treatment of prostatitis may prevent edema of the prostate with resultant obstruction of the urethra. If severe urinary retention occurs, suprapubic needle aspiration is safer than urethral straight or indwelling catheterization that would increase the risk of epididymitis. Prostatic massage to eliminate residual pus pockets is contraindicated during the acute phase, since it may cause bacteremia; however, it may be used after the acute attack subsides.

Recurrent episodes of acute prostatitis may cause fibrotic tissue to form. The fibrosis causes a hardening of the prostate, which may initially be confused with carcinoma. In the granulomatous form of prostatitis, the enlargement may take 3 to 6 months to resolve.

Inadequate treatment of acute infection can result in chronic prostatitis. A subacute infection may also develop into a chronic prostatitis that remains asymptomatic. Therefore prostatic secretions should be examined routinely to detect infection and to prevent complications such as acute or chronic cystitis, pyelonephritis, or epididymitis. It is believed that inflammation permits entry of antibiotics that normally do not diffuse into the prostatic fluid. Although they may be used during an acute infection, they are ineffective in a chronic condition. Trimethoprim is the only antibiotic that diffuses into the prostatic fluid and is therefore the drug of choice in chronic prostatitis.[10] Occasionally *prostatic abscesses* complicate the clinical course and may have to be drained surgically. If prostate calculi are present, they may be infected. Antibiotics are ineffective, and surgical excision is required. Prostatectomy may be necessary to eradicate the infection.

#### Nursing Management

Nursing management consists of teaching the patient how to reduce the effects of swelling of the prostate. The patient is taught how to perform warm sitz baths, use antiinflammatory medications, and avoid allergy-producing foods that may be exacerbating the inflammation.

The patient should refrain from sexual activity until the antibiotic medication has started to work, approximately 2 weeks into therapy. The antibiotic therapy must be taken for the entire prescribed time, even if the symptoms have been relieved sooner. Avoiding the use of alcohol and over-the-counter drugs (e.g., decongestants) can help prevent exacerbation of the symptoms of urinary obstruction. The use of stool softeners can decrease irritation to the inflamed prostate during defecation.

## BENIGN PROSTATIC HYPERTROPHY (HYPERPLASIA)

### Etiology/Epidemiology

The prostate gland, located below the bladder, surrounds the urethra and is responsible for contributing to ejaculatory fluid. During puberty, the prostate grows rapidly. After puberty, growth tapers off by age 30 years. Changes in the size of the gland next occur after age 50, when the gland begins to atrophy and become nodular. **Benign prostatic hypertrophy** (hyperplasia, BPH) is an enlargement of portions of this gland that eventually causes problems with urination. Parts of the gland may atrophy, whereas other parts become large and nodular. BPH is a common problem in men over age 50.

The exact cause of these changes in the size and shape of the prostate are associated with increased androgen levels. There is a greater concentration of dihydrotestosterone in males with BPH. Studies have shown that BPH is not seen in males castrated before puberty and that BPH does not progress after castration. Males without the enzyme 5-alpha-reductase cannot convert testosterone to dihydrotestosterone and consequently also do not develop BPH.[17] It is estimated that as many as 75% of men over age 50 have enlargement of the prostate producing symptoms of urinary difficulties. Symptoms may develop in men as young as age 30. Men that live to be 80 have a 10% chance that they will require some form of treatment to correct symptoms of BPH.[7]

### Pathophysiology

The changes in the prostate gland of older men can create a number of problems with the associated urinary system. When the enlarged nodular tissue of the prostate impinges on the urethra, the urethra elongates and compresses, causing obstruction of urinary flow. This can result in a compensatory hypertrophy of the bands of bladder muscles. This in turn increases the trabeculation (contouring) of the bladder wall, providing pockets for urinary retention. These trabeculated areas show up on ultrasound. Because of the muscular thickening, the bladder has less capacity. Muscle tone can diminish over time. Consequently, the bladder cannot empty completely at each voiding (residual urine); the urine becomes alkaline from stasis and is a fertile medium for bacterial growth.

These changes to the urethra and bladder can result in symptoms of urinary obstruction and irritation. Often the symptoms of obstruction are gradual and not noticed by the male until acute urinary retention takes place. Symptoms of gradual obstruction include a decrease in the urinary stream with less force on urination and often dribbling at the end of voiding. Other related symptoms include hesitancy, a difficulty in starting the stream, intermittency, and not being able to maintain a constant stream. The patient may also complain of a sense of incomplete emptying of the bladder. Straining and urinary retention are the symptoms that often influence the patient to seek medical attention.

**BOX 53-2 Clinical Manifestations of Benign Prostatic Hypertrophy**

- Prostate gland enlarges, becomes more nodular
- Straining on urination
- Hesitancy in starting urine flow
- Decreased urine stream
- Postvoid dribbling
- Nocturia
- Dysuria
- Blood in urine
- Urgency

Symptoms of irritation often accompany the obstructive problems. Nocturia from incomplete emptying is common. Dysuria, urgency, and urge incontinence are symptoms associated with loss of muscle tone in the bladder and changes in the angle of the bladder neck. The patient may also have symptoms of UTI because of incomplete emptying and the increased risk of infection. Blood in the urine is also a symptom. As the prostate enlarges, so does the vasculature, and when straining takes place, these vessels break and cause bleeding into the urinary stream. Urinalysis and culture and sensitivity tests are routinely done to screen for occult blood and possible UTIs. Box 53-2 summarizes the typical clinical manifestations of BPH.

Other problems that can stem from BPH are kidney disorders caused by backflow of urine. Hydronephrosis and pyelonephritis are possible sequelae to urinary obstruction. Anemia may also occur if blood loss is severe or as a result of secondary renal insufficiency.

### Prevention

#### Primary prevention

No specific preventive measures exist for BPH. Castration is the only known means of avoiding BPH, and this method of prevention is not acceptable to most males.

#### Secondary prevention

Early detection and adequate follow-up can prevent complications that would result from obstruction if left untreated. Yearly physical examination of all men over age 40 should include palpation of the prostate via rectal examination. The individual should avoid certain drugs and alcohol if symptoms of urinary obstruction are evident.

Some researchers believe a pattern of regular or frequent ejaculation helps prevent BPH. However, the studies pertaining to frequency of sexual activity and how it affects the prostate are still inconclusive.[17]

## Medical Management

The expected length of stay of patients with BPH as determined by diagnosis-related group (DRG) is 3 days. Common medical therapies for management of BPH are described next.

### Diagnostic tests

Common medical therapy for management of BPH includes diagnostic tests that are associated with analyzing renal function. These include monitoring changes in blood urea nitrogen (BUN), creatinine, proteinuria, hematuria, and increases in WBC. Other disease entities that result in outflow obstruction symptoms should be ruled out. Prostate cancer, bladder neck contracture, urethral stricture, bladder calculi, bladder cancer, inflammatory prostatitis, and neurogenic bladder are all problems that have similar symptoms.

Besides the urinary and blood tests already mentioned, endoscopic procedures may be performed. Cystourethroscopy is used to assess for outflow obstruction, measure the length of the urethra, and visualize the extent of bladder involvement. Uroflowmetry is a noninvasive procedure that can evaluate bladder emptying. An intravenous pyelogram (IVP) is a test that requires the infusion of dye into the bloodstream to outline the urinary tract. Sequential x-ray films are performed to assess the anatomy of the upper urinary tract, check for calculi (stones), and evaluate the degree of bladder emptying. (IVPs are not routinely ordered for evaluation of BPH unless hematuria is present.) Obtaining postvoid residual urine is an easy but invasive technique that can also assess bladder emptying.

### Medication

Medications used in the treatment of BPH attempt to decrease the production of dihydrotestosterone. Finasteride (Proscar) inhibits the activity of 5-alpha-reductase so that it cannot turn testosterone into dihydrotestosterone and consequently can reduce the prostate size.[7] Often the therapeutic effects of finasteride are not noticed for several months because of the time required to demonstrate an appreciable difference in the size of the prostate. Even though this drug actually changes the size of the prostate, it may not always help the symptoms of possible urinary retention. The urethra may remain compressed because the nodular growth in that immediate area may not shrink sufficiently to affect the flow of urine positively. Adverse drug effects include decreased libido, impotence, and ejaculation disorders.

Other drugs are used to relax muscles and reduce straining on urination. These drugs are selective or nonselective alpha blockers. Selective blockers are prazosin (Minipress), doxazosin, and terazosin (Hytrin). Nonselective alpha blockers such as phenoxybenzamine (Dibenzyline) tend to have more severe side effects. The main side effects of all these drugs are orthostatic hypotension and fatigue. These drugs are usually taken in the evening to reduce nocturnal symptoms of BPH.

### Treatment

Usually, no specific treatment exists for mild BPH besides medication and some dietary restrictions. Clients are routinely monitored for signs of subtle changes in kidney function, which may initially be diagnosed by the use of blood tests. The phrase "watchful waiting" is often used to describe the monitoring of the condition with regular checkups.

### Diet

No special diet will prevent BPH. However, certain beverages and medications can exacerbate the symptoms of urinary retention because of their effects on the muscles of the bladder and urethral sphincter. Alcohol should be avoided. Other drugs that impair muscle function include anticholinergics and antidepressants. Tranquilizers and nasal decongestants often have a side effect of urinary retention and should be avoided if the patient experiences symptoms of irritation.

### Activity

The man with BPH does not need to restrict his normal activity in any way. Frequent emptying of the bladder and avoiding bladder distention are important to prevent hypertrophy of the bladder. Avoiding straining and lifting heavy weights will help prevent hemorrhage resulting from strain on the increased vasculature in the prostate.

### Referral/Consultation

In some settings the nurse assumes responsibility for making referrals to other services. Referrals for persons with BPH are rarely needed because of the temporary nature of any complications associated with the therapies.

## Surgical Management

For patients with recurrent and obstructive problems caused by BPH, surgery is often the treatment of choice. The decision for surgery is also based on the degree of urinary symptoms, presence of UTI, and the degree of physiologic changes. Surgery for BPH often ranges from minimally invasive to extensive invasion of tissue with increased risks and long-term effects. Immediate consequences of surgery can be hemorrhage and fluid imbalances. Potential long-term effects of these surgeries are prolonged incontinence and retrograde ejaculation of semen into the bladder, causing cloudy urine and diminished fertility. During these surgeries, the capsule of the prostate gland is left intact, and the nodular gland tissue is removed by one of several surgical routes. Males who undergo one of these therapies are typically symptom free for at least 8 years, after which there is a 5%

**TABLE 53-4 Comparison of Types of Prostate Surgery**

| REASON FOR SURGERY | LOCATION OF INCISION | DRAINAGE TUBES | BLADDER SPASMS | DRESSING | COMPLICATIONS |
|---|---|---|---|---|---|
| **TRANSURETHRAL RESECTION** | | | | | |
| Enlargement of medial lobe surrounding urethra | No incision; removal by way of urethra | Three-way Foley catheter with 30 ml bag in urethra; constant irrigation for 24 hr | Yes | None | Hemorrhage; water intoxication; incontinence |
| **SUPRAPUBIC RESECTION** | | | | | |
| Extremely large mass of obstructing tissue | Low midline abdominal incision through bladder to prostate gland | Cystotomy tube or drain through incision; Foley catheter with 30 ml bag in urethra | Yes | Abdominal dressing easily soaked with urinary drainage | Hemorrhage; wound infection |
| **RETROPUBIC RESECTION** | | | | | |
| Large mass located high in pelvic area | Low midline abdominal incision into prostate gland (bladder not incised) | Foley catheter with 30 ml bag in urethra, constant irrigation for 24 hours | Few | Abdominal dressing; no urinary drainage | Hemorrhage; wound infection |
| **PERINEAL RESECTION** | | | | | |
| Large mass located low in pelvic area | Incision between scrotum and rectum | Foley catheter with 30 ml bag in urethra | Few | Perineal dressing; no urinary drainage | Hemorrhage; wound infection |
| **RADICAL PERINEAL RESECTION** | | | | | |
| Cancer of prostate gland | Large perineal incision between scrotum and rectum | Foley catheter with 30 ml bag in urethra; drain in incision | Few | Perineal dressing; urinary drainage | Urinary incontinence; wound infection; impotence; sterility |

to 15% retreatment rate.[7] Discussion of the surgical techniques follows, and Table 53-4 compares the different approaches.

### Transurethral prostatectomy

**Transurethral prostatic resection (TURP)** is performed when the major glandular enlargement exists in the medial lobe that directly surrounds the urethra. There must be a relatively small amount of tissue requiring resection so that excess bleeding will not occur and the time required to complete the surgery will not be prolonged. A resectoscope (an instrument similar to a cystoscope but equipped with a cutting and cauterization loop attached to an electric current) is passed through the urethra. The bladder and urethra are continuously irrigated during the procedure. Tiny pieces of tissue are cut away, and the bleeding points are sealed by cauterization (Figure 53-5). A TURP may be performed with the patient under general or spinal anesthesia.

After a TURP, a large three-way Foley catheter is often inserted into the bladder. (The decision by the physician to insert a Foley catheter depends on the amount of bleeding that is expected after the procedure.) After the retention balloon of the catheter is inflated, the catheter is pulled down so that the balloon rests in the prostatic fossa and provides hemostasis. Traction may be applied to the Foley catheter to increase pressure on the operative area to control bleeding. The large-size catheter is used to facilitate removal of clots from the bladder. Because the catheter balloon exerts pressure on the internal sphincter of the bladder, the patient may continually feel the urge to void. If the catheter is draining properly, the strongest of these sensations usually passes momentarily. Attempting to void around the catheter causes the bladder muscles to contract and results in a painful "bladder spasm." As the nerve endings become fatigued, the frequency and severity of spasms decrease. This usually occurs after 24 to 48 hours.

If a Foley catheter is inserted, the bladder is constantly

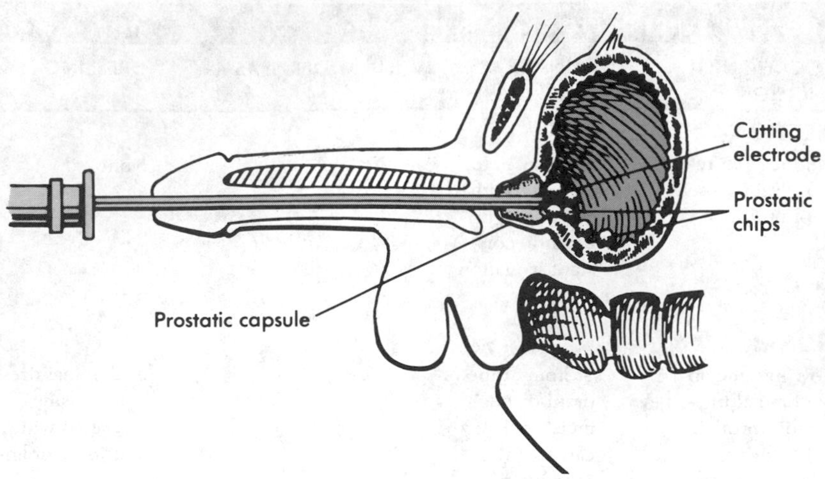


**FIGURE 53-5** Transurethral resection of prostate gland by means of resectoscope. Note enlarged prostate gland surrounding urethra and tiny pieces of prostatic tissue that have been cut away.

irrigated by a three-way drip apparatus with normal saline or another solution prescribed by the surgeon. The purpose of the constant irrigation is to keep the bladder free of clots that would block the drainage of urine.

Persistent bladder discomfort, bladder spasms, or failure of a catheter to drain properly usually signifies one of the following serious complications, which requires immediate medical attention: (1) hemorrhage and clot retention, (2) displacement of the catheter, or (3) unsuspected perforation of the bladder during surgery.

Sometimes patients develop *water intoxication,* formerly known as transurethral resection (TUR) syndrome, as a result of excessive irrigating solution being absorbed into the venous sinusoids during surgery. Cerebral edema may result. Confusion and agitation may be the first signs of this condition.

Constant bladder irrigation is usually discontinued after 24 hours if no clots are draining from the bladder. After catheter removal, the patient should measure and record the time and amount of each voiding. The patient may not be able to void after removal of the catheter because of urethral edema. When this occurs, the catheter may need to be reinserted. Continence is also assessed, since the internal and external sphincters lie above and below the prostate, close to the operative area, and may have been disturbed during surgery.

About 2 weeks after TURP, when desiccated tissue is sloughed out, a secondary hemorrhage may occur. The patient, who probably is home at this time, must contact the physician immediately if there is any bleeding.

### Suprapubic prostatectomy

The alternate methods of prostatectomy are open procedures (Figure 53-6). In the *suprapubic resection,* the prostate gland is removed from the urethra by way of the bladder; this type of resection is performed when a large mass of tissue must be resected. Some type of hemostatic agent is placed in the prostatic fossa, and urine is drained by Foley catheter or cystotomy tube or both.

*Hemorrhage* is a possible complication, and the precautions are the same as those taken after TURP. Since some oozing of blood from the prostatic fossa occurs, continuous bladder irrigations are usually ordered for the first 24 hours.

Cystotomy tubes are usually removed 3 to 4 days postoperatively; urethral catheters generally remain until the suprapubic wound is well healed. After the urethral catheter has been removed, the nursing care of the patient is similar to that for the patient undergoing TURP. If the suprapubic wound should reopen and drain, a urethral catheter is usually reinserted.

### Retropubic prostatectomy

In a retropubic prostatectomy, a low abdominal incision similar to that used for suprapubic prostatectomy is made, but the bladder is not opened. The bladder is retracted, and the prostatic tissue removed through an incision in the anterior prostatic capsule. A large-diameter Foley catheter is inserted, and hemorrhage and infection are potential complications, but the sphincter muscles are not damaged, and the patient rarely has difficulty voiding.

### Trial surgical procedures

Other surgical procedures being evaluated for efficacy include balloon dilation of the urethra. This is similar to the procedure done for coronary arteries. The procedure is intended to dilate the lumen of the urethra by pushing the impinging prostate gland back. This pro-

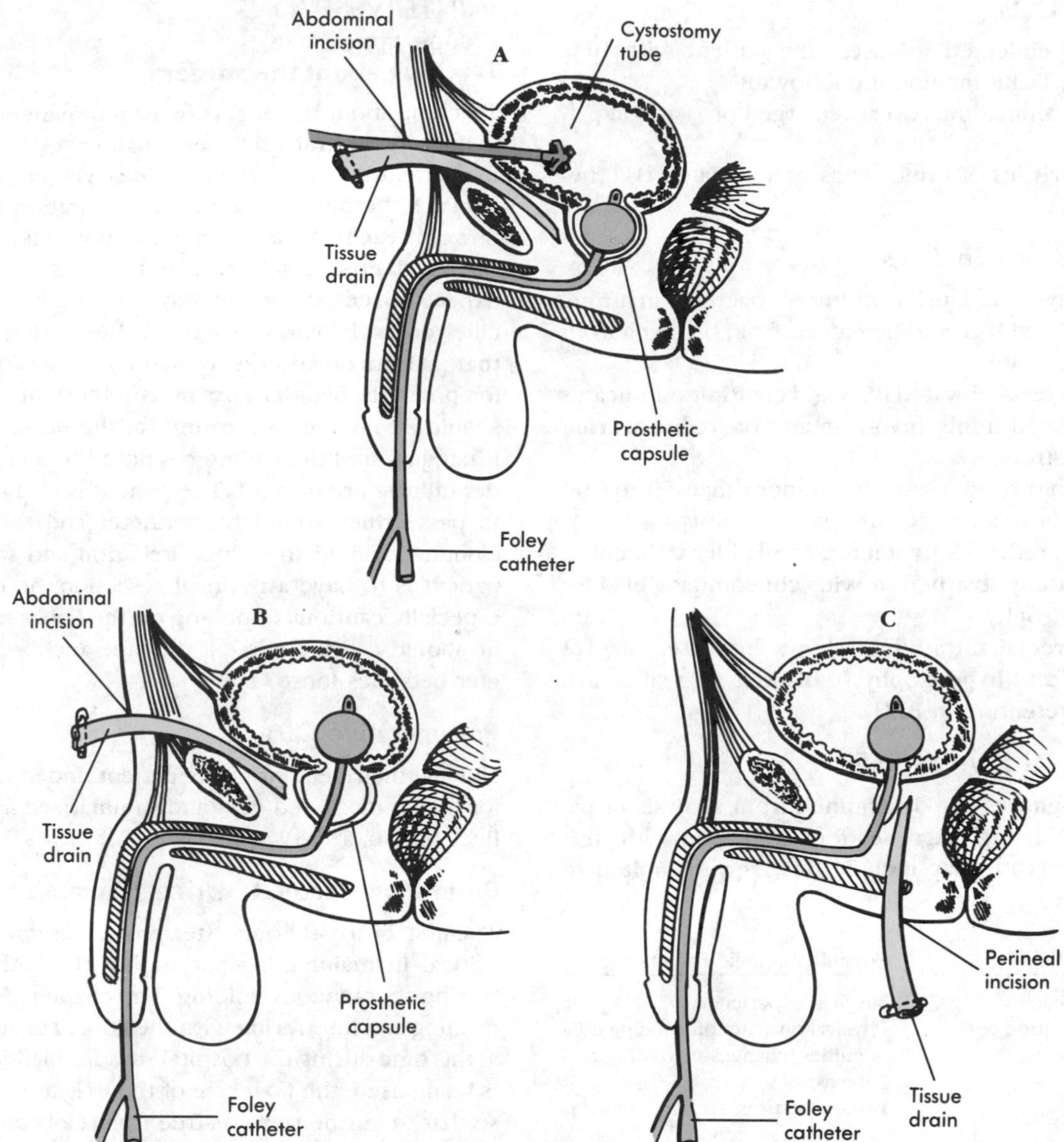


**FIGURE 53-6** Three types of prostatectomies. **A,** Suprapubic: note placement of inflated Foley catheter in prostatic fossa. **B,** Retropubic. **C,** Radical perineal: note tissue drain placed in incision between scrotum and rectum.

cedure is of controversial efficacy.[7] Another procedure being tried is a microwave technique that burns the area. The tissue sloughs, creating a larger lumen in the urethra. Care after these procedures is similar to that for cystoscopy or sometimes that of a TURP if a catheter is left in place. Nursing management of patients with surgery of the prostate is included in the following discussion.

# NURSING MANAGEMENT

## ♦ ASSESSMENT

### Subjective Data

Data to be collected to assess the patient with BPH undergoing TURP include the following:

Pattern of urination: frequency, number of times voiding per night, urgency, acute urinary retention

Characteristics of voiding: difficulty starting or stopping stream, dribbling, hesitancy

Sensations: a feeling of incomplete emptying of bladder, need to strain, pain on urination, bladder spasms

Medication use and associated voiding symptoms (recent colds with the use of decongestants may trigger an acute urinary retention episode)

Age: usually see signs in men 40 years or older

Knowledge of the purpose and function of the prostate gland, effects of TURP on sexual functioning and fertility

## Objective Data

Data to be collected to assess the patient with BPH undergoing TURP include the following:

Rectal examination: reveals enlarged prostate on palpation

Characteristics of urine: signs of associated UTI, hematuria

## Diagnostic Test Findings

1. Urinalysis and urine cultures: bacteria in urine, associated UTI, and hematuria from bleeding from the prostate
2. Blood tests; elevated BUN and creatinine: indicates associated kidney involvement from reflux of urine or obstruction
3. Postvoid residuals of urine: more than 50 to 100 ml indicates inadequate bladder emptying
4. Cystourethroscopy: increased bladder trabeculae, indicating obstruction with concomitant bladder hypertrophy
5. Transrectal ultrasound: shows increased size of gland and hypertrophy of bladder as well as urinary retention in BPH

# ♦ NURSING DIAGNOSES

Nursing diagnoses are determined from analysis of patient data. Nursing diagnoses for the person with BPH undergoing TURP may include but are not limited to the following:

| Diagnostic Title | Possible Etiologic Factors |
|---|---|
| Knowledge deficit | Surgical experience |
| Urinary elimination pattern, altered | Physical obstruction, voiding difficulties, changes in voiding patterns |
| Pain | Bladder spasms, straining with voiding, surgery |
| Infection, high risk for | Urinary stasis, surgical manipulation |
| Anxiety | Fears of complications of surgery, including incontinence and infertility |

# ♦ EXPECTED PATIENT OUTCOMES

Expected patient outcomes for the patient with BPH undergoing TURP may include but are not limited to the following:

1. Describes nature of surgery and postoperative care.
2. Demonstrates complete bladder emptying; no problems with urinary stream or voiding patterns.
3. States methods of relieving pain from bladder spasms and surgical procedure. Demonstrates effective use of pain-reducing technique and verbalizes reduction in pain.
4. Lists methods of preventing UTIs and urinary stasis.
5. States risks involved with surgery; lists methods of coping with functional changes.

# ♦ INTERVENTIONS

## Preoperative Care

### Teaching about the surgery

Teaching about the effects of local or general anesthesia is done preoperatively (see Chapter 23 for details). If the patient is to undergo a perineal resection, the nurse explains the need for a bowel preparation to clear the bowel. Teaching also includes information about the specific drains, irrigations, and dressings the patient may expect to see postoperatively (see Table 53-4 for specifics on each type of surgery). Reassuring the patient that pain medication is available for incisional pain or for potential bladder spasms is important. The patient should be encouraged to inform the nurse promptly if leaking around the catheter is noted or feelings of bladder fullness are present. The patient is told not to strain to pass urine around the catheter and to drink large amounts of fluid to reduce irritation and spasm. If the patient is to have a perineal resection, he needs to be especially cautious of pulling on the Foley catheter, and he should call the nurse if the tape anchoring the catheter becomes loose.

## Postoperative Care

Nursing management of the patient undergoing surgery for BPH is discussed next and summarized in the Guidelines box, p. 1793.

## Promoting Adequate Urine Elimination

The first 24 to 48 hours after prostatectomy surgery are critical in maintaining patency of the catheter or restoring spontaneous voiding. The chance of blood clots forming and interfering with the flow of urine is greatest at this time during the hospital stay. If a bladder irrigation is being used, the flow rate of the irrigation must be set so that the urine remains free from clots and remains a cherry red to pink color. If a dark-red color is noted, the flow of the fluid needs to be increased. The nurse is responsible for regulating the flow of the irrigation in response to the color and consistency of the urine output.

An accurate intake and output record of the urine flow compared with the flow of the irrigation solution should be documented. The output should be at least 50 ml per hour greater than the hourly flow of the irrigation. Less urine output indicates a possible obstruction. All tubing should be checked for patency first, and if no equipment cause can be determined and rectified, irrigations using a 50 ml syringe may be ordered to help clear the catheter of any clots.

Because irrigation solutions may be used in large quantities, there is a potential risk for water intoxication. The patient may absorb much of the irrigation fluid and problems of hyponatremia, and other electrolyte imbalances may occur. The nurse assesses the patient for symptoms of elevated blood pressure, decreased pulse rate, confusion, and nausea. The nurse prepares for and administers treatment ordered by the physician for

### Guidelines for Postoperative Care for the Person Undergoing Prostatic Surgery

1. Maintain patency of catheter system.
2. Monitor appearance of urine: red to light pink (24 hours) to amber (3 days).
3. Monitor patient for signs of water intoxication after TURP (confusion, agitation, warm moist skin, anorexia, nausea, vomiting).
4. Instruct patient not to try to void around catheter; explain feeling of needing to void from pressure of catheter.
5. Avoid use of enemas and rectal temperature.
6. Give prescribed medications (analgesics, antispasmodics) as needed; tell patient spasms will decrease in intensity and severity within 24 to 48 hours.
7. After catheter removal:
    a. Monitor output for signs of urinary retention.
    b. Monitor for continence; teach perineal exercises if dribbling occurs.
    c. Encourage increased fluid and frequent voiding.
8. Change dressings frequently around suprapubic wounds after suprapubic prostatectomy to prevent skin maceration.
9. Give patient opportunities to discuss feelings about sexuality and possible incontinence.
10. Teach patient to:
    a. Avoid vigorous exercise, heavy lifting (over 20 pounds), and sexual intercourse for at least 3 weeks after returning home.
    b. Avoid driving for 2 weeks.
    c. Avoid straining with defecation; use stool softeners or mild laxatives if needed.
    d. Drink at least 2500 ml fluids/day to prevent urinary stasis and infection and to keep stools soft.
    e. Notify physician if urinary stream diminishes or if bleeding occurs.
    f. Report for medical postoperative visit; urinary stream will be checked at this time.

hyponatremia, which often include infusions of hypertonic saline and the use of diuretics such as furosemide (Lasix).

## Controlling Pain From Bladder Spasms and Straining

Narcotics are given to lessen the pain sensation of bladder spasms. Belladonna and opium (B & O) suppositories are most often prescribed to reduce bladder spasm. These are soft suppositories that will not cause pain or damage to the fragile tissue around the rectum, which may have been involved in the surgical procedure. Encouraging fluids, at least 8 to 10 full glasses of fluid per day, helps to flush the system and reduce irritation that causes spasms. Frequent voiding after the catheter has been removed also decreases irritation that causes spasms.

To prevent straining during defecation, which can put pressure on the recently traumatized tissues of the perineum, the patient is encouraged to take mild laxatives and, again, maintain a well-hydrated state. Stool softeners are also frequently used to promote painless defecation.

## Preventing Infection

Intravenous antibiotics are often administered in the first few days after surgery. The patient is placed on oral antibiotics as soon as the parenteral antibiotics are discontinued. The patient is also encouraged to increase his fluid intake to promote flushing of the system and help prevent urinary stasis and decrease the chances of infection.

## Relieving Anxiety

The patient should be told that most men have some temporary difficulty with continence after any type of prostatectomy. The man should understand that this is normal for a time but will improve. Teaching perineal exercises such as Kegel's exercises (see Chapter 49) can be helpful in controlling voiding. Frequent voiding can help reduce problems of dribbling. Specific suggestions about absorptive devices and specialty underwear products used for the temporary control of incontinence may be helpful to the patient.

The surgeries used to treat BPH do not physically affect the man's ability to have an erection. The patient needs to be reassured that there is a difference between infertility and impotence. Depending on the extent of prostate removed, fertility can be minimally or greatly reduced. Also, if the patient has continued retrograde emission of prostatic fluid even after several months, fertility will remain diminished.

The nurse must not assume that because males with BPH routinely are older, fertility is not an issue. Even if the man is not planning on having additional children, fertility is often closely associated with sexuality. The nurse may need to provide opportunities for the patient to express these concerns. Reminding the patient that an erection is still possible is often helpful. The ability to feel an orgasm is also intact. The patient should be cautioned that he may still be fertile, and use of birth control may still be necessary to prevent unwanted pregnancies.

# ♦ EVALUATION

To evaluate the effectiveness of nursing interventions, compare patient behaviors with those stated in the expected patient outcomes. Successful achievement of patient outcomes for the patient with BPH undergoing surgery is indicated by the following:

1. Correctly describes the surgical procedure, postoperative care, and discharge restrictions.
2. Achieves complete bladder emptying, no problems with clotting, voiding patterns, or urine stream.
3. Avoids straining around the catheter, requests pain medication in a timely manner, drinks fluids, and demonstrates methods of softening stools and promoting defecation.
4. Finishes the course of oral antibiotic medications, drinks 2500 ml of fluid daily, and recognizes signs of infection and appropriate actions.

# NURSING CARE PLAN

## PERSON WITH TUR PROSTATECTOMY FOR BENIGN PROSTATIC HYPERTROPHY

**DATA:** Mr. J. is a 67-year-old retired married automobile mechanic. He has been diagnosed by his physician as having benign prostatic hypertrophy. Mr. J. has undergone medical examinations on an outpatient basis and has never been admitted to the hospital. He is slightly obese. On admission his blood pressure is 140/90. He denies any history of hypertension. Mr. J. takes aspirin three to four times a day for control of what he describes as chronic headaches. He had a TURP performed today.

### ■ NURSING DIAGNOSIS
Altered urinary elimination pattern related to surgery

| Expected Patient Outcome | Nursing Interventions | Rationale |
|---|---|---|
| Urine output is greater than 50 ml per hour | 1. Monitor urine output and characteristics.<br>2. Maintain constant bladder irrigation (CBI) as prescribed during first 24 hours.<br>3. Maintain patency of indwelling urinary catheter:<br>a. Irrigate manually as prescribed to keep catheter free of clots.<br>b. Maintain straight-line closed drainage system<br>4. Encourage high fluid intake (2500 to 3000 ml/day) to promote increased urine flow.<br>5. After catheter is removed, monitor for signs of retention. | Ensure adequate bladder emptying. There is a potential for reabsorption of water from the bladder, so output must be carefully assessed. Clots may also obstruct drainage catheter and must be detected early. |

### ■ NURSING DIAGNOSIS
Pain related to bladder spasm

| Expected Patient Outcome | Nursing Interventions | Rationale |
|---|---|---|
| States feeling more comfortable. | 1. Teach patient not to try to void around catheter.<br>2. Monitor patient at regular intervals for 48 hours to identify early signs of bladder spasms.<br>3. Give prescribed medications (analgesics, antispasmodics).<br>4. Tell patient spasms will decrease in intensity and frequency within 24 to 48 hours. | Bladder spasm frequently follows urologic procedures. Forcing voiding will encourage spasms. Antispasmodics may offer best relief by elimination or reduction of spasm. |

### ■ NURSING DIAGNOSIS
High risk for fluid volume excess related to irrigating fluid

| Expected Patient Outcome | Nursing Interventions | Rationale |
|---|---|---|
| Does not exhibit signs of water intoxication. | 1. Monitor patient for signs of water intoxication during first 24 hours: confusion, agitation, warm moist skin, anorexia, nausea, vomiting, and low serum $Na^+$ level.<br>2. Monitor fluid intake (oral, IV, CBI) and output. | Irrigation fluid may be reabsorbed through bladder wall, resulting in water intoxication. |

# NURSING CARE PLAN

## PERSON WITH TUR PROSTATECTOMY FOR BENIGN PROSTATIC HYPERTROPHY—cont'd

### ■ NURSING DIAGNOSIS

High risk for infection/injury (hemorrhage) related to surgery

| Expected Patient Outcome | Nursing Interventions | Rationale |
|---|---|---|
| Does not exhibit signs of infection or hemorrhage. | 1. Monitor vital signs; report signs of shock or fever.<br>2. Monitor appearance of urine for persistent bright-red color rather than expected light red/pink color beyond first few hours postoperatively.<br>3. Teach patient to avoid Valsalva's maneuver, which may initiate prostatic bleeding.<br>4. Avoid use of rectal thermometers, rectal examinations, or enemas for at least 1 week.<br>5. Maintain strict asepsis of urinary drainage system; irrigate only when necessary.<br>6. Encourage high fluid intake. | Change in vital signs may alert nurse to infection. Bleeding is common after TURP but must be closely monitored. |

### ■ NURSING DIAGNOSIS

High risk for stress or urge incontinence related to catheter use

| Expected Patient Outcome | Nursing Interventions | Rationale |
|---|---|---|
| Achieves urinary continence. | 1. Assess patient for dribbling after catheter is removed.<br>2. If dribbling occurs:<br>a. Tell patient this is a common occurrence but that continence will return.<br>b. Teach patient perineal exercises.<br>3. Explain use of devices and pads for temporary incontinence. | Dribbling may occur after TURP but should resolve. Perineal exercises strengthen sphincter tone. |

### ■ NURSING DIAGNOSIS

High risk for sexual dysfunction related to surgery

| Expected Patient Outcome | Nursing Interventions | Rationale |
|---|---|---|
| Describes effects of TURP on sexual functioning. | 1. Give patient opportunities to discuss feelings about the effects of prostatectomy on sexual intercourse.<br>2. Provide information as necessary:<br>a. Probable return of previous level of functioning.<br>b. Occurrence of retrograde ejaculation (first urine after intercourse may have a milky appearance).<br>c. Avoid sexual intercourse for 3 to 4 weeks after surgery. | Sexual functioning usually returns to presurgical level. Patients often need to be encouraged to discuss their feeling about sexual intercourse. |

*Continued.*

## NURSING CARE PLAN

### PERSON WITH TUR PROSTATECTOMY FOR BENIGN PROSTATIC HYPERTROPHY—cont'd

#### ■ NURSING DIAGNOSIS

Knowledge deficit (activity restriction, prevention of complications) related to lack of information

| Expected Patient Outcome | Nursing Interventions | Rationale |
|---|---|---|
| Describes activity restrictions and medical follow-up. | 1. Teach patient:<br>a. Avoidance of heavy activities for 3 to 4 weeks.<br>b. Avoidance of straining at stool for 4 to 6 weeks; use stool softeners or laxatives as necessary. | By adequately educating patient about postsurgical routine and restrictions, the nurse can help ensure compliance with the medical regimen. |

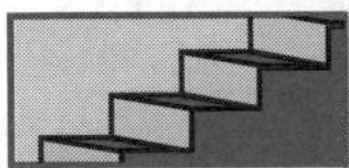

## CRITICAL PATHWAY TURP Without Complications

**DRG #: 336; expected LOS: 4 days**

| | Day of Surgery<br>Day of Admission<br>Day 1 | Day 2 | Day 3 | Day of Discharge<br>Day 4 |
|---|---|---|---|---|
| **Diagnostic Tests** | Preoperative: Chest x-ray film, CBC, UA, PT/PTT, ECG, SMA/18,* acid phosphatase<br>Postoperative: CBC, electrolytes | CBC, electrolytes | | |
| **Medications** | Preoperative: IV antibiotic<br>Postoperative: IVs, IV antibiotic, IV or IM analgesic, B & O suppository PRN, stool softener | IV to saline lock, IV/PO antibiotic, PO analgesic, B & O suppository PRN, stool softener | Disc saline lock, PO analgesic, PO antibiotics, B & O suppository, stool softener | PO analgesic, PO antibiotics, stool softener |
| **Treatments** | I & O q8hr including Foley catheter and continuous GU irrigation; ? tension on Foley catheter, VS q4hr; assess neurocirculation to legs q2hr; elastic leg stockings (ELS) | I & O q8hr including Foley catheter; disc GU irrigation; Foley catheter to DD; VS q6hr; ELS | I & O q8hr; disc Foley catheter; VS q8hr; ELS; 7-bottle urine assessment | Disc I & O; VS q8hr; ELS; 7-bottle urine assessment |
| **Diet** | NPO, advance to regular diet as tolerated | Regular diet, force fluids | Regular diet, force fluids | Regular diet, force fluids |
| **Activity** | Flat for 6-8 hr after spinal anesthesia, then bedrest; assist with arising | Assist with arising | Assist with arising | Arise ad lib |
| **Consultations** | | Social service, home health | | |

*Serum calcium, phosphorus, triglycerides, uric acid, creatinine, BUN, total bilirubin, alkaline phosphate, aspartate aminotransferase (ALT, formerly serum glutamic oxaloacetic serum glutamic oxaloacetic transaminase [SGPT]), lactic dehydrogenase (LDH), total protein, albumin, sodium, potassium, chloride, total $CO_2$, glucose.

5. Discusses anxieties about sexuality and incontinence, is able to list devices to reduce effects of incontinence, and describes sexual systems that were not affected by surgery.

See Nursing Care Plan and Critical Pathway, p. 1794-1796.

## SPECIAL CONSIDERATIONS FOR CARE OF THE GERONTOLOGIC PATIENT

Spinal anesthesia may be the choice for the more elderly patient if surgery is necessary for BPH. Often the less aggressive surgery is performed on the elderly patient to avoid complications of prolonged procedures.

## HOME CARE CONSIDERATIONS

After any prostatectomy surgery, the patient is instructed to avoid heavy lifting and walking more than two flights of stairs. The patient should avoid sexual activity for at least 3 weeks. Driving should not be done for 2 weeks.

The patient should watch for and report any sign of infection at any incision site. The patient should also watch for blood or clots in the urine and any change in urine stream. If the catheter must remain in when the patient is discharged from the hospital, the nurse provides instructions for cleansing around the catheter with mild soap once a day.

Analgesics are often prescribed, and information on their use and side effects is provided. The patient is often given a return appointment to the urology clinic, usually in 2 to 3 weeks.

For the patient with mild BPH, teaching about avoiding the use of alcohol and over-the-counter medications such as antihistamines is helpful in reducing the risk of urinary retention. The man is reminded to void at regular intervals and avoid straining and physical activity that create excessive abdominal or perineal pressure. It is also important to teach the patient the indications and side effects of the androgen antagonist medications. These side effects include reports of impotence, hot flashes, loss of libido, gynecomastia, tender nipples, and heat intolerance. The alpha-blocker drugs frequently cause side effects such as fatigue and dizziness.

### Complications

Complications of surgery for BPH include but are not limited to the following: hemorrhage, water intoxication from continuous bladder irrigation, UTI, incontinence, and decreased fertility.

## CANCER OF THE PROSTATE

### Etiology/Epidemiology

Cancer of the prostate often starts as a discrete, localized hard nodule in an area of senile atrophy. It is most often caused by an adenosarcoma that arises in the peripheral regions of the gland. Seventy-five percent of prostate cancers arise in the peripheral zone (outer area of gland, contiguous with the capsule), 20% in the transitional zone (midportion of gland), and 10% in the central zone surrounding the urethra. Because the growth is generally on the outer portion of the gland, compression and subsequent voiding symptoms are not common until late in the disease. Nonurinary symptoms are often so ambiguous that this disease is often not diagnosed until it is well advanced.[19]

Factors that may affect the development of prostate cancer include hormonal changes and viral infections. Hormonal influences have been clinically proved to be a cancer risk factor, since men castrated before puberty do not develop prostate cancer. Hormonal changes during aging are the reason that prostate cancer is seen almost exclusively in men over age 40. A direct viral etiology has not been proved, but a strain of cytomegalovirus isolated from the prostate gland can produce malignant transformation in prostate tissue in the laboratory setting.[17] In addition, positive antibody titers to herpes simplex and cytomegalovirus have been found in men with prostate cancer.

Environmental influences may increase the risk for prostate cancer. Immigrants from countries with a low incidence of prostate cancer have demonstrated an increased incidence after living in a country with a high incidence of prostate cancer.[19] Other risk factors include a history of multiple sexual partners, episodes of STDs, the presence of cervical cancer in sexual partners, and industrial exposure to cadmium.

The prostate gland is the most common site of cancer in American men. Prostate cancer is the second leading killer from cancer in American men.[3,7] Prostatic cancer rarely occurs before age 40, the incidence increases sharply with age, and there is an increased familial risk. African-Americans have the highest incidence of prostate cancer in the world. Although white men in the United States have a lower incidence compared with black men, they have a rate higher than men in other parts of the world.[2,19]

### Pathophysiology

Prostate cancer may be confined to the gland and surrounding capsule. This limited extension of the tumor usually causes no symptoms. Sixty percent of men have a form of localized prostate cancer. However, the cancer can be found outside of the capsule boundaries and can spread to the lymphatic system and be disseminated through the vascular system. The most common sites of metastasis are the bones of the pelvis; lumbar and thoracic spine; femur; and ribs. Organ involvement (lung, liver, kidneys) is seen primarily in the late stages of terminal disease.

Because the prostate gland is adjacent to the rectal wall, growth can often be detected by rectal examination before symptoms appear. On examination, prostate can-

**BOX 53-3 Clinical Manifestations of Prostate Cancer**

- Often no symptoms if cancer is confined to the gland.
- Symptoms of urinary obstruction.
- Symptoms of urinary tract infection.
- Low back pain, malaise, aching in legs, and hip pain if cancer has metastasized.

cer may present as a discrete or diffuse area of increased firmness. Unfortunately, however, up to 40% of cancers may arise anterior to the midline of the prostate gland and consequently cannot be felt on rectal examination.[19]

The prostate secretes a glycoprotein that increases with inflammation, benign growth, and cancer. Prostate-specific antigen (PSA) measures the elevation of this glycoprotein and is used to help identify possible cancers. Epithelial cells in the ductal system of the prostate gland secrete acid phosphatase. If acid phosphatase is found in serum blood tests, it usually indicates that prostatic tissue has spread beyond the capsule of the gland.

This cancer can spread at a very slow rate or be very aggressive. The biologic aggressiveness of malignant tumors depends at least in part on the degree of differentiation of the cells (see Chapter 16). Most of the prostatic malignancies are defined as adenocarcinomas or sarcomas. Pathologic grading of the tumors is difficult because there are often multiple tumor sites and often a variety of cell differentiation at different sites in the prostate gland. The Gleason grading scale is used to rank the correlation between the extent of tissue differentiation and the patient's prognosis. The Gleason system of grading has total scores ranging from 2 to 10. Two biopsy sites are used in testing, and the scores of each (which range from 1 to 5) are added together to obtain the total score of 2 to 10. The lower the score, the less aggressive is the cancer and the better the prognosis.

Clinical manifestations of prostate cancer may include complaints of stiffness, back pain, and occasionally pathologic fractures. The symptoms may also mimic those of BPH, with urinary outflow obstruction or severe bladder irritation with no signs of infection. Often there are no symptoms in the initial stages of prostate cancer (Box 53-3).

## Prevention

### Primary prevention

No true primary prevention exists for prostate cancer.

### Secondary prevention

Because symptoms are often ambiguous, regular screening for prostate cancer is very important. It is recommended that men over age 40 have an annual rectal examination. In addition, a combination of diagnostic tests is now used to improve the accuracy of detection.

**RESEARCH**

Millon-Underwood S: Factors influencing early detection of prostate cancer, *Appl Nurs Res* 5(1):30-31, 1992.

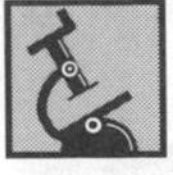

This study was undertaken to determine why many men never have rectal examinations or other forms of screening done for prostate cancer. Millon-Underwood hypothesizes that interest in prostate screening was influenced by the man's belief that he was susceptible to prostate cancer and/or to his belief that screening was beneficial. A questionnaire that measured the beliefs and attitudes about screening and susceptibility was administered to a sample of 90 males, ranging in age from 39 to 78 years.

Of the 90 subjects, 88% believed that screening would help prevent advanced prostate cancers, and 61% thought that rectal examinations for screening were important but too embarrassing. Less than half the subjects had a rectal examination for prostate cancer. Thirty-six percent of the subjects believed that the screening could cause needless worry.

Millon-Underwood also found that men who believed that health screening was important were more likely to have prostate screening done. The men who thought that their health was too good to worry about screening were less likely to have screening done.

Because there was a significant correlation between the men's beliefs of susceptibility to prostate cancer and their willingness to be screened, Millon-Underwood believes that attitudes and beliefs need to be addressed by nurses to help the patient take advantage of health screening.

Blood screens, rectal examination, and ultrasound techniques all help in early detection. High-risk patients, with histories of multiple sexual partners, STDs, and certain viral infections, should be given special attention in screening routines.[2] See Research box above.

## Medical Management

The expected length of stay for a patient who has had surgical intervention (radical prostatectomy) for prostate cancer as determined by DRG is 4 days. Common medical therapies for the management of prostate cancer are described next.

### Diagnostic tests

Even before disease is noted on the rectal examination, the blood screening test for PSA may show that there is a possible prostatic cancer. PSA screening is done before the rectal examination so that manipulation of the prostate does not give false-positive readings. Blood screening is often done serially because a rise in PSA or consistently high PSA is more reliable than a single assay. Because PSA levels can rise with inflammation, benign hypertrophy, or irritation as well as a response to cancer,

**TABLE 53-5 Diagnostic Tests for Prostate Cancer**

| PROCEDURE | SCREENING VALUE | STAGING VALUE |
|---|---|---|
| Digital rectal examination (DRE) | +++ | + |
| Prostate-specific antigen (PSA) | ++++ | +++ |
| Transrectal ultrasound (TRUS) | ++ | ++ |
| Prostatic acid phosphatase (PAP) | | |
| Automated radioimmunoassay | – | – |
| Enzymatic method | – | +++ |
| Radionuclide bone scan | – | +++ |
| Pelvic computed tomography (CT) | – | ++ |
| Endorectal magnetic resonance imaging (MRI) | – | +++ |
| Lymphadenectomy | – | +++++ |

Data courtesy Gerald L. Andriole, Jr, MD.

screening is done in conjunction with other diagnostic procedures. Knowledge of prostate size, along with PSA levels, provides a more definitive diagnosis than PSA alone. PSA is now routinely drawn before and after biopsies or surgery on the prostate gland. Serial levels can be followed after the test or treatment to detect recurrence of the cancer. The laboratory parameters for significant PSA values are still being studied. Table 53-5 compares efficacy of diagnostic tests.

Transrectal ultrasound (TRUS) aids in the screening of nonpalpable tumors. It may also be used in helping to direct the physician in biopsy of palpable tumors. TRUS allows greater accuracy in tumor localization and needle placement than just using digital rectal examinations alone to help guide the biopsy. Biopsy of any firm or nodular areas is necessary to confirm the diagnosis of prostate cancer. The biopsy procedure may be done in a clinic setting or minor surgery operating rooms. The biopsy can be done with the patient under local anesthesia or light general anesthesia. If done with ultrasound, a probe is placed in the rectum; otherwise, the surgeon uses a digital technique to guide the procedure. The needle biopsy can be performed by transperineal or transrectal route, depending on the physician's choice.

Typical patient preparation for prostate biopsy focuses on providing an optimal environment for visualization, preventing complications, and baseline data gathering for follow-up. Rectal cleansing by enema or oral laxative is often done before the procedure as a means of preventing potential infection. Preprocedural antibiotics are used and may be continued for several days after the procedure. The patient may have nothing by mouth or allowed to eat a light breakfast before the study. The extreme vascularity of the gland increases the risk of bleeding, and coagulation profiles are usually drawn before the procedure. Patients are also taken off

**BOX 53-4 Staging of Prostatic Neoplasia**

| | |
|---|---|
| Stage I/A | Microscopic lesions found in prostate gland removed because of benign hypertrophy |
| Stage II/B | Nodules confined to prostate gland: no capsular adherence or urethral involvement; normal serum acid phosphatase level |
| Stage III/C | Carcinoma involving prostatic capsule, seminal vesicles, urethra, bladder, and pelvic lymph nodes, or a malignant tumor of a lesser extent with elevated serum acid phosphatase level |
| Stage IV/D | Findings as in stage III plus evidence of extrapelvic lesions or osseous involvement |

any anticoagulants and drugs such as aspirin before the test.

**Staging.** A system of staging prostate cancer has been developed to classify the location, size, and spread of the tumor and guide treatment decisions. For example, a tumor that is confined to the capsuled gland and is very small is termed a stage A. If the tumor is confined to the gland but is a larger size, it may be staged as an A1 (Box 53-4). The use of staging helps in determining the prognosis and provides the basis for treatment recommendations. Higher numeric values and/or letter values of C or D have a poorer prognosis.

Staging is done by gathering information from blood tests, diagnostic imaging procedures, and lymph node biopsies. An elevated serum acid phosphatase and PSA blood test usually indicates metastatic disease. Bone scans of the femur, pelvis, and spine are frequently done, and regional lymph nodes are removed for microscopic examination. If biopsy results are negative, node involvement can usually be ruled out.

Treatment decisions by the physician are based on the results of the staging and the Gleason scale rating. Prostate cancer that is detected in the very beginning stages may not be treated at all. Instead, the patient is placed on a schedule of frequent clinical checkups to monitor possible changes in the cancer and the potential need for therapeutic interventions. Two other options used for stages A and B prostate cancers are radiation and/or radical prostatectomy.

### Medication

**Hormone therapy.** When cancer of the prostate gland is inoperable or when signs of metastasis occur after surgery, pharmacologic treatment is given. Relief with hormonal therapy is quite dramatic in many patients and may last for 10 years or more in some instances. Usually, the response is quite good for about 1 year, and then the patient's condition begins to deteriorate.

Huggins' treatment may be used for inoperable cancer of the prostate gland to cause atrophy of the local lesion, control metastases, and relieve pain. It is based on the elimination of androgens by removal of the testes or the administration of estrogenic hormones or both. The estrogen given is usually stilbestrol, 3 mg/day for 1 to 2 weeks. The dosage is then reduced to 1.5 to 3 mg/day. Stilbestrol causes engorgement and tenderness of the male breasts (gynecomastia); it may also cause nausea. Severe side effects should be reported to the physician so that the dosage or type of estrogenic preparation can be adjusted.

Estrogen preparations also result in fluid retention and dependent edema, which may be controlled with salt restriction and diuretics. Other problems include cardiovascular complications and increased risk of stroke. If a large tumor does not diminish in size with this treatment, some of the prostate gland may be resected to relieve obstruction. The use of hormone therapy provides a longer symptom-free period but makes palliation more difficult when symptoms recur. If endocrine therapy is delayed, symptoms recur earlier, but longer palliation is possible.

When symptoms of obstruction begin to recur or when the diagnosis of cancer is first made, a bilateral orchiectomy (castration) may be performed. This procedure is technically minor and is often performed using local anesthesia, but it may cause the patient considerable psychologic distress. The man's permission for sterilization must be obtained. If he is married, he is usually urged to discuss the procedure with his wife. This surgery eliminates the testicular source of male hormones and seems to cause regression of the cancer or at least slow its growth. Very seldom, a hypophysectomy may be performed to further reduce hormonal stimulation.

### Treatment

**Radiation therapy.** Radiation may be delivered by external beam or by implant. The testes are shielded during external radiation. Iodine retropubic prostatic implantation may be used initially or after failure of external radiation therapy. The mortality and morbidity of internal irradiation when coupled with lymphadenectomy are less than for radical prostatectomy. Complications of $^{125}$I implantation include blood loss from multiple needle punctures during implantation, deep vein thrombosis, pulmonary emboli, hematomas, and abscesses.[11] Impotence from radiation may deveop over time as a result of scar tissue formation. There is a greater risk of complications if radioactive implants are used after external beam radiation. Irritability of the bladder caused by radioactive implants can produce urinary symptoms.

### Diet

No therapeutic diet exists for patients with prostate cancer. A high-fiber, low-fat diet is recommended because men from countries that routinely eat this type of diet have a lower incidence of prostate cancer. However, there is no clinical evidence that diet plays any role in preventing or slowing the growth of prostate cancer. Diets are routinely modified if the patient is to have surgery.

### Activity

If the patient has undegone radiation therapy or prostatic surgery, he should limit heavy lifting or straining on urination. The patient should not drive a vehicle for 2 weeks after surgery. If the Foley catheter has been left in place at the time of discharge from the hospital, the patient should be cautioned not to engage in any activity that could pull or put strain on the catheter.

### Referral/Consultation

Because many of the therapeutic interventions affect the patient's fertility and ability to have an erection, a specialist in sexual therapy or counseling may be helpful to the patient. Sometimes patients are also interested in family-planning counseling for alternative means of conceiving children. If persistent urinary incontinence is a problem, nurses specializing in the care of incontinent patients (enterostomal therapy nurses) may be consulted. The American Cancer Society can help the patient deal with the emotional issues related to the diagnosis of cancer, as well as provide information on a variety of helpful resources.

## Surgical Management

A radical resection of the prostate gland usually is curative for patients with stage A or B prostate cancer. The entire prostate gland, including the capsule and the adjacent tissue, is removed. The remaining urethra is then anastomosed to the bladder neck. The surgery is accomplished by using a perineal, retropubic, or suprapubic approach. The retropubic approach makes it possible to spare the nerves around the urethra to preserve urinary continence. Nerve-sparing surgeries are the treatment of choice if the patient has less invasive cancer.[16] The retropubic approach uses a low midline incision, and the perineal approach uses a perineal incision. The patient has a Foley catheter in place for a period of days to several weeks, depending on the approach used by the physician, and if he is at risk for delayed healing because of previous radiation therapy. Figure 53-6 compares different surgical methods of placing drains and incisions. Nursing management of the patient undergoing perineal prostatectomy is discussed next.

# NURSING MANAGEMENT

## ♦ ASSESSMENT

### Subjective Data

Data to be collected to assess the patient with prostate cancer include the following:

History of STDs, sexual partners with cervical cancer, and viral infections such as herpes

Urinary symptoms: similar to those of BPH
Generalized complaints: low back pain, hip joint pain, arthritic type pain in hip and back area
Knowledge of normal prostatic function, purpose of blood tests, purpose of scans, and biopsies; purpose of treatments, surgery, radiation, and hormonal therapy; expected postoperative care routines

### Objective Data

Data to be collected to assess the patient with prostate cancer include the following:

Rectal examination (nurse practitioner): nodular or diffuse areas of firmness, enlarged prostate
Age: usually seen in men over 40

### Diagnostic Test Findings

1. Elevated PSA
2. Elevated prostatic acid phosphatase (PAP)
3. Enlarged prostate with possible areas of metastasis seen on ultrasound
4. Gleason scale showing nondifferentiated cells in at least two sites
5. Staging showing tumor localized to the gland or extending beyond the gland

## ♦ NURSING DIAGNOSES

Nursing diagnoses are determined from analysis of patient data. Nursing diagnoses for the patient with prostate cancer may include but are not limited to the following:

| Diagnostic Title | Possible Etiologic Factors |
|---|---|
| Knowledge deficit | Surgical experience |
| Incontinence, functional; bowel incontinence | Side effects of prostate surgery |
| Sexual dysfunction | Impotence |
| Grieving, anticipatory | Diagnosis of cancer |

## ♦ EXPECTED PATIENT OUTCOMES

Expected patient outcomes for the patient with prostate cancer may include but are not limited to the following:

1. Describes nature of surgery and postoperative care.
2. Reestablishes urinary/bowel continence.
3. Lists alternative methods of sexual activity; discusses sexual concerns and needs with professional staff and partner.
4. Addresses grieving process

## ♦ INTERVENTIONS

### Preoperative Care

If the patient is to have a perineal approach in surgery, he is given a bowel preparation, which includes enemas, cathartics, and sulfasalazine (Azulfidine) or neomycin preoperatively and only clear fluids the day before surgery to prevent fecal contamination of the operative site.

### Postoperative Care

The care of the perineal wound consists of monitoring for possible urine leaks, hemorrhage, and signs of infection. Often the patient wears a Fuller shield or briefs-type underwear to support the dressing on the perineal incision. The use of a "donut" or "Life Saver" cushion may be used to relieve pressure on the incision site while sitting. The use of rectal thermometers, rectal tubes, and hard suppositories is avoided to prevent injury to the fragile perineal area.

When solid food is permitted, a low-residue diet may be given until wound healing is well advanced. Camphorated tincture of opium may be prescribed to inhibit bowel action in the first postoperative week to prevent contamination of the incision.

### Restoring Urinary and Bowel Continence

Regardless of the surgical approach, the patient returns from surgery with a urethral catheter inserted. A large amount of urinary drainage on the dressing for a number of hours is not unusual. This can be managed by the use of an ostomy bag around the dressing. The urinary drainage should decrease rapidly. The amount of bleeding in the urine should not be the same as after other prostatic surgery. Since the catheter is not being used for hemostasis, the patient usually experiences less bladder spasm. The catheter is used both for urinary drainage and as a splint for the urethral anastomosis; therefore, care should be taken that it does not become dislodged or blocked. Clinically, the risk of blockage from clots is greatest during the first hour. The catheter may be irrigated intermittently or continuously as ordered by the physician. The catheter is usually left in the bladder for 2 or 3 weeks or longer.

Temporary urinary incontinence is often a problem with patients that have had any type of radical prostatectomy. The patient needs to be encouraged, and provisions should be made to keep him dry so that he will feel able to be up and to socialize with others without fear of incontinence. (See Chapter 49 for ways to manage incontinence.)

If voluntary urinary control has not been regained within 6 months to a year, a prostatic prosthesis is available to control urinary incontinence. The prosthesis consists of a silicone gel–filled sac placed at the base of the penis.[9] Four tapes of polypropylene mesh are stapled to the pelvic rami or sutured to the periosteum to secure the prosthesis in place. This puts pressure on the urethra, and if the pressure is too great, urethral erosion can occur. Therefore intraurethral pressure is measured during surgery. If the pressure decreases within the prosthesis, injections may be used to increase it. There is a 60% success rate.

Because of their suppressed immune response, patients who have undergone radiation therapy have a greater risk of osteomyelitis and wound complications; therefore they are not candidates for prostatic prosthesis. The prerequisite for surgery is a sterile urine sample and a normal WBC count.

Since perineal surgery causes relaxation of the perineal musculature, the patient may suddenly also have fecal incontinence. It is disturbing to the patient and sometimes can be avoided by starting perineal exercises within a day or two after surgery. Control of the rectal sphincter usually returns readily. Perineal exercises should be continued even after rectal sphincter control returns, since the exercises also strengthen the bladder sphincters, and unless the bladder sphincters have been permanently damaged, the patient will regain urinary control more readily on removal of the catheter.

### Promoting Sexual Function

Total prostatectomy, which includes bilateral pelvic lymphadectomy, can result in physiologic sexual dysfunction as a result of disruption of genital innervation. The patient may be temporarily impotent for several months even after a nerve-sparing prostatectomy has been performed. Ninety-five percent of patients that undergo the nerve-sparing prostatectomy regain potency within 1 year.[16] The patient needs to know that return of erectile capability may be delayed and that alternative sexual interactions may be used until function returns. (See the following section on impotence for further information.)

The patient should understand that he is no longer fertile after any radical prostatectomy and that the loss of the prostate gland interrupts the flow of semen and there will be no ejaculation. However, the patient can still experience the sensations of orgasm.

### Dealing with Grief

Patients who have stage A or B prostate cancer have an excellent survival rate. It is important to remind patients that prostate cancer is very different from many other forms of cancer, since even men with stage C prostate cancer have a long survival rate. Prostate cancer is usually slow growing, and many elderly men do not die of prostate cancer but from other causes. The fear of cancer must be acknowledged, however, and the patient needs time and encouragement to express these fears. (For more information on the grieving process related to cancer, see Chapter 16.)

## ♦ EVALUATION

To evaluate the effectiveness of nursing interventions, compare patient behaviors with those stated in the expected patient outcomes. Successful achievement of patient outcomes for the patient with prostate cancer is indicated by the following:

1. Correctly describes the surgical procedure, postoperative care, and discharge restrictions.
2. Is continent of urine and stool or controls incontinence using effective, safe methods.
3. Understands the changes in sexual functioning and is able to express concerns about sexual function.
4. Discusses concerns about the diagnosis of cancer and is aware of prognosis.

## ✹ SPECIAL CONSIDERATIONS FOR CARE OF THE GERONTOLOGIC PATIENT

Because prostatic cancer is often slow growing, treatment options for elderly patients may be more palliative in nature. Radical prostatectomies have not been known to prolong life for elderly patients. Consequently, radiation or measures to decrease the size of the prostate (e.g., TUR) to relieve symptoms of urinary obstruction may be the treatment of choice rather than the radical prostatectomy.

If surgery is done, healing times are prolonged. The perineal muscles of the elderly patient are weaker, and problems of urinary incontinence and bowel incontinence may take longer to be controlled. Perineal muscle exercises may be started before surgery to help the elderly client regain muscle tone sooner.

## HOME CARE CONSIDERATIONS

If the patient had a radical perineal prostatectomy, the perineal wound may still be open when the patient is discharged from the hospital. Cleansing the wound after defecation should consist of simple cleansing with water and possible use of a douche bottle as a means to provide low-pressure irrigation to the area. Many physicians allow showers within the first week of surgery. The dressing to the incision site is held in place with the use of briefs-type underpants, just as in the hospital. The dressing should remain dry, and the patient should be encouraged to change the pads whenever drainage on the dressing becomes irritating, often twice a day or more.

The patient is taught how to use a urinary leg bag and how to connect and disconnect the Foley catheter from the bedside drainage bag into the leg bag. Signs of UTI are taught to the patient, and he is told to notify his physician if any signs of infection occur. The insertion site of the catheter at the penis should be washed once a day with water and/or a mild soap if desired. The catheter needs to remain firmly anchored to the thigh or abdomen. Perineal exercises to promote the return of urinary continence when the catheter is removed should be practiced on a regular basis at home.

Reminding the patient that bowel incontinence may still be a problem for a few days when he returns home is important. The patient should have easy access to a bathroom. Instructing the patient to use the commode a few hours after meals may help to promote bowel continence.

## COMPLICATIONS

Complications of radical prostatectomy for prostate cancer include, but are not limited to, the following: hemorrhage, urinary and bowel incontinence, infertility, impotence, and leakage at the anastomotic site of the urethra and bladder. Prostate cancer may metastasize to local organs such as the lymph nodes, bowel, and bladder. Sites of distant metastasis include but are not limited to the liver, spine, and lungs.

# PROBLEMS OF THE PENIS

Structural problems of the penis are typically related to the head of the penis and the foreskin. The head of the penis is susceptible to diseases caused by irritations, cancer, and trauma. The foreskin can also be a source of structural difficulties that can affect urination, cause pain, and interfere with blood flow to the penis. The anatomy of the penis is illustrated in Figure 53-7.

Functional abilities of the male reproductive system include erection, ejaculation, and fertility. The later portion of this section focuses on the ability of the male to have an erection (potency) and the procedure used to render the male infertile (vasectomy). STDs are discussed in Chapter 55.

## PHIMOSIS AND PARAPHIMOSIS

### Etiology/Epidemiology

**Phimosis** is a condition in which the opening of the prepuce or foreskin is unable to be retracted behind the glans. It may be congenital or acquired as a result of inflammation or infection.

**Paraphimosis,** conversely, is a condition in which the prepuce is retracted over the glans and forms a constriction at the base of the glans. This is usually a result of manipulation of the foreskin over the glans and failure to return it to cover the glans. This condition is most often seen in children or in men with changes in mental status that predispose them to memory loss or with decreased sensation in the penis (Figure 53-8).

### Pathophysiology

With phimosis the inability to retract the foreskin may interfere with adequate hygiene. Consequently, urine and smegma may be trapped in the preputial sac, resulting in irritation and predisposing the glans to infection. Chronic irritation may be a cause of penile carcinoma. Healing of the irritation or infection causes scar tissue formation, which can worsen the acquired phimosis. If the constriction of the foreskin at the head of the penis is severe enough, it causes urinary obstruction and painful urination.

Constriction is also a major problem with paraphimosis. This constriction at the base of the glans usually results in swelling of the glans. If the swelling is not

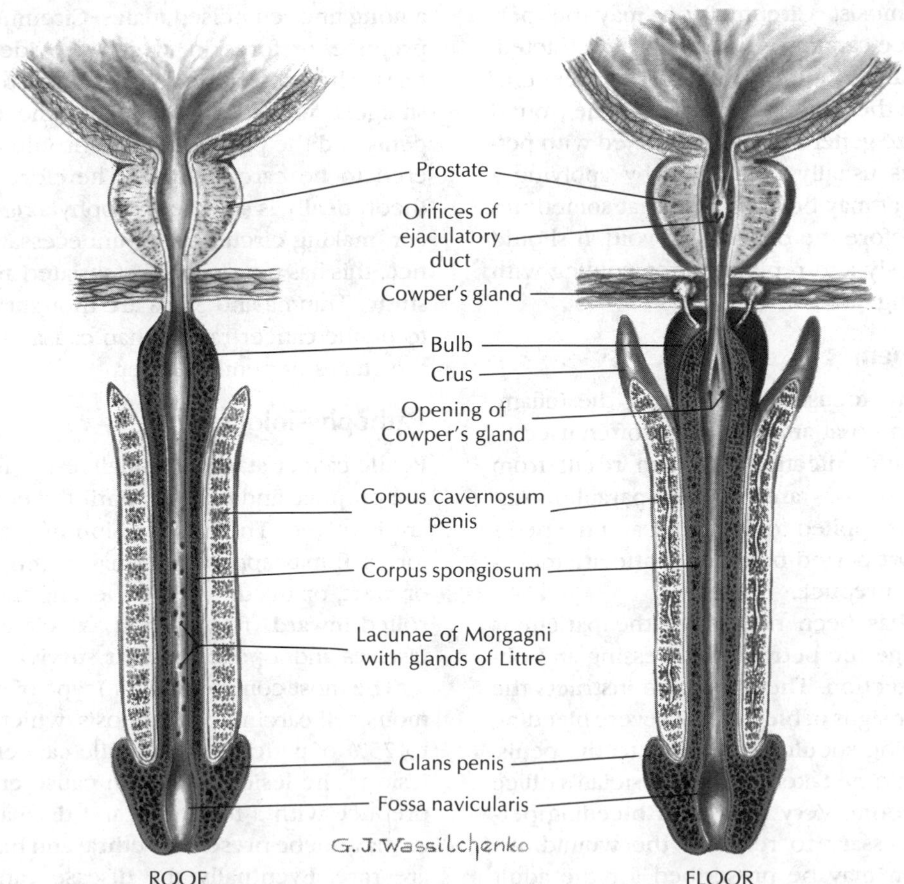


**FIGURE 53-7** Anatomy of the penis. (From Bobak IM, Jensen MD: *Maternity and gynecologic care,* ed 5, St Louis, 1993, Mosby.)

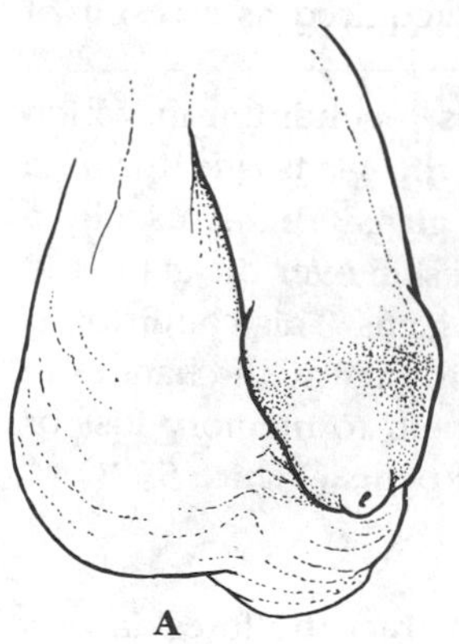


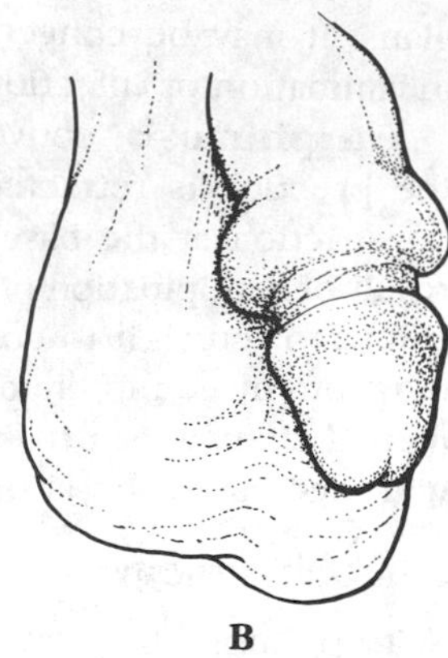


**FIGURE 53-8** **A,** Phimosis; note pinpoint opening of foreskin. **B,** Paraphimosis; note foreskin is retracted but has become constricting band around penis.

reduced, blood vessels to the glans are compressed, reducing flow. Inadequate blood flow can result in necrosis of the glans.

### Medical Management

Treatment for severe cases of phimosis may consist of incisions in the foreskin to reduce the contracture and widen the opening. Stretching of the foreskin by repeated retraction behind the glans may be the treatment for congenital phimosis. Circumcision may be performed if the prepuce cannot be satisfactorily retracted.

Circumcision is also done to prevent recurrence of paraphimosis. When the penis is circumcised, the wound is covered with gauze generously impregnated with petrolatum. Bleeding is usually controlled by applying a pressure dressing that may be bulky and that sometimes must be removed before the patient can void. It should be removed cautiously and replaced after voiding with a petrolatum dressing.

### Nursing Management

Nursing management focuses on reducing the inflammation. Hot soaks and oral antibiotics are often used to treat the swelling and infection that can result from phimosis. Cool compresses are used for paraphimosis. The cool compress is applied to the penis, and the penis is elevated for a short period before a gentle attempt is made to reduce the prepuce.

If circumcision has been necessary, the patient is taught how to change the petrolatum dressing and observe for signs of infection. The nurse also instructs the patient to be alert for signs of bleeding. If severe bleeding occurs, a firm dressing should be applied to the penis, and the patient should be taken to the physician's office or the emergency room. Very seldom, if bleeding persists, it may be necessary to resuture the wound. An estrogen preparation may be prescribed for the adult patient for several days after surgery to prevent painful erections.

**BOX 53-5 Stages of Penile Cancer**

| | |
|---|---|
| Stage A: | Lesions confined to glans or foreskin |
| Stage B: | Shaft or corpora cavernosa invaded by tumor |
| Stage C: | Shaft involvement; lymph nodes involved but operable |
| Stage D: | Shaft involvement; lymph nodes inoperable; metastases to distant sites |

## CANCER OF THE PENIS

### Etiology/Epidemiology

In America, penile cancer accounts for 0.5% to 1.5% of all male malignancies. It is most common between ages 50 and 70, but it can occur in younger men and has been reported in children.[1] There is a higher incidence in blacks than whites, possibly because of a lower incidence of circumcision. Penile cancer accounts for 10% to 20% of all male malignancies among African and Asian peoples.[3]

The incidence of penile cancer depends greatly on hygienic standards and cultural and religious practices. It almost never occurs in a male who was circumcised at birth. Circumcision after puberty does not decrease the risk of cancer when compared with the incidence among uncircumcised males. Circumcision removes the prepuce, or foreskin, which provides a haven for bacteria. The bacteria act on desquamated cells, producing smegma, which is irritating to the tissue of the glans penis and the prepuce. This chronic irritation is considered to be carcinogenic. Therefore adequate hygiene theoretically is sufficient prophylaxis against penile cancer, making circumcision unnecessary. In clinical practice, this has not been substantiated and requires further study. Trauma and STDs are thought to be coincidental to penile cancer rather than causative. Box 53-5 shows the stages of penile cancer.

### Pathophysiology

Penile cancer starts as a small lesion usually on or under the prepuce and extends until the entire glans and shaft are involved. The initial lesion may assume a variety of forms. It may appear as a small bump, resemble a pimple or wart, or occur as a nonhealing ulcer with the edges rolled inward. The latter is associated with earlier metastases and a poorer 5-year survival.

The most common (95%) type of malignancy is squamous cell carcinoma. Phimosis, which is present in 25% to 75% of patients with penile cancer, may obscure the lesion. The lesion may then cause erosion through the prepuce with a foul odor and discharge. Bleeding may or may not be present. Urethral and bladder involvement are rare. Eventually the disease can become autoamputative. If left untreated, death occurs in 2 to 3 years.

Clinical manifestations of penile cancer include weakness, fatigue, malaise, and weight loss. Men may complain of itching and burning under the prepuce and an occasional foul discharge. A delay of 1 year before seeking treatment is common in 15% to 50% of cases. Biopsy is performed to establish the diagnosis; however, benign penile lesions occur infrequently.

Metastasis usually occurs at the regional femoral and iliac nodes and is associated with a significantly worse prognosis. Five-year survival with inguinal node involvement is 20% to 25%.

### Medical Management

Treatment is usually surgical. Radiation therapy is indicated only in younger patients in whom preservation of sexual function is important and who have small superficial lesions.

If the lesion is confined to the prepuce, circumcision may be adequate. If the lesion is on the glans, partial penectomy or amputation of the penis is required. If the shaft of the penis is involved, total amputation may be necessary. The decision is based on the amount of penis remaining after excision with an adequate tumor-free margin. The remaining penis must be long enough for the patient to void standing, direct the stream, and not void on himself. If this is possible, sexual function will probably be retained. If total amputation is required, a perineal urethrostomy is performed, in which the urethra is redirected to an opening between the scrotum and the anus. With spread of the cancer to the scrotum, radical removal is required, either hemipelvectomy or hemicorporectomy.

Approximately one third of men with penile cancer have metastatic nodal disease at the time of the initial diagnosis. Radiation therapy is used as adjuvant therapy at all stages.

Lymphadenectomy is indicated for lymph node involvement. Accurate detection of metastases is difficult, since enlarged lymph nodes may be free of cancerous tissue, whereas normal-sized lymph nodes may contain metastatic lesions.

Chemotherapeutic agents have been used with some success, particularly in patients with stages A and B disease. Agents that have been used include high-dose methotrexate, bleomycin, and cisplatin. Because of the rarity of the disease, large-scale clinical studies to evaluate chemotherapeutic agents are lacking. Methotrexate given intravenously has been somewhat successful. Other chemotherapeutic agents have not been effective. If the disease is confined to the penis, 5-year survival is 80% to 85% with amputation. With metastasis to the lymph nodes, it is only 20%.

### Nursing Management

The nurse teaches the patient about the potential side effects of radiation in the perineal area. Radiation in this location can affect the skin so that it becomes dry, itchy, and sensitive. Special gels to apply to the skin that are safe to use during radiation may be applied to the affected area.

Urethral strictures can develop several months to years after radiation therapy. The nurse informs the patient of symptoms of urethral stricture, which include difficulty starting or stopping the urine flow, frequent UTIs, and nocturia. Bowel patterns may change during radiation therapy and for up to several weeks after the treatments. Affects of chemotherapy and nursing interventions are discussed in Chapter 16.

Sexual counseling is indicated for the patient with total penectomy. Some patients with a urethrostomy have experienced orgasm and ejaculation after stimulation of the perineal, scrotal, and testicular regions.

## IMPOTENCE

### Etiology/Epidemiology

**Impotence** is the inability for a man to have an erection firm enough or sustain an erection long enough for satisfactory intercourse. The term *satisfactory* is defined by the couple involved and may vary from couple to couple. The ability to have an erection depends not only on a healthy psychologic state, but also on adequately functioning neurologic, vascular, and hormonal systems. The brain is the controlling organ for sexual arousal. The brain perceives sexual stimuli and controls the physiologic changes that occur during arousal. There are two fundamental causes of impotence: physical and psychologic.

Physical causes include changes in blood flow to the penis and neurogenic dysfunctions. Diseases such as diabetes, lupus, and rheumatoid arthritis can cause obstruction of blood flow in the penis from damaged vessels. Anemia and dehydration can cause insufficient blood volumes to maintain an erection. Cardiac diseases and antihypertensive drugs can interfere with the capillary blood pressure.

Neurologic problems can be caused by spinal cord injuries, diseases that cause neurogenic damage (e.g., diabetes), and renal failure. Many neurologic disorders, such as multiple sclerosis and Parkinson's disease, also can interfere with erectile function. Hormonal changes in testosterone levels can affect the male sex drive. Aging affects the level of testosterone, and sexual function usually declines somewhat with advancing age.

Other causes of impotence include medical interventions. Some surgical procedures interfere with both blood engorgement and neurogenic innervation of the penis. Many prescription drugs produce the side effect of impotence.

Psychologic impotence can be attributed to many factors, such as long-term stressors, fears, anxiety, anger, and frustrations. "Performance anxiety," a fear of not performing well during sexual intercourse, is common. Fatigue also influences the ability to have an erection.

Most men experience impotence on occasion. Short-term impotence is often caused by fatigue, stress, anx-

**BOX 53-6 Clinical Manifestations of Impotence**

- Inability to have an erection
- Inability to sustain an erection
- Inability to have an erection firm enough for penetration (incomplete erection)

iety, or the use of alcohol or other drugs. Until recently, psychologic problems were considered to be the cause of 90% of impotence cases. Now, physical causes have been found in 80% of cases. One in every 10 males in the United States has continuing or chronic impotence.[14]

## Pathophysiology

Inability of the brain to respond to sexual stimuli can interrupt the signals to the parasympathetic nervous system that release a transmitter substance causing the small arteries in the penis to dilate. The result is insufficient blood flow to fill the network of sinusoids inside the corpora cavernosa (erectile chambers) that cause the penis to enlarge and become firm. If inadequate blood flow and blood volume exist in the erectile chambers, they cannot create enough pressure within the chambers to block blood return. Blood then drains from the penis, and an erection cannot be maintained.

The sympathetic nervous system controls both orgasm and ejaculation. These two functions therefore can occur without an erection. After ejaculation, or when sexual stimulation diminishes, the arteries in the penis constrict, reducing blood flow, and the veins need to expand to allow disengorgement. Box 53-6 summarizes the clinical manifestations of impotence.

## Prevention

### Primary prevention

Reducing stress, maintaining a healthy diet, avoiding alcohol, getting adequate rest, and having a positive attitude toward sex can help prevent problems of temporary impotence.

### Secondary prevention

Closely adhering to medical therapy to reduce sequelae of various disease states can help prevent problems of chronic impotency.

## Medical Management

The expected length of stay in the hospital for patients with impotence being treated with a surgical implant as determined by DRG is 3 days. Common medical therapies for the management of impotence are discussed next.

### Diagnostic tests

Diagnostic tests for the initial work-up of impotence include complete blood count, urinalysis, BUN, creatinine, and fasting blood sugars. These tests help rule out disease entities such as anemia, renal disease, and diabetes as possible causative factors. Other blood tests include cholesterol levels and hormonal studies.

Nocturnal monitoring of penile tumescence is also performed. These tests involve the male wearing a device around the penis at night that can gauge if there is normal nocturnal engorgement of the penis. These are simple, noninvasive devices that indicate the ability of the penis to enlarge and become firm.

Psychologic testing is also usually done. Often this testing includes the partner as well.

Invasive studies are ordered only when other testing measures are inconclusive. Arteriograms (dye injections to study blood flow) and cavernosometry, which measures pressures and blood vessel responses in the erectile chambers, are sometimes performed.

### Medication

Medications used to treat impotence are few. One possible medication is yohimbine, an oral medication that acts as a mild aphrodisiac and vasodilator. It is a selective alpha-adrenergic blocker that improves sympathetic outflow. The usual dose is 6 mg per day with a 30% response rate from patients. Yohimbine is often prescribed in combination with other therapies and may be a temporary intervention until other, more definitive treatments can be found.[8]

Hormonal therapy is prescribed for the 2% of the impotent population who have a low serum testosterone or an elevated serum prolactin level. Testosterone is given either intramuscularly or transdermally to avoid the hepatotoxicity of the oral preparations. Testosterone can stimulate growth of normal prostatic tissue, promote metastasis of prostatic cancer, stop sperm production, and cause fluid retention and therefore must be used with caution.

Injecting a vasodilator into the penis induces penile erections by means of increased arterial blood flow, sinusoidal relaxation, and increased venous resistance. The drugs generally used are a papaverine and phentolamine combination injected by the patient into the corpus carvernosum of the penis. Other drug combinations may also include the use of prostaglandin E (PGE). A delivery method of introducing these drugs into the urethra is also being studied. Once injected, the penis becomes turgid within 5 to 10 minutes, and the erection may last up to 2 hours. Response rate is about 100% for those with neurogenic impotence and 60% to 70% for those with vascular problems.[8] Test doses are given initially to determine the appropriate amount for each patient. Dosages range from 0.1 to 1.5 ml of the combination drug. Side effects include dizziness, facial flushing, hypotension, and priapism (an erection that lasts longer than 4 to 6 hours).

Many medications have side effects that inhibit erectile function (see Chapter 11). Modifying the dosage, changing the brand, or trying an alternative medication to limit side effects that cause sexual dysfunction may be therapeutic for many patients.

### Treatment

External vacuum devices are sometimes used to achieve an erection for a short time. These devices are cylinders that fit over the penis and use a suction pump to pull blood into the penis. A band is applied to the proximal aspect of the penis when an erection is achieved to impede the venous return of blood. The erection may be maintained for approximately 30 minutes. These devices can be used daily and have minimal side effects if used properly.

Counseling and sexual therapy classes may be suggested for clients who have identified psychologic impotence. They may also be suggested for those men dealing with the problem of impotence and the need to find alternative measures for sexual fulfillment.

Therapies for alterations in sexual arousal include decreasing anxiety about the problem and correcting or transcending the physiologic problems if possible. Anxiety can be reduced through desensitization exercises, in which the person is instructed to use erotic imagery to approximate sexual situations evoking anxiety. Structuring sexual encounters so that they are not demanding is another strategy. Exercises that emphasize pleasure rather than pressure to perform often begin by refocusing the person's attention on the sensual aspects of touch without genital touching for a time. After the person has pleasure in sensual experiences without anxiety, sexual activity is gradually reintroduced.

### Diet

A well-balanced diet is recommended for men with impotence. No studies have proved that any vitamin or mineral supplements specifically enhance the male's ability to have an erection. However, some foods are considered to be aphrodisiacs in various cultures, including oysters, avocados, and bull testicles. Obesity can interfere with erectile functioning. Low-fat reduction diets are recommended for patients who are overweight.

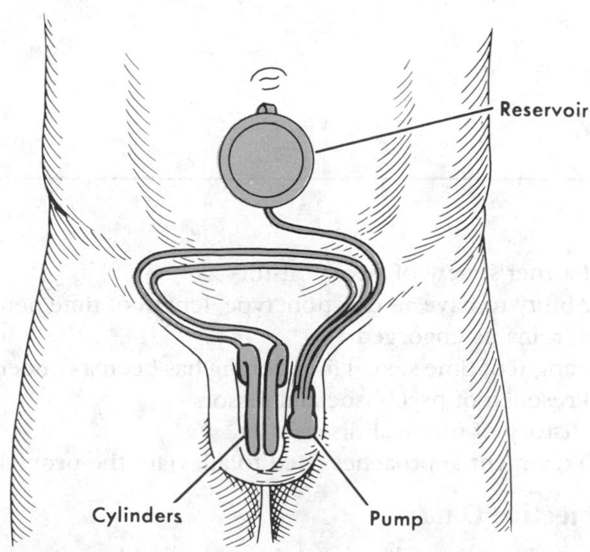


FIGURE 53-9 Inflatable penile prosthetic implant.

### Activity

Men who are in better physical condition often have more endurance and may fatigue less quickly when engaging in sexual activity. However, there are reports that men who routinely train for and run long-distance marathons have a reduced interest in sexual activity.

### Referral/Consultation

In some settings the nurse assumes responsibility for making referrals to other services. Common referrals for a person with impotence include certified sex therapists, social workers, and family counselors.

## Surgical Management

Vascular reconstructive surgery may be helpful for the approximately 5% of the impotent population who have problems with venous leakage. *Venous leakage* is defined as the inability to maintain an erection for more than about 2 minutes. The surgery may include the microscopic reconstruction of arterial vessels or removal of some veins to slow the draining of blood from the penis. These surgeries have a limited success rate of only 30% to 50%. There is also a high rate of relapse because of arteriosclerosis and the continued development of incompetent veins. Complications of vascular surgery include numbness of the penile skin, shortened length, curvature, and hematoma formation.

A penile prosthesis may be implanted in men as a method of treatment for organic erectile dysfunction. There are two types of penile prostheses. The older type consists of two sponge-filled silicone rods, which are implanted in the corpora cavernosa. This maintains the penis in a constant semierect position. The newer method, which more closely imitates an actual erection, is the inflatable penile prosthesis (Figure 53-9). This consists of two inflatable rods inserted into either side of the penis. The rods are connected to a reservoir that allows fluid to flow in or out of the rods when the man presses on a pump device inserted in the thigh or scrotum.

Both types of prostheses are implanted surgically and do not interfere with normal urinary elimination. The silicone implants are inserted through perineal or penile incisions and the inflatable prostheses through perineal and abdominal incisions. Penile edema is minimal, but scrotal edema may occur with the inflatable type. Pain may be severe during the first week, and mild pain may continue for several weeks after surgery. As with any prosthetic device, there is a need for the man to integrate

**TABLE 53-6 Treatment Options for Male Sexual Dysfunction**

| ADVANTAGES | DISADVANTAGES |
|---|---|
| **NONSURGICAL** | |
| **Oral Medications (yohimbine)** | |
| Increases libido<br>Inexpensive<br>Minimal side effects<br>Can be used with other options | Must be taken on long-term basis<br>Limited effectiveness (25%)<br>Side effects include dizziness, nausea |
| **Hormonal Therapy (testosterone)** | |
| Increases libido<br>Inexpensive<br>Does not interfere with other treatment options<br>Widely available | Limited effectiveness (10% to 15%)<br>Contraindicated with prostate cancer<br>Must be taken on long-term basis<br>Side effects include fluid retention, liver damage |
| **External Vacuum Devices** | |
| Easy to understand<br>Inexpensive<br>Safe, reversible<br>Can be used with other treatment options | Requires preparation<br>Long-term effects not known<br>Side effects include bruising, pain<br>Requires manual dexterity |
| **Sexual Devices** | |
| Inexpensive<br>Easy to understand<br>May enhance foreplay/orgasm | Does not produce satisfactory erection<br>May not fit into value system<br>Inaccessibility |
| **Counseling** | |
| Involves partner<br>Can be used with other treatment options<br>May improve other psychosocial issues | Limited effectiveness<br>Long-standing problems may be difficult to treat |
| **Penile Injections** | |
| Use only when desired<br>Produces rapid, natural-appearing erections<br>Can be used with other treatments<br>Minimal pain | Requires close monitoring<br>Moderately expensive<br>Not effective with severe blood flow problems<br>Side effects include priapism, fibrosis<br>Patient may have aversion to needles |
| **SURGICAL** | |
| **Vascular Reconstructive Surgery** | |
| Possibility of restoration to normal function<br>Natural appearance | Expensive<br>Technically difficult surgery<br>Low long-term success rate (30% to 50%)<br>High relapse rate |
| **Inflatable Prosthesis** | |
| Natural-looking erection<br>No preparation time<br>Use as desired<br>Increases girth of penis<br>No concealment problem | Device failure<br>Requires manual dexterity<br>May require removal/reimplant<br>Expensive<br>Risk of infection, erosion |
| **Self-contained Inflatable Prosthesis** | |
| Natural-looking erection<br>No preparation time<br>Use as desired<br>No concealment problem<br>Simpler surgery than that for full inflatable prosthesis | Device failure<br>Requires manual dexterity<br>May require removal/reimplant<br>Expensive<br>Risk of infection, erosion<br>Does not increase girth |
| **Semirigid/Malleable Prosthesis** | |
| Simple surgery<br>No moving parts<br>Least expensive implant<br>Use as desired | May be difficult to conceal<br>Does not increase girth of penis<br>Expensive<br>Risk of infection/erosion<br>May require removal/reimplant |

the device successfully into his body image and sexual relationship. Table 53-6 compares treatment options for erectile dysfunction.

## NURSING MANAGEMENT

### ♦ ASSESSMENT

#### Subjective Data

Data to be collected to assess the patient with impotence include the following:

- History of sexual dysfunction
- Partner's view of sexual history
- Ability to have an erection: type, length of time penis remains engorged
- Length of time sexual functioning has been a concern
- Presence of psychosocial stressors
- History of physical diseases
- Treatment approaches tried to alleviate the problem

#### Objective Data

Data to be collected to assess the patient with impotence include the following:

Sensory deficits: manual dexterity and visual acuity needed for many treatment options

### Diagnostic Test Findings

1. Blood tests: sickle cell trait, low hematocrit and hemoglobin, clotting times
2. Results of nocturnal tumescence test

## ♦ NURSING DIAGNOSES

Nursing diagnoses are determined from analysis of patient data. Nursing diagnoses for the patient with impotence may include but are not limited to the following:

| Diagnostic Title | Possible Etiologic Factors |
|---|---|
| Sexual dysfunction (impotence) | Difficulty in attaining or maintaining an erection |
| Anxiety | Sexual performance |

## ♦ EXPECTED PATIENT OUTCOMES

Expected patient outcomes for the patient with impotence may include but are not limited to the following:

1. Identifies alternative methods of sexual intimacy that will provide a positive sexual interaction.
2. Demonstrates the effective use of devices to obtain an erection.
3. Demonstrates a relaxed positive attitude about sexual performance.

## ♦ INTERVENTIONS

### Identifying Alternatives

Helping the patient choose sexual therapy options by providing accurate and up-to-date information is an important part of caring for the patient with impotence. Myths and erroneous information are common obstacles in sexual rehabilitation. The patient needs to be informed of the physiologic and psychologic aspects of erectile function. The use of external devices and medications needs to be reviewed, including their modes of action, side effects, and contraindications.

#### Penile injections

The nurse may be responsible for teaching the patient how to administer penile injections. These patients need to be followed in an office or clinic on a regular basis. Systemic complications of the injections include orthostatic hypotension and dizziness. Local complications include pain, hematoma, edema, decreased glandular sensation, fibrosis, and priapism. Priapism may be reversed by application of ice, manual masturbation, injection of epinephrine, or the use of antihistamines. If priapism persists longer than 4 to 6 hours, the patient should notify his physician.

Injection sites should be rotated, and injection into the urethra should be avoided. Applying pressure to the injection site can help decrease the possibility of fibrosis. The patient should not use injections more than twice a week. Liver enzyme levels should be monitored about every 3 months. If liver function studies are elevated or fibrosis is noted on the penis, it is usually recommended that the injections be discontinued. The drug should be kept in the refrigerator to avoid degeneration of the solution. Dosages can be altered if initial results are not satisfactory.

#### External vacuum devices

Vacuum devices come in one size with ring seals at the end that are different diameters to accommodate individual erection size. The patient needs to be taught how to use the device and make sure that the seals are the appropriate size to ensure sufficient vacuum to the penis. The vascular ring is slipped on once the penis is engorged and should only be left on for approximately 30 minutes to prevent possible vascular damage. Teaching both sexual partners the use of the device is appropriate. Couples need to discuss how sexual activity may be modified with the use of the device so that they can feel more comfortable with this change in routine.

The vacuum device may be used every day if desired. Complications include pulling of scrotal tissue, hematoma, inability to achieve or maintain the erection, and discomfort with the vascular ring. These complications may be remedied by adjusting the user's procedure, schedule changes, and possibly different brands of the device. Blocked or retrograde ejaculation may also be a side effect. Orgasm should not be affected. The patient should receive ongoing medical support to help him cope with this altered sexual pattern. The device is contraindicated in patients with bleeding disorders, sickle cell anemia, and severe circulatory compromise.

#### Penile implants

Infection rates are generally low with penile implant surgery. Often, antibiotics are administered a few days before surgery and for a week after surgery to prevent the possibility of infection. The patient may also be told to perform a Hibiclens prewash 7 days before surgery, again to decrease the chance of infection. Patients should be instructed to take all antibiotics and report any symptoms of infection, such as unusual swelling, redness, excessive pain or redness around the incision sites, and drainage.

To prevent the possibility of erosion of the device through the penile skin, the patient should be instructed to avoid sexual intercourse for at least 6 to 8 weeks after returning home. When sexual activity can resume, the patient should be instructed to use a water-soluble lubricant. The patient needs to avoid wearing tight-fitting clothing and avoid sitting with the legs crossed and in other positions that put pressure or cause friction to the penis.

The nurse teaches the patient that his erections will not be any larger than before and most likely will be somewhat smaller. Partners should be included in teaching sessions if possible and counseled on expectations related to the functioning of the device. The implant will not affect a man's sex drive or interfere with penile sensation. The patient should be able to have an orgasm and ejaculate after the implant has been placed. Patients with inflatable implants need to be instructed on how to inflate and deflate the prosthesis properly.

### Reducing Performance-Related Anxiety

Sexual counseling is usually done in conjunction with other forms of surgical or prosthetic type of interventions for the impotent patient. The nurse is often the person to encourage patients to avail themselves of counseling opportunities. The nurse helps the patient to understand his needs and explains the goals and some of the methodologies used in sexual counseling. Often, patients have misconceptions concerning the treatment modalities used in sexual counseling. The nurse provides some specific examples of exercises used during sexual counseling and explains how partner communication can be enhanced with counseling.

## ♦ EVALUATION

To evaluate the effectiveness of nursing interventions, compare patient behaviors with those stated in the expected patient outcomes. Successful achievement of patient outcomes for the patient with impotence is indicated by the following:

1. Is capable of having sexual intimacy with a significant other that is a positive experience for both partners; statements by both partners that indicate personal growth and closeness.
2. Is able to use devices to obtain an erection correctly and safely.
3. States he feels more relaxed and more positive about sexual performance.

## ✸ SPECIAL CONSIDERATIONS FOR CARE OF THE GERONTOLOGIC PATIENT

The nurse should not assume that elders do not have sexual needs. Impotence in the elderly patient is often caused by narrowing of the blood vessels and consequently decreased blood flow to the penis. Most healthy males can obtain an erection even at an advanced age. Often the elderly male needs more and prolonged stimulation than his younger counterpart to have an erection. The nurse can inform patients and their partners of the need for longer "foreplay" with the older male.

## ❦ HOME CARE CONSIDERATIONS

If the patient had surgical treatment for impotence, any signs of infection or erosion of the penile implant should be immediately reported to the physician.

Often, when the patient uses the penile erectile devices for the first few times in the home, questions arise. Patients need to be sent home with explicit instructions and phone numbers for resource persons.

## COMPLICATIONS

Complications of penile implant surgery include infection and erosion of the prosthesis through the penis. Complications of injections and mechanical erectile devices include possible priapism and circulatory occlusions to the penis, causing tissue necrosis.

# VASECTOMY: MALE STERILIZATION

## ETIOLOGY/EPIDEMIOLOGY

Voluntary sterilization has become increasingly acceptable to both men and women as a method of preventing pregnancy. It is the most frequently used method of fertility control for married couples over 30 years of age and is the most widely used contraceptive method worldwide, protecting approximately 100 million couples. It has been estimated that more than 13.7 million adults have been sterilized in the United States and 100 million worldwide. Each year, 500,000 to 1 million American men have vasectomies.

A profile of men and women seeking sterilization indicates that they come from all strata of society, are between 25 and 50 years of age, are married, have large families, and are likely to be white and of the Protestant faith. The primary reason given by both men and women for wishing sterilization is a desire to limit family size. Other reasons include financial inability to support a large family, concern over population growth, problems with other methods of contraception, and age, with some couples preferring personal freedom from the risk of childbearing with advancing age. More frequently than women, men give as an important reason for sterilization their wish for an effective contraceptive that does not interfere with sexual pleasure. Also, men express concern over the health of their sex partners. Some men whose sexual partners (including wives) use oral contraceptives believe that the "pill" is actually or potentially harmful to the woman.

Medical indications for sterilization include any condition or situation in which pregnancy would be attended by risks to the life or health of the woman or her infant. Included in this category are severe heart disease, diabetes, and probable genetic defects in the infant.

The laws governing sterilization vary from state to state and have undergone many changes. In general, if the surgery does not violate specific state provisions and if written informed consent is given by a man or woman legally capable of giving permission, the surgery can be performed by a physician. Since sterilization is a permanent method of contraception, it is absolutely necessary that informed consent be ensured before the procedure.

## PATHOPHYSIOLOGY

Bilateral **vasectomy** is the surgical procedure used for male sterilization. Vasectomy interrupts the continuity of the vas deferens, and sperm are prevented from being ejaculated with other components of the semen. However, sperm are still produced, and the ejaculate is not noticeably diminished in amount. Residual fertility may be present for a variable period because of existing sperm in the semen beyond the point of occlusion of the vas deferens. Sperm *gradually* disappear from the ejaculate; thus conception is possible in the immediate postoperative period.

After vasectomy, antibodies to sperm develop in about 50% to 66% of men. No relationship has been found in humans between the presence of sperm antibodies and any systemic pathologic condition. In some studies with samples of 5 to 10 monkeys, atherosclerosis has developed more extensively in vasectomized monkeys. It is hypothesized that antisperm antibodies formed after vasectomy may result in circulating immune complexes that exacerbate atherosclerosis. A relationship between vasectomy and atherosclerotic changes in humans has not been found.

## MEDICAL MANAGEMENT

At least 11 different techniques for vasectomies exist to accomplish what is generally considered to be a safe, simple procedure. Two reasons probably account for the variety of techniques developed. The first is the tendency of the vas deferens to rejoin spontaneously, a distressing long-term complication. The second reason centers around developing techniques that have the potential for reversal.

Bilateral partial vasectomy is the surgical method used most often. Because of its safety and simplicity, the procedure can be performed on an outpatient basis in a clinic or a physician's office using a local anesthetic. A small incision is made in the scrotum to expose the sheath of the vas deferens. The sheath is opened, the vas deferens is exposed, and a segment measuring 0.63 to 1.27 cm is removed. The severed ends of the vas deferens are then ligated. Some physicians prefer to coagulate the severed ends of the vas deferens to ensure sterility. The incision is then closed by suturing.

Complications after vasectomy are rare and usually minor. Most complications are preventable by using proper anesthetic doses, aseptic technique, and counseling against strenuous exercise for 1 to 2 days after the procedure. Bruising, mild edema, and mild discomfort are common and usually subside without treatment. Infection of the wound occurs in about 3% of patients. Hematoma, epididymitis, and granuloma formation may occur. The incidence of failure as a result of recanalization is reported to be 0% to 6%. The cause of spontaneous recanalization (reanastomosis) is unknown, but duplication of the vas deferens has occasionally been noted. The literature does not report any occurrences of mortality from vasectomy.

## STERILIZATION REVERSAL

A surgical attempt to restore male fertility after vasectomy is called a *vasovasotomy.* An attempt is made to rejoin the severed ends of the vas deferens. Success is measured by the presence of sperm in semen specimens after reconstruction. Reports of success in restoring fertility range from 29% to 85%.

Considerable research is now in progress for the development of a reversible vasectomy device. Ideally, reversible vasectomy devices would effectively block the vas deferens, permit simple and safe insertion and removal of the device, could be turned on and off to provide for timing of conception, would not cause discomfort when in place, and would not cause complications. The ideal vasectomy device has not been developed, and the incidence of pain and tissue reaction is presently a major problem with the current procedures.

## NURSING MANAGEMENT

### Preoperative Counseling and Care

Most men are satisfied with the results of vasectomy, but some have experienced emotional difficulties after sterilization. There is a need to recognize that vasectomies can affect women partners as well as men. The findings of studies about the psychologic aspects of sterilization indicate a need to identify men and women before surgery who may later have strong regrets and emotional problems. One aim of counseling before surgery is to confirm that the decision for sterilization has been made as objectively as possible. Asking hypothetic questions about the possibility of divorce, loss of the spouse, or loss of a child can assist in estimating whether the decision to be sterilized has been treated as a serious step.

Previous experience with other methods of contraception can be explored and reasons for dissatisfaction with the methods determined. An individual or couple may lack knowledge about contraceptive methods and with adequate information might choose something other than sterilization. Care must be taken, however, that persons who are knowledgeable and have made a firm, objective decision are not made to think that their decision is a poor one or is unacceptable.

The discussion of sterilization methods should be based on the federal government's informed consent guidelines (see Box 52-7 in Chapter 52). The nature and consequences of the surgery must be explained to the patient. It is important to emphasize that the sterilization procedure does nothing to increase or decrease sexual performance or enjoyment, but simply removes the chance of pregnancy. Lay people typically equate sterilization with castration and loss of femininity or masculinity. Even those patients who know the difference need reassurance. Visual aids and models can be of great value in giving explanations about the surgery to patients.

The facts concerning reversibility, including current success rates, are discussed. In the case of vasectomy, the chance of recanalization and return of fertility should be pointed out. The man or couple must also be informed of progressive rather than immediate sterility after vasectomy, and alternate methods of protection until sterility occurs should be discussed.

For men having vasectomies, a preoperative specimen of semen is examined to serve as a baseline for interpreting sperm disappearance after surgery. The patient is instructed to shave the scrotal hair and to take a shower the night before surgery. He is advised to bring briefs-type underpants with him on the day of surgery to hold the postoperative dressing in place.

### Postoperative Care

After vasectomy, men are advised to expect slight swelling of the scrotum, minor pain, and a small amount of bleeding. Ice to the scrotal area, sitz baths, time, and rest will ameliorate these discomforts. After a vasectomy, it is important for the man to report for semen analysis as advised. A sperm count is usually taken 4 weeks after vasectomy. Two consecutive sperm-free specimens are usually considered necessary before the man can be considered sterile. Reanastomosis of the vas deferens is suspected if sperm fail to disappear from the ejaculate, if there is an increase in sperm in the semen after two successive sperm counts, if motile sperm are found in the semen beyond 3 months after vasectomy, and if, of course, pregnancy occurs.

In the postoperative period, men need opportunities to express their feelings about having been sterilized. The nurse repeats and reinforces previously given information about sexual performance. If the patient expresses feelings of regret or guilt, a review of the reasons for the sterilization may be of assistance in recognizing that the decision was made as objectively as possible.

## QUESTIONS TO CONSIDER

- What factors predispose men to infections of the reproductive system? What can men do to decrease their risk of reproductive tract infection?
- What areas should nurses cover in explaining to men the consequences of structural changes in the reproductive system?
- How would the sexuality of a 35-year-old with penile cancer be affected? What sexual options exist for him?

## CRITICAL THINKING ACTIVITIES

- Mr. Charles is a 40-year-old patient who is post orchiectomy and radical node dissection for a nonseminomatous neoplasm. The nurse identifies hemorrhage, atelectasis, thrombosis, and paralytic ileus as potential complications of the surgery. Discuss preventative nursing measures for these potential complications specifically with regard to activity.
- As a community health nurse in an industrial company, Marian is designing a program to teach men in the company about reproductive health. Develop an outline depicting the *priority* diseases and preventative measures she might teach.
- Dean, 59, is admitted to the hospital complaining of difficulty urinating. The ER physician orders routine urinalysis, CBC, and chemistry profile. Outline questions designed to help differentiate the cause of these symptoms.

## CHAPTER SUMMARY

Men's reproductive health care is an important aspect of the new nursing specialty in men's health.

#### PROBLEMS OF THE TESTES AND RELATED STRUCTURES

- Epididymitis is the most common intrascrotal inflammation. It affects men between ages 19 and 35 and is typically caused by an ascending infection acquired sexually.
- Epididymitis causes acute scrotal pain and swelling and produces a distinctive waddling gait. Treatment involves antibiotics, antiinflammatories, and supportive care with bedrest and scrotal elevation.
- Orchitis involves infection of a testicle by a bacteria or virus or as a complication of mumps. Infertility is a potential complication; therefore prompt diagnosis and treatment are critical.
- Testicular torsion occurs when testicular circulation is acutely impaired by a sudden twisting of the spermatic cord. If not diagnosed and treated within hours, torsion results in gangrene and testicular destruction.
- Testicular cancer is the leading cause of cancer death in men ages 15 to 35. It is 90% to 100% curable if diagnosed early, but more than half the cases are in advanced stages at diagnosis.
- Curative treatment of testicular cancer is surgical orchiectomy. Regular testicular self-examination should be taught to all young adult men.

#### PROBLEMS OF THE PROSTATE

- Prostatitis may be bacterial or nonbacterial. It is a common inflammation in young and middle-aged adults. Treatment is conservative with antibiotics and supportive care.
- The prostate gland undergoes both atrophy and hyperplasia during midlife. The changes are associated

with increased androgen levels. Symptoms are classically urinary: hesitancy, urgency, decreased stream, straining, and dysuria.

- Classic treatment of benign prostatic hypertrophy (BPH) involves surgery by transurethral prostatic resection (TURP). Early BPH may be treated by finasteride, which blocks conversion of testosterone and shrinks the gland.
- Care after a TURP involves managing the continuous bladder irrigation to keep the drainage light in color and free of clots and to control painful bladder spasms. The irrigation and catheter are discontinued after 24 to 48 hours.
- Postdischarge care after TURP involves encouraging a liberal fluid intake, preventing straining at stool, restricting activity, and reassuring the patient that potency is rarely affected by the surgery, although sterility is common.
- Prostate cancer is the most common cancer site in men and the second leading cause of cancer death.
- Prostate cancer is associated with aging and frequently starts as a discrete hard nodule that may be asymptomatic.
- Prostate cancer tends to grow slowly in elderly men. Treatment options include curative radical prostatectomy or radiation therapy by implant or external beam. Both approaches can result in sterility and impotence, and surgery causes temporary problems with incontinence.

### PROBLEMS OF THE PENIS

- Phimosis and paraphimosis involve the inability to move the foreskin freely across the glans penis. Treatment involves relieving constriction and may involve circumcision.
- Penile cancer is rare but typically develops in the late middle-age years. It is rare in circumcised men and is believed to be associated with chronic bacterial irritation. The treatment is surgical.
- Impotence may have psychologic, neural, vascular, and drug-related causes. Treatment involves vasodilator injections, medication adjustments, external vacuum devices, and penile prostheses. Sex therapy is used for psychogenic causes.

### VASECTOMY: MALE STERILIZATION

- Sterilization is the most common method of contraception for married couples over age 30. One-half to 1 million vasectomies are performed a year. The procedure is simple, carries few risks, and is performed on an outpatient basis. Research is ongoing to address issues related to both reversibility and unplanned reanastomosis.

## REFERENCES


1. American Cancer Society: *Report on the cancer-related health check-up,* New York, 1980, The Society.
2. American Cancer Society: *Cancer facts and figures for minority Americans,* New York, 1983, Springer.
3. American Cancer Society: *1989 cancer facts and figures,* New York, 1989, The Society.
4. Babaryan R: When to refer: evaluation of scrotal masses, *Hosp Pract* 20(3):51-53, 1985.
5. Blank B, Schneider R: Acute scrotal problems, *Patient Care* 24(11):152-155, 158, 1990.
6. Bozett F, Forrester D: A proposal for a men's health nurse practitioner, *J Nurs Schol* 21(3):158-161, 1989.
7. Bruskewitz R, Cassel C: Benign prostatic hyperplasia: intervene or wait? *Hosp Pract* 27(8):99-115, 1992.
8. Bryant R, Boarini J: Treatment options for men with sexual dysfunction, *JET* 19(4):131-142, 1992.
9. Confer DJ, Beall ME: Evolved improvements in placement of the silicone gel prosthesis for post-prostatectomy incontinence, *J Urol* 126:605-608, 1981.
10. Crawford E: Diagnosis and treatment of prostatitis, *Hosp Pract* 20(9):77-80, 1985.
11. Cumes DM et al: Complications of $^{125}$iodine implantation and pelvic lymphadenectomy for prostatic cancer with special reference to patients who had failed external beam therapy as their initial mode of therapy, *J Urol* 126:620-622, 1981.
12. Higgs D: The patient with testicular cancer: nursing management of chemotherapy, *Oncol Nurs Forum* 17:243-249, 1990.
13. Kaler S: Epididymitis in the young adult male, *Nurse Pract* 15(5):10-16, 1990.
14. Kaplan HS: *Disorders of sexual desire,* New York, 1979, Simon & Schuster.
15. Lasater S: Testicular cancer, a perioperative challenge, *AORN* 51(2):513-526, 1990.
16. Moore S et al: Nerve sparing prostatectomy, *Am J Nurs* 92(4):59-64, 1992.
17. Paulson D: Diseases of the prostate, *Clin Symposia* 4(2):2-32, 1989.
18. Tonetti J, Tonetti J: Testicular torsion or acute epididymitis? Diagnosis and treatment, *J Emerg Nurs* 16(2):96-98, 1990.
19. Trump D: How to screen—and what the results mean, *Consultant* 32(8):7-30, 33, 36, 1992.

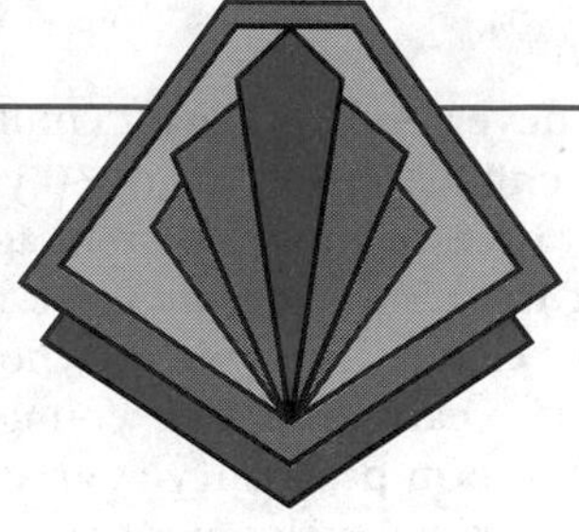

C H A P T E R 54

# Management of Persons With Problems of the Breast

*Gladys E. Deters*

## CHAPTER OBJECTIVES

***After studying this chapter, the learner should be able to do the following:***

1 Recognize the differences between benign breast conditions and breast cancer.
2 Analyze the patient's risk factor profile for developing breast cancer.
3 Describe early detection approaches to and diagnostic tests for breast evaluation.
4 Explain the rationale for breast self-examination, and describe the proper technique for performing the procedure.
5 Explain the most frequently used treatment modalities for breast cancer, including surgery, chemotherapy, radiation, and hormonal therapy.
6 Describe the types of breast preservation and reconstruction procedures available.
7 Explain the rationale for postmastectomy rehabilitation exercises and how they are performed.
8 Discuss the role of Reach to Recovery volunteers in the adjustment to mastectomy surgery.
9 Discuss common benign breast conditions and their treatment.

## KEY TERMS

autogenous tissue flap
breast reconstruction
breast self-examination (BSE)
fibroadenoma
fine-needle aspiration
gynecomastia
implant
lumpectomy
lymphedema
mammary duct ectasia
mammogram
mastectomy
mastitis
postmastectomy arm exercises
prosthesis

## MALIGNANT CONDITIONS OF THE BREAST

### ETIOLOGY

For more than 30 years breast cancer has been the most prevalent, the most feared, and the malignant disease with the highest mortality rate in women. Although the yearly incidence of breast cancer continues to rise and remains the number-one cancer found in women today, mortality rates appear to have leveled off in recent years. At present breast cancer ranks second only to lung cancer as the major cause of death as a result of cancer in women.[1] The continued rise in incidence is the result in part of improved detection methods that can diagnose breast cancer in an earlier, localized state. In addition, treatment modalities are more successful and long-term survival is being achieved.

The underlying cause of breast cancer is still unknown. A number of risk factors have been identified as potential causes of breast cancer development. Each risk factor is addressed in the ensuing discussion. At present, however, these risk factors account for only about 21% of the breast cancer risk in women aged 30 to 54 years and 29% in women 55 to 84 years of age.[33] It is hoped that ongoing research efforts will reveal other as yet unidentified risk factors that have a role in the cause of breast cancer.

#### Age and Gender

Women today have a 1:9 chance of developing breast cancer in their lifetime. The American Cancer Society (ACS) predicted that in 1993, of the 183,000 new cases of breast cancer expected to be diagnosed, only 1000 would be in men.[1] As is the case with most malignant conditions, the incidence rate of breast cancer increases with age. The disease is diagnosed most frequently in women older than 50 years. The reason for this age-related increase is thought to be the increased probability of mutagenic changes occurring over a longer life span rather than any instability inherent in aging cells.[31] Another reason that elderly women are at greater risk is related to present population figures. Elderly women outnumber younger women, and the gap is expected to widen.[55]

### Genetic Factors

Breast cancer occurring within family members has been recognized for centuries, but the first documented cases were recorded only in 1866. The mode of transmission for hereditary breast cancer is complex but is thought to be through an autosomal dominant gene.[40] Noninherited breast cancer is considered to be a two-step process, the first step being a change in cell structure or function, followed by a second event that promotes another change in the cell and causes it to become malignant. In hereditary breast cancer the inherited cell may already be in an altered state (first step) and require only one event to change it to a cancer cell.[57]

The presence of inherited breast cancer is demonstrated by the incidence in first-degree relatives: mother, daughter, or sister. The risk increases if the first-degree relative had a history of premenopausal breast cancer or bilateral disease. When both conditions occur (premenopausal and bilateral disease), the risk to a first-degree relative increases ninefold, including the risk of also developing bilateral disease.[40] In hereditary breast cancer the age at the time in which breast cancer develops is earlier than the age when it occurs in the noninherited type of disease. The characteristics of inherited breast cancer are listed in Box 54-1.

### Menstrual and Reproductive History

The risk of breast cancer is increased when menstruation begins at an early age and extends to about 55 years of age. The risk lessens when menopause occurs before age 45 years or is induced early for medical reasons (ablative or surgical oophorectomy).[31] The probability of mutagenic changes taking place from an intermediate phase to a malignant phase is more likely when the menstrual cycle spans more than 30 years.

**BOX 54-1 Characteristics of Inherited Breast Cancer**

- Occurs at an early age (premenopausal)
- Incidence of bilateral disease increased
- First-degree relative (mother, daughter, sister) with the disease
- Personal history of breast cancer in one breast, which increases the risk of developing it in the second breast

Modified from Smith P: *Semin Oncol Nurs* 8(4):258-264, 1992.

Women who have never been pregnant (nulliparity) or who had their first child after the age of 30 years are at an increased risk of breast cancer. Women age 30 to 35 years in their first full-term pregnancy are at three times the risk for breast cancer than women who deliver for the first time at 18 years of age or younger. The implication is that a full-term pregnancy at an early age promotes changes in breast development that protect the breast from cancer. Breast development begins at menarche; however, full differentiation of mammary gland epithelium is not complete until a full-term pregnancy completes the developmental process. In addition, the longer the menstrual history (15 years or more), the greater is the possibility that ductal cells, which had undergone the first phase of cell transformation, will progress to the malignant state.[31] Pregnancy itself is not considered a risk factor for breast cancer development.

### Hormones and Oral Contraception

Hormonal replacement therapy at menopause has created a great deal of concern and controversy because of the increased incidence of breast cancer associated with it. Some reports indicate a 40% increased risk, especially in older women who have been on a medication regimen such as Premarin for many years. Combining estrogen with progesterone to alleviate the risk of endometrial cancer has not diminished the breast cancer risk and may, in fact, have increased it.[26]

An association between the use of oral contraceptives (OC) and the risk of breast cancer is not clear at this time. The report from a nationwide, case-controlled study by the Cancer and Steroid Hormone Study (1983) concluded that women 20 to 54 years of age who had used OC compared with women who had never used OC had the same breast cancer risk.[47] Other more recent findings indicate that nulliparous women 20 to 44 years of age have a breast cancer risk that correlates with the length of contraceptive use. For example, use for 10 years doubles the chance of breast cancer occurring.[43] More research is needed to settle this issue.

### Diet and Body Weight

The consumption of a high-fat diet with large amounts of animal fat has long been considered a breast cancer risk. This claim is largely unproved. Some large cohort studies indicate that there is no relationship between the total amount of fat intake and breast cancer in premenopausal and postmenopausal women.[63] Although a diet high in fat is not thought to be a causative factor in breast cancer development, some animal studies suggest that fat may be a *promoter* of cells being transformed from a normal to a malignant state.[11]

Obesity also has been considered a factor in breast cancer development. Although no positive correlation has as yet been established, obesity can have a stimulating effect on breast cancer growth. Estrogen is stored in body adipose tissue. Some breast cancers are estrogen receptor positive (ER+), meaning that estrogen will stimulate breast cancer cell growth. Therefore the more body adipose tissue present, the more estrogen will be available to attach to ER+ cancer cells. In the postmenopausal woman, androgens in adipose tissue can be converted to estrogen and become the source for stimulating cancer growth and spread. Recent studies have shown that the pattern of body-fat distribution (high waist-to-hip ratio) in postmenopausal women can influence their risk for breast cancer. In fact, there is a high correlation of breast cancer associated with obesity that has a high waist-to-hip ratio, low parity, and greater age at first pregnancy in postmenopausal women with a family history of breast cancer.[56]

## Benign Breast Disease

Fibrocystic disease, a benign condition, is considered to be a risk for breast cancer but usually only when it is related to hyperplasia (increased cellular proliferation). The risk for women with this condition, with no evidence of hyperplasia, rests in the fact that unless a woman performs monthly breast self-examination and knows the normal feel of her own breast, new lesions or hyperplastic changes may go undetected.[31]

## Radiation Hazard

The survivors of the atomic bombing at Nagasaski and Hiroshima have provided data on the effects of radiation exposure and breast cancer development. Young women who were exposed to the radiation effects show an increased incidence of breast cancer compared with older women (older than 39 years of age) exposed to the same degree of radiation.[31] Women who have had repeated fluoroscopic examinations of the chest or radiation as a treatment for mastitis also have demonstrated an increased incidence of breast cancer later in life. Table 54-1 reviews the risk factors associated with breast cancer development.

**TABLE 54-1 Risk Factors Associated With Breast Cancer**

| FACTOR | DEGREE OF RISK | COMMENTS |
|---|---|---|
| Female gender | Increased | 99% of all breast cancers occur in women and 1% in men. |
| History of a previous breast cancer | Increased | The risk of developing a cancer in the opposite breast is five times greater than for the average population at risk. |
| Age >40 | Increased | Incidence increases with age and peaks in the fifth decade. |
| *Menstrual history:* | | |
| Early menarche or late menopause or both | Increased | The risk of breast cancer rises as the interval between menarche and menopause increases; shortening the interval by castration reduces the risk, especially if performed in women younger than 35 years of age. |
| *Reproductive history:* | | |
| Nulliparity<br>First child born after 30 years of age | Increased | Childless women have an increased risk as do women who bear their first child near or after the age of 30 years. |
| *Family history:* | | |
| Mother or sister or both | Increased | Risk increases two to three times if a mother or sister has had breast cancer and is further increased if the relative was diagnosed during the premenopausal state and if the cancer was bilateral. |
| Diet | Controversial | Animal data and description epidemiology of breast cancer incidence strongly suggest an association of dietary factors, specifically a high fat diet, with an increased risk of breast cancer. The National Academy of Science recommends decreasing total fat intake to 30% of available calories. |
| Alcohol | Unknown | A suggested small increase in risk with moderate alcohol consumption has been reported, although limitations in methodology have been cited, and results require confirmation. |
| Obesity | Controversial | Weight, height, obesity, and increased body mass have been reported to be associated with an increased risk of breast cancer. |
| Ionizing radiation | Increased | Three groups of women who received low-level radiation exposure demonstrated an increased breast cancer risk, which was particularly notable if the exposure occurred in the early years (<30 years). |
| Benign breast disease | None | Fibrocystic breast disease is not associated with breast cancer. However, biopsy-proven atypical hyperplasia is associated with an increased risk. |
| Oral contraceptives | None | There is no evidence yet to suggest a causal relationship between oral contraceptives and incidence of and survival from breast cancer. |
| Exogenous hormones | Controversial | Several studies report no link with replacement hormones and breast cancer, and those that do appear to identify only subsets of patients at risk: those who have taken replacement estrogens for very long periods of time and those who have taken large cumulative doses. |

Modified from Baird SB et al: *Cancer nursing: a comprehensive textbook*, Philadelphia, 1991, WB Saunders.

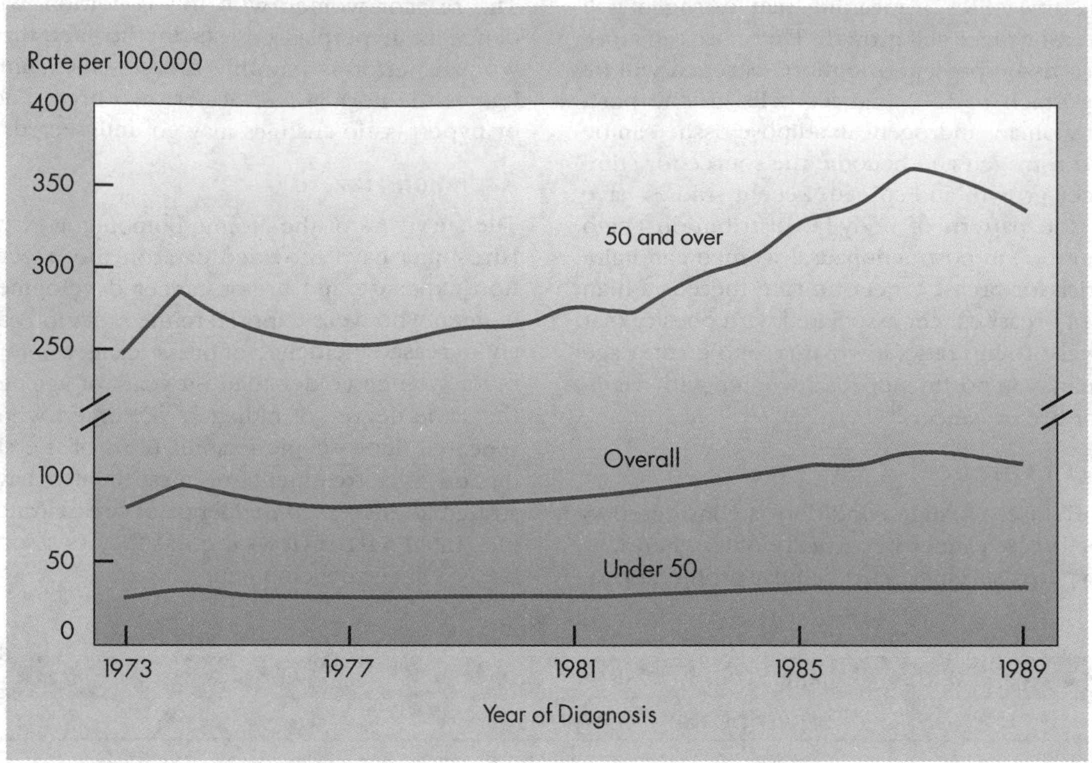


**FIGURE 54-1** Breast cancer incidence, 1973-1989. (From Hankey BF: *Natl Cancer Institute* 84[19]:1467, 1992.)

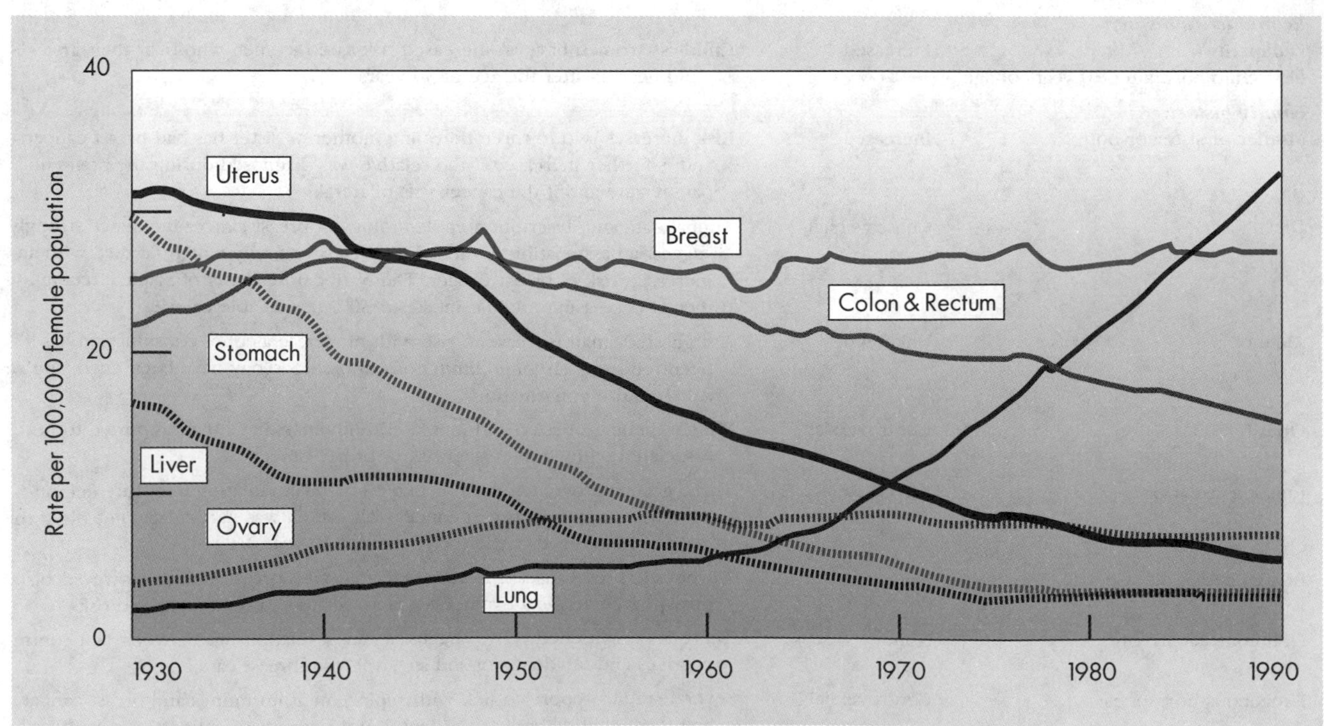


**FIGURE 54-2** Cancer death rates by site, females, United States, 1930-1989. (From American Cancer Society: *1993 cancer facts and figures,* New York, 1993, The Society.)

## EPIDEMIOLOGY

Breast cancer recognizes neither national boundaries nor racial/ethnic groups. It is a worldwide problem, especially in the United States and Western Europe, where breast cancer incidence and mortality rates are the highest. The reason for this occurrence has been debated without any consensus. One theory often put forth is that these countries are highly industrialized and therefore more economically and socially advantaged than some of the emerging third-world countries. As a consequence of this affluence, the dietary pattern of ingesting more expensive animal food (red meat high in fat) may be implicated as a causative factor[38] (see preceding discussion of diet and obesity). Although this theory is merely speculative, it is known that when women emigrate from third-world countries and the Far East to the United States and other Western countries, their rate of breast cancer incidence rises, possibly because of changes in eating patterns. Statistics from the National Cancer Institute's Surveillance, Epidemiology, and End-Results (SEER) program, which collects data on cancer, reveal that the incidence of breast cancer in the United States has shown a steady increase since 1973 when the program was initiated. This trend can be seen in Figure 54-1. A comparison of the estimated 1993 cancer incidence and death rate figures revealed that breast cancer was to account for about one third (32%) of all cancers detected in women and 18% of all cancer-related deaths.[1] Despite advances in detection and treatment the annual death rates as a result of breast cancer have changed little since 1930, as seen in Figure 54-2.

Although breast cancer is predominantly a disease of white women, the incidence and mortality among African-American women have been increasing. The underlying reason for the rise is not genetic but related to the fact that more black women live at or near the poverty level, have less basic education and educational opportunities, and have limited access to health care programs such as early screening and detection programs.[9] Black women have poorer survival rates than do white women, even when stage of disease is adjusted for. Black women are more frequently diagnosed at a later stage of disease because they neither participate in nor are encouraged to participate in early detection and treatment programs.[61]

### Prognostic Factors

Several factors are used to determine the overall prognosis at the time of diagnosis of breast cancer. These include the number of axillary nodes involved, tumor size, and hormone receptor status.

#### Axillary node involvement

Because metastasis to the lymph nodes is common, the number of axillary nodes involved has long been used as a predictor in breast cancer outcome. When axillary nodes are not involved in the disease process, the expected outcome is good, with a low risk for recurrent disease.[51] As the number of nodes involved increases, the chance of distant metastasis increases and prognosis worsens. If more than 10 nodes are involved, each additional node adds to the risk of relapse after initial treatment.[27,42]

**BOX 54-2 Staging of Breast Cancer**

**T—PRIMARY TUMOR SIZE**

| | |
|---|---|
| TX | Primary tumor cannot be assessed |
| T0 | No evidence of primary tumor |
| Tis | Carcinoma in situ: intraductal carcinoma, lobular carcinoma in situ, or Paget's disease of the nipple with node |
| T1 | Tumor 2 cm or less in greatest dimension |
| T2 | Tumor more than 2 cm but not more than 5 cm in greatest dimension |
| T3 | Tumor more than 5 cm in greatest dimension |
| T4 | Tumor of any size with direct extension to chest wall or skin |

NOTE: Paget's disease associated with a tumor is classified according to the size of the tumor

**N—REGIONAL LYMPH NODES**

| | |
|---|---|
| NX | Regional lymph nodes cannot be assessed (e.g., previously removed) |
| N0 | No regional lymph node metastasis |
| N1 | Metastasis to movable ipsilateral axillary lymph node(s) |
| N2 | Metastasis to ipsilateral axillary lymph node(s) fixed to one another or to other structures |
| N3 | Metastasis to ipsilateral internal mammary lymph node(s) |

**M—DISTANT METASTASIS**

| | |
|---|---|
| MX | Presence of distant metastasis cannot be assessed |
| M0 | No distant metastasis |
| M1 | Distant metastasis (includes metastasis to ipsilateral supraclavicular lymph node(s) |

**STAGE GROUPING**

| | | | |
|---|---|---|---|
| Stage 0 | Tis | N0 | M0 |
| Stage I | T1 | N0 | M0 |
| Stage IIa | T0 | N0 | M0 |
| | T1 | N1 | M0 |
| | T2 | N0 | M0 |
| Stage IIB | T2 | N1 | M0 |
| | T3 | N0 | M0 |
| Stage IIIA | T0 | N2 | M0 |
| | T1 | N2 | M0 |
| | T2 | N2 | M0 |
| | T3 | N1 | M0 |
| | T3 | N2 | M0 |
| Stage IIIB | T4 | Any N | M0 |
| | Any T | N3 | M0 |
| Stage IV | Any T | Any N | M1 |

From Beahrs OH, Hutter RV, Kennedy BJ, editors: *Breast manual for staging of cancer,* ed 4, Philadelphia, 1992, JB Lippincott.

#### Tumor size

Smaller tumor size at diagnosis is associated with fewer positive nodes involved and less metastasis. Tumors less than 2 cm with no node involvement have the best predicted outcome. Recent investigations into breast cancer cell kinetics indicate that the percentage of tumor cells in the synthesis (S) phase of the cell cycle suggests a fast-growing tumor and a poorer prognosis.[51] (See Chapter 16 for a more detailed discussion on cell kinetics.)

#### Hormone receptor status

Estrogen receptors (ER+) and progesterone receptors (PR+) are well-recognized predictors of long-term survival in women with breast cancer. The presence of these receptors on cells indicates that the cell has retained its regulatory control over the mammary epithelium, thus reflecting a more well-differentiated tumor.[20] An ER+ or PR+ tumor is associated with a more favorable prognosis and a longer disease-free survival time.[24] Survival for patients who have a negative ER or PR status is 40% to 50% less than for those whose status is ER or PR positive. About 30% of those with a negative status will experience a relapse of breast cancer within 10 years.[51]

### Staging of Breast Cancer

Staging of malignant breast disease incorporates the TNM (tumor, node, metastasis) classification as shown in Box 54-2. Treatment decisions are based on the stage of the breast cancer, as well as those factors already discussed.

## PATHOPHYSIOLOGY

### Normal Breast

The breasts are mammary glands, which in the female have the primary function of producing milk for the newborn infant. The internal composition of the breast consists of glandular, fibrous, and adipose tissue. Glandular tissue comprises lobes that contain lobules situated around the nipple. Milk is produced in the lobules. The lobes are imbedded in adipose tissue and drain into lactiferous ducts that converge at the nipple and serve as storage compartments for milk.[30] Fibrous bands of tissue, known as *Cooper's ligaments,* support the breast tissue and attach it to the chest wall. The amount of each type of tissue depends on the woman's age, stage of the menstrual cycle, whether she is pregnant or lactating, and her overall nutritional status.

The breast is divided into four quadrants, as shown in Figure 54-3. The quadrants are used to describe the location of changes found on breast examination. The breast is served by an extensive lymphatic drainage system: central axillary nodes, pectoral (anterior), subscapular (posterior), and lateral nodes. The ipsilateral axillary nodes drain up to 75% of lymph from the breast. Additional drainage flows upward to the infraclavicular and supraclavicular lymph nodes.[30] The normal lymphatic system and directional flow are shown in Figure 54-4.

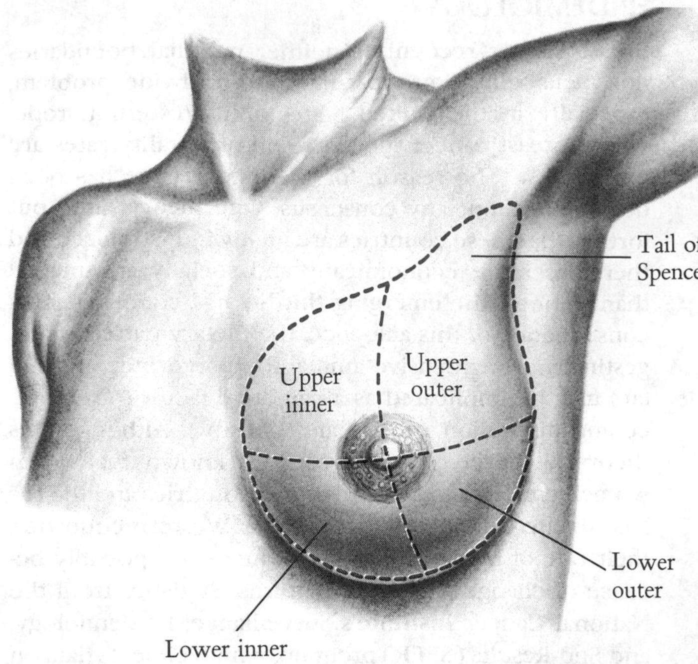


**FIGURE 54-3** Quadrants of left breast and axillary tail of Spence. (From Seidel HM et al: *Mosby's guide to physical examination,* ed 3, St Louis, 1995, Mosby.)

### Breast Changes Related to Tumor Development

#### Histologic cell types

Tumors of the breast arise in the epithelial cells of either ductal or lobular tissue and are referred to as *carcinomas.* A number of histologic subtypes also have been identified but are not as commonly seen, nor are they as invasive as ductal and lobular carcinomas. When the tumor is confined within a duct or a lobule and has not invaded surrounding tissue, it is considered localized or in situ carcinoma of the breast. *Infiltrative* ductal or lobular carcinomas are tumors that have spread directly into surrounding tissue and may have distant metastasis if they have penetrated the axillary or internal mammary nodes or the systemic circulation. Most breast tumors are located in the upper outer quadrant but can occur in any area of the breast.

Paget's disease, an eczema-like inflammatory process affecting the nipple and aerola, may progress from an epidermal condition to an intraductal carcinoma of the breast. It can be accompanied by a palpable lump. Paget's is characterized by pain, itching, burning, and nipple discharge. Short-term treatment with topical steroids should clear the lesions and thus help with differentiation of a skin disorder from a potential malignant condition. Paget's disease of the breast accounts for less than 5% of breast cancers.[5]

Of the invasive breast tumors, infiltrative ductal car-

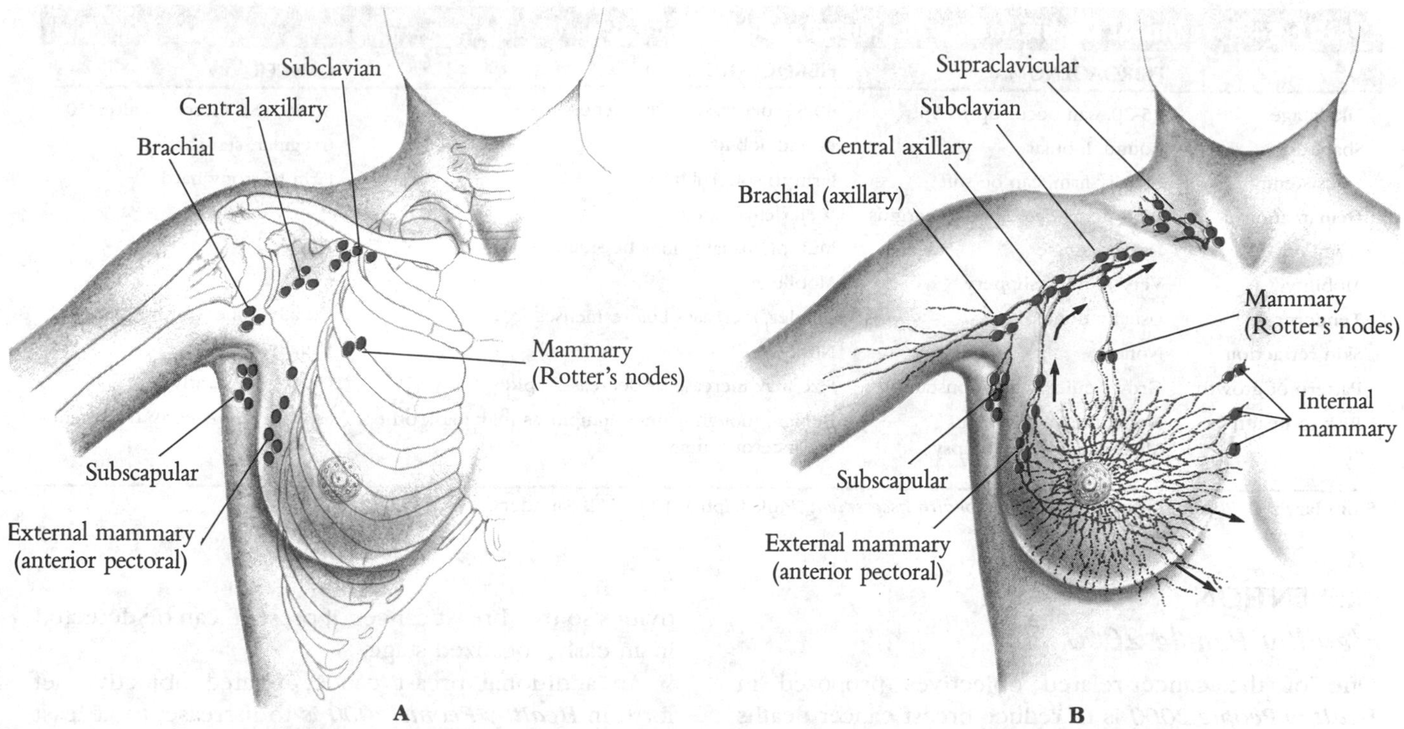


**FIGURE 54-4** A, Lymph nodes of the axilla. **B,** Lymphatic drainage of the breast. (From Seidel HM et al: *Mosby's guide to physical examination,* ed 3, St Louis, 1995, Mosby.)

**TABLE 54-2 Invasive Breast Carcinomas**

| HISTOLOGIC CELL TYPE | % OF CASES | PRESENTATION | METHOD OF METASTASIS | COMMON SITES OF METASTASIS |
|---|---|---|---|---|
| Ductal | 75% | Well defined "lump" | Axillary lymph nodes | Bone and intraparenchyma of the lung, liver, brain |
| Lobular | 5%-10% | Poorly defined "thickening" of breast "Multicentric" tumors present in same or opposite breast | Axillary lymph nodes | Meninges and other serosal tissue |

From Entrekin N. In Clark JC, McGee RF: *Oncology Nursing Society core curriculum for oncology nursing,* ed 2, Philadelphia, 1992, WB Saunders.

cinoma is the most prevalent histologic cell type, followed by infiltrating lobular carcinomas. Subtypes of each of these histologic cell types comprise the remainder of breast tumors. Table 54-2 reviews the common characteristics of these invasive cell types of breast carcinoma.

## Clinical Manifestations

Early-stage tumors of the breast (symptomless) can be detected only on physical examination of the breast or by mammogram. With more advanced tumors a variety of signs and symptoms are helpful in differentiating a benign tumor from a malignant tumor. Benign tumors generally have well-defined edges, are encapsulated, and are freely movable. The shape of a malignant tumor is more difficult to define and is less mobile on palpation, usually the result of the tumor becoming "fixed" and adhering to the chest wall. As the tumor infiltrates into surrounding tissue, it can cause retraction of the overlying skin and create what is referred to as *dimpling.* The nipple also may be retracted or deviated at an odd angle from the same growth pattern. A peau d'orange breast sign indicates lymphatic obstruction from tumor growth with resulting edema. The breast resembles an orange peel with large prominent pores. These signs are more ominous, and their appearance should alert the examiner to investigate further for a possible malignant condition. These signs and symptoms, as well as others, related to both benign and malignant tumors are found in Table 54-3.

**TABLE 54-3 Clinical Manifestations of Benign and Malignant Breast Tumors**

| | FIBROADENOMA | FIBROCYSTIC DISEASE | CANCER |
|---|---|---|---|
| Likely age | 15-20, can occur up to 55 | 30-55, decreases after menopause | 30-80, risk increases after 50 |
| Shape | Round, lobular | Round, lobular | Irregular, star-shaped |
| Consistency | Usually firm, can be soft | Firm to soft, rubbery | Firm to stony hard |
| Demarcation | Well demarcated, clear margins | Well demarcated | Poorly defined |
| Number | Usually single | Multiple usually, may be single | Single |
| Mobility | Very mobile, slippery | Mobile | Fixed |
| Tenderness | Usually none | Tender, increases before menses | Usually none, can be tender |
| Skin retraction | None | None | Usually |
| Pattern of growth | Grows quickly and constantly | Size may increase or decrease rapidly | Grows constantly |
| Risk to health | None; they are benign. Must diagnose by biopsy | Benign, though general lumpiness may mask other cancerous lump | Serious, needs early treatment |

From Jarvis C: *Physical examination and health assessment,* Philadelphia, 1992, WB Saunders.

## PREVENTION

### *Healthy People 2000*

One of the cancer-related objectives proposed in *Healthy People 2000* is to reduce breast cancer deaths to no more than 20.6 per 100,000 women by the year 2000.[59] Because the mortality rate from breast cancer has shown little decline during the past 60 years even with improved detection and treatment methods (see Figure 54-2), this is an objective well worth achieving.

### Primary Prevention

The ultimate goal of primary prevention is to prevent the incidence of a disease occurring. It implies that the etiology of the disease is known and has proved therapeutic interventions. In the case of breast cancer many risk factors have been identified (see Table 54-1), but the specific cause is unknown, even though therapies are available to treat it and, in some cases, even to achieve complete cure of the disease. Women, even with knowledge of their own personal risk factors, cannot control such factors as age, gender, family, and menstrual or reproductive history. Thus *secondary prevention* is more appropriate in discussing breast cancer prevention.

### Secondary Prevention

Secondary prevention is used to detect a disease process in its early stage so that, with appropriate and timely intervention, the condition can be successfully treated and complete cure is a distinct possibility. Areas in which secondary prevention efforts might be used to decrease the risk of breast cancer include diet control, weight reduction, and avoidance of prolonged use of oral contraceptives and exogenous hormones. Other important measures are monthly **breast self-examination (BSE)** and mammographic examination as directed by a physician or as part of a mammography screening program. All health care professionals should promote these activities so that breast cancer, if present, can be detected in an early, localized stage.

An additional breast cancer–related objective set forth in *Healthy People 2000* is to increase, to at least 80%, the proportion of women 40 years of age and older who have had a clinical breast examination and mammogram and to at least 60% those aged 50 and older who have received them within the preceding 1 to 2 years.[59] The American Cancer Society (ACS) has stated that physical examination of the breast and use of mammography are the approved basic detection methods for breast cancer[19] (Table 54-4).

Although BSE is recommended by the ACS, its true value in detecting breast cancer at an early stage and decreasing breast cancer mortality has not been fully determined. Although 90% of all breast lesions are first detected by the woman herself, the practice of BSE has not resulted in more women performing the examination on a regular schedule. Some studies reveal that even though women recognize the importance of BSE and can perform it accurately, only about 25% of women practice

**TABLE 54-4 American Cancer Society Guidelines for Breast Cancer Screening: Asymptomatic Clients**

| TEST OR EXAMINATION | AGE | RECOMMENDATION |
|---|---|---|
| Breast self-examination | Over age 20 | Monthly |
| Breast physical examination | 20-40 | Every 3 years |
| | Over 40 | Yearly |
| Mammogram | 35-40 | One baseline mammogram |
| | 40-49 | Every 1-2 years |
| | Over 50 | Yearly |

From Dodd DG: *CA* 42(3):177-180, 1992.

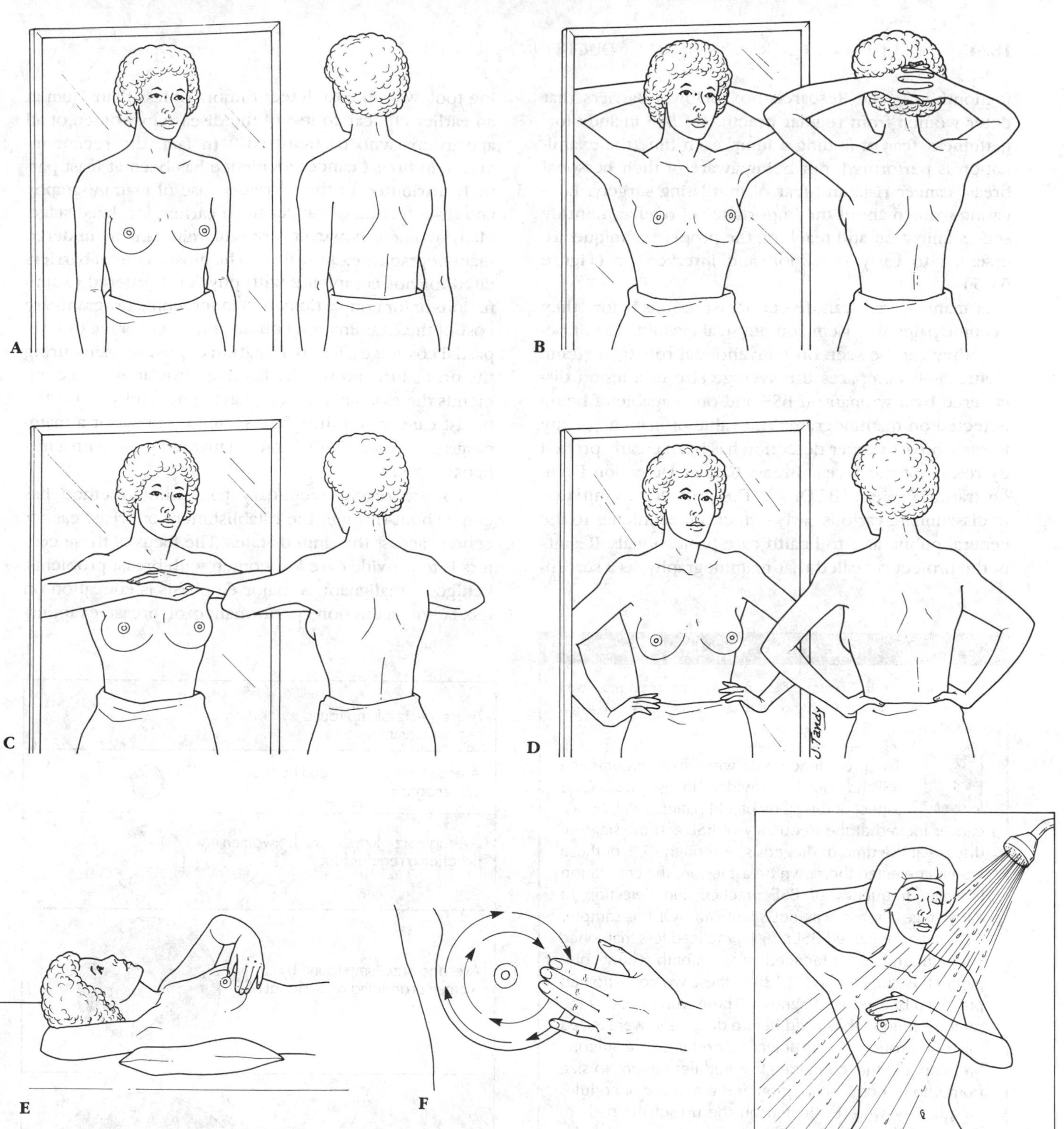


**FIGURE 54-5** Breast self-examination (BSE). **A,** Stand in front of a mirror where you can see yourself from head to waist in good light. Observe your breasts from the front, then from the right and left sides, in each position described as follows. With arms at your side, notice the normal size, shape, color, contour, veins, nipple, and other characteristics of each breast. **B,** Raise your arms above your head; both breasts should rise when the arms are lifted. **C,** With your hands in front of you at shoulder height, press your palms firmly against each other to contract the chest wall muscles. Notice the manner in which your breasts move during position changes. **D,** Put your hands on your hips, squeeze your shoulders inward, and lean slightly forward and down. Look to see that the breasts appear normal for you. **E,** Lie down with one hand under your head and a pillow or folded towel under the scapula of the side you will be examining. **F,** Bring your middle three fingers of the other hand together, and using the flat part of the fingers, move in small, concentric circles. It usually takes three circles to cover all breast tissue. Include the tail of the breast and axilla. Palpate areola; inspect and gently squeeze nipples to check for discharge. Move the nipples from side to side for mobility. Repeat for other breast. **G,** Repeat this technique during bath and shower, when soap and water allow fingers to glide easily over skin.

it monthly.[16] (See Research box below.) Barriers that deter women from regular practice of BSE include forgetfulness, fear of finding a lump each time the examination is performed, not being aware of their personal breast cancer risk, and fear of mutilating surgery. Educating women about the importance of regular monthly self-examination and teaching the proper technique are essential to early detection and intervention (Figure 54-5).

A mammogram can detect breast lesions before they become palpable (1 cm) on physical examination or before they can be seen on conventional roentgenogram. Figure 54-6 compares the average size of a lesion discovered by a woman on BSE and one capable of being detected on mammogram. The value of mammography in early breast cancer detection has been clearly proved by results of the 5-year Breast Cancer Detection Demonstration Project (BCDDP). The project was initiated to disseminate various early-detection techniques to the general public and to health care professionals. Results of the project revealed that mammography, as a screening tool, was able to detect tumors of less than 1 cm at an earlier clinical course of the disease in women of all age-groups who participated.[55] In fact, the recent increase in breast cancer incidence has been at least partially attributed to the increased use of mammography and its detection of cancer in an earlier, localized stage. Many women, however, are still reluctant to undergo mammographic examination. The most frequent barriers cited for not complying with physician-ordered examinations or for nonparticipation in screening programs are cost of the examination (no insurance coverage or only partial coverage), fear of radiation exposure, pain during the procedure, no regular family physician who recommends the examination, and having no family history of breast cancer and therefore seeing no need for a mammogram.[44] Figure 54-7 depicts a mammogram with a malignant lesion.

A more recent secondary prevention method has come about through the establishment of breast cancer centers across the United States. The focus of these centers is to provide care for women with breast problems, benign or malignant. A major emphasis is education on risk-factor reduction, performance of breast examina-

## RESEARCH

Haughey BP et al: Breast self-examination: reported practices, proficiency, and stage of disease at diagnosis, *Oncol Nurs Forum* 15(3):315-319, 1988.

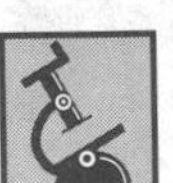

The proficiency with which women practice BSE has not been widely investigated. One aspect of this study of 334 patients with breast cancer looked at the frequency of BSE and the stage of disease at the time of diagnosis. Although 87% of these women detected their own breast lesion, the correlation between frequency of BSE practice and detection of early-stage disease was not significant. Of this sample, 36% never practiced BSE; 26% practiced less than once a month; and 38% practiced once a month. The second part of the study looked at 130 of these women who had practiced BSE before diagnosis. These women, using the same technique they used before diagnosis, were tested for their proficiency in detecting nodules in a silicone breast model that contained five nodules ranging in size from 4 to 0.5 cm. In addition to the number of nodules found, they were evaluated on the use of the pads of fingers while performing the examination and the duration of the total examination. These findings were correlated with the stage of the women's disease at diagnosis. Findings revealed that 41% of those who practiced BSE did not detect any lesions in the model; average length of examination was 30 seconds, and there was no significant correlation between frequency of practice and stage of disease. The results of this study indicate that proficiency and frequency of BSE were not significantly related to the pathologic stage of disease at diagnosis. Nurses teaching BSE technique should include an evaluation of proficiency as a component of BSE education.

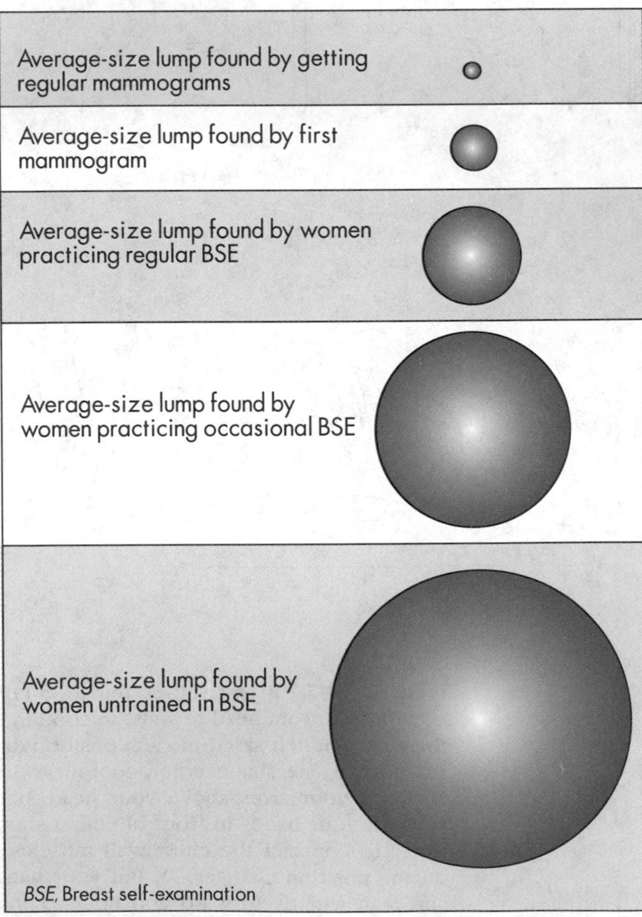


**FIGURE 54-6** Relative sizes of tumors detected by various detection methods, as reported by the Breast Health Program of New York.

tions, teaching BSE techniques, and initiating referrals for screening, diagnosis, and treatment consultations.[15] Ultimately these centers hope to detect more breast cancer in the early localized stage. Another positive outgrowth of the centers is the empowerment and education of a woman to take a more active role in promoting her own personal breast health care.

Last, the National Surgical Adjuvant Breast and Bowel Project (NSABP), a cooperative group that carries out research on breast and bowel cancer, is conducting clinical trials with the drug tamoxifen for women who are at high risk for breast cancer. Tamoxifen is a nonsteroidal antiestrogen drug that has demonstrated antitumor effects. The clinical trials will help answer (1) whether long-term use of tamoxifen will prevent cancer in high risk women, (2) whether tamoxifen can decrease the mortality from breast cancer, and (3) whether tamoxifen can decrease the incidence and mortality from cardiovascular disease in the women participating in the study.[25]

# MEDICAL MANAGEMENT

The management of breast cancer is complex and controversial. Treatment options are ever changing and influenced by new and better surgical techniques, more accurate knowledge of breast cancer growth and dissemination, and new cytotoxic drugs and drug combinations.

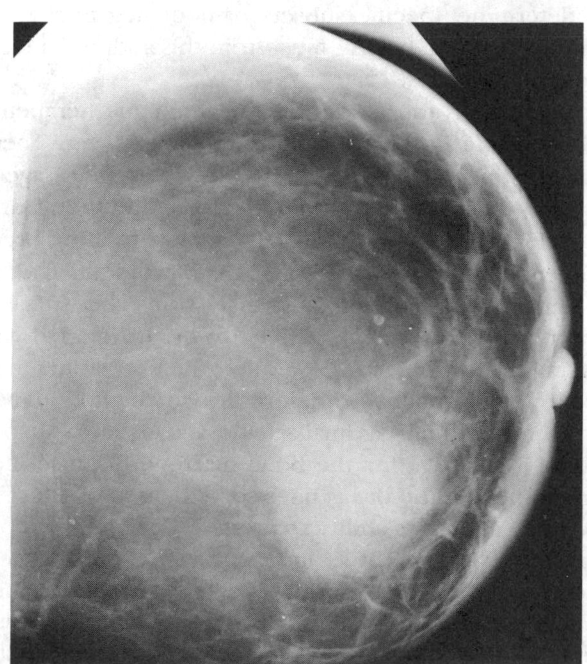

**FIGURE 54-7** Mammogram of patient with area of density indicating carcinoma. (From Cramer LM, Lapayowker MS. In Masters FW, Lewis JR Jr, editors: *Symposium on aesthetic surgery of the face, eyelid, and breast,* vol 4, St Louis, 1972, Mosby.)

The goal for discharge of patients with breast cancer as determined by DRGs is 3.3 days. Common medical therapy for management of breast cancer includes the following measures.

## DIAGNOSTIC TESTS

When a lump has been found, the exact nature of the lesion, benign or malignant, must be determined. Regardless of how the lesion was initially discovered, the physician will follow up with a complete history and physical examination. The physician will look for signs and symptoms that can assist in differentiating a malignant lesion from a benign process, such as observing for skin dimpling, nipple retraction, discharge, eczematous symptoms, and peau d'orange appearance and determining mobility of the tumor.

The presence of a benign lesion, such as a fibroadenoma, cyst, or fibrocystic breast disease, must be ruled out. *Fibroadenomas,* which generally occur in women younger than 30 years, are nontender and mobile on palpation. A *cyst* is the most common form of solitary breast lesion in women older than 30 years. The size of cysts is known to change with the menstrual cycle, becoming more tender and enlarged just before menses. *Fibrocystic* breast disease usually is found in premenopausal women who complain of bilateral breast tenderness with lesions that increase in size with the menstrual cycle.[6] Most breast lesions are benign; however, only histologic examination of tissue from the lesion will determine the true nature of the disease process.

### Noninvasive Diagnostic Tests

A two-view **mammogram** is the most important noninvasive diagnostic tool to detect breast tumors. When performed accurately and read by an experienced radiologist, a mammogram can detect the presence of a lesion 2 to 4 years before it is large enough to be detected by conventional x-ray film or palpated on physical examination.[2]

*Ultrasound* also can be used as a noninvasive test that is capable of determining the size of a lesion and differentiating a fluid-filled cyst from a solid lesion. Although a useful test, ultrasound examination cannot equal the diagnostic capability of mammography.

### Invasive Diagnostic Tests

Most breast tumors are not malignant; however, a diagnosis cannot be made accurately until tissue from the tumor is examined for histologic cell type. Therefore when a tumor mass is discovered, whether on physical examination or mammogram, an invasive procedure, such as *needle biopsy* or *excisional* or *incisional biopsy,* is required.

**Fine-needle aspiration** can be diagnostic for a cyst versus other solid tumor masses. The contents of a cyst range from clear aspirate to bloody or even black fluid. The fluid generally is sent for *cytologic* examination and may be helpful in the identification of cell histology. A cytologic examination is never used alone as a diagnostic tool for cancer because of the chance of both false-positive and false-negative reports.

*Tru-cut needle biopsy* is a useful diagnostic test. When performed correctly, it can provide a central core of tissue from a tumor that can be examined by a pathologist. This type of biopsy is helpful in differentiating the presence of a fatty necrosis or localized infection from tumor.[6]

*Excisional* or *incisional biopsies* can be performed with the patient under local anesthesia in an outpatient department or a physician's office. Biopsies of deep lesions in a large breast are better performed in an operating suite. Tissue specimens are examined for cell type. If the lesion is malignant, the estrogen and progesterone receptor status should be determined at the same time. This information is important because the ER and PR receptor status helps determine treatment choices.

### Other Diagnostic Tests

Breast cancer has a predilection to metastasize to the bone; therefore a *bone scan* and *bone marrow biopsy* may be ordered. Positive findings on these tests indicate the presence of widespread disease and a poorer prognosis. A *liver scan* may be indicated when results of *liver function tests* are abnormal. A *chest x-ray film* reveals lung status before any surgical intervention and also shows the presence of metastasis.[28]

## MEDICATION

The role for adjuvant systemic therapy in the treatment of breast cancer (chemotherapy and endocrine therapy) is to either eradicate or impede the growth of micrometastatic disease.

### Chemotherapy

#### Stages I and II disease (localized)

As a result of improved diagnostic tests, breast cancer is being discovered earlier and in a more localized stage, frequently without nodal involvement. It is estimated that more than 90% of women with tumors 1 cm or less without nodal involvement can be expected to achieve a long-term disease-free survival time.[12] However, because the tumor cells of breast cancer are heterogenous in nature—meaning there is no uniformity of cells and the cells are subject to changes with each cell generation—even localized, node-negative tumors can and frequently do recur. The presence of micrometastasis may go undetected at the time of initial treatment. It is known that when micrometastasis is present, changes (mutations) can occur to the tumor cells making them resistant to the effects of chemotherapeutic agents even though tumor sensitivity to drug therapy is greatest when the tumor burden is small. Thus it is not always possible to predict with confidence that *all* tumors 1 cm or less without node involvement are "cured" with initial locoregional treatment. The early introduction of drug protocols is now being advocated. These regimens, which can shrink tumor size, include cyclophosphamide, methotrexate, and fluorouracil (CMF); fluorouracil, Adriamycin (doxorubicin), and cyclophosphamide (FAC); and fluorouracil, epirubicin, and cyclophosphamide (FEC). These drugs can be administered at the time of diagnosis, before surgery, permitting in many cases surgical lumpectomy as initial treatment rather than the more extensive mastectomy procedure. Preoperative chemotherapy also can make larger inoperable tumors more amenable to surgical removal. An additional advantage to the early use of combination drug therapy when the tumor is small is that this therapy may reduce the number of drug-resistant cells present.[12]

The National Cancer Institute (NCI) issued a drug update in 1989 encouraging physicians to treat *all node-negative* breast cancer regardless of the woman's age with combination chemotherapy or hormonal therapy of tamoxifen for 2 years after initial treatment with mastectomy or lumpectomy and radiation therapy. The reluctance of physicians to follow this recommendation is based on data that suggest that not all women with a node-negative status need additional systemic therapy because they are already "cured." It is feared that the additional systemic therapy will expose these patients to unnecessary side effects and to long-term sequelae of the therapy that are as yet not fully known. As a result of this controversy, clinical trials are being conducted to determine specific subsets of node-negative breast cancers that will benefit most from this additional treatment modality.

At present there are few new chemotherapeutic agents useful in the treatment of breast cancer. Therefore treatment approaches that use established agents in new ways are being investigated. Alternating drug combinations may be more effective in treating breast cancer than the use of a single drug protocol. The use of various combinations also may prove beneficial in improving tumor-cell sensitivity to drug therapy by reducing drug resistance. Another new treatment approach is to administer the prescribed chemotherapeutic agents at their maximal safe dosage levels while providing a "rescue" for the bone marrow. Because most chemotherapeutic drugs have some degree of effect on the bone marrow's ability to produce vital cellular components (WBCs, RBCs, and platelets), hematopoietic growth factors such as granulocyte colony-stimulating factors (G-CSF) and granulocyte-macrophage colony-stimulating factors (GM-CSF) are given to stimulate and hasten bone marrow recovery after high-dose therapy. The use of *Taxol,* an anticancer agent approved for the treatment of ovarian cancer, is now in clinical trials to determine its activity in treating breast cancer.[62] Results are hopeful but nonconclusive to date.

**Stages III and IV disease (advanced)**

Chemotherapy with multiple drug combinations has been used in the treatment of recurrent and advanced breast cancer for many years with positive results. From the preceding discussion, it can be seen that chemotherapy will not prevent disease recurrence when used after conservative surgery alone or after conservative surgery and radiation therapy. Many of the new treatment modalities useful in treating localized breast cancer are being used to treat recurrent and advanced disease. The use of chemotherapy continues to generate many unanswered questions, such as optimal drug combinations, optimal dosage, and length of treatment. These are just a few of the treatment concerns being addressed in clinical trials. (See Chapter 16 for a more detailed discussion of chemotherapy drugs and nursing care.)

## Hormonal Therapy

**Stages I and II disease**

Hormonal therapy has been a useful treatment modality for breast cancer for many decades. Whereas chemotherapy acts on rapidly dividing cells to achieve its effects, hormonal therapy targets cells that are estrogen-dependent for growth. The underlying reason for the success of hormonal therapy was not known until the development of bioassay methods that revealed the presence of estrogen receptors on the cell surface. Before this discovery it was known only that surgical removal of the ovaries interfered in some way with breast cancer growth. One in three premenopausal women with advanced breast cancer who had their ovaries removed showed a delay in cancer growth or a disease-free interval.[32] Research into this phenomenon revealed that tumors that are estrogen-receptor (ER) rich (>10) are considered ER+ and estrogen-receptor poor (<10) are ER−, meaning that estrogen can stimulate the growth of tumors that are high in positive estrogen receptors. It was surmised that if the level of circulating estrogen was removed or decreased, the growth of ER+ tumor could be impeded and disease-free interval and survival time increased. The unfortunate outcome of estrogen ablation was induced menopause, inasmuch as the primary source of estrogen is the ovaries. Hot flashes, vaginal dryness, rise in plasma lipids, atherosclerosis, and osteoporosis resulted. To counteract these menopausal side effects, antiestrogen drug research commenced and led to the development of the antiestrogen drug tamoxifen. Tamoxifen is a nonsteroidal drug that competes for the estradiol-binding site on the ER+ cell, thus removing the stimulus (estrogen) for tumor growth. Although tamoxifen is most effective on ER+ breast cancer, it also affects (but to a lesser degree) ER− tumors as well. Tamoxifen is now considered the hormonal therapy of choice for both premenopausal and postmenopausal women.[32]

Tamoxifen is now being used in early-stage breast cancers in both node-negative and node-positive cases. Data indicate that both groups have a decreased recurrence rate that increases with length of time on the drug regimen—5 years versus 10 years.[32] Although recent research controversy has temporarily halted several major studies on the use of tamoxifen for prevention of breast cancer, it is clear that its usefulness will continue to be explored in both treatment and prevention. Centers are exploring its ability to prevent breast cancer in women at high risk and to prolong survival time in all age-groups with both ER+ and ER− status. Tamoxifen also is being tested with the drug cyclosporine to evaluate whether this drug combination can overcome drug resistance by altering the tumor cell membrane so that the chemotherapy agents can enter the cell but not escape, thus destroying more tumor cells.[62]

**Stages III and IV disease**

Hormonal therapy as just described is a mainstay of treatment for advanced breast cancer, especially ER+ tumors with involved lymph nodes. The higher the estrogen level, the better the response to the drug. Tamoxifen has been used either alone or in combination with chemotherapeutic agents. When used alone, it has fewer of the side effects such as hair loss and nausea that often accompany chemotherapy drugs.

The size of the tumor and histologic grade are factors that presently are being researched, which will shed light on more efficient use of this drug. The length of treatment with tamoxifen is still a debatable question that needs to be addressed.

Until more data become available and standard treatment protocols can be agreed on for both chemotherapy and hormonal manipulation, the patient and her physician will need to discuss each for its known advantages and disadvantages and select the modality that meets each woman's individual needs and concerns.

## TREATMENT

## Radiation Therapy

**Stages I and II disease**

Radiation to the breast after preservation surgery (lumpectomy) is accepted therapy for tumors of 4 cm or less.[48] Radiation to the breast will eradicate tumor cells left behind after manipulation and handling of the tumor during surgery. The total recommended radiation dose is 4500 to 5000 cGy over 6 to 7 weeks. A booster dose of up to 1000 cGy may be prescribed with use of either implants or external beam irradiation. The risk of local recurrence is minimal after this protocol. Tumors of less than 1 cm generally are not treated with radiation after breast-preservation surgery because the risk of metastasis is minimal and prognosis is considered excellent (see discussion under Medications on early-stage breast cancer). Although radiation after conservative surgery is widely used, some large breast tumors may be irradiated before surgery to facilitate easier surgical removal. Close medical follow-up is important after conservative surgery and radiation (CS + RT). Guidelines recommended include a breast physical examination every 3 to 4 months for 3 years, twice a year for 7 years after CS + RT, and then yearly. A mammogram is recommended every 6 months for the first year and thereafter on an annual basis.[48]

When the breast is irradiated, the side effects include skin reactions (redness, dryness, itching), edema, mild tenderness, and fatigue. Fatigue is the result of bone marrow suppression from radiation to the thorax. The adult sternum, ribs, and thoracic vertebrae contain more than one third of the total body bone marrow (sternum 3%, ribs 16%, thoracic vertebrae 16%). When these areas are within the treatment port, even when shielding devices are in place, some bone marrow function will be destroyed and full recovery takes up to 6 months or more.[50] Patient instruction in dealing with the side effects of anemia and increased vulnerability to infection is vital to achieve patient compliance in completing treatment with the total prescribed radiation dose.

### Local recurrence

Local recurrence of breast cancer usually occurs within 2 to 8 years after the initial diagnosis and treatment. Approximately 80% occur within 3 years.[45] Generally the earlier the recurrence, the graver the prognosis. When recurrence follows conservative surgery and radiation therapy, mastectomy alone or with adjunct systemic therapy is the recommended intervention.

Tissue subjected to radiation therapy given at a dose intended for a "cure" does not respond well to repeated radiation exposure. This is because of the changes that occur in the vascular bed after initial radiation treatment, which results in a reduced blood and oxygen supply to the irradiated tissue. Radiation therapy works best on tissue with a good blood supply and a high oxygen saturation content. Therefore previously irradiated tissue may not respond well a second time. Complications of such therapy include fibrotic changes to the lung, tissue necrosis, and rib fractures.

### Stages III and IV disease

The role of radiation therapy in advanced breast cancer usually is palliative. Breast cancer has the propensity to metastasize to bone, which is a major source of pain and discomfort. Bone involvement can result in pathologic fractures and fractures to the vertebrae of the spine, causing compression on nerve roots and on the spinal cord. Radiation therapy can help to alleviate the discomfort from these complications. Metastasis from breast cancer often results in lymphatic obstruction as evidenced by the presence of a pleural effusion. In addition, metastasis frequently involves other vital organ systems such as the lung and liver. Radiation therapy frequently is used to treat these metastatic lesions. When radiation is prescribed, the patient requires information and instruction on the rationale for the therapy and any specific care measures that will be necessary during treatment. It is important that the patient be made aware that the radiation treatments will not cure her disease but can provide pain relief and improve her quality of life. (See Chapter 16 for a more thorough discussion of radiation therapy in the treatment of cancer.)

Critical pathways (also referred to as *collaborative necessary paths* or *care maps*) have been developed in some inpatient and outpatient settings to guide both medical and nursing management. (See Critical Pathway, p. 1831, and Nursing Care Plan, p. 1829, for the person undergoing lumpectomy and radium implantation.) In some settings the nursing care plans are combined with the critical pathway document.

## Surgery

### Stages I and II disease

Surgery is the mainstay of breast cancer treatment, especially when the disease is localized without distant metastasis. The surgical removal of breast cancer has evolved over the past 100 years from the mutilating radical mastectomy to the more conservative surgical approaches in use today. Halsted introduced the radical procedure (removal of the entire breast, skin, chest wall muscles, and axillary lymph nodes) in the mistaken belief that as a breast tumor grows, it will spread in an orderly manner from the tumor core outward to all adjacent tissue and lymph nodes in its path. Unfortunately, this surgical procedure became the standard form of treatment for breast cancer for more than 70 years. Today, after years of clinical trials, surgery employing less extensive tissue removal is now the rule.

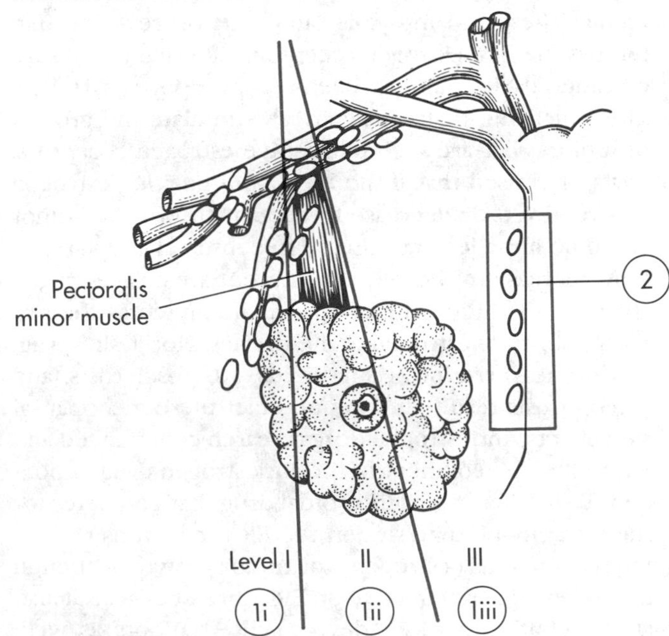


**FIGURE 54-8** Regional axillary lymph nodes demonstrating levels I, II, and III node dissection. (From Beahrs OH, Hutter RV, Kennedy BJ, editors: *Breast manual for staging of cancer,* ed 4, Philadelphia, 1992, JB Lippincott.)

## NURSING CARE PLAN

### PERSON WITH LUMPECTOMY AND RADIUM IMPLANT FOR BREAST CANCER

**DATA:** Mrs. C. is a 46-year-old premenopausal white woman who discovered a lump in her left breast while showering 3 days before admission. She is married and the mother of two teen-age daughters, ages 18 and 15 years. She is employed as a real estate agent for a local agency. Mrs. C. was seen by her primary care physician who on physical examination was able to palpate a small indiscrete mass in the upper outer quadrant of her left breast. Axillary nodes were nontender and normal in size on examination. A bilateral, two-view mammogram confirmed the presence of a 3-cm lesion. The right breast appeared normal. A fine-needle aspiration and biopsy of the mass were performed in the physician's office. Pathology report revealed invasive intraductal carcinoma of the left breast. Treatment options were discussed with the patient and her husband. Mrs. C. has decided to have breast-preservation surgery (lumpectomy) followed by radiation therapy. Iridium-192 will be implanted to provide the initial radiation source, which will be followed by external radiation treatments once the wound has healed.

The nursing history identified the following:

- Mrs. C. is anxious but cooperative. States she wants to "get this thing over with as soon as I can. I'm really scared about what is going to happen."
- Cancer history reveals maternal grandmother died of breast cancer at age 53 years of age. Mother died of injuries sustained in an automobile accident at 25 years of age. Has no siblings.
- Practices BSE monthly but states she never thought she needed to get a baseline mammogram.
- Good nutritional state. Weight has not fluctuated over past 6 months; states that she is 15 pounds above weight for height and age.
- Denies taking any prescribed or OTC drugs. Has never smoked; takes an occasional alcoholic cocktail when socializing.

Collaborative nursing actions include those to prepare for postoperative care expectations and radiation implant, care during "implant boost," and home care management. Nursing actions include *monitoring* for the following:

- Indications of neurovascular and lymphatic complications—increased or decreased wound drainage, swelling of affected arm and hand, decreased peripheral pulse, cool, pale skin, and decreased movement ability
- Understanding and compliance with radiation safety guidelines and limitations in personal activities and contact with staff members and visitors

#### ■ NURSING DIAGNOSIS

Knowledge deficit related to inadequate understanding of expected postlumpectomy care routine

| Expected Patient Outcomes | Nursing Interventions | Rationale |
|---|---|---|
| Assumes an active role in own recovery:<br>■ Requests analgesic prn.<br>■ Performs respiratory toilet measures as directed.<br>■ Uses correct method of getting out of bed.<br>■ States reason for neurovascular checks on affected arm.<br>■ Performs exercises to minimize postoperative lymphedema. | Administer prescribed analgesic to provide maximum level of comfort. | Freedom from pain promotes patient cooperation and compliance with ROM exercises and increasing physical activity. |
| | Assist patient with performing deep breathing, turning q 2 hr, incentive spirometer q 2 hr, and ambulation. | Prevents inadequate respiratory efforts and pooling of secretions, which cause respiratory infection. |
| | Assist patient to get out of bed on unaffected side. | Reduces strain on incision. |
| | Elevate affected extremity on pillows so that arm, hand, elbow are positioned above shoulder. | Promotes lymphatic and venous return and prevents lymphedema. |
| | Monitor dressing/Hemovac function; change dressing prn; and check wound and saline lock for signs and symptoms of infection. | Increased drainage may indicate that drain is improperly placed or obstructed, leading to lymphedema; wet dressings are potential source of infection; and fresh dressing increases patient comfort. |
| | Perform neurovascular assessment on affected side q 4 h. | Presence of lymphedema causes pressure on peripheral nerves, leading to cool, pale extremity, diminished pulse, poor movement. |
| | Monitor ability to take and retain fluids and solid food; increase diet from IVs to liquids to regular food; record I & O. | Promotes return to normal eating patterns necessary for energy needs and wound healing. |
| | Post sign in room alerting staff *not* to use affected arm for *blood pressures, injections,* or *venipunctures.* | Lymph node dissection disrupts lymphatic function; inflated blood pressure cuff can obstruct lymph flow through channels and increase damage; injections and venipunctures cause breaks in skin and provides source for infection. |

## NURSING CARE PLAN

### PERSON WITH LUMPECTOMY AND RADIUM IMPLANT FOR BREAST CANCER—cont'd

#### ■ NURSING DIAGNOSIS

Anxiety related to radioactive implant placement, the effects of internal radiation, and inadequate knowledge of postimplant restrictions on activities and self-care

| Expected Patient Outcomes | Nursing Interventions | Rationale |
|---|---|---|
| Describe iridium implant procedure.<br>Relates rationale for "booster" radiation dose.<br>Verbalizes own limitations while implant is in place<br>Describes precautions necessary for staff and visitors | Instruct regarding advantages of RT implant (can cure stages I and II disease). | This instruction provides confidence in therapy. |
| | Provide rationale for "booster" radiation dose to tumor bed immediately after lumpectomy surgery. | Procedure performed at initial surgery eliminates need for second hospital admission, and second exposure to anesthesia, as well as less expense to patient. |
| | Explain need for external-beam radiation for 5-6 weeks after wound healing is complete. | Prepares patient for the need to continue therapy as an outpatient. |
| | Instruct on radiation implant procedure: hollow plastic catheters are placed during surgery and then filled with iridium needles when patient returns to private room. | Afterloading technique prevents unnecessary radioactive exposure to health care personnel (Figure 54-13). |
| | Instruct on postimplant care: confined to private room. | Patient is radioactive and a danger to staff and visitors. |
| | Ambulate patient as tolerated. | Increased activity promotes more rapid physical and mental recovery. |
| | Assist with sponge bathing only (no tub or showering); keep area dry. | Prevents contamination of implant area and potential infection at site. |
| | Avoid touching/moving catheter. | May change positioning and displace catheter, resulting in irradiation to wrong tissues. |
| | Provide patient with isolation tray although no dietary restrictions are needed. | Isolation tray alerts dietary staff that special precautions should be taken with patient. |
| | Limit time staff members spend caring for patient. | Radiation safety precautions regarding time and distance criteria prevent overexposure of staff members. |
| | Instruct visitors that they must follow radiation safety guidelines and avoid close contact such as hugging. | See preceding. |
| | MD removes catheter and iridium at designated time (no more than 3 days). | Once iridium is removed, patient no longer is radioactive. |
| | Tell patient she may feel breast fullness/heaviness. | Feelings of fullness/heaviness are expected. |
| | Discharge teaching: | |
| | ■ Encourage 8 hours' sleep and rest periods throughout day. | Fatigue is a common side effect of radiation and recent surgery. |
| | ■ Skin care: wash gently with plain soap and water. | Dryness and crusting at insertion site are common; cleansing prevents infection. |
| | ■ Breast will feel heavy and full; advise to wear firm brassiere. | Result of local tissue reaction secondary to radiation effects. |
| | ■ Reinforce need for ROM and positioning measures to affected arm/shoulder, and remind patient to avoid heavy lifting. | Prevents complications and facilitates successful rehabilitation. |
| | ■ Provide dates for follow up for RT start date and surgical checkup, as well as rationale for each. | Promotes compliance with treatment plan. |
| | ■ Review precautions for affected arm: *no blood pressures, injections, venipunctures.* | Prevents complications. |

## CRITICAL PATHWAY Lumpectomy With Radium Implant for Breast Cancer

**DRG #: 258 Expected LOS: 4**

| | Day of Surgery Day of Admission Day 1 | Day 2 | Day 3 | Day of Discharge Day 4 |
|---|---|---|---|---|
| **Diagnostic Tests** | *Preoperative:* CBC, UA, SMA/18*; radiologic needle localization | | | |
| **Medications** | IVs, IV/IM analgesic, Rx for rest/sleep | IV to saline lock, PO analgesic, Rx for rest/sleep | IV saline lock, PO analgesic, Rx for rest/sleep | Disc saline lock, PO analgesic |
| **Treatments** | I & O q8hr including incisional Hemovac; VS q4hr; neurocirculatory assessment of affected side q2hr; elevate affected arm on pillow; T, C, & DB q2hr; incentive spirometry q2hr; check dressing | I & O q8hr; VS q6hr; neurocirculatory assessment of affected side q4hr; elevate affected arm on pillow; T, C, & DB q2hr; incentive spirometry q2hr | Disc I & O; VS q6hr; neurocirculatory assessment of affected side q8hr; elevate affected arm on pillow; T, C, & DB q2hr; incentive spirometry q4hr | VS q8hr; neurocirculatory assessment of affected side q8hr; elevate affected arm on pillow |
| **Diet** | NPO; clear liquids when nausea stops | Advance diet as tolerated; regular diet | Regular diet | Regular diet |
| **Activity** | Up in room with help; *no BP, IVs, injections, etc., in affected arm* | Up in room *only* with help; *no BP, IVs, injections, ect., in affected arm; est and maintain radiation safety measures for patient, staff, visitors* | Up ad lib in room only; *no BP, IVs, injections, etc., in affected arm; maintain radiation safety measures for patient, staff, visitors* | Up ad lib in room only until radiation removed; *no BP, IVs, injections, etc., in affected arm; maintain radiation safety measures until radiation disc* |
| **Consultations** | | Radiation &/or medical oncologist, phy therapist | | |

*CBC,* Complete blood cell count; *disc,* discontinue; *est,* estimate; *SMA,* sequential multiple analysis; *T, C, & DB,* turn, cough and deep breathe; *UA,* urinalysis; *VS,* vital signs.

*Serum calcium, phosphorus, triglycerides, uric acid, creatinine, BUN, total bilirubin, alkaline phosphate, aspartate aminotransferase (AST) (formerly serum glutamic-oxaloacetic transaminase [SGOT]), alanine aminotransferase (ALT) (formerly serum glutamate pyruvate transaminase [SGPT]), lactic dehydrogenase (LDH), total protein, albumin, sodium, potassium, chloride, total $CO_2$, glucose.

When primary, localized breast cancer (less than 2 to 5 cm and no metastasis) is diagnosed, two surgical options may be offered: modified radical **mastectomy,** with or without breast reconstruction, or breast preservation (**lumpectomy**) procedures. Both procedures include axillary lymph-node dissection because metastatic dissemination takes place primarily through these nodes. The number of diseased nodes (three to four) directly correlates with the risk of recurrent disease after initial treatment and with overall prognosis.[23] The level of lymph node dissection (sampling versus levels I, II, and III dissection) has been debated for many years. *Sampling* involves the removal of one to several nodes from the lower axilla without any defined boundary. Low axillary dissection *(level I)* is the removal of an entire bloc of nodes in the area from the latissimus dorsi muscle laterally to the medial pectoralis muscle. *Levels II and III* dissection removes en bloc nodes from the middle to the entire axillary node chain, respectively (Figure 54-8). There is now general agreement that when axillary nodes are negative for cancer, a level I to II dis-

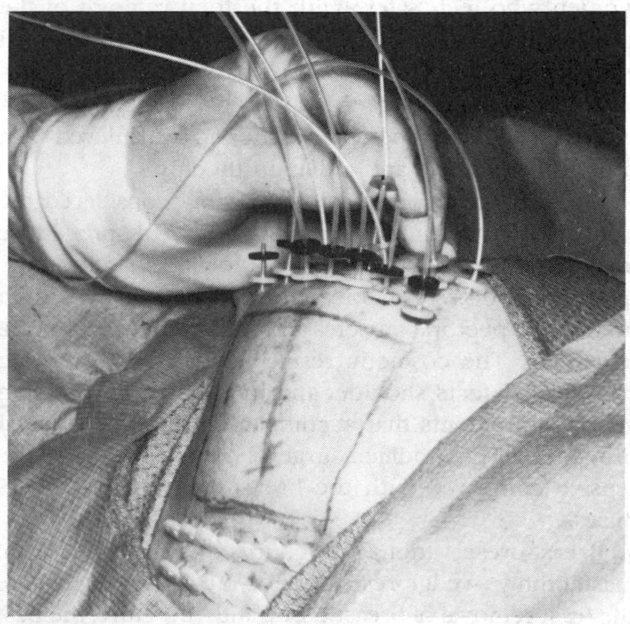

**FIGURE 54-9** Interstitial "booster" radiation therapy for breast cancer using iridium needles.

**BOX 54-3 Contraindications for Use of Breast-Preservation Procedures**

Pregnancy: first and second trimester preclude the use of radiation therapy
Multiple lesions located in separate quadrants of the breast or diffuse malignant or indeterminate-appearing microcalcifications
Prior irradiation of the breast
History of collagen-vascular disease, which is recognized as having poor tolerance to the effects of radiation therapy
Tumor size: large tumor in a small breast will not allow adequate resection of tumor
Breast size: large pendulous breasts are difficult to irradiate adequately
Location of tumor: tumors located beneath the nipple necessitate removal of the nipple-areola complex, which has questionable value compared with mastectomy

**TABLE 54-5 Factors Influencing Type of Surgery for Primary Breast Cancer**

| FACTOR | LUMPECTOMY | MASTECTOMY |
|---|---|---|
| Tumor size | Small | Large |
| Breast size | Average | Very small or very large |
| Tumor location | Upper outer quadrant | Near nipple |
| Type of cancer | Less aggressive | More aggressive or extensive intraductal |
| Number of tumors | One tumor present | More than one tumor present |

From Ellerhorst-Ryan JM: *Innovations Oncol Nurs* 5(1):5, 1988.

section is adequate. If nodes are positive for disease, a complete level III dissection is advised.[34] The goal of both surgical options is to control local/regional disease, to accurately stage the disease so that patients at high risk for recurrence are identified, and to provide the best chance for long-term survival, in addition to achieving the best cosmetic result.[34] The overall long-term survival rates, comparing the two surgical methods, are approximately the same.[64]

A major consideration in choice of surgical option relates to patient preference. After the advantages and disadvantages of both procedures are thoroughly explained, the patient is in a position to make a more informed choice and one that best suits her own needs. Selection of mastectomy over conservative surgery and radiation therapy (CS + RT) often is preferred by women who feel "safer" with the total removal of the affected breast. Also, some patients prefer not to deal with radiation therapy on a daily basis for 6 to 7 weeks. For those who are concerned with body image and self-esteem, a better cosmetic outcome can be achieved with breast preservation and radiation therapy.

Modified radical mastectomy is now considered the standard form of mastectomy surgery. This procedure involves the removal of the whole breast, some fatty tissue, and dissection of some of the axillary lymph nodes. The pectoral muscles and surrounding nerves are left intact. The cosmetic result avoids the devastating chest wall defects, shoulder and arm limitations, and skin graft requirements that accompanied the more radical procedure. The modified surgery, however, is more extensive compared with the breast-preservation procedures.

Breast-preservation procedures, known as partial mastectomy, wedge resection, or lumpectomy, involve the least removal of breast tissue and, therefore, the best cosmesis. The tumor is removed, including a margin of normal tissue. The pathologist usually examines the specimen immediately to be sure that the margins around the tumor are cancer-free. If not, a wider excision is required. A separate incision is used to determine axillary node involvement. Breast-conservation treatment for local disease is followed in 2 to 4 weeks by radiation therapy when wound healing is complete. The decision to include irradiation after breast-conservation procedures is a result of studies that showed that in up to 50% of cases some residual tumor cells were still present after tumor removal.[23] Breast preservation is not advised for all stage I and II disease. Contraindications are listed in Box 54-3. Table 54-5 reviews the major factors that influence which type of breast surgery provides the best outcome.

**Mastectomy and breast reconstruction.** The female breast, although not essential to life, has considerable impact on body image, self-esteem, sexual attractiveness, and intimacy and love.[37] When a woman is faced with the loss of a breast because of cancer, she can be overwhelmed by the fear and anxiety that result from unknown outcome, the threat of death, and uncertain future. The decision to undergo immediate or delayed breast reconstruction often needs to be made during this time of fear and confusion—sometimes without sufficient knowledge to make an informed decision. It is important that options be clearly outlined regarding the length of hospital stay, time frame for treatment, expected outcome, and the complications that may be encountered. Of equal importance is the determination of how the loss of a breast will affect sexuality, marital adjustment, and expectations.

Mastectomy with reconstruction requires 1 to 2 days of additional hospitalization. Recovery and rehabilitation time also are increased. Mastectomy with or without breast reconstruction will not change the ultimate long-term survival time but may determine how well the woman adjusts to the loss of a breast.

When mastectomy without breast reconstruction is chosen as the option, a breast **prosthesis** always is necessary. For many elderly women this may not be viewed as a problem. Younger women often find the need for prostheses an uncomfortable nuisance and a constant reminder of their breast cancer experience. Some women describe feeling "out of balance" when wearing the prosthesis compared with the weight of the opposite normal breast. They also may feel confined in their choice of clothing or participation in physical activities. Frequently these kinds of concerns prompt women to undergo breast reconstruction many months to years after selecting mastectomy alone. Some surgeons believe that a wait of 3 to 6 months is beneficial before reconstruction surgery. This delay permits recovery from initial surgery and recovery from potential postoperative complications such as infection, hematoma formation, and lymphedema.

Two types of procedures are available for **breast reconstruction:** implants and autogenous tissue flaps. **Implants,** in their simplest form, are soft sacs filled with silicone gel that are placed in a pocket beneath the pectoralis major muscle and held in place by the pectoralis major, anterior serratus, and upper rectus abdominis muscles. The size and shape of the implant are matched to the size of the remaining breast. A second type of implant is called a *tissue expander* prosthesis. The expandable implant is placed in the manner just described by means of a single empty sac or a double-lumen sac with two compartments: a small one with silicone gel and a larger compartment for saline.[6] The expander sac is filled with 100 to 200 ml of sterile saline at the time of surgery and then with 30 to 100 ml weekly until the desired size of breast is reached. The sterile saline is added to the expander sac through a needle inserted into a subcutaneous access port. The gradual expansion of the implant stretches the size of the pocket, thus giving size and shape to the new breast.[37] Maximal expansion takes several months to achieve, at which time the prosthesis is removed and replaced by a silicone-filled implant. Newer expander sacs are available that do not need to be replaced unless a complication such as infection requires their removal. No activity restrictions are necessary during the expansion period. Pain and discomfort are usually within tolerable limits.

The use of silicone implants is not without complications or dispute. Complications include fibrous capsular contractions around the implant, causing pain, tenderness, and fixation of the implant to the chest wall. Massaging the area several times daily is helpful in breaking up these constrictions.[6] Infection is a rare cause for implant removal. Debate about the effects of silicone on a woman's health resulted in 1992 in the Food and Drug Administration restricting its use temporarily to those women undergoing breast reconstruction for cancer. Although silicone is not believed to be a health risk, this restriction is in place until more definitive data are available on its safety.

Nipple reconstruction, using tissue obtained from the opposite nipple-areola complex or skin from the upper portion of the inner thigh, requires a second surgical procedure after breast reconstruction. The use of a dermal tattoo that can match normal breast pigment is an alternative method of nipple formation.[37]

The use of **autogenous tissue flaps** is a second means of breast reconstruction that can be performed at the time of mastectomy or at a later date. Tissue flaps eliminate the need for an implant unless insufficient tissue is available to form a breast of dimensions equal to the remaining normal breast. Performing immediate breast reconstruction avoids the cost of a second hospitalization and surgery and loss of time from normal activities.[37] Flaps include use of latissimus dorsi musculocutaneous tissue from the upper portion of the back to create a breast or the transverse rectus abdominis myocutaneous (TRAM) tissue from the lower portion of the abdomen. A major disadvantage of the latissimus dorsi flap is the visible scar left on the back. A TRAM flap has the advantage of using tissue that is similar in elasticity to normal breast tissue and is available in sufficient quantity to reconstruct a new breast of equal size and shape of the uninvolved breast. An additional advantage is that the abdominal scar can be easily hidden.[39] Nipple reconstruction is performed in the same manner as already described. Figure 54-10 shows the three types of breast-reconstruction methods.

#### Stages III and IV disease

Surgery for advanced breast cancer includes mastectomy in combination with systemic chemotherapy or hormonal therapy.

### Bone Marrow Transplantation as a New Treatment for Breast Cancer

The use of bone marrow transplantation (BMT), a therapy traditionally reserved for treatment of hematologic cancers, is now being investigated for its usefulness in treating solid malignant tumors. At the present time, BMT is considered experimental therapy for breast cancer and the long-term outcome of this therapy is still in question. Most health insurance providers are withholding coverage for the procedure until more definitive data have been obtained. (See Chapter 16 for further discussion of bone marrow transplantation.)

## Diet

Maintenance of good nutrition is essential for all patients with cancer. Dietary requirements include an increase in calories, carbohydrate (CHO), and protein. Body energy demands are known to increase with cancer, and more energy is necessary to withstand the potentially debilitating side effects of treatment. A diet high in calories and CHO spares body protein, necessary for tissue and wound repair, from being broken down for energy needs.

Good dietary management and patient education are especially important for the person with breast cancer. This diagnosis can evoke great emotional stress, and its treatment can affect appetite and nutrition in many ways.

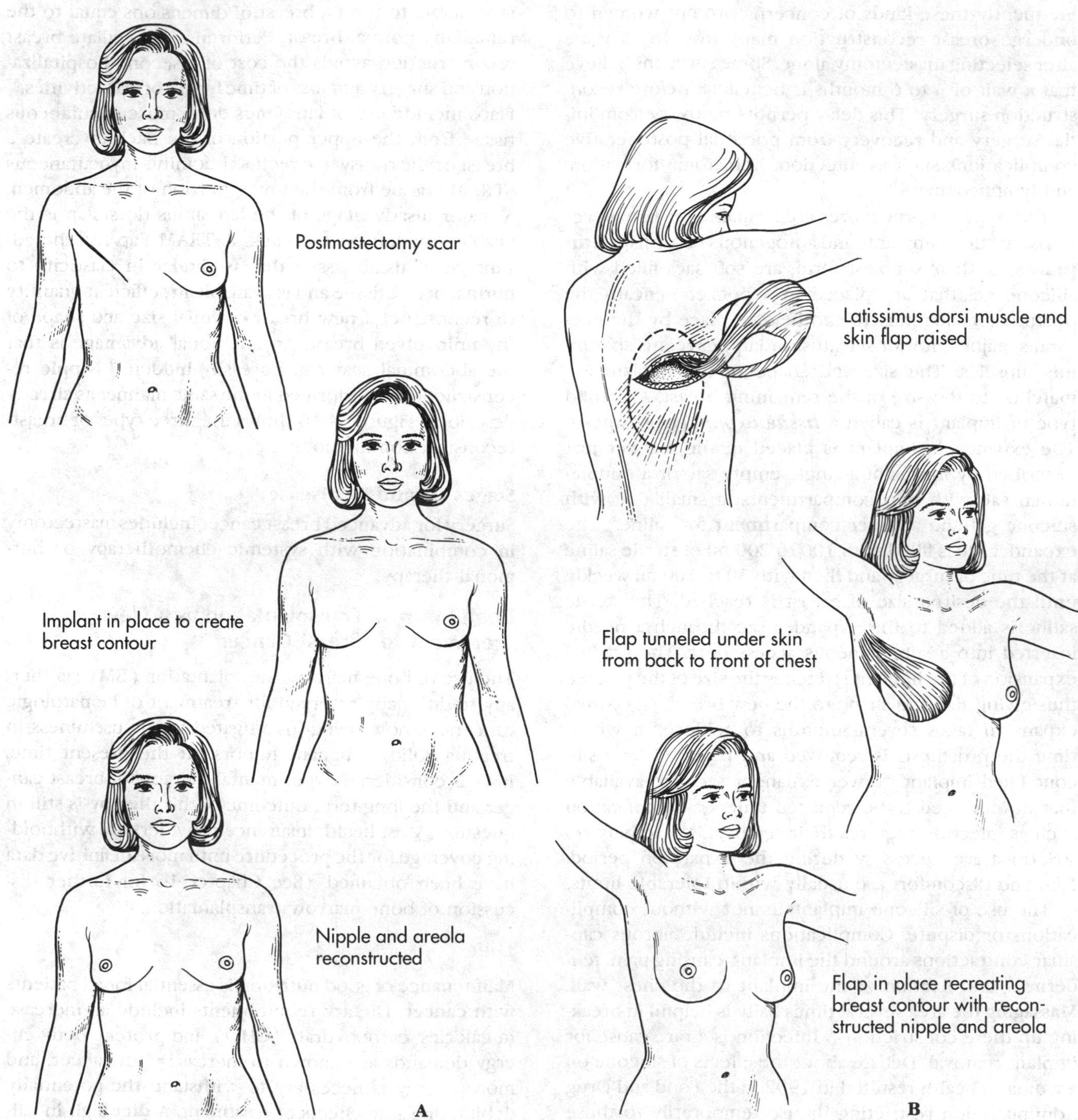


**FIGURE 54-10** Three types of breast reconstruction procedures. **A,** "Simple" implant placement. **B,** "Latissimus dorsi" reconstruction. (From US Department of Health and Human Services: *Breast reconstruction,* NIH Pub No 91-2151, Washington, DC, 1990, US Government Printing Office.)

At the time of diagnosis, fear and anxiety regarding the outcome of tests can lead to anorexia and poor nutritional intake. Family and marital concerns, worry over treatment option decisions, and an uncertain future add to the problem. Once treatment is under way, the patient requires dietary assistance and direction to cope with treatment side effects.

All of the prescribed treatment options—surgery, radiation therapy, chemotherapy, and hormonal therapy, as well as adjunct medication and activity restrictions—affect body nutritional needs and maintenance to some degree. The patient and family members require instruction on how to manage these problems that can and often do occur after discharge from the hospital. Table 54-6 provides an overview of nutritional problems generated by various cancer treatment options and the interventions commonly used to treat them.

## Activity

The activity level of the patient with breast cancer depends on several factors: the extent of the disease process, type of treatment employed, phase within the treat-

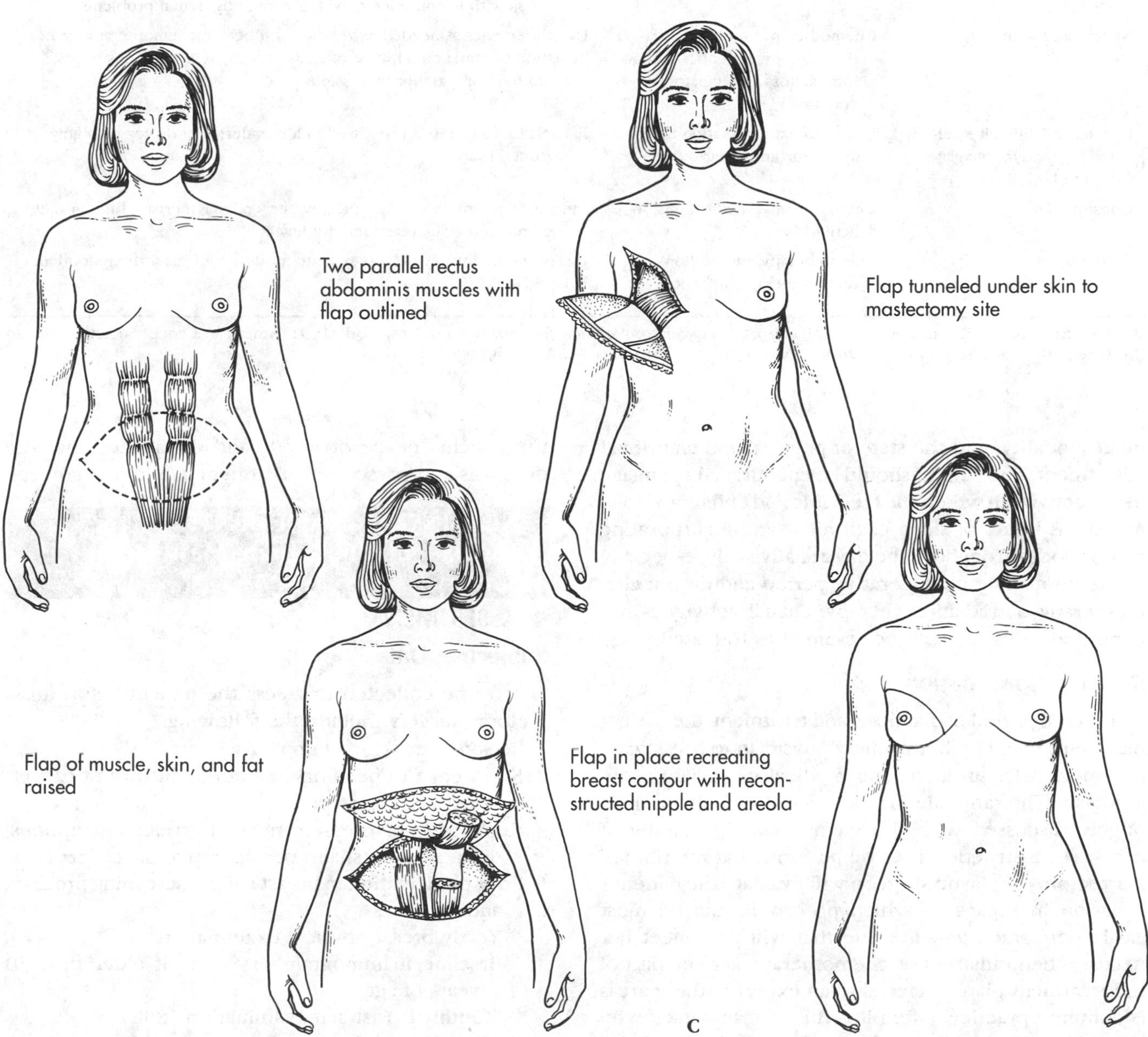


**FIGURE 54-10, cont'd** C, "Rectus abdominis" reconstruction.

**TABLE 54-6 Plan of Care for Treatment-Induced Nutritional Problems**

| NUTRITIONAL PROBLEM GENERATED | TREATMENT OPTIONS INVOLVED AND STRESS-RELATED FACTORS | INTERVENTIONS |
|---|---|---|
| *Oral:* | | |
| Stomatitis (mouth sores) | Chemotherapy, radiation therapy | Eliminate acidic, salty, and spicy foods; abstain from alcohol and tobacco; use good oral hygiene. |
| Anorexia | Chemotherapy, radiation therapy, emotional distress | Provide small, frequent high-caloric meals; make meal time an enjoyable occasion; avoid noxious odors. |
| Xerostomia (dry mouth) | Chemotherapy, radiation therapy, medications; mouth breathing | Ensure adequate fluid intake; suck on hard candies; use artificial saliva; moisten mouth with water, using a dropper or syringe if necessary. |
| Abnormal taste | Chemotherapy, radiation therapy, medications | Avoid offensive foods (red meat); mask bad taste by adding wine/beer to soups and sauces; marinate meats; use more and stronger seasonings; serve cold or room-temperature food; drink more liquids; add tartness with lemon juice or vinegar; remedy dental problems. |
| Nausea and vomiting | Chemotherapy, surgery, radiation therapy, narcotics; behavioral factors (anticipatory vomiting) | Use antiemetics as needed; withhold food before chemotherapy or radiation treatment: eliminate offensive foods; avoid noxious odors; avoid food preparation if possible. |
| Dysphagia (difficult swallowing), odynophagia (painful swallowing) | Chemotherapy, radiation therapy; neuromuscular defects | Eat soft foods or foods processed in a blender; avoid spicy or highly seasoned foods. |
| Constipation | Chemotherapy, medications; inactivity | Increase fluid intake (prune juice, water, coffee); increase bulk in diet; use bran cereal; increase activity level. |
| Diarrhea | Chemotherapy, medications, radiation therapy; infection | Increase fluid intake; use low-residue foods; avoid gas-forming food and liquids. |

Modified from Baraie KV. In Baird SB et al, editors: *A cancer source book for nurses,* ed 6, New York, 1991, American Cancer Society; Casciato DA, Lowitz BB, editors: *Manual of clinical oncology,* ed 2, Boston, 1992, Little, Brown & Co.

ment modality, and the state of physical and emotional adjustment. The patient should be encouraged to engage in any activity in which she feels able and finds enjoyable. At least 8 hours of sleep each night and incorporating rest periods throughout the day are advisable, especially in the immediate postoperative period and during chemotherapy or radiation therapy. Sexual activity is not contraindicated and can be resumed as tolerated.

### Referral/Consultation

During the period of diagnosis and treatment, the patient may be referred by her primary physician to breast cancer specialists: surgeons and medical or radiation oncologists. The rationale for the referrals should be thoroughly discussed with the woman and her family. If breast reconstruction is to be performed at the time of mastectomy, a plastic surgeon will evaluate the patient's situation in regard to which procedure can be most easily performed and the one that will best meet her needs. When radiation or chemotherapy is to be part of the treatment plan, a referral to an expert in these areas is common practice. Often it is the woman herself who initiates a referral or consultation in the effort to obtain a "second opinion" regarding her breast cancer diagnosis. Second opinions should be encouraged and names of appropriate medical experts provided. This ensures the patient "peace of mind" and confidence that the diagnosis and prescribed treatment are in fact correct.

## NURSING MANAGEMENT: The Patient Undergoing Mastectomy Surgery

### ♦ ASSESSMENT

#### Subjective Data

Data to be collected to assess the patient before mastectomy surgery include the following:

- Personal report of "lump" discovery
- Knowledge of personal and family history of cancer, especially breast cancer
- Knowledge of breast cancer, its treatment options, diagnostic tests, and perioperative procedures
- Prior participation in breast cancer screening program and practices:
  - Yearly breast physical examination
  - Baseline mammogram or yearly if older than 50 years of age
  - Monthly breast self-examination (BSE)
- History of oral contraception use or hormonal replacement therapy
- Concerns about loss of breast on femininity, sexuality, and self-esteem

### Objective Data

Data to be collected to assess the patient before mastectomy surgery include the following:

- Breast physical examination
  - Inspection—breast symmetry, size, discharge, edema, skin signs (dimpling), nipple retraction
  - Palpation—size and location of lesion within quadrant, cutaneous nodules, enlarged lymph nodes in axillary, infraclavicular, and supraclavicular areas
  - Signs and symptoms of discomfort
- Age and menopausal status
- Presence of other physical or emotional conditions that may influence successful surgical outcome and rehabilitation
- Understanding of treatment options and ability to make an informed choice
  - Mastectomy with or without breast reconstruction
  - Breast preservation surgery followed by radiation therapy

### Diagnostic Test Findings

1. Noninvasive test findings:
   a. Mammogram demonstrating presence of single lesion
   b. Breast physical examination revealing
      (1) Solitary, immobile, fixed lesion
      (2) Skin signs (dimpling, edema, eczema)
      (3) Nipple retraction, discharge, tenderness
      (4) Lesion in upper outer quadrant
2. Invasive tests: findings from needle aspiration, incisional or excisional biopsy that are positive for malignant disease:
   a. Cell histology and cytology—invasive infiltrative ductal or lobular carcinoma or inflammatory breast cancer
   b. Stages I and II local disease to stages III and IV regional to distant metastasis
   c. Enlarged and infiltrated lymph nodes in axillae, infraclavicular, and supraclavicular areas
3. Blood tests:
   a. Elevated alkaline phosphatase—bone and/or liver metastasis
   b. Elevated calcium and decreased phosphorus levels—bone metastasis
   c. Increased carcinoembryonic antigen (CEA)—presence of cancer or evidence of recurrence after initial treatment
   d. Elevated liver enzymes: asparate aminotransferase (AST) (formerly SGOT); alanine aminotransference (ALT) (formerly SGPT); lactic dehydrogenase (LDH)—liver metastasis
4. Positive liver and bone scan findings—liver and bone metastasis
5. Positive results of bone marrow biopsy—marrow involvement in malignant process
6. Chest x-ray film—infiltrates with lung metastasis
7. Positive results of estrogen and progesterone receptor assay tests—positive assay results indicate the tumor will be more responsive to hormonal therapy if required in future

## ♦ NURSING DIAGNOSES

Nursing diagnoses are determined from analysis of patient data. Nursing diagnoses for the patient with breast cancer undergoing mastectomy surgery may include but are not limited to the following:

| Diagnostic Title | Possible Etiologic Factors |
|---|---|
| Conflict decisional: appropriate diagnostic and treatment option | Insufficient knowledge of breast cancer, breast cancer treatment, diagnostic procedures; unknown surgical outcome, future health state; available financial resources |
| Self-esteem disturbance | Loss of breast(s); body-image change; altered role performance; lack of adequate support systems (family/community); misconceptions about possible surgical "mutilation" |
| Coping, ineffective (individual) | Misunderstanding and confusion about personal participation in postoperative care measures; pain, infection, muscle weakness, and immobility (arm/shoulder); sensory changes |
| Grieving, anticipatory | Actual, perceived, or anticipated losses associated with surgical outcome; loss of part or total breast, feelings of anger, depression, and denial; adaptation and rehabilitation concerns |
| Home maintenance management, impaired | Insufficient knowledge or motivation to perform arm/shoulder exercises; wound care; reportable signs and symptoms of complications; prevention strategies to protect affected arm; need for follow-up care; availability and use of support services and groups |

## ♦ EXPECTED PATIENT OUTCOMES

Expected patient outcomes for the patient with breast cancer undergoing mastectomy may include but are not limited to the following:

1. Diagnosis and treatment
   a. Discusses each diagnostic test/procedure as it relates to achieving a definitive diagnosis.
   b. Describes each treatment option, including advantages, disadvantages, and expected long-term outcomes.
   c. Expresses positive feelings about treatment option chosen.
2. Self-esteem
   a. Discusses feelings about loss of a breast and how it will affect her feelings of self-worth and sexuality.
   b. Verbalizes strategies to be used to enhance feelings of self-esteem.

3. Participation
   a. Demonstrates readiness to participate in self-care activities.
   b. Asks pertinent questions about rationale for each care intervention.
   c. Appropriately positions and exercises arm/shoulder to reduce postoperative edema.
   d. Describes correct equipment and procedure for wound care, including care and emptying of drainage device.
   e. Demonstrates skill and understanding of aseptic technique necessary for wound care.
4. Feelings
   a. Freely discusses grief about loss of breast and changes in body image.
   b. Discusses adaptive coping strategies successfully used in past stressful situations.
   c. Identifies community resources and support groups available to assist in adjustment to physical and life-style changes.
5. Home management
   a. Discusses factors that contribute to lymphedema.
   b. Describes activities hazardous to affected arm.
   c. Discusses strategies that will be employed to protect affected arm.
   d. Provides rationale for continued close medical follow-up care.
   e. Describes the available support persons and services within the family and community.
   f. Describes signs and symptoms to report for infection, sensory deficits, and edema.

## ♦ INTERVENTIONS

### Preoperative Management

#### General measures

The nurse provides general preoperative teaching measures in regard to what the patient can expect after surgery. Instruction for the patient undergoing mastectomy and lymph node dissection should cover information that is specific for this procedure. The nurse reviews the expected incision line and the type of dressing, drains, and drainage collection device anticipated. If breast reconstruction is to be performed immediately, the location of the donor tissue is indicated (upper back area or lower abdomen). The use of pictures or diagrams similar to those shown on pp. 1834-1835 will facilitate patient understanding. If an implant is to be used, the nurse clarifies position and placement guidelines. The patient should be informed that movement of the arm and shoulder on the affected side will be limited for the first 24 hours and that the arm and hand will be elevated on a pillow to facilitate lymphatic and venous drainage. Return demonstration of breathing exercises and turning techniques prepare the patient for a greater understanding of and participation in postoperative recovery. (For a more extensive discussion of preoperative patient preparation see Chapter 23.)

#### Resolution of conflict related to treatment decision

The discovery of a breast "lump" elicits one of the most powerful and distressing emotional reactions that a woman of any age can experience. Studies of the diagnostic and presurgical phase of treatment indicate this to be the most stressful period for a woman because of uncertainty of the diagnosis, surgery scheduling problems, inadequate information, and the necessity to make a complex treatment choice in a relatively short time span.[60] Anxiety level has, in fact, been found to be greater during the breast biopsy phase than at the time of the definitive surgical intervention. Nurses caring for patients during this critical time of treatment need to be cognizant of the impact these events have on a woman's normal coping abilities and decision-making processes. The nurse must be ready to provide emotional support in a caring and informative manner.

Once a definitive diagnosis of breast cancer has been established, a complete explanation of treatment options must follow. Most patients come to this situation with some prior knowledge about breast cancer, either from media exposure or through friends or relatives who have had breast cancer. Their knowledge base may be accurate or laden with misconceptions and false information. Because treatment of breast cancer is ever evolving, it is essential for the nurse, in conjunction with the physician, to determine what the patient knows and to provide accurate information so that a more informed treatment choice can be made. Inclusion of family and especially the spouse or partner in all discussions about treatment is vital to a successful outcome.

The physician will discuss the stage of the disease process and the treatment option in detail so that the patient is aware of the advantages and disadvantages of each, as well as the immediate and long-term outcome expectations. The information is often complex and confusing even to the most intelligent and well-informed patient. Women are no longer pressured to select a surgical procedure without knowledge of the final biopsy report. Delay between breast biopsy and definitive treatment provides time in which to consider the options available, review the one that is most personally suitable, and choose the option that permits a feeling of personal control and involvement over a major health decision. The nurse should plan to be present, if possible, when treatment options are presented. This allows assessment of patient and family understanding and time to clarify misinformation and misconceptions.

It is important that the physician and nurse provide unbiased and accurate information on each option. Studies have revealed that the manner in which information is presented can influence the patient's final decision. The option that is presented in a positive manner regarding prognosis in terms of survival rather than in terms of disease recurrence may be chosen over an equally appropriate option. Even when physician treatment preference is not indicated or solicited, the patient may perceive that one exists and make her choice accordingly.[29]

Contrary to past reports, patients who choose mastectomy do so not because they were uninformed about breast conservation surgery but because they may not wish to go through an additional 6 to 7 weeks of radiation therapy. Radiation may be perceived as decreasing quality of life and thus rejected. Mastectomy surgery allows the patient to have definitive surgery, recover, and return more readily to previous activities and lifestyle.

Financial concerns also can influence treatment decisions. The most recent information on the cost of a modified radical mastectomy in the United States, including hospital costs and physician fees, is about $6000.[3] If the patient is covered by health insurance, generally she can be assured that costs for surgery and, especially breast-reconstruction surgery, usually are covered.

Most patients report receiving adequate information to make an informed choice for treatment. Recent studies, however, indicate that 2 months after surgery, recall of specific information and treatment risks is extremely poor.[29] Thus it may be that patients select their treatment on the basis of a combination of previously held opinions and beliefs, as well as on information presented by the health care team during a time of high emotional stress.

**RESEARCH**

Northouse L: A longitudinal study of the adjustment of patients and husbands to breast cancer, *Oncol Nurs Forum* 16(4):511-516, 1989.

Past studies have shown that spouses of cancer patients report more anxiety, depression, distress, and helplessness than do spouses of patients with cardiac disease. Both the patient and spouse experience considerable distress at the time of diagnosis, but little was known regarding the duration of the distress or the time required for adjustment. The purpose of this three-part longitudinal study was to assess the ongoing adjustment to breast cancer by 41 couples at 3 days, 30 days, and 18 months after modified radical mastectomy. Psychosocial adjustment was evaluated by means of three instruments: Affects Balance Scale (mood), Brief Symptom Inventory (psychologic distress), and Psychosocial Adjustment to Illness Scale (role function). The study revealed that, although mood and role function data indicated few significant adjustment problems at 18 months, distress scores for both the patient and spouse were in the mild to severe levels. Data analysis showed that there was no change in the *average* levels of distress across the three assessment times and that the level of distress at 18 months was comparable to levels at 3 days and 30 days after surgery. The study's implications for nursing is that psychosocial adjustment is an ongoing process not confined to the early phase of illness but persisting over time for both patients and their husbands.

### Promoting self-esteem

It has been thought that patients who select breast-conservation surgery are more concerned with their body image and sexual well-being. However, regardless of which surgical option is chosen, psychologic, sexual, and marital concerns are the same for all women. Therefore, during the presurgical phase of treatment, it is essential for the nurse and physician to determine what the impact of breast cancer and total or partial loss of a breast will be on the patient's self-esteem and perceived sexuality. Schover[54] reports that contrary to common belief, most women cope well with surgery and loss of a breast. Other investigators have reported that psychosocial adjustment to breast cancer and surgical treatment continues for many months after initial treatment. Husbands, especially, have been noted to have stress levels at 18 months that equal what they experienced at 3 days and 30 days after surgery. This may be attributable to the fear they have of cancer recurrence and to their spouses' ongoing distress and adjustment problems.[46] See Research box below.

The nurse must assess each patient for indications of potential sexuality concerns and intimate relationship problems in the preoperative time period. Identification of problems and referral for counseling may facilitate a more rapid sexual adjustment and a more positive self-concept. Characteristics of women at highest risk for poor sexual adjustment and self-esteem problems are listed in Box 54-4. Unmarried women also may benefit from sexual counseling or referral to a support group of women similar to themselves. Women older than 65 years of age should not be excluded as having no sexual or self-esteem concerns. They too will benefit from the aforementioned measures.

## Postoperative Management

### General postoperative information

The focus of postoperative care after breast surgery is to provide physical comfort, maintain nutritional support, prevent complications, and prepare the patient for discharge and successful home management. Adequate information must be provided so that the patient has full understanding of each intervention and staff expectations regarding her involvement and cooperation throughout hospitalization.

Pain and discomfort are expected after mastectomy

**BOX 54-4 Women at Risk for Sexual and Self-Esteem Problems Following Loss of Breast**

1. Reported lack of support from a loving spouse or partner
2. Existence of an unhappy, unstable intimate relationship
3. Desire to conceive more children if still in the childbearing years
4. Past sexual problems
5. History of sexual abuse such as rape or incest

From Schover LR: *CA* 41(2):112-120, 1991.

surgery but can be controlled effectively with analgesics and comfort measures. Surgical pain results from the transverse incision that usually extends from the sternum to the axilla. In addition, discomfort may result from either trauma or transection of thoracic and intercostal nerves from fluid collection in the chest wall or at the site of the lymph node dissection. The fluid collection can be a source of infection in both areas, whereas fluid buildup in the axillary area can result in neurovascular complications. Lymphedema is always a concern after mastectomy and lymph node dissection. The lymphatic system (nodes, vessels, and tissue) is a one-way vascular system whose function is the transport of interstitial tissue fluid and plasma protein back to the venous vascular system from which it originated. Lymph depends on gravity, muscle contraction, and arterial pulsations to squeeze it along its channels. The lymphatic system is involved in the removal of foreign substances in the lymph, destruction of bacteria, and production of lymphocytes and antibodies.[41] When lymph nodes are removed, edema can occur in the immediate postoperative period. It usually is a transitory event until collateral lymph channels are formed. When measures are not implemented to increase lymphatic flow, fibrosis can occur within the system and lymphedema becomes an irreversible condition. The chronic collection of fluid and any subsequent injury to the involved extremity can result in infection.[41]

### Promoting comfort/rest/nutrition

Pain relief is managed after mastectomy surgery by the administration of prescribed analgesics and comfort measures. The amount of discomfort experienced varies with the individual patient and her degree of pain tolerance. Most patients are relatively pain-free by the time of discharge, requiring only a mild analgesic to obtain relief of symptoms. Thorough assessment of the patient's pain level and prompt administration of analgesic can not only achieve surgical pain relief but also ensure that the patient has adequate sleep and rest. Maintaining physical comfort also will help diminish the high emotional stress level seen in the immediate postoperative period. Medicating the patient before activities such as turning or getting out of bed for the first time is advisable. Instructing the patient to get out of bed from the unaffected side will lessen pain and tension on the operative site. Providing support to the affected side for the first few days after surgery is necessary because movement of muscles of the affected arm and shoulder is restricted for at least the first 24 hours. The patient should be informed that on initial ambulatory efforts she may feel "out of balance" because of the weight and bulkiness of the dressing. This will lessen after the dressing size is reduced. Temporary use of a sling to the affected arm during early ambulation, if approved by the physician, will provide comfort and support by lessening strain on the shoulder and will prevent the accumulation of dependent lymphatic and venous stasis.

When nerves are cut or traumatized within the operative field, the patient may experience sensory changes such as numbness, tingling, changes in skin sensitivity of the chest wall, and even phantom breast sensations. The patient should be informed that these changes are common and expected outcomes after surgery. The nurse can assure the patient that these nerve-related discomforts gradually will decrease and usually cease within 12 months of surgery.[36]

Nutritional problems usually are minimal. The patient is encouraged to resume her normal eating patterns as soon as possible. A diet high in calories and protein is required for proper wound and tissue repair and for supplying energy needs. Fatigue is a common complaint. Assisting the patient with meals may be necessary in the early postoperative period. Some assistance in bathing also may be required, but the performance of as many activities of daily living during hospitalization is good preparation for meeting these needs after discharge.

### Promoting mobility of the arm and shoulder

One of the priority nursing interventions after mastectomy surgery is to maintain elevation of the affected arm and hand on pillows so that they are higher than the elbow and the elbow is higher than the shoulder. This strategy must be carried out while the patient is in bed or sitting in a chair so that venous and lymphatic pooling will be averted.[21] The nurse monitors for lymphatic and venous stasis by measuring the circumference of the affected arm 6 inches above and below the elbow and comparing results with a preoperative baseline measurement and with the unaffected arm. The affected arm is kept immobile for 24 hours to decrease any strain on the incision line. Hand exercises may then be started, consisting of squeezing on a ball, opening and closing the fist, and flexing and extending the wrist and elbow several times each hour. These exercises help facilitate lymphatic flow. More rigorous full range of motion exercises for the arm and shoulder are initiated at the discretion of the physician, some of which may be delayed 7 to 10 days until the sutures and drains have been removed. Figure 54-11 presents an overview of exercises prescribed after mastectomy surgery (see also Box 54-6).

### Preventing infection

After the initial dressing change by the physician, the nurse performs wound care and dressing changes as needed, noting the condition of the wound and observing for signs of infection (redness, swelling, drainage, odor, increased discomfort, and fever). Maintaining strict asepsis is essential. Infection at the site of fluid collection in the chest wall or at the node dissection site may occur. Proper placement of drains and drainage collection devices usually prevent this postsurgical problem. The nurse assesses the devices (Hemovac, Jackson-Pratt) for placement and for the amount and type of drainage. When the drain and drainage-collection

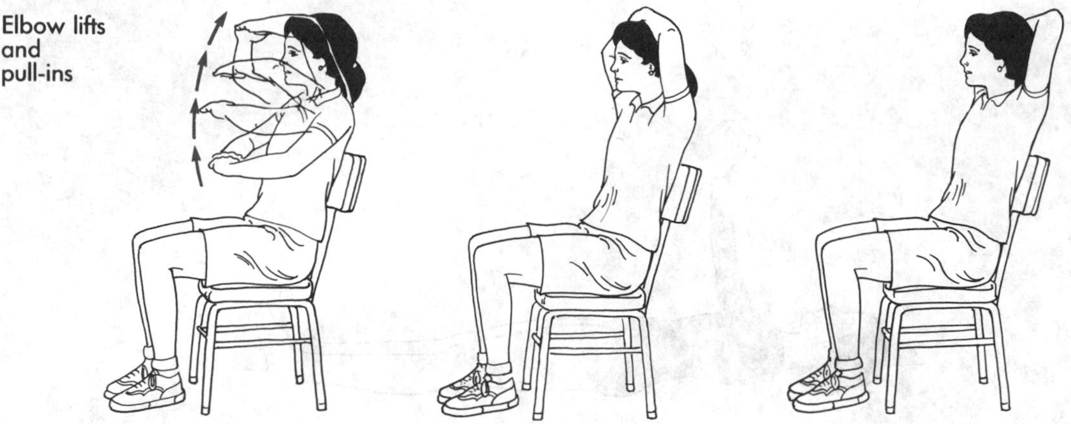


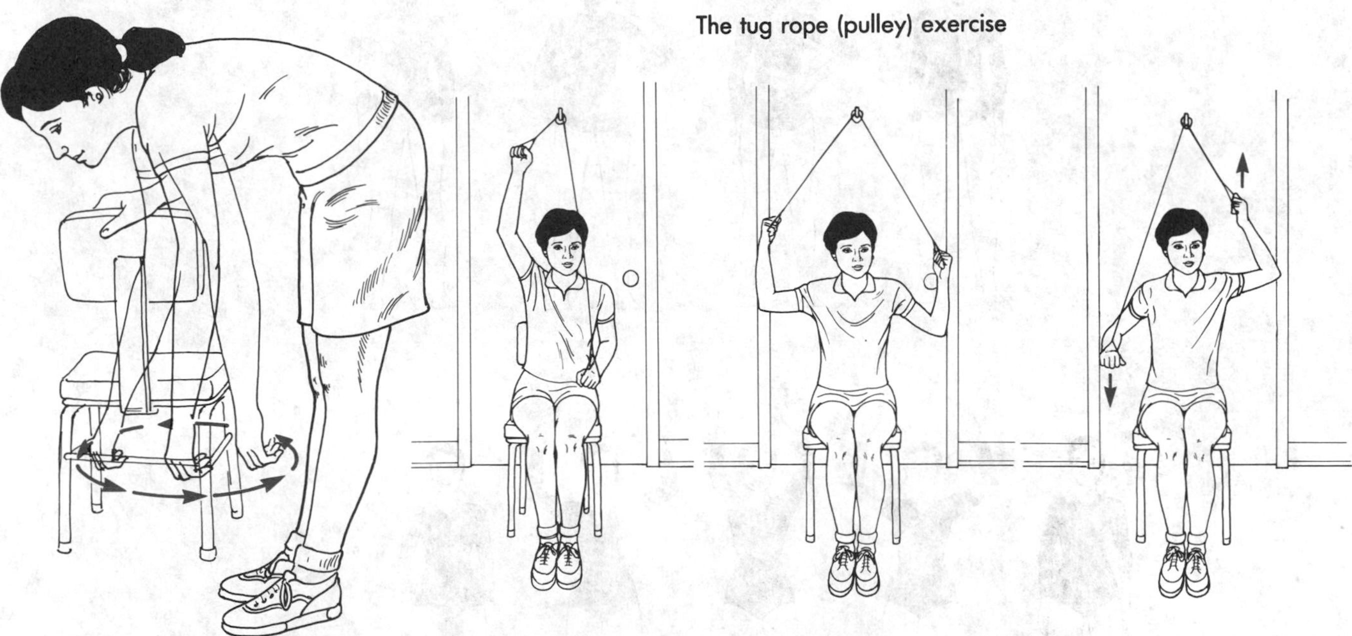


**FIGURE 54-11** Arm and shoulder exercises commonly prescribed for patients after breast cancer surgery. (From *Reach to recovery exercises after mastectomy patient guide,* No 4624-PS, Atlanta, 1983, American Cancer Society.) *Continued.*

device are functioning properly, the amount of fluid around the incision is minimal. The patient should be instructed to avoid touching the dressing and drainage device unnecessarily, unless she is actively involved in the dressing change or measuring output.

**Assisting with the grief and adaptation process**

The loss of a breast can be compared with the emotions engendered by limb amputation. Reactions include anger, depression, denial, and withdrawal. Grieving the lost body part is normal, and the patient should be permitted time to work through her grief. The nurse should offer reassurance that the expression of grief is "OK" behavior, one that is accepted and understood by staff members. It also is important that family members be made aware of the grieving process and encouraged to provide emotional support until feelings have been resolved.

The nurse pays close attention to comments that reflect concerns about body image or self-esteem. The nurse should attempt to have the patient share her concerns before discharge. The spouse or partner should be present if at all possible during these discussions so that his concerns also can be addressed. The patient should be encouraged to look at the incision and become involved in learning how to change the dressing as soon as possible. This is often one of the first steps taken on

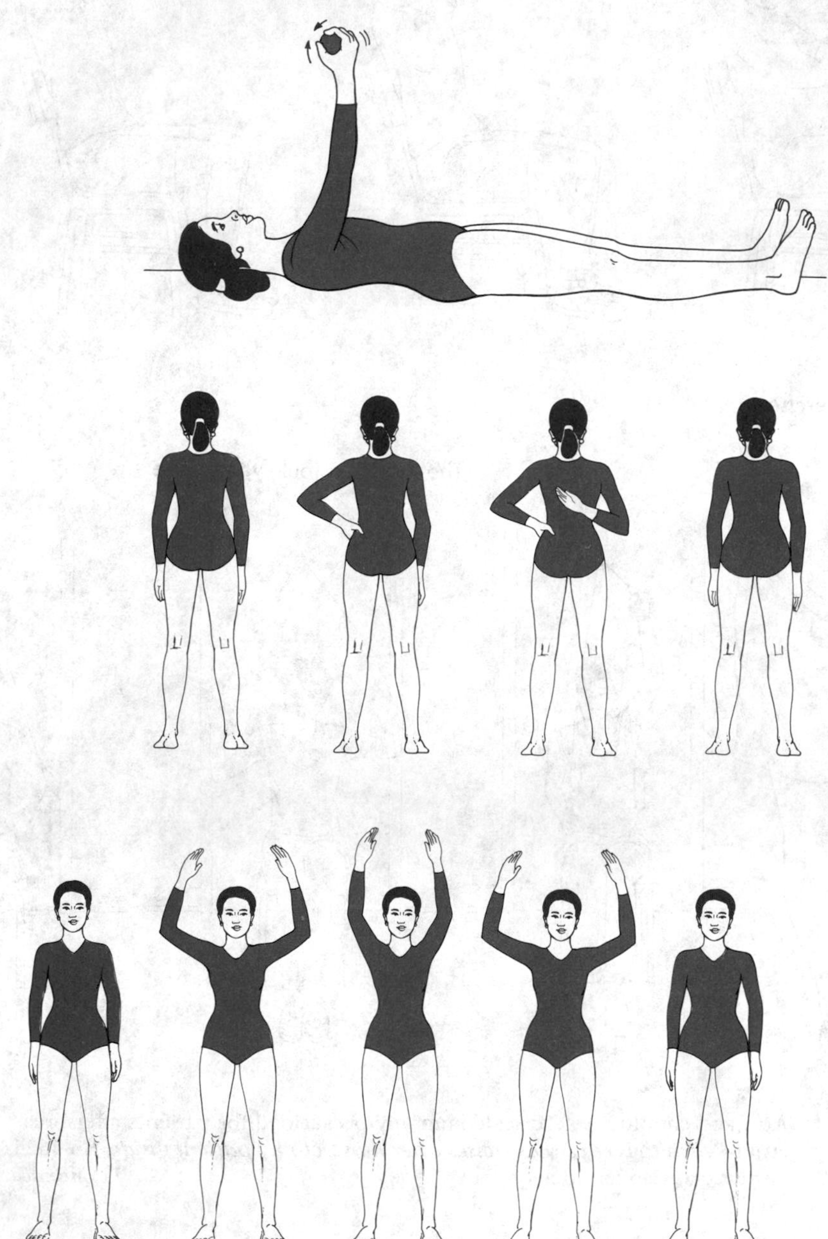

**FIGURE 54-11, cont'd** Arm and shoulder exercises commonly prescribed for patients after breast cancer surgery. (From *Reach to recovery exercises after mastectomy patient guide,* No 4624-PS, Atlanta, 1983, American Cancer Society.)

the road to successful adaptation and full recovery.

Referral to the ACS's Reach to Recovery program provides another means of assisting the patient to work through her grief and anxieties after breast cancer surgery. A Reach to Recovery volunteer is a woman who has had breast cancer and has undergone successful surgery and rehabilitation. These volunteers have personal knowledge of the problems and fears faced by the patient. If possible, the volunteer is matched to the patient by age and type of surgery undergone. The volunteer is able to answer questions about rehabilitation, as well as types of prostheses and brassieres and where these items can be purchased. If the patient has not yet undergone breast-reconstructive surgery, the volunteer will provide the patient with a temporary breast prosthesis and will demonstrate how to use it for the first time. In addition, the volunteer will provide pamphlets that demonstrate the prescribed rehabilitative exercises, as well as a rope and ball used for some of these activities. If breast reconstruction has been performed at the time

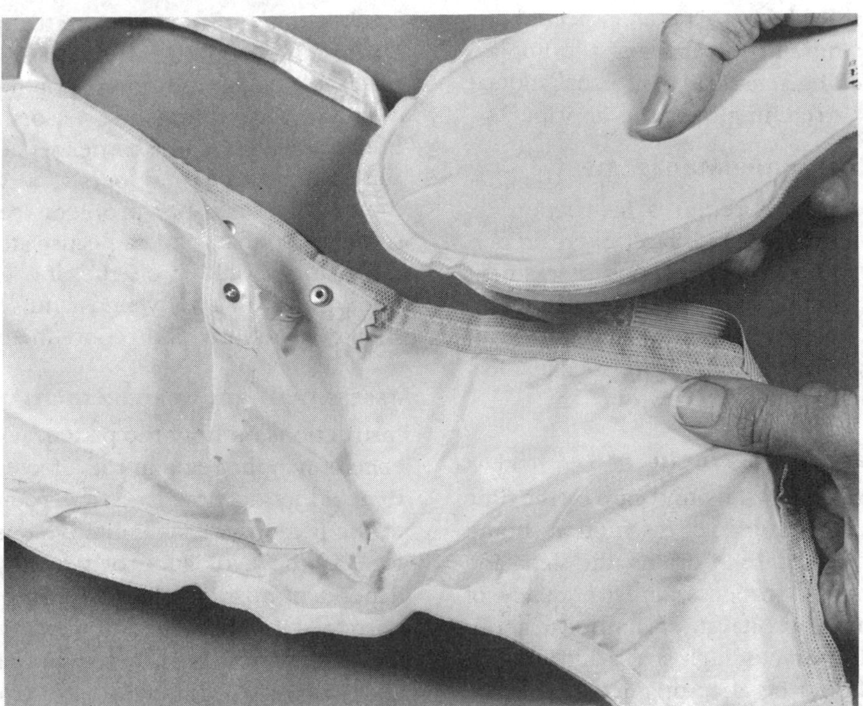

**FIGURE 54-12** Placement of breast prosthesis into brassiere. Inner pocket that will hold padding or breast prosthesis securely can be made in patient's own brassiere. Note snaps that simplify removal of padding.

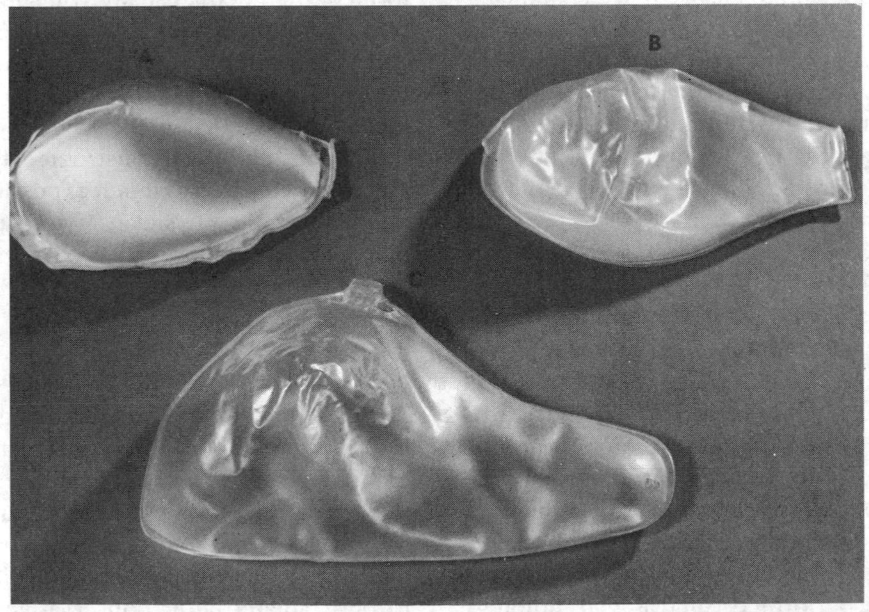


**FIGURE 54-13** Three types of available breast prostheses. **A,** Foam rubber prosthesis. **B,** Prosthesis containing fluid. **C,** Prosthesis containing air.

of mastectomy, the volunteer will be able to address the expected cosmetic outcome and any rehabilitation concerns expressed by the patient. Figure 54-12 shows the placement of a breast prosthesis into a special brassiere or the patient's own brassiere, and Figure 54-13 shows some common types of breast prostheses available.

After breast reconstruction, it is important that the flap used for reconstruction be observed closely for color and capillary refill in the first 2 days after surgery. If reconstruction with use of an implant has been performed, the implant itself may appear higher on the chest wall than the remaining breast and feel quite firm. The patient should be reassured that this is an expected outcome and that softening and lowering of the implant will occur in time. Pulling sensations are usual and are caused by the muscle stretching over the implant.[53]

## Teaching for Effective Home Management

Before discharge, the patient requires instruction regarding the management of wound care, exercise performance and sensory change precautions, assessment and management of lymphedema, and prevention of trauma and infection. Box 54-5 provides an overview of some general discharge instructions. More specific measures are discussed next.

### Teaching wound care management

Having the patient perform total wound care by the time of discharge is a major nursing goal. Instruction should include aseptic technique, care of drains, the signs and symptoms of an infectious process, and frequency of dressing change. Because hospital stay is limited to about 4 days and is generally a time of high stress and anxiety, all verbal teaching should be accompanied by simple, clearly written instructions at the time of discharge. At least one return demonstration of the care will ensure that there is full understanding of the procedure and the skill necessary for correct performance. Dressing change is necessary at least once a day to examine the incision site for signs of infection and to ensure that the drainage is working satisfactorily. The wound should be kept dry inasmuch as an infection is more prone to develop in a warm, moist environment. The patient should be instructed that once the sutures and drains are removed, usually in 7 to 10 days, the physician will indicate that either a continuous sterile dressing is needed or the wound can be left uncovered.

### Instruction for arm/shoulder exercises

At the time of discharge the patient will still have restrictions on the type and amount of exercise permitted to the affected arm and shoulder. Squeezing on a ball and bending and flexing the wrist and elbow of the affected arm should be continued at home. The more rigorous exercises meant to restore full range of motion to the shoulder are delayed until the patient returns to the clinic for suture and drain removal. The physician will then prescribe a gradual increase in the amount and type of exercises to be performed (such as wall climbing, combing hair). Some of the exercises are described in Box 54-6. Performance of these exercises several times daily helps to restore full range of motion to the arm and shoulder, thus preventing a "frozen shoulder" as a result of lack of normal movement. The exercises will, in addition, facilitate the development of collateral lymphatic channels and the prevention of lymphedema.

If the patient has had reconstructive surgery, she should be cautioned to avoid heavy lifting for up to 6 weeks and to wear a brassiere that provides support and normal alignment of the breast. Increasing exercises to reach full range of motion should be done gradually.

When the patient has sensory changes because of transection or trauma to nerves at the time of surgery, some side effects may persist well after discharge. Although most sensory problems resolve within 1 year, some may persist and can cause atrophy of muscles that move the shoulder on the affected side. The patient should be alert to any signs and symptoms of impaired shoulder mobility and report them immediately.

### Assessment and management of lymphedema

Instructions on how the patient will assess for the presence of lymphedema in the affected extremity and how to avoid its occurrence are very important. Adherence to the prescribed rehabilitative exercises is stressed, as well as the avoidance of keeping the extremity in a dependent position for extended periods of time. Compliance with these instructions will help prevent the chronic form of **lymphedema,** which can occur soon after discharge or many months afterward. Some edema may be present at discharge, especially if lymph node dissection was performed at the time of surgery. The greater the number of nodes removed at surgery, the greater the chance of some edema being present. As the wound heals and the prescribed exercises are performed, the edema usually will subside. Demonstration of the proper technique to measure arm circumference and a method to record arm measurements will enable the patient to quickly recognize the presence of a problem and report it immediately. When edema is present, the patient should be instructed to keep the affected extremity elevated as much as possible. If edema persists or increases, the physician should be notified. Treatment may include the application of an elastic bandage to the entire extremity, as well as continued elevation and range of motion exercises.

### Strategies to prevent trauma and infection

The patient who has had breast surgery involving a level II or III lymph node dissection must be vigilant in avoiding trauma and infection to the affected arm. Protecting the arm and hand is essential because lymphatic circulation has been compromised by the removal of nodes from the axillary lymph node chain. When the axilla is to be irradiated after conservative surgery, damage to the cells within the nodes can occur, which interferes with their normal function of removing foreign substances and destroying bacteria. Thus infectious agents can easily enter the compromised lymphatic system from the trauma of cuts, scratches, or burns. Special instructions to avoid these complications are listed in Box 54-7. It is important that the patient understand the rationale for these precautions and comply completely because she will be at risk for the rest of her life.

## BOX 54-5 Patient Discharge Instructions After Breast Cancer Surgery

### DRESSINGS

**Incision**

There will be a dry gauze dressing over the incision when you leave the hospital. It is not necessary to change this dressing until you return to see the doctor.

**Drain Site**

A small dry dressing will be around the site where the drain is placed. Often there is some leakage of fluid around the drain. Check the gauze dressing for drainage and change if soiled. Some leakage is normal, but if the dressing becomes soaked more than once a day, call your doctor.

**Drains**

Your nurse has shown you how to empty the reservoir from your drain and how to measure the volume of drainage. You should empty the drain twice a day and record the measurements.

Drains are generally removed when drainage is about 30 ml in 24 hr.

Drains are often removed at the same time as the stitches, generally 7 to 10 days after surgery.

### BATHING

Sponge baths or tub baths, making certain that the area of the drain and incision stay dry, are permitted. You may shower after the stitches and drains are removed.

### HAND AND ARM CARE

You can begin using your arm for normal activities such as eating or combing your hair. Exercises involving the wrist, hand, and elbow such as flexing your fingers, circular wrist motions, and touching hand to shoulder are very good. More strenuous exercises can usually be resumed after the drains have been removed.

### COMFORT

Some discomfort or mild pain is expected following surgery, but within 4 to 5 days, most women have no need for medication or require something only at bedtime.

Numbness in the area of the surgery and along the inner side of the arm from the armpit to the elbow occurs in virtually all patients. It is a result of injury to the nerves that provide sensation to the skin in those areas. Women have described sensations such as heaviness, pain, tingling, burning, and "pins and needles." These sensations change over the months and usually resolve by 1 year.

### SUPPORT AND INFORMATION

Pamphlets on exercises, hand and arm care, and general facts about breast cancer are available from your nurse or volunteer visitor. The American Cancer Society has volunteers who have had surgery similar to yours and are available to visit you.

---

**From Knobf MT. In Baird SB: *Cancer nursing: a comprehensive textbook*, Philadelphia, 1991, WB Saunders.**

## BOX 54-6 Postmastectomy Arm Exercises

### EXERCISE: BALL SQUEEZING

1. Lying in bed, hold a rubber ball in your hand.
2. Lift arm straight up and alternately squeeze and relax the ball.
3. Do this exercise as often as recommended by your physician.
4. If it is uncomfortable to hold arm straight up, support it using several pillows.

### PULLEY MOTION

1. Toss the rope over the top of the door with unaffected arm.
2. Sit with legs hugging both sides of the door closely, and keep soles firmly planted on the floor.
3. Hold the ends of the rope in each hand with knots between third and fourth fingers.
4. Slowly raise affected arm as far as comfortable by pulling down on the rope with unaffected arm; the raised arm close to your head. Reverse the motion to raise unaffected arm by lowering affected arm. Rest and repeat.

### HAND WALL CLIMBING

1. Start in standard position, with toes 6 to 12 inches from and facing wall.
2. Bend elbows and place palms against the wall at shoulder level.
3. Work both hands up the wall parallel to each other until incisional pulling or pain occurs. Mark spot so progress can be checked.
4. Work hands down to shoulder level. Move feet and body closer to wall as comfort allows and reach requires.
5. Return to standard position. Rest and repeat.

### BACK SCRATCHER

1. Start in standard position.
2. Place hand of unoperated side on hip for balance.
3. Bend elbow of arm on operated side, placing back of hand on small of your back. Gradually work hand up your back until fingers reach the opposite shoulder blade.
4. Slowly lower arm and return to standard position. Rest and repeat.

### ELBOW PULL-IN

1. Stand in standard position.
2. Extend arms sideways to shoulder level.
3. Bend elbows, clasping fingers at back of neck.
4. Pull elbows in toward each other until they touch.
5. Return to position 3, with elbows bent and fingers clasped at back of neck.
6. Unclasp fingers and extend arms sideways at shoulder level.
7. Return to standard position. Rest and repeat.

---

**From *Reach to recovery, excercises after mastectomy patient guide*, No 4624-PS, Atlanta, 1983, American Cancer Society.**

**BOX 54-7 Precautions for the Person After Mastectomy**

Ensure that the affected arm is never used for blood pressure, injections, or venipunctures.
Wear no constricting clothing or jewelry, including wrist watch, on affected arm.
Do not carry heavy objects (pocketbook, packages) in affected arm.
Wear rubber gloves when washing dishes.
Use unaffected arm when removing items from hot oven, or protect by wearing a padded glove pot holder.
Use a thimble when sewing; wash needle pricks and cover as necessary.
Take care when trimming finger nails and cuticles; avoid using scissors.
Use softening lotions or creams to keep skin in soft, supple condition.
Outdoor activities:

- Wear gloves when gardening.
- Avoid sunburn—wear protective clothing or use sunscreen liberally.
- Use insect repellent when in an area where biting or stinging insects may be located.
- Tend to cuts and scratches immediately by washing and applying protective covering.

## ♦ EVALUATION

To evaluate the effectiveness of nursing interventions, compare patient behaviors with those stated in the expected outcomes. Successful achievement of patient outcomes for the patient undergoing mastectomy for breast cancer is indicated by the following:

1. Diagnosis and treatment
   a. Reports understanding of diagnostic tests and procedures.
   b. Reports understanding of rationale for available treatment options.
   c. States "I want to be sure they get it all; I believe I have the best chance with mastectomy and lymph node dissection. I'll have breast reconstruction in a few months."
2. Self-esteem
   a. Shares feelings about loss of breast with husband or partner.
   b. States "I'm sure I can live without a breast. I have lots of family support."
3. Participation
   a. Performs self-care with a minimum of assistance on the second postoperative day.
   b. Keeps affected arm elevated on pillows when in bed or sitting up in chair.
   c. Asks for written instructions for wound care procedure and handling of drainage-collection device.
   d. Is able to identify signs and symptoms for infection.
4. Feelings
   a. Welcomes the meeting with the Reach to Recovery volunteer and reads pamphlets on breast reconstruction and use of temporary breast prosthesis.
   b. Lists names of local department stores that sell breast prostheses.
   c. Discusses with husband the information and support offered by Reach to Recovery volunteer.
5. Home management
   a. States she will be more careful when gardening by "wearing gloves and a long sleeve shirt."
   b. Describes why venipunctures and blood pressure readings cannot be taken on the arm with the "node dissection."
   c. Describes feelings of phantom breast pain, numbness and tingling, and decreased sensitivity at the mastectomy site as signs of nerve deficits.
   d. States a commitment to performing monthly BSE and having a yearly mammogram.
   e. Describes rehabilitation exercises she will perform after the sutures and drains are removed.

## ✸ SPECIAL CONSIDERATIONS FOR CARE OF THE GERONTOLOGIC PATIENT

A comprehensive review of cancer and elders is beyond the scope of this discussion. However, a few pertinent facts related to breast cancer and the elderly woman are relevant. Nearly one half of all breast cancer cases occur in women older than 65 years of age. Advanced-stage breast cancer is more often detected in elderly women than in their younger counterparts. One reason for this unfortunate occurrence may be that elderly women tend to receive less instruction on BSE technique and less encouragement to perform it on a regular schedule. Many older women are reluctant to touch and examine their breasts even with appropriate teaching. In addition, the elderly woman may not be aware of her increased vulnerability to cancer, especially breast cancer, nor know the suspicious signs and symptoms she should report to her physician.

Among the many bodily changes that occur with the aging process, changes in vision (accommodation), cataracts, and glaucoma can prevent the detection of breast tissue changes. Women with arthritis may not be able to perform BSE and may discontinue the practice altogether. Changes occurring in the breast as a result of aging—such as fibrosis, calcification, shrinkage, and loss of subcutaneous fat—may cause confusion regarding what is normal for aging and which changes may indicate a possible malignant condition. Diminished hearing acuity with age may result in the elderly woman following inaccurate information because of misunderstanding what was said or not requesting clarification because of embarrassment.

Other factors that affect early diagnosis of cancer and successful treatment may be related to the socioeconomic status of elders. Retirement with reduced financial resources and the lack of health insurance beyond Medicare/Medicaid may deter elderly women from seeking medical care for a breast lump or other suspicious signs and symptoms of breast cancer. Financial concerns about ability to pay for long-term chemotherapy or radiation therapy may cause elders to terminate treatment. Becoming a burden, both physically and financially, on their significant others is always of great concern to the elderly patient with cancer.

Another distressing situation that has occurred, more in the past than at present, is in the area of treatment options offered to the elderly woman with breast cancer. Mastectomy, rather than the conservative surgical lumpectomy procedure, was the only surgical treatment advised for elderly women, even those with early, localized disease and negative nodes. Although elders take longer to recover from surgery and often encounter more side effects and complications of therapy, age should never be a factor that determines whether they receive the best possible treatment available.

The elderly population (older than 65) is increasing in numbers each year; makes up the majority of hospital admissions; and is the age-group with more chronic illnesses, cancer being one of them. Nurses will be working with this age-group throughout their career and will, therefore, need to be more informed about the normal aging process, be able to perform a more thorough physical and psychosocial assessment examination, and know how to detect abnormal change indicative of cancer. The nurse must encourage the elderly woman to participate in cancer screening and detection programs, have a yearly mammogram, and perform monthly BSE. The nurse should also act as a patient advocate when treatment options are being presented and advised.

## ❦ HOME CARE CONSIDERATIONS

Patients who require further therapeutic medical management after mastectomy should be provided with information about what the therapy will be, when it will begin, and why it is necessary to keep all follow-up appointments. Unfortunately, no assurances can be made that breast cancer will never recur or that malignant disease will never develop in the remaining breast. The nurse should determine the patient's knowledge and skill level in the performance of BSE. If necessary the proper procedure should be demonstrated and a pamphlet on BSE provided. Because breast cancer has a tendency to recur at the incision line, the nurse instructs the patient on how to assess this area. Follow-up mammograms are prescribed as an integral part of long-term care. The necessity and rationale for these examinations cannot be overstressed.

The ACS is an important resource for all cancer patients undergoing rehabilitation. Reach to Recovery volunteers are always available to meet with patients after discharge to answer questions and concerns. Some will make home visits, accompany the patient in purchasing a permanent prosthesis and brassiere, and talk about breast-reconstruction issues. Other ACS volunteer groups, such as I Can Cope, are helpful for persons who have gone through a cancer experience and are successfully coping with life after cancer. Family members of a patient with cancer frequently find needed support from this group as well.

## COMPLICATIONS

The woman who has undergone treatment for breast cancer will always live with the fear of *recurrent disease* even when the cancer was found and treated in an early, localized stage. In some women recurrent disease will develop within months of initial treatment or many years later. It is important that all women, regardless of age or stage of disease, be constantly reminded to report the presence of symptoms such as bone pain or changes at the incision site, which could be indications of disease recurrence or the presence of distant metastasis.

A *chronic form of lymphedema* may occur at any time after breast surgery, especially when large numbers of lymph nodes were removed. These women must always be on guard for signs of increasing edema. When the affected arm circumference exceeds the unaffected arm by 10% or more, the beginning of the irreversible and chronic form of the condition may have occurred. This is a serious problem that may require hospitalization and the use of a compression sleeve with intermittent pressure to force the edema fluid along. These sleeves permit a uniform circumferential progression of the fluids that cannot be achieved with an elastic wrap. Antibiotics, salt and fluid restrictions, and in some cases, diuretic therapy have been used to treat chronic lymphedema.

The threat of *trauma and infection* after mastectomy and node dissection is ever present and requires that the woman always comply with the aforementioned precautions. If signs and symptoms of trauma or infection occur, the woman should be advised to inform her physician immediately so that appropriate measures can be instituted.

# NONMALIGNANT CONDITIONS OF THE BREAST

## CYSTIC BREAST DISEASE

The presence of benign breast disease is common and accounts for about 90% of all breast problems. Because there is no universally accepted classification system for benign disorders, the term *fibrocystic disease* has been used as an umbrella category into which most benign disorders are placed. This has resulted in confusion in diagnosing and treating benign conditions.[52] A more acceptable classification system may be one that is based on symptoms and clinical findings. Terms such as *benign mastopathy, chronic cystic mastitis, mammary dysplasia, epithelial* and *fibrocystic mastopathy* have been used to diagnose cystic breast disease.[49]

### Etiology/Epidemiology

The underlying cause of cystic breast disease is not fully known at this time. Changes in the breast are cyclic and thought to be caused by hormonal imbalance or the exaggerated response of breast tissue to ovarian hormones. Breast tenderness is more painful during or before menstruation. Cystic breast disease is most common in nulliparous women between the ages of 40 and 50 years but can occur at any age. Occurrence is least frequent after menopause.

### Pathophysiology

A number of commonalities are seen in cystic disease regardless of the diagnostic name used. Changes once thought to be abnormal such as microcysts, apocrine change, adenosis, fibrosis, and varying degrees of hyperplasia are now recognized to be a part of the involutional process of the breast.[17] These changes include the presence of lumps of varying size, nipple discharge, and breast pain (mastodynia). Cystic lesions are soft, well demarcated, and freely movable. The process is almost always bilateral, with most lesions located in the left breast. The cysts may contain clear, milky, straw-colored, or yellow to dark brown fluid. Occasionally the contents may be blood-tinged.

### Medical Management

The woman who discovers a mass or masses in her breast should seek the advice of a physician, who will decide whether aspiration or biopsy should be considered. A needle aspiration generally confirms the presence of a cyst. Only blood-stained fluid should be sent for cytologic examination.[17] Because the presence of nodular tissue in the breast makes the early detection of malignant lesions more difficult, some physicians suggest periodic mammograms to detect any changes. There is no evidence to suggest that cystic disease predisposes the woman to the development of a malignant lesion, but these women are at more risk than those without cystic disease. (See Table 54-3 for a comparison of signs and symptoms of benign and malignant breast tumors.)

Methylxanthines, a class of chemicals found in coffee, tea, cola, and chocolate, have been excluded from the diet as a means of controlling cystic disease. Although some women have been treated successfully with this approach, there has been no widespread beneficial response for all women. At present it has not been proved that methylxanthines cause benign or malignant breast disease.[22] Vitamin therapy, especially vitamin E, may have some anticancer properties, but again, no conclusive evidence is available that it can reduce the risk of cancer or relieve the distress of cystic breast disease. The drug danazol, an attenuated androgen, has some demonstrated therapeutic properties that have decreased breast pain, feelings of heaviness, and tenderness in patients with cystic disease.[22] Studies of tamoxifen are ongoing. Some women with cystic disease have reported results that range from some regression of lesions to the complete disappearance of breast pain with its use. The appropriateness of tamoxifen for cystic breast disease will be determined more fully by data gleaned from current clinical investigations.

### Nursing Management

Hospitalization is seldom required in the treatment of cystic breast disease. The nurse should teach BSE to those women who are not familiar with it and stress its use every month. Women should be taught to recognize through touch their normal breast tissue and the location and size of lesions present. They should report significant changes that differ from the normal cyclic fluctuations or that appear at a different time in the menstrual cycle. The use of a mild analgesic and wearing a firm supportive brassiere may provide comfort and reduce pain on movement. The use of warm, moist heat also may be beneficial to relieve aching pain. Eliminating caffeine consumption and decreasing salt content before menstruation to relieve bloating and weight gain can be recommended to women willing to try dietary means of gaining relief from symptoms. The woman should be advised to consult her physician before attempting vitamin E as a therapeutic intervention. Although side effects are few, it is best to have the physician prescribe therapy so that the beneficial effects, if any, can be monitored.

## FIBROADENOMA

### Etiology/Epidemiology

**Fibroadenoma,** or adenofibromas, are the most common benign breast neoplasm. Approximately 10% to 25% of women have one or more of these tumors.[49] The tumors occur most often in women younger than 25 years of age; some become evident by age 15. Fibroadenomas usually are firm, rubbery, round, freely movable, nontender, and encapsulated; they may be multiple and bilateral. Tumor size ranges from 1 to 3 cm. A "giant" fibroma is the most common lesion seen in the adolescent breast.

### Pathophysiology

Fibroadenomas are tumors of fibroblastic and epithelial origin thought to be caused by hyperestrinism. They are estrogen-dependent and associated with menstrual irregularities.[49] Tumors are slow growing and often are stimulated by pregnancy and lactation. Regression may occur after delivery. Fibroadenomas tend to regress at menopause and become hyalinized. "Giant" fibroadenomas grow very rapidly to 10 to 12 cm in diameter but are not more prone to malignant change.

### Medical Management

Standard treatment for fibroadenomas is surgical removal. Some are amenable to removal with only local anesthesia in an outpatient setting. Although the tumor is examined for definitive pathologic characteristics, the association between fibroadenomas and cancer is very weak.

### Nursing Management

When the woman discovers a breast mass, her primary concern is always a diagnosis of cancer. Reassurance that most breast lesions are not malignant should be avoided. Only the final pathology report will provide this reassurance. Before the surgical removal of the fibroadenoma, the nurse prepares the woman for the type of surgery to be performed, what to expect during the procedure, and how to care for the incision afterward. Practice of BSE should be encouraged, as well as the reporting of any unusual changes found during the examination.

## INFLAMMATORY LESIONS

### Mammary Duct Ectasia

#### Etiology/Epidemiology

**Mammary duct ectasia,** also referred to as *plasma cell mastitis,* is a benign condition of unknown etiology. Some investigators believe an anaerobic bacteria may be implicated. Another causative factor may be bacterial infection that results from stasis of fluid in the large ducts of the breast. The primary risk factor for development of duct ectasia is age, with a mean ranging from 45 to 55 years of age. Breast pain and a palpable mass are typical symptoms in premenopausal women; nipple discharge predominates in perimenopausal women; and nipple retractions secondary to periductal fibrosis are more often noted in postmenopausal women.

#### Pathophysiology

Mammary duct ectasia involves inflammation of the ducts behind the nipple, duct enlargement, and a collection of cellular debris and fluid in the involved ducts. As the inflammatory response resolves, the ducts become fibrotic and dilated. Nipple discharge usually is bilateral and ranges from serous to thick, sticky, or pastelike. Drainage may be green, greenish brown, or blood-stained. Nipple itching, suggestive of Paget's disease, may accompany transient pain in the subareolar and inner quadrant areas of the breast. On palpation, the areolar area may feel wormlike; the nipple may be red and swollen or flat and retracted.

#### Medical management

Treatment plans vary depending on the severity of the problem. Because of the chronic nature of this problem, most women are periodically followed up with routine physical examination of the breast. The symptoms of mammary duct ectasia may engender the fear of malignant disease in the patient. Once the benign nature of this chronic condition is affirmed, fears generally are dispelled and most women are able to deal with their symptoms.[14] Although there is no cure for mammary duct ectasia, antibiotics are prescribed in the event of acute inflammatory episodes, such as the development of an abscess. When the chronic discharge can no longer be tolerated, surgical excision of the retroareolar ducts is the treatment of choice. This therapy corrects the nipple retraction; however, reduced nipple sensation may be an outcome.[14]

#### Nursing management

The nurse must be cognizant of the chronic yet benign nature of this condition and offer support and understanding care. The woman should be taught how to cleanse the breast to minimize the risk of infection. Teaching good handwashing technique and personal hygiene measures is stressed. Suggestions on wearing a supportive yet nonconfining brassiere padded with sterile gauze and changing the bra daily or as necessary will help to prevent abscess formation. Signs and symptoms indicative of abscess should be provided, and the woman is taught to report them immediately.

### Acute Mastitis and Abscess

#### Etiology/Epidemiology

There are two forms of **mastitis:** acute and chronic. The *acute* form is a rare condition almost always found in breast-feeding mothers during the first 4 months of lactation.[30] It occurs most frequently from *Staphylococcus aureus* or *S. epidermidis* infection that spreads from a break in the skin surface of the nipple to underlying breast tissue. It may be confined to only one quadrant of the breast. Symptoms include a fissured nipple, fever, localized tenderness, and erythema. Purulent discharge may be present.

The *chronic* form of mastitis can follow acute mastitis or have a slow and insidious onset. Both acute and chronic mastitis are caused by the same bacterial agents. The chronic form occurs more often in older women, and the symptoms can mimic inflammatory breast cancer. The infection usually arises in the sweat or sebaceous glands and spreads to the breast. Symptoms of chronic mastitis include a painful breast mass that involves the nipple and areola and that causes a low-grade fever.

#### Pathophysiology

In both acute and chronic mastitis there are edema and congestion of the periductal and interlobular stromata.

The ducts are distended from the accumulation of neutrophils and retained secretions. If an abscess forms, its central core may be necrotic and contain creamy, yellow exudate. Fibrosis of the involved tissue can develop after treatment. Both acute and chronic forms of mastitis can mimic inflammatory breast carcinoma, but recent lactation usually excludes the acute form and the need for further evaluation. Fibrosis of the involved tissue can develop after treatment.[49]

#### Medical management

Acute mastitis is easy to diagnose in a nursing mother after pregnancy. Treatment with antibiotics will resolve the infectious process. In older women, because the condition has similarities to inflammatory breast carcinoma, aspiration of the inflammatory exudate should be performed to determine the cause. Antibiotics can then be prescribed.

#### Nursing management

When acute mastitis is the result of an infection during lactation, most women will immediately stop breast-feeding. Women should be informed that discontinuing breast-feeding is not always necessary or advisable. It is believed that continued breast-feeding reduces the pain and lessens the volume of milk that can be a source for bacterial growth. If breast-feeding is discontinued, however, the woman should be instructed to keep her breasts as empty as possible by pumping. If the breast is not emptied, it will become engorged and pain will increase. Instruction on antibiotic therapy includes stressing that the total prescribed dose must be completed—7, 10, or 14 days—and not discontinued when symptoms seem to be relieved. Because the infection in this type of mastitis generally does not originate in the breast, teaching about personal hygiene measures is important. The older woman with mastitis may be anxious about a diagnosis of carcinoma. Emotional support and frank discussion and answers to her questions should be offered until the aspiration biopsy results are known.

Both acute and chronic mastitis will resolve with antibiotic therapy, rest, and application of local heat to the involved breast.[30] Discomfort generally is relieved by analgesics.

# MALE BREAST PROBLEMS

## GYNECOMASTIA

### Etiology/Epidemiology

**Gynecomastitis** is a common disorder of the male breast. It is estimated that this condition develops in up to 70% of pubertal boys during the time of rapid testicular growth, between the ages of 12 to 15 years. Symptoms include a firm, circular, disklike, circumscribed, tender mass beneath the areola, usually bilateral at onset. In adolescent boys the condition is transient and lasts for approximately 12 to 24 months. A second-occurrence period of gynecomastia is seen in men aged 45 years and older, with 40% of elderly men having some degree of the condition.[8] Gynecomastia is seen in obese men because obesity increases the rate of conversion of androgens to estrogen. It also occurs commonly in patients with cirrhosis of the liver, a condition in which there is incomplete hepatic clearance of estrogen. Gynecomastia also develops in men who are receiving estrogen for treatment of prostate cancer.

### Pathophysiology

Gynecomastia is caused by hormonal imbalance. As a result of the large estrogen secretion, hyperplasia (overdevelopment) of the stromata and ducts in the mammary glands occurs. The primary cause of gynecomastia in the older man is the aging process. As men age, the plasma testosterone concentration declines at the same time that the plasma testosterone-estrogen level increases. Thus less free testosterone is available.

### Medical Management

When gynecomastia occurs and the condition cannot be attributed to rapid testicular growth (teen-age boys), to treatment with estrogen therapy (middle-aged men), or to hepatic dysfunction, a human chorionic gonadotropin–beta subunit (HCG-β) level should be obtained. This finding assists in ruling out a malignant testicular germ cell condition, which can manifest with gynecomastia and an elevated HCG-β level. Chest and mediastinal roentgenograms, as well as a careful testes examination, also should be included in the evaluation. In older men the physician may suggest obtaining a breast biopsy specimen because this age-group is more prone to male breast cancer.

### Nursing Management

The nurse who cares for men with gynecomastia must offer sympathetic understanding. Most men are intensely anxious about the condition, a tension that is little reduced by the information that the condition is benign. Enlarged breasts constitute serious assault on the male self-image. The freedom to be "topless" in the sun, at home, in construction work, and in recreational activities makes the developing and existent condition visible and joke-provoking. Similarly the man with breast cancer (unrelated to the dysplasia) who undergoes primary surgical therapy has a publicly visible mastectomy, and the asymmetry is apparent. The problems and needs of this patient still have not been fully recognized.

Patients who will be treated with hormonal therapy for prostate cancer should be warned that one of the side effects of treatment is gynecomastia. Treatment of this malignant condition usually takes priority over breast enlargement, but it may still constitute a psychologic stress the man will need to deal with. Elderly men should be informed that with normal aging, breast enlargement may occur. If the man is obese and elderly, the enlargement may be more pronounced. The nurse should be aware that a variety of drugs, other than hormones, can increase male breast size. These include digitalis, thiazides, and spironolactone. Men should be forewarned of this side effect.

## MALE BREAST CANCER

### Etiology/Epidemiology

The incidence of breast cancer in men is relatively uncommon, accounting for approximately 1% (1000) of the 183,000 new cases of breast cancer that were predicted for 1993.[10] The presentation, use of diagnostic measures, and response to treatment are similar to those factors for women with the disease.

The epidemiologic characteristics of male breast cancer reveal an incidence rate that increases with age, usually occurring 5 to 10 years later than breast cancer found in women. The average age at the time of diagnosis is 60 to 66 years of age.[35] A family history places men at increased risk for breast cancer.

### Pathophysiology

Approximately 80% of breast cancers in men are estrogen receptor positive, with ductal infiltrating carcinoma being the predominant histologic cell type.[18] Bioassay for the presence of estrogen and progesterone receptors is performed at the time of biopsy. Tumor staging is based on the primary tumor, regional nodes, and metastasis (TNM) system.

Physical examination, mammography, fine-needle aspiration, and incisional or excisional biopsy are standard diagnostic procedures. The presence of advanced disease at the time of initial diagnosis is common, largely a result of delays in seeking medical evaluation that average 10 to 18 months.[18] Gynecomastia caused by drug, alcohol, or hormone ingestion can be differentiated from a malignant lesion by both physical examination and mammogram. Gynecomastia generally is bilateral, whereas a malignant lesion generally occurs in a single breast.

The symptoms commonly seen at the time of diagnosis involve a firm mass directly beneath the nipple in the subareolar area, most frequently in the left breast. A lesion in the upper outer quadrant is the next most frequent location for tumor growth. Bloody nipple discharge with nipple inversion is common. Evidence of Paget's disease of the nipple (eczema), itching, ulceration, and local tenderness also may be seen at diagnosis. Some reports indicate that axillary nodes are positive for disease in about 55% of cases.[35] As is seen in women with breast cancer, metastasis may occur in bone, the lungs, and the liver.[18]

### Medical Management

Treatment for a primary localized tumor is modified radical mastectomy with node dissection. Breast-conservation procedures are not often used because men do not appear to have the psychologic need for this body image–sparing procedure. In addition, the typical location of the lesion in the subareolar area requires that the nipple be removed along with a tumor-free margin of tissue. Thus breast-preservation procedures cannot be safely employed. Radiation therapy may be prescribed before or after surgery for control of micrometastasis or to prevent local recurrence, but radiation has no value in increasing long-term disease-free survival time.[18] When axillary nodes are involved in the disease process, systemic adjuvant therapy (chemotherapy or hormonal) is advised.

Recurrent or advanced disease is highly amenable to palliative therapy with hormonal manipulation inasmuch as most tumors are ER+. In the past orchiectomy or adrenalectomy followed by hypophysectomy was used to eliminate the source of estrogen in the body. Today the antiestrogen drug tamoxifen is the treatment of choice because it eliminates the need for surgical intervention. Chemotherapy in the treatment of male breast cancer does not have a long history of use. Protocols such as cyclophosphamide, methotrexate, and 5-fluorouracil (CMF) and 5-fluorouracil, Adriamycin (doxorubicin), and cyclophosphamine (FAC) may be prescribed. Chemotherapy has the advantage of shorter treatment cycles, lower cost than the long-term use of hormone therapy, and effectiveness against ER+ tumors. Chemotherapy, however, is less well tolerated, has more physically disabling side effects, and does not have a history of long-term responses. Therefore hormone therapy appears to be the more accepted treatment at present. Antiandrogenic drugs such as flutamide and cyproterone acetate (CPA) are under investigation for their usefulness in treating male breast cancer.[18]

### Nursing Management

The nursing management of male breast cancer reflects the basic principles outlined beginning on p. 1836. However, a man diagnosed with breast cancer faces unique psychosocial stressors that the nurse needs to address on an individual basis. The long delays in diagnosis may reflect in part a basic disbelief that this "female problem" can be occurring. A subtheme of embarrassment needs to be identified, if present, and acknowledged. The threats of cancer remain present, however, and the treatment is aggressive. The use of tamoxifen has reduced the need for palliative surgeries such as orchiectomy, with their accompanying assault on male self-concept and body image. The male patient treated for breast cancer will not be a common challenge, but the nurse will need to be sensitive to his unique needs and tailor the standard surgical care routines to the individual situation.

## QUESTIONS TO CONSIDER

- How would you help a woman who has a high risk for breast cancer—specifically in alleviating her anxiety and helping her understand the significance of a regular breast examination?
- What approaches might you consider for a woman who has great difficulty accepting her diagnosis of cancer?
- How would you respond when a woman tells you, "Most of our sex life has centered on my breasts. What am I going to do now that I will need a mastectomy?"
- When do you consult home care agencies to help a woman and her family live with her diagnosis of breast cancer?
- How do you care for a woman who is fatigued and weak from weekly chemotherapy treatments and ready to quit when therapy includes 6 more months of treatment?

## CRITICAL THINKING ACTIVITIES

- Given that mammography is able to detect 1-centimeter lesions and that recent research suggests breast self-examinations are not significantly correlated to stage of disease at the time of diagnosis, provide a convincing argument why women should perform regular breast self-examination.
- Alice, 50, is recovering from a modified radical mastectomy for stage II ductal carcinoma. All lymph nodes were negative. The physician is recommending a combination of chemotherapy and tamoxifen therapy. Discuss the ethical implications of adjuvant therapy for node-negative patients.

## CHAPTER SUMMARY

### MALIGNANT CONDITIONS OF THE BREAST

- Factors placing the woman at high risk for breast cancer include age, personal or family history of breast cancer, parity, and environmental agents.
- Breast cancers can be detected early with regular breast self-examination (BSE), physical examination, and mammograms.
- It appears that BSE skills are regularly practiced by women who are taught to look and feel for what is *normal* for them. This approach lessens their anxiety about finding "cancer" (pathology) each month, which discourages many from doing BSE regularly.
- Therapy for breast cancer depends on various factors, including histopathology, hormonal status, location and size of tumor, local or regional metastasis, and the woman's life-style.
- In the rehabilitation phase after breast cancer, women are working through the loss of a breast and its significance, learning to do wound care, initiating post-mastectomy/lumpectomy exercises, mobilizing support systems, and pursuing prosthesis and clothing styles and possibly reconstruction options, if appropriate.
- Radiation therapy for women with breast cancer can last up to 6 weeks. Teaching includes mechanisms of radiation therapy's effect on cells, common side effects, and management of side effects and symptoms. Interstitial therapy requires additional support and teaching on the isolating aspects imposed by radiation policies.
- Teaching the woman with breast cancer about chemotherapy includes information on medications and mechanisms for managing side effects and suggestions on managing and monitoring side effects and symptoms.

### NONMALIGNANT CONDITIONS OF THE BREAST

- Common benign conditions of the breast include cystic breast disease, fibroadenoma, inflammatory breast conditions, and male gynecomastia.

## REFERENCES


1. American Cancer Society: *1993 Cancer facts and figures,* New York, 1993, The Society.
2. Andolina VF, Lille SL, Willison KM: *Mammographic imaging: a practical guide,* Philadelphia, 1992, JB Lippincott.
3. Anonymous: Average charges for modified radical mastectomies, *Oncology* 5(3):51-58, 1991.
4. Bacon F: Rarer problems. In Fentimen I, editor: *Detection and treatment of early breast cancer,* Philadelphia, 1990, JB Lippincott.
5. Baker RR, Niederhuber J: Clinical management of a palpable breast mass. In Baker RR, Niederhuber J, editors : *The operative management of breast disease,* Philadelphia, 1992, WB Saunders.
6. Barale KV: Nutritional support. In Baird SB et al, editors: *A cancer source book for nurses,* ed 6, New York, 1991, American Cancer Society.
7. Beahrs OH, Hutter RV, Kennedy BJ, editors: *Breast manual for staging of cancer,* ed 4, Philadelphia, 1992, JB Lippincott.
8. Bland KI, Page DL: Gynecomastia. In Bland KI, Copeland EM, editors: *The breast: comprehensive management of benign and malignant diseases,* Philadelphia, 1991, WB Saunders.
9. Boring CC, Squires TS, Heath CW: Cancer statistics for African Americans, *CA* 42(1):7-17, 1992.
10. Boring CC, Squires TS, Tong T: Cancer statistics, *CA* 43(1):7-26, 1993.
11. Boyd NF: Nutrition and breast cancer, *J Natl Cancer Institute* 85(1):6-7, 1993.
12. Brylawski R: Studies raise fresh questions about breast cancer treatment: is chemo always needed? *Oncol Times* 13(1):3-21, 1991.
13. Casciato DA, Lowitz BB, editors: *Manual of clinical oncology,* ed 2, Boston, 1992, Little, Brown & Co.

14. Chetty U: Nipple discharge. In Smallwood JA, Taylor I, editors: *Benign breast disease,* Baltimore, 1990, Urban & Schwarzenberg.
15. Coleman C: Breast cancer team: roles, conflicts, interfaces, *Innovations Oncol Nurs* 8(3):2-6, 1992.
16. Cope DG: Self-esteem and the practice of breast self examination, *West J Nurs Res* 14(5):618-631, 1992.
17. Dixon JM: Cystic disease of the breast. In Smallwood JA, Taylor I, editors: *Benign breast disease,* Baltimore, 1990, Urban & Schwarzenberg.
18. Dodd DG: American Cancer Society guidelines on screening for breast cancer: an overview, *CA* 42(3):177-180, 1992.
19. Donegan WL: Cancer of the breast in men, *CA* 41(6):339-354, 1991.
20. Dow KH: Newer developments in the diagnosis and staging of breast cancer, *Semin Oncol Nurs* 7(3):166-174, 1991.
21. Entrekin N: Breast cancer. In Clark JC, McGee RF: *Oncology Nursing Society core curriculum for oncology nursing,* ed 2, Philadelphia, 1992, WB Saunders.
22. Farber M, Chhibber G, Hewlett G: Medical management of benign breast disease. In Mitchell GW, Bassett LW, editors: *The female breast and its disorders,* Baltimore, 1991, Williams & Wilkins.
23. Fentimen IS: Breast conservation. In Fentiman IS, editor: *Detection and treatment of early breast cancer,* Philadelphia, 1990, JB Lippincott.
24. Goodman M: Adjuvant systemic therapy of stage I and II breast cancer, *Semin Oncol Nurs* 7(3):175-186, 1991.
25. Gulick AV: The NSABP breast cancer prevention trial, *Innovations Oncol Nurs* 9(1):9-10, 1993.
26. Harris JR et al: Breast cancer, *N Engl J Med* 327(5):319-328, 1992.
27. Harris JR et al: Breast cancer, *N Engl J Med* 327(6):390-398, 1992.
28. Haskell CM, Lowitz BB, Casciato DA: Breast cancer. In Casciato DA, Lowitz BB, editors: *Manual of clinical oncology,* Boston, 1988, Little, Brown & Co.
29. Hughes KK: Decision making by patients with breast cancer: the role of information in treatment selection, *Oncol Nurs Forum* 20(4):623-628, 1993.
30. Jarvis C: Breast and regional lymphatics. In Jarvis C, editor: *Physical examination and health assessment,* Philadelphia, 1992, WB Saunders.
31. Johnson S: The causes of breast cancer. In Fentiman IS, editor: *Detection and treatment of early breast cancer,* Philadelphia, 1990, JB Lippincott.
32. Jordan VC: Targeted hormone therapy for breast cancer, *Hosp Pract,* pp 55-62, March 15, 1993.
33. Kelsey JL, Gammon MD: The epidemiology of breast cancer, *CA* 41:146-165, 1991.
34. Kinne DW: The surgical management of primary breast cancer, *CA* 41(2):71-84, 1991.
35. Kinne DW: Management of male breast cancer, *Oncology* 5(3):45-47, 1991.
36. Knobf MT: Breast cancer. In Baird SB, editor: *Cancer nursing: a comprehensive textbook,* Philadelphia, 1991, WB Saunders.
37. Knobf MT, Stahl R: Reconstructive surgery in primary breast cancer, *Semin Oncol Nurs* 7(3):200-206, 1991.
38. Kritchensky D: Diet and cancer, *CA* 41(6):329-333, 1991.
39. Kroll SS: Mastectomy with immediate autogenous tissue reconstruction (Nursing Interventions in Oncology), *MD Anderson Case Rep Rev* 5:8-10, 1993.
40. MacKay J, Steel M: Genetic aspects of human breast cancer. In Ragaz J, editor: *High-risk breast cancer: diagnosis,* New York, 1989, Springer-Verlag.
41. McGrath EB: Lymphedema. In Dow KH, Hilderly LJ: *Nursing care in radiation oncology,* Philadelphia, 1992, WB Saunders.
42. Merkel DE, Osborne CK: Prognostic factors in breast cancer, *Hematol Oncol Clin North Am* 3:641-651, 1989.
43. Miller BA, Feuer EJ, Hankey BF: Recent incidence trends for breast cancer in women and the relevance of early detection: an update, *CA* 43(1):27-41, 1993.
44. Morra ME, Blumberg BD: Women's perceptions of early detection, *Semin Oncol Nurs* 7(3):151-160, 1991.
45. Nicholson GI, Hug V: Breast cancer growth and metastasis (Nursing Interventions in Oncology), *MD Anderson Case Rep Rev* 3:16-20, 1991.
46. Northouse L: A longitudinal study of the adjustment of patients and husbands to breast cancer, *Oncol Nurs Forum* 16(4):511-516, 1989.
47. Peterson HB, Wingo MS: Breast cancer and the pill, *Patient Care,* pp 67-82, Nov 30, 1992.
48. Pierce SM, Harris JR: The role of radiation therapy in the management of primary breast cancer, *CA* 41(2):85-96, 1991.
49. Ramzy I: Pathology of benign breast disease. In Mitchell GW, Bassett LW, editors: *The female breast and its disorders,* Baltimore, 1991, Williams & Wilkins.
50. Recht A, Hayes DF, Harris JR: The use of adjuvant therapy in patients treated with conservative surgery and radiotherapy. In Henderson IC, editor: *Adjuvant therapy of breast cancer,* Boston, 1992, Kluwer Academic Publishers.
51. Robert NJ: Biologic indicators of prognosis in breast cancer, *Hosp Pract,* pp 93-102, Oct 15, 1990.
52. Sauba WW: Evaluation and treatment of benign breast disorders. In Bland KI, Copeland EM: *The breast: comprehensive management of benign and malignant disease,* Philadelphia, 1991, WB Saunders.
53. Sawaya MB: Nursing care of the patient with breast reconstruction post mastectomy, *Plast Surg Nurs* 4(3):80-83, 1984.
54. Schover LR: The impact of breast cancer on sexuality, body image, and intimate relationships, *CA* 41(2):112-120, 1991.
55. Seidman H et al: Survival experience in the Breast Cancer Detection Demonstration Project, *CA* 37(5):258-290, 1987.
56. Sellers TA et al: Effect of family history, body-fat distribution, and reproductive factors on the risk of postmenopausal breast cancer, *N Engl J Med* 326(20):1323-1329, 1992.
57. Silliman RA et al: REVIEW breast cancer care in old age: what we know, don't know, and do, *J Natl Cancer Institute* 85(3):190-196, 1993.
58. Smith P: Familial breast and ovarian cancers, *Semin Oncol Nurs* 8(4):258-264, 1992.
59. US Department of Health and Human Services, Public Health Service: *Healthy people 2000: Summary report,* Boston, 1992, Jones & Bartlett.
60. Wainstock JM: Breast cancer: psychosocial consequences for the patient, *Semin Oncol Nurs* 7(3):207-215, 1991.
61. Wells BL, Horn JW: Stage at diagnosis in breast cancer: race and socioeconomic factors, *Am J Public Health* 82(10):1383-1385, 1992.
62. Whendon MB: New frontiers in breast cancer: emerging treatments, *Oncol Patient Care* 3(3):8-9, 1993.
63. Willett WC et al: Dietary fat and fiber in relation to risk of breast cancer: an 8-year follow-up, *JAMA* 268(15):2037-2044, 1992.
64. Winchester DP, Cox JD: Standards for breast conservation treatment, *CA* 42(3):134-162, 1992.

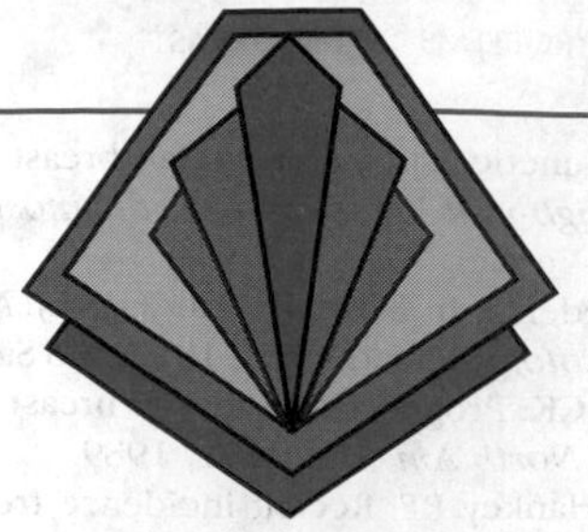

C H A P T E R 55

# Management of Persons With Sexually Transmitted Diseases

*Wilma J. Phipps*

## CHAPTER OBJECTIVES

***After studying this chapter, the learner should be able to do the following:***

1. Define sexually transmitted diseases (STDs).
2. Describe the transmission, prevention, and control of STDs.
3. List the causative agent, incubation period, signs and symptoms, medical therapy, and long-term effects of gonorrhea, syphilis, herpes genitalis, and chlamydia infection.
4. Describe the subjective and objective data to be collected from a person suspected of having an STD.
5. Write a teaching plan for a unit on the prevention of STDs for a sex education course for adolescents.

## KEY TERMS

bacterial vaginosis
chancroid
chlamydial infection
cluster suspect
genital warts
gonorrhea
granuloma inguinale
hepatitis B
herpes genitalis
latent infection
lymphogranuloma venereum
partner notification
pediculosis pubis
scabies
sexually transmitted disease (STD)
syphilis
trichomoniasis

## ETIOLOGY/EPIDEMIOLOGY

**Sexually transmitted diseases (STDs)** are diseases that usually are or can be transmitted from one person to another with heterosexual or homosexual intercourse or intimate contact with the genitalia, mouth, or rectum. Until the 1980s, only five venereal diseases (syphilis, gonorrhea, chancroid, lymphogranuloma venereum, and granuloma inguinale) were regularly monitored. In the 1980s several diseases were added to the list of STDs. These include *Chlamydia trachomatis,* genital herpes, human papillomavirus, genital mycoplasmas, cytomegalovirus, hepatitis B, vaginitis, enteric infections, and ectoparasitic disease.[19]

Early in the 1980s the human immunodeficiency virus (HIV) was identified, and acquired immunodeficiency syndrome (AIDS) emerged as a major STD. Because of AIDS's profound effect on the immune system, Chapter 71 is devoted to its discussion.

The diseases classified as STDs and their causative organisms are listed in Table 55-1. Because of improved laboratory and epidemiologic methods, the prevalence, modes of transmission, and clinical consequences of these newer STDs are better understood than in earlier decades. In addition, many of the newly recognized STDs have become epidemic or hyperendemic as a consequence of changing sexual behavioral patterns. Not only has the incidence of many STDs increased, but also, for agents with multiple modes of transmission (e.g., hepatitis B virus, enteric pathogens), the proportion of infections that are transmitted sexually has increased. In addition to the immediate consequences of STDs there are the recognized effects on maternal and infant morbidity as well as on human reproduction and fertility.

All states require that each case of syphilis and gonorrhea be reported to the state or local health officer. Most states also require the reporting of chancroid, granuloma inguinale, and lymphogranuloma venereum. Herpes genitalis, trichomoniasis, and candidiasis do not need to be reported in any state. The true incidence of STDs is not known because of variable reporting re-

**TABLE 55-1 Sexually Transmitted Diseases**

| TYPE OF ORGANISM | DISEASE |
|---|---|
| Bacteria | Gonorrhea, chancroid, granuloma inguinale, *Gardnerella vaginalis* |
| Spirochete | Syphilis |
| *Chlamydia* | Nongonococcal urethritis, epididymitis, cervicitis, pelvic inflammatory disease (PID), lymphogranuloma venereum |
| Virus | Herpes genitalis, hepatitis B, cytomegalovirus, AIDS, genital warts |
| Protozoa | Trichomoniasis |
| Yeast | Candidiasis |
| Parasites | Pediculosis pubis, scabies |

quirements and also because many cases are not reported by the clinicians who treat them.

In the United States almost 12 million cases of STDs occur yearly, 86% of them in persons ages 15 to 29 years. By 21 years of age, approximately one out of every five young persons has undergone treatment for an STD. Because only some teenagers are sexually active, this amounts to an effective rate of at least 25% among those who are sexually active.[19]

In addition to the immediate consequences of STDs, there are serious complications, most of which have the greatest impact on women and children. The most serious complications are pelvic inflammatory disease (PID), sterility, ectopic pregnancy, blindness, cancer associated with the human papillomavirus, fetal and infant deaths, birth defects, and mental retardation. The proportion of the population most affected are medically underserved persons, poor persons, and racial and ethnic minorities.[19] The total societal costs of STDs exceed $315 billion annually, with the cost of PID and PID-associated ectopic pregnancy and infertility alone exceeding $2.6 billion.

In explaining the trends of reported cases of STDs in the United States, *three changes* occurring since the 1960s are often referred to in the literature. The *first* of these concerns the use of antibiotics and changes in the antibiotic susceptibility of pathogenic organisms. The widespread, perhaps indiscriminate, use of penicillin and other antibiotics between the late 1940s and early 1950s parallels the decline in both syphilis and gonorrhea. It is said that the organisms developed a greater resistance to antibiotics over time and that antibiotics have therefore become less effective than previously. No firm evidence indicates a decrease in effectiveness of penicillin against syphilis. However, the gonococcus tends to develop resistance to antibiotics, and this has been increasing.

A *second* explanation for the rise in incidence of STDs is that they are more likely to occur if a social system is permissive. During times of war and other catastrophes, it is easier for agencies to control interpersonal behavior, whereas in times of peace and absence of national crisis, civil liberties tend to flourish. The incidence curve of syphilis and gonorrhea after the years of World War II seems to support this thesis.

The *third* explanation centers around sexual behavior patterns and includes permissiveness. Concern has been expressed particularly about the prevalence of gonorrhea among adolescents and young adults who are considered to be promiscuous. In fact, rates for gonorrhea show young adults of 20 to 24 years of age accounted for 40% of reported cases of gonorrhea, whereas persons 15 to 19 years of age accounted for 25% of cases. The highest morbidity for males was in the 20- to 24-year age group; for females it was in the 15- to 19-year age group.

The above discussion makes an assumption of sexual promiscuity and, in doing so, requires acknowledgment of advances in contraceptive technology, especially "the pill." These social changes are often termed the three Ps (permissiveness, promiscuity, and the pill).[9] The underlying idea is that, with the advent of antibiotics and the pill, people began to lose fear of untreated venereal disease and pregnancy and that sexual promiscuity increased significantly, leading to increased exposure to infection.

If the definition of promiscuity is that sexual relations are not restricted to one partner, studies show that patients diagnosed in clinics as having STDs are not promiscuous. In one study 66.4% of patients having an STD named only one sexual contact. It must be realized, however, that persons may hesitate to admit to having more than one sex partner for any number of reasons.

In the past, prostitution has been considered a major force in the transmission of STDs. Before World War II it was estimated that approximately 75% of all STDs could be traced to prostitutes and that at least 10% of all prostitutes had contracted an STD at least once. Today less than 5% of patients with syphilis can be classed as prostitutes. Also, most persons with gonorrhea are single and under 25 years of age, and most clients of prostitutes are usually older, married men. *Chlamydia trachomatis* and herpes are two STDs that are common in middle-class America.

Before 1960 homosexuals were rarely mentioned in the literature as carriers of STDs. Since the early 1970s much more attention has been given to the risk of STDs among homosexual and bisexual men. Homosexual men carry pathogens in the rectum and colon, including gonococcus, *Giardia*, ameba, *Shigella*, and *Campylobacter*. Although lesbians are at low risk for contracting STDs and gay males are at higher risk, it is important to note that sexual orientation does not prescribe individual forms of sexual behavior.

The condom was the main method of contraception used before the advent of antibiotics and oral contraceptives. Use of the condom may have prevented the spread of STDs by providing a mechanical barrier to the organisms. The pill revolutionized contraceptive practices, and it is known that neutralization of the vaginal and cervical environment by estrogenic substances predisposes to infection.

Several events during the 1980s and early 1990s bear mentioning:

1. The designation of AIDS as an STD put other STDs in competition with it for attention and resources.[18]
2. Studies of the sociodemographic and geographic distribution of gonorrhea clearly indicate that the transmission of gonorrhea is predicated on the existence of small groups of persons who share common sociodemographic, behavioral, and geographic characteristics of a so-called "core group." This concept was verified empirically in such diverse locations as New York state; Colorado Springs, Colorado; Dade County, Florida; and Liverpool, England. With the understanding of a core group pattern comes the opportunity to design intervention programs tailored to the group at risk.[11]
3. A recent analysis of the trends of sexually transmitted infections among adolescents, ages 10 to 19 years, from 1981 to 1991 revealed the following[8]:
   a. During this time period, 24% to 30% of reported cases of gonorrhea and 10% to 12% of the cases of syphilis were in this age group. Some of the highest rates of gonorrhea were among 15- to 19-year olds. Gonorrhea rates among adolescents remained the same from 1981 to 1991, whereas rates among older age groups decreased.
   b. Gonorrhea rates decreased among all age and sex groups except for 10- to 14-year-old males, 10- to 14-year old females, and 15- to 19-year-old males. Gonorrhea rates increased 41% for 10- to 14-year-old males, 51% for 10- to 14-year-old females, and 1.6% for 15- to 19-year-old males.
   c. Gonorrhea rates among 15- to 19-year-old Whites were highest in the South (325.0 cases per 100,000 population for White females and 124.4 cases per 100,000 population for White males). Rates among Hispanic 15- to 19-year-olds were highest in the Northeast. In the Northeast the rates were 749 cases per 100,000 for females and 720.7 per 100,000 for males. The reported gonorrhea rates for African-Americans were high in all regions of the United States. The proportion with infections was approximately 3.5% to 7.3% among 15- to 19-year old African-American females and 4.0% to 7.0% among 15- to 19-year-old African-American males.
   d. From 1981 to 1991 approximately 10% to 12% of the cases of primary and secondary syphilis were among adolescents. The rates of primary and secondary syphilis among 15- to 19-year-old males were similar to rates among males 30 years of age and older. For example, the rate among 15- to 19-year-olds in 1991 was 18.1 cases per 100,000 population, compared with a rate of 19.6 for males 30 years of age and older.
   e. Primary and secondary syphilis rates among 15- to 19-year-old females were lower than the rates among 15- to 19-year-old males from 1981 to 1983. However, rates among females increased 112% from 1984 to 1991. By 1991 the primary and secondary syphilis rates for 15- to 19-year-old females was double that of 15- to 19-year-old males.
4. Although the incidence of gonorrhea decreased, the incidence of syphilis increased dramatically (Figure 55-1). In 1990 the 50,223 reported cases of primary

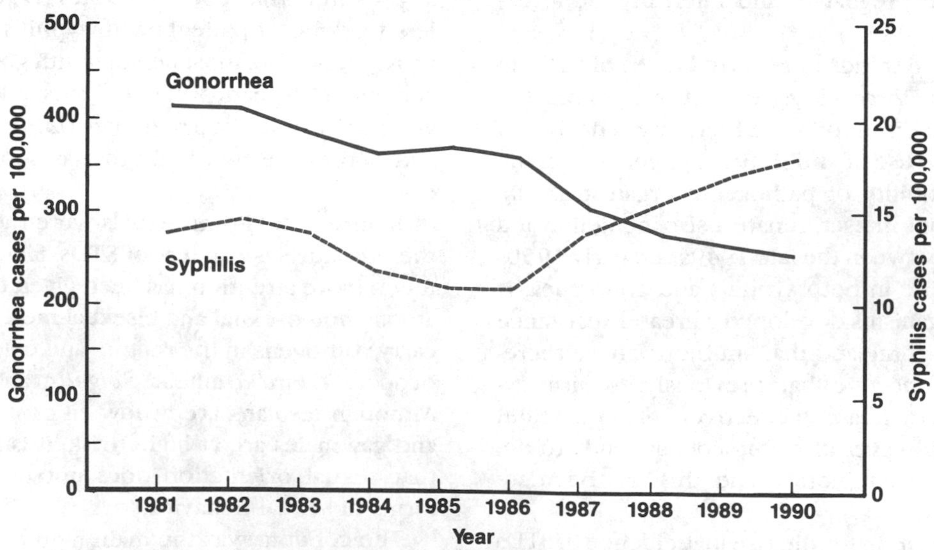


**FIGURE 55-1** Trend in the incidence of gonorrhea and primary and secondary syphilis, 1981 to 1990. (From Centers for Disease Control: Summary of notifiable diseases 1990, *MMWR* 39[53]: 1990.)

and secondary syphilis were the single largest yearly total since 1948. This epidemic is occurring primarily among young, heterosexual, minority populations and may be related to cocaine use and exchange of sex for drugs, especially crack cocaine.[18]

# SEXUAL TRANSMISSION

The STDs are contagious diseases spread almost exclusively by contact during sexual intercourse; that is, when mucous membrane surfaces come in contact during genital, oral, or anal sexual activity. Because the causative organisms survive only very briefly outside a warm, moist environment, there is almost no way to contract STDs from toilet seats, towels, or bed linens. Although STDs are not usually transmitted in public restrooms, conditions caused by fungi, bacteria, and lice can be transmitted from water in unclean toilet bowls. Women using a conventional toilet expose the vaginal and anal area to pathogens that can be introduced by the back splash of contaminated toilet water.

There are some notable exceptions to sexual transmission. During pregnancy the fetus may become infected in utero by placental transmission, and the infant may acquire congenital syphilis or be stillborn. Infants of mothers with gonorrhea may contract an infection of the eyes (ophthalmia neonatorum) during birth, and unless treated, it can lead to permanent blindness.

## PREVENTION AND HEALTH EDUCATION

Prevention and control measures for STDs include three levels of prevention. *Primary prevention* is directed at preventing the disease. This includes educating uninfected persons so that they can take responsibility for their own health and not expose themselves to an infected person; identification and treatment of exposed persons who are asymptomatic; interviewing persons with infection for identification of contacts, examination and preventive treatment of contacts; educational programs for the public; and active involvement of professionals in programs of control. The goal of these efforts includes eradication of the reservoir of disease in the population. *Secondary prevention* is directed toward prevention of complications. *Tertiary prevention* focuses on the following: (1) prevention of complications, (2) supporting and counseling infected persons to receive treatment, and (3) asking infected persons to notify their sexual partners so that they can be examined and treated if infected.

### Partner Notification (Contact Investigation)

In the prevention and control of STDs, especially gonorrhea, emphasis was once placed on interviewing for information regarding sexual contacts. The named contacts were sought out for examination and treatment. Lay people knowledgeable about the required reporting to the local health department of some of the diseases were very hesitant to name their sexual contacts. Young people often feared that their parents and the parents of the sexual partner(s) would find out about their infection. Minors need to know that they can probably obtain treatment without parental consent. Presently most states permit health care providers to treat minors for STDs without obtaining parental consent, and several states are proposing changes in existing legislation restricting treatment of minors. People also may perceive reporting of STDs as a threat from an official agency and may hesitate to name their contacts out of a sense of protection if they do not know that no punishment is involved.

Interviewing the patient for contacts is done at the time of the initial visit in the event that the patient does not return for follow-up. It is probably best that this interview take place after the patient is examined, the type of infection is determined, and the treatment is prescribed. If assessment is accompanied by information giving, the person should be better informed about STDs and how they are treated and be more willing and able to give information about sexual contacts.

Interviewing for contacts involves two aspects. The patient is first asked to name sexual contacts. Second, the patient is interviewed for **cluster suspects,** who are friends or acquaintances who may have been exposed to the same contacts or who have symptoms of an STD.

Because one focus of STD control is increasing self-referrals, the patient is asked to inform known contacts **(partner notification)** and cluster suspects to come in for examination and treatment. Confidentiality is stressed. There is reason to believe that patients do not name all their contacts at the time of the first interview and that a reinterview will usually result in additional names of contacts. Because of the understandable reluctance of many people to name their sexual contacts, the patient may be given the responsibility of informing the contacts and advising them of their need for treatment. (The contacts are not named, but instead cards that permit both examination and treatment without identification are given to the contacts by the patient.) Local health departments cooperate in locating, examining, and treating these contacts as necessary.

Whenever possible, the contacts of the infected person are located and advised to have an examination and tests as soon as possible. If the sexual partner or partners do not have symptoms of infection at the time of the first examination, treatment is instituted to abort infection. Giving preventive treatment to named contacts who have no clinical evidence of infection has gained popularity and acceptance in the United States, and there are indications that this same approach is being used more often in management of patients having the "minor" STDs.

**BOX 55-1 Estimated STD Threats**

1.4 million cases of gonorrhea
130,000 cases of syphilis
4 million cases of chlamydia
500,000-1,000,000 cases of human papillomavirus
200-500,000 cases of genital herpes
3 million cases of trichomoniasis
270,000-300,000 cases of hepatitis B
1.2 million cases of urethritis (nongonococcal, non–*Chlamydia trachomatis*)
1 million cases of mucopurulent cervicitis (MPC) (nongonococcal, non–*Chlamydia trachomatis*)

## CURRENT NEEDS

In its Annual Report for 1990, the Division of STD/HIV Prevention of the Centers for Disease Control defined the problem as follows:

> Sexually transmitted diseases continue as one of the nation's most serious public health problems. Not only is HIV infection the most devastating public health problem of this century, but also infectious syphilis has continued an unprecedented increase since the advent of penicillin therapy; resistant gonococcal infection is steadily increasing; chlamydial infections account for twice as many cases as gonorrhea; studies of human papillomavirus associate it with the development of cervical dysplasia; and trichomoniasis and other vaginal infections are being recognized as potentially major contributors to premature birth.

In addition, the CDC lists estimated STD threats to the health of Americans, primarily adolescents and young adults (Box 55-1).

## PREVENTION

### *Healthy People 2000*

*Healthy People 2000* established several goals to be attained by the year 2000.[19] These are listed below.

1. Reduce gonorrhea to an incidence of no more than 225 cases per 100,000 people, as compared with a baseline of 300 per 100,000 in 1989.
2. Reduce *Chlamydia trachomatis* infections, as measured by a decrease in the incidence of nongonococcal urethritis, to no more than 170 cases per 100,000 people, compared with a baseline of 215 cases per 100,000 cases in 1988.
3. Reduce primary and secondary syphilis to an incidence of no more than 10 cases per 100,000 people, as compared with a baseline of 18.1 per 100,000 in 1989.
4. Reduce congenital syphilis to an incidence of no more than 50 cases per 100,000 live births from a baseline of 100 per 100,000 live births in 1989.
5. Reduce herpes and genital warts, as measured by a reduction to 142,000 and 385,000, respectively, in the annual number of first-time consultations with a physician for these conditions. The baseline for 1988 was 167,000 and 451,000 cases per 100,000 persons, respectively.
6. Reduce the incidence of PID, as measured by a reduction in hospitalizations for PID, to no more than 250 per 100,000 women aged 15 to 44 years. The baseline was 311 per 100,000 in 1988.
7. Reduce sexually transmitted hepatitis B infection to no more than 30,500 cases from a baseline of 58,300 cases in 1988.

Risk reduction objectives to help achieve the above goals include the following[19]:

1. Reduce the proportion of adolescents who have engaged in sexual intercourse to no more than 15% by age 15 years and no more than 40% by age 17 years. The baseline was 27% of girls and 33% of boys by age 15 years; 50% of girls and 66% of boys by age 17 years; as reported in 1988.
2. Increase to at least 50% the proportion of sexually active, unmarried people who used a condom at last sexual intercourse. The baseline was 19% of sexually active, unmarried women aged 15 to 44 years who reported that their partners used a condom at last intercourse in 1988.

The special population targets for this last objective appear in Table 55-2.

**TABLE 55-2 Special Population Targets for Condom Use**

| USE OF CONDOMS | 1988 BASELINE | 2000 TARGET |
|---|---|---|
| Sexually active young women aged 15-19 yr (by their partners) | 25% | 60% |
| Sexually active young men aged 15-19 yr | 57% | 75% |
| Intravenous drug abusers | — | 60% |

To achieve these important goals, changes need to occur in agencies that deliver primary care, such as family planning clinics, maternal and child health clinics, drug treatment centers, and primary care clinics that screen, diagnose, treat, counsel, and provide (or refer for) partner notification services for HIV infection and bacterial STDs (gonorrhea, syphilis, and chlamydia). The CDC wants the goals to occur in at least 50% of the health care providers as compared with 40% of family planning clinics for 1989.

Another need to achieve the objectives relates to education of the young. The CDC recommends that instruction in STD prevention be included in the curricula of all middle and secondary schools, preferably as part of quality school health education.

In addition, the CDC wants to increase to at least 90% the proportion of primary care providers treating

**TABLE 55-3 Selected Sexually Transmitted Diseases**

| INCUBATION PERIOD | SIGNS AND SYMPTOMS | MEDICAL THERAPY |
|---|---|---|
| **GONORRHEA** | | |
| Men: 3-30 days<br>Women: 3 days to an indefinite period | Men: purulent urethral discharge, dysuria, epididymitis, prostatitis<br>Women: asymptomatic in early stages: cervicitis with purulent discharge, bartholinitis, salpingitis | Ceftriaxone, 125 mg IM in a single dose, plus doxycycline, 10 mg PO bid for 7 days, or Cefixime, 400 mg PO, plus doxycycline, 10 mg PO bid for 7 days, or ciprofloxacin, 500 mg PO, plus doxycycline, 10 mg PO bid for 7 days, or Ofloxacin, 400 mg PO, plus doxycycline, 10 mg PO bid for 7 days |
| **SYPHILIS** | | |
| 3 wk (9 days to 3 mo) | Positive serologic tests, chancre in stage I | Benzathine penicillin G, 2.4 million units IM |
| **HERPES GENITALIS** | | |
| 3-14 days | Vesicles that rupture and form ulcerations, pain, inguinal lymph node enlargement, dysuria, flulike symptoms | Symptomatic; topical acyclovir |
| ***CHLAMYDIA*** | | |
| 5-10 days or longer | Women: painful or difficult urination, abnormal vaginal discharge or bleeding, pain or bleeding with coitus, irregular menses; one third are asymptomatic<br>Men: testicular pain, nonspecific urethritis or epididymitis | Doxycycline, 100 mg PO bid for 7 days, or azithromycin, 1 g PO in a single dose |
| **CONDYLOMATA ACUMINATA (GENITAL WARTS)** | | |
| 1-6 mo | Horny papules on vulva, vagina, cervix, perineum, anal canal, urethra, glans penis | Cryotherapy (see Table 55-7 for pharmacologic therapy) |

patients with STDs who correctly manage cases, as measured by their use of appropriate types and amounts of therapy. The baseline was 70% in 1988. The success of this objective will be monitored by the number of women treated for gonorrhea and PID. For example, one study found that only 10% of primary care providers assessed the sexual behavior of their patients. Also, a large proportion of providers did not prescribe combination antibiotics to treat polymicrobial PID.

Another need to achieve the goals relates to counseling services. It is recommended that at least 75% of primary care and mental health providers provide age-appropriate counseling on the prevention of HIV and other STDs. As mentioned above, baseline figures for 1987 indicate that only 10% of physicians reported that they regularly assessed the sexual behaviors of their patients in 1987.[19]

The goals for the year 2000 also recommend an increase to at least 50% for the proportion of all patients with bacterial STDs (gonorrhea, syphilis, and chlamydia) who are offered provider referral services. The baseline was 20% of those treated in STD clinics in 1988.

Provider referral services (previously called *contact tracing*) is the process by which health department personnel notify the sexual partners of infected individuals that they have been exposed to an infectious disease. The goal of provider referral is to find other persons who may be infected and to get them under treatment so that they can be adequately treated and the transmission of the STD is stopped within the community. Proper treatment also helps prevent complications among those already infected.[19]

Even though the provider may be involved in the notification process, it is crucial that infected persons be supported and coached so that they can do partner notification themselves. This is especially so because provider referral is labor intensive and current resources (budget constraints) may not allow health departments to notify all persons named by infected persons. Partner notification should help the infected person internalize the need to assume more responsibility for his or her health and for the well-being of sexual partners.[19]

## SIGNS AND SYMPTOMS

Vaginitis, cervicitis, lower abdominal pain, urethritis, epididymitis, pharyngitis, proctitis, and skin or mucous membrane lesions are common in persons with STDs (Table 55-3). Some people may be asymptomatic.

## MEDICAL MANAGEMENT

Treatment depends on the causative organisms identified through the history, physical examination, and laboratory tests and is discussed in detail in the following pages. It is not unusual for an individual to harbor two or more organisms simultaneously. Medical therapy for each STD is discussed under the specific diseases.

## NURSING MANAGEMENT

### ♦ ASSESSMENT

#### Subjective Data

Data to be collected to assess the patient suspected of having an STD include the following:

- Exposure to STD contact including HIV
- Prior STD history, treatment
- Sexual orientation: "Have you been having sex with men, women, or both?"
- Time of last sexual activity
- Number of sexual partners in the past 2 months
- Women are questioned about:
  - Vaginal discharge
  - Vulvar itching
  - Dysuria
  - Urinary urgency
  - Lower abdominal pain
  - Rectal symptoms
  - Sore throat
  - Genital lesions
  - Skin rashes or itching
  - Menstrual periods
- Heterosexual men are questioned about:
  - Urethral discharge
  - Dysuria
  - Genital lesions
  - Skin rashes
  - Itching
  - Testicular pain
  - Sore throat
- Gay or bisexual men are asked the same questions as heterosexual men plus the following:
  - Rectal symptoms such as pain, bleeding, discharge, and diarrhea
- If hepatitis is also suspected, the person is questioned about:
  - Dark-colored urine
  - Clay-colored stools
  - Fatigue
  - Jaundice

#### Objective Data

Data to be collected to assess the patient suspected of having an STD include the following:

- Inspection and palpation of the integumentary system, reproductive system, and anorectal area
- Examination for women includes the following:
  - Inspection of skin of lower abdomen, inguinal area, hands, palms, and forearms
  - Inspection of pubic hair for lice and mites
  - Inspection and palpation of external genitalia, including perineum and anus
  - Speculum examination of vagina and cervix
  - Bimanual pelvic examination
  - Palpation for inguinal and femoral lymphadenopathy
  - Inspection of mouth and throat, including tonsils
- Examination of heterosexual men includes the following:
  - Inspection of the skin and pubic hair
  - Inspection of the penis, including the meatus, with retraction of the foreskin and "milking" of the urethra
  - Palpation of the scrotum
- Examination of homosexual or bisexual men is the same as for heterosexual men plus the following:
  - Inspection of the mouth, throat including the tonsils, and anorectal area
  - Anoscopic examination if there are rectal symptoms

#### Diagnostic Tests

Specific diagnostic tests are used to establish the diagnosis of each of these diseases. Diagnostic tests will be discussed under the specific disease later in this chapter.

### ♦ NURSING DIAGNOSES

Nursing diagnoses are determined from analysis of patient data. Nursing diagnoses for the person with an STD may include but are not limited to the following:

| Diagnostic Title | Possible Etiologic Factors |
|---|---|
| Knowledge deficit | Lack of exposure/recall, information misinterpretation, lack of familiarity with information sources about STDs |
| Health maintenance, altered | Lack of knowledge, cultural practices, lack of material recources |

### ♦ EXPECTED PATIENT OUTCOMES

Expected patient outcomes for the person with an STD may include but are not limited to the following:

1. Person and/or partner can explain the etiology and factors contributing to the STD.
2. Person and/or partner can state the name, dosage, and schedule of administration of drug therapy, as well as its possible side effects.
3. Person and/or partner can explain the need for adherence to the entire treatment regimen.
4. Person and/or partner can state the reasons for abstaining from sexual activity during the infectious stages of the STD.
5. Person and/or partner can state effects of the STD on the reproductive system of oneself and one's partner.
6. Person and/or partner can state indications for seeking immediate health care if signs and symptoms reappear.
7. Person and/or partner can explain necessity for treatment of sexual partner or partners.

**BOX 55-2 Recommendations From the CDC for the Use of Condoms**

The following recommendations for proper use of condoms to reduce the transmission of STD are based on current information:

1. Latex condoms should be used, because they offer greater protection against viral STD than natural membrane condoms.
2. Condoms should be stored in a cool, dry place out of direct sunlight.
3. Condoms in damaged packages or those that show obvious signs of age (e.g., those that are brittle, sticky, or discolored) should not be used. They cannot be relied on to prevent infection.
4. Condoms should be handled with care to prevent puncture.
5. The condom should be put on before any genital contact to prevent exposure to fluids that may contain infectious agents. Hold the tip of the condom and unroll it onto the erect penis, leaving space at the tip to collect semen, yet ensuring that no air is trapped in the tip of the condom.
6. Adequate lubrication should be used. If exogenous lubrication is needed, only water-based lubricants should be used. Petroleum- or oil-based lubricants (e.g., petroleum jelly, cooking oils, shortening, and lotions) should not be used, because they weaken the latex of the condom.
7. Use of condoms containing spermicides may provide some additional protection against STD. However, vaginal use of *spermicides* along with condoms is likely to provide greater protection.
8. If a condom breaks, it should be replaced immediately. If ejaculation occurs after condom breakage, the immediate use of spermicide has been suggested. However, the protective value of postejaculation application of spermicide in reducing the risk of STD transmission is unknown.
9. After ejaculation, care should be taken so that the condom does not slip off the penis before withdrawal; the base of the condom should be held while withdrawing. The penis should be withdrawn while still erect.
10. Condoms should never be reused.

From Center for Disease Control: Condoms for the prevention of sexually transmitted disease, *MMWR* 37(9):133-137, 1988.

8. Person and/or partner can accept the occurrence of the STD.
9. Person and/or partner can explain how to prevent the transmission of STDs by using safer sex practices, including the type of condom to use, when and how to apply it, and how to remove it.[3] Recommendations on the proper use of condoms to prevent transmission of STDs can be found in Box 55-2.

## ♦ INTERVENTIONS

Interventions will be discussed under the specific diseases.

### Facilitating Learning

The nurse's first responsibility in STD control is to educate patients who have a sexually transmitted infection or may develop one. Nurses must be knowledgeable about the most prevalent diseases, the signs and symptoms, methods used in diagnosis, treatments used, and where individuals can obtain help and information. They also can influence the knowledge and attitudes of their colleagues and peers toward STD and its control. Nurses can exert influence in the community by taking an active role in education programs. Perhaps the best way to reduce the risk of STD is for persons who are sexually active to know their sexual partners. Sexual activity with different partners increases the risk of infection.

Preventive measures such as washing or showering with soap and water and using a condom are recommended but are no guarantee against STD. Good laundry and personal hygiene practices also may help reduce risk.

Before nurses can be effective in working with patients who have STDs, they must confront their own feelings and attitudes about STDs. The patient is often young, fearful of pain, and unaccustomed to surroundings in a clinic or physician's office. Young patients especially fear that their families and friends may learn they have an STD.

Once the diagnosis, tentative or conclusive, is made, focus should first be placed on obtaining a cure and preventing complications and reinfection. Many lay people know that the treatment for syphilis and gonorrhea is penicillin, but they may not be fully informed about this and other aspects of treatment. Because some of the diseases respond to penicillin or other antibiotics, many people believe that all genital infections can be cured easily, and this is not so. Some people believe that antibiotics not only cure an infection but also produce immunity against reinfection. Persons receiving an antibiotic or other medications for STDs must be informed of the action of the drug, its duration of effectiveness, side effects, chances of cure, and the need for follow-up. *They need to be advised that treatment failures do occur and that reinfection rates are high.* Return visits should be encouraged whenever possible, because adequacy of treatment of all of the STDs is evaluated best by laboratory analysis for the specific organism.

### Providing Social and Emotional Support

Many patients focus on how the diseases are spread rather than on the consequences of having an infection. For single persons, contracting an STD and securing help mean they must admit to sexual activity, and some of them may feel guilty. Their self-esteem may be threatened by what has happened to them. Patients with an STD have not only a physical but also a social, an emotional, and perhaps an economic problem. They need constructive and comprehensive help. The nurse who is successful in working with persons who have an STD is one who can create an atmosphere of trust in which the person feels free to discuss all aspects of the problem.

Persons who seek help recognize they have a problem; they want to get better and stay well. Because of this they are highly motivated to do what is necessary, receptive to information and advice, and attentive when advice is given. Nurses can take advantage of the patient's readiness to learn and motivation to improve and maintain health.

### Promoting Self-Care

Persons treated for sexually transmitted infections need information about self-care. To understand their therapy and to responsibly engage in self-care, they must be informed about the sexual nature of the infection, how it is transmitted, and the *possibility of reinfection and infection of their sexual partner or partners.* The patient needs to know that it is important for sexual partners to be checked for signs of infection, to be advised of what the signs are, and to have a culture for asymptomatic infection. Patients should be advised to abstain from intercourse until cured. *It also should be stressed that condoms should be used to prevent infection or reinfection if persons persist in engaging in intercourse even when advised not to.*

Teaching about hygiene and personal health practices is beneficial in reducing the chances of secondary infection, recurrence, and infections of various types in the future. Frequent bathing and hand washing are indicated. It is known that many of the organisms causing STDs are destroyed by soap and water. *For women, douching is contraindicated unless it is prescribed for the purpose of applying heat or applying medication.* All women should be informed that, for personal cleanliness, frequent douching at any time is *not* advisable, because this may disturb the vaginal and cervical environments and predispose the woman to infection. If douching is prescribed by the physician, the patient should be instructed in the procedure.

If the lesions are present on body surfaces, the patient should be instructed in their care. Unless contraindicated, a hot bath is taken two to three times per day; and lesions are kept as dry as possible between baths. Both men and women should be advised to wear cotton underwear, and women should be advised to avoid wearing pantyhose, because they tend to trap moisture and prevent circulation of air to the genitalia. Unless lotions, creams, or ointments are specifically prescribed as local medications, the patient should not apply them to any of the lesions associated with an STD.

Self-examination is important for sexually active people, especially those with more than one partner. Inspecting skin, mouth, genitalia, and perianal areas for lesions and discharges is recommended. In addition, people can learn to casually inspect their partners during the initial period of lovemaking to identify any signs of STDs. Urinating after sexual activity can be helpful in cleansing the urethra of organisms.

### Promoting Healthy Sexual Attitudes

Opportunities for promoting healthy attitudes about sexual activity and STDs frequently arise. These topics are approached tactfully and with consideration of the patient's feelings. Adolescents especially require an approach that indicates understanding balanced with the ability to help them set limits. They need to understand that they are responsible for their own bodies and they do not have to give in to sexual pressures. It is well documented, however, that the strongest influence on teenagers comes from their peer group. For this reason, discussion with groups of teenagers about their sexual responsibilities may be helpful. In the climate of the 1990s there should be no doubt that abstinence is the only absolute way to prevent STD. If a teen elects to be sexually active he or she needs to understand that the consequences of unprotected sex may include unwanted pregnancy and STD. Monogamous relationships and the proper use of condoms should be stressed for those who are sexually active.

Another problem among teenagers and young adults is serial monogamy. When questioned about their sexual activities, most of them consider themselves to be monogamous, but the monogamy lasts for only a few weeks or months. Thus they are not having sex with more than one person in a time span, but are going from one short-term relationship to another without concern about their partners' sexual histories.

## ♦ EVALUATION

Evaluation is based on the expected patient outcomes. Questions to be asked include the person's and/or partner's ability to do the following:

1. State the factors that contributed to the present infection with STD (multiple sexual partners; not using a condom).
2. State the drug therapy to be followed, including name of drug, dosage, schedule of administration, and side effects.
3. Explain why the therapy must be taken without interruption (to prevent resistant strains of organisms from developing).
4. State why he or she should not engage in sexual activity while the STD is infectious.
5. State effects of STDs that may develop in the reproductive system of either partner.
6. State signs and symptoms (fever, pain, discharge) that indicate the need for immediate health care.
7. Verbalize understanding of the necessity of treatment for his or her sexual partner or partners.
8. Verbalize that she or he has an STD, and identify ways to prevent further STD infections.
9. Explain what is meant by practicing "safer sex," including what type of condom to use, when and how to apply it, and how to remove it.

# GONORRHEA

## ETIOLOGY

**Gonorrhea,** often referred to as GC or *the clap* by lay people, is caused by *Neisseria gonorrhoeae.* Gonorrhea is of great concern, because persons with it often have another STD such as chlamydia or HIV. They also have a high reinfection rate and serious residual effects. The incubation period is 3 to 30 days in men and 3 days to an indefinite period in women.

## EPIDEMIOLOGY

The incidence of gonorrhea in the United States decreased dramatically in the 1980s (Figures 55-2 to 55-4). Since 1981, cases of gonorrhea decreased 29% in males and 24% in females. There is concern, however, that the rates will not continue to decrease because of an increase in the number of cases caused by antibiotic-resistant organisms. Despite these decreases the CDC estimated that there would be 1.4 million cases of gonorrhea in 1991. The proportion of antibiotic-resistant gonococcal organisms increased from 0.8% in 1985 to 7% in 1989 (Figure 55-5). The incidence of gonorrhea is accepted to be much higher than shown, because it is known that the cases of many patients treated by private physicians are never reported to public health authorities and therefore are not reflected in the statis-

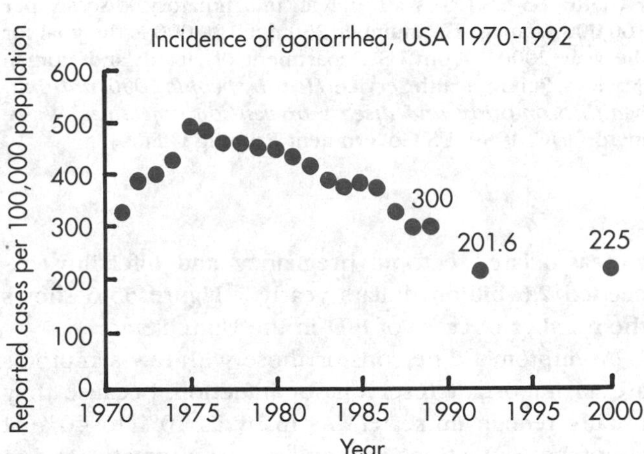


**FIGURE 55-2** Incidence of gonorrhea in the United States from 1970 to 1990. The rates are per 100,000 population. The number 225 is the goal for year 2000. (From US Dept of Health and Human Services, Public Health Service: ***Healthy people 2000: national health promotion and disease prevention objectives,*** Washington, DC, 1990, US Government Printing Office.)

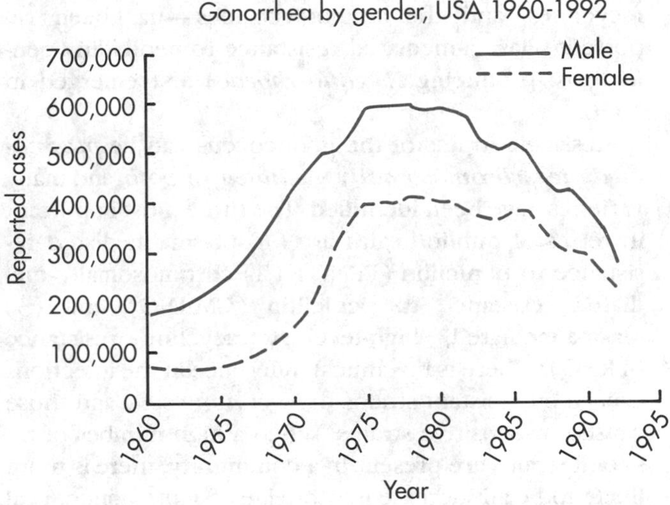


**FIGURE 55-3** Incidence of gonorrhea in the United States by gender, 1960 to 1992. (From Centers for Disease Control: Graphs and maps for selected notifiable diseases in the United States, *MMWR* 41[55]:13-64, 1993.)

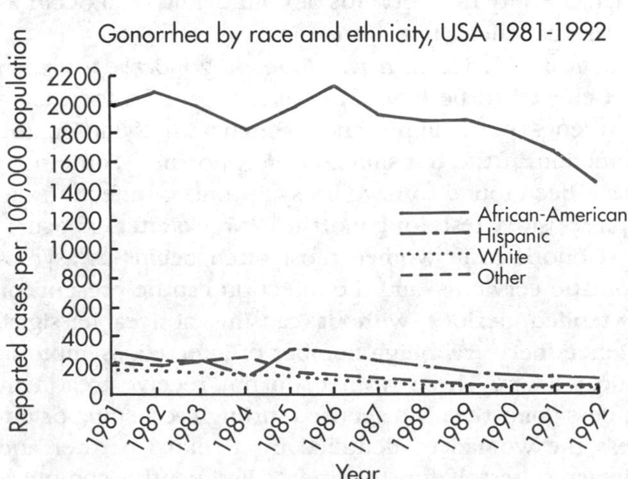


**FIGURE 55-4** Incidence of gonorrhea in the United States by race and ethnicity, 1981 to 1992. (From Centers for Disease Control: Graphs and maps for selected notifiable diseases in the United States, *MMWR* 41[55]:13-64, 1993.)

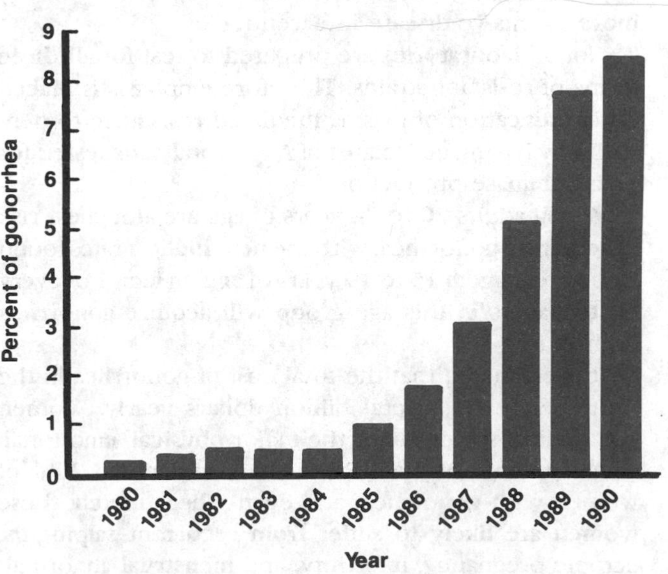


**FIGURE 55-5** Percentage of antibiotic-resistant strains of gonorrhea in the United States, 1980 to 1990. (From Centers for Disease Control: Summary of notifiable diseases 1990, *MMWR* 39[53]:24, 1990.)

tics. It is generally accepted that only 25% to 50% of cases treated by private physicians are reported. In addition, women have few if any signs or symptoms of gonorrhea and thus are often not diagnosed. For this reason it is commonly believed that the actual number of cases per year in the United States is probably more than 2 million.

## PATHOPHYSIOLOGY

Compounding the problem is the rapid increase of cases of gonorrhea caused by resistant strains of *N. gonorrhoeae.* Clinically significant resistance to the three widely used classes of drugs—the penicillins, the tetracyclines, and the aminoglycosides—has been reported.[2] Plasma-mediated resistance to penicillin (penicillinase-producing *N. gonorrhoeae*) first emerged in 1976.

Resistant strains of the gonococcus can be *plasma-mediated, chromosomally mediated,* or *both,* and many varieties have been identified. The three most important in terms of public health are (1) plasma-mediated resistance to penicillin (PPNG); (2) chromosomally mediated resistance to penicillin (CMRNG); and (3) plasma-mediated, high-level tetracycline resistance (TRNG).[2] There is no clinical difference in the infections caused by resistant strains of *N. gonorrhoeae* and those caused by sensitive strains. When a high number of resistant strains are present in a community, there is more likely to be an increase in sequelae of acute gonococcal infections such as PID, gonococcal ophthalmia, and disseminated gonococcal infection (DGI).[2]

The costs of patient management in communities with a high rate of resistant strains of *N. gonorrhoeae* are increased because of (1) additional laboratory tests, (2) added drug costs, (3) extra clinic visits, and (4) more extensive disease intervention.

Not all laboratories are prepared to test for all three forms of resistant strains. Therefore emphasis is placed on identification of plasma-mediated resistance to penicillin by having all isolates of *N. gonorrhoeae* tested for beta-lactamase production.[2]

Young adults 20 to 24 years of age are at highest risk of acquiring gonorrhea, with the next highest rates found among teenagers 15 to 19 years of age. In fact, 1 of every 30 teenagers in this age group will acquire gonorrhea each year.

It is estimated that the total cost of gonorrhea in the United States is several billion dollars yearly. Women and their offspring suffer the major physical, emotional, and economic burden. PID occurs in 10% to 20% of women with gonorrhea; and even when treated, these women are likely to suffer from recurrent salpingitis, ectopic pregnancy, infertility, and menstrual abnormalities and may face surgical removal of the pelvic organs, as well as fetal loss.

More than 1 million cases of PID are diagnosed and treated yearly. According to one report the cost of PID

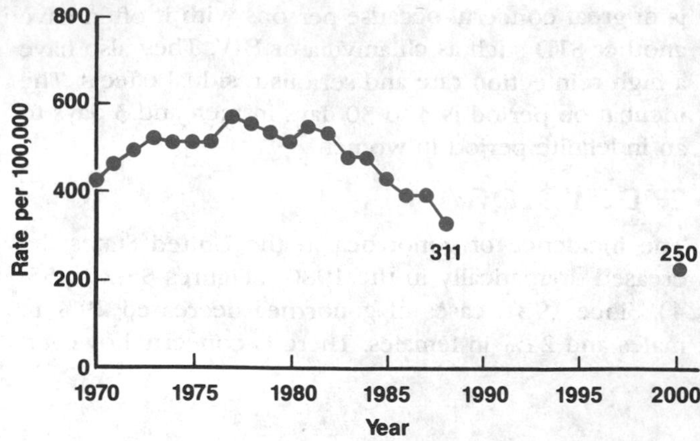


**FIGURE 55-6** Cases of pelvic inflammatory disease per 100,000 women. The number 250 per 100,000 is the goal for the year 2000. (From US Department of Health and Human Services, Public Health Service: *Healthy people 2000: national health promotion and disease prevention objectives,* Washington, DC, 1990, US Government Printing Office.)

and associated ectopic pregnancy and infertility exceeded 2.6 billion dollars yearly.[19] Figure 55-6 shows the number of cases of PID in the United States.

Asymptomatic persons or those with few symptoms are an important reservoir for infection, because they usually remain untreated. As many as 10% to 40% of gonorrheal infections in men are asymptomatic, and in women as many as 80% of infections are asymptomatic. Homosexual men can harbor reservoirs of anorectal and pharyngeal infections.

The most common signs and symptoms are listed in Box 55-3. In men the gonococcus is introduced into the anterior urethra during sexual activity. Because most men are diagnosed and treated early, complications and residual effects of gonorrhea are uncommon among men. Sterility from orchitis or epididymitis can occur as a residual effect, but this is rare.

The incidence of *asymptomatic gonorrhea* in men is believed to be low; however, there is an increasing awareness of the importance of men with asymptomatic infection in the transmission of gonorrhea. Some men have been found to have no symptoms of infection despite positive tests for gonorrhea 2 weeks after exposure.

Gonorrhea in women most often begins as asymptomatic cervicitis, and the infection can be present for extended periods without causing noticeable signs. Hence there are a high number of infected, asymptomatic women. These women do not receive treatment unless gonorrhea is diagnosed through screening or unless the woman is identified by a sexual partner and presents herself for treatment. Frequently, complications are the first indicators of gonorrhea in women. *Salpingitis is the most common complication, with 10% to 20% of women presenting themselves with symptoms of salpingitis as the first sign of gonorrhea.*

**BOX 55-3 Signs and Symptoms of Gonorrhea**

**HETEROSEXUAL MEN**

1. Urethritis—often first symptom
2. Severe dysuria—especially with first voiding in morning
3. Purulent discharge from urethra
4. Swelling of the penis and balanitis—rare symptoms

**HOMOSEXUAL AND BISEXUAL MEN**

1. Rectal gonorrhea is common—usually asymptomatic and discovered by rectal culture
2. Pharyngeal gonorrhea—usually asymptomatic

**WOMEN**

Women rarely have early, distressing symptoms such as men have. When symptoms are present, they include the following:

1. Slight purulent vaginal discharge
2. Vague feeling of fullness in pelvis
3. Discomfort or aching in abdomen
4. If bladder is involved—burning, frequency, and urgency, which usually cause the person to seek medical attention

The first three symptoms are so slight that they may be ignored by the person.

During the course of treatment for salpingitis, many women are surgically sterilized. In cases of untreated gonorrhea, the residual effects of chronic PID, infertility, and ectopic pregnancy are well known.

Other complications of untreated gonorrhea in both men and women include dermatitis, carditis, meningitis, and arthritis. The incidence of these complications is higher among women because of the prolonged period of infection without symptoms.

## PREVENTION

Prevention of gonorrhea and its complications can be achieved in three stages. The *first* and most crucial *stage, primary prevention,* is prevention of the disease. The *second stage, secondary prevention,* involves prevention of complications of the disease such as PID. The *third stage, tertiary prevention,* is reversal of the damage caused by the disease, such as by tubal reconstruction.

Early treatment of infected persons is the most effective method to prevent new infection of sexual partners. Mechanical barrier methods such as condoms used with spermicides may reduce but not prevent gonorrhea.[16] Education to acquaint people with the symptoms of gonorrhea, the efficacy of condoms, and the availability of diagnostic and treatment resources is also important. Early detection through partner notification and screening can reduce the serious complications of gonorrhea. There is no effective vaccine for gonorrhea, although clinical trials have been attempted.[16]

Some physicians believe that all persons with gonorrhea should be treated for chlamydia even though there are no signs and symptoms of it. No therapy for both diseases is effective when given in a single dose. This will be discussed further under treatment. It is generally accepted that all patients with gonorrhea should be offered testing and counseling for HIV.

## NURSING MANAGEMENT

### ♦ ASSESSMENT

Subjective and objective data to be collected are the same for all STDs and are discussed on p. 1860.

#### Diagnostic Tests

Gonorrheal infection may be suspected on the basis of history, symptoms, and clinical evidence obtained by physical examination. However, ***identification of the organism is necessary to confirm the diagnosis*** and to rule out other problems. In men the diagnosis is confirmed by gram-stained smear of the discharge from the penis. Culture of the discharge from the penis is usually reserved for those whose smears are negative in the presence of strong clinical evidence.

Gram-stained cervical smears are inadequate for diagnosing gonorrhea in women. These smears are negative in about 50% of women having gonorrhea and are falsely positive in some cases. Therefore cultures from the cervix, urethra, throat, and anus are usually taken. Because of the great length of time required to obtain reports of cultures for gonorrhea, treatment is usually begun on a presumptive basis.

### ♦ NURSING DIAGNOSES

The nursing diagnoses are the same for all STDs and are discussed on p. 1860.

### ♦ EXPECTED PATIENT OUTCOMES

See p. 1860 for a discussion of the patient outcomes for any of the STDs.

### ♦ INTERVENTIONS

#### Administering Medications

Therapy for gonorrhea presents a greater problem than for syphilis, because the gonococcus tends to develop resistance to antibiotics. It also is believed that *inadequate therapy is common in the United States.* Several drug regimens are in use. Emphasis is on single-dose treatment, because it avoids the need for follow-up and patient cooperation.

The treatment regimen recommended by the CDC[6] is as follows:

1. Ceftriaxone (Rocephin), 125 mg IM in a single dose
2. Alternative therapy: spectinomycin, 2 g IM once; ciprofloxacin, 500 mg by mouth once; or ofloxacin, 400 mg by mouth once

Spectinomycin is recommended by the CDC for the treatment of persons with resistant strains of *N. gonorrhoeae.*

Because of the inconvenience of IM injections and concern about the possible needle-sticks associated with IM injections in persons who may also have HIV, a recent study using oral medication was undertaken.[6] As a result of the study, the following recommendations were made by the CDC for the treatment of uncomplicated gonococcal infections: ceftriaxone, 125 mg IM in a single dose, or cefixime, 400 mg orally in a single dose, or ciprofloxacin, 500 mg orally in a single dose, or ofloxacin, 400 mg orally in a single dose, plus a regimen effective against possible coinfection with *C. trachomatis,* such as doxycycline, 100 mg orally twice daily for 7 days.

### Other Interventions

Facilitating learning, providing emotional and social support, promoting self-care, and promoting healthy sexual attitudes are important interventions. They are discussed earlier in the chapter (see p. 1861).

## ♦ EVALUATION

The questions to be answered in evaluation are the same for all STDs (see p. 1862).

# SYPHILIS

## ETIOLOGY

**Syphilis** is caused by a spirochete, *Treponema pallidum,* that gains entry into the body through either the mucous membrane or skin during intercourse. The organism is readily destroyed by physical and chemical agents, including heat, drying, and mild disinfectants such as soap and water.

The incubation period for syphilis is usually 3 weeks. However, symptoms can appear as early as 9 days or as long as 3 months after exposure, which is the case for rectal infections in homosexual men.

## EPIDEMIOLOGY

Reported cases of syphilis reached an all-time high during World War II, with 575,593 cases being reported in 1943. The number of cases dropped sharply in the 1950s and began to rise again in the 1960s. There was a steady yearly increase in the number of cases until 1977, when the total number of cases leveled off, until 1986, when the number of cases increased.

Recently there has been a dramatic increase in the number of cases of infectious syphilis (primary and secondary) reported to the CDC. The number of cases increased more than 55% between 1986 and 1989. In 1990 there were 50,223 reported cases of syphilis, which was the single largest yearly total since 1948[5,11] (Figures 55-7 and 55-8).

As mentioned earlier in the chapter, the current syphilis epidemic is occurring primarily among young, heterosexual minority populations and is believed to be related to cocaine use and the exchange of sex for drugs. This same population is at risk for HIV infection, and treatment of syphilis is more problematic in the presence of HIV infection.[11]

The incidence of syphilis went down among homosexual/bisexual men, especially White males. This decrease in incidence is believed to result from safer sexual practices by this population because of education about how to prevent HIV infection.

The cause of the increase in syphilis is unknown but

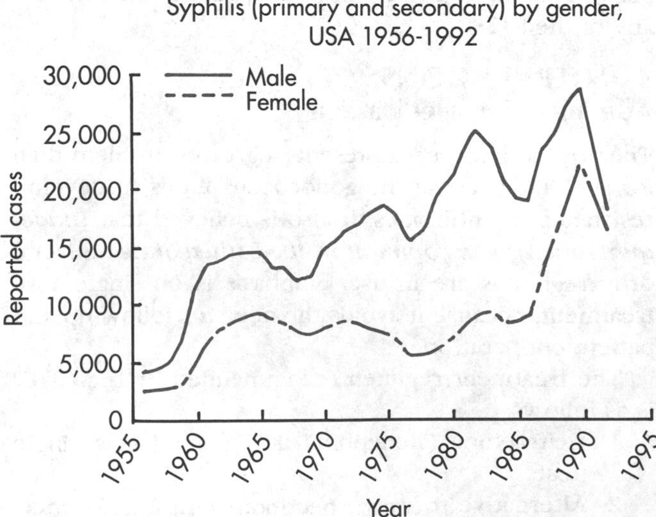


**FIGURE 55-7** Incidence of primary and secondary syphilis in the United States by gender, 1956 to 1992. (From Centers for Disease Control: Graphs and maps for selected notifiable diseases in the United States, *MMWR* 41[55]:13-64, 1993.)

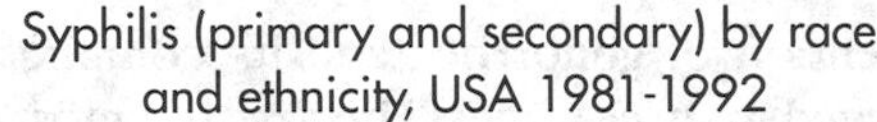


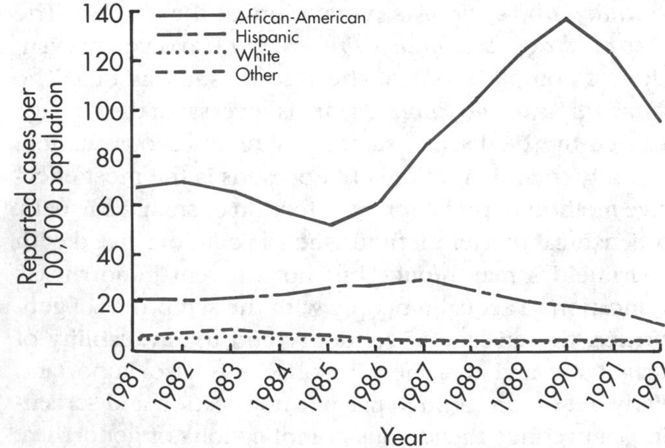


**FIGURE 55-8** Incidence of primary and secondary syphilis in the United States by race and ethnicity, 1981 to 1992. (From Centers for Disease Control: Graphs and maps for selected notifiable diseases in the United States, *MMWR* 41[55]:13-64, 1993.)

suggests a shift in epidemiology of the disease in the United States. Possible reasons for this increase identified by the CDC include the following:

1. Anecdotal reports from persons interviewing syphilis patients and their sexual partners indicate that prostitution that involves *nonintravenous* drugs (especially "crack" cocaine) may be partially responsible.
2. Routine use of spectinomycin to treat gonorrhea in areas where resistant strains of *N. gonorrhoeae* are common may have contributed to the increase in syphilis *because spectinomycin does not appear to cure incubating syphilis.* This is supported by data from New York City, Florida, and Los Angeles, where spectinomycin was widely used to treat resistant strains of *N. gonorrhoeae.* However, it does not explain the nationwide increase in syphilis.[11]
3. In some of the high-incidence areas there had been a decrease in the amount of money allocated to syphilis control programs, and fewer interviewers were available in six of the high-incidence areas. However, the relationship between the number of interviewers and the increase in the incidence of syphilis was *not* statistically significant.[11]

The increases in infectious syphilis among females and heterosexuals are causing concern for three reasons:

1. An increase in syphilis in females will probably be followed by increased incidence of and deaths from congenital syphilis.
2. The marked increase in syphilis among inner-city, heterosexual minority groups indicates that *high-risk sexual activity is increasing despite the risk of HIV infection.* This is especially alarming, because among these groups risks are already increased because of the high prevalence of intravenous drug abuse in their communities.
3. Studies in Africa and in the United States suggest that genital ulcer diseases such as primary syphilis increase the risk of HIV transmission.[4]

The trends for early congenital syphilis have paralleled the trends for primary and secondary syphilis among women. Factors thought to contribute to the sustained level of early congenital syphilis are (1) an increase in the incidence of early infectious syphilis among pregnant women, (2) lack of available prenatal care, and (3) failure of the prenatal system to provide timely serologic testing and prompt follow-up.

In addition, it is believed that the greatest percentage of cases of syphilis go unreported, and thus the incidence is much greater than the figures indicate.

## PATHOPHYSIOLOGY

The signs and symptoms of the four stages of syphilis are listed in Table 55-4. If syphilis is adequately diagnosed and treated during the primary stage, the other stages can be prevented.

## PREVENTION

As with gonorrhea, three levels of prevention are important. *Primary prevention* is prevention of the initial infection by finding and treating those with the disease so that they cannot spread it to others. *Secondary prevention* is directed at early treatment of cases to prevent

**TABLE 55-4 Stages of Syphilis**

| PRIMARY | SECONDARY | LATENT | LATE |
|---|---|---|---|
| **DURATION** | | | |
| 2-8 wk | Appears 2-4 wk after chancre appears; extends over 2-4 yr | 5-20 yr | Terminal if not treated |
| **SIGNS AND SYMPTOMS** | | | |
| Hard sore or pimple on vulva or penis that breaks and forms painless, draining chancre; may be a single chancre or groups of more than one; may be present also on lips, tongue, hands, rectum, or nipples; chancre heals, leaving almost invisible scar | Depends on site; low-grade fever, headache, anorexia, weight loss, anemia, sore throat, hoarseness, reddened and sore eyes, jaundice with or without hepatitis, aching of joints, muscles, long bones; sores on body or generalized fine rash; condylomata acuminata (venereal warts) on rectum or genitalia | No clinical signs | Tumorlike mass (gumma) on any area of body; damage to heart valves and blood vessels; meningitis; paralysis; lack of coordination; paresis; insomnia; confusion; delusions; impaired judgment; slurred speech |
| **COMMUNICABILITY** | | | |
| Exudates from lesions and chancre are highly contagious | Exudates from lesions highly contagious; blood contains organisms | Contagious for about 2 yr; not contagious to others after that; blood contains organisms; may be transmitted placentally to fetus | Noncontagious; spinal fluid may contain organisms |

late syphilis or congenital syphilis. Finally, as *tertiary prevention,* efforts can be made to treat the complications of syphilis when they occur. Contact investigation, which is necessary for all STDs, is discussed on p. 1857.

## NURSING MANAGEMENT

### ♦ ASSESSMENT

The subjective and objective data to be collected from a person suspected of having any STD are discussed on p. 1860.

### Diagnostic Tests

Syphilis is most often diagnosed by standard serologic tests. Massive screening programs in the past made serologic diagnosis of syphilis very common. Mass screening with the VDRL test is no longer practiced except in high-risk populations, pregnant women, sexually active women, and couples who are applying for a marriage license. Dark-field microscopic examination of tissue scrapings from lesions or material obtained by aspiration of regional lymph nodes also reveals the presence of the spirochete, especially during the primary and secondary stages. A presumptive diagnosis is made on the basis of suspicious lesions, positive serologic tests, known exposure to infection, and involvement of regional lymph nodes. False-positive VDRL reactions are common among persons previously treated for syphilis, but fluorescent treponemal antibody (FTA) and absorption (ABS) tests are more specific (Table 55-5). *Also, once a VDRL test is positive, it remains so and is not useful for identifying reinfection.* Infectious mononucleosis; hepatitis; pregnancy; viral pneumonia; malaria; chickenpox, measles, and smallpox vaccination; narcotic addiction; and terminal malignancy have also been associated with false-positive VDRL results.

**TABLE 55-5 Serologic Tests for Syphilis (STS)**

| DESCRIPTION | EXAMPLES | COMMENTS |
|---|---|---|
| **FLOCCULATION** | | |
| Antibody-antigen reaction produces a precipitation (flocculation) | VDRL<br>RPR | Used primarily for screening; performed in standard laboratories |
| **COMPLEMENT FIXATION** | | |
| Complement is used up in antigen-antibody reaction (fixed); hemolysis occurs | Reiter (Wasserman outdated) | Nonspecific; used less frequently; performed in standard laboratories |
| **FLUORESCENT ANTIBODY** | | |
| Antigen of killed *Treponema pallidum* is labeled with a fluorescent dye | FTA<br>FTA-ABS | More specific than flocculation or complement-fixation test; differentiates false-positive from true-positive results; performed in special laboratories |
| ***T. PALLIDUM* IMMOBILIZATION** | | |
| Serum is mixed with live *T. pallidum*; presence of antibody decreases organism mobility | TPI | Most sensitive test; performed only at CDC laboratory in Atlanta |

### ♦ INTERVENTIONS

#### Administering Medications

Syphilis can be successfully treated at any stage of the disease, although treatment may have to be more prolonged in latent and late syphilis. Even though syphilis can be cured in late stages, the damage to the body is much more difficult to manage.

Because penicillin continues to be effective in the treatment of syphilis, it remains the drug of choice. All types of penicillin are effective, but penicillin G benzathine is preferred because it is long acting and can be given in a limited number of injections.

Patients with primary, secondary, and latent syphilis (and their sexual partners) are usually given 2.4 million units of penicillin intramuscularly in one dose. Patients with late syphilis are generally given 2.4 million units intramuscularly at 7-day intervals until a total of 7.2 to 9.6 million units has been given. When the use of penicillin is contraindicated because of drug sensitivity, doxycycline, 100 mg orally twice per day for 2 weeks, or tetracycline, 500 mg orally four times per day for 2 weeks, is given. For persons who cannot take tetracycline, erythromycin, 500 mg four times per day for 2 weeks, may be given. Compliance with any oral treatment regimen can be difficult, especially when the person is a chronic drug abuser and engages in other high-risk behaviors. The patient will need follow-up reminders to take the drug as prescribed.

If there is a question of whether or not the person is allergic to penicillin, penicillin skin tests and desensitization should be considered (see Chapter 70).[14]

Pregnant women with penicillin sensitivity pose problems for treatment. In the large dosage required to treat syphilis, tetracycline produces mottling and staining of fetal teeth and possible abnormal bone formation. If the woman is given the usual adult dose, inadequate placental transfer of tetracycline is likely, and congenital syphilis would probably develop. Erythromycin in a dose of 30 g over a period of 15 days seems to be the best alternative treatment for pregnant women with syphilis. Neurosyphilis is treated with intravenous penicillin. Sexual partners are treated with 2.4 million units of penicillin G benzathine.

### Other Interventions

The nurse's role in the care of patients with syphilis is the same as for other STDs and includes facilitating learning, providing social and emotional support, promoting self-care, and promoting healthy sexual attitudes. All of these are discussed earlier in this chapter (see p. 1861).

## ♦ EVALUATION

The outcomes to be evaluated are the same as for any patient with an STD (see p. 1862).

# HERPES GENITALIS

## ETIOLOGY

**Herpes genitalis** (genital herpes, HSV-2) is caused by infection with *Herpesvirus hominis* type 2 (HSV-2).

## EPIDEMIOLOGY

Herpes genitalis was the most important STD of the 1970s. Its chronicity, frequent recurrences, and difficult treatment and prevention distinguish it from other STDs. It is estimated that about 400,000 to 600,000 new cases occur annually.[6] It is believed that at least one in six Americans now suffer from genital herpes and that because of poor control measures the number of cases is increasing dramatically. Its peak incidence parallels the young age groups affected by other STDs. Once acquired, herpes genitalis is a lifelong disease and carries with it not only intense and recurrent discomfort, but also anxieties about future childbearing, malignancy, and sexual and marital function. In early pregnancy, women infected with herpes have an increased chance of miscarriage. Because genital herpetic lesions endanger the fetus during delivery, cesarean delivery is often necessary. Genital herpes has also been associated with cervical cancer. It is now generally accepted that HSV-2 is spread by sexual contact.[5]

## PATHOPHYSIOLOGY

The incubation period is 3 to 7 days. The primary lesion appears as a vesicle on the external genitalia in men; often in the rectum in homosexual men; and on the vagina, cervix, or external genitalia in women. These lesions often ulcerate, especially when located on moist surfaces. Following primary herpes, the virus persists in a *latent* or *unrecognized* form in most patients. It is believed that **latent infections** are localized in the ganglia of sensory nerves to the genitalia. When the host factors favor it, the *latent infection* becomes clinically apparent as *recurrent herpes*.

The common signs and symptoms of primary herpetic infection follow:

1. Local inflammation
2. Pain
3. Enlargement of inguinal lymph nodes
4. Generalized signs of infection
   a. Photophobia
   b. Headache
   c. Flulike symptoms

Although primary herpetic lesions begin as single or multiple reddish papules, they then develop into clear, fluid-filled vesicles. Once they rupture they form ulcerations that may fuse with other lesions to form large ulcerated areas. The disease tends to be more extensive in women than in men. In some women cervical infection accompanies the external lesions, and in certain cases it may be the only infected site. Cervical involvement may be mild or severe with extensive ulceration and pus. Genital lesions often worsen during the first 10 to 15 days but usually heal within 3 to 4 weeks. These symptoms usually lead the individual to seek medical attention.

Vaginal discharge is common among women, and discharge from the urethra is usual in men having primary infections. Urinary tract involvement may occur and is reflected in symptoms of dysuria or urinary retention. The lesions can cause severe pain, requiring hospitalization for parenteral analgesia. Subclinical infections in which patients are unaware of any problem occur in only about 10% of the cases of genital herpes. Unfortunately, about 75% of all patients have at least one recurrence. Fortunately, recurrent infections are usually milder and of shorter duration than primary infections and usually produce local rather than systemic reaction. The patient experiencing a recurrent infection often has prodromal signs of paresthesia and burning at the site where the lesion will erupt. Factors known to predispose to recurrent infection include fever, emotional upsets, premenstrual states, and overexposure to heat and sunshine. Although the mode of recurrent infection is not clear, it has been theorized that during primary infection the virus ascends sensory nerve sheaths, localizing in corresponding nerve ganglia, and that when the environment becomes favorable, the virus is reactivated. Recurrent herpes usually begins with an abnormal sensation or itching of a localized genital area. Lesions of recurrent infections usually occur at the site of the primary infection. Herpes encephalitis may also occur.

## PREVENTION

### Primary Prevention

Primary prevention of herpes depends on limiting sexual contact between infected individuals and uninfected partners. Evidence indicates that the herpes virus may survive on towels for up to 20 minutes; therefore it is important to use separate linens. *Refraining from sexual intercourse while lesions are present and for 10 days after they heal is essential.* Sexually active young persons should be taught to examine themselves and prospective partners for such lesions. In some communities, groups of individuals with herpes have chosen to restrict themselves to sexual contact only with others who already have been exposed to herpes. Condoms may be helpful. Transmission to the fetus may be prevented by cesarean delivery. Infected neonates may develop subsequent mental retardation or die. If drug therapy for HSV-2 is effective, it will help limit new infections by eradicating at least some of the reservoir of infected individuals by preventing reactivation of HSV-2.

### Secondary Prevention

Secondary prevention is aimed at reducing or eliminating complications such as cervical cancer. A yearly Pap smear is recommended. Another important complication of herpes genitalis is its ability to create great psychologic pain and anxiety, to disrupt normal social and sexual relationships, and to stigmatize its victims. In the event that secondary prevention is not possible, efforts to detect and treat cervical cancer in its early stages are essential.

## NURSING MANAGEMENT

### ♦ ASSESSMENT

The subjective and objective data to be collected from any person suspected of having an STD are discussed on p. 1860.

### Diagnostic Tests

Diagnosis of herpes genitalis is made by isolation of the virus from specimens obtained from lesions. Pap smears or fluid from the vesicles collected in transport medium demonstrates cellular characteristics of viruses.

### ♦ INTERVENTIONS

### Providing Symptomatic Therapy

Treatment for genital herpes has most often been symptomatic, because there is no known cure for the disease. Acyclovir appears capable of inhibiting the replication of herpetic viruses. For primary herpetic infection, acyclovir is prescribed, 200 mg orally every 4 hours (while the patient is awake) for 10 days. It should be started as soon as prodromal signs appear. If severe constitutional symptoms develop, the person may need to be admitted to the hospital for intravenous acyclovir, 10 mg per kg per day in three divided doses. If recurrences of genital herpes occur six or more times per year, prophylactic or suppressive therapy may be recommended. In this case acyclovir, 200 mg orally three times daily for 1 year or 400 mg orally twice daily, is the dose ordered.[12] The acyclovir treatment reduces viral shedding and the duration of the disease in patients with primary initial infections who are treated within 6 days of the onset of symptoms. It does not prevent recurrences. No effective treatment prevents recurrences or shortens their duration.

Symptomatic treatment consists of using Burow's solution or hydrogen peroxide and soap and water to cleanse the lesions. The involved areas are blown dry with a hair dryer. Women are advised to use a mirror to examine the vulva, vagina, and cervix for hidden lesions.

### Facilitating Learning

Persons with herpes should *abstain from sexual contact while the lesions are present and for 10 days after the lesions heal.* Risk of transmission during asymptomatic periods is unknown. Some experts advise using condoms to prevent transmission of the disease.

### Providing Social and Emotional Support

Because herpes genitalis is a recurrent disease with no cure, patients infected with the virus require considerable support. Some infected persons withdraw from an active social life rather than face the possibility of making a commitment that will require them to share knowledge of their disease with another person. For this reason, in some communities support groups have been formed for persons who have herpes genitalis.

## CHLAMYDIAL INFECTION

### ETIOLOGY

*Chlamydia trachomatis* is caused by the gram-negative obligate *C. trachomatis.*

### EPIDEMIOLOGY

**Chlamydial infection** is recognized as the most prevalent of the STDs in the United States. Because it is not a reportable disease, the actual number of cases is unknown. It is estimated, however, that each year more than 4 million Americans experience epidemic chlamydial infections.

Chlamydial infections are responsible for about 20% to 30% of diagnosed PID cases, and it is estimated that about 11,000 women each year become involuntarily sterilized and 36,000 suffer ectopic pregnancies as a result of this organism.[17] Chlamydial infections can be transmitted to infants during delivery, causing conjunctivitis and pneumonia in many.

*C. trachomatis* is the leading cause of pneumonia in infants less than 6 months of age. The rate of infection with pneumonia is 3 to 10 per 1000 live births and may go as high as 50 to 60 per 1000 in areas where *C. trachomatis* is epidemic. The organism has superseded *N. gonorrhoeae* as a cause of neonatal conjunctivitis.[10]

The incidence of chlamydia is highest in young, promiscuous, indigent, unmarried women who live in the inner city and in those who have had a prior history of STD.

### PATHOPHYSIOLOGY

*C. trachomatis* is a parasite that has specific requirements for adenosine triphosphate (ATP) and amino acids. There are two stages in the life cycle of the organism. In *stage 1,* the *infective stage,* the *elementary body attaches* to the host cell and is ingested by phagocytosis. In *stage 2,* the *elementary body undergoes metamorphosis* to become a *reticulate or initial body.* This is the *metabolic phase* of the life cycle. The initial body duplicates by binary fission and changes into the

**TABLE 55-6 Chlamydia Trachomatis Infections**

| MALES | FEMALES | INFANTS |
|---|---|---|
| **TRANSMISSION** | | |
| Males ⟷ | Females → | Infants |
| **INFECTIONS** | | |
| Urethritis | Cervicitis | Conjunctivitis |
| Postgonococcal urethritis | Urethritis | Pneumonia |
| Proctitis | Proctitis | Asymptomatic pharyngeal carriage |
| Conjunctivitis | Conjunctivitis | Asymptomatic gastrointestinal carriage |
| Pharyngitis | Pharyngitis | |
| Subclinical lymphogranuloma venereum | Subclinical lymphogranuloma venereum | |
| **COMPLICATIONS** | | |
| Epididymitis | Salpingitis | |
| Prostatitis | Endometritis | |
| Reiter's syndrome | Perihepatitis | |
| Sterility | Ectopic pregnancy | |
| Rectal strictures* | Infertility | |
| | Vulvar/rectal carcinoma* | |
| | Rectal strictures* | |

From Centers for Disease Control: Chlamydia trachomatis infections, policy guidelines for prevention and control, *MMWR* 35(suppl):54, 1985.

*Associated with lymphogranuloma venereum.

elementary body. The host cell, which contains the elementary bodies, undergoes lysis, liberating infectious organisms that are capable of reinfecting new cells.[10]

Serotypes L1, L2, and L3 are responsible for lymphogranuloma venereum, which is common in South America and the far East.

Serotypes D through K cause chlamydial infections. It is estimated that between 20% and 40% of sexually active women have been exposed to the bacterium and have antibody titers to *C. trachomatis.*[10] Table 55-6 shows how the infection can be transmitted between male and female sexual partners and from females to infants. It also lists the various ways the disease is manifested in males, females, and infants.

## PREVENTION

*Primary prevention* of chlamydial infections consists of limiting sexual contact with infected partners. *Secondary prevention* requires early diagnosis and treatment.

Risk assessment factors require special attention. Age, number of sex partners, socioeconomic status, and sexual preference are predictors of infection with *C. trachomatis*[1]:

1. Age—Infection rates are two to three times higher in sexually active women under age 20 years than in those over age 20 years. The rates for women between 20 and 29 years of age are considerably higher than for women over age 30 years. The rates of urethral infection are higher for teenage males than for adult men.
2. Number of sex partners—Persons with several sex partners are at higher risk of infection.
3. Socioeconomic status—Some studies have shown that persons of lower socioeconomic status are at increased risk for infection with *C. trachomatis.*
4. Sexual preference—The prevalence of urethral chlamydial infection among homosexual men is one third that among heterosexual men. However, 4% to 8% of homosexual men seen in STD clinics have rectal chlamydia infection.

**BOX 55-4 Clinical Clues Used to Diagnose Chlamydia in Women**

- Purulent discharge
- Endocervical mucus
- Spotting after intercourse
- Spotting between periods
- Vague lower abdominal pain
- Cervical atypia (not normal)
- Infertility
- *C. trachomatis* should be looked for when there is premature rupture of amniotic membranes

Data from Faro S: *Chlamydia trachomatis* infection. In Rakel RE, editor: *Conn's current therapy 1991,* Philadelphia, 1991, WB Saunders.

**BOX 55-5 Clinical Findings With Chlamydial Infection**

- Presence of mucus in the endocervical canal
- Microscopic examination
  - Presence of WBCs
  - Absence of bacteria on Gram stain
  - Decrease of 10 squamous epithelial cells per high-powered field
- Hypertrophy of columnar epithelium of endocervix
- Pyuria but no bacteria on Gram stain or culture of urine

From Faro S: *Chlamydia trachomatis* infection. In Rakel RE, editor: *Conn's current therapy 1991,* Philadelphia, 1991, WB Saunders.

## NURSING MANAGEMENT

### ♦ ASSESSMENT

#### Subjective and Objective Data

The clinical clues used to diagnose chlamydia in women are presented in Box 55-4. Men usually have nonspecific urethritis or may seek treatment for epididymitis. However, up to 80% of women and 25% of men may be asymptomatic.

Box 55-5 lists the clinical findings in women with *C. trachomatis* infection.

### Diagnostic Tests

*C. trachomatis* infection may be diagnosed by traditional tissue culture or by one of the new rapid tests listed below.

1. Enzyme immunoassay (EIA) (chlamydiazime or test patch [Abbott])
2. Direct immunofluorescence—several of which are commercially available.
3. If none of the above are available, a tentative diagnosis can be made by microscopic examination of an endocervical specimen.

## ♦ INTERVENTIONS

### Administering Medications

1. Doxycycline, 100 mg orally twice per day for 7 days, or
2. Azithromycin, 1 g orally in a single dose
3. During pregnancy, erythromycin, 500 mg orally four times per day for 7 days, or
4. Erythromycin ethyl succinate, 400 to 800 mg orally four times per day for 7 days

Because neonatal infection rates of infants of untreated women approach 50%, all women diagnosed during pregnancy should receive treatment. Their sexual partners must be treated simultaneously; otherwise the women can be reinfected. The follow-up culture should be performed 7 to 14 days after treatment is completed.[7,10]

Patients with PID being treated with cephalosporin must also be given an agent effective against chlamydia, such as doxycycline or erythromycin.

### Facilitating Learning

It is important that the patient encourage sexual partner(s) to seek care as soon as possible to avoid reinfection of the patient and complications in the partner. Patients who are sexually active should be advised to wear condoms or use spermicides to reduce reinfection.

### Providing Social and Emotional Support

Social and emotional support of these patients is as important as it is with any person with an STD (see p. 1861).

# LYMPHOGRANULOMA VENEREUM

## ETIOLOGY

**Lymphogranuloma venereum** is a systemic STD caused by serotypes $L_1$, $L_2$, and $L_3$ of *C. trachomatis*. Other species of *Chlamydia* are the causative organisms of trachoma and psittacosis. The disease is contracted by vaginal, anal, or oral intercourse; primary inoculation with the organism may occur at any site involved in close contact. The incubation period is 7 to 12 days. Lymphadenitis of regional lymph nodes draining the site of primary infection occurs, and the disease spreads by way of the lymphatic system.

## EPIDEMIOLOGY

Lymphogranuloma venereum is most prevalent in the tropics. In the United States it is found most often in the southern states, but epidemiologic studies are needed to determine its true incidence. Reports of the incidence of lymphogranuloma venereum indicate that there are less than 500 cases annually. The symptoms of lymphogranuloma venereum resemble those of other STDs, and its reported incidence may be influenced by this fact.

## PATHOPHYSIOLOGY

The three clinical phases of infection in lymphogranuloma venereum are (1) inoculation and appearance of the primary lesions, (2) lymphatic spread and generalized symptoms, and (3) late complications. In individual cases any one of the phases may be absent or go unnoticed.

The primary lesion, which is transient, appears as a papule, small erosion, or vesicle. The most common sites of the primary lesion are the prepuce and glans in men and the vagina and cervix in women. Because it is painless, the primary lesion may go unnoticed, especially in women. Localized edema may be present. If the rectum is infected, a bloody discharge is followed by a mucopurulent discharge, diarrhea, and cramping.

Involvement of the lymphatics occurs 1 to 4 weeks after the appearance of the primary lesion. If the primary lesion is on the penis, anal margin, clitoris, or upper vulva, the superficial inguinal lymph nodes are involved. Infection of the vagina or cervix as the primary site produces involvement of the deep iliac and anorectal lymph nodes. The large lymph nodes or *buboes* that appear are firm and lobular. The skin over the superficial nodes is bluish red and adheres to the nodes.

# NURSING MANAGEMENT

## ♦ ASSESSMENT

### Subjective and Objective Data

The first indication of infection in most patients is a feeling of stiffness and aching in the groin followed by swelling in the inguinal area. Symptoms of nongonococcal urethritis may be present. Constitutional symptoms of infection may or may not appear at this time. The involved lymph nodes may suppurate, causing extensive scarring. Obstruction of the lymphatics may result, leading to chronic edema and ulceration. Lymphatic spread of the infection is accompanied by generalized symptoms. Mild to severe fever, malaise, nausea, and vomiting may occur. Abdominal pain, symptoms of cystitis, and urinary retention are common when pelvic lymph nodes are involved. Acute proctocolitis is common in homosexual men.

Among the most severe complications of lymphogranuloma venereum are development of perianal abscesses, rectovaginal or rectovesical fistulas, and rectal strictures. In the last clinical phase, generalized infection is indicated by blood values showing anemia, leukocytosis, and an elevated sedimentation rate.

### Diagnostic Tests

Lymphogranuloma venereum is isolated from aspirate from an affected lymph node. The lymphogranuloma venereum complement-fixation test (LGV-CFT) is a test for antibodies. A positive LGV-CFT test along with a careful history and physical examination affords the best chances for diagnosing lymphogranuloma venereum.

## ♦ INTERVENTIONS

### Administering Medications

Early antibiotic therapy is essential for controlling and reducing morbidity from lymphogranuloma venereum, and it is generally agreed that treatment should not be delayed until diagnostic test results are obtained. Doxycycline, 100 mg twice daily for 21 days, is given. Alternative regimens are erythromycin, 500 mg orally four times per day for 21 days, or sulfisoxazole, 500 mg orally four times per day for 21 days.

Patients should be observed clinically until signs and symptoms are resolved. Sexual partners should receive the same therapy. If lymphadenopathy does not respond to therapy in 1 to 2 weeks, an alternate drug may be required. In some patients therapy must be continued for as long as 6 weeks. Sexual partners should also receive the therapy for the same period of time.

### Other Interventions

Fluctuant lymph nodes may be aspirated with a large-bore needle and syringe to prevent tissue breakdown and the formation of draining sinuses.[20] If rectal stricture occurs, rectal dilation at 2-week intervals may be attempted. Development of fistulas is especially distressing and requires surgical repair. Lymphogranuloma venereum is characterized by remissions and exacerbations; thorough surveillance is important. Antibiotics should be reinstituted as soon as symptoms of reactivation occur. *Biopsy of lesions and lymph nodes is advised in chronic lymphogranuloma venereum, because cancer may develop in the ulcerative lesions and may be overlooked because of similarity in appearance.*

### Providing Support

These patients may require much counseling and teaching as they deal with their disease. Because the fluctuant lymph nodes may be disturbing to the patient's self-image, social and emotional support is very important. See p. 1861 for more discussion of these topics.

---

# CHANCROID

## ETIOLOGY

**Chancroid** is an STD caused by a gram-negative bacillus, *Haemophilus ducreyi.* Before 1980 fewer than 1000 cases were reported yearly in the United States. Since then the number of reported cases has increased to 4000 to 5000 cases yearly.[15]

## EPIDEMIOLOGY

Since the early 1980s epidemics associated with prostitutes have occurred in Boston, New York City, Dallas, Florida, and Orange County, California.

Although it is found worldwide, chancroid is most prevalent in tropical and semitropical areas in the Orient, the West Indies, and North Africa. The disease occurs more often in men and more often among non-White people. It is possible that returning military personnel may have introduced the disease into areas where it did not previously exist. The incubation period varies from 1 to 14 days and averages 4 to 5 days.

Chancroid has been established as a cofactor for HIV transmission, and a high rate of HIV infection among patients with chancroid has been reported in the United States and other countries. As many as 10% of patients with chancroid may be coinfected with *Treponema pallidum* or HSV.[8]

## PATHOPHYSIOLOGY

The initial lesions are acutely tender genital ulcers, lymphadenopathy, and tender buboes. The buboes may suppurate and lead to abscesses. Exudate from the ulcers or aspirate from the buboes is stained, and a "school-of-fish" pattern may be noted on microscopic examination by someone experienced in interpretation.[15]

## NURSING MANAGEMENT

## ♦ ASSESSMENT

### Subjective and Objective Data

In women the lesions of chancroid are most often found on the labia, anus, clitoris, vagina, and cervix. A few women do not have any lesions but may have signs of mild vaginitis. In men the lesions appear on the prepuce, glans, or shaft of the penis.

The ulcers found in chancroid are typically ragged and irregular. They are highly infectious, and autoimmunity may occur, resulting in multiple lesions. The ulcers appear excavated; have a granulating, purulent surface; and are painful. Often, edema of the surrounding tissues is present. Involvement of the inguinal lymph nodes occurs in about 50% of all cases of chancroid within 2 weeks after appearance of the primary lesion. The buboes are most often unilateral, painful, and spheric in shape. The skin over the buboes is inflamed. The buboes tend to become softer as abscesses form. These abscesses in turn may suppurate and rupture, further spreading the infection. Generalized symptoms of infection usually appear when inguinal abscesses form.

### Diagnostic Tests

Diagnosis of chancroid depends on growth of the organism on special media. A specimen is collected by aspiration of a vesicle, pustule, or lymph node or from the margin of an ulcer. Sensitivity testing has become more important, because antibiotic resistance is increasing.

### ♦ INTERVENTIONS

#### Administering Medications

The treatment of choice is erythromycin, 500 mg orally four times daily for 7 days, or ceftriaxone, 250 mg IM once, or Azithromycin 1 g orally in a single dose. Other antimicrobial therapies are available but are not considered to be as effective. Plasma-mediated resistance to tetracycline has been documented in the United States and in other countries where chancroid is endemic.

#### Other Interventions

Suppurative buboes are aspirated, preferably through normal skin. Warm saline compresses may be helpful for ulcerations.

#### Facilitating Learning

Patient follow-up is essential, because treatment failure can occur. The patient is taught to report any signs or symptoms that persist or worsen during treatment. Patients should be advised to abstain from sexual activity until all lesions are healed. Proper use of a condom should also be stressed (see Box 55-2).

## GRANULOMA INGUINALE (DONOVANOSIS)

### ETIOLOGY

**Granuloma inguinale**, or granuloma venereum, is believed to be most often transmitted by sexual contact, although nonsexual transmission has been reported. The infection is caused by a gram-negative bacillus, *Calymmatobacterium (Donovania) granulomatis*, widely referred to as *Donovan bacillus*. The organism is related to *Klebsiella*. The incubation period is uncertain but is about 8 to 12 weeks.

### EPIDEMIOLOGY

Donovanosis is common in tropical and subtropical areas and rarely occurs in the United States. It is very common in New Guinea, India, and the Caribbean. The disease is mildly contagious and probably requires repeated exposures for spread of infection. Predisposing factors are poorly understood. The disease is more common in men than women and is especially common among homosexual men. The incubation period varies from several days to several months.

### NURSING MANAGEMENT

### ♦ ASSESSMENT

#### Subjective and Objective Data

Lesions appear on the genitalia and in the perianal area. The most common sites of lesions are the prepuce and glans in men and the vagina and labia in women. The infection first appears with development of subcutaneous nodules. These elevated areas eventually ulcerate, producing sharply defined, painless lesions. The ulcers enlarge slowly and bleed on contact. With ulceration the infection tends to spread along the pubic region. Involvement of the lymph nodes is uncommon but can occur and produce occlusion of the lymphatics, resulting in elephantiasis.

#### Diagnostic Tests

Smears of exudates taken from the lesions do not always demonstrate the causative organism, even when donovanosis is present. Therefore a sample of tissue is taken from the lesion, crushed between two slides, and stained with Wright's or Giesma stain. The specimen is examined for the presence of Donovan bodies, which represent the intracellular stage of the causative organism. Examination of a tissue sample also makes it possible to differentiate between donovanosis and cancer.

### ♦ INTERVENTIONS

#### Administering Medications

There is no standard treatment. Tetracycline, 500 mg four times per day for 14 to 21 days, is the treatment of choice. If tetracycline fails, streptomycin or gentamicin may be prescribed.

## TRICHOMONIASIS

### ETIOLOGY

A protozoan, *Trichomonas vaginalis*, is the causative organism of **trichomoniasis.** Evidence suggests that the incubation period ranges between 4 and 28 days.[13]

### EPIDEMIOLOGY

Trichomoniasis may well be the most frequently acquired STD in the United States, with an estimated incidence of 3 million cases occurring annually. *T. vaginalis* organisms are found in 3% to 15% of women under the care of private physicians, 13% to 23% of women attending gynecologic clinics, and 50% of women who have gonorrhea. It is most often sexually transmitted. The parasite commonly exists in vaginal and cervical secretions and in seminal fluid. It is estimated that one of five females will have a trichomonal infection during her lifetime.

### PATHOPHYSIOLOGY

Trichomoniasis is frequently viewed as an innocuous infection, yet there are serious implications for health. During the postpartum period in women who have trichomoniasis, the rate of persistent fever, prolonged vaginal discharge, and endometritis is twice as high as in women who do not harbor the organism. About 90% of patients with trichomoniasis have cervical erosions and leukorrhea, and it has been suggested that chronic irritation may predispose to cervical cancer. Interpretation of cervical cytology, as in the Pap test, is unreliable in the presence of trichomoniasis, because the infection produces atypical cervical cells. Unless repeated cervical smears are taken, cancer of the cervix may be missed. Trichomoniasis results in urethritis; it also causes prostatitis in men 40% of the time; and, finally, reversible sterility can occur as a result of inhibition of sperm motility by toxins produced by the organism.

## NURSING MANAGEMENT

### ♦ ASSESSMENT

#### Subjective and Objective Data

Only 25% of women harboring the organism are asymptomatic. Pruritus of the vulva and vagina is the predominant symptom among women. The itching may be so severe as to awaken the patient from sleep, and excoriation from scratching is common. Secondary infection of the broken skin may result.

Classically, the symptoms of trichomoniasis in women are a copious, frothy, green or greenish yellow vaginal discharge, inflammation of the labia minora and lower vagina, and a red-speckled appearance of the vaginal canal and cervix known as "strawberry patches." Only a small number of patients present this classic picture that is usually described in texts.[13] Most patients have a vaginal discharge, but it is small in amount and white and watery, and there is some inflammation of the labia and vagina. Itching is almost universally present, however; and dyspareunia, dysuria, and urinary frequency may also occur.

In men, urethritis and its symptoms of purulent discharge, itching, burning, and inflammation are the signs of trichomoniasis most often seen. Prostatitis, epididymitis, and urethral stricture may occur as complications among men. However, these consequences of trichomoniasis have not been extensively studied and are not well documented.

#### Diagnostic Tests

Diagnosis of trichomoniasis is most often made by preparing a hanging drop slide containing a specimen of the discharge and observing the motile organism under the microscope. Serologic and skin tests are currently being investigated but lack reliability so far. Because of the high incidence of coexisting gonorrhea, smears or cultures for gonococci should also be taken.

### ♦ INTERVENTIONS

#### Administering Medications

The recommended treatment is metronidazole (Flagyl), 2 g by mouth in a single dose. An alternative regimen would be metronidazole increased to 500 mg orally two times per day for 7 days.

The CDC recommends that both partners be treated simultaneously to prevent reinfection by the untreated partner at a later date. Vaginal inserts of metronidazole are less effective. The drug is known to cross the placental barrier. For this reason it is not given to pregnant women until after the first trimester.

# BACTERIAL VAGINOSIS

## ETIOLOGY

**Bacterial vaginosis** can be cultured from 23% to 96% of women with vaginitis and is recovered from up to 50% of asymptomatic women.

## NURSING MANAGEMENT

### ♦ ASSESSMENT

#### Subjective and Objective Data

Bacterial vaginosis infection is characterized by a small amount of homogeneous gray or grayish white discharge. The discharge usually has a disagreeable odor, and because it is less irritating than discharges caused by other organisms, pruritus is mild or absent. On inspection the vaginal walls are slightly reddened, and the discharge appears to adhere to the mucosal lining. Some women are asymptomatic despite positive cultures.

#### Diagnostic Tests

The diagnosis is confirmed by microscopic examination of a smear or culture of the vaginal discharge.

### ♦ INTERVENTIONS

#### Administering Medications

Treatment of bacterial vaginosis consists of oral metronidazole, 250 to 500 mg twice per day for 7 days. The CDC *does not* recommend treating the patient's sexual partner at the same time.

# HUMAN PAPILLOMAVIRUS (GENITAL WARTS)

## ETIOLOGY

**Genital warts** caused by the human papillomavirus (HPV) are important because of their possible role in the development of cervical cancer.

## EPIDEMIOLOGY

Between 500,000 and 1 million cases of genital warts occur per year in the United States. They are the leading cause of office visits. Genital warts occur in or around the vulva, vagina, cervix, perineum, anal canal, urethra, and glans penis. They enlarge during pregnancy and may cause hemorrhage or obstruction during delivery. The disease is most common in adolescent girls and young women. The HPV can remain dormant for decades before recurrences appear.

## NURSING MANAGEMENT

### ♦ ASSESSMENT

Diagnosis is made by clinical appearance or histologic examination.

**TABLE 55-7 Comparisons of Three Methods Used to Treat External Genital/Perianal Warts**

| METHOD | ADVANTAGES | EFFICACY |
|---|---|---|
| Cryotherapy with liquid nitrogen or cryoprobe | Relatively inexpensive and does not result in scarring | Efficacy of 63%-88% in randomized trials with recurrence in 21%-39% of patients |
| Podofilox, 0.5% solution, for self-treatment for genital warts only; contraindicated during pregnancy | Relatively inexpensive, simple to use, and safe for patients who are able to see and reach the warts easily | Efficacy in randomized trials of 45%-88% with recurrence in 33%-60% of patients |
| Podophyllin, 10%-25% in compound tincture of benzoin; application should be limited to less than 0.5 ml or less than 10 cm² per treatment | Relatively inexpensive, simple to use, and safe | Efficacy in recently randomized trials of 32%-79% with recurrences among 27%-65% of patients |

From US Department of Health and Human Services, Public Health Service: 1993 Sexually transmitted diseases treatment guidelines, *MMWR* 42 (RR-14):1-102, 1993.

### ♦ INTERVENTIONS

Table 55-7 summarizes current therapy.

#### Facilitating Learning

Prevention of HPV should be stressed. It includes (1) avoiding sexual relationships with persons in known high-risk groups, (2) using latex condoms if having sexual intercourse, and (3) avoiding anal intercourse.

The CDC does not recommend a cesarean birth to prevent transmission of HPV to newborns. Cesarean delivery may be indicated for warts obstructing the pelvic outlet or if a vaginal birth would cause excessive bleeding of the warts. Because genital warts sometimes undergo malignant change, the patient is advised to have an annual Pap smear. Malignant changes, especially in the cervix, may not be apparent for 5 to 40 years.[21]

## HEPATITIS B

### ETIOLOGY

Etiology is established by serologic testing. Most persons with acute viral hepatitis are asymptomatic. Because there is no specific treatment for **hepatitis B,** emphasis is placed on prevention.

### EPIDEMIOLOGY

In the United States, hepatitis B is most frequently transmitted by sexual contact. Persons at high risk for sexual transmission of hepatitis B include homosexual/bisexual men, heterosexual men and women with multiple sex partners, and sexual partners of intravenous drug users.

### PREVENTION

#### Primary Prevention

The CDC recommends *vaccination* for all the persons identified above as being at high risk. In addition, residents of correctional or long-term care facilities, persons seeking treatment for an STD, and prostitutes should be vaccinated. *Vaccination is also recommended for health care workers because of the possibility of needlesticks.*

#### Secondary Prevention

The CDC recommends that *postexposure prophylactic treatment* with hepatitis B immune globulin (HBIG) should be considered in the following situations: sexual contact with a person who has active hepatitis B or who contracts hepatitis B and sexual contact with a hepatitis B carrier (blood test positive for hepatitis B surface antigen). The prophylactic treatment should be given within 14 days of sexual contact.

Because pregnant women can transmit hepatitis B virus to their infants at delivery, HBIG and hepatitis B vaccine are given to the infant after birth. All pregnant women should be screened during their first obstetric visit for the presence of HBsAg. If they are HBsAg positive, their newborns should be given HBIG as soon as possible after birth and subsequently immunized with hepatitis B vaccine. HBIG is also given to health care workers who suffer a needle-stick. For more information about hepatitis see Chapter 42.

## OTHER SEXUALLY TRANSMITTED DISEASES

In addition to those diseases already discussed, pediculosis pubis and scabies are considered to be STDs.

**Pediculosis pubis,** also known as "crabs," is caused by pubic lice. Although lice can be transmitted by bedding or clothing, they are often transmitted during sexual contact. They produce erythematous, itchy papules. The lice adhere to hair around the pubic area, anus, abdomen, and thighs. Diagnosis is made by observation of lice or microscopic observation of nits at the base of pubic hairs. Recommended treatment is 1% Kwell lotion or shampoo. One treatment per episode is necessary, but itching may persist.

**Scabies,** caused by mites known as *Sarcoptes scabiei,* is transmitted by close body contact, bedding, and clothing. Diagnosis is made from linear burrows, often characterized by a reddened papule containing the mite. Common sites are finger webs, wrists, elbows, ankles, and the penis. Nocturnal itching is common. A one-time use of 1% Kwell shampoo is recommended. Family, household, and sexual contacts should also be treated.

## QUESTIONS TO CONSIDER

- What is the incidence of STDs in your community?
- How does the incidence in your community compare with the incidence in other parts of the country?
- What services are available in your community for detection and treatment of STDs?
- Are human sexuality and prevention of STDs taught in your local schools?
- Are similar teaching programs available for adults in the community in which you reside?
- Describe the nurse's role in working with persons with a newly diagnosed STD.

## CRITICAL THINKING ACTIVITIES

- You have been requested to give a presentation on STDs to several health education classes at a local high school. What information should you be prepared to discuss? If you are limited to 45 minutes, what information do you think is most important to cover and why?
- Explain why the incidence of STDs is growing among American teens. How might the care of a teenager who has an STD differ from that of an adult with the same disease?

## CHAPTER SUMMARY

### ETIOLOGY/EPIDEMIOLOGY

- The term *sexually transmitted diseases* refers to diseases that are usually transmitted by heterosexual or homosexual intercourse.
- The five classic venereal diseases are gonorrhea, syphilis, chancroid, lymphogranuloma venereum, and granuloma inguinale.
- In the 1980s chlamydia trachomatis, genital herpes, human papillomavirus, genital mycoplasmas, cytomegalovirus, hepatitis B vaginitis, enteric infections, and ectoparasitic disease were added to the list of STDs.
- Three changes have affected the incidence of STDs in the United States since World War II: (1) antibiotics and antibiotic resistance, (2) social permissiveness, and (3) sexual behavior patterns.
- The highest incidence of STDs is in young adults and adolescents. This is believed to be because of permissiveness, promiscuity, and "the pill."

### SEXUAL TRANSMISSION

- Partner notification (formerly called *contact investigation*) is important to identifying persons who may have been exposed to an STD and in trying to identify the source of the infection.

### NURSING MANAGEMENT

- Latex condoms are recommended to prevent the transmission of STDs. They are recommended because they provide greater protection against viral STDs than natural membrane condoms.

### GONORRHEA

- During the 1980s there was a decline in the incidence of gonorrhea except in adolescents between 10 and 19 years of age. It remains an important risk for young minority populations who practice unprotected sex.
- A major concern in the treatment of gonorrhea is the increased resistance of the organism to penicillin and other antibiotics.
- Gonorrhea in women is often asymptomatic and is only diagnosed when complications such as salpingitis occur.

### SYPHILIS

- The incidence of syphilis increased dramatically in the late 1980s, and in 1990 the reported cases of primary and secondary syphilis were the highest they had been since 1948.
- The increase in syphilis has been in young, heterosexual, minority populations and may be related to cocaine use and the exchange of sex for crack cocaine. The drug of choice in the treatment of syphilis is penicillin G benzathine (2.4 million units IM).

### HERPES GENITALIS

- Herpes genitalis is a lifelong disease with no cure. It can be transmitted to the fetus during delivery, and thus cesarean delivery is often recommended.
- Treatment for herpes genitalis is symptomatic, and acyclovir is prescribed, 200 mg orally every 4 hours. It does not prevent recurrences.

### CHLAMYDIAL INFECTION

- *Chlamydia trachomatis* infections are recognized as the most prevalent STD in the United States.
- *C. trachomatis* can be spread between sexual partners during intercourse and from mothers to infants.
- Chlamydial infections are most common in women under the age of 20 years. They are also more common in persons who have several sex partners.
- The treatment of choice for chlamydial infections is doxycycline, 500 mg twice daily for 7 days, or azithromycin, 1 g orally in a single dose.

### HUMAN PAPILLOMAVIRUS

- Condylomata acuminata (genital warts) is caused by the papillomavirus; it is most common in adolescent girls and young women.
- Genital warts are of particular concern, because they

can undergo malignant changes after a latent period of 5 to 40 years.

### HEPATITIS B

- In the United States hepatitis B is most often transmitted by sexual contact.
- The CDC recommends that all persons at high risk for hepatitis B be vaccinated. This includes health care workers because of the possibility of needle-sticks.

## REFERENCES


1. Centers for Disease Control: *Chlamydia trachomatis* infections, policy guidelines for prevention and control, *MMWR* 34(3S):54S-73S, 1985.
2. Centers for Disease Control: Antibiotic-resistant strains of *Neisseria gonorrhoeae*: policy guidelines, *MMWR* 36(5S):1S-18S, 1987.
3. Centers for Disease Control: Condoms for the prevention of sexually transmitted diseases, *MMWR* 37(9):133-137, 1988.
4. Centers for Disease Control: Continuing increase in infectious syphilis—United States, *MMWR* 37(3):35-38, 1988.
5. Centers for Disease Control: Graphs and maps for selected notifiable diseases in the United States, *MMWR* 41(55):13-64, 1993.
6. Centers for Disease Control: 1993 Sexually transmitted diseases treatment guidelines, *MMWR* 42(RR-14):1-102, 1993.
7. Centers for Disease Control: Recommendations for prevention and management of *Chlamydia trachomatis* infections, *MMWR* 42:1-39, 1993.
8. Centers for Disease Control: Special focus: surveillance for sexually transmitted diseases, *MMWR* 42:1-39, 1993.
9. Darrow WW: Changes in sexual behavior and venereal disease, *Clin Obstet Gynecol* 18:255-267, 1975.
10. Faro S: Chlamydia trachomatis infection. In Rakel RE: *Conn's current therapy 1991,* Philadelphia, 1991, WB Saunders.
11. Gersham KA, Rolfs RT: Divergent gonorrhea and syphilis trends in the 1980s: are they real? *Am J Public Health* 81(10):1263-1267, 1991.
12. Krusinski PA: Viral diseases of the skin. In Rakel RE, editor: *Conn's current therapy 1993,* Philadelphia, 1993, WB Saunders.
13. Maberry MC: Vulvovaginitis. In Rakel RE: *Conn's current therapy 1991,* Philadelphia, 1991, WB Saunders.
14. Noble RC: Syphilis. In Rakel RE: *Conn's current therapy 1991,* Philadelphia, 1991, WB Saunders.
15. Schulte JM, Schmid G: Chancroid. In Rakel RE: *Conn's current therapy 1993,* Philadelphia, 1993, WB Saunders.
16. Smith CE, McAllister CK: Gonorrhea. In Rakel RE: *Conn's current therapy 1991,* Philadelphia, 1991, WB Saunders.
17. Thompson SE, Washington AE: Epidemiology of sexually transmitted *Chlamydia trachomatis* infections, *Epidemiol Rev* 5:96-123, 1983.
18. Those other STDs, *Am J Public Health* 81(10):1250-1251, 1991 (editorial).
19. US Department of Health and Human Services, Public Health Service: *Healthy people 2000: national health promotion and disease prevention objectives,* Washington, DC, 1990, US Government Printing Office.
20. Wilms NA: Lymphogranuloma venereum. In Rakel RE: *Conn's current therapy 1991,* Philadelphia, 1991, WB Saunders.
21. Zurowski SM: Warts *(verruca vulgaris).* In Rakel RE: *Conn's current therapy 1993,* Philadelphia, 1993, WB Saunders.

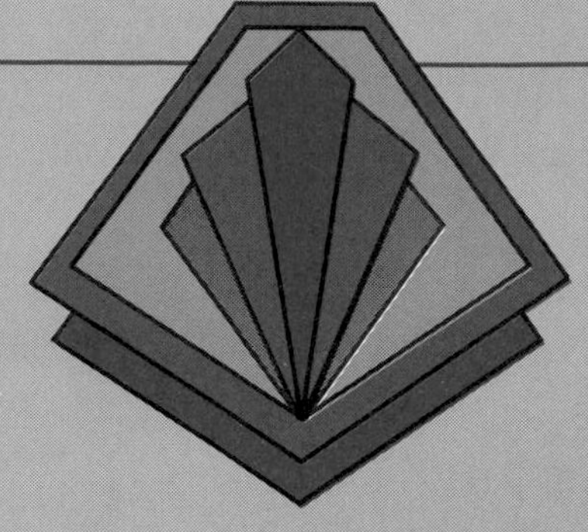

UNIT X

# Alterations in Cognition, Sensation, and Motion

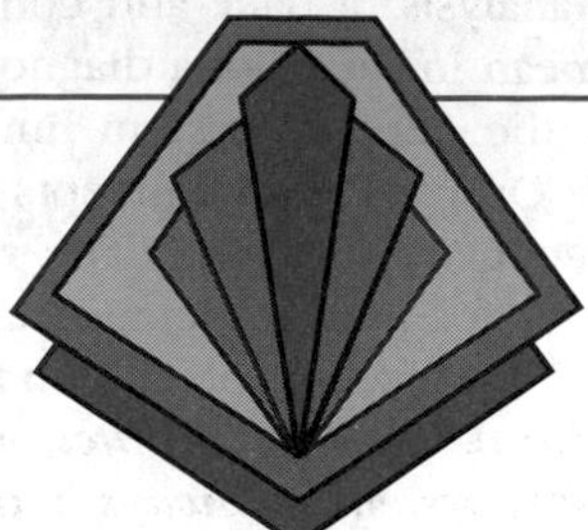

CHAPTER 56

# Assessment of the Nervous System

***Elizabeth Anne Schenk***

## CHAPTER OBJECTIVES

***After studying this chapter, the learner should be able to do the following:***

1. State the four general kinds of functions of the nervous system.
2. Name the three parts of the neuron and explain the function(s) of each part.
3. Define the following terms: *differential permeability, excitability, polarization, depolarization, action potential,* and *synapse.*
4. Name the two major divisions of the nervous system.
5. Name the three main areas of the brain and at least two functions of each part.
6. Name the four parts of the cerebral cortex and at least one function of each.
7. Explain what symptoms a patient may manifest with pathology in the frontal lobe.
8. Name at least two special characteristics of circulation in the brain.
9. Name the three meningeal layers and the three potential spaces associated with the meninges.
10. Name at least four physiologic changes that occur in the nervous system with aging.
11. Describe the parts of the neurologic assessment that are assessed through the history.
12. Explain how aphasia is different from dysarthria.
13. Name the 12 cranial nerves and the function of each.
14. List and describe at least six diagnostic procedures used to evaluate neurologic disease.

## KEY TERMS

action potential
aphasia
aproxia
areflexia
ataxia
arteriography
circle of Willis
computed tomography
cranial nerves
depolarization
differential permeability
dysarthria
dysphagia
effector organs
excitability
gnosia
hyperkinesia
hyperreflexia
hyporeflexia
meninges
motor system pathways
myelography
myoclonus
neuron
pneumoencephalography
receptor neurons
repolarization
synapse
tremor
ventriculography

Many systemic diseases have neurologic manifestations; thus individuals may have their first neurologic assessments performed during a routine physical examination. Consequently, the physician generalist often is the first medical professional to document the neurologic problems. However, on referral to a physician specialist (neurologist), the individual will undergo a more detailed assessment to localize the particular lesion and to identify its pathophysiology. To enable the specialist to determine the specific diagnosis, the neurologist's examination will be more detailed, exact, and comprehensive than that of the generalist.

Persons with neurologic deficits require skilled assessment by both physician and nurse. Neurologic assessment may be performed by generalists and specialists in both fields, and data collected will be used both collaboratively and independently to permit these professionals to provide their distinct services to the individual.

Professional nurses are involved in initial and ongoing assessments of a patient's neurologic status. The nurse's role is that of an independent professional, as well as that of a collaborator.

The nurse generalist may become involved in baseline and continuing assessments early in the patient's course of therapy. Although data collected also will be useful to the physician, the primary purpose is to enable the nurse to identify the degree to which the patient is able to perform self-care activities and to assess how such activities are limited by the identified deficits in sensory, motor, affective, or intellectual capacities. With these problem areas identified, the nurse then is able to select appropriate strategies to maximize the patient's capabilities.

Because of additional experience and preparation in the speciality, the neurologic nurse specialist has developed skills beyond those of the generalist. Like the physician specialist, the neurologic nurse's assessments are more comprehensive and detailed in nature and, as such, they are more likely to overlap with those of the neurologist.

Again, although these data will be useful to the neurologist, the primary purpose is to enable the neurologic nurse specialist to formulate more comprehensive analyses of patient conditions. Problems identified may provide more thorough descriptions of deficits observed, patient responses to these deficits, and the effects of such deficits on the patient's family and life-style. This thorough analysis will lead to more comprehensive plans of care extending from the acute phase through rehabilitation. Also, the neurologic nurse specialist serves as a consultant to nurse generalists caring for patients with neurologic problems.

The purposes of this chapter are to review selected neuroanatomy and physiology, to discuss aspects of history taking, to present the components and methods of and the observations to be made during the neurologic examination, and to discuss selected tests and procedures used to assist in the diagnosis of neurologic problems.

## ANATOMY AND PHYSIOLOGY

Neurologic assessment depends on the examiner's knowledge of normal neurophysiology and neuroanatomy and ability to interpret the degree of change in status from what is considered to be normal. The attainment of a logical diagnosis (nursing or medical) begins with a recognition of abnormality followed by grouping of the data, analysis of data, and conclusions about what the data mean in terms of a diagnosis.

The complexity of the nervous system limits what can be presented here. Only selected concepts relevant to neurologic assessment are included. The reader is referred to current texts for a more detailed and comprehensive coverage.[7,10] Emphasis is placed on key concepts including the *neuron, synapse, conduction, motor system pathways, sensory system pathways,* and *effector organs.*

### FUNCTION

Functionally, the nervous system, like an electrical conductance system, coordinates and controls all activities of the body. Broadly, the nervous system carries out four general kinds of functions as related to informational processes:

1. Receives stimuli or information from the internal and external environments over varied *afferent,* or *sensory, pathways*
2. Communicates information between distant parts of the body (periphery) to the central nervous system
3. Computes or processes the information received at various *reflex* (spinal cord) and *conscious* (higher brain) levels to determine responses appropriate to existing situations
4. Transmits information rapidly over varied efferent or *motor pathways* to effector organs for body action control or modifications.

Whereas the basic structural and functional unit of the nervous system is the neuron, neuroglia cells serve as an adjunct. They provide nourishment, support, and protection for the neurons. Neuroglia cells make up almost half of the microscopic structures of the spinal cord and brain. Four different types of neuroglia cells have been found.[16] Most arise from the embryonic ectoderm. Because they can divide and multiply by mitosis, they serve as a source for tumors of the nervous system. See Table 56-1 for these types of cells and their functions.

#### Neuron

The single **neuron** is the basic structural and functional unit of the nervous system. It shares all of the basic biologic and biochemical properties of other body cells. It also is a highly specialized and differentiated cell. The

**TABLE 56-1 Neuroglia Cells**

| TYPE OF CELL | FUNCTION |
|---|---|
| Astrocyte | Maintain chemical environment for conduction and transmission of impulses |
| Ependyma | Produce cerebrospinal fluid |
| Microglia | Part of process of phagocytosis |
| Oligodendroglia | Produce lipid-protein complex that forms myelin |

single neuron acts as a miniature nervous system and has properties specialized for its electrical function.

Microscopically, the neuron consists of a cell body, or *soma,* with two extensions that project from it: a *dendritic tree* and an elongated *cylindric axon.* A *cell membrane* encloses the outer boundary of the soma, dendrites, and axon, thus separating the inside from the outside of the cell. The presence of a large surface area of cell membrane makes it suitable to receive a large number of synaptic contacts at one time (Figure 56-1). The *axon* is specialized for the transmission of information along its extension *away from* the cell body to adjacent neurons; the *dendrite* or *dendrites* are specialized for receiving information from axon terminals at special sites called **synapses.** (It should be noted that the word *axon* is used in various ways. It may be used to describe the extension of one cell or the extension of several cells making up a nerve.) See Figure 56-2 for types of neurons.

### Cell membrane

Many of the most important *functional* properties of the neuron lie within the *cell membrane* itself. Structurally, the membrane is made up of lipids and proteins

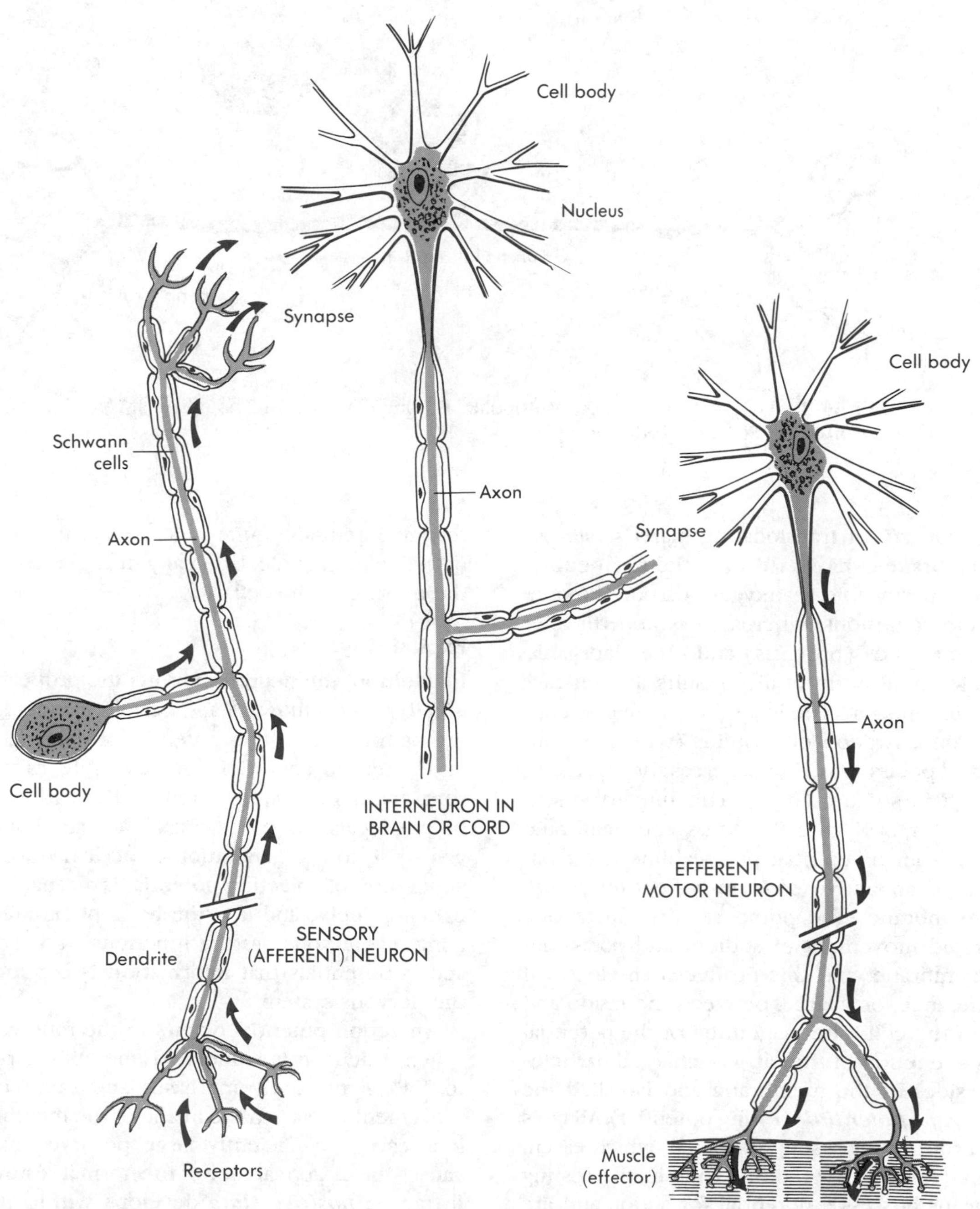


**FIGURE 56-1** Diagram of neurons showing the cell body (soma), dendrites, and axon. Direction of impulse conduction indicated by arrows.

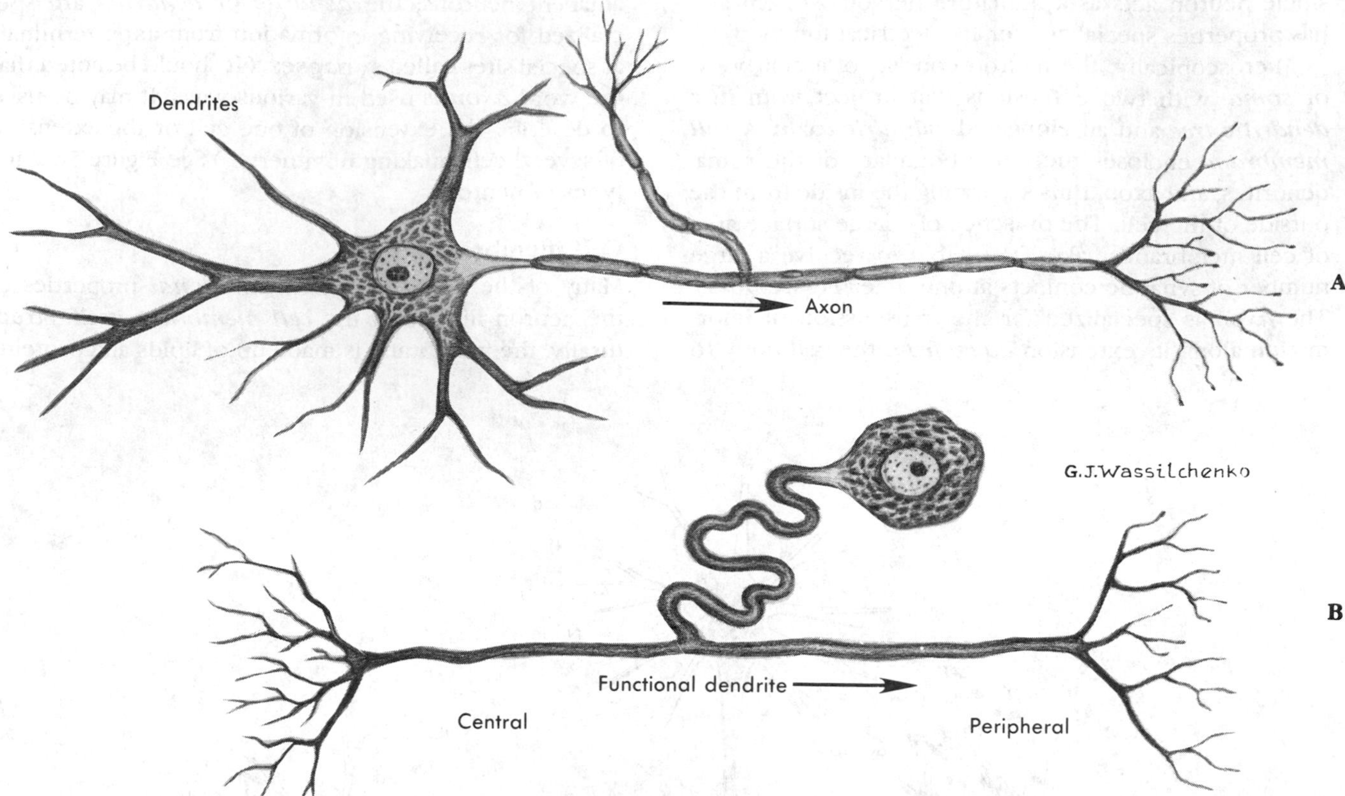


**FIGURE 56-2** Types of neurons. **A,** Multipolar. **B,** Unipolar. (From Thompson JM et al: *Clinical nursing,* St Louis, 1986, Mosby.)

and has the property of translocating materials across itself. The membrane exhibits **differential permeability** in that it is permeable to oxygen, carbon dioxide, and certain inorganic ions, whereas it is impermeable to organic compounds (proteins) and other inorganic ions. This differential permeability results in a characteristic ionic distribution. The inside of the neuron contains a high concentration of proteins (which are impermeable) and potassium ($K^+$), whereas the outside of the cell is high in sodium ($Na^+$). This unequal distribution, or gradient, of $K^+$ and $Na^+$ across the membrane results in part from differential permeability and from the presence of an active *sodium-potassium pump* within the membrane. The pump requires metabolic energy for rapid movement of sodium and potassium across the membrane, and this produces an electrical potential difference, or charge, between the inside and the outside of the cell. The magnitude of the potential difference is a function of the ratio of charged particles on opposite sides of the membrane and is called the *resting membrane potential* (resting potential). All cells exhibit this property of resting potential, which essentially remains constant over time. Thus in the resting state all neurons possess a potential for action and are said to be *polarized* (a difference in voltage charge between inner and outer cell membrane or surface). This resting potential is quite small, −60 mV, with the inside of the cell being electronically negative compared with the outside of the cell.

### Excitability

In addition, the neuron exhibits the property of *"excitability,"* as do muscles and certain glands. **Excitability** means that the resting potential of neurons is unstable under certain conditions, for example, as when a neuronal membrane is subjected to stimulation, application of chemicals, or mechanical damage. This instability gives rise to the generation of **action potentials.** The generation of an action potential is a capacity unique to excitable cells, and it is the basic phenomenon underlying all nervous system functions. It is by means of action potentials that information is conducted within the nervous system.

An action potential occurs in the following manner: When a neuron is stimulated, membrane permeability to $Na^+$ significantly increases and there is a sudden movement of $Na^+$ to the inside of the membrane. These ions carry a sufficiently large positive charge, which causes the disappearance of the normal resting potential. In fact, a *positive state* develops within the cell and **depolarization** occurs.

Almost instantaneously the membrane pores return

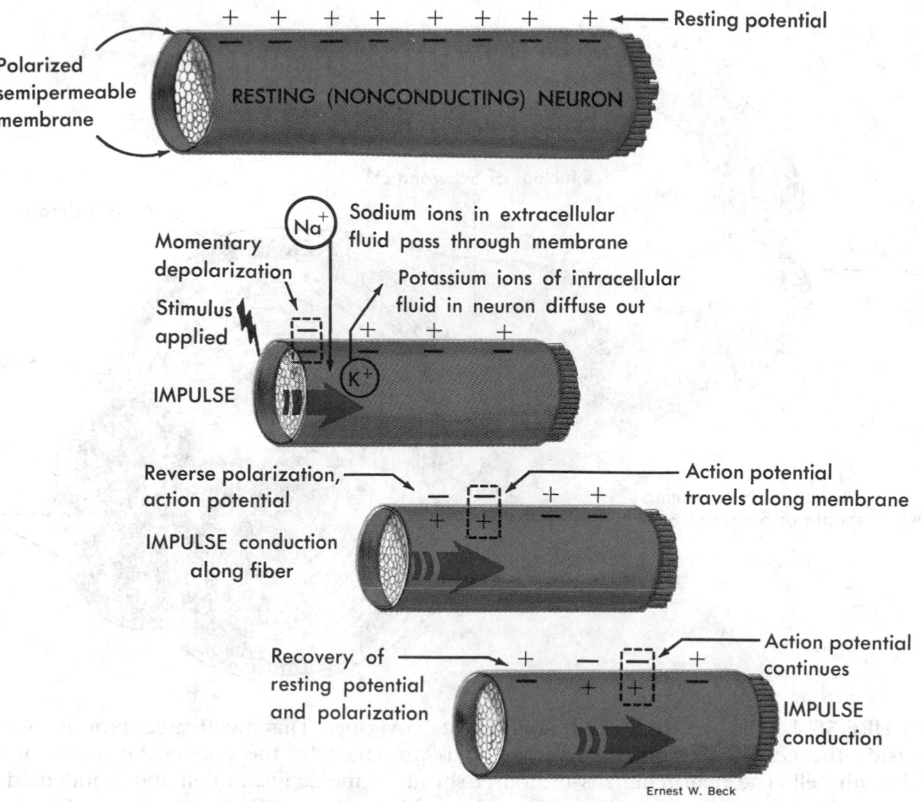


**FIGURE 56-3** Upper diagram represents polarized state of membrane of nerve fiber when it is not conducting impulses. Lower diagrams represent nerve impulse conduction: a self-propagating wave of negativity or action potential travels along membrane. (From Thibodeau GA: *Anthony's textbook of anatomy and physiology,* ed 13, St Louis, 1990, Mosby.)

to the state of being virtually impermeable to $Na^+$ while $K^+$ moves to the outside of the cell. The $K^+$ movement also quickly returns to normal, and active transport brings $Na^+$ and $K^+$ movement back to the original state. These mechanisms result in the disappearance of the internal positive state and a return to the normal resting potential. This phase is called **repolarization.** These two phases together form the *action potential.* An entire AP occurs within 1 to 2 msec (Figure 56-3).

When an action potential is generated it proceeds *automatically to completion,* independent of the property of the stimulus that initiated the depolarization; that is, a strong stimulus does not give rise to a larger action potential but does cause it to proceed to completion in an "all-or-none" fashion. The action potential is also spread, or propagated, over the entire membrane without a decrease in its velocity. The propagation velocity is related to the size of the axon (the larger the diameter, the higher the velocity) and to the presence or absence of myelin.

## Myelin

Myelin is an excellent insulator of axons. The myelin sheath is deposited around the axons by Schwann's cells, and this layer may be as thick as the axon itself. Myelin prevents almost all ion flow across the axon and its membrane. However, at distances approximately 1 mm apart the sheath is interrupted by nodes of Ranvier. At these small, uninsulated areas, ions can flow easily between the extracellular fluid and the axon. In fact, at these nodes the axonal membrane is 500 times more permeable than the membranes of some nonmyelinated fibers. Thus impulses are conducted from node to node (Figure 56-4).

The presence of myelin causes such fibers to be called *large* fibers; those without myelin are called *small* fibers. Large fibers have a greater conduction velocity because (1) the jumping effect allows depolarization to proceed quickly and (2) energy is conserved, since only the nodes depolarize. Large fibers appear white because of the myelin; the "white matter" of the nervous system is made up of myelinated fibers.

Many action potentials of neurons originate in a receptor neuron where internal and external stimuli are normally received. A receptor is like a transducer and can change one form of energy into another form. A receptor, however, responds or depolarizes to *only one* type of stimulus. For example, the retina of the eye responds only to the stimulus of light, which is converted to electrical energy and travels over the optic

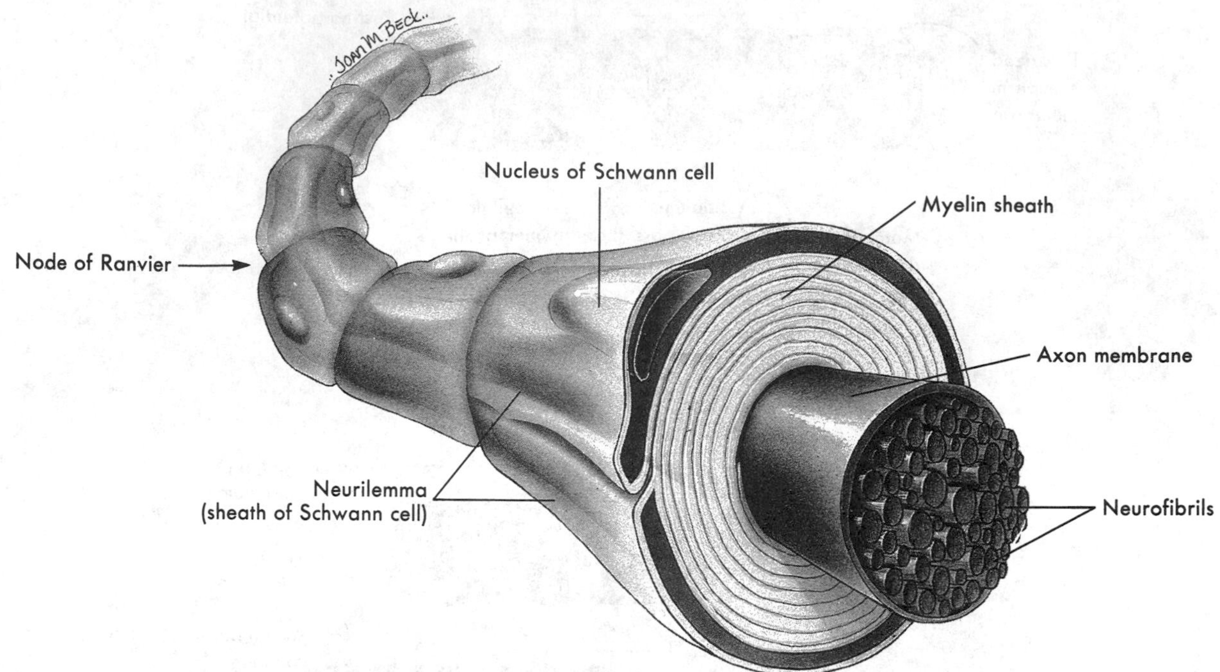


**FIGURE 56-4** Diagram of a nerve fiber and its coverings. This myelinated axon is located outside the central nervous system. Myelin is produced by the concentric layers of the Schwann cell. The neurilemma is the outer sheath of the Schwann cell and is indented by successive nodes of Ranvier. (From Christensen BL, Kockrow EO: *Foundations of nursing,* St Louis, 1991, Mosby.)

nerves to the visual cortices for perception. In this way the receptor neuron may initiate the depolarization. It does, however, limit what the neuron responds to, although the receptor neuron does obey the all-or-none theory; a strong stimulus does make the receptor neuron fire more action potentials per unit of time within its time limitations than does a weak stimulus.

### Synapse

Neurons make functional contact with one another at specialized sites called *synapses.* Whenever an action potential is generated in one neuron that invades a synapse site, a sequence of processes results in the action potential affecting the second neuron. Transmission across a synapse is essentially a *chemical process.* The end of the axon contains a chemical substance located within its vesicles. When an action potential reaches the vesicle, it releases a transmitter substance, which depends on the influx of calcium. It then diffuses across the synapse to the adjacent neuronal cell membrane. *Synaptic transmission* is both *excitatory* and *inhibitory* in nature. Inhibition means that the dendritic membrane becomes hyperpolarized because of the release of the specific neurotransmitter. The membrane potential shifts toward $K^+$ equilibrium, thus stabilizing the membrane and taking the potential further from threshold. Each neuron only acts when its membrane is *depolarized to threshold.* Thus whether a neuron fires depends on the sum of excitatory and inhibitory inputs. *Chemicals* allowing *excitatory transmission* are *acetylcholine, norepinephrine, dopamine,* and *serotonin.* Those that *inhibit transmission* include *gamma aminobutyric acid (GABA) in brain tissue* and *glycine* in the *spinal cord.*

In summary, each single neuron contains all the structural and functional building elements of an electrical conductance system that also makes interconnections with adjacent neurons at synapses. Collectively, the neurons are in turn organized into larger and larger units of function that serve to coordinate all the activities of the body. All neurons function basically in the same manner. There is, however, a major difference in the functions carried out by sensory and motor neurons.

In neurologic assessment the examiner should appreciate that any disruption in the conductance system results in dysfunction distal to the break. The degree of change in status of a particular function or functions depends on the location and nature of the stressor or lesion causing the disruption.

## DIVISIONS OF THE NERVOUS SYSTEM

Macroscopically, the nervous system is divided into two major divisions: the central nervous system and the peripheral nervous system.

## Central Nervous System

The central nervous system (CNS) is made up of collections of neurons and their connections organized within the brain and spinal cord. All of the basic informational processes as summarized on p. 1888 occur within the CNS. Areas of the brain and spinal cord are distinguished where cell bodies are concentrated into *nuclei* and groups of axons running in *tracts* that interconnect the parts. Collections of neurons are connected in complex ways. The *connections* determine the capability of each collection of neurons. The neurons are organized into circuits: some are simple and made up of relatively few neurons; others are very complex. A single neuron may be a component of a number of different neuronal circuits and thus play a role in different functions.

Structurally, the brain and spinal cord are continuous. They are protectively housed within the skull and vertebral column, respectively. When injured, centrally located neurons are unable to reproduce themselves because most cell bodies are located centrally and nerve cell bodies cannot reproduce. However, *nerve endings can regenerate* because of the presence of *neurilemma.* Neurilemma covers all peripheral nerves; it is theorized that the living neurilemma contains openings through which axonal growth occurs proximally to distally. This growth seems to occur at a rate of 1 to 4 mm/day. Rarely, however, is there 100% regrowth.[7] In the nervous system a phenomenon exists that limits the free movement of substances from the blood to the brain tissue. Passage of substances into the brain is slower in comparison with passage into other body organs. The neurologic sheath, as well as capillaries that have thickened basement membranes, slows the process of diffusion in between the blood and the brain.

The barrier is selective, allowing entry of fluid, gases, and small molecular substances, while preventing the entry of toxic substances, plasma protein, and large molecules. The ability to overcome this barrier has proved instrumental in chemotherapy of brain lesions.

### Meninges

The **meninges** are the coverings of the nervous tissue in the brain and spinal cord. These fibrous coverings help support, protect, and nourish the brain and spinal cord. Outermost is the *dura mater,* a very tough membrane consisting of two layers. This meningeal layer is significant in that it sends four processes deep into the

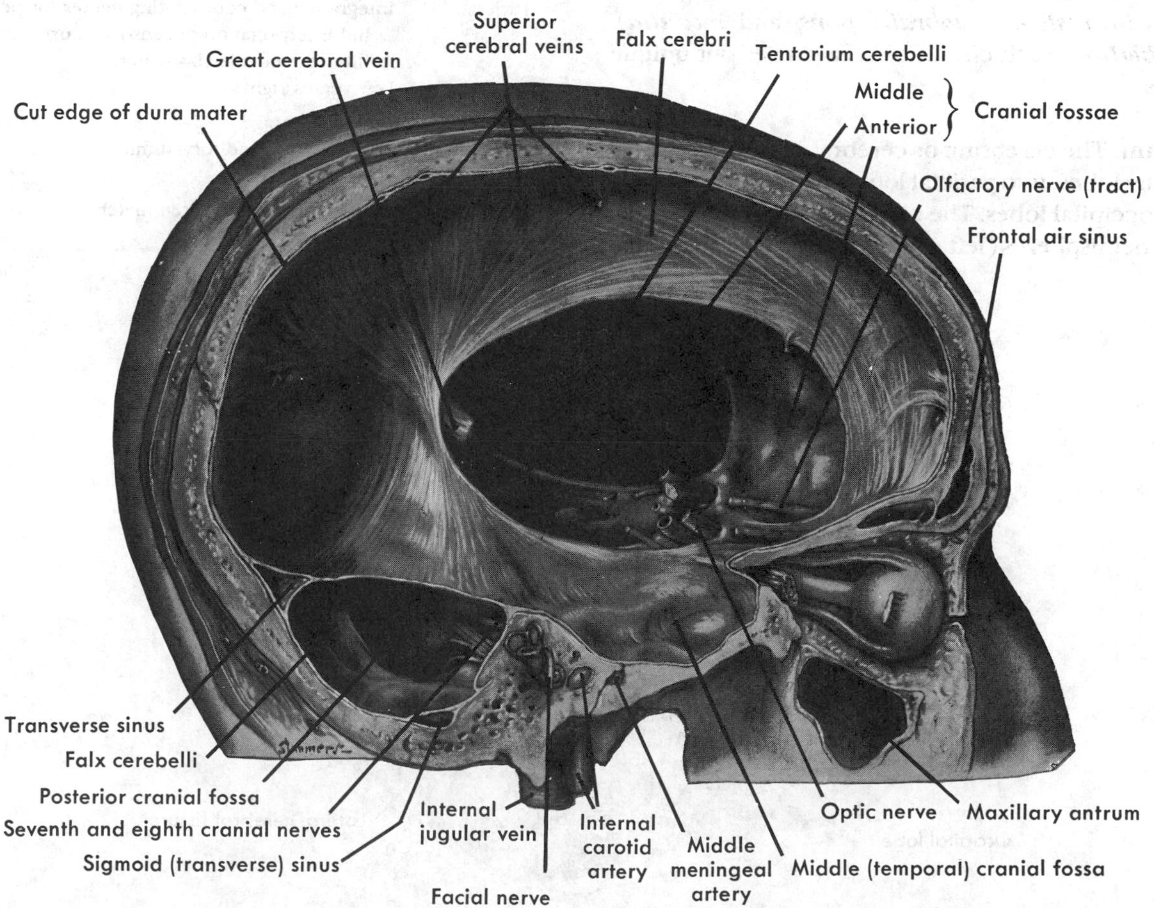


**FIGURE 56-5** The brain and the meningeal layers. The subdural space and subarachnoid space are also shown. (From Mettler FA: *Neuroanatomy,* ed 2, St Louis, 1948, Mosby.)

cranium and these processes form fibrous compartments for portions of the brain. These are the *falx cerebri,* the *tentorium cerebelli,* the *falx cerebelli,* and the *diaphragma sellae* (Figure 56-5).

The *arachnoid,* the delicate membrane lying beneath the dura, covers the brain more loosely. Projections called the *arachnoid villi* extend into the overlying dura. The *pia mater,* innermost of the meninges, is a vascular membrane having many small plexuses of blood vessels. The pia mater follows the course of the penetrating blood vessels as they dip into the substance of the brain.

These three coverings with only minor variations are also found in the spinal cord. For example, the spinal cord arachnoid expands to surround the cauda equina; thus the subarachnoid space ends at S2 in the adult and is most wide caudally. Also, the spinal cord pia mater is thicker and less vascular than that of the cranium.

It should be noted that three potential spaces are associated with the meninges: *epidural* (external to the dura); *subdural* (between dura and arachnoid); and *subarachnoid* (between arachnoid and pia mater).

### Brain

The brain (encephalon) is grossly divided rostrally to caudally into three main areas: the *cerebrum,* diencephalon *brainstem (midbrain, pons,* and *medulla),* and *cerebellum.* Each circuit or area carries out unique functions.

**Cerebrum.** The cerebrum or cerebral cortex comprises two frontal lobes, two parietal lobes, two temporal lobes, and two occipital lobes. The cerebral cortex is separated into two hemispheres (left and right) by the *falx cerebri,* a tough dural tissue. Each of the hemispheres is further divided into the respective lobes by folds in the cerebral cortex called *fissures* or *sulci.* The frontal lobe is separated from the parietal lobe by the *fissure of Rolando* (also called the *central sulcus*) and from the temporal lobe by the *sylvian fissure.* It is separated from the occipital lobe by the *parieto-occipital fissure.* The temporal lobe lies below the *sylvian fissure.*

The *cortex* of the cerebrum is approximately ¼ inch thick. It controls over 14 billion neurons, receives and analyzes all impulses, controls voluntary movement, and stores knowledge of all impulses received.

Each cerebral lobe is named from overlying cranial bones (Figure 56-6) and carries out one or more functions as listed in Table 56-2.

Important to note is that speech is a function of the

**TABLE 56-2 Specific Functions of Cerebral Cortex**

| LOBE | FUNCTION |
|---|---|
| Frontal | Conceptualization<br>Abstraction<br>Motor ability<br>Judgment formation<br>Ability to write words |
| Parietal | Integrative and coordinating center for perception and interpretation of sensory information<br>Ability to recognize body parts<br>Left versus right |
| Temporal | Memory storage<br>Integration of auditory stimuli |
| Occipital | Visual center<br>Understanding of written material |

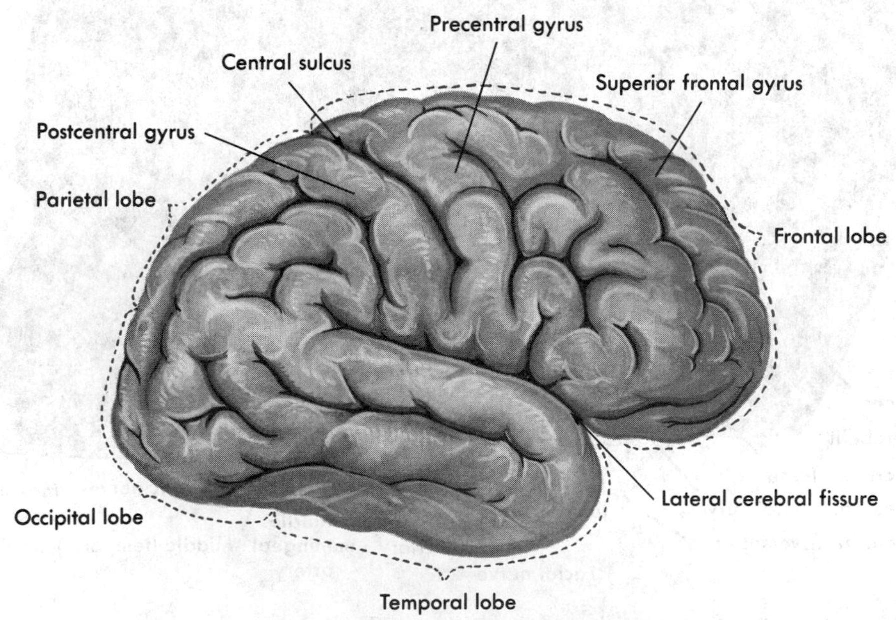


**FIGURE 56-6** Lobes, sulci, and gyri of the brain.

*dominant hemisphere,* which for all right-handed people and most left-handed people is the left side. The two identified speech centers are *Broca's area* and *Wernicke's area* (Figure 56-7). Broca's area is located in the lateral, inferior portion of the frontal lobe adjacent to the motor cortex and its projections. This area appears to control verbal, expressive speech. Wernicke's area is located in the posterior part of the superior temporal convolution and may extend to adjacent portions of the parietal lobe. This area is responsible for the reception and understanding of language. Other areas of the brain that also are involved in speech include an area in the frontal lobe, which governs the ability to write words, and an area in the occipital lobe, which governs the ability to understand written material (see Figure 56-4 for important cortical areas).

Finally, deep within the cerebrum are structures called the *basal ganglia.* These are masses of gray matter (cell bodies) and include such structures as the *caudate nucleus, putamen,* and *globus pallidus.* In general, the basal ganglia function as part of the *extrapyramidal* system and are responsible for postural adjustments and gross volitional movements.

**Diencephalon.** The diencephalon consists of the hypothalamus, thalamus, metathalamus, and epithalamus. It surrounds and includes most of the third ventricle of the brain. The diencephalon often is called the *interbrain* because it lies directly beneath the cerebrum. The thalamus composes four fifths of the diencephalon and acts as a relay station for some sensory impulses, while interpreting other sensory impulses. (See Table 56-3 for a more detailed explanation of the functions of the structures and functions of the diencephalon.)

**TABLE 56-3 Diencephalon and Brainstem Structures and Functions**

| STRUCTURE | FUNCTION |
|---|---|
| **DIENCEPHALON** | |
| Thalamus | Serves as end station for all sensory impulses<br>All sensory fibers synapse for final relay to appropriate portion of sensory cortex<br>General sensation perceived (meaning and locality imparted by cortex)<br>Houses pain threshold |
| Epithalamus | Contains pineal body or epiphysis (thought to be endocrine gland whose secretion retards sexual development and growth) |
| Subthalamus | Receives fibers from globus pallidus, is part of afferent descending pathway |
| Hypothalamus | Contains cell bodies mediating most autonomic functions, endocrine functions, and emotional responses; contains stalk of pituitary |
| **BRAINSTEM** | |
| Midbrain | Relays impulses from cerebral cortex above and subcortical structures below<br>Origin of righting and postural reflex located here |
| Pons | Connects medulla, midbrain, and cerebrum<br>Contains pneumotaxic center—controls rhythmic quality of respirations |
| Medulla | Connects with central canal or spinal cord<br>Vital centers of cardiac, respiration, vasomotor control, as well as swallowing and hiccoughing; gag and cough reflex |

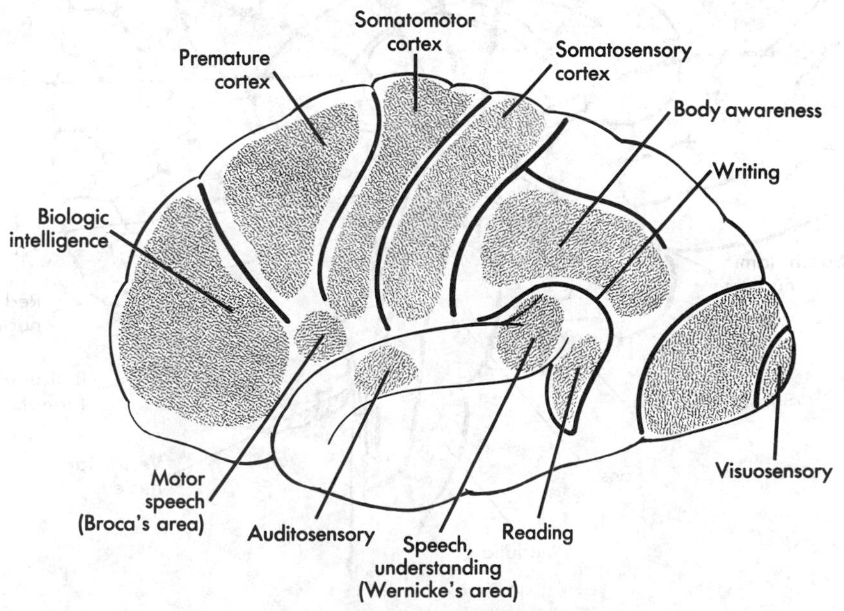


**FIGURE 56-7** Lateral view of cerebral cortex with identification of major cortical areas.

**Brainstem.** The brainstem is located deep in the center of the hemispheres and is not visible when the intact brain is viewed. It includes a series of parts making connections with the spinal cord at the level of the medulla (Figure 56-8), and it carries all nerve fibers passing between the hemispheres and the cord. All cranial nerves except the olfactory nerve (I) arise from it (Figure 56-9).

The brainstem is made up of several structures. These include the *midbrain, pons,* and *medulla oblongata.* (See Table 56-3 for a more detailed explanation of the functions of the various structures and functions of the brainstem.)

Of special importance is the core of tissue extending throughout the entire brainstem. This is called the *reticular formation* (see Figure 56-8). This interconnected network of cells has important integrating centers for respiration, cardiovascular function, afferent and motor systems, and states of consciousness. Increased stimulation leads to wakefulness, and decreased stimulation (as in anoxia caused by increased intracranial pressure) results in sleepiness.

**Cerebellum.** The *cerebellum* is located in the posterior cranial fossa, just below the posterior cerebrum. It contains *short* and *long tracts.* The short tracts act as connections of nuclei with the cerebellum, whereas the long tracts enter and exit through *peduncles.* There are three peduncles—*inferior, middle,* and *superior.* The inferior peduncle connects the cerebellum with the medulla, the middle peduncle connects it with the pons, and the superior peduncle connects it with the midbrain (see Figures 56-10 and 56-11).

The cerebellum has the following three main functions, all of which are related to monitoring and making corrective adjustments of body movements:

1. To keep persons oriented in space and to maintain truncal equilibrium
2. To control antigravity muscles
3. To check or halt volitional movements

**Circulation of the brain and spinal cord.** The blood supply for the brain derives from the aortic arch via the right innominate, left common carotid, and left subclavian arteries (Figure 56-7). It includes the conducting and penetrating vessels. The conducting arteries are (1) the internal carotids, which supply most of the cerebral hemispheres, basal ganglia, and the upper two thirds of the diencephalon, and (2) the vertebral arteries, which supply the brainstem, the lower one third of the dien-

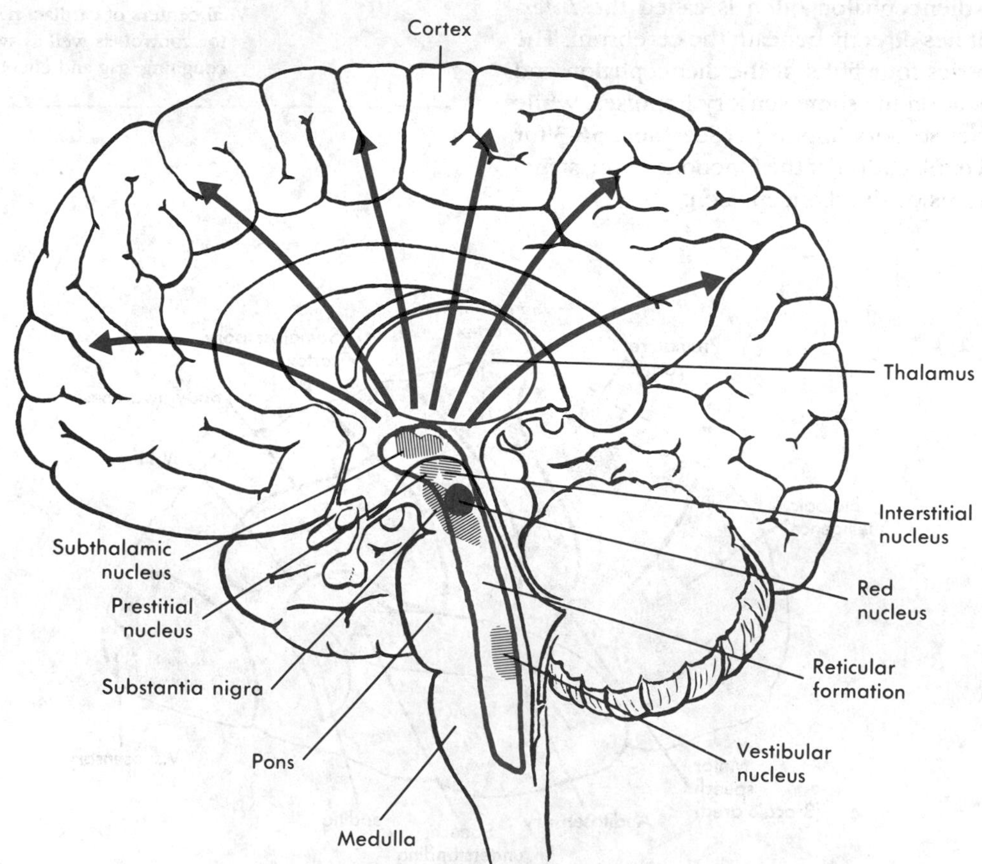


**FIGURE 56-8** Reticular activating system (RAS). (From Thompson JM et al: *Mosby's manual of clinical nursing,* ed 2, St Louis, 1989, Mosby.)

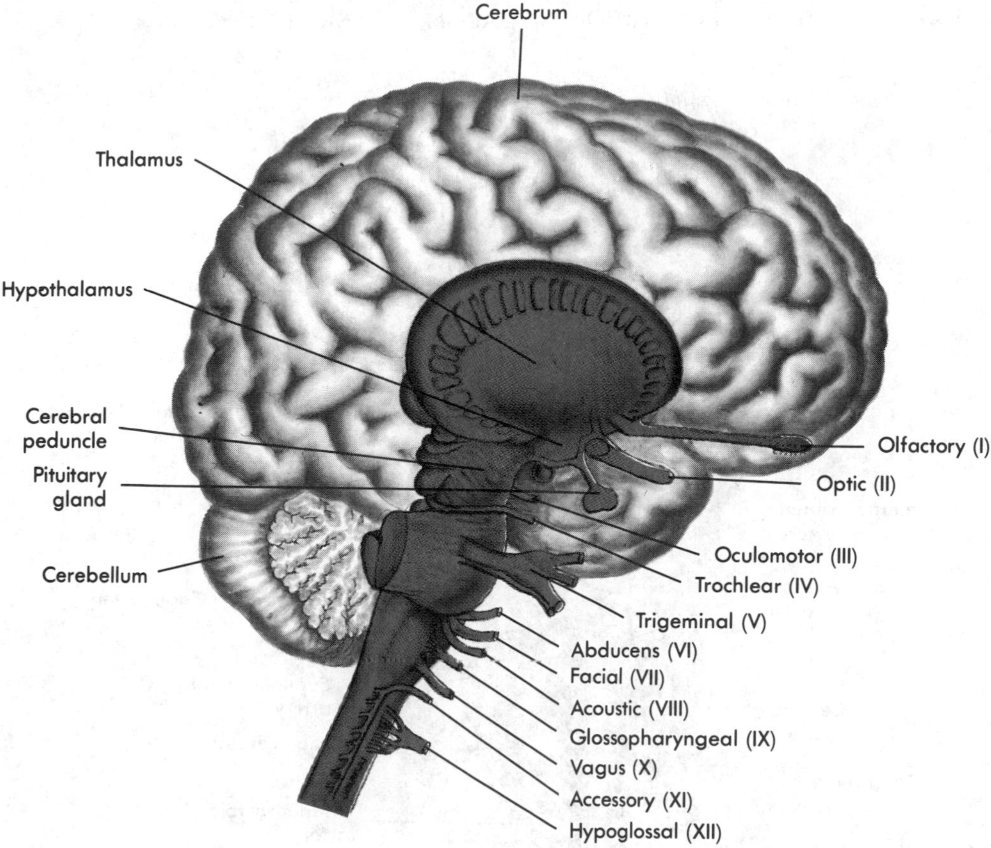


**FIGURE 56-9** Lateral view of the brain, showing the brainstem. Also shown are the cranial nerves, which arise from it. (From Rudy EB: *Advanced neurological and neurosurgical nursing,* St Louis, 1984, Mosby.)

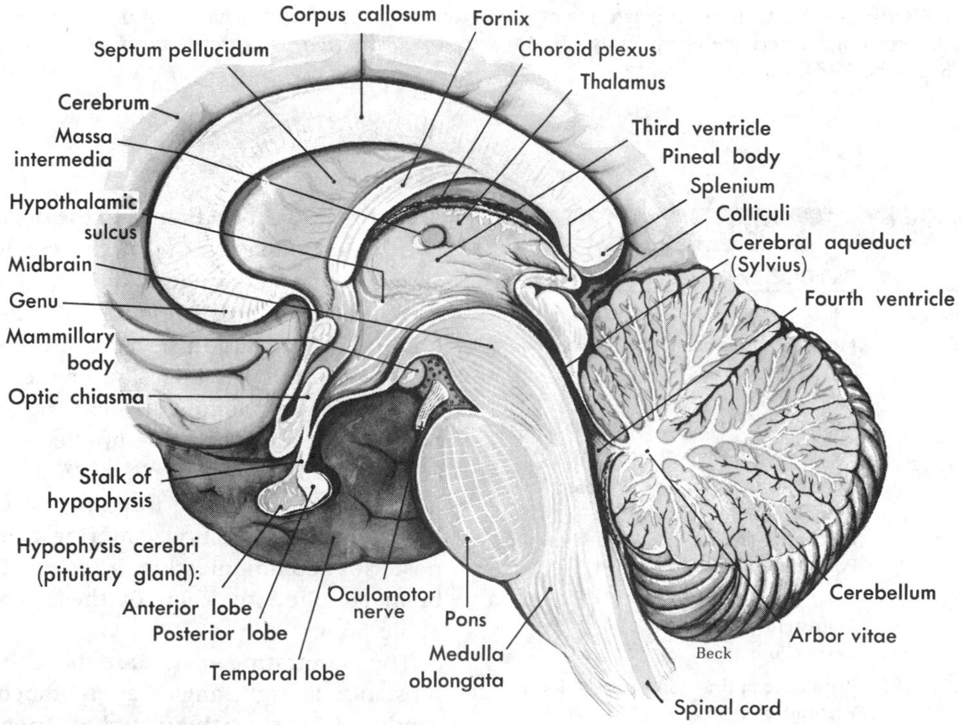


**FIGURE 56-10** Sagittal section through midline of brain showing continuity of brain and spinal cord. (From Anthony CP, Thibodeau GA: *Textbook of anatomy and physiology,* ed 11, St Louis, 1983, Mosby.)

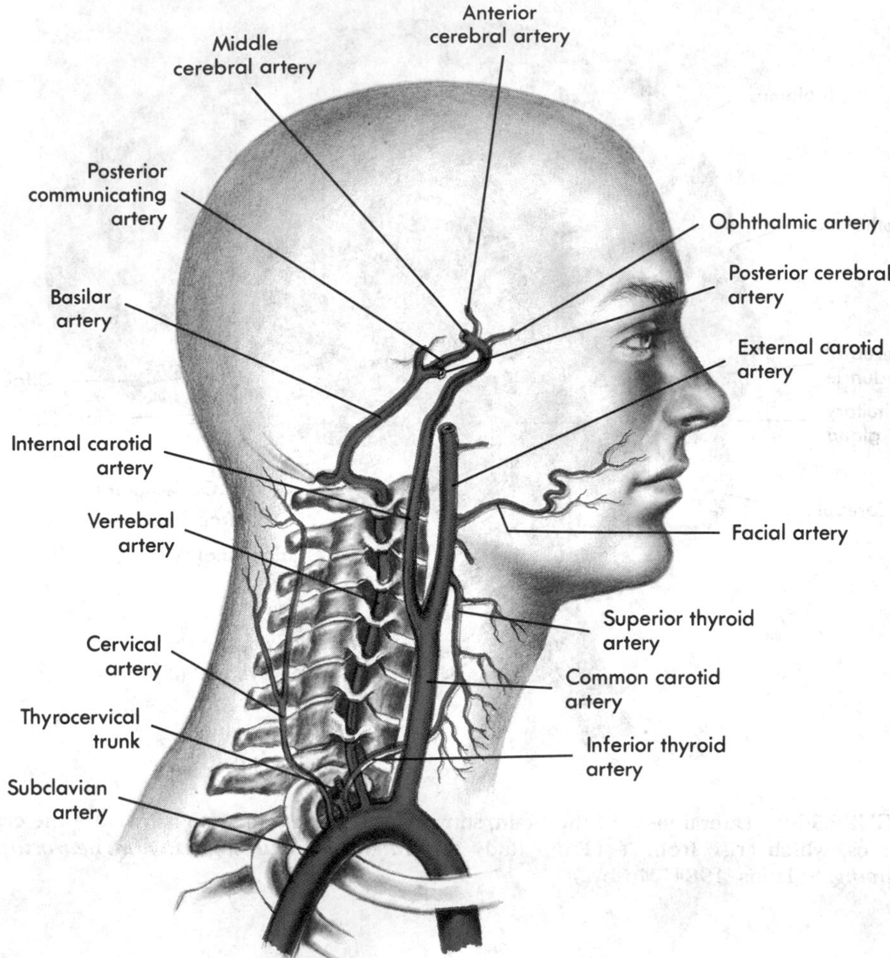


**FIGURE 56-11** Conducting arteries of the brain, including the internal carotid arteries and the vertebral arteries. (From Rudy EB: *Advanced neurological and neurosurgical nursing,* St Louis, 1984, Mosby.)

**TABLE 56-4 Circulation of the Brain**

| VESSEL | PART OF BRAIN SUPPLIED |
|---|---|
| Internal carotid arteries | |
| Anterior cerebral | Medial surface of the frontal and parietal lobes<br>Basal ganglia<br>Parts of the internal capsule and corpus callosum |
| Middle cerebral | Lateral surface of parietal, frontal and temporal lobes<br>Precentral (motor) gyri<br>Postcentral (sensory) gyri |
| Vertebral arteries | |
| Basilar | Brainstem<br>Cerebellum |
| Posterior cerebral | Parts of temporal and occipital lobe<br>Vestibular organs<br>Cochlear apparatus |

cephalon, the cerebellum, and the occipital lobes. These two systems anastomose at the **circle of Willis.** This allows them to compensate for alterations in blood flow and blood pressure. The circle of Willis is important to total brain circulation because it provides equal circulation bilaterally. If one side of the circle of Willis is unable to supply adequate blood, the other side provides blood to the area normally supplied by the damaged side (Figure 56-12). The circle of Willis is formed by the interconnection of the internal carotid, anterior cerebral, posterior cerebral, anterior communicating, and posterior communicating arteries. The parts of the brain supplied by each of these vessels is found in Table 56-4.

The penetrating vessels are those that enter the brain substance at right angles after branching off from the conducting vessels; they supply nutrients to the neurons.

The venous system draining the brain is divided into vertebral veins that receive blood from the cerebrum and the cerebellar veins that receive blood from the

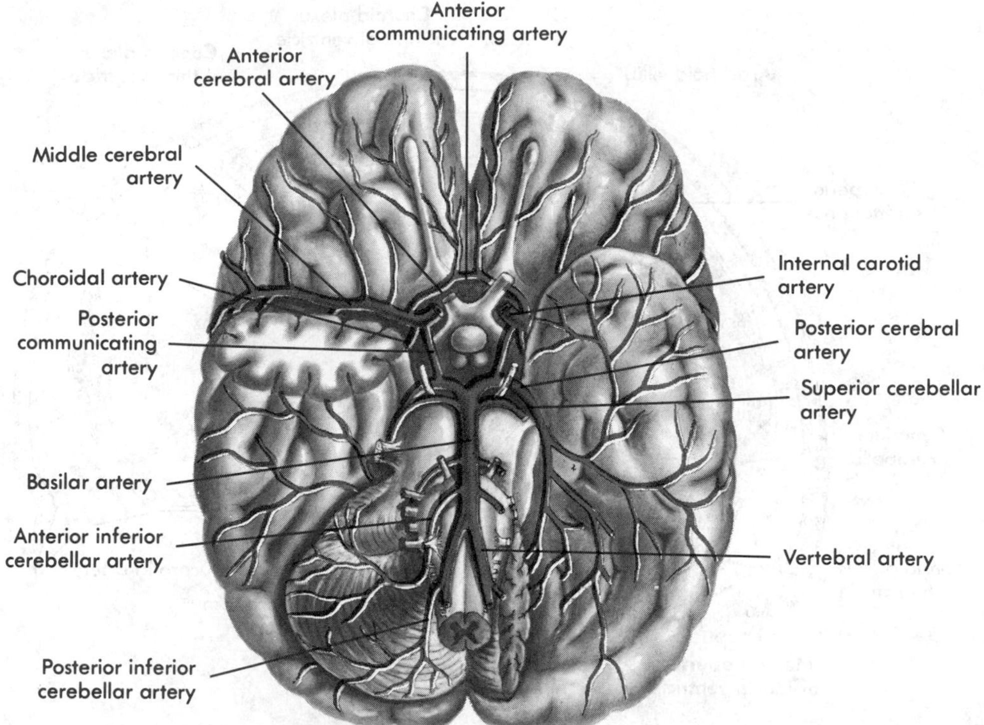


**FIGURE 56-12** Blood supply of the brain showing the penetrating vessels and the circle of Willis. The internal carotids and the vertebral arteries anastamose at the circle of Willis. (From Rudy EB: *Advanced neurological and neurosurgical nursing,* St Louis, 1984, Mosby.)

cerebellum. The venous system of the brain is unique in that the cerebral veins have no valves. Also, all the veins of the brain terminate in dural sinuses or reservoirs, which eventually empty into the superior vena cava by means of the jugular veins.

Circulation in the brain possesses special characteristics. For example, systemic circulation favors the central nervous system over all other body parts. This helps provide a constant supply of nutrients (glucose and oxygen) to nervous tissue. The brain's vessels themselves also possess capabilities that allow them to assist in achieving a constant blood flow. The brain is able to autoregulate its blood flow to respond to changes in intraluminal pressure. In the presence of increased blood pressure, cerebral vessels constrict so as to decrease flow and possible tissue damage. Conversely, in the presence of decreased intraluminal pressure, cerebral vessels dilate to increase flow. Cerebral vessels also react to biochemical changes. For example, elevated carbon dioxide content causes notable vasodilation of cerebral vessels; hypoxia and elevated hydrogen ion concentration also cause vasodilation. However, these autoregulatory mechanisms become less responsive with increasing age and in the presence of arteriosclerosis.

The blood supply to the spinal cord comes from the spinal artery and two radicular arteries. The spinal artery arises from the vertebral arteries, whereas the radicular arteries arise from the aorta.

### Cerebrospinal fluid

Another fluid in the nervous system is *cerebrospinal fluid* (CSF). CSF is found in the ventricles of the brain, in the central canal of the spinal cord, and in the subarachnoid space. It serves as a fluid cushion for nervous tissue and helps to support the weight of the brain. It also carries nutrients to the brain and removes metabolites. CSF is continually formed by vessels of the *choroid plexus* at a rate of 18 ml/hr. In the adult there is 90 to 150 ml of CSF.

After circulating around the brain and spinal cord, CSF returns to the brain and is absorbed through the arachnoid villi. From here, CSF enters the venous system and follows its pathway through the jugular veins to the superior vena cava and into the systemic circulation (Figure 56-13).

### Spinal cord

The spinal cord weighs about 1 ounce and is approximately 1½ inches wide. It is elliptical in shape and appears wider from right to left than from anterior to posterior. Cervical and lumbar enlargements are areas of nerve origin to the upper and lower limbs.

The spinal cord forms a continuous structure with the medulla oblongata. It extends 42 to 45 cm from the foramen magnum through the spinal foramina of the vertebral column to the upper border of the second lumbar vertebra.

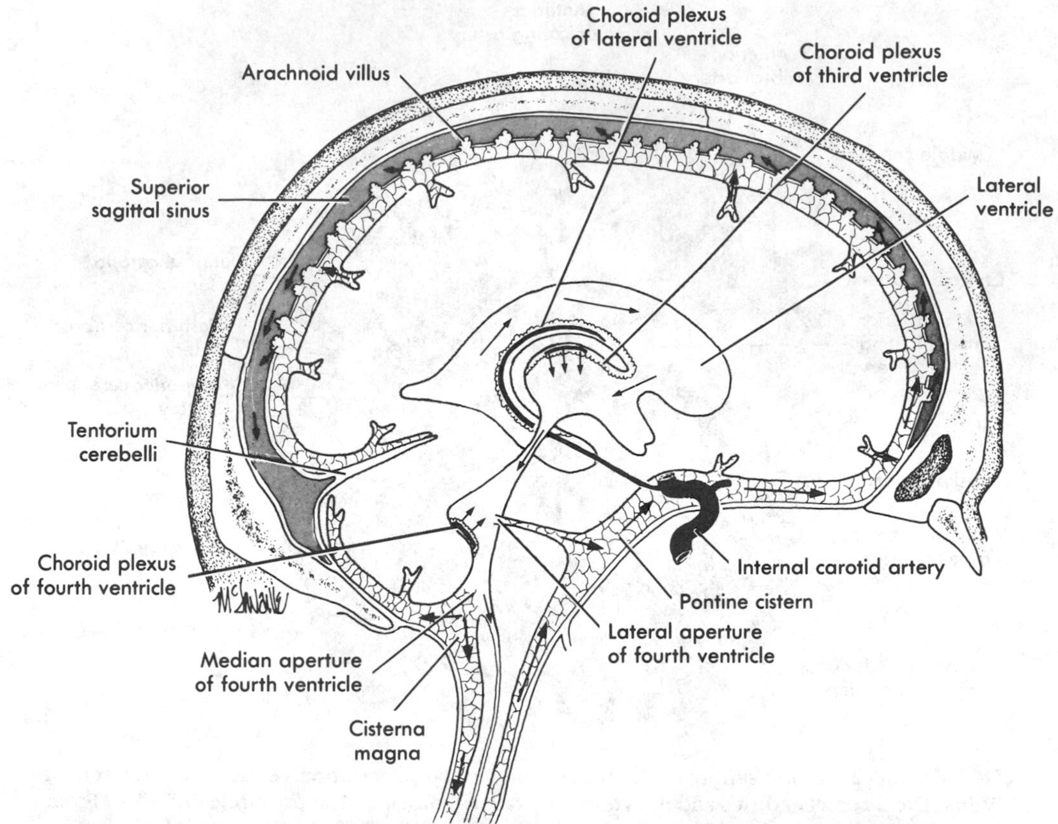


**FIGURE 56-13** Path of circulation of cerebrospinal fluid from its formation in the ventricles to its absorption into the superior sagittal sinus. (From Nolte J: *The human brain,* St Louis, 1981, Mosby.)

The spinal cord structurally includes H-shaped central gray matter (nerve cell bodies surrounded by white matter) that is divided into three columns or *funiculi* according to their location (*anterior, ventral, lateral,* and *posterior* or *dorsal columns).* Each contains ascending and descending tracts that will be described in more detail later in the chapter (Figure 56-14). These tracts connect different segments of the spinal cord to each other and connect the spinal cord with the brain. The names of the tracts usually show the point of origin by the first part of the name, and the end point by the last part of the name (see Table 56-5).

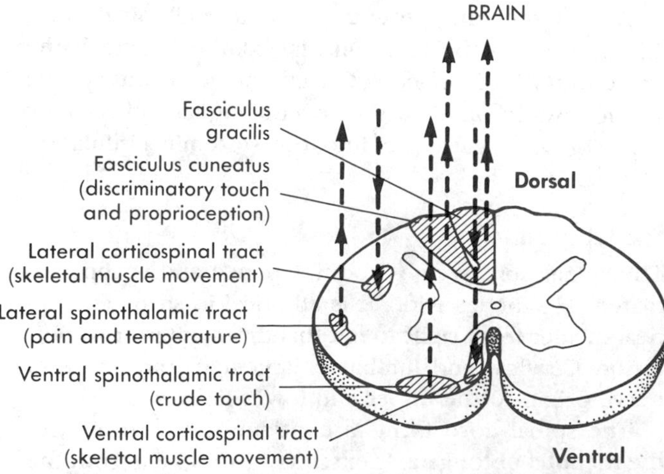


**FIGURE 56-14** Nerve pathways arise from white matter of the spinal cord. Impulses travel to and from the spinal cord and brain along these pathways.

The spinal cord is also the site of reflex pathways. Reflexes are an example of the simplest neuronal circuit. They *do not* require relay to the brain level for action. A reflex action consists of a *specific stereotyped motor response to an adequate sensory stimulus.* The response may involve skeletal muscle movement or glandular secretion. It may involve only two neurons as in a simple monosynaptic reflex arch such as occurs with the myotactic knee jerk reflex. In the knee jerk reflex, a brisk tap over a partially stretched knee tendon stimulates sensory nerve endings within the tendons, and the stimulus travels over a sensory nerve fiber within a peripheral nerve toward the spinal cord where it synapses with a central motor neuron (anterior horn cell). Following this, the impulse is transmitted down the motor nerve (over the anterior nerve root of the spinal nerve or peripheral nerve) and across the neuromuscular junction to stimulate the muscle to contract. Figure

**TABLE 56-5 Tracts of the Spinal Cord**

| TRACT | COLUMN | DIRECTION | FUNCTION |
|---|---|---|---|
| Ventral corticospinal | Anterior | Descending | Voluntary motion |
| Vestibulospinal | Anterior | Descending | Balance reflex |
| Tectospinal | Anterior | Descending | Sight and vision reflex |
| Reticulospinal | Anterior | Descending | Muscle tone |
| Ventral spinothalamic | Anterior | Ascending | Light touch |
| Spinoolivary | Anterior | Ascending | Proprioception reflex |
| Lateral corticospinal | Lateral | Descending | Voluntary movements |
| Rubrospinal | Lateral | Descending | Synergy and muscle tone |
| Olivospinal | Lateral | Descending | Reflex |
| Dorsal spinocerebellar | Lateral | Ascending | Reflex proprioception |
| Ventral spinocerebellar | Lateral | Ascending | Reflex proprioception |
| Lateral spinothalamic | Lateral | Ascending | Pain and temperature |
| Spinotectal | Lateral | Ascending | Reflex |
| Fasciculus interfascicularis | Posterior | Descending | Integration and association |
| Septomarginal fascicularis | Posterior | Descending | Integration and association |
| Fascicularis gracilis | Posterior | Ascending | Vibration, passive movement, joint, and two-point movement |
| Fascicularis cuneatus | Posterior | Ascending | Vibration, passive movement, joint, and two-point movement |

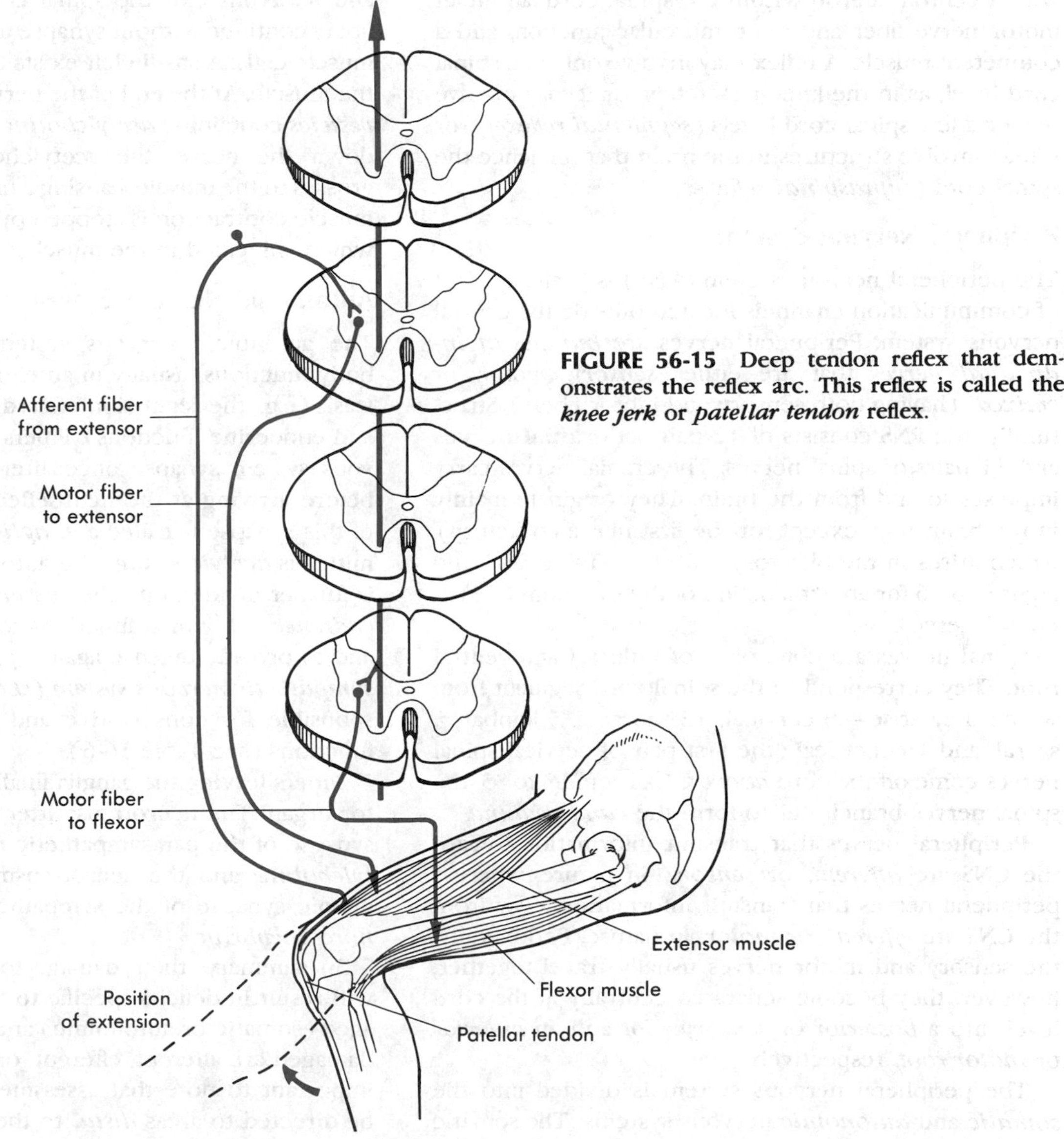


**FIGURE 56-15** Deep tendon reflex that demonstrates the reflex arc. This reflex is called the ***knee jerk*** or ***patellar tendon*** reflex.

**TABLE 56-6 Parasympathetic and Sympathetic Nervous System Influence**

| ORGAN SYSTEM | PARASYMPATHETIC INFLUENCE | SYMPATHETIC INFLUENCE |
|---|---|---|
| Heart | Decreases rate | Increases rate |
| Blood vessels | Dilates visceral and brain vessels | Constricts |
| Lung | Constricts bronchi | Dilates bronchi |
| Gastrointestinal | Increases peristalsis | Decreases peristalsis |
| Anal sphincter | Opens | Closes |
| Urinary | Contracts bladder | Relaxes bladder |
| | Opens sphincter | Closes sphincter |
| Eye | Constricts pupil | Dilates pupil |
| | Accommodates for near vision | Accommodates for far vision |
| Skin | Not applicable | "Goose flesh" |
| Gastric and salivary secretions | Increases | Decreases |
| Liver | Not applicable | Stimulates glycogen |
| Adrenal medulla | Not applicable | Stimulates production of epinephrine |

56-15 shows the reflex arc. In summary, a reflex arc depends on an intact sensory nerve, a functional synapse with a central neuron within the spinal cord, an intact motor nerve fiber and neuromuscular junction, and a competent muscle. A reflex may involve only one spinal cord level, as in the knee jerk reflex, or it may involve one or a few spinal cord levels *(segmental reflexes),* or it may involve structures in the brain that influence the spinal cord *(supraspinal reflexes).*

## Peripheral Nervous System

The peripheral nervous system (PNS) is basically a set of communication channels located outside the central nervous system. Peripheral nerves are *bundles of individual nerves* that are either *sensory, motor,* or *"mixed"* (having both sensory and motor fibers). Structurally, the PNS consists of 12 pairs of **cranial nerves** and 31 pairs of spinal nerves. The cranial nerves carry impulses to and from the brain. They originate mainly in the brainstem, except for the first nerve (olfactory), which arises in the olfactory bulb (see Table 56-9 and Figure 56-16 for an explanation of the functions of each cranial nerve).

Spinal nerves are composed of a dorsal and ventral root. They correspond to the spinal cord segment from which they arise—8 cervical, 12 thoracic, 5 lumbar, 5 sacral, and 1 coccygeal (the first pair of cervical spinal nerves come off the cord *above* C1). From L3 to S5, the spinal nerves branch out to form the *cauda equina.*

Peripheral nerves that transmit information toward the CNS are *afferent,* or *sensory,* in nature, whereas peripheral nerves that transmit information away from the CNS are *efferent,* or *motor,* in nature. Peripherally, the sensory and motor nerves usually travel together; however, they become separated centrally at the cord level into a *posterior* or *sensory root* and an *anterior* or *motor root,* respectively.

The peripheral nervous system is divided into the *somatic* and *autonomic* nervous systems. The somatic nervous system innervates skeletal (striated) muscles. Its neuronal cell bodies lie in groups within the CNS, and its axons exit the spinal cord at all levels. These fibers continue without synapse until they reach skeletal muscle cells. A small cleft exists between the nerve and the muscle. At the end of the nerve terminal are located *vesicles* containing *acetylcholine.* As the impulse moves down the nerve, the acetylcholine is released and crosses to the muscle, causing a muscle contraction. The muscle contraction is stopped by *acetyl cholinesterase,* which is located in the muscle.

### Autonomic Nervous System

The autonomic nervous system regulates automatic body functions, usually in an effort to preserve homeostasis (e.g., the regulation of cardiovascular, respiratory, and endocrine functions). Fibers of the autonomic nervous system synapse once after leaving the CNS and before arriving at the neuroeffector junction. The site of this synapse is called a *ganglion,* and its neurotransmitter is *acetylcholine.* The autonomic nervous system is further divided into the *sympathetic nervous system (adrenergic),* which functions to maintain homeostasis and to provide defense against stressors, and the *parasympathetic nervous system (cholinergic),* which is responsible for conservative and restorative vegetative functions (see Table 56-6).

Fibers leaving the ganglia finally synapse at the effector organ. The neurotransmitter for the postganglionic synapse of the parasympathetic nervous system is *acetylcholine;* and the neurotransmitter for the postganglionic synapse of the sympathetic nervous system is *norepinephrine.*

In summary, then, damage to any peripheral nerve will result in deficits specific to the type of nerve damaged (somatic or autonomic) and to whether the fibers damaged are afferent, efferent, or mixed in nature. It is important to note that assessment of dysfunction will be directed to areas *distal* to the injury.

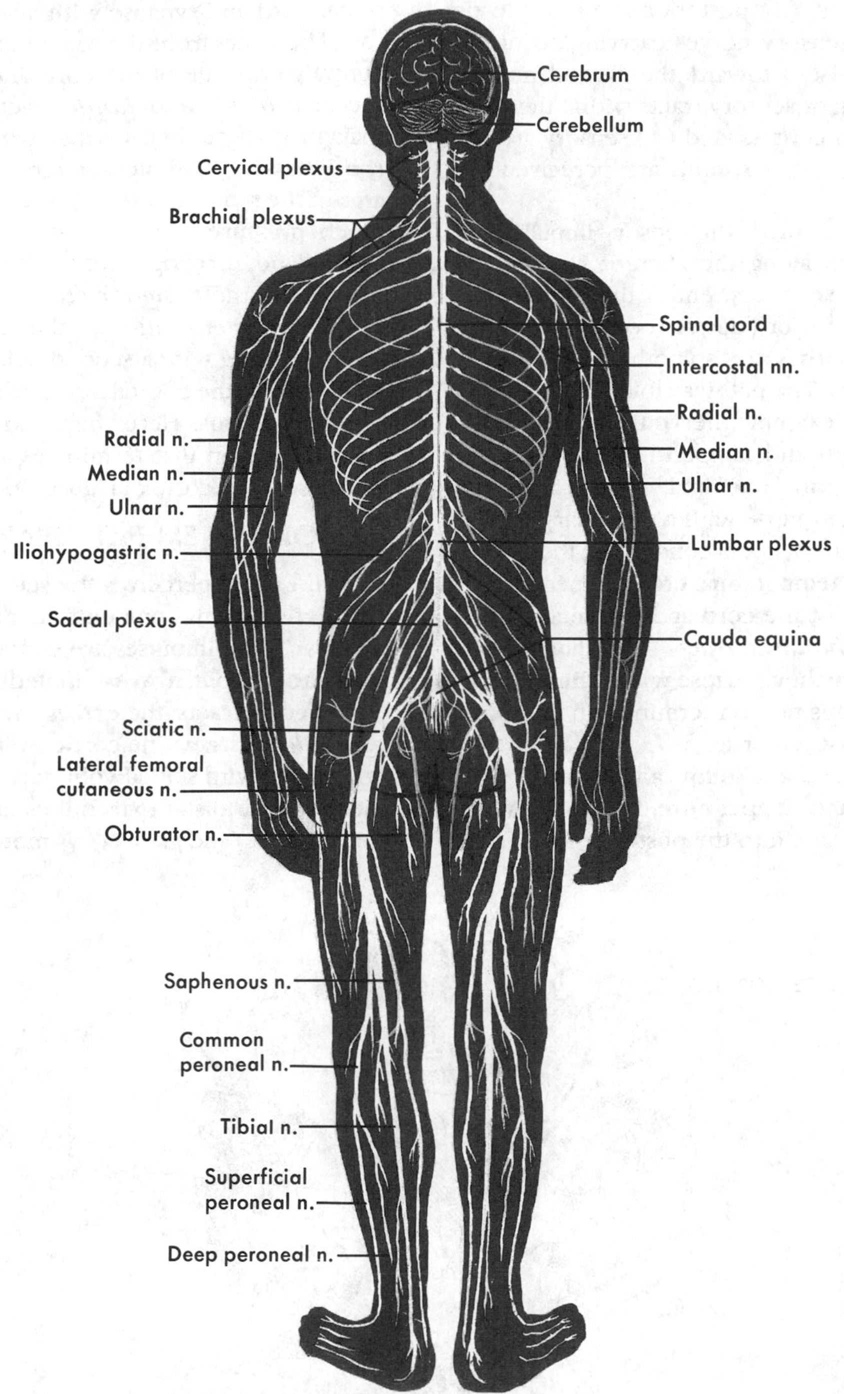


**FIGURE 56-16** The central and peripheral divisions of the nervous systems. The central nervous system (CNS) consists of the brain and spinal cord. The peripheral nervous system is composed of the cranial and spinal nerves. (From Christensen BL, Kockrow EO: *Foundations of nursing*, St Louis, 1991, Mosby.)

## SENSORY SYSTEM PATHWAYS

Sensation as perceived by the individual is initiated by stimulation of **receptor neurons** located throughout the body. Receptor neurons function to provide the brain with information about the condition and composition of both the internal environment (e.g., position *[proprioception]* and action *[enteroception]* of body parts) and the external environment *(exteroception)*. The latter is achieved through the eyes, ears, nose, skin, and tongue. The general sensory system by which this information is conveyed includes (1) receptor neurons responsive to special stimuli from both the internal and external environments, (2) posterior roots of the peripheral or afferent sensory nerves carrying action potentials (nerve impulses) toward the central nervous system, (3) ascending or sensory tracts within the spinal cord and upper brain centers, and (4) sensory areas of the cerebral cortex where stimuli are perceived and localized.

From the receptor neuron, the sensory impulse travels to the spinal cord along the afferent fibers of the nerve involved. These fibers enter the spinal cord through the posterior root (dorsal root ganglion) and may proceed along either the spinothalamic tracts or the posterior columns. The pathway followed is specific to the sensation. For example, nerve fibers conducting the sensations of *pain* and *temperature* pass into the posterior horn of the spinal cord and, within a few spinal segments from entry, synapse with a secondary sensory neuron. From this neuron, fibers conducting the sensory impulses of pain and temperature cross immediately to the contralateral side of the cord and continue upward as the *lateral spinothalamic tract.* These fibers arrive at the thalamus, where they synapse with a third sensory neuron. Fibers from this neuron terminate in the appropriate area of the sensory cortex.

Sensations for crude touch follow a very similar pathway to that for pain and temperature. Nerve fibers conducting the impulses pass into the posterior horn of the spinal cord and synapse with a secondary sensory neuron. The fibers from the secondary neuron cross to the contralateral side of the cord and continue upward as the *ventral spinothalamic* tract. These travel to the thalamus where they synapse with a third sensory neuron. Fibers from this neuron terminate in the appropriate area of the sensory cortex. Sensations of fine touch, deep touch/pressure, vibration, and proprioception, on the other hand, arriving at the spinal cord are conducted directly by the *posterior columns (fasciculus gracilis* or *fasciculus cuneatus*) to the level of the medulla before synapsing with a second neuron. These fibers then cross over to the contralateral side, where they continue to the thalamus. Here they also synapse with a third sensory neuron that terminates at the appropriate area of the sensory cortex (Figure 56-17).

## MOTOR SYSTEM PATHWAYS

After the brain perceives the state of the body's internal and external environments, it may initiate corrective actions. These impulses are conveyed by the **descending motor pathways**—including the *corticospinal* (pyramidal) tracts, the *extrapyramidal system,* and the *cerebellar system.* The corticospinal system is primarily concerned with skilled voluntary skeletal muscle movements of the distal extremities and, in particular, with the alpha ($\alpha$) and gamma ($\gamma$) motor neurons. Fibers that

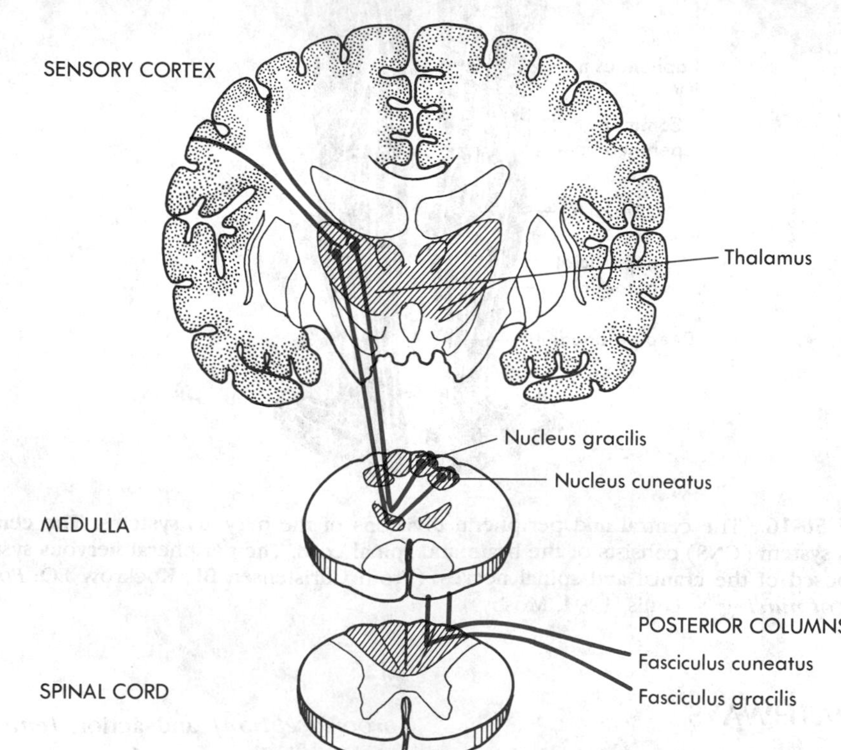


**FIGURE 56-17** Pathways for fine touch, deep touch and pressure, vibration, and proprioception. Note how stimuli entering through dorsal route (posterior) travel on the same side as posterior columns to medulla where they cross to the opposite side, ascend to the thalamus, and end in somasthetic area where perception occurs.

combine to form the corticospinal *tracts* arise from the *upper motor neurons.* Their cell bodies are located in the primary motor area of the cerebral cortex in the precentral gyrus of the frontal lobe and in the premotor cortex in the frontal lobe.

After fibers leave the cerebral cortex, they descend through the posterior limb of the internal capsule, middle of the cerebral cerebri, break up into bundles in the basilar portion of the pons, and then collect into discrete bundles within the pyramids of the medulla. In the medulla, the majority of the fibers cross over, or *decussate,* to the opposite side of the medulla and become the *lateral corticospinal tract,* which then passes to all spinal cord levels in the lateral funiculus and terminally synapse in the lateral aspect of laminae IV through VIII (Figure 56-18). The remaining fibers descend directly from the medulla (do not decussate) and synapse directly with α- and γ-neurons in lamina IX of the spinal cord. The latter is known as the *anterior corticospinal tract.* The *left* cerebral motor strip of the primary motor area controls the muscular movement of the right side of the body.

Eventually these fibers synapse with large *anterior horn cells* located in the spinal cord, as well as in the

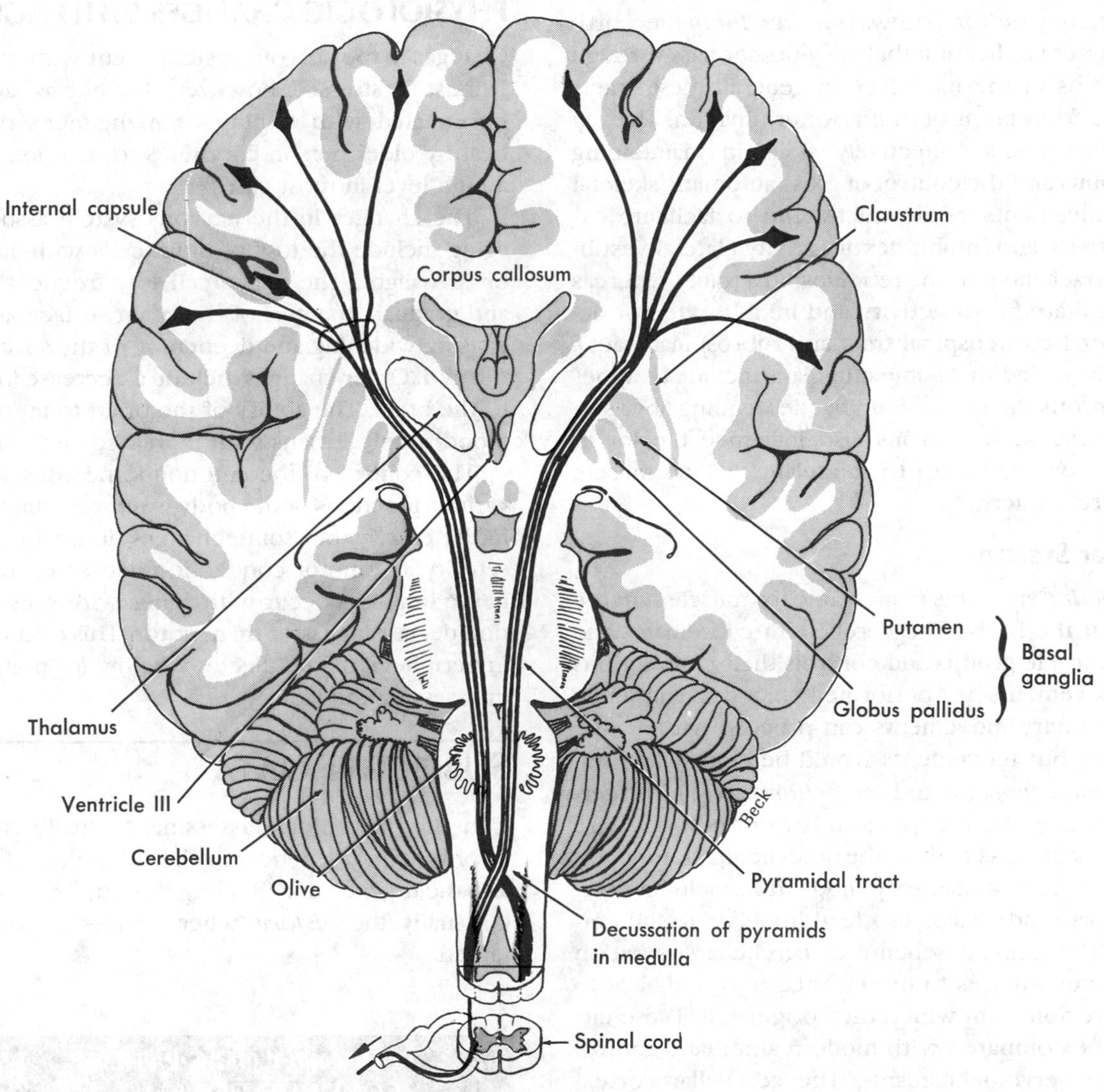


**FIGURE 56-18** Crossed corticospinal (pyramidal) tracts. Axons that compose pyramidal tracts (corticospinal) come from neuron cell bodies in cerebral cortex. After they descend through the internal capsule of the cerebrum and white matter of the brain stem, about three fourths of fibers decussate (cross over from one side to the other) in the medulla, as shown. Then they continue downward in lateral corticospinal tract on opposite side of cord. Each crossed corticospinal tract, therefore, conducts motor impulses from one side of the brain to interneurons or anterior horn motoneurons on the opposite side of the cord. Therefore impulses from one side of cerebrum cause movements of opposite side of the body. (From Anthony CP, Thibodeau GA: *Textbook of anatomy and physiology,* ed 11, St Louis, 1983, Mosby.)

motor cranial nuclei in the brainstem. These cells are called the *lower motor neurons* and are responsible for providing the final direct link or *final common pathway* with muscles via the myoneural (neuromuscular) junction at the motor end plates. Thus skeletal muscle activity is the result of the net influence of upper motor neurons on the α- and γ-motor neurons through the anterior horn cells (lower motor neurons) in the spinal cord and motor cranial nuclei.

### Extrapyramidal Tracts

The *extrapyramidal tracts* are complex and provide separate pathways between the cortex, the basal ganglia, the brainstem, and the cord. In general, these include all descending motor pathways *other than* the corticospinal tract (indicating that they do not pass through the pyramids of the medulla). In general, these tracts are named from point of origin to termination. The extrapyramidal tracts collectively assist in maintaining muscle tonus and the control of gross automatic skeletal muscle movements. Some tracts tend to facilitate extensor activity and inhibit flexor activity (lateral vestibulospinal tract and pontine reticulospinal tract), whereas others facilitate flexor activity and inhibit extensor activity (lateral corticospinal tract and rubrospinal tract). It should be noted that some clinicians include as upper motor neurons the extrapyramidal descending fiber systems because such neurons also influence the lower motor neurons and help to modulate skeletal muscle tone and reflex activity.

### Cerebellar System

The *cerebellar system* is responsible for muscle synergy throughout the body. The cerebellum coordinates the action of muscle groups and controls their contractions so that movements are performed smoothly and accurately. Voluntary movements can proceed without the cerebellum, but movements would be clumsy and uncoordinated (*asynergia* and *cerebellar ataxia*). The cerebellum receives both *sensory* and *motor inputs.* There are feedback circuits with all the descending motor pathways. In addition, all sensory modalities, including tactile, auditory, and visual, also feed impulses to the cerebellum. The general scheme of cerebellar operation allows nerve impulses to be returned to or fed back to the same region from which they originated. These circuits can be compared with modern automatic control devices, or servomechanisms. The cerebellar cortex, similar to a computer, can detect any errors in muscle synergy and return the proper messages to adjust muscular control within the body.

Visceral efferent motor pathways from the spinal cord mediate the action of *involuntary,* or *smooth, muscles* located within walls of tubes, hollow organs, the heart, and the glands. *Most viscera are supplied by both excitatory and inhibitory fibers.*

## EFFECTORS

Effectors may be thought of as the cells of the body that "do something." They in turn interact with the internal and external environments in some way and carry out the commands of the nervous system. The two classes of effectors are *muscles* and *glands.* They are both transducers and capable of converting one form of energy into another. Effectors, like nerve tissue, are excitable tissues and are able to generate action potentials. The nervous system controls muscles and glands by directly turning them on or by altering their level of spontaneous activity through a neuron-to-effector chemical communication system.

## PHYSIOLOGIC CHANGES WITH AGING

Changes in the nervous system occur with normal aging. It must be stressed, however, that normal aging cannot be equated with senility or Alzheimer's disease. The healthy older person continues to function mentally at a high level in most cases.

The changes in the nervous system associated with aging include the loss of brain cells with actual loss of brain weight. The nerve cell loss frequently is diffuse and gradual. The gyri of the brain surface also atrophy, causing widening and deepening of the spaces between the gyri. Other changes include a decrease in blood flow to the brain. The ability of the brain to autoregulate its blood supply lessens with increased age.

The control of the autonomic nervous system over various functions of the body is unpredictable and labile in the elderly, but some changes do occur. In addition, sensory and motor conduction decreases in velocity of nerve impulses occur with aging, with sensory conduction decreasing faster than motor. This occurs especially in peripheral nerves. See box below for points to check in assessing the elderly.

# SUBJECTIVE DATA

Complete neurologic assessment usually is completed in phases and depends on the condition of the person and the urgency in collecting the data.[3,4,9] The first phase is usually the *history,* where *subjective data* are obtained.

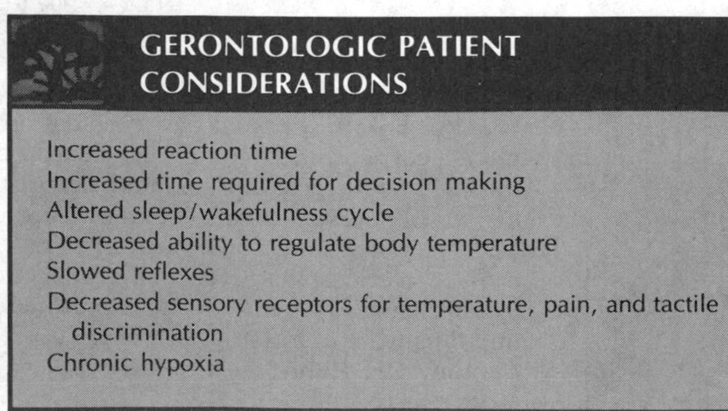

GERONTOLOGIC PATIENT CONSIDERATIONS

- Increased reaction time
- Increased time required for decision making
- Altered sleep/wakefulness cycle
- Decreased ability to regulate body temperature
- Slowed reflexes
- Decreased sensory receptors for temperature, pain, and tactile discrimination
- Chronic hypoxia

Several aspects of the neurologic examination contain largely subjective data. These are the assessment of *mental status, level of consciousness, language and speech, perceptual status,* and *sensory status.* Levels of consciousness are discussed in Chapter 57. The others are discussed in this chapter.

The reader is reminded that often it is difficult to separate subjective from objective data in the neurologic examination. One example of this is the testing of the cranial nerves. These are discussed under objective data to prevent confusion, although many of these nerves have sensory components.[5]

## HISTORY

As in other specialties, a careful history precedes physical examination of the nervous system. In the course of history taking, the person's chief complaints are elicited through an interview. The person is asked to give a timewise account of the illness. The onset and progression of the condition, as well as the nature of symptoms, should be determined. As the person describes the onset of symptoms, note particularly the *speed of onset, frequency of remissions* (if any), and any *diurnal patterns* or *intensity changes in symptoms.* Symptoms often reported with vagueness and thus requiring sophisticated analyses are complaints of pain, headache, seizures, vertigo, numbness, visual changes, and weakness. Identification of specific patterns of these common neurologic manifestations may provide pertinent diagnostic information about the pathologic process and the person's perception of limitations. Ongoing collection of psychosociocultural data is of special importance. Information is collected about family members and their relationships and interactions, ethnic background, housing, recreational interests, occupation, education, coping mechanisms, dependence-independence characteristics, and how usual activities of daily living are correctly managed by the person. Particular attention should be paid to reports of any *recent changes in the person's usual behaviors;* for example, *increased irritability, memory loss,* or *complaints of increasing job-related pressure* or *tension.* A family health history and developmental history also are included. During the course of the neurologic or physical examination, some of the observations made during the history may be confirmed. A skillfully taken history with accurate analysis and interpretation of the collected data often holds the key to diagnosis. Some observations made during the history that are validated during the examination will require further study through special neurodiagnostic procedures.

### Mental Status

Specific abnormalities to higher cerebral function are particularly significant in determining the presence of organic brain disease; therefore clinical observation of mental function is important.[5]

Along with level of consciousness, the patient is tested for *orientation* to time (day, month, week), place, and person. Disorientation to place and person indicates a more profound cerebral disorder. It is helpful to remember that orientation depends on the ongoing sensory impressions and involves the cerebral cortex. The nurse must be aware of the patient's access to sensory information before deciding the patient is disoriented.

The identification of *mood* and *behavior* also is included in a mental examination, because a particular mood may be associated with a specific disease. For example, *emotional lability* often is seen in *bilateral* (diffuse) *brain disease,* where the mood shifts easily and quickly from one extreme to the other. *Euphoria is a superficial elevation of mood* accompanied by unconcern even in the presence of threatening events. It needs to be determined if the person's mood is appropriate to the topic of conversation. *Personality changes* with the appearance of violent temper and aggressive behavior may occur with destructive lesions of the inferior frontal parts of the limbic system. Such behaviors can be validated by family and friends.

The individual's *knowledge* and *vocabulary* are tested in reference to common knowledge of current events. The ability to think abstractly may be tested by asking the person to explain the meaning of a proverb. Calculation is tested by examining the ability to subtract serially 7 from 100. *Dyscalculia* is the inability to solve simple problems. *Recent memory loss* is more common in brain disease than is remote memory loss. The findings of these gross tests may indicate the need for more definitive tests of mental function. Thus it can be seen that much data concerning mental status can be collected through a careful and thoughtful patient history.

### Language and Speech

In assessing language and speech, one must first distinguish between aphasia and dysarthria. **Aphasia** is the general term for impairment of language function; it is a disorder of symbolic language. **Dysarthria,** on the other hand, is an indistinctness in word articulation or enunciation resulting from *interference* with the *peripheral speech mechanisms* (e.g., the muscles of the tongue, palate, pharynx, or lips).[12]

Gross assessment of speech and language is made while the examinee's history is being taken. To further assess language, one must recall that language ability is concentrated in a cortical field that includes parts of the temporal lobe, the temporoparietal-occipital junction, the frontal lobe of the dominant (usually the left) hemisphere, and the occipital lobes. Lesions in any of the above areas will produce some impairment of language ability.

#### Aphasia

Several different types of aphasia have been identified: (1) fluent, (2) nonfluent, and (3) global. Although one

**TABLE 56-7 Types of Aphasia**

| TYPE | DEFINITION | SITE OF LESION | CLINICAL MANIFESTATIONS | PATIENT AWARENESS |
|---|---|---|---|---|
| Wernicke's | Type of fluent aphasia | Wernicke's area of left hemisphere | Fluent speech with normal and rapid rate; grammar and rhythm are intact, but with little content to speech.<br>Paraphasias, neologisms, and verbal nonwords occur | Not aware of mistake |
| Anomic | Type of fluent aphasia | Area of angular gyrus | Speech is fluent but patient cannot name objects or places; may define or describe what he is trying to name | Is aware |
| Conduction | Type of fluent aphasia | Arcuate fasciculus | Speech characterized by literal paraphasia, but comprehension is intact | Is aware |
| Fluent | Impairment of ability to comprehend spoken language or written language | | | |
| Nonfluent | Loss of ability to express one's thoughts in speech and/or writing (motor, Broca's, expressive) | Motor cortex at Broca's area | Problems in selecting, organizing, and initiating motor speech patterns<br>Speech halting, with effort to produce each word<br>Limited vocabulary<br>Telegraphic speech—omission of small grammatic words | Knows what he or she wishes to say and comprehends disability<br>Often frustrated |
| Global | Occurs with extensive left damage and involves several speech areas<br>Few intact language skills | Several sites | Nonfluent speech, poor comprehension, limited ability to name objects or repeat words | Cannot comprehend world around him or her |

type often predominates, often one or more of the other types will be detected to some degree. (See Table 56-7 for further information on the aphasias.)

Aphasic problems can be detected by assessing spontaneous speech and by asking the examinee to follow simple commands, written and oral, to read and interpret newspaper stories, or to write down thoughts. Once a problem is identified, referral may be made to a speech pathologist for a definitive diagnosis and suggestions for treatment.

### Dysarthria

The ability to produce speech is tested through the detection of weakness or incoordination of muscles used in articulating speech. Limitations are observed during *cranial nerve testing* and particularly in reference to cranial nerves V, VII, IX, X, and XII. As previously discussed, involvement of the motor component of these nerves may produce alterations in phonation, resonance, and articulation. The examiner asks the individual to produce different speech sounds to localize the problem.

*Dysarthrias* are usually noticed during ordinary conversation or by having the examinee repeat a difficult phrase such as "Methodist Episcopal" or "third riding artillery brigade." Dysarthrias may be manifested by a single alteration or a variety of alterations. There are characteristic changes in particular diseases. For example, in cerebellar disease, speech is often thick and explosive with a prolongation of speech sounds occurring at intervals (scanning). In parkinsonism, speech is referred to as being hyperkinetic and is characterized by a decrease in loudness and in vocal emphasis patterns that makes sounds seem monotonous to the listener.

*Apractic speech* is a rare, yet interesting, disorder in which there is difficulty in the production of speech volitionally in the absence of motor programming through cortical integration. (Apraxia is a general term that also relates to motor acts other than speech.)

## Perception

All sensation is integrated and interpreted in the sensory cortex, especially in the parietal lobe. It is important for the nurse to recognize *perceptual problems,* for they can be more difficult to deal with than changes in the patient's ability to move or sense. Disorders of percep-

TABLE 56-8 Apraxia

| TYPE | IMPAIRMENT PRODUCED | LESION SITE |
|---|---|---|
| Constructional | Impairment in producing designs in two or three dimensions<br>Involves copying, drawing, or constructing | Occipitoparietal lobe of either hemisphere |
| Dressing | Inability to dress oneself accurately<br>Makes mistakes, as putting clothes on backwards, upside-down, inside-out, or putting both legs in the same pant leg | Occipital or parietal lobe usually in nondominant hemisphere |
| Motor | Loss of kinesthetic memory patterns, which results in patient's inability to perform a purposeful motor task although it is understood | Frontal lobe of either hemisphere, precentral gyrus |
| Idiomotor | Inability to imitate gestures or perform a purposeful motor task on command<br>May be able to do task spontaneously | Parietal lobe of dominant hemisphere, supramarginal gyrus |
| Ideational | Inability to carry out activities automatically or on command because of inability to understand the concept of the act | Parietal lobe of dominant hemisphere or diffuse brain damage as in arteriosclerosis |

tion frequently involve *spatial-temporal relationships* or the *perception of self.*[1,11]

The special ability to recognize objects through any of the special senses is known as **gnosia.** Lesions involving a specific association area of the cortex produce a specific type of gnosia (absence of this ability). One type of ability often tested is *stereognosis,* the ability to perceive an object's nature and form by touch. This is assessed by asking the examinee to identify familiar objects placed in the hand one at a time.

*Apraxia* is another perceptual problem often seen. This is the inability to perform skilled, purposeful movements in the absence or loss of motor power, sensation, or coordination. (See Table 56-8 for examples of the different types of apraxia.)

## Sensory Status

Accurate assessment of sensory function depends on the person's cooperation, alertness, and responsiveness. The examinee should be relaxed and have the eyes closed during all portions of the sensory examination to avoid receiving visual clues. Also, sensation should be tested side to side and distally to proximally.

General sensory function of the trunk and extremities is tested for both superficial and deep sensations. Areas of sensory loss or abnormality are mapped out on a body diagram with a red pencil according to the distribution of the *spinal dermatomes* and peripheral nerves (see Figure 56-16). A dermatome, or skin segment, may be thought of as the area of skin supplied by one dorsal root of a cutaneous nerve. An area in which sensation is absent *(anesthesia)* is differentiated from areas in which a sensation is intensified *(hyperesthesia)* or lessened (*hypesthesia* or *hypoesthesia*). *Paresthesia* is an abnormal sensation that is perceived as burning, prickly, or itching.

### Pain, temperature, and touch

*Superficial pain* perception is assessed by stimulating a suspected area by pinprick and asking the examinee to report discomfort. One can alternate sharp with dull objects for increased discrimination. *Deep pain* may be assessed by multiple means, some of which have the potential of causing tissue injury. It is necessary to assess deep pain only when the person being examined has a decreased level of consciousness. The method used should be chosen carefully, and the reader is directed to use the expertise of a nurse specialist to learn the correct techniques. Some ways that deep pain may be assessed are by applying pressure over the nailbeds or supraorbitally. Pressure may be applied also over bone areas, such as the sternum. Nailbed pressure is accomplished by placing a pen or similar object on the nailbed and squeezing it between the examiner's thumb and forefinger (Figure 56-19). Deep pain may be elicited also by squeezing the trapezius muscle. Pinching and pricking may damage tissues and are avoided whenever possible.[10]

*Crude touch* may be assessed by touching a suspected area with cotton and requesting that the examinee indicate when the touch is felt. *Temperature* is tested by touching particular areas with warm to hot and cool to cold objects and asking the person to state the sensations felt. ***Because pain and temperature have the same nerve pathway*** (lateral spinothalamic), ***testing for temperature can be eliminated in the routine examination if the tests for pain perception are normal.***

### Motion and position

Proprioceptive fibers (fascicularis gracilis and fascicularis cuneatus) transmit sensory impulses from muscles, tendons, ligaments, and joints. This results in an awareness of the position of one's limbs in space (kinesthetic

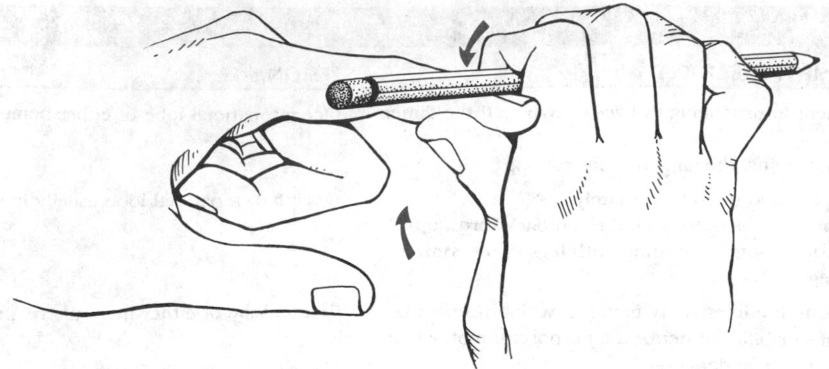

**FIGURE 56-19** Nailbed pressure stimulation using pencil.

sense). *Proprioception* is tested by the examiner's grasping the sides of the examinee's distal phalanx and moving it up and down without assistance from the examinee. If proprioception is intact, the examinee will report correctly the direction in which the joint is being moved. One also can assess proprioceptive abilities by the Romberg test in which the person being tested is asked to stand erect with the feet together and the eyes closed. A positive test occurs when the person loses balance, which indicates a pathologic condition of the brain.

*Vibration* is tested by placing a low-frequency tuning fork on a bony prominence of each extremity and assessing the examinee's ability to feel it.

## OBJECTIVE DATA

The sequence in performing the neurologic examination varies with the examiner, but it should be one that ensures completeness and thoroughness without exhausting the person being examined.[13,14,15] Throughout the examination the examiner attempts to localize the site of any abnormality. Using knowledge of normal neuroanatomy and neurophysiology, combined with a series of tests, the abnormal findings with reference to their *distribution* and *symmetry* of both sides of the body are noted.

The examination depends largely on inspection and palpation and only occasionally on percussion. Auscultation may be used to detect related vascular abnormalities. Varied instruments are used. Initially, functions may be tested grossly, followed by definitive testing should an abnormality be identified.

Equipment required to perform a neurologic examination (in addition to materials used for a general physical examination) is often assembled for convenience on a neurologic tray (see Box 56-1).

**BOX 56-1 Equipment Needed to Perform a Neurologic Examination**

1. Compass
2. Cotton applicators
3. Diagram of dermatomes
4. Dynamometer
5. Flashlight
6. Miscellaneous items of varied shapes and sizes (coin, key, marble)
7. Ophthalmoscope
8. Otoscope
9. Colored pencil
10. Pins with sharp and blunt ends
11. Printed page
12. Reflex hammer
13. Tape measure
14. Tongue depressors
15. Tuning fork
16. Snellen chart
17. Stoppered vials containing:
    a. Peppermint, oil of cloves, coffee, soap (smell)
    b. Sugar, salt, vinegar, quinine (taste)
    c. Cold and hot water (temperature)
18. Watch with second hand

### CRANIAL NERVES

A general description of cranial nerve testing is included at this point. It is helpful to recall from anatomy the number of the nerve (the sequence of the nerve along the rostrocaudal axis of the brain) and the name (explains the function or distribution) and to be able to express in a few words the function or functions of each cranial nerve so that it has practical meaning. Knowledge of the brainstem anatomy assists in relating the cranial nerve locations (see Figure 56-9).

The 12 cranial nerves may be tested in numbered sequence as presented on the following pages.[2] Some nurses prefer to test at the same time those cranial nerves that have similarity of function, such as voluntary motor function and visceral motor function and special sensory and general sensory functions. It should be recalled, however, that some cranial nerves have both motor and sensory functions, whereas others are purely

**TABLE 56-9 Cranial Nerves**

| NERVE | ORIGIN | FUNCTION | ASSESSMENTS |
|---|---|---|---|
| Olfactory (I) | Olfactory | Sensory—smell | Identification of odors |
| Optic (II) | Lateral geniculate body | Sensory—vision | Visual acuity; inspection of fundi; determination of visual fields |
| Oculomotor (III) | Midbrain | Motor—pupil constriction, elevation of upper eyelid, extraocular movements | CN III, IV, and VI are tested together for extraocular movements (Figure 56-22); also pupil reflex for CN III |
| Trochlear (IV) | Midbrain | Motor—downward/inward eye movements | |
| Trigeminal (V) | Pons | Motor—jaw movement<br>Sensory facial sensation | Jaw strength; facial sensation; corneal reflex |
| Abducens (VI) | Pons | Motor—lateral eye movements | |
| Facial (VII) | Pons | Motor—facial muscles<br>Sensory taste on anterior two thirds of tongue | Facial movements; identification of tastes |
| Acoustic (VIII) | Pons | Hearing—cochlear division<br>Balance—vestibular division | Whisper; caloric test |
| Glossopharyngeal (IX) | Medulla | Sensory—pharynx and posterior tongue, with taste<br>Motor—pharynx | Identification of tastes<br>Gag reflex; uvula motion; soft palate movement; hoarseness |
| | | Sensory—pharynx and larynx | |
| Vagus (X) | Medulla | Motor—palate, pharynx, and larynx | |
| Spinal accessory (XI) | Medulla | Motor—sternocleidomastoid; upper part of trapezius | Shoulder and neck motion |
| Hypoglossal (XII) | Medulla | Motor—tongue | Tongue motion |

Modified from Bates B: *A guide to physical examination,* ed 2, Philadelphia, 1979, JB Lippincott.

motor or sensory. It also should be recognized by the examiner that data collected from sensory testing are subjective. To counteract this, the person should be retested several times and in a random order to avoid memorization by the examinee (Table 56-9).

## Cranial Nerve I (Olfactory)

The function of cranial nerve I is purely *sensory,* namely, smell. Special receptors located within the superior or uppermost part of each nasal chamber, when stimulated by odors, transmit neural impulses over the olfactory bulbs to the olfactory nerves terminating in the area of the central cortex concerned with olfaction. When testing this cranial nerve, it is first determined whether an odor is perceived. If so, identification of the specific odor is requested by name. Data are collected in relation to the ability to perceive odor and identify substances by their odor. The ability to be aware of an odor must be differentiated from the ability to name a specific substance. *Anosmia* (absence of smell) or *hyposmia* (decreased sensitivity of the sense of smell) is often associated with complaints of lack of *taste,* even though tests may demonstrate that sense to be intact. Anosmia is caused by varied lesions involving any part of the olfactory pathways. Neoplasia at the base of the frontal lobe and trauma are the common causes of neurogenic anosmia. Intranasal disease affecting the epithelium containing the receptors should be excluded before a diagnosis is made.

## Cranial Nerve II (Optic)

The function of cranial nerve II is purely *sensory,* namely, *sight or vision.* Rods and cones, the special receptors sensitive to light, are located within the retina of the eye. When the retina is stimulated, nerve impulses are transmitted over the optic nerves (extending from the optic disc to the chiasm), over the optic tracts with the radiations terminating in the visual cortex of the occipital lobes. It should be noted, as shown in Figure 56-20, that the medial (nasal) fibers of each optic nerve cross at the chiasm to the opposite side of the brain, whereas the lateral (temporal) fibers remain uncrossed. Thus fibers of the *left optic tract* contain fibers from only the left half of each retina and carry impulses to the left occipital lobe; fibers of the right optic tract contain fibers from only the right half of each retina and carry impulses to the right occipital lobe. Vision depends on the intactness of the visual pathways described previously. Optic nerve function is assessed in relation to visual acuity, visual fields, and the appearance of the fundus (inner eye posterior to the lens). Each eye is tested separately.

### Visual acuity

Visual acuity is mediated by the *cones* of the retina. Central vision is grossly tested by reading fine newspaper print. Distant visual acuity is assessed through the use of the Snellen chart (see Chapter 59). Individuals with vision less than 20/20 are tested to determine light

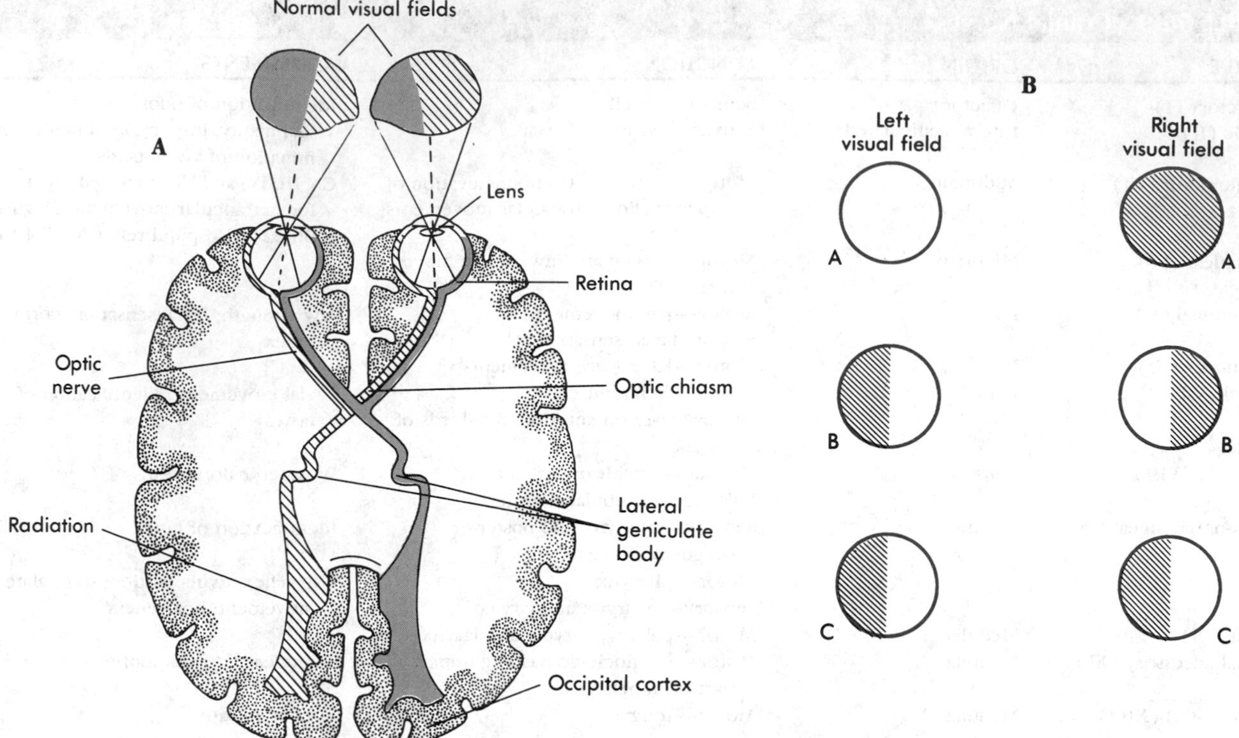


FIGURE 56-20 **A,** Visual pathways showing partial decussation at optic chiasm. Normal visual fields show reversal of light rays from the temporal and nasal sides to receptors in the retina. **B,** Abnormal visual fields. *A,* Normal left field of vision with loss of vision in right field as a result of complete lesion off right optic nerve. *B,* Loss of vision in temporal half of both fields as a result of lesion of optic chiasm (bitemporal hemianopia). *C,* Loss of vision in nasal field of right eye and temporal field of left eye caused by lesion of right optic tract (homonymous hemianopia).

perception (LP), hand movement (HM), and finger count (FC).

### Visual fields

Field of vision is defined as that portion of space in which objects are visible during the fixation of vision in *one* direction. The field of vision thus relates to peripheral vision, or indirect vision. As in visual acuity, normality depends on the intactness of all parts of the visual pathway of the eye. The receptors for peripheral fields are the *rod* neurons of the retina. These are efficient for detection of form and movement but are poor for vision and color. Visual acuity and color are functions of the central field. The visual fields are tested grossly by *confrontation techniques.* This is a method of assessing the visual field of a patient by moving an object into the periphery of each of the quadrants of the eye. The test is conducted while one eye is covered and the vision of the other is fixed on a point straight ahead. The patient reports when the moving object is first detected at the edge of each visual field. The examiner's finger may be the moving finger. Visual fields may be altered in a variety of central nervous system diseases, such as neoplasia and vascular disease. Ocular disease such as glaucoma is a major cause. Damage to one optic nerve anterior to the chiasm affects only the field of the involved eye. Lesions at the chiasm or posterior to it produce bilateral visual field defects of a wide variety. For example, a pituitary gland tumor compressing the optic chiasm damages the crossing fibers from the nasal retina and classically causes bitemporal hemianopsia, or the loss of vision in the temporal halves of each eye. Loss of vision in the corresponding halves of both visual fields produces *homonymous hemianopsia* and can be further designated as right or left. For example, patients with *right* cerebrovascular accidents often experience hemianopsia with left visual field loss.

### Ocular fundus

The fundus is examined through the *ophthalmoscope.* The ocular fundus is defined as that portion of the interior of the eyeball that lies posterior to the lens. It includes the optic disc, blood vessels, retina, and macula. Examination, although painless in the normal eye, does require cooperation from the person being examined.

#### Examination and interpretation of ophthalmoscopic findings

The optic disc (papilla) is normally the most prominent structure visible; *it is the center of observation from*

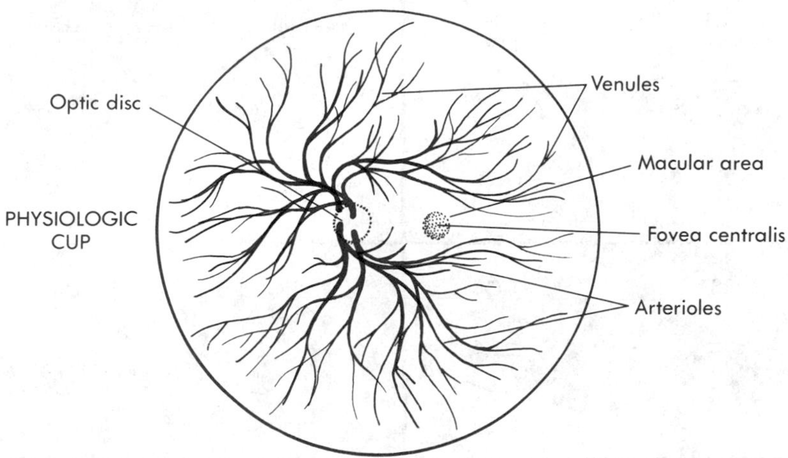


**FIGURE 56-21** Structures of the left eye as visualized through the funduscope.

**TABLE 56-10 Normal Characteristics of the Optic Disc**

| | |
|---|---|
| Size | 1.5 mm |
| Shape | Flat round or vertically oval |
| Margins | Sharply defined |
| Color | Creamy red with a small whitish depression in the center (physiologic cup) |

*which the funduscopic* examination proceeds. The fundus is the area where the blood vessels and nerve fibers enter and exit from the eyeball (Figure 56-21). The normal characteristics of the optic disk are presented in Table 56-10.

The disc is examined in detail to assess size, shape, margins, and color. There can be excessive pallor or redness. Swelling of the optic disc, or *papilledema*, may be caused by active inflammation or passive congestion. Papilledema because of passive congestion and edema from increased intracranial pressure is called *choked disc* (see Chapter 57). The neurologist is most interested in differentiating between early and late papilledema. *Optic atrophy* indicates partial or complete destruction of the optic nerve. It is associated with decreased visual acuity and with a change in the color of the disc to a lighter pink or gray. The recognition of advanced papilledema is relatively easy, but differentiation of physiologic variations is difficult.

The largest blood vessels just visible in the fundus, the central retinal artery and central retinal vein, branch throughout the retina. The retina is the only site in the human body where microcirculation can be viewed directly.

## Cranial Nerve III (Oculomotor), Cranial Nerve IV (Trochlear), and Cranial Nerve VI (Abducens)

Cranial nerves III, IV, and VI are *motor nerves* that arise from the brainstem and innervate the six *extraocular muscles* attached to the eyeball. These muscles function as a group in the coordinated movement of each eyeball in the six cardinal fields of gaze (straight, up, and down on both nasal and temporal sides). The motor nerves control the ocular muscles so that the eyes remain parallel throughout all ranges of motion and thus maintain *binocular* (stereoscopic) vision. The oculomotor nerves, in addition, send parasympathetic autonomic fibers to the constrictor muscles of the iris and to the levator palpebrae muscles of the upper eyelids.

### Extraocular movements

Individual eye movements are tested by covering one eye and following the examiner's finger in all fields of gaze with the uncovered eye while keeping the head stationary. Limitations of movement in all directions are observed, as well as actual paralysis *(ophthalmoplegia)*. If one of the extraocular muscles is paralyzed by damage to the nerve, the eye is unable to deviate fully into the corresponding field of gaze.

*Conjugate movements of the eyes* also are tested by asking the person to look with both eyes as far possible to either side and then up and down. The examiner observes for parallel movements of the eyes in each direction or any deviation from normal (Figure 56-22).

Double vision *(diplopia)*, squint *(strabismus)*, and involuntary rhythmic movements of the eyeballs *(nystagmus)* may indicate weakness of some of the extraocular muscles because of deficits of the motor nerves. These nerves may be involved singly or in unison in some neurologic diseases. *Ptosis*, or dropping of the upper eyelid over the globe, may be caused by damage to the oculomotor nerve. Normally, the upper lid minimally overlaps the iris as the examinee moves the eyes downward. The person with ptosis is unable to raise the lid voluntarily.

### Pupils

Each pupil should be inspected first as to size and then as to shape and equality. *Argyll Robertson* pupils, for

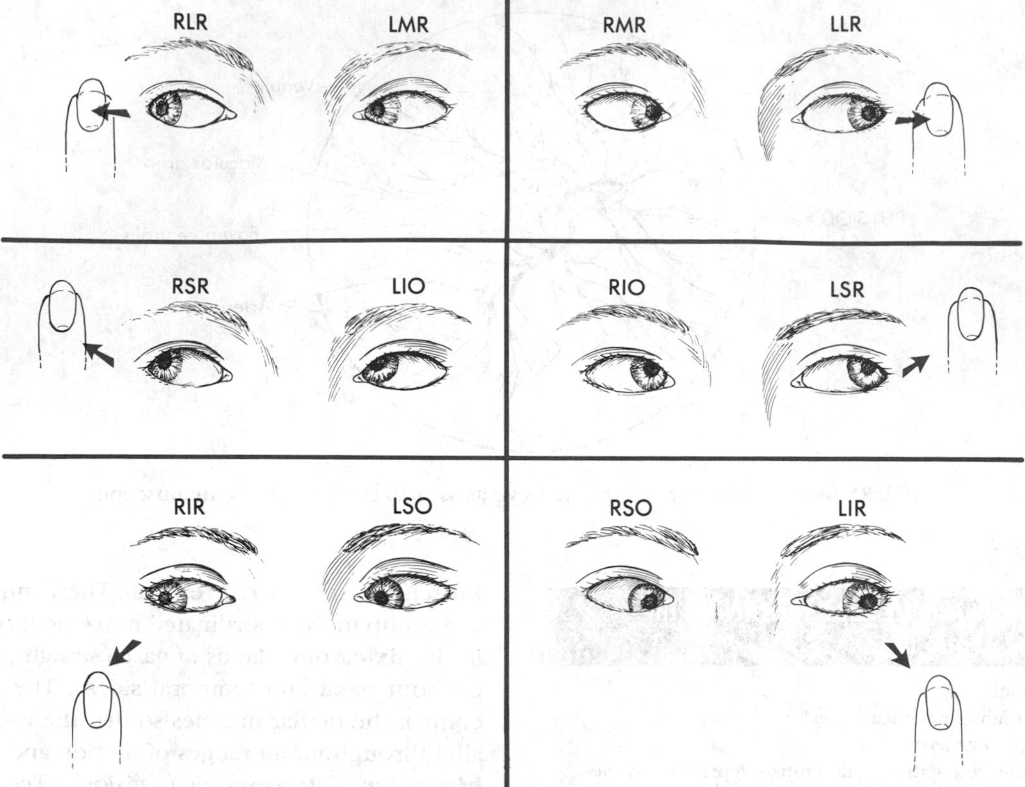


**FIGURE 56-22** Examination of extraocular muscles. Note that two muscles are involved in each cardinal direction. *R,* right; *L,* left; *LR,* lateral rectus; *MR,* medial rectus; *SR,* superior rectus; *IO,* inferior oblique; *IR,* inferior rectus; *SO,* superior oblique.

example, are constricted and do not react to light, although they react to accommodation for near objects. Pupil inequality, or *anisocoria,* may assist in diagnosis of some neurologic diseases (Figure 56-23). The pupil is normally round, centrally placed, regular in outline, and equal in size to the other pupil. However, unequal pupils are found in approximately 25% of the normal population. Thus it is more significant to assess briskness of the pupillary response.

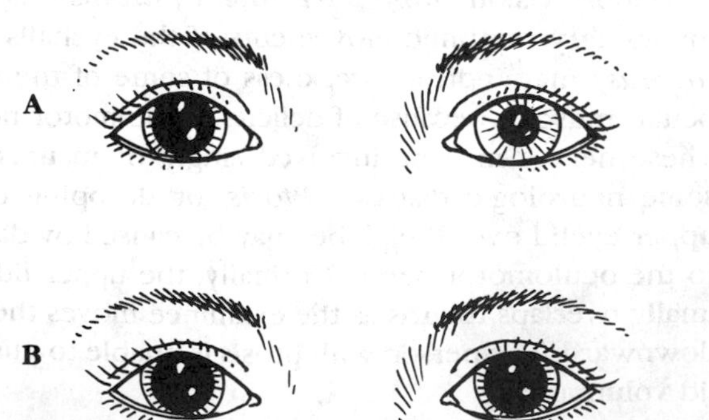


**FIGURE 56-23** **A,** Unequal pupils, also called *anisocoria.* **B,** Dilated and fixed pupils, indicative of severe neurologic deficit.

### Pupillary reflex

The examiner darkens the room before examination. A small beam of light is focused directly into each eye in turn. The examiner avoids shining the light into both eyes simultaneously and instructs the person not to focus on the light beam, thus producing an accommodation reaction. Normally, the pupil constricts quickly when a light is focused on the homolateral retina. Constriction is reported to be especially brisk in young people and those with blue eyes. After a head injury, for example, a *dilated, fixed* pupil may be observed on the side of the cranial injury (Fig. 56-23, *B*). A slow or sluggish pupil occurs as the pupil contracts slowly or imperfectly and relaxes immediately.[8]

### Consensual light reflex

Observations include inspection for constriction of the pupil *opposite* to the one directly stimulated. As a result of the decussation (crossing) of nerve fibers both in the optic chiasm and in the pretectal area, the homolateral pupil, as well as the contralateral pupil, normally reacts to light.

## Cranial Nerve V (Trigeminal)

Cranial nerve V is a *mixed* nerve with motor and sensory components. It is the largest cranial nerve. The motor part innervates the temporal and masseter muscles; the sensory part supplies the cornea, face, head, and mucous membrane.

In muscle weakness the opened jaw tends to deviate to the opposite side of the weakened muscles. The sensory components supplying the face are tested for touch, pain, and temperature and for any deficits noted as to distribution.

Next, bilateral *corneal reflexes* may be assessed if they are in question. Normally, the examinee will blink bilaterally. This is an especially important reflex to assess in persons with *decreased levels of consciousness* because corneal damage may result in its absence.

## Cranial Nerve VII (Facial)

Cranial nerve VII is a *mixed nerve* that is concerned with facial movement and the sensation of taste. The inability to smile, close both eyes tightly, look upward and wrinkle the forehead, show the teeth, purse the lips, and blow out the cheeks constitutes weakness or paralysis of facial muscles innervated by this nerve. Distinction must be made between central and peripheral neurologic involvement. Special attention in examination is given to asymmetry. Peripheral involvement as in *Bell's palsy* is caused by compression of this cranial nerve and is a common *lower motor neuron* type of facial paralysis. (This means the lesion affects the facial nerve or its nucleus.) Lesions affecting the facial nerve produce paralysis of half of the entire face including the eyelids, forehead, and lips. Forehead function, by contrast, remains intact in *central* or *upper motor neuron* lesions. This suggests that the lesion lies somewhere on the path from the contralateral cerebral cortex to the nucleus of the facial nerve. The sensation of taste is tested by placing in turn, salty, sweet, bitter, and sour substances on the side of the protruded tongue for identification. A loss of taste over the anterior two thirds of the tongue is present when this nerve is diseased, as occurs in mastoid canal lesions.

## Cranial Nerve VIII (Acoustic)

Cranial nerve VIII is composed of a *cochlear* division related to hearing and a *vestibular* division related to equilibrium. The cochlear portion is tested grossly by having the examinee listen and identify whispered words. It is recommended that the ticking of a watch not be used routinely because it produces a high-pitched tone and such tones are not heard very well by the elderly. A more complete examination, including bone and air conduction of sound, involves testing with a tuning fork and audiometric testing (Chapter 61). The vestibular portion of the acoustic nerve may be tested in a variety of ways. In the *past-pointing test,* the examinee is asked to raise the arms and to bring the index finger down on the examiner's finger with the arm outstretched, first with the eyes open and then with the eyes closed. Normally, the examinee's finger touches the examiner's without difficulty. In vestibular disease, the finger points to one side or the other consistently. The vestibular portion also is tested by looking for the presence of *nystagmus,* "to-and-fro" movements of the eyeballs on horizontal and vertical planes, as the examinee looks to one side and upward. True nystagmus is characterized by sustained movement of the eyeball including a fast jerk to the side of the deviation and a slow jerk back to the midline. Additional tests can include caloric tests and electronystagmography (see Chapter 61).

Disease of the *cochlea* is characterized by nerve deafness (perception deafness). There is loss or impairment of hearing. Nerve deafness usually is the result of disease of the peripheral nerve. It also may occur from central lesions involving *acoustic nerves* and *nerve pathways* in the brainstem and their *termination within the temporal lobe. The vestibular portion frequently is affected in diseases of the central nervous system, and the most important symptom is vertigo.*

## Cranial Nerve IX (Glossopharyngeal) and Cranial Nerve X (Vagus)

Cranial nerves IX and X are tested together. The chief function of cranial nerve IX is *sensory* to the pharynx and taste to the posterior third of the tongue. Both nerves supply the posterior pharyngeal wall, and normally when the wall is touched there is prompt contraction of these muscles on both sides, with or without gagging. This test is thus unreliable in regard to either nerve alone. Because cranial nerve X is the chief *motor nerve* to the soft palatal, pharyngeal, and laryngeal muscles, the detection of abnormalities is made through testing of voice sounds and cough sounds. In unilateral involvement of the motor portion of the vagus nerve there is harshness and nasality of the voice. When the person says "ah," the soft palate does not stay in the midline but deviates to the intact side. Bilateral involvement produces more severe effects in speech; also, swallowing is difficult **(dysphagia),** and fluids regurgitate through the nose because of palatal and pharyngeal involvement. Sensory function usually is not tested in the vagus nerve.

## Cranial Nerve XI (Spinal Accessory)

Cranial nerve XI is a motor nerve that supplies the sternocleidomastoid muscle and upper part of the trapezius muscles. Weakness or paralysis of these muscles constitutes abnormality of this nerve.

## Cranial Nerve XII (Hypoglossal)

Cranial nerve XII is a purely *motor* nerve. To begin, the examinee's tongue should first be inspected at rest in the mouth. Any asymmetry, unilaterality, decreased bulk, deviations, or fasciculations (fine twitching) should be noted. When this nerve is involved, the tongue deviates toward the side of the lesion. Atrophy of the tongue is shown through wrinkling and loss of substance on the affected side. In an upper motor neuron lesion there is involvement of the tongue on the side opposite (contralateral) the lesion.

## MOTOR STATUS

Function of the motor system is assessed as to gait and stance, muscle strength, muscle tonus, coordination, involuntary movements, and muscle stretch reflexes.

### Gait and Stance

Gait and stance should be recognized as complex activities that require muscle strength, coordination, balance, proprioception, and vision. Gait, or walking, and associated movements give considerable information about motor status. Changes in gait may be characteristic of a specific neurologic disease. **Ataxia** is a general term meaning lack of coordination in performing a planned, purposeful motion such as walking. It can be caused by disturbance of position sense or by cerebellar or other diseases. In evaluation of gait the person is asked to walk freely and naturally. A request may be made to walk *heel to toe* in a straight line, since this exaggerates any abnormalities. To evaluate stance, the person may perform the *Romberg test.* In this test the individual stands with feet close together, first with eyes open and then with eyes closed. Patients with problems of proprioception have difficulty maintaining balance with their eyes closed; patients with cerebellar disease have difficulty even with their eyes open.

The *hemiparetic gait* seen in upper motor neuron disease is characterized by circumduction of the affected leg and inversion of the foot. Persons with Parkinson's disease walk with a slow, shuffling gait and as they start walking, there is an increase in rapidity until they are almost running *(propulsive).* They also have difficulty stopping, and deviation in the center of gravity causes retropulsion or lateropulsion. In addition, there is loss of associated movements of the arms in walking. Persons with cerebellar disease, on the other hand, walk with a wide-based, *staggering gait.*

*Muscle strength,* or power, is assessed systematically, including trunk and extremity muscles. One common assessment of muscle strength is asking the patient to grasp both hands of the examiner and to squeeze both at the same time. The examiner compares the squeezing ability of one hand with the other. This can be done also with the feet, including planter flexion and dorsiflexion. During manual testing of each muscle group the examinee attempts to resist the examiner in moving the muscles when placed in fixed positions. Weakness of a specific muscle is identified by the examiner as to distribution and degree of muscle weaknesses. The examinee also may be tested for *drift.* This test is performed by asking the person to hold the arms straight out for 20 to 30 seconds with palms supine and eyes closed. *Hemiparesis* is suggested when there is pronation of one forearm or when there is a downward drift of the arm with elbow flexion. Evaluation may include all major muscles. *Hemiplegia* is complete paralysis of one half of the body (linear), whereas *hemiparesis* is weakness or incomplete paralysis in the same distribution. *Paraplegia* is paralysis of the lower extremities, and *quadriplegia* is paralysis of the four extremities. The reader should note the distribution of peripheral motor nerves to skeletal muscles. (The distribution varies from that of sensory nerve distributions.)

### Muscle Tonus

*Muscle tonus* is tested by the examiner passively moving the examinee's limbs through a full range of motion. An increase *(hypertonia)* or a decrease *(hypotonia)* can be differentiated by the skilled examiner. In hypertonia extremities tend to stay in fixed positions and feel firm; in hypotonia the extremities assume a position governed by gravity. Overextension and overflexion are found in hypertonia; resistance to passive movement increases rapidly and then suddenly gives way to *pyramidal spasticity,* or *clasp-knife rigidity.* A steady, passive resistance throughout the full range of motion is characteristic of *parkinsonian rigidity;* the combination of passive resistance and parkinsonian tremor with small regular jerks is called *cogwheel rigidity.* In *decorticate rigidity* the upper limbs are flexed and pronated and the lower limbs are extended. In *decerebrate rigidity,* on the other hand, the upper limbs are extended.

### Coordination

*Coordination of muscle movements,* or the ability to perform skilled motor acts, may be impaired at any level of the motor system. However, the cerebellum is primarily responsible for control, so that movements take place in a smooth and precise manner. Disturbance in cerebellar function may result in ataxia (as discussed relative to gait), difficulty in controlling the range of muscular movement *(dysmetria),* and an inability to alternate rapid opposite and successive movements *(adiadochokinesia).* Simple motor activities are evaluated on command of the examiner to perform rapid and rhythmic movements. For example, the nose-finger-nose test requires the individual to alternately touch the nose and the tip of the examiner's finger with variation in rate and level. Other tests include the knee pat (pronation-supination) and heel-knee or shin test, during which the examinee slides his or her heel over the shin toward the dorsum of the foot. There are many such tests, often modified by the examiner.

### Involuntary Movements

*Involuntary movements* also need to be observed and described during neurologic examination. Description of abnormal movements **(hyperkinesia)** is difficult but necessary. Observation of the following is helpful: location of muscles involved, amplitude of movement, speed of onset, duration of contraction and relaxation, and rhythm. The effects of posture, rest, sleep, diversion of attention, voluntary movements, and emotional stress on involuntary movement are determined. Involuntary movements usually are increased by emotional stress and may subside during sleep. They can be the result of organic disease, or they may be psychosomatic in origin. A few of the more common types of involuntary movements are considered next. **Tremor** consists of rhythmic to-and-fro movements that are usually of small amplitude. They are the result of alternate contractions of opposing groups of muscles; they are continuous while the patient is awake and may or may not be present during sleep. *Chorea* consists of short, sharp, rapid movements, usually of small excursion and irregular; movements occur in different parts of the body and persist during sleep. *Hemiballismus* is a variation of chorea in which movement is confined to one side of the body and affects the limbs to a great extent. *Athetosis* consists of slow, sinuous, and more sustained movements that may be of considerable amplitude; movements occur within the neck and trunk, as well as the extremities, and may be called *torsion spasms*. **Myoclonus** consists of irregular, abrupt, and arrhythmic contractions of a muscle or a group of muscles. Myoclonus may involve the extremities, the trunk, or the face and may be consistent in site.

## Reflexes

Although all muscles can be made to contract reflexly, only a few reflexes are tested clinically. The *muscle stretch reflexes* (MSRs) (also called *myotactic* and *deep tendon reflexes*) that are tested more routinely include the biceps, triceps, brachioradialis, quadriceps, and gastrocnemius and soleus muscles. (Superficial reflexes are omitted in this discussion.) Because the muscle reflexes are simply monosynaptic reflexes, they may be diminished in normal response **(hyporeflexia)** or lost completely **(areflexia)** because of interruption of afferent sensory fiber transmission or extensive destruction of efferent motor fibers of the anterior horn cells (lower motor neurons). On the other hand, release of the monosynaptic reflex from the influence of suprasegmental fibers (pyramidal and supplementary motor systems) (upper motor neuron influence) produces an increased muscular response **(hyperreflexia).**

**TABLE 56-11 Grading of Muscle Stretch Reflexes (MSR)**

| SCALE | INTERPRETATION |
|---|---|
| 0 | Areflexia |
| ± | Hyporeflexia |
| 1+ to 3+ | Normal |
| 3+ to 4+ | Hyperreflexia |

The degree of response of the reflex above or below normal is noted and graded on a scale. The most important feature of any reflex pattern is not the absolute value on the scale but the difference between one side of the body and the other (asymmetry). Stick figures are commonly used to record the bilateral values (scale may range from 0 to 4+). See Table 56-11 for one example of how reflexes are graded on a scale. Because the threshold for muscle stretch reflexes has a normal range of variability, some individuals with generalized hyporeflexia or hyperreflexia will not have pathologic conditions but will rank at the end of the normal range. On the other hand, areflexia is usually a pathologic condition.

One *pathologic reflex* often referred to clinically is the *plantar reflex*. This reflex when present in adults results in extension of the great toe (moves toward dorsum) with fanning (abduction) of the other toes when pressure is applied to the plantar surface of the foot laterally from the heel toward the toes. This response is known as *Babinski's sign* and is associated with upper motor neuron disease (Table 56-12). Other reflexes may also be classified as pathologic. These are reflexes that are present in infancy for variable periods. They are thought to be released in adults by acquired diseases of the cerebrum. Examples include the sucking, pouting, and grasp reflexes.

A reflex when present may assist in localizing a lesion, as does the presence of a unilateral Babinski's sign. Reflex findings, however, are used only in relation to total assessment data and are not used alone. (Refer to neurology tests for techniques on eliciting specific reflexes.) Variations of grading-scale values used should be noted. It also should be recognized that grading is somewhat subjective.

**TABLE 56-12 Clinical Syndromes of Upper Motor Neuron and Lower Motor Neuron Lesions**

| MOTOR COMPONENT | UPPER MOTOR NEURON CHARACTERISTICS | LOWER MOTOR NEURON CHARACTERISTICS |
|---|---|---|
| Reflex | Hyperreflexia, extensor toe sign (Babinski's sign) | Hyporeflexia or areflexia |
| Muscle tonus | Hypertonia, clasp-knife spasticity, clonus | Hypotonia, flaccidity |
| Muscle movement | Paralysis or paresis of movements in hemiplegic distribution | Paralysis or paresis of individual muscles in peripheral nerve distribution |
| Muscle wasting | Late atrophy from disuse | Early atrophy from denervation |
| Muscle fasciculations | Not present | Present |

### Meningeal Irritation

To test for meningeal irritation, or stiff neck, the head is passively flexed sharply toward the chest while the person is in a recumbent position. In the presence of meningeal irritation there is marked resistance to flexion, accompanied by rigidity of the neck (nuchal), spasm, and pain. There is also resistance to extension and rotary movements of the neck. *Brudzinski's sign,* indicating meningeal irritation, is also elicited by passive neck flexion. When the neck is flexed, the hips and legs flex involuntarily. *Kernig's sign* is a classic test used in the diagnosis of meningitis. In this test the examiner flexes one of the patient's thighs to a right angle and then attempts to extend the leg on the thigh (there are many variations of this test). A positive Kernig's sign is present when there is spasm of the hamstring muscles with resistance to extension of the leg and with neck and head pain.

# DIAGNOSTIC TESTS

Relevant diagnostic tests can be an important source of data in making a diagnosis of neurologic disease.

## LABORATORY TESTS

### Blood

A normal part of the neurologic assessment includes obtaining blood for screening. This usually includes electrolytes, as well as a complete blood count. Serology screening is used to rule out syphilis, which in the tertiary form of the disease may yield neurologic symptoms. Arterial blood gases may be obtained, especially if the patient is critically ill or comatose. One particular form of blood test that can be very helpful is the obtaining of drug levels, especially the level of anticonvulsants. The actual blood level can give the practitioner a sense not only of the way a person metabolizes the drug but also of how compliant the person is about following the prescribed medication regimen.

Abnormalities in any of the blood studies may be indicative of neurologic disease. (See Table 56-13 for some specific abnormalities that may be found.)

**TABLE 56-13 Blood Abnormalities**

| ELEMENT | ABNORMALITY SEEN | POSSIBLE REASON |
|---|---|---|
| Potassium | Decreased | Poor dietary intake |
| White blood cells | Increased | Infection such as meningitis<br>Common steroid effect |
| $Po_2$ | Decreased | Increased intracranial pressure |
| Red blood cells | Increased | Dehydration |
| | Decreased | Anemia |
| Hematocrit and hemoglobin | Increased | Dehydration |
| | Decreased | Anemia |
| Anticonvulsant drug | Increased | Toxicity or patient overdose |
| | Decreased | Patient not taking drug |
| Plasma cortisol | Increased | Acute head injury |
| Sodium | Decreased | Inappropriate antidiuretic hormone |

### Urine

Urinary output, as well as excretion of electrolytes, is easily influenced by cranial surgery and/or trauma. This is especially true if the pituitary gland has been traumatized by injury or surgery. (See Table 56-14 for possible alterations in urinary results.)

### Cerebrospinal Fluid

Cerebrospinal fluid (CSF) is obtained either through a lumbar or cisternal puncture. These will be discussed later in this chapter. CSF is examined for an increase or decrease of its normal constituents; it is examined also for foreign substances such as pathogenic organisms and blood. CSF normally is a clear fluid that is formed in the lateral ventricles of the brain.

Spinal fluid normally is under slight positive pressure; 75 to 180 mm of water is considered normal. It is measured on a manometer when a spinal puncture is performed.

Normally each milliliter of spinal fluid contains up to

**TABLE 56-14 Urine Abnormalities**

| ELEMENT | ABNORMALITY SEEN | POSSIBLE REASON |
|---|---|---|
| Urinary output | Decreased amount | Metabolic problem<br>Kidney failure |
| | Increased amount | Diabetes insipidus |
| Specific gravity | Decreased | Diabetes insipidus |
| | Increased | Dehydration |
| Sugar and acetone | Present | Steroid effect—possible chemical diabetes |
| Sodium | Increased amount | Inappropriate antidiuretic hormone<br>Diabetes insipidus |

**TABLE 56-15 Normal Values of CSF**

| | |
|---|---|
| Pressure | 75 to 180 mm $H_2O$ |
| Glucose | 50 to 80 mg/dl |
| Chloride | 118 to 132 mEq/L |
| Protein | 20 to 50 mg/dl |
| Gamma globulin | 3% to 9% |
| Lymphocytes | 0 to 5/ml |

eight lymphocytes. An increase in the number of cells may indicate an infection. Tuberculosis and viral infections may cause an increase in lymphocytes, whereas pyogenic infections may cause an increase in polymorphonuclear leukocytes, which may be in large enough numbers to make the fluid cloudy. Bacterial infections, such as tuberculosis meningitis, often lower the blood sugar levels. They also may reduce the chloride level. In the presence of degenerative diseases and when a brain tumor is present, the spinal fluid protein usually is increased. (See Table 56-15 for normal values of CSF.)

Other tests of CSF that may be helpful include the colloidal gold test that can be used to diagnose neurosyphilis or multiple sclerosis. CSF is abnormal in about 90% of patients with multiple sclerosis, including CSF pleocytosis and abnormal gamma globulins as demonstrated by electrophoresis. Cultures of CSF may indicate the actual organism causing disease. The spinal fluid serologic test for syphilis may be positive even when the blood serologic test is negative.

Blood in the spinal fluid indicates hemorrhage into the ventricular system. It may be caused by a fracture at the base of the skull that has torn blood vessels, or it may be caused by the rupture of a blood vessel, which may occur, for example, with a congenital aneurysm. Occasionally the first specimen of spinal fluid contains blood from slight bleeding at the point of puncture. For this reason the specimens of fluid are numbered and the first one is not used to determine the cell count.

## RADIOLOGIC TESTS

The multiple radiologic procedures of the brain and spinal cord are best carried out and interpreted by a neuroradiologist. These include plain radiographs, special contrast studies of the ventricular system (including the cisternal and subarachnoid space) and the cerebral vessels, and computed tomography.

### Routine or Plain Radiographs

Routine or plain radiographs of the brain and spinal cord are usually taken first, using varied projections to detect any developmental, traumatic, or degenerative bone abnormalities. These films are still used frequently because of safety and easy availability.

### Computed Tomography (CT Scan)

One of the most significant technologic advances in radiographic equipment is the electromagnetic imager (EMI) scanner, which is capable of providing as much as 100% more information than conventional radiographic techniques. The EMI scanner is also referred to as CT scan and **computerized axial tomography.** This technique offers increased versatility, efficiency, and enhanced image detail. The CT scanner is based on a technique of scanning the brain without isotopes in which series of images using the principles of tomography are x-rayed and each of the images is derived from a specific layer of brain tissue. The brain is thus scanned in successive layers by a very narrow beam of x-rays. The total system includes a scanning unit that houses the x-ray tube, two scintillation detectors, an x-ray control unit, a computer and magnetic disk unit, viewing unit, a line printer, and a teletyper. Data are thus collected in x-ray form and printout form, and information is also stored for future use. (See Guidelines box below for further information about this procedure.)

By comparing tissue densities found with the CT scan with norms, abnormalities can be detected. Tumor masses, infarctions, displacement of bone, and ventricles can be accurately detected. The CT scan is particularly efficient in detecting brain neoplasia and cerebrovascular lesions (Figure 56-24).

#### Nursing care

After the completion of the CT scan, the nurse should monitor the patient for any signs of increased intracranial pressure (if dye was used). If the patient has become disoriented as a result of the test, as may occur with elders, reassurance should be given and the patient protected from injury. The patient may need rest after the test.

### Brain Scan

Another radiologic test is the brain scan. The purpose of this test is to detect cerebral pathology using radioactive isotopes and a scanner (Figure 56-25). It is generally used as an adjunct to routine radiographs and CT.

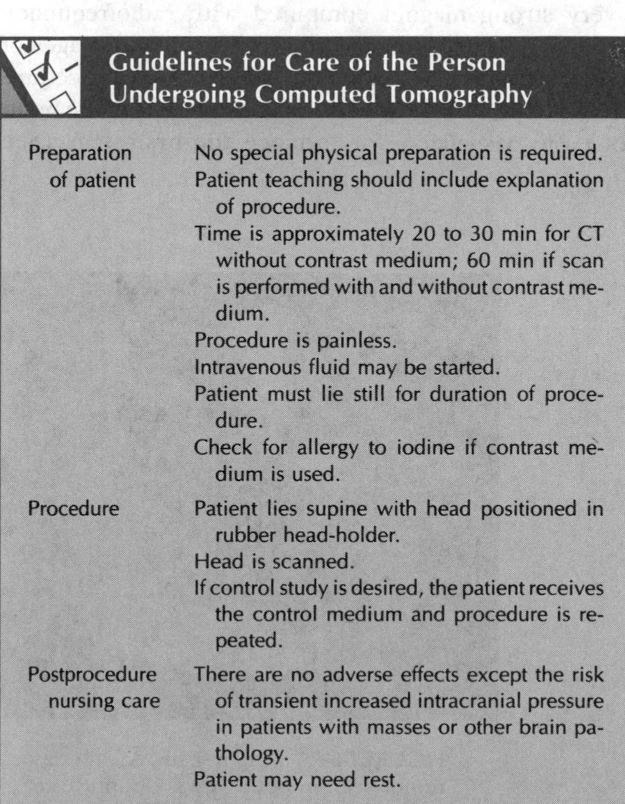

**Guidelines for Care of the Person Undergoing Computed Tomography**

| | |
|---|---|
| Preparation of patient | No special physical preparation is required.<br>Patient teaching should include explanation of procedure.<br>Time is approximately 20 to 30 min for CT without contrast medium; 60 min if scan is performed with and without contrast medium.<br>Procedure is painless.<br>Intravenous fluid may be started.<br>Patient must lie still for duration of procedure.<br>Check for allergy to iodine if contrast medium is used. |
| Procedure | Patient lies supine with head positioned in rubber head-holder.<br>Head is scanned.<br>If control study is desired, the patient receives the control medium and procedure is repeated. |
| Postprocedure nursing care | There are no adverse effects except the risk of transient increased intracranial pressure in patients with masses or other brain pathology.<br>Patient may need rest. |

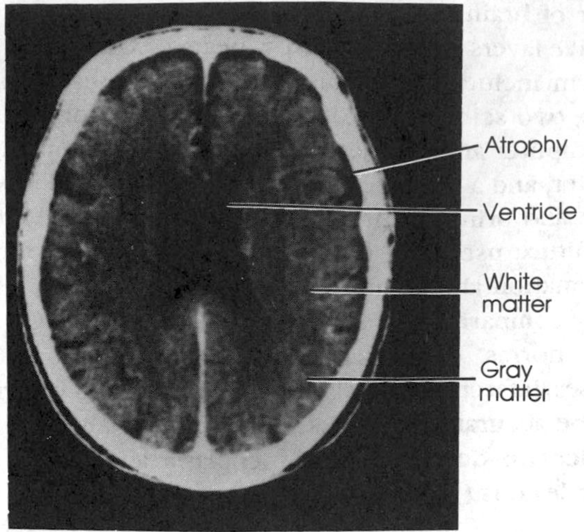


**FIGURE 56-24** CT scan printouts. CT brain scan differentiates between gray and white brain matter. (From Ballinger PW: *Merrill's atlas of radiographic positions and radiologic procedures,* ed 5, St Louis, 1982, Mosby.)

(See Guidelines box, p. 1915, left-hand column, for a description of the brain scan.) The nurse may need to reassure and support the patient during the procedure. The injection site should be monitored for bleeding, and the patient may need rest after the procedure.

## Magnetic Resonance Imaging (MRI)

One of the newest methods of scanning the brain is magnetic resonance imaging (MRI). This procedure uses a very strong magnet combined with radiofrequency waves and a computer to produce x-ray–like images of body chemistry. No radiation is used. This procedure often is extremely helpful in visualizing areas of the brain not easily visualized, for instance the brainstem. (See Guidelines box, p. 1915, right-hand column, for a description of this procedure.) As with CT and brain scan, the patient who has undergone an MRI may need rest. The disoriented patient may have been frightened by the noises the machine makes during the scan and may need reassurance and monitoring for agitated behavior.

## Pneumoencephalography

**Pneumoencephalography** (air encephalography) is a special contrast study of the ventricular and cisternal systems that permits accurate localization of brain lesions. It provides greater visualization of the posterior fossa than ventriculography. It combines a spinal or cisternal puncture with x-ray examination (Figure 56-26).

Pneumoencephalography is not used as frequently today because of the availability of other diagnostic measures, including CT and MRI. It is contraindicated when there is increased intracranial pressure because of the danger of herniation of the temporal uncus and the cerebellar tonsils, resulting in compression of the brainstem and possible death. Also, the procedure itself is extremely uncomfortable and may produce severe, life-threatening reactions. (See Guidelines box, p. 1916, left-hand column, for a description of this procedure.)

## Ventriculography

**Ventriculography** is similar to pneumoencephalography except that air is introduced directly into the lateral ventricles through trepine openings (burr holes) into the skull. This procedure is always performed in the operating room. It may be used when the suspected diagnosis contraindicates performing a spinal or lumbar puncture because of the extreme pressure within the skull or because the spinal canal is blocked. (See Guidelines box, p. 1916, right-hand column, for additional information about the procedure.)

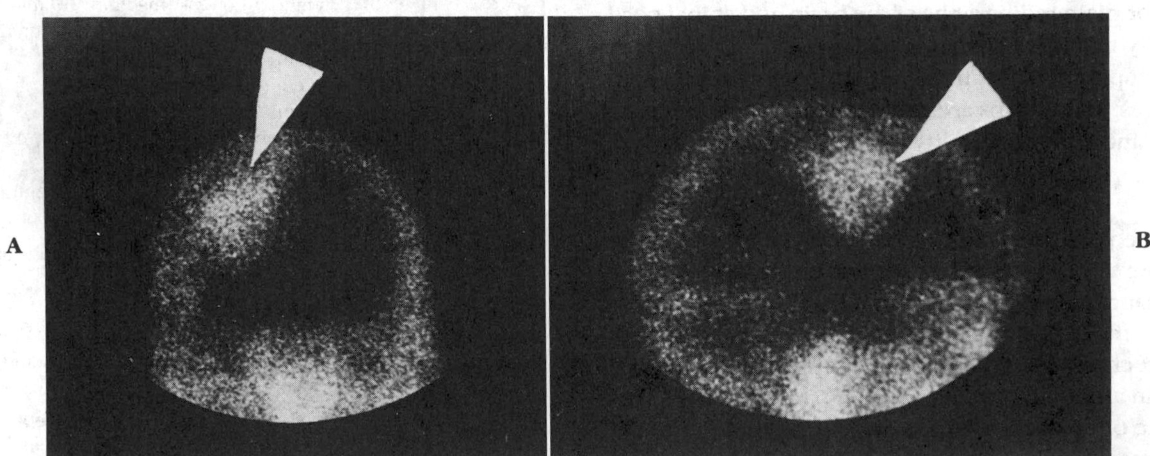


**FIGURE 56-25** Brain scans. **A,** Anteroposterior view. **B,** Lateral view. White pointers indicate tumor seen in both views. (From Pagana K: *Diagnostic testing and nursing implications: a case study approach,* St Louis, 1982, Mosby.)

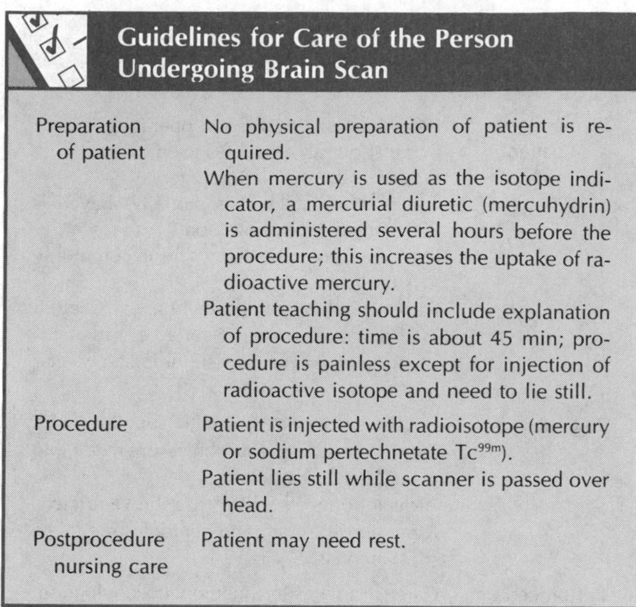

### Guidelines for Care of the Person Undergoing Brain Scan

| | |
|---|---|
| Preparation of patient | No physical preparation of patient is required.<br>When mercury is used as the isotope indicator, a mercurial diuretic (mercuhydrin) is administered several hours before the procedure; this increases the uptake of radioactive mercury.<br>Patient teaching should include explanation of procedure: time is about 45 min; procedure is painless except for injection of radioactive isotope and need to lie still. |
| Procedure | Patient is injected with radioisotope (mercury or sodium pertechnetate $Tc^{99m}$).<br>Patient lies still while scanner is passed over head. |
| Postprocedure nursing care | Patient may need rest. |

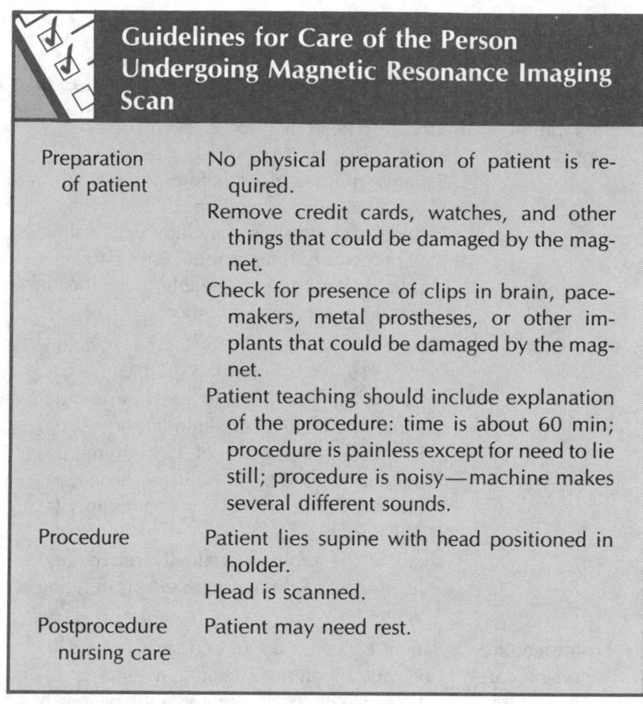

### Guidelines for Care of the Person Undergoing Magnetic Resonance Imaging Scan

| | |
|---|---|
| Preparation of patient | No physical preparation of patient is required.<br>Remove credit cards, watches, and other things that could be damaged by the magnet.<br>Check for presence of clips in brain, pacemakers, metal prostheses, or other implants that could be damaged by the magnet.<br>Patient teaching should include explanation of the procedure: time is about 60 min; procedure is painless except for need to lie still; procedure is noisy—machine makes several different sounds. |
| Procedure | Patient lies supine with head positioned in holder.<br>Head is scanned. |
| Postprocedure nursing care | Patient may need rest. |

A

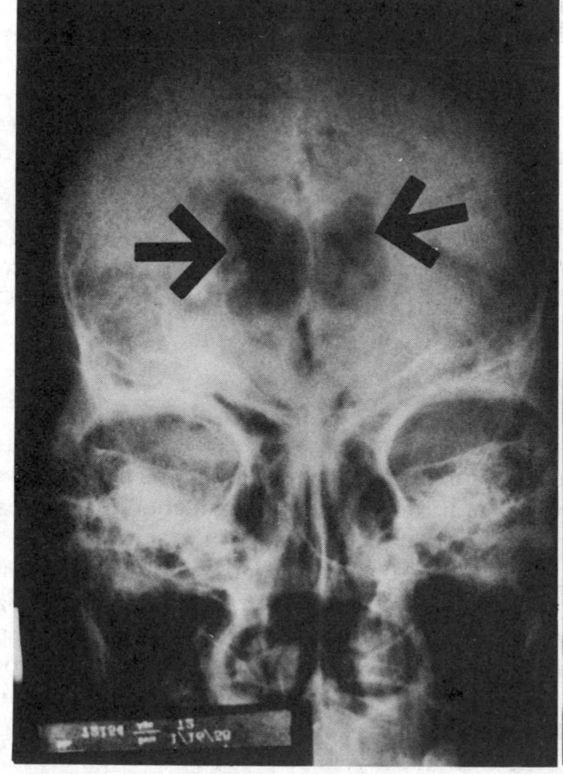

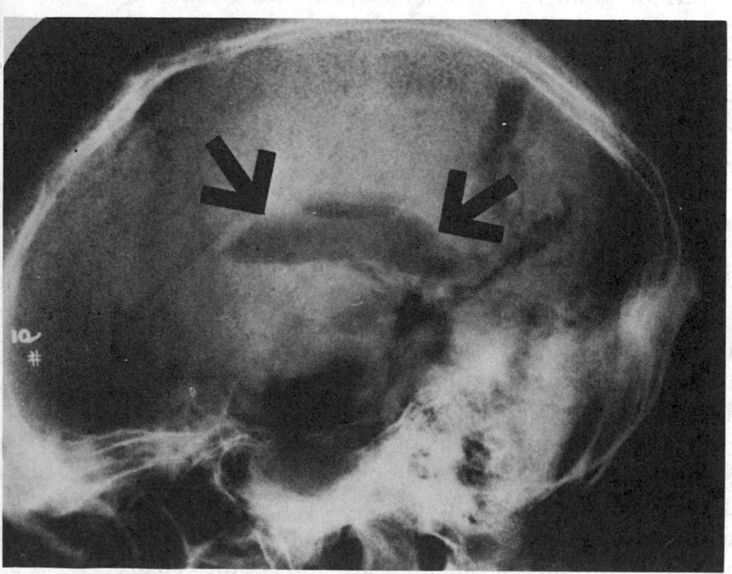

B

**FIGURE 56-26** Pneumoencephalograms. **A,** Anteroposterior view. **B,** Lateral view. Black arrows indicate normal lateral ventricles. (From Pagana K: *Diagnostic testing and nursing implications: a case study approach,* ed 2, St Louis, 1990, Mosby.)

### Guidelines for Care of the Person Undergoing Pneumoencephalogram

| | |
|---|---|
| Preparation of patient | Prepare patient as if for surgery.<br>Make sure permit is signed.<br>Sedative may be given before procedure.<br>General anesthesia may be used.<br>Patient teaching should include explanation of procedure: time is about 2 hr; patient is usually very uncomfortable, with headache, nausea, or vomiting. |
| Procedure | Patient is positioned as for lumbar puncture (p. 1919) or cisternal tap (p. 1920).<br>After the tap is done and pressure is measured, the contrast medium (air or oxygen) is injected in amounts of 25 to 30 ml; patient is watched carefully for headache, nausea, vomiting, or any change in vital signs or color.<br>Head of the table is gradually raised, and head may be rotated to assist air in filling ventricles. |
| Postprocedure nursing care | Patient is placed flat in bed for 24 to 48 hr.<br>Constant attention to vital signs and neurologic checks is important until patient is awake and alert.<br>Severe headache is common and may last 48 hr (until air is absorbed).<br>Seizure precautions should be maintained if patient has history of seizures.<br>Observe for respiratory difficulty.<br>Reactions to procedure may be severe and include vomiting, shock, respiratory difficulty, and increased intracranial pressure. |

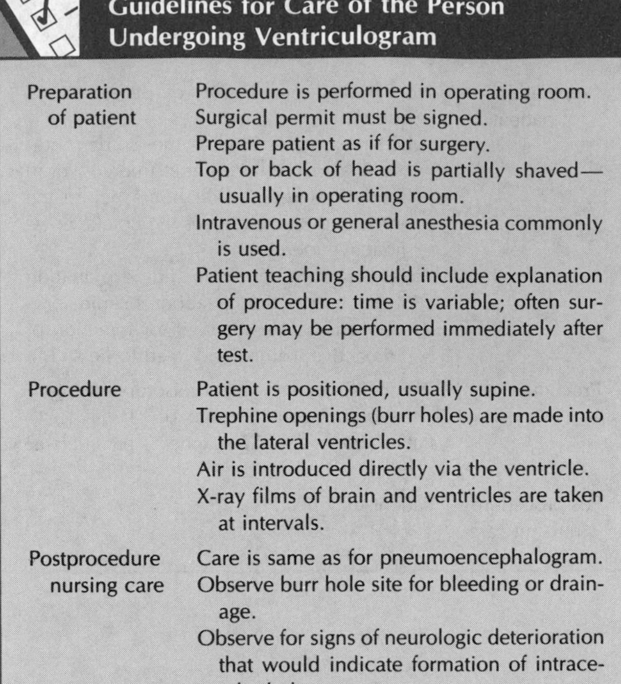

### Guidelines for Care of the Person Undergoing Ventriculogram

| | |
|---|---|
| Preparation of patient | Procedure is performed in operating room.<br>Surgical permit must be signed.<br>Prepare patient as if for surgery.<br>Top or back of head is partially shaved—usually in operating room.<br>Intravenous or general anesthesia commonly is used.<br>Patient teaching should include explanation of procedure: time is variable; often surgery may be performed immediately after test. |
| Procedure | Patient is positioned, usually supine.<br>Trephine openings (burr holes) are made into the lateral ventricles.<br>Air is introduced directly via the ventricle.<br>X-ray films of brain and ventricles are taken at intervals. |
| Postprocedure nursing care | Care is same as for pneumoencephalogram.<br>Observe burr hole site for bleeding or drainage.<br>Observe for signs of neurologic deterioration that would indicate formation of intracerebral clot. |

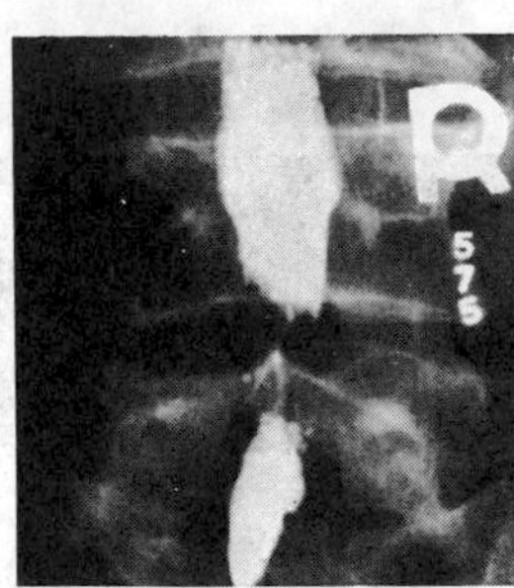


**FIGURE 56-27** Myelogram showing almost complete block of interspace between fourth and fifth lumbar vertebrae. (From Moseley HF, editor: *Textbook of surgery,* ed 3, St Louis, 1959, Mosby.)

### Nursing care

The nurse must closely monitor a patient who has had a ventriculogram or pneumoencephalogram for complications such as respiratory difficulty and seizures. Comfort measures, such as analgesics or a cold cloth to the forehead, may help relieve the headache that almost always occurs after the procedure. Because the patient will be on bedrest for a period of time after the test, the nurse will need to assist the patient with activities of daily living.

## Myelography

In **myelography,** either a gas or a radiopaque liquid is injected into the spinal subarachnoid space by way of a lumbar or cisternal puncture and radiographs are taken. It is useful in the identification of lesions in the intradural or extradural compartments of the spinal canal. Observations of the flow of the radiopaque dye fluoroscopically through the subarachnoid space provides valuable information. Lesions in the spinal cord in the subarachnoid space produce a blocking at some point (Figure 56-27).

The blockage may be complete or incomplete. The exact configuration of the defect causing the block may be helpful in determining whether the lesion is intramedullary or extramedullary. Turning the patient in varied positions throughout the examination assists in securing a more complete visualization.

Another contrast medium, *metrizamide,* may be used in myelograms. However, it may precipitate seizure activity after the procedure, and special precautions must be taken. Side effects of metrizamide are nausea, vomiting, and seizures, and they are most likely to occur 4 to 8 hours after the procedure. However, the advantages of the metrizamide myelogram often outweigh the risks. Major advantages are that the metrizamide is water soluble, and thus the dye does not need to be removed. Also, metrizamide is less viscous than the iodine-based

### Guidelines for Care of the Person Undergoing Myelogram (Metrizamide and Pantopaque)

| | |
|---|---|
| Preparation of patient | Permit must be signed.<br>If patient is to have metrizamide dye, the following medications should be restricted for 24 to 48 hours before the test: phenothiazines, tricyclic antidepressants, and CNS stimulants, amphetamines.<br>With metrizamide dye, fluids are encouraged.<br>Lower extremity strength and sensation should be assessed for baseline.<br>Patient teaching should include how procedure is performed: time is approximately 2 hours; slight pain and pressure may be felt as dura is entered; varied positions that must be assumed during procedure may be uncomfortable. |
| Procedure | Patient is positioned on the side with both knees and head flexed at acute angle (as for lumbar puncture).<br>Puncture is in lumbar region, or cisternally.<br>Dye is instilled and needle may be removed or left in place.<br>Patient is turned to varied positions to visualize spinal cord while fluoroscopic and radiologic films are taken.<br>After procedure, Pantopaque dye is removed; leaving it in will cause serious irritation to meninges.<br>With metrizamide dye, patient usually has CT scan of spinal cord 4 to 6 hours after the myelogram. |
| Postprocedure nursing care | For Pantopaque myelogram, patient lies flat overnight.<br>For metrizamide myelogram, head must be elevated 30 to 50 degrees for at least 8 hours and then elevated 30 degrees for 24 hours.<br>Fluids are encouraged.<br>Strength and sensation of lower extremities must be assessed.<br>Site of puncture should be assessed for leakage of CSF.<br>Headache is common with both types of myelogram.<br>With metrizamide dye, nausea and vomiting may occur.<br>For metrizamide procedure, avoid previously listed drugs. |

dye and therefore permits better visualization of small areas.[6] (See Guidelines box above for a further description of the procedure.)

#### Nursing care

Patients who have undergone myelography should be assessed for leakage from the puncture site. Drinking fluids is encouraged after the procedure, and the patient

### Guidelines for Care of the Person Undergoing Cerebral Arteriogram (Angiogram)

| | |
|---|---|
| Preparation of patient | Patient is given clear liquids the morning of procedure.<br>Assess patient for allergy to iodine.<br>If femoral approach is to be used, assess and mark locations of bilateral pedal pulses.<br>If carotid artery is used, assess neckline circumference.<br>Sedation may be given before procedure.<br>Check vital signs and baseline neurologic examination immediately before procedure.<br>Patient teaching should include explanation of test: time is 2 to 3 hours; lying still is uncomfortable; patients usually complain of hot feeling as dye is injected. |
| Procedure | Patient is positioned supine on x-ray table.<br>Local anesthetic is used to anesthetize puncture site.<br>Catheter is inserted percutaneously.<br>Each vessel is injected as films are taken.<br>Catheter is withdrawn and pressure is applied to puncture site for at least 5 minutes. |
| Postprocedure nursing care | Patient is kept on bedrest overnight.<br>Vital signs are checked frequently, along with neurologic checks.<br>Site of puncture is assessed frequently for presence of hematoma.<br>With carotid site, check for difficulty in breathing or swallowing—check neck girth.<br>Dye used in angiogram may raise intracranial pressure and cause decreased extremity strength or change in level of consciousness. |

is assessed for headache or loss of strength in the lower extremities. If metrizamide dye has been used, the patient may be nauseated and vomiting may occur. The patient should be medicated with a drug that does not lower the seizure threshhold.

## Cerebral Angiography (Angiogram)

**Cerebral arteriography** is a method of radiologic visualization of the cerebral arterial system during the injection of radiopaque material. The carotid or vertebral vessels or the femoral artery is the usual source of entry for the catheter. Vessels are injected with dye as serial films are taken. The selection of needle puncture site is determined by the clinical problem under study. The large vessels of the *circle of Willis* and the large penetrating vessels can be visualized through arteriography (Figure 56-28). This test is effective in detecting arterial aneurysms, vessel anomalies, ruptured vessels, and displacement of vessels by mass lesions. (See Guidelines box above for a further description of this test.)

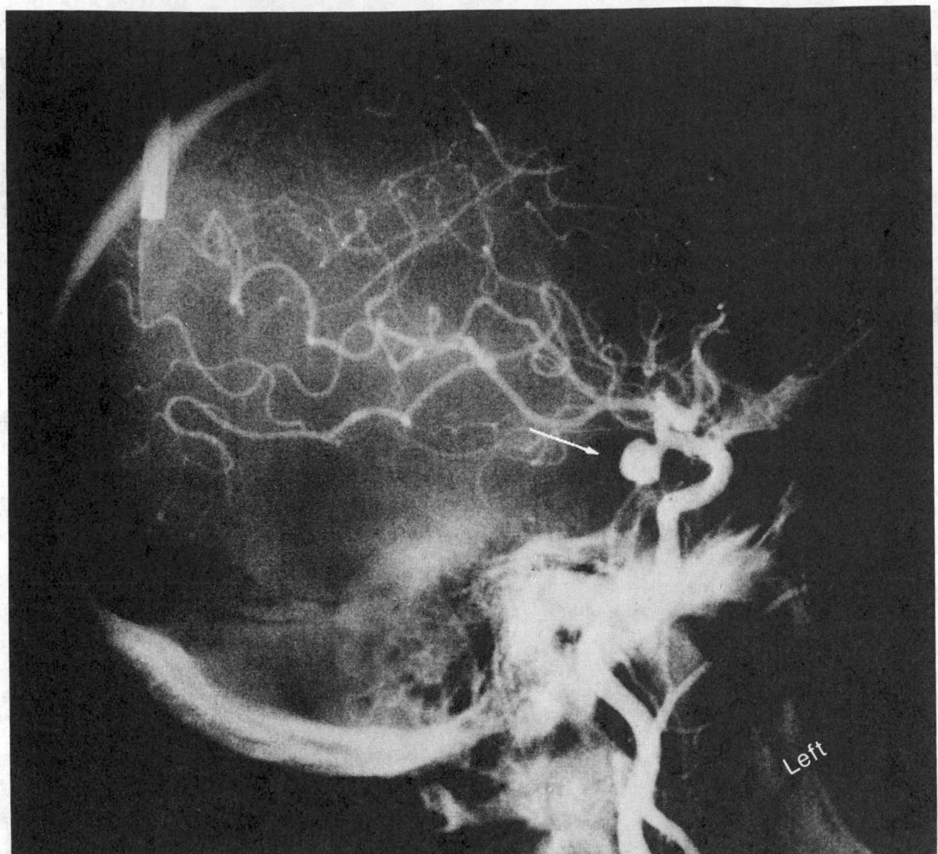


**FIGURE 56-28** Cerebral angiography showing location of aneurysm at posterior communicating artery. (From Tortorici M: *Fundamentals of angiography,* St Louis, 1982, Mosby.)

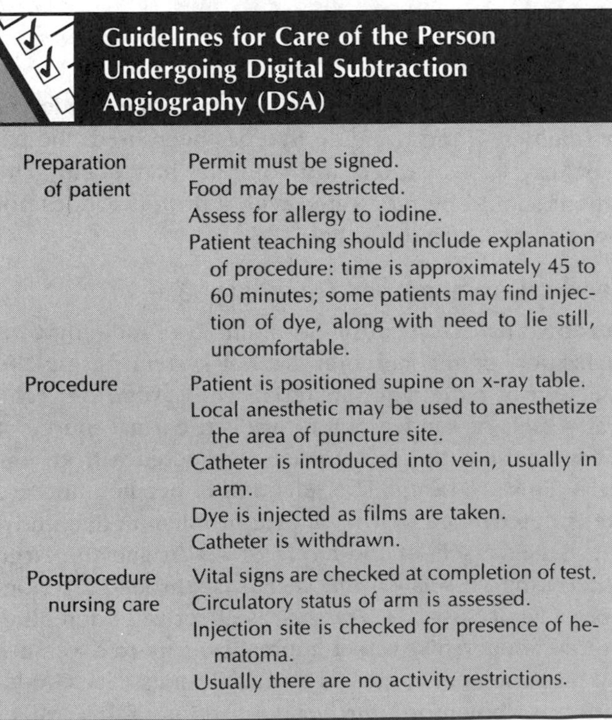

**Guidelines for Care of the Person Undergoing Digital Subtraction Angiography (DSA)**

| | |
|---|---|
| Preparation of patient | Permit must be signed.<br>Food may be restricted.<br>Assess for allergy to iodine.<br>Patient teaching should include explanation of procedure: time is approximately 45 to 60 minutes; some patients may find injection of dye, along with need to lie still, uncomfortable. |
| Procedure | Patient is positioned supine on x-ray table.<br>Local anesthetic may be used to anesthetize the area of puncture site.<br>Catheter is introduced into vein, usually in arm.<br>Dye is injected as films are taken.<br>Catheter is withdrawn. |
| Postprocedure nursing care | Vital signs are checked at completion of test.<br>Circulatory status of arm is assessed.<br>Injection site is checked for presence of hematoma.<br>Usually there are no activity restrictions. |

## Digital Subtraction Angiography

A digital subtraction angiogram (DSA) may be performed instead of the angiogram. The purpose is to identify abnormalities of the cerebrovascular system, using a process that removes overlying structures in an image so that the clinically significant details can be displayed with enhanced visibility. It is generally considered to be much safer than the angiogram, because it uses venous rather than arterial access. It can be performed on an outpatient basis. (See Guidelines box at left for a further description of this test.)

### Nursing care

After the arteriogram or DSA, the patient should be monitored for any bleeding at the site of the puncture. A pressure dressing is usually left in place for at least 6 to 8 hours. With the femoral approach, the pulses in the lower extremities should be assessed; with the brachial approach, the radial pulse should be assessed. With the carotid approach, the ability of the patient to breathe and swallow without difficulty is important to assess. Because the dye used may raise intracranial pressure, the patient should be assessed for any change in level of consciousness.

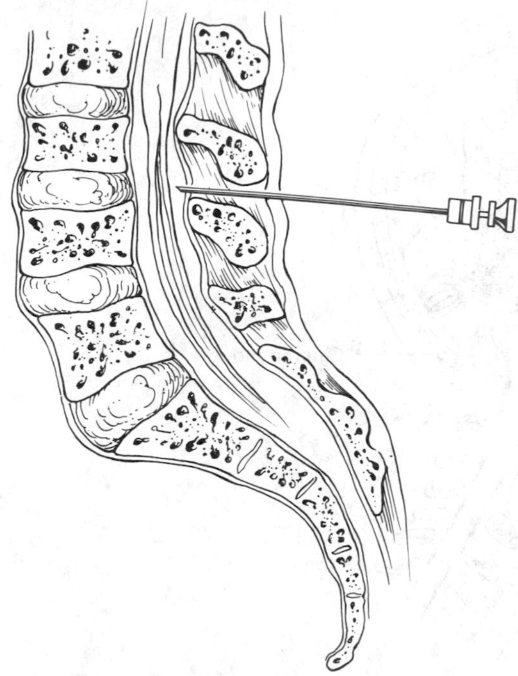

**FIGURE 56-29** Position and angle of the needle when lumbar puncture is performed. Note that the needle is in the fourth lumbar interspace below the level of the spinal cord.

## Positive Emission Tomography (PET Scan)

One of the newest developments in the assessment of neurologic conditions is the positive emission tomography (PET). This scan involves use of radioactive substances that emit positive electrons (positrons) while CT scanning is performed. It provides a metabolic profile by revealing the rate at which tissues metabolize glucose. The patient either inhales a radioactive gas or is injected with a radioactive substance. This material emits positrons, which combine with negatively charged electrons in body cells. Gamma rays are then given off, which can be seen by the scanning device. The computer translates the patterns of gamma ray emissions.

# SPECIAL TESTS

Other tests can be important in determining the nature of neurologic symptoms. These include the lumbar puncture, cisternal puncture, electroencephalogram, electromyogram, and evoked potentials.

## Lumbar Puncture

The lumbar puncture is performed to obtain CSF for examination (Figure 56-29). The importance of examining the constituents has already been described. A lumbar puncture may be performed also to relieve intracranial pressure in carefully selected cases. In most cases, a lumbar puncture is not performed in the presence of signs of increased intracranial pressure or when a brain tumor is suspected because the quick reduction in pressure produced by removal of spinal fluid causes the brain structures to herniate into the foramen magnum, which would put pressure on vital centers in the medulla and might cause sudden death.

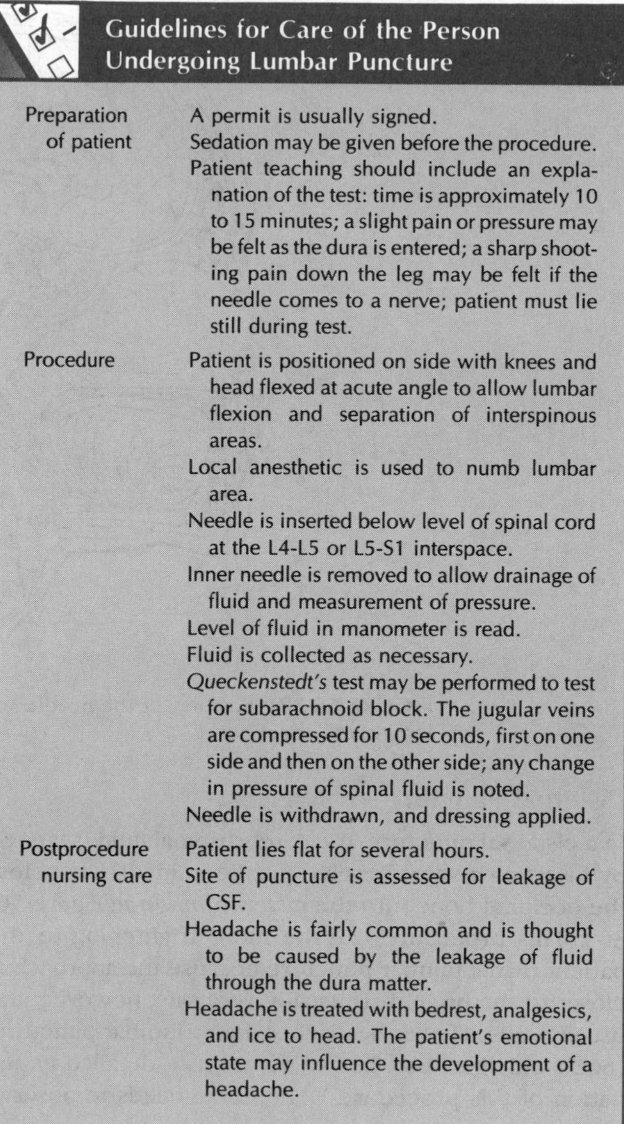

**Guidelines for Care of the Person Undergoing Lumbar Puncture**

| | |
|---|---|
| Preparation of patient | A permit is usually signed.<br>Sedation may be given before the procedure.<br>Patient teaching should include an explanation of the test: time is approximately 10 to 15 minutes; a slight pain or pressure may be felt as the dura is entered; a sharp shooting pain down the leg may be felt if the needle comes to a nerve; patient must lie still during test. |
| Procedure | Patient is positioned on side with knees and head flexed at acute angle to allow lumbar flexion and separation of interspinous areas.<br>Local anesthetic is used to numb lumbar area.<br>Needle is inserted below level of spinal cord at the L4-L5 or L5-S1 interspace.<br>Inner needle is removed to allow drainage of fluid and measurement of pressure.<br>Level of fluid in manometer is read.<br>Fluid is collected as necessary.<br>*Queckenstedt's* test may be performed to test for subarachnoid block. The jugular veins are compressed for 10 seconds, first on one side and then on the other side; any change in pressure of spinal fluid is noted.<br>Needle is withdrawn, and dressing applied. |
| Postprocedure nursing care | Patient lies flat for several hours.<br>Site of puncture is assessed for leakage of CSF.<br>Headache is fairly common and is thought to be caused by the leakage of fluid through the dura matter.<br>Headache is treated with bedrest, analgesics, and ice to head. The patient's emotional state may influence the development of a headache. |

Strict aseptic technique is mandatory in all procedures in which the cerebrospinal fluid system is entered. (See Guidelines box above for a further description of this procedure.)

### Nursing care

After a lumbar puncture, the patient is instructed to lie flat in bed and not lift the head up off of a thin pillow, because such movement may cause a headache. If a headache occurs, the patient is given an analgesic. While the patient lies flat, assistance with care may be necessary. Some lumbar punctures are performed on an outpatient basis. In this case, the patient lies flat for 1 to 2 hours before being discharged. The patient is taught about signs and symptoms to watch for.

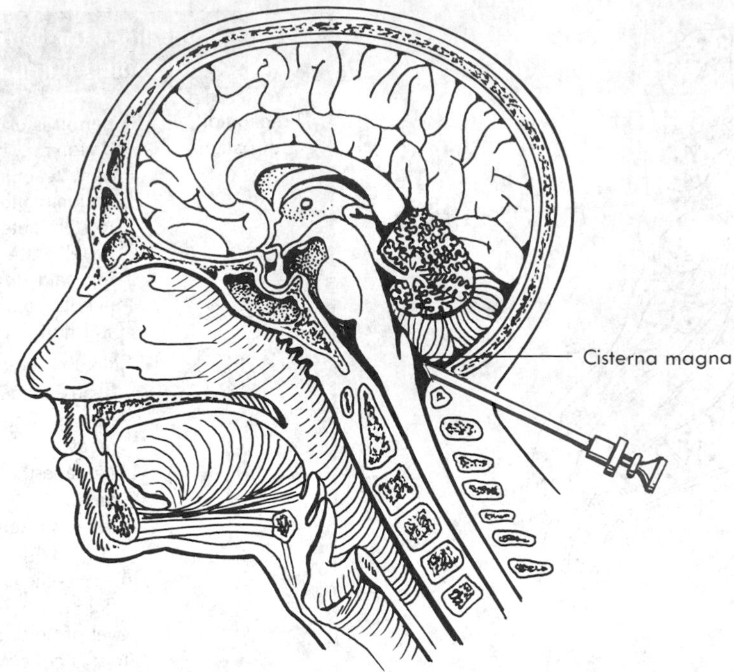


**FIGURE 56-30** Position of the needle when cisternal puncture is performed. Note needle length and short bevel.

## Cisternal Puncture

In a cisternal puncture, the cerebrospinal fluid is tapped by inserting a short-beveled needle immediately below the occipital bone into the *cisterna magna* (Figure 56-30). This procedure may be more frightening to the patient than a lumbar puncture because the approach is closer to the brain. It is usually very safe, however, and usually causes fewer headaches than a lumbar puncture. (See Guidelines box below, for a more detailed explanation of this procedure.) The nurse needs to observe the patient for any respiratory difficulties such as dyspnea, apnea, or cyanosis. The site of the puncture should be assessed for leakage.

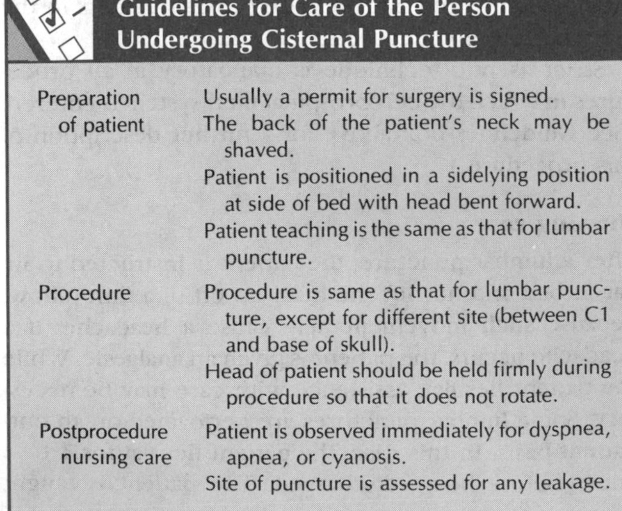

**Guidelines for Care of the Person Undergoing Cisternal Puncture**

| | |
|---|---|
| Preparation of patient | Usually a permit for surgery is signed.<br>The back of the patient's neck may be shaved.<br>Patient is positioned in a sidelying position at side of bed with head bent forward.<br>Patient teaching is the same as that for lumbar puncture. |
| Procedure | Procedure is same as that for lumbar puncture, except for different site (between C1 and base of skull).<br>Head of patient should be held firmly during procedure so that it does not rotate. |
| Postprocedure nursing care | Patient is observed immediately for dyspnea, apnea, or cyanosis.<br>Site of puncture is assessed for any leakage. |

## Electroencephalography (EEG)

An electroencephalograph measures the electrical impulses of the brain. The electroencephalogram (EEG) is a pictured recording of the electrical activity of the brain amplified many times and recorded in a manner similar to that of the electrocardiogram. The recording represents the synthesis of collective neurons. Certain characteristic patterns in the recordings are normal, and by study of the recordings of brain action, areas of abnormal action can be detected. This test is nonspecific and is only an adjunct to other diagnostic tests, but it may be helpful in locating the site of a lesion. (See Guidelines box, p. 1921, left-hand column, for further information about EEG.) Most patients who return from an EEG require rest. The patient may need assistance in washing the hair to remove the collodion used to apply the electrodes. The EEG is often performed as an outpatient procedure.

## Electromyography (EMG)

The electromyography measures the electrical activity of muscles; the electromyogram (EMG) is a recording of the variations of electric potentials (voltage) detected by a needle electrode inserted into skeletal muscles. The electrical activity can be heard over a loudspeaker and viewed on an oscilloscope and on a graph at the same time. No electrical activity can be detected in muscles

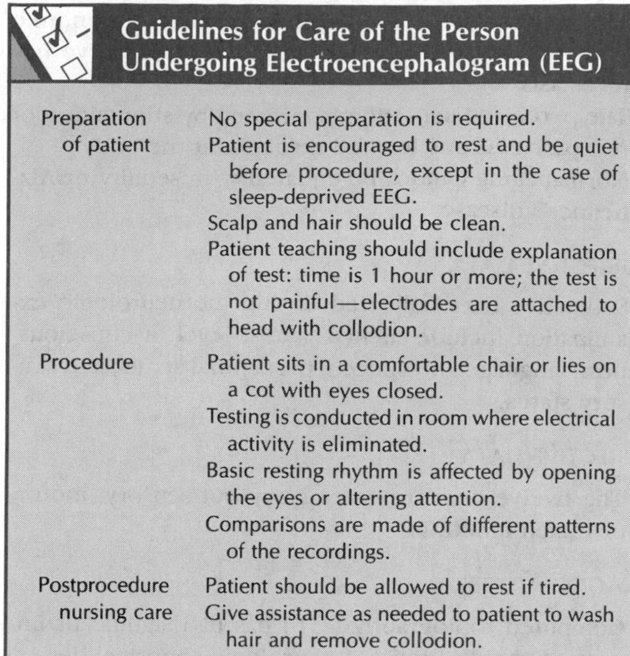

**Guidelines for Care of the Person Undergoing Electroencephalogram (EEG)**

| | |
|---|---|
| Preparation of patient | No special preparation is required.<br>Patient is encouraged to rest and be quiet before procedure, except in the case of sleep-deprived EEG.<br>Scalp and hair should be clean.<br>Patient teaching should include explanation of test: time is 1 hour or more; the test is not painful—electrodes are attached to head with collodion. |
| Procedure | Patient sits in a comfortable chair or lies on a cot with eyes closed.<br>Testing is conducted in room where electrical activity is eliminated.<br>Basic resting rhythm is affected by opening the eyes or altering attention.<br>Comparisons are made of different patterns of the recordings. |
| Postprocedure nursing care | Patient should be allowed to rest if tired.<br>Give assistance as needed to patient to wash hair and remove collodion. |

**Guidelines for Care of the Person Undergoing Electromyogram (EMG)**

| | |
|---|---|
| Preparation of patient | No special preparation is required.<br>Patient teaching should include explanation of procedure: time is approximately 45 minutes for one muscle; some discomfort is experienced when electrodes are inserted; patients with sensory neuropathies may experience more intense pain; electrical current is uncomfortable; muscles may ache for a period of time after procedure. |
| Procedure | Electrodes are inserted into skeletal muscles.<br>Electrical current is passed through electrodes.<br>Machine graphs the variations of muscle potentials (voltage). |
| Postprocedure nursing care | Observe for signs of bleeding at electrode insertion sites.<br>Patient may need rest period.<br>Medicate patient as needed for discomfort. |

at rest, but during volitional movement action potentials can be detected. However, in motor disease, electrical activity of various types of abnormal patterns appears in resting muscles. An EMG provides direct evidence of ***motor dysfunction*** and can be used to some extent to detect a dysfunction located in the motor neuron, the neuromuscular junction, or muscle fibers. This is particularly helpful in the detection of lower motor neuron disease, primary muscle disease, and defects in the transmission of electrical impulses at the neuromuscular junction. (See Guidelines box, above, right, for an explanation of EMG.)

### Nursing care

After the EMG the patient should be assessed for bleeding at the needle insertion sites. Medication may be needed for discomfort. The patient may also require rest, even when the procedure is performed on an outpatient basis.

## Echoencephalography

Echoencephalography is a rapid and simple diagnostic procedure. Information provided is supplementary to an EEG and complementary to radiologic studies as to the nature and location of brain lesions.

Ultrasonic pulses (capable of reflection or refraction at cerebrospinal fluid and brain tissue surfaces) are delivered to the head in such a way that the beam intersects the site under study at a perpendicular angle, transverses the area, and is then reflected back. The returning echoes are then coverted back to electrical impulses and recorded on a screen. This procedure provides a right, left, and lower trace or picture that gives reliable information as to the position of the midline of the brain. Shifts from midline, as caused by right or left hemispheric brain masses, can be inferred. Estimation of ventricular size can also be made from the traces.

## Evoked Potentials

Evoked potentials are electrical measurements of physiologic maturation of the human nervous system. Used diagnostically, they can provide information about the maturational development of all the primary sensory areas of the cortex. Most commonly used are ***auditory evoked potentials*** and ***visual evoked potentials.*** Evoked potentials aid in the diagnosis of multiple sclerosis.

## CRITICAL THINKING ACTIVITIES

- Explain why an individual with a hemisection of the cord would experience ipsilateral loss of proprioception and contralateral loss of pain and temperature.
- Trish 68, is admitted to the hospital with signs and symptoms of cerebrovascular compromise. She is scheduled for a digital subtraction angiogram. Before the procedure, Trish asks, "How is this test different from the cerebral angiogram I had several months ago?" In terms that Trish can comprehend, explain the main differences between these two procedures.

# CHAPTER SUMMARY

## ANATOMY AND PHYSIOLOGY

- Neurologic assessment depends on the examiner's knowledge of normal neurophysiology and neuroanatomy and the ability to interpret the degree of change in status from normal.
- The nervous system coordinates and controls all activities of the body.
- The four general kinds of function carried out by the nervous system include receiving stimuli or information, communicating information, computing or processing the information, and transmitting information.
- The basic structural and functional unit of the nervous system is the neuron.
- The neuron is composed of a cell body (soma), a dendritic tree, a cylindric axon, and the cell membrane.
- The axon transmits information away from the cell body to adjacent neurons, whereas the dendrites communicate information to the cell body.
- The neuron cell membrane transmits information through properties called *differential permeability* and *excitability.*
- The myelin sheath is deposited around axons and assists in transmission of impulses.
- Synapses are specialized sites in the nervous system where neurons make functional contact with each other.
- The nervous system is divided into two major divisions: the central nervous system (CNS) and the peripheral nervous system (PNS).
- The CNS is made up of collections of neurons and their connections organized within the brain and spinal cord.
- The parts of the brain include the cerebrum, the brainstem (diencephalon, midbrain, pons, and medulla), and the cerebellum, each of which carries out specific functions.
- Speech is a function of the dominant hemisphere, usually on the left side of the brain.
- The blood-brain barrier is a phenomenon that limits the free movement of substances from the blood to the brain tissue.
- Cerebrospinal fluid serves as a fluid cushion for nervous tissue, helps to support the weight of the brain, and carries nutrients to the brain and removes metabolites.
- The meninges are the coverings of the nervous tissue in the brain and spinal cord that help support, protect, and nourish the brain and spinal cord.
- Three potential spaces are associated with the meninges: epidural, subdural, and subarachnoid.
- The PNS is a set of communication channels located outside the CNS.
- The autonomic nervous system regulates autonomic body functions, usually in an effort to preserve homeostasis.
- The perceived sensation is initiated by stimulation of receptor neurons located throughout the body.
- Normal aging cannot be equated with senility or Alzheimer's disease.

## SUBJECTIVE DATA

- Subjective data collected during the neurologic examination include mental status, level of consciousness, language and speech, perceptual status, and sensory status.

## OBJECTIVE DATA

- The twelve cranial nerves carry out sensory, motor, or mixed functions.

## DIAGNOSTIC TESTS

- Computed tomography (CT) has had significant impact on the diagnosis of neurologic abnormalities.
- A lumbar puncture is not performed in the presence of signs of increased intracranial pressure or when a brain tumor is suspected because of the danger of brain herniation.

# REFERENCES


1. Baggerly J: Sensory perceptual problems following stroke: the invisible deficits, *Nurs Clin North Am* 26(4):997-1005, 1991.
2. Barker E: Cranial nerve assessment, *RN* 55(5):62-69, 1992.
3. Barker E, Moore E: Neurological assessment, *RN* 55(4):28-35, 1992.
4. Dykes P: Minding the five P's of neurovascular assessment, *AJN* 93(6):38-39, 1993.
5. Jess L: Investigating impaired mental status: an assessment guide you can use, *Nurs '88* 18(6):42-50, 1988.
6. Jones A et al: Side effects following metrizamide myelography and lumbar laminectomy, *J Neurosci Nurs* 21:290-294, 1987.
7. Long B et al: *Medical-surgical nursing: a nursing process approach,* ed 3, St. Louis, 1993, Mosby.
8. Lord-Feroli K, Maguire-McGinley M: Toward a more objective approach to pupil assessment, *J Neurosurg Nurs* 17:309-312, 1990.
9. Lower J: Rapid neuro assessment, *Am J Nurs* 92(6):38-45, 1992.
10. *Mosby's medical, nursing, and allied health dictionary,* ed 3, St. Louis, 1990, Mosby.
11. Olson E: Perceptual deficits affecting the stroke patient, *Rehabil Nurs* 16(4):212-213, 1991.
12. Phipps MA: Assessment of neurologic deficits in stroke: acute-care and rehabilitation implications, *Nurs Clin North Am* 26:(4):957-970, 1991.
13. Stevens S, Becker K: A simple, step-by-step approach to neurological assessment—part 1, *Nurs '88* 18(9):53-61, 1988.
14. Stevens S, Becker K: A simple, step-by-step approach to neurological assessment—part 2, *Nurs '88* 18(10):51-58, 1988.
15. Sullivan J: Neurologic assessment, *Nurs Clin North Am* 25(4):795-809, 1990.
16. Tortora G, Anagnostakos N: *Principles of anatomy and physiology,* New York, 1990, Harper & Row.

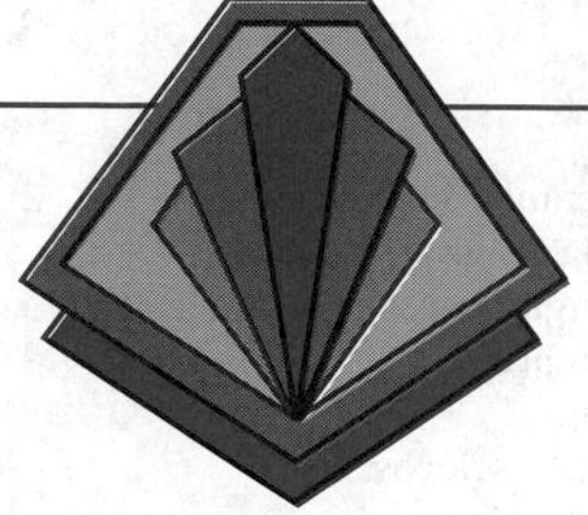

C H A P T E R 57

# Management of Persons With Problems of the Brain

***Elizabeth Anne Schenk***

## CHAPTER OBJECTIVES

***After studying this chapter, the learner should be able to do the following:***

1 Name at least five causes of headache.
2 Differentiate among migraine, cluster, and tension headaches.
3 List at least six key points in assessing headache.
4 Name at least one nursing intervention for each type of headache discussed.
5 List at least five symptoms of increased intracranial pressure.
6 Explain the mechanism of increased intracranial pressure.
7 Explain how nursing interventions can decrease intracranial pressure, and give two examples of these interventions.
8 Describe the difference between sensory, motor, and global aphasia.
9 Name the six levels of consciousness, and describe characteristics of each.
10 State two ways that brain death is determined.
11 Describe the usefulness of the Glasgow coma scale and the Rancho Los Amigos scale in caring for patients with altered levels of consciousness.
12 Explain three ways in which the comatose patient should be stimulated.
13 State at least five nursing interventions that are important for persons with a decreased level of consciousness.
14 Give examples of at least three different types of seizures.
15 Explain the observations that must be made about a person having a seizure.
16 Compare and contrast two neurologic degenerative diseases.
17 List at least six nursing diagnoses for the patient with multiple sclerosis, and describe at least three nursing interventions for each.
18 Define the term *catastrophic reaction* as related to patients with Alzheimer's disease.
19 Correlate the stages of Alzheimer's disease and the symptoms and behaviors seen in each.
20 Distinguish among the causes of a cerebrovascular accident.
21 List at least three infections that can occur in the nervous system.
22 Define the following terms in relation to craniocerebral trauma: contusion, coup, contrecoup, concussion, and laceration.
23 List at least three diagnostic tests that can be used to rule out head injury.
24 List at least three different types of intracranial tumors.
25 Discuss the preoperative and postoperative care of the patient undergoing a craniotomy.
26 Describe at least two complications that can occur as a result of brain surgery.
27 Explain why neurologic symptoms often develop in patients with AIDS.

## KEY TERMS

acquired immunodeficiency syndrome (AIDS)
Alzheimer's disease
amyotrophic lateral sclerosis (ALS)
apneustic breathing
ataxic breathing
aura
Brudzinski's sign
central neurogenic hyperventilation (CNHV)
cerebrovascular accident (CVA)
Cheyne-Stokes respiration
cluster breathing
cluster headache
coma
concussion
contusion
craniocerebral trauma
craniotomy
decerebrate posturing
decorticate posturing
delirium
depressed breathing
disorientation
Eaton-Lambert syndrome
encephalitis
epilepsy
gasping breathing
Glasgow coma scale (GCS)
glioma
grand mal seizure
headache
hemiplegia
hydrocephalus
increased intracranial pressure (ICP)
intracranial hemorrhage
Kernig's sign
meningioma
meningitis
migraine
multiple sclerosis
myasthenia gravis
papilledema
Parkinson's disease
petit mal seizure
Rancho Los Amigos level of cognitive functioning
seizure
status epilepticus
stroke
tension headache
transient ischemic attack (TIA)

This chapter discusses the care of persons with clinical manifestations that result from common neurologic problems. The first part of this chapter includes manifestations of (1) altered levels of consciousness, (2) headache, (3) increased intracranial pressure, (4) alterations in communication, and (5) alterations in sensory and perceptual function. The second part of the chapter examines specific neurologic problems.

# CLINICAL MANIFESTATIONS OF NEUROLOGIC PROBLEMS

## ALTERED LEVELS OF CONSCIOUSNESS

Consciousness is an ongoing process of awareness of the self and the environment; it is the mental ability to evoke feelings and provide meaning for that awareness based on previous experience. One infers awareness in others on the basis of their observed behaviors.

Impaired consciousness may be the result of the following three general types of pathologic processes:

1. Conditions that widely and directly depress the function of the cerebral hemispheres
2. Conditions that depress or destroy the brainstem-activating mechanisms that lie in or near the central core of the gray matter of the diencephalon, midbrain, and rostral pons
3. Conditions that involve combined bilateral cortical and brainstem failure (the latter are seen most commonly in cases of metabolic encephalopathy and intoxication in which the relative amount of the brain's impairment varies)

The two aspects of consciousness that must be considered are arousal and awareness. *Arousal* is a physiologic function associated with wakefulness. It involves a primitive set of responses that are located entirely within the brainstem and are synchronized by a network of tracts and nuclei. The network is located in the core of the brainstem and extends from the medulla to the thalamus. *Awareness* is the sum of all cognitive and affective functions. It involves a higher level integration of multiple sensory input that allow meaningful understanding of self and environment.

### ETIOLOGY

There are multiple causes of impaired consciousness, many of which are not primarily neurologic. For this reason, a detailed history, extensive neurologic examination, and laboratory screening often are needed. These factors are discussed later in the chapter. Generally, causes of impaired consciousness can be categorized into two broad categories: (1) primary brain injury or disease (usually a structured lesion) or (2) a systemic condition that secondarily affects the brain. (See Box 57-1 for a more complete listing of the possible causes of coma.)

The *conscious* person is able to respond to sensory stimuli, has subjective experiences, exercises will, and is capable of thought and reasoning. Consciousness also can be defined as self-awareness—ability to function mentally and physically in a manner appropriate to the level of one's normal ability and to experience life to the fullest degree. All body activities are controlled and coordinated by the nervous system. The cerebrum plays the central role in the higher functions. Rather than experiencing sensory input individually and discretely, the components are integrated into a single consciousness, a perception; for example, one can identify items by touch that one has seen but not touched before.

In contrast, to be *unconscious* implies that there is no response to sensory stimuli—no thinking and no feelings or emotions. The conscious person is aware of

**BOX 57-1 Possible Causes of Decreased Levels of Consciousness**

1. Resulting from primary brain injury or disease
   a. Trauma (concussion, contusion, laceration, traumatic intercerebral hemorrhage, subdural hematoma, epidural hematoma)
   b. Vascular disease (intracerebral hemorrhage, subarachnoid hemorrhage, infarction)
   c. Infections (meningitis, encephalitis, abscess)
   d. Neoplasms (primarily intracranial, metastatic, or nonmetastatic complication of malignant tumor)
   e. Seizures
2. Resulting from systemic conditions that secondarily affect the brain
   a. Metabolic encephalopathies (hypoglycemia, diabetic ketoacidosis, hyperglycemic nonketotic hyperosmolar states, uremia, hepatic encephalopathy, hyponatremia, myxedema, hypercalcemia, and hypocalcemia)
   b. Hypoxic encephalopathies (severe congestive heart failure, chronic obstructive pulmonary disease with decompensation, severe anemia, and hypertensive encephalopathies)
   c. Toxicity (heavy metals, carbon monoxide, and drugs—especially opiates, barbiturates, and alcohol)
   d. Physical causes (heat stroke and hypothermia)
   e. Deficiency states (Wernicke's encephalopathy)

what is going on in the environment. To differentiate these two ends of the continuum are many levels of awareness and mental ability not so easily defined or precisely described.

Because consciousness is a complex expression of the mind and not just a single function, a wide spectrum of levels of consciousness exists between the two ends of the continuum: consciousness and coma. Although it is better to avoid labels, the nurse must have an understanding of terms and criteria commonly used to facilitate communication about states of consciousness. The levels of consciousness can be divided into the following six levels of cerebral function:

1. Alert
2. Confused
3. Drowsy
4. Stupor
5. Light coma
6. Deep coma

See Table 57-1 for behaviors that reflect degrees of decreased levels of consciousness.

Other terms also have been identified. These are *obtunded* and *locked-in states.*[35] The term *obtunded* implies a reduction in alertness and a decreased interest in the surroundings. *Stupor* has been described as unresponsiveness from which the subject can be aroused only by vigorous and repeated stimuli; *coma* is unarousable responsiveness. Various clinical pictures of coma have been described. The most common one is a *sleeplike condition* with *eyes closed;* the closed eyes are not seen in the chronic state. Second is a *hypersomnia* state very much like *normal sleep* because patients can be aroused, but they return to sleep immediately. The third state is one in which the person's *eyes are open,* but *no movement or speech* can be elicited.

The chronically brain-damaged comatose patient may have periods during which the eyes are open, alternating with closed-eye periods, and may seem to be making some response to environmental stimuli. This is referred to as a *vegetative* state. Brainstem function may be intact and respirations remain normal, yet forebrain damage is too extensive to permit any awareness.

The *locked-in* state refers to the condition of persons

**TABLE 57-1 Common Terms Used to Describe Levels of Consciousness and Associated Behaviors**

| CONSCIOUS | AWARE | SEMICONSCIOUS | SEMICOMATOSE | UNCONSCIOUS | COMATOSE |
|---|---|---|---|---|---|
| **LEVEL** | | | | | |
| Alert | Confused | Obtunded, drowsy | Stupor | Light coma | Deep coma |
| **BEHAVIORS** | | | | | |
| Normal activity<br>Aware, mentally functional | Poor coordination<br>Delirium<br>Hallucinations<br>Restlessness<br>Excitable<br>May be combative<br>Short attention span<br>Inappropriate actions and judgments<br>Decreased awareness<br>Disorientation | Sleepy<br>Very short attention span<br>Ready arousal<br>Responds appropriately when aroused<br>Ability to respond verbally<br>Fends off painful stimuli with purposeful movement | Apathetic<br>Slow-moving<br>Blank expression<br>Drooping head<br>Staring<br>Arousal only to vigorous stimuli<br>Incomplete arousal to painful stimuli<br>No verbal response or moaning<br>Response to verbal communication is inconsistent and vague | Not oriented to time, place or person<br>Response is only by grimace or withdrawing limb from pain<br>Primitive and disorganized response to painful stimuli | Absence of response to even the most painful stimuli |

who may be awake and alert, completely able to think and reason, yet who, because of a metabolic or structural disease in the nervous system, are unable to realize any motor expression of the cerebral function. Some of these patients have the ability to move their eyes in an up-and-down direction. Most commonly this state is caused by lesions in the brainstem. Three categories of events can produce this state: (1) supratentorial masses or lesions that secondarily compress or damage both cerebral hemispheres, (2) subtentorial lesions or masses damaging the reticular activating system (RAS), which normally activates the cerebral hemispheres, and (3) metabolic disorders that interrupt function of supratentorial and subtentorial brain structures.[35]

## Pathologic Motor Responses

Damage to the central nervous system may be demonstrated by pathologic motor responses in the comatose patient. These include decorticate and decerebrate posturing. **Decorticate posturing** includes flexion of the arms, wrists, and fingers, with adduction of the upper extremities. This indicates a lesion that involves large portions of the sensorimotor cortex, both anterior and posterior to the primary motor area. **Decerebrate posturing** also is called *extensor spasm.* In this pattern, all four extremities are rigid in extension, with hyperpronation of the forearm and extension of the feet. This response indicates a lesion at the level of the brainstem. With this response, the prognosis is grave. It is possible that a person may demonstrate both of these responses concurrently. These responses often are accompanied by deep coma, rapid breathing, and dilation of both pupils (Figure 57-1).

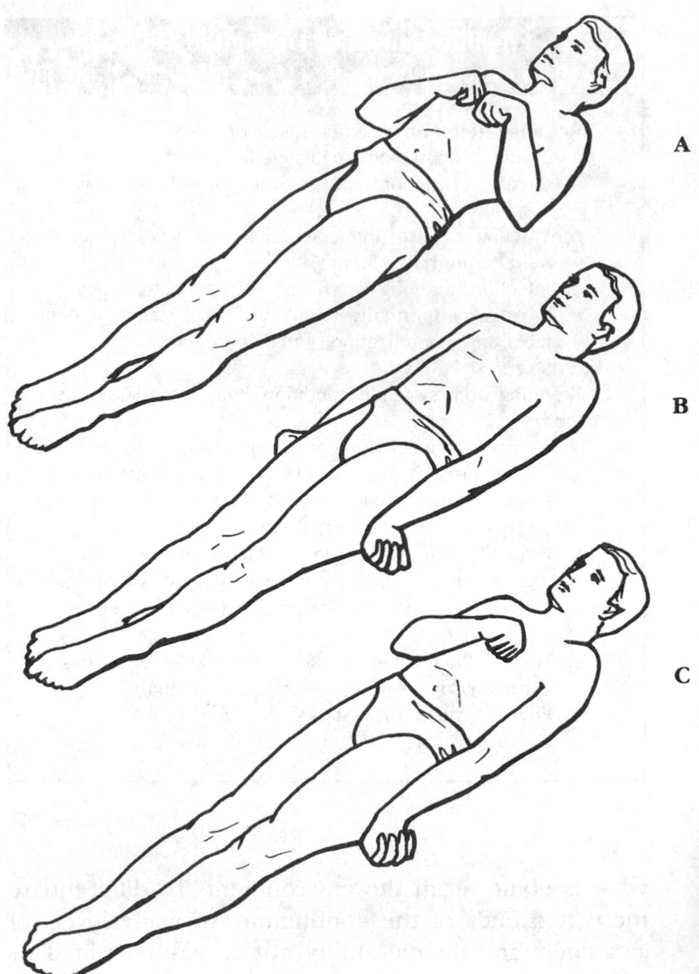


FIGURE 57-1 Decorticate and decerebrate responses. **A,** Decorticate response. Flexion of arms, wrists, and fingers with adduction in upper extremities. Extension, internal rotation, and plantar flexion in lower extremities. **B,** Decerebrate response. All four extremities in rigid extension, with hyperpronation of forearms and plantar extension of feet. **C,** Decorticate response on right side of body and decerebrate response on left side of body. (From Zschoche D: Mosby's comprehensive review of critical care, ed 2, St Louis, 1981, Mosby.)

## Brain Death

With advanced means of prolonging life, the issue of when death occurs has arisen. From this has come debates about the nature of brain death. If a person is receiving artificial means of ventilation, it is possible to sustain breathing and circulation in the absence of brain activity. It is necessary in these cases to determine that all functions of the brain have ceased, including those of the cerebrum and brainstem. Usually one or more electroencephalograms (EEG) are necessary to substantiate brain death. In addition, the following should be absent:

1. All cerebral responses to light, noise, motion, and pain
2. All reflex activity (except of spinal cord origin) and muscle activity
3. Spontaneous respirations
4. Cranial nerve reflexes and responses

## Confused or Disoriented Patient

With disturbed consciousness—rather than a decrease in the level of consciousness (LOC)—the person is said to be experiencing a confused or disoriented state. It is the *content* of the consciousness that is altered. The disoriented person may experience hallucinations or have illusions or delusions or become agitated. With **disorientation** the patient is awake but perceives phenomena incorrectly. Thinking and reasoning are inappropriate, and remembering is difficult.

**Delirium** is a response often encountered in an intensive care unit. It is characterized by progressive disorientation first to time, then place, then person. *Illusions, hallucinations,* and *delusions* also commonly occur. Patients become agitated and combative or secretive and withdrawn. Sleep deprivation is implicated as a causative factor when it is impossible for the patient to complete even one sleep cycle because of frequently interrupted sleep. Either too much stimulation (constant pain) or too little stimulation (eye patches) can initiate delirium. Microemboli in the postcardiotomy patient have been suggested as a possible cause. Analgesic and antipsychotic agents, metabolic imbalance, and shock are contributory factors. High fevers, drug overdose, alcoholism, and strong fears also can lead to delirium.

An *illusion* is a sensory experience based on fact but misinterpreted. This may happen when one of the senses is faulty or when environmental conditions prohibit a true interpretation of what is sensed. For example, the older person who has failing vision may think there is someone present in the room when a shadow moves.

A *hallucination* is an impression on any of the senses in the absence of a stimulus. The patient believes he or she sees, hears, tastes, feels, or smells something; but the source of this occurrence is within the patient's thinking rather than in reality. Confusion and hallucinations may be caused by injury, drugs, psychologic problems, or organic problems. Organic causes may be acute infections with high fever, drug toxicity from alcohol or psychedelic drugs, withdrawal from drugs, brain tumor, senility, or exhaustion.

*Agitation* refers to a state of psychomotor excitement that is characterized by purposeless, restless activity. The person may pace, cry, and laugh without appropriate cause. Agitation may occur as a result of stress, fear, or anxiety.

## EPIDEMIOLOGY

The incidence of those who experience altered levels of consciousness is not known. It can be said, however, that it is a common manifestation in patients for whom nurses provide care. Patients of all ages may experience altered levels of consciousness.

## PATHOPHYSIOLOGY

Although it is not known precisely what the neural mechanisms are that make awareness possible, it is known that many different parts of the nervous system work together to determine the nature of a person's awareness. To date, our knowledge of brain mechanisms is insufficient to explain the functioning of the mind as we experience it. No unified representation of one's environment exists in any single cortical area. The necessary conditions for consciousness, such as perception, memory, and language, depend on cortical functions. The presence of consciousness depends on a normally functioning interplay among certain neurons, the brain, and the reticular activating system (RAS).

The RAS, or deep central core of gray matter beginning in the brainstem, extends into the hypothalamus and thalamus either directly or indirectly, transmitting stimuli to the cerebral cortex and influencing arousal or wakefulness. Conscious behavior depends on an intact functioning cerebrum. The organization of the reticular network is vague; however, it does contain some distinct nuclei with long overlapping fibers and dendrites. Anatomic and physiologic details of brainstem nuclei are not yet fully understood. Impulses from the RAS keep us active and serve as an alerting system.

The RAS mediates responses such as eye opening to painful stimuli, as well as corneal reflexes, pupillary reaction, and ocular motility. The RAS acts as a relay to the cerebral cortex and functions like an on-off switch for the cortical awareness system. It is the cycling of this system that accounts for the sleep-wake cycle.

When the effects of an insult impinge on the RAS, the state of consciousness can be altered. As the severity of the insult or dysfunction increases, there is increasing impairment of responsiveness to events in the internal and external environment. If the dysfunction is great enough, unconsciousness or coma will result. Any impairment, reduction, or absence of consciousness indicates a serious dysfunction of the brain.

Cerebral function is most commonly affected by lack of oxygen or glucose. The brain is extremely sensitive to hypoxia, and only a few seconds of anoxia can lead to loss of consciousness. The amount of oxygen available to cells of the cerebral cortex depends on adequacy of blood flow, blood oxygen tension, hemoglobin concentration, and serum pH. ***Delirium usually results with a $PO_2$ level below 55 mm Hg and coma*** when the level falls below 25 mm Hg. Oxygen saturation usually is measured by pulse oximetry.

Cerebral cells are affected by the same conditions that affect cellular metabolism elsewhere in the body. Thus altered levels of consciousness can result from conditions such as fluid and electrolyte imbalances or toxins that interfere with metabolism of cerebral cells. (See Box 57-1 for possible causes of decreased levels of consciousness.)

## PREVENTION

*Primary prevention* of decreased levels of consciousness involves avoidance of those factors that can contribute to it (such as carbon monoxide, drugs, or alcohol), as well as control of chronic diseases such as diabetes and chronic obstructive pulmonary disease (COPD). Avoidance of situations that can lead to head injury and subsequent trauma is important. With coma that results from vascular problems, it is important to avoid factors that can lead to decreased levels of consciousness. These include the following:

1. Cigarette smoking
2. Hypertension
3. Hypercholesterolemia
4. Obesity
5. Stress-related occupations and hectic pace of life

*Secondary prevention,* or early detection, is of the utmost importance in dealing with patients with a decreased level of consciousness. Many initial symptoms are so vague that it is easy to deny or minimize their importance. In addition, *tertiary prevention,* or prevention of complications, is vitally important in this type of patient. The dependence on nursing care that these patients usually exhibit makes it extremely important for the nurse to prevent *iatrogenic* problems. These problems are discussed in more detail later in this chapter.

## MEDICAL MANAGEMENT

The goal for discharge of patients with altered states of consciousness is determined by DRGs that are linked to the causative factor. The nurse works collaboratively with the physician for implementation of prescribed medical therapy. Because the nurse has a major role in discharge planning and patient teaching, these are discussed under nursing management.

### Diagnostic Tests

Diagnostic testing can be very important for the patient with a decreased level of consciousness (LOC). Routine laboratory tests should be performed as indicated in Box 57-2.

A toxicology screen also should be obtained on blood, urine, and gastric aspirate for opiates, barbiturates, sedatives, antidepressants, and alcohol. Other studies that are helpful to determine the cause and nature of decreased LOC include the following:

1. Skull roentgenogram
2. Brain scan
3. EEG
4. Computed tomography scan
5. Cerebral angiography
6. Lumbar puncture (if there is a suspicion of intracranial infection such as meningitis or encephalitis)
7. Evoked potentials

See Chapter 56 for a description of these tests.

### Medication

If there is some evidence that the decreased LOC is the result of an opiate overdose, naloxone should be given intravenously. The usual dosage is 0.4 to 2 mg, repeated every 2 to 3 minutes.[4] Naloxone is a narcotic antagonist that reverses the effects of opioids. In patients with an opiate addiction, it might provoke an acute withdrawal state that will require treatment with narcotics.

The nurse should observe the patient for symptoms of narcotic withdrawal, which include abdominal cramping, diarrhea, goose flesh, and anxiety. Medications such as clonidine or hyoscyamine (Levsin) may be needed to control these symptoms.

In patients in coma who are found to have increased intracranial pressure (ICP), hyperosmolar agents, such as mannitol, and steroids, such as dexamethasone, usually are given. With these medications the nurse should monitor the patient closely for urinary output, especially when mannitol is given. The output is often large, and catheter insertion may be needed to prevent bladder distention. It is important to monitor the neurologic status of the patient at frequent intervals.

When other methods of controlling the increased ICP are ineffective, intravenous barbiturates may be used to place the patient in a barbiturate coma to reduce the brain's need for oxygen. This requires both experienced personnel and a setting in which internal intracranial monitoring can take place. The patient in a barbiturate coma is totally dependent and thus requires total nursing care.

The patient who is agitated may be treated with medications such as haloperidol (Haldol) or lorazepam (Ativan). When administering these medications, the nurse should monitor the patient for adequate respiratory status and proper elimination. Efforts to orient the patient should continue. Monitoring the safety of both the patient and staff members is part of the nurse's responsibility.

### Treatment

There is no specific treatment for the patient with an altered level of consciousness inasmuch as treatment depends on the cause. The reader is referred to other sections of this text for appropriate treatment of the various disorders that can cause coma.

### Diet

There is no special diet for the patient with decreased level of consciousness. Dietary considerations are based on the patient's state of awareness.

### Activity

The activity level of the patient depends on the level of alertness and awareness. Mobility of the patient is encouraged unless there is danger of increased intracranial pressure.

### Referral/Consultation

In some settings the nurse assumes responsibility for making referrals, for example, to a social worker.

**BOX 57-2 Important Laboratory Tests for Patients in Coma**

| | |
|---|---|
| Complete blood count | Calcium |
| Urinalysis | $Po_2$ |
| Electrolytes | Liver function studies |
| Blood urea nitrogen | Enzymes |
| Creatinine | Osmolality |
| Blood glucose | |

## NURSING MANAGEMENT

### ♦ ASSESSMENT

Both subjective and objective data about patients with decreased LOC should be collected.

## Subjective Data

It may be impossible to obtain accurate information from the patient with a decreased level of consciousness. Data for the history should always be obtained from the family or significant other, as well as the patient. Subjective data to be collected to assess the patient with decreased LOC include the following:

When the decreased LOC started
Concomitant symptoms
Patient's awareness of condition
Ability to think, calculate, and abstract
Presence of pain or discomfort, including stiff neck
Presence of visual symptoms
History of trauma

## Objective Data

Objective data to be collected to assess the patient with decreased level of consciousness include the following:

Vital signs
Pupillary signs—size, equality, and reactivity
Focal motor or sensory signs—presence, symmetry, and character of movements, including eye movements
Presence of vomiting or hiccoughing
Eye changes, including papilledema
Speech patterns
Odor of breath (a clue to diabetic ketoacidosis)
Abnormal reflexes

The respiratory rate is helpful in localizing and, in certain instances, determining the nature of the process. These patterns include the following:

Cheyne-Stokes respiration
Central neurogenic hyperventilation (CNHV)
Apneustic breathing
Cluster breathing
Ataxic breathing
Gasping breathing
Depressed breathing

See Table 57-2 for characteristics of each of these types of breathing.

The reflex eye movements often used to evaluate brainstem functioning in the comatose patient include the oculocephalic reflex response (doll's eyes) and the oculovestibular reflex response. The *oculocephalic reflex* is demonstrated by holding the person's eyelids open and rotating the head from side to side. If the brain's pathways to the eye muscles are intact, the eyes will move to the left as the head is rotated to the right. This parallel or conjugate gaze is called *positive* or *normal doll's eyes* (Figure 57-2).

The *oculovestibular reflex* refers to reflex conjugate eye movements or *nystagmus* that is caused by stimulating the semicircular canals of the ear with ice water. This is an accurate method of assessing brainstem functioning. The reflex is evaluated by the caloric ice water test. What should be seen is horizontal nystagmus with

**TABLE 57-2 Altered Respiratory Patterns in Coma**

| CHARACTERISTICS | INDICATIONS |
|---|---|
| **CHEYNE-STOKES** | |
| Periods of hyperventilation that gradually diminish to apnea of variable duration; respirations then resume and gradually build up to hyperventilation | Bilateral deep hemispheric and basal ganglionic dysfunction; the upper brainstem may be involved |
| **CENTRAL NEUROGENIC HYPERVENTILATION (CNHV)** | |
| Continuous rapid and deep respirations at a rate of 25/min | Systemic acidosis and hypoxemia should be excluded; has no segmental localizing influence; increasing regularity correlates with increasing depth of coma |
| **APNEUSTIC BREATHING** | |
| Prolonged inspiratory phase followed by apnea (inspiratory cramp) | Indicates lower pontine damage |
| **CLUSTER BREATHING** | |
| Closely grouped respirations followed by apnea | Indicates lower pontine damage |
| **ATAXIC BREATHING** | |
| Chaotic respirations | Indicates damage to medullary centers; can precede respiratory arrest |
| **GASPING BREATHING** | |
| Characterized by gasps followed by apnea of variable duration | Indicates damage to medullary centers; can precede respiratory arrest |
| **DEPRESSED BREATHING** | |
| Shallow, slow, and ineffective breathing | Usually caused by medullary depression |

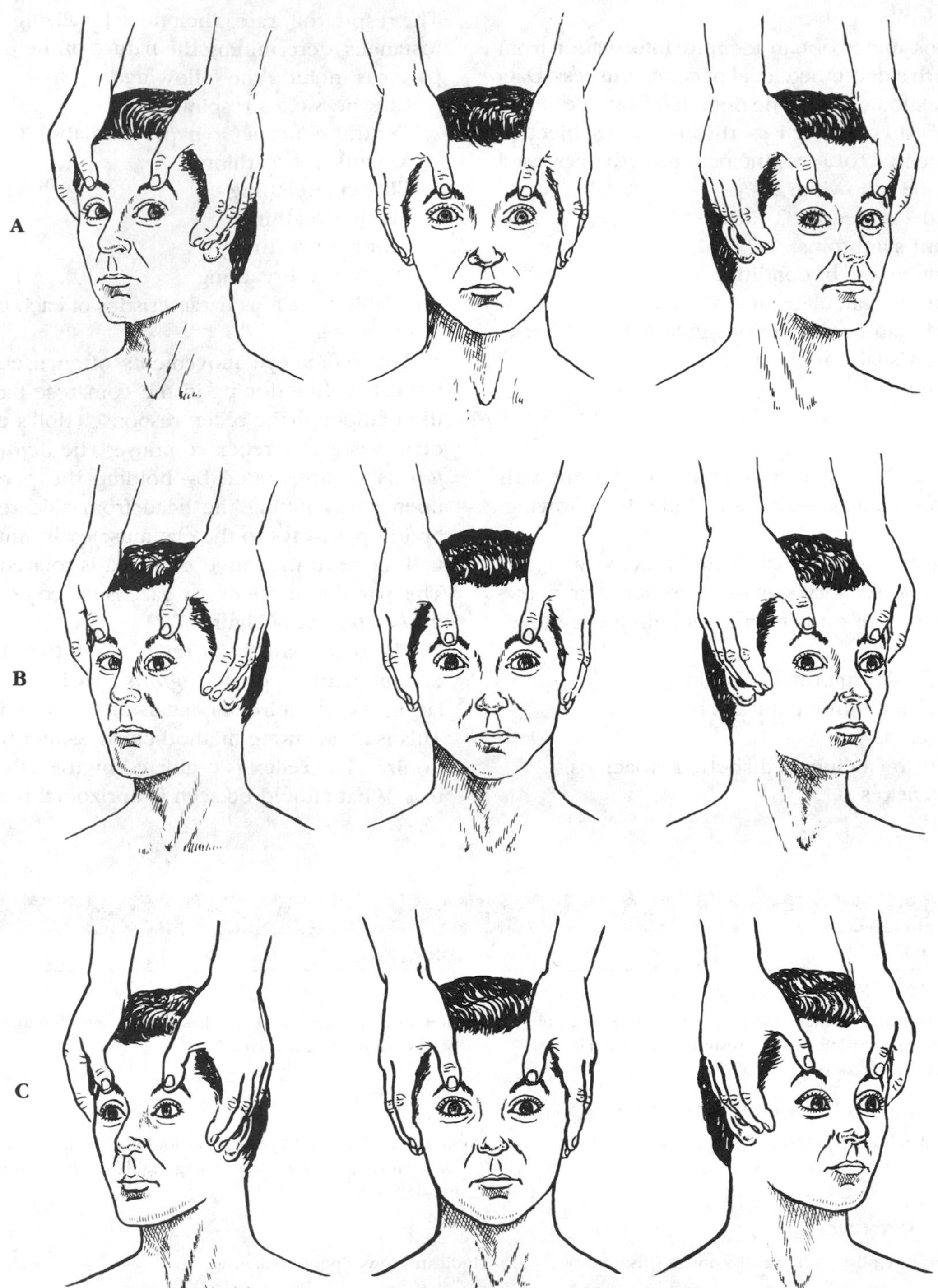


**FIGURE 57-2** Test for oculocephalic reflex response (doll's eyes phenomenon). **A,** Normal response—eyes turn together to side opposite from turn of head. **B,** Abnormal response—eyes do not turn in conjugate manner. **C,** Absent response—eyes do not turn as head position is changed. (From Rudy EB: Advanced neurologic and neurosurgical nursing, St Louis, 1984, Mosby.)

slow eye movement toward the irrigated ear and rapid eye movement away. If warm water is used, the normal eye movements will be reversed (Figure 57-3).

Accuracy is best attained when a systematic approach is used by all persons involved in the continuing assessments. Although some efforts have been made to develop scales to measure LOC, there is a paucity of tools. What is vital is that all persons in a facility consistently use a single technique. The clues or evidence that might lead to the use of a descriptive term are recorded or reported as opposed to the descriptive term itself.

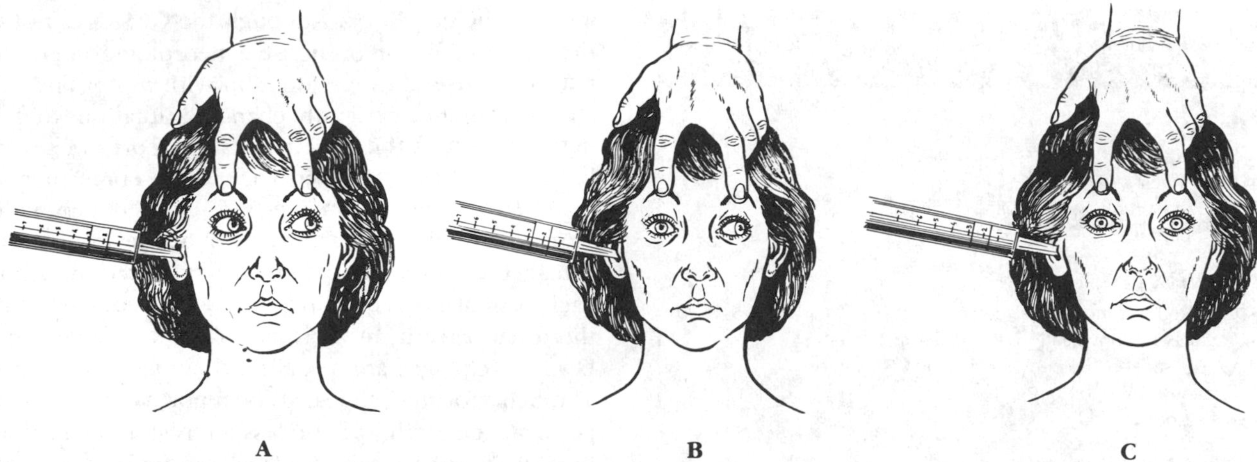


**FIGURE 57-3** Test for oculovestibular reflex response (caloric ice water test). **A,** Normal response—conjugate eye movements. **B,** Abnormal response–dysconjugate or asymmetric eye movements. **C,** Absent response—no eye movements. (From Rudy EB: Advanced neurological and neurosurgical nursing, St Louis, 1984, Mosby.)

**BOX 57-3 Levels of Cognitive Functioning (Rancho Los Amigos Scale)**

**I. NO RESPONSE**
Patient is completely unresponsive to any stimuli.

**II. GENERALIZED RESPONSE**
Patient reacts inconsistently and nonpurposefully to stimuli in nonspecific manner.

**III. LOCALIZED RESPONSE**
Patient reacts specifically but inconsistently to stimuli.

**IV. CONFUSED—AGITATED**
Patient is in heightened state of activity with severely decreased ability to process information.

**V. CONFUSED—INAPPROPRIATE**
Patient appears alert and is able to respond to simple commands fairly consistently.

**VI. CONFUSED—APPROPRIATE**
Patient shows goal-directed behavior but depends on external input for direction.

**VII. AUTOMATIC—APPROPRIATE**
Patient appears appropriate and oriented within hospital and home setting, goes through daily routine automatically, with minimal to absent confusion and has shallow recall of actions.

**VIII. PURPOSEFUL—APPROPRIATE**
Patient is alert and oriented, is able to recall and integrate past and recent events, and is aware of and responsive to culture.

From Malkmus D et al: *Rehabilitation of the head-injured adult—comprehensive cognitive management,* Downey, Calif, 1980, Professional Staff Association of Rancho Los Amigos Hospital, Inc.

### Ranchos Los Amigos scale

One scale that is widely used is the **Ranchos Los Amigos** levels of cognitive functioning (Box 57-3). It was developed as a behavioral rating scale to aid in assessment and treatment of the head-injured person. It represents the progression of recovery of cognitive abilities as demonstrated through behavioral change. The tool is used to assess the patient and to give some structure to interventions.

For purposes of patient management, eight levels of cognitive functioning are grouped in the following four basic recovery phases and intervention strategies:

| Level | Recovery Phase | Approach |
|---|---|---|
| II, III | Decreased response | Stimulation |
| IV | Agitated response | Structure |
| V, VI | Confused response | Structure |
| VII, VIII | Automatic response | Community |

**BOX 57-4 Glasgow Coma Scale Scoring**

**EYES OPEN**
- **4** Spontaneously
- **3** On request
- **2** To pain stimuli (supraorbital or digital)
- **1** No opening

**BEST VERBAL RESPONSE**
- **5** Oriented to time, place, person
- **4** Engages in conversation, confused in content
- **3** Words spoken but conversation not sustained
- **2** Groans evoked by pain
- **1** No response

**BEST MOTOR RESPONSE**
- **5** Obeys a command ("Hold out three fingers.")
- **4** Localizes a painful stimulus
- **3** Flexes either arm
- **2** Extends arm to painful stimulus
- **1** No response

### Glasgow coma scale

An objective measure to describe LOC is the **Glasgow coma scale (GCS),** which has been shown to be reproducible by professional and other health personnel.[57] The scale is simple; it is based on the patient's response in three areas: eye opening, motor response, and verbal response. Numbers are assigned to the best performance in each of the three areas (Box 57-4), and the total score provides an overview of the patient's LOC. When a sequence of the numbers for each of the three categories is plotted on a graph over time, a visual picture of the direction of progress evolves (Figure 57-4). It may show stability, or it may indicate deterioration or improvement in the condition. Although the GCS does not take the place of a comprehensive neurologic check, it is extremely useful in conjunction with motor and brainstem assessment in rapidly changing situations to detect deterioration in the patient's status. Scores of seven or less (but not scores of nine or more) represent **coma.**

When the onset of unconsciousness is *not* immediate, as it is with fainting or extreme shock or trauma, there usually is a consistent pattern of deterioration, although each patient is unique and may depart somewhat from the usual pattern. In the early stages of a deteriorating LOC the changes are so subtle they may not be noted. The behavior may appear to be a normal mood change. For instance, there may be less interest in the surroundings or in events taking place; the patient may seem bored or drowsy, inattentive or irritable, and restless. If these behaviors are noted and if there is any history that could lead one to suspect altered brain function, further exploration is necessary (see Chapter 56).

Another procedure for assessing level of consciousness is outlined in Figure 57-5. One begins by determining the patient's orientation by means of several questions about time, place, and person. The month and year are more readily recalled than days and dates. One can be satisfied if patients know they are in a hospital even if they cannot recall the name of the institution. Persons can be asked their name and occupation.

Next the person is requested to respond to simple commands such as blinking the eyes or touching the nose or ear with the fingers. Lack of symmetry can be noted by testing both sides of the body. This is important in localizing some lesions. The person can be asked to squeeze the examiner's hand with first the right and then the left hand or to lift both feet simultaneously. If the person cannot perform in response to these commands, then the response to pain is assessed.

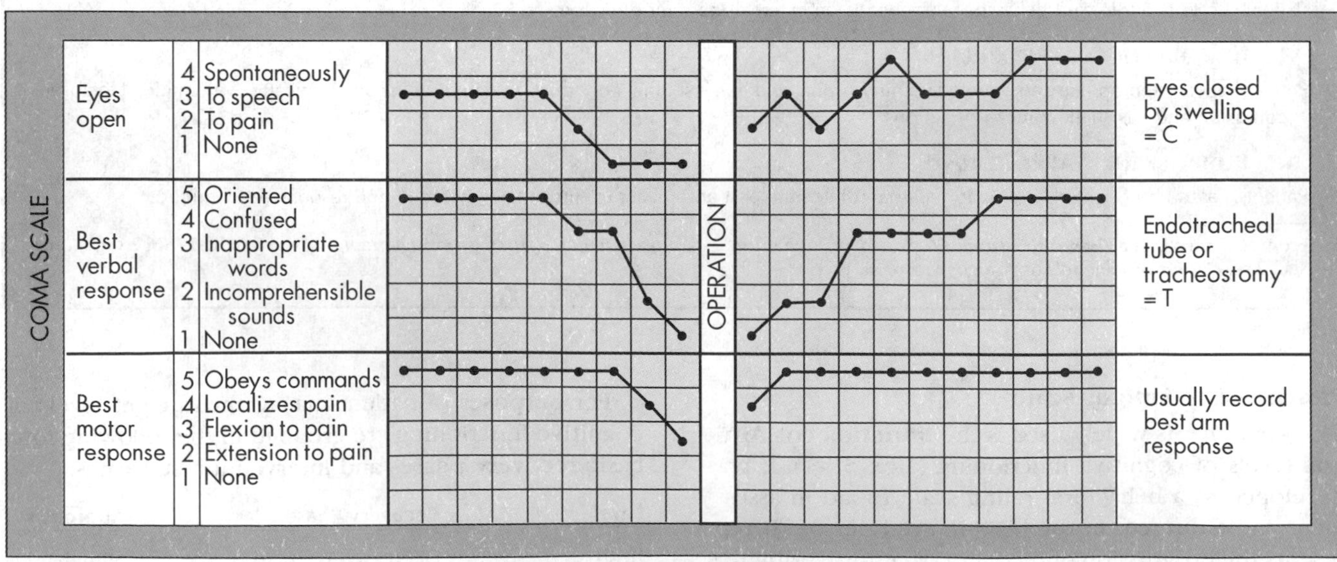


**FIGURE 57-4** Glasgow coma scale, demonstrating measurement of level of consciousness. Notice change in patient's condition just before and after surgery.

There are several techniques for checking response to pain that do not cause trauma to the patient. Pinching and pricking may damage tissues and are avoided when possible. The two preferred methods of delivering a pain stimulus are nailbed pressure and supraorbital pressure. Nailbed pressure is accomplished by placing a pen or similar object on the nailbed and squeezing it between the examiner's thumb and forefinger (see Figure 56-19). If there is no response to nailbed pressure, supraorbital pressure is used.

To perform the supraorbital pain maneuver, the examiner places the thumb on the upper edge of the bony groove of the eye socket about one third the distance from the inner aspect of the orbit and presses. One can also apply pressure to the trapezius by pinching it between the patient's neck and the shoulder. (Practice on yourself to see how much pressure is necessary.) The response showing the highest level of consciousness is for the patient to withdraw from the stimulus or try to push it away. If the response is indicated by grimaces or by moving or thrashing around but in a nonpurposeful manner, the level of awareness is lower. Finally, with very deep coma there may be no response at all. Regardless of the response, the examiner records the type of stimulus and the patient's response behavior (see Research box above, right).

To further assess brainstem function and to determine indications for nursing care, the integrity of the brainstem at the level of the pons can be assessed by checking the ***lash reflex*** or the ***corneal reflex***. The lash reflex is checked by stroking the eyelashes with a finger. An intact reflex is indicated by immediate blinking (the eyes can be open or closed to do this). The corneal reflex is checked by holding the eyelid open and gently stroking the cornea with a thin wisp of cotton. An intact reflex is indicated by immediate blinking. The lash reflex is preferred over the corneal reflex because the cornea can be easily damaged. If no blink response is seen, the nurse must ensure protection of the cornea. If the response was present before, absence of the response may indicate deterioration of the patient's condition. The integrity of the medulla can be assessed by the ***gag reflex***. The gag reflex is checked by touching both sides of the posterior pharynx with a tongue depressor. Absence of a gag reflex indicates danger of aspiration of food and secretions.

If the neurologic status deteriorates, assessments may need to be made more frequently. Likewise, if the patient's status improves, assessments may be made less frequently. The nurse independently institutes more frequent observations when the patient's status so indicates.

**RESEARCH**

Grant J, Kinney M: Validity of a nursing diagnosis, *Res Nurs Health* 13(6):403-410, 1990.

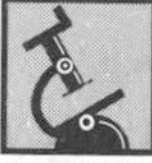

The purpose of this three-phase study was to examine the validity of the nursing diagnosis *altered level of consciousness (ALC)*. Twenty-six content experts in neuroscience nursing completed four rounds of a Delphi survey to ascertain identifying characteristics and operational definitions for this nursing diagnosis. Study results supported altered levels of consciousness as a nursing diagnosis appropriate for use in neuroscience nursing.

## Diagnostic Test Findings

Significant or abnormal findings on diagnostic tests may include positive results on the drug toxicology screen, as well as bacteria and red or white blood cells in the spinal fluid obtained by lumbar puncture. The EEG may

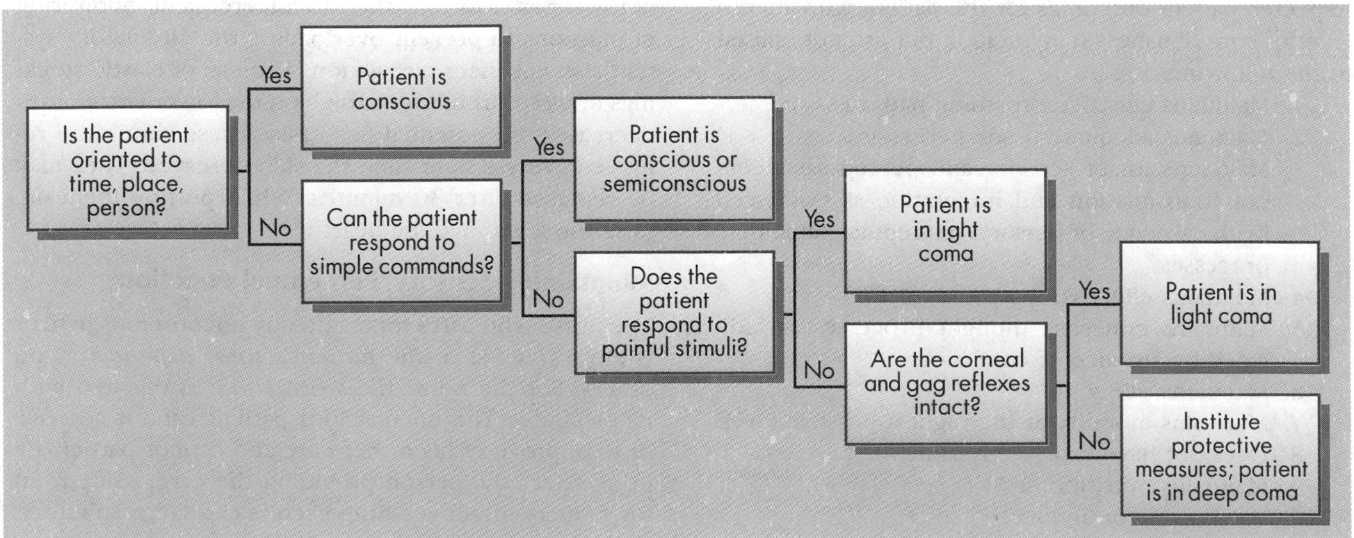


**FIGURE 57-5** Procedure for assessing level of consciousness.

show slowed brain waves, and the CT scan, brain scan, skull films, and cerebral angiogram may indicate the presence of a tumor or hemorrhage.

## ♦ NURSING DIAGNOSES

Nursing diagnoses are determined from analysis of patient data. Nursing diagnoses for the patient with altered level of consciousness may include but are not limited to the following:

| Diagnostic Title | Possible Etiologic Factors |
|---|---|
| Breathing pattern, ineffective | Neuromuscular impairment, perception/cognition impairment |
| Tissue perfusion, altered (cerebral) | Decreased blood flow (arterial) |
| Sensory/perceptual alterations | Altered sensory reception/transmission, integration |
| Thermoregulation, ineffective | Trauma/illness |
| Thought processes, impaired | Neurologic disorders, hypoxia |
| Injury, high risk for | Sensory/motor deficits |
| Mobility, impaired physical | Perceptual/cognitive impairment, neuromuscular impairment |
| Disuse syndrome, high risk for | Immobility, weakness |
| Nutrition, altered: less than body requirements | Chewing or swallowing difficulties |
| Incontinence, bowel | Neuromuscular impairment |
| Urinary elimination pattern, altered | Sensorimotor impairment |
| Self-care deficit: feeding, bathing/hygiene, dressing/grooming, toileting | Cognitive/perceptual impairment, neuromuscular impairment |
| Skin integrity, impaired, or high risk for | Mechanical forces (pressure or shearing forces, restraint), immobility |
| Coping, family: compromised | Inadequate or incorrect information or understanding |

## ♦ EXPECTED PATIENT OUTCOMES

Expected patient outcomes for the patient with altered level of consciousness may include but are not limited to the following:

1. Maintains effective breathing pattern.
2. Maintains adequate tissue perfusion.
3. Maintains intact sensory and perceptual reception/transmission and integration as evidenced by the absence of sensory/perceptual pathologic processes.
4. Maintains effective thermoregulation.
5. Maintains coherent thought processes as indicated by absence of confusion.
6. Maintains safety.
7. Maintains mobility at the highest possible level.
8. Does not have disuse syndrome.
9. Maintains nutrition.
10. Has bowel continence.
11. Has urinary continence.
12. Performs activities of daily living independently.
13. Maintains skin integrity.
14. Family demonstrates effective coping processes.

## ♦ INTERVENTIONS

### Maintaining Breathing Patterns

It is important for the nurse to closely monitor the breathing patterns of the patient with an altered level of consciousness. The patient may require assistance in keeping the airway clear, including the use of suctioning when warranted. Positioning the patient on the left side and keeping the head of the bed elevated to at least 30 degrees may help facilitate an open airway. It may be necessary to provide the patient with supplemental oxygen or mechanical ventilation. The need for both approaches can be assessed through the use of pulse oximetry, which indicates the oxygen saturation level of the blood. Arterial blood gas determinations yield the same results but are more invasive. It is important for the nurse to realize that hypoxia in these patients may result in increased intracranial pressure.

### Maintaining Tissue Perfusion

Circulation can be assisted in several ways. Conscientiously turning the patient from side to side at least every 2 hours will enhance circulation because muscle movement stimulates circulation. Careful attention to positioning so that there are no constricted areas, as would be caused by twisted clothing, tight bedclothes, or a poorly positioned limb, will allow for maximum circulation. Joints bent at sharp angles slow circulation and should be avoided. Passive range of motion exercises planned into the nursing care regimen at least every 8 hours will increase blood flow. Padding of dependent bony prominences when they are being lain on decreases pressure and helps to maintain good circulation. A commonly overlooked area is the ear. If it is folded over, circulation to the outer area is occluded and tissue necrosis occurs quickly. Always check the lower portion of the ear after turning the patient. Frequent monitoring of infusions to prevent overloading the circulatory system also enhances circulation. The use of elastic stockings or wraps from toe to thigh on the lower extremities decreases the potential for stasis. These should be removed every 8 hours and the skin observed. They may be replaced after 30 minutes. When putting them on, raise the leg above the heart level.

### Maintaining Sensory/Perceptual Function

The nurse who cares for an already unconscious patient is always aware of the *patient's total dependency* on others. For the nurse the word *coma* is equated with helplessness. The unconscious patient cannot approve or disapprove of his or her care and cannot participate in or select the person providing the care. Aside from involuntary motor activities such as cardiac, respiratory, and gastrointestinal actions, the patient is unresponsive. It then becomes paramount for others to provide for additional life-sustaining requirements, including nourishment, elimination, and protection of tissues.

Such a comatose state may lull the nurse into thinking that nothing is taking place in the patient's social world. We can only speculate about receptiveness. *Meaningful stimuli can be introduced* into the comatose patient's environment. To do this, the nurse must first learn as much of the patient's life-style as possible: social activities, work, friends, family. Key factors in the patient's former 24-hour routine are then selected, and the care should approximate previous habits. As an example, tube feedings should be scheduled about the same time of day as the patient was accustomed to eating so that stomach distention is closely related to former habits. If the patient worked in a noisy factory, provide sound during the former working hours. Record familiar sounds and play them at appropriate times, for example, table talk when the family has dinner. For the long-term unconscious patient, this approach appears to have merit in keeping the focus of care from becoming too oriented to body functions to the exclusion of social factors.

Because *hearing is probably the last sense to be lost,* the monitoring of what is said in the presence of the unconscious person is vitally important. At present there is no sure device to assess when patients no longer are able to hear; therefore, even when patients appear incapable of receiving messages, they may still understand what is said. Grave prognoses or flippant comments are best kept outside a patient's range of hearing. In fact, positive and hopeful comments made in the patient's presence may give the patient motivation to struggle back to consciousness. Thus the nurse speaks to the patient and explains what is being done as if the patient were fully aware of what is going on.

Another factor to consider is the *therapeutic effect of touch.* The patient is spoken to before being touched and is handled with gentleness. Because there is no pain response to remind care providers when stress is increased, the tendency is to move the unconscious patient without consideration of soft tissue. Touch is one of the first sensations experienced by the human organism, and without proper touch, normal development would not take place. Touch is a medium for communication. Holding and cuddling infants seem to make them more tranquil and content. Research has shown positive results from the use of touch with disoriented

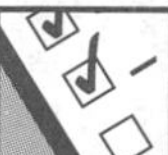

### Guidelines for Care of the Person With Decreased Level of Consciousness or Coma

1. Maintain stimulation
   a. Introduce meaningful stimuli
   b. Monitor what is said around patient
   c. Speak to patient before touching
   d. Use gentleness in handling patient
   e. Maintain low-key environment
2. Maintain nutrition
   a. Monitor intravenous fluids
   b. Administer tube feedings with patient in high Fowler's position
   c. Administer tube feedings at room temperature
   d. Change feeding tube every 5 to 7 days
   e. Cleanse and lubricate naris to prevent breakdown
   f. Begin oral feedings as soon as patient is able
3. Maintain elimination
   a. Institute suppository regimen, considering patient's normal bowel routine
   b. Administer enemas only as last resort
   c. Stool softeners as ordered
   d. Give adequate fluids—use prune juice
   e. Regular toileting to institute regimen
   f. Use of condom catheter for male
   g. Adequately care for indwelling catheter
4. Maintain circulation
   a. Reposition frequently
   b. Avoid positioning joints at acute angles
   c. Use elastic stockings or Ace wraps to legs
5. Maintain normal body temperature
   a. Hyperthermia
      (1) Remove excess bedclothes and clothing
      (2) Lower room temperature
      (3) Ice bags to groin or axilla
      (4) Tepid water sponge baths
      (5) Use of hypothermia blankets
      (6) Use of antipyretics
   b. Hypothermia
      (1) Add additional clothing or blankets
      (2) Increase room temperature
      (3) Warmed blankets
6. Promote safety
   a. Side rails up at all times
   b. Pad rails as necessary
   c. Keep supplies and equipment out of reach of patient
   d. Use restraints only when absolutely necessary
   e. Remove contact lenses
   f. Cleanse eyes at least daily and check for redness or other signs of irritation or infection
7. Promote activity
   a. Position properly at least every 2 hours
   b. Use prone position if patient is able to tolerate
   c. Range of motion exercises at least twice a day
   d. Mobilize patient into chair as soon as possible
8. Maintain skin integrity
   a. Cleanse skin daily using warm water
   b. Judicious use of lotion to prevent dryness
   c. Keep linen pulled tight and free of crumbs or other residue
   d. Use air or water mattresses as necessary
   e. Inspect skin frequently
9. Maintain good hygiene
   a. Wash hair every 1 to 2 weeks, or more often if needed
   b. Braid or arrange long hair to prevent matting
   c. Give good mouth care at least three times a day

and some mentally ill persons. It is highly possible that some of the same positive responses can be elicited in the unconscious patient. Using a firm hand grasp while talking to the patient about the day or the environment, smoothing the hair away from the face with the full palmar surface of the hand, or tucking the bed covers snuggly around the patient may stimulate the feeling of being cared for or encompassed.

Another factor relates to the patient's environment. The *environment should be low key,* with loud noises kept to a minimum. Soft music may be beneficial, but unnecessary sounds should be eliminated. The unconscious person with improving awareness often has an overly excitable nervous system response and is unable to attend to multiple stimuli. To facilitate the patient's ability to focus on any stimulus, eliminate all but necessary noises.

When a patient begins to recover, the first response often is to a familiar voice or face, and this may be in the form of a verbal comment. The patient needs the security of knowing that family, friends, and staff are concerned and will need much support and encouragement, as well as explanation (see Guidelines box, p. 1937, and Research box below).

## Maintaining Normal Body Temperature

Normal body temperature generally is considered to range from 36° C (97° F) to 37.2° C (99° F). Because the comatose patient is unable to express being too cold or too warm, it becomes the nurse's responsibility to monitor the body temperature at least every 4 hours and more frequently if a problem arises. If the heat center in the hypothalamus is disturbed, as it often is by trauma or by certain medical problems, the temperature may change rapidly. An excessively elevated temperature is called *hyperthermia*. An elevated temperature also may indicate an infection or dehydration. When a patient is experiencing hyperthermia, the nurse can assist in maintaining the temperature within a normal range by removing bedclothes and lowering the room temperature. If necessary, remove all of the patient's clothes except enough to protect modesty and the family's sense of propriety. Antipyretics may be given via the nasogastric or gastrostomy tube or by suppository. Ice bags covered with protective wraps to prevent tissue damage may be placed on the groin and axilla where there is a large blood supply. This helps to hasten body cooling. Sponging the body with tepid water causes evaporation and subsequent cooling. The use of a fan to blow over the patient while the patient is being sponged further enhances cooling. Electrically controlled hypothermia blankets often are used to reduce fever when a patient suffers from hyperthermia. The patient should not be allowed to get chilled and shiver because shivering increases body metabolism and produces heat, thus raising the temperature. Continued hyperthermia will result in brain damage and ultimately death; thus the temperature is kept as near normal as possible. On the other end of the continuum, a subnormal temperature (hypothermia) may be experienced. Additional clothing and covers and increased room temperature are helpful. Warmed blankets may help elevate temperature in the hypothermic patient.

### RESEARCH

Ackerman L: Interventions related to neurologic care, *Nurs Clin North Am* 27(2):325-335, 1992.

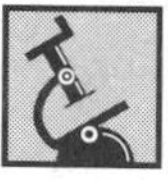

This study examined more than 300 activities that are used in the planning and delivery of care to neuroscience patients with intracranial disease processes. Nurses were asked to rate activities on a questionnaire. These were then grouped into 13 neurologic intervention categories: (1) surveillance: neurologic, (2) cerebral edema management, (3) ICP monitoring, (4) tube care: ventriculostomy/lumbar drain, (5) subarachnoid hemorrhage precautions, (6) aspiration precautions, (7) seizure precautions, (8) seizure management, (9) environmental management, (10) behavior management, (11) cognitive stimulation, (12) body alignment: neurologic, and (13) eye care. It is hoped that these categories will encourage additional study and research and that they can be helpful in forming a taxonomy of neuroscience nursing care.

## Promoting Thought Processes

The care of the *confused* patient begins with a thorough assessment to determine the cause of the confusion and the patient's needs. Establish communication with the patient. A good way to get the patient's attention is through touch. Once the contact is made, use a calm, quiet, unhurried voice. To keep the patient oriented, explain in advance what you will do. Include the patient in planning and discussions. See that the room is well lighted. Keep a large calendar and clock in view. Introduce yourself each time you care for the patient. Talk slowly and distinctly and use short statements. Face the patient and stay within a conversational distance of 4 feet. When speaking to the patient, eliminate extra stimuli such as the radio and television, which would tend to clutter the sensory field and might prevent a clear communication between the nurse and patient. When it is possible, provide consistency by having the same staff members care for the patient every day. It is advisable to keep decision making at a minimum for the confused person.

The nurse can minimize effects of confusion by recognizing environmental areas likely to precipitate delirium and teaching the patient what to expect before placement there. When emergency placement is required, discussion and explanation should take place as soon as possible after the crisis situation. Emphasize that physical and environmental factors are contributing to the confusion, fears, and memory loss; reassure the patient that the state eventually will pass. Other interventions include keeping the environment simplified and well organized. Place noisy machines as far from the patient's head as possible. Dim lighting to facilitate sleep. Organize care to provide the longest possible rest periods. Place familiar personal objects within view. Use touch judiciously. Treatment directed at known causes such as fever, shock, and drug overdose will result in decreasingly confused responses.

Regardless of the specific treatments, the nurse provides safety for the patient and protection from self-injury. This may include keeping the environment quiet and nonstimulating or using side rails if the patient is to be left alone. If the presence of side rails disturbs the patient, as they sometimes do, a judgment must be made whether to use them and risk increased agitation or not use them and risk a fall. Occasionally it becomes necessary to restrain the patient.

One also monitors the physiologic processes, ensures the adequate intake of fluid and food, and monitors and supports elimination. Speak slowly and clearly. This facilitates communication with the person who is experiencing delirium. Recognizing that the patient cannot control behavior fosters acceptance and patience.

Help family members or significant others to understand what is happening and what such behavior might imply. Let them know that their presence provides a familiar stabilizing force. Let them make plans for the patient's care in the hospital and at home. Support them as much as possible in whatever they decide. (See Guidelines box below for a summary of care for the confused or disoriented patient.)

## Promoting Safety/Preventing Injury

Numerous nursing activities are geared toward providing a safe environment for the comatose patient experiencing a changing level of consciousness. Side rails are kept up at all times for the unconscious patient unless the nurse is present. When the patient is restless and likely to be thrashing about, the railing should be padded. Equipment is placed far enough from the bed that a confused patient would be unlikely to interfere with its operation. Any prosthetic device such as false teeth, an artificial eye, or contact lenses should be removed and carefully stored in a safe place until the patient is lucid enough to use them appropriately. Restraint should be avoided unless the patient is agitated enough to do harm. When any type of restraint is used, caution should be taken to put it on properly and not too tightly. Periodic checks should be made for tissue damage.

When a person becomes unconscious, one of the first interventions is to remove contact lenses (see Chapter 60). When properly done, there is little likelihood of causing damage. The cornea receives its oxygen supply primarily through exchange of gases in the atmosphere. When eyes are closed during sleep, the metabolic rate of the cornea decreases and the oxygen supply from the blood system is adequate to maintain health. When contact lenses are worn, however, the metabolic rate of the cornea increases. If the eyes are closed for a long time with the contact lenses in place, the cornea cannot remain healthy. The damage will be directly related to the time the lenses have been in place and the extent of interference with metabolic rate of the tissue. Contact lenses should be stored either in saline solution or distilled water, keeping the right and left lens separated and labeled.

Because the eyes are very precious and cannot be replaced, precautions should be taken to prevent their damage. Pull the lid back and check the eyes several times a day. Make sure they do not become dried out. Cleanse them with clear water or one of the commercial lubricants. Keep the eyelids closed. *If there is any problem with keeping the eyelid closed, place a shield to cover the eye to prevent irritation from scratching or from dryness.*

### Guidelines for Care of the Person With Confusion or Disorientation

1. Promote communication
   a. Touch may be useful to establish communication
   b. Use calm, quiet, and unhurried voice to talk to patient
   c. Talk slowly and distinctly and use short sentences
   d. Face patient when talking and stay within conversational range
2. Promote orientation
   a. Explain procedures in advance
   b. Environment should be well lighted
   c. Keep large calendar and clock in view
   d. Introduce self when caring for patient
   e. Keep sensory stimulation to a minimum
   f. Provide consistency in staff caring for patient
   g. Keep decision making to a minimum
3. Support family

## Promoting Mobility/Preventing Disuse Syndrome

### Positioning

Numerous interventions and aids are available to protect musculoskeletal integrity. Perhaps the most crucial is positioning. Improper positioning can lead to contractures, foot drop, wrist drop, and other deformities. The preferred position for the comatose patient is the *side-lying position*[40] (Figure 57-6).

The comatose patient is at risk for pulmonary complications. Therefore frequent changes of position are essential. Turning the patient from side to side at frequent intervals prevents pooling of pulmonary secretions. In some instances, tracheal suctioning may be necessary because of the patient's inability to cough. Unless neurologic complications contraindicate it, postural drainage may be initiated.

Comatose patients may be placed in a prone or supine

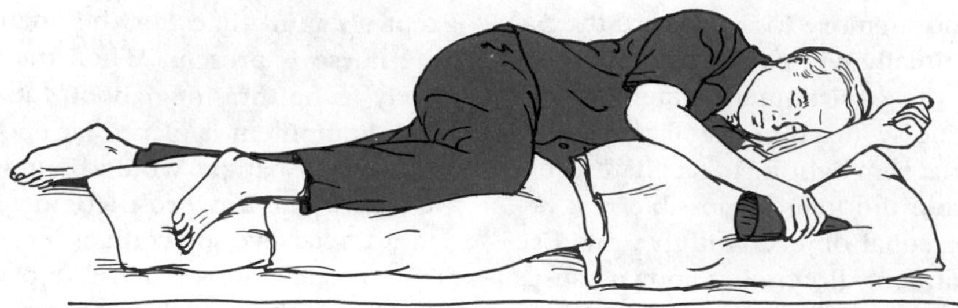

**FIGURE 57-6** Lateral position with hand cone to prevent flexion contracture of hand. (From Dittmar SS: *Rehabilitation nursing: process and application,* St Louis, 1989, Mosby.)

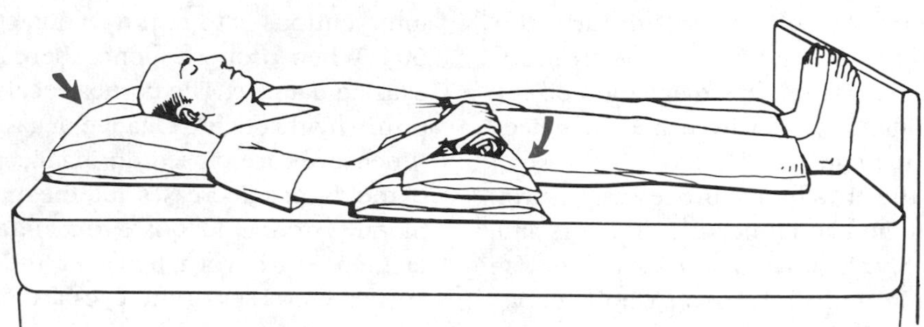

**FIGURE 57-7** Patient lying supine with feet against foot board. Note that the lower part of arm is elevated on a small pillow and hand is flexed over a rolled towel.

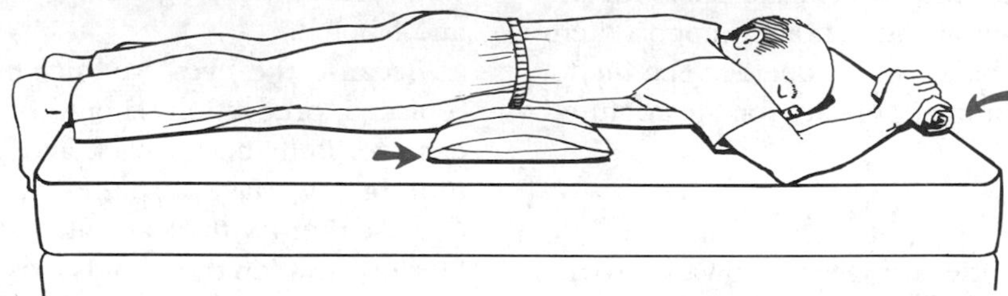

**FIGURE 57-8** Patient lying prone with feet extending over end of mattress. Note that small pillow is positioned under patient's midsection and that hand is flexed around rolled towel.

position; however, care must be taken to ensure a patent airway (Figures 57-7 and 57-8).

Patients who are comatose may be positioned without significant risk of increasing intracranial pressure.

### Exercise

Passive range-of-motion (ROM) exercise is performed a minimum of twice daily and ideally several times a day. One way to accomplish this is to put the upper side of the body through complete ROM each time the patient is turned. Doing it systematically helps ensure that it is not postponed and subsequently overlooked. ROM exercises increase circulation and decrease the likelihood of thrombi.

When the physical condition is stable and consciousness returns, the patient should sit in a chair at least once and preferably twice a day. The upright posture fosters weight bearing on the long bones, thus limiting calcium loss, and enhances pulmonary expansion, circulation, and digestive motility. Unless the patient is small enough for two persons to manage, use a mechanical lift. Position the patient so that he or she is seated squarely on the buttocks with the spine straight and feet flat on the floor or foot rest. Support the arms and head with pillows.

## Maintaining Nutrition

When a patient is experiencing rapidly decreasing awareness, nutrition is not a primary concern; however, if the patient becomes comatose and remains so for an extended period of time, nutritional support becomes a major concern. For the first few days of unconsciousness

## RESEARCH

Ozuna J, Friel P: Effect of enteral tube feeding on serum phenytoin levels, *J Neurosurg Nurs* 16(6):289-291, 1984.

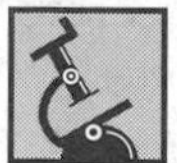

This study examined the relationship of timing of phenytoin (Dilantin) administration, delivery of tube feedings, and increasing the serum levels of phenytoin. Seven patients were studied. Tube feedings were stopped 2 hours before and 2 hours after administration of the phenytoin. No increase in levels was found. The study indicated that when increased phenytoin serum levels in patients receiving tube feedings are desired, the dose of phenytoin should be increased.

the patient probably will be maintained on intravenous fluids, as prescribed by the physician. Close observation of the needle site for inflammation or infiltration, as well as attention to flow rate to prevent excessive fluid intake, is essential. After 2 or 3 days a nasogastric tube, which will supply nourishment in liquid form, may be inserted into the stomach. Feedings usually are prescribed every 2 to 3 hours in small amounts to decrease the possibility of regurgitation and aspiration. The tube should be changed every 5 to 7 days unless it becomes clogged sooner, but the naris through which the tube is placed should be cleaned daily with warm water and lubricated with a water-soluble lubricant to decrease the formation of crusts.

The presence of a tube in the nostril is irritating and may cause tissue damage. Thus, if coma lasts for an extended period, a gastrostomy tube may be needed to provide a means for feeding. The *gastrostomy tube* is inserted through the abdominal wall into the stomach. A catheter with an inflatable tip (to prevent the tube from slipping out of the stomach) is then sutured in place. This tube remains clamped or plugged except during feedings, and the area around the tube is cleaned daily and covered with a dry dressing. It has been found that patients receiving tube feedings often have decreased phenytoin levels (see Research box above).

## Maintaining Elimination

### Bowel

Measures must be taken to assist in elimination and to maintain the tone of the bowel muscles. Without intervention, the tendency is for the comatose patient to become constipated, with possible impaction. Routinely palpate the abdomen to determine when a fecal mass is present. This palpation also may serve to stimulate peristalsis and induce a bowel movement. If possible, determine the patient's normal elimination schedule and place the patient on a bedpan at that hour. If a suppository is needed, administer it about 30 minutes before the regular elimination schedule. Bisacodyl (Dulcolax) is an effective suppository to use for bowel training. When laxatives are needed, a mild one such as milk of magnesia often is used and can be administered via the nasogastric tube.

Unconscious patients should be placed on a bowel program to ensure regular evacuation of stool (see Chapter 47).

Sometimes it becomes necessary to give a cleansing enema. Usual techniques for administering an enema are used; however, it may be necessary to hold the patient's buttocks together to prevent expulsion of the solution before the enema contents should be expelled. The enema also may be administered through a Foley catheter placed in the rectum. The balloon is inflated before the fluid is introduced, thus preventing the expulsion of the fluid until the desired amount has been administered. The balloon is deflated (before removing the catheter) to allow expulsion of the enema. When the patient is placed on the bedpan, care is taken to align the body correctly and to protect the skin. Gentle massage of the abdomen along the path of the transverse and descending colon will assist in the expulsion of the fecal mass. Stool softeners such as docusate sodium (Colace) administered via the nasogastric tube also helps facilitate elimination. Ensuring an adequate liquid intake helps keep the fecal mass soft, and juices that have a laxative effect, such as prune juice, may be included in the diet. In the event that an impaction does occur, a retention enema is administered. If this is unsuccessful, the impaction may require manual removal, that is, the use of a gloved, lubricated finger to remove small pieces of the fecal material until the mass is eliminated.

The need for communication among health care providers is especially important with reference to bowel function. Only if bowel movements are carefully recorded as to time, amount, and consistency can the nurse make competent judgments about laxatives and enemas.

### Bladder

A condom catheter connected to a urinary elimination bag may be placed on the male patient. The condom is unrolled on the penis and secured by an elasticized piece of tape around the penis. Care should be taken that the tape is placed not on the skin but on the condom and that it is wrapped around the penis snugly enough to prevent the condom from slipping, but not so tight as to interfere with circulation. Tactile stimulation may cause a temporary engorgement of the penis. When the size of the penis diminishes, the condom may slip off unless it has been securely attached. The condom is removed and the penis cleaned with soap and water daily.

An indwelling catheter with closed drainage may be needed for the female patient. While the catheter remains in place, continual observation for signs of infection, chills, or fever is required. Accurate monitoring of intake in relation to output is essential. *Irrigation of the*

***bladder through an indwelling catheter increases the possibility of introducing organisms; therefore, irrigate only when absolutely necessary.*** Scrupulous sterile technique is indicated. Infections from prolonged use of an indwelling catheter cause the urine to become alkaline. This, in turn, causes inorganic materials such as phosphorus and calcium to settle out, and as a result bladder stones may form. A fluid intake of at least 3000 ml/day will keep the urine diluted enough to lessen the risk of bladder stones.

The catheter should be changed before mineral deposits plug the lumen or tip of the catheter. If no manufacturer's information is available about how frequently the catheter must be changed, a safe estimate is every 7 to 10 days.

## Maintaining Skin Integrity

The integument of the comatose patient is prone to many assaults: being pulled across bed linens, lying too long on bony prominences, dryness or moisture, and increased bacteria from urinary and bowel incontinence. A warm-water bath daily is recommended. Although it is not always possible to give a tub bath, the patient can be placed in a tub or shower when consciousness returns if adequate personnel are present to prevent injury. Until such time, a daily bed bath should include a brisk rub (except when the skin is fragile) with sparing use of soap and a thorough rinse. Soap residue causes dryness and skin irritation, and moisture increases the potential for skin breakdown.

To prevent dryness, place a lotion (such as Alpha-Keri oil or Jeri-Bath) in the bath water. If this is not sufficient, rub the body with a lanolin preparation or other cream. A family member may suggest a lotion the patient has used routinely.

The skin of the feet is especially prone to drying, and the nails harden with decreased circulation. Rub the feet daily with a lubricant such as Vaseline. Never use alcohol unless specially indicated, because it makes the skin extremely dry. Comatose patients perspire just as alert patients do. If talcum powder is used, it tends to hold perspiration. Because moist skin is more prone to necrosis, avoid using talcum.

Linens are kept dry. Keep them pulled taut to avoid wrinkles underneath the patient that might cause decubitus ulcers. Protect the patient's skin from the shearing effect of sliding on the sheets by positioning the head of the bed at not more than a 10-degree angle unless otherwise ordered so that the patient will not constantly be sliding down in bed. The use of sheep skin under pressure areas also helps prevent decubitus ulcers. A water or air mattress to equalize pressure can be used, although if the patient is turned carefully, this is not necessary. Be sure never to use a doughnut or rubber ring, which causes a circle of pressure and decreases the blood supply to the area within that circle, making skin breakdown more likely.

## Maintaining Daily Care

### Hair

Shampoos are indicated every 1 or 2 weeks unless contraindicated by the patient's underlying problems. The scalp of the comatose patient continues to secrete oils and perspiration, and the hair becomes sour-smelling and difficult to manage when not properly cleansed. Comb hair daily, and braid or arrange long hair to prevent matting. Take care that there are no clumps of hair on the part of the head on which the patient lies.

Hair care for black persons differs from that recommended for white persons. For the black person, cleansing the hair with a warm solution of one part alcohol with four parts of mineral oil is followed by an application of warm olive oil, baby oil, or Vaseline oil to the scalp and hair. Excess oil may be removed with a towel. Long hair can be braided; very short hair can be left loose after combing. Afro combs or picks make combing less uncomfortable for the patient.

Hair care is important to the patient's sense of well-being and is comforting for the family because a well-groomed patient conveys that he or she is "cared about" as well as "cared for."

### Mouth and teeth

The unconscious patient often is a mouth breather and therefore has a dry mouth. Regardless of how he or she breathes, the patient experiencing a decreased LOC requires mouth care. When not cleansed, the mouth becomes inflamed and more prone to infection. Mucus and bacteria form plaque. Plaque, tartar, and food debris collect in gingival crevices around the teeth and cause mechanical and bacterial irritation. The tissue becomes swollen and inflamed. In time, gingival tissue will separate from the teeth and form pockets where still more debris can accumulate. Teeth may be lost and bone may become involved. Elderly persons have thinner oral membranes and less flow of saliva to help wash the mouth, so that their problem is compounded. (See Chapter 44 for oral care guidelines.)

### Nose

The nares are cleansed daily to help keep them patent. Inspect for secretions and note the type. If crusts are forming, gently remove with a moist applicator unless the patient's condition contraindicates. A thin application of a water-soluble lubricant helps decrease accumulation of debris. This is especially important when a nasogastric tube is in place because it causes some trauma to the tissues, and inflammation may ensue if the naris is not kept cleaned.

### Ears

The folds of the ears are cleansed and dried carefully. The area behind the ear is easily overlooked when drying but is prone to skin irritation when soap or moisture is not removed. Check the ears for wax while bathing the patient. Over a period of time large amounts of wax may accumulate; this is easily removed with a small wire loop. When head trauma is the basis of coma, be very cautious about introducing anything into the ear until it has been ascertained that there is no damage within the ear.

### Facilitating Family Coping

The unconscious patient has no awareness of the severity of the situation, but the alert family does. This awareness creates great anxiety and stress. During the initial phase of injury or onset of disease when consciousness is being affected, the family has many decisions to make about the patient's care. If the outcome of those decisions is not positive, family members may feel guilty for having made them. In addition, they will experience feelings of loss and grief. As time passes, the family members remain in limbo, unable to complete the grieving process, yet equally unable to sustain the high pitch of grief initially experienced. Guilt feelings may be expressed as anger and hostility toward those who are providing care. It is difficult for family members to understand what is going on, and it is very frightening to stand by feeling inadequate and unable to help. The family members then become part of the responsibility of the nurse. From the beginning, they need special understanding and special consideration. For them the patient's condition may precipitate a crisis. They can be helped to cope by being encouraged to participate in the patient's care.

A good way to involve family members in the care of the patient is by asking for help with positioning the patient. They usually are capable of doing an excellent job of monitoring and maintaining position and often are with the patient for extended periods when the nurse cannot be. Their involvement not only ensures more consistent care for the patient but is beneficial in giving them a sense of accomplishment and purpose. The hours of waiting are lessened for significant others when they feel they are needed and involved. For this reason, carefully explain what is to be done and the principles underlying the actions; then allow them to help you, not only with positioning but in other aspects of care as they desire. Acknowledge the value of their contributions.

Family members often will wish to stay at the bedside. If they do, share with them that their talking is providing sensory stimulation to the patient. The assumption is made that some of this talking may be filtering through to the awareness of the patient even though the patient is unable to respond to it.

The nurse conveys to the family a willingness to listen, to be involved, and to help them explore their thoughts. Keeping the family informed of what is being done, what is planned, and changes in the patient's condition is crucial. Provide the family with a comfortable environment. An expression of the nurse's willingness to help is frequently all that is required to comfort the family.

## ♦ EVALUATION

To evaluate effectiveness of nursing interventions, compare patient behaviors with those stated in the expected patient outcomes. Successful achievement of patient outcomes for the patient with altered level of consciousness is indicated by the following:

1. Has respirations in range of 14 to 20/min and pulse oximetry above 90%.
2. Is awake, alert, oriented to time, place, and person and has no signs or symptoms of ICP.
3. Appropriately recognizes sensory clues and has no sensory/perceptual abnormalities.
4. Has body temperature within a range of 97.5° to 99° F.
5. Shows no signs of confusion.
6. Has no injuries.
7. Can ambulate, transfer, and/or move freely in wheelchair.
8. Does not have signs of joint contractures, pressure sores, thromboembolic events, or loss of muscle mass.
9. Maintains usual body weight and has laboratory values (hematocrit, hemoglobin, and protein) within normal limits (WNL).
10. Has no impaction, constipation, or diarrhea; has formed stools on a regular schedule; and is continent, with or without bowel program.
11. Has bladder continence, with or without bladder training program and can completely empty bladder.
12. Can perform activities of daily living independently.
13. Has no signs of skin breakdown.
14. Family verbalizes willingness to assist in patient care.

## COMPLICATIONS

The patient with altered level of consciousness is prone to many complications. Most are connected to immobility. These are discussed under the nursing management section for headache (see p. 1944).

# HEADACHE

## ETIOLOGY

Headache from a neurologic perspective may have many causes, including the following:

1. Expanding masses, such as a neoplasm
2. Intracranial bleeding
3. Inflammation of the meninges
4. Other infections of the brain and spinal cord
5. Dilation of cerebral vessels
6. Head trauma
7. Cerebral hypoxia
8. Psychologic factors, such as stress
9. Systemic disease of the eye, ear, or sinus

**TABLE 57-3 Comparison of Migraine, Cluster, and Tension Headaches**

| ONSET | FREQUENCY | DURATION | NATURE | PRODROMAL SYMPTOMS/ ASSOCIATED SYMPTOMS | TREATMENT |
|---|---|---|---|---|---|
| **MIGRAINE HEADACHES** | | | | | |
| Occur at any age<br>Strongly hereditary<br>More common in women than men | Episodic; tend to occur with stress or life crisis | Hours to days | Occur slowly; pain becomes severe, with one side of head affected more than other | Prodromal: vision field defects, confusion, paresthesias<br>Associated: nausea, vomiting, chills, fatigue, irritability, sweating, edema | Ergotamine tartrate<br>Propranolol<br>Nonnarcotic analgesics<br>Relaxation techniques |
| **CLUSTER HEADACHES** | | | | | |
| Early adulthood; precipitated by alcohol or nitrates<br>More common in older men | Episodes clustered together in quick succession for few days or weeks with remissions that last for months | Few minutes to few hours | Intense, throbbing, deep, often unilateral pain; begin in infraorbital region and spread to head and neck | Prodromal: uncommon<br>Associated: flushing, tearing of eyes, nasal stuffiness, sweating, swelling of temporal vessels | Narcotic analgesics during acute phase, often intramuscularly |
| **TENSION HEADACHES (MUSCLE CONTRACTION)** | | | | | |
| Often in adolescence; related to tension or anxiety<br>No family history | Episodic; vary with stress | Variable; can be constant | Dull, constant, uncommon aggravating pain; vary in intensity; usually bilateral and involve neck and shoulders; pain may be poorly defined | Prodromal: uncommon<br>Associated: sustained contraction of head and neck muscles | Nonnarcotic analgesics<br>Relaxation techniques<br>Amitriptyline (Elavil) |

Generally, headaches can be divided into three categories: vascular, tension, and combinations of vascular and tension. This chapter discusses two types of vascular headaches, *migraine* and *cluster,* as well as tension headaches. See Table 57-3 for a comparison of these three types of headaches.

## EPIDEMIOLOGY

**Headache,** or head pain, is a common symptom experienced by many persons. As a symptom of an underlying disease, it varies in degree of severity from being relatively unimportant and transient to a very serious prognosis. This symptom clearly originates in many different pathologic processes.

Each type of headache has certain characteristics. For instance, **migraine** has a high hereditary influence, usually begins in persons between ages 16 and 30 years, and affects more women than men. **Cluster headaches,** on the other hand, usually begin in early adulthood and occur most often in middle-aged men.

## PATHOPHYSIOLOGY

The pathophysiology of head pain is not fully known. The skull and brain tissues, from a neurophysiologic standpoint, are not capable of sensing pain. Rather the pain arises from the scalp, its blood vessels, and muscles; from the dura mater and its venous sinuses; and from the blood vessels at the base of the brain. All these structures have pain receptors. Pain most often originates in muscles (face, neck, head), blood vessels, and the dura mater. The blood vessels dilate and become congested with blood extracranially and intracranially. The pain is thought to result from tension on or stretching of these tissues.

With migraine, chemical changes in and around the cranial blood vessels seem to have a causative role.

### Migraine Headache

Prodromal signs and symptoms *(aura)* that occur before the acute attack may include the following:

1. Visual field defects
2. Confusion
3. Paresthesias
4. Paralysis in extreme cases

The usual signs and symptoms that occur at the attack are severe and vary in intensity and duration. The pain usually is intense and starts gradually. The headache often is present when the person awakens, and one side of the head usually is more affected than the other. Pain may be most severe over the temporal area but may occur anywhere in the head, including the face. Signs and symptoms that may occur at the attack, in addition to the pain, include the following:

1. Nausea and/or vomiting
2. Chilliness
3. Fatigue
4. Irritability
5. Diaphoresis
6. Edema
7. Associated autonomic signs
8. Temporary paralysis or paresis as well as aphasia

### Cluster Headache

In cluster headache, pain episodes are clustered or spaced together in quick succession for a few days or weeks and with relatively long remissions that may last for months. The frequency of the attacks is a unique characteristic. The duration of the pain usually is a few minutes to a few hours. The pain often is described as very intense, throbbing, and deep. It is abrupt in onset and also stops abruptly. The pain, which is unilateral, most often starts in the face, usually in the infraorbital region, and spreads to the head and neck as it increases. The pain usually reaches its peak in 1 to 3 hours. Prodromal signs are uncommon, but associated signs may include the following:

1. Flushing
2. Lacrimation (tearing)
3. Nasal stuffiness
4. Diaphoresis
5. Swelling of temporal vessels

### Tension Headache

**Tension headaches** vary in frequency and duration and are related to fatigue and stress. There is no aura. The pain usually is constant, bandlike, and bilateral and involves the occipital region, neck, and shoulders. The headache may be intermittent and transitory or may persist for days, weeks, and months. It may spread to all parts of the head and be poorly defined. (See Table 57-3 for comparison of types of headaches.)

## PREVENTION

### Primary Prevention

The key to prevention of headaches is the identification of triggering factors, if these can be found. An ongoing assessment of personality, habits, and activities of daily living (ADL) is helpful. The nurse should help the patient identify what purpose, if any, the headache serves. Internal conflicts and anxiety are frequent causes. Once identified, these causes can be decreased or eliminated. Clues to the source of headaches may be obtained by understanding the person's goals and aspirations, work habits, family relationships, coping mechanisms, and relaxation patterns. The person may be asked to keep a diary of ADL and the occurrence of the headaches, as well as their nature and treatment. Triggering factors that have been identified include fatigue, alcohol ingestion, stress, and hunger. Preventing these can prevent many headaches.

Prevention of migraines may include the avoidance of certain foods, such as chocolate, nuts, and onions. Persons with cluster headaches may need to avoid the ingestion of alcohol.

### Secondary Prevention

The source of recurring headache should be determined through careful physical examination and neurologic testing. Persons have been known to self-treat a headache for months in the belief that it was not significant, only to learn later that it was caused by a more serious problem such as a brain tumor or hypertension. Because of the site of some tumors in the brain, headache may be the only overt symptom for many months.

## MEDICAL MANAGEMENT

The nurse works collaboratively with the physician for implementation of prescribed medical therapy. Because the nurse has a major role in discharge planning and patient teaching, these are discussed under Nursing Management.

### Diagnostic Tests

It is important to evaluate severe and chronic headaches. Usual testing consists of a neurologic examination, including a computed tomography (CT) scan (see Chapter 56 for description). A lumbar puncture also may be performed but not if there is evidence of increased intracranial pressure (ICP) or if a brain tumor is suspected, because the quick reduction in pressure produced by removal of the spinal fluid may cause brain herniation.

### Medication

Treatment for headache often includes the use of selected medications. These are described in terms of their use for persons with migraines and cluster and tension headaches.

#### Migraine headache

Acetylsalicylic acid (aspirin) may be helpful in the treatment of migraine headaches after the headache has developed. The drug of choice is ergotamine tartrate. If it is taken early in an attack, it may prevent the migraine from developing. The success of this drug in relieving the headache often is considered diagnostic of migraine. This medication acts by constricting cerebral blood vessel walls, thus reducing cerebral blood flow. It usually is administered orally, but it can be given rectally or sublingually in dosages of 2 to 4 mg or by injection in dosages of 0.25 to 0.5 mg. Ergot preparations are also available in combination with other drugs such as caffeine, phenobarbital, and belladonna. Side effects to watch for include nausea, vomiting, numbness and tingling, muscle pain, and changes in heart rate. This drug cannot be taken by pregnant women because it stimulates contraction of uterine smooth muscle.

Other medications that may be prescribed for migraine include the following:

1. Phenacetin
2. Acetaminophen
3. Propoxyphene (Darvon)
4. Narcotics such as codeine
5. Propranolol (Inderal)

#### Cluster headache

Narcotic analgesics often are prescribed for use during an acute attack of a cluster headache. Because the pain is so severe, it may be necessary to give these medications intramuscularly for optimal relief. Patients with cluster headaches usually feel no pain between attacks; thus analgesia is not needed during these times.

#### Tension headache

Nonnarcotic analgesics often are prescribed for tension headaches. These include acetaminophen, propoxyphene, phenacetin, and acetylsalicylic acid. It is far better for the patient to learn to control the headaches with other means than to prescribe narcotics or sedatives to control tension and stress.

### Treatment

Treatment of headaches generally is pharmacologic. No specific treatment has been found to be effective in alleviating the discomfort other than medications. Patients with chronic headaches may respond to psychotherapy. If the cause of the headache can be determined (e.g., if sinus problems exist), appropriate medical care usually alleviates the headache.

### Diet

A special diet is not necessary in dealing with headaches. However, as discussed under Prevention, some persons may find that certain foods such as chocolate, nuts, and onions may lead to or worsen migraine. Also, alcohol may bring on a cluster headache.

### Activity

The patient with a headache is encouraged to be as active as possible. However, with migraine and cluster headaches, rest during an acute attack may be helpful in alleviating the pain.

### Referral/Consultation

In some settings the nurse assumes the responsibility for making referrals to other services, which may include a referral to a psychiatric nurse practitioner or clinical specialist for counseling on stress management.

## NURSING MANAGEMENT

### ♦ ASSESSMENT

The collection of both subjective and objective data is important in the diagnosis of headache.

### Subjective Data

Subjective data to be collected to assess the patient with headache include the following:

- Patient's understanding of headache and possible causes
- Awareness of any precipitating factors such as stress
- Measures that relieve symptoms, including medications
- Location, frequency, pattern, and character of head pain, including site of return, time of day, and intervals between headaches
- Initial onset of headache
- Presence of any prodromal symptoms
- Presence of associated symptoms
- Family history of headaches (especially important with migraine)
- Situations that worsen headaches

### Objective Data

Objective data to be collected to assess the patient with headache include the following:

- Behavior that indicates presence of stress, anxiety, or pain
- Change in ability to carry on normal daily activities
- Abnormalities found on neurologic examination
- Elevated temperature or painful flexion of neck (may be present with meningitis)

Other key points to consider in assessing headache are listed in Box 57-5.

### Diagnostic Test Findings

Often with headache the results of the diagnostic testing are normal. However, if the headache is caused by a brain tumor or other pathologic condition, the abnormality will be visualized on the CT scan. The presence

**BOX 57-5 Key Points in Assessing Headache**

- Localized type of head pain usually is associated with migraine or an organic disorder.
- Generalized headache usually is related to psychologic causes or the presence of increased ICP.
- Migraine may change from one side of the head to the other.
- Headaches that occur with increased ICP usually are present on awakening and may awaken the person from sleep.
- Sinus headaches typically occur early in the morning and increase in intensity as the day progresses.
- Pain described as dull, nagging, aggravating, and continuous, often occurs with psychogenic headaches.
- Organically caused pain tends to be constant and progressive.
- Migraine may be associated with menstruation.
- Sleeping too long, fasting, or inhaling toxic fumes in work situations with inadequate ventilation may cause headaches.
- Oral contraceptives may exacerbate migraine headaches.

of blood in the spinal fluid also may indicate a pathologic condition of the brain that could cause headache.

## ♦ NURSING DIAGNOSES

Nursing diagnoses are determined from analysis of patient data. Nursing diagnoses for the patient with headache may include but are not limited to the following:

| Diagnostic Title | Possible Etiologic Factors |
|---|---|
| Pain | Headache |
| Sleep-pattern disturbance | Pain/discomfort |
| Knowledge deficit: cause of headache and needed medications, as well as dietary restrictions | Lack of exposure, unfamiliarity with information sources |

## ♦ EXPECTED PATIENT OUTCOMES

Expected patient outcomes for the patient with headache may include but are not limited to the following:

1. Will have decreased headache pain.
2. Will sleep at least 6 hours per night.
3. Medications. Will be able to explain prescribed medications and follow-up:
   a. Dosage, action, side effects, and frequency
   b. Reason for adequate and early treatment with prescribed drugs
   c. Need for continued medical supervision
4. Can state necessary dietary modifications.
5. Can state probable cause of headache.

## ♦ INTERVENTIONS

### Promoting Comfort

Treatment for headache often includes the use of selected medications (already described in the medical management section). In addition, cold packs applied to the forehead or base of the skull may be helpful in decreasing pain. Some patients describe relief when pressure is applied to the temporal artery area. Patients with migraine generally find it more comfortable to be in a darkened room with minimal auditory stimulation.

### Promoting Rest and Relaxation

Because tension and stress are triggering factors for headaches, nursing measures for persons with headache include those that facilitate relaxation and rest (see Guidelines box above). Relaxation techniques, the use of biofeedback, regular sleeping patterns, and provisions for rest are important. Regular physical exercise may help the patient relax.

### Facilitating Learning

Patient teaching for the person with a headache should include the following:

1. Avoidance of factors found to increase the headache
2. Use of relaxation measures, including biofeedback when appropriate
3. Maintenance of regular sleep patterns

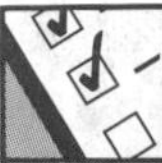

**Guidelines for Care of the Person With Headache**

1. Promote rest and relaxation:
   a. Relaxation techniques, including biofeedback and meditation
   b. Regular sleeping patterns
   c. Provision for rest periods
2. Promote comfort:
   a. Cold packs to forehead or base of the skull
   b. Pressure applied to temporal artery area
   c. Rest in darkened room with minimal sensory stimulation
   d. Judicious use of medication

4. Importance of taking medication as prescribed and knowledge of expected action and side effects
5. Importance of follow-up medical care
6. Structuring of home and work environment to keep stressors at a reasonable level

## ♦ EVALUATION

To evaluate the effectiveness of nursing interventions, compare patient behaviors with those stated in the expected patient outcomes. Successful achievement of patient outcomes for the patient with headache include but are not limited to the following:

1. States that no pain is present and evidences lack of grimacing, shallow breathing, holding head, or other behaviors indicative of pain.
2. Has sleep pattern that includes at least 6 hours of sleep per night.
3. Medications. Correctly explains prescribed medications and follow-up:
   a. Dosage, action, side effects, and frequency
   b. Need to use of drugs early in course of headache
   c. Need for continued medical supervision
4. Correctly describes any dietary modifications.
5. Correctly explains probable cause of headache.

## COMPLICATIONS

Complications of headache include the loss of income and ability to manage ADLs. Many persons with severe headache suffer psychologic problems because of the severe pain.

# INCREASED INTRACRANIAL PRESSURE

## ETIOLOGY

**Increased intracranial pressure (ICP)** is a complex manifestation that is caused by multiple neurologic conditions and often requires surgical intervention.

The cranial contents, including the brain tissues, vascular tissues, and cerebrospinal fluid (CSF), are contained within a bony vault for protection. Any increase in the volume of any of the cranial contents, singly or in combination, results in increased ICP because the

**BOX 57-6 Space-Occupying Lesions**

Cerebral contusions
Hematomas
Infarctions
Abscesses
Intracranial tumors

cranial vault is rigid, closed, and nonexpandable. Several neurologic lesions, either by their nature of by causing cerebral edema, increase the volume of tissue within the cranium. Any lesion that increases tissue volume is known as a *space-occupying* lesion. Common examples are found in Box 57-6.

Intracranial tumors arising from all types of brain tissue increase cell mass and thus increase ICP. An increase in the production of CSF, blockage of the ventricular system, or decreased absorption of CSF can likewise increase tissue fluid volume. Activities such as coughing, sneezing, or straining at stool or other Valsalva maneuvers also increase ICP for a short time. After activity ceases, the pressure then returns to its baseline.

It is also important to note that contrast dye used with cerebral angiography and CT scans may result in irritation to cerebral blood vessels, with resulting cerebral edema and increased ICP. Patients who have had either of these tests should be observed carefully for deterioration in neurologic status.

## EPIDEMIOLOGY

There are no data concerning the incidence or distribution of this condition.

## PATHOPHYSIOLOGY

According to the *box theory* of the brain, an increase in any one of the contents of the cranium usually is accompanied by a reciprocal change in the volume of one of the others. Brain tissue cannot expand without serious effects on the flow and amount of CSF and cerebral circulation. Space-occupying lesions must displace and distort the brain and vascular tissues as pressure increases (Table 57-4). Pressure may build up slowly over days or months or rapidly over minutes or hours. This process usually depends on the cause. At first one hemisphere is more involved, depending on the lesion site, but eventually both hemispheres may become involved if the pressure continues to increase.

As pressure increases within the cranial cavity, it is initially compensated for by venous compression and CSF displacement. Although the brain has autoregulatory mechanisms to maintain a normal cerebral blood flow with some increase in ICP, as the pressure continues to rise, the cerebral blood flow decreases and *inadequate perfusion* occurs. The inadequate perfusion initiates a vicious cycle, causing the partial carbon dioxide pressure ($P_{CO_2}$) to increase and the partial oxygen pressure ($P_{O_2}$) and pH to decrease. These changes cause vasodilation and cerebral edema. The edema further increases ICP, causing increased compression of neural tissue and an even greater increase in ICP.

When the pressure within the cavity exceeds the compensatory mechanisms, the only escape for the brain hemisphere is to be displaced caudally or by downward herniation. The *falx cerebri* oppose medial shift of the

**TABLE 57-4 Normal Function, Primary Pathophysiology, and Clinical Manifestations of Increased Intracranial Pressure**

| NORMAL FUNCTION | PATHOPHYSIOLOGY | CLINICAL MANIFESTATIONS |
|---|---|---|
| Vasomotor center controls blood pressure and pulse | Compression by herniating brain | Changes in blood pressure: rise in systolic blood pressure, decrease in diastolic blood pressure; widened pulse pressure; slowed pulse |
| Control of body temperature | Compression by herniating brain | High, uncontrolled body temperature |
| Cerebral perfusion adequate | Inadequate perfusion of the brain | Increasing $P_{CO_2}$ and decreasing $P_{O_2}$ and pH; vasodilation of cerebral vessels with resulting cerebral edema |
| Control of diaphragm by vagus nerve | Compression of vagus nerve | Hiccuping |
| Control of body movements by upper motor neuron pathways | Compression of upper motor neuron pathways | Decerebrate rigidity, decorticate rigidity; seizures; progressive muscle weakness |
| Pupils that react to light consensually | Compression of cranial nerves affect vision | Dilated ipsilateral pupil, bilateral fixed and dilated pupils; visual disturbances such as diplopia and decreased acuity |
| Absent headache | Venous congestion and tension in intracranial blood vessels | Headache that usually increases in intensity with coughing, straining at stool, or stooping; pain usually present in early morning |

hemispheres, and the *tentorium cerebelli* oppose downward shift to some extent. Structures that allow internal herniation are the cingulate gyrus, which permits medial subfacial herniation (under the falx); the uncus, which permits downward transtentorial herniation (across the free edge of the tentorium); and the cerebellar tonsil, which permits transforaminal herniation (through the foramen magnum). Because of the herniation, the brainstem is compressed at variable levels, which in turn compresses the vasomotor center, posterior cerebral artery, oculomotor nerve, corticospinal nerve pathways, and fibers of the ascending reticular activating system (RAS). Internal herniation in this way represents the critical state of decompensation. The life-sustaining mechanisms for consciousness, blood pressure, pulse, respirations, and temperature regulation fail.

Increased ICP produces multiple signs and symptoms. One of the first is a decreasing level of consciousness (see p. 1924).

## Pupillary Signs

Pupillary responses are controlled by the oculomotor nerve (cranial nerve III), which carries sensory, motor, and parasympathetic fibers as well as sympathetic fibers. The oculomotor nerve is compressed by the herniating tissue and specifically by the downwardly displaced posterior cerebral artery. The pupilloconstrictor fibers of the oculomotor nerve run in a group in the top part of this nerve and are the first to be compressed. Consequently the ipsilateral pupil (when the lesion is in one hemisphere) remains dilated and is incapable of constricting. The pupil appears larger than in the other eye and does not react to light. Eventually, as cerebral pressure increases and both hemispheres are affected, bilateral pupil dilation and fixation occur. Inequality of the pupils may appear earlier than fixation when the nerve is only stretched. The pupil may respond to light slowly rather than with the usual brisk response. In examining the pupils, the nurse should note the size and equality first and then test the reaction of each pupil to light in a darkened room. Dilating pupils are a sign of impending tentorial herniation. When pupils dilate or change in their ability to react, the physician should be notified immediately. A pupil that is fixed and dilated sometimes is referred to as a "blown pupil" (see Figure 56-23, *B*).

## Blood Pressure and Pulse

The effect of cerebral pressure on blood pressure and pulse is variable. Compensatory changes occur in the cerebral vasculature relative to hypoxia or diminished blood flow. When the compensatory changes are no longer effective, however, compression of the brainstem occurs, and ischemia in the vasomotor center will be present. This excites the vasoconstrictor fibers, causing an increase in systolic blood pressure. If the ICP continues to increase, the ability of the vasomotor center to stimulate the vasoconstrictor fibers decreases and the blood pressure may fall. An increased systolic blood pressure with a widening pulse pressure followed by a sharp drop in blood pressure often is seen as the patient's condition deteriorates.

Pressure on the vasomotor center also increases the transmission of parasympathetic impulses via the vagus nerve to the heart, and the pulse rate is slowed. As the ICP continues to rise, however, the heart rate may sharply increase. *Slowing of the pulse rate in conjunction with a rising systolic blood pressure is a significant observation to be made and reported.* For consistency, blood pressure readings should be taken in the same arm, and the pulse should be taken for a full minute in the same location each time.

## Respiration

Herniation produces respiratory dysrhythmias that are variable and related to the level of brainstem compression or failure. The breathing pattern may be deep and stertorous or Cheyne-Stokes (periodic); fatal respiratory paralysis may follow. The beginning of periodic episodes of apnea is significant. The usual manifestation is slowing of respiration, a slow pulse, and a rising systolic blood pressure. The nurse should learn to look for variability in vital signs and detect trends as they occur. It is important to remember that the patient with a decreasing LOC requires assistance in keeping the airway clear. Consequently, respiratory difficulty is further aggravated by this problem. Hypoxia also causes increased ICP. Persons who are experiencing increased ICP require supplemental oxygen.

## Temperature Regulation

Failure of the thermoregulatory center because of compression occurs later and gives rise to high uncontrolled temperatures. The nurse must understand that hyperthermia needs to be controlled because it increases the metabolic needs of the already compromised brain tissues. Temperatures are taken rectally unless otherwise ordered.

## Focal Motor and Sensory Signs

Compression of upper motor neuron pathways (corticospinal tract) interrupts the transmission of impulses to lower motor neurons, and progressive muscle weakness results. For example, a contralateral weakened hand grasp may progress to hemiparesis and hemiplegia; a weak hand, however, is not always a good indicator of motor weakness. More accurate is the observation and testing for *drift,* which requires the patient to close the eyes and extend the arms out straight in front for 30 seconds. If one arm is weakened, it will drift downward without the patient being aware of it. This can be tested in patients with increased ICP as long as they are capable of cooperating. Testing of the lower extremities include the patient's ability to do straight leg raises, as well as push and pull against the examiner. Ability to perform plantar flexion and dorsiflexion of the feet also can be evaluated.

When the patient is comatose, the response to tactile or painful stimuli is important. The nurse should note whether the person responds appropriately to pain or touch or whether the response is *decorticate* or *decerebrate posturing.*

The presence of Babinski's sign, hyperreflexia, and rigidity are additional motor signs that provide evidence of decreasing motor function from upper motor neuron involvement. *Transtentorial herniation* of the upper or rostral part of the brainstem produces decerebrate rigidity. The motor inhibitory fibers are blocked, and the person involuntarily assumes a fixed posture with arms, legs, and trunk extended and with flexion of the palmar and plantar joints. Seizures also may occur. Decorticate rigidity may be present (see Figure 57-1). This consists of a fixed posture with flexion of the arm, wrist, and fingers, with adduction of the arms and extension and internal rotation of the legs. Decorticate and decerebrate posturing both may be seen in the patient with herniation. The nurse should use gross tests or more definitive tests to determine motor changes. *The worsening of existing motor deficits is significant.*[4,37]

### Visual Acuity and Papilledema

The blind spot of the retina measures the size and shape of the optic papilla, or optic disc. As venous congestion and ICP increase, the resulting pressure is transmitted to the eyes through the CSF and to the optic disc (choked disc). Inasmuch as the meninges of the brain reflect out around the eyeball, they permit the direct transmission of pressure along the subarachnoid space through the CSF. As the optic disc swells, the retina adjacent to it also is compressed. The damaged retina cannot detect light rays. As the size of the blind spot enlarges, visual acuity decreases. The ability of the nurse to detect papilledema depends on skill in examination of the fundi (see Figure 56-21).

Many nurses will not have learned to observe for papilledema and must rely on other means to assess ICP. Decreasing visual acuity can be detected through the confrontation technique (see Chapter 60). Papilledema occurs most often when the increased ICP develops slowly. A rapid rise in ICP may not be reflected by papilledema.

### Headache

Headache may occur as an early symptom. It is thought to result from venous congestion and the tension on the intracranial blood vessels as the cerebral pressure rises. The onset of the headache should be noted along with its location and duration. It increases in intensity with cough, straining, and stooping.

### Vomiting

The occurrence of projectile vomiting often is associated with increased ICP. Its frequency and character should be noted. The significance of vomiting and headache needs to be associated with other clinical signs, such as papilledema and vital signs.

## PREVENTION

### Primary Prevention

Because many of the sources of increased ICP involve trauma, certain actions are important in prevention, including the following:

1. Use of seat belts
2. Use of helmets while riding motorcycles, snowmobiles, or bicycles
3. Safe use of firearms
4. Minimal use of drugs and alcohol
5. Not driving after taking drugs or drinking alcohol
6. Safe use of motor vehicles

### Secondary Prevention

Prevention of increased ICP involves the early detection of signs and symptoms so that corrective actions can be taken. This requires skill in nursing assessment (see assessment discussion).

## MEDICAL MANAGEMENT

The goal for discharge of patients with increased ICP as determined by DRGs depends on the underlying cause of the increased pressure. The nurse works collaboratively with the physician for implementation of prescribed medical therapy. Because the nurse has a major role in discharge planning and patient teaching, these are discussed under nursing management.

### Diagnostic Tests

The diagnosis of increased ICP can be made with the CT scan, which can show the actual structural herniation, as well as shifting of the brain. Most often, however, acute increased ICP is a medical emergency, and the diagnosis must be made on the basis of observation and neurologic testing alone.

The frequency of "neurologic checks" of the patient often is ordered by the physician. However, with significant deteriorating changes in the aforementioned signs, the nurse should decide when more frequent assessments and recordings are indicated. On the basis of the results obtained from observations and the patient's medical history, the nurse must make a decision concerning the frequency of monitoring. Tools used for assessing the patient's neurologic condition may vary from institution to institution. The important point is that the patient's condition is regularly compared with an established baseline through continuous monitoring.

Various methods for measurement of ICP have been devised. One of the most frequent methods requires placement of a hollow screw through the skull into the subarachnoid space. The screw is attached to a 3-way stopcock, which is connected to a transducer and oscilloscope for continued monitoring. The transducer is fastened to the head of the bed and must be level with

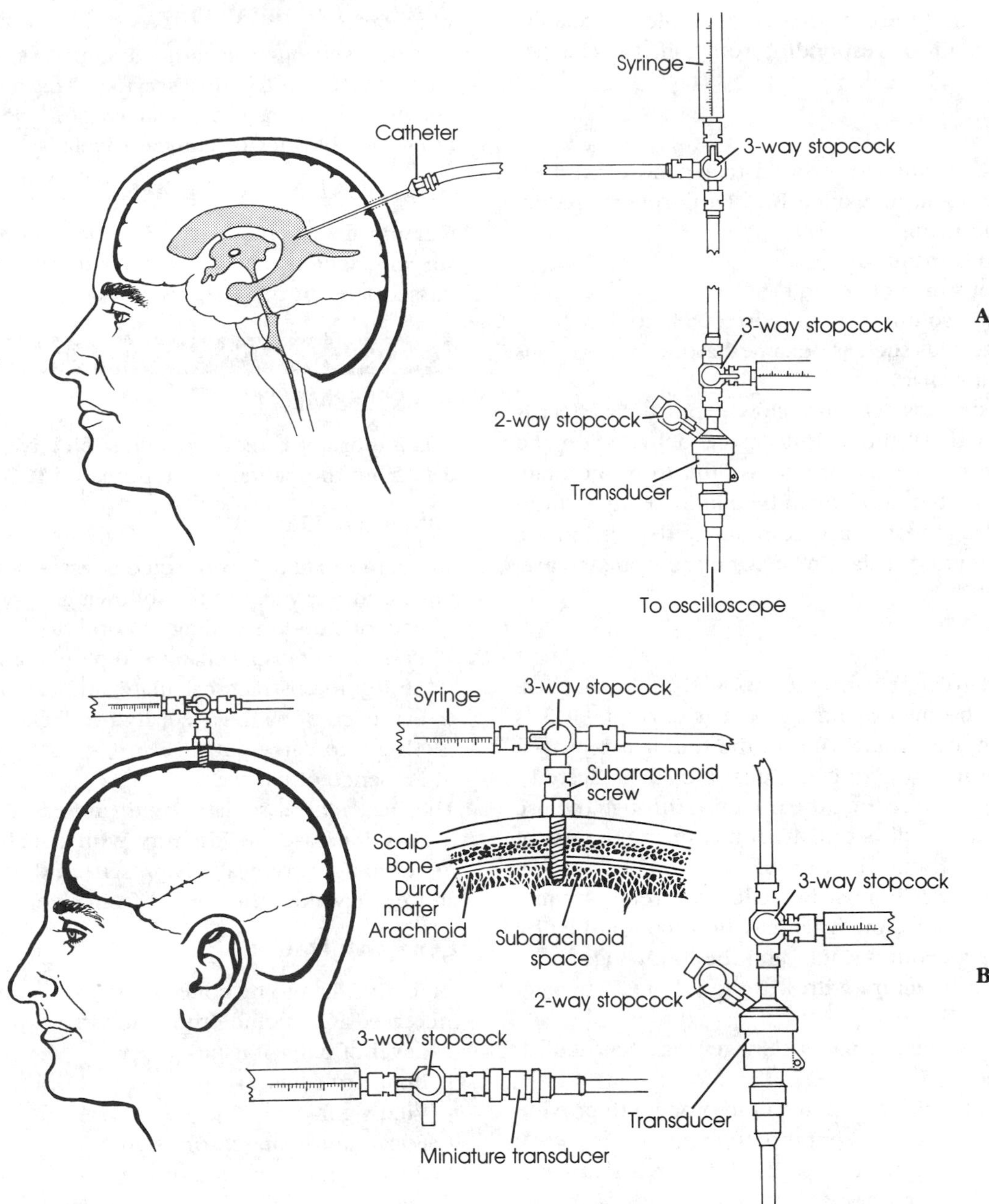


**FIGURE 57-9** Equipment for ICP monitoring. **A,** Ventricular pressure monitoring. Catheter is inserted through a burr hole in the skull into the lateral ventricle and attached to a transducer and oscilloscope to monitor ICP. **B,** Subarachnoid screw pressure monitoring. Subarachnoid screw is inserted through a burr hole in the skull and attached to a transducer and oscilloscope for continuous monitoring. (From Rudy EB: *Advanced neurological and neurosurgical nursing,* St Louis, 1984, Mosby.)

the screw for accurate monitoring. The screw may be attached to a manometer for intermittent readings. Directions for the use of this measurement device can be found in the literature[33,54] (Figure 57-9).

Experience with the use of continuous internal intracranial monitoring has shown that the traditional clinical signs of increased ICP do not always correlate with the actual pressure changes seen on the monitor. Studies have found that many of the classic signs of increased ICP do not appear until the pressure has reached extremely high levels and the opportunity to reverse the rising pressure and prevent permanent brain damage has already passed.

It is important to note that ICP is not constant and unchanging. The nurse can significantly alter pressure depending on the interventions carried out. Intracranial monitoring of patients with increased ICP indicates that the pressure is in constant flux. When performing such monitoring, the nurse is responsible for reading the monitor and for responding to significant changes as they occur.

### Medication

Medications usually are ordered to promote rapid osmotic diuresis and to reduce ICP. Drugs often used include the following:
1. Intravenous mannitol
2. Intravenous urea (Ureaphil)
3. Hypertonic solutions of glucose (25% to 50%)
4. Corticosteroids such as dexamethasone (intravenous or intramuscular)

The corticosteroids act more slowly, but their effect is more sustained. All these drugs cause dehydration and promote the movement of excess fluid from the brain tissues into the blood so it can be eliminated. Narcotics and other drugs that cause respiratory depression are avoided. Phenytoin (Dilantin) may be prescribed to prevent seizures.[56]

### Treatment

The medical treatment of patients with increased ICP depends on the underlying cause. For example, if it is caused by an intracranial tumor, the tumor is removed surgically. When surgery is not possible (or indicated), efforts are made to reduce the pressure through the use of drug therapy or direct physical measures. The use of medications is discussed later.

Rapidly rising ICP must be relieved directly by mechanical decompression. This may be accomplished by a variety of procedures, including the following:
1. Ventricular puncture with withdrawal of CSF by needle or cannula
2. Continuous ventricular drainage via ventriculostomy tube
3. Removal of a piece of skull (craniotomy) to provide room for the cranial contents to expand
4. Burr holes made in the skull with or without evacuation of subdural hematoma
5. Continuous drainage of subdural hematoma via subdural drain

Each of these measures requires careful monitoring by the nurse for signs of increased ICP and the maintenance of asepsis at the entrance site into the skull.

### Diet

No specific diet is prescribed for the patient with increased ICP. The patient's ability to eat and the LOC determine to a large extent what diet is appropriate. The patient who is in coma will be maintained on intravenous or enteral feedings.

### Activity

The activity of the patient with increased ICP may be kept to a minimum to prevent further increases in the pressure. This is discussed in the section pertaining to nursing management, p. 1952.

### Referral/Consultation

In some settings the nurse assumes responsibility for making referrals to other services. This may include the hospital chaplain, the social worker, or a psychiatric nurse practitioner or clinical specialist.

## SURGICAL MANAGEMENT

Nursing management of the patient undergoing brain surgery, which may be needed to relieve ICP, is discussed later in the chapter, p. 2002.

## NURSING MANAGEMENT

## ♦ ASSESSMENT

It is important to collect both subjective and objective data from the patient with increased ICP.

### Subjective Data

Subjective data to be collected to assess the patient with increased ICP include the following:

Patient's understanding of condition
Presence of visual changes: diplopia or blurred vision
Ability to abstract, calculate, and reason
Presence of pain, especially headache
Ability to carry out ADL
Presence of nausea

The headache associated with increased ICP pressure usually increases in intensity with coughing, straining, or stooping. It typically is present in the early morning and may awaken the patient from sleep.

### Objective Data

Objective data to be collected to assess the patient with increased ICP include the following:

Level of consciousness
Pupillary signs
Vital signs
Focal motor or sensory signs
Presence of vomiting or hiccuping
Eye changes, including papilledema
Speech patterns

The detection of increased ICP must occur early, when it is reversible and before the stage of decompensation. The ability to make accurate observations, to interpret observations intelligently, and to record observations carefully is the most important part of nursing care of the patient experiencing increased ICP (see Research box, p. 1951).

### Diagnostic Test Findings

The CT scan of the patient with increased ICP often shows evidence of a brain tumor or hemorrhage. As with many other neurologic disorders, there may be evidence of blood in the spinal fluid and a slowed EEG.

## ♦ NURSING DIAGNOSES

Nursing diagnoses are determined from analysis of patient data. Nursing diagnoses for the person with in-

**RESEARCH**

Turner H et al: Comparison of nurse and computer recording of ICP in head injured patients, *J Neurosci Nurs* 20:236-239, 1988.

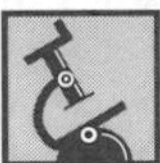

This study tested the ability of the nurse to describe the ICP course by a manual record and compared these results with an on-line computerized ICP monitoring system. The nurse recorded one value of ICP from the bedside monitor at the end of an hour, whereas the computer averaged 720 data samples of ICP during the hour. Data were collected from five patients who had suffered a head injury. Comparison of the two sets of scores showed that the nurse's "end-hour" value was a reasonable estimate of the patient's mean ICP for the entire hour as measured by the computer.

creased ICP are the same as those discussed in the section on altered levels of consciousness.

### ♦ EXPECTED PATIENT OUTCOMES

Expected patient outcomes for the patient with increased ICP may include but are not limited to those identified in the section on altered levels of consciousness.

### ♦ INTERVENTIONS AND EVALUATION

The reader is referred to the appropriate sections under altered levels of consciousness. See also Box 57-7 and Guidelines box at right.

**BOX 57-7 Intracranial Pressure Monitoring**

- Intraventricular (catheter)
- Subarachnoid/subdural (screw or bolt)
- Epidural (sensor)
- Intraparenchymal (catheter)

**Guidelines for Care of the Person With Increased Intracranial Pressure**

1. Decrease ICP:
   a. Elevate head of bed 15 to 30 degrees.
   b. Avoid flexion of hips, waist, and neck.
   c. Avoid rotation of head, especially to the right.
   d. Space out nursing activities to maintain lower pressure levels.
   e. Avoid Valsalva type of movements.
   f. Perform suctioning only as necessary.
2. Monitor fluid balance:
   a. Restrict fluids.
   b. Carefully monitor urinary output, often have indwelling catheter. Catheter is always used if mannitol is being used.
   c. Use minidripper with intravenous fluids.
   d. Encourage use of normal saline as intravenous fluid.
3. Maintain oxygenation:
   a. Provide oxygen before and after performing suctioning.
   b. Administer oxygen via mask or cannula.
   c. Intubation may be necessary.
   d. Controlled respirations may be implemented to lower $P_{CO_2}$ (thus causing a slightly alkaline pH and decreased vasodilation of cerebral vessels).

# ALTERATIONS IN COMMUNICATION

## ETIOLOGY/EPIDEMIOLOGY

*Aphasia* is a disorder of language caused by damage to the speech-controlling areas of the brain. It is a general term used to describe organic disturbances in language. It includes all areas of language, including speech, reading, writing, and understanding.

Cerebral hemorrhage and cerebral thrombosis are the most common causes of cortical damage, but tumors, multiple sclerosis, and trauma also can lead to aphasia. Aphasia caused by cerebral edema after trauma usually is temporary. Occasionally a person cannot speak after a cerebrovascular accident (CVA) because motor function of the vocal cords is affected, not because of damage to cortical speech centers. Defective innervation of the muscles of speech articulation, such as those in the vocal cords, tongue, cheeks, and palate, results in *dysarthria.*

## PATHOPHYSIOLOGY

Communication problems are the result of damage to the speech centers of the brain (Broca's region and Wernicke's area) or damage to the nerves that innervate muscles required for speech. A variety of abnormalities in communication can occur. The patient may be unable to comprehend the spoken word *(sensory aphasia)* or may comprehend and yet be unable to use the symbols of speech *(motor aphasia).* The patient may have both disorders at the same time *(global aphasia).* Writing may be possible even though speaking is not. Some patients may be able to speak but use the wrong words. A selective loss of words may occur, or the patient may be able to read but be unable to speak or write.

## PREVENTION

Because many patients who suffer a CVA also experience aphasia or dysphasia, the elements concerning prevention of CVAs also apply here.

## MEDICAL MANAGEMENT

The medical management of aphasia and dysphasia usually involves the referral of the person to a speech therapist, who can evaluate the disorder and institute necessary actions.

### Diagnostic Tests

Many sophisticated tests are used to assess the degree and characteristics of a language problem. These are administered by a speech pathologist in most cases. The reader is referred to a more specific text on language and communication disorders for a description of these tests.

## NURSING MANAGEMENT

## ♦ ASSESSMENT

Both objective and subjective information are important factors in assessment of the patient with a language disorder.

### Subjective Data

Subjective data to be collected to assess the patient with a language disorder include the following:

Patient's understanding of problem
Other sensory deficits
Onset of problem
Ability to think clearly

### Objective Data

Objective data to be collected to assess the patient with a language disorder include the following:

Change in level of consciousness
Ability to verbalize
Ability to write
Ability to name objects

Gross tests can be performed to determine which specific language abilities have been lost. These include the following:

1. Spread several familiar objects, such as keys, a pencil, and coins, before the patient.
2. Ask the patient to do the following:
   a. Name each object.
   b. As the nurse names each object, point to it.
   c. Write the name of each object as it is pointed to.
   d. Write the name of each object as it is stated aloud.
   e. When shown a card containing the printed name of each object, read the word aloud and point to the object.

## ♦ NURSING DIAGNOSES

Nursing diagnoses are determined from analysis of patient data. Nursing diagnoses for the patient with alterations in communication include but are not limited to the following:

| Diagnostic Title | Possible Etiologic Factors |
|---|---|
| Communication, impaired verbal | Aphasia |
| Knowledge deficit: alternate ways to communicate | Lack of exposure, unfamiliarity with information sources |

## ♦ EXPECTED PATIENT OUTCOMES

Expected patient outcomes for the person with alterations in communication may include but are not limited to the following:

1. Demonstrates the ability to communicate within the constraints of the disease process.
2. Uses assistive devices correctly.
3. Uses compensatory techniques correctly.
4. Uses alternative techniques of communication.
5. Can state how to obtain assistance from community resources.
6. Can state plans for follow-up care.

## ♦ INTERVENTIONS

### Facilitating Communication

Each person reacts to language problems differently. Most persons with aphasia become tense and anxious. They may be irritable and emotionally upset because they are unable to evoke the words they need, and they become discouraged easily in their efforts to speak. Some may quickly refuse to attempt to communicate; others feel ashamed and withdraw from people, including their family and close friends. Yet desire to communicate and persistence in efforts to do so are the essential ingredients in speech rehabilitation.

Care is taken to reduce tension so that patients with aphasia can make satisfactory adjustments to their loss. The environment should be relatively free of excess stimuli. These patients are not deaf, and they should be spoken to in a normal voice. Procedures are explained to them in the same manner as that used with other patients. Recreational activities should be soothing and nonstimulating. Music is often relaxing, and some patients enjoy listening to the radio. If the patient is able to read and comprehend the written captions, watching television may be gratifying. Some patients do not enjoy listening to the radio or watching television when they cannot follow what is going on. Being alert to the patient's facial expressions often gives clues to the activities that are most satisfying.[29]

Specific interventions are based on whether the patient's aphasia is primarily one of *comprehension* or *expression*. Some approaches for patients with comprehension deficits are (1) to keep distractions to a minimum (i.e., clear the patient's visual field of extraneous stimuli before initiating conversation), (2) to face the patient when speaking and speak simply and slowly, and (3) if the patient miscomprehends the message, to slow down the rate of speech and reword the message, using gestures to emphasize points. If the message is still not comprehended, go on to another topic after supplying the correct response.

Although the nurse does not initiate the formal speech therapy program with the patient, the nurse's cooperation is needed to reinforce the program. As the nurse cares for the patient, common objects should be named; the patient should be encouraged to handle them, to speak their names, and to write or copy their names. Family members can supply these words and others that are particularly important for the patient. Speech retraining should be given for short periods because it is exceedingly trying, and fatigue tends to increase difficulty in speaking. Praising patients for each small improvement and encouraging them to take their mistakes good-naturedly helps to make this difficult problem more bearable. A patient's progress in language retraining depends on the level of intelligence, the age (older patients have more difficulty), the severity of the damage, and whether the brain lesion is progressive. Complete language rehabilitation may require months of painstaking work on the part of skilled pathologists.* *A Guide to Clinical Services in Speech Pathology and Audiology*† lists clinics in the United States where speech and hearing services are available. Some of these clinics offer specialized help to persons with aphasia and dysphasia.

### Facilitating Learning

The patient should be helped to understand that speech may be relearned. In the interim, gestures, pointing to objects, pointing to pictures or words on communication boards, or writing may be used to improve communication. After the most effective approach to communication is determined, it is shared with all who interact with the patient, including the family and other members of the health care team.

## ♦ EVALUATION

To evaluate the effectiveness of nursing interventions, compare patient behaviors with those stated in the expected patient outcomes. Successful achievement of patient outcomes for the patient with alterations in communication is indicated by the following:

1. Can communicate needs to caregivers and significant others.
2. Uses assistive devices correctly.
3. Uses compensatory techniques correctly.
4. Can explain alternative techniques of communication.
5. Can describe how to obtain assistance from community resources.
6. Can explain plans for follow-up care.

# ALTERATIONS IN SENSORY AND PERCEPTUAL FUNCTION

## ETIOLOGY

The presence of a lesion anywhere within the sensory system pathways—from the receptor to the sensory cortex—alters the transmission or perception of sensory information (Figure 57-10). The parietal lobe cortex is of major importance for interpretation of sensation with the exception of sight, hearing, smell, taste, and thermoregulation. A loss, decrease, or increase in the sensation of pain, temperature, touch, and proprioception, singly or in combination, results in difficult problems in daily living for the person. Because these sensations normally help the person to be aware of alterations in the internal and external environments, any alteration in sensibility lessens the ability to be completely and accurately protected. As a consequence, there is a need to adapt to the alteration and plan for safety and comfort.

## EPIDEMIOLOGY

There are no definitive statistics as to the occurrence of problems with sensory and perceptual function. These disorders, however, accompany many neurologic problems, such as traumatic head injury and stroke. Therefore they are a common problem for those hospitalized with these conditions.

## PATHOPHYSIOLOGY

Some specific losses deserve to be mentioned. The loss of *proprioception,* or the ability to know the position of the body and its parts without looking directly at the part, is a serious loss that requires considerable adaptation. Lack of control of body temperature, or *hyperthermia,* occurs because of a malfunction in the thermoregulatory center in the brain, such as occurs after brain surgery near the hypothalamus or from head injury, brain tumors, and other cranial conditions. Hyperthermia is believed to occur as a result of hypoxia of the thermoregulatory center. Affected persons also often complain of *dysesthesia* or *paresthesia* (abnormalities of the sensation of touch), which typically are associated with peripheral neuropathies.

### Sensory Losses

Figure 57-11 presents common patterns of sensory alteration. The clinical manifestations of sensory alterations are listed in Table 57-5.

### Perceptual Problems

*Apraxia* and *agnosia* are *perceptual deficits* that occur quite often in neurologic conditions (see Chapter 56 for details). They may occur in association with each other or separately. Research concerning perceptual problems is still in the early stages. Even though the perceptual deficits and their corresponding lesion sites have been described in the literature, the neurologist is still concerned about how to rehabilitate the person.

## PREVENTION

The prevention of sensory and perceptual problems is related to prevention of the causative problem. The reader is referred to these sections in other parts of the text.

*Some institutions that specialize in working with patients who have aphasia are ICD Rehabilitation and Research Center, New York, N.Y.; The Institute of Logopedics, Wichita, Kan.; and Vanderbilt University Hospital Clinic, Nashville, Tenn.

†American Speech-Language-Hearing Association, 10801 Rockville Pike, Rockville, MD 20852.

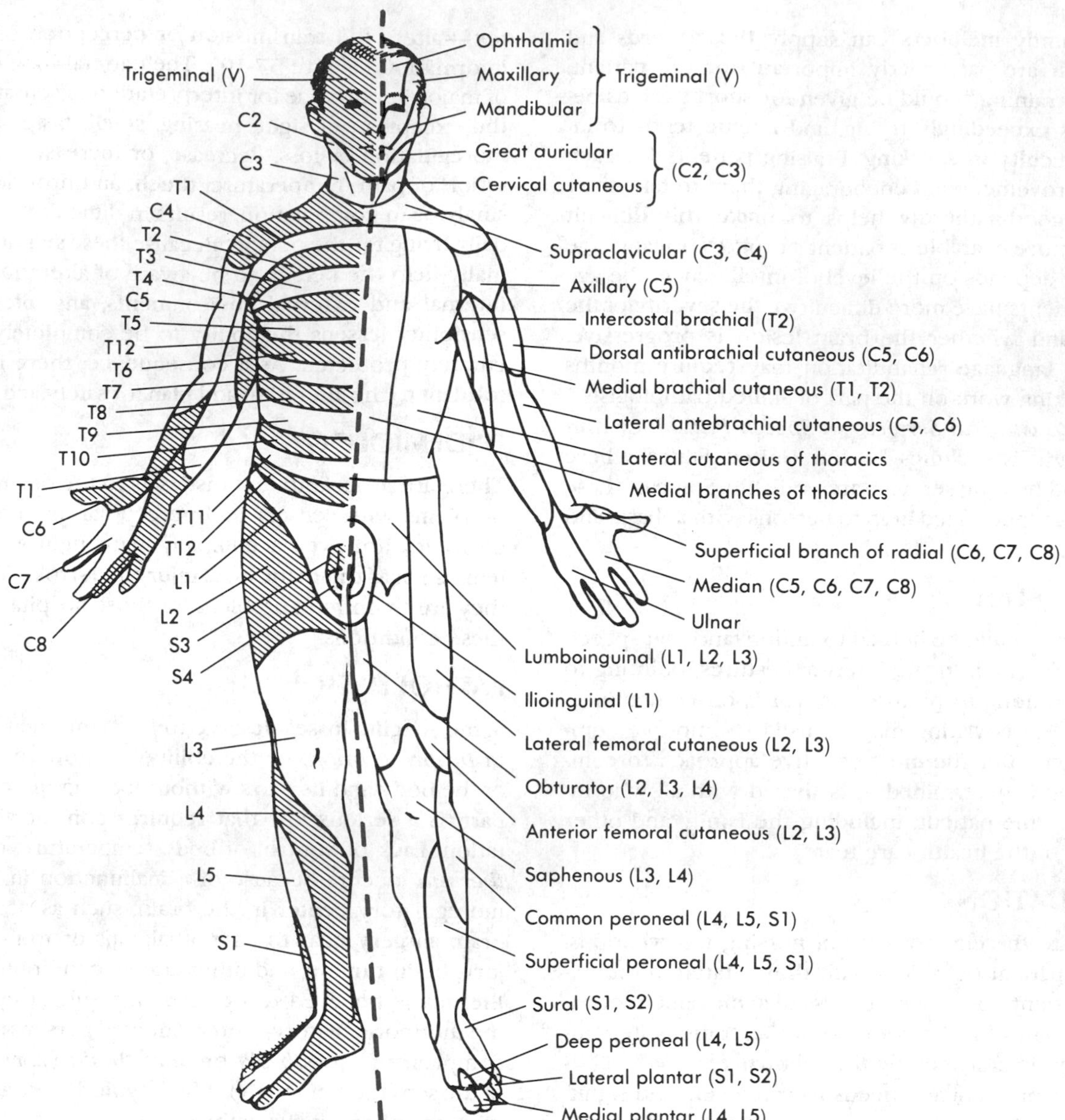


**FIGURE 57-10** Peripheral distribution of sensory nerve fibers, anterior view. *Right,* Distribution of cutaneous nerves. *Left,* Dermatomes *(shaded areas)* and segmental distribution of cutaneous nerves.

## MEDICAL MANAGEMENT

The nurse works collaboratively with the physician for implementation of prescribed medical therapy. Because the nurse has a major role in discharge planning and patient teaching, these are discussed under nursing management. (See section on the person with altered levels of consciousness, p. 1934.)

## NURSING MANAGEMENT

### ♦ ASSESSMENT

The sensory and perceptual parts of the neurologic examination are very difficult to assess, but are important.

#### Subjective Data

Subjective data to be collected to assess the patient with sensory and perceptual problems include the following:

- Patient's understanding of the problem
- Measures that relieve symptoms, including medications
- Site of sensory abnormality
- Onset of problem
- Presence of associated symptoms
- Alteration in sensation
  - Pain
  - Temperature
  - Touch

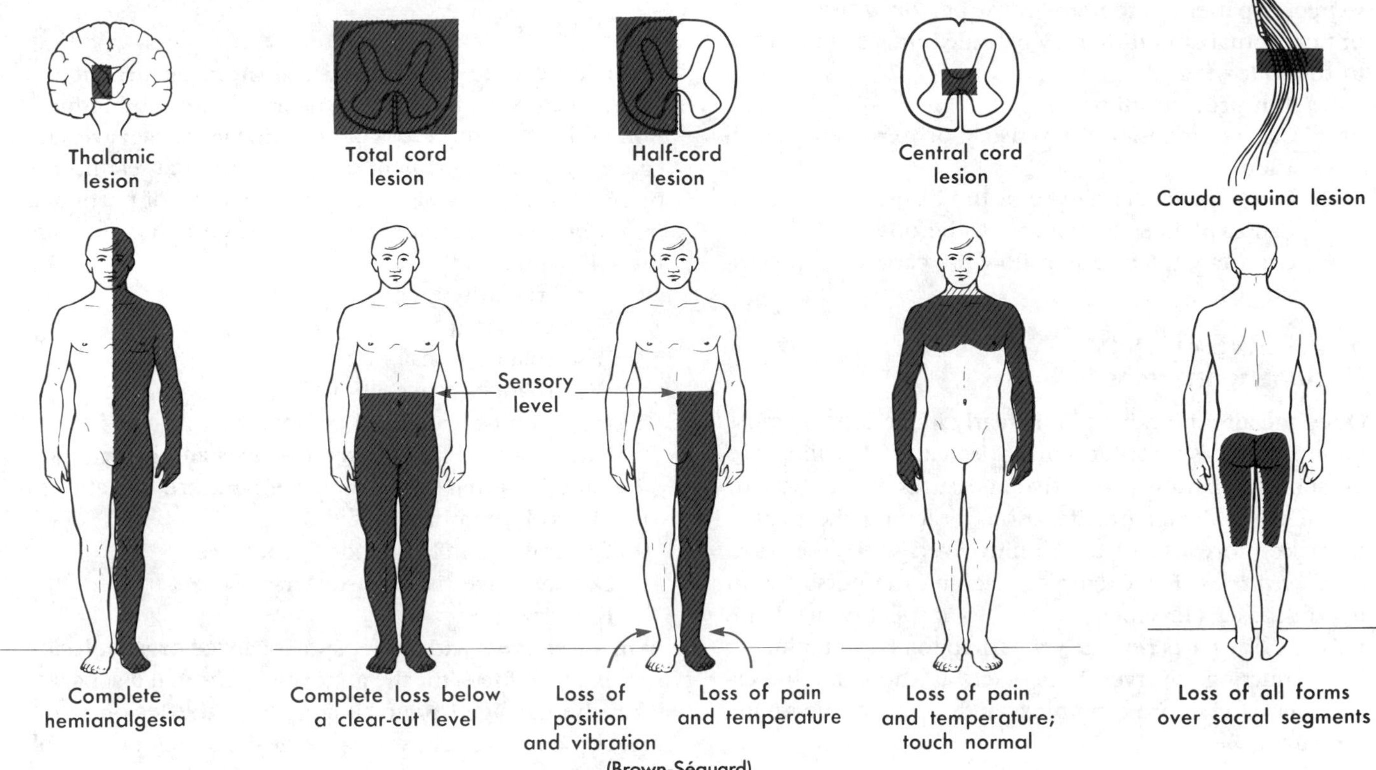


**FIGURE 57-11** Common patterns of sensory abnormality. Upper diagrams show site of lesion; lower diagrams show distribution of corresponding sensory loss. (Modified from Bickerstaff ER: *Neurology for nurses,* ed 2, London, 1971, English Universities Press Ltd, and Hodder & Stoughton Ltd.)

Proprioception
Stereognosis (object recognition by touch)

## Objective Data

Objective data to be collected to assess the patient with sensory and perceptual problems include the following:

Ability to perform purposeful movements in the absence of motor power, sensation, or coordination
Ability to recognize familiar objects

## ♦ NURSING DIAGNOSES

Nursing diagnoses are determined from analyses of patient data. Nursing diagnoses for the patient with a sensory or perceptual alteration may include but are not limited to the following:

| Diagnostic Title | Possible Etiologic Factors |
|---|---|
| Injury (trauma), high risk for | Sensory/motor deficits, lack of awareness of environmental hazards |
| Knowledge deficit: prevention of injury | Lack of exposure, unfamiliarity with information sources |
| Sensory/perceptual alterations: visual, tactile | Altered sensory reception/integration |

**TABLE 57-5 Clinical Manifestations of Alteration in Sensory Function**

| PATHOLOGIC CONDITION | MANIFESTATIONS | CAUSE |
|---|---|---|
| Cerebral lesion | Alterations in sensation contralateral to lesion | All sensory fibers decussate before reaching sensory cortex of cerebrum |
| Transection of spinal cord | Bilateral sensory loss distal to the lesion | All pathways have been severed |
| Hemisection of cord (Brown-Séquard syndrome) | Ipsilateral loss of proprioception and vibratory sense | Posterior column decussates in the medulla |
| | Contralateral loss of pain, temperature, and crude touch sensation | Spinothalamic tracts decussate in the cord |

## ♦ EXPECTED PATIENT OUTCOMES

Expected patient outcomes for the person with a sensory or perceptual alteration may include but are not limited to the following:

1. Can prevent injury.
2. Can compensate for sensory or perceptual alterations.
3. Can explain the nature of the disorder.
4. Can explain safety factors to be observed.
5. Can state plans for follow-up care with professionals.

## ♦ INTERVENTIONS

### Facilitating Learning

Once the alteration has been clearly identified, the most important nursing intervention is that of teaching the person and family protective measures in relation to the sensory deficit or alteration. Teaching the person to make more use of the noninvolved senses helps *to avoid injuries.* For example, teaching the person with hypoesthesia (lessened touch) to inspect visually involved body parts regularly will help to prevent injuries. Some nursing interventions, such as those for hyperthermia, are more complex and require life-saving measures.

## ♦ EVALUATION

To evaluate the effectiveness of nursing interventions, compare the patient behaviors with those stated in the expected patient outcomes. Successful achievement of patient outcomes for the patient with alterations in sensory and perceptual function include but are not limited to the following:

1. Uses other senses and/or compensatory devices to avoid injury.
2. Can describe the nature of sensory/perceptual problem and changes necessary in life-style.
3. Describes adaptations in home to provide for safety (use of night lights, removal of throw rugs, rearrangement of furniture, painting of steps and door jambs in contrasting colors to surrounding area).
4. Describes schedule for follow-up care with physician, physical and occupational therapists, and speech pathologist as necessary.

# SPECIFIC NEUROLOGIC PROBLEMS

The second part of this chapter discusses the care of the patient with specific neurologic problems. These include (1) epilepsy, (2) degenerative diseases (multiple sclerosis, Parkinson's disease, and Alzheimer's disease), (3) cerebrovascular accident and intracerebral hemorrhage, (4) infections and inflammations, (5) traumatic brain injury, (6) intracranial tumors, and (7) AIDS.

# CONVULSIVE DISORDERS: EPILEPSY

## ETIOLOGY

**Epilepsy** can be defined as a transitory disturbance in consciousness or in motor, sensory, or autonomic function with or without loss of consciousness. Seizures are caused by uncontrolled electrical discharges in the brain. Seizures as a sign and symptom are of particular importance in neurologic diseases. Causes may include the following:

1. Cerebral anoxia
2. Hypoglycemia
3. Disturbance of calcium balance
4. Disturbance in hydration
5. Ingestion of drugs and poisons
6. Numerous metabolic disturbances and disorders
7. Infections that cause high temperature elevations
8. Electrolyte imbalances
9. Generalized inflammatory processes
10. Degenerative tissue disorders
11. Hysteria

In many patients with epilepsy, a localized organic lesion serves as the focus for the abnormal neuronal discharges from the damaged brain tissue. Often the lesion is microscopic in size. These organic lesions include the following:

1. Neoplasms
2. Inflamed areas or abscesses
3. Sclerosis
4. Vascular formations or hematomas
5. Congenital malformations
6. Trauma
7. Other space-occupying lesions

The role of heredity in the causation of epilepsy has not been completely clarified. The disease is not directly inherited, although abnormal brain waves, as shown on the electroencephalogram (EEG), are found in many relatives of persons who have seizures.

## EPIDEMIOLOGY

Epilepsy (convulsive disorders) is one of the oldest diseases known to human beings. It was described in detail by Hippocrates, as well as noted in the Bible. It has come to be defined as "seizure" or "convulsion." For purposes of this chapter, the terms *epilepsy, seizure disorder,* and *convulsive disorder* are used interchangeably.

At one time epilepsy was thought to be of divine origin, and perhaps for this reason it has been linked in the public mind with the occult, the strange, and the unmentionable. No disease has been more carefully concealed within families, and many attitudes toward the disease have persisted from early times to the present. Attitudes also may be affected by the following:

1. The frightening experience of seeing a person during a severe seizure
2. The belief that mental deterioration occurs with epilepsy

3. The possibility that the tendency to develop epilepsy is inheritable

The incidence of epilepsy is believed to be 1 in every 200 to 300 persons. This means that more than 1 million persons in the United States are subject to seizures. Seizures occur in all races and affect both genders equally. There seems to be no geographic distribution. Epilepsy can begin at any age, but many persons have seizures before 20 years of age. The life expectancy of persons with seizures is somewhat less than that for the population as a whole because these persons may die of an injury accidentally incurred during a seizure.

## PATHOPHYSIOLOGY

Convulsions or **seizures** are brief cerebral storms. These are associated with sudden, excessive, and disorderly electrical discharges in the neurons of the brain. The patterns or forms of seizures vary and depend on the area of the brain from which the seizure arises. The pattern is stereotyped in the individual, although variations may occur with progression of the cerebral lesion. Seizures can involve essentially all parts of the brain at once, as in the generalized type, or only a minute focal spot.

In the generalized type, the excessive neuronal discharges are thought to originate in the brainstem portion of the reticular activating system (RAS); these then spread throughout the central nervous system (CNS), including the cortex and the deeper parts of the brain. The process may last from a few seconds to as long as 3 to 5 minutes, or it may stop immediately, as in a **petit mal seizure.** It is not known what stops the seizure at a given time, but it is believed to result from fatigue of the neurons involved in precipitating the seizure or by inhibition of certain structures within the brain. Focally, the excessive neuronal discharges may result in a *tonic convulsion,* with the contraction of all muscles at once, or a *clonic convulsion,* with alternate contraction and relaxation of opposing muscle groups and characteristic jerking movements of the body.

The seizure, regardless of origin or type, is always inappropriate to the immediate situation. It is followed by an inhibition of cerebral function, the length of which may last longer than the seizure itself. The inhibition of function is often incomplete and depends on the area of the brain from which the seizure arises.

### Classification of Seizures

There are numerous ways to classify seizures. One frequently used method is the International Classification of Epileptic Seizures, which identifies them as partial, generalized, unilateral, or unclassified.

Most experts find it useful to classify seizures according to the clinical features. In this schema the following five groups can be identified:

1. Grand mal (major or generalized)
2. Petit mal
3. Psychomotor
4. Jacksonian, or focal
5. Miscellaneous

Table 57-6 shows the characteristics of each type of seizure.

### Types of Seizures

#### Grand mal seizures

The **grand mal seizure** is by far the most common and dramatic type. It is generalized and characterized by a loss of consciousness for several minutes and tonic and clonic convulsions. The seizures follow a typical course that includes the aura, cry, loss of consciousness, the fall, tonic and clonic convulsions, and incontinence.

**Aura.** The symptoms that occur during the prodrome are called an *aura.* Prodromal symptoms occur in about 50% of all patients and usually include a change in sensation or a change in affect. The exact character of the aura varies from person to person but may include any of the following:

1. Numbness
2. Flashing lights
3. Dizziness
4. Tingling of the arm
5. Smells
6. Spots before the eyes

The patient may find it difficult to describe the aura precisely, but it gives warning of the actual seizure activity. This serves a useful purpose in that it allows the person to seek safety and privacy before the onset of the seizure. Occasionally the aura occurs as much as a day before the actual seizure. The aura represents the local "signature" of the attack and is the result of an abnormal stimulation of the cortical area.

Almost at the same time that loss of consciousness occurs there is the so-called epileptic cry. It is caused by the spasm of the thoracic and abdominal muscles, which expels air through the glottis. Another type of cry results from an inspiratory effort. The loss of consciousness is sudden and variable in duration. It usually lasts several minutes.

The person slumps or falls, depending on his or her position at the time. This is followed immediately by bilateral *tonic contraction* of all muscles: the legs are extended and the arms are flexed; the jaw is clenched and the tongue frequently is caught between the teeth; the eyes roll upward and pupils dilate and become fixed. Respiration ceases and cyanosis occurs. The tonic spasms may occasionally be so violent that a joint, such as the shoulder, hip, or temporomandibular, is dislocated. Fractures also may result. As the tonic phase ends, it is replaced by a series of *clonic contractions.* As the clonic movements continue, the contractions become stronger. Breathing returns and is shallow and irregular at first. There is often frothing at the mouth, which may

**TABLE 57-6 Characteristics of Seizures**

| ETIOLOGY | CHARACTERISTICS | CLINICAL SIGNS | AURA | POSTICTAL PERIOD |
|---|---|---|---|---|
| **GRAND MAL** | | | | |
| Most common type | Generalized, characterized by loss of consciousness for several minutes | Aura<br>Cry<br>Loss of consciousness<br>Fall<br>Tonic-clonic movements<br>Incontinence | Present<br>Flashing lights<br>Smells<br>Spots before eyes<br>Dizziness | Present<br>Need for sleep for 1-2 hr<br>Headache common |
| **PETIT MAL** | | | | |
| Usually occurs during childhood and adolescence<br>Frequency decreases as child gets older | Sudden impairment in or loss of consciousness with little or no tonic-clonic movement<br>Occurs without warning<br>Has tendency to appear a few hours after arising or when person is quiet | Sudden vacant facial expression with eyes focused straight ahead<br>All motor activity ceases except perhaps for slight symmetric twitching about eyelids<br>Possible loss of muscle tone<br>Consciousness returns | None | None |
| **PSYCHOMOTOR** | | | | |
| Occurs at any age | Sudden change in awareness associated with complex distortion of feeling and thinking and partially coordinated motor activity<br>Longer than petit mal | Behaves as if partially conscious<br>Often appears intoxicated<br>May perform antisocial acts such as exposing self or carrying out violent acts<br>Autonomic complaints may occur:<br>Chest pain<br>Respiratory distress<br>Tachycardia<br>Gastrointestinal distress<br>Urinary incontinence | Present<br>Complex hallucinations or illusions | Present<br>Confusion<br>Amnesia<br>Need for sleep |
| **JACKSONIAN, OR FOCAL** | | | | |
| Occurs almost entirely in patients with structural brain disease | Depends on site of focus<br>May or may not be progressive | Typically begins in hand, foot, or face<br>May end in grand mal seizure | Present<br>Numbness<br>Tingling<br>Crawling feeling | Present |
| **MYOCLONIC** | | | | |
| May antedate grand mal by months or years | May be very mild or may cause rapid, forceful movements | Sudden involuntary contraction of muscle group, usually in extremities or trunk<br>No loss of consciousness | None | None |
| **AKINETIC** | | | | |
| Uncommon | Peculiar generalized tonelessness | Person falls in flacid state<br>Unconscious for 1 or 2 min | Rarely present | None |

be streaked with blood if the tongue and lips have been bitten during the convulsion. Fecal or urinary incontinence often occurs during the clonic phase or earlier. As the clonic phase subsides, within a few minutes the muscles relax. Partial consciousness is regained and color improves.

**Postictal period.** During the *postictal period* (postseizure) the person appears groggy and confused. Complaints of headache or muscular pain are common. A deep sleep usually follows. During this phase the pupils may remain dilated and abnormal plantar reflexes may occur. After a variable period the patient awakens and frequently is unaware of the occurrence of the seizure. A dull headache and depression are common. The depression may be caused in part by knowledge that a seizure has occurred.

General fatigue may last 1 or 2 days. In addition to the injuries that may occur, the violent activity during a grand mal seizure may result in ruptures of blood vessels with the production of corneal and subconjunctival hemorrhages.

In some persons seizures occur during sleep. In such instances the occurrence of the seizure is recognized on awakening by the presence of blood on the pillow or by soiled linen resulting from fecal or urinary incontinence.

### Petit mal seizures

Petit mal seizures are characterized by a sudden impairment in or loss of consciousness with little or no tonic-clonic movement. They usually occur without warning, and the arrest of voluntary activity is very brief, usually 10 to 20 seconds. The attacks have a tendency to appear a few hours after arising or when the person is quiet. In the classic petit mal seizure there is a sudden vacant facial expression with the eyes focused straight ahead. All motor activities cease except perhaps for a slight symmetric twitching about the eyelids or of the face and arms, or a loss of muscle tone. Consciousness returns as quickly as it left, and the person may resume speaking at the point interrupted, unaware that the seizure occurred. The individual may learn to recognize when a few seconds of time have been lost. Petit mal seizures usually occur many times a day and have no aura, falling, or tonic and clonic phases.

This type of seizure usually occurs during childhood and adolescence, particularly at puberty. The frequency of the episodes usually diminishes as the child grows older. Although petit mal seizures do not have the dramatic and frightening aspects of grand mal seizures, they are disconcerting, and the momentary loss of consciousness presents safety problems.

### Psychomotor seizures

Psychomotor seizures are more complex and bizarre than either grand mal or petit mal seizures. They can occur at any age and are characterized by a sudden change in awareness or consciousness, associated with a complex distortion of feeling and thinking and partially coordinated motor activity. Any aura present is usually a complex hallucination or illusion. The length of the seizure is longer than that of petit mal. Persons with these seizures often behave as though they were partially conscious and perform antisocial acts such as exposing themselves or committing acts of violence. They often appear intoxicated. Talking with them during this type of seizure shows that they are out of contact with their environment. Smacking of the lips and chewing movements may take place. Visceral symptoms with autonomic complaints of chest pain, respiratory distress, tachycardia, urinary incontinence, and gastrointestinal distress also may occur. Abnormal smell and taste sensations are common.

These persons are likely to be confused and amnesic for a time and often fall asleep at the end of the seizure activity. A relationship has been found between psychomotor epilepsy and lesions in the temporal lobe of the brain. Because of the crimes that may occur during this type of seizure, the diagnosis is of interest not only to physicians but to law enforcement officials, lawyers, and judges as well.

### Focal, or jacksonian, seizures

Focal, or jacksonian, seizures arise initially in the motor or sensory areas of the brain adjacent to the rolandic fissure or any localized part of the cerebral cortex. These seizures occur almost entirely in patients with structural brain disease and often occur as a symptom in persons with brain tumor, vascular malformations, scars, or infections. The clinical manifestations seen in this type of seizure thus depend on the site of the focus and differ from the generalized motor seizure (grand mal). If, for example, the abnormal neuronal discharge is initiated in the *precentral,* or *motor region* of the cortex for the thumb, the person will experience a tonic contracture of the thumb muscles. If the abnormal neuronal discharge spreads to adjacent parts of the motor strip, there is progressive involvement of associated musculature with a progression (march) of movements from thumb to hand, arm, face, and so forth. The discharge may or may not progress. The localized seizure that does spread progressively to other muscles after initiation is known as a *jacksonian seizure.*

Focal motor seizures typically begin in the hand, face, and foot but may arise in any part of the motor strip. The seizure may end in a shower of clonic movements, or it may end in a generalized convulsion. Consciousness is retained unless the opposite half of the body is involved. When abnormal neuronal discharges arise in the lower part of the motor strip, which controls salivation and mastication, seizures then manifest by chewing, smacking of the lips, and swallowing movements. Salivation may be profuse. Other seizures may begin with a forced turning of the head and eyes. Such attacks are termed *adversive* and originate in the eye-turning fields of the brain; the head turns away from the side of the lesion, or focus. When the abnormal neuronal discharges arise in the *postcentral,* or *sensory, strip* of the cortex, the seizure is initiated with complaints of disturbed sensations such as a numbness, tingling, prickling, or crawling feeling. As in a focal motor seizure, a march of sensations may or may not occur. The neuronal discharge also may spread from the sensory area to the motor area.

### Miscellaneous seizures

The category of miscellaneous seizures includes many different types, two of which are described here.

**Myoclonic seizures.** Myoclonic seizures are characterized by the sudden involuntary contraction of a muscle group, usually in the extremities or trunk. These contractions may be very mild, or they may result in rapid, forceful movement of the part. No loss of consciousness occurs. Some experts see myoclonus as a variant of petit mal seizures. The myoclonus may be found in some petit mal conditions. Myoclonus sometimes antedates grand mal seizures by months or years.

**Akinetic seizures.** Akinetic seizures are characterized by a peculiar generalized tonelessness. An aura rarely occurs, but the person falls in a flaccid state and is unconscious for a moment or two. Recovery comes quickly, with no postictal phase.

### Status epilepticus

When recurrent generalized seizure activity occurs with such frequency that full consciousness is not regained between seizures, it is referred to as **status epilepticus.** Although this condition is relatively rare, it can lead to death from brain damage secondary to prolonged hypoxia and exhaustion. *Status epilepticus is a medical emergency requiring intensive medical and nursing care.*

The person with status epilepticus is often in a coma for 12 to 24 hours or longer, during which time recurring seizures occur. The seizures may cease spontaneously with return of consciousness, or death may result from the repeated attacks. The attack usually is related to failure to take prescribed medication.

## PREVENTION

*Primary prevention* of epilepsy is limited. Preventing problems such as electrolyte imbalances or other causes previously listed can prevent some seizures. *Secondary prevention* or early diagnosis is important, especially with the adult who experiences a first seizure after 21 years of age. This almost always heralds an organic lesion that needs prompt attention.

## MEDICAL MANAGEMENT

The nurse works collaboratively with the physician for implementation of prescribed medical therapy. Because the nurse has a major role in discharge planning and patient teaching, these are discussed under nursing management. A sample Nursing Care Plan and Critical Pathway are included at the end of this section.

### Diagnostic Tests

By far the most common test used to evaluate seizure activity is the EEG. It is a safe and noninvasive test that allows for more specific diagnosis. It may be performed with the patient in a sleep-deprived state. (See Chapter 56 for a description of this test.)

### Medication

Treatment of patients with a seizure disorder almost always includes the use of one or more of the anticonvulsant drugs (Table 57-7). The choice of medications depends on the type of seizure. Anticonvulsant medications act on the cerebral cortex generally and are not selective in acting on the part of the brain involved in abnormal neuronal discharges.

The dosages of anticonvulsant drugs are difficult to establish and regulate because of the high incidence of side effects and the toxicity of the drugs. The drug of choice is introduced in an average therapeutic dose and then increased until control of seizures is obtained. If

**TABLE 57-7 Anticonvulsants Used to Prevent Seizures**

| DRUG | USE RELATED TO SEIZURE TYPE | AVERAGE DAILY DOSE | TOXIC EFFECTS |
|---|---|---|---|
| Phenytoin sodium (Dilantin) | Grand mal, focal, psychomotor | 0.4-0.6 g (often at hs) | Ataxia, vomiting, nystagmus, drowsiness, rash, fever, gum hyperplasia, lymphadenopathy |
| Phenobarbital (Luminal) | Grand mal, focal, psychomotor (adjunctive) | 0.1-0.4 g (divided dose) | Drowsiness, rash |
| Primidone (Mysoline) | Grand mal, focal, psychomotor | 0.5-2.0 g | Drowsiness, ataxia |
| Mephenytoin (Mesantoin) | Grand mal, focal, psychomotor | 0.3-0.5 g | Ataxia, nystagmus, pancytopenia, rash |
| Ethosuximide (Zarontin) | Petit mal, psychomotor, myoclonic, akinetic | 750-1500 mg | Drowsiness, nausea, agranulocytosis |
| Trimethadione (Tridione) | Petit mal | 0.3-2.0 g (divided dose) | Rash, photophobia, agranulocytosis, nephrosis |
| Diazepam (Valium) | Status epilepticus, mixed | 8-30 mg | Drowsiness, ataxia |
| Carbamazepine (Tegretol) | Grand mal, psychomotor | 0.3-2.0 g | Rash, drowsiness, ataxia |
| Valproic acid (Depakene) | Petit mal, absence of seizures | 5-35 mg/kg body weight (at least tid dosage) | Nausea, vomiting, indigestion, sedation, emotional disturbance, weakness, altered blood coagulation |
| Clonazepam (Clonopin) | Petit mal, akinetic, myoclonic | 5-20 g | Grand mal seizures, drowsiness, ataxia, hypotension, respiratory depression |

toxicity is reached before control of the seizures, the dose is decreased to the previous nontoxic or tolerated dose. Additional secondary drugs may be introduced at this time to aid in control of the seizures.

Corticosteroids are used occasionally to treat myoclonus. Bromides are used less frequently than in the past and have been largely replaced by the anticonvulsant drugs. Occasionally a ketogenic diet may be prescribed for patients with petit mal seizures. The diet is not easy to follow, and the effectiveness of available medication has led to its decline in use.

Failure to take the prescribed medication or an adequate dose is often the cause of a failed treatment. Blood tests to determine the level of drugs in the blood are helpful to ensure compliance and prevent toxicity.

### Treatment

Aside from medications and surgery (see relevant sections of text) there is no specific treatment for seizures. Sometimes psychologic counseling helps the person with a seizure disorder accept the condition.

### Diet

No special diet is needed for persons with a seizure disorder, unless mandated by the side effects of medications. The use of alcohol should be avoided, however. The person should be taught the importance of good mouth care if on long-term phenytoin (Dilantin) therapy because gingival hyperplasia is a common side effect.

### Activity

There is no prescribed activity pattern for the patient who has a seizure disorder. The person is encouraged to live a full and active life, which is discussed further under nursing management.

### Referral/Consultation

In some settings the nurse assumes responsibility for making referrals to other services. For the patient with a seizure disorder a referral to a local support group or to the local chapter of the Epilepsy Foundation is important.

## SURGICAL MANAGEMENT

Surgical treatment of seizures is used in some cases when medical therapy is not effective. *Cortical resection* is one surgical approach. It involves removal of the brain tissue where the focus of electrical discharge is located. The localization of tissue must occur in a part of the brain that is easily accessible to surgery or that can be removed without leaving the person with a serious disability. A *temporal lobectomy* is the most common resection. Data have shown a cure from seizure activity or a drastic reduction in the number of seizures in 60% to 90% of patients undergoing this procedure.[24]

A *corpus callostomy* sometimes is used. This procedure was first performed in the 1930s after it was observed that patients who suffered a CVA of the corpus callosum had fewer seizures. A *hemispherectomy* has been performed in children with unilateral hemispheric disease and refractory epilepsy. Although often associated with significant morbidity, it has been found to improve the quality of life for some children.[24]

Another surgical approach involves *stereotactic* procedures with the use of electrical stimulation. This technique is used in an attempt to interrupt the pathways of seizure activity, to destroy the foci, or to alter the actions of the cortical nerve cells.

## NURSING MANAGEMENT

### ♦ ASSESSMENT

Both subjective and objective data are important to assess in the patient with seizures.

### Subjective Data

Subjective data to be collected to assess the patient with seizures include the following:

- Understanding of the seizure disorder and what may be causing it
- Awareness of precipitating factors
- Presence of aura
- Postictal feelings

**BOX 57-8 Observations To Be Made About a Person Having a Seizure**

**AURA**
Presence or absence, nature of if present; ability of patient to describe it (somatic, visceral, psychic)

**CRY**
Presence or absence

**ONSET**
Site of initial body movements, deviation of head and eyes, chewing and salivation, posture of body, sensory changes

**TONIC AND CLONIC PHASES**
Movements of body as to progression, skin color and airway, pupillary changes, incontinence, duration of each phase

**RELAXATION (SLEEP)**
Duration and behavior

**POSTICTAL PHASE**
Duration, general behavior, ability to remember anything about the seizure, orientation, pupillary changes, headache, injuries present

**DURATION OF ENTIRE SEIZURE**
Number of minutes

**LEVEL OF CONSCIOUSNESS**
Length of unconsciousness if present

### Objective Data

Objective data to be collected to assess the patient with seizures include the following:

Number of seizures occurring within a specific time
Behavior: signs of stress or fatigue
Results of EEG
Character of seizures (see Box 57-8 for observations to be made about a person having a seizure)

### Diagnostic Test Findings

Abnormal findings will appear on the EEG of patients with a seizure disorder. Other tests usually do not reveal abnormalities. In an adult experiencing a first seizure, however, further diagnostic testing will be necessary. A CT scan or angiogram often identifies a brain tumor or other pathologic condition.

## ♦ NURSING DIAGNOSES

Nursing diagnoses are determined from analysis of patient data. Nursing diagnoses for the patient with a seizure disorder may include but are not limited to the following:

| Diagnostic Title | Possible Etiologic Factors |
|---|---|
| Aspiration, high risk for | Decreased consciousness |
| Injury (trauma), high risk for | Sensory/motor deficits |
| Activity intolerance, high risk for | Immobility |
| Adjustment, impaired | Disability requiring change in life-style |
| Knowledge deficit: cause of seizures and care needed | Lack of exposure to information |

## ♦ EXPECTED PATIENT OUTCOMES

Expected patient outcomes for the patient with a seizure disorder may include but are not limited to the following:

1. Will have fewer seizures or at least will avoid increase in severity or number.
2. Aspiration will not occur.
3. Injury will be prevented.
4. Can explain schedule to carry out ADLs that includes a balance of rest and activity and avoidance of excesses in exercise, stress, or fatigue.
5. Verbalizes a positive adjustment to seizure disorder.
6. Medication
    a. Can explain any medications to be taken or treatment program to be carried out at home: action, side effects, toxic effects, and dosage schedule for each anticonvulsant drug.
    b. Understands importance of taking medication even when seizure-free.
    c. Acknowledges need to seek medical assistance if side effects occur.
    d. Understands incompatibility of anticonvulsant drugs with alcohol and other drugs that counteract the anticonvulsants.
7. Can explain how to secure professional and community resources.
8. Will state plans for follow-up care.
9. Significant other can demonstrate precautions to be followed during and after a seizure.

## ♦ INTERVENTIONS

### Managing Critical Care

**Status epilepticus**

With status epilepticus, vigorous therapy is directed toward arrest of the seizures. The first priority is ensuring an adequate airway, which may be compromised by the seizure and complications of certain drug therapy. The type of drugs used to stop status epilepticus may lead to pulmonary complications. Drug therapy is given intravenously. Medications used include sodium phenobarbital, diazepam (Valium), phenytoin (Dilantin), and paraldehyde. Optimal results appear to result from large or full (not divided) therapeutic dosages. At times it may be necessary to give a general anesthetic.

Constant monitoring of vital signs is necessary to assess for respiratory depression and cardiac changes. The responsibilities pertaining to the observation and recording of seizure activity are the same as those described in Box 57-8. It may not be possible to note the separate seizure phases because of the frequency of seizures. A safe environment is essential. See Guidelines box below, for care of the person with status epilepticus.

### Maintaining the Airway

It is important to observe the patient for airway problems, which sometimes are caused by aspiration. If time is available, the nurse should insert an airway before the patient's mouth is clenched. The nurse should never attempt to insert anything into the clenched mouth because injury may result to both patient and nurse.

It may be helpful to position the person on the left side to encourage drainage of any secretions. A suction

**Guidelines for Care of the Person With Status Epilepticus**

1. Promote oxygenation:
    a. Ensure patent airway.
    b. Prepare for possible need to intubate or assist ventilation.
    c. Oxygenate.
2. Promote cessation of seizures:
    a. Provide quiet and nonstimulating environment.
    b. Give medications as ordered intravenously.
3. Promote safety:
    a. Lower head of bed.
    b. Turn patient to side-lying position.
    c. Put side rails up.
    d. Constantly observe vital signs and neurologic status.

machine should be kept at the bedside or within easy access to the patient in the hospital. Oxygen may be administered. If the seizure is prolonged, it may be necessary to provide intubation or ventilation assistance.

## Preventing Injury

The primary goals of the nurse and the family caring for a patient having a seizure are to protect the person from injury and observe and record the seizure activity. Specific actions are listed in the Guidelines box below.

Accurate observation of the seizure from the beginning, when possible, is important because it provides needed information that may assist the physician in locating the site or focus of a cerebral lesion. It is more important to describe the seizure activity and sequence and determine where it started than to name or classify the seizure. (See Research box below, right.)

## Promoting Adjustment

Because most persons with seizures are without symptoms between attacks and most seizures can be controlled by medication, the person with seizures should be encouraged to lead as normal a life as possible. The person should not be made to feel that he or she is a chronic invalid. With treatment the person can live a useful, normal, and happy life. Until seizures are controlled, the person should avoid dangerous activities such as driving a car, working on or about machinery, or swimming. Once the seizures are controlled with medications and the person has learned the importance of taking the medication regularly and avoiding alcoholic beverages, these restrictions can be relaxed. Achieving adequate rest and maintaining nutritional intake also are important.

The issue of driving a car often poses a problem. Epilepsy is one condition that imposes driver limitations. Usually a waiting period of one seizure-free year should elapse before the person is eligible to drive and then *only* if seizures are completely controlled.

No special diet is needed for persons with a seizure disorder, unless mandated by the side effects of medications. The use of alcohol should be avoided, however. The person should be taught the importance of good mouth care if on long-term phenytoin (Dilantin) therapy because gingival hyperplasia is a common side effect.

The person with seizures should use all resources to cope with feelings of self-consciousness and inferiority resulting from attacks. Adults should be encouraged to lead normal, productive lives. Children should be kept in school unless the frequency of attacks disturbs the activities of the classroom. Family members need to be assisted to discuss their attitudes and feelings about the person's illness. Excessive attention to the overprotection of the person with seizures is to be avoided. The family needs to understand the problems resulting from seizures and the prescribed therapy but should not make a chronic invalid of the person.

## Changing Public Attitudes

One of the most important aspects in epilepsy therapy is changing the public's attitude toward the disease. The person subject to seizures and the public must view seizures not as bizarre catastrophes but as relatively normal events that can be dealt with rationally. Many persons with epilepsy lead normal, productive lives. Many outstanding figures in world history had seizures (Julius Caesar, Lord Byron, Napoleon). Studies do not bear out the popular assumption that mental deterioration occurs with epilepsy. Cognitive abilities vary among persons with epilepsy as with the population generally. Also, no evidence exists that personality changes are the result of pathologic processes; when they occur, they probably are the result of society's attitude toward the person with epilepsy.

For example, until recently some persons who were found to have epilepsy were dismissed from their jobs even though they were not dangerous to themselves or others. In addition, some employers refused to hire a

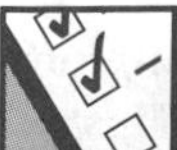

### Guidelines for Care of the Person During a Seizure

- Never leave person alone.
- If person is standing, lower to floor or bed and move adjacent articles and equipment away to prevent injury.
- Loosen constrictive clothing, especially around neck.
- Turn head or body to one side to aid with airway.
- Do not restrain, either manually or with restraints.
- Do not pry jaw open to place padded tongue blade. Oral airway may be inserted after seizure to aid in suctioning during postictal phase.
- Pad side rails for patient who is confined to bed or has seizures during sleep. *Pillows should not be used* because of the danger of suffocation.
- Observe seizure and make relevant recordings.

### RESEARCH

Tucker C: Safety assessment for the postictal confusional phase following complex partial seizure, *J Neurosurg Nurs* 17(3):201-209, 1985.

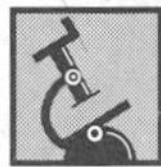

This study examined the behavior of patients after a complex partial seizure (one in which consciousness is lost). All subjects who suffered seizures (20) were observed in a safe environment for at least 30 minutes after the seizure. They were asked a series of six questions that included orientation questions of name, year, month, day, place, and city. The results indicated that persons who responded to the six questions could safely leave their rooms after the seizure.

person known to have epilepsy, even though at least 80% of all persons with epilepsy are employable. The Epilepsy Foundation has been active in trying to improve state laws concerning the hiring of persons with epilepsy. The Foundation's efforts, as well as the efforts of other organizations and disabled persons, resulted in the passage of the federal law guaranteeing the rights of persons with disabilities in employment and public accommodations. With the passage of the Americans With Disabilities Act by Congress in 1990, employers may not refuse to hire or promote a person with a disability (see Chapter 8 for additional information on the Act).

Children with epilepsy have been segregated to separate schools, and only recently have some major cities passed laws ensuring children with epilepsy the right to attend the public schools if they are under adequate medical care. In many schools children are barred from the classroom according to the inclination of the teacher. Limitation of environment and of educational opportunity often limits the child's knowledge, but this does not mean that learning capacity is poor.

Interest in epilepsy and in the problems of the epileptic person has been increased by various organizations, such as the National Association to Control Epilepsy, Inc.,* National Epilepsy League, Inc.,† Epilepsy Foundation of America,‡ and United Epilepsy Association.§

The care of the person with a seizure disorder is summarized in the Guidelines box at right.

### Facilitating Learning

Teaching is an important part of the care of the person with seizures. This includes the patient as well as the members of the family who need to learn about care during and after seizure. Teaching needs to include the following points:

1. Use of medication, including side effects, dose, timing, and reporting side effects to physician
2. Importance of avoiding use of alcohol if taking anticonvulsants
3. Safety measures to avoid injury in case of a seizure
4. Good oral hygiene for persons taking phenytoin (a side effect is gingival hyperplasia)
5. Importance of adequate rest
6. Importance of taking medication even when seizure-free
7. Available community resources
8. Restrictions concerning driving
9. Importance of follow-up care

## ♦ EVALUATION

To evaluate the effectiveness of nursing interventions, compare patient behaviors with those stated in the expected patient outcomes. Successful achievement of patient outcomes for the patient with a seizure disorder is indicated by the following:

1. Has decreased or constant number of seizures.
2. Avoids aspiration during seizure.
3. Experiences no seizure-related injury.
4. Describes schedule to carry out ADL that achieves balance between rest and activity and avoids fatigue.
5. Indicates a positive adjustment to seizure disorder.
6. Medication
   a. Correctly describes medications to be taken, including the action, side effects, toxic effects, and dosage schedule for each anticonvulsant drug.
   b. Correctly explains importance of taking medication even though seizure-free.
   c. Explains importance of seeking medical assistance if side effects occur.
   d. Correctly describes incompatibility of anticonvulsant drugs with alcohol and other drugs.
7. Explains how to secure professional and community resources.
8. Describes plans for follow-up care.
9. Significant other demonstrates correct precautions to be followed during and after a seizure.

*Headquarters: 22 East 67th St, New York, NY 10021.
†Headquarters: 203 Wabash St, Chicago, IL 60604.
‡Headquarters: 1828 L St, NW, Washington, DC 20036.
§Headquarters: 113 West 57th St, New York, NY 10019.

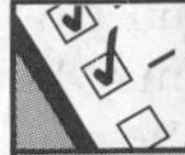

### Guidelines for Care of the Person With a Seizure Disorder

1. Prevent seizures:
   a. Take medication on regular basis.
   b. Avoid alcoholic beverages and other drugs that lower seizure threshold.
   c. Achieve adequate rest.
   d. Eat well-balanced diet.
2. Promote activity:
   a. Until seizures are controlled, avoid dangerous activities
      (1) Driving car or other vehicle
      (2) Operating machinery
      (3) Swimming
   b. Once seizures are controlled, patient can lead normal life.
3. Promote mental health:
   a. Encourage to lead active life.
   b. Teach family not to overprotect patient.
   c. Patient and family should discuss concerns and feelings openly.

# DEGENERATIVE DISEASES

The term *degenerative diseases* as used here refers to those neurologic diseases in which there is a premature senescence of nerve cells, a known or suspected metabolic disturbance exists, or the cause is unknown. See Table 57-8 for a comparison of these degenerative neurologic diseases.

# NURSING CARE PLAN

## PERSON WITH SEIZURES

**DATA:** Mrs. B. is a 25-year-old married secretary admitted with a diagnosis of a seizure disorder. The seizures began approximately 4 months after surgery for a brain aneurysm. She was admitted yesterday from the emergency room after having experienced a grand mal seizure. Intravenous fluids were initiated, and she was given Dilantin 1000 mg by IV push. She also has been started on oral Dilantin. A CT scan documented no new pathologic condition of the brain. Mrs. B. initially was very lethargic, with a postictal period of about 15 minutes, but she is now awake and alert. She is embarrassed by the seizures, especially because they began while she was at work. She suffered no injury during the seizure, and she has no memory of the event.

The nursing history revealed the following:

- Mrs. B. had made a complete recovery from the aneurysm surgery without any apparent neurologic deficit.
- She was not placed on anticonvulsants after brain surgery.
- The patient has a cocktail before dinner several times a week.
- Mrs. B. has been "pushing herself" at work in the past month.

Collaborative nursing actions include those to prevent further seizures and to protect the patient from danger if a seizure does occur. Nursing actions include monitoring for the following:

- Any neurologic deficit: weakness, confusion, aphasia
- Any seizure activity

### ■ NURSING DIAGNOSIS

High risk for aspiration related to decreased consciousness

| Expected Patient Outcome | Nursing Interventions | Rationale |
|---|---|---|
| Does not experience aspiration. | If seizure occurs, turn onto left side. | Position will facilitate airway. |
| | During any seizure activity, monitor airway. | Help will be available as needed. |
| | Insert airway only before seizure activity begins or after seizure ends. | Insertion of airway during active seizure can damage mouth or teeth of patient and/or can cause injury to nurse. |

### ■ NURSING DIAGNOSIS

High risk for injury (trauma) related to seizure activity

| Expected Patient Outcome | Nursing Interventions | Rationale |
|---|---|---|
| Avoids injury. | If seizure begins while patient is walking, lower to floor. | Lowering to floor protects her from falling and injuring self. |
| | Give Dilantin as prescribed. | Dilantin acts in the motor cortex of the brain to reduce the spread of electrical discharges from the rapidly firing epileptic foci in this area—thus reducing seizures. |
| | Keep padded side rails on bed up at night and when Mrs. B. is in bed. | Seizure activity may occur during sleep. |

### ■ NURSING DIAGNOSIS

High risk for activity intolerance related to seizures and immobility

| Expected Patient Outcome | Nursing Interventions | Rationale |
|---|---|---|
| Will complete ADL without difficulty. | Assist to plan activities so that there is a balance between rest and activity. | Fatigue may increase the frequency of seizures. |
| | Assist to plan activities to avoid excesses in exercise, stress, or fatigue. | Excesses may increase number of seizures. |

### ■ NURSING DIAGNOSIS

Impaired adjustment related to disability requiring change in life-style

| Expected Patient Outcome | Nursing Interventions | Rationale |
|---|---|---|
| Demonstrates a positive adjustment to diagnosis of seizures. | Encourage to discuss her feelings about seizure disorder. | Ventilation of feelings is important for acceptance. |
| | Inform of local support group or a contact person. | Group support can make life-style adjustment easier. |

*Continued.*

## NURSING CARE PLAN

### PERSON WITH SEIZURES—cont'd

■ **NURSING DIAGNOSIS**
Knowledge deficit related to lack of recall of exposure

| Expected Patient Outcomes | Nursing Interventions | Rationale |
|---|---|---|
| Describes nature of and therapy for seizure disorder. | Review nature of seizure disorder and possible recurrence. | Recall or reinforcement of earlier teaching will help promote retention. |
| States importance of not drinking alcohol while on Dilantin therapy. | Review relationship of interaction between alcohol and Dilantin. | Alcohol may inhibit absorption of Dilantin and increase possibility of seizure. |
| Describes importance of good mouth care. | Review side effects of Dilantin. | Dilantin may cause gingival hyperplasia. |

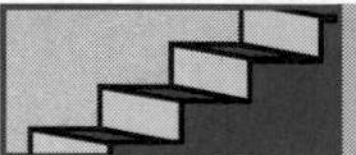

## CRITICAL PATHWAY Seizure Disorder

**DRG #: 024 Expected LOS: 5**

| | Day of Admission Day 1 | Day 2 | Day 3 | Day 4 | Day of Discharge Day 5 |
|---|---|---|---|---|---|
| **Diagnostic Tests** | CBC, UA, SMA/18,* drug screen, ?MRI, ?CT head | EEG | Dilantin level | CBC | |
| **Medications** | IV & TKO, Dilantin | IV & TKO, Dilantin | If no seizures, IV to saline lock; Dilantin | IV saline lock; Dilantin | Disc saline lock; Dilantin |
| **Treatment** | I & O q8hr; VS q4hr; neurologic assessment q1hr; skin and mouth assessment and special care q2hr | I & O q8hr; VS q4hr; neurologic assessment q4hr; skin and mouth assessment and special care q2hr | I & O q8hr; VS q8hr; neurologic assessment q8hr | Disc I & O; VS q8hr; neurologic assessment q8hr | VS q8hr; neurologic assessment q8hr |
| **Diet** | NPO until seizures controlled; ice chips | If no seizures diet as tolerated | Regular diet | Regular diet | Regular diet |
| **Activity** | Bed rest; to BR with help; patient safety considerations (bed in lowest position, suction ready, etc.) | Up in room; continue with patient safety considerations | Up ad lib; continue with patient safety considerations | Up ad lib; continue with patient safety considerations | Up ad lib |
| **Consultations** | Neurologist | | ?Psychologist, ?Career counselor | | |

*BR,* Bathroom; *Disc,* discontinue; *SMA,* sequential multiple analysis; *TKO,* to keep open; *UA,* urinalysis.
*Serum calcium, phosphorus, triglycerides, uric acid, creatinine, BUN, total bilirubin, alkaline phosphate, aspartate aminotransferase (AST) (formerly serum-glutamic oxaloacetic transaminase [SGOT]), alanine aminotransferase (ALT) (formerly serum glutamate pyruvate transaminase [SGPT]), lactic dehydrogenase (LDH), total protein, albumin, sodium, potassium, chloride, total $CO_2$, glucose.

**TABLE 57-8 Comparison of Neurologic Degenerative Diseases**

| PATHOLOGIC SIGNS | EFFECT |
|---|---|
| **MULTIPLE SCLEROSIS** | |
| Multiple foci (patches) of nerve degeneration throughout brain and spinal cord | Demyelination causes nerve impulse to be interrupted (blocked) or distorted (slowed) |
| **MYASTHENIA GRAVIS** | |
| Decreased secretion of acetylcholine or an increase of cholinesterase enzyme at myoneural junction | Interference of nerve impulse across myoneural junction |
| **AMYOTROPHIC LATERAL SCLEROSIS** | |
| Destruction of myelin sheath of motor neurons of lateral tracts in spinal cord and brain | Demyelination causes nerve impulse to be interrupted (blocked) or distorted (slowed) |
| **PARKINSONISM** | |
| Destruction of nerve cells of basal ganglia of brain | Decreased dopamine (neurotransmitter substance with anticholinergic effect) |
| **SYRINGOMYELIA** | |
| Destruction of gray and then white matter of spinal cord by development of "syrinx" (cysts filled with cerebrospinal fluid) | Destruction of nerve pathways in spinal cord—interruption of nerve impulses |
| **MUSCULAR DYSTROPHY** | |
| *Not a neurologic disease;* atrophy of voluntary muscles | Effect is a wasting away of the voluntary muscles; no nerve effect |
| **ALZHEIMER'S DISEASE** | |
| Degeneration of neurofibrils and presence of plaques in brain | Destruction of neurons leading to impairment in intellectual functioning |

## MULTIPLE SCLEROSIS

### Etiology

**Multiple sclerosis** is a common neurologic disease in northern climates. The exact prevalence of this disease is not known because in many instances the diagnosis is not made, but probably at least 250,000 persons in the United States are known to have multiple sclerosis. The onset of symptoms usually occurs between 20 and 40 years of age. The course of the disease is estimated to be 12 to 25 years. Multiple sclerosis has serious implications for family life inasmuch as it affects both men and women in the active productive years when their responsibilities are greatest. Women are affected twice as often as men. Several studies have demonstrated that an increased incidence of multiple sclerosis seems to occur among siblings and even distant relatives. No evidence has been found to suggest a conjugal relationship.

### Epidemiology

During the past 15 years, major advances have occurred concerning knowledge of the cause, pathology, diagnosis, and treatment of multiple sclerosis. The cause, however, remains unknown despite new findings and the numerous hypotheses that have been advanced as to cause. Mineral deficiency, toxic substances, disturbance of blood-clotting mechanism, viruses, and autoimmunity are a few of the causes studied. The last two are currently the most favored. Experimental allergic encephalomyelitis has been produced in animals by the injection of the basic protein from a homologous neuron sheath. Despite the resemblance to multiple sclerosis, it is not yet clear to what extent this disease represents a human model for multiple sclerosis. The recent discovery of slow viruses (those with a long latent period) in association with the frequent findings of an increase of gamma globulin ($\gamma$-globulin) and immunoglobulin (IgG) in the spinal fluid of patients with multiple sclerosis gives support to these theories. What constitutes an elevation of $\gamma$-globulin or of IgG is not clear. Whether the $\gamma$-globulin and IgG get into the spinal fluid by transudation or by increased permeability of the blood-brain barrier is still controversial.

### Pathophysiology

Multiple foci of demyelination are distributed randomly in the white matter of the brainstem, spinal cord, optic nerves, and cerebrum. During the demyelination process (primary degeneration) the myelin sheath and the sheath cells are destroyed, but early sparing of the axon cylinder occurs. The outer myelin sheath in the spinal cord neuronal pathways often is compared with the insulation on an electric wire. Its destruction causes interruption or distortion of the impulse so that it is *slowed* or *blocked.* This type of demyelination differs from that of *wallerian degeneration* in that damage is always primary to the myelin sheath or sheath cells. There is evidence of partial healing in areas of degeneration, which accounts for the transitory nature of early symptoms. In late stages the degeneration may extend to gray areas of the cord and limit healing.

Because of the wide distribution of areas of degeneration, *a greater variety of signs and symptoms in multiple sclerosis occurs than in other neurologic diseases.* The scarring that occurs at the degenerative lesions, as well as the increasing number of lesions, provides the name *disseminated sclerosis.*

Multiple sclerosis is a *chronic, remitting,* and *relapsing disease* although the clinical course may vary widely. Most persons recover from their early episodes. Usually acute exacerbations and remissions may last for a year or more, although eventually exacerbations will recur. There is no record of any patients having recovered from the disease, although many have lived for 20 years or more and have died of other causes. Exacerbations may be aggravated or precipitated by fatigue, chilling, and emotional disturbances. In some cases the disease may terminate in death within a few months of onset. This so-called malignant multiple sclerosis is rare.

Early symptoms usually are transitory and may include double vision *(diplopia),* spots before the eyes *(scotomas),* blindness, tremor, weakness or numbness of a body part such as the hand, fatigue, susceptibility to upper respiratory infections, emotional instability, or problems with the bowel or bladder. Many persons with early multiple sclerosis may be considered neurotic by their associates and sometimes by their physicians because of the wide variety and temporary nature of symptoms and because of the person's emotional instability. As the disease progresses, symptoms may include nystagmus, disorders of speech *(scanning),* urinary frequency and urgency, constipation, and changes in muscular coordination and gait. Other symptoms may include urinary incontinence, difficulty in swallowing, severe muscle spasm and contractures, and spastic ataxic gait.

A sense of optimism and well-being *(euphoria)* also seems to be characteristic of persons with multiple sclerosis, especially during remissions. It is suspected that this reaction is largely a result of patients' attempts to reassure themselves that their condition is not so serious. This response is helpful to patients in many ways, but sometimes it may lead them to overdo and thus increase symptoms. This euphoria may also be an indicator of involvement of selected areas of the brain.

Motor signs have upper motor neuron characteristics. Pain is not a common symptom of multiple sclerosis except when there is severe muscle spasm. Death generally is caused by infection, usually developing in the respiratory or genitourinary system.

## Prevention

The cause of multiple sclerosis remains unclear; therefore no primary prevention for this disease is available. Again, the secondary and tertiary preventive aspects are important.

## Medical Management

The nurse works collaboratively with the physician for implementation of prescribed medical therapy. Because the nurse has a major role in discharge planning and patient teaching, these are discussed under nursing management.

### Diagnostic tests

Because multiple sclerosis involves multiple parts of the nervous system, it is often characterized by exacerbations and remissions, and frequently includes transient and bizarre signs and symptoms, it is difficult to diagnose with certainty. Because there is no specific diagnostic test, diagnosis is often a clinical judgment. The determination of cerebrospinal fluid (CSF) $\gamma$-globulin by chemical or electrophorectic methods or of CSF fluid IgG by electroimmunodiffusion appears to be the most valuable single laboratory test when used with the history and neurologic examination. Testing of *visual-evoked potentials* is now being performed to assess optic nerve integrity. Evidence of early damage has been closely linked with the diagnosis of multiple sclerosis.

### Medication

At present no specific treatment exists for multiple sclerosis. Many physicians achieve favorable results from symptomatic treatments and the judicious use of adrenocorticotropic hormone (ACTH) or corticosteroids. Psychotherapy, social rehabilitation, physical therapy, patient education, and much compassion also are indicated. Although ACTH or the steroids are widely used, their efficacy remains controversial. These drugs have been shown to prevent experimental allergic encephalomyelitis. At present some clinicians prefer oral prednisone; others prefer intramuscular ACTH; still others prefer intravenous ACTH. Dexamethasone (Decadron), administered intramuscularly or orally, has become popular. Its demonstrated antiedema effect may explain the favorable results in acute attacks of multiple sclerosis. The effects of ACTH and the steroids on the demyelinating activity per se are not known. Testing has shown that (1) nothing is gained from long-term treatment with either steroids or ACTH and (2) some gain may result from taking high doses of steroids at the start of a fresh episode, inasmuch as the episode tends to resolve itself more rapidly if patients are treated with intensive courses of these drugs. The mood-elevating drugs are used to relieve depression, which often is present in multiple sclerosis. Chemotherapy (low-dose cyclophosphamide [cytoxan] and interferon) is now being used to treat exacerbations of the disease.

Persons with multiple sclerosis react similarly to others with a chronic illness. Their reactions include fear, guilt, grief, denial, and depression (see Research box below).

**RESEARCH**

Wineman N: Adaptation to multiple sclerosis: the role of social support, functional disability, and perceived uncertainty, *Nurs Res* 39(5):294-299, 1990.

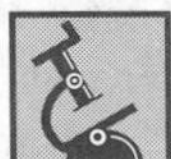

This study attempted to depict a relationship among special support, functional disability, perceived uncertainty, and psychosocial adaptation in 38 women and 80 men with multiple sclerosis. Results showed that the perceived supportiveness of interactions was directly related to purpose in life but not to depression. Functional disability also was found to have a direct effect on adaptation.

**Treatment**

Treatment of multiple sclerosis is based mainly on symptom relief. At one time ice water baths were suggested, but the efficacy of this approach was never validated.

**Diet**

There is no specific diet for the patient with multiple sclerosis. The emphasis is on a well-balanced diet that provides the needed requirements without additional calories.

**Activity**

Persons with multiple sclerosis should have a daily routine for rest and activity. Rest must be balanced with adequate exercise. Patients usually are advised to exercise regularly but never to the point of extreme fatigue. Because persons with multiple sclerosis almost always feel tired, they must look for some special sign that tells them that they have exercised enough. If they exercise more, they may suffer ill effects. For example, a tight feeling in the chest may indicate that the person must rest or else have severe discomfort. During the acute exacerbation, many physicians keep the patient as quiet as possible, limit all activities, and place the patient on bed rest. After an exacerbation, it may be difficult to resume exercises, but it usually is best that the person resume an established schedule as soon as possible. The person must conserve energy for priority activities.

**Referral/Consultation**

In some settings the nurse assumes responsibility for making referrals to other services. In the case of the patient with multiple sclerosis these referrals may include a social worker, psychiatric clinical nurse specialist, dietitian, or recreational therapist. Referring the patient to a local support group is very important.

## NURSING MANAGEMENT

### ♦ ASSESSMENT

Subjective and objective data are important in establishing the diagnosis.

#### Subjective Data

Data to be collected to assess the patient with multiple sclerosis include the following:

- Patient's understanding of disease
- Presence of eye problems
  - Diplopia
  - Scotomas
  - Blindness
- Presence of weakness or numbness of part of the body such as the hand
- Presence of unusual fatigue
- Presence of tremor
- Presence of emotional lability
- Presence of bowel and bladder problems
- Presence of impotence in men

#### Objective Data

Data to be collected to assess the patient with multiple sclerosis include the following:

- Documented abnormalities on neurologic examination:
  - Nystagmus
  - Scanning speech
  - Muscle weakness and spasms
  - Changes in coordination
  - Spastic ataxic gait
- Behavior: presence of euphoria
- Urinary incontinence, frequency, or urgency
- Difficulty in swallowing

#### Diagnostic Test Findings

The diagnosis of multiple sclerosis often involves the elimination of other causes for the symptoms experienced. Visual evoked potential testing may reveal abnormalities, and protein electrophoresis of the cerebral spinal fluid may provide fairly positive indications of a probable diagnosis.

### ♦ NURSING DIAGNOSES

Nursing diagnoses are determined from analysis of patient data. Nursing diagnoses for the patient with multiple sclerosis may include but are not limited to the following:

| Diagnostic Title | Possible Etiologic Factors |
|---|---|
| Disuse syndrome, high risk for | Immobility, weakness |
| Nutrition, altered: less than body requirements | Chewing/swallowing difficulties, inability to obtain food |
| Pain | Immobility, improper positioning, overactivity |
| Self-care deficit: feeding, bathing/hygiene, dressing/grooming, feeding, toileting | Intolerance to activity; fatigue, neuromuscular impairment |
| Mobility, impaired physical | Intolerance to activity; neuromuscular impairment |
| Coping, ineffective (individual) | Situational crises |
| Communication, impaired verbal | Physical impairment |
| Skin integrity, high risk for impaired | Prolonged immobility |
| Incontinence, functional | Sensory/cognitive/mobility deficits |
| Constipation | Immobility |
| Fatigue | Muscle weakness |
| Knowledge deficit (medications and daily care) | Lack of exposure/recall, unfamiliarity with information sources |

### ♦ EXPECTED PATIENT OUTCOMES

Expected patient outcomes for the patient with multiple sclerosis may include but are not limited to the following:

1. Prevents disuse syndrome as evidenced by the absence of contractures and the presence of normal range of motion.

2. Maintains nutritional status.
3. Has no complaints of pain or discomfort.
4. Maintains mobility.
5. Shows positive coping as evidenced by ability to stay active and maintain positive attitude.
6. Maintains communication and can express needs.
7. Maintains intact skin.
8. Has no urinary or bowel incontinence.
9. Does not complain of fatigue.
10. Can verbalize knowledge of medications (dose, effects and side effects, time to take, when to report to physician), as well as daily routine and care needed.

## ♦ INTERVENTIONS

### Preventing Disuse Syndrome

The patient with multiple sclerosis is at high risk for the development of disuse syndrome. Thus the nurse must constantly be aware of incorporating rehabilitation nursing concepts into the patient's care. Range-of-motion exercises are important, as well as positioning to prevent any contractures or skin breakdown. Each feature of the remaining discussion of nursing intervention has relevance in maintaining function and preventing disuse syndrome.

### Promoting Adequate Nutrition

A well-balanced diet with plenty of high-vitamin foods and fluids is important. Obesity must be avoided because it is more difficult for the obese person to maneuver, and this makes it more difficult to meet daily needs. High-fiber foods and prune juice may help to reduce constipation.

### Promoting Comfort

*Diplopia* can be relieved by an eye patch. Peripheral neurectomies, rhizotomies, and cordotomies often are used for the relief of *spasticity, pain,* and *parathesias.* Relief from severe spasticity often is obtained from intrathecal injections of phenol. In more severe cases of spasticity when contractures have developed, surgical release of tendons may be necessary, followed by application of a cast for a time.

### Maintaining Activities of Daily Living

The patient with multiple sclerosis is assisted with ADL. Often the patient is able to manage if activities are spaced throughout the day. The patient is cautioned against becoming too fatigued. Assisting the patient in learning to use energy-conservation techniques and aids can make a real difference. The occupational therapist often is helpful in assisting the patient with managing daily living activities.

### Maintaining Mobility

One side of the body usually is affected more than the other, and the person may learn to stabilize gait by leaning toward the uninvolved side. The annoyance of having the foot slap forward in taking a step sometimes can be overcome by putting the heel down in a pronounced fashion and rolling the weight forward on the side of the foot.

Effort is made to maintain activity and work for as long as possible, and many persons have worked for 5 to 10 years and even longer after the onset of the first symptoms. Women at home can be helped to plan their shopping, housework, and other duties so that they may continue to function as wives and mothers even when the disease is advanced.[12] Many persons with multiple sclerosis remain mobile with only mild to moderate disability.

### Facilitating Coping

Persons with multiple sclerosis need a peaceful, relaxed environment. They should never be hurried and should not be expected to respond quickly either physically or mentally. They may be slow in speaking and in responding, and this difficulty should be ignored by persons around them. Family members and friends need help in understanding this problem and in meeting it calmly. The person may have sudden, explosive emotional outbursts of crying or laughing brought on by such simple acts as putting something hot into the mouth. Close family members must protect both patient and visitors from the embarrassment of prolonged emotional outbursts. Reminding the patient of something sad may stop the laughing, and holding the mouth open will sometimes stop the crying.

### Promoting Communication

Problems in verbal communication may develop in persons with multiple sclerosis who nevertheless should be encouraged to express themselves through talking, even if this is difficult. The speech most often is described as scanning in nature. If the patient loses the ability to talk, compensatory measures should be instituted. These include the use of a communication board or a letter alphabet board. Sophisticated computers are available to patients who can afford them.

### Promoting Skin Integrity

Many persons with multiple sclerosis have motor involvement that prevents them from moving about and changing position easily. Also, they may experience sensory disturbances that affect how they sense pressure. As a result, these patients are especially prone to the development of decubiti. They must be taught the importance of turning at least every 2 to 3 hours. Air mattresses or other devices may be used to help prevent pressure, but it is important to note that no substitute exists for regular turning.

### Preventing Bladder Problems

Problems with urinary frequency and urgency, often the source of social disability, may respond to timed doses of propantheline bromide (Pro-Banthine). Prevention of urinary tract infection remains a problem, and such infections are a major cause of death. Cholinergic drugs such as bethanechol (Urecholine) may be of help in the patient with an atonic bladder. Oxybutynin chloride (Ditropan) is a newer drug used to treat neurogenic bladder. It acts by exerting a direct antispasmodic effect on smooth muscles. Some patients are placed on prophylactic doses of medications such as trimethoprim and sulfamethoxazole (Bactrim, Septra) or nitrofurantoin (Macrodantin) indefinitely. Cystometrographic study is important to detect the specific bladder problem.

### Preventing Bowel Problems

The most common bowel problems are constipation and incontinence. Constipation may be minimized with the use of a fiber-rich diet and adequate fluid intake (at least eight glasses of water per day). If needed, prunes or prune juice may be helpful. The use of a stool softener may be necessary. Suppositories can be used to train the bowel and encourage evacuation of stool. Enemas may be used as a last resort, but their chronic use may lead to loss of bowel tone and dependency on them.

If incontinence of the bowel occurs, a bowel training program should be started. The use of suppositories, as well as the other measures just mentioned, can help the patient develop a regular pattern of evacuation and prevent incontinence. A good nursing assessment should include the time the patient usually has a bowel movement. This knowledge is incorporated into the bowel training program.

### Preventing Fatigue

Hot baths should be avoided because the heat can increase weakness in the person with multiple sclerosis. (In some centers, patients have been treated with ice water baths.) Traveling in hot weather should be carefully planned to prevent travel during the warmest part of the day. It is essential that the patient and family members understand the importance of checking the skin routinely and taking measures to relieve tissue pressure.

### Facilitating Learning

Teaching is important for both patient and significant others. In the later stages of multiple sclerosis, all aspects of care may have to be assumed by someone other than the patient. The teaching needs include the following:

1. Use of medications, including side effects, dosage, timing, and desired effects
2. Importance of reporting side effects to the physician
3. Importance of good fluid intake
4. Importance of balancing activities to include relaxation and fun activities
5. Need for balanced diet
6. Range of motion (ROM) exercises
7. Safety factors to prevent injury
8. Positioning to prevent contractures and decubiti
9. Importance of skin inspection and how to do it
10. Importance of avoiding temperature extremes
11. Community resources and how to obtain them
12. Education about the disease, what can bring on symptoms, and how to manage them[12]

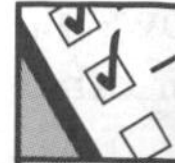

**Guidelines for Care of the Person With Multiple Sclerosis**

1. Promote activity:
   a. Maintain daily routine for rest and activity.
   b. Avoid fatigue.
   c. Maintain work and activity as long as possible.
   d. Conserve energy for priority activities.
2. Provide comfort:
   a. Use eye patch for diplopia.
   b. Take prescribed medications to relieve spasticity.
3. Prevent bladder problems:
   a. Take medications as prescribed.
   b. Drink adequate fluids.
   c. Provide intermittent catheterization if needed.
4. Prevent bowel problems:
   a. Eat fiber-rich diet
   b. Drink adequate fluids.
   c. Use stool softeners or suppositories if needed.
5. Promote adequate nutrition:
   a. Eat well-balanced meals.
   b. Encourage foods high in fiber.
   c. Avoid excessive fiber.
6. Control environment:
   a. Avoid extremes in temperature.
   b. Avoid stressful situations.
7. Promote communication:
   a. Encourage patient to talk.
   b. Use compensatory measures if needed.

The National Multiple Sclerosis Society* is a national voluntary, nonprofit organization founded in 1946. Its functions are to encourage and finance research, to gather statistics, and to act as an information center for patients and for the public. Some local chapters also supply equipment to patients. Membership is open to healthcare and welfare workers and to patients and their families. Local organizations can be found in many large cities. The care of the patient is summarized in the Guidelines box above.

## ♦ EVALUATION

To evaluate effectiveness of nursing interventions, compare patient behaviors with those stated in the expected patient outcomes. Successful achievement of patient outcomes for the patient with multiple sclerosis is indicated by the following:

1. Absence of contractures of any joints of the body and of thromboembolic events or loss of muscle mass.
2. Maintenance of usual body weight, with results of laboratory work (protein, hematocrit, and hemoglobin values) within normal limits.

*257 Park Ave South, New York, NY 10010.

3. States that pain is not present and shows no guarding, shallow breathing, grimacing, or other behaviors that indicate pain.
4. Maintains ability to ambulate, to transfer, and/or move freely in wheelchair.
5. Indicates a positive attitude and remains active.
6. Can communicate needs.
7. Has neither skin breakdown nor sustained redness of skin.
8. Experiences no bowel or bladder incontinence, with urination and defecation maintained on a regular schedule.
9. States that fatigue is not a problem; does not look tired.
10. Correctly describes medications, including dose, effects, side effects, and time to take; correctly explains when to report symptoms to physician; and correctly explains daily routine and care needed.

## COMPLICATIONS

The patient with multiple sclerosis is prone to many complications, especially infections and pressure sores. Bladder infections are common, especially with the presence of an indwelling catheter. Prevention of complications is discussed in the earlier part of this section.

## PARKINSON'S DISEASE (PARALYSIS AGITANS)

### Etiology/Epidemiology

**Parkinson's disease** is one of the more common diseases of the nervous system. It was first described in 1817 by James Parkinson. It affects both men and women in their middle and late years (50 to 60 years old) and is seen in all races and classes of persons. It is estimated to affect 100 to 150 persons per 100,000 population.

The cause is not known, but the cluster of symptoms was first observed in many patients after the 1916-1917 worldwide epidemic of encephalitis.

The characteristic symptoms of Parkinson's disease sometimes are found in patients with arteriosclerosis, leading some researchers to believe that arteriosclerosis may be a causative factor. Viral infections also have been suggested as a cause. Drug-induced parkinsonian syndromes have been linked with the phenothiazines, reserpine (Serpasil), and butyrophenones (e.g., haloperidol).

### Pathophysiology

The pathologic process that occurs with Parkinson's disease is basically a *depigmentation* of the *substantia nigra* of the basal ganglia. The loss of neurons in the substantia is severe. Also, selective depletion of dopamine occurs and can be correlated with the degree of striatal degeneration. Without dopamine, loss of inhibitory influence occurs and excitatory mechanisms are unopposed.

Parkinson's disease begins with a faint tremor and progresses so slowly that the person is seldom able to recall its onset. No true paralysis and no loss of sensation occurs. Tremor (pill rolling of the fingers or resting tremor) is the outstanding sign of the disease. Two other frequent signs are muscular weakness (with rigidity) and loss of postural reflexes. Parkinson's disease has some characteristics of upper motor neuron involvement (see Chapter 58). It is essentially a problem with motion. Muscle rigidity prevents normal response in frequently performed acts and leads to characteristic changes that make the diagnosis almost unmistakable to persons who have observed patients with the disease.

There is a masklike appearance to the face and slowed, monotonous speech. Drooling may occur because of difficulty in swallowing saliva. This may cause skin irritation, which is best prevented or treated by frequent sponging followed by protecting the skin with an emollient such as cold cream. There is a characteristic shuffling gait in which patients tend to walk on their toes. The trunk is bent forward, and the arms fall rigidly to the sides and do not swing in normal rhythmic gait. Neuromuscular control may be altered so that the patient is unable to stop this propulsive gait until an obstruction is met. The patient usually has moist, oily skin. Defects in judgment and emotional instability may occur, but intelligence is not impaired. The appetite may be increased, and heat intolerance occurs. A decrease in blinking is seen. Fatigue is a common complaint, and pain in the arms or shoulder may be present. All signs and symptoms increase with fatigue, excitement, and frustration. As the disease progresses, the severity of symptoms increases. More and more symptoms develop. Patients with Parkinson's disease usually die of other causes, most often pulmonary or renal disease.

### Prevention

Because the cause of Parkinson's disease is not known, primary prevention is difficult to achieve. With patients who have drug-induced symptoms, the judicious use of these drugs along with the use of anticholinergic drugs, such as benztropine mesylate (Cogentin) and trihexyphenidyl hydrochloride (Artane), may be helpful in preventing worsening symptoms.

Early detection (secondary prevention) is important, as is prevention of complications (tertiary prevention).

### Medical Management

#### Diagnostic tests

No test is diagnostic of Parkinson's disease. The clinical examination and history, along with the patient's response to administration of medication used to treat the disease, confirm the diagnosis.

#### Medication

Treatment for Parkinson's disease is palliative and symptomatic and depends on the pharmacologic manipulation of the pathophysiologic state. The severity of symptoms and presence of associated disease processes determine the drugs to be used. Anticholinergic alkaloids such as scopolamine hydrobromide and related drugs (hyoscyamine) have been used for more than a century. They act against cholinergic excitatory effects and are more effective in lessening muscle rigidity than in controlling tremor. Many synthetic anticholinergic drugs of varied chemical structure also are available. There is little to recommend one over the other, aside from personal preference, but each has some degree of central nervous system (CNS) anticholinergic action. However, they are incapable of restoring striatal balance. The preferred anticholinergic agents are trihexyphenidyl, benztropine, procyclidine (Kemadrin), and biperiden (Akineton). These drugs have some selectivity of action in that they have greater central than peripheral anticholinergic activity. Optimal results from these drugs depend on a dosage that provides a compromise between the limited symptomatic improvement given by these drugs and the disagreeable symptoms of central and peripheral cholinergic blockade (blurring of vision, dryness of mouth and throat, constipation, urinary urgency or retention, ataxia, dysarthria, mental disturbances). Antihistaminic drugs such as diphenhydramine (Benadryl), which are not primarily anticholinergic, exert mild central anticholinergic properties when used alone or in combination with other drugs.

Some patients with severe Parkinson's disease for whom anticholinergic drugs provided little relief have experienced dramatic benefits from levodopa. Levodopa assists in restoring striatal dopamine deficiency because it is a precursor of dopamine. This drug does not affect the underlying process of parkinsonism. In this way, levodopa acts more as replacement drug than a cure. Once benefits are obtained for levodopa, they are likely to be sustained. After prolonged periods of treatment, side effects may increase, and the effectiveness of the medication may decrease. The dosage usually is increased gradually but cannot be increased indefinitely. It has been found helpful to admit some patients into the hospital for a "drug holiday" during which all medications are withdrawn for 7 to 10 days. The medications are then restarted, and often much smaller doses can produce favorable results. This drug holiday must take place within the hospital setting, however, because of the danger of aspiration pneumonia or other complictions that can occur, because the immobility, rigidity, and other signs and symptoms will return when the drugs are withdrawn. Usually patients remain on anticholinergic drug therapy, or these may be added as an adjunct. Most persons experience side effects from levodopa, such as nausea and vomiting, orthostatic hypotension, insomnia, agitation, and mental confusion, but these lessen with continued medication and dosage modification.

Kidney and liver damage have occurred in some patients taking levodopa. Candidates for levodopa should be selected carefully. Amantadine hydrochloride (Symmetrel), an antiviral agent, is known to have antiparkinsonian activity. It acts by blocking the reuptake and storage of catecholamines and allowing the accumulation of dopamine in extracellular or synaptic sites. This drug may not sustain its effectiveness for more than 3 months in some patients. Side effects, although infrequent, include mental confusion, visual disturbances, and seizures.

Carbidopa-levodopa (Sinemet) is being used more often in neurologic practice. It is a combination of levodopa with an inhibitor of the enzyme dopa decarboxylase, which limits the metabolism of levodopa peripherally and provides more levodopa for the brain. Reduction in peripheral metabolism by the enzyme dopa decarboxylase results in more levodopa being available to be converted to dopamine in the brain. Therefore more beneficial effects occur with fewer side effects.

Table 57-9 lists the drugs used to treat Parkinson's disease.

#### Treatment

There is no specific treatment for the patient with Parkinson's disease.

#### Diet

There is no special diet for the patient with Parkinson's disease. The emphasis is on a well-balanced diet in the consistency that the patient can tolerate.

#### Activity

Special attention should be paid to *posture*. Lying on a firm bed without a pillow during rest periods may help to prevent the spine from bending forward, and lying in the prone position also helps. Holding the hands folded behind the back when walking may help to keep the spine erect and prevent the annoyance of the arms falling stiffly at the sides. The tremor often is less apparent when persons are sitting in an armchair, because they can grip the arms of the chair and partially control the tremor in their hands and arms. (See Chapter 65 for a discussion of alterations of movement and posture.)

The patient with Parkinson's disease should continue to work as long as possible. Most physicians advise this unless the occupation is such that continued work is dangerous.

#### Referral/Consultation

In some settings the nurse assumes responsibility for making referrals to other services. For the patient with Parkinson's disease this may include a referral to a social worker or dietitian. Referral of the patient and the significant other to a local support group is helpful.

### Surgical Management

In most cases, medical care of the patient with Parkinson's disease involves the use of medication. However,

**TABLE 57-9 Medications Used in Parkinson's Disease**

| MEDICATION | ACTION/EFFECTS | SIDE EFFECTS | COMMENTS |
|---|---|---|---|
| Levodopa | Assists in restoring striatal dopamine deficiency | Kidney, liver damage<br>Nausea, vomiting<br>Orthostatic hypotension<br>Insomnia<br>Agitation and mental confusion | Side effects common |
| Carbidopa-levodopa (levodopa with inhibitor of the decarboxylase) (Sinemet) | Inhibitor limits metabolism of levodopa peripherally and provides more levodopa to brain | Same as for levodopa | Fewer side effects than with levodopa used alone |
| Amantadine hydrochloride (Symmetrel) | Acts by blocking the reuptake and storage of catecholamines and allowing accumulation of dopamine in extracellular or synaptic sites | Mental confusion<br>Visual disturbances<br>Seizures | May not be effective for longer than 3 months |
| Synthetic anticholinergic drugs<br>Trihexyphenidyl (Artane)<br>Benztropine mesylate (Cogentin)<br>Procyclidine (Kemadrin)<br>Biperiden (Akineton) | Some degree of CNS anticholinergic action, but incapable of restoring striatal balance | Same as for anticholinergic drugs | Same for anticholinergic drugs |
| Antihistamine drugs<br>Diphenhydramine (Benadryl) | Exert mild central anticholinergic properties | Sleepiness<br>Dry mouth | Does not affect underlying process of Parkinson's disease |
| Anticholinergic drugs<br>Scopolamine hydrochloride<br>Hyoscyamine | Act against cholinergic excitatory effects<br>More effective in lessening muscle rigidity than in controlling tremor | Central and peripheral cholinergic actions<br>Blurring of vision<br>Dryness of mouth and throat<br>Constipation<br>Urinary retention or urgency<br>Ataxia<br>Dysarthria<br>Mental disturbances | Optimal results depend on dosage that provides compromise between improvement and development of side effects |

a surgical procedure has been used with some success in the treatment of selected patients. Descriptions of successful surgery in popular magazines have led some patients and their families to believe that a cure for all patients has been found. Many patients cannot be treated surgically. Results seem to be best in younger patients who have unilateral involvement and who have severe tremor and rigidity. Treatment consists of destroying portions of the ***globus pallidus*** (relieves rigidity) or the ***thalamus*** (relieves tremor) in the brain by stereotactic methods through the use of cautery, removal, or injection of alcohol. Surgical techniques involving cooling or freezing with liquid nitrogen (cryogenic surgery) have been attempted with good results in selected patients and with fewer complications than when cautery or alcohol was used. Medications used to control rigidity and tremor are discontinued several days before surgery so that symptoms will be at their peak during surgery. Preoperative nursing care includes seeing that nutrition is adequate, as well as other preoperative care.

Postoperative care includes the most careful attention

## RESEARCH

Freed C et al: Survival of implanted fetal dopamine cells and neurologic improvement 12 to 46 months after transplantation for Parkinson's disease, *N Engl J Med* 327(22):1549-1555, 1992.

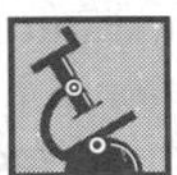

In an effort to modify the disability of persons with advanced Parkinson's disease, embryonic mesencephalic tissue containing dopamine cells was implanted into the caudate and putamen of seven patients. In six of the seven patients the fetal tissue was obtained from a single embryo with a gestational age of 6 to 7 weeks. On the basis of activities of daily living scale all patients reported improvement 3 to 12 months after surgery. Results of neurologic examination according to the unified disease rating scale showed that five of the seven patients improved 6 months after surgery. Fluctuations in the patients' clinical state had moderated, and periods of dyskinesia and "off" episodes, which occur in patients on levodopa, were shorter and less severe than before implantation. Both immunosuppressed and nonimmunosuppressed patients improved, and drug dosages were reduced by an average of 33%.

to the vital signs; use of side rails to prevent accidents in the event of convulsions, disorientation, or temporary hemiplegia; and frequent turning and moving to prevent respiratory and circulatory complications. Excessive salivation and difficulty in blinking the eye on the surgically treated side may be problems requiring nursing attention.

A relatively new and still experimental treatment for Parkinson's disease is the adrenal medullary transplant (see Research box, p. 1974). In this procedure tissue from the adrenal medulla is placed in contact with the substantia nigra with the hope of restoring the balance of dopamine and acetylcholine. The procedure is difficult because the patient undergoes three major surgeries at the same time: (1) stereotactic localization of the caudate nucleus, (2) craniotomy, and (3) laporotomy for the adrenalectomy. Results so far have been somewhat encouraging.[8]

## NURSING MANAGEMENT

### ♦ ASSESSMENT

#### Subjective Data

Subjective data to be collected to assess the patient with Parkinson's disease include the following:

- Patient's understanding of disease
- Complaints of fatigue
- Presence of incoordination
- Defects in judgment and emotional instability
- Heat insensitivity

#### Objective Data

Objective data to be collected to assess the patient with Parkinson's disease include the following:

- Presence of tremor (pill-rolling motion of the fingers or resting tremor)
- Muscular response to movement
- Postural reflexes
- Appearance of face, including skin
- Presence of drooling
- Gait disturbances
- Abnormal findings on sensory testing
- Inability to carry out daily activities

#### Diagnostic Test Findings

The diagnosis of Parkinson's disease is made on the basis of the CT scan, which may indicate atrophy of the brain. A trial on medication with an improvement in the symptoms also is indicative of the disease. The presence of physical symptoms such as cogwheel rigidity and pill-rolling movements is used primarily to make the diagnosis. Results of diagnostic tests rule out other pathologic conditions.

### ♦ NURSING DIAGNOSES

Nursing diagnoses for the patient with Parkinson's disease are the same as those for patients with multiple sclerosis, with the addition of the following:

| Diagnostic Title | Possible Etiologic Factors |
|---|---|
| Aspiration, high risk for | Upper motor neuron lesion |

### ♦ EXPECTED PATIENT OUTCOMES

The reader is referred to the patient outcomes for the patient with multiple sclerosis on p. 1969 with the following additional outcome:

Will not experience aspiration.

### ♦ INTERVENTIONS

#### Preventing Aspiration

*Feeding* the patient becomes a real problem when the disease is far advanced because of the *danger of choking* in attempts to swallow; eventually, aspiration pneumonia may terminate the patient's life. Unless the patient's condition is well controlled by medication, drooling can be a problem and increases with general excitement. A bib can be used to protect the clothing during napping hours. When patients are dressed, garments with generous pockets that are well supplied with soft tissues will help them be less conspicuous and more comfortable. Speech pathologist, nutritionist, nurses, and/or dysphagia team may be consulted to evaluate and assist with determining techniques to reduce dysphagia (difficulty swallowing).

### ♦ EVALUATION

To evaluate the effectiveness of interventions, the behavior of the patient with Parkinson's disease is compared with expected outcomes. Successful achievement of the outcome is indicated by the patient not experiencing aspiration.

## MYASTHENIA GRAVIS

### Etiology/Epidemiology

**Myasthenia gravis** is a relatively rare disease of unknown cause. It usually occurs in young adults and is thought to have a link with autoimmune reactions. It affects about 1 in 20,000 persons. In young persons, women are more often affected than men, but among older persons the distribution between the genders is about equal. Occurrence within families is rare; however, infants of affected mothers may have symptoms at birth, but these symptoms usually disappear within several weeks.

### Pathophysiology

With myasthenia gravis, no observable structural change occurs in the muscle or nerve. Nerve impulses fail to pass to muscles at the *myoneural junction.* It is not known specifically why the motor nerve impulses fail to pass the muscle and cause it not to contract. Suggested causes include (1) the inability of the motor end plate to secrete adequate acetylcholine, (2) excessive quantities of the cholinesterase enzyme at the nerve ending, and (3) nonresponse of the muscle fibers to acetylcholine. Relative to the third theory, myasthenia gravis may be considered a primary muscle disease; relative to the first two theories, it is a neuromuscular disease with lower motor neuron characteristics. About 25% of patients with myasthenia gravis have been found to have thymoma, and almost 80% have changes in the cellular structure of the thymus gland. Myasthenia gravis is considered a serious disorder because the respiratory muscles and the bulbar cranial nerves may be involved. During periods of exacerbation or lack of drug control, the patient may have to be cared for in a respiratory intensive care unit.

The outstanding symptoms of myasthenia gravis are muscle weakness and severe generalized fatigue. These symptoms come on quickly and are usually more evident in the evening. In the early stages of the disease, the symptoms disappear quickly with rest.[46] Weakness of arm and hand muscles first may be noticed when the person shaves or combs the hair. Facial muscles innervated by the cranial nerves often are affected, and it may not be possible for the person to hold the eyelids open (ptosis), to keep the mouth closed, or to chew or swallow. Diplopia (double vision) is also common. As the disease progresses, the trunk and lower limbs are affected, leading to difficulty with walking and sustained sitting. Usually the distal muscles are not as affected as the proximal muscles. Muscle weakness may become so severe that the person cannot breathe without assistance. Exacerbations of the disease may be initiated by upper respiratory infections, emotional tension, and menstruation.

#### Eaton-Lambert syndrome

The **Eaton-Lambert syndrome** is a condition associated with cancer that has many of the same symptoms as myasthenia gravis. It is important to differentiate between the two diseases. *The Eaton-Lambert syndrome is a special form of myasthenia that is found almost invariably in persons with oat cell carcinoma of the lung.* In this syndrome the muscles of the trunk, as well as those of the pelvic and shoulder girdles, are the ones most frequently affected by weakness, fatigue, and atrophy. Visual symptoms occur less frequently. Increasing weakness occurs after exertion, but muscle power may increase temporarily at first.

The onset of the Eaton-Lambert syndrome usually is insidious and the course progressive. Because the myasthenia may precede discovery of the lung tumor by months or years, it is important that a thorough check for a malignancy be performed at regular intervals. In addition to oat cell carcinoma of the lung, the syndrome has occurred with carcinoma of the rectum, stomach, prostate, and breast.

Table 57-10 compares myasthenia gravis and Eaton-Lambert syndrome.

**TABLE 57-10 Comparison of Myasthenia Gravis and Eaton-Lambert Syndrome**

| MYASTHENIA GRAVIS | EATON-LAMBERT SYNDROME |
|---|---|
| **ONSET** | |
| Slow and insidious | Slow and insidious |
| **VISION** | |
| Diplopia common | Diplopia not as common |
| **MUSCLE INVOLVEMENT** | |
| Cranial nerves, arms and hands, trunk and lower limbs affected (difficulty with walking and sitting); distal muscles not as affected as proximal muscles | Muscles of trunk, as well as those of pelvic and shoulder girdle, are most often involved |
| **WEAKNESS** | |
| Weakness and generalized fatigue that comes on quickly | Increased weakness with exertion, but temporary increase in muscle power may occur initially |

### Prevention

No known form of primary prevention exists for patients with myasthenia gravis. As noted, some patients have been found to have a thymoma. Surgical removal may decrease the symptoms of the disease or result in almost complete recovery.

As with all neurologic diseases, secondary and tertiary prevention is important.

### Medical Management

Medical management involves the use of medication. In persons who have thymomas, surgical removal of the thyoma often decreases the symptoms.

During acute exacerbations of the disease, and when the respiratory status is compromised, the patient may require intubation and mechanical ventilation. A tracheostomy may be necessary (see Chapter 36).

#### Diagnostic tests

Because of the slow, insidious onset and occurrence of symptoms with stress, myasthenia gravis sometimes is misdiagnosed as hysteria or neurosis. The diagnosis can be made partly on the basis of electromyography (EMG). A specific diagnostic test is the edrophonium chloride (Tensilon) test. In this test, Tensilon (a very short–acting anticholinesterase drug) is injected intravenously. When increased strength in a predetermined muscle group is seen, test findings are considered positive. To obtain true results, it is important that the patient not know when the medication is being given.

The procedure for the test is as follows:

1. Edrophonium and normal saline are drawn up in separate syringes.

2. Each is injected intravenously separately.
3. It is important that the patient not know which solution is being administered.
4. Increased strength in a predetermined muscle group with the administration of edophonium is a positive test reaction.

### Medication

No known cure exits for myasthenia gravis. However, great improvement follows the use of neostigmine (Prostigmin) or pyridostigmine (Mestinon). These drugs block the action of cholinesterase at the myoneural junction and allow acetylcholine, a chemical necessary for transmission of impulses to the muscles, to act. Acetylcholine is the neurotransmitter between postganglionic parasympathetic fibers and receptor organs. Atropine or some other anticholinergic agent that blocks these *muscarinic effects* of acetylcholine may be used to treat the side effects of neostigmine and pyridostigmine. Treatment is planned so that the patient can continue to receive the amount of drug that can be tolerated without side effects and yet carry out activities essential for normal living. Usually the patient is permitted to adjust the dosage. *The nurse should teach the importance of taking medications at the time prescribed.* If the drug is delayed, dyspnea may result, followed by severe respiratory depression, which, if untreated, can cause death.

It is important also to teach that (1) dosage is individually determined and related to the person's activity, (2) dosage needs to be adjusted to maintain muscle strength, and (3) the effects of drugs need to be monitored. The nurse and family must understand that it is often difficult to distinguish between *myasthenic crisis* (too little drug) and *cholinergic crisis* (too much drug) inasmuch as both conditions cause severe muscle weakness. Tensilon administered intravenously is used to differentiate between the two conditions. A positive test result (increase in strength) usually indicates underdosage of medication. An increase in weakness when Tensilon is administered may be a sign of overdosage. Drugs to be avoided are listed in Box 57-8. Because of the effects of these drugs on the myoneural junction, they can potentiate the weakness associated with myasthenia gravis.

**BOX 57-8 Drugs To Be Avoided by Persons With Myasthenia Gravis**

- Muscle relaxants
- Barbiturates
- Morphine sulfate
- Tranquilizers
- Neomycin (potentiates muscle weakness because of effect on myoneural junction)

## NURSING MANAGEMENT

## ♦ ASSESSMENT

Both subjective and objective data are important to collect from the patient with myasthenia gravis.

### Subjective Data

Subjective data to be collected to assess the patient with myasthenia gravis include the following:

Patient's understanding of disease
Fatigue—when it occurs and where it occurs
Profound muscle weakness
Presence of diplopia
Difficulty in keeping eyelids open and mouth closed or difficulty in chewing and swallowing
Effect of stress on symptoms
Patient's perception of muscle weakness

### Objective Data

Objective data to be collected to assess patient with myasthenia gravis include the following:

Documented muscle weakness on neurologic testing
Presence of ptosis of eyelids
Documented weight loss
Breath sounds that are diminished
Muscle atrophy

### Diagnostic Test Findings

A positive finding on the Tensilon test indicates a diagnosis of myasthenia gravis. Results of the EMG also may be abnormal.

## ♦ NURSING DIAGNOSES

Nursing diagnoses are determined from analysis of patient data. Nursing diagnoses for the patient with myasthenia gravis may include but are not limited to the following:

| Diagnostic Title | Possible Etiologic Factors |
|---|---|
| Gas exchange, impaired | Ventilation/perfusion imbalance |
| Activity intolerance, high risk for | Immobility, generalized weakness |
| Knowledge deficit: importance of preventing respiratory infections, taking medications | Lack of exposure/recall, unfamiliarity with information sources |

## ♦ EXPECTED PATIENT OUTCOMES

Expected patient outcomes for the patient with myasthenia gravis may include but are not limited to the following:

1. Maintains gas exchange as evidenced by a pulse oximetry reading of at least 90%.
2. Maintains activity levels as evidenced by the ability to carry out daily routines for as long as possible.
3. Will be able to state knowledge of health that includes importance of preventing respiratory infections and taking medications on schedule.

## ♦ INTERVENTIONS

### Promoting Adequate Ventilation

Respiratory problems typically occur in patients with myasthenia gravis. For this reason they usually are advised not to live alone. Upper respiratory infections occur because patients may not have the energy needed to cough effectively and pneumonia or airway obstruction may develop. Aspiration often occurs. Many patients keep airway equipment at their bedside at home.

During acute episodes of the disease, the patient will require hospitalization. The following are important measures to be taken:

1. Tracheostomy equipment at bedside because respiratory status may change suddenly
2. Serial determinations of vital capacity, minute volumes, and tidal volumes
3. Suction as necessary
4. Nasogastric tube if swallowing is too dangerous

Care must be taken that the nasogastric tube is in the stomach before fluid is introduced, because the patient cannot cough to indicate presence of fluid in the trachea.

### Promoting Mobility/Activity

Persons with myasthenia gravis may have to change daily patterns of activity. The nurse can help the patient and family plan so that minimal energy is used in activities that are essential to remaining relatively self-sufficient and yet allow energy for activities in which the patient wishes to take part.

### Facilitating Learning

The patient with myasthenia gravis usually is able to adjust the medication depending on the symptoms. Also, the patient can have much control over preventing respiratory complications. Therefore teaching is very important and should include the following:

1. Importance of taking medication at time prescribed
2. How to adjust dose to maintain muscle strength
3. Side effects and how to monitor
4. Medications to avoid
5. Importance of seeking medical attention at first sign of upper respiratory infections
6. Importance of eating only when sitting up
7. Avoiding crowds in flu and cold season
8. How to adjust to daily activities to allow for activities and rest periods
9. Planning to use minimal energy in activities that are essential, so that energy may be conserved for activities that patient enjoys

## ♦ EVALUATION

To evaluate effectiveness of nursing interventions, compare patient behaviors with those stated in the expected patient outcomes. Successful achievement of patient outcomes for the patient with myasthenia gravis is indicated by the following:

1. Shows no signs of respiratory distress, has pulse oximetry readings of at least 90%, and maintains regular rate and rhythm of respirations.
2. Indicates ability to carry out ADL and is observed in maintaining daily routines.
3. Correctly describes importance of (a) preventing respiratory infections, (b) receiving timely medical care for upper respiratory infections, (c) practicing health habits to minimize infections, and (d) taking medications on schedule, providing description of medications, including dosage, effects, and side effects.

## AMYOTROPHIC LATERAL SCLEROSIS

**Amyotrophic lateral sclerosis (ALS)** is a motor neuron disease that affects upper or lower motor neurons lying within the brain or spinal cord or a combination of the two.

### Etiology/Epidemiology

ALS sometimes is called Lou Gehrig's disease because the famous New York Yankee ballplayer died of the disease. It affects men more than women. It usually occurs in middle age but may occur in younger persons. Some believe a familial or genetic component to ALS exists. The cause is unknown, but a slow viral infection has been suggested as the causative agent.

### Pathophysiology

Myelin sheaths are destroyed and are replaced by scar tissue in ALS. The lateral tracts of the spinal cord are directly involved, with possible eventual involvement of the medulla and the ventral tracts. The nerve impulses are distorted or blocked. Symptoms depend on whether lower or upper motor neurons are affected.

Early symptoms of ALS include fatigue and awkwardness of fine finger movements and muscle wasting. Dysphagia may be the first symptom in many persons. *Progressive muscle weakness, atrophy,* and *fasciculations* occur. Spasticity of flexor muscles is typically present. With involvement of the brainstem and medulla, dysphagia, dysarthria, jaw clonus, tongue fasciculations, and respiratory difficulty are present. As the disease progresses, disability is relative to both upper and lower limbs, and one side of the body becomes more involved than the other. The person remains alert. No sensory loss occurs with the disease. Death usually ensues within 5 to 10 years, generally from respiratory or bulbar paralysis.

### Prevention

No cause for ALS is known; thus primary prevention cannot be implemented. However, prompt diagnosis (secondary prevention) and prevention of complications (tertiary prevention) remain extremely important.

### Medical Management

The goal for discharge of patients with amyotrophic lateral sclerosis is determined in part by the reason for hospitalization. The nurse works collaboratively with the physician for implementation of prescribed medical therapy. Because the nurse has a major role in discharge planning and patient teaching, these are discussed under nursing management.

The medical management of ALS is mainly directed toward symptom relief. As the disease progresses, surgical intervention to place a gastrostomy tube may be necessary.

#### Diagnostic tests

Initial testing for ALS may include an EMG (see Chapter 56) to rule out other muscle diseases. No definitive test exists for ALS.

## NURSING MANAGEMENT

### ♦ ASSESSMENT

#### Subjective Data

Subjective data to be collected to assess the patient with ALS include the following:

- Patient's understanding of the disease
- Presence of fatigue
- Presence of dysphagia
- Difficulty with tasks involving finger movement

#### Objective Data

Objective data to be collected to assess the patient with ALS include the following:

- Inability to carry out ADLs
- Muscle abnormalities on testing
- Evidence of involvement of brainstem and medulla
- Weight loss

### ♦ NURSING DIAGNOSES

Nursing diagnoses are determined from analysis of patient data. Nursing diagnoses for the patient with ALS include those for the patient with multiple sclerosis (see p. 1969), as well as the following:

| Diagnostic Title | Possible Etiologic Factors |
|---|---|
| Airway clearance, ineffective | Decreased energy/fatigue, tracheobronchial infection |

### ♦ EXPECTED PATIENT OUTCOMES

Expected patient outcomes for the patient with ALS may include but are not limited to the following:

1. Will maintain an effective airway clearance.
2. Will not experience respiratory distress.

### ♦ INTERVENTIONS

#### Promoting Effective Airway Clearance

As ALS progresses, the patient typically experiences increased difficulty in maintaining a clear airway. Aspiration often occurs. The patient should be taught to use a tucked chin position while eating or drinking to encourage more effective swallowing. Because the cough is weak, the person may not be able to clear the airway by coughing. A suction machine may be necessary. Many patients learn to suction themselves using a tonsillar suction tip.

#### Facilitating Adjustment

Emotional support is extremely important. Patients with ALS and their families should be involved in making decisions about the types of interventions that will be used as the disease progresses. Some patients will decide to use ventilators at home as respiratory muscles become involved, whereas other patients will decide not to use any supportive devices. Patients and families need help and support in making decisions about how they are going to live their lives from the time the diagnosis is made until the disease causes the patient's complete dependency on others. Referral to local support group of ALS patients and families may be helpful. Whatever decisions the patient and family make must be supported by the health care team. Because the patient remains alert until the end, nurses should not forget that they are caring for a person who is probably very afraid of what lies ahead. Patients should be helped to retain some control over their treatment as long as possible.[30]

Treatment is directed toward relieving the symptoms of the disease. Nursing interventions include assistance with ADL as limb deficits increase. Prostheses often are applied to support the weakened muscles. Providing adequate nutrition can be a real challenge. As swallowing becomes more difficult, a nasogastric or gastrostomy tube may be necessary.[50]

### ♦ EVALUATION

To evaluate the effectiveness of nursing interventions, compare patient behaviors with those stated in the expected patient outcomes. Successful achievement of patient outcomes for the patient with ALS is indicated by the following:

1. Clears airway by coughing or self-suctioning.
2. Has no respiratory distress.

## ALZHEIMER'S DISEASE

### Etiology/Epidemiology

**Alzheimer's disease** is a degenerative disorder that affects the cells of the brain and causes impairment of intellectual functioning. According to the Alzheimer's Disease Association, it is the fourth leading cause of death among elderly persons in the United States, resulting in more than 10,000 deaths annually. It affects an estimated 4 million persons each year. Most cases occur in persons over age 60 years; however, some persons in their 40s and 50s are affected. The incidence of Alzheimer's disease greatly increases with age. About 10% of persons aged 65 years and older have the disease.

The incidence increases to 20% in those aged 75 to 84 years and to nearly 50% in those aged 85 years and older. It affects all segments of the population and is not restricted to any one race, gender, or socioeconomic class.

The cost of treatment for those affected with Alzheimer's disease in the United States has reached $90 billion a year. The care of patients at home costs the average family $18,000 to $20,000 per year. Nursing home care often costs $3000/month or $36,000/year.

The cause of Alzheimer's disease is not known. Genetic factors, viral agents, and environmental toxins are all under investigation for the role they might play in causing onset of the disease.

## Pathophysiology

The changes in the brain of the patient with Alzheimer's disease are visible in the cerebral cortex. The first change is the presence of microscopic "plaques" found in brain tissue. These plaques consist of a core surrounded by strands of fiberlike material. In addition, there is degeneration of some of the small fibers (neurofibrils) that run through the body of the nerve cells. These changes were first discovered in 1907 by the German neurologist Alzheimer. It is now known that these plaques are made up of a number of substances, one component of which is a fibrous protein called *beta-amyloid.* Researchers in the United States, Canada, and Japan are studying beta-amyloid and its relationship to Alzheimer's disease.

The diagnosis of Alzheimer's disease usually is made after other conditions in which memory loss occurs have been ruled out, such as the following:

- Pernicious anemia
- Drug reactions
- Hormonal imbalances
- Depression
- Drug or alcohol abuse
- Brain tumor
- Chronic meningitis
- Head trauma
- Pick's disease
- Parkinson's disease with dementia

The patient with Alzheimer's disease goes through rather distinct clinical stages (see Box 57-9 for details of a three-stage model).

Also cited is a *four*-stage progression of Alzheimer's disease:

Stage 1—mild memory lapses, difficulty with attention span, little interest in immediate surroundings or personal affairs

Stage 2—obvious short-term memory lapses, great hesitancy in verbal responses with confabulation to hide memory problems, disoriented to time, frequent losses of objects

Stage 3—disintegration of personality; disoriented to self, time, and place; apraxia; wandering behavior

Stage 4—terminal stage with severe physical and mental deterioration, incontinence, loss of ability to communicate, no recognition of family or self, swallowing problems

**BOX 57-9 Clinical Stages of Alzheimer's Disease**

**STAGE ONE**

Mild mental impairment
Forgetfulness
Impairment in judgment
Lessening of initiative
Lack of spontaneity

**STAGE TWO**

Confusion
Agitation
Irritability
Extreme restlessness
Incontinence of urine and stool
Need for constant supervision

**STAGE THREE**

Total inability to care for self
Inability to communicate
Total incontinence

Although the signs and symptoms of Alzheimer's disease occur progressively, the rate at which they occur varies from person to person. A few patients have a very rapid decline, but usually many months pass with little change. As the condition progresses, pneumonia or other illnesses are more likely to develop and may cause death.

## Prevention

No known preventive measure or practice exists for Alzheimer's disease. Much of the focus of research includes finding a cause so that prevention can be implemented.

## Medical Management

The care of the patient with Alzheimer's disease can be frustrating for the physician because the treatment options are so limited. Often, medication makes the problem worse. No currently known medical treatment will improve the condition of the patient with Alzheimer's disease.

### Diagnostic tests

No diagnostic test is specific for Alzheimer's disease. A computed tomography (CT) scan often is obtained to rule out other abnormalities. Neuropsychologic testing usually can reveal characteristic changes in the ability to think.

### Medication

Tacrine is one drug currently being evaluated in the treatment of Alzheimer's disease. It was first used in the

## RESEARCH

Davis K et al: A double-blind, placebo-controlled multicenter study of tacrine for Alzheimer's disease, *N Engl J Med* 327(18):1253-1259, 1992.

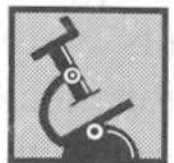

Tacrine, a cholinesterase inhibitor (1, 2, 3, 4-tetrahydro-9-acridinamine monohydrochloride monohydrate) was given to a sample of patients with probable Alzheimer's disease. The 215 patients were randomly assigned to receive either a placebo or their usual dose of tacrine in a 6-week, double-blind study. At the end of the 6 weeks the patients who had received tacrine had a smaller decline in cognitive function and in ADL than did the control group. The primary measures used to assess the changes were the cognitive subscale of the Alzheimer's Disease Assessment Scale and the Clinical Global Impression of Change Scale, as well as the Mini-Mental State Examination and the assessment of activities of daily living.

1940s in Australia in combination with morphine to lessen respiratory depression without affecting the analgesia.[14] (See Research box above, for results of a study of tacrine.)

## NURSING MANAGEMENT

### ♦ ASSESSMENT

#### Subjective Data

Subjective data to be collected to assess the patient with Alzheimer's disease include the following:

Patient's understanding of the disease
Change in mental status noticed by patient or family
Onset of symptoms

#### Objective Data

Objective data to be collected to assess the patient with Alzheimer's disease include the following:

Inability to carry out ADL
Behavior—evidence of agitation or restlessness
Presence of incontinence
Demonstrated change in mental status assessment

#### Diagnostic Test Findings

There is no specific test that indicates the presence of Alzheimer's disease. Research is ongoing in this area. At this time conclusive proof exists only at the time of autopsy when brain tissue can be examined. The diagnosis of Alzheimer's disease in the live patient is made by ruling out other pathologic conditions and by examining the family history for other cases of Alzheimer's disease. Many family members of patients with Alzheimer's disease are cooperating with research centers. This cooperation may include an autopsy at the time of the patient's death.

### ♦ NURSING DIAGNOSES

Nursing diagnoses are determined from analysis of patient data. Nursing diagnoses for the patient with Alzheimer's disease include those for the patient with multiple sclerosis (see p. 1969), as well as the following:

| Diagnostic Title | Possible Etiologic Factors |
|---|---|
| Injury, (trauma), high risk for | Sensory/motor deficits, lack of awareness of environmental hazards |
| Sleep-pattern disturbance | Anxiety, environmental changes |
| Violence, high risk for: self-directed or directed at others | Inability to control behavior, sensory/perceptual alterations |

### ♦ EXPECTED PATIENT OUTCOMES

Expected patient outcomes for the patient with Alzheimer's disease may include but are not limited to the following:

1. Will experience no injuries.
2. Will sleep at least 6 hours per night.
3. Will not harm others.

In many cases the person with Alzheimer's disease is mentally incompetent; thus the caregiver must be closely involved in planning for the outcomes. The patient may not be able to have real input in the outcomes.

### ♦ INTERVENTIONS

#### Preventing Injury

It is important to protect the patient with Alzheimer's disease from injury. It may be necessary to install double locks on doors and windows to prevent the patient from wandering when there is no supervision; for example, this often occurs during the middle of the night. Controls on stoves may need to be removable to prevent the person from turning them on and possibly causing a fire. Matches should be stored in an inaccessible place, as should any poisonous fluids. The patient should be supervised at all times.[3]

The Research box, p. 1982, left, indicates the relationship between cognitive impairment and wandering.

Patients with Alzheimer's disease may seem to have unlimited energy. They engage in many repetitive behaviors, such as walking for long periods or folding linens over and over. This activity should be somewhat encouraged because it keeps affected persons healthy for a longer time and tires them out, helping them sleep for longer periods at night. Walking can be an excellent activity for the patient, as well as for the caregiver.

As the disease progresses, the person becomes more and more physically disabled. The nurse must then be aware of the need to turn the patient regularly to prevent skin breakdown and other complications of immobility. Range of motion should be performed to prevent the development of contractures. Restraints used indiscriminately can hasten the person's physical decline.

At times patients are so active that, for example, it is difficult for them to sit long enough to eat. Finger foods

**RESEARCH**

Algase D: Cognitive discriminants of wandering among nursing home residents, *Nurs Res* 41(2):78-81, 1992.

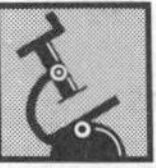

This study examined which dimensions of cognitive impairment best discriminated between wandering and nonwandering ambulatory subjects. Cognitive impairment was measured along four dimensions: abstract thinking, language, judgment, and spatial skills. Wanderers were found to have higher overall levels of cognitive impairment and poorer performance on all cognitive dimensions. The dimension of language was the most important higher-order cognitive skill that differentiated wanderers from nonwanderers.

**RESEARCH**

Hurley A et al: Assessment of discomfort in advanced Alzheimer patients, *Res Nurs Health* 15(5):369-377, 1992.

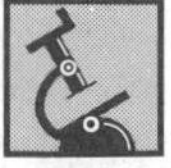

Perspectives of nursing staff members practicing on special care Alzheimer units were used to develop an objective scale for measuring discomfort in noncommunicative patients with advanced Alzheimer's disease. On the basis of a pilot test, the discomfort scale was reduced to nine items. After a rater training program was completed and a quantitative scoring procedure was developed, the scale was tested for 6 months on 82 subjects at two sites. The nine factors were (1) noisy breathing, (2) negative vocalization, (3) content facial expression, (4) sad facial expression, (5) frightened facial expression, (6) frown, (7) relaxed body language, (8) tense body language, and (9) fidgeting.

that can be eaten while walking may be necessary. Patients should be encouraged to sit, and at times a soft waist restraint can help them do this at mealtime.

## Promoting Sleep

The tendency of patients with Alzheimer's disease to sleep for short periods can be very frustrating for caregivers. It may be helpful to structure bedtime at the same time each night. Caffeine should be restricted in the late afternoon and evening, and activities in the evening should be quiet if possible. Patients should be encouraged to exercise during the day to help tire them. At times the use of medications may be helpful in encouraging the patient to sleep, thus enabling the caregiver to rest as well.

## Preventing Agitation/Violence

When persons are diagnosed with the disease, they face the beginning of many experiences, feelings, and fears. As the disease progresses, memory functions continue to deteriorate and patients become increasingly frustrated with their deficits. Significant depression, anxiety, and attempts at denial and rationalization occur as they observe their own brain failure. Patients are able to recognize that they are not reacting in a normal or predictable way. When asked, they can state that they are not thinking as well as they once did.

Self-esteem is fostered by allowing and encouraging the patient to be as independent as possible. It is vital to avoid unnecessary frustrations so that complex tasks can be broken down into simpler components. Predictable routines are important. The caregiver must be aware of the patient's *stress threshold* and attempt to minimize stress to avoid angry, aggressive behavior.

Five basic groups of stressors that can produce dysfunctional behaviors include *fatigue, change of routine, excessive demands, overwhelming situations,* and *physical stressors* such as illness or pain.[26] In the early stages of the disease, patients can be taught to structure their schedule and environment to maintain function. Memory aids can be helpful. As the disease becomes more disabling, the caregiver must assume more responsibility for monitoring and structuring the environment. Patients function best in predictable, known routines and environments.

When patients with Alzheimer's disease are put in situations where they cannot cope, overreaction to the stress may occur. This is described as a *catastrophic reaction.*

Patients are aware of the feelings of those around them. Presenting care in a calm, unhurried manner helps reduce stress. It is important to treat these persons with dignity and allow them to make whatever choices they are capable of making. Making decisions and choosing among the alternatives, however, requires higher-level cognitive processes and can be frustrating. If a decision or task precipitates a catastrophic reaction or if the patient becomes more agitated, decision making must be limited.[25]

The patient should never be scolded or embarrassed. Arguing or reasoning with the patient increases patient resistance and escalates dysfunctional behavior. Reality-orientation techniques usually only increase confusion in these patients. If the patient is found to be depressed or distressed, counseling and possibly antidepressant medications may increase function.

As the patient becomes more and more noncommunicative, it is difficult for the patient's caregivers to determine if the patient is uncomfortable. A recent nursing research study identified factors associated with patient discomfort (see Research box above).

Support groups for family members can be vital in supporting their care of the patient with Alzheimer's disease.[18] Some areas also conduct groups for the patients themselves. The Alzheimer's Disease and Related

Disorders Association,* which has chapters in many cities, may offer support groups for caregivers. Respite care services may assist the caregiver to cope (see Chapter 8).

## ♦ EVALUATION

To evaluate effectiveness of nursing interventions, compare patient behaviors with those stated in the expected patient outcomes. Successful achievement of patient outcomes for the patient with Alzheimer's disease is indicated by the following:

1. Is not injured and maintains calm behavior.
2. Has sleep pattern that includes at least 6 hours of sleep per night.
3. Causes no harm to others, for example, hitting, kicking, or biting.

## COMPLICATIONS

Complications in Alzheimer's disease are related to the occurrence of infections and injury. These are common as the disease progresses and often are a cause of death. Prevention of injury is addressed under nursing interventions.

# VASCULAR DISEASES

## CEREBROVASCULAR ACCIDENT

### Etiology

In this chapter the term **cerebrovascular accident (CVA)** is discussed as a general term. It should be recognized, however, that most neurologists and neurosurgeons more specifically refer to the disturbance in cerebral circulation as either a *thrombus, embolus, hemorrhage,* or *transient ischemic attack.* The nursing and medical care may differ depending on the specific cause. These differences are discussed in each relevant section. **Hemiplegia** and **stroke** also are terms used referring to CVA. Clinically, stroke refers to the sudden and dramatic development of focal neurologic deficits, and hemiplegia is one neurologic deficit that is typically seen.

The major causes of CVA are a thrombus, an embolus, or a hemorrhage, which can be precipitated by many underlying factors (Box 57-10) frequently associated with other chronic diseases that cause vascular problems. These include heart disease, kidney disease, peripheral vascular disease, hypertension, and diabetes mellitus.

**BOX 57-10 Conditions Causing Cerebrovascular Accident**

**THROMBUS**

- Atherosclerosis in intracranial and extracranial arteries
- Adjacency to intracerebral hemorrhage
- Arteritis caused by collagen (autoimmune) disease or bacterial arteritis
- Hypercoagulability such as in polycythemia
- Cerebral venous thromboses

**EMBOLI**

- Valves damaged by rheumatic heart disease (RHD)
- Myocardial infarction
- Atrial fibrillation (this dysrhythmia causes variable emptying of left ventricle; blood pools and small clots form; and then at times the ventricle is emptied completely with release of small emboli)
- Bacterial endocarditis and nonbacterial endocarditis, causing clots to form on endocardium

**HEMORRHAGE**

- Hypertensive intracerebral hemorrhage
- Subarachnoid hemorrhage
- Rupture of aneurysm
- Arteriovenous (A-V) malformation
- Hypocoagulation (as in patients with blood dyscrasias)

**GENERALIZED HYPOXIA**

- Severe hypotension, cardiopulmonary arrest, or severe depression in cardiac output caused by dysrhythmias

**LOCALIZED HYPOXIA**

- Cerebral artery spasms associated with subarachnoid hemorrhage
- Cerebral artery vasoconstriction associated with migraine headache

### Epidemiology

CVA is the most common disease of the nervous system and is the third highest cause of death in the United States; 500,000 Americans each year have an acute CVA. In recent years there has been a decline in stroke mortality in the United States. This is thought to result from the use of medications to lower high blood pressure, as well as to population-wide decreases in levels of blood pressure, cigarette smoking, and coronary heart diseases.[27,45]

### Pathophysiology

The brain depends greatly on oxygen and has no reserve oxygen supply. Thus, when anoxia occurs, cerebral metabolism is promptly altered and cell death and permanent damage can occur within 3 to 10 minutes. Any condition that alters cerebral perfusion will cause hypoxia or anoxia. Hypoxia first leads to cerebral ischemia. Short-term ischemia (less than 10 to 15 minutes) causes temporary deficits but no permanent deficits. Long-term ischemia causes permanent cell death and results in a cerebral infarction. Cerebral edema accompanies the infarction and worsens the neurologic deficits seen in the patient.

The permanent focal deficits may be unknown when the patient is first seen because generalized cerebral dysfunction (coma) may be present. The generalized dysfunction may be a result of generalized ischemia af-

*Alzheimer's Disease and Related Disorders Association, 360 N. Michigan Ave, Suite 601, Chicago IL 60641.

**TABLE 57-11 Deficits Resulting From Disruption of Blood Flow in the Brain**

| AREAS OF BRAIN SUPPLIED* | DEFECTS WITH DISRUPTION OF FLOW |
|---|---|
| **INTERNAL CAROTID ARTERY** | |
| Retina by its branch to retinal artery; lateral and medial surfaces of cerebral hemispheres by their branches to middle cerebral artery and anterior cerebral artery; portions of hypothalamus | Occasionally asymptomatic if good collateral circulation present<br>Most frequently find the following:<br>Intermittent ipsilateral visual impairment or blindness caused by retinal artery insufficiency<br>Impairment similar to that seen with disruption of flow through middle cerebral artery<br>Impairment caused by disruption of flow in anterior cerebral artery not frequently seen because both anterior cerebral arteries can be fed by one internal carotid artery<br>Ipsilateral Horner's syndrome (ptosis, miosis, absence of sweating on same side of face) from hypothalamic damage |
| **ANTERIOR CEREBRAL ARTERY** | |
| Medial and superior surfaces of cerebral hemispheres; contains motor and sensory cortex for foot and leg and supplementary motor cortex; feeds large portion of frontal lobe | Contralateral hemiparesis or hemiplegia and contralateral sensory loss of lower extremities<br>Upper extremities and face usually spared<br>Confusion, dementia, and personality changes |
| **MIDDLE CEREBRAL ARTERY** | |
| Lateral portion of cerebral hemispheres, which contain motor and sensory areas for face and upper extremities and speech areas | Contralateral paralysis of paresis<br>Contralateral sensory loss<br>Sensory and motor loss are most noticeable in face, neck, and upper extremities<br>Dysphasia or aphasia; may be global aphasia or only difficulty with expression without loss of comprehension; aphasia or dysphasia occurs if dominant hemisphere affected (left hemisphere in right-handed persons and most left-handed persons)<br>Spatial perceptual problems (inability to judge distances, rate of movement, form and relationship of body parts); changes in judgment and behavior; neglect of paralyzed side; and inability to recognize paralyzed extremity as own (anosognosia) if nondominant hemisphere affected<br>Contralateral homonymous hemianopia |
| **POSTERIOR CEREBRAL ARTERY** | |
| Posterior lateral and posterior medial surfaces of cerebral cortex, which contain primary visual receptive areas and internal structures; multiple branches that feed parts of optic pathway and diencephalic structure (thalamus and midbrain) | Paralysis usually absent<br>Homonymous hemianopic field defects<br>If dominant side, difficulty with visual learning, visual recognition, and visual spatial orientation<br>If branch to midbrain affected, can have ipsilateral oculomotor palsy and contralateral hemiparesis (Weber's syndrome) because of effect on cerebral peduncle; may have ataxia and choreoatherosis<br>If bilateral occlusion to midbrain, will have quadriparesis (because all tracts pass through midbrain as they leave cortex); impaired consciousness; divergent gaze; and dilated, unresponsive pupils<br>Patients in coma have unusual appearance in that they seem to be awake but do not communicate and do not respond; this has been termed *akinetic mutism*<br>If thalamus affected, may have major sensory disturbances such as abnormal pain and dysesthesia, which are increased with emotional distress; the patient also may have emotional lability (crying, laughing without motivation); these symptoms are sometimes called *thalamic syndrome* |
| **VERTEBROBASILAR ARTERIES** | |
| Multiple branches supply medulla oblongata, pons, midbrain, and cerebellum; no one structure receives all its blood supply from one branch; blood supply to ventral paramedian, ventrolateral, and dorsal brainstem structures all originate from different groups of arteries | Many different signs and symptoms depending on area of brainstem affected (pons, midbrain, or medulla) and what part of that area affected<br>Because motor and sensory tracts pass through this area, paresis and sensory deficits affecting one to all four extremities may occur<br>All cranial nerve nuclei are in this area; thus disruption of their function may be present as visual impairment, focal paralysis, loss of sensory innervation to face, difficulty in swallowing, dysarthria, deafness, and so on |

*Only major areas identified.

**TABLE 57-11 Deficits Resulting From Disruption of Blood Flow in the Brain—cont'd**

| AREAS OF BRAIN SUPPLIED* | DEFECTS WITH DISRUPTION OF FLOW |
|---|---|
| | Interference with cerebellar function can occur, causing ataxia, tremors, choreoatherosis, and so on<br>Interference with reticular activating system causes alteration in consciousness<br>Partial or complete Horner's syndrome caused by hypothalamic problem (ptosis of eyelid, constriction of pupil, absence of sweating on same side of face)<br>Respiratory difficulty, syncope, nausea, and vomiting caused by dysfunction of major vital centers in brainstem |

fecting larger areas of the brain than the area of infarction and cerebral edema alone.

The type of permanent focal deficits depends on the area of the brain that has been affected. The area of the brain affected depends on which cerebral vessels are involved. Table 57-11 lists the major vessels of the brain, the major areas of the brain perfused by each vessel, and the resultant deficits that occur when blood flow is disrupted.

The *vessel most frequently affected is the middle cerebral artery.* The *second most frequently affected vessel is the internal carotid artery.* Other vessels are more rarely affected.

Because major differences exist in the clinical manifestations and care of the patient who suffers a CVA caused by hemorrhage, this is discussed in a separate section. The onset, pathologic process, and incidence of CVA from thombosis and embolism are different, and thus each is described before discussing care of the patient.

### Cerebral thrombosis

Thrombosis is the most frequent cause of a CVA; in one study of nonhemorrhagic causes of CVA it accounted for 92% of all CVAs. The most frequent cause of cerebral thrombosis is atherosclerosis. CVA secondary to thrombosis is seen most frequently in the 60- to 90-year age-group, and many of these persons have a history of hypertension or diabetes mellitus.

It is important for nurses to be aware of the relationship between CVA and (1) atherosclerosis, (2) hypertension, and (3) diabetes mellitus so that they can be involved in appropriate preventive care.

The onset of symptoms of CVA secondary to thrombosis tends to occur during sleep or soon after arising. This may be related to elderly persons having decreased sympathetic activity and recumbency causing a lowering of blood pressure, which can lead to ischemia of the brain. In addition, these persons frequently have *postural hypotension and poor reflex response to changes in position,* which can cause hypotension on arising. Neurologic signs and symptoms frequently deteriorate or worsen during the first 48 hours.

Cerebral arteriosclerosis also may lead to deterioration of brain tissue, even though CVAs do not occur. This condition, which usually is associated with high blood pressure, may occur in persons in their 50s, although it usually is considered a disease of old age.

Multiple small thrombi may occur in persons whose blood pressure is normal or even below normal if atheromatous changes have occurred in the lining of arteries. This condition causes frequent small, barely perceptible strokes. Both cerebral arteriosclerosis and multiple small strokes from thrombi may produce personality changes. The person who has arteriosclerosis is likely to have a more consistent downward course, whereas the one suffering from multiple small thrombi may have periods of apparently normal physical and mental episodes of confusion.

Cerebral arteriosclerosis, multiple small thrombi, and atrial fibrillation may cause slowly progressive changes that are particularly distressing to members of the person's family. Complete brain deterioration may occur. The person may feel irritable and unhappy with apparently little cause, and no amount of reassurance can make him or her feel better. The family must be prepared for gradual deterioration of the person's condition and should make provision for the person's safety and for the results of poor judgment. For example, the person may forget to dress appropriately, may give away family possessions, and may enter into unwise business dealings. The family needs help in learning how to treat the patient as an adult and yet deal with his or her limitations. The physician, the social workers, and the nurse can help family members care for the patient in such a way that their own lives are not completely disrupted and yet they are not plagued by guilt feelings when the patient dies. Institutional care sometimes is necessary, and the family needs encouragement and help in arriving at joint decisions that serves the best interests of all its members.

### Cerebral embolism

Embolism is the second most common cause of CVA. Patients who have CVAs secondary to embolism are usually younger, and most often the emboli originate from a thrombus in the heart. The myocardial thrombus most frequently is caused by rheumatic heart disease with mitral stenosis and atrial fibrillation. Therefore nurses can help to decrease the incidence of CVA from emboli by instituting the *preventive care measures* for persons with *rheumatic heart* disease described in Chapter 31. In addition, because cerebral embolism can originate from emboli in infarcted myocardium, another set of preventive measures that nurses should be practicing are those described for the *prevention of myocardial infarctions* (see Chapter 30). Symptoms may occur at any time and progress rapidly. Emboli that originate from infected material can produce abscesses or other types of infections.

#### Transient ischemic attacks

CVA has just been discussed in relation to the causative agent or the vessel involved. CVA also can be described according to the temporal (time) character of the total clinical episode. Three profiles have been defined: transient ischemic attacks, stroke in evolution (progressive stroke), or completed stroke.

The term **transient ischemic attacks (TIAs)** refers to transient cerebral ischemia with temporary episodes of neurologic dysfunction. The neurologic dysfunction can be profound, with complete loss of consciousness and loss of all sensory and motor function, or there may be only focal deficits of some sensory and motor functions. Focal deficits that occur depend on the area of the brain involved. The most *common deficit is contralateral weakness of the lower portion of the face, fingers, hands, arms and legs; transient dysphagia; and some sensory impairment.* Ischemic attacks may occur many times over days, weeks, months, or years. The neurologic deficit resolves, and between attacks results of the neurologic examination are normal.

TIAs may be caused by any of the conditions listed for CVA but most often precede cerebral thrombosis.

*Stroke in evolution* refers to development of a neurologic deficit over several hours to days. The clinical manifestation is the same as for a completed stroke; only the time course is different. *Completed stroke* refers to a permanent neurologic deficit.

The major importance of TIAs is that they warn the patient and health care provider of the existence of an underlying pathologic condition. At least one third of the patients who have TIAs will have a CVA within 2 to 5 years. Some patients are treated with vasodilators, anticoagulant therapy, or drugs that inhibit platelet aggregation after they experience a TIA. The use of anticoagulants decreases the number of attacks. Aspirin (which prevents platelet aggregation) also has been shown to decrease subsequent attacks. The dose is 300 mg per day. If an isolated, extracranial arterial lesion is found, surgical correction is possible.

The clinical manifestations of a CVA vary depending on the area of the brain affected. The most common focal neurologic signs and symptoms are those caused by disruption of flow through the midcerebral artery (see Table 57-11).

Frequently the patient is unconscious and may experience convulsions. Both unconsciousness and convulsions result from generalized ischemia and the brain's response to abrupt hypoxia.

Depending on the amount of cerebral edema present, the patient may have increased intracranial pressure (see earlier section for a description of signs and symptoms of this condition).

### Prevention

Neurovascular disease can at times be prevented, or at least the results can be minimized. Many of the cerebrovascular diseases are thought to occur as a result of certain risk factors, which include the following:

- Cigarette smoking
- Hypertension
- Hypercholesterolemia
- Obesity
- Stress-related occupations and a hectic-paced lifestyle

*Secondary prevention* is important with cerebrovascular disease because it is hoped the disease can be arrested before it causes irreversible results. The prevention of complications (tertiary prevention) also is important.

### Medical Management

The goal for discharge of patients with a CVA as determined by DRGs is 6 days. The nurse works collaboratively with the physician for implementation of prescribed medical therapy. Because the nurse has a major role in discharge planning and patient teaching, these are discussed under nursing management. A sample Critical Pathway and Nursing Care Plan are included at the end of this section.

#### Diagnostic tests

A lumbar puncture usually is performed and may reveal elevated spinal fluid pressure. If hemorrhage has occurred, there will be blood in the spinal fluid. In almost all instances a CT scan will be used to visualize the infarcted areas. If the patient is in a coma and it is uncertain how severe the increase in pressure is, CT may be used before the lumbar puncture. Lumbar puncture can precipitate tentorial or foraminal herniation when an expanding intracranial mass is present.

After a TIA a cerebral angiogram or digital subtraction angiogram may be obtained to discover blocked or occluded vessels.

#### Medication

In an attempt to prevent further thrombosis or emboli, bishydroxycoumarin (dicumarol) and heparin may be given in the hospital if it is certain that the cause is cerebral thrombosis or emboli and not cerebral hemorrhage. The use of anticoagulants is controversial. Some patients may be treated with various types of vasodilating agents, although the effectiveness of this type of therapy is not well established.

### Treatment

A CVA may occur when the person is at work or elsewhere outside the home and may be confused with convulsive seizures, diabetic coma, or drunkenness. Emergency care at the scene consists of turning the person carefully onto the affected side (determined by the puffiness of the cheek on this side) and elevating the head without tilting the neck forward, because tilting may constrict blood vessels and in turn cause congestion of blood within the cerebrum. Turning the person to the affected side permits saliva to drain out of the mouth and lessens the danger of aspiration into the lungs. Elevation of the head may help to prevent edema of the brain. Clothing should be loosened about the throat to aid further in preventing engorgement of blood vessels in the head, which may lead to cerebral edema. The person should be kept quiet, moved as little as possible, and protected from chilling. Medical assistance is sought at once.

### Diet

Fluids may be restricted for the first few days after a CVA in an effort to prevent edema of the brain. Patients are fed intravenous fluids, or the physician may insert a nasogastric tube and order tube feedings. When patients are no longer comatose, small amounts of fluid, 5 to 10 ml, can be given several times daily to determine patients' ability to swallow and to help them regain this function. Returning as soon as possible to a regular diet and a normal fluid intake is desirable.

### Activity

Rest and quiet are important even if the CVA has not been serious enough to cause complete loss of consciousness. Some neurologists may prescribe that the head of the bed be kept flat for several days. This is believed to assist cerebral perfusion. No attempt should be made to rouse the patient from coma, although respiratory and circulatory stimulants may be prescribed by the physician if depression of these systems is present.

The time the patient remains in bed depends entirely on the type of CVA suffered and the judgment of the physician in regard to early mobilization. Some physicians prescribe fairly long periods of rest after CVAs, whereas others believe in *early mobilization of the patient with cerebral thrombosis.* Mobilization sometimes begins a day or two after the CVA has occurred.

### Referral/Consultation

In some settings the nurse assumes responsibility for making referrals to other services. These may include referrals to a social worker or dietitian. It is important to refer both the patient and significant other to a local support group for stroke survivors.

### Surgical Management

After the patient's condition is stable, or after the acute or rehabilitation phase, surgery may be used for selected patients. If the CVA is associated with a distinct atherosclerotic lesion in the extracranial system (internal carotid artery or common carotid artery), a carotid endarterectomy may be performed.

A carotid endarterectomy involves the reaming out of the diseased vessel with the patient under either local or general anesthesia. Postoperative care includes the following:

1. Close attention to neurologic signs (changes in muscle strength, mentation, speech, and level of consciousness)
2. Observation for bleeding in incisional area
3. Observation for swelling of the neck or complaints of dysphagia
4. Keep tracheostomy set in patient's room in case of severe respiratory distress

*Revascularization procedures* are now possible with the use of stereoscopic microscopes. Usually the superficial temporal artery is anastomosed to an artery within the brain such as the midcerebral artery. Other vessels can be used. The purpose is to provide for greater blood flow. The surgery usually does not resolve any permanent deficits but may prevent further problems. The preoperative and postoperative care of the patient is similar to that for any patient with cranial surgery but also includes the following:

1. Checking for pulse in anastomosed vessel
   a. Use of Doppler to detect pulse
   b. Gentle palpation
2. Keeping graft areas free of pressure
   a. Eyeglass frames bent out so as not to occlude vessel
   b. No other constricting bands around head

A postoperative angiogram is obtained to assess the patency of the vessel.

## NURSING MANAGEMENT

### ♦ ASSESSMENT

### Subjective Data

Subjective data to be collected to assess the patient who has had a CVA include the following:

- Patient's understanding of disease or symptoms
- Characteristics of onset of symptoms
- Presence of headache—nature and location
- Any sensory deficits
- Visual ability—presence of diplopia, blurred vision
- Ability to think clearly
- Any other concomitant symptom

### Objective Data

Objective data to be collected to assess the patient who has had a CVA include the following:

Motor strength—paresis or paralysis common
Change in level of consciousness, including coma
Signs of increased intracranial pressure
Respiratory status
Ability to verbalize—presence of aphasia

### Diagnostic Test Findings

The CT scan often shows the occurrence of a CVA but not until several days after the onset of the stroke. Other abnormalities include areas of occlusion and hemorrhage that can be detected on angiographic examination.

## ♦ NURSING DIAGNOSES

Nursing diagnoses are determined from analysis of patient data. Nursing diagnoses for the patient with a CVA may include but are not limited to the following:

| Diagnostic Title | Possible Etiologic Factors |
|---|---|
| Tissue perfusion, altered: cerebral | Decreased blood flow (arterial) |
| Nutrition, altered: less than body requirements | Chewing/swallowing difficulties |
| Sensory/perceptual alterations: visual, auditory, kinesthetic, gustatory, tactile, olfactory | Altered sensory reception/transmission/integration |
| Mobility, impaired physical | Perceptual/cognitive impairment, neuromuscular impairment |
| Self-care deficit: feeding, bathing/hygiene, dressing/grooming, toileting | Perception/cognitive impairment, neuromuscular impairment |
| Body image disturbance | Loss of body function |
| Communication, impaired verbal | Aphasia |
| Incontinence, total | Neurologic disease |
| Adjustment, impaired | Disability requiring change in lifestyle |
| Disuse syndrome, high risk for | Immobility, weakness |
| Health maintenance, altered | Perceptual/cognitive impairment |

## ♦ EXPECTED PATIENT OUTCOMES

Expected patient outcomes for the patient with a CVA may include but are not limited to the following:

1. Maintains cerebral perfusion as indicated by the absence of signs or symptoms of increased intracranial pressure.
2. Maintains nutrition at optimal level as indicated by a weight that is within 5 pounds of usual body weight and by normal serum protein, hematocrit, and hemoglobin values.
3. Verbalizes ways to compensate for sensory/perceptual alterations.
4. Maintains mobility at optimal level.
5. Is able to carry out ADL, with or without assistance.
6. Verbalizes a positive body image.
7. Is able to communicate to express needs.
8. Is continent of urine and stool, with or without training programs.
9. Demonstrates and verbalizes a positive adjustment to the CVA.
10. Prevents disuse syndrome as shown by the absence of contractures and pressure sores.
11. Can state ways to maintain health status.

## ♦ INTERVENTIONS

### ➠ Managing Critical Care

Goals are directed toward survival needs and preventing further brain damage. Care by the nurse is directed toward the unconscious state, if present (see p. 1924). Neurologic assessment is performed at regular intervals to detect changes in status and complications. The vital signs should be carefully checked, and the nurse should observe for such signs as a rise in temperature within the first day or two, slowing of pulse and respiration, and deepening of the coma, all of which indicate pressure on the vital centers and poor prognosis. Drugs to reduce intracranial pressure, such as dexamethasone (Decadron), may be given.

After the patient's physical condition is stabilized as just described, the nurse has the greatest influence of all health caregivers on the patient's recovery. Goals for care in the acute phase are directed toward preventing complications from the original CVA, from the immobility and dependency it causes, and from the loss of function caused by focal deficit.

### Maintaining Nutrition

It is important to maintain the nutritional status of the patient who has experienced a CVA. If the patient is obtunded, it usually is necessary to feed the patient intravenously. Because swallowing and chewing problems are common with CVA, a feeding tube may be necessary to sustain nutrition. If the patient continues to have difficulty, the nasogastric feeding tube is removed and a gastrostomy tube is placed.

It is important to assess the patient carefully for any signs of aspiration or choking. A videofluoroscopic examination is performed to determine the nature and degree of any aspiration. The patient is carefully begun on feedings, with close supervision by the nurse or another member of the health care team. As the patient's ability to eat improves, progression to the next level of diet consistency is effected.[15]

### Compensating for Perceptual Difficulties

After a stroke, patients may have difficulty relating to themselves and to their environment.[21,38] After the acute stage a multibed environment is advocated because the

## NURSING CARE PLAN

### PERSON WITH CEREBROVASCULAR ACCIDENT

**DATA:** Mr. W. is a 68-year-old married man with a history of hypertension and non–insulin-dependent diabetes mellitus. He awoke on the morning of admission unable to move one side of his body or to talk. He was taken to the hospital where he was admitted with the probable diagnosis of a cerebral vascular accident. On admission he was noted to be lethargic and to have a paresis of his right arm and leg. He also was aphasic, although he seemed to be able to understand some commands. Diagnostic testing confirmed the presence of the stroke. His blood pressure was 184/106 mm Hg on admission. He was noted to have slight difficulty with swallowing. He was continent of bowel and bladder. Admitting laboratory work showed a blood glucose of 130 mg/dl and a cholesterol level of 290 mg/dl.

The nursing history, obtained from both Mr. W. and his wife, revealed the following:

- Mr. W. had stopped taking his blood pressure medication because he felt so good.
- Mr. W. was taking an oral hypoglycemic and his blood glucose levels were reported to be in good control.
- Mr. W. was employed at the time of his stroke as an insurance agent.
- Mr. W. knew that his cholesterol levels were elevated and tried to watch his diet. Both Mr. and Mrs. W. were unsure of recent results.

Collaborative nursing actions include interventions to monitor for worsening of the stroke, as well as to maintain cerebral perfusion and to prevent complications. Nursing actions include monitoring for the following:

- Any change in neurologic deficit: increased paresis or paralysis, decreased level of alertness, change in pupil response, presence of signs or symptoms of increased intracranial pressure
- Increased blood pressure
- Increased confusion or aphasia
- Increased difficulty in swallowing
- Respiratory difficulty
- The need for rehabilitation beyond the acute hospitalization

#### ■ NURSING DIAGNOSIS

Altered cerebral tissue perfusion related to compromised blood supply to the brain

| Expected Patient Outcome | Nursing Interventions | Rationale |
|---|---|---|
| Will remain alert with no signs or symptoms of increased intracranial pressure. | Perform neurologic assessment q 1 hr × 4, then q 2 hr × 4, then q 4 hr until day 3 or 4, then q 6 or q 8 hr. | Will indicate change in cerebral perfusion quickly when interventions may be effective. |
| | Maintain bed rest with HOB elevated 30 degrees. | Will aid in cerebral perfusion. |
| | Provide anticoagulation as ordered. | |

#### ■ NURSING DIAGNOSIS

Altered nutrition: less than body requirements related to difficulty in chewing and swallowing

| Expected Patient Outcome | Nursing Interventions | Rationale |
|---|---|---|
| Will maintain usual body weight. | Assess swallowing ability. | Will prevent aspiration. |
| | Refer to speech consultant as required. | Treatment of dysphagia involves team approach. |
| | Begin diet with clear liquids and advance as tolerated. | Allows for adaptation to stroke. |
| | Alter consistency of diet as needed. | Compensates for any difficulty in chewing. |
| | Supervise meals as indicated. | Will prevent aspiration. |

#### ■ NURSING DIAGNOSIS

Impaired physical mobility related to hemiparesis

| Expected Patient Outcome | Nursing Interventions | Rationale |
|---|---|---|
| Will maintain mobility at highest level. | Turn q 2-4 hr. | To prevent complications. |
| | Supervise progressive mobility starting at day 3 (up in chair with assistance and then progress as able). | Allows patient to adapt to change and to remain free of complications. |
| | Assess for safety needs. | Safety concerns are common as a result of perceptual and sensory impairments. |
| | Provide physical therapy consultation as indicated. | Allows for input of team members. |

*Continued.*

## NURSING CARE PLAN

### PERSON WITH CEREBROVASCULAR ACCIDENT—cont'd

#### ■ NURSING DIAGNOSIS

Self-care deficit: feeding, bathing/hygiene, dressing/grooming, toileting related to lethargy and weakness

| Expected Patient Outcome | Nursing Interventions | Rationale |
|---|---|---|
| Will perform ADL independently. | Assist as needed, but allow patient to do what he can. | Having patient do as much as possible fosters sense of independence and positive self-esteem. |
| | Provide equipment as needed. | Compensates for neurologic deficit. |
| | Arrange occupational therapy consultation. | Provides for input of team. |

#### ■ NURSING DIAGNOSIS

Impaired verbal communication related to aphasia

| Expected Patient Outcome | Nursing Interventions | Rationale |
|---|---|---|
| Will be able to communicate needs. | Encourage patient to attempt to verbalize. | Will increase his feelings of control and allow staff to better care for him. |
| | Provide communication aids as needed (e.g., communication board). | Facilitates communication. |
| | Arrange speech therapy consultation as indicated. | Will involve team members in care. |

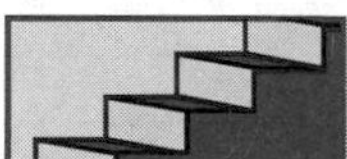

## CRITICAL PATHWAY Cerebrovascular Accident

**DRG #: 014 Expected LOS: 6**

| | Day of Admission Day 1 | Day 2 |
|---|---|---|
| **Diagnostic Tests** | CBC, UA, SMA/18,* ABGs, PT/PTT, ECG, CT scan, chest film | PT/PTT, ?ECHO, carotid Doppler |
| **Medications** | IVs, heparin; antihypertensive drugs if necessary | IVs, heparin |
| **Treatment** | I & O q8hr; VS and neurologic assessment q1hr × 4, then q2hr × 4, then q4hr; telemetry, wt, $O_2$; assess skin and mouth and special care q2hr; ROM to all extremities; assess for safety needs; ELS | I & O q8hr including % of nutrition consumed; VS and neurologic assessment q4hr; telemetry, $O_2$; assess skin and mouth and special care q2hr; ROM q2hr; ELS; initiate bowel/bladder training if needed |
| **Diet** | NPO; assess swallowing ability, if unaffected clear liquids | Clear liquids; if tolerated, advance to full liquids |
| **Activity** | Bed rest; HOB elevated 30 degrees while in bed; T & DB q2hr | Bed rest, HOB elevated 30 degrees while in bed, T & DB q2hr |
| **Consultations** | Rehabilitation team | Physical therapy; occupational and speech therapy, dietary, social services |

*ABGs,* Arterial blood gases; *Disc,* discontinue; *ECHO,* echocardiography; *ELS,* elastic leg stockings; *HOB,* head of bed; *LOS,* length of stay; *PT,* prothrombin time; *PTT,* partial thromboplastin time; *ROM,* range of motion; *SMA,* sequential multiple analysis; *SNU,* skilled nursing unit; *T & DB,* turn and deep breathe; *UA,* urinalysis; *VS,* vital signs; *wt,* weight.

## NURSING CARE PLAN

### PERSON WITH CEREBROVASCULAR ACCIDENT—cont'd

#### ■ NURSING DIAGNOSIS

Impaired verbal communication related to aphasia—cont'd

| Expected Patient Outcome | Nursing Interventions | Rationale |
|---|---|---|
| | Encourage family and patient to be patient with attempts to communicate. | Will decrease frustration. |

#### ■ NURSING DIAGNOSIS

High risk for disuse syndrome related to weakness and lethargy

| Expected Patient Outcome | Nursing Interventions | Rationale |
|---|---|---|
| Will not experience disuse syndrome. | Provide range of motion exercises. | Will prevent loss of muscle mass and contractures. |
| | Use antiembolism stockings. | Will prevent deep vein thrombosis. |
| | Turn patient every 2 to 4 hours. | Will prevent skin breakdown. |
| | Encourage progressive mobility as above. | Will encourage strength and movement. |

| Day 3 | Day 4 | Day 5 | Discharge to Home/Rehabilitation Day 6 |
|---|---|---|---|
| PT/PTT, ?Arteriogram | PT/PTT | SMA/6,† PT/PTT, CT scan | PT |
| IV to saline lock; heparin | IV saline lock; heparin titrated; Coumadin | IV saline lock; Disc heparin; Coumadin | Disc saline lock; Coumadin |
| I & O q8hr including % of nutrition consumed; VS and neurologic assessment q6hr; telemetry, wt, $O_2$; assess skin and mouth q2hr; ROM q4hr; ELS | I & O q8hr; VS and neurologic assessment q8hr; disc telemetry, disc $O_2$; ROM q4hr; ELS | I & O q8hr; VS and neurologic assessments q8hr; wt, ROM q4hr; ELS | Disc I & O, VS and neurologic assessment q8hr; ROM q4hr |
| Full liquids; advance to soft diet as tolerated | Soft diet | Regular diet | Regular diet |
| Bed rest; up in chair with assistance × 1, HOB elevated 30 degrees; T & DB q2hr | Up in chair with assistance × 2; HOB elevated 30 degrees; T & DB q2hr | Ambulate with assistance × 2; up in chair × 4 | Up ad lib |
| Continue with rehabilitation; SNU/home health | Continue with rehabilitation | Continue with rehabilitation | Continue with rehabilitation |

*Serum calcium, phosphorus, triglycerides, uric acid, creatinine, BUN, total bilirubin, alkaline phosphate, aspartate aminotransferase (AST) (formerly serum glutamic-oxaloacetic transaminase [SGOT]), alanine aminotransferase (ALT) (formerly serum glutamate pyruvate transaminase [SGPT]), lactic dehydrogenase (LDH), total protein, albumin, sodium, potassium, chloride, total $CO_2$, glucose.

†Serum sodium, potassium, chloride, total $CO_2$, glucose, BUN.

## Guidelines for Care of the Person With Cerebrovascular Accident

1. Promote nutrition:
   a. Use intravenous or tube feeding until patient is able to eat.
   b. Begin attempts to feed as soon as patient is no longer comatose.
2. Promote activity:
   a. Position affected limbs to prevent contractures.
   b. Turn frequently.
   c. Perform ROM exercises.
   d. Begin mobilization as soon as medically possible.
3. Promote elimination:
   a. Monitor intake and output to check for urinary retention.
   b. Start bladder program early.
   c. Avoid urinary catheters.
   d. Start bowel program.
4. Provide emotional support:
   a. Reassure patient of progress.
   b. Explain what is being done.

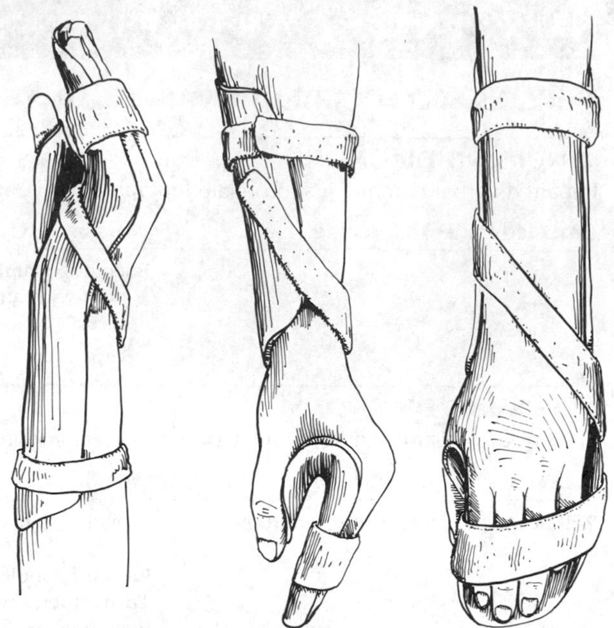

**FIGURE 57-12** Volar resting splint provides support to wrist, thumb, and fingers of patient following CVA, maintaining them in position of extension. (From Dittmar SS: *Rehabilitation nursing: process and application,* St Louis, 1989, Mosby.)

sensory input from others is helpful. In the initial stage, bringing familiar articles into the patient's environment can be a helpful stimulus. Examples are a clock, watch, family picture, or a Bible. *Hemianopsia,* or decreased visual field, occurs quite frequently. Approaching patients from the side of intact vision and teaching them to scan will not only make them more aware of stimuli but can help prevent injury. Diminished awareness or denial of the affected side (anosognosia) can occur and could be a safety hazard. This possibility should be considered when the patient runs into objects with the wheelchair or allows the affected arm or leg to drag behind during transfer from chair to bed.[25]

The nurse's observations regarding the patient's mental status are important. The patient may be disoriented and have decreased judgment or poor memory. A consistent environment and routine are helpful in improving orientation and the ability to function. Poor judgment and impulsiveness can be major safety hazards. Such behavior is brought to the attention of the physician. The family also must be aware of this if they are to care for the patient at home (see Guidelines box above).

### Promoting Mobility/Ambulation

*Active exercise* of the affected side may be started early. In the hospital it may be directed by the physical therapist or nurse. In consultation with the physical therapist, the nurse plans the exercises while the patient is in the hospital, and the nurse or the physical therapist may teach the exercises to the family in preparation for the patient's return home.

Because the patient who has had a CVA will greatly depend on the unaffected arm and leg when moving about, the unaffected part of the body needs attention to prevent contractures and preserve muscle strength (Figure 57-12). Even while in bed, the patient should exercise the unaffected arm and use it in all normal positions. The unaffected leg should be in a position of slight *internal rotation* most of the time while the patient is in bed, and the knee should be bent several times each day. Exercises to strengthen the quadricep muscles should be performed because the quadriceps is the most important muscle in providing stability to the knee joint, which is needed for walking (see Chapter 65).

Early *ambulation* facilitates vasomotor tone and has positive psychologic effects on the patient and family. Ambulation usually is started by the physical therapist by having the person walk between parallel bars. Transfer techniques also are taught to the patient and family (see following discussion).

When patients begin to move about and to try to help themselves, they may have several problems that can alter their ability to proceed. They may have loss of position sense, so that it is awkward for them to handle their bodies normally even when they have the muscular coordination to do so. They may have dizziness, spatial-perceptual deficits, diplopia, and alteration of skin sensation. They also may have to work harder than other persons to receive a normal amount of air on inhalation, because the involved side of the chest does not expand easily. This difficulty may lead to excessive fatigue unless those caring for the patient plan activities so that the patient's effort is not wasted.

Before standing or walking, patients may practice raising themselves up in bed and may sit on the side of the bed while holding firmly to an overbed table or to a strap with their good hand and pressing their feet on a chair or stool. The patient benefits from wearing shoes because it is good for morale and keeps the paralyzed foot in good position.

If preparation for walking has been adequate, the patient usually needs only one crutch when walking begins; then a cane will be used as walking progresses. When walking first begins, the nurse must remain close to allay the fear of falling. Balancing may be practiced by standing between parallel bars or by leaning on the backs of two chairs (provided the chairs are heavy enough to support weight safely). Good walking patterns must be established early because incorrect patterns are difficult and sometimes impossible to change. A sideward shuffle should be watched for and avoided. The patient should begin by leaning rather heavily on the crutch or cane and lifting the body sufficiently to bring the leg and foot forward so that the toes point straight ahead and not inward. The cane or single crutch is held in the hand opposite the paralyzed or weakened side of the body. Pivot transfers may be the easiest way to transfer the patient from bed to chair, and vice versa. When a pivot transfer is used, the chair always is placed so that the unaffected side leads the transfer.

## Promoting Activities of Daily Living

The patient is evaluated on ability to carry out the usual ADL and is assisted by the occupational therapist or nurse in becoming independent in each activity to the extent possible. Assistive devices may be used (Figures 57-13 to 57-17). Rehabilitation in this way is essentially a teaching-learning process in which the patient is actively involved. Motivation is absolutely essential to rehabilitation but unfortunately is not found to the same degree in all patients. Some patients devote all their energies to their rehabilitation, whereas others just seem to "give up." *If there is return of hand function in 2 to 3 weeks, fecal incontinence has disappeared, and no contractures, decubiti, or other complications have developed, there is reason to believe that the patient can be independent in care.*

Patients need preparation for each new step in learning to move and care for themselves. Each new activity must be demonstrated by the nurse and then practiced by patients; supervision and encouragement must be given by the nurse. Careful and detailed instruction on how to hold and support the body will save patients much embarrassment, discomfort, and confusion. By using the unaffected hand, the patient may, for example, straighten out the flexed fingers on the affected side and move the affected arm to a position in which, with the weight of gravity, the elbow will be straightened. Most patients can relearn to do ADL such as those pertaining to personal hygiene and dressing.

## Providing Emotional Support

If the patient survives the first few days, consciousness may begin to return and some of the paralysis may disappear. It is then that the greatest understanding is needed by persons attending the patient. The patient will become aware of the aphasia, drooling, paralysis, and unsteadiness and will be very upset by the awareness. It is at this point that the nurse's active part in rehabilitation begins. By quiet assurance a nurse can help the patient feel that progress toward recovery and self-sufficiency has begun and will continue. See Research box, p. 1995.

## Promoting Communication

The nurse can help promote communication by explaining what is going to be done even though the person may not be able to respond by speaking. If the patient has *aphasia* and also is unable to use the dominant *hand*, an additional problem of trying to write with the nondominant hand occurs. The nurse should try to anticipate the patient's needs and should make every effort to understand indistinct speech, because repeated attempts to be understood only increase misery and frustration. Usually, if partial speech is present at the time of return to consciousness, speech probably will improve and the patient is heartened by this knowledge. Speech also may be affected because of involvement of the tongue, mouth, and throat muscles.

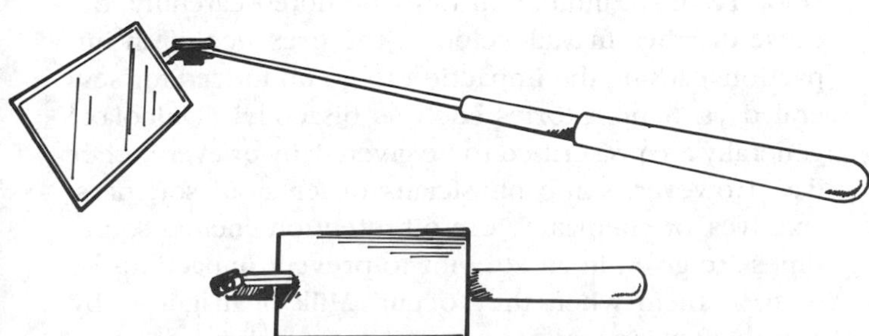

**FIGURE 57-13** Long-handled skin inspection mirror. (From Dittmar SS: *Rehabilitation nursing: process and application,* St Louis, 1989, Mosby.)

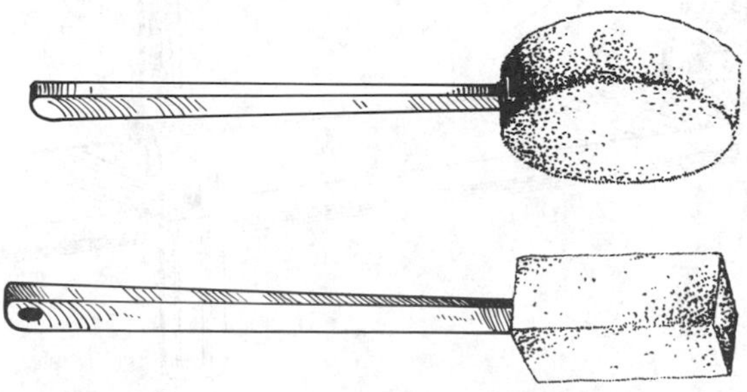

**FIGURE 57-14** Long-handled bath sponges. (From Dittmar SS: *Rehabilitation nursing: process and application,* St Louis, 1989, Mosby.)

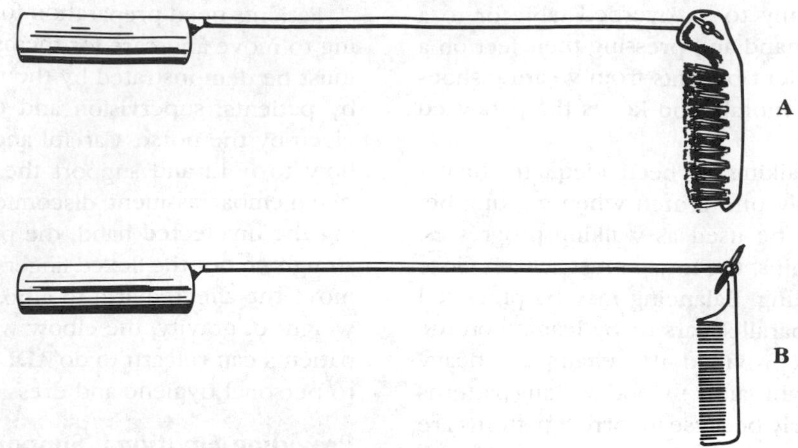


**FIGURE 57-15** Adapted hairbrush **(A)** and comb **(B)**. (From Dittmar SS: *Rehabilitation nursing: process and application,* St Louis, 1989, Mosby.)

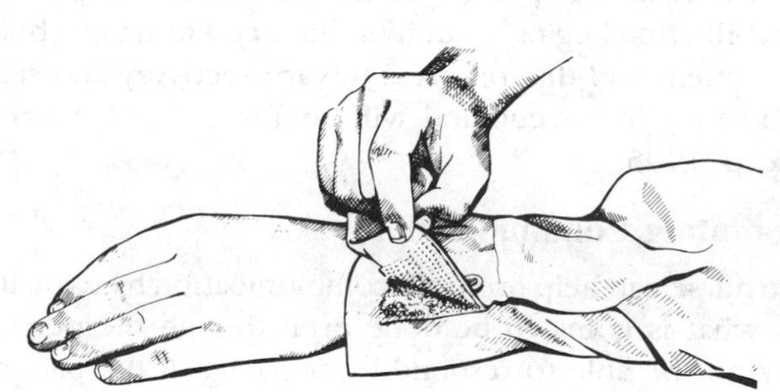

**FIGURE 57-16** Velcro shirtsleeve to facilitate closure. (From Dittmar SS: *Rehabilitation nursing: process and application,* St Louis, 1989, Mosby.)

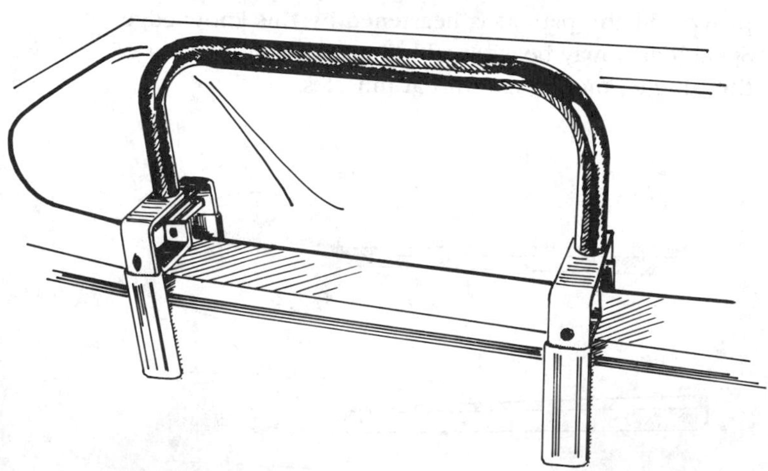

**FIGURE 57-17** Bathtub with grab bars. (From Dittmar SS: *Rehabilitation nursing: process and application,* St Louis, 1989, Mosby.)

The patient who has sustained a CVA may be overly emotional. This reaction, combined with the fear and frustration on becoming aware of his or her condition, is upsetting to the family. Crying is common, and sometimes family members believe that they are responsible for this sadness when this is usually not true. Family, staff, and other patients need reassurance that they are not the cause of the reaction.

## Promoting Bowel and Bladder Function

Urinary output should be noted carefully and recorded for several days after a CVA. Retention of urine may occur, but it is more likely that the patient will be incontinent. If urinary incontinence occurs, the patient who is not comatose may be told that control of excretory function probably will improve day by day. Offering a bedpan or a urinal immediately after meals and at other regular intervals helps to overcome incontinence. A retention catheter may be used for the first few days for female patients.

Fecal incontinence is fairly common after a CVA, and again the patient must be assured that as general improvement occurs, this condition will be overcome. Some patients develop constipation, and impactions develop readily. Elimination must be noted carefully, because diarrhea may develop in the presence of an impaction, causing the impaction to go unnoticed for several days. Suppositories such as bisacodyl (Dulcolax) generally are prescribed to be given daily or every other day. However, some physicians order stool softeners, laxatives, or enemas. Warm oil-retention enemas sometimes are given in an attempt to prevent impactions or to treat them when they occur. Milk of magnesia by mouth often is given because straining during defecation increases ICP. The patient must be cautioned not to strain and must be assured that the suppositories can easily be repeated if no results are obtained. The patient

RESEARCH

Williams A: Self-report of indifference and anxiety among persons with right hemispheric stroke, *Res Nurs Health* 15(5):343-347, 1992.

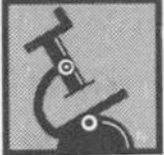

This study compared seven persons with right hemispheric stroke with ten persons with left hemispheric stroke. Both groups were queried concerning social indifference and lack of anxiety. Persons with right hemispheric stroke reported themselves as substantially less anxious and somewhat more indifferent than those with left hemispheric stroke. It was thought that lack of appropriate anxiety may contribute to the clinical descriptions of indifference, failure to make expected recovery, and difficulty in relationships with others.

usually needs assistance in getting on and off the bedpan. Side rails that can be held onto while turning or a trapeze that can be reached with the unaffected arm and hand help the patient to move independently and to get on and off the bedpan if this activity is allowed.

## Promoting Adjustment

General care and the pattern of living that should be followed after a CVA vary for each patient and are determined by the circumstances, the amount of recovery, and the guidance given in the early stages of the illness. Despite all efforts, the patient may, for example, never be able to negotiate stairs. The social worker and the community health nurse are indispensable in helping to arrange the patient's home so that the greatest possible degree of self-sufficiency and independence is possible. Family members often need help in assisting the person to accept limitations, both physical and emotional. The family also must make adjustments to actual circumstances. Almost all persons who have CVAs need health supervision for the rest of their lives. Whether the patient will be able to return home or must go to a nursing home will depend a great deal on the family's understanding and acceptance of the patient and his or her limitations when maximal rehabilitation has been achieved.[13] (See the Research box above, right.)

## Promoting Rehabilitation

The greatest challenge for the nurse in care of the patient who has had a CVA comes after the patient is past the point of danger. Then the long, slow process of learning to use whatever abilities remain or can be relearned must be faced, and adjustments to limitations must be made if the patient and family are going to have fulfilling lives.

The nurse is an important member of the rehabilitation team, which functions in terms of three basic rehabilitation goals[41]:

RESEARCH

Davidson A, Young C: Repatterning of stroke rehabilitation clients following return to life in the community, *J Neurosurg Nurs* 17(2):123-128, 1985.

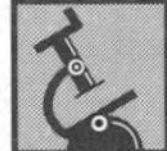

This study explored problems that stroke patients experience after rehabilitation and how they perceive and interact with their environment. Subjects, all of whom had experienced a CVA and completed the same rehabilitation program, were interviewed in their homes by means of a 16-question interview form developed and pretested by the investigators. The results indicated that although most subjects had gained some physical return of function, most energy was consumed with accomplishing ADL. To do pleasurable activities involved complex planning and timing. The study indicated that nurses need to consider individual life patterns, current patient goals, and the resources of the home and community in planning interventions.

1. Prevention of further impairment
2. Maintenance of existing abilities
3. Restoration of as much function as possible

## Facilitating Adjustment

Although CVAs may recur, the person may go for years with no further difficulty and eventually die of some other cause. The physician usually explains the prognosis to the person and to the family. The nurse should know what explanation has been given by the physician and sometimes must help in interpreting it to the family.

The person who has sustained a CVA and who has high blood pressure usually is advised to take prescribed antihypertensive medications as ordered, to get sufficient rest, and to avoid strain and excitement. Persons involved in strenuous work may be advised to reduce their work schedule and take more frequent vacations. Those who are overweight are advised to bring their weight within normal limits, and those who smoke are advised of the hazards of vasoconstriction caused by nicotine. ADL may be modified; sitting while shaving or doing other similar activities helps conserve energy.

Before discharge to the home or to another health care setting, certain outcomes should be achieved. The major emphasis is on maintaining structural and body integrity consistent with pathologic involvement. The parameters involved in achieving this are intact skin, normal range of joint motion with no contractures, loss of muscle tone confined to that which is consistent with pathologic condition, and maintenance of bladder and bowel function. When these outcomes are achieved at the highest degree possible, the person is ready for discharge. Obviously, some persons' conditions will limit their ability to become completely sufficient in ADL, and

**BOX 57-11 Recovery Stages After Cerebrovascular Accident**

**FLACCIDITY**

No voluntary motion and no muscle tone are present.

**PARTIAL SYNERGY**

Muscle tone develops, and muscles contract either voluntarily or with spasticity. Patient can move extremities in part of synergy pattern.

**SYNERGY**

Spasticity is moderate to severe. Patient can move joints through all or most of synergy pattern.

**BREAKING OUT**

Spasticity decreases. Patient can perform combinations of movements that are out of synergy.

**PARTIALLY ISOLATED**

Spasticity has less influence. Movement combinations bear less resemblance to stereotyped patterns.

**ISOLATED**

Almost normal movement is present, with good control of voluntary movement and little spasticity.

some persons will benefit from long-term rehabilitation either in a rehabilitation hospital or through regular outpatient follow-up care.

## Preventing Disuse Syndrome

Return of motor impulses and subsequent return of function are evidenced by a tightening and spasticity of the affected part. The return occurs in stages. These stages can last from hours to months. Recovery also may halt at a specific stage and progress no further. The recovery stages have been defined in terms of degrees of synergy. *Synergy* has been defined as muscles acting together as a bound unit in stereotyped movement patterns. See Box 57-11 for these stages in recovery.

Return of motor impulses is significant for the future use of the affected part but presents new problems for the patient, nurse, and all others who may be involved in care. Muscles that draw the limbs toward the midline become very active, and the arm may be held tightly adducted against the body. The affected lower limb may be held inward and adducted to, or even beyond, the midline. Muscles that draw the limbs into flexion also are stimulated, with the result that the heel is lifted off the ground, the heel cord shortens, and the knee becomes bent. In the upper limb, flexor muscles draw the elbow into the bent position, the wrist is flexed, and fingers are curled in palmar flexion. This is often seen after a CVA because the adductor and flexor muscles are stronger than opposing muscles.

Persistent nursing efforts must be directed toward prevention of further impairment and keeping any part of the body from remaining in a position of flexion long enough for the occurrence of muscle shortening and joint changes that might interfere with free joint action. If a physical therapist is not available, the total responsibility for preventive measures may rest with the nurse. *Every minute counts in prevention, and the nurse must not miss one opportunity to move the patient's adducted or flexed limbs back to the correct position.*

*Passive exercise* stimulates circulation and may help to reestablish neuromuscular pathways. No difficulty is encountered with these procedures until tightening of the muscles begins to appear. Then other physical measures are needed, and at this point, if not earlier, a physical therapist should be involved in the patient's treatment. The occupational therapist also may be involved and may provide various kinds of splints (see Figure 57-12).

The Bobath technique has been found useful to assist in the functional recovery of the patient who has had a CVA. The Bobath technique is a treatment approach that attempts to make muscle tone more normal. This is accomplished by providing as many sensations of normal muscle tone, posture, and movement as possible. The goal of treatment is to redirect short-term memory toward an appreciation of normal movement of the paralyzed side by using techniques of weight bearing, counterrotation, and protraction of the shoulder girdle and pelvis.[9] (The reader is referred to a rehabilitation nursing text for a further description of this technique.)

## Facilitating Learning

The teaching for a patient with a CVA is the same as that for the patient with a motor problem (see Chapter 57).

# ♦ EVALUATION

To evaluate effectiveness of nursing interventions, compare patient behaviors with those stated in the expected patient outcomes. Successful achievement of patient outcomes for the patient with a CVA is indicated by the following:

1. Has no signs or symptoms of increased intracranial pressure.
2. Maintains usual body weight and shows laboratory values (hematocrit, hemoglobin, and protein) that are within normal limits.
3. Is aware of (a) sensory/perceptual deficits and (b) how to compensate for sensory/perceptual alterations; and (c) how to use compensatory techniques such as scanning.
4. Has the ability to ambulate, to transfer, and/or to move freely in wheelchair.
5. Has the ability to perform ADL, including feeding, dressing, bathing, grooming, and toileting, with or without assistive devices.

6. Indicates a positive body image and cooperates with therapies.
7. Has ability to communicate needs.
8. Maintains bowel and bladder continence, with or without training programs, and experiences no constipation, diarrhea, or impaction.
9. Indicates adjustment to CVA and limitations that are present.
10. Experiences none of the following: contractures of joints, skin breakdown, thromboembolic events, or loss of muscle mass.
11. Explains ways to maintain health status: correctly describes needed medications, including dosage, route, effects, and side effects, and correctly explains care required.

## COMPLICATIONS

Prevention of joint deformity is initiated during the acute stage. This includes positioning of affected limbs in anatomic position and ROM exercises. There should be a regular schedule for turning the patient to avoid the danger of circulatory stasis, hypostatic pneumonia, and decubitus ulcer.

## INTRACRANIAL HEMORRHAGE

**Intracranial hemorrhages** include *bleeding into the subarachnoid space or into the brain tissue itself.* Unlike cerebral thrombosis or cerebral embolism, *intracranial hemorrhages cause damage to the brain by destroying and replacing neighboring brain tissue.* Nursing and medical treatment of patients with aneurysms and intracranial hemorrhage can be significantly different from that of patients with CVAs caused by embolism or thrombosis. Because of this, intracranial hemorrhages are considered separately.

### Etiology

Bleeding may be from a vessel on the surface of the brain, and the bleeding may be limited to the subarachnoid space. This is called a *subarachnoid hemorrhage with intracerebral hemorrhage.*[34] Bleeding from a vessel in the brain substance is called an *intracerebral hemorrhage* and may form a cerebral hematoma. Intracerebral hemorrhages may extend through the brain tissue to the ventricles and the subarachnoid space.

The most common causes of cerebral hemorrhage are listed in Box 57-10. *Berry aneurysms* can result from congenital deficits. *Fusiform aneurysms* can develop from atherosclerosis. *Mycotic aneurysms* are caused by *necrotic vasculitis* occurring in the vessel at a site where septic emboli have lodged. The necrosis causes thinning of the vessel wall and aneurysm formation.

Hypertension causes thickening and degeneration of cerebral arterioles, making the small arteries vulnerable to rupture. Arteriovenous (A-V) anomalies are tangled, interconnected vessels that allow blood to pass directly from the artery to the vein without passing through the capillaries. These vessels may be fed by one or several normal cerebral arteries and usually are malformed. Arterial pressure distends and eventually ruptures these vessels.

### Epidemiology

Intracranial hemorrhages are the third most frequent cause of CVAs.

### Pathophysiology

Any of these problems (aneurysms, hypertensive vascular disease, A-V malformation) can result in a subarachnoid hemorrhage, intracerebral hemorrhage, or a combination of the two. The most common site for berry aneurysms is the anterior portion of the circle of Willis at the junction between the internal carotid and posterior communicating arteries. Other common sites are the middle cerebral artery or the anterior communicating artery. A small number of intracranial hemorrhages occur in the vertebrobasilar artery system. Multiple aneurysms are found in many persons. The rupture of a vessel causes disruption of the blood flow to a selected area, as well as focal ischemic changes and infarction of brain tissue. In addition, the sudden release of blood acts as a concussion and unconsciousness results. It also causes a rapid rise in cerebrospinal fluid (CSF) pressure with displacement of the brain. *Bleeding into brain tissue itself can cause brain damage by dissecting the brain along the fiber tracts.* The blood itself is a noxious agent, and as it is hemolyzed, it irritates the blood vessels, the meninges, and the brain. The blood and the release of vasoactive substances promote arterial spasms, which can further decrease cerebral perfusion.[16]

Symptoms of an intracranial hemorrhage include sudden explosive headache, photophobia, and neck rigidity (if subarachnoid), nausea and vomiting, loss of consciousness (usually), convulsions, signs and symptoms of increased intracranial pressure, respiratory distress, and shock.

The following system of grading has been developed to classify the clinical state of the patient with intracranial bleeding by level of consciousness and neurologic deficit.

**grade I** Minimal bleeding, alert, no neurologic deficit
**grade II** Mild bleeding, alert, minimal neurologic deficit such as third nerve palsy and stiff neck
**grade III** Moderate bleeding, drowsy or confused, stiff neck with or without neurologic deficit
**grade IV** Moderate or severe bleeding; semicoma with or without neurologic deficit
**grade V** Severe bleeding, coma, decerebrate movement

Additional grades are added for patients older than 50 years of age and those with major heart, lung, kidney and liver conditions that increase risk for procedures.

### Prevention

Prevention of intracranial hemorrhage is similar to prevention of CVA. Many of the same risk factors also apply.

## Medical Management

### Diagnostic tests

The diagnostic tests used for intracranial hemorrhage are the same as those used for cerebrovascular accidents.

Laboratory findings include an abnormal CT scan, increased CSF pressure, and blood and white blood cells in the CSF. Lumbar puncture may not be performed if there is evidence of extensive brain damage for fear of precipitating *tentorial herniation*. An arteriogram is used to identify the exact cause of the problem.

### Medication

Medications are at times given to sedate the patient who has suffered an intracranial hemorrhage. This occurs especially when there is a delay in surgical management. Dexamethasone (Decadron) often is administered, as well as aminocaproic acid (Amicar), which is given to seal the clot. Phenytoin (Dilantin) may be given for the prevention of seizures.

### Treatment

Not all aneurysms can be treated surgically at the site of the lesion. If such surgery is not feasible, an alternate procedure may be used to reduce the chances of hemorrhage. The aneurysm may be wrapped[47] or the common carotid artery in the neck may be completely or partially obliterated to lessen the blood flow to the site of the aneurysm, *provided* enough blood can be supplied from collateral vessels to preserve vital brain function. The procedure usually is performed in stages of several days.

A clamp (Silverstone or Salibi) that has a detachable screw stem and can be tightened gradually is used. Usually the surgeon adjusts it each day, and the nurse who attends the patient watches closely and is instructed to release the clamp at once if evidence of inadequate blood supply exists. The nurse completes regular neurologic checks relative to placement of the clamp in the dominant or nondominant hemisphere. Any signs of muscle weakness in the face or in either extremity on the side opposite the incision or any changes in the level of consciousness, vital signs, or sensory or muscular coordination or control should be reported to the neurosurgeon at once. Immediate removal of the clamp may prevent irreversible complications such as hemiplegia, aphasia, and loss of consciousness.

If symptoms of inadequate blood supply appear, further surgical treatment cannot safely be performed, although the clamp may be left indefinitely to partially obliterate the vessel. If complete occlusion can be tolerated, the vessel may be permanently ligated. Serial embolizations of blood vessels that "feed" the aneurysm also may be accomplished via the femoral or axillary route.

The procedure is similar to that for a cerebral angiogram, and the postoperative care is the same. Thrombus formation with resultant cerebral embolism may complicate the patient's postoperative course after any surgery for a cerebral aneurysm. It is a feared and often fatal complication.

### Diet

No special diet is prescribed for the patient with an intracranial hemorrhage. If the patient is unconscious, intravenous feedings are carried out.

### Activity

The immediate treatment for intracranial hemorrhage is to keep the person absolutely quiet to prevent additional bleeding. Many of these patients are unconscious and require care as described earlier in this chapter. In addition, because the bleeding causes an elevation in the intracranial pressure, they need care for this problem as well. An antifibrinolytic agent (aminocaproic acid [Amicar]) may be used to seal the clot. (See the Guidelines box below, for further details of the nursing care of the patient with an intracranial hemorrhage.)

### Referral/Consultation

The reader is referred to this section under care of the patient with a CVA.

## Surgical Management

The only satisfactory treatment for congenital aneurysm is surgery. If an intracerebral hematoma has formed, it may be evacuated after the patient's condition is stable. Before surgery can be performed, however, the location of the aneurysm must be determined by arteriography (angiography). The time after the acute rupture when arteriograms are taken and when surgery is performed varies with the person, age, the intensity and kind of symptoms present, and the surgeon's judgment. Because angiography may increase symptoms, it may be followed by immediate surgery.

Before surgical treatment of an aneurysm is attempted, the surgeon usually explains the hope for cure

**Guidelines for Care of the Person With an Intracranial Hemorrhage**

Use gentleness in moving patient.
Keep room darkened.
Keep patient on bed rest; head of bed usually is elevated 30 degrees. Occasionally bathroom privileges are allowed.
Give patient no ice water.
Initiate a bowel program to prevent straining at stool.
Only allow a few visitors.
Decrease stimuli in room; no TV or radio in severe cases.
Take no rectal temperatures; give no enemas or suppositories.

and the risks involved to the patient's family. The nurse must appreciate how distressing the situation is for family members and should realize that the time spent waiting to know whether the outcome will be favorable seems interminable to them. The nursing care the patient will receive postoperatively should be explained to family members if they are to be with the patient. For example, it is important that both the patient and the family know that blood pressure, pulse rate, respiratory rate, and other pertinent observations will be taken frequently, because these procedures can be most upsetting if their purpose and the need to check them so frequently are not understood. Some patients may spend the initial postoperative period in the intensive care unit. The family should be prepared for this possibility.

Surgery consists of a *craniotomy* and *location of the aneurysm.* When found, the aneurysm may be obliterated by ligation at its neck with the application of a silver clip. If the base of the aneurysm is too large for ligation to be practical, it may be wrapped or it may be coated with a liquid, adherent, plastic substance that hardens to form a firm support about the weakened vessel wall and thereby prevents rupture.[47] If the aneurysm has not ruptured but has produced symptoms, attempts may be made to produce thrombosis within the aneurysm by use of an electric current and other means. Both before and after surgery the nurse should observe the patient for signs of increased intracranial pressure.

If the surgery is successful, patients will be cured, although usually they will be advised to avoid strenuous exercise and emotional stress for the remainder of their lives. Occasionally, they may have a severe physical or mental handicap resulting from damage to brain tissue during surgery. If so, they need the same type of care as discussed for patients with a CVA (see p. 1988).

### Nursing Management

The nursing management of the patient with an intracerebral hemorrhage is the same as that for the patient with a CVA, except in the cases in which surgery is performed. The reader is referred to the appropriate sections in this chapter. See the Guidelines box, p. 1998, for a description of key points of care for a patient who requires aneurysm precautions.

# INTRACRANIAL TUMORS

## ETIOLOGY

***Primary intracranial tumors,*** or ***neoplasms,*** arise from the intrinsic cells of brain tissues and from the pituitary and pineal glands. *Secondary* or *metastatic* tumors are also a frequent contributing type of intracranial tumor. Intracranial tumors are only one example of intracranial lesions. Variable intracranial lesions occur, such as hemorrhage, abscess, and trauma, and cause similar signs and symptoms as a neoplasm, depending on the site of the lesion.

## EPIDEMIOLOGY

Tumors occur in great variety; produce neurologic symptoms because of their size, location, and invasive qualities; usually destroy the tissues in which they are situated and displace tissues around them; and are a frequent cause of increased intracranial pressure.

## PATHOPHYSIOLOGY

The symptoms of intracranial tumors result from both local and general effects of the tumor. Locally, the effects are from infiltration, invasion, and destruction of brain tissues at a particular site (Box 57-12). There is also direct pressure on nerve structures, causing degeneration and interference with local circulation. Local edema develops, and if it is long-standing, it often is sufficient to interfere with the function of nerve tissues.

A brain tumor of any type situated anywhere in the cranial cavity may cause an increase in intracranial pressure. The increased intracranial pressure is then transmitted throughout the brain and the ventricular system. Eventually the ventricular system is distorted and displaced sufficiently to cause partial ventricular obstruction at some site, even though the tumor is some distance from the ventricular system. A tumor may directly obstruct a particular ventricle early when it grows adjacent to the ventricle. A tumor of the cerebrum can distort the lateral ventricles. A tumor that presses on the third ventricle, the aqueduct of Sylvius, or the fourth ventricle can result in obstruction of CSF flow into the central canal of the spinal cord. Cerebral edema forms even at some distance from the tumor and generally adds to the increasing pressure. As the edema increases, the blood supply to the brain is compromised and carbon dioxide is retained. The vessels dilate in an effort

**BOX 57-12 Symptoms of Tumors Found in Specific Brain Lobes**

**FRONTAL LOBE**

Personality disturbances (range from subtle personality changes to obvious psychotic behavior)
Inappropriate affect
Indifference of bodily functions

**PRECENTRAL GYRUS**

Jacksonian seizures

**OCCIPITAL LOBE**

Visual disturbances preceding convulsions

**TEMPORAL LOBE**

Olfactory, visual, or gustatory hallucinations
Psychomotor seizures with automatic behavior

**PARIETAL LOBE**

Inability to replicate pictures
Loss of right-left discrimination

to increase blood oxygen supply. Unfortunately, this also increases edema, and the situation can deteriorate rapidly.

**Papilledema** results from the general effects of the increased intracranial pressure and often is a relatively late sign. Death usually is caused by brainstem compression resulting from herniation. The mechanism for the occasional acute focal symptoms that occur is thought to be caused by rapidly increasing cerebral edema or by functional decompensation of edematous tissues.

Common clinical circumstances in which intracranial tumors are present, or are likely to be found, include those persons with (1) general impairment of cerebral function or a seizure, (2) evidence of increased intracranial pressure, and (3) specific or focal intracranial tumor syndrome.

### Types of Tumors

Brain tumors are named for the tissues from which they arise. The more frequently encountered ones include gliomas, meningiomas, pituitary adenomas, and acoustic neuromas. In addition, the brain is a frequent site for secondary tumors from other organs.

**Gliomas** account for about one half of all brain tumors. They arise in any part of the connective tissue of the brain. As a rule, in adults they primarily infiltrate the cerebral hemisphere tissues and are not so well outlined that they can be completely excised surgically. They grow rapidly, and most persons do not live longer than a year after diagnosis. The less malignant gliomas are the *astrocytomas* and the *oligodendrogliomas. Ependymomas* arise from the walls of the ventricular system. They cause death in about 3 years. The most malignant and rapidly growing forms are the *glioblastoma multiforme* and *medulloblastoma.* Gliomas sometimes start as one type and develop into more malignant forms if untreated.

The **meningiomas,** which account for 13% to 18% of all primary tumors in the intracranial cavity, arise from the meningeal coverings of the brain.[7] They occur most frequently in the meninges over the cerebral hemispheres in the parasagittal region along the ridge of the sphenoid bone and in the anterior fossa in relation to the olfactory groove or the sella turcica. When located in the posterior fossa, they arise from the cerebellopontine angle, from the tentorium, or rarely in the region of the foramen magnum. Meningiomas vary widely as to size and histologic findings. They usually are benign, but many undergo malignant changes. The neurologic signs and symptoms produced by meningiomas relative to these sites may include anosmia, optic atrophy, extraocular palsies, visual defects, papilledema, pituitary disturbances, and cerebellar dysfunction. Meningiomas frequently cause seizures and involvement of the limbs as related to their presence in the convexity of a cerebral hemisphere.

*Acoustic neuromas* constitute about 8% of all primary intracranial tumors.[11] Neuromas may arise from any cranial nerve. The tumor affecting the acoustic nerve generally arises from its sheath but usually extends to affect the nerve fibers. The signs and symptoms resulting from these slowly growing tumors are related to compression of adjacent cranial nerves (trigeminal and facial), cerebellum, and the brainstem. Pituitary tumors are another intracranial tumor.

Metastatic tumors that arise primarily in the lung, kidney, breast, colon, and other organs account for about one fifth of all intracranial tumors. Primary brain tumors, conversely, rarely metastasize to other organs. (See Table 57-12 for review of types of brain tumors.)

## PREVENTION

No known primary prevention exists for intracranial tumors, except in cases in which the tumor results from metastatic disease. Cigarette smoking is directly linked to brain tumors because neoplasms of the lung often metastasize to the brain. In fact, a significant number of malignant lung tumors are discovered subsequent to signs and symptoms of brain metastasis.

## MEDICAL MANAGEMENT

The nurse works collaboratively with the physician for implementation of prescribed medical therapy. Because the nurse has a major role in discharge planning and patient teaching, these are discussed under nursing management.

### Diagnostic Tests

No one procedure is entirely diagnostic for brain tumors, but the CT scan certainly has revolutionized the ease of diagnosis with minimal danger and discomfort to the patient. If the patient's condition is stable, an EEG, brain scan, or echoencephalogram may be used to help determine the exact site and nature of the tumor. Patients with increased intracranial pressure but with no evidence of specific neurologic deficits are evaluated as rapidly as possible. In emergency situations, arteriography or ventriculography may be used to locate the tumor.

A lumbar puncture may be helpful in assessment of patients suspected of having a brain tumor. As mentioned previously, it is not undertaken in patients with symptoms of increased intracranial pressure except in special circumstances because of the danger of herniation.

Brain scans are particularly useful in screening patients for suspected brain tumors by demonstrating the size and site of the tumor. A negative brain scan result does not, however, exclude a tumor, because a small tumor may not be visualized. Conversely, positive scan findings may be caused by a cranial lesion other than a tumor. An EEG is particularly useful in the detection of abnormal brain waves, generally or focally, within the cerebral hemispheres or their coverings. The encephalo-

**TABLE 57-12 Types of Brain Tumors**

| TYPE | INCIDENCE | PATHOLOGY |
|---|---|---|
| Glioma<br>Astrocytomas<br>Oligodendrogliomas<br>Ependymomas<br>Medulloblastoma<br>Glioblastoma multiforme—most malignant | Accounts for one half of brain tumors | Arises in any part of brain connective tissue; infiltrates primarily cerebral hemisphere tissue; not so well outlined as to be incised completely; grows rapidly—most persons live months to years; tumors assigned grade from 1 to 4, with 4 the most malignant |
| Meningioma | 13% to 18% of all primary tumors in intracranial cavity | Arises from meningeal coverings of brain; usually benign but may undergo malignant changes; usually encapsulated, and surgical cure possible; recurrence possible |
| Pituitary tumor | Occurs in all age groups, but more often in women | Arises from various tissues; surgical approach usually successful; recurrence possible |
| Neuroma (schwannoma, neurofibroma) | Acoustic neuroma is most common | Arises from Schwann's cells inside auditory meatus on vestibular portion of third cranial nerve; usually benign but may undergo cellular change and become malignant; will regrow if not completely excised; surgical resection often difficult because of location |
| Metastatic tumors | From 2% to 20% of all patients with cancer have metastasis to the brain | Cancer cells spread to brain via circulatory system; surgical resection very difficult; even with treatment, prognosis is very poor; survival beyond 1 or 2 years is uncommon |

gram is helpful in identifying displacement of the ventricular system and the pineal gland from their normal midline positions. Displacement to the right of the midline or to the left may indicate a tumor within the respective hemisphere. This so-called displacement also is referred to as a *brain shift* and is a relatively late stage of increased intracranial pressure. Radiographic studies of the skull are obtained initially and may reveal increased intracranial pressure and abnormal calcifications.

Other tests that may be helpful in locating the tumor are arteriographic and ventriculographic examination. The ventriculogram is used when the suggested diagnosis is such that a spinal or lumbar puncture is contraindicated. Two newer procedures that can help with diagnosis of a brain tumor are the magnetic resonance imaging (MRI) and positron emission tomography (PET) scans. These are described in Chapter 56.

## Treatment

With the development of newer diagnostic techniques, modern surgical and radiologic methods, more effective chemotherapeutic agents, and an increased understanding of functional anatomy of the cerebrum, the prognosis for patients with intracranial tumors is more favorable today than in the past. The prognosis, however, depends on early diagnosis and treatment because as the tumor grows within the cranial cavity, it exerts pressure on vital brain centers and causes irreparable brain damage and death. Although approximately one half of all brain tumors are benign, they also may cause death by exerting pressure on vital brain centers. It is important to remember that although cells of the CNS can regain function, even after cerebral edema, dead cells cannot regenerate. Early treatment is thus necessary to preserve cerebral functions. Early treatment also becomes important as newer techniques have been developed that improve surgical risks and postoperative prospects for patients with intracranial tumors. These techniques include *hypothermia,* the establishment of *controlled hypotensive states during surgery* by means of appropriate drugs; *hyperthermia to destroy tumor cells*[55]; and *dehydration of cerebral tissues* by the administration of osmotic diuretics such as urea compounds or mannitol before, during, and after surgery.

The nurse's attitude about the treatment of brain tumors cannot help but be communicated to the patient and family. The nurse should make an effort to communicate a positive attitude while stressing the importance of early diagnosis and treatment of intracranial tumors.

## Diet

No special diet is prescribed for the patient with a brain tumor. Rather the diet is modified in terms of the patient's mental status.

## Activity

The patient is encouraged to be as active as possible. The only contraindication to normal activity is the presence of increased intracranial pressure in which case the patient is kept as quiet as possible.

## SURGICAL MANAGEMENT

Intracranial surgery typically is used for all types of pathologic conditions of the brain, including tumor removal.

A surgical opening through the skull is known as a **craniotomy.** It is a basic preparatory procedure for intracranial surgery. A series of burr holes are made first, and then the bone between the holes is cut with a special saw (Gigli) to permit removal of the bone. Bone is then removed in such a way that it can be replaced if desired. The opening depends on the lesion site. Brain surgery may be performed under hypothermia to lessen bleeding during the procedure. Drugs such as norepinephrine bitartrate (Levophed) may be used to maintain blood pressure. *Patients also may be placed in a barbiturate coma during the surgery and for several days afterwards to lessen brain activity, metabolism, and oxygen needs.* This may help to prevent worsening of deficits because of hypoxia.

When the brain lesion is in the *supratentorium* (above the tentorium or in the cerebrum), the incision usually is made behind the hairline. When the incision is into the *infratentorium* (below the tentorium or in the brainstem and cerebellum), it is made slightly above the nape of the neck. Neither of these incisions is apparent when the hair has regrown.

Tumors involving the pituitary gland that do not extend outside the sella turcica usually are removed by means of a transphenoidal approach. After the surgery, packing is placed inside the nose and remains for 3 to 4 days. A muscle graft from the thigh is used to close the defect in the dura. With this type of surgery, recovery is rapid and the patient has no loss of hair or external cranial incision.

After craniotomy and removal of the bone, an incision is made into the meninges and the tumor is removed or other cranial surgery performed. The removed bone is carefully saved or preserved. After brain surgery, *the bone may be replaced immediately (as in a bone flap with muscle attachment) when no evidence of infection or increased intracranial pressure exists.* At times the bone is left out for variable periods to prevent postoperative pressure from cerebral edema or to permit expansion of an inoperable tumor. In this instance the preserved bone is used as a mold for a bone prosthesis, which is inserted with wire at a later date, or the preserved bone is reinserted. Sterile acrylic is the material presently used to make the bone prosthesis. The acrylic can be molded directly into the skull opening after the dura mater is covered with a thin plastic sheet at surgery, or it can be molded from the preserved bone at a later time. The removal of part of the skull without replacement is called *craniectomy.* When a tumor cannot be removed because of its location and nature, a subtemporal decompression is made by leaving an opening in the dura and skull. *Cranioplasty* is the repair of a cranial defect through use of substitute bone materials.

Limitation of some functions may necessarily follow the complete removal of brain tumors occurring in the cerebral hemispheres. Portions of the frontal lobe are removed in some instances with little residual damage. Patients with tumors located where they are rapidly accessible to removal, such as meningiomas and tumors of the outer cerebrum, have the best prognosis. Today the decision to operate on persons with large tumors is weighed carefully by the neurosurgeon. If the surgery is likely to leave the patient with much permanent disability, the decision not to operate often will be made.

## NURSING MANAGEMENT

### ♦ ASSESSMENT

It is important to assess both subjective and objective data in the patient with an intracranial tumor.

#### Subjective Data

Subjective data to be collected to assess the patient with intracranial tumor include the following:

- Patient's understanding of the diagnosis
- Changes in personality or judgment
- Presence of abnormal sensation (paresthesia or anesthesia)
- Visual problems—loss of visual acuity or diplopia
- Complaints of unusual odors (especially with temporal lobe tumors)
- Headache
- Hearing loss
- Inability to carry out ADL

Headache is an early symptom in about one third of patients with brain tumors and is variable in nature. The pain can be either slight or severe, dull or sharp, and transitory or intermittent. Possible characteristics of the headache is its nocturnal occurrence or its presence on first awaking and its deep nonpulsatile quality; however, these are not specific attributes because they occur in headaches from other causes. The mechanism for the headache is not known. In most patients the intracranial pressure is normal for the first weeks when headache is present. The headache may be caused by local swelling of tissues and distortion of blood vessels in and around the tumor. Later, headache seems to be related to increased intracranial pressure. Tumors above the tentorium cause headache on the side of and in the vicinity of the tumor. Those on the posterior fossae usually cause ipsilateral, retroauricular, or occipital headache. With elevated intracranial pressure, the headache becomes bilateral regardless of location of the tumor.

#### Objective Data

Objective data to be collected to assess the patient with intracranial tumor include the following:

- Motor strength
- Gait
- Level of alertness and consciousness

Orientation
Pupils: size, equality, and reactivity
Vital signs
Funduscopic examination for evidence of papilledema
Seizures
Speech abnormalities
Cranial nerve abnormalities
Symptoms of increased intracranial pressure

### Diagnostic Test Findings

The tumor can be visualized on the CT scan, the MRI, or a brain scan.

## ♦ NURSING DIAGNOSES

Nursing diagnoses are determined from analysis of patient data. Nursing diagnoses for the patient with a brain tumor may include but are not limited to the following:

| Diagnostic Title | Possible Etiologic Factors |
|---|---|
| Tissue perfusion, altered (cerebral) | Decreased blood flow (arterial) |
| Injury (trauma), high risk for | Sensory/motor deficits |
| Skin integrity, impaired | Surgery |
| Nutrition altered: less than body requirements | Chewing/swallowing difficulties |
| Fluid volume excess or deficit | Compromised regulatory mechanism |
| Constipation | Immobility |
| Pain | Immobility, trauma of surgery |
| Mobility, impaired physical | Neuromuscular impairment, decreased strength or endurance |

## ♦ EXPECTED PATIENT OUTCOMES

Expected patient outcomes for the patient with a brain tumor may include but are not limited to the following:

1. Maintains cerebral perfusion as indicated by the absence of signs and symptoms of increased intracranial pressure.
2. Remains free of injury.
3. Has intact skin, with no areas of breakdown.
4. Maintains adequate nutritional status as evidenced by usual body weight and normal laboratory values.
5. Has no edema or dehydration.
6. Maintains bowel continence.
7. Is relieved of pain or discomfort as indicated by the absence of subjective or objective symptoms.
8. Maintains mobility.

## ♦ INTERVENTIONS

### Facilitating Surgery

#### Preoperative care

Baseline data of neurologic and physiologic status should be recorded by the nurse before surgery. Written permission for surgery on the brain must be given by the nearest relative unless the patient is able to sign. Even when the patient has given consent, close relatives usually are consulted, and the neurosurgeon obtains their consent before surgery. The patient and family usually feel extremely threatened by the prospect of brain surgery and should be encouraged to express their fears. Specific fears may be related to a permanent change in appearance, dependency, or death. Psychologic support of the patient and family is a priority intervention. The nursing staff should provide time for this part of essential nursing care of the patient. The patient also may wish to see a spiritual advisor before surgery.

Treatments and procedures should be explained to the patient even though the person *may not* seem to understand fully. Enemas may not be given before surgery because of the danger of increasing intracranial pressure further by exertion and by the absorption of fluid. Narcotics, except codeine, rarely are ordered preoperatively because they may cause further depression of cerebral function. Any order for their use should be carefully verified by the nurse. If the head is to be shaved, the procedure may be delayed until the patient is in the operating room. Hair should not be discarded but should be returned to the patient unit because the patient may wish to have it made into a wig. Synthetic wigs are a good alternative for many patients. In many hospitals it is the practice to shave only the portion of the patient's head necessary to do the surgery. Hair along the front hairline often can be left so that after surgery it can be drawn backward to cover the scar. The hair is shampooed, and the condition of the scalp is noted.

**Preparation of the family.** Family members need to be prepared for what they will face when they see the patient after surgery. They need to know that the patient will have a head dressing and that edema may distort facial features. They also need to know that the patient may have discolored areas about the eyes (ecchymosis). If the patient is unconscious or has a limitation such as aphasia, this should be discussed with family members before they see the patient. If the patient is alert, the family will be advised to sit quietly at the bedside because talking will tire the patient.

The Guidelines box, p. 2004, summarizes preoperative care.

#### Postoperative care

**Postanesthesia care.** Whether in the patient unit or in the recovery room, the nurse should be certain that the following are readily available: side rails for the bed, suction machine or wall suction with disposable suction catheters, an airway, a lumbar puncture set, and an emergency medication tray (cardiac and respiratory stimulants, amobarbital sodium [Amytal], anticonvulsive drugs), syringes, intravenous and hypodermic needles, and a tourniquet. An emergency tracheostomy tray should be also readily available on the unit.

The patient is observed regularly during the early

### Guidelines for Preoperative Care of the Person Having Intracranial Surgery

Baseline data of neurologic and physiologic status should be recorded.
Patient and family should be encouraged to verbalize fears.
Treatments and procedures are explained fully, even if unsure whether patient understands.
If head is shaved, it usually is done in the operating room.
Antiseptic shampoo may be ordered night before surgery and may be repeated in morning.
If hair is shaved, it is saved and given to patient or family.
Prepare family for appearance of patient after surgery:
- Head dressing
- Edema and ecchymosis of face common
- Temporarily decreased mental status (possible)

postoperative period for signs of increased intracranial pressure. Frequency of making and recording specific observations depends on the patient's condition.

Any change in the patient's *vital signs, state of consciousness, pupillary response,* or *ability to use muscles* is reported at once. Restlessness, often secondary to tissue hypoxia; forewarnings of hemorrhage or irritation to the brain; or other symptoms of increased intracranial pressure should be watched for and reported immediately to the surgeon. These changes are described earlier in this chapter.

**Maintaining cerebral perfusion.** Immediately after surgery the patient is placed on the side to ensure an adequate airway. To facilitate change of head dressings and other treatments after surgery, the patient may be placed in bed "head to foot." If a large brain tumor has been removed, the patient must not be turned on the affected side because this position may cause displacement of brain structures by gravity. Otherwise, turning to either side is permitted. The primary objective is to eliminate pressure on the operative site. Handling of the brain tissues and surgical trauma cause cerebral edema, which contributes to increased intracranial pressure.

If there has been *supratentorial* surgery (above the cerebellum), *the head of the bed is elevated at least 45 degrees and a large pillow is placed under the patient's head and shoulders.* This position should lessen the possibility of hemorrhage, provide for better circulation of the CSF, and promote venous return. All these measures assist in decreasing cerebral edema and in preventing increased intracranial pressure. Internal bleeding would also contribute to a rise in intracranial pressure. If an *infratentorial* tumor has been removed, *the bed should be kept flat with only a small pillow under the nape of the neck and the patient turned to either side.* Any *flexion* of the neck should be avoided, either midline or laterally. Because infratentorial incisions are made adjacent to the medulla, vital centers, and ninth and tenth cranial nerves, there is more danger of respiratory complications and brainstem compression.

*Coughing* and *vomiting* are to be avoided because these increase intracranial pressure. Suctioning, if permitted, should be performed gently and cautiously to avoid initiating coughing. Suctioning through the nose also is avoided. Deep breathing exercises should not be followed by coughing.

**Preventing injury.** Some patients must be protected from injuring themselves after surgery. Patients who pull at dressings or catheters or scratch or hit themselves must be attended constantly. Occasionally some type of hand restraint such as a large mitten made of dressings, bandages, and stockinette fastened at the wrist with adhesive tape may be used. Mittens usually upset patients less than arm restraints, because with mittens they can move their arms freely. The fingers should be separated with gauze to prevent skin irritation and should be curled around a large bandage roll in the palm to prevent hyperextension of the fingers. The hand is then well covered with dressings held in place with a bandage. A piece of stockinette is closed at one end and everted so that the tied end cannot cause injury to the eye. It is then slipped over the bandaged hand and fastened securely at the wrist with adhesive tape. The wrist should be shaved and the skin protected with tincture of benzoin before adhesive is used. At least every other day the mitten must be removed, the hand washed in warm water, and passive exercise given to the fingers before the mitten is reapplied.

**Caring for the wound.** Usually the wound is covered with gauze dressings, and a special head dressing (neurosurgical roll) is then applied in a recurrent fashion from the back to the front of the head and anchored. The head *dressing* is inspected regularly for amount and type of drainage. Serosanguineous drainage on the dressings should be measured and marked, as is done with other dressings, so that it can be accurately checked for an increase in amount. Yellowish drainage should be reported immediately to the physician because it probably indicates loss of spinal fluid. If the head dressing appears to be soaked with drainage, the dressing should be reinforced. It may be necessary to apply a pressure dressing. Dressings that become wet should be removed by the neurosurgeon and replaced. It is not unusual for dressings to be removed the day after surgery and the incision left open to the air.

When the final dressings are removed, the scalp can be gently cleansed with hydrogen peroxide to remove dried blood. Crusts can be loosened with mineral oil. Patients usually are advised to wait 7 to 10 days after the surgery before the head is shampooed. A head covering usually is worn to protect the wound, to help remind the patient not to scratch, and for cosmetic reasons until the hair has grown back. A cap can be made by tying one end of a 10-inch piece of tubular stockinette. Head scarves or wigs usually are preferred by women, and wigs also can be worn by men. Many patients prefer to wear disposable paper caps such as those worn by the operating room staff. The patient who has had a piece of bone left out will have a depression in the scalp and should be warned of the danger of bumping the head in this area.

**Promoting nutrition.** Fluid intake and output should be accurately recorded. Fluids can be resumed when the person has good bowel sounds, is awake enough to swallow, and has a stable neurologic status. If no orders exist to the contrary, 2500 to 3000 ml of fluid should be given each day. Some neurosurgeons routinely restrict fluids to 1500 ml/day for the first 3 days after a craniotomy.

Because the gag and swallowing reflexes may be depressed or absent after *infratentorial* brain surgery, fluids by mouth usually are withheld for at least a day and intravenous fluids are substituted. They should be run very slowly to prevent increased intracranial pressure. If reflexes are present, water is carefully given by mouth. The patient should be placed in a semisitting position. Fluid should never be forced on a patient who is still neurologically depressed because of the danger of aspiration. If after several days the gag and swallowing reflexes are still absent, a nasogastric tube may be inserted. A regular diet is given to all neurosurgical patients as soon as it can be tolerated.

**Promoting elimination.** Care must be taken to see that the patient voids sufficiently. Urinary output must be carefully recorded, and the specific gravity of most specimens should be measured. Sometimes an indwelling catheter may be used for a few days after surgery. A *decrease* in output must be reported because it may indicate the onset of a metabolic disorder of CNS origin. Correspondingly, an *increase* in urine output with low specific gravities also should be reported because it may herald the onset of *diabetes insipidus.* Although this condition occurs most frequently after hypophysectomy for pituitary tumor, it also can occur after trauma to the head or intracranial surgery (especially involving areas near the pituitary).

Because most patients who have intracranial surgery will be given some type of steroids, it is important to test the urine for glucose and acetone. Patients who develop diabetes mellitus as a sequela of steroid treatment may require active treatment of the diabetes until the steroids are discontinued.

Laxatives or stool softeners should be used liberally to prevent constipation and straining during defecation. The patient should be instructed not to strain. Bowel function should be monitored by the nurse to prevent fecal impaction. If an impaction does develop, enemas or manual evacuation may be necessary. Suppositories also may be used after the initial postoperative period to promote bowel regularity.

**Promoting comfort.** Patients who are conscious after intracranial surgery may complain of a severe ***headache*** for 24 to 48 hours. CNS depressants, such as opiates and sedatives, are avoided. Codeine sulfate often is prescribed and is given parenterally. Acetylsalicylic acid (aspirin) or acetaminophen (Tylenol) may be given by rectum, or by mouth if fluids can be swallowed. An ice cap may be placed on the head, and sudden movement

**Guidelines for Postoperative Care of the Person With Intracranial Surgery**

1. Perform monitoring:
   a. Assess neurologic status, including ability to move, level of orientation and alertness, and pupil checks.
   b. Assess degree and character of drainage.
      (1) Amount of drainage and bleeding should be minimal.
      (2) Initial head dressing can be reinforced as necessary.
      (3) Often incision is left open to air after first several days.
2. Promote mobility:
   a. Turning to either side is permitted except when large brain tumors have been removed. If this is the case, patient is not turned to affected side because gravity may cause displacement of brain structures.
   b. If supratentorial surgery was performed, the head of the bed is elevated at least 30 degrees.
   c. If infratentorial surgery was performed, the bed is flat or elevated only slightly and a small pillow is placed under the nape of the neck. Neck flexion is avoided.
   d. Early ambulation is encouraged to prevent complications of bed rest. Observe carefully for signs of postural hypotension; raise head of bed gradually; patient should always sit on edge of bed before standing.
3. Promote decreased intracranial pressure:
   a. Space nursing activities to allow patient to rest between them.
   b. Coughing and vomiting should be avoided.
   c. Suctioning should be performed only as necessary, and then gently and cautiously.
4. Protect safety of patient:
   a. Use soft hand restraints if restraints are necessary.
   b. Use mittens as alternative to restraints; make sure fingers are separated and fingers are placed around large roll. Change mitt at least daily—give range of motion to hand at this time.
   c. Keep side rails up at all times.
5. Promote electrolyte balance:
   a. Perform accurate intake and output with measurement of specific gravity. Do frequent testing for glucose and acetone if patient is taking steroids.
   b. Have patient resume diet as soon as possible; assess for difficulty in swallowing or absence of gag reflex.
   c. Monitor electrolytes for evidence of abnormalities.
6. Promote comfort:
   a. Medicate for comfort with codeine sulfate or nonnarcotic analgesic.
   b. Ice cap to head for headache may be helpful.

and jarring are avoided. The patient should be protected from loud noises and bright lights. The patient may need assistance with turning and other ADL.

**Promoting early mobility.** The patient who has had surgery for a *supratentorial* lesion usually is allowed out of bed on the second to third postoperative day. If the surgery was extensive or complications develop, bed rest may be prescribed for longer periods. Activity is increased gradually, and the patient is watched carefully for signs of increased intracranial pressure. First the head of the bed should be elevated to high Fowler's position, and then the patient should sit on the edge of the bed with the feet dangling over the side. If this is tolerated, 4 to 6 hours later, with the help of two persons, the patient may be assisted to a chair and usually may sit up for a half hour. It is important to check the patient for postural hypotension while progressive activity is begun. Any drop in blood pressure of more than 20 points or complaints of dizziness by the patient should delay ambulation for several hours before another attempt is made. Patients then progress to normal activity as quickly as they desire and are able.

The patient who has had surgery for an *infratentorial* lesion usually is not permitted up for a much longer time. The trend is toward getting up earlier, depending on the patient's condition. Initial progress may be slower because patients who have been kept flat in bed for some time may be dizzy and experience orthostatic hypotension when arising until the circulatory system readjusts to the change in position.

The Guidelines box, p. 2005, contains a summary of postoperative care.

## ♦ EVALUATION

To evaluate the effectiveness of nursing interventions, compare patient behaviors with those stated in the expected patient outcomes. Successful achievement of patient outcomes for the patient with a brain tumor is indicated by the following:

1. Has no signs or symptoms of increased intracranial pressure.
2. Remains free of injury.
3. Has intact skin, with no sustained redness.
4. Maintains usual body weight and has laboratory values (hematocrit, hemoglobin, and protein) within normal limits.
5. Has no edema or signs of dehydration such as decreased skin turgor or abnormalities in laboratory values.
6. Maintains continence, has bowel pattern that includes soft, formed stool at least every other day without undue straining, and experiences no constipation, diarrhea, or impaction.
7. Has no pain and shows no behavior that indicates pain, such as grimacing, shallow breathing, or restlessness.
8. Is able to ambulate and to transfer.

## COMPLICATIONS

### Hydrocephalus

Occasionally a catheter is placed in a ventricle of the brain to drain excess spinal fluid and prevent increased intracranial pressure. The catheter usually is attached to a drainage system, and the collection bottle frequently is attached to the bed. The tubing and drainage receptacle should be sterile, and care must be taken to prevent kinking of the tubing. If drainage appears to stop, the neurosurgeon should be notified. The catheter usually is left in place for 24 to 48 hours and is then removed by the surgeon.

**Hydrocephalus** of a more permanent nature also occurs in the presence of intracranial tumors and is manifested by symptoms of increased intracranial pressure. Treatment consists of a shunting procedure. The different types of shunting procedures are named for their point of origin and termination and include the following:

1. Cyst to peritoneal
2. Lumbar-peritoneal
3. Ventricular-jugular
4. Ventricular-peritoneal

In this type of surgery, excessive CSF is shunted away from the CNS and into either the peritoneal cavity

**Guidelines for Postoperative Care of the Person With a Shunt**

1. Perform monitoring:
   a. Assess neurologic status frequently for any decrease in mental status.
   b. Observe for symptoms of subdural hematoma, one of the possible side effects of the surgery.
   c. Monitor for symptoms of overdrainage, as evidenced by headache, especially when patient is sitting upright or standing.
   d. Assess degree and character of drainage:
      (1) Amount of drainage and bleeding should be minimal.
      (2) Reinforce dressing as needed.
      (3) Often incisional areas are left open to air after several days.
2. Maintain gastrointestinal status:
   a. Check frequently for signs of paralytic ileus; manipulation of the bowel that occurs with the placement of the shunt's peritoneal part can predispose the patient to this.
   b. Patient usually is given nothing by mouth for first day, and then clear liquids are started.
   c. Regular diet is resumed as soon as good bowel sounds are present and patient tolerates liquids.
3. Maintain comfort:
   a. Patient may need more frequent pain medication because of involvement of abdominal area.
   b. Keep pressure off incisional sites.
4. Promote mobility:
   a. Turning to either side is permitted.
   b. Raise head of bed gradually when mobilizing patient.
   c. Patient is encouraged to ambulate as much as possible to encourage adaption to decreased intracranial pressure.

(where it is absorbed) or the jugular vein. At times, a Ryckham reservoir is placed through a burr hole into the ventricle. This device can easily be palpated through the skin. Some of the shunts have an on-off valve, as well as a part that may be pumped to facilitate drainage. Valves that are inserted can be set for a certain pressure, with some control over the amount of fluid drained.

See the Guidelines box, p. 2006, for key elements of the care of the patient having a shunt.

### Meningitis

Meningitis is a relatively rare complication of brain surgery but can result from infection acquired during or after surgery. After supratentorial surgery, the nurse should watch for any clear, watery drainage from the nose. This drainage may be present if there has been a tear in the meninges, which causes subsequent loss of CSF. The treatment consists of keeping the patient very quiet, avoiding suctioning the nose or blowing it, and administration of appropriate antibiotics. The leakage usually subsides spontaneously. Because of the danger of causing damage that might be followed by the drainage of CSF through the nose, many surgeons request that the nose never be suctioned when supratentorial surgery has been performed. A sign with this caution may be placed at the head of the bed.

### Respiratory Problems

*Respiratory collapse* may follow infratentorial surgery. It is caused by edema of the brainstem or edema above the brainstem, which causes herniation of the brainstem into the foramen magnum and pressure on the respiratory center. Any irregularity of respiration, dyspnea, or cyanosis should be reported at once. Equipment should be ready for administering oxygen, performing a ventricular tap, and inserting an endotracheal tube if one is not already present. (For details of nursing care of the patient with an endotracheal tube, see Chapter 36.) Occasionally a ventilator is necessary.

### Convulsions

Convulsions are not unusual after a craniotomy. Side rails should be used even if the patient is unconscious and it is believed that movement is not possible. Phenytoin sodium (Dilantin) often is ordered prophylactically to prevent convulsions. It *should not* be given intramuscularly because of its poor absorption via this route. If the patient has a history of seizures before surgery or if convulsions occurred in the postoperative period, this drug may be given for several months.

### Corneal Abrasions

*Loss of the corneal reflex* may follow surgical removal of brain tumors. If the eye appears inflamed or if the patient does not seem to blink when objects approach the open eye, the neurosurgeon should be notified. Special eye care such as that given to patients who have had CVAs or who have had surgery for trigeminal neuralgia may be necessary (see earlier discussion, p. 1937).

The patient may complain of ***diplopia*** after brain surgery. This condition is often temporary, and the patient should know that it will probably improve. It can be relieved by placing an opaque eye shield over one eye. The eye covered usually is alternated each day to prevent atrophy of eye muscles through disuse.

# CRANIOCEREBRAL TRAUMA

## ETIOLOGY

Craniocerebral trauma may result in injury to the scalp, skull, and brain tissues, either singly or collectively. Variables that may modify the extent of the injury to the head include the location and direction of the impact, rate of the energy transfer, the surface area of energy transfer, and the status of the head at the time of the impact. Injuries vary from minor scalp wounds to concussions and open fractures of the skull with severe damage to the brain. The amount of obvious damage is not indicative of the seriousness of the injury.

Contusions, abrasions, and lacerations of the scalp may occur. Lacerations of the scalp bleed profusely because of the scalp's large blood supply. Most bleeding is minor and controlled readily. An internal hematoma of the scalp may form as a result of the bleeding and resemble a depressed fracture. Infection of the scalp may result from the presence of foreign debris. It should be stressed that the absence of external scalp injury does not preclude serious craniocerebral damage.

The skull indents and deforms when a physical impact occurs. Fractures often result and are classified as in other parts of the body. Skull roentgenograms may detect the fractures; a negative finding on x-ray film does not exclude the presence of a hairline fracture. Fractures can occur distal to the point of impact. A compound and depressed fracture causes serious complications. *The presence of a skull fracture does not necessarily indicate that brain injury has occurred.* A reverse correlation often exists between skull damage and brain damage. Complications of skull damage may include injury to cranial nerves, epidural hemorrhage, and brain contusion.

## EPIDEMIOLOGY

**Craniocerebral trauma,** or head injury, causes death and serious disability in persons of all ages. In the United States, head injuries result in about 80,000 deaths yearly. Morbidity and mortality are higher in males. Primary traumatic lesions result from industrial, motor vehicle, and military accidents. Head injury is the second most common cause of major neurologic deficits and the major cause of death between ages 1 and 35 years. It is estimated that 70% of motor accidents result in head injury. Brain injury causes more deaths than does injury to any other organ. In some states the repeal of laws requiring motorcyclists to wear helmets has resulted in an estimated threefold increase in death and injury resulting from damage to the brain sustained in motorcycle accidents.

No data for exact numbers of traumatic brain injuries exist. An estimated 70,000 persons annually incur moderate-to-severe head injuries and require long-term rehabilitation. Children and young persons are disproportionately affected by traumatic brain injuries that often require lifelong rehabilitation services.[45]

Motorcycle accidents cause approximately 11% of all motor vehicle deaths. Many motorcycle crash injuries are due to lack of operator skill, intoxication of the operator, and absence of protective headgear.[45]

Older adults account for a larger share of motor vehicle injuries each year. They have a greater risk of a crash per mile driven than younger adults, and once in a crash, they are much more vulnerable to injury and death.

## PATHOPHYSIOLOGY

Damage to brain tissues per se may include concussion, contusion, or laceration. Each is discussed briefly here to differentiate them in terms of their degree of damage and significance. The dura may remain intact in brain damage (a *closed injury*), or the dura may be opened from a direct blow or from penetrating objects such as bone fragments or knives (an *open injury*).

A **concussion** is characterized by an immediate and transitory impairment of neurologic function caused by the mechanical force. No structural alteration is demonstrable. There may be loss of consciousness that is instant or delayed and is usually recovered. The effect of a blow on the cranium to the soft brain tissues contained within the closed cavity is one of sudden movement. This effect can be likened to what happens as one stops suddenly when moving quickly with an open dish of fluid—some of the fluid spills. The only difference is that instead of spilling in the closed cavity, the brain tissues strike the bony coverings forcibly. The damage sustained is variable in degree. Damage may occur to the brainstem centers and the cerebral hemispheres. There can be loss of consciousness, the cause of which is not clearly understood. Any person who exhibits an alteration in consciousness after a blow on the head should be under constant observation for a time inasmuch as damage is not always immediately apparent.

A **contusion** is a structural alteration characterized by extravasation of blood cells. It can be likened to bruising without tearing of the tissues. The contusion may be at the site of the impact or on the opposite side. A concussion or contusion site may be classified as a *coup* (at the site), *contrecoup* (opposite the site), or *intermediate*. Contusions often damage the cortex.

*Laceration* of the brain tissues and blood vessels is a tearing of the tissues that may be caused by a sharp fragment or object or a shearing force. It is obvious that hemorrhage may be a serious complication.

In summary, when the head receives a direct blow or injury, the brain moves in the skull and suffers varying degrees of damage not always at the site of the injury. In addition, the brain swells to a great extent, and the capacity of the brain to swell may exceed the capacity of the closed cranial cavity to expand. Most deaths from head injury are from the brain swelling rather than from the actual primary destruction of vital centers. Brain edema is thus a major cause of increased intracranial pressure and its consequences. Along with the swelling, local and systemic disturbances in circulation occur with resulting anoxia. The brain damage may be minor or severe. A great disparity often exists between functional neurologic derangement and structural damage that can be demonstrated.

Table 57-13 compares the effects seen with the different types of head trauma.

Hemorrhage resulting from craniocerebral trauma may occur at the following sites: scalp, epidural, subdural, subarachnoid, intracerebral, and intraventricular. Epidural and subdural hematomas are discussed because of the need for careful and continuing observations by the nurse.

An *epidural hematoma* forms as blood collects between the dura and the skull. Because bleeding in this area usually is caused by laceration of the middle meningeal artery, it is capable of producing rapid clot formation. ***If lethargy or unconsciousness develops after the patient regains consciousness, an epidural hematoma may be suspected.*** Bleeding needs to be controlled promptly and the blood evacuated. Common sites for bleeding include basal and temporal skull fractures. The nurse should be alert for potential epidural hematomas when it is known that fractures exist in these sites.

A *subdural hematoma* forms as venous blood col-

**TABLE 57-13 Damage of Brain Tissue Caused by Trauma**

| CHARACTERISTICS | STRUCTURAL ALTERATION | EFFECTS |
|---|---|---|
| **CONCUSSION** | | |
| Characterized by immediate and transitory impairment of neurologic function caused by mechanical force | No | May be loss of consciousness that is instant or delayed; usually reversible |
| **CONTUSION** | | |
| Likened to bruising with extravasation of blood cells | Yes | Injury may be at site of impact or at opposite site; often damage is to cortex |
| **LACERATION** | | |
| Tearing of tissues caused by sharp fragment or shearing force | Yes | Hemorrhage is serious complication |

lects below the dural surface. Because the bleeding is under venous pressure, the hematoma formation is relatively slow. However, the clot formation will cause pressure on the brain surface and eventually may displace brain tissue. If this expanding clot is not evacuated, it can contribute to a rise in intracranial pressure and its sequelae. Thus a subdural hematoma can become serious because of its location and compression of vital areas. If a patient who has been conscious for several weeks or months after a head injury becomes unconscious and develops neurologic symptoms, a subdural hematoma should be suspected. *Nurses need to be aware of the delayed signs of head injury as well as the immediate and more obvious ones. The focal neurologic signs from clot formation can be related to the site of the clot.*

Fractures of the *base of the skull* usually are serious because of the site. When one is sustained, *vital centers, cranial nerves, and nerve pathways may be permanently damaged.* Trauma and the resulting edema may obstruct CSF flow directly or indirectly, with resultant increased intracranial pressure. If the injury has caused a direct communication between the cranial cavity and the middle ear or the sinuses, meningitis or a brain abscess may develop. Bleeding from the nose and the ears suggests a basal fracture. Serosanguineous drainage from these orifices may contain CSF and should be noted. Intracranial bleeding as a result of trauma may cause the same signs and symptoms as nontraumatic hemorrhage.

## PREVENTION

### Healthy People 2000

Traumatic head injuries often result from motor vehicle accidents and falls. The following goals have been identified for both areas in *Healthy People 2000*[53]:

- Reduce deaths caused by motor vehicle crashes to no more than 1.9 per 100 million vehicle miles traveled and 16.8 per 100,000 persons. (Baseline: 2.4 per 100 million vehicle miles traveled [VMT] and 18.8 per 100,000 persons [age-adjusted] in 1987)
- Reduce deaths from falls and fall-related injuries to no more than 2.3 per 100,000 persons. (Age-adjusted baseline: 2.7 per 100,000 in 1987)
- Reduce nonfatal head injuries so that hospitalizations for this condition are no more than 106 per 100,000 persons. (Baseline: 125 per 100,000 in 1988)

### Primary Prevention

Much can be done in terms of primary prevention of head injuries. Factors that can influence the outcome include the following:

1. Use of seat belts in automobiles
2. Use of helmets when riding motorcycles, snowmobiles, or bicycles
3. Practice of firearm safety
4. Minimal use of alcohol and drugs
5. Not driving after taking drugs or drinking alcohol
6. Use of precautions while swimming and especially not diving into shallow water or where depth unknown

### Secondary Prevention

Secondary prevention of injury to the patient with a head injury includes rapid and accurate diagnosis and treatment. These patients often are life-flighted to a trauma center, where the best in emergency care is available.

## MEDICAL MANAGEMENT

The patient who has a skull fracture or other serious head injury *must be attended constantly.* The major aims of medical and nursing management are as follows:

1. To be constantly alert for changes in the patient's condition, especially changes that indicate any increase in intracranial pressure
2. To sustain patient's vital functions until they can be resumed on their own
3. To minimize complications that will be life threatening or interfere with full recovery

Because many persons with head injury, especially from motor vehicle accidents, have sustained other injuries, the intrathoracic and intraabdominal areas are checked carefully. The limbs are examined for fractures and injuries to nerves or arteries.

The nurse works collaboratively with the physician for implementation of prescribed medical therapy. Because the nurse has a major role in discharge planning and patient teaching, these are discussed under nursing management.

### Diagnostic Tests

Diagnostic procedures are performed as necessary and most often include CT scans, skull roentgenograms, and possibly cerebral angiography. When a hematoma is suspected, a trephine of the skull (burr holes) may be performed. It is important to remember that the contrast media used during the CT scan and angiography will increase intracranial pressure.

Many neurosurgeons believe that alert and intelligent nursing care often is the decisive factor in determining the outcome for the patient. Side rails should always be used on the bed because restlessness may come on suddenly and convulsions may occur. Usually the bed is kept flat, although some neurosurgeons believe that the danger of edema to the brain may be reduced by slight elevation of the head of the bed.

### Medication

Medications for the patient with a head injury depend on the symptoms the patient is experiencing. They may include those used to prevent seizures or those to decrease intracranial pressure.

### Diet

No special diet is prescribed for the patient with a head injury. It is determined largely by the patient's condition.

### Activity

The level of activity of the patient with a head injury is determined by the neurologic status. At times the patient may be sedated to facilitate healing. With minor head injuries there may be no activity restriction.

### Referral/Consultation

In some settings the nurse assumes responsibility for making referrals to other services. For the patient with a head injury, this may include a dietitian and social worker. The family often is aided by a referral to the local chapter of the Head Injury Foundation or another support group.

## SURGICAL MANAGEMENT

If the head injury causes hematoma formation, the best medical approach may be surgery. The surgical treatment for extradural hematoma consists of making a burr hole in the skull to relieve the pressure caused by the bleeding and to attempt to control the bleeding. Sometimes a craniotomy, removal of a large bony window, is necessary. Occasionally the patient has so much damage to the soft tissue of the brain that death occurs despite relief of pressure caused by the bleeding. Usually such a patient is unconscious after the accident and is taken to the hospital at once.

## NURSING MANAGEMENT

### ♦ ASSESSMENT

### Subjective Data

Subjective data to be collected to assess the patient with a head injury who is conscious include the following:

- Patient's understanding of injury and resulting pathologic consequences
- Patient's ability to understand
- Information about nature of injury—how it happened
- Presence of headache, nausea, or vomiting
- Presence of diplopia or other visual problems
- Unusual sensations (paresthesias, ringing in ears)
- History of bleeding from ear, nose, eye, or mouth
- History of loss of consciousness

### Objective Data

Objective data to be collected to assess the patient with head injury include the following:

- Respiratory status (presence of patent airway, need for suctioning, need for intubation and mechanical ventilation)
- Arterial blood gases
- Level of consciousness and alertness
- Pupils—size, equality, reactivity
- Orientation
- Motor status
- Vital signs
- Presence of bleeding
- Presence of vomiting
- Presence of discharge from ears or nose
- Speech pattern abnormalities

### Diagnostic Test Findings

The nature of diagnostic findings can vary to a great extent in the patient who has experienced a head injury. Evidence of a fracture may appear on x-ray examination or obvious pathologic findings may be present on the CT scan or MRI. Battle's sign and raccoon eyes occur in a basilar skull fracture. At other times, however, pathologic findings are not significant enough to explain the patient's serious symptoms.

### ♦ NURSING DIAGNOSES

Nursing diagnoses are determined from analysis of patient data. Nursing diagnoses for the patient with a head injury may include but are not limited to the following:

| Diagnostic Title | Possible Etiologic Factors |
|---|---|
| Ventilation, inability to sustain spontaneous | CNS disturbance trauma |
| Tissue perfusion, altered (cerebral) | Decreased blood flow (arterial), pressure |
| Thermoregulation, ineffective | Trauma, illness |
| Fluid volume excess or deficit | Hypermetabolic states |
| Infection, high risk for | Sensory/motor deficits |
| Activity intolerance | Generalized weakness |
| Coping, family: comprised | Crisis |
| Knowledge deficit (knowledge of head injury) | Lack of exposure/recall |

### ♦ EXPECTED PATIENT OUTCOMES

Expected patient outcomes for the patient with a head injury may include but are not limited to the following:

1. Maintains ventilation as indicated by pulse oximetry readings above 90%.
2. Maintains cerebral perfusion as indicated by the absence of signs or symptoms of increased intracranial pressure.
3. Maintains temperature within the range of 97.5° to 99.5° F.
4. Does not develop edema or dehydration.
5. Remains free of infection.
6. Maintains activity at preinjury level.
7. Family member or significant other of the patient verbalizes adequate coping.
8. Patient or family members are able to verbalize knowledge of head injury.

### ♦ INTERVENTIONS

### Promoting Adequate Ventilation

One of the most common complications of severe head injury is respiratory failure. Cerebral anoxia, which is a sequela of respiratory failure, is a leading cause of death in these patients. The patient with respiratory failure may have hypoxia, hypercapnia, hypotension, and dyspnea. Usually intubation and respiratory assistance with a mechanical respirator are ordered for these patients.

Arterial blood gas levels and pH are checked frequently to determine whether respiratory exchange is adequate. Suctioning must be performed as necessary to maintain a patent airway. (See Chapter 37 for further nursing care of the patient undergoing intubation and mechanical ventilation.)

## Controlling Cerebral Edema

Cerebral edema and increased intracranial pressure are common problems in patients with head injuries. Osmotic diuretics that penetrate the brain slowly, such as 30% solution of urea in 10% invert sugar or 20% mannitol, may be given intravenously for several days. When the patient's condition is deteriorating because of cerebral edema, dexamethasone usually is administered intravenously. The usual dose is 10 mg initially, followed by 4 mg intramuscularly or intravenously every 4 hours thereafter. Steroids also are useful in combatting shock associated with head injury. Usually they are employed only during the acute phase because of their side effects (rebound effect).

The patient should be kept as quiet as possible. No vigorous effort should be made to "clean the patient up" during the first few hours after an accident. Rest and constant observation are much more important. Sudden noises, flashes of light, and the clatter of equipment can increase the patient's restlessness and should be avoided. Portable equipment should be used to obtain roentgenograms. Nurses must remain in the room with patients to help them move and to protect them from exertion. Restlessness may be caused by the need for a slight change of position, the relaxation of a limb, or the need to empty the bladder. If nursing measures fail to allay extreme restlessness, the physician may order sodium amytal intramuscularly or paraldehyde. Morphine is not given to relieve pain because it will depress the patient's responsiveness and cause pupillary constriction, thus interfering with the necessary observation of pupillary change. Codeine or other mild analgesics may be necessary, however.[40,49,56]

Twitching or convulsive movement of a body part is recorded in detail and reported at once. In some medical centers, anticonvulsants are given prophylactically when seizures are anticipated; they are always given once seizures occur.

## Maintaining Vital Signs and Temperature Control

Usually the blood pressure, pulse, and respiratory rate are taken and recorded every 15 minutes until they become stabilized and remain within safe limits. Leaving the deflated blood pressure cuff on the arm helps to prevent disturbing the patient unduly when the pressure must be taken often. Developing the habit of not forcing the mercury column much above the expected reading also can facilitate taking the blood pressure with less disturbance to the patient. The eyes are observed for inequality of the pupils and the lips and fingernails for cyanosis. A sudden sharp rise in temperature, which may go to 42° C (106° F) or higher, and a sudden drop in blood pressure indicate that the regulatory mechanisms have lost control and the prognosis is poor. When temperature is elevated, measures need to be instituted to reduce it to normal. Although hypothermia has been used in the treatment of patients with severe brain contusions, it is being used less often because of some of the undesirable side effects. Instead, the nursing measures usually employed to reduce temperature are used, such as the administration of aspirin, tepid sponges, ice bags to the groin and axillae, and reduction of the temperature in the patient's room. Electrically controlled cooling mattresses are frequently used (Figure 57-18).

## Monitoring Fluid Volume

Intake and output should be carefully measured and recorded. The specific gravity of the urine also is measured and recorded. These measurements may be performed hourly when the patient's condition is acute.

Fluid intake may be restricted to 1500 to 2500 ml daily, and it is the nurse's responsibility to see that this is spread over the 24-hour period. Fluids may be given parenterally, by nasogastric tube, or by mouth, depending on the condition of the patient. The nurse must use caution in administering fluids orally because the patient may have difficulty with vomiting and aspiration. The urinary output should be approximately 0.6 to 1 ml/kg of body weight/hour. This means that a person weighing 175 pounds (79 kg) should eliminate between 45 and 80 ml/hr, and if osmotic diuretics have been given, this amount may be greater. An indwelling catheter is essential when giving mannitol because of the large amounts of urine produced and the need to measure output exactly. The presence of an indwelling catheter increases the risk of urinary tract infection and should be removed as soon as possible.

## Monitoring Electrolyte Balance

Careful monitoring of electrolytes is necessary. Several types of sodium imbalance are known to occur in head injury. *Natriuresis,* or increased urinary excretion of sodium, is common. More recently this has been attributed to the syndrome of inappropriate secretion of antidiuretic hormone (SIADH) (with an increased plasma level of ADH, serum hyponatremia, and hypotonicity). This aggravates cerebral edema. *Hypernatremia,* or cerebral sodium retention, also may occur. No specific variations in potassium or chloride levels have been noted. Plasma cortisol levels also are elevated in acute head injury. Plasma, blood urea nitrogen (BUN), pH, electrolytes, and urinary electrolyte levels are checked frequently.

## Monitoring Drainage From Ears and Nose

The patient's ears and nose are observed carefully for signs of blood and serous drainage, which may indicate

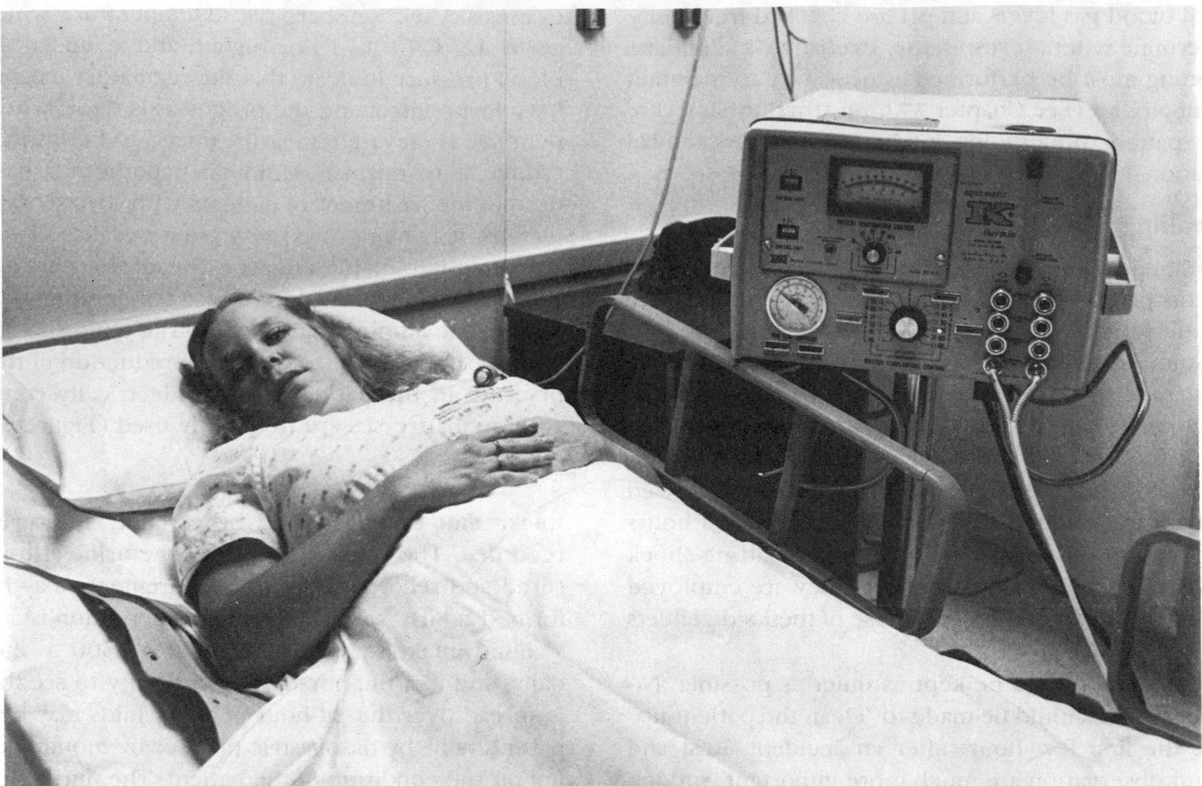

**FIGURE 57-18** Patient lying on cooling mattress connected to hypothermia machine.

that the meninges have been torn (common in basal skull fractures) and that spinal fluid is escaping. No attempt should be made to clean out these orifices. Loose, sterile cotton may be placed in the outer openings only. This procedure must be performed with caution so that the cotton does not in any way act as a plug to interfere with free flow of fluid. The cotton should be changed as soon as it becomes moistened. Usually the flow of fluid subsides spontaneously. Antibiotics usually are given when a basal fracture has been sustained. Because of the danger of causing further damage, suction is never used to remove nasal secretions in any patient who has a head injury or who has undergone brain surgery. *Meningitis is a possible complication when communication with the nose and ears occurs.* If evidence of drainage of spinal fluid from the nose exists, the patient should not cough, sneeze, or blow the nose. These activities may, in addition to contributing to the development of meningitis, enable air to enter the cranial cavity, where it may increase symptoms of intracranial pressure. Sometimes it is difficult to determine whether drainage from the nose is mucus or CSF. A Tes-Tape will give a positive glucose reaction to spinal fluid and a negative reaction to mucus.

## Resuming Activities

The length of convalescence depends entirely on how much damage has been done and how rapid recovery has been. Patients usually are urged to resume normal activity as soon as possible. Headache and occasional dizziness may be present for some time after a head injury. These difficulties should disappear within 3 to 4 months.[23] Loss of memory and initiative also may persist for a time. Occasionally, convulsions develop because of the formation of scar tissue in injured brain substance or in its coverings. Such scar tissue often may be surgically removed to effect a complete cure. Loss of hearing and strabismus (cross-eye) sometimes complicate basal skull fractures and require a long period of rehabilitation. Sometimes corrective surgery can be performed for the strabismus.

Some persons require intensive rehabilitation in a rehabilitation center. Recovery from head injury is most likely in those younger than 20 years of age. Persons between the ages of 20 and 50 years who remain in a coma longer than 2 weeks rarely recover.

## Providing Emotional Support

The patient with a head injury may manifest loss of memory and initiative. Behavioral problems associated with lack of judgment and restlessness also may occur. These patients need firm but gentle care, with specific guidelines for what behavior is allowed. The patient and family need to have gains in functioning pointed out because it is easy to become frustrated and depressed when progress is slow.[59]

### Guidelines for Care of the Person With a Head Injury

Patient should be awakened periodically through the first 24 hours to be sure he or she can wake up easily.

Also, for the first 24 to 48 hours, the family should watch carefully for the following warning signs:

1. Vomiting, often with force behind it
2. Unusual sleepiness, dizziness and loss of balance, or falling
3. Complaint of seeing two of everything or blurry objects; jerking movements of the eyes
4. Bleeding or discharge from nose or eyes
5. A slight headache may be expected; however, if it worsens and the patient complains of feeling even worse when moving about, it should be reported
6. Convulsions (fits)—any twitching or movements of arms or legs that the patient is not able to stop
7. Any behavior or symptom that is not normal for the individual

*Call a physician at once* if any of these signs are observed by the family. Call either your personal physician or the emergency services.

Courtesy Department of Nursing, University Hospitals of Cleveland, Cleveland, Ohio.

## Facilitating Learning

A patient with a head injury may be seen in the emergency room but not admitted to the hospital. These patients need teaching about observations for complications. A sample set of instructions is presented in the Guidelines box above.

Teaching for the patient with a head injury who is left with deficits severe enough to require extended rehabilitation is similar to that for the patient with a motor problem. In addition, the following points are important:

1. Causes of increased intracranial pressure
2. Factors that increase or decrease intracranial pressure
3. Signs and symptoms to report to the physician

## Facilitating Planning With Patient's Family

Few illnesses tax the entire physical and emotional resources of the patient's family as do chronic neurologic diseases. It is imperative that the family participate in long-term plans for the patient. Family members may have severe emotional reactions and difficulties in adjustment that may require the assistance of a specially trained person such as a psychiatrist. Both patient and family need time to work through their feelings. Sometimes the enormity of the diagnosis cannot be grasped for weeks or even months by either patient or family members. Toxic polyneuritis in a young husband and father and multiple sclerosis in a young mother are examples of problems of such magnitude that long-term plans cannot be made quickly.

If the patient with neurologic disease has severe personality changes, aphasia, or convulsions, the family may even be afraid of the patient. Because family members are unaware that the patient may fully understand what is being said, they may make tactless remarks in front of the patient. When the patient is admitted to the hospital, it is often desirable to take family members aside to ascertain their insight into the situation. This interview provides an opportunity to help interpret the patient's actions and responses so that the family may better understand and be more supportive of the patient.

See Chapter 8 for more information about the general care of persons with prolonged illness.

## Coping With Behavioral Problems

Even the person who has suffered a mild head injury may experience long-term effects. These most often include cognitive problems such as difficulty with concentration and loss of memory. Recovery of intellectual functioning often is delayed, as frequently manifested in an inability to keep a job, with increasing periods of unemployment.[23]

## ♦ EVALUATION

To evaluate the effectiveness of nursing interventions, compare patient behaviors with those stated in the expected patient outcomes. Successful achievement of patient outcomes for the patient with a head injury is indicated by the following:

1. Has pulse oximetry readings above 90%, with regular and unlabored respirations.
2. Lacks signs and symptoms of increased intracranial pressure.
3. Has body temperature between 97.5° and 99.5° F.
4. Has neither edema nor signs of dehydration (i.e., elevated BUN and electrolyte levels, decreased skin turgor) and has an intake of at least 1500 ml of fluid per day.
5. Is free of infection.
6. Has the ability to ambulate, transfer, and/or move freely in a wheelchair.
7. A family member or significant other states ability to cope with injury of loved one: absence of excessive crying, inability to sleep, appetite disturbances, and other signs of increased stress.
8. Family member or significant other correctly explains pathology of head injury and care needed by patient.

## COMPLICATIONS

Patients with severe head injuries are vulnerable to several complications, some of which are discussed in this section. As with any other patient who is seriously ill, *atelectasis, pneumonia,* or a *urinary tract infection* (secondary to an indwelling catheter) may develop. These infections are treated with a suitable antibiotic. *Stress ulcers* of the stomach and duodenum also typically

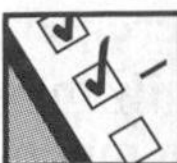

## Guidelines for Care of the Person With a Closed Head Injury

1. Promote rest and control convulsions:
   a. Provide quiet environment.
   b. Observe constantly.
   c. Give anticonvulsants.
   d. Medicate for pain as necessary.
2. Maintain temperature:
   a. Give tepid sponge baths.
   b. Administer aspirin as ordered.
   c. Use hypothermia blanket if ordered.
   d. Apply ice bags to groin and axilla.
   e. Reduce temperature in patient's room.
3. Promote adequate respiration:
   a. Suction only as necessary to provide adequate airway.
   b. Elevate head of bed to 30 degrees.
   c. Administer supplemental oxygen if ordered.
4. Observe for drainage from ears or nose:
   a. Make no attempt to clean out orifice.
   b. Use cotton in outer opening.
   c. Change cotton as soon as it is moistened.
   d. Do not suction nose if drainage is present.
   e. Use Tes-Tape to verify presence of CSF.
   f. Have patient avoid coughing, sneezing, or blowing nose.
5. Control cerebral edema:
   a. Administer diuretics as ordered.
   b. Elevate head of bed to 30 degrees.
6. Maintain electrolyte balance:
   a. Observe for inappropriate ADH.
   b. Monitor electrolytes.
7. Maintain elimination:
   a. Keep accurate intake and output record.
   b. Restrict fluid if ordered.
   c. Monitor output.
   d. Remove catheter as soon as possible.
8. Provide emotional support:
   a. Give firm but gentle care.
   b. Give specific guidelines for appropriate behaviors.
   c. Give positive feedback.
   d. Allow patient adequate time to complete tasks.

occur after a head injury and apparently are caused by autonomic imbalances associated with the injury. Cimetidine (Tagamet) can be given intravenously and acts to decrease the acid production of the stomach. Antacids can be given when the patient is able to take oral fluids. Antacids are especially important if the patient is taking steroids such as prednisone, which is ulcerogenic.

See Guidelines box above, for care of the patient with a closed head injury.

### Prolonged Unconsciousness

General nursing care, as described on p. 1934, is necessary for the patient with a head injury who remains unconscious for some time. Patients may be unconscious for long periods and yet make a satisfactory recovery, provided good supportive care has been given.

### Extradural Hematoma

Because of the danger of extradural hematoma, as discussed previously, many physicians believe that any patient who has sustained any injury to the head with loss of consciousness should be hospitalized for at least 24 hours. If patients are asleep during this time, they should be awakened hourly to determine the state of consciousness. Some physicians believe that fluids should be restricted to 1000 to 1500 ml for the first day or two and that an osmotic diuretic should be given. If patients remain at home, the families should be told to watch them closely for signs of increased intracranial pressure, to awaken them hourly during the night after injury, and to bring them to a hospital at once if drowsiness, stupor, paralysis, convulsions, or inequality of the pupil size should occur. A written handout with appropriate instructions about head injury can be extremely helpful to families of patients who are sent home instead of hospitalized. It not only alerts them about signs to observe in the patient but also may help to allay their anxiety. (See Guidelines box, p. 2013.)

## INFECTIONS/INFLAMMATIONS

The nervous system may be attacked by a variety of organisms and viruses and may develop a toxic reaction to bacterial and viral disease. Sometimes the infection becomes walled off and causes an abscess; sometimes the meninges, or coverings of the brain and spinal cord, are involved; and sometimes the brain itself is affected most. Organisms and viruses may reach the nervous system by various routes. Untreated chronic otitis media and mastoiditis, chronic sinusitis, and fracture in any bone adjacent to the meninges may be the source of infection. Some organisms, such as the tubercle bacillus and probably the pneumococcus, reach the nervous system by means of the blood or the lymph system. Meningitis also can occur as a complication of invasive procedures such as lumbar puncture or procedures involving the use of contrast media. The exact route by which some infectious agents, such as the meningococcus in epidemic meningitis and the viruses that cause encephalitis, reach the central nervous system is not known.

Meningococcal meningitis (epidemic) and poliomyelitis are reportable communicable diseases. Because they are becoming less common and because they are discussed in specialized texts, they are mentioned only briefly here.

Several conditions that occur as a result of infection or inflammation of the nervous system are discussed in this section. These conditions include meningitis, encephalitis, and AIDS.

### MENINGITIS
### Etiology

**Meningitis** is an acute infection of the meninges usually caused by pneumococci, meningococci (epidemic), staphylococci, streptococci, *Haemophilus influenzae,* or aseptic agents (usually viral). Any other pathogenic organism, such as the tubercle bacillus, that gains access to the subarchnoid spaces also can cause meningitis. Mild forms of the disease do occur and may be referred to as *meningism.* They may be caused by viruses. A common form of the disease is lymphocytic meningitis, which in many instances is believed to be associated with a virus.

## Epidemiology

The incidence of bacterial meningitis is higher in fall and winter when upper respiratory tract infections typically occur. Children are affected more often than adults because of frequent colds and ear infections. Disease caused by the enteroviruses is more common in the summer and early fall than in other seasons of the year.

## Pathophysiology

As previously stated, organisms and viruses reach the nervous system by many routes. Once organisms reach the brain, the CSF in the subarachnoid spaces and in the pia-arachnoid membrane becomes infected. The infection then spreads rapidly throughout the meninges and eventually invades the ventricles. Pathologic alterations include hyperemia of the meningeal vessels, edema of brain tissue, increased intracranial pressure, and a generalized inflammatory reaction with exudation of white blood cells into the subarachnoid spaces. An associated hydrocephalus may be caused by exudate blocking the small passages between the ventricles.

Meningitis can be a medical emergency. The onset (except when caused by tubercle bacilli) usually is sudden and characterized by severe headache, stiffness of the neck, irritability, malaise, and restlessness. Nausea, vomiting, delirium, and complete disorientation may develop quickly. **Kernig's sign** (the inability of the patient to extend the legs completely without extreme pain) usually is present with meningitis. When the neck of the patient with meningitis is flexed, the hip and knee also flex; this is known as **Brudzinski's sign.** Temperature, pulse rate, and respirations are increased. The diagnosis usually is confirmed by examination of spinal fluid obtained from a lumbar puncture. Usually the offending organism can be isolated from the spinal fluid; if a pyogenic organism is the cause, the fluid is cloudy. The CSF pressure usually is elevated, the protein level is elevated, and the glucose content is decreased.

Residual damage from meningitis includes deafness, blindness, paralysis, and mental retardation. These complications usually are the result of chronic arachnoiditis or subdural effusion. Hydrocephalus also may develop. These complications are now less common because the infection is effectively treated with antibiotics before permanent damage to the nervous system occurs.

## Prevention

Because meningitis is linked closely with upper respiratory and ear infections, prevention of these can help prevent meningitis. Prevention includes avoiding crowds during peak seasons for colds and other viral infections and receiving prompt treatment for ear or upper respiratory infections.

The prompt diagnosis and treatment of meningitis can prevent morbidity and mortality.

## Medical Management

### Diagnostic tests

Most of the infections involving the nervous system can be diagnosed by examining the CSF. A CT scan and an EEG also may be performed. (These procedures are discussed in Chapter 56.)

### Medication

Treatment consists of massive doses of the antibiotic specific for the causative organism. Culture and sensitivity studies determine the most effective antibiotic. Usually a course of at least 10 days of parenteral administration is needed. The antibiotic may be given directly into the spinal canal (intrathecally). The use of hyperosmolar agents or steroids also may be necessary to decrease cerebral edema. Anticonvulsants may be administered to prevent seizures.

### Treatment

If the patient develops hydrocephalus as a result of the meningitis, medical management may include the insertion of a shunt to facilitate movement of the CSF.

### Diet

No special diet is prescribed for the patient with meningitis. The consistency of the diet is determined by the patient's mental status.

### Activity

Respiratory isolation is required until the pathogen can no longer be cultured from the nasopharynx. This usually is accomplished after 24 hours of effective antimicrobial therapy. Therapy is continued until the patient has been afebrile for 5 days or after 7 days of therapy (whichever is longer).

### Referral/Consultation

In some settings the nurse assumes responsibility for making referrals to other services. In the case of the patient with meningitis the referral may involve the family, depending on the condition of the patient.

## NURSING MANAGEMENT

### ♦ ASSESSMENT

Subjective and objective data are important with any patient with an infection of the nervous system. This assessment includes common characteristics of all infections/inflammations discussed in this section.

### Subjective Data

Subjective data to be collected to assess the patient with infection of the nervous system include the following:

- Patient's understanding of process and possible causes
- Any history of infection, such as upper respiratory infections
- Initial onset of symptoms
- Measures that relieved symptoms
- Presence of discomfort, including headache or stiff neck
- Presence of difficulty in thinking
- Presence of muscle weakness, soreness, or incoordination

### Objective Data

Objective data to be collected to assess the patient with infection of the nervous system include the following:

- Behavior—signs indicating discomfort or disorientation
- Change in ability to carry out ADL
- Abnormalities on physical assessment part of neurologic examination
- Temperature elevations
- Presence of vomiting
- Pulse and blood pressure
- Respirations
- Level of consciousness

## ♦ NURSING DIAGNOSES/EXPECTED PATIENT OUTCOME

The nursing diagnoses and expected outcomes for the patient with meningitis are the same as for the patient with altered levels of consciousness. The reader is referred to p. 1934.

## ♦ INTERVENTIONS

Nursing care for the patient with meningitis includes the general care given a critically ill patient who may be irritable, confused, and unable to take fluids and yet is dehydrated because of elevation of temperature. The room is kept darkened, noise is kept at a minimum, and care is taken not to jar the bed because any increase in sensory stimulation can cause a seizure. The patient must be observed very carefully and must be constantly attended if disorientation is present. Padded side rails should be placed on the bed. The patient should be observed for symptoms of inappropriate secretion of antidiuretic hormone (see Chapter 20), which can occur readily in patients with meningitis.

## ♦ EVALUATION

To evaluate effectiveness of nursing interventions, compare patient behaviors with those stated in the expected patient outcomes.

## COMPLICATIONS

See appropriate discussion under the care of the patient with a CVA for prevention of complications.

## ENCEPHALITIS

### Etiology

**Encephalitis** is inflammation of the brain tissues and its coverings. Occasionally the meninges of the spinal cord also are involved. Encephalitis can have a variety of causes. A generalized inflammation of the brain can be caused by syphilis, and encephalitis can follow exogenous poisoning, such as that following the ingestion of lead or arsenic or the inhalation of carbon monoxide. It can be caused by reaction to toxins produced by infections such as typhoid fever, measles, and chickenpox, and occasionally it follows vaccination.

### Epidemiology

Encephalitis caused by a virus and occurring in epidemic form was first described by von Economo in Austria, and the name von Economo's disease is still used to identify the widespread epidemic in the United States that followed the influenza epidemic in 1918. This form of the disease has not recurred since 1926. Von Economo's disease also was called *encephalitis lethargica,* as well as *sleeping sickness,* a term still used by lay persons. The demonstration that viruses can affect the central nervous system after a prolonged incubation period has resulted in considerable search for viral agents in many chronic neurologic diseases.

The death rate from encephalitis varies with epidemics but is generally fairly high. The most common sequela for patients who do recover from the acute disease is *paralysis agitans,* which may come on suddenly or develop slowly. Other residual neurologic symptoms also may occur and occasionally incapacitate the patient completely.

### Prevention

Prevention of arboviral infections consists of eradication of the mosquito or tick vector, including destruction of larvae and elimination of breeding places. Infection is controlled by avoiding mosquito or tick bites. Avoiding the substances that cause exogenous poisoning also helps decrease the occurrence of encephalitis. Accurate, timely diagnosis is necessary for successful treatment.

### Acute Viral Encephalitis

#### Etiology/Epidemiology

Viral encephalitis appears to be caused by several viruses, some of which may be interrelated. Acute viral encephalitis can be classifed into epidemic and sporadic forms. The primary causes of acute epidemic encephalitis are members of the *arbovirus* (those transferred by a biting arthropod to human beings) or *togavirus* group (named after properties of the virus). About 80 viruses of the arbovirus group cause disease in humans. Six of the viruses cause infections of the central nervous system (Table 57-14).

Clinical features of acute epidemic encephalitis,

**TABLE 57-14 Arbovirus Infections of the Central Nervous System Occurring in the Western Hemisphere**

| DISEASE | CAUSAL AGENT | LOCATION | INCUBATION PERIOD (Days) | CLINICAL MANIFESTATIONS |
|---|---|---|---|---|
| California encephalitis | Arbovirus of California virus (mosquito-borne) | United States, Canada, Alaska, Yukon, Northwest Territories | 5-15 | Aseptic meningitis, encephalitis |
| Eastern equine encephalitis | Eastern equine encephalitis virus (mosquito-borne) | Eastern seaboard and Gulf states, Caribbean | 5-15 | Severe encephalitis (usually infants and children) |
| Powassan encephalitis | Powassan virus (tick-borne) | Canada, northeastern and north-central United States | 4-8 | Encephalitis |
| St. Louis encephalitis | St. Louis encephalitis virus (mosquito-borne) | Central, southern, northwestern, western, and central United States; southern Ontario; Caribbean | 4-21 | Encephalitis aseptic meningitis |
| Venezuelan equine encephalomyelitis | Venezuelan equine encephalomyelitis virus (mosquito-borne) | Texas, Florida, Mexico, Central and South America | 2-5 | Fever, headache, myalgia, malaise, cough, encephalitis |
| Western equine encephalomyelitis | Western equine encephalomyelitis virus (mosquito-borne) | Central and western United States and Canada, Central and South America | 5-10 | Encephalitis (infants), fever, aseptic meningitis |

caused by the arboviruses that infect humans, are similar. The eastern equine form is more severe than the western form. The onset is abrupt, with a high fever, headache, meningeal signs, nuchal rigidity, and vomiting. Drowsiness or coma and focal or generalized convulsions develop within 24 to 48 hours after onset. Focal neurologic signs occur, such as hemiplegia and cranial nerve palsies. There are typical findings in the CSF. Fatality rates may be as high as 60%. Those who survive usually have no sequelae.

## Acute Encephalitis (Nonepidemic)

Acute encephalitis occurs sporadically and is caused by the herpes simplex virus (HSV). It occurs at any age, but more than half the persons are at least 15 years of age. Upper respiratory complaints often precede the onset of neurologic symptoms by at least 24 hours or longer. Headache and focal or major convulsions are the common early signs of cerebral involvement. A persistent high fever and coma typically occur. Spinal fluid proteins may be moderately elevated, and red blood cells often are present when spinal fluid is examined. Herpetic skin lesions (cold sores) do not usually occur.

### Medical management

Medical management of acute encephalitis involves the use of antibiotics to eradicate the virus. Other measures to reduce increased intracranial pressure may be necessary.

### Nursing management

**Assessment/diagnoses/outcomes.** The reader is referred to the section on meningitis for subjective and objective data, nursing diagnoses, and expected patient outcomes.

Nursing care consists mainly of symptomatic or supportive care and careful observation. Any change in appearance or behavior must be reported at once, because the progress of this disease can be extremely rapid. The patient is kept in bed, and side rails are used if disorientation develops.

## Brain Abscess

### Etiology/Epidemiology

A brain abscess is almost always secondary to foci of infection somewhere else in the body. Common sites include the ear, sinus or mastoid, lung, heart, pelvic organs, teeth, or skin. The three most common organisms involved are streptococci, staphylococci, and pneumococci. Brain abscesses occur most often in older children and young adults but may be seen at any age. At times no organism is found, and the abscess is called a *sterile abscess.*

### Pathophysiology

In the first stage of brain abscess, a localized inflammation of the brain occurs with formation of exudate. Septic thrombosis of some vessels develops, and the surrounding brain tissue becomes edematous and necrotic. After days to weeks the inflammatory reaction decreases as the area is walled off. "Satellite" abscesses may occur, and the abscesses may rupture into the ventricles. Brain abscesses are most often found in the temporal lobe and the cerebellum.

There may be a history of infection, although the person may not recall an infection. The most common symptom is a constant or intermittent headache that is not relieved by medication and that worsens with straining. There may be drowsiness, confusion, and mental slowness. Focal or generalized seizures may occur. Fever with bradycardia is often present. There may be signs and symptoms of increased intracranial pressure (see p. 1945). The evolution of symptoms is variable. In some patients a rapid progression of symptoms may end in death, whereas in others the course is more benign. Generally, however, the mortality is high with brain abscess; residual disability often results. Brain abscess also may recur.

#### Medical management

**Diagnostic tests.** The diagnosis of brain abscess is made primarily on the basis of the history and examination of the CSF. EEG changes are present, and areas of increased uptake of dye are seen on the CT scan.

**Treatment.** Treatment consists of administering the appropriate antibiotics, often for extended periods. Because it may take some time to isolate the causative organism, broad-spectrum antibiotics or combined antibiotic therapy may be used. Appropriate agents to reduce intracranial pressure may be necessary.

#### Nursing management

Nursing care is supportive and directed toward ongoing assessment for signs and symptoms of increased intracranial pressure, seizures, and spread of the infection. Measures to prevent permanent damage from neurologic deficits that might be present should be instituted. The long hospitalization, length of treatment, neurologic deficits, and chance for recurrence all are major sources of stress. The nurse must be prepared to spend time with the patient and significant others to help them cope with these stressors.

## ACQUIRED IMMUNODEFICIENCY SYNDROME

### ETIOLOGY

**Acquired immunodeficiency syndrome (AIDS)** is associated with several abnormalities in the body's immune system, including decreased numbers of lymphocytes as well as impaired lymphocyte function. The result is an immunosuppressed patient. In these patients the cellular response of the CNS also is decreased, enabling neurologic dysfunction to occur. Because the blood-brain barrier in some way protects the CNS from the systemic immune system, the CNS is relatively unable to resist organisms that do cross the blood-brain barrier, and they can increase rapidly.

### EPIDEMIOLOGY

A significant number of patients with AIDS develop neurologic problems as the disease progresses.[19,36] At times subtle neurologic signs and symptoms may go unnoticed in patients with systemic illness. The incidence of patients with neurologic components to AIDS is increasing steadily. (See Chapter 71 for a more complete discussion of AIDS.)

### PATHOPHYSIOLOGY

The patient with AIDS can suffer neurologic disturbances as a result of three mechanisms, as follows[48]:

1. Frank infiltration of the CNS by specific organisms
2. Encephalopathy as a result of profound metabolic disturbances
3. Systemic peripheral neuropathy

The infiltration of the CNS may occur as a result of latent or inactive organisms in the CNS. Organisms that have been found to be particularly dangerous to the CNS include *Toxoplasma gondii, Cryptococcus,* and cytomegalovirus (CMV).[36]

Patients with AIDS also have been found to be at high risk for certain malignant tumors. Several of these have a high occurrence in the CNS. Primary CNS lymphoma or systemic lymphoma with CNS infiltration is common in patients with AIDS.

The neurologic manifestations of AIDS are listed in Box 57-13.

### PREVENTION

The prevention of AIDS is of extreme importance to the nurse working in neurologic nursing (see Chapter 71).

### MEDICAL MANAGEMENT

#### Diagnostic Tests

The diagnostic tests used to determine if a neurologic problem is related to AIDS include the following:

1. Serologic studies
2. Lumbar puncture

**BOX 57-13 Neurologic Manifestations of Acquired Immunodeficiency Syndrome**

- Neuropathies
- Minor personality changes
- Mild forgetfulness
- Hemiparesis
- Blindness
- Seizures
- Dementia

3. CT scan

At times cerebral biopsy may be necessary to make the differential diagnosis.

### Treatment

The treatment for patients with AIDS-related neurologic problems differs according to the actual pathologic process. Various methods used have included antiviral, antifungal, and antibacterial agents. Radiation to the specific part of the brain affected also has been used. Experimental therapies, including interferon, have been attempted. The mortality rate remains high despite aggressive therapy.

### Diet

No special diet is prescribed for the patient with AIDS-related neurologic problems. However, the presence of sores in the mouth may make eating difficult. The emphasis is on providing a nutritional diet that is appealing and able to be tolerated by the patient with AIDS.

### Activity

The patient with AIDS is encouraged to be as active as possible for as long as he or she is able. Activity may be impeded by neurologic complications or by diarrhea, along with other symptoms.

### Referral/Consultation

In some settings the nurse assumes responsibility for making referrals to other services. For the patient with AIDS this may include a referral to a social worker or dietitian. The patient should be referred to a support group or network, if one is not in place. Referral to a psychiatric clinical nurse specialist may be helpful in assisting the patient to cope with the diagnosis of AIDS.

## NURSING MANAGEMENT

### ♦ ASSESSMENT

The nursing assessment of the AIDS patient with neurologic manifestations varies. It is based on the specific pathologic process.

### ♦ NURSING DIAGNOSES/EXPECTED PATIENT OUTCOMES

The nursing diagnoses and expected patient outcomes are related to the underlying problem caused by neurologic symptoms. The reader is referred to other parts of this chapter for information on the care needed.

### ♦ INTERVENTIONS

Care of the patient with AIDS will differ and depends on the underlying problem causing the neurologic symptoms. The reader is referred to other parts of this chapter for the necessary care of patients with neurologic involvement and to Chapter 71 for more information about care of the person with AIDS.

## QUESTIONS TO CONSIDER

- ► A patient is admitted to your unit with a Glasgow Coma Scale score of 3 and a Rancho Los Amigos scale of level II. What does this tell you about the care needs of this patient?
- ► How is brain death determined?
- ► Why is the diagnosis of many neurologic diseases difficult?
- ► How would your care of the head-injured patient differ from that of the patient with a brain tumor?
- ► Why is a work-up for cancer important in patients who have symptoms of myasthenia gravis?
- ► Your patient with amyotrophic lateral sclerosis decides not to become dependent on a ventilator. What issues and nursing implications does this raise?

## CRITICAL THINKING ACTIVITIES

- ► The physician orders Dilantin 400 mg/day for Mr. Yarbo. Three days after initiation of the medication, Mr. Yarbo's Dilantin level = 9 g/ml (below therapeutic blood level). Mr. Yarbo is exhibiting breakthrough seizures. Evaluate the effectiveness of Dilantin therapy, and offer your hypothesis regarding its use in this patient.
- ► Mr. Yarbo develops a red area on his sacrum/coccyx. Nurse X suggests an air mattress to prevent skin breakdown as a whole. Nurse Y suggests a doughnut focusing on the sacral area with cost containment in mind. Critique each nurse's line of reasoning.
- ► Discuss the potential positive and negative consequences of using or not using restraints for patients with altered levels of consciousness.

## CHAPTER SUMMARY

### ALTERED LEVELS OF CONSCIOUSNESS

- Level of consciousness may be defined by the terms *confusion, drowsiness, stupor, light coma,* and *deep coma.*
- The Glasgow Coma Scale and the Rancho Los Amigos scale are two tools that are helpful to the nurse in assessing behaviors seen in the patient with an altered level of consciousness.
- Stimulation of the comatose patient is important.

### HEADACHE

- Headache is a common symptom that varies in degree of severity from relative unimportance to serious prognosis.
- Identification of triggering factors may help prevent headache.
- Prevention of migraine headaches may include avoiding certain foods (e.g., chocolate, nuts, onions).
- Headache pain arises from the scalp and its blood vessels and muscles, from the dura mater and its ve-

nous sinuses, and from the blood vessels at the base of the brain.

- The aura that occurs before an acute migraine attack may include visual field defects, confusion, paresthesias, and in extreme cases paralysis.
- With cluster headaches, the pain episodes are clustered together in quick succession for a few days or months with relatively long remissions that may last for months.

## INCREASED INTRACRANIAL PRESSURE

- Increased intracranial pressure (ICP) is a complex manifestation that results from multiple neurologic conditions.
- An increase in the volume of any of the cranial contents, singly or in combination, results in increased ICP and a reciprocal change in the volume of the other contents because the cranial vault is rigid, closed, and nonexpandable.
- Prevention of increased ICP involves the early detection of signs and symptoms so that corrective actions can be instituted.
- One of the first symptoms of increased ICP is a decreasing level of consciousness.
- Slowing of the pulse rate in conjunction with a rising systolic blood pressure is a significant observation related to increased ICP.
- The medical treatment of increased ICP depends on the underlying cause.
- Rapidly rising ICP must be relieved by mechanical decompression.

## ALTERATIONS IN COMMUNICATION

- Aphasia is a disorder of language (speech, reading, writing, understanding) caused by damage to the speech-controlling areas of the brain.

## CONVULSIVE DISORDERS

- Epilepsy may be defined as a transitory disturbance in consciousness or in motor function, sensory function, or autonomic function, with or without loss of consciousness, and may be caused by neoplasms, abscesses, and trauma.
- Seizures or convulsions are associated with sudden, excessive, and disorderly electrical discharges in the neurons of the brain.
- The grand mal seizure is the most common and dramatic type of seizure and is characterized by a loss of consciousness for several minutes and by tonic and clonic convulsions.
- An aura is a set of symptoms that occurs before a seizure; the exact nature of the aura varies from person to person.
- The period after a seizure is called the *postictal period.*
- Status epilepticus is recurrent, generalized seizure activity that occurs with such frequency that full consciousness is not regained between seizures and can lead to death from hypoxia and exhaustion.
- Observations to be made about a person having a seizure include those associated with the aura, cry, onset, tonic and clonic phases, relaxation, postictal phase, duration of entire seizure, and level of consciousness.
- The primary goals of the care of the patient with a seizure disorder are to protect the person from injury, observe and record the seizure activity, and treat the seizure with one or more anticonvulsant drugs.
- The person with seizures should be encouraged to lead as normal a life as possible.

## DEGENERATIVE DISEASES

- Degenerative diseases are those neurologic diseases in which a premature senescence of nerve cells occurs and there is a known or suspected metabolic disturbance or the cause is unknown.
- Multiple sclerosis, the cause of which is unknown, is a common neurologic disease in northern climates that is chronic, remitting, and characterized by relapses.
- With multiple sclerosis, multiple foci of demyelination are distributed randomly in the white matter of the brainstem, spinal cord, optic nerves, and cerebrum. Because of the randomness of the degeneration, a greater variety of signs and symptoms is seen in multiple sclerosis than in other neurologic diseases. The treatment is symptomatic.
- The pathologic process that occurs in Parkinson's disease is basically a depigmentation of the substantia nigra of the basal ganglia, which leads to multiple problems with motion.
- Treatment for Parkinson's disease is palliative and symptomatic and depends on the success of the drug used to treat it.
- Myasthenia gravis is a neurologic disease in which nerve impulses fail to cross the myoneural junction.
- Respiratory problems are common in persons with myasthenia gravis.
- Alzheimer's disease, the most frequent cause of dementia in the older adult, is a degenerative disorder that affects the cells of the brain and causes impairment in intellectual functioning. No diagnostic test is specific for Alzheimer's disease.
- Nursing care of the patient with Alzheimer's disease is directed toward maintaining nutrition, continence, hydration, and safety.

## VASCULAR DISEASES

- Cerebrovascular accident (CVA) is the most common disease of the nervous system and a major cause of death in the United States.
- The major causes of CVA are thrombus, embolus, and hemorrhage, all of which can be precipitated by many underlying factors. The blood vessel most frequently affected by a CVA is the middle cerebral artery.

- A transient ischemic attack (TIA) is a transient cerebral ischemia that warns the patient of an underlying pathologic condition.
- Care of the patient with a CVA includes prevention of further impairment, maintenance of existing abilities, and restoration of as much function as possible.
- Intracranial hemorrhages include bleeding into the subarachnoid space or into the brain tissue itself.

### INTRACRANIAL TUMORS

- The treatment of brain tumors includes radiation, chemotherapy, and surgery.
- The symptoms of a brain tumor are determined by the size and location of the tumor in the brain.
- Primary intracranial tumors, or neoplasms, arise from the intrinsic cells of brain tissues and the pituitary and pineal glands and include gliomas or astrocytomas, meningiomas, pituitary tumors, and neuromas.
- Hydrocephalus may occur in the presence of a brain tumor and is treated by a shunting procedure.

### CRANIOCEREBRAL TRAUMA

- Craniocerebral trauma, or head injury, causes death and serious disability in persons of all ages.
- Damage to brain tissue by trauma can include concussion, contusion, and laceration.
- The results of cerebral trauma often are devastating to deal with and if the patient is a child can present a challenge for many years.

### INFECTIONS/INFLAMMATIONS

- The brain may be affected by infections/inflammations that are caused by a variety of organisms and viruses and also may be affected by toxic reactions to bacterial and viral disease.
- Infections that can affect the brain include meningitis and encephalitis.

### ACQUIRED IMMUNODEFICIENCY SYNDROME

- Many patients with acquired immunodeficiency syndrome (AIDS) develop neurologic problems as the disease progresses.
- Neurologic problems in the patient with AIDS can occur because of infiltration of the central nervous system by specific organisms, encephalopathy, or systemic peripheral neuropathy.

## REFERENCES


1. Ackerman L: Interventions related to neurologic care, *Nurs Clin North Am* 27(2):325-335, 1992.
2. Ake J, Perlstein L: AIDS: impact on neuroscience nursing practice, *J Neurosci Nurs* 19:300-304, 1987.
3. Algase D: Cognitive discriminants of wandering among nursing home residents, *Nurs Res* 41(2):78-81, 1992.
4. Andrus C: Intracranial pressure: diagnosis and nursing management, *Neurosci Nurs* 23:85-92, 1991.
5. Aumick J: Head trauma: guidelines for care, *RN* 54(4):27-31, 1991.
6. Baggerly J: Sensory perceptual problems following stroke: the invisible deficits, *Nurs Clin North Am* 26(4):997-1005, 1991.
7. Berkshire J, Watson-Evans H: Meningioma: a nursing perspective, *J Neurosci Nurs* 18:86-89, 1986.
8. Berry P, Ward-Smith P: Adrenal medullary transplant as a treatment for Parkinson's disease: perioperative considerations, *J Neurosci Nurs* 20:356-361, 1988.
9. Borgman M, Passarella P: Nursing care of the stroke patient using Bobath principles: an approach to altered movement, *Nurs Clin North Am* 26(4):1019-1035, 1991.
10. Burns E, Buckwalter K: Pathophysiology and etiology of Alzheimer's disease, *Nurs Clin North Am* 23(1):11-30, 1988.
11. Campbell C: Acoustic neuroma: nursing implications related to surgical management, *J Neurosci Nurs* 23:50-56, 1991.
12. Csesko P: Sexuality and multiple sclerosis, *J Neurosci Nurs* 20:353-355, 1988.
13. Davidson A, Young C: Repatterning of stroke rehabilitation clients following return to life in the community, *J Neurosurg Nurs* 17(2):123-128, 1985.
14. Davis K et al: A double-blind, placebo-controlled multicenter study of tacrine for Alzheimer's disease, *N Eng J Med* 327(18):1253-1259, 1992.
15. Emich-Herring B, Wood P: A team approach to neurological based swallowing disorders, *Rehabil Nurs* 15:242-247, 1990.
16. Fode N: Subarachnoid hemorrhage from ruptured intracranial aneurysm, *Am J Nurs* 88:673-680, 1988.
17. Freed C et al: Survival of implanted fetal dopamine cells and neurologic improvement 12 to 46 months after transplantation for Parkinson's disease, *N Eng J Med* 327(22):1549-1555, 1992.
18. Given C et al: Source of stress among families caring for relatives with Alzheimer's disease, *Nurs Clin North Am* 23(1):69-82, 1988.
19. Grabbe L, Brown L: Identifying neurologic complications of AIDS, *Nursing '89* 19(5):66-73, 1989.
20. Grant J, Kinney M: Validity of nursing diagnosis, *Res Nurs Health* 13(6):403-410, 1990.
21. Hahn K: Left vs. right: what a difference a side makes in stroke, *Nursing '87* 17(9):44-48, 1987.
22. Hickey J: Myasthenic crisis—your assessment counts, *RN* 54(5):54-59, 1991.
23. Hinkle J: Nursing care of the patient with minor head injury, *J Neurosci Nurs* 20(1):8-14, 1988.
24. Hodges K, Root L: Surgical management of intractable seizure disorder, *J Neurosci Nurs* 23:93-100, 1991.
25. Holt J: How to help confused patients, *Am J Nurs* 93(8):32-36, 1993.
26. Hurley A et al: Assessment of discomfort in advanced Alzheimer patients, *Res Nurs Health* 15(5):369-378, 1992.
27. Jacob D et al: The U.S. decline in stroke mortality: what does ecological analysis tell us? *Am J Public Health* 82(12):1596-1599, 1992.
28. Kalbach L: Unilateral neglect: mechanism and nursing care, *J Neurosci Nurs* 23:125-129, 1991.
29. Keller C et al: Psychological responses to aphasia: theoretical considerations and nursing implications, *J Neurosci Nurs* 21:290-294, 1989.
30. Kim T: Hope as a mode of coping in amyotrophic lateral sclerosis, *J Neurosci Nurs* 21:341-347, 1989.
31. Larsen P: Psychosocial adjustment in MS, *Rehabil Nurs* 15:242-247, 1990.
32. Long BC, Phipps WJ, Cassmeyer VL: *Medical-surgical nursing: a nursing process approach,* St Louis, 1993, Mosby.
33. Luchka S: Working with ICP monitors, *RN* 54(3):34-37, 1991.
34. MacDonld E: Aneurysmal subarachnoid hemorrhage, *J Neurosci Nurs* 21:313-321, 1989.
35. Mauss-Clum N et al: Locked in syndrome: a team approach, *J Neurosci Nurs* 23:273-86, 1991.

36. Mocsny N: Toxoplasmic encephalitis in the AIDS patient, *Rehabil Nurs* 18(1):20-22, 1993.
37. Muswaswes M: Increased intracranial pressure and its systemic effects, *J Neurosurg Nurs* 20:217-222, 1988.
38. Olson E: Perceptual deficits affecting the stroke patient, *Rehabil Nurs* 16(4):212-3, 1991.
39. Ozuna J, Friel P: Effect of enteral tube feeding on serum phenytoin levels, *J Neurosurg Nurs* 16(6):289-291, 1984.
40. Palmer M, Wyness M: Positioning and handling: important considerations in the care of the severely head-injured patient, *J Neurosci Nurs* 20:42-49, 1988.
41. Phipps MA: Assessment of neurologic deficits in stroke: acute-care and rehabilitation implications, *Nurs Clin North Am* 26(4):957-970, 1991.
42. Plylar P: Management of the agitated and aggressive head injury patient in an acute care setting, *J Neurosci Nurs* 21:353-356, 1989.
43. Deleted in proofs.
44. Rankin J: The nursing diagnosis: swallowing, impaired and bedside assessment of swallowing in neurologically involved cases, *J Neurosci Nurs* 24:117-118, 1992.
45. Rehabilitation of persons with injuries, *MMWR* 41(RR-6): 35-38, 1992.
46. Rhynsburger J: How to fight myasthenia's fatigue, *Am J Nurs* 89:337-341, 1989.
47. Rutledge B: Aneurysm wrapping: principles applicable to the neuroscience nurse, *J Neurosci Nurs* 19:158-165, 1987.
48. Scherer P: How AIDS attacks the brain, *Am J Nurs* 90(1):44-53, 1990.
49. Sherman D: Managing an acute head injury, *Nursing '90* 20(4):44-51, 1990.
50. Stone N: Amyotrophic lateral sclerosis: a challenge for constant adaptation, *J Neurosci Nurs* 19:166-173, 1987.
51. Tucker C: Safety assessment for the postictal confusional phase following complex partial seizures, *J Neurosurg Nurs* 17(3):201-209, 1985.
52. Turner H et al: Comparison of nurse and computer recording of ICP in head injured patients, *J Neurosci Nurs* 20:236-239, 1988.
53. US Dept. of Health and Human Services, Public Health Services: *Healthy people 2000: national health promotion and disease prevention objectives,* Washington, DC, 1990, US Government Printing Office.
54. Vos H: Making headway with intracranial hypertension, *Am J Nurs* 93(2):28-35, 1993.
55. Welsh D, Zumwalt C: Volumetric interstitial hyperthermia: nursing implications for brain tumor treatment, *J Neurosci Nurs* 20:229-235, 1988.
56. White R, Likavec M: The diagnosis and initial management of head injury, *N Engl J Med* 327(21):1507-1511, 1992.
57. Williams A: Self report of indifference and anxiety among persons with right hemispheric stroke, *Res Nurs Health* 15(5):343-348, 1992.
58. Wineman N: Adaptation to multiple sclerosis: the role of social support, functional disability, and perceived uncertainty, *Nurs Res* 39(5):294-299, 1990.
59. Zasler N, Kreutzer J: Family and sexuality after traumatic brain injury. In Williams J, King T, editors: *Impact of head injury on the family system: an overview for professionals,* Baltimore, 1990, Paul H Brookes.

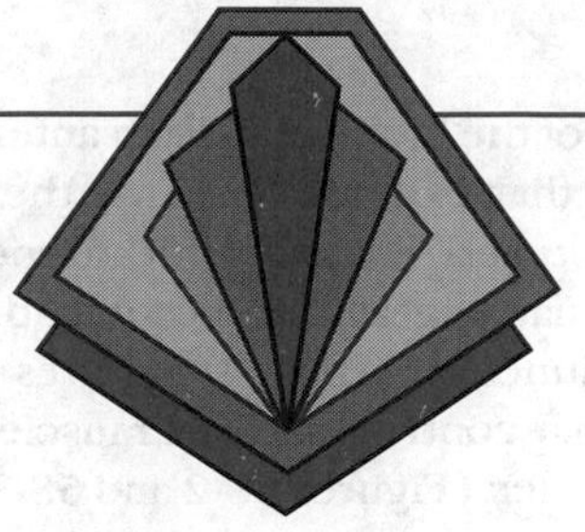

CHAPTER 58

# Management of Persons With Problems of the Spinal Cord and Peripheral Nerves

*Elizabeth Anne Schenk*

## CHAPTER OBJECTIVES

***After studying this chapter, the learner should be able to do the following:***

1 State at least three nursing interventions to assist the patient with neurologic pain.
2 Differentiate between upper motor neuron and lower motor neuron disease.
3 Describe the pathophysiology of Guillain-Barré syndrome.
4 Explain the difference between an incomplete and a complete spinal cord injury.
5 Describe the motor losses with cervical, thoracic, lumbar, and sacral levels of spinal cord injury.
6 List at least three symptoms of autonomic dysreflexia, and give examples of at least four nursing interventions in this emergency situation.
7 Define the differences among neuropathy, mononeuropathy, polyneuropathy, neuritis, and neuralgia.
8 List at least three nursing actions important for the patient with trigeminal neuralgia.

## KEY TERMS

analgesia
autonomic dysreflexia
causalgia
clonus
dysesthesia
electromyography
fasciculation
flaccidity
Guillain-Barré syndrome
herpes zoster
hyperalgesia
hypalgesia
intractable pain
LMN lesion
local pain
mononeuropathy
neuralgia
neuritis
neuropathy
paralysis
paraplegia
paresis
paresthesia
polyneuritis
polyneuropathy
quadriplegia
referred pain
root pain
shingles
spinal shock
tic douloureux
trigeminal neuralgia
UMN lesion

This chapter discusses the care of persons with neurologic problems affecting the spinal cord or peripheral nervous system. These include manifestations of (1) alterations in muscle tone and motor function, (2) alterations in movement and posture, and (3) neurologic pain. Common neurologic problems or disorders are also discussed, including (1) Guillain-Barré syndrome, (2) herpes zoster, (3) spinal cord trauma, (4) intravertebral tumors, (5) peripheral nerve trauma, and (6) trigeminal neuralgia.

## ALTERATIONS IN MUSCLE TONE AND MOTOR FUNCTION

### ETIOLOGY/EPIDEMIOLOGY

Disturbances of motor function probably surpass all other clinical neurologic symptoms in frequency and importance. Because the nervous system is designed primarily for movement of the body in space and of the various parts in relation to each other, damage to the nervous system often causes serious problems in mobility.

## PATHOPHYSIOLOGY

The term **paralysis** refers to a loss of function, either motor or sensory. When applied to motor function, it means loss of voluntary movement because of interruption of the descending efferent motor pathways. A lesser degree of paralysis is called **paresis.** Damage to sensory pathways that are intimately concerned with motor function may occur concomitantly with the loss of motor function. Loss of sensory function is described later in this chapter.

Injury or disease of motor neurons and their extensions at any level results in alterations of muscle strength, tone, and reflex activity. The specific clinical manifestations differ according to whether the lesion involves an upper motor neuron or a lower motor neuron (Figure 58-1).

### Lower Motor Neuron Lesion

Recall that *lower motor neurons* (LMNs) consist of the large anterior horn cells located in the anterior gray matter of the spinal cord. They are also located in the motor cranial nuclei of the brainstem. Each anterior horn cell has a long axon that exits the cord via the anterior (ventral) spinal root and extends out to peripheral nerve, eventually synapsing at the motor end plate of the neuromuscular junction. These structures together form a *motor unit* that controls skeletal muscle activity, both voluntary and reflex (Figures 58-2 and 58-3). When a lesion selectively involves some part (cell body, motor root, isolated peripheral nerve) of the LMN, it characteristically results in flaccid muscle weakness or paralysis, loss of reflex activity, loss of muscle tone, and atrophy confined to the involved muscle or muscles.

The *degree* of muscle weakness occurring in the involved muscle or muscles in an **LMN lesion** is directly related to the extent and severity of the lesion. Since each anterior horn cell innervates several separate muscle fibers and since several anterior horn cell columns exist at each spinal level, a lesion confined to *one* spinal segment may not damage all the anterior horn cells innervating an entire muscle. Thus such a lesion will cause muscle *weakness* (paresis) rather than paralysis of the

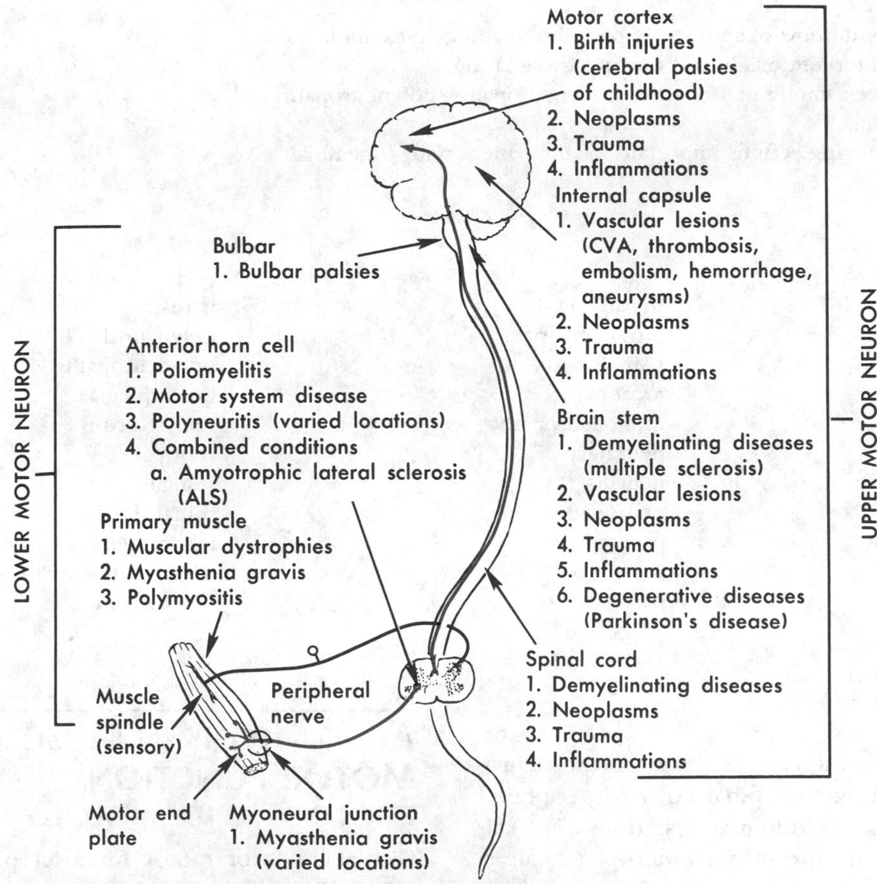


**FIGURE 58-1** Disturbances in motor function are classified pathologically along upper motor neuron (UMN) and lower motor neuron (LMN) structures. It should be noted that the same pathologic condition occurs at more than one site in UMN area shown on right. A few pathologic conditions involve both UMN and LMN structures, as in amyotrophic lateral sclerosis. Other lesion sites include myoneural junctions and primary muscles, making it possible to classify conditions as neuromuscular and muscular, respectively.

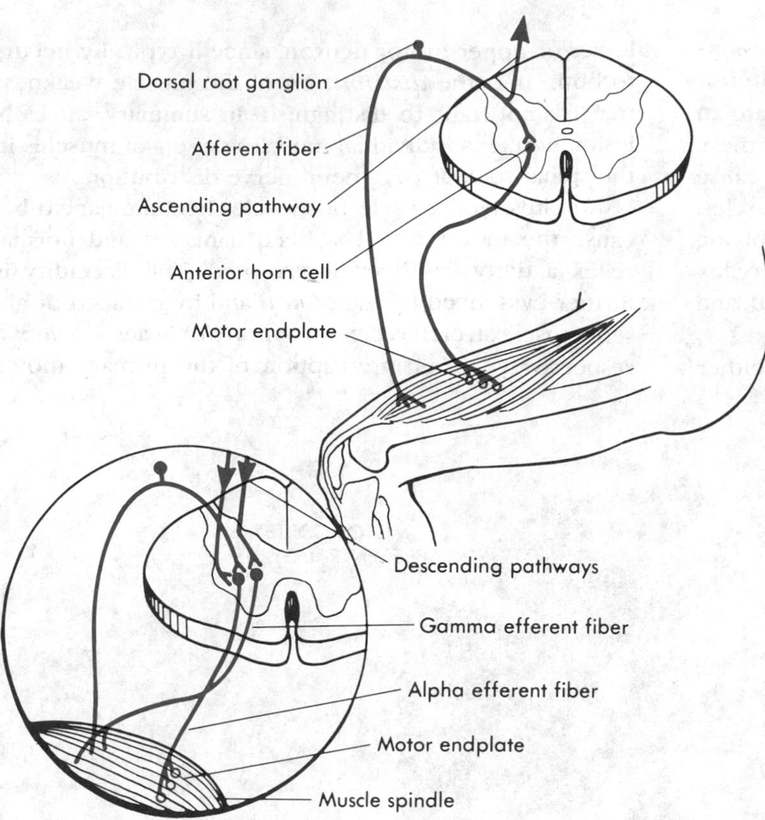


**FIGURE 58-2** Structures making up LMN, including motor (efferent) and sensory (afferent) elements. Shown on left is anterior horn cell in anterior gray column of spinal cord and its axon, which terminates in motor end plate as it innervates extrafusal muscle fibers in the quadriceps muscle. Detailed in enlargement are sensory and motor elements of gamma-loop system. Gamma-efferent fiber is shown innervating polar or end region of muscle spindle (sensory receptor of skeletal muscle). Contraction of muscle spindle fibers stretch central portion of spindle and cause afferent spindle fiber to transmit impulse centrally to cord. Muscle spindle afferent fibers in turn synapse on anterior horn cell and are transmitted by way of alpha-efferent fibers to skeletal (extrafusal) muscle, causing it to contract. Muscle spindle discharge is interrupted by active contraction of extrafusal muscle fibers.

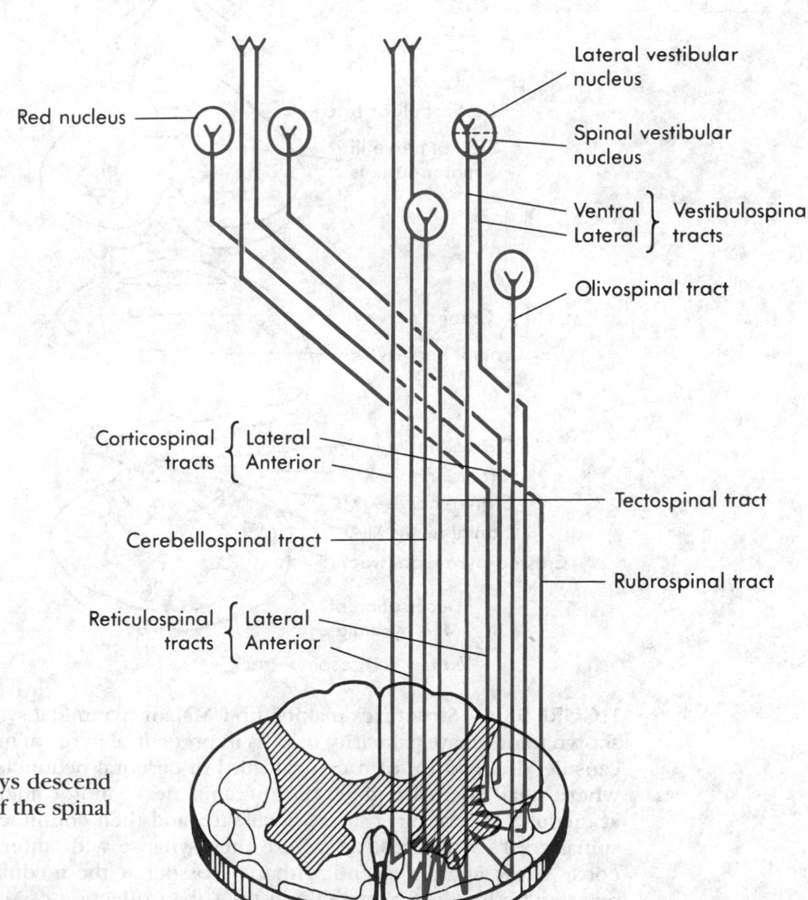


**FIGURE 58-3** Nuclei and their respective pathways descend and terminate around LMN in the ventral column of the spinal cord.

entire muscle. Complete paralysis occurs in LMN lesions only when the lesion involves the column or anterior horn cells in several spinal segments that innervate an entire muscle or the ventral roots arising from these cells. A lesion in a single motor nerve root will cause varying degrees of muscle weakness in several muscles. If *all* or almost all the peripheral motor fibers supplying a muscle are destroyed, all voluntary postural and reflex movements are lost. The entire muscle becomes lax and soft, a condition known as **flaccidity.**

Muscle weakness itself cannot be classified as either lower or upper motor neuron, since it typically occurs to both. It is the *distribution* of the muscle weakness that is important to distinguish. In summary, an LMN lesion weakens individual muscles or sets of muscles in the spinal root or peripheral nerve distribution.

The involved muscle or muscles become flaccid because the motor unit has been damaged and normal reflex activity has been interrupted. This flaccidity is further evidenced by *hypotonia* and by reduced or absent muscle stretch reflexes (*hyporeflexia* and *areflexia,* respectively). This interruption of the primary motor

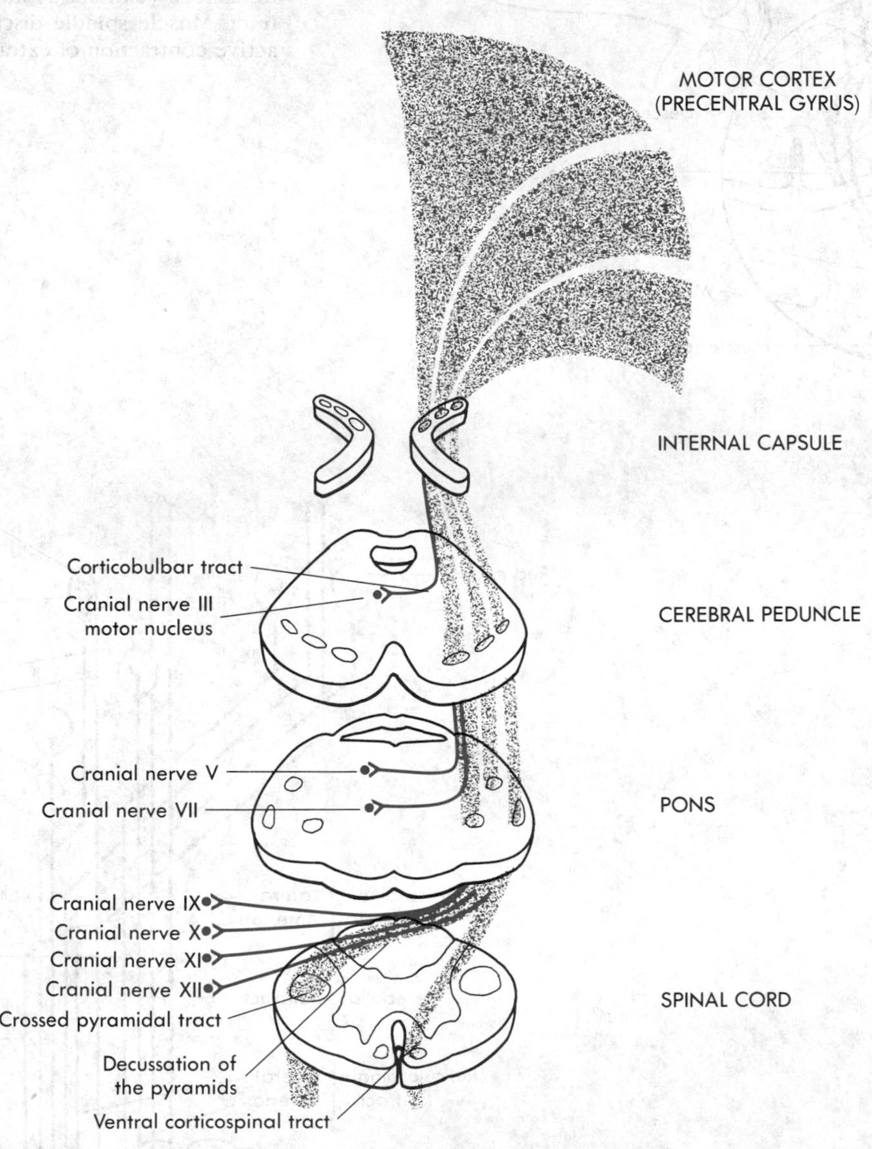


**FIGURE 58-4** Structures making up UMN, or pyramidal system. Pyramidal system fibers are shown to originate primarily in cells in precentral gyrus of motor cortex; converge at internal capsule; descend to form central third of cerebral peduncle; descend further through pons, where small fibers are given off to cranial nerve motor nuclei along the way; form pyramids at medulla, where most fibers decussate; and then continue to descend in lateral column of spinal cord's white matter, where they synapse with anterior horn cells at all segments of cord. A few fibers descend without crossing at the medulla level. (Modified from original painting by Frank H Netter. From the Ciba Collection of Medical Illustrations, Copyright by Ciba Pharmaceutical Co, division of Ciba-Geigy Corp. All rights reserved.)

unit results in localized muscle atrophy, or wasting, corresponding to the spinal segmental distribution of the anterior horn cells involved.

Atrophy also increases with nonuse of the muscle. In some LMN lesions, the affected muscle bundle or unit exhibits small, localized, spontaneous, and involuntary contractions known as **fasciculations.** These are visible through the skin and should not be confused with fibrillation. The fasciculations are thought to represent the discharge of isolated muscle fibers arising from a single-functioning LMN unit. Fasciculations are coarse in large motor units but may be fine in smaller motor units, as in the hands.

The criteria for an LMN lesion site or disease include segmental or localized muscle weakness and atrophy in the same distribution, with absent or decreased muscle stretch reflexes in the affected muscles.

In summary, when a lesion involves the LMN, the following signs are present:

1. Flaccid muscle weakness or paralysis
2. Loss of reflex activity
3. Loss of muscle tone
4. Atrophy confined to the involved muscle or muscles

## Upper Motor Neuron Lesion

Recall that *upper motor neurons* (UMNs) originate in the motor strip of the cerebral cortex and in multiple brainstem nuclei. From the cortex, these axons pass through the internal capsule and brainstem, cross over (decussate) in the medulla, and continue descending in the spinal cord via the corticospinal tracts. These fibers eventually synapse with LMNs in the spinal cord (Figure 58-4).

The corticospinal tracts are thought to be primarily responsible for the execution of precise, fine, voluntary muscle movements. However, together with the extrapyramidal tracts descending to the LMNs, they assist in modulating muscle tone and reflex activity to some degree. Thus all descending systems collectively combine their influences on the LMNs so that efferent neural impulses are modified. This results in fine, orderly, and smooth muscle movements.

Any lesion that destroys UMNs or interferes with their influences over LMNs therefore is called a **UMN lesion.** When a UMN lesion is *rostral* to the medulla, as in a cerebrovascular accident (CVA), deficits are contralateral to the lesion and are demonstrated as a hemiplegia. The distribution or degree of paralysis is not always equal or the same within the hemiplegic distribution. For example, the face and arm may be weak or the weakness may involve the leg alone, depending on the part of the motor cortex involved. The following may be considered *UMN signs* following CVA: weakness of the mouth muscle associated with eye muscle weakness (forehead muscle is intact), weakness of forearm and wrist extensors, and weakness of the hip flexors and foot dorsiflexors. These muscle weaknesses result in the characteristic gait and appearance of the patient with a CVA. Circumduction of the affected leg occurs with inversion of the foot, which drags. The arm is held semiflexed at the elbow and wrist. The facial muscles around the eye and mouth droop.

Initially and for a variable period, the muscles affected by the lesion are flaccid (hypotonic) and hyporeflexic. Gradually the flaccidity recedes, and the reflex arcs become increasingly hyperreactive in the absence of UMN modulation. Eventually, paresis or paralysis of voluntary muscle movement occurs with increased muscle tone and spasticity. The spasticity is characterized by increased resistance to passive movement, hyperreflexia, clasp-knife phenomenon, and **clonus.** Clonus is related to the hyperreflexia, in which the contraction of one muscle group is sufficient to stretch the antagonistic muscles and perpetuate the contractions. A unilateral Babinski's sign is present on the hemiparetic side. Atrophy of the muscle results from disuse and occurs late and to a lesser extent than in LMN disease.

UMN lesions within the brainstem also produce the characteristic motor manifestations just described and also cause involvement of the cranial nerve nuclei and sensory pathways near the midbrain lesion site. The problem of localizing the site of a UMN brainstem lesion is made more difficult by the proximity of the descending fiber systems and cranial motor nuclei in the brainstem area.

UMN lesions that are caudal to the medulla (as in spinal cord trauma) produce deficits ipsilateral to the lesion. If the cord is transected or the lesion extends into both halves of the spinal cord, deficits are demonstrated as a quadriplegia or paraplegia. A complete transection of the spinal cord immediately produces loss of motor function, muscle tone, and reflex activity as well as somatic and visceral sensations below the level of the injury. Usually, when examined after a year, voluntary motor losses remain, but there is increased spasticity of extensor muscles and hyperreflexia of *all* cord reflexes (muscle stretch, autonomic, nociceptive). Thus any stretch on the spastic muscles may result in extreme contraction. Likewise, contact with a noxious stimulus may cause flexion withdrawal of the limb along with variations of autonomic activity. Occasionally, all three types of reflex activity may occur simultaneously as a response to a single stimulus. For example, a full bladder or decubitis irritation may cause flexion of the lower extremities, reflex bladder or bowel emptying, and altered vasomotor response to that area. A bilateral, positive Babinski's sign is also present.

Table 58-1 summarizes and compares the characteristic clinical syndromes seen in UMN and LMN lesions.

In summary, when a lesion involves the UMN, the following signs are present:

1. Paresis or paralysis of voluntary muscle tone and spasticity
2. Hyperreflexia

**TABLE 58-1 Clinical Syndromes of UMN and LMN**

| MOTOR COMPONENT | UMN CHARACTERISTICS | LMN CHARACTERISTICS |
|---|---|---|
| Reflex | Hyperreflexia, extensor toe sign (Babinski's sign) | Hyporeflexia or areflexia |
| Muscle tonus | Hypertonia, clasp-knife spasticity, clonus | Hypotonia, flaccidity |
| Muscle movement | Paralysis or paresis of movements in hemiplegic and other distributions | Paralysis or paresis of individual muscles in peripheral nerve distribution |
| Muscle wasting | Late atrophy from disuse | Early atrophy or denervation |
| Muscle fasciculations | Not present | Present |

3. Late atrophy from disuse
4. Increased muscle tone

## PREVENTION

As with many neurologic diseases, often little can be done to prevent them. Much of the focus is on secondary prevention (early diagnosis) and tertiary prevention (prevention of complications). Some muscle injuries related to trauma and the preventive aspects (primary prevention) are discussed under the care of the comatose patient in Chapter 57.

## MEDICAL MANAGEMENT

The goal for discharge of patients with alterations in muscle tone and motor function is determined by diagnosis-related groups (DRGs) that are defined by the cause of the alteration. The nurse works collaboratively with the physician for implementation of prescribed medical therapy. Because the nurse has a major role in discharge planning and patient teaching, these are discussed under nursing management.

### Diagnostic Tests

One of the most common diagnostic procedures used to evaluate muscle dysfunction is **electromyography.** In motor disease, electrical activity of various types and abnormal patterns appears in resting muscle. The electromyogram (EMG) provides direct evidence of motor dysfunction and can be used to detect a dysfunction located in the motor neuron, the neuromuscular junction, or muscle fibers. (See Chapter 56 for a description of this procedure.)

### Medication

Patients experiencing ongoing problems with spasticity may receive one or more skeletal muscle relaxants to decrease tone and involuntary movements and to help relieve anxiety and tension. In general, the centrally acting preparations specifically affect the spinal polysynaptic reflexes and, at the same time, depress the central nervous system (CNS). Common side effects include drowsiness and dizziness; these become intensified when combined with alcohol, barbiturates, sedatives, hypnotics, or tranquilizers. Some frequently prescribed drugs include the following:

1. Baclofen (Lioresal), a derivative of gamma aminobutyric acid (GABA) (an inhibitory neurotransmitter), acts on the spinal cord.
2. Dantrolene (Dantrium) acts directly on skeletal muscle. Effects from the drug become apparent about a week after it is started. It acts by impairing $Ca^{++}$ release from the sarcoplasmic reticulum. Additional side effects include muscle weakness, slurred speech, drooling, and anuresis.
3. Diazepam (Valium) is a centrally acting muscle relaxant and antianxiety agent.

### Treatment

No specific treatment exists for patients with alterations in muscle tone and motor function. Other treatments that may be useful in patients with spasticity who do not respond to medications include intrathecal phenol (to alleviate painful spasm in lower extremities), individual peripheral nerve blocks, and physical therapy.

### Diet

There is no specific diet for patients with alterations in muscle function or tone.

### Activity

The patient with an alteration in muscle function or tone is encouraged to be as active as possible. Keeping the person active may slow any adverse results from muscle weakness.

### Referral/Consultation

In some settings the nurse assumes responsibility for making referrals to other services. For the patient with alterations in muscle function or tone, this might include a referral to a physical therapist or to the social worker for help in discharge planning.

## NURSING MANAGEMENT

### ♦ ASSESSMENT

Both subjective and objective data are important in determining more about abnormal muscle movements.

### Subjective Data

Data to be collected to assess the patient with alterations in muscle function or tone include the following:

Patient's understanding of the problem and possible causes

Initial onset of problem

Measures that improve symptoms
Presence of clumsiness or incoordination
Presence of any abnormal sensation

Often, subjective symptoms occurring early in an illness involving muscle movements or sensations are ignored.

## Objective Data

Data to be collected to assess the patient with alterations in muscle function or tone include the following:

Coordination
Muscle strength
Muscle tone
Any atrophy of muscles
Presence of clonus or fasciculations
Ability to move muscles; abnormal gait
Reflexes
Change in ability to carry out activities of daily living (ADL)

# ♦ NURSING DIAGNOSES

Nursing diagnoses are determined from analysis of patient data. Nursing diagnoses for the patient with alterations in muscle function or tone may include but are not limited to the following:

| Diagnostic Title | Possible Etiologic Factors |
|---|---|
| Injury trauma, high risk for | Sensorimotor deficits |
| Skin integrity, high risk for impaired | Prolonged immobility |
| Disuse syndrome, high risk for | Immobility, weakness |
| Nutrition, altered; less than body requirements | Chewing/swallowing difficulties |
| Incontinence, total | Neurologic dysfunction/disease |
| Self-feeding, bathing-hygiene, dressing-grooming, and toileting deficits | Neuromuscular impairment |
| Adjustment, impaired | Disability requiring change in lifestyle |
| Knowledge deficit (medication and care required) | Lack of exposure/recall |

# ♦ EXPECTED PATIENT OUTCOMES

Expected patient outcomes for the patient with alterations in muscle tone or function may include but are not limited to the following:

1. Remains free of injury.
2. Skin remains intact.
3. Disuse syndrome does not develop, as indicated by the absence of (a) contractures, (b) skin breakdown, (c) immobility, (d) thromboembolic events, and (e) muscle mass.
4. Nutritional status is optimal, as evidenced by (a) maintenance of usual body weight and (b) normal laboratory work (protein, hematocrit, hemoglobin).
5. Is continent or has elimination controlled by a bowel and bladder program.
6. Is able to perform ADL as independently as possible.
7. Verbalizes positive adjustment to the disability.
8. Verbalizes knowledge of the following: (a) safety needs, (b) skin care, (c) activity needs, (d) medications, (e) nutrition/diet, and (f) techniques to perform ADL.

# ♦ INTERVENTIONS

## Promoting Safety

Patients who are paralyzed need to be protected from falling. The person with hemiplegia must have the side rail of the bed raised on the affected side when unattended. If permitted up in a chair, a chair restraint is used.

The *eye on the affected side* should be protected if the lid remains open and there is no blink reflex. Otherwise, damage to the cornea can lead to corneal ulcers and blindness. Irrigations with a physiologic solution of sodium chloride, followed by drops of sterile mineral oil, sterile castor oil, sterile petroleum jelly, or artificial tears solution (methylcellulose), are sometimes used. After the lid is gently closed, an eye pad may be taped over the affected eye. If a pad is used, it must be changed daily, and the eye cleansed and carefully examined for signs of inflammation or drying of the cornea. Eye shields are preferable to pads because they lessen the danger of lint entering the eye.

## Promoting Skin Integrity

The skin of the paralyzed person needs to be inspected for signs of pressure. These patients are at risk for decubitus formation. The following factors account for this:

1. Muscles are not being used.
2. Interference with autonomic reflexes that monitor and maintain vasomotor tone may result in altered circulation in the paralyzed areas.
3. Sensory loss may prevent the patient from perceiving pain and pressure (the usual warning signs of tissue injury).

In monoplegic, hemiplegic, and quadriplegic distributions, successively larger areas of skin surface must be protected.

## Promoting Activity

The limbs of a person with acute hemiplegia, as with those of the person with paraplegia, are often flaccid at first. Spasticity with a tendency to muscle contracture develops gradually. The joints then become flexed or extended and fixed in useles positions with deformity *unless preventive measures are taken by the nurse.* Shortening of joint capsules and ligaments occurs around the immobile joint, and the limb may be drawn into flexure or extensor contracture with or without muscle spasm.

Through assessment, the nurse determines the specific joints that are vulnerable to contracture and deformity formation as related to the existing degree and type of paralysis. For example, greater contracture vulnerability occurs with quadriplegia than with paraplegia or hemiplegia, since the amount of muscle and joint involvement is greater. Assessment includes free range of motion (ROM) to determine the level of motion in all joints. On the basis of assessment, the nurse carefully positions the limbs in normal anatomic positions to prevent deformity. By having knowledge of the distribution patterns of paralysis in UMN or LMN lesions, *counter-positioning* can also be initiated. In hemiplegia, for example, the neglected upper limb is pulled inward at the shoulder joint and the wrist drops; in the lower limb the knee flexes and the foot drops. In counterpositioning the nurse plans for the shoulder and upper arm to be in abduction, the elbow slightly flexed, the wrist in dorsiflexion, the knee in neutral position, and the foot in dorsiflexion. If the person is supine, a pillow can be placed between the upper arm and body to hold the arm in abduction. A roll made of one or two washcloths or a styrofoam cup serves as a good support to prevent flexion of the fingers, and a splint made from a padded tongue blade may be used to ensure straightening of the thumb or other fingers for periods during the day. Some question the common use of soft devices to prevent hand deformity and believe that one should experiment with hard devices to improve hand functioning after a UMN lesion such as a CVA.

A firm box at the foot of the bed holds the feet at right angles and prevents contractures in the drop-foot position (see Figure 57-7). Some physical therapists believe that footboards used in the prevention of footdrop contribute to increased spasticity and that their use should *not* be a routine practice for persons with UMN lesions (also true for high-topped tennis shoes).

Positioning is equally important as related to paraplegic and quadriplegic distributions. Knee flexion and footdrop are severe complications that must be prevented. The development of a flexion contracture at the knee joint interferes with the ability of the person to bear weight later in an upright position and to transfer unaided from one place to another. As a consequence, the person's level of self-care and independence may be greatly diminished when a joint deformity occurs. Subluxation of a shoulder joint in a person with hemiplegia, related to inadequate support of the joint when in an upright position, causes pain and limits therapy of the limb. In addition, keeping the paralyzed person in a semi-upright position for long periods, whether in or out of bed, results in hip deformities. Positioning in the prone position helps to counteract the formation of this type of deformity (see Figure 57-8). (See Guidelines box at left.)

In summary, most joint deformities in a paralyzed person are *preventable* with early and continuing nursing interventions.

In addition to positioning, interventions for the person with paralysis include ROM exercises to all joints. Passive ROM exercises are indicated at least *twice daily* for all joints that the person cannot voluntarily move. The individual must perform frequent active ROM of the unaffected joints. The regularity of ROM is most important so that limitations do not develop.

### Guidelines for Care of the Person With Motor Dysfunction

1. Promote safety.
   a. Always keep side rail up on affected side of hemiplegic patients.
   b. Use restraints judiciously as needed.
   c. Protect affected eye if there is no blink reflex.
      (1) Irrigate eye with normal saline solution as needed.
      (2) Use artificial tear solution if ordered.
      (3) Use eye shield to keep eye closed. Change daily and inspect eye for dryness, redness, or other signs of infection. (Eye shield is preferable to eye pad because of no lint.)
2. Promote integrity of skin.
   a. Change position frequently; patient should do so if able.
   b. Shift weight for patients in chairs.
   c. Inspect skin at least daily.
   d. If sensory loss is present, avoid use of hot water bottles, heating pads, or hot water.
3. Promote activity.
   a. Position or counterposition as necessary.
   b. Use hand splints as needed.
   c. Use measures to protect from footdrop, such as footboards.
   d. Use sling for shoulder subluxation.
4. Promote nutrition.
   a. Give positive feedback to patient when progress is made.
   b. Turn patient on back or unaffected side to help swallowing.
   c. Avoid foods that cause choking, such as mashed potatoes.
   d. Check affected side of mouth for accumulated food and poor mouth care.
   e. Encourage patient to feed self as soon as possible.
   f. Use dentures if patient has them.

## Promoting Nutrition

Patience and persistence are necessary in giving foods and fluid to the person with hemiplegia. So much difficulty may be encountered in swallowing food and fluids because of the paralysis that the patient may become easily frustrated.[7,15] The Guidelines box (at left) lists important nursing measures.

## Promoting Elimination

The person with paralysis from a UMN or LMN lesion may experience problems with bowel and bladder control (see Chapters 47 and 49).

### Promoting Activities of Daily Living

During the acute and rehabilitative phases, patients with paralysis are taught how to carry out ADL to the extent they are able. A variety of self-help devices are available that assist, for example, with dressing with one hand. The occupational therapist becomes involved in many of these activities, including homemaking tasks. It is important to stress the concept of the rehabilitative *team* in managing these patients.

### Promoting Psychologic Adjustment

The person with paralysis will need assistance in adjusting to the change in the body. The loss of the ability to function independently when paralyzed is traumatic. The person may also have fears about the future and loss of self-esteem. A grief reaction similar to that described for the stages of death and dying may occur. At times, persons may relate to the paralyzed portion of the body as though it were not a part of them. Nursing interventions to help the patient cope with the loss of function and change in body image are essential.[12]

### Facilitating Learning

Teaching is an extremely important part of caring for the patient with motor problems. Relevant points include the following:

1. Safety needs
   a. Always lock wheelchair when transferring patient
   b. Check condition of affected eye frequently
   c. Be aware of placement of affected extremities before movement
   d. Protect paralyzed limbs from injury
   e. Stress the importance of wearing well-fitting shoes for ambulation
2. Skin care
   a. Regular inspection of skin surfaces using mirror or other device as necessary
   b. Need to turn frequently
   c. Need to shift body weight from one position to another
   d. No use of heating pads, hot water bottles, or excessively hot water for bathing
3. Activity needs
   a. ROM exercises
   b. Proper positioning
   c. Frequent changes in position
4. Medications
   a. Use of medication, side effects, dosage, and timing
   b. Importance of reporting side effects to physician
   c. Importance of not combining medication with other mood-altering chemicals
5. Nutrition/diet
   a. Foods that can easily be tolerated
   b. Measures to decrease swallowing difficulty
   c. Use of special appliances to assist with eating
6. ADL
   a. Teaching techniques of bathing, grooming, and dressing
   b. Importance of having meaningful recreational activities
   c. Bowel and bladder care
7. Other teaching
   a. Importance of good fluid intake
   b. Follow-up care such as where to procure equipment and supplies
   c. Methods of relieving or handling feelings of frustration

## ♦ EVALUATION

To evaluate the effectiveness of nursing interventions, compare patient behaviors with those stated in the expected patient outcomes. Successful achievement of patient outcomes for the patient with alterations in muscle tone or function is indicated by the following:

1. No injury occurs to the patient.
2. Skin is intact with no sustained redness.
3. Disuse syndrome does not occur, as evidenced by (a) absence of contractures of any joints of the body; (b) no skin breakdown; (c) ability to ambulate, transfer, and/or move freely in a wheelchair; (d) absence of thromboembolic events; and (e) absence of loss of muscle mass.
4. Usual body weight is maintained, and laboratory work (protein, hematocrit, hemoglobin) is within normal limits.
5. Is continent of bowel and bladder, whether naturally or as the result of a bowel or bladder training program.
6. Is able to perform ADL, including feeding, dressing, bathing, grooming, and toileting with or without assistive devices.
7. States positive adjustment to disability.
8. Correctly describes the following: (a) safety needs; (b) skin care; (c) activity needs; (d) medications, including route, time, side effects, and desired action; (e) nutritional needs; and (f) techniques to perform ADL.

## COMPLICATIONS

The patient with an alteration in motor function or tone is at risk for various complications (see Interventions section).

# ALTERATIONS IN MOVEMENT AND POSTURE

## ETIOLOGY/EPIDEMIOLOGY

Various neurologic lesions of the extrapyramidal motor system result in alterations of movement and posture.

Clinically, this is seen most often in paralysis agitans, or *parkinsonism.* In this condition, degeneration of various parts of the basal ganglia occurs (see Chapter 57). Other conditions that produce alterations in movement and posture include the following:

1. Drug-induced extrapyramidal syndromes
2. Idiopathic dyskinesias and dystonias
3. Huntington's chorea
4. Wilson's disease
5. Myoclonus
6. Tic
7. Cerebral palsy

The reader is referred to a neurologic text for a further description of these disorders.

In contrast to UMN syndrome with the loss of volitional movement and spasticity, extrapyramidal lesions involve characteristic muscle rigidity, involuntary movements, and bradykinesia without loss of voluntary movement. Muscle rigidity, or *hypertonus,* is present in all muscle groups, both flexor and extensor, but appears to be more prominent in those muscles that maintain a flexed posture. The smaller muscles of the face, tongue, and even the larynx become involved, with consequent difficulty in chewing, swallowing, and speech. The muscles remain continuously or intermittently firm and tense. Hypertonus is present even when the person is relaxed. There is an even or uniform quality to the hypertonus throughout the passive ROM of a limb. The rigidity is often described as "plastic." In addition, a superimposed rhythmic contraction of the muscle may be felt as the joint is moved through its ROM. This is termed *cogwheel rigidity.*

Strength of muscle is not significantly decreased in bradykinesia. *Bradykinesia,* or *hypokinesia,* refers to slowness rather than lack of movement *(akinesia);* the actual time in carrying out a movement is longer than normal. There is also an extreme poverty of movement. The semiautomatic or habitual movements observed in the normal state, such as putting the hands to the face, folding the arms, or crossing the legs, are absent or greatly reduced. In looking to the side, the eyes move but not the head. In arising from a chair, the necessary adjustments such as putting the feet back and the hands on the arm of the chair are not made, although the person can do it with effort or will. The muscle is not paralyzed or apraxic. Various involuntary movements occur, such as static tremor or pill rolling of the fingers, as seen in parkinsonism; rest tremors that decrease when the limb is used; and chorea, athetosis, and dystonia. In all basal ganglia disorders, stress and nervous tension worsen motor performance; relaxation improves it.

### PREVENTION

As with many of the neurologic diseases, the focus of prevention is on secondary and tertiary care. Because many of these diseases are genetically transmitted, appropriate genetic counseling may prevent their transmission.

### MEDICAL MANAGEMENT

The medical management of motor problems is mainly pharmacologic and aimed at the relief of symptoms. No cures exist for most of the diseases that cause alterations in movement and posture.

### NURSING MANAGEMENT

The nursing assessment (subjective and objective data) is the same as that for the patient with motor problems. The nurse should also ask about family members who may have the same symptoms. The reader is referred to the section on motor dysfunction for appropriate nursing diagnoses, expected patient outcomes, and evaluation.

#### Interventions

Muscle rigidity may be relieved by physical therapy. It is important that the person remain physically active to prevent the complications of immobility. It requires great patience and understanding on the part of the family not to take over physical activities that the individual can perform, even though they will be performed slowly and with much effort. Nursing interventions are planned to assist with feeding problems related to swallowing, with ambulation, and with speech. Often the person with parkinsonism is viewed as unintelligent because of the dysarthria produced by the rigid and bradykinesic muscles of articulation and phonation. Education of the patient and family is a nursing priority. They must understand the need to reduce stress and nervous tension to improve rigidity.

## NEUROLOGIC PAIN

### ETIOLOGY

The causes of pain are many and varied. Although in practice pain may be viewed from the standpoint of neural transmissions, the transmission of pain impulses is not fully understood. However, what is known about the neuroanatomy of pain transmission can serve to explain sources of neurologic pain and some of the interventions used (Table 58-2).

Receptors for temperature and touch are adaptable, whereas pain receptors are not. The pain impulses continue at the same rate as long as the stimulus is present. These receptors are considered specific for pain only and are present in layers of the skin, the periosteum, the adrenal walls, and the falx and tentorium of the dura. Factors that can activate pain receptors include the following:

1. Cellular damage
2. Certain chemicals, including histamine
3. Heat

**TABLE 58-2 Site of Problem and Resulting Neurologic Pain**

| SITE/RESULTS | CHARACTERISTICS OF PAIN |
|---|---|
| **PERIPHERAL CUTANEOUS NERVES** | |
| Pain usually limited to anatomic area supplied by affected nerve or nerves | Often described as burning sensation but may be sharp or dull and aching<br>May be constant or permanent<br>Often described as severe<br>Also called local pain |
| **ROOT PAIN** | |
| Limited to dermatomes supplied by affected sensory nerve roots (pain from lesion arising from deep somatic and visceral stimuli may radiate beyond dermatomes) | Aggravated by anything that causes direct or indirect movement of spinal cord (sneezing, coughing, or straining) |
| **CENTRAL LESION WITHIN THALAMUS** | |
| Pain confined to contralateral side of body | Pain described as burning, pulling, and swelling<br>Often aggravated by emotional stress and fatigue |
| **CENTRAL SPINOTHALAMIC TRACT** | |
| Pain sensation distributed to level of tract involved<br>Hemisection of spinal cord produces loss of pain and temperature sensation on contralateral side at a level one or two segments below injury | May be similar to thalamic pain, but less disturbing |

4. Ischemia
5. Muscle spasms
6. Sensations of heat, cold, and itching that go beyond a specific level of intensity

## EPIDEMIOLOGY

Pain other than headache is one of the most common symptoms seen in neurology. It is sometimes difficult to distinguish between pain produced by lesions within the nervous system that cause objective sensory abnormalities and peripherally produced somatic pain in a distant organ. The nurse working with the patient in pain must appreciate the individuality of the pain experience and understand the multiple factors that influence the patient's perception and expression of pain.

## PATHOPHYSIOLOGY

The quality of neurologic pain may vary from mild to excruciating. The sources of neurologic pain also vary, as described next.

The pain resulting from peripheral nerve lesions occurs as a direct result of stimulation of the pain receptors. The location and distribution of these pain receptors can be compared with charts showing the distribution of peripheral sensory fibers (Figure 58-5). Table 58-2 describes the site of the problem, the resulting neurologic pain, and the sensations accompanying the pain.

All peripheral nerves are mixed nerves (sensory and motor). Damage to a nerve at its periphery results in loss of both sensation and muscle function. An occasional sequela of peripheral injury is **causalgia.** An attack may arise spontaneously, in response to touch, or even as a result of emotions and stress. The quantity and quality of pain are disproportionate to sensory intake.

**Root pain,** or *radicular pain,* is limited to the dermatomes supplied by the affected sensory nerve roots (Figure 58-5). However, pain from lesions arising from deep somatic and visceral structures may radiate beyond the dermatomes. It should be remembered that sensory (posterior) nerve roots are fixed directly to the spinal cord, and lesions in this area may extend to include the motor (anterior) nerve roots and may cause motor signs and symptoms.

Pain resulting from central lesions within the thalamus is confined to the contralateral side of the body, since the thalamus receives sensory pain impulses from the opposite side of the body. In massive thalamic lesions, only contiguous portions of the body may be affected. This type of pain is described as pulling, burning, and swelling.

Lesions that involve the central spinothalamic tract produce pain sensations distributed to the level of the tract involved. Hemisection of the spinal cord involving the spinothalamic tract usually produces loss of pain and temperature perception on the contralateral side at a level one or two segments below the injury. The pain is similar to thalamic pain.

Pain may also be called **referred pain;** that is, it occurs in a site other than its origin. This often occurs with visceral pain. Perhaps the most common example is chest pain that is referred to the left arm, shoulder, neck, or jaw.

## PREVENTION

As with headache, little can be done to prevent neurologic pain unless the actual triggering factors are identified. With other types of pain, however, factors that make it worse can be addressed.

Primary prevention may include protection from injury, such as a back injury. Workers are now being taught proper body mechanics and may also wear special support belts to decrease the chance of injury. Secondary prevention is also important in detecting the source of neurologic pain early in the course so that complications may be prevented.

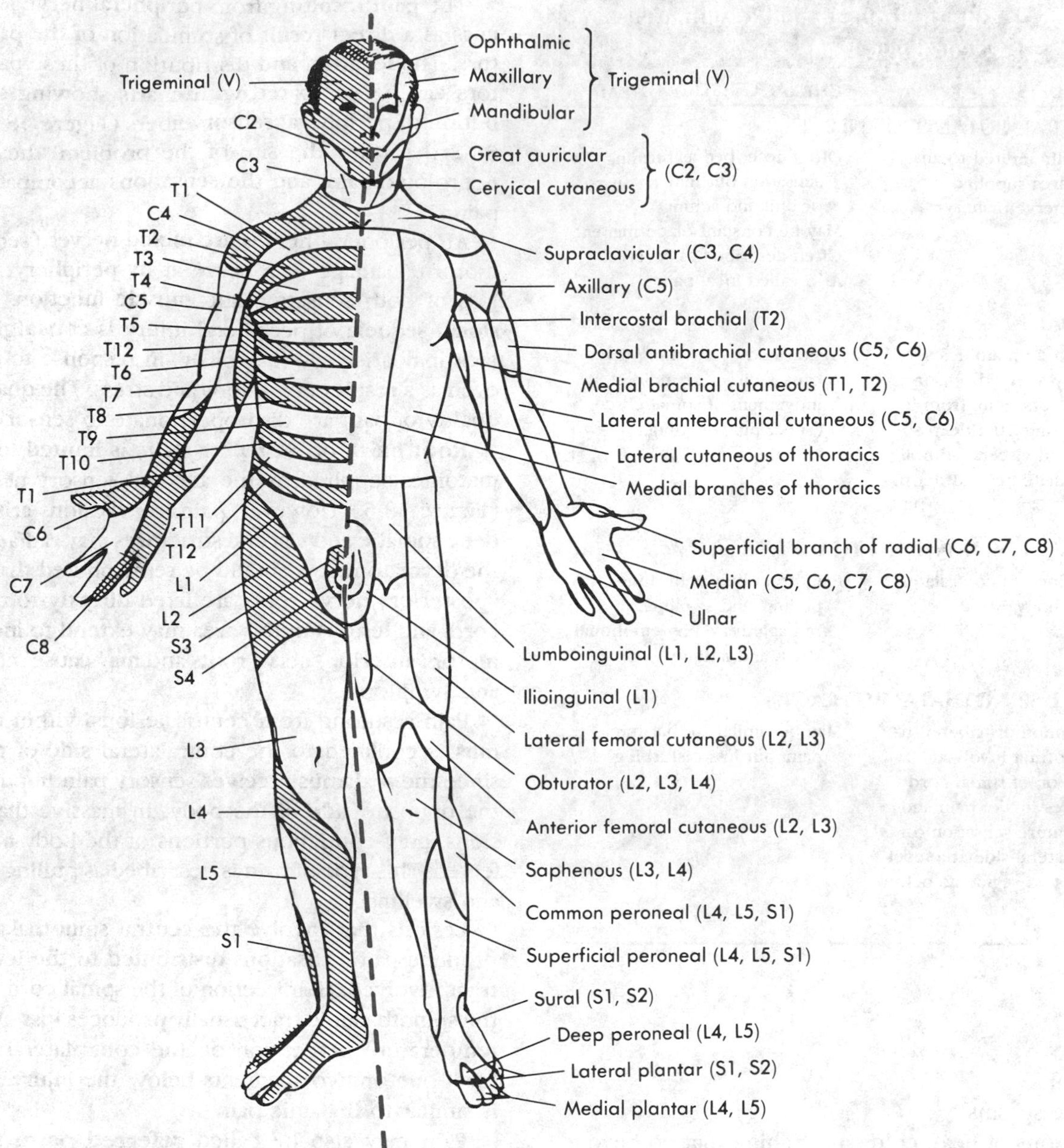


**FIGURE 58-5** Peripheral distribution of sensory nerve fibers, anterior view. *Right,* Distribution of cutaneous nerves. *Left,* Dermatomes *(shaded areas)* and segmental distribution of cutaneous nerves.

## MEDICAL MANAGEMENT

The goal of discharge of patients with neurologic pain is determined by the DRGs assigned to the underlying disorder. The nurse works collaboratively with the physician for implementation of prescribed medical therapy. Because the nurse has a major role in discharge planning and patient teaching, these are discussed under nursing management.

### Diagnostic Tests

It is extremely difficult to evaluate pain objectively. Electrical stimulation may be used to define the pain to a greater extent. Psychologic testing also may be done as part of the work-up. Other tests to rule out the cause of the pain may be helpful. One example is the myelogram, which is often done when the patient has back pain (see Chapter 56).

### Medication

Treatment for patients with neurologic pain may include the use of medications. These often include nonnarcotic analgesics such as acetaminophen, propoxyphene, phenacetin, ibuprofen, and acetylsalicylic acid. Narcotics may be prescribed, but they should be used with discretion because of the potential for abuse. Diazepam (Valium) and amitriptyline (Elavil) are often used as adjuncts for pain control. The emphasis generally should be on helping the patient learn other measures to control pain. Medications may be given via the epidural route.[9]

### Treatment

The treatment of neurologic pain is determined by the specific cause of the pain. No universal treatment exists for pain.

The medical management for patients with neurologic pain is mainly symptomatic. If the source of the problem can be identified, medical or surgical intervention may be possible to cure the source. Psychotherapy may be used as a primary treatment or as an adjunct to palliative treatment.

Unbearable pain that does not respond to the definitive treatment of the causative lesion is classified as **intractable pain.** The pain is chronic and often disabling. It is usually possible to alleviate intractable pain surgically through deafferentation at varied sites by nerve block, neurectomy, rhizotomy, and cordotomy.[11] Electrical stimulation may also be used. These techniques and the care required when instituted are described in Chapter 17.

### Diet

No special diet is prescribed for patients with neurologic pain. Any dietary modifications are determined by the specific disorder causing the pain. In some instances, obesity may be an aggravating factor, as in back pain. For these persons, a weight reduction diet may be prescribed.

### Activity

The patient with neurologic pain may need to restrict activity levels for a time. As the pain lessens, activity is progressively increased. With back pain, strengthening exercises may be used, as well as teaching the person about proper body mechanics.

**BOX 58-1 Common Terminology to Describe Types of Pain Sensation**

**Paresthesia**—abnormal sensation
**Hyperalgesia**—increased pain sensation
**Hypalgesia**—decreased pain sensation
**Analgesia**—blocked pain sensation
**Dysesthesia**—pain sensation caused by stimulus that normally would not be painful
**Referred pain**—pain that occurs in a site other than its origin
**Causalgia**—intense, continuous, burning pain
**Local pain**—caused by direct stimulation of pain receptors
**Intractable pain**—unbearable pain that does not respond to treatment

### Referral/Consultation

In some settings the nurse assumes responsibility for making referrals to other services. For the patient with neurologic pain, this may include a referral to a physical therapist or to a pain center.

## NURSING MANAGEMENT

### ♦ ASSESSMENT

Both subjective and objective data are important to assess in the patient with neurologic pain. Because pain is a highly subjective experience, few objective data may accompany the subjective complaints.

### Subjective Data

Data to be collected to assess the patient with neurologic pain include the following:

- Patient's understanding of the pain
- Any precipitating factors
- Measures that relieve pain, including medication
- Site, frequency, and nature of pain
- Usual coping patterns when under stress
- Presence of associated symptoms
- Measures that worsen pain
- Description of the pain (see Box 58-1)

### Objective Data

Data to be collected to assess the patient with neurologic pain include the following:

- Behavior, including signs to indicate pain or stress
- Change in ability to perform ADL
- Muscle weakness or wasting
- Vasomotor responses, including flushing
- Spinal reflexes and sensory examination

### Diagnostic Test Findings

Often, diagnostic test findings for the patient with neurologic pain are normal. If the pain is caused by damage to the nerves innervating the area, the EMG often indicates this. (See Chapter 56 for a description of this test.)

### ♦ NURSING DIAGNOSES

Nursing diagnoses are determined from analysis of patient data. Nursing diagnoses for the patient with neurologic pain may include but are not limited to the following:

| Diagnostic Title | Possible Etiologic Factors |
|---|---|
| Pain, chronic | Chronic physical disability |
| Sleep pattern disturbance | Pain/discomfort |
| Self—bathing-hygiene, dressing-grooming, feeding, and toileting defects | Pain/discomfort |
| Knowledge deficit (cause of pain and needed treatment) | Lack of exposure/recall, unfamiliarity with information sources |

**Guidelines for Care of the Person With Neurologic Pain**

1. Promote rest and relaxation.
   a. Relaxation techniques, including biofeedback and meditation
   b. Regular periods of rest
   c. Regular sleeping patterns
   d. Structuring of environment to reduce stress
2. Promote comfort.
   a. Assume position of comfort
   b. Judicious use of medication
3. Promote ADL.
   a. Development of plan to manage ADL
   b. Frequent rest periods interspersed with periods of activity

## ♦ EXPECTED PATIENT OUTCOMES

Expected patient outcomes for the patient with neurologic pain may include but are not limited to the following:

1. Pain is decreased.
2. Is able to sleep at least 6 hours at night.
3. Performs ADL better.
4. Explains the following: (a) methods to control discomfort or pain; (b) prescribed analgesics or alternatives as to action, side effects, and dosage schedules; (c) positioning methods and relationships to occurrences of pain; (d) general health practices, such as maintenance of sleep and rest patterns; (e) relationship between pain and emotional upsets; (f) plan for follow-up care; and (g) physical methods that can be used to relieve pain.

## ♦ INTERVENTIONS

### Promoting Comfort, Rest, and ADL

It is important for the nurse to promote comfort, rest and relaxation, and the ability to carry out ADL in the patient with neurologic pain. (See Guidelines box above for a summary of the nursing care.)

Root pain is often aggravated by anything that causes direct or indirect movement of the spinal cord, leading to increased spinal pressure. Valsalva maneuvers such as sneezing, coughing, or straining at stool increase intrathoracic and intraabdominal pressure and indirectly produce distention of veins in the epidural space, thus affecting the dura mater surrounding the nerve roots. (See Guidelines box above, right, for care of the patient with root pain.)

### Facilitating Learning

Teaching for the person with neurologic pain is important and should include the following:

1. Avoid factors that increase pain.
2. Use relaxation measures when emotional tension is present.
3. Maintain regular rest and sleep pattern.

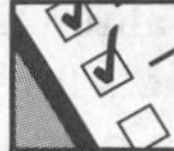

**Guidelines for Care of the Person With Root Pain**

1. Avoid sharp flexion of the neck and extension of the leg.
2. Patient should not lie on horizontal plane for long periods.
3. Use stool softeners as indicated.
4. Sitting may relieve tension on nerve roots.

4. Take medication as prescribed.
5. Be aware of physical methods to control pain and use them appropriately.
6. Follow up with medical care as appropriate.
7. Structure home and work environment to keep stressors to a minimum.
8. Obtain help to complete ADL if needed.

## ♦ EVALUATION

To evaluate the effectiveness of nursing interventions, compare patient behaviors with those stated in the expected patient outcomes. Successful achievement of patient outcomes for the patient with neurologic pain is indicated by the following:

1. States that pain is at 2 or less on pain scale and does not exhibit splinting, grimacing, shallow breathing, or other behaviors indicative of pain.
2. Sleeps at least 6 hours per night.
3. Has no or decreased difficulty when performing ADL, including bathing, dressing, feeding, toileting, and grooming.
4. Correctly describes the following: (a) methods to control discomfort or pain; (b) prescribed analgesics or alternative medications as to action, side effects, route, and dosage schedules; (c) positioning methods and their relationships to occurrences of pain; (d) importance of adequate rest and sleep; (e) correlation between pain and emotional upsets; (f) plans for follow-up care; and (g) methods that can be used to relieve pain.

# SPINAL CORD INFECTIONS/ INFLAMMATIONS

## GUILLAIN-BARRÉ SYNDROME (POLYNEURITIS)

### Etiology

**Guillain-Barré syndrome,** known also as acute inflammatory polyradiculoneuropathy and postinfectious **polyneuritis,** is often serious because of the extent to which the nervous system may be affected. The cause is unknown, but two theories are emerging: (1) that it is caused by a viral agent or (2) that it is an autoimmune reaction.

### Epidemiology

This condition has become better known to the public since it was identified as a sequela of swine flu immu-

# NURSING CARE PLAN

## PERSON WITH GUILLAIN-BARRÉ SYNDROME

**DATA:** Mr. D. is a 45-year-old married auto mechanic with a history of progressive weakness that began in his feet and legs. For the past day, he has not been able to walk. He is also complaining of shortness of breath. He gives a history of an upper respiratory tract infection 2 weeks before admission. On admission he demonstrated weakness of all four extremities. His tidal volume was decreased, and his respiratory rate was 32. He complained of discomfort in his lower extremities. The sensory examination was WNL. He was alert and oriented ×3. He was admitted to the neurologic unit for observation. He started receiving corticosteroids, and his respiratory rate was closely monitored. The day after admission the patient demonstrated paralysis of muscles below the waist.

The nursing history identified the following:
- He is unsure about what has happened to him and the reason for his weakness.
- He expresses anxiety about what to expect.
- He seems to have a close relationship with his wife.
- Leisure activities are mainly sports activities.

Collaborative nursing actions include those to prevent further complications caused by muscle weakness and respiratory weakness. Immediate reporting may prevent serious effects (respiratory arrest, clot formation). Nursing actions include monitoring for the following:
- Signs of respiratory compromise: decreased tidal volume, increased shortness of breath, tachypnea, cyanosis, restlessness
- Signs of pulmonary embolism: chest pain, hemoptysis
- Signs of DVT (deep vein thrombosis): difference in leg girth, positive Homans' sign, leg pain, difference in temperature of legs

### ■ NURSING DIAGNOSIS
Anxiety related to change in health status

| Expected Patient Outcome | Nursing Interventions | Rationale |
|---|---|---|
| Verbalizes minimal anxiety. | Explain to patient procedures being done. | Explanations help minimize anxiety. |
| | Allow him time to verbalize feelings. | Expression of fears lessens anxiety. |
| | Encourage his wife to spend time with him. | Family members are an important source of support. |

### ■ NURSING DIAGNOSIS
Ineffective breathing pattern related to neuromuscular impairment

| Expected Patient Outcome | Nursing Interventions | Rationale |
|---|---|---|
| Has adequate breathing pattern. | Assess respiratory rate, tidal volume, and color frequently. | Ongoing assessment will detect critical changes. |
| | Notify physician of any changes immediately. | Changes in respiratory status can occur quickly. |
| | Keep head of bed at 30 degrees. | Position helps respiratory effort. |
| | Give supplemental oxygen as ordered. | Lowered oxygen levels in blood are common with impaired respiratory efforts. |

### ■ NURSING DIAGNOSIS
Pain in legs related to Guillain-Barré syndrome

| Expected Patient Outcome | Nursing Interventions | Rationale |
|---|---|---|
| States that leg pain is improved. | Position for comfort. | Positioning may relieve pain. |
| | Administer mild analgesic such as acetaminophen. | Pain relief is provided. |
| | Teach relaxation measures as appropriate. | This promotes rest and eases pain. |

*Continued.*

# NURSING CARE PLAN

## PERSON WITH GUILLAIN-BARRÉ SYNDROME—cont'd

### ■ NURSING DIAGNOSIS

High risk for injury related to possible trauma

| Expected Patient Outcome | Nursing Interventions | Rationale |
|---|---|---|
| Contractures do not develop. | Position patient with limbs in normal anatomic position. | Such positioning will prevent flexion contractures. |
| | Change position q 2 hr. | |
| | Perform passive or active ROM to all extremities several times a day. | Activity stretches muscles and keeps joints movable. |
| | Assist out of bed at least daily. | Change in position helps prevent complications of immobility. |
| | Apply elastic stockings and keep legs elevated when up in chair. | This assists with venous return and helps prevent stasis. |

### ■ NURSING DIAGNOSIS

Knowledge deficit related to lack of exposure to information

| Expected Patient Outcome | Nursing Interventions | Rationale |
|---|---|---|
| Describes nature of disease and possible complications. | Review nature of disease with frequent reinforcement. | Teaching can raise patient's level of cooperation. |
| | | Reinforcement of earlier teaching helps promote retention. |

### ■ NURSING DIAGNOSIS

Impaired physical mobility related to neuromuscular impairment

| Expected Patient Outcome | Nursing Interventions | Rationale |
|---|---|---|
| Has minimal impairments in mobility. | Allow patient to do as much for self as possible. | Active exercise has positive effect on patient. |
| | See actions under "High risk for injury." | |

### ■ NURSING DIAGNOSIS

Self—bathing/hygiene, dressing, toileting deficits related to neuromuscular impairment

| Expected Patient Outcome | Nursing Interventions | Rationale |
|---|---|---|
| Carries out ADL at highest ability level. | Provide basic ADL needs as necessary but encourage patient to do what he can. | Self-care will promote positive self-concept. |
| | Provide sufficient time to do ADL. | Doing ADL when patient has deficits often takes more time. |
| | Work with therapists to optimize patient's learning needs. | Team work can accentuate care. |

### ■ NURSING DIAGNOSIS

Body image disturbance; disturbance in role performance related to loss of body functions and immobility

| Expected Patient Outcome | Nursing Interventions | Rationale |
|---|---|---|
| Verbalizes positive self-concept. | Provide information about disease and expected progress. | Understanding of disease improves self-concept. |
| | Provide privacy. | Patient may be embarrassed by need for physical care. |
| | Provide care but encourage patient to do as much for self as possible. | Ability to care for self improves self-concept. |

## NURSING CARE PLAN

### PERSON WITH GUILLAIN-BARRÉ SYNDROME—cont'd

| Expected Patient Outcome | Nursing Interventions | Rationale |
|---|---|---|
| | Encourage family to visit. | Visitors cheer patient. |
| | Give family chance to share their concerns. | If family concerns are met, they can be more supportive of patient. |
| | Encourage family to maintain previous role relationships, if possible. | There is comfort in knowing that role in family is intact. |
| | Identify patient's strengths and weaknesses. | This can assist nurse in planning care with patient. |

■ **NURSING DIAGNOSIS**

High risk for impaired skin integrity related to mechanical forces and pressure

| Expected Patient Outcome | Nursing Interventions | Rationale |
|---|---|---|
| Skin remains intact. | Monitor pressure areas for signs of skin breakdown. | Early detection of pressure can allow time for measures to prevent breakdown. |
| | Use turning sheet when turning patient to prevent shearing effect. | Shearing forces lead to skin breakdown. |
| | Turn patient q 2 hr. | Turning prevents pressure areas. |
| | Keep skin clean and dry. | Moisture leads to skin breakdown. |
| | Use air mattress or water mattress or special bed. | Can assist with relief of pressure areas. |

nization. The disease occurs most often in persons 30 to 50 years of age and is seen equally in men and women.

### Pathophysiology

Patchy demyelination occurs in the peripheral nerves, nerve roots, and root ganglia and spinal cord in Guillain-Barré syndrome. For this reason, it may be classified as a neuritis. Axons are generally spared so that recovery may occur early; in severe forms, *wallerian degeneration* occurs with involvement of the axons, making recovery slow. In the severe form, protein in the cerebrospinal fluid (CSF) is elevated.

If the seventh, ninth, and tenth cranial nerves are involved, the patient may have varying degrees of difficulty in swallowing, speaking, and breathing. The vital centers in the medulla oblongata may be affected, and the patient may die of respiratory failure. Patients with less severe involvement may recover fully, although complete recovery may take a year or more.

The patient with Guillain-Barré syndrome has symmetric muscle weakness and lower motor paralysis characteristics (flaccidity). The paralysis usually starts in the lower extremities, and it ascends upward to include the thorax, upper extremities, and face. Selected cranial nerves may also be affected, as previously mentioned. Other symptoms that may be assessed clinically are paresthesias and sensory alteration as the sensory roots and nerves may also become involved. Respiratory failure may occur as intercostal muscles are affected, and without mechanical ventilation, there is a 10% to 20% mortality. The bowel and bladder are rarely affected. Autonomic symptoms, such as a fluctuating blood pressure, may occur.

Variations may exist in the pattern of onset of weakness, as well as in the rate of progression of symptoms. The progression may stop at any point.

### Medical and Nursing Management

A priority goal for the nurse and the patient with Guillain-Barré syndrome is the maintenance of respiratory function. Close observation of respiratory function is necessary. This should include serial measurements of the patient's vital capacity, tidal volume, and minute volume. Urine retention occurs in about 5% of patients. Patients who develop respiratory failure require mechanical ventilation and are usually placed in an intensive care unit (See Chapter 37 for nursing care of patients with respiratory failure.) Adrenocortical steroids are used empirically to treat symptoms. Convalescence may require several months. Attention to the prevention of iatrogenic complications, such as contracture, decubitus ulcers, muscle atrophy, and loss of ROM, is imperative. Recovery is usually complete.

The nursing diagnoses, patient outcomes, and nursing interventions for the patient with Guillain-Barré syndrome are found in the accompanying nursing care plan.

## HERPES ZOSTER

### Etiology

The causative organism of **herpes zoster** is the varicella-zoster virus (VZV), which also causes varicella (chickenpox).

### Epidemiology

Herpes zoster, also known as **shingles**, is a common disease that occurs at higher rates among elderly persons and in patients with decreasing cell-mediated immunity, Hodgkin's disease, and acquired immunodeficiency syndrome (AIDS).

### Pathophysiology

Herpes zoster occurs as a result of reactivation of the viral infection that lies dormant in the ganglion after a primary case of chickenpox. It is not communicable, except in persons who have not had chickenpox. An acute inflammatory reaction develops in the spinal or cranial sensory ganglions, the posterior gray matter of the cord, and the meninges.

The rash in herpes zoster consists of a vesicular, cutaneous eruption within one to three adjacent dermatomes. It may be preceded by severe itching, pain in the area, fever, and malaise. The Tzanck smear is positive in approximately 80% of the skin lesions.[10] There may be segmental weakness and atrophy in the same area as the sensory changes. A small percentage of patients are seen with ophthalmic herpes, with the rash and pain occurring along the distribution of the trigeminal nerve.

### Medical Management

Treatment for herpes zoster consists mainly of supportive care with medication for control of pain. The pain may persist for some time after the rash disappears. Pain lasting 3 months or more after clearing of the rash is called *postzoster neuralgia.* It is more likely to occur in elderly persons and may be severe. Some patients are incapacitated by the pain. It is treated with topical 0.075% capsaicin cream (Zoster-HP) four to six times daily and/or oral doses of tricyclic antidepressants.[10] Special emphasis on rest, nutrition, and hydration during the acute period is important.

Isolation precautions may be necessary, especially to protect staff who have not had chickenpox and most especially to protect pregnant women. Also, patients who have decreasing cell-mediated immunity, Hodgkin's disease, or AIDS or who have not had chickenpox should be protected from exposure to the patient.

Because the virus is spread by direct contact and airborne routes, strict isolation is often necessary, at least until any drainage from the lesions stops. Box 58-2 lists isolation measures for herpes zoster.

**BOX 58-2 Isolation Measures for Herpes Zoster**

- Private room with private toilet facilities
- Gown, masks, and gloves required of caregivers
- Strict handwashing
- Linen handled as isolation linens
- Double-bagging of dressings
- Disposable dishes if possible
- Transport of patients out of room only as necessary
- Isolation procedure for all visitors

## SPINAL CORD TRAUMA

### ETIOLOGY

The spinal cord may be damaged by lesions arising outside the cord or by intramedullary lesions. The latter are a less common cause and usually the result of intramedullary tumors (see Chapter 57). Various types of lesions arising *outside* the cord eventually cause damage within it. (The term *lesion* as used here includes both disease and injury.) For example, there may be direct extension of an extramedullary vertebral tumor to the cord, protrusion of a ruptured intervertebral disk into the spinal canal, or a fracture of the spine from direct trauma with resultant tearing of the spinal cord (Figure 58-6). All such lesions may produce compression of the cord. The anatomy and size of the spinal cord subject the cord to compression with even minimal inward encroachment by extramedullary lesions. Edema then forms and contributes even more to cord compression. With damage to any part of the vertebral column, the

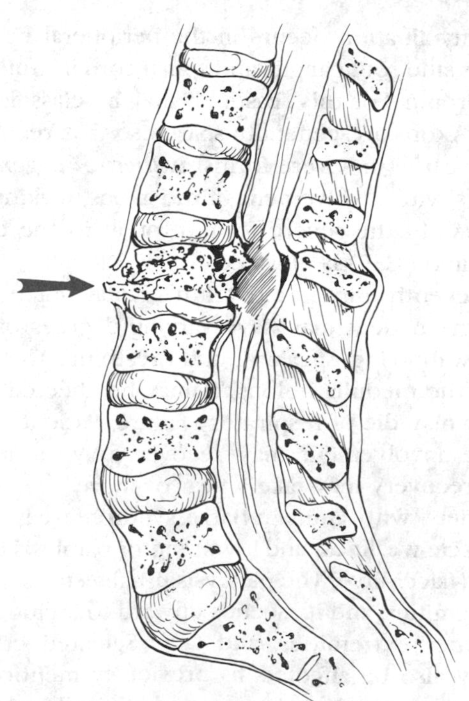

**FIGURE 58-6** Damage to spinal cord and distortion of adjacent structures may occur in traumatic injuries to spine.

cord itself becomes more vulnerable to damage. Recognition of the function of the spinal cord as the only conducting system of nerve impulses to and from the brain makes one realize the seriousness of spinal cord damage from any cause.[2]

## EPIDEMIOLOGY

Spinal cord injuries are catastrophic health crises that result in tremendous economic costs. Estimates of spinal cord injury in the United States range from 2.8 to 5 per 100,000 people. Of these, about 40% all prove to be fatal. Males sustain about 80% of all spinal cord injuries. Adolescents and young adults ages 15 to 24 have the highest incidence of injury, which results in lifelong needs for care. The total number of people with spinal cord trauma in the United States ranges from 177,000 to 200,000. The cost is estimated at $6.2 billion annually.

The primary cause of spinal cord injuries is motor vehicle accidents, and falls are the second leading cause. The third cause is diving accidents, with firearms and assaults also causing significant numbers of injuries, especially in urban areas. An estimated 8000 to 20,000 people experience a spinal cord injury each year.[16]

## PATHOPHYSIOLOGY

Important variations exist in the neuroanatomy of the vertebral column at the cervical, thoracic, and lumbar areas, and important segmental variations occur in the spinal cord itself. In the cervical area the vertebrae are unstable (to permit movement of the neck), and the cord at this level houses the most important neural structures in a copious dural tube. The anterior horn cells innervating the diaphragm (above C4) and the upper extremities are located in the cervical cord segments as well as in the long motor tracts to the remainder of the body. In the thoracic area, by contrast, a stable bony column is supported by the rib structures. The thoracic spinal cord fills the subarachnoid space almost completely, and injuries in this area produce bony malalignments and are often associated with serious neurologic deficits. Finally, in the lumbar area the vertebrae are heavier and are supported by massive lumbar paraspinal muscles. The lumbar vertebrae thus have more stability than the cervical vertebrae but less than the thoracic vertebrae. The lumbar spine is more apt to be injured at the junction between the thoracic and lumbar area. The cauda equina, rather than the spinal cord, is housed below L1. The tip of the spinal cord, or the conus, houses the micturition center.

Severe traumatic lesions of the spinal cord, as from accident, may result in total *transection* of the spinal cord or a tearing of the cord from side to side at a particular level (see Figure 57-11). This represents the most serious damage to the cord, with a complete loss of spinal cord functions. This total transection injury is also referred to as a *complete cord injury.* With the complete injury, there is a *loss of all voluntary movement and loss of all sensations below the level of the lesion.* A partial transection, or *incomplete injury,* involves a partial transection or injury of the cord. The symptoms of incomplete injuries can vary depending on the nature of the injury and the resultant syndrome. Possibilities include the anterior cord syndrome, central cord syndrome, Brown-Séquard syndrome, conus medullaris syndrome, and cauda equina syndrome. (See Chapter 57 and Figure 57-11 for further information about these syndromes and their respective symptoms.)

Initially in most spinal cord injuries, a period of flaccid paralysis and a complete (or almost complete) loss of all reflexes occurs. This is called **spinal shock,** *neural shock,* or *areflexia* and is a transitory event. After the injury, afferent impulses are unable to ascend from below the injured site to the brain, and efferent impulses are unable to descend to points below the site. Because transection represents an acute form of spinal cord damage, it is used as an example to relate and discuss the symptoms of spinal cord damage. *Considerable variation exists in the extent to which signs and symptoms are manifest in the individual patient.* The baseline assessment of the person with acute spinal cord injury should include the data listed in Box 58-3.

### Sensorimotor Function

The signs and symptoms of cord transection and of lesser cord lesions depend on the level at which the lesion occurs and the degree of the damage (Table 58-3). In the *immediate stage of a transection,* there is a complete loss or deficit of motor and sensory functions as well as somatic and visceral sensations below the level of the tear (areflexia). The individual has flaccid paralysis, areflexia, and hypotonia caused by the disruption of nerve impulses as related to the injury level. During this period, persons may require temporary respiratory assistance until the body begins to recover.

Within hours, days, or weeks, the involved muscles gradually become spastic and *hyperreflexic* with the characteristic signs of an UMN lesion. These changes are

**BOX 58-3 Baseline Assessment of the Person With Acute Spinal Cord Injury**

Respiratory status
Level of alertness and consciousness
Orientation
Pupil size, equality, and reactivity
Proper positioning of body in neutral alignment
Motor strength
Absence of sensation-sensory level
Temperature, blood pressure, pulse
Bowel and bladder status; distention
Skin integrity
Pain control

**TABLE 58-3 Muscle Function After Spinal Cord Injury**

| SPINAL CORD INJURY | MUSCLE FUNCTION REMAINING | MUSCLE FUNCTION LOST |
|---|---|---|
| Cervical | | |
| Above C4 | None | All including respiration |
| C5 | Neck<br>Scapular elevation | Arms<br>Chest<br>All below chest |
| C6-C7 | Neck<br>Some chest movement<br>Some arm movement | Some arm, fingers<br>Some chest movement<br>All below chest movement |
| Thoracic | Neck<br>Arms (full)<br>Some chest | Trunk<br>All below chest |
| Lumbosacral | Neck<br>Arms<br>Chest<br>Trunk | Legs |

reflexes from the inhibitory influence of the damaged pyramidal tract, resulting in hyperactive responses. Another theory is that damage of the extrapyramidal descending fibers, in proximity to the pyramidal fibers, permits unmodified excitatory impulses to reach the LMNs via the muscle spindles. Thus the LMNs have increased sensitivity to afferent stimulation from the muscle spindles. Nurses need to be able to explain spinal cord damage to patients and their families so that involuntary movements are not confused with voluntary movements.

*Damage at the cervical cord level is the most critical level for an injury to occur.* It causes paralysis of all four extremities and the trunk **(quadriplegia).** The sparing of any one muscle movement of the shoulder, arms, and fingers depends on the specific cervical level of the injury. At the C5 level, for example, only scapular elevation movements would remain. All other muscle movements in the arms, chest, trunk, and legs are lost. In the immediate stage, muscles of internal organs such as the bladder and bowel are atonic. Perspiration is diminished, as is touch sensation. Because the diaphragm and intercostal muscles are affected, respiratory failure and death may result unless the patient receives adequate respiratory assistance. Respiratory assistance is sometimes necessary during transportation of the patient to the hospital. Pain is not usually an early problem.

*Injury at the thoracic level* results in chest, trunk, bowel, bladder, and lower extremity muscle losses. The amount of remaining function varies in this area relative to the specific level. Fortunately, the individual has use of the upper extremities; the lower extremities are not functional **(paraplegia).**

*Injury at the lumbar and sacral levels* results in paralysis of the lower extremities. When injury occurs in the lower sacral area and the cauda equina nerve roots, away from the cord, the signs are variable and less severe. Paraparesis and scattered LMN signs often occur.

## Voiding

The center for micturition is located in the conus medullaris (S2 to S4) and is linked to the detrusor muscle of the bladder by parasympathetic sensory and motor fibers that run in the pelvic nerves. Levels above the conus result in a bladder that is capable of emptying itself reflexly or involuntarily after the spinal shock phase. The bladder is hypertonic and is variously known as an *upper motor neuron bladder* and *reflex neurogenic bladder.* The emptying occurs spontaneously or automatically. The patient has no control over the act of micturition. Voiding may occur at intervals of 3 to 4 hours; there may be frequency, urgency, and incontinence. The reflex arc is intact in this type of bladder. When the cord lesion is at or below the micturition center, destruction of the center or the sacral nerve roots occurs; the reflex arc is no longer intact. This type of bladder condition is known as a *lower motor neuron bladder* or *autonomous neurogenic bladder.* Contractions of the bladder muscle are the result of impulses transmitted though a mechanism within the bladder wall but are not of sufficient strength or duration to empty the bladder. Abdominal straining or manual compression is necessary for this to happen. Retention of urine and infection typically occur.

## Autonomic Dysreflexia

One result of spinal cord injury that is extremely important to understand is **autonomic dysreflexia** (see Figure 58-7). It occurs in patients with cord lesions above T6, most often those with cervical injuries. Clinical signs and symptoms include the following:

1. Bradycardia
2. Paroxysmal hypertension
3. Sweating
4. "Goose flesh"
5. Severe headache
6. Nasal stuffiness

Patients tend to develop individual signs and symptoms of this condition and are soon able to recognize it.

The most common cause of autonomic dysreflexia is *visceral distention,* which may include a *distended bladder* or *impacted rectum. It is a medical emergency that requires immediate treatment because it can lead to CVA, blindness, or death.*

## Sexual Function

Most men with spinal cord injury experience impotence, decreased sensation, and difficulties with ejaculation. Impairment of fertility typically occurs. The act of erection is under the control of sensory and parasympathetic fibers, whereas ejaculation requires sympathetic and parasympathetic innervation. Lesions above S2 leave the parasympathetic reflex arc intact; patients may be able to have an erection, but ejaculation is usually not possible. Lesions in the S2 to S4 region usually prevent erection and ejaculation. The higher the level of injury, the more likely a man with complete cord injury is able to perform sexually. The experience of orgasm is described as different than before the injury.

Women with spinal cord injury can continue to perform sexually, although perception of sexual orgasm is usually altered. Usually, fertility does not decrease.

## PREVENTION

The reader is referred to the section on preventive care during head injury in Chapter 57.

### Healthy People 2000

A goal in *Healthy People 2000* is to reduce nonfatal spinal cord injuries and resultant hospitalizations to no more than 5 per 100,000 people (baseline: 5.9 per 100,000 in 1988).[17] Other objectives include the following:

- Increase use of occupant protection systems, such as safety belts, inflatable safety restraints, and child safety seats, to at least 85% of motor vehicle occupants (baseline: 42% in 1988).
- Increase use of helmets to at least 80% of motorcyclists and at least 50% of bicyclists (baseline: 60% of motorcyclists in 1988 and an estimated 8% of bicyclists in 1984).
- Extend to the 50 states laws requiring safety belt and motorcyle helmet use for all ages (baseline: 33 states and the District of Columbia in 1989 for automobiles; 22 states, the District of Columbia, and Puerto Rico for motorcycles).
- Enact in the 50 states laws requiring that new handguns be designed to minimize the likelihood of discharge by children (baseline: 0 states in 1989).

## MEDICAL MANAGEMENT

The goal for discharge of patients with a spinal cord fracture as determined by DRGs is 6 days. The nurse works collaboratively with the physician for implementation of prescribed medical therapy. Because the nurse has a major role in discharge teaching and patient teaching, these are discussed under nursing management. A sample critical pathway for the patient undergoing a lumbar laminectomy can be found on p. 2054.

### Diagnostic Tests

It is most important to determine first if a cervical vertebra fracture or dislocation has occurred. Roentgenograms are usually taken to detect fracture-dislocation, which can occur when the patient is moved from the backboard or stretcher. Myelography may also be used to detect any blockage. It can be carried out without moving the patient if the dye is injected at the junction between C1 and the base of the skull. Computed tomography (CT) scanning may also be very helpful in ruling out spinal cord injury. (See Chapter 56 for details of these tests.) Further diagnostic measures are often delayed until any cervical fractures have been corrected. The presence of spinal compression in the thoracic, lumbar, and sacral spine areas must be determined, but the need for treatment is not as compelling as with a cervical injury. Both the lumbar and the cervical spines are prone to flexion and extension movements that result from severe trauma.

### Medication

Adrenocorticosteroids are prescribed for the prevention and alleviation of spinal cord edema. The efficacy of steroids in the reestablishment of membrane stability and in the control of CNS tissue edema has been documented clinically. Methylprednisolone (Solu-Medrol), 60 to 80 mg/day (or equivalent dosage of other corticosteroids), may be used for the first week or longer after injury.

### Treatment

*Immediate medical care* after spinal cord injury with fracture is ***directed toward realignment of the cervical column.*** The following measures may be used to realign the cervical column:

1. Simple immobilization
2. Skeletal traction
   a. Crutchfield tongs
   b. Vinke tongs
   c. Virginia tongs
   d. Stryker or Foster frame
3. Surgery for spinal decompression[3]
4. Halo apparatus[13]

Often, surgical decompression is not performed until after a period of skeletal traction. This allows the patient's condition to stabilize and some initial swelling of the cord to subside. The beginning spontaneous healing of the fracture sites provides more stability.

### Diet

No special diet is prescribed for the patient with a spinal cord injury. The patient is not fed, however, while spinal shock continues. A functioning gastrointestinal (GI) tract is needed for oral feedings. Before this, the patient is maintained on intravenous (IV) feedings.

### Referral/Consultation

In some settings the nurse assumes responsibility for making referrals to other services. For the patient with a spinal cord injury, this may include referrals to the dietitian, the social worker, or to a psychiatric clinical specialist. Facilitating patient contact with a support group is extremely helpful.

## SURGICAL MANAGEMENT

Sometimes, despite skeletal traction, extruded cervical disk materials produce continued compression of the cord. *With the introduction of the anterior surgical approach to the cervical spinal column, surgical intervention is safer and can be attempted earlier* in the hospitalization. The primary advantage of the anterior surgical approach (or anterior diskectomy or laminectomy) is that it provides immediate stabilization of the spinal column by techniques of interbody cervical fusion and the direct removal of any extruded disk materials. If evidence of spinal cord compression is demonstrated early, surgery may be warranted by the anterior approach.

Less immediate attention to *thoracic* fracture immobilization is necessary for the patient *with limited neurologic deficits.* The patient is often treated later with simple bedrest, hyperextension, and bracing (see Chapter 64). Diagnosis is necessary, however, to determine the presence or absence of spinal cord compression at this level. Patients who show subarachnoid blockage and have associated neurologic deficits are treated through early surgical decompression. The onset of instantaneous paraplegia after direct thoracic trauma is often reversible through spinal cord decompression.

An early to an intermediate laminectomy may be performed in the presence of even severe *lumbar* neurologic deficits. Stabilization of the spine is done at the time of the primary surgical intervention or delayed until later in the posttraumatic period. Long delays in lumbar laminectomies or explorations in patients who show early partial recovery are reported to be beneficial for recovery of some neurologic function. If the patient has surgery for spinal cord decompression, the nurse has an important role in making this a safe procedure. (See Guidelines box at left.)

### Guidelines for Care of the Person Undergoing Spinal Cord Decompression

1. Provide preoperative care.
   a. Clarify patient's knowledge of surgery and expected changes.
   b. Explain expected postoperative measures (including positioning, bedrest).
   c. Encourage patient and family to verbalize fears.
   d. Assess and record baseline neurologic and physiologic data.
2. Provide postoperative care.
   a. Perform monitoring.
      (1) Assess ability to move legs, arms, and hands.
      (2) Assess degree and character of drainage on dressing (amount of drainage and bleeding should be minimal).
      (3) Assess ability of patient to swallow; observe neck for swelling (with anterior cervical fusions).
   b. Promote mobility.
      (1) Turn patient from side to side and onto back.
      (2) If decompression is in lumbar region, do not permit sitting.
      (3) If decompression is in thoracic area, patient should not use arms to pull or push; a trapeze *cannot* be used.
      (4) Assist with active ROM and quadriceps setting as well as other leg exercises.
   c. Promote psychologic comfort.
      (1) Encourage patient to verbalize fears and reactions.
      (2) Spend time with patient other than when giving direct care.
      (3) Share information about daily activities, tests, and procedures with patient.
      (4) Medicate as needed for pain.
   d. Prevent infections.
      (1) Keep area of incision clean and dry.
      (2) Check temperature frequently for several days.
      (3) Report any redness, drainage, or hardness of wound to physician.
      (4) Note that incision is often left open to air after the first few days.

## NURSING MANAGEMENT

### ♦ ASSESSMENT

Assessment of the patient with a spinal cord injury includes both subjective and objective data.

#### Subjective Data

Data to be collected to assess the patient with a spinal cord injury include the following:

- Patient's understanding of injury and the resulting deficit
- Information about nature of injury—how it happened
- Presence of shortness of breath
- Unusual sensations (paresthesias, etc.)
- History of loss of consciousness
- Presence of pain
- Absence of sensation-sensory level

#### Objective Data

Data to be collected to assess the patient with a spinal cord injury include the following:

- Respiratory status
- Level of alertness and consciousness
- Orientation
- Pupil size, equality, and reactivity
- Proper alignment of body in neutral position
- Motor strength
- Temperature, blood pressure, pulse
- Skin integrity
- Bowel and bladder status; distention
- Presence or absence of anal wink reflex

The patient with a spinal cord injury should be assessed carefully for the presence of other injuries, especially head injuries or fractures.

#### Diagnostic Test Findings

The presence of a spinal fracture can usually be visualized on roentgenograms. A positive finding on a CT scan of the spine or on the myelogram is also indicative of pathology in the spinal cord.

## ♦ NURSING DIAGNOSES

Nursing diagnoses are determined from analysis of patient data. Nursing diagnoses for the patient with a spinal cord injury may include those covered under care of the patient with altered muscle tone and motor function, with the addition of the following:

| Diagnostic Title | Possible Etiologic Factors |
|---|---|
| Ventilation, inability to sustain spontaneous | Neuromuscular weakness |
| Dysreflexia | Distended bladder, impacted rectum |
| Mobility, impaired physical | Neuromuscular impairment |
| Disuse syndrome, high risk for | Immobility, weakness |
| Incontinence, total or reflex | Neurologic impairment and disease |
| Sexual dysfunction | Physiologic limitations |
| Knowledge deficit (medications and care required) | Lack of exposure/recall |

## ♦ EXPECTED PATIENT OUTCOMES

Expected patient outcomes for the patient with a spinal cord injury may include but are not limited to the following:

1. Resumes spontaneous ventilation.
2. Does not develop autonomic dysreflexia.
3. Maintains mobility to the greatest extent possible.
4. Does not develop disuse syndrome, as evidenced by the absence of contractures, pressure sores, and thromboembolic events.
5. Manages incontinence by a bladder program, as shown by voiding not interfering with daily activities.
6. Maintains the ability to express self sexually.
7. Verbalizes knowledge of medications and care required.

## ♦ INTERVENTIONS

### ➡ Managing Critical Care

#### Maintaining ventilation

Intubation and respiratory assistance with a ventilator may be required in the immediate stage following upper cervical cord injury. In the conscious quadriplegic patient with a spinal cord lesion below C5, respiratory function generally is not compromised unless it is associated with acute blunt trauma to the chest. A lesion at the C5 level produces paralysis of the intercostal muscles, leaving only the diaphragm to function for respiration. The nerve roots C3, C4, and C5 innervate the diaphragm and make up the phrenic nerves. C4 supplies roots mainly to the phrenic nerves. Therefore any patient who has a cord lesion at the C4 level with quadriplegia probably will require *permanent ventilatory support.*

Respiratory complications are common after injury of the spinal cord. Any patient with a cord injury level at C4 or above can be expected to need assistance to maintain respiration, often on a long-term or permanent basis. In addition, patients with lower cervical fractures often have temporary respiratory difficulties until the spinal shock phase subsides.

Respiratory assistance may include intubation with ventilator assistance. Long-term ventilator assistance will require a tracheotomy. After the initial period, these patients need continued respiratory support, including postural drainage and clapping. Deep breathing and coughing, if medically approved, are essential. At times the rocking bed, a bed that rocks on a central axis, is used. It alternately raises the head and then the foot of the bed. The bed assists in inspiration and expiration. Inspiration occurs as the diaphragm moves down as the head of the bed tilts up. With the reverse movement, the patient exhales as the head is tilted down and the abdominal contents push upward against the diaphragm. If the patient is able to maintain respiration for a time, the bed may be turned off for eating and nursing care.

Persons who have injury at the cervical level may need respiratory assistance to prevent respiratory arrest. Those who have injury at the thoracic level tend to splint their chests and have shallow breathing; therefore measures to facilitate deep breathing and aeration of the alveoli are carried out (see Chapter 37). Because coughing can increase spinal pressure, the physician should be consulted before urging the patient to cough. Good nursing assessment of respiratory status in the patient with spinal cord injury is essential to prevent respiratory complications.

#### Preventing dysreflexia

Autonomic hyperreflexia or autonomic dysreflexia (mass reflex) occurs in patients with cord lesions above T6; most often it occurs in cervical injuries. The clinical signs are bradycardia, paroxysmal hypertension, sweating, "goose flesh," and severe headache (Figure 58-7). Patients tend to develop individual symptoms of this condition. They soon are able to recognize this complication when it occurs. For instance, some patients feel flushed but never develop a headache. The wise nurse learns to listen to what the patient says is happening to him or her.

The most common cause is visceral distention (distended bladder, impacted rectum). If the patient complains of these symptoms, the patency of the catheter should be checked for kinking and a new catheter inserted *immediately* if the catheter is plugged. The patient should be placed in a sitting position to decrease blood pressure. The rectum should be checked for impaction. If it is necessary to remove stool, dibucaine (Nupercaine ointment) should be instilled in the rectum for its anesthetic effect. At times, urinary infections can lead to symptoms of autonomic dysreflexia. If no other

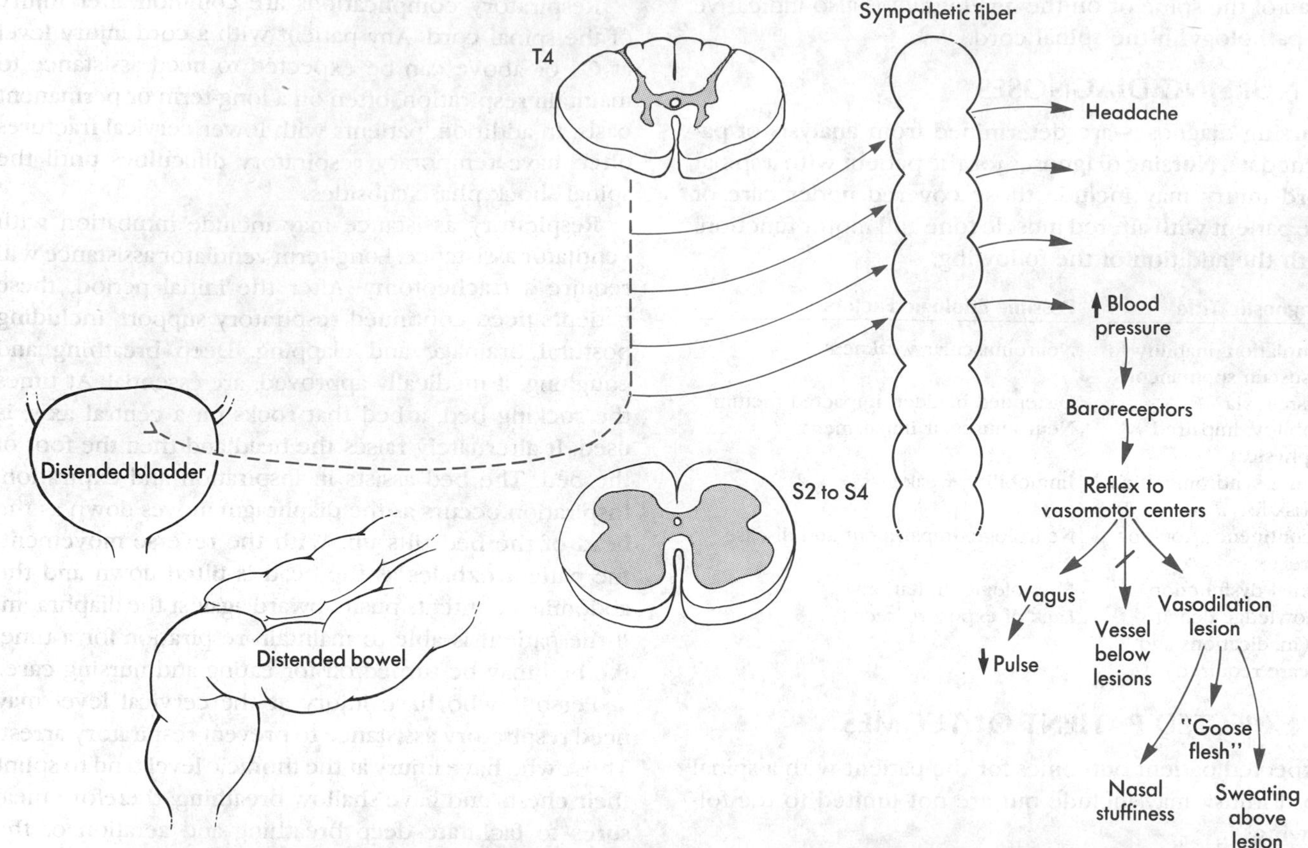


**FIGURE 58-7** Pictorial diagram of cause of autonomic hyperreflexia (dysreflexia) and results.

obvious cause is found, a urine specimen is sent for culture.

Autonomic dysreflexia is a medical emergency (Figure 58-7). The hypertension can lead to CVA, blindness, or even death. If conservative measures are not effective, a ganglionic blocking agent such as hexamethonium chloride or a vasodilator such as nitroprusside (Nipride) is given intravenously. (See Guidelines box, below, for details of care.)

## Guidelines for Care of the Person With Autonomic Dysreflexia

1. Place patient in a sitting position to decrease blood pressure.
2. Check patency of catheter. Be sure it is not kinked. If catheter is plugged, insert new catheter immediately.
3. Check rectum for fecal impaction.
4. If it is necessary to remove an impaction, dibucaine (Nupercaine ointment) should be instilled in the rectum for anesthetic effect.
5. Send urine for culture if patient has elevated temperature and no other cause is found. A urinary tract infection may cause symptoms.
6. Administer ganglionic blocking agent such as hexamethonium chloride or a vasodilator such as nitroprusside (Nipride) if conservative measures are not effective.

The major focus is to prevent such attacks. Before any bladder and bowel procedure such as cystoscopy or proctoscopy, the patient is given a local anesthetic. If autonomic dysreflexia is a continual problem, the patient may need long-term therapy to block sympathetic impulses.

■ ■ ■

Throughout all stages of hospitalization of the spinal cord–injured person, nursing and medical interventions are directed toward restoration of structural or body integrity consistent with the pathologic condition present. This means that all efforts are taken to ensure (1) that the skin is intact, (2) that contractures do not develop, (3) that ROM is maintained to the greatest degree possible, (4) that muscle tone is consistent with pathologic condition, and (5) that bladder and bowel functions are maintained. The following sections discuss specific interventions to achieve these outcomes. (See Guidelines box, p. 2047, for nursing care of the patient with a spinal cord injury.)

## Maintaining Mobility

Before moving a patient with acute spinal cord injury onto a bed from the stretcher, the physician should be consulted about the type of bed desired. The selection

## Guidelines for Care of the Person With a Spinal Cord Injury

1. Maintain mobility and function.
   a. Keep in neutral alignment when moving patient.
   b. Provide good skin care
   c. Assist with ROM exercises.
   d. Position in good body alignment at frequent intervals.
2. Maintain elimination.
   a. Reflex bladder
      (1) Provide stimulation of bladder.
      (2) Check for residual urine.
      (3) Use external catheters for males.
   b. Areflexic bladder
      (1) Use Credé's maneuver if effective.
      (2) Provide intermittent catheterization.
      (3) Check for residual urine.
   c. Encourage adequate fluids.
   d. Give cranberry juice to prevent medium conducive for infection.
   e. Place patient on bowel program.
3. Relieve pain.
   a. Use narcotics judiciously.
   b. Teach alternative methods of pain control, such as relaxation techniques or biofeedback.
4. Provide emotional support.
   a. Realize that patient probably will be very frustrated with limitations.
   b. Allow patient to vent feelings.
   c. Give patient positive feedback.

will depend on the physician's preference, the type of injury, the size of the patient, and the equipment available. If a regular bed is to be used, a full-length fracture board should be placed on top of the bedspring under the mattress. This board prevents sagging of the mattress and motion of the spine. If the bed is to be gatched, the board must be hinged, or two or more boards with correctly placed breaks can be used. Mattresses containing springs should not be used. Instead of springs and one mattress, some physicians prefer two air mattresses placed on top of the fracture board. Some use the knee gatch to provide hyperextension to the spine in selected thoracic and lumbar fractures; the bed must then be made up "head to foot." Sponge rubber mattresses are widely recommended and, when available, are often used when the patient may be moved very little and with extreme difficulty for some time. If available, an alternating air-pressure mattress often is used. Because the patient has loss of sensation and paralysis of part of the body, pressure areas develop easily. The mattress and entire bed foundation must be well protected with plastic sheeting so that incontinence will not cause damage.

To prevent injury when moving the patient, the bed foundation should be completely adjusted, with gatches raised as ordered, bolsters placed in the desired positions, and a turning sheet available so that minimal motion will be necessary. Three to five people are needed to move the patient from the stretcher to the bed, depending on the patient's weight and the location of the spinal injury. The physician may supervise moving the patient and may support the head and neck during the transfer. The body should be supported in proper alignment, and if necessary, manual hyperextension should be applied to the spine as the patient is moved.

***The nurse must carefully observe the patient with a spinal fracture, a cord tumor, or a ruptured intervertebral disk for signs of cord compression.*** The motion, strength, and sensation in the extremities should be tested at least every few hours for the first 24 to 36 hours and then at least four times a day. Any change in motion or sensation should be reported at once as related to level, because immediate surgery may be needed to relieve pressure on the cord. Some of the laminae may be removed to prevent pressure from edema.

During the intermediate stage of treatment, rehabilitation and nursing care measures are focused on mobilization and patient-family education. Quadriplegic and paraplegic patients need to learn to live with the sequelae of paralysis. ***The two goals of rehabilitation of these patients are to minimize the disability and to assist them toward independence to the extent possible.*** Rehabilitation depends on the extent and level of the cord injury, the patient's emotional reactions, his or her age, and other factors.[14]

***Early mobilization*** of the patient is important regardless of the level of injury. At first, mobilization includes active or passive turning movements and ROM exercises to prevent pressure sores and contractures and to develop independence in bed activities. Later, mobilization is usually progressively effected through wheelchair activities. Most patients with spinal cord injury find it impractical to walk because of the energy required. Patients with very low cord injuries may be able to ambulate with braces. If ambulation is not possible, the patient may still use the braces to stand at intervals throughout the day. This helps to decrease $Ca^{++}$ mobilization. Mat exercises and resistive exercises are initiated to increase muscle strength and endurance in remaining muscles.

When patients, especially quadriplegic patients, begin to sit up, it may be necessary to wrap their legs with Ace wraps to encourage venous return. Slowly increasing the angle of sitting is essential to prevent hypotension. For this reason, the patient who has recently become a quadriplegic should use a recliner wheelchair until he or she is able to sit at 90 degrees for several hours.

The patient with paraplegia and the family are taught proper methods of transfer from bed to wheelchair or commode (Figures 58-8 and 58-9). Physical therapy activities facilitate learning to transfer. The patient also learns how to do weight shifts if able. Even patients who are not able physically to do weight shifts can take responsibility in obtaining others' help.

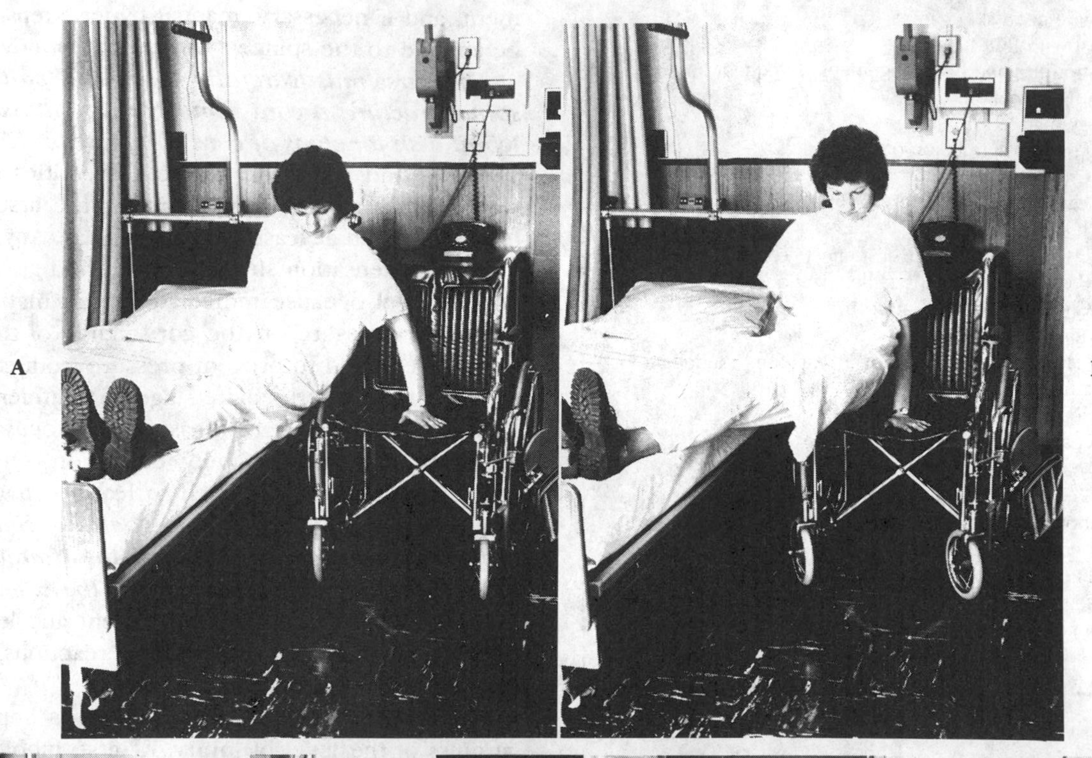


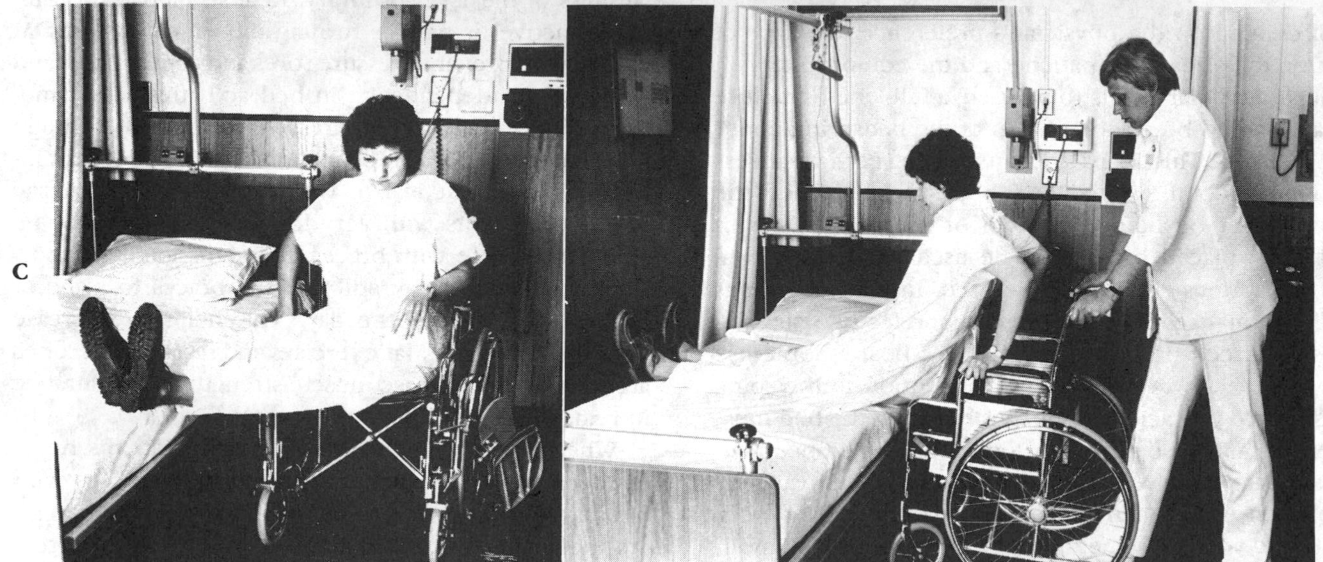


**FIGURE 58-8** Two methods for patient with paraplegia and strong upper extremities to transfer from bed to chair. With one method: **A,** patient moves sideways (note wheelchair, with right armrest removed, placed next to bed); **B,** then patient uses her arms to lift trunk into chair seat; and **C,** patient settles her hips comfortably into chair; she will then swing footrests into place and lift her legs from bed. **D,** Second method involves patient pushing backward off bed into chair.

Before the patient is permitted to be up after a spinal injury, a brace may be prescribed. All braces and corsets must be custom made and are quite expensive. The cost of a back brace varies according to the materials used in construction. *The brace or corset should be applied before the patient gets out of bed.* Help is needed in putting it on. The patient should wear a thin, knitted undershirt next to the skin to keep the brace clean and to protect the skin. Correct use so that the brace fits contours of the buttocks and chest as designed makes a great difference in the patient's comfort. The patient's emotional reaction to wearing a brace or a corset is important because it vitally affects ultimate rehabilitation. Attention to small details that help in initial acceptance of this somewhat uncomfortable and unfamiliar piece of "clothing" is important. The patient should practice putting the brace on while in the hospital if it must be worn for some time after discharge. A significant other may visit the hospital and learn to assist the patient. Patients who live alone and are unable to care for their braces themselves may require a community health nurse to help them in the home or to teach someone else to assist the patient.

In addition to instruction about mobilization techniques, the patient is trained to be *functional in ADL,* with or without equipment and as related to his or her life-style. The patient needs to know how to obtain bowel and bladder automaticity and how to prevent bladder infection. One must understand how to prevent decubitus ulcers when one sits in a wheelchair most of the day and must know how to manage the wheelchair itself. *The patient's family or significant others are included in instruction, because many quadriplegic patients may require some supervision or assistance in ADL following discharge from the hospital.* The reaction of family members to spinal cord injury is often great. The family as well as the patient needs help in coping. In addition to medical and physical rehabilitation measures, psychologic, emotional, sociologic, and vocational rehabilitation is equally important. The trauma of spinal cord injury may result in numerous interpersonal problems and make adjustment to one's environment difficult. (See Research box below.)

*Orthotics,* or the application of external appliances to support a paralyzed muscle or to promote a specific motion required in ADL, may require further follow-up care. Patients who have a ruptured cervical disk may need to use a neck brace. The brace extends well up under the chin and prevents flexion of the neck. Leg braces may be ordered for the patient with paraplegia who is able to ambulate or stand.

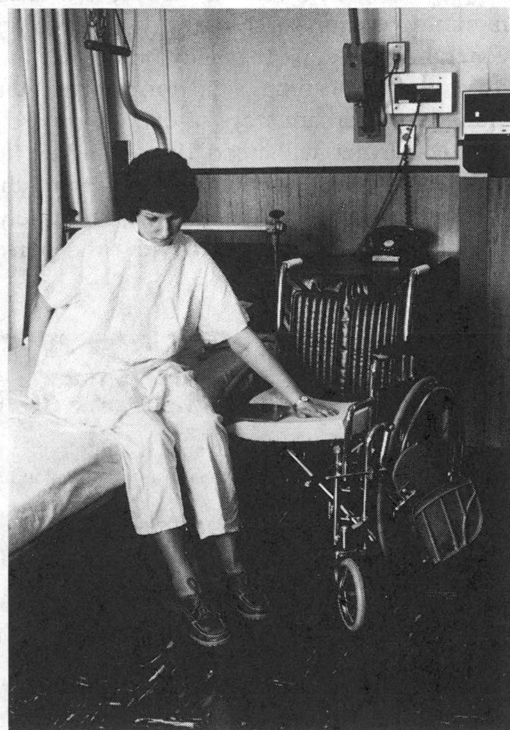

**FIGURE 58-9** Paraplegic patient whose upper extremity strength is not yet developed can use a sliding board to transfer from bed to chair. Board provides a firm surface on which to move, and trunk is supported by board through the move.

## Preventing Complications

If cord damage has occurred, nursing care will depend on the level of the injury. Patients with cervical lesions, for instance, will be unable to do anything for themselves. Meticulous skin care, maintenance of correct body alignment, preservation of joint ROM, and attempts to preserve muscle tone are imperative nursing measures, as in the care of any paralyzed person. (See Chapter 57 for a discussion of the care of the person with paralysis.)

## Maintaining Elimination

The patient may have urinary retention because of injury to lumbar and sacral spinal nerves. Since the patient may

**RESEARCH**

DeJong G et al: Independent living outcomes in spinal cord injury: multivariate analysis, *Arch Phys Med Rehabil* 65:66-72, 1984.

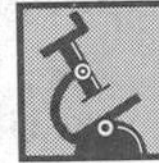

This study examined what factors could best predict the ability of a person with spinal cord injury to live independently. Seventy-five patients were studied with the use of a variety of variables. The most important predictors of overall independent living were found to be marital status, transportation barriers, education, work disincentives, and severity of the disability. Being married and well educated positively correlated with independent living, whereas the other variables had a negative effect on independence.

have no sensation of needing to void, ***the nurse should check carefully for voiding and for distention of the bladder.*** A Foley catheter may be inserted into the bladder, or a cytostomy may be performed.

Most persons with spinal cord injuries have a reflex (autonomic or spastic) bladder, which occurs when the spinal cord reflexes are still present but the inhibiting influences from the higher cortical centers are lost. Reflex bladder is seen in persons with spinal cord injury or disease above the level of the sacral cord after the initial spinal shock phase. Because the pathways for motor and sensory impulses to the cord are still present, the reflex arc is intact. Any stimulation from the bladder wall leads to contraction of the detrusor muscle and relaxation of the internal and external sphincters, resulting in involuntary bladder emptying. The spastic bladder often responds to even a minor stimulus such as touching or stroking the genitalia, thighs, or lower abdomen. Small, frequent voidings are common and demonstrate that the bladder empties long before it has reached normal capacity.

Some patients can be taught to recognize the stimulation for voiding and use it to induce voiding. Male patients often need to wear an external catheter for incontinence. Females, unfortunately, may have to wear disposable pads and waterproof pants. One important measure that will help decrease incontinence is the prevention of urinary tract infections.

Damage to the sacral cord or the peripheral nerves produces an atonic or areflexic bladder. Patients with spinal shock also have an atonic bladder. Any contraction from the bladder wall fails to stimulate the motor neurons in the cord. Because the reflex arc is disrupted, no sensations reach the brain. The person has no awareness of the need to void and no voluntary control.

## Maintaining Sexuality

Persons with cord injuries need assistance in learning about the effects of their injury on sexual functioning.[5,8] The important thought to keep in mind is that most patients with a cooperative partner are able to engage in satisfying sexual activity. The limitation depends on the site of the lesion and whether the cord injury is complete or incomplete. Generally, the higher the lesion, the more normal sexual function is likely to be. Patients with sacral lesions are the only spinal cord–injured men who are not able to have an erection and to ejaculate.

In men, erections are *reflexogenic* (secondary to stimulation) or *psychogenic* (response to sexual pictures, etc.). Most men with spinal cord injury are not able to have psychogenic erections but are capable of reflexogenic erections. These occur not only as a result of direct stimulation of the genitalia but may also result from stroking the inner thigh, stimulating the rectum with a finger, or manipulating the catheter. The nursing staff can help point out these "trigger" points to the patient.

The ability to ejaculate usually is not present with complete injuries. With incomplete injuries, ejaculation may be possible. Even when patients have lost sensation, many report that there is increased intensity of feeling in other body parts, such as the breasts. Orgasms may be experienced, with release of tension.

Male patients with indwelling catheters can either remove the catheter just before sexual activity or turn it back on the penis, where it provides extra support. The bowels should be emptied before intercourse; otherwise, bowel incontinence typically occurs.

Because many male patients who are able to ejaculate do so into the bladder (retrograde ejaculation), they are usually infertile. Without sperm counts, however, infertility cannot be guaranteed.

The spinal cord–injured woman is able to participate fully in sexual activity. She may not experience orgasm but can enjoy the sexual experience. Women who have a Foley catheter can keep it in place if desired.

Most spinal cord–injured women maintain their ability to conceive; for some reason, many of these women do not realize this. All such sexually active women should have access to family-planning information. If pregnancy is desired, the woman can usually have a normal vaginal delivery. However, she is at increased risk for autonomic dysreflexia and hydronephritis.

The nurse can be supportive and helpful to cord-injured patients by making it comfortable for them to discuss sexual matters. Nurses not prepared for sexual counseling need to be aware of resources available in the community to help the spinal cord–injured person. Some general suggestions that may be helpful include: (1) sex has many meanings, and for persons with no genital function, alternate ways of expression are available; (2) the partner will need time to adjust to the situation; openness in communication is helpful; and (3) it is sometimes difficult for a partner who routinely provides bladder and bowel care to view the person as

**BOX 58-4 Sexual Functioning in Persons With Spinal Cord Injury**

1. Reflexogenic erections occur not only as a result of stimulation of the genitalia, but also as a result of stimulation of the following "trigger points":
   a. Stroking the thigh
   b. Stimulating the rectum with a finger
   c. Manipulating the catheter
2. Males with catheters can either remove the catheter just before sexual activity or turn it back on the penis to provide extra support.
3. Bowels should be emptied before intercourse to prevent incontinence.
4. Women with a catheter can keep it in place during intercourse if desired.
5. Women maintain the ability to conceive; birth control should be used to avoid pregnancy.

sexually desirable; it may be helpful in this situation if this care can be provided by a community nurse or part-time attendant. Box 58-4 outlines sexual functioning in patients with spinal cord injury.

### Facilitating Learning

Teaching the patient with spinal cord injury encompasses all the points covered under teaching the patient with altered muscle tone and motor function. In addition, the patient needs to be taught about the effects of injury on sexual functioning, as just discussed.

### Research

Research data on spinal cord injuries continue to be gathered (see Research box at right). Interestingly, electrostimulation of muscles of the bladder through remote control to regain micturition control in the paraplegic patient has been tested clinically. Success of this electronic spinal neuroprosthesis will assist in preventing urinary complications, which are often a cause of death. Functional intramuscular electrostimulation of paralyzed upper extremity muscles is also currently being tested. Because little or no external splinting is required in the latter orthosis, it will be cosmetically appealing to the quadriplegic person if successful.

*In summary, although most complications of paralysis are now preventable, it is regrettable that complications do occur during and after hospitalization.*

## ♦ EVALUATION

To evaluate the effectiveness of nursing interventions, compare patient behaviors with those stated in the expected patient outcomes. Successful achievement of patient outcomes for the patient with a spinal cord injury is indicated by the following:

1. Maintains spontaneous and adequate ventilation and has no dyspnea or hypoxia.
2. Does not develop autonomic dysreflexia.
3. Is able to be in wheelchair for functional periods and can move self in chair.
4. Has no contractures, pressure sores, or thromboembolic events.
5. Completely empties bladder, with no reflux voiding that interferes with daily activities.
6. States that he or she is still a sexual being and has sexual contact with partner.
7. Correctly explains physical care needed and describes medications, including dose, route, and side effects.

## COMPLICATIONS

The patient with a spinal cord injury is very prone to complications, including bladder and urinary tract infections, pressure sores, and respiratory tract infections. Although these are not usually fatal, they prove expensive, require increased length of stay, and result in impaired ability to live independently.

**RESEARCH**

Borkowski C: A comparison of pulmonary complications in spinal cord–injured persons treated with two modes of spinal immobilization, *J Neurosci Nurs* 21:79-85, 1989.

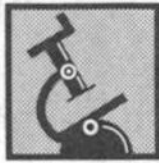

This study investigated two modes of spinal immobilization, the Kinetic Treatment Table and the traditionally used wedge turning device and their relationship to the development of pulmonary complications in two groups of patients with acute spinal cord injury. The following parameters were examined: incidence of pulmonary infection, length of need for mechanical ventilation, length of intensive care unit (ICU) stay, and length of hospitalization. Those clients turned with the Kinetic Treatment Table had a lower incidence of pulmonary infection and required less time on the ventilator. The length of ICU stay and the length of hospital stay did not differ.

# INTRAVERTEBRAL TUMORS

## ETIOLOGY/EPIDEMIOLOGY

Primary intravertebral tumors, or neoplasms, occur either extramedullary (involving tissues outside the cord) or intramedullary (involving tissue cells within the cord). Secondary or metastatic tumors may also involve the spinal cord, its coverings, and the vertebrae.

## PATHOPHYSIOLOGY

Extramedullary tumors of the intradural type at first may cause subjective nerve root pain. With tumor growth, this will include motor and sensory deficits relating to the level of the root and spinal cord involvement. As the tumor enlarges, it compresses the cord. Eventually the patient loses all motor and sensory function below the level of the tumor.

An intramedullary tumor, beginning within the spinal cord, often appears as a central cord syndrome, including segmental loss of pain and temperature function. In addition, loss of anterior horn cell function often occurs, especially in the hands. Most of the central long tracts of the nervous system become dysfunctional. There is gradual, progressive, and descending loss of pain and temperature sensations and motor weakness. Caudal motor and sensory functions are the last to be lost, including bowel and bladder function.

## MEDICAL MANAGEMENT

The medical care of the patient with an intravertebral tumor may involve surgery. Radiation therapy may be used as an adjunct to surgery or as primary treatment when the tumor is considered to be inoperable. Chemotherapy also may be used.

A spinal decompression is typically done even when complete removal of the tumor is not considered pos-

# NURSING CARE PLAN

## PERSON UNDERGOING A LAMINECTOMY

**DATA:** Mr. S. is a 45-year-old single man who was admitted to the emergency room with a diagnosis of a ruptured disk at L3-L4 with no displacement of the vertebrae. The patient is neurologically intact, except for some tingling in his left leg. The tingling began about 2 days ago but became worse an hour before admission. He was not able to ambulate without pain. After being admitted for testing, the decision is made to do a laminectomy.

The nursing history revealed the following:

- Mr. S. had no significant past medical history.
- Mr. S. lived alone.
- He expressed concern about the chance of becoming paralyzed.
- He had a good understanding of the pending surgery.

Collaborative nursing actions include those to prepare Mr. S. for surgery and to provide postoperative care and promote mobility. Nursing actions include monitoring for the following:

- Any change in neurologic deficit: increased tingling, pain
- Level of anxiety
- Pain and discomfort

### ■ NURSING DIAGNOSIS

Knowledge deficit related to lack of recall or exposure

| Expected Patient Outcomes | Nursing Interventions (Preoperative) | Rationale |
|---|---|---|
| Explains surgery and activities after procedure. | Review nature of surgery and activities after surgery. | Recall or reinforcement of earlier teaching helps promote retention. |
| Explains reasons not to sit. | Review relationship of sitting and stress on lumbar area. | Sitting is contraindicated for a time after surgery. |
| Explains follow-up care. | Review follow-up care with patient. | Understanding of follow-up care assists with compliance. |

### ■ NURSING DIAGNOSIS

Impaired physical mobility related to back pain

| Expected Patient Outcome | Nursing Interventions | Rationale |
|---|---|---|
| Maintains mobility. | Begin to ambulate in room on day of surgery. | Early mobilization leads to decreased complications from surgery. |
| | Ambulate in hallway, at first with assistance and then independently. | Progressive ambulation increases strength. |
| | Do not allow sitting. | Sitting puts stress on lumbar area. |
| | Refer to physical therapy. | Therapy helps patient learn good body mechanics and build strength. |

### ■ NURSING DIAGNOSIS

Pain related to back surgery

| Expected Patient Outcome | Nursing Interventions | Rationale |
|---|---|---|
| Has relief from pain. | Medicate with analgesic as needed. | Relief of pain is priority. |
| | Assist with positioning. | Change in position may relieve pain or discomfort. |

### ■ NURSING DIAGNOSIS

High risk for disuse syndrome related to surgery and pain

| Expected Patient Outcomes | Nursing Interventions (Preoperative) | Rationale |
|---|---|---|
| Does not develop deep vein thrombosis. | Assist in performing leg exercises. | Exercises increase circulation to lower extremities. |
| | Provide antiembolism stockings. | |
| Does not have atelectasis. | Provide incentive spirometry q 2 hr. | Interventions decrease postoperative complications. |
| | Have patient cough and deep-breathe q 2 hr. | |
| Skin breakdown does not occur. | Assist with turns q 2 hr. | This decreases chance of skin breakdown. |

## NURSING CARE PLAN

### PERSON UNDERGOING A LAMINECTOMY—cont'd

■ **NURSING DIAGNOSIS**
Altered peripheral tissue perfusion related to trauma of surgery

| Expected Patient Outcome | Nursing Interventions | Rationale |
|---|---|---|
| Maintains circulation to legs. | Assess for neurocirculatory changes initially q 2 hr. | Circulation may be impaired as a result of swelling from surgery. |
| | Assess wound q 2 hr for first 24 hours. | Bleeding could occur. |

sible. As much of the tumor as possible (and possibly bone) is removed to reduce the obstruction for a time. It can be performed at any level of the vertebral column and may include several vertebrae. The procedure is sometimes palliative.

### NURSING MANAGEMENT

Convalescent care and rehabilitation of the patient depend on the type of tumor and whether it has been successfully removed. The decompression procedure may give relief of symptoms for years, if the tumor is a slow-growing one. The reader is referred to the previous section on spinal cord injury for further relevant care.

## PERIPHERAL NERVE TRAUMA

### ETIOLOGY

Traumatic causes of peripheral nerve injury typically include gunshot and knife wounds, fragmented fracture wounds, and surgical transections, as in denervation surgery and amputations. They variously result in stretching, laceration, and compression of the peripheral nerve; great variation also exists in the degree of injury. Fortunately, the axons of peripheral nerves are capable of regeneration under favorable conditions.

### EPIDEMIOLOGY

The peripheral nerves that lie outside the brain and spinal cord include the cranial and spinal nerves and their branches and plexuses. The disorders involving the peripheral nerves are similar to those that affect the CNS and are the result of traumatic, degenerative, vascular, inflammatory, neoplastic, and metabolic causes. **Neuropathies,** noninflammatory disorders, may involve one peripheral nerve (mononeuropathy) or multiple nerves (polyneuropathies). **Neuritis** refers to an inflammatory disorder, whereas **neuralgia** means a painful nerve disorder. Although discussion in this section is limited to neuropathies caused by trauma, it should be clear that regardless of cause, the resulting nerve dysfunction will be similar and will be related to the site of the lesion. Some of the more common neuropathies (other than trauma) include nutritional, alcoholic, diabetic, lead, arsenic, hereditary, and infectious.

### PATHOPHYSIOLOGY

After trauma (or disease), the axon undergoes *secondary* or *wallerian degeneration* distal to the lesion (i.e., distal to the cells of origin) and for several segments proximal. The axon and the myelin sheath (secondary) degenerate and immediately undergo fragmentation; the fragmented particles are completely ingested within several weeks; and the axis cylinder remains. Schwann cells and fibroblasts begin to proliferate along the degenerated fibers. (Myelin in *peripheral fibers* is formed by Schwann cells.) During the regenerative phase, new axoplasm forms at the proximal edge of the injury, and the regenerating fibers now grow distally and enter the empty neurolemmal sheath, which since has proliferated. Myelin then forms around the regenerated axon. When a nerve has been severely damaged and fibrous tissue is abundant, regeneration is interfered with by a tangled mass known as a *traumatic neuroma;* this may have to be removed surgically.

The clinical signs and symptoms resulting from peripheral nerve lesions depend on the exact location of the lesion and the specific function of the involved nerve or nerves. Since peripheral nerves contain both sensory and motor components, deficits may exist in both components distal to the site. Alterations occur in pain, touch, temperature, proprioception, and stereognosis. Motor alterations include LMN signs such as flaccid paralysis and muscle wasting in those muscles innervated by the affected nerves.

### PREVENTION

The same measures taken to prevent head injury are applicable to peripheral nerve trauma (see p. 2009).

### MEDICAL MANAGEMENT

#### Diagnostic Tests

The electromyogram (EMG) may be helpful in diagnosing peripheral nerve injuries. (See Chapter 56 for a description of this test.)

## CRITICAL PATHWAY Laminectomy Without Complications or Fusion

**DRG #: 214 Expected LOS: 6**

| | Day of Surgery<br>Day of Admission<br>Day 1 | Day 2 | Day 3 |
|---|---|---|---|
| **Diagnostic Tests** | Preoperative: Chest x-ray film, CBC, UA, SMA/6,* PT/PTT, creatinine, MRI, myelogram, ECG, lumbar spinal x-ray films<br>Postoperative: CBC, electrolytes | | |
| **Medications** | Preoperative: IV antibiotic<br>Postoperative: IVs, IV analgesic, stool softener | IV @ TKO, IV or IM analgesic, stool softener | IV to saline lock, PO analgesic, stool softener |
| **Treatments** | Preoperative: Wt, VS<br>Postoperative: I & O q8hr, VS q4hr, assess neurocirculatory systems to legs q2hr, T-C-DB q2hr, incentive spirometry q2hr, elastic leg stockings (ELS) | I & O q8hr, VS q6hr, assess neurocirculatory systems to legs q4hr, T-C-DB q2hr, incentive spirometry q2hr, ELS | I & O q8hr, VS q8hr, T-C-DB q4hr, incentive spirometry q4hr, ELS |
| **Diet** | NPO; advance to full liquids after nausea | Advance to regular diet | Regular diet |
| **Activity** | Bedrest, to BR with assistance; ambulate in room with assistance, no sitting | Ambulate in hallway with assistance, no sitting | Ambulate in hallway with assistance, no sitting |
| **Consultations** | | Physical therapy | Physical therapy |

*Serum sodium, potassium, chloride, total $CO_2$, glucose, BUN.

### Treatment

Medical care of the patient with a peripheral nerve trauma depends on the nature of the individual nerve involved. Surgical intervention may be necessary.

## NURSING MANAGEMENT

Nursing care is specific to the areas of the body affected by the sensory and motor deficits. Plans for care are based on the nurse's understanding of the distribution and function of the involved peripheral nerves. The flaccid muscles demand attention to prevent deformities. *Because of the atonia or hypotonia of the paralyzed muscles, they are pulled excessively by the muscles that normally oppose them into abnormal or contracted positions.* When associated tendons shorten, the contracture is permanent. Positioning of extremities in neutral or counter positions helps in preventing joint deformities. Those areas of the body with a loss of sensation need to be protected from injury. These patients must be taught *protective measures,* such as not staying in one position too long, since they cannot sense that damage is occurring in an area served by a damaged nerve. When positional sense is lost, patients must also be taught to protect themselves when walking and in other activities. Pain is usually localized, and more paresthesia may occur than pain. The painful areas need to be protected from external stimulation when present. After surgical intervention, careful positioning of the operative area, as prescribed, is important. Finally, the promotion of good health measures assists in the creation of conditions favorable to nerve regeneration. See Box 58-5 for peripheral nerve trauma terminology.

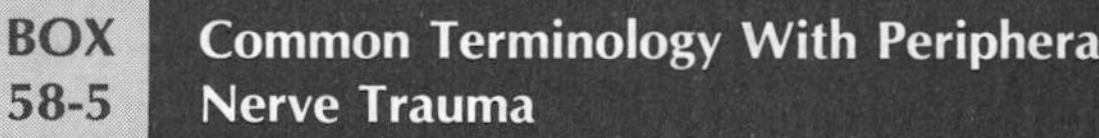

**BOX 58-5 Common Terminology With Peripheral Nerve Trauma**

**Neuropathies**—noninflammatory disorders
**Mononeuropathy**—disorder affecting one peripheral nerve
**Polyneuropathy**—disorder involving multiple nerves
**Neuritis**—inflammatory disorder
**Neuralgia**—painful nerve disorder

# TRIGEMINAL NEURALGIA

## ETIOLOGY

**Trigeminal neuralgia** is one specific type of peripheral nerve problem. It is also called **tic douloureux.** In most cases, no etiology for this disorder can be found. When it is associated with hypesthesia in the distribution of the fifth cranial nerve, with onset before age 40, or is associated with other cranial nerve palsies, a work-up to rule out multiple sclerosis or a posterior fossa brain tumor is necessary.

| Day 4 | Day 5 | Day of Discharge Day 6 |
|---|---|---|
| IV saline lock, PO analgesic, stool softener | Disc saline lock, PO analgesic, stool softener | PO analgesic, stool softener |
| I & O q8hr, VS q8hr, ELS | I & O, VS q8hr, ELS | VS q8hr, ELS |
| Regular diet | Regular diet | Regular diet |
| Ambulate in hallway with assistance, no sitting | Ambulate in hallway | Ambulate in hallway |
| Physical therapy | Physical therapy | |

## EPIDEMIOLOGY

More than 90% of cases of trigeminal neuralgia occur in persons over age 40. Women are affected somewhat more frequently than men.

## PATHOPHYSIOLOGY

Trigeminal neuralgia is characterized by *excruciating, burning pain* that radiates along one or more of the three divisions of the fifth cranial nerve (Figure 58-10). The pain typically extends only to the midline of the face and head, because this is the extent of the tissue supplied by the offending nerve. Areas along the course of the nerve are known as *trigger points,* and the slightest stimulation of these areas may initiate pain. Persons with trigeminal neuralgia try desperately to avoid "triggering" the pain. It is not unusual to see them lying in bed with the covers over their heads in an effort to avoid drafts. They frequently have been unable to eat properly for some time because chewing causes pain. They may therefore be undernourished and dehydrated. They may have slept poorly and have not washed, shaved, or combed their hair for some time. Oral hygiene may often be neglected because of pain.

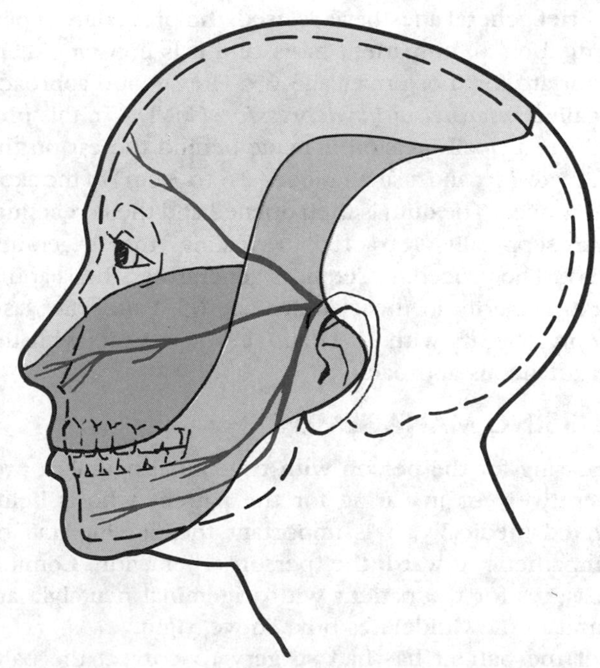

FIGURE 58-10 Pathway of trigeminal nerve and facial areas innervated by each of the three main divisions of this nerve.

## MEDICAL MANAGEMENT

### Medication

Carbamazepine (Tegretol) currently is the drug of choice for the treatment of the pain (also used for convulsions). The initial dose is 100 mg twice a day, increasing over time to 800 to 1000 mg daily. The inhalation of trichloroethylene (10 to 15 drops on cotton) has been tried with variable success for relieving pain. Drugs such as nicotinic acid, thiamine chloride, cobra venom, and analgesics have all been tried, but usually they offer the person little if any relief. Sedatives may be given for sleep.

Two other drugs that may be helpful in treating the patient with trigeminal neuralgia are baclofen (Lioresal) and phenytoin (Dilantin), which is used when both carbamazepine and baclofen are ineffective.

The peripheral branches of the trigeminal nerve may be injected with absolute alcohol.[1] This provides relief for weeks or months, and the procedure may be repeated as necessary. Permanent relief can be obtained only by surgery, but this is not always successful.

### Diet

When the *lower branch* of the fifth cranial nerve is interrupted, hot foods must be avoided because the person is not aware if the mucous membrane is burned. The patient may have difficulty chewing and swallowing at first.

## SURGICAL MANAGEMENT

Several surgical procedures have been used to treat trigeminal neuralgia. Currently, two major approaches are used. In *percutaneous* procedures, a needle or trochar is inserted at the corner of the mouth and guided into the ipsilateral foramen ovale under fluoroscopy. Local or brief general anesthesia is used; the procedure is performed on an outpatient basis; and it is considered appropriate for those over age 65. The second approach is called *microvascular depression* (MVD). In this procedure, a small incision is made behind the ear on the affected side, and a small piece (2.5 to 3 cm) of the skull is removed. The dura is then opened and the cerebellum microscopically retracted, revealing the trigeminal nerve. The procedure requires general anesthesia and is used primarily in those under age 65. Pain relief lasts about 15 years with MVD and 1½ to 4 years with the percutaneous approach.[4]

## NURSING MANAGEMENT

In caring for the person with trigeminal neuralgia preoperatively or in caring for the patient who is being treated medically, it is important the nursing staff be sympathetic toward the person's behavior. Comfort measures for the patient with trigeminal neuralgia are found in the Guidelines box, above, right.

If the patient has had surgery to correct the pain, certain nursing measures are important. Postoperatively, it is important to know which branches of the nerve have been cut or destroyed in the procedure so that necessary protection can be accomplished. If the *upper branch* is completely severed, the corneal reflex on that side will be lost. Usually an attempt is made to preserve a few of the fibers of the first division of the fifth nerve, because even a few intact fibers seem to preserve this vital function. Until the physician has tested the corneal reflex and verified its presence, an eye shield is used to prevent dust or lint from getting onto the cornea and causing injury.

Within 24 hours after a fifth nerve resection, many patients develop herpes simplex (cold sores) about the lips. Phenol and camphor (Campho-Phenique) applied frequently seems to give more relief than any other treatment. Usually the lesions heal in about 1 week. (See Guidelines box above for postoperative care involved.)

The assessment, nursing diagnoses, and expected outcomes for the patient with trigeminal neuralgia are the same as those for the patient with peripheral nerve trauma (see p. 2054).

### Guidelines for Comfort Measures for the Person With Trigeminal Neuralgia

1. Keep room free of drafts.
2. Avoid walking briskly to bedside of patient.
3. Place bed out of traffic area to prevent jarring of bed.
4. Avoid touching patient's face.
5. Advise patient *not* to wash or shave the affected area or to comb hair.
6. Avoid hot or cold liquids that trigger pain.
7. Note that food may have to be pureed and lukewarm and taken through a straw.

### Guidelines for Postoperative Care of the Person With Trigeminal Neuralgia

1. Preserve eye function.
   a. If upper branch of nerve was cut, corneal reflex is lost.
   b. Eye shield is used to prevent dust or lint from getting onto cornea.
   c. Avoid contact with eye when washing face.
   d. Bathe eye with methylcellulose solution.
   e. Inspect eye several times a day.
2. Promote mouth function when lower branch of fifth cranial nerve is interrupted.
   a. Avoid hot food because of loss of sensation.
   b. Food should be placed on unaffected side of mouth because of difficulty in swallowing.
   c. Perform mouth care after each meal to remove retained food.
3. Promote safety (e.g., electric razor should be used for shaving of face).

## QUESTIONS TO CONSIDER

- What nursing actions may be helpful in alleviating spasticity in a patient with spasticity?
- A patient you are caring for is experiencing intractable pain. The patient states, "There's no hope, I just want to end it all." What would you say in response?
- How would you differentiate between an upper motor neuron lesion and a lower motor neuron lesion?
- Your patient with Guillain-Barré syndrome expresses that his wife may "catch" the disease from him. How would you answer him?
- How would you respond to another staff member who says, "Just leave her alone; after all, she's paralyzed, and won't know if we turn her"?
- How would your care of a person with quadriplegia at the C5 level differ from that of a person with paraplegia at the L5 level?

## CRITICAL THINKING ACTIVITIES

- Brent, 19, sustained a spinal cord injury during an automobile accident. Physical assessment reveals the following findings: hyperreflexia and positive Babinski's sign, spastic paralysis of the lower extremities. His roommate Brian has polyneuritis and exhibits flaccid paralysis of the lower extremities. Analyze each situation and determine which patient suffers from an upper motor neuron lesion and which has a lower motor neuron lesion. List data that support your decision.
- Given the level of spinal cord injury, predict what muscle function will be remaining in the following situations: (1) 29-year-old man with transection of the cord at C3; (2) 34-year-old woman with injury at C6; (3) 18-year-old man with transection of the cord at T10; and (4) 22-year-old woman with injury at L2.

## CHAPTER SUMMARY

### ALTERATIONS IN MUSCLE TONE AND MOTOR FUNCTION

- Damage to the nervous system often causes serious problems in mobility.
- Injury or disease of motor neurons and their extensions at any level results in alterations of muscle strength, muscle tone, and reflex activity.
- Lower motor neurons (LMNs) consist of large anterior horn cells located in the anterior gray matter of the spinal cord, whereas upper motor neurons (UMNs) originate in the motor strip of the cerebral cortex and in multiple brainstem nuclei.
- Patients experiencing ongoing problems with spasticity may be treated with one or more skeletal muscle relaxants to decrease muscle tone and involuntary movements.
- In persons with paralysis, the joints become flexed and fixed in useless positions with resulting deformity unless the nurse takes preventive measures.

### NEUROLOGIC PAIN

- The experience of pain depends on the individual, and many factors influence the patient's perception and expression of pain.
- Pain receptors may be activated by cellular damage, certain chemicals (including histamine), ischemia, muscle spasm, or sensations of heat, cold, and itching that go beyond a specific level of intensity.
- The quality of neurologic pain may vary from mild to excruciating.
- Referred pain occurs in a site other than its origin.
- Unbearable pain that does not respond to the definitive treatment of the causative lesion is called intractable.
- Techniques to relieve pain surgically include neurectomy, rhizotomy, and cordotomy.

### SPINAL CORD INFECTIONS/INFLAMMATIONS

- Infections and inflammations that may affect the spinal cord include Guillain-Barré syndrome and herpes zoster.

### SPINAL CORD TRAUMA

- Automobile accidents, motorcycle accidents, diving and other athletic accidents, and gunshot wounds are major causes of spinal cord injuries.
- In a complete cord injury, total transection of the spinal cord occurs with a complete loss of spinal cord functions, whereas an incomplete injury involves a partial transection or injury of the cord.
- Autonomic dysreflexia is a complication associated with spinal cord injury above the level of the sixth thoracic vertebra. It requires immediate nursing intervention.

### INTRAVERTEBRAL TUMORS

- The symptoms of an intravertebral tumor often mimic those of an incomplete spinal cord injury.

### PERIPHERAL NERVE TRAUMA

- Symptoms of peripheral nerve trauma may vary greatly.

## REFERENCES


1. Adler R: Trigeminal glycerol chemoneurolysis: nursing implications, *J Neurosci Nurs* 21:337-341, 1989.
2. Barker E, Higgins R: Managing a suspected SCI, *Nursing '89* 19(3):52-59, 1989.
3. Borkowski C: A comparison of pulmonary complications in spinal cord–injured patients treated with two modes of spinal immobilization, *J Neurosci Nurs* 21:79-85, 1989.
4. Burchiel KJ: Trigeminal neuralgia. In Rakel RE, editor: *Conn's current therapy 1993,* Philadelphia, 1993, Saunders.

5. Chicano L: Humanistic aspects of sexuality as related to spinal cord injury, *J Neurosci Nurs* 21:326-329, 337, 1989.
6. DeJong G et al: Independent living outcomes in spinal cord injury: multivariate analysis, *Arch Phys Med Rehabil* 65:66-72, 1984.
7. Emich-Herring B, Wood P: A team approach to neurological based swallowing disorders, *Rehabil Nurs* 25:242-247, 1990.
8. Goddard L: Sexuality and spinal cord injury, *J Neurosci Nurs* 20:240-244, 1988.
9. Hansberry J et al: Managing chronic pain with a permanent epidural catheter, *Nursing '90* 10:53-57, 1990.
10. Krusinski PA: Viral diseases of the skin. In Rakel RE, editor: *Conn's current therapy 1993,* Philadelphia, 1993, Saunders.
11. Lamb S, Barbaro N: Neurosurgical approaches to the management of chronic pain syndromes, *Orthop Nurs* 6(1):23-29, 1987.
12. Morgan S: A passage through paralysis, *Am J Nurs* 92(4):54-58, 1992.
13. North B et al: Living in a halo, *Am J Nurs* 92(4):54-58, 1992.
14. Pettibone K: Management of spasticity in spinal cord injury: nursing concerns, *J Neurosci Nurs* 19:269-299, 1988.
15. Rankin J: The nursing diagnosis: swallowing, impaired and bedside assessment of swallowing in neurologically involved cases, *J Neurosci Nurs* 24:117-118, 1992.
16. Rehabilitation of persons with injuries, *MMWR* 41(RR-6):35-38, 1992.
17. US Department of Health and Human Services, Public Health Service: *Healthy people 2000: national health promotion and disease prevention objectives,* Washington, DC, 1990, US Government Printing Office.

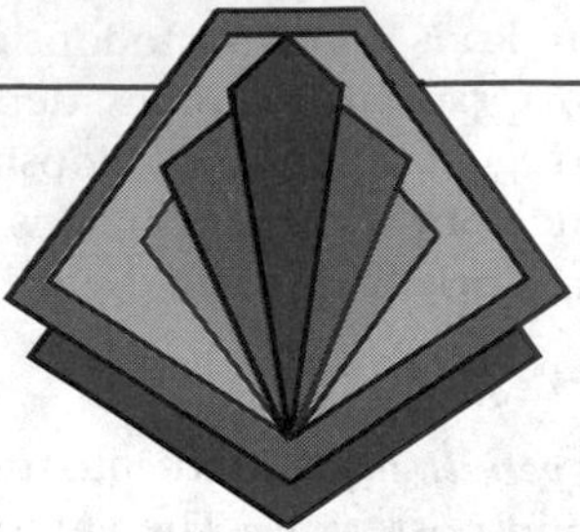

CHAPTER 59

# Assessment of the Visual System

*Marion Allen*

## CHAPTER OBJECTIVES

***After studying this chapter, the learner should be able to do the following:***

1 Describe the structure and function of the eye.
2 Identify the normal physiologic and anatomic changes that occur with aging.
3 Identify the subjective and objective data that should be obtained when assessing the eye.
4 Describe the purpose of the diagnostic studies used to assess the eye and its visual function.

## KEY TERMS

astigmatism
dermatochalasis
ectropion
enophthalmos
entropion
exophthalmia
exophthalmos
hyperopia
hyphema
hypopyon
myopia
presbyopia
refracted
scotoma

Orientation to our world is primarily visual. We learn much about our environment and ourselves through our eyes. Practically no behavior is not affected by the visual sense. One hears a noise and looks in the direction from which it came. Something touches our body and we look to see what it was. Vision contributes meaning and pleasure to the human experience. Our eyes reflect the pleasure, sorrow, or pain that we feel in relation to human experiences. A world without the sight of children playing, the esthetic pleasure of the museum, or the beauty of the rainbow would be, to some, bleak indeed or almost unimaginable.

Assessment of the visual system is an integral part of the nurse's role. Visual screening is conducted with persons of all ages and in all settings, including homes, schools, industries, and health care institutions. In fact, persons with eye disorders usually are identified by nurses and physicians in outpatient clinics or ophthalmologists' offices. Admission to the hospital usually indicates a need for more extensive investigation of an eye problem or for medical or surgical treatment that cannot routinely be accomplished on an outpatient basis.

Because persons with eye problems usually are seen on an outpatient basis, visual impairment may not be the initial problem or the major diagnosis of persons for whom the nurse is providing care. However, visual impairment is frequently present. As a consequence, nurses should routinely assess visual ability, especially in those persons who have systemic diseases that affect vision or who are taking medications with known visual side effects.

Nursing assessment focuses on the status of the patient's vision, the degree to which any vision loss affects the person's ability to carry out activities of daily living, the meaning that the person attaches to his or her visual impairment, the person's support systems, and the coping skills that have been used successfully in the past. Nursing interventions are designed to help people meet or learn to meet their basic needs, to strengthen existing support systems, and to encourage the use of successful coping mechanisms.

# ANATOMY AND PHYSIOLOGY OF THE EYE

## LAYERS OF THE EYE

The eyeball has three main coats or layers (Figure 59-1). The tough *outer layer* consists of the *opaque sclera* (white) and the *transparent cornea.* These structures are joined at the *corneoscleral sulcus* or *limbus.* The *middle vascular layer* or *uvea* is composed of three parts: the *choroid,* the *ciliary body,* and the *iris,* which contains an opening in its center that is called the *pupil.*

The *retina,* the *third* and *innermost layer* of the eye, is composed of *two parts: a sensory portion* and a layer of *pigmented epithelium. The sensory portion contains the photoreceptors (rods and cones).* These photoreceptors synapse in the retina with bipolar neurons and then with ganglion neurons, and these become the fibers of the optic nerve that pass visual information to the brain.

The cones, which are less numerous than the rods, are concentrated near the center of the retina in an area termed the *macula* (Figure 59-2). They are considered to be the receptors for bright daylight and color vision and allow us to see sharp images. The *rods,* which are found mostly in the periphery of the retina, are receptors for dim or night vision. Rods contain rhodopsin, a photosensitive protein that rapidly becomes depleted in bright light. The slow regeneration of rhodopsin, which depends on the presence of vitamin A, explains the time needed to adjust from a bright to a dim light.

## CHAMBERS OF THE EYE

The interior of the *eyeball* is divided into two *compartments* (anterior and posterior). The anterior compartment includes the space from the back of the cornea to the lens, and the posterior compartment is the space from the posterior surface of the lens to the retina.

The anterior compartment is further subdivided into an *anterior chamber* (between the cornea and the iris) and a *posterior chamber* (between the iris and the lens). This compartment is filled with a clear liquid called *aqueous humor,* which is produced by the ciliary body in the posterior chamber and flows through the pupil into the anterior chamber. *Aqueous humor* leaves the eye through the filtration structures at the junction of the iris and cornea (anterior chamber angle). The filtration structures consist of a structure called the *trabecular* meshwork and an encircling tubular channel that the aqueous humor drains into (Schlemm's canal).

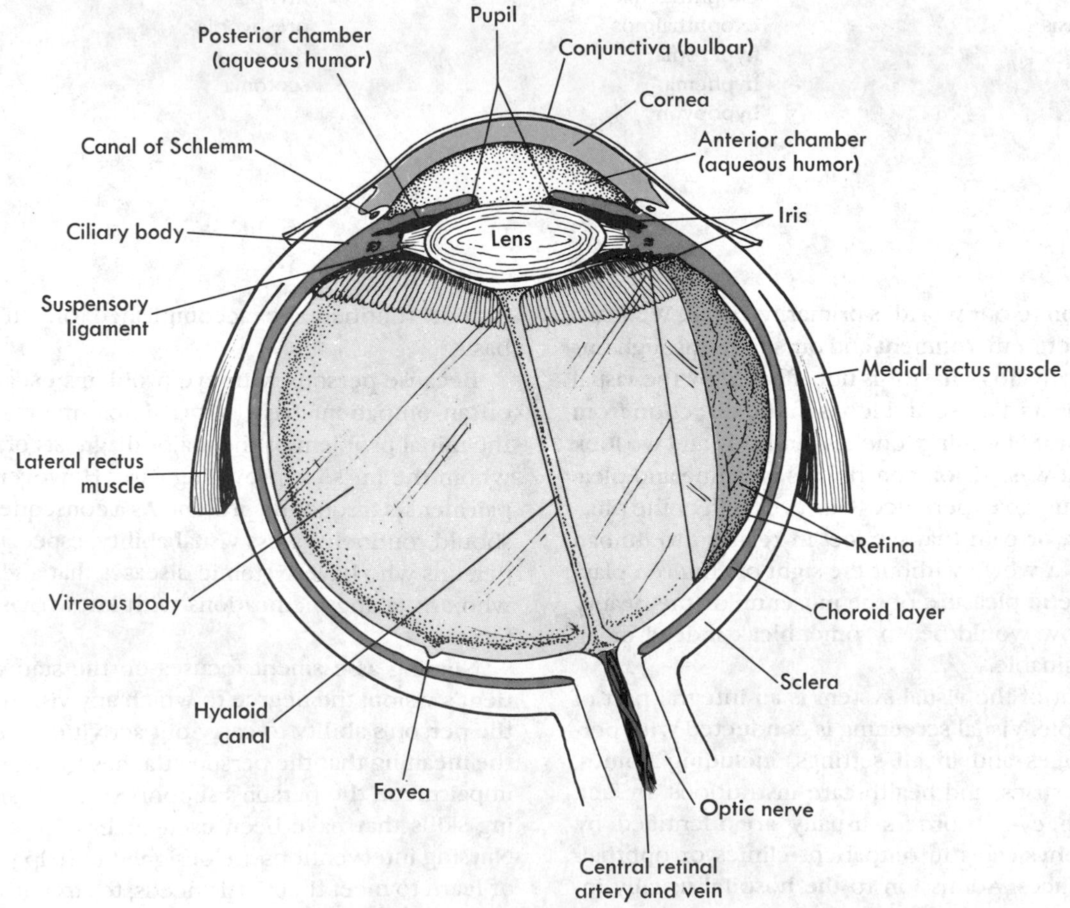


**FIGURE 59-1** Horizontal section through left eyeball.

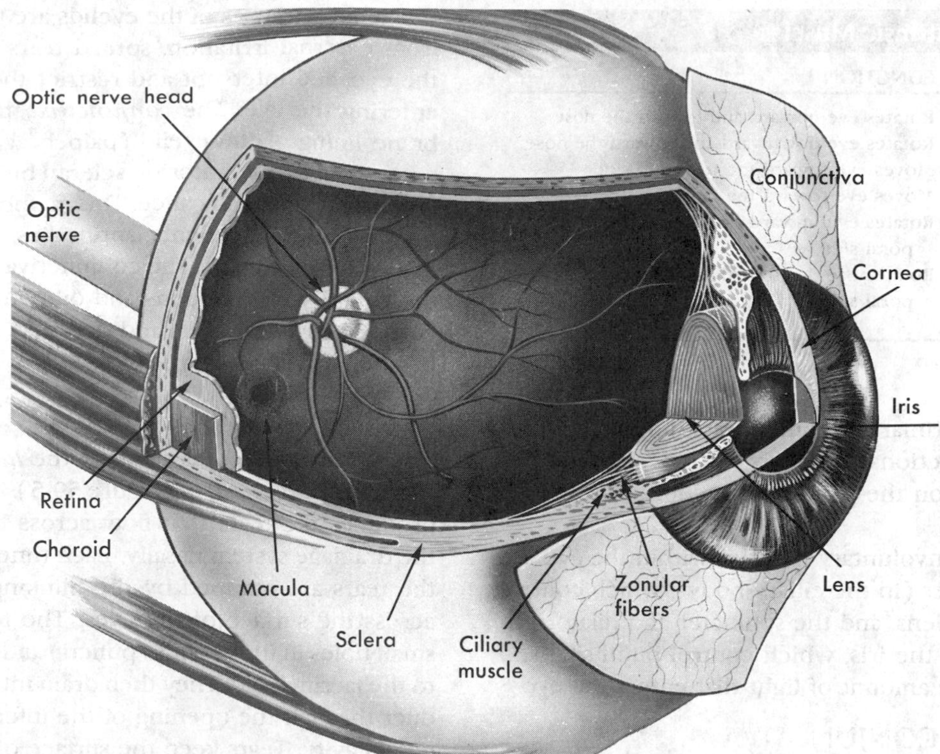


**FIGURE 59-2** Cutaway section of the eye. (From Stein HA, Slatt BJ, Stein RM: *Ophthalmic terminology: speller and vocabulary builder,* ed 3, St Louis, 1992, Mosby.)

Schlemm's canal has several exit channels that empty into the scleral and episcleral veins. Aqueous humor passes through these exit channels and eventually is absorbed into general circulation (Figure 59-3).

The *posterior* compartment is the larger of the two and is filled with a clear gel-like substance called the *vitreous humor.* The structure of the vitreous humor can be pictured as fine collagen fibers crossing one another to form a scaffolding that helps to maintain the shape of the eyeball. This fibrous network becomes more dense toward the outermost portion of the vitreous humor, particularly in the areas of strong attachment between the vitreous humor and retina. These attachments occur at the anterior edge of the retina, the optic disc, the equator of the eye, and the macula. The vitreous humor is clear, thus allowing proper transmission of light posteriorly to the retina.

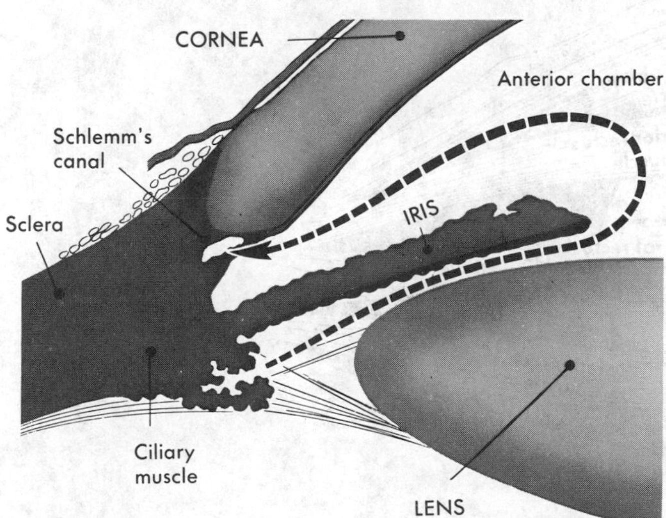


**FIGURE 59-3** Flow of aqueous humor. Aqueous humor is largely produced by the ciliary processes in the posterior chamber; it flows into the anterior chamber and leaves the eye through Schlemm's canal. (From Stein HA, Slatt BJ, Stein RM: *Ophthalmic terminology: speller and vocabulary builder,* ed 3, St Louis, 1992, Mosby.)

## LENS

The lens is a transparent biconvex structure located directly behind the iris and pupil. It is attached to the ciliary body by multiple suspensory ligaments called *zonules.* The lens, which is the fine-focusing mechanism for the eye, allows a clear image to be focused on the retina.

## EYE MUSCLES

*Eye muscles* consist of *two types: extrinsic* and *intrinsic.* The extrinsic voluntary muscles outside the eyeball control extraocular movement (Table 59-1 and Figure 59-4). Six extraocular muscles control the movement of each eye. The muscles of each eye are controlled simultaneously by the brain. The lateral and medial rectus muscles control outturning (abduction) and inturning (adduction), respectively, with the remaining four

**TABLE 59-1 Extrinsic Muscles**

| NAME | FUNCTION |
|---|---|
| Superior rectus | Rotates eye upward and toward the nose |
| Inferior rectus | Rotates eye downward and toward the nose |
| Lateral rectus | Moves eye toward the temporal side |
| Medial rectus | Moves eye toward the nose |
| Inferior oblique | Rotates eye upward and toward the temporal side |
| Superior oblique | Rotates eye downward and toward the temporal side |

muscles having primary, secondary, and tertiary actions. The combined actions of all six extraocular muscles vary, depending on the person's direction of gaze (see Table 59-1).

The intrinsic involuntary muscles within the eye are the ciliary muscles (in the ciliary body), which control the shape of the lens, and the sphincter and dilator pupillae muscles in the iris, which control pupil size and consequently the amount of light that enters the eye.

## EYELIDS AND CONJUNCTIVA

The *eyelids* (palpebrae) are made up of *thin layers of skin, muscle, fibrous tissue, and mucous membrane.* The main purposes of the eyelids are to protect the eye from external irritation, spread tears over the front of the eye, and interrupt and restrict the amount of light entering the eye. The *conjunctiva,* the mucous membrane lining of the eyelid (palpebral conjunctiva) that extends over the anterior sclera (bulbar conjunctiva), is of particular significance. This membrane and its blood vessels provide nutrients, antibodies, and leukocytes to the avascular cornea. The conjunctiva and glands within the eyelid secrete mucus and oil, which help keep the cornea moist and clear and decrease friction when the lids blink over the cornea.

## LACRIMAL SYSTEM

The lacrimal system consists of the *lacrimal gland* and a *tear drainage system* (Figure 59-5). The lacrimal gland produces the tears that flow across the eye and enter the drainage system nasally. Each time the eyelids blink, the tears are pumped by the blinking action and flow across the surface of the eyes. The tears flow through small holes in the eyelids (puncti) and ducts (canaliculi) to the lacrimal sac. They then drain into the nasolacrimal duct through the opening of the inferior meatus of the nasal cavity. Tears keep the surface of the eye and conjunctiva moistened and lubricated. Tears also contain an enzyme that functions as an antibacterial agent.

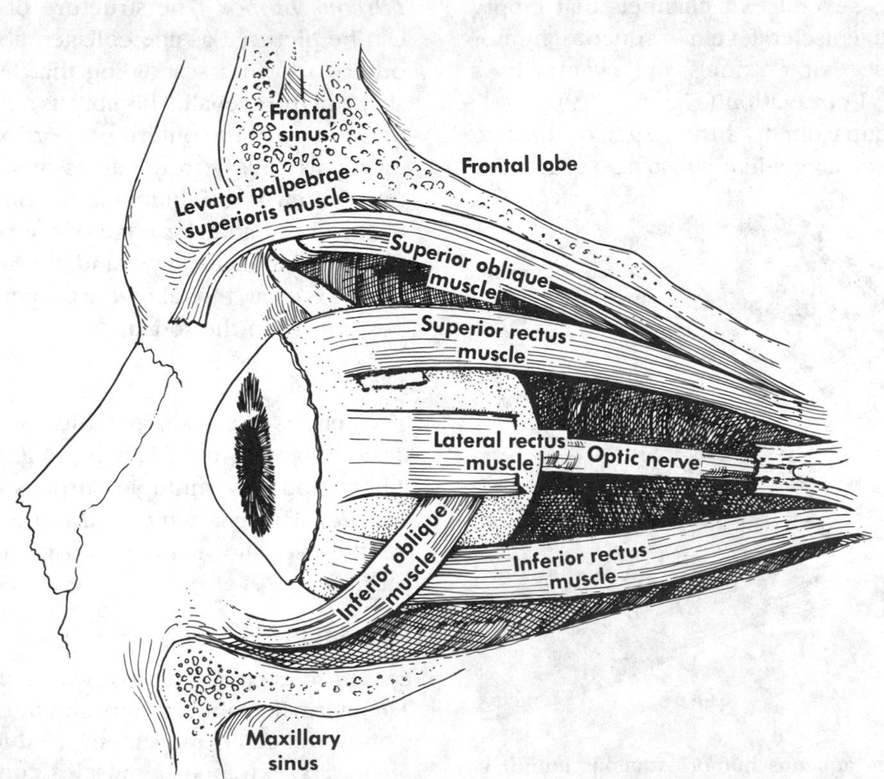


**FIGURE 59-4** Extrinsic muscles of the eye. Both oblique muscles insert behind the equator of the globe. The inferior oblique muscle passes inferior to the body of the inferior rectus muscle but beneath the lateral rectus muscle. (From Newell FW: *Ophthalmology: principles and concepts,* ed 7, St Louis, 1992, Mosby.)

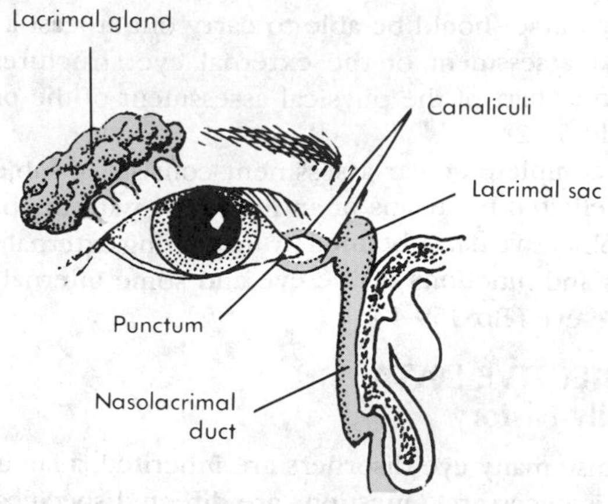


**FIGURE 59-5** Lacrimal system.

## ORBIT

The eye rests within the confines of the bony orbit. This orbit is a cone-shaped cavity formed by the *union of cranial and facial bones.* The eyeball itself occupies only about one fifth of the space of the orbit. The remainder is filled with the lacrimal gland, muscles, blood vessels, nerves, and fatty tissue. This fatty tissue serves as a protective cushion for the eye. The optic nerve exits the orbit posteriorly, transmitting visual information from the eye to the brain.

## PHYSIOLOGY OF VISION

Light rays entering the eye are bent **(refracted)** as they pass over the curved surfaces of the cornea and through the various (more posterior) structures of the eye (aqueous humor, lens, vitreous humor)—which have varying densities—to focus on the retina. The cornea provides the major refractive change for light entering the eye, with the lens providing the fine focus for light transmitted posteriorly to the retina.

The eye can adjust *(accommodation)* to *seeing objects at various distances* by the *flattening or thickening of the lens.* Near vision requires contraction of the ciliary body, which decreases the distance between the edges of the ciliary body, thus relaxing the zonules attached to the lens. The lens then bulges to bend the light rays more acutely so that the rays will focus on the retina. Accommodation also is facilitated by changing the size of the pupil. With near vision the iris constricts the pupil to force light rays to pass through the shortened but thicker lens. The pupils also constrict with bright lights to protect the retina from intense stimulation.

Light rays are absorbed by the photoreceptors on the retina, changed to electrical activity, and transmitted via the optic nerve to the visual cortex areas of the brain for processing. The fibers of the optic nerve (cranial nerve II; see Chapter 56) divide at the optic chiasm; the medial portion of each nerve crosses to the opposite side (see Figure 56-20), and the impulses are then transmitted to the visual cortex. In this way, visual information received by each eye is transmitted simultaneously to both sides of the brain. *Bilateral vision provides depth perception.*

## CHANGES WITH AGING

Aging affects many aspects of visual function, both physiologic and anatomic. Decreased flexibility and elasticity of the lens lead to one of the first noted signs of aging—the decreased ability of the eye to focus (accommodate) for near and detailed work (presbyopia).

The lens also yellows with age. This causes greater difficulty in distinguishing among colors at the blue end of the spectrum. A smaller pupil (senile miosis) adds to this distortion of color. It also affects the amount of light that reaches the retina and the ability of the person to adapt to dim light and darkness. Persons older than 60 years of age need about twice as much light to see as they did when they were 20.[3]

This needed increase in light for close work can cause another aging problem—glare. Glare, a veil-like luminance superimposed on the retinal image, masks and reduces the brightness of objects in the visual field.[8] Glare is related to increased light scatter in the eye caused by corneal, scleral, lens, and vitreal changes.

The field of vision also begins to decrease, affecting the breadth of vision that is possible. It is uncertain whether this decrease is caused by retinal changes, decreased pupil size, or loss of lens transparency.

*The decrease in lens transparency, which begins to appear in the fifth decade of life, is not fully understood.* The compression of lens fibers, the yellowing of the lens, and the efficiency of aqueous humor may all play a part in the increased opaqueness of the lens, leading to cataract formation.

*Aqueous humor production drops off sharply in the sixth decade.* This compensates for the reduced drainage and shallowness of the anterior chamber. This combination of events enables the eye to maintain a relatively stable intraocular pressure.[5]

The quantity and quality of tears decrease with age, and the tears tend to evaporate more readily. The eyes take on a duller appearance, and there is a feeling of tightness, scratchiness, or dryness. Instillation of artificial tears may relieve these symptoms. The drainage system for the tears also is less efficient. This may lead to a block in the system, with tearing as a result.

One of the more common eye changes that results from aging is *arcus senilis.* This *hazy gray ring around the periphery of the cornea is a result of fat deposits through the layers of the cornea.* Another important change in the cornea is its change in shape. It tends to flatten, resulting in an irregular curvature in the corneal surface. Light entering the eye tends to be refracted at varying angles, leading to a distorted and blurred image (astigmatism).

# ASSESSMENT OF EYES AND VISION

Examination of the eyes can be one of the most rewarding aspects of a physical examination. It is relatively easy to measure both the stimulus and the response of the entire visual system by the measurement of visual acuity. The tissues of the eye are for the most part transparent, making *abnormalities easily detectable.* Ocular manifestations of systemic disease also can be identified. In addition, the vascular system (retinal vascular system) and cranial nerve (optic nerve) of the eye can be visualized on examination.

Assessment of the eye's structure and functioning is performed by ophthalmologists, other physicians, nurses, optometrists, and paraprofessional health workers. Nurses often are trained to conduct vision screening tests with preschool children. Assessment includes inspection of the external structures and gross measures of visual acuity. More complete eye examinations, such as electrophysiologic studies of the retina and other fundus examinations, are performed by physicians in conjunction with specially trained nurses or technicians.

The nurse's role in assessment of the eye and vision depends on the place of employment, the nurse's preparation, and the patient's age and health. For instance, a nurse working in a community health agency may have the need and opportunity to do more extensive eye assessment than a nurse in a teaching hospital where physicians need an opportunity to learn these skills.

**TABLE 59-2 Basic Assessment of the Eye and Vision**

| | |
|---|---|
| Facial and ocular expression | Prominence of eyes; alert or dull expression |
| Eyelids and conjunctiva | Symmetry, presence of edema, ptosis, itching, redness, discharges, blinking, equality, growths |
| Lacrimal system | Tears, swelling, growths |
| Sclera | Color |
| Cornea | Clarity |
| Anterior chamber | Depth, presence of blood/pus |
| Iris and pupils | Irregularities in color, shape, size |
| Pupillary reflex | |
| Light | Constriction of pupil in response to light in that eye (direct light reaction); equal amount of constriction in the other eye (consensual light reaction) |
| Accommodation | Convergence of eyes and constriction of pupil as gaze shifts from far to near object |
| Lens | Transparent or opaque |
| Peripheral vision | Ability to see movements and objects well on both sides of field of vision |
| Acuity with and without glasses | Ability to read newsprint, clocks on wall, and name tags and to recognize faces at bedside and at door |
| Supportive aids | Glasses, contact lenses, prosthesis |

Every nurse should be able to carry out at least a basic ocular assessment of the external eye structures and vision as part of the physical assessment of the patient (Table 59-2).

A complete ocular assessment consists of subjective data elicited by means of an interview with the patient and objective data obtained by inspecting external structures and functions of the eye and some internal parts of the eye (Box 59-1).

## SUBJECTIVE DATA

### Family History

Because many eye disorders are inherited, a family history is necessary. Questions are directed specifically to family history of cataracts, glaucoma, diabetes mellitus, poor vision that could not be corrected by glasses, or blindness.

### Symptoms Associated With Eye Disorders

In addition to any current complaints, the person's previous eye problems, diagnoses, and treatment are recorded. Also, the patient's general state of health, presence of systemic diseases such as diabetes and hypertension, and ocular and systemic medication history should be determined. The nurse should ask if the person perceives any of the following: changes in visual acuity; abnormal signs and symptoms such as burning, tearing, or blurred vision; and events surrounding onset of symptoms, duration of symptoms, and sources of relief.

## OBJECTIVE DATA

### Inspection of External Structures

The nurse will first inspect the general appearance of the face and eyes of the patient, observing for the type of expression (dull or alert) and prominence of the eyes. The presence of an abnormal protrusion or bulging of an eye is called **exophthalmia** or **exophthalmos.** In elderly persons the eyes tend to sink into the orbit **(enophthalmos).** This is caused primarily by the loss of orbital fat.

The appearance of the *eyelids* is noted in relation to color, texture, mobility, and position. The lids should be able to close completely to prevent drying of the conjunctiva and cornea. Any swelling, redness, or dis-

**BOX 59-1 Ocular Assessment**

- Recording of history
- Assessment of vision
- Assessment of ocular movement
- Assessment of pupillary reflexes
- Assessment of visual fields
- Inspection of external structures
- Inspection of internal structures
- Estimation of intraocular pressure

charge is noted. If one upper lid seems to be in a position lower than the other, or "droops," the condition may be *ptosis* of the eyelid. If ptosis is present in both eyes, the upper lid is noted to be in an abnormally low position, covering the upper portion or more of the iris. Ptosis of the upper lids may be the result of extreme debility or neuromuscular disease. Extreme ptosis can interfere with vision by covering the pupil.

As the person ages, the eyelids become thinner and less elastic and positional defects may occur. In addition to ptosis, ectropion, entropion, and dematochalasis may be present. Ectropion is eversion of the lower lid. It is usually bilateral, and symptoms include tearing and irritation. Entropion is the turning in of the eyelids. The person experiences a foreign body sensation caused by the eyelashes rubbing against the cornea. Dermatochalasis is a redundancy of upper or lower lid tissues. This usually occurs from loss of elasticity and results in wrinkles and drooping folds.

The *conjunctiva* of the lower lid is examined by pulling downward on the lid as the person looks upward (Figure 59-6). To examine the conjunctiva of the upper lid, the lid must be everted (Figure 59-7).

The lacrimal gland normally is not observable. Enlargement of the gland may occur in certain disorders such as inflammation. This may be most evident when the upper lid is everted. The lacrimal sac may be palpated on the temporal side of the nasal bone for patency of the lacrimal puncta.

Small blood vessels normally are visible in the conjunctiva. The *sclera* shows through the conjunctiva and has a shiny porcelain-like appearance. Dilation of blood vessels of the conjunctiva may indicate disease of the cornea or disease within the eye. Spontaneous small hemorrhages may occur beneath the conjunctiva in the normal eye. A yellow discoloration of the sclera indicates jaundice.

The *cornea,* which is normally visible except for surface reflections, must be smooth and transparent for good vision. It should look shiny and bright when examined with a penlight. Moving the light and directing it from the side, the examiner looks for abrasions and opacities. If the cornea is clear, the iris and pupils should be clearly visible.

Defects in the epithelium of the cornea may be demonstrated with the use of topical dyes. Before instilling the topical dye, the nurse should first ask the person to remove contact lenses, if present, because the dye tends to stain soft contact lenses. The dye is put in the conjunctiva by drops or by touching the conjunctiva with a moistened strip of filter paper that has been impregnated with the dye. Because the injured tissue remains stained, visualization of foreign bodies, abrasions, and inflammation of the cornea is possible.

Fluorescein is the most commonly used dye, although rose bengal and methylene blue also are available. The latter two dyes stain more deeply than does fluorescein

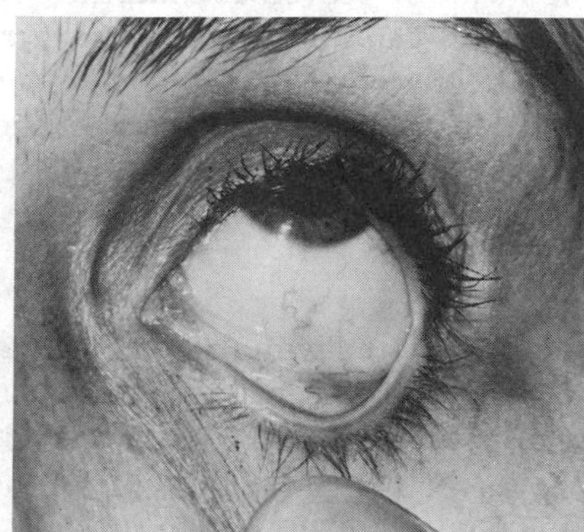

**FIGURE 59-6** Eversion of lower eyelid by drawing the margin downward as subject looks upward. (From Newell F: *Ophthalmology: principles and concepts,* ed 7, St Louis, 1992, Mosby.)

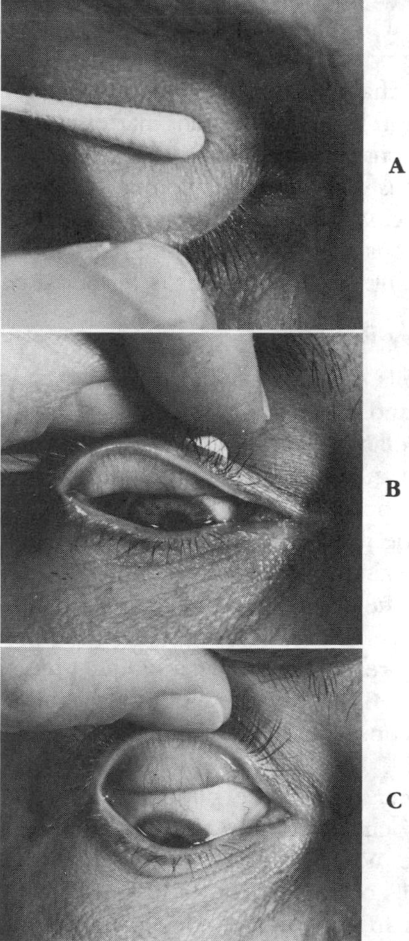


**FIGURE 59-7** Eversion of upper eyelid. Patient is instructed to look downward, and lashes of upper eyelid are grasped between thumb and index finger. **A,** Cotton-tipped applicator is placed at level of tarsal fold. **B,** Eyelid is folded back on applicator while patient continues to look downward. **C,** Applicator is removed. (From Newell FW: *Ophthalmology: principles and concepts,* ed 7, St Louis, 1992, Mosby.)

but are more irritating. After the test, the nurse should cleanse the dye from the patient's face with a moist tissue.

Occasionally, a physician may have the nurse perform a *tear test (Schirmer).* This tear test usually is performed to verify abnormal tear production *(dry eyes).* The nurse should explain the procedure to patients and inform them that the test may be uncomfortable but is not painful. The quantity of tears is measured with a strip of filter paper, 5 × 35 mm, that is folded 5 mm from the end. The folded end is hooked over the lower lid and is left in place for approximately 5 minutes. The extent to which the filter paper is soaked with tears beyond the fold is then measured. Tear formation generally is considered normal if 10 to 15 mm or more of the filter paper is moistened. More than 25 mm of moistened paper indicates excessive tear formation.

The anterior chamber, the dome-shaped space between the back of the cornea and the front of the iris, should be examined. The anterior chamber is bathed in aqueous humor and has a normal depth of 3 to 3.5 mm. Blood and purulent matter in the anterior chamber may interfere with vision. When blood is observed in the anterior chamber, the condition is called a **hyphema; hypopyon** is when purulent matter accumulates in the anterior chamber.

The *iris* of each eye is compared for color, pattern, and shape. When looking through the pupillary opening, the nurse is also inspecting the *lens,* which is normally transparent. An opaque lens is termed a *cataract.*

## Pupillary Reflexes

The pupils normally should be equal, round, and react to light and accommodation (PERRLA). When assessing the pupillary reflexes, the nurse approaches from the side and quickly shines a light into one eye, causing constriction of the pupil in that eye (direct light reaction). The pupil of the other eye also should constrict the same amount (consensual light reaction) (see Chapter 56). The other eye is then tested in the same manner.

A light shining into a blind eye will not produce a pupillary response; however, a light shining into a normal eye will produce a pupillary response in the blind eye by consensual reaction if the oculomotor nerve is intact.[2]

Another test of the pupillary reflex is to have the person focus on an object that is moved directly toward the nose. When the person focuses on the near object, the pupils of both eyes should constrict (near reaction, reaction in accommodation). The examiner looks for the presence of a response and whether the response is equal in both eyes. Loss of pupillary reflexes when sight is present is caused by neurologic disease.

## Assessment of Vision

Visual acuity means acuteness or sharpness of vision and includes measurement of distance and near vision. Visual acuity can vary with attention, intelligence, and physical conditions such as lighting.[7] The nurse who works in a clinic, an ophthalmologist's office, or a school must know how to perform vision screening tests and how to teach others to do them.

### Distance vision

Distance vision usually is determined by the use of a *Snellen* chart (Figure 59-8, *A*), with the person standing 20 feet (6 m) from the chart. The chart consists of rows of letters, numbers, or other characters arranged with the larger ones at the top and the smaller ones at the bottom. The uppermost letter on the chart is scaled so that it can be read by the normal eye at 200 feet, and the successive rows are scaled so that they can be read at 100, 70, 50, 40, 30, 20, 15, and 10 feet, respectively (see Figure 59-8, *A*, for distances in meters). Visual acuity is expressed as a fraction, and a reading of 20/20 (6/6) is considered normal. The upper figure refers to the distance of the person from the chart, and the lower figure indicates the distance at which a normal eye can read the line. The distance from the chart to where the patient stands must be carefully measured. The nurse indicates the line to be read so that no mistake occurs. Each eye is tested separately, and its performance is carefully recorded. The person is tested with and without distance lenses. When vision is tested, a piece of stiff paper or a plastic occluder is placed over one eye while the other eye is tested.

For preschool children, illiterate adults, and others unable to read the English alphabet, a modified Snellen chart may be used (Figure 59-8, *B*). A block E is shown in varying positions, and the person is asked to indicate in which direction the "legs" or "fingers" of the E point. In addition to the modified Snellen chart, a variety of other visual acuity testing charts are available for measuring visual acuity in preschool children (Figure 59-8, *B*). For example, the Allen charts have various silhouetted pictures, such as a telephone, that the child is asked to identify. It can be difficult to measure visual acuity in the infant or preverbal child. However, three objective measures can be used to assist in estimating visual acuity. These are the optokinetic nystagmus test, the preferential-looking test, and visual evoked potentials.[4] Specialized training is required to perform these three tests of visual acuity.

### Near vision

Near vision can be tested with the use of a *Jaeger* chart or newsprint. The Jaegar chart is a card containing varying sizes of print and is held 35 cm (14 inches) from the eye. The score obtained can be expressed in Snellen, metric, and percentage figures.

For persons unable to read the letters on the charts, another method of assessing visual acuity is for the examiner to hold fingers in front of their eyes and ask them to count the number of fingers that they can see. Other

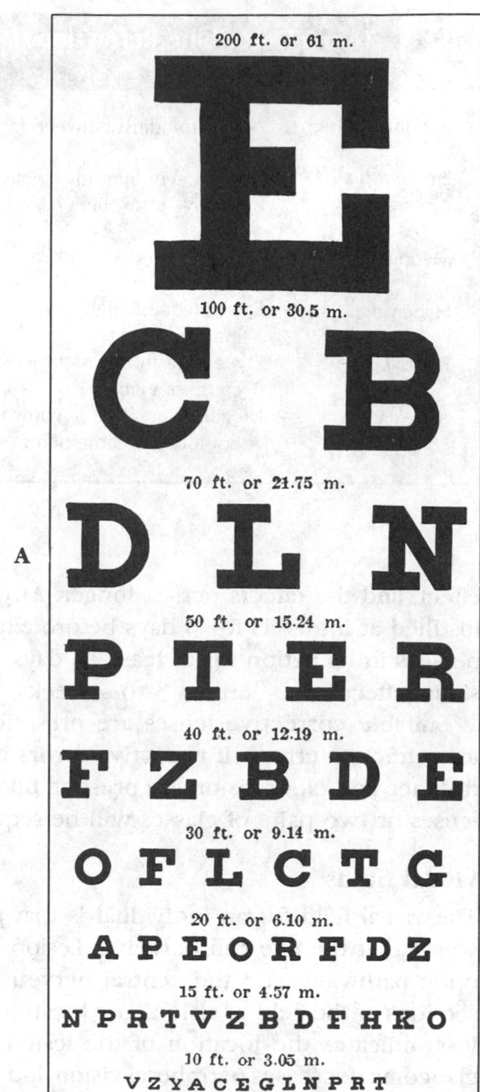


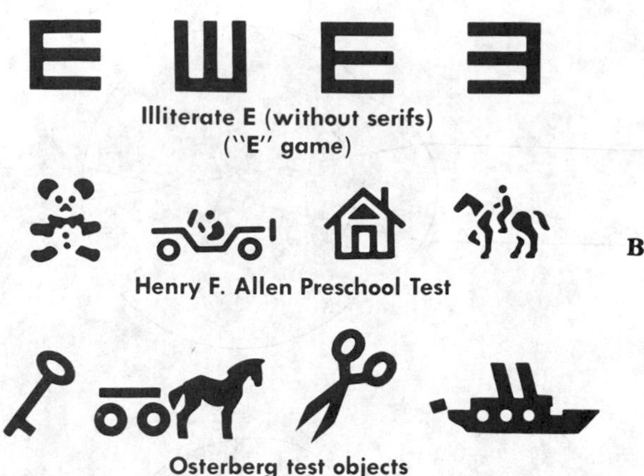


**FIGURE 59-8** **A,** Snellen chart used in testing vision. **B,** Symbols used in testing distance vision in children and illiterate adults. (Modified from Newell FW: *Ophthalmology: principles and concepts,* ed 7, St Louis, 1992, Mosby.)

**TABLE 59-3 Examples of Visual Acuity Measurement**

| MEASUREMENT | MEANING |
|---|---|
| 20/20 | Normal |
| 20/40-2 | Missed two letters of the 20/40 line |
| 10/400 | At 10 ft, reads line that normal eye sees at 400 ft |
| CF/2 ft | Counts fingers at 2 ft |
| HM/3 ft | Sees hand movement at 3 ft |
| LP/Proj. | Light perception with projection |
| NLP | No light perception |

persons may not be able to count fingers but can see hand movement. Still others may be able to tell only the direction from which light is coming (light projection) or just respond to light flashed in their eyes (light perception). Table 59-3 outlines some examples of visual acuity measurements.

Any person with vision less than 20/30 OD (right eye) or OS (left eye) or with a two-line difference between eyes should be referred to an ophthalmologist for further testing and treatment. The Snellen, block E, or Jaegar chart examinations provide only basic screening test data. Additional detailed procedures are used to test for nearsightedness, astigmatism, color blindness, and many other abnormalities.

## Refraction

A ray of light entering the eye passes through the various transparent refractive media and is bent (refracted) to focus on the retina. The bending of the light rays and the location of the image depend on the shape and condition of the eye. The eye has the ability to adjust to near or far objects *(accommodation)* by means of the ciliary muscles, which contract or relax, causing the lens to flatten or thicken as the need arises. If the anteroposterior dimension of the eye is abnormally long, the light rays will focus in front of the retina **(myopia)** (Figure 59-9, *A*). Conversely, if the anteroposterior dimension is abnormally short, the rays will focus behind the retina **(hyperopia)** (Figure 59-9, *B*). When the lens becomes less elastic and responds less to the need for accommodation, as occurs in persons past the age of 40 years, blurring of near objects **(presbyopia)** results. The curvature of the cornea also may be asymmetric or irregular so that rays in the horizontal and vertical planes do not focus at the same point **(astigmatism).**

When the image is not clearly focused on the retina, *refractive error* is present (Box 59-2). Refractive errors account for the largest number of impairments of good vision. The refractive error is tested by means of trial lenses and the Snellen chart (see Figure 59-8, *A*). A simple means to determine whether a refractive error is present is to have the person look at the Snellen chart

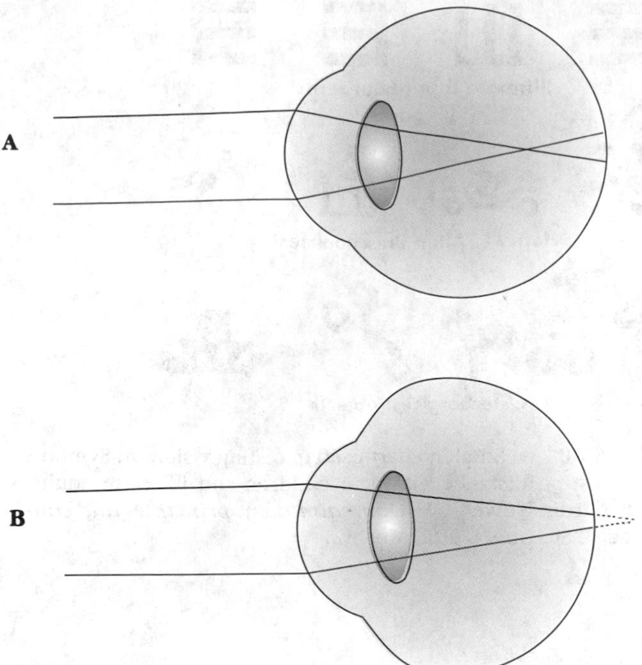


**FIGURE 59-9** Two major types of refractive errors. **A,** Myopia. Parallel light rays come to a focus in front of the retina. **B,** Hyperopia. Parallel light rays come to a focus behind the retina.

**BOX 59-2 Terms Describing Refraction**

| | |
|---|---|
| Accommodation | Ability to adjust between far and near objects |
| Emmetropia | Normal eye; light rays focus on retina |
| Ametropia | Refractive error; light rays do not focus on retina |
| Myopia | Nearsightedness; light rays focus in front of retina |
| Hyperopia | Farsightedness; light rays focus behind retina |
| Presbyopia | Hyperopia from loss of lens elasticity because of aging |
| Astigmatism | Irregular curvature of cornea; light rays do not focus at same point |

through a small opening in an opaque shield (pinhole shield). Vision usually is improved if a refractive error is present. This occurs because only light rays that are nearly parallel to the visual axis are seen.

In situations in which formal acuity testing equipment is not available, estimates of refractive error can be made. For instance, the person can be asked to read print or identify pictures at varying distances. The person's visual acuity can be compared with that of the examiner's.

To obtain a more definitive refractive error measurement in children and adults, a *cycloplegic* drug often is instilled before the examination. A cycloplegic drug temporarily dilates the pupil and paralyzes the ciliary muscle (placing it at rest), thus paralyzing accommodation. This is called a *cycloplegic refraction.* Cyclopentolate (Cyclogyl), 1% or 2%, usually is used because it is effective in 30 minutes and the effect generally wears off completely by the end of 6 hours. The duration of effect will vary, however, lasting longer than 6 hours in persons with a light-blue iris. A blue-eyed person's iris will dilate more rapidly and remain dilated longer than that of a brown-eyed person because more of the drug is absorbed into an iris with less pigmentation.

When the appointment is made for an eye examination with the use of a cycloplegic drug, the person is told that blurred vision will be present after the examination. It should be explained that driving or reading will not be possible until the effect of the drug subsides. Atropine occasionally is used for younger children to achieve cycloplegia, but this drug requires longer to take effect, and the effects persist longer. Atropine must be instilled at intervals for 3 days before examination and persists in its action for at least 10 days with some residual effect for as long as 3 to 4 weeks.

Suitable corrective lenses are prescribed if needed for refractive errors. If refractive errors involving both distance and close vision are present, bifocal or trifocal lenses or two pairs of glasses will be required.

### Visual fields

The visual field for an individual is that portion of the world that the eye can perceive. Lesions of the retina, optic pathways, and the central nervous system affect sections of the field of vision. The location of visual field loss indicates the location of the lesion. For instance, glaucoma decreases peripheral vision, indicating damage to the optic nerve at its head or the optic disc. A rough measurement of the visual fields can be made with the confrontation test (see Chapter 56). If there appears to be any abnormality in the field of vision, more precise testing should be performed with precision instruments by an ophthalmologist or a specially trained technician. One precise method by which the patient's peripheral vision can be plotted is the perimeter, an instrument that measures the visual fields in degrees of arc. The tangent screen is the simplest perimeter, in which peripheral vision is plotted as a test object is moved against a black screen. Also, several automated and computer-assisted perimeters, such as the Octopus, are used to measure a patient's visual field.

Another method used to measure the visual field is the *Amsler grid.* The Amsler grid is a 20-cm square that is divided into 5-mm squares with a dot in the center (Figure 59-10). The grid is employed to detect and follow a *central area of blindness* **(scotoma).** It most commonly is used at home by the patient to detect progression of a macular disease (central visual area).

With glasses on and one eye closed, the person holds the grid at the customary reading distance (12 inches).

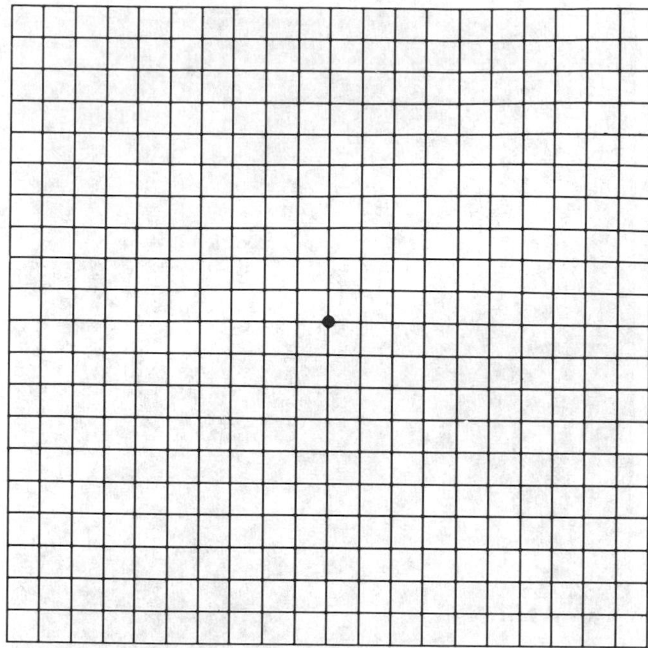

**FIGURE 59-10** The Amsler grid.

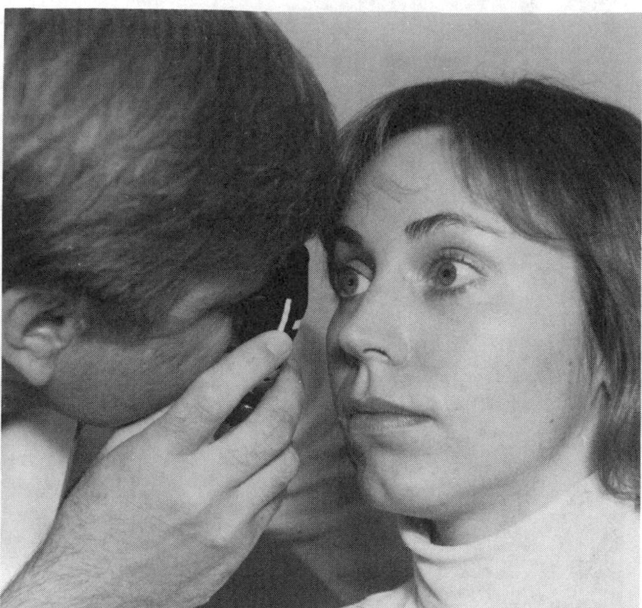

**FIGURE 59-11** Direct method of ophthalmoscopic examination. (Photo by Stephen M. Beazley.)

While fixating at the central dot, the person describes and outlines any area of distortion or absence of the grid. Distortions or "blind spots" are abnormal and imply dysfunction of the central retina (macula) or diseases of the optic nerve. The patient who is performing the test at home should be taught to call the physician immediately if there are any changes.

#### Color vision testing

Color vision testing is not always part of the normal eye examination. It is used most frequently to test for color blindness in those persons seeking motor vehicle licenses or jobs in which color discrimination is important.

There are both gross and sensitive measures of color vision. A common test consists of color plates on which numbers are outlined in primary colors and surrounded by confusion colors. The person with a color vision problem is unable to recognize the figure. The more sensitive tests involve hue discrimination. One such test consists of 84 chips of color that are matched in terms of increasing hue.

Color vision deficiencies occur as a hereditary defect in both men (7%) and women (0.5%). Nutritional deficiencies, drug toxicities, and various disorders of the optic nerve and fovea centralis also can alter color perception.

### Assessment of Ocular Movements

Ocular movements are evaluated to determine whether the eyes are moving in a synchronous manner. Muscle imbalances and cranial nerve damage also can be detected.

To test ocular muscles the nurse and patient being tested are seated facing each other. While the patient looks straight ahead at a target, a penlight is shined on the cornea. The corneal light reflex should be in exactly the same position on each pupil. The nurse then covers one of the person's eyes while the person looks at the light. When the cover is quickly removed, the nurse notes whether that eye moves to regain fixation on the light. Movement may indicate a drift of the eye behind the cover, which can indicate muscle imbalances.

To evaluate possible weaknesses of individual extraocular muscles, muscle balance testing can be performed in six cardinal fields of gaze, as well as straight ahead. The reader is referred to Chapter 56 for more detailed information about assessment of ocular movements.

### Inspection of Internal Structures

#### Ophthalmoscopy

The fundus of the eye is examined with a hand-held instrument called an *ophthalmoscope,* which magnifies the view of the back of the eye so that the optic nerve, retina, blood vessels, and macula can be seen through the pupil. The examiner may use either the ***direct*** (Figure 59-11) or the ***indirect*** (Figure 59-12) ***method of ophthalmoscopic examination.*** The indirect ophthalmoscope allows the examiner to view the retina stereoscopically, thus allowing a wide-angle, three-dimensional view. This method provides visualization of the ocular fundus as far as the ora serrata (anterior margin of the retina). The indirect method, which requires a great degree of skill, normally is performed by an ophthalmologist. Nurses trained to perform an ophthalmoscopic examination use the direct method, which is

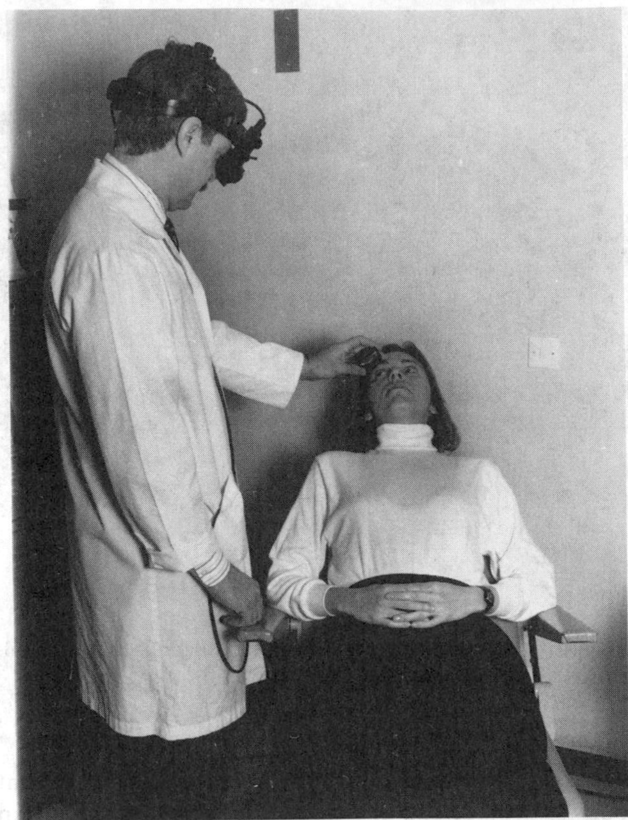

FIGURE 59-12 Indirect method of ophthalmoscopic examination. (Photo by Stephen M. Beazley.)

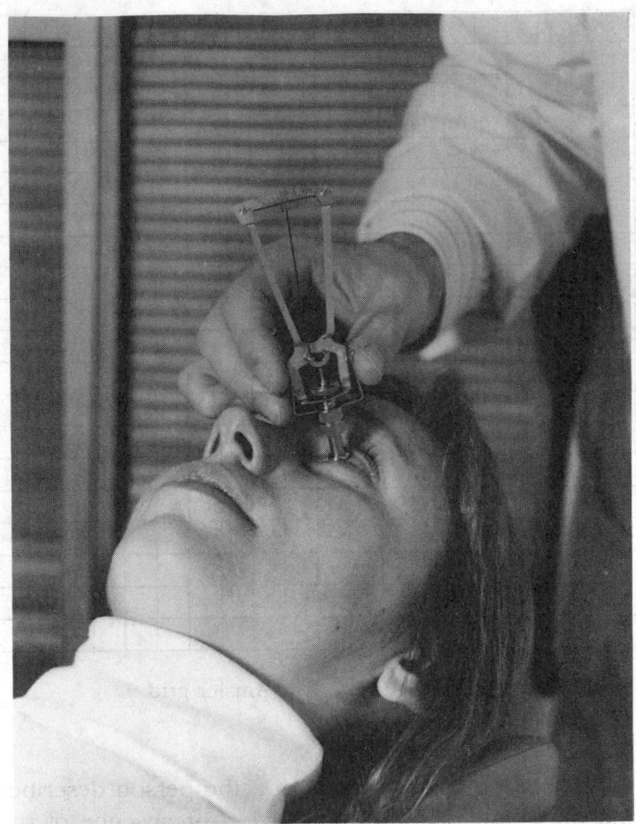

FIGURE 59-13 Measurement of intraocular pressure with Schiøtz tonometer. (Photo by Stephen M. Beazley.)

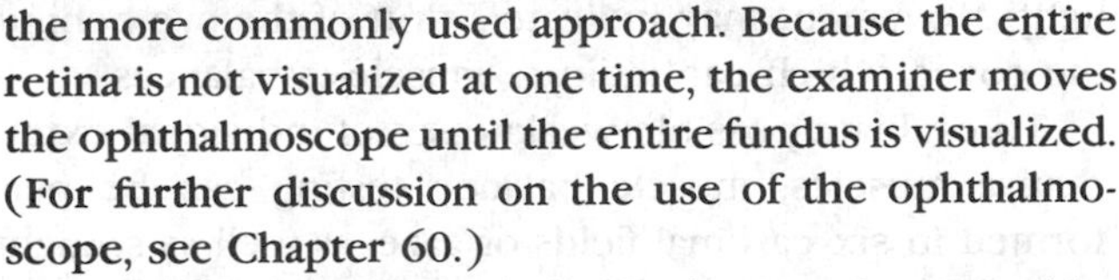

the more commonly used approach. Because the entire retina is not visualized at one time, the examiner moves the ophthalmoscope until the entire fundus is visualized. (For further discussion on the use of the ophthalmoscope, see Chapter 60.)

Difficulty in perceiving the fundus may be caused by interference with the light penetrating the eye as a result of intraocular inflammation, corneal scarring, or cataract. Data obtained from visualization of the fundus may indicate eye disease (cupping of the disc in glaucoma) or systemic disease (arteriosclerosis or hypertension). Hemorrhages in deep retinal layers occur in advanced hypertension, severe renal disease, certain collagen diseases, advanced diabetes, and blood dyscrasias.

### Slit-lamp examination of the fundus

The ophthalmologist can examine the interior of the eye with a slit-lamp microscope in a darkened room. The slit-lamp is an instrument that combines a microscope and a light source and is used to examine the anterior segment of the eye. By adjusting the lens, the examiner can test the person's eye for such changes as corneal ulcerations, lens changes, foreign bodies in the vitreous, or retinal changes. With the use of a contact lens on the surface of the cornea, the slit-lamp also can be used to examine the retina.

## Estimation of Intraocular Pressure

An instrument known as a *tonometer* is used to measure ocular tension and is helpful in detecting early glaucoma. Some ophthalmologists suggest that tonometric readings be taken by the medical internist or the family physician as part of a regular annual physical examination. The most common indentation tonometer in clinical use is that of Schiøtz. The procedure is performed with the patient lying down or in the chair with the head back and looking upward at some fixed point. The eye may be anesthetized with one or two drops of proparacaine hydrochloride (Ophthaine), 0.5%, after which the tonometer is placed on the cornea (Figure 59-13). While the weight of the tonometer is supported by the cornea, the amount of indentation that the plunger of the instrument makes in the cornea is measured on the attached scale. This reading is used to determine the pressure within the eye. Readings over 24 torr (Schiøtz) may suggest glaucoma, but tests usually are repeated because temporary increases sometimes may be caused by such things as emotional stress. The applanation tonometer (Goldmann) is more accurate in estimating intraocular pressure (Figure 59-14). The most commonly used *applanation tonometer* is attached to the slit-lamp, although hand-held models are available. Instead of indenting the eye, a small area of the cornea is flattened

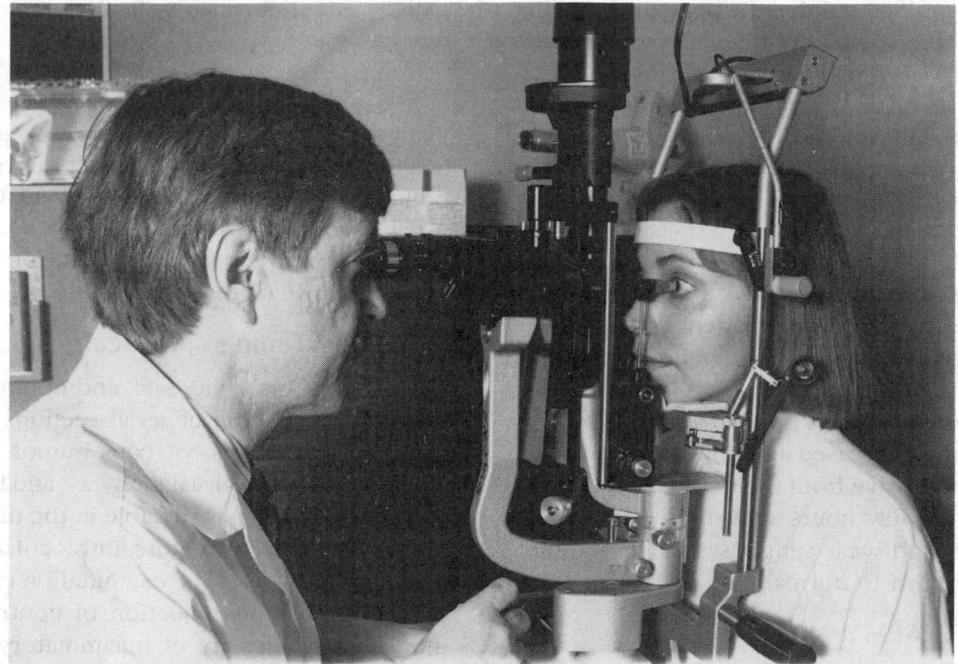

**FIGURE 59-14** Measurement of ocular tension with applanation tonometer. (Photo by Stephen M. Beazley.)

to counterbalance a spring-loaded measuring device and the pressure is measured directly.

The noncontact tonometer also is available for measuring intraocular pressure. This applanation instrument uses a puff of air to flatten a circular area of the cornea, thus bypassing the necessity for physical contact between the tonometer and the eye. This test does not require the eye to be anesthetized.

# DIAGNOSTIC TESTS

## FLUORESCEIN ANGIOGRAPHY

Fluorescein angiography is a specialized procedure used in the diagnosis, monitoring, and treatment of eye diseases. After the pupil is dilated, fluorescein dye is injected into the antecubital fossa of the patient's arm. The retinal and ciliary arteries transmit the dye into the eyes, and the *retinal arteriovenous circulation* is visualized. The dye reaches the retinal arteries 10 to 16 seconds after the injection, and the veins are filled within 25 seconds. To provide a permanent record of this circulation, photographs are taken with a specially designed camera called a *fundus camera*. The fundus camera is equipped with an optical system for viewing the retina, a 35-mm camera with a film advance mechanism, and a light flash system for illumination. The fundus camera is mounted on a stand similar to that for a slit-lamp. The patient sits in a chair with the chin placed in the chin rest and the forehead against a bar while a rapid series of photographs are taken to capture the movement of the dye through the retinal arteriovenous circulation. This test may take as long as 1 hour to complete. When the photographs are assessed, they provide definitive information about any avascular obstruction, the growth of new vessels (neovascularization), microaneurysms, abnormal capillary permeability, and defects in the pigmented layer of the retina.

Fluorescein angiography is a relatively safe procedure with few untoward effects. Before administering the fluorescein dye, the nurse asks if the patient has any allergies or has had any previous reactions to dyes. Those with a history of hay fever or asthma may be given a small test dose before the entire dose is injected.[1] Although rare, a severe allergic reaction can occur; therefore epinephrine and emergency resuscitation equipment should be readily available. This test is contraindicated for those who are pregnant or have a history of an allergic reaction to the dye.

### Pretest

Before the procedure, the nurse explains the procedure and obtains an informed consent. The nurse also explains the need to keep the head still and move just the eyes as the photographer indicates. It also can be explained that the worst thing the patient is likely to experience is a dazzle effect caused by the frequent camera flashes. Before the test, mydriatic eyedrops (phenylephrine hydrochloride 2.5% and tropicamide 1%) will be instilled to dilate the pupils, facilitating visualization of the fundus (back of the eye). The dye is administered by the nurse or other specially trained ophthalmic personnel, and the photographs are taken by an ophthalmic photographer. Some patients may experience transient nausea or vomiting. Care must be taken when the dye is injected because it can cause intense burning at the injection site if leakage into subcutaneous tissue occurs.

### Posttest

Patients should be told that they may be unable to see for a few minutes after the test because of the *dazzle effect*.[2] The nurse also informs the patient that yellowing of the skin, especially in persons with fair complexions, and a fluorescent orange or green discoloration of the urine usually is present for 24 hours. Patients should be encouraged to drink increased amounts of fluids to promote excretion of the dye from their system. The pupils remain dilated for a few hours, and the patient should avoid bright light and wear sunglasses when outdoors until the pupils return to normal.

## ULTRASONOGRAPHY

Ultrasonography provides a noninvasive test that uses high-frequency sound waves to pass through soft tissues and fluid *to outline and detect intraocular and orbital structures,* as well as to measure the distance between them. Various abnormalities, such as *retinal masses* and *detachments, intraocular foreign bodies,* and *changes in the orbit,* can be easily delineated by this test. Two types of ultrasonography, A-scan and B-scan, are used in ophthalmology. The A-scan is useful in differentiating between benign and malignant tumors and measuring the axial length of the eyeball. The axial length of the eyeball is needed to calculate the power of an intraocular lens for implantation after a cataract extraction. The B-scan provides a two-dimensional image that helps visualize tumors, retinal detachments, swollen muscles, or inflamed tissue. The nurse gives the patient information about the procedure itself and any sensory effects. In both the A- and B-scan, a probe attached to a machine that delivers sound waves is placed on the front of the eye (or on the closed eyelid) and measurements are recorded on the screen of the oscilloscope. If the probe is applied directly to the eye, anesthetic drops may be instilled. The patient should be informed that the test is not uncomfortable. Specific information relating to the sensations the patient can expect include the feeling on the eyelids of the gel-like contact medium used on the transducer and feeling and hearing the vibration of the transducer on the eyelid.[6]

## RADIOLOGIC TESTS

Several radiologic procedures are used to aid in the diagnosis of eye conditions. These include plain x-ray films, computed tomography (CT) scans, and magnetic resonance imaging (MRI). The nurse's responsibility in all radiologic tests is to explain the procedure to the patient. Such information facilitates understanding and decreases anxiety.

### Plain X-Ray Films

Plain x-ray films of the orbit are used to assist in the diagnosis of orbital fractures and tumors. Right and left oblique views and a lateral view of the affected side usually provide the needed information. These views are obtained with the person lying face down with the forehead and nose or the chin resting on the table.

### Computed Tomography Scan

The CT scan is a rapid, safe, and noninvasive technique for the investigation of serial sections of the orbit and eye. The globe, lens, vitreous humor, optic nerve, extraocular muscles, visual pathway, and brain can be evaluated. The CT scan is valuable in the diagnosis of orbital disease, retrobulbar tumors, intraocular eye masses, and intracranial disease. The examination can be augmented by the intravenous injection of contrast material that increases the density of inflammatory or vascularized orbital lesions.[7] Therefore the nurse must first explain the procedure and then obtain an informed consent. The nurse should ask the patient about any previous reactions ("allergies") to the contrast material.

### Magnetic Resonance Imaging

MRI is a noninvasive technique of medical imaging that uses a high magnetic field to evaluate the brain, orbit, and eye. Pulses of energy alter the alignment of protons in the body (hydrogen, sodium, and phosphorus), releasing energy. The energy released varies from tissue to tissue in the brain and can be processed by a computer that generates a detailed picture. The test can provide a direct comparison with the results of a CT scan. However, MRI provides better definition of tissues and fluids in the brain and eye. It is particularly helpful in identifying edema (e.g., from trauma or brain tumors).[9] This test is contraindicated in pregnancy, and it should not be used in patients who have a cardiac pacemaker or who may be retaining metallic foreign bodies that could be dislodged by the magnetic field created during an MRI scan. Therefore the nurse will explain the procedure and ask about the presence of anything metallic in the patient's body, in which case another test, such as a CT scan, may be substituted.

## ELECTRODIAGNOSTIC EXAMINATION

Two of the electrodiagnostic examinations performed in ophthalmology are electroretinography and visual evoked potential.

### Electroretinography

Electroretinography (ERG) is a process of graphing the electrical response from the retina that occurs as a consequence of light stimulation. In this test the pupil is dilated, a topical anesthetic is applied, and a corneal electrode is placed on the cornea using a contact lens. A grounding electrode is placed on the ear. Lights at various intensities and intervals are then flashed and the nervous response graphed.

ERG is a test of the function of the rods and cones and is helpful in evaluating widespread retinal disease such as *retinitis pigmentosa.* The visual potential of an eye that has a dense cataract or other opacification also can be assessed with ERG. However, normal results do not rule out the presence of macular or optic nerve disease. The patient needs to be told the nature of the test and the steps of the procedure. A demonstration of the flashing lights often is helpful. Before insertion of the contact lens, it is necessary to explain that the patient will feel a little pressure against the lids as the lens is positioned in place. The test does not require any special follow-up care.

### Visual Evoked Potential

Visual evoked potential (VEP) is a measurement of visual function, which is monitored at the level of the occipital cortex with scalp electrodes, which evaluates the integrity of the visual pathways from the optic nerve to the occipital cortex. Stimulation of the retina with light changes the electrical activity of the cortex. Through various computer activities, the electrical activity that is synchronized with this stimulation of the retina is summed and shown as a measurable electrical wave. ***Optic neuritis, demyelinating disease, and optic atrophy can alter this wave.*** The nurse explains the procedure, indicating that it is pain-free and requires no special follow-up.

## CRITICAL THINKING ACTIVITIES

- You are giving a workshop on eye/visual changes encountered with aging. Your audience is primarily elderly individuals. Outline aspects of visual alterations that you would teach the group to expect as normal age-related changes.
- Compare and contrast the following refractory conditions: myopia, hyperopia, and presbyopia.

## CHAPTER SUMMARY

### ANATOMY AND PHYSIOLOGY OF THE EYE

- The eye has three main layers: the outer layer, made up of the sclera and cornea; the uvea, consisting of the choroid, ciliary body, and iris; and the innermost layer, or the retina.
- Visual changes that occur with aging include presbyopia, decreased ability to tolerate glare, decreased peripheral fields, decreased ability to adapt to dim light and darkness, and a decrease in the quantity and quality of tears.

### ASSESSMENT

- A complete history—including a family history of eye problems and the presence of any systemic diseases—is necessary in assessing a person's eyes and vision.
- Objective data required when doing an ocular nursing assessment include assessment of visual acuity, visual fields, pupillary reflexes, and ocular movement, as well as inspection of internal structures and an estimation of intraocular pressure.

### DIAGNOSTIC TESTS

- Radiologic tests used to aid diagnosis of eye problems include x-ray films, CT scans, and MRIs.
- Electrodiagnostic examinations are used mainly to evaluate retinal and optic nerve diseases.
- The main nursing responsibility is to explain diagnostic tests, including any discomfort or alteration in vision that may be experienced.

## REFERENCES

1. Anand R: Fluorescein angiography. I. Technique and normal study, *J Ophthalmic Nurs Technol* 8:48-52, 1989.
2. Bates B, Heokelman RD, Thompson JB: *A guide to physical examination and history taking,* ed 5, Philadelphia, 1991, JB Lippincott.
3. Ebersole P, Hess P: *Toward healthy aging: human needs and nursing response,* ed 3, St Louis, 1990, Mosby.
4. Jakobiec FA, Azar D, editors: *International ophthalmology clinics: pediatric ophthalmology,* Boston, 1992, Little, Brown & Co.
5. Kapperud MJ: *The aging eye: a guide for nurses,* St Paul, 1983, The Minnesota Society for the Prevention of Blindness and Preservation of Hearing.
6. Mrochuk J: Introduction to diagnostic ophthalmic ultrasound for nurses in ophthalmology, *J Ophthalmic Nurs Technol* 9:234-239, 1990.
7. Newell F: *Ophthalmology: principles and concepts,* ed 7, St Louis, 1992, Mosby.
8. Sullivan N: Vision in the elderly, *J Gerontol Nurs* 9:228-235, 1983.
9. Wirtschafter JD, Berman EL, McDonald CS: *Magnetic resonance imaging and computed tomography: clinical neuro-orbital anatomy,* San Francisco, 1992, American Academy of Ophthalmology.

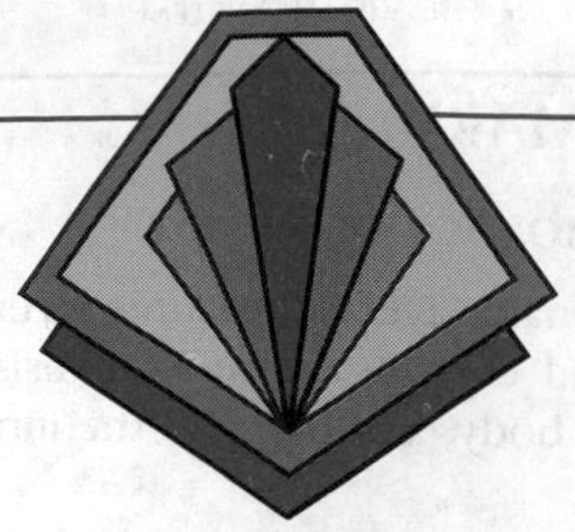

# CHAPTER 60

# Management of Persons With Problems of the Eye

*Marion Allen*
*Barbara Astle*

## CHAPTER OBJECTIVES

***After studying this chapter, the learner should be able to do the following:***

1. Describe the care of healthy eyes, including safety and first aid measures.
2. State the common types of eye medications and their role in diagnosing and treating eye diseases.
3. Outline three common systemic diseases that have manifestations in the eyes.
4. State the correct methods for carrying out nursing procedures related to eye care, including instillation of eye medications, eye irrigations, and eye compresses, and insertion and removal of contact lenses and a prosthetic eye.
5. Discuss the epidemiology and etiology, pathophysiology, clinical manifestations, and medical and nursing management of cataracts and glaucoma.
6. Describe the nursing assessment, nursing diagnoses, expected patient outcomes, and preventive, acute, and long-term care for persons with diabetic retinopathy.
7. Discuss the demands and the factors that facilitate or hinder adjustment to a visual impairment.
8. Describe the nurse's role in assisting a person to learn to live with visual impairment.

## KEY TERMS

amaurosis fugax
aphakia
blepharitis
blepharospasm
cataract
chalazion
conjunctivitis
cycloplegics
enucleation
glaucoma
hordeolum
keratitis
macular degeneration
miotics
mydriatics
retinal detachment
retinopathy
sympathetic ophthalmia
trachoma
uveitis
visual impairment

Eye disease and blindness cause suffering, disability, and loss of productivity for millions of people throughout the world. In the United States alone nearly 11.5 million persons have some degree of visual impairment. Of these 11.5 million, approximately 1.5 million either cannot read the newspaper with corrective lenses or do not have useful vision in one or both eyes.[6] The incidence of blindness is likely to continue to increase because the number of persons 65 years of age and older is increasing yearly.

The major causes of visual impairment and blindness are different in developing and industrialized countries. In developing countries, a high incidence of blindness occurs from preventable causes such as eye infections and malnutrition. Although inflammatory disorders of the eyelids, conjunctiva, cornea, and uveal tract are frequently seen in the United States and Canada, the incidence of blindness from these infectious disorders has declined. However, blindness from diseases that occur more frequently among older persons, including diabetic retinopathy, glaucoma, cataract, and retinal degeneration has increased.

## PREVENTION

### *Healthy People 2000*

***Healthy People 2000*** has set the following goal for the year 2000: reduction of visual impairment to no more than 30 cases per 1000 persons from a baseline of 34.5 per 1000 during 1986 to 1988. The special target population for this goal is people age 65 and older. The year 2000 target for this age-group is 70 per 1000 as compared with 87.7 in 1986 to 1988.[8]

To decrease the problem of visual impairment and meet the *Healthy People 2000* goals, health care professionals need to focus on primary prevention of eye injuries and secondary prevention including early detection of eye disease, as well as on adequate treatment. Because of the involvement with persons of all age-groups, nurses have a unique opportunity to be active in the promotion of health care of the eyes.[5] Health care includes health education and care of the healthy eye, including eye safety measures, first aid for eye injuries, and eye examination. Each of these is discussed below.

## HEALTH EDUCATION ABOUT CARE OF THE EYES

The education of individuals, families, and the public about the care of healthy eyes, prevention of eye disease, and impairment is an important nursing function. Nurses can carry out this function by doing the following:

1. Teaching and promoting eye safety measures
2. Teaching and providing first aid for eye injuries
3. Promoting regular eye examinations by an eye specialist
4. Detecting evidence of disease or impaired acuity
5. Explaining and administering treatments used to improve sight or prevent further loss of sight (for example, medications)

To implement these actions, nurses should have knowledge about common eye diseases and their treatment, ophthalmic drugs, corrective lenses, methods of assessment, and first aid for eye injuries. In addition, the nurse should recognize signs and symptoms suggestive of eye problems and teach them to others (Table 60-1).

**TABLE 60-1 Signs and Symptoms Suggestive of Eye Disorder**

| SIGNS AND SYMPTOMS | EYE DISORDER |
|---|---|
| Conjunctival redness | Conjunctivitis, blepharitis, sty |
| Crusting discharge | Conjunctivitis, blepharitis, sty |
| Ocular pain | Foreign body, sty, acute lid infection, glaucoma, keratitis, uveitis |
| Foreign body sensation ("something in the eye") | Foreign body, corneal erosion, blepharitis, chronic conjunctivitis |
| Blepharospasm | Keratitis, corneal ulcer |
| Multiple spots ("floaters") | Retinal detachment, intraocular hemorrhage, diabetic retinopathy |
| Photophobia | Uveitis, keratitis, glaucoma, corneal abrasions |
| **VISION CHANGES** | |
| Blurred vision | Refractive error, cataract, glaucoma, uveitis, retinal detachment |
| Double vision | Strabismus |
| Halos around lights | Glaucoma |
| Blind spots | Hemorrhage, choroiditis |
| Sudden vision loss | Central retinal artery or vein occlusion |

## CARE OF HEALTHY EYES

The eye is a remarkably resilient organ. It cleans itself through the constant production and excretion of tears and the secretions from the conjunctivae, which also are protective. As a consequence, normal healthy eyes do not need special local treatment. The numerous over-the-counter preparations recommended to cleanse the eye are usually unnecessary. Although these preparations are generally harmless, some proprietary solutions contain substances that may cause allergic reactions in sensitive persons.

People frequently treat eye ailments with over-the-counter remedies or with eye medications that they or others have used in the past. Self-treatment of the eyes is dangerous not only because it may lead to eye injury, but also because it may delay necessary treatment. There are many disorders that can affect the eyes for which many different drugs are used, each of which has a specific purpose. A patient may be receiving two drugs with completely opposite effects. Ophthalmic drugs may deteriorate, become more concentrated from evaporation of liquid, or become contaminated with bacteria or fungi; therefore, using preparations that a family member or friend has on hand can actually contribute to eye damage.

Boric acid solution, like other ophthalmic solutions, may present the problem of drug crystals precipitating on the tip of the dropper and irritating the eye. Preparations having mydriatic properties, such as phenylephrine hydrochloride 0.8%, have the potential to produce sufficient dilation of the pupil to cause an attack of narrow-angle glaucoma in susceptible persons. Contamination of ophthalmic solutions may also be a problem. It is best to *discard* any ophthalmic solution that is cloudy, is discolored, has been opened for 3 months, or contains particles.

Many people believe erroneously that eyestrain causes permanent eye damage. Eyestrain actually refers to strain of the ciliary muscles when there is difficulty in accommodation. It causes a sense of fatigue but does not produce serious damage to the eyes. To avoid eyestrain, a good light should be used when reading and doing work that requires careful visual focus, and extremely fine work should not be done for long periods of time without giving the eye muscles periodic rest. Looking at distant objects for a few minutes helps to rest the eyes after close work. Besides the belief about eyestrain, many other myths are held about the eye. Some of these are outlined in Box 60-1. For each eye myth stated, the exact opposite is true.

Care should be taken not to irritate the eyes or introduce bacteria into the eyes by rubbing them. Rubbing

**BOX 60-1 Common Eye Myths**

Children will outgrow crossed eyes.
Night vision will improve by eating more carrots.
Reading in dim light for long periods can harm the eyes.
Watching TV is bad for the eyes.
Older persons who may have trouble seeing should not use their eyes too much, because they will wear out sooner.
Wearing glasses causes dependence on them.
Persons with weak eyes should rest their eyes often to strengthen them.

the eyes may be a natural response of many persons who are nervous, are fatigued, or wear contact lenses. It also may be the result of eczematous scaling, infection of the lids from contaminated eye makeup, or occasionally louse attachment on the lashes. The cause of severe or chronic irritation should be investigated.

Adequate nutrition is as important for eye health as it is for maintaining other body functions. Nutrition-related eye disorders are rare in developed countries but are common in many underdeveloped countries. Vitamin deficiencies can cause night blindness (vitamin A), corneal damage (vitamin A), optic neuritis (vitamin B), and other disorders. Although a sufficient vitamin intake is necessary, an excessive amount is wasted and may actually do more harm than good. For example, too much vitamin A can damage the optic nerve.

### Eye Safety Measures

Two to three million persons each year in the United States will sustain an injury to their eyes. Of these, 4000 will have permanent blindness as a result. Most of these injuries are preventable through the use of simple measures (Box 60-2). Prevention of accidental injury to the eyes should be stressed in child and adult education. Slingshots, BB guns, and even seemingly harmless rubber bands and paper wads can be dangerous. In addition, misuse in cooking some foods and improper handling of food containers from the microwave oven can cause eye injuries.[10] For example, sustained corneal injuries have occurred from steam released too rapidly from microwave popcorn bags.[5]

Protective goggles and break-resistant corrective lenses are available for persons engaging in active sports and selected occupations. The eyes should be protected by goggles or special dark glasses from prolonged exposure to very bright light such as sunlight on snow. They also need special protection from sudden flashes of light and heat that occur in some industrial occupations. Contact lenses may be prohibited for some industrial occupations because of concern for corneal irritation from particles or chemicals trapped under the lens.

**BOX 60-2 Rules of Eye Safety**

1. Spray aerosols away from eyes.
2. Wear protective glasses during active sports such as racquetball.
3. Slowly release steam from ovens, pots, pressure cookers, and microwave popcorn bags.
4. Gaze at solar eclipses only through adequate filters.
5. Wear safety goggles whenever hazardous work is being done or you are in a work place area where such hazards exist.
6. Fit all machinery with safeguards.
7. Keep dangerous items and chemicals away from children.
8. Store sharp objects safely.
9. Pick up rocks and stones rather than going over them with a lawn mower.

### First Aid for Eye Injuries

First aid measures necessary for eye injury should be known by everyone; these measures can be taught in schools and industry. The sight of many persons could be saved each year if everyone understood the need for immediate copious flushing of the eye with water when an acid, alkali, or other irritating substance has been accidentally introduced (see Guidelines box, p. 2077).

Much damage is done by the layperson's well-intentioned efforts to remove foreign bodies from the eye. It is essential to know that a person who has a foreign object lodged on the cornea must be referred to a physician; the layperson should never attempt to remove it. The eye should be kept closed to prevent further irritation and the lid loosely covered with a dressing or patch anchored with a piece of transparent or adhesive tape. The person should be advised not to squeeze the eye and should be taken at once to an ophthalmologist or an emergency room.

### Regular Eye Examinations

The eyes should be examined by an ophthalmologist at regular intervals throughout life. Many authorities believe children should have their eyes examined at birth, at age 3 or 4, at approximately age 10, and in early adolescence. The young adult should consult an ophthalmologist at least every 3 to 5 years. Medical specialists recommend an eye examination every 2 years after the age of 35, especially with a family history of glaucoma.

Because the eyes are often profoundly affected by conditions within other areas of the body, they cannot be considered alone. In fact, many diseases cause some eye changes that are diagnostically important. The nurse who is teaching eye health must be aware of *total health.* When apparently minor disease or abnormality of the eyes occurs, the nurse must be particularly alert for other signs of disease. Many serious medical conditions such as diabetes, renal disease, neurologic disease, and generalized arteriosclerosis may be diagnosed through

## Guidelines for Eye Irrigations

**PURPOSE**

1. Remove chemical irritants, foreign bodies, and secretions.
2. Cleanse the eye postoperatively (may be done preoperatively).

**PROCEDURE**

1. Prepare solution. Physiologic solutions of sodium chloride or lactated Ringer's solution are most commonly used.
2. Position person comfortably toward one side so that fluid cannot flow into the other eye.
3. Use appropriate means (e.g., kidney basin, large towel) to catch irrigating fluid.
4. Use appropriate amounts of solution.
   a. If small amounts are needed (to cleanse eye postoperatively) sterile cotton balls moistened with solution can be used.
   b. If moderate amounts of fluid are needed (removing secretions) a plastic squeeze bottle is used to direct irrigating fluid along the conjunctiva and over the eyeball from inner to outer canthus (Figure 60-1).
   c. If copious amounts of fluid are needed (that is, for removing chemical irritants), bags of solution such as intravenous bags along with the tubing to direct the flow onto the eye can be used (Figure 60-2).
5. Avoid directing a forceful stream onto the eye.
6. Avoid touching any eye structures with the irrigating equipment.
7. If there is drainage, wrap a piece of gauze around the index finger to raise the lid and ensure thorough cleansing.

**FIGURE 60-1** Irrigating the eye. Fluid is directed along conjunctiva and over eyeball from inner to outer canthus. (From Long BL, Phipps WJ: *Medical-surgical nursing: a nursing process approach,* ed 3, St Louis, 1993, Mosby.)

early recognition of eye symptoms and examination of the eyes by an ophthalmologist.

There is widespread confusion and misunderstanding on the part of the public as to the proper specialist to consult about visual problems (Table 60-2). People who demand the best care when other medical and surgical problems arise may fail to seek help from an ophthalmologist when they have eye problems. The ophthalmologist is a physician and surgeon who can diagnose and treat diseases of the eye. The optometrist does not treat eye diseases but assesses vision and prescribes corrective lenses or exercises.

In their search for help, some people may purchase glasses from stores or use glasses originally prescribed for friends or relatives. Nurses can explain that eye conditions cannot always be remedied simply by the purchase of a pair of glasses or a change of lenses. A serious disease process such as glaucoma or cataract formation could be the cause of the problem.

## Lenses

### Eyeglasses

Acceptance of glasses seems to be influenced by the improvement in vision that they afford, the age and personality of the wearer, and current fashion trends. Because some stigma may be attached to wearing glasses, the young child will have a period of adjustment after receiving glasses. Acceptance of glasses may increase when children start school and realize that the glasses are needed to see the blackboard. The vogue for attractive frames makes the wearing of glasses more acceptable to teenagers and adults. All persons should be en-

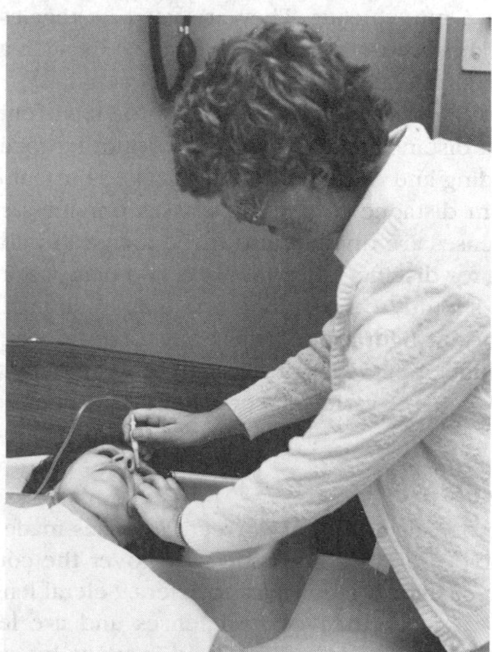

**FIGURE 60-2** Eye irrigation using an intravenous bag and tubing.

**TABLE 60-2 Persons Who Specialize in Eye Problems or in Visual Prostheses**

| | |
|---|---|
| Ophthalmologist | Physician who specializes in the diagnosis and treatment of eye diseases; may also prescribe lenses |
| Oculist | Same as ophthalmologist |
| Optometrist | Professional person with special preparation in assessment of vision and in treatment of visual problems (for example, prescribes lenses, visual training, or orthoptic exercises); is not a physician and does not treat eye diseases |
| Optician | Person who grinds and fits lenses according to prescriptions written by ophthalmologist or optometrist |

couraged to wear their glasses as prescribed and to have periodic examinations of their eyes by an ophthalmologist or an optometrist. Instructions for persons who wear glasses include how to clean their glasses, how to protect them from being scratched or broken, and how to care for them when they are removed.[11]

Federal law now requires that all prescription glasses be made with impact-resistant lenses. Each finished lens must pass an impact test before it is dispensed. *Plastic* lenses weigh less than half of equivalent glass lenses but cost more and scratch more easily. They are useful for persons who wear thick lenses that are heavy when made of glass and for those who are active in sports. *Hardened* lenses have been exposed to a tempering process that makes them extremely hard and resistant to impact and breakage. *Safety* lenses are similar to hardened lenses but are 1 mm thicker. They are used in goggles worn by workers whose eyes may be injured by such articles as chips of metal or glass.

*Bifocal* lenses consist of an upper portion of one focus used for distance and a lower part of another focus used for reading and close work. They make constant changing from distance to reading glasses unnecessary. *Trifocal* lenses are divided into three focuses to give correction for distance, intermediate, and near vision. *Sunglasses* should be carefully ground, large enough to exclude bright light around their edges, and dark enough to exclude about 30% of the light. The amount of light filtered can be varied according to the needs of the person.

### Contact lenses

Contact lenses are small corrective lenses made of different types of ground plastic worn over the cornea of the eye or over the cornea and sclera. Scleral lenses are harder to wear than corneal lenses and are less frequently used. The lenses are held in place by capillary attraction and the upper lid. Conjunctival secretions provide the lubrication needed for the lenses to be worn in comfort. The lenses are used mainly for cosmetic reasons or by persons who engage in sports, because the lenses do not fog or break easily. In some cases they provide better vision correction than can be achieved with glasses. This may be seen in *keratoconus,* a cone-shaped deformity of the cornea, which can prevent satisfactory fitting with conventional glasses. Also, persons who have had a cataract extraction and are not candidates for intraocular lenses achieve better vision wearing contact lenses than they would with conventional glasses.

Contact lenses may be rigid, soft, gas permeable (rigid), extended-wear (soft) or disposable (soft). *Rigid* (hard) lenses are easy to care for, are relatively inexpensive, and correct vision efficiently, particularly if there is significant astigmatism. However, they are generally more uncomfortable than soft lenses and require adaptation by progressive increases in wearing time, which does not usually exceed 12 to 14 hours.

*Soft* lenses are very flexible and have been used successfully by many persons who cannot tolerate hard lenses. The disadvantages of soft lenses may include a higher initial cost and more frequent replacement. They are also more difficult to clean and maintain. *Extended-wear* (soft) *contact lenses* can be left in place for as long as a month. However, the current trend is to limit wear to 1 week before removal for cleaning and disinfection. Those persons who use extended-wear lenses must be educated in and prepared for the extra care required by these lenses.

Disposable soft contact lenses look similar to the standard soft contact lenses or extended-wear lenses. The primary advantage of these lenses is that they can be inexpensively manufactured and can be discarded after 1 week, thus eliminating cleaning and disinfecting. There is concern that any extended-wear contact lens, including disposable lenses, will increase the risk of *ulcerative keratitis* (inflammation of the cornea). In a recent study, investigators discovered that extended-wear contact lens users had a 10 to 15 times higher risk of developing ulcerative keratitis than wearers who removed and cleaned their lenses every day.

*Gas permeable contact lenses* have the optical qualities of the hard lenses and the comfort of the soft lenses. Because they are permeable to oxygen and other gases, some of the complications associated with both the hard and soft lenses are avoided. Gas permeable lenses are generally used on a daily-wear basis but can be used on an extended-wear basis if absolutely necessary.

Successful wearing of contact lenses requires careful personal hygiene and cleansing of the lenses. Patients should receive instructions for proper cleansing and storage of their lenses. Hands should be washed before insertion and removal of the lenses. Lenses should also not be worn longer than the prescribed length of time. Overwearing can cause edema and abrasion of the cornea. All contact lenses can cause problems. Most are minor and can be handled by changes in routine or in lenses. However, problems should not be ignored, because they may lead to or be indicative of more serious difficulties.

Persons interested in wearing contact lenses are encouraged to consult an ophthalmologist, who will make recommendations regarding their use. The person who dispenses the contact lens may be an ophthalmologist, optometrist, or technician supervised by the ophthalmologist. Persons with high astigmatic refractive errors are not good candidates for contact lenses. Other persons may never be able to physiologically or psychologically tolerate the presence of a foreign object in the eye, even for a short time.

### Guidelines for Removal of Contact Lenses

**RIGID LENS**

*Method 1:*

a. Wash hands.
b. Place finger at outer canthus of eye.
c. Pull skin obliquely upward, then straight down.
d. Lens will appear on lower lashes as the upper lid moves downward.
e. If lens moves off center, reposition it by gentle pressure on lid or lens itself and repeat steps b, c, and d.

*Method 2:*

a. Wash hands.
b. Place finger or thumb of each hand at base of eyelashes (upper and lower).
c. Bring eyelids together, trapping the lens (the lens will eject).
d. If lens moves off center, reposition it by gentle pressure on lid or lens itself and repeat steps b, c, and d.

*Method 3:*

a. Wash hands.
b. Using eye irrigation set, gently flush eye with sterile normal saline.
c. Retrieve lens in curved basin.

*Method 4:*

a. Wash hands.
b. Use small suction device shaped like a miniature "plumber's helper."
c. Place over center of lens and pull lens off gently.

**SOFT LENS**

a. Wash hands.
b. Ensure that lens is in place before attempting removal.
c. Pull upper lid up with one thumb.
d. Move lens over conjunctiva before grasping it, if possible. If lens does not move freely, put several drops of sterile saline in eye, close lid, and wait 1 min before trying again.
e. Grasp lens with thumb and forefinger of other hand and pinch the soft lens (it will pop off the cornea).

**SCLERAL LENS**

a. Wash hands.
b. Spread eyelids with both thumbs.
c. Exert slight downward pressure on upper lid (the lower edge of the lens will lift above the lid margin).
d. Slide thumbs to outer canthus to eject lens.

Badly injured or unconscious persons should be checked for the presence of contact lenses, which must be removed (see Guidelines box below). The lenses are stored separately in suitable containers such as capped test tubes filled with sterile normal saline. It is important to note that the risk of human immunodeficiency virus (HIV) or hepatitis B virus (HBV) from tears is extremely low or nonexistent. Universal precautions apply to tears when they contain visible blood.

*Soft contact lenses* must be kept wet at all times; drying causes the soft lens to deteriorate. If a soft lens does become dry, add sterile saline to soften it before handling. Label the lens storage containers with the patient's name and label compartments for the right and left lens. Place the containers in a safe location and record this in the appropriate record.

## ADMINISTERING MEDICATIONS

Accuracy in the administration of medications and treatments is essential. Irreparable damage can follow instillation of unprescribed or deteriorated preparations into the eyes. Solutions that have changed color, that are cloudy, that contain sediment, or whose expiration date has passed should not be used. All medications bottles must be checked frequently for smearing or obliteration of labels so as to avoid instilling the wrong medication. Eye medications in the home are discarded when the course of the treatment is completed unless otherwise indicated by the nurse or physician. The nurse must know the usual dosage and strength, desired action, and side effects of medications being used, as well as signs of toxicity.[13] For example, osmotic agents that reduce intraocular pressure by increasing plasma osmolarity are contraindicated in patients with poor kidney function. Steroids may cause an exacerbation of an already existing herpes corneal ulcer or increase the intraocular pressure.[19] Children and elderly persons are particularly susceptible to side effects of medications.

### OPHTHALMIC DRUGS

A large variety of drugs are used for treatment of eye diseases (Tables 60-3 and 60-4). Most of the drugs are applied as drops, irrigations, or ointments.

**Mydriatics** are drugs that ***dilate the pupil*** by acting on the dilator muscle of the eye. Mydriasis is necessary for thorough examination of the back of the interior of the eye (fundus). An example of a mydriatic drug is phenylephrine (Neo-Synephrine).

**Cycloplegics** are drugs that not only ***dilate the pupil*** but also ***block accommodation*** by paralyzing the ciliary muscles. These drugs are used to keep the pupil dilated as part of the treatment for diseases of the cornea and for inflammatory diseases of the iris and ciliary body, after certain operations, and for eye examination. Commonly used cycloplegics are cyclopentolate (Cyclogyl), tropicamide (Mydriacyl), and atropine. Cycloplegic and

**TABLE 60-3 Mydriatic and Cycloplegic Drugs**

| DRUG | FORM AND CONCENTRATIONS | DURATION OF EFFECT |
|---|---|---|
| **MYDRIATIC ACTION** | | |
| Phenylephrine hydrochloride (Neo-Synephrine, Mydfrin) | Eyedrops, 2.5%, 10% | 2-3 hrs |
| Hydroxyamphetamine hydrobromine (Paredrine) | Eyedrops, 1% | 2 hrs |
| **CYCLOPLEGIC AND MYDRIATIC ACTION** | | |
| Atropine sulfate (Atropisol, Isopto-Atropine) | Eyedrops, 0.5%, 1%, 3%<br>Ointment, 0.5%, 1% | up to 2 wks |
| Cyclopentolate hydrochloride (Cyclogyl) | Eyedrops, 0.5%, 2% | 24 hrs |
| Homatropine hydrobromide (Isopto-Homatropine) | Eyedrops, 2%, 5% | 1-2 days |
| Scopolamine hydrobromide (Isopto-Hyoscine) | Eyedrops, 0.25%, 0.5% | 1-2 days |
| Tropicamide (Mydriacyl) | Eyedrops, 0.5%, 1% | 4-6 hrs |

mydriatic drugs are contraindicated in persons with acute angle glaucoma. These medications can prevent drainage of the aqueous humor, thus increasing intraocular pressure to levels at which eye damage can occur.

**Miotics** are drugs that constrict the pupil and stimulate ciliary muscle pull on the trabecular meshwork, permitting the aqueous humor to flow out more readily, thus reducing intraocular pressure. Miotics such as pilocarpine are the drugs most often used in the *treatment of glaucoma. Osmotic agents* may also be used to reduce intraocular pressure. These drugs—for example, urea and mannitol— are given intravenously in the treatment of acute glaucoma or to reduce intraocular pressure during eye surgery. β-Blockers may be prescribed to help control intraocular pressure (IOP). Timolol maleate (Timoptic), the prototype drug in this class, is used widely in the treatment of glaucoma.

***Secretory inhibitors*** decrease intraocular pressure by reducing aqueous humor production. Drugs in this classification inhibit the enzyme carbonic anhydrase, which is necessary for the production of aqueous humor. These drugs are given orally and include acetazolamide (Diamox). They have several side effects, including nausea and vomiting, anorexia, diuresis, and abdominal cramping. These side effects are mostly related to the inhibi-

**TABLE 60-4 Other Ophthalmic Drugs**

| DRUG | FORM | DOSE |
|---|---|---|
| **ANTIBIOTICS AND ANTIVIRAL DRUGS** | | |
| Polymyxin B, bacitracin (Polysporin) | Ointment or eyedrops, 0.1%-0.5% | As directed |
| Polymyxin B, neomycin, bacitracin (Neosporin) | Ointment | As directed |
| Bacitracin | Ointment, 500-1000 U | As directed |
| Idoxuridine (IDU) | Eyedrops, 0.1% solution<br>Ointment, 0.5% | As directed |
| Gentamicin sulfate (Garamycin) | Eyedrops, 3 mg/ml<br>Ointment, 3 mg/g | 2-4 drops q 6 hr<br>2-3 times daily |
| Chloramphenicol (Chloromycetin, Chloroptic) | Oral, IV, subconjunctival<br>Eyedrops, ointment | 50 mg/kg/day<br>As directed |
| **STEROIDS** | | |
| Prednisone | Topical, 0.25%-0.5% suspension<br>Oral, 5-15 mg | As directed<br>1 tablet q 6 hr |
| Prednisolone acetate | Eyedrops, 0.12-1% solution | 1-2 drops q 6-12 hr |
| Methylprednisolone (Depo-Medrol) | Subconjunctival, 0.5 mg | q 2-4 wk |
| Triamcinolone (Aristocort) | Solution or ointment, 1%, subconjunctival | As directed |
| Dexamethasone (Decadron, Maxidex) | Solution, 0.1%, ointment,<br>Injection, 4 mg | As directed |
| Fluorometholone (FML) | Eyedrops, 0.1% or 0.25% suspension<br>Ointment, 0.1% | As directed |
| **ANESTHETICS** | | |
| Proparacaine (Ophthaine, Ophthetic, Alcaine) | Eyedrops, 0.5% solution | 1-2 drops |
| Lidocaine (Xylocaine) | Local infiltration, 0.5%-2%, 4% solution | As directed |
| **LUBRICANTS AND TEAR SUBSTITUTES** | | |
| Methylcellulose, gonioscopic | Eyedrops, 1% solution | As needed |
| Methylcellulose | Eyedrops, 0.1% solution | As needed |

tory effect on the carbonic anhydrase systems found throughout the body.

*Local topical anesthetics* such as proparacaine and tetracaine are used frequently for diagnostic and therapeutic purposes. Local injectable anesthetics (lidocaine, procaine) are used frequently for eye surgery and treatments. Epinephrine (Adrenalin), 1:50,000 or 1:100,000, may be used in combination with local anesthetics to prolong the duration of anesthetics by constricting blood vessels so that the anesthetic remains longer in the injected area and its absorption is delayed. Hyaluronidase (Wydase), which makes cell membranes more permeable, often is mixed with local anesthetic solutions to increase the diffusion of the anesthetic through the tissues.

Antibiotics such as bacitracin, polymyxin B, gentamicin, and neomycin may be prescribed for ocular instillation, because bacteria are less likely to be resistant to them. Because penicillin causes ocular allergy in about 5% of adult patients, it is not often prescribed.

If the patient is being treated for an active infection, individual medicine bottles, droppers, tubes of ointment, and other equipment are mandatory. This precaution is also necessary when an infected eye is being treated with an antibacterial drug such as bacitracin, and the same medication is ordered prophylactically for the other eye. In this situation, the unaffected eye is treated first.

A *lubricant* such as methylcellulose (artificial tears) may be used for dryness of the cornea and conjunctiva caused by deficiency in production of tears or faulty lid closure as a result of nerve involvement or unconsciousness.

*Antiinflammatory drugs* such as prednisolone, dexamethasone, and hydrocortisone as drops or ointment are used to control inflammatory and allergic reactions postoperatively, as well as for a variety of conditions involving the eyelids, the conjunctiva, and the cornea. Steroids also may be given systemically for the treatment of acute or subacute infections such as those of the iris and choroid.

*Astringents* such as zinc sulfate preparations are often useful in treating chronic conjunctivitis. The *dye* fluorescein is used for applanation tonometry and to stain and thereby outline superficial injuries and infections of the external globe of the eye. Strips of filter paper impregnated with the dry dye are used in place of prepared solutions, because the solution is easily contaminated by *Pseudomonas aeruginosa.*[17]

## SYSTEMIC EFFECTS OF OPHTHALMIC DRUGS

Drugs applied topically to the eye can be absorbed and may cause systemic side effects. Systemic reactions may occur when anticholinergic drugs are instilled into the eye to produce mydriasis. Atropine is the anticholinergic drug that most frequently causes systemic reactions. Signs and symptoms of systemic atropine toxicity include flushing, dryness of mouth and skin, fever, rash, tachycardia, and confusion, but rarely progression to coma and death.

Topically instilled miotic drugs can also cause unwanted systemic effects, most frequently with the long-acting anticholinesterase drugs such as echothiophate. Signs and symptoms include hypersalivation, sweating, gastrointestinal tract disturbances, decrease in heart rate and blood pressure, and bronchoconstriction. These drugs should be used with caution in patients with intestinal obstruction or bronchial asthma.

To avoid undesired systemic reactions, the nurse should take care with topically applied medications to give exactly what is ordered and no more. Pressure applied at the inner canthus, including the puncta, after instillation will minimize drainage into the nose and throat, thereby decreasing systemic absorption.[4]

## INSTILLATION OF MEDICATIONS

*Solutions* such as eyedrops are the most commonly used preparations in the local treatment of eye disease. Advantages of solutions are that they (1) are easily instilled, (2) do not interfere with vision, (3) cause few skin reactions, and (4) do not interfere with the mitosis of the corneal epithelium.

The major disadvantage of eyedrops is that they do not remain in contact with the eye very long. Approximately 90% of aqueous solutions are eliminated from the eye within the first minute of application. It is sometimes necessary to instill the solution at frequent intervals to achieve therapeutic results.

Eyedrops and eyedroppers must be sterile. Each patient should have his or her own bottle or vial of medication. If the bottle is small, it may be warmed slightly by holding it in the hands for a few moments. Blunt-edged eyedroppers are available and may be used for children. The dropper is held downward so that medication does not flow into the rubber bulb, because foreign material from the bulb can contaminate the solution. Most eyedrops are packaged in small plastic bottles with an attached dropper (Figure 60-3, *A*).

If a patient requires instillation of eyedrops, the following procedure is followed. The nurse explains the procedure to allay anxiety and gain cooperation. Hands must be washed before administration and, in some hospitals and doctors' offices gloves are worn. If crusting or discharge is present, or if the patient has an eyepad or dressing, the eye is cleaned before instillation of medication. Before administering the eyedrops, the correct medication is checked for strength and expiration date. When eyedrops are instilled, the patient is instructed to tilt the head backward and look up with both eyes toward the ceiling. The lower lid is pulled *gently* down and out, exposing the lower palpebral conjunctiva and forming a pocket to instill the eyedrop. The dropper should approach the patient's eye from the side and not

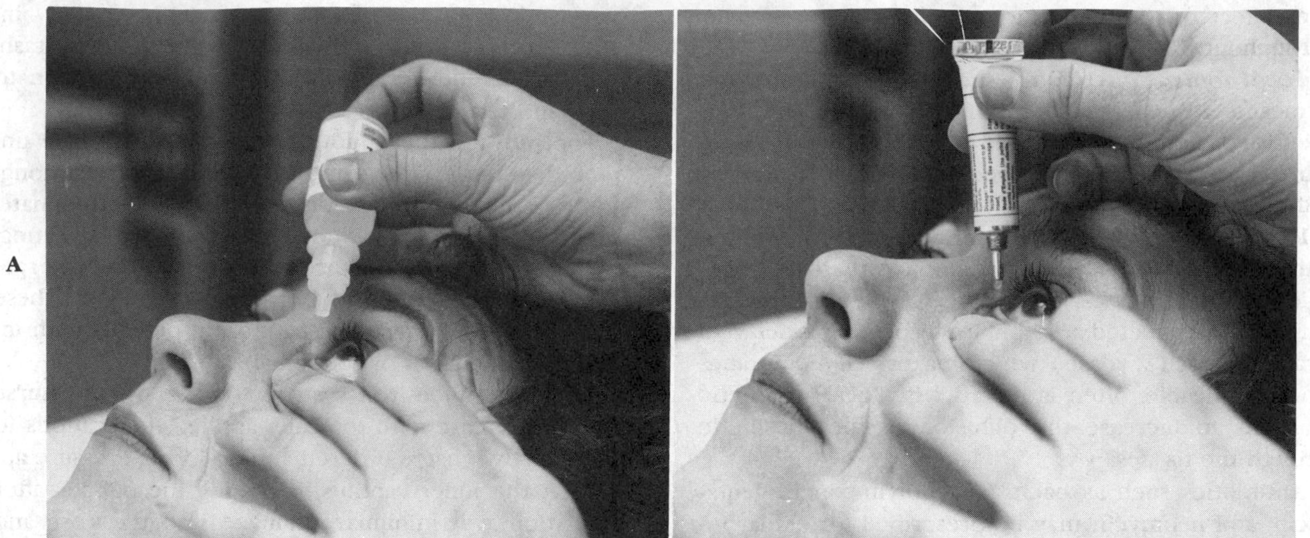

**FIGURE 60-3 A,** Ophthalmic solution is dropped onto conjunctiva of lower lid. **B,** Ophthalmic ointment is squeezed onto conjunctiva of lower lid.

directly from the front (Figure 60-3, *A*). Care must be taken not to touch the eyelashes, the conjunctiva, or the surface of the eyeball with the dropper to prevent contamination of the eyedrops or ocular injury. Eyedrops should not be instilled directly on the cornea because this is the most sensitive surface of the eye. The patient is instructed to close both eyes gently and is reminded not to squeeze the eye shut because this causes the medication to escape. Absorbent tissues or cotton held against the cheek just below the eye will prevent the drops from running down the cheek.

*Ophthalmic ointments* remain in contact with the eye much longer, providing a prolonged effect. They usually do not cause discomfort when instilled. There is less absorption into lacrimal passages than with eyedrops. Ointments, particularly those containing antibiotics, are more stable than solutions. Disadvantages of ointments are that they (1) produce a film in front of the eye that may blur vision, (2) cause contact dermatitis reaction more frequently, and (3) may inhibit mitosis of the corneal epithelial cells.

Before instilling an ophthalmic ointment, the nurse follows the same procedure used for instilling eyedrops. The patient is instructed to tilt the head backward and look up with both eyes toward the ceiling. The lower lid is *gently* pulled down and the ointment is expressed directly onto the exposed palpebral conjunctiva from inner to outer canthus (Figure 60-3, *B*). Care is taken not to touch the eyelashes or the surface of the eye with the tip of the tube to prevent contamination of the ophthalmic ointment and ocular injury to the cornea. The patient is instructed to close both eyes gently. Also, the patient is told that vision may be blurred because the ointment smears the cornea.

Often patients are receiving multiple topical medications, including both eyedrops and ointments. *If more than one drop is to be instilled, even if it is the same medication, the nurse should wait at least 30 seconds before instilling the second drop.*[4] Eyelids should be kept closed between instillations to prevent blinking, which pumps drug into the nose, thereby increasing systemic absorption.[25] Because ointments smear the cornea and blur vision, they should be applied after the prescribed eyedrops have been instilled, or at bedtime.

## EYE MANIFESTATIONS OF SYSTEMIC DISEASES

Diseases and infections that affect other parts of the body also affect the eye. The eye has been described as the most important square inch of body surface, both diagnostically and functionally. By examining the back portion of the interior of the eyeball (fundus) with an ophthalmoscope, many major diseases can be recognized. Some of the diseases and pathologic states that can be identified through their typical fundus picture and other eye assessment include metabolic diseases, vascular and hematologic disorders, neurologic disorders, connective tissue disease, and nutritional deficiencies. Assessment of the eye often will indicate the severity of the disease.

### METABOLIC DISEASES

Of the metabolic diseases affecting the eye, *diabetes* is the most common. Diabetes may affect any of the structures of the eye. *Senile cataracts occur earlier in persons who have diabetes* and progress more rapidly than in most elderly people. *Diabetic retinopathy* produces characteristic changes in the retina that can cause severe visual damage and eventually result in blindness. Diabetes also causes the growth of new blood vessels on the surface of the retina and optic disc that later extend into the vitreous humor *(retinitis proliferans)*. This condition often causes *blindness* because of recurrent *vitreous hemorrhages* and *retinal detachment*.

## VASCULAR AND HEMATOLOGIC DISORDERS

*Vascular disorders* such as persistent systemic hypertension will eventually produce changes in the retina (hemorrhage, edema, and exudates) that may result in the loss of sight. If the cause of the elevated blood pressure is pregnancy-induced hypertension and is of short duration, the **retinopathy** (any disorder of the retina) usually subsides when the pregnancy ends. Retinopathy caused by hypertension resulting from renal arteriosclerosis or diffuse glomerulonephritis is usually progressive and irreversible. Severe hypertension causes narrowing of the retinal arteries; and the blood flow through the retina and choroid is diminished, resulting in degenerative changes in the retina and loss of vision.

Visual loss may result from vascular accidents to vessels anywhere in the eye or in the main blood vessels outside the eye. A *cerebrovascular accident* may cause hemianopia (blindness for one half of the field of vision in one or both eyes) or total blindness, depending on its location. Arteriosclerosis and atheromatosis, particularly involving the carotid and cranial arteries, may release emboli that lead to occlusion of the retinal vessels. Fleeting or transient loss of vision **(amaurosis fugax)** is often associated with carotid occlusive disease but can occur with any microembolic arthrombotic disorder such as cardiac or valvular disease.

*Hematologic disorders* such as acute leukemia, polycythemia, and sickle cell disease cause characteristic retinal hemorrhages, arterial occlusions, or neovascularization, as in the case of sickle cell disease. The retinal changes may be reversed in hyperviscosity syndromes (polycythemia) if there is reduction in the abnormality that produced this condition.

## NEUROLOGIC DISORDERS

Neurologic disorders include a wide range of problems. Eye examination aids in evaluation of seven of the twelve cranial nerves (II through VIII) and provides information about the sympathetic and parasympathetic pathways (see Chapter 56). Demyelinating disorders (for example, multiple sclerosis) cause typical nerve damage to the eye. Increased intracranial pressure causes swelling of the optic disc (papilledema). Through eye examination (such as perimetry studies), lesions of the brain can be pinpointed to a specific lobe in the brain (temporal, parietal, or occipital). Unilateral dilation of the pupil helps diagnose severity and location of head injury.

## CONNECTIVE TISSUE DISEASES

Persons with connective tissue diseases commonly have eye involvement. One of the more frequent eye manifestations is dry eyes. Patients complain of a scratchy burning sensation, with possible redness of the eye and photophobia (sensitivity to light). Any eye structure can be involved; the tissues of the eye that are affected are, in general, of the same type as the tissue involved in the primary manifestation of the disease. For example, rheumatoid diseases most commonly affect the cornea, sclera, and uveal tract, whereas systemic lupus erythematosus usually involves the vasculature of the eye.

## NUTRITIONAL DEFICIENCIES

Nutritional deficiencies can cause pathologic changes in the eye. There seems to be a direct relationship between good nutrition and eye health. *A lack of vitamins A and B* in the diet *can cause changes in the conjunctiva, corneal epithelium, and retina*. The lack of vitamins available for body use may also be caused by interference with absorption, storage, or transport capacities. Tears are reduced, and eyes and lid margins become reddened and inflamed. Sensitivity to light is often present, and some loss of visual acuity is noticed at night. Significant difficulty is called night blindness *(nyctalopia)*. If night blindness is nutritionally caused, it may respond favorably to ingestion of a nutritious diet and vitamin A. On the other hand, *excessive* amounts of vitamin A can damage the retina. Vitamin B deficiency may cause *bilateral optic neuritis,* especially in individuals who drink large quantities of alcohol. When damage to the optic nerve has been severe and prolonged, a diet high in vitamin B and other essential nutrients can accomplish only partial recovery. Fortunately, eye problems from nutritional deficiency are rarely found in the developed countries.

# EYE TRAUMA AND INJURY

## PREVENTION

Although the eye is vulnerable to trauma, natural protective mechanisms can prevent or minimize injury (Table 60-5).

In addition to the body's natural defenses against injury, *protective equipment* such as goggles, shields, and shatterproof safety lenses are advised for certain occupations and sports activities. Knowledge of safety precautions and first-aid techniques are valuable in preventing serious damage from trauma.

Prompt and appropriate care of the injured eye may prevent serious vision impairment or loss of the eye (Table 60-6). The two major categories of trauma are *burns* and *contact* (mechanical) *trauma*.

## BURNS

*Chemical burns* such as those caused by acid or alkali must be treated immediately to prevent the possibility of permanent visual impairment from damage to the

**TABLE 60-5 Protective Mechanisms of the Eye**

| PROTECTIVE FEATURE | FUNCTION |
|---|---|
| Bony orbital rim | Prevents many mechanical injuries |
| Orbital fluids and tissues | Cushion direct blows |
| Eyelashes and eyelids | Quickly close reflexively (blink) from visual or mechanical stimuli |
| Bell phenomenon | Eyes reflexively rotate upward with lid closing to protect cornea |
| Lacrimal secretions | Can flush away chemicals or foreign bodies |

cornea. For chemical trauma of any nature, prompt immediate irrigation is the essential action that may result in salvaging an otherwise irrevocably lost eye. Irrigation after chemical trauma should be performed immediately after the injury and continued for a prolonged period of time, a minimum of 15 minutes. Although cool tap water is excellent for irrigation, any nontoxic solution can be used. After irrigation, and *only* after irrigation, is the patient transported to a physician. After transportation, the nurse irrigates the eye further and removes all particles from the eye and conjunctiva. Topical antibiotics may be used to prevent infection.

*Ultraviolet burns* of the cornea may occur from exposure under a sunlamp or from exposure to the sun (outdoor workers, sunbathers, skiers). The individual becomes aware of painful eyes several hours after exposure. In fact, the eyes may be so painful that a topical anesthetic may be required in order to examine the eyes. Treatment consists of cold compresses, analgesics (for example, aspirin, acetaminophen, or codeine), and topical ophthalmic anesthetics. Topical antibiotics may also be used to prevent infection. Most patients are comfortable within 24 hours after treatment begins. Rarely is the cornea scarred permanently. Ultraviolet burns may also occur from the use of germicidal lamps, electric flashes, and arc welding.

*Thermal burns* of the eyelids can cause lid contracture. Skin grafting may be necessary to prevent severe contractures and exposure of the eye. Full-thickness grafts can be taken from the uninjured eyelid, the inner aspect of the forearm, or behind the ear.

## CONTACT TRAUMA

### Lacerations of Eyelid

Lacerations of the eyelid require treatment by an eye specialist, because there is danger of scar formation as healing occurs. Although lid lacerations may bleed freely, pressure against the lid to stop bleeding can cause damage to the eye beneath. Cuts or tears in the eyelid may need to be sutured after bleeding is controlled and any foreign material is removed. Antitetanus serum usually is given to all patients who sustain eye wounds.

**TABLE 60-6 First Aid for Eye Injuries**

| INJURY | INTERVENTIONS |
|---|---|
| Burns: chemical, flame | Flush eye immediately for 15 min with cool water or any available nontoxic liquid; seek medical assistance |
| Loose substance on conjunctiva: dirt, insects | Lift upper lid over lower lid to dislodge substance, produce tearing; irrigate eye with water if necessary; do not rub eye; obtain medical assistance if above interventions fail |
| Contact injury: contusion, ecchymosis, laceration | Apply cold compresses if no laceration present; cover eye if laceration present; seek medical assistance |
| Penetrating objects | Do not remove object; place protective shield over eye (for example, paper cup); cover uninjured eye to prevent excess movement of injured eye; seek medical assistance |

### Injuries to Ciliary Body, Sclera, Globe, and Orbit

Injuries to the ciliary body and sclera and injuries involving the globe and orbit are critical, because adjacent tissues usually are injured also and contents of the eyeball may escape and possible infection of the interior of the eye may occur. If these injuries result in wounds that are small and clean, treatment consists of antibiotics given systemically and topically, suturing the wound, instilling atropine to put the iris and the ciliary body at rest, and a firm dressing. If the injury is extensive and if sight is lost, **enucleation** (removal of the eyeball) may be necessary.

Contusion of the globe is frequently followed by frank bleeding into the anterior chamber (hyphema). This blood settles at the most dependent portion of the anterior chamber and may or may not be visible. Spontaneous recovery usually occurs if bleeding is not excessive. Bed rest may be prescribed and cycloplegic drugs instilled if more than 5% of the anterior chamber is filled with blood.[25] Close observation is required, since the original hyphema may be followed by a more severe bleeding 2 to 3 days after the initial injury. The use of oral aminocaproic acid to stabilize clot formation may reduce the risk of rebleeding.[25] A secondary glaucoma may occur immediately or several years later. If secondary bleeding occurs, bed rest may be prescribed and the injured eye protected with a shield.

### Ecchymosis

Persons with ecchymosis of the eyelid and surrounding tissues (black eye) should be examined to rule out coexisting skull fractures and intraocular bleeding or other eye damage. Initially, cold compresses will help to control the bleeding. Subsequent warm compresses after 48 hours will speed up the reabsorption of blood from the tissues. The discoloration, which lasts about 2 weeks, can be covered to some extent with cosmetics.

## Penetrating Injury

Penetrating injury of the eye requires immediate medical care. The most important goal is to prevent further damage before reaching the ophthalmologist. It is easy to convert a minor corneal laceration without iris prolapse into the loss of an eye when applying even gentle pressure on the eye during transportation of the patient. It is very important that *no* attempt be made to remove or wash the object out of the eye.[5] To protect the eye against pressure, a shield can be used. A cardboard cone or a paper cup can be taped securely over the patient's eye to prevent anyone or anything from touching it. Tears, blood, and other discharges cannot be wiped away without risking dangerous pressure changes. Also, covering the *uninjured* eye prevents excessive movement of the *injured* eye. Although the patient may walk or be transported sitting up in an automobile, *unnecessary exertion such as bending over or carrying heavy objects should be avoided.* These activities could *increase the intraocular pressure* and cause *more damage to the eye.*

## Corneal Injuries

Corneal injuries are serious, because resistance to infection is low in the cornea and scarring can impair vision. It has been estimated that foreign bodies on the surface of the cornea constitute about 25% of ocular injuries.[17] Tearing, photophobia, and a sensation of "something in the eye" warn a person that a foreign body is present if neuromuscular networks are functioning properly. If an abrasion of the cornea occurs, there may be considerable pain. For those persons with impaired sensorimotor function, the nurse must assess for corneal damage.

Sterile fluorescein solution instilled in the eye will demarcate the foreign body and aid in its removal. The foreign body must be entirely removed to permit epithelization and relieve pain. Following removal of the object, sulfonamide or antibiotic drops may be administered. In addition, a dressing may be applied to prevent blinking, thereby decreasing discomfort.

## SYMPATHETIC OPHTHALMIA

**Sympathetic ophthalmia** is a serious inflammation of the uveal tract (ciliary body, iris, and choroid) in the *uninjured* eye that follows a penetrating injury or retained foreign body to the other eye. Although the cause of this condition is unknown, it may be the result of an *autoimmune inflammatory response to uveal pigment.* This inflammation spreads from the uvea to the optic nerve. Children are especially susceptible to sympathetic ophthalmia; however, it may occur at any age. The uninjured eye becomes inflamed; photophobia, lacrimation, dimness of vision, and pain in the eye may be experienced. *Sympathetic ophthalmia may appear 3 to 8 weeks after the eye injury or months or years later.* A severely injured blind eye may be removed soon after the injury in an attempt to prevent the development of sympathetic ophthalmia. Because of increased medical skill in treating perforating wounds and the administration of cortisone at the earliest suggestion of inflammation, sympathetic ophthalmia has become rare in recent years.

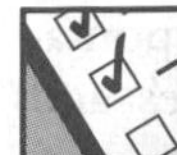

**Guidelines for Application of Warm Moist Compresses**

1. Use sterile technique when infection or ulceration are present; clean technique may be used for allergic reactions.
2. Use separate equipment for bilateral eye infections.
3. Wash hands before treating each eye.
4. Temperature of compress should not exceed 49° C (120° F).
5. Change compresses frequently every 5 minutes as ordered.[26] Always wash hands first.
6. Do not exert pressure on the eyeball.
7. Sterile petrolatum may be used on skin around eyes, if desired, to protect the skin.
8. If sterility is not required, moist heat may be applied by means of a clean face cloth.

# INFECTIONS AND INFLAMMATION

Infections and inflammation can occur in any of the eye structures and may be caused by microorganisms, mechanical irritation, or sensitivity to some substance. Inflammation of the eye accounts for more than one half of the total incidence of acute disease conditions, with more than 1 million cases per year. Conjunctivitis represents about two thirds of the total.

## HORDEOLUM

### Etiology and Management

**Hordeolum** (stye) is a relatively mild but extremely common infection of the small glands of the lid margins. Staphylococci are often the infecting organisms. Poor hygiene and excessive use of cosmetics may be contributing causes. Patients should be taught not to squeeze styes, because the infection may spread and cause cellulitis of the lids. Warm moist compresses (see Guidelines box above) are used, and styes usually open and drain without surgery. A topical ophthalmic antibiotic may hasten healing.

## CHALAZION

### Etiology and Management

A **chalazion** is a sterile granulomatous inflammation of the sebaceous glands (meibomian glands) located in the connective tissue in the free edges of the eyelids. The cysts present a hard, shiny, lumpy appearance as viewed from the inner side of the lid. They may cause pressure on the cornea. Small chalazions may disappear spontaneously or after massage and use of hot compresses, and topical antibiotics. If they are large or become infected, they usually require surgical incision and curettage. Chalazions usually are removed in the physician's office or in the clinic using local anesthesia. An antibacterial ointment (for example, neomycin sulfate) may be applied to the conjunctiva; and an eyepad is worn for a few hours.

## CONJUNCTIVITIS AND BLEPHARITIS

### Etiology/Epidemiology

**Conjunctivitis** (inflammation of the conjunctiva) and **blepharitis** (inflammation of the eyelids) are common infections that can occur from a variety of causes. They may result from mechanical trauma such as that caused by sunburn or from infection with organisms such as *staphylocci, streptococci,* or *Haemophilus influenzae.* Two sexually transmitted agents that cause conjunctivitis are *Chlamydia trachomatis* and *Neisseria gonorrhoeae.* Inflammation is often caused by allergic reactions within the body or by external irritants (e.g., poison ivy or cosmetics). Viral agents that cause conjunctivitis include most human adenovirus strains and herpes simplex viruses.

### Acute Bacterial Conjunctivitis

Acute bacterial conjunctivitis is often called *pinkeye.* Common in school children, pinkeye is highly infectious. Conjunctival redness and crusting discharge deposited on the lashes and corners of the eye are the characteristic findings. Treatment includes cleansing of the lids and lashes, use of topical antibiotics, and precautions to prevent the spread to others. Firm adherent crusts may be softened by use of warm moist compresses. Because the material is infectious it should be disposed of in a sanitary manner. Fortunately, acute bacterial conjunctivitis is usually self-limited and leaves no permanent scars.

### Seborrheic Blepharitis

Seborrheic blepharitis often begins in childhood and continues frequently throughout life. The lid margins of upper and lower lids are reddened with scales attached to the base of the lashes. The scalp, eyebrows, and lid margins must be kept clean with water and a mild shampoo. Scales should be removed daily with a moistened cotton applicator and baby shampoo. Frequently, some degree of conjunctivitis is present. Application of local antibiotics is helpful if infection occurs. The condition can be kept under control if treated effectively before any serious eye involvement (e.g., keratitis) develops.

## TRACHOMA

### Etiology/Epidemiology

**Trachoma** (a form of conjunctivitis) is one of the most common chronic diseases, with approximately 600 million people in the world affected. Although rare in North America, trachoma is endemic among low-income persons living in the dry, hot Mediterranean countries, and in Africa, Brazil, and the Far East, and is a major cause of blindness in these areas. It is caused by a strain of the virus *Chlamydia trachomatis.* Highly contagious in the early conjunctivitis state, trachoma is spread by direct contact with the ocular discharge. Insect vectors may also play a role in transmission. Following the acute conjunctivitis stage, the eyelids become scarred, and granulations form on the inner surface of the lids and invade the cornea. The entire cornea may eventually become involved, with subsequent loss of vision. Secondary bacterial infection is common.

### Medical Management

Trachoma can be arrested in the early stages with topical and oral tetracycline or erythromycin. Eyelid granules may be removed surgically.

## KERATITIS

### Etiology/Epidemiology

Inflammation of the cornea is called **keratitis.** It may be acute, chronic, and superficial, or deep (interstitial). Acute epithelial keratitis commonly occurs in association with bacterial conjunctivitis caused by *Staphylococcus aureus* or *epidermatitis, Streptococcus pneumoniae,* or *Streptococcus viridans, Moraxella liquefaciens, Pseudomonas aeruginosa* or *Serratia marcescens,* as well as various coliform and proteus organisms. Viruses such as herpes simplex may also cause a type of keratitis. Keratitis may be associated with a corneal ulcer or be caused by diseases such as tuberculosis and syphilis. Allergic reactions, vitamin A deficiency, or viral diseases (e.g., mumps, measles, and herpes simplex) may contribute to its development in children.

### Pathophysiology

The cornea has many pain fibers; therefore any inflammation causes pain. The pain is increased by movement of the eyelid over the cornea and usually persists until healing occurs. Photophobia (sensitivity to light), tearing, and **blepharospasm** (spasm of the eyelids) are also common. Uncontrolled keratitis can result in loss of vision caused by impairment of corneal transparency or destruction of the eye by corneal perforation.

### Medical Management

If possible, the systemic cause is found and treated. Steroids may be used cautiously to control the inflammation. Except for cases of herpes simplex, topical antibiotics are given to treat the infection. Cycloplegic agents, which will keep the iris and ciliary body at rest, and hot compresses will help promote healing. Medications such as idoxuridine (IDU) applied locally are effective in helping to clear keratitis caused by herpes simplex in 80% of cases. The eyes may be covered to limit eye movements, and bed rest may be prescribed.

### Surgical Management

When the cornea is so damaged that severe visual impairment occurs, a corneal transplant may be required. See Chapter 72 for information on corneal transplants and the nursing management of patients having this procedure performed.

## CORNEAL ULCER

### Etiology/Epidemiology

Because of its location, the cornea is vulnerable to trauma and contamination with microorganisms. Infections of the cornea are not common occurrences. When present, however, they *can lead to scarring, perforation, extensive intraocular infection, and loss of the eye.* The ulcer may be caused by trauma, by contact lenses, or by infections of the conjunctiva that have spread to the cornea. Prompt treatment of ocular injuries can usually prevent the complication of infection. Persons at risk for infection may develop ulcers from little apparent cause (e.g., the individual whose immune system is compromised).

### Pathophysiology

Persons with a corneal ulcer may complain of pain, photophobia, tearing, and spasms of the eyelid (blepharospasm). Reduced vision may also occur.

Assessment of the corneal ulcer is accomplished with the use of the slit lamp or with a bright movable light such as a small flashlight. With oblique illumination from a flashlight, directed from the side rather than straight on, details are seen more clearly. A greyish-white to yellowish-white opacity on the cornea may be seen. The shape, size, and depth of the ulcer can be outlined by instilling sterile fluorescein. *Hypopyon* (pus in the anterior chamber) may also be noted. If pain and blepharospasm interfere with examination, a drop of an anesthetic such as 0.5% proparacaine may be used.

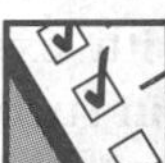

**Guidelines for Care of the Person With an Eye Inflammation**

1. Promoting comfort
   a. Apply compresses as prescribed to decrease pain and promote healing
   b. Dim lights and encourage use of dark glasses if patient is photophobic
   c. Administer analgesics as prescribed
   d. Apply eye patch as recommended
2. Teaching, as appropriate
   a. Self-care techniques
      (1) Instilling eyedrops or ointment
      (2) Applying compresses, eye patch
   b. Prevention of spread of infection
      (1) Wash hands before and after treatment of eye
      (2) Use separate medicine bottles or tubes for each eye
      (3) Use compresses one time only if infection is present

### Medical Management

1. Culture and sensitivity, as required
2. Antibiotics, antiviral, and antifungal agents (depending on the causative agent) (Some given topically or subconjunctivally)
3. Cycloplegic agent
4. Steroid therapy, with caution
5. Cleansing of deep ulcers with an antiseptic solution, cauterization, and covering with a firm patch
6. Corneal transplant, if the ulcer causes permanent impaired vision

### Nursing Management

Nursing interventions are similar to those for persons with eye inflammation (see Guidelines box below, left). Nursing management of the patient who has had a corneal transplant is discussed in Chapter 72.

## UVEITIS

### Etiology/Epidemiology

Inflammation of the uvea is referred to as **uveitis.** Inflammatory disorders of the uveal tract, usually unilateral, are common principally in the young and in middle aged adults.[25] Uveitis is caused by a wide variety of factors and infectious agents that may involve the choroid, the ciliary body, the iris, or all three simultaneously. Classification by cause includes *infection, allergy, trauma, toxic agents, noninfective systemic diseases such as diabetes, and unknown factors.* The specific cause of most cases of uveitis cannot be determined.

### Pathophysiology

Uveitis produces pain in the eyeball radiating to the forehead and temple, photophobia (sensitivity to light), lacrimation, and interference with vision. There is edema of the upper lid, the iris is swollen because of congestion and exudation of cells and fibrin, and the pupil is contracted and irregular as a result of the formation of adhesions. The clinical picture may vary somewhat depending on the portion of the uveal tract involved.

### Medical and Nursing Management

In self-limited acute inflammations, the cause is frequently not actively sought. In chronic uveitis, attempts are made to discover the possible cause, such as sarcoid, histoplasmosis, toxoplasmosis, or connective tissue disease.

The instillation of a cycloplegic agent such as atropine or cyclopentolate in the eye puts the iris and ciliary body at rest, relieves pain and photophobia, and diminishes congestion. By keeping the pupil dilated, the cycloplegic drug prevents adhesions from forming between the anterior capsule of the lens and the iris and tends to cause those already formed to regress. Moist, warm compresses may be applied several times each day to help diminish pain and inflammation. The eyes usually are covered, and in the convalescent period dark glasses are prescribed. Systemic analgesics are given as necessary for pain. Cortisone preparations are of great value in controlling the inflammation in many persons, but the inflammation in others resists almost all forms of treatment. Complications of uveitis include the formation of adhesions, keratitis, secondary glaucoma, and the loss of vision.

# CATARACT

## ETIOLOGY

A **cataract** is a clouding or opacity of the lens that leads to gradual painless blurring of vision and eventual loss of sight (Figure 60-4). In general, cataracts are classified as *senile,* those associated with aging; *traumatic,* those associated with injury; *congenital,* those present at birth; or *secondary,* those that occur following other eye diseases.

Cataracts occur so often in elderly persons that the term *senile cataract* is used. Of persons 52 to 85 years of age, 15% have cataracts that reduce visual acuity to 20/30 or less, and at 80 years of age, about 85% of all persons have some clouding of the lens.[17] Senile cataracts are listed as the most common cause of blindness in older persons, yet the response of the condition to surgery often is excellent.

After aging, the next most common cause of cataract is injury to the eye. The transparency of the lens may be destroyed by either a penetrating wound or a contusion. Cataracts may result from the ingestion of injurious substances such as dinitrophenol or naphthalene. Some researchers report that cataracts may result from systemic absorption of hair dyes.

Cataracts may also occur secondary to eye diseases, such as uveitis or eye trauma; or with systemic diseases, such as diabetes mellitus, galactosemia, or sarcoidosis.

## EPIDEMIOLOGY

In the United States, cataracts are the third most likely cause of preventable blindness. The prevalence of cataracts increases with age. Epidemiologic studies indicate that for persons over 65 years of age, incidence of cataracts increases in geographic areas where there are long periods of sunlight.

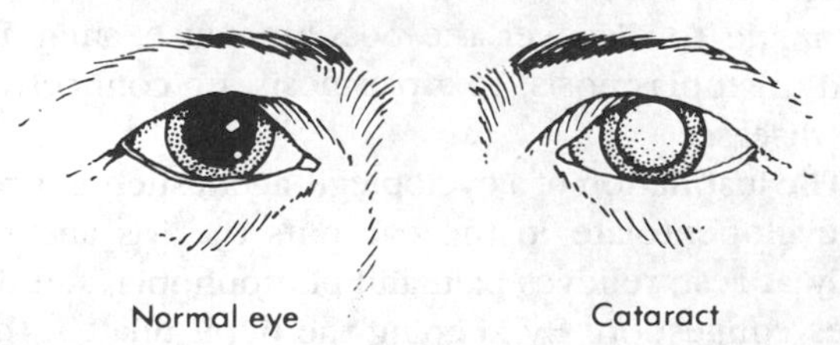


**FIGURE 60-4** Cataract, visible in left eye as white opacity of lens, is seen through pupil.

## PATHOPHYSIOLOGY

Cataract formation is characterized chemically by a reduction in oxygen uptake and an initial increase in water content, followed by dehydration. Sodium and calcium content is increased, and potassium, ascorbic acid, and protein content is decreased.

Cataracts resulting from aging or disease usually develop gradually. Both eyes may develop cataracts, but they usually develop at different rates. Blurring of vision may occur immediately following trauma. The predominant symptom is progressive loss of vision. The degree of loss depends on the location and extent of the opacity. Persons with an opacity in the center portion of the lens can generally see better in dim light when the pupil is dilated. The person with *presbyopia* may find that reading without glasses is possible in the early stage of cataract formation because of artificial myopia caused by the greater convexity of the lens. To diagnose cataract(s), the pupil is dilated and the lens of the eye is examined with the ophthalmoscope and the slit lamp. See Table 60-7 for a comparison of normal function, pathophysiology, and clinical manifestations found with cataract.

## PREVENTION

### Primary Prevention

Senile cataracts are part of the normal aging process; therefore their occurrence is not preventable. Recently, some evidence suggests that ultraviolet radiation may be a significant contributing factor to cataract formation.[25] This finding requires more study. If this evidence is supported, *primary prevention* may include protective sunglasses to decrease absorption of ultraviolet rays. Many agents are frequently advertised to delay, prevent, or reverse cataract formation. None has proved successful.

The incidence of most traumatic cataracts is *preventable.* Persons working in environments with exposure to heat or metals or those participating in such sport activities as racquetball should be encouraged to wear protective safety goggles.

### Secondary Prevention

Because cataracts can occur in conjunction with systemic disorders, such as diabetes mellitus, hypoparathyroidism, and galactosemia, persons with these conditions should have their disease closely monitored to prevent cataract formation.

## SURGICAL MANAGEMENT

Operative treatment is the only method for treating cataracts. Unlike most other damaging diseases of the eye, vision loss from cataract can be restored by surgical removal of the cataract. Even patients who are in their

**TABLE 60-7 Normal Function, Pathophysiology and Clinical Manifestations in Cataract Formation**

| NORMAL FUNCTION | PATHOPHYSIOLOGY | CLINICAL MANIFESTATIONS |
|---|---|---|
| Lens fibers continuously produced, with older fibers being compressed toward center of lens | With aging, nuclear portion of lens becomes increasingly dense; normal transparency of lens decreases | Gradual decrease in vision |
| Focuses light on retina | Light rays that strike opacity scatter | Glare, halos around lights |
| | Opacity filters out blue end of visible light spectrum | Ability to discriminate hues decreases; vision "rosier" |
| | Trauma to lens leads to rupture or break in lens capsule, causing rapid swelling and opacification of lens | Sudden decrease in vision |

90s can often be operated on with good results. Between 90% and 95% of all cataract operations are successful. The decision as to when to remove the cataract depends on the general health of the patient and how much the cataract interferes with the person's activities.

It was previously thought that a cataract had to become mature or "ripe" before it could be extracted, that is, separated easily from the lens capsule. Now cataracts are removed whenever the decreased vision interferes with the person's activities of daily living or when the cataract may lead to other eye complications such as glaucoma.

Cataracts are usually removed using a local anesthetic. The most popular method of cataract removal is the extracapsular cataract extraction (ECCE). In this method, only the anterior portion of the lens capsule plus the capsule contents are removed, using techniques such as irrigation and aspiration or phacoemulsification (ultrasonic vibration to break up the lens). Cataracts can also be removed within their capsule (intracapsular cataract extraction) using a freezing (cryo) probe that adheres to the surface of the lens.

## Corrective Lenses

Because the lens or lens content has been removed, something is needed to replace the lost focusing power. The *intraocular lens* is most commonly used. When this is not possible, cataract glasses or contact lenses are necessary. The intraocular lens, made of polymethylmethacrylate, is implanted within the eye at the time of surgery. It can also be secondarily implanted months or years after cataract extraction. The intraocular lens is the primary form of lens replacement today because it restores vision to near 20/20 (Figure 60-5).

There are two types of intraocular lens implants being used. The *anterior chamber lens* is placed in front of the iris and is supported by it. This type of implant is used following an intracapsular cataract extraction or when the lens capsule cannot support a lens. The *posterior chamber lens* is placed behind the iris and is supported by the posterior portion of the lens capsule that was left in place (extracapsular technique). This type of implant is not dependent on the pupil or iris for support and rarely moves out of position. It is the most frequently used type of lens implant, because it is believed that the lens position most closely approximates the natural lens and magnification is minimized. Fewer postoperative complications are associated with posterior chamber lenses as compared with anterior chamber lenses.

If an intraocular lens is not inserted during surgery, the person must wear an external lens. Cataract glasses

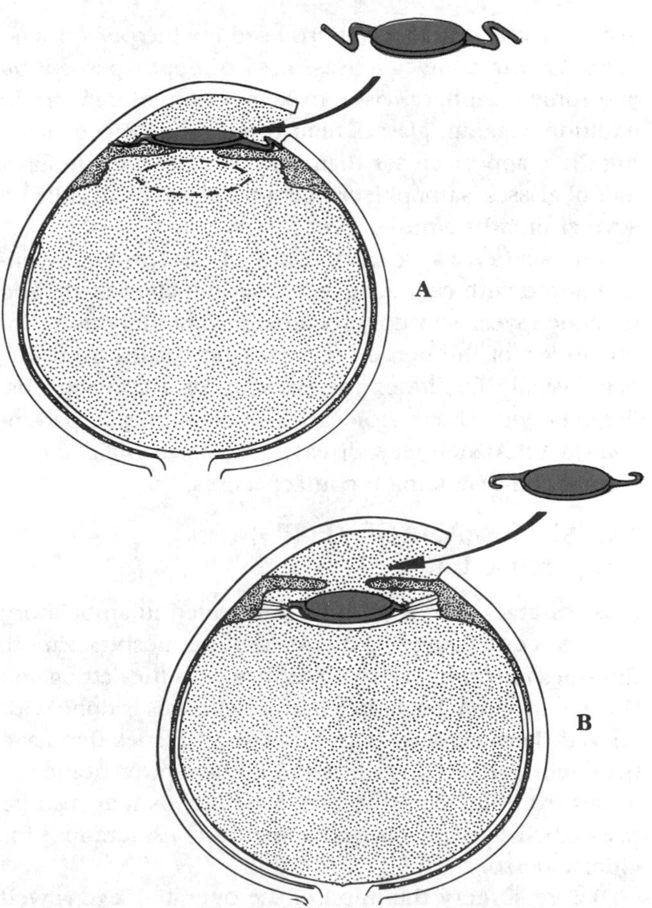


**FIGURE 60-5** Intraocular lens. **A,** Anterior lens implant in front of iris. **B,** Posterior lens implant behind iris. (From Long BL, Phipps WJ: *Medical-surgical nursing: a nursing process approach,* ed 3, St Louis, 1993, Mosby.)

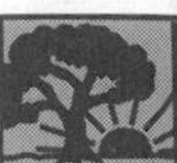

## GERONTOLOGIC PATIENT CONSIDERATIONS

**ASSESSMENT**

Assess all older patients for problems with distance and close vision, seeing in dim light, color perception, and glare.

Check on availability and cleanliness of vision aids.

**INTERVENTIONS**

Obtain low-vision aids for visually impaired older patients: large-print instructional materials, magnifying glasses, and talking books.

Set up meal tray according to clock face and instruct patient accordingly.

Provide plenty of light during meals, toileting, and ambulation because vision is decreased in dim light.

Post a sign at bedside of older patient alerting other personnel of patient's visual impairment.

Provide nonambiguous large signs at eye level with important instructions and names; for example, TOILET.

**COMMON DISORDERS IN ELDERS**

Cataracts
Glaucoma
Diabetic retinopathy

## Guidelines for Care of the Person After Cataract Surgery

1. Position patient on *unoperative* side to prevent pressure on operated eye.
2. Keep side rails up as necessary for protection.
3. Place bedside table on side of unoperated eye (patient then turns toward unoperated side).
4. Place call light within reach.
5. Stress avoidance of actions that increase IOP (for example, sneezing, coughing, vomiting, straining, or sudden bending over with the head below the waist).

are the least desirable but are used for the person who cannot wear contact lenses. Loss of depth perception and some peripheral vison make adjustment difficult. In addition, cataract glasses tend to magnify objects, making them appear closer than they actually are. The final pair of glasses is not prescribed until vision has stabilized several months after surgery.

Contact lenses correct some of the problems encountered with cataract glasses, but not all of them. The extended-wear soft contact lens is commonly used. Interruption of the nerve supply to the cornea from surgery usually facilitates the wearing of a contact lens. Persons with rheumatoid arthritis, hemiplegia, parkinsonism or Alzheimer's disease may have difficulty inserting and maintaining contact lenses.

## NURSING MANAGEMENT

### Preoperative Care

Most cataract surgery is now performed in ambulatory surgery centers; few patients require hospitalization. Routines for preoperative care vary with the setting and the eye surgeon. Eyelashes may be cut; this is done with curved sharp scissors with fairly short blades that have been lubricated with petrolatum to help prevent the cut lashes from entering the eye. Face scrubs may also be prescribed. See box above for special considerations for elderly persons.

Before surgery the pupil of the operative eye is well dilated. The medications must be given at the prescribed times so that the eye is prepared at the time of surgery. Sedation may also be given, particularly for persons who are apprehensive.

Surgery is generally performed using a local anesthetic injected behind the eyeball and in and around the eyelids. The patient usually can go home within 1 to 3 hours after surgery. General anesthesia may be necessary for patients who cannot hold still during surgery.

### Postoperative Care

The general goals of postoperative care are to prevent increased IOP, stress on the suture line, hemorrhage into the anterior chamber, and infection. Immediate postoperative care is described in the Guidelines box above.

After any cataract operation, a dressing is applied to the eye and covered with a metal shield to protect the eye from injury. The dressing is usually removed the day of or a day after surgery, but a metal eye shield is worn at night for a few weeks until the eye is healed to avoid accidental bumping of the eye during sleep.

As mentioned previously, most patients have their cataracts removed in day surgical units and are discharged in a few hours. Because of advancements in the techniques of lens extraction, activities of daily living are resumed as the patient feels able. The patient is cautioned not to sleep on the operated side for 3 to 4 weeks to prevent pressure on the operated eye. Depending on the techniques used to implant the lens, some patients will be cautioned not to bend over with the head lower than the waist for about 2 weeks. Other patients will have no restrictions on bending over. The nurse instructing the patient will need to clarify with the surgeon whether such restrictions are necessary.

Care should be taken in washing the face and hair to prevent any soap or water from entering the operated eye. Restrictions on activities such as heavy lifting may continue until complete healing has occurred (6 to 8 weeks). Patient teaching about follow-up care includes activity restrictions, the use of eye medications, and the eye shield. Patients should be given written instructions and a phone number to call if they have any questions (see the Nursing Care Plan, p. 2091). A research study describing effective discharge planning of elderly cataract patients undergoing day surgery[8] can be found in the Research box, p. 2093.

# NURSING CARE PLAN

## PERSON WITH A CATARACT

**DATA:** Mrs. W. is a 75-year-old woman who has had gradually decreasing vision in her right eye from a cataract. She states that it hasn't interfered too much with her activities until the past year. She remarks that now she can no longer drive at night because the car lights bother her; also, she has found it increasingly difficult to read even large print books. She comments that she is still able to look after herself and her home, although she occasionally misses some of the dust. Mrs. W. has been admitted to the day surgery unit for an extracapsular cataract extraction with intraocular lens implant.

The nursing history identified the following:

- Mrs. W. is widowed and lives alone.
- She defines her cataract as a "growth on my eye" and thinks the physician needs to take "my eye out to fix it and then put it back in."
- Mrs. W. perceives herself as healthy except for some osteoarthritis in her hip.
- She states that she is anxious about the surgery because she depends on her eyes for everything.

### ■ NURSING DIAGNOSIS

Anxiety related to surgical procedure and possible loss of vision

| Expected Patient Outcomes | Nursing Interventions | Rationale |
|---|---|---|
| Shows decreased signs of anxiety. | Give patient an opportunity to explore concerns about possible loss of vision. | Talking may help decrease anxiety and identify specific fears. |
| Verbalizes feelings of anxiety. | Explore knowledge of cataracts and preoperative and postoperative events; correct any misunderstandings; answer questions honestly. | Information decreases uncertainty and helps patient to gain control and feel less anxious. |

### ■ NURSING DIAGNOSIS

High risk for infection related to invasive procedure (cataract extraction)

| Expected Patient Outcome | Nursing Interventions | Rationale |
|---|---|---|
| Shows no signs or symptoms of infection. | Observe patient for signs and symptoms of infection. | Allows for early detection. |
| | Use sterile technique when performing eye care and changing dressings. | Decreases possibility of introducing pathogens. |
| | Administer antibiotic/steroid drops. | Helps prevent infection. |
| | Stress importance of not touching or rubbing operated eye. | Prevents contamination and disruption of operative site. |

### ■ NURSING DIAGNOSIS

High risk for injury related to increased intraocular pressure, vitreous humor loss, hemorrhage

| Expected Patient Outcomes | Nursing Interventions | Rationale |
|---|---|---|
| Describes factors that increase risk of injury. | Discuss postoperative course: pain, activity restrictions, and use of shield. | Information enhances cooperation with necessary restrictions. |
| Demonstrates behaviors to protect self from injury. | Keep bed at lowest position and side rail up on right side. | Ensures safety. |
| | Assist patient when first getting up after surgery. | Ensures safety (strange environment). |
| | Instruct patient to avoid sneezing, coughing, straining, and vomiting | Helps avoid increasing intraocular pressure (IOP). |
| | Administer cough medicine, antiemetics as required. | Controls cough and vomiting as they occur. |
| | Instruct patient to wear eye shield at night or when taking a nap during 6 weeks following surgery. | Prevents accidental bumping of the eye. |
| | Instruct patient not to put pressure on eye when administering eye medications. | External pressure can increase IOP, causing rupture of the sutures. |
| | Observe for flat anterior chamber, pear-shaped pupil, or bulging of wound. | Indicates wound rupture, prolapse of iris related to loose sutures or pressure on eye. |

# NURSING CARE PLAN

## PERSON WITH A CATARACT—cont'd

### ■ NURSING DIAGNOSIS

Knowledge deficit regarding condition, surgery, preoperative and postoperative care, self-care at home related to lack of exposure to information

| Expected Patient Outcomes | Nursing Interventions | Rationale |
|---|---|---|
| Can describe a cataract and explain the basis for the symptoms experienced. | Teach about the eye and the role of the lens in vision. Explain why patient experienced decreased vision and difficulty driving at night. | Increases understanding and promotes cooperation with postoperative routine. |
| Verbalizes or demonstrates knowledge of surgery, preoperative and postoperative care, and self-care at home. | Teach about preoperative routine, surgery. | Increases understanding and promotes cooperation with postoperative routine. |
| | Instruct patient in permitted activities postoperatively:<br>1. May climb stairs, watch TV, read, carry out ADLs as long as eye is comfortable<br>2. Avoid heavy physical activity for 6 weeks (lifting heavy objects, heavy house or yardwork, sports, shovelling)<br>3. Should not lift any object over 10 lbs<br>4. May bathe in tub or take shower; avoid splashing eyes when washing face<br>5. Protect eye with patch and shield when washing hair; tilt head backward | Activities that cause eyestrain or increase IOP may compromise surgery. |
| | 6. Should not bend so that head is below waist; avoid sudden movements | Prevents increasing IOP. |
| | Demonstrate proper technique in cleaning eye from inner to outer canthus using clean cotton ball for each wipe. Stress handwashing before and after cleaning eye. | Good technique reduces risk of spread of bacteria within eye. |
| | Demonstrate proper technique to put in drops and ointment, apply shield. Stress handwashing as above. | Good technique reduces risk of introducing infection. |
| | Instruct patient to call doctor if these occur:<br>1. Eye pain is severe or persistent<br>2. Redness of eye or lid increases<br>3. Quantity of discharge from eye increases or drainage changes to greenish color<br>4. Vision decreases | These are early signs of infection and require immediate attention. |

### ■ NURSING DIAGNOSIS

Pain related to inflammation, increased intraocular pressure

| Expected Patient Outcome | Nursing Interventions | Rationale |
|---|---|---|
| States eye feels comfortable. | Assess the level of discomfort. | Mild discomfort is expected postoperatively; acute pain suggests increased IOP or hemorrhage. |
| | Administer analgesics as required. | Promotes comfort. |

## NURSING CARE PLAN

### PERSON WITH A CATARACT—cont'd

**■ NURSING DIAGNOSIS**

Pain related to inflammation, increased intraocular pressure

| Expected Patient Outcome | Nursing Interventions | Rationale |
|---|---|---|
| | Instruct patient to avoid rapid head movements and not to bend head below waist to put on shoes, pick things up from floor, feed pet and so on. A long-handled reacher may be helpful in reaching things on floor. Stooping with knees bent is acceptable. | Avoids increasing IOP and pain. |

**■ NURSING DIAGNOSIS**

Sensory alteration: visual related to altered sensory reception/transmission

| Expected Patient Outcome | Nursing Interventions | Rationale |
|---|---|---|
| Understands that minimal alteration in normal sensory perception will be experienced. | Orient patient to physical surroundings and prepare her for the sensations and sounds she will feel and hear during surgery. | Provides for increased comfort and familiarity. |
| | Approach patient from unoperated side. | Aids orientation. |
| | Explain that vision will not be "normal" until the eye heals and glasses may be necessary in some cases (astigmatism). | Increases awareness of expected sensory alterations. |

### RESEARCH

Jairath N, et al: Effective discharge preparation of elderly cataract day surgery patients, *J Ophthalmic Nurs Technol* 9:157-160, 1990.

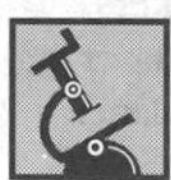

Knowledge regarding postdischarge recovery and safe and appropriate health care practices during early convalescence of elderly unilateral cataract patients was investigated. Sixteen women and four men, ranging in age from 66 to 82, participated in the study. All subjects received individualized educational interventions before hospitalization from their physician/designate, and on admission, before surgery, and at discharge from nurses. Patient knowledge was determined by a short true-or-false test before surgery, before discharge, and 24 hours after discharge. Total knowledge scores were high at all three times of testing but they increased significantly from before surgery to before discharge. The high scores before surgery suggest that most knowledge was acquired before admission to the hospital. However, less than perfect scores indicated that some knowledge deficits existed. The significant increase in scores after surgery signifies that hospital teaching partially rectified gaps in knowledge. Therefore, in-hospital teaching was effective, and knowledge acquisition was not precluded by the short length of stay on the day surgery unit.

# GLAUCOMA

## ETIOLOGY

The term **glaucoma** designates eye disease characterized by increased intraocular pressure associated with progressive loss of peripheral visual fields. Glaucoma is generally classified into two types: open angle and angle closure (closed angle). It is also classified as primary or secondary. When the cause is known, the glaucoma is designated as *secondary;* when it is not known, it is called *primary.* Secondary glaucoma can result from contracture of fibromuscular membranes in the anterior chamber, pupillary block interfering with the flow of aqueous humor from the posterior to the anterior chamber, or closure of the anterior chamber angle as a result of forward shift of the peripheral iris.

## EPIDEMIOLOGY

Glaucoma is responsible for 12% to 15% of all blindness in the United States today.[17] About 2% of persons over the age of 40 years have glaucoma. In African-American persons between 45 and 65 years of age, the prevalence of glaucoma is 15 times that of whites in the same age-group. It has been estimated that nearly 1 million persons in the United States have glaucoma that has not

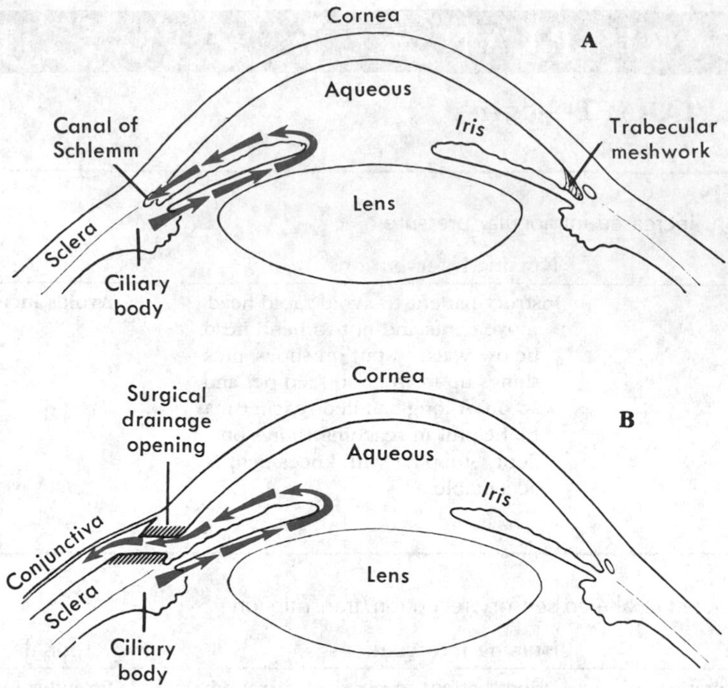


**FIGURE 60-6** **A,** Originating from ciliary processes, aqueous humor flows through pupil into anterior chamber and normally leaves eye by way of canal of Schlemm. **B,** In glaucoma, normal aqueous humor outflow is blocked. Purpose of glaucoma surgery is to create new channel through which aqueous humor can leave eye. (From Havener WH: *Synopsis of ophthalmology,* ed 5, St Louis, 1979, Mosby.)

**TABLE 60-8 Types of Glaucoma**

| TYPE | CHARACTERISTIC | MANIFESTATIONS | TREATMENT |
|---|---|---|---|
| Primary open-angle (chronic, simple) | Most common type (90%)<br>Usually caused by obstruction in trabecular meshwork | Frequently no signs or symptoms in early stages<br>Slow loss of vision<br>Peripheral vision lost before central (Figure 60-7)<br>Tunnel vision<br>Persistent dull eye pain<br>Difficulty adjusting to darkness<br>Failure to detect color changes<br>Later: headache, pain, blurred vision, halos around lights | Medical: miotics, carbonic anhydrase inhibitors, β-blockers<br>Surgical: trabeculectomy, laser trabeculoplasty, seton implants (Moltemo) |
| Primary angle closure (narrow angle, acute) | Outflow impaired as result of narrowing or closing of angle between iris and cornea<br>Intermittent attacks—pressure normal when angle open; if persistent, acute ocular emergency | Acute: severe prostrating pain, decreased vision, pupil enlarged and fixed, colored halos around lights, eye red, steamy cornea<br>Permanent blindness if marked increase in IOP for 24-48 hours | Medical: osmotic diuretics, carbonic anhydrase inhibitors, miotics<br>Surgical: peripheral iridectomy, laser iridotomy |
| Congenital | Abnormal development of filtration angle; can occur secondary to other systemic eye disorders<br>Rare (0.05%) | Enlargement of eye, lacrimation, photophobia, blepharospasm | Goniotomy (incision into region of trabecular meshwork)<br>Trabeculotomy<br>Seton implants<br>Cyclocryotherapy |
| Secondary | Can result from ocular inflammation, blood vessel changes, trauma | May be similar to open angle and angle closure, depending on cause | Directed at cause as well as at decreasing IOP |

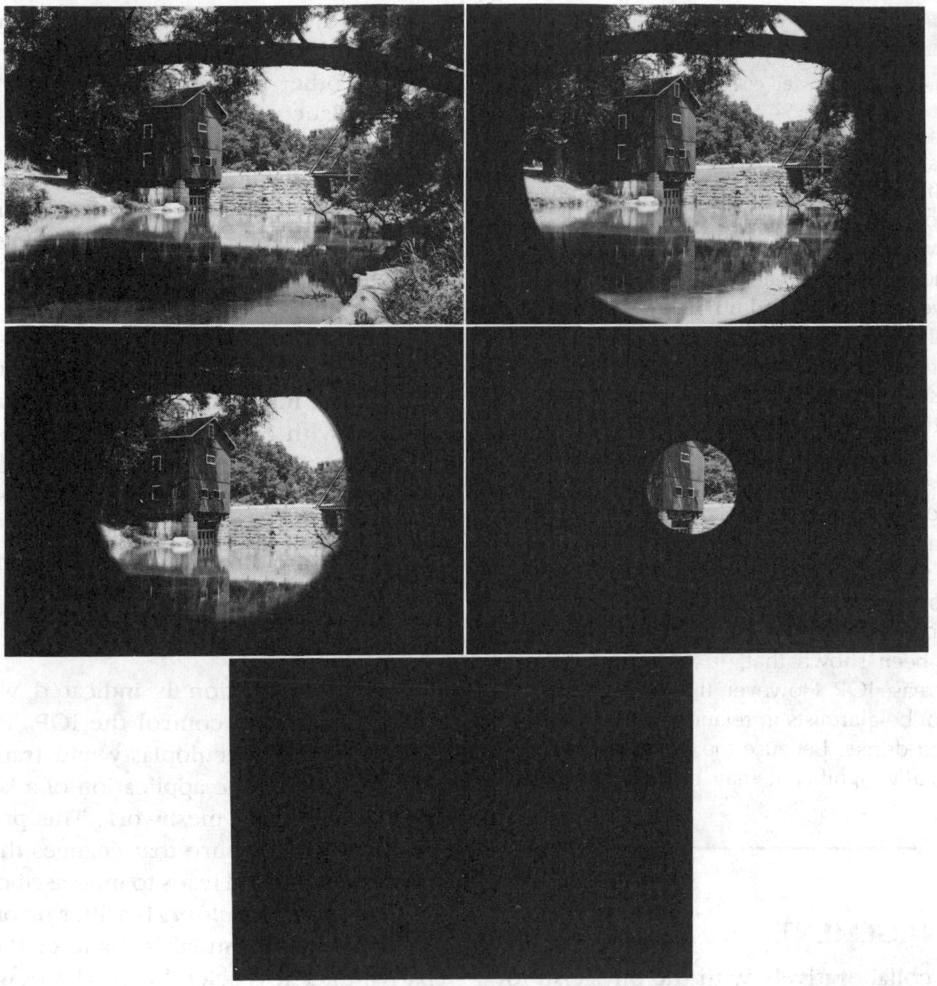

**FIGURE 60-7** Gradual loss of sight from glaucoma so insidiously destroys vision that person is unaware of impending blindness until extensive and irreversible damage is present. Note loss of peripheral vision. (From Saunders WH et al: *Nursing care in eye, ear, nose, and throat disorders,* ed 4, St Louis, 1979, Mosby.)

been diagnosed. The incidence of glaucoma is increasing as the number of older persons in our population increases. Glaucoma is the greatest threat to vision in older persons. Although it is seldom seen in persons under 35 years of age, it does occur in infancy.

## PATHOPHYSIOLOGY

Glaucoma results when the IOP is increased sufficiently to produce damage to the optic nerve. Normally there is a balance between production and drainage of aqueous humor, permitting the IOP to remain relatively constant (Figure 60-6). The normal range of IOP is 10 to 21 mm Hg, with a mean of 16 mm Hg. The pressure may vary by as much as 5 mm Hg as a result of diurnal changes. Obstruction in any part of the outflow channels results in backup of fluid and increased pressure. This may occur as a primary condition or it may be secondary to infection or trauma. Most rarely, glaucoma results from abnormal placement of the iris against the angle of the anterior chamber, thus blocking the outflow of aqueous humor (acute angle closure glaucoma). Table 60-8 outlines the different types of glaucoma along with their characteristics and treatment.

## PREVENTION

In either chronic or acute glaucoma, early diagnosis and treatment are mandatory to prevent destruction of nerve fibers on the optic disk that is caused by increased IOP. Those persons with a family history of glaucoma should have their eyes examined, including measurement of intraocular pressure, every 2 years after the age of 40. Mass screening programs are important in detecting possible glaucoma in persons who do not have periodic medical eye examinations. It is important to detect and treat this disease because the *permanent vision loss* it causes is usually *preventable.* A research study in which the effect of caffeine on IOP was investigated[18] is presented in the Research box, p. 2096.

**RESEARCH**

Okimi PH et al: Effects of caffeinated coffee on intraocular pressure, *Appl Nurs Res* 4(2):72-76, 1991.

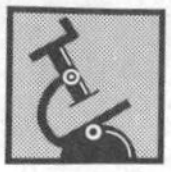

In this first phase of a larger study, the effects of caffeinated coffee on the intraocular pressure of nonglaucomatous subjects were investigated. Twelve subjects, all under the age of 50, were randomly assigned to receive each of three treatments: caffeinated coffee, hot water, and no fluid. All subjects were given the three treatment conditions over a 3-day period. Blood pressure, pulse, and intraocular pressure (IOP) were measured hourly for 3 hours after the treatment. The investigators discovered that intraocular pressure was significantly higher after ingesting caffeinated coffee than it was after the other two treatment conditions. It was also established that increased intraocular pressure was maintained at significant levels over a 3-hour period. No significant changes were found in pulse rate, and blood pressure findings were inconclusive. The investigators recommend that patients with glaucoma be told that it has been shown that, in some instances, caffeine may increase IOP. However, they also note that nurses should not be alarmists in relation to the normal use of caffeinated drinks, because the increase in IOP, although *statistically* significant may not be *clinically* significant.

## MEDICAL MANAGEMENT

The nurse works collaboratively with the physician for implementation of prescribed medical therapy. Because the nurse has a major role in patient teaching, this is discussed under Nursing Management.

### Diagnostic Tests

Several diagnostic tests are used to diagnose and monitor glaucoma. These include (1) tonometry, measurement of IOP; (2) ophthalmoscopy, evaluation of color and configuration of the optic cup; (3) perimetry, measurement of visual function in the central field of vision; and (4) gonioscopy, observation of the anterior chamber angle by the use of a contact lens combined with either a mirror or a prism.

### Medications

Persons with glaucoma may be taking medication for the rest of their lives. The goals of medication therapy are to provide better drainage of aqueous humor and to decrease the amount of aqueous humor produced. It is important that patients understand the necessity of taking the medication when prescribed to control the IOP and thus help prevent vision loss. The patient and family should know specifically what to do if essential eyedrops are accidentally spilled; for example, they should know which local drugstore is open at night and on holidays. The person often is advised to have an extra bottle of medication in the home and to carry one when away from the home. It is advisable for the person to carry a card or other information that identifies him or her as having glaucoma in case an accident occurs.

Drugs used in the treatment of glaucoma are outlined in Table 60-9. Pilocarpine, a miotic, and timolol maleate, a β-blocker, are two of the most common drugs used. Caution must be exercised in administering β-blockers to patients with asthma, chronic obstructive pulmonary disease, and cardiac disease.[25]

Angle-closure glaucoma is an emergency situation, because vision will be lost permanently unless IOP is controlled. Intravenous and oral acetazolamide, supplemented with osmotic agents and topical β-blockers, is usually effective in lowering IOP. Pilocarpine 4% will then be used intensively (1 drop every 15 minutes for 1 to 2 hours) along with topical steroids. Steroids in high doses are thought to be helpful in reducing damage to the iris and trabecular meshwork.

## SURGICAL MANAGEMENT

Surgical intervention is indicated when conservative treatment fails to control the IOP. Two common procedures are trabeculoplasty and trabeculectomy. ***Trabeculoplasty*** is the application of a laser beam (argon) on the trabecular meshwork. This produces a nonpenetrating thermal burn that changes the configuration of the meshwork and leads to increased outflow of aqueous humor. ***Trabeculectomy*** is a filtering procedure in which an opening, or fistula, is made at the limbus under a partial-thickness scleral flap. The new opening circumvents the obstruction, and aqueous humor flows into the subconjunctival spaces.

Trabeculectomy usually requires overnight hospitalization. Trabeculoplasty, however, is frequently performed on an ambulatory basis, and the person usually remains for 3 to 4 hours after the procedure so that IOP can be checked. A complication of the procedure is a sudden rise of IOP 8 to 12 hours after surgery. IOP control is achieved in about 85% of all patients, but most (75%) continue to require glaucoma medications. Nursing care for the person after trabeculectomy is summarized in the Guidelines box below.

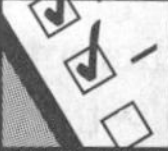

**Guidelines for Care of the Person After Trabeculectomy**

Nursing care for the patient following trabeculectomy includes the following:

1. Routine postanesthesia care
2. Protection of operative eye with patch, shield, positioning patient on back or unoperative side, and safety measures
3. Maintaining comfort in the operative eye
4. Assessment, as appropriate, of the IOP, appearance of the bleb, and anterior chamber depth
5. Administration of medications such as a cycloplegic, a mydriatic, and a combination antibiotic and steroid

**TABLE 60-9 Drugs Used in Treatment of Glaucoma**

| DRUG | FORM AND DOSAGE | ACTION |
|---|---|---|
| **CHOLINERGIC DRUGS (MIOTICS)** | | |
| Pilocarpine | 0.5%-10% solution: 1 drop q 6-12 hr<br>Ocular insert: replace weekly | Increased outflow of aqueous humor due to ciliary muscle pull on trabecular meshwork |
| Carbachol (Carbacel) | 0.75%-3% solution: 1 drop q 6-12 hr | |
| **CHOLINESTERASE INHIBITORS (MIOTICS)** | | |
| Physostigmine (Eserine) | 0.25%-1% solution: 1 drop q 6-8 hr or ointment h.s. | Increased outflow of aqueous humor due to ciliary muscle pull on trabecular meshwork |
| Isoflurophate (Floropryl) | 0.01%-0.1% solution: 1 drop q 12-24 hr or 0.25% ointment h.s. | |
| Demecarium bromide (Humorsol) | 0.125%-0.25% solution: 1 drop q 12-24 hr | |
| Echothiophate iodide (Phospholine iodide) | 0.03%-0.25% solution: 1 drop q 12-24 hr | |
| **ADRENERGIC AGENTS** | | |
| Epinephryl borate (Eppy) | 0.25%-1% solution: 1 drop q 12 hr | Reduces aqueous humor formation and increases outflow facility |
| Epinephrine hydrochloride (Glaucon) | 0.5%-2% solution: 1 drop q 12 hr | |
| Epinephrine bitartrate (Epitrate) | 2% solution: 1 drop q 12 hr | |
| Dipivefrin (Propine) | 0.1% solution: 1 drop q 12 hr | |
| **CARBONIC ANHYDRASE INHIBITORS** | | |
| Acetazolamide (Diamox) | 250 mg tablets: 1 tablet q 6-8-12 hr; 500 mg. capsules, sequential: 1 capsule q 12-24 hr<br>500 mg vials for IM or IV use if patient vomiting | Decreases aqueous humor production (inhibition of carbonic anhydrase in ciliary processes) |
| Ethoxzolamide (Cardrase) | 125-250 mg tablets: 1 tablet q 6-12 hr | |
| Dichlorphenamide (Daranide) | 50 mg tablets: 1 tablet q 8-12 hr | |
| Methazolamide (Neptazine) | 50 mg tablets: 1 tablet q 8-12 hr | |
| **OSMOTIC AGENTS** | | |
| Glycerin (Osmoglyn) | 1.0-1.5 g/kg body wt (usually 4-6 oz) | Moves water from the intraocular structures, resulting in a marked ocular hypotonic effect, thereby decreasing IOP |
| Mannitol (Osmitrol) | 2 g/kg body wt or 25-50 ml of 20% solution IV | |
| Isosorbide (Ismotic) | 1.5-3.0 g/kg body wt | |
| **β-ADRENERGIC BLOCKER** | | |
| Timolol maleate (Timoptic) | 0.25%-0.5% solution: 1 drop q 12 hr | Decreases aqueous humor production |
| Betaxolol (Betoptic) | 0.25%-0.5% solution: 1 drop q 12 hr | |
| Levobunolol (Betazan) | 0.5% solution: 1 drop q 12 hr; qd | |

Cyclodestructive procedures such as *cyclotherapy* and *YAG laser thermal procedures* attempt to lower IOP by direct permanent damage to the ciliary body.[25] These procedures are not always predictable in their effects and may have to be repeated. Patients receiving these treatments often have eyes that are prone to severe inflammation, retinal detachments, hemorrhaging, and phthisis. Therefore they must be closely followed by an ophthalmologist.

Molteno implants and other seton implants provide a new surgical approach for patients with glaucoma that is resistant to other forms of surgery.[12] In implant surgery, a polymethylmethacrylate plate is implanted against the sclera. A tube is then surgically implanted directly into the anterior chamber. The aqueous humor then drains out of the eye through the tube, collecting under the plate posteriorly. The plate is designed to block scar tissue from affecting aqueous reabsorption and from physically blocking the outflow tube. If the implant is overdraining, potential complications such as retinal detachments and choroidal and vitreous hemorrhages may occur. However, if the implant is functioning properly, vision can be restored.

In acute closure, once the IOP is under control, a *peripheral iridectomy* is frequently performed to form a permanent connection between the anterior and posterior chambers, thus preventing the iris from occluding the anterior chamber. A surgical peripheral iridectomy can be performed if laser treatment is unsuccessful.

## NURSING MANAGEMENT

### ♦ ASSESSMENT

#### Subjective Data

The symptoms of angle-closure glaucoma are related to a sudden increase in intraocular pressure. Patients may complain of sudden onset of severe blurring of vision, excruciating pain, halos around lights, and nausea and vomiting. There may be repeated attacks of pain and blurred vision occurring after a prolonged time in darkness or prolonged emotional upset. Open-angle glaucoma is usually asymptomatic until late in the disease, when vision loss is noted.

## Objective Data

Assessment in glaucoma includes monitoring the patient's IOP, visual fields, and optic disk. The nurse can also identify any change in vision.

### Diagnostic test findings

Measurement of IOP will indicate an increase in pressure. Once medication has been initiated, the IOP should return to within normal limits, although careful monitoring is required to assess the ongoing effectiveness of the medications. The increased IOP will cause destruction of the ganglion cells of the retina and atrophy of the optic disk. Assessment of visual fields will demonstrate increasing loss of vision, which starts at the periphery and can proceed to total blindness (see Figure 60-7). Examination of the optic disk will reveal loss of disk substance detectable as enlargement of the optic disk cup and disk pallor, particularly in the area of cupping.

## ♦ NURSING DIAGNOSES

Nursing diagnoses are determined from analysis of patient data. Nursing diagnoses for the patient with glaucoma may include but are not limited to the following:

| Diagnostic Title | Possible Etiologic Factors |
|---|---|
| Pain | Increased IOP |
| Knowledge deficit (about glaucoma) | Lack of exposure/recall of information or misinterpretation of information |
| Health maintenance, altered | Impairment in vision, difficulty in doing ADLs independently |
| Sensory alteration: visual | Altered sensory reception/transmission |

## ♦ EXPECTED PATIENT OUTCOMES

Expected patient outcomes for the patient with glaucoma may include but are not limited to the following:

1. States discomfort is decreased.
2. Can describe the following:
   a. Need for lifetime use of eye medications
   b. Prescribed medication therapy
   c. Preventive measures
   d. Signs and symptoms requiring immediate medical attention
3. Can maintain health despite alteration in vision.
4. Vision not decreased further.

## ♦ INTERVENTIONS

### Promoting Comfort

The eye usually becomes more comfortable when the IOP decreases. Analgesics may be prescribed (see Guidelines box, p. 2096). Cold eye compresses may also increase comfort.

**Guidelines for Teaching the Person With Glaucoma**

1. Lifetime eye medication required
2. Preventive measures
   a. Have reserve bottle of eyedrops at home.
   b. Carry eyedrops when away from home.
   c. Carry identification for glaucoma and the prescribed eyedrop solution.
   d. Be aware of location of local drugstore open nights, weekends, and holidays.
3. Name, dosage, frequency, and side effects of prescribed eye medications
4. Signs and symptoms requiring immediate reporting to physician (for example, eye pain, sudden change in vision, halos around lights)

### Facilitating Learning

Glaucoma is a chronic condition, and the person with newly diagnosed glaucoma needs help in understanding and learning to live with the disease. Despite explanations from the physician, the person frequently hopes that an operation will cure the condition, that no further treatment will be necessary, and perhaps that lost sight will be restored. It should be explained that the lost vision cannot be restored, but that further loss can usually be prevented and life can be quite normal if the person continues under medical care. Usually no restrictions are placed on the use of the eyes. Fluid intake generally is not curtailed, and exercise is permitted. Bright lights or darkness are not harmful to the eyes of the person with glaucoma. Patient teaching is summarized in the Guidelines box above.

## ♦ EVALUATION

To evaluate the effectiveness of nursing interventions, compare patient behaviors with those stated in the expected patient outcomes. Successful achievement of patient outcomes for the patient with glaucoma is indicated by the following:

1. Looks comfortable and gives no verbal or physical indications of being in pain.
2. States his or her role in posthospital care:
   a. Describes medication therapy (name of eyedrops, dose, frequency).
   b. Demonstrates correct way to instill eyedrops.
   c. States that eye medications must be taken for the remainder of his or her life.
   d. Discusses need to have reserve bottle of eyedrops at home and to carry eyedrops on person (not in luggage) when traveling.
   e. Displays identification card or wears Medic-Alert bracelet that identifies the person as hav-

ing glaucoma and lists prescribed eyedrop solution.
   f. States need to call physician immediately if eye pain, sudden change in vision, or halos around lights occur.
3. Demonstrates ability to carry out own ADLs.
4. States that vision is not decreasing, and demonstrates this by performing ADLs and walking about independently.

# DETACHMENT OF THE RETINA

## ETIOLOGY/PATHOPHYSIOLOGY

**Retinal detachment** occurs when the two retinal layers (outer pigmented epithelium and inner sensory layer) separate as a result of a full-thickness break in the sensory retina, with subsequent passage of liquefied vitreous humor through the break into the subretinal space (rhegmatogenous detachment), accumulation of fluid beneath the sensory retina (serous or hemorrhagic detachment), or traction produced by contraction of the vitreous body (traction detachment) (Figure 60-8). As the detachment extends and becomes complete, blindness results because the macula detaches. Myopic degeneration, trauma, and **aphakia** (absence of the crystalline lens) are the most frequent causes of retinal detachment. It may also result from hemorrhage, tumor, or exudates in front of or behind the retina. Detachment of the retina may follow sudden severe physical exertion, especially in persons who are debilitated. Most often, however, no apparent cause is identified.

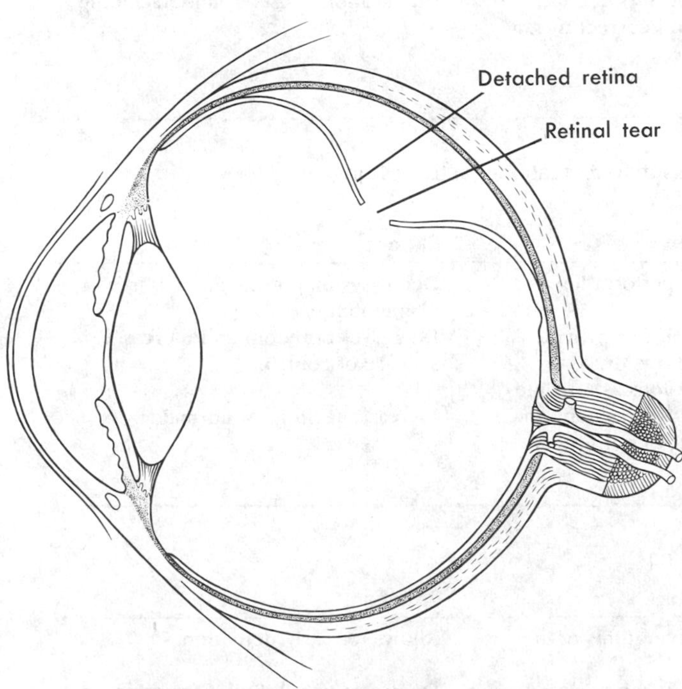


**FIGURE 60-8** Retinal detachment.

Retinal detachment may occur suddenly or may develop slowly. Symptoms include floating spots or opacities before the eyes, flashes of light, and progressive loss of vision in one area. The floating spots are blood and retinal cells that are freed at the time of the tear; they cast shadows on the retina as they seem to drift about the eye. The flashes of light are caused by vitreous traction on the retina. The area of visual loss depends entirely on the location of the detachment. When the detachment is extensive and occurs quickly, the patient may have the sensation that a curtain has been drawn before the eyes. The diagnosis of retinal separation is based on the ophthalmoscopic appearance of the retina.

## PREVENTION

Preventive measures are directed toward early detection. Persons at risk for retinal detachment, such as those with a high degree of myopia and diabetic retinopathy, should have routine eye examinations that include ophthalmoscopy. Regular monitoring will help identify degenerative changes in the retina that will increase the risk for retinal detachment.

## SURGICAL MANAGEMENT

### Preoperative Care

Immediate care for the detachment depends on its degree and site. There may be moderate to little restriction on activity, as well as bilateral to no patching of the eyes. If the macular region is threatened or a large detachment has occurred, care may include keeping the patient quiet in bed with the eyes covered to try to prevent further detachment and aid absorption of subretinal fluid. The head is positioned so that the retinal hole is in the lowest part of the eye so there is less chance of the detachment worsening. Activity may also be restricted (see Nursing Care Plan, p. 2100).

### Surgical Procedures

Surgery is primarily performed using general anesthesia. Cyclopentolate or phenylephrine is used to keep the pupils widely dilated so that tears in the retina may be identified during the operation. The surgical procedure may include draining the fluid from the subretinal space so that the retina returns to its normal position, thereby closing the opening in the retina. To drain the fluid from the subretinal space, the sclera and choroid are perforated at the time of the operation.

The retinal breaks are sealed off by various methods that produce an inflammatory reaction *(chorioretinitis)* in the area of the tear so that adhesions will form between the edges of the break and the underlying choroid to obliterate the opening. When the tears are small or of recent origin, *diathermy* may be applied through the sclera with needlepoint electrodes to produce the inflammatory process. An intense beam of visible light directed to the area by means of an argon laser may be used to close a retinal tear when the retina is not ele-

# NURSING CARE PLAN

## PERSON WITH RETINAL DETACHMENT

**DATA:** Mr. A. is a 56-year-old warehouse clerk who complains of decreasing vision in his left eye over the past few days, like "a curtain coming over my eye." He comments that he began to notice spots floating in front of his eye about 2 weeks ago and flashes of light out of the corner of his eye a week ago. He states that he did not get concerned about these, because he thought they were just normal aging changes. He remarks, "I began to get scared when I started to go blind in that eye, and then it didn't take me long to get to my eye doctor." He continues, "I got more scared when the doctor sent me straight to the hospital." Mr. A. states that, except for nearsightedness, he has had no trouble with his eyes. He is generally healthy except for high blood pressure, which is well controlled with medication and diet. Examination of his left eye revealed a superior retinal detachment with inferior visual loss. His visual acuity is 20/80. He is scheduled for retinal detachment surgery (scleral buckling). His left eye is patched, and his orders are for bedrest with bathroom privileges.

The nursing history identified the following:

- He and his wife have little understanding of what has happened to his eye or what the physician is going to do to his eye in the hospital.
- The loss of vision is very frightening to Mr. and Mrs. A. They are also concerned about whether Mr. A. will get any vision back in the eye and whether it will spread to the other eye.
- Mr. A. has not had any accidents or injuries to his eyes that he can remember.
- Mr. A. is a very active man, swimming and jogging regularly. He comments that he has to do some "good" activity every day so he can feel his best.

### ■ NURSING DIAGNOSIS

Anxiety/Fear related to surgical procedure and possible loss of vision

| Expected Patient Outcomes | Nursing Interventions | Rationale |
|---|---|---|
| Shows decreased signs of anxiety. | Give patient and spouse an opportunity to explore concerns about possible loss of vision. | Talking may help decrease anxiety and identify specific fears. |
| Verbalizes fears and feelings of anxiety. | Answer questions honestly. | Information decreases uncertainty and helps person to gain control and feel less anxious. |
| | Encourage realistic hope about maintaining vision. | Helps relieve their anxiety. |
| | Explore knowledge of disorder and planned therapy, and correct misunderstandings. | Clarification assists in understanding. |

### ■ NURSING DIAGNOSIS

Diversional activity deficit related to inability to participate in routine recreational activities (jogging, swimming)

| Expected Patient Outcome | Nursing Interventions | Rationale |
|---|---|---|
| Participates in activities to decrease boredom and maintain sense of fitness. | Encourage patient to perform leg exercises. | Decreases monotony and hazards of immobility. |
| | Vary patient's daily routine; provide tapes, and radio. Allow Mr. A. to make as many decisions as possible. | Decreases boredom and increases sense of control. |
| | Encourage postoperative resumption of normal activities, as permitted. | Increases feelings of normalcy. |

### ■ NURSING DIAGNOSIS

High risk for infection related to surgical repair of detached retina

| Expected Patient Outcome | Nursing Interventions | Rationale |
|---|---|---|
| Shows no signs or symptoms of infection. | Assess for signs and symptoms of infection. | Allows for early detection. |
| | Use sterile technique when performing eye care and changing dressings. | Decreases possibility of introducing pathogens. |
| | Administer antibiotic drops. | Helps prevent infection. |

## NURSING CARE PLAN

### PERSON WITH RETINAL DETACHMENT—cont'd

#### ■ NURSING DIAGNOSIS

High risk for injury related to sensory deficit, lack of awareness of environmental hazards

| Expected Patient Outcomes | Nursing Interventions | Rationale |
|---|---|---|
| Sustains no injury. | Orient patient to physical surroundings. | Increases awareness of potential hazards. |
| Experiences no decreased vision. | Keep bed at lowest position and side rail up on left side. | Ensures safety when patient has eyes patched and is in strange environment. |
| | Assist patient when first getting up after surgery. | Ensures safety. |
| | Instruct patient to avoid sneezing, coughing, and vomiting. Administer cough medicine, antiemetics, if required. | Helps avoid increasing IOP. |
| | Instruct patient to wear eye shield at night or when taking a nap during 2 weeks following surgery. | Prevents accidental bumping of the eye. |

#### ■ NURSING DIAGNOSIS

Knowledge deficit regarding condition, surgery, preoperative and postoperative care, and self-care at home related to lack of exposure

| Expected Patient Outcomes | Nursing Interventions | Rationale |
|---|---|---|
| Patient and his wife can describe retinal detachment and explain the basis for the symptoms experienced. | Teach about the eye and the role of the retina in vision. Explain why flashing lights, spots appear before the eyes, and decreased vision occurs. | Increases understanding and promotes cooperation with postoperative routine. |
| Patient and wife can verbalize or demonstrate knowledge of surgery, preoperative and postoperative care, and self-care at home. | Teach about preoperative routine and surgery. Instruct patient in permitted postoperative activities:<br>1. Ask physician when a return to work can be made<br>2. May climb stairs, watch TV, read, carry out ADLs as long as eye is comfortable<br>3. Avoid driving, heavy house or yard work, or sporting activities before checking with physician<br>4. May bathe in tub; avoid splashing eyes when washing face<br>5. Do not bend head below waist: avoid sudden movements | Activities that cause eyestrain, or increase IOP, may compromise surgery. |
| | Demonstrate proper technique in cleaning eye from inner to outer canthus using clean cotton ball for each wipe. Stress handwashing. | Good technique reduces risk of spread of bacteria. |
| | Demonstrate proper technique to administer drops and ointment and apply shield. Stress handwashing. | |
| | Instruct patient and spouse to call doctor if:<br>1. New flashing lights, floaters, or shadows appear<br>2. Eye pain is severe or persistent<br>3. Redness of eye or lid increases<br>4. Quantity of discharge from eye increases or changes to greenish color | Early intervention can prevent development of complications. |

## NURSING CARE PLAN

### PERSON WITH RETINAL DETACHMENT—cont'd

■ **NURSING DIAGNOSIS**

Pain related to inflammation, increased intraocular pressure

| Expected Patient Outcome | Nursing Interventions | Rationale |
|---|---|---|
| States eye feels comfortable. | Assess the level of discomfort. | Postoperative discomfort is expected, but acute pain suggests increased IOP or hemorrhage. |
| | Apply cool, moist compresses. | Reduces swelling and promotes comfort. |
| | Administer analgesics as required. | Promotes comfort. |
| | Instruct patient to avoid rapid head movements and not to bend head below waist. | Avoids increasing IOP and pain. |

■ **NURSING DIAGNOSIS**

Sensory alteration: visual related to altered sensory reception/transmission

| Expected Patient Outcomes | Nursing Interventions | Rationale |
|---|---|---|
| Experiences no further decrease in vision. | Maintain prescribed activity and position restrictions. | Restricted eye movement helps decrease risk of further detachment. |
| | Place bedside table within patient's reach without need to turn head. | Gravity is used to help keep the retina in its proper position. |
| ADLs are met. | Assist with ADLs as necessary. | Decreased vision and restrictions in activity alter or interfere with familiar ways of doing things. |
| Can describe physical surroundings. | Orient patient to physical surroundings. | Provides for increased comfort and familiarity. |
| | Place bed so patient is not facing wall and can see others approaching. Approach patient from unaffected side. | Offsets isolation and aids orientation to surrounding environment. |
| | Encourage diversional activities such as radio and conversation. | Provides sensory input and feelings of normalcy. |

vated *(photocoagulation).* The *laser beam* is used as a source of intense energy to produce chorioretinitis. Subfreezing temperatures (−40° to −60° C) may be applied to the surface of the sclera in the area of the hole to produce the inflammatory reaction *(cryotherapy).* Nitrous oxide or carbon dioxide under pressure, flowing through a tube attached to a delicate instrument, is used to produce these low temperatures.

For most retinal detachments, *scleral buckling* procedures are used. In this procedure, the sclera and choroid are indented (buckled) toward the retinal break. Buckling is accomplished by placing silicone of various shapes and sizes in the region of the break (Figure 60-9). In addition an encircling tape of silicone can be placed around the entire eye. By these procedures, the choroid is pushed into contact with the retinal tear during healing, and vitreous adhesions that have exerted traction, or pull, on the retinal break are relaxed as the size of the scleral shell is decreased.

Retinal detachments can also be repaired by pneu-

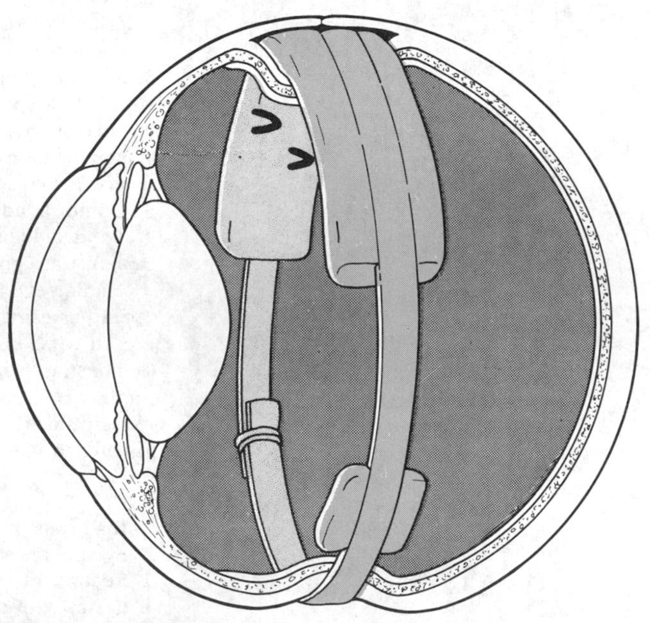

**FIGURE 60-9** Scleral buckle.

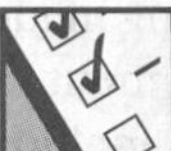

**Guidelines for Care of the Person After Retinal Detachment Surgery**

The postoperative care for the person with retinal detachment includes the following:

1. Position and ambulate the patient as ordered.
2. Assist with ADLs as required.
3. Administer eye medications as ordered (mydriatics, cycloplegics, and combination steroid/antibiotic).
4. Apply cold compresses as ordered to reduce swelling and promote comfort.
5. Implement safety measures such as use of side rails.
6. Instruct the patient to avoid jerking motions of the head (sneezing, coughing, vomiting)
   a. Administer antiemetics, as required.
   b. Administer cough medication, as required.

matic retinopexy. This surgical procedure involves the intraocular injection of air or an expandable gas, for example, $SF_6$ (sulfurhexafluoride) or perfluorcarbon, to tamponade the retinal tear and allow healing to occur.[24]

## NURSING MANAGEMENT

Specific nursing interventions for the patient undergoing retinal detachment surgery are outlined in the nursing care plan (see p. 2100). Preoperative and postoperative interventions are directed toward promoting safety, counseling, and patient teaching. Specific teaching is outlined in the Guidelines box above.

### Promoting Safety

Although most surgeons do not patch both eyes (binocular), some do so preoperatively and for 2 or 3 days postoperatively. Safety precautions such as side rails are essential if binocular patching is used. Call signals need to be kept within reach. Explanation of the immediate environment is also indicated.

### Providing Emotional Support

Patients are usually anxious and apprehensive when admitted to the hospital. Generally there has been a rapid loss of vision, and patients fear losing more vision. Restoration of sight will depend on the extent and duration of the detachment and the success of the surgery. Opportunity to discuss concerns needs to be provided. Nurses can do much to allay apprehension by answering questions honestly and instilling realistic hope.

### Facilitating Learning

Patient teaching for persons with retinal detachment includes the following:

1. Report to ophthalmologist any signs of redetachment (increase in floaters, flashes of light, decreased vision, increased eye pain).
2. Use appropriate techniques for administration of eye medications.
3. Limit activities to sedentary work for 1 to 2 weeks.
4. Check with physician about resumption of activities such as sports or heavy lifting.
5. Discuss plan for medical follow-up (appointment with physician and so on).

# DIABETIC RETINOPATHY

The quality of health and the life expectancy of the person with diabetes have improved as a result of the use of insulin and regulated exercise and diet. Because of the longer life span, however, some of the complications associated with diabetes, such as pathologic conditions of the retina, have increased.

## ETIOLOGY/EPIDEMIOLOGY

Diabetic retinopathy is a disorder of the blood vessels of the retina, which usually appears about 10 years after onset of diabetes mellitus. The incidence seems to depend mainly on the duration of the diabetes. Retinopathy can be detected in approximately 65% of persons who have had Type I diabetes for 15 years and in about 60% of older persons with Type II diabetes.[20] Diabetic retinopathy is responsible for at least 10% of cases of newly reported blindness each year and 20% of cases in persons 45 to 75 years of age.[6,15,23]

## PATHOPHYSIOLOGY

In the initial phase of diabetic retinopathy, which usually lasts several years, the retinal capillary walls thicken and develop tiny pouchings (microaneurysms), and the retinal veins widen and become tortuous. Small hemorrhages develop, which may eventually disappear, leaving small scars that decrease vision in those areas. Protein leaks from the vessels as a result of increased capillary permeability, causing retinal edema, especially in the area of the macula, with subsequent decreases in visual acuity level.

In advanced disease, small blood vessels develop on the retina and grow out into the vitreous humor *(neovascularization)* in response to retinal ischemia. These vessels frequently rupture, causing decreased vision. Some of the blood may be reabsorbed, and vision will increase until the next hemorrhage, but the continuing hemorrhagic process eventually leads to marked visual loss. Resolution of the hemorrhagic products may create a pull (traction) on the retina, leading to tearing and detachment of the retina.

The *signs of diabetic retinopathy—tortuous vessels, small dots (microaneurysms), "fluffy wool" exudates on the retina,* and *new vessel formation—can be identified only by* examining the retina through *ophthalmoscopy* and *fluorescein angiography.* As the disease progresses, the person describes increasing loss of vision and sees multiple spots (floaters). The floaters are minute hemorrhagic products in the vitreous humor.

## PREVENTION

### Primary Prevention

It is recommended that persons with Type I diabetes be referred to an ophthalmologist within 3 years of diagnosis and annually thereafter. Persons with Type II diabetes should be examined at diagnosis and annually thereafter. Because diabetic retinopathy can become particularly aggressive during pregnancy, diabetic women who are pregnant should be examined in the first trimester and every 3 months until the end of the pregnancy.

### Secondary Prevention

Early detection and treatment can help reduce the risks of massive retinal hemorrhage and retinal detachment.

## MEDICAL MANAGEMENT

The nurse works collaboratively with the physician for implementation of prescribed medical therapy. Because the nurse has a major role in patient teaching, this is discussed under Nursing Management.

Several methods of treatment are being used and studied for effectiveness. These include the following:

1. *Photocoagulation.* In this therapy an intense beam of light from a laser (argon) is directed into the eye and focused on a small spot on the retina. The light energy is transformed into heat energy. The laser therapy damages and scars the peripheral retina in order to decrease the ischemia, which induces neurovascularization. The process should resolve without subsequent retinal hemorrhages or retinal detachments. At present, the *panretinal* or *scatter type* of treatment is the preferred approach. The physician scatters 200 to 2000 laser burns around the retina. Recent research indicates that retinal photocoagulation reduced, at least temporarily, the risk of blindness by about 60% in those persons with moderate to severe retinopathy.[20]
2. *Vitrectomy.* Eyes that cannot be treated by photocoagulation can sometimes be treated surgically by a *vitrectomy.* The vitrectomy procedure allows proper visualization of the retina so that photocoagulation and other surgical retinal detachment procedures can be performed. Although the effectiveness has steadily improved, this still is a difficult procedure, and complications occur. In this procedure the surgeon removes (a) the opaque bloody fluid (from hemorrhage) in the vitreous and replaces it with a saline solution, (b) the fibrous or scar tissue that could pull on the retina causing it to detach, and (c) the tissue that could serve as a scaffold for the growth of new vessels between the retina and vitreous. Retinal reattachment procedures, such as scleral buckling and injection of air or gases into the eye may be performed at the same time.
3. *Methods under investigation.* Because of the limitations of surgical methods to preserve vision in diabetic retinopathy, efforts are continually being made to find medical means of preventing development of the condition. Methods being investigated include (1) better metabolic control of blood sugar, (2) aldase reductase inhibitors, and (3) laser and aspirin therapy.

## NURSING MANAGEMENT

Nursing management of the person with diabetic retinopathy includes the following:

1. Teaching the patient about the importance of regular eye examinations.
   a. All diabetics should have their visual acuity and fundi checked yearly. More frequent examinations may be required if positive findings develop.
   b. Children should be examined 3 to 5 years after the onset of diabetes or at puberty.
   c. Those persons with mild forms of retinopathy are urged to have three to four examinations a year.
   d. Better long-term diabetic control is important to decrease the incidence of severe diabetic retinopathy over time.
2. Teaching the patient about photocoagulation, as appropriate.
   a. Procedure usually is done on outpatient basis.
   b. There may be mild to moderate discomfort.
   c. Analgesia will be prescribed as necessary.
   d. Vision may be blurred following the procedure.
3. Assessing knowledge of diabetes, and teaching as required.
4. When vision is impaired, assessing ability to administer own insulin and test own blood sugar.
5. Altering patient's self-management techniques as required (see discussion of diabetes in Chapter 40).
6. Providing opportunity for patients to discuss concerns and fears about disease and visual impairment.
7. If patient admitted for vitrectomy, carrying out routine preoperative and postoperative nursing care for persons having eye surgery. The nurse should remember that many of these patients have poor vision.

# MACULAR DEGENERATION

## ETIOLOGY/EPIDEMIOLOGY

The exact cause of macular degeneration is not known, although the incidence increases after age 50. **Macular degeneration,** a disease of the aging retina, is the leading cause of blindness in the elderly.

The prevalence of macular degeneration increases markedly in persons over 65, and approximately 25% to 30% of individuals between the ages of 75 and 85 years are affected. Other factors associated with macular degeneration include gender (females affected slightly more often), family history, cigarette smoking, and race (usually white). There also appears to be an association between macular degeneration and arteriosclerosis, stroke, and ischemic attacks.

## PATHOPHYSIOLOGY

Macular degeneration results from degenerative changes in the *choriocapillaris, Bruch's membrane,* or the *retinal pigment epithelium.* The choriocapillaris is a thin layer of blood vessels originating in the retina and extending into the choroid. Bruch's membrane separates the choriocapillaries from the retinal pigment epithelium.

The two types of macular degeneration generally seen are the exudative (wet) and nonexudative (dry) types. The *wet type* is characterized by a sudden growth of new vessels in the macular region. These vessels are fragile and tend to leak blood and fluid that displaces and damages the macula by interfering with its blood supply. Scarring occurs, and the function of the macula is destroyed, frequently very quickly. The *dry type* is the most common and is caused by degenerative processes other than neovascularization. Scattered round spots (drusen) begin to appear in the macular region of the retina. Drusen are discrete deposits that may in fact be waste products that could not be properly eliminated from the pigment epithelium. Sometimes following the appearance of drusen, there is a slow atrophy of the choroid, pigment epithelium, and retina in the macular region.

The most common form of macular degeneration is called *involutional macular degeneration,* which is associated with aging. This form of macular degeneration accounts for 70% of all cases and can be of either the wet or dry type. The main manifestations of macular degeneration are the following:

1. Varying degree of central vision loss in one or both eyes
2. Decreased ability to distinguish colors

## PREVENTION

Although there is no primary prevention for macular degeneration, early signs or changes in existing disease can be detected with the Amsler grid (see Figure 59-10 in Chapter 59). Distorted lines, dark spots, or areas that are completely missing will be noted by persons with macular degeneration. This test should be done two to three times a week by those at risk and may be performed daily by those with existing disease. Any changes should be reported immediately to the ophthalmologist.

## MEDICAL MANAGEMENT

No generally acceptable treatment is available for the dry type of macular degeneration. Some evidence suggests that supplemental oral zinc may reduce the progression of the disease in patients already diagnosed with macular degeneration.[25] Laser therapy using the argon and/or krypton lasers is used to coagulate the abnormal vessels in a small percentage of persons with the wet type. This is usually an outpatient procedure and is possible only if the person is treated before the abnormal blood vessels have begun to grow into the center of the macula.[27] Treatment *must* begin as soon as possible after the onset of symptoms. Each day that elapses before treatment is sought significantly decreases the chance of preserving vision.

## NURSING MANAGEMENT

### Providing Emotional Support

Fear of blindness is a frequent concern. Opportunity to discuss this fear, along with the frustration of changing vision, must be provided. Support and help are also needed as the person learns new and different ways to carry out normal routines.

### Facilitating Learning

It is difficult to predict the degree of vision loss for each person. However, the disease, type of vision loss, and prognosis can be discussed. Optical aids such as magnification spectacles, magnifying glasses, and special reading lights may be helpful. The fact that peripheral vision will be maintained needs to be emphasized, because only the central (macular) area of the retina is involved. Teaching includes preparation for diagnostic testing (fluorescein angiography and retinal photographs).

# TUMORS

## ETIOLOGY

Both *benign* and *malignant* tumors may occur in the eye or related structures such as the eyelid. Neoplasms may originate in the retina or the uveal tract or may metastasize to the eye from a primary site. Orbital neoplasms include *benign hemangiomas, pseudotumors, lymphomas, mucoceles* from the sinuses, *malignant melanomas, retinoblastomas,* and others. If tumors are malignant, both vision and life are endangered. Tumors within the eyeball are often silent except for a bloodshot appearance of the eye. As in all malignant tumors, the prognosis depends on early diagnosis and prompt treatment.

## TUMORS OF THE EYELIDS

The eyelids are subject to the usual tumors of the skin such as *nevi, xanthelasma* (lipid deposits seen as yellow, wrinkled patches on the anterior surface of the eyelid near the corner of the eye), and *verrucae* (warts). Carcinoma of the lids is a common type of ocular malignancy, with basal and squamous cell carcinoma being the most common. Any warty growth in the eyelids should be removed for histologic examination. Treatment consists of surgical excision of the growth.

## RETINOBLASTOMA

***Retinoblastoma* is a *highly malignant intraocular neoplasm.*** The neoplasm arises from mutations in the retinal cells (noninheritable form) or in the germinal cells (inheritable form). It is the most frequent ocular malignancy in childhood, occurring in 1 of every 23,000 to 34,000 births.[17] It is transmitted in an autosomal dominant fashion. The diagnosis is made in 90% of patients by the age of 4 years. Signs and symptoms may include decreased vision, strabismus, retinal detachment, white pupillary reflex, and secondary glaucoma. In about one third of patients, the tumors invade both eyes. Retinoblastomas grow rapidly and spread backward along the optic nerve and invade the brain. Retinoblastomas can also metastasize to distant sites by way of the bloodstream and lymphatics.

Treatment of large retinoblastomas consists of enucleation, with removal of as much of the optic nerve as possible. Treatment modalities such as cobalt, plaque irradiation, photocoagulation, and cryotherapy may be used for selected small retinoblastomas. Frequent examination of the remaining eye is recommended. When the tumor is bilateral, the more involved eye is removed. An attempt is made to save the other eye by using radiation, chemotherapy, or both. If the tumor is very advanced, removal of both eyes may be necessary to save the child's life. When the tumor is unilateral and diagnosed and treated early, there is a 90% survival rate.

When normal parents have one child with retinoblastoma, there is a likelihood of less than 4% that a subsequent child will have such a tumor. There is a 50% chance that children of the individual who has survived a proved hereditary retinoblastoma will also be so affected. Persons who survive the tumors should receive *genetic counseling* to alert them to the danger of transmission to their offspring.

## MALIGNANT MELANOMAS

Malignant melanomas are neoplasms that occur in the choroid, ciliary body, and iris of adults. They grow slowly, but because of the vascularity of the choroid, they metastasize early to the liver and lungs. Vision may not be affected until the tumor is very large or until it affects the macula.

## SURGICAL MANAGEMENT

Treatment of tumors of the eye may include enucleation, forms of radiation treatment consisting of brachytherapy, proton beam therapy, and external beam radiation,[22] and tumor excision with eyeball resection and photocoagulation.

The emotional response to a tumor of the eye is perhaps even greater than that to malignancies elsewhere. The surgeon may advise immediate enucleation in the hope of saving the patient's life. Both the patient and family need to be encouraged to talk about their feelings and concerns and to be helped to adjust their lives when confronted by this serious situation. The nurse has a key role in supporting the patient and family during these difficult times.[21]

### Removal of an Eye

An eye, with or without its supportive structures, may be removed surgically for four reasons: (1) to attempt to save a life when a malignant tumor has developed, (2) to save sight in the other eye when *sympathetic ophthalmia* is feared or threatens, (3) to control pain in an eye blinded by disease such as chronic glaucoma or chronic infection, or (4) for cosmetic reasons after blindness from trauma or disease.

Three types of surgery may be performed. *Enucleation* is surgical removal of the entire eye including the sclera. *Evisceration* is removal of the contents of the eye with retention of the sclera. *Exenteration* involves removal of the entire eye and all other soft tissues in the bony orbit.

If feasible, the eyeball alone is removed, leaving the surrounding layers of fascia (Tenon's capsule) and the muscle attachments. A *silicone, plastic,* or *tantalum implant* is inserted into the eye socket, the cut ends of the muscle attachment are overlapped and sutured around it, and the Tenon's capsule and the conjunctiva are closed. This procedure provides a stump that supplies both support and motion for an artificial eye and therefore gives the patient whose eye has been removed a more normal appearance. The ball-shaped implant is left in place permanently. A plastic conformer is placed in the socket until edema subsides and an artificial eye (prosthesis) can be inserted. A new implant called *hydroxyapatite* may provide better movement of an ocular prosthesis.[1] This implant has the same consistency as human bone, thus allowing the extraocular muscles to strongly anchor to it. The result is superior motion of an ocular prosthesis and improved cosmetic appearance.

#### Postoperative care

*Hemorrhage, thrombosis of blood vessels,* and *infection* are possible complications after enucleation, exenteration, or evisceration of an eye. Pressure dressings are used for 1 or 2 days to help control possible hemorrhage. Headaches or pain in the operated side of the head should be reported at once, because meningitis occasionally occurs as a complication after thrombosis of adjacent veins. The patient is usually allowed out of bed the day after surgery. Antibiotic or steroid ointment or both may be prescribed until the patient receives the ocular prosthesis.

When a person has lost one eye, the preservation of sight in the other eye becomes crucial. Wearing impact-resistant glasses provides some protection from injury. Because binocular vision is gone when there is only one functioning eye, depth perception is affected. The individual needs to be taught about the adjustments necessary in learning to carry out normal activities with one eye and about the potential safety hazards. Driving a car, for example, is potentially dangerous for the person who suddenly must use only one eye and is not accustomed to the alteration in depth perception. With patience and practice, however, almost all normal activities are possible; for instance, surgeons who have had an eye removed have been able to operate successfully.

#### Prosthetic eye

A prosthetic eye can be used as soon as healing is complete and edema has disappeared, usually 4 to 8 weeks after surgery, although many patients begin to wear a prosthetic eye after only 2 to 3 weeks.

### Factors Associated With Adjustment

Many factors are associated with adjusting to a visual impairment. The ability to maintain the give and take in a relationship, especially with those who provide some form of service, helps to counteract some of the feelings of dependence on that person. Other factors that are associated with adjustment include age, amount of residual vision, gradual loss of vision, self-concept, previous coping patterns, and social support.

### Factors Hindering Adjustment

There are factors that do not help in the adjustment process. Other health problems, especially if they also limit or alter normal functioning, make learning to live with the visual impairment more difficult. Lack of social support can lead to a sense of isolation and loneliness. Insufficient information about the impairment in terms of diagnosis, prognosis, and aids and strategies to help live with the impairment may affect their ability to cope. Blind persons relate experiences of being ignored, "yelled at" as if deaf, and not addressed directly when with companions (see the Guidelines box below, for guidelines in communicating). These unhelpful or negative behaviors of others do not help adjustment. Blind persons are sensitive to being treated differently at the onset of their blindness. Helen Keller observed that the attitudes of the seeing toward the blind rather than blindness itself was the hardest burden for her to bear.

**Guidelines for Communicating With the Blind Person**

1. Talk in a normal tone of voice.
2. Do *not* try to avoid common phrases in speech, such as "See what I mean."
3. Introduce yourself with each contact (unless well known to the person). If in a hospital, knock on the door before entering.
4. Explain any activity occurring in the room or what you will be doing.
5. Announce when you are leaving the room so the person is not put in the position of talking to someone who is no longer there.

## NURSING MANAGEMENT

Newly blind persons, and those with deteriorating vision need an opportunity to talk about their feelings and their fears and concerns about the future and their ability to cope. Nurses can provide this opportunity along with the support that persons need as they reorganize their lives or come to terms with the need to change life goals or priorities. Social support is a key factor in adjusting to visual impairment. Assistance may be needed from nurses to help in the establishment and maintenance of social networks that include both sighted and visually impaired persons.

Integration of blindness and decreasing vision into one's self-concept can take a long time. It may be difficult to accept such things as the white cane; or being labeled as "blind" and consequently "different." The stigma related to blindness still exists. Patience and understanding are required.

Fear of many of the aspects and consequences of visual impairment frequently occurs within the process of adjustment. The specific fears and the context in which they occur need to be elicited by the nurse. This can lead to development of appropriate interventions to alleviate or decrease these fears.

Today artificial eyes are made of plastic instead of glass. They can be bought in shades that closely match the normal eye or they can be specifically made by the ocularist. The ocularist will take an impression of the socket and paint the prosthesis to match the person's own eye. The majority of patients have custom made eyes, with stock eyes used for temporary fitting following surgery.

Follow-up care is provided by the ocularist, who polishes the eye to remove buildup of salt and protein and assesses fit and appearance. At one time it was recommended that the prosthetic eye be removed and cleaned on a regular basis. It was discovered that this frequent removal kept the eye socket mildly irritated. Because of improved fitting and polishing techniques, some patients do not need to remove their artificial eye between yearly visits to the ocularist. For those who clean the eye more frequently, removal and cleansing is an easy process (see Guidelines box, p. 2108, left).

General tips on care of the the artificial eye are outlined in the Guidelines box, p. 2108, right.

Instead of a regular prosthetic eye, a scleral cover shell may be prescribed. In general, scleral cover shells are indicated for blind and disfigured eyes. The cover shell is made of the same material as hard contact lenses

**Guidelines for Removal and Cleaning of a Prosthetic Eye**

1. Remove prosthesis: gently depress the lower lid and exert a small amount of pressure under lower edge of prosthesis.
2. Wash prosthesis with soap (for example, Ivory) and water. Soap is less irritating than detergents. Rinse thoroughly.
3. Irrigate socket with water, if necessary.
4. Reinsert prosthesis: place upper portion under upper lid, pull down lower lid and slip lower edge behind lower lid. With finger or thumb, gently pull down on lower lid and slide prosthesis in place.

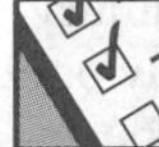

**Guidelines for Care of Prosthetic Eyes**

1. If the eye is left out of the socket, store it in water or contact lens solution.
2. Do not expose the plastic eye to alcohol, ether, chloroform, or any other solvent; they can damage the eye beyond repair.
3. If rubbing the eye, rub toward the nose. Wiping away from the nose may cause the eye to fall out.
4. Wear a protective patch or goggles when swimming, diving, or water skiing—or remove the eye and store it.

and is customarily made to match the color of the other eye. Wearing time of the shell is increased until it can be worn all day. It is usually removed at night to rest the eye. The shell is stored in water, hard contact lens solution, or saline. Cleansing is the same as for a plastic prosthetic eye (see Box 60-11).

# VISUAL IMPAIRMENT

A person is considered legally blind when either of the following conditions exist: (1) the person's visual field is no greater than 20 degrees or (2) central distance vision in the better eye is 20/200 or worse with use of corrective lenses. In the United States there are an estimated 1 million legally blind persons. Annually, more than 46,000 persons become blind. Most blind people are 65 years or older, and in this older population more women than men are blind.

There is a broad diversity of characteristics in persons classified as legally blind. Loss of visual acuity may range from profound to slight; visual field loss may be peripheral or central; or there may be other visual functions affected such as "dark adaptation." Thus many persons classified as legally blind do have useful vision. Of the total blind population, only 25% have no useful vision, that is, they are totally blind or have light perception or light projection only.[15]

The visually impaired population does not include only those who are legally blind. There are well over a million people who, although unable to see well enough to read a newspaper, have vision better than 20/200. Also, over 3 million are monocularly blind, with a small proportion having a defective but not blind second eye.[15] Most persons in this visually impaired but not legally blind population are between the ages of 25 and 64.

## CONSEQUENCES OF VISUAL IMPAIRMENT

Blindness imposes limitations in the range and variety of experiences, in mobility, and in orientation to the environment. Limitations in the range and variety of experiences are related to the fact that a person who cannot see must use touch and kinesthetic experience to gain knowledge of the world. Objects too large or too small to handle are not perceivable.

Many blind persons feel that the restriction in mobility resulting from blindness is its most serious effect. Blind persons cannot move about as quickly, as securely, or as easily as sighted peers. They need to rely on aids or other persons, particularly in unfamiliar areas.

Vision is the sense that permits persons to control their environment and themselves in relation to that environment. Loss of vision can limit the interaction between persons and their environment. It may be that blind persons withdraw from others or that others pull away from the blind. Limitations in social interaction may also be related to difficulties in nonverbal communication. Glances, smiles, and frowns, for example, are missed.

Not only are blind persons restricted in nonverbal communication, but they are also limited in the ways they can process information. Decreased ability to read and communicate in conventional ways can lead to decreased opportunities for learning experiences and may alter established careers.

Visual impairment can cause more than just difficulty in mobility and communication. Difficulties also arise in carrying out personal care, housework, cooking, and home maintenance. These limitations in activities may be even greater in older persons who tend to have more severe impairments.

## ADJUSTMENT TO VISUAL IMPAIRMENT

Visual impairment requires a major life adjustment. Persons need to adjust to both the initial impact of the loss and the subsequent changes that will occur in their life because of the loss of vision. The initial reaction is often characterized by disbelief and then depression, withdrawal, self-pity, and, at times, embarrassment over changed abilities. In time, most persons make a decision, consciously or unconsciously, to live with their impairment (see Research box, p. 2109). They learn new ways or adapt their present ways of doing things to carry out their normal activities. Most recognize that there are some things that they will never be able to do again on their own or that they can do only with help.

Adjustment is an ongoing process. New situations occur, to which the blind person must adjust. These new situations can cause frustration and annoyance. How-

## RESEARCH

Gallagher, CM: The young adult with recent vision loss: a pilot case study, *Insight* 16(6):8-14, 1991.

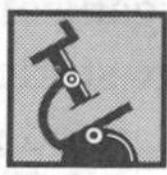

Through a single subject case study, the recent loss of vision of a 25-year-old woman was explored to discover what she was experiencing and how she adjusted to and coped with her blindness. The subject had been blind for 24 months from Leber's optic neuropathy at the time of the interviews. The Jalowiec Coping Scale, a measure of coping methods, and three tape-recorded interviews were the methods used to collect data. The investigator found that learning to live with a visual impairment was an ongoing process. The person goes through several phases of reaction before moving to acceptance of the loss. It is at the time of acceptance that the person decides to learn to adapt and adjust to the impairment. Coping strategies included such things as information seeking, seeking purpose and meaning, hoping, and praying and trusting God. Nurses can assist the visually impaired person to learn to live with vision loss by giving information about the eye disease and strategies to aid self-care, providing emotional support, and assisting the person to utilize available rehabilitation programs.

## Guidelines for Facilitating Independence in ADLs for Blind Persons

1. Place clothing in specific locations in drawers and closets.
2. Place food and cooking utensils in specific locations in cupboards and/or refrigerator.
3. Encourage use of cane when walking.
4. Keep furniture and household objects in specific places.
5. When assisting a blind person in walking, let the person take your arm (Figure 60-10).
6. Provide descriptions of food on the plate using clock placement of food; for example, put the peas at "7 o'clock." Cut food as appropriate.
7. Always permit blind persons to pull out their own chairs and seat themselves.

ever, these feelings do not occur as frequently, nor do they last as long, as they did initially.

The key variable in this process of adjustment is time. Time is needed to grieve for the lost sight and to recognize and come to terms with the implications of the loss. Time is also needed to master many of the difficult tasks and the work associated with adjustment to a visual impairment.

### Difficult Areas in Adjusting

For many blind persons the dependence on others for help in carrying out normal routines and the necessity to ask for help are two of the most difficult things to which they must adjust. The inability to carry out tasks or role obligations in the usual way and the inability to recognize friends and acquaintances are also difficult areas. Fluctuating vision, a common occurrence for many visually impaired persons, leads to frustration and difficulties in planning or implementing tasks. Fears and uncertainties about the progression of visual impairment can lead to concern about the ability to cope with further deterioration of vision or the necessity of preparing for the future.

## INTERVENTIONS

### Assisting with Activities of Daily Living

Although most visually impaired persons develop ways of carrying out their activities of daily living, they do need ongoing assistance in learning techniques that can help them to maintain or regain this ability. Nurses can provide specific guidance to aid patients in this process of relearning (see Guidelines box above).

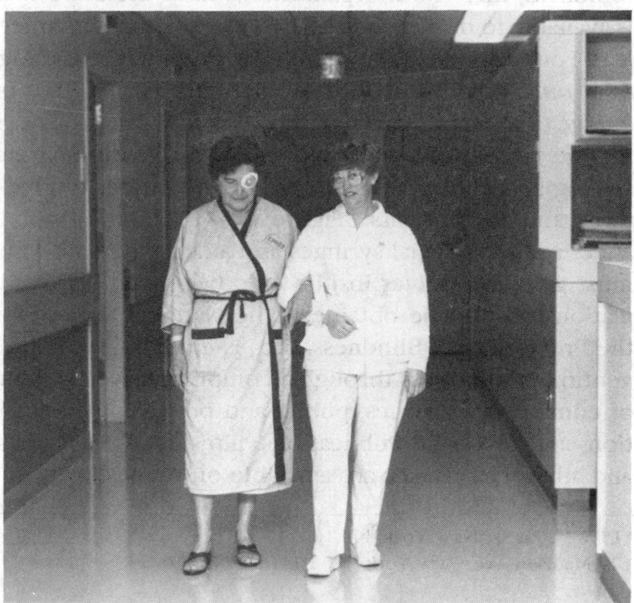

**FIGURE 60-10** Ambulation of person who cannot see. Note that patient is holding nurse's arm and is led without being held.

### Providing Information

Information is needed by blind persons, not only about their particular disease and prognosis, but also about aids and strategies to help them live with a visual impairment. Nurses, working in collaboration with other health team members and rehabilitation centers for the blind, can help provide this needed information. An example of a new device to assist with reading is the Kursweil Personal Reader. This reader allows the visually impaired person to hear printed texts. The user runs a hand-held scanner over the text or lays the text on a portable scanner. The device then "reads" the text in one of nine different voices.[16]

## COMMUNITY SERVICES

Many federal, state, and local agencies provide services to persons with severe visual impairment. It is imperative that nurses be aware of the resources in their region so that they can refer these persons and their families to the services and facilities in their home area. Services available to visually impaired persons include mobility training, personal counseling, vocational rehabilitation, relearning independent self-care, special education, and, in some instances, financial compensation.

### National Voluntary Organizations

In the United States there are two national voluntary health agencies concerned with blindness and the prevention of blindness: The American Foundation for the Blind* and the National Society for the Prevention of Blindness, Inc.† Both organizations have literature that is available to nurses and patients on request. The American Foundation for the Blind distributes a free catalog, ***Aids and Appliances*** (also available in braille, free of charge to blind persons), which contains a list of devices for the visually impaired person. The catalog includes sewing and kitchen utensils as well as various kinds of tools and instruments (Figure 60-11). Medical appliances such as special syringes and aids for persons who must give themselves insulin or other parenteral medication can also be obtained. The National Society for the Prevention of Blindness, Inc., is engaged in the prevention of blindness through a comprehensive program of community services, public and professional education, and research. Publications, films, lectures, charts, and advisory services are available on request.

*15 W. 16th St., New York, NY 10011.
†79 Madison Ave, New York, NY 10016.

Recording for the Blind, Inc.* is a national, nonprofit voluntary organization that provides audiotapes or records free on loan to anyone who cannot read normal printed material because of visual or physical impairments. "Talking" books produced by this organization are fundamental aids to high school and college students and persons who require educational or specialized material in the pursuit of their occupations. These recordings also may be obtained from many local and state libraries. Tape players or record players are loaned free to persons who are legally blind. Information can be obtained from public libraries or organizations for blind persons.

### Government Assistance

Persons who are legally blind are entitled to certain federal assistance. An amendment to the Social Security Act made provision for assistance to blind persons, and now all 50 states and all U.S. territories have approved plans for such aid. Assistance through this program is based on need. The Internal Revenue Act of 1948 permits blind persons to claim an extra personal deduction in reporting income. In 1943 the federal government established a counseling and placement service for the blind in the Vocational Rehabilitation Administration. This agency, now called the Social and Rehabilitation Service (SRS), shares rehabilitation costs with the states. The Veterans Administration provides a substantial pension for the veteran who has had an enucleation of both eyes.

The Americans with Disabilities Act, passed in 1990, should improve job opportunities for persons with limited vision. The law ensures that employers cannot dis-

*20 Roszell Rd, Princeton, NJ 08540.

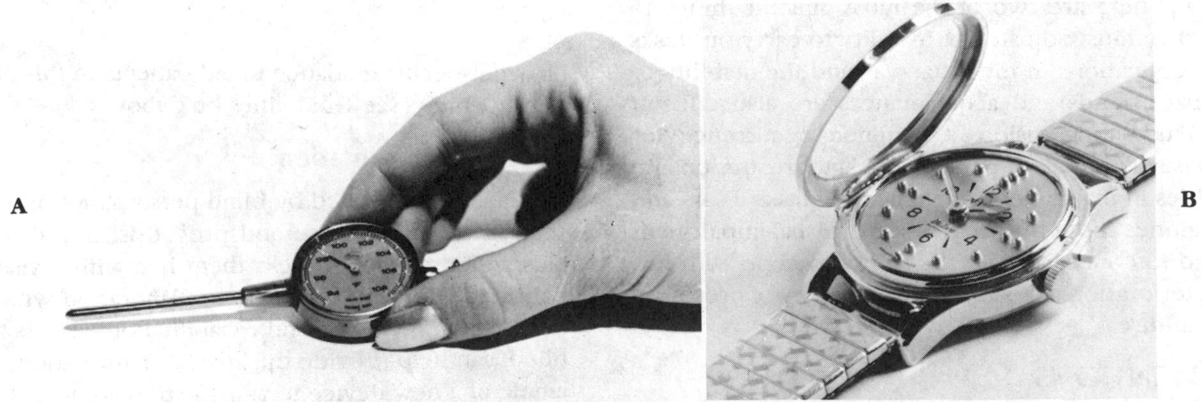


**FIGURE 60-11** **A,** Dial-type clinical thermometer with unbreakable stem. Braille (raised) dots mark scale, one dot at odd numbers and two at even numbers. Raised line is at 98.6° F. Button is pushed to register temperature, which remains set until button is released. Needle then returns to zero. **B,** One of many models of watches available in both braille and ink print. (Courtesy American Foundation for the Blind, New York.)

**criminate in the hiring of qualified individuals with disabilities.**

## QUESTIONS TO CONSIDER

- ► How would your care differ if the patient who suddenly went blind were 20 years of age versus 70 years of age?
- ► What areas would you include in a class that you are teaching on the care of the eyes for nurses working in occupational health care fields?
- ► How would you teach a visually impaired person who is using three different types of eye drops to identify the correct drops?
- ► What approaches might you consider for a person with glaucoma who refuses to administer eye drops four times a day as prescribed by the physician?

## CRITICAL THINKING ACTIVITIES

- ► Charlotte, 20, has an eyelash floating on the surface of her left eye. The nurse has Charlotte lie on her right side and begins irrigating the left eye with a syringe filled with normal saline. She directs the fluid from the outer to inner canthus. Critique this irrigation procedure.
- ► Juan sustains a chemical splash into an eye. The nurse has him close his eye and then covers the eye with a light patch, applies cool compresses, and transports Juan to a physician or ER. Is this emergency procedure appropriate? Why or why not?

## CHAPTER SUMMARY

### EYE DISEASES AND BLINDNESS

- **Normal healthy eyes do not need special treatment.**
- **The eyes should be examined by an ophthalmologist or optometrist at regular intervals throughout life.**
- **When administering more than one eye drop at a time, wait 5 minutes between instillations.**
- **Many systemic diseases have eye manifestations.**
- **Following any chemical burn, the eye must be irrigated immediately, before transportation to a physician.**
- **Acute bacterial conjunctivitis (pinkeye) is highly contagious.**
- **Teaching the person who has a corneal transplant includes instruction about medications and assessment for corneal graft rejection.**

### CATARACT

- **A cataract is an opacity of the lens. Cataracts most commonly occur as a result of the aging process.**

### GLAUCOMA

- **In glaucoma, IOP is increased because of obstruction to the outflow of aqueous humor. The person with glaucoma may need help to adhere to a lifetime of medication therapy.**

### DETACHMENT OF THE RETINA

- **Common factors placing the person at risk for a retinal detachment include myopia, trauma, and aphakia.**

### DIABETIC RETINOPATHY

- **Diabetic retinopathy occurs in about 90% of persons who have had diabetes for 30 years.**

### MACULAR DEGENERATION

- **Macular degeneration causes loss of central vision and decreased ability to distinguish colors.**

### VISUAL IMPAIRMENT

- **Blindness imposes limitations on mobility, interaction with the environment, and the range of experiences readily available to the sighted person.**
- **Loss of social supports is a major factor hindering adjustment to a visual impairment.**
- **Nursing care of the person with a visual impairment includes support and counseling, instruction about the aids and strategies that facilitate living with a visual impairment, and referral to appropriate community agencies.**

## REFERENCES


1. Albiar E: Hydroxyapatite implants—a new trend in enucleation and orbital reconstructive surgery, *Insight* 17(1):25-28, 1992.
2. Allen MN: Adjusting to visual impairment, *J Ophthalmic Nurs Technol* 9:47-51, 1990.
3. Allen MN, Birse E: Stigma and blindness, *J Ophthalmic Nurs Technol* 10:147-152, 1991.
4. Boyd-Monk H, Steinmetz CG: *Nursing care of the eye,* Norwalk, Conn, 1987, Appleton & Lange.
5. Burlew JA: Preventing eye injuries—the nurse's role, *Insight* 16(6):24-28, 1991.
6. Department of Health and Human Services: Vision research: a national plan 1983-1987—the 1983 report of the National Advisory Eye Council, NIH Pub. No. 83-2469, 1983, Washington, DC, Author.
7. Gallagher CM: The young adult with recent vision loss: a pilot case study, *Insight* 16(6):8-14, 1991.
8. US Department of Health and Human Services, Public Health Service: *Healthy people 2000: national health promotion and disease prevention objectives,* Washington, DC, 1990, US Government Printing Office.
9. Hunt L: Eyeglasses and common complaints, *Insight* 17(3):20-22, 1992.
10. Hunt L: Microwave ovens and eye injuries, *Insight* 17(4):23,25, 1992.
11. Jairath N et al: Effective discharge preparation of elderly cataract day surgery patients, *J Ophthalmic Nurs Technol* 9:157-160, 1990.
12. Kruse MR: Nursing management of uncontrolled glaucoma

with the Molteno filtering implant, *Ophthalmic Nurs Forum* 4(2):1-7, 1988.

13. McCoy K: Ophthalmic drug use in the OR, *Insight* 17(4):10-21, 1992.
14. National Advisory Eye Council (US): Vision research: a national plan 1983-1987, vol 1, The Report of The National Eye Council, Bethesda, Md, 1983, National Institutes of Health.
15. National Society to Prevent Blindness, Operational Research Department: *Vision problems in the United States: a statistical analysis,* New York, 1980, Author.
16. New product for seniors, *The Futurist,* July-August, 19, 1992.
17. Newell FW: *Ophthalmology: principles and concepts,* ed 7, St Louis, 1992, Mosby.
18. Okimi PH et al: Effects of caffeinated coffee on intraocular pressure, *Appl Nurs Res* 4(2):72-76, 1991.
19. Pavan-Langston D, Dunkel EC: *Handbook of ocular drug therapy and ocular side effects of systemic drugs,* Boston, 1991, Little, Brown.
20. Roach VG: What you should know about diabetic retinopathy, *J Ophthalmic Nurs Technol* 7:166-169, 1988.
21. Servodidio CA: Teaching aids for patients diagnosed with choroidal melanoma, *Insight* 16(6):21-23, 1991.
22. Servodidio CA, Abramson DH: Choroidal melanoma, *Nurs Clin North Am* 27(3):777-790, 1992.
23. Smith S: Diabetic retinopathy, *Insight* 17(2):20-25, 1992.
24. Spires R: Perfluorcarbon liquid in the management of complex retinal detachments, *J Ophthalmic Nurs Technol* 11(4):157-160, 1992.
25. Vaughan DE, Asbury T, Riordan-Eva P: *General ophthalmology,* ed 13, Norwalk, Conn, 1992, Appleton & Lange.
26. Williams MB: Nurse-client management of skin and tissue integrity. In Berger KJ, Williams MB: *Fundamentals of nursing: collaborating for optimal health,* Norwalk, Conn, 1992, Appleton & Lange.
27. Woods S: Macular degeneration, *Nurs Clin North Am* 27:761-775, 1992.

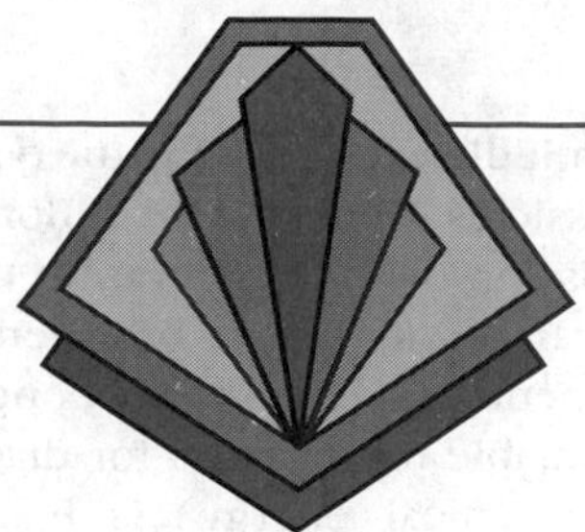

C H A P T E R 61

# Assessment of the Ear

*Linda T. Schuring*

## CHAPTER OBJECTIVES

***After studying this chapter, the learner should be able to do the following:***

1 Describe the basic structure and function of the temporal bone and ear.
2 Describe behavioral clues suggesting loss of hearing.
3 Perform a nursing assessment of the ear for hearing and balance.
4 Recognize normal findings in the ears.
5 Identify specific diagnostic tests for hearing and balance.
6 Describe the role of the nurse in the detection of hearing and balance problems.

## KEY TERMS

nystagmus
ossicles
otolaryngology
otology
Valsalva maneuver

Nurses are involved in every aspect of the care of the patient with ear problems, including prevention, detection, and treatment of hearing and vestibular disorders. Ear problems are common, can occur at any age, and often require immediate attention.

The ear and hearing are recognized together as one of the five senses of the human body. Hearing and balance are important in our activities of daily living. Sound helps us to be in touch with our environment, adding aesthetic pleasure, as well as warnings of danger. The sense of hearing is essential for normal development and maintenance of speech. The ability to communicate with others depends on the ability to hear. The ear also contains the organs of balance that relay information about the body's position and direction of body motions to the brain.

The nurse must be able to look holistically at the patient with ear problems. Ear problems can interfere with the patient's activities of daily living, such as working, talking on the telephone, or walking. The patient may have to cope with the temporary or permanent loss of hearing or balance.

**Otolaryngology** is the sum of knowledge concerning the ears, nose, and throat, or the head and neck. An *otolaryngologist* is a physician who *treats diseases of the ear, nose, and throat.* A subspecialty of otolaryngology is **otology,** the branch of medicine dealing only with the ear and its diseases. An otologist is a physician who has specialized in studying and treating the ear and its diseases. A nurse may choose to focus the practice of nursing on patients with ear problems. The Society of Otorhinolaryngology and Head-Neck Nurses, Inc., a specialty organization, provides education and growth opportunities.

However, every nurse, regardless of education or focus of care, should be prepared to both examine the outer ear and grossly assess the patient's hearing and equilibrium. Very often nurses participate in case findings of persons with hearing and balance disorders, as well as in the rehabilitation of these individuals.

The nurse can help direct the person with a hearing loss or balance problem and the family to the appropriate agencies for assistance. There might be ways of improving hearing through medical or surgical therapy. If the loss is irreversible, aural rehabilitation can make it possible for the person with a hearing loss to understand and communicate with others. The detection of some degree of hearing impairment and/or a balance problem in patients is an important nursing responsibility. Often the nurse is the first member of the health team to be approached by the patient regarding problems with the ear.

# ANATOMY AND PHYSIOLOGY

## THE EAR AND COMMUNICATION

Personal communication involves two aspects of hearing. Hearing is used not only to receive information but also to monitor one's own voice. Therefore a person who is deaf from birth will have difficulty learning to speak distinctly and to regulate voice volume. In addition, any level of hearing impairment will alter both aspects of communication.

Behavioral clues are useful in the assessment of hearing difficulties, as seen in Box 61-1. Persons who exhibit any of these behavioral clues should have their ears examined by an otolaryngologist, who will perform a hearing test. Thus a complete evaluation of the hearing problem can be made to determine the extent and cause of the hearing loss, as well as treatment options.

The ears are a pair of complex sensory organs located in the middle of both sides of the head. The position of the ears is important because the use of both ears simultaneously produces binaural hearing, allowing us to detect the direction of sound and aiding in maintaining equilibrium. A person detects the direction from which a sound comes in two ways: (1) by the time lag between the sound entry into one ear compared with the sound entry into the other ear, and (2) by the intensities of sounds in both ears. Each ear is also responsible for sending signals to the brain for the maintenance of equilibrium. Therefore the *two major functions* of the ears are *hearing* and *balance*.

Nerve impulses are transmitted between the ear and the brain by way of the eighth cranial nerve, called the acoustic or vestibulocochlear nerve. The acoustic portion of the ear responsible for hearing is innervated by the cochlear branch, and the vestibular portion responsible for equilibrium and posture is innervated by the vestibular branch.

Sound is transmitted from the external ear to the inner ear by two routes, *air conduction* and *bone conduction*. Air conduction is the transmission of sound vibration through the middle ear, involving the tympanic membrane and the ossicles (Figure 61-1). Bone conduction is the transmission of sound vibration through the skull to the inner ear. A comparison between the air conduction measurement and the bone conduction measurement gives valuable information for diagnosis.

Sound energy (mechanical energy) is first transformed into neural energy (electrical energy) and is then decoded by the brain for hearing. In a similar way, the inner ears send impulses to the brain that are decoded to maintain normal balance.

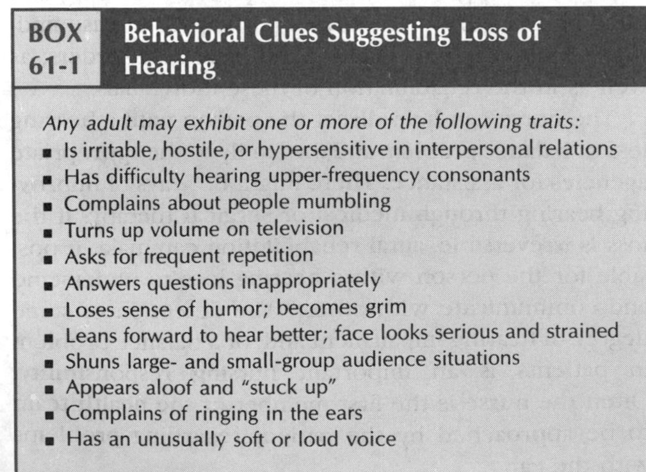

**BOX 61-1 Behavioral Clues Suggesting Loss of Hearing**

*Any adult may exhibit one or more of the following traits:*

- Is irritable, hostile, or hypersensitive in interpersonal relations
- Has difficulty hearing upper-frequency consonants
- Complains about people mumbling
- Turns up volume on television
- Asks for frequent repetition
- Answers questions inappropriately
- Loses sense of humor; becomes grim
- Leans forward to hear better; face looks serious and strained
- Shuns large- and small-group audience situations
- Appears aloof and "stuck up"
- Complains of ringing in the ears
- Has an unusually soft or loud voice

## STRUCTURE, FUNCTION, AND ASSESSMENT OF THE EAR

The ears are housed in the temporal bones of the skull. Each ear is divided into three parts. The first part is the *external ear,* which contains a sound-collecting portion (a short conducting tube with a membrane at its deepest end) (Figure 61-2). The second part is the ***middle ear,*** which is an air-containing cavity in the petrous portion of the temporal bone. Three small bones traverse this cavity, and a small (eustachian) tube connects the middle ear to the pharynx. The third part is the ***internal ear,*** which consists of membranous sacs and ducts encased in bony canals. The cochlea, which is specific for hearing, and the vestibular canals, which help to maintain equilibrium, are found in the internal ear.

### The Temporal Bone

Understanding the structure and function of the temporal bone is necessary not only for physical assessment, but also as a basis for understanding the hearing and balance tests and the normal hearing and balance process.

The human skull is composed of 22 bones: 13 facial bones, 8 cranial bones, and the mandible. The temporal bones (2 of the 8 cranial bones) house the ears. The

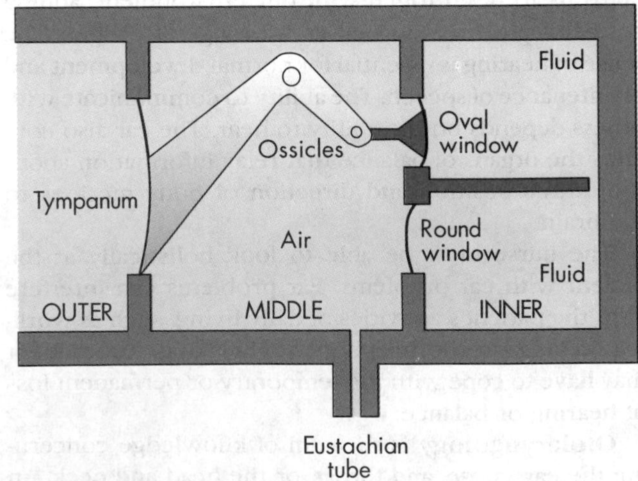


**FIGURE 61-1** Diagrammatic representation of transmission of sound impulses from outer to inner ear.

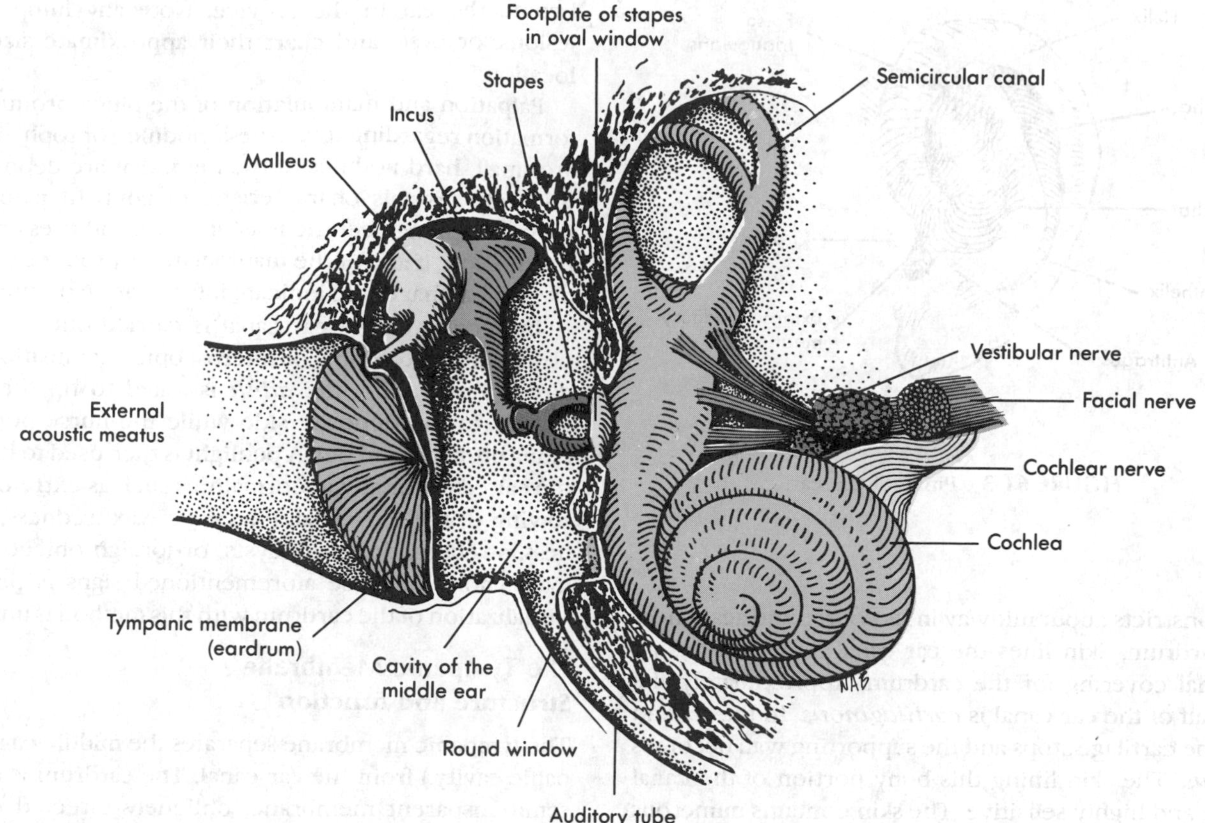


**FIGURE 61-2** Structures of the ear.

paired temporal bones are part of both the base and the lateral wall of the skull. Each of the *temporal bones* can be *divided* into *four parts: squamous, mastoid, petrous,* and *tympanic.* If the external opening of the ear canal is used as a reference point, the squamous part is upward, the mastoid part is backward, the tympanic part is forward and downward, and the petrous portion is forward toward the face. The temporal bone interfaces with the sphenoid, parietal, and occipital bones.

The temporal bone is the hardest bone in the human body and provides adequate protection for the organs of hearing and balance. The function of the temporal bone is to house the external and internal auditory canals, the mastoid air cells, the blood vessels and nerves, the labyrinth, and the cochlea.

## The External Ear

### Structure and function

The external ear, or auricle, consists of the *pinna* and the *external auditory canal,* or the ear canal. The ears are located on each side of the head at approximately eye level. An imaginary line drawn from the outer canthus of the eye to the top of the ear should be straight and almost parallel to the floor. The pinna is attached to the side of the head at approximately a 10-degree angle.

The pinna is composed of cartilage covered by skin. There is little fat except in the lobule. Hair covers most of the ear but is usually rudimentary except in the region of the tragus and the antitragus. Sebaceous glands also are found on the surface.

The pinna is attached to the side of the head by skin, ligaments, and muscles. Muscles of the pinna are innervated by a branch of the facial nerve.

The parts of the pinna are illustrated by Figure 61-3. The *concha* is the deepest part and leads to the ear canal. The *helix* is the outmost rim of the ear and leads inferiorly into the lobule. The concha is bounded anteriorly by a prominent process called the tragus, which projects posteriorly over the entrance to the ear canal.

In human embryology, the ears are formed at the same time as the renal system. Therefore abnormalities in the shape and form of the pinna might be found in conjunction with renal abnormalities. In addition, in the sixth month of fetal life, the human ear possesses a small tubercle, a downward protrusion of the helix (close to the resemblance of the ears of some adult monkeys) named Darwin's tubercle. If present, Darwin's tubercle is a normal finding.

The ear canal extends from the concha of the pinna at one end to the eardrum at the other end, in a path inward, forward, and downward in an adult. It is an S-shaped curve through the temporal bone, approximately 2.5 cm (1 in) in length. The lumen is irregular in outline

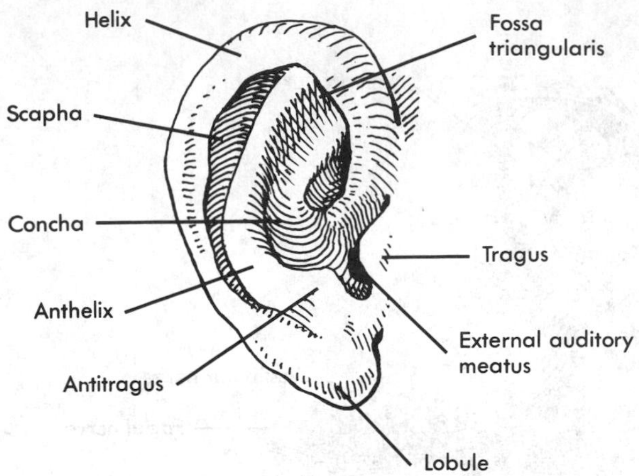


**FIGURE 61-3** Pinna of the ear.

and constricts about midway in its course and again near the eardrum. Skin lines the ear canal and furnishes an external covering for the eardrum. Approximately the first half of the ear canal is *cartilaginous.* In the second half, the cartilage stops and the supporting wall becomes *osseous.* The skin lining this bony portion of the canal is thin and highly sensitive. The skin contains numerous fine hairs and sebaceous glands. *Ceruminous glands* (modified sweat glands) produce *cerumen* or *ear wax.* The openings of these ducts appear as dark points to the unaided eye.

The funnel shape of the external ear provides for collection and direction of sound. Together with the head, the pinna and ear canal act as an integrated system that transforms sound on its way to the eardrum. For example, the external ear actually amplifies certain frequencies.

The secretion of wax functions as a protective mechanism. Wax is to the ears what tears are to the eyes. The sticky consistency of wax, along with the fine hairs of the ears, help to cleanse the ear canal of foreign matter. At times the wax must be mechanically removed from the ear.

### Objective data

*Inspection* and *palpation* are the two methods used to assess the external ear. The external ear should be inspected for size, configuration, and angle of attachment to the head. An imaginary line is drawn from the greatest protuberance on the occiput to the outside corner (lateral canthus) of the eye. When the top of the pinna falls below the eye-occipital line, the angle of attachment is significantly more than 10 degrees. The configuration of the pinna is observed for gross deformity. Whether the ears protrude and the degree of protrusion, the color of the skin of the ear, and whether any additional skin tags are present is noted. The skin of the ear should be smooth and without breaks or inflammation, especially behind the ear in the crevice. Note any lumps, skin lesions, or cysts and chart their approximate size and location.

Palpation and manipulation of the pinna produce information regarding tenderness, nodules, or tophi. *Tophi* are small, hard nodules in the helix that are deposits of uric acid crystals characteristic of gout. In palpation, move the pinna, feel the mastoid area, and press on the tragus. Note if any of the manipulations produce pain or discomfort that could indicate inflammation or infection.

Inspection of the ear canal is carried out by direct observation, otoscopy, or microscopic examination. For direct observation, the *adult* is asked to tip the head slightly to the opposite side while the nurse pulls the pinna up, back, and out. A penlight is then used to inspect the ear canal for any abnormalities such as extreme narrowing of the ear canal, excessive wax, redness, scaliness, swelling, drainage, cysts, or foreign objects. Normally, none of these aforementioned signs is present. Visualization of the eardrum with this method is unlikely.

## The Tympanic Membrane

### Structure and function

The tympanic membrane separates the middle ear (tympanic cavity) from the ear canal. The eardrum is a thin, semitransparent membrane, obliquely directed downward and inward. Nearly oval in shape, this membrane is approximately 9 mm in diameter and pearly gray in color.

A few distinguishing landmarks of the normal eardrum are the *annulus,* which is the thickened border that attaches the eardrum to the temporal bone; the *umbo,* the most depressed point where the first ossicle attaches to the eardrum, almost in the center; the *pars flaccida,* a small triangular area above the short process of the malleus; and the largest portion of the tympanic membrane, the *pars tensa* (Figure 61-4).

The *tympanic membrane* is formed by three layers: an outer skin layer continuous with the skin of the external ear canal, a fibrous supporting middle layer, and an inner mucosal layer continuous with the mucosal lining of the middle ear cavity. The pars tensa (about four fifths of the eardrum) contains all three layers, whereas the pars flaccida is composed of only two layers. The fibrous middle layer is missing and allows the pars flaccida to be more vulnerable to negative pressure, causing pathologic disorders.

The tympanic membrane serves as a common membrane between the external ear canal and the middle ear cleft. The tympanic membrane protects the middle ear and conducts sound vibrations from the external ear to the ossicles. The sound pressure applied to the *stapes* in the oval window connecting to the inner ear is 22 times greater than the pressure exerted by the sound pressure on the eardrum. The force of the sound vibrations increases after transmission from a larger area to a smaller area.

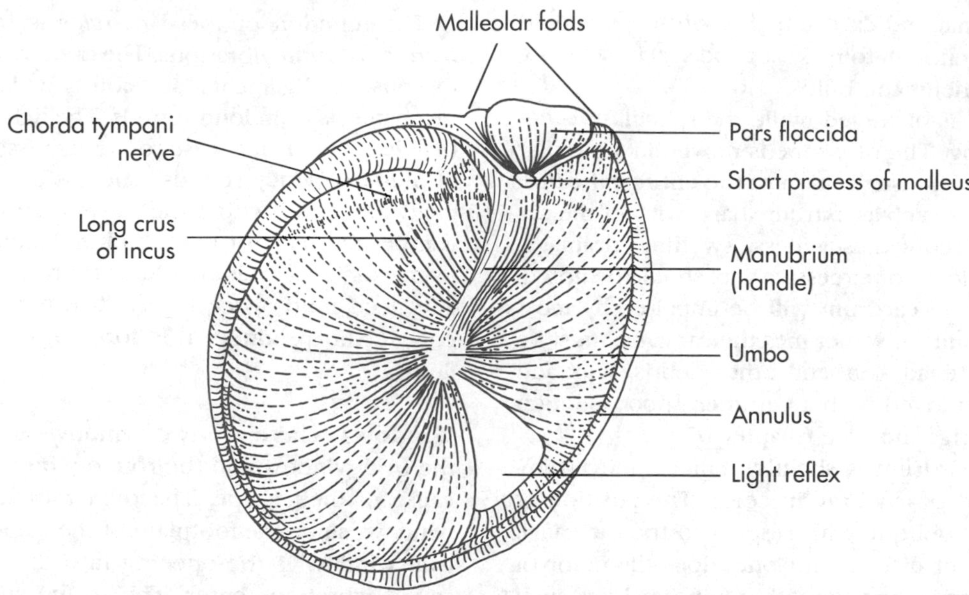


**FIGURE 61-4** Right tympanic membrane. (From Prior JA, Silberstein JS: *Physical diagnosis: the history and examination of the patient,* ed 5, St Louis, 1977, Mosby.)

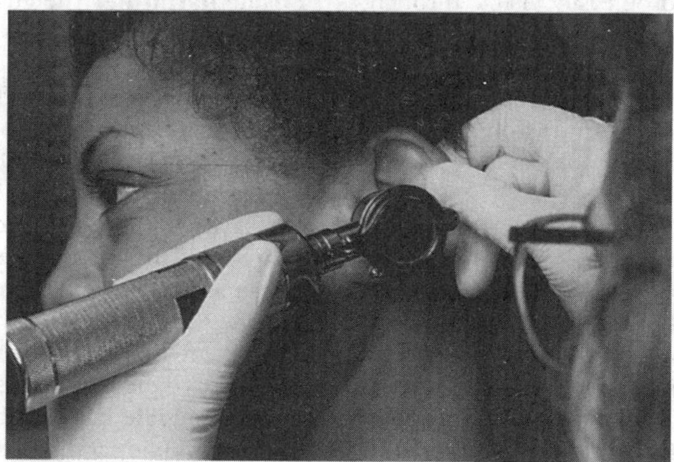

**FIGURE 61-5** Otoscopic examination. (From Sigler B, Schuring L: *Ear, nose, and throat disorders,* St Louis, 1993, Mosby.)

## Objective data

The eardrum is located within the head at the end of the only skin-lined canal in the body, the ear canal. Therefore visualization is difficult and requires illumination. The addition of magnification also allows a more accurate assessment of the ear. An otoscope is a device consisting of a handle, a light source, a magnifying lens, and an attachment for visualizing the ear canal and eardrum (Figure 61-5). Some otoscopes have a pneumatic device for injecting air into the ear canal to test the mobility and integrity of the eardrum.

Specula for the otoscope come in a variety of sizes. The diameter of the meatus and the length of the ear canal vary; thus the one with the largest diameter that fits comfortably into the ear canal should be chosen. The light source must be checked for brightness. If the light appears yellowish or dim (like a flashlight with weak batteries), the batteries must be recharged or replaced.

The otoscope is held with the dominant hand, with the hand resting against the patient's head. In this manner, should the patient move suddenly, the otoscope will move also, so that the nurse will be less likely to damage the external canal. With the nondominant hand, the pinna is pulled up, back, and out, thus straightening the ear canal. While doing this, the patient's head should be gently tilted away from the nurse and the speculum inserted slowly and carefully into the ear canal. The nurse's eye is brought close to the magnifying lens to view the ear canal and eardrum. The otoscope should be advanced far enough to make a good seal to facilitate the use of the pneumatic bulb.

The ear canal is observed while the speculum is entering and exiting. The otoscope is moved in a circular fashion to allow for visualization of the entire ear canal. Any abnormalities such as extreme narrowing of the ear canal, nodules, redness, scaliness, swelling, drainage, cysts, foreign objects, or excessive wax should be noted. Visualization of the eardrum will be impaired by most of these abnormalities. Sometimes the ear canal must be cleaned of wax, dead skin, and other debris. Wax and debris can be removed with a cerumen spoon, suction aspirator, and irrigation (see Chapter 62).

The normal eardrum is slightly conical, quite shiny and smooth, and pearly gray in color. The position of the drumhead is oblique with respect to the ear canal. In the presence of disease, not only does the color of the eardrum change, but also other abnormalities such as retraction, bulging, or perforation of the eardrum, or a white plaque in the eardrum may exist.

Carefully inspect the entire eardrum, including the border or the annulus. The umbo and the long and short process of the malleus should be easily visible through the eardrum.

The mobility of the eardrum is tested by using the pneumatic device on the otoscope to inject a small puff of air into the ear canal. The eardrum is observed for gentle movement that normally accompanies the procedure.

## The Middle Ear

### Structure and function

The middle ear consists of the middle ear cleft and its contents, the *ossicles,* the *oval* and *round windows,* and the *eustachian tube.* The middle ear cleft or tympanic cavity is an air-filled space located within the petrous bone of the temporal bone. If the middle ear is viewed in relationship to surrounding structures, the middle ear is above the jugular fossa, behind the carotid canal, and in front of the mastoid air cells. The external auditory canal is external to the middle ear, and the labyrinth is internal. The middle ear is traversed by a chain of three movable bones that connect the tympanic membrane to the labyrinth (see Figure 61-2).

**Ossicles.** The three smallest bones in the body are called the *malleus* (hammer), the *incus* (anvil), and the *stapes* (stirrup). The **ossicles** have been given these common names because of their appearance. The outermost ossicle is the malleus, which is firmly attached to the tympanic membrane and is the largest of the auditory ossicles. The innermost ossicle is the stapes, which is fixed in the oval window, in direct contact with the perilymph of the inner ear, and the smallest of the auditory ossicles. The incus lies between the other two and has the same shape as a tooth with two roots.

The function of these *ossicles* is to *mechanically transmit sound* vibrations. The ossicles are held in place by muscles, ligaments, and joints and offer protective mechanisms from loud sounds. The light weight of these ossicles allows for ease of transmission, particularly of high-frequency sounds. The ossicles provide an efficient means by which the movement of air molecules can be transferred to the fluid molecules that circulate in the inner ear. Liquids offer more resistance than air and need more force to produce movement; the ossicular chain produces this force against the inner ear fluids.

**Windows.** There are two windows in the middle ear, the oval window and the round window, so named because of their shape. The *oval window* is not a true window, since the footplate of the stapes covers it. The oval window is the opening into the inner ear where sound vibrations enter. The *round window* is a true window and provides an exit for sound vibrations from the inner ear. The windows are discussed more fully in a later section.

**Eustachian tube.** The eustachian tube is a channel approximately 35 mm (1½ in) in length through which the middle ear communicates with the nasopharynx. The structure is mostly bone, cartilage, and fibrous tissue and extends downward, forward, and inward from each middle ear. The lining of the eustachian tube is mucous membrane continuous with that which lines the middle ear cavity at one end and that which lines the nasopharynx at the opposite end. Only a small segment at the superior end remains open permanently; otherwise the walls are in direct contact with each other. This is to prevent the sound of normal nasal respiration and one's own voice from passing up the eustachian tube into the middle ear. A failure of normal function leads to many middle ear disorders. However, during yawning, swallowing, and sneezing, the eustachian tube is opened by the tensor veli palatine muscle. The tube can be *forcibly opened by increasing nasopharyngeal pressure,* a technique called the **Valsalva maneuver.**

The eustachian tube normally allows air to enter and leave the middle ear. This tube is responsible for both ventilation and pressure regulation, which are necessary for normal hearing. Malfunction of the eustachian tube can lead to many middle ear disorders.

### Objective data

Assessment of the middle ear involves both measuring hearing and inspecting the middle ear through the tympanic membrane with the otoscope or other ear microscopes. Gross assessment of hearing can be accomplished by the presentation of a sound (whisper or watch tick) and the comparison of one ear to the other, as well as the comparison of the nurse's hearing and responses (provided the nurse has normal hearing) to the patient's

**TABLE 61-1 Subjective Data to be Collected**

| SYMPTOMS | CHARACTERISTICS |
|---|---|
| Pain (earache) | Onset, severity, radiation |
| Itching | Site, intensity, duration |
| Drainage | Onset, occurrence, consistency, type |
| Fullness (pressure) | Duration, association with other symptoms |
| Loss of hearing | Onset, location, duration |
| Ringing in the ear (tinnitus) | Onset, frequency, loudness, location, duration |
| Dizziness (vertigo) | Onset, frequency, sensation, duration |
| Facial weakness | Onset, extent, pain |

responses. Tuning forks are also used to assess hearing. Typical tuning fork tests are the *Weber* and *Rinne* tests (p. 2120). *Behavior clues* (p. 2114) may indicate a hearing loss. Table 61-1 lists *subjective data* to be collected.

## The Mastoid

### Structure and function

The term *mastoid* (which means breastlike) pertains to the mastoid bone, part of the temporal bone; the mastoid process, which is conical-shaped and part of the mastoid bone; the mastoid antrum, a large cavity that is continuous with the middle ear; and the mastoid air cells that branch off of the mastoid cavity. The mastoid cavity and cells are within the mastoid bone, which is located directly posterior to the pinna or external ear. The mastoid process can be felt as a bony protuberance behind the lower portion of the pinna.

The system of air-filled cells and cavity of the mastoid bone aids the middle ear in adjusting to changes in pressure. Therefore the mastoid system is a buffer to the middle ear. Equally important, this system of cavities and air cells lightens the mastoid bone. Because humans stand erect and have a slender neck, the weight of the skull is important. The denseness of the temporal bone is necessary for inner ear protection, and the mastoid air system lightens the weight of this protective bony structure.

### Objective data

The assessment of the mastoid bone and process is performed by palpating the bone behind the pinna. A normal mastoid bone is smooth, hard, and not tender. In comparing the mastoid bone on either side, the mastoid process is not always equal in size. This fact is sometimes mentioned by a patient but is not of pathologic significance. Inspection of the mastoid area should show normal skin.

## The Inner Ear

### Structure and function

The *inner ear* is located in the petrous part of the temporal bone and is the *organ for hearing* and *equilibrium.* The inner ear is a complex system of intercommunicating chambers and connecting tubes composed of two major structures: the *bony labyrinth* and the *membranous labyrinth,* which lies within but does not completely fill the bony labyrinth.

**Bony labyrinth.** The bony labyrinth is the rigid capsule in which the membranous labyrinth lies and consists of the vestibule, the three semicircular canals, and the cochlea (Figure 61-6). The *vestibule* is the connecting chamber between the semicircular canals posteriorly and the cochlea anteriorly. The *cochlea* looks like a snail shell and has two compartments. In cross section, the upper compartment is called the *scala vestibuli* and leads from the oval window to the apex of the cochlea. The lower compartment is called the *scala tympani* and continues from the apex of the cochlea to the round window. This system allows sound vibrations to enter at the oval window and exit at the round window. The main function of the cochlea is hearing. There are three semicircular canals: the superior, the lateral (horizontal), and the posterior. These canals provide the sense of balance.

**Membranous labyrinth.** The membranous labyrinth within the bony labyrinth is bathed in a fluid called *perilymph.* The membranous labyrinth consists of the utricle, saccule, three semicircular ducts, the cochlear duct, and the end organ for hearing called the organ of Corti. The membranous labyrinth contains a fluid called *endolymph.* The utricle, saccule, and the three semicircular canals are the sense organs responsible for position and balance. The semicircular canals are arranged to sense rotational movement, whereas the utricle and saccule are involved with linear movements. The cochlear duct is located in the cochlea between the scala vestibuli and the scala tympani. Membranes separate the cochlear duct from the scala vestibuli, and the scala tympani (called the vestibular membrane) from the basilar membranes. As sound vibrations enter the perilymph at the oval window and travel along the scala vestibuli, they pass through the vestibular membrane, enter the cochlear duct, and cause movement of the basilar membrane.

The organ of Corti is located on the basilar membrane and stretches from the base to the apex of the cochlea. This structure transforms mechanical sound vibrations into neural activity and separates sound into different frequencies. This electrochemical impulse travels via the acoustic nerve to the temporal cortex of the brain and is interpreted as meaningful sound.

### Objective data

The inner ears are inaccessible to direct examination. However, some inferences concerning their condition can be made by testing auditory and vestibular function. A gross assessment of the patient's hearing can be made

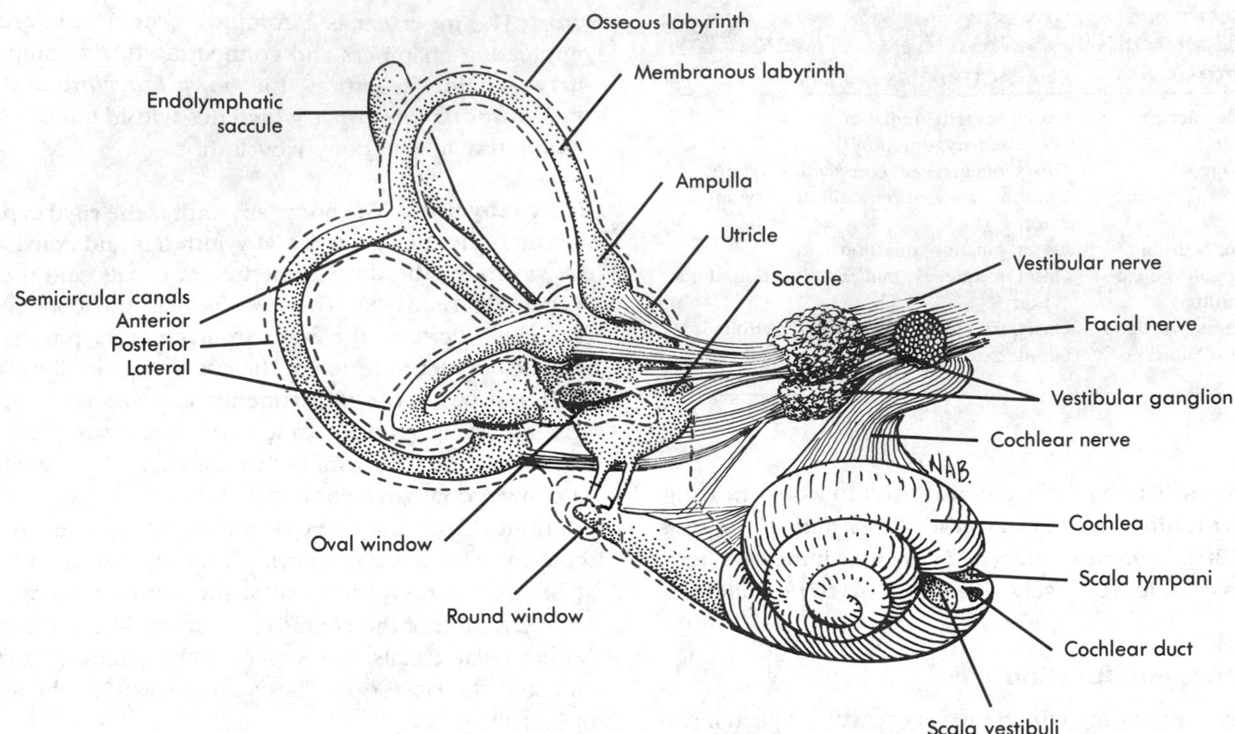


**FIGURE 61-6** Structures of the inner ear.

simply through conversation and by evaluating the logical sequences of replies. Assessment of the inner ear is divided into two sections: tests for auditory acuity and tests for balance.

# DIAGNOSTIC TESTS

## DIAGNOSTIC TESTS FOR AUDITORY ACUITY

### Whisper Voice Test

Each ear must be tested separately to estimate the hearing. One of the patient's ears is occluded with a finger. While standing 1 to 2 feet away, the nurse whispers two-syllable numbers softly toward the unoccluded ear, and the patient is asked to repeat the numbers. The intensity of the nurse's voice can be increased from a soft, medium, or loud whisper to a soft, medium, or loud voice. If the nurse suspects that the patient is lip reading, the nurse's face should be turned away. The patient is asked if hearing is better in one ear than in the other ear. If the auditory acuity is different, the ear that hears better should be tested first. Then, noise is produced in the better-hearing ear by rapidly but gently moving the finger in the patient's ear canal while testing the other ear.

A watch tick can also be used to test hearing. However, a watch tick is a higher-pitched sound and less relevant to functional hearing than the voice test.

### Tuning Fork Tests

The tuning fork also provides a general estimate of hearing loss. The three major tuning fork tests date from the nineteenth century and are named after their originators: Rinne, Weber, and Schwabach.

#### Rinne test

The vibrating tuning fork is shifted between two positions: against the mastoid bone (bone conduction) and 2 inches from the opening of the ear canal (air conduction) (Figure 61-7). As the position is changed, the patient is asked to indicate which tone is louder (in front of the ear or behind the ear) or is asked to indicate when one of the tones is no longer heard (Table 61-2). The Rinne test is useful to differentiate between conductive and sensorineural hearing losses.

With conductive hearing loss, the pathways of normal sound conduction are blocked. However, vibrations against the mastoid bone can bypass the obstruction; therefore bone conduction lasts longer than air conduction. With sensorineural hearing loss, the acoustic nerve has decreased ability to perceive vibrations from either route; therefore normal patterns (i.e., air conduction heard longer than bone conduction) are reported by the patient.[1]

#### Weber test

The tuning fork is set into vibration by striking the tines on the examiner's knuckles or knee. The rounded tip of the handle is placed on the patient's forehead or teeth (Figure 61-8). Placement on the teeth (even if the patient has false teeth) is generally more reliable. The pa-

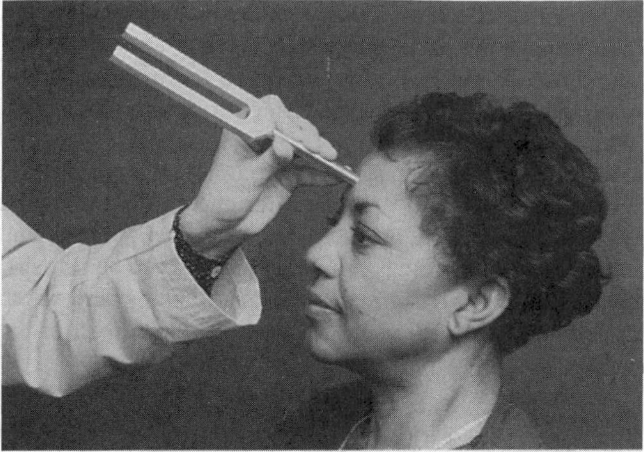

FIGURE 61-8 Weber test. The tuning fork is placed on the midline of the skull. (From Sigler B, Schuring L: *Ear, nose, and throat disorders,* St Louis, 1993, Mosby.)

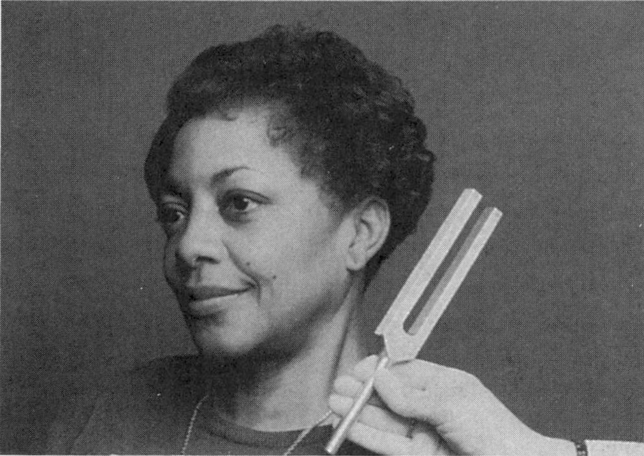

A

B

**FIGURE 61-7** Rinne test. **A,** The tuning fork is placed on the mastoid bone for bone conduction. **B,** The tuning fork is placed in front of the ear for air conduction. (From Sigler B, Schuring L: *Ear, nose, and throat disorders,* St Louis, 1993, Mosby.)

**TABLE 61-2 Tuning Fork Tests for Auditory Acuity**

| SITE OF PROBLEM | WEBER TEST | RINNE TEST |
|---|---|---|
| **NORMAL HEARING** | | |
| No problem | Tone heard in center of head | Air conduction lasts longer than bone conduction |
| **CONDUCTIVE LOSS** | | |
| External or middle ear | Tone heard in poorer ear because ear not distracted by room noise | Bone conduction lasts longer than air conduction |
| **SENSORINEURAL LOSS** | | |
| Inner ear | Tone heard in better ear because inner ear less able to receive vibrations | Air conduction lasts longer than bone conduction |

tient is asked whether the tone is heard in the middle of the head, the right ear, or the left ear (see Table 61-2). The Weber test is useful in cases of *unilateral loss.*

### Schwabach test

This test is also used to differentiate between a conductive and sensorineural hearing loss. The Schwabach test compares the hearing of the examiner (who must have normal hearing) with that of the patient by alternately placing a tuning fork on the mastoid process of the patient and the examiner. However, the Rinne test has replaced this test.

■ ■ ■

The aforementioned tests can be performed at the bedside by the nurse to give some indication of the level of hearing. More elaborate and specific hearing tests are performed in a soundproofed room.

## DIAGNOSTIC TESTS FOR BALANCE

Balance and equilibrium depend on *four systems* being intact: the *vestibular* (the labyrinth or inner ear), the *proprioceptive* (somatosensors of joints and muscles), the *visual* (the eye), and the *cerebellar* (coordination). The sensations transmitted from the joints (that is, the somatosensors) and the inner ears are integrated in the brainstem and cerebellum and perceived in the cerebral cortex. *Dizziness* is most likely to occur when *two* or *more systems* are *impaired simultaneously* or when they transmit sensory information that is contradictory.

Assessment of the inner ear for balance should be accomplished by a thorough *history, observation of gait, gaze test for nystagmus,* and the *Romberg test.* The importance of the history and interview cannot be overemphasized. All patients bring some degree of anxiety regarding the illness to the interview and examination. Dizziness can have devastating effects on the patient's quality of life. The disruption of the patient's routine, the severity of the attacks, and the fear of the unknown can all make the patient agitated, anxious, and depressed. The nurse must be aware of these feelings and demonstrate self-confidence, patience, courtesy, consideration, and gentleness.

*Gait* is tested by asking the patient to walk in one direction away from the examiner and then to turn and walk back. Posture, balance, swinging of the arms, and movement of the legs should be observed. Normally, balance is easy; the arms swing at the sides, and when the patient turns, the face and head lead the rest of the body.

**Nystagmus** is the involuntary, rhythmic oscillation of the eyes. It occurs normally when a person watches a rapidly moving object. Nystagmus is essentially a disorder of ocular posture but is associated with vestibular dysfunction. To check for *gaze nystagmus,* the finger of the examiner is placed directly in front of the patient at eye level. The patient is asked to follow the finger without moving the head. The finger is moved slowly from the midline toward the ear in each direction. The eyes should be observed for any jerking movements. For example, if the eyes jerk quickly to the left and drift slowly back to the right, the patient has a left nystagmus. Nystagmus can be horizontal, vertical, or rotary.

For a *Romberg test,* the patient stands with feet together, without arm support, and with eyes open (Figure 61-9). Note ability to maintain an upright posture. Perform the same test with the eyes closed. Normally only a minimal amount of swaying exists. If the patient loses balance (positive Romberg test), this might indicate an inner ear problem (vestibular problem) or cerebellar ataxia.

Other noninvasive tests include hyperventilation, Valsalva maneuver, neck twist, and fistula test. Because these tests may simulate dizziness comparable to that which the patient is experiencing, more knowledge and special training is necessary to perform and interpret them.

A series of tests for the vestibular system that assess balance by electrophysiologic means is also available. In some settings the tests are performed by audiologists, because audiometry is also used secondarily to assess balance problems. The physical proximity of the vestibular and cochlear systems in the labyrinth mirrors the juxtaposition of the clinical tests. Although the physical assessment of balance is important, the most common objective measurement of balance is accomplished by *electronystagmography* (ENG). The ENG instrument was developed to measure nystagmus in response to stimulation of the vestibular system. This stimulation includes testing the patient at rest in different positions for both the eyes and the head and with different temperatures in the ear canals, thus stimulating the semicircular canals. The different test results give an *electronystagmogram* that reflects the status of each labyrinth and can point to central nervous system disorders.

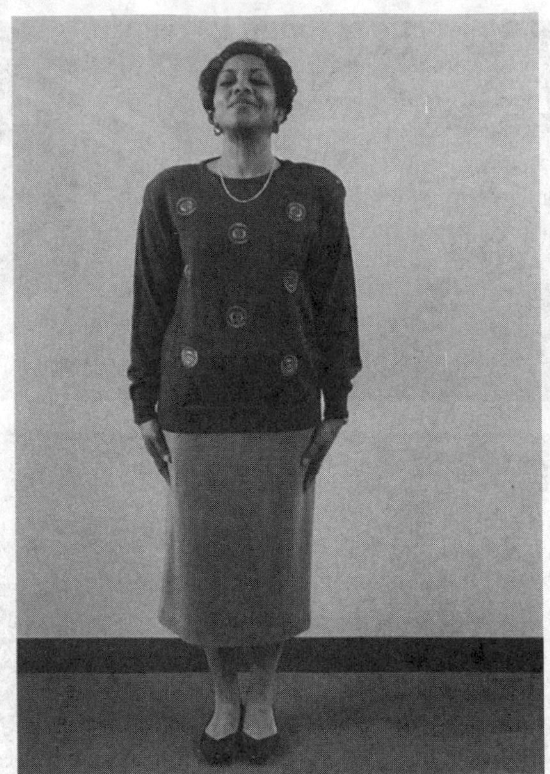

**FIGURE 61-9** Evaluation of balance with the Romberg test. (From Sigler B, Schuring L: *Ear, nose, and throat disorders,* St Louis, 1993, Mosby.)

Other means of testing the balance system, mostly research tools, include stimulation by rotary chair, pendulum swings, and postural changes. *Platform posturography* is a computerized test performed while the person is standing. This test can separate the balance problem into inner ear, visual, and muscle stretch origins. The platform test helps to identify, quantify, and localize the source of balance disorders.

## PHYSIOLOGIC CHANGES WITH AGING

As in any other organ system, the ear is affected by changes that occur over the years. The most common cause of hearing loss in elderly persons is *presbycusis.* Most individuals develop presbycusis as they age. The amount of hearing loss is affected by familial differences and can begin in middle age. Presbycusis is not curable, but some persons will find a hearing aid helpful. Other physiologic changes with aging are found in Table 61-3.

## DIAGNOSTIC OTOLOGIC TESTS

### Laboratory Tests

Four laboratory tests are useful for assessment of ear problems: (1) blood tests, (2) ear cultures, (3) cerebrospinal fluid identification, and (4) pathologic tissue examination.

*Blood tests* that are diagnostic for systemic abnor-

**TABLE 61-3 Physiologic Ear Changes With Aging**

| PROBLEM | ETIOLOGY |
|---|---|
| Impacted cerumen | Decreased secretion and increased amounts of keratin, which make cerumen harder and more easily impacted |
| Conductive hearing loss | Problems of external or middle ear:<br>Build-up of cerumen<br>Otosclerosis (osseous growth leading to fixation of the stapes in the oval window)<br>Atrophy, sclerosis, or rupture of tympanic membrane<br>Recurrent otitis media |
| Sensorineural hearing loss | Problems of inner ear:<br>Loss of efficiency<br>Presbycusis (degeneration of cells of auditory nerve leading to initial loss of ability to hear high-frequency sounds, followed eventually by loss of ability to hear sounds in all ranges)<br>Vascular changes<br>Diabetes<br>Tumors<br>Prolonged exposure to excessive noise<br>Ototoxic drugs such as aspirin and many antibiotics |

malities are only secondarily significant for ear disease. For example, an elevated white blood count points to an infection but is not diagnostic of ear disease. However, in the face of possible ear infection and in the absence of other infection, blood tests may be helpful.

Drainage from the ear canal or a surgical incision is usually *cultured* to identify the organism. This is especially necessary in acute infections to choose the appropriate antibiotic. When long-term drainage is present, such as in chronic otitis media, cultures are less helpful because gram-negative bacilli cover up the original pathogen. In these cases many surgeons do not culture the drainage but rather begin treatment with broad-spectrum antibiotics.

When drainage is found in the ear, a dilemma is presented. Is this clear fluid *cerebrospinal fluid?* A fistula from the inner ear to the middle ear and external ear can produce cerebrospinal fluid. This pathway also can lead to meningitis by retrograde contamination. Therefore an analysis of clear fluid is often helpful in diagnosing the problem.

*Pathologic examination of abnormal tissue* from the ear canal or from other tissue harvested during surgery is necessary to both rule out a malignancy and identify unusual problems. In an infected ear, affected tissue is readily identified with pathologic assessment. If the surgeon is in doubt as to the findings, then a tissue sample (biopsy) is taken for examination. The surgical finding of *cholesteatoma* is usually documented by a pathologic examination.

## Radiologic Tests

### Computed tomography

Computed tomography (CT) scanning involves sending an x-ray beam through the body at various angles. The images that are created by the x-ray beam are passed through a computer to produce cross-sectional images. The temporal bone can be evaluated in thin sections, or slices, producing more and smaller components than a plain film x-ray. The CT scan can also be done with a contrast medium, an iodinated dye that is useful in imaging vascular lesions and increasing the clarity of the images. An enhanced CT scan is most commonly ordered to rule out retrocochlear pathologic conditions.

### Magnetic resonance imaging

Magnetic resonance imaging (MRI) uses a large magnet rather than ionizing radiation to emit energy. The patient is placed in a tube or tunnel containing a large magnet equipped with radiofrequency coils, which transmit radio waves into the body part being imaged. The patient's own atoms (mainly hydrogen atoms) are given additional bursts of energy by these radiofrequency waves and in turn emit signals that are processed and displayed as computer-generated images of the body part. The advantage of MRI is that soft tissue is detailed rather than bony structures. Therefore the membranous organs, nerves, and blood vessels of the temporal bone can be examined.

### Arteriography and venography

Adjuncts to radiography are *arteriography* and *venography* in which contrast dye is injected into blood vessels. These studies are especially useful for diagnosing vascular abnormalities in the temporal bone. Compression of the vessels can be recognized, and tumors of the temporal bone and related structures can be recognized in greater detail.

# DIAGNOSTIC AUDIOMETRIC TESTS

## Hearing Tests

Hearing tests are conducted in a soundproof booth by an *audiologist. Hearing* is *measured* in a special unit named the *decibel,* a logarithmic function of sound intensity. The sound is presented through an audiometer. The patient wears earphones and signals the audiologist when a tone is heard. These responses are plotted on a graph called the audiogram. By varying the loudness of the pure tones or speech, a hearing level is established. The use of earphones results in a pure tone level or air conduction. The earphones are also used to measure the *level* of speech hearing (speech reception threshold) and the *understanding* of speech (discrimination). By presenting the sound through a bone conduction oscillator placed on the mastoid bone, the middle ear structures are bypassed, and a bone conduction level is established. This is a level at which the cochlea can hear and is commonly referred to as the nerve hearing level.

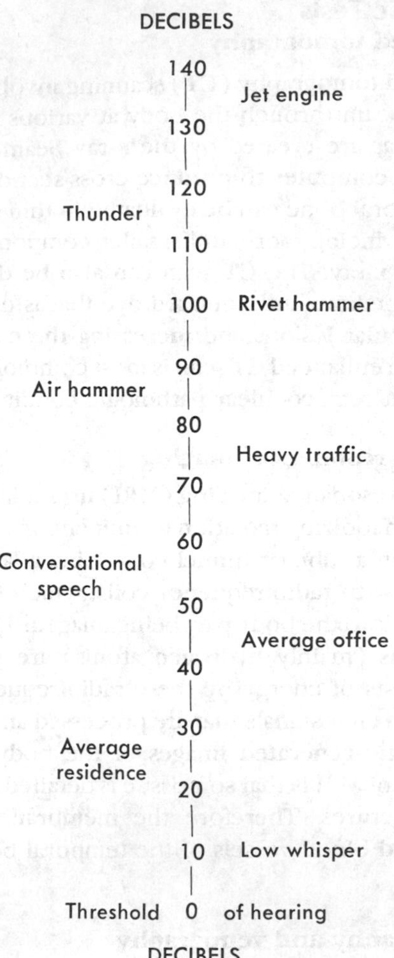


**FIGURE 61-10** Intensity range of human hearing. Intensity levels of various environmental sounds and situations. (From Saunders WH et al: *Nursing care in eye, nose, and throat disorders,* ed 4, St Louis, 1979, Mosby.)

A person with *normal* hearing would have the same air conduction as bone conduction hearing levels. Normal hearing is a range that was established nationally by measuring the hearing levels of the population, including all ages. Figure 61-10 relates normal hearing to other common noises.

Because the middle ear structures serve as a transformer that enhances sound and transfers sound to the inner ear (cochlea), a difference in hearing levels between air conduction and bone conduction results in a *conductive hearing loss.* A patient with a conductive hearing loss has a problem with the tympanic membrane, middle ear, or mastoid. Fortunately, most disorders causing a conductive hearing loss can be corrected by microsurgery. If the air and bone conduction levels are equal but not within the normal range, a sensorineural nerve hearing loss has occurred. Surgery cannot correct the problems that cause a *sensorineural hearing loss,* although a hearing aid is very useful if the discrimination of speech is adequate. A distinction is made between the sensory (cochlea) and neural (acoustic nerve) portions of a sensorineural hearing loss. It is quite common for a patient to have a conductive and sensorineural hearing loss; this combination is called a *mixture hearing loss* (see Chapter 62).

## Tympanometry and Impedance Audiometry

A popular test used for differentiating problems in the middle ear is *tympanometry or impedance audiometry.* This automatic test of applying pressure to the tympanic membrane and measuring the result creates a distinctive tracing on a graph called a *tympanogram.* Abnormalities of the tympanogram indicate problems of the middle ear, eustachian tube, and/or the ossicles. Tympanometry can also be used to measure the stapedial muscle reflex and its decay. This test measures the status of the acoustic nerve. With pathologic conditions of the cochlea, acoustic reflex thresholds often are obtained at less intense stimulation levels. With a retrocochlear lesion, the reflex thresholds often are elevated and may demonstrate abnormal decay or absence of the reflex. With conductive hearing loss, the reflexes may be elevated but usually are absent.

## Auditory Brainstem Response

Brainstem auditory evoked potential testing is one approach to assessment of the auditory nervous system for evaluating dysfunction at the level of the eighth cranial nerve (acoustic nerve), pons, or midbrain. Evoked potentials measure and record changes in brain electrical activity that occur in response to auditory sensory stimulation; that is, the evoked potential measures and records brain electrical activity along the central auditory pathways of the brainstem in response to clicking sounds. The test involves placing electrodes on the vertex, mastoid process, and/or earlobes while the patient is seated in a comfortable chair. The data are fed into a computer. Abnormal findings suggest dysfunctions at the various levels in the auditory nervous system. For example, abnormal test results may suggest a lesion of the acoustic nerve or brainstem.

In addition to the tests of the eighth cranial nerve discussed above, mention of seventh cranial nerve (facial nerve) testing is necessary. Tests of the seventh cranial nerve are related to audiometric tests because the facial and acoustic nerves share the internal acoustic canal. The facial nerve is tested in the same way as other motor nerves with nerve conduction tests and muscle excitability tests. The auxiliary functions of the facial nerve (taste and tearing) can also be measured. The facial and acoustic nerves are usually both involved in lesions of the temporal bone.

## CRITICAL THINKING ACTIVITIES

- You are admitting a patient for suspected acute myocardial infarction and note that he speaks very loudly and looks at you intensely when you ask him questions. Occasionally he answers inappropriately or asks you to repeat the question. He has no complaints of ear problems or ringing in his ears and denies hearing loss. What is your analysis of this patient?
- Compare and contrast bone conduction and air conduction.

## CHAPTER SUMMARY

### ANATOMY AND PHYSIOLOGY

- Detection of patients with a hearing impairment or a balance problem is an important nursing responsibility.
- Behavior can alert the nurse to the possibility of hearing impairment.
- The ear is housed in the temporal bone and divided into the external, middle, and inner ear.
- Sound vibrations reach the inner ear by mechanical energy through air conduction and bone conduction.
- The tympanic membrane is a common membrane between the external ear canal and the middle ear cleft.
- The otoscope is the most common instrument used to examine the ear.
- The functions of the eustachian tube are ventilation and pressure regulation, both of which are essential for normal hearing.
- The functions of the mastoid bone include helping the middle ear to adjust to pressure changes and lightening the weight of the skull.
- The inner ear transforms mechanical energy into electrochemical impulses that travel via the acoustic nerve to the temporal cortex of the brain. The brain interprets these impulses as meaningful sound and as balance.
- Nystagmus can be an objective sign of a vestibular problem.

### DIAGNOSTIC TESTS

- Electronystagmography is the test used to measure nystagmus.
- Audiometric tests, usually performed by audiologists, are used to evaluate the ear for hearing.

## REFERENCE

1. Bates B: *A guide to physical examination,* ed 5, Philadelphia, 1991, JB Lippincott.

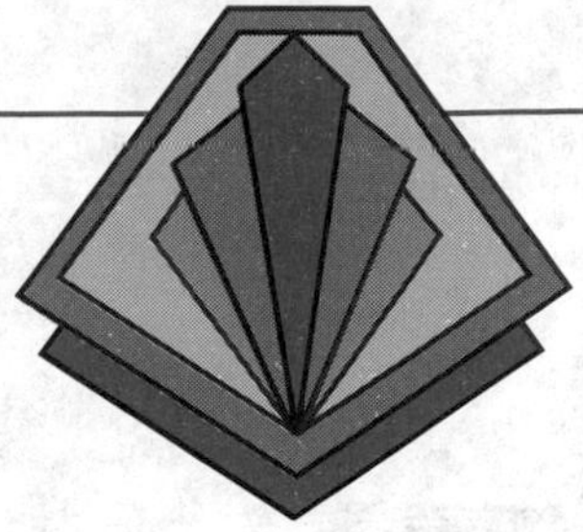

C H A P T E R 62

# Management of Persons With Problems of the Ear

*Linda T. Schuring*

## CHAPTER OBJECTIVES

***After studying this chapter, the learner should be able to do the following:***

1 Discuss three measures that are important in preventing hearing loss.
2 Differentiate between conductive and sensorineural hearing loss and describe methods for assessing each.
3 Describe the pathophysiology and nursing requirements of the patient with otitis media.
4 Describe the preoperative and postoperative care of the patient undergoing ear surgery.
5 Discuss the signs and symptoms and nursing care of the person with Ménière's disease.
6 Describe methods of aural rehabilitation and communication with hearing-impaired persons.
7 Describe the pathophysiology and nursing care of the person with a balance disorder.

## KEY TERMS

acoustic neuroma
barotrauma
bullous myringitis
central deafness
cholesteatoma
cochlear implants
conductive hearing loss
endolymphatic sac procedures
exostosis
external otitis
functional hearing loss
hearing impairment
labyrinthectomy
labyrinthitis
mastoidectomy
mastoiditis
Ménière's disease
mixed hearing loss
myringoplasty
noise-induced hearing loss
ossiculoplasty
otitis media
otosclerosis
ototoxicity
perichondritis
presbycusis
sensorineural hearing loss
stapedectomy
stapedotomy
tinnitus
tympanoplasty
tympanosclerosis
vertigo

## HEARING LOSS

Hearing loss has become the nation's number one disability, affecting 1 of 15 Americans. Approximately 28 million people in the United States (including 29% of persons age 65 or older) have some kind of hearing impairment.[3] By the year 2050, approximately 1 of every 5 persons in this country will be 55 years of age or older. Of these estimated 58 million persons, 26 million are expected to have a hearing impairment. **Hearing impairment** ranges from difficulty in understanding words or hearing certain sounds, such as ringing or buzzing, to total deafness.

Nurses have a responsibility not only to communicate with the hearing impaired and provide the necessary information regarding health care but also to develop ways to relate to persons with hearing impairments. Very often, persons with hearing problems must be motivated to seek professional help. Although some diseases of the ear canal can be helped with medicine or surgery, the vast majority of persons with a hearing impairment cannot be treated effectively. Of all hearing impairments, 80% are caused by nerve deafness for which, at present, there is no known cure.

Hearing impairment and dizziness (a major symptom of inner ear problems) can hinder communication with

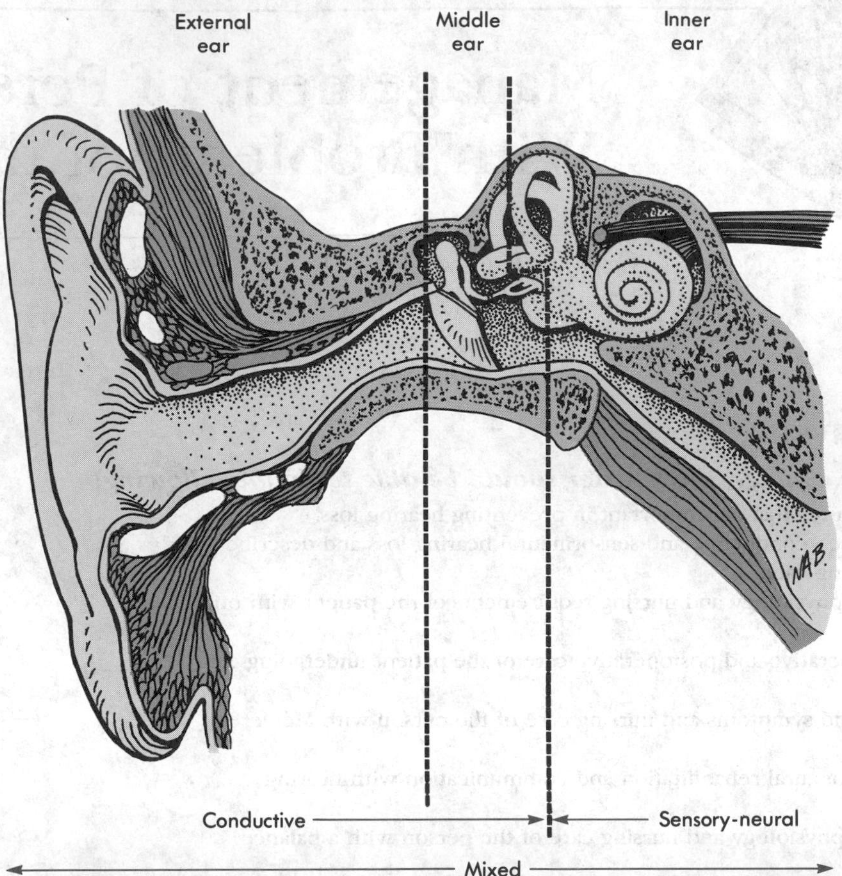


**FIGURE 62-1** Three types of hearing loss. Conductive loss results from interference with conduction in the external and middle ear; sensorineural loss results from interference with conduction in the inner ear; and mixed hearing loss results from interference with conduction in all three areas.

others, limit social activities, and reduce constructive use of leisure time. Career options, job opportunities, and financial security may be affected negatively. These problems may influence the ability to remain independent or to feel able to be a contributing member of society. Finally, the aesthetic enjoyment of that which is pleasurable or beautiful may be decreased, and the ability to share the human experience is temporarily or permanently diminished. All of these variables can affect the person's quality of life. Hearing impairment diminishes the quality of life for one third of U.S. adults who are between 65 and 75 years of age.

## CLASSIFICATION OF HEARING LOSS

### Conductive Hearing Loss

Any interference with the conduction of sound impulses through the external auditory canal, the eardrum, or the middle ear results in a **conductive hearing loss,** or transmission deafness. The inner ear is not involved in a pure conductive loss, and sound amplification will reach the inner ear (Figure 62-1).

Conductive hearing loss may be caused by anything that blocks the external ear, such as wax, infection, or a foreign body; a thickening, retraction, scarring, or perforation of the tympanic membrane; or any pathophysiologic changes in the middle ear affecting or fixing one or more of the ossicles.

### Sensorineural Hearing Loss

**Sensorineural hearing loss** results from disease or trauma to the *inner ear,* neural structures, or nerve pathways leading to the brainstem. Some of the causes of "nerve" deafness are infectious diseases (measles, mumps, and meningitis), arteriosclerosis, ototoxic drugs (Box 62-1), neuromas of cranial nerve VIII, otospongiosis (form of progressive deafness caused by the formation of new abnormal spongy bone in labyrinth), trauma to the head or ear, or degeneration of the organ of Corti occurring most commonly from advancing age (presbycusis).

### Central Deafness

**Central deafness** is also known as central auditory dysfunction. With this phenomenon, the central nervous

**BOX 62-1 Selected Ototoxic Drugs**

**AMINOGLYCOSIDE ANTIBIOTICS**
Streptomycin
Neomycin
Kanamycin
Gentamycin
Tobramycin
Netromycin
Amikacin

**OTHER ANTIBIOTICS**
Vancomycin
Viomycin
Polymyxin B (Aerosporin)
Polymyxin E (Colistin/Coly-Mycin)
Erythromycin
Minocycline
Capreomycin

**DIURETICS**
Ethacrynic acid (Edecrin)
Furosemide (Lasix)
Acetazolamide (Diamox)

**OTHER DRUGS**
Quinine
Chloroquine
Nitrogen mustard
Bleomycin
Quinidine
Cisplatin
Salicylates

system cannot interpret normal auditory signals. Therefore hearing ability test results are normal, although the patient is "deaf." Diseases that alter the central nervous system, such as cerebrovascular accidents and tumors, are the cause of this rare form of sensorineural hearing loss.

## Other Types of Hearing Loss

Different types of hearing loss are listed in Box 62-2. A person is considered to have a **mixed hearing loss** when both a conductive and a sensorineural hearing loss are present simultaneously (Figure 62-1). A **functional loss** is a hearing loss for which no organic lesion can be found. A hearing loss may also be congenital or acquired. *The majority of persons with ear problems have some degree of hearing loss.*

# HEARING RESEARCH

Hearing and balance research is conducted at the National Institute of Deafness and Other Communication Disorders (NIDCD). This division of the National Institutes of Health will vastly improve the care of patients with hearing impairments. Research grants are available to nurses as well as to other health care providers.

**BOX 62-2 Types of Hearing Loss**

**Central hearing loss** Loss of hearing from damage to the brain's auditory pathways or auditory center
**Conductive hearing loss** Loss of hearing from a mechanical problem
**Fluctuating hearing loss** A sensorineural hearing loss that varies with time
**Functional hearing loss** Loss of hearing for which no organic lesion can be found
**Mixed hearing loss** Elements of both conduction and sensorineural hearing loss
**Neural hearing loss** A sensorineural hearing loss originating in the nerve or brainstem
**Sensorineural hearing loss** Loss of hearing involving the cochlea and hearing nerve; bone and air conduction are equal but diminished
**Sensory hearing loss** A sensorineural hearing loss originating in the cochlea and involving the hair cells and nerve endings
**Sudden hearing loss** A sensorineural hearing loss with a sudden onset

# PREVENTION

## *Healthy People 2000*

Goals of *Healthy People 2000* that pertain to hearing loss include the following[3]:

1. Reduce to no more than 15% the proportion of workers exposed to average daily noise levels that exceed 85 decibels (dB).
2. Reduce significant hearing impairment to a prevalence of no more than 82 per 1000 people, as measured by self-reported hearing impairment.

## Primary Prevention

To maintain normal ear function, adequate protection of the ears is important and includes the following activities: care of the healthy ear, prevention of ear trauma, and monitoring of noise pollution.

### Care of healthy ears

The external ear may be washed with soap and water daily while bathing or showering. The ear canal is generally "self-cleaning." Wax is to the ears what tears are to the eyes; it serves as a protective mechanism. Earwax lubricates the skin and traps foreign material that enters the canal. Therefore wax should not be cleaned out of the ear routinely. Although recommendations have been made that the ear should be cleaned only with a wet washcloth over the tip of a finger, cotton-tipped applicators can be used. The applicator should be moistened with alcohol and inserted into the canal only the length of the cotton tip. The ear canal in an adult is approximately 1 to 1½ inches long from the external opening to the eardrum, which is long enough to safely clean with a cotton-tipped applicator.

#### Preventing ear trauma

People should be taught to avoid inserting hard articles into the ear canal, obstructing the ear canal with any object, inserting unclean articles or solutions into the ear, or swimming in water that has been identified as polluted. These practices can lead to damage to the tympanic membrane or to ear infections. Adults often traumatize the ear by inserting hard articles into the outer ear in an attempt to remove cerumen or to scratch an itch in the ear canal.

#### Monitoring noise pollution

Occupational noise is a primary cause of hearing loss in our society. The most common type of occupational hearing loss is caused by loud noise. **Noise-induced hearing loss** is caused from progressive destruction of sensory cells in the ear and cannot be medically or surgically repaired. Therefore prevention is the key to reducing noise-induced hearing loss.

Sound intensity is measured in decibels (dB). In the United States, the Occupational Safety and Health Administration (OSHA) has established acceptable levels of noise in work environments. The protocols regarding noise protection are complex; but in general, *exposure to noise levels in excess of 90 dB over an 8-hour day is considered excessive* and should be avoided. Ordinary speech level is about 50 dB and heavy traffic about 70 dB; above 80 dB, noise becomes uncomfortable to the human ear. Exposure to levels greater than 85 dB to 90 dB for months or years can cause cochlear damage. OSHA now requires yearly audiometric tests for noise-exposed workers. The nurse must participate in teaching the proper use of protective ear devices or earplugs for persons working in areas of high-decibel noise. Courses are available to educate nurses about industrial hearing conservation requirements.

Other causes of noise-induced hearing loss include the use of firearms and high-intensity music. A person firing guns who notices tinnitus (ringing in the ears), a sensation of fullness in the ear, or a temporary hearing loss should stop firing guns or wear suitable ear protection. Noise from a rock band can exceed 120 dB, and hearing losses have been measured in some members of rock bands. If proximity to the high noise level cannot be avoided, earplugs should be worn during exposure.

*Earplugs* are inserted into the external auditory canal and are capable of reducing the noise that reaches the middle ear by 10 dB to 30 dB. Usually standard plugs are effective, but custom-made plugs molded to the individual's ear canal can be purchased. For noise levels reaching 140 dB and above, such as around jet airplanes, individuals must wear earmuffs.

### Secondary Prevention

Methods of secondary prevention include early detection of hearing losses, periodic ear examinations, monitoring side effects of ototoxic drugs, and early adequate treatment of ear diseases.

#### Early detection of hearing loss

Because the hearing (auditory) nerve does not regain function, early detection of hearing loss is important so that the cause of the loss can be diagnosed and, it is hoped, the problem can be corrected or arrested. However, the signs of a small loss of hearing are elusive and are often ignored.

A hearing loss in both ears may first be detected by a family member rather than the affected person. The earliest sign is not hearing what was once heard. Another common sign is asking for a repetition of what was said. Usually the request is in the form of a question such as "What did you say?" Sometimes the hard of hearing person may repeat the information, even incorrectly, to evoke a response and thus a repetition of the information.

A hearing loss in one ear is more difficult to detect. The person may notice the loss only when using a telephone or when having difficulty determining the direction of sounds.

#### Periodic ear examinations

Periodic (every 2 to 3 years) ear examinations for evaluation of hearing are important in the adult because aging frequently causes degenerative changes in the ear, as well as in other body tissues.

#### Monitoring side effects of ototoxic drugs

Some drugs may affect the cochlea, the vestibule of the ear, or the eighth cranial nerve (see Box 62-1). Persons taking ototoxic drugs need to know the signs and symptoms of side effects of these drugs to prevent hearing loss from developing. If these symptoms (dizziness, decreased hearing acuity, tinnitus) occur, the next dose of the drug is omitted, and the physician is consulted. Audiometric testing (see Chapter 61) may be necessary.

#### Early, adequate treatment of ear diseases

Any disease that causes prolonged symptoms of the ear such as pain, swelling, drainage, "plugged" feeling, or decreased hearing should be promptly assessed and treated by a physician. The nurse must encourage persons with these symptoms to seek professional help. Many chronic problems such as perforations and necrotic ossicles could be prevented with prompt and adequate medical attention.

During upper respiratory infections (colds), the nose should be blown with both nostrils open. Excessive pressure occurs when one nostril is closed and can force infected secretions up the eustachian tube into the middle ear.

## TYPES OF EAR DISORDERS

The same types of disorders that occur in other parts of the body also occur in the ear; these include *obstructions* or *blockage; trauma; inflammation, infection,* and *scarring;* and *skin disorders.* Some disorders that only affect the ear include hearing loss, dizziness and balance (disorders of the inner ear), and tinnitus (ringing in the ears).

In this chapter, the discussion of ear problems is divided into three parts: (1) problems of the external ear; (2) problems of the tympanic membrane, middle ear, and mastoid; and (3) problems of the inner ear.

# PROBLEMS OF THE EXTERNAL EAR

## ETIOLOGY/PATHOPHYSIOLOGY

### Congenital Ear Problems

The auricle and external ear canal develop separately embryologically, resulting in two types of potential congenital disorders of the external ear. The pinna can be deformed or absent with a normal external ear canal, or the pinna and ear canal together can show congenital changes. External ear canal abnormalities result in different degrees of incomplete development or *canal atresia.* Congenital findings of the external ear do not necessarily mean that the middle or inner ear is involved. A minor congenital finding is protruding ears, in which the auricle has a greater than normal angle to the head. Also, cysts and skin tracts that develop from incomplete formation of the pinna are quite common.

### Infections

The most common problems found in the external ear are infections, primarily bacterial or fungal. The most frequent infection, called **external otitis,** involves the external ear canal (Table 62-1). This infection begins in the skin lining of the ear canal and can occlude the canal. External otitis occurs more frequently in the summer than in the winter. A localized form of this infection is seen as an *ear canal furuncle* or *abscess.* When a systemic disease such as diabetes is present, the external otitis can spread wildly through cartilage and bone and is then named *malignant external otitis.* The most common form of external otitis is called *swimmer's ear,* because it is prevalent when water remains in the ear canal. In addition, opportunistic fungal infections are common. Occasionally, infection involves only the cartilage of the auricle **(perichondritis),** resulting in necrosis of the cartilage and loss of the distinctive shape of the auricle if not treated quickly.

*Pain* in the external ear is the *most common symptom* of infection. Painful sites are also tender because of the close proximity of bone (a hard surface) when palpating the ear. A clue to early external otitis is tenderness when gently pulling on the pinna. A *forerunner of pain* in external otitis is *itching in the ear canal. Inflammation (redness)* is easily identified with an otoscope. At different stages of infection, *drainage* is found exiting the ear canal. In early infectious disorders, the drainage may be clear and not discolored by pus.

### Masses

Benign masses of the external ear canal are usually cysts arising from a sebaceous gland, rarely from the cerumen (earwax) glands. Cysts can also be congenital. Bony protrusions seen in the lower bony portion of the ear canal are called **exostosis.** The skin covering the exostosis is normal. If the skin is red, the mass is usually an abscess. *Infectious polyps* found in the ear canal arise from either the tympanic membrane or, more commonly, the middle ear through a hole in the tympanic membrane. Malignant tumors are also found in the external ear. The *cutaneous carcinomas* are most often *basal cell carcinoma* on the pinna and *squamous cell carcinoma* in the ear canal. These carcinomas can invade the underlying tissue if not treated, and squamous cell carcinoma may spread throughout the temporal bone. Rare tumors of the cerumen glands are of the *adenoma* cell type.

### Cerumen

On inspection of the external canal, the most frequent problematic finding is *impacted cerumen* (wax). Although the ear canal is self-cleaning, cerumen may become impacted from a disorder or from improper cleaning. Removal of cerumen must be performed carefully and may be necessary before the tympanic membrane can be examined.

### Trauma

Trauma, either sharp or blunt, is becoming a more common finding. A residual finding of repeated blunt trauma is a hypertrophic scar formation known as a *cauliflower ear,* an occupational hazard for boxers. With prompt treatment, traumatic injuries can be corrected successfully.

A wide array of *foreign bodies* fit into the ear canal. The most common foreign body found in adults is a piece of cotton; probably the most annoying is an insect.

**TABLE 62-1 Normal Function, Pathophysiology, and Clinical Manifestations in External Otitis**

| NORMAL FUNCTION | PATHOPHYSIOLOGY | CLINICAL MANIFESTATIONS |
|---|---|---|
| The pinna of the external ear channel acts like a funnel into the ear canal. The ear canal is 1-1½ in long and is lined with epithelium that contains modified sweat glands, cerumen glands, and hair. | Exposure to moisture, contamination, or local trauma produces an environment conducive to the overgrowth of normal flora. | Tenderness on pulling the pinna, whitish drainage, inflammation of the ear canal including redness, swelling, itching, decreased hearing because of debris, and narrowing of the ear canal. |

**BOX 62-3 Complications of External Ear Problems**

Abscess
Cellulitis
Discoloration
Disfigurement of pinna
Hearing loss
Infection of middle ear
Ischemia or necrosis of pinna
Keloid
Lymphadenopathy
Metastasis
Osteitis
Septicemia
Stenosis

In children, the most common is a small toy. The difficulty encountered in removing a foreign body can be tremendous. The least traumatic method of removing a foreign body is with the aid of a *microscope.* For removal of a live insect, the ear canal is filled with mineral oil, *NOT WATER.* Water causes the insect to swell, and it becomes difficult to remove.

Finally, an allergic reaction involving the pinna can occur. This reaction is usually generalized and does not involve the ear canal.

A common complaint of patients with occlusion of the ear canal is a *loss of hearing.* Both infection and cerumen can cause a sudden hearing loss. Accompanying the loss of hearing may be the complaint of a *blocked* ear. Complications commonly associated with problems of the external ear are listed in Box 62-3.

## MEDICAL MANAGEMENT

The most common external ear problems are infections; these are treated with antibiotics in the form of drops and ointments, as well as systemically. However, the first rule of treating infection is meticulous cleaning of the site so that the local antibiotic can reach the infected area. Then external otitis must be treated by microscopic cleaning before applying antibiotic drops or ointments. If the ear canal is swollen shut, a *wick* must be inserted to allow the drops to penetrate the canal. If the infection is not localized, systemic antibiotics are standard. And if debris that cannot be removed accumulates in the ear canal, irrigations (with an ear syringe) can be used. Because external otitis is one of the most painful disorders of the ear, use of appropriate analgesics is in order.

The removal of cerumen by medicinal means often leads to minor complications caused by irritation resulting from mild caustic commercial products. An infection that involves cartilage has to be treated aggressively and quickly with systemic antibiotics to avoid complications.

**TABLE 62-2 Diagnostic Tests**

| DIAGNOSTIC TEST | PURPOSE |
|---|---|
| Culture of discharge | Identify specific microbe (bacteria, fungus, virus) |
| Otoscopic and/or microscopic examination | Diagnose specific external ear disorder or infection or to remove cerumen and/or foreign body |
| Audiometric testing | Identify hearing loss |
| Biopsy | Rule out malignancies and identify tissue |
| Complete blood cell count | Detect a systemic infection |
| Imaging studies | Diagnose tumors, osteitis, or exostosis |

## SURGICAL MANAGEMENT

The surgical treatment of infections involves *incision and drainage* in the acute phase for abscesses and, at times, for perichondritis. Chronic infection can also require surgical treatment. The most common surgical treatment is *excision of cysts and cutaneous carcinomas.* For the most part, the surgery involved is minimal. For conditions that occlude the ear canal, more extensive surgery involving skin grafting *(canalplasty)* is performed. Extensive surgery of the external ear is usually necessary to repair congenital defects. The correction of protruding ears is called *otoplasty.*

# NURSING MANAGEMENT

## ◆ ASSESSMENT

### Subjective Data

The most frequent problems of the external ear seen by the nurse are *inflammation* and *infection. Pain* is the *chief symptom,* followed by a *sense of fullness* in the ear, *hearing loss,* and *itching.* Data to collect include onset, duration, and degree of severity of symptoms.

### Objective Data

When assessing the external ear, manipulation of the ear is important. If the patient complains of pain when any part of the ear is palpated, a *furuncle, lesion,* or some kind of *inflammatory process* of the ear canal is suspected. If an otoscopic examination is performed, care must be taken not to cause the person unnecessary pain. A furuncle may be close to the opening of the canal, causing increased pain from the pressure of the speculum. Water in the ear canal from showering or swimming may aggravate the symptoms.

The external ear is inspected for signs of drainage, either serous or purulent. The auricle is also inspected for signs of redness, scaliness, and crusting.

### Diagnostic Test Findings

Diagnostic tests and their purposes can be found in Table 62-2.

## ♦ NURSING DIAGNOSES

Nursing diagnoses are determined from analysis of patient data. Nursing diagnoses for the person with an external ear problem may include but are not limited to the following:

| Diagnostic Title | Possible Etiologic Factors |
|---|---|
| Pain | Infection, buildup of fluid in small bony ear spaces, swelling, trauma |
| Infection, high risk for | Damage to skin or ear canal conducive to bacterial or fungal growth |
| Sensory/perceptual alteration: auditory | Debris or infection blocking ear canal |
| Knowledge deficit | Lack of exposure to information |

## ♦ EXPECTED PATIENT OUTCOMES

Expected patient outcomes for the person with an external ear problem may include but are not limited to the following:

1. States pain is decreased by a lower rating on scale of 1 to 10 (1 = no pain).
2. Exhibits no sign of infection: negative culture, lack of ear drainage; ear canal is clean and healing.
3. Able to hear as well as before external ear problem.
4. Explains or demonstrates prescribed treatment.
5. Explains signs and symptoms indicating need to call health care provider (otorrhea, itching of ear, erythema or edema of ear canal or pinna, pain in ear or pinna).

## ♦ INTERVENTIONS

### Promoting Comfort

1. Monitor ear pain using pain scales and flow sheets (see Chapter 17).
2. Assess for nonverbal signs of ear pain, and ask patient to be specific about location and type of pain.
3. Assess for factors that increase or decrease ear pain.
4. Assist with nonpharmacologic measures for pain relief, such as music, massage, distraction, relaxation, imagery.
5. Identify optimal pain relief schedule, and administer prescribed analgesics; assess for response and side effects, and consult physician as necessary.

### Reducing Infection and Restoring Hearing

Guidelines for care of the external ear are described in the Guidelines box above.

#### Administering eardrops

Antibiotics and antiinflammatory agents are usually administered locally rather than systemically for infections of the external ear. The procedure and directions for administration of eardrops are as follows:

1. Wash hands before and after the procedure.
2. Warm the eardrops to body temperature by holding vial in the hand for a few minutes or by placing it in a dish of warm water. (Dizziness may occur from insertion of drops that are too warm or too cold.)
3. Patient should tilt the head so that the ear to be treated is up.
4. Straighten the ear canal by pulling up and back.
5. Instill prescribed number of drops to run along ear canal.
6. Press gently several times on the tragus of the ear to ensure proper instillation, or hold the head in position for 2 to 3 minutes.
7. Wipe the external ear with a cotton ball or tissue to prevent skin irritation.
8. A cotton ball may be placed in the ear but is not necessary.

A wick may have been inserted by the physician to allow the drops to penetrate if the canal is swollen shut. In this case, the prescribed number of eardrops are placed directly on the wick. The wick serves not only as a bandage but also as an excellent vehicle to medicate the ear canal.

**Guidelines for Ear Care**

The following guidelines are imperative when caring for a patient with a problem of the ear:

1. Teach patients how to care for their ears, whether lessons are preventive, therapeutic, or rehabilitative in nature.
2. Wash hands before and after caring for the patient's ear and between procedures for both ears to prevent cross-contamination.
3. Observe sterile technique when the middle ear or inner ear has been opened traumatically or surgically.
4. Be aware that certain conditions make the ear extremely sensitive. Be gentle when manipulating the external ear.
5. Have an adjustable light source for good visualization.
6. Place *nothing* in the ear canal without a physician's order—especially not water.
7. Solutions for instillation or irrigation should be at body temperature.

#### Inserting and removing earwicks

Commercially prepared wicks or single pieces of ¼-inch-wide gauze are used in the ear to promote drainage or to provide a pathway for the instillation of eardrops. The wick is gently inserted into the ear canal by means of bayonet forceps while gently pulling upward and backward on the external ear. The wick is usually slightly less than 1 inch in length. Frequently, a wick is inserted for swollen ear canals, commonly seen in acute external otitis.

#### Applying ear ointment

To apply ointment to the ear canal, use a cotton-tipped applicator. Care must be taken not to damage the ear canal or eardrum. Insert the cotton applicator no farther than the cotton end, remembering that the adult ear canal is approximately 1 inch in length. Instruct the patient not to move the head during the procedure and to use a new applicator each time the ointment is applied.

**Removing cerumen**

Wax that is visible in the ear canal can be removed with a cotton-tipped applicator. *Do not put more than the cotton portion in the ear.* Impacted accumulations of earwax may be softened and loosened for removal by alternate instillation of glycerine and hydrogen peroxide. Three drops of glycerine are used at bedtime to soften the wax, and three drops of hydrogen peroxide are used twice a day to loosen the wax. The eardrops are warmed to body temperature and used daily as directed for 1 to 2 weeks. The ear is then irrigated with warm water to remove the softened wax or cleaned under magnification with a cerumen spoon. Wax that is on the tympanic membrane must be removed by a physician or a clinical nurse specialist in otology.

**Irrigating the ear**

The ear is commonly irrigated either to cleanse the external auditory canal or to remove impacted wax. Irrigations are not used for persons with a history of a perforated eardrum. The irrigating solution (usually water) is warmed to body temperature and placed in the irrigating syringe. The patient's clothes are protected with a plastic drape, and a kidney-shaped basin is placed below the ear to catch the irrigating solution. The patient sits with the ear to be syringed toward the nurse and with the head tilted toward the opposite ear. The external ear is pulled upward and backward for the adult, and the tip of the syringe is directed along the upper wall of the ear canal (Figure 62-2). The canal should not be completely obstructed by the syringe to allow for the backflow of solution. When charting the ear irrigation, record the nature of returned solution including amount, texture, and color of cerumen.

### Facilitating Learning

Patients with inflammations or infections of the external ear may be diagnosed and treated on an ambulatory basis. These problems are not life-threatening or life-shortening and are usually easily treated with topical antibiotic solutions. During the infection, patients should avoid getting water in the ear by using earplugs or cotton with Vaseline on it. If earplugs are used, thorough cleansing with alcohol or a mild detergent between uses is recommended to prevent reinfection. No swimming is permitted during this time. Signs and symptoms to be reported to a health care provider include otorrhea (ear discharge), itching of the ear, erythema or edema of the ear canal or pinna, and pain in the ear canal or pinna.

## ♦ EVALUATION

To evaluate the effectiveness of nursing interventions, compare patient behaviors with those stated in the ex-

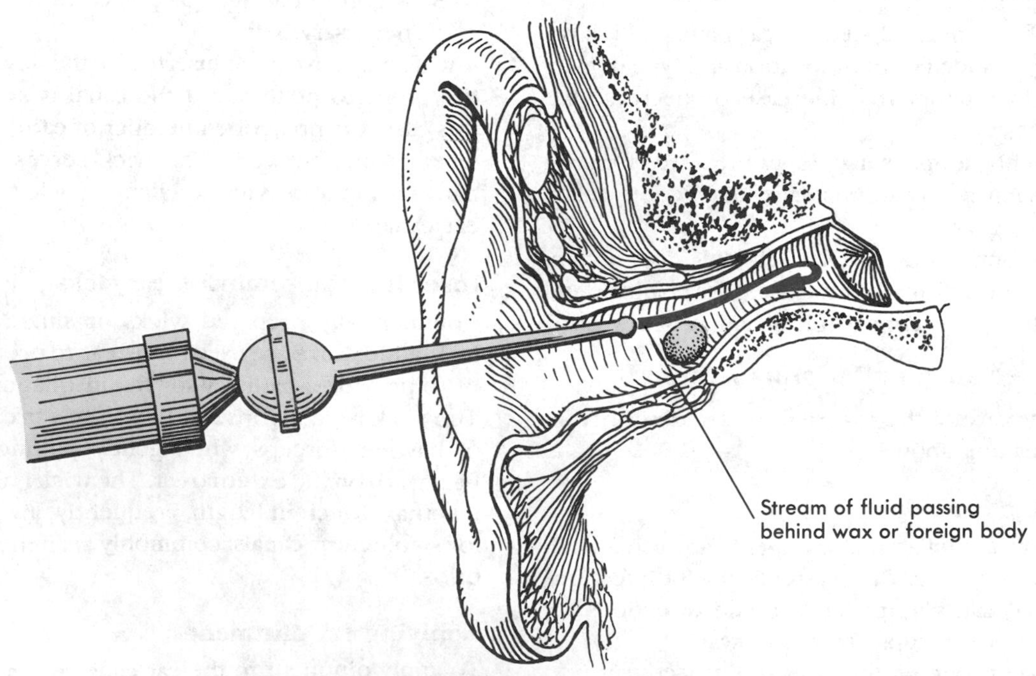


**FIGURE 62-2** Ear irrigation. Note that fluid is directed toward the upper canal wall so that the stream will pass behind the wax or object.

pected patient outcomes. Successful achievement of patient outcomes for the patient with external ear problems is indicated by the following:

1. States that no pain is present (1 on a scale of 1 to 10).
2. Has no ear drainage or cerumen in canal and no redness or edema of ear canal or pinna; ear canal is clean and healing.
3. Responds appropriately to auditory cues indicating improvement of hearing.
4. Correctly explains and demonstrates prescribed treatments.
5. Correctly describes signs and symptoms indicating need to call health care provider (otorrhea; pain, itching, edema or erythema of ear canal or pinna).

# PROBLEMS OF THE TYMPANIC MEMBRANE

## ETIOLOGY/PATHOPHYSIOLOGY

### Congenital Disorders

The tympanic membrane is the end of the external ear canal and the beginning of the middle ear and thus is involved with problems of both structures. Therefore congenital problems of the tympanic membrane are also problems of the adjacent structures.

### Infections

Infections of the external ear canal can involve the surface of the tympanic membrane, and the tympanic membrane will be a "window" for infection of the middle ear. Infection can cause hard deposits in the tympanic membrane known as **tympanosclerosis,** which is discussed in the section on the middle ear. A specific viral infection of the tympanic membrane is **bullous myringitis.** In this inflammatory disease blisters or bullae form on the tympanic membrane. Holes or *perforations* of the tympanic membrane can be caused by infection or trauma.

### Tumors

Both benign and malignant tumors can involve the tympanic membrane but seldom arise from it. However, an infectious glandular polyp can be isolated to the tympanic membrane.

### Perforation

The major finding in tympanic membrane disorders is a perforation. A *perforation* may be either *acute,* as seen in trauma and acute infection, or *chronic,* as seen in repeated infection. *An acute perforation has a better chance of healing spontaneously than does a chronic perforation.* A perforation that is located away from the annulus of the tympanic membrane is a *central perforation.* A perforation involving the annulus is a *marginal perforation.* A marginal perforation has less chance of spontaneous closure and a greater chance of invasion of skin from the external ear, thus causing a cholesteatoma (see p. 2139). A perforation causes a hearing loss, depending on its size and location. The largest hearing loss found with a perforation is approximately 35 dB (one third of the hearing). If a perforation is present, damage to the ossicles should be suspected, which will cause an even greater hearing loss.

Because the tympanic membrane is a semitransparent membrane, it can reveal what lies underneath it, as well as discoloration and displacement of the membrane. Therefore both fluid in the middle ear and infection can be seen. The normal color is pearly grey; dullness or redness indicate an infection. Bulging of the membrane is a result of positive pressure in the middle ear; the tympanic membrane may rupture, causing drainage. Negative pressure in the ear causes a retraction of the tympanic membrane, outlining the ossicles. Any alteration of the membrane can cause a hearing loss. The major clinical manifestations of a tympanic membrane problem are summarized in Box 62-4.

## MEDICAL AND SURGICAL MANAGEMENT

The medical management of tympanic membrane disorders involves both systemic and local antibiotics. Local antibiotics are used in the form of eardrops.

Surgical treatment involves using a surgical microscope to enlarge the tympanic membrane; the power of magnification most commonly used is 6 to 25 times normal. The major surgical procedure performed is closure of a perforation. This procedure is called a **myringoplasty** if only the perforation is in the surgical field or a **tympanoplasty** if more of the middle ear is involved. Sometimes the ossicles must also be reconstructed, altering the type of tympanoplasty performed (types I through IV). A tympanoplasty may also be performed in conjunction with surgery involving the mastoid. The most common material that is used as a free graft to close the perforation is fascia taken from the temporalis muscle. Less commonly used tissue is perichondrium or vein. At the present time, *tympanoplasty is a common surgical procedure of the ear with a high rate of success.*

Nursing management of the patient with surgery of the tympanic membrane is discussed on p. 2142.

**BOX 62-4 Clinical Manifestations of Tympanic Membrane Problems**

- Pain in the ear
- Visible changes of the tympanic membrane with otoscopic examination
  - Bubbles in the middle ear
  - Color change to red or white, and dullness
  - Bulging or perforations
  - Drainage
- Sensation of aural fullness
- Hearing loss

**TABLE 62-3 Normal Function, Pathophysiology, and Clinical Manifestations in Otitis Media**

| NORMAL FUNCTION | PATHOPHYSIOLOGY | CLINICAL MANIFESTATIONS |
|---|---|---|
| The middle ear is separated from the external ear by the tympanic membrane. The middle ear is transversed by ossicles that transmit sound from the eardrum to the inner ear.<br>The middle ear is aerated by the eustachian tube, which connects the nasopharynx to, and equalizes pressure in, the middle ear. | Blockage of the eustachian tube from allergic swelling, throat infection, or adenoiditis produces negative pressure and fluid in the middle ear. This fluid can become infected. | Throbbing pain, drainage, fever, decreased hearing, inflammation, and bulging of the eardrum, with a possible perforation. |

# PROBLEMS OF THE MIDDLE EAR

## ETIOLOGY/PATHOPHYSIOLOGY

### Congenital Disorders

Congenital malformations of the ear include incomplete development of the ossicles, causing the absence or deformity of the ossicles. Another common congenital finding is the absence of the bony canal covering the facial (seventh) nerve or, very rarely, an abnormal course throughout the middle ear. Congenital disorders of the middle ear usually involve the tympanic membrane and, more often than not, the external ear canal and the auricle.

### Infections

The most prevalant diseases of the middle ear are infections and are known as **otitis media.** Otitis media is caused by various types of bacteria, depending on the age of the patient and type of infection. When the infection is sudden in onset and short in duration, the diagnosis is *acute otitis media.* (See Table 62-3 for a comparison of normal function, pathophysiology, and clinical manifestations of otitis media.) When the infection recurs, usually causing drainage and perforation, the problem is called *chronic otitis media.* In between bouts of otitis media, fluid may form in the middle ear *(serous otitis media).* This fluid is formed by a vacuum in the middle ear caused by a blocked eustachian tube. Infection causes swelling of the mucosa throughout the middle ear and eustachian tube. When the swelling subsides, the remaining fluid can be too thick to drain. At times, serous otitis media is found in conjunction with upper respiratory infections or allergies. If the fluid remains over a period of years, causing tympanic membrane retraction, *adhesive otitis media* becomes the diagnosis. Infection present over a long period of time can cause necrosis of the tympanic membrane (perforations) or of the ossicles. Both problems create a conductive hearing loss. Necrosis of the bony covering of the facial nerve may cause facial paralysis. *Because of the extraordinary anatomy of the temporal bone, middle ear infection can also lead to a brain abscess that is life-threatening if not treated properly.*

*Tympanosclerosis* is a result of repeated infection and deserves special emphasis. Tympanosclerosis is a deposit of collagen and calcium within the middle ear that can harden around the ossicles, causing a conductive hearing loss. Tympanosclerosis can also be found mounded up in the middle ear or as plaque on the tympanic membrane.

**Cholesteatoma** is a complication from otitis media but is primarily a problem of the mastoid (see p. 2139).

### Otosclerosis

**Otosclerosis,** or "hardening of the ear," which involves the stapes, is important in middle ear disorders. A summary of the normal function, pathophysiology, and clinical manifestations in otosclerosis appears in Table 62-4. This bony disease of the otic capsule causes excess bone to form, impeding normal movement of the stapes. *The conductive hearing loss that results is the second most common correctable middle ear disorder following an infection of the ear.* Another form of otosclerosis that does not involve the stapes is *cochlear otospongiosis,* which can cause a toxic sensorineural hearing loss.

### Tumors

The *most common benign* growth in the middle ear is an *infectious polyp.* Next in frequency is a *cholesteatoma.* The rarest forms of benign middle ear tumors involve either the blood vessels or the facial nerve. Arising from the jugular vein is a *glomus jugulare,* known as a *glomus tympanicum* when limited to the middle ear. A *facial nerve neuroma* is found along the course of the facial nerve. Malignant tumors involving the middle ear can be primary or secondary in nature.

### Trauma

Trauma to the tympanic membrane from a blast or blunt injury can involve the middle ear, causing a fracture or dislocation of the ossicles and tearing the tympanic membrane. The facial nerve is also vulnerable to trauma. A *basal skull fracture* involves the temporal bone and, depending on the fracture site, causes ossicular damage as well as facial nerve paralysis.

**TABLE 62-4 Normal Function, Pathophysiology, and Clinical Manifestations in Otosclerosis**

| NORMAL FUNCTION | PATHOPHYSIOLOGY | CLINICAL MANIFESTATIONS |
|---|---|---|
| The stapes articulates with the incus and oval window and transmits sound from the other ossicles to the inner ear. | Progressive loss of stapes movement is caused by the formation of sclerotic bone, which fixes the stapes footplate. The stapes becomes immobile, causing a conductive hearing loss. | Normal ear canal, normal eardrum, progressive conductive hearing loss, or mixed hearing loss. |

## Eustachian Tube Disorders

The eustachian tube is part of the middle ear but presents separate problems. Because the eustachian tube connects the middle ear to the nasopharynx, pharyngeal disorders cause eustachian tube dysfunction and thus secondary middle ear problems. For example, the most common disorder is blockage of the eustachian tube by enlarged adenoid tissue in children. The most common blockage in adults is swelling of the mucosa in the eustachian tube during an upper respiratory infection that can lead to serous otitis media. In a unilateral blocked eustachian tube, a malignant tumor must be ruled out as the cause. Acute blockage from **barotrauma** (altitude changes) caused by flying or underwater diving also causes middle ear problems. *Any long-term blockage of the eustachian tube leads to a serous otitis media and a hearing loss.*

Because the middle ear is the transformer for hearing (that is, it transmits the sound vibrations from the tympanic membrane to the inner ear), a *hearing loss is the most frequent middle ear finding.* Fortunately, a conductive hearing loss is found in 95% of problems and is correctable by either medical or surgical treatment. *Pain is also quite common because of pressure from infection or fluid behind the tympanic membrane.* Once a perforation is caused by infection, drainage of pus, blood, and other material is often found. In chronic middle ear and mastoid problems, a thick yellow pus discharge is common. *With an acute otitis media, all three findings (hearing loss, pain, and discharge) can be present.*

## MEDICAL MANAGEMENT

With any form of otitis media, appropriate antibiotic therapy may be necessary. If drainage is present, a culture and sensitivity should be performed. However, most episodes of acute otitis media do not produce a drainage, and the most probable bacterial cause must be identified. In chronic ear discharge, the normal contaminants of the ear abound and unfortunately do not respond to the common antibiotics. Thus local treatment such as ear irrigations, drops, and powders are used.

Blood in the ear canal usually points to a minor problem such as a scratch and not a major disease. Persistent hemorrhage must be checked by an otologist.

Because the eustachian tube is an integral part of middle ear disorders, decongestants and antihistamines are used to decrease the swelling and open the eustachian tube. Pain medication is used appropriately when necessary.

The medical therapy for otosclerosis is a hearing aid (see Aural Rehabilitation, p. 2151).

## SURGICAL MANAGEMENT

Repairing the damage from middle ear infection is the most challenging microscopic surgical procedure facing the surgeon. But removing fluid from the middle ear is the easiest and most common procedure. A simple incision in the tympanic membrane is a *myringotomy,* through which fluid is removed by suction. To keep the incision open and prevent a recurrence of fluid, various types of *transtympanic tubes* can be inserted into the incison (Figure 62-3). These tubes extrude in 3 to 12 months by themselves and rarely have to be removed.

Reconstruction of the necrotic ossicles is not yet an exact science. Various methods of repositioning these tiny ear bones are now in use, although the surgery is difficult to perform and unfortunately is not always successful over the long term. Various prostheses have been used to reconnect the ossicles to carry sound. Extrusion of prostheses through the eardrum has also plagued the surgeon during the past few decades. In an attempt to solve this problem, the tissue is combined with a prosthesis to connect the ossicles and prevent extrusion. This method is now used in different forms by the majority of otologic surgeons.

The surgical procedure of ossicular reconstruction is called **ossiculoplasty** (Figure 62-4). But many surgeons use the term *tympanoplasty,* meaning to make a new eardrum, to include ossiculoplasty.

Surgery of the facial nerve in the middle ear is limited. In the past, facial nerve decompression for idiopathic facial paralysis (Bell's palsy) was routine, but not today. *A controversy is raging, with physicians who advocate no surgery for Bell's palsy in the forefront.* Other middle ear lesions are excised often in combination with other recognized middle ear procedures. For example, tympanosclerosis is removed routinely during tympanoplasty or ossiculoplasty without recognition in the procedures' names.

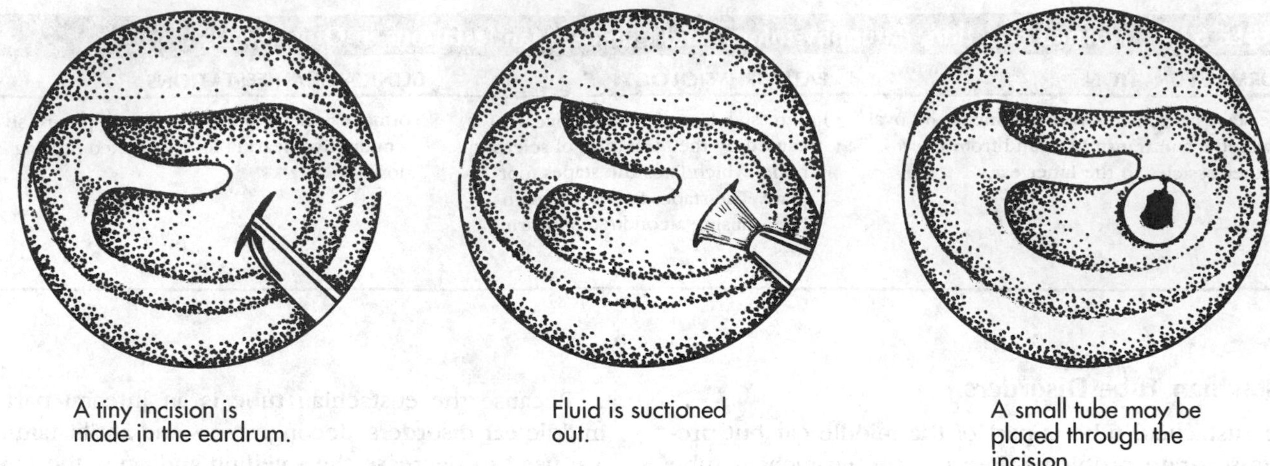


**FIGURE 62-3** Myringotomy and transtympanic tube placement to prevent chronic serous otitis media. (From Sigler B, Schuring L: *Ear, nose and throat disorders,* St Louis, 1993, Mosby.)

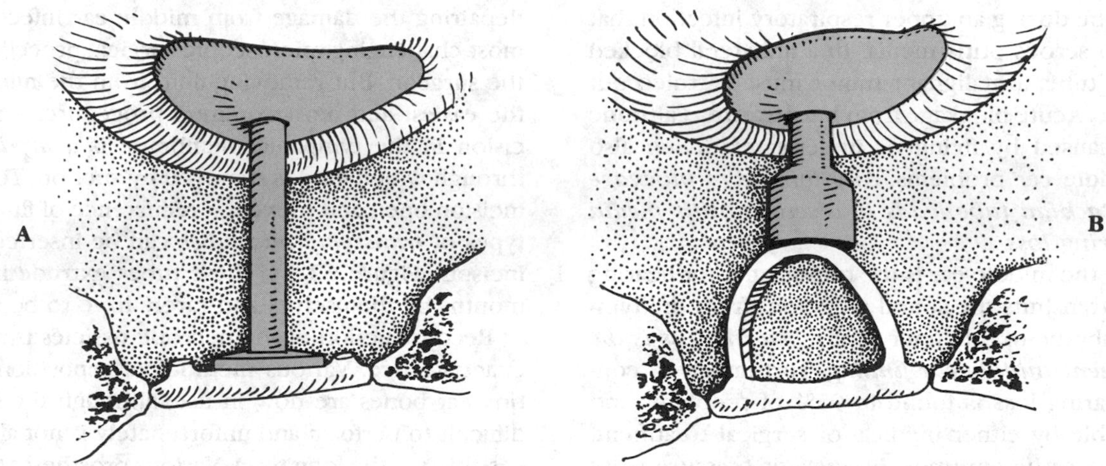


**FIGURE 62-4** Middle ear prostheses. **A,** Schuring ossicle columnella prosthesis for total ossicular replacement surgery. **B,** Schuring ossicle cup prosthesis for incus replacement surgery.

*Stapes replacement surgery* is the treatment of choice for otosclerosis. Either the traditional *stapedectomy* or the *stapedotomy* is performed. Both procedures are performed through the canal aided by a microscope. The superstructure of the stapes is fractured from the otosclerotic footplate and removed. The stapes footplate is also removed in a **stapedectomy;** a graft is placed over the oval window, and a prosthesis is positioned between the incus and covered oval window (Figure 62-5). Prostheses are made of various materials, and every surgeon has a preference.

In **stapedotomy,** a laser is used to create a hole in the footplate of the stapes and a Teflon piston prosthesis with a diameter of 0.4 or 0.6 mm is placed in the hole and crimped over the incus. Stapes replacement surgery has a high success rate, and the patient notices improved hearing while in the operating room.

# PROBLEMS OF THE MASTOID

## ETIOLOGY/PATHOPHYSIOLOGY

### Congenital Disorders

Because the mastoid cavity is irregular in dimensions and is often influenced by infection early in life, congenital irregularities are less significant. Of more significance are the structures directly surrounding the mastoid cavity. For the surgeon, the congenital abnormality of the course of the facial nerve is of primary concern in avoiding injury during surgery. Likewise, knowledge of a congenital change in the brain or sigmoid sinus is

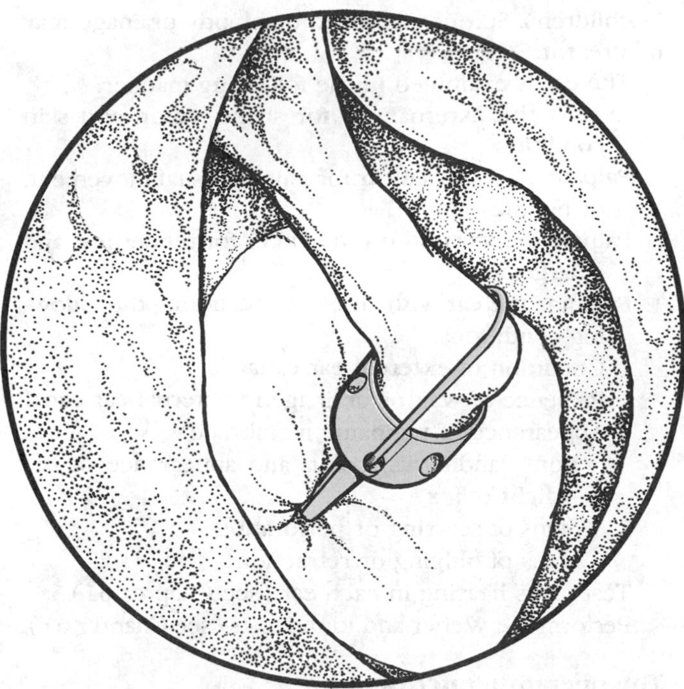

**FIGURE 62-5** Stapedectomy with Robinson stainless steel prosthesis in place. (From Sigler B, Schuring L: *Ear, nose and throat disorders,* St Louis, 1993, Mosby.)

very important and mastoid x-ray films are obtained before surgery.

### Tumors

The same kinds of tumors that arise in the middle ear can be found in the mastoid cavity. Because the mastoid cavity is connected to other air cells throughout the temporal bone, malignant tumors in the mastoid carry a poor prognosis.

### Infections

Before the discovery of antibiotics, a mastoid infection was a life-threatening event. Now with the use of antibiotics, ***acute mastoiditis*** is rare. On the other hand, ***chronic mastoiditis*** is still seen. With repeated middle ear infections, the mastoid cavity becomes part of the problem, increasing the amount of drainage.

Drainage from the mastoid cavity is the most common sign of **mastoiditis.** The drainage courses through the middle ear and out of the tympanic membrane through a perforation. Tenderness over the mastoid cavity behind the ear points to an infection but usually is caused by an acute exacerbation of chronic rather than an acute mastoiditis. The protrusion of the pinna as a result of swelling over the mastoid may be part of this process, especially in children. Clinical manifestations of mastoiditis are listed in Box 62-5.

**BOX 62-5 Clinical Manifestations of Acute Mastoiditis**

- Ear drainage
- Tenderness over mastoid process
- Pain in the ear
- Protrusion of the pinna
- Hearing loss
- Perforation of the tympanic membrane

### Cholesteatoma

Cholesteatoma is a complication of chronic otitis media in the middle ear, as well as the mastoid. Squamous epithelium of the external ear canal and outer layer of the tympanic membrane grows into the middle ear cleft through a perforation. This skin can form a sac that fills with debris such as degenerated skin and sebaceous material. The sac destroys structures in the middle ear and mastoid by pressure necrosis. In the past, cholesteatoma has given rise to the stories of brain abscesses, dizziness, and facial paralysis. These conditions are still seen today but, like acute mastoiditis, are becoming less frequent. Often infection is present in the mass of the cholesteatoma. These chronic changes produce cholesterol granules from which the term *cholesteatoma* was coined. Other complications of mastoiditis are listed in Box 62-6.

## MEDICAL MANAGEMENT

Antibiotics are the most common medical therapy for an infection of the mastoid. Because infection starts in the middle ear, the problems in the mastoid cavity are avoided by early treatment with antibiotics. Various irrigations of the mastoid and middle ear are used in chronic infections, along with antibiotic eardrops or powders.

## SURGICAL MANAGEMENT

At the turn of the century, a **mastoidectomy** was used as an incision and drainage of a mastoid infection, thus

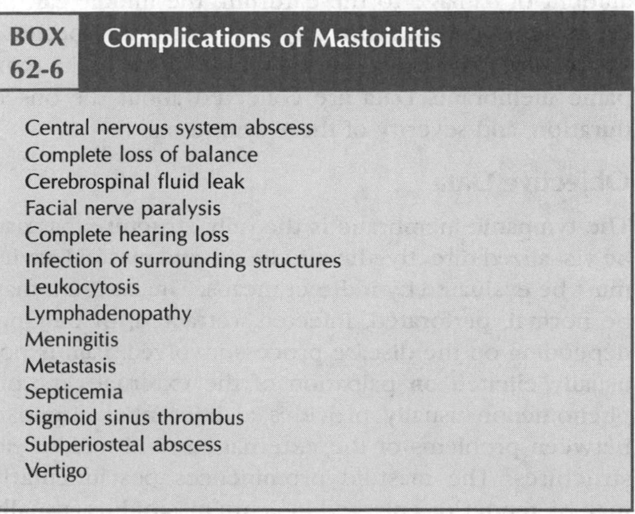

**BOX 62-6 Complications of Mastoiditis**

- Central nervous system abscess
- Complete loss of balance
- Cerebrospinal fluid leak
- Facial nerve paralysis
- Complete hearing loss
- Infection of surrounding structures
- Leukocytosis
- Lymphadenopathy
- Meningitis
- Metastasis
- Septicemia
- Sigmoid sinus thrombus
- Subperiosteal abscess
- Vertigo

saving the life of the patient. Also around this time, the radical removal of the mastoid bone was first advocated and is even used today for both infection and cholesteatoma. Since the *radical mastoidectomy* sacrificed hearing, a *modified radical mastoidectomy* was advocated that saved the remaining middle ear structures. At the onset of the period of antibiotics, a *simple mastoidectomy* was performed, maintaining a normal appearing ear. Because the radical and modified mastoidectomies exteriorize the mastoid cavity to the external ear canal, they are known as *open mastoidectomies.* Closed mastoidectomies are simple mastoidectomies with modifications in conjunction with tympanoplasty and ossiculoplasty. Today, even the open mastoidectomy is performed with various tympanoplasties.

The excision of cholesteatoma by mastoidectomy is still in controversy. The historic and safe procedure is to perform an open mastoidectomy and to ignore the hearing. The advocates of the closed mastoidectomy point out that the cholesteatoma can be removed safely and better hearing can be achieved if a *staged mastoidectomy* is peformed after the original procedure to check for reforming cholesteatoma. *Because of the recurrence of cholesteatoma, a universally accepted surgical procedure is not yet available.*

## NURSING MANAGEMENT

### ♦ ASSESSMENT

The nursing assessment of the person having problems with the *tympanic membrane,* the *middle ear,* or the *mastoid cavity* is the same, regardless of the need for surgery.

#### Subjective Data

A thorough history should precede the ear examination. *Hearing loss* is the most frequent symptom of blockage of the tympanic membrane or the ossicles. The amount of conductive hearing loss is directly proportional to the amount of damage to the eardrum, the middle ear, or the mastoid cavity. *Pain* may also be present because of pressure from infection or fluid behind or in the tympanic membrane. Data are collected about the onset, duration, and severity of these symptoms.

#### Objective Data

The tympanic membrane is the only structure that can be visualized directly; the middle ear and mastoid cavity must be evaluated by indirect means. The eardrum may be normal, perforated, infected, retracted, or bulging, depending on the disease process involved. Pain is not usually elicited on palpation of the external ear; this phenomenon usually provides a differential diagnosis between problems of the external ear and middle ear structures. The mastoid prominences postauricularly may be tender or enlarged in acute mastoiditis (usually in children). Serous, purulent, or bloody drainage may be present.

The ear is examined in the following manner:

- Inspect the external ear for shape, color, and skin condition.
- Palpate the external ear for pain, unusual movement, or nodules.
- Palpate the mastoid prominences for tenderness and enlargement.
- Examine the ear with an otoscope, noting the following conditions:
  - Condition of external ear canal
  - Presence of wax or drainage in external ear canal
  - Appearance of tympanic membrane
    - Bony landmarks, color, and appearance of the light reflex
    - Signs of scarring or perforation
    - Signs of bulging or retraction
- Test gross hearing in each ear (see Chapter 61).
- Perform the Weber and Rinne tests (see Chapter 61).

**The operating microscope**

The binocular operating microscope is found in the offices and clinics of most otologists. With specialized instruction the nurse may learn to use the microscope and manipulate instruments inserted through a speculum into the external ear. The speculum holds open the outermost portion of the external ear canal and allows the passage of both light and instruments. The appropriate speculum size for adults is from 4 to 7 mm in diameter. The microscope provides the examiner with excellent illumination, increased depth perception, and three-dimensional vision. Most operating microscopes allow changes in magnification to be made. The nurse can use the microscope to differentiate normal from abnormal, remove cerumen, and suction out drainage.

**TABLE 62-5 Diagnostic Tests for Middle Ear and Mastoid**

| DIAGNOSTIC TEST | PURPOSE |
|---|---|
| Otoscopic or microscopic examination | Examine tympanic membrane, remove debris of infection, perform minor surgery |
| Ear culture | Identify specific infection microbe |
| Biopsy of lesion | Identify tissue and rule out malignancy |
| Audiometric testing | Determine amount of hearing loss and middle ear impedence |
| Imaging | Diagnose tumors, infection, fluid osteitis, and metastasis |
| Complete blood cell count | Detect a systemic infection |
| Facial nerve testing | Determine extent of damage to facial nerve and prognosis for paralysis |
| Electronystagmography | Determine extent of damage to labyrinth |

### Diagnostic Test Findings

The diagnostic tests commonly used for middle ear or mastoid infection and the purpose of each are listed in Table 62-5.

## ♦ NURSING DIAGNOSES

Nursing diagnoses are determined from analysis of patient data. Nursing diagnoses for the patient with a middle ear problem may include but are not limited to the following:

| Diagnostic Title | Possible Etiologic Factors |
|---|---|
| Sensory/perceptual alteration: auditory | Infection, drainage, or fixation of ear bones in middle ear |
| Infection, high risk for | Inadequate primary defenses, pressure necrosis, broken skin, chronic disease |
| Pain | Infection, inflammation, swelling |
| Knowledge deficit: ear infection | Lack of exposure to information, unfamiliarity with information sources |

## ♦ EXPECTED PATIENT OUTCOMES

Expected patient outcomes for the person with a tympanic, middle ear, or mastoid problem may include but are not limited to the following:

1. Hearing is improved or stabilized.
2. Ear infection does not occur or shows signs of healing (no drainage from ear, no tenderness over mastoid, negative culture).
3. States pain is decreased or absent as evidenced by a lower rating on scale of 1 to 10 (1 = no pain).
4. Describes measures to prevent further infection and to avoid getting water in ear, and describes signs requiring medical consultation, such as decreased hearing, pain in ear, or drainage from ear.

## ♦ INTERVENTIONS

Hospitalization is rarely necessary for the patient who does not require surgery and usually does not exceed 2 days for patients having ear surgery. Surgical intervention follows unsuccessful attempts to treat the problem medically.

### Facilitating Hearing

1. Assess and document recent changes in hearing acuity; assess audiogram and/or tympanogram for hearing impairment or improvement.
2. Speak distinctly without shouting (shouting distorts speech).

### Reducing Infection

**Medications**

Eardrops and ear ointment may be prescribed for patients with problems of the tympanic membrane, middle ear, or mastoid. Oral antibiotics may also be required. The patient is instructed as to the amount, frequency, and duration of medication.

**Guidelines for an Ear Wash**

1. Wash hands before and after procedure.
2. Warm solution to body temperature by placing bottle in a pan of hot water. Do *not* warm solution on the stove. Solution that is too warm or too cold may cause dizziness.
3. Fill ear syringe with warmed solution.
4. Have patient lie down with affected ear uppermost.
5. Pull external ear up and out, and place tip of ear syringe in ear canal. Do not be afraid to put it down into the ear, but a return flow should occur; if not, pull syringe out slightly.
6. Pump warmed solution vigorously and repeatedly from syringe back and forth into ear by squeezing and releasing bulb of syringe. The ear wash must be forced back and forth, in and out of ear canal.
7. Have patient lean over and let solution run out of ear into a basin.
8. If solution burns too much at first, dilute solution (mix 2 ounces of water with 2 ounces of solution).
9. Use the wash twice a day for 2 weeks and then until the ear stops running or becomes dry. Dryness can be checked by putting a cotton-tipped applicator down into ear canal. If cotton-tipped applicator is wet or if there is an odor, continue using the wash until applicator comes out dry.

**Ear wash**

In addition to other treatment, the patient may be asked to use ear wash. The most common solution for ear wash is boric acid and alcohol, which is obtained by prescription at the drugstore. This solution cleanses the ear of debris and infection and provides a drying agent. A 2- or 3-ounce ear syringe, which also can be purchased at the drugstore, will be needed. A family member performs the ear wash for the patient (see Guidelines box above). Usually the ear wash is followed by the use of eardrops.

### Promoting Comfort

1. Monitor pain using pain scales and flow sheets (Chapter 17); assess for nonverbal signs of pain. Ask the patient to be specific about location and type of pain.
2. Assess for factors that increase or decrease pain.
3. Implement measures to reduce pain:
   a. Assist with nonpharmacologic measures for pain relief.
   b. Assist patient to identify optimal schedule for prescribed analgesics.
4. Encourage patient to consult physician if pain-reducing measures fail to provide adequate pain relief.

### Facilitating Learning

Teaching persons with an infection of the tympanic membrane, middle ear, or mastoid cavity includes the following:

1. Prevent further infection:
   a. Provide adequate treatment of allergic or persistent upper respiratory infections by seeking medical attention and taking medications as prescribed.
   b. Persons with a tympanic perforation should avoid getting water in the ear (such as while showering, shampooing the hair, or swimming).
2. During treatment for infection, avoid getting water in the ear. If the possibility exists, place two pieces of cotton in the ear: the first piece dry and the second piece saturated with petrolatum.
3. Seek medical attention for signs of decreased hearing, pain in the ear, or drainage from the ear.
4. Teach the patient about medication therapy: name, purpose, dosage, side effects, and signs and symptoms to report immediately; provide written instructions.
5. Assess the patient's ability to perform skills of prescribed regimen, and provide opportunities for practice and return demonstrations.
6. Refer the patient to community agencies as needed to provide necessary information (such as for decreased hearing).
7. Clarify patient and family understanding about the need and plans for follow-up care.

### ♦ EVALUATION

To evaluate the effectiveness of nursing interventions, compare patient behaviors with those stated in the expected patient outcomes. Successful achievement of patient outcomes for the patient with tympanic membrane, middle ear, or mastoid cavity problems is indicated by the following:

1. Responds appropriately to auditory cues indicating improvement of hearing.
2. Does not have ear drainage or pain over mastoid; has negative culture.
3. States that no pain is present (1 on a scale of 1 to 10).
4. Correctly explains and demonstrates prescribed treatments.
5. Correctly describes ways to prevent further infection, (avoid water in the ear), describes signs requiring medical attention (decreased hearing, pain or drainage from ear), and describes medical regimen.

## NURSING MANAGEMENT OF THE PATIENT HAVING EAR SURGERY

### PREOPERATIVE CARE

The responsibilities of the nurse begin in the preoperative phase when the decision for surgical intervention is made. The scope of nursing activities for the patient having ear surgery can be as broad as a preoperative assessment performed in an office or clinic or as limited as an assessment performed in the holding area of the surgical suite. Data are collected to assess the following about the patient: (1) knowledge of events that are going to occur, (2) mental readiness for surgery, and (3) physiologic status.

The person undergoing ear surgery should be told what to expect in surgery because frequently the patient is given only local anesthesia. The patient is awake but sedated during surgery. The patient is instructed about the length of the procedure and the estimated length of hospital stay. Immediate postoperative instructions should also be discussed. Very often, fear of the unknown can be decreased by an understanding of events that will occur.

### POSTOPERATIVE CARE

Immediate postoperative instructions include the following:

1. Lie with the operative ear in the specified position after surgery.
2. If necessary, blow nose gently one side at a time.
3. Sneeze or cough with mouth open.
4. Normal occurrences in the initial period may include the following:
   a. Decreased hearing in the operated ear from the packing (possibly, like the sound of talking in a barrel)
   b. Noises in the ear such as cracking or popping
   c. Minor earache and discomfort in the cheek and jaw
   d. Swelling of the ear

Most persons having ear surgery have a short hospitalization. For reconstructive ear surgeries such as sta-

**Guidelines for Teaching the Person After Ear Surgery**

1. Blow the nose gently one side at a time and to sneeze or cough with mouth open for 1 week after surgery.
2. Avoid physical activity for 1 week and exercises or sports for 3 weeks after surgery.
3. Return to work 1 week after surgery (3 weeks if work is strenuous).
4. Change cotton ball in ear daily as prescribed.
5. Keep ear dry for 6 weeks after surgery.
   a. Do not shampoo hair for 1 week after surgery.
   b. Protect ear when necessary with two pieces of cotton (outer piece saturated with petrolatum).
6. Avoid airplane flights for first week after surgery. For sensation of ear pressure, hold nose, close mouth, and swallow to equalize pressure.
7. Wear noise defenders such as ear muffs for loud noise environments.
8. Report any drainage other than a slight amount of bleeding to the physician.

pedectomy or ossiculoplasty, hearing is increased in the operating room. However, packing, swelling, and bleeding diminish hearing until healing occurs. Pain is not usually a major problem. Dizziness or light-headedness may occur when ambulating for the first time. Patients require supervision when ambulating on the day of surgery to protect them from falling. Some persons who are quite dizzy exhibit nystagmus from stimulation of the inner ear. The dizziness usually passes very quickly and seldom requires medication.

The ear rarely bleeds after surgery. Small amounts of serosanguinous drainage on a cotton ball is expected. Most ear surgeries require only a cotton ball in the ear postoperatively, although a dressing over the ear may be necessary following a *tympanomastoidectomy.* Postoperative patient teaching is listed in the Guidelines box, p. 2142.

# Problems of the Inner Ear

## ETIOLOGY/PATHOPHYSIOLOGY

### Congenital Disorders

Incomplete development of the cochlea is the most frequent congenital disorder of the inner ear and results in a sensorineural hearing loss. In contrast, congenital disorders of the vestibular system do not usually cause dizziness or equilibrium problems.

### Infections

An infection of the inner ear called **labyrinthitis** can be either viral or bacterial in origin. Viral labyrinthitis is usually isolated to the inner ear, whereas the rarer bacterial labyrinthitis is associated with infection in the middle ear and mastoid.

### Tumors

Both benign and malignant tumors of the temporal bone can involve the inner ear. The most common *benign tumor* is an **acoustic neuroma** of the eighth nerve, arising in the internal ear canal. Spread of this tumor out of the internal ear canal toward the brainstem causes other neurologic problems and can be life-threatening. Other tumors in the *cerebellar-pontine angle* likewise involve the seventh (facial) and eighth (acoustic) cranial nerves as they enter the internal acoustic meatus.

### Balance Disorders

Disorders of the vestibular structures arc lumped under the term *vertigo.* In the true sense, vertigo is only a symptom, but it is commonly used to describe an illness. The most common balance disorder is a ***viral labyrinthitis*** or viral neuronitis; other problems include toxic reactions from drugs, trauma causing fractures of bones of the ear, and tumors such as an acoustic neuroma. A specific balance disorder called **Ménière's disease** is characterized by a triad of symptoms, including *vertigo, hearing loss,* and *tinnitus* (see Table 62-6 for normal function, pathophysiology, and clinical manifestations). The cause is unknown but is thought to be from a virus. Recurring episodic bouts of incapacitating vertigo and hearing loss characterize this disorder. Because of the violent nature of Ménière's disease, the diagnosis is usually dreaded. However, control of the episodes is possible in about 80% to 90% of patients. Various treatments are used, including tranquilizers, vagal blockers (such as atropine), antihistamines, vasodilators, diuretics, and avoidance of alcohol, caffeine, and tobacco.[1]

### Hearing Disorders

A *sensorineural hearing loss* is the most common inner ear disorder. This hearing loss may occur in conjunction with a known disorder but is usually an isolated finding. Factors that influence the type and amount of hearing loss include hereditary disease, toxic substances, and noise-induced hearing loss. At times, the hearing loss may fluctuate, usually ending in progressive hearing loss.

*Noise-induced hearing loss* accounts for the major proportion of hearing impairment among people between the ages of 35 and 65. This hearing loss can be traumatic, for example, a sudden loud noise such as a blast injury. More commonly, a hearing loss occurs over time from repeated injury from noise. The major cause is industrial noise; the use of firearms is a distant second cause. Whatever the cause, noise-induced hearing loss is characterized by a greater loss in the higher frequencies. The only treatment is to prevent the injury by avoiding noise or by wearing ear protection.

*Sudden or fluctuating hearing loss* is recognized as a separate hearing disorder because of the isolated findings and dramatic outcome. Although the exact cause

**TABLE 62-6 Normal Function, Pathophysiology, and Clinical Manifestations in Ménière's Disease**

| NORMAL FUNCTION | PATHOPHYSIOLOGY | CLINICAL MANIFESTATIONS |
|---|---|---|
| The vestibular labyrinth contains fluid and hair cells that convert mechanical energy into neural impulses to maintain balance. The fluids of the inner ear are perilymph and endolymph, which are separated by a thin membrane. | Tissue changes in the labyrinth cause an excess of endolymph, which distorts the membranous labyrinth. The cause is thought to be a virus, but this has not been definitely established. | Episodic attacks of incapacitating vertigo, fluctuating hearing loss, tinnitus, and ear fullness occur, often accompanied by nausea and vomiting. Symptoms are relieved by rest and medications (see text on p. 2146). |

# NURSING CARE PLAN

## PERSON WITH MÉNIÈRE'S DISEASE

**DATA:** Mrs. B. is a 59-year-old schoolteacher. During the past 6 months, she has had three attacks of "whirling in space" or vertigo, fluctuating hearing in the left ear, noise in the left ear or tinnitus, nausea and vomiting, and a sense of fullness or pressure in the left ear. Two attacks have occurred during class, and one attack occurred at home where she lives alone. Embarrassment, fear, anxiety, and uncertainty are some of her feelings. Mrs. B. made an appointment at an otology office where diagnostic tests were performed. These tests included an audiogram, tympanometry, electronystagmography, electrocochleography, a nursing assessment, and physical examination. A diagnosis of Ménière's disease was made. A 1500 mg sodium restricted diet, hydrochlorothiazide (HCTZ) PO qd, labyrinthine compensatory exercises, and niacin 100 mg tid were prescribed to control the incapacitating attacks of vertigo.

### ■ NURSING DIAGNOSIS
Anxiety (related to effects of disorder)

| Expected Patient Outcome | Nursing Interventions | Rationale |
|---|---|---|
| Signs of anxiety are decreased. | Encourage Mrs. B. to explore concerns about decreased hearing and effects of dizziness attacks and to take action in relation to the concerns.<br>Explore Mrs. B.'s knowledge of the disorder and correct misunderstandings.<br>Encourage realistic hope about expected hearing ability as described by physician.<br>Refer Mrs. B. to necessary support services, such as social worker or audiologist. | Expressing concerns and receiving realistic counseling and support reduces helplessness and apprehension. |

### ■ NURSING DIAGNOSIS
Sensory/perceptual alteration (vestibular, auditory)

| Expected Patient Outcomes | Nursing Interventions | Rationale |
|---|---|---|
| Describes actions to avoid dizziness.<br>Interacts with others accurately. | Help Mrs. B. identify avoidable actions that precipitate dizziness attacks.<br>Encourage Mrs. B. to move slowly and not turn head suddenly when dizziness is present. | Understanding cause of dizziness and measures to reduce it may lessen occurrence. |
| | If tinnitus is distressing, increase background noises such as music. | Use of distraction may lessen effects of tinnitus. |
| | If hearing is decreased:<br>1. Use measures to facilitate communication with hearing impaired (see Box 62-8).<br>2. Refer Mrs. B. to an audiologist, if appropriate. | |

### ■ NURSING DIAGNOSIS
Injury, high risk for

| Expected Patient Outcome | Nursing Interventions | Rationale |
|---|---|---|
| Is not injured from falls. | Explore pattern of dizziness with Mrs. B. | Knowledge of pattern of attacks can be used in planning. |
| | Reinforce need to take prescribed medications. | Therapy may help prevent dizziness, which leads to falls. |
| | Explore home environment to decrease risk for injury if falls do occur. | Knowledge of safety measures reduces possibility of injuries. |

## NURSING CARE PLAN

### PERSON WITH MÉNIÈRE'S DISEASE—cont'd

■ **NURSING DIAGNOSIS**
Fluid volume deficit, high risk for

| Expected Patient Outcomes | Nursing Interventions | Rationale |
|---|---|---|
| Fluid intake is >2500 ml/day. | Explain need for fluids. | Dehydration may occur from vomiting and from diuretic (HCTZ). |
| Mucous membranes are moist. | Help Mrs. B. plan ways to maintain a fluid intake >2500 ml/day. | Use of a variety of fluids (juices, soups, soft drinks) will increase probability that Mrs. B. will drink >2400 ml/day. |
| Does not experience thirst. | | |

■ **NURSING DIAGNOSIS**
Coping, ineffective (individual)

| Expected Patient Outcomes | Nursing Interventions | Rationale |
|---|---|---|
| Identifies coping pattern and resultant effects. | Make decisions regarding safety of Mrs. B. and others when patient is unable to do so. | Support and understanding by caregivers improves coping. Discussing possible coping behaviors assists the patient to choose behaviors that are most functional for her. |
| Describes alternative coping behaviors. | Assist Mrs. B. to identify usual coping behaviors and the consequences of the behaviors. | |
| | Assist Mrs. B. to identify personal strengths. | |
| | Teach Mrs. B. alternative coping behaviors (see Chapter 7). | |

■ **NURSING DIAGNOSIS**
Knowledge deficit (about pathophysiology of Ménière's disease related to lack of exposure to information)

| Expected Patient Outcome | Nursing Interventions | Rationale |
|---|---|---|
| Describes nature of disorder, therapy, and safety measures. | Teach Mrs. B. about the disorder, therapy, and need for medical follow-up (see text). | Need for information regarding disease increases learning that assists the patient to care for herself and to live as independently as possible. |
| | Teach Mrs. B. ways to protect herself from injury and to prevent dizziness attacks when possible. | |

of the disorder is not known, it is thought to be vascular in nature. Therefore attempted treatments are made to alter the vascular system in some way. Occasionally, the hearing may return to normal without apparent reason. However, most patients do not regain normal hearing. One cause that is becoming better recognized is a fistula from the inner ear to the middle ear via the oval or round window. If this is suspected, the fistulas are closed by a tissue graft.

*Presbycusis* is a hearing loss associated with aging that becomes more common after age 50. Changes in the delicate labyrinthine structures over the decades causes a ***hearing loss predominantly in the higher frequencies.*** The amount of the hearing loss will have familial differences. Tinnitus usually accompanies presbycusis. The vast majority of persons eventually suffer from presbycusis during the aging process (Table 62-7). In some of these persons, the amount of hearing loss warrants the use of a hearing aid. Presbycusis cannot be cured. Furthermore, the presence of coexisting visual problems, so prevalent among older adults, further exacerbates the limitations of not only hearing (decreased speech reading) but also balance.

Most inner ear disorders are accompanied by a sensorineural hearing loss. The hearing loss is usually incomplete but can be progressive in some illnesses. A characteristic of a severe hearing loss is the *loss of discrimination* (understanding of words).

**TABLE 62-7 Relationship Between Age and Percentage of Persons With Presbycusis**

| AGE | PERCENTAGE |
|---|---|
| 65-74 | 23 |
| 75-84 | 33 |
| 85 and older | 48 |

**BOX 62-7 Complications of Inner Ear Problems**

Central nervous system abscess
Complete loss of balance
Loss of cerebrospinal fluid
Dehydration
Complete hearing loss
Falling
Inability to ambulate
Septicemia
Meningitis

### Tinnitus

Ringing, or any other noises, in the ear are called **tinnitus.** Tinnitus accompanies most sensorineural hearing losses and is very annoying. In some patients, the tinnitus becomes the problem, and the underlying cause may be forgotten. Unfortunately, the only cure for tinnitus is correction of the underlying cause; however, new and unproven cures are still advertised for this chronic ailment. The best treatment is to mask the tinnitus with background sounds such as music, which may help the patient adjust to the ear noise.

### Vertigo

Vertigo also is associated with inner ear problems. The close anatomic relationship between the balance and hearing systems sometimes, but not always, causes the sensation of vertigo in conjunction with a hearing loss. However, in most instances, vertigo is present without a hearing loss.

**Vertigo,** or spinning, is the medical term for dizziness, but specific descriptions of vertigo are not helpful in diagnosing the vestibular abnormality. Dizziness is described in such varied terms that it is almost impossible to define the symptom. All descriptions should be accepted as the symptom caused by a disorder of the balance system. Because the balance system can compensate, *dizziness is usually* not present consistently but is *episodic.* Dizziness, like pain, is subject to psychologic influences. *Dizziness is second only to headache as the most common symptom currently found in America.*

For the patient with vertigo, the differential diagnosis may be accomplished by a thorough medical assessment, including audiometry, vestibular tests, radiologic evaluation, and laboratory studies (see Chapter 61). The nurse may be involved in any or all of these procedures, depending on the setting, and must be able to explain the procedures to the patient to promote understanding and trust. The complications of inner ear problems are listed in Box 62-7.

## MEDICAL MANAGEMENT

Although patients have been hospitalized for medical treatment of dizziness in the past, this trend is decreasing for three reasons: (1) increased use of prophylactic treatment, (2) increased specialization in the care of the person with dizziness by physicians and nurses, and (3) economic pressures such as diagnostic related groups (DRGs). Other than antibiotics for infections, medical treatment of hearing loss is lacking. General modalities include steroids and vasodilators, but specific therapy is still to be determined. Vertigo can be helped by labyrinthine suppressants and other medicines, but a specific medicinal cure does not exist. Likewise, treatment for Ménière's disease consists of more than 50 different medicines. Usually a combination of medical therapy will control the vertigo, but no cure has been found.

### Hearing Aids

Because most hearing losses are permanent, the use of a hearing aid should always be considered. A patient should undergo a trial period to establish its benefit before purchasing the aid. Bilateral or binaural aids are desirable.

The technology of aided hearing is part of the current electronic explosion (see Aural Rehabilitation, p. 2151). The evolution in hearing aid development has led to smaller and more effective aids. Small hearing aids currently are available that fit into the ear canal; however, the greater the hearing loss is, the larger the hearing aid. Hearing aids also are available for placement within the ear concha or behind the ear. Special hearing aids can transmit sound by radio waves to the opposite ear or by vibration to the inner ear through the skull. In the future, hearing aids will be semi-implantable and finally totally implantable within the middle ear and mastoid.

### Implantable Hearing Devices

Three types of implanted hearing devices are either available for use or in the investigation stage. They are cochlear implants, bone conduction devices, and semiimplantable hearing devices.

**Cochlear implants** for those patients with no aidable hearing are currently available (Figure 62-6). This device incorporates a small computer that changes the spoken word to electrical impulses. The impulses are transmitted across the skin to an implanted coil that carries the impulse to the hearing nerve endings in the cochlea by an electrode introduced through the round window. The best of the cochlear implants use multichannels and are able to return about half of the patient's hearing and understanding. Cochlear implants are available for both children and adults.

In some cases of hearing loss, sound can be transmitted through the skull to the inner ear by *bone conduction devices.* Patients with a conductive hearing loss can use a device in which an orthopedic screw is implanted under the skin into the skull. The external device transmits the sound through the skin. This device is worn above the ear and not in the ear canal.

Patients who already use a hearing aid will gain the most from the implantable device. Clinical research has shown that a magnet implanted in the middle ear can be stimulated by an ear canal driver, which changes sound to a magnetic force. This system eliminates several bothersome problems of hearing aids, such as feedback and difficulties with hearing in noisy environments. A *semiimplantable hearing device* is the first step to a totally implantable device that would eliminate any external device. However, many challenges have yet to be met before a workable device is available.

## SURGICAL MANAGEMENT

The delicate inner ear does not lend itself to surgical treatment, except for destructive procedures. Nonetheless, surgeons have gingerly approached surgical methods involving the inner ear in an attempt to alleviate vertigo. The ideal surgery would relieve the vertigo safely while preserving hearing. Any surgery performed on the vestibular system carries a high risk of damage to the auditory system. The **endolymphatic sac procedures** include decompression and various forms of shunts. The intent of these procedures is to reduce the fluid pressure within the labyrinth and control vertigo. Other attempts to do the same are performed through the oval or round windows. A destructive procedure to remove the membranous labyrinth, either subtotally through the oval window or totally through the mastoid bone, is called **labyrinthectomy.** Also, *vestibular nerve section* can be performed to alleviate vertigo; this may provide immediate relief. Because of the compensation by all of the other structures related to maintaining balance, a person can function with only one labyrinth. However, any surgery directed toward destroying the vestibular system also carries a high risk of residual or recurring vertigo.

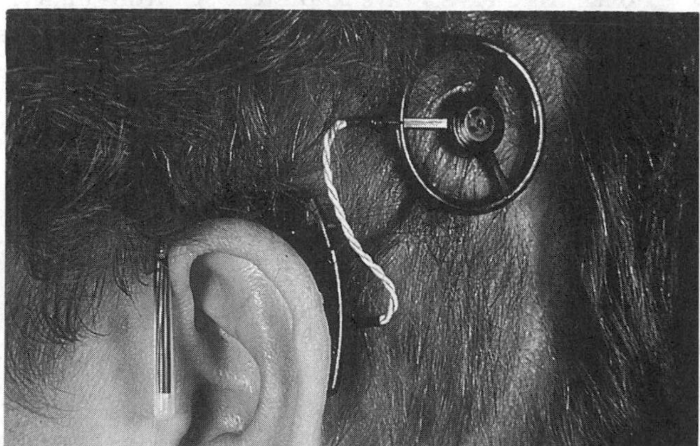

**FIGURE 62-6** Cochlear implant in place. (From Sigler B, Schuring L: *Ear, nose and throat disorders,* St Louis, 1993, Mosby.)

The necessity of removing tumors of the inner ear and internal auditory canal has led to various approaches through and around the temporal bone. These procedures are sometimes performed in cooperation with a neurosurgeon. As time passes, a greater number of patients will undergo this surgery and thus retain facial nerve function and, rarely, hearing function. Because of the limited exposure of the central nervous system by the new techniques, the mortality and morbidity of the surgery are lessened. Facial nerve disorders are also treated by the same surgical approaches. Malignant tumors in this area can be excised by a *temporal bone resection.* However, surgery of the inner ear is still in a pioneering stage. The care of the person having inner ear surgery is the same as that described on p. 2142.

## NURSING MANAGEMENT

Because vertigo is only a symptom, the diagnosis and treatment of the underlying disease is frustrating to both the patient and the health care providers. The nurse's role becomes even more important as psychologic factors, such as social isolation or fear of participating in activities because of the possibility of dizziness, complicate the illness. The nurse's ability to understand and to assess the person with vertigo will aid in providing care that will contribute to the patient's recovery.

Balance and equilibrium depend on four systems being intact: the *vestibular* (labyrinth of the inner ear), the *proprioceptive* (somatosensors of joints and muscles), the *visual* (eye), and the *cerebellar systems.* The sensations transmitted from the eyes, the somatosensors, and the inner ears are integrated in the brainstem and cerebellum and perceived in the cerebral cortex. Dizziness is most likely to occur when two or more systems are impaired simultaneously or when they transmit sensory information that is contradictory.

### ♦ ASSESSMENT

#### Subjective Data

Dizziness is a common vague symptom with a wide variety of unpleasant meanings and with multiple individual interpretations. Spinning, or vertigo, may be the most common form of dizziness. Other "feelings" include light-headedness, giddiness, imbalance, veering in one direction while walking, unsteadiness, or a vague feeling of uncertainty during changes in body position.

Nursing assessment of dizziness may include the following:

1. A patient interview obtaining a health history and specific data about the following:
   a. Onset and characteristics of the dizziness
   b. Description of attacks and any associated symptoms
   c. History of falls
   d. Disability in relation to activities of daily living
   e. Concerns or fears related to the illness
   f. Hearing acuity, history of hearing loss, and occurrence of tinnitus
   g. Patient's cognitive appraisal of illness and factors that may be contributing to inability to cope
2. An interview with the family to identify the effect of the person's dizziness on others

The importance of the history and interview cannot be overemphasized. All patients experience some degree of anxiety regarding the illness, and dizziness can have devastating effects on the person's behavior. The disruption of the person's routine, the severity of the "attacks," and the fear of the unknown may make the patient agitated, anxious, and depressed. The nurse must be aware of these feelings and demonstrate self-confidence, patience, courtesy, consideration, and gentleness.

## Objective Data

Data to be collected to assess the patient with vertigo include the following:

Physical examination, with specific emphasis on eyes, ears, thyroid, heart, and lungs, and a neurologic examination

Review of laboratory tests

## Diagnostic Tests

The purposes of common diagnostic tests performed for problems of the inner ear are listed in Table 62-8.

# ♦ NURSING DIAGNOSES

Nursing diagnoses are determined from analysis of patient data. Nursing diagnoses for the patient with balance problems may include but are not limited to the following:

| Diagnostic Title | Possible Etiologic Factors |
|---|---|
| Injury, high risk for | Dizziness leading to falls |
| Anxiety | Vertigo as a threat to self-concept and to successful role functioning |
| Fear | Uncertainty of attacks, decreased quality of life, and sensory impairment |
| Fluid volume deficit, high risk for | Vomiting, diaphoresis, diarrhea, and inadequate oral intake that accompany ear balance problems |
| Sensory/perceptual alteration: vestibular, auditory | Damage to inner ear |
| Coping, ineffective (individual) | Personal vulnerability from attacks of dizziness |
| Knowledge deficit | Lack of exposure to information |

**TABLE 62-8 Diagnostic Tests of the Inner Ear**

| DIAGNOSTIC TEST | PURPOSE |
|---|---|
| Audiometric testing | Determine amount and kind of hearing loss |
| Automatic brainstem response test | Determine site of lesion and extent of involvement |
| Imaging studies | Identify tumors, masses, retrocochlear disorders, and necrosis |
| Electronystagmography | Determine extent of labyrinth damage |

# ♦ EXPECTED PATIENT OUTCOMES

Expected patient outcomes for the person with balance problems may include but are not limited to the following:

1. Remains free of any injuries associated with imbalance and/or falls.
2. States less or no anxiety.
3. States feeling less fearful.
4. Is hydrated (fluid intake equals fluid output, good skin turgor, moist mucous membranes, no thirst).
5. Regains or maintains hearing.
6. Demonstrates coping skills necessary to decrease vulnerability and unmet needs.
7. Describes nature of the disorder, purposes of the diagnostic tests, ways to protect self from injury, therapeutic regimen, and symptoms requiring medical attention.

# ♦ INTERVENTIONS

## Promoting Safety

Loss of balance places the person with vertigo at high risk for falls. The patient needs to explore the living environment for potential hazards. It is important that the person follow the prescribed vestibular/balance therapy (antivertiginous or vestibular sedation medication).

## Reducing Anxiety and Fear

1. Encourage the patient to discuss anxieties and fears and to explore concerns about vertigo.
2. Dispel distorted perceptions and misinformation about vertigo.

3. Provide information about vertigo and its treatment (see p. 2146).
4. Encourage use of comfort measures, such as music, religious practices, and enhancing relations with family and friends.
5. Teach stress management techniques as needed.

### Promoting Fluid Balance

1. Weigh daily before breakfast; weight should return rapidly to predeficit level.
2. Monitor every 8 hours for return of signs to normal: skin turgor, moistness of mucous membranes, no complaints of thirst; laboratory tests within normal limits (serum osmolality, serum sodium, hematocrit, and urine specific gravity).
3. Encourage fluid intake of 2500 to 3000 ml per day unless contraindicated.

### Promoting Hearing

1. Face the patient when speaking.
2. Speak distinctly without shouting.

### Improving Coping Skills

1. Encourage and assist with patient participation in the decision-making process regarding adjustments in life-style.
2. Help the patient identify personal strengths and develop coping strategies based on personal strengths, previous positive experiences with stress, and situational supports.
3. Refer the patient to support groups or counseling as indicated.

### Facilitating Learning

Teach the patient about the nature of the disorder and therapeutic regimen:

1. Reason for the dizziness
2. Circumstances that may precipitate an attack of dizziness and what to do when one occurs
3. Safety precautions during episodes of dizziness
4. Symptoms requiring medical intervention
5. Dosage and side effects of medications
6. Need for increased fluid intake if vomiting, diaphoresis, or diarrhea occur

## ♦ EVALUATION

To evaluate the effectiveness of nursing interventions, compare patient behaviors with those stated in the expected patient outcomes. Successful achievement of patient outcomes for the patient with vertigo is indicated by the following:

1. Sustains no injuries associated with balance problems.
2. Offers statements of feeling less anxiety or fear; demonstrates no signs of anxiety.
3. Fluid intake is equal to fluid output; skin turgor is good, mucous membranes are moist, no thirst is sensed.
4. Hearing is maintained.
5. Demonstrates control over life, with verbalizations of positive feelings about the ability to achieve a sense of power and control over vertigo.
6. Describes the nature of vertigo and the therapeutic regimen, safety precautions, and symptoms requiring medical intervention.

# NURSING MANAGEMENT

## ♦ ASSESSMENT

The sensorineural hearing loss is assessed by history, physical examination, and audiometry. The diagnosis is usually reached quickly in the physician's office or in a clinic. On occasion, laboratory, radiologic, and vestibular examinations are necessary. In an otology office, the nurse may have the responsibility for obtaining the history and performing otologic examination and screening audiometry (see Chapter 61).

### Subjective Data

People with hearing losses may experience fears of inadequacy, feelings of inferiority, depression, and varying degrees of stress and isolation. Some people withdraw from social situations and become anxious and insecure because of the decreased hearing. The history is often the most important part of the clinical assessment. The following questions are included in the history for a person with a sensorineural hearing loss:

What was the age at onset of the hearing loss?
Was the hearing loss progressive?
Is there a fluctuation in hearing loss?
Is the hearing loss in one ear or both?
Is there a family history of hearing loss?
Is there pressure in the ears?
Is there ringing in the ears?
Is there any dizziness?
What medications are currently being taken? (Determine whether a possibility of ototoxicity from medication exists.)
Has there been any head trauma?
What is the person's exposure to noise (present and past)?
Has the person experienced any other neurologic disturbances?
Has the person experienced any speech or visual disturbances?
Is there any ear pain or drainage?

### Objective Data

A physical examination and audiometry are part of the objective data. The extent of physical assessment of the sensorineural hearing loss by the nurse depends on the setting and the nurse's educational preparation. All nurses, however, should be able to inspect the outer ear and grossly assess auditory acuity (see Chapter 61).

Additional data include observing the person for the following indications of a hearing loss:

Failure to respond to oral communication
Inappropriate response to oral communication
Excessively loud speech
Abnormal awareness of sounds
Strained facial expressions
Tilted head when listening
Constant need for clarification of conversation
Faulty speech articulation
Behavioral clues (see Chapter 61)

## ♦ NURSING DIAGNOSES

Nursing diagnoses are determined from analysis of patient data. Nursing diagnoses for the patient with sensorineural hearing loss may include but are not limited to the following:

| Diagnostic Title | Possible Etiologic Factors |
|---|---|
| Sensory/perceptual alteration: auditory | Ear disorder, toxic substance, noise, trauma, age |
| Anxiety | Threat to self-concept and successful role functioning |
| Diversional activity deficit | Decreased social activities because of loss of hearing, environmental lack of such activity |

## ♦ EXPECTED PATIENT OUTCOMES

Expected patient outcomes for the person with sensorineural hearing loss may include but are not limited to the following:

1. Communicates adequately with the help of aural rehabilitation, hearing aids, or other devices for the hearing impaired.
2. States feeling less or no anxiety.
3. Takes more interest in social, leisure, and recreational activities.

## ♦ INTERVENTIONS

### Facilitating Communication

Fewer than 1% of all persons with a sensorineural hearing loss require surgery of the inner ear. However, the hearing loss may be the secondary diagnosis of many hospitalized patients. The nurse must therefore understand the nursing interventions for this common health problem and facilitate communication for persons with hearing loss. The suggestions listed in the Guidelines box below can apply to communicating with all persons, regardless of the type or severity of hearing loss.

### Reducing Anxiety

Facing life with dimunition of sound and decreased ability to communicate with others can be anxiety-provoking. The person needs opportunities to explore concerns and to know what can be done to improve hearing. Learning about ways to improve communication, use of devices to improve hearing, and available resources can help decrease the anxiety.

### Encouraging Diversional Activity

As cited earlier, people with diminished hearing may experience fears of inadequacy and depression and may therefore withdraw from social interactions. Actions to encourage diversional activity may include:

1. Encourage the patient to talk about anger and limitations resulting from diminished hearing.
2. Assist the patient in identifying desirable activities that could be pursued.
3. Facilitate participation in group social events.
4. Facilitate opportunities for friends and family to visit.

### Guidelines for Communicating With the Hearing Impaired Person

1. Get the person's attention by raising an arm or hand.
2. Stand with the light on your face; this will help the person speech (lip) read.
3. Talk directly to the person, facing him or her.
4. Speak clearly, but do not overaccentuate words.
5. Speak in a normal tone; do not shout. Shouting overuses normal speaking movements and may cause distortion and be too loud for the person with sensorineural damage. If the person has conductive loss only, sometimes making the voice louder without shouting is helpful.
6. If the person does not seem to understand what is said, express it differently. Some words are difficult to "see" in speech reading, such as *white* and *red*.
7. Move closer to the person and toward the better ear if he or she does not hear you.
8. Write out proper names or any statement that you are not sure was understood.
9. Do not smile, chew gum, or cover the mouth when talking to a person with limited hearing.
10. Inattention may indicate tiredness or lack of understanding.
11. Use phrases to convey meaning rather than one-word answers. State the major topic of the discussion first and then give details.
12. Do not show annoyance by careless facial expression. Persons who are hard of hearing depend more on visual clues for acceptance.
13. Encourage the use of a hearing aid if the person has one; allow him or her to adjust it before speaking.
14. If in a group, repeat important statements and avoid asides to others in the group.
15. Avoid the use of the intercom when communicating with the patient. The intercom may distort sound and cause poor communication.
16. Do not avoid conversation with a person who has hearing loss. It has been said that to live in a silent world is much more devastating than to live in darkness, and persons with hearing loss appear, in general, to have more emotional difficulties than those who are blind.

Modified from Conover M, Cober J: *Nurs Clin North Am* 5:497, 1970.

5. Provide information on community resources that would be helpful to the patient in facilitating interactions with others.

## ◆ EVALUATION

To evaluate the effectiveness of nursing interventions, compare the patient behaviors with those stated in the expected patient outcomes. Successful achievement of patient outcomes for the patient with a hearing impairment is indicated by the following:

1. Demonstrates knowledge of the cause of the hearing impairment and options for medical or surgical treatment.
2. Responds appropriately to the spoken word with or without amplification; uses alternative means of communication appropriately.
3. States there is less or no anxiety; demonstrates reduced anxiety with less tension, apprehension, and uncertainty.
4. Participates in diversional activities.

## ✹ SPECIAL CONSIDERATIONS FOR CARE OF THE GERONTOLOGIC PATIENT

Of the 10 million people in the United States with a hearing loss who are 65 years of age or older, 90% have some sensorineural hearing loss and 29% have a handicapping loss of hearing.[2] Because of fear, misinformation, lack of information, or vanity, many of them do not admit that they have a hearing problem. *Presbycusis,* which is a progressive, bilaterally symmetric perceptive hearing loss that occurs with age, is discussed on p. 2145. Important considerations for the care of persons with presbycusis include the following:

1. Assessment
   a. Assess all elderly persons for hearing loss of *high-pitched* sounds, sensitivity to background noise, and loss of sibilant consonants.
   b. Assess the patient's knowledge of hearing aids.
   c. Assess function of the patient's hearing aid, and identify availability of extra batteries.
2. Intervention
   a. Modify communication skills when speaking to the patient.
      (1) Face the patient with light on your face.
      (2) Get the person's attention; touch the patient lightly on the arm, if necessary.
      (3) Speak slowly and distinctly, but do not exaggerate lip movements; do not shout.
      (4) Use short phrases, and punctuate them with body language.
      (5) Be aware that vision may also be diminished.
   b. Place a note at the nurses' station intercom that the patient is hard of hearing.
   c. Post a sign at the bedside alerting personnel that the patient is hard of hearing.
   d. Try to obtain a pocket amplifier for the patient if a hearing aid is not available.
   e. Determine if the patient sees an otologist regularly so that ears are checked for wax.

## AURAL REHABILITATION

If hearing loss is irreversible or not amenable to surgical intervention or if the person elects not to have surgery, aural rehabilitation can increase communication. The purpose of aural rehabilitation is to maximize the hearing-impaired person's communication skills.

The auditory sense is our primary mode of communication, and rehabilitation is directed toward teaching the person more effective use of the senses of vision, touch, and vibration plus maximizing the use of any remaining hearing ability. Rehabilitation is affected by the person's background and by the severity of impairment. As with other forms of rehabilitation, success depends on the degree of the patient's motivation.

Aural rehabilitation includes auditory training, speech reading and speech training, and hearing aids. The use of instruments and training are involved.

### Auditory Training

Auditory training is an approach to enhance listening skills. The hearing-impaired person is initially exposed to gross differences in sound and then gradually "fine tuned" so that subtle differences in discrimination of two similar sounds can be made. The primary purpose of auditory training exercises is to help the person concentrate on the speaker. For some persons, only gross differences between sounds may be recognized.

### Speech Reading and Speech Training

*Speech reading* is the current term used for lip reading and is an important means of communication. *Speech training* is the process of understanding vocal communication by the integration of lip movements with facial expressions, gestures, environmental clues, and conversation contexts. Speech reading is very difficult, however, without auditory cues. Many movements for speech are very rapid, many sounds are very similar (b, m, p), and certain sounds of any language are invisible (the h in English). A high percentage of the words have

**BOX 62-8 Types of Hearing Aids**

**In-the-ear aid** For hearing loss of 25-65 dB; worn in ear concha
**In-the-canal aid** For hearing loss of 25-50 dB; worn in ear canal
**Postauricular aid** For hearing loss of 25-80 dB; worn behind ear

to be guessed at by the hearing-impaired person. Knowledge of this fact alone will help the nurse be more understanding of the person who is speech (lip) reading.

Because of reduced auditory feedback (the inability of hearing-impaired persons to monitor their own speech), the clearness, pitch quality, or rate of their speech may deteriorate. These abnormal effects alter the efficiency of communication and reduce the intelligibility of speech. The goal of *speech training* is to conserve or develop speech skills, or to prevent deterioration of speech skills.

## Hearing Aids

Hearing aids are instruments made up of miniature parts working together as a system to amplify sound in a controlled manner. They are used by both hard-of-hearing persons (slight or moderate hearing loss) and deaf persons (severe or profound hearing loss). Hearing aids make sound louder but *do not improve the ability to hear.* Therefore persons with decreased discrimination (the ability to understand what is spoken) benefit less from a hearing aid. Appropriate aural rehabilitation will ensure successful adjustment of most problems. The hearing aid amplifies all background noises such as hospital machinery, footsteps, and department store noises, as well as speech. These noises may mask conversation or confuse the hearing-impaired person, especially the elderly.

Several types of hearing aids exist according to size and location to be worn (see Box 62-8 and Figure 62-7). Regardless of the type of aid, the hearing aid consists of the following parts:

1. Microphone to receive sound waves from the air and change sounds into electrical signals
2. Amplifier to increase the strength of the electrical signals
3. Battery to provide the electrical energy needed to operate the hearing aid
4. Receiver (loudspeaker) to change the electrical signals back into sound waves

The person with a hearing aid should know how to care for the aid (see first Guidelines box, p. 2153) and what to do if the aid does not work (see second Guidelines box, p. 2153). The nurse must also have a basic knowledge of the hearing aid to assist the person who is unable or unwilling to do this when ill. The person is encouraged to use the hearing aid and to store it safely in its case when it is not in use.

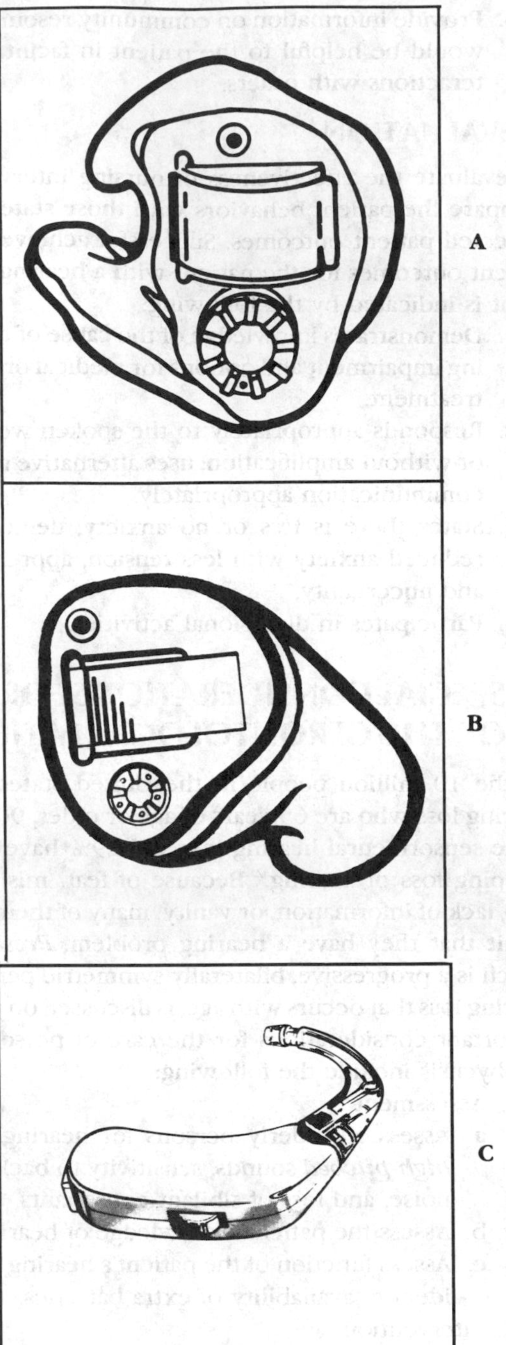


**FIGURE 62-7** Types of commonly used hearing aids. **A,** Canal aid. **B,** In-the-ear aid. **C,** Behind-the-ear aid. (From Sigler B, Schuring L: *Ear, nose and throat disorders,* St Louis, 1993, Mosby.)

## COMMUNITY SERVICES

Many agencies and associations exist for the hearing-impaired person. Services are offered by *audiology clinics* sponsored by universities, hospitals, community programs, state or local departments of health, or the Veterans Administration. *National organizations* are available to give information and counseling and include the following:

1. Acoustic Neuroma Association, P.O. Box 398, Carlisle, PA 17013; provides materials and support for acoustic neuroma patients.
2. American Academy of Otolaryngology–Head and Neck Surgeons, 1 Prince St, Alexandria, VA 22314; a professional society for physicians specializing in diseases of the ear and related areas; it can provide information on hearing and balance disorders.

### Guidelines for Care of a Hearing Aid

1. Turn the hearing aid off when not in use.
2. Open the battery compartment at night to avoid accidental drainage of the battery.
3. Keep an extra battery available at all times.
4. Wash the earmold frequently (daily if necessary) with mild soap and warm water with the use of a pipe cleaner to cleanse the cannula.
5. Do not wear the hearing aid if an ear infection is present.

### Guidelines for What to Do if a Hearing Aid Fails to Work

1. Check the on-off switch.
2. Inspect the earmold for cleanliness.
3. Examine the battery for correct insertion.
4. Examine the cord plug for correct insertion.
5. Examine the cord for breaks.
6. Replace the battery, cord, or both, if necessary. The life of batteries varies according to amount of use and power requirements of the aid. Batteries last from 2 to 14 days.
7. Check the position of the earmold in the ear. If the hearing aid "whistles," the earmold is probably not inserted properly into the ear canal, or the person needs to have a new earmold made.

3. American Annals of the Deaf, 5034 Wisconsin Ave., NW, Washington, DC 20016. The April issue every year lists a directory of programs and services for the deaf available by state and includes information about the type of facilities.
4. American Federation of the Physically Handicapped, Inc., 1370 National Press Building, Washington, DC 20004; provides counseling and information.
5. American Neurotology Society, Michigan Ear Institute, 27555 Middlebelt, Farmington Hills, MI 48334; a society for physicians specializing in diseases of the ear and brain; provides information on hearing and balance.
6. American Speech-Language-Hearing Association, 10801 Rockville Pike, Dept AP, Rockville, MD 20852. This association can answer questions or mail information on hearing aids or hearing loss and communication problems in the elderly and provide a list of certified audiologists in each state.
7. Gallaudet College, 7th and Florida Ave, Washington, DC 20002; the only liberal arts college for the deaf in the world.
8. National Association of Hearing and Speech Agencies, 919 18th St NW, Washington, DC 20006; provides counseling and information.
9. National Institute on Deafness and other Communication Disorders (NIDCD), 225 Haverford Ave #1, Narbeth, PA 19072; a focal point for research on hearing loss and other communication disorders. (Pamphlet: "Hearing loss: hope through research.")
10. Self-Help for Hard-of-Hearing People (Shhh), 4848 Battery Lane, Dept E, Bethesda, MD 20814; a nationwide organization for the hard-of-hearing; publishes a bimonthly magazine that includes experiences of the hard-of-hearing and new developments in the field of hearing loss; publications and reprints available.
11. Society of Otorhinolaryngology and Head–Neck Nurses, Inc., 116-A Canal St., New Smyrna Beach, FL 32168; a professional nursing society for nurses specializing in caring for patients with problems of the ear, nose, or throat; information on hearing and balance disorders.
12. State office of vocational rehabilitation (in each state); provides vocational training and placement services.
13. Veterans Administration; provides audiology clinics and rehabilitation services for veterans.

## QUESTIONS TO CONSIDER

- Walk around for a day with earplugs in your ears. Describe your reactions. How do you think you would feel if you were told you would never hear well again?
- What changes do you think you would have to make in your life-style if you had recurrent vertigo?
- What is the importance of the tympanic membrane? What information does an inspection of it provide?
- How does a conductive hearing loss differ from a sensorineural hearing loss in terms of predisposing factors and treatment methods?

## CRITICAL THINKING ACTIVITIES

- Describe how you think you might feel if you were told that you have a significant and permanent hearing loss.
- Compare and contrast the pathophysiology, clinical manifestations, and assessment parameters for conductive and sensorineural hearing loss.
- What measures or precautions could you suggest to the patient who is at risk for hearing loss?

## CHAPTER SUMMARY

### HEARING LOSS

- Disorders that plug the outer ear, add fluid to the middle ear, make the ossicles unmovable, destroy the hair cells of the organ of Corti, or interfere with nerve stimulus transmission over the acoustic nerve will lead to decreased hearing.

- Hearing can be preserved by preventing infection or trauma of the ear, by using ototoxic drugs with caution and seeking medical attention if symptoms occur, and by preventing frequent exposure to loud noises (or using ear protection for constant loud noises).

### PROBLEMS OF THE EXTERNAL EAR

- Ear infections are the most common disorders of the external and middle ears; pain results from pressure from fluid buildup within the enclosed spaces.
- Serous otitis media develops from collection of serous fluid in the middle ear when the eustachian tube becomes blocked. Purulent otitis media develops from bacteria entering the middle ear through the eustachian tube; pus collects in the middle ear.
- Ear infections are treated with antibiotics, which are given by eardrops, ear ointments, or systemically. Treatments to remove drainage may include ear wash, ear irrigation, or surgery of the eardrum.
- The person with an ear infection should avoid getting water in the ear (care during showering and shampooing and avoiding swimming).

### PROBLEMS OF THE MIDDLE EAR

- *Tympanosclerosis* and *cholesteatoma* are both complications from repeated otitis media.
- Any long-term blockage of the eustachian tube leads to *serous otitis media* and a hearing loss.
- Otosclerosis is the *hardening of the ear* that involves the stapes bone and causes a conductive hearing loss. *Stapedectomy* is the surgical procedure that removes and replaces the stapes.
- *Cochlear implants* are used for patients with no usable hearing at all in either ear.

### PROBLEMS OF THE INNER EAR

- *Sensorineural hearing loss* results from interference with hearing in the inner ear or neural pathways; it may result from a known disorder or may be idiopathic. Presbycusis (hearing loss resulting from aging) is a form of sensorineural hearing loss. The hearing loss is primarily that of sound discrimination, and amplification may further distort the sound. It is the most common inner ear disorder for which there is no present cure.
- Vertigo is the major symptom of disorders (such as labyrinthitis, Ménière's disease, acoustic neuroma) affecting the semicircular canals of the inner ear. Tinnitus (ringing in the ears) often accompanies vertigo. Potential for injury is a major problem for the person with vertigo. The uncomfortable sensation of vertigo can be minimized by lying down and holding the head still.
- Dizziness, like pain, is subject to psychologic influences and is second to headache as the most common symptom currently found in the United States.

### SENSORINEURAL HEARING LOSS

- The nurse's ability to understand and assess the person with dizziness will aid in providing care contributing to the person's recovery.
- The purpose of aural rehabilitation is to maximize the hearing-impaired person's communication skills.
- Aural rehabilitation includes auditory training, speechreading (lip-reading), speech training, (improving speech clarity) and the use of hearing aids.

## REFERENCES

1. Gardner G: Ménière's disease. In Rakel RE, editor: *Conn's current therapy 1993,* Philadelphia, 1993, WB Saunders.
2. Nodol JB, Jr: Hearing loss, *N Engl J Med* 329(15):1092-1102, 1993.
3. US Department of Health and Human Services, Public Health Service: *Healthy people 2000: national health promotion and disease prevention objectives,* Washington, DC, 1990, US Government Printing Office.

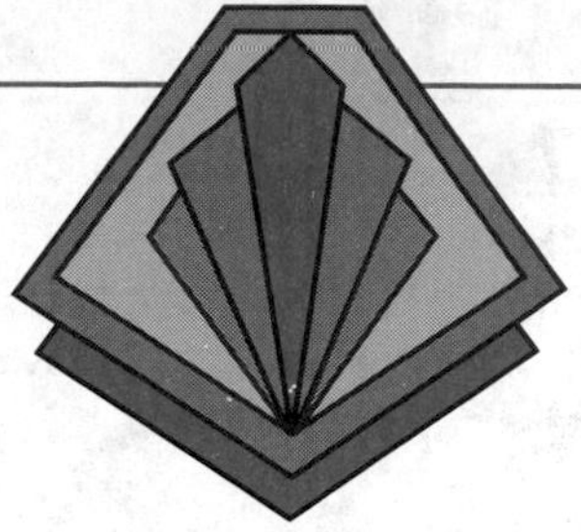

CHAPTER 63

# Assessment of the Musculoskeletal System

*Jane F. Marek*

## CHAPTER OBJECTIVES

***After studying this chapter, the learner should be able to do the following:***

1 Describe the structure and function of the tissues that compose the musculoskeletal system.
2 Explain the interrelationship of the tissues of the musculoskeletal system to the overall functioning of the system.
3 Describe the physiologic changes that occur in the musculoskeletal system with aging.
4 Explain the nature of pathologic conditions that can occur within the musculoskeletal system.
5 Describe the subjective data that should be obtained during initial nursing assessment of the person who has a musculoskeletal problem.
6 Describe the components of objective assessment to be carried out with the person who has a musculoskeletal problem.
7 Describe the diagnostic tests that could be performed for the patient with a musculoskeletal problem, and explain the rationale for each test.
8 Describe appropriate nursing interventions for persons with musculoskeletal problems who are undergoing diagnostic tests.
9 Identify the relevance of subjective and objective data and results of diagnostic tests in planning care for persons with musculoskeletal problems.

## KEY TERMS

arthrography
arthroscopy
computed tomography
contracture
crepitus
diskogram
electromyogram (EMG)
magnetic resonance imaging
manual muscle test (MMT)
myelogram
range of motion

The eagle that cannot fly will starve to death. The deer that cannot run becomes the easy prey of its enemies. And if humans could not move, they too would surely die. The musculoskeletal system enables humans to move about freely. Thus illnesses and disorders that deprive persons of this ability can be very serious.

Planning appropriate interventions for individuals who have locomotor disabilities requires that the disabilities and the individual's reaction to them are carefully assessed. Such assessment is made on the basis of knowledge and understanding of the anatomy and physiology of the musculoskeletal system, as well as of the diagnostic studies involved and what the results of these studies mean.

The muscles, bones, joints, supportive structures, and sensory and motor nerves all work together to provide controlled movement and to maintain posture. However, any problem that causes interference or disturbance at any level—innervation, contractility, articulation, or support—of this well-integrated system results in musculoskeletal dysfunction. Problems can occur as a result of the interruption of blood supply to the involved structures; from disease affecting the contour of bones or joints, or disease affecting the nerves that innervate the musculoskeletal system; or the result of trauma, of any origin that interrupts the integrity of any of the involved structures.

This chapter discusses the anatomy and physiology of the musculoskeletal system, methods and rationale for obtaining subjective and objective data about patients and their disabilities, and the pertinence of selected diagnostic studies.

# ANATOMY AND PHYSIOLOGY

## BONES

The human skeleton is made up of the axial and appendicular *skeletons,* which consist of 206 bones (Figure 63-1). The *axial skeleton* contains 80 bones, including the hyoid bone and those of the skull, vertebral column, and thorax. The remaining 126 bones make up the *appendicular skeleton,* which contains the bones of the upper and lower extremities, pectoral girdle, and pelvic girdle (os coxae). The skeleton makes up 14% of the weight of the adult body.

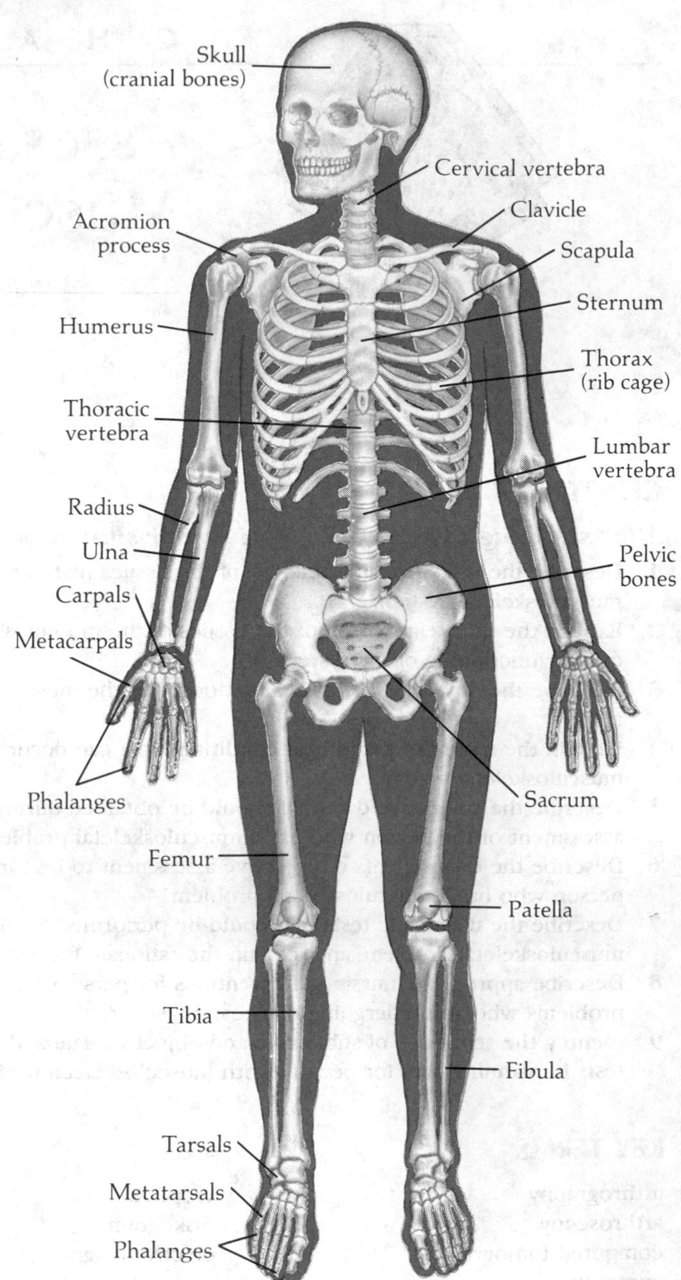


**FIGURE 63-1** Axial and appendicular skeleton. (From Thompson JM et al: *Mosby's clinical nursing,* ed 3, St Louis, 1993, Mosby.)

### Types

Bones are divided into four types, according to their shape:

1. *Long* (femur, humerus)
2. *Short* (carpals): often cuboidal in shape (see Figure 63-1)
3. *Flat* (skull)
4. *Irregular* (vertebrae)

Long bones are made up of a *diaphysis, metaphysis,* and *epiphysis.* The *diaphysis* (midportion) is made of thick cortical bone and contains the medullary cavity where the marrow is stored. The diaphyseal cavity comprises primarily fatty tissues and contains yellow marrow, which is not capable of hematopoiesis. The marrow cavity of the diaphysis connects to the cancellous bone of the *metaphysis,* or broad neck of the long bone. The *epiphysis,* or broad end of the bone, contains the red marrow, which is responsible for hematopoiesis. The *endosteum* lines both yellow and red marrow cavities. The epiphysis is made up of spongy bone covered with a thin layer of cortical bone. Its broad end allows weight to be distributed over a greater surface area. A cartilaginous *growth plate* or *epiphyseal plate* separates the metaphysis from the epiphysis in children. The epiphysis and metaphysis merge after puberty when the epiphyseal plate calcifies. This growth plate, easily seen on x-ray examination in children, is undetectable in adults (Figure 63-2).

Each bone is composed of *cancellous* (spongy) and *cortical compact* bone. In the long bones the cancellous portions are found in the ends of the bones and cortical bone in the shaft (see Figure 63-2). The short and irregular bones have an inner core of cancellous bone with an outer layer of cortical bone. Flat bones have two outer plates of cortical bone with an inner layer of cancellous bone. *Cancellous bone is also found in the ends of long bones and in the iliac crests, tibias,* and *sternum.*

### Structure

Bone, like other connective tissue, is made up of cells, fibers, and ground substance. In addition, unlike other connective tissue, it contains crystallized minerals (Table 63-1).

Both cancellous bone and cortical bone contain the same structural elements, but they differ in the organi-

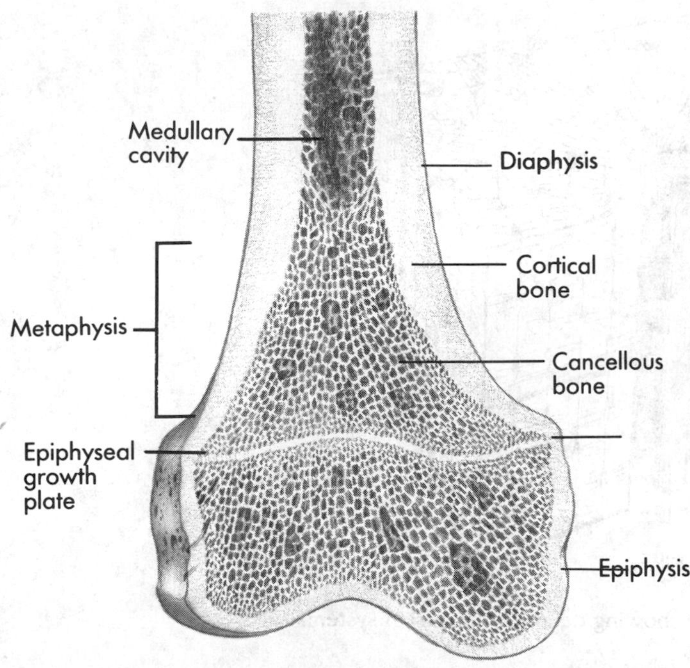


**FIGURE 63-2** Cross section of a long bone. (Modified from Thompson JM et al: *Mosby's clinical nursing,* ed 3, St Louis, 1993, Mosby.)

**TABLE 63-1 Structural Elements of Bone**

| STRUCTURAL ELEMENT | FUNCTION |
|---|---|
| **BONE CELLS** | |
| Osteoblasts | Synthesize collagen and proteoglycans |
| Osteocytes | Maintain bone matrix |
| Osteoclasts | Resorb bone |
| **BONE MATRIX** | |
| Collagen fibers | Lend support and tensile strength |
| Proteoglycans | Control transport of ionized materials through matrix |
| Glycoproteins | |
| Sialoprotein | Promotes calcification |
| Osteocalcin | Inhibits calcium-phosphate precipitation; promotes bone resorption |
| Albumin | Transports essential elements to matrix; maintains osmotic pressure of bone fluid |
| Alpha glycoprotein | Promotes calcification |
| Minerals (elements) | |
| Calcium | Crystallizes to lend rigidity and compressive strength |
| Phosphate | Regulates vitamin D and thereby promotes mineralization |

From McCance KL, Huether SE: *Pathophysiology: the biological basis for disease in adults and children,* ed 2, St Louis, 1994, Mosby.

zation of the bone matrix. Concentric layers of bone matrix are called *lamellae.*

The basic unit of cortical bone is the *haversian system* (Figure 63-3). At the center of this arrangement of concentric rings is the *haversian canal,* which runs through the long axes of bones. It contains blood vessels (capillaries, arterioles, or venules), nerve fibers, and lymphatics. Blood vessels in the canal communicate with blood vessels in the periosteum. *Lacunae* are small spaces between the rings of the lamellae and contain osteocytes. *Canaliculi* are very small canals that connect the *lacunae* and the *haversian canal.* They run parallel to the long axis of the bone. This connection allows the osteocytes access to the nutrient supply. *Haversian units* (lamellae, haversian canal, lacuane, canaliculi) fit closely together in cortical bone. The hardness and density of cortical bone give it strength and rigidity.

In contrast, *cancellous bone lacks haversian systems.* The lamellae are arranged not in concentric layers, but in connecting plates or bars called *trabeculae,* which form an irregular meshwork. The pattern of the trabecular bone depends on the direction of stress in the particular bone. Red marrow fills the spaces between the trabeculae. Lacunae, rich in osteocytes, are distributed among the trabeculae and connected by canaliculi. Capillaries flowing through the marrow provide nutrients to the osteocytes. The fine thready structure of trabecular bone provides strength to cancellous bone, while reducing its weight.

The outer, nonarticulating surfaces of long bones are covered with a white fibrous membrane called the *periosteum.* The outer layer of the periosteum contains blood vessels and nerves that reach the inner bones through *Volkmann's canals.* Nutrient arteries in the periosteum communicate with the haversian system. Collagenous fibers (Sharpey's fibers) anchor the inner layer of the periosteum to the bone.

Surfaces of bones contain grooves or ridges for nerves and blood vessels, prominences for muscular attachments, and openings for blood vessels and muscles. Articulating surfaces are covered with hyaline cartilage (Figure 63-4).

Blood supply to bone is maintained through the haversian canals, periosteal vasculature, and vessels located in the marrow and ends of bones. Bones are supplied with sensory nerve endings in the periosteum that connect with the central nervous system.

## Function

Bones have five functions:

1. *Support*—of body tissues as provided by the skeletal framework; they also give form and shape to the body.
2. *Protection*—of body organs; for example, the bony casing of the skull that protects the brain and the bones of the thorax and pelvis that protect the heart, lungs, and reproductive organs.
3. *Movement*—by muscular attachments to bone and by joint movement.

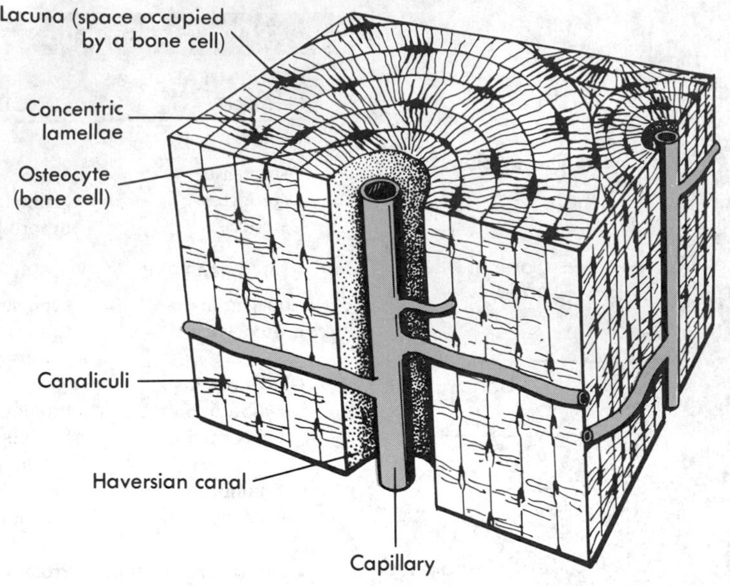


**FIGURE 63-3** Section of compact bone showing details of haversian system.

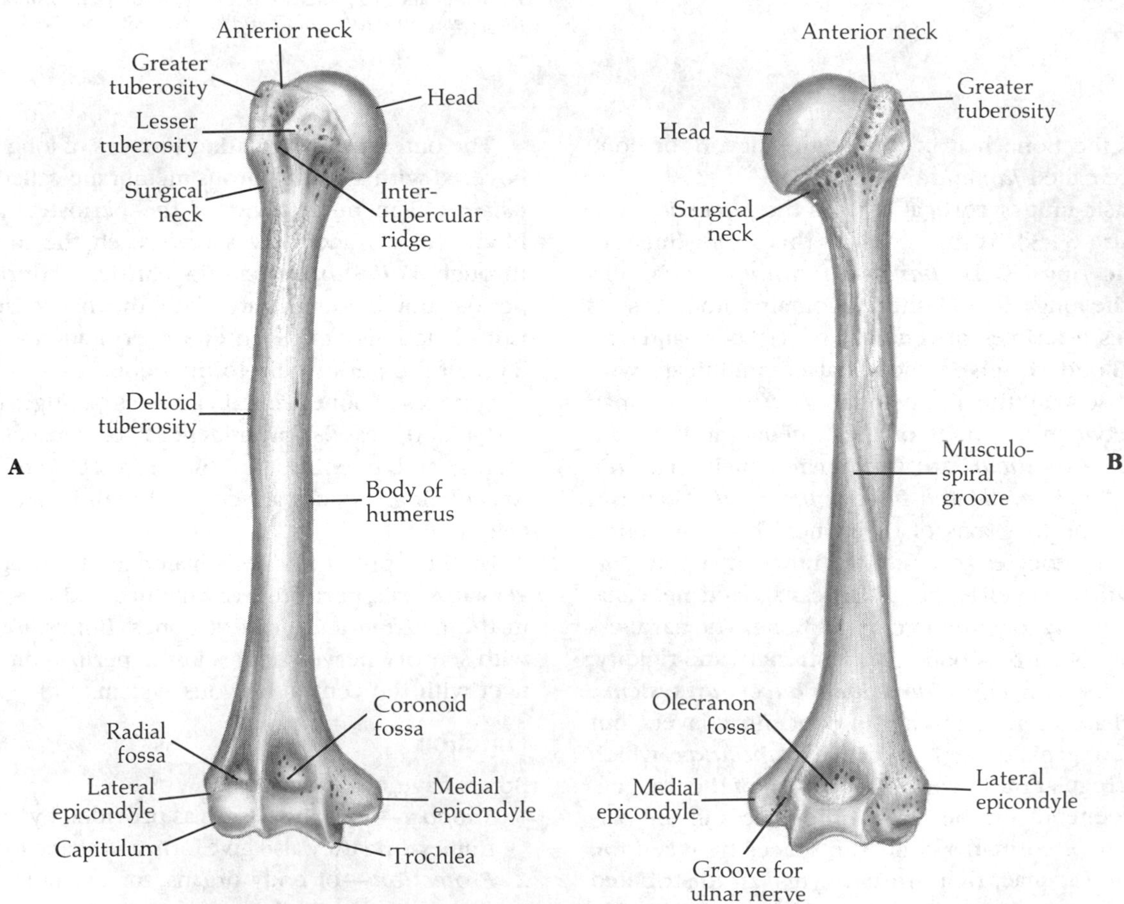


**FIGURE 63-4** **A,** Anterior view of right humerus. **B,** Posterior view of right humerus. Note groove for ulnar nerve, tuberosities for muscular attachments. (From Thompson JM et al: *Mosby's clinical nursing,* ed 3, St Louis, 1993, Mosby.)

4. *Hematopoiesis*—the marrow of some bones has a hematopoietic function. Normally, after birth red blood cell (RBC) production occurs only in the bone marrow (medullary hematopoiesis). Extramedullary hematopoiesis is usually a sign of disease. In adults, the marrow in the bones of the skull, vertebrae, ribs, sternum, shoulders, and pelvis produces RBCs. The hematopoietic function of bone continues throughout life. Blood cells are produced to replace those lost through disease, bleeding, and cellular aging. An increase in RBC production can be triggered by anemia, hemorrhage, infection, stress, and other disorders that deplete their stores. Medullary hematopoiesis is accomplished by conversion of yellow marrow to red, increased differentiation of daughter cells, and/or increased growth of stem cells.
5. *Mineral homeostasis*—bones store calcium, phosphate, carbonate, and magnesium, which are necessary for normal cellular function; approximately 99% of the body's calcium is stored in the skeleton.

## Growth

There are three types of bone cells. The primary function of *osteoblasts,* or bone-forming cells, is to lay down new bone. Once this is accomplished, osteoblasts become osteocytes. *Osteocytes* maintain the mineral content and organic elements of bone matrix. *Osteoclasts* resorb bone during growth and repair.

Longitudinal growth of the long bones emanates from the epiphyseal cartilage, which thickens because of rapid proliferation of the cartilage, which undergoes ossification *(endochondral ossification).* Growth in the diameter of the bone is accomplished as osteoblasts in the periosteum produce new bone at the outside of the bone *(membranous ossification).*

Bone formation begins in utero with the growth of cartilage. Bone growth and resorption continue throughout life. Bone has the capacity to remodel or reshape itself in response to alterations in its mechanical function. This response is in accordance with *Wolff's law: "Every change in form and function of bones or their function alone is followed by definite changes in their external configuration in accordance with mathematical laws."*

This process of formation and resorption depends on many factors including the following:

1. *Serum calcium and phosphate levels:* A primary component of bone matrix is calcium phosphate crystals. If serum levels are below normal, bone formation may be delayed.
2. *Vitamin D levels and activation:* Adequate serum levels of vitamin D are necessary for calcium to be absorbed from the intestine. Vitamin D must be activated in the liver and kidneys through the action of parathormone from the parathyroid gland to take part in calcium absorption. Vitamin D deficiencies can manifest themselves as rickets in children and *osteomalacia* in adults.
3. *Infection and inflammation:* These conditions can cause bone resorption.
4. *Hypophosphatasia:* Alkaline phosphatase is necessary for the utilization of mineral salts, necessary for bone formation.
5. *Activity and weight bearing:* Trabeculae within the bone develop and align themselves along lines of stress, and osteogenesis occurs along those lines. If the bone is not stressed, bone resorption occurs. The paraplegic or quadriplegic individual often experiences a reduction in bone mass *(atrophy)* as a result of inactivity and non–weight bearing status (lack of stress) on the bone. Conversely, a marathon runner or trained athlete may experience an increase in bony mass *(hypertrophy)* as a result of increased stress on bones. In older or inactive individuals, degeneration and resorption occur more rapidly than bone growth, which may lead to *osteoporosis.* Osteoporosis is characterized by thin, weakened cortices and trabeculae. Osteoporotic bones are more susceptible to fractures.

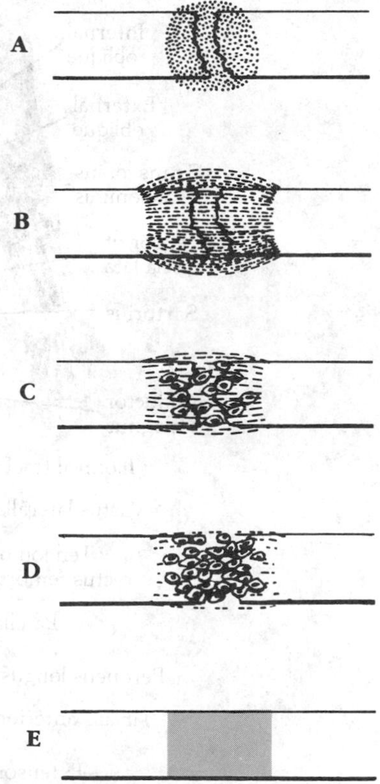


**FIGURE 63-5** Bone healing (schematic representation). **A,** Bleeding at broken ends of the bone with subsequent hematoma formation. **B,** Organization of hematoma into fibrous network. **C,** Invasion of osteoblasts, lengthening of collagen strands, and deposition of calcium. **D,** Callus formation: new bone is built up as osteoclasts destroy dead bone. **E,** Remodeling is accomplished as excess callus is reabsorbed and trabecular bone is laid down.

## Physiology of Bone Healing

Bone heals by a process known as *callus formation.* New growth of bone is called a *callus.* Callus formation proceeds in five general stages (Figure 63-5):

1. *Hematoma formation:* Because bone is highly vascular, bleeding occurs at both ends of the fractured bone. Increased capillary permeability permits further extravasation of blood into the injured area. Blood collects in the periosteal sheath or adjacent tissues and fastens the broken ends together.
2. *Fibrin meshwork formation:* Fibroblasts invade the hematoma, causing it to become organized into a fibrin meshwork. White blood cells (WBCs) wall off the area, localizing the inflammation.
3. *Invasion by osteoblasts:* As osteoblasts invade the fibrous union to make it firm, blood vessels develop from capillary buds, thereby establishing a source of supply for nutrients to build collagen. Collagen strands become longer and begin to incorporate calcium deposits.
4. *Callus formation:* Osteoblasts continue to lay the network for bone build-up as osteoclasts destroy

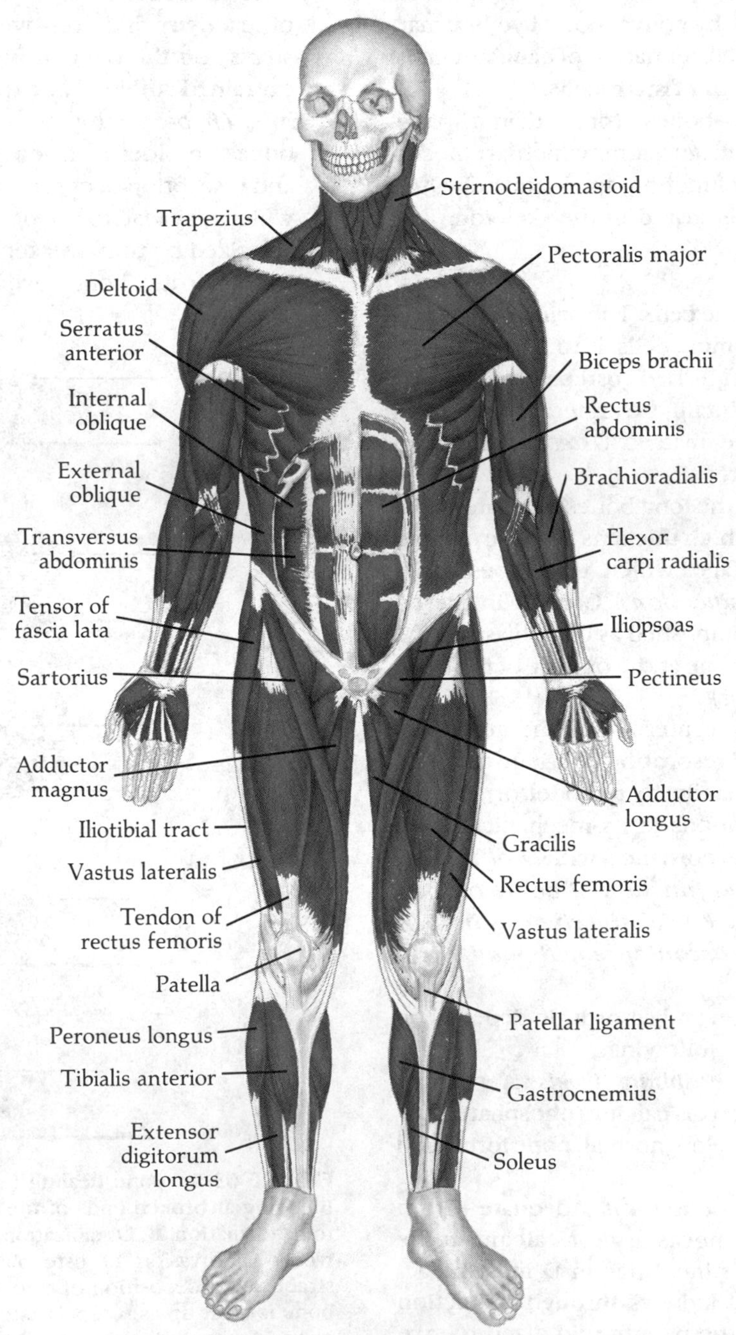


**FIGURE 63-6** Skeletal muscles, anterior view. (From Thompson JM et al: *Mosby's clinical nursing,* ed 3, St Louis, 1993, Mosby.)

dead bone and help synthesize new bone. Collagen strengthens and becomes further impregnated with calcium.

5. *Remodeling:* Excess callus is reabsorbed, and trabecular bone is laid down along lines of stress in accordance with Wolff's law.

Factors impeding good callus formation are (1) inadequate reduction of the fracture (see Chapter 64), (2) excessive edema at the fracture site impeding the supply of nutrients to the area, (3) too much bone lost at the time of injury to permit sufficient bridging of the broken ends, (4) inefficient immobilization, (5) infection at the site of injury, (6) bone necrosis, (7) anemia or other systemic conditions, (8) endocrine imbalance, and (9) poor dietary intake. If callus formation does not occur normally and efficiently, the resulting lack of repair is termed *nonunion,* or an *ununited fracture.*

## MUSCLES

### Types

Muscles are divided into three major groups:

1. Visceral (smooth, involuntary)

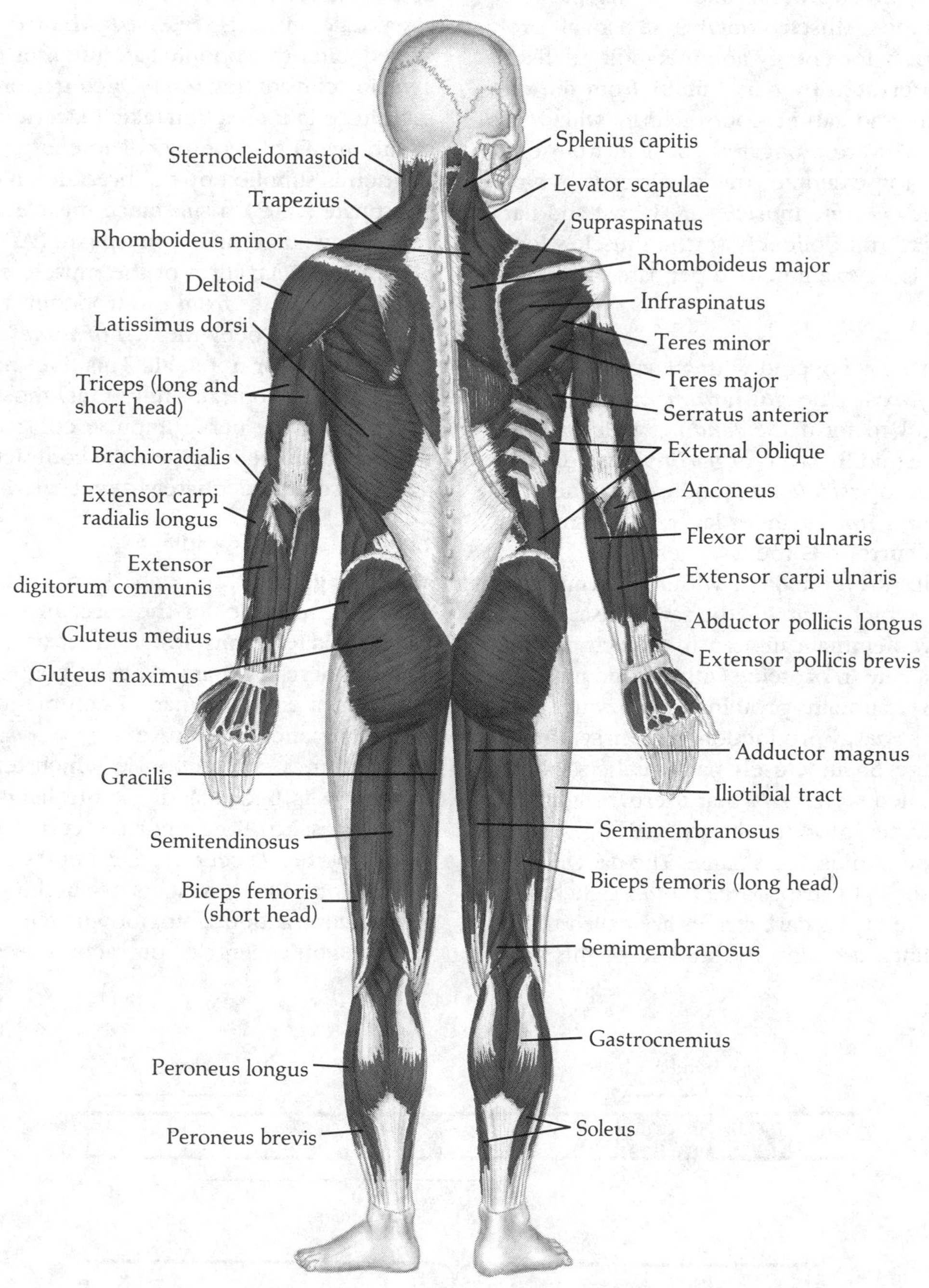


**FIGURE 63-7** Skeletal muscles, posterior view. (From Thompson JM et al: *Mosby's clinical nursing,* ed 3, St Louis, 1993, Mosby.)

2. Cardiac
3. Skeletal (striated, voluntary)

Visceral muscle, such as that in the blood vessels, stomach, and intestines, is innervated by the autonomic nervous system and therefore cannot be controlled at will.

The *cardiac muscle* found in the myocardium has the properties of automaticity, rhythm, and conductivity. It is controlled by the cardiac conduction system and the autonomic nervous system.

*Skeletal muscle* accounts for 45% to 50% of an average adult's body weight (Figures 63-6 and 63-7). Muscle is 75% water, 20% protein, and 5% organic and inorganic compounds. Muscle contains 32% of all protein stores necessary for energy and metabolism.[3] Skeletal muscle is innervated by nerve fibers from the cerebrospinal system and can be controlled by will.

*Fusiform muscles* are elongated and run from one joint to another, for example, the quadriceps, which extends the knee. *Pennate* muscles are broad and flat. Their muscle fibers run obliquely to the muscle's long axis. The deltoid is an example of a pennate muscle.[3]

## Structure

Each skeletal muscle is covered with a layered connective tissue called *fascia*. The *epimysium*, or outer layer, tapers at each end to form the *tendon*, which allows joint mobility. The middle layer, or *perimysium*, divides the muscle fibers into *fascicles*, or bundles of connective tissue. The *endomysium*, or inner layer, is the smallest unit of fibers and surrounds the fascicles.[3]

Skeletal muscles are contained within a membrane, the *sarcolemma*, which contains the sarcoplasm or cytoplasm. The sarcolemma can transmit electrical impulses and plays a role in protein synthesis and nutrient supply. *Sarcoplasm* contains proteins and enzymes necessary for the cell's energy production, protein synthesis, and oxygen storage. Small, closely packed fibers within the sarcoplasm, called *myofibrils*, that alternate light and dark horizontal stripes, produce the striated appearance that lends this type of muscle its name. The dark stripes are *A bands*, and the light stripes are *I bands*. Light bands crossing the middle of the dark stripes are called the *H zone*, and dark lines crossing the middle of the light stripes are called *Z lines*. Myofibrils consist of several sections called *sarcomeres* that contain actin and myosin, which are contractile proteins. Each sarcomere is a section that extends from one Z line of a myofibril to the next (Figure 63-8).[6] Bundles of muscle fibers (cells) make up the muscle itself.

## Function

Skeletal muscle provides controlled movement and maintains posture. This is accomplished by muscle contractions and work production, the end result being muscle movement. Muscular contraction is a complex process triggered by nerve impulses arriving at the muscle fiber. Calcium ions, released when the impulse is received, bind to troponin (an inhibitor of the molecular myosin-actin interaction). Once troponin is bound, the myosin-actin interaction takes place, and the sarcomeres of the myofibrils contract. The energy for muscle contraction is supplied by the breakdown of adenosine triphosphate (ATP), a substance muscle cells produce by combining adenosine diphosphate (ADP) with creatine phosphate. Relaxation of the muscle occurs when the calcium separates from the troponin[6] (Figure 63-9).

Muscle cells obey the "*all or none" law;* that is, they contract fully or not at all. This does not mean that the entire muscle contracts fully. Only those individual cells that receive the nerve impulse contract. Muscle fibers that are adequately oxygenated contract more forcefully than those not adequately oxygenated.

## Types of Contractions

The arrangement of the fibers within the muscle determines the capacity of the forceful contraction of the muscle. Skeletal muscles contract only if they are stimulated. There are many types of contractions[6]:

1. *Tonic:* a continual partial contraction that is vital in maintenance of posture
2. *Isotonic:* a contraction in which tension within the muscle is unchanged but the length of the muscle changes; can either shorten (concentric contraction) or lengthen (eccentric); examples of concentric contractions: lifting weights or climbing upstairs; eccentric contraction: going down stairs or putting down a weight; eccentric contraction uses less energy

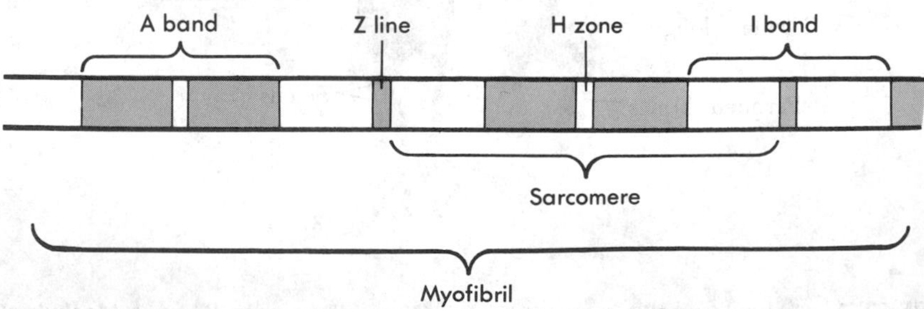


**FIGURE 63-8** Schematic drawing of structure of myofibril.

3. *Isometric:* tension within the muscle increases, but the muscle does not shorten
4. *Twitch:* a jerky reaction to a single stimulus
5. *Tetanic:* a more sustained contraction than the twitch, produced by a series of stimuli in rapid succession
6. *Spasm:* an involuntary contraction caused by stimulation of an entire motor unit
7. *Treppe:* stronger twitch contractions in response to regularly repeated, constant strength stimuli
8. *Fibrillation:* a synchronous contraction of individual fibers
9. *Convulsive:* abnormal uncoordinated tetanic contractions occurring in varying groups of muscles

### Mechanism of Muscle Movement

Movements of the body are produced by muscles pulling on bones; the bones serve as levers, and the joints serve as fulcrums for the levers. Most movements depend on several muscles acting in a coordinated manner. To produce movement a muscle acts as a *prime mover,* or *agonist,* as its reciprocal muscle, or *antagonist,* relaxes. Synergistic muscles contract at the same time as the prime movers, either to produce the movement or to stabilize a body part so contraction of the prime movers is more efficient.[6]

### Muscle Metabolism

Energy for a muscle contraction can be generated both aerobically and anaerobically. The two anaerobic processes are called the ATP-PC system and *anaerobic glycolysis.* The ATP-PC system is used for extremely short, explosive activities not lasting longer than 3 seconds. Anaerobic glycolysis is used at the beginning of sustained activity before the onset of aerobic metabolism and lasts for 2 to 3 minutes. During anaerobic glycolysis lactic acid accumulates within the muscle. When 60 to 70 g of lactic acid has accumulated, the muscle reaches exhaustive levels. The rate of lactic acid accumulation is directly proportional to exercise intensity. These two methods of energy production are very rapid and are valuable for quick bursts of energy to be used during intense activity. The aerobic method of energy production involves the burning of food stuffs. *Aerobic glycolysis* depends on the presence of oxygen and relies on the production of ATP from the oxidation of carbohydrates, fat, and protein. This method of energy production is used during prolonged activity.

Efficient muscle contraction depends on an adequate blood supply to and from the muscle fibers. Therefore skeletal muscle is highly vascular. Waste products resulting from the chemical changes that occur during muscle contraction must be transported to the liver to be resynthesized. When waste products are not adequately carried off, muscle fatigue and pain result. Conversely, oxygen must be transported to the muscle fibers to support the work of muscle contraction. Poor muscle work occurs when the oxygen supply is inadequate, for example, in conditions such as anemia, in which the amount of oxygen-carrying hemoglobin is reduced, or trauma, in which circulation to the muscle fibers is interrupted.

### Muscle Innervation

Adequate muscle contraction also depends on effective innervation. The cerebellum is primarily responsible for control of muscle movement (see Chapter 56). Every muscle cell is supplied with the axon of a nerve cell. Nerve cells that transmit impulses to skeletal muscles are known as *somatic motor neurons.* The neuron and the muscle cell it activates are called a *motor unit.* The axon of one somatic motor neuron may be divided into any number of branches and therefore innervates a like number of muscle cells. The fewer muscle cells innervated, the more precise (or fine) are the resultant movements. The actual contraction of the muscle is set off by the release of *acetylcholine,* a chemical contained in small vesicles in the axon terminal. When acetylcholine contracts the sarcolemma, it stimulates the contraction. This reaction takes place across a structure known as the *motor end plate,* or *neuromuscular junction,* where the muscle and the nerve are in contact. Damage to the nervous system at the cerebrospinal level or at any point in the nerve's course through the local motor neuron level will result in muscular dysfunction.

## CARTILAGE

Cartilage is a material composed of fibers embedded in a firm gel. It is a strong but flexible material and is avascular. Nutrients must reach the cartilage cells by the process of diffusion through the gel from capillaries located in the *perichondrium* (fibrous covering of the cartilage) or, in the case of articular cartilage, through the *synovial fluid.* The number of collagenous fibers found in the cartilage determines its type: *fibrous, hyaline,* or *elastic.* Fibrous cartilage (or fibrocartilage) composes the intervertebral disks. *Hyaline* cartilage is composed of chondrocytes (cartilage cells), type II collagen fibers in the matrix, and protein polysaccharide complexes and water between the matrix and fibers. Its composition gives hyaline cartilage its spongy and elastic qualities, which are crucial to preventing injury to the bone during weight bearing. Articular cartilage reduces friction in the joint and helps distribute weight bearing. Elastic cartilage has the fewest fibers and may be found in areas such as the external ear.

## LIGAMENTS

Ligaments are parallel bands of dense fibrous connective tissue that are flexible and tough. They connect the articular ends of bones and provide stability. Ligaments permit movement in some directions but limit movement in others, preventing injury to the joint. Examples are the medial and lateral collateral ligaments of the knee

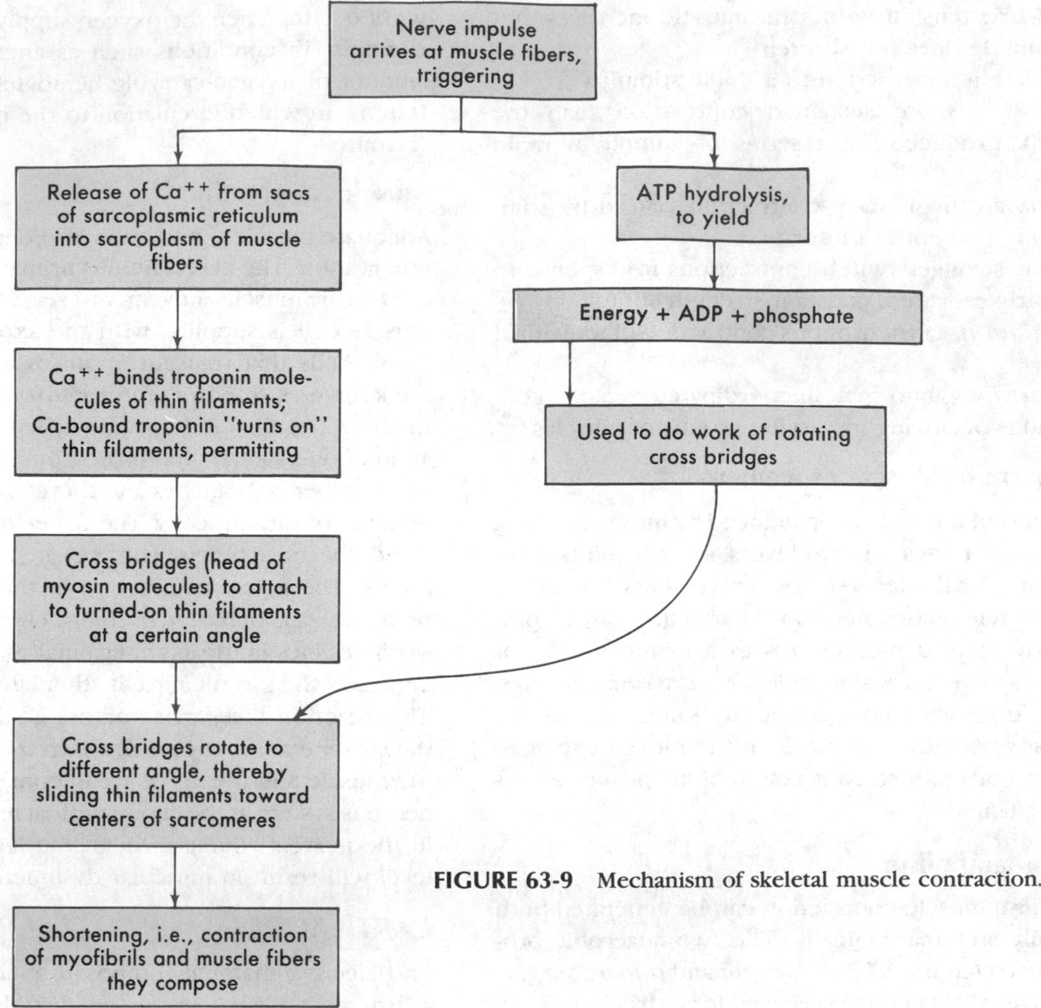


**FIGURE 63-9** Mechanism of skeletal muscle contraction.

that provide mediolateral stability to the knee joint, and anterior and posterior cruciate ligaments within the joint capsule of the knee that provide anteroposterior stability (Figure 63-10). Ligaments may also attach to soft tissue to suspend structures, for example, the suspensory ligament of the ovary that passes from the tubal end of the ovary to the peritoneum.

## TENDONS

Tendons are bands of dense fibrous tissue that form the origin and insertion of a muscle to a bone. The longitudinal arrangement of fibers gives tendons their tensile strength, while preventing damage to the tendon. The tendon is an extension of the fibrous sheath that envelops each muscle and is continuous with the periosteum at its other end. *Tendon sheaths* are tubular structures of connective tissue that enclose certain tendons, especially in the wrist and ankle. These sheaths are lined with a synovial membrane, that provides lubrication (synovial fluid) for each movement of the tendon (Figure 63-11). Ligaments and tendons may add extra stability to the capsule. The synovial membrane or synovium lines the nonarticulating surfaces of the joint capsule. The synovium is capable of repair because of its rich blood and lymph supply. Synovial membrane secretes *synovial fluid* into the joint capsule to lubricate the joint (Figure 63-12). Synovial fluid is plasma derived from blood vessels in the synovium. In addition to joint lubrication, it provides nourishment to articular cartilage. It also contains leukocytes that have a phagocytic action on bacteria and debris in the joint. A decrease in synovial fluid can lead to destruction of the articular cartilage.

## FASCIA

Fascia is a sheet of loose connective tissue that may be found directly under the skin as *superficial fascia* or as a sheet of dense, fibrous connective tissue making up the sheath of muscles, nerves, and blood vessels. The latter is known as *deep fascia.*

## BURSAE

Bursae are small sacs of connective tissue located wherever pressure is exerted over moving parts. They may, for example, occur between skin and bone, between tendons and bone, or between muscles. Bursae are lined

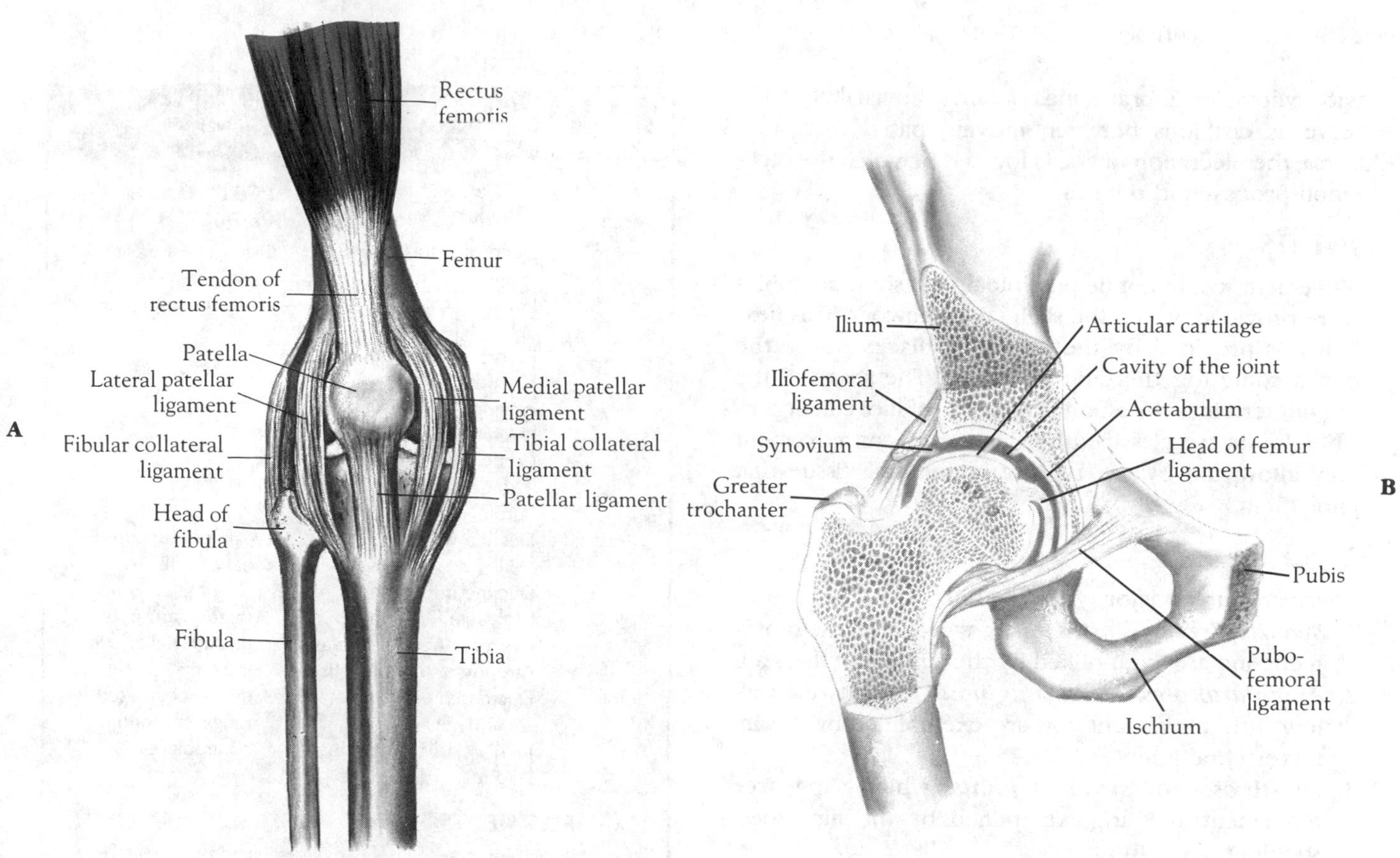

A
Rectus femoris
Femur
Tendon of rectus femoris
Patella
Lateral patellar ligament
Medial patellar ligament
Fibular collateral ligament
Tibial collateral ligament
Patellar ligament
Head of fibula
Fibula
Tibia
Ilium
Articular cartilage
Cavity of the joint
Iliofemoral ligament
Acetabulum
Synovium
Head of femur ligament
Greater trochanter
B
Pubis
Pubo-femoral ligament
Ischium

**FIGURE 63-10** A, Ligaments of knee joint. B, Ligaments of hip joint. (From Thompson JM et al: *Mosby's clinical nursing,* ed 3, St Louis, 1993, Mosby.)

Rectus femoris
Vastus lateralis
Vastus medialis
Quadriceps tendon
Patella
Tendon of sartorius
Tibia
Tibialis anterior
Gastrocnemius
Peroneus longus
Peroneus brevis
Soleus

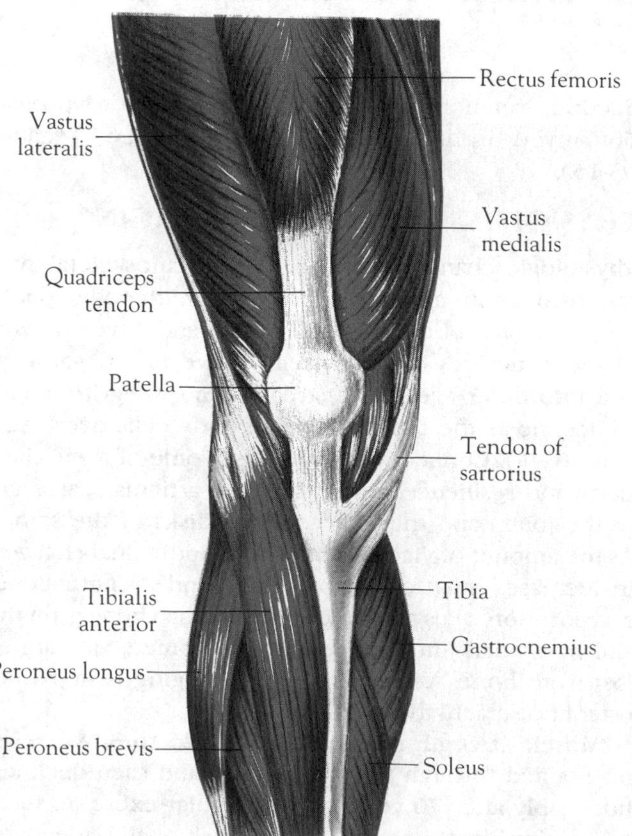

**FIGURE 63-11** Anterior view of tendons around knee joint. (From Thompson JM et al: *Mosby's clinical nursing,* ed 3, St Louis, 1993, Mosby.)

Joint capsule
Synovial membrane
Articular cartilage
Synovial (joint) cavity

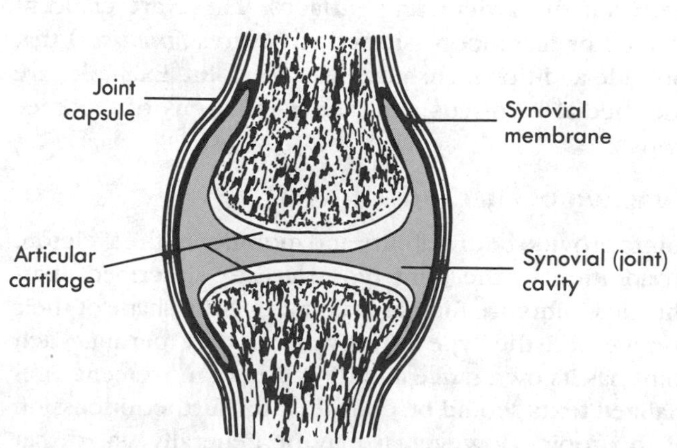

**FIGURE 63-12** Structure of diarthrodial joint, including joint capsule.

with synovial membrane and contain synovial fluid. They serve as cushions between moving parts. One such bursa, the olecranon bursa, is located bewteen the olecranon process and the skin.

## JOINTS

Movement would not be possible unless some flexibility were provided within the skeletal framework. This flexibility is provided by the joints, or places where the bones come together and articulate. The shape of the joint determines the amount and type of movement possible. Joints are classified by the amount of movement they allow and by the type of connective tissue that joins them.

### Types

There are three major types of joints:

1. *Synarthroses,* or *fibrous joints,* which allow no movement and are exemplified by the sutures of the skull
2. *Amphiarthroses,* or *cartilaginous joints,* which allow little movement and are exemplified by the intervertebral joints
3. *Diarthroses,* or *synovial joints,* which allow free movement and are exemplified by the hip, knee, shoulder, and elbow

The synarthroses and amphiarthroses may also be classified together as synarthroses, designating that both have no joint cavity but rather tissue (fibrous, cartilaginous, or osseous) grows between their articular surfaces. Because diarthroses are the joints that permit movement, they are discussed in the most detail.

### Structure of Diarthordial Joints

Each diarthrodial joint contains a small space, or *joint cavity,* between the articulating surfaces of the bones that make up the joint. Articular hyaline cartilage covers the articulating surfaces of both bones, allowing for the smooth, gliding motion of the joint. A *joint capsule,* or sleeve of fibrous tissue, encases the joint (see Figure 63-12).

Small pieces of dense cartilage may also be interposed between the articulating surfaces. These are crescent shaped or half moon–shaped structures *(menisci)* that provide additional cushioning of the joint. Examples are the medial meniscus and lateral meniscus of the knee joint.

### Function of Diarthrodial Joints

Joints provide both stability and mobility to the skeleton. In addition to the joint types already described, diarthrodial joints are further classified by the shape of their surface and the type of movement they permit. Each joint has its own range and direction of movement. Specialized texts should be consulted for further discussion of this topic. However, it may be generally stated that the diarthrodial joints permit one or more of the following movements: flexion, extension, adduction, abduction, rotation, circumduction, supination, pronation, inversion, and eversion (Figures 63-13, 63-14, and 63-15).

**BOX 63-1 Physiologic Changes with Aging**

| TISSUE | CHANGE | POTENTIAL PROBLEM |
|---|---|---|
| Bone | Decreased total bone mass<br>Impaired osteoblastic activity<br>Resorption exceeds growth<br>Erosion of haversian systems<br>Cortical bone changing to cancellous bone<br>Porous cortical bone | Osteoporosis, pathologic fracture, delayed healing |
| Muscles | Decline in strength past 70 years<br>Decline in number of muscle fibers<br>Decrease in muscle mass<br>Atrophy of muscle cells | Weakness, uncoordination, disuse atrophy, slow unsteady gait, poor posture, falls, contractures |
| Joints | Decreased elasticity of cartilage<br>Increased susceptibility to tears in cartilage | Arthritis, decreased range of motion, contractures |

**EXAMPLES OF ASSOCIATED NURSING DIAGNOSES**

- Activity intolerance
- High risk for impaired skin integrity
- Impaired physical mobility
- Self-care deficit
- Disuse syndrome
- Body image disturbance
- Alteration in comfort
- High risk for injury
- Ineffective breathing pattern

## PHYSIOLOGIC CHANGES WITH AGING

Physiologic changes occur in the musculoskeletal system throughout a person's life span. Childhood and adolescence are a time of rapid growth and development of the structures of the system. However, at maturity and into older age, tissue strength and integrity begin to decline as the total number of body cells decreases (Box 63-1). Connective tissues lose some of their elasticity and resilience, particularly the articular cartilage of the joints and the intervertebral disks of the spine. As the amount of vigorous activity an individual engages in decreases, muscles lose bulk, tone, and strength. Bone reabsorption takes place more rapidly than bone growth; and particularly in postmenopausal women, calcium is lost from bone. A universal effect of aging is impaired osteoblastic activity.[5]

Muscle strength reaches a peak at 25 to 30 years, is maintained through the fifth decade, and then declines noticeably after 70 years of age. Regular exercise, such as walking or swimming, and a nutritionally adequate

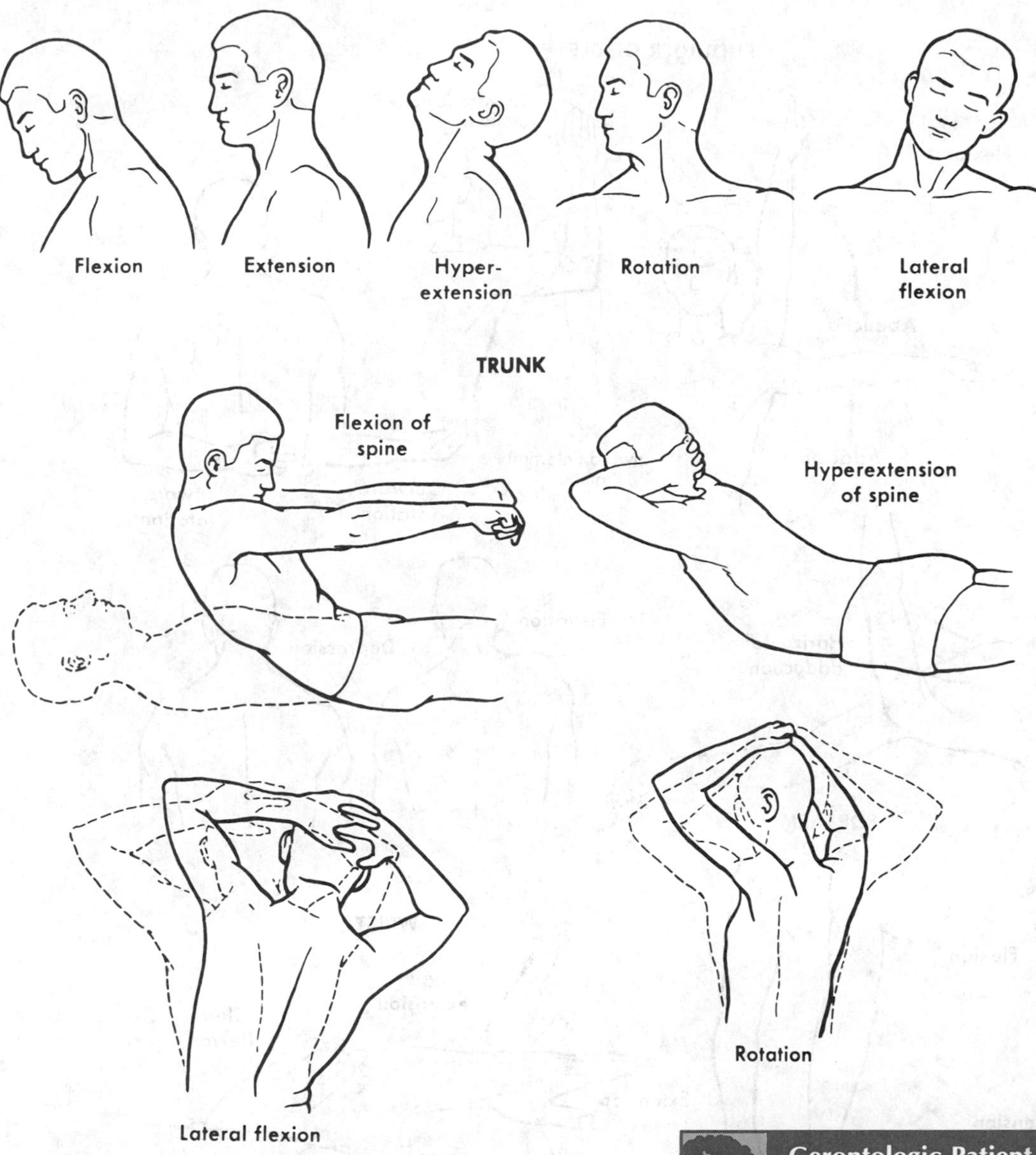


**FIGURE 63-13** Range of motion for neck and trunk.

diet can help reduce the loss of muscle mass and bone density associated with aging. With age the shoulders may become stooped and narrower. The knees and hips may be slightly flexed when standing or walking, because of pain associated with joint degeneration. Posture becomes stooped as the body attempts to compensate for changes in the center of gravity caused by lower extremity joint flexion and forward thrusting of the head, neck, and shoulders. With these changes, height decreases from 6 to 10 cm. Gait may become unsteady because of loss of muscle strength and coordination, and the individual is more susceptible to falls. (See Gerontologic Patient Considerations box for assessment of the elderly.)

### Gerontologic Patient Considerations

| OBSERVATION | RATIONALE |
|---|---|
| **General** | |
| Stooped posture | Change in center of gravity |
| Kyphosis | Osteoporosis of vertebral column |
| **Gait** | |
| Unsteady | Muscle weakness |
| Use of assistive devices | Loss of balance |
| Pain with palpation of spinous process | Possible compression fracture |
| **Joints and Extremities** | |
| Tenderness, erythema | Inflammation |
| Body enlargements, deformities | Osteoarthritis, rheumatoid arthritis |
| Flexion of knees, hips | Joint degeneration |
| Muscle atrophy | Loss of lean muscle mass, decreased activity |

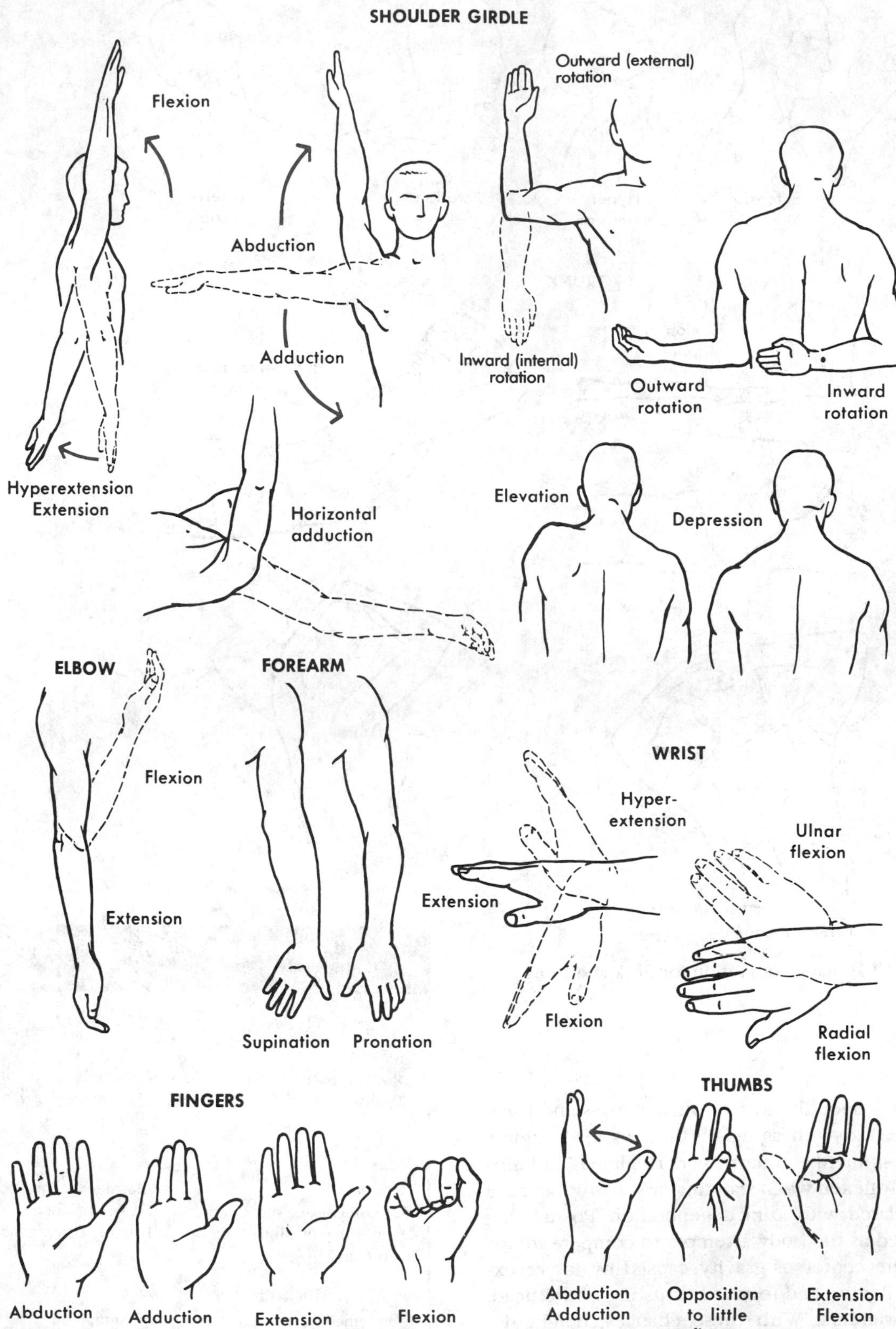


**FIGURE 63-14** Range of joint motion for shoulder and shoulder girdle, elbow, forearm, and wrist.

# ASSESSMENT

## SUBJECTIVE DATA

Plans for the care of any person with a musculoskeletal problem are based on a systematic assessment of needs, capabilities, and resources. A thorough assessment includes subjective data gathered from interviews with the person and family.

### General History

Interview the person, gathering the following data:

1. Age
2. Height, weight: any changes? If so, were they intentional?
3. Nutrition: dietary intake of calcium, vitamin D, minerals, total calories

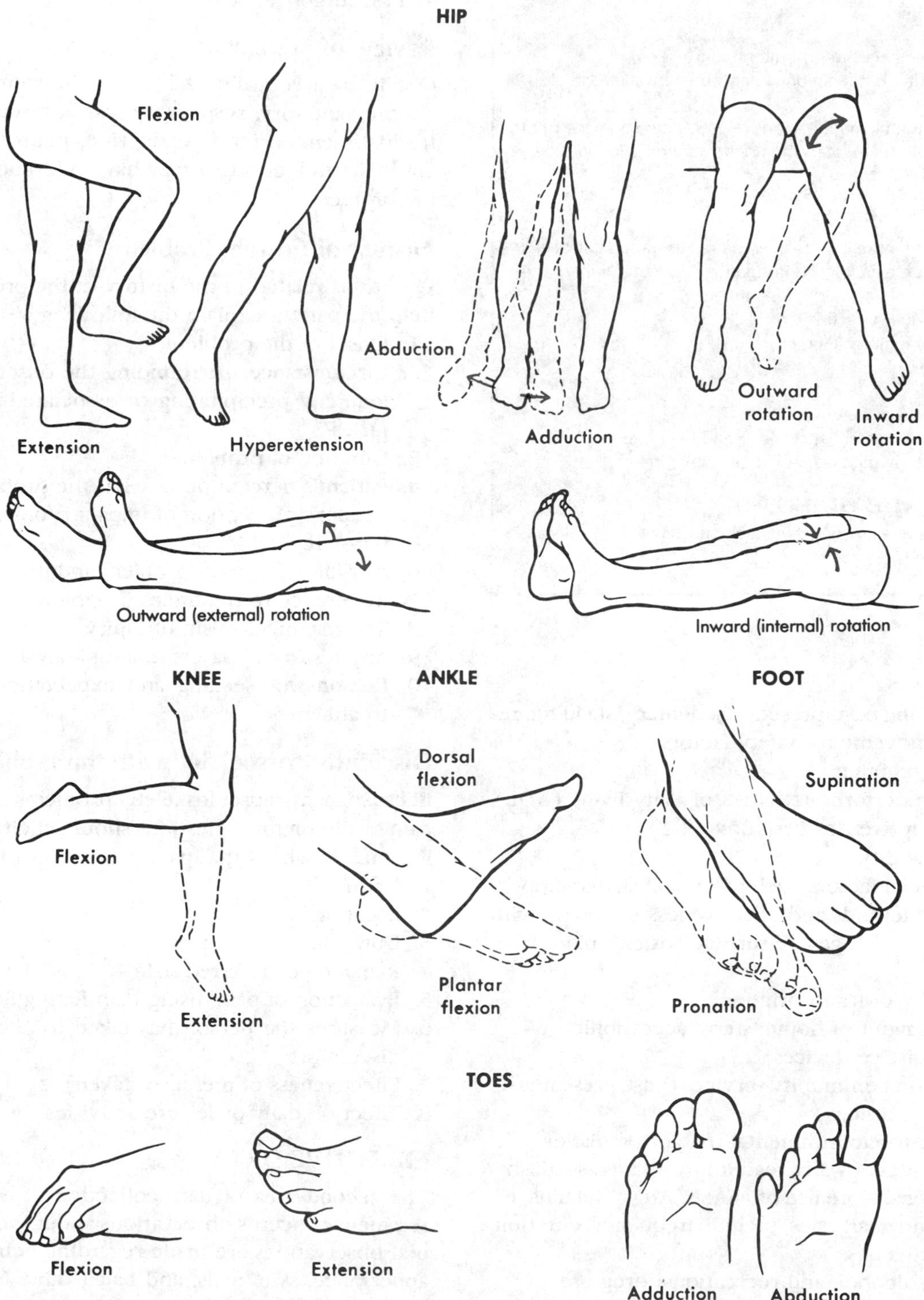


**FIGURE 63-15** Range of joint motion for hip, knee, ankle, foot, and toes.

**BOX 63-2 Assessment of Activities of Daily Living (ADL)**

**BATHING**
Independent
Uses assistive devices
Possesses ability, but function is performed by someone else
Lacks ability
Style of bathing—tub, shower, sponge, bed

**DRESSING**
Independent
Uses assistive devices (e.g., buttonhook)
Possesses ability, but function is performed by someone else
Lacks ability
Type of clothing or modifications (e.g., Velcro fasteners, front opening, split seam to accommodate cast, elastic shoelaces)

**TOILETING**
Independent
Special equipment (e.g., bedside commode, raised toilet seat)
Functional problems (e.g., constipation, diarrhea, urinary frequency, bowel or bladder incontinence)
Recurrent bladder infections
Special bowel maintenance programs

**SLEEP**
No problem, usual sleep schedule
Medications used to enhance sleep and their effect
Interfered with by pain or inability to move freely

**RELATING WITH OTHERS**
Note both positive and negative interactions with hospital staff, family, friends

4. Occupation (past, present): sedentary, standing, repetitive movements, safety factors
5. Exercise regimen
6. Ability to perform activities of daily living (ADL), use of adaptive devices (Box 63-2)
7. Transfer ability
8. Psychosocial factors such as marital status, support systems, methods and effectiveness of coping with stress, role changes, leisure activities, cultural beliefs
9. Availability of transportation
10. Physical layout of home: steps, accessibility
11. Use of assistive devices
12. Reliance on community services (past, present; usefulness of services)
13. Exposure to environmental irritants, radiation
14. Allergies: Record any reaction to iodine, shellfish
15. Medications: Note use of ASA, NSAIDs, vitamins, estrogen, and analgesics. Include frequency, duration, and effectiveness
16. Smoking, alcohol, and recreational drug use
17. Dominant hand

### Family History

1. Genetic disorders, abnormalities
2. Congenital abnormalities
3. Family history of arthritis

### Past Medical and Surgical History

1. Developmental abnormalities
2. Childhood diseases, illnesses, trauma
3. Chronic illnesses, hospitalizations
4. Past surgeries

### Review of Systems

Obtain data regarding history of integumentary, ophthalmic, auditory, respiratory, cardiovascular, gastrointestinal, genitourinary, endocrine, neurologic, or psychologic problems that may have relevance to presenting problem.

### History of Current Problem

Questions related to the history of the problem should help the patient explain the following:

1. Onset of the problem
2. Circumstances surrounding the onset of the problem: any precipitating or associated events or injuries?
3. Duration of problem
4. Patient's perception of what the problem is
5. Patient's perception of impact problem has had on life-style, ADL
6. Any efforts to treat problem and their effectiveness
7. Adherence to treatment programs
8. Trauma, mechanism of injury
9. Any history of paresthesias, paralysis
10. Reasons for seeking and expectations of current treatment

### Discomfort Associated with the Problem

Because many musculoskeletal problems are marked by pain or discomfort, questions should elicit the following information about that pain or discomfort:

1. Nature
2. Location
3. Duration
4. Radiating or referred pain
5. Evaluation of pain, using Pain Rating Scale
6. Measures the person has taken to alleviate pain or discomfort
7. Effectiveness of measures taken
8. Effect on daily or leisure activities

## OBJECTIVE DATA

The second area of data collection of a thorough assessment concerns observations about the person. General observations are made regarding behavior, general appearance, skin, nails, and hair (Table 63-2). In addition, data are collected regarding deformities, strength

**TABLE 63-2 Objective Data (Behavior, Appearance, Skin)**

| OBSERVATIONS | RATIONALE |
|---|---|
| **BEHAVIOR** | |
| Mental status<br>Orientation to time, place, person<br>Ability to understand directions<br>Capacity to retain information<br>Span of attention | Interventions must be based on the person's:<br>Ability to relate to reality<br>Ability to act on and retain instruction |
| Ability to relate to others<br>Is the person's attitude quiet, talkative, tense, guarded, negative, appropriate, inappropriate? | Ability to relate to instruction/intervention in a positive way |
| **GENERAL APPEARANCE** | |
| Age, sex | May relate to a specific disorder or attitude toward the disorder |
| Posture | May be characteristic of a specific problem, for example, kyphotic posture in ankylosing spondylitis (see Figure 65-19); guarding of head, neck, and shoulders following whiplash |
| Nutritional status | |
| Overweight | May indicate diminished ability to perform regular exercise or activity |
| Underweight | May indicate inability to secure or prepare nutritional meals or to carry out feeding activities adequately<br>May relate to specific systemic condition causing anorexia, nausea, vomiting, or malabsorption of food |
| **SKIN** | |
| Turgor (fullness) | Thin papery skin may indicate systemic connective tissue disease or long-term steroid use; skin is easily broken |
| Texture (feel) | Thick leathery patches over forearms, hands, chest, and face indicate scleroderma; ulcerates easily, especially over joints |
| Integrity | |
| Breaks in skin, ulcerations, reddened areas | Individuals with limited mobility are subject to skin breakdown from pressure over skin areas, which interferes with circulation; consequent breakdown is known as *decubitus ulcer;* possibility of shearing forces against sheets, chair surfaces, bedpans, or other surfaces tearing or abrading skin; accurate assessment of potential for skin breakdown is vital in planning for prevention |
| Impaired circulation to extremities | Increased risk of skin breakdown in distal extremities |
| Temperature | Warmth, especially over painful joints, indicative of presence and degree of inflammatory or infectious process within joint |
| Erythema over joints | Indicates inflammation and the need to keep joint at rest |
| Rash | May be present in systemic connective tissue disorders (psoriasis, scleroderma, dermatomyositis); initial observations provide useful baseline to determine effectiveness of treatment |
| Color change on exposure to cold | Change from *white* (resulting from arteriolar spasm) to *blue* (cyanosis caused by stagnation of blood) to *red* (warming and reactive vasodilation) present in some connective tissue disorders *(Raynaud's phenomenon);* requires specific interventions |
| Bruising | Often present following trauma and consequent to long-term treatment of connective tissue disease with corticosteroids; areas may slough easily and become infected (Figure 63-16) |
| Swelling of extremities or joints | In extremities, may denote prolonged dependent position, lack of activity, circulatory or renal impairment<br>In joints, may indicate presence of *effusion* (serous, purulent, or bloody fluid in the joint capsule); inflamed synovium (feels boggy): indication of need to rest joints involved |
| Bony enlargements | Indicative of disease process, for example, *Heberden's nodes* in osteoarthritis (hard, irregular swellings over the distal interphalangeal joints of the fingers) |
| Subcutaneous nodules | Indicative of rheumatoid arthritis: hard, mobile swellings commonly found in the subolecranon area |
| Bursal swelling | Indicative of bursal inflammation: felt as soft swelling over the bursa |
| Synovial cyst | Indicative of hypertrophy of synovial tissue, for example, *Baker's cyst* (swelling in the popliteal area, often extending into the calf) |
| Tophaceous deposits | Indicative of gout: hard translucent swellings over joints or in cartilage such as that of the ear |

*Continued.*

**TABLE 63-2 Objective Data (Behavior, Appearance, Skin)—cont'd**

| OBSERVATIONS | RATIONALE |
|---|---|
| Tenderness | |
| May be elicited by direct pressure, and graded by the amount of pressure required to produce discomfort | Degree of tenderness is usually in direct proportion to severity of inflammation or trauma, for example, in joint inflammation or injured soft tissue or overlying fracture |
| General hygiene | |
| Evidence of uncleanliness of body, clothing | May indicate inability to adequately carry out hygienic requirements (because this may be embarrassing for the individual, plans must be made to introduce self-help devices or to provide assistance in ways that will not be demeaning) |
| **NAILS AND HAIR** | |
| Poorly kept or diseased nails | May indicate lack of strength or inability to reach nails to care for them<br>Change in nail structure may indicate presence of connective tissue disease |
| Poorly kept hair | May indicate inability to lift arms to comb hair |
| Alopecia, scaling of scalp | May indicate connective tissue disease |

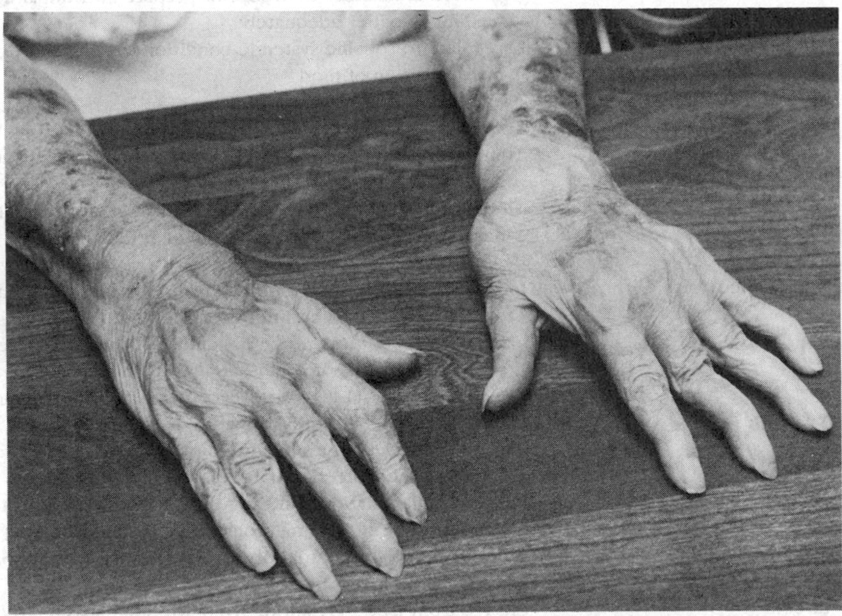

**FIGURE 63-16** Hands and forearms of an elderly woman with advanced rheumatoid arthritis. Note areas of bruising on forearms. Such ecchymoses are common in individuals who have rheumatoid arthritis and who take steroids for treatment. Handling of such individuals must be extremely gentle to avoid both bruising and potential sloughing of these areas.

and range of motion, ability to transfer and ambulate, and ability to perform other ADL.

## Inspection

Much information can be gathered even before the examination begins. Observe the patient's gait entering the examining room. Note the person's ability to stand, sit, and rise from a chair. If the patient uses assistive devices for ambulation or transferring, observe if they are being used properly. While ensuring patient privacy, assess the person's ability to dress and undress. These data will be useful in determining the individual's functional status. Observe the person's posture while standing erect, noting any abnormal curvatures of the spine. A gentle *lordotic (convex)* curve in the lumbar spine is normal, and a gentle ***kyphotic (concave)*** curve in the thoracic spine is also normal (Figure 63-17). Any exaggeration of these normal curves is considered abnormal such as a *lateral curvature* or *scoliotic curve* of the spine.

*Gait* (Box 63-3) is the manner or style of walking. An altered gait pattern indicates a pathologic process. Have the patient walk 20 to 25 feet. This distance is usually adequate to make an accurate assessment of gait. While ambulation is being observed, note the presence and type of limp, involved joints, ability to bear weight, balance, and the degree of deformity in the lower ex-

**BOX 63-3 Normal Gait Cycle**

| | |
|---|---|
| Stance phase | Begins with heel strike and ends with toe-off |
| Swing phase | Begins with toe-off and continues through heel strike |
| Double support | Brief period when both feet are on ground |

NOTE: Stance phase and swing phase are usually rhythmic and symmetric. When they are markedly asymmetric, alteration in gait is called a limp.

**BOX 63-4 Common Musculoskeletal Deformities**

**Swan neck deformity**—Flexion contracture of the metacarpophalangeal joint, hyperextension of the proximal interphalangeal joint, and flexion of the distal interphalangeal joints of the fingers (Figure 63-18); found in advanced rheumatoid arthritis

**Ulnar deviation or drift**—Fingers deviate at the metacarpophalangeal joints toward the ulnar aspect of the hand

**Valgus deformities**—Distal arm of the angle of the joint points away from the midline of the body
- **Hallux valgus**—Great toe turns toward the other toes
- **Genu valgum**—"Knock-knees" (Figure 63-19)
- **Talipes valgus**—Eversion of the foot

**Varus deformities**—Distal arm of the angle of the joint points toward the midline of the body
- **Genu varum**—Bowing of the knees (see Figure 65-23)
- **Talipes varus**—Inversion of the foot

**Scoliosis**—Lateral curvature of the spine

**Kyphosis**—Thoracic spinal curvature, the convexity of the curve being posterior

**Atrophy**—Reduction in size of an extremity or body part, for example, wasting of muscles so that they appear to lack the bulk of normal muscle; can result from lack of use or disease process, for example, polymyositis

**Hypertrophy**—Abnormal enlargement of an organ or body part; limitation of function may be associated with enlargement

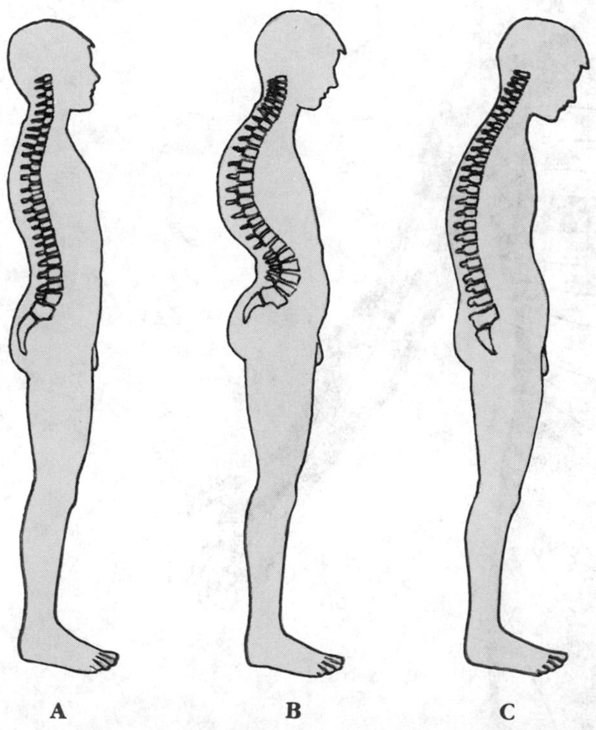


**FIGURE 63-17** **A,** Curves of spine in good posture. **B,** Curves of spine in slumping posture. **C,** Obliteration of spinal curves such as in early spondylitis.

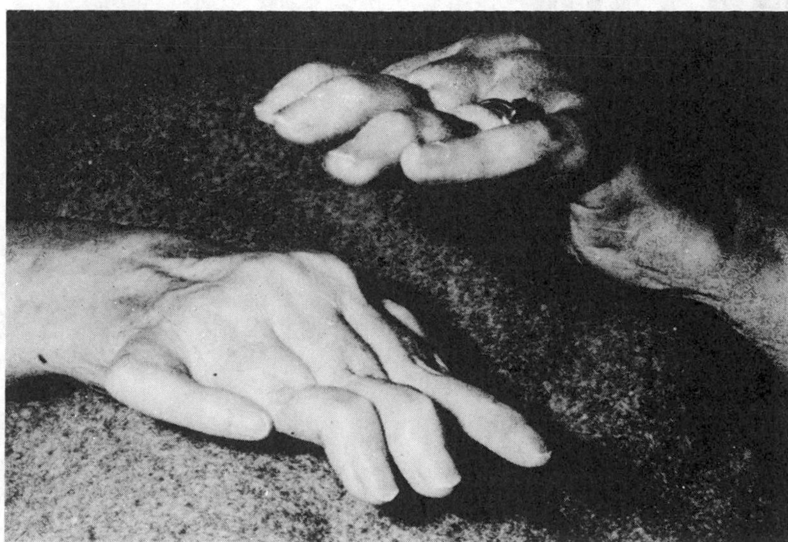

**FIGURE 63-18** Swan neck deformities of fingers in rheumatoid arthritis.

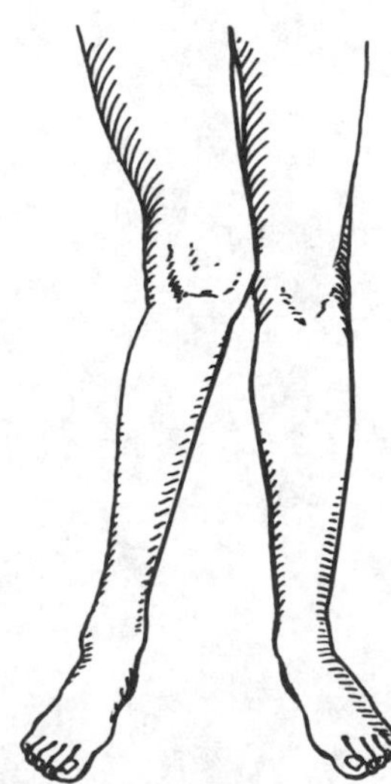

**FIGURE 63-19** Valgus deformity of knee.

tremities. Deformity of the lower extremities (genu varum, talipes varus, and so on) may not be as apparent when the joint is examined at rest as when weight-bearing forces are exerted across the joint. Further, in persons with significant upper extremity involvement, some consideration must be given both to the amount of weight bearing that might be expected from the arms and hands and to the type of assistive device that would be appropriate. For example, the individual with severe rheumatoid involvement of the hands might need a device that permits weight bearing on the forearms.

Other problems such as cardiovascular disease, res-

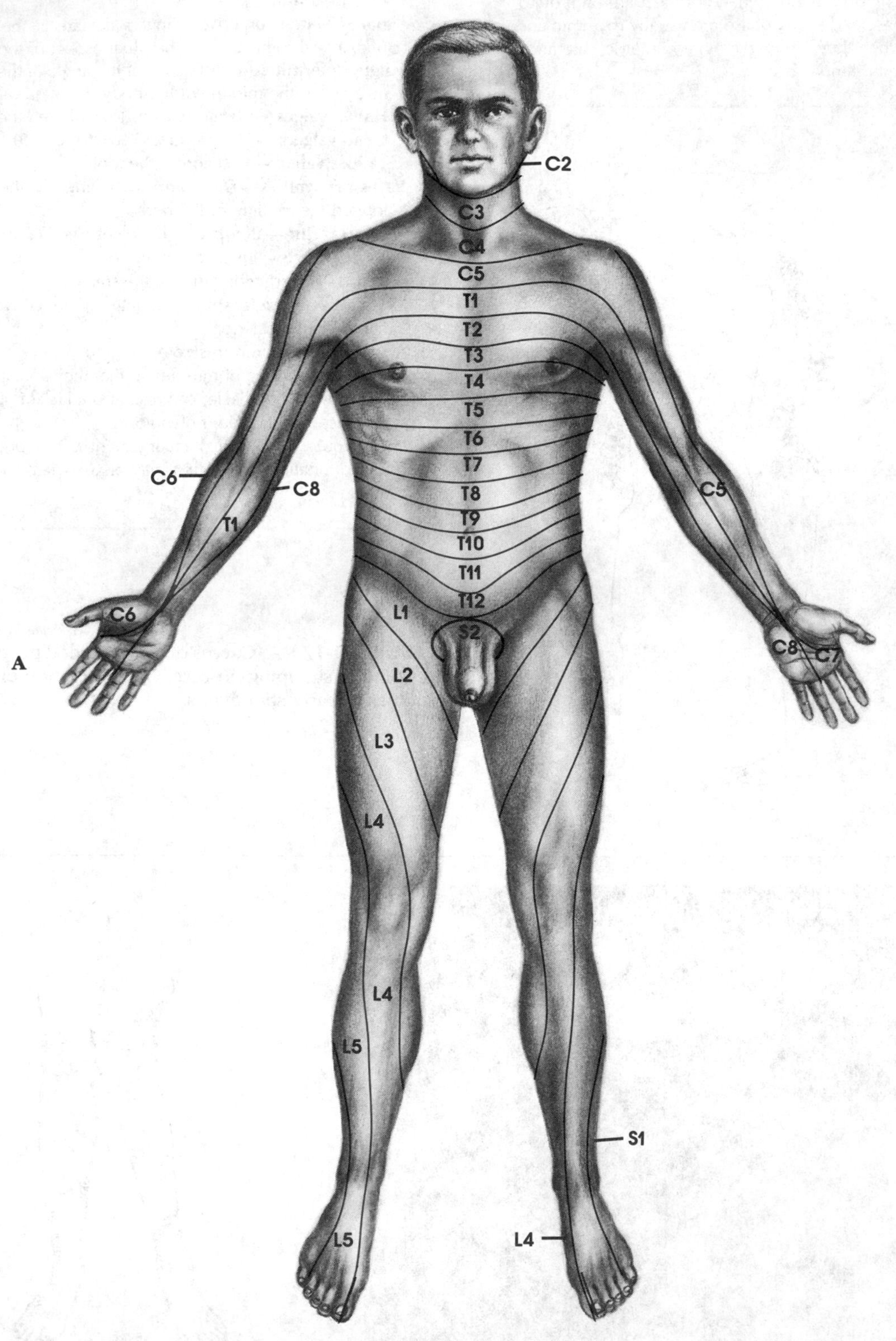


**FIGURE 63-20** **A,** Dermatomes, anterior view. (From Seidel HM et al: *Mosby's guide to physical examination,* ed 3, St Louis, 1995, Mosby.)

piratory impairment, or anemia may also affect ambulatory ability and must be taken into consideration during the assessment of ambulation. Assessment of transfer ability and ambulatory ability will help to determine a suitable level of activity for the patient. Observe all extremities for overall muscle mass, deformities, asymmetry, and masses. See Box 63-4 for a list of common musculoskeletal deformities.

## Palpation

In a head-to-toe fashion, palpate all bones, joints, and soft tissue for temperature, swelling, tenderness, pain,

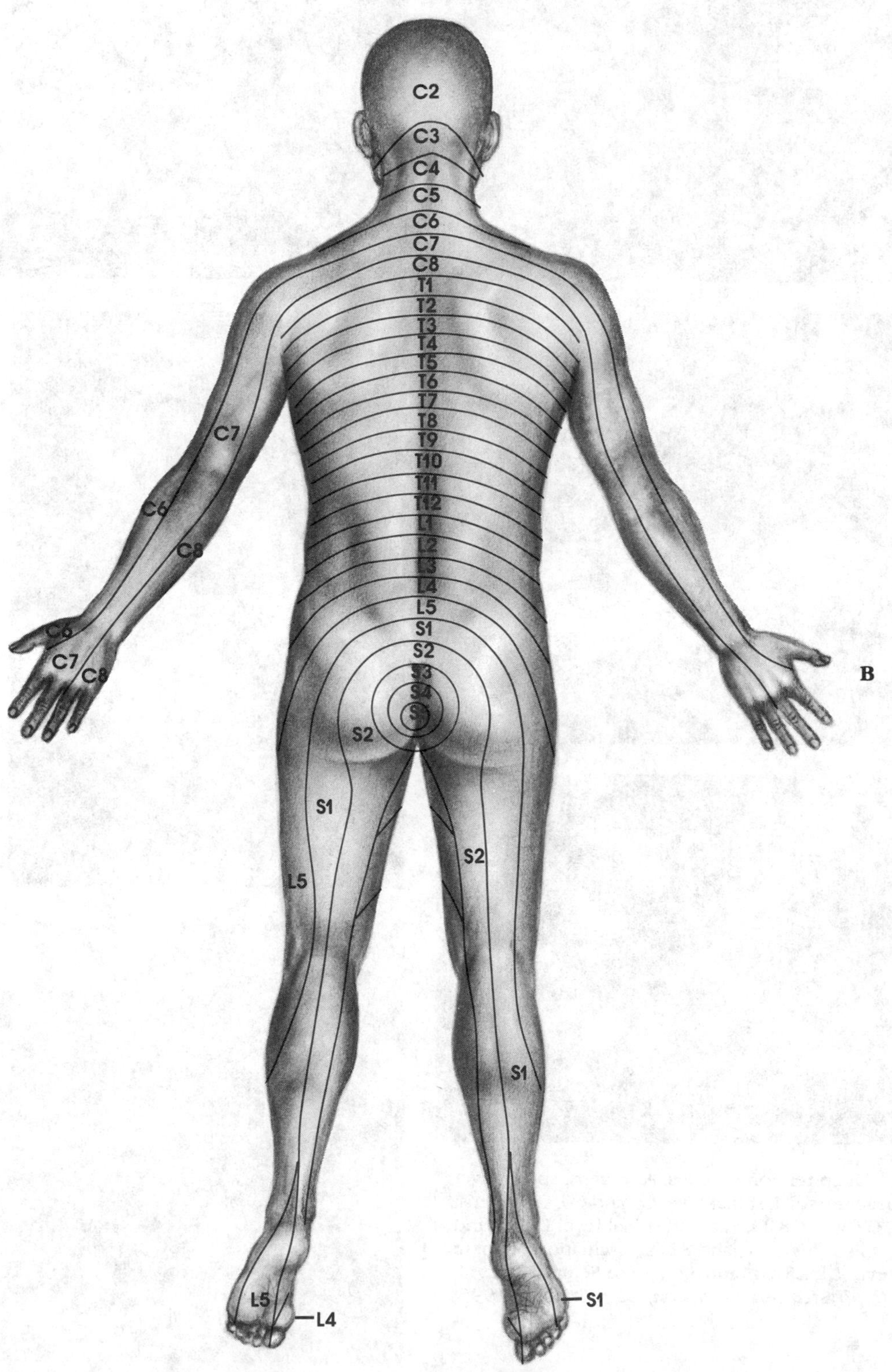


**FIGURE 63-20, cont'd B,** Dermatomes, posterior view.

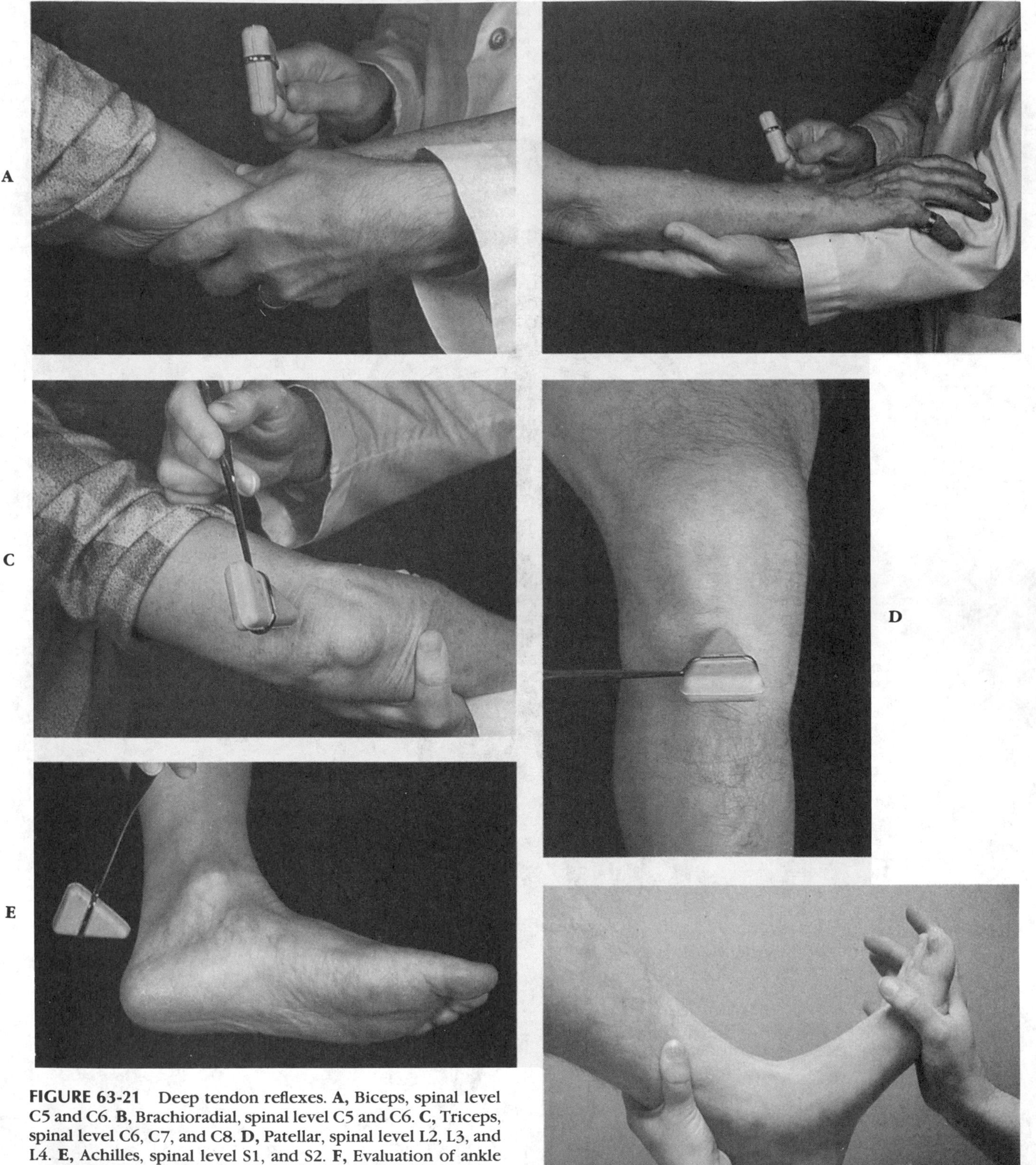


**FIGURE 63-21** Deep tendon reflexes. **A,** Biceps, spinal level C5 and C6. **B,** Brachioradial, spinal level C5 and C6. **C,** Triceps, spinal level C6, C7, and C8. **D,** Patellar, spinal level L2, L3, and L4. **E,** Achilles, spinal level S1, and S2. **F,** Evaluation of ankle clonus, spinal level L4, L5, S1, and S2. (From Seidel HM et al: *Mosby's guide to physical examination,* ed 3, St Louis, 1995, Mosby.)

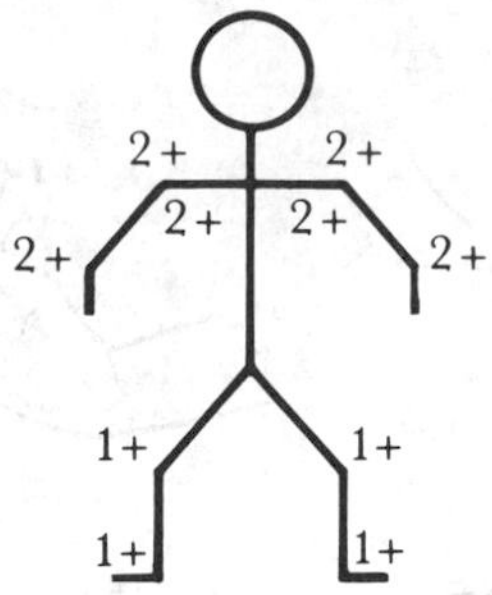


**FIGURE 63-22** Deep tendon reflex response. (From Seidel HM et al: *Mosby's guide to physical examination,* ed 3, St Louis, 1995, Mosby.)

**TABLE 63-3 Scale of Responses Used to Score Deep Tendon Reflexes**

| GRADE | DEEP TENDON REFLEX RESPONSE |
|---|---|
| 0 | No response |
| 1+ | Sluggish or diminished |
| 2+ | Active or expected response |
| 3+ | More brisk than expected, slightly hyperactive |
| 4+ | Brisk, hyperactive, with intermittent or transient clonus |

From Seidel HM et al: *Mosby's guide to physical examination,* ed 3, St Louis, 1995, Mosby.

or masses. Palpate the spinous processes and intervertebral spaces for tenderness.

## Assessment of Sensory Function

Assess the person's ability to discern light touch, gentle pressure, pain, and temperature, which will evaluate sensory innervation. Perform each test bilaterally and compare results. Check sensation in the *dermatomes,* which will show abnormalities in spinal nerve innervation (Figure 63-20). Also evaluate the person's sense of proprioception (position sense) in the extremities.

## Deep Tendon Reflex Activity

Absent reflexes may indicate neuropathy or a lower motor neuron lesion, whereas brisk reflexes indicate an upper motor neuron lesion. Again, be sure to compare bilateral responses. Figure 63-21 shows the location of tendons and their corresponding spinal level, and Figure 63-22 illustrates deep tendon response. The grading of responses and documentation of findings is shown in Table 63-3.

## Range of Motion

**Range of motion** is defined as the normal arc of movement provided for by the structure of a joint. Active range of motion is motion performed independently. Passive range of motion is accomplished with the assistance of someone else or with a mechanical device.

Before testing the muscle strength or range of motion of a joint, some assessment of the position of the person's extremities must be made. Positions that vary from the normal and that have had an acute onset may indicate the presence of fractures, dislocations, or ruptures of supporting structures. Typical of this kind of sudden change is the marked external rotation and shortening of the leg following a hip fracture; the inability to extend a "dropped" finger following rupture of an extensor tendon in the hand; or postoperative "drop foot," a complication that may occur following surgical procedures to the back, hip, or knee because of pressure on or stretching of the sciatic or peroneal nerve.

*Subluxation,* or partial dislocation of a joint, should also be noted. This is often a chronic problem, as in the shoulder of the hemiplegic person or in the wrist of the arthritic person. Its presence is usually accompanied by some loss of function or need for support. Subluxation of the shoulder may be detected by examination: a space can be felt between the head of the humerus and the glenoid cavity of the scapula.

Loss of strength or limitation of joint motion will result in some degree of loss of function. Loss of strength or joint range may be the result of a neurologic, skeletal, muscular, or traumatic disorder.

*Range of motion* is tested by having the person actively perform with each joint those motions that particular joint is capable of performing (see Figures 63-13, 63-14, and 63-15). In some instances when the person cannot actively move a joint, as with the person who has some form of paralysis, the joint may be passively moved. (Refer to Chapter 65 for discussion of passive range of motion and joint instability). When passive range of motion is performed, support must be given proximal to the joint being moved (Figure 63-23). Comparing the limitation of movement or instability present in one joint with its contralateral joint is helpful in differentiating normal from abnormal findings.

If a joint cannot be moved beyond a certain point in its range (e.g., a knee that does not extend beyond 30 degrees of flexion), it is said that the joint is contracted, or that a contracture is present. Contractures may exist because of soft tissue limitation (following immobilization for treatment of a fracture) or because of bony limitation (Figure 63-24). The location and nature of contractures can significantly limit function. For example, a person who can flex one knee only 15 degrees must climb stairs one at a time.

Crepitus, or a crunching or grating sound when the joint is actively or passively moved, is a significant indicator of a pathologic condition within the joint. This sound will also be heard if the two broken ends of a bone move against one another. *In the presence of a possible fracture, no attempt should be made to elicit*

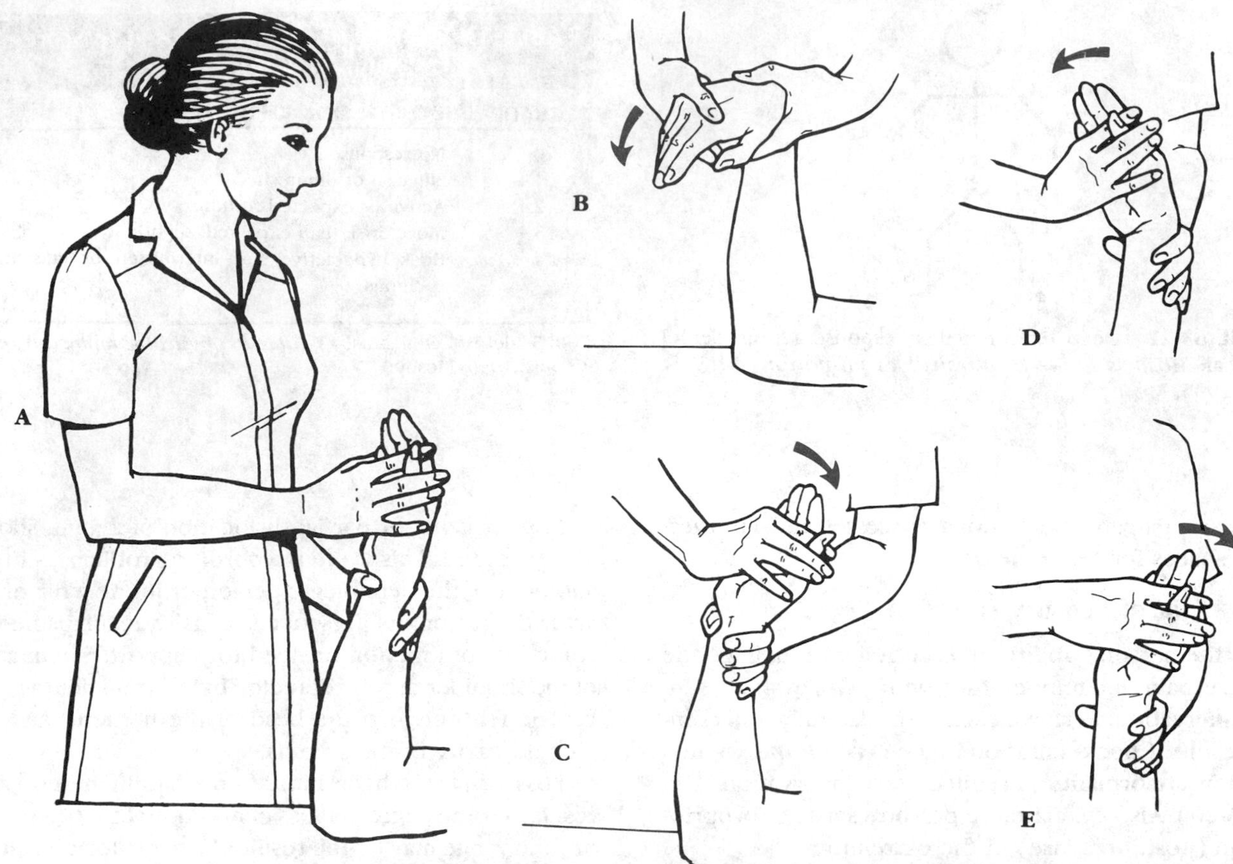


**FIGURE 63-23** Techniques of passive range of motion. With patient in supine position, upper arm is supported on bed. **A,** Forearm is supported with nurse's hand; hand is supported with nurse's other hand. **B,** Wrist is flexed forward. **C,** Wrist is extended. **D,** Wrist is moved to ulnar side. **E,** Wrist is moved to radial side.

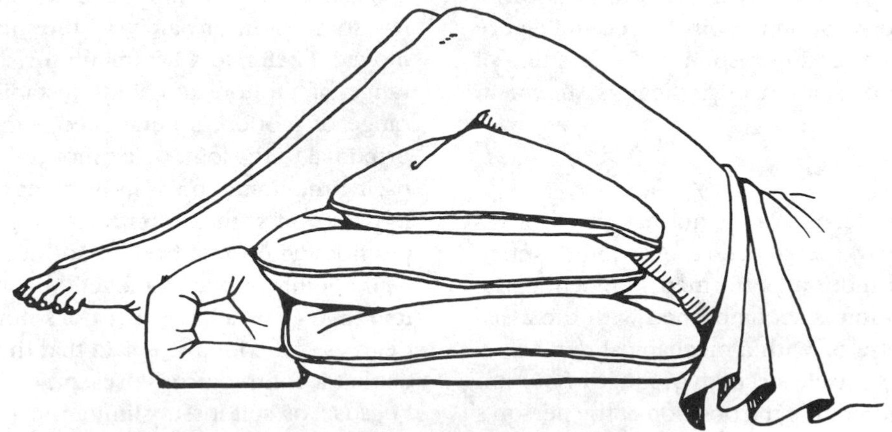

**FIGURE 63-24** Contractures of hips and knees in patient with rheumatoid arthritis caused by continuous use of pillows to support knees in flexed position.

*crepitus.* At times, grating within a joint may be felt, rather than heard, by placing a hand over the joint as it moves.

A *goniometer* can be used to measure degrees of joint movement, comparing findings with expected normal findings. It is important to remember not to forcefully move a joint if pain is encountered (Figure 63-25).

## Muscle Strength

The **manual muscle test (MMT)** is performed to determine the degree of muscular weakness resulting from disease, injury, or lack of use. The MMT rates the strength of muscles by their performance in relation to gravity and manually applied resistance. Factors such as gravity, stabilization of the tested part, proper position-

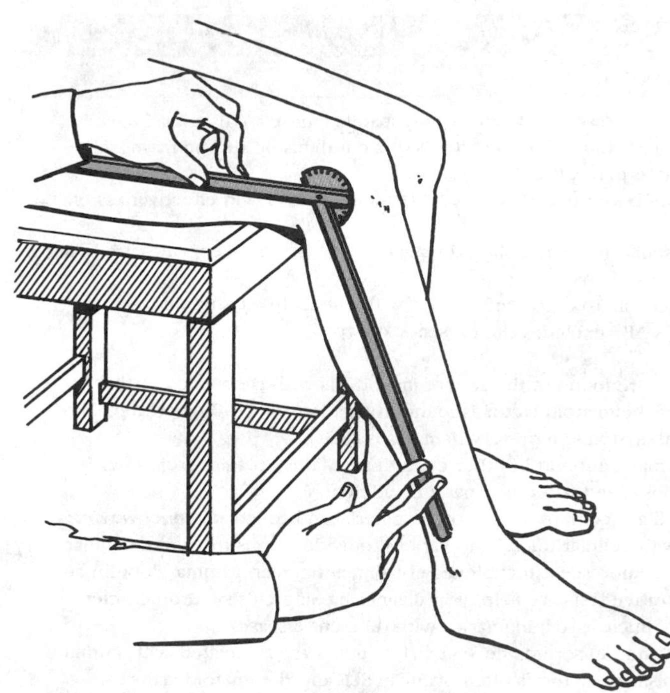

FIGURE 63-25 Use of goniometer in measuring joint range of motion.

ing, amounts of resistance, range of the joint, pain, and abnormal muscle tone must be considered in the performance of the test and can influence the test's objectivity.

Assessment of muscle strength can be accomplished by asking the person to contract a certain muscle group and resist while the examiner exerts an opposing force. Responses are compared bilaterally. If pain occurs, the joint is not forced past the point of pain. The presence of spasms is noted, and muscles are evaluated for *flaccidity* (lack of tone) *hypotonicity* (decreased tone), or *hypertonicity* (increased tone). *Atrophy* or *hypertrophy* of muscle mass is also noted. Findings are documented using a standard scale of measurement (Table 63-4).

Muscle testing is particularly helpful in determining on which muscle biopsy should be performed when confirmation of the diagnosis of myopathic disorders is required. Further, the initial test is used as a baseline examination against which later test results can be compared to determine progress or lack of progress in the treatment of myopathic and other musculoskeletal diseases. When muscle-strengthening exercises are indicated, the test will indicate the group of muscles that requires the most therapy.

The preceding tests of strength, dexterity, and range of motion are simple to perform; however, it must be noted that the person's ability to perform the movements described may be limited by pain rather than by weakness, lack of coordination, or joint limitation. It is often difficult to differentiate these factors. Although the effect of the pain is quantitatively the same as the effect of the weakness or limitation (i.e., diminished function), it is qualitatively different because treatment measures will be geared to relief of pain rather than to muscle strengthening. To further confuse the situation, the person with pain may have actual muscle weakness because of long-standing pain and consequent lack of use of muscles. It must be remembered that in performing these kinds of tests the person *must not be moved beyond the point of pain.* Pain indicates that something is wrong. Injudicious testing techniques can produce untoward results, for example, the fracture of an osteoporotic bone. The desired result of such testing is the establishment of a baseline of strength, motion, and dexterity from which interventions to assist the person to gain strength, regain lost motion, and increase functional capacity may be planned and evaluated. The reader is referred to a text on physical examination for a more in-depth description of these tests.

**TABLE 63-4 Grading of Manual Muscle Test (MMT) Scales**

| MUSCLE FUNCTIONAL LEVEL | GRADE | PERCENTAGE OF NORMAL | LOVETT SCALE |
|---|---|---|---|
| No evidence of contractility | 0 | 0 | 0 (zero) |
| Slight contractility, no movement | 1 | 10 | T (trace) |
| Full range of motion, gravity eliminated* | 2 | 25 | P (poor) |
| Full range of motion with gravity | 3 | 50 | F (fair) |
| Full range of motion against gravity, some resistance | 4 | 75 | G (good) |
| Full range of motion against gravity, full resistance | 5 | 100 | N (normal) |

Modified from Malasanos L et al: *Health assessment,* St Louis, 1990, Mosby.
*Passive movement.

## DIAGNOSTIC TESTS

As with other illnesses, diagnostic tests are employed to provide information to assist in diagnosing a patient's musculoskeletal illness and to aid in devising a treatment program for the patient. Elements of the patient's care may depend on the outcome of diagnostic studies. Some of the principal studies that may be performed on the person who has a musculoskeletal problem are described in the following sections.

### LABORATORY EXAMINATIONS

Laboratory examinations consist of two major categories of study, serologic and urinary, as described in Tables 63-5 and 63-6.

**TABLE 63-5 Serologic Tests**

| TEST | RATIONALE FOR PERFORMING TEST |
|---|---|
| Serum muscle enzymes<br>SGOT (serum glutamic-oxaloacetic transaminase)<br>Aldolase<br>CPK (creatine phosphokinase) | Enzymes can be elevated in the presence of primary myopathic (muscle) diseases. Elevated levels may result from degeneration of muscle fibers or from diffusion through a muscle membrane that has increased permeability.<br>Enzyme levels are an index of both progress of the myopathic disorder and effectiveness of treatment.<br>NURSING PRECAUTION: Intramuscular injections should be avoided when these enzymes are being monitored. |
| STS (serologic test for syphilis)<br>FTA-ABS (fluorescent treponemal antibody absorption) | False-positive STS results occur in 10%-15% of persons with connective tissue diseases, so test may aid diagnosis. FTA-ABS excludes the presence of syphilis. |
| Rheumatoid factor or latex fixation (reaction of rheumatoid factor antibodies with IgG [7S] gamma globulin) | Rheumatoid factor antibodies are found in the sera of individuals with rheumatoid arthritis. Test considered positive if rheumatoid factor is found in titrations of 1:40 or greater. May be positive in persons with systemic lupus erythematosus (SLE).<br>CAUTION: Rheumatoid factor may be found in other conditions, that is, in aging, scleroderma, acute pulmonary tuberculosis, and parenteral narcotic addiction. |
| Antinuclear antibodies (ANA) | Circulating antibodies, which are composed of protein material and called *antinuclear antibodies* and which react with cellular nuclei and various individual constituents of cellular nuclei, can be identified by fluorescent techniques utilizing antihuman gamma globulin labeled with fluorescein. Positive tests are helpful in diagnosing Sjögren's syndrome, scleroderma, and SLE. Pattern of nuclear staining varies with different diseases. |
| Serum complement | Protein substances that are found in serum and synovial fluid and are associated with immune and inflammatory mechanisms; low levels often occur in SLE and rheumatoid arthritis. |
| Erythrocyte sedimentation rate (ESR) | Increased rate of settling of erythrocytes is an important index of the presence of inflammation. *Normal values:* men, 1-3 mm/hr; women, 4-7 mm/hr |
| Hematocrit | Individuals with systemic connective tissue disease often have normocytic (normal RBCs), normochromic (normal amount of iron carried by RBCs) anemia, in the absence of any abnormal bleeding.<br>Individuals who suffer trauma or undergo major surgery to the musculoskeletal system sustain significant blood loss.<br>Symptoms of anemia (i.e., extreme tiredness, fatigue, weakness) are experienced when hematocrit drops quickly; acute symptoms may be absent if anemia develops gradually or is chronic. Individuals with acute anemia should not be physically stressed.<br>*Normal values:* men, 45-50 vol/dl; women, 40-45 vol/dl |
| Calcium | Immobility and bone demineralization (bone cancers, multiple myeloma) will show increase in serum levels. Rickets, vitamin D deficiency, will show decrease in levels. Malnutrition also results in decreased levels.<br>*Normal value:* 3.9-4.6 mg/dl |
| Alkaline phosphatase | Bone tumor and infections, fractures, Paget's disease, rickets, and other conditions that cause an increase in osteoblastic activity will cause an increase in alkaline phosphatase levels.<br>*Normal value:* 30-85 ImU/ml<br>In hypophosphatasia (characterized by a defect in bone formation), levels are decreased. |
| Phosphorus | Together with calcium, plays a vital role in bone metabolism. Conditions that cause an increase in calcium levels will cause a decrease in serum phosphates.<br>*Normal values:* 2.5-4.5 mg/dl |

## RADIOLOGIC EXAMINATIONS

### Bones and Joints

Radiologic examinations of bones and joints is imperative for the identification and treatment of fractures. It is also most helpful in determining the presence of disease (e.g., rheumatoid arthritis, spondylitis, avascular necrosis, and tumor), as well as the progress and effects of treatment on these disorders. Specialized texts should be consulted for an in-depth explanation of the variety of views that are obtained in such examinations and for the specific findings that are present in the various disorders.

It is important for nurses to remember that many patients are not able to lie on x-ray examination tables for long periods of time. In particular, persons with arthritis develop joint stiffness and pain if their ability to move about is restricted. Because radiologic examinations for individuals with rheumatic diseases are often quite extensive, careful thought should be given to the scheduling of these examinations. Very few of these patients can tolerate having all the required views of all the involved joints taken in a single session. Instead, 1 or 2 days of rest between shorter sessions may be re-

**TABLE 63-6 Urinary Tests**

| DIAGNOSTIC TEST | RATIONALE FOR TEST |
|---|---|
| 24-hour urine for creatine-creatinine ratio | In the presence of muscle disease, the ability of muscle to convert creatine is decreased, the amount of creatine excreted by the kidneys increases, and the ratio of urinary creatine to creatinine increases. Periodic studies are helpful in diagnosis and evaluation of progress of treatment of primary myopathies. |
| Urinary uric acid levels (24-hour collection)* | Helpful in diagnosis and decisions regarding treatment modalities for gout.<br>*Normal value:* should not exceed 900-mg uric acid excretion per day |

*NOTE: 24-hour urine collections must be accurate to facilitate proper diagnosis and treatment.

quired. Analgesics or local heat applications for relief of joint pain following x-ray examinations may be necessary for some patients.

## Systemic Radiologic Studies

Systemic radiologic studies such as the barium enema, upper gastrointestinal series, esophagram, and intravenous pyelogram are helpful in determining the extent of involvement of various internal organs (bowel, kidneys) in systemic rheumatic diseases. Discussion of these examinations can be found in Chapters 43 and 48.

## Myelography

A **myelogram** is a radiologic examination of the spinal canal. A radiopaque solution, (or less frequently, air) is injected into the arachnoid space. It is an extremely useful and frequently used test to identify lesions such as *herniated nucleus pulposus, nerve root involvement, spinal stenosis, tumor,* or other lesions that may encroach on the spinal canal. It can be performed on the cervical or thoracic spine but is most frequently performed on the lumbar spine.

The contrast medium used is either an oil- or a water-based solution. The viscosity of the oil-based solution (iophendylate [Pantopaque]) provides a good contrast medium for visualization of the spinal structures. However, its major disadvantage is that it must be removed as completely as possible following the examination or it may cause *arachnoiditis* or severe headaches.

These limitations led to the development of the water-soluble, nonionic solutions that are widely used today (metrizamide [Amipaque] and iohexol [Omnipaque]). Water-based dyes are less viscous and fill the canal and narrow spaces easily, allowing good visualization of the structures. They are absorbed into the cerebrospinal fluid and need not be removed following the procedure. Major adverse effects are seizures, nausea, and vomiting following the procedure.

Patient education is vital before the procedure. A thorough explanation of what will happen before, during, and after the procedure may help allay fears and clarify any misconceptions regarding myelography.

Myelography is an outpatient procedure done in the radiology department by a radiologist with the assistance of a radiology technician. The patient is admitted to the hospital the morning of the procedure. Following a clear liquid breakfast, the patient may have nothing by mouth. A careful history should be taken, noting any previous allergic reactions to other contrast agents, iodine, or shellfish. If a water-based solution is being used, the patient may not take amphetamines, phenothiazides, or tricyclic antidepressants for 12 hours before the procedure. These drugs lower the seizure threshold.

If necessary, a sedative may be prescribed before the procedure. In the radiology department, the patient is transferred to the x-ray table and placed in the prone position. Local anesthetic is injected first, and then a needle is introduced into the spinal canal. Approximately 10 ml of cerebrospinal fluid (CSF) is withdrawn and sent to the laboratory for analysis. The contrast medium is then injected, and the x-ray table is moved and tilted, allowing the dye to fill the canal as films are taken, The procedure may take up to 1 hour. Frequently, a computed tomography (CT) scan follows the myelography.

Following myelography, the patient is returned to his or her room. Fluids are encouraged to replace the removed CSF and to aid in the excretion of the contrast medium. If an oil-based dye was used, the patient is kept flat in bed for approximately 8 hours. When a water-soluble dye was used, bedrest is maintained, with the head of the bed elevated 30 degrees for 24 hours. Diet is resumed as tolerated, and fluids are encouraged, regardless of which dye was used. The patient should be observed for any reactions to the contrast agent. Headaches, nausea, and vomiting are the most common side effects. *Neurovascular checks* are performed hourly. The lumbar puncture site will be covered with a small adhesive strip and should be observed for any bleeding. The patient can be discharged the afternoon of the procedure and can gradually resume normal activities. Lifting or strenuous activity should be avoided for 24 hours.

The patient should be taught to observe the puncture site for any drainage, swelling, or signs of infection. Anticonvulsants or other medications withheld before the procedure may be resumed in 48 hours. The patient should be instructed to contact the physician if persistent nausea or vomiting develops.

## Arthrography

**Arthrography** permits visualization of structures within the joint that are not normally seen on routine radiographic films. The joint cavity is injected with radiopaque dye, air, or both. The latter is called a *double-contrast arthrogram.* The dye or air serves as a contrast medium against which the outlines of soft tissue components of the joint may be seen. *Tears of the menisci* and internal *derangements of the joint* such as *ligament disruption* and *synovial cysts* can be diagnosed with the aid of arthrograms. Before the examination, the patient should be checked for allergies to iodine or seafood. Patients may experience pain while the joint is expanded by the dye or air, and local anesthetic may be injected before the examination. Analgesics are prescribed after the examination. The patient should be instructed to watch for *redness, edema,* or *unusual pain in the joint* after the procedure.

## Radioisotope Bone Scans

Radioisotope *bone scans* are performed primarily to demonstrate the presence of metastatic disease, tumors, infection (osteomyelitis), and other conditions with increased bone activity. Intravenously injected sodium pertechnetate $^{99m}$Tc (technetium) is the isotope most frequently used in this study. The $^{99m}$Tc concentrates in areas of osteoblastic activity involved in the exchange of calcium. *Hot spots* on the scan indicate areas of increased bone turnover, as in the case of fractures, bone healing, and inflammatory responses. *Cold spots* show areas where there is no bone activity, as in lytic lesions. Lesions may be visualized on bone scans as early as 6 months before there is evidence of the lesions on routine x-ray films. Bone scans are frequently used to rule out bony metastases from the prostate, breast, and lung.

Technetium scans are also of some use in determining the degree of parotid gland involvement in Sjögren's syndrome. The uptake, concentration, and excretion of the isotope by the major salivary glands are measured by a technique called *sequential scintiphotography.*[4]

Persons being prepared for these procedures should know that the procedures will not cause them pain and that the isotopes will not harm them but that they may have to remain quietly in one position for 1 hour or more. The radioisotope will be injected intravenously about 2 hours before scanning. The patient is encouraged to drink fluids before the scan and is assessed for seafood or iodine allergies before the examination. Procedures using barium or iodine are not scheduled before bone scan, because these substances interfere with scanning. The radioisotope is excreted by the kidneys.

## Computed Tomography

*Tomography* is an x-ray technique by which detailed images of "slices" of tissue are obtained by focusing x-ray beams at predetermined planes or depths of the tissue being studied. Detailed images of the structures at that level are produced, while details of structures surrounding that level are blurred or eliminated. **Computed tomography** (CT scanning) is tomography employing a computer to compose a picture of the tissue being studied. A series of x-ray beams is rotated; 1 degree at a time, around the specific area being examined. With each rotation, a picture is generated that depicts the difference in tissue density. These pictures are very clear and detailed.

The scan picks up disruptions in normal structures. The procedure can be used in diagnosing *spinal pathologic conditions* and *tumors* and in *evaluating the hip before custom joint replacement.* The procedure is noninvasive and does not require repositioning of the patient as does conventional tomography. CT frequently follows myelography in diagnosing spinal pathologic conditions. Patients who are claustrophobic may have some difficulty tolerating the procedure, because it does require lying in a cylindric metal scanner for up to 1 hour.

## Magnetic Resonance Imaging

**Magnetic resonance imaging** (MRI) is a scanning technique that produces tomographic images by using magnetic forces rather than x-ray beams. The patient lies on a nonmagnetic scanning table that slides, head first, into a giant cylindric magnet. The magnet causes the body's atomic protons to line up and spin in the same direction. A radio frequency signal is beamed into the magnetic field, causing the protons to move out of alignment. When the signal stops, the protons move back into alignment and release energy. A receiver coil measures the energy released by the movement of the protons and the time it takes for the protons to return to their aligned position. These measurements provide information regarding the type of tissue in which the protons lie, as well as the condition of the tissue. A computer uses this information to construct an image on a television screen, showing the distribution of protons of certain atoms (usually hydrogen); and the television image can be recorded on film or magnetic tape. The images obtained by MRI are exquisitely clear, more so than CT images. Some physicians prefer MRI to myelography because of its clarity and precision.

Patients being prepared for MRI should know that the procedure is painless and that there is no special preparation for the test. However, because a magnetic field is used, the patient will be asked to remove any metallic objects, such as jewelry, hairpins, credit cards, and nonpermanent dentures. Patients who have cardiac pacemakers or intracranial vascular aneurysm clips are excluded from MRI. Persons who have metal implants cannot have that area scanned. As with CT scanning, patients who are claustrophobic may have difficulty being placed in the scanner. Sometimes medication such as diazepam (Valium) is prescribed to help the patient relax. During the scan, the patient will hear the hum of the machine, a loud thump when the radio waves are turned on and off, and other machinelike noises. The thumping can be particularly annoying to patients, and many are frightened by it if they are not told it will happen. Scanning time is usually 30 to 90 minutes.

### Diskography

A **diskogram** is a radiologic procedure using contrast medium to evaluate the integrity of the intervertebral disks. It is performed on an outpatient basis in the operating room, with the use of fluoroscopy. The patient is placed in the prone position, and local anesthetic is administered. The patient may require additional sedation as well, because the procedure can be quite uncomfortable. Needle position is confirmed by fluoroscopy; then contrast medium and saline are injected into the disk space. If a pathologic condition is present, injection of the saline reproduces the patient's back and/or leg pain. Despite the accuracy of myelography, CT, and MRI, the diskogram is still a useful diagnostic tool because the ability to reproduce the patient's symptoms may aid the surgeon in differential diagnosis, especially when several vertebral levels are involved.

## SPECIAL TESTS

### Electromyography

Electromyography measures the electrical activity of muscles; and an **electromyogram (EMG)** is a recording of the variations of electrical potentials (voltage) detected by a needle electrode inserted into skeletal muscle. The electrical activity can be heard over a loud speaker and viewed on an oscilloscope and on a graph at the same time. No electrical activity can be detected

**TABLE 63-7 Types of Biopsies**

| ORGAN | TEST(S) PERFORMED | POSITIVE RESULTS | NURSING CONSIDERATIONS |
|---|---|---|---|
| Skin (punch biopsy) | Immunofluorescent staining—tissue is washed with solution of fluorescein-labeled antihuman gamma globulin antibody | Band of immunofluorescence at epidermal-dermal junction, indicating presence of rheumatic disease (that is, scleroderma, SLE, psoriatic arthritis) | Biopsy site kept clean and dry with small adhesive bandage until scab develops; hydrogen peroxide (3%) used to cleanse open area prn; only very mild discomfort experienced by patient |
| Muscle (operative procedure) | Histochemical staining | Tissue reveals features of LMN disease, degeneration, inflammatory reaction as in polymyositis, or involvement of specific fibers indicating primary myopathic disease | Patient instructed and prepared for surgery; patient monitored per postanesthesia routine (local or general); mild to moderate pain and stiffness in biopsy area; routine activity encouraged within 24 hours to avoid undue stiffness; dressings changed as necessary |
| Synovium (closed—performed with needle; open—performed in surgery) | Histologic examination—synovial fluid obtained at the same time; may be cultured to determine presence of infection | Differentiates various forms of arthritis | Patient instructed about procedure; patient may require postanesthesia monitoring; strict asepsis observed throughout procedure and in caring for the wound; small compression dressing applied to joint, and joint rested for 24 hours to prevent hemorrhage or effusion |
| Buccal mucosa (punch biopsy) | Histologic examination of tissue from inside lower lip | Helpful in diagnosing Sjögren's syndrome | Patient instructed about procedure; generally minor discomfort experienced; diet altered to avoid rough and very hot foods (they will irritate the site) |
| Bone (operative procedure) | Microscopic analysis | Can confirm presence of infection or neoplasm | Patient instructed and prepared for surgery; patient monitored per postanesthesia routine; mild to severe discomfort may be experienced; activity restricted dependent on location and extent of surgical procedure; dressings changed as necessary |

in normal muscles at rest, but during volitional movement, action potentials can be detected. In both primary myopathic and neuropathic disorders, specific variations exist in the size of individual motor unit potentials. In neurogenic atrophy, fibrillations may be present in the resting muscle. An EMG provides direct evidence of motor dysfunction and can be used to some extent to detect a dysfunction located in the motor neuron, the neuromuscular junction, or the muscle fibers. Thus it is particularly helpful in the diagnosis of lower motor neuron (LMN) disease, primary muscle disease, and defects in the transmission of electrical impulses at the neuromuscular junction, such as myasthenia gravis. However, electromyography *cannot* be used to differentiate *specific* disease entities in either the myopathic or neuropathic categories. No special preparation is required for

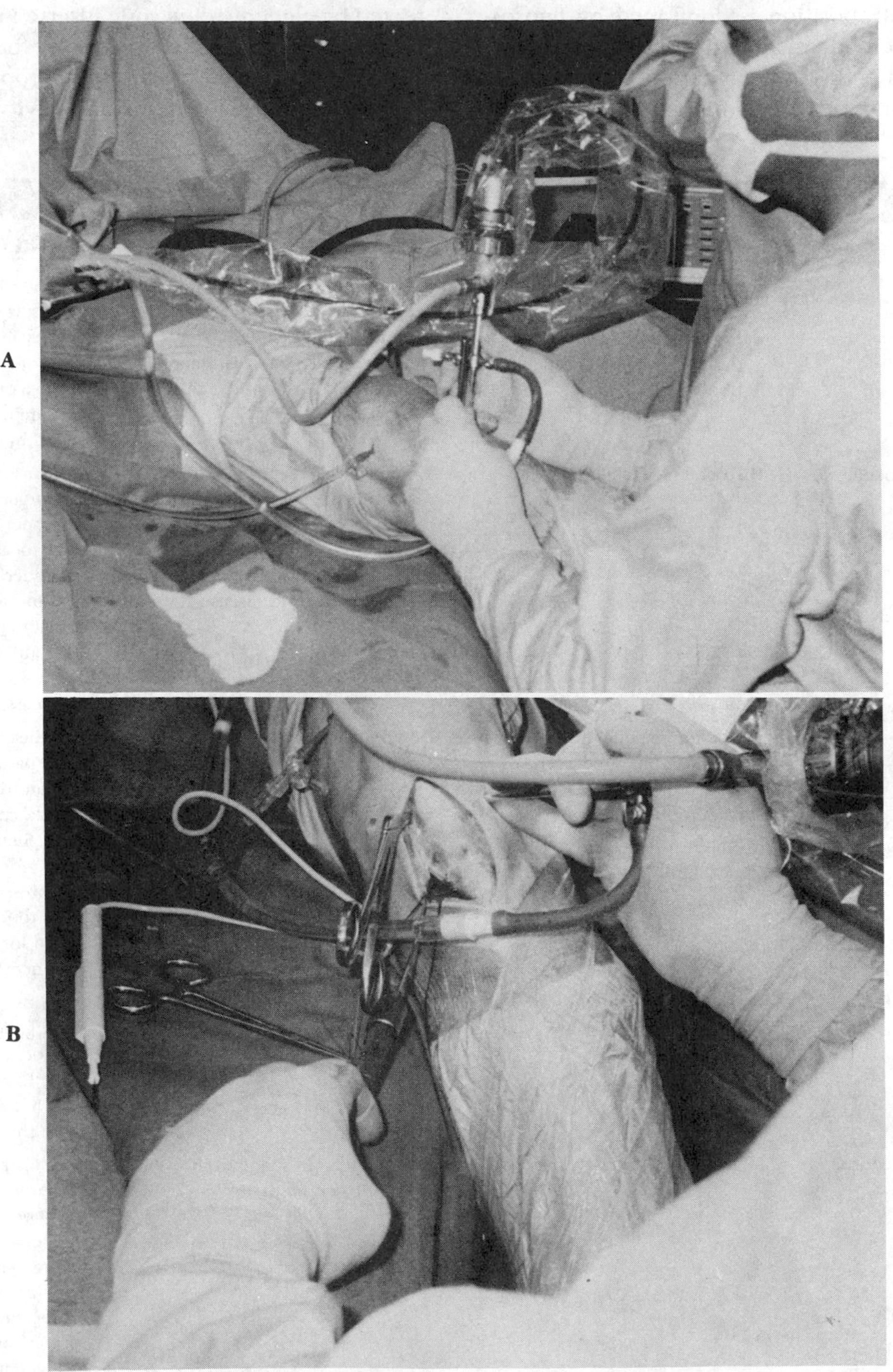

**FIGURE 63-26** **A,** Arthroscopy of knee. **B,** Arthroscopically aided reconstruction of anterior cruciate ligament.

this procedure. The patient may fear that insertion of electrode needles will be painful or that electrical stimulation of the needles will cause severe shock. Although the patient may be reassured that the procedure is not dangerous, it should be noted that some individuals do experience mild to moderate discomfort. Therefore nurses preparing patients for this test should not refer to the test as "painless."

### Biopsy

Biopsies of tissue from a variety of organs are helpful in the diagnoses of disease or disorders affecting the musculoskeletal system. Table 63-7 lists the organs that may be biopsied, the test(s) performed on the biopsied tissue, what a positive result of testing indicates, and general nursing considerations in caring for the patient on whom the biopsy is performed.

### Joint Aspiration

Joint aspiration is performed to obtain a sample of synovial fluid from within the joint cavity. This procedure (performed by introducing a needle into the joint cavity and withdrawing fluid) aids in determining the presence of an aseptic inflammatory process such as rheumatoid arthritis or a septic process such as bacterial arthritis. Samples of synovial fluid are cultured and examined both microscopically and chemically.

The synovial fluid is normally straw colored and clear. Its viscosity resembles that of motor oil. In the presence of inflammation it becomes turbid and watery. The *mucin clot test* is performed by mixing synovial fluid with glacial acetic acid. Normal synovial fluid will form a white, ropey mucin clot. When inflammmation is present, the clot breaks apart easily and becomes flaky (flocculent). The degree of flocculence increases with the degree of inflammation. Also, when inflammation is present, the number of WBCs, the protein content, and the number of polymorphonuclear cells in the synovial fluid are increased; glucose content is decreased.

A local anesthetic is usually administered before the procedure. Strict asepsis is observed during the procedure. After the procedure the joint is often wrapped in a small compression (Ace) dressing. The joint may be rested for 8 to 24 hours. Drainage should be managed in accordance with universal body substance isolation techniques.

### Scoliosis Screening

Scoliosis screening programs, particularly for school-age children, are effective in identifying early indications of scoliosis. Such indications include "wing" (or protrusion) deformity of one scapula, uneven shoulder height, one arm hanging closer to the body than the other when standing erect, demonstrable curve of the spine, and rib hump (elevation of the rib cage posteriorly and laterally in the thoracic area) on forward bending. If scoliosis is detected early, nonsurgical treatment may be effective in arresting the progression of the curvature.

### Arthroscopy

**Arthroscopy** (visualization of a joint) is a procedure performed in the operating room. A specially designed endoscope (arthroscope) is inserted through a small incision into the joint cavity, enabling the physician to visualize the structure and contents of the joint (Figure 63-26). Most arthroscopic procedures are performed on the knee, although the wrist, ankle, hip, and shoulder are also examined and treated with this technique.

The procedure is used to diagnose and treat such conditions as chondromalacia of the knee, ligamentous disruption, meniscal tears, carpal tunnel syndrome, osteoarthritis, rheumatoid arthritis, and impingement syndrome. Most recently, endoscopy has been used to perform lumbar diskectomy. Arthroscopy is performed in an operating room, usually as an ambulatory surgical procedure. Local or regional anesthesia is most often used. Analgesics are prescribed postoperatively. The patient is taught to observe the operative site for swelling and signs of infection. The period of time the joint is rested and the use of any immobilizing device is determined by the extent of the procedure. The surgeon should be consulted regarding the activity the patient is permitted following the procedure so that damage to the joint may be avoided.

Endoscopy may have indications for further use. It is currently being researched as a method to directly visualize branches of the sciatic nerve and to aid in the implantation of percutaneous intramuscular electrodes used in functional electrical stimulation (FES).[1] The goal of this FES research is to restore standing, walking, and transfer capabilities to persons with quadriplegia and paraplegia.

## CRITICAL THINKING ACTIVITIES

- Compare the musculoskeletal structure of a 20-year-old with the musculoskeletal structure of a 70-year-old. How do such structural changes affect the functioning of the musculoskeletal system?
- Discuss the essential assessment data that should be collected on an individual who has a musculoskeletal problem or disease.

## CHAPTER SUMMARY

#### ANATOMY AND PHYSIOLOGY

- Support, protection, and movement are the three mechanical functions of bones. Bones also store calcium and produce RBCs.
- Bone is produced by the process of osteogenesis or endochondral ossification. The bone-building cells are known as osteoblasts; bone cells are osteocytes. Calcium salts in the matrix give bone its characteristic "hard" quality.
- Bones are classified into four groups based on shape: long, short, flat, and irregular.

- Bone is composed of cancellous (spongy) and compact cortical (dense) bone. Lamellae are concentric cylindric layers of calcified matrix. The arrangement of lamellae within bone differentiates cancellous and compact bone. The haversian canal is at the center of the lamella.
- Periosteum is a white, fibrous membrane that covers bone except on the articular surface, which is covered with hyaline cartilage. The inner layers of the periosteum contain osteoblasts; thus the periosteum is considered a growth organ.
- Epiphyses are the ends of bone; the diaphysis is the shaft. Longitudinal bone growth begins in the epiphyseal cartilage between the diaphyseal and epiphyseal centers of ossification. Cartilage cells rapidly proliferate and the cartilage undergoes ossification. Growth in the diameter of bone is accomplished through the simultaneous processes of bone destruction, by osteoclasts enlarging the medullary cavity, and bone production, by osteoblasts in the periosteum.
- Bone reshapes itself in response to alterations of its mechanical function. Osteogenesis occurs along lines of stress. This explains why a person who regularly exercises may have some increase in bone mass (hypertrophy), whereas a sedentary person may experience loss of bone substance (atrophy).
- Circulation of blood to bone is supplied by three routes: through arterioles in the haversian canals, through Volkmann's canals (located in the periosteum), and through vessels in the marrow and the ends of bone. Blood supply to the bone can be interrupted by injury to an artery, the periosteum, or the bone itself. Because bones are supplied with sensory nerve endings, pain will result if bone is damaged.
- Callus formation is the process of bone healing and proceeds in five general stages: hematoma formation, fibrin meshwork formation, invasion by osteoblasts, callus formation, and remodeling. Good callus formation can be impeded by inadequate reduction of a fracture, excessive edema at a fracture site, too much bone loss at the time of injury, inefficient immobilization, infection, bone necrosis, anemia or other systemic conditions, endocrine imbalance, and poor dietary intake. Nonunion, or an ununited fracture, is the resulting lack of repair or of abnormal or inefficient callus formation.
- The three major types of muscle are skeletal, visceral, and cardiac. Skeletal muscle is innervated by nerve fibers from the cerebrospinal system and can be controlled at will. It provides controlled movement, maintains posture, and produces heat.
- Skeletal muscle cells are long and narrow and are made up of bundles of muscle fibers. Myofibrils are small, closely packed fibers within the sarcoplasm. They consist of several sections called sarcomeres.
- The function of muscles is to contract. The triggering of nerve impulses at the muscle fiber accomplishes this complex process. Calcium ions released when the impulse is received bind to troponin. Once calcium ions are bound, the sarcomeres contract. Energy is supplied by the breakdown of ATP. Relaxation occurs when calcium ions separate from troponin.
- Body movement is produced by muscles pulling on bones, with bones serving as levers and joints serving as fulcrums for the levers. Muscles act in a coordinated manner, involving prime movers, antagonists, and synergists.
- Skeletal muscle is highly vascular because efficient muscle contraction depends on an adequate blood supply *to and from* the muscle fibers.
- Effective innervation is necessary for adequate muscle contraction. Somatic motor neurons transmit impulses to skeletal muscles. Contraction of the muscle is set off by the release of acetylcholine across the motor end plate or neuromuscular junction.
- Cartilage is a material composed of fibers embedded in a firm gel. It is strong, flexible, and avascular. The type of cartilage (fibrous, hyaline, or elastic) is determined by the number of collagenous fibers.
- Ligaments connect the articular ends of bones and provide stability. They also may attach to soft tissue to suspend structures. Ligaments consist of dense fibrous bands of connective tissue.
- Tendons are dense fibrous tissue bands that form the termination of a muscle and attach it to a bone. They are extensions of the fibrous sheaths that cover each muscle and are continuous with the periosteum at the other end. Tendon sheaths are tubular structures that enclose certain tendons, especially at the wrist and ankle.
- Small sacs of connective tissue are called bursae. They are located wherever pressure is exerted over moving parts.
- Joints, or the places where bones come together, provide flexibility within the skeletal framework. The type and amount of movement possible are determined by the shape of the joint. There are three major classifications of joints: synarthroses, or fibrous joints, provide no movement; amphiarthroses, or cartilaginous joints, allow little movement; diarthroses or synovial joints, allow free movement.
- Diarthroidal joints contain a joint cavity between the articulating surfaces of the bones that compose the joint. The articulating surfaces of both bones are covered by articular hyaline cartilage, allowing smooth motion. The joint is encased in a joint capsule, and the capsule is lined with a synovial membrane. Lubrication is provided by synovial fluid secreted by the synovial membrane. Ligaments may be present to provide internal stability to the joint. Menisci (small

pieces of dense cartilage) may also bc present to provide additional cushioning.

- Physiologic changes with aging occur as the total number of body cells decreases, resulting in the decline of tissue strength and integrity. Connective tissues lose elasticity; muscles lose bulk, tone, and strength; bone reabsorption is more rapid than bone growth; and, particularly in postmenopausal women, calcium is lost from bone, making it softer and more prone to fracture.
- The musculoskeletal, circulatory, and nervous systems are interrelated. Any problem that causes interruption of innervation, contractility, articulation, circulation, or support results in musculoskeletal dysfunction.

### ASSESSMENT

- Assessment of any person with a musculoskeletal problem must include subjective data elicited from the person and family. This includes a description of the present problem, such as onset and duration, associated pain or discomfort, current medications, and effect on performance of ADL; the persons's perception of the problem or dysfunction; and the family's perception of the person's problem.
- Objective data involve observations of the person. Observations are made regarding behavior, general appearance, and the condition of skin, nails, and hair. Data also are collected about deformities, strength and range of motion, ability to transfer and ambulate, and ability to perform ADL. (Refer to the text and boxes for specifics.)

### DIAGNOSTIC TESTS

- Some of the principal diagnostic studies that may be performed on a person with a musculoskeletal problem include laboratory examinations (e.g., serologic and urinary tests); radiologic examinations (e.g., radiographs of bones and joints, systemic radiologic studies [to determine the extent of internal organ involvement], myelography, diskography, arthrography, radioisotope scans, CT scans, and MRI); and special tests (e.g., EMG, MMT, biopsies, and joint aspiration).
- Arthroscopy is a surgical procedure that provides visualization of a joint via a specially designed endoscope. Biopsy, diagnosis, repair of torn meniscus or ligament, and removal of loose bodies from the joint space can be accomplished with this approach.

## REFERENCES


1. Doyle J, Scheiner A, Marsolais EB: Augmentation of the accuracy of percutaneous electrode implantation by using a modified arthroscope to guide insertion, *Arthroscopy* 8(2):162-165, 1992.
2. Hilt NE, editor: *Arthroscopy of the knee.* Monograph Library, National Association of Orthopaedic Nurses, Feb 1983, Anthony J Janetti, Inc.
3. McCance KL, Huether SE: *Pathophysiology the biologic basis of disease in adults and children,* ed 2, St Louis, 1994, Mosby.
4. Moskowitz RW: *Clinical rheumatology: a problem oriented approach to diagnosis and management,* ed 2, Philadelphia, 1982, Lea & Febiger.
5. Mundy GR: New concepts in bone metabolism: clinical implications, *Hosp Prac* 26(suppl 1):7-12, 1991.
6. Thibodeau GA, Patton KT: *Anatomy and physiology,* ed 2, St Louis, 1994, Mosby.

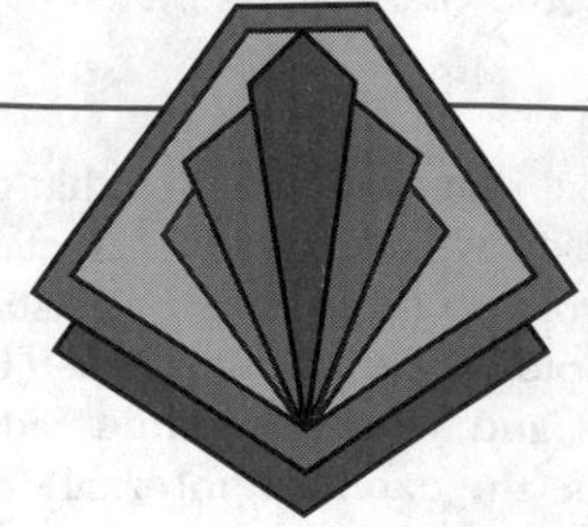

CHAPTER 64

# Management of Persons With Trauma to the Musculoskeletal System

*Jane F. Marek*
*Patricia S. Buergin*
*Kyle M. Paskert*

## CHAPTER OBJECTIVES

***After studying this chapter, the learner should be able to do the following:***

1 Describe three causes of bone fracture and four measures that can be taken to prevent fracture.
2 Define the three mechanisms of immobilization by which fractured bone can heal.
3 Discuss the medical management of fractures, including definitions of the terms *closed reduction* and *open reduction.*
4 List three major complications of bone fracture and explain how they are treated.
5 Describe what subjective and objective data the nurse should collect when assessing the person who has a fracture.
6 Describe the nursing measures that can be used in relation to the following:
  a Patient teaching
  b Pain management
  c Positioning
  d Neurocirculatory monitoring
  e Preservation of strength and mobility
  f Maintenance of skin integrity
7 Discuss four systemic complications that might occur after a fracture and the nursing measures that can be used to help prevent them.
8 Discuss the special nursing care measures required for the patient who has (1) a cast, (2), traction, and (3) an internal fixation device.
9 Describe the special nursing care measures required for the person whose hip fracture has been treated with a prosthetic implant.
10 Discuss the special nursing considerations in caring for the patient with a spine fracture.
11 Discuss the various types of trauma that can occur to ligaments, tendons, and muscles and the nursing care associated with each of these.
12 Discuss the various types of injuries that can occur to joints and the nursing care that is required.
13 Discuss the special care considerations required by the patient who has sustained multiple trauma.

## KEY TERMS

avascular necrosis
avulsion
balanced suspension
bivalved cast
braces
Buck's extension
callus formation
closed reduction
comminuted fracture
compartment syndrome (CS)
compound fracture
countertraction
crepitus
decompression fasciotomy
delayed union
epimysiotomy
external fixation devices
extracapsular fracture
fat embolism syndrome (FES)
fatigue or stress fracture
greenstick fracture
Ilizarov external fixation
internal fixation devices
intertrochanteric fracture
intracapsular fracture
Kirschner wire
logrolling
malunion
neurocirculatory compromise
nonunion
oblique fracture
open reduction
osteoporosis
pathologic fracture
Pearson attachment
physiologic splintage
prosthetic implant
reduction fracture
RICE
Russell traction
skeletal traction
skin traction
spiral fracture
splints
sprain
Steinmann pin
strain
Thomas splint
traction
transverse fracture

The person with trauma to the musculoskeletal system has sustained an interruption in the integrity of one or more components of the system. Musculoskeletal trauma is most frequently manifested as bone fracture, but it may also include injury to soft tissue, muscle, ligament, meniscus, tendon, or joint.

The National Center for Health Statistics estimates that annually an average of 1 of 10 persons suffers acute injury to the musculoskeletal system. The most common injuries are fracture, dislocation, and sprain.

# TRAUMA TO BONE

## FRACTURE OF BONE

### Etiology/Epidemiology

Fracture of bone usually occurs as a result of a blow to the body, a fall, or another accident. However, fracture may occur during normal activity or after a minimal injury, if the bone has been weakened by a disease such as primary or metastatic cancer or osteoporosis. This is called a **pathologic fracture,** or collapse of the bone. Bone may also fracture when the muscles associated with it are unable to absorb energy as they usually do. This type of fracture is called a **fatigue** or **stress fracture. Avulsion** fractures occur when a strong ligamentous or tendinous attachment pulls a fragment of bone away from the rest of the bone.

The highest incidence of fractures is in males 15 to 24 years old and in elderly persons, especially women, aged 65 years and older. Fracture can occur at any age, although older persons, persons with balance or mobility problems, persons who work at high-risk occupations (e.g., steelworkers and race car drivers), and persons with chronic degenerative or neoplastic diseases are at higher risk for injury.

### Pathophysiology

#### Definition and types of fractures

A bone is fractured when there is a complete or partial interruption of the osseous tissue. A fracture is *complete* when there is complete separation of the bone, producing two fragments; it is *incomplete* when only part of the bone is broken. The part of the bone nearest the body is referred to as the *proximal fragment;* the part more distant from the body is called the *distal fragment.* The proximal fragment is also called the *uncontrollable fragment,* because its location and muscle attachments prevent it from being moved or manipulated when attempting to bring the separate fragments into alignment. The distal fragment is called the *controllable fragment,* because it can usually be moved to bring it into correct relationship to the proximal fragment. Fractures in long bones are designated as being in the proximal, middle, or distal third of the bone.

If the skin over the fracture is intact, the fracture is classified as *simple* or *closed.* A fracture is classified as *compound* or *open* when there is a direct communication between a skin wound and the fracture site. An open or compound fracture has a high risk of contamination, and this is an important factor in its treatment. When the two bone fragments are in good alignment with no change from normal position despite the break in continuity of bone, the fracture is referred to as a *fracture without displacement.* If the bone fragments have separated at the point of fracture, it is referred to as a *fracture with displacement.* Displacement may be slight, moderate, or marked.

The *line of fracture* as revealed by x-ray film or fluoroscopy is usually classified according to type. It may be **greenstick,** with splintering on one side of the bone (this occurs most often in young children); **transverse,**

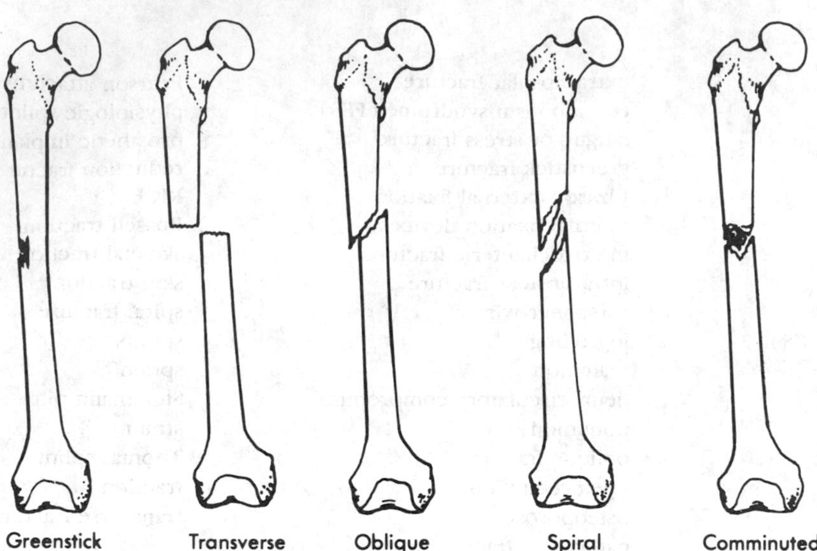


**FIGURE 64-1** Types of fractures.

**BOX 64-1 Types of Fractures**

**TYPICAL COMPLETE FRACTURES**

Closed (simple) fracture—Noncommunicating wound between bone and skin
Open (compound) fracture—Communicating wound between bone and skin
Comminuted fracture—Multiple bone fragments
Linear fracture—Fracture line parallel to long axis of bone
Oblique fracture—Fracture line at 45-degree angle to long axis of bone
Spiral fracture—Fracture line encircling bone
Transverse fracture—Fracture line perpendicular to long axis of bone
Impacted—Fracture fragments are pushed into each other
Pathologic—Fracture occurs at a point in the bone weakened by disease, for example, with tumors or osteoporosis
Avulsion—A fragment of bone connected to a ligament breaks off from the main bone
Extracapsular—Fracture is close to the joint but remains outside the joint capsule
Intracapsular—Fracture is within the joint capsule

**TYPICAL INCOMPLETE FRACTURES**

Greenstick fracture—Break on one cortex of bone with splintering of inner bone surface
Torus fracture—Buckling of cortex
Bowing fracture—Bending of bone
Stress fracture—Microfracture
Transchondral fracture—Separation of cartilaginous joint surface (articular cartilage) from main shaft of bone

From McCance KL, Huether SE: ***Pathophysiology: the biological basis for disease in adults and children,*** ed 2, St Louis, 1994, Mosby.

with the break being straight across the bone; **oblique,** with the line of the fracture being at an oblique angle to the bone shaft; or **spiral,** with the fracture lines partially encircling the bone. The fracture may be referred to as *telescoped* or *impacted* if the distal fragment is forcibly pushed against and into the proximal fragment. If there are several bone fragments, the fracture is called **comminuted.** (See Figure 64-1 and Box 64-1 for examples of fractures.)

Because bones are firmer than their surrounding structures, any injury severe enough to cause bone fracture may also cause injury to adjacent muscles, nerves, connective tissue, and blood vessels. The force that causes the fracture is dissipated through the surrounding soft tissue, and small fragments of bone may become embedded in muscle, blood vessels, or nerves.

### Healing of fractures

Immobilization of a fractured bone is necessary for healing to take place. Immobilization may be effected in any of the following three ways:

1. **Physiologic splintage,** a naturally occurring phenomenon related to pain in the affected area that causes guarding, muscle spasm, and avoidance of use; further, there will be a desire to rest the whole body until some repair has occurred
2. *External orthopedic splinting* with devices such as casts
3. *Internal fixation* with screws, plates, or rods to hold the opposing ends of the fracture in place

Once immobilization is accomplished, the bone heals by the process of **callus formation** (see Chapter 63). Factors that impede healing are described in Table 64-1. Failure of a fracture to consolidate in the time usually required is called **delayed union,** and failure to form

**TABLE 64-1 Major Factors That Impede Bone Healing**

| PROBLEM | CAUSE |
|---|---|
| Poor approximation of fracture fragments | Inaccurate reduction or malalignment of fracture fragments<br>Inadequate immobilization, resulting in movement of fragments<br>Excessive bone loss at time of fracture, preventing sufficient bridging of broken ends<br>Excessive fragmentation of bone, allowing soft tissue to be interposed between bone ends<br>Inability of patient to comply with restrictions imposed by immobilizing/fixation device(s), resulting in movement of fragments |
| Excessive edema at fracture site | Tissue swelling impedes supply of nutrients to area of fracture |
| Bone necrosis | Injury to blood vessels impedes supply of nutrients to involved bone |
| Infection at fracture site | Infection disrupts normal callus formation |
| Metabolic disorders or diseases (cancer, diabetes) | Retard osteogenesis |
| Soft tissue injury | Disruption of blood supply |

**BOX 64-2 Clinical Manifestations of Fractures**

1. Pain (caused by swelling at the site, muscle spasm, damage to periosteum)
   a. Immediate
   b. Severe
   c. Aggravated by pressure at the site of injury
   d. Aggravated by attempted motion
2. Loss of normal function (the injured part incapable of voluntary movement)
3. Obvious deformity resulting from loss of bone continuity
4. Excessive motion at site (i.e., motion where motion does not usually occur)
5. **Crepitus*** or grating sound if limb is moved gently
6. Soft tissue edema in area of injury resulting from extravasation of blood and tissue fluid
7. Warmth over injured area resulting from increased blood flow to the area
8. Ecchymosis of skin surrounding injured area (may not be apparent for several days)
9. Loss of sensation or paralysis distal to injury resulting from nerve entrapment
10. Signs of shock related to severe tissue injury, blood loss, or intense pain
11. Evidence of fracture on x-ray film

*No attempt should be made to elicit this sign when fracture is suspected, because it may cause further damage and increase pain.

a stable union after 6 to 9 months is called **nonunion.** Of the estimated 2 million cases of long bone fractures that occur annually, there will be approximately 100,000 (5%) cases of nonunion. The incidence of nonunion of tibial fractures is higher than in other long bones, especially when fracture occurs as a result of a high-energy injury, such as a motor vehicle accident.[15]

Healing with angulation or deformity is called **malunion.** If a fracture is nonunited, there will be excessive mobility at the fracture site, creating a false joint. This is called a *pseudarthrosis.*

The signs and symptoms of fracture vary according to the location and function of the involved bone, the strength of its muscle attachments, the type of fracture sustained, and the amount of related soft tissue damage. Box 64-2 gives the clinical manifestations of fractures.

## Prevention

One approach to preventing fracture is to make the environment safer. Examples of measures that can be taken include the following:
1. Mounting grab bars on the wall next to a tub or toilet
2. Attaching safety arms around a toilet
3. Removing throw rugs and obstacles from areas used by individuals with locomotor difficulties
4. Ensuring that wheelchairs have adequate locking devices
5. Teaching individuals who must use ambulatory devices and wheelchairs how to use them properly

A second approach is to continue to educate the public regarding the following:
1. The dangers of drinking and driving
2. The advisability of using seat belts while driving
3. Attending to safety precautions when climbing ladders and using power tools or heavy equipment
4. Wearing recommended protective clothing (e.g., steel-toed shoes and hard hats for hazardous work at home or on the job)
5. Wearing proper protective clothing while engaging in sports (e.g., protective padding and well-fitting running shoes)

A third approach is to continue to educate women about the problem of **osteoporosis.** Individuals most at risk to develop osteoporosis are small-framed, nonobese, menopausal White females. Contributing factors are diets low in calcium, smoking, excessive coffee intake, too much protein in the diet, and a sedentary lifestyle. Measures that can be taken to retard osteoporosis include the following:
1. Increasing calcium intake
2. Refraining from smoking
3. Decreasing coffee intake
4. Decreasing excess protein in the diet
5. Engaging in some regular moderate activity such as walking
6. Exploring with a physician the advisability of estrogen replacement at menopause

## Medical Management

### Diagnostic tests

Diagnosis is confirmed by x-ray.

### Medication

1. Analgesics are given prn to treat pain.
2. Antibiotics (initially intravenously and then orally) are given when there is an open fracture or surgical intervention.
3. Tetanus toxoid may be necessary in the case of an open fracture.

### Treatment

Management objectives include the following:

1. Reduction of fracture by approximating the fracture fragments
2. Maintenance of fragments in correct alignment through immobilization
3. Prevention of excessive loss of joint mobility and muscle tone

**Immediate management.** Immediate management objectives include the following:

1. Splinting of fracture to prevent movement of the injured part
2. Preservation of body alignment
3. Elevation of body part to limit edema
4. Application of cold packs (during first 24 hours) to reduce hemorrhage, edema, and pain
5. Observation for changes in color, sensation, or temperature of injured part
6. Observation for signs of shock

**Secondary management.** Secondary management goals include the following:

1. For simple fracture
   a. Optimal reduction (replacing bone fragments in their correct anatomic position)
      (1) Manual manipulation, or *closed reduction* (moving bone fragments into position by applying traction and pressure to distal fragment)
      (2) Traction
      (3) *Open reduction* (surgical intervention that may incorporate use of an internal fixation device)
   b. Immobilization
      (1) External fixation—cast or splint
      (2) Traction
      (3) Internal fixation such as pins, plates, screws, wires, and prostheses
      (4) Combinations of the above
2. For compound fracture
   a. Surgical debridement of wound to remove dirt, foreign material, devitalized tissue, and necrotic bone
   b. Culture of wound
   c. Packing of wound
   d. Observation for signs of osteomyelitis, tetanus, and gas gangrene
   e. Closure of wound when there is no sign of infection
   f. Reduction of fracture
   g. Immobilization of fracture
3. Use of bone growth stimulators that use low-voltage electrical impulses to enhance healing in cases of nonunion

### Maintaining immobilization of the reduced fracture

The purpose of immobilization is to hold the broken bone fragments in contact with each other (or in very close approximation) until healing takes place. ***Immobilization can be accomplished externally with external fixation devices (cast, splint, brace, cast brace), traction, or external fixators; or internally with metal plates, pins, screws and nails, alone or in combination with bone grafts, or prosthetic implants.*** Both external and internal methods can be used, with combinations of the above.

### Management of persons with external fixation devices

***Casts.*** Probably the most common external fixation device is the cast. Materials used for casts include plaster of paris, fiberglass, and plastic. All three of these materials are available in the form of rolled bandages and are applied over the body part to be immobilized in much the same manner as an Ace bandage is wrapped. *Plaster,* which has to be moistened before application, dries very slowly, is heavy, and will lose its strength and integrity if it becomes wet after initial drying. If a plaster cast requires revision, it usually must be removed and a new one applied. However, plaster is less expensive than fiberglass or plastic. *Fiberglass* and *plastic* dry quickly, are lightweight, and may be immersed in water without losing their strength. Plastic casts may be reheated and remolded if revision is necessary. Disadvantages include the fact that some types of fiberglass require drying under special ultraviolet lights, and persons wearing fiberglass or plastic casts may suffer maceration of the skin unless they dry the skin thoroughly with a warm-air dryer after bathing or showering. Specific advantages or disadvantages of various cast materials are discussed in orthopedic texts.

A cast may incorporate (1) all or a portion of an extremity (Figure 64-2), (2) all or a portion of the trunk and cervical area, or (3) all or a portion of the trunk with all or a portion of one or more extremities. The latter type of cast is called a *spica* cast (Figure 64-3). *Splints* are made from cast material, but they may be thought of as half-casts because they do not encompass a body part. They are applied anteriorly, posteriorly, medially, and/or laterally and are wrapped in place with

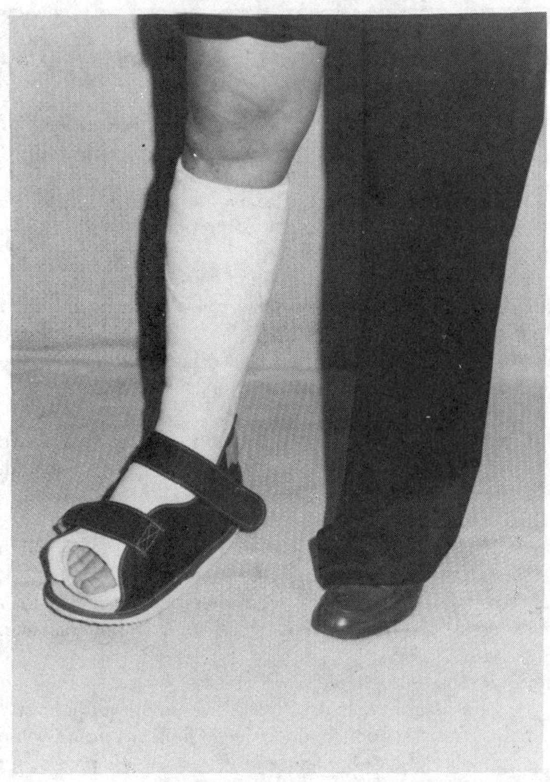

**FIGURE 64-2** Short leg walking cast with cast shoe.

bandages, usually Ace bandages. ***Cast braces*** are made of two separate casts, one applied above a joint and the other below the joint. The two casts are joined by metal or heavy polyethylene hinges that are incorporated into the cast material. Cast braces are applied to permit the patient joint mobility below the fracture while still providing immobilization for the fracture fragments.

Casts are applied over skin that has been cleansed and inspected for cuts or abrasions that may become infected. Skin lesions are treated with disinfectant before cast application. Also, before the cast is applied, the skin may be treated with tincture of benzoin and wrapped with cotton padding or stockinette. Bony prominences are padded with material—sheet wadding or felt—to protect them from pressure. For specific techniques of cast application, consult specialized texts.

***Cast removal*** is accomplished by splitting the cast with an electric cast saw. The saw is very noisy, but if used properly, it will not damage the skin beneath the cast. Skin enclosed in a cast for a time will be covered with an exudate of built-up secretions and dead skin. To remove this exudate, mineral oil is applied, followed by numerous soaks with warm water. This process may take several days, but attempts to remove the exudate more rapidly may result in uncomfortable skin irritation. Special guidelines for caring for the patient in a cast are described in the Guidelines box, p. 2194.

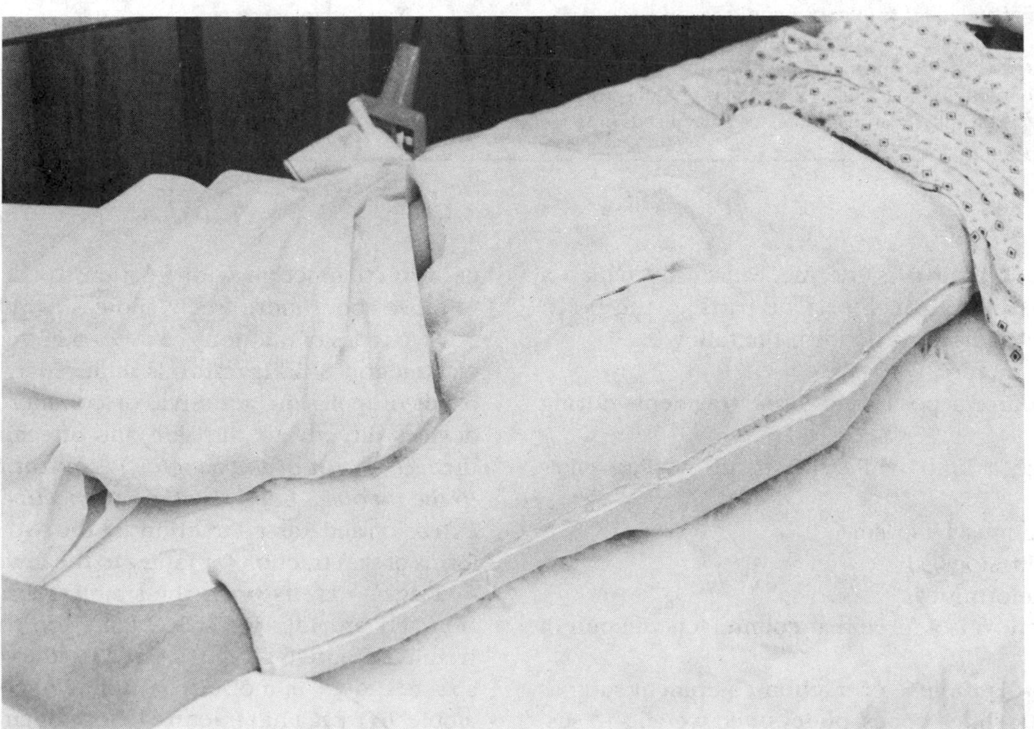

**FIGURE 64-3** Hip spica cast, applied to provide immobilization of left femoral fracture, was bivalved when patient developed severe pain and swelling of left leg several hours after cast was applied. Ace bandages wrapped over cast to provide support have been removed for purposes of this picture.

## Guidelines for Care of the Person in a Cast

1. Patient education
   a. Before cast application, explain why and how the cast will be applied.
   b. Advise the patient that the plaster cast will feel warm as it dries.
   c. Explain the extent to which the patient will be immobilized.
   d. Following cast application, explain care of the cast and expectations after discharge.
   e. Instruct patient not to insert sharp objects (coat hangers or pencils) under the cast, because these may abrade the skin and lead to infection.
2. Handling the new cast
   a. Support wet cast with the flat of the hands or on pillows to avoid indentations that will cause pressure on underlying skin.
   b. Place cotton blankets or other absorbent material under the cast to aid the drying process.
   c. Expose the cast to air as much as possible to aid the drying process.
   d. Turn the patient frequently to aid the drying process.
   e. Use a fan to circulate air over the cast.
   f. *Do not apply paint, varnish, or shellac to the cast; plaster is a porous material that allows air to circulate to the skin.*
3. Skin care
   a. Inspect skin at edges of cast and underlying the cast for redness or irritation; apply petal-shaped strips of adhesive tape or moleskin around rough edges of cast.
   b. Remove plaster crumbs from skin with a washcloth moistened with warm water.
   c. Use creams and lotions sparingly, since they may soften the skin and cause the cast to stick to the skin.
   d. Apply waterproof material around perineal area to prevent soiling of and damage to cast and irritation of the skin.
   e. Attend to patient's complaint of pain under the cast, particularly over bony prominences, since this may indicate pressure on the skin. If discomfort is not relieved by repositioning, report to physician. Cast pressure may need to be relieved by windowing or bivalving (cutting cast into two halves).
4. Turning
   a. Turning to any position is generally permitted, as long as the integrity of the cast is not compromised and the patient is comfortable.
5. Toileting (for a long leg or hip spica cast)
   a. Use a fracture pan with blanket roll or padding as support under the small of the back
   b. Elevate the head of the bed, if permitted; or place the bed in reverse Trendelenburg's position.
6. Abdominal discomfort
   a. Cast may be "windowed" (an opening cut into it) to provide relief of abdominal distention or a port for checking bladder distention.
7. Mobilization
   a. Weight bearing is at the discretion of the physician, and the amount of weight bearing will be prescribed.
   b. A cast shoe or a walking heel incorporated into a lower extremity cast will permit weight bearing without damaging the cast.
8. Prevention of neurocirculatory problems
   a. Perform neurocirculatory checks every hour for at least 24 hours after cast application to detect difficulty from swelling or pressure of cast on nerves or vessels. Notify physician of color changes, alterations in sensation, or motion unrelieved by position change; cast may need to be bivalved to relieve pressure.
   b. Elevate affected extremity on pillows until danger of swelling is over (usually 24 to 48 hours).
   c. After mobilization of patient with lower extremity or upper extremity cast, avoid keeping extremity in dependent position for prolonged periods.
   d. After lower extremity cast is removed, encourage patient to wear elastic stocking and elevate affected leg at rest until full mobility is regained.

***Traction.*** **Traction** is the mechanism by which a steady pull is placed on a part or parts of the body. Traction may be used to perform the following:

1. Reduce a fracture
2. Maintain correct position of bone fragments during healing
3. Immobilize a limb while soft tissue healing takes place
4. Overcome muscle spasm
5. Stretch adhesions
6. Correct deformities

**Countertraction** is a force that counteracts the pull of traction.

*Suspension* is the use of traction equipment such as frames, splints, slings, ropes, pulleys, and weights to suspend but not exert a "pull" on a body part. To suspend the part correctly and continuously, the suspension must be balanced by weights. Suspension is often referred to as **balanced suspension.** Balanced suspension is often used in conjunction with traction to allow the patient to move about more freely and easily in bed.

Two types of traction are used: skin traction and skeletal traction. **Skin traction** is achieved by applying wide bands of moleskin, adhesive, or commercially available devices directly to the skin and attaching weights to them. *The pull of the weights is transmitted indirectly to the involved bone or other connective tissue.* Buck's extension and Russell traction are the two most common forms of skin traction for injury to the lower extremities.

**Buck's extension** is the simplest form of skin traction and provides for straight pull on the affected extremity (Figure 64-4). It is often used to relieve muscle spasm and to immobilize a limb temporarily, for example, to treat a hip fracture before open reduction and internal fixation. If adhesive substances are to be used, the skin of the leg is shaved and tincture of benzoin is applied to protect the skin. Adhesive tape or moleskin is then placed on the lateral and medial aspects of the

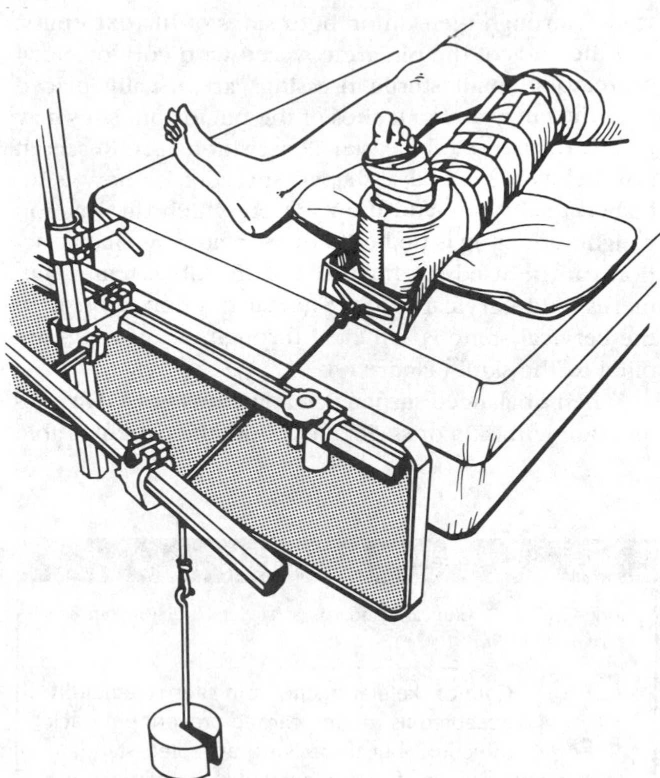

FIGURE 64-4 Buck's extension. Heel is supported off bed to prevent pressure on heel, weight hangs free of the bed, and foot is well away from footboard of bed. The limb should lie parallel to the bed unless prevented, as in this case, by a slight knee flexion contracture.

leg and secured with a circular gauze or elastic bandage. The adhesive material should not cover the malleoli, because the skin would break down over these bony prominences. The tapes are attached to a spreader bar wide enough to pull the tapes away from the malleoli. Rope is attached to the spreader, passed through a pulley on a crossbar at the foot of the bed, and suspended with weights. The maximal weight that should be applied by skin traction is 2-4 kg (5-10 lb).[9] Greater amounts of weight can cause skin damage. Commercial foam rubber Buck's extension splints are widely used and are applied with Velcro straps. Contraindications to placing a patient in Buck's extension are stasis dermatitis, arteriosclerosis, allergy to adhesive tape, severe varicosities or varicose ulcers, diabetic gangrene, or marked overriding of bone fragments that would require more than 3.6 kg of weight to reduce the fracture.

**Russell traction** is sometimes used, because it permits the patient to move somewhat freely in the bed and permits flexion of the knee joint (Figure 64-5). It requires an overhead frame attached to the bed and preparation of the leg as for Buck's extension. A foot plate with pulley attachments is used instead of a spreader bar. The knee is suspended in a sling to which a rope is attached. The rope is directed up to a pulley that has been placed on the overhead frame directly above the tibial tubercle of the affected extremity. The rope is then passed down through a pulley on a crossbar at the foot of the bed, back through a pulley on the

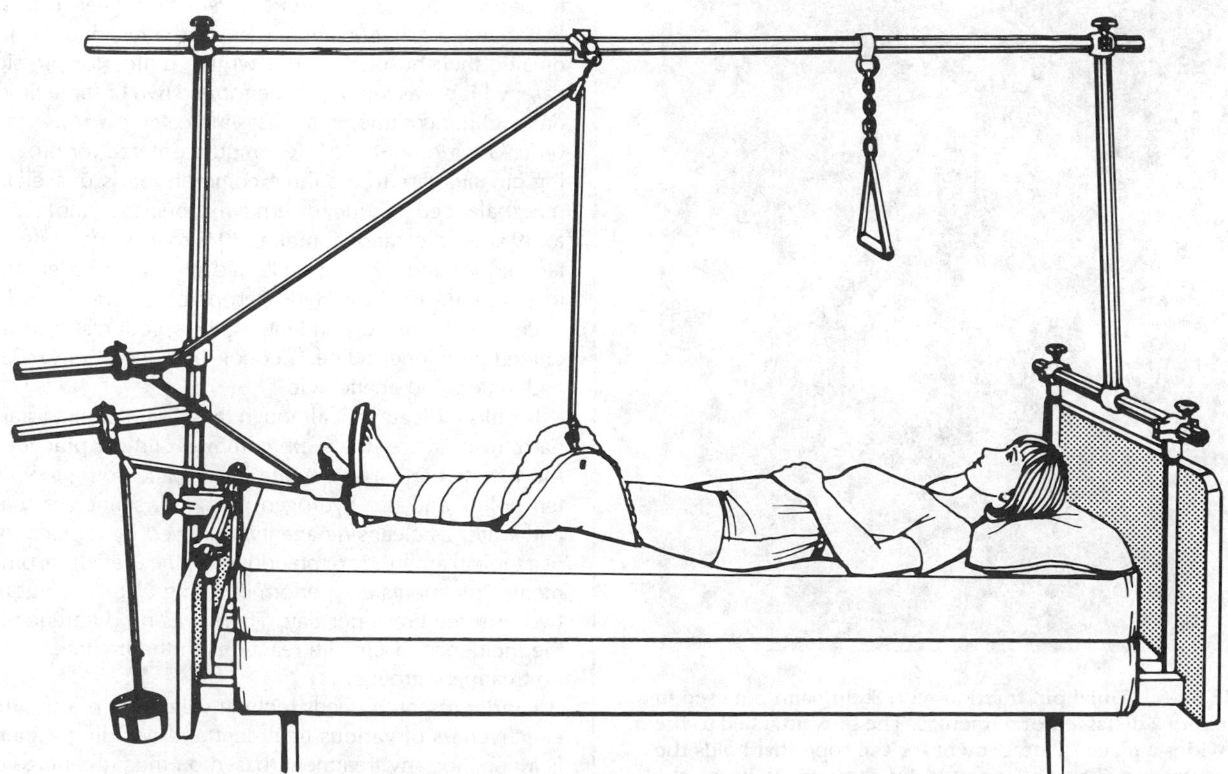

FIGURE 64-5 Russell traction. Hip is slightly flexed. Pillows may be used under lower leg to provide support and keep the heel free of the bed.

footplate, back again to another pulley on the crossbar, and then suspended with weights. This arrangement effects a double pull from the crossbar to the footplate, so the traction is approximately double the amount of weight used. Usually the foot of the bed is elevated on blocks (or the bed put in Trendelenburg's position) to provide **countertraction.**

Russell traction is used in the treatment of intertrochanteric fracture of the femur when surgery is contraindicated. Either bilateral Russell traction or Buck's extension may be used to treat back pain, because both partially immobilize the patient and reduce muscle spasm.

**Skeletal traction** is traction applied directly to bone. With the patient under local or general anesthesia, a **Kirschner wire** or **Steinmann pin** is inserted through bone distal to the fracture; the site of insertion varies with the type of fracture (Figure 64-6). The pin protrudes through the skin on both sides of the extremity, and the ends of the pin are covered with cork or metal protectors. Small sterile dressings are usually placed over the entry and exit sites of the pin, or pin sites may be left uncovered for easier observation (see Research box below). A metal U-shaped spreader or bow is attached to the pin, and the rope on which the traction weights are hung is tied onto the spreader. Skeletal traction can be used for fractures of the tibia, femur, humerus, and cervical spine. Skeletal traction applied to the cervical spine is achieved through use of tongs applied to the skull (Figure 64-7).

When a balanced suspension apparatus is used in conjunction with skin or skeletal traction, the patient is able

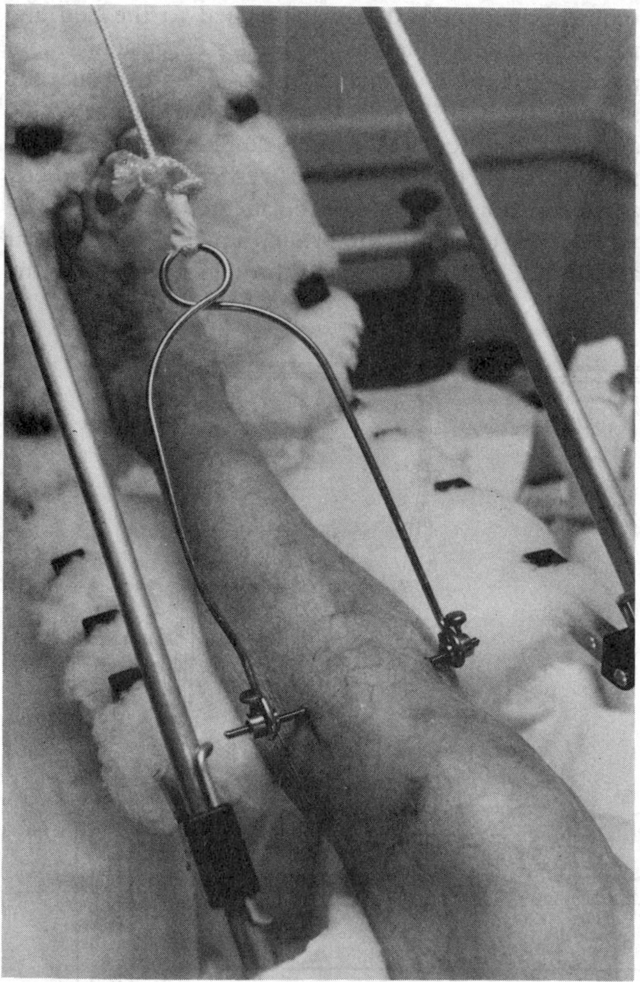

**FIGURE 64-6** Tibial pin traction with Steinmann pin used in treatment of a distal femoral fracture. The bow attached to the pin provides a place of attachment for the rope that holds the traction weights. The pull exerted by the weight keeps the fracture fragments aligned. Pin sites must be inspected at least daily to detect signs of pin reaction or infection.

## RESEARCH

Jones-Walton P: Clinical standards in skeletal traction pin site care, *Orthop Nurs* 10(2):12-16, 1991.

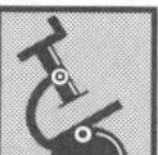

Care of skeletal traction pin sites is generally accepted as routine care to prevent pin track infection, but there is no accepted standard for the performance of care. Uncertainty exists regarding the type of products to be used, the frequency of treatment, and the effectiveness of care. This study gathered data related to pin site care in the acute care setting.

The Jones-Walton Pin Care Survey was administered to 804 subjects randomly selected from the National Association of Orthopaedic Nurses. The majority of participants in the study were RN direct-care givers or first-line managers. Fifty-eight percent of the respondents indicated their hospitals had a written policy for pin site care, which was reportedly performed two or three times daily. Other common responses indicated care "per MD order" or "do not treat." Techniques differed for providing pin site care to the three common forms of skeletal pins (balanced traction, external fixators, and halo): 55% to 59% used clean technique, 39% to 43% used sterile technique, and 27% to 44% had physician orders not to treat the pin sites. Hydrogen peroxide was used by over 91% of the respondents. Other products used included povidone-iodine, alcohol, petroleum jelly, soap and water, and acetic acid.

Results indicate that although there is no clinical standard for pin care, there are common clinical practices. Most study participants treat pin sites according to written policy and use hydrogen peroxide, saline, or soap and water as cleansing agents, followed by application of a topical antibiotic or povidone-iodine (Betadine) ointment. Treatments are performed using clean technique two or three times per day. There was no difference in the incidence of pin site reactions in the treatment and no treatment groups.

Further research needs include validation of both the effectiveness of various treatment and deciding if there is a need for any treatment (based on the percentage of "do not treat" orders).

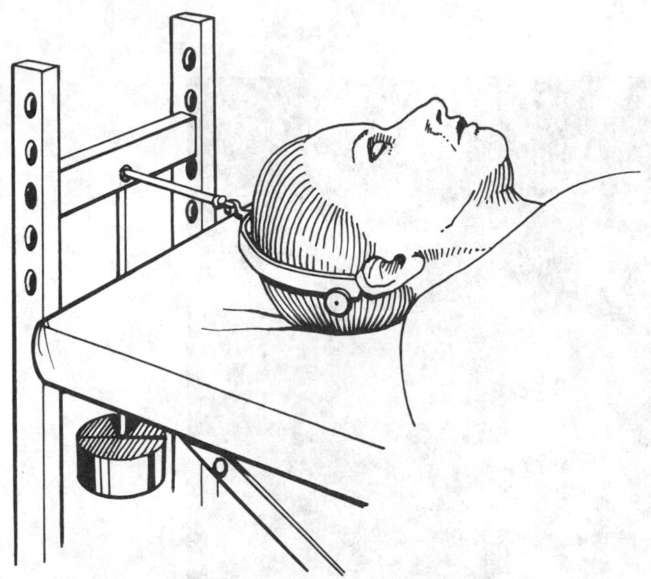

**FIGURE 64-7** Traction to the cervical spine can be maintained through the use of Crutchfield tongs inserted into the skull.

to move about in bed more freely without disturbing the line of pull of the traction. The use of a balancing apparatus facilitates nursing measures such as bathing, skin care, and positioning the bedpan. A full or half-ring **Thomas** or Hodgen **splint** (Figure 64-8) is frequently used for suspension of the lower extremity. Straps of canvas, muslin, or synthetic lamb's wool are placed over the splint and secured to provide a support for the leg. The areas under the popliteal space and heel are left open to prevent pressure on these parts. If it is desirable to have the knee flexed or to permit movement of the lower leg, a Pearson attachment is clamped or fixed to the Thomas splint at the level of the knee. Special guidelines for caring for the patient in traction are described in the Guidelines box, p. 2199.

***Other types of external immobilization.*** Other devices for external immobilization of fractures include the following:

1. Braces made of rigid plastic material
2. Plaster or plastic braces that incorporate metal struts attached to pins inserted into bone, such as a halo brace (Figure 64-9)
3. **External fixation devices** consisting of metal struts attached to pins inserted into bone (Figure 64-10)

External fixators such as the Hoffman or Synthes devices may be used in conjunction with plaster or alone. All of

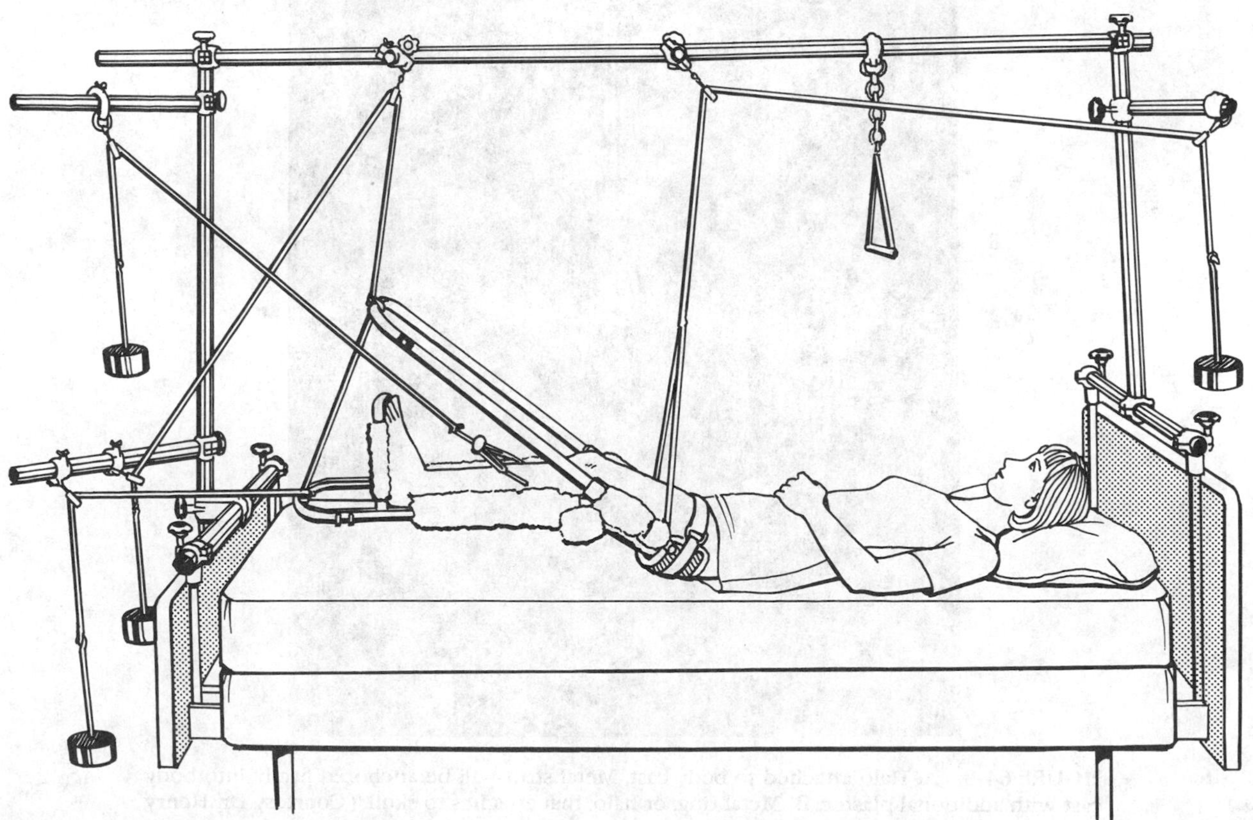

**FIGURE 64-8** Balanced suspension with Thomas splint and Pearson attachment. This apparatus can be used alone or, as in this case, with skeletal traction.

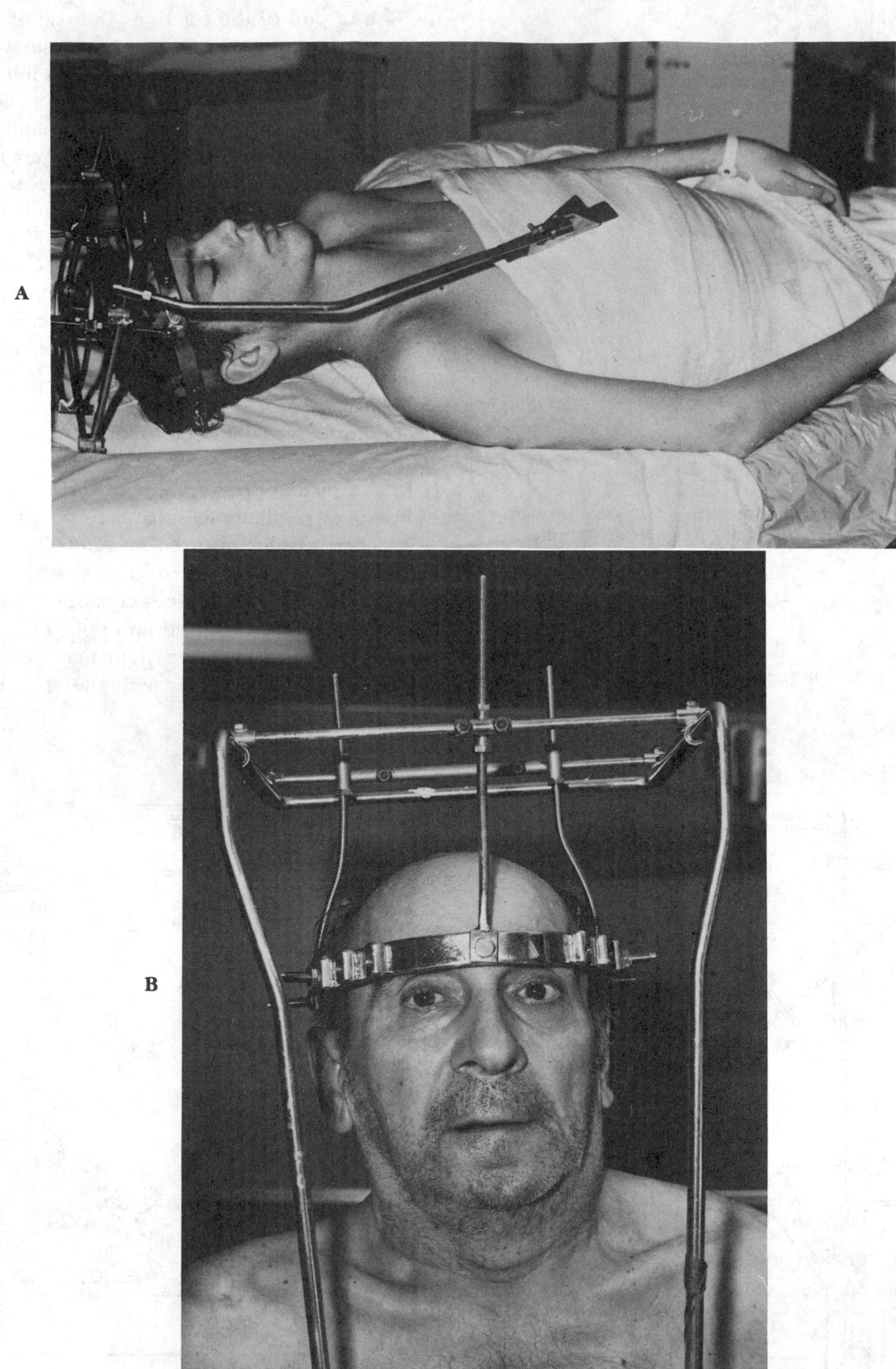


**FIGURE 64-9** **A,** Halo attached to body cast. Metal strut will be anchored firmly into body cast with additional plaster. **B,** Metal ring, or halo, that attaches to skull. (Courtesy Dr. Henry Bohlman, Cleveland.)

## Guidelines for Care of the Person in Traction

1. Patient education
   a. Explain traction in relation to fracture and physician's plan of treatment.
   b. Explain amount of movement permitted and how to achieve it (e.g., how trapeze can be used to assist with movement).
   c. Explain correct body positioning.
2. Maintaining the traction
   a. Inspect traction apparatus frequently to ensure that ropes are running straight and through the middle of the pulleys; that weights are hanging free; that bedclothes, the bed, or the frame and bars on the bed are not impinging on any part of the traction apparatus.
   b. Check ropes frequently to be sure they are not frayed.
   c. Avoid releasing weights from or altering the line of pull of the traction.
   d. Avoid adding weight to the traction.
   e. Check the position of the Thomas splint frequently; if the ring slides away from the groin, readjust the splint to its proper position without releasing traction.
   f. Avoid bumping into or jarring the bed or traction equipment.
   g. Be sure weights are securely fastened to their ropes.
   h. Avoid manipulation of pins.
3. Skin care
   a. Encourage the patient to turn slightly from side to side and to lift up on the trapeze to relieve pressure on the skin of the sacrum and scapulae; have the patient lift up for routine skin care.
   b. Avoid padding the ring of the Thomas splint, since this will create dampness next to the skin. Bathe the skin beneath the ring, dry it thoroughly, and powder the skin lightly.
   c. Inspect skin frequently to be sure it is not being rubbed, contused, or macerated by traction equipment; readjust splints or the extremity in the splint to free the skin from pressure.
   d. Keep skin areas around pin sites clean and dry; direct care to pin sites (e.g., cleansing with cotton applicators and hydrogen peroxide or alcohol) is controversial, so check with patient's physician to determine if pin care is to be done routinely and what method the physician prefers (see Research box, p. 2196).
4. Toileting
   a. Use a fracture pan with blanket roll or padding as support under the small of the back.
   b. Protect the ring of the Thomas splint with waterproof material when female patients are using the bedpan.

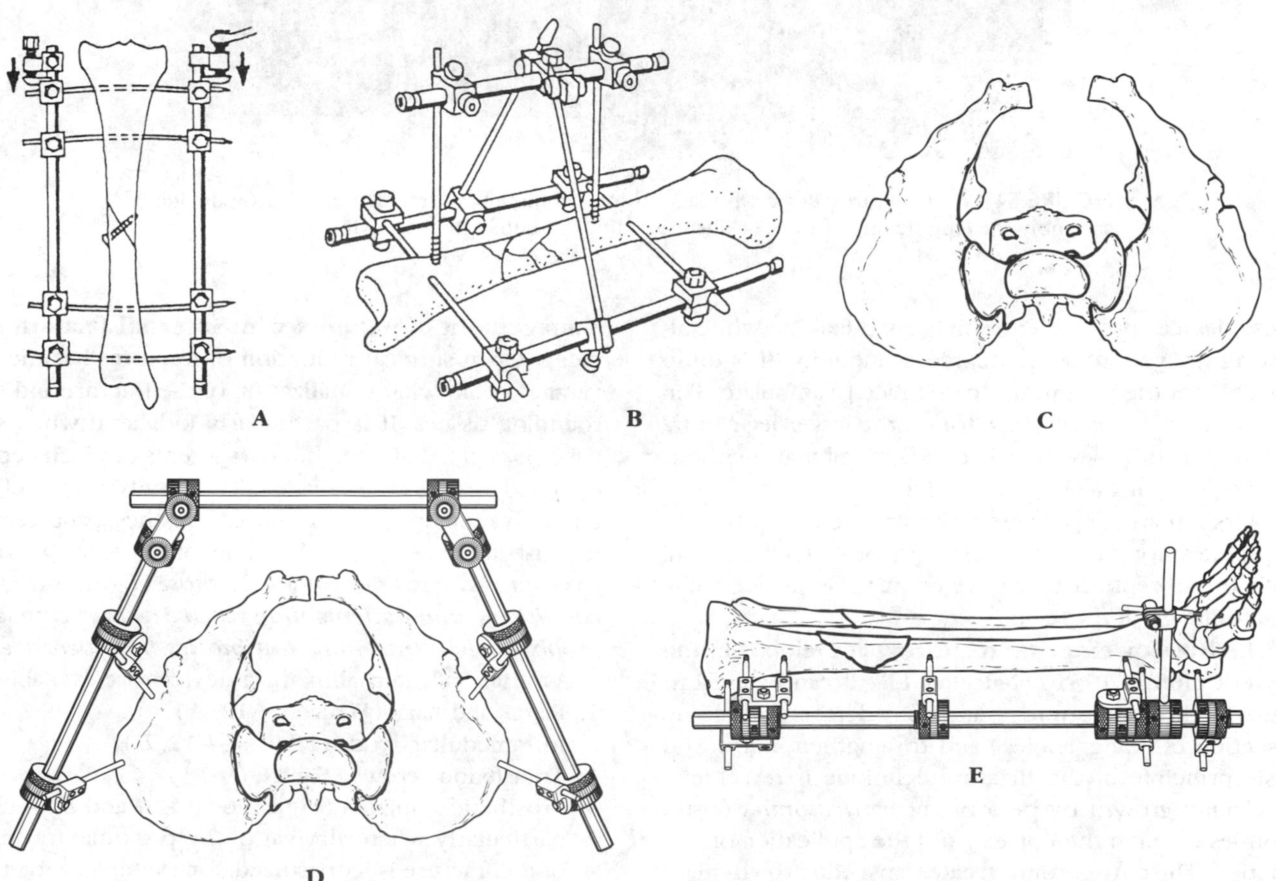


**FIGURE 64-10** **A,** Tibial fracture with simple AO external fixation with lag screw at fracture site. **B,** AO external fixator with three-dimensional or triangular fixation of comminuted fracture of the tibia. **C,** Pelvic diastasis (dislocation). **D,** Hex-Fix™ external fixator in place, showing reduction of pelvic fracture. **E,** Hex-Fix™ external fixator used to treat tibial fracture. Immobilization of ankle and foot allows soft tissue healing. (Courtesy Smith & Nephew Richards, Inc.)

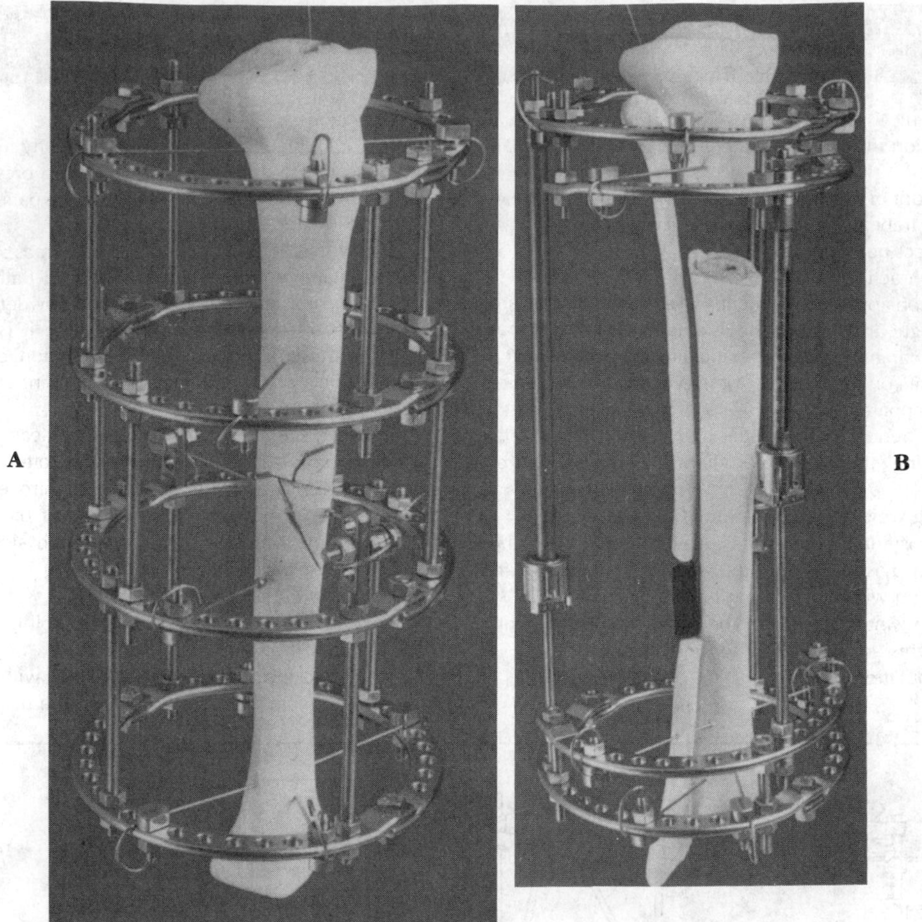


**FIGURE 64-11** **A,** Ilizarov device in place to treat comminuted fracture. **B,** Ilizarov device assembly for lengthening of tibia. (Courtesy Smith & Nephew Richards, Inc.)

these devices provide extremely rigid fixation while allowing the patient some degree of mobility. It is quite possible for the patient in a halo brace to ambulate. The patient with an external fixator on the lower leg can be out of bed in a wheelchair or even ambulate without bearing weight on the affected leg.

Nursing care for patients in these devices is essentially the same as for patients in casts and/or skeletal traction, with the exception that patients in these devices may be mobile earlier.

The **Ilizarov external fixator** was developed in the Soviet Union in 1951 (Figure 64-11). It can be used to treat fractures, deformities, and bony defects (caused by resection of malignancies) and to lengthen limbs. The basic principle of the Ilizarov technique is to achieve new bone growth by performing *corticotomies* (osteotomies through the cortex) and the application of distraction. The corticotomy creates a pseudo growth plate without disrupting the medullary cavity, thereby preserving blood supply and allowing new bone to fill in the distraction gap.[10] The application of gentle traction on the bone stimulates growth. Weight bearing, which also stimulates new bone growth, is usually encouraged.[17]

**Management of patients with internal fixation devices.** Open surgical reduction of fractures has the advantage of allowing visualization of the fracture and surrounding tissues. It is particularly indicated when soft tissue is caught between bone fragments or when nerves or blood vessels are damaged. The disadvantages of internal fixation are that it requires anesthesia and carries the risk of infection at the time of surgery. *Internal fixation is carried out under the most vigorous aseptic conditions, and patients may receive a short course of prophylactic intravenous antibiotics postoperatively.*

A variety of internal fixation devices are available:

1. Plates and nails (Figure 64-12, *A*)
2. Intramedullary rods (Figure 64-12, *B*)
3. Transfixion screws (Figure 64-13)
4. Prosthetic implants (Figure 64-14, *A* and *B*)—used particularly when survival of the proximal fragment of the fracture is jeopardized, for example, a fracture through or immediately below the femoral head

*Bone grafts,* either *autograft* (the patient's own bone) or *allograft* (human donor bone), may be used either in conjunction with internal fixation devices when excessive bone is lost at the fracture site or alone, as in

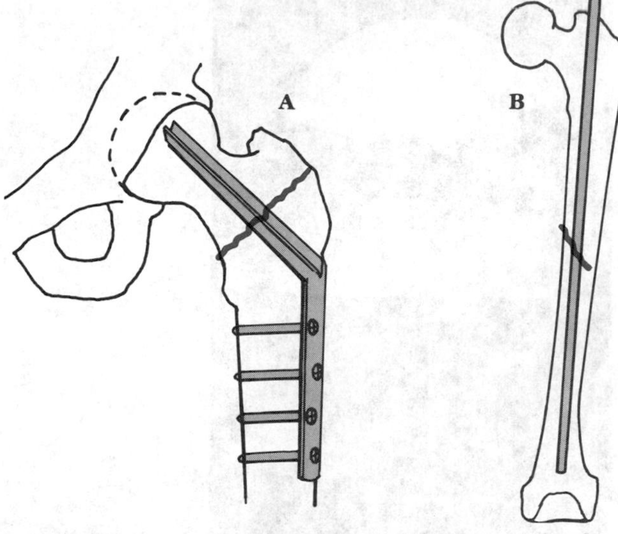


**FIGURE 64-12** **A,** Neufeld nail and screws, used in repair of intertrochanteric fracture. **B,** Küntscher nail (intramedullary rod) used in repair of midshaft femoral fracture.

### Guidelines for Care of the Person with an Internal Fixation Device

1. Patient education
   a. Prepare the patient for general anesthesia
   b. Explain the surgical procedure and general nursing care after surgery
   c. Postoperatively, explain the limits of motion and weight bearing to the affected part
2. Promoting mobility
   a. Determine, in consultation with the physician, the limits of motion and weight bearing permitted
   b. Instruct and assist the patient to turn within the prescribed limits
   c. Assist the patient to transfer and ambulate within the prescribed limits (mobilization may begin as early as the first postoperative day)
   d. Instruct and assist the patient to use an appropriate ambulatory aid if the fracture is of a lower extremity
3. Prevention of neurocirculatory problems
   a. Perform neurocirculatory checks every hour for the first 24 to 48 hours; notify the physician of any change from preoperative status, since this may indicate pressure from swelling, constricting bandages, or damage to nerves or vessels at surgery
   b. Maintain elevation of the affected extremity in bed
4. Maintenance of immobilization of fracture; considerations for care would be the same as for patients in cast/traction if those devices are used (see pp. 2194 and 2199)

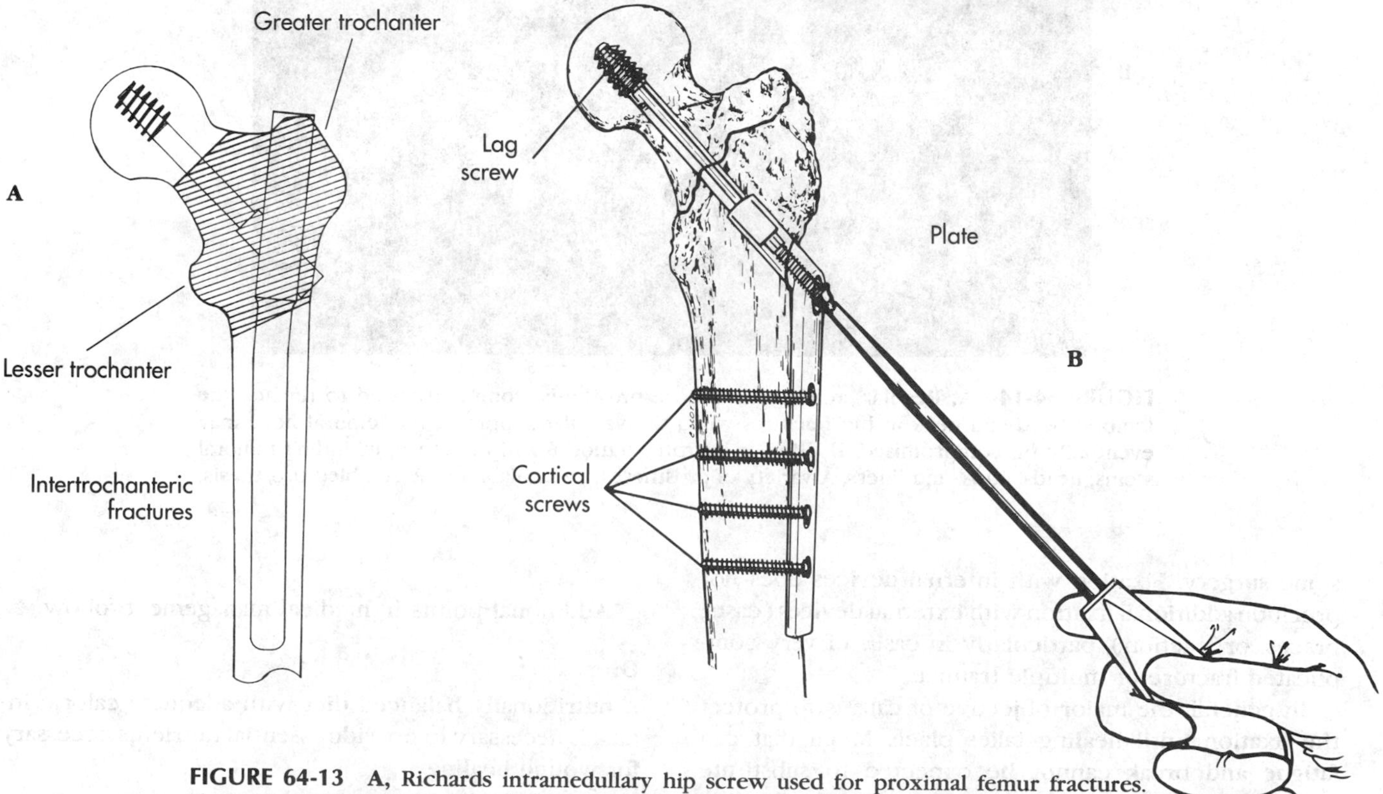

A

Greater trochanter

Lesser trochanter

Intertrochanteric fractures

Lag screw

Plate

B

Cortical screws

**FIGURE 64-13** **A,** Richards intramedullary hip screw used for proximal femur fractures. Shown here for management of intratrochanteric fracture *(shaded area)*. The device consists of intramedullary nail, lag screw, bone screws, compression screw, centering sleeve, and set screw. **B,** Richards compression screw and plate for hip fracture. Compression screw (shown at end of screwdriver) threads into the distal end of the lag screw and draws the fracture fragments together. The sliding feature of the nail and plate assembly reduces the risk of acetabular penetration and allows weight-bearing forces to be transferred to the bone, rather than to the device. (Courtesy Smith & Nephew Richards, Inc.)

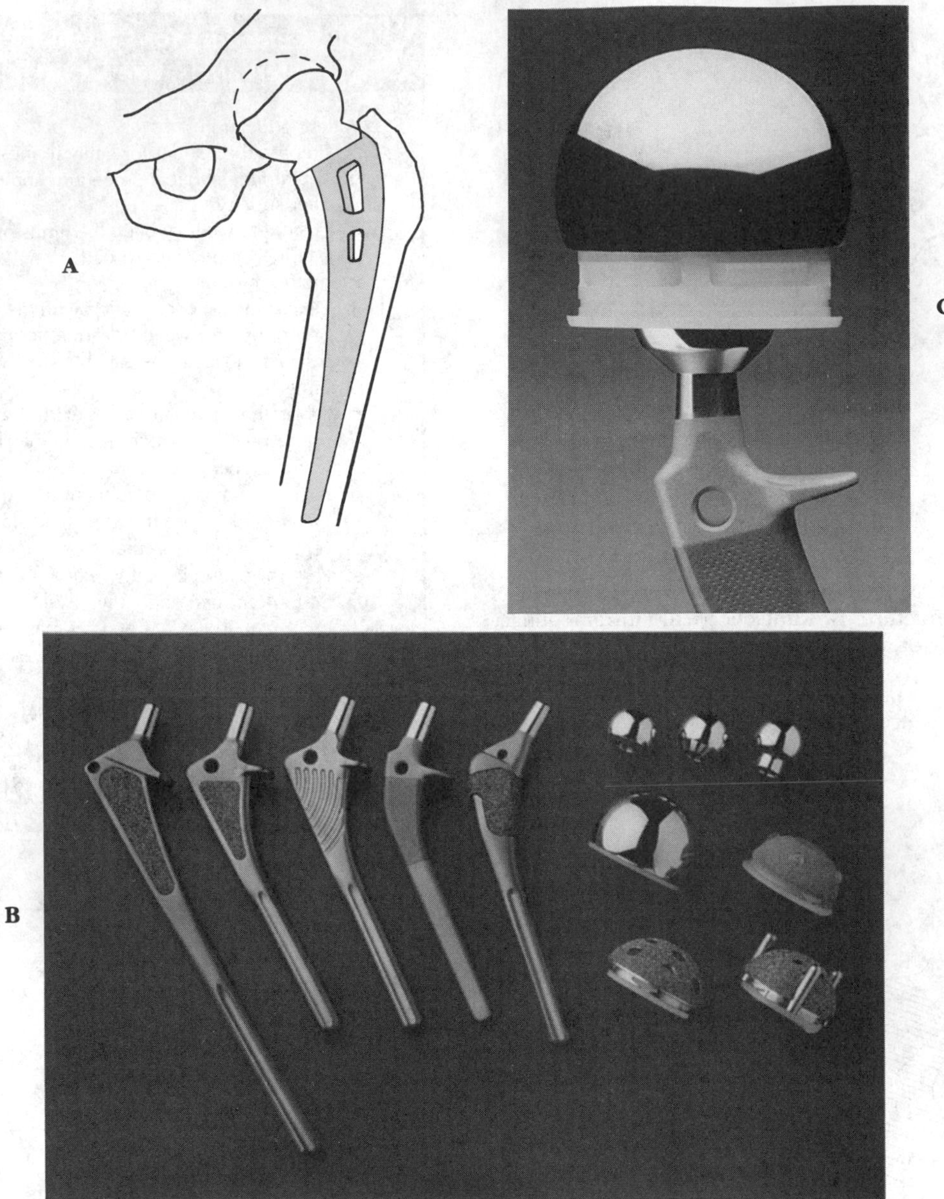


**FIGURE 64-14** **A,** Regular stem Austin Moore prosthesis, commonly used to replace the femoral head and neck in hip fractures when the vascular supply to the femoral head may eventually be compromised. **B,** Bipolar instrumentation for hip fracture, including femoral stems, heads, cups, and liners. A variety of prostheses are available. **C,** Assembled prosthesis.

spine surgery. Fixation with internal devices does not preclude additional fixation with external devices (casts, braces, or traction), particularly in cases of very complicated fracture or multiple trauma.

In general, the major objective of care is to protect the fixation until healing takes place. Metal that can fatigue and break cannot be expected to substitute for intact bone. If the fixation device breaks, healing of the fracture will be disrupted. However, ***mobilization of patients who have had internal fixation is usually much faster than for those who have had external fixation.*** Nursing care of patients with internal fixation devices is summarized in the Guidelines box, p. 2201.

■ ■ ■

Additional points in medical management follow:

### Diet

A nutritionally balanced diet with adequate caloric intake is necessary to provide essential nutrients necessary for wound healing.

### Activity

Activity is limited, depending on the individual patient, type and location of fracture, and method of reduction. The degree of ambulation, activity, and weight-bearing status will be determined by the physician. Specific exercises will also be prescribed by the physician.

**Referral/Consultation**

In some settings the nurse assumes responsibility for making referrals to other services. Common referrals for persons with fractures include physical therapy and occupational therapy for instructions regarding exercises and proper use of assistive and/or support devices.

# NURSING MANAGEMENT

## ♦ ASSESSMENT

### Subjective Data

Subjective data to be collected include the patient's complaint concerning, or description of, the following:

- Pain at site of injury
- Loss of sensation or movement of affected part
- How trauma occurred
- Understanding of injury sustained (may report having heard bone snap)

### Objective Data

Objective data to be collected include the following:

- Warmth, edema, and/or ecchymosis over and surrounding the injured part
- Obvious deformity
- Loss of normal function in the injured part
- Immobilization device(s) applied to the injured part
- Signs of systemic shock
- Signs of circulatory, motor, or sensory impairment to the injured part (Table 64-2)
- Indicators of apprehension or fear

**TABLE 64-2 Signs and Symptoms of Neurocirculatory Impairment**

| SIGNS AND SYMPTOMS | INTERPRETATION |
|---|---|
| Tissue color white | Decreased arterial blood supply |
| Tissue color blue | Venous stasis and poorly oxygenated tissue |
| Color slow to return to nail bed after application of moderate pressure | Decreased arterial blood supply |
| Edema | Fluid accumulating in tissues; poor venous return |
| Tissue cold or cool to touch | Decreased arterial blood supply |
| Patient unable to move parts distal to injury or external fixation device | Pressure on nerves innervating parts distal to injury or underlying external fixation device |
| Patient complaint of extreme pain unrelieved by elevation, analgesic, or repositioning | Pressure on nerves innervating parts distal to injury or underlying external fixation device |
| Patient complaint of heightened or decreased sensation or paresthesia in part distal to injury or underlying external fixation device | Pressure on nerves innervating parts distal to injury or underlying external fixation device |

Comparison of tissue should be made with uninvolved limb to determine the extent of the deviation from normal.

## ♦ NURSING DIAGNOSES

Nursing diagnoses are determined from analysis of patient data. Nursing diagnoses for the patient with a fracture may include but are not limited to the following:

| Nursing Diagnoses | Possible Etiologic Factors |
|---|---|
| Knowledge deficit: fracture | Lack of experience with fracture |
| Injury, high risk for | Sensorimotor deficits |
| Mobility, impaired physical | Musculoskeletal impairment, decreased strength and endurance, pain |
| Pain | Injury to bone, injury to soft tissue at fracture site, muscle spasm, immobility, improper positioning, pressure points |
| Neurovascular dysfunction, high risk for peripheral | Pressure, restrictive envelope, trauma, casts, traction |
| Tissue perfusion, altered, peripheral | Immobility, anesthesia, pressure sites |
| Infection, high risk for | Tissue trauma, surgical intervention |
| Self-care deficit | Musculoskeletal impairment, pain/discomfort, intolerance to activity |
| Home maintenance management, impaired | Surgery, altered mobility, activity restrictions |
| Skin integrity, high risk for impaired | Decreased mobility, pressure, shearing forces |
| Nutrition, altered: less than body requirements | Fatigue, pain, chewing or swallowing difficulties |
| Powerlessness | Health care environment, decreased mobility |

## ♦ EXPECTED PATIENT OUTCOMES

Expected patient outcomes for the patient with a fracture may include but are not limited to the following:

1. Patient and/or significant others can explain rationale and course of treatment including:
   a. Nature of injury and course of treatment that must be followed to prevent injury or infection and to achieve desired result
   b. Limitations of motion and restrictions of activity to be observed and for how long
   c. How to perform or modify activities of daily living (ADL) within the limitations of activity and motion that must be observed
   d. How to care for cast, pins, or other immobilization devices if applicable
   e. Safe use of an ambulatory or other ADL assistive device if necessary
   f. Safe technique in carrying out wound care if necessary
   g. Techniques appropriate to prevent skin breakdown, swelling, and neurocirculatory impairment
   h. Measures that can be taken for relief of pain or discomfort
   i. How to use prescribed medications
   j. Plans for follow-up care

2. Patient avoids injury by using adaptive or assistive devices correctly
3. Patient participates in a program of progressive activity
4. Patient states that pain is decreased with a lower rating on a scale of 1 to 10 (1 = no pain, 10 = most severe pain imaginable)
5. Patient maintains intact peripheral neurovascular status in all extremities
6. Patient maintains adequate tissue perfusion
7. Patient does not develop an infection
8. Patient demonstrates ability to do self-care
9. Patient adapts home environment to meet his or her needs
   a. Removes scatter rugs
   b. Positions furniture to provide clear pathway when ambulating with walker or crutches
   c. Places safety devices in bathroom (grab bars, elevated toilet seat, tub rails)
10. Patient maintains skin integrity
11. Patient stabilizes weight at an acceptable level
12. Patient verbalizes sense of power and control of life

## ♦ INTERVENTIONS

### Facilitating Learning

Treatment of the acute fracture is usually carried out in the hospital's emergency room or in the operating room before the patient is admitted to the general hospital unit. Patients will have had little or no opportunity to become oriented to the hospital or to the care they will be receiving. In addition, they will probably be frightened or overwhelmed by what has happened to them, be experiencing pain, and possibly be groggy from pain medication or anesthesia. Careful and often repeated explanation and direction regarding the following will be necessary:

1. Nature of injury and course of treatment, including follow-up care
2. Positioning
3. Skin care routines
4. Deep breathing and coughing
5. Pain relief measures
6. Exercises to be performed to prevent complications

Direction, explanation, and physical handling must be accomplished gently but efficiently during the initial stages of hospitalization. Patients must be given time to adjust to their situation before they can begin to understand how they can cooperate in their care.

### Preventing Injury/Promoting Self-Care

As healing progresses and pain diminishes, patients will be more receptive to learning what will be necessary for a safe return home. The following instructions should be included:

1. How to move comfortably in bed
2. How to transfer safely in and out of bed
3. What weight-bearing restrictions to observe and for how long
4. What activity limitations to observe and for how long
5. How to properly use ambulatory or other ADL assistive devices
6. What assistance will be needed to perform ADL
7. What equipment will be needed and how it can be obtained
8. How to use and/or care for immobilization devices (slings, casts, and pins)
9. How to avoid swelling in the affected part by proper elevation
10. How to control pain or discomfort in the affected part
11. What exercises to perform to maintain strength and enhance circulation

The easiest and most effective way to teach patients how to manage themselves is to have them function as independently as possible within their prescribed limitations and with whatever assistive aids they need while they are in the hospital.

### Maintaining Strength and Mobility/Promoting Activity

One objective in the care of the patient who has sustained a fracture is to prevent loss of mobility and muscle tone. This is true for the fractured part, as well as for the rest of the body. The nurse can use the following interventions to maintain mobility, muscle tone, and strength:

1. Allow and encourage the patient to move about to the greatest extent possible within the restrictions of the fracture reduction and the immobilizing devices.
2. Allow and encourage the patient to accomplish as much self-care as possible.
3. Encourage the patient to perform muscle toning (isometric) exercises on a regular basis, for example, quadriceps setting, gluteal setting (see Chapter 23).
4. Encourage and assist the patient to follow through with exercise programs (including ambulation) prescribed by the physician and taught by the physical therapist.
5. Encourage and assist patient to resume normal functioning for all ADL (within limits of immobilization or fixation device) as soon as possible, for example, using bedside commode or toilet instead of bedpan.

### Promoting Comfort

The person with a fracture will most often have severe pain at the fracture site, pressure from edema in the damaged soft tissues adjacent to the fracture, and spasm of the muscles in the fracture area. Continued pain and the muscle spasm accompanying it can put undue stress on the fracture fragments and retard efforts both to reduce and to maintain reduction of the fracture. Patients who are in severe pain will resist efforts to help them carry out measures designed to prevent complications. If the fracture is repaired by **open reduction** and **internal fixation,** the patient will have operative pain.

Measures the nurse can take to help reduce pain include the following:

1. During initial stages of treatment, administer prescribed narcotic and nonnarcotic analgesics in appropriate doses at timely intervals.
2. Administer prescribed agents such as diazepam (Valium) to reduce muscle spasm.
3. Apply ice compresses, as ordered, to the affected part to reduce swelling.
4. Reposition patient frequently within prescribed position or activity limitations to avoid prolonged pressure over bony prominences and to prevent stiffness.
5. Instruct patient how to use relaxation techniques (deep breathing, imagery) to reduce tension.
6. As pain subsides, negotiate with the patient a reduction in the strength and/or frequency of analgesic administration.

With the use of analgesics, it is important to try to maintain a balance of having the patient comfortable enough to perform required exercises and other activities but not so overly medicated as to risk potential damage through overextending activity or heavy sedation. Devices that allow patients to self-administer intravenous narcotics (*patient-controlled analgesia* [PCA] pumps) are extremely effective in managing posttraumatic and postoperative pain, because they eliminate the highs and lows of drug concentrations characteristic of intermittent parenteral dosing.[13]

Positioning is a measure that promotes comfort, provides for adequate ventilation and mobilization of pulmonary secretions, enhances circulation, and relieves pressure on skin areas. However, there is certain knowledge the nurse must have before positioning a patient with a fracture:

1. Where is the fracture?
2. What is the nature of the fracture?
3. Has the fracture been reduced?
4. What method was used to reduce the fracture?
5. What are the tolerances of the method used to reduce the fracture?
6. Is the fracture stable?
7. Has the orthopedist requested special precautions?

After this information is obtained, positioning should be done with careful attention to avoid the following:

1. Altering the alignment of the fracture
2. Changing the direction of the pull of traction (if used)
3. Compromising the integrity of the cast (if used)
4. Placing undue stress on the internal fixation device (if used)

Generally, nurses should avoid changing the position of patients with unreduced, unsplinted fractures.

Once the parameters for safe positioning are defined, the nurse should assist the patient to change position at least every 2 hours until the patient can independently perform this function. Providing an overhead frame with a trapeze will assist the patient to move about in bed.

## Maintaining Intact Neurovascular Status and Tissue Perfusion

*Monitoring for* **neurocirculatory compromise** *must be carried out every hour in the initial stages of fracture.* Damage to blood vessels and/or nerves may occur at the time of the fracture or subsequent to the fracture or its reduction. Some swelling of a fractured extremity may be expected and is often well controlled by elevating the extremity. However, unrelieved swelling of an extremity that is confined in a cast or compression dressing causes undue pressure on vessels and nerves and can result in circulatory and/or neurologic impairment. *Evidence of impaired circulation or sensation must be reported to the physician immediately.* Frequency of neurocirculatory checks can usually be reduced if there is no evidence of compromise within 48 hours of the fracture or reduction (see Table 64-2). Observations of the involved extremity should be compared with observations of the uninvolved, or normal, extremity to validate deviations from "normal."

Monitoring neurocirculatory status of the injured part includes the following:

1. Palpating for warmth
2. Observing color
3. Applying moderate pressure to nail bed and observing speed of capillary refill
4. Questioning patient about pain and paresthesias in injured part
5. Touching injured part to test patient's ability to discriminate sensation
6. Observing patient's ability to voluntarily move body part distal to fracture
7. Instituting measures to promote venous blood flow:
    a. Elevate extremities to level slightly above the heart
    b. Apply elastic stockings
    c. Use proper positioning techniques
    d. Avoid external compression on pressure sites
    e. Encourage range of motion (ROM) exercises
8. Assessing for presence of positive Homans' sign
9. Encouraging ambulation if possible
10. Obtaining baseline and ongoing measurements of circumference of both calves for comparison

## Preventing Infection

Interventions to promote wound healing include the following:

1. Carefully attending to aseptic technique during dressing changes to prevent infection

2. Attending to drains to maintain their placement and patency to prevent the development of hematoma
3. Observing pin sites regularly and caring for them as ordered to prevent infection
4. Providing and encouraging patient to eat a well-balanced diet to provide the essential nutritional elements necessary for tissue healing

## Facilitating Return to Home Environment

In preparation for the patient's discharge the following should be determined:

1. Assess probable level of functioning at time of discharge and determine type of assistance and equipment that will be needed.
   a. As necessary refer to home care team, community health nurse, or other agency that will meet with patient and family to determine what help (aide, homemaker) may be needed. This is especially important for persons who live alone or who will be alone from long periods of time while family members are at work.
   b. Most patients will need a walker and/or crutches, and should be taught to use these before discharge. It should be reinforced that scatter rugs need to be removed so that the patient will not trip on them when walking with an assistive device. Low-pile bathroom carpets that completely cover the bathroom floor are available and may be an option for patients not on a limited income.
   c. Furniture should be positioned to provide a clear pathway in areas where the patient will be walking, especially between bedroom and bathroom.
   d. Safety devices such as an elevated toilet seat and grab bars and tub rails should be in place before the patient arrives home. Elevated toilet seats with arms on each side can be rented from a medical supply store.
2. Provide guidance about the availability of community resources such as Meals on Wheels and exercise pools.
3. Assess the patient's support system, and encourage its use.
4. Support the patient's and family's decision-making abilities.
5. Teach and supervise correct use of adaptive devices. In many institutions much of this teaching is done by physical and occupational therapists. However, the nurse needs to reinforce the teaching and supervise the patient in the correct use of these devices.

## Maintaining Skin Integrity

When determining interventions to maintain skin integrity, the nurse must consider ways to prevent skin breakdown, as well as ways to promote wound healing. Measures to prevent skin breakdown include the following:

1. Identifying skin areas at risk, particularly areas over bony prominences (e.g., heels, sacrum, elbows, and ischial tuberosities)
2. Applying a skin-toughening agent such as tincture of benzoin two or three times per day to areas identified as being at risk
3. Inspecting skin (at least every 8 hours) for signs of pressure, for example, erythema or induration
4. Turning (at least every 2 hours) within limits of system of fracture immobilization using a turning sheet
5. Moving patient from one surface to another with a pull sheet or roller board
6. Rolling patient onto side or lifting patient to place him or her on a bedpan rather than sliding pan under patient
7. For patient who cannot be fully turned because of traction apparatus or other limiting factors, possibly using one or more of the following pressure-relieving devices:
   a. Sheepskin pads
   b. Flotation pads
   c. Alternating air pressure mattress, or alternating air pressure system such as Lapidus system
   d. Foam mattress
   e. Foam heel and/or elbow pads
   f. Special bed such as the Clinitron, Mediscus, or Biodyne
   g. Turning frames such as the Foster or Stryker frames
8. Regularly inspecting skin areas in contact with cast edges or traction apparatus and taking appropriate measures to eliminate chafing or rubbing in those areas (see pp. 2194 and 2199)
9. Assisting patient to keep skin clean and dry, especially under casts, slings, and traction apparatus

## Promoting Nutrition/Stabilizing Weight

The essentials of a nutritious diet, which includes fruits, vegetables, proteins, and vitamins, are as important for the individual after a fracture as for anyone else. *If mobility is restricted, catabolic activity is accelerated,* producing a rapid breakdown of cellular materials, leading to *protein deficiency* and *negative nitrogen balance.* Decalcification and demineralization of bone take place during immobility, regardless of the quantity of calcium intake. Therefore increasing calcium in the diet above normal requirements is not recommended, because the excess calcium cannot be used. However, a diet high in protein is indicated to overcome protein deficiency and to return the body to a state of positive nitrogen balance. Patients who have had fractures have increased needs for iron, protein, and vitamins if bone repair is to progress normally. Weight gain is to be avoided, especially if the patient is in a cast or molded brace.

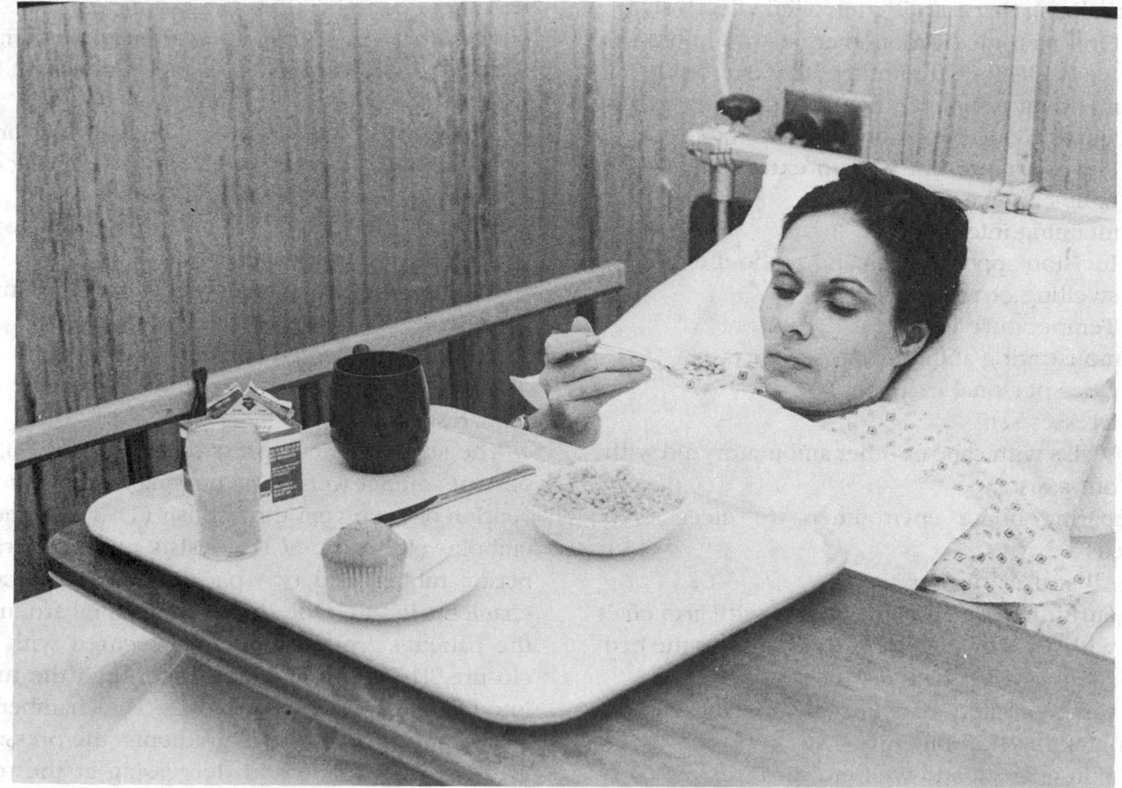

**FIGURE 64-15** Patient who can neither sit up nor lie on one side to eat meals can still be made comfortable with some elevation of the head and shoulders on pillows. Additional means of elevating patient to a more upright position is to put frame of bed in reverse Trendelenburg's position.

Interventions the nurse can use to ensure adequate nutrition for the patient include the following:

1. Encourage the patient to eat regular meals.
2. Allow the patient adequate time to eat.
3. Encourage self-feeding, but help the patient or provide special assistive utensils as necessary.
4. Attend to the patient's need for roughage and fluid as noted and encourage protein intake of 150 to 300 g per day.
5. Position the patient to facilitate comfortable intake of food and fluid (Figure 64-15).

## Promoting Autonomy and Sense of Control

To prevent the patient from feeling powerless, the following interventions may be helpful:

1. Explain course of treatment to patient and family.
2. Provide opportunities for decision making when possible.
3. Incorporate patient preferences into daily plan of care.
4. Allow the patient to manipulate the environment whenever possible.

# ♦ EVALUATION

To evaluate the effectiveness of nursing interventions, compare patient behaviors with those stated in the expected patient outcomes. Successful achievement of patient outcomes for the patient with a fracture is indicated by the following:

1. Describing the nature of the injury and course of treatment correctly
   a. Explaining the limitations of motion and the restrictions to be observed and for how long
   b. Explaining how to perform ADL correctly
   c. Describing how to care for cast, pins, or other immobilization devices
   d. Explaining correct way to walk with cane, walker, or crutches
   e. Explaining how to cleanse wound and apply sterile dressings if applicable
   f. Explaining how to prevent skin breakdown, swelling, and neurocirculatory impairment
   g. Explaining how to take NSAIDs: always with food and never on an empty stomach
   h. Explaining plans for follow up care
2. Ambulating safely using a cane, walker, or crutches
3. Participating in a program of progressive exercise
   a. Goes to physical therapy twice daily to practice prescribed exercises
   b. Performs exercise program in bed before going to sleep
   c. Gets up to use bathroom by self
   d. Prepares self for bed

4. Verbalizing that pain is controlled effectively by:
   a. Oral pain medication every 4 to 5 hours
   b. Ice packs for 20 minutes after exercising
5. Maintaining peripheral neurovascular status and adequate tissue perfusion
   a. Pulses are present in both extremities
   b. Limbs are warm and pink
6. Maintaining infection-free status
   a. Incision appears clean and without excessive swelling or redness
   b. Temperature is normal
7. Demonstrating ability to do self-care
   a. Does personal care
   b. Dresses self
   c. Walks with cane or other ambulatory aid without assistance
8. Preparing home environment to meet safety needs
   a. All scatter rugs taken up
   b. Furniture placed conveniently with firm chair with arms in areas most used, such as the bedroom and kitchen
   c. Has two safety bars in stall shower
9. Maintaining skin integrity
   a. Skin is clean and well moisturized
   b. Skin is free of abrasions
10. Maintaining weight at acceptable level
    a. Weight is 5 lb less than before surgery
    b. Is eating a varied diet with adequate calories to return weight to presurgery level
11. Verbalizing feeling in control of own life

## COMPLICATIONS OF FRACTURES

Complications can arise as a result of the initial trauma, treatment, or the resulting loss of mobility. Systemic complications usually are a result of immobility or surgical intervention and include *circulatory, respiratory, gastrointestinal,* and *urinary* complications.

### Preventing Systemic Complications

#### Preventing circulatory complications

Individuals who have sustained trauma and are wholly or partially immobilized are at risk to develop circulatory complications because of the following:

1. Failure of blood vessels in the legs to achieve and maintain a state of vasoconstriction
2. Pooling of venous blood and decreased venous return
3. Decreased cardiac output
4. Increased prothrombin time and platelet adhesiveness

These factors contribute to decreased ability to adapt to an erect posture, increased incidence of deep-vein thrombosis and pulmonary embolus, increased workload on the heart, and decreased tolerance to exercise or activity.

Interventions the nurse can use to help offset or prevent these complications are as follows:

1. Encourage and assist the patient to perform routine active or active-assisted ROM exercises (at least four times per day).
2. Teach and encourage the patient to perform active dorsiplantar flexion and quadriceps setting exercises every 1 to 2 hours.
3. Position the patient so that pressure is not exerted over major vessels.
4. Mobilize the patient slowly and increase activity gradually.
5. Elevate the affected extremity for the first 48 hours; thereafter, elevate the extremity when the patient is at rest.

The sequential compression device (SCD) is an important adjunct to routine nursing measures in the prevention of deep vein thrombosis (DVT) and pulmonary embolus (PE). The SCD consists of an electric motor, plastic tubing, and two plastic leg sleeves containing chambers for air. One sleeve is wrapped around each of the patient's legs, and each is secured with a Velcro closure. The motor pumps air through the tubing and into the chambers in the sleeves. The chambers fill with air at controlled pressure gradients, the pressure being greater at the ankle and decreasing at the top of the thigh. The SCD promotes venous return by filling and then decompressing, thus "pumping" blood through the veins and substituting for the pumping effect of the muscles in the person who is ambulatory. This device can be applied before a fracture is reduced and should be continued for 72 hours after reduction or until the patient is ambulatory.

#### Preventing respiratory complications

Factors that contribute to pooling of secretions in the bronchi and bronchioles are pain on movement or deep breathing, decreased movement, decreased stimulus to cough, and decreased depth of respiration.

Unless interventions are used to facilitate movement and removal of secretions, hypostatic pneumonia can result. Nursing interventions include the following:

1. Turning patient frequently to mobilize secretions
2. Encouraging patient to perform active or active-assisted ROM exercises to increase depth of respiration
3. Using appropriate pain control measures to improve respiratory effort
4. Teaching and encouraging patient to take maximal sustained inhalations and to cough to mobilize and clear secretions every 2 hours
5. Encouraging patient to move independently as much as possible to solicit improved respiratory effort

#### Preventing gastrointestinal complications

Individuals who sustain trauma to the spine, fracture one or more of the lower extremities, or undergo surgery for spine or lower extremity fracture fixation will frequently experience a slowing or temporary cessation of bowel function. If these persons eat or drink, they are at risk to develop paralytic ileus (see Chapter 45). Therefore nurses must withhold food and fluid until the presence of bowel sounds is established or, preferably, until the patient is passing flatus.

In addition, individuals with fractures who are wholly are partially immobilized are frequently constipated. Contributing factors are changes in normal dietary habits and fluid intake, lack of activity, and use of a bedpan. Interventions the nurse can use to promote gastric motility and prevent constipation include the following:

1. Turning the patient frequently
2. Elevating the head of the bed (as permitted)
3. Administering stool-softening agents, laxatives, or suppositories
4. Encouraging the patient to incorporate in the diet bulk-building foods such as bran
5. Encouraging a fluid intake of 2000 to 3000 ml per day
6. Assisting the patient to use a bedside commode or toilet instead of a bedpan when possible

**Preventing urinary complications**

Patients with fractures, particularly if immobilized, are at risk to develop bladder infections and renal stones for the following reasons:

1. Increased serum calcium, because of bone destruction
2. Increased urinary pH (alkaline)
3. Increased citric acid (which precipitates calcium salts)
4. Stasis of urine in bladder, because of difficulty emptying bladder when using a urinal or bedpan in bed

Nursing interventions to decrease risk of these problems include the following:

1. Encouraging a fluid intake of 2000 to 3000 ml per day
2. Encouraging patient to decrease calcium intake
3. Encouraging patient to limit intake of citrus fruits and juices
4. Assisting patient to use a bedside commode or toilet when possible to facilitate emptying bladder

## FAT EMBOLISM SYNDROME

*Fat embolism syndrome (FES)* is a potentially fatal complication associated with fractures, crush injuries, total hip arthroplasty, and total knee arthroplasty. Fat emboli may lead to *adult respiratory distress syndrome (ARDS),* with an associated mortality of 50%, especially if the onset is more than 5 days after trauma.

### Etiology/Epidemiology

FES is most common following fractures of the *pelvis, femur, and tibia.* Persons with total hip and knee arthroplasties are at risk for FES because of surgical reaming of the intramedullary canal to allow seating of the prosthesis, which may cause fat to enter the venous system. The incidence of FES following long bone fractures is reported to be 0.5% to 2% and 5% to 10% following multiple fractures or pelvic fracture. An increase in serum glucose and beta lipoprotein levels may increase the incidence of FES.[8] FES usually occurs within 24 hours of injury in 60% of patients and within 48 hours after injury in 85% of cases.

### Pathophysiology

Following fracture, fat globules are released from the bone marrow and local tissue into circulation. The fat molecules enter the venous circulation, travel to the lungs, and embolize the small capillaries and arterioles. Lipase is produced to break down fat molecules into fatty acids. These chemical changes are irritating to pulmonary tissue and result in increased permeability of the alveolocapillary membrane, interstitial hemorrhage, edema, and atelectasis. Eventually, hypoxemia and ARDS may develop. Refer to Chapter 37 for a discussion of ARDS. Fatty acids attract red blood cells (RBCs) and platelets, forming an aggregate, which can lead to disseminated intravascular coagulation (DIC) and emboli to the brain and other vital organs.

Symptoms of FES include hypoxemia, tachypnea, tachycardia, petechiae, fever, lipuria, chest pain, and altered mental status. Alteration in mental status is an important clinical indicator of FES. Seventy-five percent of persons with FES will develop significant neurologic symptoms, which may manifest as restlessness, confusion, lethargy, or coma. Petechiae, considered a "classic" symptom of FES, occur in only 50% to 60% of persons with FES. They are usually found on the conjunctiva, axilla, chest, and neck and are thought to be caused by capillary occlusion with fat and fibrin. The rash does not blanch with pressure but usually disappears within 48 hours of onset. The *presence of unexplained fever,* especially when *accompanied by a change in mental status and petechiae, should alert the caregiver to the possibility of FES.* This is a medical emergency, and the physician should be notified immediately.

### ➠ Managing Critical Care

The patient is transferred to the intensive care unit because of the need for constant monitoring. Treatment consists of oxygen therapy, mechanical ventilation with *positive end-expiratory pressure (PEEP),* fluid replacement, and administration of steroids (their use is controversial).[8,14] Preventive measures include early immobilization (within 24 hours of injury) of patients with long bone fractures. Patients who undergo early stabilization of fractures experience shorter hospital stays and less incidence of respiratory complications than those with late stabilization (more than 48 hours after injury) of fractures.

**TABLE 64-3 Comparison of Fat Embolism and Pulmonary Embolism**

| FAT EMBOLISM | PULMONARY EMBOLISM |
|---|---|
| **PATHOPHYSIOLOGY** | |
| Fat globules released from marrow following fracture(s) enter bloodstream and obstruct pulmonary circulation | DVT dislodges and obstructs pulmonary circulation |
| **ONSET OF SYMPTOMS** | |
| Usually 1-4 days after injury | Usually 4-10 days after trauma or development of thrombophlebitis but can occur much later |
| **SIGNS AND SYMPTOMS** | |
| Altered mental status<br>Dyspnea<br>Tachypnea<br>Tachycardia<br>Petechial rash<br>Fever<br>Restlessness<br>Agitation | Dyspnea<br>Chest pain<br>Apprehension<br>Anxiety<br>Cough<br>Hemoptysis<br>Tachypnea<br>Tachycardia<br>Fever |
| **RISK FACTORS** | |
| Hypovolemia<br>Shock<br>Delayed immobilization of fracture<br>Multiple fractures | Venous stasis<br>Immobility<br>Obesity<br>Trauma<br>Major surgery<br>History of heart disease<br>Age >40 yr<br>History of DVT, PE |

## Diagnostic Tests

Arterial blood gases are obtained to determine the amount of hypoxemia. Fat may be found in the blood and urine, although *lipuria* is a *normal finding after fracture* and therefore is not of clinical significance in FES. *Blood analysis* will reveal a *decreased hemoglobin* and *platelet count.* Chest x-ray films will detect changes related to fat embolus in only one third of patients. If ARDS develops, chest films will show areas of consolidation. A lung scan (VQ scan or ventilation/perfusion scan) may be used to rule out pulmonary embolus (Table 64-3).

## Nursing Management

The most important nursing interventions are the recognition of patients who are at risk for developing FES and careful monitoring for early detection of clinical indicators of FES. Careful handling of the fractured extremity, especially when turning and positioning the patient, will decrease manipulation of the fracture site, decreasing the risk of fat emboli. Other nursing interventions are those that pertain to the care of persons with ARDS (see Chapter 37).

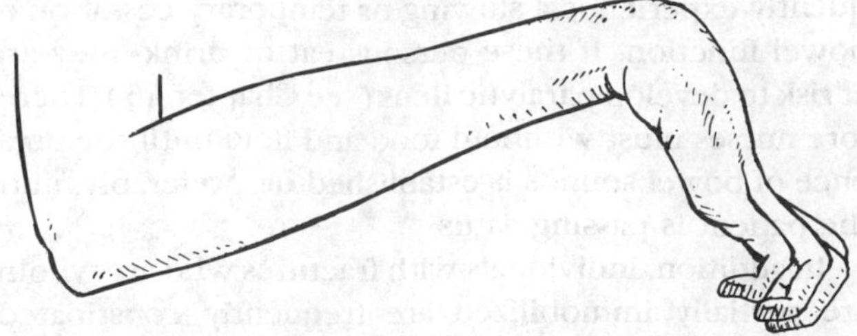

**FIGURE 64-16** Volkmann's ischemic contracture.

# COMPARTMENT SYNDROME

*Compartment syndrome (CS)* is a complication following trauma in which *increased pressure* within a *limited anatomic space compromises the circulation, viability,* and *function of the tissues within that space.*[12,14] CS was first recognized more than 100 years ago. In 1881 Volkmann described an upper extremity contracture that he attributed to trauma, swelling, and restrictive dressings[12] (Figure 64-16). If unrecognized, CS can lead to loss of function, deformity, and possibly amputation. Failure to recognize CS has been cited as the most common cause of medical litigation in the United States.[12]

## Etiology/Epidemiology

For CS to occur, there must be a *space-limiting sleeve surrounding the tissue* and *increased tissue pressure.* The *space-limiting sleeve* can be a *restrictive dressing, splint, cast, fascia, or epimysium.* Increased pressure within the compartment results from anything that either increases the contents of the compartment or decreases its size. Compartments consist of muscles, nerves, and blood vessels surrounded by a nonelastic covering. The body contains 46 compartments, 38 of which are found in the extremities, which are the most vulnerable to the development of CS. The most common sites are the four compartments of the lower leg (deep posterior, superficial posterior, lateral, and anterior) (Figure 64-17), the dorsal and volar compartments of the forearm, and the interosseous compartments of the hand.

Although CS usually occurs as a result of trauma, there are several other causes (Box 64-3). Shock can also increase the risk of CS.

## Pathophysiology

Following trauma, fluid accumulates in the compartment and fascia cannot expand to accommodate the excess fluid, causing compartment pressure to rise. Increases in tissue and venous pressures result in a decreased arteriovenous gradient. The end result is decreased blood supply and tissue hypoxia. In an attempt to correct

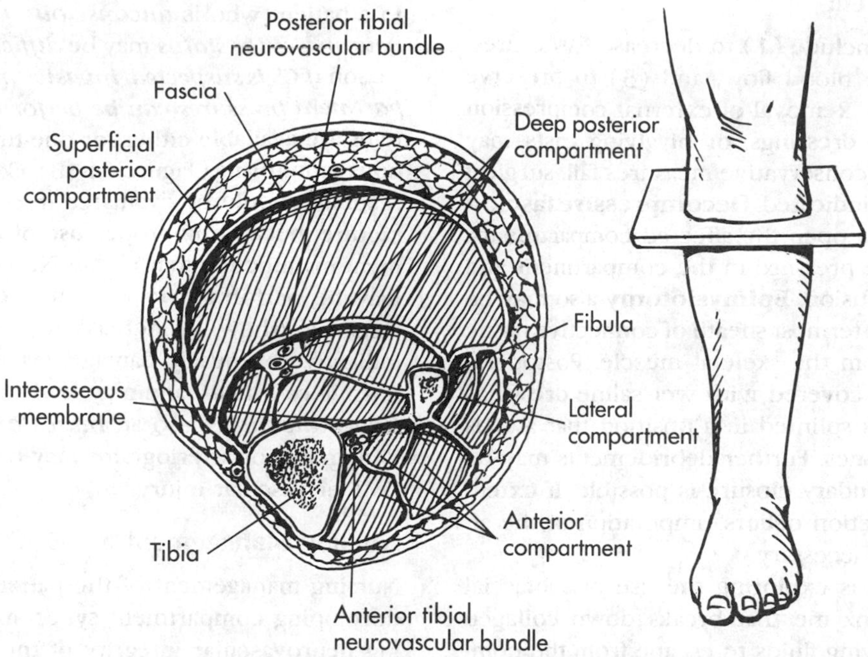


**FIGURE 64-17** Compartments of lower leg.

the hypoxia, histamine is released, causing vasodilation and increased capillary permeability, which causes compartment pressure to continue to rise. Rising pressures lead to *tissue ischemia* and eventually *necrosis. Muscle tissue* will undergo *ischemic changes* within 4 to 12 hours after injury. *Neuropathy* can develop within 12 to 24 hours and *contracture (ischemic paralysis)* begins to develop within 12 hours of ischemia. If extensive ischemic muscle damage occurs, *myoglobinuria* may occur, leading to systemic *complications* that include *renal failure, metabolic acidosis, hyperkalemia,* and *sepsis.* Normal tissue compartment pressure is 1 to 10 mm Hg. Sustained pressure readings of 40 to 60 mm Hg usually require prompt treatment, but this varies with the individual patient.

Early recognition of symptoms and prompt treatment may preserve the function of the limb. Pain is the most common symptom of compartment syndrome. The patient may report severe, unrelenting pain, unrelieved by analgesia and increased by elevation of the extremity. The intensity of pain is usually greater than expected for the extent of the injury. Passive movement or stretching of the digits will increase pain.

Motor and sensory function will also be affected. *Hypoesthesia, paresthesias,* and *muscular weakness* or *paralysis* are *common.* Skin color, temperature, capillary refill, and quality of peripheral pulses are not reliable clinical indicators for the presence of CS. If *pallor, coolness, slow capillary refill,* and *diminished* or *absent pulses* are present, *extensive* and probably *irreversible damage* has probably already occurred.

**BOX 64-3 Causes of Compartment Syndrome**

**BLEEDING**
- Vascular injury
- Coagulation defect (hemophilia, anticoagulant therapy)

**NEPHROTIC SYNDROME**

**EXCESSIVE MUSCLE USE**
- Exercise
- Seizures
- Tetany
- Eclampsia

**TRAUMA**
- Fractures
- Crush injuries
- Hypothermia, frostbite
- Burns
- Snake or spider bites

**INFILTRATED INFUSIONS**

**SURGERY**

**EXTERNAL PRESSURE**
- Positioning (lying on limb)
- Surgical tourniquets
- MAST trousers
- Circumferential restrictive dressings
- Tight cast
- Splints

**DECREASED COMPARTMENT SIZE**
- Excessive traction
- Closure of fascial defects

## Medical Management

Goals of treatment include (1) to decrease tissue pressure, (2) to restore blood flow, and (3) to preserve function of the limb. Removal of external compression devices by splitting dressings, or bivalving casts may alleviate early CS. If conservative measures fail, surgical intervention may be indicated. **Decompressive fasciotomy** is performed to open the affected compartments, which decreases the pressure in the compartment and restores normal perfusion. **Epimysiotomy** also may be necessary, and the outermost sheath of connective tissue will be removed from the skeletal muscle. Postoperatively the wound is covered with wet saline dressings and the extremity is splinted in a position that avoids stretching of the tissues. Further debridements may be necessary until secondary closure is possible. If extensive damage or infection occurs, amputation of the affected limb may be necessary.

Current research is exploring the use of subfascial hyaluronidase, an enzyme that breaks down collagen fibers in fascia, allowing fluids to escape from the compromised compartment.[12] As yet, this method has not been demonstrated to be effective.

If contractures develop, splints and physical and occupational therapy may be indicated. In some cases, additional surgery such as joint fusion, tenotomy, or tendon transfers may be performed.

### Diagnostic tests

As mentioned earlier, recognition of early signs and symptoms may lead to prompt diagnosis and treatment. In a patient who is *unconscious, pain and changes in neurovascular status* may be *difficult to assess.* For this reason *if CS is suspected, invasive measurement of compartment pressures can be performed.* A variety of systems are available either for one-time use or for continuous monitoring (Figure 64-18). Compartment pressure readings should be evaluated in relation to the clinical picture, because improper use of the device or instrument malfunction may occur. Nerve conduction studies may be performed to evaluate nerve function. Blood tests may show an increase in CPK, LDH, and SGOT, indicative of muscle damage. *Myoglobinuria* indicates *muscle cell death* and may lead to *acute renal failure. Hyperkalemia* is also an *indicator* of *muscle damage.* Venograms or arteriograms may be ordered to rule out DVT or vascular injury.

## Nursing Management

Nursing management of the patient with or at risk for developing compartment syndrome includes maintaining neurovascular integrity of the extremities. Careful monitoring of the neurovascular status of the extremities is crucial in the detection and prevention of CS. The nurse obtains baseline data and always assesses both limbs. Knowledge of innervation to the extremities is useful when assessing for deficits. Hourly assessments should be performed and recorded, noting any reports of increased pain, pain that occurs with passive stretching, and alterations in sensory or motor function. The patient should be assessed for the ability to extend, flex, abduct, adduct, and oppose the fingers and thumbs and

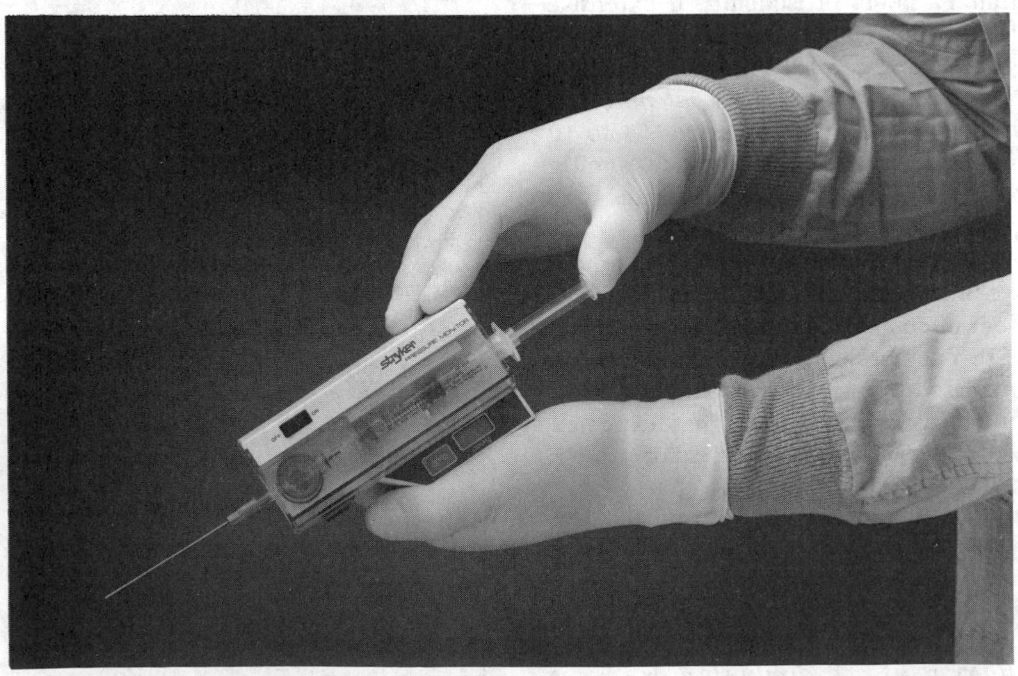


**FIGURE 64-18** Compartment pressure monitor. (Courtesy Stryker Instruments, Kalamazoo, Mich.)

flex the wrist. If the lower extremities are involved, the ability to extend and flex the toes, perform plantar flexion and dorsiflexion, and to invert and evert the foot should be assessed.

An adequate fluid intake is encouraged. Active ROM to other extremities and ambulation are performed if possible. Isometric exercises are taught and encouraged. Dressings, splints, and casts are checked for excessive pressure, and compartment pressures are monitored and recorded. Any significant changes are reported to the physician.

Reports of pain are monitored, and the effectiveness of pain relief measures is assessed.

If CS is suspected, the physician is notified, restrictive dressings are loosened, and the extremity is lowered to the level of the heart. If ice packs are being used, they are removed because the application of cold and elevation of the limb may further impair the circulation.

## HIP FRACTURE

### Etiology/Epidemiology

Hip fractures are a serious problem, especially for elderly persons. The incidence of hip fracture increases with age, doubling every 5 years over 50 years of age.[1] It is estimated that one third of the female and one sixth of the male population over 90 years of age will experience a hip fracture.[1] Currently it is estimated that more than 200,000 hip fractures occur annually and the health care costs associated with them exceed 7 billion dollars.[16] Repair of a hip fracture is probably the most common surgical procedure for persons over 85 years. As the incidence of osteoporosis increases, the incidence of fracture of the femoral neck may increase by 40% with an estimated occurrence of 500,000 hip fractures annually by the year 2000.[1] Risk factors commonly associated with hip fracture include osteoporosis, advanced age, being female and white, decreased estrogen levels (because of postmenopausal changes or bilateral oophorectomy), and sedentary life-style.[16] Other risk factors include an inadequate dietary intake of calcium and vitamin D, excessive dietary protein, caffeine intake, smoking, alcohol use, and use of psychotropic drugs. Although the incidence of hip fracture is most commonly associated with women, the risk of hip fracture in elderly men has increased as well.[16] Black persons past 45 years of age are less likely to experience hip fractures because of the increased mineral content and increased mass of their bones.

The hospital stay of elderly persons with hip fractures is often complicated and prolonged and may result in chronic disability, transfer to an extended care facility, or death. It is estimated that approximately 15% of persons hospitalized with a hip fracture die within a short period of time, 30% die within 1 year, and 30% to 50% never return to their prior level of functioning.[3] The greater the individual's age, the less chance there is of regaining prefracture functional status. Factors that negatively influence recovery and increase mortality following hip fracture include being male, preexisting medical problems, cognitive impairment, and the development of postoperative complications.

### Pathophysiology

Fractures of the hip may be classified in the two following general categories (Figure 64-19):

1. **Intracapsular**—occurring within the hip joint and capsule; these include the following types:
   a. Subcapital fracture
   b. Transcervical fracture
   c. Basal neck fracture
2. **Extracapsular**—occurring outside the hip joint and capsule to an area 5 cm (2 inches) below the lesser trochanter; called *intertrochanteric* fractures

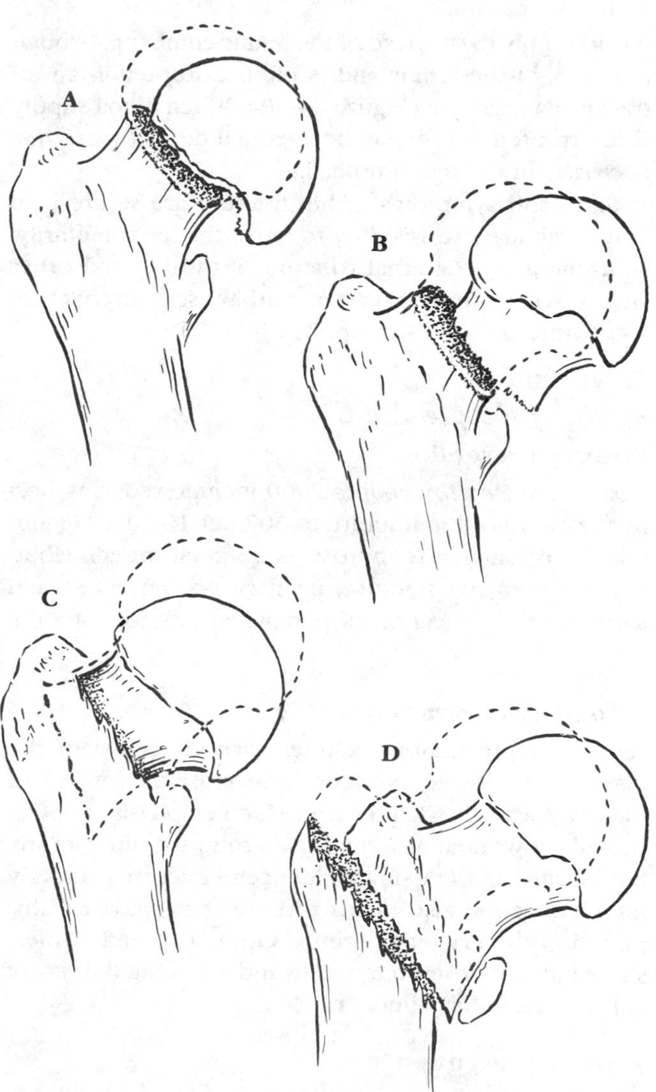


**FIGURE 64-19** Fractures of the hip. **A,** Subcapital fracture. **B,** Transcervical fracture. **C,** Impacted fracture of base of neck. **D,** Intertrochanteric fracture.

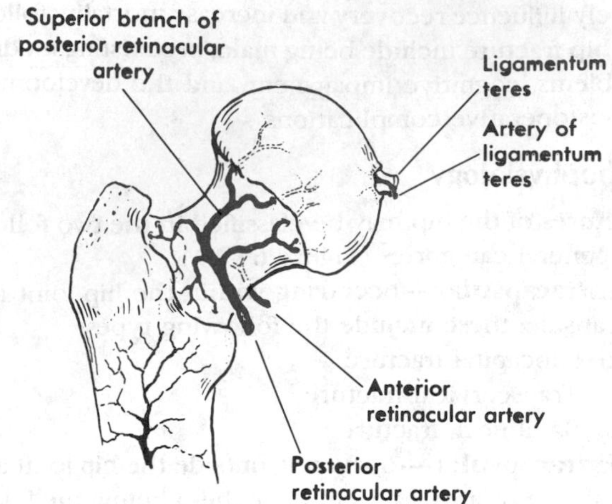


**FIGURE 64-20** Posterior view of blood supply to head of femur.

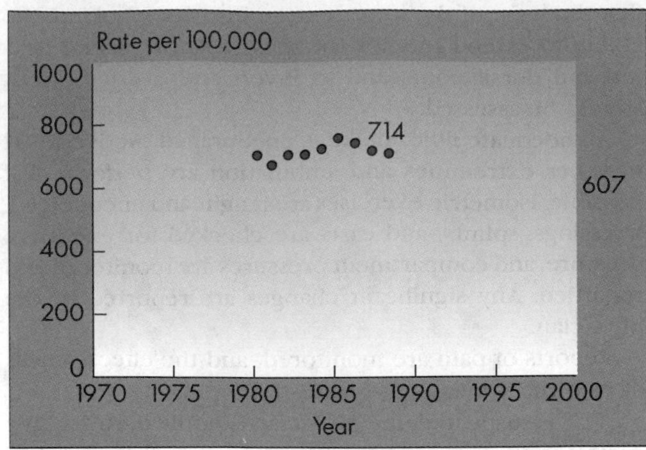


**FIGURE 64-21** Hip fracture rate among people aged 65 years and older. Note case rate of 714 in 1985 and target goal of 607 cases per 100,000 in the year 2000. (From US Department of Health and Human Services, *Healthy people 2000: national health promotion and disease prevention objectives,* Washington, DC, 1990, US Government Printing Office.)

Blood supply to the head of the femur comes up through the neck of the femur and is often disrupted in an intracapsular fracture (Figure 64-20). When blood supply is interrupted, there may be eventual death *(avascular necrosis)* of the femoral head.

Signs and symptoms of hip fracture are severe pain at the fracture site, inability to move the leg voluntarily, shortening and external rotation of the leg, and other signs and symptoms consistent with those of any fracture (see Nursing Care Plan, pp. 2215-2217).

## Prevention

### *Healthy People 2000*

#### Primary prevention

Goals from *Healthy People 2000* include reducing hospitalizations for hip fracture to 607 per 100,000 (Figure 64-21). Because osteoporosis is a significant contributing factor to hip fracture, primary prevention should focus on the education of persons at risk for osteoporosis.

#### Secondary prevention

Secondary prevention includes early detection of the disease process and methods to decrease the severity of the disorder (see Chapter 65). Much emphasis has been placed on women as a high-risk group for hip fracture, but because of the rising incidence of fracture in elderly men, education also needs to be directed toward this previously overlooked group. Other preventive measures include promoting safety and reducing the risk of falls among elderly persons.

#### Tertiary prevention

Tertiary preventive measures are focused on maintaining or restoring the individual to prefracture levels of functioning and preventing further disability. Improving the general medical condition of the elderly patient before surgery, which includes the stabilization of preexisting medical problems and the correction of fluid and electrolyte imbalances, will increase the chances for functional recovery.[1] This includes nursing interventions to prevent the most common postoperative complications such as thromboembolism, pneumonia, decubitus ulcers, and voiding dysfunction.

## Medical Management

The expected length of stay of patients with hip fractures as determined by DRG is 7 days.

Medical management, including diagnostic tests, medications, and diet of persons with hip fracture, is the same as for persons with other fractures (see p. 2192).

## Treatment

Treatment of hip fracture includes both conservative measures and surgery. Surgical intervention is usually preferred, unless the general medical condition of the patient precludes it. Conservative management involves prolonged immobility with the associated complications but avoids the risks associated with anesthesia. The risks and benefits of both modalities should be discussed by the patient, family, physician, and nurse.

## Surgical Management

Surgery involves reduction and stabilization of the fracture and insertion of an internal fixation device. A variety of fixation devices are available. The choice of fixation device depends on the location of the fracture, potential for avascular necrosis of the femoral head, and the personal preference of the surgeon. An **impacted intracapsular fracture** without displacement may be treated

# NURSING CARE PLAN

## PERSON WITH AN INTRACAPSULAR HIP FRACTURE, OPEN REDUCTION, AND INTERNAL FIXATION WITH A PROSTHETIC IMPLANT

**DATA:** Mrs. W. is an 81-year-old widowed, retired secretary. This evening she tripped and fell on an icy step when leaving her niece's home. She complained of immediate, severe pain in her left hip and was unable to move her leg. Emergency Medical Services was phoned, and Mrs. W. was accompanied to the hospital by her niece and her niece's husband. In the emergency room it was noted that her left leg was shorter than her right, and it was externally rotated. Her vital signs were stable, and the neurocirculatory status of the left leg was intact. An x-ray examination revealed an intracapsular femoral neck fracture. Intravenous fluids were initiated. An ECG, a urinalysis, a CBC, and a serum electrolyte study were obtained. She was transferred to the nursing unit with physician's orders for morphine sulfate, 4 to 6 mg every 3 to 4 hours as necessary for pain. Buck's extension was applied. Consent was obtained for surgical repair in the morning. Replacement of the femoral head and neck with a regular stem Austin Moore prosthesis is planned.

The nursing history identified the following:

- Mrs. W. lives alone in her own apartment in a senior citizen complex.
- Mrs. W. has no children but has nieces and nephews in the area who see her regularly. They assist with shopping and other errands.
- Mrs. W. would like to return to her own apartment after being discharged from the hospital, but she worries that she might need help at home. Her family is considering hiring a home health aide.
- She takes no medications other than aspirin for occasional "stiffness" on awakening.
- She has never been hospitalized and last saw a physician 2 years ago for "the flu."

### ■ NURSING DIAGNOSIS

Knowledge deficit related to lack of exposure to surgery and treatment protocols

| Expected Patient Outcomes | Nursing Interventions | Rationale |
|---|---|---|
| Can explain the teaching provided by the nurse about preoperative and general postoperative care.<br>States that she is experiencing less anxiety related to fear of the unknown and/or misconceptions about surgery and the recovery period. | Assess need for instruction and provide as necessary.<br>Provide written materials pertaining to the surgery, if available in the institution.<br>Review preoperative instruction with patient and family before the surgery.<br>Evaluate patient's understanding of the information taught. | Understanding the surgical procedure and postoperative care should lessen anxiety and promote participation in postoperative routine. |
| | Reinforce information taught. | Reinforcement of information previously taught will improve retention. |
| Will actively participate in plan of care. | Keep patient and family informed of plan of care and rationales for treatment. | Encourage family support and participation in care routines while the patient is hospitalized and after discharge. |
| Will verbalize understanding of need for follow-up care and activity restrictions. | Provide information and rationale for discharge activity restrictions.<br>Collaborative nursing actions include those to identify possible complications of surgery and immobility. Nursing actions include monitoring for the following: | Understanding the rationale for activity restrictions may promote compliance and avoidance of complications. |
| Performs active dorsiflexion, plantar flexion, isometric quadriceps setting, and gluteal and active ROM of unaffected limbs q 12 hr until ambulatory. | 1. Neurocirculatory compromise: Perform neurocirculatory checks q 2 hr for the first 24-48 hours. Notify physician of any changes from preoperative status. | Exercising promotes venous return, prevents thrombus formation, and helps to maintain muscle tone. |

*Continued*

# NURSING CARE PLAN

## PERSON WITH AN INTRACAPSULAR HIP FRACTURE, OPEN REDUCTION, AND INTERNAL FIXATION WITH A PROSTHETIC IMPLANT—cont'd

| Expected Patient Outcomes | Nursing Interventions | Rationale |
|---|---|---|
| | 2. Dislocation of the prosthesis: Notify physician if patient complains of sudden onset of increased pain, especially groin pain, particularly if accompanied by deformity or external rotation. | |
| | 3. Impaired skin integrity and/or impaired wound healing: Monitor pressure areas for signs of redness, monitor temperature, and assess incision for signs or symptoms of infection or excessive drainage. | |
| | 4. Atelectasis/respiratory infection: Monitor breath sounds until patient is ambulatory. Have patient deep breathe and cough every hour until fully ambulatory. | If carried out correctly and at appropriate intervals, pulmonary exercises can effectively prevent atelectasis and pneumonia. Frequent monitoring and early detection of complications can speed recovery and increase functional status. |
| | 5. Urinary retention: Assess for urinary retention or stasis. | |
| | 6. Constipation: Assess bowel status each day until patient is able to have a bowel movement. | |
| | 7. Fluid and electrolyte imbalance: Monitor intake and output until patient is taking oral fluids without difficulty, monitor IV fluid rates, and assess patient for fluid volume excess or deficit. | |
| | By discharge the patient should be instructed in and be able to explain or demonstrate the following:<br>1. Independent ambulation on level surfaces and stairs with appropriate ambulatory aid.<br>2. Activity restrictions to be observed for approximately 2 months or until follow-up with physician, for example, limiting flexion of the affected hip to 90 degrees, avoiding adduction of the affected leg beyond midline, avoiding extreme internal and external rotation of the affected hip, and maintaining partial weight-bearing status with the walker or crutches.<br>3. Independent ADL with assistive devices. | |

### ■ NURSING DIAGNOSIS

Pain related to surgical procedure

| Expected Patient Outcomes | Nursing Interventions | Rationale |
|---|---|---|
| Reports decrease or absence of pain after the use of pain relief measures. | Assess patient's pain, and evaluate response comfort measures provided. | Subjective and objective data are important in ascertaining the nature of patient's postoperative pain and determining its management. |

## PERSON WITH AN INTRACAPSULAR HIP FRACTURE, OPEN REDUCTION, AND INTERNAL FIXATION WITH A PROSTHETIC IMPLANT—cont'd

### ■ NURSING DIAGNOSIS

Pain related to surgical procedure

| Expected Patient Outcomes | Nursing Interventions | Rationale |
|---|---|---|
| Can perform necessary postoperative routine and exercises. | Administer analgesics (usually narcotic) as prescribed during initial postoperative period. | It usually is necessary to administer narcotics in the first 48 to 72 hours after surgery. Analgesics have a greater effect if they are administered before pain becomes severe. |
| Reports decreasing levels of pain. | Teach relaxation techniques as appropriate. | Relaxation facilitates rest and may modify the response of pain. |
| | Use other pain-relieving techniques as appropriate, for example, back rubs, repositioning. | A change in type of cutaneous stimulation may result in pain relief. |
| | As pain decreases, use milder analgesics as prescribed. | Pain may be controlled by less potent analgesics (with fewer untoward side effects) as pain lessens in severity. |

### ■ NURSING DIAGNOSIS

Impaired physical mobility related to alteration in lower limb status after surgical repair of hip fracture

| Expected Patient Outcomes | Nursing Interventions | Rationale |
|---|---|---|
| Will demonstrate optimal level of mobility with adaptive devices within prescribed limitations of activity by time of discharge. | | |
| Will be free from complications associated with immobility. | Determine from surgeon the limits of motion and weight bearing permitted, keeping in mind the following guidelines:<br>1. Hip flexion is usually to 90 degrees for 2 to 3 months.<br>2. Adduction beyond midline is prohibited for 2 to 3 months.<br>3. Extreme internal or external rotation is prohibited for 2 to 3 months.<br>4. Partial weight bearing on affected body part with the aid of a walker or crutches is usually observed for 2 to 3 months. | Restrictions on positioning are designed to avoid dislocating the prosthesis. |
| | Turn patient from back to unoperated side q 2 hr and PRN. Avoid positioning patient on operative sides, and observe flexion restrictions when elevating the head of the bed. | Turning and repositioning frequently promote circulation, respiratory effort, and muscle activity. |
| | When turning the patient, hold the operative leg in abduction; use pillows to maintain 30-degree abduction when turning is accomplished. | Prevents adduction of leg. |
| | Assist patient to walk using the appropriate ambulatory aid. Begin walking the first or second postoperative day and increase the frequency and distance of ambulation as tolerated. | Early postoperative activity, including walking, can hasten recovery and prevent postoperative complications. |
| | Begin sitting when patient demonstrates sufficient control of the affected leg to sit within flexion restriction. | Prepare patient for discharge while assuring the patient functions safely within prescribed limits on flexion. |
| | Elevate sitting surface with pillows to keep angle of hip within prescribed limits. | Limits hip flexion to 90 degrees. |

## CRITICAL PATHWAY Fractured Hip, Repair by Prosthetic Device*

DRG #: 236 Expected LOS: 7

| | Day of Admission Day 1† | Day 2 | Day of Surgery Day 3 |
|---|---|---|---|
| **Diagnostic Tests** | Hip and chest x-rays, CBC, UA, SMA/18,‡ T & X match, PT/PTT, ECG | | Preoperative: CBC, SMA/8,§ ECG Postoperative: CBC, electrolytes, PT/PTT daily until discharge if sodium warfarin (Coumadin) prescribed |
| **Medications** | IVs; IV/IM analgesic; IV antibiotic | IVs; IV/IM analgesic; IV antibiotic | IVs; IV analgesic; IV antibiotic; anticoagulant |
| **Treatments** | I & O q8hr; VS q4hr; Buck's extension to affected leg; neurocirculatory checks to both legs q2hr; skin assessment and special care q2hr; elastic leg stocking (ELS) to unaffected leg; pneumatic intermittent (ICD) compression devices to both lower extremities | I & O q8hr; VS q4hr; neurocirculatory checks to both legs q2hr; skin assessment and special care q2hr; ELS; ICD | I & O and drain q8hr, including Foley; VS q4hr; disc traction postoperatively; neurocirculatory checks to both legs q2hr; check drainage on dressing q2hr; ELS; ICD |
| **Diet** | As tolerated | NPO p̄ MN for morning of surgery; diet as tolerated | NPO; clear liqs post nausea or on return of bowel sounds |
| **Activity** | Bedrest; pillow splint; trapeze on bed; C-DB q2hr | Bedrest; pillow splint; trapeze on bed; C-DB q2hr | Bedrest; trapeze with abductor pillow; C-DB q2hr; hip flexion limited to 90 degrees; no adduction beyond midline, minimal internal/external rotation |
| **Consultations** | PT; social service; other specialists as needed for other medical problems; medical clearance for surgery | | PT‖ |

*Type of prosthesis will affect postoperative course. Critical pathway is based on bipolar type of prosthesis.
†Some patients may be admitted to hospital and undergo surgery the same day, which will decrease LOS to 5 days.
‡Serum calcium, phosphorus, triglycerides, uric acid, creatinine, BUN, total bilirubin, alkaline phosphatase, aspartate aminotransferase (AST) (formerly serum glutamic oxaloacetic transaminase [SGOT]), alanine aminotransferase (ALT) (formerly serum glutamic pyruvic transaminase [SGPT]), lactic dehydrogenase (LDH), total protein, albumin, sodium, potassium, chloride, total $CO_2$, glucose.
§Serum Sodium, Potassium, Chloride, total $CO_2$, Glucose, BUN.
‖ORIF (open reduction, internal fixation) with nail, plate does not require abduction pillow or positioning restrictions.
¶Weight-bearing status depends on type of implant and use of methylmethacrylate.

with bedrest alone. The following treatments are often chosen for other types of hip fractures:

1. Stable plate and screw fixation; implies non-weight-bearing status for 6 weeks to 3 months
2. Telescoping nail fixation; implies minimal to partial weight-bearing status for 6 weeks to 3 months
3. Prosthetic implant, usually Austin Moore prosthesis or Bi-Polar prosthesis, to replace femoral head and neck; implies some *position restrictions* for 2 weeks to 2 months and *partial weight-bearing restrictions* for up to 2 months

### Referral/Consultation

In some settings the nurse assumes responsibility for making referrals to other services. Common referrals for persons with hip fracture include physical and occupational therapy as described under the general management of fractures. Special emphasis is placed on discharge planning. Social service referrals are initiated to aid in placement in an extended care or rehabilitation facility or to arrange for home health services or equipment.

Critical pathways (also referred to as collaborative care paths or care maps) have been developed in some inpatient and outpatient settings to guide both medical and nursing management. These critical pathways are collaboratively developed along time lines and include the information described above for specific hours, days, or visits. Pertinent information about discharge planning and patient teaching to be implemented at specified times also is included. Because the nurse has a major role in these two aspects of care, they are discussed under Nursing Management.

A sample of a critical pathway for the six areas of care discussed in this medical management section is presented above, and a nursing care plan for the same type of patient is on pp. 2215-2217. In some settings these are combined within the critical pathway document.

| Day 4 | Day 5 | Day 6 | Day of Discharge Day 7 |
|---|---|---|---|
| PT/PTT | PT/PTT | CBC, PT/PTT | PT/PTT |
| IV to saline lock if tolerating PO fluids, IV/IM analgesic; IV antibiotic; anticoagulant; stool softener | IV saline lock; IM/PO analgesic; disc antibiotic and anticoagulant; stool softener | Disc saline lock; analgesic; disc antibiotic; stool softener | PO analgesic; stool softener |
| I & O and drain q8hr including Foley; VS q6hr; neurocirculatory checks to both legs q4hr; check drainage on dressing q4hr; ELS; ICD | Disc drain at 48 degrees; I & O q8hr; disc; Foley; VS q8hr; neurocirculatory checks to both legs; ELS; ICD | I & O q8hr; VS q8hr; ELS; Disc ICD | Disc I & O; VS q12hr; ELS |
| Advance diet as tolerated | Regular diet | Regular diet | Regular diet |
| Bedrest, up with help & walker × 1; minimal wt bearing; ROM to unaffected side | Up with help and walker × 3, minimal weight bearing; ROM to unaffected side; up in chair as tolerated | Up with help and walker × 4, minimal weight bearing; ROM to unaffected side | Up with walker × 4, minimal weight bearing; ROM to unaffected side |
| PT¶; dietary | Rehabilitation/SNU/home health PT | PT | |

## Nursing Management

Nursing management should include those interventions already noted for general care of patients with fractures, with specific attention to interventions for persons with internal fixation. *Special consideration should be given to persons who have had a* **prosthetic implant,** *because there will be specific position restrictions, unless they have external fixation as well.* These include the following:

1. Avoidance of hip flexion beyond 60 degrees for up to 10 days
2. Avoidance of hip flexion beyond 90 degrees from day 10 to 2 months
3. Avoidance of adduction of the affected leg beyond midline for 2 months
4. Maintenance of partial weight-bearing status for approximately 2 months

Suggestions for nursing management are the following:

1. Instruct the patient on the limits of motion to be observed.
2. Avoid positioning the patient on the operative side in bed.
3. Assist patient to maintain abduction of hip (Figures 64-22 and 64-23).
4. Carefully monitor the patient's position during transfer (while patient is standing and sitting).
5. Provide a chair with a firm, nonreclining seat and arms; elevate the sitting surface as necessary with pillows or foam cushions to keep the angle of the hip within the prescribed limits when the patient is sitting.

In general, patients who have had *any* kind of internal fixation for fractured hip should avoid elevation of the operated leg when sitting in a chair, because this puts excessive strain on the fixation device.

## FRACTURE OF THE SPINE

### Etiology/Epidemiology

Spine or vertebral fractures can occur as the result of falls, motor vehicle or diving accidents, or blows to the head or body by heavy objects. With increasing frequency, fractures of the spine are also occurring as the result of osteoporosis and metastatic lesions of the spine. Spinal fracture can occur at any age.

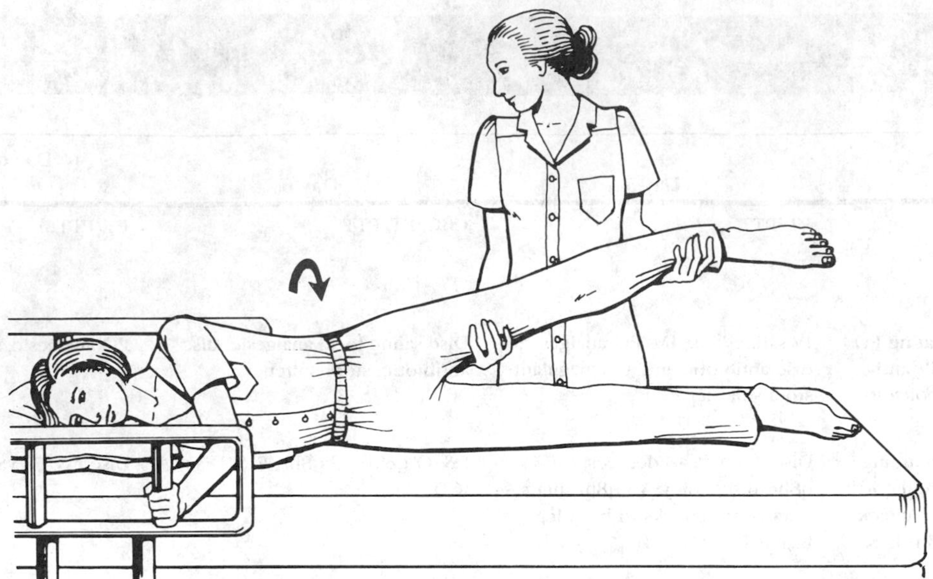

**FIGURE 64-22** Assisting patient to turn while maintaining *abduction of the hip.* Leg is supported at the thigh and just above the ankle to avoid putting undue stress on the hip.

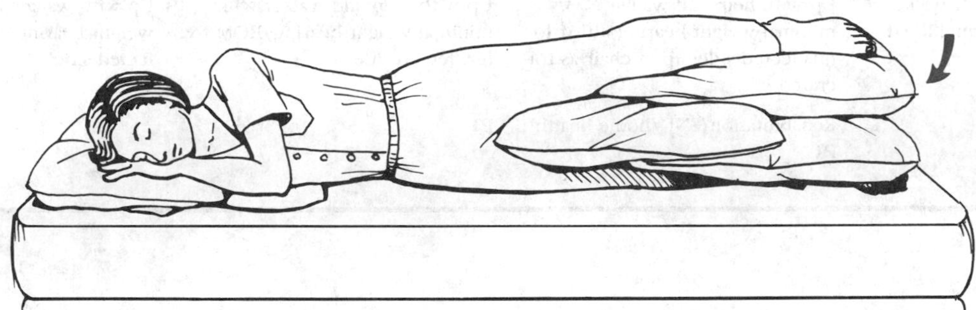

**FIGURE 64-23** Pillows are staggered in a wedge-shaped arrangement to maintain *abduction of the hip.*

## Pathophysiology

Vertebral fracture may occur with or without displacement. If fracture fragments are displaced, they may place pressure on spinal nerves or injure the spinal cord itself. Such pressure will result in partial or complete dysfunction of the body parts innervated from the level of injury. Depending on the extent of injury to the nervous system, dysfunction may be permanent or temporary. Fracture can occur at any level of the spine, from occiput through the sacrum.

Signs and symptoms of vertebral fracture include *pain at the site of injury, partial or complete loss of mobility or sensation below the level of injury, and evidence of fracture/fracture dislocation on routine x-ray examination, myelography, CT scan, and/or MRI scan.*

## Medical Management

Objectives in management will be stabilization and reduction of the fracture and decompression (i.e., removal of pressure from spinal nerves or the spinal cord).

### Emergency management at site of injury

Immediate management objectives are (1) immobilization of the patient with backboard and cervical collar and (2) immediate transport to a hospital.

## Surgical Management

Objectives of surgical management are as follows:

1. Decompression of nerve structures through laminectomy (see Chapter 65) or appropriate reduction of the fracture and removal of fracture fragments
2. Reduction of the fracture through operative procedures or, in some cases, traction (e.g., cervical traction through application of tongs to the skull)
3. Stabilization of the fracture with bone grafting and/or internal fixation devices such as pedicle screws and plates, TSRH, or Harrington, or Luque rods (see Chapter 65)
4. Maintenance of stabilization with external fixation devices such as casts, corsets, or braces as necessary

If there is no displacement of fracture fragments and no

pressure on spinal nerves or the spinal cord, *compression fractures may be treated with bedrest until the patient's pain subsides.* Then the patient is gradually mobilized, sometimes with stabilization by a corset or brace.

### Nursing Management

Many of the nursing interventions required by the patient with spinal fracture are identical to those outlined for the patient with spinal cord injury in Chapter 58. Of special concern are interventions designed for the following:

1. Maintaining the stability of the fracture fixation
   a. Pay strict attention to "**logrolling**" the patient for position changes (see Figure 65-27) to avoid twisting the spine and placing stress at the fracture site.
   b. Position the patient with pillows between the legs and behind the back when patient is side lying to prevent strain on the back.
   c. Changes of position can be accomplished with the use of special beds that rotate 45 degrees from side to side. *Recent literature indicates that when the spine is unstable, logrolling and/or the use of turning frames is contraindicated because they can stress the fracture site.*
   c. Avoid elevating the head of the bed beyond the prescribed level (usually only 30 degrees and only on the physician's order).
   d. When the patient is to be mobilized, apply prescribed corsets or braces *before* getting the patient out of bed.
2. Preventing neurocirculatory problems
   a. Perform neurocirculatory checks every hour in the first 24 to 48 hours postoperatively; report decrease in neuromotor function to the physician, because this may indicate displacement or pressure at the fracture site.
   b. Perform passive ROM to involved extremities at least four times daily to maintain joint motion.
   c. Encourage patient to actively move noninvolved extremities to the fullest extent possible as frequently as possible to maintain joint motion and promote circulation.
3. Promoting comfort—in addition to usual comfort measures
   a. Reposition the patient frequently.
   b. Wait a few minutes to ascertain the patient's comfort, because small adjustments may be necessary and may not be immediately recognized.
4. Promoting psychologic comfort
   a. Recognize that the patient may have feelings of powerlessness, anger, and/or fear about the situation, particularly if there is neuromotor deficit.
   b. Encourage the patient to express his or her feelings.
   c. Encourage the patient to take advantage of psychologic and/or social counseling, when it is available.
   d. If long-term rehabilitation is indicated, prepare the patient for care in a rehabilitation setting.

Other nursing interventions are similar to those for any patient who has a fracture, including interventions for individuals in casts or traction, which are discussed earlier in this chapter.

# TRAUMA TO SOFT TISSUE STRUCTURES

## TRAUMA TO LIGAMENTS AND TENDONS

### Etiology/Epidemiology

Trauma to ligaments and tendons is usually seen in connection with injury to a joint caused by a blow, twisting, or severe stretching. The most common site of ligament damage is the knee, often resulting from a sports injury, because of the anatomy, location, and complex motions of the joint. The Achilles tendon is susceptible to partial or complete tears, usually caused by a sports injury. See Table 64-4.

### Pathophysiology

The most common ligamentous or tendon injuries are partial or complete tears. In the knee there may be damage to the medial, lateral, and posterior ligaments and to the anterior and posterior cruciate ligaments. Injuries may be classified as mild, moderate, or severe:

| | |
|---|---|
| Mild (class I) injuries | A few ligament fibers are torn |
| Moderate (class II) injuries | Several ligament fibers torn with a partial loss of function |
| Severe (class III) injuries | Severe or complete disruption of the ligament with resulting instability |

Signs and symptoms of class I injuries are mild pain and swelling. Class II injuries are associated with moderate pain and swelling, and persons with class III injuries typically report severe pain, swelling, joint instability, and disability or loss of function.

The clinical manifestations of trauma to the knee are listed in Box 64-4.

### Medical Management

Immediate first aid measures for soft tissue injuries of the musculoskeletal system can be easily remembered by the mnemonic **RICE:**

**R** Rest of the injured part

**I** Ice for at least 48 to 72 hours to decrease bleeding and edema

**C** Compression by the utilization of elastic bandages, splints, or casts (Be sure to monitor for signs of compartment syndrome.)

**E** Elevation of the extremity to slightly above the level of the heart to increase venous return and decrease edema

**TABLE 64-4 Common Soft Tissue Injuries**

| MECHANISM OF INJURY | SYMPTOMS | TREATMENT |
|---|---|---|
| **MENISCAL** | | |
| Medial and lateral tears usually occur with rotary or extension/flexion injuries of knee | Joint pain<br>Swelling<br>"Locking" | Splint, bracing, or cast<br>Surgical treatment by meniscectomy via arthroscopy or arthrotomy |
| **ANTERIOR CRUCIATE LIGAMENT (ACL)** | | |
| Valgus stress applied to knee while in hyperextension and external rotation<br>Associated with deceleration and changes in direction | Audible "pop" or "snap"<br>Pain<br>Joint effusion<br>Hemarthrosis<br>Joint deformity<br>Joint instability<br>"Giving way" of knee | Treatment depends on age and lifestyle of patient<br>Conservative treatment: quadriceps and hamstring strengthening, bracing, and avoidance of high risk activities<br>Surgical reconstruction of anterior cruciate ligament (ACL) either open or arthroscopically aided, using autologous or synthetic graft followed by extensive rehabilitation program |
| **ROTATOR CUFF** | | |
| Strain or tear of rotator cuff muscles or tendons of shoulder (supraspinatus, infraspinatus, teres minor, subscapularis)<br>Usually results from falling on an outstretched hand, throwing objects (baseball pitchers), or chronic or excessive use | Severe pain with loss of ability to flex and abduct shoulder | Rest, sling and swath for immobilization, physical therapy, NSAIDs<br>Surgical repair for complete rupture, disability, or chronic pain, followed by physical therapy |

**Diagnostic tests**

Diagnosis is made by evaluation of the history and physical examination, including specialized tests to detect ligamentous instability. X-ray films are used to rule out the presence of fracture. Arthrography and arthroscopy may be performed to visualize the extent of the injury. It is especially important to elicit a complete history of the specific mechanism of injury, which aids in differential diagnosis.

**BOX 64-4 Clinical Manifestations of Knee Trauma**

- Tenderness
- Swelling
- Pain
- Hematoma
- Disability; "knee gives way"
- Abnormal motion at joint
- Audible pop

**Treatment**

1. Mild injuries
   a. Rest
   b. Compression dressing
2. Moderate injuries
   a. Rest
   b. Possible aspiration of excess fluid
   c. Compression dressing to control swelling and further effusion
   d. Support—splint or brace
   e. Strengthening exercises
3. Severe injuries
   a. Surgical repair to prevent disability and instability; possible knee surgery performed through an *arthroscope*
   b. Modified compression dressing to prevent effusion
   c. Immobilization of the joint for a prescribed time
   d. Remobilization of the joint, sometimes with the aid of a continuous passive motion machine; appropriate strengthening exercises through a program of physical therapy

## Nursing Management

Postoperative nursing interventions for the patient with a ligamentous or tendon tear include the same considerations as for the partially immobilized patient after fracture reduction and application of an external fixation device. Of particular importance is patient teaching. The following information should be included:

1. Information about the nature of the injury and the general nursing care after surgery
2. Use of the brace/cast postoperatively (see p. 2192)
3. Limitations of motion and weight bearing
4. Use of appropriate ambulatory aids
5. Exercises to perform and frequency of exercising
6. Plans for follow-up with the physician

## TRAUMA TO MUSCLE

### Etiology/Epidemiology

Muscle strains result from using muscles beyond their intended or functional ability. **Strain** *may result from a one-time occurrence or as a cumulative effect of overuse.* Common strains are back strains. Muscle may rupture as the result of severe overuse.

### Pathophysiology

Acute strain may disrupt tissue surrounding the involved muscle, and there may be localized hemorrhage. Chronic strain may produce the same symptoms but with a more gradual onset. Signs and symptoms of muscle strain may include *mild aching to severe pain, (depending on severity of the injury), disability, swelling, and tenderness.*

### Medical Management

Medical management includes immediate *application of ice to control swelling, rest, application of heat after 24 to 48 hours to control pain, and surgical intervention and immobilization of the part to repair ruptured muscle.*

### Nursing Management

Individuals who sustain only mild to moderate strain of a muscle seldom require hospitalization. Those who require surgical intervention (e.g., a person with a ruptured quadriceps muscle) will need such nursing interventions as pain management and preservation of strength and mobility, similar to those for the patient who has sustained a fracture that requires surgical repair and external immobilization. Additionally, the nurse should explain the following:

1. The nature of the injury and what nursing care to expect postoperatively
2. How to modify ADL within the limitations of activity and motion that must be observed
3. How to keep the involved muscle at rest until the physician permits activity of the muscle; for example, no active movement of the involved part, no isometric exercise of the involved muscle
4. How to use and care for the immobilizing device being used

## TRAUMA TO JOINTS AND JOINT STRUCTURES

Injuries to joints and joint structures may occur as a *sprain* (tearing of the capsule or ligaments surrounding a joint, including disruption of the synovial membrane), meniscus tears, joint dislocation, or joint subluxation.

### ETIOLOGY/EPIDEMIOLOGY

**Sprains** *are almost always the result of twisting injuries, as are meniscus tears.* Dislocation and subluxation (partial dislocation) of a joint occur as the result of excessive stress being applied to the joint, forcing it in an abnormal direction. Many of these injuries are incurred in running or contact sports such as football. Cervical sprains (whiplash) may result from rear-end automobile collisions.

**BOX 64-5 Clinical Manifestations of Joint Trauma**

**SPRAIN**
Pain
Limitation of motion
Edema
Superficial bruising
Tenderness over the involved joint
Cervical sprain, possibly accompanied by dizziness, visual disturbance, headache, and nausea

**MENISCUS TEARS**
Pain
Swelling
Limited motion, especially flexion/extension
"Locking" or "slipping" of the joint
Evidence of tissue tear on arthrography or arthroscopy

**TEAR OF LIGAMENTS WITHIN THE JOINT**
Pain
Swelling
Instability of the joint
Evidence of tissue tear on arthrography or arthroscopy

**DISLOCATION**
Pain
Loss of function
Obvious deformity
Possible impairment of neurovascular status
Evidence of loss of articulation on x-ray film examination

**SUBLUXATION:** Signs and symptoms are similar to dislocation but less severe

### PATHOPHYSIOLOGY

When a sprain occurs, the ligaments and capsule surrounding the joint are partially torn, producing *hemorrhage and swelling.* Function may not be limited. A meniscus tear results in decreased ability of the meniscus to absorb shock and stabilize the joint. With a *dislocation, contact is lost between the articulating bones of the involved joint, whereas a subluxation causes a partial loss of contact between the articulating bones of the involved joint.* The clinical manifestations of trauma to joints and joint structures are listed in Box 64-5.

### MEDICAL MANAGEMENT

Medical management includes the following:

1. *Sprain*
   a. Application of ice to retard swelling and relieve pain

b. Possible immobilization of joint with cast or splint
c. Isometric exercises for involved joint
d. Cervical collar for whiplash

2. *Meniscus tears*
   a. Strengthening exercises; for example, quadriceps setting, straight leg raising, progressive resistive exercises
   b. Surgical repair as necessary, often through arthroscope
3. *Tears of ligaments within the joint*
   a. Strengthening exercises
   b. Surgical repair or reconstruction of the ligament, often through arthroscope
4. *Dislocation*
   a. Reduction, either closed (by manipulation) or open (surgical)
   b. Immobilization for a specified period of time
5. *Subluxation*
   a. Reduction
   b. Immobilization for a specified period of time

## NURSING MANAGEMENT

Individuals who require surgical intervention for repair of joint injury may require short-term hospitalization or may be managed on an ambulatory surgery basis. Nursing interventions are essentially the same as for the person with severe strain, except that the emphasis will be on maintaining and improving muscle strength around the involved joint instead of resting the muscles. The joint may be immobilized for a relatively short period (1 to 5 days depending on the nature and extent of the injury) and gradually mobilized, either with a continuous passive motion machine in combination with a program of physical therapy exercises or with a program of physical therapy exercises alone. Programs of physical therapy may be extensive and rigorous; for example, *programs for anterior cruciate ligament reconstruction may last up to 6 months.* The nurse will want to concentrate on patient teaching, with special emphasis on prescribed exercises and following through with the prescribed program of physical therapy.

## TRAUMATIC HIP DISLOCATION

### Etiology/Epidemiology

Traumatic hip dislocation usually occurs as a result of a motor vehicle accident, especially if a frontal impact is sustained. This type of force can drive the victim's knees into the dashboard, forcibly dislocating the hip. *Traumatic dislocation of the hip is considered an orthopedic emergency because of the risk of* **avascular necrosis** *of the femoral head.* Research indicates that if reduction occurs within 6 hours of injury, there is less risk of persistent pain, decreased range of motion, and avascular necrosis.[11]

### Pathophysiology

As the hip is forcibly dislocated, the blood supply to the femoral head can be disrupted (Figure 64-20). Damage to the sciatic nerve is also possible and can result in partial to complete motor and sensory loss in the affected extremity. Another potential problem is fracture of the femoral head, acetabulum, and/or pelvis. The articular surface of the femoral head may be eroded by bone fragments. Clinical manifestations of traumatic hip dislocation can be found in Box 64-6.

**BOX 64-6 Clinical Manifestations of Traumatic Hip Dislocation**

- Pain
- Deformity
- Decreased range of motion
- Decreased sensation
- Diminished or absent pulses
- Anterior dislocation
  Hip in extension and external rotation
- Posterior dislocation
  Hip in flexion and internal rotation; may be a visible leg length discrepancy when compared with unaffected leg

### Medical Management

#### Diagnostic tests

Diagnosis is made on the basis of history, physical examination, and evidence of dislocation on x-ray film.

#### Treatment

If possible, the hip is reduced immediately. The patient is given intravenous sedation, and the physician uses manual traction to relocate the hip **(closed reduction).** If closed reduction is not feasible, or in the presence of acetabular or pelvic fracture, skeletal traction may be used to reduce the hip until surgery is possible. If there is no fracture, **open reduction** is accomplished by opening the hip capsule and relocating the head. For pelvic and acetabular fractures, internal fixative devices are usually used. If *avascular necrosis results, prosthetic replacement of the hip is required.*

### Nursing Management

Nursing management of a person with a traumatic hip dislocation is the same as for a patient with a hip fracture. The major emphasis is on keeping the limb in alignment by proper positioning. In addition, some patients will have a brace applied either in surgery (if orthotist is available) or the next day.

## MULTIPLE TRAUMA

### ETIOLOGY/EPIDEMIOLOGY

The leading cause of death in the United States for persons under the age of 45 is trauma. Causes of trauma include falls, crushing, vehicular (including airplane) accidents, and gunshot wounds. The nature of the injuries sustained in trauma are often extensive, involving multiple organ systems and multiple sites of injury. *Fifty percent of trauma deaths occur at the scene of injury, before medical help can arrive.* Death usually results from brainstem trauma, spinal cord injury, hemorrhage, or major organ injuries. *The second peak of trauma deaths occurs within 2 hours after injury,* as a result of head, chest, and abdominal injuries, or hemorrhage. *Death during the third peak occurs within days to weeks after initial injury,* usually because of sepsis or multisystem failure.[5]

The fact that many individuals who sustain such extensive injuries are able to survive and reach treatment facilities is related to improvements in scene-of-the-accident treatment and methods of transport to hospitals (including airlift by helicopter), as well as to increasing knowledge and skill in the field of emergency medicine. Regional trauma centers have been established across the country and, when possible, patients are transported there. Personnel in any hospital may be confronted with a multiply injured patient and should be prepared to treat the patient. Often the patient is stabilized and then airlifted to a trauma center.

The most common orthopedic injuries that occur as a result of multiple trauma are *pelvic fracture and crush injuries. Approximately 30% of persons involved in multiple trauma will sustain a pelvic fracture.*[6] Fractures of the pelvis usually occur as a result of *motor vehicle accidents, falls,* and *crush injuries.* Depending on the type of fracture and coexisting injuries, pelvic fracture has an associated mortality of 8% to 50%.[6] Hemorrhage is usually the cause of death. *Shearing forces* from the impact of trauma cause rupture of blood vessels surrounding the pelvic ring, causing hemorrhage and hypotension. Damage to internal organs can occur from shearing forces, bone fragments, and compression. The retroperitoneal space can accommodate up to 4 L of blood before tamponade results.[6] Coagulopathy is a significant problem because of loss of clotting factors and because of continued bleeding at the fracture site.[7] Pelvic fractures are classified by the mechanism of injury and degree of instability.[2]

*Crush injuries* may result from *falls, motor vehicle accidents,* and *blunt trauma,* such as being trapped under heavy fallen objects. *Multiple fractures* and *internal bleeding* may result, with *hemorrhage being the usual cause of death.*

**BOX 64-7 Pelvic Fractures**

**SIGNS AND SYMPTOMS**

Pain with compression of iliac crests
Asymmetry of iliac crests
Abnormal rotation of femurs
Leg length discrepancy
Lacerations of perineum, vagina, or rectum
Hematuria
Neurologic deficits
Hypotension

**DIAGNOSTIC TESTS**

X-ray
CT scan*
Peritoneal lavage to determine presence of intraabdominal bleeding*
Arteriogram: intravenous pyelogram may be done if the patient is stable to determine extent of internal injury

**MANAGEMENT**

Pelvic sling
Skeletal traction
Spica cast
Open reduction and internal fixation
External fixators are the treatment of choice

**ASSOCIATED INJURIES**

Vascular
Genitourinary
Abdominal
Intestinal and rectal

*Controversial.

## MEDICAL AND NURSING MANAGEMENT

*Treatment of victims of multiple trauma is based on the ABCs of airway management with cervical spine control, breathing, and circulation.*[4] The pelvis and abdomen must be evaluated for fractures and hemorrhage (Box 64-7). Fractures of the ribs and spine may cause life-threatening neurologic and cardiovascular injuries.

Obvious fractures are immobilized and splinted and sterile dressings are applied to open fractures until surgical reduction is feasible. The goals of medical management are to correct or stabilize any life-threatening problems (e.g., obstructed airway, pneumothorax, bleeding) and then to reestablish the continuity of injured tissues. Musculoskeletal injury may require reduction of fractures and repair of related soft tissue injury. *Because life-threatening problems must be addressed first, musculoskeletal injuries are usually not repaired until the patient has been stabilized.* However, sites of fracture or potential fracture must be splinted or otherwise protected until reduction can be effected.

The principles of nursing management are as follows:

1. *Before reduction,* protection of all actual or potential sites of fracture through maintaining splints, traction, and/or positioning precautions
2. *After reduction,* observation of all the previously discussed principles of nursing management of the patient with a fracture

The challenge for the nurse is to devise a plan of care that will take into account the demands of the variety of fixation techniques, fracture sites, and mobilization/immobilization requirements for that patient. The psychosocial needs and the rehabilitation requirements for individuals who have sustained multiple trauma are often long-term and very extensive. Consideration of rehabilitation requirements must occur early in the patient's hospital course and be reviewed frequently (see Chapter 8).

## QUESTIONS TO CONSIDER

- Name three causes of bone fracture, and describe some measures that can be taken to prevent fracture.
- Define bone fracture. Include an explanation of the terms *complete, incomplete, simple, closed, compound,* and *open*. Name several of the various classifications of bone fracture.
- List three ways a fractured bone can be immobilized.
- Discuss the process by which bone heals, and list some factors that might impede bone healing.
- Describe the five most common signs and symptoms of fracture, and explain why they occur.
- Discuss immediate and secondary medical management of the patient with a fracture. Define the terms *closed reduction* and *open reduction*. What additional special treatment is required in the treatment of a compound fracture?
- Identify three major complications of fracture, and discuss how those complications are treated.
- Identify what subjective and objective data the nurse should collect about the person with a fracture. List four possible nursing diagnoses that can be identified for the patient, based on this assessment.
- Identify four potential *systemic* complications of fracture and the nursing measures carried out to help prevent them.
- Describe the nursing measures for the patient who has the following: (1) a cast, (2) traction, (3) internal fixation device.
- Explain why hip fractures are more common in women than men. Define the two general categories of hip fracture, explain the pathophysiology of each, and describe the signs and symptoms of hip fracture.
- List three methods for reducing a hip fracture, and identify factors that the surgeon considers in choosing a fixation device.
- Describe the specific position restrictions and nursing care requirements for the patient with a prosthetic hip implant.
- What are some of the common causes of spinal fractures?
- Discuss the clinical significance of vertebral fractures without displacement versus fracture with displacement.
- Describe the signs and symptoms of vertebral fracture.
- What are the primary objectives of medical management for the patient with vertebral fracture? Discuss immediate versus surgical management.
- Discuss the nursing interventions of special concern for the patient with spinal fracture.
- Describe the types of injuries that can occur to joints and joint structures and how they are usually incurred. What are the signs and symptoms?
- What are the primary goals of both medical and nursing management for the person who has sustained multiple trauma?
- Discuss the special challenges the nurse encounters when caring for the multiple trauma patient. Include considerations of acute and long-term care needs.

## CRITICAL THINKING ACTIVITIES

- What aspects of care for a patient with a bone fracture can be generalized to the care of other patient populations?
- Explain how the care of an individual undergoing an open reduction differs from the care of a patient undergoing a closed reduction of a fracture.
- Discuss the essential assessment parameters used by the nurse to detect four systemic complications from a bone fracture.

## CHAPTER SUMMARY

### TRAUMA TO BONE

- Musculoskeletal trauma is most frequently manifested as bone fracture but may include injury to other structures of the system.
  a. Fracture of bone is usually the result of a blow to the body, a fall, or accident, but it may occur during normal activity if the bone is weakened by disease (pathologic fracture). A fatigue or stress fracture results when muscles associated with the fractured bone are unable to absorb energy as they usually do.
  b. Making the home and work environment safer, educating the public about safety hazards, and teaching women about the problem of osteoporosis are all measures to prevent fracture.
  c. A bone is fractured when there is a complete or partial (incomplete) interruption of the osseous tissue. Fractures may be further classified as simple (closed) or compound (open), depending on whether the skin over the fracture remains intact. If fracture fragments are moved away from the normal alignment of the bone, the fracture is “displaced”; if the fragments are not moved out of alignment, the fracture is “nondisplaced.”
  d. Greenstick, transverse, oblique, spiral, telescoped (impacted), and comminuted are terms that describe the line of the fracture.
  e. Immobilization of fractured bone is necessary for healing to take place. This can be accomplished through physiologic splintage, external orthopedic splinting, or internal fixation. Bone heals by the process of callus formation. Complications of bone healing, such as delayed union, nonunion, malunion, and pseudoarthrosis can occur.
  f. The most pronounced signs and symptoms of fracture usually include pain, loss of normal function, obvious deformity, edema, and ecchymosis.

g. Medical management of the patient with a fracture focuses on reduction of the fracture, maintenance of correct alignment of the bone fragments, and prevention of excessive loss of joint mobility and muscle tone.
h. Nursing management is planned in collaboration with the medical plan. Nursing interventions emphasize promoting knowledge, controlling pain, maintaining safety; preserving strength and mobility; maintaining skin integrity; preventing systemic complications (circulatory, respiratory, gastrointestinal, and urinary); promoting nutrition; and maintaining immobilization of the reduced fracture. A major objective of nursing care is to protect external or internal fixation devices until healing takes place.
i. Internal fixation is carried out with the patient under anesthesia in the operating room. The result is open surgical reduction of the fracture. Fixation with external devices may be used in conjunction with internal devices.
j. Nursing care of the patient with internal fixation will be similar to that for patients with external fixation, except that mobilization is usually much faster.

- Fractures of the hip are common; they occur more commonly in women than in men.
- *Intracapsular fractures* occur within the hip joint and capsule. *Extracapsular fractures* occur outside the hip joint and capsule. *Avascular necrosis* may result if blood supply to the head of the femur is disrupted as a result of the fracture.
  a. The signs and symptoms of hip fracture include severe pain, inability to move the leg, and shortening and external rotation of the leg.
  b. Medical management of the patient with a hip fracture focuses on reduction and fixation of the fracture. Choice of fixation device depends on the location of the fracture, potential for avascular necrosis of the femoral head, and personal preference of the surgeon.
  c. Nursing management of the patient with a hip fracture includes the same considerations and interventions as for any patient with a fracture. Special considerations relate to specific position restrictions for persons who have had a prosthetic implant. Patients who have had any kind of internal fixation for fractured hip should avoid elevation of the operative leg when seated in a chair, because this puts excessive strain on the fixation device.
- Spinal fracture can occur at any age, usually as a result of trauma or, with increasing frequency, as the result of osteoporosis and metastatic lesions.
  a. Fracture can occur at any level of the spine. If fracture fragments are displaced, they may injure the spinal nerves or spinal cord, resulting in partial or complete dysfunction of the body parts innervated from the level of injury. Dysfunction may be permanent or temporary, depending on the extent of the injury.
  b. The signs and symptoms of vertebral fracture include pain, loss of sensation or mobility below the level of injury, and evidence of fracture/dislocation on x-ray film or other radiologic studies.
  c. Immediate medical management of the patient with suspected spinal fracture includes immobilization with backboard and cervical collar and transport to a hospital. The general medical management objectives are stabilization and reduction of the fracture, and decompression (i.e., removal of pressure from spinal nerves or the spinal cord). This may be accomplished surgically or with traction. Surgical intervention often requires bone grafting and/or internal fixation devices.
  d. Nursing management of the patient with spinal fracture may include both interventions required by any patient who has a fracture and those for a patient with a spinal cord injury.

## TRAUMA TO SOFT TISSUE STRUCTURES

- Trauma to ligaments and tendons is usually seen with injury to a joint. The most common site of ligament damage is the knee. Ligament and tendon injuries may be classified as mild, moderate, or severe depending on the extent of the tear.
  a. The signs and symptoms of ligament and tendon injury may include tenderness, swelling, pain, effusion, hematoma, disability, and abnormal joint motion. These are not always present and may vary in intensity.
  b. Medical management of trauma to ligaments and tendons is determined by the extent of the damage and may range from rest and immobilization for mild injuries to surgical repair for severe injuries.
  c. Specific nursing management takes into consideration all the principles that are observed in the care of the patient who has a fracture.
- *Trauma* to muscle is manifested as *muscle strain,* which results from using muscles beyond their capacity. The signs and symptoms of muscle strain include pain, disability, swelling, and tenderness.
  a. Medical management of strains includes control of swelling and pain and rest. Surgery and immobilization are warranted if muscle is ruptured.
  b. Nursing management of patients with muscle strain is similar to that for patients who have sustained a fracture and require surgical repair and/or external immobilization.

## TRAUMA TO JOINTS AND JOINT STRUCTURES

- *Injuries to joints* and their structures may occur as *sprains, tears of the capsule surrounding the joint, meniscus tears, joint dislocations, or subluxation.* Joint sprains and meniscus tears are almost always the result of twisting injuries. Dislocation and subluxation occur as the result of extreme stress applied to the joint, forcing it in an abnormal direction.

a. The signs and symptoms of trauma to the joints and their structures are specific to the type of injury and include pain, swelling, limitation of motion, instability of the joint, and possible impairment of neurovascular status.
b. Medical management for sprains includes treatment of swelling, possible immobilization, and isometric exercise. Joint dislocation and subluxation require reduction and immobilization.
c. Nursing management of the patient with trauma to joints and joint structures is the same as for the person with severe strain, except there will be emphasis on maintaining and improving muscle strength around the injured joint. Patient teaching is a priority and emphasizes performing the prescribed exercises and following through with physical therapy regimens.

### MULTIPLE TRAUMA

- *Trauma is the leading cause of death in the United States for persons under 45 years of age.*

a. Causes of trauma include falls, crushing injuries, vehicular accidents, and gunshot wounds. These injuries are often extensive and involve multiple organ systems and multiple sites of injury.
b. Pelvic fracture and crush injury are the most common injuries resulting from polytrauma.
c. The goals of medical management in multiple trauma are to *correct or stabilize any life-threatening problems and to repair injured tissues.* This would include reduction of fractures and repair of related soft tissue injury. Because attention to life-threatening problems is the priority of immediate care, musculoskeletal injuries may not be repaired until after the patient has been stabilized. Fracture sites must be splinted until this can be accomplished.
d. Immediate nursing management of the patient with musculoskeletal trauma focuses on protection of actual and potential sites of injury until they can be repaired. After repair, nursing interventions are similar to those carried out for the patient with a fracture.
e. Nursing care takes into account a variety of challenging considerations, for example, fracture sites, fixation devices, and mobilization/immobilization requirements. Planning for long-term and extensive rehabilitation begins early in the patient's hospitalization.

## REFERENCES


1. Barangan JD: Factors that influence recovery from hip fracture during hospitalization, *Orthop Nurs* 9(5):19-28, 1990.
2. Dunwoody CJ: Pelvic fracture care: reflections on the past, implications for the future, *Nurs Clin North Am* 26(1):65-72, 1991.
3. Hay EK: That old hip: the osteoporosis process, *Nurs Clin North Am* 26(1):43-51, 1991.
4. Herron DG, Nance J: Emergency department nursing management of patients with orthopedic fractures resulting from motor vehicle accidents, *Nurs Clin North Am* 25(1):71-83, 1990.
5. Huggins B: Trauma physiology, *Nurs Clin North Am* 25(1):1-10, 1990.
6. Johnson L: Operative management of unstable pelvic fractures, *Orthop Nurs* 8(4):21-25, 1989.
7. Keitz JE: *Orthop Nurs* 8(6):29-32, 1989.
8. Mims BC: Fat embolism syndrome: a variant of ARDS, *Orthop Nurs* 8(3):22-25, 1989.
9. Mourad LA, Droste MM: *The nursing process in the care of adults with orthopaedic conditions,* ed 3, Albany, NY, 1993, Delmar Publishing.
10. Newschwander GE, Dunst RM: Limb lengthening with the Ilizarov external fixator, *Orthop Nurs* 8(3):15-21, 1989.
11. Nussman DS, Poole RC: Rescue and recovery in traumatic hip dislocation, *Am J Nurs* 91(11):34-38, 1991.
12. Ross D: Acute compartment syndrome, *Orthop Nurs* 10(2):33-38, 1991.
13. Sheidler V: Patient-controlled analgesia, *Curr Concepts Nurs* 1(1):13-16, 1987.
14. Slye DA: Orthopedic complications: compartment syndrome, fat embolism syndrome, and venous thromboembolism, *Nurs Clin North Am* 26(1):113-132, 1991.
15. Sneed NV, VanBree KM: Treating ununited fractures with electricity: nursing implications, *J Gerontol Nurs* 16(8):26-31, 1990.
16. US Department of Health and Human Services, Public Health Service: *Healthy People 2000: national health promotion and disease prevention objectives,* Washington, DC, 1990, US Government Printing Office.
17. Valentine WA, Williams PA, Tafoya WL: Ilizarov external fixation, *AORN J* 51(6):1530-1545, 1990.

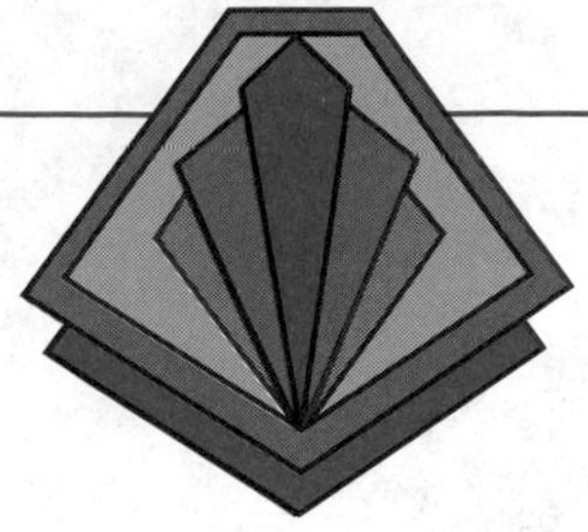

C H A P T E R 65

# Management of Persons With Inflammatory and Degenerative Disorders of the Musculoskeletal System

*Jane F. Marek*
*Patricia S. Buergin*
*Kyle M. Paskert*

## CHAPTER OBJECTIVES

***After studying this chapter, the learner should be able to do the following:***

1. Explain the five physiologic problems commonly experienced by persons who have disorders of the musculoskeletal system.
2. Discuss at least five interventions used in the management of physiologic problems experienced by persons with musculoskeletal disorders and give rationales for each.
3. Discuss the five psychosocial problems commonly experienced by persons with musculoskeletal disorders and explain the interventions that can be used in managing those problems.
4. Discuss both nonpreventable and preventable factors related to musculoskeletal disorders.
5. Explain the etiology/epidemiology, pathophysiology, and clinical manifestations of rheumatoid arthritis.
6. Explain the medical management and nursing management of persons who have rheumatoid arthritis.
7. Discuss the orthopaedic surgeries commonly employed to treat persons with rheumatoid arthritis and the nursing care associated with each of the surgeries.
8. Discuss the etiology/epidemiology, pathophysiology, and clinical manifestations of systemic lupus erythematosus (SLE).
9. Explain the medical and nursing interventions used in the care of persons with SLE.
10. Discuss the etiology/epidemiology, pathophysiology, and clinical manifestations of polymyositis, and explain the medical and nursing interventions used in the care of persons who have polymyositis.
11. Discuss the etiology/epidemiology, pathophysiology, and clinical manifestations of ankylosing spondylitis and explain the medical and nursing interventions used in the care of persons who have the disease.
12. Describe three forms of nonarticular rheumatism and describe the medical and nursing interventions used in the care of each.
13. Explain the etiology/epidemiology, pathophysiology, and clinical manifestations of degenerative joint disease and discuss its preventable aspects.
14. Describe the medical and nursing management of persons who have degenerative joint disease, including surgical intervention and postoperative nursing interventions.
15. Discuss the incidence, pathophysiology, and clinical manifestations of osteoporosis.
16. Identify risk factors associated with osteoporosis and explain nursing management of persons with osteoporosis.
17. Explain the pathophysiology and clinical manifestations of degenerative disease of the spine.
18. Discuss the medical management of persons who have degenerative joint disease of the spine and explain the nursing care required for individuals being treated (a) conservatively and (b) surgically.

19 Explain the pathophysiology and clinical manifestations of scoliosis.
20 Describe the medical management of persons who have scoliosis and explain the nursing care required for individuals being treated (a) conservatively and (b) surgically.
21 Give four examples of other disorders that can affect the musculoskeletal system, describe how they differ from disorders previously discussed, and explain the essential medical and nursing management required for persons affected by them.
22 Explain the etiology and epidemiology of tumors of the musculoskeletal system.
23 Describe the characteristics and treatment for common tumors of the musculoskeletal system.
24 Describe the medical, surgical, and nursing management of the patient with an osteosarcoma.
25 Compare and contrast potential complications after limb salvage surgery and amputation.

## KEY TERMS

allograft
ankylosing spondylitis
arthrodesis
autograft
carpal tunnel syndrome
degenerative disk disease
degenerative joint disease (DJD)
degenerative or rheumatoid involvement
dermatomyositis
Dupuytren's contracture
gout
herniated intervertebral disk
joint replacement
limb salvage surgery (LSS)
orthoses
osteomyelitis
osteophyte formation
osteoporosis
osteosarcoma
polymyositis
replacement arthroplasty
rheumatoid arthritis
rheumatoid factor (RF)
scoliosis
spinal stenosis
spondylolisthesis
systemic lupus erythematosus (SLE)
xenograft

The essence of nursing individuals with musculoskeletal problems lies in helping them to make the physiologic and psychosocial adaptations necessary to minimize their temporary or permanent disability. This chapter defines some of the common problems (both physiologic and psychosocial) experienced by individuals with motor disabilities and discusses specific methods that may be used in managing these problems.

# PHYSIOLOGIC DISABILITIES

## COMMON PROBLEMS

Five major problems must be considered in the area of physiologic disability: (1) pain, (2) stiffness, (3) decrease in muscle strength, (4) loss of dexterity, and (5) loss of locomotor ability. Most patients with a motor disability will have one or more of them.

### Pain

Pain is the priority problem that must be dealt with in planning care. Regardless of its intensity, unrelieved pain can become so all consuming a concern that the individual's entire attention is focused on relieving it. Pain prevents activity, predisposes the patient to the complications of immobility, and dulls receptiveness to care and teaching. In the extreme, it can affect the individual's attitude toward life. Therefore pain must be relieved to the greatest extent possible before other needed interventions can be implemented.

### Stiffness

Stiffness (decreased flexibility) can be a result of pain or of disuse (as in the case of persons who are immobilized), or it can be a result of pathophysiologic changes (as in degenerative joint disease). Stiffness cannot be defined as pain; however, an attempt to use an extremity that is stiff may cause pain. Stiffness may discourage activity, thereby affecting the person in much the same manner as pain.

### Decrease in Muscle Strength

Decrease in muscle strength is sometimes a primary problem, as with some myopathic and neuropathic disorders, or it can result from prolonged bedrest or immobility. Interventions designed to improve strength (e.g., increasing mobility or exercising) can be implemented when some progress is made with treatment of the primary problem. When it is not possible for the person to regain muscle strength, some means of modifying activity to maintain function must be provided.

### Loss of Dexterity

Loss of dexterity (skillful use of the hands or body) is another problem encountered either as a result of a primary pathophysiologic process (e.g., rheumatoid arthritis or ataxic neurologic disorders) or as a result of pain, stiffness, or enforced immobility. Again, the primary problem must be treated before measures to improve dexterity can be implemented. If the primary problem cannot be controlled, measures can be taken to provide alternative methods of performing activities so that function can be maintained.

## Loss of Locomotor Ability

Perhaps the most threatening component of many musculoskeletal disorders is the temporary or complete loss (or potential for loss) of the ability to move freely from one place to another or care for one's self. Although some problems present only short-term immobility, others, such as spinal cord damage, can cause lifelong disability.

Various groups of handicapped persons throughout the United States have been active socially and politically to inform the general public of the architectural barriers encountered by individuals with limited mobility. As a result, federally funded building projects must now be equipped with facilities to accommodate the handicapped individual. All new public buildings must have wheelchair ramps, special toilet facilities, and easy-access parking spaces.

The concern of those caring for hospitalized persons with activity or motor restrictions must be directed toward preventing complications, helping them work through their feelings about and adapt to restricted mobility, providing them with alternative means for moving about or performing activities of daily living (ADL), and helping them plan for adaptations they will have to make in their home environments and life-styles.

### Complications of immobility

Immobility may be accompanied by a number of potential or actual complications that can involve any or all of the major systems of the body (Table 65-1).

# COMMON INTERVENTIONS

Some interventions are common to a number of musculoskeletal disorders. They will be discussed generally here and will be referred to under specific interventions later in this chapter.

## Rest, Activity, Joint Protection, and Energy Conservation

### Rest

Rest is a therapeutic measure used in many inflammatory and traumatic conditions of the musculoskeletal system. However, too much rest can at times be as detrimental as too much activity. There are two forms of rest:

1. *Absolute rest or no activity*
   a. May be required for the whole body or for a specific part of the body
   b. Is accomplished through avoidance of use of the part
   c. Is possibly enhanced by some method of external immobilization (splint, cast, traction) to ensure inactivity
2. *Partial rest or limited activity*
   a. Some activity permitted, but other activities (e.g., weight bearing, certain movements) are limited

The nurse's responsibility in helping the patient rest is as follows:

1. Help patient understand the meaning of "rest" as it applies to him or her
2. Take over functions for the patient that would require use of body part beyond limits prescribed
3. Teach the patient how to effectively use body parts not required to rest
4. Gradually return functions to the patient when rest is no longer required

### Balancing activity and rest

Activity, particularly in chronic conditions, must be balanced with adequate rest. Individuals who have pain with certain activities or increased pain and stiffness following certain activities must learn to recognize their tolerances and adapt their ADL accordingly. This does not mean stopping all activity; it means *modifying* activity. For the individual with degenerative arthritis of the hips, for example, it may mean walking 1 mile each day instead of 2 miles.

Nurses can help patients determine their activity needs in the following ways:

1. Teach the patient the advantages of continuing, but modifying, activity
2. Help the patient identify his or her own activity tolerances
3. Help the patient work out an activity schedule approximating rest/activity requirements at home
4. Help the patient work through concerns about not being able to perform all activities he or she believes are necessary or desired

### Joint protection and energy conservation

Individuals with joint involvement and/or activity intolerances can learn to protect their joints and themselves from overuse, misuse, and stress by becoming aware of and practicing joint protection and energy conservation techniques (Table 65-2). External pressures that put stress on joints in the wrong direction and internal pressures from muscles can produce deformities in joints that have been affected by chronic inflammatory processes. Fatigue and an increase in pain are symptoms of overactivity and overuse or misuse of joints. Nursing interventions are as follows:

1. Teach patient to recognize the symptoms of overactivity.
2. Teach patient appropriate energy conservation and joint protection techniques.
3. Encourage patient to use these techniques in ADL.

## Assistive, Supportive, and Safety Devices

Many assistive devices are available for individuals who have impairment of upper and/or lower extremity func-

**TABLE 65-1 Complications of Immobility**

| MECHANISM | POTENTIAL COMPLICATION | INTERVENTION |
|---|---|---|
| **CARDIOVASCULAR** | | |
| Failure of vessels in legs to assume or maintain a state of vasoconstriction, resulting in pooling of venous blood | Deep vein thrombosis (DVT)<br>Pulmonary embolism (PE)<br>Increased work load on heart<br>Diminished cardiac output<br>Decreased ability to adapt to erect posture | Active and passive range of motion (ROM)<br>Frequent turning<br>Slow mobilization<br>Positioning to avoid pressure over major vessels |
| **RESPIRATORY** | | |
| Decreased movement<br>Decreased stimulus to cough<br>Decreased depth of ventilation | Pooling of secretions in bronchi, bronchioles<br>Hypostatic pneumonia | Active and passive ROM<br>Stimulation to take maximal sustained inhalations and cough<br>Frequent turning |
| **SKIN** | | |
| Pressure or shearing forces (two or more tissue layers sliding on each other or tissue sliding on another surface) disrupting or decreasing circulation to an area | Skin breakdown (abrasion or decubitus ulcer) | Early indentification of areas at risk<br>Turning on regular schedule<br>Pressure-relieving pads, mattresses, flotation devices, special beds |
| **GASTROINTESTINAL** | | |
| Decreased bowel motility<br>Change in dietary habits<br>Disadvantageous positioning for defecation | Constipation<br>Impaction | Increase fluid intake<br>Add roughage to diet<br>Encourage use of bedside commode or toilet when possible |
| **MUSCULOSKELETAL** | | |
| **Muscles** | | |
| Disuse | Atrophy<br>Weakness | Active ROM<br>Exercise |
| **Joints** | | |
| Limited motion leads to muscle, tendon shortening | Contracture<br>Fibrosis or bony ankylosis around joints | Active and passive ROM<br>Exercise<br>Encourage to perform own ADL as possible |
| **Bones** | | |
| Disruption of balance of osteoblastic/osteoclastic activity with destruction of bone matrix and release of calcium | Osteoporosis | Isometric and active exercise to tolerance |
| **URINARY** | | |
| Increased urinary pH, increased citric acid | Renal stones | Increase fluid intake<br>Decrease calcium intake |
| Poor bladder emptying | Urinary stasis | Improve position for bladder emptying (i.e., bedside commode or toilet when possible) |
| **NEUROLOGIC** | | |
| Loss of normal stimuli | Confusion, restlessness, forgetfulness | Provide stimulation and diversionary material |

tion (Box 65-1). Although the occupational therapist is generally the person who evaluates the patient's disability, recommends specific assistive devices, and teaches the patient how to use them, the nurse is often the person who recognizes the need for referral to the occupational therapist and encourages the patient to use devices appropriately in the hospital or at home. For example, it is nontherapeutic and time consuming to feed persons who can feed themselves independently with aids that have been provided.

Supportive devices or ambulatory aids (walkers, canes, crutches) are usually recommended for persons who cannot bear weight on one or more joints of the lower extremities. Other indications for their use are instability, poor balance, or pain on weight bearing. The physical therapist evaluates the patient to determine the

**TABLE 65-2 Joint Protection and Energy Conservation Techniques**

| TECHNIQUE | EXAMPLES |
|---|---|
| Avoid positions of possible joint deformity | Avoid keeping joints in positions of flexion for prolonged periods of time<br>Avoid twisting motions such as turning a jar lid with small joints |
| Avoid holding muscles or joints in one position for a long time | When working at a desk, stand up and walk about for a few minutes every half hour |
| Use the strongest joints for all activities | Use the knees, not the back, when lifting heavy objects<br>Push a door open with the shoulder, not the wrist<br>Use a shoulder strap, not a hand-held strap, to carry a heavy purse |
| Use joints in their best position, maintaining good standing and sitting posture | Avoid reaching or bending when another approach would work as well<br>Work at a comfortable height |
| Conserve energy | Avoid trying to accomplish difficult tasks in a single time period<br>Take breaks during work periods<br>Slide rather than lift objects<br>Use a wheeled cart to move objects from one place to another |

FIGURE 65-1 Utensils with built-up handles.

specific device that will match the patient's needs and abilities. Some considerations regarding choice of device include the following:

1. Axillary crutches
   a. Require dexterity and a good sense of balance
   b. Permit faster ambulation than walkers
   c. Can be used on stairs
2. Walkers
   a. Provide solid support

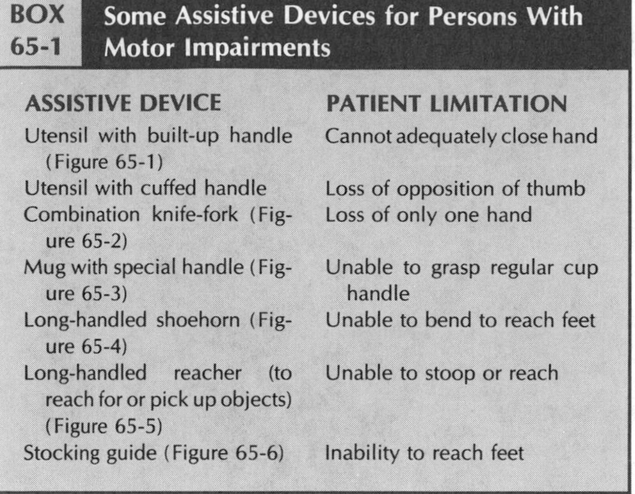

**BOX 65-1 Some Assistive Devices for Persons With Motor Impairments**

| ASSISTIVE DEVICE | PATIENT LIMITATION |
|---|---|
| Utensil with built-up handle (Figure 65-1) | Cannot adequately close hand |
| Utensil with cuffed handle | Loss of opposition of thumb |
| Combination knife-fork (Figure 65-2) | Loss of only one hand |
| Mug with special handle (Figure 65-3) | Unable to grasp regular cup handle |
| Long-handled shoehorn (Figure 65-4) | Unable to bend to reach feet |
| Long-handled reacher (to reach for or pick up objects) (Figure 65-5) | Unable to stoop or reach |
| Stocking guide (Figure 65-6) | Inability to reach feet |

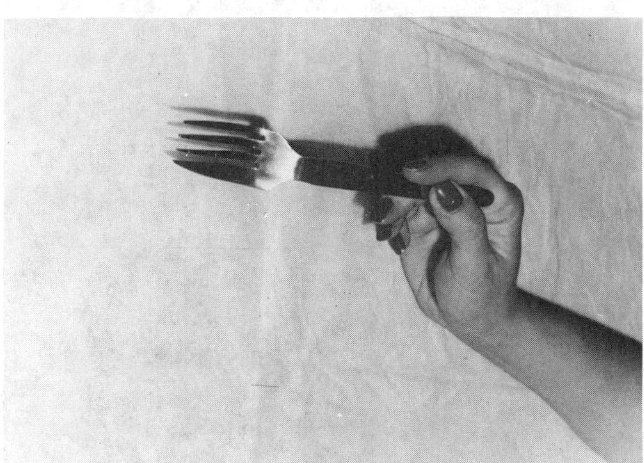

FIGURE 65-2 Combination knife-fork.

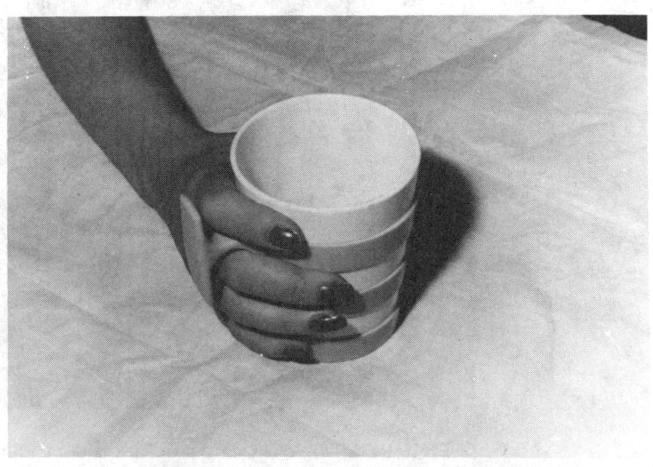

FIGURE 65-3 Mug with special handle.

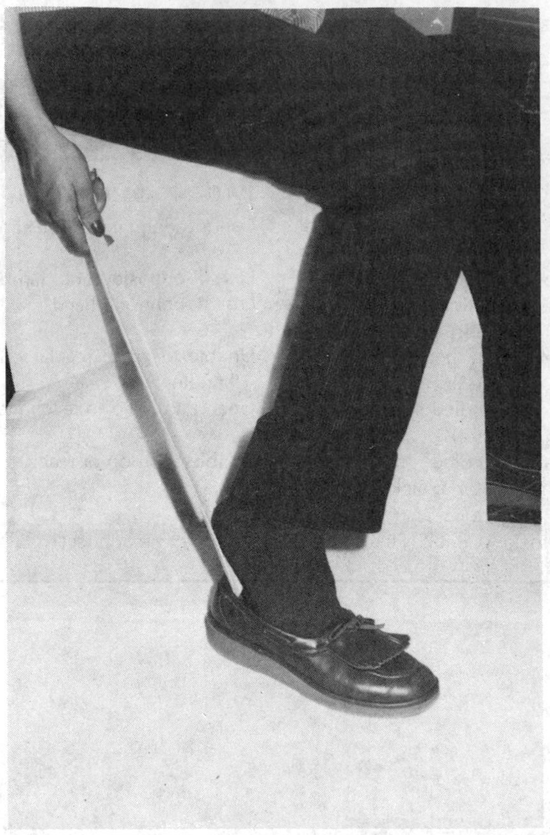

**FIGURE 65-4** Long-handled shoehorn.

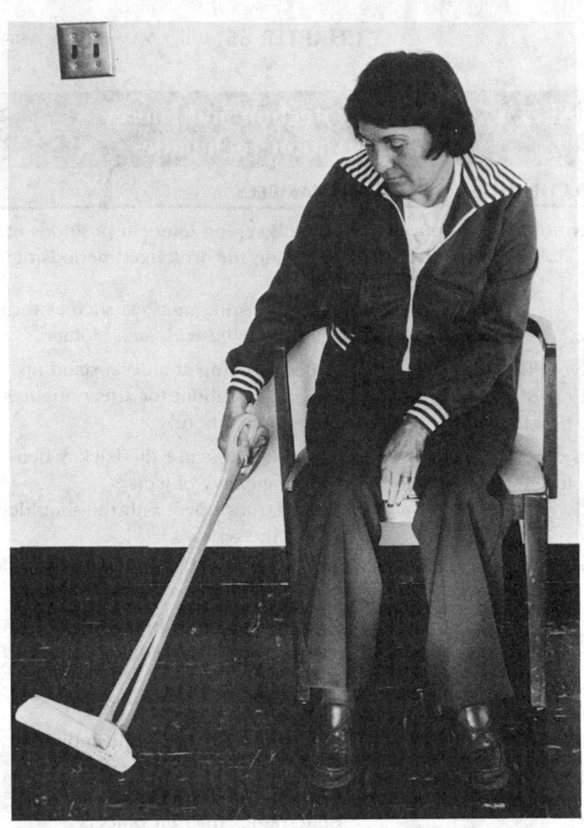

**FIGURE 65-5** Long-handled reachers are handy for picking things up off floor if person is not to bend or stoop.

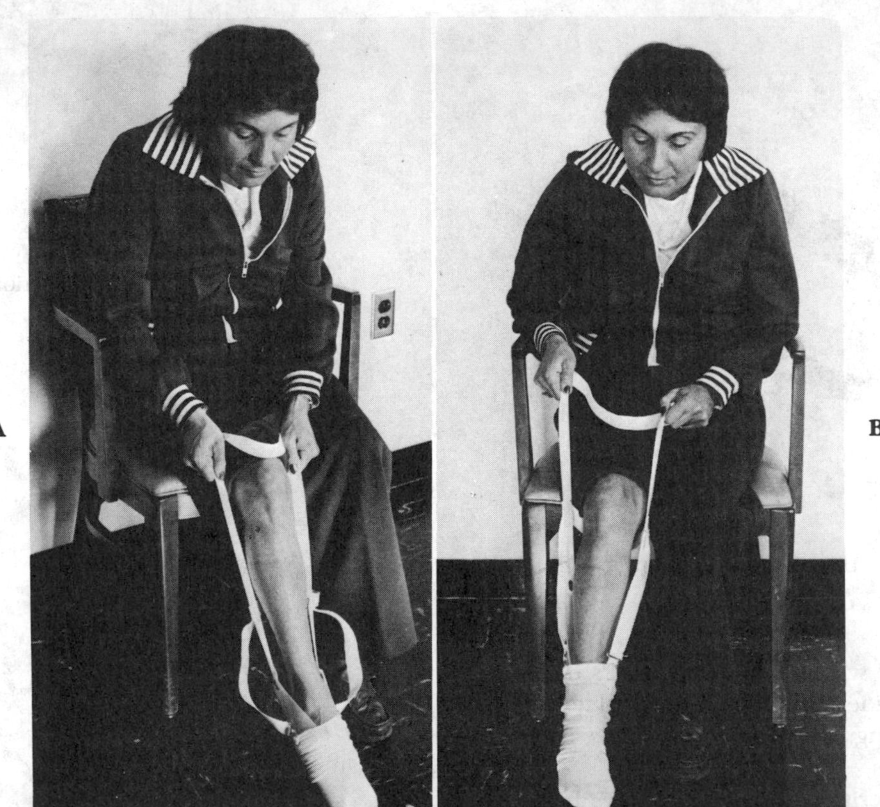

A

B

**FIGURE 65-6** **A,** Using stocking aid. Stocking has been placed over plastic guide; garter clips at ends of strap have been attached to top of stocking. Woman then places her foot into stocking. **B,** Straps are used to pull stocking over foot and up leg; when top of stocking is at knee, patient can release garters. This apparatus is useful for persons who cannot bend over to reach feet.

**TABLE 65-3 Techniques of Walking with Ambulatory Aids***

| DEVICE | GAIT |
|---|---|
| Single-support device (cane, quad cane, single crutch) | Device is held in the hand opposite the involved leg<br>Device and involved leg are advanced first, followed by the uninvolved leg |
| Double-support device | |
| Walker | Walker is advanced first, then the involved extremity, then the uninvolved extremity |
| Crutches | 3-point gait—the same as walker gait<br>4-point gait—crutch, opposite leg, opposite crutch, other leg<br>2-point gait—both crutches, both legs (one leg may be non–weight bearing) |

*SPECIAL NOTE: Climbing up stairs is accomplished by moving the uninvolved leg first, then the device and the involved leg; to descend stairs, the involved leg and the device are moved first, then the uninvolved leg. The device and the involved leg always move together.

b. Can be used by individuals with balance problems
c. Limit speed of ambulation
d. Are hazardous on stairs or uneven ground

3. Canes
   a. Are less cumbersome than crutches or walkers
   b. Do not permit as effective unloading of weight as a double support

Nurses are expected to supervise patients in their use of these devices and encourage patients to use their walking aids correctly. Techniques of walking with aids are outlined in Table 65-3.

Safety devices are items that can be used by the patient to enhance function and prevent accidents when normal function, balance, or dexterity is compromised. Examples of safety devices include safety arms around toilets, grab bars mounted at tubs or showers, elevated toilet seats, adhesive strips on tub or shower floors, hand rails along staircases, and nonskid wax applied to floors. Nurses need to be familiar with the various devices available, help patients learn to use them, and if necessary, advise patients where they may be obtained.

## Applying Heat and Cold

Heat and cold have a variety of uses for individuals with musculoskeletal problems. Heat, particularly moist heat, is used for relieving stiffness and relaxing muscles and for analgesic effect and sedative effect. Heat may be applied in a variety of ways:

1. Dry heat
   a. Electric heating pad
   b. Warm towels
   c. Aqua-K pads
2. Moist heat
   a. Hydrocollator packs (packs containing chemical filler that expands in water and retains heat; may be heated in pot of water or special machines that maintain a constant temperature of 80° C [174° F])
   b. Paraffin baths
   c. Electric heating pads that are approved for use with moist towels
   d. Electric heating pads that produce moisture
   e. Warm soaks, tub soaks, or showers

Application of cold or ice packs is helpful in reducing or preventing swelling (especially after trauma), reducing pain, and relieving stiffness. Cold packs may take the form of plastic bags containing ice, commercially available gel packs that can be refrozen and reused, or large bags of frozen vegetables (especially for home use).

Whenever heat or cold is applied, it should be left on for 15 to 20 minutes to achieve maximum effect. Cold packs and moist heat packs should be wrapped in protective towels to prevent burns to the skin, and the skin should be checked 5 minutes after application for any evidence of tissue damage. Heat or cold should be applied with caution to any individual with decreased sensation, because that person will not be able to determine if damage is occurring.

Nursing interventions with heat or cold therapy include:

1. Helping patient determine which type of application works best
2. Instructing patient about safety precautions to be observed with that method
3. Instructing patient about timely application of heat or cold (e.g., before activity or exercise or before going to bed at night) depending on patient's particular needs
4. Assisting the patient with application

## Traction

Traction can be used to help reduce contractures or to relieve pain in the presence of muscle spasm. It can be applied intermittently or constantly and usually in the form of skin traction, that is, Buck's extension, Russell traction, or pelvic traction. Patients who are receiving this form of therapy can usually be taken out of traction if the traction itself is causing discomfort, and the traction can be reapplied when the patient believes it can be tolerated. The principles of maintaining the patient's comfort and safety while in traction are discussed in Chapter 64.

## Splints and Braces

Splints and braces (orthoses) are used for the following purposes:

1. Stabilize or support a joint
2. Protect a joint or body part from external trauma
3. Mechanically correct dysfunction such as footdrop by supporting the joint in its functional position
4. Assist patients to exercise specific joints

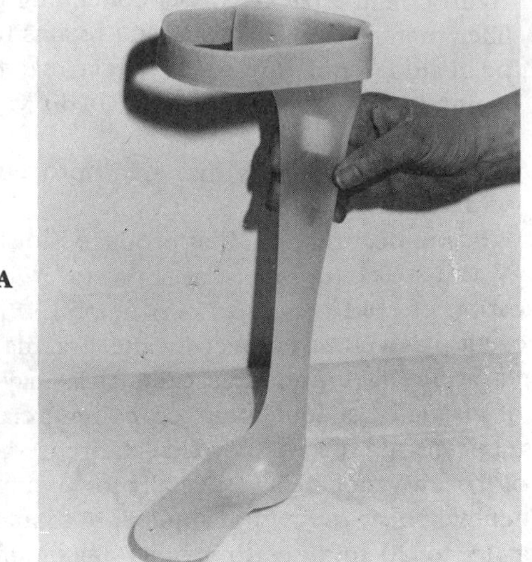


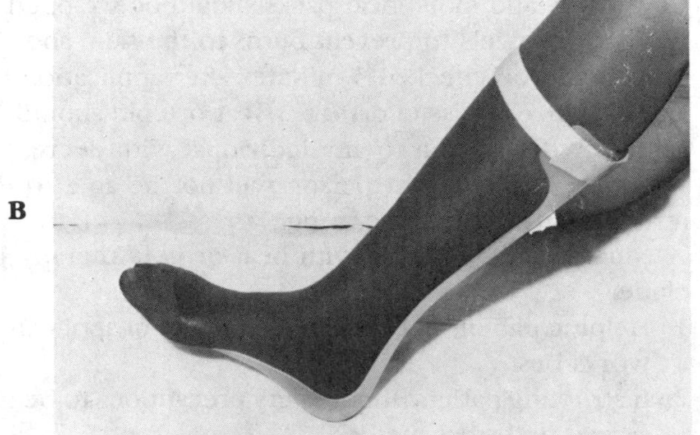


**FIGURE 65-7** **A,** Molded footdrop brace. **B,** Brace in place on foot.

**TABLE 65-4 Types of Splints and Braces and Their Function**

| TYPE | FUNCTION |
|---|---|
| Spring-loaded braces | Oppose the action of unparalyzed muscles and act as partial functional substitutes for paralyzed muscles (Figure 65-8) |
| Resting splints | Maintain a limb or joint in a functional position while permitting the muscles around the joint to relax (Figure 65-9) |
| Functional splints | Maintain the joint or limb in a usable position to enable the body part to be used correctly |
| Dynamic splints | Permit assisted exercise to joints, particularly following surgery to finger joints (Figure 65-10) |

Splints and braces (Table 65-4) are designed to be as lightweight and cosmetically acceptable as possible. Advances have been made in this area by orthotists (brace makers) who have developed plastic molded braces made out of lightweight materials; these braces are custom fitted to the patient (Figure 65-7). In many instances these have replaced the cumbersome metal and leather braces that are often obvious, even though worn under loose-fitting clothing. *Shoes* may be modified, or corrective shoes may be prescribed, to provide special support for the feet.

When patients need to use braces or splints, nurses need to do the following:

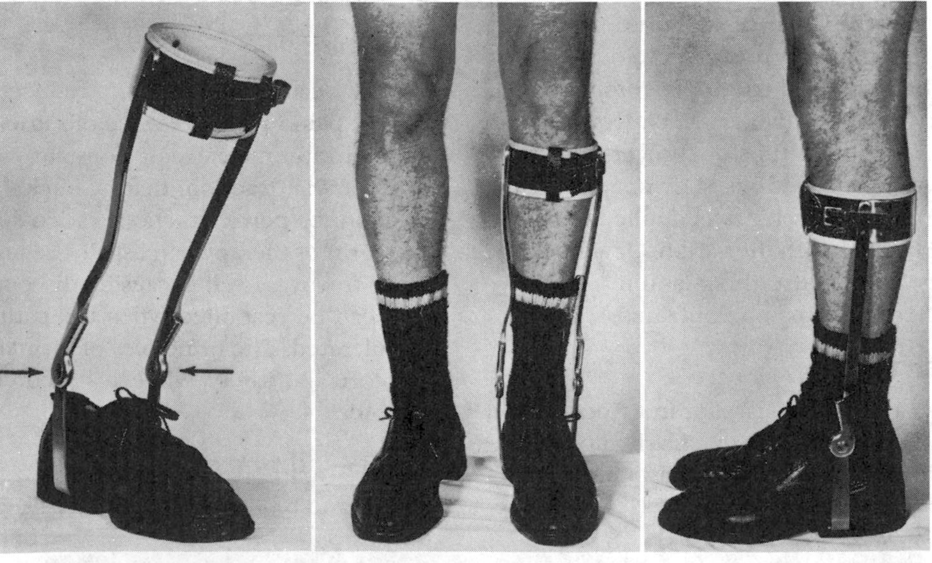

**FIGURE 65-8** Spring footdrop brace. When weak dorsiflexor muscles are overbalanced by stronger plantar flexors, adjustable spring at ankle hinge of each upright (Klenzak joint, Pope Foundation, Inc.) is used to supply passive dorsiflexion and thus prevent footdrop and an equinus limp. (From Brashear H, Raney R: *Shand's handbook of orthopaedic surgery,* ed 9, St Louis, 1978, Mosby.)

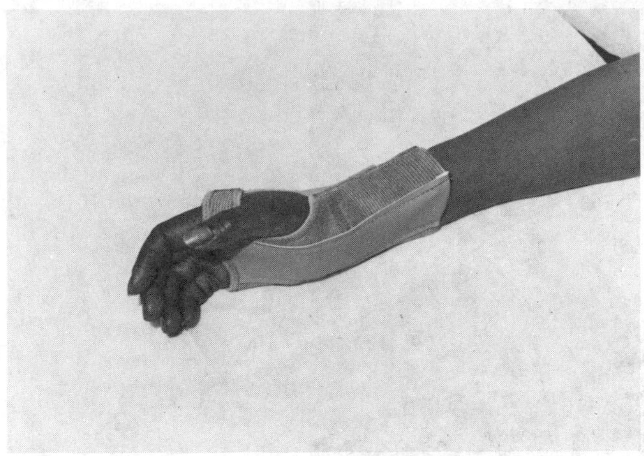
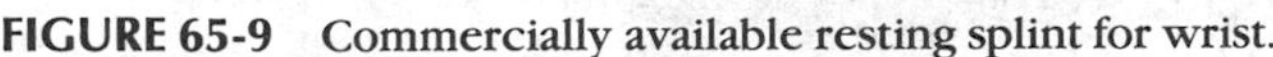

**FIGURE 65-9** Commercially available resting splint for wrist.

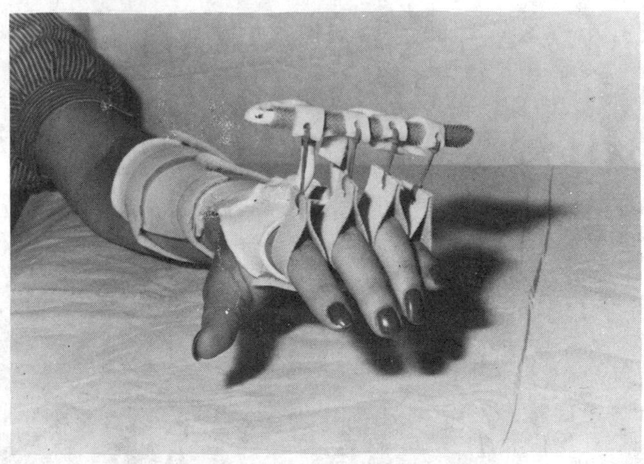

**FIGURE 65-10** Dynamic hand splint.

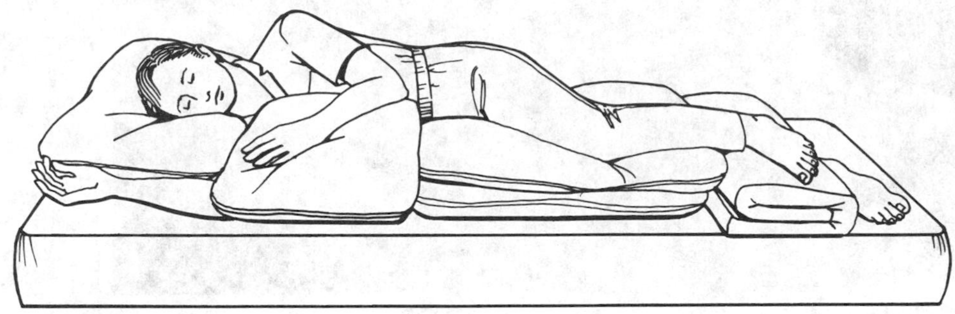

**FIGURE 65-11** Side-lying position with extremities properly supported with pillows and rolled blankets.

1. Inspect patient's skin after the orthosis has been applied for a short time to be certain it has caused no skin irritation.
2. Notify the orthotist if adjustments in the orthosis need to be made to make it more comfortable or relieve chafing.
3. Instruct the patient in the proper application and care of the orthosis.
   a. Metal braces should be stored upright.
   b. Leather materials should be treated occasionally with Neatsfoot Compound or other leather preservative to prevent cracking and drying.
   c. Orthoses fabricated of molded materials should be stored away from sources of heat.
   d. Patients fitted with molded orthoses should avoid gaining or losing weight, because the brace would have to be adjusted or refabricated.
4. Assist the patient to make the psychologic adjustment to wearing the orthosis.

## Positioning and Transfer

Principles of positioning (Figure 65-11) can be found in most fundamentals of nursing texts. However, because pain accompanies nearly all musculoskeletal problems, preventing or minimizing pain must be taken into consideration when positioning the patient. Nurses should be aware that patients in the acute stages of their disorders require the greatest care and gentleness when they must be moved. Fear of pain often causes irritability and can lead to muscular resistance, which increases pain. Care must be taken not to jar the bed. Heavy bedclothes over painful extremities may cause added pain. If bed cradles are used to support linen, caution must be taken not to accidentally bump an involved part of the body when adjusting or removing the cradle. Placing a very painful joint or extremity on a pillow or pillows to move it can reduce pain. Moving patients off the bed using a pull sheet (Figure 65-12) or a roller board (Figure 65-13) also facilitates comfort through the move. Frequently, patients would prefer to move themselves rather than risk pain from having someone else move them; when it is safe for the patient to do so, the nurse should permit it.

If the patient must use a wheelchair, it should be adjusted to fit that individual. No wheelchair should be purchased for permanent use by a patient unless someone knowledgeable about wheelchairs, preferably a physical therapist, has evaluated the patient and deter-

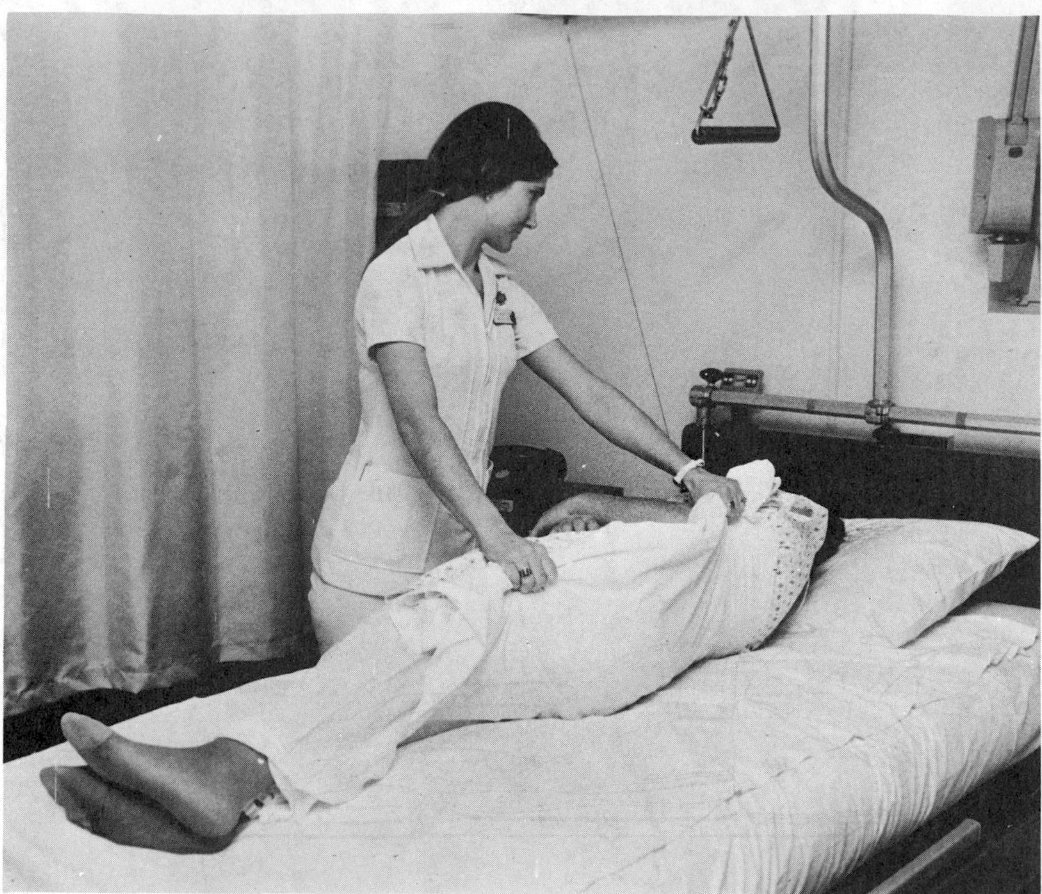

**FIGURE 65-12** Use of turning sheet. Sheet is held taut with one hand at level of patient's shoulder and other hand below patient's buttocks, providing patient with a sense of support and control. A sheet so placed may also be effectively used as a pull sheet when moving patient from bed to cart.

**FIGURE 65-13** Use of a roller board, effective in moving patients comfortably from one surface to another, such as from bed to stretcher and stretcher to bed.

**Guidelines for Transfer**

The patient should always be moved toward his or her strong side.
The person assisting supports the *strong* side.
If there is any question regarding the patient's ability to cooperate with the transfer, a second person should be standing by for assistance.
If the person assisting with the transfer has any doubt about his or her ability to do so safely, a second person should be asked to help.
The transfer should be accomplished using the strong muscles of the legs rather than the weak muscles of the back.
If lifting is required, adequate help should be available. If help is not available, the transfer should not be attempted at that time.

mined what special equipment is needed. Chairs poorly fitted to the patient's needs can be unsafe and encourage poor posture. Principles of transfer are summarized in the Guidelines box above.

## Exercise

Exercise is a prescribed form of activity designed to accomplish the following:

1. Preserve joint mobility (active and passive range of motion)
2. Maintain muscle tone (active range of motion and isometrics)
3. Strengthen selected muscle groups (resistive exercises performed against resistance provided by another person or by weights)

Exercise may be facilitated by the application of heat or cold or the administration of an analgesic before the exercise period. Exercise is contraindicated in the presence of acute joint or muscle inflammation until the inflammatory process subsides.

Exercise programs should be tailored to the patient's specific needs and capabilities. Nurses need to be aware of the specific exercise program the patient is following and be prepared to provide support and assistance in performing the exercises as needed and reinforcing the purpose, technique, frequency, and duration of the exercises.

## Medication

Many of the medications used in the treatment of musculoskeletal problems are antiinflammatory analgesics. Specific drugs are addressed in Table 65-5 and in conjunction with discussion of specific disorders. Nurses caring for patients taking these drugs should be prepared to teach patients the expected effects of the drugs, how to use them appropriately, and how to recognize side effects or toxic effects. In addition, nurses should be aware that use of narcotic analgesics in chronic inflammatory musculoskeletal conditions is generally contraindicated, because they are not antiinflammatory and the patient will develop a tolerance to them. Narcotic analgesics do have their place in the treatment of acute injuries and postoperative pain.

## Nutrition

The essentials of good nutrition are as important for individuals with musculoskeletal problems as for anyone else. Special diets, however, are usually not recommended except where other medical conditions require them. Patients should pay particular attention to avoiding weight gain. Added weight increases the patient's energy consumption and causes weight-bearing joints to be abnormally stressed. For many individuals with mobility problems, however, the problem of weight and mobility becomes a vicious circle. Mobility is impaired, therefore activity is limited, calories are not used in activity, more weight is added, and further immobility results as the individual finds it harder to move the weight. This cycle can be broken only by weight loss through a properly supervised reduction diet.

Nurses can help in the following way:

1. Teach patients the importance of a well-balanced diet
2. Teach patients the importance of restricting weight gain
3. Encourage patients to select food wisely
4. Encourage the patient's family to bring home-cooked food if the patient is not eating hospital food, particularly following surgery when the patient needs to maintain a positive nitrogen balance

## Surgical Interventions

### Indications for surgery

Individuals who have surgery to the musculoskeletal system usually fall into one of two categories: those who have suffered trauma such as a fracture (see Chapter 64) or those who require an elective orthopedic procedure for correction of deformity, relief of pain, or restoration of musculoskeletal function. The four major objectives of orthopedic treatment are as follows:

1. Restoration or maintenance of function of a body part
2. Prevention of deformity
3. Correction of deformity if it already exists
4. Development of the patient's powers of compensation and adaptation if loss of function or permanent deformity is not preventable

Before performing surgery, the orthopedist considers what procedure is best suited to achieve the desired objectives for the individual patient. It is important that those caring for the patient know and understand what the expected outcomes are so that care may be adapted to achieving them. ***Orthopedic care is highly individualized to the patient being treated, and those who work with orthopedic patients must not lose sight of the practical aspects of the treatment rationale.***

## TABLE 65-5 Medications Prescribed in the Treatment of Rheumatoid Arthritis*

| MEDICATIONS | ACTION | SIDE EFFECTS/TOXIC EFFECTS | PRECAUTIONS |
|---|---|---|---|
| **SALICYLATES** | | | |
| Examples: acetylsalicylic acid, choline salicylates | Analgesic, antipyretic, antiinflammatory | Gastric irritation; dose-related salicylism; skin rash; hypersensitivity | Take with food, milk, or antacid; space q 4-6 hr to maintain antiinflammatory effect |
| **NONSTEROIDAL ANTIINFLAMMATORY AGENTS (NSAIAs)†** | | | |
| Indomethacin (Indocin) | Analgesic, antiinflammatory | Headache; dizziness; insomnia; confusion; gastrointestinal irritation | Take with food, milk, or antacid; discontinue if CNS symptoms develop and notify physician |
| Ibuprofen (Motrin) | Same as indomethacin | Same as indomethacin but believed less irritating to gastrointestinal tract; fluid retention | Absorption delayed if taken with food |
| Tolmetin sodium (Tolectin) | Same as ibuprofen | Same as ibuprofen | Take with food or milk |
| Naproxen (Naprosyn) | Same as ibuprofen | Same as ibuprofen; also drowsiness | Take with food, milk, or antacid; avoid driving until dosage effect is established |
| Fenoprofen (Nalfon) | Same as ibuprofen | Same as naproxen | Delayed absorption if taken with food; avoid driving until dosage effect established |
| Sulindac (Clinoril) | Same as ibuprofen | Same as ibuprofen; also skin rash | Take with food, milk, or antacid; do not use with acetylsalicylic acid |
| Diflunisal (Dolobid) | Analgesic, antiinflammatory | Gastric irritation; headache; dizziness; skin rash; tinnitus; fluid retention | Take with food or milk; do not use with salicylates or other antiinflammatory medications |
| Piroxicam (Feldene) | Analgesic, antiinflammatory | Gastric irritation; anemia; skin rash; fluid retention; dizziness; headache | Take with food or antacid |
| Diclofenac sodium (Volteran) | Analgesic, antiinflammatory | Possible gastrointestinal irritation, headache, drowsiness, fatigue | Enteric coated; may be taken with food or milk |
| **POTENT ANTIINFLAMMATORY AGENTS** | | | |
| Adrenocorticosteroids (e.g., prednisone) | Interfere with body's normal inflammatory response | Fluid retention, sodium retention, potassium depletion; hypertension; decreased healing potential; increased susceptibility to infection; gastrointestinal irritation; hirsutism; osteoporosis; fat deposits; diabetes mellitus; myopathy; adrenal insufficiency or adrenal crisis if abruptly withdrawn | Take with food, milk, or antacid; dosage not to be increased or decreased without physician supervision; take in morning if taken once per day |
| Phenylbutazone (Butazolidin) | Antiinflammatory; analgesic at subcortical site in brain | Gastrointestinal irritation; hematologic toxicity; hypertension; impaired renal function | Used for a short term (7-10 days); take with food or milk |
| **SLOW-ACTING ANTIINFLAMMATORY AGENTS‡** | | | |
| **Antimalarials** | | | |
| Hydroxychloroquine (Plaquenil) | Antiinflammatory (mechanism unknown); effect not expected to be noted for 6-12 mo after beginning therapy | Gastrointestinal disturbances; retinal edema that may result in blindness | Eye examination before beginning therapy and every 6 mo thereafter |
| Chloroquine (Aralen) | Same as nydroxychloroquine | Same as hydroxychloroquine | Same as hydroxychloroquine |

*NOTE: Adjunctive therapy, at any level of the pyramid of management, may include the use of intraarticular steroids, therapy with analgesic agents that do not have antiinflammatory effects (e.g., acetominophen [Tylenol], propoxyphene [Darvon], surgery, and/or antidepressant drugs).

†Acetylsalicylic acid (aspirin) is the drug of choice in the initial treatment of rheumatoid arthritis. Nonsteroidal antiinflammatory drugs are aspirin-like drugs. Many patients prefer the NSAIAs over aspirin, because they tend to produce less gastric irritation and some of them need be taken only once or twice per day.

‡It should also be noted that the immunosuppressive agents azathioprine (Imuran), cyclophosphamide (Cytoxan), and chlorambucil (Leukeran) have been used on an investigational basis in patients with severe disease that has not responded to conventional medications. These are used with great care because of their severe side effects and the attendant risks of the development of neoplasms. The drug methotrexate has recently received Food and Drug Administration (FDA) approval for use in rheumatoid arthritis.

**TABLE 65-5 Medications Prescribed in the Treatment of Rheumatoid Arthritis*—cont'd**

| MEDICATIONS | ACTION | SIDE EFFECTS/TOXIC EFFECTS | PRECAUTIONS |
|---|---|---|---|
| Quinacrine (Atabrine) | Same as hydroxychloroquine | Same as hydroxychloroquine but may be better tolerated; yellow discoloration of skin | May be stopped periodically to prevent deepening of skin discoloration |
| Gold salts (IM)<br>Gold sodium Thiomalate (Myochrysine)<br>Gold thioglucose (Solganol)<br>Gold (oral)<br>Auranofin (Ridaura) | Antiinflammatory; effect not noted for 3-6 mo after beginning therapy | Renal and hepatic damage; corneal deposits; dermatitis; ulcerations in mouth; hematologic changes | Urinalysis and complete blood count (CBC) before each injection; report dermatitis, metallic taste in mouth, or lesions in mouth to physician<br>Oral gold may produce fewer side effects than injectable, but periodic laboratory tests are required |
| Penicillamine (Cuprimine) | Antiinflammatory (mechanism unclear); effect not expected to be noted until several months after beginning treatment | Fever; skin rash; nephrotic syndrome; hematologic changes; gastrointestinal irritation; lupuslike syndromes; allergic reactions (33% probability if allergic to penicillin); retarded wound healing | Urinalysis, CBC, differential, hemoglobin, and platelet count at least weekly for 3 mo, then monthly; report skin rash, fever to physician; food interferes with absorption—take on empty stomach between meals |

**Types of surgery**

Table 65-6 defines the common types of surgery that are performed on the musculoskeletal system and the reasons they are performed. Specific interventions for these surgeries will be discussed under the appropriate disorder.

# PSYCHOSOCIAL PROBLEMS

## COMMON PROBLEMS

### Reaction to Disfigurement, Disability, or Immobility

A major problem faced by many individuals who have musculoskeletal problems is that the disorder may be disfiguring as well as disabling. Not only must they adapt to functional disability, but they also may have to adapt to "looking different" from other people. (For further information on body image, see Chapter 9.) Loss or alteration of function or the need to use an assistive device or prosthesis can also cause them to view themselves as different from others. Depending on the nature and strength of pressures from family, social, or work situations, or the individual's degree of self-esteem, the individual may attempt to cover up the disability so as not to lose support, esteem, or a livelihood. If the disability cannot be covered up, some persons may withdraw or limit their contact with others.

### Dependence, Independence, and Interdependence

Most people want to be able to live their lives independently. In the sense of this discussion, independence would mean freedom from having to make demands on others for personal and social activities of daily living (ADL). However, persons with musculoskeletal problems may be unable to manage one or more activities for themselves. If help from another person is needed to perform a certain function, such as buttoning buttons, the individual is dependent in that area. If an assistive device (e.g., button hook, Velcro closures) can be made available and the use of it can be mastered, the individual can again be independent in that function.

Very few people live truly independent lives. As a society, we depend on the farmer to grow our food, the lawyer to attend to our legal affairs, the mechanic to repair our automobile. We are interdependent. Families are also structured around interdependent functions. Persons with motor disability may at some time be faced with losing their interdependent role; that is, they may no longer believe they are useful or needed by anyone else.

### Adaptation to Assistive, Supportive, and Corrective Devices

Walkers, canes, crutches, wheelchairs, splints, braces, and feeding aids often have negative connotations in our society. Individuals may have great difficulty overcoming their aversion to such devices and accepting them as a means of maintaining their independence and safety.

### Socioeconomic Impact

Many disorders that affect motor function occur at an age when wage earning, child rearing, and other functions can be seriously impaired. Loss of income and self-esteem, the inability to maintain one's standard of living, and increased stress on the family can all result. By no

**TABLE 65-6 Surgical Procedures of the Musculoskeletal System (Except Spine Surgery)**

| DEFINITION OF PROCEDURE | REASON FOR PERFORMING |
|---|---|
| **ARTHROTOMY** | |
| Opening of a joint | Exploration of joint<br>Drainage of joint<br>Removal of damaged tissue or foreign body |
| **ARTHROPLASTY** | |
| Reconstruction of a joint | Restore motion<br>Relieve pain<br>Correct deformity |
| **Interposition** | |
| Replacement of part of a joint with a prosthesis or with soft tissue | |
| **Replacement** | |
| Replacement of both sides of a joint with prosthetic implants | |
| **SYNOVECTOMY** | |
| Removal of part or all of the synovial membrane | Delay the progress of rheumatoid arthritis |
| **OSTEOTOMY** | |
| Cutting a bone to change its alignment | Correct deformity<br>Alter the weight-bearing surface of diseased joint to relieve pain |
| **ARTHRODESIS** | |
| Causing the bones of a joint to grow together by removing articular hyaline cartilage, introducing bone grafts, and stabilizing with internal or external fixation | Stabilize a joint<br>Relieve pain |
| **TENDON TRANSPLANTS** | |
| Moving a tendon from its usual position | Substitute one tendon for another that is not working<br>Realign tendon function; for example, for stability |

means, however, is motor impairment less of a problem for the older person. Living alone or on a fixed income and faced with the possibility of not being able to maintain independence, the person can become very frightened, depressed, or withdrawn. Nursing homes are costly, as are persons who are hired to help in the home, if they are even available in a community. The idea of giving up one's home and way of life can be very threatening and demoralizing.

### Family Relationships

Reference has already been made to the fact that family roles and relationships (social and economic) may be changed because of a patient's restricted motor function and areas of dependency. It is important that those caring for the patient recognize when those relationships are destructive and help the patient and family obtain appropriate guidance. Whenever it is possible, support should be given to "healthy," caring relationships that are identified.

## COMMON INTERVENTIONS

Interventions for psychosocial problems should relate to the following outcomes:

1. Patients can maintain or achieve a state of independence consistent with their physical abilities.
2. Patients can define and share with their families or significant others the areas in which they are dependent.
3. Patients can return to their living situations able to resume interdependent roles with their families.
4. Patients will be able to name and utilize resources within their communities to assist them in maintaining their optimum level of function.

These outcomes may be achieved through support, teaching, and counseling.

### Providing Support

The nurse can provide support in the following ways:

1. Recognizing that the patient does have a problem
2. Defining with the patient what the problem is
3. Allowing the patient to do what he or she can do independently
4. Devising methods to help the patient achieve independent function in impaired areas
5. Assisting the patient, to the extent necessary, in areas where independent function cannot be achieved
6. Involving family or significant others in care so they know what the patient can and cannot do and so thus can provide positive encouragement

If individuals are not allowed to perform functions that they are capable of performing, they can quickly become angry and discouraged and lose motivation. Losing the desire to be independent and subjecting oneself to a state of dependence can be the most destructive elements of a musculoskeletal disorder.

### Facilitating Learning

Teaching may take the form of demonstrating the positive advantages of physical interventions. The individual who resists taking medication or using a walking device may be positively influenced to continue therapy once the effectiveness of therapy in relieving pain or eliminating dependence in an area of functioning is demonstrated. Teaching may also include making the patient or family aware of community resources, for example,

Visiting Nurse Association, Meals on Wheels, job retraining programs, community housing programs, or community-responsive transport systems for handicapped persons. For individuals with economic limitations, suggestions for inexpensive modifications in their living environment may influence their ability to continue living in their present circumstances. An example would be teaching the patient how to bathe while sitting on a chair in the bathtub and using a shower hose extension on the faucet. This is much less expensive then purchasing a hydraulic tub lift and is more satisfying than a sponge bath. Such teaching requires that nurses be inventive and innovative and possess a working knowledge of community resources available to help patients to continue to function satisfactorily in settings that they can afford.

### Providing Counseling

Counseling by members of the health team concerning the nature of the patient's disability and areas of independence and dependence may be helpful in assisting patients and their families to define new roles for themselves, that is, roles in which patients can have an active part in their families' lives and concerns. Individuals with severe difficulties in adaptation may benefit from psychiatric counseling or spiritual support. Recognition of the need for counseling and the type of counseling the patient is most likely to respond to are important assessment factors in determining the correct intervention.

## PREVENTION

Whatever the nature of the musculoskeletal disability, certain factors of prevention and teaching must be considered.

### PRIMARY PREVENTION

Many of the diseases that affect the musculoskeletal system have at this time an unknown cause. Rheumatoid arthritis and the systemic connective tissue diseases are but a few examples. Although these diseases are not now preventable, some complications of the diseases are preventable (e.g., contractures, atrophy, skin breakdown). In these instances, prevention depends on teaching the patient to understand the disease process and to use measures that prevent complications.

### SECONDARY PREVENTION

Polio vaccine, screening of school-aged children for scoliosis, community programs for education of women in the prevention of osteoporosis, and screening tests for streptococcal infections with early treatment of the infection to prevent rheumatic fever are examples of preventive measures that can be employed on a community-wide basis to combat illnesses that cause musculoskeletal disability. Early attention to posture; good dietary habits; regular exercise; maintenance of optimal body weight; genetic counseling for individuals with sickle cell anemia and hemophilia; teaching of good body mechanics for individuals whose jobs entail lifting or carrying heavy objects; and concern and attention to the recommendations of the governmental agencies and community action groups to help avoid accidents at home, on the job, and on the road are all examples of preventive measures that may be used to decrease musculoskeletal disability within the general population.

#### Promoting Safety

For those individuals who have limitations of motion or mobility, a variety of precautions and protective or safety devices can be employed in the hospital or the home.

Examples would include the following:

1. Grab bars mounted on a wall near a tub or toilet
2. Safety arms fitted around a toilet
3. Elevated toilet seats
4. Removal of throw rugs and obstacles from areas used by individuals with ambulatory difficulties
5. Adequate, easy to operate locking devices on wheelchairs
6. Handrails on staircases

Although some of these measures may seem to be common knowledge, patients are frequently not aware of them or their need for them. One of the most important functions nurses can perform is to assess the safety requirements of their patients and then teach the patient

**BOX 65-2 Principles to be Observed in Maintaining Correct Posture**

**FOR THE GENERAL PUBLIC**

Standing erect decreases strain on the back, hips, and knees.

Sitting erect decreases strain on the back and hips.

Holding the head erect with the chin in relieves strain from the joints of the upper spine.

Stooping with the knees and hips flexed (Figure 65-14) prevents strain on the back.

Using the strong muscles of the legs instead of the weak muscles of the back when lifting heavy objects prevents injury to the back.

**FOR THE HOSPITALIZED PATIENT**

Using a firm mattress and bed board for the individual for whom prolonged bedrest has been ordered lessens pull on painful joints and helps keep the spine in good alignment.

Lying prone (when possible) relieves supine pressure areas (inferior scapular areas and ischial tuberosities) (Figure 65-15).

Using pillows to support extremities: pillows should not be placed in such fashion or for such periods of time that they promote flexion contractures of joints.

Bracing or supporting extremities or the trunk with pillows, trochanter rolls, and bath blankets: they must be placed with care to avoid compression of nerves or arteries.

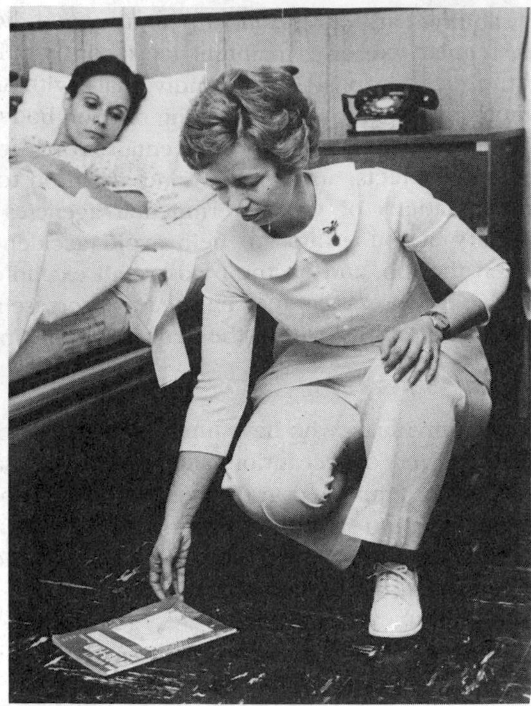

**FIGURE 65-14** Good body mechanics being used to pick up object from floor. Note that nurse's back is straight while her knees and hips are flexed sharply.

or family what steps are necessary to ensure safety. It is helpful if nurses know where in the community needed equipment can be obtained. Often the hospital social worker or physical therapist provides this information and assists the patient or family in obtaining the equipment. By the time of discharge from the hospital, arrangements should be made for the patient to have the equipment and instruction required for safe functioning at home.

### Maintaining Good Posture

Although maintenance of good posture (Box 65-2) is important for all persons, it is especially important for individuals with chronic musculoskeletal disease. Poor posture exerts further strain on already damaged joints and supportive structures, and it not only may cause pain and fatigue, but also may predispose the individual to increased deformity.

# INFLAMMATORY DISORDERS OF THE MUSCULOSKELETAL SYSTEM

The disorders and injuries of the musculoskeletal system are vast in scope. They range from those that cause the patient minor discomfort and inconvenience to those that are life threatening. Among the more troublesome are the inflammatory or rheumatic diseases. These diseases, although they may involve many systems, very often have an arthritic component. There are more than 100 arthritic diseases. One in every seven people in the United States has some form of arthritis. One in every three families in the United States is somehow affected by arthritis.

## RHEUMATOID ARTHRITIS

### Etiology

**Rheumatoid arthritis** is a chronic *systemic* disease. The disease process, although most prominent as a nonsuppurative inflammation in the diarthrodial joints, may also be manifested by lesions of the vasculature, lungs, nervous system, and other major organs of the body. The disease may shorten life expectancy by 3 to 18 years. Although the cause of this disease is unknown, several theories of causation are under investigation. Areas of study include (1) immune mechanisms, such as the interaction of the IgG class of immunoglobins with the rheumatoid factor that appears to play a role in perpetuating rheumatoid inflammation; (2) genetic and metabolic factors; and (3) infection, with particular attention to viruses.

One theory states that the disease probably occurs in a genetically susceptible host as a result of an altered immune response to an unknown antigen. Possible causative antigens being studied include bacteria, mycoplasmas, and viruses, especially the Epstein-Barr virus. After prolonged exposure to this antigen, normal antibodies (immunoglobin [Ig]) become autoantibodies and attack host tissues (self-antigen). These autoantibodies are called rheumatoid factors (RFs). RFs bind with self-antigens in the blood and synovial membrane, forming immune complexes (Figure 65-16).

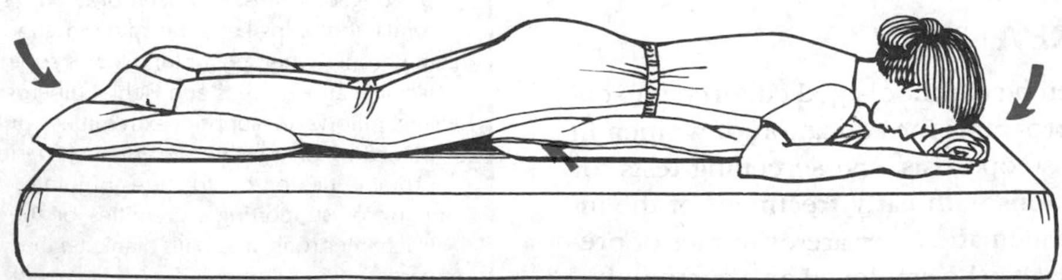

**FIGURE 65-15** Good prone lying posture, with head, abdomen, and lower legs supported on pillows to keep body in good alignment.

## Epidemiology

Rheumatoid arthritis is more prevalent in women than men by a ratio of 2:1 or 3:1. It affects 1% to 3% of the population in the United States, with an estimated 200,000 cases diagnosed annually.[23] Usually it appears during the productive years of life when career and family responsibilities are greatest.

## Pathophysiology

The disease process within the joints (intraarticular) begins as an inflammation of the synovium with edema, vascular congestion, fibrin exudate, and cellular infiltrate. The inflammatory process is set off by some sort of irritation or damage to joint tissue. This is called a "triggering" event. White blood cells rush into the area,

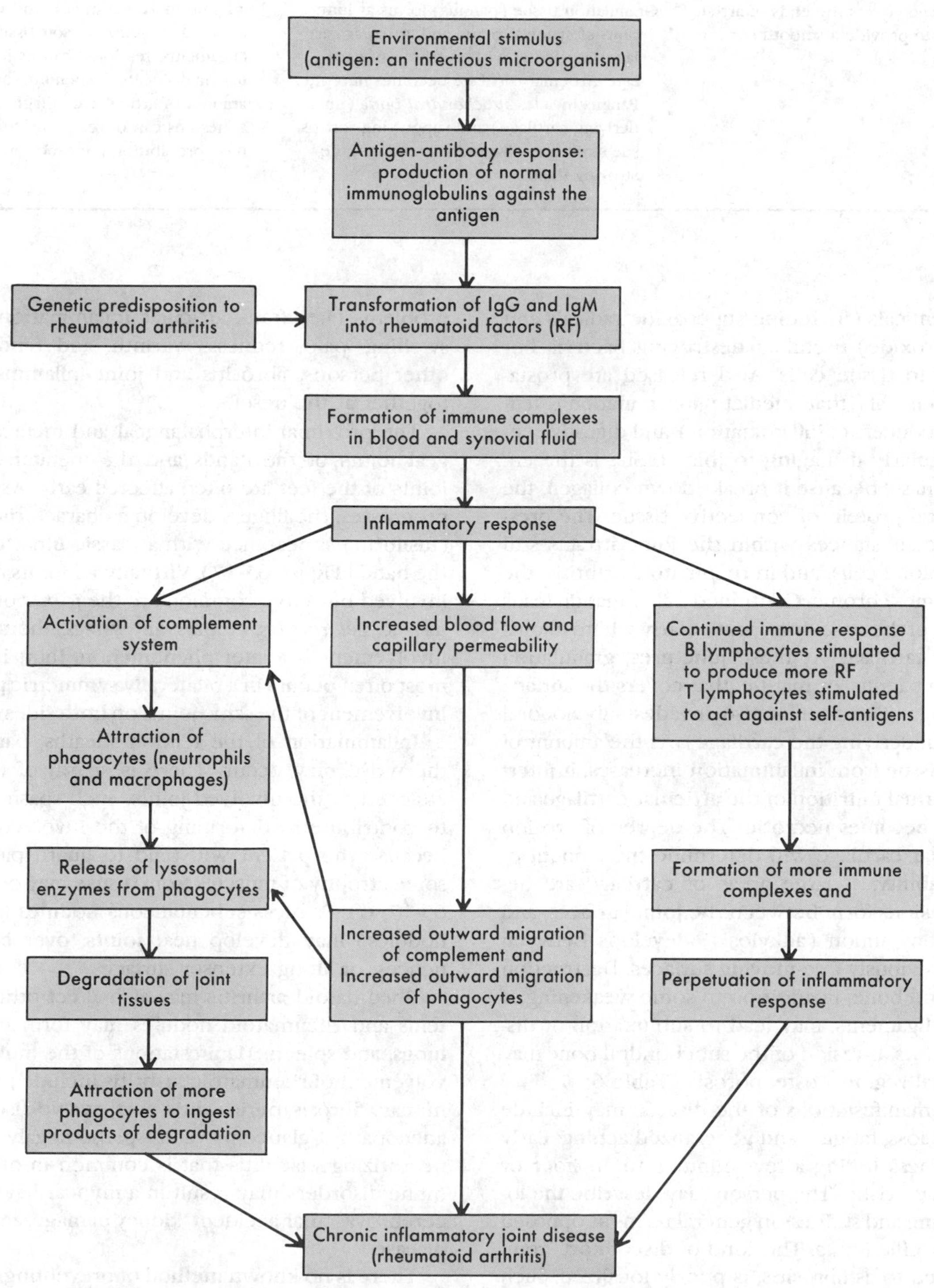


**FIGURE 65-16** Probable pathogenesis of rheumatoid arthritis. (From McCance KL, Heuther SE: *Pathophysiology: the biologic basis for disease in adults and children,* ed 2, St Louis, 1994, Mosby.)

**TABLE 65-7 Normal Function, Primary Pathophysiology, and Clinical Manifestations of Rheumatoid Arthritis**

| NORMAL FUNCTION | PATHOPHYSIOLOGY | MANIFESTATIONS |
|---|---|---|
| Synovial tissue secretes synovial fluid that both lubricates the joint and is the medium through which nutrients are supplied to the articular cartilage. | Inflammation causes edema, vascular congestion, fibrin exudate, and cellular infiltrate to build up around synovium. WBCs move into the synovium, releasing superoxide radicals, $H_2O_2$, prostaglandins, leukotrienes, and collagenase. | Synovium thickens, particularly at articular junctions. Symptoms of inflammation occur within and overlying the joint (pain, swelling, erythema, warmth). Joint mobility is limited by pain. |
| Articular cartilage covers the ends of articulating bones to provide a smooth surface for movement. | Granulation tissue (pannus) forms at junctions of synovial tissue and articular cartilage, interfering with nutrition of cartilage. Articular cartilage becomes necrotic. Pannus invades *subchondral bone* (underlying cartilage) and supporting soft tissue structures (ligaments, tendons), destroying them. | Joint pain increases at rest and with movement. Destruction of soft tissue structures (ligaments, tendons) causes joint to sublux or dislocate. Depending on the amount of articular cartilage destroyed, adhesions can develop and the joints can fuse, prohibiting joint motion. |

releasing chemicals (including superoxide radicals and hydrogen peroxide) useful in destroying bacteria but also harmful to tissue cells. Also released are prostaglandins (chemicals that mediate inflammation), leukotrienes (producers of inflammation), and digestive enzymes. Particularly damaging to joint tissue is the enzyme collagenase, because it breaks down collagen, the main structural protein of connective tissue. The presence of these substances within the joint attracts still more white blood cells, and in rheumatoid arthritis, the process becomes chronic. Continued inflammation leads to thickening of the synovium, particularly where it joins the articular cartilage. At these junctures, granulation tissue forms a pannus, or mantle, that covers the surface of the cartilage. The pannus also invades subchondral bone (bone underlying the cartilage). As the amount of granulation tissue from inflammation increases, it interferes with normal nutrition of the articular cartilage and the cartilage becomes necrotic. The degree of erosion of the articular cartilage will determine the amount of articular disability. If large areas of cartilage are destroyed, adhesions form between the joint surfaces, and fibrous or bony union (ankylosis) develops between what were previously free-moving surfaces. Destruction of cartilage and bone, in addition to some weakening of tendons and ligaments, may lead to subluxation or dislocation of joints. Invasion of the subchondral bone may cause eventual regional osteoporosis (Table 65-7).

The early manifestations of the disease may include fever, weight loss, fatigue, and generalized aching. Early morning stiffness lasting a few minutes to an hour or more is characteristic. The person may describe the location of aching and stiffness in general terms as opposed to naming specific joints. This kind of discomfort, commonly referred to as fibrositis, is poorly localized. Such discomfort may be the patient's earliest complaint. These symptoms may be present for some period of time before they are replaced by more specific, or localized, problems (i.e., frank articular inflammation with joint swelling, pain, redness, warmth, and tenderness). In other persons, fibrositis and joint inflammation occur together at the onset.

The proximal interphalangeal and metacarpophalangeal joints of the hands and the metatarsophalangeal joints of the feet are often affected early. As the disease progresses, the fingers develop a characteristic tapering (fusiform) appearance with a classic ulnar deviation of the hand (Figure 65-17). Virtually all joints can become involved but most common are the *joints* of the ***hands, wrists, feet, ankles, elbows,*** and ***knees.*** Shoulder and hip involvement is a later phenomenon. Joint involvement most often occurs in a bilaterally symmetric pattern with involvement of the same joints on both sides of the body.

Inflammation of the tendon sheaths, particularly in the wrist, may occur. There is spasm of the muscles attached to the involved joints. Such spasm is believed to contribute to deforming of the involved joints, and because the patient will tend to guard painful joints, some atrophy of muscles from disuse may occur (Figure 65-17, *C*). Painless subcutaneous nodules (rheumatoid nodules) may develop near joints, over bony prominences, or along extensor surfaces.

Rheumatoid arthritis may also affect other body systems and rheumatoid nodules may form in the heart, lungs, and spleen. Manifestations of the multisystem involvement of rheumatoid arthritis include pleuritis, pulmonary fibrosis, pericarditis, aortic valve disease, lymphadenopathy, glaucoma, and splenomegaly. The acute necrotizing vasculitis that is common in other autoimmune disorders may result in a myocardial infarction, a cerebrovascular accident, kidney damage, and Raynaud's disease.

There is no known method of preventing rheumatoid arthritis. The course and severity of the disease are unpredictable. It is marked by periods of exacerbation and remission. Some individuals have been known to recover

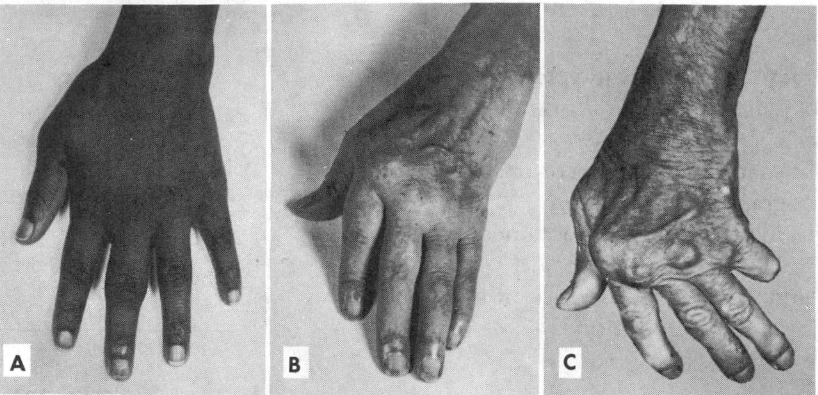


**FIGURE 65-17** Rheumatoid arthritis of hand. **A,** Early stage. Note fusiform swelling of proximal interphalangeal joints, especially that of middle finger. **B,** Moderate involvement. Note swelling form chronic synovitis of metacarpophalangeal joints and early ulnar drift. **C,** Advanced stage. Note marked ulnar drift and subluxation of metacarpophalangeal joints with extension of proximal interphalangeal joints and flexion of distal joints. Note also deformed position of thumb. Hand has wasted appearance. (From Raney R, Brashear H: *Shand's handbook of orthopaedic surgery,* ed 8, St Louis, 1971, Mosby.)

from a first attack and never suffer a recurrence. For others, particularly those in whom the rheumatoid factor is found (seropositive rheumatoid disease), the disease tends to be chronically progressive. In a small number of individuals the disease may be rapidly progressive, marked by unremitting joint destruction and diffuse vasculitis. This form of the disease is referred to as *malignant rheumatoid disease.* The length of time between exacerbations varies greatly with individuals. Some evidence suggests that exacerbations can be triggered by mental stress such as worry or grief, by overexertion, and at times by physical trauma such as surgery. The likelihood that the patient will enter a complete remission after 3 years of sustained disease activity is very slight.

If it is not treated, rheumatoid arthritis has a tendency to relapse and to recur in a more severe form. Continued competent medical care is of the utmost importance for anyone who has rheumatoid arthritis. Some individuals, when having a remission of their symptoms, believe they are cured and discontinue their therapy, only to have a later and more severe exacerbation of the disease. Even with careful management, approximately 10% of patients with rheumatoid arthritis progress to a crippling state of complete incapacity.[30]

## Medical Management

The expected length of stay of patients with rheumatoid arthritis as determined by DRG is 7 days. A discussion of common medical therapy for management of rheumatoid arthritis follows.

### Diagnostic tests

Diagnosis is made by evaluating the results of history and physical examination, radiographic studies, and laboratory analysis. ***History taking is especially important when evaluating a patient with joint pain.*** More than 100 conditions may be responsible for producing joint symptoms, many with multisystem involvement. The American Rheumatism Association has devised a system for the diagnosis of rheumatoid arthritis (Box 65-3).

Diagnostic test results usually include the following:

1. An elevated erythrocyte sedimentation rate

**BOX 65-3 Diagnostic Criteria for Rheumatoid Arthritis**

1. Morning stiffness
2. Motion pain or tenderness in at least one joint
3. Swelling (soft tissue or fluid) of at least one joint
4. Swelling of at least one other joint
5. Symmetric joint swelling (same joint on each side of the body, excluding the terminal phalangeal joint)
6. Subcutaneous nodules
7. X-ray changes (must include decalcified areas of at least one bone near joint margins, usually hands or wrist)
8. Positive rheumatoid factor (RF)
9. Poor mucin precipitate in synovial fluid
10. Characteristic histologic changes of synovium (chronic inflammatory infiltrate)
11. Characteristic histologic changes of nodules (granulomatous foci)

*Classic rheumatoid arthritis:* seven or more criteria observed
*Definite rheumatoid arthritis:* five criteria with joint signs or symptoms continuous for at least 6 weeks
*Probable rheumatoid arthritis:* three criteria with joint signs or symptoms continuous for at least 6 weeks
*Possible rheumatoid arthritis:* two criteria with joint signs or symptoms continuous for at least 6 weeks

Modified from McDuffie FC. In Cohen AS, editor: *Laboratory diagnostic procedures in the rheumatic diseases,* Orlando, Fla, 1985, Grune & Stratton.

2. Mild leukocytosis
3. Anemia
4. Positive rheumatoid factor or latex fixation test (present in 50% to 90% of patients, depending on disease duration and severity)
5. Narrowing of the joint spaces and erosion of articular surfaces on roentgenographic examination
6. Inflammatory changes in synovial tissue obtained by biopsy
7. Increased turbidity and decreased viscosity of synovial fluid obtained by needle aspiration

### Medication

Inflammation is controlled with the use of salicylates. Medications are progressively added based on the patient's response to basic therapy and with regard to the toxicity of the medications. Adjunctive therapy may include the use of intraarticular steroids, therapy with analgesic agents that do not have antiinflammatory effects (e.g., acetaminophen [Tylenol], propoxyphene [Darvon]), surgery, and/or antidepressant drugs. Specific drugs are listed in Table 65-5.

### Treatment

Treatment consists of hot and cold packs to affected joints.

### Diet

A nutritionally adequate diet is recommended. The patient is advised to maintain ideal body weight and to avoid weight gain, which will increase stress on the weight-bearing joints.

### Activity

The patient is advised to take frequent rest periods, avoid fatigue, and rest the affected joints.

### Referral/Consultation

In some settings the nurse assumes responsibility for making referrals to other services. Common referrals for persons with rheumatoid arthritis include physical therapy and occupational therapy. The goal of physical therapy is to maintain joint mobility and prevent deformity. Occupational therapy may be used to fit the patient for splints or to provide assistive devices for ADL. Supportive devices may be necessary for ambulation. A social service consult may be initiated to assist the patient with discharge needs.

Medical management is generally described as a pyramid of therapy. The pyramid is usually represented as having its foundation in a good history and physical examination, prescription of rest and appropriate exercise, education of patient and family, and control of inflammation with the use of various medications.

Goals of therapy include the following:

1. Relief of pain
2. Maintenance of joint function
3. Prevention and correction of deformity by application of orthopaedic principles
4. Correction of other health factors

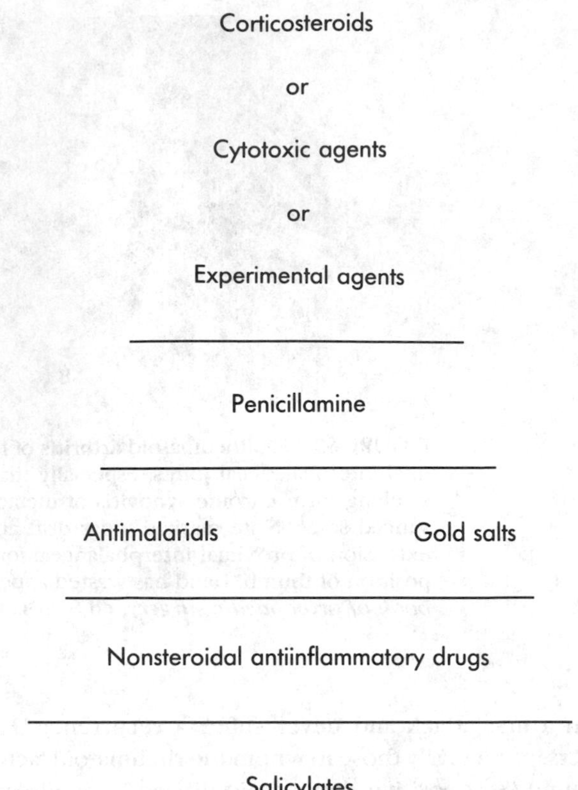


**FIGURE 65-18** Pyramid of therapy used to treat rheumatoid arthritis.

The pyramid of therapy is illustrated in Figure 65-18.

Critical pathways (also referred to as *collaborative care paths* or *care maps*) have been developed in some inpatient and outpatient settings to guide both medical and nursing management. These critical pathways are collaboratively developed along time lines and include the information described above for specific hours, days, or visits. Pertinent information about discharge planning and patient teaching to be implemented at specified times also is included. Because the nurse has a major role in these two aspects of care, they are discussed under Nursing Management.

## NURSING MANAGEMENT

### ♦ ASSESSMENT

#### Subjective Data

Early in the disease, the patient may complain of chronic tiredness, aching and stiffness in the arms or legs, and weight loss. As the disease progresses, the patient will be able to identify particular joints that are painful; will complain of loss of strength and ability to move joints freely, early morning stiffness lasting up to 2 hours, and fatigue (see Research boxes, on right and on p. 2251); and will express concern that pain interferes with normal ADL. The patient will also note that affected joints are changing in appearance. Many patients will express fear or despair over what is happening to them. (For a comprehensive assessment, see Chapter 63.)

#### Objective Data

Specific objective data to be gathered by the nurse include the following:

1. Inspection and palpation of the same joints on both sides of the body for symmetry, skin color, size, shape, tenderness, heat, and swelling
2. Limitation of active joint range of motion
3. Evidence of pain with active range of motion
4. Evidence of atrophy or loss of tone or tenderness in muscles associated with involved joints

The results from diagnostic tests commonly performed on persons with rheumatoid arthritis are discussed under Medical Management.

### ♦ NURSING DIAGNOSES

Nursing diagnoses are determined from analysis of patient data. Possible nursing diagnoses for the person with rheumatoid arthritis may include but are not limited to the following:

| Diagnostic Title | Possible Etiologic Factors |
|---|---|
| Knowledge deficit (related to arthritis) | Lack of exposure to information |
| Pain | Inflammation and swelling in joints |
| Self-care deficit (related to bathing/hygene, dressing/grooming, feeding, toileting) | Pain and musculoskeletal impairment |
| Fatigue | Chronic systemic disease |
| Self-esteem disturbance | Change in body appearance |
| Injury, high risk for | Loss of muscle strength and joint motion |
| Sleep disturbance | Chronic systemic disease, pain |

### ♦ EXPECTED PATIENT OUTCOMES

Expected patient outcomes for the person with rheumatoid arthritis may include but are not limited to the following:

1. The patient can explain the disease process, the applicability of treatment measures, and plans for follow-up with the physician.

## RESEARCH

Crosby LJ: Factors which contribute to fatigue associated with rheumatoid arthritis, *J Adv Nurs* 16(8):974-981, 1991.

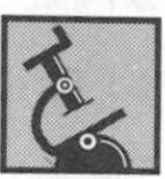

Fatigue has been identified as a clinical feature of rheumatoid arthritis and defined as "a feeling of overall unpleasantness." Chronic fatigue must be differentiated from acute fatigue, which is episodic and usually situational. Chronic fatigue is persistent, not alleviated by rest, and generally associated with illness. The purpose of the study was twofold: first, "to identify the factors which people with rheumatoid arthritis believed contributed to their fatigue" and, second, "to examine the relationships among identified factors and the sensation of fatigue." One hundred persons with rheumatoid arthritis were asked to identify factors that contributed to their fatigue. *Rheumatoid arthritis disease activity, disturbed sleep,* and *increased physical effort* were the three most commonly identified factors. These factors were operationalized using the following methods: rheumatoid arthritis disease activity was measured as joint pain using the Modified McGill Pain Inventory, fragmented sleep was recorded by overnight electroencephalographic sleep studies, and decreased physical ability was measured by walking time and grip strength.

For the second part of the study 15 of the original 100 subjects and 12 age- and gender-matched control subjects were used. Subject ages ranged from 29 to 63 years, with a mean of 44 years of age. Of the 15 subjects with rheumatoid arthritis, 5 were experiencing a disease flare at the time of the study, whereas the remaining 10 were either in remission or experiencing mildly active disease. The rheumatoid arthritis subjects with a disease flare had significantly more joint pain, more fragmented sleep, and reduced physical abilities when compared to the nonflare and control subjects. Fatigue levels were measured using a 10 cm vertical visual analog scale ranging from 0% (no fatigue) to 100% (extreme fatigue). Fatigue levels of the flare subjects positively correlated with the measured variables, whereas the fatigue levels of the nonflare and control subjects exhibited a negative correlation. The findings of the nonflare and control groups were very similar. Disease activity, measured as joint pain, emerged as a salient characteristic of fatigue. Sixty-four percent of the subjects identified disease activity as the primary cause of their fatigue. Although the physiologic basis of the fatigue associated with rheumatoid arthritis remains unknown, it is both a presenting and a persistent symptom of the disease. The results of this study indicate that assessing the impact of fatigue on the individual is an important consideration when caring for a person with rheumatoid arthritis. Nurses and other health care providers need to identify pain-relieving measures that improve the quality of sleep and increase physical abilities by reducing fatigue. Pain-relieving measures include the use of medications, rest, and splinting of affected joints, which alone or in combination ultimately reduce fatigue levels in persons with rheumatoid arthritis.

2. The patient states pain is decreased and verbalizes ways to control pain.
3. The patient demonstrates improved ability to perform self-care activities and participates in usual activities to fullest extent possible.
4. The patient can state factors that lead to fatigue and how fatigue might be avoided.
5. The patient verbalizes a more positive self-concept.
6. The patient maintains active joint range of motion within limits of disease to strengthen muscles and prevent injuries.

## ♦ INTERVENTIONS

### Facilitating Learning

As for any chronic illness, patient teaching is perhaps the most important aspect of nursing care of patients with rheumatoid arthritis. It is, after all, the patient who will have to recognize response to prescribed therapy, who will have to follow the prescribed therapy correctly, and who will have to report the effectiveness of therapy to the physician. It is estimated that hundreds of millions of dollars are spent each year on gadgets, programs, and "medicines" allegedly able to "cure" arthritis. This money is spent by persons with arthritis who often can ill afford the expense. It should be recognized that in some instances, the disease and disability associated with it may increase in spite of all legitimate efforts to control them; this is extremely discouraging for the patient, family, and members of the health team. But many more persons are able to live reasonably normal, productive lives while managing their arthritis. Their ability to do so partially depends on their knowledge of the disease and its treatment.

Nurses teaching persons about rheumatoid arthritis (and other rheumatic diseases) may find it helpful to use some of the patient teaching material prepared by the Arthritis Foundation. Booklets such as *Arthritis: The Basic Facts* are written in such a way that most patients can understand and learn from them.

Patient teaching should include information about the following:

1. Proper balance of rest and activity
2. Joint protection and energy conservation techniques
3. Proper use of medications (i.e., names of drugs, dosages, precautions in administration, and side effects or toxic effects)
4. Plans for implementation of the exercise program prescribed by the physician or physical therapist
5. Proper application of heat and/or cold packs
6. Proper use of walking aids and other assistive devices
7. Safety measures to prevent injury
8. Application of, appropriate use of, and care of splints and braces
9. Basics of good nutrition and the importance of avoiding weight gain
10. Importance of regular follow-up with the physician
11. Risks of following programs that promise a "cure"
12. Information about local arthritis support groups and programs and services of the Arthritis Foundation

### Promoting Comfort

1. Evaluate the type, amount, and duration of pain.
2. Assess intensity of pain using pain rating scale.
3. Administer medications as ordered.
4. Teach relaxation techniques and alternate methods of pain control.
5. Evaluate effectiveness of pain relief measures.
6. Observe patient for nonverbal signs of pain.
7. Provide heat or cold treatments as appropriate.
8. Promote frequent changes of position (patients are often more comfortable changing position themselves rather than having someone handle their sore joints).
9. Provide for adequate periods of rest.
10. Encourage use of resting splints.

### Promoting Independence

1. Assess patient's level of functioning and ability to perform self-care activities.
2. Assist with ADL as needed.
3. Provide frequent rest periods to maximize patient participation.
4. Encourage use of supportive and/or assistive devices.

### Reducing Fatigue

1. Encourage patient to discuss factors that cause fatigue (see Research boxes, pp. 2249 and 2251).
2. Assess times of greatest fatigue, and structure activities accordingly.
3. Provide for frequent rest periods.
4. Promote comfort by use of medications and other comfort measures.
5. Instruct patient regarding energy conservation techniques. (See Table 65-2.)
6. Assist patient in modifying daily routines to accommodate decreased abilities.

### Promoting A Positive Self-Concept

1. Establish a trusting relationship with patient.
2. Encourage verbalization of feelings regarding appearance and disease process.
3. Encourage verbalization of positive attributes of self.
4. Support positive coping mechanisms and decision-making abilities.
5. Institute referral to community resources if needed.

## RESEARCH

Belza BL et al: Correlates of fatigue in older adults with rheumatoid arthritis, *Nurs Res* 42(92):93-99, 1993.

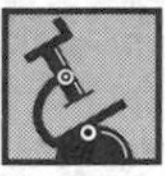

The purposes of this study were (1) to describe the prevalence of fatigue in older adults with rheumatoid arthritis, (2) to examine the relationship between fatigue and office visits, and (3) to identify correlates of fatigue in individuals with rheumatoid arthritis.

A review of the literature found pain to be one of the best indices of general health. Pain may also contribute to fatigue. Persons with rheumatoid arthritis usually have decreased activity levels because of pain and fatigue. Sleep patterns in persons with rheumatoid arthritis are often disturbed by pain, depression, and medications. Several psychosocial factors may be related to fatigue, including depression, learned helplessness, and social support. Persons with rheumatoid arthritis consistently exhibit increased levels of depression that may be accompanied by fatigue and decreased energy. Learned helplessness is a behavior that may be utilized in response to unpredictable and uncontrollable events (e.g., the uncertain and unpredictable course of rheumatoid arthritis) and is associated with behavioral changes (e.g., depression) and decreased ability to problem solve. Social support, defined as "the availability of people upon whom the individual can rely and who value him or her as a person" plays an important role in an individual's ability to manage and cope with a chronic illness.

The sample included 133 adults aged 56 to 86 years, with a mean age of 67 years and an average length of disease of 18 years. Of the sample 75% were female, 84% were White, and over 50% had at least a high school education. Of the respondents 62% were taking prednisone and 75% were taking either NSAIDs or other antirheumatic drugs. Subjects also reported the presence of an average of one other health problem in the last year, the most common being hypertension, lung disease, gastric ulcers, and genitourinary problems.

### INSTRUMENTS

Function, disability, and pain were measured by the Health Assessment Questionnaire. Pain intensity was measured on a scale of 0 (no pain) to 100 (severe pain). The Multidimensional Assessment of Fatigue Scale was used to evaluate fatigue, its severity, distress, timing, and interference with ADL. Subjects also received a physical activity and exercise index, sleep survey, Geriatric Depression Scale, and Social Support Scale. The Arthritis Helplessness Index measured subjects' perceived ability to control their rheumatoid arthritis. Demographic data were obtained through a telephone interview.

### RESULTS

The majority (86% to 94%) of the sample reported frequent waking at night, feeling tired during the day, and unsatisfactory sleep. Fatigue was a daily occurrence for 40% of the subjects. Fatigue frequently remained constant throughout the week and affected the ability to walk, complete housework, and shop. Only 7% reported no fatigue. Of the subjects 73% attributed their fatigue to their rheumatoid arthritis. Additional factors affecting fatigue included "doing too much," pain, stress, decreased physical activity, and poor sleep.

The results of this study indicate that the older adults in this sample with a long history of rheumatoid arthritis experience a high level of fatigue that occurs daily, remains constant throughout the week, causes moderate distress, and affects both ADL and leisure activities. Those who experience more fatigue made more visits to the rheumatologist than those who experienced less fatigue.

The sample was predominantly female, and global fatigue has been significantly related to gender. Previous findings indicate women have 1.5 times more risk of fatigue than men. Sleep disturbances and decreased activity also contribute to significant levels of fatigue. In this sample the variables of depression, age, and education did not significantly contribute to fatigue, which is in contrast to previous research.

Findings indicate that interventions to effectively manage pain, improve the quantity and quality of sleep, effectively balance rest and activity, and increase functional ability may be effective in reducing fatigue levels in adults with similar characteristics to those in this sample.

### Promoting Mobility and Preventing Injury

1. Assess all joints for signs of inflammation and deformity.
2. Assess and record range of motion of all joints.
3. Encourage active range of motion exercises.
4. Provide passive range of motion if needed.
5. Encourage use of splints to rest joint and provide proper alignment.
6. Avoid positions that may produce contractures—for example, pillows under knees when supine; pillows forcing neck into forward flexion.
7. Encourage patient to perform prescribed exercises on a regular basis.
8. Provide appropriate ambulatory devices and supervise patient in their use.
9. Encourage patient to wear shoes, not slippers, for ambulation.

## ♦ EVALUATION

To evaluate effectiveness of nursing interventions, compare the patient's behaviors with those stated in the expected patient outcomes. Successful achievement of patient outcomes for the patient with rheumatoid arthritis is indicated by the following:

1. The patient's explantion of the relationship of his or her signs and symptoms and the disease process in rheumatoid arthritis

# NURSING CARE PLAN

## PERSON WITH TOTAL KNEE REPLACEMENT

**DATA:** Mr. K. is a 59-year-old married office manager with osteoarthritis of the right knee. Over the past 8 months, he has had increased pain in his knee with only minimal relief from nonsteroidal antiinflammatory medications prescribed by his internist. He reports that he must now ambulate with a cane when his pain is severe. He can no longer participate in many activities he used to enjoy because of his discomfort and limited mobility. After consulting his internist and an orthopaedic surgeon, he has decided to undergo elective total knee replacement. Mr. K. is admitted to the nursing division on the morning of the day he is scheduled for surgery. Collaborative nursing actions include those to identify possible complications of the surgery.

The nursing history identified the following:

- Mr. and Mrs. K. reside in a two-story colonial house with the bedroom upstairs.
- Mr. K. plans to return home after this hospitalization and has received a 6 weeks' leave of absence from his job.
- He is not prescribed any medications other than his "arthritis pills" and has no other preexisting medical problems
- Mr. K. was last hospitalized 18 years ago for a cholecystectomy.
- He attended a total knee replacement class 2 weeks ago as part of his preadmission screening.

Immediate reporting of and treatment of early signs and symptoms may prevent serious complications. Nursing actions to prevent complications include monitoring for the following:

- Neurocirculatory compromise: Perform neurocirculatory checks every 2 hours for the first 24 to 48 hours; notify physician of any changes from preoperative status.
- Impaired skin integrity and/or wound healing: Monitor pressure areas for signs of redness, monitor temperature, assess incision for signs or symptoms of infection or excessive drainage.
- Atelectasis/respiratory infection: Monitor breath sounds until ambulatory, encourage deep breathing and coughing until ambulatory.
- Problems with elimination: Assess for urinary stasis and constipation.
- Fluid and electrolyte imbalance: Monitor intake and output until patient is taking oral fluids comfortably, monitor IV fluid flow, assess patient for fluid volume excess or deficit.

### ■ NURSING DIAGNOSIS

Knowledge deficit related to lack of exposure to total knee replacement surgery

| Expected Patient Outcomes | Nursing Interventions | Rationale |
|---|---|---|
| States he understands the teaching provided.<br>Will have less anxiety related to fear of the unknown and/or misconceptions regarding the surgery and recovery period. | Preoperatively:<br>1. Assess need for further instruction and provide as necessary.<br>2. Review preoperative instruction with patient and family before surgery. Use written materials if they are available.<br>3. Evaluate patient's understanding of the information taught.<br>Postoperatively:<br>1. Ensure that patient can explain or demonstrate the following:<br>a. Independent transfer and ambulation with appropriate ambulatory aid.<br>b. Exercises to be performed at home (straight leg raising and active flexion) and with what frequency.<br>c. Activity restrictions, including avoidance of kneeling and jarring activities, that are to be observed for 2 mo or until follow-up with the surgeon.<br>2. Evaluate patient's understanding of the need for antibiotic prophylaxis in the future, and reinforce as necessary. | Understanding the surgical procedure and postoperative recovery should lessen anxiety and promote behaviors that will enhance recovery from surgery. |

## NURSING CARE PLAN

### PERSON WITH TOTAL KNEE REPLACEMENT—cont'd

#### ■ NURSING DIAGNOSIS

Pain related to knee replacement surgery

| Expected Patient Outcomes | Nursing Interventions | Rationale |
| --- | --- | --- |
| States is feeling comfortable. | Assess patient's pain and evaluate response to comfort measures provided. | Subjective and objective data are important to ascertain the nature of the patient's postoperative pain and how to manage it. |
| Is able to perform necessary postoperative routines/exercises because pain is adequately managed. | Administer prescribed narcotic analgesics at timely intervals throughout postoperative course, particularly before exercise periods.<br>Patient may be taking patient-controlled analgesia (PCA). | It is usually necessary to administer narcotic analgesics the first 48-72 hr after surgery. Analgesics have a greater effect if they are administered before pain becomes severe. |
| | Teach relaxation techniques as appropriate. | Relaxation facilitates rest and may modify the patient's response to pain. |
| | Use other pain-relieving measures as pertinent (e.g., back rubs, repositioning, ice to knee for 30 min before and after active flexion exercises). | A change in type of cutaneous stimulation may result in pain relief. Ice is analgesic and retards swelling. |
| | As pain decreases, use milder analgesics. | Pain, as it lessens in severity, can be controlled by less potent analgesics that have fewer side effects. |

#### ■ NURSING DIAGNOSIS

Impaired physical mobility related to alterations in lower limb following total knee replacement surgery

| Expected Patient Outcome | Nursing Interventions | Rationale |
| --- | --- | --- |
| Will demonstrate optimal level of mobility with adaptive devices by time of discharge from hospital. | Turn patient side to back to side every 2 hr and as necessary while bed rest is ordered. | Turning and repositioning frequently provide for better ventilation of the lungs. |
| | Encourage patient to perform active dorsiplantar flexion, isometric quadriceps setting exercises, and, after drain is removed, straight leg raises every 2 hr until fully ambulatory, then 4 times/day. | Exercises of the lower extremities will prevent venous stasis and promote muscle strengthening. |
| | Elevate operative leg on pillows in bed and when patient is up in chair for the first 24-48 hr. Place pillows so that passive flexion of the knee is avoided. | Elevation of the operative leg on pillows enhances venous return. Flexion contracture is to be avoided. |
| | Assist patient to transfer out of bed on first postoperative day. Light weight bearing on the operated leg is generally permitted using an assistive device. | The exercise of getting in and out of bed is one means of increasing activity in the early postoperative period. The patient accrues numerous physiologic benefits from such activity. |
| | Assist patient to walk as tolerated, increasing the frequency and the distance walked each day. | Early ambulation is a significant factor in hastening recovery and preventing postoperative complications. |

*Continued.*

## NURSING CARE PLAN

### PERSON WITH TOTAL KNEE REPLACEMENT—cont'd

| Expected Patient Outcome | Nursing Interventions | Rationale |
|---|---|---|
| | Encourage patient to sit up in a chair as tolerated, especially for meals. | |
| | If continuous passive motion machine is used, patient's leg should be in the machine a minimum of 8-12 hr/day and can be in the machine up to 22 hr/day if tolerated. Advance the degrees of flexion being obtained in the machine according to the surgeon's prescription. | Passive flexion of the knee may prevent excessive swelling and bruising at the site of the surgery, and it may promote more even healing of the involved joint tissues. |
| | Begin active flexion exercise of the knee on the second postoperative day, and encourage flexion 4 times/day. | Active flexion of the knee is necessary to promote return of function. It is desired that the patient achieve approximately 90 degrees of active flexion before discharge from the hospital. |
| | A knee immobilizer may be worn at night as a night resting splint. | The knee immobilizer splints the resting knee, helping to prevent painful muscle spasm. |

#### ■ NURSING DIAGNOSIS

Impaired home maintenance management related to discharge needs

| Expected Patient Outcome | Nursing Interventions | Rationale |
|---|---|---|
| Patient and family will express satisfaction with arrangements made to manage self-care at home. | Discuss with patient and family any problems they anticipate with management of self-care at home. | Adequate discharge planning will foster safe, successful completion of rehabilitation at home. |
| | Determine the type of equipment needed, for example, crutches, walker, elevated toilet seat; consult appropriate department or agency for assistance in procuring these supplies. | |
| | Assure that the patient can climb stairs. If not, help the patient to arrange for first floor sleeping arrangements. | |

2. The patient's description of:
   a. Plans for balancing rest periods and exercises
   b. How to use 7-day pill dispenser to ensure that NSAIDs are taken with meals as prescribed
   c. How to use cold packs after exercising
3. Patient's description of pain and indicating on pain scale that pain is reduced
4. Patient performing own ADL independently
5. Patient listing factors that cause fatigue such as standing for long periods or skipping rest periods when involved in other activities
6. Plans for preventing fatigue: sitting in a firm chair with arms to do as many tasks as possible
7. Demonstrating a positive self-concept by dressing in attractive clothing and paying attention to personal hygiene
8. Demonstrating active range of motion exercises to preserve function and strengthening exercises such as straight leg lifts and quadriceps sets

■ ■ ■

### Surgical Management

When rheumatoid arthritis is relentless in its progression or has caused severe joint destruction, patients may achieve relief of pain and improve functions through selected surgical intervention.

Common surgical procedures performed for the person with rheumatoid arthritis are described in Table 65-8. Nursing management of the patient who has under-

**TABLE 65-8 Surgical Procedures and Postoperative Care for the Patient with Rheumatoid Arthritis**

| PURPOSE | POSTOPERATIVE CARE |
|---|---|
| **SYNOVECTOMY** | |
| Commonly performed on the wrist or knee to arrest the course of rheumatoid arthritis in that joint, to maintain joint function, and to prevent episodic inflammation (Synovium does grow back, so the disease process may recur; however, relief from discomfort will persist for a prolonged period.) | Joint is maintained at rest for 3-5 days or is passively exercised in CPM machine to ensure even healing of tissue.<br>Active motion of joint is permitted 3-5 days after surgery.<br>For the knee:<br>Patient is instructed to perform quadriceps setting exercises in repetitions of 10 every 1-2 hr from the time of surgery.<br>Patient is assisted to perform straight leg raising exercises four times per day until able to perform them independently.<br>Patient begins partial weight-bearing ambulation with appropriate assistive devices when able to demonstrate independent straight leg raising and active flexion to at least 45 degrees. |
| **ARTHROTOMY** | |
| Performed to explore or drain a joint or remove damaged tissue or foreign bodies (most often performed on the knee) | Care is essentially the same as for synovectomy, but motion and weight-bearing restrictions may not be observed for as long. *(CPM machine is not likely to be used.)* |
| **ARTHRODESIS** | |
| Surgical fusion of joint performed to eliminate painful motion and provide stability; commonly performed on knee, wrist, and ankle | Joint is immobilized in cast and/or with external fixation device until healing (fusion) is accomplished.<br>If joint is the knee, quadriceps setting and straight leg raising are taught as for synovectomy; partial weight bearing may be permitted after 10-14 days. If joint is the ankle, weight bearing will not be permitted for 1-3 mo. |
| **ARTHROPLASTY** | |
| Resurfacing of one or both sides of diseased joint to eliminate pain and improve motion | Refer to pp. 2268 and 2271 for special postoperative care. |

gone a total knee arthroplasty is discussed on p. 2268. Total joint arthroplasty is most commonly performed on the hip and knee but can also be used on the shoulder, elbow, ankle, and wrist. Diseased joints of the fingers and toes may be replaced with Silastic implants.

## SYSTEMIC LUPUS ERYTHEMATOSUS

### Etiology

Systemic lupus erythematosus (SLE) is a chronic inflammatory disease of autoimmune origin that affects primarily the skin, joints, and kidneys, although it may affect virtually every organ of the body. The disease was named after the characteristic rash, the erosive nature of the rash being "likened to the damage wrought by a hungry wolf."[26]

Three major areas are currently being researched as possible causes of SLE:

1. *Genetic factors* may contribute to the development of the disease. Family members of persons with SLE have an increased chance of developing the disease.
2. *Environmental factors* have been associated with cases of SLE. For example, exposure to ultraviolet light is known to cause exacerbations. Some drugs, notably procainamide (Pronestyl), isonicotinic acid hydrazide (INH, Isoniazid), and penicillin are known to induce lupus-like syndromes.[22] Other areas being considered include a viral origin and disturbances in estrogen metabolism.
3. *Alterations in the immune response* that cause immune complexes containing antibodies to be deposited in tissue, causing tissue damage.

### Epidemiology

SLE affects women, particularly adolescents and young adults, 8 to 10 times more often than men. It is estimated that the occurrence of SLE is 2.9 to 400 per 100,000 people.[6] The frequency for African-American women is 1 in 245. During the reproductive years the incidence of SLE is 10 times greater in females than males. Menses and pregnancy can cause an exacerbation of the disease. Although SLE was once thought to be relatively rare, better techniques for its recognition have demonstrated it to be fairly common. Although there is no cure, its course can usually be controlled by corticosteroids. Some patients may die as a result of lesions affecting major organs or from secondary infections.

### Pathophysiology

The exact mechanism of pathogenesis is unknown. However, several alterations in the immune system are associated with SLE. Numerous cellular antibodies have been identified in persons with the disorder. *The pres-*

## CRITICAL PATHWAY Total Knee Replacement

DRG #: 209 Expected LOS: 7

| | Day of Surgery Day of Admission Day 1 | Day 2 | Day 3 |
|---|---|---|---|
| **Diagnostic Tests** | Preoperative: CBC, UA, SMA/18,* PT/PTT, ECG, chest x-ray, type and screen autologous blood, knee x-rays<br>Postoperative: CBC | CBC, SMA/6,† PT/PTT q d until discharge, if coumadin prescribed | CBC<br>SMA/7 |
| **Medications** | Preoperative: IV antibiotic<br>Postoperative: IVs; give autologous blood if necessary; IV antibiotic, IV analgesic | IV to saline lock; IV antibiotic; IV analgesic; stool softener; Rx for sleep; prophylactic anticoagulant | IV saline lock; IV antibiotic; PO analgesic; stool softener; Rx for sleep; anticoagulant |
| **Treatments** | Postoperative: vital signs; check dressing and neurocirculatory checks q hr × 4, then q2hr × 4, then q4hr; skin assessment and special care q2hr; empty and record drain output q8hr; I & O q8hr; elastic leg stocking (ELS) to unaffected leg; incentive spirometry q2hr; intermittent compression device (ICD) on both legs | Vital signs; check dressing and neurocirculatory checks q4hr; skin assessment and special care q2hr; I & O and drain output q8hr; ELS; incentive spirometry q2hr; ICD on both legs | Vital signs; discontinue drain; check dressing and neurocirculatory checks q8hr; I & O q8hr; change dressing; ELS both legs; ICD on both legs |
| **Diet** | NPO; clear liquids after nausea and/or if positive bowel sounds | Clear liquids; advance diet as tolerated | Regular diet |
| **Activity** | Bedrest at 40-degree flexion; trapeze; CPM‡ on affected leg at least 8 hr/day; ankle exercise q2hr; T/tilt-C-DB q2hr | Bedrest, CPM on affected leg; ankle exercise q2hr; T/tilt-C-DB q2hr; advance CPM 5 degrees bid | Ambulate in room with help × 2; CPM on affected leg; ankle exercise q2hr; advance CPM by 5 degrees bid |
| **Consultations** | | Physical therapy; up in chair as tolerated | Physical therapy, social service, rehab/SNU/home health; up in chair as tolerated; encourage knee flexion |

*Serum calcium, phosphorus, triglycerides, uric acid, creatinine, BUN, total bilirubin, alkaline phosphate, aspartate aminotransferase (AST; formerly serum glutamic oxaloacetic transaminase [SGOT]), alanine aminotransferase (ALT; formerly serum glutamic oxaloacetic transaminase [SGPT]), lactic dehydrogenase (LDH), total protein, albumin, sodium, potassium, chloride, total $CO_2$, glucose.
†Serum, sodium, potassium, chloride, total $CO_2$, glucose, BUN.
‡Continuous passive motion.

***ence of antinuclear antibodies, antibodies to DNA, antihistones, and antibodies to ribonucleoprotein (Smith antigen) all are strongly associated with SLE.***

Abnormalities in both B cells and T cells have also been identified in persons with the disease. The appearance of B cells is thought to cause an increase in production of antibodies to self and nonself antigen.[7] These antibodies are responsible for the tissue injury seen in SLE. Most visceral lesions are mediated by type III hypersensitivity, and antibodies against red cells are mediated by type II hypersensitivity.[7] An acute necrotizing vasculitis can occur in any tissue. Most lesions are found in the blood vessels, kidney, connective tissues, and skin.

Because of the multisystem involvement and characteristic remissions and exacerbations, the clinical manifestations of SLE can be overwhelming. The American Rheumatism Association has developed criteria for the diagnosis of SLE (Table 65-9). The initial manifestation of SLE is often arthritis, typically a nonerosive synovitis without deformity. In many instances the joint symptoms are transient and respond to treatment. Weakness, fatigue, and weight loss may be present. The patient may complain of sensitivity to the sun, development of a rash, and at times fever or arthritis on exposure to sunlight. *Erythema,* usually in a *butterfly pattern,* appears over the *cheeks and bridge of the nose.* The margins of these lesions are bright red, and the lesions may extend beyond the hairline with partial alopecia (loss of hair) above the ears. Lesions may also occur on the exposed part of the neck. Lesions spread slowly to the mucous membranes and other tissues of the body, or they may originate there. These lesions do not ulcerate but cause degeneration and atrophy of tissues.

*Depending on the organs involved,* the patient may have findings of *glomerulonephritis, splenomegaly, hepatomegaly, pleuritis, pericarditis, lymphadenopathy, peritonitis, neuritis, or anemia. Renal and neurologic*

| Day 4 | Day 5 | Day 6 | Day of Discharge Day 7 |
|---|---|---|---|
| CBC SMA/7 | | | |
| Disc saline lock; disc antibiotic; PO analgesic; stool softener; Rx for sleep; anticoagulant | PO analgesic; stool softener; Rx for sleep; anticoagulant | PO analgesic; stool softener; Rx for sleep; anticoagulant | PO analgesic; anticoagulant |
| Vital signs and neurocirculatory checks q8hr; I & O q8hr; ELS; dressing change PRN, ICD on both legs | Vital signs and neurocirculatory checks q8hr; disc I & O; ELS; disc ICD | Vital signs q8hr; ELS | Vital signs q8hr; ELS |
| Regular diet | Regular diet | Regular diet | Regular diet |
| Ambulate in room with help × 4; CPM on affected leg; ankle exercise q2hr; advance CPM 5 degrees bid | Ambulate in hallway with help × 2; CPM on affected leg; ankle exercise q2hr; advance CPM 5 degrees bid | Ambulate in hallway with help × 4; advance CPM by 5 degrees bid | Ambulate in hallway with help × 4 |
| Physical therapy; occupational therapy if self-care help needed | Physical therapy; occupational therapy if self-care help needed | Physical therapy; occupational therapy | Physical therapy; occupational therapy |

***manifestations are among the more serious manifestations of the disease.***

## Medical Management

### Diagnostic tests

Diagnosis is made after evaluation of the history and physical examination and results of laboratory tests. Refer to Table 65-9 for selected laboratory findings.

The immunofluorescence test for DNA is positive in more than 95% of patients with SLE. However, it is considered to be of little clinical value in the definitive diagnosis of SLE, because it is also positive in many other autoimmune disorders, such as systemic sclerosis (both CREST syndrome and diffuse), Sjögren's syndrome, and polymyositis. It is also positive in 10% of the normal population. As mentioned earlier, antibodies against double-strand DNA and anti-Smith antigen are positive in 20% to 60% of patients with SLE. The LE cell test is positive in 70% of patients with SLE. The LE cell is any phagocytic leukocyte that has engulfed the nucleus of an injured cell.

### Medication

1. Antiinflammatory analgesics to control arthritic pain
2. Antimalarial drugs, particularly if rash is extensive
3. Corticosteroids for severe neurologic and renal involvement
4. Cytotoxic agents if other drugs fail
5. Ointments or skin creams for rash

### Treatment

1. Kidney dialysis or transplant for uncontrolled lupus nephritis
2. Total hip replacement for avascular necrosis consequent to high-dose steroid therapy

### Diet

No special diet is required.

### Activity

1. Rest when the disease is active
2. Exercise to maintain mobility
3. Avoidance of exposure to the sun

**TABLE 65-9 The 1982 Revised Criteria for Classification of Systemic Lupus Erythematosus***

| CRITERION | DEFINITION |
|---|---|
| 1. Malar rash | Fixed erythema, flat or raised, over the malar eminences, tending to spare the nasolabial folds |
| 2. Discoid rash | Erythematous raised patches with adherent keratotic scaling and follicular plugging; atrophic scarring may occur in older lesions |
| 3. Photosensitivity | Skin rash as a result of unusual reaction to sunlight, by patient history or physician observation |
| 4. Oral ulcers | Oral or nasopharyngeal ulceration, usually painless, observed by a physician |
| 5. Arthritis | Nonerosive arthritis involving two or more peripheral joints, characterized by tenderness, swelling, or effusion |
| 6. Serositis | *(a)* Pleuritis—convincing history of pleuritic pain or rub heard by a physician or evidence of pleural effusion, or |
| | *(b)* Pericarditis—documented by electrocardiogram or rub or evidence of pericardial effusion |
| 7. Renal disorder | *(a)* Persistent proteinuria greater than 0.5 g/dl or greater than 3+ if quantitation not performed, or |
| | *(b)* Cellular casts—may be red blood cell, hemoglobin, granular, tubular, or mixed |
| 8. Neurologic disorder | *(a)* Seizures—in the absence of offending drugs or known metabolic derangements, e.g., uremia, ketoacidosis, or electrolyte imbalance, or |
| | *(b)* Psychosis—in the absence of offending drugs or known metabolic derangements, e.g., uremia, ketoacidosis, or electrolyte imbalance |
| 9. Hematologic disorder | *(a)* Hemolytic anemia—with reticulocytosis, or |
| | *(b)* Leukopenia—less than $4.0 \times 10^9$/L (4000/mm$^3$) total on two or more occasions, or |
| | *(c)* Lymphopenia—less than $1.5 \times 10^9$/L (1500/mm$^3$) on two or more occasions, or |
| | *(d)* Thrombocytopenia—less than $100 \times 10^9$/L ($100 \times 10^3$/mm$^3$) in the absence of offending drugs |
| 10. Immunologic disorder | *(a)* Positive lupus erythematosus cell preparation, or |
| | *(b)* Anti-DNA antibody to native DNA in abnormal titer, or |
| | *(c)* Anti-Sm—presence of antibody to Sm nuclear antigen, or |
| | *(d)* False-positive serologic test for syphilis known to be positive for at least 6 months and confirmed by negative *Treponema pallidum* immobilization or fluorescent treponemal antibody absorption test |
| 11. Antinuclear antibody | An abnormal titer of antinuclear antibody by immunofluorescence of an equivalent assay at any point in time and in the absence of drugs known to be associated with drug-induced lupus syndrome |

*From Tan EM et al: The revised criteria for the classification of systemic lupus erythematosus, *Arthritis Rheum* 25:1271, 1982.
The proposed classification is based on 11 criteria. For the purpose of identifying patients in clinical studies, a person shall be said to have systemic lupus erythematosus if any 4 or more of the 11 criteria are present, serially or simultaneously, during any interval of observation.

## Nursing Management

### Facilitating learning

Guiding and teaching the patient and family to understand and manage the disease are perhaps the most important functions the nurse performs in relation to SLE. Teaching should include the following:

1. Nature, course, and treatment of disease
2. Appropriate balance of rest and activity
3. Appropriate exercise
4. How to avoid exposing skin to sunlight; for example, wearing long-sleeved blouses or dresses, slacks, broad-brimmed hats, and cotton gloves
5. Appropriate use of prescribed medications (i.e., dosage, frequency, precautions in administration, potential side effects)
6. Application of cosmetics (e.g., hypoallergenic, approved by physician) to mask skin lesions and/or wigs to mask hair loss
7. Information about lupus support groups (if available in patient's area)
8. Measures to decrease fatigue (see p. 2250)

### Promoting comfort and ADL

The nurse can promote comfort by the following:

1. Administering prescribed medications for control of joint pain
2. Providing appropriate periods of rest
3. Assisting patient to gradually resume independence in ADL
4. Providing appropriate nursing care following renal transplant (see Chapter 72) or total hip replacement (p. 2271), or during kidney dialysis (see Chapter 72)

## POLYMYOSITIS AND DERMATOMYOSITIS

### Etiology

**Polymyositis** is an inflammatory disease involving striated (voluntary) muscle that occurs two times more frequently in women than men. **Dermatomyositis** is polymyositis accompanied by skin lesions.

### Epidemiology

Polymyositis may occur at any age and is believed to affect 5 in every 1 million people in the United States. The cause of the disease is unknown; however, it is thought that some reaction of the autoimmune system is involved, perhaps triggered by a virus.

### Pathophysiology

Both polymyositis and dermatopolymyositis are characterized by inflammation of muscle fibers and connective tissue resulting in extensive tissue necrosis and destruction of muscle fibers. Both cell-mediated and humoral immune mechanisms are associated with the diseases.

Histologic studies of biopsied muscle are variable, but the pathologic alterations found, in order of their frequency, are as follows:

1. Primary degeneration of muscle fibers, either focal or extensive
2. Basophilia of some fibers with central migration of the sarcolemmal nuclei
3. Necrosis of parts or entire groups of muscle fibers
4. Inflammation of blood vessels supplying the muscles
5. Interstitial fibrosis varying in severity with the duration and, to some extent, the type of the disease[32]
6. Variation in the cross-sectional diameter of fibers

The initial symptoms of both disorders are similar to those associated with any inflammatory response: *fever, swelling, malaise, and fatigue.* The diseases, which run a *course of exacerbations and remissions,* are usually *first noted in proximal muscles, in particular the pelvic and shoulder girdles.* The weakness is symmetric. Climbing stairs, rising from a chair, and other activities that involve lifting the body become increasingly difficult or impossible. Lifting the arms becomes progressively more difficult, and hair combing may be impossible. Other muscles such as the neck flexors and the muscles of swallowing may also become involved. Muscle pain or tenderness is present in some instances in the early stages.

Clinical manifestations common to both polymyositis and dermatomyositis include dysphagia, decreased esophageal motility, cardiomyopathy, and Raynaud's phenomenon. Involvement of the skin in the form of a rash marks the disease as *dermatomyositis.* A *dusky red lesion* may be found *in the periorbital region,* along *with periorbital edema.* This dusky red rash may extend over the face, forehead, neck, upper shoulders, chest, and upper back. Lesions on the arms and legs commonly affect the extensor surfaces. These patches are sometimes scaly. Calcinosis (serum calcium deposits in the subcutaneous tissue) can also occur in dermatomyositis.

The *weakness of myositis, if it persists, can lead to contractures and atrophy. Individuals with the dermatomyositis* form of the disease, particularly if they are *over 50 years of age, have a 40% to 50% greater chance of* having evidence *of a malignant neoplasm found during the first 5 years of illness than the population at large.* Some physicians believe that routine yearly examinations should be performed to define or exclude the presence of neoplasms in these patients during that 5-year period.

## Medical Management

### Diagnostic tests

1. History and physical including manual muscle test to delineate weakness in specific muscles
2. Electromyogram to delineate a specific pattern of findings to differentiate polymyositis from other types of muscle disease
3. Muscle biopsy to define specific pathologic changes in muscle
4. Serum enzymes (SGOT, CPK, aldolase) are elevated in presence of active disease
5. 24-hour urine tests to determine abnormal creatine/creatinine ratio

### Medication

Administration of immunosuppressant drugs in sufficient doses to effect remission of symptoms and reversal of abnormal laboratory values. Steroids are most frequently chosen, but azathioprine, methotrexate, and cyclophosphamides have been reported to be as effective.

### Diet

No special diet is required.

### Activity

The patient should rest in bed but can get up as able.

### Referral/Consultation

In some settings the nurse assumes responsibility for making referrals to other services, such as physical therapy.

## Nursing Management

Nursing management is as follows:

1. Facilitating learning
   a. Instruct patient and family in nature and course of disease.
   b. Instruct patient in appropriate balance of rest and activity.
   c. Instruct patient in use of selected ADL devices to enhance function (e.g., long-handled comb).
   d. Instruct patient in appropriate use of prescribed drugs (how to take them, dosage, side effects, precautions).
2. Promoting comfort
   a. During acute episodes, assist with frequent changes of position.
   b. Administer prescribed analgesics.
   c. Assist with ADL.
   d. Provide adequate rest.
3. Promoting mobility
   a. Elevate sitting surfaces to facilitate transfer.
   b. Provide appropriate ambulatory device to facilitate comfortable walking.
   c. Provide for frequent changes of position and range of motion to prevent contractures.
   d. Encourage patient to gradually resume independent ADL as symptoms subside.
4. Preventing skin breakdown
   a. Reposition patient frequently.

b. Avoid pressure over bony prominences with appropriate protective devices (see Chapter 64).

## ANKYLOSING SPONDYLITIS

### Etiology

**Ankylosing spondylitis** *is a chronic inflammatory disorder affecting the sacroiliac joints and spine that occurs 9 times more frequently in men than women, usually between the ages of 10 and 40 years. The peak incidence occurs at 20 years.* The cause of the disease is unknown, and its progression cannot be stopped by any treatment now known.

### Epidemiology

The histocompatibility antigen HLA-B27 is present in 90% of persons with the disease, whereas it occurs in only 8% of the normal population. There is a strong genetic link with the genetic marker HLA-B27, and it is thought that a link between the marker and some form of trigger (perhaps an infection) sets off a reaction in the immune system that leads to the inflammatory process. *Klebsiella* is thought to be the causative organism.[22] African-Americans have a lower incidence of the disease, whereas the incidence in Native Americans is 18% to 50%.[7]

### Pathophysiology

Spondylitis means inflammation of the spine. As a result of inflammation, the bones of the spine grow together, or ankylose (fuse). The primary site of pathologic findings is the *enthesis.* This is where ligaments, tendons, and joint capsule insert into bone. In ankylosing spondylitis, fibrous ossification and eventually fusion of the joint occur. The joint capsule, articular cartilage, and periosteum are invaded by inflammatory cells that trigger the development of fibrous scar tissue and growth of new bone. The bony growth changes the contour of the vertebrae and forms a new enthesis called a *syndesmophyte* on top of the old one. As the spinal ligaments continue to undergo progressive calcification, the vertebral bodies lose their original contour and appear square, which gives the spine the classic *"bamboo"* appearance of ankylosing spondylitis. Inflammation usually begins around the sacroiliac joints and progresses up the spine, eventually resulting in fusion of the entire spine. As the inflammatory process involves the costosternal and costovertebral cartilage, it can cause chest pain, which is worse on inspiration.

Initial symptoms may include low back pain or aching; pain and swelling of the hips, knees, or shoulders; mild fever; loss of appetite; and fatigue. Low back pain flares and subsides intermittently. Over a period of time, pain subsides and motion of the back becomes restricted. Fusion of the sacroiliac joints and spine up through the cervical vertebrae may occur over a period of 10 to 20 years; as a result, the spine loses its normal lordotic curve and the patient may have either a "poker back" deformity or a kyphosis at the cervicodorsal junction (Figure 65-19). Knees are flexed as the person attempts to move the head upright.

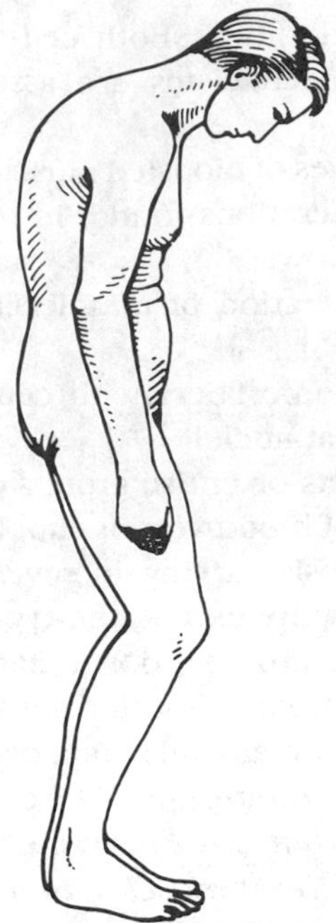

**FIGURE 65-19** Characteristic posture in advanced ankylosing spondylitis.

## Medical Management

### Diagnostic tests

Diagnosis is made by history and physical examination and the following findings:

1. Presence in the serum of HLA-B27
2. X-rays showing presence of syndesmophytes and "bamboo" spine
3. Elevation of the erythrocyte sedimentation rate

### Medication

The following antiinflammatory analgesics are used:

1. Salicylates
2. NSAIDs
3. Potent antiinflammatory agents on a short-term basis (phenylbutazone)

### Treatment

Goals of treatment are to relieve pain, achieve and maintain the best possible alignment of the spine, strengthen the paraspinal muscles, and maintain maximal breathing capacity. Following are the most common interventions:

1. Physical therapy to maintain mobility and reduce severity of deformity; for example, ROM exercises and lying prone (extension) 3 to 4 times per day for 15 to 30 minutes and deep breathing exercises to promote maximum chest expansion
2. Heat
3. Use of TLSO (thoracic lumbar sacral orthosis)

4. Cervical head halter traction to decrease muscle spasms and distract the spine
5. Spinal osteotomy and fusion, usually cervical
6. Hip arthroplasty

**Activity**

Extra rest is recommended.

### Nursing Management

Nursing management focuses on the following:

1. Facilitating learning
   a. Nature and course of disease
   b. Prescribed exercises
   c. Appropriate use of prescribed medications
   d. Methods of applying heat to back and hips
2. Promoting maximum mobility and reducing severity of deformity
   a. Provide firm mattress and bed board
   b. Encourage patient to sleep without pillow under the head to maintain extension of spine
   c. Supervise and encourage regular exercises; assist as necessary
   d. Encourage participation in ADL and usual activities to the fullest extent possible
   e. Occupational therapy referral for adaptive or supportive devices
3. Promoting comfort and relieving pain
   a. Provide heat applications/hydrotherapy, especially before exercises
   b. Administer prescribed medications on time
   c. Assess effectiveness of pain relief measures
4. Promoting acceptance of body image (see Chapter 9)

# NONARTICULAR RHEUMATISM

Nonarticular rheumatic diseases include those disorders in which the supportive structures and structures located near the joints are inflamed, but the joints themselves are not involved except by the limitations imposed by the supportive structures. *Some of these disorders are fibrositis, tenosynovitis, bursitis, and carpal tunnel syndrome.*

## BURSITIS

### Etiology/Epidemiology

Bursitis, or inflammation of the bursa, may be acute or chronic. It is usually caused by trauma, strain, and overuse of the joint with which the bursa is associated. The shoulder bursa is most often affected.

### Pathophysiology

The synovial lining of the bursal sac becomes inflamed, more fluid is secreted, and the bursa swells. Occasionally, large calcium deposits are present. The swelling is accompanied by pain and limited ability to move the associated joint or the entire extremity.

The area may be reddened and warm to the touch. *Point tenderness,* or ability to locate a specific area of increased pain, may be present.

### Medical Management

Medical management includes the following:

1. Rest for the involved area
2. Antiinflammatory agents
   a. Salicylates
   b. Phenylbutazone
   c. Indomethacin
   d. Injection of adrenocorticosteroids into bursa
3. Application of cold during early acute phase (heat is avoided, because it increases fluid exudate in the bursa during early inflammatory period)
4. Surgical removal of calcium deposits

### Nursing Management

Nursing management includes the following:

1. Patient teaching regarding rest, appropriate use of cold applications and prescribed medications
2. Promoting comfort through provision of rest, cold applications, and assistance with ADL

## CARPAL TUNNEL SYNDROME

### Etiology

**Carpal tunnel syndrome** is caused by pressure exerted on the median nerve of the wrist. The condition is *most common in women 30 to 50 years of age.* It usually affects the dominant hand. Many conditions can cause an increase in pressure in the carpal tunnel, thereby producing symptoms of median nerve compression. Symptoms are usually consistent, regardless of etiology.

### Epidemiology

Inflammatory processes such as rheumatoid arthritis, flexor tenosynovitis, and gout can cause thickening of the flexor synovium, which leads to elevated pressure in the tunnel. Patients receiving long-term hemodialysis for chronic renal failure may be at risk for developing carpal tunnel syndrome because of synovial edema and amyloid deposits.

Previous trauma may contribute to the development of carpal tunnel syndrome. Fractures and dislocations of the wrist and burns can cause constriction of the tunnel because of contractures or bony deformities.

Repetitive motion of the wrist may also contribute to the development of carpal tunnel syndrome. Work-related carpal tunnel syndrome is a cumulative trauma disorder caused by job-related tasks that involve certain motions or actions, listed below:

1. Forceful grasping or pinching of objects (e.g., tools)
2. Awkward positions
3. Direct pressure over carpal tunnel
4. Repetitive motions
5. Use of vibrating handheld tools

Other conditions that contribute to the development of carpal tunnel syndrome include diabetes, myxedema, pregnancy, abnormalities of the median artery and flexor muscle, ganglions, and lipomas. Alcoholism has also been associated with the development of carpal tunnel syndrome. Certain occupations put workers (typists, computer operators, assembly line workers, and truck drivers) at risk for developing the syndrome.

## Pathophysiology

The median nerve passes through a tunnel bounded by the carpal bones dorsally and the transverse carpal ligament volarly (Figure 65-20). Flexor tendons run through the tunnel parallel to the median nerve. Inflammation and swelling of the synovial lining of tendon sheaths narrow the space available and cause compression of the median nerve; with continued compression, median nerve neuropathy develops.

The patient will complain of *dysesthesia, paresthesia, and hypesthesia of the thumb and index and middle fingers.* Symptoms may be worse at night, perhaps caused by sleeping with the wrists in a flexed position. Complaints will usually increase when there has been forced flexion of the wrist for long periods, such as when knitting or typing. The patient may feel that the hand is "swollen" and may complain of clumsiness when using the hand, especially when grasping or holding onto small objects. Referred pain to the upper extremity and base of the neck is common. Atrophy of the thenar eminence (the padded area of the palm below the base of the thumb) may be present in late disease. Treatment is usually sought as symptoms worsen.

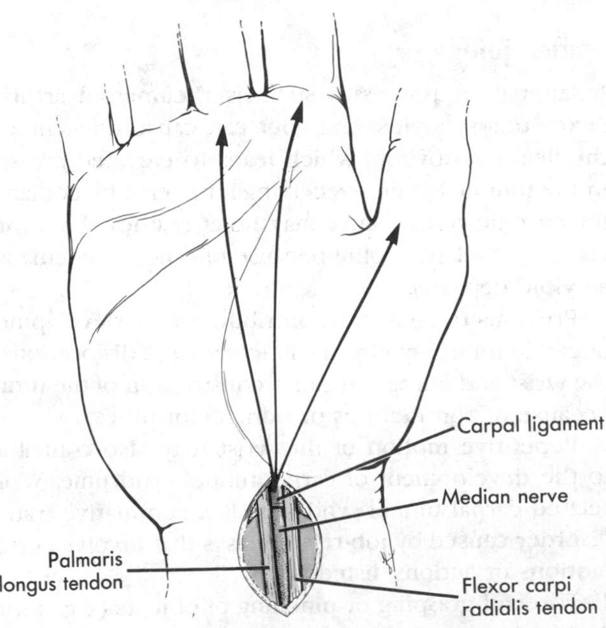


**FIGURE 65-20** Carpal tunnel syndrome. Volar aspect of wrist retracted to demonstrate position of median nerve. Distribution of median nerve is to thumb and first two fingers. (Modified from Compere EL: *Orthopaedic surgery,* Chicago, 1974, Year Book Medical Publishers, Inc.)

## Diagnostic Tests

Diagnosis is made by history, physical examination, and evaluation of diagnostic tests. Other conditions with similar symptoms must be eliminated, including cervical radiculopathy and thoracic outlet syndrome. Symptoms can be reproduced by tapping the median nerve at the wrist *(positive Tinel's sign). Phalen's test* is also used to diagnose carpal tunnel syndrome. The examiner holds the wrist in acute flexion for 60 seconds; if symptoms are reproduced or increased, the test is considered positive. Direct compression of the median nerve at the wrist for 30 seconds will also reproduce or increase symptoms in the presence of carpal tunnel syndrome. Nerve conduction studies and electromyography are used to evaluate nerve function and muscle abnormalities.

## Medical Management

Medical management of carpal tunnel syndrome includes the following:

1. Rest
2. Splinting of the wrist
3. Local steroid injections
4. Administration of NSAIDs
5. Decompression of the median nerve (usually an ambulatory procedure)

## Surgical Management

Surgical correction is performed by open release or more recently, endoscopic release and decompression. Endoscopic release decreases postoperative pain, reduces scarring, and decreases recovery time. Arthroscopic release is contraindicated in patients with rheumatoid arthritis and flexor synovitis.

## Nursing Management

Nursing management includes the following:

1. Patient teaching
   a. Instruct patient regarding rest, splinting of wrist
   b. Provide preoperative instruction if surgery is planned
   c. Occupational history and job counseling: if occupational factors such as wrist flexing and repetitive tasks contributed to development of the condition, job retraining may be indicated
2. Postoperative care and instruction
   a. Promoting comfort and circulation
      (1) Elevating hand and arm for 24 hours
      (2) Encouraging active thumb and finger motion within limits imposed by dressing
      (3) Administering prescribed analgesic as necessary
   b. Promoting safety
      (1) Check fingers for circulation, sensation, and movement every 1 to 2 hours for 24 hours
   c. Promoting self-care
      (1) Encourage patient to use hand in normal ADL 2 to 3 days following surgery

d. Postoperative teaching
 (1) Instruction of patient regarding follow-up care
 (2) Life-style modification if repetitive motions (workplace or leisure) contributed to disease process

## DUPUYTREN'S CONTRACTURE

### Etiology

**Dupuytren's contracture** *is a condition marked by hypertrophic hyperplasia of the palmar fascia that results in a flexion deformity of the distal palm and fingers* (Figure 65-21). The cause of Dupuytren's contracture is unknown. A familial tendency has been noted.

### Epidemiology

White men, middle aged or older, are affected by a ratio of 7 : 1. It is estimated that 1.5% of the total population over 60 years of age is affected to some extent with the disorder.[35] When affected, women seem to experience only mild deformity. Dupuytren's deformity is associated with epilepsy, alcoholism, and penile lesions. Although occupation does not contribute to the development of the disease, repetitive occupational trauma may increase the severity of preexisting disease.[35]

### Pathophysiology

Dupuytren's contracture may take up to 20 years to reach maximum deformity. *It often occurs bilaterally and symmetrically. Hyperplasia and progressive fibrosis of the palmar fascia on the ulnar side of the hand cause progressive shortening of the pretendinous bands to the ring and sometimes the small fingers.* The bands shorten, and the fingers are pulled into fixed flexion. The skin of the palm is drawn down, forming tight puckers and nodules.

Depending on the severity of the deformity and hand dominance, the patient may experience difficulty in grasping objects. Burning pain may accompany attempts at grasping. Usually, the main complaints are deformity and mild interference with hand function.

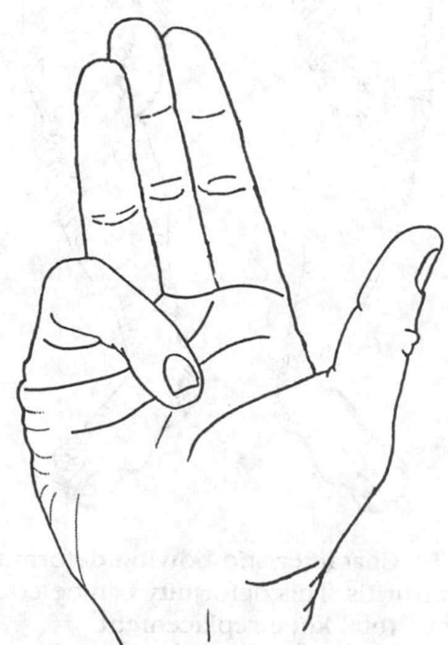

**FIGURE 65-21** Dupuytren's contracture.

### Medical Management

Medical management includes the following:

1. Avoiding activities that require grasping an object, for example, a hammer
2. Soaking hand in warm water while actively performing finger extension exercises
3. Surgically removing the involved palmar fascia (usually an ambulatory procedure)

### Nursing Management

Nursing management usually focuses on postoperative care:

1. Elevating hand to control swelling for at least 24 hours
2. Checking fingers for circulation, sensation, movement every 1 to 2 hours for 24 hours
3. Administering prescribed analgesics as necessary to maintain comfort
4. Encouraging active extension of fingers
5. Avoiding passive extension of fingers
6. Encouraging patient to begin using hand in self-care activities after 2 to 3 days

# DEGENERATIVE DISORDERS

## DEGENERATIVE JOINT DISEASE

### Etiology

**Degenerative joint disease,** also known as *osteoarthritis, hypertrophic arthritis, osteoarthrosis, or senescent arthritis, is an extremely common disease that is probably as old as civilization.* Almost everyone past 40 years of age has hypertrophic changes in the joints. Although symptomatic degenerative joint disease is usually seen in the 50- to 70-year age group, it has been observed as early as 20 years of age.

### Epidemiology

Women are more severely affected by the disease, although the incidence rates are the same for males and females. *It is estimated that 17 million people in the United States have osteoarthritis serious enough to cause pain.* The two forms of osteoarthritis are *primary* and *secondary.*

Primary joint disease is the most common type of noninflammatory joint disease. Primary degenerative joint disease is distributed throughout the central and peripheral joints of the body, usually affecting the joints of the hand, wrist, neck, lumbar spine, hips, knees, and ankles. The etiology is unknown, but age is an important factor in the development of the disease. The quantity and quality of proteoglycans decrease with the aging process and predispose the cartilage to break down and degenerate. Research indicates there may be a genetic component to the development of osteoarthritis.

**BOX 65-4 Clinical Manifestations of Degenerative Joint Disease**

| | |
|---|---|
| Pain | Worse with weight bearing, improves with rest, may be accompanied by paresthesias |
| Swelling and joint enlargement | May be from inflammatory exudate or blood entering joint capsule causing an increase in synovial fluid or from fragments of osteophytes entering synovial cavity |
| Decreased range of motion | Depends on amount of destroyed cartilage |
| Muscular atrophy | From disuse, joint instability, and deformity |
| Crepitus | May be present on movement |
| Joint stiffness | Worse in the morning ("early morning stiffness") and after a period of rest or disuse |

***Secondary joint disease is caused by any condition that damages cartilage, subjects the joints to chronic stress, or causes joint instability.*** Secondary joint disease is usually limited to the specific joints that were subjected to stress. Causes of secondary disease include trauma; long-term mechanical stressors (e.g., those associated with obesity, athletics, dancing, or the performance of repetitive tasks); infection; neurologic disorders that may alter pain and proprioceptive responses, thereby increasing the risk of abnormal movement or weight bearing; skeletal deformities; hemophilia; hyperparathyroidism; and the use of medications that stimulate collagen digesting enzymes in the synovium.

## Pathophysiology

Both primary and secondary degenerative joint diseases affect the articular cartilage. Characteristic pathologic changes include the following:

1. Erosion of articular cartilage
2. Thickening of bone underneath the cartilage
3. Formation of osteophytes or bone spurs

Normal articular cartilage is white, translucent, and smooth. When affected by the disease, it becomes yellow and opaque. Areas of cartilage soften, and the surface becomes rough, frayed, and cracked. This process is thought to occur as a result of digestion of the cartilage by enzymes and alteration of the nutrition of the cartilage. Eventually the cartilage is destroyed, and the underlying subchondral bone goes through a remodeling process. *Osteophytes,* or spurs of new bone, appear at the joint margins and at the sites of attachment of supporting structures. These may break off and appear in the joint cavity as "joint mice." Unlike rheumatoid arthritis, ***degenerative joint disease affects only the joints and their surrounding tissue.*** It is not a systemic or inflammatory disease process.

**BOX 65-5 Characteristic Changes or Symptoms in Certain Joints**

1. *Heberden's nodes*—bony protuberances occurring on the dorsal surface of the distal interphalangeal joints of the fingers (Figure 65-22)
2. *Bouchard's nodes*—bony protuberances occurring on the proximal interphalangeal joints of the fingers
3. *Coxarthrosis* (degenerative joint disease of the hip)—pain in the hip on weight bearing, with pain progressing to include groin and medial knee pain and limited range of motion
4. Knee involvement—varus (Figure 65-23), valgus (knocked knees), flexion deformity, crepitus, and limited range of motion

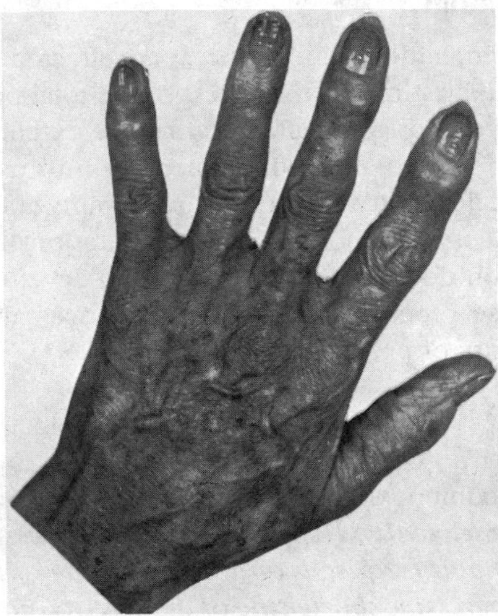

**FIGURE 65-22** Osteoarthritis of hand. Note enlargement of distal joints of index, middle, and little finger (Heberden's nodes). (From Brashear H, Raney R: *Shand's handbook of orthopaedic surgery,* ed 9, St Louis, 1978, Mosby.)

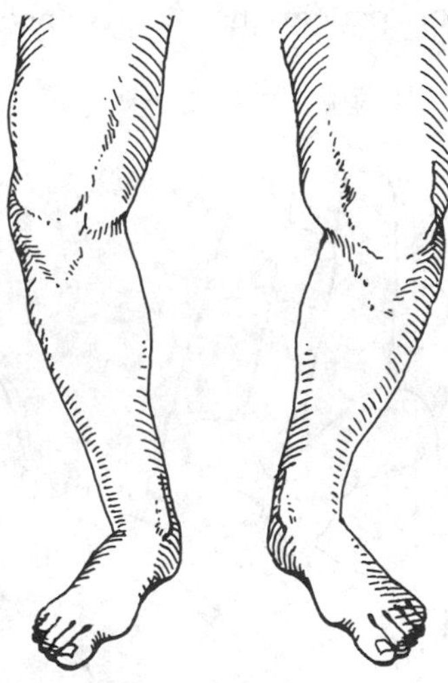

**FIGURE 65-23** Characteristic bowing deformity of knees in degenerative arthritis. This deformity can be corrected by tibial osteotomy or total knee replacement.

Clinical manifestations of degenerative joint disease are summarized in Box 65-4.

In addition to the clinical manifestations listed in Box 65-4, characteristic changes or symptoms occur in certain joints (Box 65-5).

## Prevention

Primary methods of prevention of osteoarthritis include the following:

1. Avoidance of obesity
2. Avoidance of repeated trauma to joints
3. Practice of joint protection techniques in occupations that put joints at risk

## Medical Management

The expected length of stay of patients with degenerative joint disease as determined by DRG is 5 to 7 days. Objectives in management include relief of pain, restoration of joint function, and prevention of disability or further progression of the disease. Common medical therapy for management of degenerative joint disease follows.

### Diagnostic tests

Diagnosis is made based on evaluation of history and physical assessment and the results of radiologic studies. Serologic and synovial fluid examinations will be essentially normal. However, x-ray films will reveal narrowing of the joint space, osteophyte formation, and **eburnation** (sclerosis) of subchondral bone.

### Medication

Medications used to treat degenerative joint disease are as follows:

1. Salicylates, NSAIDs
2. Intraarticular injection of steroids for severe discomfort
3. Adjunctive analgesics (Tylenol, Darvon)

### Treatment

Treatments include the following:

1. Rest
2. Exercise
3. Joint protection

### Diet

Appropriate nutritional intake is encouraged to maintain ideal body weight and avoid weight gain. Weight gain places an unnecessary stress on joints.

### Activity

Emphasis is placed on the following:

1. Unloading painful weight-bearing joints through the use of canes, walkers, crutches
2. Range of motion exercises to prevent deformities and contractures.

### Referral/Consultation

In some settings the nurse assumes responsibility for making referrals to other services. Common referrals for persons with degenerative joint disease include physical and occupational therapy.

Critical pathways (also referred to as "collaborative care paths" or "care maps") have been developed in some inpatient and outpatient settings to guide both medical and nursing management. These critical pathways are collaboratively developed along time lines and include the information described above for specific hours, days, or visits. Pertinent information about discharge planning and patient teaching to be implemented at specified times also is included. Because the nurse has a major role in these two aspects of care, these are discussed under Nursing Management.

A sample critical pathway for the six areas of care discussed in this section is presented on p. 2256. A nursing care plan for the same type of patient also is included. In some settings these are combined within the critical pathway document.

## Surgical Management

Surgical management is indicated to relieve pain, increase joint movement, correct deformity, or create a new joint. Examples of surgical procedures performed for the person with degenerative joint disease include the following:

1. Removal of bits of broken cartilage or bone (debridement, usually by arthroscopic surgery)
2. Realignment (osteotomy)
3. Fusion (arthrodesis)
4. Joint replacement (replacement arthroplasty)

# NURSING MANAGEMENT

## ♦ ASSESSMENT

### Subjective Data

Subjective data include the following:

1. Where and when does pain occur?
2. What measures give relief?
3. What modifications in ADL have been made necessary by pain? (See Gerontologic Patient Considerations box, p. 2266.)

### Objective Data

Objective data include assessing signs that are usually localized to the involved joints and are determined by inspection, palpation, and observation, including the following:

1. Limited active range of motion of involved joints
2. Enlargement; irregularity; flexion, varus, or valgus deformity
3. Crepitus on movement
4. Presence of limp, alterations in gait
5. Difficulty sitting after standing for a period of time

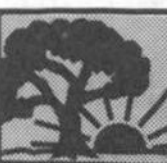

## GERONTOLOGIC PATIENT CONSIDERATIONS

### ASSESSMENT

Assess all elderly persons for muscle strength and tone, gait, painful joints or muscles, contractures, deformities, and foot problems that may interfere with ambulation and ADL.

Assess availability, condition, and use of assistive aids, such as walkers, canes, or crutches.

Assess environmental factors conducive to falls because elderly persons are at high risk for falls.

### INTERVENTION

Order assistive aids to foster independence and to increase ambulation, such as walker, cane, lift, bedside commode.

Encourage an exercise program to maintain baseline muscle and joint function.

Perform active and passive range of motion for elderly persons on bedrest.

Obtain orders for progressive ambulation as early in hospitalization as possible.

Position extremities in normal body alignment; elderly persons are highly susceptible to flexion contractures.

Teach good foot care and importance of well-fitted shoes.

Request physical therapy for patients with gait or mobility problems.

Request occupational therapy for problems with ADL and fine motor coordination.

Teach elderly persons how to transfer and ambulate safely.

Initiate a fall-prevention program that identifies risk factors and promotes an individualized plan for each patient, depending on ability and tendency to fall.

Use restraints only as a last resort; reevaluate use every 4 to 8 hours; remove them frequently for range of motion and toileting.

Be sure environment is free of clutter, bed is kept in lowest position, and night-light illuminates the floor.

### COMMON DISORDERS IN ELDERS

Degenerative joint disease (osteoarthritis)
Osteoporosis
Hip fractures

or arising from a chair after sitting for a period of time

## ♦ NURSING DIAGNOSES

Nursing diagnoses are determined from analysis of patient data. Possible nursing diagnoses for the person with degenerative joint disease may include, but are not limited to, the following:

| Diagnostic Title | Possible Etiologic Factors |
|---|---|
| Knowledge deficit (regarding degenerative joint disease) | Lack of exposure, unfamiliarity with information resources |
| Pain in affected joints | Pathologic changes in articular cartilage and stiffness in affected joints |
| Mobility, impaired physical | Pain or discomfort from degeneration of affected joints |
| Activity intolerance | Pain or discomfort and restricted mobility caused by joint involvement |
| Self-care deficit (related to ADL) | Pain and limited joint movement |
| Nutrition, altered: more than body requirements | Excessive intake in relation to ability to exercise |

## RESEARCH

Laborde JM, Powers MJ: Life satisfaction, health control orientation, and illness-related factors in persons with osteoarthritis, *Res Nurs Health* 8(1):183-190, 1985.

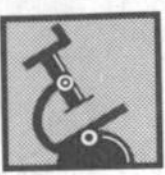

This study was based on the hypothesis that as a result of living with chronic pain, osteoarthritic persons' satisfaction with life may decrease. An earlier study by the same authors (1980) indicated that activities associated with a productive life were more compromised for arthritic persons with pain than for patients undergoing hemodialysis. The aim of this study was to explore "changes over time in levels of life satisfaction in a group of osteoarthritics and to examine the relative impact of illness-related and health belief factors on present life situation." A convenience sample of 160 osteoarthritic subjects was obtained at four different settings: an urban senior center, an outpatient clinic at a university hospital, an outpatient clinic at an urban private hospital, and two rural community centers. Cantril's Self-Anchoring Striving scale was used to assess the subjects' general sense of well-being, or life satisfaction, at three points in time: past, present, and future. The Health Locus of Control measure was administered to determine whether the subjects perceived their health-related expectations in terms of external or internal control. Additionally, subjects were interviewed for demographic and arthritis-related information. Measurements of past, present, and anticipated life satisfaction were obtained. Results indicated that past life satisfaction and present life satisfaction were viewed favorably by subjects, but "aspirations for future life satisfaction declined appreciably." The mean score for the total sample indicated "an external orientation in health beliefs for the entire group." Present life satisfaction was "found to be significantly associated with better health perception, internal health locus of control, and less joint pain." The authors suggest that "internally oriented individuals . . . engage in lifestyles that provide more satisfying experiences" than externally controlled individuals, and they conclude that osteoarthritic persons who are *"given educational programs adjunctive to therapy may become more positive about their present satisfaction with life."* These conclusions were supported by a study by Bradbury and Catanzaro (Bradbury VI, Catanzaro M-L: The quality of life in a male population suffering from arthritis, *Rehabil Nurs* 14[4]:187-190, 1989).

## ♦ EXPECTED PATIENT OUTCOMES

Expected patient outcomes for the person with degenerative joint disease may include but are not lim-

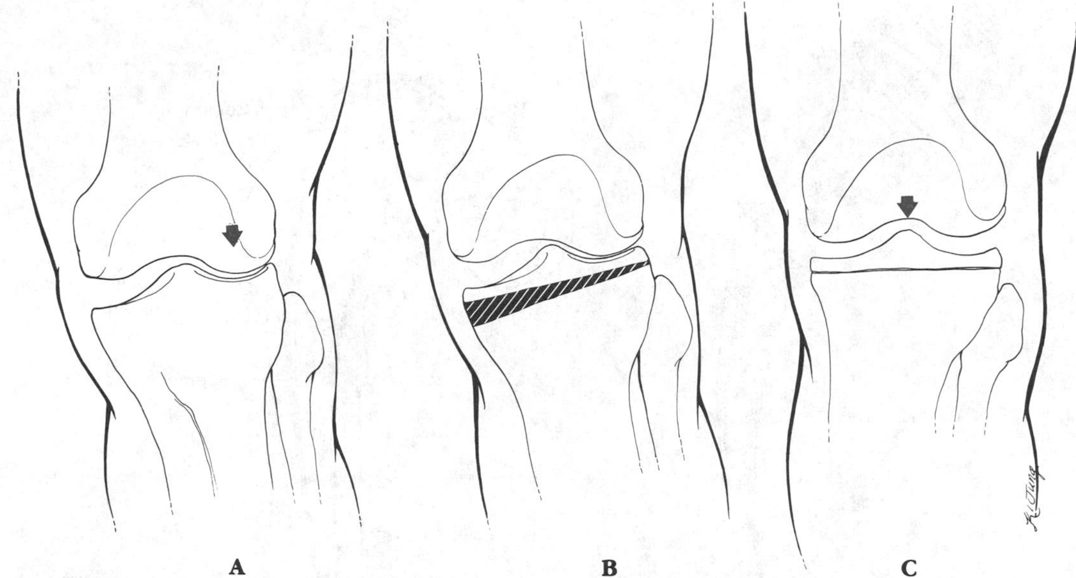


**FIGURE 65-24** Osteotomy of tibia. Genu valgum (anterior view of left knee). **A,** Weight-bearing force is concentrated on one compartment of knee. **B,** Wedge of bone is removed from tibia. Amount of bone removed is determined by how much correction in angulation is necessary. **C,** Distal portion of tibia is swung to proximal portion. Correction of angulation obtained allows weight-bearing forces to be more evenly distributed through both compartments of knee.

ited to the following:

1. Patient can explain the disease process, the applicability of treatment measures, and plans for follow-up with the physician.
2. Patient states he or she is feeling more comfortable.
3. Patient balances rest and activity appropriately.
4. Patient demonstrates improved ability to perform self-care activities.
5. Patient can state rationale for not exceeding ideal weight.

## ♦ INTERVENTIONS

As with rheumatoid arthritis, teaching the person with degenerative joint disease about the disease process and the steps to take to control that process is the most important aspect of nursing care. (See Research box, p. 2266.) Patient teaching should include the same types of information outlined on p. 2250. Other interventions are the same as those described for care of persons with rheumatoid arthritis, p. 2249.

### Special Postoperative Care

As noted above, surgical interventions may be necessary to remove damaged bone or cartilage from the joint, realign or change the weight-bearing surfaces of the joint, or resurface the joint. The objectives of surgery are to relieve pain, restore joint function (if possible), and prevent disability or further progression of the disease.

Surgery to the knee and hip is most common, but shoulder surgery is becoming more practical and effective. The following specific surgeries are performed:

1. Debridement (usually by arthroscopic surgery or arthrotomy).
   a. See Table 65-8 for postoperative nursing care.
2. Arthrodesis
   a. Through fusion of the joint, pain is relieved; joint motion is lost, but weight-bearing function is maintained. See Table 65-8 for postoperative care.
3. Osteotomy
   a. Bone is cut to change alignment, thereby correcting deformity in the bone or adjacent joint. The procedure corrects angulation or rotational deformities or alters the weight-bearing surface in a diseased joint (Figure 65-24). Osteotomy may be thought of as a surgical or intentional fracture, and the extremity is treated as following a fracture with the exception that weight bearing may be started earlier to promote healing. Immobilization of the extremity and nursing interventions are similar to those used following a fracture (see Chapter 64).
4. Two types of arthroplasty
   a. Interposition involves resurfacing of one side of the joint with metal or other inert material or soft tissue such as fascia.
   b. Replacement involves resurfacing of both sides of the joint with metal or polyethylene implants. Replacement implants are available for

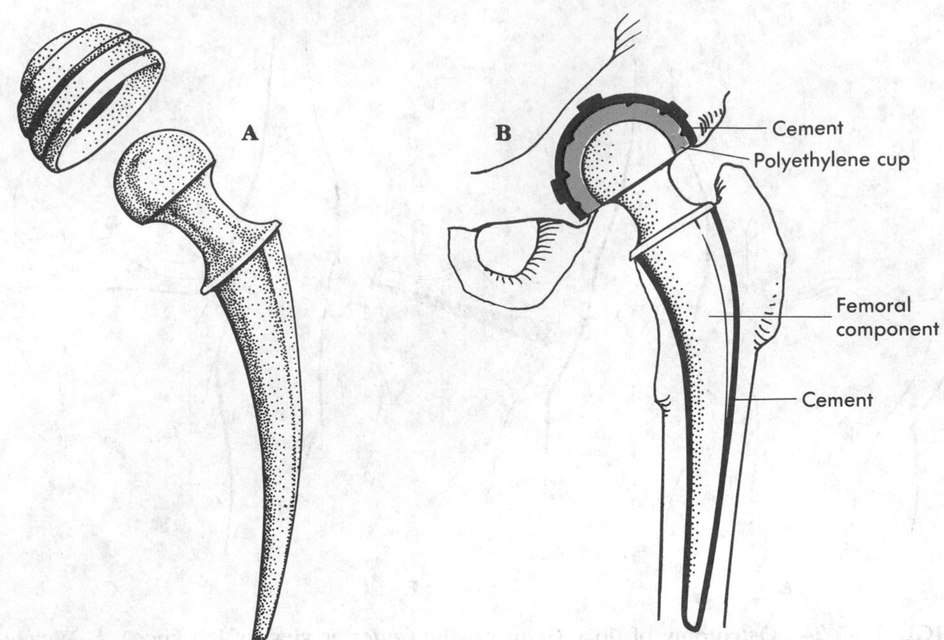


**FIGURE 65-25** **A,** Acetabular and femoral components of total hip prosthesis. **B,** Total hip prosthesis in place.

the hip (Figure 65-25), knee (Figure 65-26), shoulder, ankle, elbow, wrist, and interphalangeal joints of the fingers. Replacement prostheses may be either *cemented* (held into bone with polymethylmethacrylate) or *uncemented* (treated with a special porous coating that promotes ingrowth of bone).

The care of persons experiencing total hip or knee replacement is described in the Guidelines boxes. Understanding the mobility restrictions is of utmost importance when providing patient care (see nursing care plan on p. 2252). Of equal importance is the prevention of infection. The area of the operation must be kept free of contamination. Infection of bone implanted with prosthetic materials will require removal of the prosthesis. *Prevention of infection continues after the wound has healed; antibiotic prophylaxis must be given for future surgeries, dental work involving scraping or extraction, severe trauma or contaminated skin wounds, or systemic bacterial infection (respiratory or urinary).*

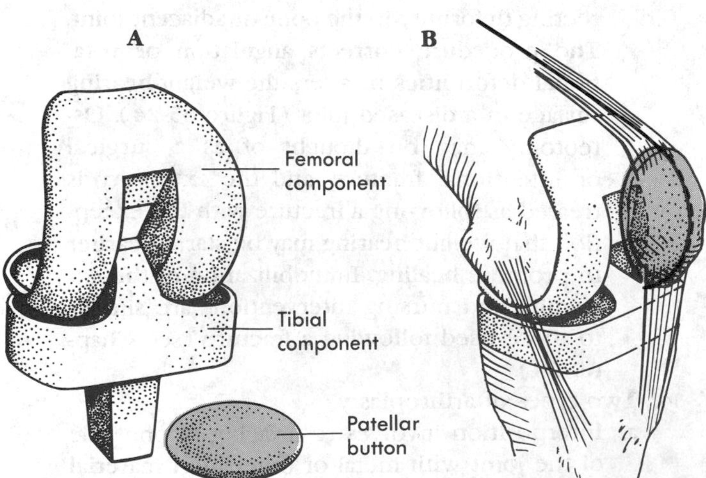


**FIGURE 65-26** **A,** Tibial and femoral components of total knee prosthesis. Patellar button, made of polyethylene, protects posterior surface of patella from friction against femoral component when knee is moved through flexion and extension. **B,** Total knee prosthesis in place.

## Nursing management of the patient with total knee arthroplasty

Postoperative management of the person with a total knee arthroplasty may include the use of a *continuous passive motion (CPM) machine* (Figure 65-28). The CPM machine supports the lower extremity while passively moving it within preset limits of flexion and extension. *Use of the CPM machine reduces postoperative swelling, prevents adhesions, decreases pain, and facilitates early mobility.* Research indicates it results in a significant increase in early and late range of knee flexion.[18] The CPM is applied immediately after surgery (usually in the operating or recovery room). Patients are encouraged to use the machine whenever they are in bed, up to 22 hours per day. Increases in the amount of knee flexion are ordered by the physician. CPM machines are also used in the postoperative management of persons with limb salvage surgery and have been beneficial in reducing pain and increasing mobility.[11]

## Complications

Complications after major orthopedic procedures such as total joint replacement include those associated with

DO

DO NOT

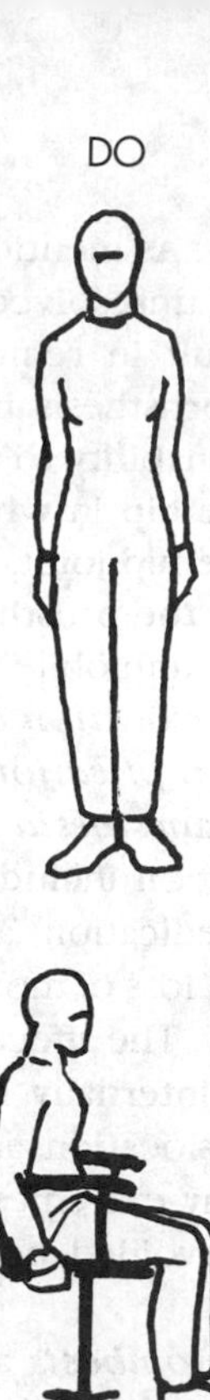

Do not cross your operated leg past the midline of the body or turn your kneecap in toward your body.

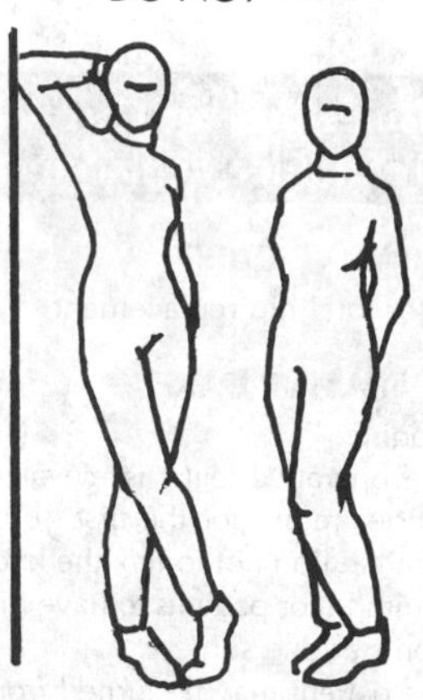

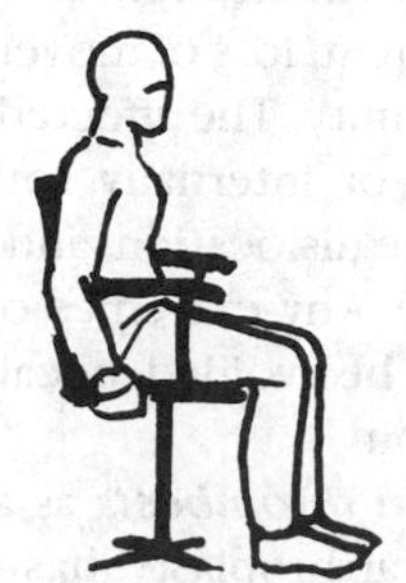

Do not sit in low chairs or cross your legs.

To sit: Use a high chair with arms or add pillows to elevate the seat.

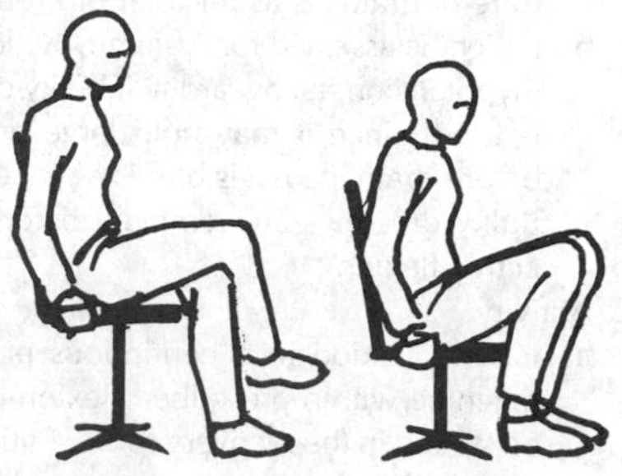

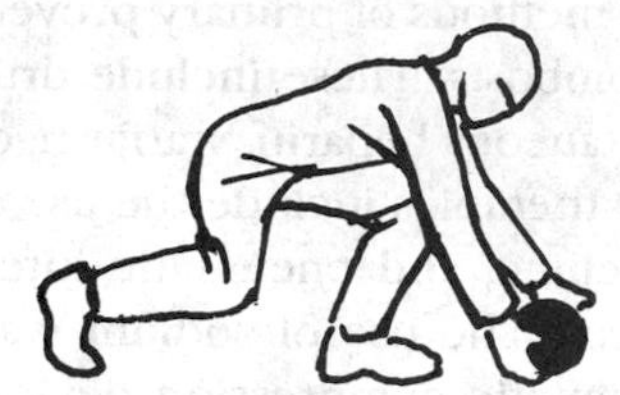

Avoid flexing your hip past 90 degrees.

To bend: Keep the operative leg behind you or as instructed by your therapist.

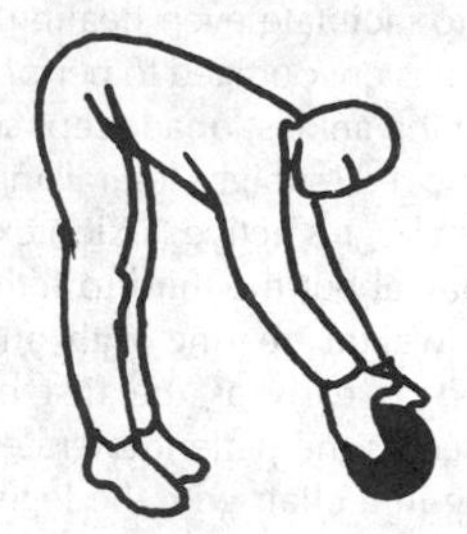

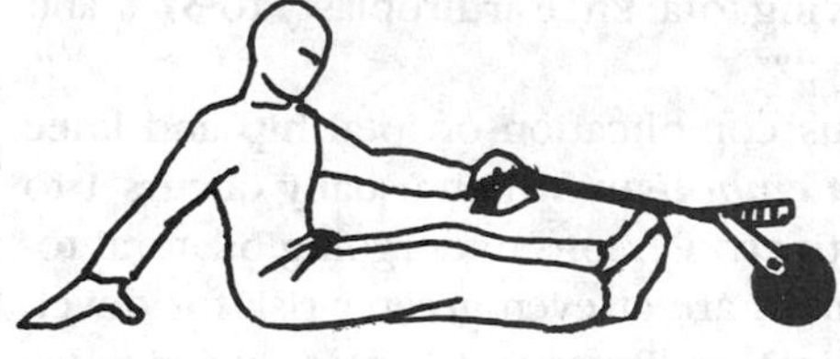

To reach: Use long-handled grabbers or as therapist advises.

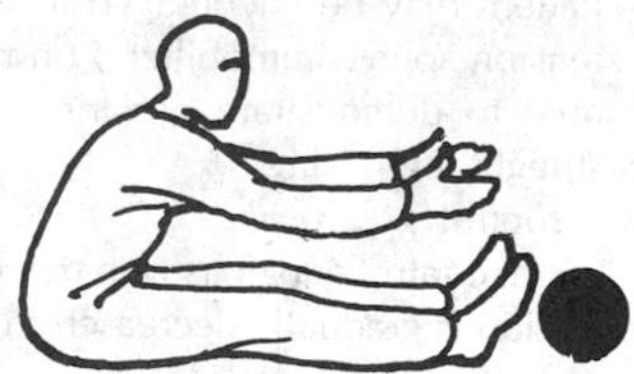

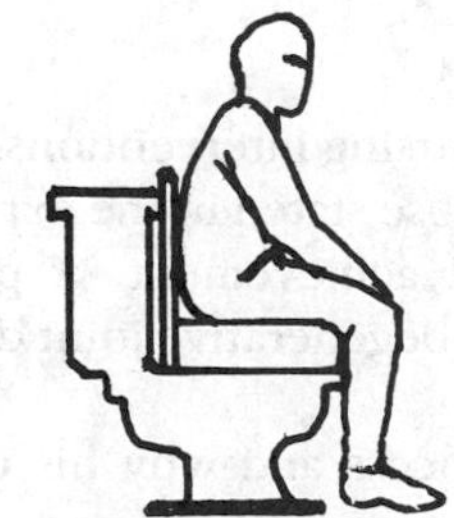

Use an elevated toilet.

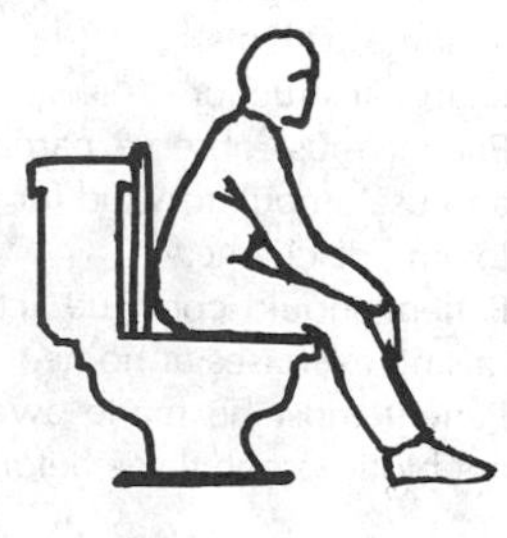

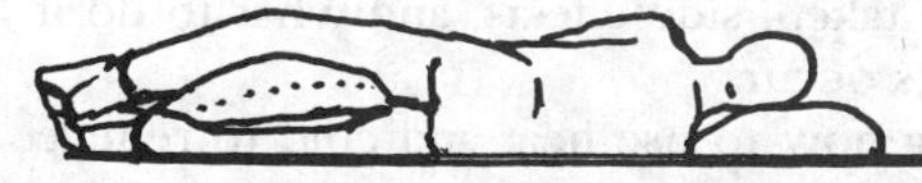

Sleep with a pillow between the legs.

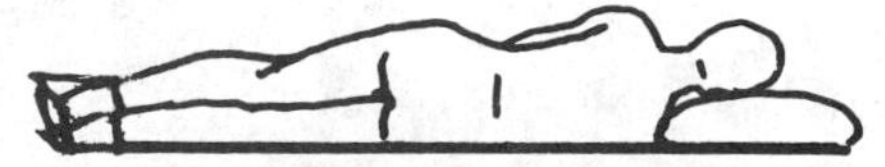

**FIGURE 65-27** Home-going instructions illustrating *DO's* and *DO NOTs* for patients with a total hip replacement. Patients are to avoid extreme flexion (past 90 degrees), adduction, and internal rotation of the operated hip—any of which may cause dislocation of the prosthesis. (Modified from Farrel J: *Illustrated guide to orthopaedic nursing*, ed 2, Philadelphia, 1982, JB Lippincott.)

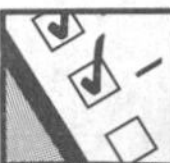

## Guidelines for Care for the Person With Total Knee Replacement

**PREOPERATIVE CARE**

Same as for total hip replacement

**POSTOPERATIVE CARE**

1. Positioning
   a. The operative leg(s) is elevated on pillows to enhance venous return for the first 48 hours. Pillows are placed with caution not to flex the knee(s). It is becoming more common for patients to have bilateral total knee replacements at one surgery.
   b. The patient may be turned from side to back to side.
2. Wound care
   a. Care of drains is as for total hip replacement.
   b. Patient is assessed for systemic evidence of loss of blood (hypotension, tachycardia) if bulky compression dressing is used, since it may hold large quantities of drainage before drainage is visible.
   c. Bulky dressings are removed before the patient begins active flexion.
3. Activity
   a. Passive flexion in a continuous passive motion (CPM) machine within prescribed flexion-extension limits may be started in the recovery room. Patient's leg may remain in machines as much as tolerated (up to 22 hours per day) to facilitate even healing of tissue.
   b. Patient is encouraged to perform active dorsiplantar flexion of the ankles, quadriceps setting, and, after the drain is removed, straight leg-raising exercises.
   c. Patient begins active flexion exercises three to four times per day about the third to fifth postoperative day.
   d. Light weight bearing with an assistive device may be started as early as the first postoperative day and increased as the patient tolerates.
   e. Sitting in a chair with the leg(s) elevated may be started on the first postoperative day.
   f. Patient may be encouraged to wear a resting knee extension splint (immobilizer) on the operated leg(s) until able to demonstrate quadriceps control (independent straight leg raising).
4. Pain control
   a. Initial control of pain is with narcotics, positioning; medication is gradually decreased to nonnarcotic analgesics as patient tolerates.
   b. Patient is encouraged to apply ice to knee(s) for 20 to 30 minutes before and following active flexion exercise.
   c. Ice may be prescribed more frequently to reduce pain in some patients.
5. Discharge instructions
   a. Patient must observe partial weight-bearing restriction and use ambulatory aid for approximately 2 months following discharge.
   b. Patient should continue active flexion and straight leg-raising exercises at home.
   c. Patient must be made aware of the lifelong need for antibiotic prophylaxis before surgery or dental work.

general anesthesia and immobility. As mentioned, infection is a serious complication. If unresolved, infection after joint replacement may result in removal of the prosthesis. Replacement of the prosthesis may not be possible. In the case of total hip, inability to replace the prosthesis results in a girdlestone hip in which fibrous scar tissue eventually replaces the hip joint. In the case of total knee, inability to replace the prosthesis results in arthrodesis of the knee and an immobile joint.

*After total hip arthroplasty, dislocation of the prosthesis is a potentially serious complication that may result in additional surgery or anesthesia to relocate the hip.* Signs of possible dislocation include a sudden onset of pain not relieved by medication, a "popping" sound associated with movement, loss of movement, leg length discrepancy, and deformity. The affected extremity may be either externally or internally rotated, depending on the direction of the dislocation, and the head of the femur may be palpable. Any extremes of flexion, adduction, or rotation should be avoided, because these motions may cause dislocation.

The incidence of *deep vein thrombosis* as a complication following total knee arthroplasty has been reported as high as 84%.[16] Pulmonary embolus can occur in 10% of patients following total knee arthroplasty. There are several accepted methods of primary prevention against deep vein thrombosis. These include drug therapy with aspirin, subcutaneous heparin, warfarin, or intravenous dextran. Other therapies include the use of elastic stockings, CPM machine, and pneumatic intermittent compression devices. The use of sodium warfarin (Coumadin) and pneumatic compression devices has been shown to decrease the incidence of deep vein thrombosis following total knee arthroplasty to 31% and 33%, respectively.[16]

Another serious complication of total hip and knee arthroplasty is *fat embolism,* which usually occurs 1 to 4 days postoperatively. Persons undergoing bilateral total joint replacement are at even greater risk for developing this complication. Refer to Chapter 64 for a discussion of fat embolism.

## ♦ EVALUATION

To evaluate effectiveness of nursing interventions, compare patient behaviors with those stated in the expected patient outcomes. Successful achievement of patient outcomes for the patient with degenerative joint disease is indicated by the following:

1. Describing disease process and why his or her joints are stiff, painful, or swollen
2. Describing prescribed medications and how they should be taken, side effects, and what to do if side effects occur
3. Describing how to use heat and cold to relieve joint pain
4. Describing rationale for activity or position restrictions

### Guidelines for Care for the Person With Total Hip Replacement

**PREOPERATIVE CARE**

1. Skin care
   a. Preparation of the skin will follow the hospital's written procedure or the physician's written orders.
   b. Patient's environment must be as free as possible from potential sources of infection.
2. Reassurance and education
   a. Patient needs to understand about the surgical procedure, postoperative care, and limitations after discharge.
   b. Both hips may be replaced at one surgery.

**POSTOPERATIVE CARE**

1. Positioning
   a. Positioning will depend on the design of the prosthesis and the method of insertion. Restrictions designed to avoid dislocation of the prosthesis usually include the following:
      (1) Flexion is limited to 60 degrees for 6 to 7 days, then 90 degrees for 2 to 3 months.
      (2) No adduction is permitted beyond midline for 2 to 3 months, therefore no side lying on operative side unless ordered by the surgeon. Leg is maintained in abduction when lying supine or on nonoperative side.
      (3) No extreme internal or external rotation is permitted (see Figure 65-27).
2. Wound care
   a. Drains are placed in wound to prevent formation of hematoma.
   b. Maintain constant suction through self-contained suction device (e.g., Porto-Vac).
   c. Note amount and types of drainage.
   d. Keep area free from contamination.
3. Activity
   a. Observe flexion restrictions when elevating head of bed.
   b. Encourage periodic elevation and lowering of head of bed to provide motion at hip.
   c. Instruct patient in use of overhead trapeze to shift weight and lift for bedpan, change of linen.
   d. Encourage active dorsiplantar flexion exercise of ankles and quadriceps and gluteal setting exercises to promote venous return, prevent thrombus formation, and maintain muscle tone (see Chapter 25).
   e. Patient may be turned to unoperative side with operative leg maintained in abduction and extension.
   f. Begin ambulation as early as the first postoperative day, if tolerated.
      (1) Observe flexion and adduction restrictions.
      (2) Observe weight-bearing restrictions prescribed by surgeon (usually partial weight bearing assisted with walker or crutches).
      (3) Increase amount of walking each day according to patient's tolerance.
   g. Begin sitting when patient demonstrates sufficient control of leg to sit within flexion restrictions (usually requires elevation of sitting surfaces, including use of raised toilet seat).
4. Medications
   a. Prophylactic anticoagulant drugs (acetylsalicylic acid, low-dose heparin, or sodium warfarin [Coumadin]) may be prescribed to decrease risk of thrombus formation.
   b. Initially, control pain with positioning; use narcotics, gradually tapered to nonnarcotic analgesics according to patient's tolerance.
5. Discharge instructions
   a. Patient must use ambulatory aid, avoid adduction, and limit hip flexion to 90 degrees for about 2 to 3 months (see Figure 65-27).
   b. A raised toilet seat is to be obtained and used at home until flexion restrictions are removed.
   c. Patient may need a long-handled shoe horn and reacher to facilitate ADL within flexion restriction.
   d. Patient must be made aware of the lifelong need for antibiotic prophylaxis to protect the prosthesis from bacteremic infection.

5. Discussing plans for follow-up care
6. Indicating on pain scale that pain is reduced to 1 or less (0 = no pain, 10 = extreme pain)
7. Appearing relaxed and giving no physical indications of being in pain
8. Resting before and after doing prescribed exercises and ADL
9. Performing ADL and other activities without assistance
10. Explaining that maintaining ideal weight will reduce stress on joints and reduce pain and immobility

## DEGENERATIVE DISORDERS OF THE SPINE

### Etiology

Back pain is the second leading cause following upper respiratory illnesses of physician office visits.[10] In the United States, 8 out of 10 people experience back problems during their life span.[13] It is estimated that 200,000 to 500,000 laminectomies are performed annually in the United States and that the cost of back problems is nearly 16 billion dollars annually.[13] The incidence of back pain in the United States is similar to the incidence in Scandinavia, Israel, and the Netherlands, but the United States has a higher rate of surgical intervention.[3]

### Epidemiology

Back problems usually present in persons between 20 to 30 years of age, adding to the expense of the disorder because of time lost from employment and because of the cost of illness and injury benefits. Of all persons experiencing back pain, only 14% have episodes exceeding 2 weeks.[10]

Risk factors associated with low back pain include occupational hazards, smoking, osteoporosis, and hyperparathyroidism. Occupational hazards include repetitive lifting, forward bending and twisting motions, and repeated prolonged exposure to vibrations.[20]

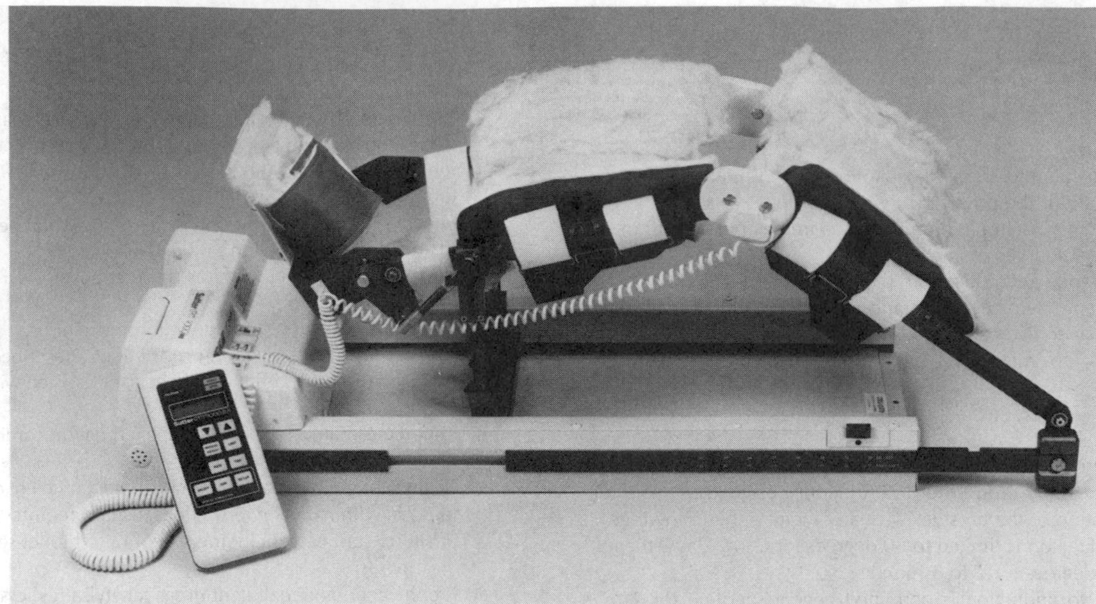

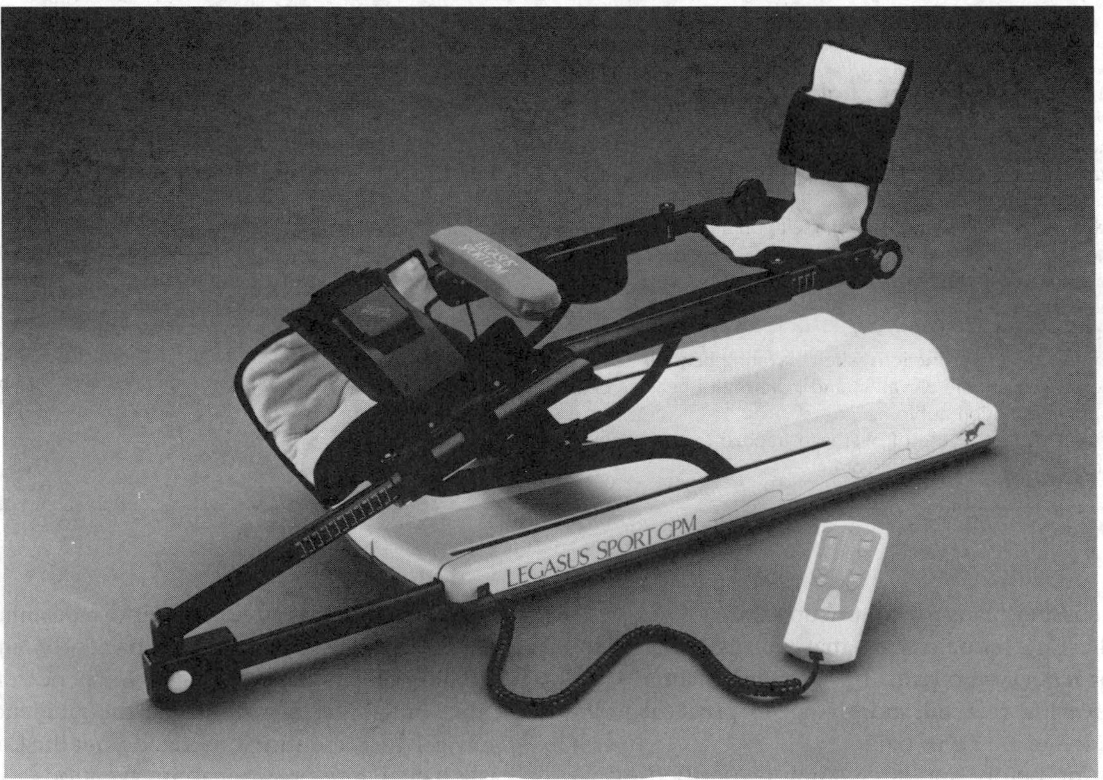


FIGURE 65-28 Examples of CPM machines. (Courtesy Sutter Corp.)

Spine surgery is performed on the cervical, thoracic, and lumbar spine for a variety of reasons. Some examples are herniated disks, intractable pain, tumors, trauma, congenital and developmental anomalies, neurologic compromise, and infections.

For approximately 85% of the people who experience back pain, there is no definitive diagnosis. In the case of some persons who undergo surgical intervention, the pain is not relieved or it recurs. When caring for persons with chronic pain, in some settings it may be appropriate to make a referral to a pain support group, such as the American Chronic Pain Association. Information may be obtained at the following address:

American Pain Society
5700 Old Orchard Rd., first floor
Skokie, IL
60077-1024
Phone: (708) 966-9418

Also refer to Chapter 17 for more information.

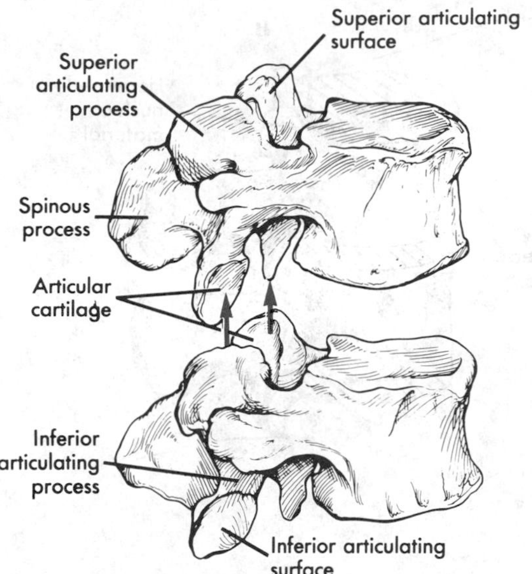


**FIGURE 65-29** Posterior facet joints of lumbar vertebrae. Each vertebra has four surfaces by which it articulates with its adjacent vertebrae: two on its superior aspect and two on the inferior. Superior articulating surfaces are medially located; the inferior, laterally. These joints are diarthrotic, having a joint capsule with a synovial lining.

**BOX 65-6 Possible Signs and Symptoms of Herniated Intervertebral Disk**

**CERVICAL**

Decreased range of motion of cervical spine
Paresthesias of upper extremities, depending on nerve root involved
Weakness or atrophy of upper extremity musculature, depending on level involved
Pain in affected nerve root distribution
Abdominal reflex activity
May have motor or sensory disturbances in lower extremities

**LUMBAR**

Tenderness or pain with palpation of disk spaces and sciatic notch
Painful and/or decreased range of motion of lumbar spine
Motor and sensory impairment in affected nerve root distribution (may note discrepancies in calf circumference, weakness in lower extremity muscle groups)
Decreased or absent reflexes
Bowel or bladder impairment
Positive straight leg raising (Lasegue's test): straight leg raising with opposite leg flat will produce leg pain or radicular symptoms
Pain in lower back and along course of sciatic nerve (sciatica)
Pain relieved by lying down

## Pathophysiology

Degenerative disease of the spine is a common but difficult problem that merits special consideration. The spine has 23 intervertebral disk joints and 46 posterior facet joints (Figure 65-29), all of which are subjected to stresses and strains in holding the human body upright and moving it about. The vertebrae in the spinal column are articulated in a series of "couplets" that are able to move through an intervertebral disk joint and two posterior facet joints. The intervertebral disks are composed of an outer layer of cartilage called the *anulus fibrosus* and an inner layer of cartilage called the *nucleus pulposus.* Several common problems arise with these structures in degenerative disease of the spine:

1. **Degenerative disk disease** occurs most commonly in individuals over 50 years of age. The normally elastic and gelatinous consistency of the nucleus pulposus is replaced by fibrocartilage. The disk space narrows with aging, losing its resiliency. The most frequent complaint is chronic low back pain.
2. **Herniated intervertebral disk** is a protrusion of the nucleus pulposus through a tear or rupture in the anulus. Herniation can occur anteriorly, posteriorly, or laterally. Extrusion of the disk material may impinge on a nerve root or on the spinal cord (Figure 65-30). Herniation may occur as a result of trauma, a sharp or sudden movement, or degeneration. In the cervical spine, herniation usually occurs at the C5-6 level. Lumbar herniations occur most frequently at L5-S1 and L4-5 (Box 65-6). Herniation of thoracic disks is rare. Symptoms may develop immediately or take years to manifest themselves. The location and size of the herniation will determine the signs and symptoms associated with the herniation. The nurse's knowledge of dermatomes and spinal nerve innervation will aid in the assessment of a patient with a herniated intervertebral disk (Table 65-10). Another consideration is the size of the patient's spinal canal. A slight herniation may cause significant symptoms in an individual with a congenitally narrow canal.
3. **Spinal stenosis** is a narrowing of the spinal canal or intervertebral foramina at any level. It creates pressure on the involved nerve root(s), resulting in neurologic symptoms. Patients may report a gradual onset of low back and leg pain that increases with walking and is relieved by sitting or lying down. A careful history and physical assessment will help to rule out vascular disorders, because the claudication type of pain the patient may report is like that seen in vascular disease. Spinal stenosis may develop as a result of aging, degenerative disk disease, spondylosis, or osteophyte formation.
4. **Spondylolisthesis** is a forward slipping of one vertebra on another. Spondylolisthesis can be a congenital abnormality or caused by degenerative changes, trauma, or bone disease. It is graded on a scale of 1 to 4, depending on the percentage of slip that is shown on x-rays of the spine. Grades 3 and 4 are usually treated surgically. Spondylolisthesis usually occurs at L5-S1 but can also occur at the L4-5 and L3-4 levels.[31] The forward slip of the vertebra can

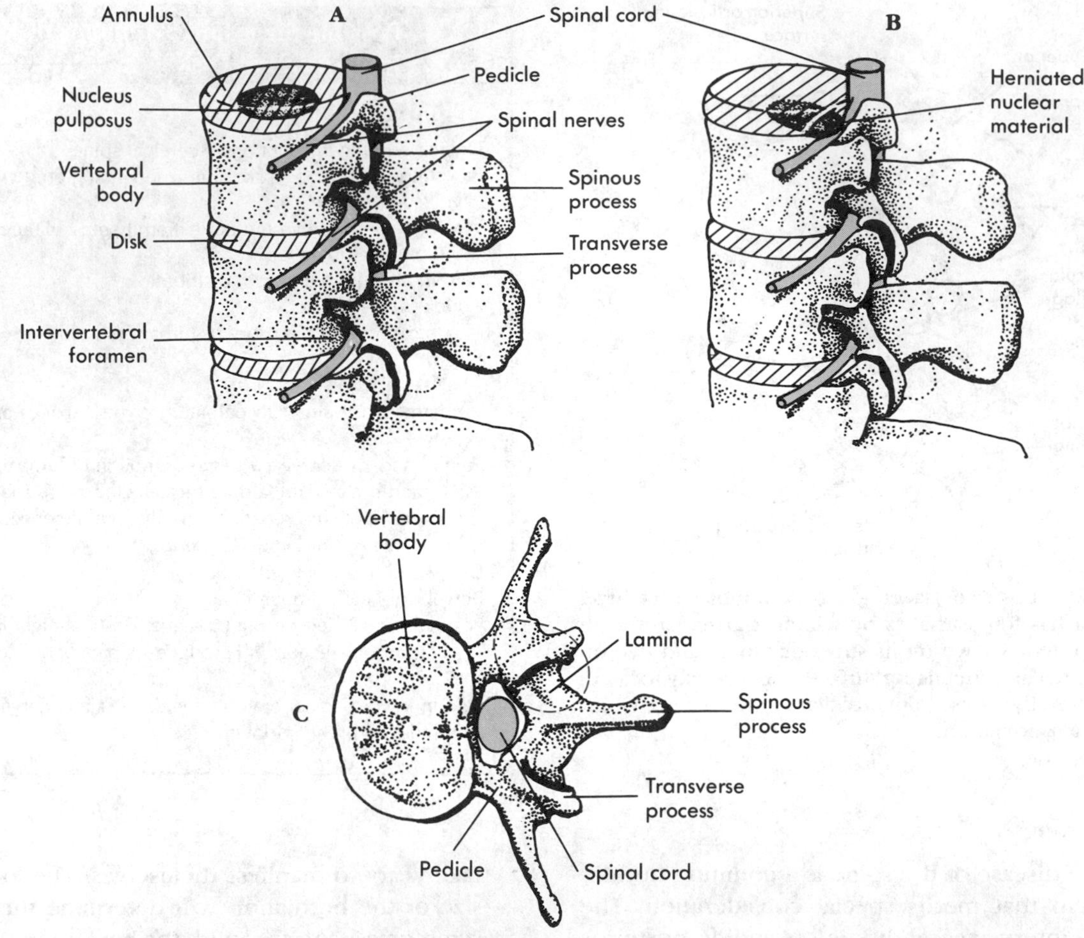


**FIGURE 65-30** Compression of spinal cord and nerve root. **A,** Disks, composed of cartilaginous outer layer (anulus fibrosus) and gellike inner layer (nucleus pulposus), lie between vertebral bodies. Spinal nerves exit the spinal cord laterally just above the pedicle. **B,** Laminae compose posterior portion of vertebrae. Each pedicle joins with a lamina *(dotted line);* the transverse and spinous processes project from laminae. **C,** When nucleus pulposus herniates posteriorly through its fibrous covering and the posterior longitudinal ligament, it may compress the spinal cord and trap the nerve root. Surgical approach to relieve this compression is through lamina, posterior to transverse process.

cause nerve impingement, manifested by motor and sensory deficits at the level(s) involved, such as pain, weakness, and/or bowel and bladder involvement. The slip may be detected when palpating the spinous processes.

5. **Osteophyte formation** along the vertebral column can cause fusion of vertebrae with consequent limitation of motion, usually in the lumbosacral region.
6. **Degenerative and/or rheumatoid involvement** of the hyaline articular surfaces of the facet joints results in pain and limited motion. Rheumatoid involvement with consequent loss of vertebral stability is particularly troublesome when it occurs in the cervical spine.

## Medical Management

The expected length of stay of patients with spinal surgery as determined by DRG is 6 days. Common medical therapy for management of spinal surgery includes the following.

### Diagnostic tests

Diagnostic tests to determine defects in the spine include x-ray films, myelography, CT scanning, and MRI. See Chapter 63 for more information.

### Medication

Conservative management of degenerative problems of the spine includes the use of antiinflammatory agents (usually nonsteroidal antiinflammatory drugs [NSAIDs]). The use of NSAIDs may cause gastric irritation or ulceration, drowsiness, headache, fluid retention, weight gain, and fatigue. The patient should be advised to take the medication with food or milk. Concomitant use of alcohol or aspirin may increase gastrointestinal irritation and bleeding tendencies and therefore should be

**TABLE 65-10 Lumbar Disk Herniation**

| LEVEL OF HERNIATION | NERVE ROOT | REFLEX | SENSATION | MUSCLE TESTING |
|---|---|---|---|---|
| L3-4 | L4 | Patellar | Medial aspects of leg and foot | Inversion of foot (tibialis anterior) |
| L4-5 | L5 | — | Lateral aspect of leg and dorsal surface of foot | Extension of toes (extensor hallucis longus) |
| L5-S1 | S1 | Achilles | Lateral aspect of foot | Eversion of foot (peroneus longus, brevis) |

avoided. Patients should be instructed to take medications as prescribed to maintain therapeutic drug levels. After the patient begins drug therapy, pain relief may not be noted for 1 week. If the patient has dental work or surgery while taking NSAIDs, the surgeon or dentist should be informed because of increased bleeding tendency. An ophthalmic and auditory examination, complete blood count (CBC), and baseline evaluation of renal and hepatic function should be performed at the initiation of drug therapy and at regular intervals thereafter for individuals receiving high doses or long-term therapy.

The use of narcotic analgesics is usually avoided, especially over a prolonged period of time, because of the risks of dependency and tolerance. If narcotic analgesics are used, the patient should be cautioned against driving or operating machinery and to avoid the use of alcohol while taking medication. Patients should also be informed of possible side effects, such as constipation and dry mouth, and measures to decrease their incidence.

Skeletal muscle relaxants may also be prescribed. The patient should be cautioned against driving or engaging in potentially hazardous activities because of drowsiness, a frequent side effect of muscle relaxants. The patient should be informed that the use of alcohol or other CNS depressants will enhance the effect of the muscle relaxant. Muscle relaxants frequently cause dry mouth, and the nurse can instruct the patient in measures to counteract this side effect.

**Treatment**

1. Heat to affected joints
2. Traction to relieve muscle spasm
   a. Bilateral Buck's traction (see p. 2193 for discussion of types of traction)
   b. Pelvic traction
3. A corset sometimes prescribed to provide external support to the spine when activity is resumed

**Diet**

Although a special diet is not indicated for the treatment of degenerative disorders of the spine, weight reduction may be advised in the case of an overweight individual. Every effort should be made to attain or maintain ideal body weight in order to decrease the mechanical stressors on the back, as well as other joints.

**Activity**

1. Encouraging rest (complete or modified, depending on the severity of symptoms)
2. Promoting comfort
   a. Encourage slight elevation of head of bed and flexion of the knees when supine (Figure 65-31).
   b. Roll patient onto bedpan rather than lifting onto bedpan.
   c. Use fracture bedpan or small bedpan.
   d. Instruct patient in logrolling (Figure 65-32).
   e. Instruct patient in good body mechanics (see Figure 65-14).
3. Promoting circulation
   a. Encourage patient to perform active dorsiplantar flexion of the ankles at regular intervals.
4. Physical therapy

The physical therapist will instruct the patient in a program to strengthen the muscles of the back and abdomen, which will increase support of the vertebral column. The patient will also be taught exercises to increase flexibility, which will enable the person to bend and move with less chance of injury. Aerobic exercises, such as swimming, may be prescribed to improve overall conditioning and to maintain or reduce weight, without placing stress on the back. The patient will be advised to avoid lifting heavy objects, participating in contact sports, and extreme twisting or bending of the spine.

**Referral/Consultation**

In some settings the nurse assumes responsibility for making referrals to other services. A referral to a back school or occupational therapist may be initiated to assist the patient and family to function effectively within the confines of the patient's disability. Emphasis is placed on body mechanics and modifications of daily routines to decrease the possibility of further injury. Job retraining may be indicated. Sometimes a referral to a pain management center is initiated, especially in the case of an individual having difficulty coping with chronic pain. In cases where back or leg pain persists longer than 6 weeks, or if a psychologic component of pain is suspected, a psychologic referral may be indicated.

## Surgical Management

Most spinal disorders are treated conservatively. Surgery is indicated when conservative modalities fail

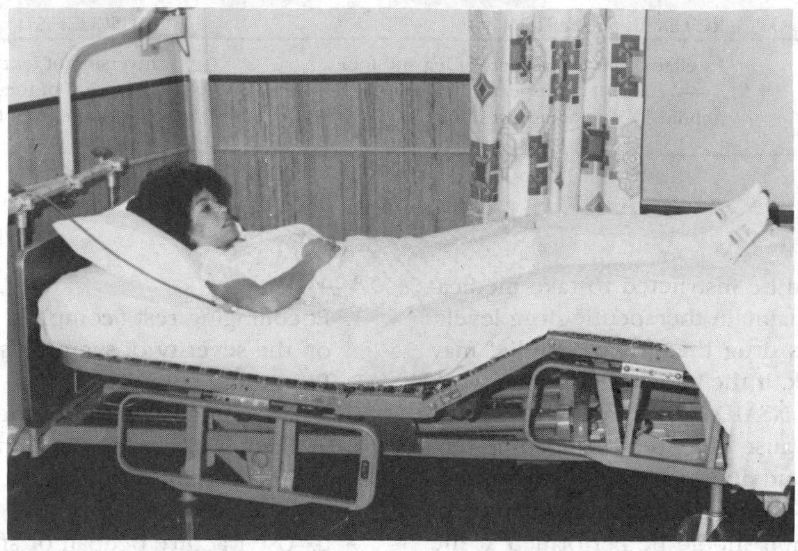

**FIGURE 65-31** Elevating head of bed 20 to 30 degrees and flexing knees provide comfortable position for patients with acute back pain.

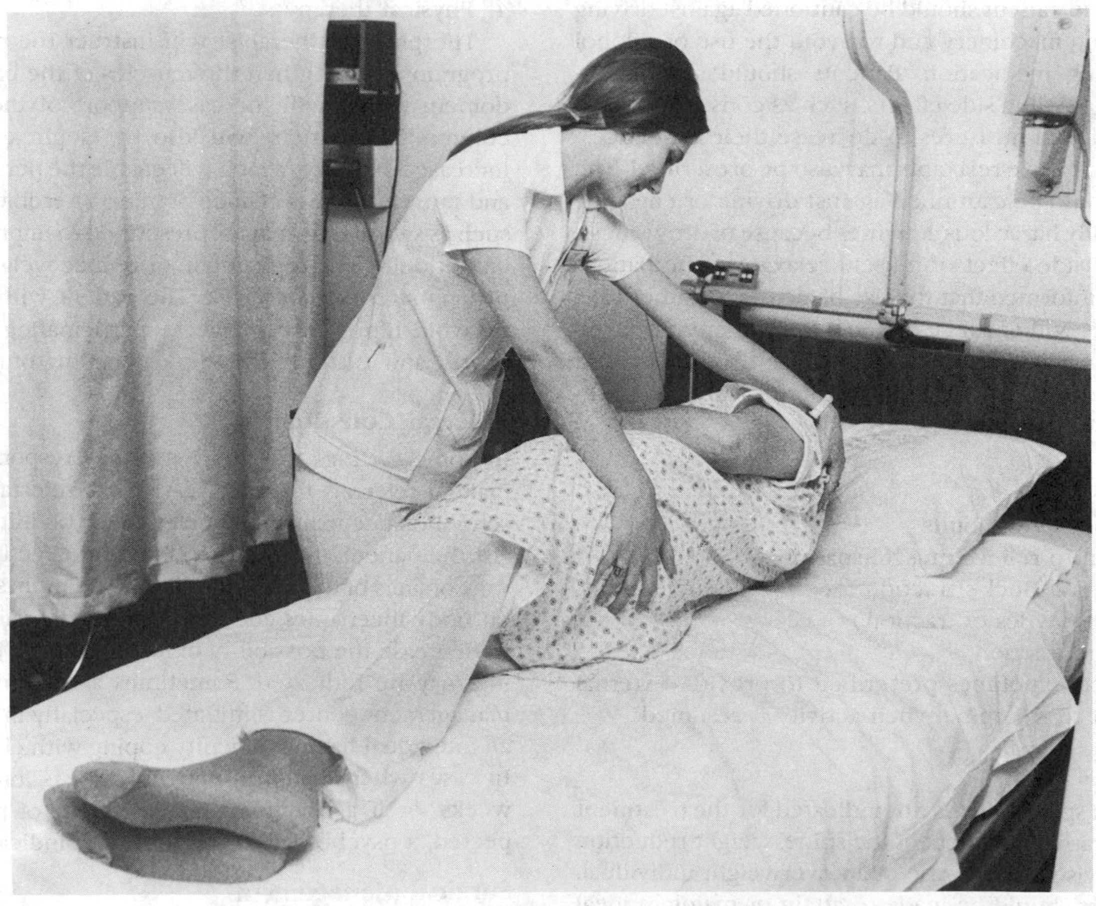

**FIGURE 65-32** Logrolling patient. Patient crosses arms over chest, holds legs in extension and feet together. Nurse supports patient at level of shoulders and buttocks.

**BOX 65-7 Types of Spinal Surgery**

**Laminectomy**—Removal of a portion of the lamina
**Diskectomy**—Removal of all or part of a herniated intervertebral disk
**Foraminotomy**—Widening of the intervertebral foramen to allow free passage of the spinal nerve
**Spinal fusion**—Fusion of two or more vertebrae by insertion of bone grafts with or without the addition of metal rods or wires to achieve vertebral stability; fusion is required when thoracic and cervical vertebrae are involved because of mobility of the spine in these areas

or for the following reasons:

1. Worsening neurologic symptoms: loss of bowel or bladder control or loss of motor function (paralysis)
2. Severe intractable pain
3. Bony instability
4. Progressive deformity with resultant loss of function

Spinal surgery is also performed for fractures and tumors, which are discussed in Chapter 64. A variety of procedures are performed on the cervical, thoracic, and lumbar spine. Surgical approaches to the spine include *anterior,* as for a *cervical diskectomy; transthoracic* or *retroperitoneal,* for *anterior spinal fusion;* and *posterior,* as for a *lumbar laminectomy.* Box 65-7 gives types of spine surgery.

In some instances, lumbar diskectomy can also be accomplished by *chemonucleolysis,* a procedure that involves injecting the disk with *chymopapain,* an enzyme that breaks down the collagen fibers in the disk, thereby lessening the pressure from the ruptured disk. There is some controversy regarding the effectiveness of this procedure.

Two newer methods of treating "contained" herniated disks, that is, disks that have not penetrated the anulus, are *percutaneous endoscopic diskectomy and microdiskectomy.* Both of these procedures involve a limited surgical exposure and faster recovery time.

Spinal surgery may involve the use of instrumentation. A number of different implants are on the market today. Instrumentation is used to maintain correction of deformity, stabilize the spine, prevent neurologic damage, enhance bony fusion, avoid external immobilization, and allow for early mobilization, thereby facilitating rehabilitation.[17] The type of instrumentation used depends on the pathologic condition, individual patient, and surgeon preference. Table 65-11 gives examples of spinal instrumentation.

Some types of spinal surgery involve the use of bone grafts. Bone grafts function as a form of scaffolding into which osteogenic cells grow and/or as a means of mechanical support. In addition to their use in spinal fusions, they are also used for patients with fractures, with tumors, and needing joint replacements. The three types of bone grafts are autograft, xenograft, and allograft. **Autograft,** or the patient's own bone or that of an identical twin, has the best result. **Xenograft** is a graft taken from a different species, for example, bovine bone. Xenografts are rarely used in the United States. **Allograft** is human bone harvested from either a cadaver or living donor. The success of the bone graft partially depends on the type of fixation of the graft and the site and condition of the host recipient.

Both cortical and cancellous bone can serve as graft material. Both allogeneic and autogenic cortical grafts initially act as weight-bearing struts to provide support until the host bone has incorporated and remodeled the graft and is able to bear weight. Freshly implanted autografts are capable of osteogenesis, the process of bone synthesis by graft or host cells. Cancellous bone, because of its larger surface area, has greater potential for osteogenesis than does cortical bone. Host bone is produced by osteoconduction, a process in which mesenchymal cells of the host differentiate into osteoblasts.

All types of bone graft are initially resorbed. Incorporation of the bone graft takes place in overlapping stages. It begins by *creeping substitution, gradual resorption of the graft, and finally replacement of the graft by new bone.* Both autografts and allografts produce an acute inflammatory response within the first week, followed by the formation of fibrous granulation tissue and an increase in osteoclastic activity. This is followed by osteoinduction, which is probably regulated by *bone morphogenic protein,* which promotes new bone production by the host.[15] Bone morphogenic protein is present in fresh autografts and in modified allografts. Autoclaving destroys bone morphogenic protein. Osteoinduction is followed by osteoconduction, characterized by capillary growth and infiltration of the graft by perivascular tissue and osteoprogenitor cells of the host. This process may last for several months in cancellous autografts and for years in cortical autografts or allografts.[15] Cancellous grafts are eventually completely replaced, whereas cortical grafts remain a mixture of necrotic graft bone and viable host bone. As remodeling takes place, the graft is resorbed and replaced by living bone, subject to Wolff's law.

Advantages of autografts are tissue compatibility and low cost. Disadvantages include a limited supply of bone, weakened donor site with a potential for fracture, and an added surgical site that can cause considerable pain for 2 to 3 years.[9,17] The most common sites for graft harvesting are the iliac crests and the fibulae.

Advantages of allograft are fewer surgical sites and thus less pain. Allografts also come in a variety of sizes and shapes. Disadvantages include a limited and costly supply and a high graft failure rate. Allografts trigger local and systemic immune responses that may affect their failure rate. Freezing and freeze-drying implants have decreased rejection, but frozen implants still have a 25% failure rate.[15] There is also a danger of transmitting dis-

**TABLE 65-11 Common Types of Spinal Instrumentation**

| INDICATIONS | APPROACH | COMPONENTS | ADVANTAGES AND DISADVANTAGES |
|---|---|---|---|
| **COTREL-DUBOUSSET (CD)** | | | |
| Idiopathic scoliosis, kyphosis, trauma | Posterior | Parallel rods<br>Hooks<br>Screws<br>C-rings<br>Cross-link plate | *Advantages:* ability to correct rib hump deformity; early mobilization; bracing not necessary<br>*Disadvantages:* time-consuming, difficult technique, difficult to revise; hook shift; expensive |
| **DWYER** | | | |
| Scoliosis<br>Kyphosis | Anterior (transthoracic retroperitoneal) | Cables<br>Staples<br>Screws<br>Bolts | *Advantages:* shorter fusion area than Harrington<br>*Disadvantages:* recurrence of deformity; loss of correction; risk to vascular structures and viscera |
| **DRUMMOND (WISCONSIN)** | | | |
| Scoliosis | Posterior | Rods<br>Hooks<br>Screws | *Advantages:* achieves segmental fixation without risks associated with sublaminar wiring<br>*Disadvantages:* increased operative time; decreased fusion area |
| **HARRINGTON** | | | |
| Thoracolumbar fracture scoliosis | Posterior | Rods<br>Hooks<br>Screws | *Disadvantages:* increased immobility postoperatively; instrument failure, breakage; loss of correction; inability to control rod; loss of lumbar lordosis; need to fuse above and below level of pathologic condition, resulting in immobile spine; requires bracing |
| **KANEDA** | | | |
| Thoracolumbar fracture<br>Kyphosis<br>Compromised spinal canal | Anterior (transthoracic retroperitoneal) | Threaded rods<br>Staples<br>Vertebral body screws<br>Nuts | *Advantages:* rigid fixation<br>*Disadvantages:* possibile damage to vascular structures |
| **LUQUE** | | | |
| Scoliosis<br>Kyphosis<br>Thoracolumbar fracture | Posterior | L-shaped rods<br>Sublaminar wires | *Advantages:* rigid stabilization; ability to contour rod<br>*Disadvantages:* risk of neural damage associated with sublaminar wiring |
| **PEDICLE SCREW AND PLATE SYSTEMS (ROY CAMILLE, AO, STEFFEE, DANEK)** | | | |
| Spinal instability<br>Spinal stenosis<br>Thoracolumbar fracture<br>Pseudarthroses<br>Failed instrumentation<br>Tumors<br>Spondylosis<br>Spondylolithesis | Posterior | Screws<br>Plates<br>Rods<br>Cables | *Advantages:* reduces deformity, restores alignment, and achieves stability while fusing fewer levels; rigid fixation; early, less painful mobility postoperatively<br>*Disadvantages:* screw breakage, failure; pseudoarthrosis; loosening of hardware; lengthy procedure; proximity of pin, screw to neural elements |
| **TSRH (TEXAS SCOTTISH RITE HOSPITAL)** | | | |
| Scoliosis<br>Spinal fracture<br>Tumor<br>Kyphosis | Anterior or posterior | Parallel rods<br>Cross-link plates<br>Hooks | *Advantages:* easily revised; can be adapted for anterior use; easily contoured rods; early ambulation<br>*Disadvantages:* pseudoarthrosis; hardware failure |
| **ZIELKE** | | | |
| Scoliosis<br>Kyphosis | Anterior (transthoracic retroperitoneal) | Threaded rods<br>Cables<br>Bone screws<br>Washers | *Advantages:* allows correction of rotational deformities; shorter fusion area than Harrington<br>*Disadvantage:* risk to vascular structures and viscera |
| **UNIT** | | | |
| Neuromuscular scoliosis | Posterior | Precontoured, continuous rod<br>Sublaminar wiring | *Advantages:* ends of rods able to be implanted in pelvis; stability: little rod migration; good correction of rotational deformities; correction of pelvic obliquity<br>*Disadvantage:* risk to neural elements associated with sublaminar wiring |

## Guidelines for Care for the Person With Lumbar Spinal Surgery

**PREOPERATIVE CARE**

1. Instruct patient in logrolling and performance of dorsiplantar flexion exercises.
2. Instruct patient about the surgical procedure, postoperative care, and expectations at discharge.

**POSTOPERATIVE CARE**

1. Positioning
   a. Head of bed is kept flat.
   b. Patient is encouraged to logroll to change position from side to back to side.
   c. Use of a turning sheet is advised until patient can assist with turning.
2. Neurologic checks to assess motor and sensory function
3. Wound care (drains placed in wound to prevent hematoma formation, if necessary)
   a. Maintain constant suction through drain as required.
   b. Maintain drain free of contamination.
   c. Monitor for excessive output from drains. Output ranges from 20 to 250 ml/8 hr for the first 24 hours, tapers for 12 hours postoperatively, and usually is removed 48 hours postoperatively. Drains that allow reinfusion of serous drainage may be used.
   d. Inspect surgical area frequently for evidence of excess drainage or formation of hematoma (bulging of tissues surrounding surgical site).
   e. If a spinal fusion has been done, inspect donor sites (usually iliac crest) for drainage, hematoma.
4. Promoting comfort
   a. Reposition patient frequently.
   b. Administer narcotic medications as needed; gradually reduce to nonnarcotic analgesics as patient tolerates.
   c. Monitor use and effectiveness of patient-controlled analgesia (PCA) pump, if ordered.
   d. Use fracture bedpan or small bedpan.
5. Promoting mobility
   a. Activity out of bed may begin as early as 1 day after surgery (laminectomy) or 3 to 5 days after surgery (laminectomy and fusion).
   b. Transfer patient out of bed with as little time spent in the sitting position as possible.
      (1) Start transfer with patient in a side-lying position at the edge of the bed.
      (2) Have the patient push off the bed with the uppermost hand and the lowermost elbow.
      (3) One person assists by guiding the patient's trunk, and another assists the patient's legs over the side of the bed.
      (4) Reverse process for return to bed.
   c. The patient may be permitted to walk as much as tolerated, with an assistive aid if necessary.
   d. Braces or corsets, if prescribed, are applied *before* the patient gets out of bed.
   e. Encourage patient to participate in ADL within prescribed limits of mobility.
6. Discharge instruction
   a. Do not lift or carry anything heavier than 2.25 kg (5 lb).
   b. Do not drive a car until permitted by surgeon.
   c. Avoid twisting motions of the trunk.

## Guidelines for Care for the Person With Thoracic Spinal Surgery

**PREOPERATIVE CARE**

Same as for lumbar surgery

**POSTOPERATIVE CARE**

Same as for lumbar surgery *with the following additions and exceptions:*

1. Positioning
   a. Head of bed may often be elevated to 30 degrees.
2. Wound care
   a. If pleural cavity is entered, a chest tube will be inserted and must be managed postoperatively (see Chapter 37).
3. Promoting comfort
   a. Assist patient to splint chest while coughing.
4. Promoting mobility
   a. Encourage and assist patient in vigorous pulmonary toileting.
   b. Assist patient to maintain bedrest for 1 week or longer with strict attention to avoidance of twisting or bending motions to prevent dislodging grafts.
   c. Discourage patient from vigorous pulling or pushing with the arms because weight bearing through the arms poses a threat to the integrity of the graft.
   d. Brace is routinely prescribed and must be applied before patient is allowed out of bed.
   e. Permit patient to perform whatever activities are comfortable within the limitations of the brace.
   f. Encourage patient to participate in ADL within prescribed limits of mobility.
5. Discharge instructions
   a. Apply and remove the brace before getting out of bed.
   b. Wear the brace whenever out of bed.

eases such as acquired immunodeficiency disease (AIDS) and hepatitis B with allograft bone. Refer to the section on bone tumor (p. 2291) for additional discussion of bone grafts.

### Nursing management of the patient with spinal surgery

Care after spinal surgery (lumbar, thoracic, or cervical) focuses on positioning and mobility, wound care, and patient comfort (see the Guidelines boxes on this page and on p. 2280 for guidelines about nursing interventions after surgery). Changing position in bed following spinal surgery must be performed by logrolling; assistance is given as necessary, but patients can learn to do this for themselves. Because patients tolerate sitting less well than walking or lying, sitting is avoided until the person can tolerate it.

Thoracic spinal surgery may involve entering the chest cavity, and if so, nursing care will include postoperative measures required following chest surgery (see Chapter 37). Mobility restrictions are more prolonged than with lumbar surgery, because the thoracic spine is more mobile; consequently, there is greater risk of dislodging grafts through improper motion.

## Guidelines for Care for the Person With Cervical Spinal Surgery

### PREOPERATIVE CARE

1. Follow general instructions as for any spine surgery.
2. If tong or halo traction or halo brace is to be used postoperatively, familiarize patient with the apparatus before surgery.

### POSTOPERATIVE CARE

1. Positioning
   a. Keep head of bed elevated 30 to 45 degrees, particularly if anterior surgical approach was used, to decrease swelling in throat.
   b. If patient is in cervical brace, position is not restricted except by patient's tolerance.
   c. If patient is in cervical traction, patient may be turned side to back to side to patient's tolerance.
2. Wound care
   a. Inspect surgical area, including iliac crest donor site, frequently for evidence of excess drainage or formation of hematoma.
   b. If *tong or halo traction* is being used, pin care may be required (see Chapter 64).
3. Promoting comfort and relieving pain
   a. Provide ice chips to soothe sore throat.
   b. Make progressive diet changes slowly; patient will have difficulty swallowing and will be afraid of choking. Full liquids (ice cream, custards, jello, nectars) are often better tolerated than clear juice or broth; however, milk products may increase mucous production.
   c. Administer analgesics as for any spine surgery. Donor sites often cause more discomfort than does neck incision.
   d. Patient may require aerosol treatments or humidification of air to loosen mucous secretions or make breathing more comfortable.
4. Promoting mobility
   a. If patient is in traction, encourage patient to perform ankle dorsiplantar flexion exercises and quadriceps setting on a regular basis to promote circulation and maintain leg strength.
   b. If patient is in brace, out-of-bed activity, including walking, may begin as soon as patient tolerates.
   c. Provide for temporary use of walker if donor site pain restricts mobility.
   d. Encourage patient to participate in ADL to greatest extent possible.
5. Promoting safety
   a. Provide suction equipment and tracheotomy set in patient's room until swelling in throat subsides and patient is swallowing and breathing normally.
   b. Check adjustment screws and straps frequently to ensure there is no loosening of the brace.
   c. Advise physician or orthotist of loosening of brace consequent to decrease in edema so brace can be readjusted.
6. Discharge instruction
   a. Wear brace at all times.
   b. Report any difficulty with brace to physician immediately.
   c. Do not drive a car during period that brace must be worn.

Persons with *cervical* spinal surgery may require tong or halo traction (see Chapter 64) or a halo brace. The person has edema of the throat in the early postoperative period, requiring attention to the person's ability to breathe and swallow.

Nursing care that is relevant to persons undergoing all types of spinal surgery will be discussed. Many persons having elective spinal surgery are admitted the morning of their surgery. Preoperative teaching and testing are completed and evaluated before admission. Preoperative evaluation may include the following: complete history and physical examination; laboratory work including complete blood count, urinalysis, SMA/18, prothrombin time, partial thromboplastin time, type, and crossmatch; chest x-ray, electrocardiogram, and diagnostics related to the spine, such as x-rays, myelography, CT, and MRI. Some patients may elect to participate in an *autologous* or *donor-directed blood program.* The optimal period for autologous donation is 4 to 6 weeks before the scheduled surgery date. The last donation must be completed at least 72 hours before surgery.[24] The patient must have a hemoglobin (HgB) of at least 11 g/dl and a hematocrit (Hct) of 33% to be eligible for autologous donation. These are recommendations of the National Blood Resource Group, and institutional policies may vary. If unable to participate in an autologous donor program, some patients may opt to obtain their own donors (designated or directed donors) in an effort to reduce chances of transmissible diseases. However, research indicates that designated donor blood is no safer than that of random volunteers[5]; in fact, it may carry more risk,[26] because donors may feel pressured to donate and conceal risk factors. Some agencies recommend that designated (directed) donor blood be irradiated to reduce graft versus host reaction.[13] The number of units requested will depend on the type of surgery planned. ***Bony fusion of multiple levels usually results in a greater blood loss because of muscle stripping required for exposure and the decortication of the host bed.*** Iron replacement therapy is usually advised for autologous donors.

If postoperative bracing will be required, the patient will be fitted for the brace and given instructions for its use preoperatively. Measurements and fabrication of the brace are done by an orthotist. Many types of braces are available, depending on the type of procedure performed. Some examples are cervical 4-poster braces, thoracic lumbar sacral orthoses (TLSO), and soft corsets.

General instructions should be given to the patient and family regarding hospital routines, visiting hours, and expected length of stay. Preoperative preparation should include an assessment of the patient's knowledge of the planned procedure and expected risks, benefits, and outcomes. Many patients are curious about the types of implants to be used. If a sample of the hardware is available, it may be helpful to show it to the patient. The patient should also be informed about the location and extent of the surgical incision(s). If a spinal fusion with autologous graft is planned, an explanation of donor site location and degree of postoperative pain is beneficial. The patient should also be informed if allograft bone is to be used. In some hospitals the information about the surgical procedure, grafts, and so on is given by a nurse from the operating room or recovery room.

The patient should be given instructions in performing logrolling, isometric exercises, incentive spirometry, and coughing and deep breathing. Instructions are also given regarding general postoperative care, such as postanesthesia care, IVs, catheters, vital sign routines, and pain management.

Perioperative care focuses on the prevention of injury and complications. The perioperative nurse can help allay the fears and anxieties frequently encountered by patients entering the operating room. After induction of anesthesia, careful attention is paid to positioning techniques, making sure that all potential pressure areas are well padded, ensuring that the thorax is supported to allow maximal chest expansion during ventilation and avoiding compression of the abdominal cavity to prevent vascular complications. Pneumatic sleeves and/or elastic stockings may be applied to avoid pooling of blood in the lower extremities. To avoid hypothermia the extremities may be covered with a heating device or warm blankets.

Postoperative care of the spinal patient includes interventions to prevent or minimize respiratory, elimination, and circulatory complications. Elastic stockings and pneumatic sleeves may be continued for postoperative care. Patients are instructed to perform isometric exercises hourly while awake. Low-dose aspirin (ASA), heparin, or sodium warfarin (Coumadin) may be used postoperatively as prophylaxis against deep vein thrombosis and pulmonary embolism.[4] The patient is evaluated daily for a positive Homans' sign. Monitoring of hemoglobin and hematocrit levels is important, especially if the patient has experienced an extensive blood loss during surgery.

With any spinal procedure, careful monitoring of neurologic function is critical. Knowledge of the patient's baseline functioning is vital when monitoring for changes postoperatively. The patient's sensory and motor function is assessed hourly in the immediate postoperative period and less frequently thereafter. The patient's ability to detect touch and discern sharp from dull is tested. Motor strength in the extremities is evaluated, and any changes are reported to the surgeon. Neurologic changes can occur up to 72 hours following surgery.[4]

Discharge planning focuses on teaching and performing ADL. Assistive devices such as long-handled brushes, shoehorns, and grabbers may be necessary to avoid extreme bending or reaching. If bracing is used, the patient and family should be able to demonstrate the proper technique when applying and removing the brace. The patient should be taught to assess the skin for evidence of pressure or breakdown, and the patient or family member should be instructed how to inspect the wound for any signs of infection.

### Complications

Posterior approaches to the spine are performed with the patient in the prone position, using a variety of frames and positioning devices. Complications can arise from positioning techniques and extremely lengthy procedures. Potential complications include pooling of blood in the lower extremities; pressure areas on the knees, forehead, chest, and other bony prominences; neuropathies as a result of local ischemia caused by prolonged pressure; blindness[36]; and infrequently, venous air embolism.[1,2,34]

Complications of the procedure and the postoperative period include dural tear and cerebrospinal fluid leakage, blood loss, hypovolemia and decreased cardiac output, hematoma formation, infection, instrument or graft failure, pseudoarthrosis, loss of correction of deformity, persistence of pain and/or deficits, neurologic impairment or loss, deep vein thrombosis, pulmonary embolism, fluid volume overload, and fat embolism.[13] Monitoring of *sensory evoked potentials* is frequently used as a method of reducing injury to the neural elements intraoperatively. Before surgery begins, electrodes are placed in the patient's scalp and extremities. Baseline data are collected, and impulse transmissions through the posterior columns of the spinal cord are monitored throughout the procedure. Any changes indicate possible injury, and the patient is given a *wake-up test.* The level of anesthesia is lightened sufficiently to allow the patient to follow commands to wiggle the toes or feet. Inability to do these tasks is considered indicative of neurologic impairment. This monitoring technique allows the surgeon an opportunity to explore, ascertain, and possibly correct the cause of neurologic loss before closing the incision.

Cell savers or autotransfusion devices are frequently used during the surgical procedure to reduce blood loss.

A complication frequently occurring in the postoperative period of spinal fusion patients is *inappropriate antidiuretic hormone secretion* (SIADH).[13] Contributing factors include decreased blood volume, the use of anesthetic agents and analgesics, and physical and emotional stressors.[13] Hyponatremia and hypoosmolality occur, accompanied by a decrease in urine output and an increase in urine osmolality and sodium. Fluid overload is caused by retention of free water, which increases plasma volume (which will cause a decrease in the hemoglobin [HgB] and hematocrit [Hct]). The increase in plasma volume is associated with three factors:

1. An increase in ADH, which is released in response to the stress of surgery, which causes retention of free water
2. The large volume of fluids given postoperatively

3. Remobilization of third-space fluid

Clinical manifestations of SIADH include the following:

1. Decreased urine output unresponsive to fluid intake
2. Decreased HgB and Hct with normal blood pressure and heart rate
3. Normal skin turgor
4. Fluid intake greater than urine output

Postoperative monitoring of spinal fusion patients should include accurate measurement of intake and output. Be suspicious of SIADH if the patient exhibits a decreased HgB and Hct (which should be normal 2 to 4 days postoperatively) and the blood pressure and pulse remain within the patient's normal range. Some experts believe that it may be advisable to withhold transfusion until diuresis occurs and blood counts can be reevaluated.[13]

Complications associated with surgical correction of thoracic spine disorders also include those associated with thoracic surgery (see Chapter 37), because the thoracic cavity is entered in an anterior approach to the thoracic spine.

Complications associated with approaches to the cervical spine include vascular injury and injury to the laryngeal nerve because of the proximity of these structures to the surgical site.

Complications associated with general anesthesia are also an important consideration following spinal surgery. These include complications such as atelectasis, paralytic ileus, and urinary retention.

# RESTRICTIVE DISORDERS

## SCOLIOSIS

### Etiology/Epidemiology

**Scoliosis** can be classified as *structural* or *nonstructural. Nonstructural scoliosis is also termed postural or functional.* This form of scoliosis is usually easily corrected, either by exercise or by removing the underlying cause. It is not a progressive disorder, and there is no vertebral rotation.

*Structural scoliosis involves a rotational deformity of the vertebrae.* It is further divided into three major categories:

1. *Congenital* (present at birth): occurs as a result of vertebral malformations in fetal life; accounts for 15% of structural scoliosis cases
2. *Neuromuscular:* results as a consequence of several diseases (cerebral palsy, poliomyelitis, myelomeningocele, muscular dystrophy, and neurofibromatosis); represents approximately 15% of cases; curves generally appear early and progress rapidly[8]
3. *Idiopathic:* unknown cause, but genetic factors have been linked to the development of disease; accounts for approximately 65% to 80% of cases.[4] It is further divided into three groups, depending on the age of onset:
   a. Infantile: 0 to 3 years of age
   b. Juvenile: 3 to 10 years of age
   c. Adolescent: older than 10 years of age

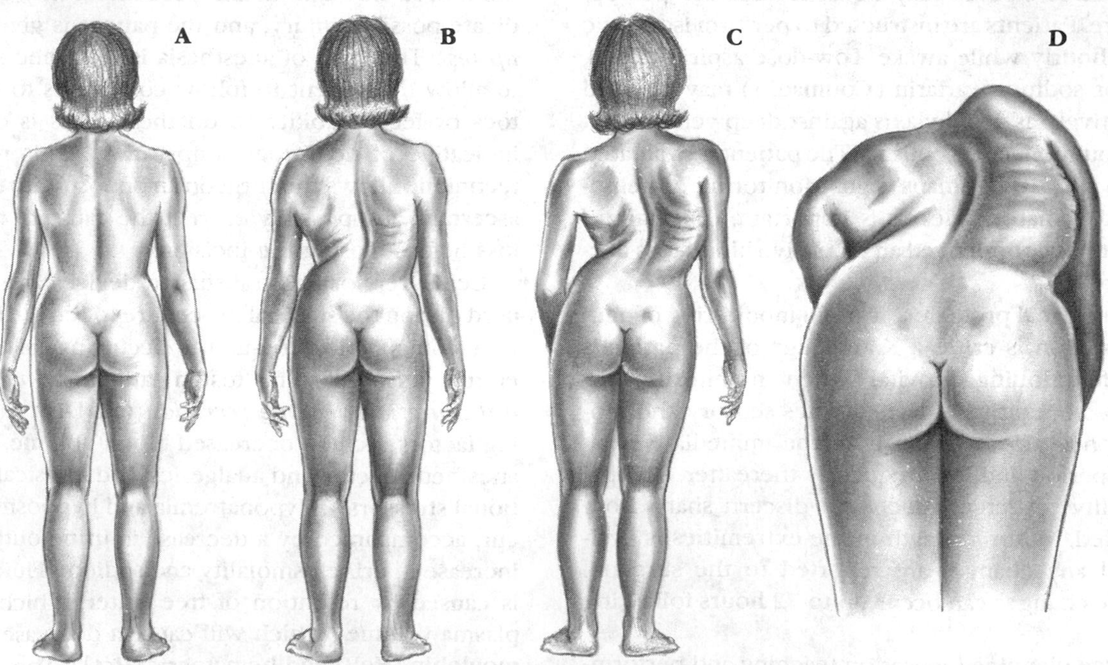


**FIGURE 65-33** Normal spinal alignment and abnormal spinal curvatures associated with scoliosis. **A,** Normal. **B,** Mild. **C,** Severe. **D,** Rotation and curvature of scoliosis. (From Thompson JL et al: *Mosby's clinical nursing,* ed 3, St Louis, 1993, Mosby.)

Girls account for 90% of persons affected with idiopathic scoliosis. Girls are also more frequently affected with curves of the spine greater than 20 degrees.[31]

## Pathophysiology

Scoliosis may develop in localized areas of the spinal column or involve the whole spinal column. Curvatures may be S shaped or C shaped (Figure 65-33).

The earliest pathologic changes begin in the soft tissues. Muscles and ligaments shorten on the concave side of the curve, progressing to deformities of the vertebrae and ribs.

The Scoliosis Research Society has devised a method of classifying curves. Deformities are classified by magnitude, direction, location, and etiology. Curve direction is designated by the convex side of the curve.[31]

The degree of rotation of the curve is important, because it determines the amount of impingement on the rib cage. The amount of vertebral compression and twisting depends on the position of the vertebrae in the curve. The forces of compression are greatest on the apical vertebrae, which become the most deformed. Deformity progresses quickly during growth and slows later in life, but the greatest increase in curvature may occur in adult life. Gravity and an increase in upper body weight may increase the deformity in adulthood.[19] In curves greater than 35 to 40 degrees, especially lumbar curves that lack rib support, the curve may continue to progress at the rate of one degree per year.

The individual can initially have slight, mild, or severe deformity. Early deformity may not be obvious except on specific examination. In the early stages, individuals may note that clothing does not fit correctly or hang evenly, because the height of the shoulders is uneven. Pain is not usually an accompanying factor.

Persons affected with structural scoliosis may exhibit asymmetry of hip height, pelvic obliquity (tilting of the pelvis from the normal horizontal position), inequalities of shoulder height, scapular prominence, rib prominence, and rib humps, which are posterior, unilateral humpings of the rib cage visible on forward bending. In severe cases, cardiopulmonary and digestive function may be affected because of compression or displacement of internal organs. Total lung capacity, vital capacity, and maximum voluntary ventilation are decreased in persons with scoliosis.[31] Cardiac output may also be compromised. Significant deviations in balance of the curve may also affect gait patterns.

## Prevention

### Primary prevention

There are no specific protective measures against scoliosis. However, attention to good posture may be effective in preventing some types of nonstructural scoliosis in both children and adults.

### Secondary prevention

Secondary prevention methods include screening of school-aged children and getting them under medical supervision.

### Tertiary prevention

There are two national support groups for persons with scoliosis.

1. Scoliosis Association Incorporated
   PO Box 811705
   Boca Raton, FL 33481-1705
   Phone: 1 (800) 800-0669
2. National Scoliosis Foundation
   72 Mount Auburn Street
   Watertown, MA 02172
   Phone: (617) 926-0397

## Medical Management

The goal for discharge of patients with scoliosis as determined by DRGs is 8.9 days. The nurse works collaboratively with the physician for implementation of prescribed medical therapy. Because the nurse has a major teaching role in discharge planning and patient teaching, these topics are discussed under Nursing Management.

### Diagnostic tests

A complete radiologic examination of the spine is completed. Curve angles, flexibility, and degree of vertebral rotation are calculated. Radiographs may also be done to determine skeletal maturity. In severe cases of thoracic scoliosis, pulmonary function studies may be completed to evaluate the degree of restrictive lung disease.

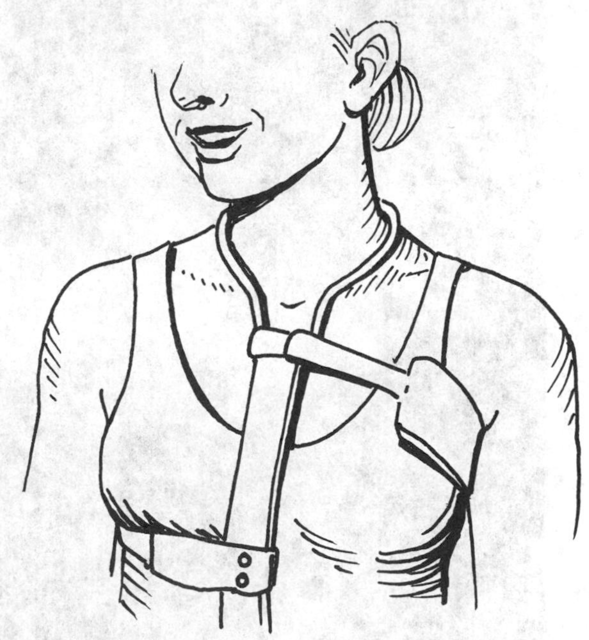

**FIGURE 65-34** Milwaukee brace.

### Medication

No medications are specific for scoliosis.

### Treatment

Treatment depends on the individual patient and the degree of lateral curvature.

1. Early or postural scoliosis may be amenable to postural exercise or exercise combined with traction. Cotrel's traction, which is a combination of cervical head halter of 5 to 7 lb and pelvic traction of 10 to 20 lb, may be used.
2. In scoliosis where the curve is flexible (less than 40 degrees) and the patient is cooperative, bracing, in combination with exercise, may be sufficient to correct the deformity (e.g., Milwaukee brace, Risser cast, or halofemoral or helopelvic traction; Figure 65-34).
3. Transcutaneous electrical muscle stimulation may be used to stimulate the muscles on the convex side of the curve. Repeated stimulation strengthens the muscles and pulls the spine into alignment. The patient usually uses the stimulator at night.

### Diet

No specific diet is indicated. However, as mentioned earlier, maintenance of ideal body weight is a consideration in reducing the stress on the spine. The patient should be advised against weight gain, especially if bracing is prescribed, because the brace is specifically fitted and contoured to the individual. The brace can usually accommodate a 10-lb gain or loss.

### Activity

No specific activities are recommended.

### Referral/Consultation

In some settings the nurse assumes responsibility for making referrals to other services. For persons with scoliosis, a physical therapy referral for exercises, myofascial release (a combination of stretch and massage techniques to lengthen soft tissue on the concave side of the curve), and electrical stimulation is common.

Critical pathways (also referred to as "collaborative care paths" or "care maps") have been developed in some inpatient and outpatient settings to guide both medical and nursing management. These critical pathways are collaboratively developed along time lines and include the information described above for specific hours, days, or visits. Pertinent information about discharge planning and patient teaching to be implemented at specified times also is included. Because the nurse has

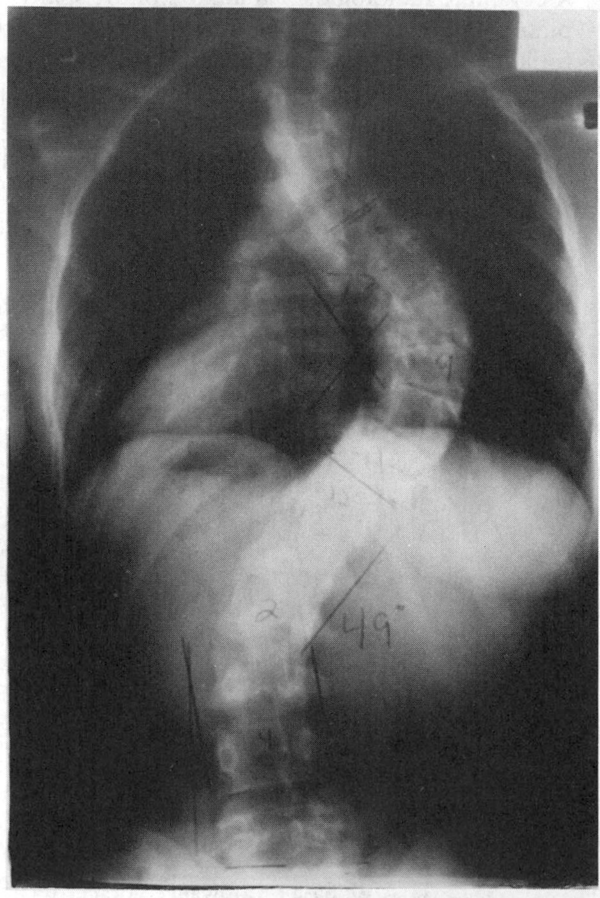


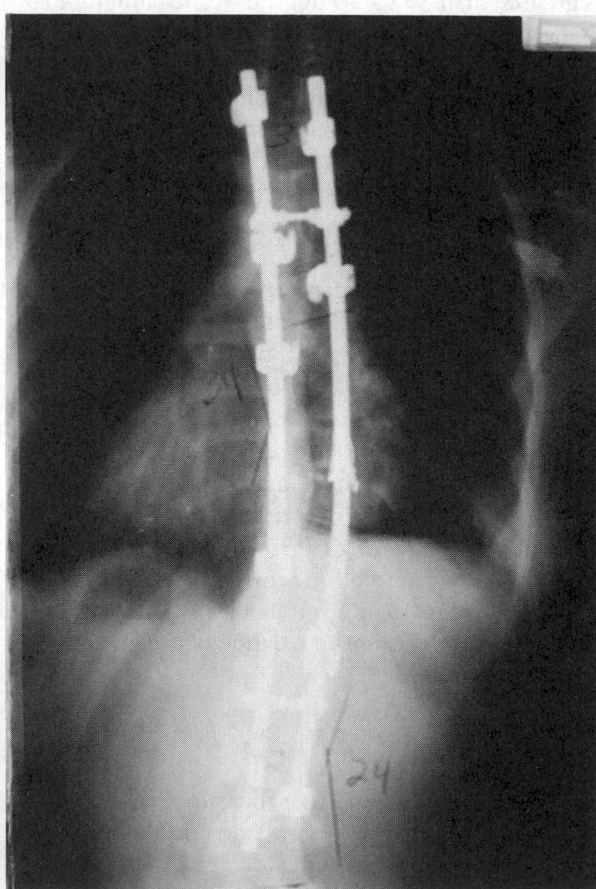


**FIGURE 65-35** **A,** Preoperative radiograph of adult with idiopathic scoliosis. **B,** Postoperative film showing correction of curve with Cotrel-Dubousset instrumentation in place.

a major role in these two aspects of care, these are discussed under Nursing Management.

### Surgical Management

Surgery is indicated in cases where conservative management has failed to halt curve progression and in cases of severe, progressing curves, intractable pain, or compromised pulmonary function or for cosmesis. Many individuals with neuromuscular scoliosis are nonambulators. Surgical correction is sometimes performed in these cases to facilitate ability to transfer or to increase sitting ability or tolerance. Surgical correction is usually performed on curves greater than 45 degrees[31] (Figure 65-35, *A*). Surgical correction usually involves a posterior approach to the spine with instrumentation and bony fusion. Patients with severe, rigid curves and pelvic obliquity frequently require a staged procedure. A transthoracic or retroperitoneal approach to the spine is performed first, followed by a posterior procedure in 1 to 2 weeks. Many types and combinations of types of instrumentation are available. The kind utilized is based on the individual patient and surgeon preference. Refer to Table 65-11 for examples of commonly used implants and see Figure 65-35, *B*.

Nursing management of the patient with surgery of the spine was discussed in the previous section on p. 2279. This nursing care is also applicable to the patient with a scoliosis fusion. Nursing management of the patient having *scoliosis fusion* is discussed below.

## NURSING MANAGEMENT

### ♦ ASSESSMENT

#### Subjective Data

Subjective data may include the following information from the patient:

1. Clothes not fitting or hanging well
2. Not being able to breathe comfortably
3. Complaints of progressive difficulty with ambulation
4. Expression of negative feelings about appearance
5. Complaints of back pain

#### Objective Data

1. Visible curvature in spine and/or a pronounced rib hump when patient bends forward from the waist
2. Palpation of spinal curve with patient in upright position
3. Notable limp
4. Shoulders uneven in height
5. One arm hanging closer to the body than the other

#### Diagnostic Test Findings

Radiographs taken of the spine will confirm the diagnosis of scoliosis.

### ♦ NURSING DIAGNOSES

Nursing diagnoses are determined from analysis of patient data. Possible nursing diagnoses for the person with scoliosis may include but are not limited to the following:

| Diagnostic Title | Possible Etiologic Factors |
|---|---|
| Mobility, impaired physical | Musculoskeletal impairment, surgical intervention, immobility |
| Knowledge deficit (related to scoliosis) | Lack of exposure |
| Pain, postoperative | Surgical intervention to correct deformity |
| Gas exchange, impaired (potential) | Surgical intervention, immobility |
| Self-esteem disturbance | Change in body apperance, use of brace |
| Skin integrity, high risk for impaired | Use of brace and/or surgical incision |

### ♦ EXPECTED PATIENT OUTCOMES

Expected patient outcomes for the patient with scoliosis may include but are not limited to the following:

1a. Demonstrates ability to perform isometrics and leg exercises after surgery
b. Verbalizes knowledge of brace or cast care; demonstrates ability to apply brace
c. Participates in ADL at maximum functional capacity
d. Ambulates to extent possible within restrictions
e. Demonstrates correct use of assistive or supportive devices to increase mobility and independence
f. Remains free of complications of immobility
2a. Verbalizes knowledge of disease process and rationale for treatment regimen
b. Actively participates in treatment program
c. Verbalizes intent to participate in follow-up care
3a. Maintains pain relief with use of prescribed analgesics
b. Utilizes knowledge of relaxation techniques to aid in pain control
c. Reports ability to effectively manage pain by time of discharge
4a. Maintains maximum lung expansion and respiratory effort
b. Maintains adequate gas exchange by demonstrating effective respiratory rate
c. Remains free of respiratory complications, such as atelectasis and pneumonia
d. Demonstrates tolerance to activity
5a. Verbalizes feelings about self and effects of disease process or surgical intervention
b. Verbalizes acceptance of appearance
c. Verbalizes positive attributes of self
6a. Demonstrates knowledge of skin care
b. Maintains intact skin, free of reddened areas and breakdown

c. Maintains surgical wound free of infection
d. Verbalizes knowledge of signs and symptoms of infection

## ♦ INTERVENTIONS

For individuals with whom conservative interventions are being employed, patient instruction is most important for achieving the desired outcomes. Points to be stressed in teaching are listed below.

### Facilitating Learning

1. Instruct patient how to apply, remove, and care for brace.
2. Instruct and supervise patient in performance of prescribed exercises and use of traction equipment.
3. Advise patient that wearing brace need not restrict normal or desired activities.
4. Instruct patient regarding disease process and rationales for treatment.
5. Explain and discuss the patient's and family's expectations of treatment.
6. Advise patient regarding the selection of loose-fitting but attractive clothing that conceals brace (particularly important for women and adolescents).
7. Inform patient and family of support groups.
8. Instruct and supervise patient in method of inspecting skin.

### Providing Postoperative Care

Postoperative care of the person following spinal fusion for scoliosis is described in the nursing management section on p. 2279 and in the Guidelines box. Postoperative considerations specific to the person with a scoliosis fusion are listed below.

**Promoting mobility**

1. Instruct patient how to apply, remove, and care for brace.
2. Assist with progressive mobilization within prescribed restrictions.
3. Teach and observe use of assistive and supportive devices if needed.

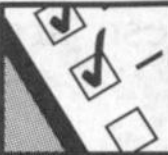

### Guidelines for Care for the Person With Scoliosis Fusion

**PREOPERATIVE CARE**

1. Instruct the patient regarding the surgery, postoperative care, and expectations after discharge.

**POSTOPERATIVE CARE**

1. Promoting comfort
   a. Administer narcotic analgesics as necessary; gradually decrease to nonnarcotic analgesics as patient tolerates.
   b. Turn and position frequently.
   c. Use a small bedpan or a fracture bedpan.
2. Positioning
   a. Bed is kept flat from 1 to 14 days, depending on the surgical technique used.
   b. Position patient side to back to side with use of a turning sheet and pillows between the legs to maintain alignment.
3. Promoting safety
   a. Monitor vital signs, motor function, and sensation in the lower extremities frequently.
   b. Monitor closely for respiratory impairment.
4. Promoting mobility
   a. Encourage leg exercises as for other spinal surgery.
   b. Encourage participation in ADL to extent possible within restrictions imposed by surgery and/or brace or cast.
   c. Begin activity out of bed, in brace or cast if prescribed, as soon as surgeon permits. (Commencement of activity depends on surgical technique.)
5. Preventing complications
   a. Encourage breathing exercises.
   b. Delay administration of oral food and fluid until patient is actively passing flatus.
   c. Monitor intravenous intake and urine output closely to prevent fluid overload until patient experiences postoperative diuresis (usually 3 to 4 days).
6. Wound care (as for any spine surgery)
7. Discharge instructions
   a. Care of brace or cast if required.
   b. Use of bed board at home.
   c. Plans for follow-up with physician.

## ♦ EVALUATION

To evaluate the effectiveness of nursing interventions, compare patient behaviors with those stated in the "Expected Patient Outcomes." Successful achievement of patient outcomes for the patient with scoliosis is indicated by the following:

1. Demonstrating isometric and leg exercises postoperatively
2. Applying own brace before getting out of bed in the morning
3. Performing own ADL with a minimum of assistance
4. Ambulating within limitations
5. Explaining what scoliosis is and rationale for treatment
6. Discussing ways she or he will participate in follow-up care
7. Utilizing relaxation techniques to assist in pain control
8. Indicating when pain medication is necessary
9. Requiring less pain medication as she or he prepares for discharge
10. Maintaining adequate gas exchange as indicated by blood gases ($P_{O_2}$ between 80 and 100 mm Hg and $P_{CO_2}$ between 35 and 45 mm Hg)
11. Remaining free of respiratory complications
12. Ability to do increasing physical activity without becoming short of breath

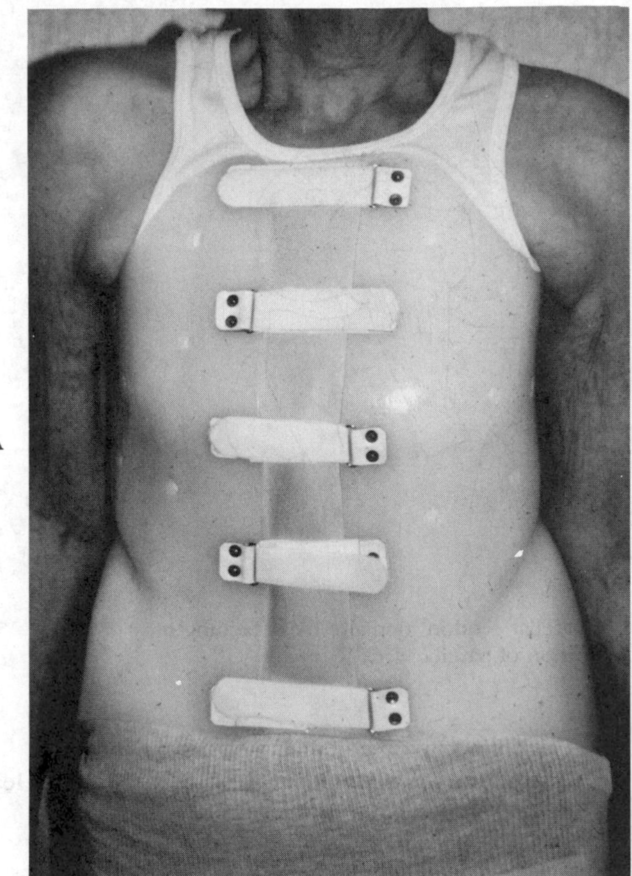


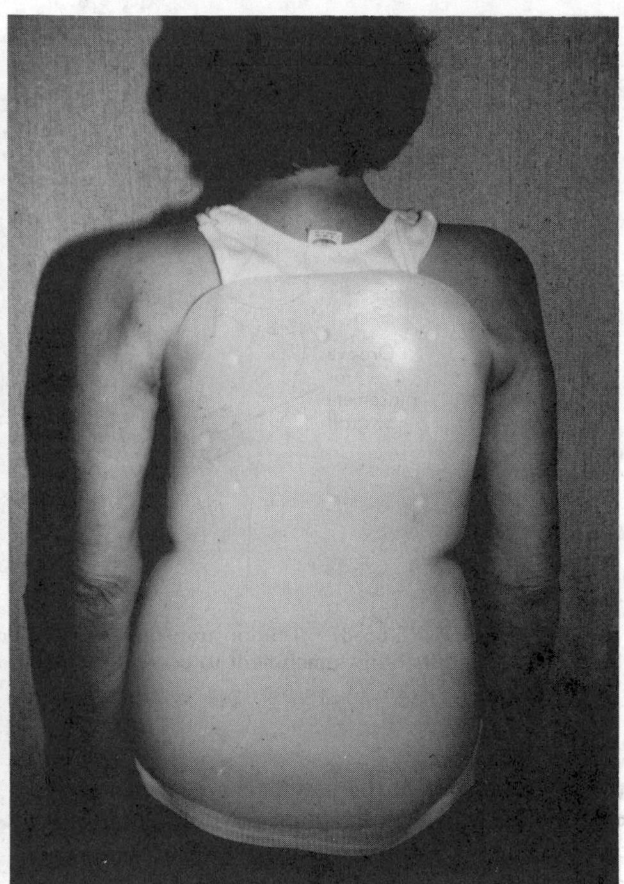


**FIGURE 65-36** **A,** Anterior view of thoracolumbar sacral orthosis (TLSO). **B,** Posterior view of TLSO. Note cotton T-shirt worn under brace.

13. Verbalizing his or her positive attributes and ways to use them after discharge
14. Demonstrating how to inspect skin, especially under the brace for reddened areas and breaks in skin
15. Discussing signs and symptoms of skin infection (redness, swelling, warmth of area, elevation in temperature, and purulent drainage)

■ ■ ■

### Complications

Complications after scoliosis fusion are discussed in the nursing management section on p. 2281. In addition, there is a high risk of postoperative pulmonary complications as a result of postoperative immobilization; therefore preventive measures are important. Paralytic ileus is also a common complication, and nasogastric suction may be used in the first 24 to 72 hours postoperatively. Patients with major spinal procedures also tend to retain fluid; therefore they are at risk for fluid overload in the early postoperative period.[30]

After surgery, a brace or cast is usually required for a period of time, and instructions are given to the person for the care of the brace or cast (Figure 65-36). A bed board is suggested for use at home to provide firm support for sleeping.

# OTHER DISORDERS

Some other disorders of the musculoskeletal system involve malposition of supportive structures, metabolic disorder, neoplasms, or problems arising as a result of infection. Five of the more common disorders (recurrent dislocation of the patella, gout, bacterial arthritis, osteomyelitis, and tumors) are examined in the following discussion.

## RECURRENT DISLOCATION OF THE PATELLA

### Etiology/Epidemiology

Patellar dislocation is usually a result of trauma to the knee. It usually occurs with the knee flexed and externally rotated. Dislocation usually occurs laterally. Recurrent dislocation is a result of ligamentous laxity. The injury frequently occurs during sports activities.

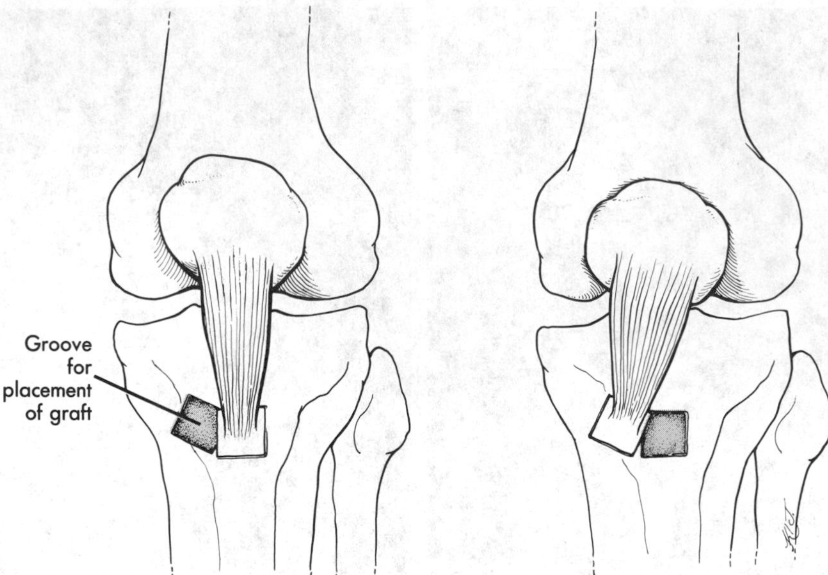


**FIGURE 65-37** Tendon transplant. Movement of patellar tendon medially by detaching it and its bony attachment to correct recurrent dislocation of patella.

### Pathophysiology

Recurrent dislocation of the patella is representative of those problems in which a tendon or other supportive structure is malplaced or not functioning in a normal fashion. In this disorder the patellar tendon is more laterally placed in its distal attachment than normal. Consequently, the patella is pulled laterally when the quadriceps contracts and it dislocates to the lateral side of the knee. The patient may complain of feelings of instability or the knee "giving way" or "going out." The knee may appear enlarged because of swelling. The disorder is painful and can restrict knee function.

### Medical Management

Patellar dislocation is usually treated surgically.

1. The distal end of the tendon is transplanted from its insertion on the tibial tubercle to a point more medial and distal to the preoperative insertion (Figure 65-37).
2. Leg is protected postoperatively with splints and a compression dressing for 3 to 5 days.
3. Cylinder cast is applied after dressing is removed.
4. Active flexion exercises are begun in about 6 weeks.

### Nursing Management

Major nursing interventions include the following:

1. Instructing the patient about the surgery, postoperative care, and expectations after discharge
2. Assessing the neurovascular status of both lower extremities
3. Encouraging the patient to perform prescribed exercises
4. Promoting mobility while observing restrictions on active flexion
5. Promoting involvement in self-care
6. Instructing the patient how to care for self after leaving hospital
   a. Care of cast
   b. Performance of exercises
   c. Use of ambulatory aid
   d. Follow-up plans with the physician and physical therapist

## GOUT

### Etiology

**Gout** *or gouty arthritis is a metabolic disorder that develops as a result of prolonged hyperuricemia (elevated serum uric acid) caused by problems in synthesizing purines or by poor renal excretion of uric acid.*

### Epidemiology

Gout affects men eight to nine times more frequently than women. It can occur at any age, with the peak age of onset occurring in the fifth decade. Eighty-five percent of all persons with gout have a genetic or familial tendency to develop the disease.

### Pathophysiology

Urate crystals form in the synovial tissue, causing severe inflammation. The inflammatory process is extremely rapid, occurring over a few hours. *Acute symptoms are extreme pain, swelling, and erythema of the involved joints.* Typically the first metatarsophalangeal joint of the great toe is involved (podagra), but other joints, such as the ankle, heel, knee, or wrists, may also be affected. Pain is so severe that the patient may not tolerate even the weight of a sheet over the joint. Renal damage may occur, especially if recurrent uric acid

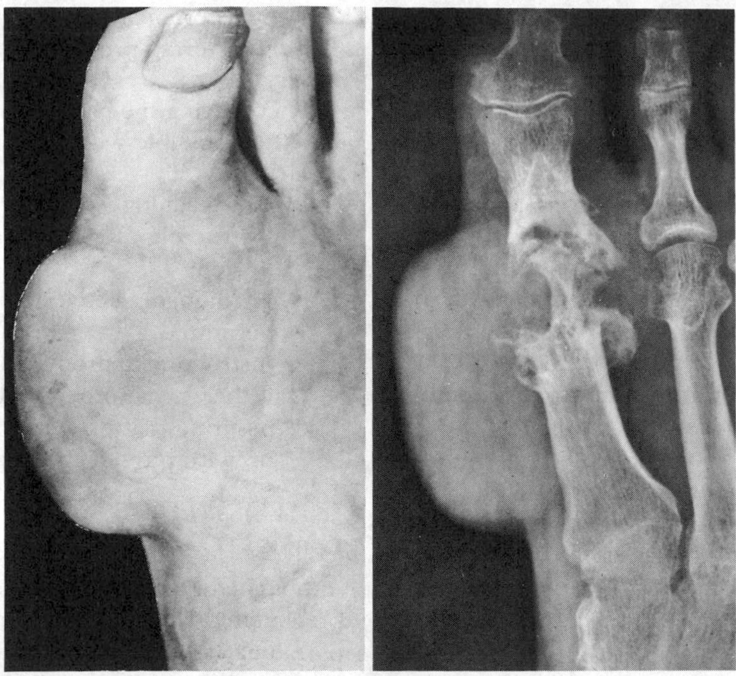

**FIGURE 65-38** Gout of long duration. Tophaceous mass at base of great toe, as well as destructive bone and joint changes shown in roentgenogram, is associated with extensive urate deposits. (From Brashear H, Raney R: *Shand's handbook of orthopaedic surgery,* ed 9, St Louis, 1978, Mosby.)

stones have been present. Between attacks of gout, the patient may be asymptomatic, but repeated attacks can occur with gradually increasing frequency if the disease is untreated. Patients with gouty symptoms may develop *tophi,* or deposits of monosodium urate in their tissues. These consist of a core of monosodium urate with a surrounding inflammatory reaction. *Patients with tophaceous deposits* (Figure 65-38) *tend to have more frequent and more severe episodes of gouty arthritis.*

Laboratory studies will indicate an *elevated serum uric acid, normal or increased urinary uric acid* over a 24-hour period, and the presence of *monosodium urate* monohydrate crystals in the synovial fluid and in the tophi.

## Medical Management

Management is directed toward control of acute attacks and prevention of recurrent attacks. Treatment of *acute* attacks includes the following:

1. Medications
   a. Colchicine (0.6 mg), oral administration of two tablets initially, then one tablet each hour until nausea, vomiting, or diarrhea develops, or joint symptoms subside; limit is 6.0 to 8.0 mg
   b. Colchicine, 1.0 to 3.0 mg in saline intravenously over a 10-minute period
   c. Phenylbutazone (Butazolidin)
   d. Indomethacin (Indocin)
2. Absolute rest of the joint

*Preventive* therapy consists of reduction of the serum urate level below 6.9 mg/dl. This is achieved by one of two methods:

1. *Enhancing uric acid excretion*
   a. Probenecid (Benemid), 0.5 g daily for 1 week, then increased by 0.5 g weekly until serum uric acid is in normal range
      (1) Daily prophylactic therapy for life (average daily dose is 1 to 2 g)
   b. Sulfinpyrazone (Anturane), used for patients who do not tolerate Benemid
      (1) Daily prophylactic therapy for life (average daily dose is 300 to 400 mg)
2. *Decreasing uric acid formation*
   a. Allopurinol (Zyloprim), 100 mg twice per day initially, increased by 100 mg every 2 to 4 weeks until serum uric acid level is normal
      (1) Daily prophylactic therapy for life (average daily dose is 300 mg)

## Nursing Management

Nursing management includes the following:

1. Patient teaching
   a. Instruct patient in nature of disease.
   b. Instruct patient in proper use of prescribed medications.
   c. Encourage patient to lose weight gradually if overweight.

d. Encourage patient to take in sufficient fluid to assure daily *output* of 2000 to 3000 ml.
e. Advise patient to avoid excessive purines (sweet breads, yeast, heart, herring, herring roe, sardines, and heavy alcohol intake).
f. Explain to patient that severe dietary purine restriction is not necessary as long as his or her hyperuricemia is well controlled by daily medication therapy.

2. Promoting comfort
   a. Provide absolute rest until pain of acute attack subsides.
   b. Avoid touching joint or moving affected extremity until acute pain subsides.

## BACTERIAL ARTHRITIS

### Etiology

Bacterial arthritis is the result of invasion of the synovial membrane by microorganisms, most often *gonococci, meningococci, staphylococci, coliforms, salmonellae,* and *Haemophilus influenzae.*

### Epidemiology

Factors that predispose to such infections are a high degree of susceptibility on the part of the patient, recent joint surgery or trauma, intraarticular injections, and rheumatoid arthritis.

### Pathophysiology

Synovial tissues respond to bacterial invasion by becoming inflamed. The joint cavity may become involved, and pus will be present in the synovial membrane and the synovial fluid. If allowed to progress, the infection will cause abscesses in the synovium and subchondral bone, eventually destroying cartilage. *Ankylosis* of the *joint* may result. The patient will complain of pain, swelling, and tenderness of the joint.

Joint aspiration is helpful in making the diagnosis if the presence of organisms can be demonstrated in the synovial fluid. White cell counts will be high, and glucose content of synovial fluid may be reduced. X-ray films taken days to weeks after onset of the infection may reveal loss of joint space and lytic changes in bone.

### Medical Management

Medical management includes the following:

1. Appropriate antibiotic therapy
2. Rest or immobilization of the joint
3. Surgical drainage or a system of irrigation and drainage if infection does not respond to antibiotic therapy or if osteomyelitis is present
4. Resumption of active range of motion when infection subsides and motion can be tolerated.

### Nursing Management

Nursing management includes the following:

1. Promoting rest of the affected joint
2. Administering antibiotics on time and as prescribed
3. Administering prescribed pain medication as necessary
4. Encouraging the patient to participate in self-care to extent possible within restrictions of prescribed rest for joint
5. Patient teaching
   a. Instructing in care of cast or other immobilizing device
   b. Encouraging active joint motion when motion is permitted
   c. Instructing in proper administration of antibiotics if therapy is to be continued after discharge
   d. Assuring that patient is aware of plans for follow-up with physician

## OSTEOMYELITIS

### Etiology

Although the development of **osteomyelitis** is often precipitated by a traumatic event or is a complication of trauma, it is included with the degenerative disorders because of its chronic and debilitating aspects. Osteomyelitis is an infection of the bone. It is most commonly caused by bacteria but can also be caused by fungi, parasites, and viruses.

### Epidemiology

The two types of osteomyelitis are classified by the mode of entry of the pathogen. *Exogenous osteomyelitis* is caused by a pathogen from outside the body, such as from an open fracture or surgical procedure, especially joint replacements or procedures involving instrumentation. The infection can also be caused by human and animal bites and fist blows to the mouth. The most common organism found in human bites is *Staphylococcus aureus* and in animal bites, *Pasteurella multocida.* The infection spreads from the soft tissues to the bone. Most susceptible to exogenous osteomyelitis are chronically ill, diabetic, alcoholic, drug-abusing, and immunosuppressed individuals.

*Hematogenous osteomyelitis* is caused by bloodborne pathogens originating from infectious sites within the body. Examples include sinus, ear, dental, respiratory, and genitourinary infections. In hematogenous osteomyelitis the infection spreads from the bone to the soft tissues and can eventually break through the skin, becoming a draining fistula. This type of osteomyelitis is more common in infants, children, and elderly persons. In elderly persons, males are more commonly affected. *Staphylococcus aureus* is the most common causative organism. Other responsible organisms include streptococcus B, *Haemophilus influenzae, Salmonella,* and gram-negative bacteria. *Salmonella* is linked with sickle cell anemia, and gram-negative organisms are associated with infections occurring in elderly and immunocompromised individuals.

### Pathophysiology

In hematogenous osteomyelitis the organisms reach the bone through the *circulatory* and *lymphatic systems.* The bacteria lodge in the small vessels of the bone, triggering an inflammatory response. The femur, tibia, humerus, and radius are commonly affected. Infections of the pelvic organs frequently spread to the pelvis and vertebrae. The pathophysiology of osteomyelitis is similar to infectious processes in any other body tissue.

Bone inflammation is marked by edema, increased vasculature, and leukocyte activity. Exudate seals the bone's canaliculi, extends into the metaphysis and marrow cavity, and finally reaches the cortex. The infectious process weakens the cortex, thereby increasing the risk of pathologic fracture. *Brodie's abscesses* are characteristic of chronic osteomyelitis. These are isolated, encapsulated pockets of microorganisms surrounded by bone matrix. They are usually found in long bones. These pockets of virulent organisms are capable of reinfection at any time.

In cases of *exogenous osteomyelitis* the infection begins in the soft tissues, *disrupting muscle* and *connective tissues* and eventually *forming abscesses.*

Chronic osteomyelitis is difficult to treat. Recurrent infection, areas of dead bone (sequestrum), and scar tissue are contributing factors to its resistance to treatment. Complications of chronic osteomyelitis include sepsis, nonunion, draining fistulas, shortening of the affected extremity, and eventual amputation.[21]

The clinical manifestations of osteomyelitis vary with the individual, type of responsible organism, precipitating event, and type of infection (acute or chronic). The patient may report fever, malaise, anorexia, and headache. The affected body part may be erythematous, tender, and edematous. There may be an opening in the skin, draining purulent material.

Blood tests reveal an increase in WBCs and in the erythrocyte sedimentation rate. A culture and sensitivity test of the drainage will reveal the causative organisms and list appropriate antibiotic therapy. Blood cultures will determine the presence or absence of septicemia. If an open debridement is necessary, pathologic examination of the tissues will confirm the diagnosis of osteomyelitis. Diagnosis can be confirmed by bone scanning, although pathologic changes may not be visible in the bone until 7 to 10 days after the infection begins.[23]

### Medical Management

Treatment is difficult and costly. The goals of treatment are as follows:

1. Complete removal of dead bone and soft tissue
2. Control of infection
3. Elimination of dead space (after removal of necrotic bone)[21]

Many modes of treatment are available. Which treatment modality is employed depends on the area of bone involved, causative organism, ability to maintain a functional limb, duration of treatment, and expected outcome. Treatment options include the following:

1. *Antibiotic therapy:* intravenous antibiotics may be prescribed for up to 6 weeks, and oral antibiotic therapy may continue for up to 6 months.
2. *Irrigation and drainage system* involving a surgical procedure in which holes are drilled into the cortex of the bone, allowing continuous infusion of antibiotic solution and drainage of inflammatory exudate. This system is usually maintained until cultures are negative.
3. *Analgesics and antipyretics* as necessary.

### Surgical Management

When conservative modalities fail to control the infection, surgical intervention is indicated. Many types of surgery are possible from simple debridement, as mentioned above, to amputation. Other options include the use of *allograft bone, Ilizarov technique* (see Chapter 64), and the *Papineau bone graft.* The Papineau technique was introduced in the 1970s as a means to treat osteomyelitis occurring in the diaphysis of long bones. It consists of removal of infected and necrotic bone, immobilization (usually achieved by an external fixator [see Chapter 64]), delayed cancellous bone grafts, and finally soft tissue closure.[23] This technique has been shown to be highly successful in the treatment of chronic osteomyelitis.[21]

### Nursing Management

Nursing management of the patient with osteomyelitis includes the following:

1. Administering antibiotics on time and as prescribed
2. Administering analgesics and/or antipyretics as prescribed
3. Promoting rest of affected joint or limb
4. Encouraging participation in ADL to fullest extent
5. Instructing the patient in correct use of assistive devices as needed
6. Teaching the patient proper administration of antibiotics if home-going therapy is prescribed; discussion of drug side effects should be included
7. Instructing the patient regarding signs and symptoms of recurring infection and potential sources of further infection
8. Providing information regarding follow-up care

## TUMORS OF THE MUSCULOSKELETAL SYSTEM

### Etiology

Tumors may arise from any of the structures of the musculoskeletal system (Tables 65-12 and 65-13). The type of tumor is determined and classified by the tissue of origin (see Figure 65-39). Tumors can be *benign* or *malignant* and can affect both adults and children. Musculoskeletal tumors comprise 3% of all malignant tumors.

**TABLE 65-12 Common Tumors of the Musculoskeletal System**

| BENIGN | MALIGNANT |
|---|---|
| **BONE** | |
| Osteoma | Osteosarcoma |
| **CARTILAGE** | |
| Osteochondroma | Chondrosarcoma |
| Enchondroma | |
| Periosteal | |
| Chondroblastoma | |
| **MUSCLE** | |
| Leiomyoma | Leiomyosarcoma |
| Rhabdomyoma | Rhabdomyosarcoma |
| **FIBROUS** | |
| Fibroma | Fibrosarcoma |
| **BONE MARROW** | |
| Giant cell | Ewing's sarcoma |
| | Myeloma |
| **UNCERTAIN CELL** | |
| Unicameral bone cyst | |
| Aneurysmal bone cyst | |

**TABLE 65-13 Muscle Tumors**

| CHARACTERISTICS | TREATMENT |
|---|---|
| **LEIOMYOMA** | |
| Affects smooth muscle, usually uterus<br>Palpable mass<br>Tenderness | Surgical excision |
| **RHABDOMYOMA** | |
| Affects striated muscle<br>Rare<br>Tenderness | Surgical excision |
| **LEIOMYOSARCOMA** | |
| Affects smooth muscle, usually uterus, stomach, or small bowel<br>Radical growth | Surgical excision with wide margins<br>Radiation<br>Chemotherapy |
| **RHABDOMYOSARCOMA** | |
| Affects striated muscle, usually in inguinal, popliteal, or gluteal areas<br>Slow-growing mass<br>Tenderness | Radiation<br>Surgical excision<br>Chemotherapy |

Generally, malignant tumors tend to cause more bone destruction, invasion of the surrounding tissues, and metastasis. Benign bone tumors tend to be less destructive to normal bone, do not invade soft tissues, and are not capable of metastasis. Common tumors of the musculoskeletal system, their characteristics, and treatment are described in Table 65-14.

The cause of bone tumors is unknown. A tumor can be defined as a new growth or *hyperplasia* of cells.[20] This growth may be in response to inflammation or trauma. Others are a result of a spontaneous, rapid, poorly differentiated proliferation of cells.

## Epidemiology

The incidence of bone tumors varies with age. Persons under the age of 20 years and over the age of 60 years have the highest incidence of bone tumor.[20]

Approximately 6000 primary bone and soft tissue tumors are diagnosed annually in the United States.[23] Osteosarcoma is the most common type of primary bone tumor, representing 20% of all cases.[22]

Other factors are associated with the development of bone tumors. A history of Paget's disease or radiation therapy increases the risk of developing a bone tumor. Bone tumors can also occur as a result of metastases

**FIGURE 65-39** Derivation of bone tumors. (From McCance KL, Heuther SE: *Pathophysiology: the biologic basis for disease in adults and children,* ed 2, St Louis, 1994, Mosby.)

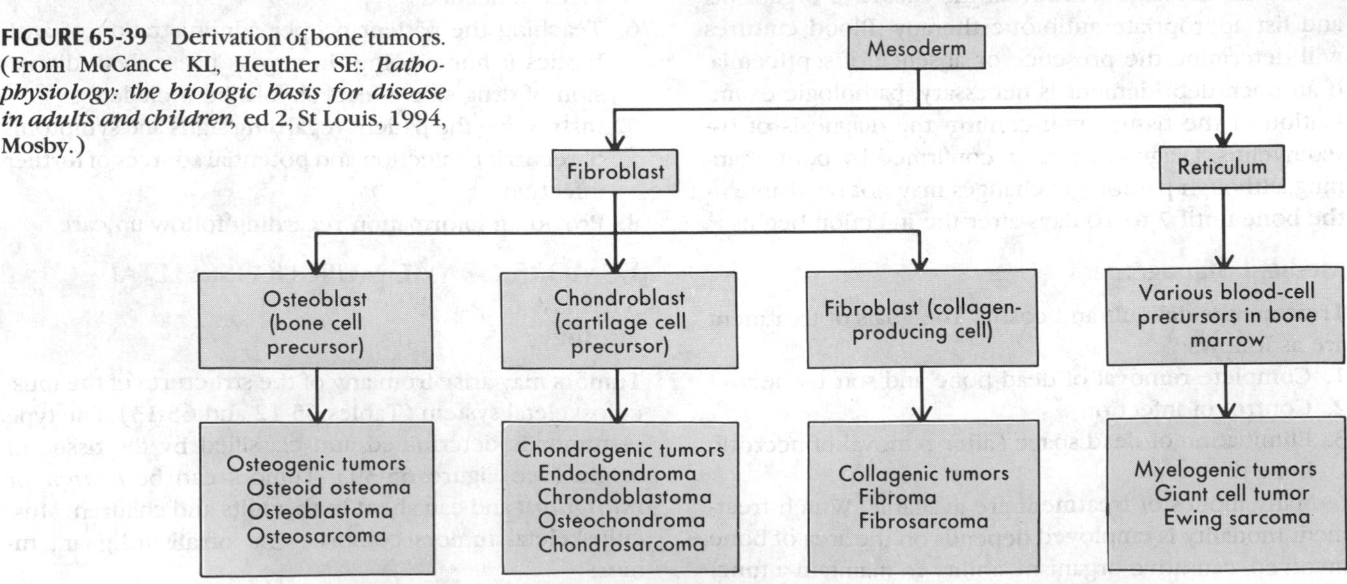

**TABLE 65-14 Other Common Tumors of the Musculoskeletal System**

| CHARACTERISTICS | TREATMENT |
|---|---|
| **OSTEOCHONDROMA** | |
| Compromise of cancellous bone with cartilaginous cap<br>Develops during growth periods at metaphysis of bone<br>Also appears in tendons<br>May limit joint motion<br>May recur | Surgical excision |
| **ENCHONDROMA** | |
| Destroys cancellous bone<br>Usually occurs in humerus or finger<br>Can cause pathologic fractures<br>May become malignant, especially in long bones or pelvis | Surgical excision with wide margins<br>Amputation |
| **CHONDROSARCOMA** | |
| Usually affects persons 50-60 yr old<br>Affects males more than females<br>Slow growing<br>Most common in humerus, femur, pelvis<br>May have palpable mass<br>Severe, persistent pain<br>May infiltrate joint space and soft tissue<br>May metastasize to lung tissue<br>May recur | Surgical excision<br>Amputation |
| **FIBROSARCOMA** | |
| Usually affects persons 40-50 yr old<br>Occurs in bony fibrous tissue of femur and tibia<br>Comprises 4% of primary malignant bone tumors<br>Night pain, swelling, possible palpable mass<br>May cause pathologic fractures<br>May metastasize to lungs | Wide surgical excision<br>Amputation |
| **GIANT CELL TUMOR (FIGURE 65-40, *A*)** | |
| Usually affects ages 20-40 yr<br>Affects females more than males<br>Comprises 4%-5% of all benign bone tumors<br>Appears in epiphyseal area, destroys bone matrix, can invade soft tissues<br>Commonly found in femur, tibia, or humerus<br>Dull, aching night pain<br>Limitation of motion<br>Swelling<br>High incidence of recurrence | Wide excision<br>May require bone graft<br>Amputation (Figure 65-40, *B*) |
| **MYELOMA, MULTIPLE MYELOMA (MULTIFOCAL)** | |
| Poor prognosis<br>Common in persons >40 yr<br>Affects males more than females<br>Comprises 27% of bone tumors<br>Higher incidence in African-Americans<br>Neoplastic proliferation of plasma cells<br>Causes cortical and medullary bone lysis and infiltrates bone marrow<br>Aching, intermittent pain in spine, pelvis, ribs, or sternum<br>Pain increased with weight bearing<br>May complain of weight loss, malaise, or anorexia<br>Causes pathologic fractures | Palliative treatment<br>Radiation<br>Chemotherapy |
| **OSTEOMA** | |
| Usually affects persons 10-20 yr old<br>Comprises 20% of benign bone tumors<br>Slow growth | Treatment only if symptomatic, then excision |

from other primary sites of neoplasias. Cancers of the breast, prostate, and lungs frequently metastasize to bone. Common sites for metastases include the spine, ribs, pelvis, hip, and humerus.

## Pathophysiology

Pathophysiology of neoplasms is found in Chapter 16. Bone tumors commonly cause bone destruction and erosion of the cortex. Benign bone tumors have a controlled growth rate. They normally compress and displace, rather than invade, normal bone tissue. This eventually leads to weakening of the normal bone. Other types of tumors destroy normal bone either by resorption or disruption of the blood supply to the bone. Three patterns of bone destruction have been identified[20]:

1. *Geographic:* characterized by slow-growing tumors; there is an identifiable margin between the normal and abnormal bone.
2. *Moth-eaten:* the margins are less defined; this type of destruction characterizes rapidly proliferating tumors and malignancies.
3. *Permeative:* tumor and normal bone are meshed with no perceivable margins.

A

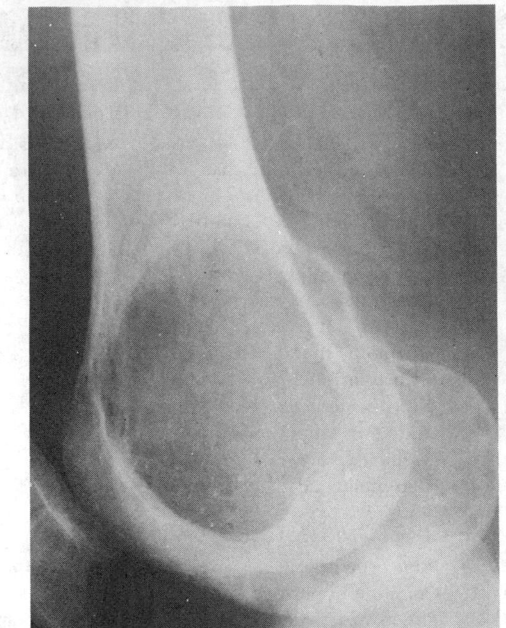

B

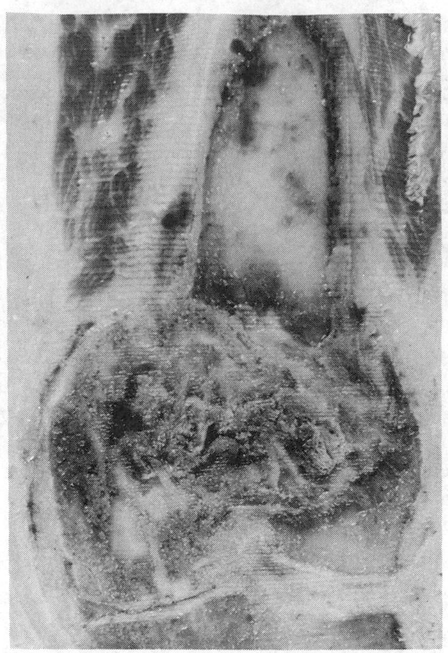

**FIGURE 65-40** Giant cell tumor. **A,** Giant cell tumor of distant end of femur. Lesion was curetted and replaced with bone chips. **B,** Giant cell tumor shown in **A** recurred, necessitating amputation. Gross specimen demonstrates bone chips still in place, with tumor replacing femur. Review of original sections showed benign giant cell tumor, but recuts of curetted material demonstrated malignant stroma. (From Rosai J: *Ackerman's surgical pathology,* ed 6, St Louis, 1981, Mosby.)

**TABLE 65-15 Surgical Staging System for Bone Tumors**

| STAGE | GRADE (G)* | SITE (T)† | |
|---|---|---|---|
| 1A | Low ($G_1$) | Intracompartmental ($T_1$) | None ($M_0$) |
| 1B | Low ($G_1$) | Extracompartmental ($T_2$) | None ($M_0$) |
| 11A | High ($G_2$) | Intracompartmental ($T_1$) | None ($M_0$) |
| 11B | High ($G_2$) | Extracompartmental ($T_2$) | None ($M_0$) |
| 111A | Low ($G_1$) | Intracompartmental or extracompartmental ($T_1$ or $T_2$) | Regional or distant ($M_1$) |
| 111B | High ($G_2$) | Intracompartmental or extracompartmental ($T_1$ or $T_2$) | Regional or distant ($M_1$) |

From Mourad LA, Droste MM: *The nursing process in the care of adults with orthopaedic conditions,* ed 3, Albany, NY, 1993, Delmar Publishers Inc.

*$G_1$ = Low-grade malignant; moderate cell differentiation; occasional distant metastasis. $G_2$ = High-grade malignant; poorly differentiated or undifferentiated cells; frequent distant metastasis.

†$T_1$ = Localized, encapsulated; intracompartmental (entirely confined in anatomic boundaries of tissues of origin). $T_2$ = Extracompartmental (spread outside of tissues of origin).

‡$M_0$ = Has no lymph node or distant metastasis. $M_1$ = Has lymph node and/or distant metastasis.

A staging system has been developed for bone tumors.[23] Malignancies are classified according to their growth patterns and sites of metastases (Table 65-15).

The rest of this section refers only to osteosarcoma.

**Osteosarcoma** exhibits a moth-eaten pattern of bone destruction with poorly defined margins (Figure 65-41). Osteoid and callus produced by the tumor invade and resorb normal cortical bone. The tumor erodes through the cortex and periosteum and eventually invades soft tissues. Metastasis to the lungs is common.

*Ninety percent of osteosarcomas occur in the metaphyses of long bones, especially the distal femur and proximal tibia.*[23] Pain and swelling are frequently reported. The initial complaint of pain is often described as dull, aching, and intermittent in nature, but the pain rapidly increases in intensity and duration. Night pain is common. Other frequent complaints include generalized malaise, anorexia, and weight loss.

## Diagnostic Tests

Bone biopsy is used to confirm the diagnosis. Because of osteosarcomas' rapid growth rate, the prognosis is

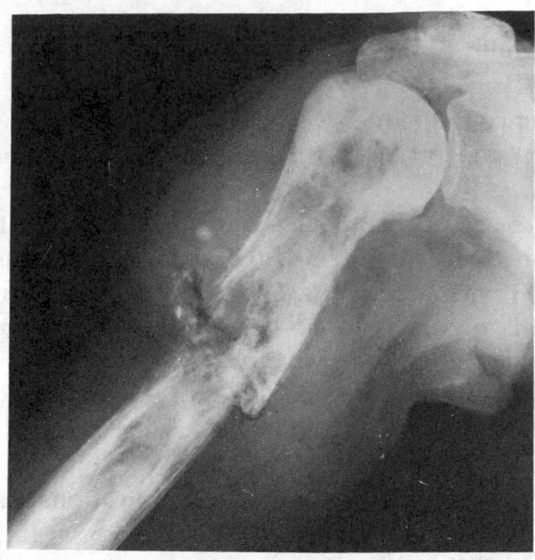

FIGURE 65-41 Osteosarcoma of proximal humerus. (From McCance KL, Heuther SE: *Pathophysiology: the biologic basis for disease in adults and children,* ed 2, St Louis, 1994, Mosby.)

poor. Death, usually from pulmonary complications as a result of metastases, may occur within 2 years of diagnosis if left untreated.

X-ray films, CT scan, MRI, and bone scans will show tumor location and size. Blood tests will reveal an elevated serum alkaline phosphatase. Chest x-ray film will confirm the presence of metastases.

## Medical Management

Treatment depends on the size and location of the tumor, presence of metastases, and the patient's age, general health, life-style, and preferences. Treatment options include the following:

1. Radiation
2. Chemotherapy
3. Surgical management
   a. Amputation
   b. Limb salvage procedures (Figures 65-42 and 65-43)

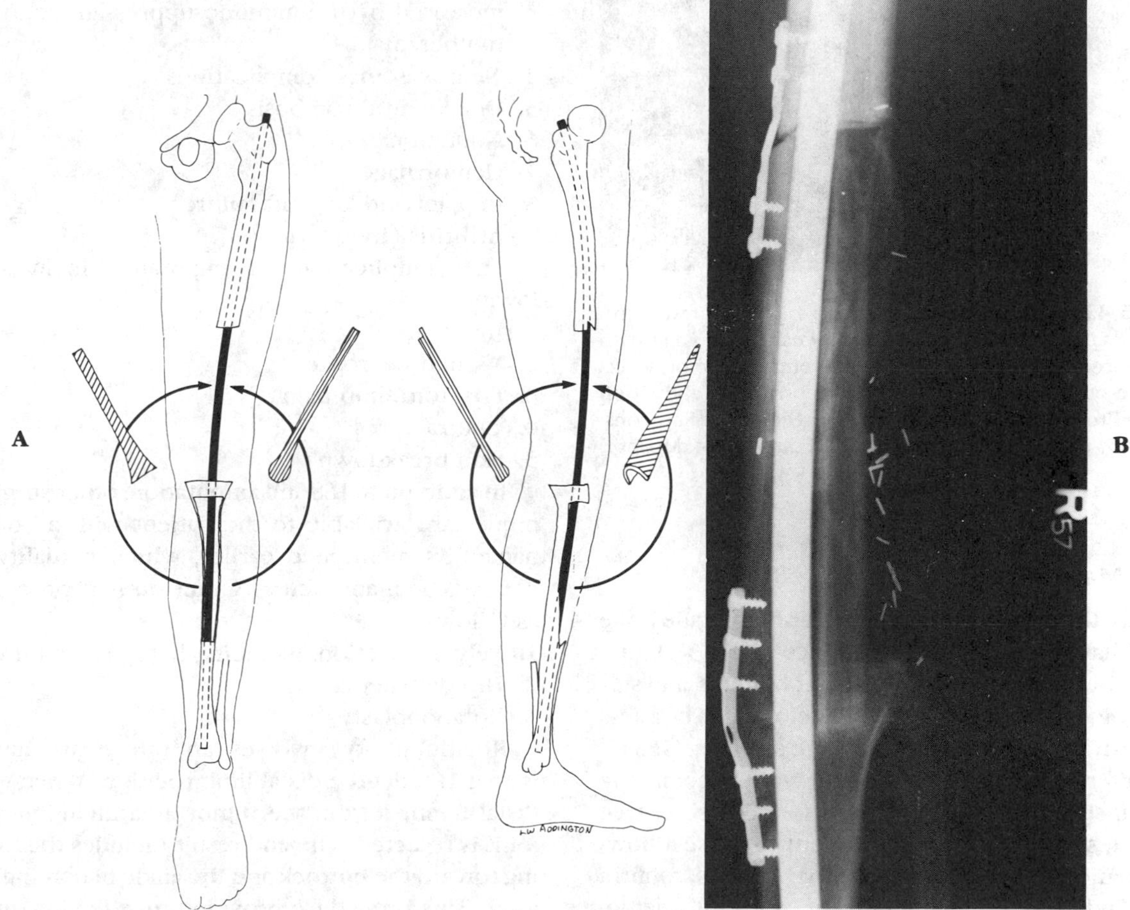


FIGURE 65-42 **A,** When distal femur has been resected and arthrodesis is desired, anterior one third of tibia and proximal fibula may be used to span defect. Extremity is stabilized with a long fluted intramedullary rod. When proximal tibia is resected, anterior one third of distal femur and a segment of fibula are used to span defect. Iliac bone graft is added to improve strength of reconstruction. Allograft segments also have proven successful in filling defect. **B,** Postoperative radiograph of patient who had resection arthrodesis for stage IIB tumor in distal femur. He uses no external aids and is fully active. (From American Academy of Orthopaedic Surgeons: *Instructional course lectures,* vol 33, St Louis, 1984, Mosby.)

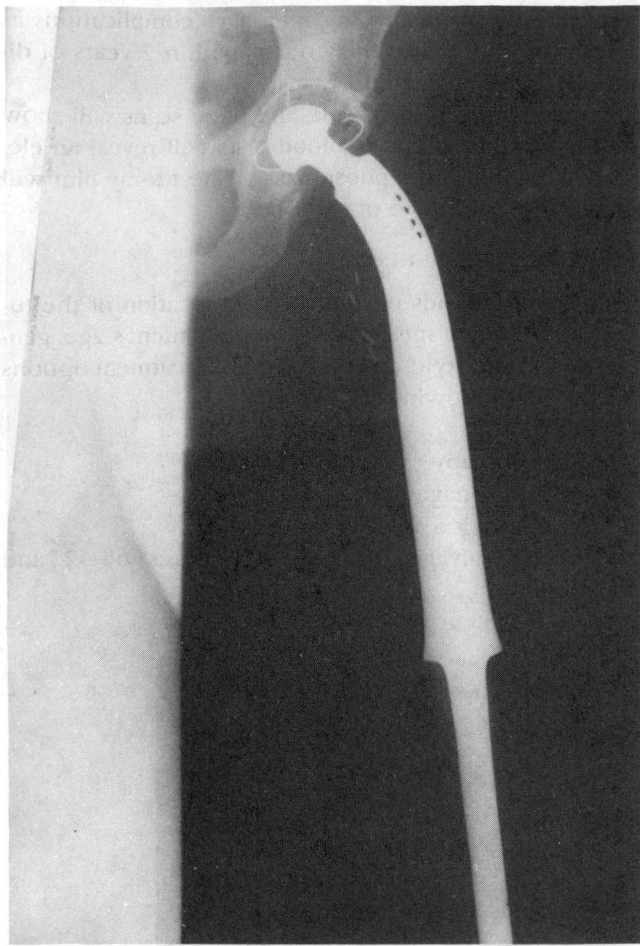

**FIGURE 65-43** This custom-made total hip was used to replace proximal femur and hip joint of 50-year-old woman with a chondrosarcoma. She has had no recurrence of tumor, walks with a cane with a modest limp, but has no active abduction of the hip. (From American Academy of Orthopaedic Surgeons: *Instructional course lectures*, vol 33, St Louis, 1984, Mosby.)

## Surgical Management

Historically the treatment of choice for high-grade bone sarcomas has been amputation. Since the 1980s advances in chemotherapy, diagnostic techniques, and surgical techniques have led to the development of a less radical treatment option: **limb salvage surgery** (LSS).[31] In 1984 after studying 2000 patients with sarcoma, the National Institute of Health (NIH) found disease-free survival rates after LSS to be equivalent to those following amputation.[25] Other retrospective studies confirm the NIH findings.[14,27,33] With current adjuvant chemotherapy protocols, the disease-free survival rate for osteosarcoma is 40% to 70%.[14] Following both limb salvage and amputation, the 5-year survival rates vary from 40% to 70%. The Musculoskeletal Tumor Society found the rate for local recurrence of tumor in the distal femur following LSS to be 10%. The reported recurrence rate was approximately the same as for patients who had undergone above-knee amputation.[14] Generally, a patient should be informed to expect a 5% to 10% (reported ranges from 3% to 25%) chance of local tumor recurrence following LSS.[27] If the tumor does recur, amputation will probably be indicated (in the absence of metastases).

There are no histologic contraindications to LSS. In addition to treatment of osteosarcoma, LSS is used to treat patients with Ewing's sarcoma, chondrosarcoma, giant cell tumor, and other tumors. Contraindications to LLS include a large invasive tumor, involvement of the neurovascular bundle, inability to achieve tumor-free margins, or a technically difficult surgical approach, such as a tumor in the distal tibia.[25,27-29]

LSS definitely results in more complications than amputation.[25,27,29] Documented complications of LSS include the following:

1. Local recurrence of tumor
2. Wound and skin necrosis: the procedure may necessitate extensive soft tissue flaps
3. Deep infection (incidence of 6% to 13%; may be increased by the immunosuppressant action of chemotherapy)
4. Neurovascular complications
5. Deep vein thrombosis
6. Nonunion
7. Hemorrhage
8. Implant and/or graft failure
9. Arthritis (long-term)

The complications of amputation include the following:

1. Infection
2. Wound necrosis
3. Phantom limb pain
4. Contractures
5. Skin breakdown

In addition to LSS and amputation, other surgical techniques are available to the patient with a bone malignancy. As mentioned earlier, which modality is used depends on many factors. Other surgical procedures are as follows:

1. Pelvic resection, including hemipelvectomy
2. Hip disarticulation
3. Rotationplasty

Rotationplasty involves an intercalary amputation with a 180-degree distal limb rotation. When used for a distal femur lesion, the tumor area including the knee joint is resected. The end result includes the foot pointing toward the buttock and the ankle becoming the knee joint. This procedure provides knee flexion and extension potential with the use of a prosthesis and also accommodates limb growth in children. It provides more function than a high level above-knee amputation or hip disarticulation. Patients may experience a disturbance of body image.

Intuitively, one might assume that patients would prefer a limb-sparing procedure to an amputation. Surprisingly enough, research does not support this hypothesis.[33] However, more research is needed to further validate these results. Data do indicate that psychologic adjustment is better following lower extremity amputation than following upper extremity amputation.[33] It has also shown that patients prefer a surgical technique that allows them knee motion.[33]

## Nursing Management

Nursing care for the patient undergoing LSS is challenging. The patient and family, who may still be trying to cope with the diagnosis of cancer, are now faced with difficult decisions regarding treatment options. Nursing interventions focus on education and support. Nursing interventions include but are not limited to the following:

1. Discussion of diagnosis, prognosis, and treatment options
2. Exploration of the patient's understanding of the risks, benefits, and expected outcomes of treatments available
3. Preoperative preparation regarding perioperative experience, including use of allograft, hardware, and possible need for transfusion
4. Explanation of potential complications
5. Exploration of the patient's expected functional abilities (Patients should understand that a "normal" limb is not a reasonable expectation following LSS and that there will be some degree of residual disability.[25,33])
6. Instruction and supervision of correct use of supportive devices
7. Support of decision-making abilities of the patient and family
8. Referral to support groups or community services
9. Promotion of independence within capabilities
10. Encouragement of effective coping strategies
11. Promotion of mobility
12. Promotion of acceptance of body image
13. Prevention of complications

## QUESTIONS TO CONSIDER

- Describe five psychosocial problems persons with musculoskeletal disorders may have. What interventions could you use to help the patient manage these problems? How would you provide support to the patient?
- What is the nurse's role when considering preventable factors of musculoskeletal disorders?
- What are some of the current theories of causation of rheumatoid arthritis?
- What are the early clinical manifestations of rheumatoid arthritis, and how do they change as the disease progresses?
- What laboratory findings usually indicate rheumatoid arthritis?

## QUESTIONS TO CONSIDER—cont'd

- What is meant by the pyramid of therapy of rheumatoid arthritis? Describe some forms of adjunctive therapy.
- What are some nursing diagnoses commonly identified for persons with rheumatoid arthritis? List their related interventions.
- List the name and purpose of some of the surgeries performed to treat persons with rheumatoid arthritis. Describe the postoperative nursing care associated with each.
- What types of treatment or surgery may be necessary for uncontrolled SLE or secondary to complications of therapy?
- Describe the etiology/epidemiology, pathophysiology, and clinical manifestations of polymyositis. What marks the disease as dermatomyositis?
- Discuss the medical and nursing management of persons with polymyositis.
- What type of deformity may develop as a result of progression of ankylosing spondylitis?
- What are the goals of treatment for persons with ankylosing spondylitis?
- What are some of the other names for degenerative joint disease? How are degenerative joint disease and rheumatoid arthritis differentiated?
- What are some of the characteristic changes or symptoms that occur in certain joints as a result of degenerative joint disease?
- Name two of the surgical procedures that may be performed for persons with degenerative joint disease.
- What are some nursing diagnoses commonly identified for persons with degenerative joint disease? List the related nursing interventions.
- What two postoperative considerations are of utmost importance when caring for a patient who has had a total joint replacement?
- Name some of the disorders that can result from degenerative changes in the spine.
- Describe the conservative treatment of degenerative joint disease of the spine. List some of the surgical procedures that may be performed on the spine. What special positioning technique will the nurse assist the patient with postoperatively?
- Explain the signs and symptoms of slight, mild, and severe deformity in scoliosis.
- Outline both conservative and surgical treatment for scoliosis. What is the importance of the degree of the curve?
- What are some nursing diagnoses commonly identified for persons with scoliosis? List their related nursing interventions.

## CRITICAL THINKING ACTIVITIES

- What aspects of nursing care will be the same or similar for all patients undergoing surgical procedures for degenerative disorders of the musculoskeletal system?
- You have cared for a postsurgical patient with bursitis. How will the care of this patient assist you in caring for patients with other nonarticular rheumatic diseases?
- In what ways can the nurse assist individuals with the prevention of musculoskeletal disorders?

## CHAPTER SUMMARY

### PHYSIOLOGIC DISABILITIES

- Most persons with a musculoskeletal disorder have one or more of five common problems: pain, stiffness, decrease in muscle strength, loss of dexterity, and loss of locomotor ability.
- A number of potential or actual complications may accompany immobility. Any or all of the major body systems may be involved.
- Rest, activity, joint protection, and energy conservation are some interventions common to a number of musculoskeletal disorders. The nurse's responsibility is to help the patient understand the meaning of these interventions and to teach the patient how to carry out these activities.
- Assistive, supportive, and safety devices are available for persons with musculoskeletal disorders. These include ambulatory, feeding, bathing, and dressing aids. Safety devices such as arms mounted around toilets are designed to help prevent falls and accidents.
- The application of heat and cold can be used for persons with musculoskeletal disorders to relieve stiffness and pain. Heat may also have a sedative or relaxing effect. Cold is helpful in reducing or preventing swelling. Caution must be used whenever heat or cold is applied to prevent tissue damage.
- Intermittent or constant traction can be used to help reduce contractures or to relieve pain. It is usually applied in the form of skin traction, such as Buck's extension, Russell traction, or pelvic traction.
- Splints and braces (orthoses) can be used to stabilize or support a joint, protect a joint or body part from external trauma, mechanically correct dysfunction by supporting the joint in its functional position, and assist patients in exercising specific joints. When patients must wear orthoses, nurses need to inspect the patient's skin for irritation, notify the orthotist when adjustments need to be made, instruct the patient in the proper application and care of the orthosis, and assist the patient in making the psychologic adjustment to wearing the orthosis.
- Principles of positioning and transfer are fundamental to most nursing care, but nurses must consider the special need for prevention or minimization of pain when moving patients with musculoskeletal problems.
- Exercise is a prescribed form of activity to preserve joint mobility, maintain muscle tone, and strengthen certain muscle groups. The ability to exercise may be enhanced by the application of heat or cold and the administration of analgesics before the exercise session. Patients should not exercise when joints or muscles are acutely inflamed. The nurse should be aware of the patient's specific exercise program and provide support and assistance to perform the exercises.
- Many of the medications used for the treatment of musculoskeletal problems are antiinflammatory analgesics. The use of narcotic analgesics in chronic inflammatory musculoskeletal conditions is generally contraindicated, although narcotics are used in the treatment of acute injuries and postoperative pain. The nurse's role when caring for patients taking antiinflammatory medications includes teaching about the action of the medication, correct dose and method of administration, and how to recognize untoward side effects.
- Special diets are usually not recommended for persons with musculoskeletal disorders, but patients should be careful about not gaining weight. Added weight increases the patient's energy consumption and causes weight-bearing joints to be overly stressed. Nurses can help promote weight loss by teaching the patient about a properly supervised reduction diet.
- Persons with a musculoskeletal problem may require elective surgery for correction of deformity, relief of pain, or restoration of musculoskeletal function. The major objectives of orthopaedic treatment are restoration or maintenance of function of a body part, prevention of deformity, correction of deformity if it already exists, and development of the patient's powers of compensation and adaptation if loss of function or permanent deformity is not preventable. The orthopaedist considers what procedure is best suited to achieve the desired objective for the patient. Orthopaedic care is highly individualized to the patient being treated. Refer to Table 65-6 for a summary of the surgical procedures to the musculoskeletal system.

### PSYCHOSOCIAL PROBLEMS

- Persons with musculoskeletal disorders may have some common psychosocial problems. These can include difficulty with their reaction to disfigurement or disability; difficulty with dependence, independence, or interdependence; adaptation to assistive, supportive, or corrective devices; the socioeconomic impact of their disorder; and their family relationships.
- Support, teaching, and guidance (counseling) are the nursing interventions employed to achieve therapeutic outcomes for psychosocial problems.

## PREVENTION

- Factors of prevention and teaching must be considered for persons with musculoskeletal disability. Preventive measures to combat illnesses that cause musculoskeletal disorders can be used on a community-wide basis. For those conditions in which the cause is unknown, attention is focused on preventing complications. General teaching on an individual basis can include early attention to good posture, body mechanics, dietary habits, and promotion of safety.

## INFLAMMATORY DISORDERS OF THE MUSCULOSKELETAL SYSTEM

- Rheumatoid arthritis is a chronic systemic disease most prominently manifested as an inflammation in the synovium of the diarthrodial joints. It is more prevalent in women than men. The cause of this disease is unknown.
- The disease process begins as an inflammation of the synovium. The inflammatory process is set off by a "triggering" event such as some sort of irritation or damage. WBCs rush into the area, releasing chemicals, prostaglandins, leukotrienes, and digestive enzymes. Collagen (the main structural protein of connective tissue) is broken down. The process becomes chronic and leads to thickening of the synovium and formation of granulation tissue. The cartilage becomes necrotic. Destruction of cartilage and bone may lead to dislocation of the joints.
- Early manifestations of the disease may include complaints of fever, weight loss, fatigue, generalized discomfort that is poorly localized (fibrositis), and morning stiffness. These symptoms may later be replaced by more specific (localized) pain and articular inflammation with swelling, redness, warmth, and tenderness.
- The joints of the hands and the feet are often affected early. The joints of the hands, wrists, feet, ankles, elbows, and knees are most commonly involved, usually in a bilaterally symmetric pattern. Shoulder involvement and hip involvement are later phenomena.
- The course of rheumatoid arthritis varies greatly from patient to patient and is marked by periods of exacerbation and remission. Some evidence suggests that exacerbations can be triggered by mental stress or physical trauma.
- Laboratory findings usually indicative of rheumatoid arthritis include an elevated erythrocyte sedimentation rate, mild leukocytosis, positive rheumatoid factor, narrowing of the joint spaces and erosion of articular surfaces on x-ray films, inflammatory changes in synovial tissue (biopsy), and increased turbidity and decreased viscosity of synovial fluid (needle aspiration).
- Medical management of rheumatoid arthritis is generally described as a pyramid of therapy. The foundation is a good history and physical examination, prescription of rest and appropriate exercise, education of patient and family, and control of inflammation with salicylates. Medications are added based on the patient's response to conservative therapy. The goals of therapy are relief of pain, maintenance of joint function, prevention and correction of deformity, and correction of other health factors.
- Nursing management consists of measures to promote comfort, promote mobility, encourage good nutrition, and promote improved self-esteem. Patient teaching is stressed.
- Surgical intervention may be warranted when rheumatoid arthritis has caused severe joint destruction. Common procedures are synovectomy, arthrotomy, arthrodesis, and arthroplasty.
- Systemic lupus erythematosus (SLE) is a chronic inflammatory disease of unknown cause. It affects women more often than men. Its course can be controlled by corticosteroids, but some patients do die as a result of lesions affecting major organs or from secondary infections.
- Pathologic manifestations of SLE include synovial involvement, severe vasculitis, renal involvement, lymph node necrosis, development of small white spots in the retina (cytoid bodies), and lesions of the nervous system.
- The initial manifestation of SLE is often arthritis, but the joint symptoms may be transient. The patient may complain of sensitivity to the sun. Erythema, usually in a butterfly pattern, can appear over the cheeks and bridge of the nose. The patient may also have findings of glomerulonephritis, pleuritis, pericarditis, peritonitis, neuritis, or anemia. Laboratory findings are specific to the organs involved.
- Medical management begins conservatively with rest, exercise, and medications. Kidney dialysis or transplant may be necessary for uncontrolled lupus nephritis, or total hip replacement may be necessary for avascular necrosis resulting from high-dose steroid therapy.
- Nursing management centers on patient teaching and promoting comfort and ADL.
- Polymyositis (dermatomyositis) is an inflammatory disease of striated (voluntary) muscle. It occurs more frequently in women than men. The cause is unknown.
- Diagnostic tests for polymyositis include manual muscle test, electromyogram, muscle biopsy, serum enzymes, and 24-hour urine tests.
- Medical management consists of rest and treatment with corticosteroids, and nursing management addresses teaching, prevention of skin breakdown, and promotion of comfort and mobility.
- Ankylosing spondylitis is a chronic, progressive disorder affecting the joints of the hips and spine. It occurs more frequently in men than women. The cause

is unknown, although there may be a genetic link. Progression of the disease cannot be stopped by any known treatment at present.

- As a result of the inflammatory process within the spine, the bones of the spine fuse (ankylose). Inflammation usually begins at the sacroiliac joints and progresses up the spine, resulting in fusion of the entire spine.
- Early symptoms may include low back pain and pain and swelling of the hips, knees, or shoulders. Mild fever, anorexia, and fatigue may also be present. Symptoms flare and subside. Eventually pain may decrease and motion of the back becomes restricted. Fusion of the sacroiliac joints and spine may occur, resulting in a kyphosis at the cervicodorsal junction.
- Presence in the serum of the HLA-B27 genetic marker and x-ray films showing bony growths (syndesmophytes) can indicate ankylosing spondylitis.
- Medical management consists of exercise, rest, heat, and antiinflammatory analgesics. Spinal osteotomy or hip arthroplasty may be necessary for persons with severe symptoms.
- Nursing management centers on patient teaching, promotion of comfort and correct posture, and prevention of complications.
- Inflammation of the supportive structures and structures located near the joints is referred to as nonarticular rheumatism. Disorders in this category include fibrositis, tenosynovitis, bursitis, and carpal tunnel syndrome.

## NONARTICULAR RHEUMATISM

- Most nonarticular rheumatic diseases are caused by trauma, strain, and overuse of the related joint. The patient will complain of swelling, pain, and limited ability to move the associated joint. With carpal tunnel syndrome, the patient will complain of dysesthesia, paresthesia, or hypesthesia of the thumb, index, and middle fingers related to pressure on the median nerve of the wrist.
- Medical management of nonarticular rheumatic diseases consists primarily of rest of the involved area, splinting, antiinflammatory agents, or local steroid injections. Surgery may be required for removal of calcium deposits (e.g., in bursitis) or release of inflamed ligaments (e.g., the carpal ligament in carpal tunnel syndrome). Nursing management focuses on patient teaching and promoting comfort. Postoperative care measures are provided for patients treated with surgical interventions.
- Dupuytren's contracture is contracture of the palmar fascia causing the ring and sometimes the little finger to flex into the palm and lose the capacity to be extended. Surgical removal of the involved palmar fascia may be required if conservative measures to relieve symptoms are ineffective. Nursing management then addresses postoperative care.

## DEGENERATIVE DISORDERS

- Degenerative joint disease is the result of degeneration of the articular cartilage of the synovial joints. Unlike rheumatoid arthritis, it is not systemic. Degenerative joint disease is also known as osteoarthritis, hypertrophic arthritis, osteoarthrosis, or senescent arthritis. It is an extremely common disease. Symptomatic degenerative joint disease is usually noted in the 50- to 70-year age group, although most persons past 40 years have hypertrophic changes of the joints.
- Two forms of osteoarthritis exist: primary, for which the cause is unknown; and secondary, which can be the result of trauma, infection, fracture, another type of arthritis, stress on weight-bearing joints from obesity, unusual wear and tear on joints associated with certain occupations, or a genetic disposition.
- The target organ of degenerative joint disease is the articular cartilage. This normally white, translucent, smooth cartilage becomes yellow and opaque with softened areas and a rough or frayed surface. The cartilage is digested by enzymes and is eventually destroyed. The underlying bone develops osteophytes (spurs of new bone) that may break off into the joint cavity.
- Persons with degenerative joint disease have pain, stiffness, and limited range of motion, particularly in the large weight-bearing joints and in the joints of the hand. Inflammation is usually not present, and tenderness is mild. The joints may become enlarged (deformed). Crepitation and changes in the alignment of the extremity may be present.
- Medical management objectives include relief of pain, restoration of joint function, and prevention of disability or further disease progression. Treatment includes medications, rest, exercise, joint protection, and the use of walking aids to decrease weight bearing on painful joints. Surgery may be indicated. Common surgical procedures include arthroscopic surgery for debridement, osteotomy for realignment, arthrodesis, and replacement arthroplasty.
- Nursing management of persons with degenerative joint disease focuses on teaching persons about the disease process and measures to exert control over their situation. Patients who undergo surgery require special postoperative care. Of particular importance are the mobility restrictions following total hip replacement, the exercise program following total knee replacement, and prevention of infection following any total joint replacement.
- Osteoporosis is a degenerative disorder of bone metabolism that is caused by a greater rate of bone resorption than bone formation. It occurs more frequently in White, postmenopausal women. The loss in bone mass predisposes the individual to pathologic fractures, especially of the vertebrae and hips.
- Medical management includes exercise, dietary supplements of calcium and vitamin D, and estrogen ther-

apy. The goal of treatment is to slow down bone loss.

- Nursing management focuses on education and identification of risk factors. Other interventions include promoting comfort, mobility, and safety to maximize independence and reduce potential for injury.
- Degenerative disease of the spine is a common but difficult problem. The intervertebral disks and facet joints of the spine are subjected to a great deal of stress in maintaining upright posture and providing mobility. Herniated nucleus pulposus, osteophyte formation, spondylolisthesis, and spinal stenosis are several conditions that result from degenerative changes in the spine.
- Degenerative diseases of the spine are clinically manifested as low back pain, sciatic pain radiating down the leg (e.g., with herniated nucleus pulposus), and neurologic signs and symptoms (e.g., with herniated nucleus pulposus, stenosis, and osteophyte formation). Conservative medical management consists of rest, heat, medications, and traction to relieve muscle spasm. Surgical interventions are carried out to decompress nerve roots and to stabilize the spine. Spinal surgery procedures include laminectomy, diskectomy, foraminotomy, and spinal fusion.
- Conservative nursing management consists of patient teaching, promoting comfort, and promoting lower extremity circulation.
- Nursing care following spinal surgery focuses on positioning (logrolling) and mobility, wound care, and patient comfort. Postoperative nursing interventions will differ depending on the level at which the spinal surgery was performed (e.g., lumbar, thoracic, or cervical).

## RESTRICTIVE DISORDERS

- Scoliosis is a restrictive disorder of the spine in which there is a lateral deviation of the spine from the midline. There are six classifications of scoliosis. Scoliosis may be present in both children and adults. Scoliosis may develop in localized areas of the spine or involve the whole spinal column. Curves may be S shaped or C shaped. The amount of impingement on the rib cage is determined by the degree of rotation of the curve. Stability of the spine and mobility of the trunk are affected by the balance of the curve.
- Scoliosis deformity can be slight, mild, or severe. Early deformity may not be easily detected but will increase with growth and age. Pain does not usually accompany scoliosis. The cardiopulmonary system can be impaired in advanced scoliosis. Medical management for early scoliosis includes exercise with or without traction, bracing in combination with exercise for curves less than 40 degrees, and corrective surgery if the curve exceeds 40 degrees and other measures have failed. Bone grafting and instrumentation are usually done to fuse the spine.
- Nursing management of persons with scoliosis consists of patient instruction for persons who are being treated conservatively. Patients who undergo surgery require special postoperative care. There is a high risk for pulmonary, gastrointestinal, and fluid balance complications following spinal fusion for scoliosis. Preventing such problems is a primary objective of the nurse. Instructing the patient about the brace he or she will be required to wear is another nursing responsibility.

## OTHER DISORDERS

- Osteomyelitis is a bone infection caused by either exogenous or internal pathogens. The most common causative organism for both types is *Staphylococcus aureus*. It is a chronic disease, treated with oral and intravenous antibiotic therapy, suction irrigation systems, and surgical debridement of infected bone.
- Other disorders of the musculoskeletal system include recurrent dislocation of the patella, gout, and bacterial arthritis. Recurrent dislocation of the patella involves malposition of the patellar tendon of the knee. Gout is a metabolic disorder that results from prolonged hyperuricemia. Urates are deposited in and around joints, usually in the knee or foot. Bacterial arthritis is a result of infection in which the synovial membrane is invaded by microorganisms.
- Recurrent dislocation of the patella is usually treated surgically. Management of gout is directed toward control of acute attacks and prevention of recurrent attacks. Medications and rest are prescribed to control joint symptoms. Medications are also used to enhance uric acid excretion or to decrease uric acid formation. Bacterial arthritis is treated with appropriate antibiotic therapy and rest (immobilization) of the joint. Irrigation and drainage may be necessary if antibiotic therapy is ineffective or if osteomyelitis is present.
- Nursing management of the above disorders is in collaboration with the medical plan of care. Patient teaching, promotion of rest or exercise as appropriate, promotion of comfort, and encouragement of participation in self-care are emphasized.
- Tumors of the musculoskeletal system include those arising from muscle, bone, cartilage, fibrous tissue, and bone marrow. Tumors can be benign or malignant.
- Some examples of benign tumors include osteoma, osteochondroma, leiomyoma, and giant cell tumor. Treatment methods include surgical excision and amputation.
- The most common primary bone tumor is osteosarcoma. It is a rapidly growing neoplasm that causes a moth-eaten pattern of bone destruction. Metastasis to the lungs is common.
- Treatment of osteosarcoma includes chemotherapy and surgical excision, either by amputation or limb salvage techniques.
- Limb salvage procedures have many potential complications but offer an alternative to amputation. The

patient must be fully informed regarding both procedures and their risks, benefits, and expected outcomes.

- Nursing interventions for patients with bone tumors focus on teaching, support, promotion of independence, and acceptance of body image.

## REFERENCES


1. Albin MS et al: Venous air embolism during lumbar laminectomy in the prone position: report of three cases, *Anesth Analges* (73):364-369, 1991.
2. Anderton JM: The prone position for the surgical patient: a historical review of the principles and hazards, *Br J Anaesthesia* (67):452-463, 1991.
3. Bauer RL: Assessing osteoporosis, *Hosp Pract* 26(suppl 1):23-29, 1991.
4. Brosnan H: Nursing management of the adolescent with idiopathic scoliosis, *Nurs Clin North Am* 26(1):17-31, 1991.
5. Brosnan H, Berda P: Pedicle screw fixation in the lumbar spine, *Orthop Nurs* 9(6):22-32, 1990.
6. Collo MCB et al: Evaluating arthritic complaints, *Nurse Practitioner* 16(2):9-20, 1991.
7. Cotran RS, Kumar V, Robbins SL: *Pathologic basis of disease,* ed 4, Philadelphia, 1989, WB Saunders Co.
8. Cotton LA: Unit rod segmental spinal instrumentation for the treatment of neuromuscular scoliosis, *Orthop Nurs* 10(5):17-23, 1991.
9. Dekker ML: Bone and soft tissue procurement, *Orthop Nurs* 8(2):31-34, 1989.
10. Deyo RA, Rainville J, Kent DL: What can the history and physical examination tell us about back pain? *JAMA* 268(6):760-765, 1992.
11. Dulin D: Facilitating early rehabilitation in limb-salvage patients, *ONF* 16(1):105, 1989.
12. Farrel J: *Illustrated guide to orthopaedic nursing,* ed 2, Philadelphia, 1982, JB Lippincott Co.
13. Feingold DJ et al: Complications of lumbar spine surgery, *Orthop Nurs* 19(4):39-57, 1991.
14. Gebhardt MC et al: The use of bone allografts for limb salvage in high-grade extremity osteosarcoma, *Clin Orthop Rel Res* 270:181-194, 1990.
15. Goldberg VM, Stevenson S: Natural history of autografts and allografts, *Clin Orthop* 225:7-16, 1987.
16. Hodge WA: Prevention of deep vein thrombosis after total knee arthroplasty: coumadin versus pneumatic calf compression, *CORR* 271:101-105, 1991.
17. Hu SS, Pashman RS: State of the art in medicine: spinal instrumentation evolution and state of the art, *Invest Radiol* 279(8):632-647, 1992.
18. Johnson DP, Eastwood DM: Beneficial effects of continuous passive motion after total condylar knee arthroplasty, *Ann R Coll Surgeons Eng* 74:412-416, 1992.
19. Liscum B: Osteoporosis: the silent disease, *Orthop Nurs* 11(4):21-24, 1992.
20. McCance KL, Huether SE: *Pathophysiology: the biological basis for disease in adults and children,* St Louis, 1990, Mosby.
21. Mosher CM: The papineau bone graft: a limb salvage technique, *Orthop Nurs* 10(3):27-32, 1991.
22. Moskowitz RW: *Clinical rheumatology: a problem oriented approach to diagnosis and management,* ed 2, Philadelphia, 1982, Lea & Febiger.
23. Mourad LA, Droste MM: *The nursing process in the care of adults with orthopaedic conditions,* ed 3, Albany, NY, 1993, Delmar Publishers Inc.
24. National Blood Resource Education Program's Nursing Education Working Group: Transfusion nursing: trends and practice for the 90's, *Am J Nurs* 91(6):42-56, 1991.
25. Piasecki PA: The nursing role in limb salvage surgery, *Nurs Clin North Am* 26(1):33-41, 1991.
26. Pigg J, Driscoll P, Caniff R: *Rheumatology nursing: a problem-oriented approach,* New York, 1985, John Wiley & Sons Inc.
27. Porth CM: *Pathophysiology: concepts of altered health states,* ed 3, Philadelphia, 1990, JB Lippincott Co.
28. Quill G et al: Complications associated with limb salvage for extremity sarcomas and their management, *Clin Ortho Rel Res* 260:242-249, 1989.
29. Racolin AA, Present DA: Osteochondral allografts for limb salvage, *Orthop Nurs* 8(2):35-39, 1989.
30. Rodts MF: Surgical intervention for adult scoliosis, *Orthop Nurs* 6(6):11-17, 1987.
31. Rothman RH, Simeone FA: *The spine,* ed 2, Philadelphia, 1982, WB Saunders Co.
32. Schlegel SI, Paulus HE: Update on NSAID use in rheumatic diseases, *Bull Rheum Dis* 36(6):1-8, 1986.
33. Simon MA: Limb salvage for osteosarcoma in the 1980s, *Clin Orthop Rel Res* 270:264-269, 1991.
34. Tempelhoff R, Williams EL, Vollmer DG: Is the "kneeling" prone position as dangerous as the sitting position for the development of venous air embolism? *Anesth Analges* 75:467-468, 1992.
35. Turek SL: *Orthopaedics: principles and their application,* vol 2, Philadelphia, 1987, JB Lippincott Co.
36. Wolfe SW, Lospinuso MF, Burke SW: Unilateral blindness as a complication of patient positioning for spinal surgery: a case report, *Spine* 17(5):600-605, 1992.

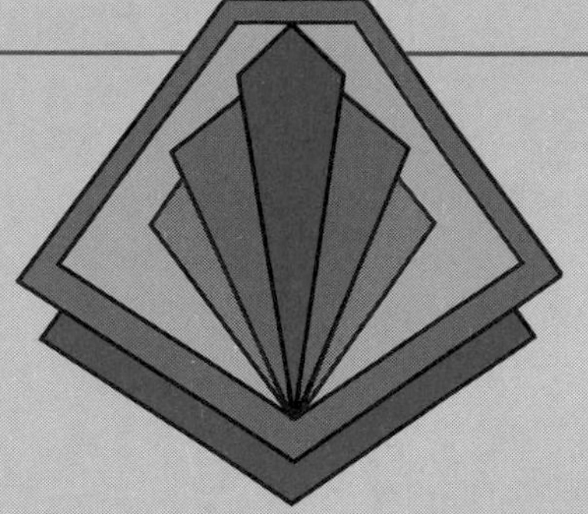

UNIT XI

# Alterations in Defense and Protection

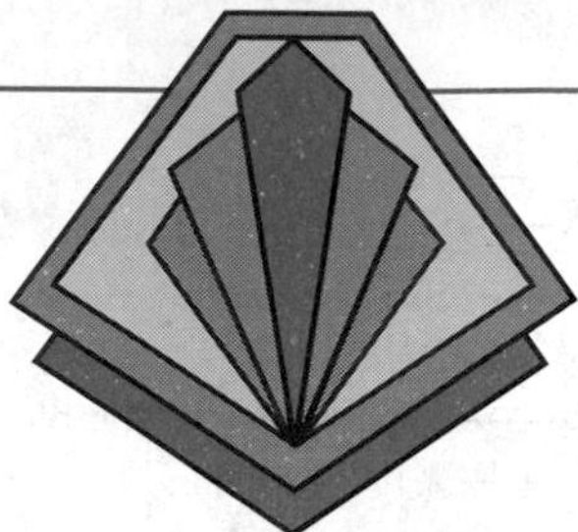

CHAPTER 66

# Assessment of the Skin

*Vickie Weaver*
*Barbara C. Long*

## CHAPTER OBJECTIVES

***After studying this chapter, the learner should be able to do the following:***

1. Identify the structures and functions of the skin.
2. Explain physiologic skin changes in elderly persons.
3. Describe guidelines and parameters for assessment of the skin and accessory structures.
4. Differentiate among various skin lesions.

## KEY TERMS

| | | |
|---|---|---|
| alopecia | melanin | sebum |
| crust | nodule | senile lentigines |
| dermis | papule | senile purpura |
| epidermis | paronychia | subcutaneous tissue |
| hirsutism | plaque | sweat glands |
| hyperpigmentation | pustule | vesicle |
| hypopigmentation | scale | vitiligo |
| macule | sebaceous glands | wheal |

## ANATOMY AND PHYSIOLOGY OF THE SKIN

The integument, or skin, is the largest organ of the body. It is exposed to the external environment and provides the first line of defense of the body; yet at the same time it is affected by changes in the internal environment. (See Chapter 13 for a review of biologic defense mechanisms.) Assessment of the integument provides data about how the person is affected by and is coping with both external and internal environments. Data obtained in the assessment provide the bases for identification of actual or potential nursing problems related to the skin, infection, fluid and electrolyte imbalances, nutritional imbalances, or inadequate oxygenation of tissues. Baseline observations are useful for identifying changes that may occur.

### STRUCTURE OF THE SKIN

The skin is composed of three major divisions: the epidermis, the dermis, and subcutaneous tissue (Figure 66-1). The **epidermis** consists of five layers. The outermost layer is a thin layer of closely packed, dead squamous cells that contain keratin, a fibrous protein, that gives skin its color. This dead cell layer is called the *stratum corneum*. The innermost layer, stratum basale or basement membrane, also is called the *stratum germinatirum* because it gives rise to new cells to renew the outermost layer that is constantly being shed and that does not have blood vessels. Between these two layers are the three other layers identified in Figure 66-1. These three layers are involved in keratin formation.

The second main layer, the **dermis,** or corium, is connected to the epidermis by the stratum basale. The dermis is composed of bundles of collagen fibers that act to support the epidermis. It is well supplied with nerves and blood vessels and contains appendages such as the sweat glands, sebaceous glands, and hair follicles.

The third layer of skin is **subcutaneous tissue,** composed of loose connective tissue filled with fat cells. Fat conducts heat only one fourth as rapidly as do other tissues and thus serves as the heat insulator of the body. It also serves as a cushion and is a storage site for energy. The subcutaneous layer also anchors the other two lay-

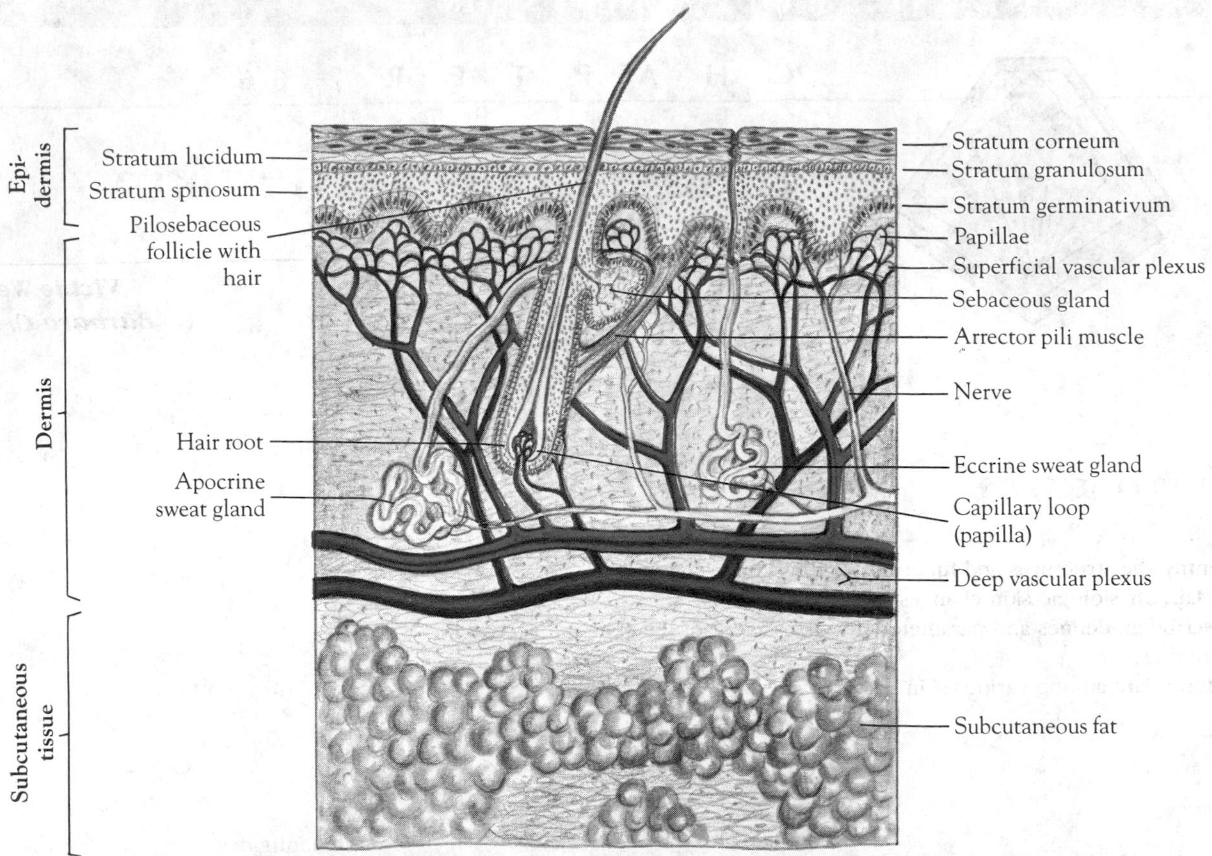


**FIGURE 66-1** Anatomy of skin and skin layers. (From Thompson JM et al: *Mosby's clinical nursing*, ed 3, St Louis, 1993, Mosby.)

ers to supportive structures (e.g., muscle, tendon, bone).

Thickness of the skin varies over different areas of the body. Exposed areas such as hands and face usually have thicker skin that contains more keratin in the epidermis. The skin on the inner aspect of the arms is thinner and therefore more sensitive to heat.

**Sweat glands** excrete directly to the surface of the skin and are under control of the sympathetic nervous system. There are two types of sweat glands—*eccrine* and *apocrine*. The eccrine glands are distributed throughout the body and are more abundant in the forehead, palms, and soles of the feet. Eccrine glands assist in the heat-regulating mechanisms of the body. The apocrine glands are found mainly in the axillary and genital regions. Some of the protoplasm of these secretory cells is secreted with the fluid, and it is bacterial decomposition of the sweat from these glands that is responsible for body odor. Sweat glands of the axilla, palms, and soles are mostly under control of the stress response.

**Sebaceous glands** secrete an oily, odorless fluid (**sebum**) into the hair follicles. Ear wax is sebum from glands in the external ear canal. Sebum protects the hair follicle from infection and lubricates the skin.

## FUNCTIONS OF THE SKIN

### Protection

The outermost layer of the epidermis, the stratum corneum, is a relatively impermeable layer of tightly packed flat cells that provide protection of the underlying tissue from the outer environment. A normal amount of nonpathogenic bacteria is present on the outer surface of the skin, but the dryness of the surface keeps the number small because microorganisms require moisture for growth. Bacteria that penetrate hair follicles usually are removed by the sebum. Fat-soluble substances such as emollient lotion can penetrate the skin by passing through the hair follicles and sebaceous glands.

An intact skin is the first line of defense against bacterial and foreign-substance invasion, slight physical trauma, heat, or ultraviolet rays. When the skin is exposed to environmental factors such as pressure, friction, and internal shearing forces, the epidermis is compressed to the depth of the supporting structures (i.e., bone). With prolonged exposure the capillary bed within the dermis and the greater vessels within the subcutaneous tissue become occluded, causing tissue ischemia to the area. If the ischemia is not reversed by removal of the source of pressure, cellular death is imminent and the skin's defensive line is in jeopardy.

The epidermis can be weakened by scraping or stripping the surface, such as by dry razors or by removal of tape. Once the barrier has weakened, permeability to bacteria, drugs, and other foreign substances is increased. Large amounts of drugs can be absorbed by extensive denuded skin areas. Epidermis that becomes overdry may crack and lead to breaks in the surface. If it remains wet for long periods of time, it becomes macerated and the moisture provides a medium for bacterial growth.

Mucous membranes, although continuous with the stratum corneum, are somewhat protected from the external environment. Fluids and other substances such as certain drugs can be absorbed through the mucous membranes.

### Heat Regulation

Body temperature is controlled by *radiation* of heat from the surface of the skin, *conduction* of heat from skin to other objects or air, removal of heat by air currents on the skin *(convection)*, or *evaporation* of water from skin surfaces. Insensible water evaporation from the skin and lungs occurs at a rate of 600 to 1000 ml/day. On a hot day the only way the body can lose heat is by evaporation, and anything that restricts evaporation under these conditions will increase body temperature. Blood vessels of the skin help control body temperature by constricting in cold environments to promote conservation of heat and dilating in warm environments to promote loss of heat by radiation. These mechanisms help maintain a constant internal body temperature.

### Sensory Perception

The skin contains receptor endings of nerves responsible for sensing pain, touch, heat, and cold. Stimulation of these nerve endings affords the person the ability to be in close communication with the immediate external environment. Distribution of the sensory endings is generalized; however, there are certain areas of the body with higher numbers. The hands, for example, have a higher concentration than the forearms.

### Excretion

Water lost through the skin is a factor in maintaining water balance in the body. Salt is lost through excessive sweating in addition to water loss. A person can become acclimatized to a continually hot environment, however, and the amount of salt lost decreases over time.

### Vitamin D Production

Synthesis of vitamin D takes place in the skin by the effect of sunlight (ultraviolet rays). Vitamin D is necessary in the metabolism of calcium and phosphorus (see Chapter 39).

### Expression

Because the skin is the part of the body that is visible to others, it is a means of communicating feelings. Also, because of its visibility, skin is largely involved in a person's *body image*. Individuals become concerned when there is fear of or presence of disfigurement. (See Chapter 9 for a discussion of body image.)

## PHYSIOLOGIC CHANGES WITH AGING

Many skin changes may be observed as the person ages (Table 66-1). These changes result primarily from loss of subcutaneous tissue, degeneration of collagen and elastic fibers, loss of melanocytes, increased capillary fragility, decreased secretion of sweat glands, hormonal changes, and overexposure to environmental elements.

The skin loses its elasticity and becomes loose and wrinkled. Exposed areas may be thickened, but in general the skin becomes thinner, drier, and more fragile. There are fewer hair follicles; therefore absorbency of fat-soluble substances is less. Lesions appear, the most common of which are **senile lentigines** (brown spots, Figure 66-2) or **senile purpura** (red to purple ecchymoses seen on exposed areas). Seborrheic keratoses (see Chapter 67) are more common than actinic keratoses. Changes in appearance of the hair and nails also occur.

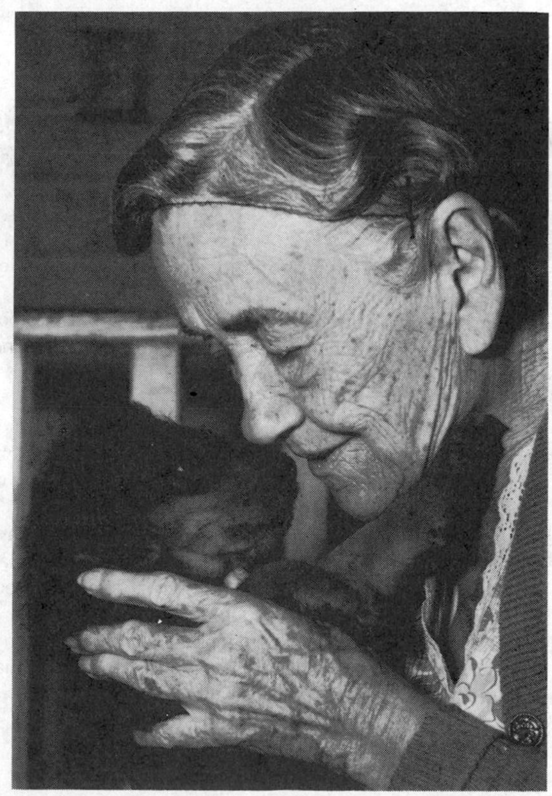

**FIGURE 66-2** Elderly patients have skin changes. Note discolored spots on skin and tiny raised area on this woman's eyelid. (VanDerMeid from Monkmeyer Press Photo Service.)

**TABLE 66-1 Changes in Skin, Hair, and Nails as a Result of Aging**

| PARAMETER | OBSERVABLE CHANGES | CAUSE |
|---|---|---|
| **SKIN** | | |
| Color | Paleness in white skin | Decreased vascularity of dermis; loss of melanocytes |
| | Brown spots (senile lentigines) | Hyperpigmentation |
| | Purple patches (senile purpura) | Blood leaking from poorly supported fragile capillaries |
| Moisture | Dry skin, decreased perspiration | Decreased sebaceous and sweat gland activity |
| Elasticity, turgor | Decreased elasticity | Loss of collagen and elastic fibers |
| | Loose folds and wrinkles | |
| | Decreased turgor | |
| Texture | Some rough areas | Environmental effects over time and less moisture |
| | Thin, more transparent skin | Thinning of epidermis from decreased vascularity of dermis; loss of underlying tissue |
| **HAIR** | | |
| Color | Grayness | Decreased number of melanocytes in hair |
| Consistency | Thinner on head and body | Decreased density and rate of hair growth |
| | Coarser in nose of men | Increased density of nasal hair |
| Distribution | Loss of hair on head and body | Decreased rate of hair growth; decreased hormones; decreased peripheral circulation |
| | Increased hair on face of women | Higher androgen to estrogen ratio |
| **NAILS** | | |
| | More brittle | Slowing of nail growth; decreased peripheral circulation |
| | Longitudinal ridges | |
| | Thickening and yellowing of toenails | |

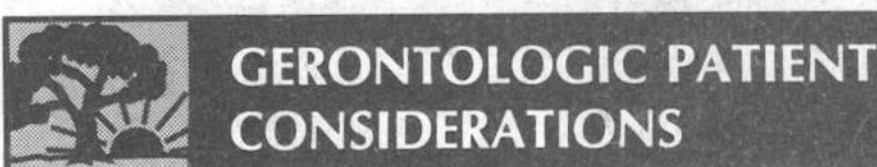

## GERONTOLOGIC PATIENT CONSIDERATIONS

### ASSESSMENT

Assess for presence of dryness and intactness of skin, skin infections, and lesions.

Identify medications currently taken by patient, and assess potential for photosensitivity (see Table 67-7). Thiazides and phenothiazides are common medications taken by elders.

### INTERVENTION

Teach patient to avoid frequent baths, especially hot baths, that cause additional skin dryness. Tell patient to apply lotion to skin immediately after bathing.

Teach patient to report early signs of skin infection to physician. The elderly person's decreased immune response may delay healing. The elderly person with herpes zoster needs protection from secondary infection such as pneumonia.

Teach patient to differentiate benign skin lesions commonly seen with aging (brown spots, bruises) from potentially malignant lesions, and to report the latter to physician.

### COMMON DISORDERS IN ELDERS

Benign skin tumors
Skin cancers
Dermatitis medicamentosa
Skin infections, especially herpes zoster
Stasis dermatitis of legs

The elderly person is also more likely to have one or more chronic diseases and to be taking medications that can cause skin changes. Dry skin may cause itching and can lead to skin breakdown if scratched. Stasis dermatitis may occur if there is marked decrease of circulation to the legs. Skin infections occur more readily because of increased epidermal permeability.

Some general principles related to assessment and health teaching and a listing of common disorders in the elderly are listed in the accompanying box.

## SUBJECTIVE DATA

The patient history is of less importance in skin disorders than is the physical assessment. If during a general history the patient describes a skin problem or skin discomfort (itching, superficial pain), then further data are obtained, including the following information[4]:

1. *Usual skin condition:* usual appearance, color, moisture, texture, integrity
2. *Onset of the problem:* initial sites: when changes were first noticed; skin appearance at onset; any other symptoms noted at time of onset, such as pain, itching
3. *Changes since onset:* changes in location of lesions; changes in appearance; new symptoms such as pain or itching
4. *Specific known cause:* for example, contact with poison ivy, exposure to a known allergen, stress

5. *If cause is unknown:*
   a. Recent exposure to sensitizing substances, such as metals, chemicals, detergents, poisonous plants
   b. New drug prescriptions such as penicillin
   c. Occupation: contact with potential skin irritants, hands constantly in water
   d. Recreational activities: for example, painting, camping, gardening
   e. Exposure to sun (burn, photosensitivity, skin cancer) or cold (frostbite)
6. *Alleviating factors:* physician-prescribed or self-prescribed
7. *Psychologic reaction to skin changes:* withdrawal from social activities; cosmetics for coverup; feelings about the problem (body image)

# OBJECTIVE DATA

## METHODS OF ASSESSMENT

The skin is an organ that can be examined by *direct inspection* and *observation* with no tools but a good light. *Palpation* also is used in gathering data about certain types of lesions. See principles related to skin assessment in the Guidelines box below.[4]

### Guidelines for Skin Assessment

1. Be prepared; have a good light available and well-controlled room temperature. If the lighting is inadequate, lesions may be missed or described inaccurately. If the room temperature is not well-controlled, vasoconstriction, vasodilation, and papillary erections occur, giving false data.
2. Be systematic: if only some parts of the skin are inspected, an important parameter may be omitted or a lesion missed.
3. Be thorough: look at all areas carefully. If the person is lying down, be sure to examine the back, especially the sacral area. Lift folds of tissue, such as under the breasts or gluteal folds. The examiner's embarrassment or anticipated embarrassment of the examinee may result in inadequate data. Do not forget to assess the mucous membranes as well.
4. Be specific: when lesions are identified, describe the lesions using metric system and established parameters (e.g., color, size, shape).
5. Compare right side with left side: when observing changes in skin color or tissue shape, always compare one side of the body with the other to differentiate structural from pathologic changes as well as symmetry of manifestation.
6. Record the data: unrecorded data are lost data. Baseline observations indicating normality or abnormality are needed for comparison with subsequent findings. Changes need to be recorded to determine progress toward achieving desired outcomes.
7. Have a metric measuring tool available; specific lesions are categorized according to size (see Table 66-3).
8. Use appropriate technique: palpation is used during physical assessment of the skin. Lesions are palpated for density, induration, and tenderness. Universal precautions (see Chapter 71) need to be observed during palpation, and the examiner should determine whether it is appropriate to use gloves.

Considerable data can be obtained from physical assessment of the skin, concerning not only dermatologic problems, but also the person's overall health status. A systematic head-to-toe skin assessment usually is conducted while gathering other significant data in the initial interview and physical assessment of the person. Specific areas of the skin are reassessed as potential or existing problems are identified.

## PARAMETERS OF GENERAL SKIN ASSESSMENT

The objective data to be collected when examining the skin for general health status include skin color, temperature, moisture, elasticity, turgor, texture, and odor.

### Color

Changes in skin color are best observed in the lips, mucous membranes of the mouth, earlobes, fingernails and toenails, and the extremities. The lips show rapid color changes. Color of the skin varies with the amount of *melanin* in the cells and with the *blood supply* (Table 66-2). Skin color may be masked by cosmetics or tanning.

#### Pigmentation

Melanin formation requires the amino acid tyrosine, the enzyme tyrosinase, and molecular oxygen. Variations of general pigmentation are seen within one individual; an increase in pigmentation usually is seen on exposed surfaces and in the areola of the nipples. Conversely, decreased pigmentation is seen on unexposed surfaces and on the palms and soles of dark-skinned persons.

**Hyperpigmentation** occurs normally in some persons as a genetic factor (dark skin). Light-skinned persons may have increased pigmentation from the effects of sunlight (tanning). Melanin is formed in the basal cells of the stratum basale and then gradually moves to the surface, where it is cast off and the tan fades. Elderly light-skinned persons may normally develop irregular brown patches. Hyperpigmentation may occur with x-ray therapy as a result of activation of tyrosinase. This type of hyperpigmentation fades slowly but may be long-lasting. Hydroquinone with salicylic acid or with retinoic acid inhibits the tyrosinase reaction. Hyperpigmentation also occurs with inflammations, acne vulgaris, drug eruptions, neurodermatitis, and pityriasis rosea.

**Hypopigmentation** occurs normally in some persons as a genetic factor (light skin). Albinos have a congenital inability to produce melanin. Severe trauma can destroy melanin-producing cells and result in hypopigmentation (scar tissue). Some healthy persons develop a condition called **vitiligo,** in which there is a failure of melanin formation in certain areas, primarily around orifices and hairy areas, producing sharply demarcated white patches. Vitiligo also can occur with hyperthyroidism, pernicious anemia, and adrenocortical insufficiency. One treatment for small patches of vitiligo is

**TABLE 66-2 Skin Color Changes**

| PHYSIOLOGY | CONDITIONS |
|---|---|
| **REDNESS** | |
| Vasodilation: more rapid blood flow, more oxygenated blood giving a reddish hue (erythema) | Blushing heat, inflammation, fever, alcohol ingestion, extreme cold (below 15° C), hot flushes, polycythemia |
| **WHITENESS (PALLOR)** | |
| Vasoconstriction: slower blood flow, less blood in capillaries | Cold, fear, shock |
| Partially obstructed blood flow: less blood in capillaries | Vasospasm, thrombus, narrowed vessels, arterial insufficiency |
| Fluid between blood vessels and skin surface | Edema |
| Decreased oxygenation of blood from decreased hemoglobin | Anemia |
| Loss of melanin | Vitiligo |
| **BLUISH** | |
| Deoxygenated hemoglobin (cyanosis) seen in earlobes, lips, mucous membranes of mouth, nail beds | Heart or lung disease, inadequate respiration, peripheral blood vessel obstruction, venous disease, cold, anxiety |
| **YELLOW** | |
| Increased bile pigment in blood eventually distributed to skin and mucous membranes and to sclera of eye | Liver disease, obstruction of bile ducts, chronic uremia, rapid hemolysis |
| **BROWN** | |
| Increased melanin deposits: normal in brown-black races | Aging, sunburn; anterior pituitary, adrenal cortex, or liver disease |
| **DULLNESS** | |
| Vasoconstriction in dark skin | Cold, fear, shock |
| Partially obstructed blood flow in dark skin | Vasospasm, thrombus, narrowed vessels, arterial insufficiency |
| Fluid between blood vessels and skin surface in dark skin | Edema |

methoxypsoralen administered orally plus exposure to sunlight or long-wave ultraviolet light.

### Dark skin

Assessment of dark-skinned persons is more difficult than that of light-skinned persons because color changes are less obvious. Often other signs and symptoms must be used to reach a conclusion. For example, when a skin area is inflamed, the erythema may not be noticeable and the involved area must be palpated for warmth and edema. Rashes may not be visible and must be determined by palpation if the rash is papular or by patient reports of pruritus.

**Melanin,** which gives skin its general color, is produced by melanocytes. The skin of darkly pigmented persons does not contain more melanocytes, but the melanocytes are larger and produce more melanin.[3] Pigmented skin offers more protection from ultraviolet radiation; hence dark skin reacts less to sunlight and skin cancers occur less frequently.

Skin color changes will be seen best in areas of lesser pigmentation, which include the lips, areas around the mouth, mucous membranes, conjunctivae, earlobes, nailbeds, palms, and soles. The sclera of many dark-skinned persons contains fatty deposits with carotene, giving the sclera a yellowish tinge.[3] In these persons, jaundice will have to be concluded by other signs, such as bile in the urine or feces.

Loss of redness provided by the blood produces grayish or dull tones rather than pallor. This sign may be difficult to observe by the untrained eye. Grayish or dull tones can be visualized best in the lips, mucous membranes, conjunctivae, and nailbeds. *Cyanosis* also gives the skin a grayish or dull tone because of loss of redness. Areas of lesser pigmentation, including the earlobes, palms, and soles, are assessed for signs of cyanosis.

## Blood Supply

The degree of blood supplied to the skin produces color changes. The rate of blood flow through the skin is highly variable because of its function in heat control. The blood vessels are innervated by the sympathetic nervous system; thus vasoconstriction occurs with the neuroendocrine response to stressors. With *vasoconstriction,* smaller amounts of blood pass through the vessels, producing decreased redness; a dark skin becomes dull and gray and a light skin whiter (pallor). *Vasodilation* increases the amount of oxygenated blood flow, and the skin acquires a reddish color (erythema). Vascular flush areas of the body are the "butterfly" band from cheek to cheek across the nose, the neck, upper portion of the chest, flexor surfaces of the extremities, and genital areas.

Changes in blood composition also can alter skin color. Excess deoxygenated hemoglobin gives a bluish tint *(cyanosis)* to the skin and mucous membranes. An excess of bile pigment results in a yellowish tint to the skin and sclera of the eyes, although the sclera of dark-pigmented persons may always have a yellowish tint.

## Temperature

The temperature of the skin is regulated by vasoconstriction or vasodilation. If an excess amount of heat is being produced within the body, such as with fever or exercise, or if heat from the external environment increases, the sympathetic centers in the hypothalamus are inhibited and vasodilation occurs. An increase in the amount of blood flow creates a sensation of warmth on the skin. This also occurs with hyperthyroidism. A local inflammation of the skin or underlying tissue also produces vasodilation; this is part of the inflammatory response. Cold skin is caused by vasoconstriction as a result of sympathetic stimulation. Diseases such as hypothyroidism also can contribute to skin coolness. To assess the temperature of the skin, the backs of the fingers, which are more sensitive than the finger tips, should be used.

## Moisture

Skin is assessed as being dry, moist, or oily. ***Dry skin*** is frequently seen in the elderly person because of decreased activity of the sebaceous glands. Dry skin and mucous membranes also are seen in persons who are dehydrated as water moves from the cells into the intravascular compartments. Persons with hypothyroidism have thick, dry, leathery skin.

***Moist skin*** is caused by the presence of water or sweat on the surface. Overheating produces sweating. Persons with hyperthyroidism have moist, smooth skin. Some persons have more effective sweat mechanisms than others. Stressors, shock, or any situation that stimulates the sympathetic nervous system will cause increased fluid loss through the sweat glands. Inasmuch as vasoconstriction also is occurring with stimulation of the sympathetic nervous system, the skin is cold and wet (clammy).

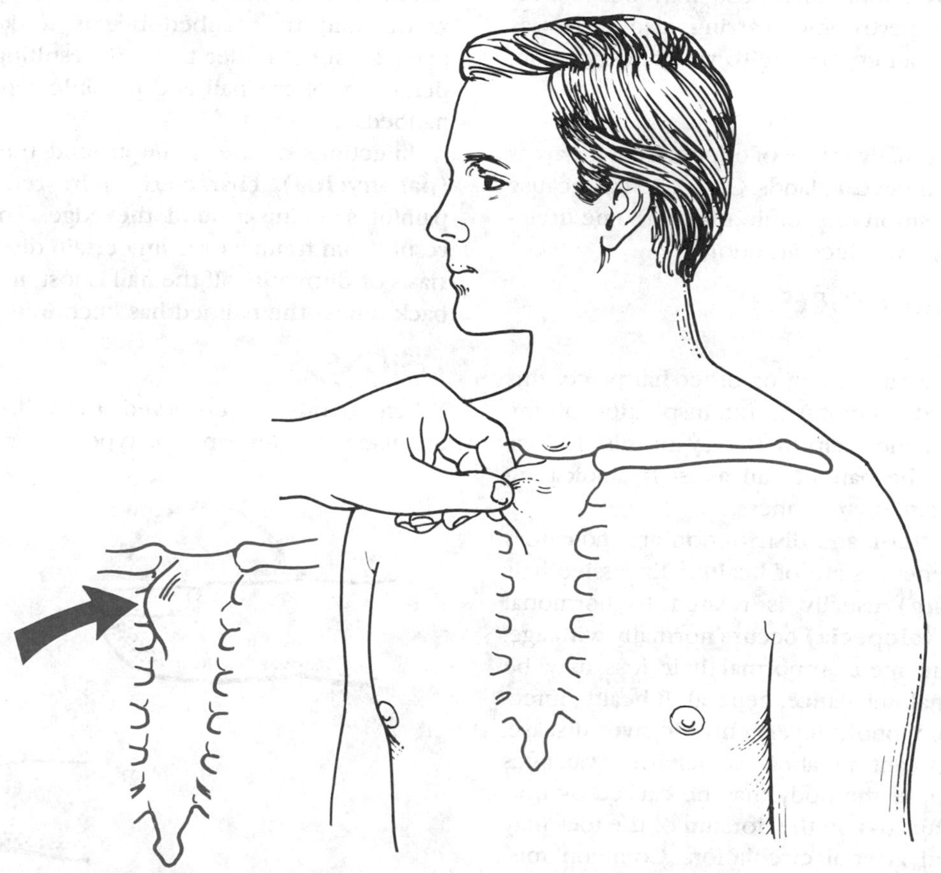

**FIGURE 66-3** Examination of skin turgor. When skin over sternum is picked up, a fold of skin remains for a few seconds when poor turgor is present.

*Oily skin* frequently is seen in the adolescent. Excess sebum formation by the sebaceous glands may lead to blocking of the follicular orifices, resulting in blackheads *(comedo),* acne, or sebaceous cysts.

### Elasticity, Mobility, and Turgor

The skin is highly elastic and moves freely over most areas. It loses its mobility when it becomes stretched; this occurs with edema, in which the interstitial spaces become filled with fluid. Skin becomes rigid in the person with scleroderma, a collagen disease, as a result of collagenous fibrosis of the tissue. *Turgor* is tissue tension and is measured by the speed of skin return to normal position of fullness after it has been stretched. Decreased turgor indicates dehydration of the tissue. To assess elasticity and turgor, a portion of skin over the sternum is picked up (elasticity) and the speed of return to normal is assessed (turgor). Skin that has decreased turgor will remain for a few seconds in a fold before returning slowly to normal (Figure 66-3).

### Texture

Roughness may occur normally on exposed areas, especially elbows and the soles of the feet. The skin of an infant is usually soft and smooth, whereas that of an elderly person may be rough and lack underlying tissue substance (atrophy). Roughness also may occur with hypothyroidism. Hypertrophic scarring, also known as *keloid formation,* can contribute to roughness of skin.

### Odor

Normal clean skin usually is free of odor except for areas that contain apocrine sweat glands. Odor occurs because of bacterial composition of protein matter. Some draining skin lesions may produce an odor.

## ACCESSORY STRUCTURES

### Hair

If the patient is wearing a wig or other hairpiece, this should be removed temporarily for inspection of any remaining hair and the scalp. It is easy to miss lesions on the scalp, and the patient can assist by indicating areas of itching, pain, or roughness.

Hair growth, pattern, and distribution are indicators of the person's general state of health.[2] Excessive hair growth **(hirsutism)** usually is related to hormonal changes. Hair loss **(alopecia)** occurs normally with age, especially in some men. Abnormal hair loss may be caused by hormonal imbalance, general ill health, infections of the scalp, typhoid fever, chronic liver disease, stressors, or drugs (antimetabolites, heparin). Changes in hair distribution of the body may be caused by hormonal changes. Hair loss on the dorsum of the toes may indicate decreased arterial circulation. Common misconceptions about hair growth include the following: shaving promotes the growth of dark, coarse hairs; singeing hair alters growth; brushing and massaging increase hair growth; and hair "turns gray overnight." None of these is true. The hair shaft is an inert structure, and changes occur over time as a result of hormonal activity and the availability of nutrients to the bulb at the base of the hair root.

Hair should be free of lice or nits. Nits are the eggs of the lice and are found embedded on hair strands behind the ears. They are observed as small, glistening, grayish specks along the hair shaft near the scalp.

### Nails

The appearance of the nails changes with age and with ill health. Changes in hardness, brittleness, roughness, or shape may indicate some metabolic diseases, nutritional imbalances including vitamin deficiencies, or digestive disturbances. Pale nailbeds and poor capillary return (slow return to normal color after the nail is pinched) may indicate hypoxia or anemia. Clubbing of the nails refers to the elimination of the small concave portion at the base of the nail by soft tissue growth; this occurs with certain diseases associated with chronic hypoxia (Figure 66-4).

The epithelial lining of the nailbed is usually inert. The nail is affixed to the nailbed, and both move outward as the nail grows. The epithelial lining of the nailbed loses its inert quality in the presence of inflammatory lesions such as those that occur with psoriasis or ringworm, and the nailbed begins to keratinize. Horny masses collect under the nail, resulting in a thickening deformity of the nail and possible separation from the nailbed.[5]

Infections of the tissue around the nail may occur **(paronychia)**, characterized by red, shiny skin and painful swelling around the edge. The infection may result from trauma or from certain diseases such as psoriasis or dermatitis. If the nail is lost, it usually will grow back unless the nailbed has been injured.

## LESIONS

When lesions are observed, the following parameters are used for description: type, color, size, shape and

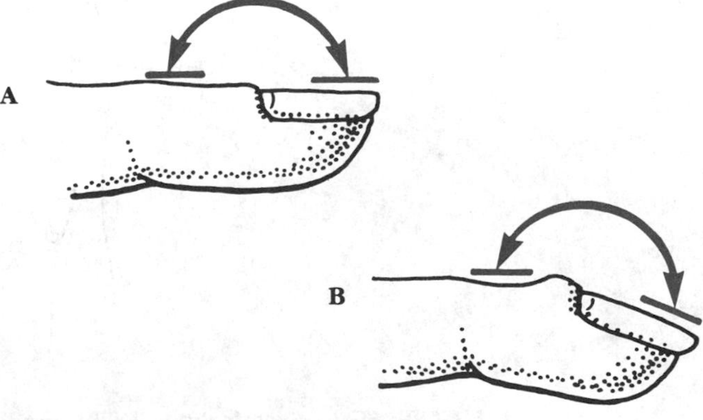


**FIGURE 66-4** **A,** Normal nail angle. **B,** Abnormal nail angle seen in clubbing.

configuration, texture, effect of pressure, arrangement, distribution, and variety.

## Type

Use of medical terminology facilitates communication (Table 66-3). For example, use of the term *vesicle* immediately establishes the lesion as a clear, fluid-filled lesion smaller than 1 cm. Figure 66-5 presents common appearance along with descriptions for **crust, macule, nodule, papule, plaque, pustule, scale, vesicle,** and **wheal.**

## Color

Color of lesions varies among pale, brown, red, normal pigmentation, and so forth. Color helps to identify whether the lesion is part of normal aging, an inflammatory process, an infection, and so forth.

## Size

The metric system is used for descriptions. A helpful hint is to measure a portion of one's own fingers, such as the distance from the tip of the right thumb to the first joint, or the width of the nail on the right little finger. This can then be used as a gauge for estimating the size of a lesion.

## Shape and Configuration

Shape can be described as round, oval, and so on. *Configuration* refers to the sharpness of demarcation of the lesion, that is, whether it is discrete or diffuse.

**TABLE 66-3 Types of Skin Lesions**

| OBSERVED SKIN CHANGES | DIFFERENTIATION | TERM | EXAMPLE |
|---|---|---|---|
| **CHANGE IN COLOR OR TEXTURE** | | | |
| Spot | Circumscribed; flat; color change | Macule | Freckle |
| Discoloration (reddish purple) | Bleeding beneath the surface; injury to tissue | Contusion | Bruise |
| Soft whitening | Caused by repeated wetting of skin | Maceration | Between toes after soaking |
| Flake | Dry cells of surface | Scale | Dandruff; psoriasis |
| Roughness from dried fluid | Dry exudate over lesions | Crust ("scab") | Eczema, impetigo |
| Roughness from cells | Leathery thickening of outer skin layer | Lichenification | Callus on foot |
| **CHANGE IN SHAPE** | | | |
| Fluid-filled lesions | Less than 1 cm; clear fluid | Vesicle | Blister; chickenpox |
| | Greater than 1 cm; clear fluid | Bulla | Large blister, pemphigus |
| | Small, thick yellowish fluid (pus) | Pustule | Acne |
| Solid mass, *cellular* growth | Less than 1 cm | Papule | Small mole; raised rash |
| | 1 to 2 cm | Nodule | Enlarged lymph node |
| | Greater than 2 cm | Tumor | Benign or malignant tumor |
| | Excess connective tissue over scar | Keloid | Overgrown scar |
| Swelling of tissue | Generalized swelling; fluid between cells | Edema | Inflammation; swelling of feet |
| | Circumscribed surface edema; transient; some itching | Wheal ("hive") | Allergic reaction |
| **BREAKS IN SKIN SURFACES** | | | |
| Oozing, scraped surface | Loss of superficial structure of skin | Abrasion | "Floor burn"; scrape |
| Scooped-out depression | Loss of deeper layers of skin | Ulcer | Pressure or stasis ulcer |
| Superficial linear skin breaks | Scratch marks, frequently by fingernails | Excoriations | Scratching |
| Linear cracks or cleft | Slit or splitting of skin layers | Fissure | Athlete's foot |
| Jagged cut | Tearing of skin surface | Laceration | Accidental cut by blunt object |
| Linear cut, edges approximated | Cutting by sharp instrument | Incision | Knife cut |
| **VASCULAR LESIONS** | | | |
| Small, flat, round, purplish, red spot | Intradermal or submucous hemorrhage | Petechia | Bleeding tendency; vitamin C deficiency |
| Spiderlike, red, small | Dilation of capillaries, arterioles, or venules | Telangiectasis | Liver disease, vitamin B deficiency |
| Discoloration, reddish purple | Escape of blood into tissue | Ecchymosis | Trauma to blood vessels |

**Lesion**

**Macule—flat; nonpalpable; circumscribed; less than 1 cm in diameter; brown, red, purple, white, or tan**
**Examples: Freckles; flat moles; rubella; rubeola; drug eruptions**
**Note: Classified as patch if greater than 1 cm in diameter**

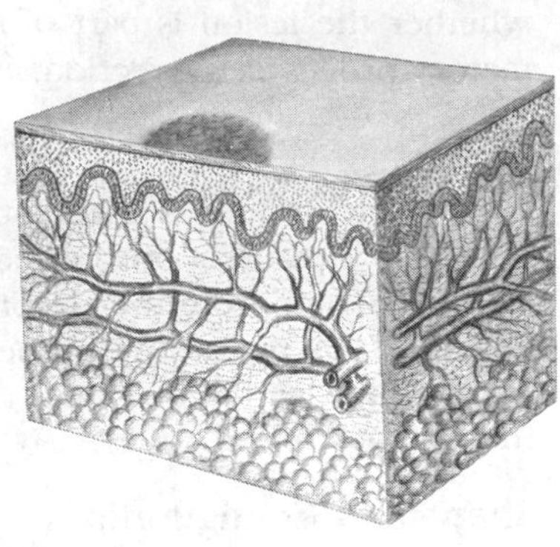

Plaque—elevated; flat topped; firm; rough; superficial papule greater than 1 cm in diameter; may be coalesced papules
Examples: Psoriasis; seborrheic and actinic keratoses; eczema

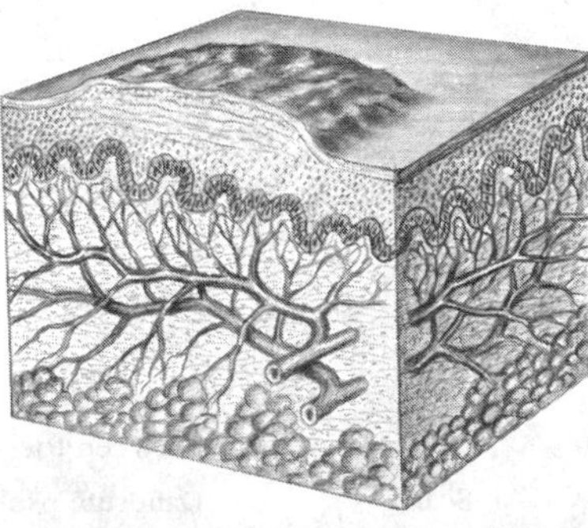

Nodule—elevated; firm; circumscribed; palpable; deeper in dermis than papule; 1 to 2 cm in diameter
Examples: Erythema nodosum; lipomas

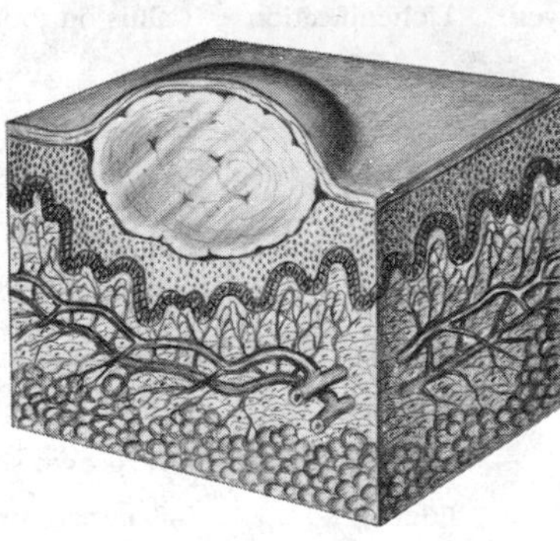

**Scale—heaped-up keratinized cells; flaky exfoliation; irregullar; thick or thin; dry or oily; varied size; silver, white, or tan**
**Examples: Psoriasis; exfoliative dermatitis**

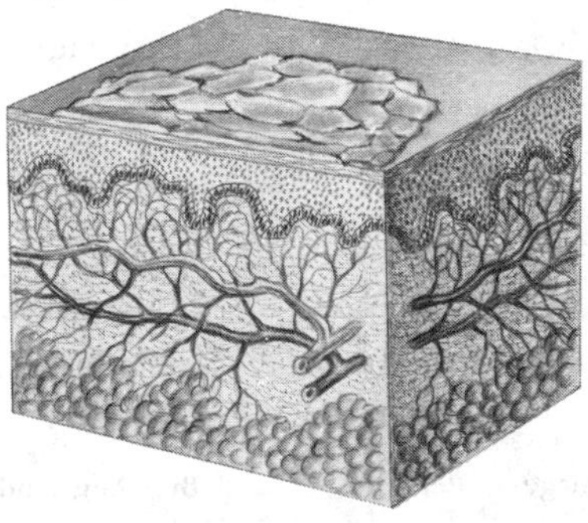

**Papule—elevated; palpable; firm; circumscribed; less than 1 cm in diameter; brown, red, pink, tan, or bluish red**
**Examples: Warts; drug-related eruptions; pigmented nevi; eczema**

Wheal—elevated, irregular-shaped area of cutaneous edema; solid, transient, changing; variable diameter; pale pink
Examples: Urticaria; insect bites

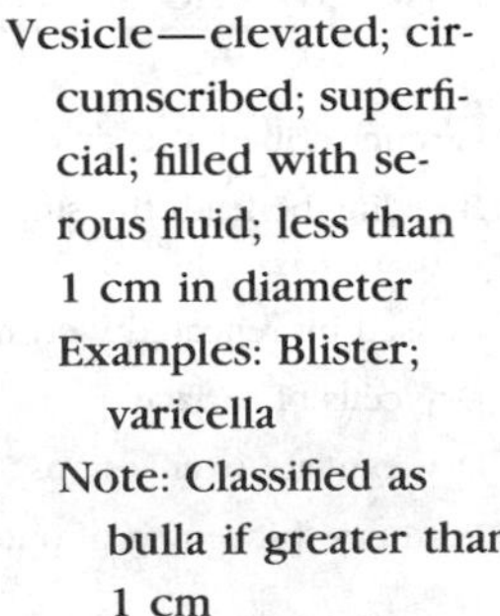

Vesicle—elevated; circumscribed; superficial; filled with serous fluid; less than 1 cm in diameter
Examples: Blister; varicella
Note: Classified as bulla if greater than 1 cm

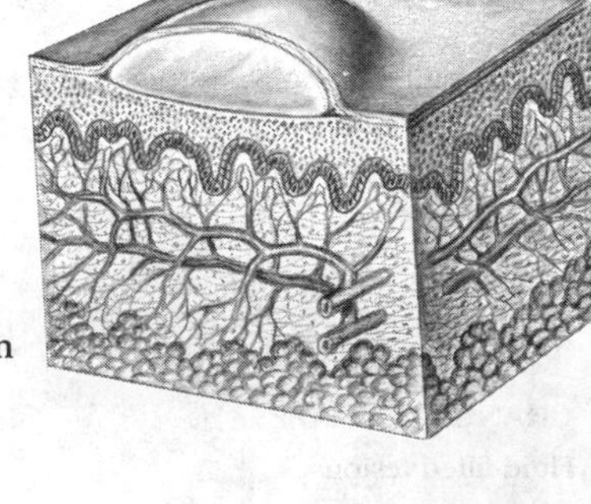

Pustule—elevated; superficial; similar to vesicle but filled with purulent fluid
Examples: Impetigo; acne; variola; herpes zoster

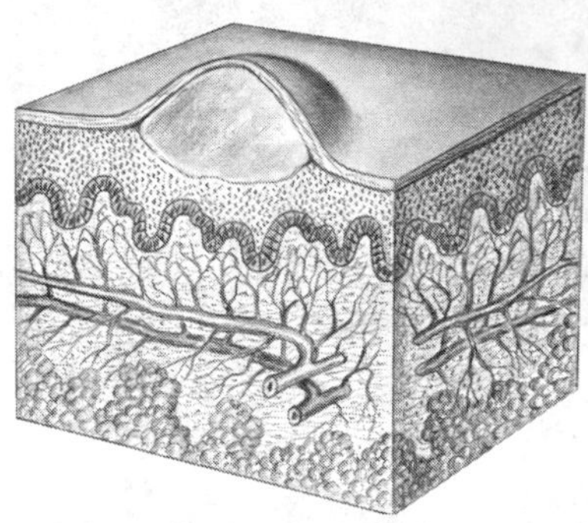

Crust—dried serum, blood, or purulent exudate; slightly elevated; size varies; brown, red, black, tan, or straw
Examples: Scab on abrasion; eczema; impetigo

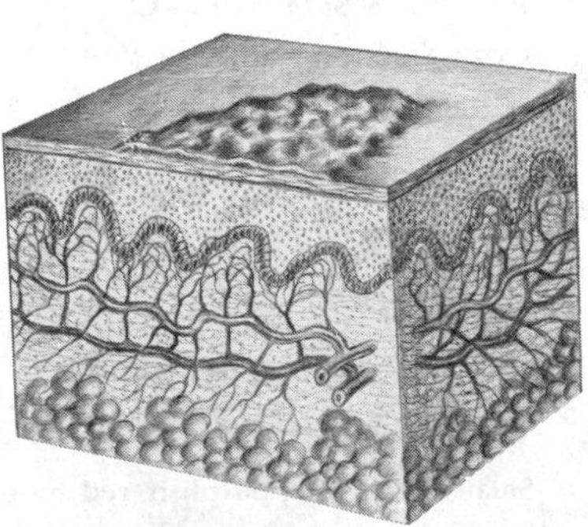

**FIGURE 66-5** Common skin lesions. (From Thompson JM et al: *Mosby's clinical nursing,* ed 3, St Louis, 1993, Mosby.)

### Texture

The lesion is described as being rough or smooth, dry or moist, and on the surface or deeply penetrating into the tissue.

### Effect of Pressure

Some vascular lesions blanch when pressure is applied and then return to their original color. Other lesions remain the same with pressure. The effects of pressure are assessed by pressing the thumb directly over the lesion and then rapidly removing it.

### Arrangement

Some lesions occur in patches, whereas others occur diffusely over the body. This is an important parameter when describing rashes.

### Distribution

Some lesions occur in certain parts of the body, such as on exposed areas as with contact dermatitis, or on main body areas as in chickenpox. The lesions may follow the area of distribution of one of the spinal nerves as in herpes zoster.

### Variety

In some diseases, such as smallpox, the lesions may all occur at the same time, whereas in chickenpox the lesions occur in crops so that there may be lesions at different stages of development at the same time.

# DIAGNOSTIC TESTS

Diagnostic tests usually are performed to confirm diagnoses of certain skin disorders. Most skin disorders, however, are diagnosed by physical assessment.

## LABORATORY TESTS

### Tzanck Smear

Vesicular disorders may be differentiated by a Tzanck smear. The top of the vesicle is cut and a smear taken from the base of the vesicle. Examination of the smear may identify a virus (herpes simplex or zoster) or acantholytic cells (pemphigus). The test shows a negative reaction for vesicles from burns, erythema multiforme, or dermatitis herpetiforme.

### Potassium Hydroxide Test

If the causative factor is believed to be a fungus, a potassium hydroxide (KOH) examination may be carried out. The lesion is scraped with a knife blade, and the scraping is placed on a slide, which is set in a KOH solution before microscopic study.

### Culture

If the primary lesion is a pustule, a culture specimen of the pustule contents may be obtained to identify the causative organism. Streptococci and staphylococci are commonly seen.

## SPECIAL TESTS

### Skin Biopsy

Biopsy specimens of skin lesions may be obtained either by incision and suturing or by punch biopsy, which does not require suturing. A punch biopsy has a sharp edge that cuts through previously anesthetized skin and removes a core from the lesion for analysis. Bleeding may be stopped by direct pressure or by electrodesiccation.

### Patch Testing

If allergic dermatitis is suspected, patch testing is performed to determine the source of the allergen. Standard concentration samples of suspected allergens are applied to the skin. Minute quantities of the products are held next to the skin by hypoallergenic tape, usually on the forearm and upper portion of the back. The patches are removed 48 hours after application, and the sites are evaluated after 20 minutes to determine redness, swelling, or vesicle formation. Because delayed reactions are possible, sites should be reevaluated in 1 week.[1]

### Diascopy

Pigmented lesions resulting from increased blood in dilated vessels (such as erythema, spider angiomas, telangiectasis) can be differentiated from other lesions resulting from blood that has escaped into the tissue (such as petechiae, ecchymoses) or from melanin changes. Diascopy consists of pressing a transparent object such as a glass slide over a pigmented lesion. The lesion caused by dilated blood vessels will whiten with pressure as the blood is pushed to other areas, whereas the other lesions will not change color.

### Wood's Light

To assist in the diagnoses of fungal infections of the hair and skin (tinea), the hair is illuminated by a special filter (Wood's filter) attached to an ultraviolet lamp. The infected hairs fluoresce brilliant green or appear luminous under the light.

## CRITICAL THINKING ACTIVITIES

- Based on the major protective functions of the epidermis, make some deductions related to specific skin care principles
- Curtis, 10, has developed crusty lesions over most of his body. His mother reports that he was recently on a camping trip with his father but neither recalled coming into contact with poison ivy. What additional data should the nurse obtain during the patient history?

# CHAPTER SUMMARY

## ANATOMY AND PHYSIOLOGY OF THE SKIN

- Functions of the skin include protection, heat regulation, sensory perception, excretion, vitamin D production, and expression.
- Skin changes in elderly persons include hypopigmented and hyperpigmented areas, dry skin, decreased perspiration, decreased elasticity and turgor, wrinkles and loose folds, and thinner skin with some roughened areas.
- Skin color changes result from changes in melanin production, vascular dilation or constriction, changes in hemoglobin and red blood cells, and increased bile pigment.
- Skin temperature changes result from vascular dilation or constriction; some causes include fever, exercise, skin inflammations, and sympathetic inhibition or stimulation.
- Elasticity of the skin is the ability of the skin to stretch; turgor is tissue tension and is measured by the ability of the skin to return to normal after being stretched.
- Hair loss results normally from aging; hair also may be lost with decreased oxygenation, general ill health, stressors, drugs, or chronic liver disease.
- Nail changes may occur from aging, metabolic diseases, nutritional deficiencies, or decreased oxygenation.

## SUBJECTIVE DATA

- Indepth subjective data are obtained if a problem is identified on a general assessment.
- Subjective data include usual skin condition, onset of problem, any changes, possible causes, alleviating factors, and psychologic responses to changes in the skin.

## OBJECTIVE DATA

- Solid tissue growths, according to size, include papules, nodules, and tumors. Fluid-filled lesions by size include vesicle and bulla; if the fluid is pus, it forms a pustule.
- Breaks in skin surfaces include abrasions, ulcers, excoriations, fissures, lacerations, and incisions.
- Vascular lesions include petechia (intradermal or submucous bleeding), telangiectasis (dilated capillaries), or ecchymosis (bruise).

## DIAGNOSTIC TESTS

- Skin diseases are primarily diagnosed by direct observation; diagnostic tests include the Tzanck smear, potassium hydroxide test, culture of a pustule, diascopy, Wood's light test, patch testing, and skin biopsy.

# REFERENCES

1. Anderson KN, Anderson LE, Glanze WD editors: *Mosby's medical, nursing, and allied health dictionary*, ed 4, St Louis, 1994, Mosby.
2. Guyton A: *Textbook of medical physiology*, ed 8, Philadelphia, 1991, WB Saunders.
3. Irwin MJ: Assessing color changes for dark skinned patients, *Adv Clin Care*, 6(6), 8-10, 1991.
4. Malasanos L, Barkauskas V, Stoltenberg-Allen K editors: *Health assessment*, ed 4, St Louis, 1990, Mosby.
5. Moschella SL, Hurley HP: *Dermatology*, ed 3, Philadelphia, 1991, WB Saunders.

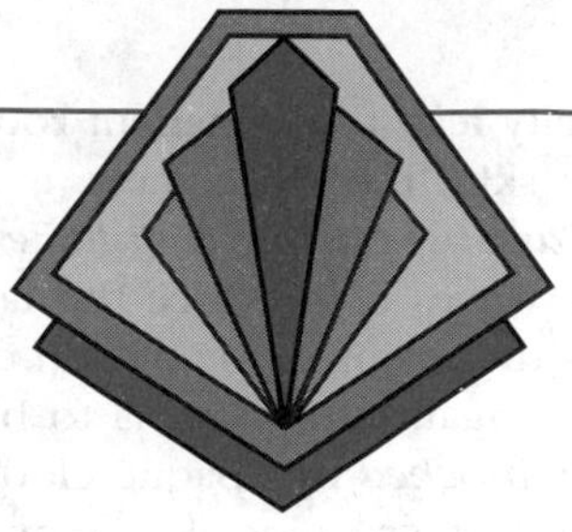

CHAPTER 67

# Management of Persons With Problems of the Skin

*Vickie Weaver*

## CHAPTER OBJECTIVES

***After studying this chapter, the learner should be able to do the following:***

1. Identify preventive measures for dermatologic disorders.
2. Describe psychologic effects of dermatologic problems.
3. Describe general nursing interventions for dermatologic problems.
4. Explain the etiology, pathophysiology, and interventions for parasitic infestations, fungal and bacterial infections, and viral diseases of the skin.
5. Describe the nature, preventive measures, and therapy for secretory disorders of the skin.
6. Compare and contrast the different types of dermatitis, preventive measures, and interventions, especially patient teaching.
7. Identify different skin reactions that may result from systemic factors.
8. Describe the nature and management of psoriasis.
9. Describe the different benign and malignant skin tumors and their management.
10. Describe preventive and early intervention measures for pressure sores.
11. Develop an individualized nursing care plan for the patient with a pressure sore.

## KEY TERMS

acne rosacea
acne vulgaris
actinic keratosis
atopic dermatitis
atopy
basal cell epithelioma
Burow's solution
calluses
candidiasis
carbuncle
contact dermatitis
corns
dermatitis
discoid lupus erythematosus
eczema
erysipelas
erythema multiforme
folliculitis
furuncle
herpes simplex
herpes zoster
herpetic whitlow
impetigo
kaposi's sarcoma
keloid
keratosis
leukoplakia
lichen planus
malignant melanoma
moles
nevi
pediculosis
pityriasis rosea
pressure sore
pruritus
pseudofolliculitis barbae
psoriasis
rhinophyma
scabies
seborrheic dermatitis
seborrheic keratosis
shingles
squamous cell carcinoma
stasis dermatitis
tinea capitis
tinea corporis
tinea cruris
tinea pedis
tinea versicolor
varicella
warts

**Prevention of dermatologic conditions not only relieves the patient of discomfort, but is cost effective, because many skin conditions are chronic. This chapter discusses methods of prevention, measures to alleviate common patient discomforts, care of skin lesions, and care of persons undergoing dermatologic surgery. This is followed by a discussion of specific problems, including their etiology/epidemiology, pathophysiology, and management.**

# PREVENTION OF DERMATOLOGIC DISORDERS

## AVOIDANCE OF CAUSATIVE AGENTS

The first step in prevention of dermatologic conditions may be directed to avoiding the causative agent. This may be a specific antigen, contact irritant, microorganism, trauma, direct sunlight, or insect. Instructing the person to avoid a known causative agent is preventive medicine; however, it may not be that simple. Many dermatologic diseases have no known cause or are hereditary; unfortunately, once the mechanism of the disease is known, it is not always possible to remove the trigger factors. Occasionally, symptoms may persist long after the agent is removed. Therefore major responsibilities of the nurse include education of the patient about measures that (1) promote rest, (2) decrease emotional stress, and (3) ensure good nutrition, and patient education about the need to closely observe sites to determine changes in skin conditions.

## CLEANSING

Bathing is an essential element of skin care. The frequency of skin cleansing should be individualized according to need and/or patient preference.[3] The outer layer of skin cells and the perspiration are acid in reaction, and their presence inhibits the life and growth of harmful bacteria. There are, however, a normal flora of bacteria that grow in acidity and act as the skin's protection. Strong soaps that are alkaline in reaction may neutralize this protective acid condition of the skin. They may also remove the oily secretion of the sebaceous glands, which lubricates the outer skin layers and contributes to their health. It is sometimes necessary to remove excess oil and scale or debris to facilitate the absorption of medication, promote healing, and enhance the appearance of the skin. In psoriasis, for example, removal of scale by mechanical means and slowing of skin metabolism are prime objectives.

Normal skin should be washed often enough to remove excess oils and excretions and to prevent odor. Care must be taken not to cause drying or irritation. Maintaining a proper degree of hydration in the skin will prevent dryness and itching, which may lead to scratching, excoriation, and further trauma. Hydrating the stratum corneum, or outer layer of skin, may be accomplished by soaking in a tub of water for 20 to 30 minutes and then immediately applying a lubricating lotion or cream. This application of a cream prevents the rapid loss of water from the skin surface.

## SUNLIGHT

Sunlight, particularly ultraviolet (UV) rays, are damaging to the skin. These rays are termed *actinic,* meaning photochemically active radiation. UV-A waves contribute to aging and carcinogenesis of the skin.[13] UV-B waves lead to burning and activation of melanin that produces tanning. Suntans eventually lead to permanent roughening and wrinkling of the skin; therefore there is no such thing as a "safe tan." *Tanning parlors should be avoided* because they use UV waves to produce the tan. Long-term sun exposure is the major cause of skin cancer.

The way to protect against UV rays is to block the rays. The rays may be *blocked* by opaque clothing, use of umbrellas, hats, or other screening aids, or by selected sunscreens. The best sunscreens have a sun-protection factor (SPF) of 15 or more.[13] Sunscreens are removed easily with water and must be reapplied after swimming or heavy sweating. Lips must be protected with sunscreens or dark lipstick. UV rays have stronger effects at high altitudes (where there is less atmosphere to absorb the rays) and at the equator (where the sun is closer to the earth); therefore additional protection is required in these places. Persons who have been diagnosed as having a skin condition that is aggravated by UV light or who are taking photosensitive drugs should avoid the sun, if possible, or ensure adequate protection.

## NUTRITION

Balanced nutrition plays an important role in preventing the occurrence of skin lesions. The nutrients considered essential to the maintenance of healthy skin include protein, vitamin C, iron, and zinc. Some skin lesions may be directly associated with dietary intake. Excessive dryness of the skin and thickening of the stratum corneum at the hair follicle openings may be caused by nutritional deficiencies. Elevated blood lipid levels caused by hyperlipoproteinemia may take the form of xanthomas on the skin surface. Restriction of sodium in patients who are receiving glucocorticoid steroids may lessen or prevent edema as a side effect.

Hypersensitive individuals may be placed on restrictive diets to exclude intake of known causative agents or as a diagnostic tool to identify causative agents. Food labels should be read carefully to determine whether the product or food additive contains the agent the hypersensitive person is to avoid. It may also be necessary to request information from the manufacturer if questions about food additives arise. The patient should know the type of diet to be followed. This includes knowledge of any restrictions; methods of preparing these foods, if necessary; and the duration of the prescribed diet.

## OBSERVATIONS OF CHANGES

Care of normal skin includes regular observation of pigmented skin areas, moles, or other apparently minor skin lesions. Any change in size, color, or general appearance should be reported to a physician at once, because a change in moles or new skin growths is one of the danger signals of cancer.

## DANGERS OF SELF-TREATMENT

People should be urged to seek competent medical help when skin conditions develop. Although skin diseases rarely cause death, they may be reflections of serious systemic illness and can account for much human discomfort and for serious interruption of work and other activities. Many persons are inclined to rely on the advice of friends or the local druggist or on medications they may have on hand. Each individual's skin reacts differently to treatment, and the skin that is already irritated or diseased may respond violently to inexpert treatment. Because of changes in the skin, medications prescribed even for a similar skin ailment in the same patient some time previously may not produce a favorable response. Medications may deteriorate, and for this reason old medications are not safe. The person may be spared much discomfort and expense by consulting a specialist when symptoms first develop and before a mild skin condition becomes a real problem.

## PSYCHOLOGIC EFFECTS OF DERMATOLOGIC PROBLEMS

There is a certain degree of "beauty orientation" in Western culture. Beauty pageants are popular, advertisements in the media use beautiful models to attract the reader, and in public groups heads turn as a good-looking person walks by. Cosmetics to enhance good looks are extensively used by women, as well as men. It is no wonder, therefore, that skin diseases or physical defects that detract from "good looks" produce psychologic reactions.

A person's emotional reaction to a deformity or defect must not be underestimated. One's pride in oneself and the ability to think well of oneself and to regard oneself favorably in comparison with others are essential to the development and maintenance of a well-integrated personality. Every person who has a defect or a handicap, particularly if it is conspicuous to others, suffers from some threat to emotional security. The extent of the emotional reaction and the amount of maladjustment that follows depend on the individual's personality and ability to cope with emotional insults. Disfigurements almost invariably lead to disturbing experiences. The child who has webbed fingers may be ridiculed at school; the adolescent girl who has acne scars may be self-conscious and avoid social situations; and the young man with a posttraumatic scar on his face may be refused a sales job. Under any of these circumstances, it is not unusual for the individual to withdraw from a society that is unkind. The defect may be used to justify failure, to avoid responsibility, or to justify striking out against an unkind society.

Skin diseases that produce marked disfigurement of visible body surfaces, therefore, can effect alterations in the person's body image, as described in Chapter 9. Feelings of decreased worth by persons with large draining lesions or with severe disfigurement are reinforced during interactions with others. Some people are repelled when viewing persons with severe skin diseases, or they may experience a threat to their own body integrity and physically withdraw to avoid interaction. Persons may also frequently experience nonverbal messages of disgust when others view them for the first time. This is markedly poignant when those nonverbal messages are sent by significant others or by health professionals.

The person with severe facial disfigurement may also experience job discrimination. One woman was moved sequentially from a large office to a smaller office to a single office and finally to the evening hours in a lonely room so that co-workers could avoid looking at her. She lived alone and was increasingly deprived of social contacts with others. It was only after her eyesight failed and she was encouraged to attend groups for the blind that she was able to develop meaningful relationships again.

In working with the person with severe skin disease, the nurse first examines his or her own feelings that could be expressed nonverbally in a negative manner. Measures to assist the patient and family to deal with and cope with their feelings are described in Chapter 9.

## GENERAL INTERVENTIONS FOR DERMATOLOGIC PROBLEMS

### RELIEF OF PRURITUS

**Pruritus** or itching is a cutaneous symptom that provokes the desire to scratch. It is caused by repetitive low-frequency stimulation of C fibers that are similar to but different from C fibers that transmit pain stimuli. Itching can be produced by mechanical stimulation of the skin or by chemical mediators, primarily the kinins.[6] Itching occurs only in the skin, certain mucous membranes, and the eyes. The areas most sensitive to itching are the nostrils, mucocutaneous junctions, external ear canals, and perineum.

Pruritus can be caused by any irritating substance that interrupts the stratum corneum layer of the skin, or it can be a result of certain systemic diseases (Box 67-1). Not all infectious diseases producing rashes cause itching. One of the most common causes is dry skin, sometimes occurring as a result of excessive bathing, particularly with "bubble bath," which has a drying effect.

**BOX 67-1 Common Causes of Itching**

- Dry skin
- Skin irritants: plastic or glass fibers, wool, plant products, insects
- Drug reactions
- Psychogenic reactions
- Infectious diseases
- Infestation: hookworm
- Systemic diseases: obstructive biliary disease, uremia, diabetes mellitus
- Neoplasia: Hodgkin's disease, leukemia, lymphoma

**TABLE 67-1 Preparations Commonly Used for Baths or Soaks**

| SUBSTANCE | EFFECT | SUGGESTED ACTIONS |
|---|---|---|
| Colloids: oatmeal, cornstarch, soybean powder | Antipruritic, drying | Tub surfaces become very slippery; support person to prevent falls. |
| Potassium permanganate $KMNO_4$ | Antifungal, drying, deodorizing | Strain pulverized tablet through cheesecloth to prevent irritation; stains surfaces and linens. |
| Burow's solution (aluminum acetate) | Antibacterial, drying | Commonly use for soaks. |
| Sulfur bath suspension | Antibacterial | Rinse body with tepid water after bath to remove residual sulfur particles. |
| Tar preparations: Balnetar, Zetar, Alma-Tar, Polytar | Antipruritic, moisturizing | Do not use soap with tar baths. |
| Bath oils: Alpha-Keri, Jeri-Bath, Domol | Antipruritic, moisturizing | Tub surfaces may become slippery. |

Factors that can intensify itching include vasodilation, tissue anoxia, and stasis of circulation. Whatever the cause, pruritus ranges from an annoyance to a severe, distressing, or exhausting problem.

Pruritus leads to the motor response of scratching. Persons with very intense itching may excoriate the skin severely by digging deeply into the skin with their fingernails when trying to alleviate the itch. Persons with generalized itching may be observed to be in almost constant motion—twisting, rubbing, and scratching.

A major step in treating pruritus is to attempt to remove the itch stimuli and break the itch-scratch cycle. Cold causes vasoconstriction and will provide some relief. Hydration in a tepid bath followed by the application of an emollient lotion is helpful. Cornstarch or oatmeal preparations may be added to the bath. Topical corticosteroids decrease inflammation leading to vasoconstriction. In some persons, antihistamines, such as diphenhydramine, or tranquilizers are of some value.

The awareness of pruritus may be more acute during the night because of a decrease in diverting stimuli. Cool, light, nonrestrictive bed clothing may help allay itching. Excessive drying of the skin caused by high room temperature and low humidity can also increase pruritus. It occurs readily in an elderly person who already has dry skin. Usually a room temperature of 20° C (68° to 70° F) and humidity of 30% to 40% are best for the person with pruritus.

## TEMPERATURE CONTROL

Temperature control is an important need in persons with dermatologic problems. The individual who has a generalized flush, or erythema, and the one who has an extensive exfoliative dermatitis may be losing body heat at an abnormally increased rate and may need a room temperature of 32.2° C (90° F) or more to maintain normal body temperature. Care must be taken to avoid chilling, particularly after baths, when compresses are used, or when parts of the body are exposed. The person with pruritus will benefit from a cool environment.

## THERAPEUTIC BATHS AND SOAKS

Baths or soaks of an affected extremity may be prescribed to remove exudates, to moisturize or dry the skin, to relieve pruritus, or to provide antibacterial or antifungal therapy (Table 67-1). Frequent baths or soaks tend to dry the skin; the application of lotion or cream immediately after a bath or soak will moisturize the skin.

Hard crusts or thickened exudates from skin disorders are often soaked with physiologic saline solution, peroxide, or mild soap in warm water. These crusts or exudates are removed only when prescribed by the physician. Unless otherwise indicated (for example, if there is a potential for infection), clean technique is used.

Tub baths may be given to cleanse the skin before therapy (such as for psoriasis), to relieve general body pruritus, or to provide therapy (for example, potassium permanganate, sulfur, or tar baths). During cleansing baths, special attention is given to intertriginous areas (that is, between skin surfaces, such as between toes or fingers or under breasts) where creams and topical medications may collect. Persons with arthropathic psoriasis may find it difficult to use a tub because of limited mobility. A lift may be used with the hospitalized patient; if a lift is not available, sitting on a chair under a gentle shower is the next best alternative to a cleansing bath. Guidelines for therapeutic baths and soaks are described in the Guidelines box below.

### Guidelines For Baths and Soaks

1. The water temperature should be of comfort to patient (usually 32° to 38° C, or 90° to 100° F).
2. Medication should be completely dissolved while tub is filled.
3. The soak should last 20 to 30 minutes.
4. To prevent patient falls when oils or colloids are added to the water, persons are assisted in and out of the water.
5. A rubber mat will help prevent slipping.
6. The skin is *patted,* not rubbed, dry to avoid skin irritation.
7. Creams or ointments are applied *immediately* after the bath to retain skin moisture.
8. After a medicated bath, cleanse tub as follows:
   a. Pour 1 cup of bleach into used tub water.
   b. Let bleach stand in water for 5 minutes.
   c. Wipe sides and bottom of tub.
   d. Drain tub and clean as usual.

**TABLE 67-2 Some Common Topical Antibiotic and Antifungal Medications**

| GENERIC NAME | TRADE NAME | VEHICLE | COMMENTS |
|---|---|---|---|
| **ANTIBACTERIAL** | | | |
| Bacitracin | Baciguent | Ointment | Effective against gram-positive organisms (nonprescription) |
| Neomycin, bacitracin, and polymyxin B | Neosporin | Cream, ointment | Broad-spectrum antibiotic effect |
| Bacitracin and polymyxin B | Polysporin | Ointment | Same as Neosporin |
| Gentamicin | Garamycin | Cream, ointment | Broad-spectrum antibiotic |
| Chloramphenicol | Chloromycetin | Cream | Broad-spectrum antibiotic |
| Clioquinol | Vioform | Lotion, cream, ointment | Has both antibacterial and antifungal effects; useful for eczema and tinea |
| Nitrofurazone | Furacin | Solution, cream, ointment | Broad-spectrum antibiotic |
| Povidone-iodine | Betadine | Solution | Kills gram-negative and gram-positive organisms, fungal, viruses, protozoa, yeasts |
| Mafenide | Sulfamylon | Cream | Effective against both gram-positive and gram-negative bacteria; used for burns |
| Silver sulfadiazine | Silvadene | Cream | Effective against bacteria and yeast; used for burns |
| **ANTIFUNGAL** | | | |
| Tolnaftate | Tinactin Pitrex | Powder, cream, solution | Useful for tinea |
| Nystatin | Mycostatin Nilstat | Powder, cream, ointment | Useful against wide variety of yeasts, especially *Candida* |
| Amphotericin B | Fungizone | Lotion, cream, ointment | Effective against *Candida* |
| Clotrimazole | Lotrimin | Cream, solution, lotion | Broad-spectrum antifungal |
| Haloprogin | Halotex | Cream, solution | Synthetic agent useful for superficial fungal infections |
| Miconazole nitrate | Micatin | Cream, lotion, powder | Synthetic agent useful for tinea |

## TOPICAL MEDICATIONS

Applications of medications to the skin surface may take many forms. Wet dressings, creams, pastes, ointments, and lotion can be used. The nurse should know the purpose for which a local application is ordered, the drugs contained in the preparation, and any toxic signs that may occur from the preparation's use.

### Types of Topical Medications

Many different topical medications are used for persons with dermatologic problems. *Antibacterial* or *antifungal* topical medications (Table 67-2) are used for bacterial or fungal infections.

*Corticosteroids* are among the most commonly used drugs for their antiinflammatory, vasoconstrictive, and antipruritic effects. There are numerous topical corticosteroids that differ in their antiinflammatory effects, ranging from low to very high potency. Hydrocortisone is of low potency. Some corticosteroids, such as triamcinolone acetonide (Aristocort, Kenalog), vary in potency depending on the dose. Greasy ointments are usually more potent and have a greater lubricating effect than creams. Fluorinated corticosteroids are powerful agents and may cause epidermal, dermal, and subcutaneous atrophy, leading to development of petechiae and ecchymoses, as well as to irritation and burning. The fluorinated corticosteroids are not used on the face where they may cause a rosacea-like dermatitis. Systemic effects are unlikely with the less potent topical corticosteroids but may occur with drugs of high potency.

Nonporous covering over corticosteroids (occlusion) potentiates the effect of topical corticosteroids. Occlusion is used primarily for (1) dermatoses of palms and soles, (2) psoriatic lesions on smooth bare skin, (3) localized patches of lichenified dermatitis, and (4) extensive, severe, steroid-responsive dermatitis.[5] The affected area should be occluded only when prescribed by the physician. Plastic wrap is good for occluding small areas. Plastic gloves may be used on hands and plastic bags on feet. Plastic garment bags or large trash bags may be used for the trunk, with holes cut for head and arms. Plastic suits are available for total body occlusion. Lesions are usually occluded at night, usually not for more than 8 hours at a time. Plastic suits are usually worn during the day for 4 hours. Persons should not exercise while wearing body suits because heat regulation is altered under plastic from inability for sweat to evaporate.

### Vehicles for Topical Medications

Topical medications can be prepared in a variety of bases (Table 67-3). *Powders* are effective in reducing friction and moisture in intertriginous areas. *Lotions* must be shaken well, because the insoluble powder may settle out. The addition of alcohol increases the cooling effect of a lotion. *Ointments* do not usually leave an oily residue on the skin unless they have a petrolatum base. A nonporous covering, such as plastic, should not be used over an ointment unless so prescribed, because the heat retention may increase percutaneous absorption of the medication.

**TABLE 67-3 Comparison of Vehicles for Topical Medications**

| BASE | EFFECT |
|---|---|
| **POWDER** | |
| Dry | Drying by absorbing moisture; cooling by evaporating moisture |
| **LOTION** | |
| Powder suspended in water or oil | Protective, cleansing, cooling, antipruritic effect depending on drug and base used |
| **CREAMS AND OINTMENTS** | |
| Emulsions of oil and water | Covering over skin to prolong contact of medication with skin—good skin penetration; warming effect |
| **PASTE** | |
| 50% or more powder in ointment base | Holds medication for long period with slower skin penetration |

## Application of Topical Medications

Gloves are worn for protection when applying topical medications. *Powders* should first be sprinkled into the gloved hand and then applied to the skin to avoid getting excess powder into the air and thus causing irritation to the mucous membrane. Powders should be used sparingly to prevent caking and should not be used on wet surfaces, because this leads to caking. Cornstarch is *not* suggested, it encourages growth of yeast, bacteria, and fungi.

*Lotions* with a water or alcohol base are applied by patting gently. A gauze pledget should be used for extremely thin lotions. Lotions with an oily base are applied thinly and evenly with the palm of the gloved hand. A small area of skin is often tested to determine whether the person will tolerate the cream or lotion over the entire body. The topical medication is applied to a small area (silver-dollar size) on the person's forearm. The time and the exact location of the trial are recorded, and the skin response to the trial medication is read 24 hours later. Crude coal tar is frequently tested in this manner.

*Ointments* may be applied with gloved hands. If a dressing is to be applied, the ointment may be spread on the dressing with a tongue blade before application to the skin. Anthralin may be caustic to normal skin, so gloves should be worn always. Crude coal tar is always applied in firm, long, *downward* strokes to prevent folliculitis, because tar is an irritant. *Creams,* as opposed to ointments, may be rubbed in.

Some topical medications, such as crude coal tar, are often removed before other treatment. Crude coal tar must be removed in the morning before ultraviolet light therapy by applying corn oil in long, downward strokes over the skin surface and then wiping with gauze pledgets, leaving only a thin film of tar. A general rule to remember is to remove only the excess ointment or ointments having a consistency of cold cream before a bath or wet dressing. Cottonseed oil or a gauze pledget may be used to remove caked, oily-based lotions.

## MEDICATED DRESSINGS

### Open Wet Dressings

Wet dressings are used frequently over various skin lesions for cooling, drying, antipruritic, vasoconstricting, or debriding effects. Plain tap water or physiologic saline may be used, or medications may be added. An astringent effect may be obtained through the use of **Burow's solution** (Domeboro, Buro-Sol, Bluboro), 1:20 or 1:40 dilution. *Potassium permanganate* ($KMnO_4$), one 300-mg tablet in 1500 ml (1:5000) or one 300-mg tablet in 3000 ml (1:10,000), has an antimicrobial and drying effect. All tablet crystals must be thoroughly dissolved to prevent chemical burning of the skin. Potassium permanganate should not be used on the face. *Silver nitrate* ($AgNO_3$), 0.5%, is also an antimicrobial and is often used in the treatment of burns. Both $KMnO_3$ and $AgNO_3$ stain skin and cloth.

The type of dressing material used for a wet dressing should be one without cotton filling, because cotton leaves particles and a residue on the skin, which may cause irritation. Several layers of fine-mesh gauze are ideal, and roller gauze or Kerlix may be used for extremities. A mask for the face may be designed by cutting out openings for the eyes, nose, and mouth from several thicknesses of gauze. At home the person can use muslintype cotton material—such as old clean sheets, handkerchiefs, cloth diapers, or muslin dish towels—that are lint free. These materials need not be sterilized but should be washed or discarded every 24 hours.

The best effects of wet dressings are obtained by several treatment periods spaced across the person's waking hours. The solution is applied at room temperature (see Guidelines box, p. 2323, on left) to prevent the marked vasoconstriction with subsequent vasodilation that occurs with cold solutions. Although the dressings can be kept wet by adding solution with the dressings in place, this practice usually leads to excessive dripping. Dressings *must* be removed, soaked, and reapplied when $KMnO_4$ or $AgNO_3$ is used, because evaporation can increase the solute on the dressings, increasing the dose and causing a chemical burn or irritation. Occlusive plastic wraps should be avoided, unless specifically ordered by the physician.

### Closed Wet Dressings

Wet dressings can be covered with a nonpermeable material, such as plastic wrap specifically to retain heat, if an early abscess is present, to soften excessive keratinized tissue, or to enhance penetration of a topical med-

### Guidelines for Applying Open Wet Dressings

1. Prepare solution to be applied at room temperature. Sterility is not required.
2. Soak dressing thoroughly in solution.
3. Protect bed or clothing with towels, bath blanket, flannel squares, etc.
4. Wring out dressings—they should be wet but not dripping.
5. Apply dressings in smooth layers (two to four layers) to involved areas. Wrap fingers and toes separately, and wrap joints so that they can bend.
6. Remove, soak, and reapply dressings *before* they dry (that is, every 3 to 5 minutes).
7. Continue treatment for 20 to 30 minutes.
8. Pat skin dry.

ication. This method is not used frequently, because interference with evaporation contributes to skin maceration.

### Wet-to-Dry Dressings

Wet-to-dry dressings are used to *debride* wounds or ulcerations. A fine-mesh gauze is moistened with the prescribed solution, placed over the lesion, and allowed to dry. The crust and debris are removed as the dressing is pulled off dry. This process is usually repeated every 4 to 8 hours. Normal saline solution is the most common solution used; however, half-strength Dakin's solution is also used for this purpose.

## PATIENT TEACHING

Many persons with dermatologic disorders are not hospitalized; therefore patient teaching is an important component of nursing care. Key points of discussion for patient teaching are described in the Guidelines box above, right. It is best to *write out* instructions specifically, because verbal instructions are easily forgotten. Preprinted teaching protocols provide an effective adjunct to adult learning. Patients commonly apply medications in excess amounts or with vigorous rubbing; these procedures may counteract all benefits or make the condition worse.

Dressing procedures may become costly and complex at times. Those patients will benefit from a home health referral to assist with teaching, as well as community financial resources.

### Guidelines for Teaching the Person With a Dermatologic Disorder

1. Nature of the disorder (cause, preventive measures, acuity or chronicity, symptoms requiring medical follow-up)
2. Treatment modalities to be carried out at home (soaks, baths, medicated dressings)
3. Special precautions to be observed during treatment, such as the following:
   a. Avoiding nonporous coverings over dressings, unless so ordered
   b. Complete dissolving of tablets or crystals in baths or soaks
   c. Avoiding excessive rubbing of medication over lesions
   d. Applying thin layers of lotions or powders
4. Prescribed medication regimens: route of administration, vehicle to be used, dose, frequency, duration of topical application, side effects, where supplies can be obtained.
5. Ways to promote socialization with others when disfiguring dermatologic lesions are present

# COMMON SKIN PROBLEMS

Skin problems may result from various causes, such as parasitic infestations; fungal, bacterial, or viral infections; reactions to substances encountered externally or taken internally; and new growths. A major skin problem is pressure sores. Many skin manifestations have no known cause, whereas others are hereditary. Specific information relevant to each problem is presented next.

## PARASITIC INFESTATIONS

The major parasitic infestations are pediculosis and scabies.

### Pediculosis

#### Etiology/Epidemiology

Pediculi (lice) are most often found among people who live in overcrowded dwellings with inadequate hygiene facilities.[14] Many children get head lice from their classmates or from people on crowded buses. Control and treatment of **pediculosis** (lice infestation) in middle- or upper-income populations can be hampered by refusal of parents to admit that their children have pediculosis. Pediculosis is rare among African-Americans and occurs mostly among children.

#### Pathophysiology

Lice obtain their nutrition by sucking blood from the skin. They leave their eggs on the skin surface attached to hair shafts, and this results in the transfer from person to person.

Three types of lice infest humans: the head louse, the body louse, and the pubic louse. The head louse *(Pediculus capitis)* attaches itself to the hair shaft, laying about eight eggs a day. The eggs, or *nits,* are firmly attached to the hair or threads of clothing. They may be viewed with a hand lens or flashlight and appear as grayish, glistening oval bodies. The head louse is usually confined to the scalp and beard.

The body louse *(Pediculus corporis)* resides chiefly in the seams of clothing around the neck, waist, and thighs. The bite causes minute hemorrhagic points and severe itching. Transmission is by direct contact or by way of clothing, bedding, and towels.

The pubic louse *(Phthirus pubis)* differs slightly from the head and body louse. It resembles a tiny crab, having clawlike pincers that attach firmly to the pubic hair. Nits are visible in the pubic hair. *P. pubis* is transmitted by sexual contact, bed clothing, towels, and occasionally toilet seats.

Diagnosis is made by finding nits or lice on a person who also has pinpoint erythema; raised macules, and a complaint of pruritus. The bite of the insect—with contamination from saliva, head parts, and feces—causes intense itching. Scratching may lead to further trauma, with the possibility of secondary infection and enlarged cervical lymph nodes.

#### Medical management

Treatment of pediculosis consists of topical application of a pediculicide, such as lindane (Kwell, Scabene), permethrin (Nix), pyrethrin (RID, A-200 Pyrinate), or malathion 0.5% (Prioderm). Directions for applications differ according to the product and body location (see Guidelines box below). Pediculicides are not used on eyebrows or eyelashes because of potential eye irritation or sensitization. If eyelashes are infested, nits are removed and petrolatum jelly is applied to smother the lice.

#### Nursing management

Patients are usually able to carry out their own treatment. The focus of nursing care is to identify infected persons and teach about the nature of pediculosis and prevention of its spread (see Guidelines box below, right).

## Scabies

### Etiology/Epidemiology

**Scabies** is caused by the female itch mite *(Sarcoptes scabiei)*. Scabies is highly prevalent during periods of overcrowding, such as occurs during wars. Since the 1960s, however, there has been a rise in the incidence of scabies worldwide. The reason for the pandemic is unknown and is thought to be multifactorial, including sexual promiscuity, increased worldwide travel, and ecologic changes.[10,12] Scabies is usually transmitted by prolonged contact, so that it is frequently observed among several members of a family. Young adults may transmit it by sleeping together, as opposed to a brief sexual contact. Scabies occurs among those in all age-groups and socioeconomic levels.

### Pathophysiology

The female itch mite penetrates the stratum corneum and burrows into the skin. Within several hours after skin penetration, the itch mite lays a large number of eggs and deposits fecal material. The larvae mature in 10 days and move to the skin surface, where the females are impregnated; then the cycle repeats itself. The incubation period varies, but often a long period elapses before symptoms are noted. Delayed hypersensitivity is thought to be a major factor.

The *classic* symptoms of scabies include lesions that resemble wavy, brownish, threadlike lines occurring most frequently on the hands (especially the interdigital webs), flexor surface of the wrists, posterior inner surface of the elbows, anterior axillary folds, nipples in the female, belt line, gluteal creases, and male genitalia. The head and neck are rarely involved. Pruritus may be severe, especially at night. Secondary infections with excoriations and pustules may result from scratching.

Diagnosis is made by identifying the itch mite. The mite is removed from the end of a burrow with a pointed scalpel blade, or the entire burrow is sliced off, placed on a slide with glycerol or mineral oil, and examined under a microscope.

#### Medical management

Medical therapy is directed to elimination of the itch mite and treatment of complications.

1. Scabies treatment (patient, all family members)
   a. Lindane (Kwell, Scabene)
      (1) Apply at bedtime in a thin layer over the *entire* body from *neck down.*
      (2) Wash off in 8 to 12 hours.

**Guidelines for Applying Pediculicides**

**HAIR**

1. Apply pediculicide shampoo to dry hair until hair is thoroughly saturated and work shampoo into a lather.
2. Allow product to remain on hair for stated period (varies with product).
3. Rinse hair and allow to dry.
4. Use a fine-toothed comb to remove dead lice and nits; rinse comb in vinegar after treatment; comb should not be shared by other family members.
5. Repeat treatment in 8 to 10 days to remove any hatched nits.

**BODY**

1. Apply pediculicide lotion or cream to affected areas.
2. Bathe after 12 hours and put on clean clothes.

**Guidelines for Teaching the Person With Pediculosis**

1. Use only the prescribed amount of pediculicide, to prevent toxicity.
2. If pediculicide accidently contacts the eyes, flush eyes immediately with water.
3. Wash brushes and combs with pediculicide.
4. Wash or dry-clean clothing and linens (garments can be stored for 1 month and will no longer be infested).
5. Vacuum carpets, mattresses, and upholstery.
6. All persons in household should use lotion or shampoo and use separate combs or brushes to decrease spread of infection.
7. Itching may continue for 4 to 6 weeks; use a menthol or phenol lotion for comfort.

(3) Give a second treatment in 24 hours if prescribed.

b. Crotamiton 10% (Eurax)

(1) Crotamiton 10% is less effective than lindane.

(2) Bathe before initial application and after each treatment.

(3) Repeat treatment as prescribed.

c. Benzyl benzoate

(1) Give two overnight treatments 1 week apart as prescribed.

(2) Not widely available; apply as directed by physician.

2. Treatment for complications from scabies
   a. Postscabies dermatitis with pruritus: topical or oral corticosteroids
   b. Secondary infections: systemic antibiotics
   c. Postscabies papules or nodules: coal tar gels

#### Nursing management

As with pediculosis, patient education is the primary intervention. Because scabies spreads within families, the patient and family members need to know the nature of the disease and the need for all family members to receive treatment, even if they are asymptomatic. Some patients experience shame and guilt feelings when they learn the diagnosis; a nonjudgmental attitude with explanations of methods of control may help these patients cope with their feelings.

Despite controversy about the potential for spread of the disease by clothing or linens, preventive measures are still being recommended. *Teaching* the patient with scabies includes the following:

1. All family members should be treated simultaneously, whether or not symptoms are present.
2. Be sure that *all* external body areas below the neck are covered by the prescribed scabicide.
3. Wash underclothing and bed and bath linens in hot water on the day of treatment; dry in dryer or iron after dry; change linens daily.
4. Signs and symptoms may not disappear until 1 or 2 weeks after treatment; pruritus of hands and feet may persist for up to 3 months.[10,13]

## FUNGAL INFECTIONS

Fungi are larger and more complex than bacteria. They may be unicellular, such as yeasts, or multicellular, such as molds. Many types are pathogenic to humans, causing common skin disorders or serious systemic diseases, such as blastomycosis. Certain types of fungi cause few symptoms, whereas others produce inflammatory or hypersensitivity reactions.

### Candidiasis

#### Etiology/Epidemiology

*Candida albicans,* a yeastlike fungus, normally inhabits the gastrointestinal tract, mouth, and vagina but not usually the skin. **Candidiasis** (moniliasis), the inflammation associated with the organism's overgrowth on the skin, is caused by the toxins that are released. Some predisposing factors causing an overgrowth of *C. albicans* are pregnancy, use of birth control pills, poor nutrition, antibiotic therapy, diabetes mellitus, other endocrine diseases, inhalational corticosteroids, and immunosuppressed conditions. Yeast thrives in a warm, moist environment, such as the perineum and intertriginous areas. The epidemiology of candidiasis is unknown.

#### Pathophysiology

Overgrowth of *C. albicans* causes candidiasis. Candidiasis of the mucous membrane is thrush. The lesions are white spots that look like milk curd on the buccal mucosa and may extend down the esophagus. Vaginal thrush causes intense itching with a cheesy vaginal discharge. Candidiasis of the skin appears as pruritic, eroded, moist, inflamed areas with vesicles and pustules, and it occurs mostly in body folds, such as beneath the breasts, in the intergluteal fold, or in the groin. Diagnosis of candidiasis at any site is made by clinical appearance and microscopic examination.

#### Medical management

Treatment is aimed at the precipitating factors. Other measures include keeping the skin dry to avoid maceration; wearing loose, absorbent clothing; and using topical medications, such as powders, that help to keep the skin dry. Nystatin (Mycostatin), an antibiotic available in tablets, powder, or vaginal suppositories; amphotericin; clotrimazole (Mycelex); ciclopirox (Loprox); and ketoconazole (Nixoral) are effective against yeast infections.

#### Nursing management

The primary focus in candidiasis is prevention by identifying candidates at high risk for the development of candidiasis and eliminating such factors as a warm, moist environment. A second focus is early detection by careful assessment of mucous membrane and skin folds. This should be done daily and all early lesions reported immediately. A last focus is patient education. Many patients, such as persons with immunosuppression, will be receiving preventive therapy. They need to be taught about the therapy, encouraged to comply, and taught self-assessment measures.

### Dermatophytoses

There are several different types of dermatophytoses (tinea) or superficial fungal infections of the skin and its appendages. The most common types are tinea capitis, tinea corporis, tinea cruris, and tinea pedis.

#### Tinea capitis

**Etiology/Epidemiology. Tinea capitis,** inappropriately called ringworm of the scalp, can be caused either

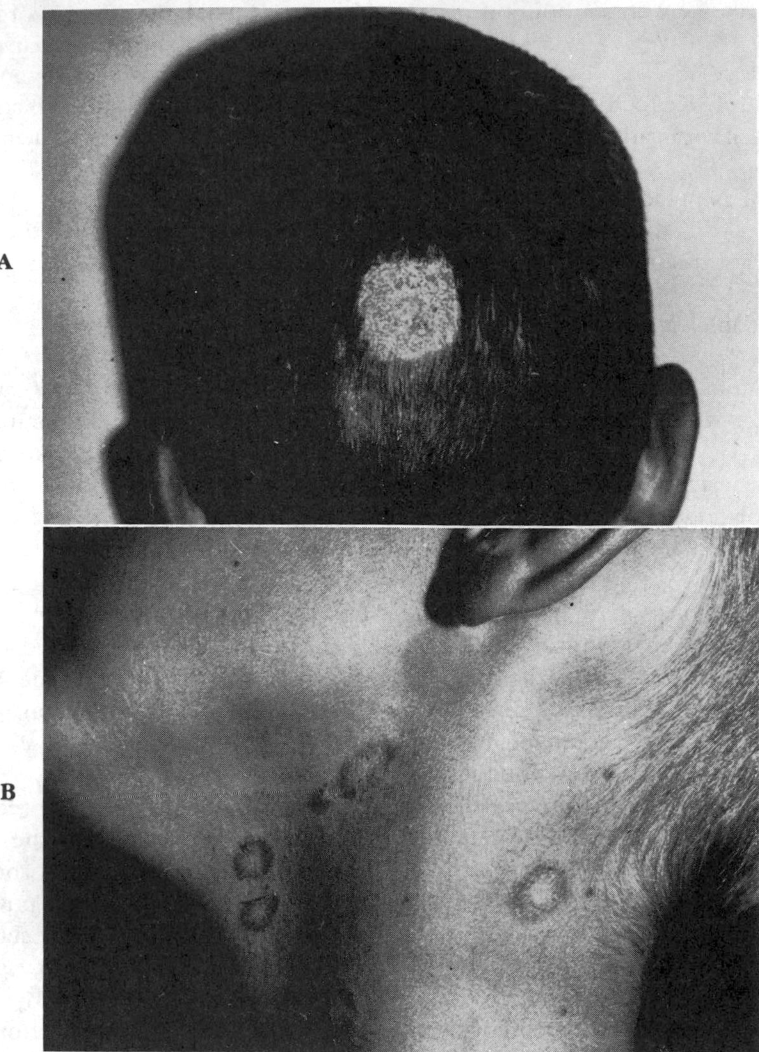


**FIGURE 67-1** **A,** Tinea capitis. **B,** Tinea corporis. (From Stewart WD, Danto JL, Maddin S: *Dermatology: diagnosis and treatment of cutaneous disorders,* ed 4, St Louis, 1978, Mosby.)

by a species of *Microsporum* or by *Trichophyton* fungi. The most common causative agent in the United States is *Microsporum audouini.* The infection is transmitted readily, especially in crowded conditions where poor hygiene exists, although many children show a high resistance. Minor scalp trauma facilitates implantation of the spores; therefore the infection can be spread by contaminated barbers' instruments, combs, or sharp brushes. Tinea capitis has a worldwide distribution, primarily among prepubertal children.

**Pathophysiology.** The characteristic lesion is round, with erythema, a slight scaling, and some pustules appearing at the edge of the lesion (Figure 67-1, *A*). Hair loss occurs, with the hair shaft broken off at skin level. The hair loss is only temporary, because the lesions usually heal without scarring. Although tinea capitis is usually noninflammatory, a painful inflammatory condition called a *kerion* may develop. Infected hairs placed under a Wood's light will fluoresce a blue-green color.

**Medical management.** Griseofulvin is an effective antifungal agent in the treatment of all the dermatophytoses. The adult dose for tinea capitis is 500 mg orally, and absorption is enhanced when the medication is administered after a high-fat meal. The infection is usually resolved within 4 to 6 weeks. A mild antifungal agent, such as tolnaftate (1%) or haloprogin, may be applied topically twice daily.

**Nursing management.** Nursing management focuses on helping the patient implement the regimen. The scalp should be shampooed at least twice a week. Cutting the hair short facilitates shampooing but may cause psychologic trauma for some children; therefore the hair is best left at an acceptable length. If inflammation occurs, the scalp is shampooed daily.

### Tinea corporis and tinea cruris

**Etiology/Epidemiology. Tinea corporis** and **tinea cruris** are dermatophytic infections. Tinea corporis oc-

**BOX 67-2 Topical Antifungal Drugs**

Miconazole (Micatin, Monistat)
Clotrimazole (Mycelex)
Econazole (Ecostatin, Spectazole)
Oxiconazole (Glaxo, Oxistat)
Ciclopirox (Loprox)
Haloprogin (Halotex)
Tolnaftate (Aftate, Pitrex, Tinactin)

curs in children living in hot, humid climates. Tinea cruris, commonly referred to as "jock itch," occurs most frequently in men, especially those who have tinea pedis and those who frequently wear athletic supporters or tight shorts. It also occurs in women who wear tight pantyhose or slacks.

**Pathophysiology.** The lesions of tinea corporis occur on nonhairy parts of the body and are flat with an erythematous scaling border and clearing center (Figure 67-1, *B*). The lesions of tinea cruris occur in the warm, moist, intertriginous areas of the groin. The lesions are bilateral and extend outward from the groin along the inner thigh. The color ranges from brown to red, scaling is absent, and pruritus is usually present.

**Medical management.** Mild infections are treated with topical fungicides (Box 67-2). Oral griseofulvin is given for severe infections.

**Nursing management.** Because the dermatophytes thrive in moist, warm environments, the affected areas should be kept clean and dry, and overbathing should be avoided. A bland dusting powder can be used to promote dryness. Loose underclothing should be worn.

### Tinea pedis

**Etiology/Epidemiology.** The most common dermatophytosis is **tinea pedis,** or athlete's foot. There are several forms of tinea pedis. Tinea pedis is rarely seen in children or women but is widespread among young men, especially those wearing shoes in hot climates. Walking barefoot in gymnasiums or around swimming pools will not necessarily lead to a tinea infection, but susceptible persons will acquire it regardless of their activities.

**Pathophysiology.** The most common form of tinea pedis is the intertriginous form. The fungus involvement usually begins in the toe webs, especially in the fourth interspace, and may extend to the undersurface of the toes or onto the plantar surface. The person may be asymptomatic or may experience itching and burning in the affected area. The nails may become discolored, thickened, or distorted (onychomycosis). It is often confused with other foot eruptions, such as simple intertrigo (chronic bacterial infection of the intertriginous areas of the toes), contact dermatitis, or psoriasis.

**Medical management.** Treatment depends on the stage of infection. Most persons have a chronic low-grade infection that is controllable with topical antifungal drugs (see Box 67-2). When thick, chronic, scaling lesions are present, the topical antifungal drugs cannot penetrate the lesion; therefore a strong peeling ointment, such as Whitfield's ointment, can be applied thinly to the lesions at bedtime, followed by an antifungal cream in the morning.[5] If the lesions become acutely inflamed, they are treated with foot soaks with a bland solution, such as Burow's solution, followed by a topical antimicrobial agent. A systemic antibacterial agent, such as penicillin or erythromycin, may be prescribed. Oral griseofulvin is prescribed only for severe infections that do not respond to local treatment.[13]

**Nursing management.** The person with tinea pedis needs to carry out meticulous foot hygiene. After the toes are dried thoroughly, a light dusting of antifungal powder is applied to promote dryness. Caking of the powder should be avoided. Socks should be of an absorbent material, such as cotton, and may need to be changed more than once daily to promote dryness. Wearing white socks does not affect the course of the infection.[11] A major focus of nursing is to initiate activities that lessen infection, such as wearing sandaltype shoes, going barefoot (to decrease tissue moisture), and using good foot hygiene, which includes washing the feet frequently and drying well between the toes. Preventive actions, such as prophylactic footbaths in public places, are not effective.

### Tinea versicolor

**Etiology/Epidemiology. Tinea versicolor** is a mild, superficial, fungal infection seen mostly in persons who perspire heavily, such as athletes or people living in warm climates. It is frequently noted during migrant health screening.

**Pathophysiology.** Patches of variable coloring and mild scaling can be observed, primarily on the trunk. The involved areas do not tan. Pruritus is mild.

**Medical management.** Treatment includes application of selenium sulfide lotion (Selsun, Exsel) daily for 10 minutes before showering. Other topical antifungal drugs may be used if selenium sulfide is ineffective.

**Nursing management.** Nursing care has two focuses. The first focus is to help in the treatment. Second, good hygiene and daily linen changes should be encouraged to assist with control.

## BACTERIAL INFECTIONS

Skin infections may result from loss of skin integrity or from altered host resistance. Most bacteria that normally inhabit the skin are nonpathogenic. Pathogenic bacteria that penetrate the outer skin layer may cause a superficial skin infection, such as impetigo or superficial folliculitis, or they may penetrate deeper, causing a deep folliculitis or a furuncle.

*General principles of treatment* for bacterial skin infections include cleansing the skin well and applying a topical antibiotic. The skin is cleansed with soap and water or with hexachlorophene. Water or saline compresses may be used to dry the horny layer of the skin, or heat may be applied. Topical antibiotics commonly used include the hydroxyquinilones, such as Vioform; neomycin, bacitracin, or polymyxin (Polysporin), either alone or in combination; and gentamicin or erythromycin. Systemic antibiotics are used only when systemic signs, such as fever and malaise, are present; when the infection is widespread; or when there is an epidemic.

### Impetigo

#### Etiology/Epidemiology

**Impetigo** is a common skin infection caused by staphylococci or β-hemolytic streptococci. Although impetigo may occur at any age, children are most often affected. It occurs more commonly in the summer or early fall. Factors that promote development of impetigo include tropical climates, uncleanliness, poor hygiene, poor nutrition, and poor health.

#### Pathophysiology

Impetigo begins as a small thin-walled vesicle that ruptures easily and leaves a weeping denuded spot. It becomes pustular and dries to form a honey-colored crust that appears stuck on the skin (Figure 67-2). The process, which is superficial, may extend below the crust. Impetigo is usually confined to the face but may occur elsewhere. If untreated, impetigo may last for several weeks with new lesions forming.

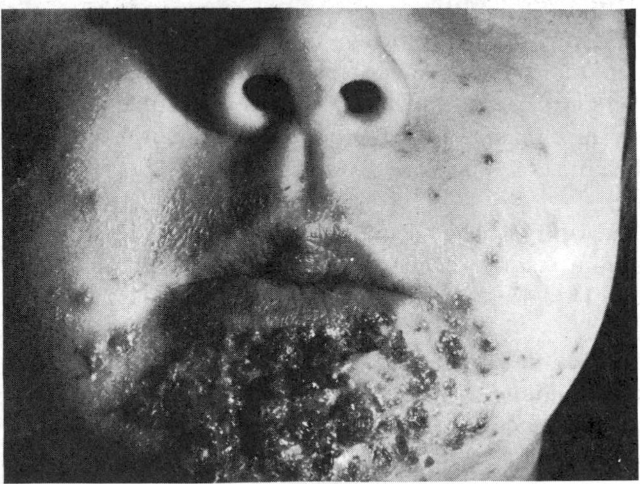

**FIGURE 67-2** Impetigo contagiosa. (From Stewart WD, Danto JL, Maddin S: *Dermatology: diagnosis and treatment of cutaneous disorders,* ed 4, St Louis, 1978, Mosby.)

#### Medical management

Treatment consists of maintaining cleanliness and applying topical antibiotics. The crusts must be removed and the lesions washed gently two or three times daily to prevent further crust formation. Warm soaks or saline compresses may be necessary to soften crusts that adhere firmly. Topical antibiotics are applied at least three times daily. Systemic antibiotics may be prescribed.

#### Nursing management

First, nursing care focuses on helping patient carry out the regimen. Second, care focuses on prevention of spread of infection. Family members or health care providers should wash their hands thoroughly with a bacteriostatic soap after contact. Patients should use personal towels. Linens should be laundered after the first day of treatment.

### Folliculitis

#### Etiology/Epidemiology

**Folliculitis** is usually caused by a *Staphylococcus* organism, but occasionally it is caused by other bacteria, both gram-negative and gram-positive. The infection may be caused by drainage from other infected lesions. Predisposing factors include uncleanliness, maceration, exposure to oils and solvents, traction of hair by tar therapy, or occlusion therapy.

#### Pathophysiology

Bacterial infections of the hair follicle may be superficial in the epidermis around the hair follicle or deep in the tissue surrounding both the lower and upper portions of the hair follicle. Deep folliculitis produces a more severe inflammatory response. *Sycosis barbae* (barber's itch) is a deep folliculitis of the beard. The hairs do not fall out or break, such as occurs with tinea barbae. *Hordeolum* (stye) is a deep folliculitis of the cilia of the eyelids. There is usually swelling of the surrounding eyelid, with crusting along the edge of the eyelid.

#### Medical management

Treatment of superficial folliculitis includes cleansing with soap and water and applying topical antibiotics. Warm compresses are applied to encourage resolution of deep folliculitis. Topical antibiotics, such as Neosporin, hasten healing.

#### Nursing management

Nursing management focuses on teaching patients about the prescribed therapy and about avoidance of predisposing factors.

## Furuncles and Carbuncles

### Etiology/Epidemiology

**Furuncles** (boils) are a deep folliculitis that originates either from a superficial folliculitis or as a deep nodule around the hair follicle. *Furunculosis* is the appearance of several furuncles. An infection that involves several surrounding hair follicles is termed a **carbuncle.** The organism causing furuncles and carbuncles is usually *Staphylococcus,* but occasionally it can be caused by other bacteria.

Both furuncles and carbuncles occur most often in obese, poorly nourished, fatigued, or otherwise susceptible persons whose hygiene may be poor; in debilitated elderly people; and in persons who have inadequately-treated diabetes mellitus.

### Pathophysiology

Local swelling and redness occur, and there is severe local pain, which is decreased by moving the involved part as little as possible. Within 3 to 5 days the lesion becomes elevated or "points up," the surrounding skin becomes shiny, and the center or "core" turns yellow. A carbuncle has several cores. The boil will usually rupture spontaneously, but it may be surgically incised and drained. As drainage occurs, the pain is immediately relieved. The drainage soon changes from a yellow purulent material to a serosanguineous discharge. All drainage usually subsides within a few hours to a few days; the redness and swelling subside gradually. Furuncles are likely to occur on the face, neck, forearms, groin, and legs, whereas carbuncles are usually limited to the nape of the neck and the back.

### Medical management

Hot, wet dressings are used to help bring the boil to a head, but these dressings are discontinued as soon as drainage occurs to prevent skin maceration and spread of infection. As the boil drains, care must be taken to keep the infected discharge off the surrounding skin, because organisms may be harbored in hair follicles and furunculosis may recur. Systemic antibiotics may be prescribed.

If the patient is hospitalized, wound isolation procedures are followed until the discharge subsides, lest the organism be carried to others. Health personnel should wash their hands thoroughly after caring for the patient and should avoid getting the discharge on their own skin.

Furuncles and carbuncles tend to recur in susceptible individuals, and the staphylococci causing them are often resistant to local treatment and to antibiotics.

### Nursing management

Nursing care focuses on the prevention of spread of the infection. Patients are cautioned to keep their hands away from the discharge to prevent spread of infection.

## Erysipelas

### Etiology/Epidemiology

**Erysipelas** is an acute febrile disease caused by a hemolytic streptococcus. Elderly people with poor resistance are most often affected.

### Pathophysiology

Erysipelas was a serious disease before the advent of antibiotics. It is characterized by localized inflammation and swelling of the skin and subcutaneous tissues, usually of the face. A bright, sharp line separates the diseased skin from the normal skin.

### Medical management

Penicillin is the drug of choice.

### Nursing management

Nursing care focuses on helping patients assume responsibility for treatment and completing the treatment.

# VIRAL DISEASES

## Warts

### Etiology/Epidemiology

**Warts** develop from hypertrophy of epidermal cells as a result of a viral infection. The infection is not highly contagious but does spread along the dermis through autoinfection. It is seen most commonly in older children and young adults.

### Pathophysiology

Warts are benign skin growths that grow in a variety of shapes. The common wart is a small, circumscribed, painless, hyperkeratotic papule usually seen on the extremities, espeically the hands. *Filiform warts* are slender fingerlike projections occurring mostly on the face and neck. *Plantar warts* grow inward from the pressure on the soles of the feet and are frequently painful. They are differentiated from calluses by lack of skin lines over the surface. Warts that develop in the anogenital region have a lighter-colored surface and a cauliflower-like appearance, and they may cause itching. Anogenital warts may be spread either by sexual activity or by other means. Some genital warts in women may predispose cancer of the cervix.

### Medical management

There are numerous treatments for warts but no one major effective method. If only a few painless warts are present, no treatment is necessary and the wart will probably disappear in time.

The most commonly used therapeutic measures for common warts are electrodesiccation and cryosurgery. In electrodesiccation the top of the wart is seared gently to soften the keratinized surface and then curetted off and the bleeding points cauterized. This method is not used for plantar warts. Cryosurgery consists of freezing the lesion with a substance, such as liquid nitrogen. Cauterant chemicals—such as formalin, phenol, nitric acid, cantharidin, salicylic acid, or podophyllum—may be used. Recalcitrant warts may respond to radiation therapy. Surgical excision is seldom used, because painful scarring may result.

#### Nursing management

Nursing care focuses on preparing the patient for treatment and assisting with treatment. Warts sometimes disappear spontaneously or under psychologic suggestion, thus creating a basis for numerous folktales on how to get rid of warts. Nurses must help patients avoid potentially dangerous home remedies.

## Herpes Simplex

### Etiology/Epidemiology

One of the most common viruses found in humans is the **herpes simplex** virus (HSV). It occurs as two similar yet serologically different strains, type 1 and type 2. HSV has a DNA-containing core surrounded by a phospholipid covering. Factors that may precipitate recurrence of herpes simplex lesions include fever, upper respiratory tract infection, exhaustion, and nervous tension. Lesions also are more common during the menses or after direct exposure to the sun's rays.

#### Pathophysiology

The type 1 virus is found primarily in lesions of the face and mouth (fever blister, cold sore), eye (keratitis), and brain (encephalitis). Type 2 is associated with a lesion of the genitalia that can be transmitted by sexual contact (see Chapter 55).

Most persons experience the initial contact with HSV (type 1) as young children. The HSV remains in the cells of the sensory nerves that supply the affected areas and causes recurrent lesions when the person is subjected to stress. The appearance of vesicles is preceded by several hours by a sensation of burning or itching. A cluster of vesicles on an erythematous base appears at the mucocutaneous junctions of the lips or nose or as an inflammation of the cornea of one eye with photophobia and tearing. The type 2 virus lesions occur in the vagina or cervix of the woman or on the penile skin of the man. The lesions are painful and frequently crack open. A crust gradually forms, and the lesions heal in about 10 days. HSV can be identified by a Tzanck smear (see Chapter 66).

#### Medical management

The development of antiviral compounds has helped in the treatment of HSV.[13,14] Topical use of acyclovir, idoxuridine, or vidarabine has been effective in preventing corneal ulceration and visual impairment in herpetic keratitis. Acyclovir is effective systemically in treating primary genital herpes simplex and preventing recurrent episodes if suppressive dosages are maintained. However, if the drug is stopped, the frequency of recurrence is not altered.

The antivirals have been found to reduce the mortality in herpes simplex encephalitis and disseminated herpetic infection of the newborn, but they do not prevent all the complications. Herpes simplex viral infections resistant to acyclovir have been found in persons with AIDS.[13] These have been treated effectively with foscarnet.[13]

#### Nursing management

Patient education is the primary nursing intervention needed for patients with herpes. Information should be given about the etiology, treatment methodology, and measures to prevent secondary infection.

## Herpetic Whitlow

### Etiology/Epidemiology

**Herpetic whitlow** is an HSV infection of the finger, occurring most commonly among nurses, physicians, and dentists. The source of infection may be direct contact with vesicular fluid of oral herpetic lesions or from viruses present in oral secretions of asymptomatic persons.[8]

#### Pathophysiology

The lesion is preceded by itching and intense pain and sometimes by fever, chills, and malaise. Vesicles form as with other HSV infections. Healing occurs within 3 to 4 weeks, but lesions will reappear.

#### Medical management

Treatment is essentially symptomatic, with elevation and immobilization of the finger and analgesics.

#### Nursing management

Nursing management focuses on prevention of spread of infection. Personal linens and utensils should be used to avoid infecting others.[8] Contact with oral secretions of persons with known HSV lesions can be prevented by using gloves when providing oral care.

## Herpes Zoster

### Etiology/Eidemiology

**Herpes zoster,** or **shingles** is caused by the same virus (V-Z) that causes **varicella** (chickenpox). Varicella is believed to be the primary infection in a nonimmune host, whereas herpes zoster is thought to be the response in a partially immune host. Although herpes zoster is far less communicable than is chickenpox, persons who have not had chickenpox may develop it after exposure to the vesicular lesions of persons with herpes zoster. For this reason, susceptible persons should not care for patients with herpes zoster. It is one of the most drawn out and exasperating conditions in elderly patients and leads to discouragement and demoralization. Herpes

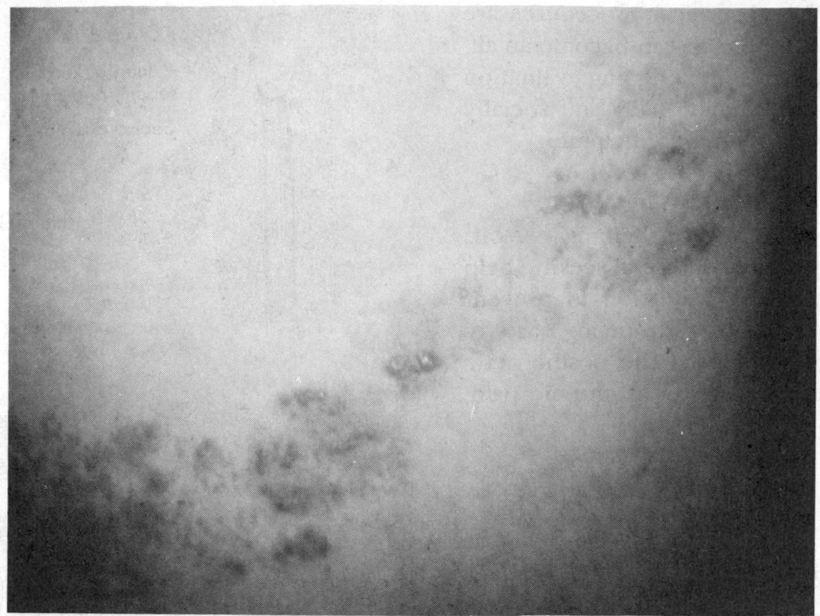

**FIGURE 67-3** Herpes zoster. (Courtesy David Bickers, MD, Cleveland, Ohio.)

zoster may recur in rare circumstances. Herpes zoster often occurs in persons with AIDS and Hodgkin's disease and in individuals with lymphoid and some bone cancers because of reduced cell-mediated immunity.

### Pathophysiology

In herpes zoster, clusters of small vesicles usually form in a line. They follow the course of the peripheral sensory nerves and often are unilateral (Figure 67-3). Because they follow nerve pathways, the lesions never cross the midline of the body. However, nerves on both sides of the body can be involved. Two thirds of persons with herpes zoster develop lesions over thoracic dermatomes, and the remainder show involvement of the trigeminal nerve with lesions on the face, eye, and scalp. The rash develops first as macules but progresses rapidly to vesicles. The fluid becomes turbid, and crusts develop and drop off in about 10 days.

Malaise, fever, itching, and pain over the involved area may precede the eruption of the lesions. If vesicles develop within 1 to 2 days after the initial pain symptoms, the lesions usually clear in 2 to 3 weeks, but if the vesicles develop over the period of a week, a prolonged course can be expected.[11]

Discomfort from pain and itching is the major problem with herpes zoster. The pain may vary from a light burning sensation to a deep visceral-type pain, and it may be intermittent or constant. It usually persists for up to 4 weeks. In approximately 50% of persons over age 60, the pain may last for months or years.[13] Enlargement of the lymph nodes may also occur with the rash.

### Medical management

For many patients, no treatment is prescribed for herpes zoster. However, for persons with immunosuppression, treatment is given. Acyclovir (Zovirax) accelerates healing and reduces acute pain and is given orally in high doses (400 mg to 800 mg, every 4 hours, five times a day for 5 to 6 days). In severe infections, acyclovir may be given intravenously; lower doses are effective intravenously. Because acyclovir may precipitate in renal tubules, drinking fluids should be encouraged. Acyclovir has no effect in preventing postherpetic neuralgia.

Analgesics are prescribed for pain relief. Aspirin, with or without codeine, is often effective; meperidine hydrochloride (Demerol) may be needed for severe pain. Herpetic pain may be decreased by systemic steroids, such as prednisone, steroid therapy may decrease the incidence of postherpetic neuralgia. However, it should not be used in immunocompromised persons. Sedatives may also be helpful, especially at bedtime. Local discomfort may be relieved by calamine lotion or by application of a vinegar solution (one-fourth cup white vinegar in 2 quarts lukewarm water.)[5] Loose clothing helps to minimize contact with the affected area. Patients should avoid exposure to highly susceptible persons (those who have not had chickenpox or who are immunocompromised).

Postherpetic neuralgia (PHN) occurs in about 10% of persons after herpes zoster infection, mostly in elderly persons.[5] The pain usually lasts less than 1 year but may persist for many years. The pain is always present with superimposed sharp pain episodes. Because the pain results from nervous system damage, it does not respond well to usual pain therapies, and thus a multimodal approach is more effective.[7] A tricyclic antidepressant is commonly prescribed. Transcutaneous electrical nerve stimulation (TENS) may be tried initially, although it usually is not effective on a long-term basis. Narcotics are avoided because of the persistence of the pain and potential for addiction. Neurosurgical procedures are usually ineffective. Because the pain can become an all-consuming part of the patient's life, ongoing evaluation of the impact on the patient functionally and socially and ongoing supportive counseling are helpful.

#### Nursing management

Nursing management focuses first on helping persons identify the onset of the problem and then seeking help as appropriate. Second, patient education to prevent spread of infection is important. Last, nursing care focuses on helping patients deal with the postherpetic neuralgia. (For a complete discussion of chronic pain, see Chapter 17.)

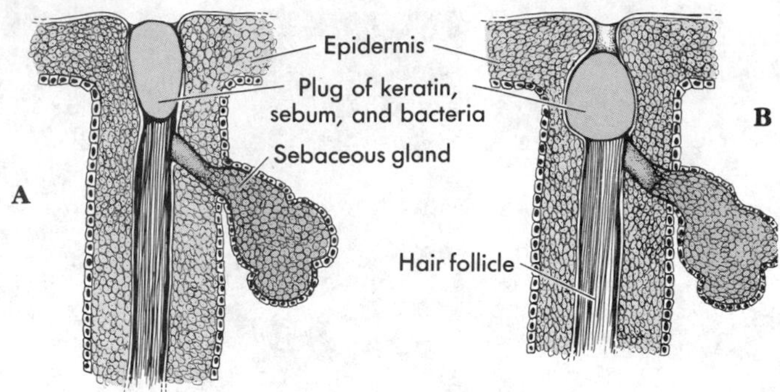


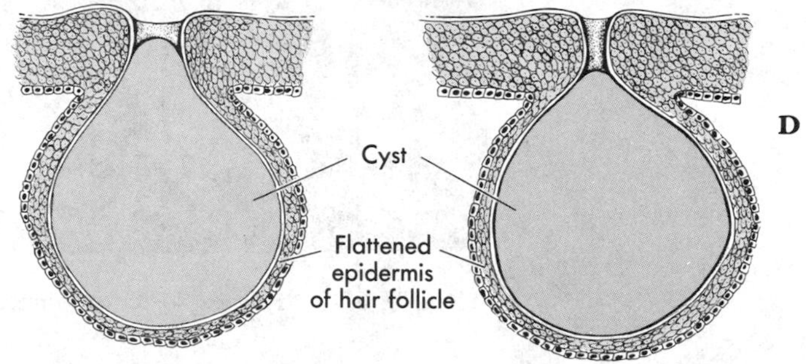


**FIGURE 67-4** Formation of lesions in acne vulgaris. **A,** Open comedo (blackhead), early stage. **B,** Closed comedo (whitehead), early stage. **C,** Cyst formation in open comedo, advanced stage. **D,** Cyst formation in closed comedo, advanced stage. (From Parrish JH: *Dermatology and skin care,* New York, 1975, McGraw-Hill Book Co. Used with the permission of McGraw-Hill Book Co.)

## ACNE

### Acne Vulgaris

#### Etiology/Epidemiology

**Acne vulgaris** is a very common skin disease seen in 80% of adolescents. It may also occur in adults. The cause of acne is still unknown but is thought to be multifactorial. Some of the common causes that have been postulated are free fatty acids, endocrine effects, stressors, diet, heredity, and infection. Diet has been essentially ruled out as a causative factor, but none of the other factors have been demonstrated conclusively. Acne occurs at puberty when the sebaceous glands are stimulated by androgens, and it is often found to be common within families. Acne is more quiescent in summer months.

#### Pathophysiology

At puberty, sebaceous glands undergo enlargement from androgen stimulation. When sebum is released, it passes through the follicular canal, where it is combined with sebaceous gland cell fragments, epidermal cells (keratin), and bacteria. At this time the triglycerides in the sebum are hydrolyzed to glycerol and free fatty acids. The sebum and debris may become plugged in the hair follicle (Figure 67-4) to form an open comedo (blackhead) if it is at the surface or a closed comedo (whitehead) if it is below the surface. The dark color of the blackhead is melanin, not dirt, and results from passage of melanin from the adjoining epidermal cells.

Inflammatory lesions apparently develop from escape of sebum into the dermis, which then serves as an irritant, causing an inflammatory reaction. Free fatty acids may also be an irritant in the follicle itself.

Acne occurs mostly on the face and neck, upper chest, and back, although the upper arms, buttocks, and thighs may also be involved. Comedones are the first visible signs, and the skin is characteristically oily. The inflammatory lesions include papules, pustules, nodules, and cysts. Superficial lesions may resolve in 5 to 10 days without scarring, but large lesions last for several weeks and often result in scarring. The typical scar resembles an old volcano (ice-pick scar); however, many other sizes and shapes may result, depending on the depth and extent of the inflammatory lesions.

There is a great variability in the extent of the lesions. Some persons have only a few small lesions. Many adolescents have several lesions that peak at ages 16 to 18 years of age and then slowly resolve. A few persons develop severe nodular acne that may not resolve for 10 to 15 years.

#### Medical management

Medical therapy may be topical, systemic, intralesional, or surgical and includes the following:

1. Topical therapy
   a. Basic method of therapy
   b. Agents: benzoyl peroxide, vitamin A acid (tretinoin), antibiotics (topical erythromycin), sulfur-zinc lotion
2. Removal of comedones with a comedo extractor
3. Systemic therapy
   a. Used with topical therapy for *severe* nodular or cystic acne
   b. Isoretinoic acid (Accutane)
      (1) A vitamin A acid analog

**Guidelines for Teaching the Person With Acne**

1. Preventive measures
   a. Keep hands and hair away from the face.
   b. Avoid constricting clothing over lesions.
   c. Shampoo hair and scalp frequently.
   d. Avoid exposure to oils and greases.
   e. Eat a well-balanced diet and avoid any foods that appear to cause skin flare-ups.
2. General skin care
   a. Keep skin clean; wash face 2 to 3 times daily.
   b. Use a medicated soap or agent prescribed by physician.
   c. Avoid vigorous rubbing of the skin.
   d. Use cosmetics that are water-based, rather than cream-based, and avoid those which contain wax esters (myristates, palmitates, stearates).
   e. Never leave cosmetics on face at night.
3. During therapy
   a. Follow the prescribed therapy even when immediate improvement is not noted for 2 to 3 weeks.
   b. Expect skin desquamation during therapy.
   c. Avoid using self-remedies during therapy.
   d. Remove cosmetics before applying topical medications.
   e. Avoid exposure to direct sunlight if using tretinoin or taking tetracycline (photosensitivity).
   f. Avoid pregnancy if taking Accutane (possiblity of birth defects).

(2) Side effects: dry lips and conjunctiva, brittle hair, tenderness of fingertips and toetips, hypertriglyceridemia, birth defects

c. Systemic antibiotics

d. Estrogens for females who have not responded to other therapies

4. Intralesional corticosteroid therapy for cysts of severe acne
5. Surgery: dermabrasion to remove scars

### Nursing management

Counseling and teaching are the major nursing strategies. Stress appears to be one of the causative factors; therefore attempts to identify and cope with stressors may be helpful. Acne, per se, can be a stressor, producing facial disfigurements and sometimes leading to behavior that is hostile, aggressive, and anxious, as well as shy and withdrawn. Psychologic counseling is often desirable.

Knowledge of the nature of acne helps the person to understand the necessary care. Teaching is directed toward general health care of the skin and guidelines for therapy (see Guidelines box above).

The lesions in acne develop when the pilosebaceous follicles become plugged; therefore activities that contribute to occlusion of the follicles are to be avoided. Hair and hands should be kept away from the face. Loose clothing prevents pressure over the follicles, and tight collars should not be worn. The skin should be kept clean. Greasy, oil-based cosmetics may be occlusive and plug up the follicles. Any food that appears to cause acne flare-ups in a given individual is best avoided.

## Acne Rosacea

### Etiology/Epidemiology

**Acne rosacea** is a skin condition that usually affects persons over 25 years of age. The actual cause is unknown. Over the years many causative factors have been suggested, including bacteria, vitamin deficiency, hormonal imbalance, alcohol, caffeine, psychologic factors, and heredity.

### Pathophysiology

Acne rosacea begins with redness over the cheeks and nose, followed by papules, pustules, and enlargement of superficial blood vessels. Years of acne rosacea lead to an irregular, bulbous thickening of the skin of the distal part of the nose **(rhinophyma),** with a red-purple discoloration and dilated follicles.

### Medical management

There is no specific treatment for acne rosacea. Some persons respond to tetracycline and topical peeling agents, but there is no specific treatment for the vascular component. Rhinophyma may be treated by plastic surgery.

### Nursing management

Nursing management focuses on teaching and support. Teaching about the disease and possible treatment is necessary. Avoiding stimuli that cause vasodilation seems appropriate.

# DERMATITIS

**Dermatitis,** a superficial inflammation of the skin, refers to several different conditions resulting in the same type of lesions. Dermatitis is often classified arbitrarily according to specific features, such as cause, pattern, age, or type of treatment required. Some of the common types of dermatitis are listed in Table 67-4 and are discussed in more detail in succeeding paragraphs. The term *eczema* is often used synonymously with dermatitis but frequently refers to the chronic type.

Regardless of the cause, the lesions in any dermatitis follow a characteristic pattern. Initially, there is erythema and local edema, followed by vesicle formation with oozing and then crusting and scaling. If the dermatitis persists, there will be evidence of excoriation from scratching and thickening of the skin, and the color becomes more brownish. Secondary infection may result.

## Contact Dermatitis

### Etiology/epidemiology

**Contact dermatitis** is caused by external agents and may affect various parts of the body (Table 67-5). There

**TABLE 67-4 Types of Dermatitis**

| TYPE | CAUSE | CHARACTERISTICS |
|---|---|---|
| Contact | External agents | Site and pattern of lesions depend on exposure pattern (linear, angular, etc.)<br>Itching a major symptom |
| Atopic | Hypersensitivity reaction, hereditary | Itching a major symptom<br>Lesions caused by scratching |
| Lichen simplex chronicus | Stasis, irritants, psychologic factors | Itching a major symptom<br>Lesions caused by scratching |
| Seborrheic | Unknown | Erythematous, scaly (e.g., dandruff) |
| Nummular | Unknown | Coin-shaped lesions<br>Severe itching |
| Stasis | Decreased circulation | Erythema, edema<br>Lesions may develop from trauma<br>Itching may be severe |

**TABLE 67-5 Common Causes of Contact Dermatitis of Different Areas**

| AREA | CAUSE |
|---|---|
| Face | Cosmetics, hair sprays and dyes, airborne contactants |
| Earlobes | Nickel |
| Ears | |
| Pinnae | Photosensitizers |
| Canals | Medications |
| Eyelids | Cosmetics, airborne sensitizers, transfer by hands |
| Nose (bridge) | Metal or plastic spectacle supports |
| Lips and perioral area | Toothpaste, lipstick |
| Neck | Perfumes, clothing (especially wool) |
| Axillae | Deodorants, clothing, perfumes |
| Scapular area | Nickel in clasps on straps |
| Breasts | Elastic and other brassiere material |
| Waist | Elastic |
| Perianal area | Dibucaine (Nupercaine) and other medications, excessive use of cleansers |
| Arms and legs | Poison ivy and other plants |
| Wrists | Nickel, etc., in watchbands |
| Hands | Detergents and other cleansers, gloves |
| Feet | Medication for "athlete's foot," shoes |

From Moschella SL, Hurley HJ: *Dermatology,* ed 3, Philadelphia, 1991, WB Saunders.

are two types of contact dermatitis, irritant and allergic. ***Irritant contact dermatitis*** can occur in any person on contact with a sufficient concentration of an irritant. Mechanical irritation may result from wool or glass fibers. Chemical irritants include acids, alkalies, solvents, detergents, or oils commonly found in cleaning compounds, insecticides, or industrial compounds. Biologic irritants include urine, fecal drainage, and toxins from insects or aquatic plants. People who are exposed to constant wetting of the hands or feet often develop irritant contact dermatitis.

***Allergic contact dermatitis*** is a cell-mediated hypersensitivity immune reaction from contact with a specific antigen. Many compounds are capable of causing sensitization under specified conditions. Typical antigens include poison ivy, synthetics, industrial chemicals, drugs (for example, sulfanilamide or penicillin), and metals (especially nickel and chromate). Once the skin has been sensitized, further contact with the sensitizing substance will produce an eczematous reaction. The sensitizing allergen may reach the site by direct contact; by indirect contact, such as transmission by animals, from one part of the body to the other by the hands, or on clothing; or by the air, as in smoke.

#### Pathophysiology

Characteristic dermatitis lesions appear sooner in irritant contact dermatitis than in the allergic type; however, the onset and appearance vary, depending on the type and concentration of the irritant. The lesions develop on the exposed areas, particularly the more sensitive areas, such as the dorsal rather than the palmar surface of the hands. If the irritant can be spread by the hands, as in poison ivy, lesions may involve other nonexposed areas.

When contact dermatitis is suspected but the agent is unknown, patch testing (see Chapter 66) may be carried out or the environment may be manipulated to exclude suspected agents.

#### Medical management

Weeping uninfected lesions respond rapidly to wet dressings with water or Burow's solution (1:40 dilution of aluminum acetate) for 20 minutes four times daily. Crusts and scales are not removed but are allowed to drop off naturally as the skin heals. Topical corticosteroids are applied to dry lesions. Systemic corticosteroids may be given in acute extensive exacerbations but are not used to treat a mild contact dermatitis. Systemic antibiotics are prescribed when infection is present. Severe pruritus may be eased by antihistamines; *plain* calamine lotion may be applied for pruritus from poison ivy.

#### Nursing management

The primary focus of nursing care is prevention. Contact dermatitis may be prevented by avoiding the irritating or sensitizing substance whenever possible. A person should know how to recognize the leaves of poisonous plants—such as poison ivy, poison oak, or poison su-

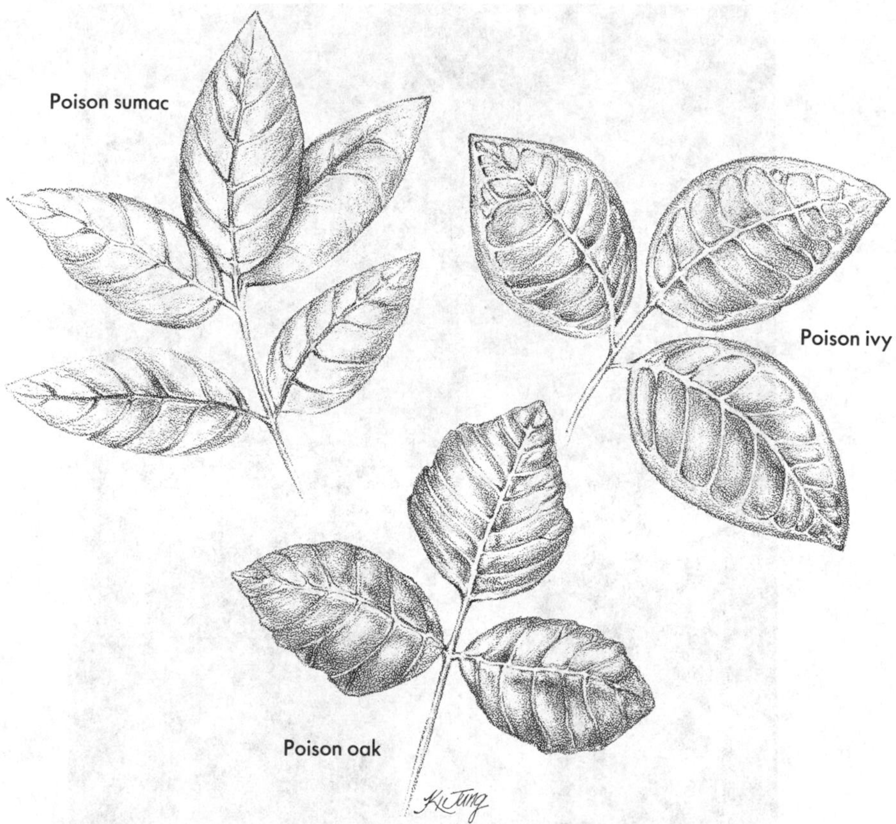


**FIGURE 67-5** Typical leaves of poison sumac, poison ivy, and poison oak.

mac—that grow where they live (Figure 67-5). Persons walking in areas where poison ivy grows need to protect the skin by clothing. If contact with poison ivy is suspected, symptoms may be averted by immediately rinsing the skin for 15 minutes with running water to remove the resin before skin penetration occurs.

The person who develops a sensitivity to material encountered in the living or working environment may need to consider a permanent change of environment if other measures are unsuccessful. Gloves may be used if the person is handling irritant or allergenic substances. Persons sensitive to detergents may need to wash their clothes and bathe with a mild soap, such as Ivory.

## Atopic Dermatitis (Eczema)

### Etiology/Epidemiology

**Atopy** refers to type I hypersensitivity, which is hereditary and includes asthma, hay fever, **eczema,** and other types of reactions (see Chapter 70 for complete discussion of hypersensitivity). Approximately 50% of persons with **atopic dermatitis** develop asthma or hay fever. The person who has inherited the tendency to eczema may not necessarily demonstrate symptoms. Exacerbating factors include sudden changes in temperature or humidity; exercise; psychologic stress; fibers such as wool, fur, or nylon; detergents; and perfumes. Atopic dermatitis in the infant is usually first noted at about the third month. It usually disappears or becomes less severe between the ages of 2 or 3 years but recurs in late childhood or adolescence in a large number of persons.

The major symptom of atopic dermatitis is *pruritus.* Chronic scratching leads to eczematous lesions and subsequent lichenification. Healing usually occurs without scarring, but hypopigmentation or hyperpigmentation may result.

### Pathophysiology

Persons with atopic dermatitis have a dry, highly sensitive skin with a lowered threshold to pruritus, so that minor stimuli cause intense itching. There is a marked tendency toward vasoconstriction of superficial blood vessels, and the skin blanches readily.[11] Cold and low humidity are poorly tolerated because of drying effects. Heat and high humidity are also poorly tolerated because vasodilation increases the inflammatory reaction, thus aggravating the dermatitis and causing increased itching and discomfort. Lesions become localized to the flexor surfaces of the neck, to the eyelids, behind the ears, in the antecubital and popliteal areas (Figure 67-6), and at the wrists. The erythema is now dusky in color, and excoriations may become secondarily infected. By the late twenties or early thirties the lesions usually disappear, but they may recur at a later date as chronic hand or foot eczema.[11]

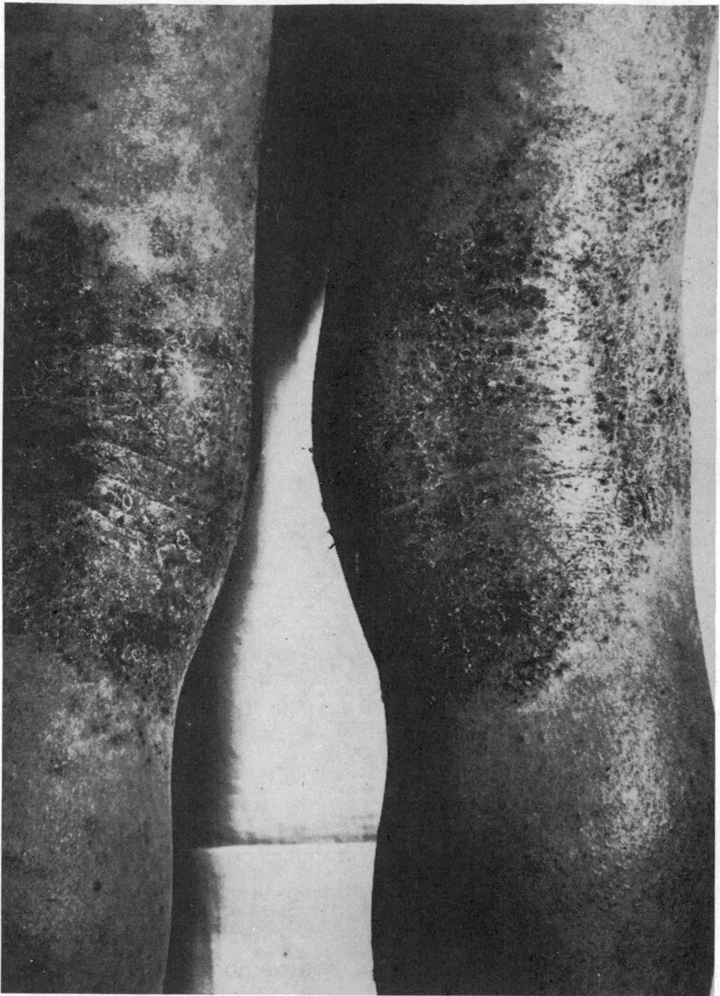

**FIGURE 67-6** Atopic dermatitis with characteristic flexural involvement and crusting. (From Stewart WD, Danto JL, Maddin S: *Dermatology: diagnosis and treatment of cutaneous disorders,* ed 4, St Louis, 1978, Mosby.)

Persons with atopic dermatitis are highly susceptible to viral infections, especially herpes, and to bacterial infections, such as those caused by staphylococcus or β-hemolytic streptococcus. There is also an increased incidence of fungal infections, such as tinea. Lymph nodes draining affected areas may be enlarged.

### Medical management

There is no cure for atopic dermatitis, but symptoms can be controlled. The focus of therapy is relief of pruritus to break the itch-scratch cycle that leads to lesions. The major form of *topical* therapy consists of corticosteroid cream or ointment. Fluorinated corticosteroids may be used for localized lesions in adults but are used less often in children and *never on the face.* An occlusion wrap over the steroid in adults may enhance the steroid effect but may lead to folliculitis. Topical antibiotics are rarely used. Cool compresses with water or Burow's solution are helpful for acute phases when weeping lesions are present.

Systemic therapy includes antihistamines, especially at night when itching is more intense. Antibiotics, such as penicillin or erythromycin, may be given systemically for bacterial infections. Systemic corticosteroids may be given for a limited period to those with severe atopic eczema.

### Nursing management

Patient education is the major focus of care and should stress prevention of hypersensitivity and then control of signs and symptoms. Patients should keep the skin hydrated and avoid temperature extremes and irritating substances (see Guidelines box, p. 2337).

## Other Types of Dermatitis

### Lichen simplex chronicus

Lichen simplex chronicus (LSC) is a chronic skin condition that results from repeated scratching. Psychologic factors are thought to be involved. Although it is more common in females and Orientals, it may occur in both

**Guidelines for Teaching the Person With Atopic Dermatitis**

1. Avoid soap over lesions (soap is an irritant); use soap minimally over nonaffected areas.
2. Soak affected areas for 15 to 20 minutes in warm water for hydration; pat skin dry, then *immediately* apply recommended lotion or cream to seal in moisture.
3. Wet wraps may be used in place of soaking; wraps permit evaporation, which cools the skin, thus decreasing pruritus.
4. Apply corticosteroids in a thin layer and rub in well; do not use fluorinated corticosteroid on the face.
5. Avoid wool, fur, or rough fibers against the skin; they act as irritants and cause itching.
6. Avoid overheating that increases sweating, leading to itching. Wear loose, light clothing in hot weather. Air conditioning promotes comfort. Sunlight is beneficial to the skin.
7. Avoid excessive cold that dries the skin.
8. Avoid anything that aggravates the eczema.
9. Rinse all garments and bed linens twice to avoid residue of cleansing agents.
10. Consult dermatologist for appropriate laundry agents to prevent irritations from clothing.
11. Seek medical care if eczema becomes worse.

genders and all races. Itching initiates the condition in normal skin and may occur as a result of stasis or an irritant, or it may occur without any known cause. LSC is more commonly found in the occipital region of the scalp, hands, perineum, and legs.

Once itching starts, the itch-scratch cycle is initiated and scratching becomes a habit. The skin becomes excoriated, and lichenified plaques result. Lesions disappear if scratching ceases, but it is difficult for the person to stop scractching. Itching is often worse at night. Topical corticosteroids are the treatment of choice. In nonhairy areas, corticosteroid tape (Cordran tape) is effective if the medicated tape covers the area, so that further excoriation is reduced.

#### Seborrheic dermatitis

**Seborrheic dermatitis** may occur primarily in areas of increased sebaceous gland activity on the face, ears, scalp, chest, and back. The cause is unknown. Mild seborrheic dermatitis is often seen in the scalp in the form of erythema and dandruff and can be controlled easily by shampooing with selenium sulfide (Selsun Blue) shampoo. More extensive seborrheic dermatitis leads to red scaly plaques and is treated with topical hydrocortisone.

#### Nummular dermatitis

Nummular dermatitis is a chronic condition of uncertain cause. It occurs most commonly in middle-aged or older men. The lesions of nummular dermatitis are coin-shaped and are found on the dorsum of the hand, the extensor surfaces of the extremities, and the buttocks.

**TABLE 67-6 Skin Reactions to Common Medications**

| REACTION | MEDICATION |
|---|---|
| Erythematous rash | Antibiotics, sulfonamides, thiazide diuretics, barbiturates, phenylbutazone |
| Purpura (ecchymosis, petechiae) | Thiazides, sulfonamides, barbiturates, anticoagulants |
| Mucocutaneous lesions (vesicles, bullae, ulcers) | Sulfonamides, penicillins, barbiturates, phenylbutazone |
| Urticaria | Penicillins, streptomycin, tetracycline, insulin, aspirin, dyes, ACTH, antiserum |

Itching is often severe. The skin is usually dry; therefore frequent bathing is inadvisable. Exposure to sunlight may be helpful. Treatment consists of topical corticosteroids and antibiotic therapy if bacteria are isolated by culture.

#### Stasis dermatitis

**Stasis dermatitis** is a common skin condition of the lower extremities in older persons. It is usually preceded by varicosities and poor circulation. With the reduction in venous return from the legs, substances normally carried away by the circulation remain in the tissues and irritate them. The skin is often reddened and edematous. Pruritus may be quite severe. Breaks in the skin are often caused by scratching, and infection then is introduced by the hands, clothing, and other sources.

The most important treatment for stasis dermatitis is prevention by careful attention to the treatment of peripheral vascular conditions and preventing the constriction of the circulation to the extremities. When acute weeping lesions are present, wet compresses and elevation of the legs are advised.

## SKIN REACTIONS FROM SYSTEMIC FACTORS

### Dermatitis Medicamentosa

#### Etiology/Epidemiology

Skin manifestations resulting from drugs may have a nonallergic or an allergic basis. Commonly seen skin reactions include erythematous rashes, purpura, vesicles, bullae, ulcers, and urticaria (Table 67-6). The reactions can appear at any time, but the onset is usually sudden.

#### Pathophysiology

Hypersensitivity reactions to drugs are the most common and may be either type I anaphylactic (urticaria, angioedema), type II cytotoxic (cellular injury), type III immune complexes (serum sickness), or type IV cell-mediated (allergic contact dermatitis, allergic photosensitivity).[9] Some drugs may have combined reactions; for example, penicillin may produce both type I and type

**TABLE 67-7 Drug Photosensitivity**

| REACTION | SYMPTOMS | DRUGS |
|---|---|---|
| Phototoxicity | Resembles sunburn (erythema, edema, vesicles) | Coal tar derivatives<br>Psoralens<br>Tetracycline<br>Nalidixic acid<br>Sulfanilamide<br>Declomycin<br>Chlorpromazine<br>Certain dyes |
| Photoallergy | Resembles eczema (exudative papules and vesicles, urticaria, lichenification) | Diuretics (thiazides)<br>Phenothiazines<br>Oral hypoglycemics<br>Griseofulvin |

III reactions. Allergic contact dermatitis is commonly seen with drugs used topically. The rash is often bright red, semiconfluent, macular and papular, generalized, and bilateral. Hypersensitivity occurs early when previous sensitization has taken place.

*Photosensitivity* may also occur with certain drugs and may take one of two forms, phototoxicity or photoallergy (Table 67-7). *Phototoxicity* may occur in any person taking a photosensitive drug and results from the reaction of the drug (chemical) with radiant energy, particularly ultraviolet light. Sunscreens are not effective in preventing photosensitivity reactions.[2] *Photoallergic* reactions are cell-mediated (type IV) hypersensitivity reactions; therefore they affect only a small group of persons after several sensitizing exposures of drug and sunlight.

#### Medical management

Treatment of dermatitis medicamentosa consists of stopping the drug and treating the symptoms with cool, moist compresses; antihistamines (for pruritus); and topical and systemic corticosteroids. Photosensitivity can be prevented by avoiding direct sunlight on the skin when taking a drug with photosensitivity effects.

#### Nursing management

Nursing care focuses first on prevention by making sure people are aware of drugs to which they are allergic and having this documented on their records. Secondary nursing care focuses on helping with treatment.

## Exfoliative Dermatitis

### Etiology/Epidemiology

Exfoliative dermatitis is a rare, generalized dermatitis. In most cases, the cause is unknown, but the disease may be associated with other types of dermatitis or with a lymphoma, or it may be the result of a drug reaction.

#### Pathophysiology

The onset of exfoliative dermatitis may be rapid or insidious and consists of an elevated temperature and a generalized erythema, followed by extensive scaling (exfoliation). Pruritus may be present, and the lesions often become infected. Loss of large amounts of water and protein from the skin leads to hypoproteinemia, weight loss, and difficulty with temperature control. Heart failure may occur in elderly patients. Death may result from overwhelming infection or circulatory collapse.

#### Medical management

Therapy consists of maintaining fluid balance and preventing infection. Methods used to prevent infection in patients with burns are applicable. All drugs are discontinued as potential causative factors, although antibiotics may be started after culture and sensitivity tests of infected lesions. Oral corticosteroids are given for severe cases. Daily baths followed by application of petrolatum to the skin promote comfort.

#### Nursing management

Nursing care focuses on promotion of comfort and management of signs and symptoms. Daily baths, followed by application of petrolatum to the skin, promote comfort.

## Erythema Multiforme

### Etiology/Epidemiology

**Erythema multiforme** is a skin condition believed to occur secondary to an underlying systemic disease, such as an infection, or to drugs.

#### Pathophysiology

The skin eruption is characterized by red to purple macules, papules, and vesicles. Most often, lesions occur on the wrists, hands (both the backs and palms), ankles, feet (both the tops and soles), knees, elbows, and face; the entire body may be involved. The skin eruption may be preceded by fever, chest pain, and arthralgia. If lesions are extensive, the manifestation is called *Stevens-Johnson syndrome* and could involve renal damage and potentially death.

#### Medical management

Treatment is to seek out the underlying cause and eliminate it if possible. Other treatment is supportive, and corticosteroids are often used.

#### Nursing management

Nursing care is supportive. Local treatment includes baths, soaks, and dressings. If lesions appear in the mouth, special mouth care is indicated, including irrigations with warm salt solution.

## Infectious Diseases

Communicable diseases—such as measles, chickenpox, smallpox, scarlet fever, and typhoid fever—produce skin reactions (Table 67-8). Nodes and hemorrhagic

**TABLE 67-8 Skin Reactions of Some Communicable Diseases**

| DISEASE | CAUSE | INCUBATION PERIOD (DAYS) | PLACE OF RASH ORIGIN | SKIN LESIONS |
|---|---|---|---|---|
| Measles (rubeola) | Rubeola virus | 11 (8-14) | Face | Pink macular-papular rash; lesions coalesce |
| German measles; 3-day measles (rubella) | Rubella virus | 14-21 | Face | Pink macular-papular rash; lesions usually discrete; may coalesce |
| Scarlet fever (scarlatina) | Hemolytic streptococcus | 1-3 | Neck, chest | Bright red (scarlet) macules (pinpoint) |
| Chickenpox (varicella) | V-Z virus | 14-21 | Back, chest | Macule, papule, vesicle, crust; lesions at different stages |
| Smallpox (variola) | Variola virus | 12 (7-21) | Face | Macule, papule, vesicle, crust; lesions all at same stage |
| Typhoid fever | *Salmonella typhosa* | 14 (7-21) | Abdomen | Macular rash |

spots in the skin also accompany severe acute rheumatic fever.

## LUPUS ERYTHEMATOSUS

One of the more common tissue diseases that may result in skin conditions is lupus erythematosus (LE), which occurs in two forms, systemic (SLE) (see Chapter 70) and discoid (DLE).

### Etiology/Epidemiology

**Discoid lupus erythematosus** is a chronic, relatively benign skin condition that has worldwide distribution among all races and that occurs most often in the fourth decade of life. It is rarely seen in children or elderly persons. Precipitating factors include physical trauma and stress.

### Pathophysiology

The lesions of DLE are well demarcated and erythematous, have a characteristic scaly border with an atrophied center, and vary in size. The most common sites are the cheeks (butterfly pattern), nose, ears, scalp, and chest, although other parts of the body—including mucous membranes—may also be involved. DLE occurs in the absence of other signs, symptoms, and serologic abnormalities of SLE. About 15% to 20% of persons with SLE will have DLE, and 5% to 10% of persons who initially have DLE will develop SLE.[13]

### Medical Management

There is no cure for DLE. Palliative measures include topical steroid therapy under occlusive wraps, intralesional steroid therapy, antimalarial therapy with chloroquine (Aralen), hydroxychloroquine sulfate (Plaquenil), or quinacrine hydrochloride (Atabrine).

### Nursing Management

Nursing care is focused on helping patients with the palliative measures and preventive care. Preventive measures include avoiding physical trauma, such as by using protective lotions to prevent sunburn, and wearing warm clothing to protect against cold and wind. If stress is a precipitating factor, measures to reduce stress can be instituted.

## PAPULOSQUAMOUS DISEASES

Papulosquamous diseases are characterized by papular, scaly lesions. Common disorders are psoriasis, pityriasis rosea, and lichen planus.

### Psoriasis

#### Etiology/Epidemiology

**Psoriasis** is a genetically determined, chronic, epidermal proliferative disease. It is not infectious or contagious and is not a nervous disorder. There are no specific precipitating factors for the majority of persons; however, some people may develop exacerbations after climatic changes, stressors, trauma, infections, or drugs (propranolol, lithium). Pregnant women often see a remission of symptoms. Approximately 1% to 2% of the population of the United States have psoriasis; 5% of this group have associated inflammatory arthritis. There is a higher incidence of psoriasis among whites and a lower incidence among the Japanese, American Indians, and people of West African origin. Men and women are equally affected. Psoriasis occurs in all ages but is less common among children and elderly persons.

#### Pathophysiology

The turnover time for normal skin is 28 days. After the basal cell divides, it normally takes 14 days to reach the stratum corneum and an additional 14 days for this cell to be sloughed off. In psoriasis the time is accelerated to 4 to 7 days.

The lesions of psoriasis are elevated, erythematous, sharply circumscribed, scaling plaques (Figure 67-7). The primary lesion is a papule; these papules then join to form plaques. In the African-American person, the plaques may appear purple. Lesions may occur over the entire body but are found more commonly on the scalp, elbows, shins, and trunk. Beefy red lesions may be observed in an acute flare-up. The nails of persons with

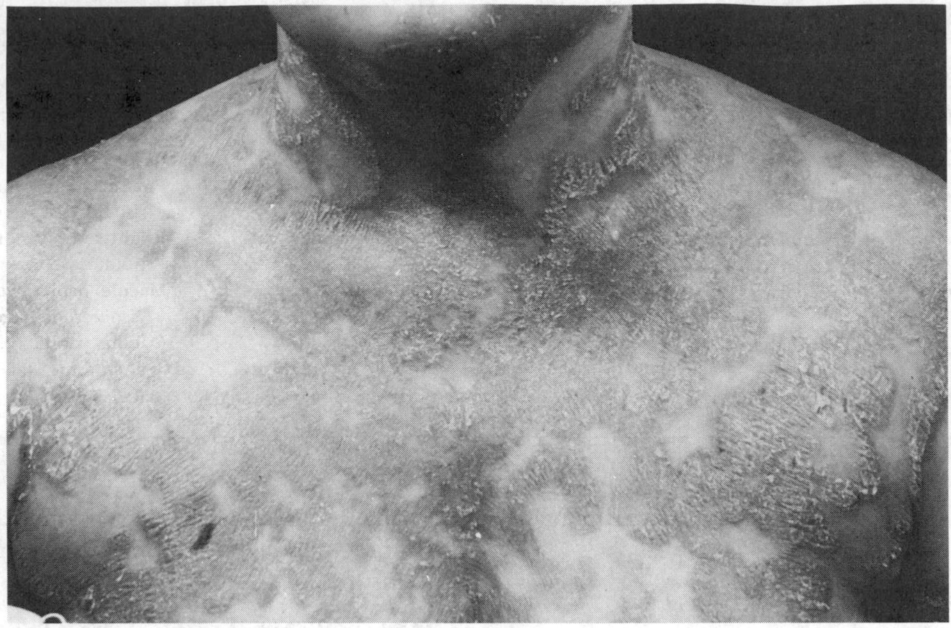

**FIGURE 67-7** Generalized psoriasis. (From Rosai J: *Ackerman's surgical pathology,* ed 6, St Louis, 1981, Mosby.)

psoriasis have characteristic involvement; there may be pitting of the nails, yellowish discoloration, and onycholysis (separation of the nail from the nail bed).

Psoriasis takes many forms. *Arthropathic psoriasis* is one of the cruelest forms and may produce crippling. The nails are always involved and show denting and pitting. *Pustular psoriasis* (von Zumbusch) may present with fever, tenderness of the skin, and sterile pustules. Fortunately, only a small percentage of persons with psoriasis have eruptions that require adaptations in lifestyles.

### Medical management

Because of the overproduction of skin in psoriasis, treatment is based on slowing mitotic activity. Initially the lesions may be treated with topical keratolytic agents or topical steroids with occlusive wraps and wet dressings to decrease inflammation (Table 67-9). If the psoriasis becomes resistant to these treatments, coal tar or anthralin therapy is used.

Ultraviolet light inhibits DNA synthesis, thus slowing the rapid skin cell growth. Ultraviolet light is divided into different waves: UVA (short), UVB (middle), and UVC (long). UVC is a potent carcinogen and can cause severe burns, so it is not used in treatment of psoriasis. Exposure to sunlamps or blacklight lamps without other therapy may benefit psoriasis. The combination of tar and ultraviolet (UVB) light, known as the *Goeckerman regimen* (see Guidelines box at left), is one of the oldest forms of therapy for psoriasis but is still effective and widely used.

Photochemotherapy (Psoralen with ultraviolet [UVA] light [PUVA]) is used for severe psoriasis when other therapies have not been effective. Etretinate (Tegison), a vitamin A derivative, and methoxsalen (Psoralen) are photosensitizing agents that react with the ultraviolet energy. The drugs are taken 2 hours before exposure to the ultraviolet light; dose is based on body weight. Moderate flare-up of psoriasis (Koebner's phenomenon) may occur after treatment. Methotrexate is reserved for persons with severe psoriasis who are recalcitrant to other treatments.

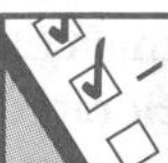

**Guidelines for Goeckerman Regimen for Psoriasis**

1. Apply crude coal tar two or three times a day over all affected areas.
2. Remove tar with corn oil before ultraviolet therapy, leaving a thin film on skin.
3. Give ultraviolet light therapy.
4. Give tub bath with soap and oil. Shampoo scalp.
5. Reapply tar to skin and lotion to scalp.
6. Have person wear pajamas to act as a dressing.

### Nursing management

Most patients with psoriasis are treated on an ambulatory basis. A new approach to therapy has been the establishment of psoriasis day care centers where patients come daily for treatments, rest, and counseling. Because the lesions are commonly found in visible skin areas, persons with psoriasis are faced with a socially disabling

**TABLE 67-9 Psoriasis Therapy**

| TYPE | ACTION | COMMENTS |
|---|---|---|
| Bland emollients (petrolatum, mineral oil) | Hydration of skin | Use for mild lesions<br>Facilitate scale removal |
| Keratolytics (salicylic acid, ammoniated mercury) | Hydration and softening of skin<br>Antimitotic | Avoid using on face<br>Cover with occlusive wraps<br>May cause skin maceration and folliculitis<br>Not applied to irritated skin |
| Corticosteroids | Antimitotic<br>Antiinflammatory | Topical use for most lesions; cover with occlusive wraps; may cause folliculitis<br>Intralesional use for plaques<br>Rarely given systemically<br>May produce rebound psoriasis when withdrawn |
| Coal tar preparations | Action unknown<br>Have keratolytic, antipruritic, and photosensitizing effects | May cause folliculitis with long-term use<br>Avoid direct sunlight for 24 hours after use<br>Avoid use on face<br>Stain skin, hair, and clothing<br>Available as cream, lotion, gel, solution, and shampoo<br>May be used with ultraviolet light therapy (Goeckerman regimen) |
| Anthralin products | Antimitotic<br>Inhibition of enzyme metabolism | May cause skin irritation<br>Not applied to open skin areas<br>Petrolatum is used to protect normal skin during therapy<br>Wear gloves during application; stain skin, hair, and clothing<br>Avoid using on face |
| Photochemotherapy with ultraviolet light | Inhibition of DNA synthesis | May cause pruritus, erythema, vesicles, flare-up of lesions, transient nausea<br>May be carcinogenic for light-skinned persons or those previously exposed to x-ray therapy<br>Avoid direct sunlight for 12 to 24 hours after ingestion of Psoralen |
| Methotrexate | Antimitotic<br>Inhibition of DNA synthesis | For severe lesions not amenable to other treatment<br>Given orally unless nausea is present<br>Requires close monitoring of hematologic, renal, and liver functioning |
| Synthetic retinoids | Correction of abnormal cell differentiation | Experimental therapy<br>Side effects: pruritus, lip edema, sore mouth, thirst, fragile skin, peeling of palms and soles<br>May be used with anthralin or ultraviolet therapies |

**Guidelines for Teaching the Person With Psoriasis**

1. Nature of psoriasis: noncurable, recurrence of symptoms
2. Reduce episodes of rapid-spreading psoriasis (flare-ups) by avoiding skin trauma (injuries, sunburn, infections), extremes of temperature, and stress.
3. Shampoo hair frequently to remove scales. If scalp has plaques, use a tar shampoo (Polytar, Sebutone) for 10 minutes before rinsing. Presoften thick plaques with mineral oil the night before a morning shampoo; use a fine-toothed comb to remove loose scales.[4]
4. Avoid self-medication, particularly when receiving prescribed therapy.
5. Apply topical medications in a thin layer for most lesions; use a thick layer over plaques.
6. Monitor for side effects of medications (see Table 67-9).
7. Seek medical follow-up during periods of exacerbation.

disease. They may need help in identifying and coping with their feelings and with changes that may occur in their life-style.

The disease is not curable and may wax and wane continuously. Lesions may fade with treatment, only to recur eventually in the same area or elsewhere. Patients who are not aware of this may lose confidence in the physician and may seek a quick cure elsewhere. Because psoriasis is so common and so stubborn in response to treatment, manufacturers of patent remedies find a lucrative field for their products among persons with the disease.

Teaching for individuals who have psoriasis is summarized in the Guidelines box at left.

## Pityriasis Rosea

### Etiology/Epidemiology

**Pityriasis rosea** is a skin condition of unknown cause but thought to be viral; the disease is not contagious. It is common, with worldwide distribution affecting all races. It occurs more commonly in women, adolescents, and young adults.

### Pathophysiology

The initial symptom is usually a single oval lesion with a thin scaly border and yellowish center, appearing most often on the trunk, upper arm, or thigh. This lesion is followed within a few hours, days, or weeks by similar smaller erythematous lesions with the long axis of the oval lesion along lines of skin cleavage and by scaling of the peripheral borders. The skin usually clears in 6 to 8 weeks, and the condition does not recur.

#### Medical management

Medical management consists of topical steroids and colloid baths. Ultraviolet therapy may be used.

#### Nursing management

Nursing care is essentially symptomatic and includes assisting patients with topical steroids and colloid baths if itching is present. Nurses will be helping patients primarily by educating them.

### Lichen Planus

**Lichen planus** is a papulosquamous eruption of unknown origin. A number of drugs (streptomycin, para-aminosalicylic acid, methyldopa, thiazides, antimalarials) may also cause lichen planus–like eruptions. Lesions occur initially as shiny, flat-topped papules on the flexor surfaces of the wrist, ankles, trunk, mucous membranes, and genitalia. The mouth is frequently involved. Bullous or hypertrophic lesions may also occur. Itching is severe, and new lesions may occur at the scratched sites. Nails may become distorted. Oral or hypertrophic lesions may become chronic. Acute lichen planus usually resolves in 6 to 18 months, but the chronic types commonly last for many years.

Colloid baths and antipruritic lotions are prescribed for itching. Benadryl or sedatives may be given at bedtime. Corticosteroids may be prescribed as topical therapy under occlusive wraps or as intralesional or systemic therapy. Psoralen with ultraviolet light (PUVA) therapy is effective. Persons with oral lesions should avoid smoking or ingesting hot or irritating foods or liquids.

## BULLOUS DISEASES

### Pemphigus Vulgaris

#### Etiology/Epidemiology

The cause of pemphigus vulgaris is unknown, but it is thought to have an autoimmune basis. It is rare and occurs worldwide, primarily in persons between the ages of 40 and 60. It has a higher incidence among Jewish persons.

#### Pathophysiology

Pemphigus vulgaris is characterized by enormous bullae that appear all over the body and on the mucous membranes. The lesions break and are followed by crusts and scarring. The disease is characterized by *acantholysis* (cells slip past one another and fluid accumulates between the cells). By placing the thumb firmly on the skin and exerting lateral sliding pressure, the upper epidermis can be dislodged, resulting in erosion or blister (Nikolsky's sign). A Tzanck test will identify acantholytic cells. Infection of the crust produces a foul odor, and toxemia occurs. If the disease is untreated, death usually ensues in about 1 year.

#### Medical management

Hospitalization is usually required for skin care and monitoring of drug effects. The treatment of choice for severe pemphigus is systemic corticosteroids in large doses; the dose is gradually reduced as improvement is noted. Immunosuppressants—such as methotrexate, cyclophosphamide, and azathioprine—may be given to reduce the corticosteroid dose. Gold therapy (gold sodium thiomalate) may be given alone or in combination with corticosteroids for chronic therapy.[14]

#### Nursing management

Nursing care of the person with severe pemphigus can be a challenge. Stryker frames may be used to help the person change position painlessly and to prevent weight bearing on raw surfaces. Air mattress or flotation systems may be used to reduce surface pressure on skin and promote comfort. Dakin's solution compresses may be applied to oozing lesions to help control odor and infection. Infection is a major concern because of the immunosuppressive effects of drug therapy. Special mouth care is required for mouth lesions, and bland diets are more easily tolerated.

Emotional support and encouragement of both patient and family are extremely important. Patients may fear rejection by others because of their appearance, and they need evidence of continued interest and attention by family and staff. The potential for altered body image and social isolation is high.

### Bullous Pemphigoid

Pemphigoid differs from pemphigus. It has an autoimmune basis. It occurs more frequently than does pemphigus, primarily in persons 60 years of age and older. Bullous pemphigoid is a benign, chronic bullous disorder. The blisters are subepidermal rather than intraepidermal, and acantholysis does not occur.

The lesions of pemphigoid are usually preceded by a pruritic or eczematous eruption. The bullae may appear anywhere but are seen mostly on the abdomen and flexor surfaces of the extremities. Lower doses of corticosteroids are required for pemphigoid than for pemphigus. Immunosuppressive drugs are combined with steroids if treatment must be long term.

## DERMATITIS HERPETIFORMIS

Dermatitis herpetiformis is a chronic skin condition of unknown cause. Many persons have an associated gluten-sensitive enteropathy. It is seen mostly in men. The lesion is a vesicular, papular, pruritic eruption. The characteristic distribution of lesions is usually symmetric, bilateral, and over the surfaces of the limbs, buttocks, and scalp. Scarring and hyperpigmentation may occur after the lesions heal.

Treatment consists of systemic sulfones, and the response is often diagnostic because of the improvement. Antipruritic drugs may or may not relieve the intense pruritus. A gluten-free diet helps to control the skin symptoms.

## TUMORS OF THE SKIN

Growths of skin cells may develop from the epidermis, from sebaceous or sweat glands, from the melanocyte system, or from mesodermal tissue (for example, connective or vascular tissue). Most skin tumors are benign, and even those which are malignant—with the exception of such tumors as malignant melanoma—are often of less serious consequence than tumors elsewhere in the body.

### Keratosis (Benign Lesion)

The term **keratosis** refers to any cornification or growth of the horny layer of the skin. There are several different types of keratosis, including corns and calluses, warts, and seborrheic and actinic (senile) keratosis.

#### Corns and calluses

Corns are caused by the pressure of ill-fitting shoes. **Corns** are thickened skin lesions, with a center core that thickens inwardly and causes acute pain on pressure. They occur on the toes. A corn is best treated by (1) placing over it a small felt pad with a hole in the center to relieve pressure and (2) wearing shoes that fit properly. As soon as the pad is removed, a new layer of skin forms unless pressure is relieved. Popular corn remedies seldom produce a cure because their active ingredient is usually salicylic acid, which dissolves only the outer layer of skin.

**Calluses** are the result of constant pressure on the bottom of the foot. Calluses, or thickening of circumscribed areas of the horny layer of the skin, appear on the plantar surface of the foot. They are often successfully treated by relief of the pressure and by regular massage with softening lotions and creams.

#### Seborrheic keratosis

The most common benign keratotic tumors seen in older persons are the **seborrheic keratosis.** African-Americans at an earlier age develop a type of seborrheic keratosis called *dermatosis papulosa nigra* with lesions that are small, pedunculated, and heavily pigmented.

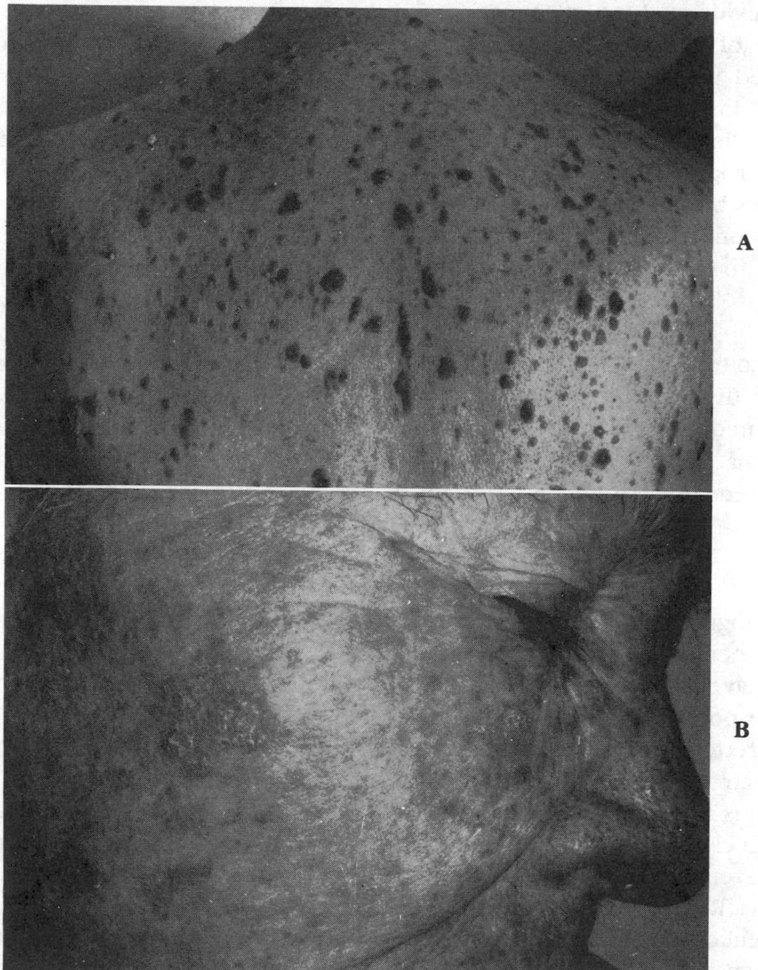


**FIGURE 67-8** **A,** Seborrheic keratosis. **B,** Actinic (senile) keratosis. (From Stewart WD, Danto JL, Maddin S: *Dermatology: diagnosis and treatment of cutaneous disorders,* ed 4, St Louis, 1978, Mosby.)

The lesions—which resemble large, darkened, greasy warts—are usually seen on the trunk but may occur also on the face, scalp, and proximal extremities (Figure 67-8, *A*). Development of malignancy from seborrheic keratosis is rare, but a sudden increase in the number and size of the lesions may indicate an internal gastrointestinal malignancy.

Most seborrheic keratosis do not require treatment, except for cosmetic reasons or at areas of frequent irritation. They may be removed with a curette followed by light electrodesiccation or by application of liquid nitrogen.

### Actinic keratosis

**Actinic** (senile, solar) **keratosis** result from exposure of the skin to irradiation, primarily solar. They are noted most often on exposed skin areas of persons who work outdoors and on older persons. Light-skinned persons are more vulnerable to skin changes from irradiation. The skin lesions are round or irregular, red-brown to gray in color, and have a dry, scaly appearance. The surrounding skin is usually dry and wrinkled from overexposure to the sun (Figure 67-8, *B*).

About 25% of the lesions become malignant (squamous cell carcinoma), evidenced by inflammation and a rapid increase in size of the lesion. The number of lesions can be restricted by the use of clothing and sunscreen lotions over skin areas frequently exposed to the sun. The lesions of actinic keratosis are removed by curettage and light electrodesiccation. Large lesions or lesions suspected of possible malignancy are removed by excision. Multiple lesions may be treated with a topical application of a 1% to 5% 5-fluorouracil cream.

## Premalignant Lesions

Skin lesions that may lead to malignancy include actinic keratosis (as previously described), leukoplakia, Bowen's disease, and pigmented moles. The term *premalignant* does not imply that all of the lesions become malignant but that the tendency to become malignant exists.

### Leukoplakia

**Leukoplakia** is a premalignant lesion that results from external irritants and other unknown causes. External irritants that appear to have an etiologic relationship to oral leukoplakia include poorly fitting dentures, cheek biting, and pipe or cigarette smoking. Chronic maceration, friction, and senile atrophy may lead to leukoplakia of the vagina. The mucous membranes of the mouth or vagina may develop a thickened white patch of keratinized cells, which may eventually develop into invasive squamous cell carcinoma. Red or red and white patches of the mouth (erythroleukoplakia) may occur also and have a higher malignancy potential than do the white patches.

Preventive measures include removal of potentially causative factors. Persons who continue to smoke need to inspect their mouths for signs of changes. Dental care should be sought for rough-edged teeth. Large lesions are usually surgically excised, and a biopsy is performed. Benign lesions may be removed by electrodesiccation.

**BOX 67-3 Differentiation of Benign and Malignant Moles**

| BENIGN MOLES | MALIGNANT MELANOMAS |
|---|---|
| Symmetric | Asymetric |
| Borders: even | Borders: uneven |
| Color: uniform | Color: multiple shades |
| Diameter: <6 mm | Diameter: >6 mm |

### Bowen's disease

Bowen's disease is related to chemical carcinogens.[11] It occurs mostly in older light-skinned men. Bowen's disease is a chronic skin disease that can be considered as squamous cell carcinoma *in situ.* The lesions are sharply demarcated brown plaques that are widely distributed, although a single lesion may be present. Persons with Bowen's disease are at high risk for developing other malignant diseases. Treatment is by surgical excision.

### Pigmented nevi

Almost all persons have some pigmented **nevi (moles),** which usually develop during childhood, becoming more raised and prominent, and often containing hair. Moles, per se, are not generally significant except for cosmetic reasons or for their potential to develop into malignant melanomas. To facilitate differentiation between benign and malignant moles, the Skin Cancer Foundation has developed the mnemonic ABCD (Box 67-3).

Small, evenly colored brown moles with hair are benign. A blue or greenish-black color does not usually indicate malignancy if the color is even. Changes in moles that should be reported immediately to the physician for further diagnosis include (1) development of a ring of new pigment around the base, (2) development of uneven pigmentation, (3) sudden growth, (4) loss of hair in a mole, or (5) bleeding in a mole.[14]

## Malignant Lesions

### Squamous cell carcinoma

**Squamous cell carcinoma** is a malignant tumor of the surface epidermis that may appear on the exposed skin surface of older persons or at areas of chronic irritation or skin damaged from irradiation or burns. If the growth developed from actinic keratosis, Bowen's disease, or leukoplakia, the lesion will be indurated and surrounded by an inflammatory base. A new lesion appears as a firm keratotic nodule with an indurated base (Figure 67-9). Lesions that develop on hair-bearing skin rarely metas-

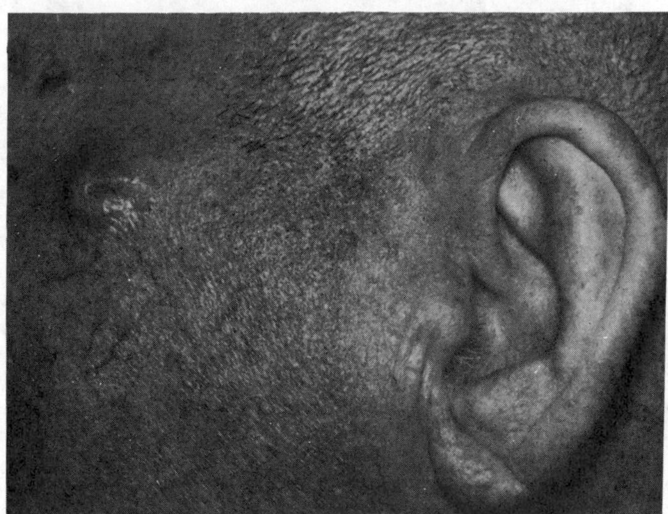

**FIGURE 67-9** Squamous cell carcinoma in infratemporal area, one of the most common sites for this tumor. (From Stewart WD, Danto JL, Maddin S: *Dermatology: diagnosis and treatment of cutaneous disorders,* ed 4, St Louis, 1978, Mosby.)

tasize, but lesions of the lip or ear frequently metastasize to regional lymph nodes.

Protection of the skin from excessive solar radiation and early detection of lesions are important preventive measures. Lesions may be removed by surgical excision, curettage with electrodesiccation, irradiation, or chemosurgery. *Chemosurgery* is used for tumors without well-defined borders. It involves application of a dressing with a fixative paste, such as zinc chloride, and then removal of the dressing with some tissue fixed to it. Reapplication is often necessary until all malignant tissue has been removed.

### Keratoacanthoma

Keratoacanthoma is a skin tumor that occurs mostly on normal skin areas exposed to sun, tar, and oils. It has microscopic characteristics similar to those of squamous cell carcinoma but is relatively noninvasive and does not metastasize. The tumor grows rapidly to a 1- to 2-cm size, remains quiescent for 2 to 8 weeks, and then begins to regress spontaneously.[11] The dome-shaped, shiny, pink lesion is filled with a keratinous plug that is expelled as the nodule shrinks. The lesion is usually excised and a biopsy performed, because of its similarity to squamous cell carcinoma.

### Basal cell epithelioma

**Basal cell epithelioma** or carcinoma is the most common malignant tumor affecting light-skinned people over 40 years of age. It is uncommon among African-Americans and Orientals. It occurs primarily over hairy areas, those containing pilosebaceous follicles. The growths initially have a characteristic translucent appearance, ranging from flesh color to a pale pink with a few telangiectatic vessels across the surface. Because the lesion grows slowly, the center becomes indurated. Basal cell epitheliomas rarely metastasize, but untreated tumors can become locally invasive with severe tissue destruction, infection, and hemorrhage.

Treatment of basal cell epitheliomas depends on the site and extent of the tumor. The four treatment modalities include curettage with electrodesiccation, surgical excision, irradiation, and chemosurgery.

### Malignant melanoma

**Etiology/Epidemiology. Malignant melanoma** is one of the most serious of malignant tumors. It may develop from a pigmented nevus or arise from healthy skin. It affects over 27,000 persons in the United States each year and has been increasing at the rate of 3.4% per year.[1] It is seen more often in whites than in African-Americans, especially those who have had frequent exposure to the sun.

**Pathophysiology.** Tumors occur most commonly on the head, neck, and lower extremities. The lesions vary considerably in appearance, some with deep pigmentation, irregular borders, and surrounding erythema, and others with irregular pigmentation (yellow, blue, black) and irregular surfaces (Figure 67-10). The rate of growth is variable. Late changes include bleeding and ulceration. The incidence of metastasis from malignant melanoma is high and depends on the depth of invasion. Metastasis occurs first to the regional lymph nodes and then by hematogenous spread to the lungs, liver, and then other areas.

**Medical management.** Early diagnosis leads to a more favorable prognosis. Treatment consists of total wide excision. Skin grafts may be needed to cover the defect. Chemotherapy by regional perfusion or systemic therapy, or immunotherapy, may be given when metastasis has occurred.

**Nursing management.** Nursing care first focuses on early detection. Second, nurses help patients cope with the diagnosis and prepare for surgery. The patient will need some of the general care of any patient undergoing surgery (see Chapters 23 to 25). After surgery the patient is followed closely, being rechecked at 3-month intervals for the subsequent 2 years and then annually.[14]

If metastasis occurs, the nursing care focuses on helping the patient understand treatment and its side effects. The patient will have to cope with many physical problems, as well as the fear of cancer, the loss of health, and the fear of dying (see Chapters 10 and 16).

### Kaposi's sarcoma

**Kaposi's sarcoma** was a rare malignant disorder in older men in the United States until recently, although

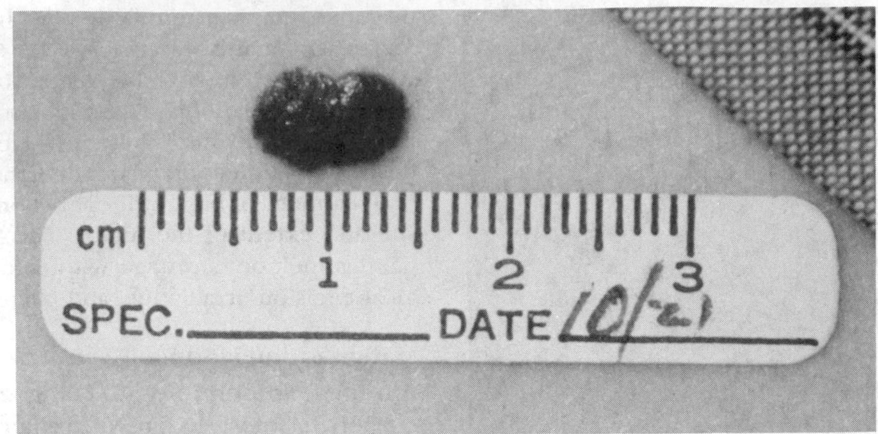


**FIGURE 67-10** Malignant melanoma. (Courtesy David Bickers, MD, Cleveland, Ohio.)

it was endemic in young men of equatorial Africa. The disorder is now commonly seen as one of the opportunistic disorders occurring in conjunction with acquired immunodeficiency syndrome (AIDS).

Persons with Kaposi's sarcoma develop discrete, red, purple, or dark plaques or nodules scattered widely over the body on the skin and mucous membranes, especially the mouth. Single lesions may occur. Some lesions may regress spontaneously. The disorder is slowly progressive, and successful treatment of the sarcoma does not affect survival. Many persons die of an associated opportunistic infection.

Treatment varies, depending on the type of Kaposi's sarcoma.[13] Radiation therapy is often effective in endemic forms of Kaposi's sarcoma. In epidemic forms, chemotherapy and immunotherapy are used. (See Chapter 71 for further discussion of Kaposi's sarcoma in persons with HIV infections and AIDS.)

## Skin Disorders in African-Americans

The reported incidence of dermatologic disorders varies among different races, and some disorders are reported to be higher among African-Americans. Socioeconomic conditions must be considered when interpreting the data, and the reported incidence may actually reflect poor diet or poor health care rather than a racial difference. Disorders commonly seen among African-Americans include lichen planus, follicular syphilis, acne, and follicular eczema. Because the pigment of dark skin screens out the sun's rays, those disorders that are affected by solar irradiation—such as squamous cell carcinoma, keratoacanthoma, and basal cell epithelioma—rarely occur.

Pigmentary changes more commonly result from dermatologic disorders in African-Americans than whites because of the greater amount of melanin present. *Hyperpigmentation* is commonly seen after acne vulgaris, drug eruptions, lichen simplex chronicus, and pityriasis rosea. *Hypopigmentation* may result from atopic dermatitis, tinea, and pityriasis alba. Some dermatologic disorders that are unique to African-Americans include traumatic alopecia, pseudofolliculitis barbae, keloids, dermatosis papulosa nigra, and perifolliculitis abscedens.

### TRAUMATIC ALOPECIA

Black hair shafts are highly susceptible to breakage, and hair loss may result from hair care practices sometimes used by blacks, such as tight hair curlers, cornrow braiding, hot combing, or the use of picks. Wetting or "softening" the hair before the use of a pick may help prevent trauma to the hair. The hair usually grows back when the specific hair practice is discontinued.

### PSEUDOFOLLICULITIS BARBAE

Hair follicles in African-Americans are curved rather than straight; therefore the hair curls back as it grows. After shaving, the sharpened point of the hair shaft (especially if a straight razor has been used) acts like a hook and reenters the skin, causing an inflammatory response called **pseudofolliculitis barbae.**

The lesions consist of papules and pustules, with some postinflammatory hyperpigmentation. The most commonly affected areas include the chin and upper anterior neck. The legs and axilla may also develop pseudofolliculitis from shaving. Treatment consists of growing a beard. As the beard is growing, a brush or rough washcloth may be used to dislodge ingrowing hairs. If shaving is done, a foil-guarded shaver is recommended. A mild depilatory may be used in place of shaving. Lesions may be treated with topical steroids or antibiotics.

### KELOIDS

Although keloids are seen in all races, they are much more prevalent in African-Americans than in whites. Keloids occur most often in young adults but may require many years to reach full growth. Highly susceptible areas for keloid growth include the sternum, mandible, ear, and neck. **Keloids** are hard, raised, shiny growths of collagen tissue that usually originate from a scar and then grow beyond the wound, often with clawlike projections. Keloids may recur after simple excision; therefore surgery is followed by intralesional steroid therapy, radiation therapy, electron beam therapy, or pressure garments.

### DERMATOSIS PAPULOSA NIGRA

Almost 35% of African-Americans develop a seborrheic keratosis consisting of small (5-mm) brown or black papules appearing in varying numbers primarily on the face but also on the neck, chest, and upper back. Pruritus may occur but is usually absent. Treatment consists of light electrodesiccation or cryotherapy.

### PERIFOLLICULITIS ABSCEDENS

Perifolliculitis abscedens is a rare, chronic skin disorder seen in African-American males. It occurs on the scalp, and the lesions consist of numerous firm or fluctuant small nodules connected by purulent sinus tracts. Alopecia and scarring occur in the affected areas. Treatment is difficult. Antibiotics are ineffective, and intralesional steroid therapy provides only temporary relief. X-ray therapy is more effective, but in severe cases scalp excision with split-thickness grafting may be necessary.[11]

## DERMATOLOGIC SURGERY

Treatment of skin lesions by dermatologists sometimes includes removal of skin lesions. Superficial skin lesions involving only the epidermis can be removed easily by various means; deep lesions involving the dermis, such as with some cancers, are removed with full-thickness skin excision.

### TYPES OF SURGERY

#### Tangential Surgery

Superficial lesions can be removed by slicing off the lesion with a sharp blade. It is especially useful for removal of flat lesions. The entire lesion may be removed for diagnosis. Hemostasis is obtained with pressure or gelatin foam.

#### Curettage

Curettage is the scraping or scooping out of a superficial lesion with a curet, which is a spoon-shaped, sharp-edged instrument. A local anesthetic is usually injected around the lesion before curettage (Figure 67-11). Hemostasis is accomplished with a chemical styptic, such as ferric chloride or Monsel's solution; with gelatin foam; or by electrocoagulation. Lesions that may be removed by curettage include seborrheic keratosis, actinic keratosis, basal cell epitheliomas, leukoplakia, warts, and nevi.

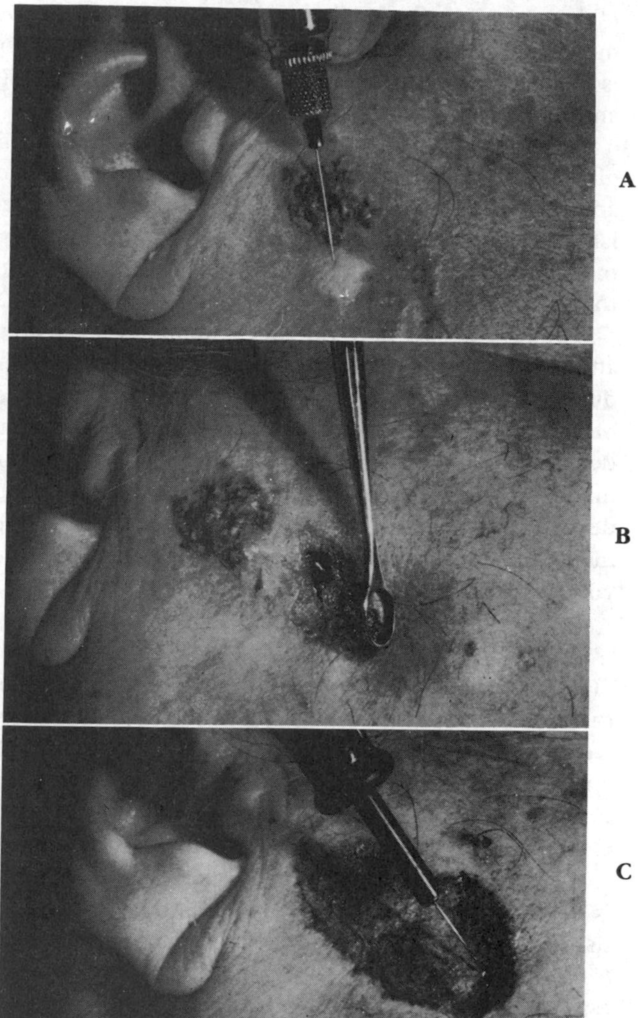


**FIGURE 67-11** **A,** Infiltration with local anesthetic. **B,** Curettage. **C,** Electrodesiccation for hemostasis. (From Stewart WD, Danto JL, Maddin S: *Dermatology: diagnosis and treatment of cutaneous disorders,* ed 4, St Louis, 1978, Mosby.)

#### Punch Biopsy

After the patient receives a local anesthetic, a punch is used to remove small, deep lesions up to 10 mm in diameter.[5] The tissue is then sent for biopsy. Small punch biopsies may be closed with a suture. Larger biopsies may be partially closed and will then heal by secondary intention. Hemostasis can be obtained with gelatin foam packing. Punch biopsies are used for identification of basal cell carcinomas and for removal of small, deep, round lesions.

#### Cryosurgery

Tissue can be destroyed by rapid freezing with such substances as liquid oxygen, carbon dioxide snow or gas, liquid nitrogen, dichlorodifluoromethane (Freon), or nitrous oxide. Carbon dioxide snow and liquid nitrogen are used most frequently. The rapid freezing causes formation of intracellular ice, which destroys the cell membranes and produces cell dehydration. Cryosurgery is frequently used for removal of skin tumors (benign and malignant), warts, and keloids.

Although the procedure usually is not painful, a tingling pain occurs when the freezing substance is applied and may be uncomfortable for some persons, particularly if multiple lesions are treated. A local anesthetic may be necessary. Analgesics may be helpful during thawing.

Tissue necrosis may not be evident until 24 hours after cryosurgery. A clear or hemorrhagic bulla forms during the first day, but inflammatory reactions and bleeding are usually absent. A serous exudate occurs during the first week, followed by eschar or crust formation. The crust drops off in 3 to 4 weeks as the underlying tissue heals. Scarring usually results. Hypopigmentation may occur, because melanocytes are highly vulnerable to freezing.

### Electrosurgery

Electric current may be used in dermatologic surgery to remove tissue and to control bleeding. *Electrodesiccation* is the drying of tissue by means of a monopolar current through the needle electrode. *Electrofulguration* is a form of electrodesiccation in which the needle electrode is held close to, rather than inserted into, the tissue, thus spraying the area with sparks. Bipolar current is used for *electrocoagulation,* which coagulates the tissue, curtailing capillary bleeding, and for *electrosection,* which cuts the tissue. Delayed bleeding may occur, especially from electrocoagulation, and may alarm the unprepared patient. The bleeding can be easily controlled by direct pressure.

Electrosurgery is usually performed after the patient has received a local anesthetic. Sedation is rarely necessary. After most uses of electrosurgery, the wound is left exposed for air drying. Dressings may be used if the area is subject to frequent trauma or rubbing or if oozing is present. The wound may be wiped with 70% alcohol to hasten drying. A hemostatic nonocclusive dressing may be made by covering the wound with Gelfoam powder and Micropore tape.[11]

## PATIENT TEACHING

After *superficial* skin surgery, the patient is instructed not to remove the crust (scab), which acts as a protection (healing occurs under the crust). The crust should be kept as dry as possible; if it gets wet, it should be patted dry. Alcohol may be applied and allowed to evaporate. Makeup may be used over the crust. The crust may be left uncovered or may be covered with an adhesive bandage. Signs of redness, edema, or pain should be reported to the surgeon.

After *deep* skin surgery, the wound is usually bandaged and the patient is given specific instructions for care by the surgeon. Aspirin should be avoided both before and after surgery because of its anticoagulant properties, which may lead to postoperative bleeding. Postoperative discomfort may be relieved with acetaminophen.

# PRESSURE SORES

## ETIOLOGY

**Pressure sores** are defined by the National Pressure Ulcer Advisory Panel (NPUAP) as lesions caused by unrelieved pressure against soft tissue, usually over bony prominences. For many years, pressure sores (also known as *pressure ulcers)* had been incorrectly termed *decubitus ulcers.* The Latin definition of the term *decubitus* implies lying flat, and *decubitus* was therefore correctly changed to *pressure* after it was ascertained that one could develop a pressure sore while assuming any body position, in any body location, and from any source of pressure (internal, as well as external). Risk factors for pressure sores include moisture, nutritional deficits, shear stress, alterations in mobility and perception, and abnormal serum albumin and hemoglobin levels.

## EPIDEMIOLOGY

Pressure sores are nonselective; that is, they can occur among those in any age-group or any ethnic population and regardless of socioeconomic status. Attempts have been made to estimate the financial burden of the pressure sore problem; however, research has been limited and inconsistent. Some studies estimate that $11.5 billion annually is expended on products for pressure sore management. Attempts to estimate the cost of an individual pressure sore also have been unsuccessful. Con-

**BOX 67-4 Stages of Pressure Sores**

**STAGE 1**

Nonblanchable erythema, redness that remains present over an area under pressure 30 minutes after pressure source is removed. Epidermis remains intact.

**STAGE 2**

Epidermis is broken, superficial lesion, no measurable depth. Partial-thickness skin loss.

**STAGE 3**

Full-thickness skin loss down through the dermis, may include subcutaneous tissue, may undermine adjacent skin.

**STAGE 4**

Full-thickness skin loss extending into supportive structures, such as muscle, tendon, and bone; may undermine and have various sinus tracts.

NOTE: If eschar (dead leathery tissue) is present, pressure sore cannot be accurately staged.

servative estimates of the cost of treatment for one pressure sore range from $5000 to $30,000.

The NPUAP reviewed over 800 available manuscripts in an attempt to define the scope of the problem and has concluded that the incidence and prevalence of pressure sores in various health care settings are high enough to warrant concern. Clinical Practice Guidelines,[3] nationally accepted standards of care, were established and reviewed for validity based on that manuscript review.

Estimates of the prevalence of pressure sores in skilled care facilities are approximately 23%; in acute care facilities, 9%; and much greater in certain high-risk populations, such as patients with a spinal cord injury. It also has been estimated that 60,000 people die annually because of complications from pressure sores.

## PATHOPHYSIOLOGY

Unrelieved pressure causes cellular necrosis. The cellular necrosis occurs from vascular insufficiency and causes tissue destruction. The cascade of events occurring to tissue under pressure is outlined in Table 67-10. Box 67-4 presents the stages of a pressure sore.

## PREVENTION

### Primary Prevention

Most pressure sores can be prevented if the nurse is diligent about assessment and appropriate interventions. Not all interventions are within the scope of nursing practice; therefore it is most important to approach the pressure sore problem from a multidisciplinary leadership fashion as recommended by the NPUAP. Prevention can be accomplished only when the nurse has identified those patients at high risk for development of pressure sores. Multitudes of "assessment tools" circulate within the literature today; however, currently only two tools are cited in the Clinical Practice Guidelines[3] as valid and research based. Most institutions incorporate information from one or both of these tools while developing their own tool.

Assessment tools consider both extrinsic and intrinsic factors that contribute to alterations in skin integrity. The Norton Scale (Figure 67-12) examines the patient's general health and mental statuses and his or her levels of mobility, activity, and continence. It is a very simple tool to use and leaves much room for nursing judgment within the specific areas. The areas listed previously are scored from one to four, and a total is calculated. The lower the total number of points, the greater the risk the patient poses for skin breakdown. The Braden Scale (Figure 67-13) is a bit more specific, with explanations for each score the patient is given, so that there is less subjective information allowed. The areas scored in this tool include the patient's levels of sensory perception, mobility, nutrition, and activity, as well as the presence or absence of moisture, friction, and shear. Once again, a number is assigned for each parameter, the total is calculated, and the lower the score, the greater the risk factor.

### Secondary Prevention

Interventions classified as secondary preventive measures are categorized according to the specific risk factor (previously discussed) they address. The Guidelines box, p. 2351, illustrates examples of nursing interventions for prevention.

## MEDICAL MANAGEMENT

Pressure sores have been identified as primarily a nursing problem, but they require collaboration with the entire health care team for effective resolution. Management includes interventions designed to control chronic disease symptomatology that affects healthy integument, such as medication regulation to keep glucose levels within normal limits and measures to promote optimal tissue perfusion and oxygenation. It is most important that the correct product for treatment of pressure sores is ordered. Products chosen inappropriately for wound management could cause more tissue damage or delay healing. The expected length of stay of patients with pressure sores as determined by DRG is 8.4 days. A discussion of common medical therapy for management of pressure sores follows.

**TABLE 67-10 Normal Function, Pathophysiology, and Clinical Manifestations of Pressure Sores**

| NORMAL FUNCTION | PATHOPHYSIOLOGY | CLINICAL MANIFESTATIONS |
|---|---|---|
| Microvasculature: capillaries supply tissue needs of oxygenated blood and nutrients | Pressure applied to soft tissue compresses capillaries, distorting structure and occluding blood flow | Ischemia at first, followed by reactive hyperemia |
| Sympathetic response | Compensation by increased shunting of capillary circulation to area under pressure; capillaries increase permeability and leak fluid into tissues | Tissue edema and inflammation |
| Capillary walls lined with endothelial cells; platelets flow smoothly through microvessels | Endothelial cells disrupted, platelets aggregate, and thrombi form in capillaries and lead to cellular death | Erythema that may or may not resolve once pressure source is removed |
| Intact skin as the body's protective mechanism | Cellular death leads to tissue necrosis | Pressure sore with visible tissue damage, described by stages (see Box 67-4) |

**Norton Scale**

| A<br>*Physical condition* | B<br>*Mental state* | C<br>*Activity* | D<br>*Mobility* | E<br>*Incontinence* | *Total score* |
|---|---|---|---|---|---|
| 4 Good | 4 Alert | 4 Ambulant | 4 Full | 4 Not | ______ |
| 3 Fair | 3 Apathetic | 3 Walks with help | 3 Slightly limited | 3 Occasional | |
| 2 Poor | 2 Confused | 2 Chairbound | 2 Very limited | 2 Usually urine | |
| 1 Bad | 1 Stupor | 1 Bedrest | 1 Immobile | 1 Double incontinence | |

**Norton Plus Scale**
(For determining high risk for pressure sores)

| *Check ONLY if YES* | *YES* |
|---|---|
| Diagnosis of diabetes | ______ |
| Diagnosis of hypertension | ______ |
| Hematocrit (M) <41% | ______ |
| (F) <36% | ______ |
| Hemoglobin (M) <14 g/dl | ______ |
| (F) <12 g/dl | ______ |
| Albumin level <3.3 g/dl | ______ |
| Febrile >99.6°F | ______ |
| 5 or more medications | ______ |
| Changes in mental status to confused, lethargic within 24 hours | ______ |
| *TOTAL Number of Checkmarks* | |
| Norton Scale Score | ______ |
| Minus total from above | ______ |
| Norton Plus Score | ______ |

**FIGURE 67-12** Norton Scale and Norton Plus Scale. (From Norton D, McLaren R, Exton-Smith AN: *An investigation of geriatric nursing problems in hospital,* Edinburgh, 1975, Churchill-Livingstone.)

## Diagnostic Tests

There are no specific laboratory tests to assist with diagnosis of pressure sores. Related laboratory examinations pertinent to risk factors have been included in the previous discussion of risk factors.

## Medication

There are no particular medications for pressure ulcers. Antibiotics are used if an infection is present.

## Treatment

More than 100 products exist as purported treatment measures for pressure sores. These are discussed in Table 67-11.

## Diet

Patients with wounds require additional protein and calorie intake to assist with tissue regeneration on a cellular level. A well-balanced diet is sufficient to maintain healthy skin; however, most patients with any identified risk factors are not eating a well-balanced diet. Protein supplementation in balanced amounts is helpful. Only a registered dietitian can determine accurately a balance of demand and replacement that will be therapeutic for the patient. Research also suggests that supplemental vitamin C and zinc, as well as a multiple vitamin with iron, are all helpful agents to stimulate wound healing on a cellular level.

## Activity

As discussed earlier, the more independently active the patient is, the lower the risk of pressure sore formation and the greater the chances of wound healing. If the patient is unable to assume an active role in mobility, it *must* be assumed by the nurse for the patient. The key factor related to wound healing is the removal of the causative agent(s). Regardless of the treatment prescribed for wound care, if the pressure is not relieved by the patient or passively by the nurse, wound healing will not occur.

## Referral/Consultation

In some settings the nurse assumes responsibility for making referrals to other services. Many disciplines have become involved with wound healing modalities. Physical therapists receive some education about wound healing. Nurses and physicians receive minimal education about products and principles of wound healing. A nursing specialty has evolved over the past 25 years called *enterostomal therapy (ET) nursing.* ET nurses are nationally recognized as leaders in the wound care arena and are an active part of the NPUAP. If your institution does not have an ET nurse on staff, the Wound, Ostomy and Continence Nurses Society in California can refer you to the closest person by calling (714) 476-0268.

## Guidelines for Prevention Based on Risk Factors Identified from Assessment

Incontinence
- Cleanse skin after each episode of incontinence is detected.
- Assess causative factors of incontinence.
- Contain urine and feces in absorbent products that control moisture and exposure to skin; plastic-lined products can contribute to the problem.
- Minimize moisture next to skin from any source.

Nutritional deficits
- Collaborate with dietitian to assess for optimal nutritional support.
- Assess for symptoms of nutritional compromise (decreased appetite and subsequently less oral intake; serum albumin level of less than 3-3.5 gm/dl; Hgb level of less than 10 gm/dl; signs and symptoms of dehydration, including thirst, poor skin turgor, and dry mucous membranes; elevated hematocrit and serum sodium levels.

Skin care and early treatment measures
- Inspect skin at regular intervals, at least daily, frequency determined by institutional policy (e.g., every shift instead of daily) and patient degree of risk. A head-to-toe inspection should be conducted, with attention to intertriginous areas and bony prominences.
- Bathing schedule should be developed according to patient preference, institutional policy, and general skin condition. Use a mild cleansing agent, and avoid water temperature extremes.
- Assess environmental factors, such as temperature and humidity, for contribution to skin condition.
- Lubricate skin with emollient lotions. Avoid lotion with scents or high alcohol contents.
- Avoid vigorous massage.

Alterations in mobility/activity
- Reposition patient at least every 2 hours.
- Use position pillows or foam wedges to separate skin areas in contact with each other or to assist with maintaining positions. Use cautiously because these devices can become an additional source of pressure if not properly placed.
- Heels should be elevated off of bed surfaces with supportive pillows. Heel protectors help reduce friction.
- Avoid positioning directly onto trochanter. Place patient more appropriately into 30-degree side-lying position.
- Elevating the head of the bed centers all body weight directly over the pelvic triangle. It is best to keep the degree of elevation to less than 45 degrees, if possible.
- To reduce friction and shear, use lifting devices to raise patient in bed, rather than dragging patient across the surface of the bed.
- A pressure reduction or relief device should be used for all patients at risk of pressure sore formation.
- Patients in wheelchairs and other chairs should be taught to shift weight and have pressure-reducing surfaces on which to sit.

Critical pathways (also referred to as "collaborative care paths" or "care maps") have been developed in some inpatient and outpatient settings to guide both medical and nursing management. These critical pathways are collaboratively developed along time lines and include the information just described for specific hours, days, or visits. Pertinent information about discharge

### TABLE 67-11 Pressure Sore Products Identified by Categories, Examples, and Manufacturers

| CATEGORY | EXAMPLE | MANUFACTURER |
|---|---|---|
| **EXUDATE ABSORPTION** | | |
| Dextronomer beads | Debrisan | Johnson & Johnson Medical, Inc |
| Copolymer starch dressings | Absorption dressing | Bard |
| | Duoderm granules | Convatec |
| Calcium alginates (absorb exudate, as well as release calcium on a cellular level—stimulates angiogenesis) | Kaltostat | Calgon Vestal Laboratories |
| | Sorbsan | Dow B. Hickam, Inc |
| | Algosteril | Johnson & Johnson Medical, Inc |
| **DEBRIDEMENT** | | |
| Enzymatic | Elase ointment | Parke-Davis |
| | Travase | Flint |
| | Santyl | Knoll Pharmaceuticals |
| | Panafil | Rystan Pharmaceuticals |
| | Biozyme C | Armour Pharmaceuticals |
| Wet-to-dry dressings* | Gauze in many forms (4×4, kerlex) | Multiple manufacturers |
| **WOUND PROTECTION, INSULATION AND MILD ABSORPTION** | | |
| Hydrocolloids (waxy pectin adhesive dressings that provide an optimal wound environment) | Duoderm | Convatec |
| | Restore | Hollister, Inc |
| | Tegasorb | 3M Health Care |
| | Ultec | Sherwood Medical |
| Transparent dressings (thin, adhesive dressings that support the microenvironment for cellular regeneration) | Tegaderm | 3M Health Care |
| | Bioclusive | Johnson & Johnson Medical, Inc |
| | OpSite | Smith & Nephew United, Inc |
| | Acu-Derm | Acme United Corp |
| | Polyskin | Kendall Healthcare |
| Polyurethane foam dressings (nonadhesive; some assist with odor control) | Allevyn | Smith & Nephew United, Inc |
| | Lyofoam | Acme United Corp |
| | EpiLock | Calgon Vestal Laboratories |
| Hydrogel dressings (nonadherent; have a topical soothing effect; varied in thickness) | Elasto-Gel | Southwest Technologies |
| | Vigilon | Bard Patient Care |
| | Second Skin | Spenco |

NOTE: Research suggests that wounds heal most effectively if there is a moist, natural environment, with a clean, debris- and necrotic-free wound area. Dressings and interventions are all designed with these principles in mind. Several have other added benefits that are discussed separately within each category.

*Solutions used vary according to preference of physician; most common solution is normal saline.

| Patient's name | | Evaluator's name |
|---|---|---|
| **Sensory perception**<br>Ability to respond meaningfully to pressure-related discomfort | **1. Completely limited:**<br>Unresponsive (does not moan, flinch, or grasp) to painful stimuli, due to diminished level of consciousness or sedation,<br>**OR**<br>limited ability to feel pain over most of body surface. | **2. Very limited:**<br>Responds only to painful stimuli. Cannot communicate discomfort except by moaning or restlessness,<br>**OR**<br>has a sensory impairment that limits the ability to feel pain or discomfort over ½ of body. |
| **Moisture**<br>Degree to which skin is exposed to moisture | **1. Constantly moist:**<br>Skin is kept moist almost constantly by perspiration, urine, etc. Dampness is detected every time patient is moved or turned. | **2. Moist:**<br>Skin is often but not always moist; linen must be changed at least once a shift. |
| **Activity**<br>Degree of physical activity | **1. Bedfast:**<br>Confined to bed. | **2. Chairfast:**<br>Ability to walk severely limited or nonexistent. Cannot bear own weight and/or must be assisted into chair or wheelchair. |
| **Mobility**<br>Ability to change and control body position | **1. Completely immobile:**<br>Does not make even slight changes in body or extremity position without assistance. | **2. Very limited:**<br>Makes occasional slight changes in body or extremity position but unable to make frequent or significant changes independently. |
| **Nutrition**<br>Usual food intake pattern | **1. Very poor:**<br>Never eats a complete meal. Rarely eats more than ⅓ of any food offered. Eats 2 servings or less of protein (meat or dairy products) per day. Takes fluids poorly. Does not take a liquid dietary supplement,<br>**OR**<br>is NPO and/or maintained on clear liquids or IV for more than 5 days. | **2. Probably inadequate:**<br>Rarely eats a complete meal and generally eats only about ½ of any food offered. Protein intake includes only 3 servings of meat or dairy products per day. Occasionally will take a dietary supplement,<br>**OR**<br>receives less than optimum amount of liquid diet or tube feeding. |
| **Friction and shear** | **1. Problem:**<br>Requires moderate to maximum assistance in moving. Complete lifting without sliding against sheets is impossible. Frequently slides down in bed or chair, requiring frequent repositioning with maximum assistance. Spasticity, contractures, or agitation leads to almost constant friction. | **2. Potential problem:**<br>Moves feebly or requires minimum assistance. During a move, skin probably slides to some extent against sheets, chair, restraints, or other devices. Maintains relatively good position in chair or bed most of the time but occasionally slides down. |

*NPO,* Nothing by mouth; *IV,* intravenously; *TPN,* total parenteral nutrition.

**FIGURE 67-13** Braden Scale for predicting pressure sore risk. (From Bergstrom N et al: 36(4):205, 1987.)

| | | Date of assessment | | | |
|---|---|---|---|---|---|
| **3. Slightly limited:**<br>Responds to verbal commands but cannot always communicate discomfort or need to be turned,<br>**OR**<br>has some sensory impairment that limits ability to feel pain or discomfort in 1 or 2 extremities. | **4. No impairment:**<br>Responds to verbal commands. Has no sensory deficit which would limit ability to feel or voice pain or discomfort. | | | | |
| **3. Occasionally moist:**<br>Skin is occasionally moist, requiring an extra linen change approximately once a day. | **4. Rarely moist:**<br>Skin is usually dry; linen requires changing only at routine intervals. | | | | |
| **3. Walks occasionally:**<br>Walks occasionally during day but for very short distances, with or without assistance. Spends majority of each shift in bed or chair. | **4. Walks frequently:**<br>Walks outside the room at least twice a day and inside room at least once every 2 hours during waking hours. | | | | |
| **3. Slightly limited:**<br>Makes frequent though slight changes in body or extremity position independently. | **4. No limitations:**<br>Makes major and frequent changes in position without assistance. | | | | |
| **3. Adequate:**<br>Eats over ½ of most meals. Eats a total of 4 servings of protein (meat, dairy products) each day. Occasionally will refuse a meal, but will usually take a supplement if offered,<br>**OR**<br>is on a tube feeding or TPN regimen, which probably meets most of nutritional needs. | **4. Excellent:**<br>Eats most of every meal. Never refuses a meal. Usually eats a total of 4 or more servings of meat and dairy products. Occasionally eats between meals. Does not require supplementation. | | | | |
| **3. No apparent problem:**<br>Moves in bed and in chair independently and has sufficient muscle strength to lift up completely during move. Maintains good position in bed or chair at all times. | | | | | |
| | **Total score** | | | | |

planning and patient teaching to be implemented at specific times also is included. Because the nurse has a major role in these two aspects of care, these are discussed under nursing management.

## SURGICAL MANAGEMENT

Some patients with wounds qualify for surgical intervention. Surgeons perform myocutaneous flaps and skin grafts of various levels, depending on the patient's physical condition, compliance level, and type of wound. Surgical interventions are discussed in Chapter 68.

# NURSING MANAGEMENT

A holistic approach to nursing management of the patient with a pressure sore contains four components: (1) controlling the contributing factors by reduction or elimination, (2) supporting the host, (3) optimizing the microenvironment based on principles of wound healing, and (4) providing education for patients and caregivers.

## ♦ ASSESSMENT

A detailed discussion about risk assessment has already been presented on p. 2349. The nursing assessment of wounds are discussed in this section. Once a wound has developed, the nurse is responsible for periodic assessments to determine whether the plan of care continues to be effective. Institutional policies differ on the frequency of assessments, so the term *periodic* has been adopted by the NPUAP to offer general guidelines while allowing flexibility for individual care settings.

### Subjective Data

Pressure sores generally do not cause subjective symptomatology, except for pain if the patient has sensation at the level of the wound. Pain management before dressing changes is a nursing consideration, as is providing restful periods for the patient to promote the optimal environment for wound healing. Cellular regeneration is slowed when the body is under stressful conditions, such as pain or fever. Management of pain is discussed in detail in Chapter 17.

### Objective Data

A staging classification system, as detailed in Box 67-4, is helpful for the nurse in determining the appropriate interventions for a particular wound; however, it is not an all-inclusive tool. Important wound characteristics—such as appearance of the wound bed, drainage, odor, and size—are not obtained using staging alone. In most cases, staging allows the nurse to determine only the depths of tissue involvement. However, if the wound is covered with necrotic tissue, the depth of tissue damage cannot be ascertained. To appropriately evaluate and document pressure sores, the nurse also must assess the size, color, and presence of exudate.

#### Size

Measure circumference of wound, diameter or length, and width if irregular shape exists. Also measure depth by inserting a sterile applicator and comparing depth with measurements on wound measuring guide. Sizing the wound not only assists with staging, but can help determine size and type of dressing(s) required.

#### Color

The color of wounds gives the examiner information about vascular supply, infection, healthy versus necrotic tissue, and nutritional status. "Healthy" wounds have a beefy-red, granular appearance. If the wound bed is pale in color, check the hemoglobin level. Necrotic tissue is white, yellow, gray, or black. Certain infections will change the color of a wound bed (*Pseudomonas* can produce greenish drainage on the wound bed).

#### Exudate

Wound drainage should be assessed for amount, color, and consistency. Odor is also an indicator for assessment. Infected wounds generally produce large amounts of odorous drainage. Be as objective as possible while documenting. Terms like *small, moderate,* and *large* are subjective. Be as descriptive as possible, such as "drainage of serosanguineous liquid, nonodorous, quarter sized on 4 × 4." Other general parameters to assess include presence of undermining or sinus tracts in wound, condition of surrounding skin, and foreign bodies in wound (e.g., sutures, orthopedic hardware).

## ♦ NURSING DIAGNOSES

Nursing diagnoses are determined from analysis of patient data. Nursing diagnoses for the patient with a pressure sore may include but are not limited to the following:

| Diagnostic Title | Possible Etiologic Factors |
|---|---|
| Skin integrity, high risk for impaired | Nutritional deficit, prolonged immobility, decreased hemoglobin and advanced age, serum albumin levels |
| Infection, high risk for | Lack of knowledge, decreased nutrition, decreased immune response, loss of skin integrity |
| Mobility, impaired physical | Intolerance to activity, decreased strength/endurance, pain/discomfort, perceptual/cognitive impairment, neuromuscular impairment, musculoskeletal impairment, depression, severe anxiety |
| Tissue perfusion, altered (skin) | Decreased blood flow, immobility, pressure |
| Self-care deficit: wound treatments | Location of wound, impaired mobility |

## ♦ EXPECTED PATIENT OUTCOMES

Expected patient outcomes for the patient with a pressure sore may include but are not limited to the following:

1. Is discharged with intact skin.
2. At discharge there is active wound healing, as evidenced by a clean, granular wound bed, minimal serosanguineous drainage, and no necrotic tissue present.
3. No clinical signs or symptoms of infection are present (pain, tenderness, fever, induration, surrounding erythema, increased drainage).
4. Shows evidence of achievement or return to maximal level of functioning.
5. No evidence of nonblanchable erythema is present.
6. The patient or caregiver states the following aspects of a continued care program: measures to reduce or relieve pressure to skin, importance of well-balanced diet, ways to manage incontinence/moisture, and treatment measures as indicated.

## ♦ INTERVENTIONS

### Preventing

1. Reduce or relieve pressure by instituting a schedule of turning the patient a minimum of every 2 hours and using available pressure relief devices for bed and chair.
2. Inspect the skin at regular intervals for signs of early breakdown.
3. Maintain skin in soft, elastic state through use of lotions; avoid massage.
4. Control incontinence and moisture next to skin.
5. Reduce or eliminate shear and friction.
6. Provide optimal nutrition; consult with dietitian.

### Protecting

1. Use of aseptic technique and universal precautions for the prevention of infection.
2. Monitor for clinical signs and symptoms of infection every shift and report as appropriate.

### Restoring

1. Involve patient in activity schedule as much as possible. Increasing activity levels assists with restoration to an optimal level of functioning.
2. Increase nutritional intake with adequate calorie, protein, and vitamins and minerals; work with dietitian.

### Teaching

1. Teach patient and caregiver about the need for continued interventions to prevent recurrence.
2. Instruct on dressing and intervention techniques.

## ♦ EVALUATION

To evaluate the effectiveness of nursing interventions, compare patient behaviors with those stated in the expected patient outcomes. Emphasis is placed throughout this discussion on early interventions for prevention of pressure sores. It remains the nurse's individual responsibility to be knowledgeable about preventive strategies and interventions in harmony with the Clinical Practice Guidelines. Adherence to national standards affords the nurse increased professional power, as well as autonomy, thus rendering feelings of professional satisfaction while maintaining high-quality patient care. If the nurse functions at the level established by the national standards, the patient will exhibit the following:

1. Intact skin or at least a decrease in the size of the pressure sore
2. A wound with no signs and symptoms of infection (e.g., the sore is clean, drainage is clear, temperature is normal)
3. Maximal functioning
4. Minimal and blanchable erythema
5. Implementation of pressure-reducing measures and measures to control moisture and incontinence
6. Awareness of a well-balanced diet

## ✸ SPECIAL CONSIDERATIONS FOR CARE OF THE GERONTOLOGIC PATIENT

Because of the numerous predisposing factors present in the elderly they are at greater risk for pressure ulcers. Predisposing factors include (1) anemia; (2) poor nutrition; (3) decreased albumin; (4) decreased mobility; (5) thinning of skin and loss of subcutaneous cushion; (6) drug therapy such as glucocorticoids; (7) incontinence; (8) comorbid conditions or use of sedatives that interfere with sensory perception, with natural shifting of body position, or with turning in bed; and (9) use of restraints.

Pressure ulcers or sores can occur not only to those confined to bed but also to those confined to a sitting position. The ulcers occur whenever pressure is allowed to be maintained. Ulcers can occur on the head, shoulders, or lower back if a recumbent position is maintained. If a side-lying position is maintained, ulcers can occur on hips, ankles, and the pinna of the ear. Sitting promotes ulcers on the buttocks. The underside of the scrotum can be injured with shearing and pressure.

Measures to prevent and treat pressure ulcers are the same for the elderly as for any person. The only difference is that tissue, because of the predisposing factors, is damaged more quickly so more frequent position changes and inspections need to be implemented. Many hospitalized elders require dietary measures to improve nutrition to prevent pressure ulcers. Also, many elderly persons require use of special beds, padding for chairs, and so forth if immobilization is required.

## ❦ HOME CARE CONSIDERATIONS

Many persons at high risk for pressure ulcerations are sent home with these same risk factors. Thus the family or other caregiver must know all the interventions including proper positioning techniqes, use of protective devices, proper nutrition, and so forth as described on p. 2351.

If a pressure ulcer has developed many times the caregiver will have to continue treatment measures after discharge. The caregiver must know how to do the treatment, the frequency of the treatment, safety precautions for self, how to dispose of used dressings, and what type of inspection to implement with each treatment. The caregiver must also know what changes need to be reported immediately.

Most patients sent home with pressure ulcers should have a referral to a home health care agency. The home care nurse can help the caregiver establish routines at home, obtain supplies most economically, and store supplies appropriately. The home care nurse can help the caregiver gain confidence in doing treatments. Additionally, the home care nurses can make sure that the patient's nutritional needs are met and an appropriate frequency and technique for change in position is maintained.

Last, most persons at home with pressure ulcers have many other physiological or psychosocial needs. The home health nurse can help the caregiver develop routines to meet these other needs and also obtain assistance to provide some respite.

## QUESTIONS TO CONSIDER

- What are the major psychosocial needs of persons with psoriasis? Why?
- What are the risk factors for pressure sores? What nursing approaches would you prescribe for an obese 60-year-old patient with diabetes mellitus who has neuropathy and is wheelchair-bound?
- Pruritus occurs in which disease states? What nursing approaches can help control pruritus?

## CRITICAL THINKING ACTIVITIES

- Compare and contrast nursing care of tinea capitis, tinea cruris, and tinea pedis.
- Discuss how a disease such as psoriasis may affect the person emotionally as compared with an individual with an ankle ulcer.

## CHAPTER SUMMARY

### PREVENTION OF DERMATOLOGIC DISORDERS

- Some dermatologic disorders may be prevented by removal of known causative agents, protecting the skin against ultraviolet rays, keeping the skin clean and hydrated, eating a balanced diet, monitoring for early signs of skin changes, and seeking medical help when skin conditions develop.

### PSYCHOLOGIC EFFECTS OF DERMATOLOGIC PROBLEMS

- Skin lesions can create changes in body image when lesions are obviously visible to others. Social interactions may be altered when there is considerable disfigurement.

### GENERAL INTERVENTIONS

- Pruritus leads to skin excoriation from scratching; it may be relieved by cold applications, hydration in a tepid oatmeal bath followed by application of emollient lotion, and maintaining room temperature at a moderate temperature with increased humidity.
- Medications used for therapeutic baths or soaks include colloids, potassium permanganate, Burow's solution, sulfur, tar preparations, and oils. These baths or soaks are given for antipruritic, antifungal, antibacterial, and moisturing or drying effects.
- The most commonly used topical medications are topical corticosteroids; the types vary in potency. Occlusion over the corticosteroid increases absorption and should be used only by prescription. Topical antibiotic and antifungal medications may also be prescribed.
- Vehicles for topical medications include powders, lotions, creams, ointments, and pastes.
- Wet dressings are used frequently over skin lesions for cooling, drying, antipruritic, or vasoconstricting effects; tap water or physiologic saline are most commonly used. The best effects are obtained by several treatment periods spaced across the person's waking hours.

### COMMON SKIN PROBLEMS

- Parasitic infestations include pediculosis and scabies; treatment includes applications of pediculicides and scabicides; patients and family members need to learn measures to prevent spread of infection.
- Fungal skin infections include candidiasis and the dermatophytoses (tinea). Treatment includes applying topical fungicides, keeping the skin dry, and wearing loose clothing or shoes, as appropriate.
- Bacterial skin infections include impetigo, folliculitis, furuncles and carbuncles, and erysipelas. Management includes cleansing the skin well and applying topical antibiotics; soaks are used to remove crusts. Heat is applied to furuncles until drainage occurs; incision and drainage may be necessary. Care must be taken to prevent spread of infection to other skin areas or to other persons.
- Viral skin infections include warts, herpes simplex (fever blister), and herpes zoster (shingles). Acyclovir may be prescribed for herpes infections. Pain is a problem with herpes infections and may persist after the lesions have healed.
- Acne results from multiple factors and is seen mostly in adolescents. The lesions result from blockage of hair follicles by sebum, leading to inflammations. Treatment may be with topical drying agents, removal

of comedones, and systemic therapy with isoretinoic acid, antibiotics, estrogens, or intralesional corticosteroids for severe acne.

- Types of dermatitis include contact (from external agents), atopic (hypersensitivity reaction), seborrheic, nummular, and stasis dermatitis and lichen simplex chronicus. Typical lesions include erythema, followed by vesicle formation with oozing, followed by crusting and scaling; itching is common. Treatment commonly includes wet dressings with water or Burow's solution and corticosteroid therapy. Antibiotics are given for superimposed infections.
- Skin reactions from systemic factors include dermatitis medicamentosa (drugs), exfoliative dermatitis, erythema multiforme, lesions of communicable diseases, and lupus erythematosus.
- Psoriasis is a genetically determined, papulosquamous disease; no cure exists. The lesions are scaling plaques. Treatment consists of bland emollients and keratolytics to hydrate and soften the skin, corticosteroids, coal tar preparations, anthralin products (antimitotic), and photochemotherapy.
- Benign skin growths are keratoses (corns, calluses, seborrheic, actinic); premalignant growths include leukoplakia, Bowen's disease, and pigmented nevi.
- Benign nevi (moles) are symmetric, with even borders, uniform color, and usually less than 6 mm in size; malignant melanomas are asymetric with uneven borders, multiple colors, and usually larger than 6 mm.
- A major contributing factor to the incidence of some skin growths (actinic keratoses, squamous cell carcinomas, keratocanthomas, malignant melanomas) is unprotected exposure to the sun. Most skin cancers, *except* malignant melanomas and some squamous cell carcinomas (on lips or ears), do not metastasize.
- Changes in moles that should be reported to the physician include change in pigmentation, sudden growth in size, loss of hair in the mole, and bleeding.
- Kaposi's sarcoma is widely scattered red, purple, or dark plaques, occurring mostly in persons with AIDS. The disorder is slowly progressive, and treatment is primarily cosmetic; the person usually dies of another opportunistic infection.

### SKIN DISORDERS IN AFRICAN-AMERICANS

- Skin disorders commonly seen in African-Americans include traumatic alopecia, pseudofolliculitis barbae, keloids, dermatosis papulosa nigra, and perifolliculitis abscedens.

### DERMATOLOGIC SURGERY

- Types of dermatologic surgeries for superficial lesions include tangenital surgery, curettage, cryosurgery, and electrosurgery. Deep lesions are removed by punch biopsy or by excision. Hemostasis is generally accomplished by gelatin foam, pressure, a chemical styptic, or electrocoagulation. The patient is taught not to remove the crust until it falls off naturally.

### PRESSURE SORES

- Pressure sores are a major health care concern for nursing.
- National Clinical Practice Guidelines were established to guide practitioners with quality preventive and management interventions.
- Nurses' primary responsibility lies with prevention of and early intervention in those with pressure sores.

## REFERENCES


1. American Cancer Society: *Cancer facts and figures,* New York, 1993, The Society.
2. Bickers DR: Treatment of selected photosensitivity diseases, *Med Clin North Am* 66:927-37, 1982.
3. Clinical Practice Guidelines: *Pressure ulcers in adults: prediction and prevention,* Washington, DC, 1992, US Dept of HHS.
4. Dunn ML: Treatment options for psoriasis, *Am J Nurs* 88(8):1082-1087, 1988.
5. Epstein E: *Common skin disorders,* ed 3, Oradell, NJ, 1988, Medical Economics Books.
6. Ganong WF: *Review of medical physiology,* ed 13, Norwalk, Conn, 1988, Appleton & Lange.
7. LeFort SM: Herpes zoster and postherpetic neuralgia: the need for early intervention in the elderly, *Nurse Pract* 14(3):30-41, 1989.
8. Lucey J: Herpetic whitlow, *Am J Nurs* 84(1):60-61, 1984.
9. Matthews KP: Clinical spectrum of allergic and pseudoallergic drug reactions, *J Allergy Clin Immunol* 74:558-566, 1984.
10. Mocsny N: Care and treatment of scabies, *Adv Clin Care* 5(5): 23-26, 1990.
11. Moschella SL, Hurley HA: *Dermatology,* ed 3, Philadelphia, 1991, WB Saunders.
12. Price SA, Wilson LM, editors: *Pathophysiology: clinical concepts of disease processes,* ed 4, St Louis, 1992, Mosby.
13. Stein JH et al: *Internal medicine,* ed 4, St Louis, 1994, Mosby.
14. Teirney L et al: *Current medical diagnosis and treatment,* ed 33, Norwalk, Conn, 1994, Appleton & Lange.

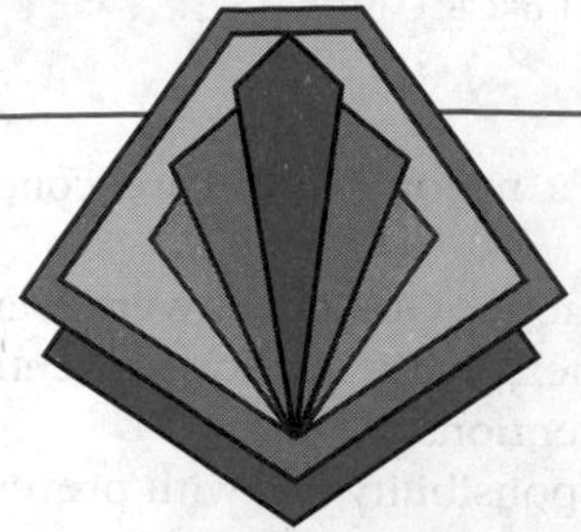

CHAPTER 68

# Management of Persons With Burns

**_Diane E. Fritsch_**
**_Lynne C. Yurko_**

## CHAPTER OBJECTIVES

***After studying this chapter, the learner should be able to do the following:***

1. Describe the assessment of the burn patient including extent, location, and etiology of the burn.
2. Differentiate among the three periods of a major burn.
3. Describe emergency care for a major burn.
4. Describe interventions for replacing body fluids, preventing infection, promoting nutrition and mobility, and providing emotional support.
5. Identify learning needs of the patient with burns.
6. Identify populations at risk for burn injury and discuss preventive measures.

## KEY TERMS

acute period
autograft
burn shock
cultured epithelium
diuretic stage
donor site
emergent period
eschar
fluid resuscitation
full-thickness burn
full-thickness graft
heterograft
hypovolemic stage
inhalation injury
major burn
mechanism of injury
minor burn
partial-thickness burn
rehabilitation period
rule of nines
split-thickness skin graft

## ETIOLOGY/EPIDEMIOLOGY

Burn injuries are in many respects the worst of all tragedies an individual can experience. An intensive burn is accompanied by an overwhelming insult to the patient physically and psychologically, and it is catastrophic in cost and suffering to the family involved.

Approximately 2.5 million people suffer a thermal injury each year in the United States. Of these victims, 70,000 are admitted to hospitals and over 7000 die as a result of burn injury. Burns are caused by flame, scald, direct contact, chemicals, electrical current, and radiation. Injury is frequently a result of the victim's own action. This is particularly true for elderly persons, whose burns frequently are caused by the ignition of clothing when cooking or smoking. Scald injuries are the most frequent type of injury, but flame injury is more serious. The direct cost of treating burn injuries is over $1 billion. Indirect costs (pain, suffering, disability) amount to several billion dollars more per year.[11] Because of the systemic effects of the burn injury, psychologic implications, and prolonged hospitalization, comprehensive nursing care is required during the acute and long-term recovery phases.

## PREVENTION

Nurses can help prevent accidental burns by participating in health education programs that stress fire prevention and the consequences of fires such as burns, deformities, and death. See Research box, p. 2359. Nurses can promote legislation that would control hazardous practices and make working and living environments safer. Community health nurses are in an unusually advantageous position to recognize unsafe practices in the home and to help families develop safe habits of living. Nurses can raise the awareness of patients and the community to the burn problem with education and burn awareness campaigns (Figure 68-1).

Prevention programs can be developed to highlight

seasonal activities that result in burn injuries (Box 68-1). Approximately 80% of accidental burns occur in the home and are caused primarily by ignorance, carelessness, and curiosity of *children*. More than 35% of all fire and burn injuries and deaths are to children. Matches and cigarette lighters are a significant factor in these fatalities. Although 75% of all homes now have smoke detectors installed, one third of these units are not functioning either because of no batteries or bad electrical connections. Children suffer permanently disfiguring and disabling injuries in preventable accidents.[11]

A high incidence of burn injuries that affect adults is related to accidents while cooking, while using microwave ovens, or while smoking or otherwise using matches. Burns commonly occur when a person is distracted while cooking or falls asleep while smoking.

Each year brings increased demand for careful inspection and regulation of places in which the *ill* and *infirm* are housed. *Aged* persons frequently are housed in old and poorly equipped structures, and many of them have been victims of fire. Nurses can bring necessary pressures to bear to ensure adequate protection and planned evacuation if a fire occurs. Basic fire prevention programs should include one mock evacuation drill each year. Attention is being focused on places where large numbers of people congregate. Laws require that doors in public buildings be hinged to swing outward, that draperies and decorations be fireproof, and that stairways with special fire doors be used in new apartment buildings and hotels. Smoke detectors and sprinkler sys-

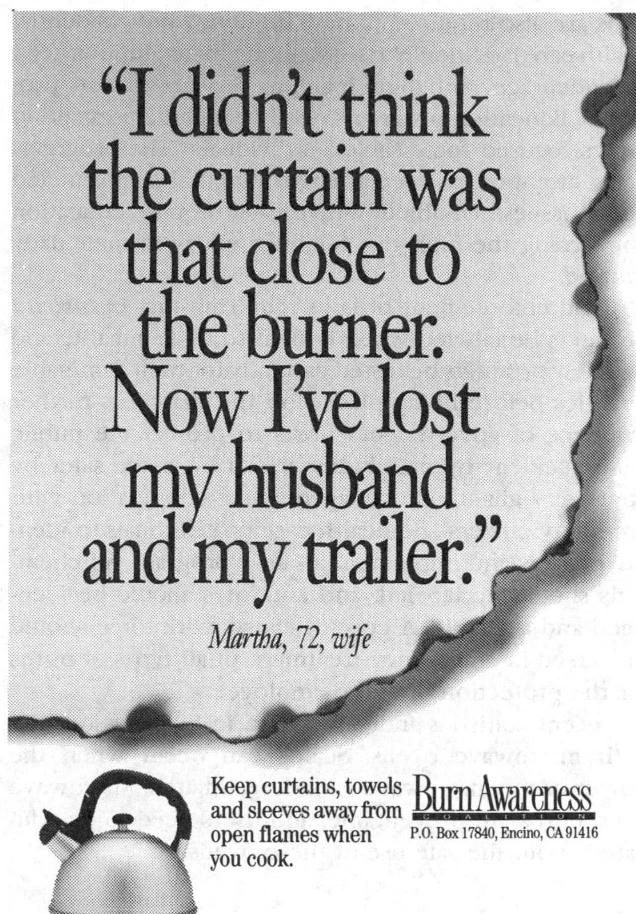


**FIGURE 68-1** Sample of a burn prevention poster.

## RESEARCH

Thompson R et al: The effect of instruction on burn prevention in eighth-grade students in preparation for babysitting, *J Burn Care Rehabil* 13:482-486, 1992.

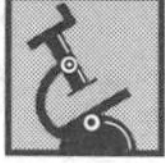

Preteens and teenagers commonly provide babysitting services to young children. Because the home (particularly the kitchen and bathroom) is the place where most burn injuries occur, children may be at risk if the babysitter is not aware of potential dangers. A pretest and posttest were used to evaluate the effectiveness of burn prevention instruction provided to eighth-grade students (N-119, ages 12-14, 83.2% were babysitters). The study concluded that students had learned burn prevention before entering the eighth grade but were not familiar with many hazards such as cigarette lighters, microwaves, bath water temperature, and insertion of objects into electrical outlets. Previous instruction on burn prevention occurred predominantly in the schools, with little occurring in Girl Scouts or Boy Scouts or by fire departments. The study indicated that burn prevention instruction may need to occur earlier than age 12, before teens begin to babysit. In addition, prevention programs could use schools and Girl Scouts and Boy Scouts as forums for instruction.

## BOX 68-1 Seasonal Activities Resulting in Burn Injuries

| | |
|---|---|
| **Spring** | Barbecuing |
| | Burning leaves |
| | Overheated radiators |
| | Gasoline |
| | Lawnmowers |
| **Summer** | Sun exposure |
| | Fireworks |
| | Beach activity |
| | Sun-heated surfaces (tar, asphalt, sand) |
| **Fall** | Hot liquids |
| | Yard clean-up |
| | Candles |
| | Halloween |
| **Winter** | Holiday activities |
| | Fireplaces |
| | Hot liquids |
| | Woodburning stoves/space heaters |
| | Electrical wires |

From Lillico S: *National burn awareness 1991*, Encino, Calif, 1991, The National Burn Awareness Task Force.

tems are also required in new buildings and residential health care facilities. Nurses working in institutions need to encourage and participate in fire prevention programs. Education programs need to include prevention topics focused for disabled individuals. The programs bring attention to special environmental supports and safety issues. Disabled individuals require education concerning the high risk for burn injury in their daily routine.

Rigid enforcement of laws requiring that *industrial* products be labeled when known to be flammable and that new products be tested carefully for their flammable qualities before being placed on the market is further evidence of government efforts to protect the public from accident by fire. Industry can be made safer by constant vigilance of management in cooperation with fire safety officers and health care professionals to identify hazards and implement a safety program. All chemicals should be labeled, and antidotes should be identified and available. A core of every work force should be versed in emergency treatment of all types of burns for the protection of every employee.

Recent statistics indicate a rise in burns associated with microwave ovens. Scalds can occur when the power of the microwave is underestimated. Microwave oven burns are preventable, and users need to be educated about the safe use of these ovens.

*Sunburn* should be avoided, because even a relatively mild burn of a large part of the body can cause change of fluid distribution and kidney damage. Camp nurses should keep this in mind in their educational programs for children and camp counselors. Many available sunscreen products are effective and should be used in times of exposure.

### Healthy People 2000

The Surgeon General's report on goals to be achieved by year 2000 includes reducing residential fire deaths to no more than 1.2 per 100,000 people from an age-adjusted baseline of 1.5 per 100,000 in 1987.[13a] Goals for special populations at high risk appear in Table 68-1.

## CLASSIFICATION OF BURNS

Traditionally, burns have been classified as *first-, second-* or *third-* degree. The terms first-, second- and third-degree are ***not descriptive*** of the injury because they are based only on the visual characteristics of the burn wound. The injury of a burn extends beyond what can be seen. A more accurate description is partial- and full-thickness, which graphically describes the burn and indicates depth and severity of the tissue injury (Figure 68-2).

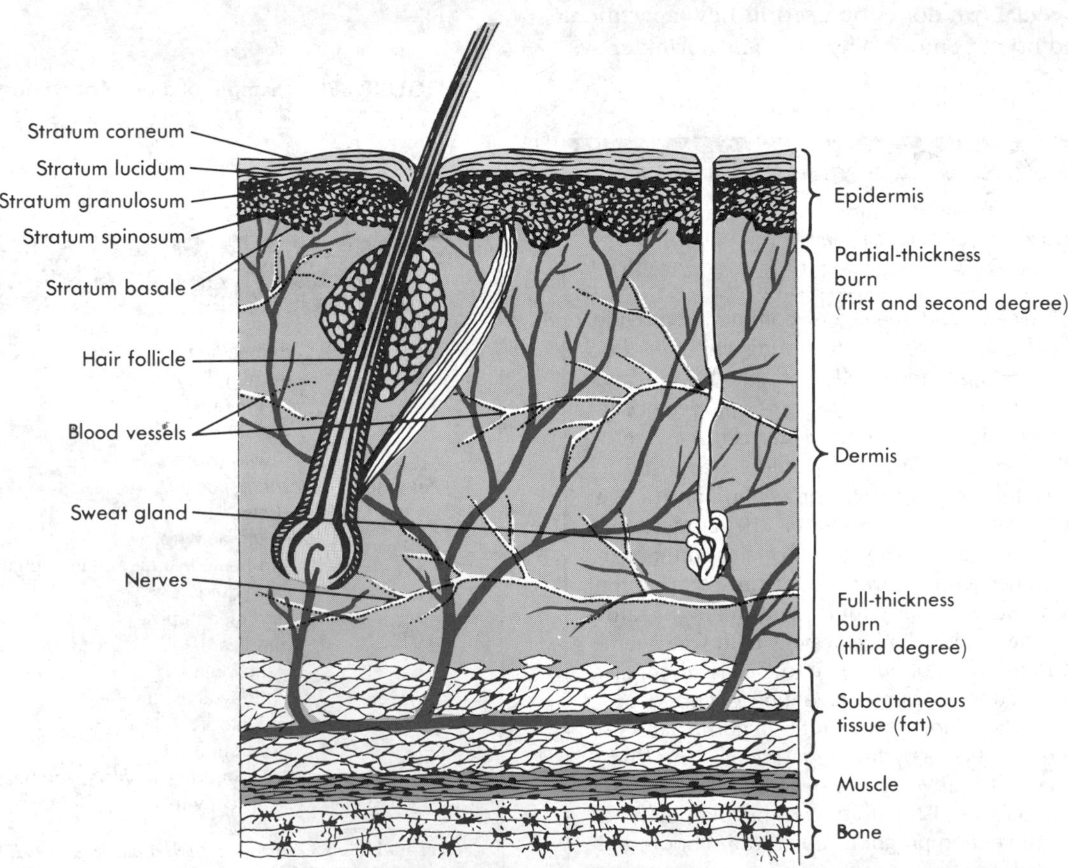


**FIGURE 68-2** Levels of human skin involved in burns.

**TABLE 68-1 Goals per 100,000 People for Reduction in Fire Deaths Among Populations at High Risk**

| POPULATIONS | 1987 BASELINE | 2000 TARGET |
|---|---|---|
| Children age 4 and younger | 4.4 | 3.3 |
| People age 65 and older | 4.4 | 3.3 |
| Black males | 5.7 | 4.3 |
| Black females | 3.4 | 2.6 |

From US Department of Health and Human Services, Public Health Service: *Healthy people 2000: national health promotion and disease prevention objectives,* Washington, DC, 1990, US Government Printing Office.

**Partial-thickness burns** are characterized by destruction in varying depths from the epidermis (outer layer of skin) to the dermis (middle layer of skin). Partial-thickness burns of the skin involve a "part" of the epidermis and dermis. The depth of tissue injury is described further as *superficial* partial-thickness, involving only the epidermis, and *deep* partial-thickness burns, which involve the entire epidermis and part of the dermis. Partial-thickness burns are likely to be painful because nerve endings have been injured and exposed, but they have the ability to heal because a portion of the epithelial cells are not destroyed. The presence of blisters often indicates deep partial-thickness injury. They may increase in size as the result of continuous exudation and collection of tissue fluid. During the healing phase, dryness and itching are common and are caused by increased vascularization of sebaceous glands, reduction of secretions, and decreased perspiration.

**Full-thickness burns** include destruction of the epidermis and the entire dermis, as well as possible damage to the subcutaneous layer, muscle, and bone. Nerve endings are destroyed, resulting in a painless wound. *Eschar,* a leathery covering comprised of denatured protein, may form as the result of surface dehydration. Black networks of coagulated capillaries may be seen. Full-thickness burns require skin grafting because the destroyed tissue is unable to epithelialize. Often a deep partial-thickness burn may convert to a full-thickness burn by infection, trauma, or decreased blood supply.

## PATHOPHYSIOLOGY OF SEVERE BURNS

As a result of burns, normal skin function is diminished, resulting in physiologic alterations. These include (1) loss of protective barriers against infection, (2) escape of body fluids, (3) lack of temperature control, (4) destroyed sweat and sebaceous glands, and (5) a diminished number of sensory receptors. The severity of these

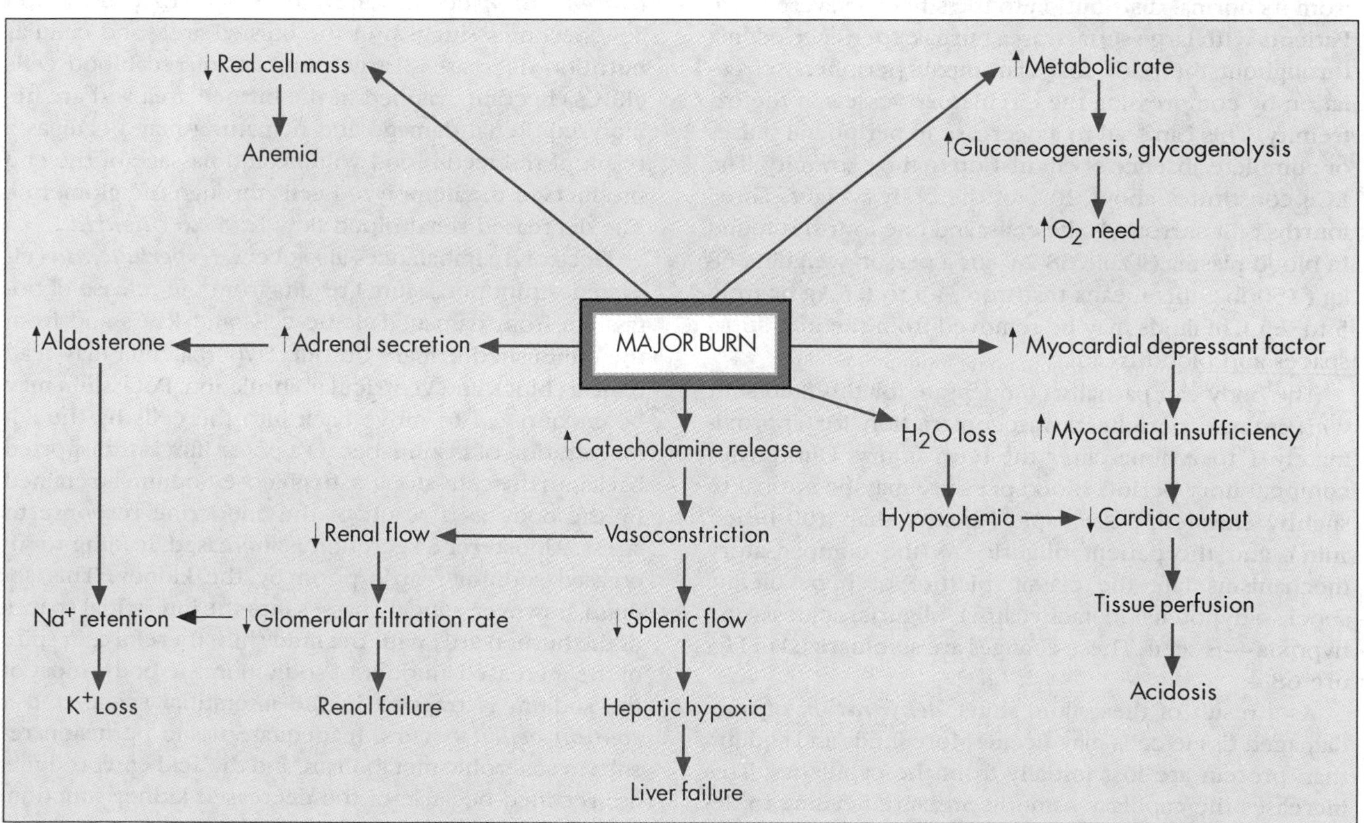


**FIGURE 68-3** Overview of pathophysiology of a major burn.

alterations depend on the extent of the burn and the depth to which damage has occurred.

Increased knowledge of the physiologic changes that occur during severe burns has led to improved outcomes. Two stages occur after severe burns: the immediate hypovolemic stage and the diuretic stage. Figure 68-3 presents an overview of the pathophysiologic changes seen in a severe burn.

## HYPOVOLEMIC STAGE

The **hypovolemic stage** begins at the time of burn injury and lasts for the first 48 to 72 hours. It is characterized by a rapid *shift of fluid* from the vascular compartments into the interstitial spaces. When tissues are burned, vasodilation, increased capillary permeability, and changes in the permeability of tissue cells in and around the burn area occur. As a result, abnormally large amounts of extracellular fluid (ECF), sodium chloride, and protein pass through the burned area to cause blister formation and local edema or escape through the open wound.

Visible fluid loss makes up only a small part of the fluid lost from the circulating blood and other essential fluid compartments. Most of the fluid loss occurs deep in the wound, where the fluid extravasates into the deeper tissues. Burns occurring in highly vascular areas such as muscle tissue or the face are believed to cause a greater fluid shift than comparable burns of other parts of the body. One half of the ECF of the body can shift from its normal distribution to the site of a severe burn. Patients with large surface area burns experience edema throughout the body that can impair peripheral circulation by compressing the circulatory vessels in the extremity. This can lead to a decrease in peripheral pulses or complete absence of circulation to the extremity. The ECF constitutes about 20% of the body weight. Three fourths of it surrounds the cells, and one fourth is found in blood plasma (Table 68-2). For a person weighing 68 kg (150 lb), this means that from 4.5 to 6.5 kg or from 5 to 7.5 L of fluids may be removed from the interstitial spaces and bloodstream.

The body can partially compensate for this fluid shift with intense peripheral vasoconstriction for approximately 1 to 2 hours after the burn injury. During this compensatory period, blood pressure may be normal to slightly elevated, pulse rapid (greater than 100 beats/min), and the patient oliguric. As the compensatory mechanisms fail, the classic picture of hypovolemic shock—hypotension, tachycardia, oliguria, acidosis and hypoxia—is seen. These changes are summarized in Figure 68-4.

As a result of these fluid shifts, *dehydration* of nondamaged tissue cells may occur. More fluids and sodium than protein are lost initially from the capillaries. This increases the capillary osmotic pressure, leading to dehydration with pronounced *edema* in the burned area.

**TABLE 68-2 Approximate Division of Total Body Fluid Into Compartments***

| BODY FLUID COMPARTMENTS | LITERS OF FLUID: LEAN ADULT WEIGHING 45 KG | LITERS OF FLUID: LEAN ADULT WEIGHING 68 KG |
|---|---|---|
| Intravascular (plasma) | 2.8 | 4.2 |
| Interstitial | 8.4 | 12.5 |
| Intracellular | 22.3 | 33.3 |
| TOTAL | 33.5 | 50.0 |

*Note that the smaller the individual, the less fluid he or she has in each compartment and that plasma is reduced most markedly with decrease in size. The normal size and body type of the individual are considered when fluid replacement is ordered.

As protein continues to be lost into the burned area because of the increased capillary permeability, *hypoproteinemia* results. The increased amount of protein in the tissue spaces is a further contributing factor to edema formation. Proteins may be lost through the open wounds. The lymphatic system, which normally functions to remove increased tissue fluid, becomes overloaded and inefficient, contributing to edema formation. Nitrogen is lost through the kidney from catabolism, leading to significant negative nitrogen balance. The BUN is elevated when oliguria is present.

With loss of fluid from the vascular system, *hemoconcentration* occurs, and the hematocrit rises. Blood flow becomes sluggish in the burned area, and cellular nutrition decreases. Large numbers of red blood cells (RBCs) become trapped in the burned area and are hemolyzed. Renal damage and hematuria may occur as a result of reduced blood volume and passage of the end products of the hemolyzed cells through the glomeruli. The decreased renal blood flow leads to *oliguria*.

Electrolyte imbalances also occur. *Hyperkalemia* (elevated serum potassium) results from the release of potassium from damaged tissue cells and RBCs and from the diminished urinary output. Hyperkalemia may lead to heart block and ventricular fibrillation. Potassium may be encouraged to move back into the cells by the administration of insulin, because potassium is transported back into the cells along with glucose. Sodium is retained by the body as a result of the endocrine response to stress. Aldosterone secretion is increased, leading to increased sodium reabsorption by the kidney. This sodium, however, quickly passes into the interstitial spaces of the burned area with the fluid shift; therefore, in spite of the increased amount of sodium in the body, most of the sodium is trapped in the interstitial space, and a *sodium deficit* occurs. Inadequate tissue perfusion results in anaerobic metabolism, and the acid end products are retained because of the decreased kidney function. *Metabolic acidosis* may then occur.

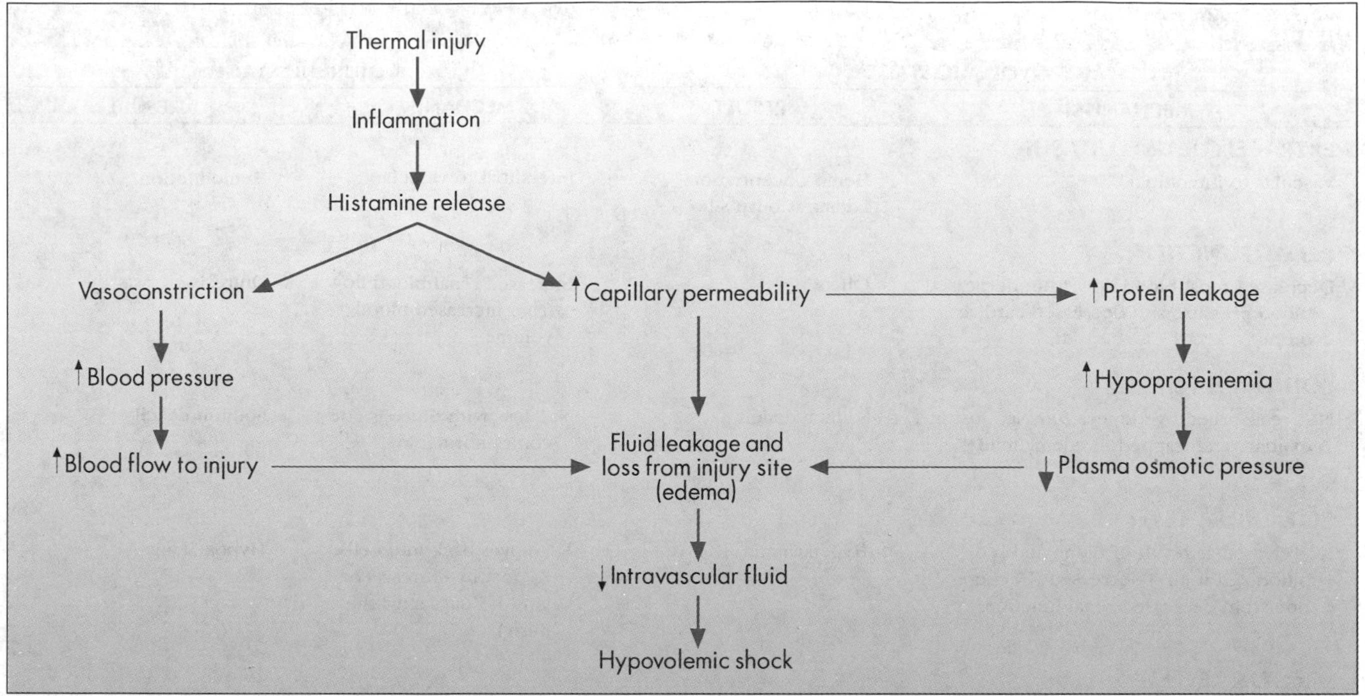


**FIGURE 68-4** Flow diagram of fluid shifts resulting in hypovolemic shock.

## DIURETIC STAGE

Return of vascular integrity begins at approximately 12 hours and rapidly progresses at 18 to 24 hours after the initial burn injury. Although full capillary integrity may not be restored for a number of days, for clinical purposes it may be considered restored at 24 hours. The **diuretic stage** begins at about 48 to 72 hours after the burn injury as capillary membrane integrity returns and edema fluid shifts back from the interstitial spaces into the intravascular space. Blood volume increases, leading to increased renal blood flow and *diuresis* unless renal damage has occurred. Serum electrolyte and hematocrit levels will be decreased because of the *hemodilution. Fluid overload* may occur as a result of the increase in intravascular volume. The patient's vital signs, breath sounds, and urinary output are used to determine the amount of intravenous fluid replacement. Dehydration may occur if rapid urinary fluid losses deplete the intravascular reserve. A *sodium deficit* continues because of the loss of sodium through the burn wound and through the increase in urine output. *Hypokalemia* results from potassium moving back into the cells or being excreted in the urine. Protein continues to be lost from the wounds. *Metabolic acidosis* remains a possibility because of the loss of sodium bicarbonate in the urine and the increased fat metabolism secondary to a decreased carbohydrate intake.

Following the period of fluid shifts, the patient remains acutely ill. This period is characterized by *anemia* and *malnutrition.* Anemia develops from the loss of red blood cells. Negative nitrogen balance begins at the onset of the burn and is the result of tissue destruction, protein loss, and the stress response. It continues throughout the acute period and is secondary to continued loss of protein from the wound, from tissue catabolism resulting from immobility, and from decreased protein intake. Special attention to the nutritional needs of the patient is an integral part of the comprehensive care during this time. Increased metabolism from loss of water and heat from the wound, loss of fluid during diuresis, and catabolism during tissue breakdown lead to *weight loss.*

Complications of the gastrointesinal system occur frequently after thermal injury. Gastric and duodenal ulceration (Curling's ulcer) has been reported in severely burned patients. Bleeding is the major clinical problem for patients with these lesions. Treatment is aimed at prevention and is best accomplished by antacids, $H_2$ blockers, and enteral feedings. Cholecystitis, pancreatitis and hepatic, dysfunction may also be seen as the result of tissue ischemia from hypoperfusion. The differences in changes between the hypovolemic and diuretic stages are summarized in Table 68-3.

## PERIODS OF TREATMENT

Management of a person with a burn injury is extensive and costly. Discharge planning starts on admission and must meet patient care needs in the time allowed under each DRG. The goal for discharge of patients with ex-

**TABLE 68-3 Physiologic Changes With Burns**

| HYPOVOLEMIC STAGE | | DIURETIC STAGE | |
|---|---|---|---|
| **MECHANISM** | **RESULT** | **MECHANISM** | **RESULT** |
| **EXTRACELLULAR FLUID SHIFT** | | | |
| Vascular to interstitial | Hemoconcentration<br>Edema at burn site | Interstitial to vascular | Hemodilution |
| **RENAL FUNCTION** | | | |
| Decreased renal blood flow from decreased blood pressure and decreased cardiac output | Oliguria | Increased renal blood flow from increased blood volume | Diuresis |
| **SODIUM LEVEL** | | | |
| $Na^+$ reabsorbed by kidneys *but* $Na^+$ lost in exudate and trapped in edema fluid | Sodium deficit | $Na^+$ loss with diuresis (becomes normal in 1 week) | Sodium deficit |
| **POTASSIUM LEVEL** | | | |
| $K^+$ released as result of tissue and red blood cell injury; decreased $K^+$ excretion from decreased renal function | Hyperkalemia | $K^+$ moves back into cells; $K^+$ lost by diuresis (begins 4-5 days after the burn) | Hypokalemia |
| **PROTEIN LEVEL** | | | |
| Protein lost into tissues by increased capillary permeability | Hypoproteinemia | Loss of protein during continued catabolism | Hypoproteinemia |
| **NITROGEN BALANCE** | | | |
| Tissue catabolism; protein loss in tissues; more nitrogen lost than taken in | Negative nitrogen balance | Tissue catabolism, protein loss, immobility | Negative nitrogen balance |
| **ACID BASE BALANCE** | | | |
| Anaerobic metabolism from decreased tissue perfusion; increased acid end products; decreased renal function (causing retention of acid end products); loss of serum bicarbonate | Metabolic acidosis | Sodium bicarbonate lost in diuresis; hypermetabolism with increased metabolic end products | Metabolic acidosis |
| **STRESS RESPONSE** | | | |
| Occurs because of trauma | Decreased renal blood flow | Occurs because of prolonged nature of injury and psychologic threat to self | Stress ulcers |

tensive burns with OR procedures as determined by DRG 472 is 21 days. The nurse works collaboratively with the physician for implementation of prescribed medical therapy. Because the nurse has a major role in discharge planning and patient teaching, these functions are discussed under nursing management.

Three periods of treatment can be identified in the care of the seriously burned patient: the emergent, acute, and rehabilitation periods. The *emergent period* refers to the first 24 to 48 hours postburn when the patient is admitted, the severity of the injury is determined, and first aid and wound care are given. The *acute period* of treatment begins at the end of the emergent period and lasts until all of the full-thickness wounds are covered with skin grafts or partial-thickness wounds are healed. The physical healing time is determined by the patient's medical condition, nutritional status, and ability to heal. A 40% injury requires a minimum of 40 days to heal. The **rehabilitation period** focuses on returning the patient to a useful place in society. There are two areas of concern during this phase: (1) the restoration of function over joint surfaces that were scarred, and (2) the emotional assistance that the patient and family will need. The rehabilitation of the patient actually begins during early hospitalization and is addressed throughout the hospital stay. After the initial discharge, the patient may require emotional assistance and counseling, and many readmissions may be necessary for reconstructive procedures. Actual emotional and social healing depends on each patient's ability to cope with physical scars and society's acceptance of the new body image. The actual time period could last the rest of the patient's life.

Comprehensive care of the burn patient can best be provided by a *multidisciplinary team approach*. The physician, nurse, pediatric and adult social workers, physical and occupational therapists, teacher, registered dietitian, vocational counselor, and others all work together to address the complex and varied needs of the patient. The nurse's role in the team is to coordinate the interactions of the various disciplines and to incorporate the team's suggestions and approaches into an effective plan of care. This plan includes referring patients to burn support groups available at hospitals with major burn units, or The Phoenix Society (an organization of burn survivors).

## EMERGENT PERIOD

The **emergent period** of therapy is defined as the time required to resolve the immediate problems resulting from the burn injury (24 to 48 hours). First aid measures are directed to treating the systemic response to trauma, concurrent injuries, and the burn wound (see Guidelines box at right).

### Medical Management

The goals of medical management during the emergent period of a burn are to: (1) secure the airway, (2) support circulation by fluid replacement, (3) keep the patient comfortable with analgesics, (4) prevent infection through careful wound care, (5) maintain body temperature, and (6) provide emotional support. The nurse and physician work collaboratively to achieve these goals. The specifics of treatment are discussed under nursing management.

### Guidelines for Initial Care of Major Burns

1. Remove victim from source of burn.
2. Douse with water and remove nonadherent smoldering clothing to stop the burning process.
3. If chemical burn, carefully remove clothing and flush wound with large amounts of water.
4. If electrical burn and victim is still in contact with electrical source, do *not* touch victim. Remove electrical source with dry nonconductive object.
5. Establish patent airway and assess for inhalation injury. Give oxygen if available.
6. Check peripheral pulses to assess circulatory status.
7. Assess and initiate treatment for injuries requiring immediate attention.
8. Remove tight-fitting jewelry or clothing.
9. Cover burn with moist sterile or clean cover.
10. Cover victim with warm, dry cover to prevent heat loss.
11. Transport victim to nearest medical facility.

## NURSING MANAGEMENT

### ♦ ASSESSMENT

Assessment of the person who has sustained a severe burn depends on the severity of the burn injury.

### Subjective Data

Knowledge of circumstances surrounding the burn injury is extremely valuable in the management of a burn victim. This information can be obtained from either the burn victim or witnesses to the event. Data should include the following:

1. How the burn injury occurred
2. When the burn injury occurred
3. Duration of contact with the burning agent
4. Location (enclosed area suggests possibility of smoke inhalation and/or carbon monoxide poisoning)
5. Presence of an explosion (suggests possibility of other injuries)

The state of health and age of the burn victim are important factors that may modify treatment. Elderly patients and very young patients have a higher mortality rate than a young adult with the same percentage burn. Preexisting endocrine, pulmonary, cardiovascular or renal disease, or a history of drug abuse will decrease a victim's ability to cope with severe burns. Because most of these patients will require topical and systemic therapy with a number of drugs, allergies and drug sensitivities must be determined and documented.

### Objective Data

Burns may be categorized as major, moderate, or minor on the basis of the size of the burn and the presence of complicating factors (Box 68-2).

#### Assessing the severity of the burn injury

**Medical history.** Identification of known and unknown disorders may prevent fatal complications in the burn victim. A prior illness, such as diabetes or renal failure, may become acute during the postburn phase. The physiologic stress seen with the burn may exacerbate a latent disease process or worsen an already active process and thus increase mortality. Diabetes and chronic obstructive pulmonary disease may be aggravated, or patients with arteriosclerotic heart disease may develop a myocardial infarction.

**Size and depth of burn.** For adults, the **"rule of nines"** is used to determine the size of the burn. The percentage of body surface area (BSA) burned is estimated with the use of charts that depict anterior and posterior drawings of the body. In adults, the body is divided into areas equal to multiples of 9% (Figure 68-5). In clinical practice, the burned area is shaded in on the drawings and the amount of body surface burned is calculated from the shaded areas. Calculations are modified for infants and children less than 10 years of age because of their relatively larger head and smaller body (consult a pediatric textbook for these figures).

**BOX 68-2 Classification of Severity of Burns**

**MAJOR BURN INJURIES**

Partial-thickness injury greater than 25% body surface area (BSA) (greater than 20% in children less than 10 years and adults more than 40 years)
Greater than 10% BSA, full-thickness (children and adults)
Involvement of face, eyes, ears, hands, feet, perineum
Electrical burns
Burns complicated by inhalation injury or major trauma
Burns in patients with preexisting disease (diabetes, congestive heart failure, or chronic renal failure)

**MODERATE BURN INJURIES**

15% to 25% BSA in adults, partial-thickness (10% to 20% BSA in children less than 10 years and adults more than 40 years)
2% to 10% BSA full-thickness
Burns with no concurrent injury
Burns in patients with no preexisting disease

**MINOR BURN INJURIES**

Less than 15% BSA in adults (10% in children or elderly persons)
Less than 2% BSA full-thickness injury
Burns in patients with no preexisting disease

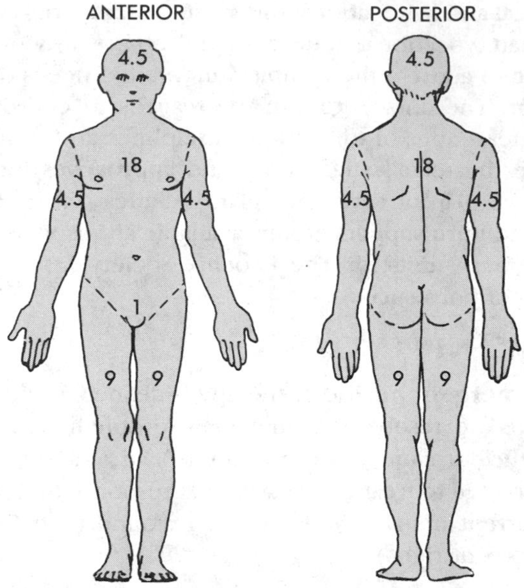


**FIGURE 68-5** Rule of nines.

**TABLE 68-4 Characteristics of Depth of Burn Injury**

| SUPERFICIAL PARTIAL-THICKNESS (FIRST-DEGREE) | DEEP PARTIAL-THICKNESS (SECOND-DEGREE) | FULL-THICKNESS (THIRD-DEGREE) |
|---|---|---|
| **SKIN DEPTH** | | |
| Epidermis | Entire epidermis, partial dermis<br>Sweat glands, hair follicles intact | Epidermis, dermis<br>Extends to subcutaneous tissue, possibly muscle and bone |
| **CAUSE** | | |
| Flash flame, ultraviolet light (sunburn) | Contact with hot liquids or solids<br>Flash flame to clothing<br>Direct flames<br>Chemicals<br>Ultraviolet light | Contact with hot liquids or solids<br>Flame<br>Chemicals<br>Electrical contact |
| **APPEARANCE** | | |
| Dry, no blisters<br>Minimal or no edema<br>Blanches with fingertip pressure and color returns when pressure removed | Large, moist blisters that will increase in size<br>Blanches with fingertip pressure and color returns when pressure removed | Dry with leathery eschar<br>Charred vessels visible under eschar<br>Blisters rare but thin-walled blisters that do not increase in size may be present<br>No blanching with pressure |
| **COLOR** | | |
| Increased redness | Mottled with dull, white, tan, pink, or cherry red areas | White, charred, dark tan, black, red |
| **SENSATION** | | |
| Painful | Very painful | No pain<br>Nerve endings dead |
| **HEALING TIME** | | |
| 2-5 days with peeling<br>No scarring<br>May discolor | Superficial: 5-21 days; no grafting<br>Deep: 21-35 days if no infection<br>May convert to full-thickness and require grafting | No healing potential<br>Requires excision and grafting<br>Healing of grafts may take months |

The depth of the burn injury is evaluated on the basis of appearance, color, and sensation (Table 68-4).

**Age of victim.** The severity of a burn also depends on the age of the victim. Infants less than 2 years of age and adults older than 60 years have a higher mortality rate than persons in other age groups with a similar size injury. The infant has a weak antibody response to infection, and in older victims the serious burn may aggravate the degenerative processes or exacerbate a preexisting health problem. See Gerontologic Patient Considerations box at right.

**Body part involved.** The body part involved is an important factor in evaluating the severity of a burn. The anatomic part of the body burned must be considered when estimating the severity of the burn: a 3% burn of the anterior surface of the thigh is not as serious as a 3% burn to the neck, face, or perineal area. Injuries that involve cosmetic and functional areas of the body require a long period of recovery because of both physical and emotional reactions to the burn injury. A burn of the face, hands, and feet requires extensive, meticulous care, and extensive physical and occupational therapy. A burn of the head, neck, and chest may also involve injury to the respiratory tract and result in severe respiratory difficulty. Burns of the perineum are difficult to manage because of the potential for contamination and infection. The circumferential, or encircling burn, of a limb, the neck, or the chest has serious consequences. This type of burn will cause *constrictive contraction* of the skin and produce a tourniquet effect that may impair breathing and/or circulation.

**Mechanism of injury.** Identifying the causative agent is of prime importance because the nature of the agent has a direct effect on prognosis and treatment. The mechanisms of burn injury are flame and flash, contact, scald, chemical, and electric.

Flame and flash injuries are the second most common types of burn injury and are commonly associated with an inhalation injury if the burn has occurred in a closed space. These injuries may occur from house fires (caused by smoking in bed, children playing with matches) or ignited gasoline or propane. Injuries may be combined-partial and full-thickness burns. The amount and duration of the flame will determine the depth of injury.

*Contact burns* occur from direct contact with a hot substance, such as hot metal, stoves, hot tar, or irons. The area of burn is usually confined to the area where the substance came into contact with the skin.

*Scald burns* are the most common burn injury, particularly in children. Scald injury may be caused by steam or hot fluids and may affect a widespread area (Figure 68-6).

*Chemical burns,* commonly seen in industry, are caused by strong acids or alkali, such as hydrochloric

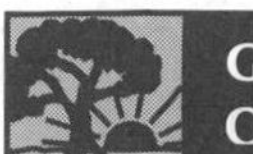

## GERONTOLOGIC PATIENT CONSIDERATIONS

### EPIDEMIOLOGY

Incidence of burn injury in the home is disproportionately higher than for younger adults.
One third of all deaths in residential fires are in elderly persons.
Elderly persons are at a higher risk for burn injury because of:
- Thinner skin, which is less resistant to heat
- Decreased mobility and reaction time
- Visual and hearing impairments that decrease ability to evaluate danger
- Living in older homes, which may have faulty wiring, poor heating systems, absence of smoke detectors

Flame injury is the most common type of burn injury.
Scald more common in younger age groups.
Inhalation injury is more common in elderly persons because of their inability to escape.

### AGING CHANGES AFFECT RECOVERY FROM BURN INJURY

Overall mortality is higher than in younger adults.
Reserve capacity of organ systems is diminished.
Cardiovascular system:
- Cardiac response to burn shock is impaired because of:
  - Lower cardiac output
  - Coronary atherosclerosis
  - Decreased baroreceptor response to volume changes
- All of these put elderly persons at risk for cardiac failure.

Pulmonary:
- Decreased elasticity of thoracic cage and decreased number and efficiency of alveoli make elderly persons more prone to hypoxia, hypoventilation, and atelectasis.

Immunologic:
- Elderly persons have diminished host resistance, impaired cell-mediated and humoral immunity.
- Elderly persons are more prone to infection and sepsis and have decreased ability to combat infection.

Wound healing:
- Diminished inflammatory response.
- Increased healing time.
- Decreased tolerance of wound excision and grafting.

### MANAGEMENT CONSIDERATIONS

Carefully assess cardiac status during burn resuscitation.
Monitor response to fluid volume administration:
- Hypotension
- Monitor breath sounds for onset of pulmonary edema
- May require the use of pulmonary artery catheter to adequately evaluate
- Urinary output

Monitor for early signs of respiratory failure.
Mobilize patient as soon as possible.
Provide pulmonary toilet.
Prevent infection.
Monitor for early signs of complications such as mental status changes, ileus, wound drainage, temperature changes (especially hypothermia).
Promote nutritional intake.
Provide thorough wound care.

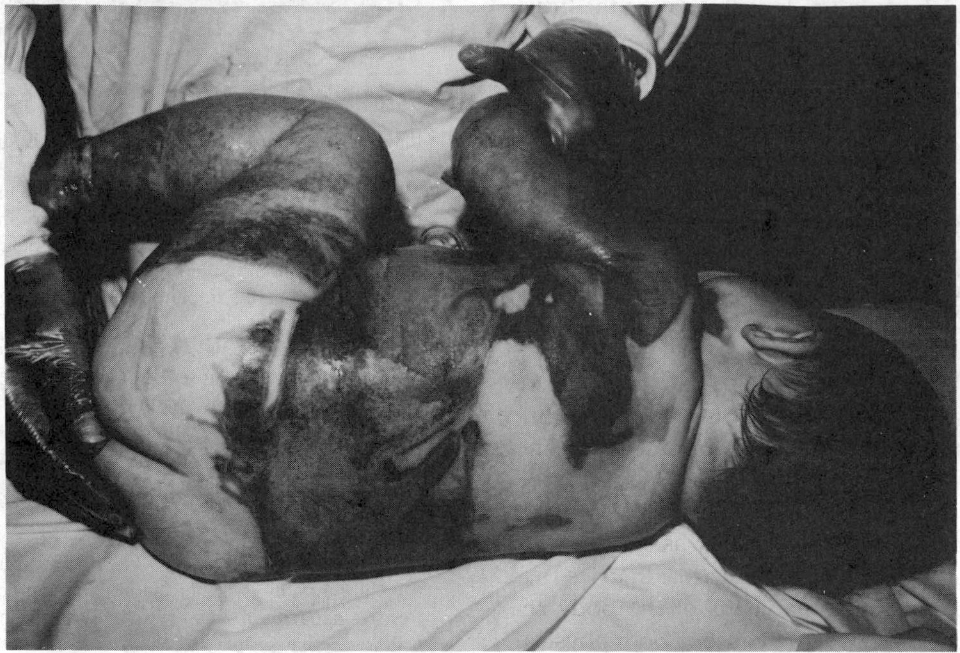

**FIGURE 68-6** Toddler with scald burn resulting from being placed in bath water that was too hot. (Courtesy Burn Center, MetroHealth Medical Center, Cleveland.)

acid and lye (Table 68-5). Household chemical burns may occur from accidental exposure to drain cleaners, paint removers, and disinfectants. Serious burns to the eye may occur when a chemical splashes onto the face. Burns to the upper gastrointestinal tract occur when a noxious chemical is ingested.

*Electrical burns* comprise a small percentage of burn injuries and may be caused by lightning, or by direct or alternating current. Injury occurs as an electrical current passes directly through the body. Tissue with the highest water content has the least resistance to electrical current and consequently, suffers the most damage. Blood, muscles, skin, tendons, fat, and bones are affected in a decreasing order of resistance. Tissue damage may appear minor at the entrance point, making electrical burns difficult to evaluate. The visual damage is referred to as the "tip of the iceberg" and does not reflect underlying tissue destruction generated as electrical current passes through the body. Victims of electrical burns must be checked frequently for signs and symptoms of hemorrhage, intestinal perforation, and cardiac dysrhythmias. The passage of current through the body may cause cardiac arrest at the time of injury.

**BOX 68-3 Factors Determining Severity of Burns**

- Size of burn
- Depth of burn
- Age of victim
- Body part involved
- Mechanism of injury
- History of cardiac, pulmonary, renal, or hepatic disease
- Injuries sustained at time of burn

Factors determining the severity of burns are listed in Box 68-3.

## ♦ NURSING DIAGNOSES

Nursing diagnoses are determined from analyses of patient data. Nursing diagnoses for the person with burns during the emergent period may include but are not limited to the following:

| Diagnostic Title |
|---|
| Airway clearance, ineffective |
| Fluid volume deficit |
| Fluid volume excess |
| Hypothermia |
| Infection, high risk for |
| Pain |
| Skin integrity, impaired |
| Anxiety |
| Knowledge |

Table 68-6 summarizes the nursing diagnoses, possible etiologic factors, and expected patient outcomes during the emergent period.

## ♦ INTERVENTIONS

### Maintaining a Patent Airway

Persons who are burned on the face and neck or those who have inhaled flame, steam, or smoke are observed closely for signs of laryngeal edema and airway obstruc-

**TABLE 68-5 Agents Associated With Chemical Burns**

| CHEMICAL AGENT | COMMON USE | CHARACTERISTICS | SYSTEMIC EFFECTS | AGENTS TO REMOVE OR DILUTE CHEMICALS |
|---|---|---|---|---|
| **OXIDIZING AGENTS** | | | | |
| Chromic acid | Metal cleansing | Ulcerates, blisters | | Water lavage |
| Potassium permanganate | Disinfectant, bleach, deodorizes | Thick, brownish purple eschar | | Water lavage<br>Eggwhite solution |
| Sodium hypochlorite (Clorox) | Disinfectants, bleach, deodorizers | Local irritation, inflammation | | Water lavage<br>Milk<br>Eggwhite<br>Starch Paste |
| **CORROSIVE AGENTS** | | | | |
| Phenol | Deodorants; sanitizers; disinfectants; manufacture of plastics, dyes, fertilizers, explosives | Soft white eschar, brown stain when eschar removed, mild to absent pain | Minor exposure: tachycardia, arrhythmias | Copious water lavage<br>Polyethelene glycol solution<br>Vegetable oil |
| | | | Significant exposure: CNS depression, hypothermia, cardiac depression, respiratory depression | Lavage with water to debride particles |
| Phosphorus (white) | Manufacture of explosives, insecticides, rodent poisons, fertilizers | Necrotic with yellowish color<br>Garlic odor<br>Glows in dark<br>Painful | Nephrotoxic<br>Hepatic necrosis | Lavage with 1% copper sulfate ($CuSO_4$)<br>Cover with castor oil |
| Pure sodium<br>Lye<br>KOH<br>NaOH<br>$NH_4OH$<br>LiOH<br>$Ba_2(OH)_3$<br>$Ca(OH)_3$ | Cleaning agents (washing powders, drain cleaners, paint removers), urine sugar reagent tablets, Portland cement | Soft gelatinous, brown eschar | | Lye; water lavage<br>Pure sodium; oil immersion |
| **PROTOPLASMIC POISONS** | | | | |
| Salt-formers<br>Tungstic<br>Picric<br>Sulfasalicyclic<br>Tannic<br>Trichloracetic<br>Cresylic<br>Acetate<br>Formic | Industrial | Thin, hard eschar | Hepatic necrosis<br>Nephrotoxicity | Water lavage |
| Metabolic competitor/inhibitor<br>Oxalic acid | Industrial | Chalky white ulcers | Hypocalcemia | Large volume calcium salts<br>Copious water lavage<br>Intravenous calcium |
| Hydrofluoric acid | Etching of glass | Painful, deep ulcerations | Hypocalcemia | Water lavage<br>Subcutaneous calcium to area<br>Subcutaneous magnesium sulfate |

tion. Data indicating potential or existing **inhalation injury** are outlined in Box 68-4.

Adequate ventilation and oxygenation may be possible on room air; however, when any inhalation injury has occurred, it is best to give oxygen. When smoke is inhaled, carbon monoxide binds with hemoglobin, displacing oxygen. High carboxyhemoglobin levels impair tissue oxygenation resulting in tissue asphyxiation. Providing the victim with 100% oxygen by mask will reverse this condition. If the victim is in respiratory distress or has a suspected inhalation injury, intubation may be necessary.

**TABLE 68-6 Nursing Diagnoses, Etiologic Factors, Expected Patient Outcomes**

| NURSING DIAGNOSES | EMERGENT PERIOD (2-3 DAYS) | ACUTE PERIOD (DAY 3 TO WEEKS, MONTHS) | REHABILITATIVE PERIOD (WEEKS TO YEARS) |
|---|---|---|---|
| **INEFFECTIVE AIRWAY CLEARANCE** | | | |
| Etiologic factors | Tracheobronchial edema, obstruction, secretions | | |
| Expected patient outcomes | The patient maintains a patent airway, adequate oxygenation, and ventilation | | |
| **FLUID VOLUME DEFICIT (HYPOVOLEMIC STAGE)** | | | |
| Etiologic factors | Abnormal fluid loss: movement of fluid from intravascular to interstitial space; evaporation | Abnormal loss via evaporation through burn wound | |
| Expected patient outcomes | The patient exhibits signs of adequate fluid balance | The patient exhibits signs of adequate fluid balance | |
| **FLUID VOLUME EXCESS (DIURETIC STAGE)** | | | |
| Etiologic factors | Movement of fluid from interstitial to intravascular space | | |
| Expected patient outcomes | The patient exhibits signs of adequate fluid balance | | |
| **HYPOTHERMIA** | | | |
| Etiologic factors | Impaired regulatory mechanisms<br>Exposure of wounds to environment | Exposure of wounds to environment during wound care | |
| Expected patient outcomes | The patient's body temperature will be greater than 37° C | The patient's body temperature will be greater than 37° C | |
| **INFECTION, HIGH RISK FOR** | | | |
| Etiologic factors | Break in skin integrity | Break in skin integrity<br>Impaired immune response | |
| Expected patient outcomes | The patient will be free from pathogenic organisms | The patient is free from pathogenic organisms | |
| **PAIN, ACUTE** | | | |
| Etiologic factors | Exposed nerve endings, trauma | Exposed nerve endings, immobility | |
| Expected patient outcomes | The patient reports decreased pain | The patient reports decreased pain | |
| **PAIN, CHRONIC** | | | |
| | | | Joint, tissue contracture |
| | | | The patient reports decreased pain |
| **SKIN INTEGRITY, IMPAIRED** | | | |
| Etiologic factors | Burn injury, impaired perfusion | Burn injury, nutritional deficit | |
| Expected patient outcomes | The patient exhibits absence of further tissue loss | The burn wound is clean and exhibits healing | |
| **SKIN INTEGRITY, IMPAIRED, HIGH RISK FOR** | | | |
| | | | Nutritional deficit, fragile new tissue |
| | | | The patient's healed tissue remains intact |
| **ANXIETY** | | | |
| Etiologic factors | Threat of death, situational crisis | Change in health status/role functioning; situational crisis | Changes in health status, role functioning, socioeconomic status |
| Expected patient outcomes | The patient verbalizes concerns and demonstrates positive coping mechanisms | The patient exhibits functional coping mechanisms | The patient exhibits functional coping mechanisms |

**TABLE 68-6 Nursing Diagnoses, Etiologic Factors, Expected Patient Outcomes—cont'd**

| NURSING DIAGNOSES | EMERGENT PERIOD (2-3 DAYS) | ACUTE PERIOD (DAY 3 TO WEEKS, MONTHS) | REHABILITATIVE PERIOD (WEEKS TO YEARS) |
|---|---|---|---|
| **KNOWLEDGE DEFICIT** | | | |
| Etiologic factors | Unfamiliarity with burn injury | Unfamiliarity with burn injury | Unfamiliarity with burn injury |
| Expected patient outcomes | The patient verbalizes understanding of injury and treatment | The patient verbalizes understanding of treatments and participates in care | The patient verbalizes understanding of treatments, demonstrates wound care, exercises |
| **NUTRITION, ALTERED: LESS THAN BODY REQUIREMENTS** | | | |
| Etiologic factors | | Increased metabolic needs, protein losses through wounds, decreased appetite | |
| Expected patient outcomes | | The patient exhibits positive nitrogen balance and wound healing | |
| **IMMOBILITY, IMPAIRED PHYSICAL** | | | |
| Etiologic factors | | Pain, splinting postgraft procedure, activity intolerance, depression, decreased strength and endurance | Pain, decreased strength and endurance |
| Expected patient outcomes | | The patient maintains full range of motion | The patient achieves full range of motion and physical activity consistent with desired levels |
| **COPING, INEFFECTIVE INDIVIDUAL** | | | |
| Etiologic factors | | Situational crisis, personal vulnerability, ineffective support systems | Situational crisis, ineffective support systems |
| Expected patient outcomes | | The patient demonstrates effective coping mechanisms | The patient demonstrates effective coping mechanism and develops realistic plan for the future |
| **COPING, INEFFECTIVE FAMILY, COMPROMISED** | | | |
| Etiologic factors | | Inadequate or incorrect information; temporary family disorganization; role changes | Inadequate or incorrect information; temporary family disorganization, role changes |
| Expected patient outcomes | | The family demonstrates effective coping mechanisms | The family demonstrates effective coping mechanisms |
| **BODY IMAGE DISTURBANCE** | | | |
| Etiologic factors | | Loss/change of body parts, function | Loss/change of body parts, function |
| Expected patient outcomes | | The patient develops a realistic image of self and makes alterations needed in daily activities | The patient develops a realistic image of self and makes alterations needed in daily activities |
| **SELF-CARE DEFICIT** | | | |
| Etiologic factors | | Intolerance to activity, pain, musculoskeletal impairment | Intolerance to activity, musculoskeletal impairment |
| Expected patient outcomes | | The patient demonstrates increased ability to perform ADLs | The patient performs ADLs |

**BOX 68-4 Factors Determining Inhalation Injury and/or Potential Airway Obstruction**

Burns to face and neck
Singed hairs, nasal hair, beard, eyelids or eyelashes
Intraoral charcoal, especially on teeth and gums
Brassy cough
Hoarseness
Copious sputum production
Carbonaceous sputum
Burn injury that has occurred in a closed space
Smell of smoke on victim's clothes or on victim
Respiratory distress

## Prehospital Care and First Aid

At the scene of a burn injury, the first action should be to remove the victim from the hazardous environment. Length of exposure to the causative agent is directly related to the severity of the injury. Initial management follows the ABCs: airway, breathing, circulation.

The most common causative agents for burn injury are fire, scalding fluids, chemicals, and electricity. Regardless of the cause, the burning process must be stopped. In the case of fire, flames should be extinguished, flammable or hot material removed from the victim, and the victim and rescuer removed from the unventilated or hazardous surroundings. If clothing is on fire, the victim's first reaction is to run, which only fans the flames. The best intervention is to stop the person, wrap him or her in a blanket, coat, sheet, or towel and roll on the ground to exclude oxygen and thereby put out the fire. The rule is stop, drop, and roll. The victim should never stand because this will cause the flames and smoke to engulf the facial area, possibly igniting the hair and causing an inhalation injury. Any water source can be used to extinguish flames, cool the burn, or dilute the chemical unless the victim is still in contact with an electrical source.

Once all flame is extinguished, clothing (excepting clothing that adheres to the burned area), jewelry, and debris are carefully removed. Any clothing removed should be saved for possible analysis of flammability. The wounds are covered with dressings dampened with normal saline to ease the pain, reduce edema, and prevent evaporation of body water. The patient is entirely wrapped in a dry cover to prevent heat loss. Ice should never be used because sudden vasoconstriction causes severe shifting of body fluids and may increase the depth of injury. Although sterile dressings are preferred, clean nonsterile dressings can be used, because all dressings will be removed at the medical facility. Oils, salves, and ointments should never be used on burns because they hamper treatment at the medical facility.

Scald injury is related to the temperature of the liquid and length of exposure. Initial care consists of cooling the skin with cool water. First aid allows the same treatment plan as for a flame burn, that is, stop the burning process.

The severity of *chemical* burns is directly proportional to the duration of exposure. Chemicals cause deep burns over a rather limited surface. The chemical should be identified, and treatment initiated quickly. The first priority is removal of the chemical agent. This is accomplished by copious flushing with water for as long as 20 to 30 minutes to ensure complete removal of the destructive agent. Although specific chemical agents have known antidotes, it is best to flood the exposed area with water to ensure removal and transport the victim to the nearest medical facility. Burns occurring about the eyes should be lavaged continuously with copious amounts of cool, clean water for up to 30 minutes.

*Electrical* burns pose a special hazard to the victim because the total body surface area of the burn is not always apparent and is often internal. Dysrhythmias and neurologic dysfunction are common in such exposure. Extreme care must be taken when removing the patient from the electrical source to prevent a similar injury to the rescuer (see Chapter 28).

### Pain Relief

In the prehospital period, pain in extensive burns is best controlled by gentle and minimal handling and by the application of dressings to exclude air from the burned surfaces. The degree of pain is usually inversely proportional to the depth of the burn injury; that is, full-thickness burns are usually painless, because nerve endings have been destroyed.

In small partial-thickness burns, cool (not cold) compresses on the burn site may provide some relief as long as the victim is kept warm. Ice packs are contraindicated because they may cause further skin injury and hypothermia.

### Transport

Burns are often more severe than they first appear; therefore, even if the burns appear superficial, all persons with burns should be seen by a physician. The hospital or burn center should be notified before transporting a severely burned victim so that preparation can be made for arrival.

For obviously small burns, fluids may be given by mouth with caution. Large burns are accompanied by decreased peristalsis; therefore, nothing should be given by mouth. Patients with large burns or smoke inhalation may vomit, so particular attention is given to preventing them from aspirating vomitus.

According to the 1991 to 1992 American Burn Association Directory, 148 hospitals in the United States reported the presence of a specialized burn care ser-

**Guidelines for Initial Treatment of Major Burns in Emergency Room**

1. Establish airway.
2. Initiate fluid therapy by intravenous catheters.
3. Insert indwelling catheter for hourly urine measurement.
4. Insert nasogastric tube to remove stomach contents and prevent gastric distention.
5. Insert central intravenous catheter, if appropriate.
6. Manage pain by intravenous narcotics in small frequent doses.
7. Provide tetanus prophylaxis.

vice.[6] This represents a 12% reduction in burn beds from 1985 to 1992. These burn units are located throughout the United States in major medical centers in urban areas. The American Burn Association publishes a list of specialized burn care services every year.

## Emergency Room Management

Rapid and efficient care is essential in the emergency room management of the victim with a **major burn** (see Guidelines box above). If any respiratory distress is present, an airway is established. Prophylactic intubation is initiated if any heat or smoke has been inhaled or if the head, neck, or face is involved. Inhalation injuries are best managed with controlled ventilation because swelling of the upper airway can progress to obstruction (Figure 68-7). Endotracheal intubation is preferred over a tracheostomy. Edema of the respiratory passages frequently subsides within a few days after the initial injury; therefore surgery of the airway should be avoided. Depending on the severity of symptoms, emergency treatment may include oxygen, suctioning, and postural drainage.

After an airway has been established, support of circulation is addressed. Burn injuries cause tremendous losses of fluid through the wound as well as into the burn wound and adjacent tissues in the form of edema. Fluid is best replaced through two large-caliber peripheral intravenous catheters. Placement of these lines is through an unburned site to prevent the introduction of infection. An indwelling urinary catheter is inserted to adequately monitor urine output. Hourly urine output measurements are used as a guide to the adequacy of fluid (plasma volume) replacement.

Almost every patient who is burned more than 15% of BSA develops thirst and an ileus. Oral fluids will not pass beyond the stomach (therefore, they will not relieve thirst), and they create a threat of regurgitation and aspiration. A nasogastric tube is inserted, and the stomach is kept empty by suction to prevent gastric distention.

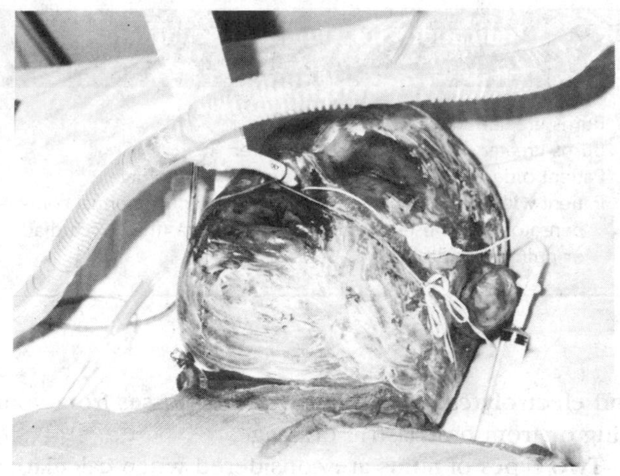

**FIGURE 68-7** Patient with severe edema 5 hours after burn occurred. Airway was managed with endotracheal intubation. Edema subsided, and patient was extubated 4 days after admission. (Courtesy Burn Center, MetroHealth Medical Center, Cleveland.)

## Promoting Comfort

Morphine sulfate is the drug of choice for pain relief and is given intravenously in small increments (2 to 4 mg). A morphine sulfate drip can be used and titrated to the patient's pain. *No medication of any kind should be given intramuscularly or subcutaneously because it may pool and be absorbed later when cardiac output and blood pressure improve.* Large doses of sedatives and analgesics are avoided because of the danger of respiratory depression and the potential of masking other symptoms.

Tetanus prophylaxis is initiated in the emergency room. Tetanus toxoid is administered if the patient has been previously immunized but has not received tetanus toxoid in the preceding 5 years. If prior tetanus immunization is not documented, a dose of human tetanus-immune globulin hormone (TIGH) is administered, and an active tetanus immunization program begun.

## Fluid Resuscitation

Replacing fluids and electrolytes (fluid resuscitation) is an essential part of the treatment of burn victims and is instituted as soon as the severity of the burn and the patient's condition is known (Box 68-5). Ideally, fluid therapy is started within an hour after a severe burn to prevent the onset of hypovolemic shock. Insertion of two large-caliber peripheral catheters or one large-caliber central venous catheter and one large-caliber peripheral catheter permits the rapid administration of fluids and electrolytes.

Fluids administered during the first 48 hours are given to maintain circulating blood volume. Additional fluids

**BOX 68-5 Indications for Fluid Resuscitation**

Burns greater than 20% BSA in adults
Burns greater than 10% BSA in children
Patient older than 65 or younger than 2 years of age
Patient with preexisting disease that would reduce normal compensatory responses to minor hypovolemia (that is, cardiac or pulmonary disease, diabetes)

and electrolytes are added to replace losses from vomiting or from nasogastric drainage.

Two types of fluids are considered when calculating the needs of the patient: crystalloids and colloids. *Crystalloids* may be isotonic or hypertonic. Isotonic solutions, such as lactated Ringer's or physiologic (0.9%) sodium chloride, do not generate a difference in osmotic pressure between the intravascular and interstitial spaces. Thus large amounts of fluids are required to restore and maintain the intravascular volume. Hypertonic salt solutions have a milliosmolar content of 400 to 600 (280 to 300 mosm is isotonic), thus creating an osmotic pull of fluid from the interstitial space back to the depleted intravascular space. The use of hypertonic solutions has helped decrease the amount of fluid a patient needs during resuscitation,[10] which helps decrease burn tissue edema and minimizes cardiopulmonary complications (pulmonary edema, congestive heart failure).

In the first three 8-hour periods (24 hours) lactated Ringer's solution (RL) is administered according to the following formula:

4 ml RL × weight (kg) × % BSA burned = ml RL for the first 24 hours

Because blood volume falls most rapidly and edema increases fastest in the first 8 hours, intravenous replacement is accomplished at a rapid rate. One half of the total amount calculated is given in the first 8 hours after the injury. *The time is calculated from the time of injury,* not from the time emergency care was initiated. In the second 8-hour period, one fourth of the total amount of calculated lactated Ringer's solution is given and in the third 8-hour period, the remaining one fourth is given. For example, if a patient weighing 75 kg has a 70% total body surface area (TBSA) burn, the fluid requirements are:

1. 4 ml lactated Ringer's × 75 Kg × 70% = 21,000 ml needed over the first 24 hours
2. one half is needed in the first 8 hours
   ½ × 21,000 = 10,500 ml in 8 hours, or 1312 ml/hr
3. one fourth is needed in each of the next two 8-hour periods
   ¼ × 21,000 = 5250 ml in 8 hours, or 656 ml/hr

*Colloids* may also be used to replace body fluids. Traditionally, the use of colloids in the first 24 hours was avoided because of the leak of protein through the capillaries into the interstitial space. The capillary permeability caused by the burn injury begins to close at 12 hours. At this time patients may receive colloids such as fresh-frozen plasma, albumin, or dextran. The oncotic pressure generated by the colloids also helps pull fluid back into the intravascular space. In addition, fresh-frozen plasma is beneficial in restoring lost clotting factors. Red blood cells are used only if the patient has had a significant loss or destruction of red cells.

Several formulas are used to calculate fluid requirements.[13] Medical authorities do not agree about the proportion of colloids and crystalloids needed. The amount of fluid administered is based on the patient's weight, age, and percentage of the body burned. The Parkland formula is a common method used to eliminate fluid requirements.

Patients may complain of moderate to severe thirst during this period. Aggressive oral hygiene may alleviate patient discomfort. If oral fluids are permitted, accurate recording of ingested fluids is important. Unlimited oral intake and failure to measure it may provide too much fluid in the circulating blood, resulting in water intoxication.

During the second 24 hours postburn, one half to two thirds of the initial 24-hour volume is required. It is also during this second 24-hour period that colloid solutions are used to replete intravascular volume once capillary permeability significantly decreases.

During fluid resuscitation, adequate volume is assessed by monitoring mental status, vital signs, peripheral perfusion, body weight, and urine output. A 15% to 20% weight gain in the first 72 hours of resuscitation is anticipated. Significant laboratory measurements include serum and urine electrolytes, serum and urine osmolality, and hematocrit. Hourly urine output is the most accessible and generally a reliable index of adequate fluid replacement. Fluid should be titrated to ensure an output of 30 to 50 ml/hr in the adult or 0.5 to 1 ml/kg/hr in the child. The most common reasons for a drop in urine output below 30 ml/hr, indicating insufficient fluid replacement, are that the calculated fluids are behind schedule and the severity of the burn has been underestimated. The urine is observed for color and analyzed for the presence of blood. The physician is notified if hematuria or a positive Hemastix reaction is present.

Other clinical criteria that indicate adequate resuscitation are pulse rate of 120 beats/min or less in the adult, CVP in low to normal range, pulmonary artery end-diastolic pressure (PAEDP) in low to normal range, and mental lucidity (see Box 68-6).

A decreasing blood pH is an indication that fluids have not been given in sufficient quantities to maximize tissue perfusion. Anaerobic metabolism ensues when the met-

**BOX 68-6 Signs of Adequate Resuscitation**

Clear sensorium
Pulse <120 beats/min
Urine output: 30 to 50 ml/hr (adult)
0.5 to 1 ml/kg/hr (child)
Systolic blood pressure: 100 mm Hg
CVP: 5 to 10 mm Hg
PAEDP: 5 to 15 mm Hg
Blood pH normal range: 7.35 to 7.45

abolic tissue requirements are not met during resuscitation.

After the first 48 to 72 hours, the patient enters the diuretic stage or phase as edema reabsorption occurs. The urinary output increases dramatically and is no longer a reliable guide to fluid needs. Fluid needs are assessed by measuring serum and urine electrolyte levels. Fluid replacement, using 5% dextrose and water, is based on individual assessment. If dehydration occurs from diuresis, fluid replacement therapy is continued until blood volume is stabilized. Potassium may be added to the intravenous fluid because of potassium losses in the urine. The patient is monitored closely for signs of water intoxication or pulmonary edema.

## Initial Wound Care

Care of the burn wound can be delayed until all first aid measures have been initiated. Wound care should be carried out carefully and with as little discomfort to the patient as possible. One of the most important factors to be considered in wound care is that the patient has lost the ability to withstand infection in the area where the skin is damaged or destroyed. The goals of the initial wound care are as follows:

1. Cleanse the wound to eliminate or decrease the dead tissue and debris that serve as the media for bacterial growth
2. Prevent further destruction of viable skin
3. Provide for patient comfort

During the admission procedure, the burn wound and the entire body are washed to remove dirt and debris as well as loose dead tissue on the burned areas. Detergents or antiseptic preparations are effective cleansing agents. Gentle cleansing with gauze is effective in removing dead tissue without causing further tissue damage.

All hair in and around the burn wound is shaved and wiped off the skin because hair attracts and shelters bacteria. Singed hair is clipped short to avoid bacterial contamination of the wound.

Firm, intact blisters can remain undisturbed because they are a natural protective and pain-free dressing. If the blisters are broken and the epidermis is separated, loose tissue must be debrided.

After the wound is cleaned and before a dressing is applied, cultures of the wound are obtained. Baseline cultures provide information about organisms present in the wounds at the time of admission. Prophylactic antibiotics are usually not indicated.

Photographs are taken on admission and at intervals during the patient's hospitalization. These pictures provide a record of the appearance of the burn wound on admission, before the application of topical therapy, and during the healing process.

The constricting effect of nonviable tissue **(eschar)** from a full-thickness injury to the chest, neck, or extremities is an early complication. Edema forming rapidly under the constricting eschar will produce a tourniquet effect that causes occlusion of venous and arterial circulation and may result in *ischemic necrosis,* especially with unburned areas distal to the constrictive eschar. Frequent monitoring of distal pulses is part of an ongoing assessment to ensure uninterrupted vascular flow to all extremities. Extremities should be monitored for signs and symptoms of circulatory compromise, including diminished peripheral pulses, decreased capillary refill, paleness or cyanosis, temperature decrease, and increase in pain or paresthesia. It may be necessary to monitor circulation every 15 minutes.

Circumferential burns of the neck and chest can lead to constriction of chest wall expansion and airway compromise resulting in respiratory distress. Monitoring chest excursions, respiratory rate, and ventilator settings, if intubated for high pressures and low tidal volume, are part of the respiratory assessment.

The treatment of the constricting effects of the eschar is the performance of an *escharotomy.* An escharotomy is a linear surgical incision through the burn eschar that releases the constriction caused by the full-thickness injury (Figure 68-8). Escharotomies are painless procedures because the nerve endings have been damaged by the burn.

## Maintaining Body Temperature

Maintenance of body temperature is a critical factor for the severely burned patient because of the loss of some of the ability to regulate body temperature. The environment must be heat controlled and kept warmer than usual. Drafts must be eliminated. A heat lamp or warming lights should be available. Prolonged exposure to air is avoided. Exposed areas of the body are covered with sterile sheets and blankets to decrease the loss of body heat through the open wounds while other areas of the burn are being cleansed.

## Providing Emotional Support

Patients with significant burn injury receive a profound insult to their body and self-image. There is fear and anxiety associated with scarring and disfigurement. There is an awareness that they may not survive, enhancing feelings of fear and helplessness. The shock and

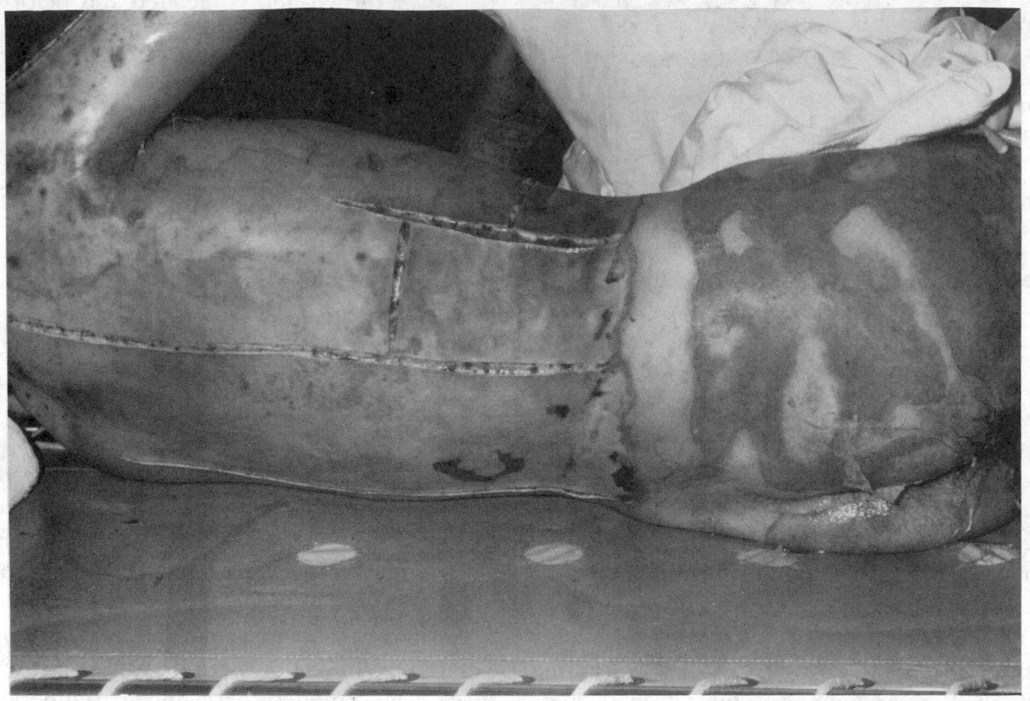

**FIGURE 68-8** Linear escharotomy used to alleviate circulatory and pulmonary constriction. (Courtesy Burn Center, MetroHealth Medical Center, Cleveland.)

pain of the accident, the chaos and rush to the hospital, and the unknown surroundings and people all intensify the emotional stress.

The nurse spends the most time with the patient and has a considerable influence on the patient's psychologic adjustment. Interventions that can be used to reassure the patient and alleviate anxiety include the following:

1. Identify self to patient.
2. Orient patient to the surroundings.
3. Describe basis of physical symptoms (skin loss, pain, cold).
4. Explain the equipment and procedures to be used in treatment.

## ♦ EVALUATION

To evaluate effectiveness of nursing interventions, compare patient's behaviors with those stated in the expected outcomes. Indications of successful achievement of patient outcomes for the patient with burns follow.

### Emergent Phase

1. Patent airway, adequate ventilation, and oxygenation.
   a. Absence of stridor and adventitious breath sounds
   b. $PO_2$ greater than 80 and $PCO_2$ less than 45
   c. Carboxyhemoglobin level <10%
2. Optimal fluid and electrolyte balance is regained and maintained.
   a. Urinary output is 30 to 50 ml/hr in adults or 1 to 2 ml/kg/hr in children
   b. Electrolytes are within normal limits
   c. Normal sensorium
   d. Systolic blood pressure >100 mm Hg
   e. Heart rate <120 beats/min
   f. pH between 7.35 to 7.45
3. Normal body temperature is maintained.
   a. Body temperature between 37 to 38.5° C

### Acute Period

#### Medical management

The acute period of treatment begins at the end of the emergent period and lasts until the burn wound is healed. The length of this period varies. If the burn is a partial-thickness injury, the acute period extends for 10 to 20 days; if the burn is a full-thickness injury over a large percentage of the body requiring surgery for skin grafting, the acute period could last for months.

During the acute period there are two main principles of management: (1) treatment of the burn wound; and (2) avoidance, detection, and treatment of complications. The most common complications are infection (septicemia and pneumonia), renal disease, and heart failure.

## NURSING MANAGEMENT

### ♦ ASSESSMENT

#### Subjective Data

Burn patients are often frightened and anxious about their injury and the associated treatments. These responses can be compounded by the intensive care unit (ICU) environment.

Burn patients experience both physical and psychologic pain. Physical pain is usually focused on specific activities such as wound cleansing and debridement, dressing changes, and physical therapy. The patient may react to physical pain in three ways: (1) by ignoring it, (2) by accepting it, or (3) by overreacting to it. The nurse should not judge whether the patient is feeling real pain; the nurse must instead assess the patient's reaction to pain and intervene appropriately.

#### Objective Data

The nurse must perform a thorough head-to-toe assessment of the burn patient every 8 hours. Data should include mental status; vital signs; breath sounds; bowel sounds; dietary intake; motor ability; intake and output; weight pattern; circulatory assessment; and observation of burn wounds, grafts, and donor site. Purulent drainage, abnormal color, foul odor, redness or swelling in surrounding normal skin, or presence of healing should be noted. Changes in these parameters from shift to shift or from day to day make further investigation necessary.

Metabolism is increased after moderate to severe burns as a result of stress, fluid loss, fever, infection, increased metabolism, and immobility. Wound healing may be prolonged if adequate nutritional support is not initiated on admission. A nutritional assessment is performed during the first days after burn injury and includes anthropometric measurements (to determine actual weight loss compared to ideal weight), serum electrolytes, liver function test, and urinalysis.

### ♦ NURSING DIAGNOSES

Nursing diagnoses are determined from analysis of patient data. Possible nursing diagnoses for the person with burns during the acute phase may include but are not limited to the following:

| Diagnostic Title |
|---|
| Skin integrity, impaired |
| Infection, high risk for |
| Altered nutrition: less than body requirements |
| Pain, acute |
| Fluid volume deficit |
| Anxiety |
| Hypothermia |
| Coping, ineffective individual |
| Coping, ineffective family |
| Body image disturbance |
| Knowledge deficit |
| Mobility, impaired physical |
| Self-care deficit |

See Table 68-6 for a summary of the nursing diagnoses, possible etiologic factors, and expected outcomes for the patient during the acute period.

### ♦ INTERVENTIONS

#### Relieving Anxiety

A burn injury is a sudden, unexpected event. Its impact on psychologic well-being is enormous, and promoting mental health is a major area of the burn-injured patient's care. The psychologic responses in the emergent period are in response to the threat of survival. During the acute period, a variety of behaviors may be seen.[4] (See Table 68-7 for a summary of psychologic responses.) As the patient becomes more aware of the extent of the injury and begins to evaluate its implications on his or her life, many problems may occur that affect the ability of both the patient and family to cope with the situation.

Nursing plays a major role in maintaining and restoring the patient to mental health. Ongoing education is imperative to assist the patient to understand the care given and to make realistic plans for the future. It is important for the patient to maintain a sense of hope for the future in order to resume a normal life after a burn injury. Without hope, the patient will have a decreased ability to cope, a sense of failure, and less gratifying interpersonal relationships.[3]

Those individuals who adjust well after burn injury have characteristics in common. Patients who have had positive coping mechanisms before injury are better able to deal with the consequences of a burn injury. In addition, they have family and social support available, can engage others in their care, and are able to revise their self-image in a realistic but positive manner.

Burn-injured patients are also at risk for the development of posttraumatic stress disorder (PTSD). This condition was first classified as a separate entity in 1980 by the American Psychiatric Association. Symptoms occur after a psychologically traumatic event that would be considered outside the range of normal human experience.[2] Symptoms of PTSD include the following:

1. Reexperiencing the trauma through dreams or intrusive recollections
2. A numbed response to the environment, such as decreased interest or detachment
3. An exaggerated startle response
4. Sleep disturbance
5. Guilt about having survived
6. Avoidance of activities that arouse recollections of the event

**TABLE 68-7 Psychologic Reactions to Severe Burns**

| DEFINITION | BEHAVIOR EXHIBITED | NURSING APPROACH |
|---|---|---|
| **CONSERVATION, WITHDRAWAL** | | |
| Decreased interaction with environment as an immediate response to serious injury<br>Occurs immediately after injury and may last for first 1-2 weeks<br>Protective value to self (may be mistaken for depression) | Decreased interaction with environment, staff, family<br>Keeps eyes closed frequently, sleeps, remains immobile | Avoid forcing patient to deal with situation<br>Supportive environment<br>Provide ongoing information on status and care |
| **DENIAL** | | |
| Protective, unconscious defense mechanism<br>Helps relieve anxiety due to threat of life, limb, self | Patient denies extent of injury, loss of limb, loss of others in accident<br>May acknowledge the loss but not the impact | Support patient<br>Avoid forcing patient to deal with fears<br>Answer questions honestly<br>Provide information in small doses over time |
| **REGRESSION** | | |
| Patient returns to earlier ways of coping with stress<br>May exhibit childlike behaviors | Assertive, demanding, temper tantrums<br>Tearful, cling to dependent relationships | Avoid attacking and responding negatively to behavior exhibited<br>Acknowledge patient's difficulty in coping<br>Encourage and reward positive behaviors and independence |
| **ANGER AND HOSTILITY** | | |
| Angry, agitated behavior in response to a perceived wrong, loss of control<br>Grieving response | Angry, agitated, hostile to staff and family | Encourage verbalization of frustration<br>Avoid responding directly to anger<br>Provide choices and control<br>Assist patient to search for meaning to injury |
| **DEPRESSION** | | |
| The extent of injury becomes distorted and impacts the patient's sense of worthiness and self-esteem | Degrading comments about self<br>Sleep disturbances, decreased appetite, generalized slowing, poor motivation | Acknowledge the loss<br>Focus patient on realistic expectations |
| **ANXIETY** | | |
| Fear and threat to self as a result of injury | Restlessness, agitation, difficulty in following instructions, poor memory, easily startled | Support patient<br>Acknowledge fears<br>Provide information in small frequent doses |

Posttraumatic stress disorder may be present in as many as one third of all burn patients, and at least 60% exhibit some of the symptoms, such as intrusive recollections of the event or dreams. Factors that influence the onset of PTSD include an extensive injury and a prolonged hospitalization.[12]

## Preventing Infection

The burn patient is at tremendous risk for infection. Measures to prevent infection begin at the time the patient is admitted to the hospital and continue until healing is complete. The break in skin integrity destroys the body's first line of defense. In addition, changes in the immune system occur as a result of the burn injury, creating a state of immunosuppression postburn. Inflammatory substances (histamine, bradykinins, leukotrienes) are released from the damaged tissue and affect both humoral and cell-mediated immunity.[8] The nutritional deficit that occurs also decreases the burn patient's ability to fight infection.

Sources of infection may be *endogenous* or *exogenous.* Bacteria that survive in the hair follicles and glands are a source of endogenous infection. In addition, after burn injury, bacteria that normally live in the intestinal tract migrate or translocate across the intestinal wall and spread to the general circulation by way of the lymphatic system.[7] Local and systemic infections (septicemia) are the most common complications of burns and are the major cause of death, particularly in burns covering more than 25% of the body. The organisms that usually infect burns are *Staphylococcus aureus, Pseudomonas aeruginosa,* and the coliform bacilli. These organisms are normally found on the skin or in the intestine and become a source of infection. Methicillin-resistant *S. aureus* has become more prevalent and affects the healing process of wounds and grafts. Fungal infections have increased in incidence because of the use of broad-spectrum antibiotics. *Candida albicans,* which normally is found in the gastrointestinal tract, accounts for the majority of the fungal infections. Cultures of the patient's nose, throat, wound, and unburned skin and a punch biopsy may be taken on admission and at biweekly intervals to determine the presence of bacteria and their sensitivity to antibiotics.

Infection is usually the cause of any deterioration of a burn patient. Signs of infection in the burn patient include increased anxiety, purulent wound drainage, and pallor of healthy viable tissue. Signs of sepsis in the burn patient are the following:

1. Change in sensorium
2. Fever
3. Tachypnea
4. Tachycardia
5. Paralytic ileus
6. Abdominal distention
7. Oliguria

To prevent the introduction of exogenous organisms into the wound, all persons who approach the patient should wear gowns, masks, caps, and gloves. Persons with upper respiratory infections should not be permitted near the patient.

Aseptic technique and sterile gloves are used during wound care and dressing changes. Thorough wound cleansing is necessary to remove the debris that acts as a media for bacterial growth. Hydrotherapy tanks and spray tables are used for aggressive cleansing of burn wounds and can be a source of infection. They need particular attention to prevent the spread of infection when the tanks are used by different patients. Care of the severely burned patient in special burn units can contribute to decreased infection because the environment is specifically geared to infection control. If the patient is cared for in a general hospital unit, a private room is essential, and all equipment needed by the patient remains in the room. *Reverse isolation precautions* are initiated.

## Promoting Skin Integrity

Wound care during the acute period is extensive and requires expert assessment skills to monitor wounds during healing and to detect any signs of infection. The wound eschar, nonviable tissue, forms after burn injury and is conducive to bacterial growth because it contains dead tissue, moisture, and warmth. Daily cleansing and mechanical debridement help remove the eschar. Washing and friction remove the buildup of debris and support healthy tissue regeneration. Hydrotherapy facilitates the removal of medications and loosens debris, sloughing eschar, and exudate. It is a more comfortable method for removal of dressings and facilitates range-of-motion exercise with minimal energy expenditure and discomfort. The solution used in a hydrotherapy tank may be plain water, normal saline, or an electrolytically balanced solution. To minimize the chance of infection, the nurse uses sterile technique during dressing care and maintains a clean environment as much as possible. The use of gowns, masks, gloves, aprons, goggles, and a plastic, disposable tub liner will decrease the chance of contamination between patients. Tubbing is usually performed once or twice daily and should not exceed 30 minutes to prevent exposure and chilling. Tubbing is initiated after the patient's vital signs and fluid balance have stabilized.

Hydrotherapy is contraindicated if the patient experiences any sudden changes in temperature, heart rate, blood pressure, or respiratory rate.

The current trend in wound cleansing is to use a spray table with the same isolation measures as with tubbings. The patient is placed on a special stretcher, which allows for drainage and has a hose system that allows the nurse to control water temperature and flow, thus maintaining patient comfort.

### Methods of treatment

Different methods of treating the burned area may be used, depending on the location of the burn, its size and depth, the facilities available, and the patient's response to therapy. One method may be replaced with another during the course of treatment. Those commonly used today include the open or exposure method, the semi-open method, and the closed or occlusive method.

**Open or exposure method.** The exposure of treatment was accidentally discovered to be effective in 1888 when, during a serious steamboat fire on the Mississippi River, those in attendance ran out of bandages and later observed that the neglected persons fared better than those who received more intensive local treatment. Today the exposure method is used most often in the treatment of burns involving the face, neck, perineum, and broad areas of the trunk. The burned area is cleansed and exposed to air (Figure 68-9). The exudate of a partial-thickness burn dries in 48 to 72 hours and forms a hard crust that protects the wound. Epithelialization occurs beneath this crust and may be complete in 14 to 21 days. The crust then falls off spontaneously, leaving a healed, unscarred surface. The dead skin of a full-thickness burn is dehydrated and converted to black, leathery eschar in 48 to 72 hours. Loose eschar may be gradually removed through hydrotherapy and/or debridement. Uninfected eschar acts as a protective covering. The danger of infection exists as bacteria proliferate beneath the eschar. Spontaneous separation, produced by bacterial action, occurs unless surgical debridement is performed first.

Isolation technique is essential when the exposure method is used. The nurse caring for the patient should wear a sterile gown, mask, apron, and goggles; sterile linen may be used on the bed. A cradle may be used on the bed because no clothing or bed clothes are allowed

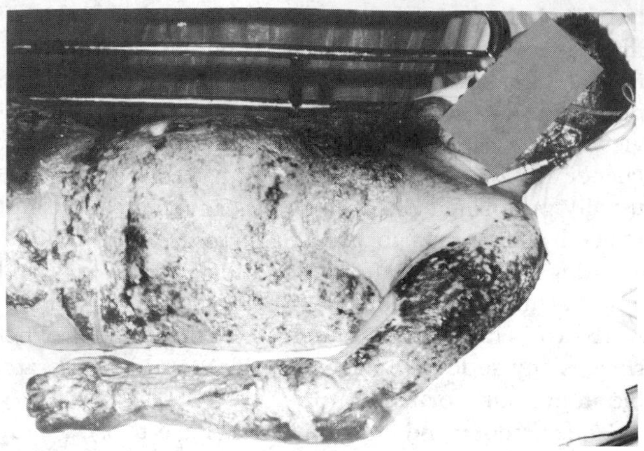

**FIGURE 68-9** Severely burned man being treated by open method. (Courtesy Burn Center, MetroHealth Medical Center, Cleveland.)

directly over burned areas. If the burn is extensive, a CircOlectric bed draped with a sheet is an ideal way to care for the patient. The patient can be kept from embarrassing exposure by wearing a halter and loin cloth. Lights or heat lamps may be used with caution to provide warmth. Advantages of the open method are that the wound is easily inspected and the patient has maximal freedom to perform exercises for the prevention of contracture and the improvement of circulation.

Patients having exposure treatment complain of pain and chilling. Pain may be controlled by administering morphine sulfate, meperidine hydrochloride (Demerol), or salicylates as ordered. Discomfort can be decreased if drafts are avoided and the temperature of the room is kept at 24.4° C (85° F). Patients lose more heat from burned surfaces than from normal skin surfaces, because the vascular bed that normally contracts and retains heat in the body is lost. The humidity of the room also should be controlled. A humidity of 40% to 50% is usually considered satisfactory. Portable electric humidifiers and dehumidifiers can be used to achieve and maintain this level.

**Semiopen method.** The semiopen wound care method consists of covering the wound with topical antimicrobial agents and a thin layer of gauze to help keep the agent in contact with the wound. This method permits the passage of wound exudate through the dressing without the loss of antimicrobial cream. The success of semiopen care depends on cleaning the wound once or twice a day, either at the bedside, in the hydrotherapy tank, or on the spray table. Meticulous semiopen wound care speeds debridement, enhances the development of granulation tissue, and makes earlier grafting possible.

**Closed method.** In the closed or occlusive method of burn treatment, the wounds are washed, and dressings changed at least once a day, or in some instances once each shift. Commonly, the dressing consists of gauze impregnated with topical ointments with a gauze wrap. Counterpressure wrappings (elastic bandages) may be applied. When a dressing is in place, nursing observation includes monitoring for signs of impaired circulation (numbness, pain, and tingling) and for signs of infection (odor on dressings, elevated temperature, and elevated pulse rate).

**Topical agents.** The application of topical agents to the burn wound can help decrease infection and hasten healing. These agents are effective because damage to the blood vessels in the burn area prevents systemic antibiotics from reaching the burn wound. Antibiotics may be given prophylactically or may be withheld until an infection occurs. The following is a description of some of the topical agents currently in use for burn patients.

***Mafenide.*** Mafenide acetate (Sulfamylon) is a white cream containing sulfonamide. It penetrates through the burn eschar and is an effective bacteriostatic against many gram-negative and gram-positive organisms. The cream is applied to the wound once or twice daily with a sterile, gloved hand in a thin layer just enough to cover the burn completely. The wound may be left open to the air, or a single layer of gauze may be used to hold the cream in place. The cream is removed from the wound, and active debriding is performed before the cream is reapplied.

Mafenide inhibits carbonic anhydrase activity, especially in patients with burns of 40% or more BSA; as a result, metabolic acidosis may occur. The patient is monitored for hyperventilation that can result from attempts to balance the increased acid load. Other side effects include pain with application of the cream and an allergic rash. *Mafenide inhibits epithelial proliferation; therefore, application should be stopped as soon as the wound is clean and there is evidence of healing.*

***Silver sulfadiazine.*** Silver sulfadiazine (Silvadene) is a white cream with bactericidal action against many gram-negative and gram-positive bacteria, as well as against *C. albicans*. It is applied directly to the wound once or twice daily on saturated gauze or with a sterile gloved hand. The wound may be covered with a dressing or left exposed. Silver sulfadiazine does not penetrate as readily as mafenide acetate; however, patients do not complain of pain with its application.

The patient is observed for side effects common with sulfonamide drugs. The wound may develop a slimy, grayish appearance simulating an infection, despite negative cultures. Silver sulfadiazine should not be used in patients with a history of kidney disease. No electrolyte imbalances are seen with its use; however, prolonged use may lead to toxic symptoms including nausea, vomiting, anemia, leukopenia, granulocytopenia, mental changes, oliguria, anuria, hematuria, jaundice, and skin rashes.

**TABLE 68-8 Topical Medications Used in Burn Therapy**

| | ADVANTAGES | DISADVANTAGES |
|---|---|---|
| **MAFENIDE ACETATE (SULFAMYLON)** | Bacteriostatic against gram-negative and gram-positive organisms<br>Penetrates thick eschar<br>Effective against *Pseudomonas* organisms | Metabolic acidosis<br>Pain on application<br>Allergic rash |
| **SILVER SULFADIAZINE (SILVADENE)** | Broad antimicrobial activity against gram-negative, gram-positive, and *Candida* organisms<br>No electrolyte imbalances<br>Painless and somewhat soothing | Repeated application may develop slimy, grayish appearance simulating an infection in spite of negative cultures<br>Prolonged use may cause skin rash and depress granulocyte formation |
| **POVIDONE-IODINE (BETADINE)** | Broad antimicrobial activity against bacteria, fungi, viruses, and protozoa | Metabolic acidosis caused by elevated serum iodine levels<br>Stains clothing and linen<br>Dry, crusting, scabbing wound<br>Skin rash in unaffected area |
| **SILVER NITRATE** | Bacteriostatic effect<br>Lessens pain and eliminates odor<br>Reduces evaporative water loss from burns | Electrolyte imbalances<br>Stains everything it comes in contact with<br>Does not penetrate eschar<br>Pain on application |
| **NITROFURAZONE (FURACIN)** | Inhibits enzymes necessary for bacterial metabolism<br>Broad spectrum of activity<br>Effective against *Staphylococcus aureus*<br>Not absorbed systemically<br>Low incidence of sensitivity | Contact dermatitis in unaffected skin<br>Urine turns a reddish color |
| **GENTAMYCIN SULFATE (GARAMYCIN)** | Broad antimicrobial activity<br>Painless | Ototoxicity<br>Nephrotoxicity<br>Development of resistant bacterial strains |
| **NEOMYCIN** | Broad antimicrobial activity<br>Causes miscoding in the messenger ribonucleic acid (RNA) of bacterial cells | Serious toxic effects<br>Ototoxicity<br>Nephrotoxicity |
| **SCARLET RED** | Nonantiseptic (applied to gauze soaked with oil-based red dye)<br>Drying agent<br>Applied to donor site<br>Promotes epithelialization | No antimicrobial effects<br>Stains and irritates skin<br>Possible infection beneath scarlet red gauze; may have systemic effects |
| **XEROFORM** | Nonantiseptic<br>Debrides and protects donor site<br>Protects graft | Removal possibly painful, because it sometimes adheres to wound<br>Neither antiseptic or antimicrobial |
| **SODIUM HYPOCHLORITE (DAKIN'S SOLUTION)** | Chlorine-based solution that is bacteriocidal<br>Aids in debriding wounds<br>Aids in cleaning and draining of "soupy" wounds | Dissolves blood clot<br>May inhibit clotting<br>May irritate the skin |
| **SUTILAINS OINTMENT (TRAVASE)** | Topical enzymatic agent<br>Dissolves necrotic tissue by proteolytic action<br>Facilitates removal of eschar and purulent drainage | Mild, transient pain on application<br>Paresthesia, bleeding, dermatitis<br>Imperative that dressing be kept moist at all times |
| **BACITRACIN** | Prevents drying of wound<br>Keeps eschar soft and pliable<br>Beneficial in facial burns to promote healing<br>Used as open technique<br>Painless on application | No major antibiotic properties<br>Oil based, difficult to wash away |
| **BIOBRANE** | Pain reduced, wound not subjected to daily dressing change<br>Water loss from skin minimized | Cannot be used on eschar or if wound is cleansed with any antiseptic before application |

***Povidone-iodine.*** Povidone-iodine (Betadine) ointment is a reddish brown germicidal preparation of 10% povidone-iodine (1% available iodine) with broad-spectrum microbial action. It is effective against gram-positive and gram-negative bacteria, fungi, yeasts, viruses, and protozoa. It is applied three times daily. Povidone-iodine can be applied either by (1) spreading it with a sterile, gloved hand onto the burned surface or (2) impregnating a single-thickness gauze with it, applying the gauze to the burned surfaces, and spreading additional ointment on top of the gauze layer.

Metabolic acidosis may be seen with the elevated serum iodine levels. Clothing and bedding need to be protected from staining. A dry, crusting wound may be seen as well as skin rashes in unaffected areas.

***Silver nitrate.*** Although silver nitrate is being used

less often than in the past, some physicians still prescribe it. In this treatment, thick gauze dressings are saturated with 0.5% solution of silver nitrate. The dressings are kept wet so that the solution remains in constant contact with the burned surfaces. If the dressing is allowed to dry, the silver nitrate can concentrate and cause tissue destruction. These dressings retain moisture and heat and reduce evaporation. Proponents of this method of treatment believe that it reduces mortality, lessens pain, eliminates odors, and has a bacteriostatic effect. The dressings are removed every 12 to 24 hours, and the patient is placed in a bath of salt solution with the temperature carefully maintained at the same level as the body. When skin grafts are applied, silver nitrate dressings are placed over the grafts and donor sites on the first postoperative day. Because the silver nitrate is hypotonic, electrolytes are lost into the wound. Therefore, throughout treatment, frequent determinations of blood sodium levels are necessary, and sodium that is lost may need to be replaced. Everything that comes in contact with silver nitrate solution is stained black, so care should be taken when applying the solution to protect skin, clothing, furniture, walls, and floors.

Other topical medications used in burn therapy are outlined in Table 68-8.

**Wound coverings.** The burn wound may be covered with dressings or grafts.

***Dressings.*** Large bulky dressings are rarely used today for large burns except in select instances because infection control is more difficult and partial-thickness burns may develop into full-thickness wounds. The purposes of applying some light covering include prevention of infection from exogenous sources, facilitation of debridement, maximal contact by topical agents, and prevention of fluid evaporation with loss of body heat. The type of dressing that is usually applied consists of a single layer of fine-mesh gauze impregnated with a topical medication and held in place by a wrapping of a coarse gauze.

The dressing change is usually a painful procedure requiring analgesics. Analgesics should be given 30 minutes before the procedure for maximal effectiveness. Most dressing changes are performed after tubbing to facilitate dressing removal and lessen pain. Additional debridement of eschar and dead tissue may be performed before the new dressing is applied.

Wet dressings may be used with silver nitrate or normal saline applications. Normal saline is applied to clean granulation tissue or to new grafts to maintain moisture or are used with fine-mesh gauze to provide for slight debridement. A single layer of fine-mesh gauze is usually placed over the wound, covered with thick gauze pads to maintain moisture, and held in place with a gauze wrapping. The dressings must be kept wet. Plastic wrap should *not* be used to cover the dressings because it prevents any fluid evaporation, causes increased heat at the wound site, and results in patient discomfort and increased tissue destruction and infection.

**TABLE 68-9 Types of Grafts**

| GRAFT | SOURCE | COVERAGE |
|---|---|---|
| Autograft | Patient's own skin removed and applied to burn | Permanent |
| Cultured skin | Patient's skin removed in small squares and grown in Petri dishes to large sizes and then grafted | Permanent |
| Homograft | Another of the same species (for example, cadaver skin obtained 6 to 24 hours after death) and applied within 5 days | Temporary |
| Heterograft | Another species (for example, pig skin) | Temporary |
| Synthetic substitute | Man-made substitute that has properties similar to skin | Temporary |

***Skin grafts.*** Skin grafts are applied to cover the burn wound and speed healing, to prevent contractures, and to shorten convalescence. Successful grafting reduces the patient's vulnerability to infection and prevents the loss of body heat and water vapor from the open wound. Grafting may be performed for cosmetic or functional purposes during the rehabilitative period. Most skin grafts are applied between the third and twenty-first day after the initial injury, depending on the depth and extent of the burn and the condition of the base.

Grafts are obtained from various sources (Table 68-9). An autograft is a graft of skin obtained from the patient's own body. A **homograft** is a graft of skin obtained from a cadaver 6 to 24 hours after death. A **heterograft** is a graft of skin obtained from another species, such as a pig. Synthetic substitutes for skin are currently being investigated.

Homografts, heterografts, and synthetic substitutes are intended to provide temporary coverage while the burn wound heals. As the wound heals, these temporary coverings are gradually rejected and are easily removed from the newly healed skin.

The advantage of a temporary graft is to reduce water, electrolyte, and protein losses at the burn surface. The covered wound is less painful and allows the patient freedom of movement. Temporary grafts may be used until the patient is ready for autografts. Often, autografting is delayed as a result of complications such as pneumonia or gastric hemorrhage.

**Split-thickness skin grafts** are used most frequently in early stages of wound treatment (Figure 68-10). The grafts include two upper layers of skin (epidermis) and part of the middle layer (dermis) but are not taken so deep as to prevent regeneration of the skin at the site

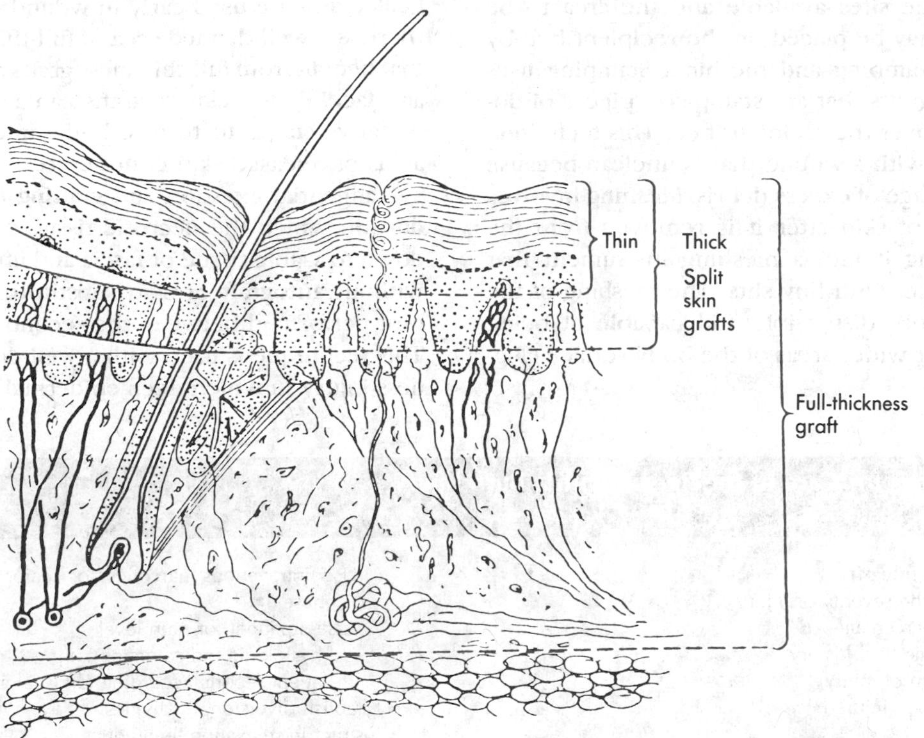


**FIGURE 68-10** Levels of the skin involved in thin- and thick-split skin grafts and full-thickness grafts.

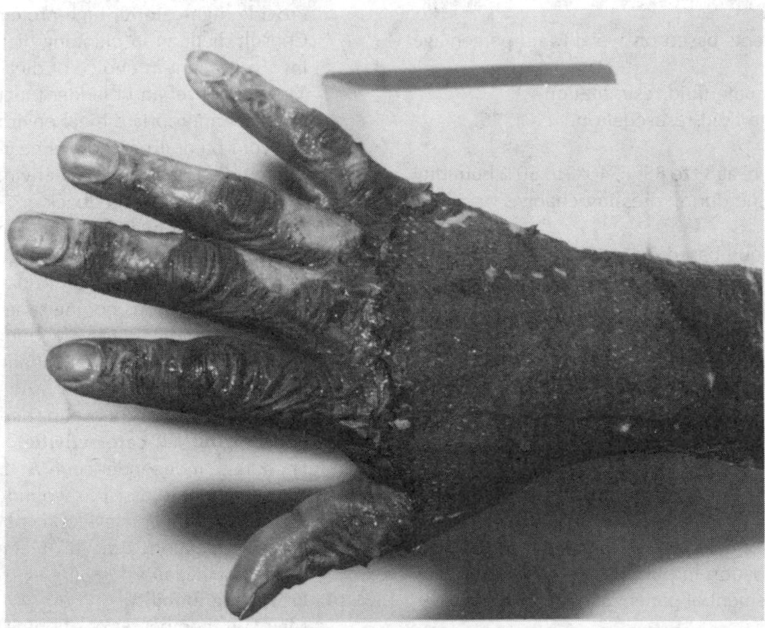

**FIGURE 68-11** Mesh graft covering a full-thickness burn to the dorsum of the hand. (Courtesy Burn Center, MetroHealth Medical Center, Cleveland.)

from which they are taken (donor site). The grafts are removed with a dermatome blade from almost any unburned part of the body. The size of these grafts are determined by the sites available and the area to be covered. Grafts may be placed on the recipient bed by two methods—stamping and meshing. Stamping uses "postage stamp" grafts that are stamp-size pieces of donor skin applied over the recipient bed. This technique is generally used with a wound that is unclean because it allows for drainage of excess debris. Meshing involves taking the sheet of skin after it is removed from the donor and feeding it into a meshing instrument that perforates the sheet with tiny slits. The meshing of the graft makes it more distensible and capable of being stretched to cover wider areas of the body surface (Figure 68-11).

**Full-thickness grafts** are composed of layers of skin down to the subcutaneous tissue. They give a better cosmetic appearance than split-thickness grafts when healed and are used early in wound management and if there is a well-defined area of full-thickness burn. Areas that benefit from full-thickness grafts are the hands, neck, and face. Full-thickness grafts can also be used in rehabilitative stages to restore body function and to repair areas of released skin contractures.

Tangential excision and grafting is a surgical procedure in which the necrotic tissue or eschar is excised down to viable tissue or fascia and immediately covered without autograft or skin substitute. The procedure is best performed between the second and fifth burn day. This technique is used with a well-defined partial-thickness injury in which deep epidermal cells remain intact

### Guidelines for Care of the Person with a Burn Injury

1. **Promoting skin integrity**
   - Assessment of the severity of injury
     - Depth and percentage
       - Age and medical history
       - Mechanism of injury
       - Area of body injured
   - Wound care
     - Hydrotherapy, cleansing, and debridement
     - Application of topical agents
     - Assessment of progression of wound healing
   - Prevention of scar formation and contractures
     - Appropriate positioning
     - Application of pressure garments
2. **Monitoring hypovolemia**
   - Calculate fluid requirements based on weight and percentage of injury
   - Monitor for signs of adequate fluid resuscitation
     - (See "Signs of adequate fluid resuscitation," p. 2375)
3. **Preventing hypothermia**
   - Maintain room temperature at 83 to 85° F, 40% to 50% humidity
   - Limit wound exposure time during dressing changes
4. **Preventing infection**
   - Establish isolation technique based on wound size
   - Control visitors and traffic
   - Follow strict wound care asepsis
   - Do routine wound, nose, throat cultures
   - Monitor for signs of wound infection/sepsis
   - Use aseptic/sterile technique with invasive lines (intravenous Foley catheters)
   - Disinfect patient care equipment thoroughly
5. **Decreasing anxiety**
   - Provide consistent information related to treatment and plan of care
   - Encourage verbalization of concerns
   - Encourage family participation in plan of care
   - Provide positive reinforcement of patient's efforts and improvement
6. **Decreasing pain**
   - Minimize wound exposure time
     - Analgesics
     - Medicate 30 minutes before dressing change
     - Use intravenous narcotics for major burns in emergent phase
     - Assess patient for pain level
       - Physiologic indicators of pain
       - Patient reports according to visual analog scale
   - Establish diversional activities
   - Instruct in relaxation techniques
7. **Providing adequate nutrition**
   - Assess preburn nutritional status
   - Instruct patient concerning current nutritional requirements
     - While in hospital
     - While on discharge
   - Maintain daily calorie counts and weights
   - Provide high-calorie, high-protein diet with supplements
   - Consult dietitian in planning diet
   - Involve patient in choice of diet
   - Monitor bowel and bladder function
   - Establish appropriate meal environment
     - Avoid painful procedures near mealtimes
     - Provide a calm, relaxed environment
     - Provide positive feedback
     - Provide oral hygiene before and after meals
8. **Promoting a positive body image and self-concept**
   - Provide emotional support to patient and family
   - Determine previous coping strategies
   - Assess for readiness to view burned area
   - Encourage expression of patient's view of his/her physical appearance
   - Provide individual counseling or refer patient to support groups
9. **Encouraging self-care activities**
   - Encourage independence in ADL
   - Allow patient to assist in wound care procedures
   - Include patient in development of plan of care concerning meal selection, time of treatments, rest periods, therapy, and socialization
10. **Promoting mobility**
    - Maintain therapeutic positioning
      - Proper splint application
      - Positioning
      - Application of continuous passive motion devices
    - Develop activity and exercise schedule
    - Adapt environment to patient's current level of mobility

for primary healing. Advantages of tangential excision and grafting are outlined in Box 68-7.

Graft sites require skilled nursing management. Autografts are delicate and should not be dislodged. The grafted area may be covered with a large, occlusive, bulky dressing to hold new skin securely in place. Splints may be applied in the operating room to provide immobilization and maintain position.

The dressing remains intact for 48 to 72 hours unless it is found to be purulent with a strong odor. The dressing is removed slowly and carefully so as not to disturb the graft.

After grafting the donor site represents a wound similar to that of a partial-thickness injury. Care of the donor site is as important as care of the graft itself, because donor sites that fail to heal result in a net enlargement of the patient's open wound surface. Donor sites may be treated by a variety of methods. One method is covering the exposed surface with fine-mesh gauze, Xeroform, or a synthetic dressing and leaving it exposed to the air. Exposing the donor site to a heat lamp also promotes healing, because, as the drainage from the wound dries, it serves as a protective covering (Figure 68-12). The site usually heals within 2 weeks. Another method is to cover the site with sterile gauze and to apply a pressure dressing.

Many patients complain of severe pain in the donor site, and the nurse should not hesitate to give medications for pain. The pain should subside in 24 to 48 hours as the wound dries. The wound is inspected daily for any signs of infection (erythema, purulent drainage, foul odor). If infection develops, antibiotics may be administered, and the wound treated with wet dressings. The guidelines for the care of the patient with a burn injury are summarized in the Guidelines box, p. 2384.

**BOX 68-10 Advantages of Tangential Excision and Grafting**

Shortened hospitalization
Prevents potential conversion of burn to full thickness by removing necrotic tissue before infection occurs
Definitive healing diminishes anxiety and lessens trauma to multiple graftings
Allows early grafting and early restoration of function
Scar formation reduced because of use of full-thickness graft

### Providing Nutrition

**Pathophysiology.** Metabolism is increased following moderate-to-severe burns as a result of stress, fluid loss, fever, infection, hypercatabolism, and immobility. Shivering plus the elevated levels of catecholamines, cortisol, and glucagon found shortly after thermal injury increase tissue oxygen consumption and heat production, de-

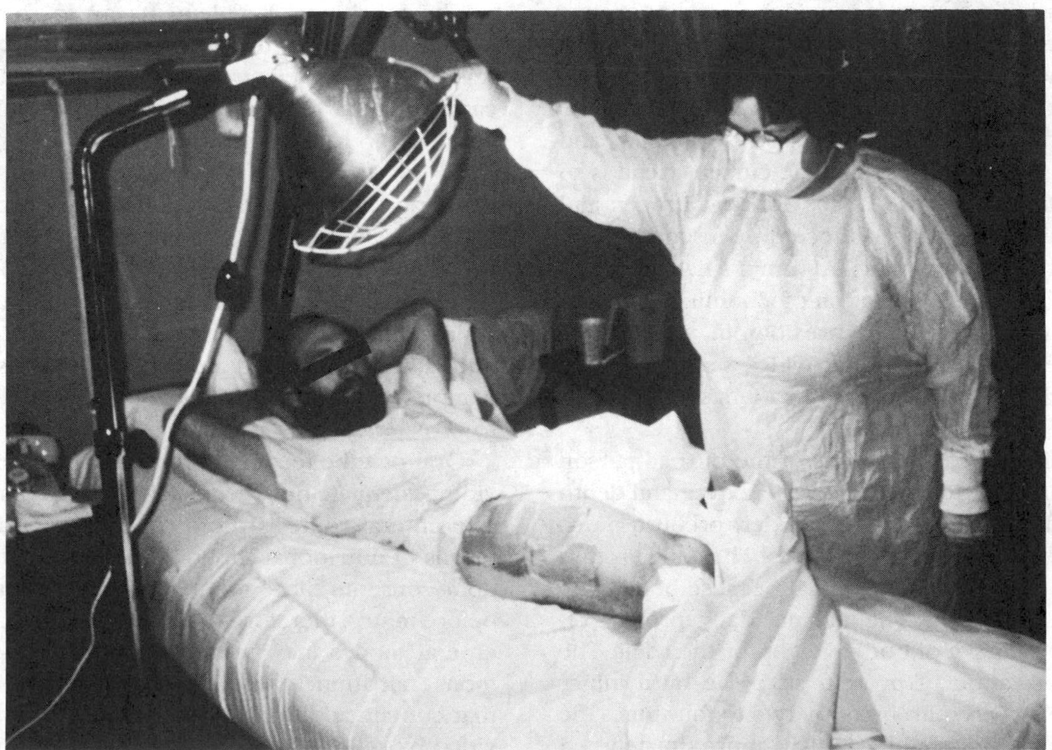

**FIGURE 68-12** Heat lamp used to dry donor site to promote epithelialization from deep layers and to prevent infection. (Courtesy Burn Center, MetroHealth Medical Center, Cleveland.)

plete liver and muscle glycogen stores and fat deposits, and lead to negative nitrogen balance and weight loss. Protein is broken down, providing amino acids for gluconeogenesis, and amino acids are prevented from incorporating into protein. The diminished rate of protein production prolongs wound healing and increases the patient's susceptibility to infection.

A burn patient remains catabolic until the caloric intake exceeds caloric expenditure. Hypermetabolism continues until the wounds are 90% healed[14] and homeostasis is restored. The patient's total energy and protein requirements become those needed for normal homeostasis plus those required to offset the catabolic state and repair the injury.

**Nutritional assessment and supplement.** Maintenance of a nutritional support program is critical to survival and is initiated on admission. The goals of the nutritional support program are to establish eating by mouth as soon as possible and to maintain sufficient caloric and protein intake to restore tissue loss. A team approach provides comprehensive input and integrates the efforts of the patient, physician, nurse, pharmacist, dietitian, and occupational and physical therapists.

A nutritional assessment is made during the first days of the burn injury and includes anthropometric measurements (to determine actual weight loss compared with ideal weight), laboratory studies (electrolytes, liver function tests, urine), and skin testing (if indicated to determine immune response) (see Chapter 6).

The admission assessment provides a baseline against which progress can be evaluated. Twenty-four-hour urine specimens and urea nitrogen tests (UUN), may be obtained two to three times a week to evaluate the patient's nitrogen balance. Evaluation of albumin and protein levels is also necessary. The current trend is to follow *prealbumin levels* (PAB). Urinary nitrogen and serum albumin levels can be affected by insensible protein loss and hydration status. Albumin's half-life of 20 days makes day-to-day evaluation of albumin difficult to interpret. On the other hand, prealbumin, which has a short half-life of 20-25 hours, provides a sensitive indicator of nutritional status and the patient's response to feeding.[5]

The protein and caloric needs of the burned person are highly variable, depending on the extent and depth of injury and the patient's age, gender, preburn nutritional status, and preexisting diseases. The daily *protein* requirement is greater than normal because of the negative nitrogen balance. The normal daily protein requirement is 0.8 g/kg of body weight for the adult. The massive mobilization of protein after the burn injury increases the daily requirement by two to four times the amount required before the injury: approximately 1.5 to 3.2 g/kg of body weight. Protein must be used for tissue repair and healing, not as a source of energy. Therefore, it is important to provide adequate carbohydrate and fat calories to satisfy energy needs. An appreciable loss of *zinc* generally accompanies a protein and weight loss. Zinc deficiency impairs wound healing, and recent data indicate that a zinc deficiency will impair cellular immunity.

The daily *caloric* requirement increases from a normal 1700 to 3000 calories to 3500 to 5000 calories. Because the demand for calories increases with a major burn, appropriate vitamin therapy is essential. *Vitamins* and *minerals* are given at two to three times the recommended daily allowances established for normal healthy adults. Vitamin C promotes healing and the daily requirement in the burn patient increases from a normal of 45 mg to 1 to 2 g. The B-complex vitamins are necessary for the metabolism of the increased protein and carbohydrate intake. Vitamins A, E, and K and folic acid are monitored and supplemented as indicated. Serum levels of calcium, phosphate, and potassium are also monitored, and therapeutic levels of iron must be maintained to prevent the ongoing threat of anemia associated with burn injury.

Weight loss and gain are monitored for evaluation of nutritional status. *Weight gain* occurs initially because of fluid retention; however, after diuresis there is a marked loss of weight. Severe *weight loss* is closely related to protein loss or the loss of body cell mass and the enormous amount of body fluid lost through the burn wound itself. As in other metabolic responses, weight loss depends on the extent of injury: the greater the burn, the greater the weight loss.

The nutritional supplements given to the severely burned patient in the emergent period are aimed at stabilization and electrolyte balance to maintain stable cardiovascular function. Patients are initially supported with 5% or 10% dextrose solution.

**Feeding methods.** Paralytic ileus or gastric dilation is frequently seen in severely burned patients because of the neuroendocrine response to stress, hypovolemia, or septicemia. This prevents enteral feeding until the gastrointestinal tract mobility is restored. Total parenteral nutrition (TPN) is indicated once fluid resuscitation is completed. TPN with supplemental fat solutions is used to provide calories (see Chapter 45).

Oral or tube feeding is the preferred method of providing adequate nutrition and is used as soon as possible. The enteral route is the most natural and convenient means of nutritional support. The burn patient will seldom consume more food from meals after injury than before injury; therefore, a combination of parenteral and enteral modes may be necessary to provide the enormous nutritional requirements. Dietary supplements that contain additional calories and protein can be provided by milkshakes that can be specially made by the hospital dietary department. Patients should be encouraged to drink supplements between meals.

Postburn lactose intolerance may occur in patients

being tube fed. Signs of bloating, flatulence, cramps, and diarrhea may be seen. A modification of the strength and type of supplement may be necessary; and starting the supplement at one-half or one-quarter strength, diluted with water, will often alleviate gastrointestinal complications.

Tube feedings provide a continuous 24-hour infusion of nutrition. Tube feedings are a high-caloric, high-protein commercially prepared supplement. These supplements, containing 1 to 1.5 kcal/ml, are hypertonic and, because of hypertonicity, diarrhea is common. The best means of administering tube feeding is a continuous, slow infusion through a small-diameter, soft, pliable tube inserted through the esophagus into the stomach or duodenum (see Chapter 45). Diarrhea, nausea, vomiting, and an uncomfortable feeling of fullness may be avoided with a slow, continuous infusion using an infusion pump to regulate the delivery. If diarrhea persists, Kaopectate or paregoric may be added to the supplement or diphenoxylate with atropine (Lomotil) may be ordered by the physician.

The patient is advanced to a regular diet as quickly as possible. However, ingenuity by the nurses and dietitian is needed to motivate the patient to eat the food necessary to meet nutritional requirements. Relatives can suggest favorite foods. All dressing changes and treatments should be timed so they don't immediately precede meals. Milkshakes can supplement the patient's diet and can be taken more easily than solid foods.

Fecal impaction is a common problem in burn patients. Bulk foods and fruit juices must be stressed. Bulk-forming laxatives such as preparations of the psyllium seed (Metamucil) or a fecal softener such as dioctyl sodium sulfosuccinate (Colace) may be ordered by the physician.

### Promoting comfort

The control of pain is a major part of the burn patient's care. Uncontrolled pain affects all aspects of recovery, including tolerance of wound care, ability to eat, mobility, and psychologic adjustment. Acute pain is most successfully managed with narcotics. The methods and routes of administration are carefully evaluated on an individual basis. Attention is paid to pain management needs during dressing changes and other activities of the day. During dressing changes, parenteral narcotics are given to achieve rapid onset of action. The use of anesthetic agents such as ketamine, fentanyl, and self-administered nitrous oxide may be beneficial for some patients. (The Guidelines box above outlines nursing interventions during dressing change.)

An around-the-clock approach to pain management is essential for the burn patient. Undermedication may occur if the patient fears becoming addicted and fails to report pain or if the nurse fails to adequately evaluate the degree of pain. The use of a numerical analog scale in which the patient rates the pain helps determine

**Guidelines for Nursing Care to Help Minimize Pain During Dressing Changes**

Provide analgesic medications 30 minutes before dressing change.
Provide clear explanations to gain patient's cooperation.
Handle burned areas gently.
Use sterile technique (infection causes increased pain).
Encourage patient to participate in treatment whenever possible.
Use distracting techniques (for example, radio, conversation) and relaxation techniques when appropriate.

whether the pain is being adequately controlled. Providing medication at frequent intervals helps to maintain ongoing comfort. Time-released morphine and patient-controlled analgesia are also viable options.[1]

Physiologic pain may be induced or aggravated by loneliness and depression. The patient's complaint of pain may be an indication of unmet emotional needs that can be addressed with the use of presence, touch, or diversional activities. Anxiety about anticipated procedures and sleep deprivation may increase the amount of pain experienced by the patient. Patients experiencing posttraumatic stress disorder report higher levels of pain.[12] Interventions may include the use of antianxiety medication and nonpharmacologic methods such as meditation or relaxation exercises. (See Chapter 17 for further discussion of pain management.)

## ♦ EVALUATION

To evaluate the effectiveness of nursing interventions, compare patient behaviors with those stated in the expected outcomes. Successful achievement of patient outcomes for the patient with burns is indicated by the following:

### Acute Phase

1. Absence of wound or systemic infection
   a. Absence of pathogenic organisms by wound culture
   b. Absence of signs of systemic infection
      (1) Fever >38.5° C
      (2) Tachypnea
      (3) Tachycardia
      (4) Paralytic ileus
      (5) Oliguria
2. Reestablishment of skin integrity
   a. Presence of wound healing
   b. Limited hypertrophic scarring
   c. Ability to perform skin care
3. Optimal nutritional status
   a. Protein and calorie intake adequate to meet calculated needs
   b. Positive nitrogen balance indicated by normal prealbumin and albumin levels

   c. Maintenance of preburn weight
   d. Absence of diarrhea or constipation
   e. Identification of foods necessary for healing
4. Adequate pain control
   a. Rates level of pain as acceptable
   b. Lacks physical signs indicative of pain, e.g., tachycardia, diaphoresis, splinting or protective movement
   c. States ability to sleep
   d. Able to perform ADL
   e. Demonstrates independence in care needs

## REHABILITATION PERIOD

Rehabilitation begins at the time of admission. However, rehabilitation as the third stage of treatment begins when the patient's burn is reduced to less than 20% BSA and the patient is capable of assuming some self-care activity. The principles of management are to return the patient to a productive place in society and to accomplish functional and cosmetic reconstruction. It is important to remember that rehabilitation does not end when the patient is discharged. It may take from 2 to 5 years after discharge for the patient to reach a maximal level of emotional and physical adjustment.

## NURSING MANAGEMENT

### ♦ ASSESSMENT

#### Subjective Data

The patient must be helped to maintain range of joint motion to prevent scars from healing in positions that will result in deformity. Complaints of pain and pressure should not be overlooked because damage may occur from an improperly applied splint or poor positioning. It is important that patients understand why ambulation or motion is necessary even though it may be painful.

The emotional impact of a severe burn is enormous. The psychologic scars last forever and affect the victim and family for the rest of their lives. The extent to which the family unit adapts depends on how the patient reacts to a new body image and feelings of self-worth.

The hospital environment and hospital personnel influence the adaptation process. In the immediate postburn period, the nurse is primarily concerned with physiologic survival of the patient. At the same time, the nurse must be able to identify psychologic problems and coping mechanisms of the patient and family.

#### Objective Data

The nurse is responsible for assessing the patient's response to positioning, splinting, exercise, and the ability of the patient and family to perform daily wound care after discharge. Correct positioning must be maintained to avoid the development of contractures. The splinted limb is assessed for adequate circulation, cyanosis, temperature, and the presence of pulses. Exercise, activities of daily living (ADL), and ambulation must be continuously assessed for patient tolerance, both physically and emotionally. Complete and comprehensive instructions followed by return demonstration of wound and dressing care are necessary before discharge.

### ♦ NURSING DIAGNOSES

Nursing diagnoses are determined from analysis of patient data during the rehabilitative period. Nursing diagnoses for the person with burns may include but are not limited to the following:

| Diagnostic Title |
|---|
| Mobility, impaired physical |
| Self-care deficit |
| Body image disturbance |
| Knowledge deficit |
| Coping, ineffective individual |
| Coping, ineffective family: compromised |
| Anxiety |
| Pain |
| Skin integrity, impaired, high risk for |
| Infection, high risk form |

Table 68-6 summarizes the nursing diagnoses, possible etiologies, and expected outcomes during the rehabilitative period.

### ♦ INTERVENTIONS

#### Promoting Mobility

As the survival rate of patients with large and deeper burns increases, so does the challenge to maintain optimal functioning and cosmetic results. Research indicates that the percentage of patients with joint limitations increases as the degree and extent of burns increase. Although these patients may be critically ill, their rehabilitative needs must be addressed immediately. A comprehensive program of positioning, splinting, exercise, ambulation, and activities of daily living must begin on the first or second day postburn and be carried through until after discharge. Any delays in initiating treatment will be detrimental to the patient's ultimate functional outcome. Contractures are among the most serious long-term complications of burns today. They result from muscle and joint stiffening, skin grafting and prolonged bedrest. Although the occupational and physical therapists are primarily responsible for addressing the patient's rehabilitation needs during all phases of the patient's recovery, the nurse is responsible for assuring that all their recommendations are followed.

**Therapeutic positioning**

Therapeutic positioning, placing body parts in antideformity positions, is vital to the prevention of burn contractures. The patient must be repositioned in bed (sidelying, supine, prone) frequently and regularly during the day and night. Correct positioning varies, depending on the area of the body burned (Table 68-10). Positioning can be enhanced by placing patients on a Stryker frame,

TABLE 68-10 Therapeutic Positioning for the Burn Patient

| AREA BURNED | DESCRIPTION OF POSITION |
|---|---|
| Neck | No pillow<br>Towel roll under cervical spine<br>Neck splint |
| Shoulder | 90-degree abduction, neutral rotation<br>Elbow splint may be used to aid in maintaining position |
| Axilla | Abduction with 10 to 15 degree forward flexion and external rotation<br>Support abducted arm with suspension from IV pole, or bedside table<br>Axilla splint |
| Elbow | Extension<br>Support extended arm on bedside table, foam trough<br>Elbow splint |
| Hand | Hand splint |
| Dorsal surface | Flexion |
| Palmar surface | Hyperextension |
| Hip | Extension with neutral rotation<br>Supine with lower extremity extended<br>Prone-lying (if medically appropriate)<br>Trochanter roll<br>Foam wedge along lateral aspect of thigh<br>Knee or long leg splint |
| Knee | Extension<br>Prone-lying (if medically appropriate)<br>Patient out of bed with lower extremities extended and elevated<br>Knee splint |
| Ankle | Dorsiflexion<br>Padded footboard with heels free of pressure<br>Ankle splint |

a Foster bed, a CircOlectric bed, or one of the many different types of low air loss beds or mattresses currently available. These beds facilitate the use of the bedpan and urinal, permit change of position with a minimum of handling, and permit larger skin surfaces to remain freer from body pressure than is possible when the patient lies on a regular mattress. These special beds are particularly useful when both the back and front of the trunk, thighs, and legs have been burned. These beds allow turning of the patient with minimal handling and thus help decrease pain.

Prolonged rest in semi-Fowler's position or with the pillow pushing the head forward must be avoided, even though many patients like this position because it enables them to see about the room better. The bed can often be turned so that the patient can look about without having to assume positions that may lead to the formation of contractures. The bedside table may be changed from one side of the bed to the other at intervals to stimulate other body positions.

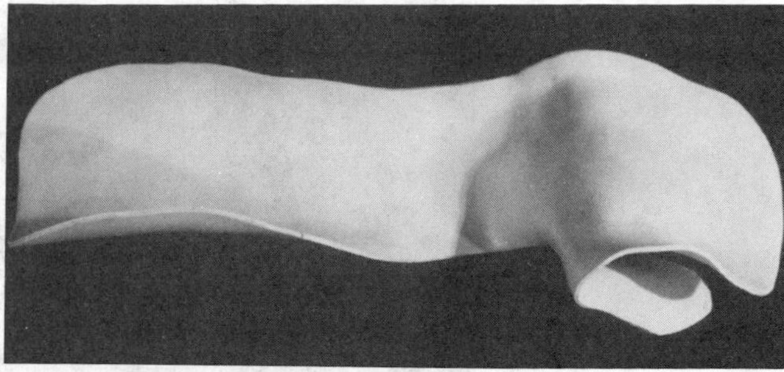

FIGURE 68-13 Orthoplast hand splint. (Courtesy Burn Center, MetroHealth Medical Center, Cleveland.)

### Splints

Splints are used to prevent or correct contractures and to immobilize joints after grafting. They are custom-made and often molded directly on the patient to assure optimal conformity (Figure 68-13). It is the responsibility of the nurse to apply the splint properly and according to an established schedule. An improperly applied splint can promote contractures and lead to additional complications. Assess the splinted limb for adequate circulation, cyanosis, temperature, and the presence of pulses. Complaints of pain and pressure should be assessed because damage may occur with an improperly applied splint. Some physicians prefer to use the open method of treatment and use frequent exercise instead of splinting to prevent contractures.

### Exercises and ambulation

Exercises for prevention and correction of contractures are begun as soon as the patient is stable. Active exercises are preferred, although active assistance and gentle pressure exercises may be more realistic. Supervision by a physical or occupational therapist is desirable. Exercises may be performed more easily in water and may be done along with dressing changes if the patient is able to tolerate the activity (Figure 68-14). Continuous passive pressure motion (CPM) devices may be used to prevent contractures of affected joints. When burns are completely covered (by healing or by graft), exercises may be performed more easily in an occupational therapy or physical therapy department where the patient may benefit from a change in environment.

Ambulation decreases the risk of thromboemboli, promotes optimal ventilation, helps maintain range of motion and strength in the lower extremities, orients the patient to the environment, and provides a sense of functional independence. Patients who have large burns have less ability to tolerate activity and will require a progressive approach to mobilization. Initially the patient may need to be transferred with maximal assistance onto a stretcher chair and progress to a sitting position. Gradually, the patient may progress to a standing pivot transfer into a nearby chair and eventually ambulate with

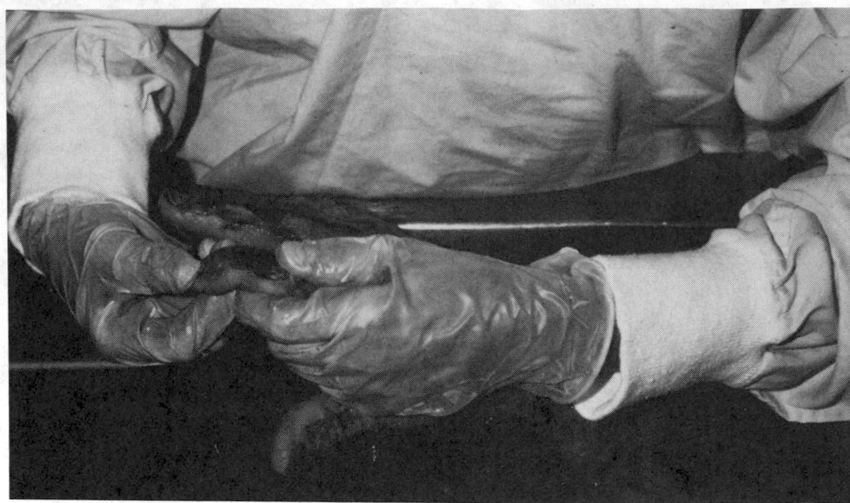

**FIGURE 68-14** Passive range-of-motion exercise during hydrotherapy. (Courtesy Burn Center, MetroHealth Medical Center, Cleveland.)

minimal assistance. Before getting out of bed, an elastic bandage support must be applied to the lower extremities to prevent venous stasis, edema, and orthostatic hypotension.

## Promoting Self-Care

One of the ultimate goals in the rehabilitation of the burned patient is to maintain or restore the patient's independence in performing ADL. The occupational therapist aids in this process by selecting activities that are appropriate to the patient's medical, physical, and mental status. Activities that the nurse can encourage are self-feeding, telephoning, reading mail, and assisting with grooming or burn wound management. The nurse must know what the patient is being taught by the physical and occupational therapist so that progress can be continued on the nursing unit.

After the initial period, the long healing process begins, accompanied by the realization of endless implications for the future. Burns on the face make adjustments particularly difficult. Different kinds of fears include the following: death, pain, disfigurement, prolonged hospitalization, job security, disruption of lifestyle, and reaction of family and friends.

To the adolescent, the thought of being different or conspicuous may be unbearable. If possible, the patient should see facial burns only after being prepared for the experience. Support and understanding will be needed for the person to cope with what will be seen in the mirror. The patient will exhibit readiness by asking to look in the mirror. Interaction with other burn patients who are further along in the healing process may help the patient feel that recovery is possible. In some cases, the recovery is incredible, and although differences in skin pigmentation remain, the redness that accompanies healed burn wounds often fades considerably within a few months. Pigmentation problems are more acute for persons with brown or black skin. Their healed skin may be a different shade, freckled, or whitish. Commercial makeup products that help blend skin tones are available.

## Promoting a Positive Body Image

Regardless of its size, a burn injury represents a change in the individual's perception of self. As the burn heals, the patient must deal with a new appearance. The patient must have the opportunity to talk about any concerns or fears. Some patients may discuss these with the nurse when they cannot express them to relatives. The nurse must be prepared to listen actively and help the patient accept changes in appearance. The patient must be allowed to grieve for the loss of the former self. However, the patient should not dwell on the negative, but focus on the positive aspects of self.

## Preventing Scarring

Whenever a wound of connective tissue heals, hypertrophic scarring will occur unless the skin adheres to the underlying structure. Hypertrophic scarring results from the overgrowth and overproduction of tissue. This occurs especially in areas of stress and movement such as the hands, legs, and chest (Figure 68-15). The thickened rigid scar that results may later cause contractures. The application of controlled constant pressure to the surface of an immature scar will reduce the scar and leave a smooth pliable tissue. If this pressure is applied to new healthy tissue, hypertrophic scarring can be prevented (Figure 68-16). The pressure garment, a specially designed elastic woven material, provides tridimensional control. It is fitted to each patient individually and then custom made (Figure 68-17). Until the garment is completed, bandages can be used for a pressure dressing.

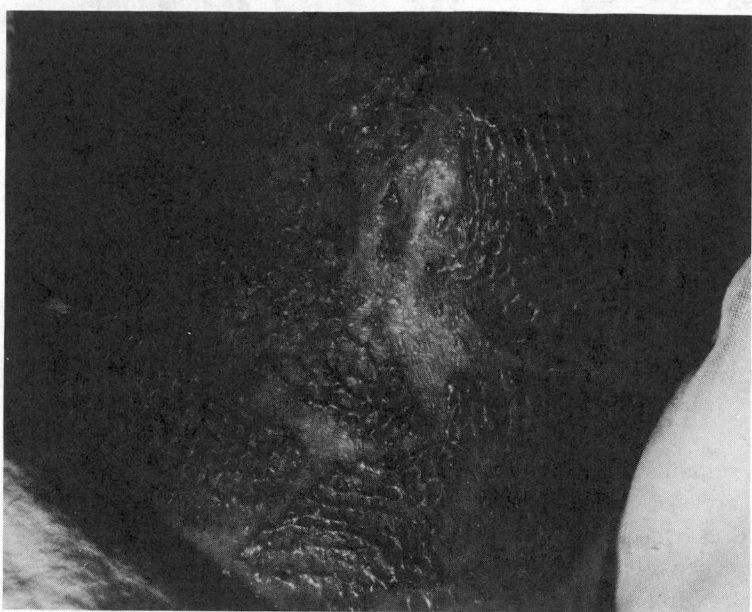

**FIGURE 68-15** Hypertrophic scarring over chest and abdomen. (Courtesy Burn Center, MetroHealth Center, Cleveland.)

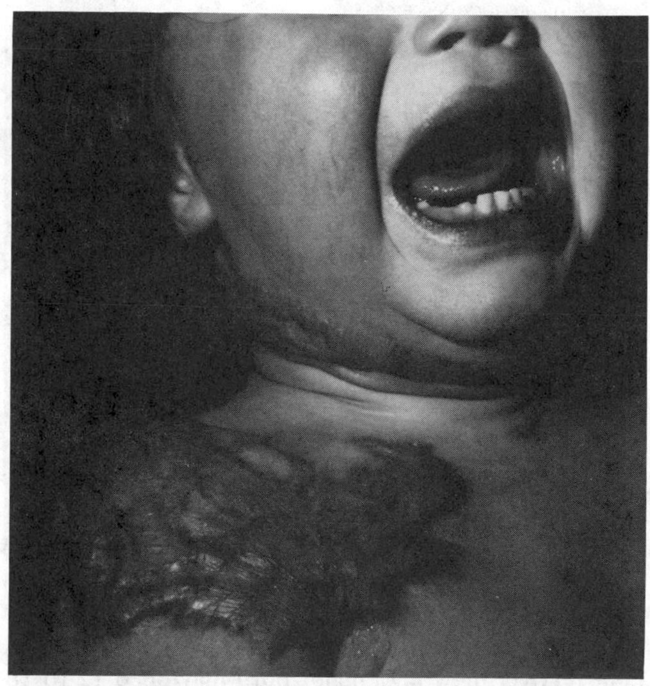

**FIGURE 68-16** Scar formation occurring from lack of pressure dressing application. (Courtesy Burn Center, MetroHealth Medical Center, Cleveland.)

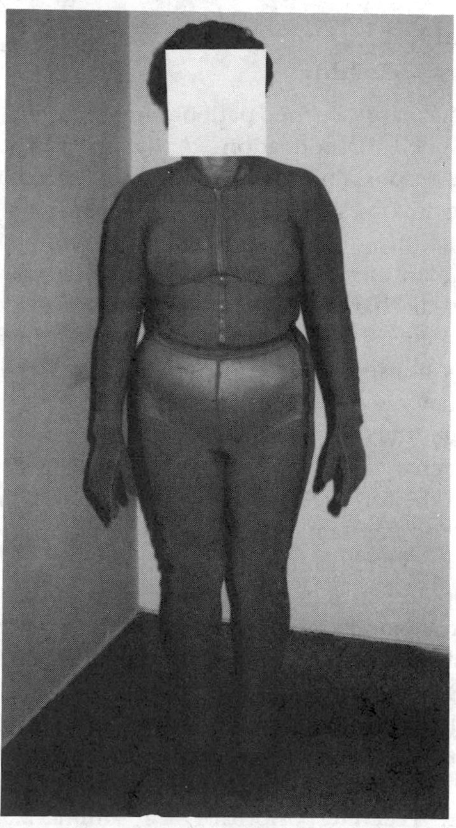

**FIGURE 68-17** Total body Jobst pressure garment consisting of three separate pieces: jacket, pants, and gloves. (Courtesy Burn Center, MetroHealth Medical Center, Cleveland.)

Even though pressure garments help decrease the formation of thick, disfiguring scars, patient acceptance is a problem. The garments are uncomfortable and make the patient warm, especially during hot weather. They must be tight enough to produce the 24 mm Hg of pressure required to exceed capillary pressure to be effective in reducing edema and scar formation. The patient must wear the garments 23 hours a day for 6 months to a year.

A plan for exercise and splinting must be established before discharge. To prevent scar contracture, daily therapy sessions may be necessary for several weeks or months. Aids can be developed by the occupational therapist to help with the activities of daily living.

## Promoting Comfort

Although less severe, pain remains a problem during the rehabilitation phase. Small areas of skin may remain open and continue to require dressing changes. In addition, newly healed skin is more sensitive. Physical and occupational therapy and increasing activity may result in discomfort. Interventions are focused on appropriate analgesics, diversional activities, and continuing to provide information about what the patient can expect. Daily hydrotherapy is beneficial in helping the patient to relax tense muscles.

## Facilitating Learning

### Discharge teaching

Before discharge, burned patients and their families have a great need for education so that they may take increasing responsibilities for their own care. Discharge teaching involves the entire burn team, and because rehabilitation is a gradual process, there should be ample time to plan the return home in every detail.

Early discharge planning accomplishes two goals. First, it helps solve problems early; for example, if the patient's house burned and needs to be repaired, the family may need to relocate. This could be done before discharge, thus preventing the added stress of moving after discharge. Second, early discharge planning emphasizes the future. If discharge is discussed, the patient and his or her family may realize more quickly that recovery and return to home is possible.

Complete and comprehensive instructions followed by return demonstrations contribute to learning the necessary skills to be independent in self-care activities after discharge. Patients should not be discharged from the hospital until they can care for themselves physically, with assistance if necessary, and are prepared to meet the stresses involved in returning to their former living patterns. Teaching priorities are summarized in the Guidelines box at right.

A major goal in discharge teaching is to prevent excessive scar formation by exercising, splinting, and applying pressure dressings. If these methods are not effective, reconstructive surgery may be necessary. A patient recovering from a major burn may need 12 to 18 months to achieve this goal.

Instructions should include how to care for the healed graft and nongrafted areas. Signs and symptoms of complications, including areas that may blister and break down, and signs of infection are also addressed.

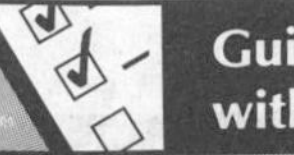

### Guidelines for Teaching the Person with a Burn

- Patient/significant other verbalizes understanding of pathophysiology of burn process
  - Depth and percentage of injury
  - Functions of the skin
  - Need for fluid replacement
- Knowledge of healing process
  - Nutritional requirements
  - Infection control measures
  - Rationale for wound management
    - Hydrotherapy and debridement
    - Topical agents
    - Grafting
  - Scar formation
    - Stages of development
    - Use of Ace bandage or pressure garments
    - Use of cosmetics and prosthetics
  - Purpose of occupational and physical therapy toward improved mobility
    - Level of activity
    - Prescribed exercises
- Pain management
  - Relation of pain to depth of injury
  - Pain control options
    - Analgesics
    - Diversional activities
    - Relaxation exercises
- Discharge needs
  - Skin care for healed areas
    - Protection from sun
    - Avoidance of chemical irritants
    - Increased sensitivity
    - Blister formation
  - Skin care for open areas
    - Prescribed dressing
    - Application
    - Abnormal conditions
  - Application and care of pressure garments
  - Home care needs
    - Care of clothing
    - Cleanliness of dressing change area, that is, shower/bathtub
    - Adaptation of home environment, that is, handicap rails
  - Nutritional needs
    - Basic four food groups
    - Relationship of dietary intake to healing process
  - Emotional readjustment
    - To new body image
    - Behaviors that may develop at home
      - Nightmares/flashbacks
      - Grief
      - Isolation
      - Depression
  - Dealing with reactions of others
  - Options for increasing social activity

## Guidelines for Discharge Instructions for the Person with a Burn

We on the burn team are happy to see that you are able to go home. To ensure you the speediest possible recovery, it is important that you are able to care for yourself and recognize problems that may interfere with your complete recovery.

If any of the following occur, please call the hospital and ask for the Burn Clinic. The nurse will be able to assist you.

1. Healed area breaking open. Cover with clean dressing.
2. Formation of blisters.
3. Signs of infection:
   a. Fever, temperature over 37.2° C (99° F).
   b. Redness, pain, swelling, hardness, or warmth in or around wound or any other part of body.
   c. Increased or foul-smelling drainage from wound.
3. Problems with your Ace bandages or Jobst garment such as improper fit, formation of blisters, or opening of healed area underneath.

Your first clinic appointment will be on ______. If a family member can come with you they can register for you and you may go to the Burn Clinic waiting room.

### BATHING

Bathing or showering daily in your usual manner cleans the wounds, especially the ones that are still open.

1. Check the water and be sure to adjust the temperature to a warm and comfortable level. Your skin is more sensitive to extra heat or cold and can be easily injured.
2. Wash gently with a clean soft washcloth, using a mild detergent soap such as Dreft or Ivory Snow, approximately 2 tsp. Be careful not to rub too hard so as not to disturb the grafted areas. Avoid harsh or deodorant soaps.
3. Rinse skin thoroughly after washing.
4. Dry thoroughly.
5. Apply specific dressing as instructed.

### CARE FOR BURN WOUND

These are your guidelines for the care of your burn wound. During this time, look at the involved areas and note if there are any changes that need to be reported.

1. Wash hands
2. Remove dressing and dispose in paper bag or wrap in newspaper.
3. Wash hands.
4. Wash open area with gauze using solution of Dreft (or Ivory Snow) and water. Add 1 tbsp Dreft to a basin of water; 2 tbsp Dreft, if you use the bathtub. Use a clean towel and washcloth with each dressing change.
5. Rinse skin well.
6. Wash hands.
7. Apply dressing as described below.
8. Wear gloves. Wash basin or bathtub with a disinfectant such as Lysol.
9. Wash hands.

### CARE OF CLOTHING

When you are discharged, you may find that healed burn areas are sensitive to harsh detergents, fabric softeners, and clothing dyes. If you are sensitive, we suggest the following:

1. Launder new clothing before use by machine or hand with Dreft or Ivory Snow.
2. Rinse clothes twice.
3. Do not use fabric softeners.
4. If you have open burns or a healed area that opens, wash all clothes separately from other family members.
5. Scarlet red ointment will permanently stain clothing.
6. If dyes used in clothing cause irritation, wear white articles.

### ACE BANDAGES

You have been taught to put on your own Ace bandages while in the hospital; but if you do have a problem with this, please notify the Burn Clinic. It is also important that you know how to care for them and understand problems that occur.

1. If they are too loose, they will be ineffective and must be rewrapped.
2. If they are too tight, they will cause discomfort, numbness, tingling, and puffiness and must be rewrapped.
3. They must be worn for a long period of time, probably 6-12 months to be effective, so please do not stop wearing them until your doctor tells you.
4. To care for your Ace bandages:
   a. Hand wash with Dreft or Ivory Snow in cold water.
   b. Towel dry.
   c. Lay flat or place over rod or clothesline.
   d. Do not use clothespins.

### PRESSURE GARMENT

You have been taught to put on your Jobst garment while in the hospital; but if you have a problem with this, please notify the Burn Clinic. It is also important that you know how to care for it and understand problems that can occur.

1. If it is too loose, it will be ineffective and you will require a new garment.
2. If it is too tight, it will cause discomfort, numbness, and tingling. Do not wear it if this occurs, but notify the Burn Clinic as soon as possible.
3. To care for your pressure garment:
   a. Hand wash with Dreft or Ivory Snow in cold water.
   b. Towel dry.
   c. Lay flat or place over rod or clothesline.
   d. Do not use clothespins.

**Courtesy Burn Service, MetroHealth Medical Center, Cleveland.**

An example of written discharge instructions is provided in the Guidelines box above. Written instructions should include the name and phone number of a physician or nurse that the patient may call with questions or problems concerning follow-up care. A referral may be made to the Visiting Nurse Association or another home health agency who may be of assistance in dressing the patient's wounds at home.

## Facilitating Individual and Family Coping

After discharge, the patient has to adjust to temporary or permanent function loss, cosmetic disfigurement, and

# NURSING CARE PLAN

## PERSON WITH BURNS

**DATA:** Mr. S. is a 54-year-old businessman, married with two children. He fell asleep while smoking in bed. He woke up after several minutes to discover his bed on fire. He was admitted to the hospital with 25% of his body burned, including his anterior arms, chest, abdomen, and scattered areas on his thighs. Six hours after admission he was receiving 40% oxygen through a face mask. Vital signs were as follows: heart rate 120 beats/min, respiratory rate 30 beats/min, blood pressure 140/80, temperature 38.8° C. Two peripheral IVs were placed, each running at 250 ml/hr. A Foley catheter has drained 50 ml the past hour. Mr. Smith has a productive cough of gray-tinged sputum and a hoarse voice. Breath sounds clear with coughing. His wounds were cleansed with Dreft and normal saline and covered with a Silvadene dressing. He complained of nausea and a nasogastric tube was inserted. Antacids were ordered to be administered every 2 hours via tube.

The nursing history identified the following:

- He smokes 1½ packs/day; he has tried several times to quit smoking.
- The same day, his wife feared that he would fall asleep while smoking.
- He owns his own business.

### ■ NURSING DIAGNOSIS

Ineffective airway clearance related to laryngeal edema and irritation from smoke inhalation and history of cigarette smoking

| Expected Patient Outcome | Nursing Interventions | Rationale |
|---|---|---|
| Maintains adequate ventilation and oxygenation. | Assess and document rate, depth, and ease of respirations; note type, amount, color of sputum; observe patient's color. | Increased respiratory effort, large amounts of tenacious, gray-tinged sputum and signs of tissue hypoxia indicate the need for endotracheal intubation.<br>Providing oxygen will increase oxygen supply to body tissues. |
| | Provide respiratory treatment and medications as ordered (pulmonary drainage and clapping, incentive spirometer, bronchodilators). | Respiratory treatments will loosen and thin secretions and will allow patient to clear his own airway. |
| | Turn patient every 2 hours. | Change in position will help mobilize secretions. |

Collaborative nursing actions include those to prevent hypovolemia from the movement of fluid from the intravascular to the interstitial compartment, to prevent respiratory distress, and to prevent gastrointestinal distress. Immediate reporting of the early signs of hypovolemia and/or respiratory distress may prevent serious effects (hypovolemic shock, respiratory failure). Nursing actions include monitoring for the following:

- Signs of hypovolemia: increased heart rate, decreased urine output, decreased blood pressure, decreased sensorium
- Signs of respiratory distress: increased respiratory rate, shortness of breath, change in patient's color, increased work of breathing, change in ABGs (decreasing pH, decreasing $Po_2$, increasing $Pco_2$)
- Signs of gastrointestinal distress: low gastric pH, heme + nasogastric aspirate, absence of bowel sounds

### ■ NURSING DIAGNOSIS

High risk for fluid volume deficit

| Expected Patient Outcome | Nursing Interventions | Rationale |
|---|---|---|
| Maintains optimal fluid balance. | Provide calculated IV fluids. | Calculated IV fluids will prevent patient from developing hypovolemic shock. |
| | Monitor and document output hourly. | Any deficit or increase in fluid intake or output must be identified quickly to avoid complications of hypovolemia. |
| | Assess for clinical signs of hypovolemia (decreased sensorium; changes in skin from pink to pale, from warm to cool). | These may be the first signs of hypovolemia. |
| | Weigh daily; compare to preinjury weight. | Weight is an accurate assessment of fluid balance. |

# NURSING CARE PLAN

## PERSON WITH BURNS—cont'd

### ■ NURSING DIAGNOSIS
Pain related to exposed nerve endings from burn injury

| Expected Patient Outcome | Nursing Interventions | Rationale |
|---|---|---|
| Experiences minimal pain. | Provide with pain medication as ordered; administer 30 minutes before dressing changes (hydrotherapy and debridement); evaluate and document effectiveness. | Decreasing pain will decrease anxiety and increase patient's cooperation during dressing changes. |
| | Assess need for other interventions that may decrease pain experience (use of the radio, relaxation therapy, hypnosis). | The pain experience is subjective; a variety of pain control techniques may decrease the pain experience. |
| | Assess pain history and response to pain. | Information about past pain experiences will aid in planning techniques for pain control. |
| | Educate patient about painful procedures and about techniques to reduce pain; encourage patient to participate in treatments whenever possible. | Information and participation may help decrease the anxiety that is often seen with pain. |
| | Use environmental comfort measures (speak in calm manner, keep warm). | Comfortable environment may decrease anxiety and pain. |

### ■ NURSING DIAGNOSIS
Anxiety

| Expected Patient Outcome | Nursing Interventions | Rationale |
|---|---|---|
| Demonstrates control of anxiety. | Gather information about background, personality, and level of coping from friends, family, and patient (as appropriate). | Information will assist the nurse in planning interventions to decrease anxiety. |
| | Offer patient and family simple explanations of his or her injury and treatments. | Too much information may overwhelm patient and increase anxiety. |
| | Assess ability to cope with illness; consult with other services. | Social services or pastoral care may be able to provide assistance to the patient. |

### ■ NURSING DIAGNOSIS
High risk for infection related to loss of skin from burn injury

| Expected Patient Outcome | Nursing Interventions | Rationale |
|---|---|---|
| Is free of pathogenic organisms. | Document initial appearance of the burn wound (color, dryness, odor). | Early changes in appearance of wound may be the first signs of infection. |
| | Monitor for signs of infection (fever, altered sensorium, increased respiratory rate, foul odor from wound). | Early detection of infection will allow appropriate antibiotics to be prescribed before serious injury occurs. |
| | Implement isolation procedures. | To protect the patient from other organisms that may cause infection. |

*Continued.*

# NURSING CARE PLAN

## PERSON WITH BURNS—cont'd

### ■ NURSING DIAGNOSIS

Impaired skin integrity related to burn injury

| Expected Patient Outcome | Nursing Interventions | Rationale |
|---|---|---|
| Demonstrates viable healing tissue. | Perform prescribed wound care (hydrotherapy and debridement); assess wound during each dressing change. | Wound care procedures may change daily, depending on assessment of wound. |
| | Assess need for equipment and supplies and have available before wound care. | Adequate supplies should be ordered ahead of time to avoid the problem of discovering halfway through the dressing change that there are not enough supplies available. |

the reactions of others. The ability to make these adjustments will depend on coping mechanisms before the burn, the severity and site of the burn, and the reaction of others. How well the patient is adapting to these changes can be evaluated during out-patient visits when the burn team and appropriate personnel are available.

Follow-up care may not take place at the institution where the patient was hospitalized if the patient lives several hundred miles away. The burn team members may need to contact their counterparts in the community to plan follow-up care. If possible, a member of the follow-up team should visit the patient in the hospital before discharge.

Job retraining may be necessary if the burn injury caused loss of joint function or other physical limitations that may prevent the patient from returning to a former job. The local office of the State Labor and Industry Board can assign a vocational counselor to help the patient return to the work force. Even if retraining cannot begin for several months, the contact with the vocational counselor and anticipation of retraining may help the patient look beyond immediate problems and think of the future.

## ♦ EVALUATION

To evaluate the effectiveness of nursing interventions, compare patient behaviors with those stated in the expected outcomes. Successful achievement of patient outcomes for the patient with burns is indicated by the following:

### Rehabilitation Phase

1. Positive coping behaviors
   a. Identifies alterations in personal or family situation and identifies strategies to adapt
   b. Develops realistic image of self and body image
   c. Reintegrates self into the community
2. Full range of motion and mobility
   a. Demonstrates exercise program for the prevention and control of contractures
   b. Able to perform ADLs
3. Maintenance of skin integrity
   a. Identifies techniques to prevent breakdown of healed areas, e.g., protection from sun, exposure to harsh chemicals, use of lotions, proper use of pressure garments

## QUESTIONS TO CONSIDER

- Discuss the differences in priorities of care during the emergent and rehabilitative phases of burn injury.
- Differentiate between a partial-thickness and full-thickness burn injury.
- How would you explain to a family member the physiologic changes following burn injury?
- Discuss the differences in fluid resuscitation in the first hours and second 24 hours after a burn injury.
- What factors would you consider in determining how aggressively to care for a healthy 80-year-old woman who suffers a 60% TBSA deep-partial and full-thickness burn?

## CRITICAL THINKING ACTIVITIES

- Two 12-year-old children are brought to the emergency room after burns from a house fire. One child has a partial-thickness burn, and the other has a full-thickness burn. What subjective data would help differentiate these two types of burns?
- Incorporating general principles of psychologic care, develop one nursing approach for each of the following patient responses to a severe burn: withdrawal; regression; anger/hostility; and depression.

## CRITICAL THINKING ACTIVITIES – cont'd

► What criteria would be used on a patient with a burn injury to determine if the physician or burn clinic should be notified or consulted during rehabilitation at home?

# CHAPTER SUMMARY

### ETIOLOGY/EPIDEMIOLOGY

- The severity of a burn injury depends on the age of the victim, body part involved, burning agent, size and depth of the burn wound, and the victim's medical history.

### NURSING MANAGEMENT

- The initial care for a burn includes removing the victim from the source of the burn and dousing the burn with water.
- The initial systemic response to a burn is the shift of fluid from the intravascular to the interstitial space, creating hypovolemia. This is treated with a calculated dose of lactated Ringer's solution. After 48 to 72 hours, the fluid shifts from the interstitial to the intravascular space and hypervolemia occurs.
- Emotional support to the victim and the victim's family is an important role for nurses.
- Burn wounds must be assessed on a daily basis.
- Correct splinting and positioning are the best methods for preventing contractures.
- There is no way to predict the appearance of a burn wound after healing.
- Nursing has a major role in identifying populations at risk for burn injury and in offering prevention programs to them.

## REFERENCES


1. Alexander L et al: Use of morphine sulfate (MS Contin) in patients with burns: a pilot study, *J Burn Care Rehabil* 13:581-583, 1992.
2. American Psychiatric Association: *Diagnostic and statistical manual of mental disorders,* ed 3, Washington, DC, 1980, The Association.
3. Bernstein NR, O'Connell K, Chedekel D: Patterns of burn adjustment, *J Burn Care Rehabil* 13:4-12, 1992.
4. Blumenfeld M, Schoeps MM: Psychological reactions. In Blumenfeld M, Schoeps MM: *Psychological care of the burn and trauma patient,* Baltimore, 1993, Williams & Wilkins.
5. Brose L: Prealbumin as a marker of nutritional status. *J Burn Care Rehabil* 11:372-375, 1990.
6. Committee on Organization and Delivery of Burn Care: *Burn care resources in North America 1991-1992,* Cincinnati, 1991, American Burn Association.
7. Deitrich EA, Berg R: Bacterial translocation from the gut: a mechanism of infection, *J Burn Care Rehabil* 8:475-478, 1987.
8. Hansbrough JF, Zapata-Sirvent R, Hoyt D: Postburn immunosuppression: an inflammatory response to the burn wound? *J Trauma* 30:671-675, 1990.
9. Deleted in proofs.
10. Horton JW, White DJ, Baxter CR: Hypertonic saline dextran resuscitation of thermal injury, *Ann Surg* 211:301-311, 1990.
11. Lillico S: *National burn awareness 1992,* Encino, Calif, 1992, The National Burn Awareness Task Force.
12. Patterson DR et al: Post-traumatic stress disorder in hospitalized patients with burn injuries, *J Burn Care Rehabil* 11:181-184, 1990.
13. Rue LW, Cioffi WG: Resuscitation of thermally injured patients, *Crit Care Nurs Clin North Am* 3:181-189, 1991.

13a. US Department of Health and Human Services, Public Health Service: *Healthy People 2000: national health promotion and disease prevention objectives.* Washington, DC, 1990, US Government Printing Office.

14. Watchel TL, Yen M, Fortune JB: Nutritional support for burned patients. In Watchel TL, Kahn V, and Frank HA, editors: *Current topics in burn care,* Rockville, Md, 1983, Aspen.

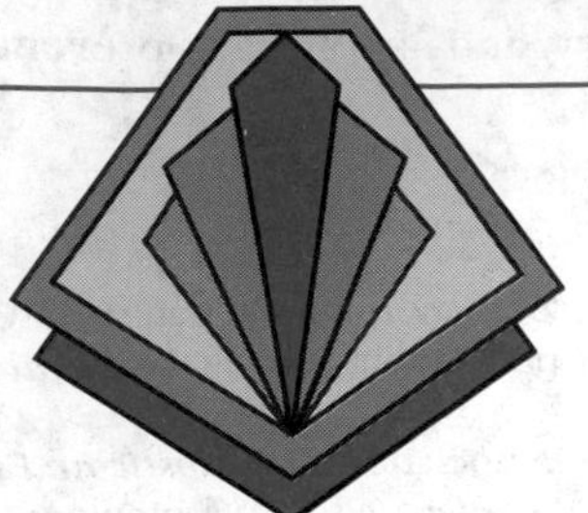

CHAPTER 69

# Assessment of the Immune System

*Katherine A. Fletcher*

## CHAPTER OBJECTIVES

***After studying this chapter, the learner should be able to do the following:***

1. Summarize the primary structures of the immune system and their role in the nonspecific and specific response of the immune system.
2. Explain the physiologic changes that occur within the immune system with aging.
3. Identify subjective and objective data that should be collected on persons with actual or potential health problems of the immune system.
4. Describe the common diagnostic tests used to identify immune dysfunction.
5. Describe the nursing implications of the diagnostic tests used to diagnose immune dysfunction.

## KEY TERMS

ABO typing
Anergic
Antinuclear antibodies (ANA)
Clusters of differentiation (CD)
Coombs' test (direct, indirect)
C-reactive protein (CRP)
Enzyme-linked immunosorbent assay (ELISA)
Erythrocyte sedimentation rate (ESR, sed rate)
Immunoelectrophoresis
Interferon
Interleukins
LE cells
Leukocytosis
Leukopenia
Lymphocytosis
Neutrophil functional assay
Protein electrophoresis
Radioallergosorbent test (RAST)
Rheumatoid factor (RF)
Shift to the left
Shift to the right
Skin tests
Total complement activity test ($CH_{50}$)
WBC count with differential
Western blot test

The chapter provides a brief review of the essential components of the immune system, related assessment data, and appropriate diagnostic tests. Disorders of the immune system are described in Chapters 70 and 71.

## ANATOMY AND PHYSIOLOGY

### REVIEW OF IMMUNE SYSTEM

The human organism exists in a world of potential biologic insults. The immune system functions to protect the body from foreign invasions by recognizing self from nonself and destroying that which is nonself. This ability allows the body to defend itself against microorganisms and to dispose of cellular debris and foreign-appearing material. The immune system also possesses the ability to remember foreign antigens so that it might mount a swifter, more effective immune response the next time the individual is exposed to particular antigens. The immune system has two levels of defense against invasion: the nonspecific and specific responses. The basic responses and their functions are described in detail in Chapter 13. These two responses are meshed together in such a way as to give individuals their own unique immunologic reaction to a particular foreign substance. This variation in immunologic response among individuals occurs because each person has a different genetic background, is exposed to different environmental conditions, and responds differently to particular stimulants.[9] In other words, what is self to one would not be recognized as self to another.

This very uniqueness of the immune system makes immune disorders difficult to treat. Nurses are unable to know how each person will respond to any new substance, and sometimes the very medical treatment modality used may put the individual at risk for pathogenic invasion. It is important for the nurse to understand the mechanisms of the immune system and its relationship to disease and health to support immune responses when appropriate, or to intervene to decrease the functioning of the immune system when it is excessive.

## Nonspecific Immune Response

The nonspecific immune response system is a collection of anatomic and chemical barriers that nonspecifically recognizes and responds to the introduction of foreign materials or damaged self-cells. The response is the same no matter what the initiating injury or material. Only the degree of response varies in relation to the extent of the damage.

### Components of the system

Body surfaces such as the *skin* and *mucous membranes* are the first line of defense. These organs are structured to provide a physical barrier against invasion from microorganisms. The surface of these organs also have built-in chemical barriers to microbial growth. If microorganisms are able to penetrate these barriers, however, a host of chemical substances within the body will further impede the progress of this foreign enemy. Chemicals such as gastric acid and lysozyme (an enzyme distributed in secretions throughout the body) cause damage to invading cells.

The *complement system of the blood* is another major factor that can be activated by antigens, antibody-antigen complexes, tissue damage, or release of endotoxins. This system is composed of inactive serum proteins that, when activated in a sequential series of steps, can initiate and modify the inflammatory response, as well as cause damage to cell membranes to produce cell lysis. The *phagocytic* cells of the body are another key component of this nonspecific response. Those cells include the *granulocytic white blood cells,* especially the *neutrophils,* and *macrophages.* In response to tissue injury or presence of infectious microorganisms in the body, chemotactic substances are carried via the blood to the bone marrow where phagocytic cells are formed and stored until they are signaled to be released in large numbers into the blood. They are then drawn by the chemotactic substances to the site of injury where they leave the vessels and move into the tissues. In the tissues they engulf and destroy foreign materials.

There are also a variety of *proteins* that are activated early in infection to help mediate the immune response. **Interferon,** a substance produced by cells damaged by viruses, protects cells in the vicinity from invasion from the same virus. Interferon also increases the macrophage's phagocytic ability that facilitates the removal of more antigens. Another group of proteins, acute phase proteins, multiply during acute infection and promote the initiation of the complement cascade.

## Specific Immune Response

The specific immune response system is designed to recognize and take action against *specific* foreign molecules known as *antigenic determinants.* These antigenic determinants elicit the formation and proliferation of specifically reactive molecules *(antibodies)* or cells *(cytotoxic lymphocytes)* that bind to the antigenic determinants to inactivate or destroy the foreign agent. The system also remembers prior contact with the antigenic material and responds faster and more efficiently to subsequent contact. Two functional components make up the specific immune response system: the ***cell mediated system,*** providing the cytotoxic lymphocytes; and the ***humorally mediated system,*** providing the circulating antibodies.

### Cell mediated immune response

*T cell lymphocytes,* responsible for provision of the cell mediated immune response, are produced in the bone marrow and mature in the *thymus* gland. From the thymus they migrate to the regional *lymph nodes* and *spleen* where they populate the medullary regions. Each mature immunosensitive T cell lymphocyte is capable of responding to a specific antigenic signal. When exposed to its specific antigen, the T cell begins to divide, increasing the number of that antigenically responsive cell in the lymph node. Some of the cells are shed into the circulation and then, carried by the blood, they seek out the antigen or antigenically labeled cells in the body. When the T cell lymphocytes encounter such cells, they attack and destroy them (cytoxic effect). They also release a number of soluble substances (lymphokines) that recruit and activate nonspecifically reactive phagocytes (LAK cells) to attack the tissues at the site.

Other T cell lymphocytes act to regulate the T cell function and production of antibodies by the B cell system. T cell lymphocytes known as ***helper T cells*** ($T_H$ or $T_4$ cells) are necessary to provide a full immunologic humoral or cell mediated response. Another type of T cell, known as *suppressor T cells* ($T_S$ or $T_8$ cells), operates to prevent or modify the function of the two systems. Additional T cells, *memory T cells* ($T_M$), remember contact with the antigen and on subsequent exposure respond immediately to its presence in the body. These T lymphocytes have an intricate communication system using a group of factors called **interleukins** (a type of lymphokine).

During embryologic development the system provides for self-tolerance. T cells that could respond to self-antigens are either destroyed or rendered nonactive so that the cell mediated system does not respond to the antigens on the body's own cells and tissues.

**Humorally mediated immune response**

***B cell lymphocytes,*** the lymphocytes providing the humorally mediated immune response, are produced in the bone marrow, and undergo maturation at a site outside of the thymus, such as in the bone marrow or mucosa-associated lymphoid tissues. They migrate to the spleen and lymphoid tissues located along the gut, bronchus, and tonsils. These are all strategic locations that are continuously exposed to antigens.[10]

As with T cells, the immunosensitive B cells are programmed to respond to a single antigen. When the antigen is present, the B cell begins to proliferate and differentiate into a ***plasma cell.*** A plasma cell is designed to synthesize and release large amounts of ***immunoglobulin*** (antibody) that will combine with the antigen that caused its production. These antibody molecules are released into the circulation where they become part of the gamma globulin fraction of the serum. The B cells producing the immunoglobulin remain in the lymphoid tissue and continue to synthesize additional molecules of the specific antibody. Note that this is different from the T cell response where cytotoxic T cells are released; in this case the B cells remain, and their product is released. Thus the level of active specific antibody begins to rise in the serum fraction ***(antibody titer),*** as well as in the level of the γ-globulin fraction in general. These antibodies are carried by the blood and other body fluids to where they encounter their specific antigen and bind to it. Upon binding, the antibody may inactivate the antigen, precipitate it, or activate other antigen-damaging processes (such as the complement cascade) to remove the antigen.

The immunoglobulins are subdivided into different classes on the basis of molecular structure and function. The generic symbol for immunoglobulins is Ig, and each of the classes is designated by a letter of the alphabet: IgG, IgM, IgA, IgE, and IgD. The predominant immunoglobulin is IgG.

The B cell system is similar to the T cell system in that it is controlled by helper and suppressor T cells, forms memory ($B_M$) cells, and is rendered self-tolerant by the same mechanisms.

## PHYSIOLOGIC CHANGES WITH AGING

The extent of immunologic changes that occur with aging varies among individuals, depending on multiple factors such as genetics, nutritional status, and presence of disorders that deplete the immune system. In general, however, the immune response decreases with aging.

Elderly persons have many physiologic changes in their body systems that increase their risk for infection by compromising the immune system. With aging, the chemical barriers within many organs decrease, increasing the person's susceptibility to microbe invasion. Many organs of elderly persons also display slower mechanical activity such as decreased ciliary action and decreased gastric emptying. These slowed processes can cause poor removal of organisms and an increase in microbe flora. The factors of decreased skin thickness, decreased "give" of aged skin, and decreased vascular flow makes the skin a less effective defense against the environment. The dermis and the subcutaneous tissue are thinner, increasing vulnerability to trauma.[3] Collagen changes within the skin of elderly persons cause the tensile strength of the skin to increase while the elasticity decreases. This can make the skin more prone to tear-type injuries because it has less "give" when exposed to trauma. Once there is a break in the skin, the healing processes are much slower because of decreased vascularity.[3] Table 69-1 lists physiologic changes in elderly persons and the consequences to the immune system.

The weight and volume of the thymus gland exhibit large variations. The thymus gland grows until the infant reaches 6 months of age and then remains constant;

**TABLE 69-1 Physiologic Changes in Elders That Affect Immune Response**

| CHANGE | EFFECT |
|---|---|
| **SKIN** | |
| Decreased thickness and elasticity<br>Increased tensile strength<br>Decreased neurosensory function | Skin more vulnerable to trauma; torn skin provides opening for microorganisms to invade body<br>Decreased awareness of injury |
| **RESPIRATORY SYSTEM** | |
| Decreased ciliary action<br>Reduced respiratory muscle strength<br>Impaired gag/cough reflexes | Decreased removal of inhaled organisms |
| **CARDIOVASCULAR SYSTEM** | |
| Decreased cardiac output<br>Increased peripheral resistance | Decreased circulation to tissues; may delay inflammatory response and increase risk of ischemic injury |
| **GASTROINTESTINAL SYSTEM** | |
| Decreased ciliary action<br>Decreased gastric emptying<br>Decreased secretion of HC1 and selected dietary enzymes | Decreased organism removal<br>Decreased digestion leading to decreased production of serum proteins |
| **GENITOURINARY SYSTEM** | |
| Decreased glomerular filtration rate<br>Relaxed musculature<br>Decreased mucosal barrier<br>Decreased estrogen | Increased risk of urinary tract infections<br>Vaginal infections |
| **LYMPHATIC SYSTEM** | |
| Decreased number and size of lymph nodes | Impaired ability to resist infection |

however, the morphologic structure of the thymus gland changes significantly with age.[10] Specific immune responses in elderly persons are altered as a result of T lymphocyte changes and include the following[10]:

1. Decreased relative proportions of $CD_4$ and $CD_8$, which affect immune system regulation. This may explain why autoantibodies are increased in this age group.
2. Low rate of T lymphocyte proliferation in response to a stimulus but not an overall decrease in the number of T cells. This would tend to cause elderly persons to respond slower to allergic stimulants.
3. Cytotoxic (killer) T cells decrease in number; therefore the normal antigen specific cytotoxicity is diminished. This produces a reduced response to foreign material.
4. Production of interleukin-2 (IL-2) by T helper cells is reduced. This further decreases the stimulation of the T lymphocytes and natural killer (NK) cells.
5. T cell function is reduced in response to certain viral antigens, allografts (from other persons such as transplants), and tumor cells.

B cell responsiveness also decreases, but is thought to be the result of a decline in helper T cell function.[10] Elderly persons experience an increased frequency of bacterial infections—possibly because of a defect in the antibody function. The total immunoglobulin concentration is not changed with age, but there is a noted increase in the level of IgA and IgG antibodies.[10]

Elderly persons frequently experience hospital stays and undergo many treatments that put them at risk for infection. They are admitted to hospitals with common medical diagnoses of heart disease, malignant neoplasm, vascular disease, fracture, pneumonia, eye disease, and prostatic hyperplasia, with an average hospital stay of 8 days.[5] These diseases cause them to be less mobile. Immobility coupled with the altered immune responses increases the risk for complications such as pneumonia and skin breakdown. Elderly persons also experience more diagnostic, nonsurgical, and surgical procedures than any other segment of the population.[5] These procedures and the use of associated invasive devices such as indwelling urinary catheters, intravenous catheters, and endoscopes put the aged at an increased risk for infection.

The end result of the immune system changes in the elderly is an increased incidence of infections. Common infections tend to be more severe, with slower recovery and less probability of developing immunity after an infection. There is also an increase in tumors and autoimmunity because of a decreased ability to recognize foreign material and regulate one's own immune system.

**BOX 69-1 Nursing History: Immunologic Data**

1. Infection history
   a. Recurrent infections: type, frequency, and any known causes
   b. Skin rash: location, itching, when rash occurs, what things make it worse, what makes it better
   c. Fever pattern: how high has the temperature been, when does it occur, how long does it last
   d. Lymph node enlargement: where, when was it noticed
   e. Fatigue and weakness: describe it, what aggravates it, what helps it, sleep patterns, changes in activities of daily living
   f. Joint pain: which joints, when does it occur, how long does it last, rate pain on scale 1-10, what aggravates it, what helps it
2. Allergy history
   a. Known allergies to medications, radiocontrast media, foods, or insect bites
   b. How the person reacts to these allergans
3. Other subjective information
   a. Concurrent disorders: autoimmune disorders (i.e., systemic lupus erythematosus [SLE], rheumatoid arthritis), HIV status, chronic systemic disorders (i.e., diabetes mellitus, renal failure), malignancies
   b. Current medication: prescription (immunosuppressive agents, NSAIDs, antibiotics), nonprescription (antihistamines, aspirin), illicit drug use
   c. Medical treatment history: radiation therapy, chemotherapy, surgery, transplant, recent diagnostic tests, blood products
   d. Diet and nutrition: actual weight and current weight, dietary restrictions, appetite, food intolerances
   e. Psychosocial status: recent stresses, changes in relationships, usual mode of coping, sexual preference, sexual habits, alcohol use, occupation
   f. Environmental history: occupational exposure, chemical exposure, smoking, animals, hobbies, home heating and cooling system

## SUBJECTIVE DATA

Persons with reduced immune responses (children, elderly, immunosuppressed persons, or those with immunodeficiency diseases) are susceptible, to varying degrees, to *infection,* especially of the upper and lower respiratory tracts. These people need to be identified so that preventive measures are taken and early treatment is initiated. Persons who have hypersensitivity disorders are highly sensitive *(allergic)* to different substances and must avoid these allergens. Therefore, assessment focuses on identification of these persons and of early signs of infection or allergy.

Much of the experience of immune dysfunction is subjective; therefore it is important to get an accurate health history (Box 69-1). Data are collected concerning recurrent infections, known allergies, history of autoimmune disorders, diet, and any therapy or environmental factors that may affect the immune system.

### INFECTION HISTORY

Recurrent infections can be a good indication that the immune system is compromised. Ask the patient what infections have occurred and when they occurred. Also investigate whether the patient has any insight into what might be causing these infections; this information provides data for future teaching, as well as assessment.

Fevers may occur with the inflammatory response, with an impaired immune system, or from rapid proliferation of white blood cells (WBCs).[8] The pattern of the fever can provide clues to the type of infective process involved. Data are collected about the fever onset, range and duration, and the presence of night sweats and chills. High fevers of 39 to 40°C may indicate serum sickness, whereas low-grade fevers may indicate allergies.[8] Fever may also be a sign of transplant rejection.

Enlarged lymph nodes usually accompany inflammation but may be seen also with Hodgkin's disease or non-Hodgkin's lymphoma, or they may be a sign of transplant rejection. Location of the enlarged nodes provides data about the source of the inflammation.

The patient may experience weakness, fatigue, and joint pain with autoimmune processes. Useful data include the pattern of these symptoms and the effect on life-style. If the patient is experiencing joint pain, a thorough assessment of the pain is required: occurrence, pattern, intensity, and aggravating factors. (See Chapter 17 for more information on pain assessment.)

### ALLERGY HISTORY

Allergic symptoms are triggered by a variety of allergens; therefore data are collected regarding allergens such as food, contrast media, medications, or other substances. The reactions to particular allergens can vary from a slight rash to life-threatening anaphylactic shock. The most common signs and symptoms of allergic disease are skin rash, difficulty hearing from obstruction of eustachian tubes, watery eyes, nasal discharge, coughing or wheezing, and gastrointestinal problems such as diarrhea or colic.[4]

### OTHER SUBJECTIVE DATA

The patient's current *medical problems* and associated *treatments* can affect the immune system. With autoimmune diseases, the patient's own antibodies attack different body organs and physicians prescribe steroids or immunosuppressant drugs, such as azathioprine (Imuran), to control this process. Patients with cancer undergo treatments such as radiation or chemotherapy, which may cause bone marrow destruction leading to increased risk of infection. In some cases diseases such as diabetes mellitus or renal failure may cause systemic changes that depress the immune response. Some medical treatments, such as surgery, or diagnostic tests can interrupt the integrity of the immune defense mechanisms.

The patient's *nutrition* and *psychosocial status* are two aspects of life-style that can greatly influence the immune system. Malnutrition is a common cause of immune deficiency (defects in cell mediated immunity, phagocytosis, and the complement system).[10] For this reason, it is important to collect data about nutritional habits. Explore with patients their usual eating habits and present appetite. *Stress* can compromise immune functioning by increased release of cortisol. If the patient has experienced recent stressors, it is important to investigate this more completely. How has the patient coped with this stressor and how has it changed relationships with others? Does the person possess any of the risk factors for HIV infection (history of blood transfusions, illicit drug use, high risk occupations such as nursing and medical technology, homosexuality, unprotected sexual intercourse, or multiple sexual partners)?

An *environmental* assessment can be helpful to identify factors in the patient's environment that might be causing allergies. Common allergens include animal dander, house dust, mold, and mites located in homes and chemicals or items used in the home, work, or with hobbies. Data about potential allergens will help to identify sources that may be controlled.

## OBJECTIVE DATA

Disorders of the immune system are more difficult to assess objectively because of less obvious physical markers. However, observations can be made about the person's general behavior, as well as the skin, lymph nodes, lungs, ears, eyes, nose, throat, and other body systems, that may suggest immune dysfunction.

### PATIENT BEHAVIOR

Some of the immune system disorders can cause problems in *cognition,* which in some cases, such as AIDS and SLE, may develop into dementia. The *facial expression* of patients with multiple sclerosis or myasthenia gravis will show facial weakness, whereas patients with scleroderma have a characteristic nonexpressive, masklike expression.

### SKIN, HAIR, AND NAILS

The skin is inspected carefully for color, skin turgor, texture, temperature, and moisture. Changes in skin color can provide information about the involved immune process; for example, jaundice of the skin may indicate an autoimmune disorder such as hemolytic anemia. The skin turgor assesses water content of the skin that can be decreased with malnutrition and dehydration. With scleroderma the texture of the skin is very thick, smooth, taut, and shiny; however, patients with Sjögren's syndrome will have scaly skin with decreased sweating. An increase in skin temperature may indicate inflammation, whereas coldness may suggest arterial insufficiency seen with Raynaud's disease (see Chapter 32).

Persons with different immune problems demonstrate different types of skin lesions. People with allergic reactions often have a maculopapular rash at the site where they were exposed to the allergen or over the whole body if the allergen was systemic. Persons with

SLE have a characteristic erythemic rash across the bridge of the nose and cheek in a butterfly pattern. Patients with AIDS may have malignant skin lesions called Kaposi's sarcoma, which are typically maculopapular and range in color from pink to bluish-purple (see Chapter 70). Patients with rheumatoid arthritis experience subcutaneous nodules located primarily over the knuckles (see Chapter 65).

Some autoimmune processes will cause notable patches of alopecia, or dry, brittle and broken hair. The nails show changes in color, configuration, or brittleness.

## EARS, EYES, NOSE, AND THROAT

The physical assessment of the ears of patients with allergies may reveal serous otitis media with retracted tympanic membranes, indicating obstruction of the eustachian tubes and fluid collection within the ear. The patient may be noted to repeat questions many times because of difficulty with hearing.

Periorbital edema may be seen in certain autoimmune disorders or hypersensitivity reactions. Dark circles, referred to as "allergic shiner," may be noted under the eyes of allergy patients because of chronic nasal obstruction resulting in venous stasis.[4] Changes in the conjunctiva, such as discoloration and vascular hemorrhage, can be caused by certain autoimmune disorders.

Nasal obstruction may cause the patient to breathe through the mouth, and the voice will have a nasal tone. Examination of the mouth and throat will identify any lesions in the mucous membrane or changes in mucosal color. Many autoimmune disorders cause oral lesions, and immunosuppressed patients may experience thrush, a white exudate that occurs over the tongue and mucous membranes.

## LYMPH NODES

Assessment of the lymph nodes includes inspection, as well as palpation, beginning at the neck and extending to the entire body. The location, size, surface characteristics, consistency, symmetry, mobility, and discomfort with palpation of the lymph nodes are documented. Inflamed, tender, or fixed nodes indicate the need for further investigation, and their location will identify the possible source of infection by the pattern of node involvement and usual drainage route.

## RESPIRATORY SYSTEM

Because persons with allergies typically show respiratory symptoms and immunosuppressed patients are particularly prone to pneumonias, it is critical that a complete respiratory assessment be made. Special attention is made to cough pattern, sputum color, skin color, the work of breathing, and lung sounds. Patients with pneumonia will display tachypnea, cyanosis, thick yellow or green sputum, and use accessory muscles to breathe. Allergic patients typically show wheezing, coughing with little sputum production, and dyspnea.

# DIAGNOSTIC TESTS

Laboratory tests, skin tests, and biopsies are the main sources of diagnostic evaluation.

## LABORATORY TESTS

Laboratory tests can measure nonspecific immune functioning, as well as specific elements of the immune process.

### Tests for Nonspecific Immune Function

This group of laboratory tests measures the nonspecific immune processes of the inflammatory response and phagocytosis. The tests include a white blood cell count with differential, erythrocyte sedimentation rate, C-reactive protein, total complement activity test, and phagocytic cell function tests.

A **white blood count with differential (WBC)** helps identify changes in bone marrow production of WBCs in response to a stimulus. Normal WBC counts are 5000 to 10,000/$cm^3$ in adults; the healthy elder range is typically lower—3000 to 9000/$cm^3$. Adults with a WBC count below the normal ranges are **leukopenic** and will have a compromised inflammatory response. A WBC count above 10,000/$cm^3$ is termed **leukocytosis** and indicates an inflammatory response to an invading organism or a disease process.

If the WBC is elevated, the *differential* count is examined to determine which specific group of WBCs (neutrophils, basophils, eosinophils, lymphocytes, monocytes) are increased or decreased. The differential is listed in such a way that the percentages of cells add up to 100%. This means that if the bone marrow proliferates one type of cell, it will increase the percentage of this cell and conversely decrease the percentage of the other cell types. The neutrophils are one of the first cells to migrate to the site of a bacterial infection, so an increase in the neutrophil percentage above 70% usually indicates a bacterial infection. Neutrophils (referred to as *bands* and *segs* or *stabs*) are usually listed first on the left side of a laboratory report. The phrase **shift to the left** means that the differential percentages have shifted to increase the number of less mature cells listed on the left side of the page, indicating a bacterial infection. The lymphocytes are one of the first cells to respond to viral infections. Lymphocytes are the largest percentage of cells listed on the right side of the laboratory report; therefore, a **shift to the right** means that the lymphocyte percentage is increased above 40% **(lymphocytosis)** indicating a viral infection. An increase in eosinophils is associated with allergic disorders.

**Erythrocyte sedimentation rate (ESR, sed rate)** is the rate at which RBCs settle and is expressed in millimeters/hour. An increased sed rate indicates that there are increased globulins, fibrinogen, or other substances in the blood, which make it clump faster than normal, usually because of infection, malignancies, or collagen vascular diseases.[2] The sed rate is frequently higher in healthy elders.[1]

Two other tests confirming inflammation are the C-reactive protein and total complement activity test. **C-reactive protein (CRP)** measures an abnormal protein found 18 to 24 hours after certain inflammatory processes. Some clinicians recommend the use of the CRP in distinguishing inflammatory from noninflammatory diseases (such as osteoarthritis from rheumatoid arthritis) and to monitor treatment effects of inflammatory diseases.[7] **Total complement activity ($CH_{50}$)** is a screening device for the complement cascade; the normal range for adults is 75 to 100 mg/dl. A positive CRP or high values on $CH_{50}$ indicate inflammation but not the source of the inflammation. Healthy elders also typically show higher values in these protein tests than younger adults.[1] Low values on the complement activity test indicate a complement deficiency.

*Phagocytic cell function tests* can be performed to evaluate the phagocytic ability of polymorphonuclear (PMN) leukocytes and macrophages. One method is observing the absolute and relative numbers of monocytes and PMN leukocytes on the WBC count. The **neutrophil functional assay** is a primary test to evaluate the motility, recognition and adhesion, ingestion, degranulation, and killing ability of the leukocytes and macrophages.[8]

## Tests for Specific Immune Function

Tests used to identify specific immune function include screening T cell and B cell functioning, antibody screening, autoantibody tests, and other tests.

### Tests for screening T cell and B cell functioning

**Protein electrophoresis** is a test that shows the relative concentrations of plasma proteins. In an applied electrical field, different proteins migrate at different rates because of their different sizes and shapes, and this property can be used to analyze plasma protein content. The plasma proteins consist of albumin and globulin, which can be further divided into $\alpha$-globulins, $\beta$-globulins, and $\gamma$-globulins (immunoglobulins). The serum proteins are subjected to electrophoresis in a medium that stabilizes the migration so that the proteins can be stained and examined. A densitometer records the color densities on graph paper. Figure 69-1 illustrates typical patterns seen in persons with normal protein levels, with decreased $\gamma$-globulin levels, and with increased $\gamma$-globulin levels. In immune disorders, the immunoglobulins may be either increased or decreased.

**Immunoelectrophoresis** identifies specific immunoglobulins. This test shows relative but imprecise quantities of immunoglobulins. Serum is separated electrophoretically and then tested for reaction with IgG, IgA, or IgM antisera. The test is useful for differentiating among various immunologic disorders (Table 69-2).

Three of the immunoglobulins, IgG, IgA, and IgM, can be measured quantitatively, whereas IgD and IgE are present in amounts too small to measure. An agar plate is impregnated with an antiserum specific to one of the immunoglobulins. A circular well is then cut in the agar, and the immunoglobulin is placed in the well. The immunoglobulin diffuses radially, forming a visible precipitate ring as it interacts with the antiserum. The radius of the ring is proportional to the immunoglobulin concentration; that is, the smaller the ring, the smaller the concentration. The diameter of the ring is compared with a standard measure to determine immunoglobulin quantity. Immunoglobulin levels vary with age. Normal adult levels are as follows: IgG, 600-1800 mg/dl; IgA, 100-400 mg/dl; and IgM, 60-150 mg/dl.

More rapid yet accurate quantitative measurement of IgG, IgA, and IgM can be done by *nephelometry*. The specific antibody is introduced into a fluid containing the specific antigen. The interaction of the antibody and antigen makes the fluid turbid; the degree of turbidity is measured by a photometric instrument.

The **radioallergosorbent test (RAST)** is a quantitative evaluation of IgE. Studies have shown that results of the RAST correlate well with skin testing for allergies.[6] This form of testing is very expensive but is useful in patients taking antihistamines that suppress skin reaction or in patients with skin diseases.[6]

### Antibody screening tests

Numerous tests are available to detect antibodies formed against specific bacteria, viruses, fungi, or parasites. Some common examples of antibody tests are streptozyme, enzyme-linked immunosorbent assay (ELISA), and Western blot test. Streptozyme is a neutralizing antibody produced after infection with Group A beta-hemolytic streptococci. Detection of this antibody titer above 166 todd units is useful in the diagnosis of rheumatic fever, scarlet fever, bacterial endocarditis, and glomerulonephritis from streptococcus group A infection.

The **enzyme-linked immunosorbent assay (ELISA)** method and the Western blot test are used for HIV (human immunodeficiency virus) antibody screening. The ELISA method is a simple screening test to determine presence of HIV antibodies. Because the ELISA method can give false-positive results, a positive result is followed by a Western blot test. The **Western blot test** identifies specific antibodies toward various fragments of the HIV and definitely confirms the presence of the virus. Antibody screening tests indicate that the patient has formed antibodies toward a particular antigenic source but does *not* necessarily mean that the patient presently has the disease. Test results can also be influenced by medication, infections, and chronic diseases.

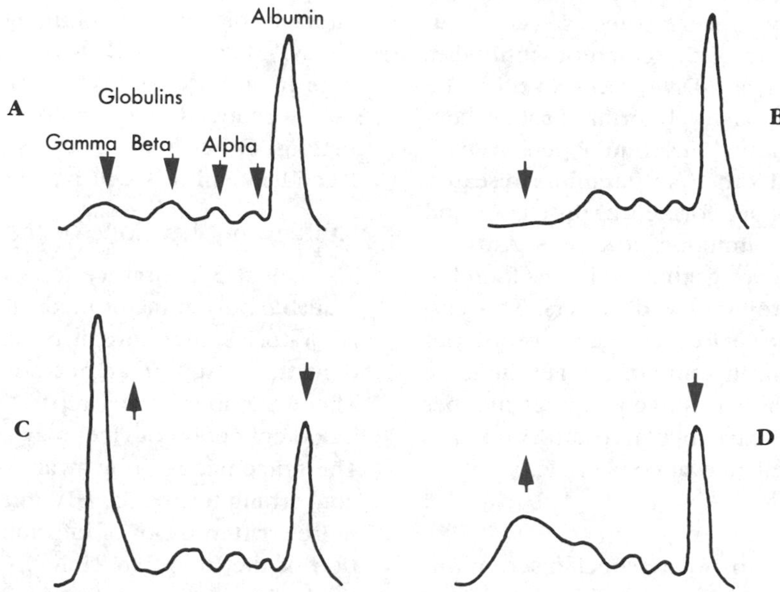


**FIGURE 69-1** Electrophoretic patterns. **A,** Normal. **B,** Hypogammaglobulinemia. **C,** Monoclonal gammopathy. **D,** Polyclonal gammopathy.

**TABLE 69-2 Clinical Significance of Changes in Immunoglobulin Levels**

| CLASS OF IMMUNOGLOBULIN | CLINICAL SIGNIFICANCE: INCREASED LEVEL | CLINICAL SIGNIFICANCE: DECREASED LEVEL |
|---|---|---|
| IgG | IgG myeloma bacterial infections, hepatitis A, glomerulonephritis, rheumatoid arthritis, SLE, AIDS | Agammaglobulinemia, IgA myeloma, IgA deficiency, chronic lymphocytic leukemia, type I dysgammaglobulinemia, lymphoid aplasia, combined immunodeficiency, common variable immunodeficiency, X-linked hypogammaglobulinemia |
| IgM | Hepatitis A and B, Waldenström's macroglobulinemia, trypanosomiasis, chronic infections, type I dysgammaglobulinemia, hepatitis, SLE, rheumatoid arthritis, Sjögren's syndrome, AIDS | Lymphoid aplasia, hypogammaglobulinemia, chronic lymphocytic leukemia, IgG myeloma, IgA myeloma, agammaglobulinemia |
| IgA | SLE, rheumatoid arthritis, IgA myeloma, glomerulonephritis, chronic liver disease | Ataxia, telangiectasia, hypogammaglobulinemia, acute and chronic lymphocytic leukemia, IgA deficiency, combined immunodeficiency, common variable immunodeficiency, X-linked hypogammaglobulinemia, agammaglobulinemia, IgG myeloma, chronic infections (especially upper respiratory type) |
| IgE | Atopic disorders: allergic rhinitis, allergic asthma, atopic dermatitis, Wiskott-Aldrich syndrome with eczema, parasitic infestation, hyperimmunoglobulin E | Associated with IgA deficiency, intrinsic (nonallergic) asthma |
| IgD | Eczema, skin disorders | Unknown |

From Mudge-Grout, CL: *Immunologic disorders,* St. Louis, 1993, Mosby.

### Autoantibody tests

Some laboratory tests will confirm the presence of abnormal antibodies produced by the body against itself (autoantibodies). The autoantibodies cause disease symptoms through injury to self tissues as seen in autoimmune processes. Some of the common antibodies include rheumatoid factor, anti-DNA, and ANA titer. The **rheumatoid factor (RF)** is an abnormal protein consisting of IgM antibodies found in serum of persons with rheumatoid arthritis and other autoimmune diseases. The anti-DNA antibodies are formed against DNA and are often elevated in autoimmune processes. **Antinuclear antibodies (ANA)** are gamma-globulins found in certain patients with autoimmune disorders. This particular group of antibodies is formed against properties of the nucleus of the cell. In some of the autoimmune diseases, such as SLE, ANA is positive in a large number of patients. Healthy elders have increased autoantibodies (ANA, RF) but the clinical relevance is unclear.[1]

### Other tests

Laboratory tests are used to isolate specific serum *antigens.* Some of these tests recognize the presence of antigens of invading organisms, whereas others isolate the antigenic properties of the patient's own tissues. Numerous tests are available that look for antigenic properties of particular organisms. For example, a positive $HB_sAG$ indicates the presence of the hepatitis B surface antigen, a specific antigenic determinant of the hepatitis B virus.

To assess the antigens on red blood cell (RBC) surfaces, the ABO blood typing, direct Coombs' test, and indirect Coombs' test (antiglobulin test) are performed. These tests monitor potential blood transfusion reactions, hemolytic anemia, and blood type compatibility. **ABO typing** identifies types of naturally occurring serum antibodies toward RBCs. The **indirect Coombs' test** indicates serum antibodies to RBCs, which are not connected to the cell. It can be used to identify the patient's Rh factor. ABO and Rh typing are used in the blood typing process and help to determine blood type compatibility; incompatible blood types lead to transfusion reactions. The **direct Coombs' test** detects antibodies coating the RBC that are not detected by ABO typing. A positive test facilitates diagnosing hemolytic disease and autoimmune disorders.[8]

Other laboratory tests commonly used to evaluate the patient's autoimmune status are the LE cell test and detection of cryoglobulins. The **LE cells** are neutrophils that contain large groups of abnormal DNA in their cytoplasm and are seen in 70% to 80% of patients with SLE.[5] The presence of LE cells helps to confirm the diagnosis of SLE. Cryoglobulins are abnormal serum proteins that precipitate at low temperatures and cause the patient to have increased sensitivity to cold. Location of these proteins in the serum are associated with immune system disorders.[8]

In patients with AIDS, there has been an increased interest in monitoring certain subsets of the T cells called **clusters of differentiation (CD).** The $CD_4$ ($T_4$ or helper T cells) level is often monitored to give the clinician information about the extent of immunodeficiency.[4] When the $CD_4$ levels fall below certain parameters, immunorestorative therapy is begun. The $CD_4$ can also be reduced in autoimmune diseases and during infections. Other T cell subsets (CD) are used to detect T cell leukemias, T cell lymphoma, or B cell tumors.[8]

## Nursing Implications of the Laboratory Testing

Many of the laboratory tests for immune diseases are available only at major medical centers or in specialized laboratories; therefore, it is necessary to inform the patient that results may not be available for some time. There are no specific preparations for testing. Different blood collection devices may be needed with each test. The nurse needs to be aware of the institutional policy concerning testing for HIV infection. Many agencies require written proof of informed consent before collection of the blood specimen. Confidentiality holds particular importance in testing for HIV infection because of the stigma that surrounds the disease.

# SPECIAL TESTS

## Skin Tests

**Skin tests** are a simple, relatively painless, and inexpensive means to diagnose particular allergies of IgE-mediated reactions. In the skin tests, the suspected allergen can be given by intradermal injection, or through a scratch, prick, or puncture of the skin. These tests are influenced by many factors such as skin reactivity to the allergen, amount of allergen administered, and the degree of sensitivity of the mast cells that produce the IgE. For instance, elderly persons have a poorer response to skin testing due to changes in mast cell reactivity.[10] Skin tests such as ***intradermal*** tests are one of the most sensitive tests but can cause a systemic reaction, such as anaphylaxis, and produce false-positive reactions. The ***scratch*** test method is difficult to standardize, and problems such as systemic reactions and false-positive results occur more commonly with this type of testing. The ***prick*** test has the ability to test more substances at one time than the other methods, but bleeding can cause false-positive results. Sites of testing can also be placed too close together to get accurate readings. ***Puncture*** methods have been used more than the other methods in recent years due to better reliability, safer administration, and better use with children.

Skin tesing may also be used to screen patients for T cell immunodeficiency. Specific antigens, including purified protein derivative (PPD), *Candida,* mumps antigen, streptokinase-streptodornase, coccidiodin, histoplasmin, and trichophyton, are injected intradermally. Reactions are read at 24-, 48-, and 78- hour intervals. The reactions determine ***hypersensitivity,*** not the presence of disease. More than 90% of healthy persons will respond to one of these antigens within 48 hours.[8] Areas of induration are carefully measured with a ruler. Indurations of 5 mm or greater are recorded as positive. A person who does not react to any of these antigens is said to be **anergic.** Anergy is associated with immunodeficiency disorders.

The nurse may be asked to administer these skin tests. The correct amount of allergen must be administered in the correct method in order for the test to be reliable and safe for the patient. For skin test reliability, it is advisable for the same person who administers the test to read the results. Because of the risk of anaphylaxis after allergen administration, emergency equipment should be available before administering the test, and the patient should be monitored for at least 30 minutes after allergen administration.

### Biopsy

A lymph node biopsy may be performed with lymphadenopathy to determine whether inflammation or malignancy is present. A synovial biopsy may be performed to obtain synovial fluid from a joint to differentiate among various types of arthritis or bone malignancies.

The nurse's role in a biopsy includes teaching the patient about the procedure and assisting the physician during the procedure. Most biopsies are completed under local anesthetic in an ambulatory setting. After anesthesia is effective, the patient should perceive only a pressure sensation; pain generally indicates insufficient anesthesia. After biopsy, the area is covered with a bandage, and the patient is instructed to monitor for bleeding and infection. Postbiopsy discomfort can be relieved by analgesics.

## CRITICAL THINKING ACTIVITIES

- How does the immune system of a young adult differ from that of an elderly adult? What consequences do differences have on the elderly individual?
- What conclusions can be drawn about the patient's condition when his/her ESR rate is elevated?

## CHAPTER SUMMARY

### ANATOMY AND PHYSIOLOGY

- The protective mechanisms of the body may be nonspecific (anatomic and chemical barriers, complement, phagocytes, interferon, acute phase proteins) or specific (T cell or B cell lymphoctyes).
- Immunologic responses generally decrease with aging, leading to increased incidence of infection. The elderly are also admitted to the hospital for longer time periods and undergo more invasive procedures than younger persons.

### SUBJECTIVE DATA

- Nursing assessment includes comprehensive subjective data about infection and allergy history.

### OBJECTIVE DATA

- Objective data are not as obvious in immunologic disorders but include general behavior, skin, ears, eye, nose and throat, and lymph node assessment.

### DIAGNOSTIC TESTS

- Laboratory tests, skin tests, and biopsies provide important data to identify the type of immune process or immune dysfunction.
- Laboratory tests include those that test the nonspecific immune functioning (WBC with differential, ESR, CRP, $CH_{50}$, phagocytic cell functioning) and specific immune functioning (qualitative and quantitative evaluation of immunoglobulins and antibody and antigen tests).
- Skin testing can aid in recognition of anergic and allergic persons.

## REFERENCES


1. Cavalieri TA, Chopra A, Bryman P: When outside the norm is normal: interpreting lab data in the aged, *Geriatrics* 45(5):66-70, 1992.
2. Corbett JV: *Laboratory tests and diagnostic procedures with nursing diagnoses,* Norwalk, 1992, Appleton & Lange.
3. Fenske NA, Lober CW: Skin changes of aging: pathological implications, *Geriatrics* 45(3):27-35, 1990.
4. Gibbs L: Assessment and management of allergic patients, *ORL-Head and Neck Nursing* 10(3):10-16, 1992.
5. *Health United States 1991 and prevention profile,* US Dept of Health and Human Services, Hyattsville, Md, 1991, DHHS Pub No (PHS) 92-1232.
6. Korenblat PE, Wedner HJ: *Allergy theory and practice,* ed 2, Philadelphia, 1992, WB Saunders.
7. Kushner I: C-reactive protein and the acute-phase response, *Hosp Pract* 25(3H):13-28, 1990.
8. Mudge-Grout CL: *Immunologic disorders,* St Louis, 1993, Mosby.
9. Patterson R et al: *Allergic diseases,* Philadelphia, 1993, JB Lippincott.
10. Stites DP, Terr AI: *Basic and clinical immunology,* ed 7, Norwalk, 1991, Appleton & Lange.

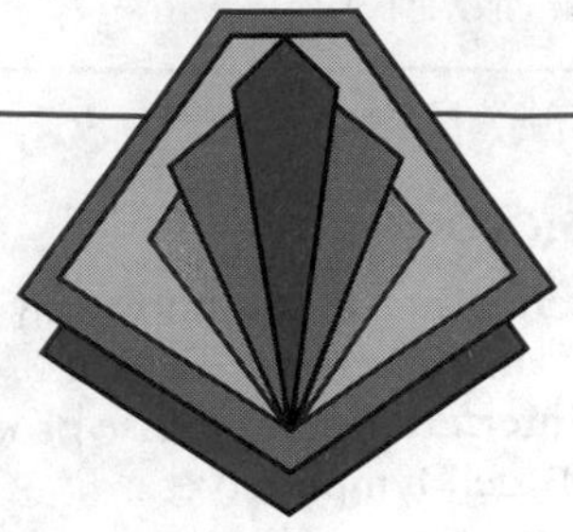

CHAPTER 70

# Management of Persons With Problems of the Immune System

*Katherine A. Fletcher*
*Barbara C. Long*

## CHAPTER OBJECTIVES

***After studying this chapter, the learner should be able to do the following:***

1. Describe the pathophysiologic difference between primary and secondary immunodeficiency disorders.
2. Develop a nursing care plan for the patient with an immunodeficiency disorder that would include teaching.
3. Describe the pathophysiologic changes that occur in a patient with monoclonal and polyclonal gammopathies.
4. Discuss the nursing problems and interventions necessary for a patient experiencing multiple myeloma.
5. Examine the differences in immunologic reactions that occur between the four classifications of hypersensitivity disorders.
6. Discuss the nursing interventions that are imperative to prevent a hypersensitivity reaction.
7. Develop a nursing plan of care that includes discharge teaching for a patient with a type I hypersensitivity disorder.
8. Describe the pathophysiologic factors involved in immunologic blood reactions and at least two safeguards to prevent immunologic blood reactions.
9. Describe the role of the nurse caring for patients with serum sickness.
10. Describe three examples of type IV hypersensitivity reactions.
11. Describe the possible etiologies of autoimmune disease.

## KEY TERMS

anaphylactic hypersensitivity (type I)
angioedema
antilymphocytic globulin (ALG)
antithymocytic globulin (ATG)
apheresis
atopy
autoimmunities
autotransfusion
Bence Jones protein
blood typing
blood crossmatching
cell-mediated hypersensitivity (type IV)
challenging dose
cytotoxic hypersensitivity (type II)
desensitization
gammopathies
hemolytic transfusion reaction
hypergammaglobulinemia
hypersensitivities
hypogammaglobulinemia
immune complex hypersensitivity (type III)
immunodeficiencies
immunotherapy
induced immunosuppression
macroglobulinemia
monoclonal antibodies (MoAbs)
monoclonal gammopathies
multiple myeloma
planned autologous transfusion
plasma cell dyscrasias
polyclonal gammopathies
posttransfusion graft-versus-host disease
Rh positive
Rh negative
sensitizing dose
systemic anaphylaxis
urticaria

Alterations in the immune system may result in deficiencies or excesses of immunocompetent cells, in altered function of these cells, or in attack against self-antigens. The biologic bases of the immune system are discussed in Chapters 13 and 69. Because immunologic factors are operative in such a wide variety of disorders, much of the information about the disorders is found elsewhere in the text. This chapter describes the various categories of immune disorders and those disorders not described elsewhere.

# CLASSIFICATION OF IMMUNOLOGIC DISORDERS

Because the immune system is such a complex, interrelated system, it can malfunction at many points. Immunologic problems reflect an immune system that may be nonresponsive or that may respond inappropriately (such as an exaggerated reaction to a stimulus, production of incompetent types of cells or an attack on self cells).

The severity of the disorders ranges from creation of a minor nuisance (e.g., mild hay fever) to an immediate life-threatening situation (e.g., anaphylactic shock) to a chronic debilitating condition (e.g., rheumatoid arthritis). The disorders may be classified into the following general categories:

1. **Immunodeficiencies**—deficiencies in the proper expression of the immune response system, parts of the system, or individual cell types within the system
2. **Gammopathies**—abnormal production of immunoglobulins
3. **Hypersensitivities**—exaggerated or inappropriate response to specific antigens
4. **Autoimmunities**—the immunologic attack on self-antigens

These four categories serve as the basis of organization for this chapter.

# IMMUNODEFICIENCIES

Protection of the host depends on an intact immune system. The four major components of the immune system (antibody-mediated immunity, cell-mediated immunity, phagocytosis, and complement) act together and independently to protect the individual from infection and disease. Deficiencies in one or more of these systems will cause an immunodeficient disorder. These disorders are characterized by chronic or recurrent infections that can lead to death.

Immune deficiencies are classified as primary or secondary. Primary immune deficiencies are congenital, whereas secondary immune deficiencies are acquired as a result of some interference with an already developed immune system. The deficiencies can be caused by many etiologic factors such as embryonic development defects, gene abnormalities, biochemical or metabolic deficiencies, nutritional deficiencies, infections, and disease processes and their medical treatments.[13]

## PRIMARY IMMUNODEFICIENCIES

### Etiology/Epidemiology

Primary immunodeficiencies are rare disorders seen mostly in infants and young children. For instance, agammaglobinemia occurs in 1:50,000 people, whereas severe combined immunodeficiency disorders occur in 1:100,000 to 1:500,000 live births. With some of the deficiency disorders, chromosomal abnormalities have been found. Despite our modern medical advances in understanding the immune system, however, the biologic errors of most deficiency diseases remain unknown.[3]

### Pathophysiology

The World Health Organization has completed a classification of primary immunodeficiency disorders (Table 70-1). These disorders are characterized by a blockage in the immunologic *cell development,* which causes the deficit (Figure 70-1). Most of the patients with these disorders are recognized because of their recurrent infections and/or history of treatment failure of infection. Without treatment, most of these patients will die of overwhelming infections very early in life.[3] Signs and symptoms depend on the site of infection and type of infecting organism. Patients with B cell deficiencies are at risk for developing infections from pyrogenic bacteria such as *Streptococcus, Staphylococcus, Pseudomonas,* and *Haemophilus influenzae.*[9]

With T cell deficiencies, the most common organisms are viruses (especially cytomegalovirus and herpes), fungi (candida), protozoa (pneumocystis), and mycobacteria. Persons with T cell deficiencies also have an increased risk for malignancies. Combined T cell- and B cell-deficient patients are at high risk for developing nearly every type of infection. Individuals with phagocytic disorders are at risk for developing mild to severe bacterial infections, whereas those with complement deficits have problems that range from recurrent infections to autoimmune diseases.

Prenatal diagnosis through fetoscopy has aided earlier detection of primary immunodeficiency disorders in infants so treatment can begin before the infection becomes too great. In some cases, identification of carriers through chromosome analysis can aid in proper counseling of at-risk parents. It is thought that gene therapy in the future may be able to correct some of these gene abnormalities.[3]

## SECONDARY IMMUNODEFICIENCIES

The most common immunodeficiencies are *acquired* disorders of depressed immunity. Any factor that can interfere with the normal growth or expression of the immune response system can lead to a secondary immunodeficiency. Major contributing factors include age

**TABLE 70-1 Selected Primary Immunodeficiencies**

| NAME OF DISORDER | BASIS OF DEFICIENCY | TREATMENT |
|---|---|---|
| **ANTIBODY DEFICIENCIES** | | |
| Bruton-type agammaglobulinemia | Sex-linked depression of all immunoglobulin classes. All serum immunogobulins are decreased. | Immune serum globulin |
| Common variable immunodeficiency (CVID) | Variable degree of ability to synthesize primarily IgA or IgM in adults or poor function of serum immunoglobulins. High concentrations of autoantibodies and abnormal immunoglobulins. | Immune serum globulin |
| **CELLULAR AND COMBINED IMMUNODEFICIENCY DISORDERS** | | |
| DiGeorge syndrome (thymic hypoplasia) | Nongenetic failure of thymic development. Normal or decreased immunoglobulins; decreased T cells. | Immune serum globulin<br>Fetal thymus transplants |
| Nezelof syndrome | Congenital failure of embryonic thymic development. Normal or increased serum immunoglobulins. Lymphopenia. | Immune serum globulin<br>Bone marrow or thymus transplants |
| **SEVERE COMBINED IMMUNODEFICIENCY DISORDERS** | | |
| Severe combined immunodeficiency disease (SCID) | Defect in stem cell differentiation and maturation of T and B cells. T and B cells are decreased or absent. | Bone marrow transplants |
| **PARTIAL COMBINED IMMUNODEFICIENCY DISORDERS** | | |
| Wiskott-Aldrich syndrome | Sex-linked IgM and T cell deficiency in males. | Immune serum globulin<br>Bone marrow transplants |
| Ataxia-telangiectasia | Autosomally recessive deficit in IgA and IgE. Decreased or normal T cells. | Immune serum globulin<br>Fetal thymus transplants |
| **PHAGOCYTIC CELL DEFICIENCY** | | |
| Chronic granulomatous disease | Sex-linked genetic disease in males producing lack of destruction of phagocytized organisms and particles. | No replacement therapy<br>Antibiotic therapy |
| Chediak-Higashi syndrome | Autosomal recessive disorder with abnormal granule formation, neutrophil chemotactic response, and intercellular killing of microorganisms. | No replacement therapy<br>Bone marrow transplant |
| **COMPLEMENT DEFICIENCY** | | |
| $C_1$, $C_3$, and $C_4$ | Develop bacterial infections. More prone to autoimmune processes (SLE; glomerulonephritis; Sjögren's syndrome). | No replacement therapy<br>Antibiotic therapy |
| Hereditary angioedema | Autosomal dominant disorder associated with $C_1$ inhibitor deficiency. Results in large amount of vasoactive peptides and increased vascular permeability. | No replacement therapy<br>Plasmin inhibitors<br>Steroids |

(see Chapter 69), nutrition, specific disorders, exposure to environmental chemicals, and induced immunosuppression. A retrovirus (HIV) causes AIDS (acquired immunodeficiency syndrome); AIDS is discussed in Chapter 71.

## Specific Disorders Affecting Immunity

Disorders can depress the immune system by the following methods:

1. Loss of serum protein: nephrotic syndrome, burns, protein-losing enteropathy
2. Decreased protein synthesis: severe liver disease
3. Severe malnutrition: cancer, alcoholism, malabsorption
4. Decrease T cell function: uremia, diabetes mellitus, infections (especially viral), autoimmune disorders
5. Alterations in B cell and T cell number and function: leukemias, lymphomas

## Exposure to Environmental Chemicals

Many chemicals have immunosuppressive effects in exposed humans. Most of these affect the T-lymphocyte system more severely. Examples of these environmental chemicals are asbestos, dioxin, insecticides, and heavy metals.[4] Much is unknown in this area, for instance, the effect of exposure to certain chemicals when coupled with the aging process.

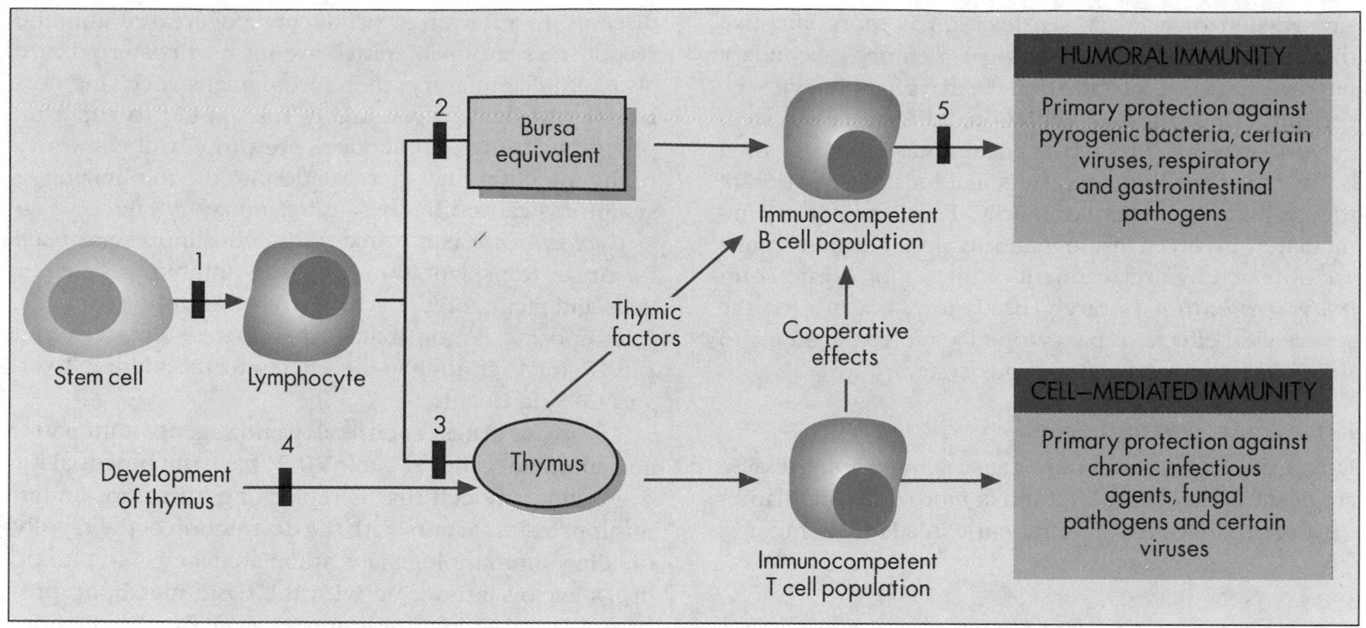


**FIGURE 70-1** Causes of immunodeficiencies. Abnormalities at *1* result in combined humoral and cell-mediated immunodeficiency. Blockage at *2* produces agammaglobulinemia. Blockage at *3* or *4* results in drastic reduction in T cell–mediated function and, because of cooperative effects on B cell system, some reduction in humoral response. Abnormalities in synthesis of specific immunoglobulin classes are reflected by blockage at *5*. Whereas some blockages result in complete deficiency, others show up as reduction in response.

## Induced Immunosuppression

**Induced immunosuppression** can be initiated to decrease unwanted immune responses, such as hypersensitivity reactions, autoimmune diseases, neoplasia, or organ rejection. There are several ways in which the unwanted immune responses can be suppressed by artificial manipulation: suppression of specific antigens causing hypersensitivities, immunologic methods of immune suppression, irradiation, and drug immunosuppression.[7]

### Suppression of specific antigens

Specific *antigens* can be administered to a hypersensitive person in small amounts over a time. The antigenic stimulation forms circulating antibodies (immunoglobulins) of the IgG class that combine with the antigen to block contact with the immunocompetent cells or IgE-coated mast cells, thus suppressing the immune response. An adaptation of this method is used by allergists to desensitize persons allergic to specific antigens such as pollens.

A slightly different method is to administer the specific *antibody,* which then combines with the antigen to block contact with the immunocompetent cell. This method has been used successfully in obstetrics to prevent the sensitive Rh-negative mother from responding to the Rh-positive fetus during pregnancy.

### Immunologic methods of immunosuppression

**Antilymphocytic globulin (ALG)** and **antithymocytic globulin (ATG)** are antisera prepared by isolating the active globulin fraction from the serum of horses, goats, or rabbits that have been immunized with human lymphocytes or thymocytes.[7] This approach is nonspecific by decreasing all lymphocytes, although T cells are more affected than B cells. Because these globulins are xenogeneic (from another species), serum sickness (p. 2432) frequently occurs and thus limits use to short-term therapy. Other adverse effects include thrombocytopenia and allergic reactions.

Common antiserum is polyclonal, because it is a collection of cells from different lymphocytes.[7] A more specific approach to immunologic immunosuppression is the administration of **monoclonal antibodies (MoAbs),** derived from a single cell, and thus directed toward specific subpopulations of lymphocytes, such as helper T cells (muromonab-CD3).[7] Monoclonal anti–T cell antibodies (e.g., $OKT_3$) have shown considerable success in reversing renal allograft rejection. Different types of MoAbs are being developed from other cell populations for other purposes such as for cancer immunotherapy (Chapter 16.)

### Irradiation

Both primary and secondary immune responses (see Chapter 13) may be suppressed by irradiation, but suppression of primary sensitization is more effective than suppression of immunologic memory (secondary immune response). Irradiation destroys lymphocytes, either directly or through depletion of the precursor stem cells. It may be directed at local areas or at the total body. *Local irradiation* results in a local destruction of the cellular elements (primarily T cell response) immediately involved in allograft rejection. The best results are obtained by pretreatment of the donor organ. *Total body irradiation* is rarely used now, because of the severe side effects of pancytopenia and toxic effects to the GI tract and central nervous system.

**Drug immunosuppression**

Drugs that most commonly cause immunosuppression are described in Table 70-2 and in more detail in Chapter 72. *Corticosteroids* are therapeutic in a large number of diseases. In addition to producing a decreased immune response as antiproliferative agents, corticosteroids are also antiinflammatory; therefore persons receiving corticosteroid therapy are highly susceptible to superimposed infections. If infections are present, the severity of the infection may increase despite the minimizing of symptoms caused by the antiinflammatory effects.

*Cyclosporine* is a primary immunosuppressant used for organ transplantation. It acts by inhibiting T-helper cells and facilitating development of T-suppressor cells. Cyclosporine is nontoxic to precursor stem cells and the GI tract, although side effects to the kidney, liver, and CNS do occur.

*Cytotoxic* drugs (such as alkylating agents, antifolates, and antimetabolites) (Table 70-2) have the potential for destroying any cell that is replicating; therefore immunosuppression occurs with the destruction of the rapidly dividing, immunologically stimulated cells. Cytotoxic drugs act by interfering with the basic metabolic processes. B cell reduction is greater than T cell reduction. Antimetabolites are frequently given with steroids for immunosuppression therapy to decrease the dosage of both antimetabolites and steroids, thereby decreasing serious side effects.

**TABLE 70-2 Major Immunosuppressive Drugs**

| IMMUNOLOGIC ACTION | INDICATIONS FOR IMMUNOSUPPRESSIVE THERAPY |
|---|---|
| **CORTICOSTEROID** | |
| Inhibits T cell proliferation. Decreases interleukin-2 production. Decreases macrophage and neutrophil function. Inhibits T helper and T suppressor cell activity. | Diseases in which immune disorder is unknown<br>Autoimmune diseases<br>Allergic disorders<br>Transplant rejection<br>Certain malignant neoplasms |
| **CYCLOSPORINE (SANDIMMUNE)** | |
| Inhibits T helper cell, lymphokine, and interleukin-2 production. Facilitates T-suppressor cell development. | Allograft rejection<br>Graft-versus-host disease |
| **ALKYLATING AGENTS (CYCLOPHOSPHAMIDE)** | |
| Interferes with DNA, RNA, and protein synthesis. Lymphocytolytic. Depresses B cell function. Decreases monocyte and macrophage function. | Autoimmune diseases<br>Lymphomas, leukemias<br>Granulomatous diseases |
| **ANTIMETABOLITE (AZATHIOPRINE)** | |
| Inferferes with RNA, DNA, and protein synthesis. Depresses bone marrow and antibody reproduction. Depresses T cell function. | Autoimmune disease<br>Organ transplantation<br>Pemphigus (skin disease)<br>Neoplasia |
| **ANTIFOLATES (METHOTREXATE)** | |
| Causes deficiency of folate coenzymes preventing synthesis of thymine and purines. | Autoimmune diseases<br>Severe asthma |

## MEDICAL MANAGEMENT

The primary goals of medical management for patients with suspected primary immunodeficient disorders are (1) to identify those at risk for the disorder, (2) to prevent infection or effectively treat already existing infections, and (3) to replace missing humoral or cellular immunologic factors.[3]

### Diagnostic Tests

The complete blood count with differential (CBC with Diff) and the erythrocyte sedimentation rate (ESR) are cost-effective ways to screen for T cell defects. An elevated ESR and a decreased absolute lymphocyte count are commonly seen with T cell defects. The *Candida* skin test is another good method to screen for T cell deficits. If the skin test is negative at 24, 48, and 72 hours, it can indicate a T cell deficiency. With B cell defects, normal antibody titers toward common proteins such as type A or type B blood cells (isohemagglutinin) are used to evaluate IgM levels, and diphtheria or tetanus titers are utilized to evaluate levels of IgG antibodies. These tests reveal decreased titers in patients with B cell types of deficiency. Immunoglobulin quantification can also be used to show which immunoglobulins are diminished. The absolute neutrophil count is decreased and the phagocytic ability of the neutrophils, as measured by the nitroblue tetrazolium test, shows defects in patients with phagocytic cell deficits. The $CH_{50}$ blood test is used to investigate the intactness of the complement pathway and is decreased in patients with complement deficits.

## Medication

For patients with already existing infections, antibiotics and fungicides are prescribed to treat the organisms responsible for the infections. For patients with antibody deficiencies **(hypogammaglobinemia)**, immunoglobulin replacement therapy is a common form of treatment. These immunoglobulin preparations are obtained from the pooled plasma of greater than 1000 donors who were screened for hepatitis and HIV antibodies. These products consist primarily of IgG antibodies with small amounts of the other serum immunoglobulins.[4] Each pool contains adequate antibodies to various vaccines (i.e., tetanus and measles) but are not standardized with antibody titers to organisms such as *Streptococcus pneumoniae* or *Haemophilus influenzae.* The half-life of IgG is highly variable among patients with hypogammaglobulinemia but usually it exceeds 70 days.

The optimal dose of IgG is maintained by monitoring the trough levels of IgG immunoglobin in the blood. It is recommended to keep these trough levels of IgG at 400 to 500 mg/dl, which is close to the lower limit of normal.[4] The immunoglobulins are given intramuscularly or intravenously. Usually patients with primary immunodeficiency diseases receive immunoglobulin infusions every 4 weeks, but this dose may have to be adjusted when the patient has lowered trough levels of IgG, rapid catabolism of IgG, or an ongoing infection. With IV immunoglobulin infusion, it is important to start the infusion slowly because the risk of reactions is greater at the beginning of the infusion. Reactions can result in back or abdominal pain; nausea and vomiting at the beginning of the infusion; or chills, fever, headache, myalgia, and fatigue at the end of the infusion. Most of these reactions are prevented by slowing the initial infusion or by pretreatment with aspirin. Anaphylactic reactions to IV immune globulin are rare. These reactions are usually noted in patients with selective IgA deficiency or common variable immune disorder.[4] Gammagard, one type of immunoglobulin product, can be given to these patients safely because it contains low levels of IgA. Immunoglobin therapy is extremely expensive; the annual cost of therapy for a 70 kg adult ranges from $25,000 to $45,000.[4]

## Treatment

Patients who are immunodeficient must be protected from infections. This may involve protective isolation in the hospital to prevent exposure to pathogens; at times when the patient becomes severely immunodeficient, laminar airflow units may be necessary (see Chapter 16). Laminar airflow rooms are specially designed rooms in which air flow crosses the unit in one-way layers to decrease the flow of microorganisms toward the patient. The air is filtered continuously through microfilters. The number of persons entering the environment is kept to a minimum, and the persons must wear a cap, mask, boot covers, and gown. All equipment and supplies are sterilized before entry into the room.

Patients with T cell deficiency syndromes may be treated with bone marrow transplantation. With this type of transplantation, the major risk to the recipient is graft-versus-host disease (GVHD).[3] (See Chapter 72 regarding bone marrow transplantation and GVHD.) Specially treated haploidentical (half-matched) bone marrow cells (from parents) have been used successfully in the treatment of severe combined immunodeficiency disorder.[3] In the case of DiGeorge syndrome, transplantation of fetal thymic tissue has been recommended.[3]

Treatment of *secondary* immunodeficiencies focuses on the underlying condition that has affected the immune response. Immunotherapy is one therapeutic mode in the treatment of cancer (Chapter 16).

## Diet

A balanced, nutritious dietary intake is necessary for patients to have an adequately working immune system. For this reason nutrition becomes an important part of the treatment for patients with immunodeficiency diseases. The diet should include all food groups, with adequate calories and protein to support tissue building. Dietary modifications may become necessary when the patient becomes severely immunodeficient. At this time, it is important to avoid the use of fresh fruits and vegetables because they contain bacteria from which the patients could not protect themselves.

## Activity

There are no specific activity restrictions for these individuals except that they should not overtire themselves and should avoid crowds because of their lowered resistance to infection.

## Referral/Consultation

Patients with immunodeficient disorders definitely need continued follow-up. With some patients, it is important to have some referrals to community health nurses regarding continued assessment and treatment of infection. Hospice care might be necessary in some cases to help family members care for those with terminal immunodeficiency disorders.

# NURSING MANAGEMENT

## ◆ ASSESSMENT

***Subjective data*** to be collected to assess the person with immunodeficiency include the following:

1. Knowledge of the immunodeficiency, the high risk for infection, and infection preventive methods
2. Occurrence of recurrent infection and, if present, types of infections
3. Nutritional data: weight changes, appetite, usual 24-hour food intake

4. Current medications
5. Medical treatments

*Objective data* include monitoring for early signs of infection (elevated temperature, nasal discharge, cough, skin lesions). Breath sounds are monitored daily for decreased sounds, indicating pulmonary infection.

## ♦ NURSING DIAGNOSES

Nursing diagnoses are determined from analysis of patient data. Nursing diagnoses for the patient with immunodeficiency may include but are not limited to the following:

| Diagnostic Title | Possible Etiologic Factors |
|---|---|
| Infection, high risk for | Decreased immune response, lack of information |
| Knowledge deficit | Lack of exposure/recall, information misinterpretation |

## ♦ EXPECTED PATIENT OUTCOMES

Expected patient outcomes for the person with immunodeficiency may include but are not limited to the following:

1. Signs of infection do not occur.
2. Describes measures to avoid infection.
3. Describes signs dictating immediate medical attention.
4. Explains the need for continued medical follow-up.

## ♦ INTERVENTIONS

### Preventing Infection

The most important factor in the care of the immunodeficient or immunosuppressed person is protection from infection. The following measures pertain to all degrees of immunodeficiency:

1. Monitor the patient's temperature at least every 8 to 12 hours; assess the skin, mucous membranes, and lungs at the same times.
2. Provide prophylactic pulmonary hygiene measures (e.g., breathing exercises, inhalation therapy, postural drainage) for persons with B cell deficiencies because they are more susceptible to bacterial infections (especially pulmonary). Monitor persons with T cell deficiencies for signs of viral and fungal infections.
3. Monitor CBC with differential.
4. Use medical asepsis including thorough handwashing.
5. Meticulously clean sources where bacteria may proliferate. No live plants should be allowed in the room when blood counts indicate that the patient is severely immunodepressed.
6. Encourage patient to complete regular personal hygiene. Assist the patient as necessary.
7. Protect patient from other persons with infections. Be sure that the other patient in a semiprivate room does not have an infection. If severe leukopenia is present, place the person in a single-occupancy room.
8. Assign only healthy staff to care for this patient.
9. Avoid injections, if possible. (Breaks in skin continuity may lead to infection.)
10. Keep invasive lines to a minimum. Monitor those needed with particular vigilance for infection.
11. Obtain cultures of any suspicious drainage.
12. Administer only CMV-negative blood products to prevent CMV infections.
13. Administer immunoglobulins as prescribed.
14. Maintain nutrition, especially protein intake, at optimal level. Remember that malnutrition significantly affects immune efficiency. If the neutrophil count decreases below 500, avoid fresh unpeeled fruits and vegetables in the diet.
15. Obtain a daily weight to monitor nutritional status.
16. Maintain adequate fluid intake of at least 1500 ml/day for hydration (prevents skin drying and flushes the urinary system to prevent infection).
17. Measure intake and output accurately.

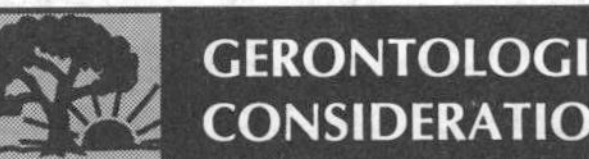

### GERONTOLOGIC PATIENT CONSIDERATIONS

#### ASSESSMENT

Assess nutritional status of all elderly persons, especially those living alone. Good nutrition is an important factor in maintenance of the immune system.

Assess carefully elderly patients in nursing homes or those entering hospital from a nursing home for signs of infection. Risk of infection in these persons is high because of high rates of immobility from neurologic or cardiovascular disorders, from high use of invasive catheters, or from malnutrition.

Assess mobility status of elderly patients; immobility may lead to skin breakdown and infection.

Assess patient for changes in mental status, anorexia, claims of "feeling poorly," or comments by family members that the elderly person looks ill. These may be early signs of infection in the elderly, as compared to signs of fever and pain in the younger adult.

#### INTERVENTION

Consider every elderly patient as partly immunodeficient and take all precautions to prevent infections, especially respiratory infections.

Monitor elderly patients' responses to antibiotic therapy; the incidence of drug reactions is greater because of the older person's greater sensitivity.

Monitor fluid and dietary intake to maintain fluid balance and good nutritional status; this is necessary for maintenance of the immune system.

#### COMMON DISORDERS IN ELDERS

Infections, especially bacteremic pneumonia, urinary tract infection, tetanus, and herpes zoster
Malignancies
Autoimmune disorders

### Guidelines for Teaching the Person With Immunodeficiency

The patient will be able to explain or perform the following:

1. Explain immunodeficiency, that is, the inability of the body to fight infection
2. Take measures to prevent infection:
   a. Avoid persons with infections (especially colds)
   b. Avoid bumping or breaking the skin
   c. Inspect skin daily for lesions
   d. Eat a balanced diet
   e. Drink at least six glasses of fluid daily
   f. Avoid fatigue and try to get a regular amount of sleep every night
   g. Avoid letting water stand unchanged around the house, such as in vases (good source for bacterial growth)
   h. Do not use cold-mist humidifiers (gram-negative organisms are often present)
   i. Do not take routine immunizations or have immediate family take them.
   j. Take prophylactic antibiotics before any manipulative or invasive procedures (e.g., dental work, biopsies, endoscopies, arteriograms)
3. Report signs of infection to physician immediately. These signs and symptoms could be an increased temperature, redness, or swelling on skin or mucous membranes; change in color of sputum; coughing; unusual looking drainage; or diarrhea.
4. See physician on a regular basis as instructed.

As noted earlier, age is a major contributing factor for secondary immunodeficiencies. Elders therefore should be considered at high risk for infection and preventive care provided (see Gerontologic box, p. 2414).

### Facilitating Learning

Immunodeficient or immunosuppressed patients and their families need to know the nature of immunodeficiency and how to avoid infection (see Guidelines box above).

## ♦ EVALUATION

To evaluate the effectiveness of nursing interventions, compare patient behaviors with those stated in the expected patient outcomes. Successful achievement of patient outcomes for the patient with immunodeficiencies is indicated by the following:

1a. Temperature is within normal range.
 b. Skin and mucous membranes are intact with no signs of redness or fungal growth.
 c. Lung sounds are clear to auscultation, and sputum is clear or white in color.
2a. Verbalizes activities to prevent recurrent infections.
 b. Verbalizes signs and symptoms that indicate they need immediate medical attention.
 c. Verbalizes the need for continued medical follow-up.
3. Has fewer incidents of infection and is managed at home without hospital admission.

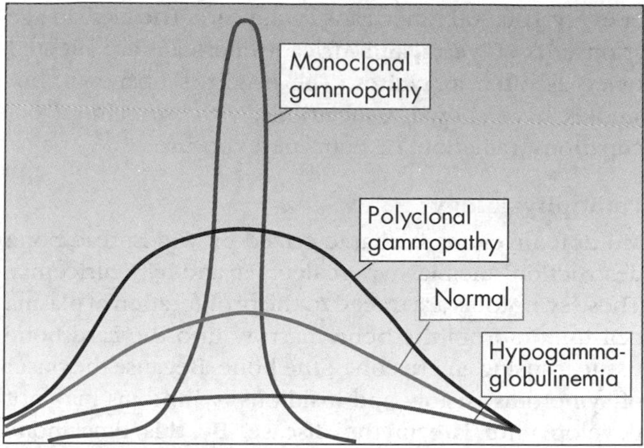


**FIGURE 70-2** Electrophoretic peaks of γ-globulin fractions in monoclonal gammopathies, polyclonal gammopathies, and hypogammaglobulinemia. Obtained by electrophoresis of γ-globulin fraction of serum.

## GAMMOPATHIES

Gammopathies, better termed **hypergammaglobulinemias,** are elevated levels of γ-globulin in serum resulting from the overproduction of whole γ-globulin or nonassociated heavy chains (H chains) or nonassociated light chains (L chains) (see Chapter 13). The normal synthesis of an immunoglobulin is the result of the proliferation and plasma cell differentiation of a single clone of B cells in response to an antigenic signal. In gammopathies, a single clone or multiple clones of plasma cells begin to overproduce immunoglobulin product. If the gammopathy involves a single B cell clone, it is termed a **monoclonal gammopathy,** and the electrophoretic pattern will be characterized by a single sharp peak in the γ-globulin region (Figure 70-2). **Polyclonal gammopathies** involve the overproduction of virtually all classes of immunoglobulins in response to inappropriate antigenic stimulation. The electrophoretic pattern of polyclonal gammopathies is characterized by a diffuse increase in the γ-globulin curve.

## MONOCLONAL GAMMOPATHIES

Monoclonal gammopathies (M-type) are commonly referred to as **plasma cell dyscrasias.** Some plasma cell dyscrasias such as multiple myeloma and macroglobulinemia have distinctive clinical patterns. In other instances, electrophoretic changes resembling the clinical forms can be identified, but no symptoms are present; these can be classified as plasma cell dyscrasias of undetermined significance (PCDUS).

### Multiple Myeloma

#### Etiology/Epidemiology

**Multiple myeloma** is the most serious and prevalent of the plasma cell dyscrasias. It affects approximately 4 of every 100,000 Americans each year.[2] The median age at onset is 60 years, and African-Americans are affected twice as often as whites. The origin is unknown, but studies have shown associations with agricultural occupations, radiation, or benzene exposure.[2]

### Pathophysiology

Multiple myeloma is characterized by widespread bone destruction, anemia, hypercalcemia, and hyperuricemia. These symptoms are traced to the proliferation of plasma cell tumors from the bone marrow into the hard bone tissue, causing an erosion of the bone. Because the onset of symptoms is slow and insidious, symptoms may not develop until late in the disease. By this time, bone lesions typically involve the skull, spine, and pelvis (Table 70-3). Painful compression fractures are one of the most common symptoms in newly diagnosed multiple myeloma patients.[2] Spinal cord compression can occur from severe spine involvement with resultant paraplegia or quadriplegia. More than 95% of multiple myeloma patients have monoclonal proteins in their serum and urine specimens called *Bence Jones protein.*[2] About 20% of the patients with multiple myeloma present with impaired renal function as a result of the hypercalcemia and hyperuricemia.[2] Frequent recurrent infections (especially of the respiratory tract) occur because of the overproduction of ineffective immunoglobulins that depress the production of normal antibodies. The median survival rate for multiple myeloma patients with treatment is 3 years.[2]

### Medical management

**Diagnostic tests.** Computed tomography (CT) scans and radiography will show punched-out type of bone lesions or generalized osteoporosis of the axial skeleton. Laboratory values may show increased serum calcium from bone demineralization and increased serum uric acid from protein breakdown. The complete blood count (CBC) with differential shows anemia, leukopenia, and thrombocytopenia, depending on the amount of bone marrow involvement. **Bence Jones protein,** an abnormal myeloma protein, is found in the serum and urine. Normal immunoglobulin levels are decreased in multiple myeloma. $B_2$ microglobin is an HLA-I complex present in high concentrations on the membrane of myeloma cells. The $B_2$ microglobin test gives a rough index of tumor burden found in multiple myeloma.[2] Values greater than 678 nmol/L are seen as advanced disease, whereas values less than 339 nmol/L are defined as early disease.

**TABLE 70-3 Pathophysiology and Clinical Manifestations in Multiple Myeloma**

| PATHOPHYSIOLOGY | CLINICAL MANIFESTATIONS |
|---|---|
| Lytic bone disease | Skull, spine, and pelvis fractures |
| Extensive osteoclast activity | Spinal cord compression<br>Paraplegia; quadriplegia<br>Hypercalcemia<br>Renal insufficiency; renal failure |
| Bone marrow infiltration by plasma cells | Anemia<br>Leukopenia<br>Thrombocytopenia |
| Proliferation of monoclonal proteins | Hyperuricemia<br>Renal insufficiency; renal failure<br>Abnormal immunoglobulin formation<br>Depressed normal immunoglobulin formation |

**Medication.** Glucocorticoids and calcitonin are prescribed to reduce the lytic destruction of the bones and to help reduce the hypercalcemia. The myeloma tumor load is treated with oral chemotherapeutic melphalan combined with prednisone. Those tumors resistant to this treatment may receive a regimen of intravenous chemotherapeutic drugs vincristine sulfate and doxorubicin. Studies have found that the use of interferon alpha between chemotherapy treatments assists in prolonging remissions.[2]

**Treatment.** The hypercalcemia is treated by promoting good hydration along with the glucocorticoids.[2] Adequate patient hydration keeps the calcium diluted, which decreases the calcium crystal formation and encourages calcium excretion. Bone plasmacytomas respond well to local radiation treatments. If the bone damage is extensive to the spine, orthopedic fixation devices may be used to stabilize these areas to prevent cord compression. Intensive chemotherapy programs supported with bone marrow transplant may be used in patients with a poor prognosis at diagnosis. Preliminary data on this intensive treatment are encouraging; remission has been seen in 50% of patients.[2] If the patient presents with renal failure, dialysis may be necessary to handle the severe azotemia, hyperkalemia, and fluid overload.

**Diet.** The diet should be balanced and nutritious. At times of hypercalcemia and hyperuricemia, a low-calcium and low-purine diet may be indicated. Good hydration is essential to avoid crystalluria and renal failure.

**Activity.** It is important to keep patients as mobile as possible because bone demineralization occurs with immobility. Keeping them on a regular exercise program and allowing rest periods because of the anemia are important aspects of treatment.

**Referral/Consultation.** At end stages of the disease, the patient becomes very debilitated, requiring comprehensive 24-hour care. At this time, home health nurses or hospice care could be consulted to help the patient and family deal with these complex emotional and physical needs.

**Nursing management**

The major problems experienced by the patient with multiple myeloma are pathologic fractures, fluid overload caused by kidney failure, and infection. The patient has extremely fragile bones because of bone destruction by the plasmacytomas. Ambulation is encouraged to prevent demineralization of the bone associated with immobility. Safety is of vital importance because of risk of fractures; a fall could be disastrous. Skeletal pain may be a deterrent to ambulation; a lightweight spinal brace, analgesics, and local radiotherapy may facilitate ambulation. If the patient is immobile, careful turning is important. At late stages, even a tug on the arm or a turn toward the bedrailing could cause a fracture. A lift sheet and the assistance of many people are necessary to facilitate moving the patient gently and safely.

Adequate hydration is necessary to prevent renal complications from the increased amounts of urates and calcium being excreted in the urine. Fluid intake should be sufficient to ensure a urinary output of a *minimum* of 1500 ml/24 hr. The patient should be weighed daily to assess fluid retention, and the blood urea nitrogen (BUN) and serum creatinine should be monitored to evaluate the patient's renal function.

Measures to prevent infection are instituted and include avoidance of persons with upper respiratory tract infections. Medical attention should be sought for any signs of infection. Good turning and deep breathing exercises should be encouraged to prevent atelectasis and pneumonia.

### Macroglobulinemia (Waldenström's Disease)

**Macroglobulinemia** is a plasma dyscrasia involving the overproduction of IgM globulins. The disease is characterized by a lymphocytic-plasmacytic proliferation in the bone marrow, lymph nodes, and spleen.

Symptoms usually begin in the fifth or sixth decade of life and include fatigue and weakness from anemia, weight loss, and bleeding (mucosal, epistaxis). Blood viscosity is increased because of the increased globulins. Disease progression is similar to a lymphoma (see Chapter 34). Medical therapy includes plasmapheresis to decrease blood viscosity and chemotherapy with chlorambucil (Leukeran) or cyclophosphamide (Cytoxan). Fludarabine phosphate is effective in 50% of patients with resistance to these chemotherapeutic agents. Interferon maintenance is important to keep the patient in remission. Median survival time is 5 years. Intensive chemotherapy supported by allogenic bone marrow transplantation is considered for younger patients.

## POLYCLONAL GAMMOPATHIES

Polyclonal gammopathies refer to a diffuse increase in antibody synthesis as a result of inappropriate antigen stimulation. The major causes of the hypergammaglobulinemia are infectious diseases (especially chronic bacterial infections such as lung abscess and osteomyelitis), connective tissue diseases such as systemic lupus erythematosus (SLE) and rheumatoid arthritis, and chronic active liver disease. IgG and IgM are the most commonly involved immunoglobulins, and the degree of immunoglobulin levels reflects the severity of the diseases.

The development of high levels of dysfunctional $\gamma$-globulins depresses the synthesis of normal immunoglobulins. This renders the person with hypergammaglobulinemia susceptible to infection; therefore carrying out measures and teaching the patient how to prevent infection are major nursing responsibilities.

# HYPERSENSITIVITY REACTIONS

The immune system is always alert to react to foreign substances to protect the body. Sometimes, given particular conditions, the response of the immune system may produce detrimental effects.

This inappropriate response is usually manifested as a tissue-damaging overreaction to the antigen; thus it is termed hypersensitivity, or allergy. The antigenic stimulants invoking the reactions are referred to as allergens. Hypersensitivities, then, are classic expressions of the immune system, but they take place in inappropriate sites, in excessive amounts, or with inappropriate involvement of nonspecific tissues. Whether an allergic response occurs and to what degree depends on a combination of interrelated factors:

1. *Responsiveness of the host to the allergen.* If sensitivity of the host is extremely high, a far greater chance exists that a tissue-damaging reaction will occur.
2. *Amount of the allergen.* Generally, the greater the amount of allergen contacted, the more severe the reaction.
3. *Nature of the allergen.* Most are complex, high-molecular-weight, multivalent proteins; but some may be low-molecular-weight nonprotein materials that exert a haptenic effect when coupled with a normal tissue protein carrier.
4. *Route of entrance of the allergen.* The greatest proportion of allergens enter through the respiratory tract; however, others may enter by epidermal or mucosal contact, injection, or through the digestive tract.
5. *Timing of exposure to the allergen.* If the host's contacts with the allergen are widely separated (for example, years apart), the immunologic mediators (antibodies or sensitized cells) may be so dilute that there will be less response.
6. *Site of the allergen-immune mediator reaction.* If certain antigen-antibody reactions occur in the tissues, there is no untoward effect; the same reaction within the bloodstream can lead to intravascular inflammation.
7. *Host's threshold of reactivity.* The host's immune system can be changed by factors such as stress, fa-

tigue, or infection, all of which could decrease the responsiveness of the immune system to potential allergens.

## CLASSIFICATION OF HYPERSENSITIVITIES

Hypersensitivities can be divided broadly into two categories based on the components of the immune system involved in mediating the hypersensitivity reaction: humoral response (B cell–mediated) or cellular response (T cell–mediated). This basic division corresponds with the older clinical symptom division of immediate and delayed, which was developed before the elucidation of the mechanisms. The terms immediate or delayed were assigned to describe the timing of the appearance of clinical symptoms and the speed of skin test reactions when a host was challenged with various allergens. This terminology is still used today, but it has taken on new significance in relation to the understanding of the basic mechanisms at work.

It is possible to subcategorize the different manifestations of the humorally mediated hypersensitivities. The most widely used scheme of classification developed by Gell and Coombs has four types of reactions (Table 70-4). As can be seen from this table, the type I, II, and III reactions are mediated by the humoral system, whereas type IV reactions are those of the cell-mediated system. Because type I, II, and III hypersensitivities are the result of interactions involving circulating antibodies, they can be transferred from a sensitized host to a nonsensitized host by serum transfer. Type IV sensitivities can be transferred by lymphocyte exchange only.

## TYPE I HYPERSENSITIVITIES

**Type I hypersensitivity (anaphylactic)** reaction classification includes a wide variety of conditions. All of these diseases are characterized by an exaggerated response directed by IgE antibodies toward some external substance. **Atopy** is the *genetic* predisposition to the production of IgE antibodies in response to some common environmental antigen. The conditions of allergic rhinitis, hay fever, asthma, atopic eczema (atopic dermatitis), venom hyperreactivity, and food allergy are examples of atopic diseases. Other diseases included in this classification which are not atopic include urticaria/angioedema and anaphylaxis. These nonatopic disorders are also mediated by IgE antibodies but lack the genetic link or the specific organ hyperresponsiveness displayed by atopic diseases. It is important to recognize the difference between the atopic and nonatopic diseases because it influences etiology, diagnostic methods of identification, prognosis, and treatment.

### Etiology/Epidemiology

The occurrence of **anaphylaxis** (life-threatening hypersensitivity reaction) is rare—0.4 cases per million a year in the general population. Researchers have not found any association of gender, race, or geographic areas with increased risk of developing anaphylaxis.

Atopic illnesses, on the other hand, are very common. More than 15% of the population react to antigens that are not antigenic for the remainder of the population. Some estimate that allergic diseases account for approximately 10% of all patient visits to physician offices.[6]

**TABLE 70-4 Summary of Hypersensitivity Reactions**

| | HYPERSENSITIVITY TYPE | | | |
|---|---|---|---|---|
| | HUMORAL (IMMEDIATE) | | | CELLULAR (DELAYED) |
| PROPERTY | I ANAPHYLACTIC | II CYTOTOXIC | III IMMUNE COMPLEX | IV CELL MEDIATED |
| Immune system mediators | IgE bound to mast cells | IgG or IgM (+ complement) | IgG or IgM (+ complement) | T cells, macrophages |
| Allergens | Exogenous antigens | Foreign cells or alteration of cell surface antigens | Soluble antigens | Infectious agent, contact allergens, foreign tissues, cancer cells |
| Response to intradermal skin test | Wheal and flare within 30 min, edema | Not done | Erythema and edema within 3-8 hr | Erythema and induration within 24-48 hr |
| Pathophysiologic effects | Release of histamines, kinins, chemotactic factors, and active products of arachidonic acid metabolism (leukotrienes, prostaglandins, and thromboxanes) from mast cells, which affect smooth muscle, mucous glands | Direct cytotoxic destruction of cells | Acute inflammatory reaction; primarily polymorphonuclear neutrophil leukocytes | Tissue destruction, primarily lymphocytes and macrophages |
| Examples | Systemic anaphylaxis, atopic allergies, hayfever, insect sting reactions | Hemolytic disease of the newborn (Rh), transfusion reactions | Serum sickness, Arthus reaction, glomerulonephritis | Tuberculin reaction, skin graft rejection, poison ivy |

This tendency to become hypersensitive is inherited as a dominant trait. If both parents are atopic, there is a high probability that the children will be atopic. What these individuals become hypersensitive to, however, is determined by the allergens to which they are exposed. A person does not inherit a specific allergy; the allergy manifests itself in response to the allergens to which the person is exposed. A sensitizing dose is necessary before allergic symptoms occur. Allergic disease can begin at any age, but the most common onset is 2 to 15 years.

## Pathophysiology

Type I hypersensitivities are mediated by the IgE class of immunoglobulins. For type I reactions to occur, the individual must initially come into contact with the allergen that eventually sensitizes the B lymphocytes to produce IgE antibodies specific to that allergen. This primary contact is known as a **sensitizing dose.** The IgE antibodies when produced have a tendency for attachment to the surface of mast cells and basophils. On subsequent contact with the allergen (termed the shocking or **challenging dose**), the individual exhibits the symptoms of type I hypersensitivity.

The mast cells are found in virtually all tissues of the body and often in close proximity to blood vessels, whereas the basophils are found circulating as one of the leukocytes within the blood. Mast cells are particularly abundant in the skin, nasal region, and lungs. Both mast cells and basophils harbor within their cells numerous, membrane-bound vacuoles containing potent, pharmacologically active substances (histamine, kinins, chemotactic factors, and active products of arachidonic acid metabolism [leukotrienes, prostaglandins, and thromboxanes]).[15] When IgE immunoglobulins bind to the surface of these cells by the Fc portion of the immunoglobulin molecule, the antigen-binding site of the molecule is left exposed to bind the allergen at the surface of the cell (Figure 70-3).

Upon second exposure to the allergen, the allergen becomes bound to the IgE causing mast cell degranulation, which releases the internal agents of this cell into the environment. These mediators then cause vasodilation, smooth muscle contraction, increased vascular permeability, and increased mucous gland secretion. The typical symptoms can include the following:

1. Respiratory: rhinorrhea, watery itching eyes, obstruction of eustachian tubes, sneezing, sinusitis with headache, facial pain, bronchospasm, dyspnea, stridor, tachypnea, wheezing, cyanosis, use of accessory muscles to breathe, flaring of nares, diaphoresis, anxiety
2. Dermal: hives, rash, angioedema
3. Abdominal: nausea, vomiting, cramping, diarrhea
4. General: fever, malaise, joint pains, hematopoietic suppression, anaphylaxis

Repeated cycles of exposure to allergens and type I responses can lead to chronic diseases. Table 70-5 lists the pathology and related clinical manifestations.

The signs and symptoms of type I hypersensitivity reactions can reflect changes in a wide variety of organs. The severity of these symptoms depends on several factors: the amount and entrance route of the sensitizing dose and of the shocking dose, and the distribution of the IgE antibodies. Figure 70-4 illustrates the way in which different allergens and their entrance routes can cause different types of symptoms. It is important to remember that the detrimental symptoms are not at the site of the antigen-antibody reaction but at the site of the organs where the pharmacologically active anaphylactic mediators exert their action. If those mediators remain confined to a local area, the tissue reactions remain localized and are referred to as local anaphylaxis. The local hypersensitivity that most people demonstrate

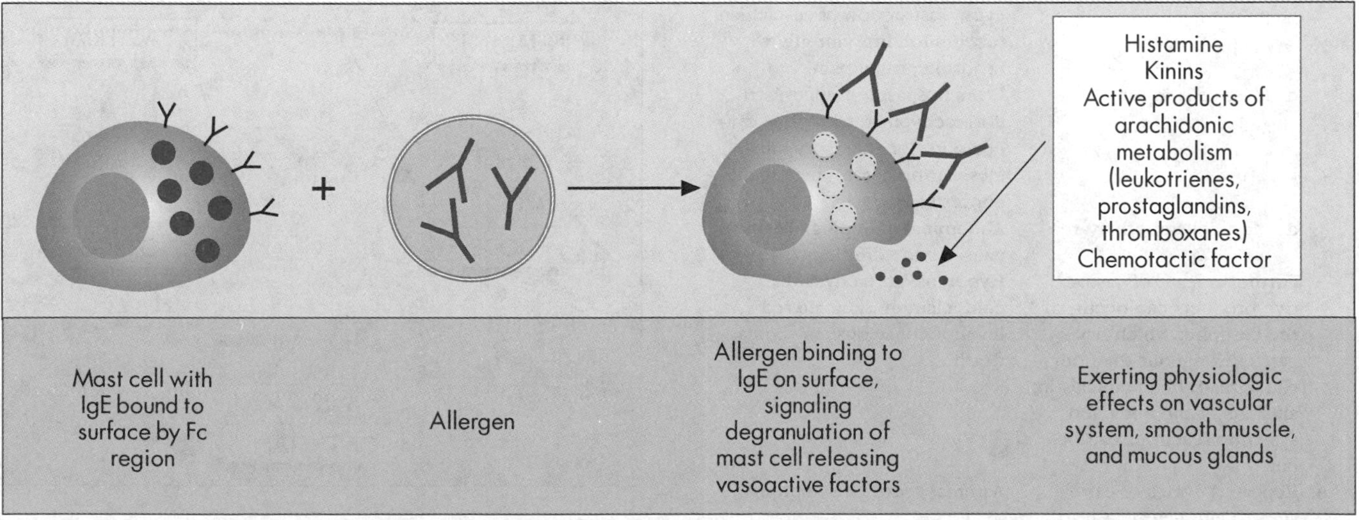


**FIGURE 70-3** Mediators of type I hypersensitivity.

**TABLE 70-5 Type I Hypersensitivity Reactions**

| PATHOPHYSIOLOGY | CLINICAL MANIFESTATIONS |
|---|---|
| 1. Individual comes into contact with allergens for first time. The macrophages pick up these allergens and present them to T lymphocytes. T lymphocytes examine the antigens of the allergen and communicate to the B lymphocytes through interleukin IV. The B lymphocytes become activated causing IgE release. IgE antibodies specific for this allergen attach to mast cells and basophils, which leaves the antigen binding portion of the immunoglobin exposed to react to the allergen. The individual is now said to be sensitized. | No signs and symptoms |
| 2. Sensitized individual comes in contact with allergen for the second time. IgE immunoglobulin on basophils and mast cells are activated and release mediators (histamine, kinins, chemotactic factors, and active products of arachidonic acid metabolsim—leukotrienes, prostaglandins, and thromboxanes). These chemicals cause vasodilation, smooth muscle constriction, increased vascular permeability, and increased mucous gland secretion. The mast cells are located in significant abundance in particular areas, and the symptoms can be very localized. | |
| a. Mast cells on skin | Hives, rash, angioedema |
| b. Mast cells in nasal region | Rhinorrhea; watery, itching eyes; obstruction of eustachian tubes; sneezing; sinusitis with headache; facial pain |
| c. Mast cells in lungs | Bronchospasm; dyspnea; stridor; tachypnea; wheezing; cyanosis; use of accessory muscles; flaring nares; anxiety; diaphoresis |
| d. Mast cells in other areas | Abdominal cramping; diarrhea; nausea and vomiting |
| 3. Further release of vasoactive products can occur; or the basophil, which navigates throughout the body, can spread the chemicals in all parts of the body and systemic reactions can occur. | Hypotension; tachycardia; cold, clammy skin; altered level of consciousness; coma; death |
| 4. Repeated cycles of exposure to allergens can lead to chronic disease. | Asthma; acute GI symptoms |

to a mosquito bite is the classic example of this type of reaction; the intradermal injection of the mosquito anticoagulants produces a wheal-flare type of reaction within a matter of minutes. On the other hand, if the mediators become released systemically, the response is known as systemic anaphylaxis, which can produce anaphylactic shock.

Atopic illnesses are typically initiated by two categories of allergens: seasonal and perennial. *Seasonal allergens* include pollens from trees, grasses, and weeds. The individual will experience symptoms whenever the pollen of that particular plant or tree is high. Every geographic area has its own specific allergens. For instance, ragweed is the most common allergen in the midwest region of the United States, whereas western United States has more allergies from olive trees and certain types of grasses such as bermuda. The season for these pollens usually begins with a brief tree season, followed by the grass and then weed seasons. *Perennial allergens* such as house dust, mites, molds, and animal dander are present throughout the year; and the individual can experience symptoms any time. Other common allergens include insect venom and certain foods.

Atopic diseases are rarely life-threatening, but symptoms can be uncomfortable. These symptoms can make the individual miss work or school and can affect the quality of his or her life.[6] Typical manifestations of atopic diseases include respiratory, skin, and abdominal symptoms. Patients with chronic allergic problems may exhibit allergic gape (open mouth caused by chronic nasal obstruction and mouth breathing), allergic "shiner" (dis-

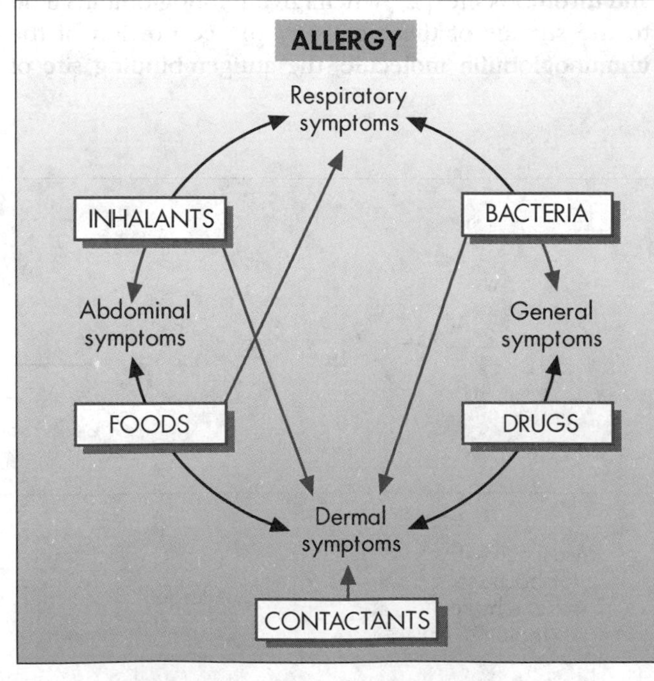


**FIGURE 70-4** Causes of allergic responses and symptoms produced.

coloration and edema around eyes caused by chronic nasal obstruction), and transverse nasal crease along the tip of the nose as a result of continual upward rubbing of the nose to relieve itching.[6]

The signs and symptoms of a nonatopic reaction can vary significantly. Nonatopic diseases can range from a local reaction such as hives or angioedema to systemic reaction such as anaphylactic shock. Hives **(urticaria)** are pruritic lesions characterized by a pale pink elevated edge (wheal) on an erythematous background (Figure 70-5). The lesions are transient and may reappear in different body areas. The allergic form of urticaria is usually caused by foods, especially eggs, fish, and nuts, or by drugs such as penicillins, sulfonamides, cephalosporins, or aspirin and other nonsteroidal antiinflammatory drugs.

**Angioedema** is a form of urticaria, but it involves the subcutaneous tissue rather than the skin. With angioedema an entire anatomic part such as the eyelid, thumb, or lip becomes swollen; there is no pruritus.

Urticaria may also occur in a chronic form from causes other than IgE-mediated hypersensitivity. Etiologic factors in the chronic form include exposure to cold, heat, or various light waves. Another form, cholinergic urticaria, occurs as a response to stress or physical exertion.

A more severe form of nonatopic reaction in humans is **systemic anaphylaxis.** The initial symptoms of anaphylaxis are edema and itching about the site of the injection, apprehension, and sneezing. These mild reactions are rapidly followed (sometimes in a matter of seconds or minutes) by edema of the face, hands, and other parts of the body; wheezing respirations; dyspnea; and signs of vascular collapse with shock (rapid and weak pulse, falling blood pressure, cyanosis). Death may ensue unless rapid action is taken.

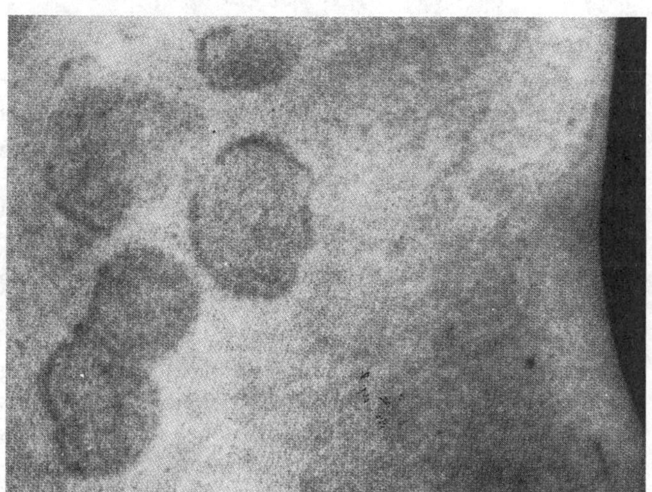

**FIGURE 70-5** Urticaria. (From Stewart WD, Danto JL, Maddin S: *Dermatology: diagnosis and treatment of cutaneous disorders,* ed 4, St Louis, 1978, Mosby.)

## Prevention

### Primary prevention

Primary prevention of type I hypersensitivities includes patient education and precautionary actions.

**Patient education.** Persons who have a type I allergy should be aware of situations in which the substance to which they are sensitized may be found. Persons who are sensitive to insect stings should learn the emergency care to take after a sting. Sting emergency medical kits are available commercially and should be readily available. If a sting occurs, the person should immediately swallow the uncoated antihistamine tablet and inject the epinephrine. The person or significant other must be taught how to use the self-injecting syringe to administer the 1:1000 epinephrine HCl. This syringe is a spring-loaded automated syringe that is simple to use and will inject through clothing. If the patient is unable to use this syringe or give the injection, an inhalation high-dose epinephrine taken from a metered-dose aerosol (found in some emergency kits) may be used. With the aerosol method, the epinephrine is rapidly absorbed through the respiratory tract and will help relieve respiratory symptoms, although it may not correct the hypotension. The aerosol method therefore is not recommended as the primary route.

**Precautionary actions.** When animal sera, allergenic extracts, or contrast media containing iodide are given, a syringe containing 1:1000 epinephrine hydrochloride should be readily available. In addition, an antihistamine, such as diphenhydramine (Benadryl), should be available. The patient is then kept under surveillance for at least 30 minutes after administration of the substance. Any reaction that occurs within a few minutes forewarns of an impending emergency.

### Secondary prevention

Secondary prevention includes identification of high-risk persons and desensitization.

**Identification of high-risk persons.** Because persons with a history of allergies are more likely to develop anaphylactic reactions to drugs than those without such a history, all patients should be questioned about allergies and sensitivities to drugs before drug therapy is initiated. Completing a nursing history as delineated in Chapter 69 is very important. If there is a positive history, the physician is consulted before a new drug is given; if a new drug is administered, the patient is monitored closely for allergic responses. High-risk persons should wear an identification bracelet or tag at all times that indicates the known allergy. These tags may be obtained commercially.* Hospitalized persons who are

*Medic-Alert Foundation, 2323 Colorado St, Turlock, CA 95380 (1-800-ID-ALERT).

sensitive to certain substances are identified, and the information is posted conspicuously outside the room and in the medical record (physician's order sheet, front of chart, medicine administration record, Kardex). Also, most hospitals use a special color identification bracelet for the person who is sensitive to certain substances.

With some medications that have a high potential for anaphylaxis (such as penicillin, streptokinase, and amphotericin B), skin testing is performed before administration. The test dose is given intradermally, and the skin is observed for induration within 30 minutes. A serum ELISA may also be obtained. A positive skin test or serum ELISA indicates potential for anaphylaxis. Informed consent must be obtained from the patient before skin testing. Measures to treat an anaphylactic reaction should be readily available.

**Desensitization.** Persons who have hypersensitivity to insect stings are recommended for immunizing injections with Hymenoptera extract. The approach is similar to hyposensitization for atopic allergies (see below).

## Medical Management

The major goals of medical intervention for type I hypersensitivities are (1) to recognize the potential for allergic reactions, (2) to maintain a patent airway, (3) to reverse the histamine response caused by IgE, and (4) to combat shock.

### Diagnostic tests

A health history is one of the most valuable diagnostic tools for the practitioner evaluating the patient with type I hypersensitivities. The history should include an environmental assessment.

With atopic patients, skin tests and the RAST (see Chapter 69) may be helpful in determining therapy. Skin tests have been used by many physicians to identify allergens responsible for the patient's symptoms. Skin tests are prone to many errors and may lead to misdiagnosis. The results of the skin tests or RAST must be correlated with the patient's history to help locate the cause of the allergic reaction.

### Medication

Drug therapy for atopic allergies is primarily for symptom relief. Prescribed drugs include the following:

1. Antihistamines: chlorpheniramine (Chlor-Trimeton), brompheniramine (Dimetane), carbinoxamine (Clistin)
2. Nonsedating antihistamines: terfenadine (Seldane), astemizole (Hismanal), cetirizine, (Zyrtec, investigational), loratadine (Claritin)
3. Decongestants (nasal sprays): phenylephrine hydrochloride (Neo-Synephrine, Duration, Sinex), oxymetazoline hydrochloride (Afrin, Allerest 12-hour nasal, Dristan long lasting), xylometazoline hydrochloride (Sine-off nasal spray, Sinex-LA)
4. Decongestants (oral: phenylephrine hydrochloride (Neo-Synephrine), pseudoephedrine hydrochloride (Sudafed, Sudrin)
5. Decongestants and antihistamines combined: Dimetapp, Triaminic, Actifed
6. Mast cell degranulation inhibitor: cromolyn sodium (Nasalcrom, Rynacrom); this is used as a nasal spray
7. Corticosteroids for severe reactions:
   a. Nasal sprays such as Decadron Phosphate Turbinaire, Vancenase, Beconase, Nasalide
   b. Oral corticosteroids such as prednisone, methylprednisolone.

Because urticaria and angioedema are usually self-limiting, treatment is often not required. Known offending agents are removed if possible. Epinephrine and antihistamines may be given to hasten resolution and to prevent further histamine reaction. Corticosteroids may be used on a short-term basis (initial dose of 40 mg, then decreased by 5 mg/day).

At the first sign of anaphylaxis, the patient is given epinephrine 1:1000 solution 0.3 to 0.5 ml subcutaneously or intramuscularly (less for children). The epinephrine opposes the action of histamine through vasoconstriction to raise the blood pressure and through relaxation of the bronchioles to facilitate breathing. Epinephrine also inhibits mast cell mediator release. An antihistamine, such as diphenhydramine, shortens the duration of anaphylaxis and prevents a relapse. Hydrocortisone is given intravenously after epinephrine and antihistamine to decrease the inflammatory effects.

Bronchodilators such as aminophylline may be given to decrease the symptoms caused by the bronchospasms. If the bronchospasms persist, ventolin administered through aerosol treatments may be administered. Vasopressors such as dopamine or metaraminol bitartrate (Aramine) may be prescribed for severe shock to assist in increasing the blood pressure and increasing the cardiac output.

### Treatment

Avoidance is the most effective treatment to decrease allergic attacks. With avoidance therapy, the patient is taught to reduce exposure to triggering allergens. This therapy appears more effective with food, drug, and allergens such as animal dander; but it also can be useful to treat seasonal allergies. For instance, limiting outdoor activities and staying in air-conditioned environments when the pollen counts are high decrease seasonal allergic symptoms.

**Immunotherapy** has been effective in diminishing symptoms of allergic rhinitis, particularly to allergies from pollens and house dusts. Hyposensitization appears to affect the immune system by two mechanisms: stimulation of T-suppressor cells specific to depression of IgE responses and stimulation of production of IgG antibodies specific to the allergen.[6] The immunotherapy program requires an individualized dose advancement and is used only in patients with atopic IgE mediated disease. Increasing amounts of allergen are injected at weekly intervals, starting with a dose to which the person has been found sensitive by skin testing. The treatment may take up to 5 years. Treatment is about 80% effective; immunotherapy is restarted if symptoms recur. Before immunotherapy is chosen as a viable treatment alternative, the physician and patient must be sure that the symptoms warrant the risk, expense, and inconvenience of the therapy regimens. Although this treatment is still widely used in allergic symptom treatment, there is still controversy over this 75-year-old therapy because of its potential for anaphylaxis and death. Safeguards are utilized during the therapy.

If large local reactions (redness, edema, pruritus, or tenderness) occur during therapy, the dose is not increased but is repeated or lowered until better tolerated. Systemic reactions, although infrequent, may occur within 30 minutes of injection. Signs of systemic reaction include nasal stuffiness, sneezing, reddening of conjunctiva, tight chest, wheezing, faintness, apprehension, and eventually anaphylactic shock. The person is placed in a supine position, and aqueous epinephrine 1:1000 (0.2 to 0.5 ml) is injected into the arm that has not received the allergen injection. An additional small amount (0.1 to 0.2 ml) may be injected in the site of the allergen injection. Short-acting corticosteroids may be prescribed to prevent recurrence.

The future of atopic disease treatment appears to lie in learning more about modulating the immune response. Possible therapies are now being explored that would include manipulating IgE response by using IgE-specific suppressor T cells, utilizing antibodies against IgE idiotopes, or cytokines that would suppress IgE synthesis.[8,11]

If the local reaction to an allergen is greater than normal, such as angioedema, application of ice and elevation of the extremity help decrease the symptoms. If the patient is showing signs and symptoms of anaphylactic shock, it is important to maintain the airway and treat the shock. Laryngeal edema is common with anaphylaxis and other allergic disorders. The physician needs to be prepared with endotracheal or tracheostomy tubes to establish an airway if necessary. The patient who experiences shortness of breath is positioned in high-Fowler's position and given oxygen therapy if the $Pao_2$ declines. However, if the patient complains of dizziness, becomes cold and clammy, or experiences a decrease in blood pressure, the patient should be placed in a recumbent position with legs elevated. IV fluids, usually normal saline, are initiated and infused rapidly to elevate the blood pressure. (See Chapter 22 for treatment of shock.)

### Diet

The diet may be altered in patients with food allergies to avoid those foods causing allergy. Common foods that cause allergies are milk, nuts, fish, egg, soy, wheat, corn, and chocolate.[6]

### Activity

The activity of the patient is not restricted. Atopic patients are encouraged to avoid activities when certain allergens or pollutants are high. Pollen counts are usually the highest between the hours of 12 midnight and 8 AM and on dry, windy days.

### Referral/Consultation

Atopic individuals who have not achieved control of their symptoms with avoidance therapy and symptom-treating drugs may be referred to allergists for testing and immunotherapy.

## NURSING MANAGEMENT

## ♦ ASSESSMENT

### Subjective Data

Nursing interventions are based on the person's knowledge about the disorder and on the source or form of allergy present. This information is obtained by taking a history.

Subjective data to be obtained might include the following:

1. History of allergic reactions in the past (e.g., type, frequency, or perceived causes)
2. Familial history of allergies
3. Recent exposure to sensitizing substances
4. Changes in living, working, or environmental conditions
5. Characteristics of present environment (house, clothing, plants, trees, or animals)
6. Increased stress in recent past (aggravates asthmatic response)
7. Types of symptoms: respiratory, dermal, gastrointestinal, or general
8. Alleviating factors, either prescribed by physician or self-prescribed

*All* persons in the health care system should be questioned about allergies and sensitivities to drugs before any drug therapy is initiated. If there is a positive history, the physician is consulted before a new drug is given; if the drug is given, the patient is monitored closely for allergic responses.

### Objective Data

The skin, mucous membranes, ears, nose, throat and lung are inspected. The skin is examined for rashes. Constant rubbing the nose upward as seen with allergic conditions can cause a crease across the lower part of the nose. Mouth breathing and difficulty hearing may indicate nasal obstruction and plugging of the eustachian tube. Venous dilation of skin beneath eyes called allergic "shiner" may make the person appear to have black eyes. Pale bluish turbinates, which are edematous and filled with clear secretions, are common with allergic conditions such as rhinitis. Tearing and scleral and conjunctival infections are common. Patients with asthma will show increased respiratory rate, audible wheezing, use of accessory muscles to breathe, flaring nares, and a look of anxiety on their face.

## ♦ NURSING DIAGNOSES

Nursing diagnoses are determined from analysis of patient data. Nursing diagnoses for the patient with a type I hypersensitivity may include but are not limited to the following:

| Diagnostic Title | Possible Etiologic Factors |
|---|---|
| *Atopy* | |
| Health maintenance, altered | Environmental changes, lack of knowledge |
| Knowledge deficit | Lack of exposure/recall, information misinterpretation |
| *Anaphylaxis* | |
| Airway clearance, ineffective | Bronchospasm, laryngeal edema, increased mucous gland secretion |
| Cardiac output, decreased, high risk for | Vasodilation, loss of vascular volume |

## ♦ EXPECTED PATIENT OUTCOMES

Expected patient outcomes for the person with a type I hypersensitivity may include but are not limited to the following:

*Atopy*

1. Symptoms decrease in intensity.
2. Describes the following:
   a. Plans to alter habits or environment, as appropriate
   b. Substances that are allergenic and approaches for avoidance
   c. Rationale for immunotherapy and need to continue regular injections (if pertinent)
   d. Need for constant availability of an anaphylaxis emergency kit for self-treatment (if anaphylaxis is a possibility)
   e. Drug therapy to relieve symptoms

*Anaphylaxis*

1. Maintains a patent airway.
2. Shows no signs and symptoms of shock or anxiety.

## ♦ INTERVENTIONS

### Patient with Atopy

#### Controlling the environment

To help maintain health, it is important to encourage the patient to control what is in the environment and to avoid allergens. Persons who are allergic to *dust* must prepare a living and working environment that is as dust free as possible. There should be a minimum of lint-producing articles (such as curtains, bedspreads, and carpets). Smooth, synthetic materials should be used in place of wool or cotton (Table 70-6). Small items such

**TABLE 70-6 Methods of Decreasing Environmental Inhalant Antigens**

| AREA | METHOD |
|---|---|
| Floors | No wool carpets or felt rug pads; washable throw rugs over wood or tile floors may be used |
| Furniture | No kapok stuffing; a minimum number of foam-stuffed furniture covered with leather or plastic is preferable |
| Clothing | No wool; place closet garments in plastic bags |
| Bedding | |
| Pillows | No feather or kapok; use polyester fiberfill |
| Mattress | Use foam mattress over a covered box spring; use allergy-free covers |
| Blankets | Washable cotton |
| Pets | No fur-bearing pets |
| Cleaning | Daily damp dusting; no shaking of articles |
| Air | Air conditioning, if possible; if not, try electrostatic filters |
| Plants | Avoid dried plants |
| Furnace | Change filters monthly |

as figurines or other small decorations that are difficult to dust are best removed or placed in glass-enclosed cabinets. Daily *damp* dusting will lessen the amount of dust in the air. Air conditioning is desirable for hot weather. ***Animal dander*** is one allergen that usually can be avoided completely. Fur-bearing pets can be removed from the environment. If total removal of a family pet is difficult because of emotional ties, the pet can be kept in an outdoor enclosure. Furniture stuffed with horsehair or feathers must be replaced with furniture stuffed with synthetic materials. It usually takes several months for symptoms from animal dander to subside.

*Seasonal inhalants* are more difficult to avoid. If financially possible, the best method is taking a prolonged vacation in an area free of the offending allergen. When the person remains at home, outside air should be avoided as much as possible during the seasonal months by the use of air conditioners. However, car air conditioners may increase the allergic reaction, because mold spores can proliferate in the moist evaporator core from the warmed car engine. To correct this problem, instruct the allergic person to start the car, turn on the air conditioner, roll down the windows, and run the air conditioner for about 10 to 15 minutes (to blow out the spores) before entering car. Mold disinfectant spray is also available.

For both pollen and spores, the highest counts (amount in the air) occur between 12 midnight and 8 AM; therefore outdoor air should be avoided during those hours. The "official" counts often cited on television or in the newspaper can be misleading, because the counts are usually from the previous day, and pollen counts differ from place to place. Being outside on dry windy days, riding in an open car, and gardening are usually reported to increase symptoms.

**Facilitating learning**

The major nursing responsibility in the care of the person with an atopic allergy is teaching the patient about the nature of the disorder and the methods that can be used to avoid the allergen and control the environment as previously described. The major points for teaching are summarized in the Guidelines box at right.

## Patient with Anaphylaxis

Death with anaphylaxis occurs from asphyxiation because of upper airway edema and congestion, irreversible shock, or a combination of these factors.[13] The primary concern of the nurse is to make sure the patient has a patent airway. Typical assessment data to observe are complaint of shortness of breath, stridor, cyanosis, use of accessory muscles to breathe, tachypnea, and edema around the facial area. Auscultation of the chest may reveal wheezing. Assess the patient's level of consciousness. A decrease in the level of consciousness might mean that the patient is experiencing hypoxia. Oxygen therapy may be given to the patient according to doctor's orders or facility protocols. Position the patient in high-Fowler's position to assist with breathing. Be alert that this patient may need an emergency intubation or tracheostomy and ensure that the necessary equipment is easily accessible. Suctioning equipment should be available and used if the patient has excessive mucus production, which compromises the airway. Secondarily, the nurse must be aware that this patient has a high risk for developing decreased cardiac output leading to shock. For care of the patient with shock, see Chapter 22.

## ♦ EVALUATION

To evaluate the effectiveness of nursing interventions, compare patient behaviors with those stated in the expected patient outcomes. Successful achievement of patient outcomes for the *patient who is atopic* is indicated by the following:

1a. Verbalizes a decrease in symptoms such as runny nose, headache, weeping eyes, difficulty hearing, and/or asthmatic attacks.
b. Hives on skin have disappeared. Does not use accessory muscles to breathe, airway is patent, and the respiratory rate is $<20$.
c. Verbalizes a decrease in the reaction to the allergen after desensitization has been completed.
2a. Verbalizes changes in environment or habits that will decrease exposure to allergens.
b. Verbalizes the purpose of immunotherapy (hyposensitization).
c. Verbalizes the need for an easily accessible anaphylaxis kit and can demonstrate the use of the medications inside.
d. Verbalizes the types of medications that are prescribed and when they will be needed.

### Guidelines for Teaching the Person With an Atopic Allergy

The person will be able to explain or perform the following:

1. Avoid allergen, if possible.
   a. Animal dander
      (1) Have no fur-bearing pets, if possible.
      (2) Keep any family fur-bearing pet in outdoor enclosure.
      (3) Avoid furniture stuffed with horsehair or feathers.
   b. Pollen spores
      (1) Vacation in selected geographic areas, such as beach or sea, that are free of specific allergen during seasonal height, if possible.
      (2) Use air conditioning if possible; keep windows closed at night; if using air conditioner in car, start car, roll down windows and allow air conditioner to run for 10-15 minutes before entering car.
      (3) Limit being outdoors between sunset and sunrise, especially when windy.
      (4) Do not hang wash outside to dry. (Pollen and molds stick to wet wash.)
      (5) Avoid gardening, raking leaves, mowing lawn, or being near freshly cut grass.
      (6) Keep car windows closed when driving.
      (7) Minimize number of indoor plants.
   c. House dust
      (1) Use synthetic materials; avoid wool and cotton.
      (2) Use a minimum of lint-producing articles.
      (3) Put away articles that are difficult to dust.
      (4) Dust with damp cloth daily.
      (5) Use air conditioner, if possible.
      (6) Change furnace filter every month during use.
2. During immunotherapy (hyposensitization)
   a. Report for regularly scheduled injections, even when symptoms subside (therapy will last for 3 to 5 months).
   b. Remain at physician's office for at least 30 minutes after receiving injection (for immediate treatment should a systemic reaction occur).
   c. Report large local reactions to physician (redness, swelling, itching, or soreness).
3. Monitor for side effects of medication taken frequently for relief of symptoms.
   a. Antihistamines: sedation, constipation, urinary retention, tachycardia; avoidance of driving or use of heavy machinery if drowsiness is present
   b. Vasoconstrictors: irregular or rapid pulse, palpitations, restlessness, dizziness
   c. Nasal corticosteroids: nasal irritation, dryness of nose and mouth
   d. Cromolyn sodium: throat irritation, headache, dizziness, rash, urticaria
4. If exposed to a known allergen and experiencing light-headedness, difficulty breathing, or swelling of the face, use the emergency anaphylaxis kit immediately. Take a pill (Benadryl) and give yourself a shot (epinephrine). This is important therapy to help prevent life-threatening complications.
5. Be careful in seeking unconventional therapy. Ask questions about the therapy and its testing.

Successful achievement of patient outcomes for the *patient who has anaphylaxis* are indicated by the following:

1a. Verbalizes no difficulty with breathing.
 b. Shows no tachypnea, stridor, use of accessory muscles, cyanosis, or flaring of nares.
2a. Maintains a systolic blood pressure >100.
 b. Has urinary output >30 ml/hr.
 c. Has no signs of third spacing (i.e., facial edema, dependent edema, ascites).
3a. Verbalizes no feelings of anxiousness.
 b. Shows no signs of anxiety (i.e., wringing of hands, eyes wide open, furrowed brow, trembling hands).

**TABLE 70-7 Types of Blood Components**

| BLOOD COMPONENT | DESCRIPTION | USAGE | COMMENTS |
|---|---|---|---|
| **RED BLOOD CELLS (RBCs)** | | | |
| Packed RBC (PRBCs) | RBCs separated from plasma and platelets | Anemia<br>Moderate blood loss | Decreased risk of fluid overload as compared to whole blood |
| Autologous PRBC | Same as packed RBC | Elective surgery for which blood replacement is expected | Units may be stored for up to 35 days |
| Washed RBCs | RBCs washed with sterile isotonic saline before transfusion | Previous allergic reactions to transfusions | Increased removal of immunoglobulins and protein |
| Frozen RBCs | RBCs frozen in a glycerol solution; cells washed after thawing to remove the glycerol | Storage of rare type blood<br>Storage of autologous blood for future use | Relatively free of leukocytes and microemboli<br>Expensive |
| Leukocyte-poor RBCs | RBCs from which most leukocytes have been removed | Previous sensitivity to leukocyte antigens from prior transfusions or from pregnancy | Fewer RBC than packed RBC; washed leukocyte-poor RBC units have more RBC than nonwashed |
| Neocytes | RBC units with high number of reticulocytes (young RBCs) | Transfusion-dependent anemias | Fewer problems with iron overload<br>Expensive |
| **OTHER CELLULAR COMPONENTS** | | | |
| Platelets | | | |
| Random donor packs | Platelets separated from RBCs by centrifuge; given in 50 ml of plasma | Thrombocytopenia<br>DIC | Plasma base is rich in coagulation factors<br>Platelet preparations can also be packed, washed, or made leukocyte-poor |
| Pheresis packs | Platelets from an HLA matched donor, separated by apheresis | Allosensitized persons with thrombocytopenia | Requires specialized techniques |
| Granulocytes | Granular leukocytes separated by apheresis | Granulocytopenia from malignancy or chemotherapy | Allergen sensitization may occur with chills and fever |
| **PLASMA COMPONENTS** | | | |
| Fresh frozen plasma (FFP) | Freezing of plasma within 4 hr of collection | Clotting deficiencies<br>Liver disease<br>Hemophilia<br>Defibrination | Preserves factors V, VII, VIII, IX, and X and prothrombin<br>Minimizes hepatitis risk<br>Administered through a filter |
| Factor concentrates VIII and IX | Prepared from large donor pools<br>Heated to inactivate HIV | VIII: Hemophilia A<br>IX: Hemophilia B | Increased risk of hepatitis (VIII, IX) and thromboembolism (IX)<br>Given in small volumes |
| Cryoprecipitate | Precipitated material obtained from FFP when thawed | Hemophilia A<br>Infection of burns<br>Hypofibrinogenemia<br>Uremic bleeding | Contains factors VIII, XIII, and fibrinogen |
| Serum albumin | Albumin chemically processed from pooled plasma | Hypovolemic shock | No risk of hepatitis |
| Normal serum albumin (NSA) | | Hypoalbuminemia<br>Burns | Does not require ABO compatibility |
| Plasma protein fraction (PPF) | | Hemorrhagic shock | Lacks clotting factors<br>Hypotension may occur if PPF is given faster than 10 ml/min |
| Immune serum globulin | Obtained from plasma of preselected donors with specific antibodies | Hypogammaglobulinemia<br>Prophylaxis for hepatitis A | Given intramuscularly |

## TYPE II HYPERSENSITIVITIES

The underlying mechanism of **type II (cytotoxic) hypersensitivities** involves the direct binding of IgG or IgM immunoglobulins to an antigen on the surface of a cell. This antibody labeling then triggers the destruction of the cell by phagocytic attack, nonspecific lymphocytic attack, or lysis of the cell through the operation of the full complement cascade (see Chapter 13).

### Blood Transfusion Reactions

Type II hypersensitivity is classically illustrated by the reactions that occur in mismatched blood transfusion reactions. Blood replacement therapy is used when there has been excessive blood loss (whole blood or blood components) or in the treatment of diseases of the hematopoietic system.

Although whole blood may be used, there has been an increased use of specific blood components. Only about 6% of blood now given in the United States is in the form of whole blood. Blood can be fractionated into red blood cells (RBCs), platelets, and plasma (Table 70-7), either by centrifuge or by automated cell separators. Blood can also be withdrawn from a donor, a portion separated from the blood, and the remainder returned to the donor **(apheresis).** Using blood components rather than whole blood provides greater use of an increasingly scarcer commodity (blood) for an increased number of recipients, prevents fluid overload, and gives the recipient only that which is required (thus decreasing possibilities of side effects).

#### Pathophysiology

There are many antigens on the surface of RBCs, but two major systems are significant clinically in terms of potential immunologic reactions: the ABO system and the Rh system. The human leukocytes antigen (HLA) system relates to leukocytes and platelets.

**ABO system.** Four major blood groups are found in humans: A, B, AB, and O (Box 70-1). Because type AB blood contains both antigens, persons with type AB may receive blood from any type (Figure 70-6). Persons with type O may donate blood to other types, but because both antigens are absent in type O, they may not receive another type without experiencing a reaction.

Erythrocyte antigens inherited from our parents give us our blood types.[12] Within 3 months of birth, the individual has formed antibodies against the other types of major erythrocyte antigens. The exact cause of this antibody formation is not clear, but it is suspected that something antigenically similar to the antibodies are found in the environment and these stimulate antibody formation.[13] For example, a person with type A blood will possess anti-B antibodies within the serum. These antibodies, called *isohemagglutinins,* are usually of the IgM class. Antibodies formed in this way are capable of cross-reacting with the A or B antigens on the surface of the "foreign" ABO types. These antibodies are naturally present in the serum; therefore mismatched blood cells from a transfusion will be immediately coated by the isohemagglutinins, causing the agglutination of the introduced cells and the rapid lysis of the cells by complement. The products released by the lysed cells are then dumped into the bloodstream.

**Rh system.** The Rh system is more complex, because there are at least 27 different antigens in this system. The D antigen is the most significant clinically, because it is more immunogenic than any other Rh antigen, and it is usually the antigen involved in hemolytic disease of the newborn. When the term **Rh positive** is used, the presence of antigen Rh-D is implied; **Rh negative** indicates the absence of antigen D. Approximately 85% of the population have Rh-positive blood.

When the Rh-negative person is first exposed to Rh-positive blood, Rh antibodies are formed. On subsequent exposures to Rh-positive blood, the Rh antibody binds to its corresponding antigen on the surface of the RBCs containing the Rh antigen. The Rh antibodies do not usually fix complement; therefore there is no immediate hemolysis as occurs in the ABO system. Instead, the Rh-antigen RBCs are rapidly broken down by macrophages in the spleen, with conversion of hemoglobin to bilirubin resulting in jaundice.

**Other erythrocyte antigens.** Another group of erythrocyte antigens that can form antibodies are grouped

**BOX 70-1 ABO Blood Groups**

| | |
|---|---|
| A | Antigen A is present |
| B | Antigen B is present |
| AB | Both antigens A and B are present |
| O | Neither antigen A nor B is present |

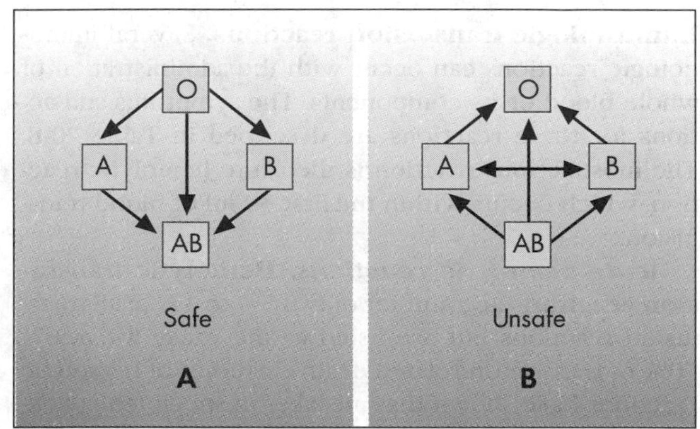


**FIGURE 70-6** Blood groups and their donor/recipient relationships. **A,** Safe. **B,** Unsafe.

**BOX 70-2 Adverse Reactions to Blood Transfusions**

**IMMUNOLOGIC**
- Acute hemolytic
- Febrile, nonhemolytic
- Mild allergic
- Anaphylactic
- Delayed hemolytic
- Graft-versus-host disease
- Noncardiac pulmonary edema

**NONIMMUNOLOGIC**
- Circulatory overload
- Sepsis
- Transmission of disease

into the Kidd, Duffy, Kell, and MNS systems.[13] The antibodies can cause hemolytic reactions if antigen-positive blood is transfused into a sensitized recipient. These antibodies cause more problems in patients who are chronically transfused.[14]

**HLA system.** Another system that has clinical significance in blood transfusions is the human leukocytes antigen (HLA) system. HLAs are found on many types of tissue cells and on blood leukocytes and platelets. The system is more complex than the RBC antigen systems, and there are literally thousands of combinations of the antigens that may occur. Sensitization may occur through pregnancy or through exposure to platelets and WBCs during transfusions. Repeated transfusions of blood cells may lead to transfusion reactions.

### Types of transfusion reactions

Although there are numerous types of adverse reactions to blood transfusions, they occur in only approximately 2% to 5% of all transfusions.[14] To facilitate the discussion of these different transfusion reactions, they are grouped into two categories: immunologic and nonimmunologic (Box 70-2).

**Immunologic transfusion reactions.** Several immunologic reactions can occur with the administration of whole blood or its components. The symptoms and actions for these reactions are described in Table 70-8. The most serious reaction is the acute hemolytic reaction, which occurs within the first 30 ml of blood transfusion.

***Acute hemolytic reactions.*** **Hemolytic transfusion reactions** account for only 0.5% to 1% of all transfusion reactions but are listed as the cause for nearly 70% of transfusion related deaths.[5] Studies of hemolytic reactions have shown that mistakes in specimen collection and labeling and inadequate patient identification, are the primary errors that lead to these reactions.[14] Acute hemolytic reactions are caused by antigen-antibody complexes on the erythrocyte membrane. These complexes activate the Hageman factor (coagulation factor XII) and the complement cascade. The Hageman factor initiates the kinin system, causing increased capillary permeability, arteriole vasodilation, and hypotension.[13] The activated complement system initiates intravascular hemolysis, as well as histamine and serotonin release from the mast cells. Hageman factor and free incompatible erythrocyte stroma (covering) activate the intrinsic clotting cascade causing disseminated intravascular coagulation (DIC).

Chills, fever, and low back pain are early signs of acute hemolytic reaction. Hemoglobin released and excreted in the urine can give the urine a red (port-wine urine) color. This hemoglobinuria can lead to tubular necrosis, oliguria, and renal failure. Hypotension, tachycardia, and tachypnea are hallmark symptoms of impending shock caused by the histamine and kinin effects on the vessels. It is important to remember that asymptomatic hemoglobinuria can occur in some patients who are not having a hemolytic reaction as a result of transfusing hemolyzed compatible cells, of giving drugs/hypotonic solutions along with the RBCs that cause RBCs to rupture, or because the patient had open heart surgery and the extracorporeal oxygenator was used. In these cases, the other signs and symptoms of hemolytic reaction would not be evident.

If the patient reports symptoms of hemolytic blood reaction, the transfusion should be stopped immediately and the patient's physician notified. The patient is monitored for signs and symptoms of shock, renal shutdown, and DIC. Make sure a large-bore, patent intravenous line is established for the patient. Be prepared to administer fluids and medications to maintain blood pressure. The best prevention of this reaction is through proper labeling of donor and recipient blood and accurate identification of the right blood type for the right patient. It is also important that all blood products be infused slowly for the first 15 to 20 minutes in case a hemolytic reaction occurs. This approach will allow less of the donor blood in the system of the recipient so the reaction will be less severe.[5]

***Febrile nonhemolytic reactions.*** Febrile nonhemolytic reactions are one of the most common transfusion reactions. They occur because the recipient becomes sensitized to the donor's WBCs, platelets, or plasma. Symptoms usually begin 30 minutes after the start of the infusion and consist of fever (usually 38° to 39° C) and chills. Although this reaction is not usually serious, it is uncomfortable to the patient. The transfusion is stopped immediately to rule out a hemolytic reaction, and the blood is sent to the laboratory for analysis. Any patient with a history of febrile nonhemolytic reaction is premedicated with Tylenol and Benadryl or receives leukocyte-poor red blood cells to prevent recurrence. (See p. 2426 for explanation of leukocyte-poor red blood cells.)

**TABLE 70-8 Immunologic Reactions to Blood Transfusion***

| CAUSE | CLINICAL MANIFESTATIONS | MANAGEMENT | PREVENTION |
|---|---|---|---|
| **ACUTE HEMOLYTIC*** | | | |
| Infusion of ABO-incompatible whole blood, red blood cells, or components containing 10 ml or more of red blood cells.<br>Antibodies in the recipient's plasma attach to antigens on transfused red blood cells causing red-blood-cell destruction. | Chills, fever, low back pain, flushing, tachycardia, tachypnea, hypotension, vascular collapse, hemoglobinuria, hemoglobinemia, bleeding, acute renal failure, shock, cardiac arrest, death | Treat shock.<br>Draw blood samples for serologic testing. To avoid hemolysis from the procedure, use a new venipuncture (not an existing central line) and avoid small-gauge needles. Send urine specimen to the laboratory.<br>Maintain BP with IV colloid solutions. Give diuretics as prescribed to maintain urine flow.<br>Insert indwelling catheter or measure voided amounts to monitor hourly urine output. Dialysis may be required if renal failure occurs.<br>Do not transfuse additional red-blood-cell-containing components until the transfusion service has provided newly crossmatched units. | Meticulously verify and document patient identification from sample collection to component infusion.<br>Transfuse blood slowly for first 15-20 minutes. |
| **FEBRILE, NONHEMOLYTIC (MOST COMMON)*** | | | |
| Sensitization to donor's white blood cells, platelets, or plasma proteins. | Sudden chills and fever (rise in temperature of greater than 1°C [2°F]), headache, flushing, anxiety, muscle pain | Give antipyretics as prescribed. Do not give aspirin to thrombocytopenic patients.<br>*Do not restart transfusion.* | Consider leukocyte-poor blood products (filtered, washed, or frozen). |
| **MILD ALLERGIC*** | | | |
| Sensitivity to foreign plasma proteins. | Flushing, itching, urticaria (hives) | Give antihistamines as directed.<br>If symptoms are mild and transient, restart transfusion slowly.<br>Do not restart transfusion if fever or pulmonary symptoms develop. | Treat prophylactically with antihistamines. |
| **ANAPHYLACTIC*** | | | |
| Infusion of IgA proteins to IgA-deficient recipient who has developed IgA antibody. | Anxiety, urticaria, wheezing, tightness and pain in chest, difficulty swallowing, progressing to cyanosis, shock, and possible cardiac arrest | Initiate CPR if indicated.<br>Have epinephrine ready for injection (0.4 ml of a 1:1,000 solution subcutaneously or 0.1 ml of 1:1,000 solution diluted to 10 ml with saline for IV use).<br>*Do not restart transfusion.* | Transfuse extensively washed red blood cell products from which all plasma has been removed. Alternatively, use blood from IgA-deficient donor. |
| **DELAYED HEMOLYTIC** | | | |
| Anamnestic immune response that occurs 7-14 days after the transfusion. Sensitization to RBC antigen not ABO system. | Fever, chills, back pain, jaundice, anemia, hemoglobinuria | Monitor adequacy of urinary output and degree of anemia.<br>Treat fever with Tylenol.<br>May need further blood transfusion. | Do more specific type and crossmatch when giving patient blood. |
| **GRAFT-VERSUS-HOST DISEASE-PT** | | | |
| Immunodeficient person receives lymphocytes and these lymphocytes begin to reject cells 4 to 30 days after the transfusion. | Anorexia, nausea, diarrhea, high fever, rash, stomatitis, liver dysfunction | No effective treatment.<br>Administer steroids. | Give irradiated blood products. |

*Adapted from the *National blood resource education program's transfusion therapy guidelines for nurses,* 1990-NIH Publication No. 90-2668.

*Continued*

**TABLE 70-8 Immunologic Reactions to Blood Transfusion—cont'd**

| CAUSE | CLINICAL MANIFESTATIONS | MANAGEMENT | PREVENTION |
|---|---|---|---|
| **NONCARDIAC PULMONARY EDEMA** | | | |
| Donor antibodies react with recipient HLA antigens, have activation of complement and histamine. Infiltration of pulmonary bed with microaggregates. | Fever, chills, hypotension, cough, orthopnea, cyanosis, shock | Stop transfusion. Continue IV saline. Give oxygen prn. Administer steroids as directed. Give furosemide (Lasix) and epinephrine as ordered. | |

***Mild allergic and anaphylactic reactions.*** Another common blood transfusion reaction is the allergic transfusion reaction. It is caused by sensitivity of the recipient to foreign plasma proteins. Common symptoms include hives, rash, and urticaria. If the symptoms are mild, the patient is treated with antihistamines and the transfusion is restarted slowly. A more severe reaction (anaphylaxis) can occur rarely, and the patient will show symptoms of bronchospasm, respiratory distress, and shock. If anaphylaxis occurs, the blood transfusion is stopped immediately and the patient is treated with epinephrine, antihistamines, steroids, vasopressors, or increased fluid resuscitation depending on the patient's blood pressure and respiratory distress. For anyone who has a mild allergic reaction, future reactions can be prevented by premedicating the patient with an antihistamine 30 minutes before the transfusion or by depleting the plasma proteins in the blood by washing before transfusion.

***Delayed hemolytic reactions.*** Delayed hemolytic reactions occur 7 to 14 days posttransfusion and are thought to be the result of sensitization of the recipient immune system of the transfused erythrocyte antigens or from an anamnestic response from a previously sensitized individual whose antibody titers are undetectable at the time of the transfusion. Typical signs and symptoms include fever, anemia, and jaundice. The treatment involves monitoring the hemoglobin, hematocrit, and renal function closely. The patient may require further transfusions if the anemia increases. A more specific type and crossmatch of the blood may be necessary on these patients to prevent this reaction from recurring.

***Posttransfusion graft-versus-host disease.*** **Posttransfusion graft-versus-host disease** (GVHD-PT) is relatively rare but recently has been reported more frequently because of increased use of purposeful severe immunodepression in certain treatments (i.e., bone marrow transplantation). With these patients, the donor lymphocytes begin to reject the host cells many days after the infusion of blood. These donor lymphocytes have become engrafted and multiply in the immunocompromised host. This type of blood reaction occurs 4 to 30 days after the transfusion and begins with a fever and rash. The rash may eventually develop into bullae, and the patient may experience severe desquamation. Gastrointestinal symptoms include anorexia, nausea and vomiting, and profuse diarrhea. The liver may become enlarged, and jaundice may be present. Treatment of GVHD-PT at present is ineffective. More than 90% die from overwhelming sepsis.[10] It is best to prevent GVHD-PT by irradiating the blood or depleting the leukocytes from the blood products before administration.[1] Irradiation of the blood products is the most common form of prevention. Persons receiving these irradiated blood products have not experienced GVHD-PT after transfusion, and no unusual transfusion reactions have been associated with the use of these irradiated blood products.

***Noncardiac pulmonary edema.*** Noncardiac pulmonary edema is thought to be caused by high titer of leukocyte antibodies in either the donor or recipient plasma. These antibody to granulocyte reactions cause granulocyte aggregates that are filtered out by the lung. The antibodies attached to the granulocytes initiate the complement cascade and promote histamine release, causing an influx of inflammatory cells into the lung. As a result, the patient will show classic signs of pulmonary edema and the transfusion should be stopped immediately. The nurse should intervene to help alleviate the respiratory distress by assisting the patient into a high-Fowler's position to facilitate breathing and should be prepared to administer treatments such as oxygen, epinephrine, furosemide (Lasix), and steroids.

**Nonimmunologic transfusion reactions.** Although there are many types of nonimmunologic blood reactions, this chapter focuses on the more common reactions of circulatory overload, bacterial contamination, and disease transmission.

***Circulatory overload.*** Circulatory overload can occur with the administration of blood when it is given too rapidly or in large quantities over a short time. Children, the elderly, and persons with congestive heart failure are particularly vulnerable to this complication. The typical symptoms include dyspnea, tightness in the chest, headache, hypertension, tachypnea, coughing, cyanosis, peripheral edema, jugular venous distention, auscultated rales in the chest, and abnormal heart sounds. The doctor should be notified and, depending on the severity of the symptoms, the blood may be stopped or slowed. Sometimes a diuretic will be given to help decrease blood volume and ease the effects of hypervolemia on the heart. Oxygen may be administered to relieve respiratory symptoms.

***Sepsis.*** Bacterial contamination of the blood can occur during blood collection or in handling the blood after collection. Reactions to contamination can occur within minutes after the blood has started to be infused. Symptoms of sepsis, including high fever (>40° C), abdominal cramps, vomiting, nausea, diarrhea, and septic shock, are caused by endotoxins being released in the blood. The blood transfusion is stopped immediately when these symptoms arise, and the physician is notified. The blood is sent back to the laboratory to be analyzed. The patient is usually treated with broad-spectrum antibiotics to treat the infection. Hypotension and other symptoms are treated with vasopressors and steroids. The best prevention of this type of reaction is use of sterile technique in phlebotomy and blood processing procedures. The blood should be observed carefully before infusion for color and consistency. If the bag appears to have gas, clots, or a dark purple color, it could mean bacterial contamination and should not be given. The blood should be infused *within 4 hours* after it is taken from the blood bank to prevent bacterial growth after being brought to the patient unit. If it cannot be infused within this time, the blood should be returned to the blood bank for proper refrigeration.

***Transmission of disease.*** Transmission of disease is another complication that can occur with the administration of blood. The most frequently reported diseases transmitted by blood transfusions in United States are hepatitis, cytomegalovirus (CMV), human immunodeficiency virus (HIV), and human T-lymphotropic virus-1 (HTLV-1). Many infectious organisms can be transmitted by blood administration, but only some can be screened for by donor-screening methods.

The incidence of developing hepatitis posttransfusion is 1% to 2%; hepatitis C comprises 95% of these reported cases.[13] Currently, the blood is screened for hepatitis antibodies before patient administration. With the increased recognition of these antibodies in the blood, it is hoped that the incidence of hepatitis transmitted by blood transfusions will decrease.

Cytomegalovirus is a type of herpes virus that causes a mild mononucleosis type of illness. A posttransfusion CMV infection can cause illness and death in patients that are severely immunosuppressed.[1] Administration of CMV seronegative blood is recommended for low-birthweight infants, CMV-seronegative pregnant women, and CMV-seronegative recipients of CMV-negative organ transplants. Donor blood is always screened for HIV antibodies by use of the ELISA and Western blot tests, which would indicate previous HIV exposure. High-risk donors are also being ruled out by community blood centers as potential donors because of their high-risk behaviors. Presently, the risk of transmission of HIV infection is between 1/40,000 and 1/100,000 for each transfused unit of blood. HTLV-1 is known to cause a form of T cell leukemia and tropical spastic paraparesis; however, it is unknown how it relates to transfusion associated disease. Although syphilis, Epstein-Barr virus, and malaria may also be transmitted by blood transfusions, the incidence is rare.

**Prevention of transfusion reactions**

***Donor prescreening.*** Prescreening of potential blood donors is essential. Blood received from volunteer donors through the American Red Cross Blood Service or hospital blood banks is preferable to that of paid donors, because paid donors may be less likely to report present or previous diseases that may affect the recipient.

Requirements have been delineated that include guidelines for persons with heart, lung, liver, or kidney disease. Persons who are not accepted as donors include those with a history of the following:

1. Infectious diseases such as hepatitis, HIV infection and AIDS, tuberculosis, syphilis, or malaria
2. Malignant disease
3. Allergies or asthma
4. Polycythemia vera
5. Abnormal bleeding tendencies
6. Hypotension (current)
7. Anemia (current)
8. Recent pregnancy or major surgery
9. Men with at least one homosexual or bisexual contact since 1975 (concern for AIDS)
10. International travel to malarial areas or high risk countries for AIDS
11. Blood transfusion during last 6 months
12. History of jaundice
13. Diseases of the heart, lungs, or liver
14. Immunizations or vaccinations with attenuated viral vaccine rubella or rabies

The donor's hemoglobin level is tested before giving blood, and the hemoglobin acceptance level is usually set at over 13.5 g/dl for men and 12.5 g/dl for women. Temperature, pulse, and blood pressure should be within normal ranges.

After the blood has been collected, it is tested for syphilis, hepatitis, HIV, and CMV. The blood group and subgroups including Rh typing are identified. The blood is typed, screened, and cross-matched again before it is given to the recipient.

***Accurate laboratory testing.*** Most of the serious reactions that now occur during transfusions are the result of human error. Type, screen, and crossmatching of the blood in the laboratory must be accurate. **Typing** is confirmed by testing the recipient's serum against commercial A and B cells to detect isoagglutinins. The recipients serum is then screened for alloantibodies that were not found in the typing. A **crossmatch** will test the compatibility between donor and recipient directly. The blood from each is mixed and are observed for hemolysis. In patients who have been sensitized to the less important antigenic systems (Kell, Kidd, Duffy, and MNS systems), it is important to obtain a more complete antibody identification to obtain a compatible donor for the RBCs. This problem tends to be more prevalent in oncology patient.[12]

***Careful blood administration.*** The unit of blood or blood components must be labeled with the name of the person for whom it is intended, and this label must be checked against the patient's wristband before the blood is administered. Always check the expiration date of the blood. Baseline vital signs should be obtained and monitored throughout the transfusion. Ask the patient to inform you if any abnormal sensations occur during this transfusion. This information may help the nurse identify transfusion reactions early.[5]

All blood products should be administered through micron mesh filters. (Consult a fundamentals of nursing text for information on care of patients during initiation and course of blood transfusions.)

***Use of autologous blood transfusions.*** One method of preventing immunologic blood transfusion reactions and disease transmission is by using the person's own blood for replacement. There are two approaches for using autologous blood: planned collection and autotransfusion. In **planned autologous transfusion,** blood is collected at regular intervals before anticipated use, such as for forthcoming surgery. The blood is then stored or frozen until needed. This method is especially useful for persons with rare blood types, for those whose religious beliefs preclude receiving donor blood, or when several units of blood are expected to be necessary during surgery (such as with selected heart surgeries or selected joint replacements).

**Autotransfusion,** which consists of collecting, filtering, and immediately reinfusing the person's own blood, may be performed in the emergency room or in the OR suite during surgery involving large blood loss. The blood is suctioned into a bag and passes through a filter to remove microaggregates. When the bag is full, it is disconnected from the system and the blood is infused into the patient with an administration set, using a standard or microembolic filter. Blood that has been contaminated by GI contents or that is close to a malignant tumor is not autotransfused.

***Use of specialized blood products.*** New developments in genetic engineering promise the manufacture of clotting factors in the laboratory.[14] This development will completely stop disease transmission for persons such as hemophiliacs requiring specific blood factors. The use of leukocyte-poor RBCs will decrease the incidence of febrile nonhemolytic reactions. Studies have shown that 70% to 99% of leukocytes can be removed by administering the blood using special leukocyte-poor filters, washing the blood before it is administered, or thawing frozen blood and removing the hypertonic preservatives.[12]

## TYPE III HYPERSENSITIVITIES

The pathogenesis of the **type III (immune complex) hypersensitivities** lies in the union of soluble antigens and immunoglobulins of the IgM and IgG classes. The complexes formed in these interactions are not properly cleared by the reticuloendothelial system (RES) because of the small size of the complexes, which tend to defy phagocytosis. The complexes can then bind complement, initiating the complement cascade causing chemotaxis, vasodilation, and cell lysis. The chemotactic factors released with the involvement of complement lead to an influx of phagocytes, which tend to intensify the inflammatory response. Complement can also aid in the phagocytosis of these immune complexes by deposition of complement protein fragments onto the complexes. Large complexes are then removed by the RES. People with complement deficiencies have increased risk of immune complex diseases. Intermediate-sized complexes, small enough to remain in circulation but large enough to activate complement, are believed to cause chronic type III disease.[15] For instance, immune complexes have been found in many diseases such as multiple sclerosis, chronic active hepatitis, primary biliary cirrhosis, idiopathic interstitial pneumonia, bacterial endocarditis, SLE, acute and chronic glomerulonephritis, rheumatoid arthritis, and some forms of vasculitis. The clinical symptoms observed are the result of the amounts and relative proportions of the antigens and antibodies and the distribution of the complexes within the body.

### Arthus Reaction

The repeated subcutaneous injection of a highly antigenic soluble antigen can lead to the formation of such *immune complexes,* which trigger a localized inflammatory response known as *Arthus reaction.* The region exhibiting Arthus reaction shows the following sequential tissue changes: reduction of blood flow, development of microthrombi in the venules, increased permeability of the venule to the point that RBCs escape into the surrounding tissues, development of edema, massive infiltration of the site by polymorphonuclear neutrophil leukocytes, and tissue destruction. Arthus reactions are not of great clinical importance, because strongly antigenic substances are not usually administered in repeated subcutaneous injections. However, a disseminated type of intravascular inflammation known as allergic vasculitis sometimes occurs in patients undergoing therapy with certain drugs (for example, sulfonamides, iodides, thioureas, and penicillin).

### Serum Sickness

#### Etiology

A type III hypersensitivity of clinical significance is serum sickness, which can develop from 1 to 3 weeks after the administration of foreign serum. This type of serum (horse or rabbit antilymphocyte antibodies) is used in the treatment of transplant rejection. Serum sickness reactions may also occur with the administration of certain drugs, particularly antimicrobials such as penicillin and sulfonamides.

### Pathophysiology

The critical factor in a type III hypersensitivity reaction is a large amount of a persisting soluble antigen, the foreign serum proteins. The antigen initiates an immune response, and the resultant antibodies appear in the blood about 1 week later where they interact with the antigen still present in the bloodstream. These antibody-antigen reactions occur in many organs. The primary organs involved are the kidneys, choroid plexus, joints, skin, and lungs. Itching and discomfort at the injection site are usually the first symptoms noted. These are followed by lymphadenopathy, fever, urticaria or erythematous rash, angioedema of the face, and joint pain. Splenomegaly, abdominal pain, headache, nausea, and vomiting may also occur. Objective signs of arthritis may be present.

### Management

Serum sickness is a self-limiting disease. Mild symptoms respond well to antihistamines and salicylates. More severe symptoms are treated with a steroid such as prednisone, with relief of symptoms often obtained within hours. Epinephrine is given if an anaphylactic reaction occurs.

## TYPE IV HYPERSENSITIVITIES

**Type IV hypersensitivities** are **cell mediated** (delayed type), involving T cells. Macrophages pick up antigens identified as "foreign" to the body. These macrophages take pieces of the antigen and present them to the T lymphocytes, which become sensitized for this type of antigen. The next time the person comes in contact with this particular antigen and the macrophages present these antigenic pieces to the T lymphocytes, the sensitized lymphocyte can form cytotoxic T cells or activate nonspecific phagocytic cells. The cytotoxic T lymphocyte can destroy the antigen directly by attaching itself to the antigen cell wall, breaking down the cell membrane, and causing lysis and cell death. The direct action approach appears to be the major factor in acute allograft rejections. The sensitized T lymphocyte can also activate nonspecific phagocytic cells (macrophages and polymorphonuclear leukocytes) through release of lymphokines (see Chapter 13).

The cell-mediated immune mechanisms function in host defense against chronic bacterial and fungal infections, in rejection of foreign tissue cells, and in surveillance for cancer cells; however, they can also produce adverse effects in the form of delayed-type hypersensitivity. Three major areas of clinical concern are (1) hypersensitivity reactions in response to infections by certain bacteria, fungi, or viruses; (2) contact dermatitis reactions; and (3) tissue transplant rejections.

### Hypersensitivity Reactions in Certain Infections

The body's reaction to the tubercle bacillus *(Mycobacterium tuberculosis)* is a classic example of a type IV hypersensitivity. The organism itself is not directly toxic to human cells or tissues. As a result, the tubercle bacillus may invade the tissues of a nonsensitized host and establish residence in the host tissues, causing virtually no damage. However, in the course of time, as the organism sheds antigenic material, the cell-mediated immune response system is triggered. The sensitized lymphocytes and the activated macrophages attack not only the organism, but also the tissues surrounding the organism. This process is aimed at destroying the foreign organism; however, in the course of the attack, tissue destruction may result. The lesions associated with tuberculosis (such as caseation necrosis cavitation) and general toxemia are results of the hypersensitivity.

After the initial sensitization with the infectious organism, subsequent contact with the tuberculosis organism or even an extract of a purified protein from the organism will elicit a hypersensitivity reaction. This is the basis of the Mantoux tuberculin skin test. The skin rashes of smallpox and measles and the lesions of herpes simplex virus and tuberculoid leprosy have all been attributed to an infectious type IV hypersensitivity.

### Allergic Contact Dermatitis

Allergic contact dermatitis is one of the most commonly encountered types of human allergic disease. Usually, both the route of sensitization and the display of symptoms are produced by direct dermal contact with the allergen. Many simple chemicals can serve as contact allergens. Among those most often implicated are industrial chemicals, topical ointments, soaps, dinitrochlorobenzene (DNCB), nickel, mercury, topical antibiotics, cosmetics, and the catecholes of poison ivy, poison oak, and poison sumac.

Many of the contact allergens are of a size (less than 10,000 molecular weight) and structure that do not allow them to serve as a complete antigen. It is most probable that the compound attaches to proteins of the skin and functions as a hapten to stimulate the proliferation of a T cell population sensitized to the compound. After sensitization, subsequent contact with the contact allergen leads to the formation of an erythematous, vesiculated (blistered) lesion. The inflamed area itches, burns, or stings. Scratching the lesion may further spread the allergen or infect the site. There is often a serous exudate. (For care of the person with contact dermatitis, see Chapter 67.)

### Tissue Transplantation Rejection

The rejection of foreign cells and tissues by the body is a beneficial function of the immune system primarily mediated by a type IV hypersensitivity. If it were not for this mechanism, the human body would be a haven for the inappropriate establishment of growth of any foreign cell that penetrated the external defense mechanisms; however, this process is regarded as a disservice when it operates to prevent the positive aspects of the exchange of tissues between hosts.

The transfer of healthy tissues and organs from one individual to replace damaged or diseased tissues of another has been surgically possible for many years. The early attempts at tissue graft failed because of the rejection process. With the growing knowledge of the immune response, the mechanisms of this rejection process became more apparent, and it is now possible to make judgments and predictions concerning the likelihood of success of such an endeavor. It is possible to control the course of the graft transfer process to favor the acceptance of the transplanted tissues (see Chapter 72).

## AUTOIMMUNE DISEASES

Autoimmunity, the formation of antibodies against self-tissues, is a natural phenomenon. Certain responses such as autorecognition and autoimmunity are necessary for removal of dead cells, cell components, aging, and response to viral and microbial infections.[10] It is when autoimmunity causes injury to host cells that it is described as pathologic. The symptoms of such a self-attack are referred to as *autoimmune disease* or *autohypersensitivity.* For the most part, these self-reactions are not immunologically initiated; the etiologic (causative) agent lies outside the immune system, but the immune response serves as the pathogenic mechanism.

The meaning of the demonstration of autoantibodies and autosensitive T cell clones is not always clear. These self-reactive immunoglobulins are often associated with certain pathologic states in the body but many times can also be isolated from the serum of "normal" individuals as well, especially in older persons. Autoantibodies have been demonstrated in high titers with autoimmune disorders. It should be remembered that low or absent titers of autoantibodies, however, cannot rule out autoimmune disease.

Autoimmunity is influenced by genetic, hormonal, viral, and environmental factors. Autoimmune disorders run in families but are not passed on by simple mendelian inheritance. HLA and non-HLA antigens have a well-documented association with certain autoimmune diseases. Many individuals with these same gene markings, however, do not have the disease so there is not a direct relationship of the disease with genetic predisposition.

The role of sex hormones is not clearly understood. Autoimmune diseases are far more common in females than in males. Experiments on mice found female mice treated with androgens had a later onset and a less severe case of SLE, whereas male mice treated with estrogen had earlier appearance and more severe form of SLE. Interactions of the host with certain environmental agents such as bacteria, viruses, drugs, and toxins have been shown to initiate autoimmune disease.

Some of the theoretical mechanisms by which the immunologic tolerance to self-antigens might be broken include the following:

1. *Release of sequestered antigens.* If an antigen does not come into contact with the immune system during fetal development when the tolerance to self normally develops (either because of anatomic site or later development), it is not registered as a self-antigen, and clones of immunoresponsive cells to that antigen remain reactive. As a result of trauma or infection, these antigens may be exposed to the immune system. If this occurs, they will elicit an immune response.

### BOX 70-3 Classification of Autoimmune Disorders

**ORGAN SPECIFIC**

**Blood**
Autoimmune hemolytic anemia
Idiopathic thrombocytopenic purpura

**Heart**
Rheumatic fever

**Central Nervous System**
Multiple sclerosis
Guillain-Barré syndrome

**Muscles**
Myasthenia gravis

**Endocrine System**
Addison's disease
Autoimmune thyroiditis (Hashimoto's disease)
Graves' disease
Hypothyroidism

**Eye**
Uveitis

**Gastrointestinal System**
Pernicious anemia
Ulcerative colitis

**Kidneys**
Glomerulonephritis
Goodpasture's syndrome

**Skin**
Pemphigus vulgaris

**NON-ORGAN-SPECIFIC**
Systemic lupus erythematosus
Rheumatoid arthritis
Progressive systemic sclerosis

2. *Activation of suppressed clones.* If one of the functions of the suppressor T cell is to suppress the activation of certain clones of potentially self-reactive T cells or B cells, it is possible through some loss of suppressor function that these "forbidden" clones are allowed to proliferate.
3. *Synthesis of cross-reactive antibodies.* Antibodies synthesized in response to certain foreign antigens may have cross-reactivity with some similar antigenic components within human tissues. Contact with antigens called heterophile antigens may trigger the production of autoantibodies. This seems to be a mechanism of rheumatic heart disease, in which the antibodies produced against certain streptococcal antigens during scarlet fever, streptococcal sore throat, or other streptococcal infections cross-react with myocardial tissue, producing a myocardial inflammation.
4. *Alteration of self-antigens.* Normal body proteins may be altered by chemicals, infectious organisms, or therapeutic drugs to present new antigenically active groups to the immune system. The autoimmune hemolytic anemia associated with α-methyldopa (Aldomet) treatment of hypertension probably results from the alteration of the Rh antigens of the RBC rendering it antigenic. Certain antibiotics such as the penicillins and cephalosporins can have the same effect.

Autoimmune disorders are grouped into categories according to the part of the body involved. Those autoimmune diseases that are organ specific are those in which chronic inflammatory changes occur in a specific organ. Non-organ-specific autoimmune disorders are characterized by chronic inflammatory changes in many different organs and tissues throughout the body. Box 70-3 indicates some of the disorders listed as autoimmune at the present time. As more knowledge is available about the etiologies of these disorders (e.g., a causative microorganism might be identified), they may be removed from the list. (The care of persons experiencing these disorders is discussed elsewhere in the text.)

## QUESTIONS TO CONSIDER

- Contrast the four mechanisms underlying autoimmune diseases and relate to at least one specific disease.
- What teaching should be done before discharging a patient from the acute care facility after treatment for a hypersensitivity reaction?
- Compare and contrast types I, II, III, and IV immunodeficiency.

## CRITICAL THINKING ACTIVITIES

- Consider the last 10 patients for whom you have provided care. To which of these patients do the concepts of immunodeficiency apply to one degree or another? (Do not forget the role of nutrition in immunodeficiency.) What measures were (or should have been) taken to prevent infection?
- Examine the chart of a patient who has received a blood transfusion. What safeguards were taken to prevent transfusion reactions? If a reaction was noted, what actions were taken?
- Mrs. K. was referred to an allergy clinic and diagnosed as allergic to pollen and grasses. She lives in a low-income housing project that faces a large park. Her husband was laid off 2 months ago. Mrs. K. cleans houses 3 days a week. What additional data would you want to collect from Mrs. K., and what would you include in your teaching plan?
- You are a nurse who works in the radiology department. What is one of the most common immune problems that occur in this area? What are the signs and symptoms of this problem? What medications and equipment would you keep on hand to treat this problem?

## CHAPTER SUMMARY

### IMMUNODEFICIENCIES

- Primary immunodeficiencies result from interference with development of immune cells; secondary immunodeficiencies are acquired disorders of depressed immunity. Major factors in the development of secondary immunodeficiencies include age, nutrition, specific disorders such as uremia and diabetes mellitus, exposure to chemicals, and drugs.
- Immunosuppression may be induced by antigen or antibody administration, immunologic methods (ALG, MoAbs), irradiation, or immunosuppressive drugs.
- Screening tests for immune deficiencies can include blood studies such as ESR, absolute lymphocyte or neutrophil counts, $CH_{50}$, antibody titers, or skin tests.
- Treatment of primary immunodeficiencies consist of identification of those at risk for the disorder, prevention of or effective treatment of infection, and replacement of missing humoral or cellular immunologic factors (bone marrow or thymus gland transplants, immune serum globulin).
- The primary approach of nursing management of the immunodeficient person is prevention of infection through good medical asepsis, removal of sources where bacteria proliferate, protecting the patient from other persons with infections, maintaining optimal patient nutrition and hydration, and teaching the patient how to prevent infection.

## GAMMOPATHIES

- Gammopathies are excessive production of immunoglobulins, the most common of which is multiple myeloma (an excess of plasma cells).
- Multiple myeloma is characterized by proliferation of plasma cells causing lytic bone disease, bone marrow infiltration, and proliferation of monoclonal proteins.
- Medical treatment of multiple myeloma is aimed at decreasing tumor bulk, preventing kidney failure, and preventing further bone demineralization.
- Nursing care of the patient with multiple myeloma includes preventing pathologic fractures, fluid volume overload, and infection.

## HYPERSENSITIVITIES

- Hypersensitivity reactions are exaggerated or inappropriate responses to specific antigens (allergens) and depend on the responsiveness of the host to the allergen, the amount, nature, route of entrance, and timing of exposure of the allergen; site of the allergen-immune mediator reaction, and the host's threshold of reactivity.
- Type I hypersensitivities are associated with reactions that are mediated by IgE immunoglobulins attached to mast cells and basophils. When the allergen binds to the IgE, histamine, kinins, chemotactic factors, and active products of arachidonic metabolism are released, producing a systemic reaction (anaphylaxis) or a local allergic reaction. There must be a primary contact with the allergen that sensitizes the individual. Repeated exposure to the allergen in a sensitized individual can lead to chronic diseases.
- Anaphylaxis is the most severe form of type I hypersensitivity; severe reactions can be prevented by identification of high-risk persons, patient education on avoiding the allergen and measures to take if sensitization occurs, desensitization, and precautionary actions when giving animal sera.
- Therapy for anaphylaxis consists of epinephrine to constrict blood vessels and dilate the bronchioles, counteracting the effect of histamine. Antihistamines are given to shorten the duration of anaphylaxis; hydrocortisone decreases the inflammatory effects. An open airway must be maintained.
- Nursing care of a patient in anaphylaxis includes maintaining an open airway and adequate cardiac output.
- Atopic illnesses are typically initiated by two categories of allergens—seasonal (trees, grasses, weeds) and perennial (house dust, mites, molds, animal dander). Symptoms are usually not life-threatening but are uncomfortable.
- Treatment of atopic illnesses include use of antihistamines, decongestants, steroids, and cromolyn sodium to treat symptoms; avoidance of exposure to triggering allergens; and immunotherapy (hyposensitization).
- Nursing care of atopic individuals includes teaching them about environmental control, hyposensitization, side effects of medications, and how to recognize and treat anaphylaxis.
- Type II hypersensitivities are cytotoxic reactions from the direct binding of IgG or IgM immunoglobulins to the surface of foreign cells to trigger cell lysis; an example is blood transfusion reactions.
- The major antigens of RBCs are AB antigens, Rh antigens, and HLA antigens. People with type AB blood may receive blood from other types because they possess both A and B antigens, but they cannot give blood to persons with other types, who possess only A or B antigens or neither antigen (type O). People with type O blood, therefore, can give blood to but cannot receive it from people with other types.
- Rh positive reactions indicate presence of antigen Rh-D; Rh negative indicates absence of antigen Rh-D.
- Immunologic reactions to blood transfusions include acute hemolytic (most serious), febrile nonhemolytic, mild allergic, anaphylactic, delayed hemolytic, graft-versus-host diseases, and noncardiac pulmonary edema. Nonimmunologic complications of blood transfusions include circulatory overload, sepsis, and transmission of diseases.
- The acute hemolytic reaction causes 70% of transfusion related deaths. Mistakes in specimen collection and labeling or inadequate identification of the patient before infusion are errors that lead to these reactions. If a hemolytic reaction occurs, as indicated by chills, fever, and backache shortly after initiation of the transfusion, the transfusion is stopped immediately, the patient is supported, and the physician notified.
- Blood transfusion reactions can be prevented by donor prescreening, accurate laboratory testing, careful administration of blood, use of autologous blood, and use of specialized blood products and equipment.
- Type III hypersensitivities are characterized by immune complexes formed by the union of IgM or IgG with soluble antigens; the small complexes get trapped in body tissues, causing an inflammatory response. An example is serum sickness, which occurs after administration of foreign serum used to treat transplant rejection.
- Type IV hypersensitivities are cell mediated (T cell reactions). T cells destroy foreign antigens directly (as in transplant rejections) or by release of lymphokines to activate phagocytic cells.

## AUTOIMMUNE DISEASES

- Autoimmune diseases are the result of an immune response to one's own antigens, usually because of an agent from outside the immune system. Mechanisms of the immune intolerance may include release of sequestered antigens, activation of suppressed clones, synthesis of cross-reactive antibodies, or alteration of self-antigens.

## REFERENCES


1. Anderson KC, Hayden GB: Specialized cell component therapy, *Semin Oncol Nurs* 6(2):140-149, 1990.
2. Barlogie B, Alexanian R, Jagannath S: Plasma cell dyscrasias, *JAMA* 268(20):2946-2951, 1992.
3. Buckley RH: *Immunologic disorders,* St. Louis, 1993, Mosby.
4. Buckley RH, Schiff RI: The use of intravenous immune globulin in immunodeficiency diseases, *N Engl J Med* 324(2):110-117, 1991.
5. Freedman S et al: Nursing considerations in the administration of blood component therapy, *Semin Oncol Nurs* 6(2):155-162, 1990.
6. Gibbs L: Assessment and management of the allergic patient, *ORL Head Neck Nurs* 10(3):10-16, 1992.
7. Hadden JW, Smith DL: Immunopharmacology, immunomodulation, and immunotherapy, *JAMA* 268(20):2964-2969, 1992.
8. Lockey RF: Future trends in allergy and immunology, *JAMA* 268(20):2991-2992, 1992.
9. Mudge-Grout CL: *Immunologic disorders,* St Louis, 1993, Mosby.
10. Nakamura MC, Nakamura RM: Contemporary concepts of autoimmunity and autoimmune diseases, *J Clin Lab Anal* 6(5):275-289, 1992.
11. Norman PS: Immunotherapy of IgE-mediated disease, *Hosp Pract* 25(4):81-92, 1990.
12. Pavel J: Red cell transfusions for anemia, *Semin Oncol Nurs* 6(2):117-122, 1990.
13. Stites DP, Terr AI: *Basic and clinical immunology,* ed 7, Norwalk, 1991, Appleton & Lange.
14. Transfusion nursing: trends and practices for the '90s, *Am J Nurs* 91(6):42-56, 1991.
15. Wener M: Basic clinical immunology, *Hosp Med* 28(1):69-82, 1992.

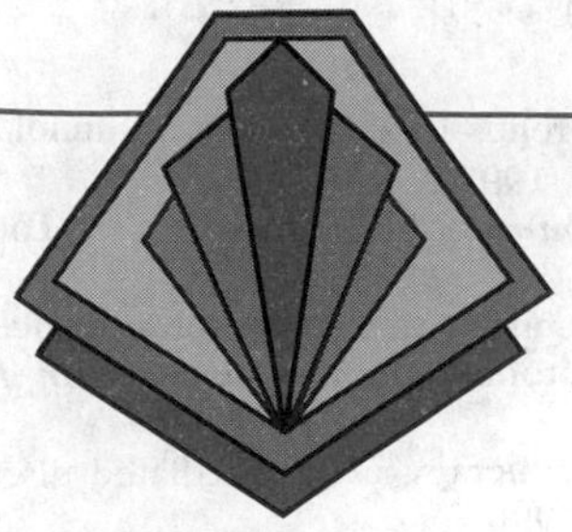

CHAPTER 71

# Management of Persons With HIV Infection and AIDS

*Cynthia F. Brogdon*
*Denise M. Kresevic*

## CHAPTER OBJECTIVES

***After studying this chapter, the learner should be able to do the following:***

1 Describe the epidemiology of HIV infection, and identify the causative virus, groups at risk, methods of transmission, and strategies for prevention.
2 Describe the continuum of HIV infection.
3 Identify the infection control guidelines recommended by the CDC to minimize transmission of HIV infection.
4 Discuss nursing problems and interventions for patients with HIV infection.
5 Describe the opportunistic infections and tumors that occur in patients with HIV infection and the medical and nursing management.
6 Discuss the role of the nurse in addressing psychosocial, legal, and ethical issues related to the HIV epidemic.

## KEY TERMS

acquired immunodeficiency syndrome (AIDS)
AIDS-related complex (ARC)
candidiasis
cryptococcosis
cryptosporidiosis
cytomegalovirus (CMV)
histoplasmosis
HIV encephalopathy (dementia)
human immunodeficiency virus (HIV)
Kaposi's sarcoma (KS)
*Mycobacterium avium* complex (MAC)
opportunistic infection
*Pneumocystis carinii* pneumonia (PCP)
retrovirus
toxoplasmosis
zidovudine (AZT)

Since the time of Florence Nightingale, nurses have provided care for individuals and families with communicable disease. One of the most dreaded communicable diseases of the twentieth century is infection with the human immunodeficiency virus (HIV). Individuals infected with this virus eventually develop acquired immunodeficiency syndrome (AIDS), which severely compromises the body's ability to fight various infections and some forms of cancer. The incidence of HIV infection and AIDS continues to increase steadily in the United States and worldwide. Therefore it is crucial that nurses have an understanding of critical concepts related to this problem.

## ETIOLOGY

On June 5, 1981, the first cases of an illness later defined as **acquired immune deficiency syndrome (AIDS)** were reported by California health care providers to the Centers for Disease Control (CDC, now the Centers for Disease Control and Prevention). This first cluster of five Los Angeles men had unusual opportunistic infections and were thought to represent a geographically localized epidemic of an unknown infectious disease. Just 4 years later in 1985, 14,049 cases of AIDS were reported in the United States. Later that same year, the **human immunodeficiency virus (HIV)** was identified as the causative agent of AIDS: 7000 Americans had already died of the disease.[2]

We are now in the second decade of this pandemic, which has claimed the lives of 1.5 million people across the globe. Although there has been scientific and clinical progress as well as development of new treatments and comprehensive models of care, HIV disease remains an incurable illness, spreading rapidly throughout the United States and worldwide.

Nurses have a pivotal role in treatment and prevention of this disease. Patient education about risk behaviors and risk reduction techniques will help prevent new infections and will undoubtedly save lives. Appropriate, compassionate nursing care for those already infected may extend survival and will most certainly improve the quality of life for those afflicted with HIV disease.

## CHARACTERISTICS OF THE ORGANISM AND THE INFECTION

Since the first description of AIDS in 1981, an extraordinary scientific adventure has ensued. In just over a decade, we have made remarkable advancements in our understanding of the disease and its causative agent, HIV. The origin of HIV is still largely unknown, although evidence appears to support the hypothesis of an African origin. The first reports of an AIDS-like illness date back to the early 1960s in central Africa. HIV in humans probably has an animal origin, most likely nonhuman primates.

The causative agent of AIDS is infection with HIV. HIV is a human **retrovirus** and belongs to the lentivirus subfamily. Currently, five human retroviruses have been identified: HTLV-1, HTLV-2, HTLV-5, HIV-$1_1$ and HIV-2. HTLV-2 has not been conclusively associated with human disease. HTLV-1 and HTLV-5 have been associated with human T-cell leukemia and lymphoma, conditions characterized by proliferation of CD4+ (T4) helper cells. HIV-1 and HIV-2 both cause depletion of T4 helper cells, resulting in loss of cellular immunity, characterized by AIDS. HIV-1 is the predominant cause of AIDS in the United States, accounting for greater than 95% of AIDS cases. HIV-2 seems to be limited in geographic distribution and is most prevalent in West Africa.[11]

The life cycle of HIV is similar to that of the other retroviruses. Mature virions interact with specific host receptors and then use the host cell for viral replication. HIV interacts with the CD4 glycoprotein, which occurs on the membrane of specific cells, primarily the CD4+ (T4) helper lymphocytes. The CD4 protein may also be found on the surface of several other cells as well, including some monocytes/macrophages, glial cells, and gastrointestinal (GI) cells. Presence of the CD4 glycoprotein allows the virus to fuse to the host cell. The viral core is subsequently injected into the cell cytoplasm, where the viral ribonucleic acid (RNA) genome is translated into deoxyribonucleic acid (DNA) by a retroviral enzyme called *reverse transcriptase.* Infection and subsequent viral replication eventually deplete the host's T4 helper cells, resulting in a dramatic loss of the protective immune response against invading microorganisms.

The routes for transmission of HIV are well documented: (1) intimate sexual contact; (2) parenteral exposure to blood, blood-containing body fluids, and blood products; and (3) from mother to child during the perinatal period. Although HIV has been identified in a variety of body fluids, those that have been consistently shown to be infectious are blood, semen, and vaginal secretions. Transmission has also been associated with breast milk, although this appears to occur relatively infrequently. HIV is transmitted directly from person to person by sexual contact; direct inoculation with contaminated blood products, needles, or syringes; or from an infected mother to her fetus/newborn. HIV is not transmitted by casual contact, including sneezing, coughing, or spitting; handshakes; or contact with potential secretions on toilet seats, bathtubs, showers, swimming pools, utensils, dishes, or linens used by an infected person. HIV disease is a blood-borne, sexually transmitted disease (STD). Although certain sexual practices may be associated with higher risks for infection than others, any practice that exposes one to infected blood, semen, or vaginal secretions has the potential for viral transmission.

## EPIDEMIOLOGY

HIV infection has occurred in approximately 1.5 million Americans and progressed to AIDS in more than 300,000 persons. More than 150,000 Americans have died from this pandemic; the numbers increase daily. Throughout the world, more than 18 million people are infected with HIV, and nearly 2 million have progressed to an AIDS diagnosis. It is estimated that more than 1 million people have died of AIDS worldwide. Although changes in risk behaviors have slowed the spread of HIV infection in some areas of the United States, HIV transmission has accelerated in others. More than 40,000 new infections are expected this year in the United States alone. Early estimates of worldwide infection rates suggested approximately 40 million infections by the year 2000. That estimate has been revised, and some sources now suggest there will be more than 110 million persons infected with HIV by the end of this decade.[13]

Throughout the pandemic, the numbers of those infected have steadily increased each year. Early in the U.S. epidemic, more than 80% of those infected were homosexual men. Currently, less than 50% of infections occur in this group. Those persons now at greatest risk for acquiring HIV infection in the United States include heterosexual women and their children and intravenous (IV) drug users. African-Americans and Hispanic-Americans are at greater risk than white Americans.[3]

Worldwide, HIV continues to ravage heterosexual

men, women, and their children. Of the more than 18 million persons infected worldwide, more than 11 million are in Africa, approximately 3.5 million in Asia, and 1.5 million in Latin America and the Caribbean. The mortality rate in the United States currently approaches 80% within 3 years of an AIDS diagnosis and may be even higher in undeveloped countries where treatment is virtually nonexistent.[13]

## PATHOPHYSIOLOGY

The natural history of HIV infection is associated with an unpredictable course of disease progression. Most patients undergo a prolonged period of clinically silent infection, often lasting more than 10 years.[11,12] Although the virus is consistently detectable throughout this time, patients typically have only subtle immunologic alterations. Once the patient becomes symptomatic, however, decreases in the number of T4 helper cells can be detected and viral replication increases.

Several potential cofactors may be associated with HIV disease progression. These cofactors, which may be viral, host, or environmental, are thought to influence directly the replication of HIV or the severity of its pathogenic effects. Viral cofactors that may influence the progression of the disease include herpes simplex, cytomegalovirus (CMV), and Epstein-Barr virus (EBV). Host cofactors may include a variety of cytokines and intracellular mediators. Environmental cofactors may include repeated exposure to HIV, which may induce hyperactivation of the immune system, resulting in an expansion of the pool of HIV-replicating cells.

As viral replication increases, depleting the body of T4 lymphocytes, the body's defense mechanisms are progressively weakened. Infections that were once disarmed by the healthy immune system are eventually able to cause serious and potentially life-threatening disease. These **opportunistic infections** include a variety of organisms, such as viruses (herpes simplex, EBV, CMV), protozoans *(Pneumocystis carinii, Toxoplasma),* mycobacteria (tuberculosis and avium complex), and fungi *(Histoplasma, Cryptococcus).* In addition to the various opportunistic infections, the profound immune dysfunction also allows for the development of several neoplasms, including non-Hodgkin's lymphoma, Kaposi's sarcoma (KS), and cervical carcinoma.

Infection with HIV, the resultant immunodeficiency, the opportunistic infections, and the related cancers result in dysfunction of almost every body system. The pulmonary, GI, neurologic, and hematologic systems; the skin; and the eyes are the most frequently affected. However, cardiac, renal, rheumatologic, and endocrine dysfunction can also occur. As survival with HIV improves, more of these later changes may be seen.

Opportunistic pulmonary infections are often the first manifestations of HIV infections. Pulmonary infection from a variety of organisms is a constant threat to the patient with HIV and AIDS. Pulmonary infections can lead to severe hypoxemia very rapidly. Decreased respiratory function may also result from pulmonary infiltration by a lymphoma.

GI dysfunction also results from a variety of organisms responsible for opportunistic infections. The patient may have difficulty eating and swallowing or may have dyspepsia, diarrhea, or weight loss resulting from the effects of the opportunistic infections on the GI tract. Loss of lean muscle mass is common. Mass lesions from lymphomas and KS are common. The hepatobiliary system also is frequently affected by HIV infections in AIDS. Hepatitis from drug toxicity, coinfection with a hepatitis virus, or granulomatous hepatitis related to opportunistic infections can occur. Cholangitis and cholestasis also may be the result of opportunistic infections. Pancreatic lesions from opportunistic infections and drugs may be present.

The nervous system is frequently affected by HIV infection. The HIV can cross the blood-brain and blood–cerebrospinal fluid (CSF) barriers and infect microglia and possibly other cells, resulting in encephalopathy. This process results in loss of cognitive and motor function. Many of the opportunistic infections can cause central nervous system (CNS) infections. Peripheral neuropathy with loss of motor function often occurs.

The initial infection with HIV may cause macular roseola eruptions that disappear. Later, seborrheic dermatitis, psoriasis, and KS lesions along with cutaneous infections result in skin changes.

The ophthalmologic manifestations result from infection with opportunistic organisms. CMV retinitis is the most common cause of visual impairment in persons with HIV. Retinal exudates associated with hemorrhage are seen. The visual loss is painless; blurring of vision and decreased acuity occur. If untreated, the lesions will progress. Therapy needs to be given indefinitely.

Hematologic problems include thrombocytopenia, anemia, and neutropenia. The causes of these problems are not known, but they may result from decreased production because of the disease or the drugs or increased destruction as a side effect of drug therapy.

The cardiovascular system may be disrupted. Pericarditis or myocarditis from the opportunistic infections is common. Right ventricular failure may result from the severe pulmonary hypertension associated with multiple episodes of *P. carinii* pneumonia.

Fluid and electrolyte imbalance and acid-base imbalance from a variety of causes, including renal, GI, endocrine, or drugs, can occur. Prerenal or acute renal failure caused by hypovolemia, interstitial nephritis caused by invasion of renal tissue by tumors or infective organisms, and glomerulosclerosis from HIV-associated nephropathy are common causes of renal dysfunction in HIV.

All endocrine glands can be infiltrated by HIV. Endocrine abnormalities, however, are not as common as other system dysfunction. The adrenal gland is most frequently affected. Adrenal insufficiency may result from invasion by infective organisms, invasion by a tumor, or drug therapy.

Rheumatologic manifestations of HIV are quite common and vary from mild to severe. Arthralgia is seen with acute infection and may also result from drug therapy. Myalgia, weakness, and wasting may also occur. The cause of these rheumatologic manifestations is unknown.

Because of the way in which HIV progresses over time, the numerous types of opportunistic infections, the related cancers, and the various types of system involvement that can be present, signs, symptoms, and diagnostic tests vary. In early HIV infection the most common finding is a positive AIDS test without other signs and symptoms. The T4 count can vary but is usually 500 cells/μL or greater. As the disease progresses, the next most common complaint is fatigue. The fatigue also varies across patients and within the same patient. Diarrhea, weight loss, and loss of lean body mass are also early symptoms. As the immunodeficiency worsens, opportunistic infections with their various manifestations and cancers with their signs and symptoms develop. Because of the effects of these infections and cancers on the body, fatigue, GI complaints, weight loss, and loss of lean body mass increase. Activity tolerance worsens as the disease progresses and is caused by loss of lean body mass, deconditioning, and anemia. Other manifestations, such as visual changes, neurologic changes, and skin lesions, vary from person to person. No specific laboratory changes are associated with $HIV_1$ except for the HIV antibody test and the changes in T lymphocytes. However, many changes may be found because of infections, treatment, and involvement of other body systems.

## PREVENTION

### *Healthy People 2000*

Because HIV is a multifaceted national and international problem that, at least now, even with treatment results

**BOX 71-1** ***Healthy People 2000*** **Objectives**

1. Confine annual incidence of diagnosed AIDS cases to no more than 98,000 cases (baseline: an estimated 44,000 to 50,000 diagnosed cases in 1989). Special populations targeted are homosexual and bisexual men, blacks, and Hispanics.
2. Confine the prevalence of HIV infections to no more than 800 persons per 100,000 population (baseline: an estimated 400 per 100,000 in 1989). Special populations targeted are homosexual men, IV drug abusers, and women giving birth to live-born infants.
3. Reduce the proportion of adolescents who have engaged in sexual intercourse to no more than 15% by age 15 and no more than 40% by age 17 (baseline: 27% of girls and 33% of boys by age 15; 50% of boys by age 17, as reported in 1988).
4. Increase to at least 50% the proportion of sexually active, unmarried people who used a condom at last sexual intercourse (baseline: 19% of sexually active, unmarried women ages 15 to 44 reported that their partners used a condom at last sexual intercourse in 1988). Special targeted populations are partners of sexually active young women, sexually active young men, and IV drug abusers.
5. Increase to at least 50% the estimated proportion of all IV drug abusers who are in drug abuse treatment programs (baseline: an estimated 11% of opiate abusers were in treatment in 1989).
6. Increase to at least 50% the estimated proportion of IV drug abusers not in treatment who use uncontaminated drug paraphernalia ("works") (baseline: 25% to 35% of opiate abusers in 1989).
7. Reduce to no more than 1 per 250,000 units of blood and blood components the risk of transfusion-transmitted HIV infection (baseline: 1 per 40,000 to 150,000 units in 1989).
8. Increase to at least 80% the proportion of HIV-infected people who have been tested for HIV infection (baseline: an estimated 15% of approximately 1 million HIV-infected people had been tested at publicly funded clinics in 1989).
9. Increase to at least 75% the proportion of primary care and mental health care providers who provide age-appropriate counseling on the prevention of HIV and other STDs (baseline: 10% of physicians reported that they regularly assessed the sexual behaviors of their patients in 1987). Special targeted populations are providers practicing in high-incidence areas.
10. Increase to at least 95% the proportion of schools that have age-appropriate HIV education curricula for students in fourth through twelfth grades, preferably as part of quality school health education (baseline: 66% of school districts required HIV education but only 5% required HIV education in each year for seventh to twelfth grades in 1989).
11. Provide HIV education for students and staff in at least 90% of colleges and universities.
12. Increase to at least 90% the proportion of cities with populations greater than 100,000 that have outreach programs to contact drug abusers to deliver HIV risk reduction messages.
13. Increase to at least 50% the proportion of appropriate clinics, including STD clinics, tuberculosis clinics, drug treatment centers, and primary care clinics that screen, diagnose, treat, counsel, and provide (or refer for) partner notification services for HIV infection and bacterial STDs (baseline: 40% of family-planning clinics for bacterial STDs in 1989).
14. Extend to all facilities where workers are at risk for occupational transmission of HIV regulations to protect workers from exposure to blood-borne infections, including HIV infection.

From US Department of Health and Human Services, Public Health Service: ***Healthy people 2000: national health promotion and disease prevention objectives,*** Washington, DC, 1990, US Government Printing Office.

in death, the first priority of care is to halt the spread of the infection. To achieve this goal, health status objectives, risk reduction objectives, and service and protection objectives have been established (Box 71-1).[20]

## PRIMARY PREVENTION

HIV infection is currently a life-threatening infectious disease with no known cure. With the continuing rapid rise in HIV infections worldwide, prevention of new infections represents the key to abolishing this devastating illness. Primary prevention efforts focus on preventing new infections.

As noted earlier, HIV disease is a blood-borne STD. As such, primary prevention efforts must be focused on techniques to avoid exposure to contaminated blood and body fluids. With less than 3% of AIDS cases attributed to exposure to contaminated blood products, the greatest exposure risk is via sexual contact. AIDS prevention efforts therefore must be focused on ways to reduce sexual transmission.

Historically, it has been difficult to talk about sexuality in American culture. The topic is laden with moral judgments and has seldom been addressed in our health care system. Nurses are in an excellent position to discuss sexuality with patients. Typically, the nurse has an intimate rapport with the patient, talking about sensitive subjects and related health concerns. The patient usually feels most at ease with the nurse, and the nurse is most accessible to patients. The nurse has a major role in the education of individuals and groups in the prevention of HIV disease.

Prevention efforts must include accurate, reliable, and clear information about risk factors for HIV disease and ways to decrease these risks. Prevention education programs must include the topics of safer sexual techniques and the use of clean drug paraphernalia as well as public health measures such as blood product screening and perinatal counseling. Prevention efforts must be focused on behaviors that put patients at risk for infection.

### Safe Sex Counseling

Any exchange of blood, semen, or vaginal secretions can potentially put an individual at risk for HIV disease. Common sexual practices that are therefore risky behaviors include vaginal or anal penetration without a condom and possibly oral sexual practices. Using barrier products such as latex condoms while engaging in these behaviors greatly reduces the likelihood of exposure to potentially infectious blood, semen, or vaginal secretions.

Prevention education must also include risk reduction techniques such as minimizing the number of sexual partners and engaging in a mutually monogamous sexual relationship. In addition, sexual practices that do not put the individual at risk for potentially infectious fluids should be discussed. Mutual masturbation, massage, and body rubbing are safe sexual practices with no exchange of body fluids.

### Intravenous Risk Reduction

The use of contaminated needles for subcutaneous (SC), intramuscular (IM), or IV injection represents a serious risk for HIV infection. Prevention education must include ways to clean needles and other paraphernalia used to inject drugs. Educational efforts may include information about substance abuse counseling and programs, but use of a bleach solution to disinfect needles and paraphernalia must also be discussed.

### Perinatal Transmission

Women who are HIV infected may pass the virus on to their newborns via three potential routes: during gestation, during delivery, and via breast-feeding. Although the exact mechanism of perinatal transmission is unknown, the current estimate of risk to the newborn from an infected mother is approximately 30% in the United States.[18] Recently, a large study at the National Institutes of Health (NIH) revealed maternal use of zidovudine (AZT) during pregnancy may reduce the risk of fetal transmission to 15%.[4,16]

### Public Health Measures

Prevention programs must also educate the public about the measures that are currently in place to screen and protect the blood supply from contamination. Currently, each unit of donated blood is tested for HIV infection as well as several other blood-borne infections, such as hepatitis B. HIV screening of blood products has been conducted since 1985 in the United States; only recipients of transfusions before that time are at significant risk for infection via the blood supply. It is possible, however, for a contaminated unit of blood to test negative for HIV if the donor has not yet formed antibodies to the virus at the time of donation. Nevertheless, the risk of exposure to HIV via the U.S. blood supply is estimated to be 1 in 400,000 units of blood.[3]

### Health Care Workers

In addition to health education strategies, infection control is one of the most important areas of concern for nurses caring for patients with HIV infection. Infection control procedures based on knowledge of disease transmission are essential.

The components necessary for transmission of blood-borne viruses such as HIV are (1) the presence of the virus in sufficient quantity to infect the host and (2) a portal of entry into the bloodstream, allowing the virus to infect host cells. HIV has been cultured from various body fluids, including blood, semen, vaginal secretions, CSF, saliva, tears, and breast milk. The fluids that contain enough viral particles to produce transmission of infection, however, are limited. Blood, semen, and vaginal secretions are the fluids most likely to produce infection. Although other body fluids such as saliva, tears, and breast milk may contain the virus, epidemiologic studies indicate that transmission via these sources is inefficient and unlikely to produce infection.

HIV is transmitted by (1) sexual contact with anyone who has the virus, (2) blood contact, and (3) perinatal transmission. The portals of entry for HIV include direct, intimate contact with mucous membrane surfaces or direct contact with a broken skin surface. No evidence indicates the possibility of casual transmission of HIV. Coughing, sneezing, touching door knobs, sharing eating utensils, swimming in public pools, and being bitten by mosquitoes are not sources of HIV infection. Transmission of HIV requires exposure to an infected fluid that comes into direct contact with mucous membranes or broken skin surfaces.

Infection control procedures therefore are based on protecting health care workers from exposure to infected body fluids, including blood, that could come into contact with a portal of entry and subsequently produce an infection. Handwashing remains the single most important principle of infection control for all diseases, including HIV disease. Washing organisms off the skin or other surfaces is an effective means of control and is the basis of good sanitation and personal hygiene.

#### Gloves and protective garments

The use of gloves and other protective garments, such as gowns, masks, and goggles, is recommended when direct contact with blood and/or other body fluids is expected. In addition, if splashing of body fluids is expected, full protective garb also should be worn. Gloves are the most often used piece of protective garb and should be used whenever it is expected that the caregiver will come into hand contact with a patient's body fluids. Examples of procedures that require the use of gloves are dressing changes, drawing blood specimens, doing fingersticks to monitor blood glucose, and starting IV lines. Activities such as feeding or ambulating patients are very unlikely to put the caregiver at risk for contact with body fluids and therefore do not require the use of gloves. Most often, the use of full protective covering is not warranted. During routine care of patients, it is unlikely that any caregiver will be exposed to body fluids. Full protective garments are usually recommended in more invasive procedures, such as bronchoscopy, surgical procedures, and delivery room procedures.

Protective garb should be worn to protect the caregiver from coming into contact with body fluids from *any* patient. Using protective gear only in situations when the patient is known to be HIV infected is extremely dangerous. Many patients may not know their HIV status; relying on self-reporting of HIV status or relying even on known medical information is simply inadequate protection for health care workers. Protective garb should be worn by all persons coming into contact with *any* patient's body fluids.

#### Needle precautions

Parenteral exposure to infected blood has been the most common means of transmitting both hepatitis B and HIV in the health care setting. Minimizing the risk of needle exposure requires the use of convenient puncture-proof needle disposal systems. In addition, needles should *never* be recapped or broken.

## SECONDARY PREVENTION

Identification of persons already infected with HIV and initiating early treatment for the disease in these persons are the targets of secondary prevention efforts. Because HIV infection may be asymptomatic for several years, many people will not know they are infected until the immune system has been compromised by the virus for several years. Early identification of infected persons allows individuals to learn about the illness and modify health habits in an effort to protect their immune function. Early initiation of treatment may extend survival and has been shown to delay onset of significant opportunistic infections. In addition, the knowledge of a life-threatening infectious disease will prompt most individuals to alter their personal behaviors to protect others from becoming infected.[6,7]

### HIV Testing

HIV antibody testing has an essential role in prevention and treatment of this disease process. The most common form of screening for HIV disease is the use of the antibody test with the enzyme-linked immunosorbent assay (ELISA) technique and the Western blot technique. The ELISA test uses spectrophotometry to detect serum antibody reactions to specific HIV viral proteins. The ELISA is highly specific with a sensitivity of 93.4% to 99.6%. A positive ELISA must be confirmed by the Western blot technique.

Both the ELISA and the Western blot techniques depend on antibody formation. Approximately 90% of the population will form antibodies in response to HIV exposure within 6 weeks to 3 months after exposure, although this period may be as long as 6 months. A negative antibody test may occur in the "window phase" between the dates of actual exposure leading to infection and development of detectable serum antibodies.

Because newborns maintain maternal antibodies for as long as 18 months, antibody testing is unreliable until the infant is 18 months of age. A newer test, the polymerase chain reaction (PCR), is now available. This test does not rely on antibody formation; instead, genetic subunits of the virus are identified, confirming infection. Although PCR is relatively new and sensitivity studies are still being conducted, it will undoubtedly prove valuable in a variety of patient populations (e.g., newborns).

Maintaining patient confidentiality is essential in HIV testing. Every measure possible should be taken to ensure that privacy is guaranteed. Unauthorized disclosure, stigmatization, and discrimination against HIV-positive individuals continue to occur with unfortunate regularity.

In 1994, the Agency for Health Care Policy and Research (AHCPR) published the clinical practice guideline, *Evaluation and Management of Early HIV Infection.*[1] This guideline is expected to become the standard of care for management of early HIV infection and will provide the guidelines for secondary prevention efforts. Three main areas of early management (secondary prevention) are identified: (1) laboratory evaluation of immune function, (2) initiation of antiretroviral therapy, and (3) initiation of *P. carinii* prophylaxis.

### Laboratory Evaluation

Because the T4 helper lymphocytes are the primary target of HIV, evaluation of this subset of white blood cells (WBCs) is critical. Most adults have a T4 helper count of about 1000 cells/μL. This count varies widely among various laboratories and can often range from 300 to 3000 cells/μL for normal adults. The T4 helper cells are also called CD4 cells; CD4 refers to the particular protein expressed on the surface of the T4 helper lymphocyte. CD4 counts should be the primary test for measuring immune function in HIV-infected individuals and should be assessed once every 6 months as long as the counts are greater than 600 cells/μL. When the counts decrease to less than 600 cells/μL, the assessment should be obtained every 3 months. If cell counts are less than 200, more frequent assessment may be desired for evaluation of a rapid decline in counts or increasing symptoms. Although the percentage of T4 helper lymphocytes may also be useful, the absolute number (CD4/T4 helper counts) is the more widely used laboratory measurement.

### Initiation of Antiretroviral Therapy

Most patients remain relatively asymptomatic as their CD4 counts decrease to about 500 cells/μL. Even with this decrease of approximately 50% of their normal CD4 counts, many patients will continue to remain asymptomatic. It is recommended, however, that **zidovudine** (also called **AZT** or azidothymidine) be offered to all asymptomatic HIV-infected individuals with CD4 counts less than 500 cells/μL. AZT is an antiretroviral therapy that is effective in delaying the onset of opportunistic infections and prolonging survival in patients with advanced HIV disease.[5] Although some more recent studies have not shown improved survival in asymptomatic patients receiving AZT, these studies have shown a delay in progression to advanced HIV disease. Currently, 500 to 600 mg/day of AZT is recommended for both symptomatic and asymptomatic individuals with CD4 counts less than 500 cells/μL.

Patients who do not tolerate AZT should be offered therapy with didanosine (ddI) or dideoxycitidine (ddC). In addition, individuals who demonstrate progression of disease while receiving AZT should be offered ddI, ddC, or a combination of AZT plus ddI or ddC. D4T (Stavudine) is a fourth antiretroviral agent currently in clinical trials and is expected to be used as an option in patients who are intolerant or unresponsive to AZT, ddI, and ddC. Table 71-1 provides an overview of AZT, ddI, and ddC.

**TABLE 71-1 Overview of Antiretroviral Agents**

| GENERIC AND TRADE NAMES | SIDE EFFECTS |
|---|---|
| **AZT** | |
| Zidovudine, ZDV, Retrovir, azidothymidine | Nausea, GI discomfort, malaise, fatigue, headache, red cell anemia, granulocytopenia |
| **ddI** | |
| Didanosine, Videx | Pancreatitis, peripheral neuropathy, liver failure, headache, diarrhea, asthenia, insomnia, nausea/vomiting, abdominal pain |
| **ddC** | |
| Dideoxycytidine, Hivid | Peripheral neuropathy, pancreatitis, esophageal ulcers, nausea, oral ulcers, abdominal pain, diarrhea, vomiting |

## TERTIARY PREVENTION

The spectrum of HIV infection ranges from asymptomatic infection to potentially life-threatening opportunistic infection. In the past, many clinicians have used an informal staging system categorizing patients as falling into one of three categories: (1) HIV positive, (2) **AIDS-related complex (ARC),** and (3) AIDS. In this staging system, HIV positive referred to those patients who were completely asymptomatic but HIV positive. Those patients classified as ARC exhibited constitutional symptoms, including persistent generalized lymphadenopathy, persistent fevers, involuntary weight loss, and/or diarrhea. Any patient who had experienced an opportunistic infection was classified as having AIDS.

### CDC Classification System for HIV Infection in Adults

Today, clinicians have become much more sophisticated about the staging of HIV disease and realize that it is a chronic, progressive illness characterized by four distinct categories. Although we usually refer to end-stage HIV disease as AIDS, most clinicians use the staging system recommended by the CDC. The CDC Classification System for HIV Infection in Adults (Table 71-2) is currently the most widely used staging system.[3]

In general, tertiary prevention efforts focus on patients with Stage IV disease, typically referred to as AIDS. These patients have profound immunodeficiency and are at risk for a variety of infections and malignancies. Tertiary prevention efforts are aimed at keeping the individual well (free of active infection) and maintaining a desired quality of life. HIV illness is currently a terminal

**TABLE 71-2 CDC Classification System for HIV Infection in Adults**

| STAGE | CHARACTERISTICS |
|---|---|
| **STAGE I** | |
| Acute infection | Occurs at time of initial HIV infection and may last from days to weeks; characterized by mononucleosis-like or influenza-like syndrome, with approximately 50% of patients reporting or recalling symptoms |
| **STAGE II** | |
| Asymptomatic infection | Occurs after Stage I and may last for several years |
| **STAGE III** | |
| Persistent generalized lymphadenopathy (PGL) | Characterized by palpable lymph node enlargement of 1 cm or greater at two or more extrainguinal sites, persisting for more than 3 months |
| **STAGE IV** | |
| Other diseases | PGL not prerequisite |
| Subgroup A | |
| Characterized by constitutional disease: fever persisting for greater than 1 month, involuntary weight loss greater than 10% of usual body weight, diarrhea persisting for greater than 1 month | |
| Subgroup B | |
| Characterized by neurologic disease, including AIDS/dementia complex | |
| Subgroup C | |
| Characterized by secondary infectious diseases, including *Pneumocystis carinii* pneumonia, yeast infections, herpes simplex infections, *Mycobacterium avium* complex | |
| Subgroup D | |
| Characterized by secondary cancer, including non-Hodgkin's lymphoma, Kaposi's sarcoma (KS), cervical cancer | |
| Subgroup E | |
| Characterized by other conditions not listed above | |

illness. Aggressive and appropriate medical and nursing management, however, may be able to prolong survival and has the ability to improve quality of life. The opportunistic infections and measures for infection prevention and treatment of active infections are discussed on pp. 2449-2463. The cancers seen in HIV infection are discussed on p. 2464.

## MEDICAL MANAGEMENT

The expected length of stay of patients with HIV and AIDS as determined by diagnosis-related group (DRG) depends on the stage of the illness and the related infections or other problem. Common medical therapy for the management of HIV and AIDS includes the following categories.

### DIAGNOSTIC TESTS

No special tests exist for HIV and AIDS, once diagnosed. T4 levels and complete blood count (CBC) with differential are monitored at 3- to 6-month intervals to check the patient's status and response to therapy. Other tests are ordered as necessary depending on the patient's symptoms and signs demonstrated and the drug therapy the patient is currently receiving.

### MEDICATION

Antiretroviral agents (see Table 71-1) are used. Many experimental drugs are being investigated to stop the progress of HIV and AIDS. Medications for prevention of opportunistic infections and treatment of active infections are described in the last section of this chapter. Other medications are to treat related cancers, neuropathy, diarrhea and other GI complaints, and skin conditions.

### TREATMENT

There are no special treatments in the early stages of HIV infections. Respiratory treatments will become necessary as the patient's disease progresses. Blood and body substance precautions will be necessary when the patient is in the hospital or when providing home care. Treatments associated with maintenance and improvement of nutritional status also will become necessary.

### DIET

No special diet exists for persons with HIV. Each patient must be carefully monitored to identify the adequacy of intake, any food intolerance, and ways to promote a high-calorie, high-protein diet.

### ACTIVITY

There are no activity restrictions for the patient with HIV infection. A pattern of rest and activity should be encouraged to help maintain lean body mass and prevent deconditioning without promoting fatigue. During acute infections, activity needs to be restricted.

### REFERRAL/CONSULTATION

In some settings the nurse assumes responsibility for making referrals to other services. Common referrals for persons with HIV and AIDS include social workers to help with financial considerations, counselors to help with adjustment and problem solving in coping with the disease, dietitians to ensure adequate nutrient intake, physical therapy and occupational therapy specialists to enhance activity level, respiratory therapy practitioners for any respiratory involvement, and professionals in many medical specialties, particularly infectious disease.

Critical pathways (also referred to as "collaborative care paths" or "care maps") have been developed in some inpatient and outpatient settings to guide both medical and nursing management. These critical pathways are collaboratively developed along time lines and include the information described previously for specific hours, days, or visits. Pertinent information about discharge planning and patient teaching to be implemented at specified times also are included. Because the nurse has a major role in these two aspects of care, they are discussed under nursing management.

## NURSING MANAGEMENT

### ♦ ASSESSMENT

Some patients may be asymptomatic; others may report nonspecific "flulike" symptoms of fever, chills, night sweats, or dry, nonproductive cough. The clinical diversity of the HIV infection (Box 71-2) can make identification and assessment of infected patients difficult. Nurses may encounter patients experiencing various clinical symptoms, including fatigue, fever, diarrhea, or confusion, depending on the continuum of illness. Patients identified at risk for HIV infection either by sexual history, drug history, or flulike symptoms should be further assessed for the presence of opportunistic infections, rashes, and neoplasms.

#### Identification of Persons at Risk

***Health assessments of all patients should include an appraisal of potential risk factors for HIV infection.*** Obtaining a complete, accurate history of sexual behavior, including past and present sexual activities, is necessary and requires skillful interviewing techniques and a professional relationship based on trust. Nurses need to be comfortable when explaining the need for information on intimate sexual activities and phrasing questions in appropriate but comprehensible terms. The sexual health history, in addition to identifying individuals at risk for possible HIV infection, may also be an opportunity for health education and disease prevention (Box 71-3).

Information on the use of mood-affecting drugs such as alcohol, marijuana, heroin, cocaine, crack, barbiturates, tranquilizers, butyl nitrate, or amphetamines should also be obtained. Frequency and routes of administration including oral, smoking, sniffing, snorting, or injecting drugs should be explored. Needle exposure through the sharing of drug paraphernalia, tattoos, or acupuncture treatment should also be assessed.

Individuals identified as being at risk for HIV infection should be counseled about the significance of testing and the necessity for follow-up. Patients with evidence of risk factors and any clinical symptoms should be referred for blood testing and medical evaluation of symptoms to diagnose exposure to the HIV infection.

#### Diagnostic Tests: HIV Seropositivity

The diagnostic tests for seroconversion are described on p. 2443.

### ♦ NURSING DIAGNOSES

Nursing diagnoses are determined from analysis of patient data. Nursing diagnoses for the person with HIV disease may include but are not limited to the following:

| Diagnostic Title | Possible Etiologic Factors |
|---|---|
| Infection, high risk for | Decreased immune response, lack of knowledge, decreased nutrition |
| Nutrition, altered: less than body requirements | Chewing/swallowing difficulties, anorexia, inability to obtain food |
| Coping, family: compromised | Inadequate or incorrect information or understanding, preoccupation by significant other with personal reac- |

**BOX 71-2 Signs and Symptoms of HIV Infection**

| | |
|---|---|
| Chills and fever | Malaise |
| Night sweats | Fatigue |
| Dry productive cough | Oral lesions |
| Dyspnea | Skin rashes |
| Lethargy | Abdominal discomfort |
| Confusion | Diarrhea |
| Stiff neck | Weight loss |
| Seizures | Lymphadenopathy |
| Headache | Progressive generalized edema |

**BOX 71-3 Sample Sexual History**

1. When did you first become sexually active? With whom? For how long? Type of sexual activity practiced:
   - Mutual masturbation
   - French kissing
   - Vaginal intercourse
   - Anal intercourse
   - Oral intercourse
   - Use of objects to enhance stimulation
   - Use of contraceptives
2. Are you currently sexually active? With whom? For how long? Type of sexual activity?
3. Do you currently have any concerns about your sexuality or sexual activity?
4. Do you suspect that any of your sexual partners have been infected with herpes, syphilis, gonorrhea, or HIV? (Patients may need further explanations of specific types of infections and symptoms.)

| Diagnostic Title | Possible Etiologic Factors |
|---|---|
| | tions, temporary family disorganization, and role changes |
| Home maintenance management, impaired | Insufficient resources, impaired cognitive status, lack of knowledge, lack of support, fear |
| Fatigue | Infections, anemia, anxiety, inadequate nutrition, inadequate rest and sleep |
| Self-care deficits: total | Intolerance to activity, fatigue, pain/discomfort, perceptive/cognitive impairment, neuromuscular impairment, musculoskeletal impairment, depression, severe anxiety |
| Social isolation | Alteration in physical appearance/mental status, unaccepted social behaviors/values, altered state of wellness, inadequate personal resources, death of significant other |
| Fear | Uncertainty of illness, fear of death, fear of abandonment |

## ♦ EXPECTED PATIENT OUTCOMES

Expected patient outcomes for the patient with HIV disease may include but are not limited to the following:

1. Secondary infections do not occur or are identified early in the disease.
2. Does not lose more weight; weight will return to within 0.5 kg of preillness weight.
   a. Verbalizes need to increase caloric intake; increases caloric intake to 3000 calories/day as tolerated.
   b. Demonstrates usual strength and activity tolerance.
3. Patient and significant others engage in communication that leads to sharing of feelings, decision making, and problem resolution as pertinent.
4. Patient and significant others can describe home maintenance program; patient and significant others state they have adequate resources.
5. Is able to sustain desired activity tolerance; states fatigue is controlled.
6. Participates in activities of daily living (ADL) at optimal level of functioning.
7. Has opportunities to interact socially with others.
8. States fear is controlled.

## ♦ INTERVENTIONS

### Preventing Infections

Monitor vital signs and laboratory results for signs of possible infection.

1. Institute a low microbial diet for patients with an absolute neutrophil count less than 500 cells/$cm^3$.
2. Perform appropriate physical assessment, including careful examination of skin integrity, respiratory, and GI status.
3. Perform appropriate mental status examinations.
4. Maintain asepsis when caring for patient, including appropriate handwashing and limiting of infectious visitors.
5. Educate patient in protective strategies such as handwashing, diet precautions such as thorough cooking of meat products, and pet care precautions.

### Improving Nutrition

Monitor daily for signs of improved nutrition: increased weight, increased blood urea nitrogen (BUN) and serum albumin, protein, hemoglobin, lymphocytes, and transferrin levels; and increased muscle strength and energy level.

1. Assess for causes of inadequate intake such as anorexia, nausea, stomatitis, impaired swallowing, and self-care deficits; develop appropriate strategies to improve intake.
2. Provide assistive/adaptive feeding equipment as appropriate; assist with feedings as needed.
3. Encourage measures to promote eating such as mouth care before meals, sitting in chair to eat, eating with others, and providing a pleasant environment.
4. Provide high-calorie, high-protein foods six times a day; incorporate foods patient likes.
5. Keep caloric/protein count or food diary for 1 week.
6. Provide diet teaching as necessary regarding normal nutrient requirements, relationship of calories required to maintian or regain weight, and distribution of nutrients and calories in foods.
7. Refer to nutritionist as needed.
8. Refer to social worker if economics are a problem.

### Promoting Communication

Establish a therapeutic nursing relationship using empathy, acceptance, and support.

1. Facilitate expression of patient's feelings.
2. Help patient identify past and current coping strategies and effective and ineffective skills.
3. Identify resources available to patient including family members, friends, clergy, and support groups.
4. Use multidisciplinary resources, including social services, clergy, and psychiatry.

### Promoting Home Maintenance

Help patient and significant others identify what knowledge, skills, and resources they need to maintain care at home.

1. Explore with patient and significant others their understanding of care needs.
2. Identify resources and support available to patient.
3. Plan educational opportunities to increase knowledge on diet, activities, medications, self-monitoring needs, prevention of infection, stress reduction (see Chapter 7), and follow-up.
4. Help patient obtain other resources.

### Decreasing Fatigue

Help patient identify importance of various activities and plan energy expenditures accordingly.

1. See Chapter 14 for discussion of fatigue.
2. Help patient plan periods of rest.
3. Use various assistive devices such as wheelchairs as needed.

### Promoting Self-Care

Encourage patient to maintain self-care to the extent possible.

1. Help patient plan energy conservation and pacing of activities.
2. Use adaptive equipment such as assistive eating devices and bedside commodes.
3. Educate patient in safety measures.
4. Refer to occupational and physical therapy as needed.

### Maintaining Social Interaction

Help patient maintain social relationships.

1. Help patient identify past, current, and future social supports.
2. Refer to social services and counseling as appropriate.
3. Educate patient about various community resources such as support groups and "buddy system."

### Decreasing Fear

Help patient control fear.

1. Identify fears.
2. Identify ways patient deals with fear.
3. Encourage use of support groups.
4. Monitor for uncontrolled fear that is interfering with care.
5. Refer to counseling as appropriate.

## ♦ EVALUATION

To evaluate effectiveness of nursing interventions, compare patient behaviors with those stated in the expected patient outcomes. Successful achievement of patient outcomes for the patient with HIV infection is indicated by the following:

1. Is free of secondary infections; temperature is normal; lungs clear; skin intact; and so forth.
2. Regains weight and maintains desired body weight.
3. Patient and family interact in a supportive manner, allowing family to help patient accomplish patient's goals.
4. Takes medicine appropriately and returns for follow-up; reports changes as necessary.
5. Is able to accomplish desired tasks; states fatigue is controlled.
6. Is able to maintain self-care in feeding, bathing-hygiene, dressing-grooming, and toileting.
7. Maintains social interactions; participates in activities.
8. Shows no signs of fear.

## SPECIAL CONSIDERATIONS FOR CARE OF THE GERONTOLOGIC PATIENT

Although much is still unknown about the immune function and aging, in general, aging is associated with depressed cell-mediated immunity, impaired antibody production, and increased autoantibody production (see Chapter 4). These aging changes often result in decreased capacity to resist infections.

Most elderly persons with AIDS to date have been traced to blood transfusions associated with common surgical procedures such as coronary bypass and valve surgery and joint replacements. Given the long incubation period, the risk of contamination from blood transfusions, and the decreased capacity of elderly persons to resist infections, the incidence of HIV in this age-group is projected to rise steadily.

Recognition of the HIV infection in elderly persons may be difficult for several reasons. A diagnosis of AIDS may be missed in elderly persons who frequently have symptoms such as pneumonia, dementia, shortness of breath, weakness, fatigue, poor nutritional intake, and weight loss. In addition, caregivers may fail to evaluate thoroughly such risk factors as IV drug use and homosexuality in this age-group.

Elderly persons with compromised immune functions or chronic illnesses such as heart and respiratory disease often have little reserve to resist or fight the multiple infections that may accompany the HIV infection. In general, this age-group exhibits more side effects from aggressive antibiotic therapy used to fight infections. Increasing numbers of acutely ill elderly persons with multiple infections associated with the HIV infection pose unique clinical challenges for nurses in all settings.

## HOME CARE CONSIDERATIONS

In the past, most HIV patients received most of their care in the hospital. With improvements in antiviral therapy as well as treatment and prophylaxis of various opportunistic infections, most patients now receive most of their care outside the hospital setting.[6,7] Although most HIV-infected patients will spend some time in the hospital, most often this will be for induction therapy for an acute opportunistic infection. Continuing therapy is most often accomplished in the home.

HIV testing is performed in the outpatient setting. If found to be HIV positive, patients first seek outpatient/clinic care, where most are followed for several years until they develop the first opportunistic infection. Even with the advent of a significant, perhaps life-threatening infection, most patients spend relatively little time in the hospital. Once induction therapy is begun and most acute symptoms are controlled, the patient is discharged and continued on induction therapy. Secondary prophylaxis may then continue lifelong.

Given this shift from hospital-based care to home care, an increasing need exists for appropriate and thorough patient education. HIV disease is a chronic illness that progresses differently among individuals. Personalized attention to the individual's health status, knowledge level, and social supports is essential to providing appropriate nursing care.

Home care referrals may be necessary to help patients with IV lines or IV medications (see Chapter 27). Meals on Wheels may be useful if the patient is unable to cook. Hospice may be used in the terminal phase of the illness.

# COMPLICATIONS

Infection prevention is one of the major needs of patients with HIV infection, even in its asymptomatic phase. This section reviews common opportunistic infections and other complications in persons with HIV.[17,19]

## BACTERIAL INFECTIONS

The two primary bacterial infections that occur in HIV-infected patients are *Mycobacterium avium* complex and *Mycobacterium tuberculosis.* Tuberculosis has increased in incidence in the last several years as the number of AIDS patients has increased. This respiratory disease represents a complex community health illness and is discussed in Chapter 37.

### Mycobacterium Avium Complex

*Mycobacterium avium* and *M. intracellulare* are closely related nontuberculous or atypical mycobacteria that are usually grouped together as **M. avium complex (MAC).** These organisms are widespread in the environment, with high concentrations found in water, soil, and aerosol droplets. Because MAC is an environmental organism, it is assumed that many persons are exposed to MAC. Despite the widespread exposure to MAC, there is low incidence of clinical disease in the normal host because of the low pathogenicity of the organism.

In normal hosts, disease caused by MAC is manifested predominantly as a tuberculosis-like pulmonary process. This presentation occurs primarily in elderly men with underlying chronic lung disease. MAC generally occurs late in the course of HIV infection and may occur in up to 50% of patients with AIDS. It is the most common bacterial infection in AIDS. Disease is most often disseminated, and infection of multiple tissues or organs may be identified.[8]

#### Medical management

**Diagnostic tests.** Disseminated MAC is usually diagnosed by blood culture. A single positive culture is considered adequate, although there have been reports of patients with transient MAC bacteremia, possibly representing fluctuating low levels of *Mycobacterium.* Most patients, however, have high-grade bacteremia, and a single blood culture is usually sufficient; repeated cultures are suggested if the first culture is negative. Diagnosis of MAC can also be confirmed by culture of MAC from other normally sterile body sites such as the liver, bone, or lymph node.

**Medication.** Use of combination therapy for the treatment of MAC has the best success. Table 71-3 lists drugs that are likely to have activity against MAC and are most widely used in various drug combinations. Because disseminated MAC is associated with significant morbidity and mortality, it is rational to attempt to prevent MAC in patients at risk. Patients at highest risk for first occurrence of MAC are those with less than 100 CD4 cells/μL. Although clinical trials are still evaluating optimal prophylaxis, rifabutin is the most frequently used agent. Clarithromycin or azithromycin may also be used in some settings.

**Treatment.** Treatments are related to associated signs and symptoms. For example, if patients have weight loss, total parenteral nutrition may be used, or if patients have bronchospasm, inhalation therapy may be administered.

**Diet.** No special diet is required for patients with MAC. Weight loss, however, is a common problem; and oral, enteral, or parenteral supplementation may be used.

**Activity.** There are no prescribed activities or activity limitations. Fatigue is usually present and may be a limiting factor in activity levels. Patients should stay as active as possible.

**Referral/Consultation.** In some settings, the nurse assumes responsibility for making referrals to other services. Because most patients with MAC are likely to have end-stage HIV disease with significant immune compromise, a variety of referrals may be used. Social services should always be consulted when an HIV-infected patient is hospitalized. This department can ensure the patient is covered by insurance or has completed the application process for Medicare/Medicaid and associated programs. In addition, a variety of services are available to HIV-infected patients, including food pantries, housing assistance, and "buddy" programs. Social services can also assist in discharge planning. Because most patients will continue some type of medical therapy at home, a referral to home nursing services is usually necessary.

A physical therapist and occupational therapist are other common referrals. Many patients will have difficulty with exercise tolerance related to the chronic illness, fevers, or weight loss. Physical and occupational therapy may assist in returning patients to their usual state of activity and may assist in improving the patient's

**TABLE 71-3 Drug Therapy for MAC**

| DRUG/DOSE | SIDE EFFECTS | NURSING CONSIDERATIONS |
|---|---|---|
| **CLARITHROMYCIN** | | |
| 1000 mg bid | Nausea, abdominal pain, diarrhea, hepatotoxicity | Assess nutritional status.<br>Monitor intake and output (I&O).<br>Monitor liver function studies. |
| **AZITHROMYCIN** | | |
| 500 mg qd | Nausea, abdominal pain, diarrhea, hepatotoxicity | Same as for clarithromycin. |
| **RIFAMPIN** | | |
| 600 mg qd | Rash, hepatotoxicity, neutropenia, orange urine | Assess skin integrity.<br>Monitor liver function studies.<br>Monitor CBC and institute neutropenic precautions if necessary.<br>Educate patient about possibility of orange urine. |
| **RIFABUTIN** | | |
| 450-600 mg qd | Rash, hepatotoxicity, neutropenia, orange urine | Same as for rifampin. |
| **AMIKACIN** | | |
| 10-15 mg/kg qd | Ototoxicity, nephrotoxicity | Monitor hearing.<br>Obtain peak and trough levels as ordered.<br>Monitor chemistries for evidence of nephrotoxicity. |
| **STREPTOMYCIN** | | |
| 15-20 mg/kg qd | Ototoxicity, nephrotoxicity | Monitor hearing.<br>Monitor I&O.<br>Assess chemistries for nephrotoxicity. |
| **CIPROFLOXACIN** | | |
| 500-750 mg bid | Nausea, abdominal pain, diarrhea, rash | Monitor nutritional status.<br>Assess hydration status.<br>Assess skin integrity. |
| **ETHAMBUTOL** | | |
| 15-25 mg/kg qd | Nausea, abdominal pain, changes in visual acuity | Monitor nutritional status.<br>Assess visual acuity and monitor for changes. |
| **CLOFAZIMINE** | | |
| 100 mg qd | Skin hyperpigmentation, nausea, abdominal pain | Educate patient about skin hyperpigmentation.<br>Assess and monitor nutritional status. |

ability to perform ADL. Psychiatry or counseling referrals may be desired or requested by patients. The nurse must assess each individual and family members for their need or willingness to participate in such an evaluation and/or program.

## NURSING MANAGEMENT

### ♦ ASSESSMENT

#### Subjective Data

Most patients with MAC have end-stage HIV disease. Because of the long-term and profound immunodeficiency associated with HIV disease, many of these patients may have constitutional symptoms caused by MAC or HIV disease. Patients may have complaints of fever, night sweats, and fatigue. Abdominal pain may also be reported.

#### Objective Data

Most people who are colonized with MAC are asymptomatic. Although symptomatic pulmonary disease is common in patients without AIDS, it is unusual to find this presentation in patients with HIV disease. Because symptomatic MAC occurs late in the course of HIV infection, many patients have symptoms that can be attributed either to MAC or to the profound immunodeficiency that is a result of HIV. Fever is the most common symptom and occurs in almost all patients. Persistent fevers may be as high as 104° F (40° C). Weight loss and diarrhea are other frequently observed symptoms. Physical examination may reveal lymphadenopathy or hepatosplenomegaly.

#### Diagnostic Test Findings

The most common laboratory abnormality associated with MAC is anemia. A sudden fall in hematocrit or the need for repeat transfusions may be associated with disseminated MAC. An elevated alkaline phosphatase level may represent direct liver involvement. Blood cultures are definitive for MAC infection.

## ♦ NURSING DIAGNOSES

Nursing diagnoses are determined from analysis of patient data. Nursing diagnoses for the patient with HIV and MAC may include but are not limited to the following:

| Diagnostic Title | Possible Etiologic Factors |
|---|---|
| Nutrition, altered: less than body requirements | Anorexia, nausea, malabsorption |
| Activity intolerance | Insufficient oxygen transport, nutritional deficiencies, diarrhea and fluid loss, prolonged immobility, lack of knowledge about rest needs and pacing ADL |
| Fluid volume deficit | Abnormal fluid loss |
| Temperature, high risk for altered body | Infection |

## ♦ INTERVENTIONS

Mycobacteria are very widely distributed and consist of approximately 19 medically important species. MAC represents two of these species, namely *intracellulare* and *avium*. Person-to-person airborne transmission is not a source of infection for MAC, and airborne precautions therefore are unnecessary. The drugs used to treat MAC are relatively toxic, and most patients have some significant side effects from therapy. Helping patients deal with the side effects is one focus of care. Treatment requires a multidrug approach, and the optimal combination is not yet known.

Nurses should educate patients early in the course of their HIV infection about strategies to reduce the risk of MAC infection. Washing fruits and vegetables well before eating, avoiding unpasteurized dairy products, and drinking bottled liquids when traveling should be considered.

## FUNGAL INFECTIONS

Fungal infections also are a common problem among HIV-infected patients. The most common fungal infections are candidiasis, cryptococcosis, and histoplasmosis.

### Candidiasis

The fungus *Candida albicans* is one of the normal organisms found in the mouth, GI tract (throat, esophagus, stomach, bowel), vagina, and skin of healthy individuals. It produces infection only when the immune system is altered. Such infections are found in people taking broad-spectrum antibiotics, people with uncontrolled diabetes mellitus, cancer patients, and patients with immunodeficiencies, including those who are HIV infected. In HIV-infected people, mucocutaneous *Candida* infections are a common problem, especially in the mouth. The esophagus, skin, rectum, and vagina are other sites where the fungus is found. Oral or vaginal **candidiasis**, although annoying, presents no significant risk or mortality to the patient. Disseminated infections occur rarely but can be associated with significant morbidity and mortality.

#### Medical management

**Diagnostic tests.** A *Candida* infection is usually diagnosed by its characteristic appearance of glistening white patches on the tongue or oral mucosal surfaces or creamy white vaginal discharge. Scrapings of the lesions from the source of infection (usually the mouth) and examination under a microscope with a potassium hydroxide preparation allow identification of the yeast organism. Candidal infections can progress to other mucocutaneous sites as well. Oral infections, when left untreated, can progress down the esophagus. Scraping of these lesions for diagnosis may then require a scoping procedure of the esophagus to obtain a sample as well as to assess the extent of infection.

**Medication.** Treatments for oral *Candida* infection include (1) nystatin, which is swished in the mouth and then swallowed; (2) clotrimazole, which is usually in the form of a lozenge that is dissolved in the mouth; and (3) fluconazole or ketoconazole, taken as tablets. Vaginal yeast infections may be treated with nystatin creams, ointments, or suppositories. For persistent or systemic infections, amphotericin may be required. Table 71-4 presents an overview of these drugs.

**Treatment.** Specific treatments depend on the patient's symptoms and signs.

**Diet.** Nutritional support is necessary. Although several studies have examined diet restrictions or therapy for candidal infections, no restriction or therapy has been identified as reducing or preventing infection. Oral candidal lesions may make it difficult for the patient to tolerate certain temperature extremes of food, and some may be unable to tolerate very spicy food. Soft foods may be better tolerated by some patients because of pain. Patients can eat what they can tolerate.

**Activity.** There are no activity restrictions. Most patients receiving amphotericin B experience fatigue, which may greatly reduce their activity tolerance. They need help to establish an activity regimen they can tolerate.

**Referral/Consultation.** A dietitian is an important referral for many patients who might have difficulty maintaining their nutrition secondary to pain from oral lesions. A gynecologist should be consulted for patients who have recurrent vaginal yeast infections and may perform routine Pap and pelvic screening as well. A dermatologist may be consulted for some patients whose lesions do not resolve. Patients with disseminated dis-

**TABLE 71-4 Drug Therapy for *Candida* Infections**

| SITE OF INFECTION | DRUG TREATMENT | SIDE EFFECTS | NURSING CONSIDERATIONS |
|---|---|---|---|
| Oral, esophageal | Nystatin suspension | Nausea, vomiting, epigastric distress, diarrhea | Assess nutritional status; refer to nutritionist as needed.<br>Educate patient about swish-and-swallow procedure. |
| Oral, topical, vaginal | Clotrimazole | Abnormal liver functions, nausea, vomiting | Monitor liver function tests.<br>Educate patient in method of medication administration.<br>Monitor nutritional status. |
| Oral, esophageal, topical, vaginal | Ketoconazole; fluconazole | Headache, nausea, vomiting, mild leukocytopenia, transient elevation in serum liver enzymes, hepatotoxicity, gynecomastia | Monitor nutritional status.<br>Assess CBC, serum chemistries, and liver function tests. |
| Disseminated, esophageal | Amphotericin B | General toxic reactions: fever with shaking chills, headache, anorexia, malaise, generalized pain | Most patients exhibit some intolerance to drug; monitor and treat symptoms and signs. |

ease require amphotericin therapy and are likely to be acutely ill. These patients will likely require social service and home nursing referrals. For prolonged illness, an occupational therapist or physical therapist also may be consulted.

## NURSING MANAGEMENT

### ♦ ASSESSMENT

#### Subjective Data

By far the most common form of candidiasis is mucocutaneous. Patients may present complaining of a coating in their mouth, anorexia, or dysphagia. Patients with vaginal candidiasis may complain of a cottage cheese–like discharge and pruritus. Patients with disseminated disease may complain of fever and fatigue.

#### Objective Data

Creamy, curdlike, yellowish patches surrounded by an erythematous base may appear on the buccal mucosa and tongue surfaces. The patches can be wiped off, leaving an erythematous or even bleeding mucosal surface. Occasionally, smooth red patches on the hard or soft palate, buccal mucosa, or dorsal surface of the tongue may be seen. Angular cheilitis may also be present. The vagina and labia usually appear erythematous with vaginal infections.

#### Diagnostic Test Findings

Scrapings of the lesions from the site of infection will identify yeast organisms. In patients with disseminated disease, cultures of blood will grow *Candida* organisms.

### ♦ NURSING DIAGNOSES

Nursing diagnoses are determined from analysis of patient data. Nursing diagnoses for the patient with candidiasis may include but are not limited to the following:

| Diagnostic Title | Possible Etiologic Factors |
|---|---|
| Mucous membrane, altered oral | Inadequate oral hygiene and/or stomatitis |
| Skin integrity, impaired | Infection |
| Pain | Mucous membrane lesions |
| Nutrition, altered: less than body requirements | Anorexia, pain, difficulty in chewing or swallowing |
| Knowledge deficit about taking medications properly | No previous exposure to the information |

### ♦ INTERVENTIONS

Candidiasis may be considered a sentinel infection, marking the beginning of significant immune decline. Mucocutaneous candidiasis is rarely cured and often becomes chronic or recurrent. Vaginal candidiasis may also be recurrent and difficult to treat. Nursing education should be directed toward prevention of severe *Candida* infections and should include oral hygiene and exposure of skin surfaces to air.

### Cryptococcosis

*Cryptococcus neoformans* is a yeastlike fungus that is ubiquitous and occurs worldwide. The organism is found in pigeon droppings and can be retrieved in nesting places, soil, fruit, and fruit juices. *C. neoformans* can remain viable for up to 2 years even in desiccated pigeon feces. Neither person-to-person nor animal-to-person transmission has been documented. The disease is naturally acquired from the environment, where the organism is aerosolized and inhaled. In patients with prolonged, severe immunodeficiency caused by HIV, the immune system may no longer be competent against *C. neoformans,* and **cryptococcosis** can develop. Cryptococcal infection usually presents as meningitis in HIV-infected patients.

#### Medical management

**Diagnostic tests.** Examination of the fungus in the CSF with an India ink stain is diagnostic in cryptococcal meningitis. The organism may also be detected by antigen testing in urine or serum. Cryptococcal antigen titers and cultures of blood or CSF are the most reliable diagnostic measures. Computed tomography (CT) of the head may be performed to rule out hydrocephalus and to look for focal lesions. Chest radiographs are helpful if cryptococcal pneumonia is suspected.

**Medication.** The primary therapy for an initial cryptococcal infection is amphotericin B. The side effects and nursing considerations of amphotericin B are reviewed in Table 71-4. In addition to the usual IV infusion of amphotericin B, intrathecal administration has been used in patients failing to respond to IV infusion.

Other medication used include flucytosine or fluconazole. Flucytosine is an oral agent and is given in combination with amphotericin B. Side effects include anemia, yellow eyes/skin, skin rash, redness, itching, sore throat, fever, unusual bleeding/bruising, confusion, sensitivity of the skin to sunlight, abdominal pain, diarrhea, loss of appetite, nausea, vomiting, dizziness, lightheadedness, drowsiness, and headache. Nursing considerations for patients receiving flucytosine therapy may include (1) patient education of the side effects; (2) monitoring of signs and symptoms of anemia, including fatigue and shortness of breath; (3) assessment for unusual bleeding or bruising; (4) mental status evaluation; (5) patient education about sun sensitivity; and (6) assessment of potential GI effects and the potential for malnutrition.

Fluconazole is less toxic than amphotericin and is better tolerated but may not be as efficacious in certain patients. The side effects and nursing implications of fluconazole are discussed in Table 71-4.

As with many of the opportunistic infections associated with HIV disease, the successful treatment of the initial acute infection does not cure the patient. Long-term suppressive therapy is necessary to prevent recurrence. Primary prophylaxis (instituted before the patient ever develops an initial infection) and long-term suppressive therapy may be accomplished with oral fluconazole therapy.

**Treatment.** There are no treatments specific to this infection other than drug therapy.

**Diet.** There are no special dietary considerations. Patients need to be encouraged to maintain a healthy diet.

**Activity.** Patients with meningitis may experience somnolence or confusion. Activity restrictions may be instituted to protect this patient.

**Referral/Consultation.** As with other serious opportunistic infections that occur in late-stage disease, patients with cryptococcal infections may require multiple referrals. Social services, home nursing services, physical/occupational therapy, and psychiatry or counseling may be appropriate.

## NURSING MANAGEMENT

### ♦ ASSESSMENT

#### Subjective Data

Patients may have a history of fever, cough, dyspnea, and pleuritic chest pain if pulmonary infection is present. Patients with CNS cryptococcosis usually have an insidious course; signs and symptoms are usually similar to other infections seen with AIDS, such as fever, chills, night sweats, and fatigue. Some patients may present with complaint of stiff neck, nausea or vomiting, photophobia, or altered mentation.

#### Objective Data

Patients with pulmonary infection may have pain on inspiration. CNS cryptococcosis may produce fevers greater than 102° F (38.8° C) as well as mental status changes, although these may be difficult to detect without family participation. Some patients may experience seizures caused by meningitis.

#### Diagnostic Test Findings

CSF positive for *C. neoformans* may be present. The organism may also be present in urine or serum. CT scan of the head may reveal hydrocephalus. Chest radiograph may reveal a pneumonia process, and bronchoscopy may reveal the cryptococcal organism.

### ♦ NURSING DIAGNOSES

Nursing diagnoses are determined from analysis of patient data. Nursing diagnoses for the patient with cryptococcosis may include but are not limited to the following:

| Diagnostic Title | Possible Etiologic Factors |
|---|---|
| Cognitive impairment, high risk for | Cerebral edema from inflammation |
| Activity intolerance | Insufficient oxygen transport, nutritional deficiencies, diarrhea and fluid loss, prolonged immobility |
| Temperature, high risk for altered body | Infection |

### ♦ INTERVENTIONS

Cryptococcal infection often has an insidious course, and patients often postpone medical evaluation. Family members and friends may be the first to notice subtle mental status changes indicative of encephalitis. Problems with short-term memory may lead to noncompliance with the medication regimen.

#### Histoplasmosis

*Histoplasma capsulatum* causes a common, usually benign fungal infection, **histoplasmosis,** and occurs primarily in the lungs. *H. capsulatum* is present in the soil where bird and bat excrement collect. The most likely sources of soil contamination in endemic areas are blackbird roosts, pigeon roosts, chicken houses, chicken manure, fertilizer, and sites frequented by bats such as caves, attics, old buildings, and hollow trees. The major endemic areas in the United States are the middle, central, and south central states. Although many individuals in endemic areas have been infected with *H. capsulatum,* the organism usually does not cause significant pulmonary disease. In immunocompromised patients, however, acute and life-threatening illness may develop. Patients may have pulmonary infection or disseminated disease. Disseminated histoplasmosis is the most common AIDS-defining opportunistic infection in many endemic areas.

#### Medical management

**Diagnostic tests.** Chest radiographs are unreliable and are normal in up to 30% of individuals with disseminated histoplasmosis. Because histoplasmosis most often presents as disseminated disease in HIV-positive patients, bone marrow biopsy and cultures, examination and culture of pulmonary tissue and secretions, and blood cultures are the most common means of establishing a diagnosis.

**Medication.** Disseminated histoplasmosis in AIDS is invariably fatal if not treated aggressively with antifungal therapy. Amphotericin B is the drug of choice in induction therapy for acute infection. Fluconazole induction therapy is being studied. These antifungal agents are discussed in Table 71-4. Because induction treatment does not cure histoplasmosis in a person with AIDS, lifelong suppressive therapy (secondary prophylaxis) is indicated. Amphotericin B[15] or ketoconazole may be used for long-term therapy. Currently, there are no recommendations for primary prophylactic therapy.

**Treatment.** No standard therapies exist other than pharmacologic.

**Diet.** There are no specific dietary recommendations.

**Activity.** No activity restrictions exist, but fatigue may greatly limit activity tolerance.

**Referral/Consultation.** As with other serious opportunistic infections that occur in late-stage disease, patients with histoplasmosis may require multiple referrals. Social services, home nursing services, dietary, physical/occupational therapy, and psychiatry or counseling may be appropriate.

## NURSING MANAGEMENT

### ♦ ASSESSMENT

#### Subjective Data

Patients usually complain of fever, weight loss, and fatigue.

#### Objective Data

Fever greater than 101° F (38.3° C) and weight loss are nearly always identified. In addition, hepatomegaly, splenomegaly, and lymphadenopathy are also common findings. In patients with fulminant disease, thrombocytopenia, leukopenia, disseminated intravascular coagulation, and even respiratory failure may be present. Less often, cerebritis, chorioretinitis, or meningitis may be found.

#### Diagnostic Test Findings

*H. capsulatum* may be identified on examination of bone marrow, pulmonary tissue, or blood cultures. Chest radiographs may reveal histoplasmosis lesions in some patients.

### ♦ NURSING DIAGNOSES

Nursing diagnoses are determined from analysis of patient data. Nursing diagnoses for the patient with histoplasmosis may include but are not limited to the following:

| Diagnostic Title | Possible Etiologic Factors |
|---|---|
| Activity intolerance | Insufficient oxygen transport, nutritional deficiencies, diarrhea and fluid loss, prolonged immobility, lack of knowledge regarding need for rest and pacing ADL |
| Nutrition, altered: less than body requirements | Anorexia, nausea |
| Gas exchange, impaired | Decreased competent alveolocapillary diffusion area |
| Temperature, high risk for altered body | Infection |

### ♦ INTERVENTIONS

Although most histoplasmosis infections occur in patients who live in endemic areas (mainly the Midwest), patients from other areas may also contract the infection, particularly if their travel history includes travel to endemic areas. Disseminated histoplasmosis causes significant fatigue and other symptoms that are often difficult to distinguish from other opportunistic infections and from progressive HIV illness. Long-term suppressive therapy is required to prevent recurrent infection.

## PROTOZOAL INFECTIONS

Protozoal infections are caused by a variety of organisms, many of which are parasitic. The organisms that most frequently cause protozoal opportunistic infections are *Cryptosporidium, Pneumocystis carinii,* and *Toxoplasma gondii.*

### Cryptosporidium

*Cryptosporidium* is a parasite present in a variety of animal species, including birds, reptiles, fish, cattle, sheep, and humans. It is a well-recognized pathogen in both immunologically intact individuals and immunocompromised hosts such as persons with HIV disease. In addition to animal-to-human transmission, person-to-person transmission has also been documented among day-care centers, household contacts, hospital patients, and health care workers. Water-borne transmission has also been documented. Chlorination does not kill *Cryptosporidium.* After ingestion of the organism, the most common site of infection is the small intestine, although the entire GI tract may be infected in immunocompromised patients.

**Medical management**

**Diagnostic tests.** *Cryptosporidium* oocytes can be identified in fresh specimens or formalin-preserved specimens.

**Medication.** No effective anticryptosporidial therapy exists. The disease is self-limited in immunocompetent individuals and therefore does not require therapy. In immunocompromised hosts, however, refractory **cryptosporidiosis** usually occurs. Death from profound malabsorption, electrolyte imbalances, malnutrition, and dehydration may occur. Octreotide may be used to reduce the volume of stool. Side effects of this medication include hyperglycemia, hypoglycemia, abdominal pain, nausea, vomiting, pain at injection site, headache, fatigue, dizziness, lightheadedness, edema, facial flushing, and hepatic dysfunction. Patient education about the use of this drug is essential. The nurse should instruct the patient to save all stool for assessment of the drug's effectiveness in reducing volume.

Several other drugs are under study to treat cryptosporidiosis, but none has thus far appeared promising. Azithromycin, diclazuril (Latrazuril), and trimetrexate are in clinical trials for cryptosporidiosis.

**Treatment.** Patients with cryptosporidiosis require IV therapy for fluid replacement and may require total parenteral nutrition (TPN) to maintain nutritional status.

**Diet.** No specific diet exists for patients with cryptosporidiosis. Some patients may find that reducing the bulk in their diet may reduce the volume of their stools. Most patients require some form of nutritional supplementation to maintain adequate nutritional status. TPN is often used to replace fluids, calories, and nutrients lost through the massive volumes of diarrhea.

**Activity.** There are no activity restrictions for patients with cryptosporidial infection. The frequency of diarrhea, however, often restricts activity patterns. Fatigue related to massive fluid volume depletion may also decrease activity tolerance.

**Referral/Consultation.** A referral to a dietitian is essential. Patients lose massive amounts of fluid and are almost always unable to maintain nutritional status. As with other opportunistic infections, other referrals may include social services, physical/occupational therapy, counseling/psychiatry, and home care.

## NURSING MANAGEMENT

### ♦ ASSESSMENT

#### Subjective Data

Patients most often complain of massive diarrhea, accompanied by nausea and fatigue.

#### Objective Data

Diarrhea volume may exceed 4 L/day. Patients may be dehydrated with poor skin turgor and electrolyte imbalances. Weight loss of greater than 20% of usual body weight is often present.

#### Diagnostic Test Findings

*Cryptosporidium* will be identified in the stool samples.

### ♦ NURSING DIAGNOSES

Nursing diagnoses are determined from analysis of patient data. Nursing diagnoses for the patient with cryptosporidiosis may include but are not limited to the following:

| Diagnostic Title | Possible Etiologic Factors |
|---|---|
| Diarrhea | Cryptosporidiosis |
| Fluid volume deficit | Abnormal fluid loss |
| Nutrition, altered: less than body requirements | Malabsorption |
| Skin integrity, impaired | Diarrhea and malnutrition |
| Activity intolerence | Nutritional deficiencies, diarrhea, fluid loss |
| Pain | Altered skin integrity, diarrhea |
| Temperature, high risk for altered body | Infection |

### ♦ INTERVENTIONS

Because palliation and symptom control are the only effective therapeutic interventions, nursing goals include measures to minimize the physical discomforts associated with continuous explosive diarrhea. Skin breakdown is common and must be assessed and treated frequently. Malnutrition, dehydration, and weight loss are also common, and patients often require emotional support to cope with significant alterations in body image.

Infection control measures are extremely important to prevent person-to-person transmission, both in the hospital and at home. Nurses and other caregivers must be sure to wear protective clothing, including gloves, during personal care and waste disposal. Meticulous handwashing is essential.

### *Pneumocystis Carinii*

*P. carinii* has been identified as both a protozoan and a fungus, although most investigators have classified the organism as a protozoan based on its morphologic structure. More recently, however, some studies of the ribosomal RNA sequences indicate that this organism bears a closer relationship to fungi than to protozoa. *P. carinii* is a ubiquitous organism with a worldwide distribution. It exists in human lungs and has been identified in the lungs of many other mammals as well. The organism can be found in the air, on food, and in water, although most transmission appears to be via airborne routes. Most healthy children have acquired *P. carinii* infection by 4 years of age. *P. carinii* is not highly virulent, and infection in a normal host is usually asymptomatic.

In the immunocompromised host, however, *P. carinii* can cause fulminant disease. The infection in the immunocompromised host is generally confined to the lungs **(P. carinii pneumonia, PCP),** although extrapulmonary pneumocystosis can occur. Since the beginning of the AIDS pandemic *P. carinii* pneumonia has been the most common life-threatening opportunistic infection in persons with AIDS. PCP has been the first AIDS-indicator opportunistic infection in 60% of persons with HIV disease. More recently, however, the use of PCP prophylaxis in the HIV population is slowing the incidence of infection.

### Medical management

**Diagnostic tests.** Bronchoalveolar and transbronchial biopsies are usually performed to identify *P. carinii* in patients with pneumonia. If unsuccessful, an open lung biopsy via thoracotomy may be performed as a last resort. Chest radiograph may reveal pneumonia, although 5% to 10% of chest radiographs in AIDS patients with PCP appear normal. Pulmonary function studies usually reveal decreased vital capacity, decreased total lung capacity, and decreased single-breath diffusing capacity of carbon monoxide. Arterial blood gas studies may reveal hypoxemia, hypocarbia, and an increase in the alveolar/arterial oxygen gradient, particularly with exercise.

Presumptive diagnosis of PCP may be made according to the following CDC guidelines: (1) history of dyspnea on exertion or nonproductive cough of recent onset; (2) chest radiographic evidence of diffuse bilateral interstitial infiltrates or gallium scan evidence of diffuse bilateral pulmonary disease; and (3) arterial blood gas analysis showing an arterial oxygen tension of less than 70 mm Hg, a low respiratory diffusing capacity, or an increase in the alveolar-arterial oxygen tension gradient; and (4) no evidence of bacterial pneumonia. *P. carinii* may present in extrapulmonary sites, although repeated biopsies may fail to yield a definitive diagnosis.

**Medication.** Current standard therapy for PCP includes either IV pentamidine isethionate or IV or oral trimethoprim-sulfamethoxazole (TMP-SMX). TMP-SMX is the preferred therapy because its efficacy is at least as good as that of pentamidine and TMP-SMX is better tolerated. Many patients, however, are sensitive to the sulfa drugs such as TMP-SMX, which may limit the medication treatment options. Other therapies that may be used include aerosolized pentamidine, trimetrexate, clindamycin/primaquine, or atovaquone. Table 71-5 summarizes information about pentamidine and TMP-SMX.

As with other ubiquitous infections, treatment of a *Pneumocystis* infection does not remove the risk of recurrence. Secondary prophylaxis therefore is recommended after a first episode of PCP. Primary prophylaxis is recommended for patients who have not developed PCP but whose T4 counts are less than 200 cells/μL. Primary or secondary prophylaxis may be accomplished by oral TMP/SMX daily or inhaled pentamidine monthly.

**TABLE 71-5 Drug Therapy for PCP**

| DRUG/ROUTE | SIDE EFFECTS | NURSING CONSIDERATIONS |
|---|---|---|
| **PENTAMIDINE ISETHIONATE** | | |
| IV | Blood dyscrasias, rapid irregular pulse, hyperglycemia, hypoglycemia, diabetes mellitus, skin rash, hypotension, pain or tenderness at site of injection, redness or flushing of the face, metallic taste in mouth | Monitor CBC.<br>Monitor vital signs during administration.<br>Monitor blood glucose.<br>Rotate injection sites. |
| Inhalation | Chest pain, congestion, coughing, dyspnea, pharyngitis, wheezing, skin rash, metallic taste in mouth, pneumothorax | Administer bronchodilators as indicated. Implement respiratory isolation precautions. |
| **TMP-SMX** | | |
| PO, IV | Hematologic: agranulocytosis, aplastic and megaloblastic anemia, hemolytic anemia.<br>Dermatologic: skin rash, itching, Stevens-Johnson syndrome<br>GI: dysphagia, nausea, vomiting, glossitis, stomatitis, hepatitis, pancreatitis<br>CNS: headache, peripheral neuritis, convulsions<br>Miscellaneous: drug fever, chills, and toxic necrosis with oliguria and anuria | Deaths associated with sulfonamides have been reported because of hypersensitivity reactions, agranulocytosis, aplastic anemia, and other blood dyscrasias.<br>Give oral preparations with full glass of water.<br>Monitor I & O.<br>Monitor blood counts.<br>Assess skin for eruptions. |

**Treatment.** Mechanical ventilation may improve the chance of survival for persons who develop respiratory failure. Aerosolized treatments with bronchodilating agents may be used for patients who develop bronchospasm. Pentamidine may be administered through inhalation therapy.

**Diet.** No special dietary restrictions or requirements exist.

**Activity.** There are no activity restrictions, although patients may be extremely short of breath, and safety precautions should be implemented to protect the patient.

**Referral/Consultation.** As with other serious opportunistic infections, patients with *Pneumocystis* infection may require multiple referrals. Social services, home nursing services, dietary, physical and occupational therapy, and psychiatry or counseling may be appropriate. Respiratory therapy also is required.

## NURSING MANAGEMENT

### ♦ ASSESSMENT

#### Subjective Data

Patients usually have a history of fever, fatigue, and weight loss for several weeks to months before respiratory symptoms develop. Patients usually complain of shortness of breath and cough.

#### Objective Data

Patients usually develop fevers greater than 101° F (38.3° C) and documented weight loss. Thrush is usually present and is indicative of significant immune system depletion. T4 cell counts are usually less than 200 cells/μL. Patients usually exhibit a nonproductive cough, although it may become productive as the pneumonia worsens. Shortness of breath is obvious, particularly on exertion.

#### Diagnostic Test Findings

Chest radiograph may reveal bilateral interstitial infiltrates, and arterial blood gas studies may reveal hypoxemia, hypocarbia, and an increase in the alveolar-arterial oxygen gradient. Bronchoscopy with biopsy reveals *P. carinii.*

### ♦ NURSING DIAGNOSES

Nursing diagnoses are determined from analysis of patient data. Nursing diagnoses for the patient with *P. carinii* pneumonia may include but are not limited to the following:

| Diagnostic Title | Possible Etiologic Factors |
|---|---|
| Gas exchange, impaired | Decreased competent alveolocapillary membrane area |
| Activity intolerance | Insufficient oxygen transport |
| Airway clearance, ineffective | Nonrelieved cough, viscous secretions |
| Pain | Muscle strain from chronic cough |
| Temperature, high risk for altered body | Infection |

### ♦ INTERVENTIONS

Zidovudine and PCP prophylaxis can greatly decrease the incidence and perhaps the severity of illness. PCP or disseminated pneumocystosis, however, may still develop, even in patients receiving primary or secondary PCP prophylaxis. Patient education therefore should include signs and symptoms of infection, including fevers, shortness of breath, and a nonproductive cough.

The effectiveness of aerosolized pentamidine therapy depends on several factors, including nebulizer used, tubing type, and the patient's ventilatory pattern. This therapy may also produce bronchospasm and/or coughing. Because tuberculosis is increasing in incidence in HIV-infected individuals, nurses must be sure to take appropriate infection control precautions during aerosol treatments. Respiratory failure may occur in patients with PCP. The nurse must address the patient's wishes regarding mechanical ventilation and other treatment choices.

#### Toxoplasmosis

*T. gondii* is a protozoan that occurs worldwide and infects both humans and domestic animals. The definitive hosts are members of the cat family, although not all cats are infected, and toxoplasmosis has been documented in locales without cats. The major means of transmission of *Toxoplasma* in humans is through ingestion of meats and vegetables containing oocysts. The prevalence of *Toxoplasma* tissue cysts in meat consumed by humans may be as high as 25%. Cockroaches, earthworms, snails, and slugs may serve as transport hosts for the oocysts. Approximately 50% of American adults have been infected with *Toxoplasma.* Human-to-human transmission is from mother to fetus, by blood transfusion, or by organ transplantation. Infection does not generally cause significant illness in healthy adult hosts. **Toxoplasmosis** is a major cause of encephalitis in persons with AIDS.

**Medical management**

**Diagnostic tests.** Because *Toxoplasma* usually causes encephalitis, definitive diagnosis generally requires brain biopsy. Presumptive diagnosis is most often accomplished by (1) brain imaging evidence of a lesion with a mass effect, (2) recent onset of focal neurologic abnormality, (3) serum antibody to toxoplasmosis or successful response to therapy for toxoplasmosis.

**Medication.** The primary therapy for toxoplasmosis in persons with AIDS is a combination of sulfadiazine and

**TABLE 71-6 Drug Therapy for Toxoplasmosis**

| DRUG/ROUTE | SIDE EFFECTS | NURSING CONSIDERATIONS |
|---|---|---|
| **SULFADIAZINE** | | |
| PO | Hematologic: agranulocytosis, aplastic anemia, thrombocytopenia, leukopenia<br>Hypersensitivity reactions: erythema multiforme (Stevens-Johnson syndrome), generalized skin eruptions, epidermal necrolysis | Monitor vital signs q 4 hr or as ordered. If fever suddenly increases or if temperature suddenly rises, inform physician immediately because this may be a sign of sensitization.<br>Hypersensitivity may be denoted by skin manifestations. |
| **PYRIMETHAMINE** | | |
| PO | Anorexia, vomiting, folic acid deficiency and megaloblastic anemia, leukopenia, thrombocytopenia, pancytopenia, and atrophic glossitis | Give with food or meals.<br>Monitor for folic acid deficiency.<br>Monitor CBC and platelet counts twice weekly.<br>Accidental ingestion by children has led to fatality. |
| **CLINDAMYCIN** | | |
| PO, IM, IV | GI: abdominal pain, esophagitis, nausea, vomiting, diarrhea, pseudomembranous colitis<br>Hypersensitivity reactions: maculopapular rash and urticaria<br>Hepatic: jaundice, abnormal liver function tests<br>Hematopoietic: transient leukopenia, eosinophilia, agranulocytosis, thrombocytopenia<br>With injections: pain, induration, and sterile abscess after IM; thrombophlebitis after IV | Single IM injections greater than 600 mg not recommended.<br>Administer deep IM injection; rotate injection sites.<br>Infuse IV over at least 10 to 60 minutes.<br>Record each bowel movement.<br>Observe for adverse effects, particularly hypersensitivity reactions and diarrhea. |

pyrimethamine (Table 71-6). Adjunctive therapy may include dexamethasone (Decadron) for cerebral inflammation associated with abscesses and phenytoin (Dilantin) for seizures induced by infection. Approximately 40% to 60% of patients may have severe adverse reactions during the initial treatment phase, however, and alternative regimens, including cessation of sulfadiazine or addition of clindamycin, may be required.[14]

As with most other opportunistic infections in patients with AIDS, long-term suppressive therapy is necessary. Pyrimethamine with or without sulfadiazine has been used for secondary prophylaxis. Primary prophylaxis may be warranted for patients with less than 100 T4 cells/μL. Primary prophylaxis is usually accomplished with pyrimethamine, 50 mg, or one double-strength TMP/SMX daily.

**Treatment.** No specific treatments exist for toxoplasmosis.

**Diet.** There are no specific dietary restrictions other than those required for appropriate medication therapy.

**Activity.** No specific activity restrictions exist. Patients with seizures or mental status changes may require safety precautions.

**Referral/Consultation.** As with other serious opportunistic infections, patients with toxoplasmosis may require multiple referrals. Referrals that may be appropriate are social services, home nursing services, dietary, physical and occupational therapy, and psychiatry or counseling.

## NURSING MANAGEMENT

### ♦ ASSESSMENT

#### Subjective Data

Complaints are often vague and nonspecific. Many patients complain of headache and altered mental status.

#### Objective Data

Mental status changes may present as confusion, lethargy, delusional behavior, frank psychosis, global cognitive impairment, or coma. Focal neurologic signs may include hemiparesis, aphasia, ataxia, visual field loss, cranial nerve palsies, dysmetria, or motor disorders. Approximately one third of AIDS patients with toxoplasmosis have seizures.[10]

#### Diagnostic Test Findings

The definitive diagnosis, neurosurgical brain biopsy, reveals the presence of *T. gondii* in the brain mass. Presumptive diagnosis, however, may utilize magnetic resonance imaging (MRI) or CT scanning, which reveals a mass effect with the appearance enhanced by injection of contrast medium. Laboratory work reveals a positive serum antibody titer to *T. gondii.*

### ♦ NURSING DIAGNOSES

Nursing diagnoses are determined from analysis of patient data. Nursing diagnoses for the patient with toxoplasmosis may include but are not limited to the following:

| Diagnostic Title | Possible Etiologic Factors |
|---|---|
| Injury (trauma), high risk for | Sensory deficit |
| Self-care deficit, total | Neurologic changes |
| Mobility, impaired physical | Limited use of extremities, hemiparesis |

## ♦ INTERVENTIONS

It is suspected that the appearance of toxoplasmosis in AIDS patients is actually caused by reactivation of a latent infection. Most patients, however, will not know whether they have been previously infected, and nurses therefore should teach patients about prevention of *Toxoplasma* infection. Key elements in prevention are (1) cooking all meats until they are well done, (2) washing fruits and vegetables thoroughly, and (3) wearing gloves when gardening or disposing of cat litter.

Toxoplasmosis generally requires brain biopsy for definitive diagnosis. Many patients refuse to undergo such procedures, and the procedure may be contraindicated in others. Presumptive diagnosis is most often used. Symptoms, however, are usually vague and often ignored, by both the patient and the caregiver. In addition, the appearance of neurologic symptoms can suggest any number of opportunistic infections and neoplastic processes.

## VIRAL INFECTIONS

Viral infections in HIV-positive patients usually involve reactivations of the various herpes viruses. Early in the course of HIV disease, reactivation of the herpes zoster virus may erupt as shingles, producing skin eruptions and fever. This infection typically responds to acyclovir therapy and is not generally considered one of the major opportunistic infections. In addition, herpes simplex infections occur with varying frequency among many patients. Patients who have had herpes simplex infections previously may notice more prolonged outbreaks and perhaps more frequent outbreaks of skin lesions. Most patients respond to acyclovir therapy, although higher doses may be used in this patient population and resistant strains may emerge. The most significant opportunistic viral infection is caused by cytomegalovirus.

### Cytomegalovirus

Infection with **cytomegalovirus (CMV)** is widely distributed throughout the world and is usually asymptomatic. Seroprevalence ranges from 30% to 100% in the general U.S. population.[9] CMV is a herpesvirus; as with other herpesviruses, it remains dormant in tissues after initial infection and is then reactivated. CMV is one of two known etiologic agents of mononucleosis (the other is the Epstein-Barr virus).

Most individuals originally contract CMV either (1) during the perinatal period, (2) throughout the preschool years, or (3) during the sexually active years. CMV can be acquired as intrauterine or congenital infection, via vaginal delivery through a contaminated cervix, from breast milk, or by transmission from child to child in day-care centers. Infected children carry the virus in the respiratory tract and urine. Among the adult population, CMV has been isolated from both semen and cervical secretions. Kissing and spread through saliva are also a probable means of CMV transmission. Transfusion of blood products and transplantation of organs or tissues may also be responsible for transmission.

CMV may destroy tissue in sites such as the brain, lungs, retina, or liver. Immunologic responses also may occur, resulting in hemolytic anemia, thrombocytopenia, or neoplastic transformation. Patients with HIV disease can remain asymptomatic or exhibit various clinical manifestations, such as chorioretinitis, pneumonitis, encephalitis, adrenalitis, colitis, esophagitis, cholangitis, and hepatitis.

#### Medical management

**Diagnostic tests.** CMV infection is present in most American adults and must be distinguished from CMV disease. The diagnosis of CMV disease is based on microscopic identification of CMV inclusion bodies or positive cultures from specific organs such as the brain, lung, liver, and adrenal glands. CMV chorioretinitis is presumptively diagnosed based on the loss of vision and characteristic ophthalmologic findings. CMV adrenalitis is also most often diagnosed based on presumptive criteria, which include adrenal insufficiency and isolation of CMV from the blood.

**Medication.** Ganciclovir is the primary treatment for CMV retinitis and is under investigation for use in other sites of infection as well. More recently, an alternative agent, foscarnet, has also become available. Other agents that have been used and are in ongoing clinical trials include acyclovir, alpha-interferon, and combination therapy with ganciclovir, foscarnet, and immune globulin. Table 71-7 reviews drugs used in CMV.

**Treatment.** No special treatments exist for persons with CMV disease.

**Diet.** There are no specific diet restrictions for persons with CMV disease.

**Activity.** No activity restrictions exist. Protective precautions must be considered in patients with impaired vision.

**Referral/Consultation.** As with other serious opportunistic infections, patients with CMV may require multiple referrals. Social services, home nursing services,

**TABLE 71-7 Drug Therapy for CMV**

| DRUG/ROUTE | SIDE EFFECTS | NURSING CONSIDERATIONS |
|---|---|---|
| **GANCICLOVIR** | | |
| IV | Hematologic: granulocytopenia, thrombocytopenia, anemia<br>CNS: mood changes, tremor, nervousness<br>GI: abdominal pain, anorexia, nausea, vomiting, abnormal liver function tests<br>Miscellaneous: skin rash, phlebitis | Monitor CBC twice weekly and liver enzymes weekly.<br>Assess for CNS effects.<br>Monitor for nutritional adequacy.<br>Monitor for phlebitis in peripheral lines. |
| **FOSCARNET** | | |
| IV | Renal insufficiency<br>Hematologic: anemia, granulocytopenia<br>GI: nausea, vomiting<br>Miscellaneous: headache, fatigue, paresthesias, hypomagnesemia, hypocalcemia | Monitor serum creatinine, calcium, magnesium, phosphorus, and potassium weekly.<br>Monitor CBC twice weekly.<br>Assess nutritional adequacy.<br>Monitor for paresthesias. |

dietary, physical and occupational therapy, and psychiatry or counseling may be appropriate. Ophthalmology services will also be required for patients with retinitis or to monitor for retinitis.

# NURSING MANAGEMENT

## ♦ ASSESSMENT

### Subjective Data

Most immunocompetent adults will have fever and fatigue caused by the mononucleosis associated with CMV. Patients with HIV disease may remain asymptomatic or have various clinical complaints. CMV retinitis is typically accompanied by complaints of visual changes such as blurred vision, decreased vision, or presence of floaters. Although infection usually affects only one eye early in disease, if left untreated, the infection will spread bilaterally. Patients with pulmonary infection may complain of shortness of breath, dyspnea on exertion, and a dry, nonproductive cough with or without fever. Virtually all parts of the GI tract, from the oral cavity to the perianal area, have been reported as sites of CMV infection. Patients with esophageal ulceration may have odynophagia and dysphagia. Weight loss and anorexia may be associated with CMV colitis.

### Objective Data

On fundoscopic examination, patients with CMV retinitis have one or many small, granular white lesions or wounds that coalesce and spread or hemorrhage in a crisscross pattern along the blood vessels. Pulmonary infection may be characterized by a nonproductive cough and wheezing or hoarseness. GI infection is usually associated with weight loss, which may be greater than 10% to 20% of the patient's usual body weight. Adrenal manifestations may include postural hypotension and sodium deficits.

### Diagnostic Test Findings

CMV retinitis is presumptively diagnosed on fundoscopic examination, as described previously. Adrenalitis reveals adrenal insufficiency on laboratory assessment (see Chapter 39) with a positive blood culture of CMV. Other organ involvement is typically diagnosed based on microscopic identification of CMV inclusion bodies or positive cultures from specific organs such as the brain, lung, liver, and gut.

## ♦ NURSING DIAGNOSES

Nursing diagnoses are determined from analysis of patient data. Nursing diagnoses for the patient with CMV may include but are not limited to the following:

| Diagnostic Title | Possible Etiologic Factors |
|---|---|
| Injury (trauma), high risk for | Sensory (visual) defect |
| Self-care deficit, total | Visual deficit, fatigue |
| Nutrition, altered: less than body requirements | Anorexia, difficulty in chewing or swallowing, inability to prepare food |
| Fluid volume deficit | Abnormal fluid loss from diarrhea |
| Activity intolerance | Insufficient oxygen transport, nutritional deficiencies, diarrhea, fluid loss |

## ♦ INTERVENTIONS

CMV retinitis can result in permanent blindness if not treated early and aggressively. For many patients with HIV disease, CMV retinitis represents one of the most feared opportunistic infections. Patients taking concurrent AZT and ganciclovir may be at significant risk for red cell destruction and anemia and granulocytopenia, specifically neutropenia, since both these agents can cause similar side effects. Before the use of growth factors, patients were often forced to make a decision about taking AZT to combat the HIV infection or taking ganciclovir to treat the CMV, which, if left untreated, would

## NURSING CARE PLAN

### PERSON WITH HIV COMPLICATIONS/AIDS

**DATA:** Mr. C. is a 32-year-old computer programmer. He was born in a small town in the Midwest but has lived on the West Coast for the past 10 years. He has had little contact with his family because of the painful situation when he left home; his family was "disgraced" because he was gay. For the last 5 years, he has been living with his lover, Mr. J. Mr. C. reveals that before moving in with Mr. J., he had multiple homosexual and heterosexual experiences. Mr. J. and Mr. C. have lived in a monogamous relationship for the last 3 years. Mr. C. describes Mr. J. as a "dependent" person who rarely "hangs onto a job for very long." Mr. C. is being admitted to the hospital for a medical evaluation of 4 months of fatigue not relieved with sleep. He has lost 20 pounds and reports night sweats that frequently awaken him, a rectal rash, and a dry cough with fevers. Mr. C.'s illness has caused him to use all his sick time from work, and he is afraid he will lose his job. He also says he is terrified that he might be dying. Mr. J. also reports that his friend has intermittent confusion.

The nursing history identified the following:

- Mr. C. has multiple risk factors for contracting the HIV infection, including multiple sexual partners, homosexual lifestyle, and anal intercourse.
- Mr. C. has several persistent clinical symptoms or evidence of new clinical symptoms indicative of HIV infection: fatigue, weight loss, dry cough, fevers, and a rectal rash.
- Mr. C. has multiple sources of stress, including his alienation from family members because of his sexual orientation, possible loss of his job because of his persistent illness, and his concern over his lover's ability to cope with stress while Mr. C. is ill.

Collaborative nursing activities include:

- Assessment of Mr. C.'s understanding of HIV testing, AIDS, and treatment regimens
- Assessment of progression of clinical symptoms or evidence of new clinical symptoms indicating complications such as infections and altered cognitive function
- Referral to a social service agency for investigation of health disability insurance and unemployment benefits
- Assessment and possible referral for mental health counseling for Mr. C. and Mr. J.

Nursing activities include monitoring the following:

- Temperature
- Daily food and fluid intake and weight
- Cognitive ability and neurologic status
- Ability to care for self
- Spread of, or drainage from, rectal rash
- Lung sounds and sputum production
- Appetite, ability to sleep, ability to discuss concerns, and other clinical indicators of anxiety or depression
- Laboratory results of ELISA, Western blot, T-cell ratios, WBCs, prothrombin time (PT), partial thromboplastin time (PTT), and serum electrolytes
- Support systems

#### NURSING DIAGNOSIS

Fear related to persistent debilitating, terminal illness; threatened loss of independence, job, and social relationships

| Expected Patient Outcome | Nursing Interventions | Rationale |
|---|---|---|
| Mr. C. and Mr. J. identify previous coping strategies for stress. Verbalize sources of fear. Identify possible coping strategies for present fears. Articulate decreased symptoms of fear such as anorexia and sleeplessness. | Acknowledge multiple sources of stress as evidenced from history.<br>Explore with Mr. C. past life crises and strategies of coping, as well as sources of support.<br>Spend time with Mr. C., explaining procedures and treatments.<br>Spend uninterrupted time with Mr. C. and Mr. J. individually to allow for empathic listening.<br>Monitor for increasing anxiety and report to physician.<br>Assess for depression and suicidal ideation. | Patterns of past successful coping are indicators of present resources and strengths.<br>Empathy as a counseling therapy utilizes realistic descriptive stressors, reflective listening, physical presence, and clarification.<br>Anxiety may increase with procedures and terminal diagnosis. |

*Continued.*

# NURSING CARE PLAN

## PERSON WITH HIV COMPLICATIONS/AIDS—cont'd

### ■ NURSING DIAGNOSIS

Knowledge deficit: HIV risk factors, disease transmission, test significance, HIV pathophysiology related to lack of exposure

| Expected Patient Outcome | Nursing Interventions | Rationale |
|---|---|---|
| Describes rationale of diagnostic tests, HIV risk factors, strategies for prevention of HIV transmission, and treatment measures. | Using discussion with repetition and printed materials, review diagnostic tests such as ELISA, Western blot, and T-cell ratios; risk factors and prevention strategies of HIV infection; clinical symptoms of HIV infection; and treatment measures. | Patients have a right to information related to health. This information will promote their ability to make decisions to prevent disease and to seek medical treatment to alleviate symptoms and complications.<br>Fear decreases ability to take in information and requires repetition and multiple learning strategies. |

### ■ NURSING DIAGNOSIS

Altered nutrition, less than body requirements, related to diarrhea

| Expected Patient Outcomes | Nursing Interventions | Rationale |
|---|---|---|
| Describes a meal plan with adequate calories and hydration.<br>Ceases to lose weight.<br>Serum albumin, potassium, and sodium remain within normal limits. | Plan with Mr. C. and nutritionist a daily schedule of six small meals, including 3000 ml of fluids and 3000 calories and excluding dairy products and raw fruits and vegetables. | Small meals prevent gastric distention and nausea; 2500-3000 ml provides adequate hydration for febrile adult; 3000 calories prevents weight loss and negative nitrogen balance.<br>Lactose in dairy products may enhance diarrhea; raw foods contain naturally occurring microorganisms that may increase infection in immunocompromised hosts. |
| | Plan routine oral care and rinses before and after meals. | Oral care before meals enhances appetite and flow of digestive juices; oral care after meals helps to prevent oral lesions and infections. |
| | Assist Mr. C. to be out of bed or sitting up. | Upright positioning prevents aspiration and pneumonia. |
| | Weigh Mr. C. daily at same time on same scale with same clothes and record. | Weight is a clinical indicator of adequate nutrition. |

### ■ NURSING DIAGNOSIS

Fatigue related to weight loss and sleeplessness

| Expected Patient Outcome | Nursing Interventions | Rationale |
|---|---|---|
| Sleeps 6-8 hours at night, is independent in ADL, and states decreased feelings of fatigue. | Plan and teach Mr. C. about pacing activity and use of energy conservation measures.<br>Include in plan uninterrupted period for sleep. | Pacing of activity and energy conservation conserves patient's energy balanced with activity. |
| | Review with Mr. C. relaxation techniques at bedtime, such as deep breathing, tepid baths, use of a radio, and meditation. | Relaxation promotes comfort and contributes to sleep. |
| | Increase nutritional intake.<br>Assist with ADL; encourage patient participation. | Increased intake provides calories for energy consumption, thereby decreasing some fatigue. |

## NURSING CARE PLAN

### PERSON WITH HIV COMPLICATIONS/AIDS—cont'd

#### ■ NURSING DIAGNOSIS

Impaired skin integrity related to genital herpes; high risk for impaired skin integrity related to malnourishment and immobility

| Expected Patient Outcomes | Nursing Interventions | Rationale |
|---|---|---|
| Rectal rash heals; reports increased comfort.<br>Herpes infection does not spread on Mr. C.'s body or to caregivers. | Assist Mr. C. to clean rectal area after each episode of diarrhea using a mild soap such as liquid Dove soap; use gloves and good handwashing after cleaning. | Herpes rashes cause local irritation and discomfort; healing is promoted by gentle cleaning, allowing regeneration of epidermis. |
| Further skin breakdown does not occur. | Assist Mr. C. to turn in bed at least every 2 hours. | Decreased pressure promotes healing and comfort by increased circulation. |
| | Assist Mr. C. with daily bathing; encourage shower, avoid tub baths. For basin baths, use clean washcloth for rash area and do not reuse. | Daily hygiene prevents secondary infections and spread of existing infections. Showers provide continued washing away of microorganisms. |
| | Apply gloves (self or Mr. C.) for cleansing or application of medications to rash. | Herpes and other rashes may be spread to patient and caregiver by skin contact. |

#### ■ NURSING DIAGNOSIS

Altered thought processes related to neurologic effects of HIV infections and the complications

| Expected Patient Outcome | Nursing Interventions | Rationale |
|---|---|---|
| Remains safe within his environment. | Assess orientation.<br>Reorient as needed.<br>Assess environmental safety, including nightlights and cues such as clocks, calendars, and newspapers.<br>Be consistent in daily routines and care.<br>Use short repetitive phrases.<br>Provide verbal reassurance. | Infections cause increased intracranial pressure, resulting in confusion or dementia. Consistency, repetition, and cues help to decrease confusion. |

almost certainly lead to blindness. Fortunately, we now have the ability to use growth factors to stimulate the neutrophils, and most patients are able to continue both ganciclovir and AZT therapy. Although ganciclovir is most widely used, foscarnet offers another option for therapy. The primary dose-limiting toxicity of foscarnet is nephrotoxicity.

## HIV ENCEPHALOPATHY

HIV itself may invade the CNS, causing **HIV encephalopathy** or **dementia.** It is believed that about 60% of all HIV-infected individuals have HIV encephalopathy. Initially, encephalopathy may be manifested by progressive loss or decline in cognitive, motor, or behavioral function. Early signs of HIV encephalopathy are subtle and may be confused with normal grieving and depression. These signs include reduced concentration, slowness of speech, and impaired memory. As HIV encephalopathy progresses, dementia results with further decline in the individual's ability to walk, control body functions, perform self-care, and make decisions. HIV encephalopathy may progress to coma. Treatment is primarily palliative and supportive. AZT has been used with some improvement in neurologic function in the early stages of the disease.

Although some patients with altered thought processes may be acutely aware of their deficits and need for assistance with ADL, others may have little insight into these needs (see Chapter 12). A major focus of nursing care for patients with cognitive impairment is the support and education of caregivers. Caregivers require instruction and supervision in patient bathing, positioning, skin care, oral care, transferring, use of assistive devices, range of motion exercises, feeding and nutrition, bowel and bladder management, and environmental safety, including infection control measures. Patients who are aware of declining cognitive abilities and the terminal nature of their HIV infection are at high risk for suicide. Therefore all patients with a diagnosis of HIV infection should be assessed for depression and suicide ideation. Referral to mental health professionals for caregivers with extreme grief and care burdens, as well as for depressed patients, can be useful in addressing quality-of-life issues despite terminal illness.

### HIV-RELATED CANCERS

*Malignant lymphomas of the CNS are common in patients with HIV infection and often indicate poor prognosis.* These lymphomas include non-Hodgkin's lymphoma and Burkitt's-like lymphomas (see Chapter 34). Clinical symptoms include malaise, myalgias, lymphadenopathy, and abdominal discomforts associated with weight loss.

**Kaposi's sarcoma (KS)** is by far *the most common neoplasm found in patients with HIV infection.* KS affects vascular epithelium and results in reddish purple cutaneous lesions (see Chapter 67). Lesions may appear on the trunk, arms, legs, head, and neck. Extracutaneous lesions may also occur in mucous membranes, lymph nodes, lungs, and the GI tract. KS tumors can block lymphatic drainage, resulting in severe edema to the face or extremities. Pulmonary lesions may result in respiratory distress and even death. Although some patients have no clinical symptoms associated with KS, others complain of malaise, weight loss, swollen lymph nodes, generalized edema, and shortness of breath. KS may be diagnosed by tissue biopsy. Radiation therapy, chemotherapy, and interferon may be used in some progressive forms of KS lesions.

Symptoms of KS depend on involved body systems. KS may invade cutaneous tissue, causing edema and skin lesions; lung tissue, causing dyspnea and a productive cough; GI system, causing diarrhea; or the brain, causing cognitive changes and gait disturbances. Radiation therapy, chemotherapy, and interferon have been used in the treatment of KS lesions, although some patients may develop additional complications of therapy.

Nursing care priorities for patients depend on the particular system affected by KS. Care considerations include skin care of lesions, promoting comfortable ventilation, and maintaining a safe environment. Prevention of the effects of edema may be a major nursing care strategy for patients with KS. Elevating the head of the bed or affected extremities may produce some relief. Facial edema may be alleviated by cool compresses. Maintaining skin integrity despite edema and radiation therapy is indeed challenging.

Gentle massages with creams and oils help promote drainage, reduce discomfort, and prevent skin breakdown. KS lesions that are dry may be left open to the air. For draining KS lesions, cleansing with mild soap and patting dry, applying normal saline wet dressings, or applying bacitracin and neomycin creams and covering with nonadhering dressings such as Telfa may provide some comfort and prevent the spread of lesions. Similar to patients with PCP, patients with pulmonary KS require nursing interventions to reduce dyspnea and promote comfortable effective airway clearance.

Cervical cancer, related in part to concomitant human papillomavirus (HPV) infection, occurs at an increased rate in women who are HIV positive. (See Chapter 52 for clinical signs and symptoms and care.)

## SOCIAL, ETHICAL, AND LEGAL ISSUES

The HIV pandemic has brought with it not only a dismal prognosis, but also severe social stigmatization, public fear, and a growing number of legal and ethical issues. Nurses providing care in a variety of settings will face many of these issues, which may jeopardize the quality of patient care. In addition, nurses caring for patients with the HIV infection will face many personal stresses, including fear of personal contamination and disease transmission to family members and burnout related to caring for terminally ill young patients with controversial life-styles. The professional commitment needed by nurses who provide care to HIV-infected patients requires clarification of personal values regarding the issues of homosexuality and drug use.

Inherent in nursing is a respect for life, dignity, and social justice. The American Nurses Association (ANA) Code of Ethics clearly reaffirms that the profession of nursing provides services with respect for human dignity and the uniqueness of each patient, unrestricted by social or economic status, personal attributes, or the nature of health problems.

The very nature of nurses' work constitutes a level of risk for various diseases that does not exist in other professions. In upholding the moral principle of justice, risks and withholding of care must be carefully balanced with potential benefits of care. In addition, individual nurses and institutions have a responsibility to take reasonable precautions to protect caregivers from harm while providing medical and nursing care to patients.

As long as the HIV infection remains a downhill continuum with multiple complications and eventual death, nurses caring for patients with progressive AIDS will be involved in decisions regarding the selective withholding of treatment while preserving the quality of life and human dignity. The role of nursing in the terminal phase of illness is a critical one. When no medical treatments can be offered to the patient, nursing has everything to offer, including providing physical care that makes the patient more comfortable, identifying values, exploring the meaning of life with the patient and significant others, supporting bonds between the patient and significant others, and providing comfort measures and support that will allow the patient to have a peaceful death.

Nurses must continually help the health care team, family, and significant others to focus on the patients' desires. This principle of autonomy, as endorsed by the ANA, is a valuable guide for many ethical decisions regarding terminally ill patients. Nurse caregivers providing such intense physical and psychologic care also need support. Peer support through informal sharing or a structured support group is an effective strategy that may alleviate feelings of helplessness.

Legal issues such as confidentiality, mandatory testing, employee screening, and school attendance of children infected with HIV remain controversial. Therefore it will be important for all nurses to keep themselves informed of policy developments and to influence, whenever possible, such decisions based on the ethical principle of justice. (For further information about ethical issues, see Research boxes.)

## RESEARCH

Flaskerud JH, Lewis MA, Shin D: Changing nurses' AIDS-related knowledge and attitudes through continuing education, *J Cont Ed Nurs* 20(4):148-154, 1989.

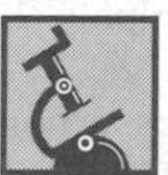

The purpose of this study was to measure changes in nurses' knowledge and attitudes following attendance at a continuing education conference. The conference topics included epidemiology of AIDS, infection control, sexual history taking, counseling, and psychosocial and institutional support for health care workers. Using a pretest, posttest, and a 3-month follow-up structured questionnaire, the researchers found significant increases in knowledge and attitude scores.

## RESEARCH

Martin DA: Effects of ethical dilemmas on stress felt by nurses providing care to AIDS patients, *Crit Care Nurs Q* 12:53-62, 1990.

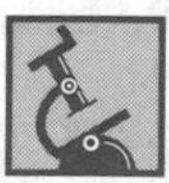

The purpose of this study was to examine the nature and prevalence of ethical dilemmas encountered by nurses who provide care to patients hospitalized with AIDS-related illnesses. Half the nurses reported a high degree of emotional exhaustion. However, a correlation existed between overall years of nursing experience and ability to cope. *The most frequent dilemmas reported were related to issues of dying and "do not resuscitate" orders. The second category of dilemmas surrounded issues of pain and symptom management.* Coping strategies ranged from venting emotions to deciding to leave the nursing unit or institution.

## QUESTIONS TO CONSIDER

- You are preparing a family to provide home care for their son with AIDS. What learning needs must you assess?
- Explain why the rate of cancers such as non-Hodgkin's lymphomas or Kaposi's sarcoma is relatively high in patients with AIDS. Are there other conditions or diseases in which you would observe this same phenomenon?
- How does infection with HIV differ from the disease AIDS?
- Explain why persons with AIDS are susceptible to infection.

## CRITICAL THINKING ACTIVITIES

- Before caring for an HIV-infected patient, what things should you consider?
- The local school has asked you to give a presentation on AIDS. What information will you include? What teaching strategies and media might be helpful?
- One of your peers confides that she is HIV positive. What ethical principles can help guide your response to her?

## CHAPTER SUMMARY

### ETIOLOGY

- The human immunodeficiency virus (HIV), a retrovirus, is the cause of acquired immunodeficiency syndrome (AIDS).

### EPIDEMIOLOGY

- The routes of HIV transmission are (1) intimate sexual contact; (2) parenteral exposure to blood, blood-containing body fluids, and blood products; and (3) from mother to child during the perinatal period.

### PATHOPHYSIOLOGY

- HIV causes gradual destruction of the immune system, targeting primarily the T4 helper lymphocytes.

### PREVENTION

- Testing for HIV is accomplished through the use of an antibody test; most individuals produce antibodies within 6 weeks to 3 months of exposure.
- Most HIV-positive individuals remain relatively asymptomatic as their T4 helper cell counts decrease to about 500 cells/µL (from an average count among the normal population of about 1000 cells/µL).
- AZT (zidovudine) therapy is usually initiated in asymptomatic patients with CD4 counts less than 500 cells/µL.
- As immune system depletion progresses, CD4 counts decrease and patients are at higher risk for opportunistic infections, cancers, and HIV encephalopathy.

## MEDICAL MANAGEMENT

- Currently, no known cure exists for HIV infection, but we have been able to extend survival with early-intervention antiretroviral therapy and appropriate primary and secondary prophylaxis against opportunistic infections.

## NURSING MANAGEMENT

- Nursing care in early stages focuses on preventing infection, maintaining adequate nutrition, helping the patient cope, promoting home maintenance management, decreasing fatigue, maintaining self-care, preventing social isolation, and controlling fear.
- Most nursing care is delivered in the outpatient setting.
- Teaching is a major intervention.
- Prevention of infections and treatment of active infections are major goals of care.

## COMPLICATIONS

- Most opportunistic infections are caused by reactivation of previous infectious organisms; most organisms are ubiquitous and are often widespread in the general population, although they typically do not cause disease with a competent immune system.
- Bacterial infections include *Mycobacterium avium* complex (MAC), which causes fever, diarrhea, and profound wasting.
- Fungal infections include (1) candidiasis, which often presents as thrush or as a vaginal infection; (2) cryptococcosis, which causes meningitis; and (3) histoplasmosis, which causes disseminated infection with fevers and weight loss.
- Protozoal infections include (1) cryptosporidiosis, which causes fulminant diarrhea and has no known therapy; (2) *Pneumocystis carinii* infection, which usually presents as pneumonia and may progress to acute respiratory failure; or (3) toxoplasmosis, which usually causes encephalitis.
- Viral infections include cytomegalovirus (CMV) infection, which most often causes retinitis; if not treated, this leads to permanent blindness.
- Most opportunistic infections are not eliminated from the body and require secondary prophylaxis to prevent recurrence.
- The HIV virus can cross the blood-brain barrier, attach to microglial cells, and cause encephalopathy or neuropathy and motor dysfunction.
- Non-Hodgkin's lymphomas, Kaposi's sarcoma, and cervical cancer occur because of the depression of T4 lymphocytes.

## SOCIAL, ETHICAL, AND LEGAL ISSUES

- HIV infection and AIDS are still associated with many social and ethical concerns.

## REFERENCES

1. Agency for Health Care Policy and Research: *Evaluation and management of early HIV infection,* Rockville, Md, 1994, US Department of Health and Human Services.
2. Centers for Disease Control: The HIV/AIDS epidemic: the first 10 years, *MMWR* 40(22):357-375, 1991.
3. Centers for Disease Control: Update: acquired immunodeficiency syndrome: United States, 1992, *MMWR* 42(28):547-557, 1993.
4. Centers for Disease Control: Zidovudine for the prevention of HIV transmission from mother to infant, *MMWR* 43(16):285-289, 1994.
5. Fischl M, Volberding P: *Antiviral therapy: clinical implications of early infection,* New York, NY, 1992, World Health Communications.

5a. Flaskerud JH, Lewis MA, Shinn D: Changing nurses' AIDS-related knowledge and attitudes through continuing education, *J Cont Ed Nurs* 20(4):148-154, 1989.

6. Flaskerud J, Ungvarski P: *HIV/AIDS: a guide to nursing care,* Philadelphia, 1992, Saunders.
7. Gee G: *AIDS: concepts in nursing practice,* Baltimore, 1988, Williams & Wilkins.
8. Gordin F: *Mycobacterium avium* complex (MAC): natural history and clinical issues, *Opportunistic Complications HIV* 2(1):1-5, 1993.
9. Ho DD: Cytomegalovirus. In Mandell GL, Douglas RG, Bennett JE, editors: *Principles and practices of infectious disease,* New York, 1990, Churchill Livingstone.
10. Israelski DM, Dannemann BR, Remington JS: Toxoplasmosis in patients with AIDS. In Sande MA, Volberding PA, editors: *The medical management of AIDS,* ed 2, Philadelphia, 1990, Saunders.
11. Lucey D: The first decade of human retroviruses: a nomenclature for the clinician, *Mil Med* 156(10):555-557, 1991.
12. Lusso P, Gallo R: Pathogenesis of AIDS, *J Pharm Pharmacol* 44(suppl 1):160-164, 1992.
13. Mann J: Global AIDS: further evolution of the pandemic and the response, *HIV Advisor* 7(3):3-8, 1993.

13a. Martin DA: Effects of ethical dilemmas on stress felt by nurses providing care to AIDS patient, *Crit Care Nurs Q* 12:53-62, 1990.

14. McCabe RE, Remington JS: *Toxoplasma gondii.* In Mandell GL, Douglas RG, Bennett JE, editors: *Principles and practice of infectious diseases,* New York, 1990, Churchill Livingstone.
15. McKinsey DS, Gupta MR: Histoplasmosis in patients with AIDS: efficacy of maintenance amphotericin B therapy, *Am J Med* 92:225-227, 1992.
16. National Institute of Allergy and Infectious Disease: *AZT reduces rate of maternal transmission of HIV,* Washington, DC, 1994, National Institutes of Health.
17. Smith D: Progress on opportunistic infections, *PI Perspect,* February, 1993, pp 15-21.
18. Tinkle M, Amaya M, Tamayo O: HIV disease and pregnancy, *Jobstet Gynecol Neonatal Nurs* 21(2):86-92, 1992.
19. Torres G, Link D: Opportunistic infections update, *Treatment Issues* 8(1):12-16, 1994.
20. US Department of Health and Human Services, Public Health Service: *Healthy people 2000: national health promotion and disease prevention objectives,* Washington, DC, 1990, US Government Printing Office.

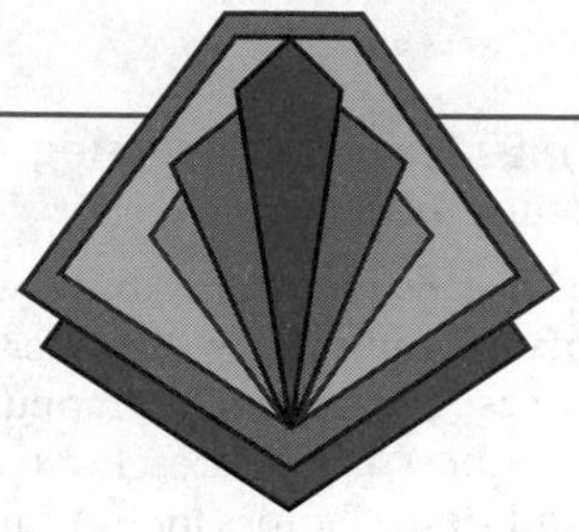

C H A P T E R 72

# Management of Persons With Organ/Tissue Transplants

*Virginia L. Cassmeyer*

## CHAPTER OBJECTIVES

***After studying this chapter, the learner should be able to do the following:***

1 Describe the criteria used to select candidates for various transplants.
2 Describe donor criteria for selected organs or tissues.
3 Discuss legislative activity that has been initiated to increase the supply of organs/tissues and to enhance fairness in the distribution of organs/tissues.
4 Describe the three types of rejections of allogenic transplants and the immunology underlying rejection.
5 Discuss the type of histocompatibility testing and matching conducted for various transplants.
6 Explain the action and major adverse effects of the five most common drugs used to prevent and treat acute rejection.
7 List the major infections for which the immunosuppressed transplant recipient is at high risk.
8 Describe the general nursing diagnoses and care needs of the potential transplant recipient, the patient before transplantation, and the patient after transplantation.
9 Design care plans that list the common needs and interventions for persons who have had corneal, renal, liver, pancreatic, heart, lung, or bone marrow transplants.

## KEY TERMS

acute rejection
alleles
allogenic bone marrow transplantation
allografts
autografts
autologous bone marrow transplantation
chronic rejection
corneal grafting (keratoplasty)
graft-versus-host disease (GVHD)
human leukocyte antigen (HLA)
hyperacute rejection
major histocompatibility complex
preformed circulating cytotoxic antibodies
rejection
xenografts

Organ transplantation has moved from being a medical experiment to being a major therapeutic intervention in selected patients. Persons with certain types of end-stage diseases can now be offered survival and improved quality of life. For many persons the term *transplantation* means whole organ transplants. However, many types of tissues are transplanted. The following are some common tissue transplants:

1. Whole blood or components
2. Cornea
3. Tendon, ligament, fascia, dura mater
4. Bone
5. Heart valve
6. Skin
7. Bone marrow
8. Pancreatic islet cells

The following are some organs that are frequently transplanted:

1. Kidney
2. Liver
3. Heart

The section on kidney transplantation has been revised by M.R. Bartucci.

**BOX 72-1 Transplant Definitions**

**AUTOGRAFTS**

Transplantation of tissue from one part of the body to another; examples include skin, bone, veins, fascia, blood, bone marrow, adrenal medulla

**ALLOGRAFTS**

Transplantation of tissue or organs from one member of a species to another member of the same species; examples include all types of tissues and organs listed; fetal tissue

**XENOGRAFTS**

Transplantation of tissue from a member of one species to a member of another species; examples include heart valves and skin; "Baby Fae case"—situation in which baboon heart was used in newborn

4. Lung
5. Heart-lungs
6. Pancreas

Although various types of transplantations can be performed, including **autografts, allografts,** and **xenografts** (Box 72-1), this chapter focuses on allograft transplantation of solid organs, corneas, and bone marrow.

# TRANSPLANTATION CRITERIA

## CRITERIA FOR RECIPIENTS

Transplantation of hearts, lungs, heart-lung in total, livers, kidneys, and pancreas and/or islet cells is considered for patients who have end-stage organ/system failure and who do not respond to conventional therapy or whose condition is worsening despite aggressive management. The patient must be free of irreversible infections, unresectable malignancies, or concurrent illnesses that make the risk of surgery unacceptably high. In addition, there should be no anatomic problems that would make transplantation impossible. Also, the therapeutic benefits of the transplantation to the recipient and the recipient's ability to pay for the transplantation are important criteria in selecting recipients.

**Allogenic bone marrow transplantation** is used not only when failure of the bone marrow occurs, such as in severe aplastic anemia or severe combined immunodeficiency disease, but also in some cases of leukemia and lymphoma to replace the bone marrow after high doses of chemotherapy or irradiation. **Autologous bone marrow transplantation** also is used after high doses of chemotherapy or irradiation. In relation to this later use of autologous bone marrow transplantations, peripherally recovered stem cells are being used in some situations. Both types of bone marrow transplantation are described in this chapter.

### Potential Factors Considered in Assessing Recipients for Transplantations

Because the supply of organs and bone marrow is limited, individual transplant centers may consider various factors besides the disease status and therapeutic benefits in deciding on the best candidates for transplantation. Some of these additional factors include age, functional ability, psychologic status, family support, perceived ability to manage postransplantation regimen, rehabilitation potential, ability to return to work, and improved quality or length of life. The citizenship of the recipient has been recommended as a consideration for kidney transplants.[14,18] The age range for recipients has been broadened considerably. In a few situations or centers, the patient's responsibility for his or her disease involvement, such as abuse of alcohol leading to liver failure, is considered.[7,16] In the past, some centers considered the patient's contributions or benefits to society, but that is not considered at this time. No one center considers all these factors. In some centers the only criteria are disease status, improved quality of life, desire and ability to handle posttransplantation regimen, and available financial reimbursement for the transplantation.

### Payment for Transplantation

A major issue in relation to transplantation is reimbursement for the procedure. At this writing, before a transplantation is undertaken, the financial reimbursement for that transplant must be clearly identified. Medicare covers the cost of kidney transplantation for anyone who meets Social Security, disability, and Medicare requirements. Also, Medicare covers the cost of liver transplantations for selected conditions at approved centers. Heart transplantations at approved centers also are covered by Medicare. A limited number of transplantations are covered by state programs and the Veterans' Administration. Many third-party payors cover the cost of selected extrarenal transplants, such as heart, liver, and heart-lung, but consider pancreatic and lung transplants experimental and will not reimburse for these. Third-party payors also cover the non—Medicare-covered aspects of renal transplantation or the total coverage if the person is not eligible for social security, disability, and Medicare. However, many persons are uninsured and therefore are not eligible for any transplantation. The issue of whether organ/tissue transplantations of all types should be available to everyone needing them without regard to ability to pay is being discussed continually at public forums as this and other health care concerns are discussed.

### Allocation of Transplant Tissue/Organs

Because of the shortage of organs for transplantation, various legislative acts have been passed to (1) increase the supply of organs and (2) ensure the fair allocation of donated tissues/organs. The present criteria for allocating extrarenal transplants are (1) blood type, (2) size, (3) medical urgency, (4) geographic location, and (5) waiting time.[9] The distribution of kidneys is based on a point system. Each patient on the waiting list for a kidney transplantation is assigned points based on the quality of the human leukocyte antigen (HLA) match, waiting time, level of sensitization, and logistic factors such as rapidity with which the transplantation can be performed. This system was designed to allow for fair distribution of kidneys. Currently, legislation requires that all families or guardians of potential donors be asked to consider donating organs and tissues.

Organ procurement organizations (OPOs) are responsible for organ recovery in the United States. These organizations have offices in major cities and provide services on a local, state, and regional basis. OPOs provide 24-hour assistance to evaluate potential donors and coordinate organ recovery. The organ transplant coordinators of the OPO assist in the recovery of organs and communicate back to donor families and hospitals about the outcomes of transplantations. Guidelines for the sharing of organs and standards for the recovery and transplantation of organs have been developed by the United Network for Organ Sharing (UNOS). UNOS operates under the U.S. Department of Health and Human Services. OPOs are members of UNOS. UNOS has a national waiting list of potential recipients and a system for computer matching potential recipients with donor organs. UNOS, through the OPO, helps to distribute organs. The Organ Procurement Transplant Network (OPTN) is operated by the UNOS and is the central repository for information about all organs procured and distributed. Although the distribution of organs has been centralized, the criteria for allocation are still controversial and subjective in some cases. Overall, the guidelines allow an organ to go to a recipient within an OPO's service area before going to someone with higher medical needs outside of the OPO's service area (except for kidney transplants, which must go to a person with a six HLA-antigen match, regardless of where they are). The philosophy behind this guideline is that keeping organs for recipients within a defined community acts as an incentive for others to donate organs and tissues.

Registered nurses can be involved in various ways with the allocation of transplant tissue and organs. They may function as organ transplant coordinators, may be involved politically on the national and state levels, may serve on advisory boards of local organ banks or OPOs, or may serve on various committees that establish policies and guidelines related to organ and tissue retrieval and transplantation within acute-care institutions.

### Guidelines for Talking with Families About Donating Organs/Tissues

Make sure that brain death or death has been discussed with the family.
Obtain permission from the primary or attending physician.
Contact the local organ procurement organization (OPO) to gain assistance.
Try to determine the beliefs of the potential donor; that is, has a donor card been signed.
Identify which of the family members to involve; in some instances this may be only the legal next-of-kin, and in other instances this may include a large extended family, stepparents, fiancee, and so on.
Approach the family after they have had some time to grieve.
Provide a comfortable, private place for discussion between the health team members and the family.
Ascertain what the family understands about brain death and the hope of recovery.
Speak slowly, be sensitive, refer to the potential donor by name, and do not be afraid to refer to the potential donor as dead.
Provide adequate, accurate information on the options available to the family related to discontinuing life support on the brain-dead person.
Provide adequate, accurate information on tissue and organ donation, including that informed consent is necessary, the other evaluation required, and that there is no cost to the family.
Ensure that the family understands that organ/tissue donation will not interfere with the timing of the funeral service or with having an open-casket service.
Provide time for the family to discuss the request and make the decision.
Present consents only after the family has had time to make the decision and has given an affirmative response.

## DONOR CRITERIA

Most organs used for transplantation are cadaver organs; for these, nurses are involved in organ donation and recovery. Nurses, particularly those in critical care, assist in identifying potential donors, approach families about donating (see Guidelines box above), provide support to families as they make their decisions, care for brain-dead persons (see Guidelines box, p. 2470), assist with laboratory studies and procedures to establish the functioning of specific organs, and assist with testing for brain death.

The typical donor of organs dies from brain death; has no preexisting disease of the organ(s) being recovered; has no transmissible diseases, sepsis, or extracranial malignancy; and has no history of death of unknown etiology. The potential donor must be hemodynamically salvageable and have relatively normal organ function.[10] Box 72-2 presents a summary of tests that may be used to assess the health status of organs for transplantation. In addition, the criteria for donors of lungs and heart-lungs include no history of smoking and no chest tubes. Potential donors of *tissues, as opposed to organs,* can have died from cardiac death. However, other specific criteria exist for donors of tissues, such as no tissue irradiation and no use of chronic steroid therapy. For

### Guidelines for Care of the Brain-Dead Person

Continuous ventilator support and care
Continuous hemodynamic monitoring (arterial blood lines (pulmonary and systemic), venous pressure lines, cardiac monitoring) with documentation of measurements at least hourly
Measurement of blood pressure, pulse, respiration, intake, output, temperature at least every hour
Measurement of blood gases every 6 hours or as ordered
Assessment of cardiac rate, rhythm, and heart sounds; breath sounds; and skin integrity every 2 to 4 hours
Collection of specimens for serum and urine electrolytes and osmolality, blood urea nitrogen (BUN), and blood, urine, and sputum cultures
Maintenance of systolic blood pressure at 100 mm Hg or greater with position, fluids, and vasopressors as ordered
Maintenance of optimal respiratory status and oxygen tension at ≥ 100 mm Hg by suctioning the airway and turning the patient as needed and manipulating the ventilator as ordered
Maintenance of urine output at 100 ml/hr by replacing fluids as ordered, assessing for presence of diabetes insipidus (see Chapter 39), and assisting with treatment as necessary; monitoring for and treating increased serum glucose; and giving fluid challenges for oliguria if necessary
Maintenance of electrolyte balance by monitoring electrolytes and renal status and administering fluid and electrolyte replacement as ordered
Prevention of infection by use of sterile technique when handling invasive lines and dressings, by providing appropriate skin and respiratory care, and by continuing or instituting antibiotic therapy as ordered
Maintenance of normal body temperature with warming or cooling blankets; aspirin is preferred for hyperthermia because acetaminophen has hepatic toxic effects; wrapping the head of the patient is helpful if hypothermia is the problem

### BOX 72-2 Additional Tests That may be Performed To Evaluate the Status of an Organ in a Potential Donor

**HEART**

Electrocardiogram (ECG)
Echocardiogram
Cardiac consultation
Cardiac enzymes and isoenzymes, including creatine kinase (CK) with MB fraction
Cardiac catheterization may be conducted if there is a questionable history of cardiac disease

**LUNG**

Chest x-ray film with measurements
Arterial blood gas analysis at baseline and after intervention with an $FiO_2$ of 100% and positive end-expiratory pressure (PEEP) of 5 mm Hg
Gram stain and culture of sputum

**LIVER**

Serum laboratory analysis of liver function, including enzymes (transaminases [AST, ALT], alkaline phosphatase, GGTP, LDH); bilirubin (total and direct); hemoglobin, hematocrit, partial thromboplastin time (PTT), prothrombin time (PT), total protein, and albumin

**KIDNEY**

Serum and urine tests, including serum electrolytes, BUN, serum creatinine, and urine culture and urinalysis

**PANCREAS**

Serum and urine tests, including serum electrolytes, BUN, creatinine, amylase, glucose and urine culture and urinalysis

potential donors of eyes, the criteria specifically identify the transmissible diseases that must not be present, including active hepatitis, acquired immunodeficiency syndrome *(AIDS)*, rabies, viral encephalitis, or Creutzfeldt-Jakob disease.[10] The age limits or requirements of potential donors vary for different organs/tissues and centers. Because of the age variation, the Midwest Organ Bank[15] recommends consulting organ procurement centers for any potential donors between the ages of birth and 70 years (Table 72-1).

To decrease the risk of transmitting human immunodeficiency virus (HIV) through transplantation, criteria for exclusion of high-risk donors have been established.[1,5,10] Those excluded, regardless of the HIV status, include the following:

1. Persons with clinical or laboratory evidence of HIV infection
2. Men who have had sex with other men one or more times since 1977
3. Persons with past or present history of intravenous (IV) drug abuse
4. Persons immigrating since 1977 from countries such as Haiti and Central Africa where HIV is thought to be transmitted mostly by heterosexual activity
5. Persons with histories of receiving clotting factor concentrates for hemophilia
6. Sexual partners of any of the persons in groups 1 to 5
7. Persons who have engaged in prostitution since 1977 and any of their heterosexual partners from the last 6 months

## IMMUNOLOGY AND TRANSPLANTATION

Successful transplantation of allografts requires manipulation of the recipient's immune system. All cells and tissues in the body have markers or antigens on the cell membrane surface. These antigens allow one cell to be recognized by other cells as either "self" or "nonself." The antigens distributed on the surface of the cells of any one person are unique for that person, except for identical twins, and are controlled by the genes of that person. These cell markers are important in protection of the body from invasion by foreign substances. Because

**TABLE 72-1 Age Criteria for Specific Donors**

| ORGAN/TISSUE | AGE |
|---|---|
| **ORGANS** | |
| Kidneys | 6 months-65 years |
| Liver | Term newborn-55 years |
| Pancreas | 1-60 years |
| Heart | Term newborn-55 years |
| Lung | 12-55 years |
| Heart-lung | Term newborn-65 years |
| **TISSUES** | |
| Bone, fascia, connective tissue, bone marrow | 15-65 years |
| Heart valves | Term newborn-55 years |
| Eyes | No age limit |
| Saphenous veins | 5-65 years |
| Skin | Maximum age 70; minimum age limited because person must be 5 feet tall and weigh at least 100 pounds |

**BOX 72-3 Inheritance of Haplotypes**

| Father haplotypes (F1) | (F2) | Mother haplotypes (M1) | (M2) |
|---|---|---|---|
| A9 | A23 | A10 | A30 |
| B5 | B27 | B35 | B8 |
| Cw7 | Cw1 | Cw5 | Cw2 |
| Dw1 | Dw2 | Dw7 | Dw8 |
| DR5 | DR7 | DR5 | DR3 |
| DQw4 | DQw3 | DQw2 | DQw3 |
| DPw1 | DPw2 | DPw3 | DPw4 |

| Father \ Mother | M1 | M2 |
|---|---|---|
| F1 | M1F1 | M2F1 |
| F2 | M1F2 | M2F2 |

foreign substances have different markers, they can be recognized as foreign (nonself) by the immune system.

The B and T lymphocytes of the immune system are the surveillance cells that can recognize the cell membrane markers as foreign (nonself) or nonforeign (self). When the markers on cell membranes are recognized as foreign (nonself), the B and T lymphocytes are activated, which means that these cells differentiate, proliferate, and clone to be able to attack and control or destroy the foreign substance.

The ability of immune cells to recognize foreign substances is the result of genetic factors on chromosome 6. The region of the chromosome is called the **major histocompatibility complex,** and codes for a class of antigens called **human leukocyte antigen (HLA).** Although these antigens are called human leukocyte antigens, the HLA genetic complex encodes cell membrane markers or antigens on almost all cells in the body. The HLA antigenic complex is classified into two groups. *Class 1 HLA* antigens are encoded by three loci on chromosome 6—loci A, B, and C. *Class II HLA* antigens are encoded at four loci—referred to as D, DR, DQ, and DP. HLA class I antigens are expressed by almost all cells, including leukocytes, platelets, and cells of most solid organs. HLA class II antigens are expressed on fewer cells; however, these antigens are found on many of the immune system cells, including B and some T lymphocytes, macrophages, monocytes, and vascular endothelium. Each of the seven loci on chromosome 6 can encode for one of many different specific antigenic factors of **alleles.** More than 118 alleles are known or suspected to exist.[13] These individual alleles are identified by a number following the specific loci. For example, *HLA-A1* refers to the specific allele numbered *1* of the *A* loci. If there is uncertainty about whether a specific allele for a loci is unique, it will be distinguished by a lower-case "w" placed before the number. For example HLA-Bw4 refers to an allele for the B loci for which some uncertainty exists.

Each person has two number 6 chromosomes, and each chromosome will encode for seven specific HLA antigens, one for each specific loci. Each person inherits one number-six chromosome and thus one set of seven HLA antigens or one *haplotype* from each parent. Therefore, using mendelian inheritance principles, two siblings have a 25% *possibility* of sharing both haplotypes, a 25% *possibility* of sharing neither haplotype, and a 50% *possibility* of sharing one haplotype (Box 72-3).

A second antigen system important to the acceptance of transplant tissue is the ABO blood typing system. The ABO antigens are on red blood cells (RBCs) and other tissues. Some minor RBC antigens, particularly the Lewis system, are important to transplantation rejection or acceptance and are assessed in recipients and donors.[4] The RHO antigen system does not seem to have a role in survival or rejection of transplant tissue or organs.

## TISSUE TYPING AND MATCHING PROCEDURES

In preparation for all transplants, some of the tests for tissue typing and matching, typing and matching RBCs, and leukocyte crossmatching will be carried out. See Box 72-4 for a description of major tests that may be used in establishing compatibility between the donor organ/tissue and the recipient.

The number of tests and the exact tests used vary for different types of transplants. Several reasons exist for this variability. First, although all the antigens discussed have some role in allowing "self" cells to be differentiated from "nonself" cells, and all antigens are on at least

**BOX 72-4 Tests Used for Tissue Typing and Matching**

**ABO COMPATIBILITY**

Tests surface antigens on RBCs and other tissues; compatibility is same as for blood transfusions; recipient would have antibodies to any ABO antigens present on donor cells and not on recipient cells.

**MINOR RBC ANTIGEN TESTING**

Test surface antigens on RBCs; transplant recipients who have had multiple transfusions may have antibodies to known minor RBC antigens.

**MICROLYMPHOCYTOTOXICITY TESTING**

Detects class I HLA antigens (A, B, C) and matches these antigens between recipient and donor.

**MIXED LEUKOCYTE CULTURE OR MIXED LYMPHOCYTE CULTURE (MLC)**

Detects class II HLA antigens (D, DR, DQ, DP); takes 4 to 5 days to complete test so only performed with living, related donors; there is a 24-hour HLA-DR typing test that may be used for cadaver kidneys.

**WHITE CELL CROSSMATCH**

Detects presence of preformed circulating cytotoxic antibodies in recipient to antigens on lymphocytes of donor; positive crossmatch is predictor of rejection.

**MIXED LYMPHOCYTE CROSSMATCH**

Also detects presence of preformed cytotoxic antibodies in recipient to antigens on lymphocytes of donor; used to test potential recipients against selected panel of donor lymphocytes; tells probability of finding crossmatch negative donor; response changes over time so potential renal transplant candidates are screened monthly.

some of the immune system cells, the individual loci of the HLA system and the RBC antigens may not be equally important in the activation of the immune system to attack the foreign "nonself" transplant tissue. Second, the immunogenicity of transplant tissue varies from most allogenic to least allogenic as follows: bone marrow, skin, islets of Langerhans, heart, kidney, and liver.[19] Last, the preservation time of many cadaver tissues and organs is too short to allow the various tests that are now available to be conducted (Table 72-2).

## Histocompatibility Testing for Different Types of Transplants

Transplantation of tissues and organs from live donors is associated with maximal histocompatibility testing. Transplantation of a kidney from a live donor requires establishment of ABO compatibility. In addition, HLA matching by use of microlymphocytotoxicity testing and mixed leukocyte (or lymphocyte) culture (MLC) must be completed. White blood cell (WBC) crossmatch and mixed lymphocyte crossmatch are also conducted. With cadaver kidneys, time does not allow for MLC testing to be performed. Compatibility of the HLA-B and HLA-DR antigens seems most important, whereas compatibility of HLA-C antigens appears to be of little value.[17]

**TABLE 72-2 Recovery and Preservation Time of Tissues and Organs**

| ORGAN/TISSUE | MAXIMAL RECOVERY TIME | MAXIMAL PRESERVATION TIME |
|---|---|---|
| Bone marrow | 6 hours | Indefinite; frozen |
| Cornea | 6 hours | 7 days |
| Heart | Immediate | 3-5 hours |
| Kidney | Immediate | 48 hours |
| Liver | Immediate | 24 hours |
| Pancreas | Immediate | 8 hours |

Data from Lifelink of Georgia, Atlanta, Ga, 1979; and Hawke D, Kraft J, Smith SL: Tissue and organ donation and recovery. In Smith SL: *Tissue and organ transplantation: implications for professional nursing practice,* St Louis, 1990, Mosby.

Successful *allograft bone marrow* transplantation requires maximal compatibility between donor and recipient. This compatibility is identified by microlymphocytotoxicity testing for class I HLA antigens and by MLC testing for class II HLA antigens. ABO and RH compatibility is not necessary. If a transplant with ABO-incompatible bone marrow is planned, the recipient must undergo plasma exchange to eliminate antibodies against the ABO group of the donor.[3]

Because of the very short preservation times of the heart, liver, lung, and pancreas, only minimal histocompatibility testing is possible. With a heart transplant, ABO compatibility is established and a mixed lymphocyte crossmatch is carried out. In liver transplants, the ideal transplant comes from an identical ABO donor. However, incompatible matches are acceptable in emergency situations. HLA typing and matching and MLC testing do not seem to be as clinically important in liver transplantation as in other types of transplantations.[22]

Histocompatibility testing, although possible for corneal transplants, is controversial. Sight is restored without HLA matching 90% of the time; and ABO compatibility has not been shown to increase the success of the transplant. However, class I HLA matching may be beneficial for patients who are at high risk for allograft rejection resulting from corneal vascularization.[2]

It is important to remember that research is ongoing to improve histocompatibility testing and to identify the most important antigen matching for the various types of transplants. As new information and technology accumulate, tissue-matching procedures for transplants may change. However, data must be collected over many years and from many recipients of transplants.

# REJECTION

The major focus of medical and nursing care after transplantation is prevention or early identification of rejection so that appropriate interventions can be initiated. The major reason for transplant failure is rejection.

**Rejection** can be classified into one of three types: *hyperacute, acute,* or *chronic.* A special type of rejection that occurs in recipients of allogenic bone marrow transplants is **graft-versus-host disease (GVHD).**

## Hyperacute Rejection

**Hyperacute rejection** occurs at the time of transplantation or within 48 hours after the transplant. It is mediated by the humoral immune system. **Preformed circulating cytotoxic antibodies** to incompatible ABO blood group antigens, to antigens on the vascular endothelium, or to histocompatibility antigens are responsible for the hyperacute rejection. The combination of the preformed antibody with the antigen causes activation of complement, entrapment of formed blood elements and clotting factors, massive intravascular coagulation, and necrosis of the graft from decreased perfusion. The degranulation of phagocytic cells causes the release of hydrolytic enzymes that also cause tissue destruction.

Currently, no data show that hyperacute rejection occurs in nonrenal transplants.[20] The liver seems to be particularly protected from hyperacute rejection, possibly because of the type of blood flow and the large cell mass of the liver. Primary prevention of hyperacute rejection is by ensuring ABO blood group compatibility and avoiding transplantation if positive lymphocyte crossmatches occur (WBC crossmatch).[20] A special type of hyperacute rejection is accelerated rejection. This type of rejection occurs over 3 to 5 days. It is treatable if caught early.

## Acute Rejection

**Acute rejection** usually occurs within 1 week to as long as 3 months after the transplantation. Acute rejection episodes may recur at any time after the first episode but decrease in frequency over time. Acute rejection is mediated by both the humoral and the cellular immune systems. In acute rejection, foreign antigens are trapped by macrophages. This macrophage-antigen interaction can stimulate differentiation and maturation of various B-cell and T-cell lines. These activated B and T cells cause destruction of the transplanted tissue directly or indirectly through activation of other immune cells. Acute rejection is treated by pharmacologic interventions. A major nursing intervention for all transplants is to assess for and assist with treatment of acute rejection.

## Chronic Rejection

**Chronic rejection** occurs from 3 months to longer after transplantation. It is mediated by both the cellular and the humoral immune systems and results in slow, progressive loss of graft function. Chronic rejection does not respond to medications currently available. Two new medications, RS-61443 and 15-deoxyspergualin, are just now being tested.[12]

Chronic rejection of a kidney means the recipient must resume dialysis, whereas chronic rejection of a pancreatic transplant requires the resumption of therapy for insulin-dependent diabetes mellitus. Chronic rejection in other nonrenal transplant recipients is potentially life-threatening unless a retransplantation is performed.

## Graft-Versus-Host Disease (GVHD)

Persons who receive allogenic bone marrow are at risk for GVHD depending on the degree to which the donor and recipient are HLA incompatible, as identified by microlymphocytotoxicity testing and MLC.[6] In the person who has an allogenic bone marrow transplant, irradiation therapy and chemotherapy are used to destroy the recipient's immunocompetent cells. The donor's immunocompetent cells, once they engraft in the recipient, recognize other cells of the recipient as foreign and attack them. The tissue and organs most affected are the skin, liver, and gastrointestinal (GI) tract.[6] GVHD can occur as an acute or chronic process. Histocompatibility testing and immune suppression are used to prevent or minimize GVHD.

# DRUG THERAPY TO PREVENT REJECTION

Survival of all types of allogenic organ grafts and bone marrow, except for the cornea, requires the use of immunosuppressive agents. The immunosuppressive agents most often used include azathioprine, corticosteroids, cyclosporine, lymphocyte immune globulin, and muromonab CD-3 (OKT-3). Each of these drugs is discussed briefly. The ideal immunotherapy regimen has not been determined. Most patients, regardless of the type of transplant, will receive over the lifetime of the transplant a combination of cyclosporine, azathioprine, and corticosteroids. Lymphocyte-immune globulin and OKT-3 are used to treat acute rejection episodes.

## Azathioprine

Azathioprine (Imuran) inhibits ribonucleic acid (RNA) and deoxyribonucleic acid (DNA) synthesis and decreases the proliferation of immune cells. It is readily absorbed from the GI tract, although it can be given intravenously. Azathioprine is metabolized in the liver, and its metabolites are excreted by the kidneys. It may take several days for its effects to be seen. The oral dosage is 1 to 3 mg/kg body weight. The major toxic effect is suppression of the bone marrow. The WBC count is used to adjust the dosage. A summary of side effects, assessment parameters, and important nursing interventions is presented in Table 72-3.

## Corticosteroids

Corticosteroids are antiinflammatory and immunosuppressive agents. This group of drugs includes the endogenous glucocorticoids, cortisol, and synthetic glucocorticoids, such as prednisone and methylprednisolone. Corticosteroids cause a decrease in lymphocytes, monocytes, eosinophils, and basophils within 4 to 6

**TABLE 72-3 Azathioprine Therapy: Summary of Side Effects, Assessment Parameters, and Nursing Interventions**

| SIDE EFFECTS | ASSESSMENT PARAMETERS | NURSING INTERVENTIONS |
|---|---|---|
| **CARDIOVASCULAR: FLUID AND ELECTROLYTES** | | |
| Fluid and electrolyte changes | Serum electrolytes<br>Urine output<br>Fluid/food intake | Monitor intake.<br>Monitor output.<br>Decrease dosage of azathioprine. |
| **GASTROINTESTINAL** | | |
| Nausea, vomiting | | Administer oral dose with meals. |
| Anorexia | Appetite | Consult with dietitian. |
| Diarrhea | Elimination pattern | Institute enteral or parenteral nutrition. |
| Hepatotoxicity<br>Pancreatitis | Serum transaminases, phosphatases, bilirubin, coagulation factors, amylase, lipase, calcium | |
| **HEMATOLOGIC** | | |
| Leukopenia<br>Thrombocytopenia<br>Macrocytic anemia | WBC count with differential<br>Platelet count<br>RBC count<br>Bleeding (oozing, hemorrhage)<br>Signs/symptoms of infection<br>Inspection of mucous membranes for opportunistic infections | Increase attention to infection control measures.<br>Administer platelets.<br>Administer packed RBCs.<br>Administer oral antifungal agent.<br>Administer antibiotics.<br>Decrease dosage of azathioprine. |
| **NEUROLOGIC** | | |
| None | None | |
| **PSYCHOLOGIC** | | |
| None | None | |
| **DERMATOLOGIC** | | |
| Stomatitis | Inspection of mucous membranes | Maintain good oral hygiene. |

From Hooks MA: Immunosuppressive agents used in transplantation. In Smith SL: *Tissue and organ transplantation: implications for professional nursing practice,* St Louis, 1990, Mosby.

hours after administration. These decreases are the result of a redistribution of these cells from circulatory to noncirculatory sites. Of the lymphocytes, T lymphocytes are affected. Corticosteroids cause an increase in neutrophils because of increased release from bone marrow and decreased migration from the circulation. However, corticosteroids inhibit the ability of neutrophils to adhere to vessel walls, which is necessary for migration to sites of inflammation. Thus the accumulation of neutrophils at the graft site is actually decreased. Corticosteroids decrease production of interleukin I (IL-I) and interleukin 2 (IL-2), which are necessary for full functioning of the immune system. They also decrease production of prostaglandins and leukotrienes.

Corticosteroids are readily absorbed from the GI tract. They also may be given parenterally. Corticosteroids are metabolized in the liver and excreted by the kidneys. Many side effects occur; these are listed in Table 72-4, along with assessment parameters and nursing interventions.

## Cyclosporine

Cyclosporine is an immunosuppressive agent that is selective for lymphocytes, mainly T lymphocytes. It is not myelotoxic. It acts by inhibiting the expression of receptors for IL-2 on T lymphocytes. Of importance, if T lymphocytes are activated to express IL-2 receptors before immunosuppression is started, cyclosporine is not effective. Cyclosporine also affects macrophage activation.

Cyclosporine is given orally and parenterally. It is eliminated by hepatic mechanisms. Cyclosporine has many adverse effects, the most important of which is nephrotoxicity. The side effects, assessment parameters, and appropriate nursing interventions are presented in Table 72-5.

## Lymphocyte Immune Globulin

Antilymphocyte sera (ALS) and globulin (ALG) are products from animals that contain heterogeneous antibodies to lymphocytes in general or to T lymphocytes in particular. ALS/ALG induces immunosuppression by depleting small lymphocytes from lymph nodes and lymphoid organs. It also coats and opsonizes the lymphocytes so that they can be phagocytized by macrophages. ALS/ALG is given by slow IV infusion. Because it is a foreign substance, the patient is monitored closely for an allergic reaction. An antipyretic, steroids, and an anti-

**TABLE 72-4 Corticosteroid Therapy: Summary of Side Effects, Assessment Parameters, and Nursing Interventions**

| SIDE EFFECTS | ASSESSMENT PARAMETERS | NURSING INTERVENTIONS |
|---|---|---|
| **CARDIOVASCULAR: FLUID AND ELECTROLYTES** | | |
| Sodium retention | Serum electrolytes | Administer low-sodium, high-potassium diet. |
| Potassium wasting | Serum calcium, phosphorus | Administer oral or parenteral electrolyte replacement. |
| Calcium and phosphorus wasting | Serum albumin | Administer oral or parenteral calcium, phosphorus replacement. |
| | Intake and output | |
| Metabolic alkalosis | Acid-base status | Administer antihypertensives. |
| Fluid retention | Peripheral edema | Instruct patient about side effects. |
| Systemic arterial hypertension | Blood pressure | Decrease dosage. |
| | Body weight | |
| **PULMONARY** | | |
| Infection | Breath sounds | Deep breathing exercises. |
| | | Ambulation. |
| | | Avoid persons with respiratory infections. |
| **GASTROINTESTINAL** | | |
| Peptic ulceration (esophagus, stomach, duodenum) | Guaiac stools and vomitus | Administer oral corticosteroids with food. |
| | Serum amylase, lipase | Administer antacids, $H_2$-receptor blockers. |
| | Serum calcium | Consult dietitian. |
| Pancreatitis | Serum transaminases, phosphatases, bilirubin | Decrease dosage. |
| Hepatitis | | |
| Increased appetite | Coagulation factors | |
| Diarrhea | Abdominal status | |
| **ENDOCRINE** | | |
| Impaired glucose tolerance | Serum glucose | Administer insulin. |
| Diabetes mellitus | Polydipsia, polyuria | Provide thyroid hormone replacement. |
| Cushing syndrome | Cushingoid characteristics—"moon face," truncal obesity, buffalo hump, striae | Instruct patient about consequences of sudden corticosteroid withdrawal. |
| Hypothyroidism | $T_3$, $T_4$, TSH | |
| Impaired carbohydrate tolerance | | |
| Hypothalmic-pituitary-adrenal suppression | During period of steroid withdrawal or increased stress: headache, lethargy, weakness, hypotension | Avoid sudden withdrawal from corticosteroids. |
| Osteoporosis | Assessment of patient complaints of back or limb pain | Administer calcium and vitamin D supplements. |
| **HEMATOLOGIC** | | |
| Neutrophilia, decreased eosinophils, decreased basophils | WBC count with differential count | Increase attention to infection control measures. |
| Lymphocytopenia | Inspection of mucous membranes for opportunistic infection | Administer oral antifungal agents. |
| Opportunistic infections | | Administer antibiotics. |
| Impaired wound healing | Signs/symptoms of infection | |
| Aseptic necrosis of femoral and humoral heads | Wound healing | |
| **NEUROLOGIC/MUSCULOSKELETAL** | | |
| Headache | Neurologic status | Administer analgesics for headaches. |
| Insomnia | Sleep periods | Provide environment conducive to sleep. |
| Vertigo | Muscle mass/strength | Initiate seizure precautions in susceptible patient. |
| Seizures | | Consult physical therapy. |
| Increased intracranial pressure | | Decrease dosage of corticosteroids. |
| Muscle weakness/wasting | | Give dose in the morning if possible. |
| | | Encourage ambulation. |
| **PSYCHOLOGIC** | | |
| Psychosis | Mental status | Consult psychiatrist if necessary. |
| Euphoria | Behavior | Instruct patient about side effects. |
| Depression | | Decrease dosage. |

From Hooks MA: Immunosuppressive agents used in transplantation. In Smith SL: *Tissue and organ transplantation: implications for professional nursing practice,* St Louis, 1990, Mosby.

*Continued*

**TABLE 72-4 Corticosteroid Therapy: Summary of Side Effects, Assessment Parameters, and Nursing Interventions—cont'd**

| SIDE EFFECTS | ASSESSMENT PARAMETERS | NURSING INTERVENTIONS |
|---|---|---|
| **DERMATOLOGIC** | | |
| Thin, fragile skin<br>Petechiae, ecchymoses<br>Erythema<br>Acne<br>Hirsutism<br>Stomatitis | Inspection of skin<br>Inspection mucous membranes | Administer topical antiacne medication.<br>Avoid adhesive tape.<br>Avoid skin trauma.<br>Counsel regarding options for dealing with hirsutism.<br>Instruct about mouth care. |
| **OTHER** | | |
| Blurred vision<br>Cataracts | Visual acuity | Consult ophthalmology department. |

**TABLE 72-5 Cyclosporine Therapy: Summary of Side Effects, Assessment Parameters, and Nursing Interventions**

| SIDE EFFECTS | ASSESSMENT PARAMETERS | NURSING INTERVENTIONS |
|---|---|---|
| **CARDIOVASCULAR: FLUID AND ELECTROLYTES** | | |
| Nephrotoxicity<br>Systemic arterial hypertension<br>Hyperkalemia<br>Hypomagnesemia<br>Anaphylaxis if administered rapidly IV | Cyclosporine levels<br>Serum creatinine, BUN<br>Creatinine clearance<br>Peripheral edema<br>Blood pressure<br>Serum magnesium<br>Serum potassium | Administer diuretics.<br>Administer antihypertensives, oral or parenteral.<br>Administer magnesium.<br>Decrease dosage of cyclosporine.<br>Administer IV cyclosporine over 2-6 hours. |
| **PULMONARY** | | |
| Infections | Breath sounds | Teach deep breathing exercises.<br>Provide ambulation.<br>Avoid persons with infections. |
| **GASTROINTESTINAL** | | |
| Hepatotoxicity | Cyclosporine levels<br>Serum transaminases, phosphatases, bilirubin<br>Coagulation factors | Decrease dosage of cyclosporine. |
| **ENDOCRINE** | | |
| None | None | None |
| **HEMATOLOGIC** | | |
| Lymphocytopenia<br>Lymphoma<br>Opportunistic infections | Cyclosporine levels<br>Complete blood count (CBC) with differential count<br>Inspection of mucous membranes for opportunistic infection<br>Bacterial, viral, and fungal cultures | Decrease dosage of cyclosporine.<br>Increased attention to infection control measures.<br>Administer oral antifungal agent.<br>Administer antibiotics. |
| **NEUROLOGIC** | | |
| Tremors<br>Paresthesias<br>Muscle weakness<br>Increased sensitivity to temperature changes | Cyclosporine levels<br>Neurologic status | Ensure patient that tremors and paresthesias are dose related.<br>Decrease dosage of cyclosporine.<br>Provide physical therapy.<br>Administer analgesics for headaches.<br>Initiate seizure precautions in susceptible patient.<br>Instruct patient about side effects. |

From Hooks MA: Immunosuppressive agents used in transplantation. In Smith SL: *Tissue and organ transplantation: implications for professional nursing practice,* St Louis, 1990, Mosby.

histamine are given first to inhibit allergic reactions. ALS/ALG is used to both prevent allograft rejection and to treat acute rejection. In both instances, it is given for 10 to 14 days in fixed doses based on body weight.

## Muromonab CD-3

Muromonab CD-3 (Orthoclone, OKT-3) is a monoclonal antibody against mature T lymphocytes. It decreases the level of T lymphocytes by making them incompetent as immune cells. OKT-3 is used primarily to treat acute rejection episodes, most frequently rejection that has not responded to steroids. However, it also is being used as a first-line agent and for induction of immunosuppression. It is given intravenously for 10 to 14 days. The effectiveness of therapy is monitored by the T-lymphocyte count and by serum levels of OKT-3.

OKT-3 is a foreign protein and can result in development of antibodies after one course of therapy. Antibody testing is necessary before a second course of the drug. Adverse reactions to OKT-3 include chills and fever lasting for up to 1 hour. Respiratory symptoms may occur and be life-threatening if the patient is fluid overloaded. Aseptic meningitis and infection with cytomegalovirus or herpes simplex virus can occur. Other adverse effects include headache and flulike symptoms. Most side effects occur during the first few doses, if they are going to occur. To decrease some of the side effects, patients may be given methylprednisolone, acetaminophen, and an antihistamine before OKT-3 is administered. The patient needs intensive monitoring of vital signs (every 15 minutes for 4 hours is recommended) during the first two doses because of the increased risk for an allergic reaction. If no problems occur during the first few doses, less frequent monitoring is required for subsequent doses. Because of the side effects, OKT-3 routinely has been used only in the hospital. However, since side effects subside after 3 to 5 days, one transplant center initiated outpatient administration after side effects subsided. This was well tolerated and resulted in decreased cost (see Research box at right).

### RESEARCH

Hrick DH et al: *Outpatient use of OKT-3 for the treatment of acute renal allograft rejection,* University Hospitals of Cleveland.

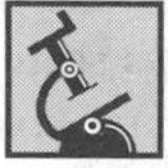

Orthoclone (OKT-3) is effective for treatment of acute rejection. All patients receiving OKT-3 experience side effects for the first 3 to 5 days, mandating hospital admission. Outpatient administration is feasible once side effects subside. A retrospective chart review of 79 consecutive renal transplant patients who received OKT-3 on 87 occasions over a 3-year period was done to (1) determine the percentage of patients able to receive outpatient therapy; (2) compare clinical variables in patients receiving outpatient therapy versus those hospitalized; and (3) identify conditions precluding outpatient therapy. Statistical analysis of clinical variables was performed using continuous variables and discrete variables. Forty-seven percent of patients received one to six outpatient doses; 136 of 856 total doses (16%) were administered as outpatient therapy. There were no significant differences in patient age, previous rejection episodes, or number of diabetic persons in the inpatient and outpatient groups. The decision to use outpatient therapy did not depend on ultimate rejection reversal after OKT-3 administration. Peak serum creatinine levels during treatment were higher in the inpatient group ($p < 0.05$). All patients exhibited fever for at least 1 day, but inpatients were febrile for more days ($p < 0.04$). Of the 46 patients remaining hospitalized, 17 had difficulty with transportation and/or concern about compliance with daily office visits. In conclusion, almost half the patients had decreased length of stay because of outpatient therapy. Persistent fever and renal dysfunction were the main factors precluding outpatient therapy. Home administration could further decrease length of stay.

## INFECTIONS

Immunosuppressive therapy must be taken for the lifetime of the allogenic transplant, except in experimental situations where chimerism is produced by simultaneous kidney-bone marrow transplant to induce immune tolerance.[21] This immunosuppressive therapy makes the transplant recipient a prime candidate for infections. Infections, besides occurring more frequently, spread more rapidly from localized sites to the total body and can result in sepsis. Although protective isolation may still be used in some institutions, the primary intervention to decrease exposure is good handwashing and aseptic techniques for all invasive procedures. The nurse must also provide care that protects surface barriers from organisms. This care would include mouth care after every meal, on arising, and at bedtime. The patient's back, perineum, gluteal folds, and other skin folds should be washed daily, kept well lubricated, and kept free of moisture. Additional preventive interventions, such as deep breathing every 2 hours and encouraging fluids to flush the urinary system, should be instituted as appropriate. Nutritional and fluid status should be assessed and interventions initiated to promote adequate nutrition, which will enhance the immune response; adequate fluid intake should be ensured.

Physical assessment of the skin; of insertion sites for invasive devices; of the lungs, mouth, and throat; and of the temperature and pulse should be implemented at least every 8 to 12 hours to allow for early detection of infections. At the same time, information about symptoms related to the presence of any infection should be elicited. Patients need to institute similar self-care measures to prevent infections and detect them early for as long as they are receiving immunosuppressive therapy.

Caregivers and others with active infections should

avoid contact with the patient during hospitalization or after discharge. The patient's hospital environment should be cleaned daily. Containers of water such as humidifier bottles, live flowers, and live plants should be eliminated from the environment or, if they are necessary, should be replaced daily. Box 72-8 lists some of the common organisms causing infections in persons with transplants who are receiving immunosuppressive drug therapy.

# NURSING MANAGEMENT

## PATIENT WHO IS A POTENTIAL RECIPIENT OF A TRANSPLANT

Persons with various types of end-stage organ failure, if they meet the criteria for transplantation as described on p. 2468, may have to consider whether to accept transplantation as a treatment alternative. These persons have additional nursing needs related to the evaluation of their candidacy for a transplant. The patient still has all the care needs related to the specific organ failure.

### Nursing Diagnoses

Nursing diagnoses are determined from analysis of patient data. Nursing diagnoses for the patient who is a potential recipient of a transplant may include but are not limited to the following:

| Diagnostic Title | Possible Etiologic Factors |
|---|---|
| Fear | Perceived inability to manage self-care; severity of illness |
| Coping, ineffective (individual) | Situational crises, threat of death, change in role within family unit |
| Powerlessness | Lack of control over when transplant will be performed |
| Knowledge deficit: pretransplant evaluation, transplantation process, self-care after transplant | Lack of exposure to information |

### Interventions

Choosing transplantation as an alternative is a decision that the patient and significant others make. Nurses provide information, support, and counseling.

A major need of the patient and significant others is education. The patient and significant others need to receive appropriate information about the transplantation, the evaluation necessary before being identified as a candidate, the preoperative and postoperative care requirements, and the continual care that will be required after the transplant. Information about the side effects of immunosuppressive therapy needs to be discussed.

Once the patient decides to have a transplant, an evaluation is done. The exact evaluation varies depending on the organ involved but includes an extensive physical and psychosocial evaluation. Histocompatibility studies as appropriate for the specific transplant are conducted. Underlying physical problems such as hypertension, ascites, bleeding, and infections must be treated before transplantation.

## PATIENT BEFORE TRANSPLANTATION

Once the patient has been placed on the waiting list for a transplant, nursing care focuses on three areas:

1. Helping patients cope with the waiting period
2. Helping patients manage the end-organ failure as well as possible
3. Helping patients implement self-care practices to maximize physical health so that potential complications of surgery will be minimized

### Nursing Diagnoses

Nursing diagnoses are determined from analysis of patient data. Nursing diagnoses for the patient before transplantation may include but are not limited to the following:

| Diagnostic Title | Possible Etiologic Factors |
|---|---|
| Coping, ineffective (individual) | Situational crises, threat of death, change in role within family unit |
| Knowledge deficit: transplantation process, self-care after transplant | Lack of exposure to information |

### Interventions

Counseling, helping patients identify coping mechanisms, and helping patients learn new coping mechanisms are the major interventions used to help patients during the waiting period. There should be established routine contact between the patient and the transplant team. Patients should have someone they can contact in case of an emergency or if any questions arise.

Pertinent self-care measures for the end-stage organ failure should be discussed and reviewed. These include a review of dietary restrictions, fluid needs, medications, and planned medical follow-up.

The interventions needed for the last area of care include promotion of adequate pulmonary function. Specific interventions include abstaining from smoking, as well as treatment of any underlying pulmonary infection. Because the person waiting for a transplant is chronically ill, nutritional status may be impaired and interventions to improve nutrition must be implemented. Adequate nutrition is important for adequate immunity, adequate energy to maintain an adequate level of activity before and after transplantation, and adequate wound healing.

Any active infection must be treated. The mouth is a common site of infection, and patients need to be referred for appropriate dental care to repair teeth and treat gum problems. The patient is taught proper oral care so that a healthy mouth is maintained. Other sites of infection, such as the bladder and the dialysis access site, are assessed and any infections treated promptly.

## PATIENT AFTER TRANSPLANTATION

### Assessment

Many of the nursing diagnoses and much of the care for the patient who undergoes transplantation is the same as that for a patient having any type of surgery (see Chapter 25). However, unique aspects of care include evaluating the patient for potential complications associated with the transplantation, assessing for and preventing infections, and assessing for rejection. Box 72-5 lists the major complications of specific transplanted organs other than infection, immunosuppression-related problems, or rejection and the resultant diminished functioning of the transplanted organ.

### Nursing Diagnoses

Nursing diagnoses are determined from analysis of patient data. Nursing diagnoses for the patient after transplantation, regardless of the organ or tissue, may include but are not limited to the following:

| Diagnostic Title | Possible Etiologic Factors |
|---|---|
| Infection, high risk for | Impaired immune function, poor nutritional status, loss of skin integrity, presence of invasive lines |
| Mucous membrane, altered oral | Infection from immunosuppression |
| Protection, altered | Drug therapies, inadequate nutrition |
| Home maintenance management, impaired | Recurrence of end-stage organ failure from rejection |
| Anxiety | Threat of rejection, threat of change in role function, threat of death |
| Fluid volume excess or deficit | Compromised organ function (renal, hepatic, cardiac, lung, pancreatic) from ischemia or rejection, loss of blood at surgical sites |
| Gas exchange, impaired | Ventilation-perfusion imbalance associated with infection or fluid overload |
| Cardiac output, decreased | Electrical abnormalities associated with electrolyte imbalance, ineffective contractility associated with fluid overload or deficit |
| Activity intolerance | Generalized weakness associated with fluid and electrolyte problems, poor nutrition, long-term chronic illness, corticosteroid therapy, imbalance between energy needs and supply |
| Body image disturbance | Change in physical function, change in appearance from corticosteroids, change in role within family unit |
| Knowledge deficit: self-care following transplantation, including diet, physical activity, fluid allotment; medicines; signs and symptoms of infection or rejection to monitor for and report; other monitoring requirements such as blood glucose, body weight, occurrence of dyspnea; follow-up care | Lack of previous exposure to information, large amount of information to master |

**BOX 72-5 Major Potential Complications Associated With Specific Types of Transplants**

**KIDNEY**

Acute tubular necrosis, fluid and electrolyte imbalance, hemorrhage, occlusion of renal artery or vein, leakage of urine from anastomoses sites

**HEART**

Leakage of blood at sites of anastomoses, hemorrhage, cardiac tamponade, hemodynamic instability such as arrhythmias, decreased cardiac output, hypervolemia, or hypovolemia

**LUNG**

Pulmonary infections, reperfusion edema of lung, hemodynamic instability

**LIVER**

Hypertension, hypovolemia, electrolyte imbalance, thrombosis of portal vein or hepatic artery, biliary complications, coagulopathy, pulmonary problems

**PANCREAS**

Thrombosis of vessels, respiratory problems, peritonitis

**BONE MARROW**

Acute and chronic complications related to radiation and/or chemotherapy given before transplant, including GI complications, pancytopenia, venoocclusive disease, and pulmonary complications; lack of engraftment

### Interventions

Infection is one of the most common problems facing the posttransplant patient. The patient's temperature is monitored regularly and fever reported immediately. Sources of fever are wound, pulmonary, or other nosocomial infections; rejection; hematoma; infarctions; or drug reactions. The search for the source of fever would include collecting sputum, urine, nasal secretions, blood, and wound drainage. Tracheal aspirates and bronchial washings may be collected and biopsies performed. The patient may have a chest x-ray film to assess for pulmonary infiltrate. Oral mucous membranes, the perineum and areas between skin folds are assessed for signs of candidal infection. Diagnostic tests to assess transplant organ function are also conducted to rule out rejection as the cause of the fever. Nursing care to prevent nosocomial infections must be instituted immediately after surgery and build on presurgical care. (See earlier discussion of care needs to prevent infection.) Invasive devices such as urinary catheters, arterial lines, and IV lines should be removed as soon as possible to decrease the risk of infection.

A major posttransplantation need is for the immunosuppressive therapy to be initiated as ordered to prevent rejection and the recurrence of signs and symptoms of organ failure. The various immunosuppressive agents are associated with multiple side effects. These side effects and relevant nursing interventions are discussed earlier in this chapter. Nursing care is implemented based on the drug therapy used.

The patient must be assessed for signs of rejection. Signs and symptoms of rejection include signs and symptoms of organ failure, such as increased serum creatinine (kidney), increased serum enzymes (liver), decreased cardiac output (heart), hypoxemia (lungs), increasing blood glucose levels (islet cells/pancreas), and increased serum amylase (pancreas). In addition, signs of increased immune activity are usually present. Early recognition of rejection is essential to allow for the most successful treatment.

General nursing needs of any patient after transplantation include the following:

1. Assess for signs and symptoms of infection.
2. Assess for signs and symptoms of rejection.
3. Assess for signs and symptoms of dysfunction of the transplanted organ or tissue.
4. Assess for signs and symptoms of common postoperative complications.
5. Assess for signs and symptoms of major complications associated with the specific types of transplants (Box 72-5).
6. Monitor for overall physical functioning including hemodynamic status, intake and output, daily weight, laboratory values, GI functioning, pulmonary status, and nutritional status.
7. Administer immunosuppressive therapy and other therapy as prescribed.
8. Assess for signs and symptoms of side effects of immunosuppressive therapy.
9. Initiate care to prevent infections and other complications of surgery.
10. Manage invasive lines, monitoring devices, the surgical incision, and dressings appropriately.
11. Initiate interventions to maintain nutritional status.
12. Initiate measures to control discomfort.
13. Teach about management of self-care needs:
    a. Medications and their side effects
    b. Signs and symptoms of side effects of medications that must be reported
    c. Ways to deal with the side effects of medications
    d. Signs and symptoms of rejection to monitor for and report
    e. Prevention of infection
    f. General health promotion measures
    g. Follow-up care
14. Provide counseling and support to help patients and significant others deal with the prolonged hospitalization, role changes, and other stressors.

## PATIENTS WITH SPECIFIC TYPES OF TRANSPLANTS

### Corneal Transplantation

When the cornea is so damaged that severe vision impairment occurs, **corneal grafting (keratoplasty)** may be necessary. Loss of vision caused by an opaque or destroyed cornea may be restored by replacing the damaged layers with a corneal graft obtained from a new cadaver or from an eye freshly removed by surgery. For best results, the donor cornea must be removed within 6 hours of death and should be grafted within 24 to 48 hours. Transplants preserved for longer periods may be used for lamellar grafts, which are discussed later in this section. The present practice is to keep a waiting list of persons who need grafts, because eye banks are not able to keep up with the demand. Eye Bank for Sight Restoration, Inc.,* is a nonprofit organization that collects and distributes donated eyes throughout the United States.

*210 E. 64th St., New York, NY 10021.

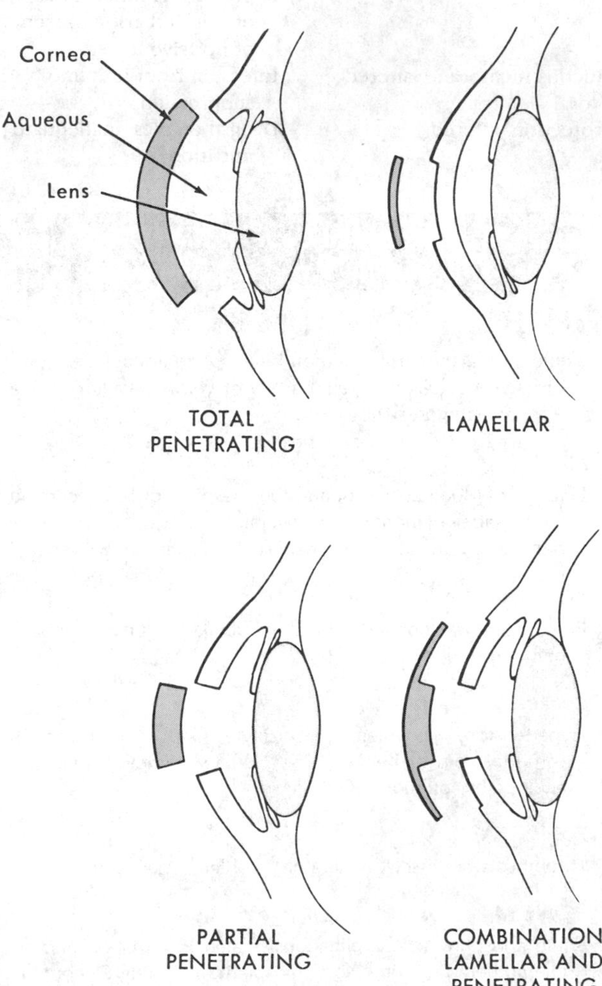


**FIGURE 72-1** Types of corneal grafts currently in use. Note that the lamellar graft defect does not penetrate the entire thickness of cornea.

Corneal transplantation cannot be performed if there is any infection. The type of corneal graft used depends on the depth and size of the damaged part that must be replaced (Figure 72-1). Corneal transplants or grafts may involve the entire thickness of the cornea (total penetrating), only part of the depth of the cornea (lamellar), or a combination of these, in which a small part of the graft involves the entire thickness of the cornea (partial penetrating). The penetrating graft establishes least well. For the penetrating graft, the eye surgeon seldom uses a donor eye that is more than 48 hours old.

#### Preoperative nursing care

Persons usually have only a short notice that they are to be admitted to the hospital for surgery. Although they have been waiting for a donor cornea, this short period for actual preparation may result in them feeling hurried and uneasy. They may be anxious about the surgical procedure itself and more specifically about its chances of success. A calm, efficient manner, along with an explanation of the routine preoperative preparation, will help ease this anxiety.

#### Postoperative nursing care

The person may be permitted out of bed following full recovery from the anesthetic. Discharge from the hospital is usually within 2 to 4 days postoperatively.

The eye is covered with a sterile eye pad. A metal or plastic shield is placed over the pad for extra protection. The patient will continue to wear the shield at night for several weeks. Corneal grafts heal very slowly because of the lack of blood vessels in the cornea and require from 12 weeks to 6 months to heal firmly.

#### Patient teaching

Patient teaching includes instructions about medications and assessment for corneal graft rejection. Patients are frequently sent home on cycloplegic, steroid, and sulfa eye drops.

Because the cornea is normally avascular, the recipient's immune cells are not exposed to the cornea and thus, immunosuppressive therapy is not used. However, patients are instructed to check for graft rejection daily for the rest of their lives. The eye is checked at the same time each day for redness or an increase in redness, irritation, discomfort, or a decrease in vision. Any symptoms that persist or increase in severity in a 24-hour period should be reported to the surgeon.

Many persons expect to see immediately after the graft. Vision, however, is sometimes poor while the sutures are in place. Once the sutures are removed, vision usually improves remarkably. The sutures may remain in place for at least a year, and the patient will be scheduled for monthly visits to the surgeon during that time.

### Kidney Transplantation

Major advances have been made in renal transplantation. In 1990 alone, more than 9000 patients with end-stage renal disease (ESRD) underwent transplantation.[23] Developments in surgical technique, tissue typing, and antirejection drug therapy have made transplantation a reasonable therapy. However, the major block to further use of transplantation as a form of treatment for chronic renal failure remains the availability of donor kidneys for transplantation. It has been estimated that of the 12,500 to 25,000 potential donors, only 10% to 15% will actually give organs.

Kidney transplants are being performed with increasing frequency in an effort to prolong the lives of persons with ESRD. At present, the ability to overcome completely the body's tendency to reject the grafted kidney has not been achieved. Persons undergoing kidney transplantation in essence exchange a program of chronic dialysis and its limitations for a new therapeutic program with new limitations and requirements. Unless the kidney has been donated by an identical twin, the body senses the graft as a foreign tissue and attempts to destroy it (rejection). Kidney allografts may be obtained from cadavers, matched family members, or an identical twin. Although more than 80% of the transplanted kidneys are from cadavers, better results are obtained from related donors. Currently, success rates 1 year after transplantation are about 75% to 85% when a cadaveric kidney is used and greater than 90% to 95% when a living related organ is transplanted.[8] The major requirement for the donated kidney is histocompatibility between the donor organ and the recipient. The important antigens are the HLA and ABO blood groups.

Living related donors must be in good general health, be highly motivated to be a donor, have good mental health, and not be receiving drugs such as barbiturates, which depress reflexes and electrical brain activity. The donor is given a complete medical evaluation and in some cases may be referred to a psychiatrist for further evaluation. Normally, the living related donor organ is harvested and immediately transplanted to the donor. Both surgeries can occur simultaneously. Cadaver donor criteria are described earlier in this chapter.

#### Surgery

During surgery, the transplanted kidney is usually placed in the iliac fossa (Figure 72-2). Generally, the peritoneal cavity is not entered. The patient's own kidneys are not disturbed unless they are infected or are the cause of significant hypertension, for which the recipient might undergo bilateral nephrectomy before transplant surgery. The recipient's kidneys are left intact whenever possible to maintain erythropoietin production, blood pressure control, and prostaglandin synthesis and metabolism. The donor ureter is used to the extent possible. If long enough, it is connected to the bladder in such a way as to prevent reflux of urine. If the donor ureter is short, a ureteroureterostomy may be performed. A catheter is placed in the surgical wound to promote drainage of any accumulating fluid.

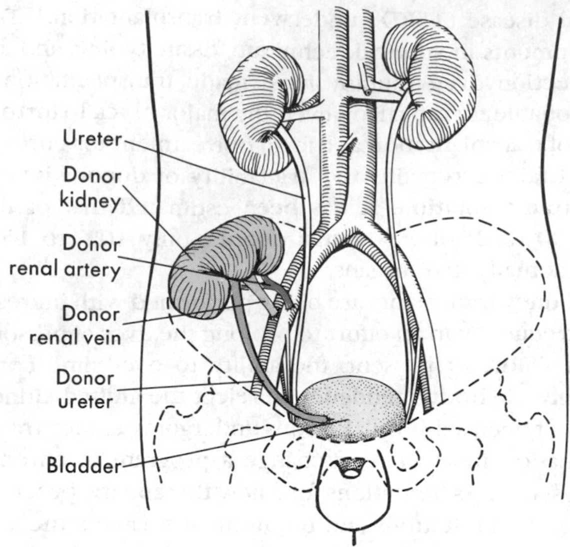


**FIGURE 72-2** Location of a transplanted kidney showing the anastomosis of the renal artery, renal vein, and ureter.

## Guidelines for Care of Renal Transplant Patient

### PREVENTION OF REJECTION, INFECTION

Maintain sterile technique in caring for wound, urinary drainage catheter, and other invasive lines.
Encourage early ambulation.
Administer medications as prescribed.
Assess patient for signs and symptoms of infection both at surgical incision and systemically.
Practice good handwashing.
Assess patient for signs and symptoms of rejection.

### FLUID AND ELECTROLYTE BALANCE

Maintain accurate intake and output.
Weigh patient daily at same time.
Monitor for signs of fluid and electrolyte imbalance.
Monitor and regulate parenteral fluid replacement as prescribed by physician (usually 1 ml replacement for each 1 ml output).
Encourage oral intake as tolerated.

### ASSISTANCE WITH COMFORT AND ACTIVITIES OF DAILY LIVING (ADL)

Promote rest periods when fatigue is present.
Administer pain medication as prescribed.
Assist with ADL as necessary but encourage independence.

### CONTROL OF ENVIRONMENT

Maintain calm, reassuring environment.
Consider use of reverse isolation while patient is immunosuppressed.
Restrict visitors with colds or other infections.
Provide diversional activities as tolerated.

### Postoperative nursing care

Immediate postoperative care includes maintaining drainage of the urinary bladder, monitoring hourly output, assessing the adequacy of fluid and electrolyte balance, protecting the patient from infection, observing for signs and symptoms of rejection and other complications (see Box 72-5), and identifying the effects of medications that have been administered throughout the entire care cycle. A free flow of communication must be maintained with the patient and significant others regarding the individual's progress.

In the operating room, a Foley catheter is inserted into the bladder to promote drainage of urine and to prevent bladder distention and pressure on the newly anastomosed ureter. If gross hematuria or clots are noted in the drainage system, the physician should be notified immediately.

As with any surgical patient, the possibility of hemorrhage and hypovolemia exists. Hemodynamic monitoring is instituted. Blood pressure and pulse are determined frequently. Because the patient may have little or no urine output for hours to days after transplantation, fluid and electrolyte balance must be monitored carefully. (See Chapter 50 for parameters indicating disturbed fluid and electrolyte balance in the patient with renal failure.) Any drainage from dressings or tubes is carefully calculated into the patient's fluid balance record. The Guidelines box above summarizes the care of the patient after renal transplantation.

### Rejection

Rejection, the leading cause of graft failure, may occur as a hyperacute event, as an accelerated event, as an acute event, or as a slow and progressive decline in renal function (chronic rejection). In a *hyperacute* event, rejection occurs immediately after surgical implantation. Instantly following arterial anastomosis, circulating cytotoxic antibodies infiltrate and infarct the foreign tissue. The kidney undergoing hyperacute rejection is usually removed immediately to prevent further complications. *Accelerated* rejection usually occurs 3 to 5 days after transplant. It presents as a sudden, severe episode of graft dysfunction, and it can sometimes be reversed with large doses of potent immunosuppressive drug therapy. *Acute* rejection typically begins within the first 2 weeks. Most transplant patients undergo at least one episode of acute rejection. The delay in occurrence of the first attack is related to the time it takes for T lymphocytes to become sensitized. Box 72-6 lists signs and symptoms indicative of acute rejection of the kidney.

*Chronic* rejection is a slow, progressive process. The signs and symptoms are similar to those that occur in acute rejection; however, they occur more slowly. In most instances the patient will eventually lose all functioning of the transplanted kidney as chronic rejection progresses.

Treatment of acute rejection usually consists of large doses of SoluMedrol (methylprednisolone) administered intravenously or the use of OKT-3.

**BOX 72-6 Signs and Symptoms of Acute Rejection in the Renal Transplant Patient**

Decrease in urine output
  Oliguria
  Anuria
Fever greater than 37.7° C (100° F); may be masked by steroid therapy
Pain or tenderness over grafted kidney
Edema
Sudden weight gain: 2 to 3 pounds in a 24-hour period
Hypertension
General malaise
Increase in serum creatinine and BUN values, proteinuria
Decrease in creatinine clearance
Evidence of rejection on renogram or other test

### Patient teaching

Thorough teaching is necessary; the following outcomes describe the teaching needs. The person who has undergone a renal transplant or the significant other can state or demonstrate the following:

1. Prescribed diet and how it will be achieved
2. Medication plan, including:
   a. Name, dose, frequency, rationale, and side effects of prescribed medications (immunosuppressives, antacids, etc.)
   b. Method of obtaining medications
3. Accurate taking and recording of oral temperature, 24-hour urine specimens, weights, fluid intake, and urine output
4. Recommended preventive health care measures
   a. Measures useful in preventing infection
   b. Plans for dental and gynecologic health care (if appropriate)
   c. Need to avoid immunization with live virus vaccines
5. Program for continued health supervision
   a. Concept of immunosuppression and relationship to health care needs
   b. Signs and symptoms requiring immediate medical attention
   c. Appropriate information regarding sexual functioning and family planning
   d. Need to preserve dialysis access
   e. Resources available for assistance with illness and rehabilitative concerns and means of contact with resources
   f. Specific plans for follow-up care

## Heart Transplantation

Heart transplantation may be considered for persons who have end-stage cardiac ischemia or cardiomyopathy. The 1-year survival rate is presently 81%, and the 5-year rate 69%. The donor heart is from a person with a comparable body weight and ABO compatibility with the recipient. Surgery consists of removal of the diseased heart (leaving the posterior walls of the recipient's atria to spare the sinoatrial node), followed by anastomosis of the atria, aorta, and pulmonary arteries.

### Postoperative nursing care

The patient who has a heart transplant needs care similar to that of any patient having open-heart surgery (see Chapter 30). In addition, the patient may have hypovolemia or hypervolemia, decreased cardiac output, rejection, or infections (see Box 72-5) and needs care to prevent these complications and to detect the early onset of any of these complications.

Hypervolemia can result from fluid replacement and corticosteroid therapy. Nursing care focuses on carrying out appropriate assessment, including hemodynamic monitoring, intake and output, daily weights, pulmonary status, and so on. The nurse administers diuretic therapy, inotropic agents, and vasodilators as ordered to treat the hypervolemia. Fluids are restricted, as is sodium. Additional care should focus on the protection of skin integrity because the hypervolemia and edema will increase the patient's risk for skin breakdown.

Decreased cardiac output can result from rejection, hypovolemia, arrhythmias, or preservation injury. Nursing interventions in the care of the patient who has undergone a heart transplant consist of monitoring the patient's cardiac output, identifying signs and symptoms of decreased output, and assisting with treatment to improve cardiac output. Treatment is the same as for other patients experiencing decreased cardiac output (see Chapter 31).

### Rejection

Rejection of the transplanted heart can be an acute or chronic process. Acute rejection occurs most frequently in the first 3 months after the transplant. To assess for rejection, an endomyocardial biopsy is the major diagnostic test used. Individual institutions use various protocols for the frequency of biopsies. The biopsies are necessary because other early signs and symptoms of rejection may not be present.

Although some patients may have rejection without early clinical signs and symptoms, the nurse monitors the patient for the early signs and symptoms listed in Box 72-7.

The patient showing signs of rejection may be treated with increasing doses of immunosuppressive agents. Additionally, methylprednisolone boluses, lymphocytic immune globulin, or OKT-3 may be given. The nurse assists with this therapy. The patient needs considerable support during rejection episodes because of the potentially life-threatening nature of rejection.

Chronic rejection is insidious and occurs more than 3 months after transplantation. The process is characterized by graft atherosclerosis, which has a different causation than other atheroscleroses. This atheroscle-

**BOX 72-7 Signs and Symptoms of Acute Rejection in the Heart Transplant Patient**

**SIGNS**

Fluid retention, peripheral edema, crackles, jugular venous distention (JVD), $S_3$ gallop
Pericardial friction rub
ECG changes: arrhythmias and decreased voltage
Decreased cardiac output
Hypotension
Cardiac enlargement

**SYMPTOMS**

Fatigue, lethargy
Dyspnea
Decreased tolerance for exercise

**BOX 72-8 Organisms Responsible for Infections in Transplant Recipients**

**BACTERIAL INFECTIONS**

Gram-negative organisms, including *Pseudomonas aeruginosa, Serratia marcescens, Proteus rettgeri, Enterobacter cloacae, Legionella pneumophila,* and various *Nocardia* species

**VIRAL INFECTIONS**

Herpesviruses, including herpes simplex viruses 1 and 2, varicella-zoster virus, cytomegalovirus, and Epstein-Barr virus

**FUNGAL INFECTIONS**

Candidal species (most often *C. albicans*) and other fungi, including *Aspergillus fumigatus, Cryptococcus neoformans, Coccidioides immitis,* and *Histoplasma capsulatum*

**PARASITIC INFECTIONS**

Include *Pneumocystis carinii* and *Toxoplasma gondii*.

rosis can result in myocardial ischemia, myocardial infarction, or cardiac failure. The ischemia and infarction may not be associated with pain because the transplanted heart is denervated. No effective treatment exists to stop the chronic rejection process or the associated atherosclerosis. Treatment focuses on interventions to improve cardiac function as much as possible. Retransplantation may be necessary.

Infection is one of the most severe complications. Pulmonary infection is the most common, but infections can occur anywhere. Box 72-8 lists the organisms causing the infections. All the care described earlier to prevent infection is necessary.

### Patient teaching

Patient and family education is an important part of nursing care. The patient will need to be able to manage all medications, administer them correctly, manage any side effects, and report those side effects that must be reported. The patient will need to manage dietary restrictions, which may include sodium, cholesterol, and calorie restrictions. A diabetic diet may be necessary for some patients who develop hyperglycemia from the corticosteroids. Sometimes the patient will have fluid restrictions. Health care measures to prevent infections and improve cardiac fitness need to be taught, and patients need to understand which signs and symptoms of infection and decreased cardiac functions need to be reported. The patient must understand the follow-up care, which includes repeat cardiac catheterizations and biopsies.

## Lung Transplantation

Lung transplantation is used to treat persons with interstitial pulmonary fibrosis, sarcoidosis, pulmonary hypertension, emphysema, cystic fibrosis, eosinophilic granuloma, and lymphangiomyomatosis. Single- and double-lung transplants may be used, as well as a heart-lung transplant.

Single-lung transplantation has been used for restrictive lung disease, because the decreased compliance and increased pulmonary resistance of the recipient's remaining lung result in preferential ventilation and perfusion of the transplanted lung. Double-lung transplants are used in persons with emphysema or cystic fibrosis. Lung transplants are still considered experimental in most instances.

### Postoperative nursing care

The patient who has undergone a lung transplantation is in the intensive care unit after surgery. The most important focuses of care are initiating appropriate immunosuppressive therapy, monitoring for infection and rejection, promoting adequate airway clearance and gas exchange, and instituting care to prevent the major complications associated with lung transplantations (see Box 72-5). Poor gas exchange is a common complication and may be caused by reperfusion edema of the lung, impaired cough, infections, or rejection.

One difference in immunosuppression in lung transplants compared with other transplants is that corticosteroids are not used for 7 to 14 days after the transplant. Because corticosteroids jeopardize the healing of the tracheal and bronchial anastomoses, OKT-3 is used instead. Once healing has occurred, corticosteroids are started.

Aggressive respiratory care is necessary. This includes frequent position change and deep breathing along with postural drainage and coughing. Supplemental oxygen is necessary. The patient with a lung transplant is prone to cardiovascular complications from hypervolemia or hypovolemia, myocardial irritability, or decreased contractility. Hemodynamic status must be carefully managed to maintain adequate cardiac output without fluid overload, which can result in pulmonary edema. Decreased cardiac output also must be managed carefully to prevent an elevation in pulmonary vascular resistance. The patient is at risk for arrhythmias because of the use of cardiopulmonary bypass. Arrhythmias are treated as they would be in any situation (see Chapter 30).

The use of anticoagulants with cardiopulmonary bypass or excessive replacement of blood products puts the patient at risk for bleeding from coagulopathy. Careful monitoring of blood loss from the mediastinal tubes and of coagulation studies is necessary. Administration of platelets or fresh-frozen plasma may be necessary. Additional needs include nutritional support, comfort measures, and promotion of adequate sleep.

#### Rejection

The patient undergoing a lung transplant is at risk for rejection and infection. Rejection may be acute or chronic. Acute rejection usually occurs before the end of the third postoperative week and is associated with increased hypoxemia, fever, malaise, desaturation with minimal activity, and pulmonary infiltrates. Pulmonary function tests will worsen. The patient needs to be monitored for any of these signs and symptoms so that appropriate therapy can be instituted. Acute rejection usually responds to bolus doses of corticosteroids. Early treatment is the key to maintaining the viability of the transplanted lung.

Infection of the lungs with any of the organisms listed in Box 72-8 is one of the most severe complications after lung transplantation. All the care for the prevention of infection described earlier is necessary.

#### Patient teaching

The patient who has a lung transplant needs education about the following:

1. Proper medication administration
2. Side effects of the medication that need to be reported and ways to deal with other side effects
3. Signs of rejection that should be monitored and reported
4. Health measures to prevent infections and promote optimal health
5. Activity regimen to enhance pulmonary functioning
6. Follow-up care

### Hepatic Transplantation

Hepatic transplantation is performed for various reasons, including biliary atresia, chronic active hepatitis, fulminant hepatitis, end-stage cirrhosis with sequelae, metabolic diseases of the liver, and hepatic malignancy. One problem with using transplants in malignancy is the excessively high recurrence rate of the malignancy.[22] Most organs are obtained from brain-dead donors, although organ transplantation from live donors has been performed in children. The recipient of a live-donor transplant is matched for HLAs and blood group. The recipient receiving a cadaver organ is usually matched for blood group, although transplants using cadaver organs have been performed despite the presence of nonidentical blood groups. Both vascular and biliary drainage system reconstruction is necessary.

#### Postoperative nursing care

The major physiologic complications postoperatively include rejection, infection, and occlusion of vessels (see Box 72-5). In addition, because of the patient's preoperative illness and the surgery itself, all patients are at increased risk for any of the common postoperative complications described in Chapter 25.

Postoperatively, the patient is in an intensive care unit. Constant monitoring of hemodynamic, cardiovascular, neurologic, and respiratory status; fluid and electrolyte balance; and liver function is necessary. Bedrest is maintained for several days. Assessment of liver function with blood tests such as serum transaminases (ALT, AST), bilirubin, albumin, and clotting factors should show improvement immediately (within 24 hours) if a complication does not occur. Immunosuppression therapy is started before surgery and must be continued on a regular schedule after the procedure.

While instituting the intensive physical care needed, the nurse must deal with the psychosocial needs of the patient and family. The patient and family must be kept aware of the status of the transplant. They have been informed of the risks of the procedure before surgery, and keeping them informed helps them deal with the uncertainty. The patient and family need time to express their fears and concerns. They also need help coping with the social isolation and the separation that can occur with the long hospitalization (several weeks to a month) that is sometimes involved.

The nurse can help the patient and family stay up to date. Short, frequent meetings between health team members and the patient and family can result in answers to many of their questions, and an established time during each day for longer meetings can be set aside as necessary. If family members cannot visit often, the nurse can decrease the patient's homesickness by encouraging telephone calls and communication via audiotapes or letters. The nurse can help the patient cope with the long separation by encouraging reading, engaging in hobbies (e.g., crossword puzzles, needlework), and watching television.

#### Rejection

Immunosuppression is usually maintained with cyclosporine and corticosteroids. Because of the nephrotoxicity of cyclosporine, various centers have examined ways to decrease the dosage of cyclosporine. One approach is to include azathioprine, which has been used with other types of transplants, so the dose of cyclosporine can be decreased.

The amount of immunosuppressive therapy is altered on the basis of the following signs of rejection:

1. Increased temperature (38° C [100.4° F] or greater), tachycardia, malaise, hypertension, fluid retention
2. Enlargement of the liver
3. Tenderness over the transplant site
4. Recurrence of abnormal liver function tests (serum transaminases [ALT, AST], bilirubin, albumin, clotting factors)
5. Altered functioning seen on hepatic scan or hepatic perfusion studies, abnormalities on liver biopsy

If signs of rejection occur, the dosage of immunosuppressive agents may be increased, or additional agents (e.g., lymphocyte immune globulin, OKT-3) are added. The nurse must always be aware that these drugs will increase the risk of infection.

#### Patient teaching

A major focus of care is on patient education. The patient and family must receive education before surgery, immediately after surgery, and in preparation for discharge. They need information about the immunosuppressive agents and must be taught how the medications are to be taken, the importance of never missing a dose, and how to monitor for signs of infection or rejection. The patient needs to learn ways to avoid infections. Follow-up care must be understood, and the patient needs to know how to contact the nurse or physician at all times.

### Pancreatic Transplantation

Pancreatic transplantations have been performed since 1966. Cadaver and live-donor pancreases, both whole and segmental sections, have been transplanted. More than 1000 transplantations were performed from 1982 to 1988. The graft and patient survival rates have increased. In transplantations performed since 1982, the 1-year patient and graft survival rates were 82% and 46%, respectively.

Pancreatic transplantation poses a unique problem: the exocrine function of the transplant is not needed, but it must be managed in some way. Digestive enzymes released from the exocrine ducts can be very irritating to tissue. Several approaches to solving this problem have been used, including injecting the exocrine duct with synthetic polymer or anastomosing the exocrine ducts to the bowel or to the bladder. The bowel anastomosis is the most physiologic because the GI tract will not be damaged by the digestive enzymes, but the transplanted pancreas is exposed to GI bacteria. The bladder anastomosis can lead to bladder damage from the exocrine secretions, but it does allow for easy assessment of graft function through assessment of urinary amylase.

The major issue about transplantation for treatment of diabetes mellitus is benefits versus risks. The documented benefits of transplantation are its favorable effects on neuropathy and progressive nephropathy. It has no influence, however, on the progression of proliferative retinopathy. The risks result from the immunosuppression necessary to prevent rejection.

Immunosuppressive therapy includes cyclosporine, azathioprine, and prednisone for long-term therapy and lymphocyte immune globulin or OKT-3 monoclonal antibodies for induction of immunosuppression or for rejection. The tremendous risk of infection, the side effects of these drugs, the cost of immunosuppression ($7000/year), the long hospitalization (2 to 3 weeks), and the frequent postdischarge clinic visits (twice a week) must be considered when risks and benefits are weighed.

Currently, some risks are eliminated because most pancreatic transplantations are performed on persons who have or are receiving a renal transplantation. Thus these patients are already undergoing immunosuppressive therapy. Transplantation in a nonrenal transplant person with insulin-dependent diabetes mellitus (IDDM) has been performed infrequently. Interestingly, persons who have a renal transplant with the pancreatic transplant have survived the longest.

Another type of transplantation that could be used in IDDM patients is islet transplantation, which is still in an experimental stage of development. Techniques have been developed to isolate islet cells from adult or fetal pancreatic tissue; the estimated 250,000 islets needed for a single transplantation can be obtained from one human pancreas. Islet cells have been transplanted into various sites, including the kidney capsule, the liver (by injection into the portal vein), and the spleen. Research about whether the site of transplant influences graft survival is ongoing.

Islet transplantation is believed to offer several advantages over pancreatic organ transplantation. One advantage is that there are no exocrine secretions to manage. However, the major advantage relates to immunosuppression needs. In animal studies, pretreatment of islet cells to destroy leukocytes on the donor tissue allowed for transplantation of the cells into a temporarily immunosuppressed recipient animal, and the graft survived after withdrawal of immunosuppressors. Transplantations of islets in humans has been limited to persons who are immunosuppressed because of renal transplantation. A clinical trial is now in progress at one center to transplant islets into persons with long-term IDDM and no kidney damage. The results of this trial and others will provide definitive information on the role of islet transplantation in persons with IDDM. Another area of experimentation in islet cell transplantation is to package the islet cells in a synthetic membrane that allows contact between the islet cells and blood but not between the islet cells and the recipient's immune cells. This type of packaging would prevent the need for immunosuppression.

#### Postoperative nursing care

Postoperatively, these patients are critically ill and need careful monitoring of hemodynamic status, fluid and electrolyte status, immune status, and graft status (see

Box 72-5). Any signs of rejection must be identified as quickly as possible so that appropriate additional immunosuppressive therapy can be initiated. The patient also needs all the care any patient would receive during the postoperative period (see Chapter 25).

The success of pancreatic and islet transplantations is assessed by analyzing blood glucose response and C-peptide levels. A successful transplantation results in normoglycemia within 2 to 3 days and increased C-peptide levels. Insulin levels can also be measured, but then the patient cannot be taking exogenous insulin. If bladder anastomosis of the exocrine pancreatic ducts is used, the success of the transplantation can be analyzed through urinary amylase levels.

Transplantation as a treatment in IDDM is still a relatively rare procedure, but as advances are made in understanding immunosuppression or with use of islet cells, more may be performed.

### Rejection

Rejection results in an elevated blood glucose level, decreased C-peptide level, and decreased urine amylase level.

### Patient teaching

A major focus of nursing care is to prepare the patient for discharge. The patient will need to perform the required self-monitoring; know signs of infection, rejection, or other complications to report; and know how to manage the immunosuppressive therapy. The patient must be aware of the follow-up care, which consists of twice-weekly visits for some time after the transplant.

## Bone Marrow Transplantation

Bone marrow transplantation (BMT) following treatment with high-dose chemotherapy or radiotherapy is being used in patients with a variety of hematologic malignancies and solid tumors. This is a "rescue" technique that allows administration of what would be toxic doses of drugs and/or radiation when best effect is achieved with high doses.

There are three types of tissue or bone marrow donors: *allogenic,* usually from a sibling who has a close HLA match; *syngeneic,* from an identical twin; or the most recent type used, *autologous bone marrow transplantation* (ABMT), in which patients serve as their own donors. ABMT has been useful because it is frequently difficult to identify a donor that has a close HLA match.[6]

In ABMT the patient's marrow is usually disease free or has been purged of tumor cells before reinfusion. The rationale for ABMT is based on the knowledge that higher doses of chemotherapy or radiation will increase the number of tumor cells killed in a logarithmic manner; that is, doubling the dose may result in 10 times or more the number of tumor cells killed. Large doses of drugs can be given because ABMT provides a rescue for bone marrow depression.

Autologous bone marrow "harvest" (the term used for donating the bone marrow) is done when the patient is in remission or when the tumor burden is small and bone marrow involvement cannot be microscopically identified. The purpose of the harvest is to collect enough stem cells (pluripotent cells) to reconstitute the hematopoietic system after therapy.

If malignant cells may be present, autologous bone marrow purging to remove the residual malignant cells may be done by one of three methods: (1) separation of malignant cells from the marrow based on density differences between malignant and normal cells (physical); (2) use of immunotoxic or monoclonal antibodies (immunologic); and (3) use of drugs such as mercocyanine 540, or 4-hydroperoxycyclophosphamide (pharmacologic).

If allogenic BMT is used, a conditioning regimen must be initiated to permit acceptance of the foreign tissue by the recipient's body. Early regimens used with allogenic BMT included total body irradiation in combination with drugs such as cyclophosphamide. New regimens include fractionated or hypofractionated irradiation, total lymphoid irradiation, busulfan, and arabinosylcytosine (cytarabine).

Most autologous or allogenic bone marrow is obtained by multiple needle aspirations from the posterior iliac crest with the patient under general or spinal anesthesia, although the anterior iliac crest and sternum may also be used. The amount of marrow extracted ranges from 600 to 2500 ml for the average adult (see the Guidelines box below).

After processing, the marrow is given to the patient intravenously through a transfusion bag, or it can be frozen at −140° C, although −196° C is preferred (cryopreservation). Marrow can be kept for 3 years or more.

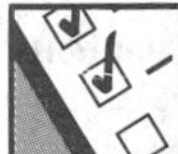

### Guidelines for Patient Teaching About the Bone Marrow Harvest Procedure

Explain that bone marrow has stem cells that are precursors to all blood cells.

Discuss special preparation, for example, showering with antiseptic soap the evening before harvest.

Describe the harvest procedure:

- General or spinal anesthesia is used.
- Needle is placed through skin in back side of hip bone.
- If transplant is autologous, filtered bone marrow is frozen until needed.
- If transplant is allogenic or syngeneic, marrow is transferred to blood transfusion bag and given immediately through an IV line

Explain what happens after recovery:

- Pain in harvest sites can be relieved by medication.
- Patient is out of bed the night of the harvest.
- Pressure dressing is removed the day after the harvest.
- Harvest sites are kept clean and covered for 3 days; on each day the sites are cleaned, Betadine ointment is applied, and the sites are covered with an adhesive bandage.

**Postoperative nursing care**

Acute complications of BMT, whether autologous or allogenic, are often caused by the high-dose chemotherapy and radiation therapy and the toxicity to the GI tract, lungs, liver, kidneys, and other organs. A second major set of problems is caused by nonfunctioning bone marrow. Another complication of BMT is venoocclusive disease (VOD) of the liver. This results from the narrowing or fibrous obliteration of the terminal hepatic venules and sublobular veins from reticulin-collagen deposits in the veins. Symptoms of VOD usually occur 1 to 4 weeks after reinfusion and include ascites; hepatomegaly; elevated alanine aminotransferase, alkaline phosphatase, and bilirubin levels; jaundice; and coagulation difficulties. Other acute complications include hemorrhagic cystitis and acute GVHD if allogenic BMT is used.

The procedure causes psychologic stress in the patient, family, and nursing staff, who should be positive about the outcome. It cannot be overemphasized that hope has a major role with BMT. The involvement of the staff and patient is intense on a BMT unit, and nurses may be placed in the paradoxical situation of providing hope to dying patients. (See Chapter 10 for a discussion of hope.)

BMTs are associated with chronic complications that are the result of the high-dose chemotherapy and radiation therapy used in the conditioning regimen and to treat chronic GVHD. Relapse of the primary disease may occur. Chronic problems from the conditioning regimen include restrictive lung disease and leukoencephalopathy.

**Rejection**

Chronic GVHD can result in changes in skin, joints, and hair growth; chronic stomatitis; caries; hepatic dysfunction; structural changes in the esophagus or other parts of the GI tract; chronic inflammation and stricture formation with adhesions in the vagina; and changes in the vaginal mucosa. The patient may also experience various types of infection resulting from bacterial, fungal, or viral organisms as a result of the immunosuppressive therapy used to treat the GVHD. The more common ones include pulmonary, sinus, oral candidal, and varicella-zoster infections. The patient is treated symptomatically for each of these problems and receives methotrexate, cyclosporine, and corticosteroids.

**Patient teaching**

The patient receiving an allogenic BMT has many educational needs. Information the patient must receive and master includes the following:

1. Medications: how to take, expected effects, side effects, and what to report
2. Health care measures to prevent infections
3. Signs and symptoms of infection that need to be reported
4. Ways to deal with the changes caused by the drug therapy and GVHD
5. Health care measures to promote optimal health
6. Planned follow-up care

## QUESTIONS TO CONSIDER

- What health care measures should be included in the daily care of posttransplantation patients to prevent candidal infections?
- Many posttransplantation patients require treatment for diabetes mellitus. Why are these patients at risk for developing diabetes mellitus?
- What are the differences in immune response, signs and symptoms, and treatment for hyperacute, acute, and chronic rejection?
- What signs of organ failure are seen with rejection of the kidney, heart, liver, lung, pancreas, or bone marrow?

## CRITICAL THINKING ACTIVITIES

- You are experiencing liver failure as a result of excessive acetaminophen use. What information would you need to know to make a decision about receiving an organ transplant?
- Given the criteria for allocating organs for transplant and guidelines offered by the United Network for Organ Sharing (UNOS), consider the following patients, each in need of a kidney transplant. The first patient lives in Colorado, the second in Wisconsin, and the third in Kansas. The patient living in Colorado is in the most life-threatening situation and therefore has the greatest need for the transplant. A donor liver becomes available in Kansas. Take a position regarding the recipient of the organ and defend your position.

## CHAPTER SUMMARY

**TRANSPLANTATION CRITERIA**

- Transplantation of tissues and organs is a major therapeutic intervention for selected patients.
- The major criteria for a recipient of transplant are the presence of end-stage disease that is unresponsive to conventional therapy or worsening despite aggressive management, ability to achieve improvement in quality and quantity of life, and financial means to cover the cost of the procedure. The age-range of potential recipients has been broadened in recent years.
- Medicare covers the cost of renal, liver, and heart transplants; some transplants are covered by state programs; and third-party payors cover some transplants. However, some persons may be ineligible for any transplant because of lack of financial means.
- Legislation has been passed to increase the supply of organs and the fair allocation of donated organs; the

family or guardians of all potential donors must be approached about donating organs.

- Donors of organs must die from brain death and have no preexisting disease of the organ(s) being recovered, no transmissible diseases or sepsis, no history of intravenous drug abuse, no extracranial malignancies, and no death of unknown etiology.
- The potential donor must have been maintained hemodynamically until the organs are recovered.
- To decrease the potential transmission of HIV, criteria for the exclusion of high-risk persons have been identified even if the HIV test is negative.

## IMMUNOLOGY AND TRANSPLANTATION

- Successful allogenic transplantation requires manipulation of the recipient's immune system with drugs to prevent rejection.
- Three types of rejections occur: hyperacute, acute, and chronic.
- Rejection results from activation of humoral and/or cellular immune responses to mismatched class I and II human leukocyte antigens, ABO antigens, and minor red blood cell antigens.
- Acute rejection is an immune response that occurs from approximately 7 days after the transplant up to 3 months after the transplant. Immunosuppressive therapy is used to prevent and treat acute rejections.
- Chronic rejection is a slow, progressive process that occurs anywhere from 3 months after the transplant and leads to loss of function of the transplant. It is not treatable.
- Azathioprine, corticosteroids, and cyclosporine are the immunosuppressive agents used in all types of transplants to prevent acute rejections.
- Bolus doses of corticosteroids, OKT-3, and lymphocyte immune globulin are used to treat acute rejection episodes.

## NURSING MANAGEMENT

- A major focus of nursing care is the prevention or early detection of infections, which the transplant patient is at risk for because of immunosuppression.
- Once the patient decides to undergo a transplant and is accepted for a transplant, nursing care needs to focus on helping the patient and family deal with the waiting period, helping the patient manage the end-stage failure carefully, and helping the patient implement appropriate preventive health practices to maintain as healthy a state as possible.
- After transplantation, all patients must be monitored carefully for rejection and infection. Rejection signs and symptoms are unique for each type of transplant but include a decrease in function of the transplanted organ.
- Other major complications after renal transplant include acute tubular necrosis, fluid and electrolyte imbalance, hemorrhage, and occlusion of the renal artery or vein.
- Heart transplants are associated with the following additional major complications: hemorrhage, cardiac tamponade, and hemodynamic instability.
- Lung transplant patients are at risk for reperfusion edema of the lung, hemodynamic instability, coagulopathy, and pulmonary infections.
- Pancreatic transplant patients are at risk for peritonitis and multiple respiratory complications.
- Patients who undergo allogenic bone marrow transplants are at risk for acute and chronic complications resulting from the conditioning radiation therapy and/or chemotherapy and acute and chronic graft-versus-host disease.
- After any organ or bone marrow transplant, all patients need consistent, detailed monitoring for signs and symptoms of infections, rejections, common complications, side effects of drugs, and overall physical functioning.
- After any organ or bone marrow transplant, all patients need extensive education about the medications and their side effects, signs and symptoms of rejection to report, general health measures, and prevention of infection.
- After corneal transplant, patients do not need immunosuppressive therapy because the cornea is normally avascular.

## REFERENCES


1. American Federation of Clinical Tissue Banks: *Operational standards,* Richmond, Va, 1989, The Federation.
2. Bennett TO et al: Histocompatibility, penetrating keratoplasty, *Acta Ophthamol* 53:403-407, 1975.
3. Bensinger WI et al: ABO-incompatible marrow transplants, *Transplantation* 33:427-429, 1982.
4. Braun WE: Histocompatibility and renal transplantation. In Garovy MR, Guttman RD: *Renal transplantation,* New York, 1986, Churchill Livingstone.
5. Brown ME: Clinical management of the organ donor, *Dimens Crit Care Nurs* 8(3):134-142, 1989.
6. Clark JC, Webster JS: Bone marrow transplantation. In Smith SL: *Tissue and organ transplantation: implications for professional nursing practice,* St Louis, 1990, Mosby.
7. Cohen C, Benjamin M, Ethics and Social Impact Committee of the Transplant and Health Policy Center, Ann Arbor, Mich: Alcoholics and liver transplantation, *JAMA* 265:1299-1301, 1991.
8. Cunningham NH, Boteler S, Windham S: Renal transplantation, *Crit Care Nurs Clin North Am* 4(1):79-88, 1992.
9. Davis FD: Organ procurement and transplantation, *Nurs Clin North Am* 24:823-836, 1989.
10. Hawke D, Kraft J, Smith SL: Tissue and organ donation and recovery. In Smith SL: *Tissue and organ transplantation: implications for professional nursing practice,* St Louis, 1990, Mosby.
11. Hooks MA: Immunosuppressive agents used in transplantation. In Smith SL: *Tissue and organ transplantation: implications for professional nursing practice,* St Louis, 1990, Mosby.

11a. Hrick DH et al: Outpatient use of OKT-3 for the treatment of acute renal allograft rejection, *Clinical Transplantation* 4:19-22, 1990.

12. Kaufman D, Jones J, Matas A: New immunosuppressive agents: FK 506, rapamycin, RS-61443, 15-deoxyspergualin, *J Transplant Coordination* 2:20-27, 1992.

13. Lancaster L: Immunogenetic basis of tissue and organ transplantation and rejection, *Crit Care Nurs Clin* 4(1):1-24, 1992.
14. Lange S: Psychosocial, legal, ethical, and cultural aspects of organ donation and transplantation, *Crit Care Nurs Clin North Am* 4(1):25-42, 1992.
15. Midwest Organ Bank: *Organ and tissue procurement manual,* Westwood, Kans, 1991, The Bank.
16. Moss AH, Siegler M: Should alcoholics compete equally for liver transplantation? *JAMA* 265:1295-1298, 1991.
17. Perryman JP, Stillerman PU: Kidney transplantation. In Smith SL: *Tissue and organ transplantation: implications for professional nursing practice,* St Louis, 1990, Mosby.
18. Prottas JM, Jonasson O, Kleinig JI: In organ transplants, Americans first? *Hastings Center Rep* 16:23-25, 1986.
19. Roitt IM, Brostoff J, Male D: *Immunology,* ed 3, St Louis, 1994, Mosby.
20. Smith SL: Immunologic aspects of transplantation. In Smith SL: *Tissue and organ transplantation: implications for professional nursing practice,* St Louis, 1990, Mosby.
21. Smith SL: The cutting edge in organ transplantation, *Crit Care Nurs Suppl,* June, pp 10-11, 26, 1993.
22. Smith SL, Ciferni M: Liver transplantation. In Smith SL: *Tissue and organ transplantation: implications for professional nursing practice,* St Louis, 1990, Mosby.
23. Workman ML, Ellerhorst-Ryan J, Hargrave-Koertge V: *Nursing care of the immunocompromised patient,* Philadelphia, 1993, Saunders.

# Bibliography

## UNIT I
## Perspectives for Health and Illness

### CHAPTER 1
### Nursing Practice With Ill Adults: Context, Structure, Process, and Outcome


#### *General*

Aiken L: *Am Nurse* 17(4):18, 1985 (editorial).

Cejka S: The changing healthcare workforce: a call for managing diversity, *Healthcare Exec* March-April 20, 1993, pp 20-23.

Kantrowitz B: Wild in the streets, *Newsweek,* Aug 2, 1993, pp 40-46.

Nursing homes' population up, *Kansas City Star,* June 28, 1993, p 6A.

*Patient Self-Determination Act,* Omnibus Reconciliation Act of 1990, Washington, DC.

Projections of the number of persons diagnosed with AIDS and the number of immunosuppressed HIV-infected persons—United States, 1992-1994, *MMWR* 41:1-29, 1992.

*Put it in writing: questions and answers on advance directives,* American Hospital Association, March 1991.

Selby T: Nurses establish clinic for the homeless, *Am Nurse* 17:1, 20, 1985.

Sherer JL: Crossing cultures: hospitals begin breaking down the barriers to care, *Hospitals* 67(10):29-31, 1993.

Turque B: Experimental states, *Newsweek,* May 17, 1993, pp 38-39.

Update: acquired immunodeficiency syndrome—United States, 1992, *MMWR* 42(28), 1993.

Update: mortality attributable to HIV infection/AIDS among persons aged 25-44 years—United States, 1990 and 1991, *MMWR* 42(25), 1993.

Weber G: Tips on implementing the Patient Self-Determination Act, *Nurs Health Care* 14:86-91, 1993.

#### *Case Management*

Alpert HB et al: 7 Gryzmish: toward an understanding of collaboration, *Nurs Clin North Am* 27(1):47-59, 1992.

Bower KA: *Case management by nurses,* Washington, DC, 1992, American Nurses Publishing.

Cohen EL: Nursing case management: does it pay? *J Nurs Adm* 21(4):20-25, 1991.

Cronin CJ, Maklebust J: Case-management care: capitalizing on the CNS, *Nurs Manage* 40(3):38-47, 1989.

del Bueno DL: Paradigm shifts—what's good and not so good for health care, *Nurs Health Care* 14:100-101, 1993.

Dunstron J: How managed care can work for you, *Nurs 90* 20(10):56-59, 1990.

Etheredge MLS: *Collaborative care: nursing case management,* Chicago, 1989, American Publishing.

Ethridge P, Lamb GS: Professional nursing case management improves quality, access and cost, *Nurs Manage* 20(3):30-35, 1989.

Fagin CM: Collaboration between nurses and physicians: no longer a choice, *Nurs Health Care* 13:354-363, 1992.

Ling K: Initiation and evolution of managed care at the Johns Hopkins Hospital, *Nurs Adm Q* 17(3):54-58, 1993.

Michelson EL: The challenge of nurse-physician collaborative practices: improved patient care provision and outcomes, *Heart Lung* 17:390-391, 1988 (editorial).

Newman M, Lamb GS, Michaels C: Nurse case management: the coming together of theory and practice, *Nurs Health Care* 12(8):404-408, 1991.

Pike AW et al: A new architecture for quality assurance: nurse-physician collaboration, *J Nurs Care Q* 7(3):1-8, 1993.

Robinson JA, Robinson KJ, Lewis DJ: Balancing quality of care and cost-effectiveness through case management, *Am Nephrol Nurs Assoc J* 19(2):182-188, 1992.

Sandrick K: Collaboration: a prerequisite to effective reform, *Healthcare Exec* 8:17-19, 1993.

Schull DE, Tosch P, Wood M: Clinical nurse specialists as collaborative care managers, *Nurs Manage* 23(3):30-33, 1992.

Simmons FM: Developing the trauma nurse case manager role, *Dimens Crit Care Nurs* 11(3):164-170, 1992.

Smith P et al: Implementing nurse case management in a community hospital, *Med-Surg Nurs* 1:47-52, 1992.

Trinidad EA: Case management: a model of CNS practice, *Clin Nurs Specialist* 7(4):221-223, 1993.

Ward-Evans S, Hodges LC, Smith J: A new role for neuroscience nurses: the case manager, *J Neurosci Nurs* 23(4):256-260, 1991.

Zander K: Nursing case management, *Nurs Clin North Am* 23(3):503-520, 1988.

Zander K: Nursing case management: strategic management of cost and quality outcomes, *J Nurs Adm* 18(5):23-30, 1988.

Zander K: Managed care within acute care settings: design and implementation via nursing case management, *Health Care Supervisor* 6(2):27-43, 1988.

Zander K: Critical pathways. In Melum MM, Simioris MK: *Total quality management,* Chicago, 1992, American Hospital Publishing.

#### *Health Care Cost and Reform*

American Nurses Association: *A national policy for health care: principles and positions,* Washington, DC, 1977, ANA.

American Nurses Association: *Nursing's agenda for health care reform,* Washington, DC, 1991, ANA.

Champlin L: Home healthcare: word to the wise for the 21st century providers, *Kansas City Health Care Times* 2(2):9, 1993.

Curtin L: Health reform: the shape of things to come, *Nurs Manage* 24(4):28-32, 1993.

Friedman E: Managed care: where will your hospital fit in? *Hospitals* 67(7):18-23, 1993.

Fries JF et al: Reducing health care costs by reducing the need and demand for medical services, *N Engl J Med* 329:321-325, 1993.

Handley T: Need for reform is in the numbers, *Kansas City Health Care Times* 2(7):5, 1993.

Hull K: Outpatient acceleration: 1992 survey traces continued ambulatory care growth, *Hospitals* 67(9):40-41, 1993.

Jaret P: Nurses—the final guardians, *Newsweek* 104:16, 1984.

Kennedy EM: Congress and the national health policy, Rosenhause lecture, *Am J Public Health* 68:241-244, 1978.

Lubitz LD, Riley GF: Trends in Medicare payments in the last year of life, *N Engl J Med* 328:1092-1096, 1993.

*Medicare: 1994 highlights,* Baltimore, 1994, US Department of Health and Human Services.

Milio N: *The storefront that didn't burn,* Ann Arbor, 1970, University of Michigan Press.

National Center for Health Statistics, Hyattsville, Md, 1992, US Public Health Service.

Olendski MC: *Cautionary tales,* Wakefield, Mass, 1973, Contemporary Publications.

One in 3 ED patients is seeking primary care, *Am J Nurs* 93(8):9, 1993.

Packard NJ: The price of choice: managed care in America, *Nurs Adm Q* 17(3):8-15, 1993.

Rakich JS, Longest BB, Darr K: *Managing health services organizations,* ed 2, Philadelphia, 1985, WB Saunders.

Sabatino F: Culture shock: are U.S. hospitals ready? *Hospitals* 67(10):23-28, 1993.

Schondelmeyer B: Home health care is a growing business, *Kansas City Health Care Times* 2(2):4, 1993.

Should health care cost concern you? *AIDE,* April 1993, pp 6-9.

Solomon J et al: Why wait for Hillary? *Newsweek,* June 28, 1993, pp 38-40.

Suzman R, Riley NW: Introducing the oldest old, health and society, *Milbank Mem Fund Q* 63:177-186, 1985.

### *Quality Care and Improvement*

Cesta TG: The link between continuous quality improvement and case management, *J Nurs Adm* 23(6):55-61, 1993.

Crosby PB: *Quality is free: the art of making quality certain,* New York, 1979, McGraw-Hill.

Deming WE: *Out of crisis,* Cambridge, Mass, 1986, Center for Advanced Engineering Study, Massachusetts Institute of Technology.

Dienemann J: *Continuous quality improvement,* Washington, DC, 1992, American Nurses Publishing.

Joint Commission on Accreditation of Healthcare Organizations: *Manual for hospitals: quality assessment and improvement,* Chicago, 1993, JCAHO.

Juran JM: *Juran on quality leadership: how to go from here to there,* Wilton, Conn, 1987, Juran Institute.

Juran JM: *Juran on planning for quality,* New York, 1988, Free Press.

Lopresti J, Whetstone WR: Total quality management: doing things right, *Nurs Manage* 24:34-36, 1993.

McCabe WJ: Total quality management in a hospital, *Q Rev Bull* 18:134-140, 1992.

Melum MM, Sinioris MK: *Total quality management,* Chicago, 1992, American Nurses Publishing.

Saldon R, Tanner FW: Quality management program boosts financial performance, *Provider* 18(10):56-57, 1992.

Update: nurse chosen to fill Joint Commission Board seat, *J Nurs Adm* 22(12):9, 1992.

Wakefield DS, Wakefield BJ: Overcoming the barriers to implementation of TQM/CQI in hospitals: myths and realities, *Q Rev Bull* 19:83-88, 1993.

### *Role of Nursing*

American Association of Colleges of Nursing: *Position statement: nursing education's agenda for the 21st century,* Washington, DC, 1993, AACN.

American Nurses Association: *The role of the clinical nurse specialist,* Washington, DC, 1986, ANA.

American Nurses Association: *Standards of clinical nursing practice,* Washington, DC, 1991, ANA.

American Nurses Credentialing Center: *Am Nurse,* July-August, 1993, p 2.

Anderson CA: Making the invisible visible, *Nurs Outlook* 41(6):246-247, 1993.

Benner P: *From novice to expert,* Menlo Park, Calif, 1984, Addison-Wesley.

Bower-Ferres S: Loeb center and its philosophy of nursing, *Am J Nurs* 75:810-815, 1975.

Cook S: Breaking with tradition, *Acad Nurs,* Summer 1993, pp 19-21.

Frik SM, Pollock SE: Preparation for advanced nursing practice, *Nurs Health Care* 14:190-195, 1993.

Griffith H: Who will become the preferred providers? *Am J Nurs* 85:539-542, 1985.

Jackson LE: Looking toward an NP/CNS merger by the year 2000, *Nurs Pract* 18(4):15-19, 1993.

Koerner J: Differentiated practice: the evolution of professional nursing, *J Prof Nurs* 8:335-341, 1992.

Kotthoff E: Current trends and issues in nursing in the U.S.: the primary health care nurse practitioner, *Int Nurs Rev* 28:24-28, 1981.

Lutz EM, Scholtfeldt RM: Pioneering a new approach to professional education, *Nurs Outlook* 33:139-143, 1985.

Manthey M et al: Primary nursing—a return to the concept "my nurse" and "my patient," *Nurs Forum* 9:65-83, 1970.

Mittelstadt PC: Federal reimbursement of advanced practice nurses' services empowers the profession, *Nurs Pract* 18(1):43-49, 1993.

Morgan WA: Using state board of nursing data to estimate the number of nurse practitioners in the United States, *Nurs Pract* 18(2):65-74, 1993.

Mundinger MO: Health care reform: nursing's vision of change, *Hospitals* 67(8):20-24, 1993.

Naisbitt J: *Megatrends,* New York, 1982, Warner.

National League for Nursing: A promising trend in the American care system, *PRISM* 1(1):3-5, 1993.

National League for Nursing: *A vision for nursing education,* New York, 1993, NLN.

National League for Nursing: Legislative initiatives: removing barriers to nursing practice, *PRISM* 1(1):6-10, 1993.

National League for Nursing: Nursing centers enter policy arena, *PRISM* 1(1):1-2, 1993.

O'Koren ML: Reflections on facilitating collaboration between nursing services and nursing education, *J Prof Nurs* 2:72-74, 1986 (editorial).

Papenhausen JL: Case management: a model of advanced practice? *Clin Nurs Specialist* 1:47-52, 1990.

Paulen A: A time for reassessment, *Cancer Nurs* 9:2, 1986 (editorial).

Pearson LJ: 1992-93 update: how each state stands on legislative issues affecting advanced nursing practice, *Nurs Pract* 18(1):23-26, 1993.

Safriet BJ: Health care dollars and regulatory sense: the role of advanced practice nursing, *Yale J Regulation* 9(2):419-487, 1992.

Sakalys JA, Watson J: Professional education: post-baccalaureate education for professional nursing, *J Prof Nurs* 2:91-97, 1986.

Scholotfeldt RM: The professional doctorate: rationale and characteristics, *Nurs Outlook* 26:302-311, 1978.

Sherer JL: Nursing education: addressing post-reform needs, *Hospitals* 67(10):25, 1993.

Spross J, Hamrick AB: A model for future clinical specialist practitioner. In Hamrick AB, Spross J, editors: *The clinical nurse specialist in theory and practice,* New York, 1983, Grune & Stratton.

US Department of Health and Human Services, Public Health Service: *Healthy people 2000: national health promotion and disease prevention objectives,* Washington, DC, 1990, US Government Printing Office.

CHAPTER 2

## Ethical Decision Making in Nursing

### *General*

Bayles MD: *Professional ethics,* Belmont, Calif, 1981, Wadsworth.

Bowie NE: *Making ethical decisions,* New York, 1986, McGraw-Hill.

Benjamin M, Curtis J: *Ethics in nursing,* ed 3, New York, 1992, Oxford University Press.

Daly BJ: Ethics in critical care. In Clochesy JM et al: *Critical care nursing,* Philadelphia, 1993, WB Saunders.

Davis GC: Nursing values and health care policy, *Nurs Outlook* 36:289-292, 1988.

Iserson KV, Mahowald MB: Acute care research: is it ethical? *Crit Care Med* 20:1032-1037, 1992.

Veatch RM, Fry ST: *Case studies in nursing ethics,* Philadelphia, 1987, JB Lippincott.

Wright RA: *Human values in health care,* New York, 1987, McGraw-Hill.

***Moral Agency***

American Nurses Association: *Code for nurses,* Washington, DC, 1985, ANA.

American Nurses Association: *Ethics in nursing,* Washington, DC, 1988, ANA.

Bandman EL, Bandman B: *Nursing ethics through the life span,* ed 2, East Norwalk, Conn, 1992, Appleton & Lange.

Barnett TJ: Are there employment risks to ethical decisions? *Nurs Forum* 28(1):17-21, 1993.

Fry ST: Autonomy, advocacy, and accountability. In Fowler M, Levine-Ariff J: *Ethics at the bedside,* Philadelphia, 1987, JB Lippincott.

Hedin BA: Nursing, education, and sterile ethical fields, *Adv Nurs Sci* 11(3):43-52, 1989.

Purtillo R: *Ethical dimensions in the health professions,* ed 2, Philadelphia, 1993, WB Saunders.

Silva MC: The American Nurses Association's code for nurses: purposes, content, and enforceability, *Health Matrix* 11(2):55-63, 1989.

Solomon MZ et al: Decisions near the end of life: professional views on life-sustaining treatments, *Am J Public Health* 83(1):14-22.

Viens DC: A history of nursing's code of ethics, *Nurs Outlook* 37(1):45-49, 1989.

Winslow GR: From loyalty to advocacy: a new metaphor for nursing, *Hastings Cent Rep* 14(3):32-39, 1984.

***Ethical Theories and Principles***

Beauchamp TL, Childress JF: *Principles of biomedical ethics,* ed 3, New York, 1989, Oxford University Press.

Chell B: Competency: what it is and what it isn't. In Monagle JF, Thomasma DC: *Medical ethics,* Rockville, Md, 1988, Aspen.

Committee on Ways and Means, US House of Representatives: *Health care resources book,* Washington, DC, 1991, US Government Printing Office.

Gorovitz S: Informed consent and patient autonomy. In Callahan JC: *Ethical issues in professional life,* New York, 1988, Oxford University Press.

Rakowski E: *Equal justice,* Oxford, 1991, Clarendon.

Veatch RM: Models for ethical medicine in a revolutionary age, *Hast Cent Rep* 2(3):5-7, 1972.

Wiens AG: Patient autonomy in care: a theoretical framework for nursing, *J Prof Nurs* 9(2):95-103, 1993.

***Resolving Ethical Dilemmas***

Fowler MD: Piecing together the ethical puzzle: operationalizing nursing ethics in critical care. In Fowler MD, Levine-Ariff J: *Ethics at the bedside,* Philadelphia, 1987, JB Lippincott.

Haggarty MC: Ethics: nurse patron or nurse advocate? *Nurs Manage* 16(5), 1985.

Halloran MC: Rational ethical judgments utilizing a decision-making tool, *Heart Lung* 11:566-570, 1982.

Holly CM: The ethical quandaries of acute care nursing practice, *J Prof Nurs* 9:110-115, 1993.

Levine-Ariff J: Preventive ethics: the development of policies to guide decision-making, *AACN Clin Iss Crit Care Nurs* 1(1):169-177, 1990.

Novak J: An ethical decision-making model for the neonatal intensive care unit, *J Perinat Nurs* 1(3):57-67, 1988.

***Common Ethical Issues in Acute Care***

Abrams FR: Advance directives: when the patient cannot communicate. In Monagle JF, Thomasma DC: *Medical ethics,* Rockville, Md, 1988, Aspen.

Badzek LA: What you need to know about advance directives, *Nurs 92* (6):58-59, 1992.

Brock D: Death and dying. In Veatch RM: *Medical ethics,* Boston, 1989, Jones & Bartlett.

Brock D: Voluntary active euthanasia, *Hast Cent Rep* 22(2):10-22, 1992.

Brody H: Assisted death—a compassionate response to a medical failure, *N Engl J Med* 327:1384-1388, 1992.

Daly BJ: Withdrawal of food and fluid, *AACN Clin Iss Crit Care Nurs* 1(1):187-195, 1990.

Emanuel L: Advance directives: what have we learned so far? *J Clin Ethics* 4:8-16, 1993.

Howe EG: The vagaries of patients' and families' discussing advance directives, *J Clin Ethics* 4(1):3-7, 1993.

Idemoto B et al: Implementing the Patient Self-Determination Act, *Am J Nurs* 93:21-25, 1993.

Jennings B: Active euthanasia and forgoing life-sustaining treatment: can we hold the line? *J Pain Sympt Manage* 6:312-316, 1991.

Lo B: The clinical use of advance directives. In Monagle JF, Thomasma DC: *Medical ethics,* Rockville, Md, 1988, Aspen.

Marsden C: "Do Not Resuscitate" orders and end-of-life care planning, *Am J Crit Care* 2:177-179, 1993.

Meisel A: The legal consensus about foregoing life-sustaining treatment: its status and prospects, *Kennedy Inst Ethics J* 2:309-346, 1992.

Meyer C: End-of-life care: patients' choices, nurses' challenges, *Am J Nurs* 93(2):40-47, 1993.

Mezey M, Latimer B: The Patient Self-Determination Act, *Hast Cent Rep* 23(1):16-20, 1993.

President's Commission for the Study of Ethical Problems in Medicine and Biomedical and Behavioral Research: *Deciding to forego life-sustaining treatment: ethical, medical, and legal issues in treatment decisions,* Washington, DC, 1983, US Government Printing Office.

Rachels J: Euthanasia. In Regan T: *Matters of life and death,* New York, 1986, Random House.

Schwarz JK: Living wills and health care proxies, *Nurs Health Care* 13(2):92-96, 1992.

Stolman C et al: Evaluation of patient, physician, nurse, and family attitudes toward Do Not Resuscitate orders, *Arch Intern Med* 150:653-658, 1990.

Veatch RM: Foregoing life-sustaining treatment: limits to the consensus, *Kennedy Inst Ethics J* 3:1-20, 1993.

***Resources for Ethical Decision Making***

Blake DC: The hospital ethics committee, *Hast Cent Rep* 22(1):6-11, 1992.

Brennan TA: Ethics committees and decisions to limit care, *JAMA* 260:803-807, 1988.

Edwards BS: When the physician won't give up, *Am J Nurs* 93(9):34-37, 1993.

Lo B: Behind closed doors: promises and pitfalls of ethics committees, *N Engl J Med* 317:46-50, 1987.

Simpson KH: The development of a clinical ethics consultation service in a community hospital, *J Clin Ethics* 3:124-130, 1992.

CHAPTER 3

## Nursing Practice With Young and Middle-Aged Adults

### *Psychosocial Development*

Sheehy G: *Passages,* New York, 1976, Dutton.

### *Health Promotion*

Hartweg DL: Self-care actions of healthy middle-aged women to promote well-being, *Nurs Res* 42(4):221-227, 1993.

Woods NF: Women's health. In Fitzpatrick JF, Taunton RL, Benoliel JQ, editors: *Annual review of nursing research,* vol 6, New York, 1988, Springer.

### *Health Risks*

Lambert VA: Arthritis. In Fitzpatrick JF, Taunton RL, Jacox AK, editors: *Annual review of nursing research,* vol 9, New York, 1989, Springer.

O'Connell KA: Smoking cessation: research on relapse crises. In Fitzpatrick JF, Taunton RL, Benoliel JQ, editors: *Annual review of nursing research,* vol 7, New York, 1989, Springer.

Pope A, Tarloff A, editors: *Disability in America: a national agenda for prevention,* Institute of Medicine, Washington, DC, 1992, National Academy Press.

### *Nursing Assessment*

Miller JF, editor: Coping with chronic illness, ed 2, Philadelphia, 1992, FA Davis.

CHAPTER 4

## Nursing Practice With Elders

### *General*

Berg R, Cassells J: *The second fifty years,* Washington, DC, 1990, National Academy Press.

Ebersole P, Hess P: *Toward healthy aging,* ed 4, St Louis, 1994, Mosby.

Lang N et al: *Quality of health care for older people in America,* Kansas City, Mo, 1990, American Nurses Association.

Miles ST, Irvine F: Deaths caused by physical restraints, *Gerontologist* 32(6):762-766, 1992.

Murray R, Zetner J: *Nursing assessment and health promotion through the lifespan,* Englewood Cliffs, NJ, 1979, Prentice-Hall.

Palmore E et al: *Normal aging III,* Durham, NC, 1985, Duke University Press.

Reed P: Implications of the life-span development framework for well-being in adulthood and aging, *Adv Nurs Sci* 6(1):18-25, 1983.

Schilke J: Slowing the aging process with physical activity, *J Gerontol Nurs* 17(6):5-9, 1991.

US Department of Health and Human Services, Public Health Service: *Healthy people 2000: national health promotion and disease prevention objectives,* Washington, DC, 1990, US Government Printing Office.

Vortherms R: Clinically improving communications through touch, *J Gerontol Nurs* 17(5):6-9, 1991.

Winogard CH, Gerety MB: Geriatrics medicine, *JAMA* 270(2):213-216, 1993.

### *Psychology and Mental Health*

Abraham IL, Smullen DE, Thompson-Heisterman AA: Geriatric mental health: assessing geropsychiatric patients, *J Psychosoc Nurs* 39(9):13-17, 1991.

Beck CK et al: Cognitive impairment in the elderly, *Nurs Clin North Am* 28(2):335-347, 1993.

Birren J, Schale K: *Handbook of the psychology of aging,* New York, 1977, Van Nostrand Reinhold.

Hogstel MO: Understanding hoarding behaviors in the elderly, *Am J Nurs* 93(7):42-45, 1993.

Heidrich SM: The relationship between physical health and psychological well-being in elderly women: a developmental approach, *Res Nurs Health* 16:123-130, 1993.

### *Medications*

Gilmore C, Whitehouse P, Wykle M: *Memory, aging and dementia,* New York, 1987, Springer.

McCaffery M, Beebe A: *Pain: clinical manual for nursing practice,* St Louis, 1989, Mosby.

Melers C: Antibiotics: old drugs, new information, *Geriatr Nurs* 12(2):61-63, 1991.

Newbern V: Beta blockers, *Geriatr Nurs* 12(2):119-121, 1991.

### *Sexuality and STDs*

Seura K, Whipple B: Older adults as an HIV positive risk group, *J Gerontol Nurs* 16(1):6-10, 1990.

Talashek M, Tichy A, Epping H: Sexually transmitted disease in elderly, *J Gerontol Nurs* 16(4):33, 1990.

Travis S: Older adults' sexuality and remarriage, *J Gerontol Nurs* 13:9, 1987.

### *Physical Problems of Elderly Persons*

Esberger K: Guide to gastrointestinal problems of elders, *Geriatr Nurs* 12(2):174-175, 1991.

Frantz RA, Ferrell-Torry A: Physical impairments in the elderly populations, *Nurs Clin North Am* 28(2):363-371, 1993.

Herr K, Mowby P: Pain assessment in the elderly, *J Gerontol Nurs* 17(4):13-19, 1991.

Kositzke J: A question of balance: dehydration in the elderly, *J Gerontol Nurs* 16(4):7-9, 1990.

Osterman H, Stuck R: The aging foot, *Orthop Nurs* 9(6):43, 1990.

Posner BM et al: Nutrition in the elderly: the nutrition screening initiative, *Am J Public Health* 83(7):972-978, 1993.

### *Racial Differences*

Ailinger RL, Dear MR, Holley-Wilcon P: Predictors of function among older Hispanic immigrants: a five-year follow-up, *Nurs Res* 42(4):240-244, 1993.

Cowie MR et al: Out-of-hospital cardiac arrest: racial differences in outcome in Seattle, *Am J Public Health* 83(7):955-959, 1993.

Escare JJ et al: Racial differences in the elderly's use of medical procedures and diagnostic tests, *Am J Public Health* 83(7):948-954, 1993.

Guralnik JM et al: Educational states and active life expectancy among older blacks and whites, *N Engl J Med* 329(2):110-116, 1993.

### *Family Caregiving*

Gregory DM, Peters N, Cameron CF: Elderly male spouses as caregivers: toward an understanding of their experience, *J Gerontol Nurs* 16(3):20-24, 1990.

Hogan S: Care for the caregiver: social policies to ease their burden, *J Gerontol Nurs* 16(5):12-17, 1990.

Pallett PJ: A conceptual framework for studying family caregiver burden in Alzheimer's-type dementia, *Image* 22(1):52-57, 1990.

### *Cultural Competence of Nurses*

Capers C: Teaching cultural content: a nursing education imperative, *Holistic Nurs Pract* 6(3):19-28, 1992.

Harris LH, Tuck I: The role of the organization and nurse manager in integrating transcultural concepts into nursing practice, *Holistic Nurs Pract* 6(3):43-48, 1992.

Leininger M: Transcultural nursing theories and research approaches. In Leininger M: *Transcultural nursing: concepts, theories, and practices,* New York, 1978, John Wiley & Sons.

Leininger M: Care facilitation and resistance factors in the culture of nursing, *Top Clin Nurs* 8(2):1-12, 1986.

Nkongho N: Teaching health professionals transcultural concepts, *Holistic Nurs Pract* 6(3):29-33, 1992.

Ogbu J: Origins of human competence: a cultural-ecological perspective, *Child Dev* 52:413-429, 1981.

Reynolds C: An administrative program to facilitate culturally appropriate care for the elderly, *Holistic Nurs Pract* 6(3):34-42, 1992.

Ruiz PM: Dominican concepts of health and illness, *NY State Nurs Assoc* 21(4):11-13, 1990.

CHAPTER 5

## Family and Cultural Influences on Illness

Harris MB, Begay C, Page P: Activities, family relationships and feelings about aging in a multicultural elderly sample, *Int J Aging Hum Dev* 29(2):103-117, 1989.

Harris M, Page P, Begay C: Attitudes toward aging a southwestern sample: effects of ethnicity, age, and sex, *Psychol Rep* 62:735-746, 1988.

Hickey M, Leske J: Needs of families of critically ill patients: state of the science and future directions, *Crit Care Nurs Clin North Am* 4(4):645-649, 1992.

McClowry S: Family functioning during a critical illness: a systems theory perspective, *Crit Care Nurs Clin North Am* 4(4):559-564, 1992.

McCool W, Tuttle J, Crowley A: Overview of contemporary families, *Crit Care Nurs Clin North Am* 4(4):549-558, 1992.

McShane R: Family theoretical perspectives and implications for nursing practice, *AACN Clin Iss* 2(2):210-219, 1992.

Osako M: Aging and family among Japanese Americans: the role of ethnic tradition in the adjustment to old age, *Gerontologist* 19(5):448-455, 1979.

Rosenthal C: Family supports in later life: does ethnicity make a difference? *Gerontologist* 26(1):19-24, 1986.

### General Readings on Culture

Bohannan P: We, the alien: an introduction to cultural anthropology. In *Anthropology, culture and society,* Prospect Heights, Ill, 1992, Waveland.

Burton L, Dilworth-Anderson P, Bengtson V: Theoretical challenges for the twenty-first century: creating culturally relevant ways of thinking about diversity & aging, *Generations,* 1991, pp 67-72.

Campinha-Bacote J: *Readings in transcultural health care,* Wyoming, Ohio, 1994, Transcultural C.A.R.E.

Ganast F, Norbeck E: *Ideas of culture,* New York, 1976, Holt, Rinehart & Winston.

Geertz C: *The interpretation of cultures,* New York, 1973, Basic Books.

Mead M: Ethnological aspects of aging, *Psychosomatics* 8(2):33-37, 1967.

### Nursing Interventions

Bushy A, Rohr K: The Plains Indians: cultural considerations in the use of apnea monitors, *Neonat Network* 8(4):59-66, 1990.

Gaskin F: Detection of cyanosis in the person with dark skin, *J Natl Black Nurses Assoc* 1(1):52-60, 1986.

Gibb J: Defensive communication, *J Communication* 11(3):141-148, 1982.

Roach L: Color changes in dark skin, *Nurs* 77(7):48-51, 1977.

Miller J: Diagnosing altered comfort states: analysis of pain expression styles of blacks and whites, *North Am Nurs Assoc* 6:360-369, 1986.

### Social and Biocultural Dimensions of Health and Illness

Anderson J: Health care across cultures, *Nurs Outlook* 38(3):136-139, 1990.

Hopper S: The influence of ethnicity of the health of older women, *Clin Geriatr Med* 9(1):231-259, 1993.

Hunter K, Linn M, Pratt T: Minority women's attitudes about aging, *Exp Aging Res* 5(2):95-108, 1979.

Mitchell AC: Black skin: an historical, psychological, and health care perspective, *J Cont Educ Nurs* 10:28-33, 1978.

Nielsen B, McMillan S, Diaz E: Instruments that measure beliefs about cancer from a cultural perspective, *Cancer Nurs* 15(2):109-115, 1992.

Reid B: "It's like you're down on a bed of affliction": aging and diabetes among Black Americans, *Soc Sci Med* 34(12):1317-1323, 1992.

Rogers R: Living and dying in the U.S.A.: sociodemographic determinants of death among blacks and whites, *Demography* 29(2):287-303, 1992.

Smith M et al: Age and health perceptions among elderly blacks, *J Gerontol Nurs* 17(11):13-19, 1991.

Torres-Gil F: An examination of factors affecting future cohorts of elderly Hispanics, *Gerontologist* 26(2):140-146, 1986.

Tran T, Wright R, Chatters L: Health, stress, psychological resources and subjective well-being among older blacks, *Psychol Aging* 6(1):100-108, 1991.

Villarruel A, de Montellano B: Culture and pain: a Mesoamerican perspective, *Adv Nurs Sci* 15(1):21-32, 1992.

White E: Giving health care to minority patients, *Nurs Clin North Am* 12:27-40, 1977.

CHAPTER 6

## Healthy Life-Styles: Nutrition, Exercise, Rest, and Sleep

### Nutrition

American Dietetic Association: Position paper on identifying food and nutrition misinformation, *J Am Diet Assoc* 88:1589-1591, 1988.

American Dietetic Association: Position paper on vegetarian diets, *J Am Diet Assoc* 88:351-355, 1988.

Cerato PL: How safe are modified fasts? *RN* 52(11):79-81, 1989.

Cerato PL: Deciphering the new food labels, *RN* 56(8):57-58, 1993.

Crist JK: Weight management. In Bulechek GM, McCloskey JC: *Nursing interventions,* ed 2, Philadelphia, 1992, WB Saunders.

Factors related to cholesterol screening and cholesterol level awareness, *MMWR* 39(37):633-637, 1990.

Fuller K: The new food labels: making it easier to eat right, *Better Homes & Gardens* 71(5):62-66, 1993.

Hospital malnutrition still abounds, *Nutr Rev* 46:315-317, 1988.

Johnson CL et al: Declining serum total cholesterol levels among US adults, *JAMA* 269(23):3002-3008, 1993.

Massachusetts Medical Society Committee on Nutrition: Fast-food fare: consumer guidelines, *N Engl J Med* 321:752-755, 1989.

McGinnis JM et al: Health progress in the United States, *JAMA* 268(11):2545-2552, 1992.

Nutrition Committee: *Position statement on dietary guidelines for healthy American adults: a statement for physicians and health professionals,* Pub No 71-1003, Dallas, 1988, American Heart Association.

Prince RL et al: Prevention of postmenopausal osteoporosis, *N Engl J Med* 325(17):1189-1195, 1991.

Robinson JI et al: Obesity, weight loss and health, *J Am Diet Assoc* 93(4):445-449, 1993.

Widdowson EM: Physiological processes of aging: are there special nutritional requirements for elderly people? *Am J Clin Nutr* 55:1246S-1249S, 1992.

### Exercise and Sleep

Astrand P: Physical activity and fitness, *Am J Clin Nutr* 55:1231S-1236S, 1992.

Cohen FL, Merritt SL: Sleep promotion. In Bulechek GM, McCloskey JC: *Nursing interventions,* ed 2, Philadelphia, 1992, WB Saunders.

Curfman GD: The health benefits of exercise: a critical reappraisal, *N Engl J Med* 328(8):574-575, 1993.

Paffenbarger RS et al: The association of changes in physical activity level and other lifestyle characteristics with mortality among men, *N Engl J Med* 328(8):538-545, 1993.

Pollock ML, Wilmore JH: *Exercise in health and disease: evaluation and prescription for prevention and rehabilitation,* ed 2, Philadelphia, 1990, WB Saunders.

Shephard RJ: Exercise and aging: extending independence in older adults, *Geriatrics* 48(5):61-64, 1993.

Singh VN: A current perspective on nutrition and exercise, *J Nutr* 132(suppl 3):758-759, 1992.

CHAPTER 7

## Stress, Stressors, and Stress Management

### General

McCance K, Huether SE: *Pathophysiology: the biologic base for disease in adults and children,* ed 2, St Louis, 1994, Mosby.

Roy C, Roberts SL: *Theory construction in nursing: as adaptation model,* Englewood Cliffs, NJ, 1981, Prentice-Hall.

Shoemaker W et al, editors: *Textbook of critical care,* ed 2, Philadelphia, 1989, WB Saunders.

Shontz F: *The psychological aspects of physical illness and disability,* New York, 1975, Macmillan.

Strauss A et al: *Chronic illness and the quality of life,* ed 2, St Louis, 1984, Mosby.

### Adaptation and Coping

Adams J, Lindemann E: Coping with long-term disability. In Coehlo GV, Hamburg DA, Adams JE, editors: *Coping and adaptation,* New York, 1974, Basic Books.

Lazarus R: *Psychological stress and the coping process,* New York, 1966, McGraw-Hill.

Lazarus RS, Folkman S: *Stress, appraisal and coping,* New York, 1984, Springer.

Levine S, Weinberg J, Ursin H: Definition of the coping process and statement of the problem. In Ursin H, Baade E, Levine S, editors: *Psychobiology of stress: a study of coping men,* New York, 1978, Academic Press.

Moos R: *Coping with physical illness,* ed 2, New York, 1985, Plenum.

Murphy LP: Coping, vulnerability and resilience in childhood. In Coehlo GV, Hamburg DA, Adams JE, editors: *Coping and adaptation,* New York, 1974, Basic Books.

Weisman A: *Coping with cancer,* New York, 1979, McGraw-Hill.

White RD: Strategies of adaptation: an attempt at systematic description. In Coehlo GV, Hamburg DA, Adams JE, editors: *Coping and adaptation,* New York, 1974, Basic Books.

### Stressors

Ballard KS: *Identification of environmental stress for patients in the surgical intensive care unit,* Unpublished master's thesis, University of Kansas School of Nursing, Kansas City, 1979.

Betrus P, Kogan H: Stressors in nursing: causes, results and interventions. In *Stressors in nursing: responses and resolutions,* Seattle, 1981, University of Washington Press.

Dixon JP, Dixon JK, Spinner J: Perceptions of life-pattern disintegrity as a link in the relationship between stress and illness, *Adv Nurs Sci* 11(2):1-11, 1989.

Hornberger CA: *Perceived stressors, perceived stress response and level of cardiac reactivity in wellness sample,* Unpublished master's thesis, University of Kansas School of Nursing, Kansas City, 1989.

Kemp VH, Hatmaker DD: Stress and social support in high-risk pregnancy, *Res Nurs Health* 12:331-336, 1989.

### Stress Response

Cannon WB: *The wisdom of the body,* New York, 1939, WW Norton.

Cox T: *Stress,* New York, 1978, Macmillan.

Frain M, Valiga T: The multiple dimensions of stress, *Top Clin Nurs* 1(1):43-57, 1979.

Gaillard RC, Al-DamLeiji S: Stress and the pituitary-adrenal axis, *Baillieres Clin Endocrinol Metab* 1:319-354, 1987.

Granner D: Hormones of the adrenal medulla. In Murray RK et al, editors: *Harper's biochemistry,* ed 21, New York, 1988, Lange.

Henry JP, Ely DL: Physiology of emotional stress: specific responses, *J SC Med Assoc* 75:501-508, 1979.

Hetzel BS et al: Changes in urinary 17-hydroxy-corticosteroid excretion during stressful life situations in man, *J Clin Endocrinol* 15:1057-1068, 1955.

Khansari DN, Murgo AJ, Faith RE: Effects of stress on the immune system, *Immunol Today* 5:170-175, 1990.

Lenox RH et al: Specific hormonal and neurochemical responses to different stressors, *Neuroendocrinology* 30:200-308, 1980.

Mason JW: A re-evaluation of the concept of nonspecificity in stress theory, *J Psychiatr Res* 8:323-333, 1971.

Mason, JW: Specificity in the organization of neuroendocrine response profiles. In Seeman P, Brown GM, editors: *Frontiers in neurology and neuroscience research,* First International Symposium of the Neuroscience Institute, University of Toronto, 1974.

Mason JW: A historical view of the stress field, *J Hum Stress* 1(1):6-12, 1975.

Munck A, Guyre PM, Holbrook NJ: Physiological functions of glucocorticoids in stress and their relation to pharmacological actions, *Endocrinol Rev* 5:25-44, 1984.

Salo M: Endocrine response to anaesthesia and surgery. In Watkins J, Salo M, editors: *Trauma, stress and immunity in anaesthesia and surgery,* London, 1982, Butterworth.

Selye H: A syndrome produced by diverse nocuous agents, *Nature* 138:32-35, 1936.

Selye H: The general adaptation syndrome and the diseases of adaptation, *J Clin Endocrinol* 6:117-230, 1946.

Selye H: *The stress of life,* New York, 1956, McGraw-Hill.

Selye H: The stress syndrome, *Am J Nurs* 65:97-99, 1965.

Selye H: *Stress in health and disease,* Sevenoaks, 1976, Butterworth.

Sikes PJ: Endocrine: responses to the stress of critical illnesses, *AACN Clin Iss Crit Care Nurs* 3:379-391, 1992.

Sutterley DC: Stress and health: a survey of self-regulation modalities, *Top Clin Nurs* 1(1):1-29, 1979.

### Stress Management

Aguilera DC: *Crisis intervention: theory and methodology,* ed 6, St Louis, 1990, Mosby.

Benson H: *The relaxation response,* New York, 1975, William Morrow.

Caplan G: *Principles of preventative psychiatry,* New York, 1964, Basic Books.

Danskin D, Crow M: *Biofeedback: an introduction and guide,* Palo Alto, Calif, 1981, Mayfield.

Guzzetta C: Effect of relaxation and music therapy on patients in a coronary unit with presumptive acute myocardial infarction, *Heart Lung* 18:609-616, 1989.

Jacobsen E: *Progressive relaxation,* Chicago, 1938, University of Chicago Press.

Kanfer F, Goldstein A: *Helping people change,* New York, 1975, Pergamon.

Kogan H et al: *Therapeutic manual for the management of stress response,* Seattle, 1980, University of Washington.

Munro BH et al: Effect of relaxation therapy on post-myocardial infarction patient's rehabilitation, *Nurs Res* 37:231-235, 1988.

Scandrett-Hibdon S, Uecker S: Relaxation training. In Bulechek GM, McCloskey JC: *Nursing interventions: essential nursing treatments,* ed 2, Philadelphia, 1992, WB Saunders.

Stevens K: Patient's perception of music during surgery, *J Adv Nurs* 15:1045-1051, 1990.

***Anxiety and Other Behavioral Responses to Stress***

Carlson CE, editor: *Behavioral concepts and nursing interventions,* ed 2, Philadelphia, 1978, WB Saunders.

Ellis A: *Reason and emotion in psychotherapy,* New York, 1962, Lyle Stuart.

James W: What is emotion? *Mind* 19:188-205, 1884.

Kadner KD: Resilience: responding to adversity, *J Psychosoc Nurs* 27(7):20-25, 1989.

Peplau H: A working definition of anxiety. In Burd S, Marshall M, editors: *Some clinical approaches to psychiatric nursing,* New York, 1963, Macmillan.

Pollock SE: The hardiness characteristic: a motivating factor in adaptation, *Adv Nurs Sci* 11(2):53-62, 1989.

Simpson GG: Behavior and evolution. In Roe AR, Simpson GG, editors: *Behavior and evolution,* New Haven, Conn, 1958, Yale University Press.

Weiss JM: Psychological factors in stress and disease, *Sci Am* 226(6):104-113, 1972.

UNIT II

# Common Concepts for Care of Ill Adults

CHAPTER 8

## Chronic Illness and Rehabilitation

***General***

Diamond M, Jones SL: *Chronic illness across the life span,* Norwalk, Conn, 1983, Appleton-Century-Crofts.

Editorial: Older Americans present a double challenge: preventing disability and providing care, *Am J Public Health* 82(3):287-288, March 1991.

Granger CV: Health accounting-functional assessment of the long-term patient. In Kottke FJ, Stilwell GK, Lehmann JF, editors: *Krusen's handbook of physical medicine and rehabilitation,* Philadelphia, 1982, WB Saunders.

Henry WF: Chronic care needs to be a higher priority, *Hospitals,* February 20, 68, 1991.

Hines-Martin VP: A research review: family caregivers of chronically ill African American elderly, *J Gerontological Nurs* 28(2):25-29, 1992.

*Institute of Medicine: The second fifty years: promoting health and preventing disability,* Washington, 1990, National Academy Press.

Kahn KL et al: Comparing outcomes of care before and after implementation of the DRG-based prospective payment system, *JAMA* 264(15):1984-1988, 1990.

Kim, MJ, McFarland G, McLane AM: *Pocket guide to nursing diagnoses,* ed 4, St. Louis, 1991, Mosby.

Lubkin IM: *Chronic illness: impact and interventions,* Boston, 1986, Jones & Bartlett.

Olson EV, editor: The hazards of immobility, *Am J Nurs* 67:780-797, 1967.

Sorensen K, Armis DB: Understanding the world of the chronically ill, *Am J Nurs* 67:811-817, 1967.

Stewart AJ et al: Functional status and well-being of patients with chronic conditions, *JAMA* 262(7):907-913, 1989.

Watson PG: The Americans with Disabilities Act: More rights for people with disabilities, *Rehabilitation Nurs* 15(6):325-328, 1990.

Woog P, editor: *The chronic illness trajectory framework—the Corbin and Strauss nursing model,* New York, 1992, Springer.

***Ethnicity and Health***

Council on Ethical and Judician Affairs: Black-white disparities in health care, *JAMA* 263(17), 2344-2346, 1990.

Schwartz E et al: Black/white comparisons of deaths preventable by medical interventions: United States and the District of Columbia 1980-1986, *Int J Epidemiol* 19(3):591-598, 1990.

Van Horne WA, Tonnoson TV, editors: *Ethnicity and health,* Madison, 1988, University of Wisconsin System Institute on Race and Ethnicity.

***Health Objectives***

McGinnis JM et al: Health progress in the United States, Results of the 1990 objectives for the nation, *JAMA* 268(18):2545-2552, 1992.

US Department of Health and Human Services: *Healthy people 2000: national health promotion and disease prevention objectives,* Washington, DC, 1990, US Government Printing Office.

US Department of Health and Human Services: *Vital and health statistics: current estimates from the national health interview surgery,* 1990, Washington, DC, 1991, US Government Printing Office.

***Health Statistics***

Centers for Disease Control: years of potential life lost before age 65—United States, 1990 and 1991, *MMWR* 42(13):252-253, 1993.

Desencios JC, Hahn RA: Years of potential life lost before age 65, by race, Hispanic origin, and sex—United States, 1986-1988, *MMWR* 41(SS-8):13-23, November 20, 1992.

National Centers for Health Statistics: *Health United States, 1991, and prevention profile,* US Department of Health and Human Services, Hyattsville, Md, 1992, US Department of Health and Human Services Publication Number PHS 92-1232.

***Home Care/Nursing Home Care***

Council on Scientific Affairs: Home care in the 1990s, *JAMA* 263(8):1241-1244, 1990.

Kahn KL et al: Comparing outcomes of care before and after implementation of the DRG-based prospective payment system, *JAMA* 264(15):1984-1988, 1990.

Kemper P, Murdaugh CM: Lifetime use of nursing home care, *New Engl J Med* 324(9):595-600, 1991.

Robertson JF, Cummings CC: What makes long-term care nursing attractive? *Amer J Nurs* 91(11):41-46, 1991.

Ryan S, Wassenberg C, editors: Community health and home care nursing, *Nurs Clin North Am* 15:2, 1980.

Shamansky SL, editor: Home health care, *Nurs Clin North Am* 23(2):305-455, 1988.

Shaughnessy PW, Kramer AM: The increased needs of patients in nursing homes and patients receiving home health care, *N Engl J Med* 322(1):21-27, 1990.

***Psychosocial***

Browning MS: An intradisciplinary approach to long term care. In Hogstel MO, editor: *Management of personnel in long term care,* Bowie, Md, 1983, Robert J Brady.

Burchardt CS et al: Quality of life of adults with chronic illness: a psychometric study, *Res in Nurs & Health* 12:347-354, 1989.

Foxall MJ, Edberg JY: Loneliness of chronically ill adults and their spouses, *Issues in Mental Health Nursing* 10(2):149-167, 1989.

Leidy NK: A structural model of stress, psychosocial resources, and symptomatic experiences in chronic physical illness, *Nurs Outlook* 34(4), 230-236, 1990.

Pollock G: The mourning liberation process in health and disease, *Psychiatric Clin North Am* 10(3):345-354, 1987.

Pollock SE: Human responses to chronic illness: physiologic and psychosocial adaptation, *Nurs Res* 36:90-95, 1986.

Primomo J, Yates BC, Woods NF: Social support for women during chronic illness: the relationship among sources and types top adjustment, *Res in Nurs Health* 13:153-161, 1990.

Raleigh EDH: Sources of hope in chronic illness, *Oncology Nurs Forum* 19(3):443-448, 1992, Raleigh.

Stotland E: *The psychology of hope,* San Francisco, 1969, Jossey-Bass.

### Rehabilitation General

American Nurses Association and Association of Rehabilitation Nurses: *Standards of rehabilitation nursing practice,* Kansas City, Mo, 1986, The Association.

Clard GS, Bray GP: Development of a rehabilitation plan. In Williams TF, editor: *Rehabilitation in the aging,* New York, 1984, Raven Press.

DeLisa JA, Jain SS: Physical medicine and rehabilitation, *JAMA* 265(23):358-359, 1991.

Dittmar S: *Rehabilitation nursing,* St. Louis, 1989, Mosby.

Golden CJ, editor: *Current topics in rehabilitation psychology,* New York, 1984, Grune & Stratton.

Halstead LS, Grabois M, editors: *Medical rehabilitation,* New York, 1985, Raven Press.

Johnson JH, editor: Rehabilitation nursing, *Nurs Clin North Am* 15:2, 1989.

Kottke F, Stillwell GK, Lehman J: *Krusen's handbook of physical medicine and rehabilitation,* ed 3, Philadelphia, 1982, WB Saunders.

Rothberg JS: The rehabilitation team: future direction, *Arch Phy Med Rehabil* 62:407, Aug 1981.

Stryker RP: *Rehabilitative aspects of acute and chronic illness,* ed 2, Philadelphia, 1977, WB Saunders.

Wahlquist G: The family in rehabilitation, *Rehabil Nurs* 12:62, March/April 1987.

Wright B: *Physical disability: a psychological approach,* ed 2, New York, 1983, Harper & Row.

Wright BA: Value-laden beliefs and principles for rehabilitation, *Rehabil Lit* 12:266-269, 1981.

### Rehabilitation Nursing

Buchanan LC: A rehabilitation clinical nurse specialist: evaluation of the role in a home health care setting, *Holistic Nurs Pract* 6(2):42-50, 1992.

Derstine JB: The rehabilitation clinical nurse specialist of the 1990s: roles assumed by recent graduates, *Rehabil Nurs* 17(3):139-140, May-June, 1992.

Doyle DL, Stern PN: Negotiating self care in rehabilitation nursing, *Rehabil Nurs* 17(6):319-322, 326, Nov-Dec 1992.

Habel M, Garland G: Rehabilitation nursing novices: changing the acute care mind set, *Rehabil Nurs* 15(2):73-76, March-April 1990.

Hoeman SP: Cultural assessment in rehabilitation nursing practice, *Nurs Clin North Am* 24(1):277-289, 1989.

Ross B: The impact of reimbursement issues on rehabilitation nursing practice and patient care, *Rehabil Nurs* 17(5):236-238, Sept-Oct 1992.

Sawin KJ, Heard L: Nursing diagnoses used most frequently in rehabilitation nursing practice, *Rehabil Nurs* 17(5):256-262, Sept-Oct 1992.

## CHAPTER 9
## Body Image and Self-Esteem

### General Self-Esteem

Burnard J, Morrison L: Body image and physical appearance, *Surg Nurs* 3(4):4-8, 1990.

Coopersmith S: *The antecedents of self-esteem,* 1967, Freeman.

Fitts W: *Tennessee self-concept scale manual,* rev 3, Los Angeles, 1983, Western Psychological Services.

Hamburg DA, Coelho GV, Adams FE: Coping and adaptation: steps toward a synthesis of biological and social perspectives, *Coping and adaption,* 127-138, 1974, Basic Books.

Kersten L: Changes in self-concept during pulmonary rehabilitation, part 1, *Heart Lung* 19(5):456-461, 1992.

McGlashan R: Strategies for rebuilding self-esteem of the cardiac patient. *Dimens Crit Care Nurs* 7(1):28-38, 1988.

Olson B, Ustanko L, Warner S: The patient in a Halo-brace: Striving for normalcy in body-image and self concept, *Orthopaedic Nursing* 10(1):44-50, 1991.

Perlow M: Validity and reliability of the PSES, *West J Nurs Res* 14(2):201-210, 1992.

Piazza D et al: Hope, social suport and self-esteem of patients with spinal cord injuries, *J Neuroscience Nursing* 23(4):224-230, 1991.

Reasoner RW: Enhancement of self-esteem in children and adolescents, *Family Community Health* 6:51-64, 1983.

Rogers C: *Client-centered therapy,* Boston, 1951, Houghton Mifflin.

Rosenberg M: *Conceiving the self,* 1979, Basic Books.

### Body Image

Brown MS: *Normal development of body image.* In Bower F, editor, New York, 1977, John Wiley & Sons.

Brown T, Cash T, Lewis R: Body image disturbances in adolescent female binge-purgers: results of a national survey, *J Child Psychol Psychiatry* 30:605-613, 1989.

Brundage DJ: Self-concept alterations: theory and assessment. In Thelan LT, Urden LD, Davies JK, editors: *Nursing diagnosis in critical care,* St Louis, 1990, Mosby.

Cooper P, Taylor M: Body image disturbance in bulimia nervosa, *Br J Psychiatry* 153(suppl 2):32-36, 1988.

Derogatis LR: The unique impact of breast and gynecologic cancers on body image and sexual identity in women: a reassessment. In Vaeth JM, editor, *Body image, self-esteem, and sexuality in cancer patients,* ed 2, Basel, 1986, Karger.

Dropkin MJ: Rehabilitation after disfigurative facial surgery, *Plast Surg Nurs* 5(4):130-134, 1985.

Esberger K: Body image, *J Gerontol Nurs* 4(4):35-38, 1978.

Faubel M: Body image and depression in women with early and late onset obesity, *J Psychology* 123(4):385-395, 1989.

Fawcett J, Frye S: An exploratory study of body image dimensionally, *Nurs Res* 29:324-327, 1980.

Fawcett J et al: Spouses' body image changes during and after pregnancy: a replication and extension, *Nurs Res* 35(4):220-223, 1986.

Fisher S: *Body experience in fantasy and behavior,* New York, 1970, Appleton-Century-Crofts.

Fowler B: The relationship of body image perception and weight status to recent changes in weight status of the adolescent female, *Adolescence* 24:557-568, 1989.

Fujita MT: The impact of illness or surgery on the body image of the child, *Nurs Clin North Am* 7:641-649, 1972.

Gardner B, Moncriefe C: Body image distortion in anorexics as a non-sensory phenomenon: a signal detection approach, *J Clin Psychology* 44(2):101-107, 1988.

Goin JM, Goin MK: *Changing the body: psychological effects of plastic surgery,* Baltimore, 1981, Williams & Wilkins.

Gruendemann BJ: Problems of physical self: loss. In Roy SC, editor: *Introduction to nursing: an adaptation model,* Englewood Cliffs, NJ, 1976, Prentice-Hall.

Hughes R: Satisfaction with one's body image and success in breast-feeding. *Issues Comprehen Nurs* 7:141-153, 1984.

Laessle R, Tuschl R, Waadt S, Pirke K: The specific psychopathology of bulimia nervosa: a comparison with restrained and unrestrained (normal) eaters, *J Consult Clin Psychol* 57(6):772-775, 1989.

Liss JL: Psychiatric issues in ostomy management. In Broadwell DC, Jackson BS, editors: *Principles of ostomy care,* St Louis, 1982, Mosby.

Murray J et al: Twenty year experience in maxillocraniofacial surgery, *Ann Surg* 190:320-331, 1979.

Noles SW, Cash TF, Winstead BA: Body image, physical attractiveness and depression, *J Consult Clin Psychol* 53(1):88-94, 1985.

Norris CM: The professional nurse and body image. In Carlson CE, editor: *Behavioral concepts and nursing intervention,* ed 2, Philadelphia, 1979, JB Lippincott.

Nortridge J: Teaching the concept of body image: use of affective and cognitive domains, *J Enterstomal Therapy* 14:255-258, 1987.

O'Brien J: Mirror, mirror, why me? *Nurs Mirror* 150(17):36-37, 1980.

Platzner H: Body image—a problem for intensive care patients (Part 1), *Int Care Nurs* 3:61-66, 1987.

Platzner H: Body image (Part 2): Helping patients to cope with changes—a problem for nurses, *Int Care Nurs* 3:125-132, 1987.

Price B: Body image: keeping up appearances, *Nurs Times,* Oct 1:58-61, 1986.

Roberts SL: *Behavioral concepts and the critically ill patient,* ed 2, Norwalk, Conn, 1986, Appleton & Lange.

Safilios-Rothschild C: *The sociology and social psychology of disability and rehabilitation,* New York, 1981, University Press of America.

Salkin J: *Body ego technique,* Springfield, Ill, 1973, Charles C Thomas.

Salter MJ: What are the differences in body image between patients with a conventional stoma compared with those who have had a conventional stoma followed by a continent pouch? *J Adv Nurs* 17:841-848, 1992.

Williamson ML: The nursing diagnosis of body image disturbance in adolescents dissatisfied with their physical characteristics, *Holistic Nurs Pract* 1(4):52-59, 1987.


### *Disturbances in Self-Esteem and Body Image*


Baxley KO et al: Alopecia: effect on patients' body image, *Cancer Nurs* 7(6):499-503, 1984.

Bernstein NR, Cope O: *Emotional care of the facially burned and disfigured,* Boston, 1976, Little, Brown.

Champion VS, Austin JK, Tzeng O: Assessment of relationship between self-concept and body image using multivariate techniques, *Issues in Mental Health Nursing* 4(4):299-315, 1982.

Diekmann JM: Measuring body image. In Frank-Stromberg M, editor: *Instruments for clinical nursing research,* Norwalk, Conn, 1988, Appleton & Lange.

Dyk RB, Sutherland A: Adaptation of the spouse and other family members to the colostomy patient, *CA* 9:123-125, 1956.

Fisher S: Influence of information about self on the body boundary. *J Pers Assess* 37:503-507, 1973.

Garrett JF, Levine ES: *Rehabilitation practices with the physically disabled,* New York, 1973, Columbia University Press.

Glockner MR: Perceptions of sexual attractiveness following ostomy surgery, *Res Nurs Health* 7(2):87-92, 1984.

Goffman E: *Stigma: notes on the management of spoiled identity,* Englewood Cliffs, NJ, 1963, Prentice-Hall.

Harris R: Cultural differences in body perception during pregnancy, *Br J Med Psychol* 52:347-352, 1970.

Hirschfield AH, Behan RC: The accident process: disability, acceptable and unacceptable, *JAMA* 197:85-89, 1966.

Kaplan SP: Some psychological and social factors present in the condition of obesity, *J Rehabil* 45(3):52-54, 1979.

Lerner RH, Brackney BE: The importance of inner and outer body parts attitudes in the self concept of late adolescents. *Sex Roles* 4:225-238, 1978.

May HJ: Psychosexual sequelae to mastectomy: implications for therapeutic and rehabilitative intervention, *J Rehabil* 46(1):29-31, 1970.

McCrea CW, Summerfield AB, Rosen B: Body image: a selective review of existing measurement techniques, *J Med Psychol* 55:225-233, 1982.

McDaniel JW: *Physical disability and human behavior,* New York, 1969, Pergamon.

Meisner A, Thoreson R, Butler A: The impact of obvious physical handicap on male and female self-concept, *Percept Motor Skills* 24:1099-1105, 1967.

Norris CM: The professional nurse and body image. In Carlson CE, editor: *Behavioral concepts and nursing intervention,* ed 2, Philadelphia, 1979, JB Lippincott.

Norris J, Kunes-Connell M: Self-esteem disturbance: a clinical validation study. In McLane AM, editor: *Classification of nursing diagnoses,* Proceedings of the Seventh Conference, St Louis, 1987, Mosby.

Rubin R: Body image and self esteem. *Nurs Outlook* 16:20-23, 1968.

Schilder P: The body image. In Bender L, editor: *Contributions to developmental neuropsychiatry,* New York, 1964, International Universities Press.

Schoenburg B et al, editors: *Loss and grief: psychological management in medical practice,* New York, 1970, Columbia University Press.

Scott DW: Quality of life following the diagnosis of breast cancer, *Top Clin Nurs* 4(4):20-37.

Secord PF, Jourard SH: The appraisal of body cathexis: body cathexis and the self, *J Consult Psychol* 17:343-347, 1953.

Slade P: Body image in anaexia nervosa, *Br J Psychiatry* 153(suppl. 2):20-22, 1988.

Smith C: Body image changes after myocardial infarction, *Nurs Clin North Am* 7:663-688, 1972.

Sultenfuss S: Psychosocial issues and therapeutic intervention. In Broadwell DC, Jackson BS, editors: *Principles of ostomy care,* St. Louis, 1982, Mosby.

Sutherland S: Burned adolescents' descriptions of their coping strategies, *Heart Lung* 17(2):150-157, 1988.

Tucker SJ: The psychology of spinal cord injury: patient-staff interaction, *Rehabilitation Literature* 41:114-121, 1980.


### *Nursing Process*


Bernado LM, Conway A, Bove M: The ABC method of emotional assessment and intervention: a new approach in pediatric emergency care, *J Emer Nurs* 16(2):70-76, 1990.

Donovan MI, Pierce SG: *Cancer care nursing,* Norwalk, Conn, 1984, Appleton & Lange.

Kim MJ, McFarland GK, McLane AM: *Pocket guide to nursing diagnoses,* ed 3, St. Louis, 1991, Mosby.

Litman TJ: The family and physical rehabilitation, *J Chronic Dis* 19:211-217, 1966.

McFarland G et al: Self-esteem disturbance. In Thompson J, McFarland GK, Hirsch J et al, editors: *Mosby's manual of clinical nursing,* ed 2, St. Louis, 1989, Mosby.

McFarland GK, McFarlane EA: *Nursing diagnosis and intervention,* ed 2, St. Louis, 1993, Mosby.

Miller KD: Body-image therapy, *Nurs Clin North Am* 26(3):727-736, 1991.

Mital MA, Peirce DS: *Amputees and their prostheses,* Boston, 1971, Little, Brown.

Nelson AL: Normalization: the key to integrating the spinal cord-injured patient into the community, *SCI Nurs* 4:3-6, 1987.

Norris J, Kunes-Connell M: Self-esteem disturbance: a clinical validation study. In McLane AM, editor: *Classification of nursing diagnoses,* Proceedings of the Seventh Conference, St Louis, 1987, Mosby.

Samond RJ, CammerMeyer M: Perceptions of body image in subjects with multiple sclerosis: Pilot study, *J Neurosci Nurse* 21(3):190-194, 1989.

Siller J: Psychosocial aspects of physical disability. In Mesilin J, editor: *Rehabilitation medicine and psychiatry,* Springfield, Ill, 1976, Charles C Thomas.

CHAPTER 10

## Loss, Grief, and Dying

### General Nursing Theory:

Captor R: *And a time to live: toward emotional well-being during the crisis of cancer,* New York, 1978, Harper & Row.

Carpenito LJ: *Nursing diagnosis: application to clinical practice,* ed 3, Philadelphia, 1989, JB Lippincott.

Donovan ML, Girton SE: *Cancer care nursing,* ed 2, New York, 1984, Appleton-Century-Crofts.

Duespohl TA: *Nursing diagnosis manual for the well and ill clients,* Philadelphia, 1986, WB Saunders.

Ebersole P, Hess P: *Toward healthy aging: human needs and nursing response,* ed 3, St. Louis, 1990, Mosby.

Haber J et al: *Comprehensive psychiatric nursing,* ed 4, St. Louis, 1992, Mosby.

Lewis S et al: *Manual of psychosocial nursing interventions: promoting mental health in medical-surgical settings,* Philadelphia, 1989, WB Saunders.

Maslow A: *Motivation and personality,* New York, 1954, Harper & Brothers.

McGoldrick M et al: *Ethnicity and family therapy,* New York, 1982, Guilford Press.

### Adaptation and Loss

Aguilera D, Messick J: *Crisis intervention: theory and methodology,* ed 3, St Louis, 1978, Mosby.

Assimacopoulos L: Realizing empathy in loss, *J Psychosoc Nurs* 25(11):26-29, 1992.

Benoliel J: Loss and terminal illness, *Nurs Clin North Am* 20(2):438-447, 1985.

Bowlby J: Attachment and loss: retrospect and prospect, *Am J Orthopsych* 52(4):664-677, 1972.

Brice C: Mourning throughout the life cycle, *Am J Psychoanalysis* 42(4):315-325, 1982.

Dufault K: *Hope and elderly persons with cancer,* Unpublished doctoral dissertation, Cleveland, 1981, Case Western Reserve University.

Engel G: A life setting conducive to illness: The giving-up given-up complex, *Ann Int Med* 69:355-365, 1968.

Flach F: Resilience: discovering a new strength at times of stress, New York, 1988, Fawcett Columbine.

Frankl V: Self-transcendence as a human phenomenon, *J Humanistic Psych* 6:97-106, 1966.

Knall K, Deatrice J: How families manage chronic conditions: an analysis of the concept of normalization, *Res Nurs Health* 9:215-222, 1986.

Miller J: *Coping with chronic illness: overcoming powerlessness,* Philadelphia, 1983, FA Davis.

Rolland J: Anticipatory loss: a family systems developmental framework, *Fam Proc* 29(3):229-243, 1990.

Selder F: Life transition theory: the resolution of uncertainty, *Nurs Health Care* 10(8):437-451, 1992.

Viorst J: *Necessary losses,* New York, 1986, Simon & Schuster.

Wortman C, Silver R: The myths of coping with loss, *Counsel Clin Psych* 57(3):349-357, 1989.

### Bereavement

Biller R, Rice S: Experiencing multiple loss of persons with AIDS: Grief and bereavement issues, *Health and Soc Work* 15(4):283-290, 1990.

Cook A, Dworkin D: *Helping the bereaved: therapeutic interventions for children, adolescents, and adults,* New York, 1992, Basic Books.

Cooley M: Bereavement care: a role for nurses, *Cancer Nurs* 15(2):125-129, 1992.

Davis B, Oberle K: Dimensions of the supportive role of the nurse in palliative care, *Oncol Nurs Forum* 17(1):87-94, 1990.

Diamond M: Bereavement and the elderly: a critical review with implications for nursing practice and research, *J Adv Nurs* 6: 461-470, 1981.

Dick L, Elmer L: *Grief in men and women: vive la différence,* Memphis, 1993, ADEC Conference.

Eliott T: The adjustive behavior of bereaved families: a new field of research, *Soc Forces* 8:543-549, 1930.

Eliott T: The bereaved family, *Ann Arbor Acad Polit Social Sciences* 160:184-190, 1932.

Elmer L: *Why her, why now?* New York, 1987, Bantam Books.

Engel G: Is grief a disease? *Psychosomatic Med* 13(1):18-22, 1961.

Freud S: *Instincts and their vicissitudes: collected papers,* New York, 1915, Basic Books.

Gifford B, Cleary B: Supporting the bereaved, *Am J Nurs* 90(2):49-54, 1990.

Glass B: The role of the nurse in advanced practice in bereavement care, *Clin Nurs Spec* 7(2):62-66, 1993.

Glick I, Weiss R, Parkes C: *The first year of bereavement,* New York, 1974, John Wiley & Sons.

Graham J: *In the company of others,* New York, 1982, Harcourt Brace Jovanovich.

Graininger R: Successful grieving, *Am J Nurs* 9:12-15, 1990.

Grassman D: Turning personal grief into personal growth, *Nurs* (April):43-47, 1992.

Houseman C, Pheifer W: Potential for unresolved grief in survivors of persons with AIDS, *Arch Psych Nurs* 2:296-301, 1988.

Jackson EN: *Understanding grief: its roots, dynamics and treatment,* Nashville, Tenn, 1957, Abingdon Press.

Kalish RA: Death and dying in a social context. In Binstock RH, Shanes E, editors: *Handbook of aging,* New York, 1976, Van Nostrand Reinhold.

Kaprio J et al: Mortality after bereavement: a prospective study of 95,647 widowed persons, *Am J Pub Health* 77:283-287, 1987.

Kübler-Ross E: *On death and dying,* New York, 1969, Macmillan.

Lennon M et al: The influence of social support on AIDS-related grief reactions among gay men, *Soc Sci and Medicine* 31:477-484, 1990.

Lev E, Munro B, McCorkle R: A shortened version of an instrument measuring bereavement, *Int J Nurs Studies* 30(3):213-226, 1993.

Lindemann E: Symptomatology and management of acute grief, *Am J Psych* 101:141-148, 1944.

Martocchio BC: Authenticity, belonging, emotional closeness, and self-representation, *Oncol Nurs Forum* 14(4):32-37, 1987.

Martocchio BC: Grief and bereavement: healing through hurt, *Nurs Clin North Am* 20(2):327-334, 1985.

Martocchio BC: Family coping: helping families help themselves, *Sem Oncol Nurs* 1(4):11-16, 1985.

Mor V, McHorney C, Sherwood S: Secondary morbidity among the recently bereaved, *Am J Psych* 143(2):158-163, 1986.

Murphy S: Preventive intervention following accidental death of a child, *Image* 22(30):174-179, 1990.

Norris FH, Murrell SA: Older adult family stress and adaptation before and after bereavement, *J Geron* 42(6):606-612, 1987.

Parkes CM: The first year of bereavement: a longitudinal study of the reaction of London widows to the death of their husbands, *Psychiatry* 33:444-457, 1970.

Parkes CM, Weiss RS: *Recovery from bereavement,* New York, 1983, Basic Books.

Pilkington F: The lived experience of grieving the loss of an important other, *Nurs Sci Quart* 6(3):130-138, 1993.

Rando T: *Grief, dying, and death,* Champaign, Ill, 1983, Research Press.

Raphael B: *The anatomy of bereavement,* New York, 1983, Basic Books.

Remondet JH, Hansson RO: Assessing a widow's grief: a short index, *J Gerontol Nurs* 13(4):30-34, 1987.

Richter JM: Support: a resource during crisis of mate loss, *J Gerontol Nurs* 13(11):18-22, 1987.

Sanders C: *Grief: the mourning after,* New York, 1989, John Wiley & Sons.

Sowell R et al: The lived experience of survival and bereavement following the death of a lover from AIDS, *Image* 23(2):89-94, 1991.

Stroebe W, Stroebe M: *Bereavement and health: the psychological and physical consequences of partner loss,* Cambridge, Mass., 1987, Cambridge University Press.

Switzer DK: *The dynamics of grief,* New York, 1970, Abingdon Press.

Temes R: *Living with an empty chair,* New York, 1992, New Horizon Books.

Vargas L et al: Exploring the multidimensional aspects of grief reactions, *Am J Psych* 146(11):1384-1488, 1991.

Weinfeld I: Help for the bereaved: the Jewish traditions, *The Forum* 2(19):3-4, 1993.

Weizman S, Kamm P: *About mourning: support and guidance for the bereaved,* New York, 1987, Human Sciences Press.

Wolfelt A: Resolution versus reconciliation: the importance of semantics, *Thanatos* (Winter):22-25, 1987.

Worden W: *Grief counseling and grief therapy,* ed 2, New York, 1991, Springer.

### *Death and Dying*

Amenta MO, Bohnet NL: *Nursing care of the terminally ill,* Boston, 1986, Little, Brown.

American Nurses Association Committee on Ethics: *Guidelines on withholding or withdrawing food and fluids,* Kansas City, 1988, ANA.

American Nurses Association: *Nursing practice in the care of the dying,* Kansas City, 1982, ANA.

American Nurses Association: *Standards and scope of hospice nursing practice,* Kansas City, 1987, ANA.

Becker E: *The denial of death,* Riverside, NJ, 1973, Free Press.

Bovee J: Nursing attitudes towards death and dying: an informal survey, *Thanatos* (Summer):5-9, 1991.

Branson J, Casebeer K: The Quinlan decision: observing the role of the physician, *Hastings Center Report* 6(1):8-11, 1976.

Curry L, Stone J: Moving on: recovering from the death of a spouse, *Am J Nurs* 6(4):180-190, 1992.

Curtin L, Flaherty MJ: *Nursing ethics: theories and pragmatics,* Bowie, Md, 1982, Robert J Brady.

Davis AJ, Aroskar MA: *Ethical dilemma and nursing practice,* ed 2, New York, 1983, Appleton-Century-Crofts.

DeSpelder L, Strickland A: *The last dance: encountering death and dying,* ed 3, Mountain View, Calif, 1992, Mayfield.

Dimond E: The oncology nurse's role in patient advanced directives, *Oncol Nurs Forum* 19(6):891-896, 1992.

Dufault K: Helping patients and families make life-sustaining treatment decisions, *AORN J* 39(7):1132-1133, 1984.

Dufault K: What is nurse's role when adults forego treatment? *Am Nurs* 16(2):5, 23, 1984.

Eakes G: Grief resolution in hospice nurses, *Nurs Health Care* 11(5):234-248, 1988.

Feifel H: *The functions and attitudes toward death and dying: attitudes of patient and doctor,* New York, 1965, Group for Advancement of Psychiatry.

Fletcher J: Ethics and euthanasia, *Am J Nurs* 73:670-672, 1973.

Grollman E: *Talking about death: a dialogue between parent and child,* Boston, 1990, Beacon Press.

Heifetz MS, Magei C: *The right to die,* New York, 1975, GC Putnam & Sons.

Hemlock Society: *Supporting the point of active voluntary euthanasia for the terminally ill,* Los Angeles, 1985, The Society.

Hull M: Coping strategies of family caregivers in hospice homecare, *Oncol Nurs Forum* 19(8):1179-1187, 1992.

Jackson EN: Grief. In Grollman E, editor: *Concerning death: a practical guide for living,* Boston, 1974, Beacon Press.

Johnson SH: The Cruzan case: who has the right to decide, *Health Prog* 89(11):22-25, 1989.

Kant I: Duties towards the body in regard to life. In Gorovitz S et al, editors: *Moral problems in medicine,* Englewood Cliffs, NJ, 1976, Prentice-Hall.

Kastenbaum R: *The psychology of death,* ed 2, New York, 1992, Springer.

Koestenbaum P: *Is there any answer to death?* Englewood Cliffs, NJ, 1976, Prentice-Hall.

Kübler-Ross E: *Death: the final stage of growth,* Englewood Cliffs, NJ, 1975, Prentice-Hall.

Lynn G et al: *The nurse's role during the living/dying interval: a self-instructional unit,* Dayton, Ohio, 1988, Community Oncology Nursing Committee of Dayton.

Martocchio BC: Agendas for quality of life, *Hosp J* 2(1):11-21, 1986.

Martocchio BC: *Living while dying,* Bowie, Md, 1982, Robert J Brady.

Martocchio BC: *The social processes surrounding the dying person.* Unpublished doctoral dissertation, Cleveland, 1975, Case Western Reserve University.

Martocchio BC, Dufault K: Dying, a part of living. In Diamond M, editor: *Advances in geriatrics, long-term care nursing,* vol. 1, New York, 1983, Pro Scienua.

Mitford J: *The American way of death,* New York, 1963, Simon & Schuster.

Mumma C: Withholding nutrition: a nursing perspective, *Nurs Admin Quart* 10(3):31-38, 1986.

Oaks J, Ezell G: *Dying and death: coping, caring, and understanding,* Scottsdale, Ariz, 1993, Gorsuch Scarisbrick.

Otte DM, Allen KS: Ethical principles in the nursing care of the terminally ill adult, *Oncol Nurs Forum* 14(5):87-91, 1987.

Pattison EM: *The experience of dying,* Englewood Cliffs, NJ, 1977, Prentice-Hall.

Petrisono BM, editor: *Nursing in hospice and terminal care: research and practice,* New York, 1986, Haworth Press.

Pine VR: Comparative funeral practices. *Pract Anthropol* 16:49-62, 1969.

Rachels J: Active and passive euthanasia. In Levine C, editor: *Taking sides: clashing views on controversial ethical issues,* Guilford, Conn, 1984, Dushkin Publishing.

Ramsey P: *The patient as a person: explorations in medical ethics,* New Haven, 1970, Yale University Press.

Rollin B: *Last wish,* New York, 1985, Simon & Schuster.

Saunders JM, Valente SM: Cancer and suicide, *Oncol Nurs Forum* 15:575-581, 1988.

Scanlon C: Creating a vision of hope: the challenge of palliative care, *Oncol Nurs Forum* 16(4):491-496, 1989.

Schneidman ES: On the deromantization of death, *Am J Psychoanalysis* 25:4-17, 1971.

Schultz R, Aderman D: Clinical research and stages of dying, *Omega* 7:137-143, 1974.

Shubin S: Offering families hope . . . or help them let go? *Nurs* (March):44-49, 1990.

Silverman P, Worden W: Detachment revisited: the child's reconstruction of a dead parent, *Am J Orthopsychiatry* 62(4):494-503,1992.

Society for the Right to Die: *Support of dying with dignity,* New York, 1985, The Society.

Steele L: The death surround: factors influencing the grief experience of survivors, *Oncol Nurs Forum* 15(5):575-581, 1990.

Thomas DC: Ethics and professional practice in oncology, *Sem Oncol Nurs* 5(2):89-94, 1989.

Ufema J: Helping loved ones say good-bye, *Nurs* (October):42-43, 1990.

Van Jennap A: *The rites of passage,* Chicago, 1960, University of Chicago Press.

Varricchio CG, Jassak P: Informed consent: an overview, *Sem Oncol Nurs* 5(2):95-98, 1989.

Waltman R: When a spouse dies, *Nurs* (July):40-51, 1992.

Zahourek R: *Relaxation and imagery: tools for therapeutic communication and intervention,* Philadelphia, 1988, WB Saunders.

CHAPTER 11

## Human Sexuality

### *Osteoporosis*

Ali NS, Bennett SJ: Postmenopausal women: factors in osteoporosis preventive behaviors, *J Gerontological Nurs* 18(12):23-31, 1992.

Blanchard DS: What women can do to protect against osteoporosis, *RN* 53(10):60-64, 1990.

Carr BR, Dawson-Hughes B, Ettinger B: A real world approach to osteoporosis, *Patient Care* 27(8):31-56, 1993.

Erickson GP, Jones JA: Osteoporosis risk assessment of mature working women, *AAOHN J* 40(9):423-428, 1992.

Fleming LA: Osteoporosis: clinical features, prevention and treatment, *J Gen Intern Med* 7(5):554-560, 1992.

Hallal JC: Back pain with postmenopausal osteoporosis and vertebral fractures, *Geriatric Nurs* 12(6):285-287, 1991.

Hay EK: That old hip—the osteoporotic process, *Nurs Clin North Am* 26(1):43-51, 1991.

Kaplan FS: Prevention and treatment of osteoporosis, *Hosp Med* 27(3):65-77, 1991.

Liscum B: Osteoporosis—the silent disease, *Orthopaedic Nurs* 11(4):21-25, 1992.

McMahon MA, Peterson C, Schilke J: Osteoporosis: identifying high risk persons. *J Geron Nurs* 18(10):19-25, 1992.

National Institute of Arthritis and Musculoskeletal and Skin Diseases: *Osteoporosis research, education, and health promotion,* (NIH Publication No. 91-3216) Bethesda, Md, 1991, US Department of Health and Human Services.

National Osteoporosis Foundation: *Physicians resource manual on osteoporosis,* ed 2, Washington, DC, 1991, The Foundation.

Tolstoi LG, Levin RM: Osteoporosis—the treatment controversy, *Nutrition Today* 27(4):6-12, 1992.

Urrows ST, Freston MS, Pryor DL: Profiles in osteoporosis, *Am J Nurs* 91(12):33-37, 1991.

### *Menopause and Estrogen Replacement Therapy*

Estok PJ, O'Toole R: The meanings of menopause, *Health Care for Women Int* 12:27-39, 1991.

Fishbein EG: Women at midlife—the transition to menopause, *Nurs Clin North Am* 27(4):951-957, 1992.

Jarrett ME, Lethbridge DJ: The contraceptive needs of midlife women, *Nurse Practitioner* 15(12):34-39, 1990.

Keresztes PA, Dan AJ: Estrogen replacement and cardiovascular disease, *Cardiovasc Nurs* 28(1):1-8, 1992.

Lichtman R: Perimenopausal hormone replacement therapy: review of the literature, *J Nurse Midwifery* 36(1):30-48, 1991.

Logothetis ML: Women's decisions about estrogen replacement therapy, *West J Nurs Res* 13(4):458-474, 1991.

Maddox MA: Women at midlife—hormone replacement therapy, *Nurs Clin North Am* 27(4):959-969, 1992.

McCraw RK: Psychosexual changes associated with the perimenopausal period, *J Nurse Midwifery* 36(1):17-23, 1991.

Quinn A: Menopause: plight or passage, *NAACOG's Clin Issues in Perinatal & Women's Health* 3(3):304-331, 1991.

Quinn AC: A theoretical model of the perimenopausal process, *J Nurse Midwifery* 36(1):25-29, 1991.

Rickert B: Estrogen replacement: making informed choices, *RN* 55(9):26-32, 1992.

Sarrel PM: Sexuality and menopause, *Obstetrics and Gynecology* 75:26S-30S, 1990.

Scharbo-DeHaan M, Brucker MC: The perimenopausal period, *J Nurse Midwifery* 36(1):9-15, 1991.

Wilbur JE, Dan A, Hedricks C, Holm K: The relationship among menopausal status, menopausal symptoms, and physical activity in midlife women, *Fam Com Health* 13(3):67-78, 1990.

Youngkin EQ: Estrogen replacement therapy and the estraderm transdermal system, *Nurse Practitioner* 15(5):19-31, 1990.

### *Sexuality and Aging*

Bates-Jenson BM: Sexuality and the elderly, *J Enterostomal Therapy* 16(4):158-163, 1989.

Butler R, Lewis M: Myths and realities of sex in the late years, *Provider* 13(10):16-18, 1987.

Dickey RM: Exploring nursing staff attitudes on sexuality and the elderly, *Nursing Homes* 38(11):15-17, 1989.

Dickey RM: Nursing staff low in sexual knowledge, *Nursing Homes* 39(12):31-32, 1990.

Glass JC, Dalton JA: Sexuality in older adults, *J Continuing Ed in Nurs* 19(2):61-64, 1988.

Kain CD, Reilly N, Schultz ED: The older adult, *Nurs Clin North Am* 25(4):833-849, 1990.

Lusky K: Elder sexuality in long term care facilities, *Long Term Care* 12(12):7-13, 1988.

McCracken AL: Sexual practice by elders: the forgotten aspect of functional health, *J Geron Nurs* 14(10):13-17, 1988.

Morrison-Beedy D, Robbins L: Sexual assessment and the aging female, *Nurse Prac* 14(12):35-45, 1989.

Rankin DJ: Intimacy and the elderly, *Nursing Homes* 38(11):10-14, 1989.

Smedley G: Addressing sexuality in the elderly, *Rehabilitation Nursing* 16(1):9-11, 1991.

## Sexuality Issues in Illness and Disability

### *General*

Chaffee MW: The missing link in nursing education: sexuality. In Ingram-Fogel CI, editor: *Sexual health promotion,* Philadelphia, 1990, WB Saunders.

Grover JW: Human sexuality—management for the primary physician, *Primary Care* 8(1):55-76, 1991.

Katzman EM: Education for sexual health care, *J Nurs Ed* 29(3):141-142, 1990.

Pryce A: Sexuality and the patient, *Nursing* 44(4):6-15, 1992.

Shah HS: Nurses views on sexuality, *J Nurs Staff Develop* 7(6): 275-279, 1991.

Waterhouse J, Metcalfe V: Attitudes toward nurses discussing sexual concerns with patients, *J Adv Nurs* 16, 1048-1054:1991.

Weston A: Challenging assumptions, *Nursing Times* 89(18):27-29, 1993.

### *Drug Effects*

Buffum J: Pharmacosexology updates: prescription drugs and sexual function, *J Psychoactive Drugs* 18:97-102, 1986.

Cole N: Drugs that influence sexual behavior, *Consultant* 3:280-291, 1990.

Steele D: Drugs causing sexual dysfunction and their alternatives, *Urologic Nursing* 9(6):10-12, 1989.

Wilson B: The effect of drugs on male sexual function and fertility, *Nurse Practitioner* 16(9):12-21, 1991.

### *Cardiovascular Disease*

Cardin S: Nursing's role in the sexual counseling of critical care patients, *Dimen Crit Care Nurs* 6(2):67-69, 1987.

Gilliss CL, Rankin SM: Social and sexual activity after cardiac surgery, *Progress Cardiovasc Nurs* 3(3):93-97, 1988.

Hook M et al: Critical care voices: including sexual counseling in clinical practice, *Dimen Crit Care Nurs* 8(12):366-369, 1989.

Kotler D: Sexual dysfunctions in patients with cardiovascular disease, *J Am Acad Physician Assist* 5(6):423-431, 1992.

McCann ME: Sexual healing after heart attack, *Am J Nurs* 89(9):1133-1138, 1989.

Relf MV: Sexuality and the older bypass patient, *Geriatric Nurs* 12(6):294-296, 1992.

### Spinal Cord Injury

Anonymous: Educational guide for SCI nurses: a sample . . . sexual function, fertility, contraception, and safe sex, *SCI Nursing* 9(1):7-11, 1992.

Anonymous: Sexual function after spinal cord injury, *Professional Nurse* 4(7):319, 1989.

Chicano LA: Humanistic aspects of sexuality related to spinal cord injury, *J Neuroscience Nurs* 21(6):366-369, 1989.

Girts C: Nursing attitudes about sexuality needs of spinal cord injury patients, *Rehab Nurs* 15(4):205-206, 1990.

Goddard LR: Sexuality and spinal cord injury, *J Neuroscience Nurs* 20(4):240-244, 1988.

Mendius RA: Female sexuality and spinal cord injury, *SCI Nursing* 6(4):68-74, 1989.

Pervin-Dixon L: Sexuality and the spinal cord injured, *J Psychosocial Nurs Mental Health Serv* 26(4):31-35, 37, 1988.

Pilsecker C: Starting out: the first six months posthospital for spinal cord-injured veterans, *Am Physic Med Rehab* 69(2):91-95, 1990.

Rieve JE: Sexuality and the adult with acquired physical disability, *Nurs Clin North Am* 24(1):265-276, 1989.

Sipski ML, Alexander CJ: Sexual function and dysfunction after spinal cord injury, *Physic Med Rehab Clin North Am* 3(4):811-828, 1992.

Spica MM: Sexual counseling standards of the spinal cord-injured, *J Neuroscience Nurs* 21(1):56-60, 1989.

Ulmer DB: Special needs of the young spinal cord injured patient in a nursing home, *SCI Nurs* 7(2):27-30, 1990.

Villeneuve MJ: Sexual function and fertility: the impact of spinal cord injury, *CONA J* 11(1):7-12, 1989.

White MJ et al: Sexual activities, concerns and interests of men with spinal cord injury, *Am J Physic Med Rehab* 71(4):225-231, 1992.

### Cancer

Frank-Stromborg M: Sexuality and the elderly cancer patient, *Sem Oncol Nurs* 1(1):49-55, 1985.

Gloeckner M: Perceptions of sexuality after ostomy surgery, *J Enterostomal Therapy* 18(1):36-38, 1991.

Lamb MA: The woman with gynecologic cancer, *Sem Oncol Nurs* 6(3):237-243, 1990.

Smith DB: Discussing sexuality, *Oncol Nurs Forum* 16(1):106-109, 1989.

Williamson ML: Sexual adjustment after hysterectomy, *JOGNN* 21(1):42-47,1992.

### Diabetes

Baum N, Neiman M, Lewis R: Evaluation and treatment of organic impotence in the male with diabetes mellitus, *Diabetes Educator* 14(2):123-129, 1988.

Conine TA, Evans JH: Sexual reactivation of chronically ill and disabled adults, *J Allied Health* 11(4):261-270, 1982.

Harward MP: Evaluation of sexual dysfunction in women, *Hospital Practice* 26(10):53-57, 1990.

Katzin L: Chronic illness and sexuality, *Am J Nurs* 90(1):54-59, 1990.

Manley G: Diabetes and sexual health, *Diabetes Educator* 12(4):366-369, 1986.

Schover LR: Women, sexuality, and diabetes, *Diabetes Forecast* 45(8):58-61, 1992.

## CHAPTER 12
## Alterations in Consciousness in the Hospitalized Adult

### General

American Psychiatric Association: *Diagnostic and statistical manual of mental disorders,* ed 4, rev, Washington, DC, 1994, American Psychiatric Association.

Bachren DF, Werman HA: Altered mental states: grappling with the unknown, *J Emerg Med Serv* 19(6):69-84, 1994.

Blazer D: *Emotional problems in later life: intervention strategies for professional caregivers,* New York, 1990, Springer.

Bosek MSD: The use of restraints: ethical considerations, *Med Surg Nurs* 2(2):154-156, 1993.

Funk SG et al, editors: *Key aspects of elder care,* New York, 1992, Springer.

Plum F, Posner JB: *Diagnosis of stupor and coma,* Philadelphia, 1980, FA Davis.

Rumble R, Morgan K: Hypnotics, sleep, and mortality in elderly people, *J Am Geriatr Soc* 40(8):787-791, 1992.

### Acute Confusion/Delirium

Favro D: Management of the schizophrenic patient on the medical-surgical unit, *Med Surg Nurs* 2(2):139-142, 1993.

Foreman MD: Acute confusional states in the hospitalized elderly. a research dilemma, *Nurs Research* 35:34-38, 1986.

Foreman MD: Confusion: incidence, onset and associated factors, *Res Nurs Health* 12:21-29, 1989.

Foreman MD: The cognitive and behavioral nature of acute confusional states, *Scholarly Inquiry for Nurs Prac* 5(1):3-16, 1991.

Foreman MD: Acute confusional states in the hospitalized elderly. In Funk SG et al, editors: *Key aspects of elder care,* New York, 1992, Springer.

Foreman MD: Adverse psychologic responses of the elderly to critical illness, *AACN Clin Issues in Crit Care Nurs* 3(1):64-72, 1992.

Foreman MD: Acute confusion in the elderly. In Fitzpatrick JJ, Stevenson JS, editors: *Annual Review of Nurs Research* 11:3-29, 1993.

Francis J: Delirium in older patients, *J Am Geriatr Soc* 40(8):829-838, 1992.

Francis J: Delusions, delirium, and cognitive impairment: the challenge of clinical heterogeneity, *J Am Geriatr Soc* 40(8):848-849, 1992.

Geary SM: Intensive care unit psychosis revisited: understanding and managing delirium in the critical care setting, *Crit Care Nurs Qtr* 17(1):51-63, 1994.

Lachs MS et al: Delusions and behavioral disturbances in cognitively impaired elderly persons, *J Am Geriatr Soc* 40(8):768-773, 1992.

Lipowski ZJ: *Delirium: acute confusional states,* New York, 1990, Oxford University Press.

Pizzi CL, Mion LC: Alcoholism in the elderly: implication from hospital nurses, *Med Surg Nurs* 2(6):453-458, 1993.

Rosen SL: Managing delirious older adults in the hospital, *Med Surg Nurs* 3(3):181-189, 1994.

Weddington WW Jr: The mortality of delirium: an underappreciated problem, *Psychosomatics* 23:1232-1235, 1982.

Williams M et al: Predictors of acute confusion states in hospitalized elderly patients, *Res Nurs Health* 8:31-40, 1985.

Williams M et al: Reducing acute confusional states in elderly patients with hip fractures, *Res Nurs Health* 8:329-337, 1985.

Williams-Russo P et al: Post-operative delirium: predictors and prognosis in elderly orthopedic patients, *J Am Geriatrics Society* 40:759-767, 1992.

Wolanin MD, Phillips LR: *Confusion: prevention and care,* St Louis, 1981, Mosby.

Yeaw EMJ, Abbate JH: Identification of confusion among the elderly in an acute care setting, *Clin Nurs Specialist* 7:192-197, 1993.

### *Chronic Confusion/Dementia*

Antai-Otong D: Cognitive and affective assessment of the geriatric patient, *Med Surg Nurs* 2(1):70-74, 1993.

Beck CK, Shue VM: Interventions for treating disruptive behavior in demented elderly people, *Nurs Clin North Am* 29(1):143-155, 1994.

Cleary BL: Alzheimer's disease: stressors and strategies associated with caregiving. In Funk SG et al, editors: *Key aspects of elder care,* New York, 1992, Springer.

Davies HD: Dementia and delirium. In Chenitz WC, Stone JT, Salisbury SA, editors: *Clinical gerontological nursing: a guide to advanced practice,* Philadelphia, 1991, WB Saunders.

Foreman MD, Gillies DA, Wagner D: Impaired cognition in the critically ill elderly patient: clinical implications, *Crit Care Nurs Qtr* 12(1):61-73, 1989.

Maas ML, Buckwalter KC: Alzheimer's disease. In Fitzpatrick JJ, Stevenson KS, editors: *Annual Review of Nurs Research* 9:19-55, 1991.

Stewart JT: Managing the care of patients with dementia, *Postgrad Med* 90(4):45-49, 1991.

Walshe III TM: Cognitive failure dementia. In Stein JH et al, editors: *Internal medicine,* ed 4, St Louis, 1994, Mosby.

### *Depression*

Abraham IL, Neese JB, Westerman PS: Depression: nursing implications of a clinical and social problem, *Nurs Clin North Am* 26(3):527-544, 1991.

Brasfield KH: Practical psychopharmacologic considerations in depression, *Nurs Clin North Am* 26(3):651-663, 1991.

Calarco MM, Krone KP: An integrated nursing model of depressive behavior in adults: theory and implications for practice, *Nurs Clin North Am* 26(3):573-584, 1991.

Fogel BS: Mood disorders. In Stein JH et al, editors: *Internal medicine,* ed 4, St Louis, 1994, Mosby.

Hauenstein EJ: Young women and depression: origin, outcomes, and nursing care, *Nurs Clin North Am* 26(3):601-612, 1991.

Neese JB: Depression in the general hospital, *Nurs Clin North Am* 26(3):613-622, 1991.

Salisbury SA: Depression. In Chenitz WC, Stone JT, Salisbury SA, editors: *Clinical gerontological nursing: a guide to advanced practice,* Philadelphia, 1991, WB Saunders.

Simpson SG, DePaulo JR Jr: Are you recognizing depression in your patients? *Postgrad Med* 94(3):85-93, 1993.

Steiner D, Marcopulos B: Depression in the elderly: characteristics and clinical management, *Nurs Clin North Am* 26(3):585-600, 1991.

US Department of Health and Human Services: *Depression in primary care: detection and diagnosis* (Clinical practice guidelines), vol 1, Number 5, 1993, US Government Printing Office.

US Department of Health and Human Services: *Depression in primary care: detection, diagnosis, and treatment* (Quick reference guide for clinicians), Number 5, 1993, US Government Printing Office.

US Department of Health and Human Services: *Depression in primary care: treatment of major depression* (Clinical practice guidelines), Number 5, 1993, US Government Printing Office.

US Department of Health and Human Services: *Depression is a treatable illness: a patient's guide,* 1993, US Government Printing Office.

### *Nursing Management*

Holt J: How to help confused patients, *Am J Nurs* 93(8):32-36, 1993.

Yeaw EMJ, Abbate JH: Identification of confusion among the elderly in an acute care setting, *Clin Nurs Spec* 7(4):192-197, 1993.

CHAPTER 13

## Inflammatory and Immune Responses

### *General*

Abbas A, Lichtman A, Pober J: *Cellular and molecular immunology,* Philadelphia, 1991, WB Saunders.

Barrett JT: Textbook of immunology, ed 5, St Louis, 1987, Mosby.

Cassileth B: Mind over body, *Cancer News,* Winter: pp 6-20, 1986.

Jaroff L: Stop that germ, *Time* 131:56-64, 1988.

National Institutes of Health: *Understanding the immune system,* No 84-529, Washington, DC, 1983, US Department of Health and Human Services.

Playfair JHL: *Immunology at a glance,* ed 2, Oxford, 1984, Blackwell Scientific Publications.

Porth CM: *Pathophysiology,* ed 3, Philadelphia, 1990, JB Lippincott.

Seeley RR, Stephens TD, Tate P: *Lymphatic system and immunity: anatomy and physiology,* St Louis, 1989, Mosby.

Stites DP et al: *Basic and clinical immunology,* ed 6, Los Angeles, 1987, Lange Medical Publications.

Workman ML, Ellerhorst-Ryan J, Hargrave-Koertge V: *Nursing care of the immunocompromised patient,* Philadelphia, 1993, WB Saunders.

### *Concept of Biologic Defense*

Ada GL, Nossal G: The clonal selection theory, *Sci Am* 257:52-69,1987.

Cohen IR: The self, the world and autoimmunity, *Sci Am* 258:52-60, 1988.

Lydyard DM, editor: *Immune response, current opinion in immunology,* vol II, London, 1988, Current Science.

Roitt I: *Essential immunology,* ed 6, London, 1988, Blackwell Scientific Publications.

Roitt I, Brostoff J, Male D: *Immunology,* ed 2, St Louis, 1989, Mosby.

### *Nonspecific Defense Mechanisms*

Nelson DS, editor: *Natural immunity,* Sydney, 1989, Academic Press.

Reynolds CW, Wiltrout RH, editors: *Functions of the natural immune system,* New York, 1989, Plenum.

Young JD, Cohn ZA: How killer cells kill, *Sci Am* 258:38-44, 1988.

Young JD, Doherty PC: Multiple mechanisms of lymphocyte-mediated killing, *Immunol Today* 9:140-144, 1988.

### *Specific Defense Mechanisms*

Alt FW et al: Development of primary antibody repertoire, *Science* 238:1079-1087, 1987.

Grey HM, Sette A, Baus S: How T cells see antigens, *Sci Am* 261:56-64, 1989.

Law SKA, Reid KBM: *Complement,* Oxford, 1988, IRL Press.

Marrack P, Kappler J: The T cell receptor, *Science* 238:1073-1078, 1987.

### *Applications and Implications of Immune Response*

Besedovsky HO, Del Ray AE, Sorkin E: What do the immune system and brain know about each other? *Immunol Today* 4:342-347, 1986.

Bolognesi D, editor: Human retroviruses: cancer and AIDS, New York, 1988, Alan R Liss.

Hall NR, Goldstein AL: Thinking well: the chemical links between emotions and health, *Ann NY Acad Sci* 34:40-45, 1986.

Matje D: Stress and cancer: a review of the literature, *Cancer Nurs* 9:339-401, 1984.

Robinson W: Clinical use of colony-stimulating factors, *Mediguide to Onc* 8(3)1-4, 1988.

Rumsey KA, Reiger PT, editors: *Biological response modifiers: a self-instruction manual for health professionals,* Chicago, 1992, Precept Press.

Truitt RL, Gale RT, Bortin MM, editors: *Cellular immunotherapy of cancer,* New York, 1987, Alan R Liss.

Vitetta ES et al: Redesigning nature's poisons to create antitumor reagents, *Science* 238:1098-1104, 1987.

Wujcik D: An odyssey into biologic therapy, *Onc Nurs Forum* 20(6):879-887, 1993.

UNIT III

# Common Problems Encountered in Care of Ill Adults

CHAPTER 14

## Fatigue

### *General*

Aaronson L (Project Director). Exploratory Center for Biobehavioral Studies of Fatigue Management, University of Kansas School of Nursing (Grant from NINR, NIH (P20NR03270), 1992-1995.

Cahill C et al: Conceptual framework for biobehavioral management of fatigue. In preparation.

Carpenito LJ: *Nursing diagnosis: application to clinical practice,* Philadelphia, 1992, JB Lippincott.

Gordon M: *Manual of nursing diagnosis: 1991-1992,* St Louis, 1991, Mosby.

Hart LK, Freel MI, Milde FK: Fatigue, *Nurs Clin North Am* 25(4):967-976, 1990.

Nelson E et al: Chief complaint fatigue: a longitudinal study from the patient's perspective, *Fam Pract Res J* 6(4):175-188, 1987.

Piper BF: Fatigue. In Carrieri-Kohlman V, Lindsey AM, West CM, editors: *Pathophysiological phenomena in nursing: human responses to illness,* ed 2, Phialdelphia, 1993, WB Saunders.

Potempa KM: Chronic fatigue. In Fitzpatrick JJ, Stevenson JS, editors: *Annual Review of Nursing Research* 11:57-76, 1993.

### *Chronic Fatigue Syndrome*

Bell DS: Chronic fatigue syndrome, *Postgrad Med* 91(6):245-252, 1992.

Calabrese L et al: Chronic fatigue syndrome, *Am Fam Phys* 45(3):1205-1213, 1992.

Gantz NM, Holmes GP: Treatment of patients with chronic fatigue syndrome, *Drugs* 38(6):855-862, 1989.

Goodnick PJ, Sandoval R: Psychotropic treatment of chronic fatigue syndrome and related disorders, *J Clin Psychiatry* 54(1):13-20, 1993.

Gupta S, Vayuvegula B: A comprehensive immunological analysis in chronic fatigue syndrome, *Scand J Immunol* 33:319-327, 1991.

Hickie I et al: The psychiatric status of patients with the chronic fatigue syndrome, *Br J Psychiatry* 156:534-540, 1990.

Holmes GP et al: Chronic fatigue syndrome: a working case definition, *Ann Intern Med* 108:387-389, 1988.

Kroenke K et al: Chronic fatigue in primary care, *JAMA* 260(7):929-934, 1988.

Landay AL et al: Chronic fatigue syndrome: clinical conditions associated with immune activation, *Lancet* 338:707-712, 1991.

Manu P, Mathews D, Lane T: The mental health of patients with a chief complaint of chronic fatigue: a prospective evaluation follow-up, *Arch Intern Med* 84:118-121, 1991.

Shafran SD: The chronic fatigue syndrome, *Am J Med* 90(6):730-739, 1991.

Sharpe MC et al: A report—chronic fatigue syndrome: guidelines for research, *J Royal Soc Med* 84:118-121, 1991.

### *Fatigue in Selected Patient Populations*

Appels A, Mulder P: Excess fatigue as a precursor of myocardial infarction, *European Heart J* 9:758-764, 1988.

Blesch KS et al: Correlates of fatigue in people with breast or lung cancer, *Oncol Nurs Forum* 18(1):81-87, 1991.

Cassmeyer VL: *Fatigue, physical activity and metabolic control in non-insulin-dependent diabetes mellitus.* A presentation to Kansas Regional Research Exchange. Wichita, Kans, Sept 1993.

Christensen T et al: Fatigue and cardiac and endocrine metabolic response to exercise after abdominal surgery, *Surgery* 105(1):46-50, 1989.

Feinstein AR, Fisher MB, Pigeon JG: Changes in dyspnea-fatigue ratings as indicators of quality of life in the treatment of congestive heart failure, *Am J Cardiology* 64(7):50-55, 1989.

Feuerstein M, Carter RL, Papciak AS: A prospective analysis of stress and fatigue in recurrent low back pain, *Pain* 31:333-344, 1987.

Friedland J, Paterson D: Potassium and fatigue. Letter to the editor. *Lancet* 2:961-962, 1988.

Goldstein V, Regnery G, Wellin E: Caretaker role fatigue, *Nurs Outlook* 29(1):24-30, 1981.

Gorensek MJ: Chronic fatigue and depression in the ambulatory patient, *Primary Care* 18(2):397-419, 1991.

Gulledge AD (Guest Editor): Depression and chronic fatigue, *Primary Care* 18(2):271-449, 1991.

Irvine DM et al: A critical appraisal of the research literature investigating fatigue in the individual with cancer, *Cancer Nurs* 14(4):188-199, 1991.

Jamar SC: Fatigue in women receiving chemotherapy for ovarian cancer. In Funk S et al, editors: *Key aspects of comfort,* New York, 1989, Springer.

King KB et al: Patients' descriptions of the experience of receiving radiation therapy, *Onco Nurs Forum* 12(4):55-61, 1985.

Kirk J et al: Chief complaint of fatigue: A prospective study, *J Fam Pract* 30(1):33-41, 1990.

Krupp LB et al: Fatigue in multiple sclerosis, *Arch Neurol* 45:435-437, 1988.

Neuberger GB et al: Correlates of fatigue in rheumatoid arthritis clients, *Arthritis Care and Research* 6(4):517 (Abstract 45), 1994.

Pickard-Holley S: Fatigue in cancer patients, a descriptive study, *Cancer Nursing* 14(1):13-19, 1991.

Pierce J, Clancy R, Trank J: *Biochemical and contractile properties of diaphragm fatigue.* A Presentation at the Midwest Nursing Research Society, 18th Annual Research Conference, Milwaukee, Wisc, April 1994.

Piper BF et al: Recent advances in the management of biotherapy-related side effects: fatigue, *Onco Nurs Forum* 16(Suppl 6):27-34, 1989.

Srivastava RH: Fatigue in end-stage renal disease patients. In Funk S et al, editors: *Key aspects of comfort,* New York, 1989, Springer.

Tack BB: Fatigue in rheumatoid arthritis: conditions, strategies, and consequences, *Arthritis Care and Research* 3(2):65-70, 1990.

Wallace PG: Epidemiology: a critical review, *Br Med Bull* 47(4):942-951, 1991.

Williams P: *Caregiver fatigue and at-risk infants at home: preliminary findings.* Fifth Annual Kansas Nursing Research Exchange, Hays, Kans, September, 1994.

### *Interventions for Fatigue*

Daiss S, Bertelson AD, Benjamin LT: Napping versus Resting: effects on performance and mood, *Psychophysiology* 23(1):82-88, 1986.

MacVicar M, Winningham M, Nickel J: Effects of aerobic interval training on cancer patients' functional capacity, *Nurs Res* 38:348-351, 1989.

Piper BF: Fatigue: current bases for practice. In Funk S et al, editors: *Key aspects of comfort,* New York, 1989, Springer.

Quested K et al: Rehabilitation program for cancer related fatigue: an empirical study, *Arch Physic Med Rehab* 63:532-538, 1982.

Rhodes VA, Watson PM, Hanson BM: Patients' descriptions of the influence of tiredness and weakness on self-care abilities, *Cancer Nurs* 11(3):1186-1194, 1988.

Smith ACW: Exercise, practical treatment for the patient with depression and chronic fatigue, *Primary Care* 18(2):271-281, 1991.

### *Measurement of Fatigue*

Barofsky I, Legro MW: Definition and measurement of fatigue, *Rev Infect Dis* 13(Suppl 1):594-597, 1991.

Bloom JR et al: Physical performance at work and at leisure: validation of a measure of biological energy in survivors of Hodgkin's disease, *J Psychosocial Oncol* 8(1):49-63, 1990.

Lee KA, Hicks G, Nino-Murcia G: Validity and reliability of a scale to assess fatigue, *Psychiatry Res* 36:291-298, 1991.

Varricchio CG: Selecting a tool for measuring fatigue, *Oncol Nurs Forum* 12(4):122-127, 1985.

### *Mechanisms of Fatigue*

Demitrack M et al: Evidence of impaired activation of the hypothalamic-pituitary-adrenal axis in patients with chronic fatigue syndrome, *J Clin Endo* 73:1224-1234, 1991.

Hultman E, Bergstrom J: Local energy-supplying substrates as limiting factors in different types of leg muscle work in normal man. In Keul J, editor: *Limiting factors of physical performance,* Stuttgart, 1971, G. Thieme.

Maclaren DP et al: A review of metabolic and physiological factors in fatigue, *Exercise and Sport Sciences Rev* 17:29-66, 1989.

Richardson JH, Palmerton T, Chenan M: The effect of calcium on muscle fatigue, *J Sports Med* 20:149-151, 1980.

Simonson E: Physiology of work capacity and fatigue, Springfield, Ill, 1971, Charles C Thomas.

CHAPTER 15

## Infection

### *General*

American Public Health Association: *Control of communicable disease in man,* ed 15, New York, 1990, The Association.

Bennett JV, Brachmann PS, editors: *Hospital infections,* Boston, 1992, Little, Brown.

Berg R, editor: *The APIC curriculum for infection control practice,* Vol III, Dubuque, Iowa, 1988, Kendall/Hunt Publishing.

Lederberg J, Shape RE, Oaks SC Jr, editors: *Emergency infections microbial threats to health in the United States,* Washington, DC, 1992, National Academy Press.

Mandell GL, Douglas RG, Bennett JE: *Principles and practice of infectious diseases,* ed 3, New York, 1990, John Wiley & Sons.

Soule BM, editor: *The APIC curriculum for infection control practice,* vol I & II, Dubuque, Iowa, 1983, Kendall/Hunt Publishing.

### *Historical Perspective*

American Hospital Association: *OSHA's final bloodborne pathogens standard: a special briefing,* Feb 1992, The Association.

### *The Infectious Disease Process*

*A clinician's dictionary of bacteria and fungi,* Indianapolis, 1986, Eli Lilly.

Bowell B: Assessing infection risk, *Nursing* (London) 4(12):12-23, 1990.

### *Infection Control in the Community*

Centers for Disease Control: Diphtheria, tetanus, and pertussis: recommendations for vaccine use and other preventive measures (ACIP), *MMWR* 40(RR-10):1-28, 1991.

Centers for Disease Control: Haemophilus b conjugate vaccines for prevention of haemophilus influenzae type b disease among infants and children two months of age and older (ACIP), *MMWR* 40(RR-1), 1991.

Centers for Disease Control: Hepatitis B virus: a comprehensive strategy for eliminating transmission in the United States through universal childhood vaccination (ACIP), *MMWR* 40(RR-13):1991.

Centers for Disease Control: Prevention and control of influenza recommendations of the immunization practices Advisory Committee (ACIP): *MMWR* 41(RR-9), 1992.

Centers for Disease Control: Recommendations of the ACIP: smallpox vaccine, *MMWR* 34(23):341-342, 1985.

Centers for Disease Control: Recommendations of the immunization practices advisory committee (ACIP): Measles Prevention: Supplementary Statement, *MMWR* 38(1):11-14, 1989.

Centers for Disease Control: Recommendations of the immunization practices advisory committee (ACIP): General recommendations on immunization, *MMWR* 38(13):205-227, 1989.

Centers for Disease Control: Recommendations of the immunization practices advisory committee (ACIP): update: pneumococcal polysaccharide vaccine usage, *MMWR* 33(20):273-281, 1984.

Conly JM, Grieves K, Peters B: A prospective, randomized study comparing transparent and dry gauze dressings for central venous catheters, *J Infectious Diseases* 159(2):310-319, 1989.

Cooper DM: Optimizing wound healing, *Nurs Clin North Am* 25(1):165-180, 1990.

Craven DE, Steger KA, Barber TW: Preventing nosocomial pneumonia: state of the art and perspectives for the 1990s, *Am J Med* 91(suppl 3B):44-53, 1991.

Doebbeling BN et al: Comparative efficacy of alternative handwashing agents in reducing nosocomial infections in intensive care units, *N Engl J Med* 327:88-93, 1992.

Garner JS, Simmons BP: Guideline for isolation precautions in hospitals, *Infect Control* 4(4):245-325, 1983.

Garner JS et al: CDC definitions for nosocomial infections, 1988, *Am J Infect Control* 16:128-140, 1988.

Gerberding JL et al: Risk of transmitting the human immunodeficiency virus, cytomegalovirus, and hepatitis B virus to health care workers exposed to patients with AIDS and AIDS-related conditions, *J Infect Diseases* 156(1):1-8, 1987.

Gerberding JL: Reducing occupational risk of HIV infection, *Hosp Prac,* June 15:103-117, 1991.

Goodman RA, Solomon SL: Transmission of infectious diseases in outpatient health care settings, *JAMA* 285(18):2377-2381, 1991.

Haley RW et al: The efficacy of infection surveillance and control programs in preventing nosocomial infections in US hospitals, *Am J Epidem* 121(2):182-205, 1985.

Haley RW: Nosocomial infections in surgical patients: developing valid measures of intrinsic patient risk, *Am J Med* 91(Suppl 3B):145S-151S, 1991.

Infection control in critical care units, *Crit Care Nurs Q* 11(4), 1989.

Jackson MM, Lynch P: Infection control: Too much or too little? *Am J Nurs* 84:208-210, 1984.

Jackson MM et al: Why not treat all body substances as infectious? *Am J Nurs* 87(3):1137, 1987.

Lynch P et al: Implementing and evaluating a system of generic infection precautions: body substance isolation, *AMJ Infect Control* 18:1-12, 1990.

***Infection Control in the Hospital***

Centers for Disease Control: Guidelines for preventing the transmission of tuberculosis in health-care settings, with special focus on HIV-related issues, *MMWR* 39(RR-17):1-29, 1990.

Centers for Disease Control: Protection against viral hepatitis: recommendations of the immunization practices advisory committee (ACIP), *MMWR* 39(RR-2), 1990.

Centers for Disease Control: Recommendations for prevention of HIV transmission in health-care settings, *MMWR* 36(2S):1987.

Centers for Disease Control: Update: universal precautions for prevention of transmission of human immunodeficiency virus, hepatitis B virus, and other bloodborne pathogens in health-care settings, *MMWR* 37(24):377-388, 1988.

Centers for Disease Control and Prevention: Public health focus: surveillance, prevention, and control of nosocomial infections, *MMWR* 41(42):783-787, 1992.

Cohen ML: Epidemiology of drug resistance: implications for a post-antimicrobial era, *Science* 257:1050-1055, 1992.

Maki DG, Botticelli JT, et al: Prospective study of replacing administration sets for intravenous therapy at 48 vs 72 hour intervals, *J Am Med Assoc* 258:1777, 1987.

Mulligan ME et al: Methicillin-resistant staphylococcus aureus: a consensus review of the microbiology, pathogenesis, and epidemiology with implications for prevention and management, *Am J Med* 94:313-327, 1993.

Nadzam DM: Infection control indicators in critical care settings, *Heart Lung* 21(5):477-481, 1992.

Nafziger DA, Wenzel RP: Catheter-related infections: reducing the risk and the consequences, *J Crit Illness* 5(8):857-865, 1990.

National Vaccine Advisory Committee: The measles epidemic: the problem, barriers, and recommendations, *JAMA* 266(11):1547-1552, 1991.

Nosocomial infection rates for interhospital comparison: limitations and possible solutions, *Infect Control Hosp Epidemiol* 12:609-621, 1991.

Petrosino BP, Becker H, Christian B: Infection rates in central venous catheter dressings, *Oncol Nurs Forum* 15(6):709-717, 1988.

Shovein J, Young MS: MRSA: Pandora's box for hospitals, *Am J Nurs* 92(2):48-52, 1992.

Simmons BP et al: CDC guidelines for the prevention and control of nosocomial infections—guidelines for the prevention of intravascular infections, *Am J Infect Control* 11(5):183-193, 1983.

Stamm WE: Catheter-associated urinary tract infections: epidemiology, pathogenesis, and prevention, *Am J Med* 91(suppl 3B):65-75, 1991.

US Department of Health and Human Services, Public Health Service: *Healthy people 2000: national health promotion and disease prevention objectives,* Washington, DC, 1990, US Government Printing Office.

Verghese A, Beck SL, editors: *Infections in nursing homes and long term care facilities,* New York, 1990, S Karger.

Wong ES: CDC guidelines for the prevention and control of nosocomial infections: guidelines for prevention of catheter associated urinary tract infections, *Am J Infect Control* 11(1):26-36, 1983.

Wysocki AB: Surgical wound healing, *AORN J* 49(2):502-518, 1989.


CHAPTER 16

## Cancer


***General***

Baird SB, McCorkle R, Grant M: *Cancer nursing: a comprehensive textbook,* Philadelphia, 1991, WB Saunders.

Carnevallil DL, Reiner AC: *The cancer experience: nursing diagnosis and management,* Philadelphia, 1990, JB Lippincott.

Groenwald SL et al, editors: *Cancer nursing: principles and practice,* ed 3, Boston, 1993, Jones & Bartlett.

Holleb AI, Finkl DJ, Murphy GP, editors: *American cancer society textbook of clinical oncology,* Atlanta, 1991, The Society.

McNally JC et al, editors: *American Nurses Association. Standards of oncology nursing practice: guideline for oncology nursing practice,* ed 2, Philadelphia, 1991, WB Saunders.

Moosa AR: *Comprehensive textbook of oncology,* vol I, ed 2, Baltimore, 1991, Williams & Wilkins.

***Aging and Cancer***

Caird FI, Brewin TB, editors: *Cancer in the elderly,* Boston, 1990, Butterworth.

McCaffrey-Boyle D et al: Oncology Nursing Society position paper on cancer and aging: the mandate for oncology nursing, *Oncol Nurs Forum* 19(6):913-933, 1992.

Simonson W: Pharmacotherapeutic consideration in the elderly patient: implications for cancer patients, *Innovations in Oncol Nurs* 8(1):2-5, 1991.

Weigle WO: Effects of aging on the immune system, *Hosp Prac* 112-120, Dec 15, 1989.

***Carcinogenesis***

Appelbaum JW: The role of the immune system in the pathogenesis of cancer, 8(1):51-62, 1992.

Cartmel B, Loescher LJ, Villar-Werstler P: Professional and consumer concerns about environment, lifestyle, and cancer, *Sem Oncol Nurs* 8(1):20-29, 1992.

***Chemotherapy***

Carey PJ et al: Appraisal and caregiving burden in family members caring for patients receiving chemotherapy, *Oncol Nurs Forum* 18(8):1341-1348, 1991.

Consensus Conference highlights: Oral complications of cancer therapies: diagnoses, prevention, and treatment, *National Institutes of Health* 8(3):1-8, 1990.

Dorr RT, Von Hoff D, editors: *Cancer chemotherapy handbook,* ed 2, Norwalk, Conn, 1994, Appleton & Lange.

Edwards JN et al: Comparison of patient-controlled and nurse-controlled antiemetic therapy in patients receiving chemotherapy, *Res Nurs Health* 14:249-257, 1991.

Reville B, Almadrones L: Continuous infusion chemotherapy in the ambulatory setting: the nurse's role in patient selection and education, *Oncol Nurs Forum* 16(4):529-538, 1989.

Travaglini J, Nevidjon B: Complications related to cancer therapy, *Clin Adv Oncol Nurs* 2(2):1-13, 1990.

***Family/Caregivers***

Laizner AM et al: Needs of family caregivers of persons with cancer, *Sem Oncol Nurs* 9(2):114-120, 1993.

Lewis FM: Psychosocial transitions and the family's work in adjusting to cancer, *Sem Oncol Nurs* 9(2):127-129, 1993.

Whitman HH, Gustafson JP: Group therapy for families facing a cancer crisis, *Oncol Nurs Forum* 16(4):539-546, 1989.

***Immunotherapy***

Caliendo G, Joyce D, Altmiller M: Nursing guidelines and discharge planning for patients receiving recombinant Interleukin-2, *Sem Oncol Nurs* 9(3)(Suppl 1):25-31, 1993.

Jackson B, Strauman J, Frederickson K, Strauman T: Long-term biopsychosocial effects of Interleukin-2 therapy, *Oncol Nurs Forum* 18(4):683-690, 1991.

Oldham RK, editor: *Principles of cancer biotherapy,* ed 2, New York, 1991, Marcel Dekker.

***Pain***

Beck SL: The therapeutic use of music for cancer-related pain, *Oncol Nurs Forum* 18(8):1327-1337, 1991.

Ferrell B et al: Effects of controlled-release morphine on quality of life for cancer pain, *Oncol Nurs Forum* 16(4):521-528, 1989.

Patt RB: *Cancer pain,* Philadelphia, 1993, JB Lippincott.

Whedon M, Shedd P, Summers B: The role of the advanced practice oncology nurse in pain relief, *Oncol Nurs Forum* 19(7) (Suppl):12-19, 1992.

### Prevention and Detection

Block G, Patterson B, Subar A: Fruit, vegetables, and cancer prevention: review of the epidemiological evidence, *Nutrition and Cancer* 17(2):18-21, 1992.

Frank-Stromberg M, Olsen SJ, editors: *Cancer prevention in minority populations: cultural implications for health care professionals,* St Louis, 1993, Mosby.

Frank-Stromberg M, Rohan K: Nursing's involvement in the primary prevention and secondary prevention of cancer: nationally and internationally, *Cancer Nurs* 15(2):79-108, 1992.

MacDonald SA: Organizational approaches to cancer program development, *Sem Oncol Nurs* 9(1):8-16, 1993.

Olsen SJ, Frank-Stromberg M: Cancer prevention and early detection in ethnically diverse populations, *Sem Oncol Nurs* 9(3):198-209, 1993.

Vranicar-Lapka D et al: Oncology patient's and their significant others response to a proposed cancer prevention/detection program, *Cancer Nurs* 15(1):47-53, 1992.

### Radiation Therapy

Campbell-Forsyth L: Patient's perceived knowledge and learning needs concerning radiation therapy, *Cancer Nurs* 13(2):81-89, 1990.

Dow KH, Hilderly LJ: *Nursing care in radiation oncology,* Philadelphia, 1992, WB Saunders.

Shenoy MA, Singh BB: Chemical radiosensitizers in cancer therapy, *Cancer Investigation* 10(6):533-551, 1992.

Strohl RA: The nursing role in radiation oncology: symptom management of acute and chronic reactions, *Oncol Nurs Forum* 15(4):429-438, 1988.

### Rehabilitation

O'Connor L, Blesch K: Life cycle issues affecting cancer rehabilitation, *Sem Oncol Nurs* 8(3):174-185, 1992.

Watson PG: Cancer rehabilitation: an overview, *Sem Oncol Nurs* 8(3):167-173, 1992.

CHAPTER 17

## Pain

### General

Angell M: The quality of mercy, *N Engl J Med* 306(2):98-99, 1982.

Copp LA, editor: *Recent advances in nursing, perspectives and pain,* New York, 1985, Churchill Livingstone.

Donovan M, Dillan P, McGuire L: The incidence and characteristics of pain in a sample of medical-surgical inpatients, *Pain* 30:69-78, 1987.

Donovan M, editor: *Pain management: nursing perspective,* St Louis, 1992, Mosby.

Fields H: *Pain,* Toronto, 1987, McGraw-Hill.

Hamilton J, Edgar L: A survey examining nurses' knowledge of pain control, *J Pain Symptom Manag* 7:18-26, 1992.

Lander J: Fallacies and phobias about addiction and pain, *Br J Addiction* 85:803-809, 1990.

McCaffery M, Ferrell B: Do you know a narcotic when you see one? *Nurs 90* 20(6):62-63, 1990.

McGuire L: Administering analgesics: which drugs are right for your patient? *Nurs 90* 20(4):34-41, 1990.

McKenry LM, Salerno E: *Mosby's pharmacology in nursing,* ed 18, St Louis, 1992, Mosby.

Watt-Watson J: Nurses' knowledge of pain issues: a survey, *J Pain Symptom Manag* 2:207-211, 1987.

Wild L, Coyne C: Epidural analgesia: the basics and beyond, *Am J Nurs* 92(4):26-36, 1992.

Wright S: The use of therapeutic touch in the management of pain, *Nurs Clin North Am* 22(3):705-714, 1987.

### Cancer Pain

Ferrell B, McCaffery M, Grant M: Clinical decision making and pain, *Cancer Nurs* 14:289-297, 1991.

Mueller R: Cancer pain: which drugs for which patient? *RN* 38-45, 1992.

Storey P et al: Subcutaneous infusion for control of cancer symptoms, *J Pain Symptom Manag* 5:33-41, 1990.

Tuttle CB: Drug management of pain in cancer patients, *Can Med Assoc J* 12:121-134, 1985.

### Patient Controlled Analgesia

Barkas G, Duafala ME: Advances in cancer pain management: a review of patient controlled analgesia, *J Pain Symptom Manag* 3(3):150-160, 1988.

Jacobs MK: Patient-controlled analgesia: who really benefits? *J Post Anesth Nurs* 3:404-407, 1988.

### Postoperative Analgesia

Lavies N et al: Identification of patient, medical and nursing attitudes to postoperative opioid analgesia: stage one of a longitudinal study of postoperative analgesia, *Pain* 48:313-319, 1992.

CHAPTER 18

## Sleep Disorders

### General

Hobson JH: *The dreaming brain,* New York, 1988, Basic Books.

Kryger MH, Roth R, Dement WB: *Principles and practice of sleep medicine,* Philadelphia, 1989, WB Saunders.

### Physiology of Sleep

Guilleminault C, editor: *Sleeping and walking disorders: indications and techniques,* Menlo Park, Calif, 1982, Addison-Wesley.

Jewett ME, Kronauer RE, Czeisler CA: Light-induced suppression of endogenous circadian amplitude in humans, *Nature* 350:59-62, March 7, 1991.

Kandel ER, Schwartz JH, Jessell TM: *Principles of neural science,* New York, 1991, Elsevier Science Publishing.

Lydic R, Biebuyck JF, editors: *Clinical physiology of sleep,* Bethesda Md, 1988, American Physiological Society.

Moore-Ede MC, Sultzman FM, Fuller CE: *The clocks that time us: physiology of the circadian timing system,* Cambridge, Mass, 1982, Harvard University Press.

### Parasomnias

Ferber R: *Solve your child's sleep problems,* New York, 1985, Simon & Schuster.

Guilleminault C, editor: *Sleep and its disorders in children,* New York, 1987, Raven Press.

### Insomnia

American Medical Association: *Straight talk, no-nonsense guide to better sleep,* New York, 1984, Random House.

Metzler DJ, Finesilver CA: When to worry if your patient can't sleep, *RN* 53(3):52-57, 1990.

### Sleep Apnea

Editorial: Sleep-Apnea a major public health problem, *NEJM* 328(17):1271-1273, 1993.

Saunders NA, Sullivan CE: Sleep and breathing. In *Lung biology in health and disease,* ed 2, New York, 1993, Marcel Dekker.

Young T et al: The occurrence of sleep-disordered breathing among middle-aged adults, *NEJM* 328(17):1230-1235, 1993.

***Narcolepsy***

Bergstrom DL, Keller C: Narcolepsy: pathogenesis and nursing care, *J Neuroscience Nurs* 24(3):153-157, 1992.

Dement WC, Mitler MM: Commentary—It's time to wake up to the importance of sleep disorders, *JAMA* 269(12):1548-1550, 1993.

Rogers AE, Aldrich MS: The effect of regularly scheduled naps on sleep attacks and excessive daytime sleepiness associated with narcolepsy, *Nurs Res* 42(2):111-117, 1993.

***Sleep in the Elderly***

Bliwise DL: Sleep in normal aging and dementia, *Sleep* 16(1):40-81, 1993.

Czeisler CA et al: Association of sleep-wake habits in older people with changes in output of circadian pacemaker, *Lancet* 340(8825):933-936, Oct 17, 1992.

Gall K et al: Night life: nocturnal behavior patterns among hospitalized elderly, *J Gerontological Nurs* 16(10):31-37, Oct 1990.

***Sleep and Shift Work***

Czeisler CA et al: Exposure to bright light and darkness to treat physiologic maladaptation to night work, *N Engl J Med* 322:1253-1559, 1990.

Gold DR et al: Rotating shift work, sleepiness and accidents related to sleepiness in hospital nurses, *Am J Public Health* 82(7):1011-1014, July 1992.

Whitehead DC, Thomas H, Slapper DR: A rational approach to shift work in emergency medicine, *Annals Emer Med* 21:1250-1258, Oct 10, 1992.


CHAPTER 19

## Substance Abuse


***General***

Abadinsky H: *Drug abuse: an introduction,* Chicago, 1993, Nelson-Hall Publishers.

American Psychiatric Association: *Diagnostic and statistical manual of mental disorders,* ed 3, Washington, DC, 1987, American Psychiatric Association.

Burns E et al: *An addictions curriculum for nurses and other helping professionals. Level A: basic knowledge and practice,* Columbus, Ohio, 1991, The Ohio State University College of Nursing.

Burns E et al: *An addictions curriculum for nurses and other helping professionals. Level B: advanced knowledge and practice,* Columbus, Ohio, 1991, The Ohio State University College of Nursing.

Johnson V: *Intervention,* Minneapolis, 1987, Hazelden Foundation.

Massachusetts Medical Society, *MMWR* 41(48):1992.

*Mosby's medical, nursing, and allied health dictionary,* ed 3, St Louis, 1990, Mosby.

Rice D et al: *The economic costs of alcohol and drug abuse and mental illness,* San Francisco, 1990, Institute for Health and Aging.

Schuckit M: *Drug and alcohol abuse: a clinician's guide to detoxification and treatment,* New York, 1989, Plenum.

Williams E: Strategies for intervention, *Nurs Clin North Am* 24(1):95, 1989.

***Prevention***

American Medical Association Board of Trustees Report: Drug abuse in the United States: strategies in prevention, *JAMA* 265(16):2102-2107, 1991.

Carnegie Corporation: Making America drug free: a new vision of what works, *Carnegie Quar* 37(3):1-7, 1992.

Eels M: Strategies for promotion of avoiding harmful substances, *Nurs Clin North Am* 26(4):915, 1991.

United States Department of Health and Human Services, Public Health Service: *Healthy people 2000: national health promotion and disease prevention objectives,* Washington, DC, 1990, US Government Printing Office.

United States Department of Health and Human Services, Public Health Service: *Health United States 1989 and prevention profile,* Washington, DC, 1990, US Government Printing Office.

***Alcoholism***

*Alcoholics anonymous,* New York, 1976, Alcoholic World Services.

Captain C: Family recovery from alcoholism: mediating family factors, *Nurs Clin North Am* 24(1):55, 1989.

Cusack J et al: Alcoholism: uncovering the hidden diagnosis, *Emerg Med* 24(7):71-73, 1992.

Flandermeyer A et al: Nursing care of women who abuse alcohol, *Med Surg Nurs Quar* 1(1):122-139, 1992.

Grinspoon L, Bakalar J: Alcohol abuse and dependence, *The Harvard Med School Mental Health Review,* 1990.

Joyce C: The woman alcoholic, *Am J Nurs* 89(10):1314-1318, 1989.

Jurkovich GJ et al: The effect of acute alcohol intoxication and chronic alcohol abuse on outcome from trauma, *JAMA* 270(1):51-56.

Krach P: Discovering the secret: nursing assessment of elderly alcoholics in the home, *J Gerontol Nurs* 16(11):32, 1990.

Mitiguy J: Alcohol and head trauma, *Addict Nurs Network* 3(2):52, 1991.

Parette H: Nursing attitudes toward the geriatric alcoholic, *J Gerontol Nurs* 16(1):26, 1990.

Perrine M et al: Epidemiological perspectives on drunk driving. In *Surgeon General's workshop on drunk driving: background papers,* Washington, DC, 1989, US Department of Health and Human Services.

Rich J: Action stat: acute alcohol intoxication, *Nurs 89* 19(9):33, 1989.

Sommers M: Alcohol intoxication and multiple trauma: a catastrophic combination, *Med Surg Nurs Quar* 1(1):110-121, 1992.

***Substance Abuse***

Amin M et al: Cocaine induced myocardial infarction: a growing threat to men in their 30's, *Postgrad Med* 90(4):50, 1991.

Bell K: Identifying the substance abuser in clinical practice, *Orthop Nurs* 11(2):29, 1992.

Dubiel S: Action stat! Cocaine overdose, *Nurs 90* 20(3):33, 1990.

Dubiel S: Drug abuse: designer drugs, *Ad Clin Care* 6(5):22, 1991.

Felblinger D: Substance abuse in women: a growing challenge for nurses, *Med Surg Nurs Quar* 1(1):101-109, 1992.

Frances R: Substance abuse, *JAMA* 265(23):3171, 1991.

House M: Cocaine, *Am J Nurs* 90(4):40, 1990.

Hughes T: Models and perspectives of addiction: implications for treatment, *Nurs Clin North Am* 24(1):1-12, 1989.

Jacques J, Snyder M: Newborn victims of addiction, *RN* 54(4):47, 1991.

Johnson L: How to diagnose and treat chemical dependency in the elderly, *J Gerontol Nurs* 15(12):22-26, 38-39, 1989.

Kinney J: *Clinical management of substance abuse,* St Louis, 1991, Mosby.

Kircus E, Brillhart B: Dealing with substance abuse among people with disabilities, *Rehab Nurs* 15(5):250-253, 1989.

Levy G, Hickey J: Fighting the battle against drugs, *RN* 54(4):44, 1991.

Lillie-Blanton M, Anthony J, Schuster C: Probing the meaning of racial/ethnic group comparisons in crack cocaine smoking, *JAMA* 269(8):993-997, 1993.

McEllen AT et al: The effects of psychosocial services in substance abuse treatment, *JAMA* 269(15):1953-1959, 1993.

Nuckols C, Greenson J: Cocaine addiction: assessment and intervention, *Nurs Clin North Am* 24(1):33-44, 1989.

Oswald L: Cocaine addiction: assessment and intervention, *Arch Psych Nurs* 3(3):134-141, 1989.

Pires M: Substance abuse: the silent saboteur in rehabilitation, *Nurs Clin North Am* 24(1):291-296, 1989.

Povenmire K: Recognizing the cocaine addict, *Nurs 90* 20(5):46, 1990.

***Eating Disorders***

Covello B: Codependency taints nursing's goals, *RN* 54(4):132, 1991.

Flood M: Addictive eating disorders, *Nurs Clin North Am* 24(1):45, 1989.

Hall S, Wray L: Codependency: nurses who give too much, *Am J Nurs* 89(11):1456, 1989.

Herrick C: Codependency: characteristics, risks, progression, and strategies for healing, *Nurs Forum* 27(3):12-19, 1992.

Klebanoff N: Caring and nursing: exploration in feminist perspectives. Codependency: caring or suicide for nurses and nursing (pamphlet), NLN Publ Center Hum Caring #14-2369: 151, 1991.

Ryan J: Codependency in nursing: healing wounds and changing patterns, *J Christ Nurs* 8(2):10, 1991.

Zerwekh J, Michaels B: Co-dependency: assessment and recovery, *Nurs Clin North Am* 24(1):109, 1989.

***Impaired Nurse***

Green P: The chemically dependent nurse, *Nurs Clin North Am* 24(1):81-94, 1989.

Lippman H: Addicted nurses: tolerated, tormented, or treated? *RN* 55(4):36, 1992.

Miller H: Addiction in a coworker: getting past the denial, *Am J Nurs* 90(5):72, 1990.

Sullivan E: Nursing and health care: the supplement: chemical dependency in the nursing profession (pamphlet), NLN Pub No 41-2365, 1990.

CHAPTER 20

## Fluid and Electrolyte Imbalance

Bowman M et al: Effect of tube-feeding osmolality on serum sodium levels, *Crit Care Nurse* 9(1):22-28, 1989.

Brocklehurst JC, Allen S: *Geriatric medicine for students,* ed 3, New York, 1987, Churchill Livingstone.

Calloway C: When the problem involves magnesium, calcium, or phosphate, *RN* 50(5):30-36, 1987.

Clark JB, Queener SF, Karb VB: *Pharmacological basis of nursing practice,* ed 3, St Louis, 1990, Mosby.

Cullen L: Interventions related to fluid and electrolyte balance, *Nurs Clin North Am* 27(2):569-597, 1992.

Ebersole P, Hess P: *Toward healthy aging-human needs and nursing response,* ed 3, St Louis, 1990, Mosby.

Epstein CDR: Adrenocortical insufficiency in the critically ill patient, *AACN's Clin Issues in Crit Care* 3(3):705-713, 1992.

Felver L, Pendarvis J: Electrolyte imbalances: intraoperative risk factors, *AORN J* 49(4):992-1008, 1989.

Gasparis L, Murray EB, Ursomanno P: IV solutions: which one is right for your patient? *Nurs 89* 19(4):62-64, 1989.

Gershan JA et al: Fluid volume deficit: validating the indicators, *Heart Lung* 19(2):152-156, 1990.

Goldberger E: *A primer of water, electrolyte, and acid-base syndromes,* ed 7, Philadelphia, 1986, Lea & Febiger.

Groer M, Shekelton ME: *Basic pathophysiology a holistic approach,* St Louis, 1989, Mosby.

Guyton A: *Textbook of medical physiology,* ed 8, Philadelphia, 1990, WB Saunders.

Handerhan B: Computing the anion gap, *RN* 54(7):30-31, 1991.

Himmelstein DV et al: Hypernatremic dehydration in nursing home patients, *J Am Geriatric Soc* 31:466-471, 1983.

Horne M, Heitz U, Swearingen P: *Fluid, electrolyte, and acid-base balance—a case study approach,* St Louis, 1991, Mosby.

Innerarity SA: Electrolyte emergencies in critically ill renal patient, *Crit Care Nurs Clin North Am* 2(1):89-99, 1990.

Kelso LA: Fluid and electrolyte disturbances in hepatic failure, *AACN's Clin Issues in Crit Care* 3(3):681-685, 1992.

Mathewson M: Intravenous therapy, *Crit Care Nurs* 9(2):21-23, 26-28, 30-36, 1989.

McCance KL, Huether SE: *Pathophysiology: the biologic basis for disease in adults and children,* St Louis, 1990, Mosby.

Mendyka BE: Fluid and electrolyte disorders caused by diuretic therapy, *AACN's Clin Issues in Crit Care* 3(3):672-680, 1992.

Metheny NM: *Fluid and electrolyte balance—nursing considerations,* ed 2, Philadelphia, 1992, JB Lippincott.

Miller L, Holloway N: Water intoxication: psychogenic hyderdipsia, *Crit Care Nurs* 9(7):74-78, 1989.

Pagana K, Pagana T: *Diagnostic testing and nursing implications—a case study approach,* St Louis, 1990, Mosby.

Porth CM, Erickson M: Physiology of thirst and drinking—implication for nursing practice, *Heart Lung* 21(3):273-282, 1992.

Sabiston DC: *Essentials of surgery,* Philadelphia, 1988, WB Saunders.

Sidebottom J: When it's hot enough to kill, *RN* 55:30-35, 1992.

Sommers M: Rapid fluid resuscitation: how to correct dangerous deficits, *Nurs 90* 20(1):52-59, 1990.

Symposium on fluid, electrolytes, and acid-base balance, *Nurs Clin North Am* 22(4):749-872, 1987.

Valle G, Lemberg L: Electrolyte imbalances in cardiovascular disease: the forgotten factor, *Heart Lung* 17(3):324-329, 1988.

Vander AJ, Luciano DS: *Human physiology: mechanisms of body functioning,* ed 5, New York, 1990, McGraw-Hill.

Vaska PL: Fluid and electrolyte imbalances after cardiac surgery, *AACN's Clin Issues in Crit Care* 3(3):664-671, 1992.

Weldy NJ: *Body fluids and electrolytes* (programmed presentation), ed 6, St Louis, 1991, Mosby.

Williams S: *Essentials of nutrition and diet therapy,* ed 5, St Louis, 1990, Mosby.

Workman ML: Magnesium and phosphorus—the neglected electrolytes, *AACN's Clin Issues in Crit Care* 3(3):655-663, 1992.

Yarnell RP, Craig MP: Detecting hypomagnesium: the most overlooked electrolyte imbalance, *Nurs 91* 21(7):55-57, 1991.

Young M, Flynn K: Third-spacing: when the body conceals fluid loss, *RN* 51(8):46-48, 1988.

CHAPTER 21

## Acid-Base Imbalance

***General***

Anderson S: Six easy steps to interpreting blood gases, *Am J Nurs* 90(8):42-45, 1990.

Brenner M, Welliver J: Pulmonary and acid-base assessment, *Nurs Clin North Am* 25:761-770, 1990.

Guyton A: *Textbook of medical physiology,* ed 8, Philadelphia, 1991, WB Saunders.

Horne M, Heitz U, Swearingen P: *Fluid, electrolyte, and acid-base balance—a case study approach,* St Louis, 1991, Mosby.

Hurray J, Saver C: Arterial blood gas interpretation, *AORN J* 55(1):180-185, 1992.

Janusek LW: Metabolic acidosis: pathophysiology and the resulting signs and symptoms, *Nurs 90* 20(7):52-53, 1990.

Janusek LW: Metabolic alkalosis: pathophysiology and the resulting signs and symptoms, *Nurs 90* 20(6):52-53,1990.

Lindell KO, Wesmiller SW: Using arterial blood gases to interpret acid-base balance, *Orthop Nurs* 8(3):31-34, 1989.

Metheny NM: *Fluid and electrolyte balance—nursing considerations,* ed 2, Philadelphia, 1991, JB Lippincott.

Middaugh R, Middaugh D, Menk E: Current considerations in respiratory and acid-base management during cardiopulmonary resuscitation, *Crit Care Nurs Q* 10(4):25-33, 1988.

Mims BC: Interpreting ABCs, *RN* 54(3):41-47, 1991.

Pagana K, Pagana T: *Diagnostic testing and nursing implications—a case study approach,* St Louis, 1990, Mosby.

Taylor DL: Respiratory acidosis: pathophysiology, signs and symptoms, *Nurs 90* 20(9):52-53, 1990.

Taylor DL: Respiratory alkalosis: pathophysiology, signs, and symptoms, *Nurs 90* 20(8):60-61, 1990.

## CHAPTER 22
## Shock

### General

Effron M, Chernow B: Shock. In *Scientific American medicine,* New York, 1992, Scientific American.

Hardaway RM: *Shock: the reversible stage of dying,* Littleton, Mass, 1986, PGS Publishing.

Rice V: Shock, A clinical syndrome: an update part I. An overview of shock, *Crit Care Nurs* 11(4):20-27, 1991.

### Etiology

Clowes GHA Jr: *Trauma, sepsis and shock: the physiological basis of therapy,* New York, 1988, Marcel Dekker.

Dickerson M: Anaphylactic shock, *Crit Care Nurs Q* 11(1):674-678, 1988.

Dislet L et al: Cardiogenic shock in evolving myocardial infarction, *Heart Lung* 16:649-651, 1987.

Goldberg RJ et al: Cardiogenic shock after acute myocardial infarction, *N Engl J Med* 325(16):1117-1122, 1991.

MacLean LD: Shock, *Br Med Bull* 44(2):437-452, 1988.

McQuillian KA, Wiles CE: Initial management of traumatic shock. In Cardona DV et al, editors: *Trauma nursing from resuscitation through rehabilitation,* Philadelphia, 1988, WB Saunders.

Weil MH, Rackow EC: Colloidal osmotic pressure and its implications for the fluid management of patients in shock. In Hardaway RM, editor: *The reversible stage of dying,* Littleton, Mass, 1986, PSG Publishing.

### Physiology

Boyle J: Cardiovascular physiology. In Bullock J, Boyle J, Wang MB, editors: *Physiology,* Pennsylvania, 1991, Harwal Publishing.

Shoemaker WC et al: Hemodynamic and oxygen transport monitoring to titrate therapy in shock, New Horizons, *The Science and Practice of Acute Medicine* 1(1):145-257, 1993.

Suhl J: Patients with shock. Critical care nursing. In Clochesy J et al, editors: *Critical care nurse,* Philadelphia, 1993, WB Saunders.

### Pathophysiology

Guyton AC: *Textbook of medical physiology,* ed 8, Philadelphia, 1991, WB Saunders.

Houston MC: Pathophysiology of shock, *Crit Care Nurse, Clin North Am* 2(2):143-149, 1990.

Jurkovich GJ, Moore EE, Eiseman B: The liver in shock. In Hardaway RM, editor: *Shock: The reversible stage of dying,* Littleton, Mass, 1986, PSG Publishing.

Littleton MT: Pathophysiology and assessment of sepsis and septic shock, *Crit Care Nurse Q* 11(2):11-20, 1988.

Rice V: Shock: *A clinical syndrome, the clinical continuum of septic shock, shock management,* Secaucus, NJ, 1985, Critical Care Nurse/Hospitals Publications.

Vincent JL et al: Oxygen uptake supply dependency, *Am Rev Resp Dis* 142:2-7, 1990.

### Clinical Manifestations

Ellerbe S: *Fluid and blood component therapy in the critically ill and injured,* New York, 1981, Churchill Livingstone.

Rice V: Shock, a clinical syndrome: an update part 2, The nursing management, stages of shock, *Crit Care Nurs* 11(5):74-82, 1991.

Summer G: The clinical and hemodynamic presentation of the shock patient, *Crit Care Nurs, Clin North Am* 2(2):161-166, 1990.

### Nursing Management

Asheervath J, Belvins D: *Handbook of clinical nursing practice,* Norwalk, Conn, 1986, Appleton-Century-Croft.

Dailey EK, Schroeder J: Techniques in bedside hemodynamic monitoring, ed 2, St Louis, 1981, Mosby.

Gawlinski A: Saving the cardiogenic shock patient, *Nurs 89* 19(12):34-41, 1989.

Holfman-Franey M: Current trends in hemodynamic monitoring of patients in shock, *Crit Care Nurs Q* 11(1):9-18, 1988.

Jeffries PR, Whelan SK: Cardiogenic shock: current management, *Crit Care Nurs Q* 11(1):48-56, 1988.

McCormac M: Managing hemorrhagic shock, *Am J Nurs* 90(8):22-29, 1990.

Rice V: Shock, a clinical syndrome: an update part 3, therapeutic management, *Crit Care Nurs Q* 11(6):41-43, 1991.

Shoemaker WC: Monitoring and management of acute circulatory problems: the expanded role of the physiologically oriented, *Crit Care Nurse, Am J Crit Care* 1(1):38-53, 1992.

Wahl S: Septic shock-How to detect it early, *Nurs 89* 19(1):52-59, 1989.

### Planning

Barone JE: Treatment strategies in shock: use of oxygen transport measurements, *Heart Lung* 20(1):81-86, 1991.

Bone RC: A critical evaluation of new agents for the treatment of sepsis, *JAMA* 266(12):1686-1691, 1991.

Calandra T et al: Treatment of gram-negative septic shock with human IgG antibody to escherichia coli J5: A prospective double-blind, randomized trial, *J Infect Dis* 58(2):312-319, 1988.

Gorelick K et al: Randomized placebo-controlled study of E5 monoclonal anti-endotoxin antibody. In Lorrick J, editor: *Therapeutic monoclonal antibodies,* New York, 1990, Stockton Press.

Hancock BG, Eberhard NK: The pharmacological management of shock, *Crit Care Nurs Q* 11(1):19-29, 1988.

Lancaster EL, Rice V: Nursing care planning overview and application to the patient in shock, *Crit Care Nurs, Clin North Am* 2(2):279-286, 1990.

Littleton MT: Prostaglandin and leukotrienes and mediators of shock and trauma, *Crit Care Nurs Q* 11(2):11-20, 1988.

MacLean LD: Shock, *Br Med Bull* 44(2):437-452, 1988.

McQuillan KA, Wiled CE: Initial management of traumatic shock. In Cardona DV et al, editors: *Trauma nursing from resuscitation through rehabilitation,* Philadelphia, 1988, WB Saunders.

McSwain NE: Pneumatic anti-shock garment: state of the art, 1988, *Am Emerg Med* 17(5):506-526, 1988.

Shumer W: Corticosteroids in the treatment of shock, *Prog Clin Biol Res* 236B:249-259, 1987.

Soulioti AM: Naloxone for septic shock, *Lancet* 2(8620):1133-1134, 1982.

## UNIT IV
## Surgery: Perioperative Nursing

## CHAPTER 23
## Preoperative Nursing

### Ambulatory Surgery

Breemhaar B, van den Born HW: Effects of education and support for surgical patients: the role of perceived control, *Patient Education and Counseling* 18:199-210, 1991.

Haicken B: Laser laparoscopic cholecystectomy in the ambulatory setting, *J Post Anesth Nurs* 6(1): 33-39, 1991.

Schirmer BD et al: Laparoscopic cholecystectomy, *Ann Surg* 213:665-677, 1991.

### High Risk Patients

Fromm CG, Metzler DJ: Preparing your older patient for surgery, *RN* Jan: 38-42, 1993.

Jackson MF: High risk surgical patients, *J Gerontol Nurs* 14(1):8-15, 1988.

### Assessment

Knight CG, Donnelly MK: Assessing the preoperative adult, *Nurs Pract* 13(1):6-17, 1988

### Preoperative Education

Kapnoullas J: Nursing interventions for the relief of preoperative anxiety, *Aus J Adv Nurs* 2:8-15, 1988

Kratz A: Preoperative education: preparing patients for a positive experience, *J Post Anesth Nurs* 8(4):270-275, 1993.

Lindeman CA: Patient education (review), *Annu Rev Nurs Res* 6:29-60, 1988

Meeker B, Rodriguez LS, Johnson JM: A comprehensive analysis of preoperative patient education, *Today's OR Nurse* March: 11-18, 1992.

Rothrock J: Preoperative psychoeducational interventions, *AORN J* 49:597-619, 1989.

Schoessler M: Perceptions of preoperative education in patients admitted the morning of surgery, *J Patient Ed Coun* 14:127-136, 1989

Stanfield V: Perioperative education: changing to meet short stay needs, *J Post Anesth Nurs* 3:74-77, 1988

Swindale J: The nurse's role in giving preoperative information to reduce anxiety in patients admitted to hospital for elective minor surgery, *J Adv Nurs* 14:899-905, 1989

Yount ST, Edgel J, Jakovec V: Preoperative teaching: a study of nurses' perceptions, *AORN J* 51:572-579, 1989

### Preoperative Skin Preparation

Garibaldi RA et al: The impact of preoperative skin disinfection on preventing wound contamination, *Infect Cont Hosp Epidem* 9(3):109-116, 1993.

Jepsen OB, Bruttomesso KA: The effectiveness of preoperative skin preparations, *AORN J* 58(3):477-484, 1993.

Kovach T: Nip it in the bud: controlling wound infection with preoperative shaving, *Todays OR Nurs* 12(9):23-26, 1990.

### Practice-Based Perioperative Research

Leske JS: Practice-based perioperative research: meeting the challenges, *AORN J* 55(2):581-587, 1992 (Feb).

### Reducing Anxiety

Moss VA: Music and the surgical patient: the effect of music on anxiety, *AORN J* 48:64-68, 1988.

Nyamathi A, Kashiwabara A: Preoperative anxiety: its effect on cognitive thinking, *AORN J* 47:164-170, 1988.

O'Connell M: Anxiety reduction in family members of patients in surgery and postanesthesia care: a pilot study, *J Post Anesth Nurs* 4:7-15, 1989.

### History of Perioperative Nursing

Pillitteri A: OR nursing 100 years ago: nursing care of President McKinley, *Todays OR Nurse* 13(12):19-24, 1991 (Dec).

OR nursing in the 1890s: operating in the home and without gloves, *Todays OR Nurse* 11(9):36-37, 1989 (Sept).

### Informed Consent

Murphy EK: Informed consent, Pt I, *AORN J* 47:1009-1016, 1988.

### Nursing Diagnoses in the Perioperative Experience

Stanfield V: Perioperative nursing diagnosis: integrating nursing diagnosis on the patient record, *AORN J* 46:699-704, 1990.

CHAPTER 24

## Intraoperative Nursing

### Types/Subspecialties of Surgery

Fairchild SS: *Perioperative nursing principles and practice,* Boston, 1993, Jones & Bartlett.

### Aseptic Technique Maintenance

Anonymous: Closed wound drainage system, *Orthopaedic Nurs* 8:32-33, 1989.

Anonymous: OSHA rules on bloodborne pathogens, *West Virginia Med J* 88:138-140, 1992.

Association of Operating Room Nurses: Recommended practices: protective barrier materials for surgical gowns and drapes, *AORN J* 55:832-837, 1992.

Association of Operating Room Nurses: Recommended practices: universal precautions in the perioperative setting, *AORN J* 57:554-558, 1993.

Association of Operating Room Nurses: Recommended practices: skin preparation, *AORN J* 55:555-562, 1992.

Association of Operating Room Nurses: Standards and recommended practices: recommended practices for aseptic technique, 105-110, 1993.

Atkinson LJ: *Berry & Kohn's operating room technique,* ed 7, St Louis, 1992, Mosby.

Ayliff GA: Role of the environment of the operating suite in surgical wound infection, *Rev Infect Dis* 10:S800-804, 1991.

Belkin NL: Barrier materials—their influence on surgical wound infection, *AORN J* 55:1521-1528. 1991.

Dealey C: Preventing surgical wound infection, *Nurs-Oxford* 4:26-27, 1991.

Fairchild SS: *Perioperative nursing principles and practice,* Boston, 1993, Jones & Bartlett.

Fay MF: Drainage systems—their role in wound healing, *AORN J* 46:442-455, 1987.

Grimes DE, Grimes RM, Hamelink M: *Infectious diseases,* St Louis, 1991, Mosby.

Hubbard MS et al: Reducing blood contamination and injury in the OR, *AORN J* 55:194-201, 1992.

Kneedler JA, Dodge GH: *Perioperative patient care,* ed 2, 1991, Jones & Bartlett.

Kovack T: Nip it in the bud: controlling wound infection with preoperative shaving, *Today's OR Nurs* 12:23-26, 1990.

Mailhot CB et al: Cover gowns—researching their effectiveness, *AORN J* 46:482-490, 1987.

Mead PB et al: Infection control in the operating room: issues for the 90's, *Asepsis* 12:2-13, 1990.

Pereira LJ, Lee GM, Wade KJ: The effect of surgical handwashing routines on the microbial counts of OR nurses, *Am J Infect Cont* 18:354-364, 1990.

Rao GG, Harman J, Pollard R: Face masks and postoperative infection, *J Hosp Infect* 20:55-57, 1992.

Rowell CC: The nosocomial wound infection report, its impact in the OR, *Today's OR Nurse* 12(1):21-23, 1990.

Wysocki A: Surgical wound healing: a review for perioperative nurses, *AORN J* 49:502-505, 1989.

### Anesthesia

Garrett N: Anesthesia pharmacology for general endotracheal anesthesia. In Phippen ML: *Sem Perioper Nurs* 2:8-12, 1993.

Lord EV: General anesthesia: what the perioperative nurse needs to know, *Sem Perioper Nurs* 2:4-7, 1993.

McSwain NE: Regional anesthesia: bier block, *Emerg Med* 21:73-74, 1989.

Minor DG: Anesthesia: the perioperative nurse's role, *Today's OR Nurse* 12:24-29, 1990.

Pasternak LR: General, regional, and local anesthesia, *Curr Opin Obstet Gyn* 2:275-279, 1990.

Quellette R: Midazolam: an induction agent for general anesthesia, *Nurs Anesth* 2:134-137, 1991.

Schiffer DH: Regional anesthesia: considerations for the perioperative nurse, *Sem Perioper Nurs* 2:23-32, 1993.

Watson DS: Safe nursing practices involving the patient receiving local anesthesia, *AORN J* 53:1055, 1058-1059, 1991.

### Assessment

DeLong DL: Preoperative holding area, personalizing patients' experiences, *AORN J* 55:563-566, 1992.

Haselfeld D: Patient assessment: conducting an effective interview, *AORN J* 52:551-557, 1990.

Johnson JC: Surgical assessment in the elderly, *Geriatrics* 43:83-90, 1988.

### Evaluation/Documentation

Association of Operating Room Nurses: Documentation of perioperative nursing care, *AORN J* 54:592-596, 1991.

Edel EM, Johnson PR, Tiller SG: Perioperative documentation: incorporating nursing diagnoses into the intraoperative record, *AORN J* 50:596-600, 1989.

Michel LL, Myrick C: Current and future trends in ambulatory surgery and their impact on nursing practice, *J Post Anesth Nurs* 5:347-349, 1990.

Pobojewski BJ et al: Documenting nursing process in the perioperative setting: continuity of care, patient evaluation, *AORN J* 56:98-112, 1992.

### Hyperthermia/Hypothermia

Blansett MT: The effects of rewarming hypothermic postanesthesia patients using thermadrape covering, heat lamps, and warmed cotton blankets, *J Post Anesth Nurs* 5:80-84, 1990.

Frederick C, Rosemann D, Austin MJ: Malignant hyperthermia: nursing diagnosis and care, *J Post Anesth Nurs* 5:29-32, 1990.

Kneedler JA, Dodge GH: *Perioperative patient care,* ed 2, 1991, Jones & Bartlett.

Moddeman G: The elderly surgical patient—a high risk for hypothermia, *AORN J* 53:1270-1272, 1991.

Thomas SD: Malignant hyperthermia, *Crit Care Nurs* 9:58-63, 65-69, 1989.

Wlody GS: Malignant hyperthermia, *Crit Care Nurs Clin North Am* 3:129-134, 1991.

Wolcott K, McDonnell A: Malignant hyperthermia—nursing implications, *Crit Care Nurs* 10:78-80, 82-85, 1990.

### Nursing Interventions for Intraoperative Patient Safety

Association of Operating Room Nurses: Recommended practices: electrosurgical safety, *AORN J* 53:744-752, 1991.

Association of Operating Room Nurses: Recommended practices: patient positioning, *AORN J,* 52:1035-1040, 1990.

Bailey SL: Electrical injuries: considerations for the perioperative nurse, *AORN J,* 49:773-778, 1987.

Biddle C, Cannady MJ: Surgical positions, their effect on cardiovascular, respiratory systems, *AORN J* 52:350-359, 1990.

Cooper DE et al: The prevention of injuries of the brachial plexus secondary to malposition of the patient during surgery, *Clin Orthopaedics and Related Res* 228:33-41, 1988.

Kemp MG et al: Factors that contribute to pressure sores in surgical patient, *Res Nurs Health* 13:293-301, 1990.

Meeker MR, Rothrock JC: *Alexander's care of the patient in surgery,* ed 10, St Lous, 1995, Mosby.

Moak E: Electrosurgical unit safety: the role of the perioperative nurse, *AORN J* 53:744-752, 1991.

Norris J: Fire safety in the operating room, *Today's OR Nurse* 14:8-10, 1992.

Parsons EC, Kee CC, Gray P: Perioperative nurse caring behaviors, *AORN J* 57:1106-1114, 1993.

Smith KA: Positioning principles, *AORN J* 52:1199-1208, 1990.

## CHAPTER 25
## Postoperative Nursing

### General Information

Reed RD: A standard of care plan in the postanesthesia care unit, *J Post Anesth Nurs* 6:255-264, 1991.

Strong NS: Assessing the postanesthesia patient, *Crit Care Nurs Q* 16:1-7, 1993.

### Respiratory Status

Berel DJ, Marz MS: SaO2 monitoring in the postanesthetic care unit, *J Post Anesth Nurs* 6:394-401, 1991.

Elmquist L: Decision making for extubation of the post-anesthetic patient, *Crit Care Nurs Q* 15:82-86, 1992.

Litwack K, Zeplin KL: Practical points in the management of laryngospasm, *J Post Anesth Nurs* 4:36-39, 1989.

McConnell EA: Preventing postoperative complications, *Nurs 91* 34-39, 1991.

Saleh KL: Practical points in understanding aspiration, *J Post Anesth* 6:347-349, 1991.

### Neurologic Status

Saleh KL: Practical points in understanding spinal anesthesia, *J Post Anesth Nurs* 6:407-409, 1991.

### Cardiovascular Status

Daleider A: Physiology and treatment of hemorrhagic shock during the early postoperative period, *Crit Care Nurs Q* 16:45-59, 1993.

Davis LA, O'Rourke NC: Pulmonary embolism: early recognition and management in the postanesthesia care unit, *J Post Anesth Nurs* 8:338-345, 1993.

Hull RD et al: Effectiveness of intermittent pneumatic leg compression for preventing deep vein thrombosis after total hip replacement, *JAMA* 263:2313-2317, 1990.

KUC J: Management of acute myocardial infarction in the post-anesthesia care unit, *J Post Anesth Nurs* 5:401-406, 1990.

### Thermoregulation

Fredrick C, Rosemann D, Austin MJ: Malignant hyperthermia: nursing diagnosis and care, *J Post Anesth Nurs* 5:29-32, 1990.

Heffline MS: A comparative study of pharmacological versus nursing interventions in the treatment of postanesthesia shivering, *J Post Anesth Nurs* 6:311-320, 1991.

Markin D et al: Comparison between two types of body surface temperature devices: efficiency, accuracy and cost, *J Post Anesth Nurs* 5:33-37, 1990.

Sessler DI, Israel D, Pozos RS: Spontaneous postanesthesia tremor does not resemble thermoregulatory shivering, *Anesth* 68:843-850, 1988.

Stevens T: Managing postoperative hypothermia, rewarming and its complications, *Crit Care Nurs Q* 16:60-77, 1993.

Summers T: Axillary, tympanic and esophageal temperature measurement: descriptive comparisons in postanesthesia patients, *J Post Anesth Nurs* 6:420-425, 1991.

Thomas SD: Malignant hyperthermia, *Crit Care Nurs* 9:58-67, 1989.

Wolcott K, McDonnell A: Malignant hyperthermia nursing implications, *Crit Care Nurs* 10:78-85, 1990.

### Comfort

Cohen B: Nonsteroidal anti-inflammatory drugs, *AORN J* 58:578-585, 1993.

Fulk C, Hadley JC: Something for pain: new trends in epidural analgesia, *J Post Anesth Nurs* 5:247-253, 1990.

Heffline MS: Exploring nursing interventions for acute pain in the postanesthesia care unit, *J Post Anesth Nurs* 5:321-328, 1990.

Hinojosa R: Nursing interventions to prevent or relieve postoperative nausea and vomiting, *J Post Anesth Nurs* 7:3-14, 1992.

Jurf B, Nirschl AL: Acute postoperative pain management: a comprehensive review and update, *Crit Care Nurs Q* 16:8-25, 1993.

Kenny G: Ketorolac tromethamine, *Br J Anesth* 65:445-447, 1990.

Lazzara MS: Patient-controlled analgesia in the intensive care unit, *Crit Care Nurs Q* 16:26-36, 1993.

### *Geriatrics*

Burden N: Handle with care: the geriatric patient in the ambulatory surgery environment, *J Post Anesth Nurs* 4:27-31, 1989.

Drevdahl D: Promoting power and control in the elderly client, *J Post Anesth Nurs* 4:22-26, 1989.

### *Psychological Status*

Cormier S, Pickett SJ, Gallagher J: Comparison of nurses' and family members' perceived needs during postanesthesia care unit visits, *J Post Anesth Nurs* 7:387-391, 1992.

Iacono MV: Precious moments of caring, *J Post Anesth Nurs* 8:26-27, 1993.

Noonan AT et al: Family centered nursing in the postanesthesia care unit: the evaluation of practice, *J Post Anesth Nurs* 6:13-16, 1991.

Poole EL: The visiting needs of critically ill patients and their families, *J Post Anesth Nurs* 7:377-386, 1992.

Redmond MC: The importance of good communication in effective patient-family teaching, *J Post Anesth Nurs* 8:109-112, 1993.

### *Ambulatory/Short-Stay Patients*

Caldwell LM: Surgical outpatient concerns: what every perioperative nurse should know, *AORN J* 53:761-767, 1991.

Llewellyn JG: Short stay surgery: present practices, future trends, *AORN J* 53:1179-1191, 1991.

Mamaril ME: Stress and the ambulatory surgical unit, *J Post Anesth Nurs* 4:172-176, 1989.

Michel LL: Current and future trends in ambulatory surgery and their impact on nursing practice, *J Post Anesth Nurs* 5:347-349, 1990.

### *Evaluation/Documentation*

Mamaril M: Standard of care: legal implications in the postanesthesia care unit, *J Post Anesth Nurs* 8:13-20, 1993.

McArdle EJ, Allain LA: A new approach to postanesthesia care unit documentation, *J Post Anesth Nurs* 6:246-254, 1991.

Miller KM, Taylor BJ: Standard care plans for the postanesthesia care unit, *J Post Anesth Nurs* 6:26-32, 1991.

Reed RD: A standard of care plan in the postanesthesia care unit, *J Post Anesth Nurs* 6:255-264, 1991.

UNIT V

# Special Environments of Care

CHAPTER 26

## Critical Care Environment

### *Environment in the Critical Care Unit*

Atkinson B: The current state of critical care, *Inten Care Nurs* 7(2):73-79, 1991.

Baker C: Discomfort to environment noise: heart rate responses of sick patients, *Crit Care Nurs Q* 15(2):75-90, 1992.

Birdsall C: *Management issues in critical care,* St Louis, 1991, Mosby.

Clochesy JM: *Advanced technology in critical care nursing,* Rockville, Md, 1989, Aspen.

Crippen D, Ermakov S: Stress, agitation, and brain failure in critical care medicine, *Crit Care Nurs Q* 15(2):52-74, 1992.

Easton C, MacKenzie F: Sensory-perceptual alterations: delirium in the intensive care unit, *Heart Lung* 17:229-337, 1988.

Henneman B: Building the model ICU, *Crit Care Nurs* 12(8):112, 1992.

Inman L, Haugen C: Six criteria to evaluate skill competency documentation, *DCCN* 10(4):238-245, 1991.

Jackson MM: Infection prevention and control, *Crit Care Clin North Am* 4(3):401-442, 1992.

Lewis DJ, Robinson JA: ICU nurses' coping measures and response to work-related stressors, *Crit Care Nurs* 12(2):18-26, 1992.

Raffin TA, Shurkin JN, Sinkler W III: *Intensive care: facing the critical choices,* New York, 1989, WH Freeman.

Riegel B, Ehrenreich D: *Psychological aspects of critical care nursing,* Rockville, Md, 1989, Aspen.

Sinclair V: High technology in critical care: implications for nursing's role and practice, *Focus Crit Care* 15(4):36-41, 1988.

Spicer JG, Robinson MA: *Managing the environment in critical care nursing,* Baltimore, 1990, Williams & Wilkins.

### *Assessment of the Critically Ill Patient*

Ahrens T: SVO2 monitoring: Is it being used appropriately? *Crit Care Nurs* 10(7):70-72, 1990.

Alspach JG: *Core curriculum for critical care nursing,* ed 4, Philadelphia, 1991, WB Saunders.

Bustin D: *Hemodynamic monitoring for critical care,* Norwalk, Conn, 1986, Appleton-Century-Crofts.

Caine RM, Bufalino PM: *Critically ill adults: nursing care planning guides,* Baltimore, 1988, Williams & Wilkins.

Carpenito LJ: Nursing diagnosis in critical care: impact on practice and outcomes, *Heart Lung* 16:595-600, 1987.

Copel LC, Stolark A: Continuous SVO2 monitoring: a research review, *DCCN* 10(4):202-209, 1991.

Daily EK, Schroeder JS: *Techniques in bedside monitoring,* ed 4, St Louis, 1989, Mosby.

Dossey BM, Guzzetta CE, Kenner CV: *Essentials of critical care nursing: body-mind-spirit,* Philadelphia, 1990, JB Lippincott.

Fulmer TT, Walker MK: *Critical care nursing of the elderly,* New York, 1992, Springer.

Gilliam EE: Intracranial hypertension: advances in intracranial pressure monitoring, *Crit Care Clin North Am* 2(1):21-27, 1990.

Hollingsworth-Fridlund P, Vos H, Daily EK: Use of fiber-optic pressure transducer for intracranial pressure measurement: a preliminary report, *Heart Lung* 17:111-120, 1988.

Holloway NM: *Nursing the critically ill adult,* Oakland, Calif, 1988, Addison-Wesley.

Hudak CM, Gallo BM, Lohr TS: *Critical care nursing, a holistic approach,* ed 4, Philadelphia, 1986, JB Lippincott.

Johanson BC et al: *Standards for critical care,* St Louis, 1988, Mosby.

Kinney ME: *AACN's clinical reference for critical-care nursing,* ed 2, New York, 1988, McGraw-Hill.

Marino PL: *The ICU book,* Philadelphia, 1991, Lea & Febiger.

Moorhouse MF, Geissler AC, Doenges ME: *Critical care plans—guidelines for patient care,* Philadelphia, 1987, FA Davis.

Parillo JE: *Current therapy in critical care medicine,* ed 2, Philadelphia, 1991, BC Decker.

Roberts SL: Physiologic nursing diagnoses are necessary and appropriate for critical care, *Focus Crit Care* 15(5):42-49, 1988.

Schermer L: Physiologic and technical variables affecting hemodynamic measurements, *Crit Care Nurs* 8(2):33-40, 1988.

Schroeder CH: Pulse oximetry: a nursing care plan, *Crit Care Nurs* 8(8):50-68, 1988.

Sommers MS: *Difficult diagnoses in critical care nursing,* Rockville, Md, 1989, Aspen.

Stillwell SB: *Mosby's critical care nursing reference,* St Louis, 1992, Mosby.

Swearingen PL, Keen JH: *Manual of critical care: applying nursing diagnoses to adult critical illness,* St Louis, 1991, Mosby.

Thelan LA et al: *Textbook of critical care nursing: diagnosis and management,* ed 2, St Louis, 1990, Mosby.

Urden LD, Davie JK, Thelan LA: *Essentials of critical care nursing,* St Louis, 1992, Mosby.

Von Rueden KT, Walleck CA: *Advanced critical care nursing,* Rockville, Md, 1989, Aspen.

Wright JE, Shelton BK: *Desk reference for critical care nursing,* Boston, 1993, Jones & Bartlett.

### Alleviation and Prevention of Physiologic and Physical Stressors

Bagby M et al: The total artificial heart, *Am J Nurs* 87:1050-1058, 1987.

Bradley RB: Adult respiratory distress syndrome, *Focus Crit Care* 14(5):48-59, 1987.

Chmielewski C, Zellers L: Continuous arteriovenous hemofiltration in the patient with hepatorenal syndrome, *Crit Care Nurs Clin North Am* 2(1):115-122, 1990.

Cohen FL: Acquired immunodeficiency syndrome research in critical care: a review and future directions, *Focus Crit Care* 15(4):30-35, 1988.

Cooper DK, Valladares BK, Futterman LG: Care of the patient with automatic implantable cardioverter defibrillator: a guide for nurses, *Heart Lung* 16:640-648, 1987.

Dillon J et al: Rapid initiation of thrombolytic therapy for acute MI, *Crit Care Nurs* 9(2):55-61, 1989.

Hoffman LA: Airway management for the critically ill patient, *Am J Nurs* 87:39-53, 1987.

Joseph DL, Bates S: Intra-aortic balloon pumping: how to stay on course, *Am J Nurs* 90(9):42-47, 1990.

Kiely MA: Type-II toxic epidermal necrolysis, *Crit Care Nurs* 7(1):34-39, 1987.

Kinney MR et al: *Comprehensive cardiac care,* St Louis, 1991, Mosby.

Koniak-Griffin D, Dodgson J: Severe pregnancy-induced hypertension: postpartum care of the critically ill patient, *Heart Lung* 16:661-669, 1987.

Konopad E, Noseworthy T: Stress ulceration: a serious complication in critically ill patients, *Heart Lung* 17:339-348, 1988.

Lovejoy NC, Rumley R: AIDS epidemiology and pathology: implications for intensive care units, *Crit Care Clin North Am* 4(3):383-394, 1992.

Metzger JT, Hoffman LA: Cardiac transplantation: the changing faces of immunosuppression, *Heart Lung* 17:414-425, 1988.

Moser SA, Crawford D, Thomas A: Caring for patients with implantable cardioverter defibrillators, *Crit Care Nurs* 8(2):52-65, 1988.

Mulford E: Nursing perspectives for the patient receiving postoperative ventricular assistance in the critical care unit, *Heart Lung* 16:246-257, 1987.

Omery A, Caswell D: A nursing perspective of the ethical issues surrounding liver transplantation, *Heart Lung* 17:626-631, 1988.

Pelter MA: Thrombolytic therapy in acute myocardial infarction, *Crit Care Nurs Q* 12(3):55-66, 1989.

Persons CB: Transcutaneous pacing: meeting the challenge, *Focus Crit Care* 14(1):13-19, 1987.

Price CA: Continuous arteriovenous ultrafiltration: a monitoring guide for ICU nurses, *Crit Care Nurs* 9(1):12-19, 1989.

Roberts SL: High-permeability pulmonary edema: nursing assessment, diagnosis, and interventions, *Heart Lung* 19:287-300, 1990.

Ross D: Acute compartment syndrome, *Orthopaedic Nurs* 10(2): 33-38,1991.

Shennib H, Adoumie R, Noirclec M: Current status of lung transplantation for cystic fibrosis, *Arch Intern Med* 152(8):1585-1588, 1992.

Smith SL, Ciferni M: Liver transplantation for acute hepatic failure: a review of clinical experience and management, *Am J Crit Care* 2(2):137-144, 1993.

Stevens LL, Redd RM, Buckingham TA: Ventricular burst pacing, *Crit Care Nurs* 9(3):38-43, 1989.

Teplitz L: Nursing diagnoses for automatic implantable cardioverter defibrillator patients, *DCCN* 10(4):188-201, 1991.

Tribett D: Immune system function: implications for critical care nursing practice, *Crit Care Nurs Clin North Am* 1(4):725-740, 1989.

Vargo RL, Whitman GR: Complications after cardiac transplantation: the role of immunosuppression, *Crit Care Nurs Clin North Am* 1(4):741-752, 1989.

Vasbinder-Dillon D: Understanding mechanical ventilation, *Crit Care Nurs* 8(7):42-56, 1988.

Vaska PL: Common infections in heart transplant patients, *Am J Crit Care* 2(2):145-156, 1993.

### Alleviation and Prevention of Psychologic Stressors

Carnevale F: High technology and humanity in intensive care: finding a balance, *Inten Care Nurs* 7(1):23-27, 1991.

Clark AP, Garry M: Legal implications of standards of care, *DCCN* 10(2):96-102, 1991.

Erickson S, Hopkins MA: Gray areas: informed consent in pediatric and comatose adult patients, *Heart Lung* 17:229-237, 1988.

Fowler MDM, Levine-Ariff J: *Ethics at the bedside: a sourcebook for critical care nurses,* Philadelphia, 1987, JB Lippincott.

Heater BS, AuBuchon B: *Controversies in critical care nursing,* Rockville, Md, 1988, Aspen.

Hickey M, Lewandowski L: Critical care nurse's role with families: a descriptive study, *Heart Lung* 17:670-676, 1988.

Hopping BL, Sickbert SF, Ruth J: A study of factors associated with CCU visiting policies, *Crit Care Nurs* 12(2):8-17, 1992.

Littrell K, Schumann LL: Promoting sleep for the patient with a myocardial infarction, *Crit Care Nurs* 9(3):44-49, 1989.

Marsden C: "Do not resuscitate" orders and end of life care plans, *Am J Crit Care* 2(2):177-179, 1993.

Morrison C: The HIV epidemic: ethical issues for the next decade, *Crit Care Clin North Am* 4(3):421-428, 1992.

Nyamathi A, Van Servellen G: Maladaptive coping in the critically ill population with acquired immunodeficiency syndrome: nursing assessment and treatment, *Heart Lung* 18:113-120, 1989.

Oermann NH, Provenzano LM: Student's knowledge and perceptions of critical care nursing, *Crit Care Nurs* 12(1):72-77, 1992.

Parillo JE: *Critical decisions: key issues in the recovery of the critically ill,* Philadelphia, 1988, BC Decker.

Pierce SF: The critical care nurse: an ethicist by trade, *Crit Care Nurs Q* 12(3):75-78, 1989.

Singleton KA, Fever R: The challenge of autonomy and respecting the patient's wishes, *DCCN* 10(3):160-168, 1991.

Wilson VS: Identification of stressors related to patients' psychologic responses to the surgical intensive care unit, *Heart Lung* 16:267-273, 1987.

Wlody GS: Ethical issues in critical care: a nursing model, *DCCN* 9(4):224-230, 1990.

### Alleviation and Prevention of Social Stressors for the Patient and Family

Hickey ML, Leske JS: Needs of families of critically ill patients: state of the science and future directions, *Crit Care Nurs Clin North Am* 4(4):645-649, 1992.

CHAPTER 27

## Home Care Environment

### Economic Aspects of Home Care

Brooten D et al: A randomized clinical trial of early hospital discharge and home follow-up of very-low-birth-weight infants, *N Engl J Med* 315:934-938, 1986.

Cronin C, Maklebust J: Case-managed care: capitalizing on the CNS, *Nurs Manage* 20(2):64-88, 1988.

Fitzgerald J, Moore P, Dittus R: The care of elderly patients with hip fracture: changes since implementation of the prospective payment system, *N Engl J Med* 319:1392-1397, 1988.

Jacobs M, Goodman G: Psychology and self-help groups, *Am Psychol* 44(3):536-545, 1989.

Maraldo P: Home care should be the heart of a nursing sponsored national health plan, *Nurs Health Care* 10(6):301-304, 1989.

National Association for Home Care: *Basic statistics about home,* National Association for Home Care, Washington, DC, 1992.

Peters D: Development of a community health intensity rating scale, *Nurs Res* 37:202-207, 1988.

Smith CE: Overview of patient education: opportunities and challenges for the twenty-first century, *Nurs Clin North Am* 24(3):583-587, 1989.

Stopfjell J: How valuable are nurses' skills? A case for fair pricing in home health care, *Nurs Health Care* 10(6):311-313, 1989.

### Family Caregiving

Archbold P et al: Mutuality and preparedness as predictors of caregiver role strain, *Res Nurs Health* 13:375-384, 1990.

Baille V, Norbeck J, Barnes L: Stress, social support, and psychological distress of family caregivers of the elderly, *Nurs Res* 37:217-222, 1988.

Corbin J, Strauss A: *Unending work and care: managing chronic illness at home,* San Francisco, 1988, Jossey-Bass.

Duvall E: *Marriage and family development,* Philadelphia, 1977, JB Lippincott.

Phillips E et al: DRG ripple and the shifting of burden of care to home health, *Nurs Health Care* 10(6):325-327, 1989.

Smith CE: Caregivers of technology dependent patients. In Fitzpatrick S, Jacox A, editors: *Annual review of nursing research* (in press).

Smith CE et al: Caregiver learning needs and reactions to managing mechanical ventilation at home, *Heart Lung* 23(2):157-163, 1994.

Smith CE et al: Financial and technological costs of high technology home care, *Nurs Econ* 10(5):369-373, 1992.

### General Home Care

Berger M: The cost and efficacy of home care for patients with chronic lung disease, *Med Care* 36(6):566-579, 1988.

Harris M: The changing scene in community health nursing, *Nurs Clin North Am* 23(3):559-568, 1988.

Johnson EA, Jackson JE: Teaching the home care client, *Nurs Clin North Am* 24(3):687-694, 1989.

Liebermann A: *Community and home health nursing,* Springhouse, Pa, 1990, Springhouse.

Lindeman C: Patient education. In Fitzpatrick JJ, Taunton RL, Benoliel JQ, editors: *Annual review of nursing research,* New York, 1988, Springer.

Lindeman C: Patient education, Part II. In Fitzpatrick JJ, Taunton RL, Benoliel JQ, editors: *Annual review of nursing research,* New York, 1989, Springer.

Martinson I, Widmer A: *Home health care nursing,* Philadelphia, 1989, WB Saunders.

Rovinski C, Zastocki D: *Home care: a technical manual for the professional nurse,* Philadelphia, 1989, WB Saunders.

Smith CE: *Patient education: nurses in partnership with other health care professionals,* New York, 1987, Grune & Stratton.

Smith CE: Technology and home care. In Fitzpatrick JJ, Jacox AK, Stevenson J, editors: *Annual review of nursing research,* New York, Springer (in press).

Smith CE, Giefer CK, Bieker L: Technological dependency: a preliminary model and pilot of home total parenteral nutrition, *J Community Health Nurs* 8(4):245-254, 1991.

Smith CE et al: Responsibilities and reactions of family caregivers of patients dependent on total parenteral nutrition at home, *Public Health Nurs* 10(2):122-128, 1993.

Stiller SB: Success and difficulty in high-tech home care, *Public Health Nurs* 5(2):68-74, 1988.

### Home Intravenous Care

Brown JM: Home care models for infusion therapy, *Caring* 9(5):24-27, 1990.

Bruera E: Ambulatory infusion devices in the continuing care of patients with advanced diseases, *J Pain Symptom Manage* 5(5):287-296, 1990.

Coker M: Teaching checklist for home infusion therapy, *Oncol Nurs Forum* 17(6):923-926, 1990.

Gorski LA: Home dobutamine therapy, *J Home Health Care Pract* 2(4):11-20, 1990.

McAbee RR: Home intravenous therapy: issues, part 1, *Home Health Care Serv Q* 12(3):59-108, 1991.

McKee J: Future dimensions in vascular access: peripheral implantable ports, *J Intravenous Nurs* 14(6):387-393, 1991.

Moeser LC: Anaphylaxis: a preventable complication of home infusion therapy, *J Intravenous Nurs* 14(2):108-112, 1991.

Moore J: Intravenous amrinone therapy at home, *Focus Crit Care* 15:32-37, 1988.

Parker GG: Chemotherapy administration in the home, *Home Health Nurse* 10(1):30-36, 1992.

Rooney A: A joint commission perspective on home infusion therapy, III. *Hospital-Home-Health* 8(8):104-106, 1991.

Santiago OL: Establishing a community-based home transfusion program, *J Home Health Care Pract* 2(4):21-28, 1990.

St. Marie B: Narcotic infusions: a changing scene, *J Intravenous Nurs* 14(5):334-344, 1991.

Streckfuss BLW: Foundation for establishing a home IV program, *Caring* 9(5):18-20, 1990.

Wood S: Extending the principle of self-care: intravenous therapy in the community, *Prof Nurs* 6(9):543-544, 546, 548-549, 1991.

### Quality Care (Quality Improvement)

Brooten D et al: Early discharge and specialist transitional care, *Image: J Nurs Sch* 20(2):64-88, 1988.

Frederick B, Sharp J, Atkins N: Quality of patient care: whose decision? *J Nur Quality Assurance* 2(3):1-10, 1988.

Joint Commission on Accreditation of Health Care Organizations: *Quality assessment in managed care organizations,* Chicago, 1993, The Commission.

Mitchell M: The power of standards, *Nurs Health Care* 10(6):307-309, 1989.

O'Hare P, Terry M: *Discharge planning strategies for assuming continuity of care,* Rockville, Md, 1988, Aspen.

Reinhard S: Case managing community services for hip fractured elders, *Orthop Nurs* 7:42-49, 1988.

Smith CE: Quality of life in long-term parenteral nutrition patients and their family caregivers, *J Parenteral and Enteral Nutrit* 17(6):501-506, 1993.

Zarle ND: Continuity of care: balancing care of elders between health care settings, *Nurs Clin North Am* 24:697-706, 1989.

CHAPTER 28

## Emergency Care Environment

### General

Bell NK: Ethical dilemmas in trauma nursing, *Nurs Clin North Am* 25(1):143-154, 1990.

Braun A: Emergency cardiac care: fine-tuning for the '90s, *RN* 56(9):50-55, 1993.

Caroline N: *Emergency medical treatment, a text for EMT-As and EMT-Intermediates,* Boston, 1991, Little, Brown.

Derlet R, Nishio D: Refusing emergency care to patients who present to an emergency department, *Ann Emerg Med* 19(3):262-267, 1990.

Diphtheria, tetanus and pertussis: guidelines for vaccine prophylaxis and other measures, *MMWR* 34:405-425, 1985.

Harrahill M, Bartkus E: Preparing the trauma patient for transfer, *J Emerg Nurs* 16(1):27, 1990.

Harwood-Nuss A et al: *The clinical practice of emergency medicine,* Philadelphia, 1991, JB Lippincott.

Headlines: *Am J Nurs* 93(8):9, 1993.

Health Security Act, 1993, United States of America, Washington, DC, 1993, US Government Printing Office.

Lamros N: *Assessment and intervention in emergency nursing,* ed 3, Norwalk, Conn, 1992, Appleton & Lange.

Lenahan G: ED noise—a legitimate patient care and staff stress issue . . . emergency department, *J Emerg Nurs* 19(3):181-182, 1993.

Missouri Department of Health: Hospital licensing rules and regulations. In *Proposed rules and regulations for hospital emergency services,* Jefferson City, Mo, 1993, The Department.

Mitchell J, Bray G: *Emergency services stress guidelines for preserving the health and careers of emergency services personnel,* Englewood Cliffs, NJ, 1990, Brady Books.

Nelson M: Critical pathways in the emergency department, *J Emerg Nurs* 19(2):110-114, 1993.

Norris MK: How to manage tissue donation, *Am J Nurs* 89(10):1294-1299, 1989.

Norwood SH: Management of the trauma patient, *Cur Rev for Post Anesth Nurs* 9(20):159-164, 1987.

Paparone P: The summer scourge: Lyme disease, *Am J Nurs* 90(6):44-47, 1990.

Rotello LC et al: Critical care management and techniques, MRI protocol for critically ill patients, *Am J Crit Care* 3(3):187-190, 1994.

Sheehy SB: *Emergency nursing principles and practice,* ed 3, St Louis, 1992, Mosby.

Stern RS et al: The emergency department as a pathway to admission for poor and high-cost patients, *JAMA* 266(16):2238-2243, 1991.

Thelan LA et al: *Critical care nursing: diagnosis and management,* ed 2, St Louis, 1994, Mosby.

US Bureau of the Census: *Statistical abstracts of the United States,* ed 108, Washington, DC, 1988, US Government Printing Office.

US Department of Health and Human Services, Public Health Service: *Healthy People 2000: national health promotion and disease prevention objectives,* Washington, DC, 1991, US Government Printing Office.

US Department of Health and Human Services, Public Health Service: *Diphtheria, tetanus, and pertussis: what you need to know,* Atlanta, 1992, Centers for Disease Control.

### Cardiac-Respiratory-Renal

Barbiere CC: Cardiac tamponade: diagnosis and emergency intervention, *Crit Care Nurs* 10(4):20-22, 1990.

Carlson R: Seattle study findings help nurses triage AMI patients . . . myocardial infarction triangle and intervention (MITI) project, *Cardiovascular Nurs* 6(1):9-11, 1993.

Carroll P: Speed—the essential response to anaphylaxis, *RN* 57(6):26-31, 1994.

Defibrillation in the emergency care setting: present and future shock, *Emerg Nurs Report* 3(3):1-8, 1988.

Emergency Cardiac Care Committee and Subcommittees of the American Heart Association: Guidelines for cardiopulmonary resuscitation and emergency cardiac care. I: introduction, *JAMA* 268(16):2289-2295, 1992.

Glanker D: Caring for the victim of near drowning, *Crit Care Nurs* 13(4):25-32, 1993.

Kuhn M: Multiple trauma with respiratory distress, *Crit Care Nurs* 14(2):68-80, 1994.

Merkley K: Assessing chest pain, *RN* 57(6):58-62, 1994.

Stark J: Acute renal failure in trauma: current perspectives, *Crit Care Nurs Q* 16(4):49-60, 1994.

Teplitz L: Action stat! hypertensive crisis, *Nurs 90* 20(4):33, 1990.

Turner JA: Cardiovascular trauma, *Nurs Clin North Am* 25(1):119-130, 1990.

### Emergency Nursing Scope of Practice

Bailey M: What the future holds for ED nursing, *Nurs 91* 21(9):56-59, 1991.

Emergency Nurses Association Emergency Nursing: Scope of practice, *J Emerg Nurs* 15(4):361-364, 1989.

Emergency Nurses Association position statement: autonomous emergency practice, *J Emerg Nurs* 17(6):30A-32A, 1991.

Nelson MS: Critical pathways in the emergency department, *J Emerg Nurs* 19(2):110-114, 1993.

Villaire M: Interview Cindy Rushton, big advocacy, little world, *Crit Care Nurs* 14(2):107-113, 1994.

### Environment-Poisons

Bauer RL, Watson WA: Clinical toxicology. In Stein JH et al, editors: *Internal medicine,* ed 4, St Louis, 1994, Mosby.

Higgins R: Cocaine abuse: what every emergency nurse should know, *J Emerg Nurs* 15(4):318-323, 1989.

Nicholson DP: The immediate management of overdose, *Med Clin North Am* 67:1279-1291, 1983.

Robey-Williams C: Hypothermia: a winter emergency. In Mlynczak-Callahan B, editor: *Case studies in emergency nursing,* Baltimore, 1990, Williams & Wilkins.

### Gastrointestinal/Abdominal

Beachley M, Farrar J: Abdominal trauma: putting the pieces together, *Am J Nurs* 93(11):25-34, 1993.

Bolton PJ, Von Rotz NP: Management of an open abdominal wound with a synthetic covering, *Crit Care Nurs* 14(2):44-51, 1994.

Greenberg L: Fast action for splenic rupture, *Am J Nurs* 94(2):51, 1994.

Kitt S: Abdominal trauma. In Kitt S, Kaiser J, editors: *Emergency nursing: a physiological and clinical perspective,* Philadelphia, 1990, WB Saunders.

Lawrence DM: Gastrointestinal trauma, *Crit Care Nurs Clin North Am* 5(1):127-140, 1993.

Mertes JE: Action stat: G.I. bleeding, *Nurs 89* 19(8):37, 1989.

Quinless FW: Emergency treatment for ruptured varices: esophagastric tamponade, *Nurs 88* 18(10):641-64n, 1988.

### Integumentary

Cantrill SV: Facial trauma. In Roseen P et al, editors: *Vol I. Emergency medicine: concepts and clinical practice,* St Louis, 1992, Mosby.

Cuzzell JZ, Stotts NA: Wound care: trial and error yields to hemorrhage, *Am J Nurs* 90(10):53-63, 1990.

Legge M, Murphy M: Human bite wounds, *J Emerg Nurs* 16:145-149, 1990.

Paul S, Lee C: Trauma case review: survival following impalement, *Crit Care Nurs* 14(2):55-59, 1994.

Simon B: Principles of wound management. In Roseen P et al, editors: *Vol I. Emergency medicine: concepts and clinical practice,* St Louis, 1992, Mosby.

### Neuromuscular-Skeletal

Ammons A: Cerebral injuries and intracranial hemorrhages as a result of trauma, *Nurs Clin North Am* 25(1):23-33, 1990.

Caplan LR: Cerebrovascular disease (stroke). In Stein JH et al, editors: *Internal medicine,* ed 4, St Louis, 1993, Mosby.

Halpern JS: Lower extremity peripheral nerve assessment, *J Emerg Nurs* 15(4):333-337, 1989.

Mlynczak B: Assessment and management of the trauma patient in pain, *Crit Care Nurs Clin North Am* 1(1):105-111, 1989.

Proehl JA: Compartment syndrome, *J Emerg Nurs* 14(5):283-292, 1988.

### *Psychosocial*

Aguilera D: *Crisis intervention: theory and methodology,* St Louis, 1990, Mosby.

George JE, Quattrone MS: Emergency department overload: how to "cya," *J Emerg Nurs* 18(2):157-158, 1992.

Gray B: The patient-driven system, *Crit Care Nurs* 14(2):95, 1994.

Hopkins A: The trauma nurses' role with families in crisis, *Crit Care* 14(2):35-43, 1994.

Johnston J: Preserving privacy and confidentiality for the emergency patient, *Emerg Nurs Reports* 3(4):1-8, 1988.

McPhee A: Let the family in, *J Emerg Nurs* 13(2):120-121, 1987.

Sommers MS: Alcohol and trauma: the critical link, *Crit Care Nurs* 14(2):82-93, 1994.

Sommers MS: The near-death experience following multiple trauma, *Crit Care Nurs* 14(2):62-66, 1994.

### *Trauma*

Cardona V et al: *Trauma nursing from resuscitation through rehabilitation,* Philadelphia, 1988, WB Saunders.

Jarosz D: The tertiary nursing survey in the assessment of trauma patients: an important addendum to survival, *Crit Care Nurs* 14(2):98-103, 1994.

Rea R: *Trauma nursing core course,* ed 3, Chicago, 1991, Emergency Nurses Association.

Sheehy SB, Marvin JA, Jimmerson CL: *Manual of clinical trauma care the first hour,* ed 2, St Louis, 1994, Mosby.

### *Violence*

Fazio J: Violence in the emergency department: strategies for survival, *Course presented at the Emergency Nurses Association Scientific Assembly,* Seattle, September 1993.

Jezierski M: Guidelines for intervention by ED nurses in cases of domestic abuse, *J Emerg Nurs* 18(10):28a-30a, 1992.

Mitchum D: Risk, hazard, danger, peril, exposure to harm, *J Emerg Nurs* 17(5):353, 1991.

Namuth T: When did he stop beating his wife? *Newsweek,* Vol CXXIII (26):21, 1994.

# UNIT VI
# Alterations in Fluid and Gas Transport

## SECTION ONE Cardiovascular System

### *General*

American Heart Association: *Heart facts,* Dallas, 1992, The Association.

American Heart Association: *Heart and stroke facts and statistics,* Dallas, 1993, The Association.

Berne RM, Levy MS: *Cardiovascular physiology,* ed 6, St Louis, 1992, Mosby.

Braunwald E: *Heart disease: a textbook of cardiovascular medicine,* ed 4, Philadelphia, 1992, WB Saunders.

Cunningham RS, Bonam-Crawford D: The role of fibrinolytic agents in the management of thrombotic complications associated with vascular access devices, *Nurs Clin North Am* 28(4):899-909, 1993.

Freedman SE, Gosserman G: Tunneled catheters: technologic advances and nursing care issues, *Nurs Clin North Am* 28(4):858, 1993.

Gullo SM: Implanted ports: technologic advances and nursing care issues, *Nurs Clin North Am* 28(4):859-871, 1993.

Hurst JW et al: *The heart,* ed 7, New York, 1990, McGraw-Hill.

Johnson GB: Nursing care of patients with implanted pumps, *Nurs Clin North Am* 28(4):873-883, 1993.

Kinney M et al: *Comprehensive cardiac care: a text for nurses, physicians, and other health practitioners,* ed 7, St Louis, 1991, Mosby.

Lewis JF, Maron BJ: Cardiovascular consequences of the aging process, *Cardiovasc Clin* 22(2):25-34, 1992.

Orr ME: Issues in the management of percutaneous central venous catheters: single and multiple lumens, *Nurs Clin North Am* 28(4):911, 1993.

Purdy RE, Boucek RJ: *Handbook of cardiac drugs,* Boston, 1988, Little, Brown.

Roberts WC: The aging heart, *Mayo Clin Proc* 63:205-206, 1988.

Sokolow M, McIlroy MB: *Clinical cardiology,* ed 6, East Norwalk, Conn, 1993, Appleton & Lange.

### *Basic Life Support*

American Heart Association: *Textbook of advanced cardiac life support,* Dallas, 1993, The Association.

Baas LS: *Nursing responsibilities during CPR,* Springhouse, Pa, 1992, Springhouse.

Bonnin MJ et al: Distinct criteria for termination of resuscitation in the out-of-hospital setting, *JAMA* 270(12):1457-1462, 1993.

Guidelines for cardiopulmonary resuscitation and emergency cardiac care, *JAMA* 268(16):2184-2198, 1992.

Niemann JT: Cardiopulmonary resuscitation, *N Engl J Med* 3287(15):1075-1080, 1992.

## CHAPTER 29
## Assessment of the Cardiovascular System

Apple S, Thurkauf GE: Preparing for and understanding transesophageal echocardiography, *Crit Care Nurse* 8:29-34, 1988.

Baita KJ, Vacek JL: Transesophageal atrial pacing with stress echocardiography, *Focus Crit Care* 16(1):12-17, 1989.

Bean LC: Cardiac imaging after acute myocardial infarction: identification of patients at continual risk, *Postgrad Med* 92(8):93-100, 1992.

Beattie S, Meinhardt L: Transesophageal echocardiograph: advanced technology for the cardiac patient, *Crit Care Nurse* 12:42-48, 1992.

Beller GA: Current status of nuclear cardiology techniques, *Curr Prob Cardiol* 7:451-535, 1991.

Darovic GO: *Hemodynamic monitoring: invasive and noninvasive clinical applications,* ed 2, Philadelphia, 1993, WB Saunders.

Feinstein SB: Myocardial perfusion: contrast echocardiography perspectives, *Am J Cardiol* 69(20):36H-41H, 1992.

Gardin JM et al: Effects of aging on peak systolic left ventricular wall stress in normal subjects, *Am J Cardiol* 63:998-999, 1989.

Gore JM et al: *Handbook of hemodynamic monitoring,* Boston, 1985, Little, Brown.

Gould KL: Positron emission tomography and interventional cardiology, *Am J Cardiol* 66:51F-58F, 1990.

Jain DJ, Zaret BL: Assessment of right ventricular function: role of nuclear imaging techniques, *Cardiol Clin* 10(1):23-39, 1992.

Tilkien A, Conover M: *Understanding heart sounds and murmurs,* ed 3, Philadelphia, 1993, WB Saunders.

Veram MS: Adenosine thallium-102 myocardial perfusion scintigraphy, *Am Heart J* 122:269-278, 1991.

Veram MS: Thallium-201 single-photon emission computed tomography (SPECT) in the assessment of coronary artery disease, *Am J Cardiol* 70(14):3E-9E, 1992.

Verdeber A et al: Preparation for cardiac catheterization, *J Cardiovasc Nurs* 7(1):75-77, 1992.

CHAPTER 30

## Management of Persons With Dysrhythmias and Coronary Artery Disease

### *Cardiac Rhythms and Dysrhythmias*


Abraham T: Arrhythmogenic mechanisms, *AACN Clin Issues Crit Care Nurs* 3(1):157-165, 1992.

Berry SL, Schleicher CA: Adjusting the beat, *Am J Nurs* 94(6):28-32, 1992.

Bharati S, Lu N: The pathologic changes in the conduction system beyond the age of ninety, *Am Heart J* 124(2):486-496, 1992.

Breithardt G, Borggrefe M: Recent advances in the identification of patients at risk of ventricular tachyarrhythmias: role of ventricular late potentials, *Circulation* 75:1091-1096, 1987.

Conover MB: *Understanding electrocardiography: arrhythmias and the 12-lead ECG,* ed 6, St Louis, 1992, Mosby.

Fleg JL et al: Age-associated changes in the components of atrioventricular conduction in apparently healthy volunteers, *J Gerontol* 45(3):M95-M100, 1990.

Hopson JR, Hopson RC, Kerber RE: The role of energy and current in successful defibrillation and cardioversion: C16 arrhythmias and conduction disturbances, *Cardiol Board Rev* 6(5):31-45, 1989.

Jones J et al: The aging electrocardiogram, *Am J Emerg Med* 8(3):240-305, 1990.

Landsdowne LM: Signal-averaged electrocardiogram, *Heart Lung* 55:329-336, 1990.

Leclerq JF et al: Long-term follow-up after sustained monomorphic ventricular tachycardia: causes, pump failure, and empiric antiarrhythmic therapy that modify survival, *Am Heart J* 121:1685-1686, 1991.

Marriott HJL: *Practical electrocardiography,* ed 9, Baltimore, 1993, Williams & Wilkins.

Merva JA: Temporary pacemakers, *RN* 55(5):29-33, 1992.

Merva JA: A closer look at the heart SAECG, *RN* 56(5):50-53, 1993.

Owens M, Zetters-Jacobs L: Adenosine: the newest drug for PSVT, *RN* 55(12):38-41, 1992.

Purcell JA, Burrows SG: A pacemaker primer, *Am J Nurs* 85:553-568, 1985.

Schactman M, Grune JS: Signal-averaged electrocardiography: a new technique for determining which patients may be at risk for sudden cardiac death, *Focus Crit Care* 18(3):202-210, 1991.

Schaeffer C et al: Care for a patient with an AICD, *Nurs 92* 22(12):48-50, 1992.

Snowberger P: Second-degree AV block, *RN* 56(2):43-45, 1993.

Solomon J: Take the ECG one step further, *RN* 55(5):56-60, 1992.

Vatterott PJ et al: Signal-averaged electrocardiography: a new noninvasive test to identify patients at risk for ventricular arrhythmias, *Mayo Clin Proc* 63:931-942, 1988.

Willens HJJ, Conover MB: *The ECG in emergency decision making,* Philadelphia, 1992, WB Saunders.


### *Coronary Artery Disease*


Alpert JS: Nitrate therapy in the elderly, *Am J Cardiol* 65:23J-27J, 1990.

Aronson MK et al: Coronary heart disease, the old old and quality of life, *Quality Life* 2:197-207, 1986.

Brannon P, Tower S: Ventricular failure: new therapy using mechanical assist device, *Crit Care Nurse* 6(2):70-85, 1986.

Cantwell JD: Exercise and coronary heart disease: role in primary prevention, *Heart Lung* 13:6-13, 1984.

Chatterjee K: Ischemia, silent or manifest: does it matter? *J Am Coll Cardiol* 13:1503-1505, 1989.

Expert Panel on Detection, Evaluation and Treatment of High Blood Cholesterol in Adults: Summary of the second report of the National Cholesterol Education Program (NCEP) (Adult Treatment Panel II), *JAMA* 269(23):3015-3023, 1993.

Gottlieb SV: Ischemia as an indicator of future adverse events in patients with coronary artery disease, *J Myocard Ischemia* 1:20-28, 1989.

Hadley SA, Saarmaneh L: Lipid physiology and nutritional considerations in coronary heart disease, *Crit Care Nurse* 11(10):28-37, 1991.

Hamilton GA, Seidman RN: A comparison of the recovery period for women and men after an acute myocardial infarction, *Heart Lung* 22(4):308-315, 1993.

Johnson CL et al: Declining serum total cholesterol levels among U.S. adults, *JAMA* 269(23):3002-3008, 1993.

Kleven MR: Comparison of thrombolytic agents and mechanisms of action, efficacy, and safety, *Heart Lung* 17:750-755, 1988.

Kloner RH: Nuclear cardiology. II. Detection of coronary artery disease, *Cardiovasc Rescus Res* 8:16-39, 1989.

Lazar EJ et al: Angina pectoris and silent ischemia in the elderly: a management update, *Geriatrics* 47(7):24-36, 1988.

Misenski M: Pathophysiology of acute myocardial infarction: a rationale for thrombolytic therapy, *Heart Lung* 17:743-750, 1988.

Mueller RT et al: Painless myocardial infarction in the elderly, *Am Heart J* 110(1):202-204, 1990.

Parker JO: Nitrate tolerance, can it be prevented? *Eur Heart J* 12(suppl A):13-15, 1991.

Penckofer S, Holm K: Hopes and fears after coronary artery bypass surgery, *Prog Cardiovasc Nurs* 2(4):139-146, 1987.

Pipilis A et al: Heart rate variability in acute myocardial infarction and its association with infarct site and clinical course, *Am J Cardiol* 67:1137-1138, 1991.

Roubin GS: Intracoronary stenting, percutaneous placement of intracoronary prostheses: new solutions and new problems, *J Invasive Cardiol* 1(1):1-6, 1988.

Runions J: A program for psychological and social enhancement during rehabilitation after myocardial infarction, *Heart Lung* 14:117-125, 1985.

Sanborn TA: New interventional techniques for atherosclerotic disease, *Prim Cardiol* 15(8):21-28, 1989.

Scaner AM: Lipoprotein(a): a genetic risk factor for premature coronary heart disease, *JAMA* 267(24):3326-3329, 1992.

Sempos CT et al: Prevalence of high blood cholesterol among U.S. adults, *JAMA* 269(23):3009-3014, 1993.

Sparks KE et al: Alternatives for cardiac rehabilitation patients unable to return to a hospital-based program, *Heart Lung* 22(4):298-303, 1993.

Tyroler HA et al: Task force: environmental risk factors in coronary heart disease, *Circulation* 76(suppl I):1139-1144, 1987.

Urban P et al: Intravascular stenting for stenosis of aortocoronary venous bypass grafts, *J Am Coll Cardiol* 13:1085-1091, 1989.

Wenger NK: Special considerations in managing coronary heart disease in the elderly, *J Crit Illness* 3(10):46-57, 1988.


CHAPTER 31

## Management of Persons With Valvular and Inflammatory Heart Disease and Congestive Heart Failure

### *Inflammatory Heart Disease*


Barlow JB: Aspects of active rheumatic carditis, *Aust NZ J Med* 22:592-600, 1992.

Giundo J et al: Recurrent pericarditis: relief with colchicine, *Circulation* 82(4):1117-1120, 1990.

Grady KL, Costazo-Norden MR: Myocarditis: review of a clinical enigma, *Heart Lung* 18:347-354, 1989.

Hehrlein FW et al: The role of pericardiectomy in pericardial disorders, *Eur Heart J* 12(suppl D):7-9, 1991.

Izor-Povenmire K, House MA: Acute crack cocaine intoxication: a case study, *Focus Crit Care* 16:112-119, 1989.

Loveys BJ: Physiologic effects of cocaine with particular reference to the cardiovascular system, *Heart Lung* 16:175-182, 1987.

Luquire R, Houston S: Cardiomyopathy: how to buy time, *RN* 56(5):29-33, 1993.

Majid AA, Amar A: Diagnosis and management of purulent pericarditis, *J Thorac Cardiovasc Surg* 102:413-417, 1991.

Marrie TJ: Infective endocarditis: a serious and changing disease, *Crit Care Nurs* 7(2):31-46, 1987.

Maze SS, Adolph RJ: Myocarditis: unresolved issues in diagnosis and treatment, *Clin Cardiol* 13:69-79, 1990.

McAllister RG: Age-related changes in drug handling in men, *Am Cardiol* 57:59C-62C, 1986.


### *Valvular Heart Disease*


Constancia PE: The Ross procedure: aortic valve replacement using autologous pulmonary valve, *Crit Care Nurs Clin North Am* 3(4):717-721, 1991.

Cosgrove D et al: Results of mitral valve reconstruction, *Circulation* 74(suppl I):182-187, 1986.

Deans K, Hartshorn J: Use of antithrombotic agents in valvular heart disease, *J Cardiovasc Nurs* 1(3):65-69, 1987.

Hioki M et al: Successful combined operation for mitral stenosis and atrial fibrillation, *Ann Thorac Surg* 55:776-778, 1993.

Kay JH: Surgical treatment of tricuspid regurgitation, *Classics Thorac Surg* 53:1132-1133, 1993.

Kretten C, Bass L: Valvular heart disease, surgery, and postop care, *RN* 50(12):38-43, 1987.

Loop FE et al: Mitral valve repair for mitral insufficiency, *Eur Heart J* 12(suppl B):30-33, 1991.

Nair CK: Ten years experience with mitral valve replacement in the elderly, *Am Heart J* 124:154-159, 1992.

Ohler L et al: Aortic valvuloplasty: medical and critical care nursing perspectives, *Focus Crit Care* 16(4):275-287, 1989.

Olsson M et al: Aortic valve replacement in octogenarians with aortic stenosis: a case controlled study, *J Am Coll Cardiol* 20(7):1512-1516, 1992.

Russell A, Blake A: Aortic valvuloplasty: potential nursing diagnoses, *DCCN* 8(2):72-82, 1989.

Tyers GRO: Mitral valve replacement: what should be the standard technique? *Ann Thorac Surg* 49:861-862, 1990.

Whitman G: Prosthetic cardiac valves, *Prog Cardiovasc Nurs* 2:116-123, 1987.


### *Cardiac Surgery*


Anderson GM et al: Use of coronary artery bypass surgery in the United States and Canada, *JAMA* 269(13):1661-1666, 1993.

Ball GB, Grap MJ: Postoperative GI symptoms in cardiac surgery patients, *Crit Care Nurse* 12(1):56-62, 1992.

Beattie S: CABG surgery: the second time around, *Am J Nurs* 93(8):42-45, 1993.

Boldt J et al: The effects of preoperative aspirin therapy on platelet function in cardiac surgery, *Eur J Cardiothorac Surg* 6:598-602, 1992.

Borders CR: When the bypass patient returns home: problems your bypass patients face after discharge, *Patient Care* 19(13):65-76, 1986.

Copeland J et al: Selection of patients for cardiac transplantation, *Circulation* 75:2-9, 1987.

Cox JL: Evolving applications of the maze procedure for atrial fibrillation, *Ann Thorac Surg* 55:578-580, 1993.

Duncan C et al: Effect of chest tube management on drainage after cardiac surgery, *Heart Lung* 16:1-9, 1987.

Howie JN: Hypothermia and rewarming after cardiac surgery, *Focus Crit Care* 18(5):414-418, 1991.

Jeffrey D et al: Results of coronary bypass surgery in elderly women, *Ann Thorac Surg* 42:550-553, 1986.

King KB et al: Coronary artery bypass graft surgery in older women and men, *Am J Crit Care* 1(2):28-35, 1992.

Ruzevich SA, Swartz MT, Pennington DG: Nursing care of the patient with a pneumatic ventricular assist device, *Heart Lung* 17:399-405, 1988.

Sakallares BR: Advances and controversies: laser therapy for cardiovascular disease, *Heart Lung* 16:464-473, 1987.

Shinnick MA: ARDS in the postoperative cardiac surgery patient: a case study, *Crit Care Nurs* 12(4):12-17, 1992.

Stradtman JC, Ballenger MJ: Nursing implications in sternal and mediastinal infection after open heart surgery, *Focus Crit Care* 16(3):178-183, 1989.

Suszbach LM, Landsdowne LM: Temporary atrial pacing after cardiac surgery, *Focus Crit Care* 17(4):308-312, 1990.


## CHAPTER 32
## Management of Persons With Vascular Problems

### *General*


Blank CA, Irwin GH: Peripheral vascular disorders, *Nurs Clin North Am* 25(4):777-794, 1990.

Bright LD, Georgi S: Peripheral vascular disease—is it arterial or venous? *Am J Nurs* 92:34-47, 1992.

Dosick SM, Hobson RW, Krosnick A: Management of ulcers on the ischemic limb, *Curative Technol* 2:1-14, 1991.

Eliopoulos C: PVD: protecting patients from complications, *Nurs 91* 21:32-34, 1991.

Ernst CB, Stanley JC: *Current therapy in vascular surgery,* ed 2, Philadelphia, 1991, BC Decker.

Fahey VA: *Vascular nursing,* Philadelphia, 1988, WB Saunders.

Hiatt WR et al: Benefit of exercise conditioning for patients with peripheral arterial disease, *Circulation* 81(2), 1990.

LaQuaglia JD, Appleton DL: Vascular disease and postoperative nursing management, *Crit Care Nurse* 5:34-42, 1985.

Lundgren F et al: Intermittent claudication—surgical reconstruction or physical training? A prospective randomized trial of treatment efficacy, *Ann Surg* 209:346-355, 1989.

Machleder HI: *Vascular disorders of the upper extremity,* ed 3, Mount Kisco, NY, 1989, Futura.

Moore WS: *Vascular surgery: a comprehensive review,* ed 3, Philadelphia, 1991, WB Saunders.

Rutherford RB: *Vascular surgery,* ed 3, Philadelphia, 1989, WB Saunders.

Siedlecki B: Peripheral vascular disease, *Can Nurse* 88:26-28, 1992.

Williams L et al: Vascular rehabilitation: benefits of a structured exercise/risk factor modification program, *J Vasc Surg* 14(3):320-326, 1991.

Young JR et al: *Peripheral vascular diseases,* St Louis, 1991, Mosby.


### *Arterial Diseases (General)*


Anderson K: Thrombolytic therapy for treatment of acute peripheral arterial occlusion, *J Vasc Nurs* 10(3):20-24, 1992.

Bergan J, Yao S: *Aortic surgery,* Philadelphia, 1989, WB Saunders.

Bergan J, Yao S: *Techniques in arterial surgery,* Philadelphia, 1990, WB Saunders.

Emma LA: Chronic arterial occlusive disease, *J Cardiovasc Nurs* 7:14-24, 1992.

Fellows E, Jocz AM: Getting the upper hand on lower extremity arterial disease, *Nurs 91* 21:34-42, 1991.

Harris KA: Graft infections, *J Vasc Nurs* 10(1):13-17, 1992.

Payne JS: Alternative for revascularization: peripheral atherectomy devices, *J Vasc Nurs* 10(3):2-8, 1992.

Robinson LC: Atherosclerotic occlusive disease of the aorta, *J Vasc Nurs* 10(4):17-23, 1992.

Rudolphi D: Limb loss in the elderly peripheral vascular disease patient, *J Vasc Nurs* 10(3):8-13, 1992.

Widlus DM, Osteman FA: Evaluation and percutaneous management of atherosclerotic peripheral vascular disease, *JAMA* 261:3148-3154, 1989.


### *Raynaud's Disease*


Adee AC: Managing Raynaud's phenomenon: a practical approach, *Am Fam Physician* 47:823-829, 1993.

Coffman JD: *Raynaud's phenomenon,* New York, 1989, Oxford University.

Davis E: The diagnostic puzzle and management challenge of Raynaud's syndrome, *Nurse Pract* 18:18-25, 1993.

### Aneurysms

Lovell MB, Harris KA: Abdominal aortic aneurysms, *J Vasc Nurs* 9:2-6, 1991.

Moore K, Moore S: Abdominal aortic aneurysm, *Top Emerg Med* 12(2):61-65, 1990.

### Hypertension

Aristizabal D, Frohlich ED: Hypertension due to renal arterial disease, *Heart Dis Stroke* 1(4):227-234, 1992.

Hart BP: Vascular consequences of smoking and benefits of smoking cessation, *J Vasc Nurs* 11:48-51, 1993.

Johannsen JM: Update: guidelines for treating hypertension, *Am J Nurs* 93:42-49, 1993.

Trottier DI, Kochar MS: Hypertension and high cholesterol: a dangerous synergy, *Am J Nurs* 92:40-43, 1992.

### Deep Vein Thrombosis

Burns D: Review of thrombolytic use in acute myocardial infarction, pulmonary embolism, and cerebral thrombosis, *Crit Care Nurs Q* 15(4):1-12, 1993.

Comerota AJ: *Thrombolytic therapy,* Orlando, Fla, 1988, Grune & Stratton.

Herzog J: Deep vein thrombosis in the rehabilitation client: diagnostic tools, prevention, and treatment modalities, *Rehabil Nurs* 18:8-11, 1993.

Kuc JA: When heparin causes clots, *RN* 56:34-38, 1993.

Mills D: When blood won't clot, *RN* 55:28-32, 1992.

Nunnelee JD, Kurgan A: Interruption of the inferior vena cava for venous thromboembolic disease, *J Vasc Nurs* 11(3):80-82, 1993.

### Venous Diseases (General)

Bergan JJ, Yao JST: *Venous disorders,* Philadelphia, 1991, WB Saunders.

Lovell MB et al: The management of chronic venous disease, *J Vasc Nurs* 11(2):43-47, 1993.

Mignor D: The unna boot makes a comeback, *Home Healthcare Nurse* 8(5):22-25, 1990.

Notowitz LB: Normal venous anatomy and physiology of the lower extremity, *J Vasc Nurs* 11(2):39-42, 1993.

### Leg Ulcers

Ciocon JO et al: Leg edema: clinical clues to the differential diagnosis, *Geriatrics* 48(5):34-45, 1993.

Krasner D: The 12 commandments of wound care, *Nurs 92* 22:34-41, 1992.

Menzoian JO, Doyle JE: Venous insufficiency of the leg, *Hosp Pract* 30:109-116, 1989.

Mulder G, Reis T: Venous ulcers: pathophysiology and medical therapy, *Am Fam Practitioner* 42(5):1323-1330, 1988.


## SECTION TWO Hematologic System

## CHAPTER 33
## Assessment of the Hematologic System


### General

American Cancer Society: *Cancer facts and figures—1994,* Atlanta, 1994, The Society.

Baird SB: *Decision making in oncology nursing,* Philadelphia, 1988, BC Decker.

Brain MC, Carbonne PP: *Current therapy in hematology-oncology,* ed 4, St Louis, 1991, Mosby.

Carnevali D, Reiner A: *The cancer experience: nursing diagnosis and management,* Philadelphia, 1990, JB Lippincott.

Daeffler RJ, Petrosino B: *Manual of oncology nursing practice,* Rockville, Md, 1990, Aspen.

Dalton W, Miller T: Multidrug resistance: principles and practice of oncology, *Updates* 5(7):1-13, 1991.

DeVita V, Hellman S, Rosenberg S: *Cancer principles and practice of oncology,* ed 3, Philadelphia, 1989, JB Lippincott.

Dodd MJ: *Managing side effects of chemotherapy and radiation therapy: a guide for patients and nurses,* East Norwalk, Conn, 1987, Appleton & Lange.

Dodd MJ et al: Self-care for patients experiencing cancer chemotherapy side effects: a concern for home nurses, *Home Healthcare Nurse* 9(6):21-26, 1991.

Goodman M: Managing the side effects of chemotherapy, *Semin Oncol Nurs* 5(2):29-52, 1989.

Groenwald SL et al: *Cancer nursing: principles and practice,* Boston, 1990, Jones & Bartlett.

Harmening DM: *Clinical hematology and fundamentals of hemostasis,* Philadelphia, 1992, FA Davis.

Morstyn G, Burgess AW: Hemopoietic growth factors: a review, *Cancer Res* 48:5624-5637, 1988.

Oncology Nursing Society: *Cancer chemotherapy guidelines,* Modules I-V, Pittsburgh, 1988, The Society.

Ratnoff OD, Forbes CD: *Disorders of hemostasis,* ed 2, Philadelphia, 1991, WB Saunders.

Rostad ME: Management of myelosuppression in the patient with cancer, *Oncol Nurs Forum* 17(suppl 1):4-8, 1990.

Wintrobe MM et al: *Clinical hematology,* ed 7, Philadelphia, 1989, Lea & Febiger.

Wyngaarden JB, Smith LH: *Cecil textbook of medicine,* ed 19, Philadelphia, 1992, WB Saunders.

Yasko J: *Guidelines for cancer care: symptom management,* Reston, Va, 1983, Reston.

Yasko J, Dudjak LA: *Biologic response modifier therapy: symptom management,* San Diego, 1990, Park Row.


## CHAPTER 34
## Management of Persons With Hematologic Problems


### Disorders of Red Blood Cells

Baum K et al: The painful crisis of homozygous sickle cell disease, *Arch Intern Med* 147:1231-1234, 1987.

France-Dawson M: Sickle cell disease: implications for nursing care, *J Adv Nurs* 11(6):729-737, 1986.

Froberg J: The anemias: causes and courses of action, *RN* 52(1):24-29, 1989.

Hickstadt A: Hemophilia: the person, family and nurse, *Rehabil Nurs* 11(3):225-228, 1986.

London F: Nursing diagnoses and caring for patients with sickle cell disease, *Adv Clin Care* 5(5):12-16, 1990.

Lusher J et al: Recombinant factor VIII for the treatment of previously untreated patients with hemophilia A, *N Engl J Med* 328(7):453-459, 1993.

Martinelli A: Sickle cell disease: etiology, symptoms, patient care, *AORN J* 53:716-724, 1991.

Piomelli S: Sickle cell diseases in the 1990s: the need for active and preventative intervention, *Semin Hematol* 28(3):227-232, 1991.

Rozzell MS, Hijazi M, Pack B: The painful episode in sickle cell disease, *Nurs Clin North Am* 18(1):185-199, 1983.

Trotta P: Nursing assessment of symptoms associated with hyperviscosity syndrome, *Oncol Nurs Forum* 14(1):21-27, 1987.

William I, Earles AN, Pack B: Psychological considerations in sickle cell disease, *Nurs Clin North Am* 18(1):215-229, 1983.

### Disorders of Coagulation

Brannan D, Guthrie T: Idiopathic thrombocytopenia purpura in adults, *South Med J* 81(1):75-80, 1988.

### Disorders of White Blood Cells

Baker LS: *You and leukemia: a day at a time,* Philadelphia, 1988, WB Saunders.

Brandt BA: A nursing protocol for the client with neutropenia, *Oncol Nurs Forum* 17(suppl 1):9-15, 1990.

Johnson J: Prevention and management of neutropenia in the cancer patient, *Oncol Nurs Forum* 17(suppl 1):3-6, 1990.

Lakhani AK: Current management of acute leukemias, *Nurs 88 (Lond)* 3:755-758, 1988.

Mauer AM: Acute lymphoblastic leukemia in a young adult, *Hosp Pract* 22(9):145-156, 1987.

Simonson GM: Caring for patients with acute myelocytic leukemia, *Am J Nurs* 88:304-309, 1988.

### Disorders of the Lymph System

Armitage JO: Treatment of non-Hodgkin's lymphoma, *N Engl J Med* 328(14):1023-1030, 1993.

Canellos G et al: Chemotherapy of advanced Hodgkin's disease with MOPP, ABVD, or MOPP alternating with ABVD, *N Engl J Med* 327(21):1478-1484, 1992.

# SECTION THREE Respiratory System

## CHAPTER 35
## Assessment of the Respiratory System

Ahrens T: The cutting edge in pulmonary critical care, *Crit Care Nurse* 13(6):45-55, 1993.

American Thoracic Society: Recommended respiratory disease questionnaire for use with adults and children in epidemiological research, *Am Rev Respir Dis* 118(1):7-53, 1978.

American Thoracic Society: Lung function testing: selection of reference values and interpretive strategies, *Am Rev Respir Dis* 144(5):1202-1218, 1991.

Bates B: *A guide to physical examination,* ed 5, Philadelphia, 1991, JB Lippincott.

Bordow R, Moser K: *Manual of clinical problems in pulmonary medicine,* ed 2, Boston, 1988, Little, Brown.

Borg G: Physical performance and perceived exertion, *Studia Psychol Paedagog* 11:1-64, 1962.

Borg G: Psychophysical bases of perceived exertion, *Med Sci Sports Exerc* 14:377-381, 1982.

Bridges EJ, Woods SL: Pulmonary artery pressure measurement: state of the art, *Heart Lung* 22:99-111, 1993.

Brown M: Selecting an instrument to measure dyspnea, *Oncol Nurs Forum* 12(3):98-100, 1985.

Brucia J: Self perception of premonitory cues signaling COPD onset, unpublished master's thesis, Cleveland, 1982, Case-Western Reserve University.

Cohen S: Pulmonary function tests in patient care: programmed instruction, *Am J Nurs* 80:1135-1161, 1980.

De Troyer A, Estenne M: Functional anatomy of the respiratory muscles, *Clin Chest Med* 9(2):175-193, 1988.

Edlund B, Wheeler E: Adaptation to breathlessness, *Top Clin Nurs* 2(3):11-25, 1980.

Ehrhardt BS, Graham M: Pulse oximetry: an easy way to check oxygen saturation, *Nurs 90* 20(3):50-54, 1990.

Finesilver C: Perfecting the art of respiratory assessment, *RN* 55(2):22-30, 1992.

Forouzesh M, Price JH, Taylor C: Pulmonary disease, *Nurs Care* 15:19-22, 1992.

Fuchs-Carroll P: Cyanosis: the sign you can't count on, *Nurs 88* 18(3):50, 1988.

Gift AG: Dyspnea, *Nurs Clin North Am* 25:955-965, 1990.

Higgins LA: Questioning capnography, *Am J Nurs* 93(4):24, 1993.

Howder C: *Respiratory care: know the facts,* Philadelphia, 1989, JB Lippincott.

Janson-Bjerklie S, Carrieri GK, Hudes M: The sensations of pulmonary dyspnea, *Nurs Res* 35(3):154-159, 1986.

Kersten LD: *Comprehensive respiratory therapy,* Philadelphia, 1989, WB Saunders.

Killian KJ: The objective measurement of breathlessness, *Chest* 88(2):84S-90S, 1985.

Killian KJ, Jones NJ: Respiratory muscles and dyspnea, *Clin Chest Med* 9(2):237-248, 1988.

Levitzsky MG: *Pulmonary physiology,* ed 2, New York, 1986, McGraw-Hill.

Mahler DA et al: The measurement of dyspnea: contents, interobserver agreement, and physiologic correlates of two new clinical indexes, *Chest* 85(6):751-757, 1984.

McCaffrey TV, Kern EB: Clinical evaluation for nasal obstruction: a study of 1000 patients, *Arch Otolaryngol* 105:542-545, 1979.

Mergaert S: S.T.O.P. and assess chest tubes the easy way, *Nurs 94* 25(2):52-53, 1994.

Murray J: *The normal lung: the basis for diagnosis and treatment of pulmonary disease,* ed 2, Philadelphia, 1986, WB Saunders.

Nicholson C, Coleman CA, Mack M: Are you ready for video thoracoscopy? *Am J Nurs* 93(3):54-57, 1993.

Pagana K, Pagana T: *Diagnostic testing and nursing implications: a case study approach,* ed 4, St Louis, 1994, Mosby.

Reischman R: Review of ventilation and perfusion physiology, *Crit Care Nurse* 8(7):24-28, 1988.

Reischman R: Impaired gas exchange related to intrapulmonary shunting, *Crit Care Nurse* 8(8):35-49, 1988.

Roach L: Skin changes: the subtle and the obvious. In *Assessing vital functions accurately,* Horsham, Pa, 1978, Intermed Communications.

Sonnesso G: Are you ready to use pulse oximetry? *Nurs 91* 21(8):60-64, 1991.

Stevens S, Becker K: How to perform picture-perfect respiratory assessment, *Nurs 88* 18(1):57-63, 1988.

Stevens SA, Becher KL: Respiratory assessment, *Nurs 88* 18(1):57-63, 1988.

Stiesmeyer JK: A four-step approach to pulmonary assessment, *Am J Nurs* 93(8):22-31, 1993.

Szaflarski NL, Cohen NH: Use of capnography in critically ill adults, *Heart Lung* 20(4):363-372, 1991.

Tampinco-Golos I: Endoscopic thoracotomy, *AORN J* 55:1167-1180, 1992.

Tasota FJ, Wesmiller SW: Assessing A.B.G.s—maintaining the delicate balance, *Nurs 94* 25:34-44, 1994.

Thompson J, Bowers A: *Clinical manual of health assessment,* ed 3, St Louis, 1992, Mosby.

West J: *Respiratory physiology—the essentials,* ed 4, Baltimore, 1990, Williams & Wilkins.

Westia B: Assessment under pressure: when your patient says "I can't breathe," *Nurs 84* 14(5):34-40, 1984.

Wilkens R, Sheldon R, Krider S: *Clinical assessment in respiratory care,* St Louis, 1985, Mosby.

Witkowski A: *Pulmonary assessment: a clinical guide,* Philadelphia, 1985, JB Lippincott.

Witta KM: When gauging respiratory status is critical, *RN* 56(11):40-45, 1993.

Zagelbaum G, Pare J: *Manual of acute respiratory care,* Boston, 1983, Little, Brown.

## CHAPTER 36
## Management of Persons With Problems of the Upper Airway

### General

DeWeese DD, Saunders WH: *Otolaryngology, head and neck surgery,* ed 7, St Louis, 1987, Mosby.

Glass C et al: Nurses' ability to achieve hyperinflation and hyperoxygenation with a manual resuscitation bag during endotracheal suctioning, *Heart Lung* 22:158-165, 1993.

Goodman MS: Head and neck malignancies. In Groenwald SL, editor: *Cancer nursing: principles and practice,* Boston, 1987, Jones & Bartlett.

Groothius JR: Viral respiratory infections. In Rakel RE: *Conn's current therapy 1993,* Philadelphia, 1993, WB Saunders.

Haffner JE, Sah SA: The technique of weaning from tracheostomy, *J Crit Illness* 2(6):74-78, 1987.

Hassard AD, Holness RO: The "crossbow" incision and nasal flap: its blood supply on clinical application, *Head Neck Surg* 7:135-138, 1984.

Hirsch JE: Ear, nose and throat. In Thompson JM et al: *Mosby's manual of clinical nursing,* ed 2, St Louis, 1989, Mosby.

Holt JE: Orbital blowout fracture, *Ear Nose Throat J* 62:346-351, 1983.

Mathews PJ, Mathews LM, Mitchell RR: Artificial airways resuscitation guidelines you can follow, *Nurs 92* 22(1):53-59, 1992.

Mulgrew B, Dropkin ML: Coping with craniofacial resection: a case study, *The Journal* (official publication of SOHN) 9(3):8-27, 1991.

Pichichero ME: Streptococcal pharyngitis. In Rakel RE, editor: *Conn's current therapy 1993,* Philadelphia, 1993, WB Saunders.

Scher RL, Richtsmeier SJ: Otolaryngology: head and neck surgery. In Sabiston DC, Lyerly KH, editors: *Sabiston essentials of surgery,* ed 2, Philadelphia, 1994, WB Saunders.

Sigler BA, Schuring LT: *Ear, nose and throat disorders,* St Louis, 1993, Mosby.

Smalley PJ: Lasers in otolaryngology, *Nurs Clin North Am* 25:645-656, 1990.

### *Sinus Conditions*

Leach JL, Schaeffer S: Sinusitis. In Rakel RE, editor: *Conn's current therapy 1993,* Philadelphia, 1993, WB Saunders.

Miller WE: The role of the outpatient nurse in endoscopic sinus surgery, *ORL—Head Neck Nurs* 10(3):20-24, 1992.

Newman LJ et al: Chronic sinusitis: relationship of computed tomographic findings to allergy, asthma, and eosinophilia, *JAMA* 271:363-367, 1994.

Williams JW, Simel DL: Does this patient have sinusitis? Diagnosing acute sinusitis by history and physical examination, *JAMA* 270:1242-1246, 1993.

Yonkers AJ: Sinusitis—inspecting the causes and treatment, *Ear, Nose, Throat J* 71:258-262, 1991.

### *Allergies*

Gibbs L: Assessment and management of the allergic patient, *ORL—Head Neck Nurs* 10(3):10-16, 1992.

Howard BA: Guiding allergy sufferers through the medication maze, *RN* 57(4):26-31, 1994.

Jaroff L: Allergies—nothing to sneeze at, *Time,* June 22, 1992, pp 54-61.

McConnell EA: How to instill nose drops, *Nurs 93* 24(7):18, 1993.

Nurse's guide to O.T.C. allergy products, *Nurs 93* 24(9):67-70, 1993.

Patten BC, Holt JA: When your patient is allergic, *Am J Nurs* 92(9):58-61, 1992.

Pope AM: Indoor allergens—assessing and controlling adverse health effects, *JAMA* 269:2721, 1993.

Rodman MJ: OTC interactions: cough, cold, and allergy preparations, *RN* 56(2):38-42, 1993.

Simons FE, Simons KJ: The pharmacology and use of $H_1$-receptor-antagonist drugs, *N Engl J Med* 330:1663-1670, 1994.

Tips for taking O.T.C. allergy products (patient teaching aid), *Nurs 93* 24(9):71-72, 1993.

### *Head and Neck Cancer*

Campos AC et al: Home enteral nutrition via gastrostomy in advanced head and neck cancer patients, *Head Neck* 12:137-142, 1990.

Dropkin MJ: Coping with disfigurement and dysfunction after head and neck cancer surgery: a conceptual framework, *Semin Oncol Nurs* 5:213-219, 1989.

Droughton ML, Krech RL: Head and neck cancer resection and reconstruction: from past to present, *Today's OR Nurs* 14(9):25-34, 1992.

Farrar WB et al: Radical neck dissection: is it enough? *Am J Surg* 156:173-176, 1988.

Grant M et al: Nutritional management in the head and neck cancer patient, *Semin Oncol Nurs* 5:195-204, 1989.

Harris LL, Smith S: Chemotherapy in head and neck cancer, *Semin Oncol Nurs* 5:174-181, 1989.

Johns ME, Niparko JK: Otolaryngology—head and neck surgery, *JAMA* 270:243-245, 1993.

Lavertu P, Droughton ML: Postoperative management following head and neck surgery. In Sviak E, Higgins T, Scivers A, editors: *The high risk patient: management of the critically ill,* Philadelphia, Williams & Wilkins (in press).

Logemann JA: Swallowing and communication rehabilitation, *Semin Oncol Nurs* 5:205-212, 1989.

Martin LK: Management of the altered airway in the head and neck cancer patient, *Semin Oncol Nurs* 5:182-190, 1989.

Mathieson CM et al: Psychosocial adjustment after laryngectomy: a review of the literature, *J Otolaryngol* 19:331-336, 1990.

Merlano M et al: Treatment of advanced squamous-cell carcinoma of the head and neck with alternating chemotherapy and radiotherapy, *N Engl J Med* 327:1115-1121, 1992.

Rook JL, Rook M: Head and neck cancer, *J Postanesth Nurs* 4:363-372, 1989.

Sawyer DL, Bruya MA: Care of the patient having radical neck surgery or permanent laryngostomy: a nursing diagnostic approach, *Focus Crit Care* 17:166-173, 1990.

Schleper JR: Prevention, detection, and diagnosis of head and neck cancers, *Semin Oncol Nurs* 5:139-149, 1989.

Schwartz SS, Yuska CM: Common patient care issues following surgery for head and neck cancer, *Semin Oncol Nurs* 5:191-194, 1989.

Sigler BA: Nursing care of patients with laryngeal carcinoma, *Semin Oncol Nurs* 5:160-165, 1989.

Strohl RA: Radiation therapy for head and neck cancers, *Semin Oncol Nurs* 5:166-173, 1989.

Trudeau MD, Schuller DE: Mechanisms for vocal communication following total laryngectomy, *Cancer Treatment Res* 52:117-131, 1990.

Williams L, Stieg F: Neck masses, *Plast Surg Nurs* 10:131-135, 1990.

## CHAPTER 37
## Management of Persons With Problems of the Lower Airway

### *General*

Ahrens T: The cutting edge in pulmonary critical care, *Crit Care Nurse* 13(6S):4-5, 1993.

American Thoracic Society: Environmental controls and lung disease, *Am Rev Respir Dis* 142:915-938, 1990.

Attfield MD, Althouse RB: Surveillance data on U.S. coal miners' pneumoconiosis, 1970-1986, *Am J Public Health* 82:971-977, 1992.

Attfield MD, Castellan RM: Epidemiological data on U.S. coal miners' pneumoconiosis, 1960-1988, *Am J Public Health* 82:964-970, 1992.

Baier H: Primary lung abscess. In Rakel RE, editor: *Conn's current therapy 1993,* Philadelphia, 1993, WB Saunders.

Bates D: *Respiratory function in disease,* ed 3, Philadelphia, 1989, WB Saunders.

Belcaster A, Middleton WS: Responding to pulmonary hemorrhage: how to prevent airway obstruction, *Nurs 93* 24(11):33, 1993.

Brown WD, Campbell GD: Histoplasmosis. In Rakel RE, editor: *Conn's current therapy 1993,* Philadelphia, 1993, WB Saunders.

Centers for Disease Control: Coccidioidomycosis—United States, 1991-1992, *MMWR* 42(2):21-25, 1993.

Centers for Disease Control: Unintentional carbon monoxide poisoning following a winter storm—Washington, January 1993, *MMWR* 42(6):109-111, 1993.

Cherniak R: *Current therapy of respiratory disease—2,* Toronto, 1986, BC Decker.

Ebersole P, Hess P: *Toward healthy aging,* ed 4, St Louis, 1994, Mosby.

Forouzesh M, Price JH, Taylor C: Pulmonary disease, *Nurs Care* 15:19-22, 1992.

Fraser RG et al: *Diagnosis of disease of the chest,* vol 3, ed 3, Philadelphia, 1990, WB Saunders.

George RB: Blastomycosis. In Rakel RE, editor: *Conn's current therapy 1993,* Philadelphia, 1993, WB Saunders.

Hill RC: Bronchiectasis. In Sabiston DC, Lyerly HK, editors: *Sabiston essentials of surgery,* ed 2, Philadelphia, 1994, WB Saunders.

Hill RC: The pleura and empyema. In Sabiston DC, Lyerly HK, editors: *Sabiston essentials of surgery,* ed 2, Philadelphia, 1994, WB Saunders.

Kataria YP, Halter JF: Sarcoidosis. In Rakel RE, editor: *Conn's current therapy 1993,* Philadelphia, 1993, WB Saunders.

Kerston LD: *Comprehensive respiratory nursing: a decision making approach,* Philadelphia, 1989, WB Saunders.

Larsen EB, Ramsey PG, editors: *Medical therapeutics,* ed 2, Philadelphia, 1992, WB Saunders.

Larsen RA: Coccidioidomycosis. In Rakel RE, editor: *Conn's current therapy 1993,* Philadelphia, 1993, WB Saunders.

Lederberg J, Shape RE, Oaks SC Jr: *Emerging infections: microbial threats to health in the United States,* Washington, DC, 1992, National Academy Press.

Rich EA, Ellner JJ: Acute bronchitis. In Rakel RE, editor: *Conn's current therapy 1993,* Philadelphia, 1993, WB Saunders.

Roberts SL: High-permeability pulmonary edema: nursing assessment, diagnosis and interventions, *Heart Lung* 19:287-299, 1990.

Schwartz LB, Sabiston DC: Pulmonary embolism. In Sabiston DC, Lyerly HK, editors: *Sabiston essentials of surgery,* ed 2, Philadelphia, 1994, WB Saunders.

Struve SW, Dean NC: Acute respiratory failure. In Rakel RE, editor: *Conn's current therapy 1991,* Philadelphia, 1991, WB Saunders.

Traver G, Mitchell JT, Flodquist-Prestley G: *Respiratory care: a clinical approach,* Gaithersburg, Md, 1991, Aspen.

US Department of Health and Human Services, Public Health Service: *Healthy people 2000: national health promotion and disease prevention objectives,* Washington, DC, 1990, US Government Printing Office.

Weinberger SE: Recent advances in pulmonary medicine. Part 1, *N Engl J Med* 328:1389-1397, 1993.

Weinberger SE: Recent advances in pulmonary medicine. Part 2, *N Engl J Med* 328:1462-1470, 1993.

West JB: *Pulmonary pathophysiology—the essentials,* ed 4, Baltimore, 1991, Williams & Wilkins.

Wright SA, Bieluch VM: Selected nosocomial viral infections, *Heart Lung* 22:183-187, 1993.

Yeaw EMJ: Good lung down? *Am J Nurs* 92(3):27-32, 1992.


### *Chest Trauma*


Fink MP: Trauma. In Sabiston DC, Lyerly LK, editors: *Sabiston essentials of surgery,* ed 2, Philadelphia, 1994, WB Saunders.

Hefts D: Chest trauma, *RN* 54(5):28-32, 1991.

Jordan K: Chest trauma, *Nurs 90* 21(9):34-42, 1990.

Rich J: Penetrating chest injury: how to stabilize the patient and prevent pulmonary collapse, *Nurs 93* 24(9):33, 1993.


### *Pulmonary Embolism*


Burns D: Review of thrombolytic use in acute myocardial infarction, pulmonary embolism, and cerebral thrombosis, *Crit Care Nurs Q* 15(4):1-12, 1993.

Goldhaber SZ, Morpurgo M: Diagnosis, treatment and prevention of pulmonary embolism, *JAMA* 268:1727-1733, 1992.

Goldhaber SZ et al: Quantitative plasma D-dimer levels among patients undergoing pulmonary angiography for suspected pulmonary embolism, *JAMA* 270:2819-2822, 1993.

Quinn DA et al: A prospective investigation of pulmonary embolism in women and men, *JAMA* 268:1689-1696, 1992.


### *Adult Respiratory Distress Syndrome*


Bone RC: The ARDS lung: new insights from computed tomography, *JAMA* 269:2134-2135, 1993.

Gattinoni L et al: Regional effects and mechanism of positive end-expiratory pressure in early adult respiratory distress syndrome, *JAMA* 269:2122-2127, 1993.

Gattinoni L et al: Lung structure and function in different stages of severe adult respiratory distress syndrome, *JAMA* 271:1772-1779, 1994.

Hunter FC, Mitchell S: Managing ARDS, *RN* 56(7):53-57, 1993.

Meyer KC, McManus DJ, Maki DG: Overwhelming pulmonary blastomycosis associated with adult respiratory distress syndrome, *N Engl J Med* 329:1231-1236, 1993.

Roberts SL: High-permeability pulmonary edema: nursing assessment, diagnosis and interventions, *Heart Lung* 19(3):287-299, 1990.


### *Lung Cancer*


American Cancer Society: *Cancer facts and figures—1994,* Atlanta, 1994, The Association.

Carroll PL: What's new in chest-tube management, *RN* 54(5):34-40, 1991.

Carroll P: Nursing the thoracotomy patient, *RN* 55(6):34-42, 1992.

D'Amico TA, Sabiston DC: Carcinoma of the lung. In Sabiston DC, Lyerly LK, editors: *Sabiston essentials of surgery,* ed 2, Philadelphia, 1994, WB Saunders.

Fontham ETH et al: Environmental tobacco smoke and lung cancer in nonsmoking women, *JAMA* 271:1752-1759, 1994.

Gift AG, Bolgiano CS, Cunningham J: Sensations during chest tube removal, *Heart Lung* 20:131-137, 1991.

Harvey JC, Beattie EJ: Lung cancer, *Clin Symp* 45(3):1993.

Ihde DC: Chemotherapy of lung cancer, *N Engl J Med* 327:1434-1441, 1992.

Lee JS, Hong WK: Prognostic factors in lung cancer, *N Engl J Med* 327:47-48, 1992.

Lin AY, Ihde DC: Recent developments in the treatment of lung cancer, *JAMA* 267:1661-1664, 1992.

Saturated fat and lung cancer, *Harvard Health Lett* 19(3):8, 1994.

Trichopoulos D et al: Active and passive smoking and pathological indicators of lung cancer in an autopsy study, *JAMA* 268:1697-1701, 1992.


### *Oxygen Transport and Hypoxia*


Carpenter KD: Oxygen transport in the blood, *Crit Care Nurs* 11(9):20-31, 1991.

Epstein CD, Henning RJ: Oxygen transport in the identification and treatment of tissue hypoxia, *Heart Lung* 22:328-348, 1993.

Openbrier DR, Fuoss C, Mall CC: What patients on home oxygen therapy want to know, *Am J Nurs* 88(2):198-202, 1988.

Ronco JJ et al: Identification of the critical oxygen delivery for anaerobic metabolism in critically ill septic and nonseptic humans, *JAMA* 270:1724-1730, 1993.

Sonnesso G: Are you ready to use pulse oximetry? *Nurs 91* 21(8):60-64, 1991.


### *Pneumonia and Influenza*


Anastasi JK: Why give corticosteroids for Pneumocystis carinii pneumonia? *Am J Nurs* 92(2):30, 1992.

Butler JC et al: Pneumococcal polysaccharide vaccine efficacy: an evaluation of current recommendations, *JAMA* 270:1826-1831, 1993.

Caruthers DD: Infectious pneumonia in the elderly, *Am J Nurs* 90(2):56-60, 1990.

Centers for Disease Control: Recommendations for prophylaxis against *Pneumocystis carinii* pneumonia for adults and adolescents infected with human immunodeficiency virus, *MMWR* 41(RR-4):1-11, 1992.

Centers for Disease Control: Update: influenza activity—United States and worldwide, 1993, *MMWR* 42(38):752-755, 1993.

Centers for Disease Control: Final results: Medicare influenza vaccine demonstration—selected states, 1988-1992, *MMWR* 42(31):601-604, 1993.

Centers for Disease Control: Prevention and control of influenza. Part 1. Vaccines, *MMWR* 43(RR-9):1-13, 1994.

Douglas RG: Prophylaxis and treatment of influenza, *N Engl J Med* 322:443-449, 1990.

Gardner P, Schaffner W: Immunization of adults, *N Engl J Med* 328:1252-1258, 1993.

Hardy WD et al: A controlled trial of trimethoprim-sulfamethoxazole or aerosolized pentamidine for secondary prophylaxis of *Pneumocystis carinii* pneumonia in patients with the acquired immunodeficiency syndrome, *N Engl J Med* 327:1842-1848, 1992.

Hoge CW et al: An epidemic of pneumococcal disease in an overcrowded, inadequately ventilated jail, *N Engl J Med* 331:643-648, 1994.

Lynch JP: Bacterial pneumonia. In Rakel RE, editor: *Conn's current therapy 1993,* Philadelphia, 1993, WB Saunders.

Masur H: Prevention and treatment of *Pneumocystis* pneumonia, *N Engl J Med* 327:1853-1860, 1992.

Piirilia P: Changes in crackle characteristics during the clinical course of pneumonia, *Chest* 102:176-183, 1992.

Rello J et al: Pneumonia due to *Haemophilus influenzae* among mechanically ventilated patients: incidence, outcome, and risk factors, *Chest* 102:1562-1565, 1992.

Zoler ML: Antibiotics: medicine's double-edged sword, *Harvard Health Lett* 18(6):4-6, 1993.

### Mechanical Ventilation

Benner KL: Terminal weaning: a loved one's vigil, *Am J Nurs* 93(5):22-25, 1993.

Bouley GH, Froman R, Shah H: The experience of dyspnea during weaning, *Heart Lung* 21:471-476, 1992.

Bridges EJ: Transition from ventilatory support: knowing when the patient is ready to wean, *Crit Care Nurs Q* 15(1):14-20, 1992.

Campbell ML: Terminal weaning, *Nurs 94* 24(9):34-40, 1994.

Carroll KC, Magruder CC: The role of analgesics and sedatives in the management of pain and agitation during weaning from mechanical ventilation, *Crit Care Nurs Q* 15(4):68-77, 1993.

Cohen IL, Lambrinos J, Fein A: Mechanical ventilation for the elderly patient in intensive care, *JAMA* 269:1025-1029, 1993.

Dettenmeier PA, Johnson TM: The art and science of mechanical ventilator adjustments, *Crit Care Nurs Clin North Am* 3:575-583, 1991.

DuPuis YG: *Ventilators: theory and clinical application,* ed 2, St Louis, 1991, Mosby.

Ferland PA: Are you ready for ventilator patients? *Nurs 91* 21(1):42-47, 1991.

Hansen-Flaschen JH et al: Use of sedating drugs and neuromuscular blocking agents in patients requiring mechanical ventilation for respiratory failure: a national survey, *JAMA* 266:2870-2875, 1991.

Jablonski RAS: Remember the person attached to the ventilator, *Nurs 92* 23(4):67-70, 1992.

Kaplow R, Bookbinder M: A comparison of four endotracheal tube holders, *Heart Lung* 23:59-66, 1994.

Knebel AR: Complications in critical care: weaning from mechanical ventilation—current controversies, *Heart Lung* 20:321-331, 1991.

Kollef MH: Do age and gender influence outcome from mechanical ventilation? *Heart Lung* 22:442-449, 1993.

Mason SG: When a ventilator patient is going home, *RN* 55(10):60-64, 1992.

Smith CE et al: Adaptation in families with a member requiring mechanical ventilation at home, *Heart Lung* 20:349-356, 1991.

Spector N: Nutritional support of the ventilator-dependent patient, *Nurs Clin North Am* 24:407-414, 1989.

Stiesmeyer JK: What triggers a ventilator alarm? *Am J Nurs* 91(10):61-64, 1991.

Tobin MJ: Mechanical ventilation, *N Engl J Med* 330:1056-1061, 1994.

Wiener C: Ventilatory management of respiratory failure in asthma, *JAMA* 269:2128-2131, 1993.

### Cystic Fibrosis

Coutelle C et al: Gene therapy for cystic fibrosis, *Arch Dis Child* 68:437-443, 1993.

Davis PB: Pathophysiology of pulmonary disease in cystic fibrosis, *Semin Respir Med* 6(4):261-269, 1985.

Davis PB: Cystic fibrosis: new perceptions, new strategies, *Hosp Pract* 27(11):79-83, 1992.

Fuchs HJ et al: Effect of aerolsolized recombinant human DNAs on exacerbations of respiratory symptoms and on pulmonary functions in patients with cystic fibrosis, *N Engl J Med* 331:637-642, 1994.

George MR: CF not just a pediatric problem anymore, *RN* 53(9):60-65, 1990.

Marx JL: The cystic fibrosis gene is found, *Science* 245:923-925, 1989.

New drug bulletin: dornase alfa, *RN* 57(4):41-42, 1994.

Ramsey BW, Smith AL: Reduced incidence of respiratory tract infections in cystic fibrosis patients using aerosolized dornase alfa, *Dornase Alfa Clin Series* 1(1):1-5, 1994.

Ramsey BW et al: Efficacy of aerosolized tobramycin in patients with cystic fibrosis, *N Engl J Med* 328:1740-1746, 1993.

### Smoking

Boyle P: The hazards of passive—and active—smoking, *N Engl J Med* 328:1708-1709, 1993.

Brownson RC et al: Demographic and socioeconomic differences in beliefs about the health effects of smoking, *Am J Public Health* 82:99-103, 1992.

Carmelli D et al: Genetic influence on smoking—a study of male twins, *N Engl J Med* 327:829-833, 1992.

Centers for Disease Control: The surgeon general's 1990 report on the health benefits of smoking cessation (executive summary), *MMWR* 39(RR-12):1-10, 1990.

Centers for Disease Control: Cigarette smoking among adults—United States, 1990, *MMWR* 41(20):354-361, 1992.

Centers for Disease Control: Cigarette smoking—attributable mortality and years of potential life lost—United States, 1990, *MMWR* 42(33):645-649, 1993.

Centers for Disease Control: Populations at risk from air pollution—United States, 1991, *MMWR* 42(16):301-304, 1993.

Centers for Disease Control: Smoking cessation during previous year among adults—United States, 1990 and 1991, *MMWR* 42(26):504-507, 1993.

Centers for Disease Control: Preventing tobacco use among young people: a report of the surgeon general, *MMWR* 43(RR-4):1-10, 1994.

Centers for Disease Control: Cigarette smoking among adults—United States, 1992, and changes in the definition of current cigarette smoking, *MMWR* 43(19):342-346, 1994.

Centers for Disease Control: Guidelines for school health programs to prevent tobacco use and addiction, *MMWR* 43(RR-2):1-15, 1994.

Escobedo LG et al: Sports participation, age at smoking initiation, and the risk of smoking among U.S. high school students, *JAMA* 269:1391-1395, 1993.

Farley CJ: The butt stops here: threatening to snuff out smoking for good, the crusade against tobacco shifts in higher gear, *Time,* April 18, 1994, pp 58-64.

Feighery E, Altman DG, Shaffer G: The effects of combining education and enforcement to reduce tobacco sales to minors, *JAMA* 266:3168-3171, 1991.

Jason LA et al: Active enforcement of cigarette control laws in the prevention of cigarette sales to minors, *JAMA* 266:3159-3161, 1991.

Macaskill P et al: Mass media–led antismoking campaign can remove the education gap in quitting behavior, *Am J Public Health* 82:96-98, 1992.

Moss AJ et al: Recent trends in adolescent smoking, smoking-uptake correlates, and expectations about the future. Advance data from *Vital and Health Statistics,* no 221, Hyattsville, Md, 1992, National Center for Health Statistics.

Warner KE, Goldenhar LM, McLaughlin CG: Cigarette advertising and magazine coverage of the hazards of smoking: a statistical analysis, *N Engl J Med* 326:305-309, 1992.

### *Asthma*

Ahmed T, Garrigo UJ, Danta I: Preventing bronchoconstriction in exercise-induced asthma with inhaled heparin, *N Engl J Med* 329:90-95, 1993.

Asthma. Part 1, *Harvard Health Lett* 16(7):5-7, 1991.

Asthma. Part 2, *Harvard Health Lett* 16(8):1-4, 1991.

Cheung D et al: Long-term effects of a long-acting $\beta_2$-adrenoceptor agonist, salmeterol, on airway hyperresponsiveness in patients with mild asthma, *N Engl J Med* 327:1198-1203, 1992.

Clinical highlights: Could you teach patients to use an inhaler? *RN* 56(5):21, 1993.

Dyer J: Drug watch: new long-lived bronchodilator knocks out albuterol, *Am J Nurs* 93(5):53-54, 1993.

Hunt LW et al: Accuracy of the death certificate in a population-based study of asthmatic patients, *JAMA* 269:1947-1952, 1993.

Janson-Bjerklie S, Shnell S: Effect of peak flow information on patterns of self-care in adult asthma, *Heart Lung* 17:543-549, 1988.

Janson-Bjerklie S, Ferketich S, Benner P: Predicting the outcomes of living with asthma, *Res Nurs Health* 16:241-250, 1993.

Janson-Bjerklie S et al: Clinical markers of asthma severity and risk: Importance of subjective as well as objective factors, *Heart Lung* 21:265-272, 1992.

Janson-Bjerklie S et al: Disappearance of eosinophils from bronchoalveolar lavage fluid after patient education and high-dose inhaled corticosteroids: a case report, *Heart Lung* 22:235-238, 1993.

Jess LW: When your patient has asthma, *Nurs 92* 23(4):48-51, 1992.

Kaliner MA: Asthma deaths: a social or medical problem? *JAMA* 269:1994-1995, 1993.

Larsen GL: Asthma in children, *N Engl J Med* 326:1540-1545, 1992.

McFadden ER, Gilbert IA: Asthma, *N Engl J Med* 327:1928-1937, 1992.

Mullen M, Mullen B, Carey M: The association between β-agonist use and death from asthma, *JAMA* 270:1842-1845, 1993.

O'Connor BJ, Airman SL, Barnes PJ: Tolerance to the nonbronchodilator effects of inhaled $\beta_2$-agonists in asthma, *N Engl J Med* 327:1204-1208, 1992.

Orsi AJ: Asthma—the danger is real, *RN* 54(4):58-62, 1991.

Pearlman DS et al: A comparison of salmeterol with albuterol in the treatment of mild-to-moderate asthma, *N Engl J Med* 327:1420-1425, 1992.

Reinke LF, Hoffman LA: How to teach asthma co-management, *Am J Nurs* 92:40-51, 1992.

Robinson DS et al: Predominant $T_{H2}$-like bronchoalveolar T-lymphocyte population in atopic asthma, *N Engl J Med* 326:298-304, 1992.

Rodman MJ: OTC interactions: asthma medications, *RN* 56(4):40-45, 1993.

Spitzer WO et al: The use of β-agonists and the risk of death and near death from asthma, *N Engl J Med* 326:501-506, 1992.

US Department of Health and Human Services, Public Health Service, National Heart, Lung, and Blood Institute: *Guidelines for the diagnosis and management of asthma,* Bethesda, Md, 1991, DHHS.

US Department of Health and Human Services, Public Health Service, National Heart, Lung, and Blood Institute: *Teach your patients about asthma: a clinician's guide,* Bethesda, Md, 1992, DHHS.

Utiger RD: Differences between inhaled and oral glucocorticoid therapy, *N Engl J Med* 329:1731-1733, 1993.

### *Tuberculosis*

American Thoracic Society: Diagnostic standards and classification of tuberculosis, *Am Rev Respir Dis* 142:725-735, 1990.

American Thoracic Society: Diagnosis and treatment of disease caused by nontuberculous mycobacteria, *Am Rev Respir Dis* 142:940-953, 1990.

American Thoracic Society: Control of tuberculosis in the United States, *Am Rev Respir Dis* 146:1623-1633, 1992.

Avey MA: TB skin testing: how to do it right, *Am J Nurs* 93(9):42-44, 1993.

Barnes P et al: Tuberculosis in patients with human immunodeficiency virus infection, *N Engl J Med* 324:1644-1649, 1991.

Barry MA et al: Tuberculosis infection in urban adolescents: results of a school-based testing program, *Am J Public Health* 80:439-441, 1990.

Beck-Sague C et al: Hospital outbreak of multidrug-resistant *Mycobacterium tuberculosis* infections, *JAMA* 268:1280-1286, 1992.

Bellin E: Failure of tuberculosis control: a prescription for change, *JAMA* 271:708-709, 1994.

Bellin E, Fletcher D, Safyer S: Abnormal chest x-rays in intravenous drug users: implications for tuberculosis screening programs, *Am J Public Health* 83:698-700, 1993.

Bellin EY, Fletcher DD, Safyer SM: Association of tuberculosis infection with increased time in or admission to the New York City jail system, *JAMA* 269:2228-2231, 1993.

Bloch AB et al: Nationwide survey of drug-resistant tuberculosis in the United States, *JAMA* 271:665-671, 1994.

Boutotte J: Protecting yourself against T.B., *Nurs 93* 24(10):64, 1993.

Boutotte J: T.B., the second time around, *Nurs 93* 24(5):42-49, 1993.

Braun MM, Cote RT, Rabkin CS: Trends in death with tuberculosis during the AIDS era, *JAMA* 269:2865-2868, 1993.

Centers for Disease Control: Update—tuberculosis elimination—United States, *MMWR* 39(10):153-156, 1990.

Centers for Disease Control: Management of persons exposed to multidrug-resistant tuberculosis, *MMWR* 41(RR-11):61-70, 1992.

Centers for Disease Control: Meeting the challenge of multidrug-resistant tuberculosis: summary of a conference, *MMWR* 41(RR-11):51-57, 1992.

Centers for Disease Control: National action plan to combat multidrug-resistant tuberculosis, *MMWR* 41(RR-11):1-48, 1992.

Centers for Disease Control: Prevention and control of tuberculosis in migrant farm workers: recommendations of the Advisory Council for the Elimination of Tuberculosis, *MMWR* 41(RR-10):1-15, 1992.

Centers for Disease Control: Prevention and control of tuberculosis among homeless persons: recommendations of the Advisory Council for the Elimination of Tuberculosis, *MMWR* 41(RR-5):1-23, 1992.

Centers for Disease Control: Initial therapy for tuberculosis in the era of multidrug resistance: recommendations of the Advisory Council for the Elimination of Tuberculosis, *MMWR* 42(RR-7):1-8, 1993.

Centers for Disease Control: Severe isoniazid-associated hepatitis—New York, 1991-1993, *MMWR* 42(28):545-547, 1993.

Centers for Disease Control: Tuberculosis among pregnant women—New York City, 1985-1992, *MMWR* 42(31):605-612, 1993.

Centers for Disease Control: Tuberculosis control laws—United States, 1993, *MMWR* 42(RR-15):1-15, 1993.

Centers for Disease Control: Tuberculosis morbidity—United States, 1992, *MMWR* 42(36):696-704, 1993.

Centers for Disease Control: Tuberculosis prevention in drug-treatment centers and correctional facilities—selected U.S. sites, 1990-1991, *MMWR* 42(11):210-213, 1993.

Centers for Disease Control: Tuberculosis—Western Europe, 1974-1991, *MMWR* 42(32):628-631, 1993.

Centers for Disease Control: Expanded tuberculosis surveillance and tuberculosis morbidity—United States, 1993, *MMWR* 43(20):361-366, 1994.

Colditz GA et al: Efficacy of BCG vaccine in the prevention of tuberculosis, *JAMA* 271:698-702, 1994.

Cynaman MH, Klemens S: Tuberculosis and other mycobacterial diseases. In Rakel RE, editor: *Conn's current therapy 1993,* Philadelphia, 1993, WB Saunders.

Daugherty JS, Hutton MD, Simone PM: Prevention and control of tuberculosis in the 1990's, *Nurs Clin North Am* 28:599-611, 1993.

Dooley SW et al: Guidelines for preventing the transmission of tuberculosis in health care settings, with special focus on HIV-related issues, *MMWR* 39(RR-17):1-26, 1990.

Dooley SW et al: Nosocomial transmission of tuberculosis in a hospital unit for HIV-infected patients, *JAMA* 267:2632-2635, 1992.

Dowling PT: Return of tuberculosis: screening and preventive therapy, *Am Fam Physician* 43(2):457-467, 1991.

Edlin BR: An outbreak of multidrug-resistant tuberculosis among hospitalized patients with the acquired immunodeficiency syndrome, *N Engl J Med* 326:1514-1521, 1992.

Frieden RT et al: The emergence of drug-resistant tuberculosis in New York City, *N Engl J Med* 328:521-526, 1993.

Gordin F: Tuberculosis control: back to the future? *JAMA* 267:2649-2650, 1992.

Iseman MD, Cohn DL, Sbarbaro JA: Directly observed treatment of tuberculosis: we can't afford not to try it, *N Engl J Med* 328:576-578, 1993.

Joseph S: Tuberculosis, again, *Am J Public Health* 83:647-648, 1993 (editorial).

Lerner BH: New York City's tuberculosis control efforts: the historical limitations of the "War on Consumption," *Am J Public Health* 83:758-766, 1993.

Mahmoudi A, Iseman MD: Pitfalls in the care of patients with tuberculosis, *JAMA* 270:65-68, 1993.

Moran JF: Surgical treatment of tuberculosis. In Sabiston DC, Lyerly HK, editors: *Sabiston essentials of surgery,* ed 2, Philadelphia, 1994, WB Saunders.

O'Brien LM, Bartlett KA: TB plus HIV spells trouble, *Am J Nurs* 92(5):28-34, 1992.

Snider DE, Roper WL: The new tuberculosis, *N Engl J Med* 326:794-795, 1992.

TB hits 500 NYC hospital workers: city strains to control outbreaks, *Am J Nurs* 92(4):103-104, 1992.

Trubo R: Conspicuous consumption, *Harvard Health Lett* 18(11):6-8, 1993.

### *Chronic Obstructive Pulmonary Disease*

Alex CG, Tobin MJ: Chronic obstructive pulmonary disease. In Rakel RE, editor: *Conn's current therapy 1993,* Philadelphia, 1993, WB Saunders.

Brandstetter RD et al: Pneumothorax after thoracentesis in chronic obstructive pulmonary disease, *Heart Lung* 23:67-70, 1994.

Breslin EH et al: Standardization of a device to measure unsupported arm exercise endurance in chronic obstructive pulmonary disease, *Nurs Res* 41:292-295, 1992.

Carrieri-Kohlman V et al: Desensitization and guided mastery: treatment approaches for the management of dyspnea, *Heart Lung* 22:226-234, 1993.

Clinical highlights: "Balloon therapy" may alleviate chronic bronchitis, *RN* 56(7):20, 1993.

Cossette S, Levesque L: Caregiving tasks as predictors of mental health of wife caregivers of men with chronic obstructive pulmonary disease, *Res Nurs Health* 16:251-263, 1993.

Della-Bella LA: Steroidphobia and the pulmonary patient, *Am J Nurs* 92(2):26-29, 1992.

Dompeling E et al: Slowing the deterioration of asthma and chronic obstructive pulmonary disease observed during bronchodilator therapy by adding inhaled corticosteroids, *Ann Intern Med* 118:770-778, 1993.

Edlund B, Wheeler E: Adaptation to breathlessness, *Top Clin Nurs* 2(3):11-25, 1980.

Ferguson GT, Cherniack RM: Management of chronic obstructive pulmonary disease, *N Engl J Med* 328:1017-1022, 1993.

Gift AG, McCrone SH: Depression in patients with COPD, *Heart Lung* 22:289-297, 1993.

Kerstjens HAM et al: A comparison of bronchodilator therapy with or without inhaled corticosteroid therapy for obstructive airways disease, *N Engl J Med* 327:1413-1419, 1992.

Killian KJ: The objective measurement of breathlessness, *Chest* 88(2):84S-90S, 1985.

Kim MJ et al: Inspiratory muscle training in patients with chronic obstructive pulmonary disease, *Nurs Res* 42:356-362, 1993.

Klinger JR, Nichols NS: Right ventricular dysfunction in chronic obstructive pulmonary disease, *Chest* 90(3):715-723, 1991.

Kuo C, Chiao G, Lee J: The effects of high-fat and high-carbohydrate diet loads on gas exchange and ventilation in COPD patients and normal subjects, *Chest* 104:189-196, 1993.

McBride S: Perceived control in patients with chronic obstructive pulmonary disease, *West J Nurs Res* 15:456-464, 1993.

Muza SR: Comparison of scales used to quantitate the sense of effort to breathe in patients with chronic obstructive pulmonary disease, *Am Rev Respir Dis* 141:909-913, 1990.

Ray JW, Robin ED: Cost-effectiveness of $alpha_1$-antitrypsin replacement therapy in treatment of congenital chronic obstructive pulmonary disease, *Am J Public Health* 81(4):427-433, 1991.

Renfroe KL: Effect of progressive relaxation on dyspnea and state anxiety in patients with chronic obstructive pulmonary disease, *Heart Lung* 17:408-413, 1988.

Small SP, Graydon JE: Uncertainty in hospitalized patients with chronic obstructive pulmonary disease, *Int J Nurs Studies* 30:239-246, 1993.

Stephenson J: Positively breathtaking, *Harvard Health Lett* 18(2):5-8, 1992.

Vale F, Reardon JZ, ZuWallack RL: The long-term benefits of outpatient pulmonary rehabilitation on exercise endurance and quality of life, *Chest* 103:42-45, 1993.

Weaver TE, Narsavage GL: Physiological and psychological variables related to functional status in chronic obstructive pulmonary disease, *Nurs Res* 41:286-291, 1992.

Whitney L: Chronic bronchitis and emphysema: airing the difference, *Nurs 92* 23(3):34-41, 1992.

# UNIT VII Alterations in Metabolism

## SECTION ONE Endocrine System

## CHAPTER 38 Assessment of the Endocrine System

### *General*

Carpenito LJ: *Nursing diagnosis: application to clinical practice,* ed 5, Philadelphia, 1993, JB Lippincott.

Chernow B et al: Critical care endocrinology. In Shoemaker WC et al, editors: *Textbook of critical care,* ed 2, Philadelphia, 1989, WB Saunders.

Civetta JM, Taylor RW, Kirby RR, editors: *Critical care,* Philadelphia, 1988, JB Lippincott.

Ebersole P, Hess D: *Toward healthy aging,* ed 4, St Louis, 1994, Mosby.

Halloran TH: Nursing responsibilities in endocrine emergencies, *Crit Care Nurs Q* 13(3):74-81, 1990.

Hyman RB et al: The effects of relaxation training on clinical symptoms: a meta-analysis, *Nurs Res* 38:216-220, 1989.

Marx SJ: Familial multiple endocrine neoplasia type 1. In the Endocrine Society: *41st Post Graduate Annual Assembly syllabus,* Bethesda, Md, 1989, The Society.

McCance K, Huether SE: *Pathophysiology: the biologic basis for disease in adults and children,* St Louis, 1990, Mosby.

Pagana KD, Pagana TJ: *Diagnostic testing and nursing implications: a case study approach,* ed 4, St Louis, 1994, Mosby.

Rose, DB: *Clinical physiology of acid-base and electrolyte disorders,* ed 3, New York, 1989, McGraw-Hill.

Streiff LD: Can clients understand our instructions? *Image* 18:48-52, 1986.

Taylor S: *Positive illusions,* New York, 1989, Basic Books.

Tepperman J: *Metabolic and endocrine physiology: an introductory text,* ed 5, Chicago, 1987, Year Book.

Wilson JD, Foster DW, editors: *Williams' textbook of endocrinology,* ed 7, Philadelphia, 1985, WB Saunders.

Wyngaarden JB, Smith LH, editors: *Cecil textbook of medicine,* ed 18, Philadelphia, 1988, WB Saunders.

CHAPTER 39

## Management of Persons With Problems of the Pituitary, Thyroid, Parathyroid, and Adrenal Glands

### *Adrenal Gland*

Chin R: Adrenal crisis, *Crit Care Clin* 7:23-41, 1991.

Cryer P: Pheochromocytoma and adrenergic dysfunction. In the Endocrine Society: *41st Post Graduate Annual Assembly syllabus,* Bethesda, Md, 1989, The Society.

Gumowski J et al: Endocrinopathies of hyperfunction: Cushing's syndrome and aldosteronism, *AACN Clin Issues Crit Care Nurs* 3(20):331-347, 1992.

Jagger P: Addison's disease, polyglandular deficiency syndrome. In the Endocrine Society: *41st Post Graduate Annual Assembly syllabus,* Bethesda, Md, 1989, The Society.

King RJB: Enlightenment and confusion over steroid hormone receptors, *Nature* 312:20, 1984.

Lee L, Gumowski J: Adrenocortical insufficiency: a medical emergency, *AACN Clin Issues Crit Care Nurs* 3(2):319-330, 1992.

Loriauy DL: Cushing's syndrome. In the Endocrine Society: *41st Post Graduate Annual Assembly syllabus,* Bethesda, Md, 1989, The Society.

Miyagawa K et al: Multiple endocrine neoplasia type 1 with Cushing's disease, primary hyperparathyroidism, and insulin—glucagonoma, *Cancer* 61:1232-1236, 1988.

Seck JR, Dunger, DB: Diabetes insipidus: current treatment recommendations, *Drugs* 44:216-224, 1992.

Shapiro B, Gross MD: Pheochromocytoma, *Crit Care Clin* 7(1):1-2, 1991.

Svec F: Steroid usage: too much of a good thing. In the Endocrine Society: *41st Post Graduate Annual Assembly syllabus,* Bethesda, Md. 1989, The Society.

Winer N: Hypertensive crisis, *Crit Care Nurs Q* 13(3):23-33, 1990.

Winer N: Pheochromocytoma, *Crit Care Nurs Q* 13(3):14-22, 1990.

### *Pituitary Gland*

Barkan A: Acromegaly and giantism. In the Endocrine Society: *41st Post Graduate Annual Assembly syllabus,* Bethesda, Md, 1989, The Society.

Barkan A et al: Preoperative treatment of acromegaly with long-acting somatostatin analog SMS 201-995: shrinkage of invasive pituitary macroadenomas and improved surgical cure rate, *J Clin Endocrinol Metab* 67:1040-1048, 1988.

Batcheller J: Disorders of antidiuretic hormone secretion, *AACN Clin Issues Crit Care Nurs* 3:370-378, 1992.

Black P, Zervas NT, Candia GL: Incidence and management of complications of transsphenoidal operation for pituitary adenomas, *Neurosurgery* 20(6):920-924, 1987.

Cagno J: Diabetes insipidus, *Crit Care Nurs* 9(6):86-93, 1989.

Chanson P, Jedynak CP, Czernichow P: Management of early postoperative diabetes insipidus with parenteral desmopressin, *Acta Endocrinol* 117:513-514, 1988.

Grumbach MM: Evaluation of treatment of the child with short stature. In the Endocrine Society: *41st Post Graduate Annual Assembly syllabus,* Bethesda, Md, 1989, The Society.

Holzman EJ et al: Brief report: a molecular defect in the vasopressin V2-receptor gene causing nephrogenic diabetes insipidus, *N Engl J Med* 328:24, 1993.

Illowsky BP, Kirch DG: Polydipsia and hyponatremia in psychiatric patients, *Am J Psychiatry* 145:675-683, 1988.

Kaplan S: The newer uses of growth hormone in adults, *Adv Intern Med* 38:287-301, 1993.

Kinzier BJ: Management of the syndrome of inappropriate secretion of antidiuretic hormone, *Clin Pharm* 6:833, 1987.

Klibanski, A: Glycoprotein hormone-producing pituitary tumors. In the Endocrine Society: *45th Post Graduate Annual Assembly syllabus,* Bethesda, Md, 1993, The Society.

Krege J, Kagtz VL, Bowes WA: Transient diabetes insipidus of pregnancy, *Obstet Gynecol Surv* 44:789-795, 1989.

Melmed S: Acromegaly, *N Engl J Med* 322:966-975, 1990.

Molitch M: Lactation and prolactinomas. In the Endocrine Society: *41st Post Graduate Annual Assembly syllabus,* Bethesda, Md, 1989, The Society.

Murty GE, Lamballe MB, Welch AR: Early inappropriate secretion of antidiuretic hormone after transphenoidal pituitary adenomectomy, *J Laryngol Otol* 104:894-895, 1990.

Poe CM, Taylor LM: Syndrome of inappropriate antidiuretic hormone: assessment and nursing implications, *Oncol Nurs Forum* 26(3):373-381, 1989.

Reasner CA: Anterior pituitary disease, *Crit Care Nurs Q* 13(2):62-66, 1990.

Riggs AT et al: A review of disorders of water: homeostasis in psychiatric patients, *Psychosomatics* 32(2):133-148, 1991.

Seck JR, Dunger DB: Diabetes insipidus: current treatment recommendations, *Drugs* 44:216-224, 1992.

Smith-Rooker JL, Garrett A, Hodges LC: Case management of the patient with pituitary tumor, *Med Surg Nurs* 2:265-274, 1993.

Snyder PJ: The myth of the nonsecreting pituitary adenoma. In the Endocrine Society: *41st Post Graduate Annual Assembly syllabus,* Bethesda, Md, 1989, The Society.

Thorner MO: A current management of hyperprolactinemia. In the Endocrine Society: *45th Post Graduate Annual Assembly syllabus,* Bethesda, Md, 1993, The Society.

Verbalis JG: SIAD and other hyponatremic states. In the Endocrine Society: *41st Post Graduate Annual Assembly syllabus,* Bethesda, Md, 1989, The Society.

Wass JSH, Popovic V, Chayvialle JA: Proceedings of the discussion, "Tolerability and safety of sandostatin," *Metabolism* 41(9)(suppl 2):80-82, 1992.

### *Thyroid Gland*

Baylin S: Familial and sporadic carcinoma of the thyroid. In the Endocrine Society: *41st Post Graduate Annual Assembly syllabus,* Bethesda, Md, 1989, The Society.

Cooper DS: Antithyroid drugs. In the Endocrine Society: *41st Post Graduate Annual Assembly syllabus,* Bethesda, Md, 1989, The Society.

Crapo LM: Thyroid function testing. In the Endocrine Society: *45th Post Graduate Annual Assembly syllabus,* Bethesda, Md, 1993, The Society.

DeGroot JL et al: *Endocrinology,* ed 2, Philadelphia, 1989, WB Saunders.

Gorman CA: Thyroid orbitopathy: the gravest problem in Graves' disease. In the Endocrine Society: *41st Post Graduate Annual Assembly syllabus,* Bethesda, Md, 1989, The Society.

Greenspan FS: Medical management of thyroid nodules and thyroid cancer. In the Endocrine Society: *45th Post Graduate Annual Assembly syllabus,* Bethesda, Md, 1993, The Society.

Harada T et al: Current treatment of Graves' disease, *Surg Clin North Am* 67:299-314, 1987.

Hershman JM: Effect of nonthyroid illness on thyroid function. In the Endocrine Society: *45th Post Graduate Annual Assembly syllabus,* Bethesda, Md, 1993, The Society.

Hetzel BS: The control of iodine deficiency. *Am J Pediatr* 83:494-495, 1993.

Isley WL: Thyroid disorders, *Crit Care Nurs Q* 13(3):39-49, 1990.

Lammon CA: Recognizing thyroid crisis, *Nurs 93* 23(4):33-43, 1993.

Mazzaferri E et al: Solitary thyroid nodule: diagnoses and management, *Med Clin North Am* 72:1177-1211, 1988.

McKenzie JM: Thyroid autoimmunity—etiologies, pathogenesis and management. In the Endocrine Society: *41st Post Graduate Annual Assembly syllabus,* Bethesda, Md, 1989, The Society.

Paul T et al: Long-term L-thyronine therapy is associated with decreased hipbone density in premenopausal women. *JAMA* 295:3137-3141, 1988.

Reasner CA II, Isley WI: Thyrotoxicosis in the critically ill, *Crit Care Clin* 7:57-73, 1991.

Sakiyama R: Common thyroid disorders, *Am Fam Physician* 38(1):227-238, 1988.

Sarsany S: Thyroid storm, *RN* 51(7):46-48, 1988.

Sawin CT: Hypothyroidism, *Med Clin North Am* 69:989-1003, 1988.

Sawin CT: Thyroid dysfunction in older persons, *Adv Intern Med* 37:223-247, 1992.

Singer FR: Calcitonin: actions and therapeutic uses. In the Endocrine Society: *41st Post Graduate Annual Assembly syllabus,* Bethesda, Md, 1989, The Society.

Spittle L: Diagnoses in opposition: thyroid storm and myxedema coma, *AACN Clin Issues Crit Care Nurs* 3(2):300-308, 1992.

Woeber KA: Iodine and thyroid disease. In the Endocrine Society: *45th Post Graduate Annual Assembly syllabus,* Bethesda, Md, 1993, The Society.

### *Parathyroid Gland*

Bilezikian JP: Therapy of hypercalcemia. In the Endocrine Society: *41st Post Graduate Annual Assembly syllabus,* Bethesda, Md, 1989, The Society.

Braverman L: Use and abuse of iodides and thyroid hormones. In the Endocrine Society: *41st Post Graduate Annual Assembly syllabus,* Bethesda, Md, 1989, The Society.

Davies M: Primary hyperparathyroidism: aggressive or conservative treatment? *Clin Endocrinol* 36:326-332, 1992.

Gladziwa U et al: Secondary hyperparathyroidism and sonographic evaluation of parathyroid gland hyperplasia in dialysis patients, *Clin Nephrol* 38:162-166, 1992.

Harris ST: Osteoporosis: pharmacologic treatment strategies, *Adv Intern Med* 38:303-321, 1993.

Heath H: Primary hyperparathyroidism: recent advances in pathogenesis, diagnosis, and management, *Adv Intern Med* 37:275-293, 1992.

Malluche HH, Monier-Faugere MC: Uremic bone disease: current knowledge, controversial issues, and new horizons, *Electrolyte Metab* 17:281-296, 1991.

### *Pancreas*

American Diabetes Association: Office guide to diagnosis and classification of diabetes mellitus and other categories of glucose intolerance (positive statement), *Diabetes Care* 16(suppl 2):4, 1993.

Wingard DL et al: Community-based study of prevalence of NIDDM in older adults, *Diabetes Care* 13(2):3-8, 1990.

CHAPTER 40

## Management of Persons With Diabetes Mellitus and Hypoglycemia

### *General*

Blevins D, Cassmeyer VL: The patient with diabetes mellitus. In Long B, Phipps WJ, Cassmeyer VL, editors: *Medical-surgical nursing: a nursing process approach,* ed 3, St Louis, 1993, Mosby.

Bloomgarden ZT: Epidemiology, diagnosis, and treatment of type II diabetes: a meeting report, *Pract Diabetol* 12(2):4-9, 1993.

Fain JA, editor: Diabetes, *Nurs Clin North Am* 28(1):1-119, 1993.

Keegan A et al: Bringing research to light, *Diabetes Forecast* 45(9): 34-43, 1992.

Krall L, Beaser R: *Joslin diabetes manual,* ed 12, Philadelphia, 1989, Lea & Febiger.

National Diabetes Data Group: Classification and diagnoses of diabetes mellitus and other categories of glucose intolerance, *Diabetes* 28:1039-1057, 1979.

Raymond M: *The human side of diabetes: beyond doctors, diets and drugs,* New York, 1992, Noble Press.

Rifkin H, Porte D, editors: *Ellenberg and Rifkin's diabetes mellitus: theory and practice,* ed 4, New York, 1990, Elsevier.

Saudek CD, Segal-Polin S: Economic aspects: insurance, employment, and licensing, In Rifkin H, Porte D, editors: *Ellenberg and Rifkin's diabetes mellitus: theory and practice,* ed 4, New York, 1990, Elsevier.

The following six journals are published monthly or bimonthly and are excellent sources of information on all aspects of diabetes mellitus.

*Clinical Diabetes,* American Diabetes Association, Inc, Alexandria, Va.

*Countdown,* The Juvenile Diabetes Foundation International, New York, NY.

*Diabetes Care,* American Diabetes Association, Inc, Alexandria, Va.

*Diabetes Forecast,* American Diabetes Association, Inc, Alexandria, Va.

*Diabetes Spectrum—From Research to Practice,* American Diabetes Association, Inc, Alexandria, Va.

*Practical Diabetology,* RA Rapaport Publishing, Inc, New York, NY.

### *Activity*

Depres JP et al: Loss of abdominal fat and metabolic response to exercise training in obese women, *Am J Physiol* 261:159-167, 1991.

Franz MJ: Exercise and diabetes. In Haire-Joshu D: *Management of diabetes mellitus: perspectives of care across the life span,* St Louis, 1992, Mosby.

Franz MJ, Norstrom J: *Diabetes, actively staying healthy: your game plan for diabetes and exercise,* Wayzata, Minn, 1990, DCI.

Graham C: Exercise and aging: implications for persons with diabetes, *Diabetes Educator* 17(3):189-195, 1991.

Horton ES: Exercise. In Lebovitz HE, editor: *Therapy for diabetes mellitus and related disorders,* Alexandria, Va, 1991, American Diabetes Association.

Pollock ML, Wilmore JH: *Exercise in health and disease: evaluation and prescription for prevention and rehabilitation,* ed 2, Philadelphia, 1990, WB Saunders.

### Complications

Ashley D: Surgery and the diabetic patient, *Post Anesth Nurs* 1:205-207, 1986.

Beaser RS, Aho C: *Fighting long term complications,* Diabetes self-manager series, Boston, 1992, Joslin Diabetes Center.

Capsaicin Study Group: Effect of treatment with capsaicin on daily activities of patients with painful diabetic neuropathy, *Diabetes Care* 15(2):159-165, 1992.

Casey C: Diabetes complications that can cripple, *RN* 55(8):36-42, 1992.

Cleveland M: *Living well, a twelve-step response to chronic illness and disability,* San Francisco, 1988, Harper/Hazelden.

Coleman W: Foot care and diabetes mellitus. In Haire-Joshu D, editor: *Managmenet of diabetes mellitus: perspectives of care across the life span,* St Louis, 1992, Mosby.

Falchuk KR, Conlin DC: The intestinal and liver complications of diabetes mellitus, *Adv Intern Med* 38:269-287, 1993.

Fleckman AM: Diabetic ketoacidosis, *Pract Diabetol* 10(3):1-8, 1991.

Genuth S: Diabetic ketoacidosis and hyperglycemic hyperosmolar coma in adults. In Lebovitz, H, editor: *Therapy for diabetes mellitus and related disorders,* Alexandria, Va, 1991, American Diabetes Association.

Gorden P: The clinical spectrum of hypoglycemia. In the Endocrine Society: *41st Post Graduate Annual Assembly syllabus,* Bethesda, Md, 1989, The Society.

Graves L III: Diabetic ketoacidosis and hyperosmolar hyperglycemic nonketotic coma, *Crit Care Nurse Q* 13(3):50-61, 1990.

Henderson G: The psychosocial treatment of recurrent diabetic ketoacidosis: an interdisciplinary team approach, *Diabetes Educator* 17(2):119-123, 1991.

Herman W: *The prevention and treatment of complications of diabetes mellitus: a guide for primary care practitioners,* US Department of Health and Human Services, Public Health Service, Centers for Disease Control, National Center for Chronic Disease Prevention and Health Promotion, Division of Diabetes Translation, Washington, DC, 1992, US Government Printing Office.

Juliano J: *When diabetes complicates your life,* Minneapolis, 1993, Chronimed.

Knighton DR: Treating diabetic foot ulcers, *Diabetes Spectrum* 3(1):51-56, 1990.

Lloyd CE et al: Psychosocial factors and complications of IDDM, *Diabetes Care* 15(2):166-172, 1992.

Lorber DL: Important considerations: acute glycemic complications, *Pract Diabetol* 11(2):33-35, 1992.

Mulcahy K: Hypoglycemic emergencies, *AACN J* 3(2):316-369, 1992.

Parillo M et al: Prevention of early-morning hyperglycemia in IDDM patients with long-acting zinc insulin, *Diabetes Care* 15(2):173-177, 1992.

Paulk LH: *Hypoglycemic reactions from the diabetic's perspective,* unpublished master's thesis, Kent, Ohio, 1983, Kent State University.

Shakir KM, Amin RM: Hypoglycemia, *Crit Care Clin* 7(1):75-87, 1991.

Ulchaker MM, Sheehan JP: Iatrogenic brittle diabetes: the hold the insulin decision, *Diabetes Educator* 17(2):111-113, 1991.

Vinicor FA: Epidemiology of diabetes complications: defining risk factors and frequency of complications, *Diabetes Spectrum* 5(2):86-121, 1992.

Zehrer J, Rode S: Hypertension and diabetes, *Drugs* 35(suppl 6): 135-141, 1988.

### Etiology/Epidemiology

American Diabetes Association: *Diabetes—1991 vital statistics,* Alexandria, Va, 1991, The Association.

American Diabetes Association: One-page handouts, Alexandria, Va, 1992, The Association.
The dangerous toll of diabetes
Diabetes among American Indians
Diabetes among Black Americans
Diabetes among Hispanics
Diabetes among seniors
Diabetes among youth
Diabetes: facts you need to know
Direct and indirect costs of diabetes in the United States

Atkinson MA, MaClaren NK: What causes diabetes? *Sci Am* 263:62-67, 1990.

Pasmantier R: Muscle cells' resistance to insulin may start decades before the diagnosis of type II, *Diabetes News* 12(2):14-16, 1993.

US Department of Health and Human Services: *Diabetes in the United States: a strategy for prevention,* Map reference, US Public Health Service, National Center for Chronic Disease Control and Prevention, Division of Diabetes Translation, Washington, DC, 1992, US Government Printing Office.

World Health Organization: WHO expert committee on diabetes mellitus, second report, *WHO Tech Rep Series* 646:1-80, 1980.

Wysocki T: SMBG: has the promise been fulfilled? *Diabetes Spectrum* 1(2):83-87, 1988.

Zimmet PZ: Challenges in diabetes epidemiology: from West to the rest, *Diabetes Care* 15(2):232-252, 1992.

### Home Care

Jackson JE, Johnson EA: *Patient education in home care: a practical guide to effective teaching and documentation,* Rockville, Md, 1988, Aspen.

### Medical Management

American Diabetes Association: *Physician's guide to insulin-dependent (type I) diabetes, diagnosis and treatment,* Alexandria, Va, 1988, The Association.

American Diabetes Association: *Physician's guide to non-insulin-dependent (type II) diabetes, diagnosis and treatment,* ed 2, Alexandria, Va, 1988, The Association.

American Diabetes Association: *Report on diabetes control and complications trial,* national meeting, June 1993.

American Diabetes Association: Clinical practice recommendations, 1992-1993, *Diabetes Care* 16(suppl 2):1-66, 1993.

Riddle MC: Strategies for non-insulin-dependent diabetes mellitus, *Hosp Pract* 28(4A):14-20, 1993.

### Medications

*Drug Facts and Comparisons,* St Louis, 1993, Wolters Kluwer.

Eli Lilly: *Characteristics of Lilly insulins,* chart, Indianapolis, 1993, Eli Lilly.

Galloway JA: Chemistry and clinical use of insulin. In Galloway JA, editor: *Diabetes mellitus,* ed 9, Indianapolis, 1988, Eli Lilly.

Laube BL et al: Preliminary study of the efficacy of insulin aerosol delivered by oral inhalation in diabetic patients, *JAMA* 269(16):2106-2109, 1993.

Lebovitz HE: Combination therapy for hyperglycemia. In Lebovitz HE, editor: *Therapy for diabetes mellitus and related disorders,* Alexandria, Va, 1991, American Diabetes Association.

Novo Nordisk: *Product reference guide,* chart, Princeton, NJ, 1992, Novo Nordisk.

***Nursing Management***

Drass J: What you need to know about insulin injections, *Nurs 92* 22(11):40-43, 1992.

Edelwich J, Brodsky A: *Diabetes: caring for your emotions as well as your health,* Reading, Mass, 1986, Addison-Wesley.

Guthrie DW, editor: *Diabetes education: a core curriculum for health professionals,* Alexandria, Va, 1988, American Association of Diabetes Educators.

Guthrie DW, Guthrie RA: *Nursing management of diabetes mellitus,* ed 3, New York, 1991, Springer.

Marrero D: *Diabetes education/a video course review/psychological factors and social support,* Alexandria, Va, 1991, American Association of Diabetes Educators.

***Nutrition***

American Diabetes Association: *Month of meals 4: a menu planner,* Alexandria, Va, 1993, The Association.

American Diabetes Association: *Healthy living catalogue,* Alexandria, Va, 1993, The Association.

American Diabetes Association and American Dietetic Association: *Exchange lists for meal planning,* Alexandria, Va, 1986, The Association.

Amick BL, Lopes GL: *Kansas diet manual,* ed 6, Topeka, 1992, Kansas Dietetic Association.

Anderson J, Clark JT: The promise of fiber, *Diabetes Forecast* 40:47-48, 50, 52, 1987.

Anderson JW et al: Dietary fiber and diabetes, a comprehensive review and practical application, *J Am Diet Assoc* 87:1189-1197, 1987.

Breckenridge BP: *Diabetes guide sheet: please tell me about what I can eat,* Princeton, NJ, 1992, Novo Nordisk.

Daly A, Arky RA: Nutritional management. In Lebovitz HA, editor: *Therapy for diabetes mellitus and related disorders,* Alexandria, Va, 1991, American Diabetes Association.

Debetz B: *Your diet coach,* New York, 1989, Prentice Hall.

Franz MJ: Evaluating the glycemic response to carbohydrates, *Clin Diabetes* 11:127-130, 1986.

Franz MJ: *Fast food facts,* Wayzata, Minn, 1990, DCI.

Franz MJ: *Fast food facts: nutritive and exchange values for fast-food restaurants,* Minneapolis, 1990, International Diabetes Center, DCI.

Franz MJ, Cooper N: Meal planning: adding flexibility. In Weiler C, editor: *Learning to live well with diabetes,* Minneapolis, 1991, International Diabetes Center, DCI.

Jameel N et al: Dietary protein intake is not correlated with clinical proteinuria in NIDDM, *Diabetes Care* 15(2):178-183, 1992.

Lyon R, Vinci DM: Nutrition management of insulin-dependent diabetes mellitus in adults: review by the Diabetes Care and Education Dietetic Practice Group, *J Am Diet Assoc* 93(3):309-317, 1993.

McDonald's: *Food exchanges for McDonald's menu items,* Oak Brook, Ill, McDonald's.

Oexmann MJ: *Total available glucose: a diabetic food system,* New York, 1989, William Morrow.

Powers MA, editor: *Nutrition guide for professionals,* Alexandria, Va, 1988, American Diabetes Associaton.

US Department of Agriculture/HNIS: *Food guide pyramid: a guide to daily food choices,* Washington, DC, 1992, USDA/HNIS.

***Pathophysiology***

Feldman JM: Pathophysiology of diabetes mellitus. In Galloway JA, editor: *Diabetes mellitus,* ed 9, Indianapolis, 1988, Eli Lilly.

Moller DE, Flier JS: Insulin resistance: mechanisms, syndromes, and implications, *N Eng J Med* (324):938-948, 1991.

Schwartz F: Obesity in adult females, *AAOHN J* 41(10):504-509, 1993.

Surwit RS et al: Stress and diabetes mellitus, *Diabetes Care* 15(10):1413-1422, 1992.

***Patient Teaching***

American Diabetes Association: *Goals for diabetes education,* Clinical education program, Alexandria, Va, 1989, The Association.

American Diabetes Association: *Meeting the standards: a manual for completing the American Diabetes Association application for recognition,* ed 3, Chicago, 1991, The Association.

Becton-Dickinson Consumer Products: *Managing diabetes at home,* Franklin Lakes, NJ, 1985, Becton-Dickinson.

Bode BW et al: *Diabetes Dek: how to control and manage diabetes mellitus,* Atlanta, 1992, Lifescan Infodek.

Deakins DA: Teaching elderly patients about diabetes, *Am J Nurs* 94(4):38-42, 1994.

Dolinar RO: *Diabetes 101: candy apples, log cabins and you,* Wayzata, Minn, 1989, DCI.

Eaks GA: *An evaluation of a self-instructional teaching package for the elderly with diabetes mellitus,* unpublished master's thesis, Kansas City, Kans, 1986, University of Kansas School of Nursing.

Eaks GA: *Diabetes: an owner's manual,* Kansas Diabetes Control Project, Kansas City, Kans, 1990, Cray Diabetes Education Center, University of Kansas Medical Center.

Eaks GA: *Professional prompter,* Kansas City, Kans, 1993, Cray Diabetes Education Center, University of Kansas Medical Center.

Eli Lilly: *Glucagon emergency kit,* Indianapolis, 1990, Eli Lilly.

Eli Lilly: *Low blood sugar,* Indianapolis, 1991, Eli Lilly.

Fox MA et al: Blood glucose self-monitoring usage and its influence on patient's perceptions of diabetes, *Diabetes Educator* 10(1):27-31, 1984.

Franz MJ: *Goals for diabetes education,* American Diabetes Association Task Group on Goals for Diabetes Education, Clinical education program, Alexandria, Va, 1989, The Association.

Funnell MM: Empowerment, *Pract Diabetol* 10(3):15-18, 1991.

Hamera E et al: Self-regulation in individuals with type II diabetes, *Nurs Res* 37:363-367, 1988.

Javonovic-Peterson L et al: *A touch of diabetes,* Minneapolis, 1991, DCI.

Kentucky Diabetes Foundation: *Personal guidelines: a guide to servings,* Basic counseling tool (card 12), Lexington, 1984, The Foundation.

Meichenbaum D, Turk D: *Facilitating treatment adherence: a practitioner's guide book,* New York, 1987, Plenum.

Novo-Care: *Hypoglycemia (low blood sugar),* Princeton, NJ, 1992, Novo Nordisk.

Poteet GW et al: Outcome of multiple usage of disposable syringes in the insulin-requiring diabetic, *Nurs Res* 36:350-352, 1987.

Pratt Pharmaceutical: *Self-monitoring, taking charge of your diabetes,* New York, 1992, Pfizer.

Stveiff LD: Do clients understand our instruction? *Image* 18(2):48-52, 1986.

Villagomez ET, Anding RH: Hispanic diabetic adults: special patient-teaching strategies, *Med Surg Nurs Q* 1(4):52-66, 1993.

***Prevention***

Dinsmoor RS: Better prediction spurs new approaches to prevention, *Juvenile Diabetes Foundation Int Countdown* 14(1):6-13, 1993.

Groop LC et al: Association between polymorphism of the glycogen synthase gene and non-insulin-dependent diabetes mellitus, *N Engl J Med* 328(10):568, 1993.

Leahy JL, Boyd AE: Diabetes genes in non-insulin-dependent diabetes mellitus, *N Engl J Med* 328(1):56-57, 1993.

Palmer JP: Predicting IDDM: use of humoral immune markers, *Diabetes Rev* 1(1):104-112, 1993.

US Department of Health and Human Services, *Healthy people 2000: national health promotion and disease prevention objectives,* Public Health Service: Washington, DC, 1991, US Government Printing Office.

# SECTION TWO Hepatic System

## CHAPTER 41
## Assessment of the Hepatic System


### General

Korniewicz DM et al: Integrity of vinyl and latex procedure gloves, *Nurs Res* 38:144-146, 1989.

Quigley EM et al: Hepatobiliary complications of total parenteral nutrition, *Gastroenterology* 104:286-301, 1993.

Rector WG Jr: *Complications of chronic liver disease,* St Louis, 1992, Mosby.

US Dept of Health and Human Services, Public Health Service: *Healthy people 2000: national health promotion and disease prevention objectives,* Washington, DC, 1990, US Government Printing Office.

Wungaarden JB, Smith LH, Bennett JC, editors: *Cecil textbook of medicine,* ed 19, Philadelphia, 1992, WB Saunders.


## CHAPTER 42
## Management of Persons With Problems of the Hepatic System


### Ascites

Lancaster S, Stockbridge J: PV shunts relieve ascites, *RN* 55(8):58-61, 1992.

Levine BA, Sirinek KR: The portacaval shunt—is it still indicated? *Surg Clin North Am* 70:361-377, 1990.

McCormick PA, McIntyre N: Pathogenesis and management of ascites in chronic liver disease, *Br J Hosp Med* 47(10):738-744, 1992.

Williams JW, Simel DL: Does this patient have ascites? How to divine fluid in the abdomen, *JAMA* 267(19):2645-2648, 1992.

### Assessment

Clouse ME: Current diagnostic imaging modalities of the liver, *Surg Clin North Am* 69(2):193-234, 1989.

Pagana KD, Pagana TJ: *Diagnostic testing and nursing implications: a case study approach,* ed 4, St Louis, 1994, Mosby.

Renkes J: GI endoscopy: managing the full scope of care, *Nurs 93* 23(6):50-55, 1993.

Waite WW: Clinical laboratories for the practicing pharmacist: liver function tests, *Am Pharm* NS28(12):51-55, 1988.

Wilkinson M: Nursing implications after endoscopic retrograde cholangiopancreatography, *Gastroenterol Nurs* 13(2):105-109, 1990.

### Cirrhosis

Arora S, Kaplan MM: Cirrhosis. In Rakel RE, editor: *Conn's current therapy,* ed 28, Philadelphia, 1989, WB Saunders.

Butler RW: Managing the complication of cirrhosis, *Am J Nurs* 94(3):46-49, 1994.

Covington H: Nursing care of patient with alcoholic liver disease, *Crit Care Nurs* 13(3):47-59, 1993.

### Esophageal Varices

Adams L, Soulen MC: TIPS: a new alternative for variceal bleeder, *Am J Crit Care* 2(3):196-201, 1993.

Burns SM et al: Evaluation and revision of a vasopressin/nitroglycerin protocol for use in variceal bleeding, *Am J Crit Care* 2(3):202-207, 1993.

Doherty MM, Carver DK: Transjugular intrahepatic portosystemic shunt: new relief for esophageal varices, *Am J Nurs* 93(4):58-63, 1993.

Kerber K: The adult with bleeding esophageal varices, *Crit Care Nurs Clin North Am* 5(1):153-162, 1993.

### Hepatic Tumors

Clouse ME: Hepatic artery embolization for bleeding and tumors, *Surg Clin North Am* 69:419-432, 1989.

Gullate MM, Foltz AT: Hepatic chemotherapy via implantable pump, *Am J Nurs* 83:1674-1678, 1983.

Nord HJ et al: Endoscopic diagnosis and therapy of hepatocellular carcinoma, *Endoscopy* 25:126-130, 1993.

Sato Y et al: Early recognition of hepatocellular carcinoma based on altered profiles of alpha-fetoprotein, *N Engl J Med* 328(5): 1802-1806, 1993.

Sitzman J, Order SE: Immunoradiotherapy for primary nonresectable hepatocellular carcinoma, *Surg Clin North Am* 89:393-400, 1989.

Tsukuma H et al: Risk factors for hepatocellular carcinoma among patients with chronic liver disease, *N Engl J Med* 328(25):1797-1801, 1993.

### Hepatic Trauma

Semonin-Holleran R: Critical nursing care for abdominal trauma, *Crit Care Nurse* 8(3):48-58, 1988.

### Hepatitis

Advisory Committee Immunization Practices (ACIP): Recommendation for protection against viral hepatitis, *MMWR* 39(S-2):1-26, 1990.

Alter MJ et al: The natural history of community-acquired hepatitis C in the United States, *N Engl J Med* 327(27):1899-1905, 1992.

Bloom BS et al: A reappraisal of hepatitis B virus vaccination strategies using cost-effectiveness analysis, *Ann Intern Med* 118(4):298-306, 1993.

Carey WD, Patel G: Viral hepatitis in the 1990s. Part I. Current principles of management, *Cleve Clin J Med* 59(3):317-325, 1992.

Carey WD, Patel G: Viral hepatitis in the 1990s. Part II. Hepatitis B and delta virus, *Cleve Clin J Med* 59(4):393-401, 1992.

Carey WD, Patel G: Viral hepatitis in the 1990s. Part III. Hepatitis C, hepatitis E, and other viruses, *Cleve Clin J Med* 59(6):595-601, 1992.

Czaja AJ: Chronic hepatitis C virus infection—a disease in waiting? *N Engl J Med* 327(27):1949-1950, 1992.

Franchis R et al: The natural history of asymptomatic hepatitis B surface antigen carriers, *Ann Intern Med* 118:191-194, 1993.

Gurevich I: Hepatitis. Part I. Enterically transmitted viral hepatitis: etiology, epidemiology, and prevention, *Heart Lung* 22:370-372, 1993.

Herrera JL: Hepatitis E as a cause of acute non-A, non-B hepatitis, *Arch Intern Med* 153:773-775, 1993.

Hsia PC, Seeff LB: Non-A, non-B hepatitis: impact of the emergence of the hepatitis C virus, *Adv Intern Med* 37:197-222, 1991.

Jackson MM, Rymer TE: Viral hepatitis: anatomy of a diagnosis, *Am J Nurs* 94(1):43-48, 1994.

Kelen GD et al: Hepatitis B and hepatitis C in emergency department patients, *N Engl J Med* 326(21):1399-1404, 1992.

Maddrey WC: Chronic hepatitis, *Dis Mon* 39(2):53-126, 1993.

Raloff J: Successful hepatitis A vaccine debuts, *Sci News* 142:103, 1992.

Seeff LB et al: Long-term mortality after transfusion-associated non-A, non-B hepatitis, *N Engl J Med* 327(27):1906-1911, 1992.

Smith JP: Hepatitis C: a major public health problem, *J Adv Nurs* 18(3):503-506, 1993.

### Hepatorenal Syndrome

Epstein M: The hepatorenal syndrome—newer perspectives, *N Engl J Med* 327(25):1810-1811, 1992.

Mudge C, Carlson L: Hepatorenal syndrome, *AACN Clin Issues Crit Care Nurs* 3(3):614-632, 1992.

### Liver Abscess

Frey CF et al: Liver abscesses, *Surg Clin North Am* 69:259-271, 1989.

Maxwell AJ, Mamtora H: Fungal liver abscesses in acute leukemia—a report of two cases, *Clin Radiol* 39:197-201, 1988.

***Liver Failure***

Kelso LA: Fluid and electrolyte disturbances in hepatic failure, *AACN Clin Issues Crit Care Nurs* 3(3):681-687, 1992.

Kucharski SA: Fulminant hepatic failure, *Crit Care Nurs Clin North Am* 5(1):141-151, 1993.

Martin FL: When the liver breaks down, *RN* 92:52-57, Aug 1992.

Reishtein J: Liver failure: case study of a complex problem, *Crit Care Nurse* 13(5):36-47, 1993.

Sherlock S: Fulminant hepatic failure, *Adv Intern Med* 38:245-267, 1993.

Young LM: Managing the patient with liver failure, *Med Surg Nurs* 2(4):275-281, 1993.

***Pharmacology***

Mycek MJ, Gertner SB, Perper MM: *Lippincott's illustrated reviews: pharmacology,* Philadelphia, 1992, JB Lippincott.

***Portal-Systemic Encephalopathy***

Anderson FP: Portal-systemic encephalopathy in the chronic alcoholic, *Crit Care Q* 8(4):40-52, 1989.

Kearns PJ et al: Accelerated improvement of alcoholic liver disease with enteral nutrition, *Gastroenterology* 102:200-205, 1992.

UNIT VIII

## Alterations in Digestion and Elimination

SECTION ONE **Gastrointestinal, Biliary, and Exocrine Pancreatic Systems**

CHAPTER 43

### Assessment of the Gastrointestinal, Biliary, and Exocrine Pancreatic Systems

Alford DM, Moll J: Gastrointestinal changes. In Esberger K, Hughes S: *Nursing care of the aged,* East Norwalk, Conn, 1989, Appleton & Lange.

Altman DF: Changes in gastrointestinal, pancreatic, biliary and hepatic function with aging, *Gastroenterol Clin North Am* 19(2):227-233, 1990.

Becker KL, Stevens SA: Performing in-depth abdominal assessment, *Nurs 88,* 18(6):59-63, 1988.

Bell JE, Dixon L, Sehy YA: Physical assessment: the breast, pulmonary, cardiovascular, gastrointestinal and genitourinary systems. In Chenitz WC, Stone JT, Salisbury SA: *Clinical gerontological nursing,* Philadelphia, 1991, WB Saunders.

Carr-Locke D et al: New frontiers in GI procedures, *Patient Care* 22:241-270, 1992.

Groth K: Age related changes in the gastrointestinal tract, *Geriatr Nurs* 9(5):278-280, 1988.

Holmgren C: Abdominal assessment, *RN* 55(3):28-33, 1992.

*Illustrated guide to diagnostic tests,* Springhouse, Pa, 1994, Springhouse.

Jarvis C: *Physical examination and health assessment,* Philadelphia, 1992, WB Saunders.

Jeffrey RB, Novelline RA, Ros PR: Fast track imaging in abdominal pain, *Patient Care* 22:107-140, 1992.

Lindsey M: Abdominal assessment, *Orthop Nurs* 8(4):34-38, 1989.

Massoni M: GI handbook, *Nurs 90* 20(11):65-80, 1990.

McConnell E: Auscultating bowel sounds, *Nurs 90* 20(6):76-79, 1990.

Morton PG: Improving your palpation techniques, *Nurs 89* 19(12):32C-32F, 1989.

O'Toole MT: Advanced assessment of the abdomen and gastrointestinal problems, *Nurs Clin North Am* 25(4):771-775, 1990.

Pagana KD, Pagana TJ: *Mosby's diagnostic and laboratory test reference,* St Louis, 1992, Mosby.

Renkes J: GI endoscopy—managing the full scope of care, *Nurs 93* 23(6):50-55, 1993.

Seidel HM et al: *Mosby's guide to physical examination,* ed 3, St Louis, 1995, Mosby.

Smith CE: Assessing bowel sounds, *Nurs 88* 18(2):42-44, 1988.

Taffet SL, Goldberg RJ, Kressner MS: Esophageal and gastric endoscopy in critically ill patients, *Postgrad Med* 89(4):123-126, 1991.

Wilkinson M: Nursing implications after endoscopic cholangiopancreatography, *Gastroenterol Nurs* 13(2):105-109, 1990.

CHAPTER 44

### Management of Persons With Problems of the Mouth and Esophagus

***Problems of the Mouth***

Bhasker SN, Lilly GE, Pratt LW: A practical high-yield mouth exam, *Patient Care* 24:53-74, 1990.

Mashberg A, Samit AM: Early detection, diagnosis, and management of oral and oropharyngeal cancer, *Cancer* 39:67-88, 1989.

***Esophageal Reflux Disease***

Castell DO: Esophageal disorders in the elderly, *Gastroenterol Clin North Am* 19(2):235-253, 1990.

Castell DO, Holtz A: Gastroesophageal reflux—don't forget to ask about reflux, *Postgrad Med* 86(5):141-148, 1989.

Ellis EH: Diaphragmatic hiatal hernias, *Postgrad Med* 88(1):113-124, 1990.

Gelfand MD: Gastroesophageal reflux disease, *Med Clin North Am* 75(4):923-935, 1991.

Hixson LJ et al: Current trends in the pharmacotherapy for gastroesophageal reflux disease, *Arch Intern Med* 152:717-723, 1992.

Kitchin LI, Castell DO: Rationale and efficacy of conservative therapy for gastroesophageal reflux disease, *Arch Intern Med* 151:448-453, 1991.

Richter JE: Gastroesophageal reflux: diagnosis and management, *Hosp Pract* 27(1):59-66, 1992.

Sutherland JE: Gastroesophageal reflux disease—when antacids aren't enough, *Postgrad Med* 89(7):45-53, 1991.

***Esophageal Cancer***

Foltz AT: Nutritional factors in the prevention of gastrointestinal cancer, *Semin Oncol Nurs* 4(4):239-245, 1988.

Kelsen D et al: Alarming trends in esophageal cancers, *Patient Care* 26:72-122, 1992.

Medvec BR: Esophageal cancer: treatment and nursing interventions, *Semin Oncol Nurs* 4(4):246-256, 1988.

***Achalasia***

Clouse RE, Abramson BK, Todorczuk JR: Achalasia in the elderly, *Digest Dis Sci* 36(2):225-228, 1991.

DiIorio C, Price ME: Swallowing: an assessment guide, *Am J Nurs* 90(7):38-46, 1990.

Ferguson MK: Achalasia: current evaluation and therapy, *Ann Thorac Surg* 52:336-342, 1991.

Meehan M: Nursing Dx: potential for aspiration, *RN* 55(1):30-34, 1992.

Sauer L, Pellegrini CA, Way LW: The treatment of achalasia, *Arch Surg* 124(8):929-932, 1989.

CHAPTER 45

### Management of Persons With Problems of the Stomach and Duodenum

***Obesity Surgery***

Black J, Mangan M: Body contouring and weight loss surgery for obesity, *Nurs Clin North Am* 26(3):777-789, 1991.

Bufalino J et al: Surgery for morbid obesity: the patient's experience, *Appl Nurs Res* 2(1):16-22, 1989.

Calloway CW et al: Obesity: a quartet of approaches, *Patient Care* 26:157-199, 1992.

Grace DM: Gastric restriction procedures for treating severe obesity, *Am J Clin Nutr* 55(suppl 2):556S-559S, 1992.

Kral JF: Overview of surgical techniques for treating obesity, *Am J Clin Nutr* 55(suppl 2):552S-555S, 1992.

Sugarman HJ et al: Gastric bypass for treating severe obesity, *Am J Clin Nutr* 55(suppl 2):560S-566S, 1992.

### Stress Ulcers and Gastrointestinal Bleeding

Ahern H, Rice K: How do you measure gastric pH? *Am J Nurs* 91:70-73, 1991.

Dudnick R, Martin P, Friedman LS: Management of bleeding ulcers, *Med Clin North Am* 75(4):947-961, 1991.

Eisenberg P: Monitoring gastric pH to prevent stress ulcer syndrome, *Focus Crit Care* 17:316-322, 1990.

Gardner SS, Messner RL: Gastrointestinal bleeding, *RN* (12):43-46, 1992.

Gervin AS, Gostout CJ, Zinner MJ: Upper GI bleeding: treatment options, *Patient Care* 25:59-77, 1991.

Konopad E, Noseworthy T: Stress ulceration: a serious complication in critically ill patients, *Heart Lung* 17:339-348, 1988.

Levinson M: Gastric stress ulcer, *Hosp Pract* 24:59-67, 1989.

Mertes JE: Action stat! GI bleeding, *Nurs 89* 19(8):37, 1989.

Neill KM, Rice KT, Ahern HL: Comparison of two methods of measuring gastric pH, *Heart Lung* 22(4):349-355, 1993.

Patras A: Managing GI bleeding: it takes a two tract mind, *Nurs 88* 18(4):68-74, 1988.

Perkins SB, Kennally KM: The hidden danger of internal hemorrhage, *Nurs 89* 19(7):34-41, 1989.

Pilchman J, Lefton HB, Braden GL: Cytoprotection and stress ulceration, *Med Clin North Am* 75(4):853-863, 1991.

Prevost SS, Oberle A: Stress ulceration in the critically ill patient, *Crit Care Nurs Clin North Am* 5(1):163-169, 1992.

Reinus JF, Brandt LJ: Upper and lower gastrointestinal bleeding in the elderly, *Gastroenterol Clin North Am* 19(2):293-315, 1990.

### Peptic Ulcer Disease

Clearfield HR: *Helicobacter pylori:* aggressor or innocent bystander? *Med Clin North Am* 75(4):815-829, 1991.

Clearfield HR, Wright RA: Update on peptic ulcer disease, *Patient Care* 24:28-40, 1990.

Feickert DM: Gastric surgery: your crucial pre and postop role, *RN* 50(1):24-35, 1987.

Feldman M et al: Treating ulcers and reflux: what's new, *Patient Care* 26:53-72, 1992.

Gilbert G, Chan CH, Thomas E: Peptic ulcer disease—how to treat it now, *Postgrad Med* 89(4):91-96, 1989.

Gilinsky NH: Peptic ulcer disease in the elderly, *Gastroenterol Clin North Am* 19(2):255-268, 1990.

Johns JL: When the patient has an ulcer, *RN* (11):44-50, 1991.

Katz J: The course of peptic ulcer disease, *Med Clin North Am* 75(4):831-839, 1991.

Marotta RB, Floch MH: Diet and nutrition in ulcer disease, *Med Clin North Am* 75(4):967-977, 1991.

Mertz HR, Walsh JH: Peptic ulcer pathophysiology, *Med Clin North Am* 75(4):799-811, 1991.

Sachdeva AK, Zaren HA, Sigel B: Surgical treatment of peptic ulcer disease, *Med Clin North Am* 74(4):999-1011, 1991.

Schindler BA, Ramchandani D: Psychologic factors associated with peptic ulcer disease, *Med Clin North Am* 75(4):865-873, 1991.

Wardell TL: Assessing and managing a gastric ulcer, *Nurs 91* 21(3):34-41, 1991.

### Gastric Cancer

Ajani JA, Ota DM, Jackson DT: Current strategies in the management of locoregional and metastatic gastric carcinoma, *Cancer* 67:260-265, 1991.

Barkin JS et al: What's new in stomach cancer? *Patient Care* 26:22-59, 1992.

Boddie AW Jr, McBride CM, Balch CM: Gastric cancer, *Am J Surg* 157:595-606, 1989.

Boeing H: Epidemiological research in stomach cancer: progress over the last ten years, *J Cancer Res Clin Oncol* 117:133-143, 1991.

Cady B, Rossi RL, Silverman ML: Gastric adenocarcinoma: a disease in transition, *Arch Surg* 124:303-308, 1989.

Feickert DM, Jillson E, Palazzo T: Gastrectomy for stomach carcinoma, *AORN J* 47:1396-1406, 1988.

Gohmann JJ, MacDonald JS: Chemotherapy of gastric cancer, *Cancer Invest* 7:39-52, 1989.

Hisamichi S: Screening for gastric cancer, *World J Surg* 13:31-37, 1989.

Kneller RW, McLaughlin JK, Bjelke E: A cohort study of stomach cancer in a high risk American population, *Cancer* 68:672-678, 1991.

Wang JF: Stomach cancer, *Semin Oncol Nurs* 4:257-264, 1988.

Wilke H, Preusser P, Fink V: New developments in the treatment of gastric carcinoma, *Semin Oncol* 17(suppl 2):61-70, 1990.

## CHAPTER 46
## Management of Persons With Problems of the Gallbladder and Exocrine Pancreas

### General

Anderson KN, Anderson LE, Glanze WD, editors: *Mosby's medical, nursing, and allied health dictionary,* St Louis, 1994, Mosby.

Beck M, Evans NG, editors for the Society of Gastroenterology Nurses and Associates, Core Curriculum Committee: *Gastroenterology nursing: a core curriculum,* St Louis, 1993, Mosby.

Cullen L: Interventions related to fluid and electrolyte balance, *Nurs Clin North Am* 27(2):569-597, 1992.

Price SA, Wilson LM, editors: Pathophysiology: clinical concepts of disease processes, ed 4, St Louis, 1992, Mosby.

### Gallbladder Disease

Adwers JR: Clinical trials of gallstone lithotripsy, *Hosp Pract* 24(7):83-90, 1989.

Apstein MD, Carey MC: Biliary tract stones and associated diseases. In Stein JH et al, editors: *Internal medicine,* ed 4, St Louis, 1994, Mosby.

Diehl AK: Laparoscopic cholecystectomy: too much of a good thing? *JAMA* 270(12):1469-1470, 1993.

Farha GJ, Beamer RL: New options for treating gallstone disease, *Am Fam Physician* 44(4):1295-1304, 1991.

Frazee RC et al: Open versus laparoscopic cholecystectomy, *Ann Surg* 213:651-653, 1991.

Grimaldi CH et al: Increased mortality with gallstone disease: results of a 20-year population-based survey in Pima Indians, *Ann Intern Med* 118(3):185-190, 1993.

Haicken BN: Laser laparoscopic cholecystectomy in the ambulatory setting, *J Post Anesth Nurs* 6(1):33-39, 1991.

Jurf JB, Clements L, Llorente J: Cholecystectomy made easier, *Am J Nurs* 90(12):38-39, 1990.

Lancaster S, Biaro-Marshall D: Gallstone lithotripsy, *Am J Nurs* 88:1629-1630, 1988.

Legorreta AP et al: Increased cholecystectomy rate after the introduction of laparoscopic cholecystectomy, *JAMA* 270(12): 1429-1432, 1993.

O'Donnell LD, Heaton KW: Recurrence and re-recurrence of gallstones after medical dissolution: a long-term follow-up, *Gut* 29:655-658, 1988.

Ostrow JD: Jaundice and disorders of bilirubin metabolism. In Stein JH et al, editors: *Internal medicine,* ed 4, St Louis, 1994, Mosby.

Rowland GA, Marks DA, Torres W: The new gallstone destroyers and dissolvers, *Am J Nurs* 89(11):1473-1478, 1989.

Southern Surgeons Club: A prospective analysis of 1518 laparoscopic cholecystectomies, *N Engl J Med* 324(16):1073-1078, 1991.

Stillman A: Laparoscopic cholecystectomy, *AORN J* 57(2):429-436, 1993.

Swazuk KJ, Mueller BG, Daly CJ: Laser cholecystectomy: a perioperative nursing view, *AORN J* 50:998-1001, 1004-1005, 1989.

Thistle JL et al: The natural history of cholelithiasis: the national cooperative gallstone study, *Ann Intern Med* 101:171-175, 1984.

Thistle JL et al: Dissolution of cholesterol gallbladder stones by methyl tert-butyl ether administered by percutaneous transhepatic catheter, *N Engl J Med* 320:633-639, 1989.

Torres WE, Baumgartner BR, Casarella WJ: Abnormalities of the gallbladder after extracorporeal shock-wave lithotripsy: imaging findings, *Am J Roentgenol* 159:325-327, 1992.

Way LW, Sleisenger MH: Cholelithiasis: chronic and acute cholecystitis. In Sleisenger MH, Fordtran JS, editors: *Gastrointestinal disease,* ed 4, Philadelphia, 1989, WB Saunders.

### *Pancreatic Disease*

Bagg AM: Whipple's procedure: nursing guidelines, *Crit Care Nurs* 8(5):34-45, 1988.

Birdsall C, Fiore-Lopez N: How do you manage pancreatic sump tubes? *Am J Nurs* 87:770-771, 1987.

Brown A: Acute pancreatitis: pathophysiology, nursing diagnoses, and collaborative problems, *Focus Crit Care* 18:121-130, 1991.

Fontham E, Correa P: Epidemiology of pancreatic cancer, *Surg Clin North Am* 69:551-567, 1989.

Greifzu S, Dest V: When the diagnosis is pancreatic cancer, *RN* 22(9):38-44, 1991.

Jeffres C: Complications of acute pancreatitis, *Crit Care Nurs* 9(4):38-48, 1989.

Krumberger JM: Acute pancreatitis, *Crit Care Nurs Clin North Am* 5(1):185-202, 1993.

Latifi R, McIntosh K, Dudrick S: Nutritional management of acute and chronic pancreatitis, *Surg Clin North Am* 71:579-595, 1991.

Marta MR: Endoscopic retrograde cholangiopancreatography: its role in diagnosis and treatment, *Focus Crit Care* 14(5):62-63, 1987.

Neoptolemos VP et al: Controlled trial of urgent endoscopic sphincterotomy virus conservative treatment for acute pancreatitis due to gallstones, *Lancet* 2:979-983, 1988.

Ranson JHC: Complications of pancreatitis. In Taylor MB, editor: *Gastrointestinal emergencies,* Baltimore, 1992, Williams & Wilkins.

Ranson JHC et al: Prognostic signs and nonoperative peritoneal lavage in acute pancreatitis, *Surg Gynecol Obstet* 143:209-215, 1976.

Regan PT, Go VLW: Pancreatic disease. In Stein JH et al, editors: *Internal medicine,* ed 4, St Louis, 1994, Mosby.

Smith A: When the pancreas self-destructs, *Am J Nurs* 91(9):38-48, 1991.

Steer ML: Classification and pathogenesis of pancreatitis, *Surg Clin North Am* 69:467-480, 1989.

Thelan LA et al: Gastrointestinal disorders and therapeutic management. In Thelan LA et al, editors: *Critical care nursing: diagnosis and management,* ed 2, St Louis, 1994, Mosby.

CHAPTER 47

## Management of Persons With Problems of the Intestines

### *Ileostomy/Colostomy Care*

Bates-Jensen B: Psychological response to illness: exploring two reactions to ostomy surgery, *Ostomy/Wound Manage* 23(3): 24-30, 1989.

Benedict P, Haddad A: Postop teaching for the colostomy patient, *RN* 52(3):85-90, 1989.

Blaylock B: Enhancing self care of the elderly client: practical teaching tips for ostomy care, *J ET Nurs* 18(4):118-121, 1991.

Hampton B, Bryant R: *Ostomies and continent diversions: nursing management,* St Louis, 1992, Mosby.

Krasner D: Six steps to successful stoma care, *RN* 56(7):32-38, 1993.

Long LV: Ileostomy care—overcoming the obstacles, *Nurs 91* 21(10):73-75, 1991.

Paulford-Lecher N: Teaching your patient stoma care, *Nurs 93* 23(9):47-49, 1993.

Turnball GB: Dealing with sexuality after ostomy surgery, *Progressions* 1(1):15-18, 1989.

### *Constipation and Diarrhea*

Brillman JC: Preparing for the diseases of travel, *Emerg Med* 22(10):56-72, 1990.

Jong EC: Travel-related infections, *Hosp Pract* 24(11):145-148, 1989.

McMillan SC: Validity and reliability of the constipation assessment scale, *Cancer Nurs* 12(3):183-188, 1989.

McShane RE: Constipation: impact of etiological factors, *J Gerontol Nurs* 14(4):31-34, 46-47, 1988.

Newman MD: Infectious diarrhea: major pathogens, *Physician's Assistant* 12(2):119-128, 1988.

Wadle KR: Diarrhea, *Nurs Clin North Am* 25(4):901-910, 1990.

Wald A: Constipation and fecal incontinence in the elderly, *Gastroenterol Clin North Am* 19(2):405-417, 1990.

### *Colorectal Cancer*

Ahlquist DA et al: Accuracy of fecal occult blood screening for colorectal neoplasia, *JAMA* 269(10):1262-1267, 1993.

Burris J, McGovern P: Mass colorectal cancer screening, *AAOHN J* 41(4):186-191, 1993.

Frogge MH: Future perspectives and nursing issues in gastrointestinal cancer, *Semin Oncol Nurs* 4:300-302, 1988.

Mandel JS et al: Reducing mortality from colorectal cancer by screening for fecal occult blood, *N Engl J Med* 328(19):1365-1371, 1993.

McVey L: A direct assault on abdominal cancers, *RN* 55(2):46-52, 1992.

Mendeloff AI: Diet and colorectal cancer, *Am J Clin Nutr* 48:780-781, 1988.

O'Connell MJ, Rich TA, Steele GD: Low rectal Ca: sphincter-sparing strategies, *Patient Care* 22:32-48, 1992.

Ransohoff DF, Lang CA: Sigmoidoscopic screening in the 1990's, *JAMA* 269(10):1278-1281, 1993.

Wallach CB, Kurtz RC: Gastrointestinal cancer in the elderly, *Gastroenterol Clin North Am* 19(2):419-431, 1990.

### *Inflammatory Bowel Disease*

Bayless TM, Harris MC: Inflammatory bowel disease and irritable bowel syndrome, *Med Clin North Am* 74(1):21-27, 1990.

Black M: Crohn's disease, pathophysiology, diagnosis and management, *Gastroenterol Nurs* 2(4):259-262, 1989.

Fazio VW: Conservative surgery for Crohn's disease of the small bowel: the role of strictureplasty, *Med Clin North Am* 74(1):169-181, 1990.

Grimm IS, Friedman LS: Inflammatory bowel disease in the elderly, *Gastroenterol Clin North Am* 19(2):361-385, 1990.

Hanauer SB, Peppercorn MA, Present DH: Current concepts, new therapies in IBD, *Patient Care* 22:79-102, 1992.

Jagelman DG: Surgical alternatives for ulcerative colitis, *Med Clin North Am* 74(1):155-167, 1990.

Kinash RG: IBD: implications for the patient, challenges for the nurse, *Rehabil Nurs* 34(12):82-89, 1989.

Meize-Grochowski AR: When the Dx is Crohn's disease, *RN* 54(2):52-55, 1991.

Rankin GB: Extraintestinal and systemic manifestations of inflammatory bowel disease, *Med Clin North Am* 74(1):39-49, 1990.

Whelan G: Epidemiology of inflammatory bowel disease, *Med Clin North Am* 74(1):1-11, 1990.

### *Enteral and Parenteral Nutrition*

Beck ML: Percutaneous endoscopic gastrostomy, *Am J Nurs* 89(6):76-78, 1989.

Bockus S: Troubleshooting your tube feedings, *Am J Nurs* 91(5):24-30, 1991.

Bockus S: When your patient needs tube feedings, *Nurs 93* 23(7):34-42, 1993.

Bruckstein DC: Percutaneous endoscopic gastrostomy, *Geriatr Nurs* 9(2):32-33, 1988.

Eisenberg P: Enteral nutrition: indications, formulas and delivery techniques, *Nurs Clin North Am* 24(2):315-337, 1989.

Hennessy KA: Now TPN therapy begins at home, *RN* 51(6):81-84, 1988.

Hennessy KA: Nutritional support and gastrointestinal disease, *Nurs Clin North Am* 24(2):373-381, 1989.

Irwin M: Managing leaking gastrostomy sites, *Am J Nurs* 88:359-360, 1988.

Johndrow PD: Making your patient and family feel at home with TPN, *Nurs 88* 18(10):65-69, 1988.

Klein S, Rogers R: Nutritional requirements in the elderly, *Gastroenterol Clin North Am* 19(2):473-489, 1990.

Kohn CL, Keithley JK: Enteral nutrition: potential complications and patient monitoring, *Nurs Clin North Am* 24(2):339-350, 1989.

Sitrin MD: Nutrition support in inflammatory bowel disease, *Nutr Clin Pract* 7:53-60, 1992.

Starkey JF, Jefferson PA, Kirby DF: Taking care of a percutaneous endoscopic gastrostomy, *Am J Nurs* 88:42-45, 1988.

Webber-Jones J: How to declog a feeding tube, *Nurs 92* 22(4):62-64, 1992.

Worthington PH, Wagner BA: Total parenteral nutrition, *Nurs Clin North Am* 24(2):355-369, 1989.

### *Diverticular Disease and Bowel Obstruction*

Bryant GA: When the bowel is blocked, *RN* 55(1):58-66, 1992.

Jess LW: Acute abdominal pain: revealing the source, *Nurs 93* 23(9):34-41, 1993.

Novak LT: Accelerated recovery technique: a new approach to abdominal surgery, *Nurs 92* 22(7):48-55, 1992.

Palmer RC: Diverticular disease: dietary and other measures that help control these lesions, *Consultant* 28(5):75-82, 1988.

Pickleman J, Lee R: The management of patients with suspected early postoperative small bowel obstruction, *Ann Surg* 210(2):216-221, 1989.

Roberts MK: Assessing and treating volvulus, *Nurs 92* 22(2):56-58, 1992.

## SECTION TWO Renal System

## CHAPTER 48
## Assessment of the Renal System

### *General*

Andreesen G: A fresh look at assessing the elderly, *RN* 52(6):28-40, 1989.

Chmielewski C: Renal anatomy and overview of nephron function, *ANNA J* 19(1):34-40, 1992.

Davidson RA, Wilcox CS: Newer tests for the diagnosis of renovascular disease, *JAMA* 268(23):3353-3358, 1992.

Guyton A: *Textbook of medical physiology,* ed 8, Philadelphia, 1991, WB Saunders.

Holechek MJ: Glomerular filtration rate and renal hemodynamics, *ANNA J* 19(3):237-248, 1992.

Massry S, Glassock R, editors: *Textbook of nephrology,* ed 2, Baltimore, 1989, Williams & Wilkins.

Newman DK et al: Restoring urinary continence, *Am J Nurs* 91(12):44-45, 1991.

Peschman P: Renal physiology. In Clochesy J et al: *Critical care nursing,* Philadelphia, 1993, WB Saunders.

Powers I, William D: Urinary incontinence, *Nurs 92* 22(12):46-47, 1992.

Preisig P: Urinary concentration and dilution, *ANNA J* 19(4):351-355, 1992.

Resnick B: Retraining the bladder after catheterization, *Am J Nurs* 93(11):46-49, 1993.

Tanagho EA, McAninch JW, editors: *Smith's general urology,* East Norwalk, Conn, 1992, Appleton & Lange.

Wiseman KC: Nephrotic syndrome: pathophysiology and treatment, *ANNA J* 18(5):469-478, 1991.

## CHAPTER 49
## Management of Persons With Problems of the Kidney and Urinary Tract

### *Renal Calculi*

Coe FL, Parks JH, Asplin JR: The pathogenesis and treatment of kidney stones, *N Engl J Med* 327(16):1141-1152, 1992.

Curhan GC et al: A prospective study of dietary calcium and other nutrients and the risk of symptomatic kidney stones, *N Engl J Med* 328(12):833-838, 1993.

### *Cancer and Urinary Diversion*

American Cancer Society: *Cancer facts and figures—1994,* Atlanta, 1994, The Society.

Benson M, Olsson C: Urinary diversion, *Urol Clin North Am* 19(4):779-795, 1992.

Bristol-Myers Squibb Company: *For a better way of living with a urostomy: the Durahesive Sur-Fit way,* Princeton, NJ, 1992, Convatec.

Bristol-Myers Squibb Company: *Living with a urostomy the easy, active life way,* Princeton, NJ, 1992, Convatec.

Faller NA, Lawrence KG: Obtaining a urine specimen form a conduit urostomy, *Am J Nurs* 94(1):97, 1994.

Hampton BG, Bryant RA: *Ostomies and continent diversions,* St Louis, 1992, Mosby.

Heneghan GM et al: The Indiana pouch: a continent urinary diversion, *J Enter Ther* 17:231-236, 1990.

Licklinder D, Mauffray D: Conventional urostomy vs continent urostomy, *Ostomy/Wound Manage* 34:26-29, 1991.

Moon S et al: Treating bladder cancer: new methods and new management, *Am J Nurs* 93(5):32-39, 1993.

Neil JV: What's wrong with this peristomal skin? *Am J Nurs* 91(1):28-34, 1991.

Smith DB, Babaian RJ: Patient adjustment to an ileal conduit after cystectomy, *Enter Ther* 16:244-246, 1989.

Tootla J, Easterling AD: Current options in bladder cancer management, *RN* 55(4):42-49, 1992.

## CHAPTER 50
## Management of Persons With Renal Failure

### *Renal Failure*

Baer C, Lancaster L: Acute renal failure, *Crit Care Q* 14(1):1-21, 1992.

Butler B: Nutritional management of catabolic acute renal failure requiring renal replacement therapy, *ANNA J* 18(3):247-259, 1991.

Flaherty JM, O'Brien ME: Family styles in coping with end-stage renal disease, *ANNA J* 19(4):345-349, 1992.

Latham D, Nichols E: Epoetin alpha: patient management issues and development through recombinant DNA technology, *ANNA J* 17(4):311-316, 1990.

Levinsky NG, Pettig RA: The medical end-stage renal disease program, *N Engl J Med* 324(16):1143-1148, 1991.

Price C: Continuous renal replacement therapy: the treatment of choice for acute renal failure, *ANNA J* 18(3):239-244, 1991.

Shusterman N et al: Risk factors and outcome of hospital-acquired acute renal failure, *Am J Med* 83:65-71, 1987.

Whittaker A: Patients with acute renal failure. In Clochesy J et al: *Critical care nursing*, Philadelphia, 1993, WB Saunders.

Yarian S: Patients with end-stage renal disease. In Clochesy J et al: *Critical care nursing*, Philadelphia, 1993, WB Saunders.

***Dialysis***

Bosworth C: SCUF/CAVH/CAVD: critical differences, *Crit Care Nurs Q* 14(4):45-55, 1992.

Counts C: Potential complications of the internal vascular access: implications for nursing, *Dialysis Transplant* 22(2):75-87, 105, 1993.

Dunn SA: How to care for the dialysis patient, *Am J Nurs* 93(6):26-33, 1993.

Graham-Macaluso MM: Complications of peritoneal dialysis: nursing care plans to document teaching, *ANNA J* 18(3):479-483, 1991.

Massry SG: Nephrology, *JAMA* 270(2):227-228, 1993.

Nissenson AR, Fine RN, editors: *Dialysis therapy*, ed 2, St Louis, 1993, Mosby.

Stark JL: Dialysis options in the critically ill patient: hemodialysis, peritoneal dialysis, and continuous renal replacement therapy, *Crit Care Nurs Q* 14(4):40-44, 1992.

Threlkeld JS: Nursing implications in kinetic modeling, *ANNA J* 19(2):178-181, 1992.


UNIT IX

# Alterations in Reproduction and Sexuality

CHAPTER 51

## Assessment of Reproduction and Sexuality


***Anatomy and Physiology***

Hamm T: Physiology of normal female bleeding, *NAACOGS Clin Issues Perinat Womens Health Nurs* 2(3):289-293, 1991.

Tortora GJ, Anagnostakos NP: *Principles of anatomy and physiology*, New York, 1990, Harper & Row.

***Assessment***

Barkauskas VH et al: *Health and physical assessment*, St Louis, 1994, Mosby.

Bates B: *A guide to physical examination and history taking*, ed 5, Philadelphia, 1991, JB Lippincott.

Blesch KS, Prohaska TR: Cervical cancer screening in older women: issues and interventions, *Cancer Nurs* 14(3):141-147, 1991.

Bowers AC, Thompson JM: *Clinical manual of health assessment*, St Louis, 1992, Mosby.

Gould D: Assessing menstrual cycle function, *Nurs Stand* 6(23):24-27, 1992.

Pritchard JA, MacDonald PC, Gant NF: *Williams' obstetrics*, ed 17, East Norwalk, Conn, 1989, Appleton-Century-Crofts.

Robie PW: Cancer screening in the elderly, *J Am Geriatr Soc* 37:888-893, 1989.

Seidel HM et al: *Mosby's guide to physical examination*, ed 3, St Louis, 1995, Mosby.

Szydlo VL: Approaching a male adolescent about a pelvic exam, *Am J Nurs* 88:1052-1056, 1988.

***Physiologic Changes With Aging***

Ebersole P, Hess P: *Toward healthy aging*, ed 4, St Louis, 1994, Mosby.

***Diagnostic Tests***

Koss, LG: The Papanicolaou test for cervical cancer detection: a triumph and a tragedy, *JAMA* 261:737-743, 1989.

Modica MM, Timor-Tritsch IE: Transvaginal sonography provides a sharper view into the pelvis, *J Obstet Gynecol Neonatal Nurs* 17:89-95, 1988.

Pagana KD, Pagana TJ: *Mosby's diagnostic and laboratory test reference*, St Louis, 1992, Mosby.

Wheat ME, Mandelblatt JS, Kunitz G: Pap smear screening in women 65 and older, *J Am Geriatr Soc* 36:827-830, 1988.


CHAPTER 52

## Management of Women With Reproductive Problems


***Infectious Processes***

Biswas MK: Bacterial vaginosis, *Clin Obstet Gynecol* 36:166-176, 1993.

Grant MM, Davidson SB: Assessment of vaginitis. In Frank-Stromborg M: *Instruments for clinical nursing research*, East Norwalk, Conn, 1988, Appleton & Lange.

Heine P, McGregor JA: *Trichomonas vaginalis:* a reemerging pathogen, *Clin Obstet Gynecol* 36:137-144, 1993.

McNeeley SG: Pelvic inflammatory disease, *Curr Opin Obstet Gynecol* 4(5):682-686, 1992.

Sobel JD: Vaginitis in adult women, *Obstet Gynecol Clin North Am* 17:851-879, 1990.

Sobel JD: Candidal vulvovaginitis, *Clin Obstet Gynecol* 36:153-165, 1993.

Stacey CM, Barton SE, Singer A: Pelvic inflammatory disease. In Studd J: *Progress in obstetrics and gynecology*, vol 9, Edinburgh, 1991, Churchill Livingstone.

Williams D, Riddle J: Understanding salpingitis: a pelvic inflammatory infection, *Prof Nurs* 6:217-220, 1991.

***Menstrual Disorders***

Ball KA: Laser endometrial ablation treatment of dysfunctional uterine bleeding, *AORN J* 48:1153-1164, 1988.

Barber HR: *Perimenopausal and geriatric gynecology*, New York, 1988, Macmillan.

Booten DA, Seideman RY: Relationship between premenstrual syndrome and dysmenorrhea, *AAOHN J* 37(8):308-315, 1989.

Bowman JA: More on lasers . . . endometrial ablation with rollerball electrode: an alternative to hysterectomy, *AORN J* 54:960, 1991.

Brinton LA: Menopause and the risk of breast cancer, *Ann NY Acad Sci* 592:357-362, 1990.

Bush TL: The epidemiology of cardiovascular disease in postmenopausal women, *Ann NY Acad Sci* 592:263-271, 1990.

Charles AG: Estrogen replacement after menopause, when is it warranted? *Postgrad Med* 85(4):99-104, 1989.

Collins J: Menopause, *Prim Care* 15:602-605, 1988.

Corson ST: Physiology of menopause and update on hormonal replacement therapy, *NAACOGS Clin Issues Perinat Women's Health Nurs* 2:483-496, 1991.

Cortese J, Brown MA: Coping responses of men whose partners experience premenstrual symptomatology, *J Obstet Gynecol Neonatal Nurs* 18:405-412, 1989.

Dawson-Hughes B et al: A controlled trial of the effect of calcium supplementation on bone density in postmenopausal women, *N Engl J Med* 323:878-883, 1990.

Doll H et al: Pyridoxime and the premenstrual syndrome: a randomized crossover trial, *J R Coll Gen Pract* 39:364, 1989.

Ensign JE et al: Premenstrual syndrome, *AORN J* 47(4):962-971, 1988.

Freeman EW, Sondheimer SJ, Rickels K: Effects of medical history factors on symptoms severity in women meeting criteria for premenstrual syndrome, *Obstet Gynecol* 72:236, 1988.

Freeman SB: Management of perimenopausal symptoms, *NAACOGS Clin Issues Perinat Women's Health Nurs* 2:429-439, 1991.

Gannon L: The potential role of exercise in the alleviation of menstrual disorders and menopausal symptoms: a theoretical synthesis of recent research, *Women Health* 14(2):105-127, 1988.

Heitkemper MN, Shaver JF, Mitchell ES: Gastrointestinal symptoms and patterns across the menstrual cycle in dysmenorrhea, *Nurs Res* 37:108-113, 1988.

Higham JM: Medical treatment of menorrhagia. In Studd J, editor: *Progress in obstetrics and gynaecology,* vol 9, Edinburgh, 1991, Churchill Livingstone.

Higham JM, O'Brien PMS, Shaw RW: Assessment of menstrual blood loss using a pictorial chart, *Br J Obstet Gynaecol* 97:734-739, 1990.

Hsia L, Long M: Premenstrual syndrome: current concepts in diagnosis and management, *J Nurse Midwife* 35:351, 1990.

Jackson KD: Endometrial ablation with rollerball electrode, *AORN J* 54:265-282, 1991.

Kronenberg F: Hot flashes: epidemiology and physiology, *Ann NY Acad Sci* 592:52, 1990.

Lichtman RC: Perimenopausal hormone replacement therapy: review of the literature, *J Nurse Midwife* 36(1):30-48, 1991.

Lindow K: Premenstrual syndrome: family impact and nursing implications, *J Obstet Gynecol Nurs* 20:135-138, 1991.

Lobo RA: Estrogen and cardiovascular disease, *Ann NY Acad Sci* 592:286-294, 1990.

Longcope C: Hormone dynamics at the menopause, *Ann NY Acad Sci* 592:21, 1990.

Maddox MA: Women at midlife: hormone replacement therapy, *Nurs Clin North Am* 27:959-969, 1992.

Mortola JF, Girton L, Yen SSC: Depressive episodes in premenstrual syndrome, *Am J Obstet Gynecol* 161:1682, 1989.

Murata J: Primary amenorrhea, *Pediatr Nurs* 15:125-129, 1989.

Murata J: Abnormal genital bleeding and secondary amenorrhea: common gynecological problems, *J Obstet Gynecol Neonatal Nurs* 19:26-36, 1990.

Rapkin AJ, Chang LI, Reading AE: Mood and cognitive style in premenstrual syndrome, *Obstet Gynecol* 74:644, 1989.

Ravnikar V: Physiology and treatment of hot flashes, *Obstet Gynecol* 75(suppl):3-8, 1990.

Saver CL: Rollerball endometrial ablation: new treatment options for women, *Today's OR Nurse* 14:11-14, 1992.

Shapiro S: Treatment of dysmenorrhea and premenstrual syndrome with non-steroidal antiinflammatory drugs, *Drugs* 36:484, 1988.

Smith S, Schiff I: The premenstrual syndrome: diagnosis and management, *Fertil Steril* 52:527, 1989.

Stevenson JC et al: Dietary intake of calcium and postmenopausal bone loss, *Br Med J* 297:15-17, 1988.

Wickes S: Premenstrual syndrome, *Prim Care* 13:480, 1988.

Youngs DD: Some misconceptions concerning the menopause, *Obstet Gynecol* 75:881-883, 1990.


### *Cancer of the Female Genital Tract*


Berger PH, Saul HM: Radical hysterectomy: treatment for advanced cervical carcinoma, *AORN J* 52:1212-1222, 1990.

Bernhard LA: Consequences of hysterectomy in the lives of women, *Health Care Women Int* 13:281-291, 1992.

Bernhard LA: Men's views about hysterectomies and women who have them, *Image* 24:177-181, 1992.

Campion MJ, Reid R: Screening for gynecologic cancer, *Obstet Gynecol Clin North Am* 17:695-727, 1990.

Cohen SM, Hollingsworth AO, Rubin M: Another look at psychologic complications of hysterectomy, *Image* 21:51-53, 1989.

Corney R et al: The care of patients undergoing surgery for gynecological cancer: the need for information, emotional support and counselling, *J Adv Nurs* 17:667-671, 1992.

Dobkin PL, Bradley I: Assessment of sexual dysfunction in oncology patients: review, critique, and suggestions, *J Psychosoc Oncol* 9:43-74, 1991.

Dulaney PE, Crawford VC, Turner C: A comprehensive education and support program for women experiencing hysterectomies, *J Obstet Gynecol Neonatal Nurs* 19:319-325, 1989.

Eriksson JH, Walczak JR: Ovarian cancer, *Semin Oncol Nurs* 6:214-227, 1990.

Graff BM et al: Development of a postoperative self-assessment form, *Clin Nurse Spec* 6:47-50, 1992.

Gurganus S, Morris J: Pelvic exenteration: the challenge of rehabilitation in a patient with multiple psychosocial problems, *J Enter Ther* 18:52, 1991.

Hubbard JL, Holcombe JK: Cancer of the endometrium, *Semin Oncol Nurs* 6:206-213, 1990.

Kaplan A: Endometrial carcinoma, *Hosp Med* 23:79, 1989.

Lamb M: Psychosexual issues: the woman with gynecologic cancer, *Semin Oncol Nurs* 6:237-243, 1990.

Lowdermilk D: Nursing care update: internal radiation therapy, *NAACOGS Clin Issues Perinat Women's Health Nurs* 1:532-541, 1990.

McKenzie F: Sexuality after total pelvic exenteration, *Nurs Times* 84:27-30, 1988.

McMullin M: Holistic care of the patient with cervical cancer, *Nurs Clin North Am* 27:847-858, 1991.

Mishel MH, Sorenson DS: Uncertainty in gynecological cancer: a test of the mediating functions of mastery and coping, *Nurs Res* 40:167-171, 1991.

Nolte S, Hanjani P: Intraepithelial neoplasia of the lower genital tract, *Semin Oncol Nurs* 6:181-189, 1990.

Piver S et al: Epidemiology and etiology of ovarian cancer, *Semin Oncol* 18:177, 1991.

Rostad ME: The radical vulvectomy patient: preventing complications, *DCCN J* 7:289-294, 1988.

Rubin SC, Sutton GP: *Ovarian cancer,* New York, 1993, McGraw-Hill.

Schultz W et al: Psychosexual functioning after the treatment of cancer of the vulva, *Cancer* 66:402-407, 1990.

Schumaker D: Preventing gynecologic cancer: every woman's guide, *Can Nurs* 87:23-24, 1991.

Seeley T: Estrogen replacement therapy after hysterectomy, *Br Med J* 305:811-812, 1992.

Shell J: Sexuality for patients with gynecologic cancer, *NAACOGS Clin Issues Perinat Women's Health Nurs* 1:479-494, 1990.

Smith D: Sexual rehabilitation of the cancer patient, *Cancer Nurs* 12:10-15, 1989.

Strohl R: External beam radiation in gynecologic cancers, *NAACOGS Clin Issues Perinat Women's Health Nurs* 1:525-531, 1990.

Strohl R: Radiation therapy: recent advances and nursing implications, *Nurs Clin North Am* 25:309-329, 1990.

Thompson L: Importance of pre-operative dialogue in pelvic surgery, *Can OR Nurs J* 6:22-23, 1988.

Thompson L: Cancer of the cervix, *Semin Oncol Nurs* 6:190-197, 1990.

Whale Z: A threat to femininity? Minimizing side-effects in pelvic irradiation, *Prof Nurs* 6:309-312, 1991.

Williamson ML: Sexual adjustment after hysterectomy, *J Obstet Gynecol Neonatal Nurs* 21:42-47, 1992.

Wolenski M, Pelosi MA: Laparoscopic hysterectomy, *Todays OR Nurse* 13:23-29, 1991.

Woods N, Lewis F, Ellison E: Living with cancer: family experiences, *Cancer Nurs* 12:28-33, 1989.

Zimny M: Ovarian cancer: a nursing overview, *Oncology* 5:147, 1991.


### *Benign Tumors of the Female Genital Tract*


Adamson GD: Surgical and medical treatment of endometriosis, *Contemp Obstet Gynecol* 36:48-63, 1991.

Moore J: Vaginal hysterectomy: its success as an outpatient procedure, *AORN J* 48:1114, 1116-1120, 1988.

Parker W: Management of ovarian cysts by operative laparoscopy, *Contemp Obstet Gynecol* 36:47-58, 1991.

Wilson E: Surgical therapy for endometriosis, *Clin Obstet Gynecol* 31:859, 1988.

### *Gynecologic Health and the Aging Process*

Blesch KS, Prohaska TR: Cervical cancer screening in older women, *Cancer Nurs* 10:141-147, 1991.

Denny MS, Koren ME, Wisby M: Gynecological health needs of elderly women, *J Gerontol Nurs* 15:33-37, 1989.

Diekmann JM: Cancer in the elderly: systems overview, *Semin Oncol Nurs* 4:169-177, 1988.

Hogstel MO: *Nursing care of the older adult,* Albany, NY, 1994, Delmar.

### *Infertility*

Cook AS, Rock JA: The role of laparoscopy in the treatment of endometriosis, *Fertil Steril* 55:663-680, 1991.

Frank DI: Factors related to decisions about infertility treatment, *J Obstet Gynecol Neonatal Nurs* 19:162-167, 1989.

Garner C: *Principles of infertility nursing,* Boca Raton, Fla, 1991, CRC Press.

Halman LJ, Abbey A, Andrews FM: Attitudes about infertility interventions among fertile and infertile couples, *Am J Public Health* 82:191-194, 1992.

Hirsch AM, Hirsch SM: The effect of infertility on marriage and self-concept, *J Obstet Gynecol Neonatal Nurs* 18:13-20, 1989.

James CA: The nursing role in assisted reproductive technologies, *NAACOGS Clin Issues Perinat Women's Health Nurs* 3:328-334, 1992.

Kuczynski HJ: The holistic health care of couples undergoing IVF/ET, *Midwives Chron Nurs Notes* 102:9-11, 1989.

Rabar FG: Gamete intrafallopian transfer, *AORN J* 53:1466-1475, 1991.

White GB: Understanding the ethical issues in infertility nursing practice, *NAACOGS Clin Issues Perinat Women's Health Nurs* 3:347-352, 1992.

Woods NF, Olshansky E, Draye MA: Infertility: women's experiences, *Health Care Women Int* 12:179-190, 1991.

Zion AB: Resources for infertile couples, *J Obstet Gynecol Neonatal Nurs* 17:255-258, 1988.

Zion AB: Unblocking fallopian tubes (clinical update), *Nurs 91* 21:70-71, 1991.

CHAPTER 53

## Management of Men With Reproductive Problems

### *Problems of the Testes and Related Structures*

Blackmore C: The impact of orchidectomy upon the sexuality of the man with testicular cancer, *Cancer Nurs* 11(1):33-40, 1988.

Blank B, Schneider R: Acute scrotal problems, *Patient Care* 24(11):152-155, 158, 1990.

Friman P, Finney J: Health education for testicular cancer, *Health Educ Q* 17(4):443-453, 1990.

Jenkins B, Carbaugh C: Action stat: testicular torsion, *Nurs 89* 19(7):33, 1989.

Lasater S: Testicular cancer, a perioperative challenge, *AORN J* 51(2):513-526, 1990.

Millon-Underwood S: Factors influencing early detection of prostate cancer, *Appl Nurs Res* 5(1):30-31, 1992.

### *Problems of the Prostate*

Andriole G, Winfield H: New options in urology, *Patient Care* 27(1):12-27, 1993.

Bruskewitz R, Cassel C: Benign prostatic hyperplasia: intervene or wait? *Hosp Pract* 26:99-115, 1992.

Fleming C et al: A decision analysis of alternative treatment strategies for clinically localized prostate cancer, *JAMA* 269(20):2650-2658, 1993.

Littrup P, Lee F, Mettlin C: Prostate cancer screening: current trends and future implications, *CA* 42(4):198-209, 1992.

Moore S et al: Nerve-sparing prostatectomy, *Am J Nurs* 92:59-64, 1992.

Stevens J, Miller J: Transrectal ultrasound, an aid to diagnosing prostate cancer, *AORN J* 53(5):1166-1178, 1991.

Taylor T: Endocrine therapy for advanced stage D prostate cancer, *Urol Nurs* 12(9):22-26, 1991.

Wozniak-Petrofsky J: BPH: treating older men's most common problem, *RN* 54(7):32-37, 1991.

### *Problems of the Penis*

Bryant R, Boarini J: Treatment options for men with sexual dysfunction, *JET* 19(4):131-142, 1992.

Cozad J: Impotence: psychosocial aspects, evaluation methods and treatment, *Urol Nurs* 9(2):10-12, 1988.

Lasater S: Cancer of the penis: perioperative interventions, *AORN J* 56(1):19-30, 1992.

Mackey V: Another look at the circumcision debate: options of nursing-home caregivers, *Nurs Practitioner* 17(3):63-73, 1992.

CHAPTER 54

## Management of Persons With Problems of the Breast

### *General*

Baird SB, McCorkle R, Grant M: *Cancer nursing: a comprehensive textbook,* Philadelphia, 1991, WB Saunders.

Clark JC, editor: *Core curriculum for oncology nursing,* ed 2, Philadelphia, 1992, WB Saunders.

Mitchell GW, Bassett LW, editors: *The female breast and its disorders,* Baltimore, 1991, Williams & Wilkins.

### *Adjuvant Therapy*

Chittoor SR, Swain SM: Adjuvant therapy in early breast cancer, *Am Fam Physician* 44(2):453-461, 1991.

Dow KM, Hilderley LJ, editors: *Nursing care in radiation therapy,* Philadelphia, 1992, WB Saunders.

Gelber RD, Goldhirsch A, Coataes AS: Adjuvant therapy for breast cancer: understanding the overview, *J Clin Oncol* 11(3):580-585, 1993.

Sparano JA: The potential role of biological agents in the management of breast cancer, *Mediguide Oncol* 12(1):1-7, 1992.

Veronesi U et al: Radiotherapy after breast-preserving surgery in women with localized cancer of the breast, *N Engl J Med* 328(22):1587-1591, 1991.

### *Diet and Breast Cancer*

Freedman LS et al: Dietary fat and breast cancer: where we are, *J Natl Cancer Inst* 85(10):764-765, 1993.

Kushi LH et al: Dietary fat and postmenopausal breast cancer, *J Natl Cancer Inst* 84:1092-1099, 1992.

### *Genetic Issues*

Biesecker BB et al: Genetic counseling for families with inherited susceptibility to breast and ovarian cancer, *JAMA* 269(15):1970-1974, 1993.

King MC, Rowell S, Love SM: Inherited breast and ovarian cancer, *JAMA* 269(15):1975-1980, 1993.

### *Prevention of Breast Cancer*

Digman D et al: Measuring the use of mammography: two methods compared, *Am J Public Health* 82(10):1386-1388, 1992.

Frank-Stromborg M, Olsen SJ, editors: *Cancer prevention in minority populations: cultural implications for health care professionals,* St Louis, 1993, Mosby.

Grier S: Breast cancer: prevention and detection, *Oncol Patient Care* 3(1):5-13, 1993.

Wells BL, Horm JW: Stage at diagnosis in breast cancer: race and socioeconomic factors, *Am J Public Health* 82(10):1383-1385, 1992.

### Psychosocial Issues

Germino BB: Quality of life for families with cancer: research issues, *Qual Life* 2(2):39-45, 1993.

Wegmann JA: Sources of anxiety: what breast cancer patients worry about most, *Oncol Patient Care* 3(1):1-16, 1993.

### Quality of Life

Caird FI, Brewin TB, editors: *Cancer in the elderly,* Boston, 1990, Butterworth.

Ferrell BR: Overview of breast cancer: quality of life, *Oncol Patient Care* 3(1):7-8, 1993.

### Sexuality and Body Image

Granai CO et al: Female sexuality and cancer, *Clin Adv Oncol Nurs* 3(2):1-9, 1991.

Kaplan HS: A neglected issue: the sexual side effects of current treatments for breast cancer, *J Sex Marital Ther* 18(1):3-19, 1992.

Mock F: Body image in women treated for breast cancer, *Nurs Res* 42(3):153-158, 1993.

CHAPTER 55

## Management of Persons With Sexually Transmitted Diseases

Aronson MD, Phillips RS: Screening young men for chlamydial infection, *JAMA* 270:2097-2098, 1993.

Bolus J: Teaching teens about condoms, *RN* 57(3):44-47, 1994.

Cates W et al: Commentary: the quest for women's prophylactic methods—hopes vs. science, *Am J Public Health* 82:1479-1482, 1992.

Cook LS et al: Circumcision and sexually transmitted diseases, *Am J Public Health* 84:197-201, 1994.

Gadde J et al: Clinical experience with penicillin skin testing in a large inner-city STD clinic, *JAMA* 270:2456-2463, 1993.

Genc M et al: An economic evaluation of screening for *Chlamydia trachomatis* in adolescent males, *JAMA* 270:2057-2064, 1993.

Greendale GA et al: The relationship of *Chlamydia trachomatis* infection and male infertility, *Am J Public Health* 83:996-1001, 1993.

Handsfield HH: A comparison of single-dose cefoxime with ceftriaxone as treatment for uncomplicated gonorrhea, *N Engl J Med* 325(19):1337-1341, 1991.

Richert CA et al: A method for identifying persons at high risk for sexually transmitted infections: opportunity for targeting intervention, *Am J Public Health* 83:520-524, 1993.

Roper WL et al: Commentary: condoms and HIV/STD prevention—clarifying the message, *Am J Public Health* 83:501-503, 1993.

Rosenberg MJ, Gollub EL: Commentary: methods women can use that may prevent sexually transmitted disease, including HIV, *Am J Public Health* 82:1473-1478, 1992.

Shafer MA et al: Evaluation of urine-based screening strategies to detect *Chlamydia trachomatis* among sexually active asymptomatic young males, *JAMA* 270:2065-2070, 1993.

US Department of Health and Human Services, Public Health Service: Decreased susceptibility of *Neisseria gonorrhoeae* to fluoroquinolones—Ohio and Hawaii, 1992-1994, *MMWR* 43:325-327, 1994.

Workowski KA et al: Long-term eradication of *Chlamydia trachomatis* genital infection after antimicrobial therapy, *JAMA* 270:2071-2075, 1993.

UNIT X

# Alterations in Cognition, Sensation, and Motion

SECTION ONE **Nervous System**

CHAPTER 56

## Assessment of the Nervous System

### General

Ackerman L: Interventions related to neurologic care, *Nurs Clin North Am* 27(2):325-335, 1992.

Boss B: Memory impairment: forgetfulness vs. amnesia, *J Neurosci Nurs* 20:151-158, 1988.

Dittmar S: *Rehabilitation nursing: process and application,* St Louis, 1989, Mosby.

Emich-Herring B, Wood P: A team approach to neurological based swallowing disorders, *Rehabil Nurs* 15:242-247, 1990.

Glick OJ: Normal thought processes: an overview, *Nurs Clin North Am* 28(4):715-727, 1993.

Grant J, King M: Validity of nursing diagnosis, *Res Nurs Health* 13(6):403-410, 1990.

Hickey J: *Neurological and neurosurgical nursing,* ed 3, Philadelphia, 1992, JB Lippincott.

Keller C et al: Psychological responses to aphasia: theoretical considerations and nursing implications, *J Neurosci Nurs* 21:290-294, 1989.

Mauser G: Neuromuscular respiratory failure—what the nurse knows makes a difference, *J Neurosci Nurs* 20:110-117, 1988.

Morgan S: A passage through paralysis, *Am J Nurs* 92(4):54-58, 1992.

Olson E et al: The hazards of immobility, *Am J Nurs* 90(3):43-48, 1990.

Rankin J: The nursing diagnosis: swallowing, impaired and bedside assessment of swallowing in neurologically involved cases, *J Neurosci Nurs* 24:117-118, 1992.

Snyder M, editor: *A guide to neurological and neurosurgical nursing,* ed 2, New York, 1991, Delmar.

St George CL: Spasticity: mechanisms and nursing care, *Nurs Clin North Am* 28(4):819-827, 1993.

US Department of Health and Human Services, Public Health Service: *Healthy people 2000: national health promotion and disease prevention objectives,* Washington, DC, 1990, US Government Printing Office.

Wilson LD: Sensory perceptual alteration: diagnosis, prediction, and intervention in the hospitalized adult, *Nurs Clin North Am* 28(4):747-765, 1993.

Zasler N: Sexuality in neurologic disability: an overview, *Sexual Disabil* 9(1):11-27, 1991.

Zasler N, Kreutzer J: Family and sexuality after traumatic brain injury. In Williams J, King T, editors: *Impact of head injury on the family system: an overview for professionals,* Baltimore, 1990, Paul Brooke.

CHAPTER 57

## Management of Persons With Problems of the Brain

### Assessment

Baggerly J: Sensory perceptual problems following stroke: the invisible deficits, *Nurs Clin North Am* 26(4):997-1005, 1991.

Baker DM: Assessment and management of impairments in swallowing, *Nurs Clin North Am* 28(4):793-805, 1993.

Barker E: Cranial nerve assessment, *RN* 55(5):62-69, 1992.

Barker E, Moore E: Neurological assessment, *RN* 55(4):28-35, 1992.

Dykes P: Minding the five P's of neurovascular assessment, *Am J Nurs* 93(6):38-39, 1993.

Jess L: Investigating impaired mental status: an assessment guide you can use, *Nurs 88* 18(6):42-50, 1988.

Jones A et al: Side effects following metrizamide myelography and lumbar laminectomy, *J Neurosci Nurs* 21:290-294, 1987.

Lord-Feroli K, Maguire-McGinley M: Toward a more objective approach to pupil assessment, *J Neurosurg Nurs* 17:309-312, 1990.

Lower J: Rapid neuro assessment, *Am J Nurs* 92(6):38-45, 1992.

*Mosby's medical, nursing, and allied health dictionary,* St Louis, 1994, Mosby.

Olson E: Perceptual deficits affecting the stroke patient, *Rehabil Nurs* 16(4):212-213, 1991.

Phipps MA: Assessment of neurologic deficits in stroke: acute-care and rehabilitation implications, *Nurs Clin North Am* 26(4):957-970, 1991.

Stevens S, Becker K: A simple, step-by-step approach to neurological assessment. Part 1, *Nurs 88* 18(9):53-61, 1988.

Stevens S, Becker K: A simple, step-by-step approach to neurological assessment. Part 2, *Nurs 88* 18(10):51-58, 1988.

Sullivan J: Neurologic assessment, *Nurs Clin North Am* 25(4):795-809, 1990.

Tortora G, Anagnostakos N: *Principles of anatomy and physiology,* New York, 1990, Harper & Row.

### Altered Levels of Consciousness

Ackerman LL: Alteration in level of responsiveness: a proposed nursing diagnosis, *Nurs Clin North Am* 28(4):729-745, 1993.

Maher M, Strong S: Organ donation: a nursing perspective, *J Neurosci Nurs* 21:357-361, 1989.

Mauss-Clum N et al: Locked in syndrome: a team approach, *J Neurosci Nurs* 23:273-286, 1991.

Tosch P: Patients' recollections of their posttraumatic coma, *J Neurosci Nurs* 20:223-228, 1988.

### Alzheimer's Disease and Dementia

Abraham IL et al: Care environments for patients with Alzheimer's disease, *Nurs Clin North Am* 29(1):157-172, 1994.

Abraham IL et al: Multidisciplinary assessment of patients with Alzheimer's disease, *Nurs Clin North Am* 29(1):113-128, 1994.

Algase D: Cognitive discriminants of wandering among nursing home residents, *Nurs Res* 41(2):78-81, 1992.

Burns E, Buckwalter K: Pathophysiology and etiology of Alzheimer's disease, *Nurs Clin North Am* 23(1):11-30, 1988.

Collins CE, Given B, Given CW: Interventions with family caregivers of persons with Alzheimer's disease, *Nurs Clin North Am* 29(1):195-207, 1994.

Davis K et al: A double-blind, placebo-controlled multicenter study of tacrine for Alzheimer's disease, *N Engl J Med* 327(18):1253-1259, 1992.

Duffey B: Demented, old and alone, *Am J Nurs* 89(2):212-218, 1989.

Finocchiaro D, Hersfeld S: Understanding Alzheimer's disease, *Am J Nurs* 90(9):56-60, 1990.

Given C et al: Source of stress among families caring for relatives with Alzheimer's disease, *Nurs Clin North Am* 23(1):69-82, 1988.

Gray-Vickrey P: Evaluating Alzheimer's patients: the importance of being thorough, *Nurs 88* 18(12):34-41, 1988.

Hall G: This hospital patient has Alzheimer's, *Am J Nurs* 91(10):45-52, 1987.

Hall GR: Caring for people with Alzheimer's disease using the conceptual model of progressively lowered stress threshold in the clinical setting, *Nurs Clin North Am* 29(1):129-141, 1994.

Holt J: How to help confused patients, *Am J Nurs* 93(8):32-36, 1993.

Hurley A et al: Assessment of discomfort in advanced Alzheimer patients, *Res Nurs Health* 15(5):369-378, 1992.

Maas ML et al: Alzheimer's special care units, *Nurs Clin North Am* 29(1):173-194, 1994.

Rocca WA: Frequency, distribution, and risk factors for Alzheimer's disease, *Nurs Clin North Am* 29(1):101-111, 1994.

Stolley JM et al: Managing the care of patients with irreversible dementia during hospitalization for comorbidities, *Nurs Clin North Am* 28(4):767-782, 1993.

Tacrine for treatment of Alzheimer's disease, *JAMA* 268(18):2564-2565, 1992 (editorial).

Treatment for Alzheimer's disease, *N Engl J Med* 327(18):1306-1308, 1992 (editorial).

Yi ES, Abraham IL, Holroyd S: Alzheimer's disease and nursing: new scientific and clinical insights, *Nurs Clin North Am* 29(1):85-99, 1994.

### Cerebrovascular Problems

Bell T et al: Transcranial Doppler: correlation of blood velocity measurement with clinical status in subarachnoid hemorrhage, *J Neuro Sci Nurs* 24:215-219, 1992.

Borgman M, Passarella P: Nursing care of the stroke patient using Bobath principles: an approach to altered movement, *Nurs Clin North Am* 26(4):1019-1035, 1991.

Doolittle N: Stroke recovery—review of the literature and suggestions for further research, *J Neurosci Nurs* 20:169-173, 1988.

Flynn E: Cerebral vasospasm following intracranial aneurysm rupture: a protocol for detection, *J Neurosci Nurs* 21:348-352, 1989.

Fode N: Subarachnoid hemorrhage from ruptured intracranial aneurysm, *Am J Nurs* 88:673-680, 1988.

Hahn K: Left vs. right: what a difference a side makes in stroke, *Nurs 87* 17(9):44-48, 1987.

Jacob D, McGovern P, Blackburn H: The U.S. decline in stroke mortality: what does ecological analysis tell us? *Am J Public Health* 82(12):1596-1599, 1992.

Kalbach L: Unilateral neglect: mechanism and nursing care, *J Neurosci Nurs* 23:125-129, 1991.

Keller C et al: Psychological responses in aphasia: theoretical considerations and nursing implications, *J Neurosci Nurs* 21:290-294, 1989.

MacDonald E: Aneurysmal subarachnoid hemorrhage, *J Neurosci Nurs* 21:313-321, 1989.

Moore K, Trifiletti E: Stroke: the first critical days, *RN* 57(2):22-28, 1994.

Rutledge B: Aneurysm wrapping: principles applicable to the neuroscience nurse, *J Neurosci Nurs* 21:370-374, 1989.

Whitney F: Relationship of laterality of stroke and emotional and functional outcome, *J Neurosci Nurs* 19:158-165, 1987.

Williams A: Self report of indifference and anxiety among persons with right hemispheric stroke, *Res Nurs Health* 15(5):343-348, 1992.

### Brain Tumors

Berkshire J, Watson-Evans H: Meningioma: a nursing perspective, *J Neurosci Nurs* 18:86-89, 1986.

Campbell C: Acoustic neuroma: nursing implications related to surgical management, *J Neurosci Nurs* 23:50-56, 1991.

Edwards D et al: Hyperthermia treatment for malignant astrocytomas: nursing implications, *J Neurosci Nurs* 23:34-38, 1991.

Hodges K: Meningioma, astrocytoma, and germinoma: case presentations of three intracranial tumors, *J Neurosci Nurs* 21:113-121, 1989.

Krause E et al: Radiosurgery: a nursing perspective, *J Neurosci Nurs* 23:24-28, 1991.

Welsh D, Zumwalt M: Volumetric interstitial hyperthermia: nursing implications for brain tumor treatment, *J Neurosci Nurs* 20:229-235, 1988.

### *Seizure Disorders*

Brewer K, Sterling M: Neurosurgical treatment of intractable epilepsy, *J Neurosci Nurs* 20:366-370, 1988.

Friedman D: Taking the scare out of caring for seizure patients, *Nurs 88* 18(2)52-60, 1988.

Hodges K, Root L: Surgical management of intractable seizure disorder, *J Neurosci Nurs* 23:93-100, 1991.

### *Parkinson's Disease*

Berry P, Ward-Smith P: Adrenal medullary transplant as a treatment for Parkinson's disease: perioperative considerations, *J Neurosci Nurs* 20:356-361, 1988.

Delgado J, Billo J: Care of the patient with Parkinson's disease: surgical and nursing interventions, *J Neurosci Nurs* 20:142-150, 1988.

Fitzsimmons B, Bunting LK: Parkinson's disease: quality of life issues, *Nurs Clin North Am* 28(4):807-818, 1993.

Freed C et al: Survival of implanted fetal dopamine cells and neurologic improvement 12 to 46 months after transplantation for Parkinson's disease, *N Engl J Med* 327(22):1549-1555, 1992.

Spencer D et al: Unilateral transplantation of human fetal mesencephalic tissue into the caudate nucleus of patients with Parkinson's disease, *N Engl J Med* 327(22):1541-1548, 1992.

Vernon G: Parkinson's disease, *J Neurosci Nurs* 21:273-284, 1989.

Widner H et al: Bilateral frontal mesencephalic grafting in two patients with parkinsonianism induced by 1-methyl-4-phenyl-1,2,3,6-tetrahydropyridine (MPTP), *N Engl J Med* 327 (22):1556-1563, 1992.

### *Amyotrophic Lateral Sclerosis*

Kim T: Hope as a mode of coping in amyotrophic lateral sclerosis, *J Neurosci Nurs* 21:342-347, 1989.

Stone N: Amyotrophic lateral sclerosis: a challenge for constant adaptation, *J Neurosci Nurs* 19:166-173, 1987.

### *Myasthenia Gravis*

Hickey J: Myasthenic crisis—your assessment counts, *RN* 54(5):54-59, 1991.

Litchfield M, Noroian E: Changes in selected pulmonary functions in patients diagnosed with myasthenia gravis, *J Neurosci Nurs* 12:375-381, 1989.

Rhynsburger J: How to fight myasthenia's fatigue, *Am J Nurs* 89:337-341, 1989.

### *Traumatic Brain Injury*

Aumick J: Head trauma: guidelines for care, *RN* 54(4):27-31, 1991.

Ferido T, Habel M: Spasticity in head trauma and CVA patients: etiology and management, *J Neurosci Nurs* 20:17-22, 1988.

Hinkle J: Nursing care of the patient with minor head injury, *J Neurosci Nurs* 20:8-16, 1988.

Mahon D, Elger C: Analysis of posttraumatic syndrome following head injury, *J Neurosci Nurs* 21:382-384, 1989.

Palmer M, Wyness M: Positioning and handling: important considerations in the care of the severely head-injured patient, *J Neurosci Nurs* 20:42-49, 1988.

Plylar P: Management of the agitated and aggressive head injury patient in an acute care setting, *J Neurosci Nurs* 21:353-356, 1989.

Rehabilitation of persons with injuries, *MMWR* 41(RR-6):35-38, 1992.

Sherman D: Managing an acute head injury, *Nurs 90* 20(4):44-51, 1990.

White R, Likavec M: The diagnosis and initial management of head injury, *N Engl J Med* 327(21):1507-1511, 1992.

### *Increased Intracranial Pressure*

Andrus C: Intracranial pressure: diagnosis and nursing management, *J Neurosci Nurs* 23:85-92, 1991.

Frange E, Beideman M: Infections related to intracranial pressure monitoring, *J Neurosci Nurs* 20:94-103, 1988.

Luchka S: Working with ICP monitors, *RN* 54(3):34-37, 1991.

Muswaswes M: Increased intracranial pressure and its systemic effects, *J Neurosurg Nurs* 20:217-222, 1988.

Turner H et al: Comparison of nurse and computer recording of ICP in head injured patients, *J Neurosci Nurs* 20:236-239, 1988.

Vos H: Making headway with intracranial hypertension, *Am J Nurs* 93(2):28-35, 1993.

### *Multiple Sclerosis*

Buelow J: A correlational study of disabilities, stressors, and coping methods in victims of multiple sclerosis, *J Neurosci Nurs* 23:247-252, 1991.

Csesko P: Sexuality and multiple sclerosis, *J Neurosci Nurs* 20:353-355, 1988.

Francabandera F: Multiple sclerosis rehabilitation: inpatient vs outpatient, *Rehabil Nurs* 13:251-254, 1988.

Larsen P: Psychosocial adjustment in MS, *Rehabil Nurs* 15:242-247, 1990.

McBride E, DiStefano K: Explaining diagnostic tests for MS, *Nurs 88* 18(2):68-72, 1988.

Morgante L et al: Research and treatment in multiple sclerosis: implications for nursing practice, *J Neurosci Nurs* 21:285-289, 1989.

Ross AP: Nursing interventions for persons receiving immunosuppressive therapies for demyelinating pathology, *Nurs Clin North Am* 28(4):829-838, 1993.

Wineman N: Adaptation to multiple sclerosis: the role of social support, functional disability, and perceived uncertainty, *Nurs Res* 39(5):194-299, 1990.

## CHAPTER 58
## Management of Persons With Problems of the Spinal Cord and Peripheral Nerves

### *Spinal Cord Injury*

Barker E: Action stat SCI, *Nurs 90* 20(11):33, 1990.

Barker E, Higgins R: Managing a suspected SCI, *Nurs 89* 19(3):52-59, 1989.

Borowski C: A comparison of pulmonary complications in spinal cord–injured patients treated with two modes of spinal immobilization, *J Neurosci Nurs* 21:79-85, 1989.

Chadwick A, Oesting H: Not for specialists only: caring for patients with spinal cord injuries, *Nurs 89* 19(11):52-56, 1989.

Chicano L: Humanistic aspects of sexuality as related to spinal cord injury, *J Neurosci Nurs* 21:336-369, 1989.

Cyr L: Sequelae of SCI after discharge from initial rehabilitation program, *Rehabil Nurs* 14:326-329, 337, 1989.

Goddard L: Sexuality and spinal cord injury, *J Neurosci Nurs* 20:240-244, 1988.

Gryfinski J: Intramedullary spinal cord abscesses, *J Neurosci Nurs* 20:34-38, 1988.

North B et al: Living in a halo, *Am J Nurs* 92(4):54-58, 1992.

Pettibone K: Management of spasticity in spinal cord injury: nursing concerns, *J Neurosci Nurs* 19:269-299, 1988.

Stenger KM: Surveillance of spinal cord motor and sensory function, *Nurs Clin North Am* 28(4):783-792, 1993.

### *Infections and Inflammations*

Ake J, Perlstein L: AIDS: impact on neuroscience nursing practice, *J Neurosci Nurs* 19:300-304, 1987.

Grabbe L, Brown L: Identifying neurologic complications of AIDS, *Nurs 89* 19(5):66-73, 1989.

Mocsny N: Slow virus diseases of the central nervous system, *Rehabil Nurs* 14(3):130-132, 1989.

Mocsny N: Toxoplasmic encephalitis in the AIDS patient, *Rehabil Nurs* 18(1):20-22, 1993.

Prendergrast V: Bacterial meningitis update, *J Neurosci Nurs* 19:95-99, 1987.

Scherer P: How AIDS attacks the brain, *Am J Nurs* 90(1):44-53, 1990.

### Pain

Hansberry J et al: Managing chronic pain with a permanent epidural catheter, *Nurs 90* (10):53-57, 1990.

Lamb S, Barbaro N: Neurosurgical approaches to the management of chronic pain syndromes, *Orthop Nurs* 6(1):23-29, 1987.

Leijon G, Boive J: Central post-stroke pain—neurological symptoms and pain characteristics, *Pain* 36:13-25, 1989.

McCaffery M, Beebe A: Giving narcotics for pain: a problem solver handbook, *Nurs 89* 19(10):161-168, 1989.

Purath J: Assessing headache pain, *RN* 54(10):26-31, 1991.

Schaefer S: Relieving pain—an analgesic guide, *Am J Nurs* 88:825-827, 1988.

Whitney C, Daroff R: An approach to migraines, *J Neurosci Nurs* 20:284-289, 1988.

Wilton L: Thalamic pain syndrome, *J Neurosci Nurs* 21:362-365, 1989.

### Peripheral Nerve Problems

Adler R: Trigeminal glycerol chemoneurolysis: nursing implications, *J Neurosci Nurs* 21:337-341, 1989.

Burchiel JK: Trigeminal neuralgia. In Rakel RE, editor: *Conn's current therapy 1993.* Philadelphia, 1993, WB Saunders.

# SECTION TWO Visual and Auditory Systems

## CHAPTER 59

## Assessment of the Visual System

### General

American Society of Ophthalmic Registered Nurses: *Standards of ophthalmic nursing practice,* San Francisco, 1992, ASORN.

Boyd-Monk H, Steinmetz CG: *Nursing care of the eye,* East Norwalk, Conn, 1987, Appleton & Lange.

Foxall MJ et al: Living arrangements, loneliness, and social support of low vision older clients, *J Ophthalmic Nurs Technol* 12:67-74, 1993.

Goldblum K: Knowledge deficit in the ophthalmic surgical patient, *Nurs Clin North Am* 27(3):715-725, 1992.

Greenberg MD: Emergency care for acute visual loss, *Emerg Med* 24(8):112-14, 117-118, 120, 1992.

Grimes MR, Scardino MA, Martone JF: Worldwide blindness, *Nurs Clin North Am* 27(3):807-816, 1992.

Hunt L: Eyeglasses and common complaints, *Insight* 17(3):20-22, 1992.

Jakobiec FA, Azar D, editors, for International Ophthalmology Clinics: *Pediatric ophthalmology,* Boston, 1992, Little, Brown.

Hunt L: Dry eye, *Insight* 16(1):5, 1991.

Hunt L: Eye risks for ventilated or unconscious patients, *Insight* 16(2):7, 1991.

Lloyd F: Eye care for ventilated or unconscious patients, *Nurs Times* 86(1):36-37, 1990.

MacInnis B: Lasers and the eye, *Med Clin North Am* 33:6045-6047, 6051, 1989.

Maerov PH: Ocular emergencies, *Med Clin North Am* 33:6004-6013, 1989.

National Advisory Eye Council: *Vision research: a national plan 1983-1987,* vol 1, Bethesda, Md, 1983, National Institutes of Health.

National Society to Prevent Blindness, Operational Research Department: *Vision problems in the United States: a statistical analysis,* New York, 1980, The Society.

Newell FW: *Ophthalmology: principles and concepts,* ed 7, St Louis, 1992, Mosby.

Stein HA, Slatt BJ, Stein RM: *Ophthalmology terminology: speller and vocabulary builder,* St Louis, 1992, Mosby.

Traynor M: Day care eye surgery, *Nurs Times* 86(39):54-56, 1990.

US Department of Health and Human Services, Public Health Service: *Healthy people 2000: national health promotion and disease prevention objectives,* Washington, DC, 1990, US Government Printing Office.

US Department of Health and Human Services: *Vision research: a national plan, 1983-1987—the 1983 report of the National Advisory Eye Council,* NIH pub no 83-2469, 1983, Washington, DC, DHHS.

Vaughan D, Asbury T, Riordan-Eva P: *General ophthalmology,* ed 13, East Norwalk, Conn, 1992, Appleton & Lange.

Williams MB: Nurse-client management of skin and tissue integrity. In Berger KJ, Williams MB: *Fundamentals of nursing: collaborating for optimal health,* East Norwalk, Conn, 1992, Appleton & Lange.

### Eye Safety

Boyd-Monk H: Spectacles . . . goggles or face shields? *J Ophthalmic Nurs Technol* 7:84-86, 1988.

Burlew JA: Preventing eye injuries—the nurse's role, *Insight* 16(6):24-28, 1991.

Farber AS: Preventing eye injuries: what to tell patients, *Postgrad Med* 89(5):121-122, 127-128, 237-238, 1991.

Gerali PS: Lifesight: growing older with good vision, *J Ophthalmic Nurs Technol* 10:181-182, 1991.

Hunt L: Eye safety: not all toy guns are toys, *Insight* 14(4):5, 1989.

Hunt L: Protected eyes make sports safer, *Insight* 14(3):13, 1989.

Hunt L: Sight-threatening hazards around the house, *J Ophthalmic Nurs Technol* 8:148-154, 1989.

Hunt L: Eye hazards for the health care worker, *Insight* 15(6):14, 1990.

Hunt L: Use caution with eye cosmetics, *Insight* 15(1):7, 1990.

Memmer MK: Preventing eye damage from the sun's ultraviolet light: what health educators should teach, *Health Educ* 20(7):42-47, 1989.

Patterson P: Eyewear policies are a major safety issue, *OR Manager* 7(5):9-11, 1991.

Turrif TW: Summer sight savers, *J Ophthalmic Nurs Technol* 10(3):129-130, 1991.

Turrif TW, Gerali PS: Don't play games with your eyes, *J Ophthalmic Nurs Technol* 10:82-83, 1991.

Vader LA: Invisible light, *Insight* 17(2):12-14, 1992.

Vader LA: Vision and vision loss, *Nurs Clin North Am* 27:705-714, 1992.

Yelland D: Personal protective equipment: a practical guide to eye protection, *Occup Health (Lond)* 41(10):280-281, 1989.

York S, Proud G: Ophthalmic triage, *Nurs Times* 86(8):40-42, 1990.

### External Structure

Bowie I: Eye structure: a functional view, *Nurs Stand* 5:54-55, 1991.

### Aging

Calvani D et al: Experiental perspectives on aging and vision, *J Visual Impair Blindness* 81(7):317-322, 1987.

Ebersole P, Hess P: *Toward healthy aging,* ed 4, St Louis, 1994, Mosby.

Kapperud MJ: *The aging eye: a guide for nurses,* St Paul, Minn, 1983, The Minnesota Society for the Prevention of Blindness and Preservation of Hearing.

Kolananowski AM: The clinical importance of environmental lighting to the elderly, *J Gerontol Nurs* 18(1):1-14, 1992.

Maise AR, Silberman R, Trief E: Aging and visual impairment, *J Visual Impair Blindness* 81:323-325, 1987.

*New product for seniors, Futurist,* July-Aug 1992, p. 19.

Roberts A, Besterman A: Systems of life no. 177, senior systems-42, *Nurs Times* 85:55-58, 1989.

Sullivan N: Vision in the elderly, *J Gerontol Nurs* 9:228-235, 1983.

### *History*

Donshik PC, Lewis RA, Singerman LJ: Eye to eye with systemic disease, *Patient Care* 23:34-41, 1989.

Larson PM: Double vision, *J Ophthalmic Nurs Technol* 11:79-83, 1992.

### *Assessment*

Bates B, Heokelman RD, Thompson JB: *A guide to physical examination and history taking,* ed 5, Philadelphia, 1991, JB Lippincott.

Best S: Visual fields in glaucoma and neuroophthalmology, *J Ophthalmic Nurs Technol* 11:45-56, 1992.

Boyd-Monk H: How to use a direct ophthalmoscope, *J Ophthalmic Nurs Technol* 10:23-27, 1991.

Boyd-Monk H: Assessing acquired ocular diseases, *Nurs Clin North Am* 25:811-822, 1990.

Garber N: Basic ocular motility assessment, *J Ophthalmic Nurs Technol* 10:215-219, 1991.

Hunt L: Ophthalmic nursing assessment, *Insight* 17:9-11, 1992.

Pruett RC: Detecting disorders in the ocular fundus, *Emerg Med* 21(17):20-24, 29-30, 32, 1989.

Soperia JD et al: The funduscopic examination: how to make the most of it, *Consultant* 30(6):22-27, 1990.

### *Visual Acuity*

Colenbrander A, Fletcher DC: Low vision rehabilitation: visual acuity measurement in the low vision range, *J Ophthalmic Nurs Technol* 11:62-69, 1992.

Neff JA: Visual acuity testing, *J Emerg Nurs* 17:431-436, 1991.

Romano PE: Changes in visual acuity tests for vision screening in preschool children, *J Ophthalmic Nurs Technol* 7:183, 1988.

Schraeder BD, McEvoy-Shields K: Visual acuity, binocular vision, and ocular muscle balance in VLBW children, *Pediatr Nurs* 17:30-33, 1991.

### *Color Vision*

Beninsger R: Color vision testing, *J Ophthalmic Nurs Technol* 11:161-163, 1992.

### *Fluorescein Angiography*

Anand R: Fluorescein angiography: technique and normal study, Part 1, *J Ophthalmic Nurs Technol* 8:48-52, 1989.

Anand R: Fluorescein angiography: technique and normal study, Part 2, *J Ophthalmic Nurs Technol* 8:102-107, 1989.

### *Magnetic Resonance Imaging*

Wirtschafter JD, Berman EL, McDonald CS: *Magnetic resonance imaging and computed tomography: clinical neuro-orbital anatomy,* San Francisco, 1992, American Academy of Ophthalmology.

### *Ultrasonography*

Affel EL: Ophthalmic ultrasonography A-scans, *J Ophthalmic Nurs Technol* 9:52-56, 1990.

Best SJ: Visual fields in glaucoma and neuro-ophthalmology, *J Ophthalmic Nurs Technol* 11:46-56, 1992.

Mrochuk J: Introduction to diagnostic ophthalmic ultrasound for nurses in ophthalmology, *J Ophthalmic Nurs Technol* 9:234-239, 1990.


CHAPTER 60

## Management of Persons With Problems of the Eye


### *Medications and Ophthalmic Drugs*

Alopecia linked to beta blocker eye drops, *Nurses Drug Alert* 14(5):39, 1990.

Angioedema reported with calcium channel blockers, *Nurses Drug Alert* 13(11):85, 1989.

Burton S: Drugs and the eyes, *Nursing (Lond)* 3(45):24-26, 1989.

Hahn K: Administering eye medications, *Nurs 89* 19(9):80, 1989.

Hunt L: A complete drug history is crucial, *Insight* 15(3):8, 1990.

Hunt L: Caution: systemic adverse reactions from eye drop medications, *Insight* 16(4):5, 1991.

McCoy K: Ophthalmic drug use in the OR, *Insight* 17(4):10-21, 1992.

Orticio LP: Confusion and the patient on an intensive topical ocular antibiotic regimen: a case analysis, *J Ophthalmic Nurs Technol* 9:145-149, 1990.

Pavan-Langston D, Dunkel EC: *Handbook of ocular drug therapy and ocular side effects of systemic drugs,* Boston, 1991, Little, Brown.

Williams A, Winfield A: Topical medication for eye patients, *Nurs Times* 86(27):42-43, 1990.

### *Eye Manifestations of Systemic Diseases*

Donshik PC, Lewis RA, Singerman LJ: Eye to eye with systemic disease, *Patient Care* 23(11):34-41, 1989.

Goldblum K: Nursing care of the patient with myasthenia gravis, *Insight* 16(1):7, 24, 1991.

Kanski JJ, Thomas DJ: *The eye in systemic disease,* ed 2, London, 1990, Butterworth-Heinemann.

Mason G et al: Sickle cell retinopathy, *Insight* 16(6):15-20, 1991.

Morris WR: The eyes give the clue: ocular manifestations of systemic disease, *Postgrad Med* 91:195-199, 202, 293-296, 1992.

Walsh JB, Bierly J: Hypertension: the ocular fundus mirrors its severity, *Consultant* 29(8):92-104, 1989.

Yeatts RP, Clontz DM: Graves' ophthalmopathy, *J Ophthalmic Nurs Technol* 9:16-21, 1990.

### *Eye Injuries*

Barker-Stotts K: Action STAT! Hyphema, *Nurs 88* 18(12):33, 1988.

Boozalis GT et al: Ocular changes from electrical burn injuries: a literature review and report of cases, *J Burn Care Rehabil* 12(5):458-462, 1991.

Bowie I: Wounds to the eye, *Nursing (Lond)* 4(15):24-27, 1990.

Boyd-Monk H: Eye trauma: a close-up on emergency care, *RN* 2(12):22-30, 1989.

Boyd-Monk H: Eye trauma in the workplace, *J Ophthalmic Nurs Technol* 10:117-123, 1991.

Burns FR, Patterson CA: Prompt irrigation of chemical eye injuries may avert severe damage, *Occup Health Safety* 58(4):33-36, 1989.

Erie JC: Eye injuries: prevention, evaluation and treatment, *Physician Sports Med* 19(11):108-112, 115-116, 119-120, 1991.

Hunt L: Microwave ovens and eye injuries, *Insight* 17(4):23, 25, 1992.

Lawlor MC: Common ocular injuries and disorders, *J Emerg Nurs* 15(1):36-43, 1989.

Ortiz JM et al: Orbital and ocular injury, *Top Emerg Med* 13(4):67-77, 1991.

Pashby T: Eye injuries in sports, *J Ophthalmic Nurs Technol* 8:99-101, 1989.

Tannen M, Marsden J: Chemical burns of the eye, *Nurs Stand* 6(6):24-26, 1991.

Tolley FM et al: Alkaline injury to the eye, *Ophthalmic Nurs Forum* 5(1):1-4, 6-8, 1989.

### *Infections and Inflammations*

Friedlaender MH et al: Ocular allergy: nuisance or hazard? *Patient Care* 24(7):60-64, 67-69, 72, 1990.

Powell MA: Conjunctivitis versus iritis . . . questions and answers, *J Am Acad Nurse Pract* 2(3):125-126, 1990.

Radzewicz PL: Nursing management of corneal ulcers, *Ophthalmic Nurs Forum* 6(1):1-4, 6-8, 1990.

Small RG: Red eye: five steps toward a differential diagnosis, *Consultant* 30(7):29-32, 1991.

### *Cataracts*

Allen MN et al: Effectiveness of a preoperative teaching program for cataract patients, *J Adv Nurs* 17:303-309, 1992.

Ascroft R: Making sense out of cataract surgery, *Nurs Times* 88(6):36-38, 1992.

Hannon VM: Cataract surgery, *J Ophthalmic Nurs Technol* 12:13-17, 1993.

Hatch D, Phillips K, Drews RC: Evaluating postoperative cataract patients using the Kowa Flare Cell Meter, *J Ophthalmic Nurs Technol* 10(5):201-203, 1991.

Jaffe NS, Jaffe MS, Jaffe GF: *Cataract surgery and its complications,* St Louis, 1990, Mosby.

Jairath N et al: Effective discharge preparation of elderly cataract day surgery patients, *J Ophthalmic Nurs Technol* 9:157-160, 1990.

Legro MW: Quality of life and cataracts: a review of patient-centered studies of cataract surgery outcomes, *J Ophthalmic Nurs Technol* 10:260-272, 1991.

Moak E. Perioperative care of the patient undergoing cataract surgery, *Today's OR Nurse* 14(4):11-17, 30-31, 1992.

Packard RBS, Kinnear F: *Manual of cataract and intraocular lens surgery,* New York, 1991, Churchill Livingstone.

Parker P: The Eyecare Group: a volunteer support group for cataract patients, *J Ophthalmic Nurs Technol* 9:240-242, 1990.

Ruehl CA, Schremp PS: Nursing care of the cataract patient: today's outpatient approach, *Nurs Clin North Am* 27:727-743, 1992.

Seery J: Phacoemulsification, an improved method of cataract removal, *AORN J* 50:1230-1234, 1989.

Woods SM: Cataract development after prolonged use of corticosteroids, *Ophthalmic Nurs Forum* 6(2):1-4, 6-8, 1990.

### *Glaucoma*

Capino DC, Leibowitz HM: Glaucoma: screening, diagnosis, and therapy, *Hosp Pract* 25(5A):73-86, 1990.

Field D: Managing chronic simple glaucoma, *Nurs Stand* 6:28-30, 1992.

Frandzel S: Ophthalmology: two new systems to treat glaucoma, *Laser Nurs* 4(4):21, 1990.

Geraldi PS, DiVerde M: Glaucoma high risk alert, *J Ophthalmic Nurs Technol* 10(1):34, 1991.

Huusko H, Viinamaki M, Krause K: Developing standards for instructions to patients with glaucoma, *Nurs Pract* 3(2):23-26, 1990.

Karlin JD: Diagnosis and therapy of open-angle glaucoma, *J Am Acad Physician's Assistants* 4(7):573-581, 1991.

Krupin T: Implanted aqueous shunt devices for glaucoma surgery, *J Ophthalmic Nurs Technol* 11:23-25, 1992.

Kruse MR: Nursing management of uncontrolled glaucoma with the Molteno filtering implant, *Ophthalmic Nurs Forum* 4(2):1-7, 1988.

Martinelli AM: Glaucoma: classification, treatment options, patient care, *AORN J* 54:743-748, 750, 752-753, 1991.

Price MJ: Glaucoma screening, *J Ophthalmic Nurs Technol* 9(5):203-205, 1990.

### *Retina*

Brown GG: Retinal vascular diseases, *J Ophthalmic Nurs Technol* 10:71-75, 1991.

Clanton C, Means ME: Retinal reattachment: quality and appropriateness of care, *J Ophthalmic Nurs Technol* 7(4):130-133, 1988.

Shakin EP, Lucier AC: Retinitis pigmentosa, *J Ophthalmic Nurs Technol* 9(1):6-9, 1990.

### *Diabetic Retinopathy*

Boyd-Monk H: Keeping an eye on diabetes mellitus, *J Ophthalmic Nurs Technol* 8:173-174, 1989.

Clinical practice recommendations, American Diabetes Association, 1989-90, Eye care guidelines for patients with diabetes mellitus, *Diabetes Care Suppl* 1:145, 1990.

Cryer TH, Cryer KS: A view of diabetic retinopathy, *J Am Acad Physician's Assistants* 4(4):327-332, 1991.

Ferris FL: How effective are treatments for diabetic retinopathy? *JAMA* 269:1290-1291, 1993.

Ghartey KN: The importance of early detection of diabetic retinopathy, *J Ophthalmic Nurs Technol* 9:193-198, 1990.

Graham C, Lasko-McCarthey P: Exercise options for persons with diabetic complications, *Diabetes Educator* 16(3):212-220, 1990.

Ponchillia SV, LaGrow S: Independent glucose monitoring by functionally blind diabetics, *J Visual Impair Blindness* 82:50-53, 1988.

Roach VG: What you should know about diabetic retinopathy, *J Ophthalmic Nurs Technol* 7:166-169, 1988.

Rosenthal JL: Timely recognition of diabetic retinopathy, *Emerg Med* 21(11):87-90, 1989.

Smith S: Diabetic retinopathy, *Insight* 17(2):20-25, 1992.

Spencer M: Screening for diabetic retinopathy, *Nurs Stand* 5(50):52-53, 1991.

Spires R: Perfluorocarbon liquid in the management of complex retinal detachments, *J Ophthalmic Nurs Technol* 11(4):157-160, 1992.

Stepien CJ, Bowbeer MA, Hiss RG: Screening for diabetic retinopathy in communities, *Diabetes Educator* 18(2):115-120, 1992.

Wakelee-Lynch J: The winding road of research: developments in blood vessel research may offer clues to new treatments for proliferative retinopathy, *Diabetes Forecast* 45(2):32-35, 1992.

Williams AS: Adaptive diabetes education for visually impaired persons: teaching nonvisual diabetes self-care, *J Home Health Care Pract* 4(3):62-71, 1992.

### *Macular Degeneration*

Brown GC: Retinal vascular diseases, *J Ophthalmic Nurs Technol* 10:71-75, 1991.

Macular degeneration: the center will not hold, *Harvard Health Lett* 17(4):4-6, 1992.

Woods S: Macular degeneration, *Nurs Clin North Am* 27:761-775, 1992.

### *Tumors*

Abramson DH et al: Visual fields in a successfully radiated retinoblastoma patient, *J Ophthalmic Nurs Technol* 11:17-19, 1992.

Karrel-Brant R: Periorbital skin cancers, *Dermatol Nurs* 3:115-116, 130, 1991.

Mercer MA: Radioactive plaque therapy for the treatment of choroidal malignant melanoma: nursing implications, *Ophthalmic Nurs Forum* 5(2):1-8, 1989.

Servodidio CA: Retinoblastoma, *Cancer Nurse* 14:117-123, 1991.

Servodidio CA: Choroidal melanoma: what is it? *Insight* 16(1):16-17, 1991.

Servodidio CA: Presenting signs and symptoms of choroidal melanoma, *Insight* 16(2):20-21, 1991.

Servodidio CA: Teaching aids for patients diagnosed with choroidal melanoma, *Insight* 16(6):21-23, 1991.

Servodidio CA, Abramson DH: Choroidal melanoma, *Nurs Clin North Am* 27:777-790, 1992.

### *Visual Impairment and Blindness*

Allen MN: The meaning of visual impairment to visually impaired adults, *J Adv Nurs* 14:640-646, 1989.

Allen MN: Adjusting to visual impairment, *J Ophthalmic Nurs Technol* 9:47-51, 1990.

Allen MN, Birse E: Stigma and blindness, *J Ophthalmic Nurs Technol* 10:147-152, 1991.

Bentz LN: Caring for and communicating with blind and visually impaired persons, *J Visual Impair Blindness* 81:472-481, 1987.

Bishop VE: Visually handicapped people and the law, *J Visual Impair Blindness* 81:472-481, 1987.

Edmonds SE: Resources for the visually impaired, *J Ophthalmic Nurs Technol* 9:14-15, 1990.

Emerson DL: Facing loss of vision: the response of adults to visual impairment, *J Visual Impair Blindess* 75(2):41-45, 1981.

Estey A, Jeremy P, Jones M: Developing printed materials for patients with visual deficiencies, *J Ophthalmic Nurs Technol* 9:247-249, 1990.

Gallagher CM: The young adult with recent vision loss: a pilot case study, *Insight* 16(6):8-14, 1990.

Keller H: *Out of the dark,* Garden City, NY, 1913, Doubleday.

Kirchner C: *Data on blindness and visual impairment in the U.S.: a resource manual on social demographic characteristics, education, employment, income, and service delivery,* ed 2, New York, 1989, American Foundation for the Blind.

Lambert RM, West M, Carlin K: Psychology of adjustment to visual deficiency: a conceptual model, *J Visual Impair Blindness* 75:193-196, 1981.

Large T: The effect of attitudes upon the blind: a reexamination, *J Rehabil* 48(2):33-34, 45, 1982.

Moore JE; Impact of family attitudes toward blindness/visual impairment on the rehabilitation process, *J Visual Impair Blindness* 78:100-105, 1984.

Norris RM: Commonsense tips for working with blind patients, *Am J Nurs* 89(3):360-361, 1989.

Peters J: After the examination: care of low vision patients beyond ocular services, *J Ophthalmic Nurs Technol* 11:13-16, 1992.

Spencer RE: Transitions: being blind in a sighted world, *J Ophthalmic Nurs Technol* 7:220-222, 1988.

### *AIDS*

Ai E, Kelly MP: Ophthalmic manifestations of the acquired immunodeficiency syndrome, *J Ophthalmic Nurs Technol* 11:148-156, 1992.

Fong ACO: AIDS and its effect in ophthalmology, *Today's OR Nurse* 13(2):21-24, 1991.

Moffatt AK: Cytomegalovirus retinitis in patients with AIDS: pathophysiology and nursing care, *ANNA J* 17(1):44-50, 66, 1990.

Plona RP, Schremp PS: Nursing care of patients with ocular manifestations of human immunodeficiency virus infection, *Nurs Clin North Am* 27:793-805, 1992.

### *Enucleation and Artificial Eyes*

Albiar E: Hydroxyapatite implants—a new trend in enucleation and orbital reconstructive surgery, *Insight* 17(1):25-28, 1992.

Barking H et al: Making sense of... artificial eyes, *Nurs Times* 86(18):40-41, 1990.

Folley FM et al: Perceived stressors during the recovery period following enucleation, *Insight* 16(3):18-19, 1991.


## CHAPTER 61
## Assessment of the Ear


### *General*

Adams R, Victor M: *Principles of neurology,* ed 3, New York, 1985, McGraw-Hill.

Alberti PW, Ruben RJ, editors: *Otologic medicine and surgery,* vol 1 and 2, New York, 1988, Churchill Livingstone.

Bulechek GM, McCloskey JC: *Nursing interventions: treatments for nursing diagnosis,* Philadelphia, 1985, WB Saunders.

Cummings CW et al: *Otolaryngology: head and neck surgery,* ed 2, St Louis, 1993, Mosby.

DeWeese DD, Saunders WH: *Textbook of otolaryngology,* ed 7, St Louis, 1988, Mosby.

Hawke M, Albertin PW: *Clinical otoscopy,* New York, 1990, Churchill Livingstone.

Hughes GB: *Textbook of clinical otology,* New York, 1985, Thieme-Stratton.

Kashima HK, Goldstein JC, Kooperman CF: *Clinical geriatric otolaryngology,* ed 2, St Louis, 1989, Mosby.

Reiner A: *Manual of patient care standards,* Rockville, Md, 1988, Aspen.

*Report of the Task Force on the National Strategic Research Plan of the National Institute on Deafness and Other Communication Disorders,* Bethesda, Md, 1989, National Institutes of Health.

Riley MAK: *Nursing care of the client with ear, nose and throat disorders,* New York, 1987, Springer.

Sigler BA, Schuring LT: *Ear, nose and throat disorders,* St Louis, 1993, Mosby.

Thompson JM et al: *Mosby's clinical nursing,* ed 3, St Louis, 1993, Mosby.

US Department of Health and Human Services, Public Health Service: *Healthy people 2000: national health promotion and disease prevention objectives,* Washington, DC, 1990, US Government Printing Office.

### *Anatomy and Physiology*

Jahn AF, Santos-Sacchi J: *Physiology of the ear,* New York, 1988, Raven Press.

Programmed instruction: patient assessment of the ear, *Am J Nurs* 75(3):457-476, 1975.

Seeley RR, Stephens TD, Tate P: *Anatomy and physiology,* ed 2, St Louis, 1991, Mosby.

Thibodeau GA, Patton KT: *Textbook of anatomy and physiology,* ed 2, St Louis, 1993, Mosby.

### *Assessment*

Bates B: *A guide to physical examination,* ed 4, Philadelphia, 1987, JB Lippincott.

Malkievicz J: The fine art of giving a physical: how to assess the ears and test hearing acuity, *RN* 45(3):56-63, 1982.

Seidel HM et al: *Mosby's guide to physical examination,* ed 3, St Louis, 1995, Mosby.

### *Diagnostic Tests*

Curtin HD: The use of magnetic resonance imaging in otolaryngology–head and neck surgery, *Adv Otolaryngol Head Neck Surg* 5:71-107, 1991.

### *Hearing*

Fountain D: Hearing aids and their care, *Geriatr Nurs Home Care* 7(2):12-14, 1987.

Glasscock ME, Stambaugh GE: *Surgery of the ear,* ed 4, Philadelphia, 1990, WB Saunders.

Mitchell VL: Cochlear implantation: a nursing perspective, *The Journal* 5(2):11-15, 1987.

Nodol JB Jr: Hearing loss, *N Engl J Med* 329(15):1092-1102, 1993.

### *Balance*

Barber HO, Sharpe JA: *Vestibular disorders,* Chicago, 1988, Mosby.

Chipps E, Clanin N, Campbell V: *Neurologic disorders,* St Louis, 1992, Mosby.

Gardner G: Meniere's disease. In Rakel RE, editor: *Conn's current therapy 1993,* Philadelphia, 1993, WB Saunders.

***Drugs***

Fairbanks DNF: *Antimicrobial therapy in otolaryngology–head and neck surgery,* ed 6, Alexandria, Va, 1991, American Academy of Otolaryngology–Head and Neck Surgery.

Karb VK, Queener SF, Freeman JB: *Handbook of drugs for nursing practice,* St Louis, 1989, Mosby.

## SECTION THREE Musculoskeletal System

## CHAPTER 63
## Assessment of the Musculoskeletal System

***General***

Carpenito LJ: *Handbook of nursing diagnosis,* ed 5, Philadelphia, 1993, JB Lippincott.

Cotran RS, Kumar V, Robbins SL: *Pathologic basis of disease,* ed 4, Philadelphia, 1989, WB Saunders.

Farrel J: *Illustrated guide to orthopaedic nursing,* ed 3, Philadelphia, 1988, JB Lippincott.

McCance KL, Huenther SE: *Pathophysiology: the biologic basis for disease in adults and children,* ed 2, St Louis, 1994, Mosby.

Metcalf EM: The orthopaedic critical path, *Orthop Nurs* 10(6):25-31, 1991.

Mosher C et al: Upgrading practice with critical pathways, *Am J Nurs* 91:41-44, 1991.

Mourad LA: *Orthopedic disorders,* St Louis, 1991, Mosby.

Mourad LA, Drosle MM: *The nursing process in the care of adults with orthopaedic conditions,* ed 3, Albany, NY, 1993, Delmar.

Porth CM: *Pathophysiology: concepts of altered health states,* ed 3, Philadelphia, 1990, JB Lippincott.

Russell IJ: NSAIDS and bone metabolism, *Hosp Pract* 26(suppl 1):13-17, 1991.

Sheildler V: Patient-controlled analgesia, *Curr Concepts Nurs* 1(1):13-16, 1987.

Thompson JM et al: *Mosby's manual of clinical nursing,* ed 3, St Louis, 1993, Mosby.

Turek SL: *Orthopaedics: principles and their application,* vols 1 and 2, Philadlephia, 1984, JB Lippincott.

***Assessment***

Arnold WJ: Arthroscopy in the diagnosis and therapy of arthritis, *Hosp Pract* 26:43-53, 1992.

Bates B: *A guide to physical examination,* ed 4, Philadelphia, 1987, JB Lippincott.

Doyle J, Scheiner A, Marsolais EB: Augmentation of the accuracy of percutaneous electrode implantation by using a modified arthroscope to guide insertion, *Arthroscopy* 8(2):162-165, 1992.

Hilt NE, editor: *Arthroscopy of the knee,* Monograph Library, National Association of Orthopaedic Nurses, Philadelphia, 1983, Anthony J Janetti.

Hoppenfeld S: Physical examination of the spine and extremities, East Norwalk, Conn, 1976, Appleton-Century-Crofts.

Hoppenfeld S: *Orthopaedic neurology: a diagnostic guide to neurologic levels,* Philadelphia, 1977, JB Lippincott.

McClennan BL: Ionic and nonionic contrast media: evolution and strategies for use, *AJR* 155:225-233, 1990.

Mundy GR: New concepts in bone metabolism: clinical implications, *Hosp Pract* 25(suppl 1):7-12, 1991.

Peters VJ, Ferkel RD: Arthroscopic surgery of the ankle, *Orthop Nurs* 8(5):12-18, 1989.

Seidel HM et al: *Mosby's guide to physical examination,* ed 3, St Louis, 1995, Mosby.

Thibodeau GA, Patton KT: *Textbook of anatomy and physiology,* ed 2, St Louis, 1993, Mosby.

## CHAPTER 64
## Management of Persons With Trauma to the Musculoskeletal System

***Spine***

Adjei-Boachie O, Bradford D: The Cotrel-Dubousset system—results in spinal reconstruction, *Spine* 16(10):1155-1160, 1989.

Albin MS et al: Venous aid embolism during lumbar laminectomy in the prone position: report of three cases, *Anesth Analg* 73;364-369, 1991.

Allison RE, Amundson G: Spinal fixation: using the Steffee pedicle screw and plate system, *AORN J* 49(4):1016-1029, 1989.

Anderton JM: The prone position for surgical patient: a historical review of the principles and hazards, *Br J Anaesth* 67:452-463, 1991.

Brosnan H: Nursing management of the adolescent with idiopathic scoliosis, *Nurs Clin North Am* 26(1):17-31, 1991.

Brosnan H, Berda P: Pedicle screw fixation in the lumbar spine, *Orthop Nurs* 9(6):22-32, 1990.

Buckham KR: Surgical bone banking: the living donor, *Orthop Nurs* 10(12):47-53, 1991.

Chase JA: Spinal stenosis: when arthritis is more than arthritis, *Nurs Clin North Am* 26(1):53-64, 1991.

Cotton LA: Unit rod segmental spinal instrumentation for the treatment of neuromuscular scoliosis, *Orthop Nurs* 10(5):17-23, 1991.

Cowan P, Lovasik, DA: American Chronic Pain Association: strategies for surviving chronic pain, *Orthop Nurs* 9(4):47-49, 1990.

Dekker ML: Bone and soft tissue procurement, *Orthop Nurs* 8(2):31-34, 1989.

Deyo RA, Rainville J, Kent DL: What can the history and physical examination tell us about back pain? *JAMA* 268(6):760-765, 1992.

Feingold DJ et al: Complications of lumbar spine surgery, *Orthop Nurs* 19(4):39-57, 1991.

Goldberg VM, Stevenson S: Natural history of autografts and allografts, *Clin Orthop* 225:7-16, 1987.

Hu SS, Pashman RS: State of the art in medicine: spinal instrumentation evolution and state of the art, *Invest Radiol* 279(8):632-647, 1992.

Krismer M, Bauer R, Sterzinger W: Scoliosis correction by Cotrel-Dubousset instrumentation, *Spine* 17(85):S263-S269, 1992.

Mayer HM, Brock M: Percutaneous endoscopic discectomy: surgical technique and preliminary results compared to microsurgical discectomy, *J Neurosurg* 78:216-225, 1993.

National Blood Resource Education Program's Nursing Education Working Group: Transfusion nursing: trends and practice for the 90's, *Am J Nurs* 91(6):42-56, 1991.

Olson B, Ustanko L, Warner S: The patient in a halo brace: striving for normalcy in body image, *Orthop Nurs* 10(1):44-50, 1991.

Preksto D: The Kaneda device: a new anterior spine stabilization system, *AORN J* 55(3);734-746, 1992.

Richardson AB, Taylor ML, Murphee B: TSRH instrumentation: evolution of a new system, *Orthop Nurs* 9(6):15-21, 1990.

Rodts MF: Surgical intervention for adult scoliosis, *Orthop Nurs* 6(6):11-17, 1987.

Rothman RH, Simeone FA: *The spine,* ed 2, Philadelphia, 1982, WB Saunders.

Tempelhoff R, Williams EL, Vollmer DG: Is the "kneeling" prone position as dangerous as the sitting position for the development of venous air embolism? *Anesth Analg* 75:467-468, 1992.

Vawter-Popkess S, Patzel B: Compounded problem: chronic low back pain and overweight in adult females, *Orthop Nurs* 11(6)31-43, 1992.

Wolfe SW, Lospinuso MF, Burke SW: Unilateral blindness as a complication of patient positioning for spinal surgery, a case report, *Spine* 17(5):600-605, 1992.

### Tumors

Dulin D: Facilitating early rehabilitation in limb-salvage patients, *Oncol Nurs Forum* 16(1):105, 1989.

Gebhardt MC et al: The use of bone allografts for limb salvage in high-grade extremity osteosarcoma, *Clin Orthop* 270:181-194, 1991.

Mosher CM: The Papineau bone graft: a limb salvage technique, *Orthop Nurs* 10(3):27-32, 1991.

Piasecki PA: The nursing role in limb salvage surgery, *Nurs Clin North Am* 26(1):33-41, 1991.

Quill G et al: Complications associated with limb salvage for extremity sarcomas and their management, *Clin Orthop* 260:242-249, 1990.

Racolin AA, Present DA: Osteochondral allografts for limb salvage, *Orthop Nurs* 8(2):35-39, 1989.

Simon MA: Limb salvage for osteosarcoma in the 1980s, *Clin Orthop* 270:264-269, 1991.

Springfield DS: Introduction to limb-salvage surgery for sarcomas, *Orthop Clin North Am* 22(1):1-5, 1991.

### Fracture

Barden RM, Sinkora GL: Bone stimulators for fusions and fractures, *Nurs Clin North Am* 26(1):89-104, 1991.

Einhorn T: Mechanisms of fracture healing, *Hosp Pract* 26(suppl 1):41-45, 1991.

Gaehle KE et al: Thoracolumbar burst fractures, *AORN J* 55(3):721-731, 1992.

Helfet DL et al: Limb salvage versus amputation: preliminary results of the mangled extremity score, *Clin Orthop* 256:80-86, 1990.

Higgins RM: Replantation of digits, *Orthop Nurs* 10(3):11-18, 1991.

Jauernig PR: Organizing and implementing an Ilizarov program, *Orthop Nurs* 9(5):47-55, 1990.

Newschwander GE, Dunst RM: Limb lengthening with the Ilizarov external fixator, *Orthop Nurs* 8(3):15-21, 1989.

Sneed NV, VanBree KM: Treating ununited fractures with electricity: nursing implications, *J Gerontol Nurs* 16(8):26-31, 1990.

Valentine WA, Williams PA, Tafoya WL: Ilizarov external fixation, *AORN J* 51(6):1530-1545, 1990.

Williamson VC: Amputation of the lower extremity: an overview, *Orthop Nurs* 11(2):55-65, 1992.

### Complications of Fracture

Good LP: Compartment syndrome: a closer look at etiology, treatment, *AORN J* 56(5):904-911, 1992.

Mims BC: Fat embolism syndrome: a variant of ARDS, *Orthop Nurs* 8(3):22-25, 1989.

Ross D: Acute compartment syndrome, *Orthop Nurs* 10(2):33-38, 1991.

Slye DA: Orthopedic complications: compartment syndrome, fat embolism syndrome, and venous thromboembolism, *Nurs Clin North Am* 26(1):113-132, 1991.

### Hip Fracture

Barangan JD: Factors that influence recovery from hip fracture during hospitalization, *Orthop Nurs* 9(5):19-28, 1990.

Jacobsen SJ et al: Race and sex differences in mortality following fracture of the hip, *Am J Public Health* 82(8):1147-1150, 1992.

Nelson L et al: Improving pain management for hip fractured elderly, *Orthop Nurs* 9(3):79-83, 1990.

Nussman DS, Poole RC: Rescue and recovery in traumatic hip dislocation, *Am J Nurs* 91:34-38, 1991.

US Department of Health and Human Services, Public Health Service: *Healthy people 2000: national health promotion and disease prevention objectives,* Washington, DC, 1990, US Government Printing Office.

### Soft Tissue Trauma

Arnoczky SP: Anatomy of the anterior cruciate ligament, *Clin Orthop* 172:19-25, 1983.

Campbell TD: Anterior cruciate ligament reconstruction, *AORN J* 51(4):944-966, 1990.

Hales AL: Arthroscopically assisted anterior cruciate ligament reconstruction, *AORN J* 49(1):234-255, 1989.

Rothenberg JR: Innovations in treating anterior cruciate ligament deficiency, *Orthop Nurs* 10(2):17-24, 1991.

Whittington CF, Carlson CA: Anterior cruciate ligament injury evaluation, arthroscopic reconstruction and rehabilitation, *Nurs Clin North Am* 26(1):149-158, 1991.

### Multiple Trauma

Dunwoody CJ: Pelvic fracture care: reflections on the past, implications for the future, *Nurs Clin North Am* 26(1):65-72, 1991.

Herron DG, Nance J: Emergency department nursing management of patients with orthopedic fractures resulting from motor vehicle accidents, *Nurs Clin North Am* 25(1):71-83, 1990.

Huggins B: Trauma physiology, *Nurs Clin North Am* 25(1):1-10, 1990.

Johnson L: Operative management of unstable pelvic fractures, *Orthop Nurs* 8(4):21-25, 1989.

Keitz JE: Emergent assessment of the multiple trauma patient, *Orthop Nurs* 8(6):29-32, 1989.

Kosmos CA: Emergency nursing management of the multiple trauma patient, *Orthop Nurs* 8(6):33-36, 1989.

Peck SA: Crush syndrome: pathophysiology and management, *Orthop Nurs* 9(3):33-40, 1990.

Rosenberg A, Wise K: Neurologic assessment of the multiple trauma patient, *Orthop Nurs* 8(6):49-55, 1989.

Schreiber ME: Cardiac complications of the Stryker frame, *Crit Care Nurse* 10(8):73-77, 1990.

## CHAPTER 65

## Management of Persons With Inflammatory and Degenerative Disorders of the Musculoskeletal System

### Inflammatory Disorders

Belza BL et al: Correlates of fatigue in older adults rheumatoid arthritis, *Nurs Res* 42(2):93-99, 1993.

Collo MCB et al: Evaluating arthritic complaints, *Nurse Practitioner* 16(2):9-20, 1991.

Crosby LJ: Factors which contribute to fatigue associated with rheumatoid arthritis, *J Adv Nurs* 16:974-981, 1991.

Moskowitz RW: *Clinical rheumatology: a problem-oriented approach to diagnosis and management,* ed 2, Philadelphia, 1982, Lea & Febiger.

Pigg J, Driscoll P, Caniff R: *Rheumatology nursing: a problem-oriented approach,* New York, 1985, John Wiley & Sons.

Schlegel SI, Paulus HE: Update on NSAID use in rheumatic diseases, *Bull Rheum Dig* 36(6):1-8, 1986.

### Carpal Tunnel Syndrome

Anderson BA: Endoscopic carpal tunnel release: a new approach to carpal tunnel syndrome, *AORN J* 57(2):413-428, 1993.

Centers for Disease Control: Occupational disease surveillance: carpal tunnel syndrome, *JAMA* 262(7):886-889, 1989.

### Osteoporosis

Bauer RL: Assessing osteoporosis, *Hosp Pract* 26(suppl 1):23-29, 1991.

Foldes J et al: Progressive bone loss during long-term home total parenteral nutrition, *J Parenter Enter Nutr* 14(2):139-142, 1990.
Hay EK: That old hip: the osteoporosis process, *Nurs Clin North Am* 26(1):43-51, 1991.
Liscum B: Osteoporosis: the silent disease, *Orthop Nurs* 11(4):21-24, 1992.
Pavlik M: Measuring bone mineral content, *Orthop Nurs* 10(2):39-42, 1991.

#### Degenerative Joint Disease

Dale KG, Orr PM, Harrell PB: Total elbow replacement, *Orthop Nurs* 11(5):23-28, 1992.
Dunajcik LM: The hip: when the joint must be replaced, *RN* 4:62-71, 1989.
Funk JR, MacBriar BR, Peterson AF: Tibial osteotomy, *Orthop Nurs* 9(2):29-34, 1990.
Hodge WA: Prevention of deep vein thrombosis after total knee arthroplasty: coumadin versus pneumatic calf compression, *CORR* 271:101-105, 1991.
Johnson DP, Eastwood M: Beneficial effects of continuous passive motion after total condylar knee arthroplasty, *Ann R Coll Surg Engl* 74:412-416, 1992.
Johnson RL: Total shoulder arthroplasty, *Orthop Nurs* 12(1):14-22, 1993.
Nolde T, Wong S, Wong J: Teaching patients to use a new hip, *Geriatr Nurs* 10(2):69-70, 1989.
Olson B et al: Variables associated with hypotension in post operative total knee arthroplasty patients receiving epidural analgesia, *Orthop Nurs* 11(4):31-37, 1992.
Orr PM: An educational program for total hip and knee replacement patients as part of total arthritis center program, *Orthop Nurs* 9(5):61-69, 86, 1990.
Schremp PS, Jeffrey JE, Paskert KM: Clinical implications of the impact of autologous blood donation on functional recovery, *Orthop Nurs* 10(4):33-37, 1991.
Selman SW, Mistretta EF: Elder care, *AORN J* 55(2):618-622, 1992.

UNIT XI

## Alterations in Defense and Protection

SECTION ONE **Integumentary System**

CHAPTER 66

### Assessment of the Skin

#### General

American Cancer Society: *Cancer facts and figures,* New York, 1993, The Society.
Epstein E: *Common skin disorders,* ed 3, Oradell, NJ, 1988, Medical Economics Books.
Habif TP: *Clinical dermatology: a color guide to diagnosis and treatment,* ed 2, St Louis, 1990, Mosby.
Moschella SL, Hurley HP: *Dermatology,* ed 3, Philadelphia, 1991, WB Saunders.

#### Age-Related Skin Changes

Newcomer V, editor: *Geriatric dermatology,* New York, 1989, Igaku-Shoin.
Young E: *Geriatric dermatology,* Philadelphia, 1993, Lea & Febiger.

#### Allergic Skin Reactions

Matthews KP: Clinical spectrum of allergic and pseudoallergic drug reactions, *J Allergy Clin Immunol* 74:558-566, 1984.

CHAPTER 67

### Management of Persons With Problems of the Skin

#### Bacterial, Viral, and Fungal Diseases

Bodey GP: Topical and systemic antifungal agents, *Med Clin North Am* 72:637-659, 1988.
Krusinski PA: Viral diseases of the skin. In Rakel RE, editor: *Conn's current therapy 1993,* Philadelphia, 1993, WB Saunders.
Lefort SM: Herpes zoster and postherpetic neuralgia: the need for early intervention in the elderly, *Nurse Pract* 14(3):30-41, 1989.
Lucey J: Herpetic whitlow, *Am J Nurs* 84(1):60-61, 1984.

#### Infestations

Mocsny N: Care and treatment of scabies, *Adv Clin Care* 5(5):23-26, 1990.
Sheahan SL: Management of common parasitic infections encountered in primary care, *Nurse Practitioner* 12(8):19-33, 1987.

#### Malignancies

Chak LY: Radiation therapy for acquired immunodeficiency syndrome related to Kaposi's sarcoma, *J Clin Oncol* 6(5):863-867, 1988.
Edwards KS: Diagnosing and treating AIDS-related Kaposi's sarcoma and carcinoma, *Ohio Med* 84(7):525-526, 1988.

#### Pathophysiology

Ganong WF: *Review of medical physiology,* ed 16, East Norwalk, Conn, 1993, Appleton & Lange.
Guyton A: *Textbook of medical physiology,* ed 8, Philadelphia, 1991, WB Saunders.
McCance K, Huether S: *Pathophysiology,* ed 2, St Louis, 1994, Mosby.
Price SA, Wilson LM, editors: *Pathophysiology: clinical concepts of disease processes,* ed 4, St Louis, 1992, Mosby.
Stein JH et al: *Internal medicine,* ed 4, St Louis, 1994, Mosby.
Tierney L et al: *Current medical diagnosis and treatment,* ed 3, East Norwalk, Conn, 1994, Appleton & Lange.

#### Photosensitivity

Bickers DR: Treatment of selected photosensitivity diseases, *Med Clin North Am* 66:927-937, 1982.
Harber LC, Bickers DR: *Photosensitivity diseases,* ed 2, 1989, BC Decker.
Rumsfield J: Sunscreens: what you and your patients should know, *Dermatol Nurs* 2(3):134-147, 1990.

#### Physical Assessment

Barakauskas V et al: *Health and physical assessment,* St Louis, 1994, Mosby.

#### Pigmentation Changes

Bridges BF: The rashes of dermatomyositis in a black patient, *Am J Med* 91(6):661-662, 1991.
Grimes A: Cosmetics in blacks, *Dermatol Clin* 9(1):53-68, 1991.
Irwin MJ: Assessing color changes for dark-skinned patients, *Adv Clin Care* 6(6):8-10, 1991.

#### Pressure Ulcers

Bryant R: *Acute and chronic wounds: nursing management,* St Louis, 1992, Mosby.
Clarke M: The nursing prevention of pressure sores in community and hospital practice, *J Adv Nurs* 13(3):365-373, 1988.
Kosiak M: Prevention and rehabilitation of pressure ulcers, *Decubitus* 4(2):60-62, 64, 66, 1991.
Krasner D: *Chronic wound care,* King of Prussia, Pa, 1990, Health Management.

Maklebust J: *Pressure ulcers: guidelines for prevention and nursing management,* Chicago, 1990, Smith & Nephew.

Maklebust J: Impact of AHCPR pressure ulcer guidelines on nursing practice, *Decubitus* 4(2):46-50, 1991.

US Department of Health and Human Services: *Clinical practice guidelines, pressure ulcers in adults: prediction and prevention,* Washington, DC, 1992, US Government Printing Office.

Vogelpohl T: What do nursing students learn about pressure ulcers? A survey of content on pressure ulcers in nursing school textbooks, *Decubitus* 6(2):48-50, 52, 1993.

### Psoriasis

Dunn ML: Treatment options for psoriasis, *Am J Nurs* 88(8):1082-1087, 1988.

Grizzard D: Understanding the pathophysiology of psoriasis: a nursing perspective, *Dermatol Nurs* 3(5), 1991.

## CHAPTER 68
## Management of Persons With Burns

### General

Caine RM, Lefcourt ND: Patients with burns. In Clochesy J et al, editors: *Critical care nursing,* Philadelphia, 1993, WB Saunders.

Demling RH, LaLonde C: *Burn trauma,* New York, 1989, G Thieme.

Dyer C, Roberts D: Thermal trauma, *Nurs Clin North Am* 25:85-117, 1990.

Mikhail JN: Acute burn care: an update, *J Emerg Nurs* 14:9-18, 1988.

Talley MA, Luterman A: Myths and facts about burns, *Nurs 89* 19(1):21, 1989.

Trofino RB: *Nursing care of the burn-injured patient,* Philadelphia, 1991, FA Davis.

### Etiology, Prevention, and Health Education

Bayley EW et al: Research priorities for burn nursing: patient, nurse, and burn prevention education, *J Burn Care Rehabil* 12:377-383, 1991.

Clark DE, Katz MX, Campbell SM: Decreasing mortality and morbidity rates after institution of a statewide burn program, *J Burn Care Rehabil* 13:261-270, 1992.

Thompson R et al: The effect of instruction on burn prevention in eighth-grade students in preparation for babysitting, *J Burn Care Rehabil* 13:482-486, 1992.

Victor J et al: A statewide targeted burn prevention program, *J Burn Care Rehabil* 9:425-429, 1988.

### Classification

Mozingo DW et al: Chemical burns, *J Trauma* 28:642-647, 1988.

Sawhney CP, Kaushish R: Acid and alkali burns: considerations in management, *Burns* 15:132-134, 1989.

Trofino RB, Orr PM: Types of burns. In Trofino RB: *Nursing care of the burn-injured patient,* Philadelphia, 1991, FA Davis.

### Pathophysiology of Severe Burns

Bert JL et al: Microvascular exchange during burn injury: IV fluid resuscitation model, *Circ Shock* 34:285-297, 1991.

Grossman AR: Impact of DRGs on a private burn care facility, *J Burn Care Rehabil* 5:314-315, 1984.

Heimbach DM: Impact of DRGs on a state-supported burn care facility, *J Burn Care Rehabil* 5:311-313, 1984.

Horton JW, Baxter CR, White DJ: Differences in cardiac responses to resuscitation from burn shock, *Surg Gynecol Obstet* 168:201-213, 1989.

Lazarus HL: Impact of DRGs on drug product selection in burn care therapy, *J Burn Care Rehabil* 5:316-318, 1984.

Marvin JA: Burn nursing and DRG reimbursement, *J Burn Care Rehabil* 5:319, 1984.

Morehouse JD et al: Resuscitation of the thermally injured patient, *Crit Care Clin* 8:355-365, 1992.

Robins EV: Burn shock, *Crit Care Clin North Am* 2:299-307, 1990.

### Periods of Treatment

Bayley EW: Wound healing in the patient with burns, *Nurs Clin North Am* 25:205-221, 1990.

Blumenfield M, Schoeps MM: *Psychological care of the burn and trauma patient,* Baltimore, 1993, Williams & Wilkins.

Burgess MC: Initial management of a patient with extensive burn injury, *Crit Care Nurs Clin North Am* 3:165-179, 1991.

Choiniere M et al: The pain of burns: characteristics and correlates, *J Trauma* 29:1531-1539, 1989.

Cioffi WG, Rue LW: Diagnosis and treatment of inhalation injuries, *Crit Care Nurs Clin North Am* 3:191-198, 1991.

Courtemanche DJ, Robinow O: Recognition and treatment of the posttraumatic stress disorder in the burn victim, *J Burn Care Rehabil* 10:247-250, 1989.

Deitch EA, Clothier J: Burns in the elderly: an early surgical approach, *J Trauma* 23:891-894, 1983.

Demling RH: Fluid replacement in burned patients, *Surg Clin North Am* 67:15-30, 1987.

Enzi G et al: Metabolic and hormonal effects of early nutritional supplementation after surgery in burn patients, *Crit Care Med* 18:719-721, 1990.

Fitzgerald KA, Gonzales McLaughlin E: Inhalation injuries, *AACN Clin Issues* 1:535-542, 1990.

Foyt MM: Does aging magnify the danger of burn injury (part 1)? *J Gerontol Nurs* 11(11):22-28, 1985.

Foyt MM: Does aging magnify the danger of burn injury (part 2)? *J Gerontol Nurs* 11(12):17-21, 1985.

Hammond J, Ward C: Decision not to treat: "do not resuscitate" order for the burn patient in the acute setting, *Crit Care Med* 17:136-138, 1989.

Hansbrough JF, Zapata-Sirvent R, Hoyt D: Postburn immunosuppression: an inflammatory response to the burn wound, *J Trauma* 30:671-675, 1990.

Horton JW, White J, Baxter CR: Hypertonic saline dextran resuscitation of thermal injury, *Ann Surg* 21:301-311, 1990.

Jerrard DA, Cappadoro K: Burns in the elderly patient, *Emerg Med Clin North Am* 8:421-428, 1990.

Keys TC, Moresi JM, Deitch EA: Thermal injury in the elderly: the limited need for nursing home care, *J Burn Care Rehabil* 10:429-431, 1989.

Kinsella J, Booth MG: Pain relief in burns: James Laing memorial essay 1990, *Burns* 17:391-395, 1991.

Kraemer MD, Jones T, Deitch EA: Burn contractures: incidence, predisposing factors, and results of surgical therapy, *J Burn Care Rehabil* 9:261-265, 1988.

Lee JJ, Marvin JA, Heimbach DM: Effectiveness of nalbuphine for relief of burn debridement pain, *J Burn Care Rehabil* 10:241-246, 1989.

Lewis JM: Prevent burn injury to older adults: develop and implement a plan that works! *J Gerontol Nurs* 11(9):8-12, 1985.

Mechanic HF, Dunn LT: Nutritional support for the burn patient, *Dimens Crit Care Nurs* 5(1):20-29, 1986.

Molter NC: Pain in the burn patient. In Puntillo KA, editor: *Pain in the critically ill,* Gaithersburg, Md, 1991, Aspen.

Morra-Martin L: Nursing implications of today's burn care techniques, *RN* 52(5):26-33, 1989.

Nowicki CR, Sprenger CK: Temporary skin substitutes for burn patients: a nursing perspective, *J Burn Care Rehabil* 9:209-215, 1988.

Patterson DR et al: Post-traumatic stress disorder in hospitalized patients with burn injuries, *J Burn Care Rehabil* 11:181-184, 1990.

Peck MD, Heimbach DM: Does early excision of burn wounds change the patterns of mortality? *J Burn Care Rehabil* 10:7-10, 1989.

Petro JA et al: Burn accidents and the elderly: what is happening and how to prevent it, *Geriatrics* 44(3):26-48, 1989.
Robins EV: Immunosuppression of the burned patient, *Crit Care Nurs Clin North Am* 2:767-774, 1989.
Rue LW, Cioffi WG: Resuscitation of thermally injured patients, *Crit Care Nurs Clin North Am* 3:181-189, 1991.
Smith GW, Savinski-Boxinko G: Giving emergency care for burns, *Nurs 89* 19:55-62, 1989.
Summers TM: Psychosocial support of the burned patient, *Crit Care Nurs Clin North Am* 3:237-244, 1991.
Ward RS: Pressure therapy for the control of hypertonic scar formation after burn injury: a history and review, *J Burn Care Rehabil* 12:257-262, 1991.
Williams J, Lewis RW, Kealey GP: Carbon monoxide poisoning and myocardial ischemia in patients with burns, *J Burn Care Rehabil* 13:210-213, 1992.

## SECTION TWO Immune System

### CHAPTER 69
### Assessment of the Immune System

#### General

Mudge-Grout CL: *Immunologic disorders,* St Louis, 1993, Mosby.
Stites DP, Terr AI: *Basic and clinical immunology,* ed 7, East Norwalk, Conn, 1991, Appleton & Lange.
Wener M: Basic clinical immunology, *Hosp Med* 28(1):69-82, 1992.

#### Immune System of Elderly Persons

Barcellini W et al: Heterogeneity of immune responsiveness in healthy elderly subjects, *Clin Immunol Immunopathol* 47:142-151, 1988.
Blair KA: Aging: physiological aspects and clinical implications, *Nurse Pract* 15(2):14-28, 1990.
Fenske NA, Lober CW: Skin changes of aging: pathological implications, *Geriatrics* 45(3):27-35, 1990.
Gillis S et al: Immunological studies aging: decreased production of and response to T cell growth factor by lymphocyte from aged humans, *J Clin Invest* 67:937-942, 1981.
Guidi L et al: Impairment of lymphocyte activities in depressed aged subjects, *Mech Ageing Dev* 60:13-24, 1991.
Hallgren HM et al: Lymphocyte proliferative response to receptor levels as biomarkers of age and health, *Mech Ageing Dev* 43:175-185, 1988.
Murasko DM et al: Immunologic response in an elderly population with a mean age of 85, *Am J Med* 81:612-618, 1986.
Nagel JE et al: Decreased proliferation, interleukin 2 synthesis and interleukin 2 receptor expression are accompanied by decreased mRNA expression in phytohemagglutin stimulated cell from elderly donors, *J Clin Invest* 81:1096-1102, 1988.
US Department of Health and Human Services: *Health, United States 1991, and prevention profile,* DHHS Pub No (PHS) 92-1232, Hyattsville, Md, 1991, DHHS.

#### Diagnostics of the Immune System

Cavalieri AT, Chopra A, Bryman P: When outside the norm is normal: interpreting lab data in the aged, *Geriatrics* 45(5):66-70, 1992.
Corbett JV: *Laboratory tests and diagnostic procedures with nursing diagnoses,* East Norwalk, Conn, 1992, Appleton & Lange.
Fischback F: *A manual of laboratory and diagnostic tests,* ed 4, Philadelphia, 1992, JB Lippincott.
Gawlikoski J: White cells at war, *Am J Nurs* 92(3):45-51, 1992.
Korenblat PE, Wedner HJ: *Allergy theory and practice,* ed 2, Philadelphia, 1992, WB Saunders.
Kushner I: C-Reactive protein and the acute-phase response, *Hosp Pract* 25(3H):13-28, 1990.
Orson RM et al: Interleukin 2 receptor expression by T cells in human aging, *Cell Immunol* 124:278-291, 1989.
Pagana KD, Pagana TJ: *Mosby's diagnostic and laboratory test reference,* St Louis, 1992, Mosby.
Rabinowich H et al: Interleukin-2 production and activity in aged humans, *Mech Ageing Dev* 32:213-266, 1985.

### CHAPTER 70
### Management of Persons With Problems of the Immune System

#### Immunodeficiencies

Buckley RH: Immunodeficiency diseases, *JAMA* 268(20):2797-2806, 1992.
Buckley RH, Schiff RI: The use of intravenous immune globulin in immunodeficiency diseases, *N Engl J Med* 324(2):110-117, 1991.
Hadden JW, Smith DL: Immunopharmacology, immunomodulation and immunotherapy, *JAMA* 268(20):2964-2969, 1992.
Parsons L, Klopovich PM: Immune globulin therapy, *Semin Oncol Nurs* 6(2):136-139, 1990.
Worley K, White JA: Primary immunodeficiencies, *J Otolaryngol* 144:497-500, 1992.

#### Gammopathies

Barlogie B, Alexanian R, Jagannath S: Plasma cell dyscrasias, *JAMA* 268(20):2946-2951, 1992.

#### Hypersensitivities

Anderson KC, Hayden GB: Specialized cell component therapy, *Semin Oncol Nurs* 6(2):140-149, 1990.
Creticos PS: Immunotherapy with allergens, *JAMA* 268(20):2834-2839, 1992.
DeJarnatt AC, Grant JA: Basic mechanisms of anaphylaxis and anaphylactoid reactions, *Immunol Allergy Clin North Am* 12(3):501-515, 1992.
Folkes ME: Transfusion therapy in critical care nursing, *Crit Care Nurs Q* 13(2):15-28, 1993.
Freedman S et al: Nursing considerations in the administration of blood component therapy, *Semin Oncol Nurs* 6(2):155-162, 1990.
Gibbs L: Assessment and management of the allergic patient, *ORL Head Neck Nurs* 10(3):10-16, 1992.
Gloe D: Common reactions to transfusions, *Heart Lung* 20(5):506-512, 1992.
Greenberger PA: Use of immunotherapy for allergic disorders, *Immunol Allergy Clin North Am* 12(3):1-12, 1992.
Herrera AM, deShazo RD: Current concepts in anaphylaxis, *Immunol Allergy Clin North Am* 12(1):517-536, 1992.
Kagen SL: Other indications for administration of allergen immunotherapy, *Immunol Allergy Clin North Am* 12(1):177-179, 1992.
Kaliner M, Lemanske R: Rhinitis and asthma, *JAMA* 268(20):2807-2829, 1992.
Kay AB, Lessof MH: Allergy: conventional and alternative concepts, *J R Coll Physicians Lond* 26(3):260-264, 1992.
Kotwas L et al: Blood collection techniques, *Semin Oncol Nurs* 6(2):109-116, 1990.
Lockey RF: Cytotoxic and immune complex reactions, *J Allergy Clin Immunol* 84(6):1032-1035, 1989.
Lockey RF: Future trends in allergy and immunology, *JAMA* 268(20):2991-2992, 1992.
Miller TP, Greenberger PA: Anaphylaxis: recognition and management, *Hosp Med* 27:70-94, 1991.
Norman PS: Immunotherapy of IgE-mediated disease, *Hosp Pract* 25(4):81-92, 1990.
Patterson R et al: *Allergic diseases,* Philadelphia, 1993, JB Lippincott.

Transfusion nursing: trends and practices for the '90s, *Am J Nurs* 91(6):42-56, 1991.

***Autoimmune Diseases***

Nakamura MC, Nakamura RM: Contemporary concepts of autoimmunity and autoimmune diseases, *J Clin Lab Anal* 6(5): 275-289, 1992.

CHAPTER 71

## Management of Persons With HIV Infection and AIDS

***General***

Centers for Disease Control: The HIV/AIDS epidemic: the first 10 years, *MMWR* 40(22):357-375, 1991.

Centers for Disease Control: 1993 revised classification system for HIV infection and expanded surveillance case definition for AIDS among adolescents and adults, *MMWR* 41(RR-17):1-19, 1992.

Centers for Disease Control: Update: acquired immunodeficiency syndrome: United States, 1992, *MMWR* 42(28):547-557, 1993.

Denenberg R: *Gynecological care manual for HIV positive women,* Durant, Okla, 1993, Essential Medical Information Systems.

Fee E, Krieger N: Understanding AIDS: historical interpretations and the limits of biomedical individualism, *Am J Public Health* 83(10):1477-1486, 1993.

Selik RM, Chu SY, Buehler JW: HIV infection as leading cause of death among young adults in U.S. cities and states, *JAMA* 269(23):2991-2994, 1993.

Vermund SH: Rising HIV-related mortality in young Americans, *JAMA* 269(23):3034-3035, 1993.

***Medical Management***

Goldsmith MF: HIV/AIDS early treatment controversy cues new advice but questions remain, *JAMA* 270(3):295-296, 1993.

Hirsch MS, D'Aquila RT: Therapy for human immunodeficiency virus infection, *N Engl J Med* 328(23):1686-1695, 1993.

Sande M, Volberding P: *The medical management of AIDS,* Philadelphia, 1992, WB Saunders.

***Nursing Management***

Beier A et al: AIDS/HIV teaching ideas, *J Health Educ* 24(1):47-49, 1993.

Bennett JA, DeMayo M, Germain MS: Caring in the time of AIDS: the importance of empathy, *Nurs Admin Q* 17(2):46-60, 1993.

Brown MA, Powell-Cope G: Themes of loss and dying in caring for a family member with AIDS, *Res Nurs Health* 16:179-191, 1993.

Flaskerud J, Ungvarski P: *HIV/AIDS: a guide to nursing care,* Philadelphia, 1992, WB Saunders.

Gee G: *AIDS: concepts in nursing practice,* Baltimore, 1988, Williams & Wilkins.

Hisgen JW: AIDS "to tell the truth" gaming activity: a teaching method, *J Health Educ* 24(1):44-46, 1993.

Lewis A: *Nursing care of the person with AIDS/ARC,* Rockville, Md, 1988, Aspen.

Lucey D: The first decade of human retroviruses: a nomenclature for the clinician, *Mil Med* 156(10):555-557, 1991.

***Opportunistic Infections in AIDS***

AIDS update: how HIV affects the eye, *Nurs 92* 22(6):26, 1992.

Anastasi JK, Rivera J: Understanding prophylactic therapy for HIV infections, *Am J Nurs* 94(2):36-42, 1994.

Bartlett J: *Recommendations for the medical care of persons with HIV infection,* Baltimore, 1992, Johns Hopkins Medical Institutions.

Girard PM et al: Dapsone-pyrimethamine compared with aerosolized pentamidine as primary prophylaxis against *Pneumocystis carinii* pneumonia and toxoplasmosis in HIV infection, *N Engl J Med* 328(21):1512-1520, 1993.

Gordin F: *Mycobacterium avium* complex (MAC): natural history and clinical issues, *Opportunistic Complications HIV* 2(1):1-5, 1993.

Henry D et al: Recombinant human erythropoietin in the treatment of anemia associated with human immunodeficiency virus (HIV) infection and zidovudine therapy, *Ann Intern Med* 117(9):739-748, 1992.

Ho DD: Cytomegalovirus. In Mandell GL, Douglas RG, Bennett JE, editors: *Principles and practices of infectious disease,* New York, 1990, Churchill Livingstone.

Hughes W et al: Comparison of atovaquone (566C80) with trimethoprim-sulfamethoxazole to treat *Pneumocystis carinii* pneumonia in patients with AIDS, *N Engl J Med* 328(21):1521-1527, 1993.

Israelski DM, Dannemann BR, Temingron JS; Toxoplasmosis in patients with AIDS. In Sande MA, Volberding P, editors: *The medical management of AIDS,* ed 2, Philadelphia, 1990, WB Saunders.

McCabe RE, Remington JS: *Toxoplasma gondii.* In Mandell GL, Douglas RG, Bennett JE, editors: *Principles and practices of infectious disease,* New York, 1990, Churchill Livingstone.

McKinsey DS, Gupta MR: Histoplasmosis in patients with AIDS: efficacy of maintenance amphotericin B therapy, *Am J Med* 92:225-227, 1992.

Newman SL: Colony-stimulating factors activate human macrophages to inhibit intracellular growth of *Histoplasma capsulatum* yeasts, *Infect Immunol* 60(11):4593-4597, 1992.

Pluda J et al: Subcutaneous recombinant granulocyte macrophage colony-stimulating factor as a single agent and in an alternating regimen with azidothymidine in leukopenic patients with severe human immunodeficiency virus infection, *Blood* 76(3):463-472, 1992.

Roilides E et al: Granulocyte colony-stimulating factor enhances the phagocytic and bacteriocidal activity of normal and defective human neutrophils, *J Infect Dis* 163(3):579-583, 1991.

Schneider MME et al: A controlled trial of aerosolized pentamidine or trimethoprim-sulfamethoxazole as primary prophylaxis against *Pneumocystis carinii* pneumonia in patients with human immunodeficiency virus infection, *N Engl J Med* 327(26):1836-1841, 1992.

Small PM et al: Exogenous reinfection with multidrug-resistant mycobacterium tuberculosis in patients with advanced HIV infection, *N Engl J Med* 328(16):1138-1144, 1993.

Smith D: Progress on opportunistic infections, *PI Perspect,* Feb 1993, pp 15-21.

Torres G, Link D: Opportunistic infections update, *Treatment Issues* 8(1):12-16, 1994.

***Other Complications in AIDS***

Agostini C et al: HIV-1 and the lung, *Am Rev Respir Dis* 147:1038-1049, 1993.

AIDS update: a quick review of neuropathies in AIDS patients, *Nurs 92* 22(1):85, 1992.

Bondmass M: The cardiac manifestations of acquired immune deficiency syndrome and nursing implications, *Med Surg Nurs* 3(1):42-48, 1994.

Grinspoon SK, Bilezikian JP: HIV disease and the endocrine system, *N Engl J Med* 327(19):1360-1365, 1992.

Grohmann GS et al: Enteric viruses and diarrhea in HIV-infected patients, *N Engl J Med* 329(1):14-20, 1993.

Loder PAW: HIV infection of the central nervous system: what are the nursing implications? *Nurs Clin North Am* 28(4):839-847, 1993.

Masharani U, Schambelan M: The endocrine complications of acquired immunodeficiency syndrome, *Adv Intern Med* 38:323-336, 1993.

Mocsny N: Toxoplasmic encephalitis in the AIDS patient, *Rehabil Nurs* 18(1):20-22, 1993.

Scherer P: How AIDS attacks the brain, *Am J Nurs* 90(1):44-53, 1990.

### *Pathophysiology and Clinical Manifestations*

Anastasi JK: Symptomatology in HIV-seropositive women, *Med Surg Nurs* 2(2):121-125, 1993.

Kessler HA et al: AIDS: part I, *Dis Mon* 38(9):634-690, 1992.

Kessler HA et al: AIDS: part II, *Dis Mon* 38(10):692-764, 1992.

Lusso P, Gallo R: Pathogenesis of AIDS, *J Pharm Pharmacol* 44(suppl 1):160-164, 1992.

Mann J: Global AIDS: further evolution of the pandemic and the response, *HIV Advisor* 7(3):3-8, 1993.

Tannenbaum I: Women and HIV, *RN* 56(5):34-41, 1993.

### *Primary Prevention (Education and Risk Reduction)*

Centers for Disease Control: Publicly funded HIV counseling and testing—United States, 1991, *MMWR* 41(34):613-617, 1992.

Centers for Disease Control: Community awareness and use of HIV/AIDS-prevention services among minority populations—Connecticut, 1991, *MMWR* 41(43):825-829, 1992.

Centers for Disease Control: HIV instruction and selected HIV-risk behaviors among high schoool students—United States, 1989-1991, *MMWR* 41(46):866-868, 1992.

Centers for Disease Control: Update: barrier protection against HIV infection and other sexually transmitted diseases, *MMWR* 42(30):589-591, 1993.

Centers for Disease Control: Zidovudine for the prevention of HIV transmission from mother to infant, *MMWR* 43(16):285-289, 1994.

Centers for Disease Control: Human immunodeficiency virus transmission in household settings—United States, *MMWR* 43(19):347-356, 1994.

de Wit JBF et al: Increase in unprotected anogenital intercourse among homosexual men, *Am J Public Health* 83(10):1451-1453, 1993.

Ehrhardt AA: Trends in sexual behavior and the HIV pandemic, *Am J Public Health* 82(11):1459-1461, 1992.

Gollub EL, Stein ZA: Commentary: the new female condom—item 1 on a women's AIDS prevention agenda, *Am J Public Health* 83(4):498-500, 1993.

Hein K: "Getting real" about HIV adolescents, *Am J Public Health* 83(4):492-494, 1993.

McCusker J et al: Behavioral outcomes of AIDS educational interventions for drug users in short-term treatment, *Am J Public Health* 83(10):1463-1466, 1993.

National Institute of Allergy and Infectious Disease: *AZT reduces rate of maternal transmission of HIV,* Washington, DC, 1994, National Institutes of Health.

Otten MW et al: Changes in sexually transmitted disease rates after HIV testing and posttest counseling, Miami, 1988-1989, *Am J Public Health* 83(4):529-533, 1993.

Richert CA et al: A method for identifying persons at high risk for sexually transmitted infections: opportunity for targeting intervention, *Am J Public Health* 83(4):520-524, 1993.

Roper WL, Peterson HB, Curran JW: Commentary: condoms and HIV/STD prevention—clarifying the message, *Am J Public Health* 83(4):501-503, 1993.

Tinkle M, Amaya M, Tamayo O: HIV disease and pregnancy, *J Obstet Gynecol Neonatal Nurs* 21(2):86-92, 1992.

US Department of Health and Human Services, Public Health Service: *Healthy people 2000: national health promotion and disease prevention objectives,* Washington, DC, 1990, US Government Printing Office.

### *Secondary Prevention (Testing and Early Intervention)*

Agency for Health Care Policy and Research: *Evaluation and management of early HIV infection,* Rockville, Md, 1994, US Department of Health and Human Services.

Baker R, Moulton J, Tighe J: *Early care for HIV disease,* San Francisco, 1991, The San Francisco AIDS Foundation.

Fischl M, Volberding P: *Antiviral therapy: clinical implications of early infection,* New York, 1992, World Health Communications.

Gogu RR, Malter JS, Agrawal KC: Zidovudine-induced blockade of the expression and function of the erythropoietin receptor, *Biochem Pharmacol* 44(6):1009-1012, 1992.

Miles S et al: Combined therapy with recombinant granulocyte-stimulating factor and erythropoietin decreases hematologic toxicity from zidovudine, *Blood* 7(10):2109-2117, 1991.

Tinkle M, Amaya M, Tamayo O: HIV disease and pregnancy, *J Obstet Gynecol Neonatal Nurs* 21(2):86-92, 1992.

### *Social Issues and AIDS*

Bayer R, Fairchild-Carrino A: AIDS and the limits of control: public health orders, quarantine and recalcitrant behavior, *Am J Public Health* 83(10);1471-1476, 1993.

Boyd KM: Institute of medical ethics: working party report. HIV infection: the ethics of anonymised testing and of testing pregnant women, *J Med Ethics* 16(4):173-178, 1990.

Hellinger FJ: The lifetime cost of treating a person with HIV, *JAMA* 270(4):474-478, 1993.

Herek GM, Capitanio JP: Public reactions to AIDS in the United States: a second decade of stigma, *Am J Public Health* 83(4):574-577, 1993.

McCarthy BD et al: Who should be screened for HIV infection? *Arch Intern Med* 153:1107-1116, 1993.

Philipson T: Economists show important role of information in AIDS epidemic, *Div Social Sci Rep,* Spring 1993, pp 10-11.

Phillips KA: Subjective knowledge of AIDS and use of HIV testing, *Am J Public Health* 83(10):1460-1462, 1993.

Stein ZA: The double bind in science policy and the protection of women from HIV infection, *Am J Public Health* 82(11):1471-1472, 1992 (editorial).

Vacalis TD, George T: Legal issues, AIDS, and the practicing physician, *Tex Med* 86(9):79-84, 1990.

CHAPTER 72

## Management of Persons With Organ/Tissue Transplants

### *General*

American Federation of Clinical Tissue Banks: *Operational standards,* Richmond, Va, 1989, The Federation.

Butkus DE, Meydrech EF, Seshadri SR: Racial differences in the survival of cadaveric renal allografts: overriding effects of HLA matching and socioeconomic factors, *N Engl J Med* 327(12):840-845, 1992.

Mandefield H: Tissue of progress, *Nurs Times* 89(16):26-29, 1993.

Midwest Organ Bank: *Organ and tissue procurement manual,* Westwood, Kans, 1991, The Organization.

Robbins RA et al: Pulmonary complications of transplantation, *Annu Rev Med* 43:425-435, 1992.

Sigal LH, Ron Y, editors: *Immunology and inflammation: basic mechanisms and clinical consequences,* New York, 1994, McGraw-Hill.

Smith SL: The cutting edge in organ transplantation, *Crit Care Nurse Suppl,* June 1993, pp 10-11, 26.

### *Donor and Recipient Issues*

Brown ME: Clinical management of the organ donor, *Dimens Crit Care Nurs* 8(3):134-142, 1989.

Cerney MS: Solving the organ donor shortage by meeting the bereaved family's needs, *Crit Care Nurse* 13(1):32-36, 1993.

Davis FD: Organ procurement and transplantation, *Nurs Clin North Am* 24:823-836, 1989.

Hathaway D, Strong M, Ganza M: Posttransplant quality of life expectations, *ANNA J* 17(6):433-440, 1990.

Hawke D, Kraft J, Smith SL: Tissue and organ donation and recovery. In Smith SL: *Tissue and organ transplantation: implications for professional nursing practice,* St Louis, 1990, Mosby.

Lange S: Psychosocial, legal, ethical, and cultural aspects of organ donation and transplantation, *Crit Care Nurs Clin North Am* 4(1):25-42, 1992.

Linde-Zwirble ME, Bishop BS, Menker JB: Management of the organ donor: a first step in transplantation, *Crit Care Nurs Q* 13(4):19-24, 1991.

Norris MKG: How to manage tissue donation, *Am J Nurs* 89(10):1300-1302, 1989.

O'Connell DA: Ethical implications of organ transplantation, *Crit Care Nurs Q* 13(4):1-7, 1991.

Porter RR et al: Stress during the waiting period: a review of pretransplantation fears, *Crit Care Nurs Q* 13(4):25-31, 1991.

Prottas JM, Jonasson O, Kleinig JI: In organ transplants, Americans first? *Hastings Center Rep* 16:23-25, 1986.

Snyder LA, Peter NK: How to manage organ donation, *Am J Nurs* 89(10):1294-1298, 1989.

Soukup M Sr: Organ donation from the family of a totally brain-dead donor: professional responsiveness, *Crit Care Nurs Q* 13(4):8-18, 1991.

Willis R, Skelley L: Serving the needs of donor families: the role of the critical care nurse, *Crit Care Nurs Clin North Am* 4(1):63-77, 1992.


### Immunology and Transplantation


Duffy MM, Nestor A: Nursing guidelines for muromonab-CD3 (OKT-3), *ANNA J* 19(5):493-495, 1992.

Holechek MJ: Medication review: FK 506, *ANNA J* 18(2):199-200, 1991.

Hooks MA: Immunosuppressive agents used in transplantation. In Smith SL: *Tissue and organ transplantation: implications for professional nursing practice,* St Louis, 1990, Mosby.

Jackson SA: The immune system: basic concepts for understanding transplantation, *Crit Care Nurs Q* 13(4):83-88, 1991.

Jahansouz F, Kriett JM: Transplantation: a review of immunosuppressive agents, *Crit Care Nurs Q* 15(4):13-22, 1993.

Kaufman D, Jones J, Matas A: New immunosuppressive agents: FK 506, rapamycin, RS-61443, 15-deoxyspergualin, *J Transplant Coordination* 2:20-27, 1992.

Lancaster L: Immunogenetic basis of tissue and organ transplantation and rejection, *Crit Care Nurs Clin* 4(1):1-24, 1992.

Payne JL: Immune modification and complications of immunosuppression, *Crit Care Nurs Clin North Am* 4(1):43-61, 1992.

Pedersen A et al: Intramuscular administration of RATG in the heart transplant patient, *Crit Care Nurse* 13(1):22-26, 29-31, 1993.

Pezze JL, Whiteman K: Orthoclone OKT 3: an overview of the monoclonal antibody and the nursing considerations it presents, *Crit Care Nurse* 11(5):98-107, 1991.

Roitt IM, Brostoff J, Male D: *Immunology,* ed 3, St Louis, 1994, Mosby.

Smith SL: Immunologic aspects of transplantation. In Smith SL: *Tissue and organ transplantation: implications for professional nursing practice,* St Louis, 1990, Mosby.

Soulillou JP: Bioreagents in allograft immunosuppression, *Adv Nephrol* 21:373-386, 1992.

Trusler LA: OKT 3: Nursing considerations for use in acute renal transplant rejection, *ANNA J* 17(4):299-303, 1990.

Workman ML, Ellerhorst-Ryan J, Hargrave-Koertge V: *Nursing care of the immunocompromised patient,* Philadelphia, 1993, WB Saunders.


### Bone Marrow Transplants


Bensinger WI et al: ABO-incompatible marrow transplants, *Transplantation* 33:427-429, 1982.

Clark JC, Webster JS: Bone marrow transplantation. In Smith SL: *Tissue and organ transplantation: implications for professional nursing practice,* St Louis, 1990, Mosby.

Freedman S et al: Bone marrow transplantation: overview and nursing implications, *Crit Care Nurs Q* 13(2):51-62, 1990.

Kernan NA et al: Analysis of 462 transplantations from unrelated donors facilitated by the national marrow donor program, *N Engl J Med* 328(9):593-602, 1993.

Wikle TJ: Bone marrow transplant today and tomorrow, *Am J Nurs* 90(5):48-58, 1990.

Wujcik D, Downs S: Bone marrow transplantation, *Crit Care Nurs Clin North Am* 4(1):149-166, 1992.


### Corneal Transplants


Bennett TO et al: Histocompatibility, penetrating keratoplasty, *Acta Ophthalmol* 53:403-407, 1975.

Heberlein D, Walsh G: Cornea transplantation. In Smith SL: *Tissue and organ transplantation: implications for professional nursing practice,* St Louis, 1990, Mosby.

Navarro VB, Tolley FM, Alcott MA: Restoration of sight by corneal transplantation, *Crit Care Nurs Q* 13(4):72-82, 1991.


### Heart Transplants


Dressler DK: Monitoring and prevention of renal dysfunction in cardiac transplant recipients, *AACN Clin Issues Crit Care Nurs* 3(3):633-639, 1992.

Laffel GL et al: The relation between experience and outcome in heart transplantation, *N Engl J Med* 327(17):1220-1225, 1992.

Mahon PM: Orthoclone OKT3 and cardiac transplantation: an overview: *Crit Care Nurse* 11(8):42-50, 1991.

Muirhead J: Heart and heart-lung transplantation, *Crit Care Nurs Clin North Am* 4(1):97-109, 1992.


### Liver Transplants


Balthazor JE: Steroid psychosis and hepatic encephalopathy in liver transplant patients: which is which and what do you do? *Crit Care Nurs Q* 14(3):51-55, 1991.

Bass PS, Bindon-Perler PA, Lewis RJ: Liver transplantation: the recovery phase, *Crit Care Nurs Q* 13(4):51-61, 1991.

Cohen C, Benjamin M, the Ethics and Social Impact Committee of the Transplant and Health Policy Center, Ann Arbor, Mich: Alcoholics and liver transplantation, *JAMA* 265:1299-1301, 1991.

Coleman JA, Mendoza MC, Bindon-Perler PA: Liver diseases that lead to transplantation, *Crit Care Nurs Q* 13(4):41-50, 1991.

Gilliam JE: Roles of the liver transplant clinical nurse specialist, *Clin Nurs Spec* 5(2):73-77, 1991.

Miller HD: Liver transplantation: postoperative ICU care, *Crit Care Nurse* 8(6):19-21, 24-31, 1988.

Moss AH, Siegler M: Should alcoholics compete equally for liver transplantation? *JAMA* 265:1295-1298, 1991.

Smith SL, Ciferni M: Liver transplantation. In Smith SL: *Tissue and organ transplantation: implications for professional nursing practice,* St Louis, 1990, Mosby.

Smith SL, Ciferni M: Liver transplantation for acute hepatic failure: a review of clinical experience and management, *Am J Crit Care* 2(2):137-144, 1993.

Spiro IJ et al: Brief report: lymphoma of donor origin occurring in the porta hepatis of a transplanted liver, *N Engl J Med* 329(1):27-29, 1993.

Whiteman K et al: Liver transplantation, *Am J Nurs* 90(6):68-72, 1990.

### *Kidney Transplants*

Beckman NJ et al: Kidney transplantation: a therapy option, *AACN Clin Issues Crit Care Nurs* 3(3):570-584, 1992.
Blanford NL: Renal transplantation: a case study of the ideal, *Crit Care Nurse* 13(1):46-55, 1993.
Braun WE: Histocompatibility and renal transplantation. In Garovy MR, Guttman RD: *Renal transplantation,* New York, 1986, Churchill Livingstone.
Cunningham NH, Boteler S, Windham S: Renal transplantation, *Crit Care Nurs Clin North Am* 4(1):79-88, 1992.
Holechek MJ, Burrell-Diggs D, Navarro MO: Renal transplantation: an option for end-stage renal disease patients, *Crit Care Nurs Q* 13(4):62-71, 1991.
Perryman JP, Stillerman PU: Kidney transplantation. In Smith SL: *Tissue and organ transplantation: implications for professional nursing practice,* St Louis, 1990, Mosby.
White M, McNatt G: Early transplantation for patients with diabetic nephropathy, *ANNA J* 19(5):457-462, 1992.

### *Lung Transplants*

American Thoracic Society: Lung transplantation, report of the ATS workshop, *Am Rev Respir Dis* 147:772-776, 1993.
Gallagher SL, Lawrence PA: Heart-lung transplantation: the patient with cystic fibrosis, *Crit Care Nurs Q* 13(4):32-40, 1991.
Kirchner SA: Living related lung transplantation: a new dimension in single lung transplantation, *AORN J* 54(4):703-714, 1991.
Runyon VD: Single lung transplantation: new treatment for end-stage pulmonary disease, *AORN J* 51(3);694-711, 1990.
Trulock EP: Lung transplantation, *Annu Rev Med* 43:1-8, 1992.

### *Pancreatic Transplants*

Bartucci MR, Loughman KA, Moir EJ: Kidney-pancreas transplantation: a treatment option for ESRD and type I diabetes, *ANNA J* 19(5):467-474, 1992.
Bass M: Pancreas transplantation: detecting rejection and patient care, *ANNA J* 19(5):476-482, 1992.
Korsgren O et al: Pancreatic islet transplantation in the human, *Adv Nephrol* 22:371-386, 1993.
Trusler LA: Simultaneous kidney-pancreas transplantation, *ANNA J* 18(5):487-491, 1991.
Trusler LA: Management of the patient receiving simultaneous kidney-pancreas transplantation, *Crit Care Nurs Clin North Am* 4(1):89-95, 1992.

### *Other Types of Tissue Transplants*

Fahn S: Fetal-tissue transplants in Parkinson's disease, *N Engl J Med* 327(22):1589-1590, 1992.
Kassirer JP, Angell M: The use of fetal tissue in research on Parkinson's disease, *N Engl J Med* 327(22):1591-1592, 1992.
Thomas P: Cell transplantation: new hope for old diseases, *Harvard Health Lett* 17(12):1-4, 1992.

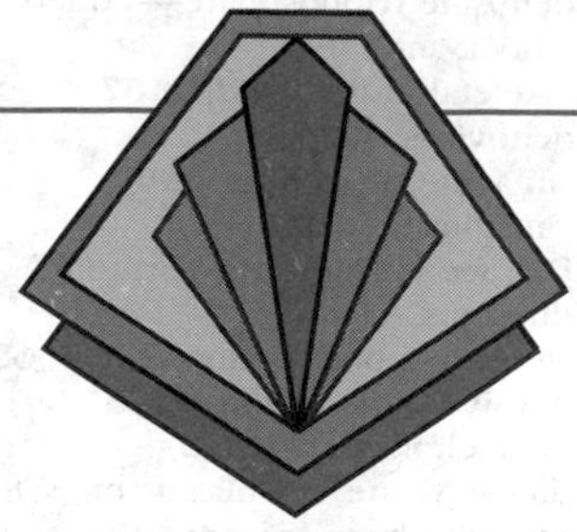

# Index

## C

G

M

## T

U

## Critical Pathways



## Guidelines for Patient Teaching





## Guidelines for Patient Teaching—cont'd



## Nursing Care Plans